Access the fully searchable text of Forfar online free when you buy this book!

www.forfarandarneil.com

. . . .

How to register

❶ Scratch off the sticker below and get your unique PIN number.

❷ Go to www.forfarandarneil.com for simple instructions for how to register. You will be asked to enter your unique PIN number.

. . . .

Important note

Purchase of this book includes a limited personal licence for the life of this edition to the online version, for use exclusively by the individual who has purchased the title. This licence and access to www.forfarandarneil.com operates strictly on the basis of a single user per PIN number. The sharing of passwords is strictly prohibited, and any attempt to do so will invalidate the password. The licence and access may not be lent, resold or otherwise circulated. Full details of the licence and terms and conditions of use are available on registration.

Book cannot be returned once panel is scratched off

Scratch off the sticker with care!

Scratch off Below
MCIN

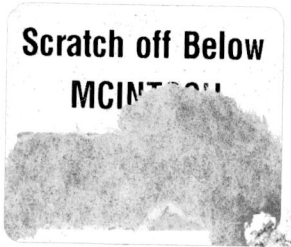

BRITISH MEDICAL ASSOCIATION

0936465

Seventh Edition

Forfar & Arneil's
TEXTBOOK
of PEDIATRICS

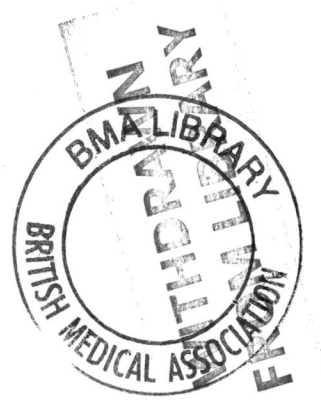

Commissioning Editor: Ellen Green, Pauline Graham
Development Editor: Janice Urquhart
Project Manager: Nancy Arnott
Design Direction: Erik Bigland
Illustrators: Tim Loughhead, Richard Prime

Seventh Edition

Forfar & Arneil's
TEXTBOOK
of PEDIATRICS

Edited by

Neil McIntosh DSc(Med) FRCP(Edin) FRCP(Lond) FRCPCH
Professor of Child Life and Health, University of Edinburgh;
Honorary Consultant Paediatrician, Lothian University Hospitals NHS Trust, Edinburgh, UK

Peter J. Helms MB BS PhD FRCP(Edin) FRCPCH
Professor of Child Health, University of Aberdeen, Aberdeen, UK

Rosalind L. Smyth MA MB BS MD FRCPCH F Med Sci
Brough Professor of Paediatric Medicine, University of Liverpool, Liverpool, UK

Stuart Logan MB ChB MSc(Epidemiology) MSc(politics) MRCP FRCPCH
Professor of Paediatric Epidemiology; Director, Institute of Health Research, Peninsula Medical Service School,
St Luke's Campus, Exeter, UK

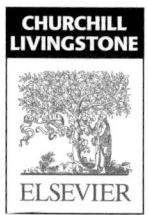

CHURCHILL LIVINGSTONE

ELSEVIER

Edinburgh   London   New York   Oxford   Philadelphia   St Louis   Sydney   Toronto   2008

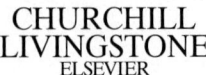

CHURCHILL
LIVINGSTONE
ELSEVIER

An imprint of Elsevier Limited

First edition 1973
Second edition 1978
Third edition 1984
Fourth edition 1992
Fifth edition 1998
Sixth edition 2003
Seventh edition 2008

ISBN 978–0–443–10396–4
IE ISBN 978–0–443–10397–1

British Library Cataloguing in Publication Data
A catalogue record for this book is available from the British Library

Library of Congress Cataloging in Publication Data
A catalog record for this book is available from the Library of Congress

Note
Knowledge and best practice in this field are constantly changing. As new research and experience broaden our knowledge, changes in practice, treatment and drug therapy may become necessary or appropriate. Readers are advised to check the most current information provided (i) on procedures featured or (ii) by the manufacturer of each product to be administered, to verify the recommended dose or formula, the method and duration of administration, and contraindications. It is the responsibility of the practitioner, relying on their own experience and knowledge of the patient, to make diagnoses, to determine dosages and the best treatment for each individual patient, and to take all appropriate safety precautions. To the fullest extent of the law, neither the Publisher nor the Authors assumes any liability for any injury and/or damage to persons or property arising out or related to any use of the material contained in this book.
The Publisher

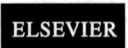

ELSEVIER your source for books, journals and multimedia in the health sciences
www.elsevierhealth.com

Working together to grow
libraries in developing countries
www.elsevier.com | www.bookaid.org | www.sabre.org

ELSEVIER   BOOK AID International   Sabre Foundation

The publisher's policy is to use **paper manufactured from sustainable forests**

Printed in China

Preface

One of the most important developments in the 21st century has been the acknowledgment that clinical practice should be embedded where possible in a sound evidence base. The editors of this new edition of *Forfar & Arneil's Textbook of Pediatrics* continue to set contributors the challenging task of ensuring that the statements and recommendations made are based on the most robust clinical research available. The objective assessment of evidence and the formulation of secure recommendations from the evidence are gathering pace. In Child Health the evidence base, with the possible exception of disciplines such as oncology and neonatology, is not as comprehensive or as well defined as we would wish. This edition of Forfar & Arneil continues to flag up the most important evidence sources for the content of each chapter. The whole book has been revised and updated and the chapter authors and editors again incorporate where possible secure evidence of therapy, diagnosis, etiology and prognosis. This evidence is incorporated into the individual chapters and in the chapter reference list is starred for easy reference. We believe that the result is the most comprehensive evidence-based general textbook of pediatrics available. Our ability to access best evidence has been greatly enhanced by the rapid advances of information technology and electronic publishing and consequently another important new feature for this edition is a website of the text in which references listed in PUBMED can be accessed via the internet. We would like to acknowledge the outstanding contributions of the many individual authors and our chapter editors, without whom this ambitious project would not have been possible. It has been a great privilege to work with them. We would also like to thank our own secretaries for their unstinting help (Elaine Forbes, Flora Buthlay, Collette Lorne and Stella Taylor) and of course our respective families for sharing the burden with us.

As with previous editions the book is produced by the Elsevier Organization. There have been many highly professional people involved. We hope that this new 7th edition with its expanded formal evidence base will be well received by you, the reader, and become as trusted a friend and guide as have previous editions.

Neil McIntosh
Peter J. Helms
Rosalind L. Smyth
Stuart Logan

Contents

Section 2

PERINATAL/NEONATAL MEDICINE

Section 3

THE SPECIALITIES

Section 4
APPENDICES AND INDEX

Contributors

Ishaq Abu-Arafeh, MBBS, MD, MRCP, FRCPCH
Consultant in Paediatrics and Paediatric Neurology, Stirling Royal Infirmary, Stirling; Honorary Consultant Paediatrician, Fraser of Allander Neurosciences Unit, Royal Hospital for Sick Children, Glasgow, UK

N. Archer, MA FRCP FRCPCH DCH
Consultant Paediatric Cardiologist, Oxford Children's Hospital, Oxford; Honorary Clinical Senior Lecturer, University of Oxford, Oxford, UK

Peter D. Arkwright, FRCPCH DPhil
Lecturer in Child Health, Department of Child Health, University of Manchester, Manchester, UK

Ian A. Auchterlonie, MB ChB FRCPCH FRCP
Honorary Consultant Paediatrician (Retired), Royal Aberdeen Children's Hospital, Aberdeen, UK

Alastair J. Baker, MB ChB FRCP FRCPCH
Consultant Paediatric Hepatologist, King's College Hospital, London, UK

Susan V. Beath, BSc MB BS MRCP DTM&H FRCPCH
Consultant Paediatric Hepatologist, The Liver Unit, Birmingham Childrens Hospital, Birmingham, UK

Thomas F. Beattie, MB MSc FRCSEd(A&E), FCEM, FRCPE, FFSEM, DCH
Consultant in Emergency Medicine, Royal Hospital for Sick Children, Edinburgh; Honorary Senior Lecturer in Paediatrics, University of Edinburgh, Edinburgh, UK

Julie-Clare Becher, MB ChB MRCPCH MD
Consultant Neonatologist, Simpson Centre for Reproductive Health, Royal Infirmary of Edinburgh, Edinburgh, UK

W. Michael Bisset, BSc MB ChB DCH MSc MD FRCPE FRCPCH
Consultant Paediatric Gastroenterologist, Department of Medical Paediatrics, Royal Aberdeen Children's Hospital, Aberdeen, UK

Peter S. Blair, PhD
Medical Statistician, Senior Research Fellow, University of Bristol, Division of Child Health, Royal Hospital for Children, Bristol, UK

Paula H.B. Bolton-Maggs, FRCPCH FRCP FRCPath
Consultant Haematologist, Manchester Comprehensive Care Haemophilia Centre, Department of Clinical Haematology, Manchester Royal Infirmary, Manchester, UK

Paul L.P. Brand, MD
Consultant Paediatrician and Director of Postgraduate Education, Princess Amalia Children's Clinic, Isala klinieken, Zwolle, The Netherlands

Colin E. Bruce, MB ChB FRCS FRCS(ORTH)
Consultant Paediatric Orthopaedic Surgeon, Alder Hey Children's Hospital, Liverpool, UK

Helen Budge, BA BM BCh PhD MRCP FRPCH
Associate Professor of Neonatology, University of Nottingham, Nottingham, UK

Neil R.M. Buist, MB ChB FRCPE DCH
Professor Emeritus, Departments of Paediatrics and Medical Genetics, Oregon Health and Science University, Portland, Oregon, USA

Nigel Peter Burrows, MD FRCP
Consultant Dermatologist and Associate Lecturer, Department of Dermatology, Addenbrooke's Hospital, Cambridge, UK

Andrew Bush, MD FRCP FRCPCH
Professor of Paediatric Respirology, Imperial College, London; Honorary Consultant Paediatric Chest Physician, Royal Brompton Hospital, London, UK

Gary Butler, MB BS MD FRCPCH
Professor of Paediatrics, Institute of Health Sciences, University of Reading and Department of Paediatrics, Royal Berkshire Hospital, Reading, UK

Catherine M. Cale, MB ChB PhD MRCP MRCPCH MRCPath
Consultant in Paediatric Immunology and Immunopathology, Department of Immunology, Great Ormond Street Hospital, London, UK

Harry Campbell, MD FRCPE FFPH FRSE
Professor of Genetic Epidemiology and Public Health Sciences, College of Medicine and Vet Medicine, University of Edinburgh, Edinburgh, UK

Andrew J. Cant, BSc MD FRCP FRCPH
Consultant in Paediatric Immunology and Infectious Diseases, Newcastle General Hospital, Newcastle upon Tyne, UK

Michael Clarke, BSc MRCP DCH FRCPCH
Consultant Paediatric Neurologist, Leeds Teaching Hospitals NHS Trust, Leeds, UK

Andrew Gavin Cleary, MB ChB BSc MSc MRCPCH
Consultant Paediatric Rheumatologist, Royal Liverpool Children's Hospital, Liverpool, UK

J. Brian S. Coulter, MD FRCP(I) FRCPCH
Honorary Clinical Lecturer in Tropical Child Health, Liverpool School of Tropical Medicine, Liverpool, UK

Jonathan Coutts, MB ChB FRCPCH FRCP(Glas)
Consultant Neonatal and Respiratory Paediatrician, The Queen Mother's Hospital and Royal Hospital for Sick Children, Glasgow, UK

Richard Coward, MB ChB MRCPCH PhD
MRC Clinician Scientist and Consultant Paediatric Nephrologist, Bristol Royal Hospital for Children, Bristol, UK

Finella Craig, BSc MBBS MRCP
Consultant in Paediatric Palliative Care, Great Ormond Street Hospital for Children, London, UK

Timothy J. David, MB ChB MD PhD FRCP FRCPCH DCH
Professor of Child Health and Paediatrics, Honorary Consultant Paediatrician, The University of Manchester, Manchester, UK

Joyce E. Davidson, BSc MBChB MRCP (UK) FRCPCH
Consultant Paediatric Rheumatologist, Royal Hospital for Sick Children, Glasgow, and Royal Hospital for Sick Children, Edinburgh, UK

E. Graham Davies, MB BChir MA FRCPCH
Consultant Paediatric Immunologist, Great Ormond Street Hospital, London, UK

Jan Dudley, BM MRCP(UK) FRCPCH PhD
Consultant Paediatric Nephrologist, Bristol Royal Hospital for Children, Bristol, UK

P. Barton Duell, MD
Associate Professor of Medicine, Division of Endocrinology, Diabetes, and Clinical Nutrition; director, Lipid-Atherosclerosis Laboratory and Metabolic Disorders Clinic, Oregon Health and Science University, Portland, Oregon

Heather Elphick, MB ChB MRCP MRCPCH MD
Specialist Registrar in Respiratory Paediatrics, Sheffield Children's Hospital, Sheffield, UK

Nicholas D. Embleton, BSc MD FRCPCH
Consultant in Neonatal Medicine and

Honorary Lecturer in Child Health, Newcastle Neonatal Service, Royal Victoria Infirmary, Newcastle upon Tyne, UK

Gregory M. Enns, MB ChB
Associate Professor of Pediatrics, Director, Biochemical Genetics Program, Division of Medical Genetics, Stanford University, Stanford, California, USA

Jeremy Farrar, FRCP DPhil OBE
Professor of Tropical Medicine Oxford University; Honorary Professor of International Health, London School of Hygiene and Tropical Medicine, London; Director, Oxford University Clinical Research Unit, The Hospital for Tropical Diseases, Ho Chi Minh City, Viet Nam

Colin D. Ferrie, BSc MB ChB MD MRCP FRCPCH
Consultant Paediatric Neurologist, Department of Paediatric Neurology, Leeds General Infirmary, Leeds, UK

Alistair R. Fielder, FRCP FRCS FRCOphth
Professor of Ophthalmology, Department of Optometry and Visual Science, City University, London, UK

Brian W. Fleck, MD FRCOph
Consultant Ophthalmologist, Edinburgh Royal Infirmary and Edinburgh Royal Hospital for Sick Children, Edinburgh, UK

Peter J. Fleming, PhD MB ChB FRCPCH FRCP FRCP(C)
Professor of Infant Health and Developmental Physiology, University of Bristol; Consultant Paediatrician, Royal Hospital for Children, Bristol, UK

Caroline Foster, MB BS MRCP
Honorary Clinical Research Fellow, Imperial College London; SPR Paediatric HIV, St Mary's Hospital, London, UK

Yvonne Freer, RGN RM RSCN BSc PhD
Research and Practice Development Facilitator, Neonatal Intensive Care, Simpson Centre for Reproductive Health, Royal Infirmary of Edinburgh, Edinburgh, UK

Vijeya Ganesan, MRCPCH, MD
Senior Lecturer in Paediatric Neurology, Institute of Child Health, University College London, London, UK

Anne S. Garden, FRCOG
Head of Department of Medicine and Director of the Centre for Medical Education, Lancaster University, Lancaster; Honorary Consultant in Paediatric and Adolescent Gynaecology, Royal Liverpool Children's Hospital, Liverpool; Honorary Consultant Gynaecologist, University Hospitals Morecambe Bay Trust, Morecambe, UK

Andrew R. Gennery, MD MRCP MRCPCH DCH DipMedSci
Senior Lecturer and Honorary Consultant in Paediatric Immunology, BMT Institute of Cellular Medicine, University of Newcastle upon Tyne, and Children's Bone Marrow Transplant Unit, Newcastle General Hospital, Newcastle upon Tyne, UK

Diana Gibb, MD FRCPCH MSc
Professor of Paediatric Epidemiology, MRC Clinical Trials Unit, University College London, London, UK

K. Michael Gibson, PhD, FACMG
Professor, Pediatrics, Pathology and Human Genetics, Division of Medical Genetics, Children's Hospital of Pittsburgh, University of Pittsburgh School of Medicine, Pittsburgh, PA, USA

Barbara Golden, BSc MB BCh BAO MD FRCPI FRCPCH DCH RNutr
Associate Dean (Medicine), Clinical Senior Lecturer, Honorary Consultant International Child Health, Child Health Institute, School of Medicine, University of Aberdeen, Royal Aberdeen Children's Hospital, Aberdeen, UK

John M. Goldsmid, BSc MSc PhD FRCPath FACTM FASM CBiol FIBiol FAIBiol HonFRCPA HonFACTM
Emeritus Professor, Discipline of Pathology, University of Tasmania, Hobart, Tasmania, Australia

John R.W. Govan, BSc PhD DSc
Professor of Microbial Pathogenicity, Centre for Infectious Diseases, University of Edinburgh Medical School, Edinburgh, UK

Stephen M. Graham, FRACP
Paediatric Research Fellow and Deputy Director Malawi-Liverpool-Wellcome Trust Clinical Research Programme, University of Malawi College of Medicine, Blantyre, Malawi; Senior Clinical Lecturer, Liverpool School of Tropical Medicine, Liverpool, UK

Anne Green, BSc MSc PhD FRCPath FRCS FIBiol FRCPCH.
Consultant Clinical Scientist, Birmingham Children's Hospital NHS Trust, Birmingham, UK

Marcus Grompe, MD
Director, Oregon Stem Cell Center; Professor, Department of Molecular and Medical Genetics, Oregon and Health Science University, Portland, Oregon, USA

Henry L. Halliday, FRCPE FRCP FRCPCH
Chair of Child Health and Welfare Research Group, Department of Child Health, Queen's University Belfast, Northern Ireland, UK

Christina Halsey, BM BCh BA MRCP MRCPath
Leukaemia Research Fund Clinical Research Fellow, Faculty of Medicine, Glasgow University, Glasgow, UK

Cary O. Harding, MD
Assistant Professor, Molecular and Medical Genetics; Director of the Biochemical Genetics Clinical Laboratory, Oregon Health and Science University, Portland, Oregon, USA

C. Anthony Hart, BScMB BS PhD FRCPCH FRCPath
Professor, Division of Medical Microbiology, School of Infection and Host Defence, University of Liverpool, Liverpool , UK

Paul T. Heath, MB BS FRACP FRCPCH
Senior Lecturer and Honorary Consultant, Paediatric Infectious Diseases, Division of Child Health, St George's University of London, London, UK

Peter J. Helms, MB BS PhD FRCP(Edin) FRCPCH
Professor of Child Health, University of Aberdeen, Aberdeen, UK

John Henderson, MD FRCP FRCPCH FRCPEd
Reader in Paediatric Respiratory Medicine, University of Bristol and Bristol Royal Hospital for Children, Bristol, UK

Tom Hilliard, MD FRCPCH
Consultant Respiratory Paediatrician, Bristol Children's Hospital, Bristol, UK

Peter Hoare, DM FRCPsych
Senior Lecturer, University of Edinburgh; Honorary Consultant Psychiatrist, Royal Hospital for Sick Children, Edinburgh, UK

Richard F. Howard, BSc MBChB FRCA
Consultant in Anaesthesia and Pain Management, Great Ormond Street Hospital for Children, London, UK

Imelda Hughes, FRCPCH
Consultant Paediatric Neurologist, Department of Paediatric Neurology, Royal Manchester Children's Hospital, Manchester, UK

Robert Hume, BSc MB ChB PhD FRCPEdin FRCPCH
Professor of Developmental Medicine, Maternal and Child Health Sciences, University of Dundee, Dundee, UK

Carol Inward, MBBCh MD FRCPCH
Consultant Paediatric Nephrologist, Bristol Royal Hospital for Children, Bristol, UK

David Isaacs, MB BChir MD FRACP FRCPCH
Senior Staff Specialist at Children's Hospital at Westmead; Clinical Professor in Paediatric Infectious Diseases, University of Sydney, Sydney, Australia

Omar Ismayl, MD MSc MRCPCH
Consultant Neurologist, Damascus University Children's Hospital, Mezza, Damascus, Syria

Huw R. Jenkins, MA MD FRCP FRCPCH
Consultant Paediatric Gastroenterologist, Department of Child Health, University Hospital of Wales, Cardiff, Wales, UK

Cheryl A. Jones, MB BS PhD FRACP
Associate Professor, and Sub Dean Postgraduate Studies, Discipline of Paediatrics and Child Health, University of Sydney; Sydney, New South Wales, Australia

Christopher J.H. Kelnar, MA MD FRCP FRCPCH
Professor of Paediatric Endocrinology,
Section of Child Life and Health, Division of
Reproductive and Developmental Sciences,
University of Edinburgh, Edinburgh, UK

Alison M. Kemp, MB BCH DCH MRCP
FRCPCH FRCP(Edin)
Reader in Child Heath, Department of Child
Health, Cardiff University, Cardiff, Wales

Alastair I.G. Kerr, MBChB FRCS(Edin & Glas)
Consultant Otolaryngologist, Ear, Nose and
Throat Department, Royal Infirmary for Sick
Children, Edinburgh, UK

Alison M. Kesson, MB BS PhD FRACP FRCPA
Virologist, Microbiologist and Paediatric
Infectious Disease Physician, The Children's
Hospital, Westmead, Sydney New South
Wales; Conjoint Associate Professor,
Paediatrics and Child Health, University of
Sydney, Sydney New South Wales, Australia

Maurice A. Kibel, FRCP(Edin) DCH(Lond).
Emeritus Professor of Child Health, School
of Child and Adolescent Health,University of
Cape Town, South Africa

Denise Kitchiner, MD FRCP FRCPCH
Consultant Paediatric Cardiologist,
Royal Liverpool Children's NHS Trust,
Liverpool, UK

Nigel J. Klein, BSc MB BS MRCP PhD FRCPCH
Professor of Infection and Immunity,
University College London; Head, Infectious
Diseases and Microbiology Unit, Institute of
Child Health; Head, Department of Infection,
University College London; Consultant in
Infectious Diseases and Microbiology,
Great Ormond Street Hospital NHS Trust,
London, UK

David M. Koeller, MD
Associate Professor, Pediatrics and Molecular
and Medical Genetics; Chief, Division
of Metabolism, Department of Pediatrics,
Doernbecher Children's Hospital, Oregon
Health and Science University, Portland,
Oregon, USA

Sailesh Kotecha, MA FRCPCH PhD
Professor of Child Health, Department of
Child Health, Wales College of Medicine,
Cardiff University, Cardiff, Wales, UK

Karen Kotloff, MD
Professor, Pediatrics and Medicine, Center
for Vaccine Development, University of
Maryland School of Medicine, Baltimore,
Maryland, USA

Ian A. Laing, MA MD FRCPE FRCPCH
Consultant Neonatologist, Simpson Centre
for Reproductive Health, Royal Infirmary of
Edinburgh, Edinburgh, UK

David G. Lalloo, MB BS MD FRCP
Reader In Tropical Medicine, Liverpool
School of Tropical Medicine, Liverpool, UK

Alison Leaf, BSc MB ChB MD MRCP FRCPCH
Consultant Neonatologist, Southmead
Hospital, Bristol, UK

Malcolm I. Levene, MD FRCPCH FMedSc
Professor of Paediatrics and Child Health,
University of Leeds, Leeds General Infirmary,
Leeds, UK

Leesa M. Linck, MD MPH
Consultant Paediatrician,
The Connty Clinic, Winthrop,
Washington State, USA.

John H. Livingston, MB ChB FRCP FRCPCH
Consultant Paediatric Neurologist,
Department of Paediatric Neurology, Leeds
General Infirmary, Leeds, UK

Stuart Logan, MB ChB MSc(Epidemiology)
MSc(Econ) MRCP FRCPCH
Professor of Paediatric Epidemiology;
Director, Institute of Health and Social
Care Research, Peninsula Medical School,
St Luke's Campus, Exeter, UK

Diana N.J. Lockwood, BSc MD FRCP
Consultant Physician and Leprologist,
Hospital for Tropical Diseases, London, UK

Andrew J. Lyon, MA MB FRCP FRCPCH
Consultant Neonatologist, Simpson Centre
for Reproductive Health, Royal Infirmary of
Edinburgh, Edinburgh, UK

Ronan Lyons, MD FFPH FFPHMI MPH DCH
Professor of Public Health, Centre for Health
Information, Research and Evaluation,
School of Medicine, Swansea University,
Swansea, UK

Anita Macdonald, PhD BSc SRD
Consultant Dietician in Inherited Metabolic
Disorders, Birmingham Children's Hospital,
Birmingham, UK, Head of Dietetics,
Birmingham Children's Hospital NHS Trust,
Birmingham, UK

Mary McGraw, FRCP FRCPCH
Consultant Paediatric Nephrologist,
Bristol Royal Hospital for Children,
Bristol, UK

Keiran McHugh, FRCR FRCPI DCH
Consultant Paediatric Radiologist, Great
Ormond Street Hospital for Children,
London, UK

Neil McIntosh, DSc(Med)
Professor of Child Life and Health,
Department of Child Life and Health,
University of Edinburgh; Honorary
Consultant Paediatrician, Lothian University
Hospitals NHS Trust, Edinburgh, UK

G.A. Mackinlay, MB BS LRCP FRCSEd
FRCSEng FRCPCH
Senior Lecturer, Department of Clinical
Surgery, University of Edinburgh; Consultant
Paediatric Surgeon, Department of Paediatric
Surgery, Royal Hospital for Sick Children,
Edinburgh, UK

Ian McKinley, OBE BSc MB ChB DCH FRCP FRCPCH
Senior Lecturer in Child Health, McKay-
Gordon Centre, Royal Manchester Children's
Hospital, Manchester, UK

Sheila A.M. McLean, LLB MLitt PhD LLD FRSE
FRCGP FMedSci FRCP(Edin) FRSA
International Bar Association Professor of
Law and Ethics in Medicine, University of
Glasgow, UK

Sabine Maguire, MB BCh BAO MRCPI FRCPI FRCPCH
Senior Lecturer in Child Health, Cardiff
University, Department of Child Health,
Cardiff, UK

Janice Main, FRCP(Edin) FRCP(Lond)
Reader and Consultant Physician in
Infectious diseases and General Medicine,
Department of Medicine, Imperial College,
St Mary's Hospital, London, UK

Guy Makin, BA BM BCh PhD MRCP FRCPCH
Senior Lecturer in Paediatric Oncology,
University of Manchester; Honorary
Consultant Paediatric Oncologist,
Royal Manchester Children's Hospital,
Manchester, UK

Timothy Martland, MB ChB MRCP MRCPCH
Consultant Paediatric Neurologist,
Department of Paediatric Neurology,
Royal Manchester Children's Hospital,
Manchester, UK

Amha Mekasha, MD MSc
Associate Professor of Paediatrics and Child
Health, Department of Paediatrics and
Child Health, Addis Ababa University,
Adis Ababa, Ethiopia

Craig Mellis, MB BS MPH MD FRACP
Head of School, Associate Dean, Central
Clinic School, Faculty of Medicine, The
University of Sydney, Sydney, Australia

Stefan Meyer, MD PhD MRCPCH
CRUK Clinician Scientist and Consultant
Paediatric Oncologist, Univeristy of
Manchester, Royal Manchester Children's
Hospital and Young Oncology Unit, Christie
Hospital, Manchester, UK, Stefan Meyer MD
PhD MRCPCH

Alan E. Mills, MA MB DCP DPath FRCPA.
FFPathRCPI FACTM
Consultant Pathologist, Dorevitch Pathology,
Bendigo, Victoria, Australia

Elizabeth Molyneux, OBE FRCP FRCPCH FEM
Professor and Head of Department of
Paediatrics, College of Medicine, Blantyre,
Malawi, C Africa.

Malcolm E. Molyneux, MD FRCP FMedSci
Director, Malawi-Liverpool-Wellcome Trust
Clinical Research Programme, College of
Medicine, University of Malawi, Malawi;
Professor of Tropical Medicine, School of
Tropical Medicine, University of Liverpool,
Liverpool, UK

Kim Mulholland, MD FRACP
Professor of Child Health, London School
of Hygiene and Tropical Medicine, London,
UK, Infectious Disease Epidemiology Unit,
London School of Hygiene and Tropical
Medicine, London, UK

Alan O. Mulvihill, FRCSI FRCSEd
Consultant Ophthalmic Surgeon, Princess
Alexandra Eye Pavilion and Royal Hospital
for Sick Children, Edinburgh, UK

Richard W. Newton, MD FRCPCH FRCP
Consultant Paediatric Neurologist,
Royal Manchester Children's Hospital,
Manchester, UK

Angus Nicoll, CBE FFPHM FRCP FRCPCH
Director, Communicable Disease Surveilaance
Centre, Centre for Infection, Health
Protection Agency, London, UK

James Y. Paton, MD, FRCPCH FRCPSG
Reader in Paediatric Respiratory Medicine,
Division of Developmental Medicine,
University of Glasgow, Royal Hospital for
Sick Children, Glasgow, UK

Michael A. Patton, MA MSc MBChB FRCPCH
Professor of Medical Genetics and Consultant
Medical Geneticist, Department of Medical
Genetics, St George's Hospital Medical
School, London, UK

Philip L. Pearl, MD
Associate Professor of Paediatrics and
Neurology, Department of Neurology,
Children's National Medical Center,
The George Washington University School
of Medicine, Washington DC, USA

Gale A. Pearson, MB BS MRCP FRCPCH
Consultant in Paediatric Intensive
Care, Birmingham Children's Hospital,
Birmingham, UK

Stavros Petrou, BSc MPhil PhD
MRC Senior Non-Clinical Research Fellow,
National Perinatal Epidemiology Unit,
University of Oxford, Oxford, UK

Ian J. Ramage, FRCPCH
Consultant Paediatric Nephrologist, Royal
Hospital for Sick Children, Glasgow, UK

John J. Reilly, BSc PhD
Professor of Paediatric Energy Metabolism,
University Division of Developmental
Medicine, Royal Hospital for Sick Children,
Glasgow, UK

J.M. Rennie, MD FRCP FRCPCH DCH
Consultant and Senior Lecturer in Neonatal
Medicine, Elizabeth Garrett Anderson and
Obstetric Hospital, University College London
Hospitals, London

Sam Richmond, MB BS FRCP FRCPCH
Consultant Neonatologist, Sunderland Royal
Hospital, Sunderland, UK

Irene A.G. Roberts, MD FRCP FRCPath FRCPCH
DRCOG
Professor of Paediatric Haematology and
Consultant Paediatric Haematologist,
Hammersmith Hospital and St Mary's
Hospitals, Imperial College, London, UK

Peter T. Rudd, MD FRCPCH
Consultant Paediatrician, Royal United
Hospital, Bath, UK

S.C. Robson, MD MRCOG
Professor of Fetal Medicine, School of
Surgical and Reproductive Sciences, Newcastle
University, Newcastle upon Tyne, UK

Jean-Baptiste Roullet, PhD
Associate Professor (Research), Division
of Metabolism, Department of Paediatrics,
Oregon Health and Science University,
Portland, Oregon, USA; Adjunct Associate
Professor of Pharmacology and Therapeutics,
University of Calgary, Calgary, Alberta,
Canada

George Rylance, MB FRCPCH
Consultant in Paediatrics, Department of
Child Health, Royal Victoria Infirmary,
Newcastle upon Tyne, UK

Moin A. Saleem, MB BS FRCP PhD
Reader and Honorary Consultant Paediatric
Nephrologist, Bristol Children's Hospital,
University of Bristol, Bristol, UK

Alison Salt, MB BS MSc FRACP FRCPCH
Consultant Developmental Paediatrician,
Neurodisability Service, Great Ormond Street
Hospital for Children NHS Trust and Institute
of Child Health, London, UK

Jenefer Sargent, MA MB BCh MSc MRCPCH
Consultant Developmental Paediatrician,
Neurodisability Service, Great Ormond
Hospital for Children NHS Trust, London, UK

Ayad Shafiq, FRCOphth MRCPPaeds DCH BM BCh
Consultant Ophthalmologist, Royal Victoria
Hospital, Newcastle upon Tyne, UK

Jonathan R. Skinner, MB ChB FRCPCH FRACP MD
Paediatric Cardiologist, Green Lane Paediatric
and Cardiac Services, Starship Children's
Hospital, Auckland, New Zealand

Alan Smyth, MA MB BS MRCP MD FRCPCH
Reader in Child Health, University of
Nottingham; Honorary Consultant in
Paediatric Respiratory Medicine,
Nottingham University Hospitals NHS
Trust, Nottingham, UK

Rosalind L. Smyth, MA MB BS MD FRCPCH
Brough Professor of Paediatric Medicine,
University of Liverpool, Liverpool, UK

Robert D. Steiner, MD
Professor, Pediatrics and Molecular and
Medical Genetics; Vice Chair for Research,
Department of Pediatrics, Doernbecher

Children's Hospital; Deputy Director,Oregon
Clinical and Translational Research Institute,
Oregon Health and Science University,
Portland, Oregon, USA

Ben Stenson, MD FRCPCH FRCPE
Consultant Neonatologist, Simpson Centre
for Reproductive Health, Royal Infirmary of
Edinburgh, Edinburgh, UK

Terence Stephenson, DM FRCP FRCPCH
Professor of Child Health; Dean,
Faculty of Medicine and Health
Sciences, Medical School, University of
Nottingham, Queen's Medical Centre,
Nottingham, UK

Stephen Stick, PhD MB BChir MRCP FRACP
Associate Professor, Department of
Respiratory Medicine, Princess Margaret
Hospital for Children, University of Western
Australia, Australia

Stephen Sturgiss, MD MRCOG
Consultant in Obstetrics and Fetal Medicine,
Royal Victoria Infirmary, Newcastle upon
Tyne, UK

David Sweet, MD FRCPCH
Consultant Neonatologist, Royal Maternity
Hospital, Belfast, Northern Ireland, UK

Angela E. Thomas, MB BS PhD FRCPE FRCPath
FRCPCH
Consultant Paediatric Haematologist,
Royal Hospital for Sick Children, Edinburgh,
UK

James Tooley, MB BS MRCPCH
Consultant in Neonatal Medicine, Neonatal
Intensive Care Unit, St Michael's Hospital,
Bristol, UK

E. Jane Tizard, MB BS, FRCP FRCPCH
Consultant Paediatric Nephrologist, Bristol
Royal Hospital for Children, Bristol, UK

Russell Viner, MB BS FRCPCH FRACP FRCP PhD
Consultant in Adolescent Medicine and
Endocrinology, Department of Paediatrics,
Middlesex Hospital, London, UK

Rachel Webster, BSc PhD DipRCPath
Clinical Scientist, Department of Clinical
Biochemistry, Birmingham Children's
Hospital, Birmingham, UK

Philip D. Welsby, FRCP(Ed)
Consultant in Infectious Diseases, Infectious
Disease Unit, Western General Hospital,
Edinburgh, UK

Johannes Wildhaber, MD PhD
Head, Division of Respiratory Medicine,
University Children's Hospital, Zürich,
Switzerland

Anthony F. Williams, BSc DPhil MB BS
FRCP FRCPCH
Reader in Child Nutrition, St George's,
University of London, London, UK

Bridget A. Wills, BmedSci BM BS MRCP DTM&H
Clinical Senior Lecturer in Paediatrics,
University of Oxford – Wellcome Trust
Clinical Research Unit, Ho Chi Minh City,
Vietnam

David C. Wilson, MD FRCP FRCPCH
Senior Lecturer in Paediatric
Gastroenterology and Nutrition, Child Life
and Health, Department of Reproductive
and Developmental Sciences, University of
Edinburgh, Edinburgh, UK

Rachael Wood, BSc MB ChB DCH MFH MFPH
Clinical Academic Fellow, Department
of Public Health Sciences and Centre for
International Public Health Policy University
of Edinburgh, Edinburgh, UK

Christopher Wren, MB ChB FRCP FRCPCH
Consultant Paediatric Cardiologist, Freeman
Hospital, Newcastle upon Tyne, UK

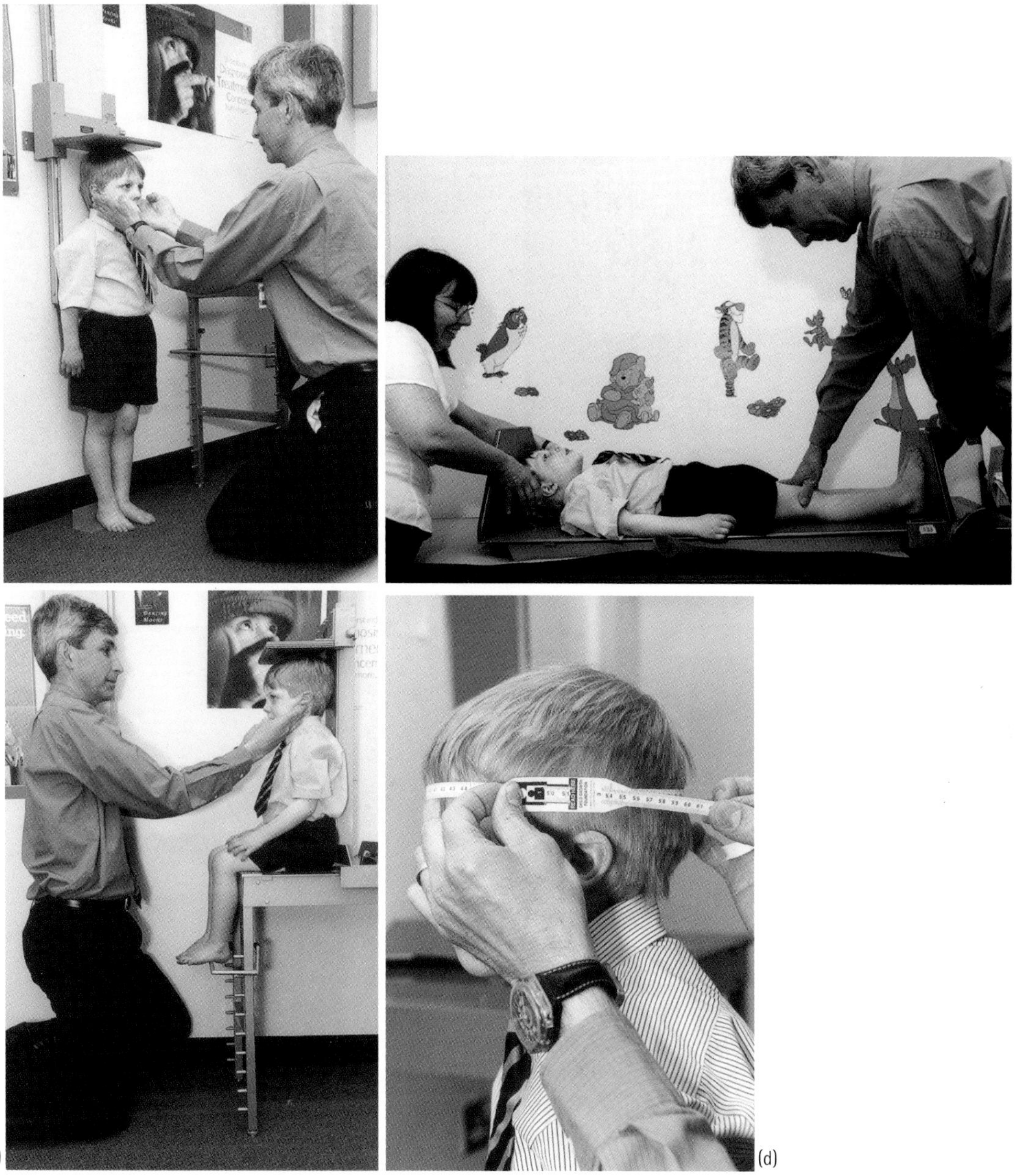

Plate 15.15 Correct positioning and technique for accurate measurement of (a) height, (b) supine length, (c) sitting height, (d) head circumference. For description see text (see p. 430).

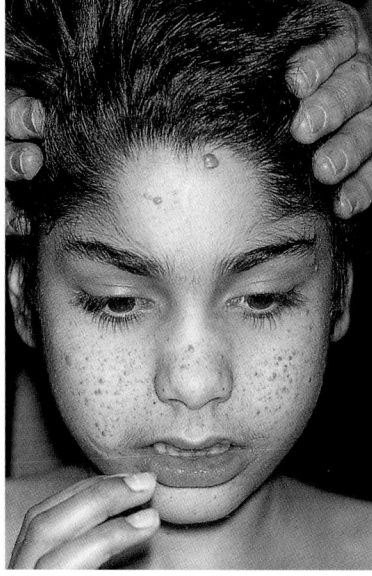

Plate 22.15 Tuberous sclerosis: adenoma sebaceum (see p. 839).

(a)

Plate 22.16 (a) Tuberous sclerosis: Shagreen patch (see p. 839).

(b)

Plate 22.16 (b) Tuberous sclerosis: depigmented patches (see p. 839).

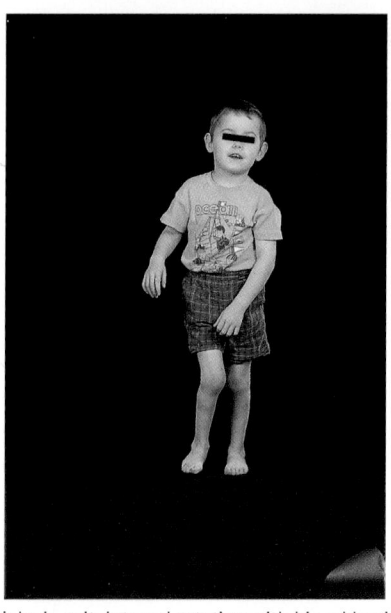

Plate 22.26 Diplegic gait. Internal rotation with hip adduction (see p. 890).

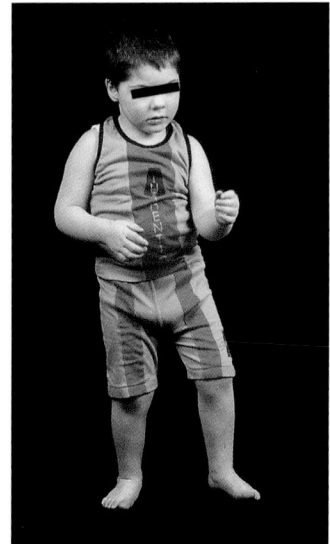

Plate 22.28 Ataxic 3-year-old child showing broad-based gait and elevated arms (see p. 891).

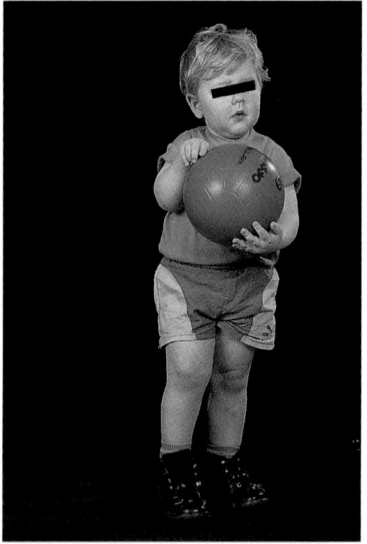

Plate 22.29 Spastic hemiplegia, right-sided – hyperpronated (see p. 892).

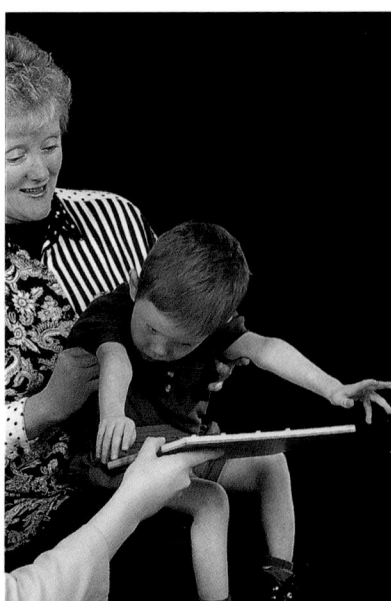

Plate 22.30 A child with dyskinetic cerebral palsy, showing uncontrolled patterns of movement and flaccid trunk, while attempting to reach out (see p. 892).

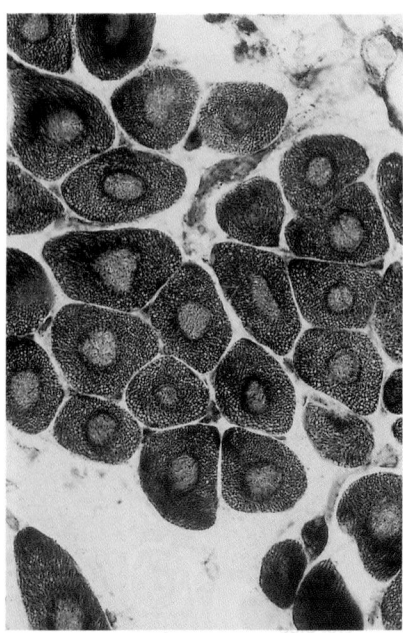

Plate 22.32 Central core disease: the cores show absence of staining with NADH (see p. 910).

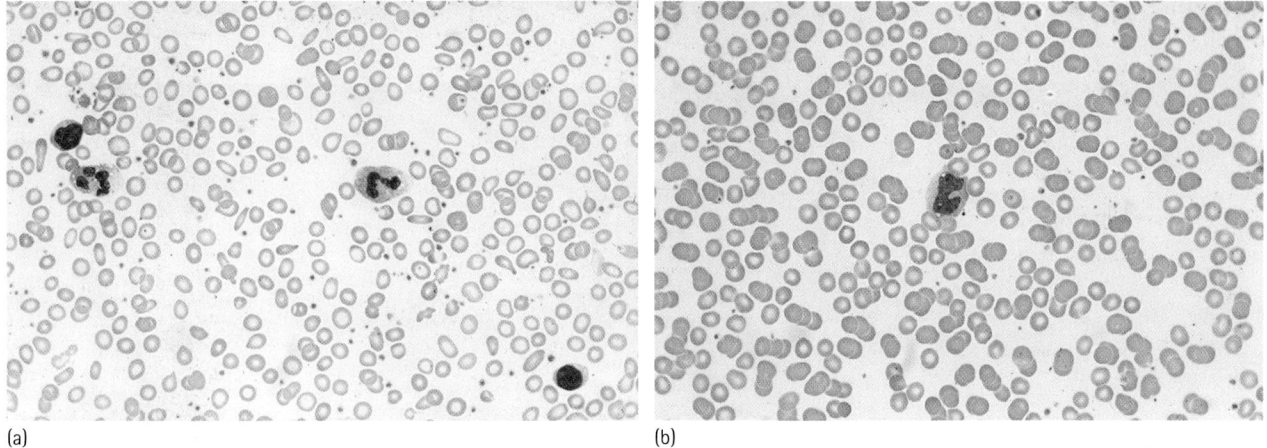

(a)　　　　　　　　　　　　　　　　　　　　　　　　　　(b)

Plate 23.4　Peripheral blood appearances in severe hypochromic iron deficiency with microcytic red cells (a) compared with a normal film (b) (same magnification) (see p. 962).

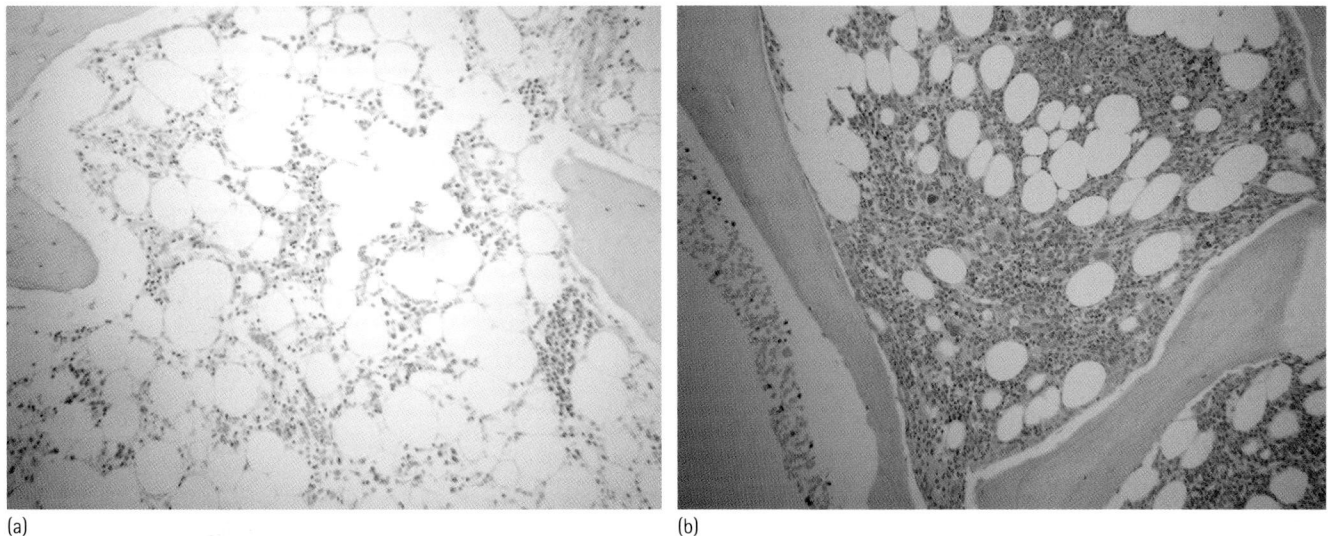

(a)　　　　　　　　　　　　　　　　　　　　　　　　　　(b)

Plate 23.7　The appearances of aplastic bone marrow (a) with a normal marrow (b) for comparison (trephine biopsy) (see p. 965).

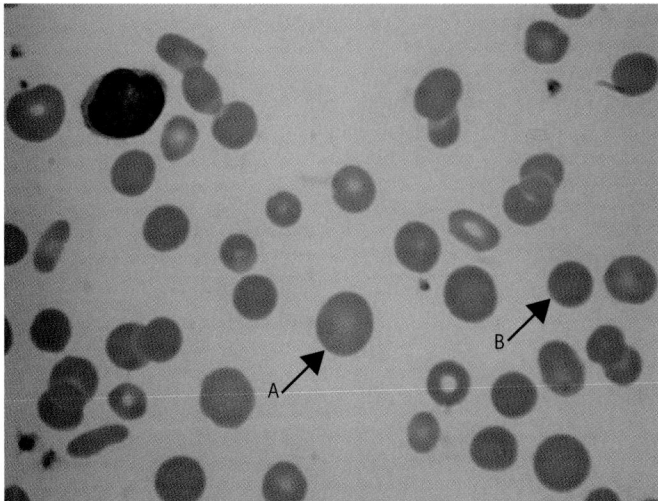

Plate 23.10　Peripheral blood appearance in spherocytosis with spherocytes and polychromasia. A, polychromatic cell; B, microspherocyte (see p. 967).

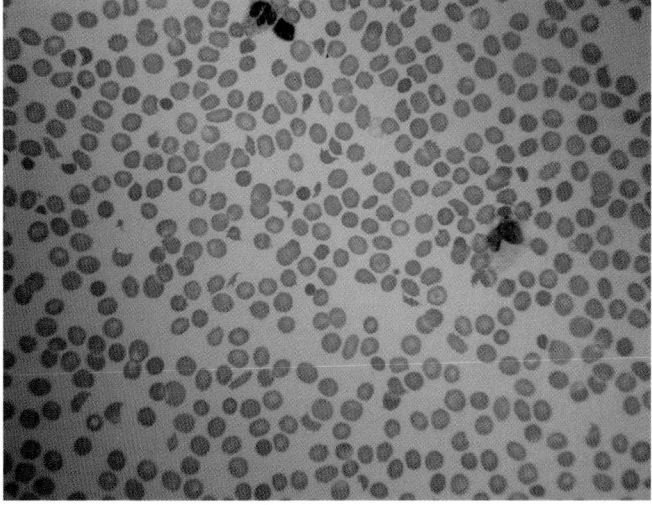

Plate 23.12　Red cell appearances in red cell fragmentation syndromes (see p. 969).

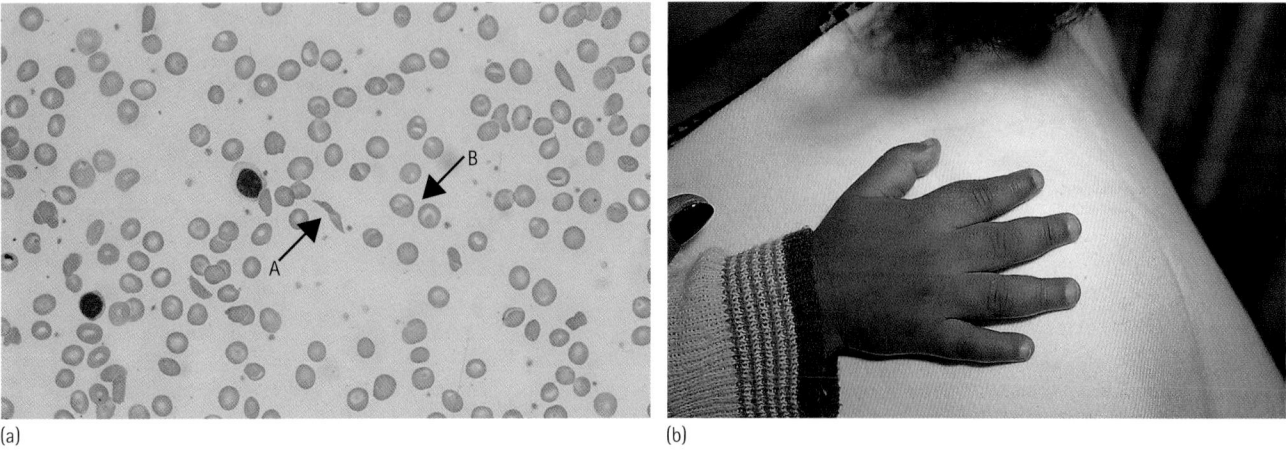

(a)   (b)

Plate 23.15 (a) Peripheral blood appearance in homozygous sickle cell disease with target cells, polychromasia and distorted red cells (A, sickle cell; B target cell). (b) Swelling of the fingers from dactylitis, a common mode of presentation of sickle cell disease in late infancy. (From Lissauer & Clayden 2001[35] with permission) (see p. 971).

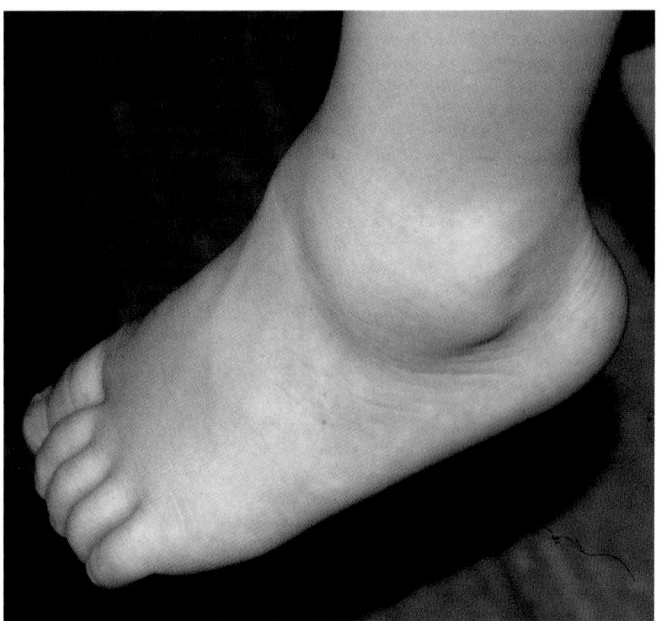

Plate 23.20 Acute ankle hemarthrosis in a child with severe hemophilia A (see p. 979).

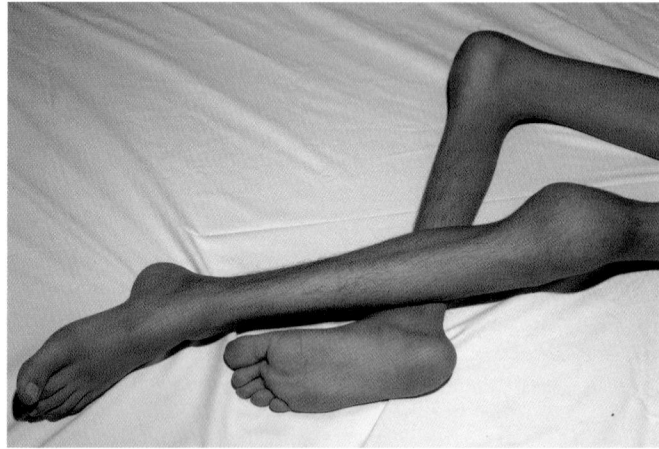

Plate 23.21 (a) Severe hemophilia in an adolescent showing fixed flexion of right knee, marked arthropathy of left knee and muscle wasting (see p. 980).

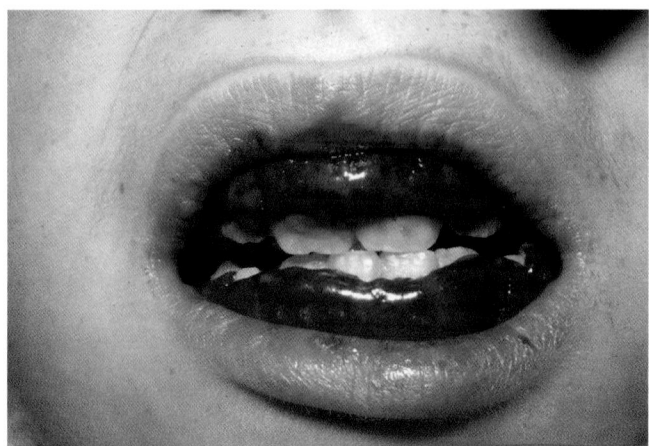

Plate 23.26 Acute monocytic leukemia causing gum infiltration (see p. 985).

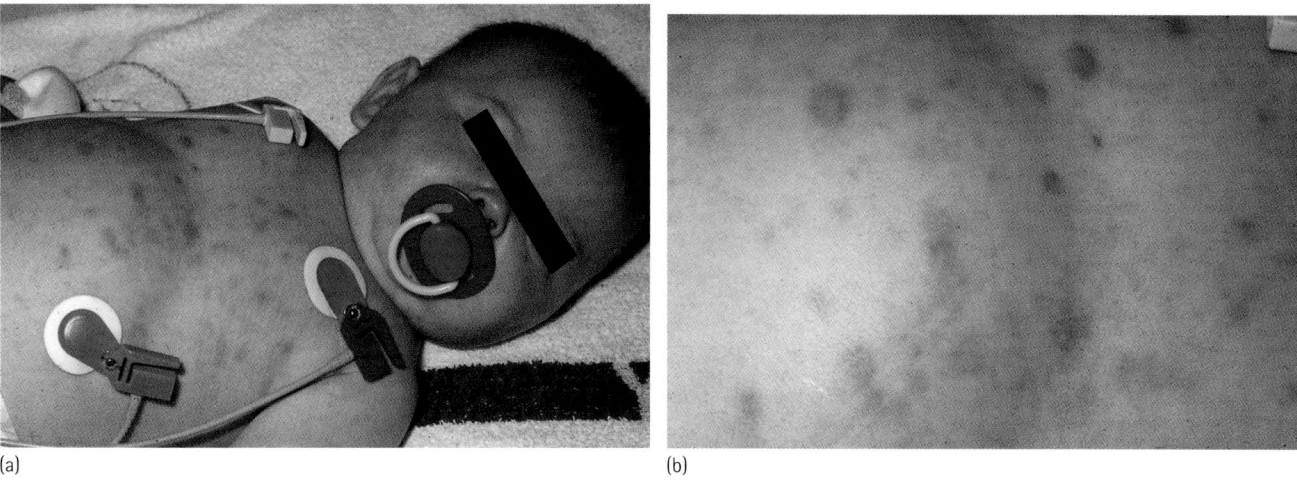

(a)

(b)

Plate 23.27 Skin infiltration in an infant with acute monocytic leukemia (see p. 985).

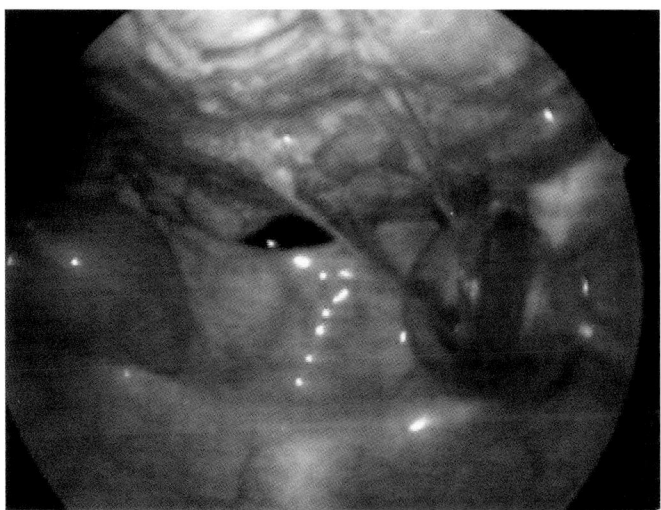

Plate 25.5 Rudimentary uterine horns in a girl with Rokitansky–Kuster–Hauser syndrome (adhesions surrounding the left horn) (see p. 1043).

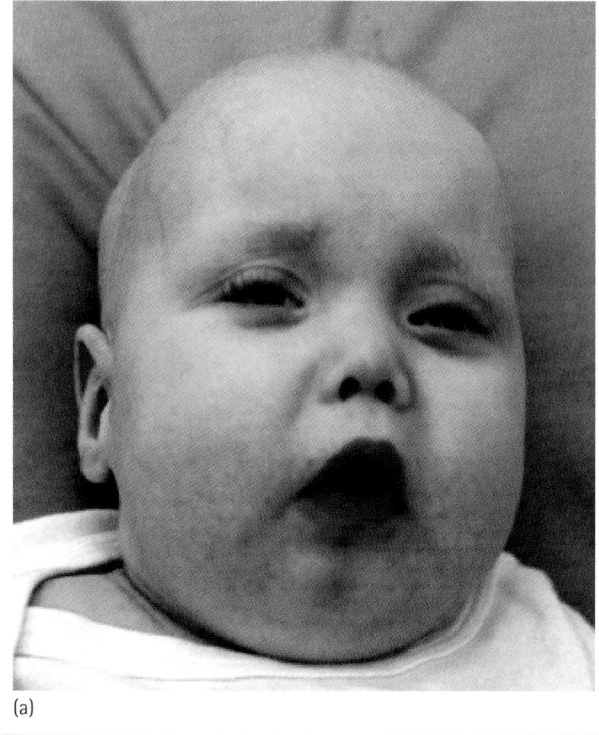

(a)

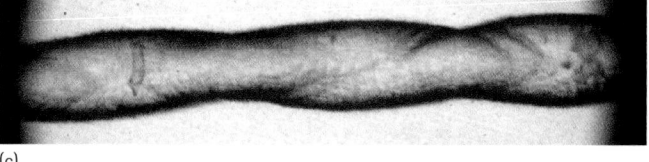

(c)

Plate 26.42 Features and typical hair of Menkes syndrome (see p. 1125).

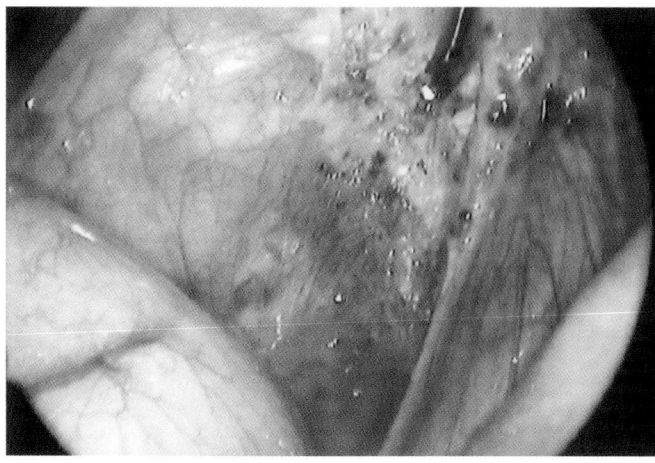

Plate 25.7 Extensive endometriosis involving the right uterosacral ligament and pouch of Douglas in an adolescent girl (see p. 1044).

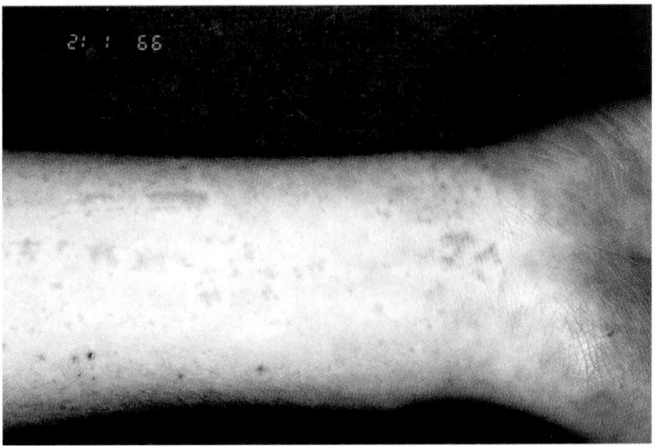

Plate 29.32 Rash of systemic juvenile idiopathic arthritis (see p. 1408).

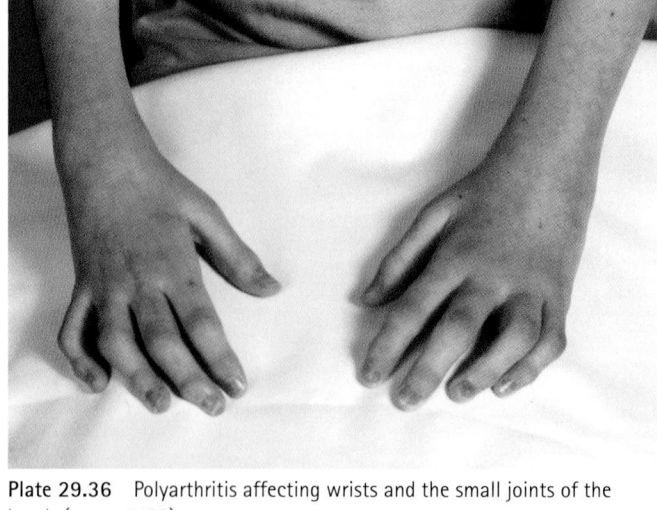

Plate 29.36 Polyarthritis affecting wrists and the small joints of the hands (see p. 1409).

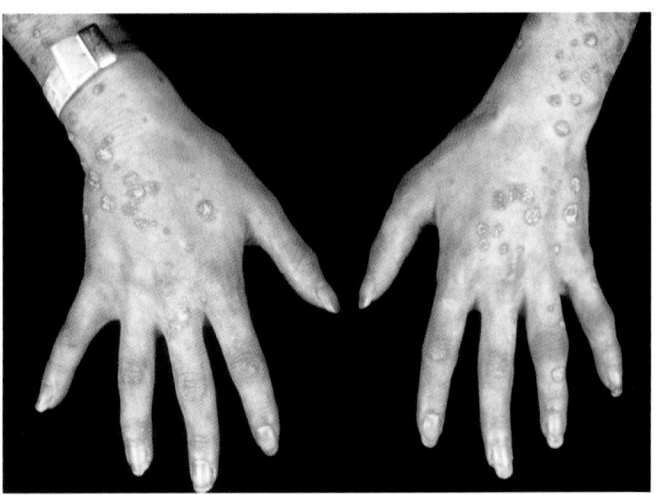

Plate 29.37 Psoriatic arthritis (see p. 1409).

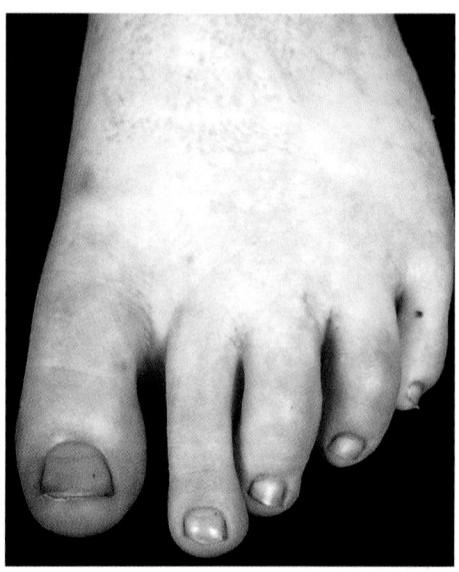

Plate 29.38 Dactylitis – swelling of third and fourth toes (see p. 1410).

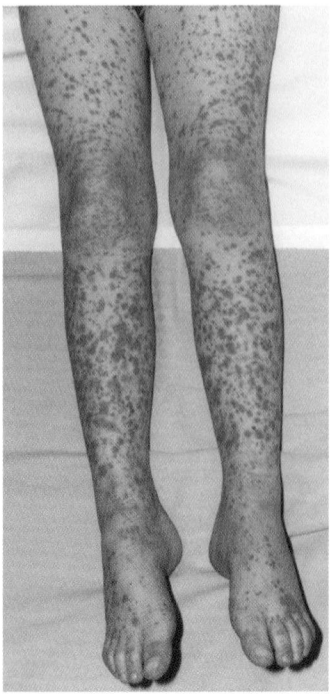

Plate 29.53 Rash of Henoch–Schönlein purpura (see p. 1424).

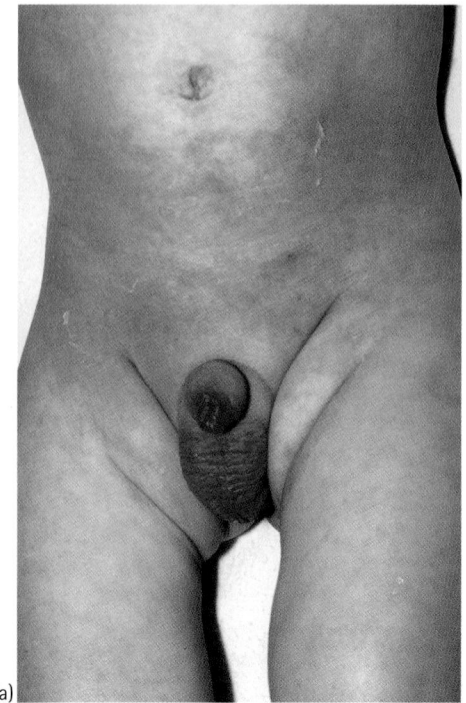

(a)

Plate 29.54 (a) Kawasaki disease: typical erythematous groin rash with peeling; (see p. 1425).

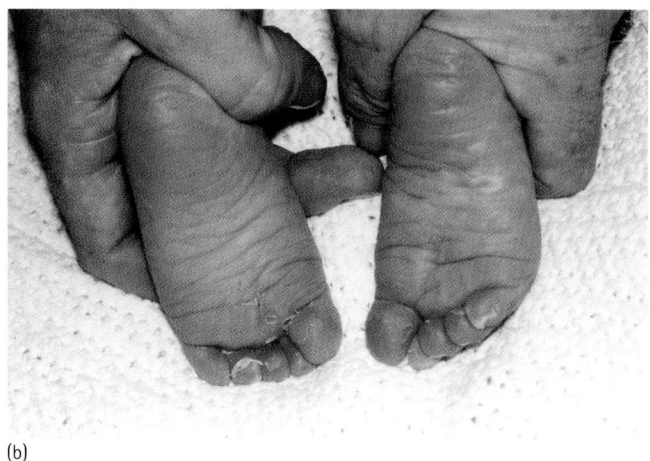

(b)

Plate 29.54 (b) Kawasaki disease: peeling of digits (see p. 1425).

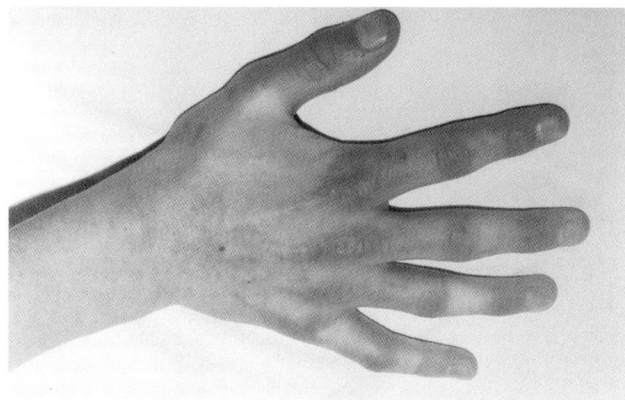

(a)

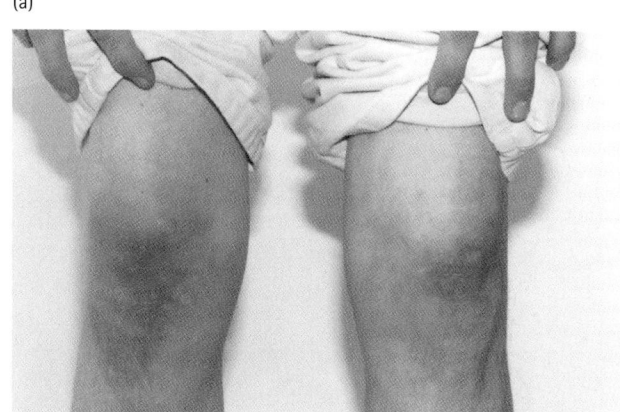

(b)

Plate 29.58 Typical rash of juvenile dermatomyositis with erythema over: (a) extensor aspects of metacarpophalangeal and proximal interphalangeal joints; (b) knees (see p. 1429).

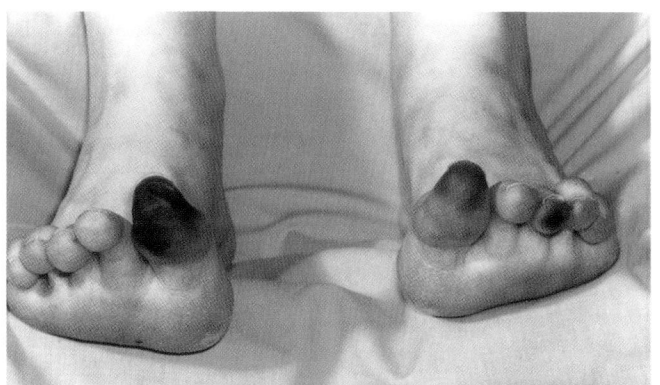

Plate 29.55 Gangrene of several toes in polyarteritis nodosa (see p. 1425).

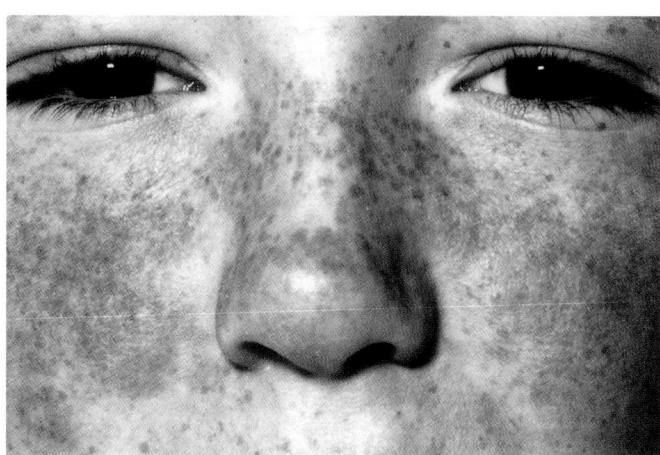

Plate 29.57 Typical facial rash in systemic lupus erythematosus – crossing the bridge of the nose and sparing the nasolabial folds (see p. 1427).

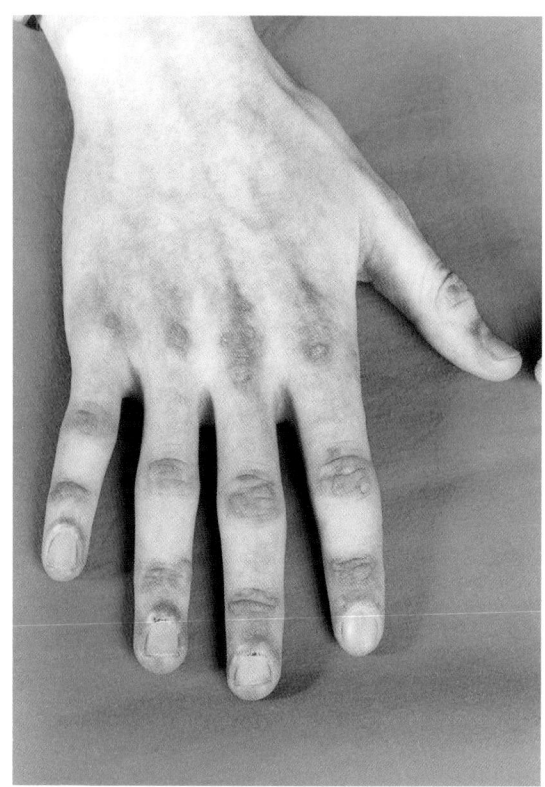

Plate 29.59 Juvenile dermatomyositis showing Gottron's papules and typical nailfold changes (see p. 1429).

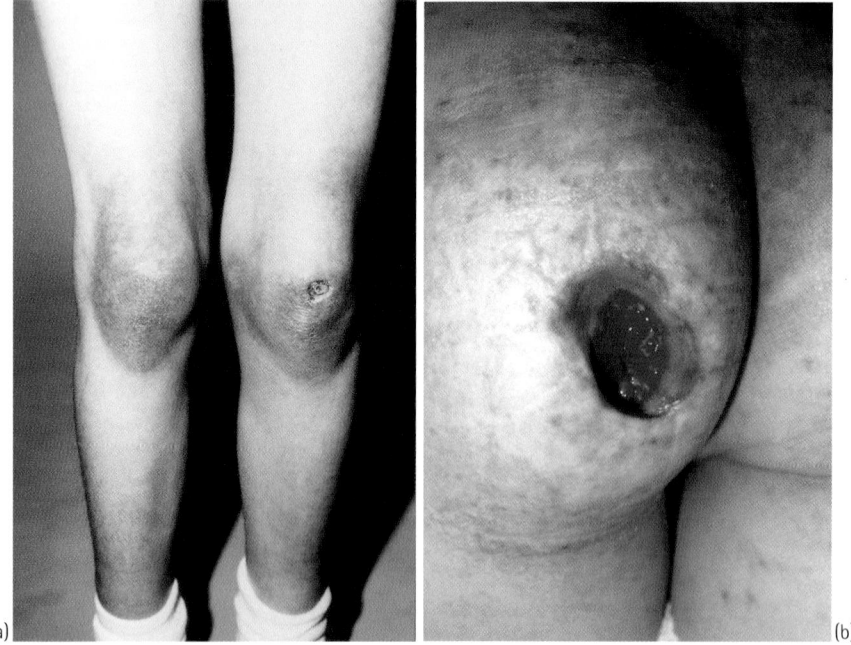

(a)　(b)

Plate 29.61　(a & b) Ulcerative vasculopathy in juvenile dermatomyositis (see p. 1430) .

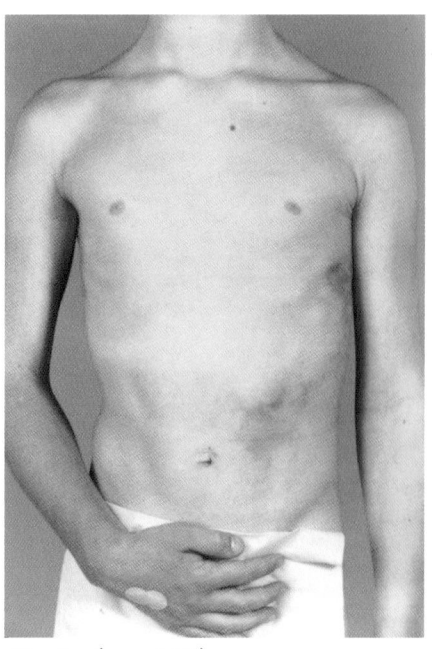

Plate 29.64　Morphea (see p. 1432).

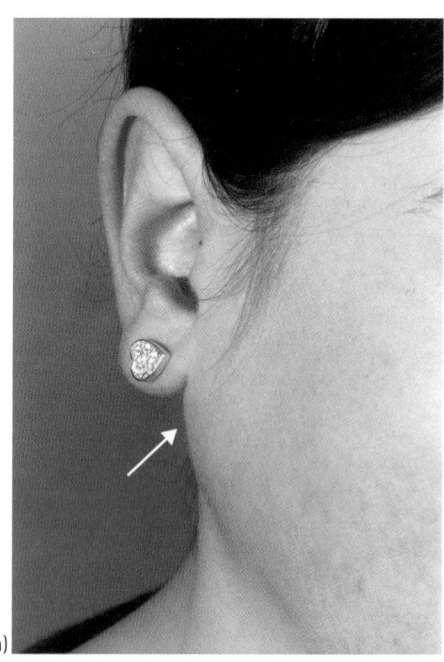

(a)

Plate 29.68　Sjögren syndrome: (a) parotid swelling (see p. 1434).

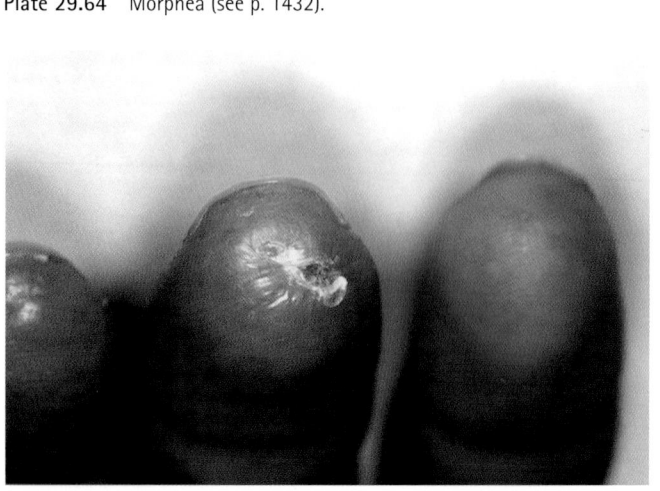

Plate 29.67　Digital pitting scars in systemic sclerosis (see p. 1433).

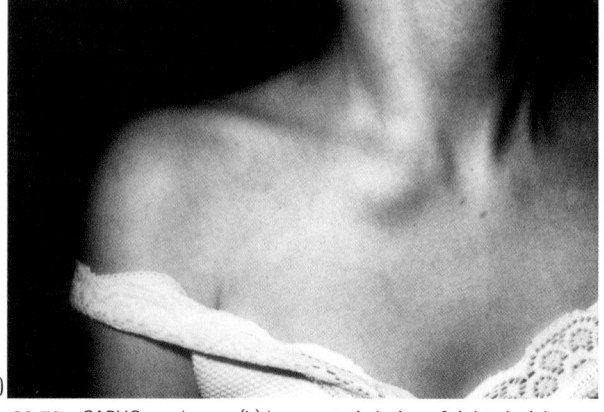

(b)

Plate 29.70　SAPHO syndrome: (b) hyperostotic lesion of right clavicle (see p. 1435).

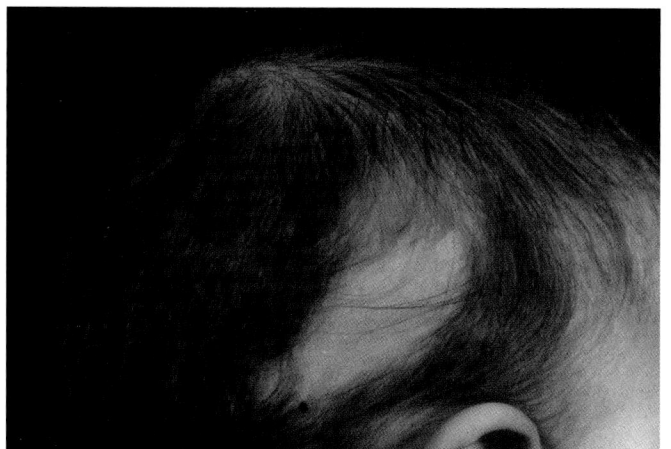

Plate 30.4 Sebaceous nevus (see p. 1450).

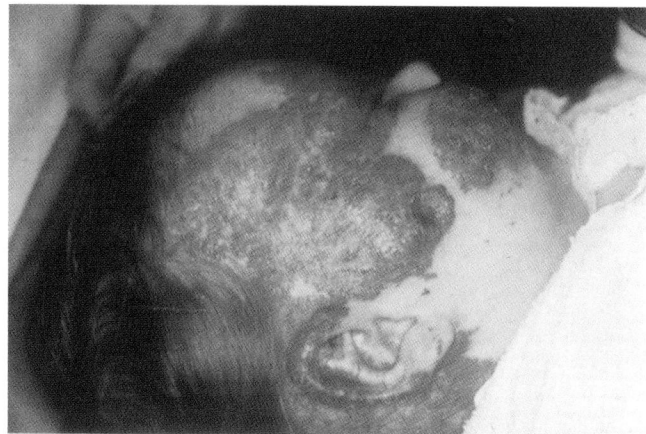

Plate 30.5 Capillary (strawberry) hemangioma (see p. 1450).

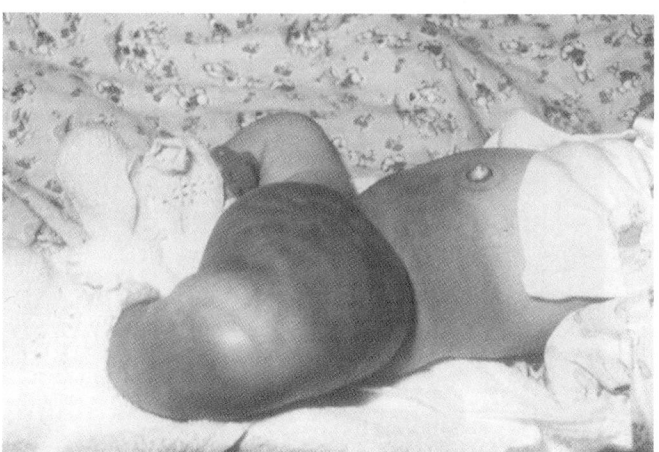

Plate 30.6 Kasabach – Merritt syndrome (see p. 1451).

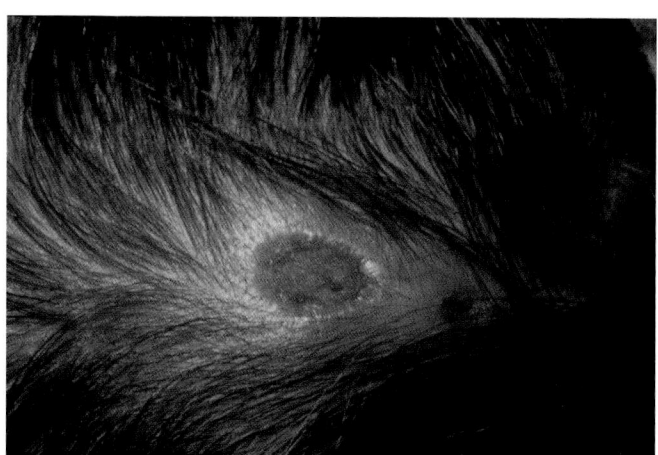

Plate 30.7 Aplasia cutis (see p. 1452).

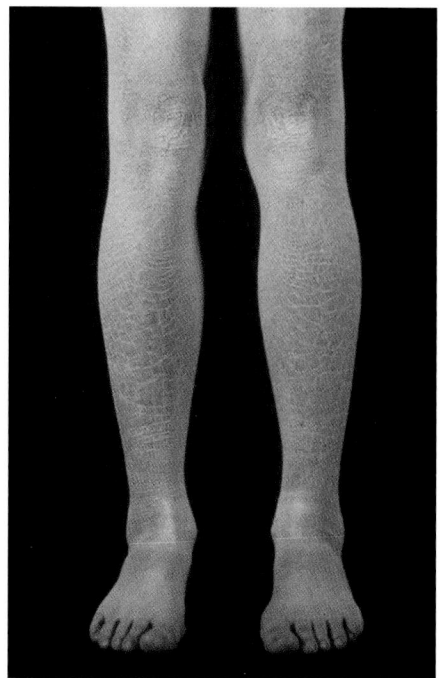

Plate 30.8 X-linked ichthyosis (see p. 1452).

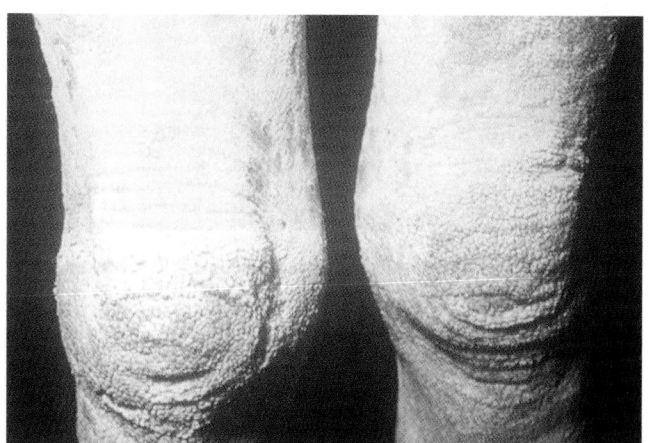

Plate 30.9 Lamellar ichthyosis (congenital ichthyosiform erythroderma) (see p. 1452).

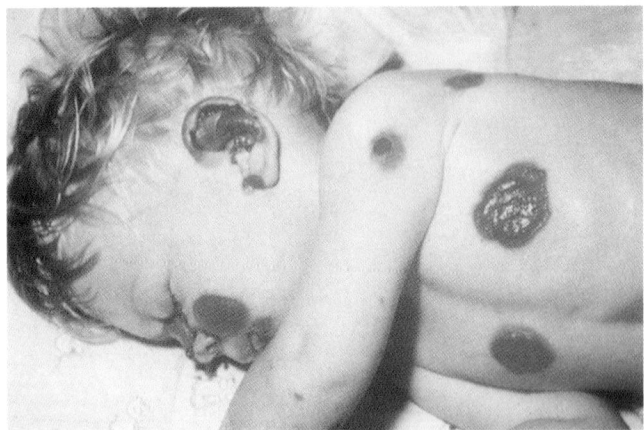

Plate 30.11 Junctional epidermolysis bullosa (see p. 1455).

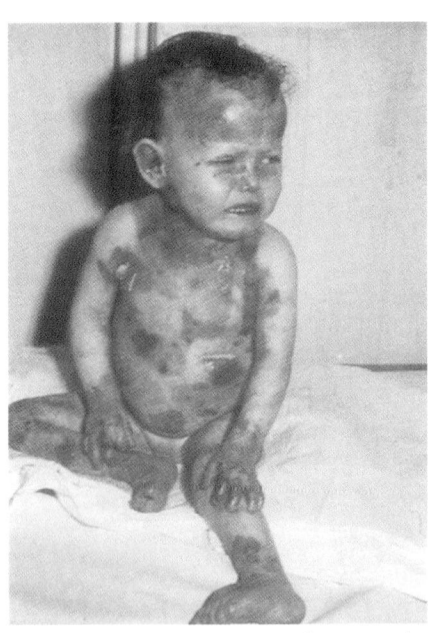

Plate 30.13 Dystrophic epidermolysis bullosa (see p. 1455).

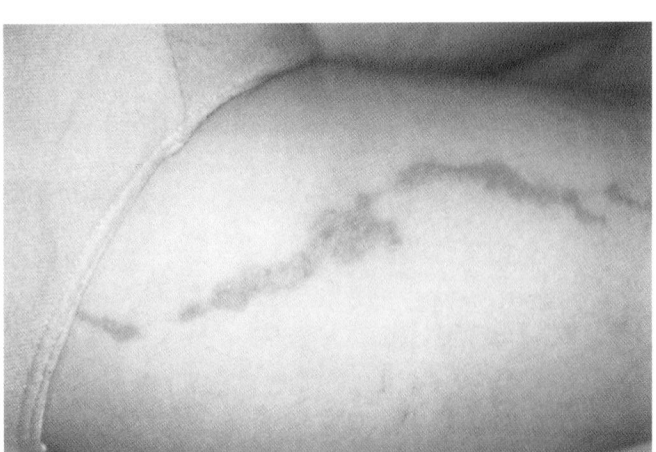

Plate 30.18 Incontinentia pigmenti: pigmented stage (see p. 1458).

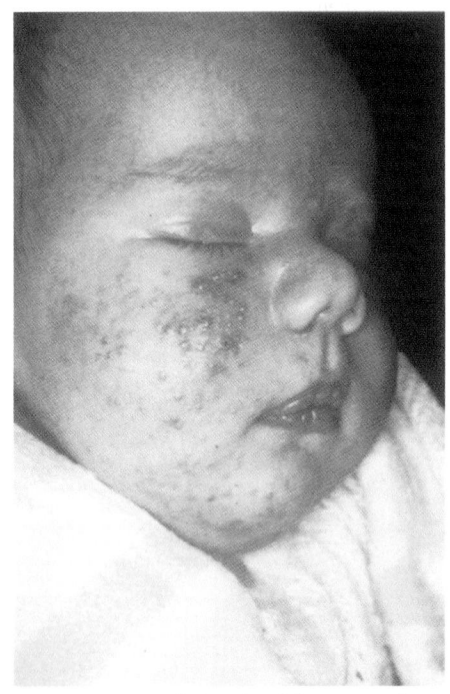

Plate 30.22 Pustular miliaria (prickly heat) (see p. 1461).

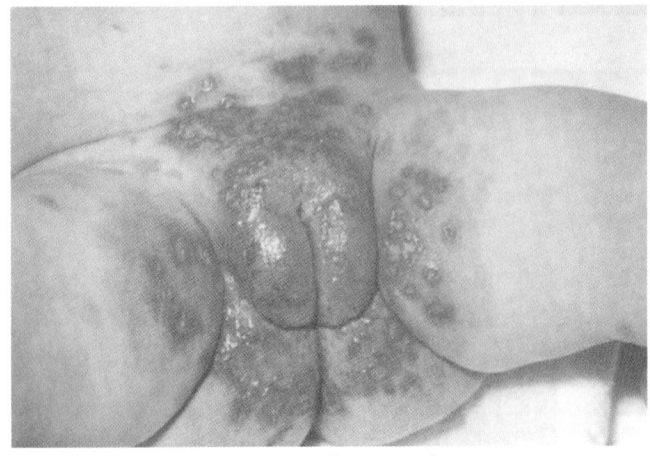

Plate 30.25 Genital herpes simplex (see p. 1461).

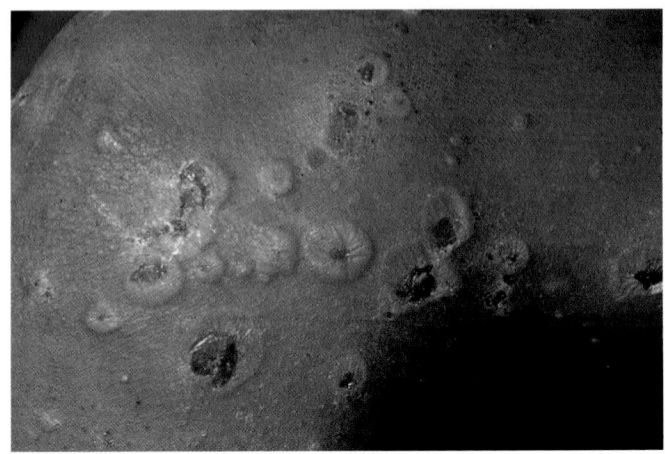

Plate 30.33 Bullous impetigo (see p. 1464).

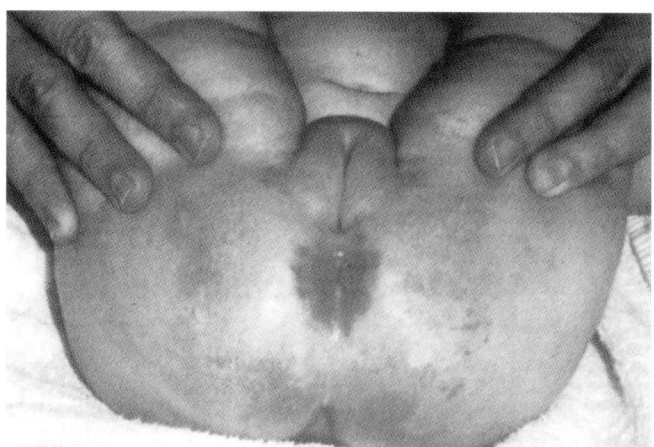

Plate 30.34 Perianal streptococcal disease (see p. 1465).

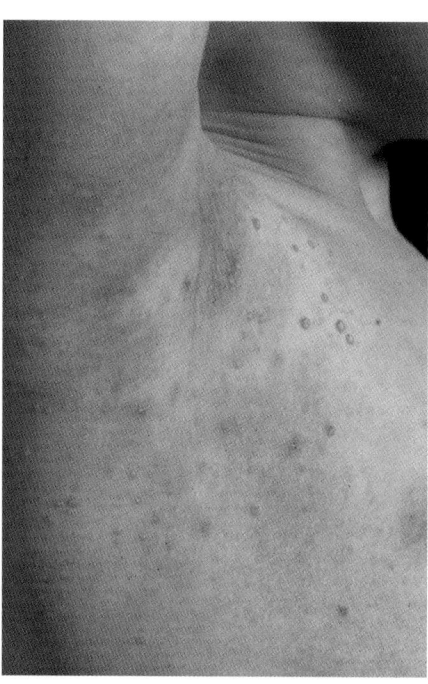

Plate 30.39 Scabies (see p. 1467).

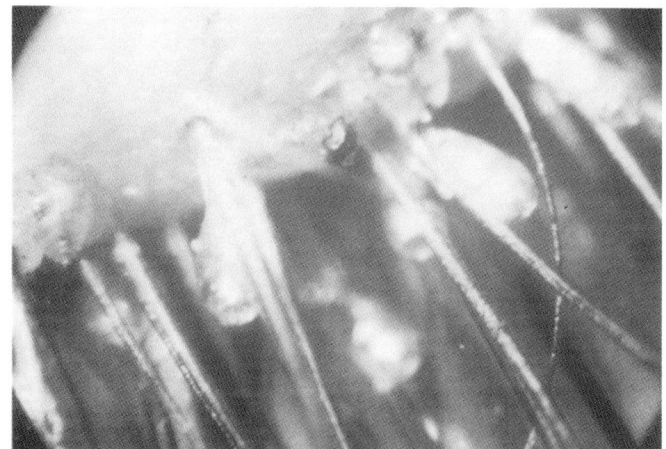

Plate 30.40 Pediculosis of eyelid (see p. 1468).

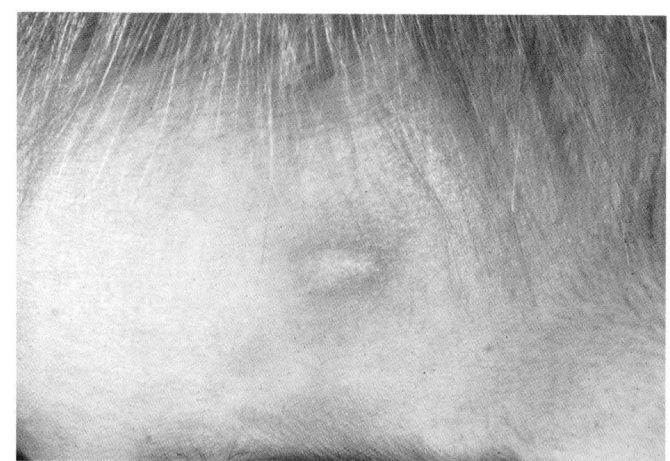

Plate 30.41 Mastocytoma (see p. 1469).

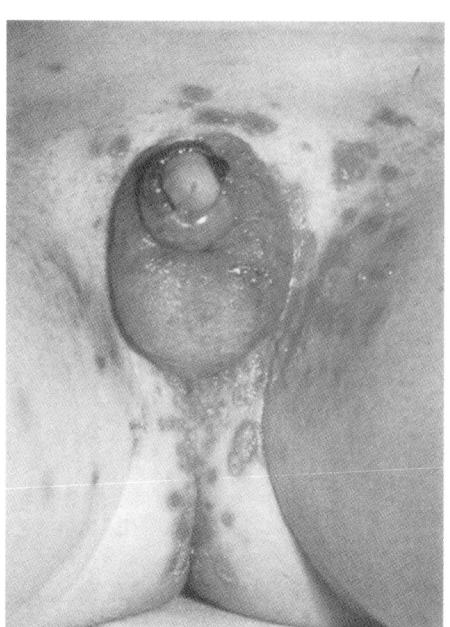

Plate 30.45 Chronic bullous disease of childhood (see p. 1471).

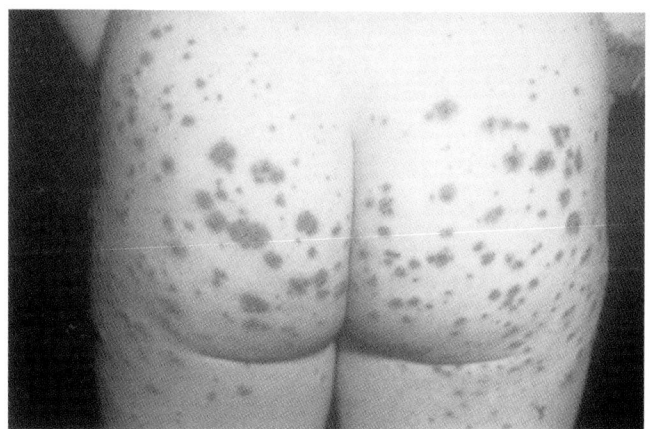

Plate 30.46 Henoch – Schönlein purpura (see p. 1471).

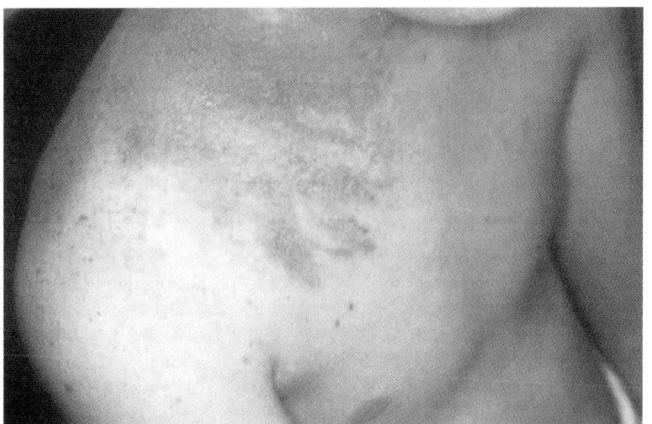

Plate 30.50 Plant (*Rhus*) dermatitis (see p. 1473).

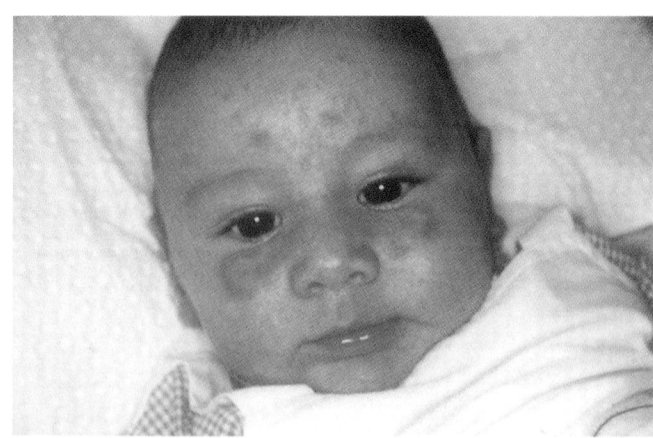

Plate 30.52 Neonatal lupus erythematosus (see p. 1474).

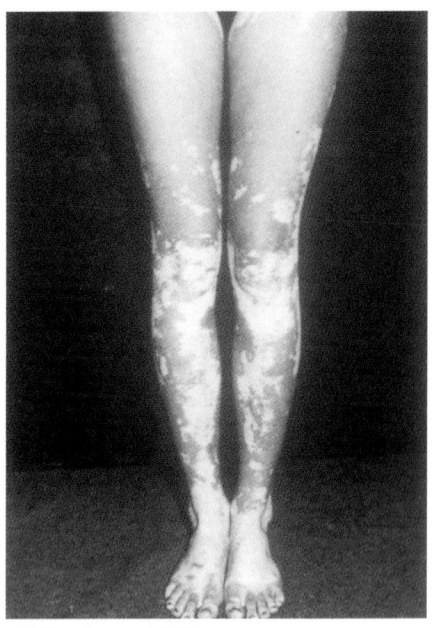

Plate 30.53 Vitiligo (see p. 1478).

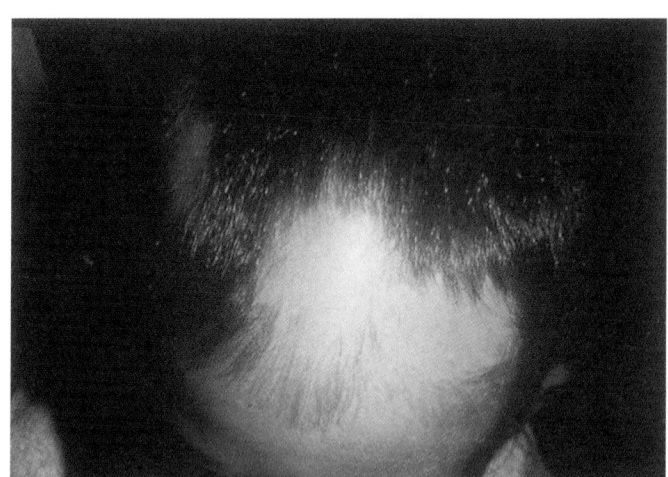

Plate 30.54 Alopecia areata (see p. 1478).

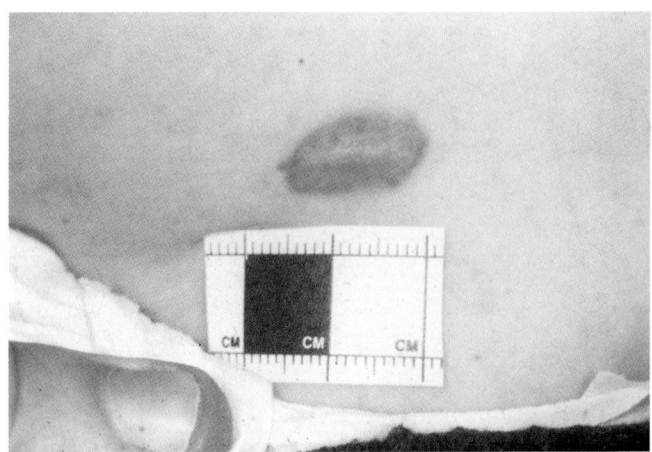

Plate 30.56 Juvenile xanthogranuloma (XTG) (see p. 1478).

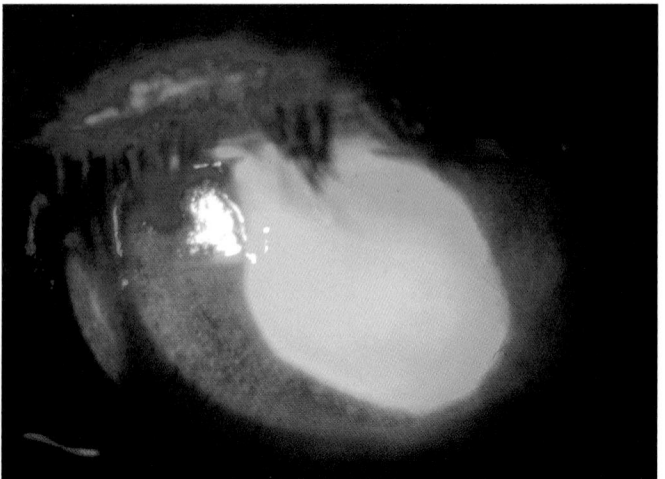

Plate 31.11 Yellow/green fluorescein staining of an area of cornea abrasion visualized using blue light (see p. 1486).

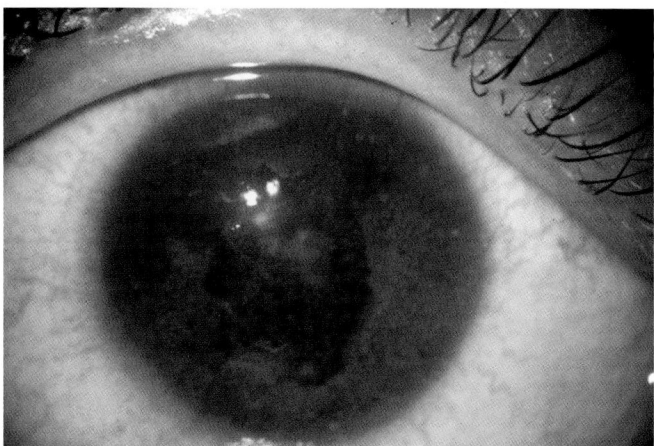

Plate 31.24 Aniridia. No iris tissue is seen. There is fibrovascular pannus covering the peripheral cornea in this case (see p. 1492).

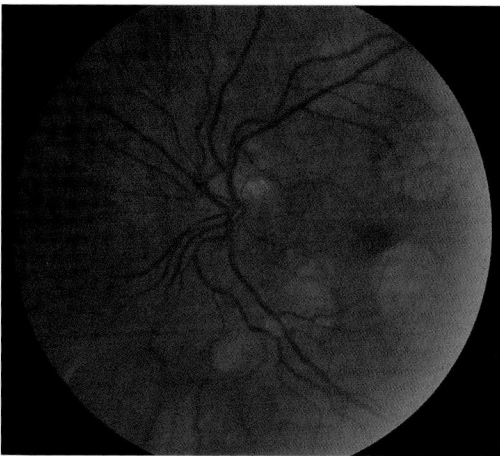

Plate 31.25 Hypoplastic disc. Optic nerve hypoplasia. The optic disc is anatomically very small in this case, with severely reduced vision (see p. 1493).

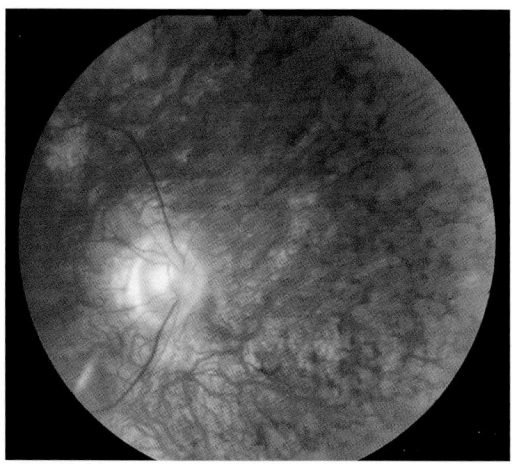

Fig. 31.26 Retinitis pigmentosa. Typical 'bone spicule' pigmentation is seen in the mid periphery of the fundus (see p. 1494).

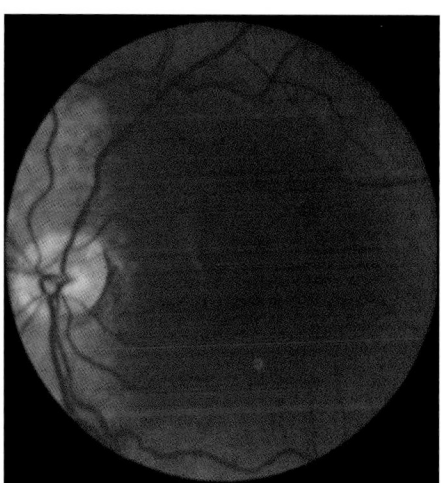

Plate 31.27 Retinal cone dystrophy with typical 'bull's eye' pigmentation at the center of the macula (see p. 1494).

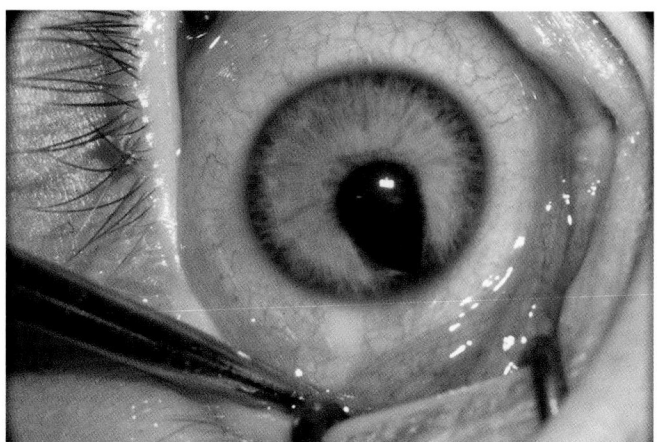

Plate 31.33 Coloboma of the inferior iris (see p. 1496).

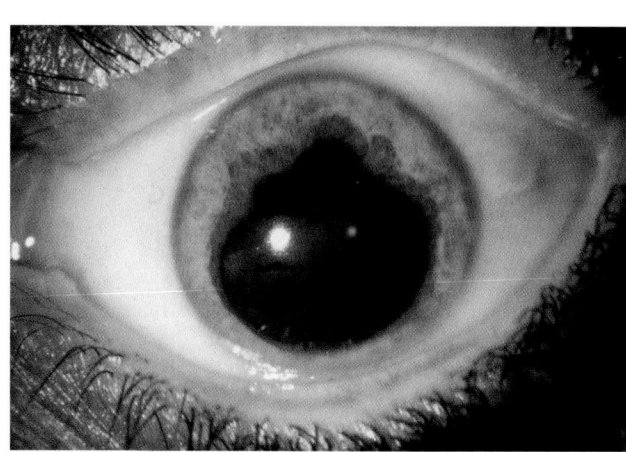

Plate 31.35 Iritis. The pupil has been dilated and adhesions between the iris and lens (posterior synechiae) are seen (see p. 1497).

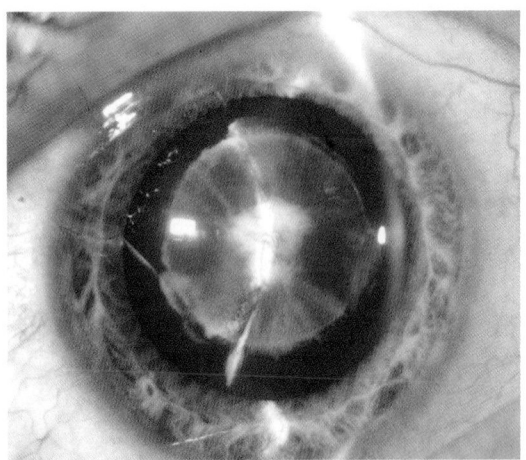

Plate 31.36   Congenital cataract. This is a partial, lamellar cataract with relatively good vision. Surgery in infancy was not needed in this case (see p. 1498).

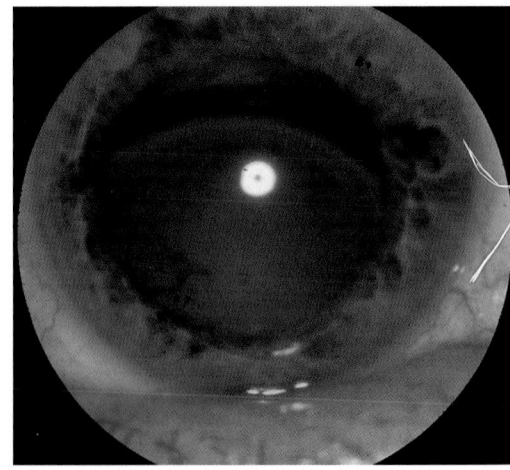

Plate 31.37   Subluxed lens (see p. 1498).

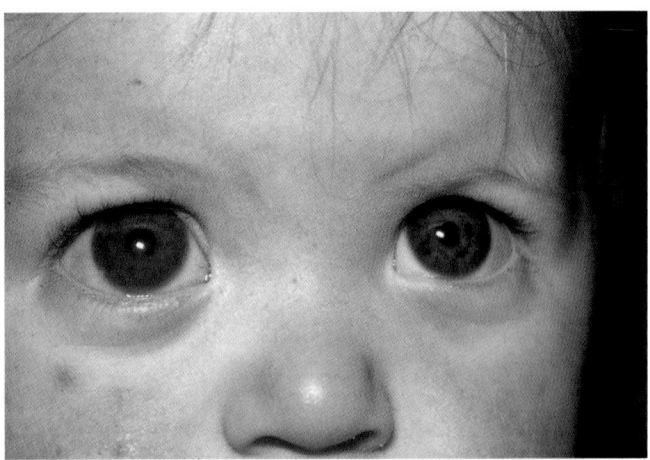

Plate 31.38   Congenital glaucoma. Note enlarged corneas. This child had goniotomy surgery performed in infancy, which satisfactorily controlled the intraocular pressures (see p. 1499).

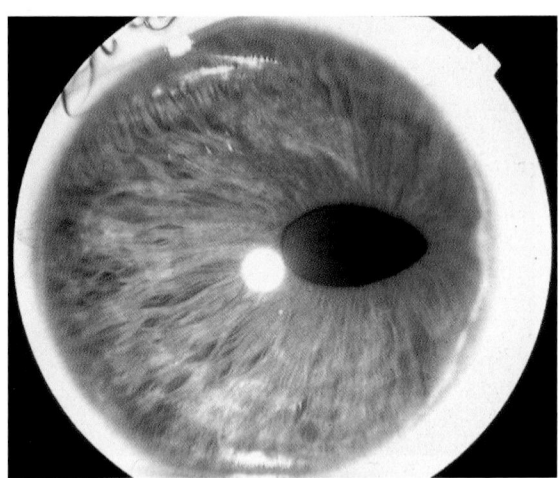

Plate 31.39   Reiger syndrome. Note posterior embryotoxon and abnormal pupil shape and position (corectopia) (see p. 1499).

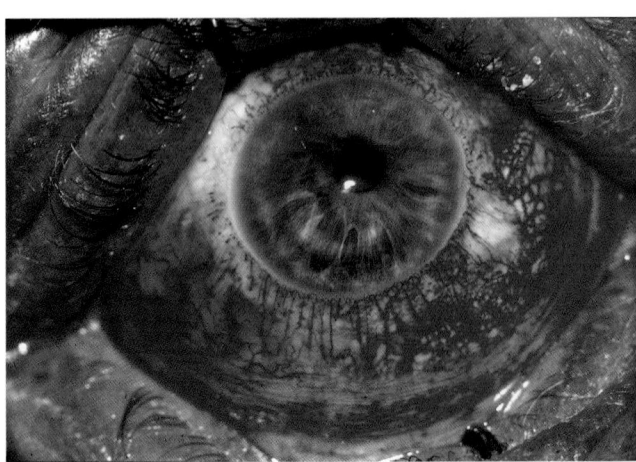

Plate 31.40   Sturge–Weber syndrome. Note eyelid port wine stain, and abnormal scleral blood vessels (see p. 1499).

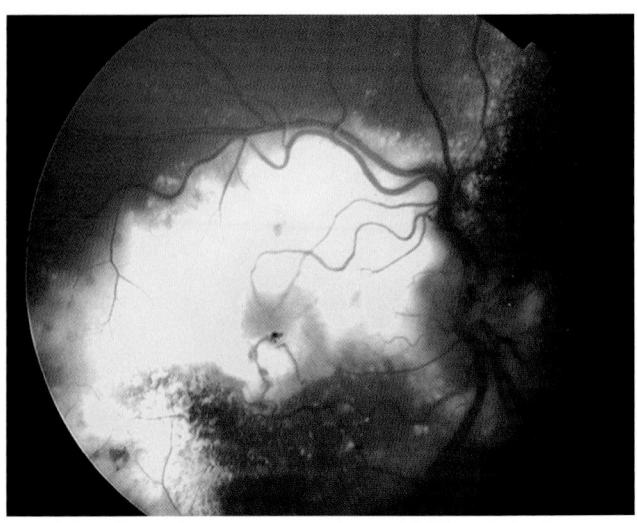

Plate 31.41   Coats disease. Massive subretinal lipid exudation is seen at the macula, with severely reduced visual acuity (see p. 1499).

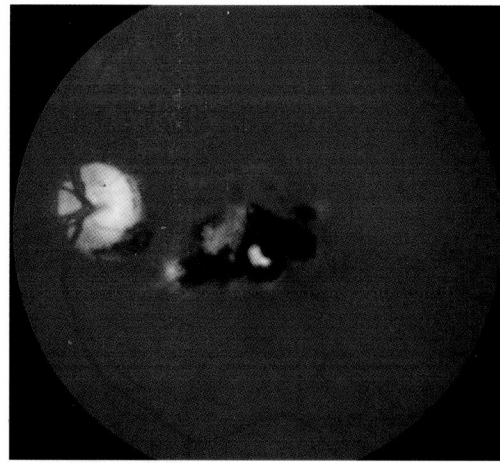

Plate 31.44 Toxoplasmosis. Pigmented scar at macula. No active inflammation present (see p. 1501).

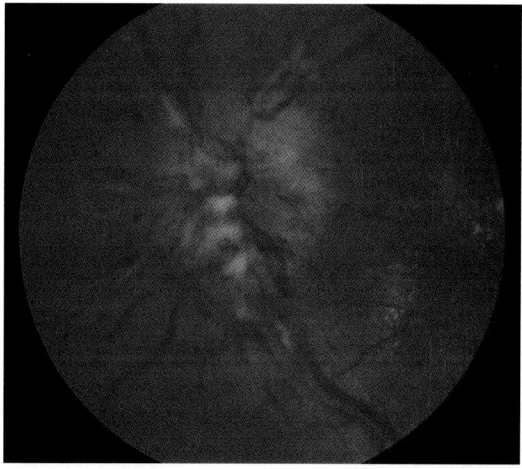

Plate 31.45 Severe papilledema with hemorrhages and exudates (see p. 1501).

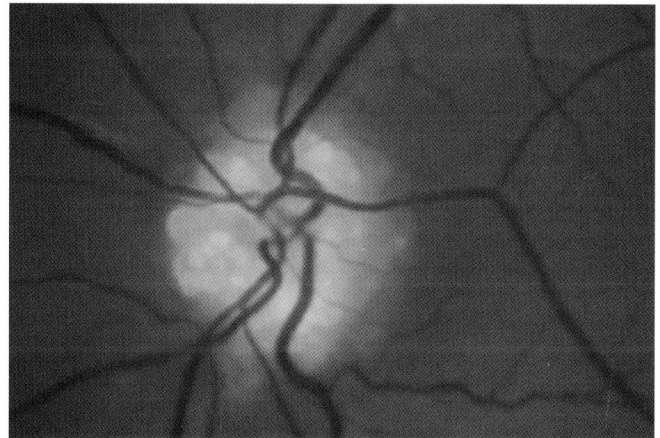

Plate 31.47 Optic disc drusen (see p. 1502).

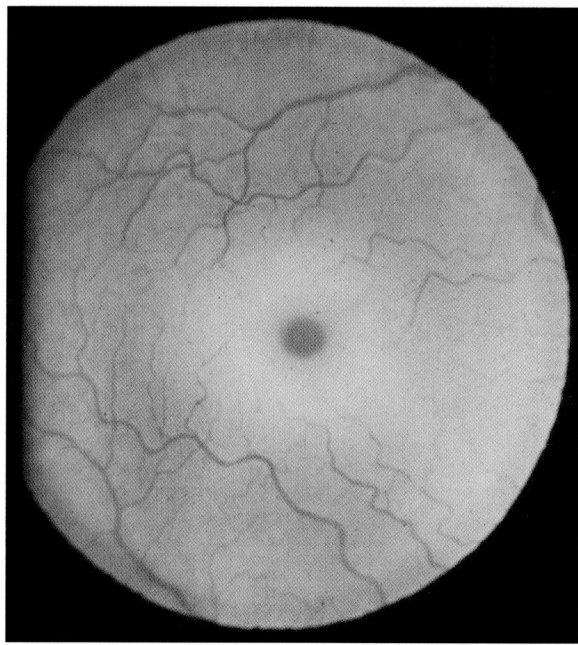

Plate 31.48 Cherry red spot due to Tay–Sachs disease (see p. 1502).

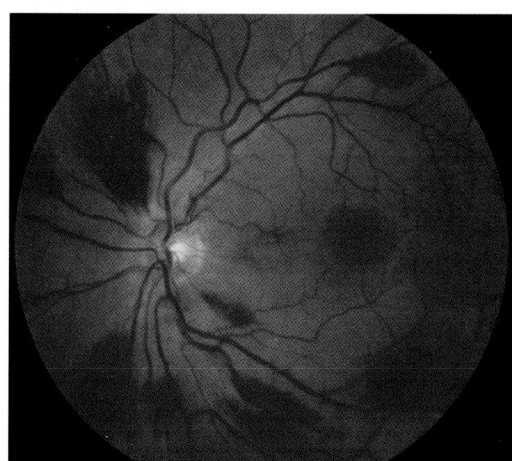

Plate 31.49 Retinal hemorrhages related to leukemia (see p. 1503).

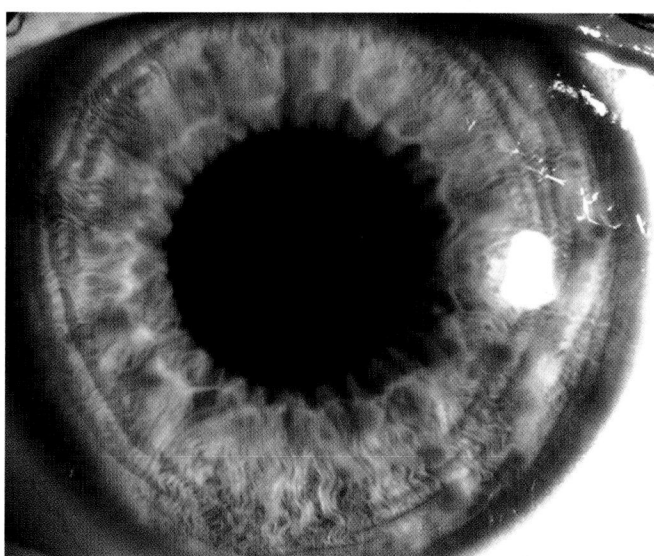

Plate 31.50 Lisch nodules of the iris. Multiple pigmented nodules are easily visualized against the background of a lightly pigmented iris in this case (see p. 1503).

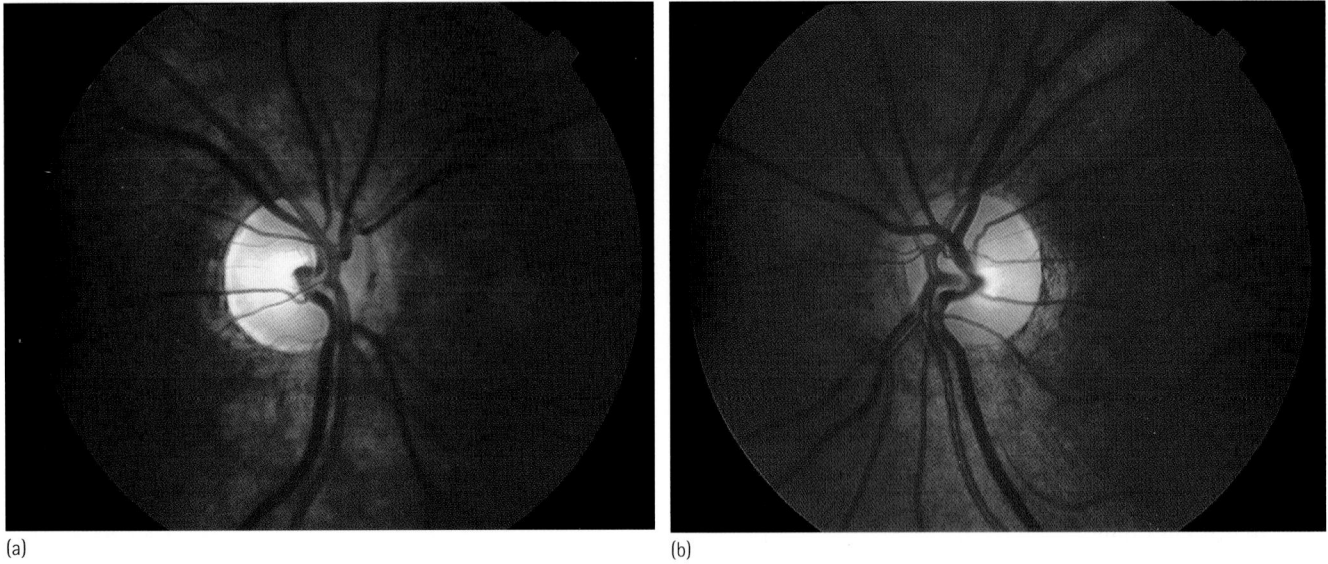

(a)   (b)

Plate 31.51   (a) Right optic disc showing pallor on the temporal side. MRI scan showed optic nerve glioma. (b) Normal left optic disc (see p. 1504).

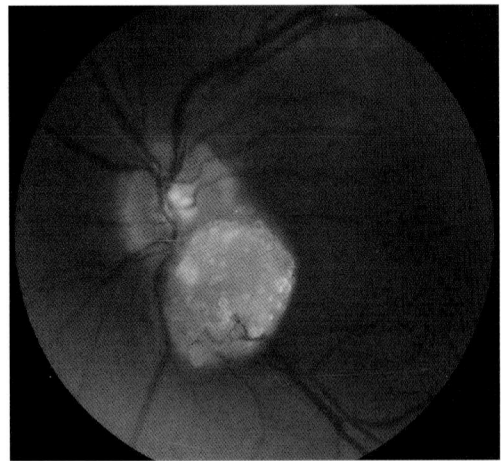

Plate 31.52   Large multinodular retinal hamartoma adjacent to optic disc in a case of tuberous sclerosis (see p. 1504).

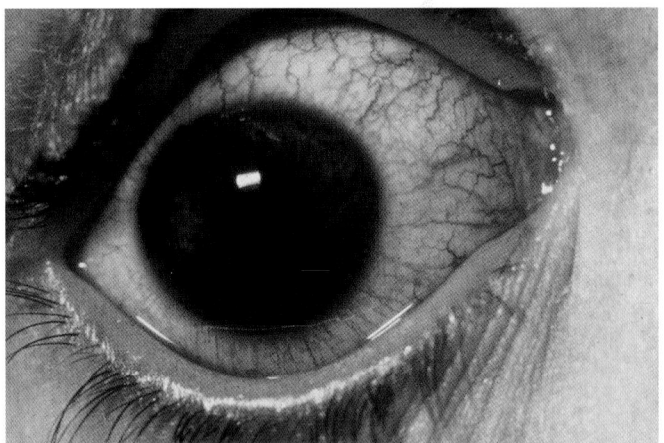

Plate 31.53   Hyphema. Blood in the anterior chamber obscures the iris (see p. 1504).

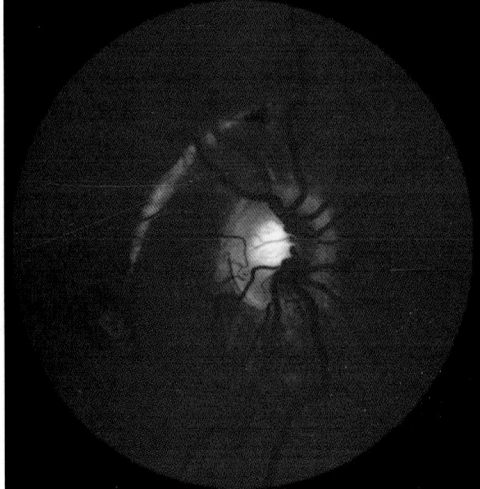

Fig. 31.54   Choroidal rupture. Blunt force has caused a curved tear in Bruch's membrane deep to the retinal pigment epithelium. There is additional pigment scarring at the macula. (see p. 1504).

Section 1
Foundations of health and practice

1

Evidence-based child health

Rosalind L Smyth

INTRODUCTION

Evidence-based pediatrics and child health has been defined as 'the integration of clinical information obtained from a patient, with the best evidence available from clinical research and experience and the application of this knowledge to the prevention, diagnosis or management of disease in that child'.[1] This definition has been adapted from an earlier one by Sackett and colleagues[2] who have consistently argued that there is an art to medicine, as well as objective scientific knowledge, and that both are essential to the clinical encounter. Within the classical clinical method, as taught in medical schools and beyond, the diagnostic approach starts with a history, leads on to a clinical examination and utilizes, if required, special investigations. In the process of history taking, the clinician integrates the case specific features of the patient's own story with their accumulated case expertise. For example, the differential diagnosis and mode of history taking in two children presenting with cough will be very different, if in one, it is elicited that she has experienced fever and night sweats and is recently returned from India, and in the other, recurrent wheeze and hay fever are accompanying symptoms. In taking a history, one constantly updates the differential diagnoses and redirects one's questioning as each new item of information is elicited. Indeed, it is this ability to take a history in a directive and efficient manner that distinguishes the experienced clinician from the new clinical student.

Sackett and colleagues have long argued that the clinical examination should be studied rigorously to establish which features are predictive of specific diagnoses. For example, they have reviewed studies that evaluated the accuracy of signs recommended for use in the diagnosis of chronic obstructive pulmonary disease.[3] They found that for all the signs reviewed, the sensitivity, specificity and likelihood ratios varied considerably between studies, and were far short of what would be required for an ideal diagnostic test.[3]

It is only the final part of the diagnostic process, the use of special investigations, for which there are many studies which meet established criteria for valid assessment of clinical evidence.[2] Conventionally, diagnostic tests are judged by their sensitivity (proportion of patients with the target disorder who have positive tests) and specificity (proportion of patients without the target disorder who have negative tests). More useful than sensitivity or specificity in understanding the performance of a test is the likelihood ratio which can be regarded as a summary of sensitivity and specificity (although it can also be used to summarize the performance of tests which have many categories where sensitivity and specificity are unhelpful). For example, suppose you are assessing a child with failure to thrive and malabsorption. You might estimate on the basis of the clinical picture that the probability of the child having celiac disease is around 10%. You might feel that this probability is too low to

justify suggesting to the parents that the child should undergo a small intestinal biopsy but also too high to allow you to dismiss the possibility. You wish to know whether a test which measures antiendomysial antibodies in the serum will, if positive, mean that the diagnosis is sufficiently likely to make the biopsy worth doing or, if negative, decrease the probability to a level where you can reasonably discount the diagnosis.

A publication from 13 European Centres has evaluated both serum antitissue transglutaminase IgA (IgA-TTG) antigliadin antibodies and serum IgA antiendomysial antibodies (IgA-EMA) and compared them with findings of subtotal or severe partial villous atrophy with crypt hyperplasia on small intestinal biopsy (the reference standard).[4] The blood samples were taken no more than 60 days before and not after the small intestinal biopsy, and were independently reviewed by two investigators, who had no knowledge of the diagnosis. So it appeared that the reference standard was applied independently of the diagnostic tests being evaluated and the reference standard was applied objectively to all patients. It is not clear from the paper whether the diagnostic tests were evaluated in an appropriate spectrum of patients or whether all patients with a possible diagnosis of celiac disease underwent small intestinal biopsy, regardless of the results of the blood tests. However, the sensitivities of IgA-TTG and IgA-EMA in the detection of celiac disease were 94% and 89%, with specificities of 99% and 98% respectively.

The likelihood ratio is the ratio of the probability of the test result in patients with the disease to the probability of the test result in patients without the disease. It enables an updated 'post-test' probability to be calculated from the pretest probability, using the results of appropriate studies. The likelihood ratio associated with a positive test result can be calculated from the sensitivity and specificity as follows:

$$LR+ = sensitivity/(1 - specificity)$$

The equation which relates post-test odds to pre-test odds, using the likelihood ratio is:

$$Post\text{-}test\ odds = pretest\ odds \times likelihood\ ratio$$

From the example of IgA-TTG provided above, the study we have found would suggest the following:

$$LR+ = 94\%/1\%,\ or\ 94$$

and for IgA-EMA:

$$LR+ = 89\%/2\%\ or\ 44.5$$

If this is applied to the estimated pretest probability, provided in the example above, of 10%, or odds of 1:9, a positive test result for IgA-TTG will convert these pretest odds to a post-test odds of 94:9, or a post-test probability of 91%. The equivalent calculation for IgA-EMA is a post-test odds of 44.5:9 or 83%. Most clinicians would consider that a small

3

intestinal biopsy should be performed in a child with these probabilities of having celiac disease.

What should the clinician do, though, if the test is negative? The likelihood ratio of a negative test result can be calculated as follows:

$$LR- = (1 - \text{sensitivity})/\text{specificity}$$

For our example, with IgA-TTG this is:

$$LR- = 6\%/99\% \text{ or } 0.06$$

and for IgA-EMA:

$$11\%/98\% \text{ or } 0.11$$

So a negative test result for IgA-TTG and IgA-EMA will convert our pretest odds of 1:9 or 10% to a post-test probability of around 0.7% and 1.2% respectively. Most clinicians would not perform intestinal biopsies in a child with the probabilities of having celiac disease.

What this example shows is that it is not only how a test works that is important in interpreting the result but also the initial likelihood of disease in the child who has the test. Imagine if you did a test for IgA-TTG on a completely well child where the probability of having celiac disease is very low (perhaps less than 0.1%). If the test was negative the likelihood of the child having celiac disease would be vanishingly small but even a positive test would mean only about an 8.5% chance that she had the condition. Using this approach to thinking about diagnostic tests lets you plan the rational use of tests and minimizes the chance of being led astray by false positive or false negative results.

For those familiar with statistical methods, it will be evident that the concept of likelihood ratios has been adopted from the Bayesian approach to statistical inference. The first step in any Bayesian analysis is to establish a prior probability distribution for the value of interest (e.g. probability of a child having a diagnosis of gluten sensitive enteropathy). The clinical evidence is then used to update the prior distribution to a posterior distribution using Bayes theorem. This is analogous to the intuitive process in clinical history taking, where the probabilities of having one of a number of different diagnoses are updated as each new piece of information is elicited. In an evidence-based medicine approach, we start with a prior view about whether, for example, a drug treatment will improve clinical outcomes for an individual patient. This view may be informed by knowledge of pathophysiology and pharmacology, the patient's preferences, cost of therapy and so on. This prior view is then updated by the results of a randomized controlled trial of the drug treatment, in a group of patients similar to our patient, which shows clear improvement in the outcomes we consider important. This evidence is integrated with our prior beliefs, to enable a clinical decision to be made. Many have argued that the natural statistical framework for evidence-based medicine is a Bayesian approach to decision making,[5] both for the individual patient and for health policy.[6]

In an article entitled 'Narrative-based medicine in an evidence-based world',[7] Greenhalgh quotes a scenario, referred to as 'Dr Jenkins's hunch', which goes as follows: 'I got a call from a mother who said that her little girl had had diarrhea and was behaving strangely. I knew the family well and was sufficiently concerned to break off my Monday morning surgery and visit immediately.' Dr Jenkins' subsequent actions resulted in the child recovering from meningococcal septicemia. To many this may seem like a fortunate fluke, and indeed meningococcal septicemia presents rarely in primary care. No guideline could have reliably prompted Dr Jenkins' action. However the doctor was integrating his clinical intuition (mothers rarely use the word 'strangely' to describe their children's behavior), his acquaintance with the family (known to be sensible and uncomplaining), with current best evidence (prognosis of meningococcal septicemia, with and without early administration of parenteral penicillin) to take a course of action which saved a child's life. Greenhalgh rejects the notion that the 'narrative of illness experience' and the 'intuitive and subjective' aspects of clinical method run counter to evidence-based medicine.[7] In making clinical decisions, either informally, by integrating new evidence with our prior views, or formally, by using Bayesian analysis, the framework exists to ensure that clinical evidence can play an explicit part in the process.

THE PRACTICE OF EVIDENCE-BASED MEDICINE

Traditionally there are four basic steps described in this approach. The first is to frame a clinically relevant question and to focus it in a way which can be answered. This is not as trivial a step as it may at first appear. The key elements of a well framed question include a description of:
1. the patient or population;
2. the intervention or exposure;
3. the comparison intervention or exposure (if relevant); and
4. the clinical outcome(s) of interest.

Such an approach can be applied whether the issue is one of diagnosis, prognosis or therapy.

For example, let us consider the following scenario. You are the clinical director of a pediatrics department in a large district hospital. An audit has demonstrated that among children who attend the pediatric clinics with a diagnosis of asthma, there appears to be a high rate of attendances at the accident and emergency department and admissions to hospital. You are interested in interventions which may improve the management of children with asthma and prevent exacerbations severe enough to require A&E attendances and admissions. It was suggested by one of your colleagues that to achieve this, the department should invest in an asthma nurse specialist, who would initiate asthma self-management programs and education programs for all children who attended outpatient clinics with asthma. The resource to provide this service has to compete with other priorities for the department and so you need to know whether or not it might be effective. To investigate this further you formulate the following question: 'in children with asthma, who attend hospital outpatients (population), does a program of education and self-management, delivered by an asthma nurse specialist (intervention), compared with no such program (comparison intervention), reduce the risk of attendances with acute asthma at the accident and emergency department and admissions to hospital (outcome)?'

Having defined the question, the second step is to undertake a comprehensive review of the best available clinical evidence. This is likely to involve searching electronic databases (e.g. Medline, EMBASE, CINAHL and *The Cochrane Library*). The development of search strategies for these databases often involves the expertise of information scientists who can adjust the search strategy to maximize finding all relevant studies (which increases sensitivity), but at the expense of identifying many irrelevant articles (decrease specificity).

Having retrieved all potentially relevant articles which address the question, the third step is to critically appraise them. Tools have been developed to appraise studies evaluating diagnostic tests, prognostic markers, treatments, adverse effects and systematic overviews.[2] In the example provided above, you will have been searching for studies which are used to evaluate the effectiveness of treatments. There are many different study designs which may address this type of question. A hierarchy of such study designs for questions about treatment effectiveness has been developed with the most rigorous at the top and the least rigorous at the bottom (Fig. 1.1). The primary research study, which is considered to be the gold standard in assessing treatments, is the randomized controlled trial. The key element in this design is that the allocation of patients to the treatment group or to the comparison group is

Systematic Review of Randomized Controlled Trials
Confirmed Randomized Controlled Clinical Trials
Single Randomized Controlled Clinical Trial
Non-Randomized Controlled Clinical Trial
Case Controlled Observational Studies
Analysis of Large Computer Databases
Case Series with Historical Controls
Case series, Literature Control
Uncontrolled Case Series
Anecdotal Case

Fig. 1.1 Research pyramid of study designs used to assess the efficacy of treatments.

done randomly, and thus the observed differences between the treatment and the comparison group(s) will be due to the experimental treatment alone rather than to biases which may be introduced by patient characteristics, physician preferences, etc. However, even given this robust study design, the methodological quality of randomized controlled trials may be subject to biases in other ways and these can be evaluated appropriately using checklists.[2]

The fourth step, which is to apply the evidence in clinical practice, is the point at which clinical expertise and patient values are integrated with the best available external evidence. To do this, clinicians need to ask two questions concerning the evidence that they have appraised. The first is 'is this evidence sufficiently robust for me to be confident in its application?' and the second is 'is this study applicable to the patient (or population) about whose care I am deciding?'

Practitioners of evidence-based medicine have long argued that it should not be conducted from ivory towers, by individuals who have little patient contact. If it is to be applicable it needs to be practiced by all clinicians, not least because the questions or question posed need to be relevant to routine practice. However, as will be apparent from the brief description above, the second and third steps of this approach can be very laborious. This has led to the development of a number of shortcuts which will enable the clinician to move easily from step one to step four. To be reliable, such shortcuts must use rigorous methods. One of the most attractive and reliable of these tools is the development of systematic reviews. As will be seen from Table 1.1, the systematic review is now regarded by many as the most rigorous study design for providing information about treatments. The term *systematic* or *scientific* review is used to distinguish them from more *traditional* or *narrative* type reviews of topic areas conducted by experts in the field.

SYSTEMATIC REVIEWS

Narrative reviews have become a regular feature of many medical journals. Such reviews may be very informative, lively and interesting and are usually well illustrated. They are popular because clinicians are busy and have limited time to try and assimilate all primary research which is relevant in a particular area. However, if judged as scientific work which provides summaries of the evidence, which can be used to guide diagnosis or treatment, they are very subject to bias and are therefore unreliable.

These deficiencies led to the concept of systematic reviews, which should adopt a rigorous scientific methodology to eliminate systematic bias or random error, as would be expected of investigators undertaking primary clinical research. The methodology for systematic reviews is outlined in Table 1.1. First the reviewer needs to state the hypothesis that they wish to investigate and then prospectively define a comprehensive search strategy to identify all potentially relevant studies. This

Table 1.1   How to conduct a systematic review

1. State objectives and hypotheses
2. Outline eligibility criteria, stating types of study, types of participant, types of intervention and outcomes to be examined
3. Perform a comprehensive search of all relevant sources for potentially eligible studies
4. Examine the studies to decide eligibility (if possible with two independent reviewers)
5. Construct a table describing the characteristics of the included studies
6. Assess methodological quality of included studies (if possible with two independent reviewers)
7. Extract data (with a second investigator if possible), with involvement of investigators if necessary
8. Analyze results of included studies, using statistical synthesis of data (meta-analysis), if appropriate
9. Prepare a report of review, stating aims, materials and methods and describing results and conclusions

Courtesy of Craig JV, Smyth RL. Evidence based practice manual for nurses. Edinburgh: Churchill Livingstone, 2002.

strategy will almost certainly include searching electronic databases but may involve other methods such as those designed to access unpublished studies, to ensure that the studies accessed are representative of all the research conducted in a particular area. The protocol for the review should state prospectively what studies will be considered eligible for inclusion, defined according to study design, type of participant, intervention, (or exposure) and comparison intervention or exposure. The outcomes of interest are stated prospectively. The protocol should also state how the quality of the included studies will be assessed.

Having determined which studies are to be included and assessed them for methodological quality, the reviewer then extracts the relevant data and analyzes it. This may involve statistical methods such as meta-analysis. This enables the data from a number of different studies to be aggregated so that a pooled effect size can be estimated. There are many examples where individual studies, usually because they are too small, fail to show that an intervention is either beneficial or harmful. By combining the results from all potentially relevant studies, such benefit or harm has been clearly demonstrated. This enables questions to be answered such as 'does this treatment have a beneficial effect?' and also 'what is the size of the effect?'

There now exists a database of systematic reviews of randomized controlled trials of interventions across the whole range of health care. This is found in *The Cochrane Library*,[8] which, at the time of writing (Disk Issue 4, 2006), contains 2905 systematic reviews. These reviews have been prepared by the Cochrane Collaboration, an international body dedicated to producing systematic reviews of the effects of health care using randomized controlled trials as the primary study design. *The Cochrane Library* is produced as a CD-ROM, is updated quarterly and is accessible on the Internet http://www.cochrane.org/ This means that systematic reviews can also be updated to take account of new knowledge.

For the question described above, 'in children with asthma, who attend hospital outpatients (population), does a program of education and self-management, delivered by an asthma nurse specialist (intervention), compared with no such review (comparison intervention), reduce the risk of attendances with acute asthma at the accident and emergency department and admissions to hospital (outcome)?', a Cochrane review, entitled, 'Educational interventions for asthma in children'[9] addresses this question. It is a systematic review of randomized controlled trials, which included children, aged 2–18 years. Studies which assessed any educational interventions targeted to children or adolescents (and/or their parents) designed to teach self-management strategies related to prevention, attack management, or social skills using any instructional strategy or combination of strategies (problem-solving, role-playing, videotapes, computer assisted instruction, booklets, etc.) presented either individually or in group sessions were included in the review. The outcomes assessed in the included studies were health care utilization outcomes, which were the main interest in our scenario, but also physiological measures, morbidity and functional status and self-perception. A number of the studies included self-management programs delivered by a specialist nurse and a high proportion of the studies took place in an outpatient setting. For the outcomes of interest in this scenario, A&E attendances and hospital admissions, 12 trials reported A&E department visits as an outcome and when the results of these trials were pooled, self-management education programs were associated with a reduction in this outcome (standardized mean difference -0.21, 95% confidence intervals -0.33 to -0.09). However, when the results, for hospital admissions, of the eight trials which reported this outcome were pooled, there was no significant benefit of educational interventions (standardized mean difference -0.08, 95% CI -0.21 to 0.05). Self-management and education was associated with improvements in lung function, days of school absence and days of restricted activity. All of this information will help informed decision-making in planning the delivery of care for children with asthma in an outpatient hospital setting.

Although well conducted systematic reviews are regarded as being at the top of the hierarchy of study designs to evaluate the effectiveness of treatments, they can be misused or be badly conducted. Therefore systematic reviews need also to be appraised and there are checklists available for doing this. Jadad et al,[10] for example, have published an evaluation of reviews and meta-analyses of treatments used in asthma. Of the 50 reviews that they considered, 40 were found to have serious methodological flaws. Included within these 40 were six reviews funded by the pharmaceutical industry. All but one of these six reviews had results and conclusions that favored the intervention related to the company which sponsored the review. Reassuringly they found that Cochrane Reviews had higher overall quality scores than reviews published in other scientific journals. The Cochrane Collaboration has made strenuous efforts to ensure that its methodology reduces bias to a minimum and has also guarded against biases which may be introduced by authors with conflicts of interest, e.g. significant support from the pharmaceutical industry. This methodology and the external appraisal by individuals such as Jadad provide reassurance that systematic reviews produced by the Cochrane Collaboration are reliable sources of information for the clinician.

EVIDENCE-BASED CHILD HEALTH

The evidence-based medicine movement was initially advanced by practitioners of internal medicine, but, more recently, pediatricians have become leading proponents. The scope of a number of Cochrane Collaborative Reviews Groups (such as the Cystic Fibrosis and Genetic Disorders Group) covers areas that deal mainly with illnesses of childhood. In addition, there is a Cochrane Child Health Field which has the goal of supporting the production of child-focused, clinically relevant, methodologically rigorous systematic reviews. However, one feature that this discipline of evidence-based health care has highlighted is that when children's health is compared to adult health care, research questions in children may have been addressed either not at all or by small, poorly designed studies.[11] This was the case when all randomized trials published during a 15-year period in a specialist pediatric journal were examined. In this review sample sizes were found to be generally small and only a small proportion of studies were multicenter.[12] Subspecialty areas within pediatrics have also been reviewed, such as cystic fibrosis,[13] pediatric rheumatology[14] and community pediatrics,[15] and the conclusions about the volume and quality of the research have been similar. The 6th edition of Forfar & Arneil was the first to ask contributors to be more explicit about the evidence that they cite and led to contributors expressing some frustration at the lack of level 1 evidence available for them to access in many different disease areas.

There are a number of reasons why it is more difficult to undertake clinical trials and other rigorous studies in children than in adults. There are obvious ethical dilemmas. For example, research on a new therapy is often conducted first in adults before studies are undertaken in children. However, if data from a study of a therapy in adults show a clear advantage for a drug over placebo, does equipoise still exist and is it ethical to repeat such a study in children? Such ethical dilemmas need to be considered clearly and dispassionately by individuals who are advocates for the interests of children. However, there are many examples of therapies which have different effects depending on the stage of the disease process or the age of the patient, including, for example, the sedative effects of phenobarbital in adults, but its frequent association with hyperactivity in children.

There are other practical problems. Generally the proportions of children affected by chronic diseases are smaller than in adults, and even for common childhood diseases such as asthma, the condition may be more heterogeneous than in adults and diagnostic criteria less precise. Outcome measures which have been developed and validated in adults, such as quality of life measures, are unlikely to be appropriate or feasible for young children and infants.

These difficulties have meant that pediatricians, wishing to practice evidence-based child health, have relatively little high quality evidence on which to base their decisions. However, there are encouraging signs that as well as identifying the deficiencies in the evidence, initiatives are being made to promote research that will meet these needs. For example, the Food and Drug Administration in the USA mandated in 1997 that new drugs brought to the market should be tested in children unless there were compelling reasons not to do so. In the European Union, the European Regulation on medicinal products for pediatric uses, which became law in early 2007, provides a system of requirements and incentives for pharmaceutical companies to agree a pediatric investigation plan for all new drugs which may have an indication in children. There is a provision, within the Regulation, for a European research network, of existing national and European networks, investigators and centres, with expertise in conducting clinical studies with children. In the UK, the Medicines for Children Research Network was established in 2005, with substantial government funding.[16]

HOW TEXTBOOKS ENSURE THAT THEY ARE EVIDENCE BASED

Most manuals written for evidence-based practitioners do not consider textbooks to be a valuable source of information. Sackett et al[2] in the relevant section in their textbook *Evidence-based Medicine* state 'we begin with textbooks only to dismiss them' later stating, 'while we may find some useful information in textbooks about the pathophysiology of clinical problems it is best not to use them for establishing the cause, diagnosis, prognosis, prevention or treatment of a disorder'. Part of the problem is that the material published in textbooks is written some time (often some years) before the book is published. Thus textbooks rapidly become out of date. Publishers have realized this and are trying to address this with strategies such as providing regular electronic updates more frequently than the published paper editions.

However, some textbooks have been found not to include information which is current at the time they are written. *The Oxford Textbook of Medicine* has been criticized for including a statement in its 2nd edition concerning the clinical benefits of thrombolysis for patients who had had a myocardial infarction, which stated that these benefits had not been established. This statement was made some years after this therapy had been shown, in a systematic review of randomized controlled trials, to reduce the risk of premature death after myocardial infarction.[17] By way of further illustration Jefferson[18] described his experience in conducting a Cochrane Review of the effects of cholera vaccine. Although much of the data available for this review concerned older, killed whole cell cholera vaccine, the reviewers were aware that the killed whole cell vaccine had been discouraged as it had become widely accepted that it had a low efficacy and short duration of effect, required multiple doses and was less effective in children under 5 than in adults. However, the systematic review found that the efficacy of the vaccine compared with placebo was over 50% in both the first 7 months and in the first year and just under 50% in the second year and that most of the trials achieved this efficacy using a single dose. Vaccine efficacy in the first year was also as great in children under 5 as in older people. The reviewers concluded that the level and duration of efficacy of the killed whole cell cholera vaccine had been underestimated in the literature and that the incidence of adverse effects had been overestimated. A further survey of journal editors and authors of reviews of cholera vaccines concluded that many narrative reviews had been written using the so called 'desk drawer method'. This involved including the evidence that was known to reviewers, but not assembling it or evaluating it systematically. Now that nearly 3000 Cochrane Reviews and 479 462 controlled trials of interventions are available on *The Cochrane Library*, there can be no excuse for the reviewer, or indeed textbook writer, not to consult *The Cochrane Library* when considering treatments for the condition or conditions they are writing about.

Many textbooks now contain the term 'evidence-based' within their title. These fall into two groups. Firstly the manuals that aim to instruct the clinician on how to practice evidence-based medicine and secondly textbooks which purport to present evidence-based information which has been synthesized in a rigorous manner and presented in an easily accessible format. Such textbooks include *Evidence-based Pediatrics and Child Health*[19] and *Clinical Evidence*.[20] *Clinical Evidence*, which states at the outset that it is 'not a textbook of medicine', is rather a handbook, or a reference guide, of topics of wide general interest in health care. In the 'Compendium of evidence', at the start of the book, the methods used are clearly presented. However, its question and answer presentation, limitation to interventions and incomplete coverage of all subjects within its scope make it rather different from a textbook such as this one. *Evidence-based Pediatrics and Child Health* describes itself as a 'melding of a textbook of evidence-based medicine and a clinical pediatric text addressing common conditions'. The first section of this book provides readers with the skills needed to practice evidence-based child health, while the second and third sections address common pediatric conditions. Again the format is in a question and answer framework, with illustration by scenarios. Within the second and third sections, only those specific questions for which evidence is available are considered and as a consequence much of clinical pediatrics is not discussed.

A large and complete textbook of pediatrics such as this one needs to provide a detailed consideration of all aspects of a condition, not just diagnosis, prognosis, prevention and treatment (which are more amenable to evidence-based approaches). Moyer and Elliott[1] refer to two sorts of questions which may be used by the reader in trying to elicit information about a topic, including background information such as: what is Cornelia de Lange syndrome, how commonly is tracheoesophageal fistula associated with esophageal atresia and what is meant by the term apoptosis? These are distinguished from 'foreground' questions relating to, for example, benefits or adverse effects of therapy. Textbooks therefore need to consider the definition, pathophysiology and clinical presentation of conditions as well as diagnosis, prognosis, prevention or treatment of the disorder.

In considering how textbook writers put this information together in a readable format it is helpful to consider how this process has evolved over decades or even centuries. Bristowe in the preface to the 1876 first edition of his *Theory and Practice of Medicine*[21] states his primary aim as 'to give in a readable form as much information as I could within a limited space'. He describes his practice of 'in every case to read the subject up carefully; to compare the knowledge thus acquired or renewed with the results of my own experience, in those cases in which I had any experience: and then, having taken a more or less definite view of the whole subject and while my mind was still full of it, and its details, to write as clear and as comprehensive an account as I was capable of'. He states that this method of procedure will partly explain 'the prevailing absence of notes, quotations and references to authorities'. This textbook, which ran to over 1000 pages, was written entirely by Bristowe and contained no references. Indeed it was unusual for textbooks to contain more than a few references per chapter until the middle of the twentieth century. The method used by Bristowe is similar to that used by many authors today, and the depth of the individual's experience contributes to the richness of the narrative and thus its readability.

So whilst retaining these traditional methods for the provision of background information we have, however, asked all authors to search for and use the best available evidence when presenting 'foreground' information. The methods that we have used to do this will be discussed in the next section.

CLINICAL EVIDENCE WITHIN THE 7TH EDITION OF FORFAR & ARNEIL

For the 6th and 7th editions of Forfar & Arneil the editors gave specific instructions to contributors to ensure that their contributions were as evidence-based as possible. The contributors were asked to identify, where possible, 'level 1 evidence'. This system of grading evidence and recommendations was chosen because it is widely used and has been developed over the last 20 years. The table which contributors were asked to use (Table 1.2) is available on the Website of the Oxford Centre for Evidence-based Medicine (http://cebm.jr2.ox.ac.uk).[22] This

Table 1.2 Oxford Centre for Evidence-Based Medicine levels of evidence (December 2006)

Level	Therapy/prevention, etiology/harm	Prognosis	Diagnosis	Differential diagnosis/ symptom prevalence study	Economic and decision analyses
1a	SR (with homogeneity*) of RCTs	SR (with homogeneity*) of inception cohort studies; CDR⁺ validated in different populations	SR (with homogeneity*) of level 1 diagnostic studies; CDR⁺ with 1b studies from different clinical centers	SR (with homogeneity*) of prospective cohort studies	SR (with homogeneity*) of level 1 economic studies
1b	Individual RCT (with narrow confidence interval⁺)	Individual inception cohort study with ≥80% follow-up; CDR⁺ validated in a single population	Validating** cohort study with good⁺⁺⁺ reference standards; or CDR⁺ tested within one clinical center	Prospective cohort study with good follow-up****	Analysis based on clinically sensible costs or alternatives; systematic review(s) of the evidence; and including multiway sensitivity analyses
1c	All or none§	All or none case-series	Absolute SpPins and SnNouts⁺⁺	All or none case-series	Absolute better-value or worse-value analyses⁺⁺⁺⁺
2a	SR (with homogeneity*) of cohort studies	SR (with homogeneity*) of either retrospective cohort studies or untreated control groups in RCTs	SR (with homogeneity*) of level >2 diagnostic studies	SR (with homogeneity*) of level 2b and better studies	SR (with homogeneity*) of level >2 economic studies
2b	Individual cohort study (including low quality RCT; e.g. <80% follow-up)	Retrospective cohort study or follow-up of untreated control patients in an RCT; Derivation of CDR⁺ or validated on split-sample§§§ only	Exploratory** cohort study with good⁺⁺⁺ reference standards; CDR⁺ after derivation, or validated only on split-sample§§§ or databases	Retrospective cohort study, or poor follow-up	Analysis based on clinically sensible costs or alternatives; limited review(s) of the evidence, or single studies; and including multiway sensitivity analyses

(Continued)

Table 1.2   Oxford Centre for Evidence-Based Medicine levels of evidence (December 2006)—cont'd

Level	Therapy/prevention, etiology/harm	Prognosis	Diagnosis	Differential diagnosis/ symptom prevalence study	Economic and decision analyses
2c	'Outcomes' research; ecological studies	'Outcomes' research		Ecological studies	Audit or outcomes research
3a	SR (with homogeneity*) of case-control studies		SR (with homogeneity*) of level 3b and better studies	SR (with homogeneity*) of level 3b and better studies	SR (with homogeneity*) of level 3b and better studies
3b	Individual case-control study		Non-consecutive study; or without consistently applied reference standards	Non-consecutive cohort study, or very limited population	Analysis based on limited alternatives or costs, poor quality estimates of data, but including sensitivity analyses incorporating clinically sensible variations
4	Case-series (and poor quality cohort and case-control studies§§)	Case-series (and poor quality prognostic cohort studies***)	Case-control study, poor or non-independent reference standard	Case-series or superseded reference standards	Analysis with no sensitivity analysis
5	Expert opinion without explicit critical appraisal, or based on physiology, bench research or 'first principles'	Expert opinion without explicit critical appraisal, or based on physiology, bench research or 'first principles'	Expert opinion without explicit critical appraisal, or based on physiology, bench research or 'first principles'	Expert opinion without explicit critical appraisal, or based on physiology, bench research or 'first principles'	Expert opinion without explicit critical appraisal, or based on physiology, bench research or 'first principles'

Produced by Bob Phillips, Chris Ball, Dave Sackett, Doug Badenoch, Sharon Straus, Brian Haynes, Martin Dawes since November 1998.

Notes – Users can add a minus-sign '–' to denote the level that fails to provide a conclusive answer because of:

• EITHER a single result with a wide confidence interval (such that, for example, an ARR in an RCT is not statistically significant but whose confidence intervals fail to exclude clinically important benefit or harm)

• OR a systematic review with troublesome (and statistically significant) heterogeneity.

• Such evidence is inconclusive, and therefore can only generate Grade D recommendations.

* By homogeneity we mean a systematic review that is free of worrisome variations (heterogeneity) in the directions and degrees of results between individual studies. Not all systematic reviews with statistically significant heterogeneity need be worrisome, and not all worrisome heterogeneity need be statistically significant. As noted above, studies displaying worrisome heterogeneity should be tagged with a '–' at the end of their designated level.

† Clinical Decision Rule (these are algorithms or scoring systems which lead to a prognostic estimation or a diagnostic category).

‡ See note #2 for advice on how to understand, rate and use trials or other studies with wide confidence intervals.

§ Met when *all* patients died before the treatment became available, but some now survive on it; or when some patients died before the treatment became available, but *none* now die on it.

§§ By poor quality *cohort* study we mean one that failed to clearly define comparison groups and/or failed to measure exposures and outcomes in the same (preferably blinded), objective way in both exposed and non-exposed individuals and/or failed to identify or appropriately control known confounders and/or failed to carry out a sufficiently long and complete follow-up of patients. By poor quality *case-control* study we mean one that failed to clearly define comparison groups and/or failed to measure exposures and outcomes in the same (preferably blinded), objective way in both cases and controls and/or failed to identify or appropriately control known confounders.

§§§ Split-sample validation is achieved by collecting all the information in a single tranche, then artificially dividing this into 'derivation' and 'validation' samples.

†† An 'Absolute SpPin' is a diagnostic finding whose Specificity is so high that a Positive result rules-in the diagnosis. An 'Absolute SnNout' is a diagnostic finding whose Sensitivity is so high that a Negative result rules-out the diagnosis.

††† Good reference standards are independent of the test, and applied blindly or objectively to all patients. Poor reference standards are haphazardly applied, but still independent of the test. Use of a non-independent reference standard (where the 'test' is included in the 'reference', or where the 'testing' affects the 'reference') implies a level 4 study.

†††† Better-value treatments are clearly as good but cheaper, or better at the same or reduced cost. Worse-value treatments are as good and more expensive, or worse and equally or more expensive.

** Validating studies test the quality of a specific diagnostic test, based on prior evidence. An exploratory study collects information and trawls the data (e.g. using a regression analysis) to find which factors are 'significant'.

*** By poor quality prognostic cohort study we mean one in which sampling was biased in favor of patients who already had the target outcome, or the measurement of outcomes was accomplished in <80% of study patients, or outcomes were determined in an unblinded, non-objective way, or there was no correction for confounding factors.

**** Good follow-up in a differential diagnosis study is >80%, with adequate time for alternative diagnoses to emerge (e.g. 1–6 months acute, 1–5 years chronic).

RCT, randomized controlled trial; SR, systematic review.

Grades of recommendation:

A. Consistent level 1 studies

B. Consistent level 2 or 3 studies *or* extrapolations from level 1 studies

C. Level 4 studies *or* extrapolations from level 2 or 3 studies

D. Level 5 evidence *or* troublingly inconsistent or inconclusive studies of any level

'Extrapolations' are where data are used in a situation which has potentially clinically important differences from the original study situation.

type of approach has been used in other evidence-based textbooks.[23] The editors appreciated that in a number of areas there may not be level 1 evidence available, but to distinguish this category of evidence from the remainder, authors were asked to identify references to level 1 evidence with an asterisk (*). This approach may be considered inadequate by some evidence-based proponents but was felt to be an important step in ensuring that the standard of information available from this textbook was as high as possible. The grading system used has some problems and a number of these are acknowledged (http://cebm.jr2.ox.ac.uk). For example, definitions of homogeneity (with respect to systematic reviews) and narrow confidence intervals (with respect to randomized controlled trials) are open to considerable interpretation and may not adequately distinguish high quality studies from those of poor quality. It is also important to realize that this particular 'hierarchy of evidence' applies only to questions about the effectiveness of interventions – other types of questions need different research approaches.

SUMMARY

Clinical decision making is a complex process. Evidence-based medicine proponents endorse the importance of clinical expertise, which uses narrative skills to integrate the information provided by the clinical method. In practicing evidence-based medicine, clinicians integrate this information with that provided by sound clinical research. When tensions arise in this approach, it is usually because the narrative/intuitive paradigm has been discarded and decision making is predicated on the 'evidence' alone. Systematic reviews are the result of rigorous research, using methodology which is designed to reduce bias. As such they can provide reliable summaries of evidence. This methodology has been most comprehensively developed for systematic reviews of randomized controlled trials, but is being developed for other study designs. By searching databases of systematic reviews, such as those contained within *The Cochrane Library*, the clinician can obtain high quality evidence rapidly and reliably and enhance his/her clinical practice.

REFERENCES (*Level 1 Evidence)

1. Moyer V, Elliott E. Preface. In: Moyer V, Elliott E, Davis R, et al, eds. Evidence based pediatrics and child health. London: BMJ Books; 2000.
2. Sackett DL, Richardson WS, Rosenberg W, et al. Evidence-based medicine: how to practice and teach EBM. London: Churchill Livingstone; 2000.
3. McAlister F, Straus S, Sackett DL. Why we need large, simple studies of the clinical examination: the problem and a proposed solution. Lancet 1999; 354:1721–1724.
4. Collin P, Kaukinen K, Vogelsang H, et al. Antiendomysial and antihuman recombinant tissue transglutaminase antibodies in the diagnosis of celiac disease: a biopsy-proven European multicentre study. Eur J Gastroenterol Hepatol 2005; 17:85–91.
5. Ashby D, Smith AFM. Evidence-based medicine as Bayesian decision-making. Stat Med 2000; 19:3291–3305.
6. Lilford R, Braunholtz D. The statistical basis of public policy: a paradigm shift is overdue. BMJ 1996; 313:603–607.

7. Greenhalgh T. Narrative based medicine in an evidence based world. BMJ 1999; 318:323–325.
8. Cochrane Library. The Cochrane Library, Issue 3, 2001. Oxford: Update Software.
9. Wolf FM, Guevara JP, Grum CM, et al. Educational interventions for asthma in children. Cochrane Database Syst Rev 2002; (4):CD000326.
10. Jadad AR, Moher M, Browman G, et al. Systematic reviews and meta-analyses on treatment of asthma: critical evaluation. BMJ 2000; 320:537–540.
11. Smyth RL, Weindling AM. Research in children: ethical and scientific aspects. Lancet 1999; 354: (suppl 2):SII21–SII24.
12. Campbell H, Surry S, Royle E. A review of randomised controlled trials published in Archives of Disease in Childhood from 1982–1996. Arch Dis Child 1997; 79:192–197.
13. Cheng K, Smyth RL, Motley J, et al. Randomized controlled trials in cystic fibrosis (1996–1997) categorized by time, design, and intervention. Pediatr Pulmonol 2000; 29:1–7.
14. Feldman B, Giannini E. Where's the evidence? Putting the clinical science into pediatric rheumatology. J Rheumatol 1996; 23:1502–1504.

15. Polnay L. Research in community child health. Arch Dis Child 1989; 64:981–983.
16. Smyth RL, Edwards D. A major new initiative to improve treatment for children. Arch Dis Child 2006; 91:212–213.
17. Chalmers I, Haynes B. Systematic reviews: reporting, updating, and correcting systematic reviews of the effects of health care. BMJ 1994; 309:862–865.
18. Jefferson T. What are the benefits of editorials and non-systematic reviews? BMJ 1999; 318:135.
19. Moyer VA, Elliott EJ, Davis RL, et al, eds. Evidence-based pediatrics and child health. London: BMJ Books; 2000.
20. Barton S. Clinical evidence. London: BMJ Publishing; 2001.
21. Bristowe J. Theory and practice of medicine. London: Smith, Elder & Co; 1882.
22. Website of Oxford Centre for EBM. Oxford Centre for Evidence-based Medicine; 2001. http://cebm.jr2.ox.ac.uk
23. Feldman W. Evidence-based pediatrics. Ontario: BC Decker; 2000.

2

Epidemiology of childhood diseases

Stuart Logan

INTRODUCTION

Children under 15 comprise about one third of the world population, with three quarters living in less developed countries. Children's health varies enormously across the world. In 2003 the under-5 mortality rate was 6 per 1000 in industrialized countries but 175 per 1000 in sub-Saharan Africa.[1]

Understanding the patterns of health and disease is important in planning health and social policies and in monitoring change over time. It is important to recognize the limitations of the data that are available. If the statistics are to be useful for comparing between areas and over time, effective systems must be in place to collect the data and there must be consistency of definitions. In many parts of the world, such systems are rudimentary, although considerable progress has been made in ensuring agreed definitions at least for the principal measures of birth and mortality. The World Health Organization is an excellent source of regularly updated health data which can be accessed on their website[1] and this chapter draws heavily on these data and can be assumed to be the source where no other reference is given.

This chapter will review the patterns of mortality and morbidity amongst children and examine the major determinants of health at a population level. These patterns vary widely between countries. This chapter will discuss mainly the extremes, with data drawn from the rich industrialized nations and the poorest nations, largely in sub-Saharan Africa. Many countries will of course have rates of mortality and patterns of disease lying between these extremes.

In describing the health of children at a population level we are usually forced to rely on measures of mortality or morbidity. Measures of health rather than disease are philosophically attractive but have proved problematic in practice. Although a number of tools have been developed to measure quality of life in childhood their application at a population level has been limited and they have mainly proved useful in clinical trials or in the investigation of the effects of specific conditions.

MORTALITY RATES

DEFINITIONS

Any infant who breathes, has a heart beat or pulsation of the umbilical cord is defined as a 'live birth', irrespective of gestation or the duration of the signs of life. It seems likely that at least some very premature infants who fulfill this definition are not in fact registered as live births and that, as the frontiers of neonatal intensive care have been pushed back over time, this proportion has changed. In the UK a stillbirth is defined now as being 'a child born at 24 or more weeks post conception who shows no signs of life', although, up until 1992, the definition required that they were born at least 28 weeks' post conception.

The definitions of the various perinatal, neonatal and infant mortality rates (IMRs) are shown graphically in Figure 2.1. The denominator for the stillbirth and perinatal mortality rates is the number of still and live births while that for the other rates is the number of live births.

The under-5 mortality rate, widely used, particularly in poorer countries, is defined as the annual number of deaths in children under 5 years of age per 1000 live births. Age-specific death rates are the number of deaths in an age group per 1000 individuals in that age group.

PATTERNS OF MORTALITY

There have been dramatic changes in life expectancy in developed countries over the last century. In 1901, the average life expectancy for women in the UK was 48 years, but by 2004 it was 81 years. Life expectancy for men in the UK, although lower than for women, at 76 years, has also risen greatly[2] (except where specifically referenced, UK data are from the Office of National Statistics, whose website gives access to an enormous range of current and historical data). Although death rates at all ages have declined, much of this change has been due to the rapid decrease in deaths in childhood, particularly in the first half of the century. Changes in death rates during childhood over time for England and Wales are shown in Figure 2.2.[2]

In Tanzania by contrast the life expectancy for women in 2004 was 49 and for men, 47. Much of the difference in life expectancy between the UK and Tanzania is driven by differences in childhood mortality, particularly mortality under the age of 5. The probability of dying between 15 and 60 years of age per 1000 population was 102 in the UK and 5.5 times higher (552 per 1000) in Tanzania. However, the under-5 mortality rate in the UK in 2004 was 6 per 1000 live births and 126 in Tanzania, 21 times higher. All these figures are for males, rates for females showing similar patterns but lower absolute rates. Not only are the relative differences larger in childhood but each childhood death contributes more to the total years of life lost and hence the life expectancy figures.

Not only are absolute mortality rates higher in poorer countries but the pattern of change over time is also different. Globally the under-5

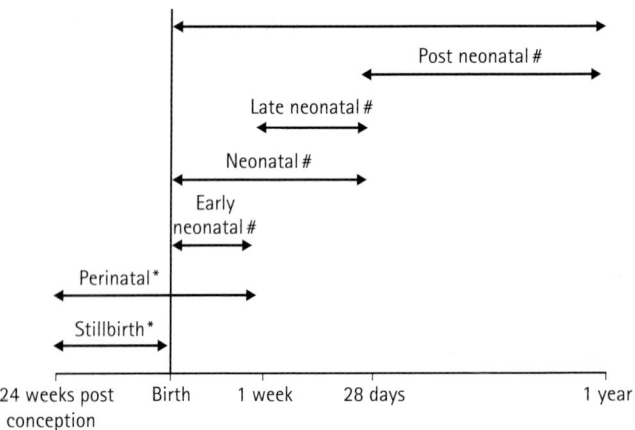

Fig. 2.1   Definitions of mortality rates in the neonatal period and infancy.

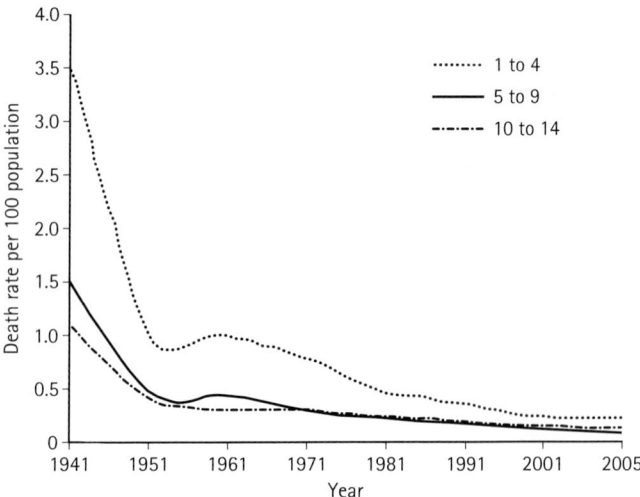

Fig. 2.2   Death rates in children in England and Wales over time.[2]

Table 2.1   Changes in under-5 and infant mortality rates per 1000 live births over time by region[1]

Region	Under-5 mortality rate		Infant mortality rate	
	1960	2003	1960	2003
Industrialized nations	39	6	32	5
Developing countries	224	87	142	60
Least developed countries	278	155	127	54
Sub-Saharan Africa*	278	175	165	104
World	198	80	127	54

*Most countries in sub-Saharan Africa are included within the category 'least developed countries' but the region is shown separately to emphasize the slow rate of improvement.

MORTALITY IN POOR COUNTRIES

The burden of mortality in children in poor countries is extraordinary. In sub-Saharan Africa some 10% of infants die in the first year of life (compared to around 0.5% in Europe) and over 15% before their 5th birthday. The proportions of deaths related to major causal groups is shown in Figure 2.3 for under-5s in Africa and in western Europe[3]. Nearly three quarters of these deaths are due to six causes: (1) pneumonia (19%), (2) diarrhea (18%), (3) neonatal sepsis or (4) pneumonia (10%), (5) preterm delivery (10%) or (6) asphyxia at birth (8%). It is estimated that undernutrition is an underlying cause in over 50% of deaths in under-5-year-olds.

The first year of life is the most dangerous period of childhood and globally 40% of under-5 deaths occur in the neonatal period. The proportion is lower in Africa (26%) because of the higher burden of deaths in the post-neonatal period, although the neonatal death rates are highest here. As in the resource rich world, the consequences of prematurity and low birth weight are important causes of neonatal deaths in resource limited countries but infections (including neonatal tetanus) are also important (Fig. 2.4).[3] The high risks related to underlying poverty are exacerbated by the lack of services. In Africa only 40% of women deliver with skilled care and in South Asia less than 30%.[4]

Communicable diseases are responsible for around half of the under-5 deaths in the world and nearly two thirds in Africa. Malaria is particularly important in Africa with 94% of all malaria deaths occurring in this region. A similar picture is seen with deaths from human immunodeficiency virus (HIV)/acquired immune deficiency syndrome (AIDS) where 89% of deaths are in Africa although this picture is likely to change as the prevalence of the infection rises in poor countries of Southeast Asia. The deaths of over 400 000 children per year due to measles is depressing considering the availability of a cheap and effective vaccine which

mortality rate fell from 198 in 1000 in 1960 to 80 in 1000 in 2003. This hides a huge variation in the rate of decline, with the least progress generally being made in countries which started with the highest rates. In 93 countries containing 40% of the world's population, < 5 mortality is declining fast, in 51 (48% of the population) progress is slow and in the remaining 43 (12% of the population), mostly clustered in sub-Saharan Africa, rates are stagnant or rising (Table 2.1).

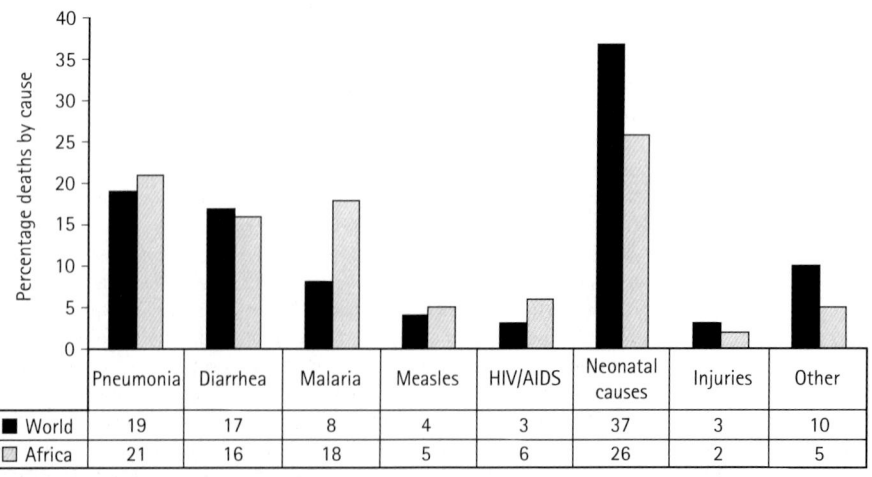

	Pneumonia	Diarrhea	Malaria	Measles	HIV/AIDS	Neonatal causes	Injuries	Other
■ World	19	17	8	4	3	37	3	10
☐ Africa	21	16	18	5	6	26	2	5

Fig. 2.3   Percentage of deaths of under-5-year-olds by cause in the world and in Africa 2000–2003.[3]

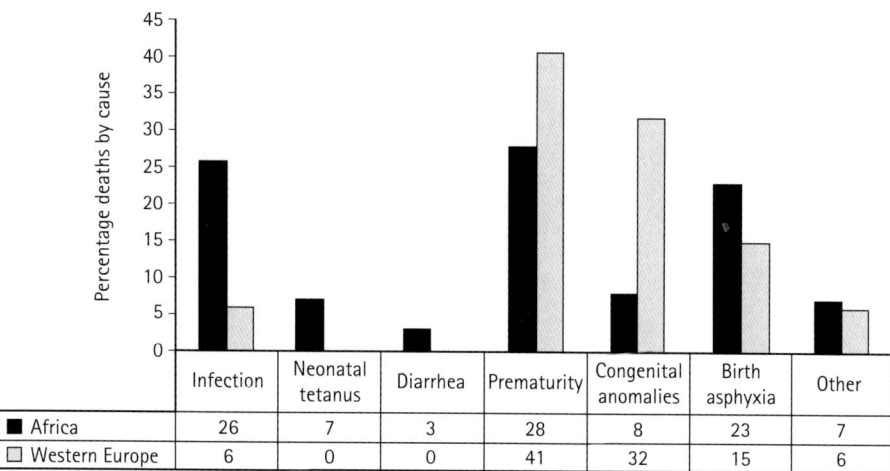

Fig. 2.4   Percentage of neonatal deaths by cause in Africa and western Europe 2000–2003.[3]

	Infection	Neonatal tetanus	Diarrhea	Prematurity	Congenital anomalies	Birth asphyxia	Other
■ Africa	26	7	3	28	8	23	7
☐ Western Europe	6	0	0	41	32	15	6

Table 2.2   Proportion < 5 deaths by cause in the 42 countries in which 90% of all < 5 deaths occur which are potentially preventable[5]

Disease or condition	% total deaths	% preventable
Diarrhea	22	88
Pneumonia	21	65
Malaria	9	91
HIV/AIDS	3	48
Measles	1	100
Neonatal disorders	33	55

has virtually eliminated deaths from this condition in countries with high vaccine coverage.

The vast bulk of these deaths are related directly or indirectly to poverty. Knowledge already exists about effective interventions for both treatment and prevention, which could substantially reduce this burden. It has been estimated that about two thirds of these deaths could be prevented by a small number of key interventions of proven effectiveness which could feasibly be introduced in low-income countries (Table 2.2).[5] The interventions considered are relatively cheap and simple including measures such as the use of oral rehydration fluid in diarrhea, insecticide treated materials for the prevention of malaria, antibiotics for neonatal sepsis and pneumonia and encouragement of high rates of breast-feeding.

CHILDHOOD MORTALITY IN THE INDUSTRIALIZED WORLD

Of all deaths in childhood in the UK (ages 0–14), 73% occur within the first year of life, 50% within the first month and 38% within the first week (Fig. 2.5).[2] The decline in the rate of stillbirths and infant mortality in England and Wales is shown in Figure 2.6. The rates for stillbirth after 1992 are not strictly comparable because of the change in definition mentioned earlier. The decline in infant mortality reflects declines in both neonatal and post-neonatal mortality rates.

In the neonatal period, a substantial proportion of deaths are related to congenital anomalies and prematurity (Fig. 2.4). Congenital anomalies are an important cause of death in the neonatal period although the birth prevalence of many anomalies appears to have declined, particularly that of anomalies of the central nervous system. While part of this decline appears to relate to the widespread introduction of screening for neural tube defects in pregnancy there has also been a substantial decline in incidence, possibly related to changes in diet or the use of periconceptual folate supplements.

Congenital anomalies remain an important cause of death after the neonatal period, accounting for 22% of all deaths between 1 month and 1 year of age in England and Wales in 2005. As with older children,

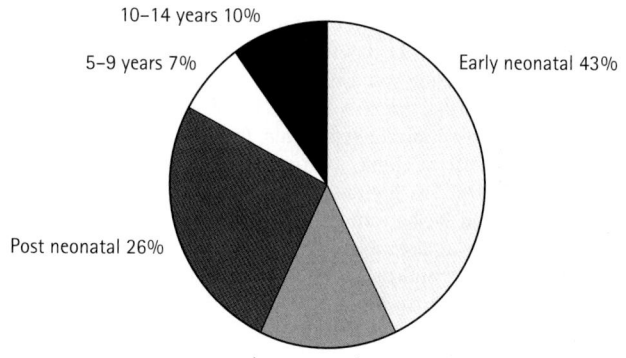

Fig. 2.5   Proportion of deaths in childhood by age of occurrence (England and Wales 2005).[2]

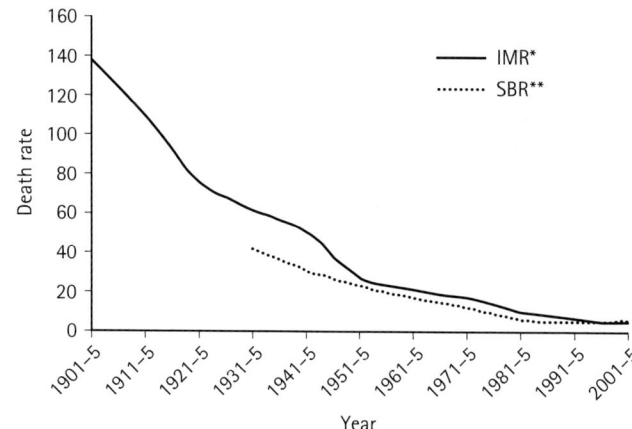

Fig. 2.6   Changes in stillbirth and infant mortality rates over time (England and Wales).[2] * Per 100 live births. ** Per 100 live and stillbirths.

injuries and poisoning are responsible for a significant number of deaths in the first year of life, but in this age group, the much higher rates of death from other conditions mean that they are responsible for a relatively small proportion of all deaths.

Even within the industrialized world there are substantial variations in IMRs (Table 2.3).[1] While there is an obvious relationship between mortality rates and wealth there are some surprising anomalies. For example, the USA has an IMR more than twice that of Sweden. To some extent, this appears to reflect differences in IMRs in different population groups within the same country. In the USA, in 2002, the IMR for infants born to non-Hispanic black mothers was 2.4 times higher than

Table 2.3 Infant mortality rates in some selected industrialized countries (2002)[1]

Country	IMR (per 1000 live births)
Sweden	3.3
Norway	3.5
Austria	4.1
France	4.1
Germany	4.2
Italy	4.5
The Netherlands	5.1
Ireland	5.1
UK	5.2
Canada	5.4
New Zealand	5.6
United States	7.0

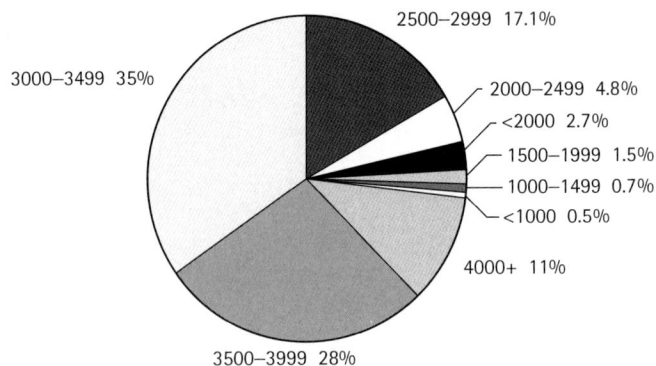

Fig. 2.8 Proportion of live births by birth weight in grams, England and Wales (2004).[2]

in non-Hispanic white, and different states reported IMRs ranging from 5.0 in New Hampshire to 11.3 in the District of Columbia.[6]

Birth weight, reflecting both gestation and intrauterine growth, is the strongest predictor of the risk of death in the first year of life (Fig. 2.7). In large part, differences in mortality between, for instance, Sweden and the UK and between different ethnic groups in the USA are accounted for by differences in the birth weight distribution. The proportion of babies by birth weight group in England and Wales in 2004 is shown in Figure 2.8. In recent decades there has been a small overall increase in mean birth weight in many industrialized countries, largely accounted for by an increase in the proportion of babies born weighing more than 3500 g. There has also, however, been an increase in the proportion of babies born weighing less than 2500 g, in the USA from 6.7% of live-born infants in 1984 to 8.1% in 2003. This partly reflects increasing numbers of twins and higher order births, which in the USA now comprise over 3% of all births.[6]

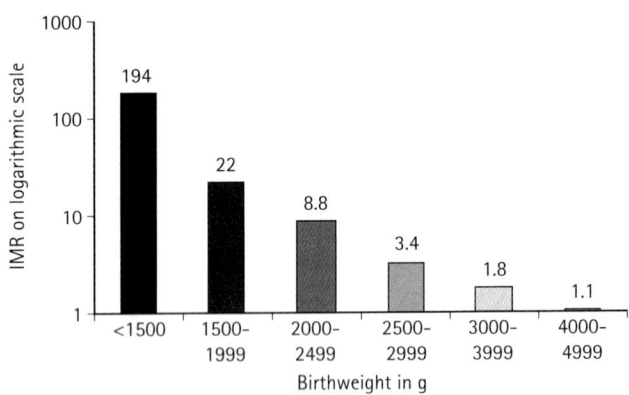

Fig. 2.7 Infant mortality rate (IMR) by birth weight (England and Wales 2004).[2]

The risk of death drops rapidly after the first year of life; in the UK to around 21 per 100 000 children aged 1–4 and to 9 per 100 000 aged 5–14 compared to a risk of death in the first year of life of 520 per 100 000 live births. Death rates then begin to rise again after the age of 15, particularly in boys and largely as a result of the increasing risk of injuries.[2]

As shown in Figure 2.2, the risk of death from all causes in childhood has been falling throughout the last 50 years. Rates of death from unintentional injury in children have also fallen, but injury and poisoning still remain responsible for the greatest proportion of deaths in older children. Table 2.4 compares the most common attributable causes of death in children aged 1–14 in 1955, 1985 and 2005, in England and Wales. Very similar patterns are seen in the USA[6] although unintentional injury rates are higher than in England and Wales and homicide is a more important cause of death in children. In 2000 in the USA, homicide accounted for some 5.8% of deaths in children aged 1–14 compared to 2.0% in England and Wales.[1] Amongst adolescents aged 15–19 in the USA in 2003, accidents were responsible for 49.7% of deaths, homicide for 13.9% and suicide for 10.9%.[6] In both the UK and USA the risks of non-intentional and intentional injuries are substantially higher in boys than in girls.

MORBIDITY IN CHILDHOOD

Morbidity data are more difficult to obtain, especially in poorer countries, and to interpret than mortality data, which are generally easily available and reasonably reliable. However such data are essential if a picture of the health of the population can be built up.

HEALTH SERVICE USE

Children are heavy users of health services and routine service data can provide useful information about patterns of morbidity. A number of different sources of health service data are available in the UK, some

Table 2.4 Percentage deaths age 1–14 by leading causes in order of frequency in 1955, 1985 and 2005 in England and Wales[2]

1955		1985		2005	
Category	%	Category	%	Category	%
Injury and poisoning	25.0	Injury and poisoning	33.6	Injury and poisoning	20.5
Respiratory disease*	13.0	Congenital anomalies	15.3	Malignant disease	20.0
Malignant disease	11.7	Malignant disease	14.0	Diseases of the CNS	13.9
Infectious disease	9.4	Diseases of the CNS	9.4	Congenital anomalies	11.3
Congenital anomalies	8.7	Respiratory disease	6.2	Respiratory disease*	8.1
Diseases of the GIT	4.1	Infectious diseases	4.0	CVS disease	6.6

derived directly from the use of services and some from special surveys such as the annual 'General Household Survey', which includes self-reported health and use of services.[7] Somewhat confusingly, these often cover different components or combinations of components of the UK. All these routine data have to be interpreted with some caution. Changes in admission rates over time for instance may reflect changes in classification either by health professionals or those who code the data, changes in thresholds for admission or real changes in incidence.

Admission of children to hospital is relatively common. In the UK, in 2002, around 11% of 0–4-year-olds and 4% of 5–15-year-olds reported being admitted to hospital at least once in the previous year.[7] There has been a steady decline in both the proportion and the average length of stay in hospital over time. The two most important reasons for admission in 5–14-year-olds are respiratory conditions, (including asthma), and injuries, each accounting for about 16% of admissions.

Children are also frequent visitors to Accident and Emergency departments and to general practitioners (GPs).[7] More than 11% of British children report going to an Accident and Emergency department over a 3-month period. Those under 5 visit a GP on average seven times per year and those between 5 and 15, three times per year. Data collected in Scotland suggest that the commonest reasons for these GP visits are upper respiratory tract infections, otitis media, coughs, sore throats and other minor conditions.

CHRONIC DISEASE AND DISABILITY

Data on chronic disease and disability are relatively poor, even in countries with highly developed health systems. In the UK, special studies generally have to be relied upon for this information. Unfortunately there are often problems with the representativeness of the samples and with the quality of the definitions used.

The General Household Survey, mentioned earlier, asks a representative group of people in the UK to report on their own and their children's health. One of the questions asks whether they have a long-standing illness and whether it limits their activities. In 2002, the parents of 20% of boys and 17% girls aged 0–14 said that their child had a longstanding illness and 7% said that this limited their child's activities.[7]

Reliable information on the prevalence of disability in childhood, except for the prevalence of a few well-defined conditions such as Down syndrome, is particularly difficult to find. Such information may also be difficult to interpret, as children's functional abilities form a continuum, and the point at which the child is labeled as 'disabled' is arbitrary. A national survey in the UK, published in 1989, reported 3% of 0–15-year-olds were perceived by their parent as disabled.[8] Clearly such reports depend on the definitions used, the way the data are collected and the population, leading to widely varying estimates. In 1994[9] Boyle et al reported that 17% of US children had developmental disabilities while in 2006[10] Blanchard et al suggested that the figure was 5%. Using multiple methods of ascertainment a study based in Atlanta (roughly 50 000 births/year) has reported on the prevalence of four specific developmental disabilities (Table 2.5).[11]

Table 2.5 Prevalence of selected developmental disabilities in Atlanta (2000)[11]

	Prevalence /1000 children
'Mental retardation'*	12.0
Mild	8.7
Moderate, severe or profound	3.3
Cerebral palsy	3.1
Hearing loss (> 40 dB)	1.2
Visual impairment (20/70 or worse corrected)	1.2

* In Europe the term more commonly used is 'learning disability'. Mental retardation was defined here as IQ <70 (mild = IQ 50–70, moderate/profound = IQ <50).

Estimates of the prevalence of cerebral palsy, the most common form of serious physical disability in childhood, are available from a number of countries. Most recent studies in industrialized countries report rates of cerebral palsy between 2 and 3 per 1000 infants surviving the neonatal period. There is conflicting evidence about trends over time. In the UK, one study reported a change between 1964–1968 and 1989–1993 from 1.68 to 2.45/1000 neonatal survivors.[12] A report combining data from five UK registers of cerebral palsy seems to suggest that rates rose during the late 1970s and then flattened thereafter but is unclear about the extent to which this represents changes in ascertainment.[13] The rate in babies born weighing > 2500 g has remained virtually constant over this period while one large study has reported that in western Europe the rate in very low birth weight babies (< 1500 g) fell from 60.6/1000 live births in 1980 to 39.5/1000 in 1996.[14] There have also been increases in the lifespan of children with cerebral palsy, which will further increase the overall prevalence of cerebral palsy in the population.

The life expectancy of children with a number of other chronic conditions has also increased in the developed world, which is again likely to raise the prevalence of such conditions in the population. A survey carried out in one health district in the UK attempted to ascertain what proportion of children suffer from nonmalignant 'life-threatening' conditions.[15] These were defined as conditions as a result of which the child had at least a 50% likelihood of dying before the age of 40 and included conditions such as cystic fibrosis, chronic renal failure and conditions causing central nervous system degeneration. The overall prevalence among children aged 0–19 was 1.2/1000, suggesting a large burden on families and services.

Mental health problems are extremely common in children and adolescents. A large population survey carried out in Great Britain in 2004 of children aged 5–16 reported that 9.6% had a mental disorder (based on ICD 10 diagnostic criteria).[16] The prevalence rises with age and rates are generally higher in boys than girls except for emotional disorders (Table 2.6). Even apparently milder psychological problems such as behavioral difficulties which would not fulfill the criteria for a mental disorder in young children can have profound effects on the quality of families' lives.

Disabling conditions in poor countries

The prevalence of disabling conditions in children is believed to be disproportionately high in poorer countries although the sources of high-quality data are few.[17] Mung'ala-Odera et al[18] reported that 61 of 1000 6–9-year-old children in one rural area in Kenya had moderate to severe neurological impairment (Table 2.7). The authors point to the relatively low prevalence of cerebral palsy in their population and suggest that this is likely to be related to a high mortality rate in these children in poor communities. The higher rates seen in girls than boys in this study are surprising and unexplained. A study of intellectual disability in children of the same age group in rural South Africa (defined as IQ < 80, mild 56–80, severe < 55) reported the more commonly observed excess in males who were 1.5 times as likely to be affected.[19] The overall reported prevalence was 35.6 of 1000 (mild 29.1 of 1000, severe 6.4 of 1000).

Poverty leads to poor nutrition, recurrent illness and inevitably deficient care as families struggle to survive. In addition to the more obvious

Table 2.6 Percentage of children with a mental disorder by age and gender in Great Britain in 2004[16]

Disorder	5–10 years		11–15 years	
	Boys	Girls	Boys	Girls
Emotional disorder	2.2	2.5	3.9	6.0
Conduct disorder	6.9	2.8	8.8	5.1
Hyperkinetic disorder	2.7	0.4	2.6	0.3
Autistic spectrum disorder	1.9	0.1	1.0	0.5
Any disorder	10.2	5.1	13.1	10.2

Table 2.7 Estimated prevalence of moderate to severe neurological impairment in 6–9-year-olds in rural Kenya per 1000 children[18]

Impairment	Boys	Girls	Total
Epilepsy	37	45	41
Cognitive impairment	27	36	31
Hearing impairment	12	15	14
Motor impairment	5	4	5
Visual impairment	2	2	2
Any impairment	52	79	61

severe forms of disability this poverty of environment means that children fail to reach their developmental potential. Grantham-Macgregor et al estimate that more than 200 million children under the age of 5 fail to reach their potential in cognitive development as a result of poverty.[20] This has serious economic and social consequences for them as individuals and for the societies in which they live.

POPULATION DETERMINANTS OF CHILD HEALTH

The health of an individual is determined by a complex interaction between genetic factors, health behaviors and environmental influences.

AGE AND SEX STRUCTURE OF THE POPULATION

Between the ages of 5 and 15 the risk of death and severe illness is at its lowest, before rising again. Death rates are higher in boys than girls at all ages in both poor and rich countries (Fig. 2.9 shows the rates by age and gender for England and Wales). The magnitude of the difference varies with age, in the UK rising from around 25% higher in boys from birth until the age of 15 and then becoming more than twice as great in adolescence and early adulthood. Much of this increasing discrepancy between the sexes is due to the much higher rates of unintentional injuries in males, particularly later in childhood and adolescence. The death rates from all injuries and poisoning (which includes the small numbers of deaths due to intentional injuries) in the UK are shown in Figure 2.10, broken down by age and gender.

GENETIC FACTORS

At an individual level there is no doubt that genetic factors play an important role in determining health status. At a population level however, there is little evidence that they have a significant effect on overall health. The genetic differences between human subpopulations are in fact small and it appears that differences in health are largely accounted for

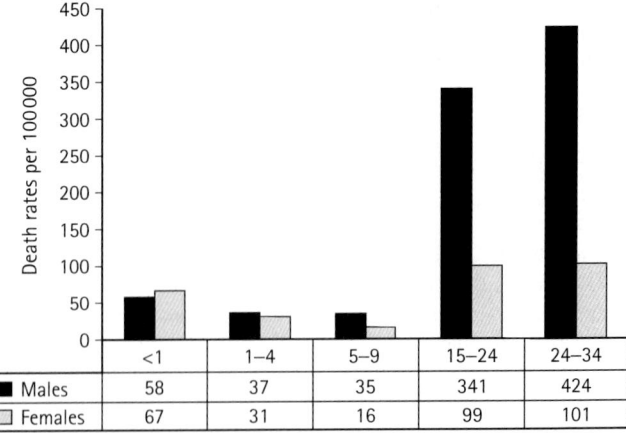

	<1	1–4	5–9	15–24	24–34
Males	58	37	35	341	424
Females	67	31	16	99	101

Fig. 2.10 Death rates form injury and poisoning per 100 000 by age and gender in England and Wales (2004).[2]

by environmental and behavioral differences. Clearly there are differences between populations in the frequency of some specific single gene disorders – for instance, sickle cell disease is uncommon in northern Europeans and cystic fibrosis is uncommon in Africans – but these contribute relatively little to the health experience on a population level. In other words, an individual's genetic makeup is important in determining their risk of ill health within a particular subpopulation who share common experiences, but not in explaining the differences between these subpopulations. This is borne out by numerous studies of immigrant populations, which suggest that the longer they spend in a new country and the more they adopt the lifestyle of that country, the more nearly their health experience comes to resemble that of the native population. Most differences that continue to exist between immigrant groups and the native population can be explained on the basis of either behavioral or socioeconomic factors.

BIRTH WEIGHT AND GESTATION

Birth weight, reflecting both gestation and intrauterine growth, is a powerful predictor of mortality (Fig. 2.7) and morbidity (e.g. cerebral palsy, Fig. 2.11)[21] in childhood. Globally 60–80% of neonatal deaths occur in low birth weight infants. In recent years it has been recognized that the effects of suboptimal birth weight may persist throughout life, with links being demonstrated between birth weight and cardiovascular and respiratory disease in adulthood. It appears that these adverse effects have a nearly linear relationship with birth weight rather than simply being associated with the lower extreme of the birth weight distribution.

Many of the determinants of both prematurity and poor intrauterine growth remain to be elucidated, although some specific conditions such as pre-eclamptic toxemia are important in individuals. Poor intrauterine

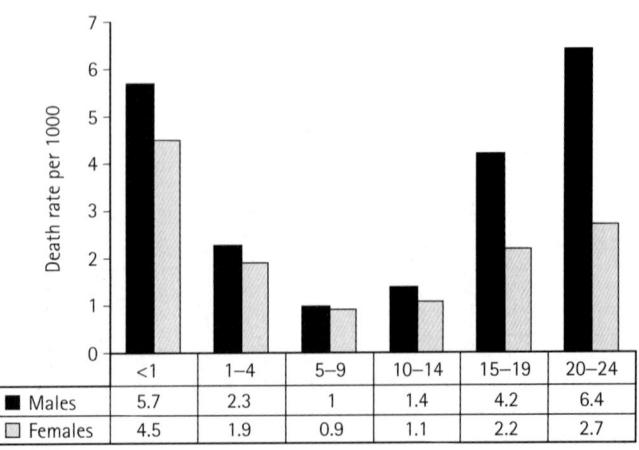

	<1	1–4	5–9	10–14	15–19	20–24
Males	5.7	2.3	1	1.4	4.2	6.4
Females	4.5	1.9	0.9	1.1	2.2	2.7

Fig. 2.9 Death rates per 1000 by age and gender in England and Wales (2005).[2]

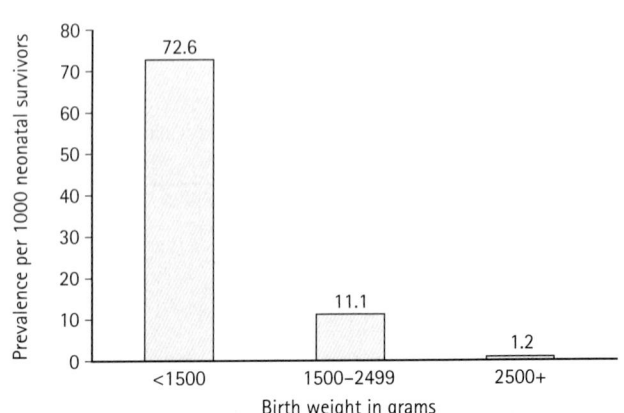

Fig. 2.11 Prevalence of cerebral palsy by birth weight in Europe.[21]

growth is associated with smoking during pregnancy and with socio-economic deprivation. Diet has often been suggested as a possible cause of intrauterine growth retardation but good evidence for this is lacking, except for the effects of extreme malnutrition.

PHYSICAL ENVIRONMENT

While some specific environmental hazards have been clearly identified, the links between others such as damp, overcrowded housing or atmospheric pollution and ill health have been difficult to determine. Many of these, possibly disadvantageous, conditions tend to occur in combination with each other and with socioeconomic disadvantage, making it difficult to disentangle their effects. Many pollutants in the environment or in food are so widespread that investigation is difficult. It is also possible that it is the interactions between such pollutants that are important, which further complicates attempts to quantify their effects. It could be argued that, in these circumstances, it may be appropriate to accept lower levels of evidence before proceeding to action, sometimes referred to as the precautionary principle, than would generally be required for reaching conclusions about causal links.

SOCIAL FACTORS

Socioeconomic status (SES) is a powerful predictor of health outcome within all societies. Within poor countries, this is unsurprising, given that SES is linked to the availability of basic necessities including food and shelter. What is perhaps remarkable is that the link remains strong even in rich industrialized countries. What may seem equally surprising is that the differences exist, not simply between the poorest members of society and the rest of the population, but, for many important health outcomes, there is something approaching a linear relationship between SES and adverse outcome.

How best to measure SES in childhood remains a source of debate. It is clearly a complicated concept and it seems likely that different aspects of disadvantage will be important for different health outcomes. In the UK, SES has traditionally been measured using an occupational classification. This scheme, first employed around the beginning of the twentieth century, assigned all occupations to six (originally five) groups based on a notion of a hierarchy of status. In 2001 this system was replaced by a new eight-group classification, the National Statistics Socio-economic Classification. Other classifications have been developed based on factors such as maternal education, income, access to material goods such as motor cars or telephones, type of housing and the nature of the area in which the family lives. Although the strength of the association between SES and a particular outcome may vary according to the measure used, the direction of effect is virtually always the same.

The effects of SES are observable from the beginnings of life, with a strong relationship between birth weight and SES. Figure 2.12 shows the proportion of infants born weighing less than 2500 g in SES deciles in one region of the UK (based on the characteristics of the small area in which they live).[22] Perhaps even more striking is the proportion of infants born weighing more than 3500 g (regarded as being an optimum birth weight) in different SES deciles (Fig. 2.13). In both figures there is a clear gradient across the different social groups. The magnitude of this effect is illustrated by the fact that this study reported that, if the whole population had the risk seen in the richest 10%, this would avoid 30% of all births below 2500 g and 32% of births below 1500 g.

In the UK in 1994–1999 the difference in life expectancy at birth between children in the 10% of most deprived areas in the UK and those in the richest 10% was 6 years for boys and 3.2 years for girls.[2]

The differences in infant mortality across social classes are shown in Figure 2.14. Particularly marked differences are seen in mortality from injuries and poisoning between social groups (Fig. 2.15).[23]

Similar differences are seen for most measures of morbidity, where figures are available, with large differences being shown between social groups for the risk of admission to hospital, for severe respiratory infections and for mental disorders (Table 2.8).[16] Finally, SES in early childhood strongly predicts the likelihood of educational achievement, which in turn predicts later job opportunities and income.

SES can of course not be said to directly cause ill health, but rather acts as a marker for various adverse circumstances and behaviors, which are the proximal causes for health outcomes. There is growing evidence that these circumstances cumulate over the life course and that the longer a child spends in adverse social circumstances, the greater the risk of poor health outcome.

HEALTH BEHAVIORS

There is considerable evidence of the deleterious effects of a number of health behaviors by parents and children on the health of children. Smoking by parents, and by children, in particular, is a major cause of many adverse outcomes including intrauterine growth retardation, sudden infant death syndrome and respiratory disease. At least in the UK and USA, smoking is much more common amongst people in poorer social circumstances and is likely to be one of the mechanisms through which SES has its effects on children's health. This close relationship between SES and smoking does, however, hamper efforts to estimate the magnitude of the effect of smoking per se as its effects may be confounded by other adverse circumstances.

Harmful effects of poor diet and lack of exercise in childhood have also been suggested. Very large increases in the proportion of children who are overweight or obese have been reported in the UK and USA. Between 1994 and 2004 in the UK the proportion of 11–15-year-old boys who were obese rose from 14% to 24% and of 11–15-year-old girls from 15% to 26%.[24] As there is substantial tracking between fatness in childhood and adulthood, this may have important implications for

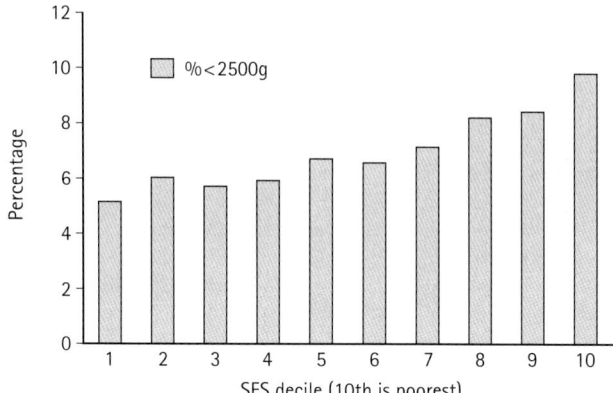

Fig. 2.12 Percentage of births < 2500 g by SES decile in the West Midlands, UK.[22]

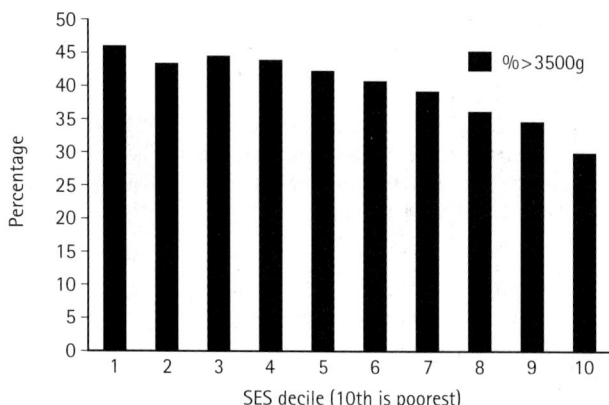

Fig. 2.13 Percentage of births > 3500 g by SES decile in the West Midlands, UK.[22]

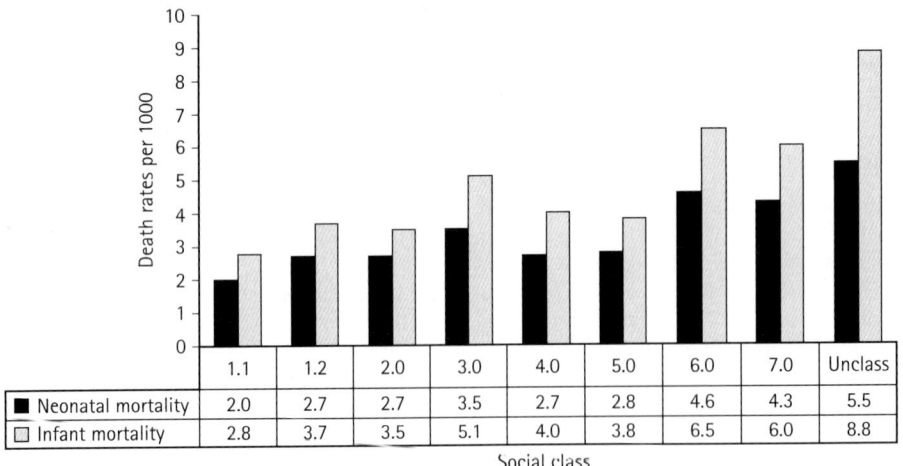

Fig. 2.14   Neonatal and infant mortality rates by parental occupational social class for jointly registered births in England and Wales (2004).[2]

Social class	1.1	1.2	2.0	3.0	4.0	5.0	6.0	7.0	Unclass
■ Neonatal mortality	2.0	2.7	2.7	3.5	2.7	2.8	4.6	4.3	5.5
□ Infant mortality	2.8	3.7	3.5	5.1	4.0	3.8	6.5	6.0	8.8

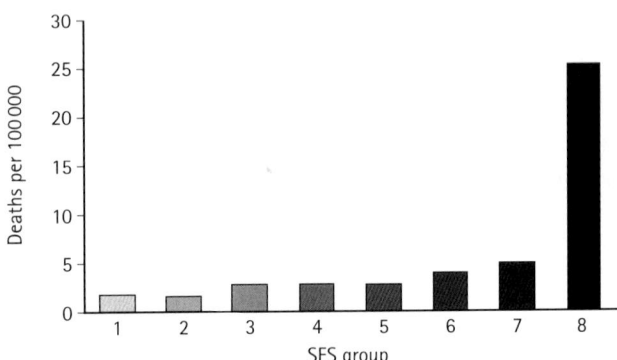

Fig. 2.15   Deaths in children aged 0–15 from injury and poisoning per 100 000 by occupational social class, England and Wales (2001–2003).[23]

Table 2.8   Percentage of children aged 5–16 with a mental disorder by gender and weekly household income in Great Britain, 2004[16]

Household income	Boys	Girls
< £100	18.4	13.4
£100–199	13.9	13.0
£200–299	17.8	11.5
£300–399	14.8	9.8
£400–499	10.2	6.8
£500–599	10.6	7.1
£600–770	6.0	3.7
>£770	6.7	3.9

the risk of cardiovascular disease and type 2 diabetes in later life. It has been suggested that these increases are likely to reflect declining levels of physical activity and the increasing consumption of convenience foods, although clear etiological evidence is lacking.

HEALTH SERVICES

Until recent years there has been surprisingly little evidence that health services are an important determinant of children's health in richer countries. The obvious exceptions are immunization and public health measures such as the provision of safe water supplies. Even for vaccine-preventable diseases, much of the decline in mortality in these countries preceded the introduction of immunization. It is nonetheless true that immunization has been associated with dramatic declines in deaths from measles, polio, meningococcal disease and other conditions which were major causes of deaths into recent times.

It is clear that the major determinants of child health lie outside the realm of curative services and are related to social and environmental factors. However, in rich societies, the rates of mortality have fallen to very low levels and the importance of the effective management of relatively uncommon conditions has become proportionately more important in determining mortality rates. For instance, the widespread use of antenatal steroids in women in preterm labor and of surfactant in premature infants has led to substantial declines in mortality from idiopathic respiratory distress syndrome in neonates. Similarly, as malignant disease accounts for an increasing proportion of childhood deaths, improvements in cure rates due to medical management can have significant effects on childhood mortality rates.

As discussed earlier, simple interventions by health services have the potential to significantly reduce deaths and morbidity in the poorest communities in the world. The difficulty has been in trying to introduce such services in the face of a shortage of resources and often weak governmental structures which are not always responsive to the needs of the poorest members of society. The 'inverse care law'[25] was first described in the UK in the 1970s and suggested that 'The availability of good medical care tends to vary inversely with the needs of the population served.' Unfortunately this law still applies between countries and between population groups, within even the poorest. For instance, in sub-Saharan Africa and Southeast Asia, amongst the 20% of richest women 86% have skilled care at the birth of their children compared to only 14% amongst the poorest 20%.[4]

While health services can significantly ameliorate the consequences of many diseases they can also lead to an increased prevalence of children with significant morbidity. Some of the children who are saved from death may survive with significant morbidity and may be kept alive for long periods in spite of their disabilities. It is important that clinicians recognize both the importance of factors outside their control in determining children's health and the potential societal consequences of advances in technology.

REFERENCES

1. World Health Organization. http://www.who. int/en/.

2. Office for National Statistics. http://www.statistics. gov.uk/default.asp.

3. Bryce J, Boschi-Pinto C, Shibuya K, et al., WHO Child Health Epidemiology Reference Group. WHO estimates of the causes of deaths in children. Lancet 2005; 365:1147–1152.

4. Lawn JE, Cousens S, Zupan J, the Lancet Neonatal Survival Steering Team. 4 million neonatal deaths: When? Where? Why? Lancet 2005; 365:891–900.

5. Jones G, Steketee RW, Black RE, et al. Bellagio Child Survival Study Group. How many child deaths can we prevent this year? The Lancet 2003; 362:65–71.

6. Hoyert DL, Mathews TJ, Menacker F, et al. Annual Summary of Vital Statistics: 2004. Pediatrics 2006; 117:168–183.

7. Office for National Statistics. Living in Britain: Results from the 2002 General Household Survey. http://www.statistics.gov.uk/lib2002/default.asp.

8. Bone M, Meltzer H. The prevalence of disability among children. OPCS Surveys of Disability in Great Britain, report 3. London: HMSO; 1989.

9. Boyle C, Decouflé P, Yeargin-Allsopp M. Prevalence and health impact of developmental disorders in children. Pediatrics 1994; 93:399–403.

10. Blanchard LT, Gurka MJ, Blackman JA. Emotional, Developmental and Behavioral Health of American Children and Their Families: A Report From the 2003 National Survey of Children's Health. Pediatrics 2006; 117:e1202–e1212.

11. Bhasin TK, Brocksen S, Avchem RN, et al. Prevalence of four developmental disabilities among children aged 8 years – Metropolitan Atlanta Developmental Disabilities Surveillance Program, 1996 and 2000. MMWR Surveillance Summaries 2006; 55:1–9.

12. Colver A, Gibson M, Hey EN, et al. Increasing rates of cerebral palsy across the severity spectrum in north-east England 1964–1993. Arch Dis Child 2000; 83:F7–F12.

13. Surman G, Bonellie S, Chalmers J, et al. UKCP: a collaborative network of cerebral palsy registers in the United Kingdom. Journal of Public Health 2006; 28:148–156.

14. Platt MJ, Cans C, Johnson A, et al. Trends in cerebral palsy among infants of very low birthweight (<1500 g) or born prematurely (<32 weeks) in 16 European centres: a database study. The Lancet 2007; 369:43–50.

15. Lenton S, Stallard P, Lewis M, et al. Prevalence and morbidity associated with non-malignant, life-threatening conditions in childhood. Child Care Health Dev 2001; 27:389–398.

16. Green H, McGinnity A, Meltzer H, et al. Mental health of children and young people in Great Britain, 2004. Office for National Statistics http://www.statistics. gov.uk/downloads/theme_health/GB2004.pdf

17. Durkin M. The epidemiology of developmental disabilities in low-income countries. Mental Retardation and Developmental Disabilities Research Reviews 2002; 8:206–211.

18. Mung'ala-Odera V, Meehan R, Njuguna P, et al. Prevalence and risk factors of neurological disability and impairment in children living in rural Kenya. International Journal of Epidemiology 2006; 35:683–688.

19. Christianson AL, Zwane ME, Manga P, et al. Children with intellectual disability in rural South Africa: prevalence and associated disability. J Intel Disabil Res 2002; 46:179–186.

20. Grantham-McGregor S, Cheung YB, Cueto S, et al. International Child Development Steering Group. Developmental potential in the first 5 years for children in developing countries. The Lancet 2007; 369:60–70.

21. Surveillance of Cerebral Palsy in Europe (SCPE). Prevalence and characteristics of children with cerebral palsy in Europe. Develop Med Child Neurol 2002; 44:633–640.

22. Bambang S, Spencer NJ, Gill L, et al. Socioeconomic status and birthweight: comparison of an area-based measure with the Registrar General's social class. J Epidemiol Community Health 1999; 53:495–498.

23. Edwards P, Green J, Roberts I, et al. Deaths from injury in children and employment status in family: analysis of trends in class specific death rates. BMJ 2006; 333:119.

24. The Health Survey for England 2004. http://www. dh.gov.uk/en/Publicationsandstatistics/PublishedSurvey/ HealthSurveyForEngland/index.htm

25. Hart JT. The inverse care law. Lancet 1971; 1:405–412.

3

Health care delivery in resource limited settings

Elizabeth Molyneux

BACKGROUND

In 1978 in Almaty Kazakstan (then Alma-Alta) a meeting on primary health care was jointly sponsored by the United Nations Children's Fund and the World Health Organization (WHO) and attended by representatives from many countries.[1] A call was made for 'health for all'. Nearly 30 years on 'health for all' is still more hope than substance.[2] In 1990 The Millennium Development Goals were defined.[3] Amongst the goals are to improve the health of both mothers and children; to reduce under 5s child mortality rate by two thirds, and maternal mortality by three quarters by 2015. At current rates these goals will not be achieved until 2165 in sub-Saharan Africa.[4] In 2003 the Bellagio child survival group (named after the place that the meeting was held) report[5] was published in which representatives of the donor communities and health services of resource constrained areas described children's health in various parts of the world and suggested that with the present state of knowledge and relatively little financial investment, 60% of the deaths in children under 5 years of age could be averted. In research too, the World Health Forum describes a 90/10 divide in which only 10% of research funding goes to poorer parts of the world where 90% of the people live.[6]

Why is the health divide so wide, and increasing, between well resourced countries and those which are financially constrained? The problems are complex.

THE PHILOSOPHY OF CARE

In the 1970s primary health was promoted as the way forward to reach the poorest and most difficult to access (often rural) population. This service was to deploy community health workers (CHWs), traditional birth attendants (TBAs) and mid-level health staff such as nurses and clinical officers. However primary care has been understood variously, as the central pivot for health systems, as a mere extension of services to underserved areas, or even as a rather second class service for the poor.[7] The first definition requires social, structural and financial investment, the other definitions diminish the value of primary care.

Funding for primary care has been inconsistent in part because it is not easy to establish clear indicators of achievements and failures and without these, financial systems do not function.[8] Primary health care is often seen as an emergency response to health disasters by international donors rather than the bedrock of health care delivery. But in the second Disease Control Priorities in Developing Countries report, it is argued that 90% of the health care demand is potentially addressable by primary care.[9] Historically most health services have been built and powered from the top down. Centrally made decisions have trickled down to primary services in the community. Urban health in resource poor countries is nearer to the health model taught in most traditional medical schools, with emphasis placed on specialization and hospital care.

The large hospitals were built, managed and staffed like those in developed countries. This tended to lead to excellent care for the politically powerful urban few, at the neglect of the rural poor. Medical students were, and are given bedside teaching which emphasizes diagnostic acumen and knowledge of diseases, but teaches little about health care delivery – for instance why did this particular child get admitted, by whom, when and why? Why were others not admitted? In the 1970s the pendulum of donor funding tipped towards primary health care and it gradually improved. The use of traditional birth attendants and village community heath workers was encouraged. Acceptance has not been universal, with some reports arguing that skilled care at delivery made the difference in maternal survival with the result that the unskilled cadre of health workers fell into some disrepute.[10,11] More recently there are many examples of the value of the CHW. They have helped improve community uptake of health services, decreasing neonatal mortality in India, and in many countries successfully run immunization services and health promotion schemes.[12-14] They work best when included as part of the health service and not made to feel outsiders, or second best.[15] A health service needs all levels of service to be effective. It is recognized that the larger hospitals have been neglected, and as these are teaching centers and service the community, there is an important swing back to seeing their improvement as equally important.

HUMAN RESOURCES

Health services are directed by policy and finance but are driven and sustained by people. In the 2006 World Health Report, the WHO highlights the crisis in human resources for health.[16] The central importance of human resources to health means that this issue deserves high international priority.[17] To achieve the Millennium Development Goals – which are wider than child and maternal health – Africa alone will need a further 1 million health personnel, and the global need is an extra 4 million health workers.[18] The ratio of health carers (nurses, doctors, midwives) to population is 10 times greater in Europe than in Africa, and yet maternal, neonatal and infant mortality are directly related to the skilled staff:patient ratio.[19]

The need for skilled health carers is at crisis point in much of subSaharan Africa and efforts are being redoubled to train as well as to deploy CHWs where possible. In Asia CHWs have worked with great effect. For instance, in the 2005 earthquakes of Pakistan 8000 female health workers were mobilized from the affected areas to assist in the camps and villages. In India there are plans to train 300 000 more CHWs while in Thailand 60 000 village health workers were trained to support 600 000 voluntary health workers; who in turn looked after 20 children each.[20] It has been suggested that a ratio of one full-time paid CHW to 500 people and one to 10–20 for local volunteers is the correct requirement.[20]

In poorly resourced settings we tend to think of resources as material needs – equipment, drugs, good buildings, transport, communications – all of which are necessary and important and which may be scarce or in poor shape. The health care team is made up of a group of people with varying backgrounds, training, skills and expectations. Each person in the team has a much bigger task in terms of quantity and breadth than their counterparts in a well-resourced system. This team may consist of a clinical officer (akin to a nurse practitioner), nurses/midwives, health care auxiliaries and health surveillance assistants. If there is a doctor he/she will be expected to lead this team.

WHAT IS EXPECTED OF THE CHILD HEALTH DOCTOR?

In such circumstances the doctor must be the leader, a teacher, a supervisor and an advocate. He/she needs to think creatively about how to deploy staff, to prioritize both their time and that of others, and to stimulate, enthuse and lead 'from the front'. In child health, whatever their own clinical interests and preferences they need to see the wider context of the health service and ensure that the team's efforts reflect the needs and demands of the community they serve.

Many doctors trained in poorly resourced countries have stayed to serve their communities for little financial or career rewards. For very many others the offers of specialization, security and financial gain have attracted them to resource rich countries.[21-23] There is much to be gained from medical exchanges, extra specialist training, sabbaticals and cross-fertilization of ideas but if these encourage a drain from settings of need to places of plenty; then the loss to poor communities is very great indeed.[24]

Government services struggle to implement health care with too few trained staff. Skill mix has become increasingly important; nurses and clinical officers have taken on many of the jobs that traditionally have been carried out by doctors, nurse auxiliaries work under the supervision of trained nurses and Health Surveillance Assistants play key roles in health promotion, disease prevention and monitoring in the community. Voluntary or paid community health workers, elected by the village community assist with bed net provision, simple treatments and health promotion. Nurses have had many tasks put upon them in the antenatal clinics beyond the monitoring of a woman's pregnancy (e.g. human immunodeficiency virus [HIV] prevention, malaria prophylaxis, nutrition teaching, advice about breast feeding, tetanus immunization, STI treatment and prevention). Similarly in the Under Fives Clinics a nurse is being asked to weigh and measure the height of a child, assess development, encourage exclusive breastfeeding for 6 months, give immunizations, give vitamin A, nutritional advice, malaria prophylaxis, co-trimoxazole prophylaxis for HIV-infected infants and children. Many of these duties can be done, and are done by less skilled but dedicated and trained staff. The World Health Report of 2006 urges health services and health training institutions to re-look at task allocations within both the professional and voluntary cadres.[16]

HEALTH CARE FINANCING

As the cost of and demand for health care has risen various ways of cost sharing have been tried. The Bamako Initiative of 1987 was an attempt to improve primary care and user fees were suggested as a key component to make improvements sustainable.[25] By raising revenue it was hoped that the quality of care, coverage and drug availability would improve without the need for persistent external inputs. User fees have been successful in some countries (Benin, Senegal, Burkino Faso) but not in others and in some places have been withdrawn as they were seen as a barrier to the poorest people accessing care.[26] They seem to help when they are part of a care package that includes insurance and good exemption schemes. Some countries (e.g. Sri Lanka) have continued successfully to provide free health at point of care while others such as Bolivia intend to provide a similar service backed up by insurance.[27] The World Health Report 2005 'Making every mother and child count'[28] rejects user fees and argues that social insurance or tax-based responses are superior.

DRUG SUPPLY – THE PHARMACEUTICAL PIPELINE

In 1975–1997, of 1325 new drugs which came on to the market only 11 were for tropical infections.[29] WHO has compiled an essential drugs list (329 drugs and 559 formulations) to help focus drug provision on basic needs.[30] Many governments have central medical stores through which bulk medical buys are made but worldwide 30% of people lack access to essential drugs. This varies from 26% in most of SE Asia, to 47% in Sub-Saharan Africa (SSA) and 65% in India.[31] UNICEF provides 40% of the global demand for vaccinations and the Global Alliance for Vaccines and Immunisation (GAVI) and the Global Fund have been very effective and active in providing a wider range of immunizations for national EPI programs as well as treatments for TB, malaria and HIV, respectively.[31-33]

Good will donations are sent to many hospitals without any clear understanding of the pharmaceutical needs or controls of a country. Lavy et al[34] gave advice to help potential donors and the WHO has come up with standards to which donated drugs must conform.[35] In some villages drug revolving schemes have been established whereby a responsible villager is chosen by the community to be custodian of a few simple medicines which he/she dispenses at cost and thus recovers the monies to buy replacement medicines.[36,37]

NATIONAL HEALTH PROGRAMS

Programs require substantial funding which is heavily dependent on donor provision.[38] Donors have, over the years, channeled funds in a variety of different ways – vertical programs, parallel programs, single disease-focused initiatives, funds targeted to one sector of the population such as reproductive health or primary care. National health services have been molded to meet the requirements of individual donor states or programs. More recently a sector-wide approach (SWAps)[39] has been introduced in which donors 'basket' (put together) funds and give them to a Ministry of Health to deliver a predetermined health program based on an assessment of needs called the Essential National Package of Health Services.[40]

HEALTH DELIVERY AND THE REFERRAL CHAIN

Health services are divided into different levels of care delivery. It is essential to provide care as near to the home as possible, but that care must be supported by a tiered system that provides support for the tier below and receives support and refers to the tier above. There must be a seamless continuum of care within which there is free and good communication at and between all tiers and appropriate use of each level of care.

THE HEALTH CENTER

At village level, health centers or mobile health clinics provide simple first-line curative treatment, immunizations and health promotion and do uncomplicated deliveries. These are ideally run by a nurse, midwife and medical assistant and Community Health Workers supervised and supported by staff from the local district hospital. These interventions collectively reduce many risk factors for ill health.

THE DISTRICT HOSPITAL

The district hospital provides first level referral care and is often staffed by clinical officers and nurses, with or without a doctor. Such a hospital will typically have about 200 beds and serve a wide catchment area. This service can be provided relatively cheaply and is reported to cost about $9/d in Kenya, $12 in Bangladesh.[41] District hospitals will refer their difficult cases to the regional or tertiary referral hospital.

This level of care is termed the first-level referral and plays a significant role in the quality of service a population can expect to receive. English et al reported on the indifferent quality of care first-level referral hospitals give in Kenya when staff members are demoralized and unsupported and equipment and structures are neglected.[42]

THE TERTIARY HOSPITAL

The tertiary hospital or regional hospital will have staff in at least the main specialties of medicine, pediatrics, surgery, obstetrics and gynecology. They are in large towns or cities and may serve as the city district hospital. They are also the teaching units for different medical and nursing cadres. Staff members of these large hospitals visit district hospitals to teach and help with problem cases. Many of these hospitals were built in the 1950s or 1960s and, when policy focused on primary care, were neglected. It is now recognized that these hospitals are where future health staff are trained and are a vital link in the continuum of care for patients.[16] The public's views of the quality of a national health service is colored by the care seen to be provided in its tertiary institutions.

VERTICAL, PARALLEL OR HORIZONTAL SERVICES?

Vertical programs may offer an effective response to address specific issues but there is a danger that programs may conflict with each other or may undermine the provision of primary health care. Maternal and child health (MCH) are interdependent but in some programs (Safe Motherhood for instance) the baby got little mention, and in some child initiatives the importance of the mother's health is unemphasized.[43] Of the 10 million children who die every year, the vast majority in resource constrained areas, 4 million are neonatal deaths.[44] Half a million mothers die every year in childbirth, which imperils infant survival and leaves many orphans, whose health and well being will inevitably suffer.[45] There are over 12 million orphans in Africa.[46,47]

In Tanzania to avoid vertical programs and strengthen subnational health systems the Tanzanian Essential Health Interventions Project (TEHIP) was started in 1997.[48] After 5 years the mix, quality, use and coverage of health services improved and there was a 40% reduction in under-fives mortality. This initiative cost $1 per person and the funding was obtained through the SWAps financing system. District health management teams set their own priorities and integrated health informatics into the plan. This experience suggests that investing in the health system can work but that it takes time. In addition to a burden of disease analysis consideration of cost effectiveness, budgeting, management, team building, mapping, transport, and communications were all necessary. Even then the effect was only seen after 5 years.[49,50]

INFORMATION, SURVEILLANCE AND RESEARCH

Comprehensive health management information is important to measure quality and coverage of health services. Poor data often leads to poor decision making and ultimately poor quality of care.[51] In many countries data is collected in too many different and uncoordinated ways and there is lack of access to information and to information research.[52–54] The importance of data and the need to rapidly cycle results back to the health care units so as to influence day-to-day decision making has become clear.[55]

Detailed country-specific epidemiological data will be available for each country from WHO so that a national health service can tailor its efforts, prioritize its needs and set goals for itself.[16]

HIGH-IMPACT HEALTH INTERVENTIONS

Some relatively simple interventions influence the health of many. Examples are immunization programs, vitamin A supplementation, zinc supplementation, infant care, simple treatments, bednet provision, improving care at first level referral hospitals and the integration of health care through the Integrated Management of Childhood Illnesses (IMCI).[56–58]

Improving inpatient care in referral hospitals and especially emergency care can make an immediate difference to inpatient morbidity and mortality. In Blantyre, improving triage and emergency care by teaching and implementing the WHO Emergency Triage Assessment and Treatment (ETAT) has led to a reduction in inpatient mortality from 11–18% to 6–8%.[59,60] Prophylactic co-trimoxazole for HIV-infected children, anti-retroviral therapy for children (and their parents) who have reached a clinical- or laboratory-based stage of the disease needing therapy, TB diagnosis and treatments gain from vertically managed programs which are not mutually exclusive and are imbedded in the health care system.

Clear consideration of evidence is important as not all apparently sensible interventions have proved as successful. For instance the blanket provision of iron and folic acid to preschool children in a highly malarial area in East Africa proved detrimental to health and outcome.[61]

SYNDROMIC MANAGEMENT OF DISEASES

Where patients are many and staff are few, supported by little or no laboratory services, a syndromic approach to the diagnosis and management of particular types of infection has been taken. A diagnosis is made on a brief history and the presence of a few key symptoms or signs. For instance in sexually transmitted diseases an appropriate history and findings elicits a treatment which covers all the common treatable bacterial causes. This leads to overtreatment but simplifies the management of large numbers of patients by relatively few staff. Clinicians are taught this approach and national programs rationalize the availability of appropriate drugs for the level of health service.

IMCI is an integrated approach to the care of children which uses flow diagrams and simple pattern recognition in signs and symptoms to treat children.[62] IMCI strategy has three main components:

1. to improve case management skills of health carers using locally adapted clinical guidelines that do not focus on a single diagnosis but rather on selected signs and symptoms which guide rational treatment
2. to provide support through the provision of appropriate therapies and referral chains

3. to see the child in the context of the family and the clinical context with the acute event used to provide not only immediate curative treatment but also attention to nutrition, immunization, counseling and other heath needs.

In Tanzania this is reported to have led to 13% reduction in cost of care and better outcomes.[63] A recent re-analysis of this data to include the quality of care given showed that the cost of using IMCI was $4.02/person per annum compared with $25.70 without IMCI.[64]

EXPANDED PROGRAM FOR IMMUNIZATION (EPI)

Immunization remains one of the most cost-effective approaches to health care but the coverage varies greatly from country to country and even between rural and urban areas. The least accessible children who are the most vulnerable in society receive least protection.

EPI programs include periodically giving vitamin A supplements to children. The included vaccines vary. While some countries (e.g. Malawi) have achieved high rates of uptake and include pentavalent vaccines (DPTHibHepB – diphtheria, pertussis, tetanus, *Haemophilus influenzae*, hepatitis B) most countries of subSaharan Africa are still using DPT. Pentavalent vaccine raises the cost of vaccination tenfold and can only be sustained with external funding such as from GAVI.[65]

HIV/AIDS – PREVENTION, DIAGNOSIS PROPHYLAXIS AND TREATMENT

Many high-burden countries with HIV/AIDS are struggling to provide for the needs of people who are living with AIDS with high proportions of the population needing care. Fixed combination drugs (FDCs) are now available and provided through the global fund, but every affected country needs a national program with registration procedures, protocols, training, stock control, prescribing controls and monitoring. The human resources required and logistical implications are huge. Children are expected to form about 10% of the total number of people on anti-retroviral therapy (ART) and their access to therapy has been slower than that of adults. In Malawi they are 5% of the total number on ART.[66] Reasons for this have been difficulty in deciding how to provide suitable doses for children with a limited variety of FDC tablets available and none of them child friendly tablets. Other difficulties include the inability to confirm a diagnosis below the age of 15 months if only HIV antibody testing is available and complex issues surrounding advice about infant feeding. What advice is best for babies whose chances of acquiring HIV infection with breast-feeding are about 14–42%,[67] but whose chances of dying of gastroenteritis in a poor family if bottle fed are much greater?[68] A Zambian study of co-trimoxazole (CoT) prophylaxis for children with HIV showed a decrease in mortality.[69] This has meant that CoT is recommended to all children (and adults) with HIV infection and HIV-exposed infants. The logistics for this provision are challenging.

PALLIATIVE CARE

Holistic care of a child and family is incomplete without palliative care, a stark reality with the HIV/AIDS epidemic. There is a steady increase in awareness of its value and national palliative care programs have started, training courses are available and oral morphine is available in some countries.[70–72] Hospital-based and home-based care must liaise to try to provide medical, moral, emotional and spiritual support to the children and their families who approach the end of the children's lives.[73] Palliative care supports the families involved and is also a great support to staff who may feel helpless when faced by the obvious needs of these families.

TB TREATMENT PROGRAMS

National TB programs have served as models for the HIV/AIDS programs. National TB drug policies, protocols, supervision and monitoring are helping to provide treatment for the increased number of TB cases with the onset of the HIV/AIDS epidemic. National control of the TB treatments also reduces the risk of poor prescribing leading to the emergence of resistant TB. The directly observed therapy (DOTs) campaign helps reduce poor compliance.[74]

Both TB and HIV/AIDS are well served by vertical national programs.

MALNUTRITION

Poor nutrition directly affects 5.6 million deaths every year in children under 5 years old. In the developing world 25% of all children (about 146 million children) are underweight, which remains unchanged since 1999. Half these children are in Bangladesh, India and Pakistan, where 45% of the children under 5 years of age are malnourished. It is particularly evident in places of rapid population growth, in areas of conflict, or with high HIV prevalence, drought or poor agricultural productivity. Diarrhea and poor feeding habits are confounding and causative factors and it is of concern that children who do not catch up with growth in the first 2 years of life may have continuing cognitive problems. Regular vitamin A supplementation and micronutrients help prevent some of the diarrheal diseases that lead to malnutrition.[75]

Malnourished children need either supplementary feeding or therapeutic feeding. This is done in a phased manner so that calorie intake and protein load are increased over a few days and high loads introduced once diarrhea and edema have started to resolve and appetite increase. This is especially important in severe kwashiorkor. Supplementary feeding is for moderately malnourished children and is provided as a nutritious porridge flour or a ready-to-use therapeutic feed (RUTF) such as plumpynut – a peanut-based high-energy food.[62,76–78] It is vital to support nutrition in all areas of health care as malnutrition has a detrimental effect on every aspect of health outcomes.

TRAINING

Training is required at many levels. University-trained doctors and nurses are needed for leadership roles and in the referral hospitals but they tend to stay in urban areas. Their training is costly and once qualified their expectations of resources and rewards are high. They are not enough to provide for a country's health needs. Other cadres of staff must be trained for different tiers of the health service. Medical assistants, clinical officers, patient attendants and community workers are trained to provide many of these services. For instance, in Malawi clinical officers receive 4 years of training, which includes 1 year's internship making them able to deal with common illness and emergencies.

DILEMMAS AND CONSTRAINTS

The means with which to meet large unresolved problems are limited. There is a dilemma in trying to provide good-quality service – service which includes kindness, courtesy and explanations – in quantity and for little cost. Rural primary health care workers in Zambia, 40% of whom worked without a doctor, identified transport, knowledge, traditional beliefs, social stigma, poorly trained health staff, poor access to drugs and user fees as barriers to good health service provision. Lack of human resources is a major problem and requires lateral and creative thinking in job allocations.

Concentrating on infectious diseases, the HIV/AIDS epidemic, TB and malaria has distracted concern from chronic medical conditions such as renal disease, hypertension, cardiac disorders and has meant that trauma has been seriously neglected. Road traffic accidents are rising in increasingly urban societies, often against a background of poor town planning, poor driving ability, poor traffic control and unsafe vehicles. Emergency care has not gained priority and is not recognized as such in many health services. Triage, resuscitation, stabilization and initial good clinical management of all acute pediatric illness will prevent many deaths and much morbidity. Reduction in hospital costs and manpower use would be considerable.

SUMMARY

Health delivery is a big subject and in this chapter a broad brush has been used to give a picture of common health themes in many countries in poorer parts of the world. The fine details are place and person specific but training, feedback of outcome, praise, constructive criticism, commitment and faithful service of members of the health team are essential to fill in the details of the picture. Without these the picture remains blurred and unfocused. It is these potent, small, personal efforts of people at the heart of the service that give it life and clarifies the picture. They identify real needs and sustain changes that really matter. Creative thinking and great ingenuity go into local health care to provide what on the surface may not look possible.

It is to these often unrewarded and unrecognized people that this chapter is respectfully dedicated.

REFERENCES

1. Primary Health Care. Report of the International Conference on Primary Health Care, Alma Alta USSR 6–12 September 1978, jointly sponsored by the World Health Organization and the United Nation's Children's Fund. Geneva: World Health Organization; 1978 (Health for All Series No 1).
2. Marcos C. The promise of primary health care [editorial]. WHB 2005; 83:322.
3. United Nations Development Programme. Human Development Report 2003 Millennium Development Goals: A compact end to human poverty. Oxford: Oxford University Press; 2003.
4. World Bank. The Millennium Development Goals for health: rising to the challenge. Washington: World Bank; 2004.
5. Jones G, Steketee RW, Black RE, et al, and the Bellagio Child Survival Group. Bellagio report. How many child deaths can we prevent this year? Lancet 2003; 362:977–988.
6. Global Forum Update on Research for Health, Vol. 2. Poverty, Equity and Health Research. Global Forum on Health Research: helping correct the 10/90 gap; 2006.
7. Werner D, Sanders D. Questioning the solution: the politics of primary health care and child survival, an in depth critique of oral rehydration therapy. Palo Alto, CA: HealthWrights; 1997.
8. Patel M. An economic evaluation of Health for All. Health Policy Plan 1986; 1:37–47.
9. English M, Lanata C, Ngugi I, et al. Disease Control Priorities in Developing Countries. Ch. 25 2nd edn. Washington DC: World Bank; 2006.
10. Kruske S, Barclay L. The effect of shifting policies on traditional birth attendant training. J Midwifery Womens Health 2004; 49:306–311.
11. Sibley L, Ann ST. What can a meta-analysis tell us about traditional birth attendant training and pregnancy outcomes? Midwifery 2004; 20:51–60.
12. Sazawal S, Black RE. Effect of pneumonia case management on mortality in neonates, infants, and preschool children: a meta-analysis of community based trials. Lancet Infect Dis 2003; 3:547–556.
13. Winch PJ, Gilroy KE, Wolfheim C, et al. Teaching mothers to provide home treatment of malaria in Tigray, Ethiopia: a randomised trial. Lancet 2000; 356:550–555.
14. Bang AT, Bang RA, Baitule SB, et al. Effect of home-based neonatal care and management of sepsis on neonatal mortality: field trial in rural India. Lancet 1999; 354:1955–1961.
15. Parry E. Volunteers can contribute to health care. Id 21 insights DFID Tropical Health Education and Training London: 2004.
16. World Health Report, 2006. Working together for health. Geneva: WHO.
17. The crisis in human resources for health. [Editorial] Lancet 2006; 367:1117.
18. Chen L, Evans T, Anand S, et al. Human resources for health: overcoming the crisis. Lancet 2004; 364:1984–1900.
19. Anand S, Barnighausen T. Human resources and health outcomes. Lancet 2004; 364:1603–1609.
20. Jamison D, Breman J, Measham A, et al. Priorities in Health. The International Bank for Development and Reconstruction. Washington DC: The World Bank; 2006:131.

21. Migration of health workers: an unmanaged crisis. [Editorial] Lancet 2005; 365:1825.
22. Hongoro C, McPake B. How to bridge the gap in human resources for health? Lancet 2004; 364:1451–1456.
23. Eastwood JB, Conroy RE, Naicker S, et al. Loss of health professionals from subSaharan Africa: the pivotal role of the UK. Lancet 2005; 365:1893–1900.
24. Davey G, Fakade D, Parry E. Must aid hinder attempts to reach the Millennium Development Goals? Lancet 2006; 367:629–631.
25. The Bamako Initiative of 1987 by African Health ministers. UNICEF.
26. Wiseman V. Reflections on the impact of the Bamako Initiative and the role of user fees. Editorial Trop Doct 2005; 35:193.
27. Regina K. Research for free heath. Real Health News 2006; 4:March.
28. The World Health Report 2005; Making every mother and child count. Geneva: 2005.
29. Jamison D, Breman J, Measham A, et al. Priorities in health. The International Bank for Development and Reconstruction. Washington DC: The World Bank; 2006: 145.
30. World Health Organization Model list of essential medicines, 14th edn. Geneva: WHO; 2005.
31. Jamison D, Breman J, Measham A, et al. Priorities in health. The International Bank for Development and Reconstruction. Washington DC: The World Bank; 2006. 145.
32. Brugha R, Starling M, Walt G. GAVI the first steps: lessons for the global fund. Lancet 2002; 359:435–438.
33. Who are we and what do we do? Investing in our future. The Global Fund to fight AIDS, Tuberculosis and Malaria. ISBN 92-9224-30-7 http://www.theglobalfund.org/en/
34. Day JH, Lavy CBD. Pills to Africa: how to donate effectively. BMJ 2001; 323:1315, Trop Doc 2004; 34:65–66
35. Medicines Crossing Borders Project WHO step by step guide to good drug donation practices. Geneva: WHO; 2002.
36. Murakami H, Phomasack B, Oula R, et al. Revolving drug funds at the front-line health facilities in Vientane Lao. Health Policy Plan 2001; 16:98–106.
37. Ghebejesus TA, Alemayehu T, Bosman A, et al. Community participation in malaria control in Tigray region, Ethiopia. Acta Trop 1996; 2:142.
38. Sall M, Sylla J. African prime ministers take a lead in child survival. Lancet 2005; 366:166–189.
39. Hutton G, Tanner M. The sector-wide approach: a blessing for public health? Bull World Health Organ 2004; 82:893.
40. Bobadilla J, Cowley P, Musgrove P, et al. Design, content and financing of an essential national package of health services. Human Development Department. Washington DC: World Bank; 1993.
41. Jamison D, Breman J, Measham A, et al. Priorities in Health. The International Bank for Development and Reconstruction. Washington DC: World Bank; 2006: 136.
42. English M, Esamai F, Wasunna A, et al. Delivery of health care at the first-referral level in Kenya. Lancet 2004; 364:1622–1629.
43. Safe Motherhood Initiative 1987 Nairobi Kenya. Safe Motherhood Inter-Agency Group. www.safemotherhood.org/reviews/publications/html

44. Lawn JE, Cousens S, Zupan J. 4 million neonatal deaths: When? Where? Why? Lancet 2005; 265:891–900.
45. Khan KS, Wojdyla D, Say L, et al. WHO analysis of causes of maternal death: a systematic review. Lancet 2006; 367:1066–1074.
46. Monasch R, Boerma JT. Orphanhood and childcare patterns in sub-Saharan Africa: an analysis of national surveys from 40 countries. AIDS 2004; 18:S55–S65.
47. Sach SE, Sach JD. Africa's children orphaned by AIDS. Lancet 2004; 364:1404.
48. Marcel T. Strengthening district health systems. Bull World Health Organ 2005; 6:403.
49. Neilson S, Smutylo T. The Tanzanian essential health intervention 'Spark': Planning and managing health resources at the district level. International Development Research Centre, Science for Humanity, Canada. TEHIP final report, 2004.
50. De Savigny D, Kasale H, Mbuya C, et al. In focus. Fixing Health Systems. IDRC; 2004.
51. Redman TC. The impact of poor data quality on the typical enterprise. Communications of the ACM 1998; 41:79.
52. Church M, Moyo C. Health Management Information System in Malawi. Ministry of Health; 1999.
53. Campbell B. Health management information systems in lower income countries: an analysis of system design, implementation and utilization in Ghana and Nepal. The Netherlands; Royal Tropical Institute; 1997.
54. Habibzadeh F. Regional associations of medical journal editors: moving from rhetoric to reality. WHO Bulletin 2005; 83:404.
55. Shibaya K, Scheele S, Boerma T. Health Statistics: time to get service. Bull World Health Organ 2005; 83:722–723.
56. Technical seminars IMCI the integrated management of childhood illness. Geneva: World Health Organization Department of Child and Adolescent Health; 2001.
57. Brooks WA, Santosham M, Naheed A, et al. Effects of weekly zinc supplements on incidence of pneumonia and diarrhoea on children younger than 2 years in an urban, low-income population in Bangladesh: randomised controlled trial. Lancet 2005; 366:999–1004.
58. Tielsch J, Khatry SK, StOltzfus RJ, et al. Effects of routine prophylactic supplementation of iron and folic acid on preschool mortality in southern Nepal: a community-based, cluster-randomised, placebo-controlled trial. Lancet 2006; 367:144–152.
59. Robertson MA, Molyneux EM. Triage in the developing world – can it be done? Arch Dis Child 2001; 85:208–213.
60. Molyneux EM, Ahmad S, Robertson A. Improved triage and emergency care for children reduces inpatient mortality in resource – constrained setting. WHO Bulletin 2006; 84:314–319.
61. Sazawal S, Black RE, Ramsan M, et al. Effects of routine prophylactic supplementation of iron and folic acid on admission to hospital and mortality in preschool children in a high malaria transmission setting: a community-based, randomised, placebo-controlled trial. Lancet 2006; 367:133–143.
62. Integrated Management of Childhood Illnesses. UNICEF and CAH (WHO). Geneva: WHO; 2001.
63. Adam T, Manzi F, Schellenberg JA, et al. Does the integrated management of childhood illness cost more

than routine care? Results from the United Republic of Tanzania. Bull WHO 2005; 83:369–377.

64. Bryce J, Cesar V, Habicht J-P, et al. The multicountry evaluation of the IMCI strategy: lessons for the evaluation of public health interventions. Am J Public Health 2004; 94:406–415.

65. Daza P, Banda R, Misoya K, et al. The impact of routine infant immunization with Haemophilus influenzae type b conjugate vaccine in Malawi, a country with high human immunodeficiency virus prevalence. Vaccine 2006; 24:6232–6239.

66. Malawi Demographic and Health Survey; 2004. Zomba, Malawi: National Statistical Office.

67. Dunn DT, Newell ML, Ades AE, et al. Risk of human immunodeficiency virus type 1 transmission through breast feeding. Lancet 1992; 340:585–588.

68. Cutting W. Breast feeding and HIV – a balance of risks. J Trop Paediatr 1994; 40:6–11.

69. Chintu C, Bhat GJ, Walker AS, et al. Co-trimoxazole as prophylaxis against opportunistic infection in HIV-infected Zambian children (CHAP): a double blind randomised placebo-controlled trial. Lancet 2004; 364:1865–1871.

70. Merriman A, Kaur M. Palliative care in Africa: an appraisal. Lancet 2005; 365:1909–1911.

71. Defippi K, Dowing J, Merriman A, et al. A palliative care association for the whole of Africa. Palliat Med 2004; 18:583–584.

72. Merriman A. Making drugs available. AIDS Action 1998; 41:8.

73. Spence D, Merriman A, Bunagwaho A. Palliative care in Africa and the Caribbean. Plos Med 2004; 1:e5.

74. Balasubramanian VB, Oommen K, Samuel R. DOT or not? Direct observation of anti-tuberculosis treatment and patient outcomes, Kerala State. Int J Tuberc Lung Dis 2000; 4:409–413.

75. Moszynski P. UNICEF warns of 'epidemic' of childhood malnutrition. BMJ 2006; 332:1051. Prognosis for children. A report card on nutrition www.unicef.org.

76. Ciliberto MA, Sandige H, Ndekha MJ, et al. Comparison of home-based therapy with ready-to-use therapeutic food with standard therapy in the treatment of malnourished Malawian children: a controlled clinical effectiveness study. Am J Clin Nutr 2005; 81:864–870.

77. Deen JL, Funk M, Guevara VC, et al. Implementation of WHO malnutrition guidelines in the management of severe malnutrition in hospitals in Africa. Bull WHO 2003; 81:237–243.

78. Ndekha MJ, Manary MJ, Ashorn P, et al. Home-based therapy with ready-to-use therapeutic food is of benefit to malnourished HIV-infected Malawian children. Acta Pediatr 2005; 94:222–225.

4

Preventive pediatrics

Harry Campbell, Rachael Wood

DETERMINANTS OF CHILD HEALTH
(see also Ch. 2)

Any child's health, development, and welfare reflect the interaction of various factors including:

- the individual's genetic endowment;
- environmental factors including aspects of the direct physical environment such as housing and 'behavioral' factors such as nutrition;
- the quality of interpersonal relationships, particularly with the child's primary caregiver;
- the wider social, political, and economic circumstances the child is living in;
- the availability of health care.

The health of the child's mother is also an important factor in determining the health of the child, whether this is, for example, in ensuring proper antenatal care of mothers with diabetes or treating and supporting mothers with psychiatric problems or alcohol addiction.

The impact of this complex web of determinants of health is reflected in the marked socioeconomic inequalities that exist in child health.[1] These inequalities are seen both between countries of the resource rich and developing worlds and also within individual countries.[2] Even within resource rich countries, almost all indicators of child health show a marked social gradient, with children living in disadvantaged circumstances having poorer health.[3] In Scotland, for example, children from the most deprived areas are more than twice as likely to die compared to children from the most affluent areas (Fig. 4.1) with some specific health problems showing particularly marked inequalities (Ch. 2).

CONTRIBUTION OF HEALTH SERVICES TO IMPROVING CHILD HEALTH

As many of the factors that influence child health are modifiable, there is considerable scope for improving children's health and reducing inequalities in child health. It is clear, however, that much of the activity required to bring about this improvement lies outwith the remit of traditional health services. The profound impact of political action, economic progress, improved education and social change on child health is shown by falling morbidity and mortality long before antibiotics, vaccines and high-technology medicine became available (Fig. 4.2). Thus improving child health has been considered to involve 'placing the health of children and their families in its full social, political and economic context' and to be 'the responsibility of decision makers in all organizations in all sectors of the economy'.[4]

Nevertheless, the organization and provision of health services can and should make a substantial contribution to improving child health.[5] This is acknowledged in the UN Convention on the Rights of the Child, which places a clear responsibility on the State to provide access to preventive care (article 24).[6] The remainder of this chapter will therefore concentrate on the actions that can be taken principally by health services to promote child health and development and prevent childhood illness and handicap, and will be considered from the perspective of health professionals working in pediatric services.

In order to maximize their potential to improve child health, health services should meet certain key criteria. Services should be:

- universal, i.e. accessible to all members of the population;
- comprehensive, i.e. focused on health promotion and disease prevention as well as curative care;
- integrated with other services that impact on the well-being of children, in particular social services and education;
- responsive to the health needs of the population;
- centered on the individual health needs of children and their families;
- evidence based and of high clinical quality.

In addition, services should be provided with the aim of reducing inequalities in health. This may mean that additional steps are taken to ensure very high coverage of essential immunizations in all sections of the population or that particularly vulnerable children (such as those in families of asylum seekers or travelers, those from economically deprived areas, or 'looked after' children) require additional special services to ensure they receive adequate preventive care. The capacity to monitor the contribution of health services to improving child health and reducing health inequalities on an ongoing basis is also important.

It is clear from the above that a focus on health promotion and disease prevention should pervade the day-to-day practice of all health professionals who work with children. This will require skilled teamwork in working with children and their families, other health workers, and colleagues outside the health services such as teachers and social workers.

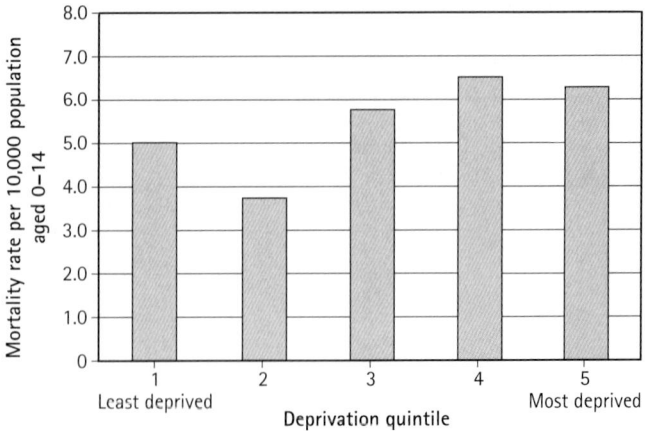

Fig. 4.1 Death from all causes by deprivation quintile, children aged under 15 years, Scotland 2004. From ISD (GRO(S) death registrations and mid-year population estimates). Deprivation quintiles based on Scottish Index of Multiple Deprivation. ISD (SMR01 and mid-year population estimates).

HEALTH PROMOTION AND DISEASE PREVENTION

Health promotion is usually thought of broadly as encompassing all activities aiming to improve health and hence incorporates specific disease prevention activities along with broader health education and lobbying for socioeconomic change.[7,8]

Disease prevention is commonly categorized into primary, secondary, and tertiary prevention.[9] Primary prevention aims to reduce the incidence of disease by controlling causes or risk factors. Examples of primary prevention interventions include vaccination against measles, the use of condoms to prevent human immunodeficiency virus (HIV) infection, antenatal folate supplementation, and fluoridation of drinking water.

Secondary prevention aims to reduce the prevalence of disease through early diagnosis and treatment that either leads to a cure or to a reduction in the more serious consequences of disease. Examples of secondary prevention interventions include screening for hypothyroidism in neonates to permit early replacement of deficient thyroxine and prevention of the disabilities of cretinism, and otoacoustic emission screening for hearing loss in neonates to improve outcomes for deaf children. The term 'secondary prevention' can also be applied to the termination of pregnancy to avoid the birth of a fetus with a recognized severe impairment.

Tertiary prevention aims to reduce the progress or complications of established disease, thus limiting its impact. It consists of measures to reduce impairments and disabilities from the disease or injury and so minimize any handicap which may result. For example, tertiary prevention through the rehabilitation of children with polio can enable them to take part in daily social life and bring about a great improvement in the well-being of these children.

CHILD HEALTH ADVOCACY

In addition to improving child health and reducing inequalities through a focus on health promotion and disease prevention in their day-to-day clinical practice, pediatricians are well placed to make a valuable contribution to child health advocacy.[10] This is advocacy that strives to promote action within society that addresses the broader determinants of child health (e.g. socioeconomic circumstances, quality of the environment, housing, nutrition and education).

Child health advocacy often begins with an individual child or family and then may extend into local, regional or even national public health action. It involves taking action to promote health beyond treatment of a medical condition. This action can be taken as an individual or collectively. Specific steps in individual pediatrician advocacy have been described by Waterston and Tonniges[11] as:
- identifying a preventable problem in one child;
- helping that child overcome the problem;
- drawing conclusions in relation to the factors that led to the problem in the first place;

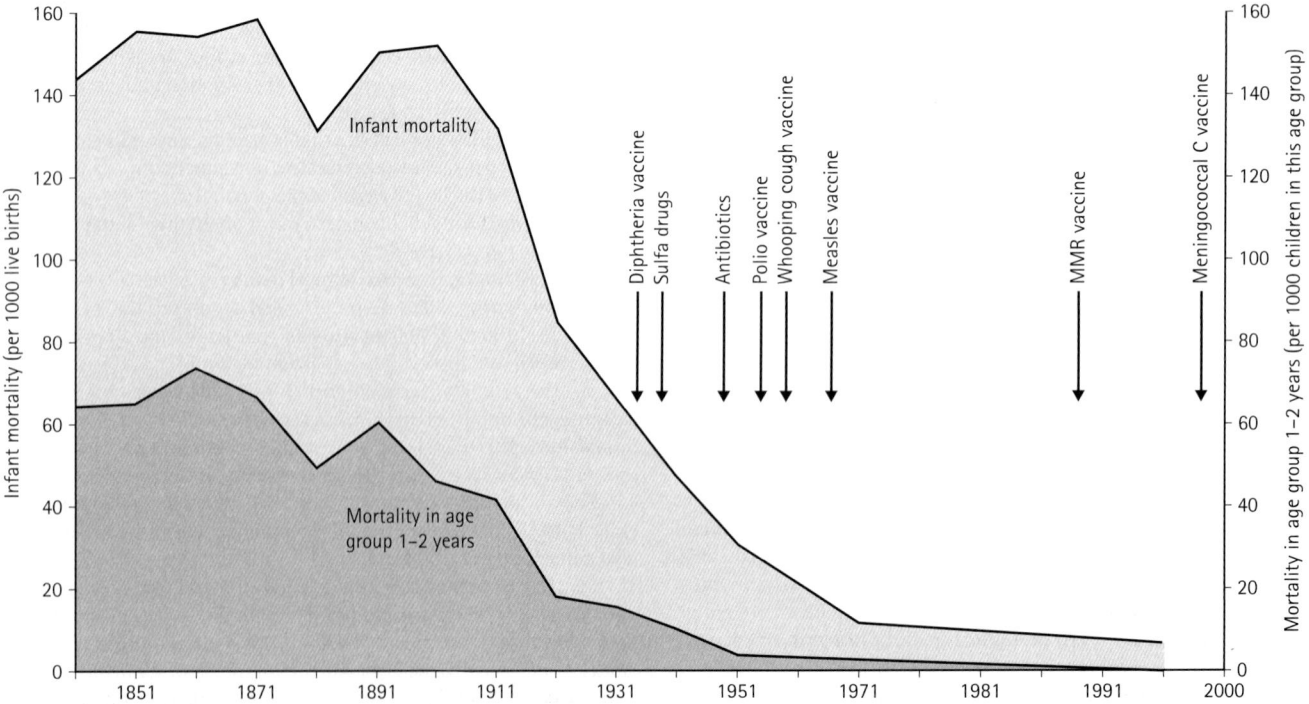

Fig. 4.2 Infant mortality in England and Wales and important developments in medicine.

- identifying the means to tackle these factors;
- influencing government or policy makers to change or reform the system that fostered these factors or introduce appropriate legislation.

Waterston gives as an example of such individual advocacy the work of Hugh Jackson, who cared for a child who died of an accidental drug overdose and whose later action led to the development of legislation requiring the use of childproof medication.[11] Collaborative action of pediatricians and other professionals involved in child health can advocate effectively against the tobacco industry, the motor industry, or baby milk manufacturers.

A LIFE COURSE APPROACH TO DISEASE PREVENTION

In this section we provide an overview of effective measures to prevent disease and improve health in childhood. In later sections we go on to consider three preventive interventions in more detail, specifically support for parenting, child health screening and surveillance, and immunization. We concentrate on measures of relevance in the developed world, as preventive actions relevant to promoting child health in developing countries are presented in Chapter 3.

Table 4.1 presents effective disease prevention measures for each stage of childhood using a 'life course' framework. Over recent decades there has been a general resurgence of interest in the life course approach to health that emphasizes the long-term health implications of the fetal and early childhood environment.[12–14] It is now widely accepted that exposure to adverse environments in early life can irreversibly program higher risk of certain diseases, in particular hypertension, diabetes and ischemic heart disease, later in life.[15–18] Thus some of the preventive actions presented here may not only lead to improvement in child health but also represent effective interventions against some of the common diseases of public health importance in the adult population.

Some of the preventive interventions presented in Table 4.1 come under the remit of the UK universal child health promotion program that is mainly delivered by midwives, health visitors and the school health service with support from GPs and specialist pediatricians (see later section on Child health screening and surveillance) however knowledge of all of the interventions listed is relevant to the day-to-day practice of pediatrics. The centrality of preventive work to pediatrics is reflected in the fact that many of the interventions presented in Table 4.1 are discussed in other chapters of this book. For this reason we have cross-referenced other chapters in addition to providing references to the evidence base for many of the interventions listed.

PREVENTION BEFORE CONCEPTION AND DURING PREGNANCY

Genetic factors in either parent, the present and past health of the mother, her age, her habits (e.g. smoking, alcohol), the frequency of her pregnancies, her previous immunizations (e.g. rubella and tetanus) and her social class are all factors which can potentially influence the health of her infant before it is conceived, and control or elimination of adverse factors will play an important part in prevention. A mother's own birth weight and growth through childhood and general nutrition during adulthood and pregnancy are being increasingly recognized as important determinants of her child's fetal growth patterns and hence subsequent risk of chronic diseases.[15–18] This developing understanding of 'biological programming' demonstrates the importance of focusing on health promotion for women and young children in order to break intergenerational cycles of poor health. It also shows how complex disease prevention interventions can be, for example it is not yet clear how best to optimize maternal nutrition.[19]

The effects of a pregnant woman's smoking or alcohol consumption on her fetus are now well recognized and demand preventive action.[20] Smoking can lead to intrauterine growth retardation, certain congenital anomalies, fetal loss, and preterm delivery.[21–23] In addition, smoking

during and after pregnancy has emerged as a major risk factor for sudden infant death syndrome (SIDS) in studies carried out after the widespread recommendations on infant sleeping position led to a reduction in the number of infants found dead in the prone position.[24–26] Reduction of smoking levels in the population requires coordinated action including increasing the cost of tobacco, banning advertising, and restricting the places where people are allowed to smoke.[27] At the individual level effective interventions to help people to stop smoking are available. Pregnant women can benefit from smoking cessation counseling and nicotine replacement therapy, and maternity services should ensure all pregnant smokers have access to specialist stop smoking care.[19,28]

Well-organized antenatal care makes a vital contribution to maternal and child health. In the UK, current recommendations suggest that routine antenatal care for healthy women should include provision of health information along with the offer of screening for anemia, red cell alloantibodies, syphilis, hepatitis B and HIV infection, immunity to rubella, asymptomatic bacteriuria, pre-eclampsia, Down syndrome, structural anomalies, and fetal growth.[20] Women with particular risk factors may require additional antenatal care, for example individuals with a family history of a genetic disorder may benefit from genetic testing. Over recent years there have been major advances in the understanding of the molecular basis of medical disorders and in the development of new techniques to identify genes associated with disease. Most of the genes for the more common inherited (single gene or 'Mendelian') disorders have now been identified (see Chapter 14). This in turn often makes prenatal detection and genetic counseling possible.[29–31] In conjunction with this there have been advances in prenatal diagnostic techniques, for example using amniocentesis or chorionic villous sampling. Secondary prevention by termination of pregnancy has therefore become more widely practiced.

In early pregnancy the avoidance of various teratogens is an important preventive measure. The following drugs and chemicals have been found to be associated with fetal defects: diphenylhydantoin (phenytoin), trimethadione, paramethadione, valproic acid, carbamazepine, thioureas, carbimazole, methimazole, isotretinoin, vitamin A, etretinate, thalidomide, warfarin, methotrexate, corticosteroids, androgens, progestins, diethylstilbestrol, iodine, lithium, mercury and chlorobiphenyls. A number of other drugs and chemicals have featured in retrospective studies or case reports but associations with fetal defects have not been confirmed by subsequent investigations (see Stevenson[32] for a further discussion). Exposure to abdominal X-rays should be avoided, but there is no evidence that ultrasound examinations are harmful to the fetus.

PREVENTION IN NEONATAL PERIOD

Good intrapartum obstetric care and subsequent effective monitoring, investigation and treatment of the many disorders from which the newborn infant may suffer are important preventive measures. Such disorders include asphyxia, birth injury, low birth weight and hyperbilirubinemia. Neonatal screening procedures are discussed in the section on Child health surveillance and screening.

The promotion of breast-feeding is a crucial preventive measure. Breast-feeding reduces the risk of necrotizing enterocolitis, diarrheal disease, lower respiratory infections, otitis media, and other serious neonatal infections.[33,34] It also appears to reduce the risk of childhood obesity, probably through better development of appetite control.[35] Recent evidence has further linked lack of breast-feeding with poorer intellectual development, possibly due to the lack of certain long chain fatty acids, essential for normal brain development, in most breast milk substitutes, although it is difficult to totally exclude the possibility of confounding from these studies.[36,37] Frequent breast-feeds given over a prolonged period also significantly reduce fertility and increase the birth interval, with indirect benefits to both mother and infant.[38]

WHO and UNICEF are coordinating a global initiative (the Baby Friendly Hospital Initiative) to promote breast-feeding and to improve health service support for breast-feeding mothers.[39,40] Hospital routines

Table 4.1 Effective preventive interventions across childhood

Intervention	Health benefits	Relevant section in Forfar and Arneil	Additional evidence (reference number)
Preconception through to infancy			
Adequate nutrition	Adequate maternal nutrition promotes a healthy pattern of fetal growth and avoids 'biological programming' of higher chronic disease risk for child throughout its life		15–19
Avoidance of smoking	Avoidance of maternal smoking reduces the risk of intrauterine growth retardation, preterm delivery, and SIDS	Ch. 6 (SIDS)	19, 21–28
Preconception			
Adequate folic acid intake	Reduced risk of neural tube defects	Ch. 22	116–120
Rubella immunization	Reduced risk of congenital rubella syndrome	Ch. 28	121–123
In pregnancy			
General antenatal care	Avoidance of preventable morbidity, e.g. maternal anemia		20
Antenatal screening, e.g. for Down syndrome	Prevention of disability through optimal management of pregnancy, delivery and child, or termination of affected pregnancies	Ch. 11	124–126
Adequate folic acid intake	Reduced risk of neural tube defects	Ch. 22	116–120
Moderate alcohol intake	Prevention of fetal alcohol syndrome		127–129
Avoidance of teratogens, e.g. drugs, infections, and radiation	Reduced risk of congenital anomalies		32
Anti D immunoglobulin if Rhesus negative	Prevention of Rhesus alloimmunization	Ch. 11	130, 131
Steroids for women at risk of preterm delivery	Reduced risk of respiratory distress syndrome in neonate	Ch. 12	132
In the perinatal/neonatal period			
General intrapartum and neonatal care	Prevention of birth injury, kernicterus, and infections including those that are health care associated, e.g. MRSA	Ch. 12	133, 134
Neonatal screening, e.g. physical examination, heel prick blood test, and hearing screening	Prevention of disability through, for example, management of congenital hip dislocation, PKU and hearing impairment	Ch. 12	135, 136
Breast-feeding	Reduced risk of necrotizing enterocolitis, gastrointestinal and respiratory infections, otitis media, and childhood obesity; increased child spacing and reduced risk of breast cancer for mother	Ch. 13	33–53
Vitamin K	Prevention of hemorrhagic disease of the newborn	Ch. 12	54–58
Interventions including medication, immunization, and management of labor and infant feeding	Avoidance of vertical transmission of infection e.g. HIV and hepatitis B	Ch. 27 (HIV)	59, 60
In infancy and childhood			
General clinical care	Prevention of a range of illness and disability through prompt and effective diagnosis, treatment, and rehabilitation		
Screening and child health surveillance	Prevention of disability associated with, for example, vision and hearing problems	Chs 7 (developmental delay), 31 (vision), and 32 (hearing)	135
Fostering of positive relationship between child and primary caregiver	Prevention of mental health problems, development of personal resilience, and increased chance of healthy behavior choices in later life		See support for parenting
Sleeping on back and avoiding overheating	Reduced risk of SIDS	Ch. 6	61–68
Immunization	Reduced risk of a range of infectious diseases and their sequelae	Ch. 28	See Immunization
Appropriate weaning	Reduced risk of iron deficiency, dental decay, and childhood obesity	Ch. 13	69–75, 79–81
Tooth brushing and fluoride provision	Reduced risk of dental decay	Ch. 13	76–78

Table 4.1–cont'd

Intervention	Health benefits	Relevant section in Forfar and Arneil	Additional evidence (reference number)
Safety promotion interventions, e.g. car seats, smoke alarms, safe toys	Reduced risk of accidental injury	Ch. 6	82–87
Adequate exercise	Reduced risk of childhood obesity	Ch. 5	88–91
Detection and treatment of child abuse	Reduced impact of abuse on mental and physical health		92–94
In adolescence			
Accessible health services	Opportunities for health promotion and disease prevention through positive interaction between health professionals and adolescents	Ch. 35	
Avoidance of development of unhealthy behaviors, e.g. smoking, unsafe alcohol intake, inadequate exercise, and use of illegal drugs	Reduced immediate adverse impact on health and prevention of establishment of damaging behavior patterns	Chs 16 (nutrition) and 35	27, 95–101, 107–111
Sexual health promotion including sex and relationships education and accessible contraceptive and GUM (Genito-urinary medicine) services	Reduced risk of unwanted teenage pregnancy and sexually transmitted infections	Ch. 35	102–105

and practices can discourage women from breast-feeding or make it difficult for them to do so successfully[41,42] hence good practice guidelines have been developed for maternity hospitals.[43] Key features of good practice include 'rooming in', i.e. allowing mother and babies to remain together, supporting skin-to-skin contact and the first breast-feed soon after birth, encouraging subsequent feeding on demand, and education of staff and mothers to promote good positioning and attachment of the baby.[44–48]

Improving hospital practices and staff skills in line with these guidelines has been shown to improve breast-feeding rates across all ethnic and socio-economic groups.[49–52] Policy statements on breast-feeding by pediatric associations have been used to raise awareness amongst pediatric staff of the need to promote breast-feeding, to promote good practice and to advocate for inclusion of breast-feeding topics in the undergraduate medical and nursing curricula and in postgraduate courses for pediatricians, obstetricians, general practitioners, midwives and maternal and child health nurses.[53]

Vitamin K should be given to all babies at birth to prevent the rare but serious disorder hemorrhagic disease of the newborn (HDN).[54] Vitamin K administered either as one intramuscular injection shortly after birth or as multiple oral doses (with more doses required for breast-fed babies) over the first few weeks of life is effective at preventing early, classic, and late HDN.[55] As compliance is higher and costs are lower with the IM route, that is the regimen that is usually preferred. This was questioned following the publication of one case–control study in 1992 that reported an association between administration of vitamin K via the intramuscular route to neonates and the subsequent development of childhood leukemia.[56] Later studies and systematic reviews have failed to replicate this finding however, and the consensus view is now that IM vitamin K does not increase the risk of cancer.[57,58] Current advice from the Department of Health for England states that all babies should be offered vitamin K but does not state which regimen should be followed.

The risks of HIV transmission are now better understood, leading to guidelines for the management of HIV-positive mothers to reduce vertical transmission of infection.[59] Key interventions include universal antenatal screening of mothers for HIV infection, antiretroviral therapy for those found to be infected along with elective Cesarian section delivery and avoidance of breast-feeding in areas where it is safe to do so.[60]

PREVENTION IN INFANCY AND EARLY CHILDHOOD

In infancy and early childhood curative medicine can have an important preventive role. Early diagnosis and effective treatment of diseases such as meningitis, pneumonia, otitis media, osteomyelitis and patent ductus arteriosus can prevent chronic illness or permanent handicap in some children following these conditions. The contribution of screening, of positive relationships between children and their primary caregivers, and of immunization to improving child health is discussed later in the sections on Child health screening and surveillance, Support for parenting, and Immunization, respectively.

Proven effective interventions to reduce the risk of SIDS include putting babies to sleep on their backs, avoiding overheating by attention to environmental temperature, not over wrapping the baby and not covering its head, and avoiding exposure to environmental tobacco smoke in the home.[61–64] Areas that are still under debate include the contribution of co-sleeping, i.e. babies sleeping with their parents in the bed and the use of pacifiers ('dummies')[65–68] (See Ch. 6 for a full discussion).

An appropriate weaning diet progressing on to a healthy diet throughout childhood is fundamental to child health. Dietary guidelines have been published by many authorities.[69,70] These combine concerns about achieving recommended daily intakes of selected essential nutrients with the need to reduce risks of chronic diseases of adulthood which are partly attributed to diet. Dental decay in childhood is a significant health problem.[71,72] Ensuring children's diets are low in free sugars, and in particular in sugary foods and drinks taken as snacks at regular intervals through the day, helps to reduce the incidence of decay.[73–75] In addition there is good evidence that twice daily tooth brushing with toothpaste containing 1000 p.p.m. fluoride from as soon as the primary teeth erupt is effective at preventing decay.[76] Fluoridation of the public water supply has also been shown to reduce decay and represents a highly clinically and cost-effective public health measure but is not routine within the UK at present.[77,78]

Care should be taken to ensure that children's diets provide adequate sources of available iron. Recent studies in the UK have shown a prevalence of iron deficiency anemia of up to 25% in young children, with particularly high rates in some ethnic minority communities.[79] Effects on mental and motor development can be reversed if treatment is prompt.[80] All premature babies should receive iron supplements. The Department of Health for England currently recommends that all children receive vitamin A, C, and D drops between ages 1 and 5 years (from 6 months for breast-fed infants).[81] Children should also receive iodine supplements where specific deficiency is endemic.

Accidents cause nearly half of all deaths at ages 1–19 years in the UK.[82,83] The cause of the accidents, and therefore the preventive action, varies with the age of the child. Important preventive measures of proven effectiveness include: area wide urban safety measures; traffic speed restrictions; child car restraints; cycle helmet wearing; road safety education; child-proof containers for drugs; and home safety devices such as stair gates and fire alarms. The use of safe playground apparatus and surfaces, the use of age-appropriate toys, and the proper supervision of children near water are also important.[84,85] Evidence also exists on effective ways to deliver safety promotion interventions, such as through targeted health visiting and provision of subsidized safety equipment to households at risk of home-based accidents.[86,87]

The health benefits of physical activity are less well defined for children than for adults. Nevertheless, there is some evidence to show that adequate physical activity in childhood helps to reduce the numbers of overweight and obese children and improve well-being and self-esteem, biological cardiovascular disease risk factors, and skeletal health.[88] Importantly also there is clear tracking of behaviors between childhood and adulthood, hence active children are more likely to become active adults and thus gain health benefits.[89] Current recommendations suggest that children should achieve at least 1 h of moderate physical activity a day. There is limited evidence available on measures to increase physical activity levels among children, although restricting television and computer viewing and developing holistic programs of health promotion with schools are likely to be important.[90,91]

All health professionals in contact with children should be alert to the possibility of child abuse, particularly in cases of repeated multiple or unusual trauma or burns, or in children with developmental delay.[92] Prompt recognition can prevent future abuse and can identify the need for counseling or specific treatment.[93,94]

PREVENTION IN LATER CHILDHOOD AND ADOLESCENCE

The prevention of poor diet, inactivity, obesity, smoking, unsafe alcohol use, abuse of drugs and related substances, unplanned and unwanted teenage pregnancy, sexually transmitted diseases including HIV, family breakdown, and child abuse and neglect is particularly challenging. Considerable medical, social, economic and, in the view of some, spiritual or moral resources are required to meet these challenges. Owing to the very close correlation between unhealthy behavior patterns in late childhood and in adulthood, prevention in childhood could make a major contribution to improving future adult health as well as the health of children.

The health risks of smoking are well recognized. The Scottish Schools Adolescent Lifestyle and Substance Use Survey (SALSUS) 2004 found that 5% of boys and 7% of girls aged 13 years were regular (i.e. at least one cigarette a week) smokers, increasing to 14% of boys and 24% of girls aged 15 years.[95] There is evidence of effectiveness for a variety of interventions designed to reduce the uptake of smoking among young people, including school-based health promotion programs, increasing the unit price of cigarettes, working with retailers to reduce sale of cigarettes to children, and mass media campaigns.[27] In addition young people who are established smokers can benefit from specialist smoking cessation support.[27,96] Health professionals should routinely ask about smoking in older children and their

parents, and provide advice and help where necessary on stopping smoking. Parents who cannot stop smoking should be encouraged not to smoke in the house or in front of their children. Health services should actively support any effective and appropriate action against the promotion of cigarettes and tobacco.[97]

Alcohol consumption among young people, in particular young girls, has increased markedly over recent years. In 2004 SALSUS found that 20% of boys and girls aged 13 years had had an alcoholic drink in the week prior to the survey compared to 40% of boys and 46% of girls aged 15 years.[95] Concern over alcohol use in adolescents is based not only on related health problems (e.g. one third of all accidental deaths in 16–19-year-olds are associated with alcohol) but also on drunkenness and its related social problems. Whilst there is evidence for effective interventions to reverse established unsafe drinking, there is very little evidence available on preventing alcohol misuse among young people.[98–100]

Experimentation with illegal drugs is common among adolescents. In 2004 SALSUS found that 11% of 13-year-olds and 31% of 15-year-olds had used drugs in the year preceding the survey, with cannabis being by far the most commonly used substance (results for boys and girls are very similar).[95] There is evidence that intensive interactive school-based health promotion programs can be effective in increasing knowledge about drugs and reducing or delaying the onset of drug use although direct effects on drug use can be small and short lived.[101]

Levels of unsafe sexual activity are worryingly high among young people. Rates of sexually transmitted infections (STIs), particularly *Chlamydia*, have increased dramatically over recent years.[102] In addition approximately 1% of girls aged 14–15 years in the UK conceive each year and over half of these pregnancies result in abortion.[103] Teenage motherhood leads to poor health outcomes for both the mother and child and contributes to intergenerational cycles of ill health.[104] There is evidence that well-organized family or school-based programs incorporating personal development, sex and relationships education, and accessible contraceptive and genitourinary medicine services do work in reducing unsafe sex, STIs, and teenage pregnancy.[105,106] Conversely there is evidence that health promotion programs that rely solely on promoting abstinence from sexual activity do not work.[105]

The dramatic increase in numbers of those overweight and obese among all age groups including children in Western societies over recent years is a major public health concern. The Health Survey for England found that in 2004 13% of boys aged 11–15 years were overweight and an additional 24% were obese: 19% of girls of the same age were overweight and an additional 26% were obese.[107] There is debate as to the precise cause of increasing levels of obesity in children but it is likely that increased consumption of high fat, energy dense foods and reduced levels of physical activity both contribute.[108] It is of note that levels of physical activity decline markedly in teenage years so that only one half of young men aged 16–24 years and one third of young women undertake recommended levels physical activity.[109] There is evidence that school-based holistic programs incorporating curricular material, nutrition education, modification of school meals and tuck shops, and physical activity promotion can prevent the development of obesity, particularly in girls.[110] There is also some evidence regarding effective interventions to promote weight loss in obese children although maintenance of reduced weight can be challenging.[110,111]

The above discussion shows the importance of holistic health promotion for young people to prevent the establishment of health damaging patterns of behavior and also the importance of the school environment in health promotion for young people. Health promotion for young people should reinforce negative views of unhealthy behaviors and promote positive views of health and of healthy behaviors such as emphasizing nonsmoking as the norm. Action needs to involve not only a wide range of health, education and social work professionals but also relevant voluntary agencies and young people themselves through peer projects, and requires to be part of an overall strategy involving both national and local action. Action can be taken in a stepped fashion with:

- broad messages or action aimed at the general population at low risk (e.g. warnings about binge drinking or the use of recreational drugs at parties);
- more focused messages or action for subgroups at higher risk;
- individual action and support for young people who are, for example, dependent on substances and at greatest risk to themselves and their community.[112]

Health professionals who care for children should maintain a high level of awareness and know where and how to seek assistance when faced with these problems. Integrated school health services could include diagnostic, treatment and health counseling services. These services operate most successfully when they are fully integrated with other community and hospital health and related social services.[113] An international network of 'health promoting schools' has developed this model further by harnessing a wide variety of school policies to promote child health within schools, for example by providing affordable and tasty healthy food options and promoting a healthy diet, by ensuring there are sufficient opportunities for physical activity such as through organized sports, adopting and enforcing no-smoking policies and making the school environment safer and more attractive.[114,115] In all these areas there is an increasing recognition of the need to adopt evidence-based action based on systematic reviews of randomized controlled trials or other evidence of effectiveness of interventions.

SUPPORT FOR PARENTING

Over recent years there has been an increasing focus on the role of parenting as a determinant of child and adult mental and physical health. Key features of 'good' parenting include consistent parental sensitivity and responsiveness to a child's needs along with positive communication, secure boundaries and positive discipline, and parental example.[137] It is therefore far more than just the absence of neglect or abuse. Good parenting is not culture dependent although specific child rearing practices vary widely between cultures.[138] Good parenting facilitates the initial establishment of secure attachment between an infant and its primary caregiver, usually its mother, and uses this as a stepping stone for broader positive relationships and increasing independence through the toddler years.[137]

Babies are highly social from birth and the quality of the social relationships they experience, in particular the provision of responsive care, influences the development of neural pathways regulating response to stressful stimuli, emotional arousal, attention, memory, and learning.[139] In practice, therefore, parenting has been shown to influence children's cognitive capacity, language development, school performance, ability to form positive social relationships, risk of health damaging behaviors, and risk of involvement in criminal activity, although clearly parenting is not the only determinant of these broad outcomes.[139-141]

Whilst almost all parents want the best for their children and work hard to provide that, unhelpful parenting is common across all sectors of society. The stresses associated with material and social deprivation make achieving good parenting even more difficult, and hence unhelpful parenting contributes to health inequalities.[142] Conversely, positive parenting has a marked protective effect on children who are living under stressful and disadvantaged circumstances and can ameliorate the adverse health consequences of social inequalities.[138]

There is reasonably robust evidence now available that specific support for parenting is both clinically and cost effective. In general terms two types of programs to facilitate helpful parenting are available: infant mental health programs and parenting education and support programs.[142,143] Infant mental health programs are based on attachment theory and generally aim to develop parental understanding, sensitivity and responsiveness to infants' needs. The programs can include elements of counseling, role play, video feedback, cognitive behavioral work, and baby massage. Parenting education and support programs can be based on either social learning theory or emotional literacy the-

ory. The former focuses more on positive discipline and improving child behavior whereas the latter focuses more on improving parent–child relationships. In practice most programs encompass elements of both approaches.

Infant mental health programs are intensive – to be most effective they should involve weekly sessions for the first 6 months of a baby's life. They can be provided either on a one-to-one basis, for example through a home visiting program, or to groups of mothers in community-based centers.[142,144] Parenting education and support programs should involve weekly sessions for around 3 months. They are most effective when provided in a group setting to parents of children aged up to 3 years.[142,145] Programs that meet these standards have been shown to improve attachment, the emotional and behavioral adjustment of young children, child language development, and maternal mental health.[142,146-149] Within the UK, infant mental health programs are uncommon but parenting programs for older children are becoming more widespread. They are often provided by nongovernmental organizations, however, and are not always well integrated with mainstream NHS services. The UK Royal College of Pediatrics and Child Health has recommended that a range of parenting programs should be universally available for expectant mothers through to parents of children aged 3, with scope to target the most intensive support to families most in need.[137] The UK system of universal health visiting for pre-school-age children provides a good setting for helping parents access available support.

Another issue closely aligned to that of helpful parenting is nonparental care for pre-school children. As more mothers of young children undertake paid work, so the requirement for nonparental care increases. The type of nonparental care used varies widely and includes informal care from friends and extended family, care from a nanny or professional childminder, and day center or nursery-based care. Nonparental care should mirror the attributes of helpful parenting and for older pre-school children should encompass high-quality early education. There is considerable evidence, mainly from the USA, that children provided with this kind of care develop better behavioral adjustment, improved school performance, and lower involvement in juvenile crime.[150,151] The availability of affordable, high-quality nonparental care for pre-school children remains a major issue in many countries.

The importance of parenting and provision of nonparental care to child health and development is being increasingly recognized in UK policy, for example in the English National Service Framework for Children, Young People, and Maternity Services (Standard 2: Supporting Parenting)[136] and the UK-wide Sure Start programme.[152] In general, pediatricians have a key role in being aware of the evidence on these topics, supporting the development of effective services in their local areas, and advocating on these issues more broadly.

CHILD HEALTH SCREENING AND SURVEILLANCE

In the UK, child health screening programs and surveillance of children's growth and development are delivered in a coordinated way within the broad child health promotion (CHP) program that is offered to all children. The CHP program also comprises the nationally agreed immunization schedule, delivery of effective health promotion advice, provision of support for parenting including advice on issues such as infant sleeping and child behavior, and identification of at-risk children and contribution to child protection procedures. Specific recommendations about the content of the program, based on a critical consideration of the published literature, are periodically published by the Royal College of Pediatrics and Child Health.[135] In addition the UK National Screening Committee publishes advice on screening programs.[153] These recommendations are then usually adopted into health policy such as the National Service Framework for Children, Young People and Maternity Services in England[136] and equivalent guidance for Scotland.[154] The current UK recommended

Table 4.2 Screening and surveillance procedures recommended for all children as part of the UK child health promotion program

Age	Intervention
Newborn	Weight and head circumference Physical examination with particular emphasis on eyes, heart, and hips
5–6 d	Newborn blood spot screening test for phenylketonuria, congenital hypothyroidism, cystic fibrosis, and sickle cell disease
Within first week	Newborn hearing screening using automated otoacoustic emissions
6–8 weeks	Weight and head circumference Physical examination with particular emphasis on eyes, heart, and hips
3 months	Weight
4 months	Weight
4–5 years	Screening for visual impairment by an orthoptist
School entry	Height and weight Screening for hearing loss by sweep test

Adapted from Health for all children, 4th ed.[135]

screening and surveillance procedures for children are summarized in Table 4.2.

Although the core content of the child health promotion program is decided centrally, the detailed decisions about how different elements of the program should be delivered remain a local responsibility. In practice a wide range of professionals are involved in delivering the program, including health visitors, school nurses, GPs, and pediatricians. It is important therefore that a local child health promotion program has clear leadership, identified responsibilities, and agreed lines of accountability.[155] A multi-agency steering group should oversee the development and implementation of local policies including detailed guidance on how the program should be delivered, staff training requirements, standards and monitoring, and use of information from the program for epidemiological purposes. Personal child health records should be made available to all families and their use by both families and health staff encouraged.[156] It is important to note the distinction between formal child health screening programs and surveillance or monitoring of child health. Screening comprises offering a test to all members of a defined population (such as all newborn babies) in order to identify those at higher risk of a particular disease or condition so that they can be offered further tests to confirm the diagnosis and then treatment or care to improve their outcome.[157,158] Screening is therefore a risk stratification process and the result of a screening test is not in itself sufficient to diagnose disease. All screening tests result in some false positives (healthy people who screen positive) and false negatives (people who have the disease of interest but screen negative). The administration of a screening test can also cause direct harm, for example by generating anxiety or causing direct complications such as a baby getting an infection following the heel prick required for blood spot testing. In addition screening programs are very resource intensive to set up and maintain. A careful consideration of the balance of potential benefits and harms of any proposed screening program is therefore required before a program is introduced,[159,160] and participation in any existing program should be on the basis of informed consent – parents should understand that a negative screening test is not a guarantee of health.

The UK National Screening Committee is responsible for reviewing the evidence for existing or proposed screening programs and recommending whether or not they should be provided. The Committee has established criteria for good screening programs which focus on the condition being screened for, the screening test, subsequent diagnostic and treatment options available, and the feasibility of providing the program as a whole.[157] All the formal screening programs included in the recommended child health promotion program, such as the newborn blood spot test for phenylketonuria, have been endorsed by the National Screening Committee. Screening is intuitively attractive and there is often considerable pressure from both health professionals and the public to provide screening for which there is little robust evidence of benefits outweighing harms. For example there is currently interest in screening newborn babies for medium chain acyl CoA dehydrogenase deficiency (MCADD) using Tandem Mass Spectrometry however the National Screening Committee has advised that this should not be provided outwith the confines of a randomized, controlled trial at present.[161]

Historically, child health promotion programs have incorporated a large element of child health surveillance or monitoring in addition to the provision of formal screening tests. Child health surveillance mainly comprises repeated assessment of a child's growth and development in order to detect abnormalities early. This type of surveillance is not formal screening and in general there is limited evidence of its clinical benefit.[162] Children with serious problems are usually identified by other means, for example by parents or nursery/playgroup workers raising concerns, and there is limited clinical value in detecting minor developmental delay of uncertain significance.[163] Surveillance may well be highly valued by parents and health care professionals however as a way of structuring contact with families, identifying vulnerable children, and providing opportunities for health promotion and reassurance.

The latest recommendations for the UK child health promotion program have moved away from formal assessment of pre-school children's growth and physical and social development at multiple fixed ages and instead suggest a more risk-based approach.[135] In Scotland all children will be allocated to varying levels of support at their 6–8-week check.[154] Whatever level of contact is agreed between health visitors and families with young children it is important that all parents are provided with information on the normal range of development and have ready access to experienced professionals at any point if they have concerns about their child. Professionals also need to take parental concerns seriously, avoid repeated unjustified reassurance, and have clear local policies for onward prompt referral of children who may have problems.

The UK Education Acts of 1981 and 1993 require health authorities to inform education departments of children who have developmental or other medical problems and who may therefore have special educational needs.[164] A full assessment of the child is then made and a statement of special educational needs produced. This system involves the parents of the child in the assessment and focuses on the needs of the child rather than on categorization of the child by diagnostic labeling. These children often require medical support and this is usually best provided by a multidisciplinary team such as those found in child development centers or 'district handicap teams'. The aim of these procedures is tertiary prevention – to limit the handicap which can result from specific impairments by early recognition of the child's medical and educational needs and then appropriate intervention.

IMMUNIZATION

IMPORTANCE AND EFFICACY OF IMMUNIZATION IN THE PREVENTION OF DISEASE

Immunity to a specific infectious disease can be acquired through natural infection or immunization.[165,166] Immunization can involve the administration of injected antibodies to generate passive immunity or the administration of a vaccine to generate active immunity. Passive immunization produces immediate protection which lasts for some weeks or months until the donated antibodies are broken down or used up by the individual. Active immunization stimulates the vaccine recipient's immune system to produce antibody and/or cell-mediated immunity and triggers immunological memory hence produces long-lasting protection.

The immediate goal of active immunization is to prevent disease in individuals, but the ultimate goal is to eliminate or even eradicate a communicable disease. Herd immunity exists if the number of people in a community who have active immunity against an infection that is spread from person to person exceeds a critical level.[167] Above this, susceptible individuals are unlikely to contact someone with the infection. In this way transmission falls or stops without universal immunity. Immunization is a simple, effective, and economic form of control for many infectious diseases.[168] The efficacy of immunization depends on the epidemiology of the pathogen, the vaccine available, the biological and social response of individuals, and the health service infrastructure for delivering the immunization.

VACCINES: PRESENT AND FUTURE

A vaccine is an antigen, originally derived from or similar to a bacterium or virus, used for active immunization. Vaccines may comprise live attenuated organisms, killed ('inactivated') organisms, isolated components of organisms (usually cell wall proteins or polysaccharides), or attenuated toxins ('toxoids').[169,170]

A live attenuated vaccine is one which produces active immunity by causing a mild 'infection'. A virulent organism is weakened, usually by multiple subcultures in unfavorable conditions, so that it produces an antigenic response without the serious consequences of a wild organism infection. Examples include the measles, mumps, and rubella components of the MMR vaccine. Cross-reacting organisms are another type of live vaccine that causes the body to produce a defense against the virulent strain. The bacillus Calmette–Guérin (BCG) vaccine is an example of this. A killed or inactivated vaccine is prepared from virulent organisms inactivated by heat, phenol, formaldehyde or some other means. Classical pertussis vaccine is an example of a whole-cell killed vaccine.

Component vaccines use parts of organisms as antigens. Examples of protein component vaccines include the newer acellular pertussis vaccines and influenza and hepatitis B vaccines. Examples of polysaccharide component vaccines include *Haemophilus influenzae* type b (Hib), meningococcal C, and pneumococcal vaccines. The response to polysaccharide vaccines is incomplete and unreliable and consequently these may be conjugated with other protein antigens to improve their immunogenicity.[171–173] An example is the linkage of Hib polysaccharide with tetanus and diphtheria toxoids to produce a vaccine conjugate capable of stimulating T cells and thus eliciting immunological memory.[174] Toxoid vaccines are used to protect against organisms such as diphtheria and tetanus, which cause damage through the release of toxins when they infect humans. Diphtheria and tetanus toxoid vaccines produce antibodies which inactivate the toxins and hence prevent the serious clinical consequences of infection but they do not kill the bacteria.

Live attenuated vaccines usually produce a lasting immune response after one dose. Multiple dose schedules incorporating an initial vaccination followed by booster doses may however be used to compensate for vaccine failures. No vaccine is 100% efficacious and some vaccine recipients will fail to generate clinically significant immunity following vaccination, for example around 10% of children fail to generate immunity following a single measles vaccine.[175] Multiple dose schedules therefore allow a second chance for children who missed their first dose for whatever reason or who received it but failed to respond. All types of nonlive vaccines usually require a course of initial vaccinations followed by later booster doses to generate and maintain adequate immunity. Nonlive vaccines may also be adsorbed onto adjuvant compounds such as aluminium hydroxide to increase their immunogenicity and reduce the risk of vaccine failure.

Despite major advances in vaccine development, major inequalities still exist in the delivery of vaccines to children around the world and large numbers of children continue to die from vaccine-preventable infections.[176,177] The Global Alliance for Vaccines and Immunization (GAVI) and the associated Vaccine Fund were established in 1999 to address these inequalities.[178] GAVI is an alliance between the World Health Organization, UNICEF, the World Bank, the Bill and Melinda Gates Foundation, governments, nongovernmental organizations, academia, and the vaccine industry. GAVI supports poor countries to develop sustainable immunization services and also fosters research of benefit to children in the developing world, for example research developing combined vaccines that do not require storage at cold temperatures or parenteral administration.[179] The development of combined vaccines, i.e. vaccines that provide protection against more than one disease, is also an issue for the industrialized world with more vaccines being adopted into childhood immunization schedules as new vaccines are developed. Combined vaccines are not simple to develop as subtle interactions that impact on the immunogenicity of the component parts can occur.[180]

ADVERSE REACTIONS AND CONTRAINDICATIONS TO IMMUNIZATION

In general, most of the routine vaccines recommended in national immunization schedules can safely be given to most children, and no child should be denied vaccination without serious thought about the consequences, both for the individual child and the community.[181] Like all medicines, however, vaccines can cause adverse reactions and the risks of these should be clearly explained to parents and set against the risks of natural infection in the absence of vaccination.

Adverse reactions following immunization may be due to faulty administration, inherent properties of the vaccines, or co-incidental.[182] Faulty administration may involve incorrect storage, reconstitution, or injection of vaccines. Co-incidental 'reactions' are those that are not directly linked to vaccination and would have occurred anyway but are linked in time to vaccination. They are important as they can be incorrectly interpreted as a direct consequence of vaccination and undermine professional and parental confidence. Adverse reactions that are due to the inherent properties of vaccines can be classified as local or generalized and they can be predictable or idiosyncratic. Local reactions comprise varying degrees of pain, swelling, and redness at the injection site, which is usually short-lived. Predictable generalized reactions include fever and rash. Unpredictable idiosyncratic reactions include anaphylaxis, idiopathic thrombocytopenic purpura (ITP), and hypotonic-hyporesponsive episodes (HHEs).[183] The range and timing of reactions varies between specific vaccines (Table 4.3).

As serious adverse reactions are rare following vaccination it is difficult to obtain precise estimates of their frequency. It is clear, however, that the risk of adverse reactions is always substantially lower than the risk of serious complications following natural infection, for example:[184]

Table 4.3 Common adverse events following vaccination

Vaccine	Adverse event	Timing
DTaP/IPV/Hib*	Local reaction**, fever, crying and irritability, loss of appetite	Within 48 h
Meningococcal C	As above plus headache in older children	Within 48 h
MMR	Measles – mild fever, rash	6–10 d
	Mumps – mild fever, swollen parotid glands	18–21 d
		7–21 d
	Rubella – mild fever, rash, joint pain in adults	

*DTaP/IPV/Hib is diphtheria–tetanus–pertussis, inactivated polio, and *H. influenzae* type b;
**Local reactions comprise pain, swelling, and redness at the injection site.
Adapted from Immunisation Against Infectious Disease.[182]

- Acute encephalitis occurs in approximately 1 in 1000 cases of measles versus < 1 in 1 000 000 recipients of MMR;
- Meningitis occurs in 1 in 10 cases of mumps versus 1 in 50 000–1 000 000 recipients of MMR;
- ITP occurs in 1 in 3000 cases of rubella versus < 1 in 30 000 recipients of MMR.

Despite this, in industrialized countries parents and professionals tend to overestimate the risks of vaccination and underestimate the risks of natural infection;[185] this is partly because successful vaccination programs ensure that cases of natural infection are rare and therefore may not be perceived as a real threat. In addition, people are generally far less willing to accept risk associated with medicines given to healthy children than treatments given to children who are already unwell.

There are relatively few genuine contraindications to vaccination and most children could and should receive the complete immunization schedule.[181,186] In practice, however, parents and professionals often withhold vaccination unnecessarily[187,188] (see Table 4.4 for a list of false contraindications to vaccination). Vaccination should be postponed for children who are acutely unwell, for example with a febrile illness, or who have an evolving neurological condition of uncertain diagnosis and/or prognosis.[189] This is primarily so that co-incidental symptoms are not incorrectly ascribed to the vaccination. A previous proven anaphylactic reaction to a specific vaccine or one of its components absolutely contraindicates further doses. The additional risks associated with live vaccines mean they are also relatively contraindicated for pregnant women and patients with significant immunosuppression, for example due to chemotherapy, post-transplant immunosuppression, or HIV infection. In the UK definitive advice on genuine contraindications to specific vaccines is available in the 'Green Book' (Immunization against infectious disease available on the Department of Health website[190]). Even when a list of specific contraindications is available, it can be difficult to interpret this for children with very complex problems and needs. Specialist advice should be sought before withholding vaccination from children with special needs as they are likely to be highly vulnerable to

Table 4.4 Situations which are *not* absolute contraindications to immunization

1	Prematurity
2	Under a certain weight
3	History of jaundice after birth
4	Breast-feeding
5	Mild self-limiting illness without fever, e.g. common cold
6	Asthma, eczema, or hay fever
7	Stable medical problems such as cardiac or renal disease
8	Stable neurological conditions, e.g. cerebral palsy or Down syndrome
9	Personal history of febrile convulsions or epilepsy
10	Treatment with antibiotics or topical or inhaled steroids
11	Recent or imminent surgery or general anesthesia
12	Previous history of the disease being vaccinated against (except for BCG)
13	Unknown immunization history
14	Over the age recommended in the routine immunization schedule
15	Contact with an infectious disease
16	Child's mother or other household member being pregnant
17	Close contact with immunosuppression
18	Family history of any adverse reactions following immunization
19	Family history of febrile convulsions or epilepsy

Note that although these situations are not absolute contraindications to immunization in some circumstances they may warrant additional precautions. Adapted from Immunisation Against Infectious Disease.[189]

the serious consequences of natural infections and hence have much to gain from vaccination.

IMMUNIZATION SCHEDULES

Immunization schedules are the basic framework for the delivery of immunizations to individuals and the community. No one schedule is applicable to all countries and communities of the world and national programs undergo frequent change in response to changing epidemiology of infection and the development of new vaccine products. The basic aim of an immunization schedule is to reach the majority of children before they become at risk of natural infection. Which vaccines are included and the ages at which they are delivered depends on the age-specific risks of disease, response to vaccines, risks of complications, potential interference from maternal antibody, cost of vaccine and health service infrastructure. The schedule should also be simple so that it can be remembered by staff and parents and should fit in with other aspects of health care such as the child health promotion program. In addition to providing comprehensive coverage of the core national immunization schedule, immunization services also need to be flexible enough to accommodate the needs of children traveling to different countries.[191] Small children now travel with their parents to every corner of the globe. Such visits may expose children to infectious diseases no longer endemic in Europe and North America and to conditions which, although preventable, are not normally covered in a routine immunization program. As the disease incidence and health regulations are constantly changing, up-to-date advice should be sought from appropriate authorities. Basic preventive measures should always be observed, in particular careful food hygiene and protection from insects which transmit infections.

The timing of the first routine immunizations is a compromise between the developing maturity of the infant's immune system and the risk of infection from virulent organisms.[192] Very young infants may not mount an adequate immune response to some vaccines and they also have residual maternal transplacental immunoglobulin G (IgG) that both offers some protection against natural infection and may interfere with the immune response to vaccination.[193] The level of protection provided to infants by maternal IgG varies between organisms, for example it is poor for pertussis but more complete for measles.

Three current immunization schedules (for the UK, the USA and that recommended for developing countries by the WHO) are set out in Table 4.5. The current UK schedule completes primary immunization by 6 months of age, minimizing the number of drop-outs. Recent changes to the UK immunization schedule include:

- the change from live oral polio vaccine to injected inactivated polio vaccine to eliminate the risk of vaccine-associated paralytic polio in 2004;[194]
- the change from whole-cell to acellular pertussis vaccines to reduce the risk of adverse reactions in 2004.[194]
- withdrawal of BCG for children aged 10–14 years and implementation of enhanced neonatal BCG immunization for at-risk infants in 2005.[195]
- introduction of pneumococcal conjugate vaccine for infants in 2006.[196]
- introduction of a booster dose of Hib vaccine in the second year of life in 2006.[196]

DEVELOPING COUNTRY SCHEDULES

In developing countries booster immunization schedules present financial and logistic problems so the main emphasis is on primary immunization as part of basic health care.[197] The priority for the WHO is to deliver the primary immunization series to over 90% of infants and thus reduce the burden of these diseases.[198] Low birth

Table 4.5   A comparison of three immunization schedules recommended for use in the UK, USA, and developing countries (the World Health Organization Expanded Program on Immunization recommendations) as at July 2006

Age	UK[201]	USA[202]	Developing countries (WHO EPI)[197]
Birth/neonatal period	BCG if higher risk Hep B if higher risk	Hep B	BCG Hep B (Scheme A for areas with high perinatal transmission) OPV if polio endemic
1 month	Hep B if higher risk	Hep B (can be given any time from 1 to 2 months)	
6 weeks			OPV DTP Hep B (Schemes A and B) Hib
2 months	DTaP/IPV/Hib PCV Hep B if higher risk	DTaP IPV Hib PCV	
10 weeks			OPV DTP Hib Hep B (Scheme B for areas with moderate perinatal transmission)
3 months	DTaP/IPV/Hib MenC		
14 weeks			OPV DTP Hep B (Schemes A and B) Hib
4 months	DTaP/IPV/Hib PCV MenC	DTaP IPV Hib PCV	
6 months		DTaP PCV Hep B (6–18 months) IPV (6–18 months) Annual influenza vaccine (6–23 months, 2 doses in first year)	
9 months			Measles Yellow fever if YF endemic
12 months	Hib MenC Hep B if higher risk	Hib (12–15 months) MMR (12–15 months) PCV (12–15 months) Varicella (12–18 months) Hepatitis A (12–23 months, 2 doses separated by ≥ 6 months)	
13 months	MMR PCV		
15–18 months		DTaP	
Pre-school/school entry	dTaP/IPV (3½–5 years) MMR (3½–5 years)	DTaP (4–6 years) IPV (4–6 years) MMR (4–6 years)	
11–12 years		dTaP Men A, C, W135, and Y	
13–18 years	Td/IPV		

BCG, bacillus Calmette–Guérin; Hep B, hepatitis B; DTP, diphtheria, tetanus and whole cell pertussis; DTaP, diphtheria, tetanus and acellular pertussis; dTaP, low dose diphtheria, tetanus and acellular pertussis; Td, tetanus and low does diphtheria; OPV, oral polio vaccine; IPV, inactivated polio vaccine; Hib: *H. influenzae* type b; PCV, pneumococcal conjugate vaccine; Men C, Meningococcal C conjugate vaccine; MMR, measles, mumps and rubella; Men A, C, W135, Y: quadrivalent meningococcal vaccine.

weight infants, whether due to premature birth or intrauterine growth retardation, or both, should generally be immunized with the same schedule as for normal weight, full-term infants.[189] In addition to the standard WHO schedule, other vaccines are available and recommended for use in specific geographic areas, for example Japanese encephalitis and pigbel vaccines. Others like Hib may not yet be affordable in some developing countries. This is a striking example of global inequity in child health care – the children at lowest risk of Hib disease receive immunization whilst the children at highest risk have no access to immunization, resulting in hundreds of thousands of child deaths each year.[199] Access to Hib vaccination is being specifically addressed by GAVI.[178] Mass immunization campaigns are an integral part of the global polio eradication strategy; they are now also recommended by WHO for use in measles elimination programs.[200] They can have a dramatic impact as the first phase of an elimination strategy, especially where health infrastructure is limited. Such campaigns should not be isolated events, but part of a long-term strategy.

In conclusion, immunization schedules should be epidemiologically relevant, immunologically effective, operationally feasible and socially acceptable. At a global level child health advocacy (see earlier) is required to promote equitable access to essential vaccines for all children in the world since immunization (with WHO Expanded Program of Immunization vaccines) represents a highly cost-effective child health promotion strategy in all world populations.

IMMUNIZATION COVERAGE

As previously mentioned, stark inequalities in access to vaccination exist within and between countries, with children living in disadvantaged circumstances having considerably lower uptake. The reasons for these inequalities are complex but ultimately they reduce population immunization coverage, prevent achievement of herd immunity, and increase the chance of continuing or re-emerging epidemics of infectious disease. Another major threat to immunization coverage is an unfounded lack of professional and parental confidence in the safety and effectiveness of immunization.[187,188,203-206] In industrialized countries this usually reflects exaggerated or erroneous fears of adverse reactions, often following media scares. In developing countries this can reflect false beliefs about infectious disease and immunization. Problems in maintaining an adequate supply of vaccine and new developments leading to frequent changes to immunization schedules also impede high coverage.

Developing and delivering an effective vaccination policy is challenging for any country. Issues to consider include having comprehensive documented policies/guidelines, clear lines of responsibility, ensuring an adequate and safe vaccine supply chain, ensuring professionals delivering vaccination are adequately trained and supported, and fostering confidence in and engagement with the immunization program. Many of these issues have been clearly set out by the World Health Organization in Immunization in Practice: A Practical Resource Guide for Health Workers.[207]

Interventions to increase vaccination coverage can be patient, provider, or system orientated. Examples of interventions of proven effectiveness include:[208-212]

- robust patient call–recall and reminder systems;
- provider prompt systems (for example computer 'pop-ups' that flag when a child attending any health care setting is overdue vaccinations);
- multifaceted education programs for professionals and parents;
- generally increasing the accessibility of immunization (including providing accessible immunization clinics and making immunization available in other settings such as hospital outpatients and Accident and Emergency departments);
- ensuring vaccination providers receive regular assessment of and feedback on their performance relative to vaccination targets;
- integrating immunization into general mother and child health programs;
- ensuring parents and providers do not incur costs associated with vaccination.

Making complete vaccination a requirement for children to enter childcare or school is effective in increasing coverage and is used in some countries. This approach has not been adopted in the UK due to the potentially damaging consequences of overriding parental choice.[213] Ensuring the availability of high-quality information on the target pop-

ulation that would benefit from vaccination is also important in developing effective recall systems and monitoring performance. Achieving and maintaining high vaccination coverage is an important effective measure to reduce health inequalities.[214-216]

SPECIFIC IMMUNIZATIONS

This section provides information on selected vaccine preventable diseases that have been the subject of recent debate in the UK or internationally.

Haemophilus influenzae *type b (Hib)*

Haemophilus influenzae type b causes a range of invasive infections including meningitis, epiglottitis, septicemia, septic arthritis, and cellulitis. It predominantly affects young children aged up to 4 years, with peak incidence at 10–11 months. Prior to immunization, Hib was the commonest cause of bacterial meningitis in pre-school-age children and around 1 in 600 children in the UK had an invasive Hib infection before their 5th birthday.[174]

Routine vaccination against Hib at 2, 3, and 4 months of age using a polysaccharide conjugate vaccine was introduced in the UK in 1992 alongside a 'catch up' campaign offering immunization to all children aged up to 4 years. The vaccination program was initially very successful with invasive Hib infections falling to very low levels.[217] From 1998, however, the enhanced surveillance program put in place to monitor the effect of vaccination noted a gradual increase in Hib disease.[218] This led to a further 'catch up' campaign in 2003[219] and the adoption of a routine booster at the age of 12 months into the UK immunization schedule in 2006.[196]

The resurgence in Hib disease was predominantly due to the use of a particular combined DTaP-Hib (acellular pertussis) vaccine and the accelerated schedule used in the UK.[220,221] When Hib vaccination was first introduced it was given as a separate injection but from 1996 it was given as a combined DTP-Hib (whole-cell pertussis) vaccine to minimize the number of injections given to infants. In 1999 there was a shortage of the DTP-Hib vaccine hence a switch to using DTaP-Hib (trivalent acellular pertussis) was made. This combined vaccine was known to result in lower Hib antibody titers but the effect was not thought to be clinically significant due to immunological memory. Experience showed however that the combined vaccine when given according to the accelerated schedule used in the UK did lead to lower protection and allowed the disease to re-emerge. The switch back to DTP-Hib vaccine (and subsequently DTaP-Hib with pentavalent acellular pertussis) and catch up campaign in 2003 was successful in reversing the re-emergence of Hib disease and the introduction of a booster dose should ensure that no further re-emergence occurs. The experience of Hib vaccination in the UK highlights the vital importance of robust surveillance mechanisms to monitor the long-term impact of vaccination on disease epidemiology.

Conjugate Hib vaccination was introduced in other developed countries around the same time as in the UK and has generally been very effective in reducing the incidence of Hib disease.[222] The problem of disease re-emergence has not been an issue in other countries that use different combination vaccines, more spaced out primary immunization courses, and/or routine booster doses of Hib vaccine in the second year of life. As previously discussed, access to Hib vaccine in developing countries is very limited despite high disease burdens and introducing sustainable Hib vaccination is a major focus of the work of GAVI.[178,199]

Poliomyelitis

Polio virus infections may be asymptomatic or, less commonly, cause mild febrile illness, aseptic meningitis, or acute flaccid paralysis. Polio infection was common in the UK prior to vaccination, with frequent large-scale outbreaks. Routine childhood immunization was implemented in 1956 initially with injected polio vaccine (IPV) and subsequently with oral polio vaccine (OPV) from 1962. The vaccination program was highly successful with the last case of wild polio infection acquired in the UK occurring in 1984. Since then 1 or 2 cases of paralytic polio have occurred in the UK per year, mainly vaccine-associated paralytic polio (VAPP) with occasional imported cases of wild polio.[223]

The World Health Assembly passed a resolution aiming for global eradication of polio in 1988 and the WHO and partners have subsequently been working towards this goal.[224] The target of globally interrupted transmission by the end of 2004 was not achieved, however by mid 2006 only four countries in the world still have endemic polio (Nigeria, India, Pakistan, and Afghanistan), with by far the majority of transmission occurring in Nigeria.[225] The relatively slow progress towards eradication in Nigeria reflects loss of confidence in the vaccination program by local leaders in 2003.[226]

As progress towards global eradication is made the benefits of continuing to use OPV become less clear.[194,223,227–230] Both OPV and IPV provide good individual protection against polio. OPV has additional benefits however in that vaccine recipients can excrete and hence transmit vaccine strain virus thus benefiting their contacts. OPV also stimulates the production of local immunity in the gastrointestinal tract as well as systemic immunity and hence reduces the risk of excretion of wild type polio virus. OPV virus strains do retain the ability to revert to virulent forms however and approximately 1 in 1 million OPV recipients develops VAAP. In areas of low population immunity OPV-derived virus can also cause outbreaks of paralytic disease. Nevertheless, the WHO continues to recommend that OPV should be used until global eradication is achieved, then there should be a coordinated switch worldwide to IPV before eventually ceasing all polio vaccination. Despite this, because of the reducing risk of imported cases of wild polio and the ongoing risk of VAPP, many resource rich countries are moving from OPV to IPV in their routine childhood schedules. The USA switched to IPV in 2000[231] and the UK followed suit in 2004.[194]

Tuberculosis and the bacillus Calmette–Guérin

Tuberculosis (TB) remains a major killer worldwide with approximately one third of the world's population infected with *Mycobacterium tuberculosis* and approximately 2 million TB deaths occurring annually.[232] Rates of TB have increased in some areas of the world over recent years, for example in sub-Saharan Africa due to the HIV epidemic and the former Soviet Union due to economic and health care infrastructure collapse. In 1993 the WHO declared TB a 'global emergency'. In the UK TB has changed from a common disease affecting all sections of society in the 1950s to a relatively uncommon disease primarily affecting certain population subgroups, specifically immigrants from areas of high endemicity and indigenous people suffering from homelessness or alcohol problems.[233]

Routine BCG immunization for 14-year-olds was implemented in the UK in the 1950s to combat the high incidence of disease in young adults. In the 1960s this was supplemented by a targeted neonatal immunization program for children of immigrants from areas of high endemicity.[233] In 2005 the adolescent program was stopped and an enhanced targeted neonatal immunization program was adopted focusing on immunizing neonates living in areas of the UK with an annual TB incidence of = 40 per 100 000 population or with family links to other countries with a similarly high incidence.[195] This change in policy reflected the changing epidemiology of TB in the UK and also growing evidence of the relative effectiveness of BCG vaccine.[234] BCG is around 70–80% effective in protecting children from severe disseminated primary disease such as military TB or TB meningitis however it has questionable effectiveness against pulmonary disease in children or reactivated disease in adults.[233]

BCG, a live attenuated strain of *Mycobacterium bovis*, is currently the only vaccine available against TB however a major international effort to develop better TB vaccines is currently underway.[235,236] Vaccines that are more effective at preventing primary disease in children are required as are vaccines that prevent the reactivation of latent infection and thera-

peutic vaccines that boost the effectiveness of treatment for active disease. Recombinant BCG or other organisms that overexpress particular *M. tuberculosis* antigens and heterologous vaccines have been developed and promising candidates are currently undergoing Phase I human trials. TB control currently focuses on active case finding and effective treatment, and concurrent HIV control, as BCG alone also does not have a significant impact on TB incidence due to its minimal effect on open pulmonary disease. It is hoped that new vaccines will contribute more to TB control.

Pneumococcus

Streptococcus pneumoniae causes a range of infections collectively known as pneumococcal disease including sinusitis, otitis media, pneumonia, bacteremia, and meningitis.[237] There are around 100 types of encapsulated pneumococci capable of causing disease in humans, although the substantial majority of infections are currently caused by 10 types. Pneumococcal infections occur in all age groups but the peak incidence is in young children and the elderly. Following the introduction of Hib vaccination, pneumococcal disease has become the commonest cause of invasive bacterial infection in young children.

Two types of vaccines are available against pneumococcal disease: polysaccharide vaccine (active against 23 serotypes) and conjugated polysaccharide vaccines (active against 7–11 serotypes). The polysaccharide vaccine is poorly immunogenic in children aged less than 2 years who are most at risk of disease, however the conjugate vaccine is effective in children from the age of 2 months.[238,239] One major randomized, controlled trial conducted in the USA showed pneumococcal conjugate vaccine (PCV7) given at 2, 4, 6, and 12–15 months was effective in preventing > 90% of invasive disease (bacteremia and meningitis) caused by the serotypes included in the vaccine in children aged up to 2 years. It was less effective against pneumonia and otitis media however, reducing all clinical diagnoses of pneumonia by 11% (but all diagnoses confirmed by consolidation seen on chest X-ray by 73%) and reducing clinical diagnoses of otitis media by 7%.[240,241]

By mid-2006, 13 countries worldwide had implemented or were planning to implement routine pneumococcal conjugate vaccination. Routine immunization of infants with PCV was implemented in the USA in 2000,[242] although vaccine shortages initially meant that many children received suboptimal schedules.[239] Enhanced surveillance of pneumococcal disease in selected areas of the USA nevertheless showed there was a 94% reduction in vaccine type invasive pneumococcal disease (IPD) in children aged under 5 during the post-vaccination period 2001–2003 compared to the pre-vaccination period of 1998–1999.[243,244] Over the same period there was a 75% reduction in all (vaccine and nonvaccine type) IPD in children aged under 5 years and a 30% reduction in all IPD in all age groups. The rate of invasive disease caused by penicillin nonsusceptible strains of pneumococcus also declined considerably following implementation of vaccination.[245] Modeling suggested that while vaccination was highly effective in preventing IPD in vaccine recipients, more cases of IPD were actually prevented in members of the general population who had not received the vaccine through the vaccine's effects on nasal carriage of the pneumococcus among young children, who are the main reservoir of infection. The enhanced surveillance did identify some replacement disease effect, i.e. disease due to nonvaccine type pneumococci did increase somewhat, although not enough to counteract the reduction of vaccine-type disease. Replacement disease is potentially a serious concern with pneumococcus due to the large number of serotypes capable of causing disease in humans and this demonstrates the paramount importance of ongoing surveillance.

The decision to introduce routine childhood immunization with PCV in the UK was taken in early 2006[196] although to date vaccine supply and funding issues have caused delays in implementation of the policy. There is currently very limited access to PCV in the developing world despite a heavy disease burden, and working towards increased access to PCV, along with rotavirus and meningococcal A and C vaccines, has been identified as a priority by GAVI.[246]

REFERENCES*

1. Inequalities in health. The Black Report and the Health Divide. 2nd edn. London: Penguin Books; 1992.
2. Spencer N. Poverty and Child Health. 2nd edn. Oxford: Radcliffe Medical Press; 2000.
3. Spencer N. Child poverty and deprivation in the UK. Arch Dis Child 1991; 66:1255–1257.
4. Kohler L. Child public health: a new basis for child health workers. Eur J Public Health 1998; 8:253–255.
5. Independent inquiry into inequalities in health report. London: The Stationery Office; 1998.
6. http://www.unicef.org/crc/
7. Downie R, Tannahill C, Tannahill A. Health Promotion: Models and Values. 2nd edn. Oxford: Oxford University Press; 1996.
8. Naidoo J, Wills J. Health Promotion: Foundations for Practice. 2nd edn. London: Bailliere Tindall; 2000.
9. Last J. A Dictionary of Epidemiology. 4th edn. Oxford: Oxford University Press; 2001.
10. Satcher D, Kaczorowski J, Topa D. The expanding role of the pediatrician in improving child health in the 21st century. Pediatrics 2005; 115(Suppl):1124–1128.
11. Waterston T, Tonniges T. Advocating for children's health: a US and UK perspective. Arch Dis Child 2001; 85:180–182.
12. Marmot ME, Wadsworth MEJ. Fetal and early childhood environment and long-term health implications. Br Med Bull 1997; 53:81–96.
13. Kuh D, Ben-Shlomo Y. A life course approach to chronic disease epidemiology. 2nd edn. Oxford: Oxford University Press; 2004.
14. Graham H, Power C. Childhood Disadvantage and Adult Health: A Lifecourse Framework. London: Health Development Agency; 2004.
15. Barker DJ. The fetal and infant origins of disease. Eur J Clin Invest 1995; 25:457–463.
16. Barker DJ. Fetal origins of coronary heart disease. BMJ 1995; 311:171–174.
17. Law CM, Barker DJ. Fetal influences on blood pressure. J Hypertens 1994; 12:1329–1332.
18. Lau C, Rogers CM. Embryonic and fetal programming of physiological disorders in adulthood. Birth Defects Research (Part C) 2004; 72:300–312.
19. Bull J, Mulvihill C, Quigley R. Prevention of low birth weight: assessing the effectiveness of smoking cessation and nutritional interventions. London: Health Development Agency; 2003.
20. Antenatal Care. Routine Care for the Healthy Pregnant Woman. Clinical Guideline 6. London: National Institute for Clinical Excellence; 2003.
*21. Castles A, Adams EK, Melvin CL, et al. Effects of smoking during pregnancy: Five meta-analyses. Am J Prev Med 1999; 16:208–215.
*22. Shah NR, Bracken MB. A systematic review and meta-analysis of prospective studies on the association between maternal cigarette smoking and preterm delivery. Am J Obstet Gynecol 2000; 182:465–472.
23. Kleinman JC, Pierre Jr MB, Madans JH, et al. The effects of maternal smoking on fetal and infant mortality. Am J Epidemiol 1988; 127:274–282.
24. Daltveit AK, Oyen N, Skjaereven R, et al. The epidemic of SIDS in Norway 1967–93: changing effects of risk factors. Arch Dis Child 1997; 77:23–27.
25. Arnestead M, Anderson M, Vege A, et al. Changes in the epidemiological pattern of sudden infant death syndrome in southeast Norway, 1984–1998: implications for future prevention and research. Arch Dis Child 2001; 85:108–115.

26. DiFranza JR, Lew RA. Effect of maternal cigarette smoking on pregnancy complications and sudden infant death syndrome. J Fam Pract 1995; 40:385–394.
27. Naidoo B, Warm D, Quigley R, et al. Smoking and public health: a review of reviews of interventions to increase smoking cessation, reduce smoking initiation and prevent further uptake of smoking. London: Health Development Agency; 2004.
28. Thorogood M, Hillsdon M, Summerbell C. Changing behaviour: cardiovascular disorders. Clin Evid 2002; 8:37–59.
29. House of Commons Science and Technology Committee. Human genetics: the science and its consequences. London: HMSO; 1995.
30. Motulsky AG. Predictive genetic testing. Am J Hum Genet 1994; 55:603–605.
31. Green JM, Hewison J, Bekker HL, et al. Psychosocial aspects of genetic screening of pregnant women and newborns: a systematic review. Health Technol Assess 2004; 8:1–109.
32. Stevenson RE. The environmental basis of human anomalies. In: Stevenson R E, Hall J G, Goodman R M, eds. Human Malformations and Related Anomalies. Oxford Monographs on Medical Genetics, number 27. Oxford: Oxford University Press; 1993: volume 1.
33. Campbell H, Jones IJ. Breastfeeding in Scotland. Scottish Needs Assessment Programme. Glasgow: Scottish Forum for Public Health Medicine; 1994.
34. Aniansson G, Alm B, Andersson B, et al. A prospective cohort study on breast-feeding and otitis media in Swedish infants. Pediatr Infect Dis J 1994; 13:183–188.
35. Arenz S, Ruckerl R, Koletzko B, et al. Breast-feeding and childhood obesity – a systematic review. Int J Obes Relat Metal Disord 2004; 28:1247–1256.
36. Lucas A, Morley R, Cole TJ, et al. Breast milk and subsequent intelligence quotient in children born preterm. Lancet 1992; 339:261–264.
37. Florey CV, Leech AM, Blackhall A. Infant feeding and mental and motor development at 18 months of age in first born singletons. Int J Epidemiol 1995; 24:S21–S26.
38. McNeilly AS. Effects of lactation on fertility. Br Med Bull 1979; 35:151–154.
39. http://www.unicef.org/programme/breastfeeding/baby.htm
40. http://www.babyfriendly.org.uk
41. Campbell H, Gorman D, Wigglesworth A. Audit of the support for breastfeeding mothers in Fife maternity hospitals using adapted baby friendly hospital materials. J Public Health Med 1995; 17:450–454.
42. Beeken S, Waterston T. Health service support of breastfeeding – are we practising what we preach? BMJ 1992; 305:285–287.
43. Saadeh R, Akré J. Ten steps to successful breastfeeding: a summary of the rationale and scientific evidence. Birth 1996; 23:154–160.
44. Taylor PM, Maloni JA, Taylor FH, et al. Extra early mother-infant contact and duration of breast-feeding. Acta Pediatr Scand 1985; 316(Supp):15–22.
45. Anderson GC, Moore E, Hepworth J, et al. Early skin-to-skin contact for mothers and their healthy newborn infants. In: Cochrane Database of Systematic Reviews. John Wiley & Sons Ltd: Chichester; 2003. Issue 2
46. Mikiel KK, Mazur J, Boltruszko I. Effect of early skin-to-skin contact after delivery on duration of breastfeeding: a prospective cohort study. Acta Paediatr 2002; 91:1301–1306.
47. Renfrew MJ, Dyson L, Wallace L, et al. Effectiveness of public health interventions to promote the duration of breastfeeding: a systematic review. London: National Institute for Health and Clinical Excellence; 2005.
48. Ingram J, Johnson D, Greenwood R. Breastfeeding in Bristol: teaching good positioning, and support from fathers and families. Midwifery 2002; 18:87–101.

49. Perez-Escamilla R, Pollitt E, Lohnerdal B, et al. Infant feeding policies in maternity wards and their effect on breastfeeding success: an analytical overview. Am J Public Health 1994; 84:89–97.
50. Phillip BL, Merewood A, Miller LW, et al. Baby-friendly hospital initiative improves breastfeeding initiation rates in a US hospital setting. Pediatrics 2001; 108:677–681.
51. Fairbank L, O'Meara S, Renfrew MJ, et al. A systematic review to evaluate the effectiveness of interventions to promote the initiation of breastfeeding. Health Technology Assessment 2000; 4:1–169.
52. Broadfoot M, Britten J, Tappin D, et al. Baby friendly hospital initiative and breast feeding rates in Scotland. Arch Dis Child Fetal Neonatal Ed 2005; 90:F114–F116.
53. Australian College of Paediatrics. Policy statement on breastfeeding. J Paediatr Child Health 1998; 34:412–413.
54. Zipursky A. Vitamin K at birth. BMJ 1996; 313:179–180.
55. Ross JA, Davies SM. Vitamin K prophylaxis and childhood cancer. Med Pediatr Oncol 2000; 34:434–437.
56. Golding J, Birmingham K, Greenwood R, et al. Childhood cancer, intramuscular vitamin K, and pethidine given during labour. BMJ 1992; 305:341–346.
57. Roman E, Fear NT, Ansell P, et al. Vitamin K and childhood cancer: analysis of individual patient data from six case-control studies. Br J Cancer 2002; 86:63–69.
58. Fear NT, Roman E, Ansell P, et al. Vitamin K and childhood cancer: a report from the United Kingdom Childhood Cancer Study. Br J Cancer 2000; 89:1228–1231.
59. Management of HIV in pregnancy. Guideline No 39. London: Royal College of Obstetricians and Gynaecologists; 2004.
60. Moore AL, Madge S, Johnson SA. HIV and pregnancy. The Obstetrician & Gynaecologist 2002; 4:197–200.
61. Department of Health. The sleeping position of infants and cot death: report of the Chief Medical Officer's Expert Group. London: HMSO; 1993.
62. Blair PS, Fleming PJ, Bensley D, et al. Smoking and the sudden infant death syndrome: results from 1993–95 case–control study for confidential inquiry into stillbirths and deaths in infancy. Confidential enquiry into stillbirths and deaths regional coordinators and researchers. BMJ 1996; 313:195–198.
63. Fleming PJ, Blair PS, Bacon, et al. Environment of infants during sleep and risk of the sudden infant death syndrome: results of 1993–5 case–control study for confidential inquiry into stillbirths and deaths in infancy. Confidential Enquiry into Stillbirths and Deaths Regional Coordinators and Researchers. BMJ 1996; 3139:191–195.
64. Fleming PJ, Gilbert R, Azaz Y, et al. Interaction between bedding and sleeping position in the sudden infant death syndrome: a population based case-control study. BMJ 1990; 301:85–89.
65. Blair PS, Fleming PJ, Smith IJ, et al. Babies sleeping with parents: case–control study of factors influencing the risk of the sudden infant death syndrome. CESDI SUDI research group. BMJ 1999; 319:1457–1461.
66. Brooke H, Gibson A, Tappin D, et al. Case–control study of sudden infant death syndrome in Scotland, 1992–5. BMJ 1997; 314:1516–1520.
67. Fleming PJ, Blair PS, Pollard K, et al. Pacifier use and sudden infant death syndrome: results from the CESDI/SUDI case control study. Arch Dis Child 1999; 81:112–116.
68. Li D, Willinger M, Petitti DB, et al. Use of a dummy (pacifier) during sleep and risk of sudden infant death syndrome (SIDS): population based case-control study. BMJ 2006; 332:18–22.

*Indicates level 1 evidence, i.e. either a randomized, controlled trial, a high-quality prospective cohort study, or a systematic review of RCT/cohort studies.

69. Kramer MS. Nutritional advice in pregnancy. Cochrane Database Syst Rev 2003; 1:1–10.

70. http://www.eatwell.gov.uk/agesandstages/pregnancy/

71. Hinds K. National diet and nutrition survey: children aged 1.5 to 4.5 years. In: Report of the Dental Survey. London: HMSO; 1995: vol 2.

72. Pitts NB, Nugent ZJ, Smith PA. Scottish Dental Epidemiological Programme: Report of the 1999–2000 Survey of 5 Year old Children. Dundee: Dental Health Services Research Unit, University of Dundee; 2000.

73. Rodrigues CS, Sheilham A. The relationships between dietary guidelines, sugar intake, and caries in primary teeth in low-income Brazilian 3 year olds: a longitudinal study. Int J Paediatr Dent 2000; 10:47-55.

74. Marshall TA, Levy SM, Broffitt B, et al. Dental caries and beverage consumption in young children. Pediatrics 2003; 112(Pt1):e184–e191.

75. Diet, nutrition, and the prevention of chronic diseases: report of a joint WHO/FAO expert consultation. Geneva: World Health Organization; 2003.

*76. Marinho VCC, Higgins JPT, Shielham A, et al. Fluoride toothpastes for preventing dental caries in children and adolescents. In: Cochrane Database of Systematic Reviews. John Wiley & Sons Ltd: Issue 1. Chichester; 2003.

77. McDonagh MS, Whiting PF, Wilson PM, et al. A systematic review of water fluoridation. York: NHS Centre for Reviews and Dissemination, University of York; 2000.

78. Water Fluoridation and Health. London: Medical Research Council; 2002.

79. James JA, Laing GJ, Logan S. Changing patterns of iron deficiency anaemia in the second year of life. BMJ 1995; 311:230.

*80. Idradinata P, Pollitt E. Reversal of developmental delays in iron deficient infants treated with iron. Lancet 1993; 341:1–4.

81. Birth to Five. London: Department of Health; 2005.

82. Jarvis S, Towner E, Walsh S. Accidents. In: Department of Health: The Health of our Children. London: HMSO; 1996.

83. Royal Society for the Prevention of Accidents. Accidents to children. Available from http://www.rospa.com/homesafety/advice/child/accidents.htm.

84. Towner E, Dowswell T, Mackereth C, et al. What works in preventing unintentional injuries in children and young adolescents: an updated systematic review. London: Health Development Agency; 2001.

85. Millward LM, Morgan A, Kelly MP. Prevention and reduction of accidental injury in children and older people. London: Health Development Agency; 2003.

86. King WJ, Klassen TP, LeBlanc J, et al. The effectiveness of a home visit to prevent childhood injury. Pediatrics 2001; 108:382–388.

87. Bull J, McCormick G, Swann C, et al. Ante- and Post-natal Home Visiting Programmes: A Review of Reviews. London: Health Development Agency; 2004.

88. Boreham C, Riddoch C. The physical activity, fitness and health of children. J Sport Sci 2001; 19:915–929.

89. Harro M, Riddoch C. Physical activity. In: Armstrong N, Van Mehelen W, eds. Paediatric Exercise: Science and Medicine. Oxford: Oxford University Press; 2000.

90. Strong WB, Malina RM, Blimkie CJ, et al. Evidence based physical activity for school aged youth. J Pediatr 2005; 146:732–737.

91. Fox KR. Childhood obesity and the role of physical activity. Journal of the Royal Society for the Promotion of Health 2004; 124:34–39.

92. Effective intervention: child abuse. Guidelines on co-operation in Scotland. Edinburgh: HMSO; 1990.

93. Green AH. Child sexual abuse: immediate and long term effects and intervention. Journal of Academic Child and Adolescent Psychiatry 1993; 32:890–902.

94. Glaser D. Treatment issues in child sexual abuse. Br J Psychiatry 1991; 159:769–782.

95. Scottish schools adolescent lifestyle and substance use survey (SALSUS). 2004 national report. Edinburgh: The Stationery Office; 2005.

*96. Brief Interventions and Referral for Smoking Cessation in Primary Care and Other Settings. Public Health Intervention Guidance No 1. London: National Institute for Health and Clinical Excellence; 2006.

97. C Power. Health related behaviour. In: Department of Health: The Health of Our Children. London: HMSO; 1996.

98. Foxcroft DR, Lister-Sharp D, Lowe G. Alcohol misuse prevention for young people: a systematic review reveals methodological concerns and lack of reliable evidence of effectiveness. Addiction 1997; 92:531–537.

99. Foxcroft DR, Ireland D, Lister-Sharp D, et al. Primary prevention for alcohol misuse in young people. In: London: Cochrane Database of Systematic Reviews. Issue 3; 2002.

100. Mulvihill C, Taylor L, Waller S. Prevention and reduction of alcohol misuse. London: Health Development Agency; 2005.

101. Canning U, Millward L, Raj T, et al. Drug use prevention among young people: a review of reviews. London: Health Development Agency; 2004.

102. The National Strategy for Sexual Health and HIV. London: Department of Health; 2001.

103. Teenage Pregnancy: report by the Social Exclusion Unit. London: The Stationery Office; 1999.

104. Botting B, Rosato M, Wood R. Teenage mothers and the health of their children. Popul Trends 1998; 93:19–28.

105. Swann C, Bowe K, McCormick G, et al. Teenage pregnancy and parenthood: a review of reviews. London: Health Development Agency; 2003.

106. Ellis S, Grey A. Prevention of Sexually Transmitted Infections (STIs): a review of reviews into the effectiveness of non-clinical interventions. London: Health Development Agency; 2004.

107. Health Survey for England 2004: Updating of trend tables to include 2004 data. London: NHS Health and Social Care Information Centre; 2005.

108. Lightening the Load: Tackling Overweight and Obesity. London: National Heart Forum and Faculty of Public Health; 2006.

109. Scottish Health Survey 1998. volume 1. Edinburgh: Scottish Executive Health Department; 2000.

*110. Mulvihill C, Quigley R. The Management of Obesity and Overweight. London: Health Development agency; 2003.

111. Management of Obesity in Children and Young People. Guideline No. 69. Edinburgh: Scottish Collegiate Guidelines Network; 2003.

112. Bonomo Y, Bowes G. Putting harm reduction into an adolescent context. J Paediatr Child Health 2001; 37:5–8.

113. American Academy of Pediatrics. School health centers and other integrated school health services. Pediatrics 2001; 107:198–201.

114. http://www.wiredforhealth.gov.uk/

115. National Healthy Schools Programme. a briefing for Directors of Public Health. London: Health Development Agency; 2004.

116. Smithells RW, Shephard S, Schorah CJ, et al. Possible prevention of neural tube defects by periconceptional vitamin supplementation. Lancet 1980; i:339–340.

*117. Laurence KM, James N, Miller MH, et al. Double blind randomised controlled trial of folate treatment before conception to prevent recurrence of neural tube defects. BMJ 1981; 282:1509–1511.

*118. MRC Vitamin Study Research Group. Prevention of neural tube defects: results of the MRC vitamin study. Lancet 1991; 338:131–137.

119. Czeizel AE, Dudas L. Prevention of the first occurrence of neural-tube defects by periconceptional vitamin supplementation. N Engl J Med 1992; 327:1832–1835.

120. Smithells D. Vitamins in early pregnancy. BMJ 1996; 313:128–129.

121. Control and prevention of rubella. evaluation and management of suspected outbreaks, rubella in pregnant women, and surveillance for congenital rubella syndrome. MMWR 2001; 50:1–23.

122. Miller E, Waight P, Gay N, et al. The epidemiology of rubella in England and Wales before and after the 1994 measles and rubella vaccination campaign: fourth joint report from the PHLS and the National Congenital Rubella Surveillance Programme. Commun Dis Rep 1997; 7:R26–R32.

123. Miller E, Cradock-Watson JE, Pollock TM. Consequences of confirmed maternal rubella at successive stages of pregnancy. Lancet 1982; 2:781–784.

*124. Wald NJ, Rodeck C, Hackshaw AK, et al. First and second trimester antenatal screening for Down's syndrome: the results of the serum, urine and ultrasound screening study (SURUSS). Health Technol Assess 2003; 7:1–88.

125. Wald NJ, Huttly WJ, Hackshaw AK. Antenatal screening for Down's syndrome with the quadruple test. Lancet 2003; 361:835–836.

126. Spencer K, Spencer CE, Power M, et al. Screening for chromosomal abnormalities in the first trimester using ultrasound and maternal serum biochemistry in a one-stop clinic: a review of three years prospective experience. BJOG 2003; 110:281–286.

127. Walpole I, Zubrick S, Pontre J. Is there a fetal effect with low to moderate alcohol use before or during pregnancy? J Epidemiol Community Health 1990; 44:297–301.

128. Abel EL. Fetal alcohol syndrome: the 'American Paradox'. Alcohol Alcohol 1998; 33:195–201.

129. Alcohol Consumption in Pregnancy. Guideline No. 9. London: Royal College of Obstetricians and Gynaecologists; 1999.

130. British Committee for Standards in Haematology: Blood Transfusion Task Force. Guidelines for blood grouping and red cell antibody testing during pregnancy. Transfus Med 1996; 6:71–74.

131. Guidance on the use of routine antenatal anti-D prophylaxis for RhD-negative women. London: National Institute for Clinical Excellence; 2002. Technology Appraisal Guidance No. 41.

*132. Crowley P. Antenatal steroids for the prevention of respiratory distress syndrome in preterm babies. In: Enkin M W, Keirse MJNC, Renfrew M J, et al. eds. The Cochrane pregnancy and childbirth database. Cochrane updates. Oxford: Update Software; 1993.

133. Intrapartum care: care of healthy women and their babies during childbirth. Final draft for consultation. London: National Institute for Health and Clinical Excellence; 2006.

134. Postnatal care: routine postnatal care of women and their babies. London: National Institute for Health and Clinical Excellence; 2006.

135. Hall DMB, Elliman D. Health for all Children. 4th edn. Oxford: Oxford University Press; 2003.

136. National Service Framework for Children, Young People, and Maternity Services. London: Department of Health; 2004.

137. Helpful Parenting. London: Royal College of Paediatrics and Child Health; 2002.

138. The Importance of Caregiver-child Interactions for the Survival and Healthy Development of Young Children. Geneva: World Health Organization (Department of Child and Adolescent Health and Development); 2004.

139. Shonkoff J, Phillips D. From Neurons to Neighbourhoods: The Science of Early Childhood Development. Washington DC: National Academy Press; 2000.

140. Gerhardt S. Why Love Matters. London: Routledge; 2004.

*141. Armstrong KL, Fraser JA, Dadds MR, et al. Promoting secure attachment, maternal mood and child health in a vulnerable population: a randomized controlled trial. J Paediatr Child Health 2000; 36:555–562.

142. Parenting and pubic health: briefing statement. London: Faculty of Public Health; 2005.

143. Marshall J, Watt P. Child Behaviour Problems: A literature review of the size and nature of the problem and prevention interventions in childhood. Perth, Western Australia: The Interagency Committee on Children's Futures; 1999.

144. Shore R. Rethinking the brain: new insights into early developments. New York: New York Families and Work Institute; 1997.

145. Wolfendale S, Einzig H. Parenting education and support: new opportunities. London: David Fulton Publishers; 1999.

*146. Barlow J, Parsons J. Group Based Parent Training Programmes for Improving Emotional and Behavioural Adjustment in 0–3 year old Children. The Cochrane Database of Systematic Reviews 2003; (Issue 2):

*147. Barlow J, Coren E. Stewart-Brown S. Parent Training Programmes for Improving Maternal Psychosocial Health. The Cochrane Database of Systematic Reviews 2003; (Issue 4):

*148. Coren E, Barlow J. Individual and Group Based Parenting Programmes for Improving Psychosocial Outcomes for Teenage Parents and Their Children. The Cochrane Database of Systematic Reviews 2001; (Issue 3):

*149. Olds D, Henderson CR, Cole R, et al. Long term effects of nurse home visitation on children's criminal and antisocial behaviour. JAMA 1998; 280:1238–1244.

150. American Academy of Pediatrics; Policy Statement. Quality early education and child care from birth to kindergarten. Pediatrics 2005; 115: 1887–1891.

*151. Zoritch B, Roberts I, Oakley A. Day Care for Pre-school Children. The Cochrane Database of Systematic Reviews. 2000. Issue 3.

152. http://www.surestart.gov.uk/

153 http://www.library.nhs.uk/screening/

154. Getting it right for Scotland's children. Health for all Children 4: guidance on implementation in Scotland. Edinburgh: Scottish Executive; 2005.

155. Blair M. Public health: the need for and the role of a co-ordinator in child health surveillance/promotion. Arch Dis Child 2001; 84:1–5.

156. Wright CM, Reynolds L. How widely are personal child health records used and are they effective health education tools? A comparison of two records. Child Care Health Dev 2006; 32:55–61.

157. Second report of the UK National Screening Committee. London: Department of Health; 2000.

158. Barratt A, Irwig L, Lasziou G, et al. Screening. In: Pencheon D, Guest C, Melzer D, Gray J A M, eds. Oxford Handbook of Public Health Practice. Oxford: Oxford University Press; 2001. 236–243.

159. Fields MM, Chevlen E. Screening for disease: making evidence based choices. Clin J Oncol Nurs 2006; 10:73–76.

160. Law M. Screening without evidence of efficacy. BMJ 2004; 328:301–302.

161. Venditti LN, Venditti CP, Berry GT, et al. Newborn screening by tandem mass spectrometry for medium-chain acyl-CoA dehydrogenase deficiency: a cost-effectiveness analysis. Pediatrics 2003; 112:1005–1015.

*162. Child health screening and surveillance: a critical review of the evidence. Sydney: National Health and Medical Research Council; 2002.

163. Dworkin PH. Developmental screening: expecting the impossible? Pediatrics 1989; 83:619–622.

164. McKinlay I. The education act 1993: working with health services to implement the code of practice. Child Care Health Dev 1996; 22:19–30.

165. Ada AL. Modern vaccines. The immunological principles of vaccination. Lancet 1990; 335: 523–526.

166. Moxon ER. Modern vaccines. The scope of immunisation. Lancet 1990; 335:448–451.

167. Anderson RM, May RM. Modern vaccines. Immunization and herd immunity. Lancet 1990; 335:641–645.

168. Immunisation against diseases of public health importance. Geneva: World Health Organization; 2005. Fact Sheet No. 288.

169. Immunity and how vaccines work. Immunisation Against Infectious Disease. 2nd edn In: London: Department of Health; 2006. Chapter 1:1–6

170. Plotkin SA. Orenstein WA, eds. 4th edn. Vaccines. 4th edn Philadelphia: WB Saunders Company; 2004.

171. Moxon ER, Rappuoli R. Modern vaccines. Haemophilus influenzae infections and whooping cough. Lancet 1990; 335:1324–1329.

172. Shann F. Modern vaccines. Pneumococcus and influenzae. Lancet 1990; 335:898–901.

173. Finn A, Heath P. Conjugate vaccines. Arch Dis Child 2005; 90:667–669.

174. Haemophilus influenzae type b (Hib). Immunisation against infectious disease. In: London Department of Health; 1996. Chapter 16:127–142.

175. Morse D, O'shea M, Hamilton A, et al. Outbreak of measles in a teenage school population: the need to immunise susceptible adolescents. Epidemiol Infect 1994; 113:355–365.

176. Shann F, Steinhoff MC. Vaccines for children in rich and poor countries. Lancet 1999; 354(SII):SII7–SII11.

177. Global immunization vision and strategy 2006–2015. Geneva: World Health Organization; 2005.

178. A promise to every child. Geneva: Global Alliance for Vaccines and Immunization; 2003.

179. Po ALW. Non-parenteral vaccines. BMJ 2004; 329:62–63.

180. Edwards KM, Decker MD. Combination vaccines. Infect Dis Clin North Am 2001; 15:209–230.

181. Lane L, Reynolds A, Ramsay M. When should vaccination be contraindicated in children? Drug Saf 2005; 28:743–752.

182. Vaccine safety and the management of adverse events following immunisation. Immunisation against infectious disease. In: London: Department of Health; 2006. Chapter 8:53–64.

183. Bohlke K, David RL, Marcy SH, et al. Risk of anaphylaxis after vaccination of children and adolescents. Pediatrics 2003; 112:815–820.

184. Childhood immunisation: a guide for healthcare professionals. London: British Medical Association; 2003.

185. Bedford H, Elliman D. Concerns about immunisation. BMJ 2000; 320:240–243.

186. De Stefano F, Chen RT, Mootry G. Safety of routine childhood vaccinations. Pediatric Drugs 2000; 2:273–291.

187. Wood D, Halfon N, Pereya M, et al. Knowledge of the childhood immunization schedule and of contraindications to vaccinate by private and public providers in Los Angeles. Pediatr Infect Dis J 1996; 15:40–45.

188. Samad L, Tate AR, Dezateux C, et al. Differences in risk factors for partial and no immunisation in the first year of life: prospective cohort study. BMJ 2006; 332:1312–1313.

189. Contraindications and special indications. Immunisation against infectious disease. In: London: Department of Health; 2006. Chapter 6:41–47

190. http://www.dh.gov.uk/PolicyAndGuidance/HealthAndSocialCareTopics/GreenBook/fs/en

191. Kirkpatrick BD, Alston WK. Current immunizations for travel. Curr Opin Infect Dis 2003; 16:369–374.

192. Routine immunisation of preterm infants. Lancet 1990; 335:23–24.

193. Siegrist CA. Immunological requirements for vaccines to be used in early life. In: Bloom B R, Lambert P H, eds. The Vaccine Book. Amsterdam: Academic Press; 2003.73–83.

194. New vaccinations for the childhood immunisation programme. London: Department of Health, Chief Medical Officer letter; 2004/3.

195. Changes to the BCG vaccination programme. London: Department of Health, Chief Medical Officer letter; 2005/3.

196. Planned changes to the routine childhood immunisation programme. Edinburgh: Scottish Executive, Chief Medical Officer letter; 2006/03.

197. Core information for the development of immunization policy 2002 update. Geneva: World Health Organization; 2002.

198. Immunization Summary 2006. New York: UNICEF; 2006.

199. Peltola H. Worldwide Haemophilus influenzae type b disease at the beginning of the 21st century: global analysis of the disease burden 25 years after the use of the polysaccharide vaccine and a decade after the advent of conjugates. Clin Microbiol Rev 2000; 13:302–317.

200. Cutts FT, Henao-Restrepo A, Olive JM. Measles elimination: progress and challenges. Vaccine 1999; 17:S47–S52.

201. Derived from information contained within Immunisation against infectious disease and Chief Medical Officer letters available on the Department of Health for England website on. www.dh.gov.uk/.

202. Recommended Childhood and Adolescent Immunization Schedule United States, 2006. MMWR 2005; 54:Q1–Q4.

203. Amanna I, Slifka MK. Public fear of vaccination: separating fact from fiction. Viral Immunol 2005; 18:307–315.

204. Mills E, Jadad AR, Ross C, et al. Systematic review of qualitative studies exploring parental beliefs and attitudes toward childhood vaccination identifies common barriers to vaccination. J Clin Epidemiol 2005; 58:1081–1088.

205. Sturm LA, Mays RM, Zimet GD. Parental beliefs and decision making about child and adolescent immunization: from polio to sexually transmitted infections. J Dev Behav Pediatr 2005; 26:441–452.

206. Yarwood J, Noakes K, Kennedy D, et al. Tracking mothers' attitudes to childhood immunisation 1991–2001. Vaccine 2005; 23:5670–5687.

207. Immunization in Practice. A Practical Resource Guide for Health Workers, 2004 update. Geneva: World Health Organization; 2000. Available on www.who.int/vaccines-diseases/epitraining/SiteNew/iip/.

208. Vaccine preventable diseases. improving vaccination coverage in children, adolescents, and adults. MMWR 1999; 48:1–15.

209. Recommendations Regarding Interventions to Improve Vaccination Coverage in Children, Adolescents, and Adults. Am J Prev Med 2000; 18:92–96.

*210. Briss PA, Rodewald LE, Hinman AR, et al. Reviews of evidence regarding interventions to improve vaccination Coverage in Children, Adolescents, and Adults. Am J Prev Med 2000; 18:97–140.

211. Increasing immunisation coverage. American Academy of Pediatrics Policy Statement. Pediatrics 2003; 112:993–996.

*212. Jacobson Vann JC, Szilagyi P. Patient reminder and patient recall systems to improve immunisation rates. The Cochrane Database of Systematic Reviews. 2005. Issue 3.

213. Salmon DA, Teret SP, MacIntyre CR, et al. Compulsory vaccination and conscientious or

philosophical exemptions: past, present, and future. Lancet 2006; 367:436–442.

214. McIntyre P, Amin J, Gidding H, et al. Vaccine preventable diseases and vaccination coverage in Australia, 1993–1998. Commun Dis Intell 2000; Sup:v–83.

215. Pegurri E, Fox-Rushby JA, Damian W. The effects and costs of expanding the coverage of immunisation services in developing countries: a systematic literature review. Vaccine 2005; 23:1624–1635.

216. Batt K, Fox-Rushby JA, Castillo-Riquelme M. The costs, effects and cost-effectiveness of strategies to increase coverage of routine immunizations in low- and middle-income countries: systematic review of the grey literature. Bull World Health Organ 2004; 82:689–696.

217. Hargreaves RM, Slack MPE, Howard AJ, et al. Changing patterns of invasive Haemophilus influenzae disease in England and Wales after introduction of the Hib vaccination programme. BMJ 1996; 312:160–161.

218. McVernon J, Trotter CL, Slack MPE, et al. Trends in Haemophilus influenzae type b infections in adults in England and Wales: surveillance study. BMJ 2004; 329:655–658.

219. Planned Hib vaccination catch-up campaign. London: Department of Health Chief Medical Officer; letter 2003/1.

220. McVernon J, Andrew N, Slack MPE, et al. Risk of vaccine failure after Haemophilus influenzae type b (Hib) combination vaccines with acellular pertussis. Lancet 2003; 361:1521–1523.

221. Heath PT, Ramsay ME. Haemophilus influenzae type b vaccine – booster campaign. BMJ 2003; 326:1158–1159.

222. Bustard KM, Kao A, Leake J, et al. Haemophilus influenzae invasive disease in the United States 1994–1995: near disappearance of a vaccine-preventable childhood disease. Emerg Infect Dis 1998; 4:229–238.

223. Poliomyelitis. Immunisation against infectious disease. In: London: Department of Health; 2006. Chapter 26:313–328.

224. Global polio eradication initiative strategic plan 2004–2008. Geneva: World Health Organization; 2004.

225. Data available on polio cases across the world from the WHO polio eradication website on. www.polioeradication.org/

226. Resurgence of wild poliovirus type 1 transmission and effect of importation into polio-free countries 2002–2005. MMWR 2006; 55:145–150.

227. Hermann DL. Polio eradication: finishing the job and protecting the investment. Bull World Health Organ 2004; 82:1–1A.

228. Sutter RW, Aceres VM, Mas Lago P. The role of routine polio immunisation in the post-certification era. Bull World Health Organ 2004; 82:3139.

229. Hayward RB, Sutter RW, Hermann DV. OPV cessation: the final step to a polio free world. Science 2005; 310:625–626.

230. Kew OM, Sutter RW, de Goreville EM, et al. Vaccine-derived polioviruses and the endgame strategy for global polio eradication. Annu Rev Microbio 2005; 59:587–639.

231. Prevention of poliomyelitis. recommendations for use of only inactivated poliovirus vaccine for routine immunisation. Pediatrics 1999; 104:1404–1406.

232. Friedens TR, Sterling TR, Massif SS, et al. Tuberculosis. Lancet 2003; 362:887–899.

233. Tuberculosis. Immunisation Against Infectious Disease. In: London: Department of Health; 2006. Chapter 32:391–408.

234. Fine P. Stopping routine vaccination for tuberculosis in schools. BMJ 2005; 331:647–648.

235. Harwinton RG. TB vaccines for the world. Tuberculosis 2005; 85:1–6.

236. Information from the WHO on TB, BCG, and potential new TB vaccines available on. http://www.who.int/vaccines/en/tuberculosis2.shtml#Administration.

237. Pneumococcal. Immunisation Against Infectious Disease. In: London: Department of Health; 2006. Chapter 25:295–311.

238. Peters TR, Edwards KM. The pneumococcal protein conjugate vaccines. J Pediatr 2000; 137:416–420.

239. Whitney CG. The potential of pneumococcal conjugate vaccines for children. Pediatr Infect Dis J 2002; 21:961–970.

*240. Black S, Shinefield H, Fireman B, et al. Efficacy, safety, and immunogenicity of heptavalent pneumococcal conjugate vaccine in children. Pediatr Infect Dis J 2000; 19:187–195.

*241. Black S, Shinefield H, Ling S, et al. Effectiveness of heptavalent pneumococcal conjugate vaccine in children younger than five years of age for prevention of pneumonia. Pediatr Infect Dis J 2002; 21:810–815.

242. Policy statement. recommendations for the prevention of pneumococcal infections, including the use of pneumococcal conjugate vaccine (Prevnar), pneumococcal polysaccharide vaccine, and antibiotic prophylaxis. Pediatrics 2000; 106:362–376.

243. Whitney CG, Farley MM, Hadler J, et al. Decline in invasive pneumococcal disease after the introduction of protein-polysaccharide conjugate vaccine. N Engl J Med 2003; 348:1737–1746.

244. Direct and indirect effects of routine vaccination of children with 7-valent pneumococcal conjugate vaccine on incidence of invasive pneumococcal disease – United States, 1998–2003. MMWR 2005; 54:893–897.

245. Kyaw MH, Lynfield R, Schnaffer W, et al. Effect of introduction of the pneumococcal conjugate vaccine on drug-resistant Streptococcus pneumoniae. N Engl J Med 2006; 354:1455–1463.

246. Information on GAVI priorities available from their website on. www.gavialliance.org/General_Information/Immunization_informa/Diseases_Vaccines/disease_info.php.

INFORMATION RESOURCES RELEVANT TO PREVENTIVE PEDIATRICS

Current UK policy and information on the health and care of British children

Department of Health for England Children's Services site
Current health policy relevant to children including a link to the National Service framework for Children, Young People, and Maternity Services
http://www.dh.gov.uk/PolicyAndGuidance/HealthAndSocialCareTopics/ChildrenServices/fs/en

National Statistics
Main source of statistics (including on health, health care, and social trends) relating to UK population
http://www.statistics.gov.uk/

Association of Public Health Observatories
PHOs across the UK provide information on the health of the population and evidence briefings on effective public health action
http://www.apho.org.uk/apho/

International resources
Centers for Disease Control and Prevention
US organization responsible for health protection and promotion; includes links to pages on infant and child health, immunization, and health promotion
http://www.cdc.gov/

World Health Organization Child Health site
Information on improving children's health in the developing world
http://www.who.int/topics/child_health/en/

Systematic reviews and evidence-based guidelines
National Institute for Health and Clinical Evidence
Evidence-based reviews of health care interventions and guidelines for clinical issues such as care of newborn infants (UK)
http://www.nice.org.uk/

Scottish Intercollegiate Guidelines Network
Evidence-based clinical guidelines (UK)
http://www.sign.ac.uk/

Cochrane collaboration
Systematic reviews of health care interventions (Int)
http://www.cochrane.org/

International Child Health Review Collaboration
Systematic reviews supporting WHO policy on child health issues in developing countries (Int)
http://www.ichrc.org/

NHS National Library for Health: Specialist Child Health Library
Evidence-based information on a range of child health and health care issues
http://www.library.nhs.uk/childhealth/

The Community Guide

CDC affiliated site providing evidence-based advice on health promotion interventions (USA)

http://www.thecommunityguide.org/

Professional associations

Royal College of Paediatrics and Child Health

UK-based professional association for paediatricians

http://www.rcpch.ac.uk/index.html

American Association of Pediatrics

USA-based professional association for pediatricians

http://www.aap.org/

Support for Parenting

Department of Health for England Birth to Five booklet

Comprehensive information for parents of pre-school children

http://www.dh.gov.uk/PublicationsAndStatistics/Publications/Public ationsPolicyAndGuidance/PublicationsPolicyAndGuidanceArticle/fs/ en?CONTENT_ID=4111315&chk=pk7lsO

Sure Start

UK-wide initiative to improve children's start in life by providing support for families including health and childcare and early education

http://www.surestart.gov.uk/

Screening and surveillance

National Screening Committee

Independent UK committee responsible for advising on national screening policy

http://www.nsc.nhs.uk/

NHS National Library for Health: Specialist Screening Library

Evidence supporting UK policy on screening programs

http://www.library.nhs.uk/screening/

Health for all Children

Web site supporting the regular Health for all Children publications that provide recommendations on the UK child health promotion program

http://www.health-for-all-children.co.uk/

Bright Futures

Comprehensive child health surveillance and promotion program produced by the AAP

http://brightfutures.aap.org/web/

Immunization

Department of Health for England 'Green Book' on Immunization

Background information and current UK immunization policy

http://www.dh.gov.uk/PolicyAndGuidance/HealthAndSocialCareTopics/ GreenBook/fs/en

Joint Committee on Vaccination and Immunization

Independent UK committee responsible for advising on national immunization policy

http://www.advisorybodies.doh.gov.uk/jcvi/

American Academy of Pediatrics site on immunization

Background information and current US immunization policy

http://www.aap.org/healthtopics/immunisations.cfm

World Health Organization site on immunization

Background information and immunization policy relevant to the developing world

http://www.who.int/topics/immunisation/en/

5

Child protection

Alison Kemp, Sabine Maguire

BACKGROUND

Identification of suspected abuse, prevention and the protection of children from abuse remain key priorities for all professional agencies who work with children. Four categories of child abuse are defined: physical, emotional, sexual abuse and neglect. The nature of what constitutes child abuse varies over time and between different cultures and ethnic groups.

HISTORICAL PERSPECTIVE

In 1895 the NSPCC described neglected children as 'miserable, vermin infested, filthy, shivering, ragged, nigh naked, pale, puny, limp, feeble, faint, dizzy, famished and dying' and those who were physically abused were battered with 'boots, crockery, pans, shovels, straps, ropes, thongs, pokers, fire and boiling water'.[1] The clinical consequences of physical child abuse were first described in the medical literature by Tardieu in 1860.[2] Caffey[3] (1946) and Silverman[4] (1953), described multiple fractures and subdural hematoma and suggested that they resulted from intentional trauma and not organic disease, as commonly thought. In a seminal paper on the 'battered child' in 1961 Henry Kempe[5] drew attention to the US problem of physical abuse, probably the first time that the issue started to gain acceptance in clinical circles.

Tardieu was also the first to describe child sexual abuse in his 1860 publication of a population study of rape in France. He stated that 80% of some 11 500 cases involved children. Following his death at the end of the century there was vociferous denial of child sexual abuse and the condition was not recognized. It was not until the beginning of 1980s that the condition was widely accepted and recognized.

Child care and parenting practices have however improved over the past century. In the UK a number of important laws came into force: in the latter part of the 19th century the Factories Acts, Coal Mines Acts and Chimney Sweeps Acts were introduced to protect children from harmful occupations while the First Children Act was introduced in 1908 at the same time as the establishment of the Juvenile Courts. The legal framework, cultural practices, tolerance and protective strategies for children vary widely between countries. At least 12 European countries have reformed their legislation to effectively ban the physical punishment of children. In England and Wales however the law permits 'reasonable chastisement' in the form of physical punishment, allowing mild smacking.

PREVALENCE

It is difficult to identify an accurate prevalence figure for child abuse. Children are abused behind 'closed doors' and only a proportion of cases are reported so there are no accurate statistics to define the extent of the problem.

In the UK, the Child Protection Register contains confidential details of children who are identified by the authorities as being at continuing risk of abuse and have a child protection plan. In 2005 the register included 32 000 children (out of a total under-16 population of roughly 10 million) under the categories of physical abuse (37%), neglect (32%), sexual abuse (26%), emotional abuse (13%) and multiple categories (9%). The UK-based National Society for Prevention of Cruelty to Children (NSPCC) completed a child maltreatment study in 2000, updated in 2002, which recorded the childhood experiences of 3000 young adults.[6] This study reported that:

- 7% of children experience serious physical harm from their carers during childhood.
- 1% of children under 16 years old experience sexual abuse by a carer and 3% by another relative; 11% by people other than relatives who are known to them and 5% by a stranger or someone that they had just met
- 6% of children experienced serious absence of care
- 6% experienced frequent and serious emotional abuse.

Children with disability are 3–4 times more likely to suffer from all types of abuse than nondisabled children.[7] It is estimated that 1–2 children die in the UK every week as a result of child abuse[8] and every year 400 will sustain permanent disability. Currently it is estimated that 79 000 children are looked after by local authorities in the UK.[9]

Child abuse is often an ongoing process rather than a one-off event. Studies quote significant recurrence rates in children who have been abused and are returned to the abusing carer.[10] This is particularly true for the youngest age group, where child abuse is most prevalent and most serious in terms of long-term morbidity and mortality. It can be argued

45

therefore that those in this age group have the greatest potential as far as prevention is concerned and justify early diagnosis and intervention.

Child abuse occurs in one form or another in all walks of life, however certain risk factors for abusive families are recognized. The strongest include: a history of previous abuse or neglect to the child or siblings, mental health problems in the carer, parental conflict or domestic violence. Weaker risk factors identified are when parents themselves were abused in childhood, parental stress, alcohol or substance abuse, a lack of social support and where the family is already in contact with social services. However in a significant number of children who are abused, there are none of these risk factors.[11]

CHILD PROTECTION PROCESS

Legislation governing child protection varies in different countries but in most, clear processes are laid out and it is the duty of all clinicians dealing with children to understand their roles in the process. In the UK, the current definitions of child abuse and child protection legislation are set out in Children Act 1989 (revised in 2004). The Act introduces the concept of significant harm as a threshold that, once breached, justifies intervention in family life to secure the best interests of the child. It establishes the principles that the welfare of the child must be the paramount consideration and that agencies must co-operate in the interests of the child to identify abuse and protect a child from further harm. The court must take the wishes of the child into consideration when making an order and ensure that the child's best interests are met. Every effort should be made to retain the family unit and the law sets out clear parental rights, duties, powers and responsibilities when caring for their child.

According to Section 47 of the Children Act, the local authority has the 'duty to investigate... if they have reasonable cause to suspect that a child who lives, or is found, in their area is suffering, or likely to suffer, significant harm.' This process involves a number of agencies including Local Authority social work and education teams, health professionals from primary care and child health teams based in the community and hospital trusts, police and family and criminal lawyers. The roles of the professionals involved and how they work together as a team are set out in Working Together.[12]

Pediatricians are primarily involved in the clinical assessment process and may call upon a wider team of clinical disciplines to inform an investigation within the Framework of Assessment of Children in Need and their families.[13]

Within each UK health organization a designated doctor and nurse take a strategic professional lead on the health service contribution to safeguarding children. All pediatricians must have the skills in the recognition of abuse, and be familiar with the procedures to be followed if abuse and/or neglect are suspected. They may be involved in difficult diagnostic situations, differentiating abuse from nonabuse and those who specialize in child protection may undertake forensic medical examinations. Pediatricians will be required to provide reports for case conferences, statements for the police, reports for civil and criminal proceedings, to appear as witnesses and to give oral evidence.

All health professionals who work with children must be able to recognize the signs of child abuse. They should be aware of the local child protection procedures and know how to contact those who have a responsibility for assessment or the named professionals for advice and support. They should receive the training and supervision needed to recognize and act upon child welfare concerns, and to respond to their needs.

Anyone who works with children may suspect child abuse and should refer their concerns to the appropriate person (the social services department in the UK). Within the health service these children may first present in Primary Care, Accident and Emergency departments, as an inpatient or to any number of health professionals during a routine investigation or procedure. However, most referrals for investigation come to the clinician via Social Services, who have received the referral from education, a member of the public, a fellow social worker or member of health services who is working in the community. If any clinician becomes concerned that a child is being abused, they should ensure that their suspicions are investigated and that an appropriate referral is made.

CLINICAL ASSESSMENT OF SUSPECTED CHILD ABUSE

When abuse is suspected, the majority of children will require a clinical assessment by a senior pediatrician (or member of the child and adolescent mental health team if emotional abuse is suspected). The clinician will be expected to take a detailed history and perform a full examination of the child detailing relevant clinical findings. Relevant investigations will be dictated by the nature of the abuse and presentation. Consideration must be given to an assessment of any siblings thought to be at risk. The examining clinician will be expected to make a clinical diagnosis, to present their findings in strategy meetings and case conferences, and to write detailed evidence-based statements for the police and reports for the relevant multidisciplinary discussion meetings. They may also be invited to Court hearings as professional witnesses.

The diagnostic process differs from other clinical areas where there may be a single confirmatory test. In this field the clinician must perform a thorough assessment and piece all of the information together to come to a decision based on a balance of probability that abuse has occurred or not. The risks of making an incorrect diagnosis are great. It is equally damaging to a family to wrongly diagnose abuse as it is when the diagnosis is missed.

PHYSICAL ABUSE

Physical abuse may involve hitting, shaking, throwing, poisoning, burning, scalding, drowning, suffocating, or otherwise causing physical harm to a child. Physical harm may also be caused when a parent or carer fabricates the symptoms of, or deliberately induces illness in a child who they are looking after.[12] The challenge for clinicians is to distinguish intentional from unintentional injuries which are common in childhood (Table 5.1).

Some features may help to make this distinction, such as:
- a history that is incompatible with the child's developmental stage (e.g. an explanation that a 6-week-old sustained their fracture by rolling off the bed). It is rare that a parent offers a full description of an abusive injury. They may be in denial, genuinely ignorant of the causal events, blame the presentation on others or propose irrelevant events as explanations;
- a history which changes as it is told to different clinicians or over time;

Table 5.1 Features that warrant investigation to exclude abuse in a child where there is no explicit and developmentally plausible explanation

- Bruising in a nonmobile child, particularly to the hands, back or areas away from bony prominences
- Rib fractures in the absence of underlying bone disease, major trauma or birth injury
- Nonsupracondylar fractures of the humerus, without clear trauma
- Femoral fractures in the nonmobile child without specific trauma
- Hemorrhagic retinopathy in a child with intracranial hemorrhage, and no history of high-impact trauma.
- Contact burns leaving a clearly demarcated imprint, particularly on back/shoulders/buttocks, without clear history
- Immersion scalds with clear upper limits, involving lower limbs with or without buttock/perineal involvement
- Unexplained oral injuries including trauma to teeth (involve dentist in interpretation)
- An adult bite on a child

- an inappropriate parental response, e.g. failure to seek medical attention for a 3-month-old who has not been using their leg for 5 d;
- history of repeated attendance with traumatic injuries which are poorly explained;
- history of an unlikely child response, e.g. a child with a scald who is said to have shown no sign of pain.

BRUISING

'Of all the physically abusive injuries that children sustain, bruising is by far the commonest'.[14] While no single injury is diagnostic of abuse in itself, certain patterns of bruising are found in accidental childhood injuries, and these are quite different from those found in abused children. Accidental bruising is very closely correlated with a child's independent mobility,[15] with bruising occurring in less than 1% of infants who are not yet crawling, rising to 17% of those who are cruising around the furniture, and 52% of those who are walking. Similarly the number of bruises increases with increasing mobility, from 1 to 5 in the children who are cruising, but up to 27 per child when they are walking.[16] However, even when bruising is as common as this, the location tends to be over the front of the body and bony prominences in more than 90% of infants.[15,17] Once children reach the age of 5 years, 90% have bruises. However, across all ages, certain sites are very rarely bruised, these include the back, buttocks, forearm, face, ears, abdomen or hip, upper arm, posterior leg, foot or hands. Indeed in children less than 2 years old, accidental bruising to the hands is hardly ever recorded in the scientific literature.[16] Contrary to popular belief, both boys and girls sustain the same amount of accidental bruising.[16]

In contrast, children who have been abused tend to have larger and more numerous bruises (up to 44 per child),[18] and these occur in quite different locations. The head is the commonest site for intentional bruises, and other sites commonly bruised are the ear, face, neck, trunk, buttocks and arms.[16] Bruises may occur in clusters, or show the negative or positive imprint of the weapon with which they were struck.[19,20] It is important to remember however, that although bruising is the commonest finding in fatally abused infants, fractures and serious intracranial injury may occur without any external bruising.[21] There is some evidence to suggest that the presence of petechiae around a bruise occurs more commonly in abuse than in accidental injuries.[22]

It is frequently stated that bruises of different ages are indicative of abuse however there is no published evidence to validate the aging of bruises with the naked eye.[23] Most people would estimate the age of a bruise by its color, but this will vary depending on the depth, location, skin color etc. of the bruised area. In addition, it is clear that we all perceive color differently, both in vivo and in photographs, and as such this becomes an unreliable indicator.[24] Considerable research is ongoing into other methods of estimating the age of a bruise at the bedside, but none are validated for clinical practice yet.[25] Clearly before deciding that a pattern of bruising is consistent with abuse, it is important to exclude other causes such as coagulation disorders, sepsis, Henoch–Schönlein purpura, idiopathic thrombocytopenic purpura, connective tissue disorders, drugs, striae, artefactual marks, or photosensitive dermatitis. When documenting bruises, it is important to record the location and dimensions of all of the bruises and to take clinical photographs with a measuring device included.

FRACTURES

Eighty percent of abusive fractures occur in children less than 18 months of age, in contrast to 85% of accidental fractures which occur in children older than 5 years.[26] Abusive fractures are consistent with a severe assault on the child. However, fractures are common accidental injuries, with up to 64% of boys and 40% of girls sustaining a fracture by their fifteenth birthday.[27] Diagnosing abusive fractures requires a careful history of the alleged accident, taking into account the weight of the child, the height fallen from and the surface on which they landed, as well as ensuring that the history offered is consistent with the child's develop-

mental ability, e.g. could they have climbed onto the surface described? It is important to establish whether there could be an underlying bony abnormality such as osteoporosis associated with prematurity, chronic disease or drugs, congenital bone fragility such as osteogenesis imperfecta, infection or mineral deficiency or whether the fracture in question could have been the result of a birth injury. Having excluded such causes, the following fracture patterns warrant investigation for possible abuse:[28]

- rib fractures, particularly in children less than 3 years old;
- multiple fractures, particularly if they show different stages of healing;
- long bone fractures in children who are not independently mobile;
- metaphyseal fractures of the femur in particular;
- spinal fractures without an adequate explanation;
- pelvic fractures where there is no history of massive trauma.

Rib fractures, in the absence of underlying bony abnormalities, birth injury or major trauma, have the highest specificity for abuse of any physical injury.[29] Abusive rib fractures are frequently multiple, predominantly anterior or posterior, in contrast to accidental fractures, which are commonly lateral.[30] Some children who present collapsed, may have undergone cardiopulmonary resuscitation (CPR), raising the question as to whether this has caused the rib fractures. CPR is an extremely rare cause of rib fractures in children, but when they do occur, they are anterior and may be multiple.[31]

Long bone fractures are recorded in abuse; the commonest site is in the shaft of the bone, especially in the premobile child.[32] Certain fracture types usually reflect accidental injuries, specifically supra-condylar humeral fractures, which are seen after falls in the increasingly mobile toddler.[33] Metaphyseal fractures although difficult to see radiologically are reported more commonly in abuse than non-abuse[26] and postmortem studies suggest that they are underdiagnosed on radiology.[34]

Skull fractures also occur in abuse, but are difficult to distinguish from accidental fractures. They are the commonest fractures in any child less than 1 year of age.[35] There is some evidence that complex or multiple/bilateral fractures or those that cross suture lines are commoner in abuse.[36,37] However, the commonest abusive and accidental fracture overall is a linear parietal fracture.[35] It is important to remember that any bone in the body may be fractured as a consequence of physical abuse.

As many abusive fractures may be occult, particularly rib fractures, which have a very high specificity for abuse, it is essential to look carefully.[38] It is recommended that all children less than 2 years with suspected physical abuse undergo a full skeletal survey (SS), including oblique views of the ribs.[39] If there is any remaining doubt as to whether fractures may be present or not, and the skeletal survey is negative, either a radionuclide bone scan may be performed or the child could be recalled for a repeat SS in 11–14 d, as each option will enhance the sensitivity of the original investigation in detecting abusive fractures.[40] In addition, repeat SS may help in clarifying ambiguous findings or dating the fractures present, although this can only be done in broad time frames in terms of weeks rather than days.[41]

BURNS

In common with head injury, abusive burns carry a high morbidity and mortality. Scalds are the commonest intentional burn injury.[42] A child can sustain a full-thickness burn in 1 s at a liquid temperature of 60°C, and the maximum household water temperature in the UK is 60°C, although in the USA it is 48.8°C. It is estimated that 2–35% of scalds in children are due to abuse.[43,44] There are certain differences however between intentional and unintentional scalds, which relate to the mechanism and agent causing the burn, and the pattern and distribution of the burn (Figs 5.1 and 5.2). Accidental scalds are predominantly caused by non-tap water, e.g. hot drinks or cooking liquids, that are usually pulled down by the child over himself.[45–47] The pattern of these burns is usually asymmetrical with irregular margins and burn depth. It typically involves the upper body, i.e. head, face, neck and trunk or

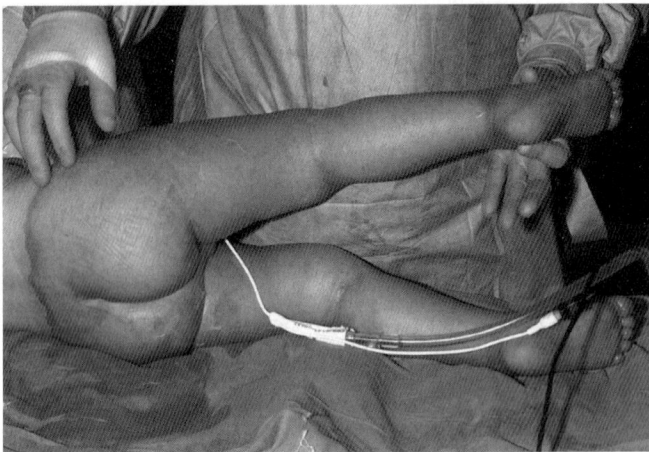

Fig. 5.1   A typical intentional scald showing clear upper margins, involving the buttocks, perineum and both lower limbs. (Printed with permission from Mr Tom Potokar, Consultant Plastic Surgeon, Welsh Centre for Burns and Plastic Surgery, Morriston Hospital, Swansea)

Table 5.2   Triage tool for identifying intentional scalds in children

Intentional scald must be excluded	Intentional scald should be considered	Intentional scald unlikely
Physical features Mechanism: Immersion	Physical features	Physical features Mechanism: Spill injury Flowing water injury
Agent: Hot tap water		Agent: Non-tap water (hot beverage)
Pattern: Clear upper limits Scald symmetry (extremities)	Pattern: Uniform scald depth Skin fold sparing Central sparing buttocks	Pattern: Irregular margin and burn depth Lack stocking distribution
Distribution: Isolated scald buttock/perineum +/– lower extremities Isolated scald lower extremities	Distribution: Glove and stocking distribution 1 limb glove/stocking	Distribution: Asymmetric involvement lower limbs Head, neck and trunk or face and upper body
Clinical features: Associated unrelated injury History incompatible with examination findings Old fractures	Clinical features: Previous burn injury Neglect/faltering growth History inconsistent with assessed development	
Historical/social features: Passive, introverted, fearful child Previous abuse Domestic violence Numerous prior accidental injuries Sibling blamed for scald	Historical/social features: Trigger, such as: Soiling / enuresis/misbehavior Differing historical accounts Lack of parental concern Unrelated adult presenting child Child known to social services	

asymmetric involvement of the upper limbs. Children can sustain accidental hot water scalds when they turn on a hot tap, which will typically cause a flowing water scald over the lower or upper limbs, which again is asymmetric.[48]

In contrast, intentional scalds are caused most commonly by immersing the child in extremely hot water. The burns have clearly defined upper limits, tend to be symmetrical, and involve upper or lower limbs with or without scalds to the perineum or buttocks.[45,46,49,50] There may be skinfold sparing, e.g. of the popliteal area if the child drew their legs up, or central sparing of the buttocks, if they were pressed firmly against the surface of the bath, which has a cooler temperature than the water (doughnut ring pattern).[45,51] There may be additional important features found in the history or on examination of the intentionally scalded child, including: an associated unrelated injury, fractures, numerous prior accidental injuries or previous abuse, a quiet or withdrawn child or a history of domestic violence. Many intentional scalds are attributed to siblings, or appear to occur following a trigger such as soiling or enuresis, or misbehavior by the child.

The triage tool shown in Table 5.2 may help clinicians to classify children with scalds into those who are at high, intermediate and low risk of having an injury that was intentionally inflicted.

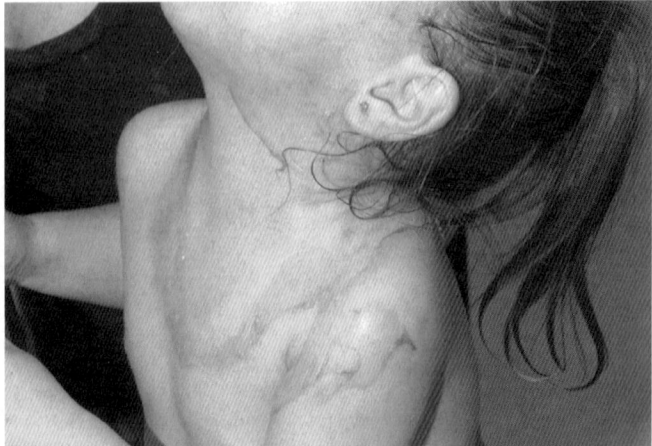

Fig. 5.2   A typical accidental scald, a spill injury showing irregular margins and burn depth, involving face, neck, and upper trunk. (Printed with permission from Mr Tom Potokar Consultant Plastic Surgeon, Welsh Centre for Burns and Plastic Surgery, Morriston Hospital, Swansea)

Contact burns may also be inflicted; examples include a child held against a hot stove, or 'branded' with an iron etc. The severity of the burn will depend on the heat of the object and the contact time. In some instances there may be a delay in presenting for medical attention. This could be interpreted as neglectful, but may simply reflect the fact that the carers have underestimated the severity of the burn initially. It is difficult to be certain if there has been delay in presentation, as there are no studies to validate how you would age a burn clinically. Clearly however, contact burns are usually deep, and as such may leave permanent scarring if appropriate treatment is not sought early.

Cigarette burns may occur accidentally, or may be inflicted. It is thought that if an infant or toddler brushes against a cigarette, they will withdraw immediately and this will either leave no mark, or an elliptical one with reddening and possible scattered small circular burns from the hot ash. An intentional cigarette burn however, although poorly defined in the literature, presents as a deep crater-like circular burn with the deepest part of the burn located in the center and corresponding to the hottest part of the cigarette end.[52,53]

Other burns such as chemical burns and flame burns have also been described, however a careful history is required to distinguish accidental causes. For example, a toddler was referred with suspicious burns when he sustained an accidental chemical burn as batteries had leaked onto his car seat and burned his buttocks.[54] Some conditions can mimic burns, particularly phytophototoxic reactions such as occur when the skin is exposed to a plant chemical, such as hogweed, and then sunlight.[55] These may appear to have occurred 'spontaneously' and often have an unusual pattern or location, so need a very careful history. In addition, certain cultural practices, such as moxibustion, where a herb, moxa, is burnt over an area of the body where there is illness, and similarly cupping or coining, may leave patterned burns or marks over the back.[56,57] Although these are inflicted injuries, they are not malicious in intent, and it is important to be aware of them.

BITES AND ORAL INJURIES

Injuries to the lips, such as bruising or lacerations are the commonest oral injuries sustained in abuse, but in themselves may not be specific. Abusive trauma to the mouth includes dental fractures, intrusions and extrusions, forced dental extractions by parents as a punishment, lacerations to the gums and foreign body insertion to the pharynx.[58] A torn labial frenum, the thin fold of mucosa between the lip and the alveolar margin, has long been held to be pathognomonic of physical abuse, but it is documented to occur accidentally in children. When an abusive torn frenum has been described in the scientific literature, the children are predominantly less than 4 years old, and the majority have suffered fatal abusive injuries, such as intra-cranial or intra-abdominal injuries. A torn frenum may result from intubation attempts,[59] and dentists commonly see young children who have accidentally torn the labial frenum by falling against a hard surface, or being hit in the mouth accidentally. When this occurs, there usually appears to be considerable bleeding, as the blood mixes with saliva, making this injury one that parents should be able to recall. A torn frenum in isolation is not diagnostic of abuse, but clearly if it occurs in a nonmobile child, there needs to be an explicit explanation.

Children are commonly bitten, but many of these are animal bites or children biting one another. However, if an adult bites a child this is an assault, and of all the physical injuries that children may sustain abusively, bites are the only one that may enable the detection of the perpetrator by use of forensic odontology or retrieval of DNA.[60] A dog bite is usually V shaped and dogs usually tear flesh, in contrast to a human, who will compress flesh when biting. A human bite leaves an oval or circular mark, measuring 2–5 cm, with or without central bruising.[61] As a general rule it is estimated that if the intercanine distance of the bite is 2.5–3.0 cm it is caused by a child or small adult, and if 3.0–5.0 cm it is caused by an adult. If you suspect a child has been bitten, it is essential to obtain good-quality clinical photographs, with a right-angled measuring device, and if the bite is on a curved surface, e.g. the arm, then obtain one photograph in each plane. Serial photographs may be beneficial. In order to confirm if this is an abusive bite, and possibly identify the perpetrator, it is essential to seek a forensic orthodontic opinion as early as possible.[62]

INTRACRANIAL AND SPINAL INJURY

Abusive head injury is the most serious form of physical abuse and carries a high morbidity and mortality. One third of children who suffer this form of abuse will die and a further third will suffer from long-term disability from central neurological damage.[63] The condition is seen most commonly in babies under 6 months old, where the estimated incidence is 35/100 000 children per year.

Abusive head injury may be caused by a direct blow to the head, or shaking, or a combination of the two. If the child has been subjected to a shaking injury, they may also suffer contusion of the spinal cord, either in the cervical or lumbar region, due to extreme hyperflexion and hyperextension.

The clinical presentation of these infants varies. The child who has suffered from extreme hyperextension whiplash-type injury may present in a moribund state. Those with significant intracranial injury are likely to be encephalopathic with altered levels of consciousness and present with a combination of apnea, seizures, vomiting and shock. More chronic symptoms of general malaise are recognized in children

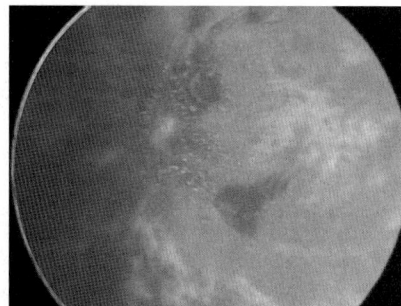

Fig. 5.3 Hemorrhagic retinopathy.

who sustain subdural hemorrhage with minimal damage to the brain itself. Thorough clinical examination and investigations reveal mixed associated signs which may include associated intentional injuries, co-existent fractures of ribs or long bones, hemorrhagic retinopathy (Fig. 5.3), anemia, subdural hematomas and intracerebral damage.[64]

The subdural hemorrhages are generally small and may be bilateral or multiple. They can be located in the interhemispheric fissure, lie along the falx or in the posterior fossa. If these children have suffered an impact injury as well as shaking, they may have a variety of additional injuries, including bruising and swelling to the head, subgaleal, or rarely extradural hemorrhage, with or without a skull fracture.

In the small number of cases who have a nonencephalopathic presentation, there may be variable combinations of subdural hemorrhages, some of which may be old at presentation. There may or may not be associated fractures of varying ages. In chronic cases, signs of raised intracranial pressure may be present, but additional findings such as hemorrhagic retinopathy may no longer be apparent. It is possible that the diagnosis is missed in these children as the clinical presentation is very similar to many childhood illnesses at this age.

It is important to have a high level of suspicion for this condition in infants with unexplained encephalopathy or other signs that suggest physical abuse. If the diagnosis is suspected, neuroimaging should be performed. Computerized tomography (CT) is widely available and currently recommended as the first-line investigation. A CT scan will show fresh bleeding and localize bleeding to the subdural or subarachnoid space. The addition of magnetic resonance imaging (MRI) may yield more information about subdural bleeds in sites not easily visualized on CT and delineate the precise pattern of intracerebral injury. Consideration should also be given to imaging the spine to exclude associated damage.[65] A further MRI study at approximately 3 months may yield further information as to the level of damage that has been caused, which may be relevant to clinical prognosis.

When taking a history, it is vital to obtain a detailed account of any alleged injury, e.g. if it was a fall, the height, surface of impact etc. Full fundoscopy by an ophthalmologist using indirect ophthalmology techniques should be performed to exclude hemorrhagic retinopathy often evident at the periphery of the retina. In a child less than 2 years of age, a skeletal survey is mandatory and will need to include a skull X-ray, as CT scanning may miss skull fractures.[66]

It is important to consider other causes of intracranial hemorrhage in infants, including coagulopathy, sepsis, and metabolic abnormalities such as glutaric aciduria type 1.[67]

VISCERAL INJURY

Abusive visceral injury, predominantly within the abdominal cavity, is rare, but can be fatal. It occurs most commonly in children under 3 years of age. It is important to remember that it is rarely accompanied by abdominal wall bruising.[68] The liver is the commonest solid organ to be injured with tears or rupture, and the duodenum is often involved. The child may present with shock/severe abdominal pain or sepsis. There may be evidence of bowel rupture, and in a number of cases co-existent head injury may be present. Investigations should include liver enzymes, amylase and full blod count (FBC). CT scanning is the most sensitive investigation to define details of injury. Other visceral injuries include pharyngeal, esophageal or cardiac rupture.

FABRICATED AND INDUCED ILLNESS

The terminology, fabricated or induced illness (FII) has replaced 'Munchausen syndrome by proxy'. The diagnosis refers to a form of abuse where the carer presents the child to the doctor with a false story of illness with or without fabricated or induced physical signs. The condition is rare and the estimated annual incidence in the UK is 0.5 per 100 000 children under 16 years of age and for children under 1 year 2.8 per 100 000. The outcome is serious with an estimated mortality rate of 10% and morbidity of 50%.[69,70]

The clinical picture may be induced by poisoning, smothering, simulation of clinical signs or interference with medical records. The perpetrator is generally the mother who is motivated by attention-seeking behavior and a form of satisfaction gained by assuming the sick role through their child. Many of the children have atypical presentations of illness which fail to resolve and they are often subjected to prolonged medical investigations which compound the attention seeking and increase the suffering.

The condition occurs mostly in young children and making the diagnosis is challenging and time consuming, and often involves an experienced pediatrician who can spot idiosyncratic issues. Factors that should alert the clinician to the condition include:

- signs that only occur in the presence of the perpetrator and disappear in their absence;
- the illness may have an unpredictable pattern and fail to respond to conventional treatment;
- the child may be seen by multiple specialists and receive many repeat investigations;
- there may be a history of unexplained death in siblings.

The diagnostic approach involves confirming symptoms and patterns of illness with other family members and the primary care team and making a detailed chronological history of events. All possible clinical causes of symptoms and signs must be considered and excluded. A trial period of observation away from the suspected perpetrator may give valuable information.

At the point in the process when the balance of probability suggests FII, the risks to the child must be considered. If the child is at risk of immediate, significant harm, social services and the police must be informed. In other cases where it is important to collect the evidence to support the diagnosis the clinician should work with the multi-agency strategy group to plan the investigation and communication strategy with parents. Careful consideration must be given to information sharing with parents or carers and should be avoided if it is likely to put the child at increased risk of harm; adequate plans must be in place for protection of the child before doing so.

Smothering is recognized as a form of child abuse and may present as alleged recurrent apneic or cyanotic attacks, recurrent seizures, an acute life-threatening event or a child who has died. This form of abuse generally occurs in infants under the age of a year. It is rare but life threatening. External signs may include facial petechiae, particularly around the eyes and conjunctiva or nasal bleeding; equally there may be none. Evidence of metabolic acidosis, hypocalcemia transient coagulation abnormalities, lymphocytosis or encephalopathic features on EEG may confirm a significant smothering event.

When this form of abuse is suspected as part of a fabricated or induced illness profile, covert video surveillance of child and carer may help to confirm or exclude the diagnosis.[71] This investigation is rarely used in current practice and has caused significant controversy in terms of potential invasion of civil liberties. In the UK this investigation must be sanctioned by senior health service management and the ultimate decision rests with the chief constable of the local police force.[70] The investigation must be conducted according to the Regulation of Investigatory Powers Act 2000, the main purpose of which is to ensure that investigatory powers are used in accordance with human rights.[72]

POISONING

Non-accidental poisoning can be seen in FII but not exclusively. It has a different profile to accidental poisoning, which is frequently seen in toddlers and preschool children. In the latter, the history is generally of a child that has been found to have ingested tablets or a domestic product. There may be evidence of an opened container and the accompanying adult can recount where the poison was kept and how the child could have accessed it. The carer will seek medical advice appropriately. The child rarely ingests much of the agent and is therefore generally asymptomatic with the exception of caustic agents, which may cause superficial oral and facial burns. Accidental poisoning is unusual in children under the age of 12 months who do not have the necessary levels of independent mobility or manual dexterity to access the poison. Deliberate self-abuse with large quantities of medication is seen in the adolescent age group.

In contrast deliberate poisoning often presents when a child has unusual symptoms and poisoning is diagnosed on clinical evaluation. The child may present acutely or with chronic indolent symptoms. Proposed explanations of accidental ingestion may be presented only when it is evident that significant quantities of drugs have been ingested and there are inconsistencies in the story given.

The commonest poisons used in intentional poisoning include prescribed medication for a family member, particularly anticonvulsants, tranquilizers, analgesics or antidepressants. Salt, iron, laxative, emetics, insulin and water poisoning are also reported. Motivations for poisoning include punitive acts, fabrication of illness or when children are included in the drug abusing activities of the parents. If poisoning is considered the clinician should identify possible agents from family prescription history and symptomatology and consult with the toxicology laboratory as to which investigatory samples are appropriate. If ingestion of a poison is confirmed, careful consultation with parents is required. There may be explanations other than intentional poisoning that explain findings. These include misguided attempts by carers to treat childhood ailments, incorrect dosage regimens or the use of alternative therapies.[69]

CHILD SEXUAL ABUSE

'Sexual abuse involves forcing or enticing a child or young person to take part in sexual activities, including prostitution whether or not the child is aware of what is happening. The activities may involve physical contact, including penetrative (e.g. rape, buggery or oral sex) or nonpenetrative acts. They may include noncontact activities, such as involving children in looking at, or in the production of, pornographic material or watching, sexual activities, or encouraging children to behave in sexually inappropriate ways'.[73]

These children may be of any age, sex or social background. The most common referrals however are girls who disclose the abuse to a trusted friend or adult. Disclosures are frequently historical and refer to ongoing abuse over a period of time. Victims may have been sworn to secrecy or threatened with reprisals and are therefore reluctant to disclose. They may only become aware that their experiences are abusive after sexual health education in the school setting. False allegations do occur but are rare and raise concerns as to whether the sexual awareness of the child is age appropriate.

The abusers are usually known to the child and are commonly male members of the household, however female abusers are recognized and female carers can be complicit in the abuse when they know what is going on but avoid intervening or protecting the child.

Sexual abuse may be associated with inappropriate sexualized behavior or sexual knowledge with respect to the child's age. Secondary effects include emotional and behavioral problems, enuresis, vaginal discharge, bleeding, or irritation, encopresis and rectal bleeding. These presentations may elicit concerns about sexual abuse, especially when associated with other worrying features, but each is associated with other clinical conditions so careful evaluation is essential.

ASSESSMENT AND INVESTIGATION OF SUSPECTED CHILD SEXUAL ABUSE

The objectives of the child protection clinical assessment are: to identify conditions that require treatment, to identify any injuries or forensic signs that support the allegations, to reassure and address the concerns of the child and family and to offer counseling or future support when needed.

Any history of sexual abuse should be taken sensitively and in consultation with the agencies involved. The clinician should be fully informed of any disclosure made to the police or social worker and consider whether it is appropriate for the child or carer to repeat a description of events, which can be extremely emotive. Repetition causes upset and potential contamination of forensic evidence that may be used in the child protection process or court. However the clinician must ensure that they have the full picture on which to base their clinical evaluation.

When the sexual abuse arises from physical contact, genital, anal or oral abuse may be involved. An examination therefore needs to be thorough and appropriate in the context of the allegation made. It is unlikely that children who have been fondled will sustain genital injury however those who have suffered penetrative abuse may have clinical signs especially if they are examined soon after the abusive event. The examination should be an integral part of a full pediatric examination to exclude other health needs and associated injury or infection. Such an assessment needs to be performed by a senior child health practitioner with expertise in the field.

Current pediatric assessment recommends a minimally invasive examination using a colposcope and providing video or photo-documentation. Small swabs are taken for sexually transmitted disease and forensic sampling. The nature and purpose of the examination and potential use of information for evidential or clinical teaching purposes must be clearly explained to the attending parent and child and detailed informed consent should be sought.

Examination should be undertaken as soon as possible after disclosure, especially if the disclosure is acute when it is more likely that signs or forensic evidence of abuse may be detected. The examination should be carefully planned with the appropriate personnel in place. Repeated examination should be avoided as far as possible but may be necessary to ensure healing or to firmly exclude infection. Forensic medical examinations are best conducted jointly between a pediatrician and trained forensic medical examiner.

Microbiology investigations after alleged penetrative sexual abuse include appropriate genital and anal swabs for *Chlamydia*, gonorrhea, and *Trichomonas vaginalis*. Serology for syphilis, herpes simplex types 1 or 2, hepatitis or human immunodeficiency virus (HIV) must be duly considered and biopsy of any anogenital warts.[74] Pregnancy should be excluded in the post pubertal female. Any evident infection must be managed appropriately and emergency contraception prescribed when there are risks of pregnancy.

Examination findings rarely provide diagnostic evidence of abuse and there are frequently no signs of injury when a child is examined, especially when this takes place some time after the most recent abusive episode. The examiner needs to be aware of the normal anatomical variants of the hymen and how it changes with puberty before they can distinguish abnormality.[75]

Findings that strongly support child sexual abuse (CSA) are semen or DNA from the alleged perpetrator on or within the genitalia or anus or pregnancy in the victim. These findings reach diagnostic significance in the pre-pubertal child who cannot be considered to have given informed consent. In the adolescent, although sexual intercourse is illegal, consensual sexual activity is now more commonly seen within relationships. Levels of force, coercion and consent need to be considered as part of the final diagnosis.

Acute genital or anal abrasions, lacerations, bleeding or bruising seen soon after an acute episode of vaginal penetration, support the diagnosis of CSA. Plausible explanations however may include an accidental straddle injury where there may be injury to the more external genital structures.

Supportive signs of previous penetrative sexual abuse include healed hymeneal lacerations through the entire hymeneal rim, often extending into the vagina (variously described in the literature as complete transections or deep clefts of the hymen). These are commonly located in the posterior part of the hymen. The significance of thinning of the hymeneal margins or partial clefts is less clear.

The diameter of the hymen is not currently thought to be relevant and may vary considerably according to the age of the child, position of examination, level of relaxation or whether the child is anesthetized.

Vaginal discharge should be swabbed for bacteriology. Nonspecific discharge is common in prepubertal girls but confirmed sexually transmitted infection (STI) is supportive of CSA, especially when it can be shown to be present in the perpetrator. It is important to exclude and treat these infections to prevent long-term morbidity.

All symptoms and signs need to be carefully considered in the context of the history and presentation of the child. The timing of onset of the symptoms may be of relevance and note should be taken of any previous examination findings that may have changed.

Labial fusion is seen in girls who have not been sexually abused as are urethral prolapse, lichen sclerosus, vaginal/perianal *Streptococcus*, seborrhea/eczema, perianal swelling, erythema, tenderness and prolapse, although they can coexist with CSA.

Boys may be sexually abused and frequently suffer from anal abuse. However traumatic injury to the male genitalia should also be carefully excluded. Signs of anal abuse seen when the child is examined soon after the abuse includes anal fissures that may extend to the perianal region, perianal swelling, erythema and sometimes venous pooling. In cases examined some time after the event anal scars and tags may be seen in up to one third of cases. In addition, reflex anal dilatation and venous congestion are reported. Children may have no abnormal signs or a combination of those listed earlier. When these physical signs are seen in association with a disclosure of anal abuse, they support the child's statement. However these signs may also occur variously in constipation, inflammatory bowel disease etc. and must be assessed in the full clinical context of the child's presentation signs and symptomatology.[76]

Sexual abuse from exploitation, witnessing sexual acts and pedophilia perpetrated over the internet opens up newer and complex risks to children. The consequences include psychological damage, risk of stalking, child trafficking and trading in pedophilic images. Challenges to prevention, diagnosis and management are vast. A recent international criminal investigation, 'Operation Orr' exposed a pedophilic pornographic website with over 75 000 paying subscribers worldwide.

EMOTIONAL ABUSE

Emotional abuse is defined as the persistent emotional ill-treatment of a child such as to cause severe and persistent adverse effects on the child's emotional development. It may involve conveying to children that they are worthless or unloved, inadequate, or valued only insofar as they meet the needs of another person. It may feature age or developmentally inappropriate expectations being imposed on children. These may include interactions that are beyond the child's developmental capability, as well as overprotection and limitation of exploration and learning or preventing the child participating in normal social interaction. It may involve seeing or hearing the ill treatment of another, causing children to feel frightened or in danger, or the exploitation or corruption of children. Some level of emotional abuse is involved in all types of ill-treatment of a child, though it may occur alone.[12]

Emotional maltreatment is increasingly recognized in conjunction with other forms of abuse. Emotional abuse is not an event but arises out of the relationship between carer and child. The earliest years of a child's life are the most important in terms of emotional stability and nurturing to secure their emotional wellbeing for the future. Attachment theory proposes that attachment is essential to human survival and relies upon infants emitting signals to the carer that elicit responses and in turn draws the child–carer pair together and secures 'attachment.' In maltreatment, carers who do not respond or respond inappropriately to the child are likely to produce children who are insecure or anxious in their attachments to them.[77] The consequences of this type of abuse in early years can be longstanding.

Emotional abuse can be confirmed in the observation of the interaction between carer and child or reflected in a carer's persistent criticism or negativity about the child. The victim may be singled out from siblings and exposed to an emotionally damaging relationship with one or both parents or a teacher or other adult. A child may be emotionally damaged by: omission, a failure to provide consistent care-giving and encouragement to foster stability; or commission, deliberate verbal harassment, ridicule, shame and threatening their emotional well-being.

An emotionally abusive relationship is pervasive and results in actual harm to the child. Five categories of emotional ill treatment are recognized. These may be mixed and occur to a varying degree:[78]

1. *Lack of interaction*: for one reason or another, carers fail to interact with their children. They may be preoccupied with their own needs through work, chronic or mental illness or substance abuse. They may also fail to respond to the child's overtures for attention.
2. *Criticism and rejection*: the carers may constantly criticize, scapegoat or ridicule the child and reject their need for affection, reassurance or conversation.
3. *Unrealistic expectations*: where the child is expected to take on roles, responsibilities or behaviors that exceed their developmental age or are overprotected and excluded from peer interaction.
4. *Projected roles*: the child is used as a vehicle to fight adult battles or a pawn in marital strife, to fulfill adult ambitions or to take on a sick role in fabricated or induced illness.
5. *Socialization*: where the child is encouraged to partake in criminal or anti-social activities or prevented from peer group social interaction or school attendance.

Parental risk factors include mental health problems, domestic violence and substance abuse.

Diagnosis requires joint assessment with the clinical psychologist and/or child and adolescent mental health team. Signs in the child include manifestations of poor functioning in terms of emotional stability, behavior, social skills, educational achievement as well as physical manifestations. The young emotionally damaged child may have an abnormal reaction to parental separation either expressed by indifference or an extreme response. They may present as unhappy children with a flat affect, depressed, frightened, anxious or withdrawn. Young children may assume habitual rocking or self-soothing behavior whilst those in the older age group may self-harm and display low self-esteem. Behavioral manifestations include attention seeking for favorable or unfavorable response, oppositional defiance, antisocial or delinquent behavior. Developmental consequences include poor school achievement or developmental delay in infants and toddlers and secondary physical symptoms include poor growth, non-organic abdominal pain or headache, encopresis or secondary enuresis. Long-term emotional–behavioral consequences include poor social relationships with peers, isolation or aggression.

NEGLECT

'Neglect is the persistent failure to meet a child's basic physical and/or psychological needs, likely to result in the serious impairment of the child's health or development. Neglect may occur during pregnancy as a result of maternal substance abuse. It may involve a parent or carer failing to provide adequate food, clothing, shelter including exclusion from home or abandonment; failing to protect a child from physical harm or danger; failure to ensure adequate supervision including the use of inadequate care-takers; or failure to ensure access to appropriate medical care or treatment. It may also include neglect of, or unresponsiveness to, a child's basic emotional needs.[73]

The definition is broad and the clinical presentation may include physical symptoms, developmental delay, illness and disease or psychological damage. A pediatrician needs to be aware of the causative events that lead to the child's clinical presentation before suspecting neglect.

Neglect may be intentional, where carers put their needs above those of the children or when their children are a low priority. In these circumstances emotional abuse is frequently associated. Factors that contribute may include domestic violence, substance abuse, mental health issues and parents who were themselves neglected. However in many cases it is seen in families where carers are suffering from health issues, mental stresses or have learning difficulties or disabilities and are unable to respond appropriately to the child's needs. The risks to the child in these circumstances may be transient and resolve with parental support.

Failure to meet a child's basic physical or psychological needs may include failure of carers to provide adequate nutrition which may result in a child with faltering growth or nutritional deficiencies. The provision of inappropriate food may result in dental caries and obesity from sugary drinks or a persistent diet of junk food. Faltering growth may arise from diets high in fiber and low in calorific content where parents impose their own weight-watching dietary practices on the child inappropriately. The levels of knowledge of carers need to be assessed in these circumstances and a judgment of omission versus commission should be made. In cases of genuine ignorance or where there is transient parental inadequacy, the situation often resolves with simple intervention. Diagnosis often relies upon a short period of admission when organic causes of weight loss can be excluded and weight gain witnessed once the child is returned to a normal diet.

Failing to meet a child's psychological needs includes failure to provide the emotional support that the child needs or to provide social interaction. This form of neglect results in many of the symptoms of emotional abuse, speech and language impairment and delay in the development of social skills.

Inadequate supervision includes the failure to protect a child from physical hazards, inappropriate contact with unsuitable people, leaving children with inappropriate carers or on their own. Failure to supervise can result in frequent injuries and visits to Accident and Emergency departments. The injuries often have the same profile as accidental injuries but are numerous and the antecedent events reflect the neglectful attention to prevention, the provision of a safe environment and appropriate adult supervision.

Medical neglect can arise when carers fail to take their children for medical assessment when they are unwell or to provide essential care or treatment. This problem may manifest as poor vaccination uptake, poor control of a chronic medical condition that is dependent upon medication or late presentation with illness. A judgment must be made as to when the threshold of significant harm has been breached and what factors influenced the carer's decisions to determine the degree of negligence involved.

Neglect may occur in any social setting but is more common in the socially deprived. It is important to distinguish failure to provide for a child through poverty, learning impairment or ignorance from a pervasive pattern of negligent parenting. The two scenarios require a different interventional approach.

EFFECTS OF DOMESTIC VIOLENCE ON CHILDREN

Domestic violence describes an ongoing abusive relationship between partners in an intimate relationship, whether the violence is physical, sexual, emotional or financial. Domestic violence and child abuse often co-exist.[79] Most domestic violence is perpetrated by men against women, and members of their family. In up to 75% of cases, children witness this violence.[80] The children themselves may develop a wide range of consequences, including depression, aggression, anxiety, post-traumatic stress disorder and behavioral problems. Sadly over the long term there is evidence for intergenerational transmission of violence. This is believed to occur as a consequence of sex-role stereotypes and the acceptance of violence against women.[81] Clearly the women who are victims of ongoing domestic abuse may themselves be unable to parent effectively or protect their children. It is important therefore to explore the possibility of domestic violence in history taking, while considering confidentiality. If the clinician is made aware of such domestic violence, they must ensure the welfare of the child first and foremost and offer support to the victim, including practical information regarding refuges, Women's Aid etc., and contribute to inter-agency processes.

ADULT MENTAL HEALTH, SUBSTANCE ABUSE AND CHILD PROTECTION

Parental mental health problems can have a significant bearing on children's welfare. 31% of children on the child protection register for emotional abuse have parents with mental health problems.[82] Adults have a one in four lifetime chance of experiencing mental health problems so the potential for problems in children is significant. Clearly not all children whose parents experience mental health problems will be affected by it, but it is important to be aware of this as a risk factor and include relevant questions in history taking. Clearly if the parent/carer is severely incapacitated by their own health problems, the child may end up as 'carer', placing a significant burden on them. It is important that the adult and children's services work together, to ensure recognition of the risks and problems experienced by parents and children.

Parental dependence on alcohol or drugs can severely impair their ability to parent effectively. This may compromise a child's health, development, and welfare at all stages from conception onwards. The dependence on alcohol or other drugs becomes a central issue when procuring such substances becomes the parents' prime objective, rendering their care of their child secondary. The influence on the child may include neglect, financial difficulties as a result of supporting their addiction, a failure on the part of the parent to recognize or place the child's need first, poor attendance at school, or recurrent episodes of injuries or abuse. It is vital that the pediatrician ensures that the child's needs are maintained as paramount and that there is effective collaboration with the other services including the drug and alcohol services.

PROTECTING THE CHILD

The UN Convention on the Rights of the Child sets out the provisions that must be realized for children worldwide to develop their full potential free from hunger, want, neglect and abuse. The Convention was developed in 1989 and recognizes the fundamental rights of children to protection from economic exploitation, harmful work, sexual exploitation and abuse, physical or mental violence. Despite near universal signature or ratification by world states, UNICEF recognizes the massive violation of children's rights in terms of their unequal access to education and legal systems; their levels of poverty, homelessness, abuse, neglect and preventable disease; their exposure and involvement in armed conflict, child trafficking, and their exploitation at every level. UNICEF has established child protection programs that include international advocacy through the mechanism of human rights, the inclusion of child protection issues in national development plans, law and community-based approaches.

On an individual level, successful child protection relies upon adequate resources and good lines of communication between the agencies and individuals involved. Identifying a suspicious bruise on an infant's face and recognizing that it may be the hallmark of a pervasively abusive household may provide the only chance for that child to be protected from an abusive future. Clinicians have an obligation to be vigilant and investigate the possibility of child abuse when suspected. Local authorities and associated agencies have an obligation to support and work with families to protect children from abuse and to contribute to the wider prevention agenda.

REFERENCES

1. Radbill SX 1987. Children in a world of violence: a history of child abuse. In: Helfer RE, Kempe RS, eds. The Battered Child, 4th edn. London: University of Chicago Press.
2. Tardieu A. Etude medico-legale sur les services et mauvais traitements exercés sur des enfants. Ann Hyg Pub Med Leg 1860; 13:361–398.
3. Caffey J. Multiple fractures in the long bones of infants suffering from chronic subdural haematoma. Am J Roentgenol 1946; 56:162–173.
4. Silverman F. The roentgen manifestations of unrecognised skeletal trauma. Am J Roentgenol 1953; 69:413–426.
5. Kempe J, Silverman FN, Steele BF, et al. The battered child syndrome. J Am Med Assoc 1962; 181:17–24.
6. Cawson et al. Child maltreatment in the United Kingdom: a study of the prevalence of child abuse and neglect. London: NSPCC; 2000.
7. Sullivan PM, Knutson JF. Maltreatment and disabilities: A population based epidemiological study. Child Abuse and Neglect 2000; 24:1275–1288.
8. Birth and death registration data: Office for National Statistics, General Register Office for Scotland, Northern Ireland Statistics and Research Agency, Central Statistics Office Ireland. UK 2002-based national population projections, 2004 to 2051: Government Actuary's Department.
9. www.nspcc.org.UK./whatwedo/aboutthenspcc/ keyfactandfigures/keyfacts-wda33645.html
10. Ranton B, Payne H, Rolfe K, et al. Do we protect abused babies from further abuse? A cohort study. Arch Dis Child 2004; 89:845–846.

11. Hindley N, Ramchandani PG, Jones DPH. Risk factors for the recurrence of maltreatment: a systematic review. Arch Dis Child 2006; 91:744–752.
12. H M Government 2006 Working Together http://www.everychildmatters.gov.uk/_files/AE53C8 F9D7AEB1B23E403514A6C1B17D.pdf.
13. DoH et al 2000 http://www.dh.gov.uk/ assetRoot/04/01/44/30/04014430.pdf.
14. Smith SM, Hanson R. 134 battered children: A medical and psychological study. BMJ 1974; 3:666–670.
15. Sugar NH, Taylor JA, Feldman KW. Bruises in infants and toddlers; those who don't cruise rarely bruise. Puget Sound Pediatric Research Network. Arch Paediatr Adolesc Med 1999; 153:399–403.
16. Maguire S, Mann MK, Sibert J, et al. Are there patterns of bruising in childhood which are diagnostic or suggestive of abuse? Arch Dis Child 2005; 90:182–186.
17. Carpenter RF. The prevalence and distribution of bruising in babies. Arch Dis Child 1999; 80:363–366.
18. Dunstan FD, Guildea ZE, Kontos K, et al. A scoring system for bruise patterns: a tool for identifying abuse. Arch Dis Child 2002; 86:330–333.
19. Brinkmann B, Püschel K, Mätzsch T. Forensic dermatological aspects of the battered child syndrome. Aktuelle Dermatologie 1979; 5:217–232.
20. Sussman SJ. Skin manifestations of the battered-child syndrome. J Paediatr 1968; 72:99–101.
21. Atwal GS, Rutty GN, Carter N, et al. Bruising in non-accidental head injured children; a retrospective study of the prevalence, distribution and pathological associations in 24 cases. Forensic Sci Int 1998; 96:215–230.
22. Nayak K, Spencer N, Shenoy M, et al. How useful is the presence of petechiae in distinguishing non-accidental from accidental injury? Child Abuse Negl 2006; 30:549–555.
23. Maguire S, Mann MK, Sibert J, et al. Can you age bruises accurately in children? Arch Dis Child 2005; 90:187–189.
24. Munang LA, Leonard PA, Mok J. Lack of agreement on colour description between clinicians examining childhood bruising. J Clin Forensic Med 2002; 9:171–174.
25. Hughes VK, Ellis PS, Burt T, et al. The practical application of reflectance spectrophotometry for the demonstration of haemoglobin and its degradation in bruises. J Clin Pathol 2004; 57:355–359.
26. Worlock P, Stower M, Barbor P. Patterns of fractures in accidental and non-accidental injury in children: a comparative study. Br Med J 1986; 293:100–102.
27. Lyons R, Delahunty AM, Kraus D, et al. Children's fractures: a population based study. Injury prevention. J Int Soc Child Adolescent Injury Prevention 1999; 5:129–132.
28. www.core-info.cf.ac.uk.
29. Barsness KA, Cha ES, Bensard DD, et al. The positive predictive value of rib fractures as an indicator of non-accidental trauma in children. J Trauma-Injury Infection Critical Care 2003; 54:1107–1110.
30. Barsness KA, Cadzow SP, Armstrong KL. Rib fractures in infants: Red Alert! The clinical features, investigations and child protection outcomes. J Paediatr Child Health 2003; 36:322–326.
31. Does cardiopulmonary resuscitation cause rib fractures in children? A systematic review. Child Abuse Negl 2006; 30:739.
32. Schwend RM, Werth C, Johnston A. Femur shaft fractures in toddlers and young children: Rarely from child abuse. J Pediatr Orthopaed 2000; 20:475–484.

33. Farnsworth CL, Silva PD, Mubarak SJ. Etiology of supracondylar humerus fractures. J Pediatr Orthopaed 1998; 18:38–42.

34. Kleinman PK, Marks SC Jr, Richmond JM, et al. Inflicted skeletal injury: A postmortem radiologic-histopathologic study in 31 infants. Am J Roentgenol 1995; 165:647–650.

35. Leventhal JM, Thomas SA, Rosenfield NS, et al. Fractures in young children. Distinguishing child abuse from unintentional injuries. Am J Dis Children 1993; 147:87–92.

36. Meservy CJ, Towbin R, McLaurin RL, et al. Radiographic characteristics of skull fractures resulting from child abuse. Am J Roentgenol 1987; 149:173–175.

37. Hobbs CJ. Skull fracture and the diagnosis of abuse. Arch Dis Child 1984; 59:246–252.

38. Merten DF, Radlowski MA, Leonidas JC. The abused child: A radiological reappraisal. Radiology 1983; 146:377–381.

39. Belfer RA, Klein BL, Orr L. Use of the skeletal survey in the evaluation of child maltreatment. Am J Emergency Med 2001; 19:122–124. Br Paediatr Radiol Society, NAI standard for skeletal surveys http://www.bspr.org.uk/.

40. Kemp A. Which radiological investigations should be performed to identify fractures in suspected child abuse? Clin Radiol 2006; 61:723.

41. Prosser I, Maguire S, Harrison S, et al. How old is this fracture? Radiological dating of fractures in children: a systematic review. Am J Roentgenol 2005; 184:1282–1286.

42. Ayoub C, Pfeifer D. Burns as a manifestation of child abuse and neglect. Am J Dis Child 1979; 133:910–914.

43. Hight DW, Bakalar HR, Lloyd JR. Inflicted burns in children: Recognition and treatment. J Am Med Assoc 1979; 242:517–520.

44. Phillips PS, Pickrell E, Morse TS. Intentional burning: a severe form of child abuse. J Am Coll Emergency Physicians 1974; 3:388–390.

45. Daria S, Sugar NF, Feldman KW, et al. Into hot water head first: Distribution of intentional and unintentional immersion burns. Pediatr Emerg Care 2004; 20:302–310.

46. Hobbs CJ. When are burns not accidental? Arch Dis Child 1986; 61:357–361.

47. Ofodile F, Norris J, Garnes A. Burns and child abuse. East African Med J 1979; 56:26–29.

48. Titus MO, Baxter AL, Starling SP. Accidental scald burns in sinks. Pediatrics 2003; 111:e191–e194.

49. Brinkmann B, Banaschak S. Verbrühungen bei einem Kleinkind: Unfall oder Kindesmißhandlung? Monatsschrift für Kinderheilkunde 1998.

50. Yeoh C, Nixon JW, Dickson W, et al. Patterns of scald injuries. Arch Dis Child 1994; 71:156–158.

51. Purdue GF, Hunt JL, Prescott PR. Child abuse by burning – an index of suspicion. J Trauma 1988; 28:221–224.

52. Hobbs CJ, Wynne JM. The sexually abused battered child. Arch Dis Childhood 1990; 65:423–427.

53. Johnson CF. Symbolic scarring and tattooing: Unusual manifestations of child abuse. Clinical Pediatrics 1994; 33:46–49.

54. Winek CL, Wahba WW, Huston RM. Chemical burn from alkaline batteries – a case report. Forensic Sci Int 1999; 100:101–104.

55. Hill PF, Pickford M, Parkhouse N. Phytophotodermatitis mimicking child abuse. J Roy Soc Med 1997; 90:560–561.

56. Asnes RS, Wisotsky DH. Cupping lesions simulating child abuse. J Pediatr 1981; 99:267–268.

57. Feldman KW. Pseudoabusive burns in Asian refugees. Am J Dis Child 1984; 138:768–769.

58. Tate RJ. Facial injuries associated with the battered child syndrome. Br J Oral Surg 1971; 9:41–45.

59. Price EA, Rush LR, Perper JA, et al. Cardiopulmonary resuscitation-related injuries and homicidal blunt trauma in children. Am J Forensic Med Pathol 2000; 21:307–310.

60. Wagner GN. Bitemark identification in child abuse cases. Pediatr Dentistry 1986; 8:96–100.

61. Kemp A, Maguire SA, Sibert J, et al. Can we identify abusive bites on children? Arch Dis Child 2006; 91:951.

62. BAFO. British Association of Forensic Odontology. Guidelines Bitemark Methodology 2001. http://www. Forensicdentistryonline.org/forensicpages/bitemarkguide. html.

63. Jayawant S, Rawlinson A, Gibbon F, et al. Subdural haemorrhages in infants: population based study. BMJ 1998; 317:1558–1561.

64. Minns RA, Busuttil A. Patterns of presentation of the shaken baby syndrome. BMJ 2004; 328:766.

65. Jaspan T, Griffiths P, McConachie N, et al. Neuroimaging for non-accidental head injury in childhood: a proposed protocol. Clin Radiology 2003; 58:44–53.

66. Saulsbury FT, Alford BA. Intracranial bleeding from child abuse: The value of skull radiographs. Pediatr Radiol 1982; 12:175–178.

67. Morris AAM, Hoffman GF, Naughten ER, et al. Glutaric aciduria and suspected child abuse. Arch Dis Child 1999; 80:404–405.

68. Barnes PM, Norton CM, Dunstan FD, et al. Abdominal injury due to child abuse. Lancet 2005; 366:234–235.

69. McClure RJ, Davies PM, Meadows S, et al. Epidemiology of Munchausen syndrome by proxy, non-accidental poisoning and non-accidental suffocation. Arch Dis Child 1996; 75:57–61.

70. Department of Health. Safeguarding children in whom illness is fabricated or induced. London: HMSO; 2002.

71. Hall DE, Eubanks L, Meyyazhagan S, et al. Evaluation of covert video surveillance in the diagnosis of Munchausen syndrome by proxy: lessons learnt from 41 cases. Paediatrics 2000; 105:1305–1312.

72. Foreman D. Detecting fabricated or induced illness in children. BMJ 2005; 331:978–979.

73. HM Government. 2006.

74. Thomas A, Forster G, Robinson A, et al. Clinical Effectiveness Group Association of Genitourinary Medicine; Medical Society for the Study of Veneareal Diseases. National Guideline for the Management of Suspected Sexually Transmitted Infections in Children and Young People. Arch Dis Child 2003; 88:303–311.

75. Heger A, Emans SJ, Muram D. Evaluation of the Sexually Abused Child. A Medical Textbook and Photographic Atlas. 2nd edn. Oxford: Oxford University Press; 2001.

76. Bruni M. Anal findings in sexual abuse of children (a descriptive study). J Forensic Sci 2003; 48:1343–1346.

77. Ainsworth MS. The personal origins of attachment theory. An interview with Mary Salter Ainsworth. Interview by Peter Rudnytsky. Psychoanal Study Child 1997; 52:386–405.

78. Glaser D. Emotional abuse and neglect (psychological maltreatment): a conceptual frame work. Child Abuse Negl 2002; 26:697–714.

79. Hughes H, Parkinson D, Vargo M. Witnessing spouse abuse and experiencing physical abuse: a 'double whammy'? J Family Violence 1989; 4:197–209.

80. NCH Action for Children 1994. The Hidden Victims: Children and domestic violence. London: NCH; 1994.

81. Geffner R, Loring MT. The effects of intimate partner violence on children: Part 2. J Emotional Abuse 2003; 3:155–157.

82. Child Protection Companion, 2006, RCPCH.

6

Accidents, poisoning and SIDS

*Ronan Lyons, John M Goldsmid, Maurice A Kibel,
Alan E Mills, Peter J Fleming, Peter Blair*

POISONING IN CHILDHOOD

Poisoning in children may be accidental, non-accidental, and iatrogenic or, in older children, deliberate.

ACCIDENTAL CHILD POISONING
Epidemiology

Accidental poisoning is predominantly seen in children under the age of 5 years but older children may be involved if they are developmentally delayed. The peak age is between 1 and 4 years. More boys than girls take poisons accidentally. Some children die from poisoning each year, but the number of deaths has fallen over recent years, probably because of better treatment and because of the child-resistant container (CRC) regulations. There are also less tricyclic antidepressants prescribed. Though the numbers of deaths are few, many more children are admitted to hospital for treatment and observation and even more present to hospital Accident and Emergency (A & E) departments. Many of these are sent home directly because they have taken relatively nontoxic substances.

Substances taken

Children may take a variety of substances accidentally. These are conveniently divided into medicines (prescribed and nonprescribed), household products and plants. The majority of children who take poisons do not have serious symptoms. Medicines may be of low toxicity, e.g. the oral contraceptive pill or antibiotics; intermediate toxicity, which may cause symptoms in young children; or potential high toxicity. Many of the household products children take may be relatively nontoxic,

but a few such as caustic soda, soldering flux and paint stripper may cause serious harm. The commonest household product that children take is white spirit and turpentine substitute. About 10% of these children have patchy chest X-ray changes. In developing countries paraffin (kerosene) poisoning is a particular problem as it is used as a cooking fuel and is often kept in open containers. These incidents are common in poor social circumstances and in summer and are probably largely related to thirst. Kerosene may cause serious aspiration pneumonitis and death.

A child may eat a poisonous plant accidentally or a group may sample a plant, such as laburnum, together. Most plants are relatively nontoxic, e.g. cotoneaster, rowan or sweet pea. However, some such as arum lily, deadly nightshade or yew can cause serious symptoms.

Etiology

Perhaps surprisingly, the availability of poisons does not appear to be a major factor in accidental child poisoning. There is evidence that family psychosocial stress and behavioral problems, such as hyperactivity, predispose towards child poisoning[1] and these family and personality findings have importance for the prevention of child poisoning.

Preventing child poisoning
Education

A campaign in Birmingham, UK, to publicize accidental child poisoning and to encourage the return of medicines concluded that 'publicity, storage and destruction of unwanted medicines have little preventive value'. A New Zealand study evaluated placing 'Mr Yuk' stickers on poisons together with a campaign to prevent child poisoning. No reduction in poisoning admissions was found. The link between accidental child poisoning and family psychosocial stress and hyperactivity make it unlikely on theoretical grounds that education will be effective. Families under stress will be unlikely to remember safety propaganda.

Child-resistant containers

CRCs were first suggested in 1959 by Dr Jay Arena in Durham, North Carolina. These containers were evaluated in a community in the US by Scherz[2] and found to be successful. They were then introduced into the US for aspirin preparations, with successful results. Following this work in the US, child-resistant closures were introduced by regulation in 1976 in the UK for junior aspirin and paracetamol preparations. This resulted in a fall in admissions of children under 5 years with salicylate poisoning.[3] In 1978 CRCs were introduced by regulation for adult aspirin and paracetamol tablets. Child-resistant containers or packaging are now a professional requirement by the Royal Pharmaceutical Society and are regulated for a number of household products (e.g. white spirit and turpentine substitute).

Other methods of preventing child poisoning

Lockable medicine cupboards have been suggested for the prevention of child poisoning. On theoretical grounds they are unlikely to be effective as parents under stress are less likely to remember to put their medicines away or lock the cabinets. Making household products unpalatable with bitter chemical agents (e.g. Bitrex – denatonium bromide)[4] is a possible preventive measure to child poisoning. Serious accidental poisoning might also be prevented by a reduction in the prescribing of toxic drugs. This has been done for barbiturates and tricyclics and might also be done for quinine and vaporizing solutions.

DELIBERATE SELF-POISONING IN OLDER CHILDREN

A number of older children take poisons deliberately. They may take medications as a response to an emotional crisis (mainly adolescent girls) or ingest excess alcohol (predominantly adolescent boys). They form one end of an age spectrum of overdose in adults.

NON-ACCIDENTAL POISONING

The recognition of non-accidental poisoning as an extended syndrome of child abuse was made in 1976. These children are deliberately poisoned by their parents and may present with bizarre or unusual symptoms rather than poisoning directly. A number of medicines or household products may be given to children including salt in feeds to babies. These cases probably form part of the syndrome of factitious illness in childhood.

TREATMENT OF CHILD POISONING
Management of accidental poisoning in childhood
General

The majority of children who present to hospital after accidental poisoning do not have serious symptoms. There are nevertheless a few children who have taken a significant poison and who are potentially ill or are ill. We should clearly like to prevent unnecessary admissions to hospital whilst maintaining safety. A way round this dilemma is to classify the substance the child has taken into one of four categories: low toxicity, uncertain toxicity, intermediate toxicity or potential high toxicity. After classification children can be either sent home, observed in the A & E department or admitted for observation or treatment. **The Poisons Information Center should be contacted if there is any doubt about the toxicity of a substance a child has taken or the treatment that is needed**. A list of some of the poisons commonly taken accidentally by children is shown in Table 6.1.

Older children who have taken poisons deliberately and cases of iatrogenic poisoning and non-accidental poisoning should all be admitted to hospital.

The parents of all children who present with accidental poisoning should be given advice regarding the storage of medicines and household products. The health visitor should be contacted in all cases, remembering that family psychosocial stress is often linked with accidental poisoning in childhood. There may be specific problems, which need medical or social help.

Emptying the stomach

It used to be standard practice to empty the stomach in cases of accidental poisoning in childhood. This has come under review and emesis using ipecacuanha pediatric mixture (ipecac) is now not used.[5] Gastric lavage was largely abandoned some years ago. It may be needed in certain cases, such as iron poisoning, for substances to be instilled into the stomach. The stomach should never be emptied in cases of hydrocarbon ingestion, such as paraffin or white spirit, or with corrosive substances such as caustic soda.

Activated charcoal

Activated charcoal is being increasingly used in the management of childhood poisoning. Activated charcoal absorbs toxic materials in the gut by offering alternative binding sites. Its routine use is limited by its poor acceptance by children. Activated charcoal may not be effective more than 1 h after ingestion.[6] Two preparations are available: Medicoal 5 g sachets and Carbomix 50 g. Activated charcoal has been used for a variety of drugs including aspirin, carbamazepine, digoxin, mefenamic acid, phenobarbital, phenytoin, quinine and theophylline. It is particularly useful in tricyclic antidepressant poisoning.

Accidental poisoning with substances of low toxicity

Children who have taken substances of low toxicity can be allowed home after assessment. Their parents should be given advice regarding storage of medicines and the general practitioner should be contacted. If there is doubt over what substance has been taken, a child should be admitted for observation.

Accidental poisoning where there is uncertainty of toxicity

If there is any doubt about the toxicity of a substance a child may have taken, the Poison Information Center should be contacted day or night:

London – Guy's Hospital   Tel. 0207 407 7600 or 0207 635 9191
Edinburgh – Royal Infirmary   Tel. 0131 536 1000
Cardiff – Llandough Hospital   Tel. 02920 709901
Belfast – Royal Victoria Infirmary   Tel. 01232 240503

Some children arrive in hospital having taken unknown tablets or household products. Often research with the pharmacist will help. If there is doubt the child should be admitted for observation.

Intermediate toxicity

Children who have taken substances of intermediate toxicity accidentally should be observed for a period in hospital (usually up to 6 h) until the practitioner can be confident that significant symptoms are not going to occur. This observation can be undertaken in many cases in an A & E department which has a section for children or for short periods in the pediatric ward or day unit. If there are adverse factors, particularly social factors, children should be admitted to hospital for longer periods.

Accidental poisoning with potentially toxic substances

Children who have taken substances of potential toxicity should be admitted to hospital for observation and treatment.

Treatment of individual poisons

Table 6.1 shows the toxicity of the substances which are most frequently taken accidentally by children under 5.

Deliberate poisoning in older children

Deliberate poisoning in older children should be treated differently from accidental poisoning in younger children. These children form one end of the age spectrum of overdose in adults and such children are more likely to take significant amounts of poison. Substances that

Table 6.1 Guide to toxicity of substances taken in accidental child poisoning

Low toxicity	*Plants*
Medicines	Berberis
Antibiotics (except ciprofloxacin, sulfasalazine and chloramphenicol)	Fuchsia
Antacids	Holly
Calamine	Pyracantha
Oral contraceptives	**Potentially toxic**
Vitamin preparations which do not contain iron	
Zinc oxide creams	*Medicines*
	Benzodiazepines
Household products	Carbamazepine
Chalks and crayons	Codeine-containing cough medicines
Emulsion paints and water paints	Clonidine
Fabric softeners	Digoxin
Plant food and fertilizers	Diphenoxylate (Lomotil)
Silica gel	Hyoscine
Toothpaste	Iron
Wallpaper paste	Mefenamic acid (Ponstan)
Washing powder (except dishwasher powder)	Metoclopramide
	Mianserin (Bolvidon)
Plants	Paracetamol tablets
Begonia	Phenytoin
Cacti	Quinine
Cotoneaster	Salicylates
Cyclamen	Theophyllines
Honeysuckle	Tricyclic antidepressants (including dothiepin and amitriptyline)
Mahonia	
Rowan	*Household products*
Spider plant	Acids
Sweet pea	Alcoholic beverages
Intermediate toxicity	Alkalis
	Bottle-sterilizing tablets
Medicines	Camphor and camphorated oil
Cough medicines (most)	Carbon monoxide
Fluoride	Cetrimide
Ibuprofen	Disk batteries
Laxatives	Essential oils (e.g. real turpentine, pine oil, citronella and eucalyptus)
Lidocaine (lignocaine) gel	Methylene chloride (paint stripper)
Paracetamol elixir	Organochloride insecticides
Salbutamol	Organophosphorus insecticides
	Paradichlorobenzene mothballs
Household products	Paraquat
Alcohol-containing colognes, aftershaves and perfumes	Petroleum distillates (white spirit, paraffin, turpentine substitute)
Bleach	Phenolic compounds
Detergents	Slug pellets (metaldehyde)
Disinfectants (most)	
Nail varnish remover	*Plants*
Paints (oil based)	Arum lily
Pyrethrins	Deadly nightshade
Rat or mouse poison	Laburnum
Talc	Philodendron
Window cleaners	Yew

can be regarded as having intermediate toxicity when taken accidentally should be regarded as potentially toxic when taken deliberately.

Poisoning in older children should be recognized as a serious symptom and an indication of child and family disturbance. Children who deliberately take poisons show more disturbed family relationships than children referred for psychiatric help for other reasons. They have a high level of psychiatric symptoms, especially depression. All children who take poisons deliberately should be admitted to hospital and should be assessed by a child and adolescent psychiatrist. Many will need educational, psychological and social work help as well as psychiatric assessment.

CHRONIC POISONING

Lead poisoning

Lead is a serious poison for children. Its toxic effects are due to its combination with sulfhydryl groups of essential enzymes resulting in disturbances in carbohydrate metabolism, cell membrane transport,

renal tubular absorption and other body processes. The blood level at which toxic effects become evident varies from child to child but in general major symptoms are unlikely if the whole blood lead level is less than 2.5 μmol/L (52 mcg/100 ml). It is probable that behavioral and learning difficulties may result from exposure to only moderately elevated lead levels between 1.4 and 2.9 μmol/L. Low-level fetal lead exposure at less than 1.4 μmol/L may also affect mental development. Children in the UK may be poisoned by sucking or chewing lead paint. Lead from burning batteries, lead shot for fishing and lead from old water pipes are other potential sources. Children from the Indian subcontinent may be poisoned by *surma*, the lead-containing eye make-up used even in young babies.

Clinical features

Children who are poisoned by lead are likely to present with pica (compulsive eating of substances other than food), anorexia, abdominal pain, irritability and failure to thrive. Severe lead poisoning may present with neurological symptoms including drowsiness, convulsions and coma from lead encephalopathy. Lead poisoning may also present as progressive intellectual deterioration.

The diagnosis is made by elevated blood lead levels and anemia with hypochromia and basophilic stippling. There may also be increased bone density with transverse bands at the ends of the long bones on radiological examination.

Treatment

The source of lead should be identified and removed. Chelating agents should be used to form nontoxic lead compounds. In mild cases D-penicillamine should be used orally in two daily doses of 10 mg/kg. In severe cases sodium calcium edetate (EDTA) should be used, 40 mg/kg by i.v. infusion over 1 h twice daily for up to 5 d. Each gram of EDTA should be diluted in 100 ml normal saline. The effectiveness of EDTA can be enhanced by the deep i.m. injection of dimercaprol 2.5 mg/kg 4-hourly for 2 d, 2–4 times on the third day, then 1–2 times daily until recovery.

Mercury poisoning

This once common disorder was called 'pink disease' because of the color of the extremities or 'acrodynia' because of the accompanying pain. It was largely due to the use of mercury-containing teething powders which have now been withdrawn. There was anorexia, loss of weight and hypotonia as well as the characteristic painful red or pink extremities. A differential diagnosis of this condition is the red extremities of neglected children. Treatment of mercury poisoning is by the deep i.m. injection of dimercaprol 5 mg/kg 4-hourly for 2 d, 2.5 mg/kg twice daily for the third day and once daily for the next 10 d.

Chronic boric acid poisoning

Chronic boric acid poisoning was a major problem in the 1940s and 1950s. It was caused by ingestion of boric acid used either as a treatment for nappy rash or as a pacifier. It presented with convulsions, vomiting and diarrhea.

NOTES ON POISONING WITH INDIVIDUAL SUBSTANCES
Intermediate toxicity
Medicines

Cough medicines. Most cough medicines do not cause serious symptoms in the doses available to children. Medicines based on antihistamines may cause drowsiness and anticholinergic effects. Drowsiness will usually not need treatment but if coma occurs resuscitative measures should be used. Medicines based on codeine should be regarded as potentially toxic.

Fluoride. Fluoride has a rapid action but is seldom toxic in the quantities taken by children. Symptoms include vomiting, nausea and abdominal pain.

Ibuprofen. Ibuprofen and other nonsteroidal anti-inflammatory agents only seldom cause symptoms in children. Symptoms may include gastrointestinal irritation, kidney and liver damage. Oral fluids should be encouraged.

Laxatives. Serious symptoms after laxative ingestion are rare. If diarrhea occurs it occurs quickly. Occasionally patients may need i.v. fluids. The child should be observed for serious symptoms for a short time.

Lidocaine (lignocaine) gel. Local anesthetics such as lidocaine are toxic in overdose, causing convulsions and circulatory collapse. Significant amounts of lidocaine gel are seldom ingested accidentally by children.

Paracetamol elixir. Paracetamol elixirs such as Calpol are sweet and sickly in large doses and serious accidental poisoning is very rare. There is insufficient paracetamol in most small bottles of elixir to cause problems. Blood levels should be checked 4 h after the ingestion if more than 150 mg/kg has been taken. Treatment (see potential toxicity section later) is only needed if the serum paracetamol level is above 200 mg/L at 4 h (or in rare delayed cases in children above 50 mg/L at 12 h). In most cases children can be discharged after a period of observation.

Salbutamol. There may be peripheral vasodilatation, muscle tremors and agitation. Serious symptoms are rare although severe hypokalemia and arrhythmias have been seen.

Household products

Alcohol-containing perfumes, cologne and aftershave. Symptomatic cases are rare. Asymptomatic children can be allowed home after a short period of observation to make certain they do not become drowsy.

Bleach. Ingestion of household bleach causes fewer problems than would be expected.[7] Ipecac or lavage should not be used. Milk or antacids can be given orally. Local lesions in the mouth can be treated symptomatically and in the few cases where significant esophageal involvement is possible, endoscopy can be undertaken.

Detergents (anionic). Dishwashing liquid and shampoo are only toxic in large doses. Vomiting occurs in large doses. A period of observation may be needed.

Disinfectants. Serious cases are unusual.

Nail varnish remover (acetone). Observation for a period should be all that is needed but nausea and vomiting may occur, going on to coma if large amounts are taken.

Paints (oil based). Unless the paint has lead in it, the only problems that occur are caused by the petroleum distillate base. The stomach should not be emptied. In practice children do not seem to take significant amounts.

Pyrethrins. These insecticides are not usually a hazard if ingested or inhaled accidentally. The child should be observed for a short period.

Rat or mouse poison. The common ingredients of rat or mouse poison (warfarin or dichlorolose) are usually nontoxic in the doses taken by children. The exact type of poison should be identified using the poisons center and in most cases the child can be sent home after a short period of observation.

If large amounts of warfarin are ingested vitamin K can be used but this is not needed in most cases.

Talc. Talc is only toxic if inhaled. It may cause retching and choking due to pulmonary edema. Cases of ingestion only need a short period of observation to make certain inhalation did not occur.

Window cleaner. Most are nontoxic unless aspirated. The cleaner should be identified using the poisons center. In most cases the child can be sent home after a short period of observation.

Plants

Berberis. Very occasionally causes confusion, epistaxis or vomiting. The child should be observed for a short period.

Fuchsia. Unlikely to cause problems although potentially toxic. Observe for a short period.

Holly. Unlikely to cause problems although potentially toxic due to ilicin and theobromine.

Pyracantha. This causes nausea and vomiting but is unlikely to cause problems. The child should be observed for a short period.

Potential toxicity
Medicines

Barbiturates. May cause coma and hypotension. Cases are becoming less common, as they are less frequently prescribed. Activated charcoal can be used.

Benzodiazepines – tranquilizers and hypnotics such as diazepam (Valium) and nitrazepam (Mogadon). These can cause drowsiness and coma, but problems are unusual in accidental ingestion. In very young children respiratory depression may need treatment with artificial ventilation.

Carbamazepine. This drug has some anticholinergic activity. Paradoxically convulsions and violent reactions may occur as well as cardiac problems such as heart block. Activated charcoal is useful to adsorb carbamazepine.

Codeine-containing cough medicines. If significant amounts are taken there can be respiratory depression, for which the antagonist naloxone can be used (10 mcg/kg i.v.)

Clonidine. Clonidine can cause bradycardia, hypotension, coma and gastrointestinal upset. The use of atropine and dopamine infusion for the hypotension is controversial and supportive treatment (including assisted ventilation) may be adequate for even the most severe cases.[8]

Digoxin. Digoxin can be a serious poison in children, with only a few tablets being fatal. Activated charcoal is useful. These children should be monitored very closely, probably in an intensive care unit, with careful ECG monitoring. Beta-blockers such as propranolol should be used in severe cases, with atropine if there is heart block. The serum potassium should not be allowed to go too low or too high. Digoxin-specific antibody fragments are now available for the reversal of life-threatening overdosage (Digibind, Wellcome).

Diphenoxylate (the active constituent in Lomotil, the antidiarrheal agent). This compound has an opiate-like action, which causes prolonged respiratory depression. Treatment is with the opiate antagonist naloxone (10 mcg/kg as i.v. bolus). There may be a transient improvement followed by relapse and cases should be observed for at least 36 h and repeated doses of naloxone given as necessary.

Hyoscine. Hyoscine may cause dilated pupils, dry mouth, tachycardia and delirium due to anticholinergic effects. Observation will be all that is needed with most patients.

Iron. Iron is a potentially very serious poison, initially causing vomiting and hematemesis, but going on to acute gastric ulceration and shock. Later convulsions and cardiac arrhythmias may occur. Iron tablets may be detected by X-ray of the abdomen. Further treatment should be aimed at preventing additional absorption of the iron, by the use of the chelating agent desferrioxamine methylate, instilled into the stomach (5–10 g in 50–100 ml of liquid). Desferrioxamine should also be used parenterally (15 mg/kg/h to a maximum of 80 mg/kg) in all cases where a potentially toxic amount of iron may have been taken. The severity of a poisoning episode can be judged by the serum iron level. Levels above 16.1 mmol/L at 4 h indicate significant poisoning.

Mefenamic acid (Ponstan). This drug rarely causes problems in young children. Activated charcoal is effective. Convulsions can be treated with diazepam.

Metoclopramide (Maxolon). In overdose this drug causes extrapyramidal signs, drowsiness and vomiting. If extrapyramidal signs develop antiparkinsonian drugs such as procyclidine can be used.

Mianserin (Bolvidon). Mianserin has milder anticholinergic effects than the tricyclic antidepressants. Serious problems are uncommon. Drowsiness is the most common symptom.

Paracetamol (acetaminophen). Serious accidental ingestion of paracetamol is rare in children because the tablets are bitter and difficult to swallow and the elixir is too sweet to take in toxic quantities. Serious paracetamol poisoning may cause hepatocellular necrosis. Patients at risk of liver damage can be identified by measurement of blood levels 4 h after the ingestion. Treatment is needed if the serum paracetamol level is above 1.32 mmol/L (200 mg/L) at 4 h (or in rare delayed cases in children, 0.33 mmol/L at 12 h). Treatment is with oral methionine (at a dose of 1 g 4-hourly) for four doses. N-acetylcysteine intravenously is an alternative particularly in children who are vomiting or who present after 12–24 h when methionine is ineffective.

Phenytoin. Phenytoin ingestion may cause ataxia and nystagmus. Activated charcoal can be used.

Quinine. Quinine is a significant poison in children and has caused several deaths. It is used for night cramps. Quinidine and chloroquine are also toxic. Activated charcoal can be used.

Salicylates. Severe poisoning is now rare as aspirin preparations are no longer used for children because of the dangers of Reye's syndrome. Hyperventilation is an early sign of significant salicylate poisoning due to stimulation of the respiratory center with resultant respiratory alkalosis. There may also be a metabolic acidosis. In severe cases there is disorientation and coma.

The severity of a poisoning episode can be judged by salicylate levels. Toxicity can occur at levels above 2.2 mmol/L (300 mg/L) in children. In asymptomatic and mild cases nothing more needs to be done apart from encouraging fluid and electrolyte replacement and giving vitamin K. Activated charcoal is useful. Forced alkaline diuresis can be used in moderate to severe cases but its use is controversial and alkalinization of the urine is the important thing rather than the induction of excessive urine flow. Peritoneal dialysis can also be effective.

Theophylline. Theophylline can cause restlessness, agitation, vomiting, convulsions, coma, hypotension, hypokalemia and ventricular tachycardia. Activated charcoal can be used. Convulsions can be treated with diazepam.

Tricyclic antidepressants. Tricyclic antidepressants such as amitriptyline are serious poisons for young children. They may cause cardiac effects such as sinus tachycardia, hypotension and conduction disorders and death by their direct effect on the myocardium. There may be blurred vision and dry mouth from the anticholinergic effects. There may also be central effects of agitation, confusion, convulsions, drowsiness, coma and respiratory depression. Activated charcoal should also be used.

There is no specific antidote for tricyclic ingestion. The ECG should be monitored for cardiac arrhythmias. No treatment is indicated if there is adequate tissue perfusion and blood pressure. Metabolic acidosis should be corrected. Convulsions should be treated with diazepam. Life-threatening arrhythmias should be treated with propranolol. As tricyclics are protein bound active methods of elimination such as hemodialysis do not remove significant amounts of the drug.

Household products

Acids. Acids tend to cause inflammation and ulceration at the pylorus rather than the esophagus. This may lead to stenosis. Emesis or lavage should not be undertaken and chemical antidotes should not be given as the heat of the chemical reaction may increase injury. The extent of the injury should be assessed by endoscopy at an early stage. Steroids should be used to suppress the inflammation (prednisolone 2 mg/kg/d).

Alcoholic beverages. These may cause severe hypoglycemia. Blood alcohol levels are useful in management. Hypoglycemia should be detected by frequent blood glucose measurements, and prevented and treated by i.v. glucose infusions.

Alkalis. Alkalis such as caustic soda and dishwasher powder can cause burns to the mouth and esophageal ulceration, leading to stricture: review by esophagoscopy and treatment with steroids have improved the outlook for this condition. Emesis or lavage should not be undertaken, nor any chemical antidotes as the heat of the reaction may increase injury. The extent of the injury should be assessed by endoscopy at an early stage. Steroids should be used to suppress the inflammation (prednisolone 2 mg/kg/d).

Bottle-sterilizing tablets. Bottle-sterilizing tablets contain a bleach-like substance (sodium dichloroisocyanurate). They effervesce with water to make a sterilizing solution. If this reaction takes place in the mouth considerable damage can take place with edema and ulceration. Cases need to be monitored for their airway patency and i.v. fluids may be needed. Monitoring for esophageal involvement by endoscopy may be needed in some cases. The use of steroids is logical in severe cases.

Camphor and camphorated oil. These are dangerous poisons for children. They are absorbed quickly and because they are lipid soluble, enter the brain causing delirium, rigidity, coma and convulsions. Convulsions should be treated with diazepam.

Carbon monoxide. Hemoglobin has an affinity for carbon monoxide over 200 times greater than for oxygen. Carboxyhemoglobin will reduce the amount of hemoglobin available to carry oxygen and also hinders oxygen release. The incidence of carbon monoxide poisoning has fallen since house gas no longer contains this substance. Carbon monoxide poisoning should be treated with 100% oxygen over a period of several hours. Hyperbaric oxygen should be considered in severe cases if it is available.

Cetrimide. Cetrimide is a cationic detergent and can be caustic when concentrated. The stomach should not be emptied. If problems with ulceration occur steroids should be used. Cetrimide may also have depolarizing muscle-relaxing effects leading to breathlessness.

Disk or button batteries. Mercury cell, alkaline manganese and silver cell batteries contain a strong alkali (usually potassium hydroxide) as a main ingredient. Mercury cell batteries contain toxic amounts of mercury. Silver cell batteries generally contain less toxic ingredients than the other types. Worn batteries are less toxic than new ones.

Disk batteries can cause problems if they lodge in the gut and become corroded and release their contents. They may cause ulceration or perforation from caustic injury if lodged in the esophagus or stomach and should be removed endoscopically if they lodge there. If they go beyond the stomach they are usually passed without problem. Their progress should be monitored by abdominal X-ray. Mercury levels should be measured when appropriate. If the battery shows signs of leaking or breaking it should be removed surgically.

Essential oils. Essential or volatile oils contain mixtures of cyclic hydrocarbons, ethers, alcohols and ketones. They include turpentine, pine oil, citronella and eucalyptus as well as such things as Karvol capsules. Their toxicity varies, with real turpentine (not to be confused with turpentine substitute) being very toxic. Symptoms of essential oils include vomiting, drowsiness and convulsions. Ipecac should not be used.

Methylene chloride (paint stripper). This is a very serious poison for children. It is caustic and may cause damage to the skin, stomach, mucous membranes and pharynx. Vomiting, dizziness, confusion, toxic myocarditis and hemoglobinuria may occur. Methylene chloride is metabolized to carbon monoxide and carboxymethemoglobin concentrations may be elevated for several days. The stomach should not be emptied. Fluids should be given to dilute the methylene chloride. High-flow oxygen should be given if carboxyhemoglobin is present.

Organochloride insecticides. These include DDT, dieldrin and lindane. Symptoms include excitability, muscle twitching and convulsions. Activated charcoal is valuable.

Organophosphorus insecticides. A wide range of compounds which include malathion. They act by inhibiting cholinesterase in the blood. Symptoms include confusion, nausea, vomiting, wheezing and convulsions. If symptoms appear atropine (i.v.) 0.05 mg/kg and pralidoxime 20–60 mg/kg as required, depending on the severity of the poisoning, should be given by slow i.v. injection and repeated if needed.

Paradichlorobenzene mothballs. Most cases of accidental ingestion do not have serious symptoms. Ingestion may cause nausea and vomiting and cyanosis may develop due to methemoglobinemia. This should be treated with methylene blue.

Paraquat. Paraquat weedkiller is available in two forms: a concentrated form (Gramoxone) available only to farmers and horticulturalists and a granular form (Weedol) which contains only 2.5% paraquat. Accidental ingestion of the concentrated form is rare and ingestion of the granular form rarely causes serious problems. Paraquat causes local ulceration and in severe cases a proliferative alveolitis. Treatment should be to prevent absorption by Fuller's earth or bentonite.

Petroleum distillates, e.g. kerosene, turpentine, white spirit and turpentine substitute. These substances may cause a pneumonitis from lung aspiration. Ipecac or lavage should not be used. Kerosene poisoning is a particular problem in the Third World. Rhonchi are the most common physical sign and X-ray changes are common. Treatment in mild cases is symptomatic, together with the use of prophylactic antibiotics. Corticosteroids are often used, but clear evidence of their effectiveness is lacking. Severe cases may need oxygen and intensive respiratory care.

Phenolic compounds. These include cresols, menthols, phenols and hexachlorophene. Coal tar vaporizing solution contains cresol. They may cause local corrosive damage and there may be cerebral symptoms. Activated charcoal can be used.

Slug pellets (metaldehyde). Slug pellets contain about 3% metaldehyde which is toxic in children and 4 g is said to be fatal for a child. Experience suggests that problems do not arise after accidental ingestion. The child should be observed for 4–6 h to check for serious symptoms such as flushing, salivation and convulsions. Convulsions should be treated with diazepam.

Plants

Arum lily. Causes gastrointestinal side-effects and later CNS manifestations.

Deadly nightshade (atropa). This plant has an atropine effect causing photophobia, visual disturbance, dryness of mouth, flushed skin, etc. If there are symptoms a slow i.v. injection of physostigmine can be used.

Laburnum. Causes vomiting, diarrhea and nausea. Although quite commonly taken, serious problems are very rare.[9]

Philodendron (Swiss cheese plant) and Dieffenbachier. This plant has a local caustic action due to oxalic acid and may cause a sore mouth and laryngeal edema. Steroids may be useful in severe cases.

Yew. Causes gastrointestinal side-effects and later CNS manifestations. There may be severe hypotension.

UNINTENTIONAL INJURY

This section deals with the nature of injury, sources of data, the magnitude of the problem, and the etiology and prevention of injuries. In many cases websites are listed where up-to-date information and evidence-based material can be found. As scientific publications often refer to data 2–3 years previously, information in the print media is always somewhat dated. Many, but not all, websites are constantly updated, and where these are available they have been included as preferential references.

DEFINING INJURIES

The first issue to determine is: what is an injury? Injury can be divided into physical injuries and psychological injuries. Physical injuries are due to tissue damage caused by excess energy transfer. When physical, radiation, or thermal energy absorbed by the body exceeds the innate capacity to deal with such forces, tissue damage results. Whether such injuries are recognized will depend on the extent of the damage and whether this causes sufficient pain or loss of function to come to the notice of the injured person. Many toddlers have bruise marks on their shins from bumping into objects but these are generally not considered to be 'injuries'. Generally, an 'injury' must reach a certain severity threshold before it is considered as such. This threshold varies between groups and cultures and depends to a considerable extent on the availability and ease of access to healthcare. The severity threshold for injury is often defined as one which leads to restricted activity for a given period (1 or 3 d are commonly used) or which leads to the injured person seeking medical attention. This leads to different methods of counting injuries, which to a large extent depend on available data sources. There are two main options: surveys and information abstracted from administrative registers, which are discussed later.

SOURCES OF DATA ON INJURY

There are a considerable number of these, including data on mortality, morbidity, and disability.

MORTALITY DATA

Mortality data are the most widely available with most countries collecting and reporting on the causes of death to their citizens. Publications on the causes of death are generally made available by national governments and some of these are summarized by bodies such as the World Health Organization (WHO). The WHO has an excellent site where it is possible to obtain a large amount of information on the scale of the burden of injuries.[10]

On this site it is possible to download major reports, such as the 2002 World Report on Violence and Health, and the 2004 World Report on Road Traffic Injury Prevention, and to access links to many useful sites and initiatives. Clicking on the research tools button brings one to a series of useful links, including the WHO mortality database.[11] Entering this site allows the downloading of data from countries and also understanding of the completeness and coverage of mortality statistics around the world. Data are missing or incomplete from many middle and low income countries, making it impossible to accurately count the global total number of deaths or the exact distribution of causes of death. The WHO site has recently been amended to include a specific area for children.[12] This area includes the WHO–UNICEF document *A Global Call to Action: child and adolescent injury prevention*, published in 2006.[13]

This report estimates that a minimum of 875 000 children under 18 years of age die from injuries each year and that 95% of these occur in low- and middle-income countries. In children aged between 1 and 15 years four mechanisms of injuries appeared in the top 15 causes of death: road traffic injuries (6th), drowning (7th), fire-related burns (11th), and poisonings (15th). The WHO has followed up this report with an action plan to reduce this enormous burden on children's health with six areas identified for improvement: data and measurement, research, prevention, treatment services, capacity development and advocacy.[14]

The WHO will publish a World report on Child and Adolescent Injury Prevention in 2008.

In the UK mortality statistics are collated by the General Register Office for England and Wales,[15] with separate offices and statistics for Scotland[16] and Northern Ireland.[17]

Table 6.2 has been compiled by abstracting data from a publication by the Office for National Statistics[18] showing the distribution of injury-related deaths in children and young adults in England and Wales in 2003.

Table 6.2 shows several interesting patterns. The absolute numbers of deaths increases across the age groups but it should be remembered that the denominators are different. Rates are required for comparisons of groups or areas but absolute numbers can also provide easily interpretable information.

From the table it can be seen that transport accidents are a major cause of injury-related deaths at all ages. Pedestrian fatalities are a problem for all age groups but become hugely outnumbered in older age groups by occupant fatalities when this becomes the dominant mode of transport. Falls account for few deaths in any of the three age groups and are substantially outnumbered by deaths due to drowning or as a result of exposure to smoke, fire and flames. Accidental poisoning fatalities are exceptionally rare in the younger age groups but would be expected to be much more frequent than in those in older age groups. It is difficult to conceive of situations in which adults mistakenly ingest a toxic substance. The low rate in the young age group is undoubtedly due to the effectiveness of child-resistant containers introduced some decades ago, one of the most effective of all injury prevention initiatives.

The much higher number of accidental poisoning deaths in the 15–24-year-old age group does not represent accidental ingestion of substances but ingestion of greater than planned amounts of recreational drugs and which result in 'accidental' deaths. The lack of quality control in the production of illegal recreational drugs produces variations in the strength and content of products. Whilst the risk is probably very low for each ingestion, the frequency of ingestion by large numbers of young people mean that even rare failures in quality control will result in frequent tragedies, both amongst new and habitual users.

Whilst the focus of this chapter is on unintentional or accidental injuries it should be noted that intentional self-harm is one of the commonest causes of death in those aged 15–24 and also that quite a few children and young adults are killed during acts of violence.

There are a limited number of studies providing international comparative data. One such study[19] compared death rates across European Union countries in the 1–4, 5–9 and 10–14 age groups. For both sexes injury deaths exceeded those due to infection of cancer at all age groups. Injury-related deaths accounted for a low of 27% of all deaths in girls aged 1–4 and a high of 51% of all deaths in boys aged 10–15. There was considerable variation between countries. The countries with the lowest injury-related death rates were Sweden and The Netherlands and the highest death rates occurred in eastern Europe.

Interpreting the meaning of variations in injury mortality across countries is not straightforward. Variations in death rates can be due to variations in exposure to certain factors or to the effectiveness of countermeasures. For example, warm countries with a lot of childhood exposure to open water, will inevitably have higher drowning rates than those which have much less open water or where the temperature is so cold that swimming is avoided. The excess deaths in the warm countries with a lot of open water will be due to a mixture of inadvertent exposure (falling in) and to difficulties encountered during planned exposure (swimming). The degree to which children are taught to swim and to which physical barriers and observation (lifeguards) protect children will also impact on the mortality rates. Generally speaking, mortality statistics are based on the place of usual residence and can mask holiday-related hazards. An analysis of childhood drowning deaths in the UK[20] demonstrated the much higher risk to UK children from unsupervised swimming pools whilst on foreign holidays than from pools in the UK. Similarly, mortality league tables for road traffic related injuries will be influenced by the degree of motorization within countries, as well as behavioral traits and investment in safety measures. Road traffic increases rapidly with industrialization and economic development and there is generally a marked rise in road traffic related deaths, which then plateau and decrease somewhat as safety measures and legislation are introduced and enforced.

MORBIDITY DATA

There are several sources of information on nonfatal injuries, although these vary across and within countries. Sources include hospital discharge or separation data, A & E department attendance data, trauma registers, survey data and data systems operated by nonhealth bodies with a focus on high-risk events such as road traffic collisions and house fires. Unlike mortality data, information from these sources is rarely reported using methods which allow direct comparison. Guidance on methodological issues in comparing injury incidence data across countries has been produced.[21] Some of the apparent differences in morbidity rates between countries are due to differences in the supply and scope of different aspects of the health service, as described in the sections dealing with hospital admission and Emergency department data. Greater or lesser proportions of trauma care are provided as inpatient, outpatient or specialized clinics in different countries and settings.

Much of the data on hospital admissions and A & E departments in this section has been derived from the Collaboration for Accident Prevention and Injury Control (CAPIC) website.[22] CAPIC is a multidisciplinary, multi-agency voluntary body which supports injury prevention initiatives in Wales.

HOSPITAL ADMISSION DATA

Table 6.3 shows hospital admission rates for all types of injury, by 5-year age groups in Wales in 2003. It can be seen that admission rates

Table 6.2 Numbers of deaths due to injury and poisoning by cause and age band to children and young adults in England and Wales in 2003 (Office for National Statistics, 2004)

Category	Age group		
	1–4	5–14	15–24
All injury and poisoning	100	172	1573
Transport accidents	18	23	221
Pedestrian	8	11	29
Motorcyclist	0	1	43
Falls	3	2	7
Drowning	11	2	6
Smoke, fire and flames	15	2	3
Poisoning (accidental)	1	0	29
Intentional self-harm	0	3	301
Assault	6	12	75

Table 6.3   Hospital admission rates for all types of injury by 5-year age groups in Wales – 2003

Age group	Number of events	Rate/1000 population
0–4	2187	13.7
5–9	1779	9.8
10–14	2574	13.1
15–19	3249	16.6
20–24	2955	16.3
25–29	2233	14.4
30–34	2454	12.8
35–39	2436	11.5
40–44	2143	10.4
45–49	1617	8.6
50–54	1487	7.7
55–59	1571	7.8
60–64	1288	8.0
65–69	1367	9.6
70–74	1735	13.8
75–79	2401	22.6
80–84	3249	40.1
85+	4915	84.1
All ages	41640	14.2

for children and young adults are higher than in middle age but not as high as in older persons, when falls and osteoporotic fractures lead to many admissions.

The data in this section reflect age-specific hospital admission rates for Welsh residents in 2003 derived from the CAPIC data. Around 1.3% of all children and young people (0–19 years) are admitted to hospital with an injury each year. Major causes of hospital admission with an injury in this age group are falls (n = 3493), accidental poisonings (n = 783), being struck by or against objects (n = 659), involvement in motor vehicle transport accidents (n = 541), and from noncollision pedal cycle injuries (n = 440). Injuries caused by glass (n = 242), knives and tools (n = 80), scalds (n = 276) and unintentional fires (n = 35) are less common but are often associated with substantial morbidity.

There are many factors which influence the probability that a person with an injury of moderate severity will be admitted to hospital. These include issues such as bed availability, variation in clinicians' propensity to treat fractures conservatively or with surgery, co-morbid conditions, uncertainty about intentionality, and social factors. These factors generally mean that it is difficult to use hospital admissions as a valid measure of the incidence of injuries of a given nature. Cryer and Langley[23] developed the most valid injury indicators to date for hospital admissions, based on a group of conditions with a probability of inpatient death of greater than 5.9%. This approach is useful for understanding national trends but the downside is that it includes a very small proportion of all injury-related hospitalizations. Generally speaking, there are insufficient numbers of these high-risk injuries to be able to use this technique for regional or local data and consequently it is not suitable for the targeting or monitoring of local preventative interventions. Guides to the evaluation of injury prevention initiatives can be found on the CAPIC website.[22]

EMERGENCY DEPARTMENT DATA

Emergency department data are increasingly being made available as electronic collection of health information grows. In many cases the information collected merely involves the administrative and diagnostic details needed to treat individuals whereas in other cases the information systems used also collect data on the location, antecedent factors and activities resulting in the injury occurrence. Both types of data collection are useful for those interested in prevention but clearly the latter are much more useful. An excellent example of the latter is the Victoria Emergency (Department) Minimum Dataset (VEMD) in use in Victoria,

Australia and exported to many parts of the world.[24] Systems such as this have provided the basis of injury surveillance which stimulated preventative interventions and the basis of much of our knowledge on the effectiveness of interventions.

Many more children are seen and treated at Emergency departments than are admitted as inpatients. Generally speaking there are 10–20 injuries treated and discharged in Emergency departments for every admission.

In the US the on-line National Electronic Injury Surveillance System (NEISS[25]) allows queries to be run on the database. In 2004 there were an estimated 13 096 983 Emergency department attendances with an injury in the US. In Europe, EuroSafe, the European Association for Injury prevention and Safety Promotion, manage the European Commission's Injury Database and collate data from Emergency departments in participating countries.[26]

Table 6.4 shows age-specific injury attendance rates in Wales in 2004. Rates in females are about one quarter or one third lower than in males at all ages. Overall, around one in four or five children and young people attend an Emergency department with an injury each year. The importance of home safety initiatives for young children is shown by the fact that 69% of all injuries to children aged 0–4 took place in the home.

Emergency department attendances are influenced by many factors other than the presence of an injury. Many less serious injuries are self-treated or treated in primary care. Distance and access can have profound effects, with one study showing a 50% reduction in injury attendance rate over a distance of 10 miles.[27] This distance decay effect was present for all injuries with the exception of fractures. Consequently fractures are frequently used as an indicator variable. The fracture rates per 1000 populations in Wales in 2004 were 16 for the 0–4 age group, and 33, 55 and 39 in the next three 5-year age groups. These are higher than any age group other than those aged 85 and over (62/1000). A further revision of the fracture indicator has been proposed, selected radiologically verifiable fractures (SRVFs), due to changes in the clinical management of different injuries. This takes into account changes in practise relating to avoiding X-ray exposure for many head and facial injuries and the likelihood that many distal radial greenstick or buckle fractures in young children do not present to Emergency departments.

Table 6.4   Estimated numbers and rates of injury for Wales, by age band, 2004

Age	Estimated numbers of injuries	Estimated rate (per 1000 population)
0–4	24560	182
5–9	27197	156
10–14	47338	241
15–19	46395	229
20–24	39104	187
25–29	29002	157
30–34	28878	141
35–39	28611	127
40–44	26306	116
45–49	19338	96
50–54	16583	85
55–59	16190	77
60–64	11706	68
65–69	9391	63
70–74	9212	72
75–79	8942	82
80–84	9371	109
85+	12493	184
Unknown	88	
Total	410704	133

SURVEY DATA

Admission and Emergency department data are often not available and even where they are, details of how and where the injury happened may not be collected. These factors are crucial to understanding the etiology and in developing preventive strategies and interventions. In such circumstances survey data can be very helpful. The World Health Organization (WHO) has developed guidelines for those carrying out community surveys on injuries and violence.[28]

Community-based surveys are particularly useful in poorer countries where access to high-quality care is often scanty and most injuries are self-treated or attended to by traditional healers. The rationale for such surveys is to implement preventive measures as outlined in the four-stage public health approach (Fig. 6.1) recommended by the WHO.

Even in wealthy countries survey data can be useful for obtaining additional information on location of injury and antecedent factors not collected at Emergency departments and also for obtaining exposure metrics.

DISABILITY DATA

There is a lack of data on the medium and long-term consequences of injuries. The Global Burden of Disease and Injuries project[29] has produced initial estimates but these are based on quite sparse data and in many cases there were no data for specific types of injury. The likely distribution of outcomes for each injury was obtained by asking the opinion of medical experts based in hospitals. This is problematic as most hospital clinicians see and treat acutely injured patients and do not have a systematic process of measuring outcomes, particularly measures of function and disability. Prospective studies and empirical data on outcomes at fixed points in time are required to answer these questions. Another issue with many of the existing studies is that the injuries included in the study were often selected using a severity measure, such as the Abbreviated Injury Scale (AIS).[30] The AIS is designed to measure the threat to life from injuries in order to improve the evaluation of counter measures. However, it is not clear how closely threat to life and threat to disability are related. A stab wound to the heart has a high threat to life but if the patient survives the probability of any physical disability is slight. Amputation of a thumb carries a very low threat to life but a very high threat to disability. One of the best studies of post injury disability in young adults was that carried out on the 1958 British National Child Development Study cohort in 1981.[31] In that study 12 537 participants were asked about unintentional injuries and disability since age 16. Two thirds of men and one third of women reported at least one injury requiring hospital treatment. Injuries requiring hospital admission carried the highest risk of disability (9.7%) but 54% of permanent disabilities reported by men and 74% reported by women resulted from injuries

treated as outpatients. Fractures accounted for one third of disabilities. Among injuries resulting in permanent disability hand injuries featured prominently (82% of disabling work injuries and 32% of disabling home injuries). The greatest gap in estimating the true burden on injuries is the lack of information on the medium- and long-term consequences of injury.

INEQUALITIES IN INJURY

Social inequalities in health were 'discovered' in the nineteenth century by seminal public health figures, such as Virchow in Germany, Villermé in France, and Chadwick in England. However, interest in social inequalities in health faded in the twentieth century until the publication of the Black Report in the UK in 1980.[32] This study compared death rates between the social classes. The largest of all the differences in death rates occurred in childhood injury deaths where the children from parents of social class 5 (unskilled workers) were several times more likely to die than those whose parents were from social class 1 (professionals). The ratio varied by a factor of 4 for all injury deaths to 7 for pedestrian deaths and 15 for deaths due to household fires.

Studies using individual level measures of socioeconomic position, such as social class, income or parental educational level show the greatest difference between the extremes. Social class scales tend to differ across countries and are not universally available. Usually several questions have to be answered to apply the scales, which prohibits their widespread use. In some countries, such as the US, concepts such as occupational social class are not commonly used and metrics such as family or individual income or educational level are preferred. Many studies use ecological or area-based measures to categorize groups by socioeconomic standing. These measures are usually obtained from official statistics taken during population censuses or the distribution of state-funded benefits. Area-based measures are attractive as they are easily applied once an address, postcode or zipcode are known. In many cases they are more suitable than individual level measures as many injury-prevention initiatives are implemented on an area or group basis. The strength of the relationship between injury deaths and ecological measures of socioeconomic position is attenuated due to the application of average measures to everybody within a community and the inevitable misclassification which results from applying an average score to a heterogeneous population.

The situation is not as simple when nonfatal injuries are considered. Some injuries show a marked socioeconomic gradient with higher rates in the less affluent groups or areas but the reverse occurring for other injuries. A population-based study of childhood fractures in Wales[33] demonstrated little overall variation in fracture rates between the most and least affluent groups. However, the most affluent group reported higher rates from sports participation, particularly notable for fractures related to horse riding and in-line skating, sports which require financial support. In contrast, assault-related fractures were substantially more common in the most deprived group. Clearly, some of the variations between socioeconomic groups related to differences in the presence and degree of exposure to hazardous behaviors, activities and environments. Childhood pedestrian injuries demonstrate substantial inequalities between affluent and deprived areas[34] as do childhood poisonings resulting in hospital admission[35] and burns.[36] These particular injuries show such a steep inequality gradient that they should be a main focus of effort to reduce inequalities in child health.

INJURY PREVENTION

Given the scale of the impact of injuries on children's lives, preventing injuries should be a major goal of society. Injuries are caused by interactions between individuals and their environments and the prevention of injuries requires an understanding of these issues. Few pediatricians or child health practitioners are taught the principles of injury prevention and how these can be applied to their everyday work environment. The World Health Organization has responded to this deficiency by

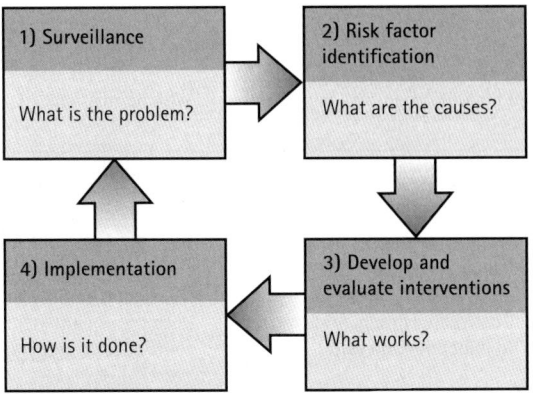

Fig. 6.1 A Public Health Perspective on injuries. (World Health Organization, p. 5 http://whqlibdoc.who.int/publications/2004/9241546484.pdf).

producing free teaching materials suitable for different circumstances. The teaching materials are suitable for three different levels of involvement: an intensive 2-day course; a 1-week short training course; and a 6-month training session. The materials are available from the WHO website.[37]

The learning objectives of the courses include:

1. to identify the basic principles of injury prevention, control and safety promotion;
2. to diagnose problems from a multidisciplinary perspective;
3. to design, implement and evaluate injury prevention and control interventions;
4. to advocate for injury prevention in communities;
5. to practice injury prevention control and safety promotion based on universally accepted ethical principles.

One important model to understand the causal chain of events involved in injuries is that proposed by William Haddon, commonly known as the Haddon Matrix (Table 6.5).

It is obvious from the matrix that injury prevention is a multidisciplinary and multi-agency task. There is scope for many different groups to become involved, either separately or in collaboration and there are many points at which preventive initiatives can be implemented. Initiatives can broadly be aimed at changing the environment, improving enforcement of safety legislation or at changing behavior through education. These are referred to as the three 'Es' of injury prevention. Clearly, each type of injury will require a tailored approach. Preventing injuries to the under fives at home will involve different groups and approaches to preventing childhood pedestrian injuries, for example. However, for almost every issue child health practitioners can play a substantial advocacy role. This is particularly the case where childhood injuries are very common or where there is social disadvantage and large inequalities in injury incidence. Advocating for those who are not in a position to protect themselves (children) and whose parents and guardians may lack the necessary information and influence to carry out this task should be a core function of child health practitioners. There are many groups which can provide assistance, including charities such as the Child Accident Prevention Trust (CAPT[38]), Royal Society for the Prevention of Accidents (RoSPA)[39] or the European Child Safety Alliance.[40]

Among the useful products produced by the European Child Safety Alliance is an 18-country Child Safety Action Plan. This action plan should help bolster support for injury prevention within participant countries and reduce the burden of injuries. Clearly, there is scope to copy this or similar initiatives in non-participant countries or with in regions and districts within countries. Child health practitioners are well placed to lead such activities but perhaps require additional training in advocacy and public health skills.

THE EVIDENCE BASE

Knowing what to implement and how to get evidence into practice are important components of the knowledge and skills framework for injury prevention practitioners. Like all aspects of health, publications relevant to injury prevention are increasing year on year and it is impossible for any practitioner or specialist to read all the published material. Several initiatives have made life easier.

For those with a need to know about latest developments SafetyLit[41] provides a weekly electronic current awareness service. This includes titles and abstracts sorted into categories from publications in over 2600 journals. For the more generalist approach to injury prevention the first source of information on effective interventions should be through systematic reviews. There are several sources of systematic reviews pertinent to injury prevention. The greatest supply of high-quality systematic reviews is produced by the Cochrane Injuries Group[42] based at the London School of Hygiene and Tropical Medicine. Their reviews are published by the Cochrane Library. Although the highest quality reviews are published by the Cochrane Group there are many others producing systematic reviews pertinent to injury prevention. Sometimes the conclusions of different groups looking at the same topics differ. This usually occurs due to differences in the thresholds set for study inclusion. The Collaboration for Accident Prevention and Injury Control (CAPIC[22]) provides a searchable database of all systematic reviews to allow the reader to identify all the relevant reviews and decide whether to focus on the most up-to-date review or read all the reviews. Some reviews focus on specific topics, such as the effectiveness of traffic calming or smoke alarms whilst others are broader ranging and cover many topics. One of the most broadly based reviews was that carried out by Elizabeth Towner and colleagues and published in two volumes,[43] in the journal Injury Prevention. These reviews cover a very wide range of topics from traffic calming to bicycle helmets to smoke alarms and educational interventions.

It is important to realize that systematic reviews only cover part of the evidence base. They are suitable for summarizing interventions which are amenable to evaluation by experimental design over a relatively short period. However, not all interventions can be evaluated using these methods. If observational studies demonstrate an intervention to be very effective then the ethical position of equipoise is lost and RCT cannot be instituted. If one considers trauma treatment as an analogy there is no trial evidence backing the use of plaster of Paris for immobilization of fractures. The evidence is based upon the principles of anatomy, physics and common sense. Nobody would ever suggest conducting a trial of immobilization versus watchful waiting to demonstrate the effectiveness of plaster of Paris although they might run trials to demonstrate the relative effectiveness of different methods of immobilization. At the other end of the spectrum it is very difficult to evaluate the effectiveness of long-term advocacy in changing cultural views in relation to the acceptability of implementing some injury prevention measures. No single mass media campaign has demonstrated effectiveness in reducing the incidence of driving whilst under the influence of alcohol. Yet, cultural attitudes to drink driving have changed over the past 30 or so years with a substantial reduction in prevalence and associated numbers of deaths.

Table 6.5   The Haddon matrix (This model is reproduced from the WHO Teach Violence and Injury Prevention course materials with permission) (http://www.who.int/violence_injury_prevention/capacitybuilding/teach_vip/en/index.html)

	Host (person)	Agent (vehicle or product)	Physical environment	Socio-economic environment
Pre-event	Is the person pre-disposed or overexposed to risk?	Is the agent hazardous?	Is the environment hazardous? Possibility to reduce hazards?	Does the environment encourage or discourage risk-taking and hazard?
Event	Is the person able to tolerate force or energy transfer?	Does the agent provide protection?	Does the environment contribute to injury during event?	Does the environment contribute to injury during event?
Post-event	How severe is the trauma or harm?	Does the agent contribute to the trauma?	Does the environment add to the trauma after the event?	Does the environment contribute to recovery?

How much of this change would have happened without mass media campaigns?

One area of evidence which is often derided is cross-national ecological comparisons. However, much can be learned from comparing practices and programs in different settings and cultures and trying to find out why some interventions seem to work in some settings and not others. One of the most useful reports on pedestrian safety in recent years is Children's Traffic Safety: International Lessons for the UK produced by Nicola Christie and colleagues for the UK Department for Transport.[44]

There were five things which distinguished the best countries, in terms of lower death rates, from the rest:

1. they had invested very widely in speed reduction measures, including environmental modification and low speed limits;
2. such measures were widely implemented outside schools;
3. there were outside play areas, such as parks and playgrounds, in most residential areas;
4. there were national publicity campaigns aimed at child pedestrian safety conducted at least once a year; and
5. they had legislation that assumes driver responsibility for accidents involving child pedestrians in residential areas.

Thus, the evidence base for injury prevention is very broad and includes systematic reviews, randomized trials, and observational, ecological and qualitative studies. Different study designs are appropriate for different questions. A comprehensive approach is usually needed to reach the correct conclusions. Providing and maintaining a broad evidence base is essential for advocacy, implementing proven strategies and developing new interventions to reduce the burden of childhood injury. The ultimate and only important aim is to have fewer dead, injured and disabled children.

POISONOUS ANIMAL BITES AND STINGS

An overview of poisonous animal bites and stings published by the World Health Organization, stated that in excess of 100 000 deaths result worldwide each year from snakes bites, scorpion stings, spider bites, marine envenomations and anaphylactic reactions to stings.[45]

SNAKE BITES

Snakes are the most widely distributed of the reptiles, and different species, often with highly individual features, predominate in different countries. Overall, there are 2.5 million snake bites each year, with a fatality rate of between 1.5 and 3%.[45,46] Tragically, in children, the mortality from snakebite is higher[47] and may reach in excess of 10% in some areas of Papua New Guinea.[48] Environmental change in some parts of the world has resulted in changes in the pattern of snakebite – as for example in parts of Africa, where prolonged drought has reduced vegetation cover, favoring the spread of *Echis ocellatus*, which has resulted in more bites.[45] Of the nearly 3000 known varieties of snake, only a minority are of medical significance and clinicians should concern themselves primarily with the characteristics and venomous effects of the poisonous snakes in their own area and importantly, have to hand details of their local supplier of antivenom.

Adder bites (Europe)

The common viper or adder (*Vipera berus*) is found throughout Europe, with the notable exception of Ireland, and its bite seldom causes death in adults, although there are reports of deaths in young children.[49] The fully grown adder may be 50–60 cm in length and is recognized by the dark zigzag band which runs along the center of the back, although rarely the snake may appear uniformly black. It is a shy creature, normally disappearing quickly on the approach of people and is only likely to bite if disturbed unexpectedly.

Clinical features

When the amount of venom injected is small, as is usual in a defensive bite, there may be few signs or symptoms, but fear often causes transient pallor, sweating or vomiting. With moderate poisoning there may be local swelling and tender enlargement of the regional lymph nodes. This swelling may increase over 1 or 2 d to involve the whole limb but usually resolves within a few weeks. A burning pain is experienced at the place bitten. Vomiting may begin within a few minutes of the bite (often followed by diarrhea) and may continue for up to 48 h. Shock is likely with weakness, sweating, thirst, coldness, absent pulse, hypotension, drowsiness and occasionally loss of consciousness. Swelling of the face, lips and tongue may occur, ecchymoses and swelling appear and may gradually extend up the limb. Bleeding may occur from gums, wound and infection sites. Other indications of envenomation include ECG abnormalities, peripheral neutrophil leukocytosis, elevated serum creatine kinase or metabolic acidosis.[49] With recovery, discoloration slowly changes from blue to green and finally to yellow before disappearing. The child generally recovers quickly from the initial collapse but in severe poisoning there may be persistent or recurrent hypotension, acute renal failure, and pulmonary or cerebral edema.[49] Full recovery may take 1–6 weeks.

Treatment

A child who is bitten by a snake should be taken to hospital as quickly as possible and, *if it can be done without causing delay and without risk of further bites*, the reptile should be killed for identification. The bite should not be incised and the patient should be kept quiet and the limb maintained at rest by splinting, helping to retard absorption of venom. Tourniquets and compression should not be used. Both the child and parents should be reassured about the expected outcome. On admission to hospital paracetamol may be given for the pain and chlorpromazine, if required, for vomiting. In hospital, blood pressure should be monitored hourly, and bleeding time should be recorded; the white cell count (raised), serum creatine phosphokinase (may be raised), serum bicarbonate (may be low) and ECG should be determined twice daily. Tetanus toxoid should be administered if there is no record of tetanus immunization within the previous 5 years, but tetanus antitoxin is not required routinely. Broad-spectrum antibiotics are required if evidence of bacterial infection develops. Antivenom (two ampoules) should be given if there is evidence of systemic poisoning, especially hypotension, bleeding or ECG changes. It should be given diluted with isotonic saline, by slow i.v. injection or infusion over a period of 30–60 min. Adrenaline (epinephrine) and i.v. antihistamine and hydrocortisone should be ready in case of anaphylaxis.[49] If the patient does not show any clinical improvement, the treatment may be repeated.[49] If there is a delay in obtaining antivenom or if a history of allergy contraindicates its use, blood transfusion or i.v. fluids may help to combat collapse.

Tropical and subtropical snakes

Morbidity and mortality from snake bites are highest in those areas where snakes have adapted to farm, plantation and village life and live in close proximity to large human populations. Examples are the Indian cobra, krait and Russell's viper in South-East Asia, some pit vipers in Latin America, the Taipan in Papua New Guinea and *Echis* species in Africa.

Land snakes may be roughly classified according to the presence or absence of poison injecting fangs, and their position when present in the snake's mouth (Table 6.6). Sea snakes, of which there are some 50 species, have characteristic flattened tails and short front fangs.

Although the Elapidae include many highly venomous varieties, these usually retreat when approached by humans and are generally non-aggressive unless cornered or molested. The large family of Colubridae contains only a few snakes of medical significance and these are rarely the cause of bites in humans. The Viperidae, on the other hand, are broad, sluggish snakes which hold their ground and may easily be trodden on (puff adder) or touched, on or in the ground or among rocks (rattlesnake, burrowing adder, berg adder). These snakes, despite their sluggishness, strike with great rapidity and power, virtually stabbing their victim with frontally situated large fangs which are swung forward during the strike.

Table 6.6   Classification of snakes

Group of snake	Features of groups	Common examples and habitat	Principal action of venom
Viperidae	Mobile front fangs	Viperinae Puff adder, widespread in Africa Gaboon viper, central and southern Africa Berg adder, southern Africa Night adder, southern Africa Rhinoceros viper, Tropical Africa Russell's viper, Asia and Indonesia Saw-scaled viper, India, Iraq, North Africa European viper (adder), Europe, Asia, Japan Crotalinae (pit vipers) Cottonmouth moccasin south-eastern United States Copperhead, N. America Fer-de-lance, Latin America; W. Indies Bushmaster, Central and South America Jaracara, South America Rattlesnakes, Mexico, southern and western United States	Cytotoxic (tropical rattlesnakes and berg adder are mainly neurotoxic)
Elapidae	Fixed front fangs	Cobras, widespread in Africa and Asia Mambas, east, central and southern Africa	Neurotoxic (king cobra also has cytotoxic effect)
Colubridae	Back fangs	Rinkhals, southern Africa Indian krait, India, Burma, Malaya, Indonesia Tiger snake, Brown snake, Australia Taipan; Death adder, Australia and New Guinea Coral snakes, southern United States; C. America Boomslang, widespread in Africa	Hematoxic
Hydrophidae (Now included in Elapidae)	Short fixed front fangs	Various species of sea snake. Mainly in the Pacific but a few species in the Indian Ocean	Neurotoxic; myotoxic
Nonvenomous	Fangless	House snake Grass snake Boas, pythons. Widespread in tropics.	Nil

Many nonvenomous snakes are capable of inflicting bites which are liable to become infected, sometimes with exotic bacteria, such as *Arizona* species.

Snake venoms broadly correspond with the families shown in the table. They are, however, complex mixtures of toxins and enzymes and effects depend upon which of these predominate. Viper (and spitting cobra) venoms are mainly cytotoxic but bleeding diatheses are common. Elapid venoms produce neurotoxic and cytotoxic effects, as do varieties of tropical rattlesnake (Crotolinae), but again microangiopathic and intravascular hemolysis may be a feature of the bites of some species. Overall, snake venoms are complex with varying mixtures of neurotoxins, myotoxins, procoagulants, anticoagulants and nephrotoxins.[46,47,49,50] The venoms may therefore also cause hemolysis, hemorrhage and coagulation disturbances.

Colubrid (e.g. boomslang) venoms are hematoxic and anticoagulant, while hydrophiid (sea snake) venoms are mainly myotoxic. Nephrotoxic properties have also been demonstrated in puff adder, sea snake and rattlesnake venoms.

Children are particularly at risk in areas where snakes are common because of their love of outdoor pursuits, together with their curiosity and carelessness. However, it is important to realize that all bites from snakes are not caused by venomous species. In the case of bites from nonvenomous snakes, two distinct puncture marks are not seen and the bites are irregular and lacerated to a greater or lesser degree, with little local swelling or pain. Even bites by venomous species do not always cause clinically significant envenomation as the bite may be deflected by clothing or the venom stores of the snake depleted. When envenomation has occurred, symptoms tend to be more severe in children because of their smaller size relative to the volume of injected venom.

Despite popular belief, while sudden collapse and death may occur (e.g. Australian brown snake, death adder), signs of systemic envenomation in even the most poisonous snake bites seldom occur before 30 min. The earliest features are often those due to fright – shock, pallor, sweating, vomiting, weak pulse and faintness. Severe pain and swelling at the site of the bite, with rapidly spreading edema, are the first signs in most viper and spitting cobra bites. Later large bullae may form around the bite and painful lymphadenopathy may develop. Sometimes there is extensive bruising in superficial and deeper tissues. Within 5 or 6 h the whole limb may be tensely swollen. There is thus a profound local cytotoxic effect and subsequent systemic disturbance is largely due to this tissue damage rather than to circulating venom. Necrosis of superficial or deep tissues may be seen. Disseminated intravascular coagulation with resultant hemolytic anemia, hemorrhagic manifestations and hemoglobinuric nephrosis, can complicate the bite.

In heavy envenomation, especially by puff adders and Gaboon vipers, bloody saliva may be expectorated, and sudden death may follow due to circulatory collapse. Notable exceptions in this family of snakes are the hemorrhagic reactions seen in bites from saw-scaled and Russell's vipers and the neurotoxic effects occurring in tropical rattlesnake and berg adder bites.

Elapid bites generally cause much less local reaction, but have profound systemic effects which are predominantly neurotoxic. Spitting cobras are however a different entity – the bites may cause significant local tissue necrosis[51] and in a review of bites from the Australian copperhead, one third showed significant local effects.[52] The first symptoms of neurotoxic snake bite are usually ptosis, rapidly followed by strabismus, slurred speech and dysphagia, with drooling saliva. There is confusion and hypersensitivity to tactile stimuli. If untreated, the victim may be completely paralyzed within minutes and respiratory paralysis may result in death within 15 h. In survivors there are no neurological sequelae. In the case of mamba bites, the first systemic symptoms are combined with a sensation of tightness and pain across the chest.

Violent abdominal pain sometimes occurs after krait and coral snake bites. Local blistering may be seen after envenomation by some cobras and a burning sensation at the site is often described. Local pain after snake bites is, however, extremely variable. Hematuria and hemoglobinuria may occur as may hemorrhage or menorrhagia.

Some elapids, such as the spitting cobra and the rinkhals of southern Africa are able to eject venom with considerable force and accuracy at the victim's head. Should this enter the eyes, a severe keratoconjunctivitis can result, which may lead to blindness if not adequately irrigated and treated.

The family Colubridae covers many snakes, including the Montpellier snakes, the red-necked keelbacks, the yamakagashis, the herald snake and the vine snake[49] but the boomslang is the only venomous snake in this large family which is a significant hazard to humans. Fortunately bites from this species are rare, usually occurring in those handling or working with snakes. There is little or no local reaction apart from mild burning pain but severe headache about 1 h after the bite is a regular and unexplained phenomenon. Colubrid venoms contain mainly fibrinolysins and hemorrhagins, which result in severe, systemic defibrination and generalized hemorrhage, widespread cutaneous bruising especially at sites of trauma, and free bleeding from fang punctures. There may be massive intestinal, urinary tract or intracranial hemorrhage leading to death. As mentioned earlier, the venom of certain vipers and also some elapids (such as the Papuan black snake) produces similar hemorrhagic effects.

Sea snakes do not attack in water if unmolested. Most bites result from handling the snake when caught in fishing nets. The bite shows no local reaction and minimal pain[53] and in most sea snake bites no envenomation occurs.[54] Initial symptoms, due to a myotoxin, are seen after a latent period of 30–120 min. There is muscular pain, stiffness and trismus followed by ptosis and progressive weakness which may threaten respiratory function. Rhabdomyolysis, myoglobinuria, renal tubular necrosis and acute renal failure may ensue.

Hadley et al,[55] in southern Africa, found thromboelastography to be a good predictor of severity in snake bite in children. They felt that, although it did not supersede clinical observation in the management of snake bite in children, it did allow stratification into high- and low-risk categories.

Treatment

The administration of antivenom, generally intravenously, is an effective treatment for a case of envenomation by a poisonous snake, but for many snake species, no antivenom may be available. The use of antivenom, especially polyvalent antivenom, carries a substantial risk of anaphylaxis and serum sickness because of its foreign protein content, but there is no doubt that the benefits of antivenom treatment far outweigh the risks.[45,51] Its administration in every case of snake bite is, however, dangerous, wasteful and unnecessary. As not all snake bites are due to poisonous snakes, it is obviously of paramount importance, as an initial step, to identify the snake accurately, or at least to decide clinically into which group it falls. Much can be deduced from the color and shape of the snake, manner and circumstances of striking, the situation of the bite and presence or absence of fang marks. For instance, the puff adder, responsible for 95% of poisonous snake bites in Africa, is encountered on paths or in grassy terrain, and almost always strikes at the feet or ankles. On the other hand, cobras often attack when they are surprised near outbuildings or chicken runs. They rear up prior to striking and bites are frequently inflicted above the knees or even on the trunk or upper limbs.

As many victims of snake bite are not within easy access of clinic or hospital, it is most important to lay down firm and easily understood guidelines which can be applied by a layman on the spot:

1. *Symptoms* developing within the first half hour of a bite are almost always due to fear and its effects – and not to envenomation. The patient should be calmed and reassured, and encouraged to lie down quietly so as not to disseminate the poison by restless body movements. The affected limb should be kept horizontal at this stage and gently splinted to avoid movement. A mild analgesic (paracetamol) should be given.

2. *Bites* from nonvenomous snakes should be thoroughly cleansed with a dilute antiseptic solution, any loose teeth removed, and a light dressing applied. Tetanus toxoid should be administered within 24 h to all cases of snake bite if there is no documented evidence that the child has received anti-tetanus immunization within the past 5 years, and broad-spectrum antibiotics should be given at the first indication of possible infection.

3. *Signs* of significant envenomation generally develop from half to 2 h after the bite. It is imperative to get the patient to a hospital, or a trained person to the patient, as soon as possible. Signs may be local in the case of viper bites, with swelling and pain, or systemic in the case of bites from snakes with neurotoxic and hematoxic venom, with varying manifestations including vomiting, abdominal pain and neurotoxic symptoms, as noted earlier.[51] They call for urgent administration of antivenom given intravenously. If this is not possible, the antivenom should be administered intramuscularly (see later). Sprivulis and Jelinek[51] advise that multiple doses of antivenom may be required. Premedication with parenteral antihistamine and low-dose subcutaneous adrenaline (epinephrine) (0.003–0.007 mg/kg) prior to administration of antivenom is advisable in sensitive individuals to prevent anaphylaxis. Sprivulis and Jelinek[51] recommend that a short course of oral steroids may reduce the incidence of serum sickness, particularly in children and in patients receiving polyvalent or multiple doses of monovalent antivenom.

4. *Tourniquets:* In many countries the use of tourniquets is generally discouraged and under no circumstances should any form of bandaging be applied in the case of bites by snakes with cytotoxic venom as the local effects and subsequent complications are aggravated by compression and such procedures waste transport time. However, where highly venomous snakes with pronounced systemic effects are incriminated (e.g. neurotoxic cobras, mambas, crotalids and sea snakes), and especially if there are already signs of systemic toxicity, it is recommended that a pressure bandage be applied to the affected limb to prevent further absorption. Australian experience with elapid bites has much to recommend it – replacing the previously recommended tourniquet for the 'pressure-immobilization method.' Thus it has been found that for this group of snakes, rather than using a tourniquet, venom movement, which occurs largely via the lymphatics, can be effectively delayed for long periods by the application of a firm crepe bandage to the length of the bitten limb combined with immobilization by a splint. The bandage is firmly applied to the bitten area and then continued to the distal end of the limb and then wound tightly back to the groin or armpit.[50] It is worth noting here that this 'pressure-immobilization' method may be used for all elapid snake bites and some other types of bites or stings such as those from bees, wasps, or ants in sensitive subjects, funnel-web spider bites and bites of the blue-ringed octopus and the cone shell.[51,56,57,58] It can also be used for sea snake bites.[53] However, exceptions when the method should *not* be applied include ant, bee and wasp stings in normal, nonsensitive subjects, red-back spider bites and jellyfish stings[56] and, as stated earlier, after viper or spitting cobra bites. Where pressure immobilization is impractical (e.g. a bite on the body), then infiltration around the bite site with diluted adrenaline (epinephrine) is suggested by Sprivulis and Jelinek.[51]

5. *Suction:* suction apparatus is available in many commercial snake bite kits but is probably of doubtful value. Suction by mouth entails a definite risk of absorption of venom through the oral or intestinal mucous membranes. In general, suction is not recommended for snake bite.[45]

6. *Incision:* Incisions over fang marks as a first aid measure is not recommended.

7. *Other local measures*, such as freezing, injection of antivenom, EDTA or other agents into the bite and application of permanganate crystals to incised wounds, have no place in the management of snake bites, and can only serve to aggravate tissue damage.

Antivenom

Some 30 centers in different countries manufacture antivenom appropriate to local snake species. Polyvalent antisera generally cover most bites encountered, but in the case of certain snakes (e.g. boomslang) monospecific antisera are required. Antivenom is preferably given intravenously. In the past it has sometimes been suggested that a small intradermal test dose of antivenom be given. However, prevailing opinion is that, to quote Eddelston et al:[59] 'There is no point giving a test dose of antivenom as it poorly predicts the individuals who will have an anaphylactoid response.' Adrenaline (epinephrine) should always be at hand to combat possible anaphylaxis. However, adrenaline may induce serious cardiovascular effects, especially in adults. It is advisable to give a corticosteroid, such as hydrocortisone, prior to antivenom as this tends to modify serum reactions as well as having anti-inflammatory and antihypotensive effects. Corticosteroids will not, however, prevent anaphylaxis. In a recent Cochrane Review[60] based upon one trial, the authors concluded that 'routine prophylactic adrenaline for polyvalent antivenom known to have high adverse event rates seems sensible' but they believed that 'antihistamine appears to be of no obvious benefit in preventing acute reactions from antivenoms.'

Once a decision to administer antivenom has been reached, it must be given in adequate dosage.[61] Pearn[62] has commented that as many as 10–12 ampoules may be required to neutralize the pro-coagulant components of bites by the Australian Brown Snake. It must be emphasized that the dosage of antivenom for children is the same as that for adults.[45] Antivenom is best given in an i.v. drip, diluted in two to four times its volume of normal saline over a period of half an hour. A recommended initial i.v. dose is 50 ml of the polyvalent antivenom and the volume of diluent can be adjusted. This should be repeated every 4 h if clinical response is not satisfactory and if necessary up to 200 ml should be given within the first 24 h. The doses of the different antivenoms differ quite substantially. When large doses are used, steroids should be continued to modify possible serum sickness reactions. Anaphylactoid reactions generally respond quickly to prompt adrenaline (epinephrine) injection. If a doctor is not available, the usual dose of antivenom that can be tolerated intramuscularly is about 20 ml.

In the case of ophthalmia due to a spitting cobra, the affected eye should be well washed with water or other bland fluid. Instillation of dilute antivenom is not recommended (G. Muller, personal communication).

ELISA kits (CSL Diagnostics, Australia), suitable for field use, are available in some countries such as Australia for venom detection and species identification in snake bite washings, blood or urine.[51,61] Thus in Australia, it is recommended that snake bite wounds are *not* washed as part of initial first aid technique.[51]

Further supportive care

Unless it has been shown with the passage of some hours that the bite is trivial all cases of poisonous snake bite require admission to hospital.

If severe bulbar or respiratory paralysis has developed, airway suction, oxygen and assisted respiration are indicated.

Management of acute renal failure should be anticipated by adequate i.v. replacement, careful monitoring of input and output, urinalysis and measurement of plasma urea and electrolytes and tests for myoglobinuria (including rhabdomyolysis).

Hemorrhagic manifestations require careful appraisal with a coagulation profile as hemorrhagins (Russell's viper), fibrin degradation products (boomslang) or intravascular clotting (puff adder) can be responsible. Antivenom administration is the only treatment modality which is effective. Other supportive measures include: i.v. vitamin K, blood transfusion, fresh plasma or fibrinogen, low molecular weight dextran, or alpha-aminocaproic acid may be required according to circumstances. The use of heparin is not recommended.[49]

In the event of severe local swelling, the limb should be kept slightly elevated on a pillow. Bullae should not be burst as this increases the likelihood of infection. Skin or fascial release to ease jeopardized circulation, debridement of necrotic tissue, and subsequent grafting or amputation are not uncommonly required, especially in untreated puff adder bites.

The prime cause of death from snake bites is delay in getting the patient to a medical facility. Sutherland[63] in Australia and Gold et al[47] in the USA have emphasized that snake bite deaths are more common in children and the elderly and result from:

1. victims not being observed for an adequate period – suspected snake bite victims should be observed for at least 12–24 h after the bite;
2. antivenom being withheld despite clear indication of systemic envenomation;
3. giving the wrong antivenom – often more than once;
4. giving too little of the correct antivenom or not giving more antivenom if signs and symptoms reoccur.

Pearn[62] has pointed out that a chronic elapid envenomation syndrome may develop in patients who have not been given antivenom for whatever reason, after a snake bite. This may involve both local and systemic effects including lassitude, weakness, loss of appetite and nausea.

Prevention

To develop a snake bite prevention strategy for a particular locality, health care workers need to understand the epidemiology of snake bites for their particular area along the lines discussed for Papua New Guinea by Williams and Winkel.[48] However, general guidelines include:

1. Establish where your closest medical facility and local poisons information center are and have their telephone numbers readily at hand.
2. Treat all snakes with respect.
3. Endeavor to know the snakes in your area.
4. Watch out in summer months, particularly after first rains. Be careful when walking at night; use a torch.
5. Wear boots and leggings or at least shoes and socks when walking in the bush (80% of human snake bites are on the legs and 55% on the ankle and foot).
6. Avoid thickly bushed country, long grass, etc.
7. Do not panic and run away when confronted by a snake; movement will attract attention whereas the snake is likely to move off if you keep still.
8. Keep an appropriate anti-snake bite kit with you.

It has also been found important in Australia to emphasize the need to believe a child who claims to have been bitten by a snake.[64]

Detailed coverage of dealing with snake bites can be found in Brent et al[65] and the publications of Warrell.[49,66,67]

INSECTS, SPIDERS, TICKS, BEETLES, SCORPIONS, CENTIPEDES AND CATERPILLARS

Hymenoptera stings

All stinging insects, such as bees, wasps, hornets and ants, are included in the order Hymenoptera. Bee venom contains many toxic fractions, the most important being mellitin, which alters capillary permeability, causes local pain, hemolyzes red cells, and lowers blood pressure. The venom also contains antigenic components which are capable of invoking an allergic hypersensitivity response in a significant proportion of the population if subjected to a subsequent challenge. Cross-antigenicity may occur between wasp and bee stings and even on occasions, the rare stings by bumblebees.

In Australia, bee stings and bee sting allergy continue to be a major cause of venom-related mortality[68] and serious clinical problems are becoming more common owing to severe allergy to jumper ant (*Myrmecia pilosula*)[69] and bull ant (*Myrmecia pyriformis*) bites and stings.

The management of insect stings has been well reviewed by Reisman.[70] In general terms, uncomplicated stings require no treatment, apart from mild analgesics. Bee sting barbs should be carefully removed with a flat blade, taking care not to express further venom, which will happen if the sting is grasped with forceps. It has been claimed that meat tenderizer, available in most homes, applied in a dilute solution (a quarter teaspoon mixed with 1 teaspoon of water), rubbed into the sting denatures the protein and relieves all pain within seconds. In sensitive individuals, however, even a single sting may result in acute anaphylactic shock with urticaria, hypotension, tachycardia and sweating, glottic edema, or bronchospasm. Prompt treatment is vital. Adrenaline (epinephrine) is indicated. In the case of laryngeal edema, hydrocortisone should be injected intravenously. Tracheostomy may be life saving in the event of severe edema of the glottis.

Skin tests to detect hypersensitivity to Hymenoptera stings are unreliable. However, children who are known to react in a hypersensitive manner should undergo desensitization with a carefully planned immunization schedule, using venom immunotherapy (VIT) – a point reiterated in a recent analysis of bee sting mortality in Australia.[68] Hymenoptera antigen immunotherapy may become more reliable with the development and use of pure venom immunization and phospholipase A, when and if it becomes available. However, children appear to exhibit considerably less frequent severe side-effects to stings than adults, which has led Valentine et al[71] to believe that immunotherapy is unnecessary for most children allergic to insect stings.

Multiple bee stings may induce a life-threatening toxic syndrome due to the cumulative effect of the toxins (short chain peptides, vasoactive amines and antigens). Bee venoms also possess hemolytic properties and multiple stings, usually in excess of 100, may result in significant hemolysis with acute anemia and subsequent renal failure, rhabdomyolysis and hepatic, respiratory and cardiac dysfunction. Cases of massive bee stings should be admitted to hospital and carefully observed for early signs of these complications, where prompt treatment can be instituted and renal failure minimized by ensuring a high urine output. Biphasic renal failure has been known to occur with early renal failure due to hemolysis and a second episode of azotemia about 10 d later, corresponding with a depressed serum complement C3 level and nephritic changes on renal biopsy – a phenomenon probably representing a serum sickness reaction caused by a large volume of foreign protein.

Studies in Australia have shown that 'Stingose' (an aqueous solution of 20% aluminum sulfate and 1.1% surfactant) is an effective, wide-acting first aid treatment to counteract the venoms of insects, marine invertebrates and plants when applied topically soon after the bite or sting.

The application of ice packs to insect stings (and platypus stings in Australia) will help to relieve local pain.[72]

Spider bites

Only a small fraction of the several hundred genera of spiders contain poisonous species and Alexander[73] has discussed these in detail. Although spiders belonging to the genera *Latrodectus* and *Loxosceles* can be dangerous to humans, most spider bites cause only minor clinical effects.[74] The topic is well covered in Brent et al.[65]

Latrodectism

Latrodectus mactans (the black widow spider of the USA), *L. indistinctus* (the button spider of South Africa), and *L. geometricus* (the brown widow spider – a cosmopolitan species) are the commonest species of the genus being widely distributed throughout the warmer areas of the world. In Australia, *L. hasseltii* (red-back spider) and in New Zealand, *L. katipo* (katipo spider) are found.[58,73]

Of the various species and subspecies of the genus *Latrodectus*, only the females are hazardous to humans. They have black or dark velvety globular bodies about 15 mm in length with orange–red markings often in the shape of an hourglass on the ventral surface of the abdomen. While they can be found under garden rocks, they tend to spin their webs in dark places, such as buildings (and especially outbuildings), garage doors, garden furniture and post boxes. Another favorite place is under lavatory seats – hence the number of bites which occur on the buttocks or genitalia. *Latrodectus* venoms (alpha-latrotoxin) possess neurotoxic properties, causing the release of peripheral neurotransmitters. Following a bite from *Latrodectus*, there is a very variable local reaction. Signs of systemic envenomation occur between 20 and 200 min later. There is often a regional lymphadenopathy within 30 min of the bite, followed by severe muscular pains involving the limbs and trunk with tightness around the chest and abdominal rigidity which may mimic an acute abdomen. Hyperreflexia is often present. Death is rare, even in untreated cases, but when it occurs, is usually due to respiratory

failure. Pressure immobilization should *not* be used as the venom is slow acting and pressure will tend to increase the pain. A cold compress can reduce pain at the site of the bite. Treatment is aimed at relieving muscular spasm. It is worth noting, however, that only about 25% of people bitten progress to systemic envenomation, depending on the species of *Latrodectus* involved.[58] Calcium gluconate 10% (5–10 ml by slow i.v. injection) is effective in temporarily depressing the excited neuromuscular junctions. However, specific *Latrodectus* antivenom is the only treatment modality which will relieve pain and is available in most endemic areas.[61] The antivenom should be given intravenously (5 ml) and if necessary repeated. If the victim shows only a mild local reaction to the bite and no systemic effects are detectable after 24 h then antivenom should not be given.[63] The possibility of adverse serum reactions although uncommon should be borne in mind and adrenaline (epinephrine) and corticosteroids should always be at hand.

The effects of untreated Redback spider bites can persist for weeks to months – a picture similar to that seen in chronic fatigue syndrome.[70]

Loxoscelism

The genus *Loxosceles* (the violin spiders) includes many long-legged spiders occurring throughout Latin America as well as in focal areas elsewhere. The venom is cytotoxic and a bite is accompanied by severe local pain and bullous skin lesions, rapidly followed by marked edema, which may progress to necrosis. It may also induce systemic effects including hemolysis, coagulopathy and sepsis. Treatment is aimed at controlling the local reaction. Parenteral antihistamines have been shown to decrease both the pain and the swelling.

Funnel web and related mouse spiders

In Australia, the Sydney funnel web spider (*Atrax robustus*), and various species of the genus *Hadronyche* are the cause of serious spider bites each year. These are large aggressive spiders which rear up before attacking when disturbed and in this group of spiders, it is the male which is the more dangerous. They have a complex venom (robustoxin, an excitatory neurotoxin) and with multiple bites being the rule, considerable pain and panic ensue. In cases where systemic envenomation develops, it may occur within about 10 min of the bite, with dry mouth, circumoral paresthesia, salivation, nausea and vomiting. Muscular fasciculation is regarded by Raven and Churchill[75] as the unique characteristic of funnel web bites. Pulmonary edema and loss of consciousness may occur, and death can result from cardiac arrest.

In management of bites from this spider, atropine and diazepam are said to help.[73] Encouraging results have been obtained in the development of a funnel web spider venom antagonist.

It is claimed that the bite of several species of spider, such as the white-tailed spider *Lampona cylindrata* in Australia can cause chronic nonhealing skin ulcers,[58,76] but definitive evidence is lacking.[74] This condition is sometimes termed 'necrotic arachnidism' or 'necrotic araneism' although Warrell[74] is not happy with this terminology and feels it is misleading. Other spiders in Australia which are sometimes claimed to be dangerous, are the wolf spider (*Lycosa* spp.) and the mouse spider (*Missulena occatoria*).[58]

Tick bites: tick paralysis

Ticks are the vectors of a number of human diseases in both tropical and temperate regions. These include the tick bite fevers, certain arbovirus diseases and Lyme disease due to *Borrelia burgdorferi*.[77] However, as well as this role in the transmission of infectious diseases, dealt with elsewhere, tick bites may cause itching, irritation, can become secondarily infected and in some species, may cause paralysis.

Engorging ticks should be encouraged to detach themselves, by applying a lubricant such as liquid paraffin, before gently extracting them. They should never be hastily pulled off, as the tick's mouthparts may be retained in the skin. This may subsequently give rise to a granuloma composed of a dense dermal granulomatous reaction associated with overlying pseudoepitheliomatous hyperplasia, which on occasions may be so marked in biopsy material that it can lead the unwary pathologist to an erroneous diagnosis of squamous carcinoma. On other occasions, the bite may lead to ulceration which is slow to heal. It remains covered by a necrotic, black eschar which takes many days to separate or the lesion may persist for months as a granuloma under the skin.[62]

Although rare, deaths from anaphylaxis following a tick bite are recorded.[62]

Certain ticks of the genera *Ixodes*, *Dermacentor*, *Haemaphysalis*, *Rhipicephalus* and *Hyalomma* produce a neurotoxin in their saliva which may cause 'tick paralysis'. The condition is commoner in children than in adults and particularly tends to afflict girls, probably because their longer hair hides the tick engorging on the scalp or neck, often with little or no local discomfort. A period of irritability starts 5–7 d after the tick has started feeding. This is followed by ascending symmetrical flaccid paralysis. Initially there is difficulty in walking and standing.[73] Within a day or two, paralysis spreads up from the legs to involve the trunk, arms and neck. Bulbar involvement causes dysphagia, slurring of speech and may result in death from respiratory failure. A local paralysis of the face, for example, may result when the tick is attached to the eardrum. Sensory changes are minimal although there may be paresthesia in the paralyzed limbs. The cerebrospinal fluid remains normal. Mortality may be significant, although death is uncommon if the engorging tick is removed.[73] Tick paralysis should be considered in the differential diagnosis of Guillain–Barré syndrome and it can mimic poliomyelitis.[73] Rapid and complete recovery usually attends the removal of the offending tick, although sometimes neuroparalysis may become transiently worse after removal of the tick. In Australia a canine tick antivenom is available[61] and has been used in children with promising results.

Beetles

Two large families of beetles, found in many parts of the world, produce urticating toxins. These are the Staphylinidae (rove beetles) and the Meloidae (blister beetles).

In Africa, and parts of Asia, America and Europe, rove beetle dermatitis due to the genus *Paederus* poses a difficult problem. When the beetles are brushed off the skin, or crushed, an irritant toxic principle, paederin, is released. This may cause blistering 1–2 d later. The blisters vesicate in 2–8 d and have a tendency to spread as a result of the release of fluid. Thereafter, the lesions flatten and dry out with subsequent peeling. On occasions the blistering is accompanied by systemic symptoms such as headache, fever, myalgia and arthralgia. A severe conjunctivitis, commonly known as 'Nairobi eye' results if paederin comes into contact with the eyes.

Several genera of Meloidae, including *Lytta vesicatoris*, the 'Spanish fly', produce a vesicant, cantharidin, which is falsely credited with aphrodisiac properties, but which is toxic if ingested or absorbed through the skin.

In the treatment of dermatitis due to rove or blister beetles topical application of compresses, such as magnesium sulfate is beneficial, and eye lesions should be bathed with isotonic saline.[73] Additionally the skin should be thoroughly washed with soap and water as should all contaminated clothing.

The condition termed 'Christmas eye' in Australia is as yet of undetermined origin. It may prove to be due to an orthopteran of some type, but a blister beetle seems more likely.

Scorpion stings

Scorpions have a single caudally placed sting with which they can inject venom. Some varieties, such as the genera *Parabuthus* (Southern Africa), *Androctonus* (North Africa; Turkey), *Centruroides* (Arizona; Texas) are dangerous especially to young children. Scorpion venoms are neurotoxins and their overall effect is hyperactivity of peripheral nerves, both somatic and autonomic. Alexander[73] notes that scorpion stings are more serious in children than in adults and that most deaths occur in children.

Serious stings are characterized by severe burning pain and local swelling at the site of the sting, hyperesthesia and myalgia in the affected limb, quickly followed by generalized weakness, muscle spasm, excessive salivation and rhinorrhea, excitement, coma, convulsions (especially in small children) and respiratory failure – often fatal.[73] Pancreatitis is a reported complication in severe cases of scorpionism. Less venomous varieties or stings in older subjects may result in only local pain and swelling, sometimes with lymphangitis.

Treatment

In many countries, it has been noted that scorpion stings in children can have a high mortality rate unless adequate symptomatic and specific therapy are given – especially respiratory support. Prompt application of a crepe bandage will slow the spread of venom but there may be problems in applying this to children because of the pain. Ice packs applied to the sting site are seldom effective and the most effective method of pain relief is infiltration of the sting area with local anesthetic (Muller, personal communication). Scorpion antivenom is available and this, together with respiratory support, can be life saving in cases of severe envenomation; 10 ml should be given intravenously, as soon as possible, keeping adrenaline (epinephrine) and corticosteroids on hand in case of anaphylaxis. When antivenom is not available, general supportive treatment is needed and subcutaneous atropine and i.v. calcium gluconate have been reported to be effective. *The need for assisted respiration must be anticipated.* In milder stings injection of a local anesthetic into the site is often the only treatment needed. The topic is covered by Brent et al.[65]

Centipedes

Centipedes are segmented arthropods with one pair of legs per segment. The first pair of legs are modified to form toxognaths with strong claws on which open the ducts from the venom glands. Bites from centipedes can cause considerable pain and swelling, and sometimes local ulceration and spreading lymphangitis result.

Caterpillars (lepidopterism/erucism)

Lepidopterism refers to a disease caused by contact with adult or larval butterflies and moths, while erucism is an illness caused by the larval and pupal stages of these insects.[78] The fine, spiny, venom-containing hairs of some species of caterpillar induce a very painful urticarial or vesicular dermatitis. This may be acquired by actual contact with the larva or from hairs blown in the wind. Where caterpillars are very prolific, severe symptoms may occasionally be induced in children, with extensive rashes, fever, vomiting and even paralysis. Hairs are best removed by applying adhesive tape to the site. Immersion in a very hot bath is soothing, and analgesics may be required. There is little evidence for the development of an allergic response from repeated exposure. Severe clinical effects including mild to severe shock and coma can follow contact with the stinging hairs from caterpillars of the genus *Megalopyge* in the southern USA and parts of Latin America.[73]

Calamine lotion applied to caterpillar hair stings helps alleviate the pain and removal of stinging hairs with sellotape stripping is suggested as a first aid measure.[73]

STINGS FROM VENOMOUS MARINE ANIMALS

Stings from venomous marine animals can be a major health problem in many parts of the world, including Australia, Papua New Guinea, South-East Asia, Asia and the Far East, the Mediterranean, North and Latin America, the Caribbean and even Russia.[79] As might be expected, the problem is greatest in tropical waters and its magnitude can be gauged by figures from Australia where, over the summer months of 1990–1991, more than 18 000 people were treated for marine stings[80] while in the USA, in Chesapeake Bay alone, about 500 000 jellyfish envenomations occur each year.[81]

Although mostly seasonal, the problem of marine stings in the waters of northern Australia is so significant that it often precludes swimming during the summer months, except in areas protected by special nets – termed 'stinger enclosures'.

Overall, the most common cause of jellyfish stings are coelenterates of the genus *Physalia*, the common blue bottle or Portuguese man-of-war. Stings from these animals occur in the water or on the beach and, especially with the short-tentacled species, can be painful for up to an hour or so, but are not usually life threatening.[72] Stings from the multiple-tentacled species, however, can be severe and rare fatalities are on record.[72,80]

The so-called 'nematocyst dermatitis' from the blue bottle jellyfish is often exacerbated by the tentacles sticking to the skin, with subsequent discharge of the nematocysts causing ongoing pain and discomfort.

Treatment of blue bottle stings consists of covering the affected area with a plastic bag containing ice to alleviate the pain.[72] The use of heat to reduce blue bottle sting pain is more controversial, needing further research but is not really practical in the first aid situation.[82]

By contrast, stings due to the seawasp or box jellyfish (*Chironex* spp.) are excruciatingly painful and are associated with a significant mortality. Thus stings by this species in northern Australia have resulted in over 300 cases between 1984 and 1994, with in excess of 80 deaths being recorded from these stings in the twentieth century in Australia – often only minutes after the sting has occurred in the water.[76,83]

The bodies of people stung by this jellyfish are often covered with long red wheals which, if the victim survives, can result in permanent scarring.[72] Reactions to the sting may, however, in some cases, be delayed for some time.[80] The toxin of this species has three modes of action – it damages the skin, attacks the red blood cells and, most importantly, can affect the heart and respiration.[76,83]

The treatment for *Chironex* stings is the immediate application of vinegar by pouring it liberally over the affected area to prevent further nematocyst discharge. Irrigation with fresh water is contraindicated as it will cause further nematocyst discharge. In severe cases, CPR can be life saving[83] and the use of a specific *Chironex fleckeri* antivenom produced by the Commonwealth Serum Laboratories in Melbourne, Australia is beneficial[53,61] but may need to be given within minutes and possibly at high doses to be effective.[82] The recommended dosage should not be reduced for children.[80] Fenner[82] has suggested that the use of antivenom with magnesium might be worth considering if the antivenom alone fails.

It is worth reiterating that vinegar is essential to inhibit the discharge of further nematocysts of *Chironex* but will not reduce pain and, paradoxically, may initially increase pain. Compression-immobilization bandaging, once thought to be helpful,[53,84] is now not recommended.[82]

In Australia, a third type of jellyfish sting is the so-called 'Irukandji sting syndrome' caused by a minute carybdeid jellyfish (*Carukia barnesi*) and a number of other species;[82] this sting can result in severe joint, low back, and trunk pains; muscle cramps; anxiety; headache; shivering; sweating; hypotension and cardiac involvement.[53,76,82,83,85] Stings usually occur in the water in the afternoon and the jellyfish, being so small, is often not seen.

In Irukandji syndrome, initial treatment with vinegar should be used to prevent further envenomation and this should be followed by treatment for the pain using ice packs.[82] The use of 20 mg i.v. furosemide (frusemide) proved beneficial in one case.[80] Immediate transfer to hospital for intensive care treatment is advisable. The use of sublingual nitrate sprays, topical analgesia (topical Fentanyl) and i.v. magnesium sulphate are all discussed by Fenner.[82]

Other jellyfish known to cause stinging of humans include the large carybdeids ('firejellies') in Tomoya or Morbakka stings; the 'hairjelly' or 'sea blubber', *Cyanea*, and *Pelagia noctiluca*, the 'mauve blubber'.[72,83]

There are, of course, a large number of other potentially dangerous marine animals, including stingrays, the blue ringed octopus, sea urchins, starfish, stonefish and lion fish amongst others.[79] The management of such a diverse range of envenomations is obviously beyond the scope of this chapter, but the topic has been well reviewed by Williamson et al,[79] Fenner,[82] Pearn,[83] Auerbach[86] and is covered in detail in Brent et al.[65]

ACKNOWLEDGEMENTS

We would like to thank Dr Gerhardus Muller for his comments, criticisms and his many constructive suggestions.

SUDDEN INFANT DEATH SYNDROME

Sudden unexpected infant deaths have been recognized since antiquity, but it was not until post-neonatal mortality rates substantially fell in the Western world during the early part of the twentieth century that greater attention was paid to the phenomenon of unexpected and unexplained deaths in apparently healthy infants.

Sudden infant death syndrome (SIDS) was proposed in 1969 as a descriptive term for those infant deaths that were unexpected and remained unexplained after thorough investigation. In 1994 a more precise definition of sudden infant death syndrome was proposed.[87]

The sudden death of an infant, which is unexplained after review of the clinical history, examination of the circumstances of death, and postmortem examination

In 1892 Templeman,[88] and in 1904 Willcox[89] noted the excess of unexpected infant deaths in the poorest families, and agreed that the majority of such deaths were due to accidental overlaying whilst bed-sharing, recommending that parents be encouraged to use cribs for their babies to sleep in. One hundred years later the American Academy of Pediatrics made a similar recommendation, though the evidence for this has been the subject of wide debate.[90–92]

EPIDEMIOLOGY OF UNEXPECTED DEATHS
Diagnosis of SIDS and subsequent decline in the SIDS rate

The diagnosis of SIDS is unique in that it is not a cause of death but rather a diagnosis of exclusion, arrived at only after thorough investigation. Only when recognized causes of infant death have been excluded can the death be labeled SIDS and there are valid concerns that such labeling could attribute too much homogeneity to what might be disparate causes of death.[93,94]

From the 1950s to the late 1980s the number of unexpected and unexplained deaths in the UK was probably between 1400 and 2000 per year, giving a rate of around 2/1000 live births.[95] In the late 1980s epidemiological evidence from several different countries[96–101] suggested that SIDS could be related to infants sleeping in the prone position. In 1991 the 'Back to Sleep' campaign was initiated in the UK to encourage parents to avoid placing their infants on their front and the SIDS rate fell from a peak of 2.3 deaths/1000 live births in 1988 to 0.7 per 1000 live births in 1994 (Fig. 6.2). Similar dramatic reductions have since been observed in many other countries following such an intervention campaign. The possibility that other modifiable risk factors might be amenable to further interventions in this mysterious group of conditions has led to multiple epidemiological studies of the residual deaths. Further identification of other unsafe infant care practices, particularly within the sleep environment have led to additional amendments and revision of the initial campaign message and probably helped to reduce the rate further over the last 10 years to 0.4 per 1000 live births. This equates to the prevention of over 10 000 infant deaths in England and Wales since the campaign was first launched, and more than 100 000 worldwide.

The fall in numbers of deaths has been accompanied by several major changes in the epidemiologic characteristics of SIDS,[102] most notably an increased proportion of the deaths occurring in deprived families and whilst bed-sharing. Some pathologists are reluctant to use the label 'SIDS', preferring to use the term 'unascertained', when parents have consumed alcohol or illegal drugs or the circumstances of death raise the unproven possibility of overlying.[103] Such practices emphasize the importance of a detailed multiprofessional review in establishing the final allocated 'cause' of unexpected infant deaths (see later).

Epidemiologic features of SIDS

Prior to the 'Back to Sleep' campaign in 1991, many epidemiologic characteristics of SIDS had been described. Unexpected, unexplained deaths of infants occurred in all cultures but the incidence varied widely. There were relatively fewer SIDS deaths in several Asian cultures but more deaths amongst certain indigenous populations such as Maoris, Australian Aborigines and Native Americans. The incidence in the UK

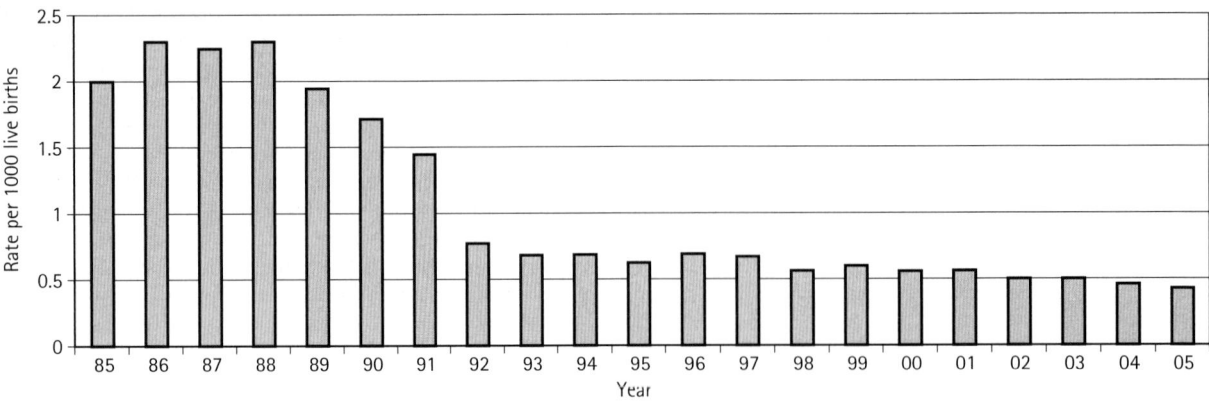

Fig. 6.2 SIDS rate in England and Wales 1985–2005 (Office for National Statistics and the Foundation for the Study of Infant Deaths).

was lower than in the white populations of New Zealand and Australia but higher than in the Nordic countries. The majority of deaths occurred within the first 6 months of life, with a peak around the third and fourth month. Many of the deaths occurred during the night-time sleep periods, and although some studies noted an excess of deaths at weekends this has not been consistent.[104–108] More deaths occurred in males and in winter months. SIDS occurred in all social strata but was more common in the socioeconomically deprived groups, particularly if parents smoked. Many of the SIDS infants had lower birth weight, shorter gestation and more perinatal problems. There was a strong correlation with young maternal age and higher parity and the risk increased with multiple births, single motherhood or a poor obstetric history.

Many of the risk factors associated with SIDS are also closely associated with other infant deaths; only the characteristic age distribution and high prevalence of tobacco exposure distinguished SIDS infants from infants who died suddenly and unexpectedly from identifiable causes.[109] Deaths from congenital malformations decrease steadily from early age whilst deaths from respiratory or infectious diseases remain relatively constant over the first year of life.[110] Overall, infant mortality rates are highest in the first month after birth, when infants are at their most vulnerable.[111,112] However few SIDS deaths occur in the first month, with a peak occurring at 3–4 months and a steady decline thereafter. Whilst smoking is most prevalent amongst mothers in the more disadvantaged socioeconomic groups, the incidence of smoking is higher amongst the mothers of SIDS infants than matched controls in all social groupings.[108,113]

It is perhaps in the infant sleeping environment that the epidemiological study of SIDS has had the most success. Prone sleeping was actively encouraged in some Western countries in the 1960s and 1970s[114] to improve infant posture and skeletal growth,[115] prevent flattening of the skull[116,117] and avoid the perceived risk of aspiration in the supine position.[118] This was also a time when neonatal intensive care units were expanding and apparent benefits of using the prone position were found amongst pre-term infants including less apnea, better gastric emptying, better oxygenation, and more effective ribcage and abdominal coupling with decreased work of breathing.[119–122] What was best in the early neonatal period for the relatively small number of pre-term infants however was not necessarily beneficial for the rest of the infant population or beyond the immediate neonatal period. Historical references to infant sleeping position in art and early medical texts suggest that very few if any infants were placed prone to sleep before the twentieth century.[123]

In the 1980s a number of population-based studies identified the prone sleeping position and heavy wrapping and/or warm environments as major risk factors associated with SIDS.[101,124–126] Gilbert found that the combination of viral infection and heavy wrapping was associated with a high relative risk[124] whilst in a study from Tasmania Ponsonby[125] found the risk from prone position was potentiated by overnight heating, swaddling, recent infection and mattress type. Williams confirmed these findings in a study from New Zealand and found a small additive effect if the mother smoked.[127]

'BACK TO SLEEP' CAMPAIGNS

Although positioning and wrapping were not sufficient to fully explain the death they could be linked to some causal chain of events and intervention campaigns to advise parents against these practices were instigated in many countries from 1990 onwards. In all countries in which risk reduction campaigns were conducted, a fall in infant prone sleeping was followed by a fall in SIDS rate. Also publicized in some campaigns was the potential risk of heavy wrapping. Studies of control infants in Avon before and after the 'Back to Sleep' campaign[124,128] showed that the thermal resistance (tog value) of bedding and clothing with which normal infants were usually covered fell by almost half after the 'back to Sleep' campaign, and the winter peaks of SIDS deaths have almost disappeared in the UK.

EPIDEMIOLOGIC CHARACTERISTICS SINCE THE FALL IN NUMBERS OF SIDS

Distal factors

A longitudinal study conducted in Avon from 1984 to 2003[102] showed that amongst SIDS families the proportion from the most disadvantaged socioeconomic groups rose from 47% to 75%. This change in the socioeconomic distribution of SIDS families was accompanied by an increased proportion of single mothers, younger mothers, mothers who smoke and lower birth weight infants. The prevalence of maternal smoking during pregnancy amongst SIDS mothers (80–90%) was twice the level expected amongst control mothers with similarly deprived socioeconomic backgrounds,[113] lending support to the hypothesis that infant exposure to tobacco smoke is some part of a causal mechanism. There is a clear increase in risk of SIDS with increasing levels of exposure to tobacco smoke, both in utero and after birth[129–131] and a recent review by Mitchell and Milerad suggests this risk has grown despite advice against smoking in almost all risk reduction campaigns.[132] In recent studies over one third of SIDS victims were preterm, compared to a UK population prevalence of 5% for preterm delivery. For such infants the effects of other risk factors in combination with the increased risk from prematurity leads to very high risk (e.g. for preterm or low birthweight infants put down on the side: OR = 9.13 [95% CI 4.93–16.90], and for those put down prone: OR = 62.8 [95% CI 12.06–327]).[133]

The previously recognized increase in risk of SIDS with increasing birth order may be changing. The longitudinal study from Avon suggests that SIDS is now most common amongst first-born infants.[102] Several studies have now shown no evidence that immunization is associated with an increased risk of SIDS, and some evidence that the risk may be reduced.[134]

Proximal factors

New evidence on risks within the infant sleeping environment has changed some of the advice now given to parents.

Risk of positioning infants on the side to sleep

Before the 'Back to Sleep' campaign few studies had looked at the use of the side sleeping position and the findings were inconclusive;[126,135–137] the side position with the lower arm extended to avoid infants rolling on their front was suggested as a safe alternative to supine sleeping. More recent studies[128,138–142] show the side sleeping position carries a significant risk, partly because the position is unstable, and some infants who roll from side to prone have difficulty extricating themselves from this position. Certain infants with abnormalities of the upper airway (e.g. Pierre Robin syndrome) may experience airway obstruction if placed supine, and some may benefit from side or occasionally prone positioning for sleep, but many can be safely placed supine. Whilst gastro-esophageal reflux is slightly reduced in the prone position compared to supine, the increased risk of SIDS means that this position should not be used to treat reflux unless this is causing severe symptoms (e.g. growth failure or recurrent aspiration) that have not responded to alternative treatments. Apart from these uncommon conditions, in most countries the only recommended sleeping position for infants is supine. In some countries use of the side position may have increased despite knowledge of its potential risks,[143,144] many parents and health care professionals citing either outdated SIDS guidelines or fear of aspiration, cyanosis or apnea when the infant is placed supine.[145–148] These concerns are not supported by findings from either pathology or epidemiology. A review of 196 infant deaths in South Australia found evidence of aspiration of gastric contents into the airways and alveoli of three infants, all of whom were found face down in the prone position.[149] Similar findings linking aspiration with the prone rather than the supine position have been found in the UK,[150] whilst a large cohort study of over 8000 surviving UK infants showed no association between the prevalence of vomiting and infant sleeping position.[151] A recent study from New Zealand[152] has linked the increase in sleeping supine with nonsynostotic plagio-cephaly, recommending that parents should vary the infant head position when putting them down to sleep and to give their infants 5 min of supervised 'tummy time' each day. This may also help reduce the risk of 'unaccustomed prone' position, when infants roll into or fall asleep in this position for the first time. In studies in Australia, the US and the UK, supine sleeping was not linked to apnea or cyanosis and no demonstrable increase in symptoms or illness amongst supine sleeping infants was found.[151,153,154]

Studies in the UK[155] and in Canada[156] have shown minor differences in gross motor skills in early infancy with infants who usually sleep supine, showing slightly slower developmental progress than those who sleep prone. In the UK study these differences had disappeared by age 18 months, but in the smaller Canadian study the differences, though small were still present at 15 months.

Both the minor developmental disadvantages and the risk of positional plagiocephaly from supine sleep position can be largely prevented by the use of periods of 'tummy time' – placing infants prone for regular periods when awake and supervised.[157]

Risk of soft sleeping surfaces

Soft surfaces for infant sleep have been associated with an increased risk of SIDS[108,158,159] and there is some evidence that this risk is even higher in combination with established risk factors such as the prone sleeping position[160,161] and heavy wrapping or warm environment.[162] Pillows, cushions and bean bags have been used not just as a sleep surface but also as a prop to maintain the body position of a sleeping infant or provide easier access to bottle feeding. This practice presents the additional risk, even to supine sleeping infants, of such objects potentially covering the external airways.[163] This includes the adult size V-shaped pillows used to facilitate breastfeeding.[164] The current advice is to sleep infants on a firm mattress and away from soft objects.

Risk of bedding covering the infant

It is not uncommon for SIDS infants to be discovered dead with bedclothes covering the head and face, indeed 'accidental mechanical suffocation' was, prior to the introduction of the term 'sudden infant death syndrome', a term commonly used to describe these deaths, despite a lack of any evidence of suffocation or asphyxia.[165–169] Uncontrolled observations from early studies[170–173] that around one fifth of SIDS infants were found with bedding covering the face or head were attributed to the agonal struggle just prior to death. Subsequent findings of reduced arousability during the sleep of SIDS infants,[174] observations of undisturbed bedding[175] and lack of such a struggle during recordings of several SIDS infants who died whilst on a monitor[176] do not support the idea that head covering is just a consequence of the terminal event. Whilst postmortem examination cannot distinguish between the possible mechanisms of airway obstruction, re-breathing or thermal stress, over 20% of SIDS victims are found with bedding over the head,[102,140,142,161,170,177–180] ten times more than the incidence amongst live age-matched controls and highly significant even after adjusting for other risk factors. Studies have linked head covering to loose bedding, infant movement down under the covers and the use of duvets or quilts.[102,108,181–183] In 1997 a 'Feet to Foot' campaign, was launched in England and Wales by the Foundation for the Study of Infant Death to encourage parents to tuck the bedding in firmly, avoid using duvets or pillows and place the feet of the infant at the foot of the cot. This approach was subsequently endorsed by the American Academy of Pediatrics.[90,184]

Risk associated with unobserved sleep

Despite a complete absence of supporting evidence, many childcare 'experts' in the 1950s to 1990s recommended that infants should sleep in a room separately from parents.[185,186] Throughout history most human infants slept in a consistently rich sensory environment with close and continual contact between mothers and babies and the solitary sleep experience of Western societies was a recent development.[187] Reports from New Zealand and the UK showed that the risk of SIDS was lower if infants shared a bedroom with parents,[188–190] and further analysis of the UK data suggests that parental supervision for day-time sleeps is equally important.[191] Parental presence during infant sleep does not guarantee the infant would be constantly observed, nor, indeed that parental intervention would prevent death from occurring. However having the sleeping infant nearby during the day may alert parents to circumstances such as young infants rolling from the side to the prone position or bedclothes covering the infant head or face.

Risk associated with bed-sharing

Unexpected infant deaths can occur in any sleep environment. Recent case–control studies show that up to half of the deaths occur whilst infants share a sleep surface ('co-sleep') with an adult,[142,161,192,193] a marked rise from studies in the 1980s. This proportional rise in co-sleeping SIDS deaths has led some authorities, including the American Academy of Pediatrics[90] to recommend against bed-sharing.

Longitudinal data from Avon over the last 20 years shows that although the *proportion* of bed-sharing deaths rose from an average of 16% of all SIDS deaths prior to the 'Back to Sleep' campaign to 34% after the campaign, the *number* of bed-sharing SIDS deaths fell (by 50%), but this is less marked than the 80% fall in deaths occurring in the cot.[102] More worrying is the rise in both prevalence and number of SIDS infants found after sleeping with a parent on a sofa, which carries a markedly increased risk.[128,142,190] At least some of these deaths occurred when mothers inadvertently fell asleep whilst feeding on a sofa during the night.

Bed-sharing is perceived to be and is treated as a risk factor in the field of SIDS epidemiology and when considered in this rudimentary way there is ample evidence to advise against such a practice. On closer inspection however there are several things to be considered. Adjusting for potential confounders specifically associated with the adult co-sleeping environment such as recent alcohol consumption, sleep deprivation, overcrowded conditions and adult-sized duvets renders bed-sharing nonsignificant as a risk factor suggesting it is not bed-sharing itself but the particular circumstances in which bed-sharing occurs that puts an infant at risk.[190] An intriguing aspect of this debate is that in certain Asian cultures where particular forms of mother–infant co-sleeping (sleeping on futons) is common such as Japan[194] and Hong Kong[195] the cot death rates are very low; corresponding to findings in the Bangladeshi[196] and other Asian[197] communities in the UK and the Pacific Island communities in New Zealand.[198] Another aspect is that of generalization: the majority of bed-sharing SIDS mothers smoke whilst the majority of bed-sharing mothers in the population do not. The magnitude of any increase in risk for nonsmoking breast-feeding mothers who are bed-sharing on a firm flat surface, and who have not taken alcohol or other drugs, is unclear, but certainly small.[142,190,199-201] There is also the wider debate beyond the field of SIDS in terms of the potential advantages associated with bed-sharing. Before the last century and in most nonWesternized cultures today the normative practice is for the mother to share a sleep surface with the infant.[202] Postulated, but largely unproven potential physiological benefits of close contact between infants and care-givers include improved cardiorespiratory stability and oxygenation, fewer crying episodes, better thermo-regulation, an increased prevalence and duration of breast-feeding, and enhanced milk production.[203,204]

It is becoming clear from recent studies that bed-sharing both for infants and mothers results in complex interactions which are completely different to isolated sleeping and which need to be understood in detail before applying simplistic labels such as 'safe' or 'unsafe'.[205-207] The unusual level of criticism and hostility generated by the recent Policy Statement by the American Academy of Pediatrics against bed-sharing[90-92] is a testament to the current polarized debate. Current advice in the UK does not advise against bed-sharing but describes particular circumstances when bed-sharing should be avoided. Co-sleeping with an infant on a sofa should always be avoided.

Apparent protective effect of infant pacifier use
The current debate on bed-sharing holds many parallels with the debate on dummy use (pacifiers). Several studies have examined the prevalence of infant dummy use and shown a reduced risk for SIDS.[142,161,193,208-213] Actively encouraging dummy use, like the advice on bed-sharing, has been met with criticism mainly concerning the potential adverse effects on breast-feeding. The evidence of a significant association is not in dispute but whether this association is causal in itself is still being debated.[91,214,215] The mechanism by which a pacifier might reduce the risk of SIDS, or by its absence increase the risk, is unknown, but several mechanisms have been postulated. These include avoidance of the prone sleeping position, protection of the oropharyngeal airway, reduction of gastroesophageal reflux through non-nutrient sucking[209] or lowering the arousal threshold.[216-218] These mechanisms however assume the presence of a pacifier in the infant's mouth but the evidence suggests pacifiers generally fall out within 30 minutes of the infant falling asleep[219] whilst many of the night-time deaths are thought to occur much later during the sleep.[191] Alternatively dummy use may be a marker for some protective factor that has eluded measurement. The physiology not only of infant dummy use, but also non-use amongst routine users and infant thumb sucking, which leads to identical physiological effects but is inhibited by pacifier use[220] deserves further investigation.

Before recommending the use of pacifiers the potential disadvantages must be considered. There appears to be a clear relationship between frequent or continuous pacifier use and a reduction in breastfeeding,[221-224] and a significantly higher risk of otitis media and oral yeast infection.[225-228] Other potential disadvantages include accidents (airway obstruction[229]), strangulation by cords tied to the dummy,[230] eye injuries[231] and dental malocclusion.[232] The current advice in the UK is no longer to discourage the use of dummies but falls short of recommending them as a preventive measure against SIDS.

INFANT PHYSIOLOGY AND PATHOPHYSIOLOGY OF UNEXPECTED DEATH

Whilst the final sequence of events leading to death is not known for the great majority of unexpected infant deaths, and there is no reason to presume that there is a single mechanism involved, a number of studies have been published of unexpected infant deaths that have occurred whilst the infant was undergoing physiological recordings.[176,233] These recordings have shown a range of physiological events leading up to the final collapse and death, but in some infants there was an initial period in which there was normal respiratory activity but a relative tachycardia. In several infants the final event was one of profound bradycardia, with respiratory activity continuing until a late stage. In many of these recordings, despite the carers having been alerted to the bradycardia by audible alarms, and having attempted resuscitation, this was not successful. This sequence of events is more suggestive of a cardiovascular rather than a respiratory event as the primary trigger for the final collapse. One possible physiological explanation for such a pattern might be a catastrophic fall in blood pressure as a consequence of sudden peripheral vasodilatation, e.g. in response to toxins or as a consequence of heat stress.[234]

Several population-based case–control studies have shown that infants who died unexpectedly were more heavily wrapped and more likely to be sleeping in warm rooms than age and community-matched controls.[108,101,201] The increased risk of SIDS from heavy wrapping was greatest for the older infants (more than 3 months of age), and was especially high for those infants with evidence of an acute viral upper respiratory tract infection.[124] In a study of the metabolic response to acute viral upper respiratory tract infection, younger infants (less than 3 months of age) commonly showed a fall in metabolic rate with infection, whilst those over 3 months usually showed an increase, commonly accompanied by fever.[235] The metabolic rate of infants during sleep rises over the first few months after birth, such that by 3 months of age healthy infants excrete up to 50% more heat per unit surface area than in the first week after birth.[236,237] Thus infants over 3 months of age might be more at risk from heavy wrapping that compromised their ability to lose heat, particularly at the time of an acute minor viral infection.

In a population-based observational study of infant thermal care at home most mothers accurately achieved conditions of predicted thermal neutrality for their infants, but younger mothers, those who smoked, and those who did not breast-feed were more likely to wrap their infants more heavily.[238] In a prospective longitudinal laboratory study of mothers and infants sharing a room or sharing a bed for overnight sleep, despite a much warmer microenvironment, infants thermoregulated more effectively, with a slightly greater diurnal fall in rectal temperature when bed-sharing with their mother than when sleeping in a cot adjacent to the mother's bed[207].

The development of the diurnal fall in core temperature occurs at ages between approximately 3 and 4 months, occurring earlier in girls and breastfed infants than in boys or bottle fed infants.[239]

Blackwell and Morris have each shown the potential importance of toxigenic Staphylococci as contributory agents to circulatory collapse and sudden death in infancy.[240,241] Toxin production by such Staphylococci increases with increasing environmental temperature and is minimal below 37 °C.[240] SIDS victims have increased nasopharyngeal colonization with staphylococci compared to healthy age and community-matched controls.[234] In the prone position, or with head covering (particularly in the presence of potential re-breathing), nasopharyngeal temperature is likely to rise above the normal value of 32 °C, with resultant increase in toxin production by any toxigenic staphylococci present on the mucosal surface.[242] Transmucosal absorption of toxin might thus lead to circulatory collapse and death without the need for invasive infection to occur.

Elevated levels of interleukin 6 (IL-6) in the cerebrospinal fluid of SIDS victims compared to age-matched controls dying of known causes raised the possibility of a vigorous pro-inflammatory response being part of the pathophysiology of SIDS.[243]

Drucker has recently shown that common polymorphisms, leading to high levels of pro-inflammatory cytokines (e.g. IL-6, VEGF) or low levels of anti-inflammatory cytokines (e.g. IL-10) are associated with increased risk for unexpected deaths in infants.[242] A high pro-inflammatory response to infection, with vigorous sympathetic activity including peripheral vasoconstriction and pyrexia might indirectly lead to further toxin production in the nasopharynx.

The relationship between the pro-inflammatory cytokine IL-1β and the risk of SIDS is complex, and Moscovis et al[244] have shown potentially important ethnic differences in the patterns of gene polymorphisms. In both Aboriginal Australian and Bangladeshi infants a particular polymorphism (TT) is found, which is uncommon in infants of European origin. This polymorphism is associated with a marked increase in IL-1β production, and increased pro-inflammatory responses on exposure to tobacco smoke. This may partially explain the major difference between Aboriginal Australian infants with high maternal smoking rates and high SIDS rate, and Bangladeshi infants, who are genetically similar with regard to IL-1β, but have very low rates of maternal smoking and very low SIDS rates.

The potential interaction between genetic and environmental factors is further exemplified by the anti-inflammatory cytokine IL-10, production of which is markedly decreased by exposure to tobacco smoke.[244]

Associations have also been described between the risk of SIDS and polymorphisms of genes involved in the development of the autonomic nervous system,[245] various cardiac channelopathies,[246] and the serotonergic system in the brainstem.[247] This latter group is of particular interest in the light of recent histological evidence of abnormalities of serotonergic neurons in the brainstem of SIDS victims.[248]

'TRIPLE RISK' HYPOTHESES AND PROSPECTS FOR PREVENTION OF SIDS

There is considerable evidence that SIDS represents a possible consequence of a wide range of genetic/developmental/environmental interactions.

The 'triple risk' hypothesis – which envisages SIDS occurring as a result of a final insult (one which is not usually fatal on its own) that affects a baby with an intrinsic vulnerability (arising from genetic or early developmental factors), at a potentially vulnerable stage of physiological development (e.g. immunological, respiratory, cardiovascular, thermal), has been proposed in various forms by a number of authors over the past 15 years.[249]

The recent developments in our knowledge of environmental, immunological, genetic and physiological factors in infants, and recognition of the changes in all these systems that occur during the first few months after birth as outlined earlier strongly support a 'triple risk' model of causation for most unexpected infant deaths, including some for which a partial or even a complete 'explanation' can be identified on thorough investigation.

This approach to understanding the pathophysiological processes that may contribute to unexpected infant deaths holds great promise for targeted interventions to further reduce the number of such deaths.

INVESTIGATION AND CLASSIFICATION OF UNEXPECTED INFANT DEATHS

The process of investigation after any unexpected infant death should seek to collect as much information as possible about factors that may have contributed to the death, in order to help understand (and in future possibly prevent) such deaths. It is essential however that the investigation is conducted with both thoroughness and sensitivity, bearing in mind that whilst the great majority of such deaths are natural tragedies it is important to identify those instances in which neglect or abuse may have caused or contributed to the death.[250,251]

The precise nature of the investigation and composition of the investigating team will vary according to the requirements of the relevant state or national legislation. In England, regulations introduced under recent legislation have defined these requirements, which will be mandatory from 2008.[252] These regulations were based upon the conclusions of the Working Party chaired by Baroness Helena Kennedy, which involved wide consultation and contributions from pediatricians, pathologists, police, coroners, social services, Government, the Judiciary and representatives of parents' organization.[251] An overview of the requirements of these regulations is given below as an example of the needs for thorough and integrated investigations.

KENNEDY PROTOCOL FOR INVESTIGATION OF UNEXPECTED INFANT DEATHS[250,251]

The protocol involves emergency first responders, clinical staff, police, pathologists, coroners, social services and other agencies working together and sharing information to minimize duplication and maximize available information to help identify contributory or causal factors. The initial investigation must include a careful and detailed medical, social and environmental history, with a thorough review of the circumstances of death, including visiting and carefully examining the scene of death. This home visit with the parents or carers should ideally be conducted jointly by a pediatrician and a child protection police officer whose combined expertise in infant physiology and development and in forensic examination respectively maximize the potential to recognize both natural and unnatural contributory factors. The pathologist (who must have appropriate pediatric training) should conduct a thorough postmortem examination to an evidence-based protocol,[108,251,253] and should be provided with as full an account as possible of the history, clinical examination of the infant and scene examination before commencing the procedure. At all stages of the investigation all agencies must continue to share information and, except in those rare instances in which criminal prosecution might be compromised by so doing, the parents must be kept fully informed. Meeting the needs of parents for care and support must be central to the process. Finally, when all investigations are completed – usually 2–4 months after the death, a multi-agency case review meeting should be convened – usually in the primary care setting. The aim of this meeting is to ensure that all professionals share information; review, and if possible come to conclusions about the cause of or contributory factors to the death; agree who is to inform the parents of the results of the investigations (usually the pediatrician plus a member of the primary health care team); and produce a report for the coroner to inform and facilitate the Inquest.

Thus the 'cause' of death as finally certified through the coroners' system reflects the full breadth of professional expertise in understanding both natural and possible unnatural contributory or causal factors.

The careful review of potentially contributory factors allows unexpected infant deaths to be separated into those for which no significant contributory factors were identified, those in which one or more factors were found that may have contributed to the death but do not in themselves give a complete explanation, and those for which a complete and sufficient explanation was found. Several classifications of unexpected infant deaths using such approaches have been published, and allow studies to distinguish varying degrees of contribution from environmental, infectious, physiological or genetically determined factors in different infants.[250,254] Table 6.7 shows the Avon Clinicopathological Classification, which is based upon this approach, and has been widely adopted in the UK.[102,108,250,251]

Most epidemiological background factors associated with unexpected but explained infant deaths (i.e. those deaths classified as III in Figure 6.3, e.g. previously unrecognized overwhelming infection) are very similar in character to those factors found amongst SIDS victims (i.e. those deaths classified as I to IIB in Figure 6.3).[109] Indeed there is some evidence that improved investigation has led to an increase in the proportion of deaths that are explained, in particular deaths due to metabolic disorders.[102,108,250] Thus it is important that similar investigation should be applied to all such deaths, and any studies of unexpected infant deaths should include all sudden unexpected deaths in infancy (SUDI), and not be restricted to those classified (either by arbitrary assignment at the beginning of the investigative process, or at the end of a full investigation) as SIDS.

Although there has been some reluctance by professionals to fully engage in such a process, on the grounds that it is demanding of both time and energy, and may not be sustainable, recent studies have shown that with minimal additional resources such an approach can be implemented and sustained over many years.[102] Certainly the savings – both financial and emotional – from avoidance of inappropriate criminal

Table 6.7 The Avon Clinicopathological Classification of Sudden Unexpected Infant Deaths[164,165]*

Classification	0	I A	I B	II A	II B	III
Contributory or potentially 'causal' factors	Information not collected	Information collected but no factors identified	Factor present but not likely to have contributed to ill health or to death	Factor present, and may have contributed to ill health, or possibly to death	Factor present and certainly contributed to ill health, and probably contributed to the death	Factor present, and provides a complete and sufficient cause of death
History: (1)						
Death–scene examination (2)						
Pathology (3)						
Other (specify)						
Other evidence of neglect or abuse?						
Overall classification (4)						

The grid is completed at the multidisciplinary case discussion meeting (usually held 8–12 weeks after the death). An entry must be made on the line of each heading line, and a score (0–III) accorded to each line as agreed by all professionals present. The overall score is generally equal to the highest score within the grid. A score of III equates to a complete and sufficient cause of death. Scores of I–IIB meet the definition of SIDS. 1, To include a detailed history of events leading up to the death, together with medical, social and family history, plus explicit review of any evidence suggesting past neglect or abuse of this child or other children in the family. 2, results of detailed review of the scene of death by the pediatrician and police child protection officer in the light of the history given by parents or carers. 3, pathological investigations to a standardized protocol, including gross pathology, histology, microbiology, toxicology, radiology, clinical chemistry, and any relevant metabolic investigations, including frozen section of liver stained for fat. 4, this will generally equal the highest individual classification listed above.

charges, together with the recognition of genuine child protection issues, whilst providing appropriate support and care to families – warrant the adoption of a robust and thorough but sensitive investigation after all unexpected infant deaths.

Bereaved parents and their organizations have spoken strongly in favor of such an approach, in which the needs of parents for help, support, information and explanations, whilst avoiding blame or unwarranted suspicion, are explicitly integrated into the practice of all professionals involved in the process.

CURRENT RECOMMENDATIONS

The scientific rigor with which data is gathered is not easily applied to the dissemination of the results and formulating advice can be a subjective exercise of weighing up the available evidence and constrained by attempts to simplify the message. The debate on the safety, advantages and disadvantages of infant care practices must be informed not just by epidemiological evidence from one narrow field but from many disciplines from different fields if it is to become more than the exchange of mere opinion. The advantages of getting the advice right are evident in the dramatic fall in SIDS deaths after advice against the prone sleeping position, but it should be remembered that adoption of the prone position was initially largely a consequence of medical advice.

REFERENCES

1. Sibert JR. Stress in families of children who have ingested poisons. BMJ 1975; ii:87–89.
2. Scherz RG. Prevention of childhood poisoning. Pediatr Clin North Am 1970; 17:713.
3. Sibert JR, Lyons RA, Smith BA, et al. Preventing deaths by drowning in children in the UK: have we made progress in 10 years? Population based incidence study. BMJ 2002; 324:1070–1071.
4. Sibert JR, Frude N. Bittering agents in the prevention of accidental poisoning: children's reactions to denatonium benzoate. Arch Emerg Med 1991; 8:1–7.
5. Krenzelok EP, McGuigan M, Lheur P. Position statement: ipecac syrup. American Academy of Clinical Toxicology; European Association of Poisons Centres and Clinical Toxicologists. J Toxicol Clin Toxicol 1997; 35:699–709.
6. Chyka PA, Seger D. Position statement: single-dose activated charcoal. American Academy of Clinical Toxicology; European Association of Poisons Centres and Clinical Toxicologists. J Toxicol Clin Toxicol 1997; 35:721–741.
7. Craft AW, Lawson GR, Williams H, et al. Accidental childhood poisoning with household products. BMJ 1984; 288:682.

8. Yagupsky P, Gorodischer R. Massive clonidine ingestion in a 9 month old infant. Pediatrics 1983; 72:500–501.
9. Bramley A, Goulding R. Laburnum 'poisoning'. BMJ 1981; 283:1220–1221.
10. http://www.who.int/violence_injury_prevention/
11. http://www.who.int/whosis/.
12. http://www.who.int/violence_injury_prevention/child_injuries.
13. http://www.who.int/violence_injury_prevention/media/news/29_11_2005/.
14. http://www.who.int/violence_injury_prevention/media/news/24_3_2006/.
15. http://www.gro.gov.uk/gro.
16. http://www.gro-scotland.gov.uk/.
17. http://www.groni.gov.uk/.
18. Statistics, LOfN. Mortality statistics injury and poisoning, SDn 2004; 28.
19. Lyons RA, Brophy S. The epidemiology of childhood mortality in the European Union. Curr Paediatr 2005; 15:151–162.
20. Sibert JR, Lyons RA, Smith BA, et al. Preventing deaths by drowning in children in the United Kingdom: have we made progress in 10 years? Population based incidence study. BMJ 2002; 324:1070–1071.

21. Lyons RA, Polinder S, Larsen CF, et al. Methodological issues in comparing injury incidence across countries. Int J Inj Contr Saf Promot 2006; 13:63–70.
22. www.capic.org.uk
23. Cryer C, Langley JD. Developing valid indicators of injury incidence for 'all injury.'. Inj Prev 2006; 12:202–207.
24. http://www.health.vic.gov.au/hdss/vemd.
25. http://www.cpsc.gov/library/neiss.html.
26. http://www.eurosafe.eu.com/csi/eurosafe2006.nsf.
27. Lyons RA, Lo SV, Heaven M, et al. Injury surveillance in children – usefulness of a centralised database of accident and emergency attendances. Injury Prevention 1995; 1:173–176.
28. http://www.who.int/violence_injury_prevention/surveillance/.
29. Lopez AD, Mathers CD, Ezzati M, et al. Global and regional burden of disease and risk factors, 2001: systematic analysis of population health data. The Lancet 2006; 367:1747–1757.
30. Des Plains, I.A.f.t.A.o.A.M., Association for the Advancement of Automotive Medicine, Abbreviated Injury Scale. 1990.
31. Barker M, Power C, Roberts I. Injuries and the risk of disability in teenagers and young adults. Arch Dis Child 1996; 75:156–158.

32. HMSO. B.R. Report of the working group on inequalities in health. London: HMSO; 1980.
33. Lyons RA, Delahunty AM, Heaven M, et al. Incidence of childhood fractures in affluent and deprived areas: population based study. BMJ 2000; 320:149.
34. Jones SJ, Lyons RA, John A, et al. Traffic calming policy can reduce inequalities in child pedestrian injuries: database study. Inj Prev 2005; 11:152–156.
35. Groom L, Kendrick D, Coupland C, et al. Inequalities in hospital admission rates for unintentional poisoning in young children. Inj Prev 2006; 12:166–170.
36. Niekerk AV, Reimers A, Laflamme L. Area characteristics and determinants of hospitalised childhood burn injury: A study in the city of Cape Town. Public Health 2006; 120:115–124.
37. http://www.who.int/violence_injury_prevention/capacitybuilding/teach_vip/.
38. www.capt.org.uk.
39. www.rospa.org.uk.
40. http://www.childsafetyeurope.org/.
41. www.safetylit.org.
42. http://www.cochrane-injuries.lshtm.ac.uk/.
43. Towner E, Hayes M, Laidman P. Contributor to Unintentional Injury Prevention Course Text. Newcastle-upon-Tyne: University of Newcastle-upon-Tyne Child Accident Prevention Trust; 2001.
44. http://www.dft.gov.uk/stellent/groups/dft_rdsafety/documents/page/dft_rdsafety_030571.pdf.
45. World Health Organization. Poisonous animal bites and stings. WHO Weekly Epidemiol Rec 1995; 44:315–316.
46. White J. How to treat snakebite. Australian Doctor 2001; March(Suppl.): Pt 1
47. Gold BS, Dart RC, Barish RA. Bites of venomous snakes. N Engl J Med 2002; 347:347–356.
48. Williams J, Winkel K. Snakebite epidemiology in Papua New Guinea. Annals of the ACTM 2005; 6:19–23.
49. Warrell DA. Treatment of bites by adders and exotic venomous snakes. BMJ 2005; 331:1244–1247.
50. Pearn J. Human snakebite – effects and first aid. In: Pearn J, Covacevich J, eds. Brisbane: Queensland Museum 1988; 97–110
51. Sprivulis P, Jelinek G. Snakebite. In: Cameron P, ed. Textbook of adult emergency medicine. Edinburgh: Churchill Livingstone; 2000.649–651.
52. Scharman E, Noffunger V. Copperhead snakebites: Clinical severity of local effects. Ann Emerg Med 2001; 38:55–61.
53. Banham NDG. Marine envenomation. In: Cameron P, ed. Textbook of adult emergency medicine. Edinburgh: Churchill Livingstone; 2000.655–657.
54. Heatwole H. Seasnakes. Sydney: University of NSW Press; 1987.
55. Hadley GP, McGarr P, Mars M. Role of thromboelastography in the management of children with snakebite in southern Africa. Trans R Soc Trop Med Hyg 1999; 93:177–179.
56. Sutherland S. Antivenom use in Australia. Med J Aust 1992; 157:734–739.
57. Tibballs J. Premedication for snake antivenom. Med J Aust 1994; 160:4–7.
58. Jelinek G. Spider bite. In: Cameron P, ed. Textbook of adult emergency medicine. Edinburgh: Churchill Livingstone; 2000.652–655.
59. Eddleston M, Pierini S, Wilkinson R, et al, eds. Oxford Handbook of tropical medicine. Oxford: Oxford University Press; 2005.
60. Nuchpraryoon I, Garner P. Interventions for preventing reactions to snake antivenom. Cochrane Database Syst Rev Issue 4. 2005.
61. White J. CSL Antivenom handbook. Melbourne: CSL Diagnostics; 1995.

62. Pearn J. Clinical contracts and chronic envenomation syndromes. Annals of the ACTM 2003; 4:10–11.
63. Sutherland S. Venomous bites and stings. Med Aust 1978; 6:402–412.
64. Sutherland S. First aid for snakebite in Australia. Parville: CSL Diagnostics; 1979.
65. Brent J, Wallace KL, Burkhart KK, et al. Critical care toxicology. Chs 101–115. New York: Mosby; 2005.
66. Warrell DA. WHO/SEARO Guidelines for the clinical management of snake bites in the Southeast Asian region. Southeast Asian J Trop Med Publ Hlth 1999; 30(Suppl.1):1–85.
67. Warrell DA. Snake bites in Central and South America: epidemiology, clinical features and clinical management. In: Campbell J A, Lammar W W, eds. The venomous reptiles of the western hemisphere. Ithaca: Comstock Cornell University Press; 2004.709–761.
68. McGain F, Winkel K. Beesting mortality in Australia, 1979–1998. [Abstract] Annals of the ACTM 2005; 6:28.
69. Wiese M. Ant sting allergy within Australia – a threat to residents and travelers. [Abstract] Annals of the ACTM 2005; 6:32.
70. Reisman RE. Insect stings. N Engl J Med 1994; 331:523–527.
71. Valentine MD, Schuberth KC, Kagey-Sobotka A, et al. The value of immunotherapy with venom in children with allergy to insect stings. N Engl J Med 1990; 323:1601–1603.
72. Sutherland S. Poisonous Australian animals. In: Victoria: Hyland House; 1992.64.
73. Alexander JOD. Arthropods and human skin. Berlin: Springer; 1984.
74. Warrell DA. Spider bites: addressing mythology and poor evidence. Am J Trop Med 2005; 72:361–364.
75. Raven RJ, Churchill TB. Funnel-web spiders. In: Pearn J, Covacevich J, eds. Venoms and victims. Brisbane: Queensland Museum 2000. 67–72.
76. Sutherland S. Venomous creatures of Australia. In: Melbourne: Oxford University Press; 1982.127.
77. Piesman J. Emerging tick-borne diseases in temperate climates. Parasitol Today 1987; 3:197–199.
78. Rosen T. Caterpillar dermatitis. Dermatol Clin 1990; 8:245–252.
79. Williamson J, Fenner P, Burkett J, et al. Venomous and poisonous marine animals. Sydney: University of NSW Press; 1996.
80. Fenner P, Williamson J, Burnett J. Some Australian and international marine envenomation reports. 1995.
81. Fischer PR. The danger of marine envenomations. Travel Medicine Adviser Update 1995; 5:32–33.
82. Fenner P. Jellyfish stings – first aid and early medical treatments revisited. Annals of the ACTM 2006; 7:3–7.
83. Pearn J. The sea, stingers, and surgeons: the surgeon's role in prevention, first aid and management of marine envenomations. J Pediatr Surg 1995; 30:105–110.
84. Beadnell CE, Rider TA, Williamson JA, et al. Management of a major box jellyfish sting. Med J Aust 1992; 156:655–658.
85. White J, Edmonds C, Zborowski P. Australia's most dangerous. Australian Geographic. Terrey Hills; 1998.
86. Auerbach PS. Marine envenomation. N Engl J Med 1991; 325:486–493.
87. Rognum TO, Willinger M. The story of the 'Stavanger definition'. In: Rognum T O, ed. Sudden infant death syndrome. New trends in the nineties. Oslo: Scandinavian University Press; 1995. 21–25.
88. Templeman C. Two hundred and fifty eight cases of suffocation of infants. Edinburgh Medical Journal 1892; 38:322–329.

89. Willcox WH. Infantile mortality from 'overlaying'. BMJ 1904 (September 24): 1–7.
90. American Academy of Pediatrics Policy Statement. The changing concept of sudden infant death syndrome: diagnostic coding shifts, controversies regarding the sleeping environment, and new variables to consider in reducing risk. Pediatrics 2005; 116:1245–1255.
91. Gessner BD, Porter TJ. Bed sharing with unimpaired parents is not an important risk factor for sudden infant death syndrome. Pediatrics 2006; 117:990–991.
92. Kattwinkel J, Hauck F, Moon RY, et al. In reply. Pediatrics 2006; 117:994–996.
93. Emery JL. Is sudden infant death syndrome a diagnosis? Or is it just a diagnostic dustbin? BMJ 1989; 299:1240.
94. Huber J. Sudden infant death syndrome: the new clothes of the emperor. Eur J Pediatr 1993; 152:93–94.
95. Limerick SR. Sudden infant death in historical perspective. J Clin Pathol 1992; 45(Suppl):3–6.
96. Beal S, Blundell H. Sudden infant death syndrome related to position in the cot. Med J Australia 1978; 2:217–218.
97. Saturnus KS. Plotzicher Kindstod – eine Folge der Bauchlage? In: Leithoff F, ed. Heidelberg: Kriminalstatistik; 1985.67–81.
98. Davies DP. Cot death in Hong Kong: a rare problem?. Lancet 1985; ii:1346–1349.
99. de Jonge GA, Engleberts AC, Koomen-Liefting AJ, et al. Cot death and prone sleeping position in the Netherlands. BMJ 1989; 298:722.
100. Mitchell EA, Scragg R, Stewart AW, et al. Results from the first year of the New Zealand cot death study. NZ Med J 1991; 71–76.
101. Fleming PJ, Gilbert R, Azaz Y, et al. Interaction between bedding and sleeping position in the sudden infant death syndrome: a population based case–control study. BMJ 1990; 301:85–89.
102. Blair PS, Sidebotham P, Berry PJ, et al. Major changes in the epidemiology of sudden infant death syndrome: a 20-year population based study of all unexpected deaths in infancy. Lancet 2006; 367:314–319.
103. Limerick SR, Bacon CJ. Terminology used by pathologists in reporting on sudden infant deaths. J Clin Pathol 2004; 57:309–311.
104. Froggatt P, Lynas MA, MacKenzie G. Epidemiology of sudden unexpected death in infants ('cot death') in Northern Ireland. Br J Prev Soc Med 1971; 25:119–134.
105. Fedrick J. Sudden unexpected death in infants in the Oxford Record Linkage area. An analysis with respect to time and space. Br J Prev Soc Med 1973; 27:217–224.
106. McGlashan ND. Sudden deaths in Tasmania, 1980–1986: A seven year prospective study. Soc Sci Med 1989; 29:1015–1026.
107. Daltveit AK, Øyen N, Skjærven R, et al. The epidemic of SIDS in Norway, 1967–93: changing effects of risk factors. Arch Dis Child 1997; 77:23–27.
108. Fleming PJ, Blair PS, Bacon C, et al. Sudden unexpected death in infancy. The CESDI SUDI Studies 1993–1996. London: The Stationery Office; 2000. ISBN 0 11 322299 8.
109. Leach CEA, Blair PS, Fleming PJ, et al. Sudden unexpected deaths in infancy: Similarities and differences in the epidemiology of SIDS and explained deaths. Pediatrics 1999; 104:e43. (electronic pages) (http://www.pediatrics.org/cgi/content/full/4/e43).
110. Bouvier-Colle MH, Inizan J, Michel E. Postneonatal mortality, sudden infant death syndrome: factors preventing the decline of infant mortality in France from, 1979 to, 1985. Paed Perinatal Epidem 1989; 3:256–267.
111. Kraus JF, Greenland S, Bulteys M. Risk factors for sudden infant death syndrome in the US collaborative perinatal project. Int J Epidemiol 1989; 18:113–119.

112. Wagner M, Samson-Dollfus D, Menard J. Sudden unexpected infant death in a French county. Arch Dis Child 1984; 59:1082–1087.

113. Fleming PJ, Blair PS, Ward Platt M, et al. Sudden infant death syndrome and social deprivation. J Paed Perinatal Epid 2003; 17:272–280.

114. Beal SM. Sleeping position and SIDS: Past, present and future. In: Rognum TO, (ed.) SIDS: New Trends in the Nineties. Oslo: Scandinavian University Press 1995;.147–151.

115. Editorial. Prone or supine? BMJ 1961; 1304.

116. Greene D. Asymmetry of the head and face in infants and in children. Am J Dis Child 1930; 41:1317–1326.

117. Abramson H. Accidental mechanical suffocation in infants. J Pediatr 1944; 25:404–413.

118. Masterson J, Zucker C, Schulze K. Prone and supine positioning effects on energy expenditure and behaviour of low birthweight neonates. Pediatrics 1987; 89:689–692.

119. Martin RJ, Herrell N, Rubin D, et al. Effect of supine and prone positions on arterial tension in the preterm infant. Pediatrics 1979; 63:528–531.

120. Yu V. Effect of body positioning on gastric emptying in the neonate. Arch Dis Child 1975; 50:500–504.

121. Schwartz FCM, Fenner A, Wolfsdrop J. The influence of body position on pulmonary function in low birth babies. S Afr Med J 1975; 49:79–81.

122. Fleming PJ, Muller N, Bryan MH, et al. The effects of abdominal loading on ribcage distortion in premature infants. Pediatrics 1979; 64:425–428.

123. Hiley C. Babies' sleeping position. BMJ 1992; 305:115.

124. Gilbert R, Rudd P, Berry PJ, et al. Combined effect of infection and heavy wrapping on the risk of sudden unexpected infant death. Arch Dis Child 1992; 67:171–177.

125. Ponsonby A-L, Dwyer T, Gibbons LE, et al. Thermal environment and sudden infant death syndrome: case–control study. BMJ 1992; 304:277–282.

126. Klonnoff-Cohen HS, Edelstein SL. A case–control study of routine and death scene sleep position and sudden infant death syndrome in Southern California. JAMA 1995; 273:790–794.

127. Williams S, Taylor B, Mitchell E. Sudden infant death syndrome: insulation from bedding and clothing and its effect modifiers. Int J Epidemiol 1996; 25:366–375.

128. Fleming PJ, Blair PS, Bacon C, et al. Environment of infants during sleep and risk of the sudden infant death syndrome: results from, 1993–5 case–control study for confidential inquiry into stillbirths and deaths in infancy. BMJ July 1996; 313:191–195.

129. Mitchell EA, Ford RPK, Stewart AW, et al. Smoking and the sudden infant death syndrome. Paediatrics 1993; 91:893–896.

130. Klonoff-Cohen HS, Edelstein SL, Lefkowitz ES, et al. The effect of passive smoking and tobacco exposure through breast milk on sudden infant death syndrome. JAMA 1995; 273:795–798.

131. Blair PS, Fleming PJ, Bensley D, et al. Smoking and the sudden infant death syndrome: results from, 1993–5 case–control study for confidential inquiry into stillbirths and deaths in infancy. BMJ July 1996; 313:195–198.

132. Mitchell EA, Milerad J. Smoking and the sudden infant death syndrome. Rev Environ Health. 2006; 21:81–103.

133. Blair PS, Ward Platt MP, Smith IJ, et al. Sudden infant death syndrome and sleeping position in pre-term and low birthweight infants: An opportunity for targeted intervention. Arch Dis Child 2006; 91:101–106.

134. Fleming PJ, Blair PS, Ward Platt M, et al. The accelerated immunisation programme in the UK & sudden unexpected death in infancy. BMJ 2001; 322:822–825.

135. Kahn A, Blum D, Hennart P. A critical comparison of the history of sudden-death infants and infants hospitalised for near-miss for SIDS. Eur J Pediatr 1984; 143:103–107.

136. Tonkin SL. Infant mortality. Epidemiology of cot deaths in Auckland. NZ Med J 1986; 99:324–326.

137. Mitchell EA, Taylor BJ, Ford RPK, et al. Four modifiable and other major risk factors for cot death: The New Zealand study. J Paediatr Child Health 1992; 28(Suppl):S3–S8.

138. Skadberg BT, Morild I, Markestad T. Abandoning prone sleeping: Effect on the risk of sudden infant death syndrome. J Pediatr 1998; 132:340–343.

139. Scragg RK, Mitchell EA. Side sleeping position and bed sharing in the sudden infant death syndrome. [Review] Ann Med 1998; 30:345–349.

140. L'Hoir MP, Engleberts AC, van Well GT, et al. Risk and preventive factors for cot death in the Netherlands, a low-incidence country. Eur J Pediatr 1998; 157:681–688.

141. Li DK, Petitti DB, Willinger M, et al. Infant sleeping position and the risk of sudden infant death syndrome in California, 1997–2000. Am J Epidemiol 2003; 157:446–455.

142. Carpenter PR, Irgens PL, Blair PS, et al. Sudden unexplained infant death in 20 regions in Europe: case control study. Lancet 2004; 363:185–191.

143. Cullen A, Kiberd B, McDonnell M, et al. Sudden infant death syndrome – are parents getting the message? Ir J Med Sci 2000; 169:40–43.

144. Kiechl-Kohlendorfer U, Peglow UP, Kiechl S, et al. Epidemiology of sudden infant death syndrome (SIDS) in the Tyrol before and after an intervention campaign. Wein Klin Wochenschr 2001; 113:27–32.

145. Rose M, Murphy M, Macfarlane JA, et al. 'Back to sleep': the position in Oxfordshire and Northampton. Paediatr Perinat Epidemiol 1998; 12:217–227.

146. Nelson EAS, Serra A, Cowan S, et al. Maternity advice survey: sleeping position in Eastern Europe. Arch Dis Child 2000; 83:304–306.

147. Hein HA, Pettit SF. Back to Sleep: good advice for parents but not for hospitals? Pediatrics 2001; 107:537–539.

148. Pastore GM, Guala A, Zaffaroni M. Back to Sleep: risk factors for SIDS as targets for public health campaigns. J Pediatr 2003; 142:453–454.

149. Byard RW, Beal SM. Gastric aspiration and sleeping position in infancy and early childhood. J Paediatr Child Health 2000; 36:403–405.

150. Fleming PJ, Stewart A. What is the ideal sleeping position for infants? Dev Med Child Neurol 1992; 34:916–919.

151. Hunt L, Fleming P, Golding J, et al. Does the supine sleeping position have any adverse effects on the child? I. Health in the first six months. Pediatrics 1997; 100:e11.

152. Hutchison BL, Thompson JM, Mitchell EA. Determinants of nonsynostotic plagiocephaly: a case–control study. Pediatrics 2003; 112:e316.

153. Ponsonby AL, Dwyer T, Couper D. Sleeping position, infant apnoea, and cyanosis: a population-based study. Pediatrics 1997; 1997:E3.

154. Hunt CE, Lesko SM, Vezina RM, et al. Infant sleep position and associated health outcomes. Arch Pediatr Adolesc Med 2003; 157:469–474.

155. Dewey C, Fleming PJ, Golding J. Does the supine position have any adverse effects on the child?: II. Development in the first 18 months. Pediatrics 1998; 101:1:e5 (electronic pages). Http://www.pediatrics.org/cgi/content/full/101/1/e5.

156. Majnemer A, Barr RG. Association between sleep position and early motor development. J Pediatr 2006; 149:623–629.

157. Kemp JS. Asymmetric heads and failure to climb stairs. J Pediatr 2006; 149:594–595.

158. Mitchell EA, Scragg J, Clements M. Soft cot mattresses and the sudden infant death syndrome. NZ Med J 1996; 109:206–207.

159. Geib LT, Nunes NL. The incidence of sudden death syndrome in a cohort of infants. J Pediatr (Rio J) 2006; 82:21–26.

160. Flick L, White DK, Vemulapolli C, et al. Sleep position and the use of soft bedding during bed sharing among African American infants at increased risk for sudden infant death syndrome. J Pediatr 2001; 138:338–343.

161. Hauck FR, Herman SM, Donovan M, et al. Sleep environment and the risk of sudden infant death syndrome in an urban population: the Chicago Infant Mortality Study. Pediatrics 2003; 111(Part 2):1207–1214.

162. Sawczenko A, Fleming PJ. Thermal stress, sleeping position, and the sudden infant death syndrome. Sleep 1996; 19(Suppl):S267–S270.

163. Scheers NJ, Dayton CM, Kemp JS. Sudden infant death with external airways covered: case–comparison study of 206 deaths in the United States. Arch Pediatr Adolesc Med 1998; 152:540–547.

164. Byard RW, Beal SM. V-shaped pillows and unsafe infant sleeping. J Paediatr Child Health 1997; 33:171–173.

165. Abramson H. Accidental mechanical suffocation in infants. J Pediatr 1944; 25:404–413.

166. Wooley PV. Mechanical suffocation during infancy. J Pediatr 1945; 26:572–575.

167. Davison WH. Accidental infant suffocation. BMJ 1945; 25:251–252.

168. Werne J, Garrow I. Sudden deaths of infants allegedly due to mechanical suffocation. Am J Pub Health 1947; 37:675.

169. Bowden K. Sudden death or alleged accidental suffocation in babies. Med J Aust 1950; I:65–72.

170. Nelson EAS, Taylor BJ, Weatherall IL. Sleeping position and infant bedding may predispose to hyperthermia and the sudden infant death syndrome. Lancet 1989; 1:199–201.

171. Nelson EAS, Taylor BJ, Mackay SC. Child care practices and the sudden infant death syndrome. Aust Paediatr J 1989; 25:202–204.

172. Bass M, Kravath RE, Glass L. Death scene investigation in sudden infant death. N Engl J Med 1986; 315:100–105.

173. Wilson CA, Taylor BJ, Laing RM, et al. Clothing and bedding and its relevance to sudden infant death syndrome: further results from the New Zealand Cot Death Study. J Paediatr Child Health 1994; 30:506–512.

174. Horne RS, Oarslow PM, Ferens D, et al. Arousal responses and risk factors for sudden infant death syndrome. Sleep Med 2002; 3(Suppl 2):S61–S65.

175. Beal SM. Sudden infant death syndrome in South Australia, 1968–97. Part 1: Changes over time. J Paediatr Child Health 2000; 36:540–547.

176. Poets CF. Apparent life-threatening events and sudden infant death on a monitor. Paediatr Respir Rev 2004; 5(Suppl A):S383–S386.

177. Dix J. Homicide and the baby-sitter. Am J Forensic Med Pathol 1998; 19:321–323.

178. Thach BT. Sudden infant death syndrome: old causes rediscovered? N Engl J Med 1986; 315:126–128.

179. Schellscheidt J, Ott A, Jorch G. Epidemiological features of sudden infant death after a German intervention campaign in 1992. Eur J Pediatr 1997; 156:655–660.

180. Nelson T, To K-F, Wong Y-Y, et al. Hong Kong case–control study of sudden unexpected infant death. NZ Med J 2005; 118:U1788.

181. L'Hoir MP, Engelberts AC, van Well GT, et al. Case–control study of current validity of previously described risk factors for SIDS in The Netherlands. Arch Dis Child 1998; 79:386–393.

182. Markestad T, Skadberg B, Hordvik E, et al. Sleeping position and sudden infant death syndrome

(SIDS): effect of an intervention programme to avoid prone sleeping. Acta Paediatr 1995; 84:375–378.

183. Ponsonby A-L, Dwyer T, Couper D, et al. Association between use of a quilt and sudden infant death syndrome: case–control study. BMJ 1998; 316:195–196.

184. Foundation for the Study of Infant deaths. BabyZone leaflet. E-mail fsid@sids.org.uk or visit the website: http://www.sids.org.uk/fsis/fsid.

185. Spock B, Rothenberg MB. Baby and child care. New York: Pocket Books; 1985:219.

186. Leach P. Baby and child. London: Michael Joseph; 1980:93–94.

187. McKenna J. An anthropological perspective on the sudden infant death syndrome (SIDS): the role of parental breathing cues and speech breathing adaptations. Med Anthropol 1986; 10:9–91.

188. Scragg RKR, Mitchell EA, Stewart AW, et al. Infant room-sharing and prone sleep position in sudden infant death syndrome. Lancet 1996; 347:7–12.

189. Tappin D, Ecob R, Brooke H. Bedsharing, roomsharing, and sudden infant death syndrome in Scotland: a case–control study. J Pediatr 2005; 147:32–37.

190. Blair PS, Fleming PJ, Smith IJ, et al and CESDI SUDI research group. Babies sleeping with parents: case–control study of factors influencing the risk of sudden infant death syndrome. BMJ 1999; 319:1457–1462.

191. Blair PS, Ward Platt M, Smith IJ, et al. Sudden infant death syndrome and the time of death: factors associated with night-time and day-time deaths. Int J Epidemiol 2006; (in press).

192. Tappin D, Brooke H, Ecob R, et al. Used infant mattresses and sudden infant death syndrome in Scotland: case–control study. BMJ 2002; 325:1007.

193. McGarvey C, McDonnell M, Chong A, et al. Factors relating to the infant's last sleep environment in sudden infant death syndrome in the Republic of Ireland. Arch Dis Child 2003; 88:1058–1064.

194. Takeda KA. A possible mechanism of sudden infant death syndrome (SIDS). Journal of Kyoto Prefecture University Medicine 1987; 96:965–968.

195. Davies DP. Cot death in Hong Kong. A rare problem? Lancet 1985; II:1346–1347.

196. Gantley M, Davies DP, Murcott A. Sudden infant death syndrome. Links with infant care practices. BMJ 1993; 16:263–282.

197. Farooqi S, Lip GYH, Beevers DG. Bed-sharing and smoking in sudden infant death syndrome. BMJ 1994; 308:204–205.

198. Tuohy PG, Counsell AM, Geddis DC. Sociodemographic factors associated with sleeping position and location. Arch Dis Child 1993; 69:664–666.

199. Wailoo M, Ball H, Fleming PJ, et al. Infants bedsharing with mothers: helpful, harmful or don't know? Arch Dis Child 2004; 89:1082–1083.

200. Fleming PJ, Blair PS, McKenna JJ. New knowledge, new insights and new recommendations: Scientific controversy and media hype in unexpected infant deaths. Arch Dis Child 2006; (in press).

201. McGarvey C, McDonnell M, O'Regan M, et al. An eight year study of risk factors for SIDS: bedsharing vs non bedsharing. Arch Dis Child 2006; 91:318–323.

202. Mosko S, McKenna J, Dickel M, et al. Parent-infant co-sleeping: The appropriate context for the study of infant sleep and implications for sudden infant death syndrome (SIDS) research. J Behavioural Med 1993; 16:589–610.

203. Anderson GC. Current knowledge about skin-to-skin (Kangaroo) care for preterm infants. J Perinatology 1991; 11:216–226.

204. Ludington-Hoe SM, Hadeed AJ, Anderson GC. Physiological responses to skin-to-skin contact in hospitalised premature infants. J Perinatology 1991; 11:19–24.

205. McKenna. Sudden infant death syndrome in cross-cultural perspective. Is infant–parent cosleeping protective? Ann Rev of Anthropol 1996; 25:201–216.

206. Ball HL, Hooker E, Kelly PJ. Where will the babies sleep? Attitudes and practices of new and experienced parents regarding co-sleeping with their new-born infant. American Anthroplogy 1999.

207. Fleming PJ, Young J, Blair PS. The importance of mother–baby interactions in determining night time thermal conditions for sleeping infants: Observations from the home and the sleep laboratory. Pediatrics and Child Health 2006; 11(Suppl):7A–11A.

208. Mitchell EA, Taylor BJ, Ford RPK, et al. Dummies and the sudden infant death syndrome. Arch Dis Child 1993; 68:501–504.

209. Fleming PJ, Blair PS, Pollard K, et al. Pacifier use and sudden infant death syndrome: results from the CESDI/SUDI case–control study. Arch Dis Child 1999; 81:112–116.

210. L'Hoir MP, Engelberts AC, van Well GT, et al. Dummy use, thumb sucking, mouth breathing and cot death. Euro J Pediatr 1999; 158:896–901.

211. Brooke H, Tappin DM, Beckett C, et al. Dummy use on the day/night of death: case–control study of sudden infants death syndrome (SIDS) in Scotland, 1996–99 [abstract] sixth SIDS International Conference, Auckland, New Zealand, February 2000.

212. Vennemann MMT, Findeisen M, Butterfaß-Bahloul T, et al. Modifiable risk factors for SIDS in Germany: results of GeSID. Acta Paediatr 2005; 94:655–660.

213. Li DK, Willinger M, Petitti DB, et al. Use of a dummy (pacifier) during sleep and risk of SIDS: population-based case–control study. BMJ 2006; 332:18–22.

214. Blair PS, Fleming PJ. Dummies and SIDS: casuality has not been established. BMJ 2006; 332:178.

215. Fleming PJ, Blair PS, McKenna JJ. New knowledge, new insights and new recommendations: Scientific controversy and media hype in unexpected infant deaths. Arch Dis Child 2006; 91:799–801.

216. Righard L. Sudden infant death syndrome and pacifiers: a proposed connection could be a bias. Birth 1998; 25:128–129.

217. Cozzi F, Morini F, Tozzi C, et al. Effect of pacifier use on oral breathing in healthy newborn infants. Pediatr Pulmonol 2002; 33:368–373.

218. Franco P, Scaillet S, Wermenbol V, et al. The influence of a pacifier on infants' arousals from sleep. J Pediatr 2000; 136:775–779.

219. Weiss PP, Kerbl R. The relative short duration that a child retains a pacifier in the mouth during sleep: implications for sudden infant death syndrome. Eur J Pediatr 2001; 160:60–70.

220. Pollard K, Fleming PJ, Young J, et al. Night time non-nutritive sucking in infants aged 1 to 5 months: relationship with infant state, breast feeding, and bed- versus room-sharing. Early Human Development 1999; 56:185–204.

221. Barros FC, Victora CG, Semer TC, et al. Use of pacifiers is associated with decreased breast-feeding duration. Pediatrics 1995; 95:497–499.

222. Righard L, Alade MO. Breastfeeding and the use of pacifiers. Birth 1997; 24:116–120.

223. Howard CR, Howard FM, Lanphear B, et al. The effects of early pacifier use on breastfeeding duration. Pediatrics 1999; 103:E33.

224. Vogel AM, Hutchison BL, Mitchell EA. The impact of pacifier use on breastfeeding: a prospective cohort study. J Paediatr Child Health 2001; 37:58–63.

225. Warren JJ, Levy SM, Kirchner HL, et al. Pacifier use and the occurrence of otitis media in the first year of life. Pediatr Dentistry 2001; 23:103–107.

226. Uhari M, Mantysaari K, Niemela M. A meta-analytic review of the risk factors for acute otitis media. Clin Infect Dis 1996; 22:1079–1083.

227. North K, Fleming PJ, Golding J. Socio-demographic associations with digit and pacifier sucking at 15 months of age and possible associations with infant infections. Early Human Development 2000; 60:137–148.

228. Mattos-Graner RO, de Moraes AB, Rontani RM, et al. Relation of oral yeast infection in Brazilian infants and use of a pacifier. J Dentistry Child 2001; 68:33–36.

229. Simkiss DE, Sheppard I, Pal BR. Airway obstruction by a child's pacifier – could flange design be safer? Euro J Pediatr 1998; 157:252–254.

230. Feldman KW, Simms RJ. Strangulation in childhood: epidemiology and clinical course. Pediatrics 1980; 65:1079–1085.

231. Stubbs AJ, Aburn NS. Penetrating eye injury from a rigid infant pacifier. Aus N Z J Ophthalmol 1996; 24:71–73.

232. Adair SM, Milano M, Lorenzo I, et al. Effects of current and former pacifier use on the dentition of 24- to 59-month-old children. Pediatr Dentistry 1995; 17:437–444.

233. Meny R, Carroll J, Carbone MT, et al. Cardiorespiratory recordings from infants dying suddenly and unexpectedly at home. Pediatrics 1994; 93:44–49.

234. Morris JA. The common bacterial toxins hypothesis of sudden infant death syndrome. FEMS Immunology and Medical Microbiology 1999; 25:11–17.

235. Fleming PJ, Howell T, Clements M, et al. Thermal balance and metabolic rate during upper respiratory tract infection in infants. Arch Dis Child 1994; 70:187–191.

236. Azaz Y, Fleming PJ, Levine M, et al. The relationship between environmental temperature, metabolic rate, sleep state and evaporative water loss in infants from birth to three months. Pediat Res 1992; 32:417–423.

237. Arkell S, Blair P, Henderson AJ, et al. Is the mattress important in helping babies keep warm? – Paradoxical effects of a sleeping surface with negligible thermal resistance. Acta Paed 2006; (in press).

238. Wigfield RE, Fleming PJ, Azaz Y, et al. How much wrapping do babies need at night? Arch Dis Child 1993; 69:181–186.

239. Lodemore MR, Petersen SA, Wailoo MP. Factors affecting the development of night time temperature rhythms. Arch Dis Child 1992; 67:1259–1261.

240. Morris JA. Common bacterial toxins and physiological vulnerability to sudden infant death: the role of deleterious genetic mutations. FEMS Immunol Med Microbiol 2004; 42:42–47.

241. Blackwell CC, Weir D. The role of infection in sudden infant death syndrome. FEMS Immunol Med Microbiol 1999; 25:1–6.

242. Dashash M, Pravica V, Hutchinson IV, et al. Association of sudden infant death syndrome with VEGF and IL-6 gene polymorphisms. Hum Immunol 2006; 67:627–633.

243. Vege A, Rognum TO, Scott H, et al. SIDS cases have increased levels of interleukin-6 in cerebrospinal fluid. Acta Paed 1995; 84:193.

244. Moscovis S, Gordon AE, Hall ST, et al. Interleukin1-β responses to bacterial toxins and sudden infant death syndrome. FEMS immunology and medical microbiology 2004; 42:139–145.

245. Weese-Mayer DE, Berry-Kravis EM, Zhou L, et al. Sudden infant death syndrome: case–control frequency differences at genes pertinent to early autonomic nervous system embryologic development. Pediatr Res 2004; 56:391–395.

246. Ackerman MJ, Siu BL, Sturner WQ, et al. Postmortem molecular analysis of SCN5A defects in sudden infant death syndrome. JAMA 2001; 286:2264–2269.

247. Kinney HC, Randall LL, Sleeper LA, et al. Serotonergic brainstem abnormalities in Northern Plains Indians with the sudden infant death syndrome. J Neuropathol Exp Neurol 2003; 62:1178–1191.

248. Paterson DS, Trachtenbert FL, Thompson EG, et al. Multiple serotonergic brainstem abnormalities in the sudden infant death syndrome. JAMA 2006; 296:2124–2132.

249. Gunteroth WG, Spiers PS. The triple risk hypotheses in sudden infant death syndrome. Pediatrics 2002; 110:e64. (electronic pages). DOI:10.1542/peds.110.5.e64 (http://www.pediatrics. org/cgi/content/full/110/5/e64).

250. Fleming PJ, Blair PS, Sidebotham P, et al. Investigating sudden unexpected deaths in infancy and childhood and caring for bereaved families: an integrated multiagency approach. BMJ 2004; 328:331–334.

251. Kennedy H, Epstein J, Fleming PJ, et al. Sudden unexpected death in infancy. A multi-agency protocol for care and investigation. The Report of a working group convened by the Royal College of Pathologists and the Royal College of Paediatrics and Child Health. London: RCPath & RCPCH; 2004. (www.rcpch.ac.uk).

252. Working Together to safeguard children. A guide to inter-agency working to safeguard and promote the welfare of children. 2006. Department for Education and Skills, UK. (http://www.everychildmatters.gov.uk/ search/IG00060/).

253. Krous HF. The international standardised autopsy protocol for sudden unexpected infant death. In: Rognum T O, ed. Sudden infant death syndrome: new trends in the nineties. Oslo: Scandinavian University Press; 1995.81–85.

254. Krous HF, Beckwith B, Byard R, et al. Sudden infant death and unclassified sudden infant deaths: a definitional and diagnostic approach. Pediatrics 2004; 114:234–238.

7

Developmental pediatrics

Alison Salt, Jenefer Sargent

INTRODUCTION

Developmental pediatrics is concerned with the processes of children's learning and competent adaptation to the environment from birth to adulthood. There are three purposes:

1. to promote optimal physical and mental health and development for all children, applying principles of prevention of impairment, wherever possible, and to reduce, where possible, disability and maximize function (Table 7.1);
2. to ensure early diagnosis and effective treatment of impairments of body, mind and personality;
3. to discover the cause and means of preventing such impairments.

Increasingly pediatricians and other clinicians caring for children will find their time spent with chronic illness, chronic physical or mental disability, learning or behavioral problems. Acute illnesses are likely to be shorter, self-limiting or more rapidly responsive to treatment. This chapter looks at the process of development, how it can be observed and how abnormalities can be identified and interpreted. The context for observing a child's development is the family, school and community. Family, educational, social, cultural, spiritual, economic, environmental and political forces act favorably or unfavorably, but always significantly, on children's health and functioning.[1]

THEORIES OF CHILD DEVELOPMENT

There is a particularly long developmental period in humans, which must be adaptive for social and cognitive competence. Childhood marks the change from the entirely dependent baby into the mature independent adult. During this period the child:

1. builds up a store of knowledge about the environment;
2. learns motor skills to survive;
3. learns a language with which to communicate and think;
4. develops a sense of self, self-regulation of emotions and behavior and the coping strategies for successful interpersonal relationships.

Philosophical views of child development (e.g. Rousseau) were replaced last century by the more empirical approach of direct observation of children's behavior and experimentation. Theories have included:

1. the 'maturational' view exemplified by Gesell (i.e. developmental progression depends upon neurological maturation);
2. 'behavioral' (i.e. changes in the environment are the most important influence in shaping the child);
3. 'psychoanalytic/psychosocial' theories of Freud and Erikson (unconscious motivations);
4. 'cognitive' theories developed by Piaget, which emphasize stages of development and the mental process of constructing knowledge from interaction with the environment that builds the next stage upon the previous one.

These theories continue to influence the ways in which we think about a child's development. Mental growth and development are dependent both on maturation of the nervous system and on experience. At 5 months the fetus has the full adult complement of 12 billion or more nerve cells. As the fetus and infant grow, the developing interconnections between these cells result in patterns of behavior that are generally similar, but the acquisition of knowledge and the refinement of skills depend on the child's opportunity to observe, copy and experiment. Neuronal maturation of the brain continues into postnatal life and myelination is completed in sensory and motor areas first and association areas last. Neural systems stabilize to optimal patterns of functioning via a process of reorganization and subtraction within neonatal architectural constraints and biases, which lead to recruitment of specific pathways. There is a capacity for plasticity, which becomes less flexible with age. At an anatomical level, the resultant brain–behavior relationships show domain specificity (e.g. specific areas devoted to language processing and learning).

There are many other theories which contribute to our understanding of child development.

1. Nativist or innate theories continue to be influential, for example in language learning[2] and motor development – theories of self-organization.[3]
2. 'Modern social learning constructivist' theories emphasize cognitive processes as mediators of environmental/behavioral influences.
3. Bronfenbrenner's 'ecological theories' emphasize the importance of the context in which children grow up, the goodness of fit and other features of the environment (i.e. the family situation, parents working, early child care and the wider cultural influences).

Table 7.1 Definitions of impairment and disability. There are many definitions and the term is used differently in different legislation

---

The Children Act 1989
'A child in need' is unlikely to achieve or maintain or to have the opportunity of achieving or maintaining, a reasonable standard of health or development without the provision for the child of services by a local authority
The health or development of 'a child in need' is likely to be significantly impaired or further impaired, without the provision for the child of such services
A disabled child is 'a child in need'

The Disability Discrimination Act 1995
This Act defines a disabled person as someone who has: 'a physical or mental impairment which has a substantial and long term adverse effect on his/her ability to carry out normal day to day activities'

The World Health Organization International Classification (ICDH)
Impairment is 'a loss or abnormality of body structure or of a physiological or psychological function'
Disability is 'the functional effect of any impairment'
Handicap is 'the limitation or prevention of fulfilment in life normal for that individual because of impairment or disability'

The new ICDH-2
The concept of disability is replaced by the 'activity' of an individual and the extent of their functioning
The concept of handicap is replaced by measure of participation

---

4. Vygotsky emphasized the immediate context for social learning, described as the 'zone of proximal development', as that area where the child cannot manage a task independently but can do more with supportive assistance. This is particularly relevant to his views of the development of language and thinking where social meaning is conferred on language and actions by the social sharing of ideas with others.
5. More mechanistic learning models and 'connectionist' theories are based on information processing and the perception, conception, storage, manipulation, transformation and retrieval of information. They are also based on the limitations that these processes place on functioning through memory capacity and attentional skills such as selection, shifting, inhibition, multi- and crossmodal functions, speed of processing, the development of automaticity and metacognitive skills, such as knowing about things and making comparisons and judgments. These are universal learning mechanisms incorporating theories of efficiency such that the mental resource and effort that is devoted to interaction with the environment and problem solving for the individual is minimized while retaining flexibility and increasing hierarchy and coherence.
6. 'Dynamic systems' theory integrates elements from all of the above. Children actively construct their understanding of the world by interacting with it, thus developing schemes and strategies that can be applied to a wide variety of situations. Intelligence reflects the child's capacity to initiate and assimilate new experiences and to profit by past experience.

FACTORS THAT AFFECT DEVELOPMENT

NATURE VERSUS NURTURE

Although there is now little disagreement that there are both genetic and environmental contributions to development of intelligence and personality, the nature/nurture debate continues. The contribution of each is complex because both the individual and the environment are continuously changing over time and the interaction between them, which molds psychological growth, is fluid and dynamic.[4] The genetic influences on a child's development extend to the environment through the parental phenotype.

ENVIRONMENTAL RISK FACTORS

Environmental factors may act in two ways:
1. by altering the child's opportunity to learn by limiting or expanding his experience – psychosocial factors;
2. by affecting the perceptual or effector organs and brain biologically at any stage from prenatally onwards.

PSYCHOSOCIAL FACTORS

In general, people rather than physical elements are the most important factors in the environment of the young child. Parents are responsible for giving the child the opportunities to enable learning, form relationships and develop social understanding. Crucially, if an infant does not develop a sense of trust in people and attachment from that first relationship with a parent then he/she is more likely to have lifelong difficulties with relationships. Various factors including material deprivation affect the parents' capacity to cope well with the task of child rearing and provision of an optimal learning environment. Resilience to life events is related to temperament as well as to family factors of warmth, cohesion and support and external support.

Temperament

Temperament is a major influence on all aspects of adaptive development as well as social–emotional development, both through the effect on the child's adaptation to the environment and his/her personal regulation, but also through the effect on the caregivers/parents and broader social context. Temperament can be seen from the earliest weeks as a mix of activity, adaptability, attention and emotional responses. Continuities of temperament over time have been well documented. For example, high reactors as infants are more inhibited in new situations at age 4 years.[5]

Most individual children do not fall simply into one particular pattern of behavior but patterns described are:
1. the easy child;
2. the slow-to-warm up child;
3. the difficult child.
Current research emphasizes both 'emotionality' and 'self-regulation' as important. Differences within children may mean that some are more sensitive than others to maternal 'sensitivity', which is thought to be an important influence on attachment in infancy.

Parenting style and parental mental illness

Depression in mothers in the postnatal period is associated with effects on children's social–emotional and cognitive development. Parental inconsistency in methods of behavioral control is linked to children's behavior problems. However, a diversity of methods of parental control of children's behavior is normal and a balance of approaches – e.g. praise and punishment – is important, providing a 'good enough' environment for most children. The emotional context is particularly important. Parental conflict can adversely affect children's performance. The social learning environment that promotes moral development is warm not punitive, emphasizes others' feelings and perspectives and models appropriate behavior. Children continue to practice skills if they are rewarded or the behavior is reinforced. A young baby hits an object during an involuntary action. If it makes a noise or looks attractive she is likely to try again and start the process of exploring the environment. If when babies wave their arms around and make a noise there is no feedback or response from their environment or they are shouted at, they are likely to stop exploring and keep quiet. It has been suggested that in this way severe deprivation in the first year of life can affect children's ability to learn for the rest of their lives. The more infants see and hear the more they want to see and hear later.

Deprivation

Material deprivation can impair parents' capacity to give time and attention to their children and increase the risk of maternal depression. Children from deprived environments (especially where neglect is prominent) may show developmental delay, particularly of language.[6,7] Children best learn the meaning of words when the word and the object are closely and frequently associated. The child deprived of simple play with adults does not have the opportunity to hear language related to the immediate environment. He/she may be surrounded by more complex visual and auditory stimuli from television or older siblings, but may be unable to interpret and learn from these stimuli because of their complexity or because of interference from background noises.

Recent studies of children who have been adopted from Romanian orphanages attest to both the resilience and the vulnerability of developmental processes. When reassessed at the age of 4 years, those children adopted within the UK by the age of 6 months had shown cognitive catch up, despite having shown severe physical and developmental retardation. Those adopted after 6 months of age showed catch up, but not to the same extent.[8,9] Social, cognitive and interactive development are particularly at risk. Age of adoption was a greater predictor of outcome than nutritional state.

BIOLOGICAL FACTORS

A child's development may be affected by abnormalities of brain function, of special senses or of effector organs such as the limbs and muscles, either as part of innate development or acquired through some damaging event.

Brain damage or dysfunction

Brain damage or dysfunction may affect all areas of function or only specific areas. Diffuse insults may produce specific dysfunction because of the vulnerability of a particular area of the brain at the time of insult (e.g. periventricular leukomalacia and basal ganglia damage due to hypoxia at term). Influences may be prenatal, through genetics, or maternal disease or postnatal, such as illness, injury or deficiencies.

Deficiencies are rare in developed countries, but iron deficiency anemia has been reported to have effects on development, and a number of studies report that the type of milk given to premature newborns affects cognitive development.[10]

The effects of certain types of brain damage (e.g. cranial irradiation) may not be immediately apparent, but only materialize when new learning is attempted. Concepts of neural plasticity are invoked in the context of damage, although some areas of differentiated function appear to show less of this (e.g. the primary motor cortex) than others.

Effects of early brain injury are often attenuated relative to later injury, for example the effects of stroke on language development in children with dominant hemisphere, but unilateral, cerebral damage. In this situation language learning is relatively unimpaired if they are under 6 or 7 years of age. In many children who have so-called 'developmental disorders', for example dyslexia and language disorder, there is no evidence of brain damage, but newer imaging techniques may identify specific areas and/or processes of dysfunction, often in the context of a strong family history.[11]

Chromosome abnormalities

Chromosome abnormalities (see Ch. 15) may affect general learning processes or have specific effects, and can result in the development of recognizable behavioral phenotypes, for example:

1. Prader–Willi: chromosome 15 deletion or uniparental disomy (early feeding difficulties and hypotonia, learning problems and later eating/hunger control disorder, see Ch. 16);
2. Smith–Magenis: chromosome 17 deletion (severe mental retardation with severe sleep disturbance, behavior problems of aggression and self-mutilation and the stereotyped behavior of upper body hugging).

Single and multiple gene disorders

The most common single gene disorder causing learning disability is Fragile X. Many developmental disorders are increasingly being recognized as having substantial genetic predisposition, but are likely to be related to the combined effects of variations within multiple genes rather than single gene defects.

Defects of special senses

Defects of special senses most commonly affect vision and hearing and can result in a severe restriction of the information a child receives, which is essential to normal development. When impairments are severe it is obvious that development will be affected. When impairments are less severe, or intermittent, as in the case of secretory otitis media, it is more difficult to assess the effect on development; however, where other impairments exist, the effect is likely to be cumulative.

Defects of effector organs – structural and movement disorders

Disorders of movement may be due to abnormality of the brain (cerebral palsy), spinal cord (paraplegia), nerves (spinal muscular atrophy) or muscles (dystrophy). These disorders have a direct effect on movement and also limit the child's experience. The child who cannot move independently does not experience space and distance and cannot reach things to manipulate them. It is important for parents and therapists to recognize this and to provide the child with compensatory experience.

Those disorders where there is no central brain involvement are less complex from the learning point of view, but some disorders that predominantly affect muscles (e.g. muscular dystrophy) have a significant effect on learning through a direct brain effect.

Other structural problems, such as facial disorders and cleft palate, influence development through direct effects (e.g. speech articulation), indirect effects (e.g. conductive hearing loss) or associated learning problems (as in chromosome 22 abnormalities: the velocardiofacial syndrome).

Sex and development

Although the mediation is unknown and texts of milestones of development do not necessarily differentiate, there are some differences between boys and girls in development. For example, in the MacArthur study of language acquisition boys were on average 1 month behind girls, but the difference accounted for less than 2% of the variation within and across ages.[12] Nearly all the developmental disorders are more common in boys than girls. One theory proposed by Geschwind and Galaburda[13] suggests that the influence of testosterone is to delay maturation of specific processes within the brain.

Gestational age

Gestational age is a relevant consideration for children under 24 months of age. Convention suggests that full correction for gestation should be made up to this time, but clinically there should be caution and some would advocate using less than the whole correction from 12 months onwards, especially in cognitive skills.

Compounding effects of impairments

Biological and social factors may interact. When there is a biological abnormality, psychosocial factors become even more important determinants of the child's future, but it is precisely in this situation that parental resources are stretched. The child with a disability may have particular characteristics that are likely to make it harder for the parents to react to her. For example, the child may not smile or may go rigid when picked up and thereby not elicit the normal parental response. This can result in a vicious cycle, with the child becoming more disabled than originally expected. The severely visually impaired child may withdraw into self-stimulation, the rarely handled child with cerebral palsy become more rigid. The child with a communication disorder such as autism may not respond as expected, so caregiver behavior changes.

The ability of parents to consciously modify their reaction and provide for the child's special needs depends on their internal and external resources.

NORMAL DEVELOPMENT

A developmental framework is essential for understanding a child's functioning and behavior and should be conceived over a life course.[14,15] Traditionally development is described as steps or stages of ages and in various fields of behavior, for example prenatal, infancy (from birth to 24 months), childhood (2–5/6 years), in areas such as physical, motor, adaptive, cognitive and language, personal, social and emotional. This should not detract from the fact that a child's development at any specific age is an integrated whole and over time is a continuous process. The integration of all aspects of development through to adolescence is shown in Table 7.2.

Descriptions of development tend to focus on universals rather than individual differences. They also tend to focus on skills acquired rather than processes of learning. Age is an ambiguous variable and is often a proxy for other processes (e.g. brain maturation). Change and continuity both need to be emphasized for individuals. At a number of time points critical periods occur with consequent disturbances to development. For example the presence of a cataract in a child's eye that prevents visual information reaching the visual cortex may result in failure to develop vision unless the cataract is removed within the first weeks of life. Whether there are other critical periods for learning social or cognitive skills remains contentious.

The following section looks at the sequence and process of development in different areas.

PHYSICAL GROWTH

Physical growth is discussed in Chapter 15. Hormones affect development and behavior but physical and mental growth may be dissociated.

MOTOR SKILLS

Figure 7.1 gives a description of motor development at different ages. The acquisition of motor skills depends on:

1. Postural control, itself depending on reflex adjustment of tone in a large number of muscles in response to visual and proprioceptive feedback, develops in a cephalocaudal direction starting with head control, then progressing with sitting, standing, walking and running.
2. The development of a body schema or image through interpretation of proprioceptive, vestibular, tactile and visual information.
3. The loss of primitive reflexes. (The fetus moves in utero and the newborn infant shows movements, some of which are reflexly determined. After birth reflex movements that initially may be useful have to disappear before purposeful controlled movements can develop. For example, the asymmetrical tonic neck reflex, most evident at 2–3 months, may contribute to the development of visually directed grasping but its persistence is abnormal, as in some children with cerebral palsy, and interferes with bimanual manipulative skills.) Primitive neonatal reflexic behavior declines as both gross and fine controlled movements increase.
4. An increasing ability to interpret the visual information in the environment in order to judge, for example, distance, depth, trajectory and weight correctly.
5. The development of movement patterns which are rapidly adjustable in response to environmental circumstances so that actions are smooth, refined and economical, and where movements are increasingly separable from each other (e.g. arm and hand reach without whole body movement – as happens in cerebral palsy).

The child cannot develop sophisticated movements without first achieving postural control. All forms of movement are sequential postural adjustments, so that without resting tone or balance movement is uncontrolled. The secondary protective reflexes of propping and saving, which develop from 20 weeks onwards, are developmental and can be absent or abnormal in motor disorders.[16] Mirror movements may be a feature of normal motor development.

Table 7.2 Integration of all aspects of development through to adolescence

	Ages (years)				
	0–1	1–2	3–5	6–12	12+
Stages	Infant	Toddler	Preschool	School	Adolescent
Motor	Sitting → Stand → Walk → Run Grasp → Finger/thumb grip →Handedness → Bimanual coordination for complex tasks				
Cognitive and play	Sensorimotor → Representational (defining by use) → Imaginative and pretence Manipulative → Matching → Categorization (conceptual) Object permanence → Concrete thinking (increasingly symbolic) → Abstract thinking Means–end → Increasing linking of events → Dual representation of ideas and theory of mind Observation → Imitation				
Communication	Joint action → Increasing sharing Joint attention (initiated and receptive) → Reciprocity and conversation				
Language	Recognizes familiar setting/shows understanding in context	Increasing understanding of meaning of words outside familiar context	Increasing understanding of abstract concepts (e.g. time, distance, motions)		
Speech	Babble → Gesture → Point → Words →Sentences → Understands and uses range of facial communicative and emotional expressions				
Social/emotional	Egocentric → Increasing awareness of other needs Dependent caregiver attachment → Explores from secure base → Peer group play → Individual friends → Extended peer group Friendly to all →Stranger awareness Fed → Feeds self →Increasing independence dressing, feeding, continence				
Moral	Aware of action/reaction → Self/other action on others → Rules → Ideals				
Attention	Distractible/single channel → Own control				
Psychosexual	Gender identity → Gender-typed behavior → Single sex play → Sexual object choice				

Position	Newborn	4 weeks	6 weeks	8 weeks	12 weeks	16 weeks	20 weeks	24 weeks
Supine	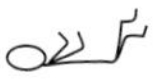	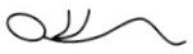			Head midline, finger play 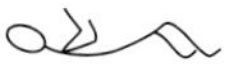		Head lifted more 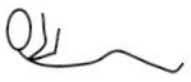	Rolls from prone to supine. Head lifted spontaneously, legs lifted, foot play 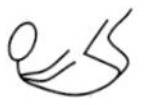
Pull to sit	No head control 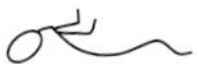	Almost complete head lag	Head lag not quite complete 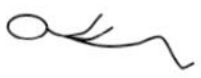		Good head control - only moderate head lag 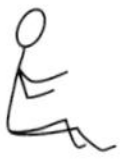		Head lifted in anticipation of being picked up 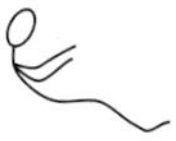	Pull to sit - head lifted off couch when about to be pulled up - hands are held up to be lifted
Sitting	Curved back 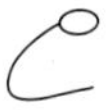	Held in sitting position may hold head up momentarily 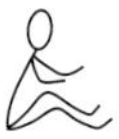		Head is held up but recurrently bobs forwards	Holds head steady and erect for several seconds, lumbar curve 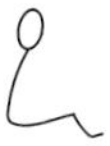	Held in sitting position - holds head well up constantly - looks actively around but head still wobbles if examiner causes sudden movement of trunk	Partial response to sideways tilt of trunk, righting but not propping with arm 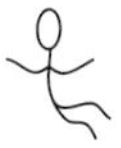	Sits in high chair for few moments (supported); sits propped forwards 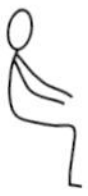
Prone	Legs tucked under 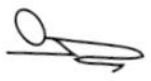	Momentarily holds chin off couch	Lifts chin off couch. Legs extended 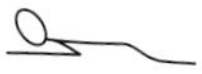		Prone - lifts head and upper chest off couch - bearing weight on forearms. 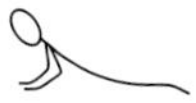 Good head control	Curvature of back - now only in lumbar region compared with rounded back of earlier weeks		Prone - weight borne on hands with extended arms - chest and upper part of abdomen being off the couch 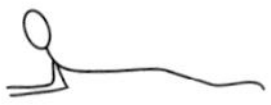
Ventral suspension in prone position with hand under abdomen	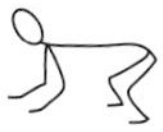		Momentary tensing of neck muscles should be noted	Ventral suspension holds head up so that its plane is in line with that of the body 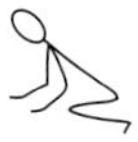				Partial forward parachute 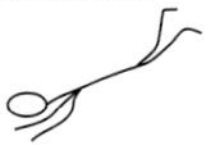
Standing	Automatic stepping 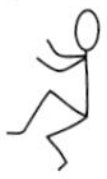				Off feet 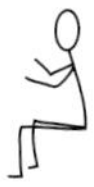			Held in standing position - bears large fraction of weight. Downward parachute response, feet meet ground plantigrade when baby held and rapidly lowered (not shufflers) 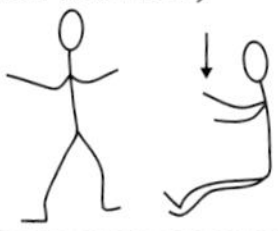

Fig. 7.1 Summary of development of spontaneous movement and posture control.

(Continued)

86 FOUNDATIONS OF HEALTH AND PRACTICE

Position	28 weeks	32 weeks	36 weeks	40 weeks	44 weeks	48 weeks	1 year	15 months	18 months
Supine	Supine - spontaneously lifts head off couch, rolls from supine to prone								
Sitting	Sits with hands forward for support	Sits for a few moments when unsupported. 90% at 8 months 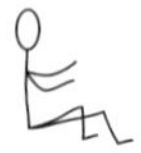	Sits steadily for 10 minutes, leans forward and recovers balance (cannot lean sideways)	Sits steadily without risk of falling over except for occasional accident Pulls self to sitting position, goes forward from sitting to prone and from prone to sitting	Sitting - can lean over sideways	Sitting - can pivot, can turn round and pick up objects 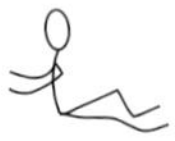			Seats itself in chair often by a process of climbing up, standing, turning round and sitting down
Prone	Prone - bears weight on one hand		Prone - in trying to crawl may progress backwards - may progress by rolling	Creeps pulling self forward with hands, abdomen on couch	Prone - crawls (abdomen off couch) 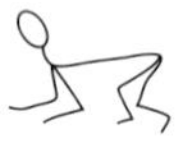		Prone - walks on hands and feet like a bear - may shuffle on buttocks and hands 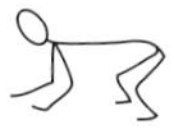	Creeps upstairs	
Evoked responses	Puts arm out to save if tilted off balance - sideways prop 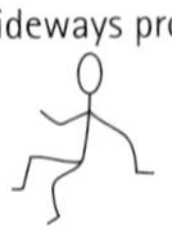	Full propping response both sides And tilt response 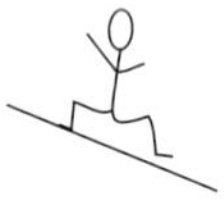		Forward parachute response, forward descent to ground, arms and hands extended 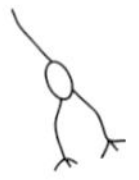	Oblique suspension. Baby held under pelvis sideways arm and leg extended 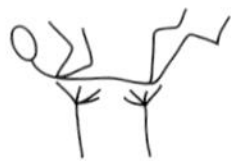				

Fig. 7.1   Continued

SENSORY AND PERCEPTUAL DEVELOPMENT

Specific domains process the perceptions of vision, hearing, smell and touch and their components (e.g. movement, form, color and dimension for vision). There are critical periods for visual information and speech sound processing. Information processing will include speed of processing, intermodal and crossmodal integration, such as the coordination of vision and hearing perception at 3 months. The meaning (conceptual understanding) of what is seen or heard probably builds on innate recognition patterns (e.g. of the face).

Vision

At birth the newborn eyeball is short and the ciliary muscles immature. The focal length for clearest vision is thus near to the baby and helped by high contrast. Movement, form and color are all perceived early. The infant scans the edges of shapes first and then internal features, showing pattern preferences (e.g. faces rather than jumbled features). By 6–7 months the baby not only recognizes faces but discriminates between facial expressions (e.g. happy or fearful). Various ingenious experiments show that by 6–7 months depth perception is present as well as an understanding that shapes stay the same whether you are close or far away (called size and shape constancy). The visual cortex appears to be highly specific and to show critical periods for its development.

Sound perception

The ear is fully developed at birth and sound perception is possible in utero. Speech perception and recognition of voices of different speakers are present shortly after birth. The capacity for smell and touch as well as the other senses are similarly developed at birth and play an important part in the perceptual learning about the environment.

Crossmodal perception

Crossmodal perception (i.e. the integration of information from different senses) is demonstrable within the first months and contributes to the conceptual development of the meaning of experiences stored in memory and the expectation of constancy of experience – shown experimentally as confusion. The 'meaning' that the child is able to attach to sensations and perceptions is the cognitive end point and this depends not only on the process of perception and conception, but also the social and cultural context, which attaches meaning as well.

Position	28 weeks	32 weeks	36 weeks	40 weeks	44 weeks	48 weeks	1 year	15 months	18 months
Standing	Standing position - can maintain extension of hips and knees for short period when supported. Bounces with pleasure having previously sagged at hips and knees	Readily bears whole weight on legs when supported	Stands holding on to furniture 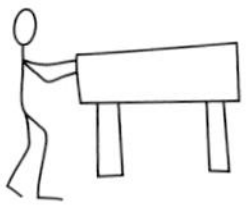	Pulls to standing position	When standing holds on - lifts and replaces one foot	Walks sideways holding on to furniture. Walks with two hands held	Walks with one hand held May stand unsupported for a moment 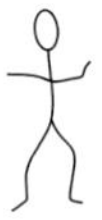 Walking alone Lower guard	Can get into standing position without support, walks without help with broad base - high stepping gait and steps of unequal length and direction. (The maturity of the gait must be noted from now onward.) The wide base decreases as balance improves and arms are released for carrying 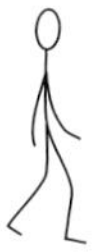	Walks well with feet only slightly apart - pulls toys as he walks - climbs stairs holding rail or helping hands. Runs rather stiffly - seldom falls. Throws ball without falling 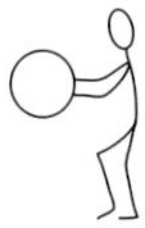 Squat and rise

Position	21 months	2 years	2.5 years	3 years	4 years	5 years	By 10 years
Walking skills	Walks backwards in imitation - picks up object from floor without falling, walks upstairs two feet per step	Goes upstairs alone, and down holding on, two feet per step	Jumps on both feet - walks on tiptoe when asked - kicks a large ball	Goes upstairs one foot per step - downstairs two feet per step Jumps off bottom step - stands on one foot for a few seconds	Runs, avoiding objects easily Goes up and downstairs one foot per step	Skips, hops, dances	Walks heel to toe backwards Can do 'fog' tests - walk on outer borders of feet with arms loose at sides
Other skills				Rides tricycle, catches well-directed ball with arms outstretched		Throws and catches a ball well enough to join in group games, but catching with one hand is not reliable until 9–10 years	

Fig. 7.1 Continued

Motor perception and manipulation skills

Figure 7.2 shows normal manipulative, visual and hearing development.

Once a child achieves reliable postural control increasingly accurate manipulative skills can be developed – integration of visual input and motor output is essential for normal acquisition of these skills. Grasping is shown in Figure 7.3.[17] Voluntary, accurate release is as essential as grasping for later manipulative skills. Handedness (which hand is dominant) is clear in many children by 24 months and is expected in the majority by 42 months. Delayed development of which hand is dominant is frequently associated with specific as well as general learning difficulties.

Manual competence can be assessed in component skills:

1. use of tools (e.g. putting a bead in a screw top jar, putting a pen together);
2. imitation of gestures (these can be miming, how to brush hair after being shown a hairbrush or a picture of one, or copying hand

Age	Manipulation	Vision	Hearing
4 weeks		Watches mother when she talks to him. Looks at a dangling toy in line of vision and follows briefly	Quiets to familiar voice
8 weeks	Hands more frequently open	Follows dangling toy from side to side past midline, eyes show fixation and convergence in focusing	
12 weeks	Watches movement of own hands, pulls at clothes, shows a desire to grasp objects and holds rattle briefly when placed in hands	Follows dangling toy from one side to the other through 180° and vertically	Turns to familiar sounds in supine
16 weeks	Hands come together, approaches objects with hands – often fails to reach. Plays for longer periods with object placed in hand	Recognizes objects, for example familiar toy	Turns head towards a sound
20 weeks	Two-handed scoop for object Arm movements increasingly better controlled to reach directly for objects	Smiles at self in mirror	Recognizes individual voices, listens to conversation
24 weeks	Manipulation – reaches and grasps objects on table surface with raking palmar grasp. Puts hands up to hold bottle, drops one object if holding when another offered	Sees and recognizes at adult distance Looks at falling objects	Turns to sounds when sitting if sounds on ear level Distraction tests used to test functional hearing
36 weeks	Has learned to transfer objects from one hand to another and can hold an object in each hand. Uses index finger approach to touch objects, can pick up small object between finger and thumb. Enjoys releasing objects over the side of cot or chair	Sees crumbs on floor Looks for fallen objects out of sight	Locates sounds made above and below ear level and at greater distance
1 year	Has mature prehension and can release object precisely. Can now hold two cubes in one hand, brings one cube in each hand together in the midline and imitates clicking and tries to build two cubes	Recognizes pictures of objects	Recognizes tunes and tries to join in Locates sounds above ear level
15 months	Can takes objects out of container and replace more precisely (e.g. pegmen in wooden boat)	100s and 1000s used for near vision	Distraction test to specific frequencies used
18–24 months	Refinement of release enables the child to build cubes to an increasing height and post objects accurately through holes. Increasing control of finger movements can be used by the child to manipulate tools (e.g. spoon, crayon) and pages of a book. Initially pencils are held with a fisted cylindrical palmar grip then a high shaft pronated grip		

Fig. 7.2 Development of manipulation, vision and hearing.

(Continued)

Age	Manipulation	Vision	Hearing
24–36 months	Learns to use a more adult grip, turn single page carefully, stack eight bricks (90% by 30 m) and take off socks 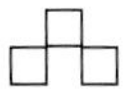 33–36 m 80% at 39 m Copies from model 36–39 m 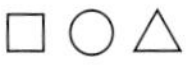 □ ○ △ Shapes inserted 24 m Insert puzzle-pieces recognized at 30 m and orientated 33 m Draws man 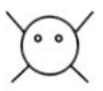	Tested with matching letters from 2+ years. Can use the Kay pictures from 24 months (naming pictures) but monocular testing difficult before 42 months Sonksen-Silver linear chart from 30 m	Hearing tested by pointing at toys/pictures from 24 months chosen for their range of component sounds (e.g. McCormick toys) and by conditioning to sounds from 30 months (to put an object in a box when a sound is heard). This leads on to pure tone audiometry; individual ears may be tested in some children at 3 years
4 years	Holds a pencil in the adult way, a dynamic tripod, is able to cut with scissors and thread beads Copies from model 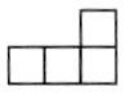 39–42 m 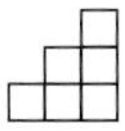 48 m 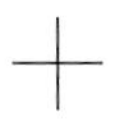 + Man 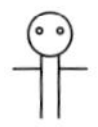	Monocular testing possible in majority	Speech/word tests and pure tone audiometry in each ear
5 years	Shows great precision in hand movements and in the use of tools. Can cut a strip of paper neatly, and when building bricks holds the cubes with the ulnar fingers tucked in and hand diagonal to get a better view. Can feed tidily with a spoon and fork, dress and brush teeth. Refinement of finger movements can be demonstrated by increasing speed at inserting pegs in a board and threading beads Copies 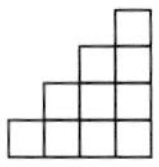 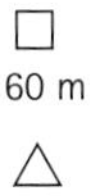 □ 60 m Man △ 66 m 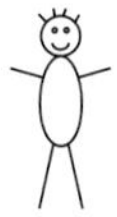 50 m+	Screening recommended by orthoptists in school	Audiometric screening recommended in school

Fig. 7.2   Continued

postures that are increasingly complex and may or may not be symbolic) – miming the use of a familiar object is a skill shown by 5 years; all others show a steady progression to the age of 12 years;[18]
3. learning a sequence of motor actions and writing/drawing.
Perceiving shapes correctly and being able to reproduce them are essential for reading and writing. The ability to match shapes can be demonstrated by the use of form boards with different shapes (e.g. circles, squares and triangles), which have to be fitted into the appropriate space on the board. The ability to copy shapes is shown by asking the child to copy a three-brick bridge (3 years) and five-brick bridge (5 years). The ability to copy shapes with a pencil starts with a vertical line (second year) and a horizontal line and circle (third year). This progresses to letters and more complex shapes requiring juxtaposition of vertical, horizontal and oblique lines (Bender Gestalt test, see p.103).

Harris[19] devised a scoring system giving age norms for the ability to draw a man. Such ability is related to control of pencil movement, ability to reproduce shapes and concept of body image. By 3 years the child has just learned to draw a circle and during the next year will add to this – vertical lines to represent legs, horizontal lines as arms and one or two features such as eyes and mouth (Fig. 7.4). It is not until 5 years that arms and legs are appropriately placed on a trunk (Fig. 7.5) At this age children can also draw a square and therefore a house with windows (some can do this at a younger age; Fig. 7.6).

LANGUAGE, SPEECH AND COMMUNICATIVE DEVELOPMENT

An essential feature of human life is the use of a system of symbols for communication and thought. The attachment of names to objects and actions is an essential prerequisite not only for language but also for thinking. If we had no such system we would need to produce the object itself each time we wished to discuss it. It is conventional to consider 'speech' separately from 'language' and both as having 'receptive' and 'expressive', or 'input' and 'output' components. The component structures of language are:

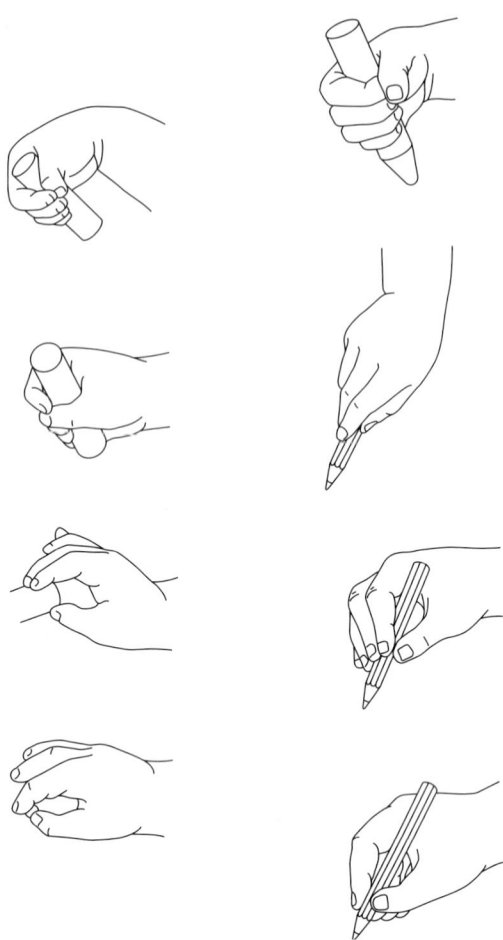

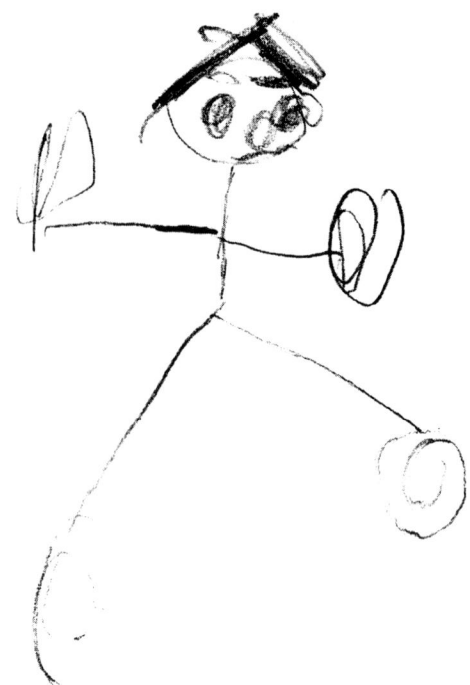

Fig. 7.5   It is not until 5 years that arms and legs are appropriately placed on a trunk.

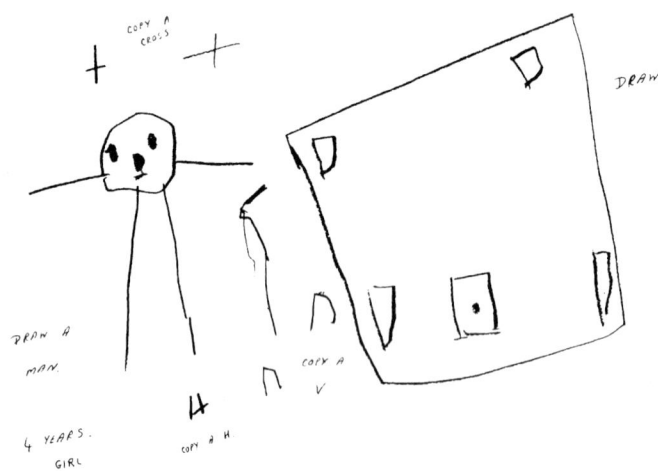

Fig. 7.6   At 5 years, children can draw a square and therefore a house with windows.

Fig. 7.3   Grasping. (Illustrations from The Erhardt Development Prehension Assessment, from Developmental Hand Dysfunction, 2nd edn. Copyright © 1994 by Rhoda P Erhardt. Published by Erhardt Developmental Products, Maplewood MN 55119, USA. Reprinted by permission.)

1. phonological (the perception and production of sounds to words and sentences);
2. semantics and syntax (words, their meaning, the small grammatical features – morphemes – and rules combining words in sentences);
3. pragmatics refers to the understanding and use of language in context.

Overview of theories applied to speech, language and communicative development

Theories of language development range from the structural linguistic to the functional social and from language as a domain-specific skill to a continuity of general cognitive processes applied to linguistic symbols.

Chomsky[2] proposed that the brain must be pre-programed to extract and master the specific grammatical structures of spoken language. He introduced the concept of the 'language acquisition device', suggesting the nativist view that language is a robust and pre-programed biological

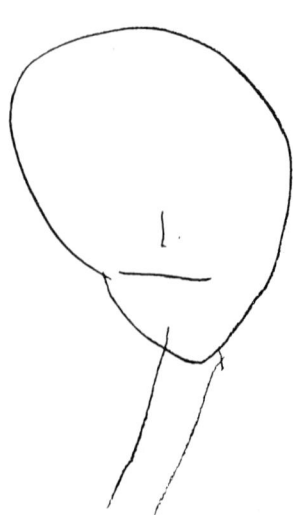

Fig. 7.4   By 3 years the child has learned to draw a circle and during the next year will add to this – vertical lines to represent legs, horizontal lines as arms and one or two features such as eyes and mouth.

function, separate, to some extent, from other intellectual functions and dependent only to a limited extent on environmental input. Some children with specific language impairments have a particular problem with acquisition of grammatical morphemes, leading to the search for particular grammatical markers of language impairment.

The psycholinguistic approach uses a language processing model of language disorder to identify the specific problem in language processing and offer remediation.

'Connectionist theories' of computer-simulated parallel processing combine sensitivity to language input with dependence on a learning architecture in the brain. Models have been described for the learning of past tenses of verbs, vocabulary, concept words and syntax. Learning takes place as the system is presented with regular and then irregular verbs and is modulated by a number of weighted activations assessing the probability of any particular ending for any particular verb stem. General learning processes, such as imitation and context bound chunk learning, followed by increasing symbolic representational development and abstraction with creativity, are thought to be important in word, verb and syntactic development.

The degree to which language and thinking are separable has taxed theorists. Vygotsky[20] conceives of language as a speech processing/word formation system developing independently and, for technical perfection and intelligibility, dependent upon a domain-specific learning system. However, the meaning of the speech processed and used depends on the social context in which it is learned and this has its basis in the social cognitive ability of the child as well as the environment and responsiveness of the parent/caregiver. Thus language acquisition is inseparable from the development of social communication, both verbal and nonverbal, and the social relationship. The meaning of communication is learned in a social cultural context and requires broader social – cognitive skills to interpret the meaning of all the coordinated forms of communication, such as body posture, facial expression, eye gaze, tone of voice, speech and gestures, which are all smoothly combined in the adult – the pragmatics of language use.

The child is an active partner in language acquisition. Babies have an innate social interest in other humans, displaying an early ability to perceive aspects of the face and the meaning of facial expressions and posture, actions and sounds in varying combinations, and are therefore programed to develop an interest in human communication. The baby responds to facial expression and tone of voice (6 months) long before she understands the meaning of words. The baby seeks the 'meaning' of social actions from a number of cues, especially emotions. Mothers reflect back certain things babies do and give them meaning. Physical actions are usually easy to interpret. The understanding that the focus of an adult's visual attention is likely to be what they are talking about is an important cognitive step. The child's understanding that objects have labels is helped by the spontaneous behavior of adults who when they see children looking at or pointing to an object will tend to name it (e.g. 'yes, that's the cat').

The child and parent develop 'joint' attention through shared actions.[21] The child learns to coordinate his attention and interest between an object and person, seen in gaze switching, facial expressions and vocalizing. The baby uses sounds in a reciprocal or turn-taking manner before they are intelligible as words. Early conversations have all the important elements of social discourse, initiating, responding and repair (i.e. making some effort if the exchange breaks down). Towards the end of the first year, the baby shows increasing awareness of self and others and becomes an intentional communicator, also showing anticipation of the parents' actions, intentions and feelings, and checking the parents' response to new situations by observing their facial expression ('social referencing').

The initiation of shared interest with an adult by the child is a good marker of normally developing social communication skills in a child of 12–18 months. Gaze switching and the frequency of this behavior in a play situation is easily observed. Communication accompanied by eye gaze has greater social meaning. The child learns to form predictions of complexes of behaviors. Early joint attention skills are deficient

in children with autism[22] and representational forms of communication may not be understood as having relevant meaning. In blind children, establishing meaning can be particularly difficult. For the deaf child in a speaking household this can also be a problem. For the learning disabled child (e.g. Down syndrome) it is a slow process needing more time for both assimilation and response.

Vocalization and speech

The development of vocalization and speech depends upon an intact motor learning system as well as hearing speech, and evolves rapidly from a limited repertoire of sounds during the first few months. From about 6 months onwards, the sound patterns take on the qualities of adult speech. By the end of the first year, the sound patterns of the child's 'native' language are established and the ability to discriminate the sounds of other languages diminishes (e.g. 9 month olds prefer to listen to native words rather than non-native). They learn to reproduce pairs of syllables by integrating the sequences in which they are presented as well as the rhythm (at 6 months babies are sensitive to the rhythm, but not the sequences of syllables). Strings of babble become more connected, intonation takes on the pattern of adult speech and the child begins to imitate phrases and words. At this stage, the words and sentences may not be analyzed into their component parts. The child may copy a whole word or phrase by the rhythm it makes.

Children vary in their rote memory capacity for memorizing chunks of speech. Constant practice in making sounds reinforces motor patterns, which become increasingly automatic. The amount of babble is correlated with early vocabulary. Abnormal or infrequent speech sounds in the first year can be a marker of later speech and language problems or deafness.

At the early stages of communicative development some children may tend to use gestures without also using spoken words, while other children use both gestures and words. Bates et al[23] suggested that this reflects individual variation in communicative style or preference. The developmental sequelae of these different early communicative styles are not known. Fenson et al[24] suggested that symbolic and communicative gestures may act as a 'bridge'[25] from word comprehension to word production.

Pointing behavior is particularly important because it indicates a precise referent on the part of the child rather than undifferentiated need and is a precursor of symbolic development.

Two reasons for pointing behaviors can be observed.
1. Proto-imperative 'indicating' behaviors represent the child's demand for needs to be met. This may be done by pointing or vocalization. Such behaviors do not necessarily involve any shared interest or attention (or mental idea of other people).
2. By contrast, proto-declarative communicative behaviors are a preverbal effort to direct the adult's attention to an event or object. This purpose of pointing is to 'share' interest with another person. Proto-declarative behaviors correlate highly with the emergence of first words and predict in normal development the vocabulary at 20 months and the sentence length at 28 months.

During the first 10-word stage words may be largely imitative or bound to context, they may be formulaic and learned in association with a particular event and may be presymbolic. The words are not necessarily securely fixed in the mental representational linguistic system.

The first words that a child utters are very dependent upon shared referents with parents: for example in the Korean culture, verbs are commoner than nouns; the opposite is true in English speakers. Children vary in the predominant types of early vocabulary they use. Some use more context-bound phrases (names of people and objects) while others begin with more communicative social words (such as 'look' or 'here y'are', or words such as 'more' and 'gone'). Most children use both styles.

Language and thinking are intimately related as the child learns to map words onto existing thoughts or concepts and the learning of a word can stimulate new concepts. While acquiring early vocabulary the child's next cognitive stage is the move from the primary and simple associative use of the sounds of language to a more symbolic, representational and decontextualized use. Overextensions are common at this stage (e.g. 'daddy' for all men).

Comprehension of language is in advance of expression in normal development. Nouns are the largest class of words in early vocabularies. When new words are used, a child tries to find a meaning for them. The development of grammar does not seem to depend on repeating adult structures; rather children seem to extract the rules of grammar and experiment for themselves, sometimes to comical effect – for example:
Lucy: Squeak, squeak – that's what mouses does.
Mother: That's what mice do.
Lucy: What do mices does?[26]

Wide normal range

As with many skills of development there is a wide normal variation in the acquisition of speech and language (e.g. in the MacArthur scales[23]). At 16 months children in the top 10% produce 154 words, those in the lowest 10% produce none; 80% of children at 16 months understand between 78 and 303 words (-1.28 SD to $+1.28$ SD). Severe delays have predictive significance, but there is no best age for determining milder speech and language delays. A child who is delayed at 18 months will not necessarily be delayed at 3 years.

SOCIAL LEARNING, SELF AND OTHERS, PLAY AND ADAPTIVE SKILLS

Social learning, self and others, play and adaptive skills include:
1. the child's social reactions to other persons and to peers through the development of attachments and social understanding;
2. development of self-awareness and self-regulation;
3. mastery of skills such as feeding, elimination and dressing.
The normal development of cognitive and adaptive skills, play, language comprehension and speech, communication and social interaction is outlined in Table 7.3.

Social learning, becoming aware of self and others, and the development of other play and adaptive skills marks the change from a dim awareness of self and mother to an understanding of the complex rules of social behavior and interaction. Even neonates are socially competent, in that they are able to elicit the attention of their parents. It has been shown that mothers respond to their babies' behavior more often than the other way round. Thus features of an infant's temperament and her potential for social communicative drive and competence will be relevant to how the parent behaves. Studies of blind babies and their mothers show how easy it is for parents to miss cues for communication when they are not conventional. The non-initiating, nonresponding, autistic child soon trains a parent not to initiate interaction. The parent of the baby with Down syndrome needs to wait for the often rather slower initiating and responding behavior so that the rhythmic turn taking of communication is not lost.

Babies respond to the human face and to objects quite differently. In response to a face their eyes widen, posture is relaxed and by 6 weeks a smile arises. This simple milestone is a very reliable indicator of abnormality if delayed beyond 8 weeks. During the latter half of the first year babies lose their indiscriminate warm response to all people and begin to recognize familiar adults and to become wary of strangers. They develop a strong attachment to their caretakers and separation at this time and during the second year of life is particularly distressing to a child. Securely attached children who are confident of their mother's warm presence are able during the second year to begin to explore and to achieve mastery of feeding and elimination.

An important stage of social cognitive development is that of joint attention (described in the language section above) shown in the transition from dyadic to triadic attention (from focus on object or focus on person to focus on object then switching focus to person and back again to object). The latter involves the sharing of focus, which is the indication of interest by the child and recognition that there is mutuality of meaning with the parent and the sharing of an idea. Such behavior appears to be the precursor of social understanding of others' feelings and perspectives, the knowing that other people have minds. Understanding other people's emotions is an important part of learning about them and sharing those feelings may lead to the development of empathy. Emotional 'knowing' and 'display' may not be the same as understanding the thinking of other minds (a connected but possibly separable skill).[27] Understanding and using the knowledge of how someone else might feel is also an important component of moral development.

In normal development, children initiate joint attention. They direct their parents to something they are interested in and respond to parental behavior that does the same, shown by gaze shifts to share looking at things and following index finger pointing. The social referencing behavior of children, in new situations, when they scan the faces of people, but especially parents, to give them cues about how they should then respond, is seen in the last trimester of the first year.

The child shows increasing independence from adults and awareness of self in relation to others during the second and third year, and this is observable both in play and language use.

During the nursery years (3–5 years) children's horizons widen as they are faced with a new social world of adults and other children. The child becomes less egocentric and learns how to play with other children, taking into account their wishes and needs, although the cognitive capacity to consider two perspectives simultaneously and reflect upon them in a judgmental way does not mature until nearer 8 or more years.

Behavior should get easier as reasoning becomes more possible and the child learns about 'deferment'. Instead of just reacting, children cognitively appraise and interpret events. The personal memories that form the basis of reflection are constructed from the experiences of the child woven into a mental schema or narrative of representations and feelings. Ideas of truth and moral rightness develop. For example, young school-age children (but not preschoolers) can accept an action by someone who is mistaken in their belief, but not where they are morally wrong. Thus it is alright to give more food to boys than girls if you believe they need more but not if it is done because it is OK to be nicer to boys![28] Moral development, the rules and conventions of interpersonal behavior, require both the behavioral opportunities for learning (i.e. example, reinforcement, rules/punishment) and the cognitive skills to be able to take perspectives and self-reflect. The environment needs to be warm, not punitive, model what is appropriate and emphasize other people's feelings and perspectives.

The child obtains final mastery of dressing and toileting self-help skills, and by 5 years of age is ready for more formal education. The child is, however, still essentially home based in outlook and influences. During the primary school years, the rules of the group become increasingly important, so that by 10 years of age they are often quoted to parents in a rather rebellious way. At this age boys and girls tend to form separate groups or gangs and the peer group social perspective becomes more important. The teenager is able to think in the abstract, work out the principles behind actions and is therefore able to become more independent. Freeing from parental authority is associated with a desire for acceptance and popularity in the peer group. However, developing sexual maturity is associated with many other concerns, which are dealt with in the chapter on adolescence (see Ch. 35).

COGNITIVE AND LEARNING DEVELOPMENT

Children learn about their world by listening, observing, copying and experimenting. The world of infants is very small and their repertoire of skills limited. They learn about their world through observation, by reaching and grasping objects and by copying sounds and actions. By contrast, toddlers are mobile and their worlds are large. Their motor skills are greater and they begin to attempt constructional tasks, thereby learning about aspects such as size, shape, the properties of objects and space.

The child is an active participant in the learning process. Progress depends upon not only the learning opportunities, but also the child's

Table 7.3 Normal development of cognitive and adaptive skills, play and nonverbal skills, personal skills, communication and social interaction, language comprehension and speech

Age	Play and nonverbal skils	Personal skills	Communication/social interaction	Comprehension	Speech
6–8 weeks			Smiles responsively when mother talks to or smiles at. Opens and closes mouth imitatively		
3 months	Interested in everything seen/ increasing intention to touch objects		Vocal turntaking, gurgles/ coos with pleasure Generally social to friendly adult but knows caregiver	Regularly localizes speaker with eyes	Often vocalizes with two or more different open vowel sounds/up to two syllables
6 months	Reaches for and grasps toys, usually both hands – takes to mouth. Watches objects disappear – no sustained searching. Excited by familiar toy	Tries to hold cup/bottle, poor tipping	Shares interest by gaze and gesture in peek-a-boo game. Makes noise to get attention. Tries to imitate (e.g. tongue protrusion). Smiles at image of self in mirror	Situational understanding of familiar phrase and angry/friendly voices. Localizes and recognizes different speakers	Occasionally vocalizes with four or more different syllables at one time. Nonspecific indication of emotion/ need etc. but tries to attract attention vocally
9 months	Persistent in getting toys. Transfers toys hand-to-hand, bangs toys (7 m) Looks for objects that disappear. Stage of 'sensorimotor' play and early 'cause and effect'. Pulls string to get toy	Interested in mirror play. Aware of different types of clothing. Finger feeds and early chewing. Some anticipation of familiar events	Responds to parental 'indicating' gesture. Beginnings of imitation of gesture (e.g. waves bye-bye, claps hands 10 months) and shows joint attention – ability to switch gaze between object and person to share interest. Understands and takes part in lap games with anticipation, demanding of repeated 'games' (e.g. peek-a-boo). Now more wary of strangers	Regularly stops activity in response to 'no'. Responds to own name and names of familiar people (e.g. 'daddy'). Understands gestures (e.g. holds out toys or other objects to a parent on verbal request with gesture, e.g. hand out) but may not yet have skills of release	Intonated babble with sequences of sounds. Babble more complete with different vowels and consonants. Imitates sounds. Attracts attention to self frequently
Around 12 months	'Container' play putting objects in and out. Interested in picture book. Finds hidden objects. Shows recognition of familiar objects (e.g. brush, telephone, cup and spoon and car). Less mouthing, may 'cast' – throw objects on floor. Imitates actions with objects (e.g. clicks bricks, rings bell, tries to build bricks)	Cooperates with dressing by putting arms up. Drinks from beaker held by self	Points to indicate need. Separation anxiety on leaving parent common. Quite distractible and switches to new dominant stimulus easily. Repeats performance to be laughed at	Generally shows intense attention and response to speech over prolonged periods of time – understands people's names and familiar words (e.g. 'shoes'/responds to familiar requests)	'Talks' to toys and people throughout the day using long verbal patterns (jargon)- protowords, or words accompanying communicative gesture. Shakes head for 'no'
Around 15 months	Early definition by use of play on self (e.g. brushes hair or mother's hair). Builds two-cube tower Uses pencil to mark paper Plays to and fro game with ball or truck	Increasing awareness of self/others shown in shift of object play from self to doll, use of me/mine pronouns and awareness of aspects of self in mirror. Increasingly persistent in attaining goals. May indicate when wet	Frequent communication initiated by child accompanied by showing and bringing of toys and pointing for interest and need. Follows adult point at object	Understands simple requests in context. Recognizes and identifies many names of objects in familiar surroundings. Points to pictures in book	More frequent use of words with meaning, final or beginning consonant often missing. Asks for objects by vocalizing and pointing

(Continued)

Table 7.3 Normal development of cognitive and adaptive skills, play and nonverbal skills, personal skills, communication and social interaction, language comprehension and speech—cont'd

Age	Play and nonverbal skills	Personal skills	Communication/social interaction	Comprehension	Speech
Around 18 months	Uses real and toy objects appropriately. Briefly imitates everyday domestic and personal activities. Shows preference in play. May use dolly/teddy to feed/put to bed. Builds a tower of three bricks. Can match circular shapes in insert puzzle	Feeds self with spoon without rotating it at mouth. Takes off hat/shoes. Alternates between clinging and resistance	Attends to own choice of activity, but attention can be caught by calling name and producing new toy. Verbally requests and comments. Watches others play and plays near them	Listens to adult and identifies two or more familiar objects on request from a group of four or more familiar objects. Generally understands more than 100 words in familiar setting	Begins repeating words overheard in conversation (mean 50–100) – uses minimum of 10–20 words spontaneously – range of vowels and m, p, b, t, d
Around 24 months	Play now more toy based linking actions (e.g. feed doll and then put to bed). Builds tower of six/seven bricks. Turns pages of book singly. Copies line with pencil. Able to play for more lengthy periods of time. Turns door knob and unscrews lids	Dry by day, pulls pants up and down. Helps with simple putting away when asked. Understands spills and tries to rectify. Behavior can be active and oppositional. Bowel control often attained	Mainly with adult still – watches other children. Simple chase games develop. Wants to please adult/shows off	Recognizes new words daily at an ever-increasing rate. Listens to conversations and responds. Carries out simple instructions. Understands objects by function (e.g. which one do we sit on). Points to several body parts	Speaks more and more new words each week, gesture used less often. Echoes some of the adult's speech. Puts words together in phrases 'me go'. Verbally very demanding
Around 36 months	Builds tower of eight cubes. Vivid make believe. Understands stories, can make plans. Beginning to draw recognizable man with head, eyes, legs. Copies circle and can do simple inset puzzle (orientate and insert all pieces) and match colors. Can unbutton buttons. Tries to cut with scissors. Able to show sustained concentration	Feeds with spoon and fork. Shows a sense of danger. Understands rules, right and wrong behavior related to self – more amenable. Can remove front opening garment and many other clothes. Attends to toilet needs without help	Can share, comfort others distressed. Plays with other children. Affectionate and confiding. Shows understanding that others can 'know' things. Shows sense of humour. Understands polite behavior	Understands on/in/under/big/little. Can give full name, age and sex. Beginning to count. Understands why, who, how many and questions such as 'what should you do when you're hungry?'	Uses sentences of three–four word phrases, personal pronouns, plurals and prepositions. Asks 'what', 'where' and beginning to ask 'why'? Relates own experiences. Able to have simple conversations. Immaturities of articulation common but mostly intelligible
Around 48 months	Able to show sustained concentration. More extended make-believe. Draws man with body. Copies cross and six brick steps	Aware of being in a group and expected behaviors		Understands concepts of number up to 3, colors, listens to a short story and can answer simple questions about it. Can listen to and answer two-part question and understand some words relating to feelings. Likes rhymes	Sentences of four–eight words, mostly grammatically correct. Counts to 10. Talks about experiences and can retell a simple story. Uses approximately 1500 words
Around 5–6 years	Copies square (5) and triangle (6) and ten-brick step from a model. Draws a man with head, body and features and a house with windows	Can care for most toilet needs independently. Can dress self except for shoe laces	Can have conversations, tell jokes and discuss emotions. Able to retell in a different way to assist others' understanding. Most children show 'first order theory of mind' (i.e. that someone else can 'know' something that is different and may be incorrect). Makes friends and has a preferred friend	Knows simple time concepts, can follow three commands together. Can define common objects in terms of use and answer 'what if' questions. Understands common opposite (e.g. hot/cold). Follows instructions given in a group. Can tell an unfamiliar story from pictures	Speech completely intelligible including consonant blends (e.g. Sh, th), rate, pitch and volume

learning strategies and processes. Information processing in infants is related to later cognitive abilities in memory and speed of processing, thus in visual recognition tasks, habituation, learning, object permanence and attention, including crossmodality.

In older children, the features of new problem solving that are linked to learning are variability, ability to shift focus, frequency of self-correction and diversity of strategies.

Problems with the learning process

In some infants, perceptual processing that depends upon innate recognition may be damaged and perceptual attributes that lead to salience may not be perceived. Perception that depends upon temporal processing may be slowed and crossmodality may be impaired. Meaning may be more easily accessed visually (i.e. what is seen may make more sense than what is heard). Infants learn from the repeated familiar and respond to difference – a learning style used in the 'habituation to repeat stimulus' in developmental experiment.

Learning from the familiar needs repeated stimulus and is enhanced if as many features as possible are fixed and what is remembered depends upon the match between context and item. This is a stage of normal development referred to as 'context bound' learning, when children recognize their own cups or shoes, for example, but not 'cupness' or a sentence said by one person in one place but not another. Some children get stuck in this stage and require a sustained high degree of contextual or environmental sameness to show a skill. This is particularly shown in autism.[29]

Children learn from 'contingency' – the event that follows within 3–5 seconds of their action. This may be disrupted by a number of mechanisms, such as:

1. failure of the adult to make the response (depressed/mentally ill caregiver);
2. the child not giving a clear enough signal (as for those who are blind or who have cerebral palsy).

Aspects of maternal or caregiver behavior that promote learning need to be sensitively adjusted to developmental level. Thus at 2 years of age, language input needs to be explicitly directive and adult actions tied to the focus of child interests. By 3 years less parental direction is needed because the child has more language and is learning to manage her own goal-setting and problem-solving skills.

Play complexity is enhanced by caregiver behaviors that maintain a child's focus of attention rather than redirect it. Children also learn more through the process of learning itself. For example, learning particular names of shapes accelerates shape learning generally, as though attention to the 'shape concept' allows noticing of 'shapeness'. The child's ability to inhibit and select responses and to try alternatives is crucial to all cognitive learning. This is seen in the progression from the 'trial and error' approach, where repeatedly forcing the square into the round hole is a less useful strategy than trying alternative placements with inset puzzles, which shows more flexibility of mental skills.

The progress from sensorimotor play, from mouthing to manipulation at 6–10 months, then to imitation and 'definition by use' play by 12 months is followed by increasing creativity in play. Make-believe play with dolls, in which the child is reconstructing events observed, is an important element of this period. It indicates early symbolic representation and concept formation. The child begins to use language to direct or describe the action of his play, and as command of language improves the need to act out the events decreases. Lack of ideas, failure of pretence and inability to play constructively are indications of a developmental problem.

The cognitive stage of mental symbolic development allows more complex thinking, including reflection and planning. Symbols (words) facilitate thinking about, and reference to, situations that are not in the 'here and now'. Answering simple questions dealing with nonpresent situations presents difficulty before 3 years and even primary and junior school children still tend to be concrete in their way of thinking (i.e. real objects, here and now). Early in school life, judgments are made intuitively on superficial appearances. With increasing experience and language at their disposal, children can imagine complex situations, think out the most appropriate solution and anticipate the outcome. This requires the ability to think abstractly and imaginatively. Thus, children develop logical thinking from assimilating experience into schemes or general laws that they can apply to a range of situations. The use of symbols also helps to inhibit prepotent responses of behaviors and allows increasing distancing from the 'here and now' (rather like the red card in football games). Children are developing skills of representation and object substitution in the second year, but the skill of mentally comparing reality with representation (dual reality) is not clearly seen in research studies until aged 3 years. For example, children shown where an object is hidden in a scale model of a room can find it in the real room at 3 years, but not at 30 months. At 3–6 years, children get increasingly skilled at knowing that others can hold particular views, even false views, and thus have what has been called a 'theory of mind'. In the classic Wimmer and Perner task, roughly half the 4- to 5-year-old children could correctly show 'knowing', whereas over 90% of 6- to 9-year-old children were correct.[30] This understanding of children's thinking is highly relevant when considering children's perceptions of events and their reporting of them.

DETECTING AND ASSESSING DEVELOPMENTAL PROBLEMS

Developmental impairments, learning and behavior problems are common. One of the aims of a child health service is to provide appropriate services for children with such problems, and their families.

An evidence based review of the UK Child Health Promotion Programme led to changes with increased emphasis on prevention at all levels, enhanced use of a parent – professional partnership model, and included active surveillance or formal screening only where there is appropriate evidence of effectiveness.

Changes to the elements of the program concerned with identification of developmental problems have not been introduced however without vigorous and continuing debate around the questions of which problems should be identified, how this should be achieved and whether early detection is beneficial.

DEVELOPMENT: NORMAL OR ABNORMAL?

Very severe developmental problems are likely to come to the attention of appropriate services. However, early identification of less severe problems presents particular difficulties. Development is a continuous process, and the cut-off for definite abnormality is not always clear. Although a majority of children walk by the age of 18 months, those who do not will be a mixture of those with biologically based disease, general learning problems and normal variants.[31] Thus, failing to acquire a particular skill by the generally accepted 'normal' age does not definitely predict a disorder. (Equally, acquiring a skill by the 'normal' age does not predict that future progress with that developmental skill will remain within normal limits.)

Information about the predictive outcome of a particular delay at any moment in time is ideally required. Thorough knowledge both of normal developmental variation, and the natural history of recognized developmental disorders is thus required. Although it is conventional to describe 'delays' of development (meaning normal but slow patterns of skill acquisition) and 'disorders' (where the pattern is abnormal), the distinction is not always logical since slow skill acquisition can be a manifestation of cognitive impairment.

Caution should also be exercised in the use of the term 'developmental delay' to describe any individual child's profile. While this may be a helpful term during initial evaluation and any investigation, its use long term can be misleading, implying, as it does to many parents, that 'catch-up' is expected at a later point. The best moment to characterize cognitive problems as 'learning difficulties' will vary according to individual and family need.

The wide variation in developmental norms means that it is unreasonable to expect that a single observation should lead to a definite conclusion. Therefore services will need to continue to include provision for observation while the child's skills unfold. For all children, there is increasing emphasis on advising and supporting parents in how to help promote developmental progress, whatever their level of developmental skill.

IDENTIFYING DEVELOPMENTAL PROBLEMS: EARLY DETECTION AND SCREENING

Enthusiasm for early detection of impairments by professionals led to a program of universal developmental checks at visits to 'well baby' clinics at multiple time points in the preschool years in the UK, the so called Child Health Surveillance programme.[32] However, aside from formal attempts to identify problems with a known adverse developmental outcome, such a 'surveillance' program rested on assuming both that early detection was possible, and that it has specific advantages. Developmental checks were effectively being used as 'quasi' screening tests, despite the difficulties discussed above in establishing normal from abnormal. These difficulties are exemplified in a systematic review of screening for primary language delay[33,34]

Screening can be defined as the identification of a condition at an early or presymptomatic stage such that treatment offered will confer greater benefit. The criteria of Wilson and Jungner[35] and Cochrane and Holland[36] need to be applied to any condition and to any screening test (Table 7.4).

Any test has to be simple, quick, easy to interpret, acceptable to parents, accurate and repeatable. It should be:
1. Sensitive – that is it should have the ability to give a positive finding if the person has the impairment.
2. Specific – that is, it should have an ability to give a negative result in a person with no impairment.

Table 7.4   The criteria of Wilson & Jungner[31] and Cochrane & Holland[32]

1. The condition being sought for should be an important health problem for both the individual and the community
2. There should be an acceptable form of treatment for those with recognized disease or some other form of useful intervention should be available (e.g. genetic advice)
3. The natural history of the condition should be adequately understood
4. There should be a recognizable latent or early symptomatic stage
5. Equity of access across a geographical area must be ensured
6. There should be a suitable test for detecting the early or latent stage that is acceptable to the population. The distribution of test value should be known with an agreed cutoff, high sensitivity, specificity and high positive predictive value
7. There must be an agreed method of diagnosis in the screen positive and there must be systems in place for adequate diagnosis and counseling. It is important to note that there are dangers to overinclusiveness in the 'at risk' group. Research has shown that the worry of a false positive screen does not disappear easily
8. There should be an agreed policy on who should be treated
9. The treatment in the presymptomatic stage should be able to favorably influence the course and prognosis of the disease
10. It is important to ensure that all the above criteria for a screening program are met before primary care groups and districts embark upon it. Experience has shown that it is much more difficult to stop than to start a widespread program
11. The cost of case finding which should include the cost of diagnosis and treatment should be economically balanced in relation to the possible expenditure on medical care as a whole and the constant treatment of the patient does not present until the disease reaches the symptomatic stage
12. Case finding should be a continuing process

In considering sensitivity and specificity the prevalence of the disease is very important. The ideal is high sensitivity and high specificity, but in practice one is usually at the expense of the other. Further scrutiny of the established 'distraction hearing test' for hearing impairment showed that, although reliable in skilled hands, it did not show adequate sensitivity when applied across the population. Introduction of universal neonatal hearing screening is expected to overcome this problem as well as result in an earlier mean age of identification, which has proven benefits for parental adjustment and for language outcomes[37].

As the previous system of developmental checks did not fulfill accepted screening criteria it is now generally believed that such a system is untenable. The reader is referred to 'Health for all Children'[32] and the American Academy of Pediatrics statement[38] for a fuller examination of this subject. In some areas there was considerable concern that time spent seeing families of normal children with no concerns diverted professional time away from families with greater needs. This has to be balanced against the findings that parents want to know about developmental problems early and that early intervention can be effective. For example, there is increasing evidence that appropriately targeted intervention improves outcomes in children with autistic spectrum disorders (reviewed by the National Research Council[39]), but a screening study of the general population showed at best moderate sensitivity.[40,41]

As research provides new information on effective interventions and appropriate screening tests, further adjustments to the program can be expected.

IDENTIFYING DEVELOPMENTAL PROBLEMS: PARTNERSHIP WITH PARENTS

Regular 'surveillance' contacts also arguably marginalized the immensely important role that parents have in detecting developmental impairments. Most very severe impairments of motor, visual or general learning skills, not detected at birth, are detected by parents. Two thirds of children with cerebral palsy had this diagnosis confirmed by 24 months, in a recent population-based study, and 89 out of 145 were detected by the parent or other family member (Baird & Scrutton, unpublished data).

When a family feels concerned about a child's developmental progress, they require a prompt response including exploration of concerns, assessment and management, if indicated. Access to health service resources is an issue and many districts have had to develop imaginative schemes to ensure that particular ethnic groups, travelers and asylum populations receive both health and developmental care. There are particular challenges attached to 'looked after' children who may change geographical location frequently yet have complex problems.

Using parental knowledge

Glascoe[42,43] has developed and evaluated a model of seeking developmental concerns and evaluating the response required using a simple series of questions, which has the advantage of being able to be used at any age in the preschool years, the PEDS – Parents' Evaluation of Developmental Status (1997). She has found that parental concerns, carefully elicited, have a 75–80% sensitivity for childhood disability and 70–80% specificity for normal development. These questions are intended to be asked of parents.
1. Do you have any concerns about your child's learning, development or behavior?
2. Do you have any concerns about how your child talks and makes speech sounds?
3. Do you have any concerns about how your child understands what you say?
4. Do you have any concerns about how your child uses his or her hands or feet to do things?
5. Do you have any concerns about how your child uses his or her arms or legs?

6. Do you have any concerns about how your child behaves?
7. Do you have any concerns about how your child gets along with others?
8. Do you have any concerns about how your child is learning to do things for him- or herself?
9. Do you have any concerns about how your child is learning preschool or school skills?
10. Do you have any other concerns?

Glascoe[42] has shown that parents who have no concerns (and where there is no literacy/language barrier) tend to have children without disabilities. Decisions about who to assess further can be based on the results of the PEDS. For example, a parent who has two or more significant concerns about the child should be referred for appropriate assessment without more screening. One significant concern should elicit a further screen in the appropriate skill and this improves specificity.

Is parental identification sufficient?

Within the child health promotion program, regular points of contact between parent and professional are retained to allow provision of a number of health-related activities (accident prevention, nutritional advice and the immunization program[32]) including discussion of developmental progress. It has been argued that leaving the onus of initiation of concern entirely to parents would lead to inequity of health care, with the likelihood that those members of society most in need would find themselves least able to access care (the so-called 'inverse care' law). The job of the professional where parental concerns are not raised is to help parents see that there is a concern, to bring the parents to the point of seeking advice, and to provide assistance and a pathway to do so.

PREVENTION OF DEVELOPMENTAL PROBLEMS

In the UK, the increasing emphasis on primary prevention is supported by the establishment of SureStart programs which aim to ameliorate the multiple disadvantages faced by children growing up in poverty. Evaluation will need to continue to ensure that local programs achieve the desired outcomes for those most in need.[44,45]

PROBLEMS WITH DEVELOPMENT
For the infant and very young child

For the infant and very young child (i.e. under 18 months), most major defects will present neonatally, at the at-risk follow-up clinic or to the family. The presenting disorders include those of motor or general development, vision and hearing. They may be static or progressive and affect more than one area of development.

After 18 months of age

After 18 months of age, problems with speech and language, learning, motor competence and behavior problems typically present.

Estimates of prevalence of neurodevelopmental problems are shown in Table 7.5.[43,46]

Developmental assessment

Developmental assessment starts with 'information gathering' from all who know the child either informally or more formally using checklists. It then encompasses the 'interview' with parents/caregivers and the 'examination' of the child. The process results in a conclusion, if possible a diagnosis with an etiological explanation, but always a plan of action to meet needs.

Knowledge of the normal patterns of child development enables us to assess the developmental level of a particular child. A major change in the examination of young children with possible developmental problems is the number of norm-based psychometrically constructed tests with standard methods of administration available that examine or test behavior in a number of areas and provide a profile of development. Choice of formal or informal assessment depends on a number of factors.

Table 7.5 Neurodevelopmental problems and estimates of their prevalence (in parentheses)[43]

Learning impairments
1. Severe learning disability (3.5/1000)
2. Moderate learning difficulties IQ 50–70 (1.8%)
3. Specific learning difficulty including dyslexia (underestimated at 2%)
4. Down syndrome (1/1000)

Motor impairments
1. Cerebral palsy (2.5/1000) – hemiplegia (30%); diplegia (20%); other types (50%)
2. Clumsy child syndrome – developmental coordination disorder (5%); deficits in attention, motor control and perception (1–3%) (overlaps with attention deficit disorder and with hyperactivity)
3. Neural tube defects (1/1000)
4. Hydrocephalus (0.1/1000)

Neuromuscular disorders
1. Duchenne muscular dystrophy (3/100 000)
2. Other neuromuscular disorders

Other chronic neurological disorders
1. Neurodegenerative disorders
2. Other chronic neurological disorders – survivors of brain infections, such as meningitis or encephalitis; damaged survivors of head injury; brain malformations
3. Epilepsy (0.8%) – usually associated with other disorders to require child development service

Speech, language and communication disorders
1. Severe speech language disorder (5/1000)
2. Autistic spectrum disorders (including Asperger syndrome) (116/10 000)[93]

Visual impairment
1. Partially sighted (0.4/1000)
2. Blind (0.3/1000)

Hearing impairment
Significant impairment (> 50 dB loss in better ear) (1.5/1000)
Many children have two or more coexisting disorders

Associated problems
1. Behavior (up to 30%)
2. Nutrition/gastroesophageal reflux/constipation
3. Recurrent respiratory infection
4. Orthopedic deformities
5. Other medical problems (e.g. asthma)
6. Social and family problems

Multidisciplinary professional assessment is the ideal, and the process should be sensitive to the family's awareness, concerns and cultural needs. The assessment process should be explained clearly in advance so that families are able to participate fully. Assessment timing and location should be according to family need rather than professional convenience.

All services should aim to:
1. enhance the parents' understanding of their child;
2. promote the relationship between parent and child;
3. support families as the most significant caregivers;
4. identify services to meet needs, provide practical help and emotional support;
5. use language that is understood by all;
6. evaluate barriers to service use by families.

The history

The general aspects of taking a history described in Chapter 8 apply to the child who presents with developmental problems. Here we comment on particular aspects of importance (Table 7.6).

Table 7.6 Topics for history taking

Growth and any medical problems
Feeding
Behavior
Vision
Hearing
Motor skills, including manipulation
Communication, speech and language
Play and interests
Social interaction and relationships
Self-help and personal skills
Drive and motivation for learning

Family history, social and family environment and the pre-, peri- and postnatal history, should all be covered, looking particularly for the risk factors as outlined below. More detailed questions follow, about the concerns in question, and other skill areas.

Certain risk factors increase the likelihood of a developmental impairment. Biological risks may be:
1. prenatal, e.g. use of drugs or alcohol, severe toxemia and viral infections, genetic disorders;
2. perinatal factors, such as prematurity, low birth weight, obstetric complications;
3. neonatal factors, such as neonatal encephalopathy, infections (e.g. sepsis or meningitis) and severe hyperbilirubinemia;
4. postnatal factors, such as injury or non-accidental injury, meningitis, encephalitis, exposure to toxins, severe continuous failure to thrive and severe epilepsy;
5. visual and hearing losses, and other specific learning difficulties.

Environmental risks, such as a parent with learning disabilities or significant mental health problems, history of abuse or neglect and concerns about parent/child interaction all increase the likelihood of a developmental impairment.

Developmental history. Although parental recall of milestones may not always be reliable, the most informative history can be obtained through the use of open-ended questions followed by requests for specific examples.

Parents are good at remembering whether or not they or other family members had concerns, and what those concerns were about. They are good at observing current behavior if the right questions are asked. Parents' interpretation of what their child does may be incorrect (e.g. he understands everything), but their observations are usually accurate (e.g. he will fetch his shoes only if they are visible). Parents find accurate estimates of comprehension difficult, as do professionals, unless a specific test is carried out.

Between 18 and 24 months is a particularly good time to note any delays of communication, for example not pointing or not using gaze to regulate communication. Between 24 and 30 months is a particularly good time to note delays in language development, because the child should move quickly from single words to putting words into simple sentences.

Some semi-structured interviews of history taking have been developed for certain situations, for example the Diagnostic Interview Schedule for Communication Disorder (DISCO 2000) developed for detailed history of both normal and abnormal patterns of development where a child might be suspected of having an autistic spectrum disorder, and the Autism Diagnostic Interview.[47] It is important to determine the rate of development of skills in order to establish whether the child has always had a problem or whether there is any possibility of regression (deterioration or loss of skills). If the latter is suspected then the exploration of etiology follows a different path from that of a static nonprogressive disorder. If there is a suggestion of regression, it is useful to inquire at what age the child was at her best and to jog memories with questions such as 'What sort of things was she doing on her last birthday that she cannot do now?'.

Past history is directed at elucidating any cause for the problems, either real or wrongly attributed by the parents. Ruling out the latter (e.g. mother working or being depressed as a cause of autism) can reduce or remove parents' guilt and help them in accepting the child's difficulties.

It is particularly important that problems are not wrongly attributed (e.g. to obstetric intervention or pertussis immunization), such that a genetic problem is overlooked. Many obstetric interventions carried out to protect the infant (e.g. forceps delivery) only very rarely cause later problems. What is of greater importance is the underlying reason for intervention, e.g. fetal distress. However, fetal distress is not always the cause of brain damage identified later, since it may in itself be a manifestation of vulnerability resulting from damage caused antenatally.[48] The condition of the baby at birth, e.g. low Apgar score (< 5 at 5 and 10 min), poor feeding, fits, may also be relevant.

General health. The child's general health and any illnesses can also be relevant.

Family history. Family history is important and inquiries must be made about first and second degree relatives. Any diagnosis, even if apparently definite, must be pursued (e.g. a reported diagnosis of spina bifida in a male cousin turned out to be muscular dystrophy).

In boys with learning disability a history of affected males on the mother's side may highlight the possibility of fragile X syndrome. The parents may need to be examined (e.g. child with hypotonia whose mother has myotonic dystrophy).

Social history. Social history is important not only because of its role in etiology, but because social factors may affect the family's capacity to cope with a child with a disability.

Examination: observations and interactive assessment

Gesell[49] stated that psychological/developmental examination should be regarded 'not as a series of achievement tests but as a means of eliciting significant behavior, which calls for diversified analysis rather than a meagre recording of success and failure'. The examiner needs to create a setting that will most easily show the spontaneous and elicited behaviors that need to be observed. Tables 7.7 and 7.8 and Figure 7.7 set the framework for observation.

The developmental examination should take place in a room with toys appropriate for the child and with one or both parents present. There should be a chair and table suitable for the child to sit at. A history is then taken, all the time observing the child's behavior and interaction with parents. This period of talking to the parents enables the child to get used to the environment and to see that the parents accept strange people. Toys and other play materials, appropriate for the age of the child, should be available (e.g. cause and effect toys, a bell, bricks, truck, doll or teddy, tea-set or other dolls' house toys for the 18 month old and for the older child, miniature toys for pretend play, crayons and pencil and paper and books with single pictures and stories). These are separate from those required for tests.

It is particularly valuable to allow time to observe how the child spontaneously makes use of toys or materials available, before moving onto adult-structured play and interaction. This is because, in certain developmental problems, children are able to function very well when a helpful adult interacts with them, as this creates structure which helps them to organize their responses. However, when left to his own devices the child may be less able to organize his environment and generate any ideas, manifesting in limited or repetitive play, or flitting attention for available activities. Such difficulties will not be apparent from the more structured assessment.

One of the cardinal rules of developmental assessment is not only to look at what the child does but also at 'how he does it'; thus all the time the quality of response is to be evaluated as well as the actual achievement. Following the history and informal observations, more structured and standardized tests for general and specific areas of

Table 7.7 Framework for making developmental observations – birth to 13 months

	Newborn	3 months	4 months	6 months	8 months	9 months	12 months	13 months
POSTURE/GROSS MOTOR MOVEMENTS AND REFLEXES								
Supine	Head to side	Head in midline Hands open Finger play		Lifts head spontaneously				
Pull to sit	No head control		Good head control	Lifts head in anticipation				
Sitting	Flopping forward	Head held up Back curved	Straight back	Sits with hands for support	Sits with no support			
Ventral suspension		Good head control			Forward parachute			
Prone		Shoulders up on forearms		Lifts chest off on hands				
Supported standing				Weight bears Downward parachute		Stands holding on	Walks hands held	Walks alone (18 months age limit)
Primary reflexes	Strong stepping, grasp and Moro reflex	Asymmetrical tonic neck reflex present (2–3 months)	Most (e.g. Moro's) markedly lessen	No primary reflexes persist beyond 6 months				
HAND FUNCTION/FINE MOTOR: Observe use of one or both hands, grasping and releasing spontaneously and on request								
	Fisting persisting beyond 2 months is abnormal		Reaches with one hand- Brings toys to mouth Transfers from hand to hand	Index finger	Pincer grasp approach Releases brick in a container	Mature grasp	Can give a toy on request	
VISUAL BEHAVIOR								
Visual fixation and following	Looks towards bright light and by 4–6 weeks looks at mother's face	Follows face beyond midline	Follows objects through 180°	Fixes on smaller objects >2.5 cm	Fixes on smaller objects >1 cm	Fixes on 1-mm sweets		
HEARING BEHAVIOR								
Response to sound	Startle	Searches for sound		Turns head toward sound (at ear level – two stage for above and below)	Turns head to sound directly up and down (above and below ear level)		Turns to sound above head	
LANGUAGE AND COMMUNICATION: Observe vocalization and gestures to attract other's attention, to indicate needs, in response to others' vocalization and to share emotions								
		Cooing		Babbling	Responds to own name	Understands words in context	First word with meaning	
PERSONAL–SOCIAL: Note awareness of parents/carers and strangers, initiation of interactions and response to others' approaches								
	Smiles responsively 6 weeks		Stranger awareness		Waves bye-bye (copies)	Points to request and show		
PLAY: Observe exploration and free play, use of real size and small toys on self and others and initiation and response to social games (e.g. peek-a-boo, pat-a-cake)								
				Bangs and mouths	Looks for fallen toy, pulls string to get toy	Plays pat-a-cake, explores with finger		Uses cup/spoon/ brush on self

Table 7.8 Framework for making developmental observations – 15 months to 5 years

	15 months	18 months	2 years	2.5 years	3 years	3.5 years	4 years	5 years
FINE-MOTOR/PERCEPTUAL COORDINATION: Note spontaneous effort, attention to directions, ability to copy from a model, response to help and praise, attention to task and quality of movements								
Construction skills with 1-inch (2.5-cm) cubes	Tower of two cubes	Tower of three cubes	Tower of six cubes	Puts three cubes in a row for a train	Makes a train with a chimney (39 months)	Three-brick bridge from a model	Steps of six cubes from a model	Steps of 10 cubes from a model
Pencil grasp and drawing	Makes a mark on paper	Straight scribble	In prone at distal end / Circular scribble	Middle of pencil / Line in imitation	Mature grasp (tripod) / Copies: O	Copies: +	Copies square	Copies triangle
Shape sorting (visuospatial skills)		Simple shapes circles and squares	Circles, squares and triangles	Six-shape sorter	Good scanning of shape sorter before putting shape in and rotating shapes to align – little or no pushing of shapes			
LANGUAGE, COMMUNICATION AND SOCIAL INTERACTION: Note speech quality, use of language: to express need, comment, describe, share interest and initiating and responding for conversation								
Understanding	Simple requests in context: give me ...	Knows two to three body parts	Gives two or more objects on requests	Prepositions: in, on. Gives objects by function	Preposition under/size big/little	Size, color		
Communication and social interaction	Initiates communication, shows, points	Many spontaneous words, repeats words	Puts two words together in phrases		Sentences of three or more words, personal pronouns. Can give full name and gender. Asks what/where questions	Joined sentences, speech mainly clear		
PLAY AND SOCIAL INTERACTION: Note initiating interactions and responding to parent/examiner/other children and use of eye contact and gestures								
	Brushes own or mother's hair	Brushes doll's hair, may feed/put to bed doll/teddy	Plays with small toys, relates two toys. Watches other children			Develops sequence with small toys. Plays with other children. Can share. Offers comfort		

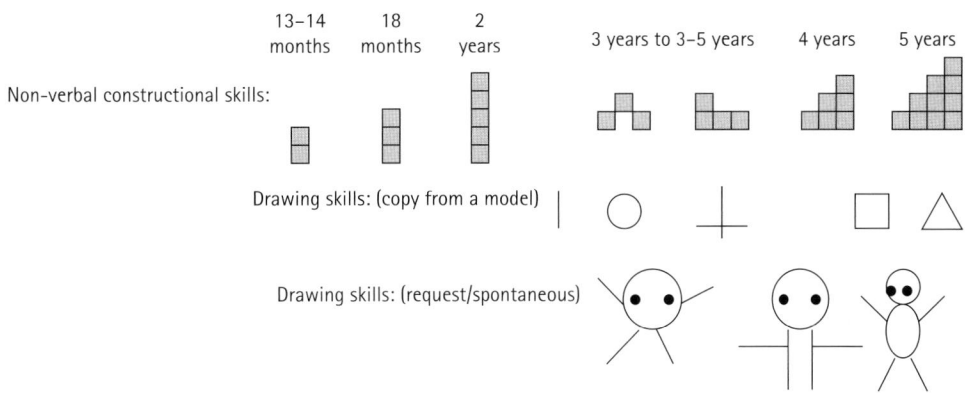

Fig. 7.7 Constructional and drawing skills.

development may be used (Table 7.9).[19,50-52] Some formal assessments deliberately include both structured and unstructured time, e.g. the play-based observation for possible autism, the Autism Diagnostic Observation Schedule.[50]

Look for patterns of development suggestive of normal variation

Some developmental patterns cause delay in the acquisition of other milestones (e.g. shuffling is associated with late walking). The mean age of walking in children who 'bottom shuffle' is 16–17 months and the 90th centile is 23 months.[53,54]

Look for patterns of development that suggest abnormal development

Besides looking for the acquisition of normal developmental skills, it is also important to look for skills that are present at an earlier stage which should have disappeared and are abnormal beyond a certain age. For example, mouthing is a normal pattern of investigation of the environment at 7–8 months, but after that hand and vision examination increasingly take the place of mouthing.

Persistent mouthing of objects beyond 18 months is indicative of a general learning problem. Persistent casting (throwing forwards or to the side) is a normal behavior at 12 months, but not at 24 months or beyond, and hand regard is a normal behavior at 3–4 months.

Some behaviors are abnormal at any age, for example the persistent visual inspection of objects out the corner of the eye seen in young children with autism. However, some of the excited arm/body actions seen persistently in older children with autism are also seen in normal development at the age of 6–9 months.

Importance of skill delays

Delays in some areas of development are more important for long term learning than others, for example:

1. Developmental delay in motor skills only is of much less long term significance than persistent significant delays in language and cognitive skills. However, cognitive difficulties frequently accompany severe motor disorders, either due to co-morbidity or because severe motor impairment limits learning through exploration.
2. Self-help competence, for example toilet training, feeding and dressing, can also be dissociated from the level of general learning.
3. Some skills (e.g. symbolic play and language) reflect understanding of the environment and are therefore better indicators of intellectual ability.
4. Make allowance for prematurity under 12 months.

Child's performance

The child may not perform at her best, and may need to be seen again, perhaps in a more familiar environment. Skills need to be developed in sharing uncertainty with parents and in negotiating a need for observa-

tions over time. It is always helpful to ask parents if the child's behaviors and responses seen are typical. Parents are more likely to accept an opinion if they think the child has behaved typically and it is based on two periods of observation.

Motor skills, vision and hearing

Make sure that the motor, vision and hearing systems are functioning normally before making judgments about the rest of the child's development.

Assessment of motor development

To assess motor development in the child under 2 years:

1. watch first;
2. then place in prone, supine, pull to sit, stand, ventral suspension and look for the secondary protective responses as illustrated (Fig. 7.8).[55] Assess tone, symmetry and spontaneous movements and then compare the motor development with other maturity milestones.

Differential diagnosis of motor problems. Problems with motor development are most likely to present concerns in the first 2 years of life, although 'clumsiness' is a common associated problem in many other developmental delays. Note, however, that early walking does not exclude other developmental problems.

The differential diagnosis of delay in motor milestones is:

1. a normal variant – e.g. shuffler, roller, asymmetrical head turner, toe walker – ask about family history; shuffling and other patterns may have a genetic predisposition;
2. global delay/general learning difficulties/mental retardation;
3. cerebral palsy/other neurological disorder;
4. early presentation of developmental coordination problems – hypotonia and delay;
5. connective tissue disorder.

Clues on examination are scissoring on downward parachute in diplegia (Fig. 7.9),[55] adopting a sitting posture on downward parachute, as in bottom shufflers (Fig. 7.10).

Definite persistent handedness at 6–9 months may indicate pathology. Headlag on 'pull to sit' after 8 months is abnormal.

Not walking by 18 months is delayed in a prone developing crawler.

An example of an evidenced-based approach to assessing motor delay is given in Case Study 1 on page 110.

Four common tests used to assess motor skills are reviewed in Wiart and Darrah.[51] As with all tests the emphasis is on knowing the tests and whether each test measures what it purports to measure and whether that is what is needed for that particular child.

Oromotor skills

A significant impairment of central origin affecting motor development will affect oral skills, as demonstrated in delayed sucking (and with a severe cerebral palsy in abnormal swallowing and breathing). Less severe difficulties may not be so obvious until solids are introduced when textures, lumps, chewing and drooling problems may present.

Table 7.9 Psychometric tests in common use

Test	Age range tested	Training required to carry out test	Areas tested[a]
Complete profile			
Bayley scales of infant development	2 months to 3 years	Professionals including pediatricians	Mental, motor and behavior
Griffiths scales	0–8 years	Clinicians trained and certified in administration	Locomotor, personal social, hearing and speech, eye–hand coordination and performance
British Ability Scales (BAS 11)	2 years 6 months to 17 years 11 months	Psychologists	Verbal and nonverbal reasoning/attainments and diagnostic scales
Wechsler Preschool and Primary Scale of Intelligence (WPPSI-III)	2 years 6 months to 7 years 3 months	Psychologists	Four core subtests (2 years 6 months to 3 years 11 months) – 2 verbal, 2 performance. Seven core subtests (4 years 0 months to 7 years 3 months) – 3 verbal, 3 performance, 1 processing speed VIQ, PIQ and IQ derived
Wechsler Intelligence Scales for Children WISC IV (WISC)	6–16 years	Psychologists	10 core subtests: 3 verbal comprehension, 3 perceptual reasoning, 2 working memory, 2 processing speed and 5 supplemental tests
Stanford–Binet intelligence scale, 4th edition	2 years to adult	Psychologist	5 subscales: verbal and nonverbal
Schedule of growing skills	0–5 years	Any professional	Profile of development in nine areas – based on Sheridan. Gives a general developmental overview
Miller assessment for preschoolers	2 years 9 months to 5 years 8 months	Any professional	Identifies developmental delays in sensorimotor and cognitive abilities in verbal and nonverbal areas
Kaufman assessment battery for children	2 years 5 months to 12 years 5 months	Psychologist	3 scales, sequential, simultaneous processing and attainments. Mental processing composite derived. There is an adolescent extension scale
Developmental neuropsychological assessment (NEPSY)	3–12 years	Psychologist	Attention/executive function; language; sensorimotor functions; visuospatial processing; memory and learning
Language			
Reynell DLS – Developmental Language Scale (RDLS111 (1997))	1–7 years	Speech therapists, psychologists, some teachers	Verbal comprehension and verbal expression
Test of Word Knowledge (TOWK)	5–17 years	Any professional, usually SLT	Detailed evaluation of semantic development and lexical knowledge; 7 subtests
Picture vocabulary test (Peabody or British)	2–8 years	Any professional	Tests single word vocabulary. The child selects picture most appropriate for the given word
Clinical Evaluation of Language Fundamentals, 4th edition (CELF)	5 years to 16 years 11 months	Any professional, usually speech therapist	Four core subtests provide a total language score, with additional composite scores in language structure, language content, language content and memory, working memory scores with supplementary subtests
Preschool CELF, 2nd edition	3–6 years	Any professional, usually SLT	Seven norm-referenced subtests in: sentence structure, word structure, expressive vocabulary, concepts and following directions, recalling sentences, basic concepts, word classes. With supplementary subtests and pre-literacy rating scale descriptive pragmatics profile
Speech/articulation tests			
Edinburgh Articulation Test (EAT)	3–8 years	Speech therapist	Picture naming task to assess English sound system
Renfrew Action Picture test (RAPT)	3–8 years	SLT	Picture description task designed to elicit specific information and grammar
Renfrew Bus Story	3–8 years	SLT	Story retelling task with pictures. Scored for information, grammar and sentence length
Preschool language scales	2 weeks to 6 years	Any professional usually SLT	A developmentally based assessment combining parental report and direct test – best for age 1–4 years
Nonverbal intelligence tests – suitable for those with impaired hearing			
Raven's Progressive Matrices and Vocabulary Scales	5 years to adult	Any professional	Assesses two complementary components of general intelligence: the ability to think clearly and make sense of complex data and the ability to store and reproduce information

Table 7.9—cont'd

Test	Age range tested	Training required to carry out test	Areas tested[a]
The Snijders–Oomen nonverbal intelligence test, revised	5 years 5 months to 17 years		Reasoning and spatial abilities subtests
Leiter International Performance Scale, revised	2 years to adult	Psychologist or appropriately trained professional	Visualization and reasoning battery, also attention and memory
Visuomotor and motor tests			
Goodenough–Harris drawing test (Harris[19])	3–15 years	Any professional	The child is asked to draw a man and a score is derived from the content and converted to a mental age
Bender Gestalt test	4 years to adult	Test of perceptuomotor function	Nine designs for the child to copy
Movement Asessment Battery for Children [47]	4–12 years	Any professional usually physiotherapist or occupational therapist	Eight items divided into three subsections: manual dexterity, ball skills, and static and dynamic balance
Frostig – Developmental Test of Visual Perception (DTVP)	4–8 years		Five areas are tested: eye motor coordination, figure ground, constancy of shape, position in space and spatial relationships
Developmental test of visuomotor integration (Beery)	3–17 years		Developmental sequence of geometric forms to be copied with paper and pencil
Test of visual perceptual skills, 3rd edition (TVPS-3)	4–19 years	Occupational therapists, psychologists, education diagnosticians, developmental optometrists, learning specialists, and other assessment professionals	Perceptual skills: visual discrimination, visual memory, visual-spatial relationships, form constancy, visual sequential memory, visual figure-ground, visual closure
Motor-Free Visual Perception Test, 3rd edition (MVPT-3)	4 years to adult	Any professional	Visual perceptual ability without any motor involvement
Test of Visual-Reasoning and Processing Skills (TVRPS)	5–14 years	Any professional	Four subtests that measure visual-reasoning and processing abilities: visual picture completion, visual–spatial relationship, visual discrimination, part–whole relationships
Matrix Analogies Test – expanded form (MAT-EF)	5–17 years	Psychologists or appropriately trained professional	Four specific subtests: pattern completion, reasoning by analogy, serial reasoning, and spatial visualization
Memory and attention tests			
Children's memory scale	5–16 years	Psychologists	A variety of memory dimensions: attention and working memory, verbal and visual memory, short- and long-delay memory, recall and recognition, learning characteristics
Rivermead behavioral memory test	Childrens version: 5–10 years 11 months Adult version can be used 11–15 years	Psychologists	Assesses memory skills related to everyday situations both episodic and prospective
Test of everyday attention for children (TEA-Ch)	6–16 years	Psychologists	Comprises nine subtests: selectively attend; sustain their attention; divide their attention between two tasks; switch attention from one thing to another; withhold (inhibit) verbal and motor responses
Play test			
Symbolic play test of Lowe & Costello	1–3 years	Any professional	Four groups of toys presented without verbal instructions. Results in an age equivalent score
Autism Diagnostic Observation Scales ADOS (Lord et al)[47]			Social interaction, communication and imaginative play observed
Tests for those with visual impairment			
Reynell Zinkin scales	Birth to 5 years	Any professional	Five subscales: social adaptation, sensorimotor understanding, exploration of environment, response to sound and verbal comprehension, expressive language and a communication subscale for children with additional problems

(Continued)

Table 7.9   Psychometric tests in common use—cont'd

Test	Age range tested	Training required to carry out test	Areas tested[a]
Behavior scales			
Vineland adaptive behavior scales	0 to adult	Any professional	Survey or interview form: semistructured carer interview for assessment of communication, daily living skills, socialization and motor skills and a maladaptive section
Strengths and difficulties questionnaire (Goodman)			Teacher and parent version summarizes behavior problems in prosocial, hyperactivity, conduct, emotional and peer group areas
Other behavior schedules (see O'Brien et al[52])			

[a] Most of these tests are available from NFER – Nelson, Danville House, Windsor 1DF, or Harcourt Assessment, Halley Court, Jordan Hill, Oxford, OX2 8EJ.
SLT, speech and language therapist.

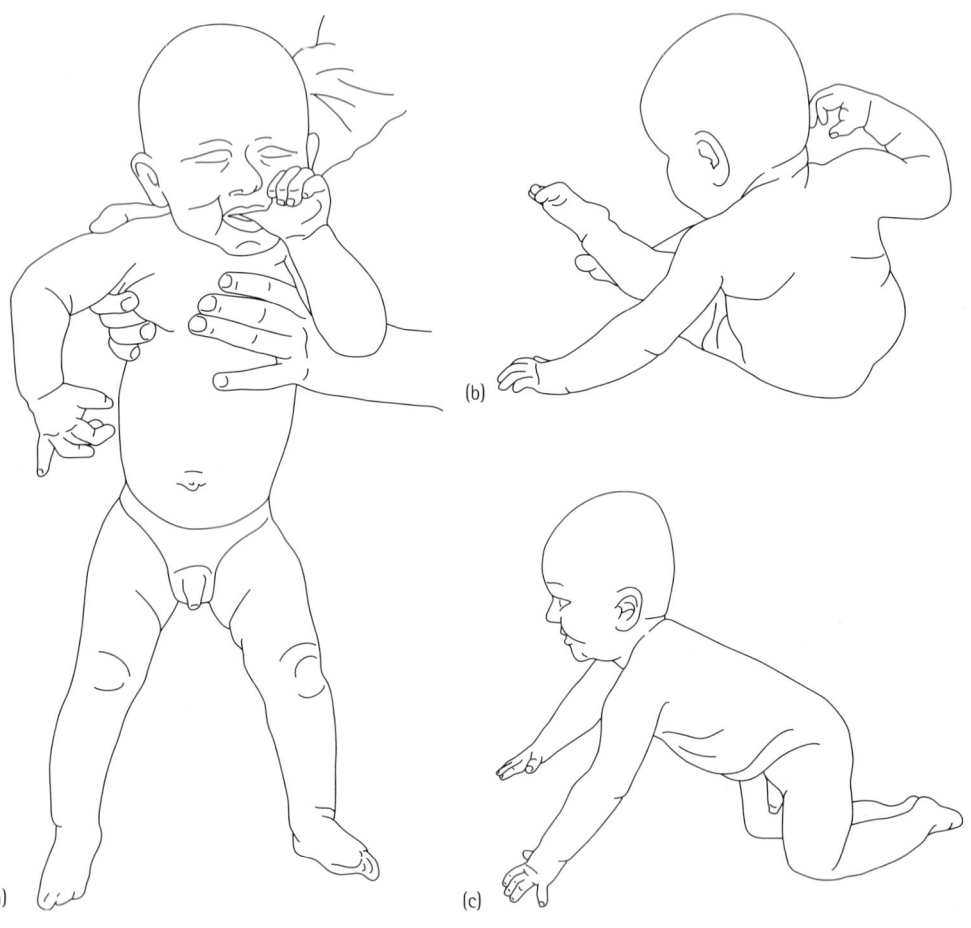

Fig. 7.8   Downward parachute (a), sideways parachute (b) and forward parachute (c). (After Milani-Comparetti & Gidoni 1967.[55])

(a)   (b)   (c)

Assessment of vision

Significant visual impairment has a potentially serious and complex impact on all areas of development, including cognition, language, social, gross and fine motor abilities. Early recognition and specialist rehabilitative support are essential. Techniques to improve vision in children with visual impairment have been shown to be successful in promoting visual development.[56] Improving vision to the level of object awareness from perception of light only in the first year of life can have a significant impact on developmental outcome.[57]

Assessment of vision in children should include history and examination. The history should cover:
1. any parental concern about the child's vision;
2. visual behavior relevant to the child's age (Fig. 7.2);
3. suspected squint.

Examination of the eyes includes assessment of:

1. any gross ocular pathology (including ophthalmoscopy);
2. the pupillary response to light;
3. eye movements (smooth pursuit and saccades);
4. squint – checking that the corneal reflection of a light is in the same position in the two eyes and by doing the cover test (in the cover test each eye is covered in turn while the child visually fixates on an object and a note is made of whether the uncovered eye moves to take up fixation).

Visual assessment includes:
1. measurement of visual acuity – ability to distinguish separation of two visual targets and therefore to distinguish detail;
2. detection vision – ability to recognize/detect individual targets;
3. electrophysiological measurement of retinal and visual pathway function.

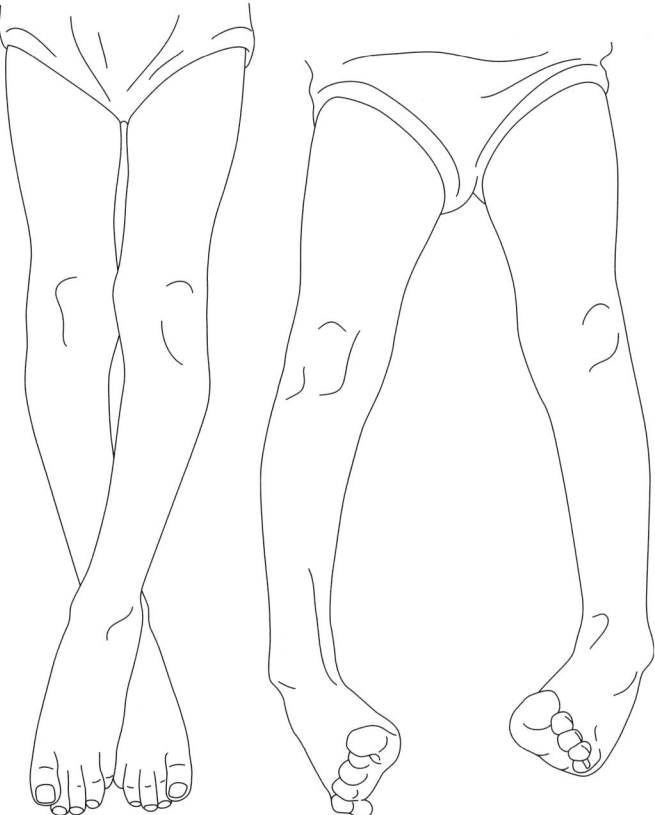

Fig. 7.9 Downward parachute in (a) spastic cerebral palsy, (b) dystonic cerebral palsy. (After Milani–Comparetti & Gidoni 1967.[55])

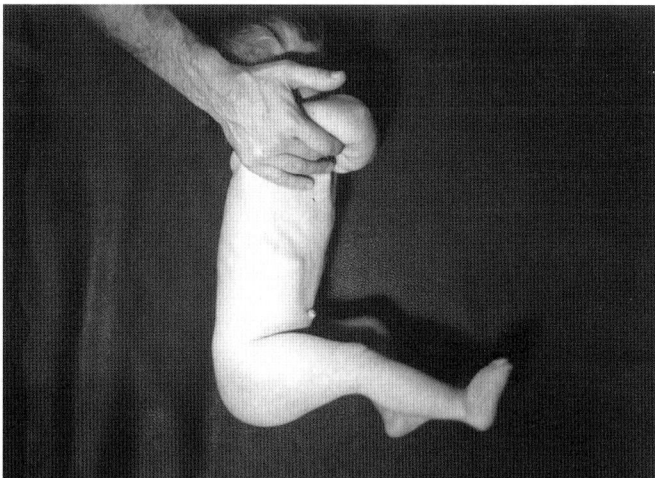

Fig. 7.10 Downward parachute in a bottom shuffler. (Courtesy of D Scrutton.)

1. Visual acuity. The Snellen letter chart was the accepted standard for measurement of acuity until recent years. The acuity is expressed as the distance at which a particular letter size is seen by a person with normal vision. The result is given as a pseudofraction – on top the distance tested at (the standard distance being 6 m or 20 feet), and below the size of the letter seen, thus 6/6 is normal vision and 6/60 very poor vision.

The logMAR (log of the Minimal Angle of Resolution) is now the increasingly accepted standard. The smaller the letters on the chart, and the further away they are, the smaller will be the angle subtended to the eye by the letters and therefore the smaller the value of the logMAR score associated with it. The logMAR scale allows more effective and precise analysis of visual acuity scores because of the equal linear steps of the scale. The progression of letter height is that any line is 1.2589 times greater than the line below. This multiplier is the root of ten or 0.1 log unit. The results are expressed as a decimal, thus the line of letters equivalent to 6/6 is 0 and 6/60 is 1.0, and each letter recognized contributes to the acuity result, as a proportion of the number of letters on each line.

Letter charts with reduced type are used for near vision in both tests. Measurement of acuity by standard adult methods is reliably possible from the age of about 5–6 years.

In younger children tests need some adaptation to allow for several developmental issues, but this does not require compromise of the adult standard after 2.5–3 years.[58]

Although young children cannot name letters, by the age of 2.5–3 years over 85% of children are able to match letters and by 3 years most children can do so.[59] Difficulties with attention control arise at a test distance of 6 m and children also have difficulty understanding the task when several lines of letters are presented simultaneously. Visual acuity should be measured if possible in each eye separately; however, a significant proportion of children under 3.5 years of age are unable to accept occlusion of one eye (46% of 2.5–3 year olds and 73% of 3–4 year olds will accept occlusion).[59] In this age group it is therefore advisable to obtain a measure with both eyes open before attempting to cover one eye.

To address these issues Sonksen devised a test of visual acuity, the Sonksen logMAR test based on the adult logMAR standard recommended by Bailey and Lovie[60] with modifications to support the developmental issues without compromising the adult standard. The adaptations were those used for the Sonksen Silver Acuity System[58] based on the Snellen standard. The test includes a booklet with several cards, each with a single row of four letters of each size (using the six letters known to be least confusing for young children[61]) surrounded by a crowding bar, a key card for letter matching and a training booklet. Seating the child at a small table and using a test distance of 3 m also improves concentration and co-operation with the test. Using this test, an acuity measure for both eyes can be obtained in 80% of 2.5 to 3 year olds, in 94% of 3 to 3.5 year olds and in 99% of children after 3.5 years.[62,63] Other tests designed for younger children include the Cambridge crowding test and the Keeler logMAR test.

Sheridan[61] devised a test (STYCAR letter test) that involved the presentation of single letters of decreasing size at 3 m. This is still widely used for young children, but these tests have been shown to significantly overestimate acuity, especially in children with amblyopia, by as much as three lines and therefore linear acuity (as above) should be measured wherever possible.

The Crowded logMar Kay Picture Test[64] uses pictograms designed to be of equivalent proportions to Snellen letters and can provide an estimate of acuity in children from 19 months to 2–2.5 years, when children are unable to match letters or in the small proportion of children from 2.5 to 3.5 years who cannot complete a letter-based logMAR test. They do then require the vocabulary to name the pictures. This test is said to be accurate to within one line of logMAR acuity tested by standard methods.[65]

Visual acuity can be measured from 2 months using forced choice preferential looking tests such as the Teller, Keeler or Cardiff Acuity Cards.[66] In this test the infant is shown two targets on a card. One is uniformly gray and the other has either black and white stripes (Teller or Keeler) or a pictogram similar to the Kay pictures (Cardiff). The stripes or pictograms become sequentially narrower or smaller on each card according to a standard scale. An infant will automatically look toward the more interesting visual target until they reach the limit of their acuity.

Opticokinetic nystagmus may also be used in very young children to estimate acuity. It can be demonstrated using an opticokinetic drum with black and white stripes of varying diameter. Nystagmus will not be elicited at the limits of the child's acuity (i.e. the stripe width is too small for the child to discriminate).

Visual acuity gradually improves with age. This has been demonstrated using grating acuity in infancy, with the Sonksen – Silver Acuity System and the Sonksen logMAR test in children aged 2.5–8 years. A large population-based study demonstrated an increase in acuity with age that is steepest in the 30 months between 2 years 9 months and 5 years 3 months and continues up to age 8 years and beyond. At 2 years 9 months 50% of children achieve binocular acuities for linear displays of 0.200 (3/4.75), by 5 years 3 months this has risen to −0.075 (3/2.6) and by 7 years 9 months to −0.175 (3/2).[63]

2. Detection vision. In the infant, evaluation of vision should begin with observation of detection vision. Near detection will include observing the child fix and follow a silent object presented at about 30 cm from the face. In the first weeks of life the infant will be most likely to follow the examiner's face and may ignore other objects (Table 7.7). Infants show little interest in small objects on a table top until 9 months. By 9–12 months, near detection vision may be tested by observing visual fixation on one small sweet (a one hundred and thousand measuring – approx 1.2 mm), placed on a dark contrasting background. In children with normal vision, immediate and sharp fixation is expected. Children with significant visual impairment (equivalent of 6/60 or greater measured with Keeler cards) may show visual awareness of this small sweet, but they show slower fixation, inexact location and peering. Inability to locate this target therefore suggests a child has severe visual impairment and is likely to meet criteria for registration for Severe Sight Impairment (previously Blind registration).

Distance detection can be measured by establishing the size of the smallest object the child can see at a particular distance. Sheridan designed a test using ten white balls of standardized diameter, which are either rolled on a dark strip horizontal to the line of the infant's gaze at 3 m from the child, or mounted on sticks for presentation from behind a dark screen (STYCAR graded balls test). This test is most appropriate in children from the age of 9 months to around 15 months because it relies on a young child's attention being drawn to the major stimulus in the environment (as in the distraction hearing test); after this age it is less reliable. It is important to note that visualization of even the smallest ball does not denote perfect vision, and rolling the ball considerably enhances its visibility. These tests can be helpful in describing a functional vision in children with severe visual impairment and for some children with learning disabilities who are not able to do acuity tests.

3. Electrophysiological Assessment. Objective measurement of vision may also be obtained by measuring the electrical response to a given visual stimulus from the retina (the electroretinogram) and the visual cortex (the visual evoked potential). The response to a simple flash and to graded check patterns can be recorded.[67]

Assessment of vision in the child with a visual impairment. In the child with visual impairment, the largest sized letters may not be recognized at 3 m and so the distance of testing is reduced until the letters are identified. In children with the most severe visual impairment, measurement of acuity at a distance may be more difficult or impossible. A methodical approach to the observation of functional (near and distance detection) vision should therefore be made. Care needs to be taken in interpretation, because the detection of small objects at near distance may lead to an overestimation of vision (see above).

A description of the size of object, the visual complexity and the distance recognized, can be used to provide advice to parents and the professionals working with them about toys and educational material that will be appropriate for learning.

A useful visual scale for near detection vision in the most visually impaired has been developed by Sonksen (personal communication) using visual targets of standardized size, ranging from a light source in a darkened room, a large, light-reflecting dangling ball through to smaller nonlight-reflecting targets. The distance from the target and the child's

ability to fixate and/or follow can then be recorded. The Stycar fixed or rolling balls, everyday objects and pictures may be shown, initially at 3 m and then moving in methodically to 2, 1, 0.5 and less than 0.5 m. The distance at which the target is recognized is then recorded. The test material should only be presented once because a child may be able to make an intelligent guess when it is re-presented.

The ability to identify pictures both near and at a distance by a child with visual impairment will vary with the level of background contrast and the level of detail required for recognition within the picture. A child may recognize a clear picture of a dog on a white background, but fail to pick out the same picture on less well contrasted background or when part of a more complex picture. Advice to teachers about this is essential, because much educational material is presented in a visually complex way and at a distance. Sonksen and Macrae[68] devised a picture recognition test using a selection of Ladybird pictures graded according to visual complexity, which provides a helpful guide to advice.

Some more complex visual disorders are outlined below.

1. Sometimes there is a delay – so called delayed visual maturation – in which the visual behaviors outlined in Figure 7.2 are all slower, often by months. A proportion of such children are later found to have other developmental impairments, which become clearer with time.[69]
2. Some children, often with more profound neurological damage, have more permanent cerebral visual problems.[70] In these children vision may show apparent variability which reflects limitations of visual attention. Damage to specific areas of the complex visual pathways and visual areas in the brain may cause very specific defects (e.g. movements may be seen, but not the level of discriminating detail that allows recognition of objects or prosopagnosia – a difficulty of face recognition, which is usually, but not invariably, an acquired brain damage deficit).
3. Visuoperceptual skills, which are particularly at risk in premature babies under 32 weeks' gestation and affect pattern recognition and topographical skills which can be assessed with specific tests.
4. Eye movement disorders, such as ocular motor apraxia may present with signs of early visual impairment, but by deploying motor control skills, with maturity the visual acuity is shown to be unimpaired.

Testing hearing

Persistent hearing loss can significantly impair speech and language development. Treatment is either by removal of the cause (in the case of middle ear effusion, or 'glue', causing conductive loss) or by aiding, either with conventional hearing aids or with a cochlear implant (in the case of sensorineural loss) and special teaching. Such interventions can change the outcome for young children and early detection is therefore a high child health priority, with 1–2 per 1000 children having sensorineural hearing loss. Even if no impairment is found on neonatal hearing screening a hearing loss may arise later due, for example, to secretory otitis media or late onset sensorineural loss.[71] Parental concerns should always be taken seriously and a hearing test should be arranged after any illness which has a high risk of hearing loss, e.g. meningitis, and should form part of the evaluation of speech delay. A history suggestive of 'risk' for hearing impairment (family history, ototoxic drugs, meningitis, NICU/SCBU experiences, structural palatal abnormality) should be elicited. Assessment of hearing in children with other developmental disorders needs particular attention as the effects of impairment on function tend to be cumulative.

Tests of hearing may be divided into objective and subjective – those reliant on child co-operation.

Objective tests

1. *Otoacoustic emissions.* This technique is applicable to the infant of any age, can be carried out in the neonatal period and has a sensitivity and specificity that makes it suitable for universal screening. However, it is only a screen of cochlear function and definitive threshold estimation requires brainstem evoked response testing.

2. *Brainstem evoked response audiometry [or auditory brainstem response (ABR) assessment].* This technique requires a still or sleeping subject, and may therefore require sedation. The stimulus sound is delivered by headphones or insert earphones. The most common stimulus is a broad-band 'click' which facilitates neural synchronicity but contains most energy in the mid- to high-frequency range, limiting threshold estimation to these frequencies. In threshold ABR assessment, responses are recorded at different stimulus intensities, allowing threshold estimation. Diagnostic ABR involves the examination of the morphology and latencies of waves recorded at higher intensities, allowing assessment of the site of lesion in cases of known impairment.

Subjective (behavioral) tests. These depend on co-operation and developmental level. They are thus also a guide to the developmental level of function of the child (Fig. 7.2). The tests can be used at any age, depending on the functional level, i.e. a child or young person with learning difficulties may still be best tested using distraction or visual reinforcement audiometry techniques (perhaps with modifications) at any age. Care needs to be taken to distinguish between hearing acuity, auditory attention and speech processing and comprehension. For example, children with autism may hear normally or even show apparent hypersensitivity to specific sounds, but may not show any attention to adult speech. Children with disorders of attention may also be able to hear normally but not show sustained attention to listening tasks (or any other tasks). Children with speech delay may be slower processors of speech and language, present as poor listeners and later be shown to have poor auditory short term memories. Therefore, even when these children hear normally, they may show apparent impairment in subjective tests.

1. *Distraction test and visual reinforcement audiometry.* The ability to locate sounds at ear level is mature by 7–8 months and prior to otoacoustic emissions was used for universal screening. The technique requires a well and alert baby who is not in an overactive or distressed state, a quiet room, two people who are trained and skilled in the technique and an adult to hold the child who is instructed to remain neutral and nonresponsive. The adult in front (the distractor) gains and controls the child's attention with an interesting toy, which may be moved or presented in such a way to attract the child's attention, and then the interest is diminished either by stopping it moving, covering or removing it. Immediately on reducing interest in the distracting object, the other adult (or a mechanical device) introduces a sound stimulus. The test stimuli should be frequency specific at a measured sound level, and include voice (both low frequency and high, e.g. a sibilant 'ss'), a specially designed rattle (high frequency) and electronically generated 'warble' tones. The usual response is a full head turn to locate the stimuli. Minimal sound levels eliciting a reliable response can be measured using a sound level meter and the stimuli are designed to test the range of frequencies needed for speech development. The location ability on ear level at 6–7 months, above and below ear level at 8 months and above the head at 12 months are markers of perceptual/cognitive maturation. However, babies of 9 months and more may also learn to play games and check who is behind them! Other common invalidators of this test are visual cues (including shadows and/or reflections visible to the baby), auditory cues (e.g. creaking shoes, floors) and even olfactory cues.

2. For this, and other, reasons *visual reinforcement audiometry (VRA)* is an important technique. In VRA the child is generally seated, again on an adult's lap, between loudspeakers. Warble tone stimuli are presented, initially at suprathreshold level, and the child's attention drawn (by a tester seated in front of the child) to a visual reward (often a bright or animated toy hidden behind smoked glass) which is illuminated briefly. Once the child has associated the auditory stimulus with the reward the stimulus level is reduced and the reward delayed until the child has begun to search for it (a positive response). In this way assessment of threshold can be performed for stimuli at different frequencies. The visual reward has been shown to elicit more responses than the social reward used in distraction testing, and the electronic stimuli used in VRA can be more accurately calibrated in terms of level and frequency. There are many reasons why these tests may not work well, but a failure to respond on the baby's part should be taken seriously as a developmental as well as a hearing concern.

3. *Behavioral tests:*
   (**a**) Speech discrimination tests. The principle is choosing toys or pictures of objects that are paired and demand careful listening and hearing to discriminate, for example cup/duck, plate/plane. Children can start to co-operate with such speech tests from 24 months but this is dependent on development of understanding of language (noun labels) and the youngest children may not manage the full 14 toys of the McCormick test (a popular example) at that age. Speech tests in the form of word lists can be used for all ages. The child sits at the table with the examiner checking that all toys can be identified at normal speaking voice and then with the voice lowered and the mouth covered, the child is asked to show each in turn. For younger children the 'co-operative test' can be performed in which the child is asked to 'give' toys to 'mummy' (or 'daddy'), 'teddy' or 'dolly', allowing assessment of speech discrimination.
   (**b**) Conditioning/performance tests. From 30 months and by 36 months children can carry out an action in response to a stimulus and have sufficient control to wait for the stimulus. The stimulus used is a machine emitting tones of a range of frequency and decibel level. The technique is a conditioning one. The child, sitting at the table, puts a brick in a box or a pegman in a boat every time the adult says 'go'. After managing this, the child listens for a tone and puts the brick in, or similar action. Once the child can do this action reliably, the child usually quickly learns to wear headphones and each ear can then be tested individually using pure tones (i.e. tones containing only one frequency), producing a pure tone audiogram – the gold standard hearing test. The ability to manage such tests can be a guide to developmental maturity.

Testing children with developmental disorders. The above tests can all be adapted for use with children with disabilities. Children with visual impairment will experience delay in sound localization and may therefore not respond by turning to sound in the distraction tests. Those with motor impairments may also have difficulty with location and/or hand actions. Objective tests are increasingly frequently employed to confirm normal hearing.

Problems with speech, language and communication

Speech and language delays. Speech and language delays are among the commonest developmental problems in children, and parental concern should always be taken seriously. A problem with speech and language may be an indicator of a broader developmental problem and all children must have their hearing tested.

Co-morbidities are common and together with severity are important in prognosis.

In general, children have significant problems if they do not babble in the first year, have less than 10 words at 2 years and are not speaking in sentences by 3 years. Most children have adult syntax and grammar by 4 years and are intelligible to most people.[72] These milestone absolutes, however, ignore the qualitative impairments in the use of speech and language for social communication, which are such a key part of social skills.

A problem affecting speech or expressive language only is generally regarded as being less severe in terms of long term significance compared with comprehension problems. However, the view that expressive disorders all have normal receptive skills is less tenable, as increasing research has shown subtle problems not previously found on cruder tests. Many children have problems in all areas of speech, language and communication.

It is helpful to think of speech and language as a means for getting needs met, sharing interests and for mental representation for thinking abstractly – an inner language. Language and communication have forms and functions. The forms (i.e. speech, gestures, facial expressions), their maturity and complexity and how well they are coordinated together, need to be assessed as well as the functions of the forms – needs met, comments, requests, frequency (both initiation and response).

Getting needs met can be verbal through words/sounds, or the written symbol/word may substitute for spoken words, or nonverbal, e.g. through gesture and facial expression which are both social and symbolic. Other nonverbal methods can be nonsocial/nonsymbolic [where there is no representation of the object (or idea)]. These include not using another person at all but going to get something, either directly, or by pulling a chair over and climbing up, bringing an object (e.g. a bottle of juice because a drink is wanted), or taking the parent by the hand or pulling/pushing them towards the object.

Concerns about reciprocity in communication and its social and symbolic function are often not noted in young children, even when quite extreme under the age of 18 months, and especially in a first child. By this age, children should show not only an increasing understanding of phrases and interest in people talking to them, but a desire to share, show and take turns with pointing used both for needs and interests. Persistent failure to do this may indicate a social communicative problem. Indeed, a lack of gaze monitoring, in combination with a lack of pointing for interest and simple pretend play, by 18 months of age was highly predictive of autism in the CHAT screening study.[41] The same study showed that over 97% of 16 000 children were able to follow an adult pointing at a distant object, were using pointing themselves to get their needs met and show things, and 93% were said by their parents to show pretend play by 21 months of age.

Some children with speech and language delays will be slow in all aspects of these skills. Those with speech/articulation problems will have better comprehension and communication but poor unintelligible speech and may have oromotor delay or disorder.

A common clinical presentation is seen in young children with language learning disability in the transition from associatively learned words to symbolic language. Parents report that the child reaches the stage of imitating word forms, but then stops progressing and may indeed lose those first words. One explanation may be that these children have not truly mastered the connection between words spoken and representational meaning and have failed to progress to the higher levels of language learning. Another common experience is for parents to say that children produce words only in situations of extreme emotional provocation or only once and never again; the explanation is likely to be that the language is attached to very particular contexts. Rapid word learning, 'fast mapping', is a skill of normal language acquisition that is significantly poorer in language impairments. A prolonged period before the child moves from single words to sentences is also more common in delayed and disordered development.

Even experts can overestimate the child's comprehension of language. Where there are any concerns, specific tests should be carried out.

Behavior

Food fads, sleep problems, night waking, problems of compliance and temper tantrums are part of normal development between 2 and 5 years of age, and show some continuity through those years. When the behaviors of normal development are functionally impairing for parent and child then they may or may not be called a disorder, but they certainly warrant assessment and intervention. Any developmental impairment puts a child at risk of psychiatric disorder, particularly severe learning and communication difficulties. Extremes of temperament also contribute to risk, as do family factors such as maternal mental ill health, family conflict, school-based difficulties and any other problem with parent – child interaction.

LEARNING IMPAIRMENTS

The terminology of neurodevelopmental impairments leading to functional disability continues to be problematical and different in the USA, the UK and Europe. For example, learning disability is the preferred term in the UK for what would be referred to as mental retardation in the USA. This is defined as an impairment in intellectual learning and adaptive skills to a degree that significantly impairs normal function and on standardized tests falls outside two standard deviations below the mean. Although the implication is that all aspects of development will be affected, in practice this is variable and within mental and adaptive skills certain strengths and weaknesses are common. In severe to profound learning difficulties a child may show normal acquisition of motor milestones, but motor development is usually slower. This may be evident in delayed achievement of milestones, but with a normal pattern of motor development with or without hypotonia (floppiness). A distinction is usually made between:

1. general learning difficulties;
2. specific learning difficulties.

It is common, however, for these distinctions to be blurred and overlap in practice.

SPECIFIC NEURODEVELOPMENTAL IMPAIRMENTS

The term 'specific' is used to mean that the skill in question is more delayed than would be expected from the overall level of cognitive ability. Although it is convenient to classify these as covering different functional domains, in practice overlaps of impairment are common.[73,74] This reflects the more common problem, seen in children, of integration of information processing in a developing brain, rather than the 'damage model' which comes from the study of adults, where brain behavior relationships may be much more specifically anatomically located. Both delay and disorder (differences in developmental pattern) occur in the problem area and often it is difficult to separate these elements. Specific neurodevelopmental impairments include:

1. specific developmental disorders of speech and language;
2. specific developmental disorders of acquired academic skills, for example reading, spelling and mathematics;
3. specific developmental disorders of motor function (developmental co-ordination disorder – clumsy child);
4. autistic spectrum disorders (also called the pervasive developmental disorders) – these disorders are usually classified in the international classification systems under the psychiatric disorders section, but can properly be considered as neurodevelopment impairments;
5. specific impairments of memory (short or long term episodic or declarative) and learning;
6. specific developmental impairments of attention (usually with impulsivity and distractibility plus or minus hyperactivity and with failure of inhibition control as the likely underlying difficulty);
7. specific developmental impairment of executive function.

Developmental impairments of attention, with or without hyperactivity, are usually classified under the psychiatric disorders, but the range of functional impairments is due not only to a failure of inhibition. Often there are additional problems with other processes of executive function (i.e. the planning, organizing and carrying through of ideas and actions) and hence these disorders are included here as a neurodevelopmental impairment.

All neurodevelopmental impairments place the child at increased risk of additional developmental impairments and behavior problems, which may be of sufficient severity for a psychiatric disorder diagnosis. All these neurodevelopmental impairments have their origin in brain function, either at a neuroanatomical or neurochemical level, and can present as behavioral or emotional problems as well as deficits in input (perception) or output functions (e.g. in speaking or recording). They are probably underdiagnosed.

Combinations of developmental impairments that are particularly common are those of attention and motor perception with or without language and learning delay. These are referred to as Delayed Attention and Motor Perception (DAMP) by Scandanavian clinicians. The autistic spectrum disorders are frequently associated with language learning difficulties and problems with motor coordination. These neurodevelopmental impairments are all described in Chapter 22.

The developmental assessment of these varying problems requires analysis and description using appropriate tools for the child's age often by a multidisciplinary team.

PHYSICAL EXAMINATION

A full examination should be carried out as described in Chapter 8. Some aspects are particularly important if the child has a developmental or neurological problem and these will be commented on. The physical examination is generally left to the end of an assessment as the child may become upset and this would interfere with the developmental examination.

Motor examination

Motor examination is best carried out by observing the child's movement patterns and posture. This can be done during the developmental examination, when the child is walking, speaking and handling material (e.g. tendency to keep the forearm pronated and rather deliberate finger movements in mild spasticity). Indeed after observing the child, one should have a good idea of the nature and extent of any motor problem and examination of tone, reflexes and power is largely confirmatory.

Compare both sides of the body

It is useful to compare the two sides of the body and to determine the child's hand preference. The motor skill, tone, reflexes or the size of the limbs may be significantly asymmetrical suggesting hemisphere dysfunction and therefore focal pathology (mild hemiparesis and visuospatial difficulties).

Head circumference

Head circumference must always be measured and plotted on a centile chart and compared with the child's height and, if there is any discrepancy, with the parents' head circumference (as this is the most common reason for a large head).[75]

Optic discs

Examination of the optic discs and fundi is difficult, but can be valuable in diagnosing particular disorders (septo-optic dysplasia) as well as raised intracranial pressure.

Appearance

Dysmorphic features and congenital malformations must be looked for because they may suggest a particular syndrome or etiology (e.g. fetal alcohol syndrome).

Skin

The skin should be carefully examined for pigmented and depigmented spots (e.g. looking for specific features of neurofibromatosis or tuberosclerosis).

Growth

Height, weight and growth rate should be determined as these may indicate a condition such as hypothyroidism.

Mental state

The child's mental state should be observed, e.g. is the child hyperactive, impulsive? Does the child concentrate well? Is the child having absence or other seizures?

Is there more than one problem?

Co-morbid neurodevelopmental conditions are common so it is important to remember that the child with one neurodevelopmental problem may have others.

EVALUATION AND INTERPRETATION

The purpose of assessment to identify an impairment in development is to make a diagnosis and seek to intervene positively to improve outcome and function for the child and family. Evaluation and interpretation of the historical, observational and test data should lead to:

1. a profile of the child – both assets and difficulties (Table 7.10);
2. a management plan to be agreed with parents and to include ways of implementing it (Table 7.11);
3. appropriate onward referrals for intervention, specific therapy, genetic advice;
4. ensuring voluntary services and social services benefits are discussed and parents are supported to access these;
5. within the UK legal framework, if the child is likely to have special educational needs there is a duty to inform the education department, with parental permission, so that they can make their own assessment (Code of Practice Guidelines in the UK[76]);
6. family support through social services, including respite as needed;
7. written record of findings and discussion to be given to parents;
8. further appointment to discuss report and plan, identify a key worker if complex neurodevelopmental disorder, further information and counseling as needed and date for further appointment.

Disclosure discussion

The sharing of information about possible impairment and disability (disclosure discussion) has been the subject of audit and research, which show how important this time is in its impact on the family both in the short and long term and how training can affect satisfaction.[77] A report by the NHS Executive Guide to Good Practice commented in 1996 that 'Despite publication of research and recommendations on good practice, this remains a subject of dissatisfaction to a significant number of families.'[78]

Important principles for disclosure are given in detail in a report by a voluntary organization SCOPE[79] and include the following key headings:

1. valuing the child;
2. respecting parents and families;
3. preparation; ensuring privacy, sufficient time;
4. who should be there; both parents;
5. tuning in to parents: effective communication;
6. next steps: practical help and information.

Table 7.10 Child profile

Diagnosis of the presenting condition
Any other specific neurodevelopmental impairments
Level of intellectual function
Medical condition, either associative or causative, to include a hypothesis about etiology that might need tests for confirmation or refuting
Associated psychosocial situations that may or may not be thought to be causative or contributory
Style of learning/motivation and needs

Table 7.11 Aims of appropriate onward referrals for intervention, specific therapy, genetic advice

Reinforcing acquired skills
Teach developmentally appropriate skills
Provide missed experience
Make use of other skills to overcome difficulties
Use learning style to promote learning

INTERPRETATION OF ABNORMAL DEVELOPMENT USING AN EVIDENCE-BASED APPROACH AND DEVELOPMENTAL ASSESSMENT FINDINGS

Case study 1: The child of 18 months who is not yet walking[80]

A boy is referred because of failure to walk independently at 18 months. Does this matter?

Not walking by 18 months places the child outside the 90th centile for British children. A literature search shows one relevant study of such children, an epidemiological survey,[31] and that less than 10% of such children had a neurological impairment, 11% had delays in other developmental areas. Bottom shuffling and a family history of late walking were common.[54] Although there is no clear evidence base to assess the yield of further physical examination or exclusion by family history of motor variants, there are two questions that are discriminatory:

1. Is the motor pattern deviant (e.g. toe walking or a pronated position of forearms suggesting spasticity) or does it look normal for a younger child? Observe the nature of the child's movement pattern and examine tone and reflexes, and look for any persistent primitive reflexes and fasciculation.
2. Is development in other areas normal or abnormal? At this age language and symbolic play should be assessed as well as adaptive competencies (e.g. building, simple shape sorting). If the child has a significant motor disorder affecting hand function the methods used to determine intellectual ability will need to be modified (e.g. eye pointing to named objects).

How likely is this to be a presentation of muscular dystrophy?

The prevalence of muscular dystrophy in male births is 1 in 3802. Of children with muscular dystrophy 50% walk by 18 months of age (although later walking than the family pattern suggests is common). Muscular dystrophy is noted because the child's motor competence falls away from the normal trajectory, even though progress continues to be made for the first few years of life (e.g. running is invariably impaired or the child presents with more general delays such as speech). The risk of muscular dystrophy because of late walking is 1 in 228 for a boy not walking at 18 months. Further information from history and examination would be required to help with your decision making about the benefits and costs of further investigation [creatine phosphokinase (CPK) estimation].

Most likely etiology in a child with:

1. A family history of bottom shuffling, no physical abnormality and no delay in other areas of development would suggest a familial pattern and reduce the likelihood of a pathological cause. Further investigation would have a low yield. You might consider review again until walking.
2. History suggesting global developmental delay and a maternal male cousin with learning disability. Likelihood of fragile X or muscular dystrophy would increase and suggest a higher yield from further investigation.
3. History of preterm delivery, 2 days' ventilation and no family history. Examination shows that the child tends to sit with a curved back and stands propped on toes with legs crossed. Tone and reflexes are increased in the lower limbs and the diagnosis is a spastic diplegia.

It is always extremely important to ascertain whether or not there is any question of regression because this would lead to another chain of inquiry and investigation.

Case study 2: The child who is saying only a few single words by 30 months

At 30 months many children will be putting two or even three words together and most will have quite large vocabularies. The possible causes of language delay are normal variation, specific language delay or disorder, general learning disability (mental retardation), deafness, autism, severe environmental deprivation.

A difficulty with speech (output unclear) may be due to specific motor disorders or other neurological disorders.

In order to discriminate between these it is necessary to determine the child's:

1. understanding of language;
2. ability in nonlanguage areas – drawing, brick building, shapes, symbolic play;
3. understanding and use of nonverbal communication and social interactive and sharing behavior (e.g. gesture, facial expression, response to and initiation of communication) – this can be observed in a play-based assessment and the peer social play assessed at nursery;
4. quality of speech – are the few words clear? – does the child speak jargon using normal speech sounds and intonation?;
5. pattern of speech development: is it following the normal lines or is it deviant in any way (e.g. use of the word rhinoceros before mum and dad)?

A persistent receptive language problem is of more global significance than an expressive problem only. From the Whitehurst and Fischel study[81] most 2-year-old children with 10 words only had caught up by 5 years of age. In another study, however, children with delays in speech and language at 4–5 years still showed impairments in language-based literacy skills in their teens[82] and children with severe receptive language disorder continue to show language and social impairments into adult life.[83] A family history of language delay might support a genetic predisposition, which is common in developmental language disorder.

Hearing should be checked in all children – even if it is not the main cause. A mild loss may be making a child with a potentially mild developmental language disorder worse.

Assessment of the language problem

Developmental profile on the Griffiths test shows that this child's ability in nonlanguage areas is normal, so he does not have a global learning disability. His symbolic play is also normal. He is a social child who understands and uses pointing and some simple gestures. His social skills with peers, play and imaginative skills show that he is not therefore autistic. His understanding of language is a little delayed, but not as much as his expressive skills. The words he has are clear and he uses normal sounding jargon. There is nothing deviant about his language development; it is simply delayed. There is a history that his father had been slow to talk and later on had reading and spelling problems. The home environment is satisfactory. Hearing is tested and found to be normal.

This child therefore has a developmental language delay for which there is probably a genetic predisposition. As his language comprehension is reasonable and he is beginning to use words he is likely to make steady progress. It is possible he will also have reading and spelling problems at school. He should be reviewed by a speech and language therapist to make sure his progress is satisfactory, and to offer parents advice on how to encourage language development and anticipate any problems with phonological awareness predictive of reading delay.

SERVICES FOR CHILDREN WITH NEURODEVELOPMENTAL DISABILITY

Children with neurodevelopmental disability require co-ordinated services between health, social services and education. Guidelines and government policy in the UK support the development of well-integrated and co-ordinated care for young children with disability. The document 'Together from the Start'[84] outlines guidance on the effective delivery of services to children with disabilities, from birth to their third birthday, and their families with the following key themes:

1. better initial assessment of need;
2. better co-ordination of multi-agency support;
3. better information and access for families;
4. improved professional knowledge and skill;
5. service review and development;
6. partnership across agencies and geographical boundaries.

This document was issued jointly by the UK Department for Education and Skills and Department of Health in May 2003.

Early Support (http://www.earlysupport.org.uk/) has become the central government mechanism to improve the quality, consistency and coordination of services for young disabled children and their families across England following the guidance of 'Together from the Start' and aims to facilitate better coordination of information and service delivery in response to the objectives set by the Government green paper 'Every Child Matters'.[85]

Health services for children with neurodevelopmental disability are often co-ordinated by child development centres or teams who provide specialist services for assessment and management of children with physical and learning disabilities, hearing, vision, speech and language and social communication problems. In the UK these services are provided on a district basis serving a population of about 250 000–300 000 people. Core members of a service for children with disability should include a pediatrician, speech therapist, physiotherapist, occupational therapist, psychologist, nurse/health visitor, teacher, social worker and administrator. The team will provide assessment, diagnosis and management of the child and team composition should be constituted according to the child and family needs. The service may be delivered in a child development centre, the child's home or in nurseries or schools.

Children with multiple disabilities, complex neurological problems or physical problems compounded by psychological and behavioral difficulties will require multidisciplinary and multi-agency assessment and management. Children with less complex or single neurodevelopmental disorders are more likely to require assessment and management by one or two disciplines.

Many services in the UK have been historically centered around the needs of children between 0 and 5 years of age.[86] However, continuity of care from preschool to school age is essential. There needs to be ongoing commitment for review and treatment of children with special educational needs in mainstream or special schools, including the provision of advice to the local education authority, contributing towards statements and reviews under the 1993 Education Act and Code of Practice (2001), together with responsibilities relating to social services under the Children Act.

Services that are family centered have been shown to promote the psychosocial well-being of children and their parents and in leading to increased satisfaction with services.[87] A standard measure of parents' perceptions of health care providers' behaviors (Measure of Processes of Care – MPOC) has been shown to be effective in evaluating the family centeredness of children's rehabilitation services.[88] The measure was developed with the participation of more than 1600 parents of children with chronic neurodevelopmental conditions throughout Ontario. It assesses five domains: enabling and partnership; providing general information; providing specific information about the child; coordinated and comprehensive care; and respectful and supportive care – domains that were most highly valued by parents.

Some essential principals of child disability services include.[89]

1. The need for co-ordinated multiagency services with local planning for provision between health, education and social services.
2. The need for comprehensive local knowledge and collaboration with primary care, education, social services, parent groups and voluntary groups in order to provide the best possible packages of care.
3. Provision of support, training and clear referral criteria and care pathways for primary health care (including general practitioners and health visitors) who will be first line in the detection and ascertainment of children with disability.
4. Access to services via 'a single front door' – a single organizational and information base for all children with special needs.
5. Children with more complex disability should have a key worker to provide a single point of contact and co-ordination for the family's care package. Research has confirmed that key workers have a positive impact on many families' lives. The factors relating to better outcomes included the management of the service, definition and understanding of the key worker role, and provision of training and supervision for key workers. This research from the Social Policy Research Unit has resulted in a number of recommendations for the management of key worker services.[90,91]
6. Parent representative involvement in planning and organization of services.
7. The client group should include children and young people with developmental disability up to the age of 19 years.
8. Transitional care plans for transfer to adult services should be drawn up in collaboration between health, social services and education. In some areas this may require support for the development of appropriate adult services.
9. Established lines of communication and referral criteria to hospital pediatric services including systems for provision of information and combined protocols for management for ward staff on how to care for and communicate with the disabled child. The needs of adolescents and young adults for appropriate inpatient accommodation should be considered both for medical needs and acute mental health issues.
10. Easy access to more specialist regional and national services for childhood disability with clear care pathways and networks supporting local services which may include combined outreach clinics.
11. Child psychiatry support should be an integral part of the service
12. Other professionals and combined clinics provide important additional services and include: a pediatric ophthalmologist, orthoptist and peripatetic teacher for the visually impaired; audiology, hearing aid service, peripatetic teacher for the hearing impaired; dietitian; a clinic for severe neurological feeding impairment; specialist dentistry; orthopedic surgery, with access to gait analysis and to a spinal unit, good orthotic support; specialist radiology (X-ray, computed tomography, magnetic resonance imaging, videofluoroscopy); specialist neurophysiology (electroencephalography, auditory and visual evoked responses); podiatry; a clinic for neuropathic bladder.
13. Respite care is for families whose children have severe/complex disability.
14. Written information for the family is essential. Early Support provides standard materials for families including: a series of booklets giving information about particular conditions or disabilities and other useful sources of information and support – publications, organizations, helplines, support groups and websites; the 'Family file' – a family-held record and a Family Service Plan which encourages all agencies working with a family to discuss the support that is being provided and to agree priorities. Advice about benefits should be readily available.
15. Sensitivity to the particular needs of ethnic and cultural minorities.
16. Clear guidelines for the management of child protection issues.
17. Regular audit to ensure best practice. Some tools available include: the MPOC.[88]

Milner et al[92] and the Early Support Service audit tool (http://www.earlysupport.org.uk/) provide tools for auditing and evaluating services for children and families with special needs.

REFERENCES (*Level 1 Evidence)

1. American Academy of Pediatrics. Committee on Community Health Services. The pediatrician's role in community pediatrics. Pediatrics 1999; 103:1304–1307.

2. Chomsky N. Language and mind. New York: Harcourt Brace Jovanovitch; 1972.

3. Thalen E, Smith L. A dynamic systems approach to the development of cognition and action. Cambridge, MA: Bradford MIT; 1994.

4. Plomin R. Genetics of childhood disorders III. Genetics and intelligence. J Am Acad Child Adolesc Psychiatry 1999; 38:786–788.

5. Kagan J, Snidman N, Arcus D. Childhood derivatives of high and low reactivity in infancy. Child Dev 1998; 69:1483–1493.

6. Culp R, Watkins RV, Lawrence H, et al. Maltreated children's language and speech development: abused, neglected, and abused and neglected. First Language 1991; 11:377–391.

7. Croft C, Andersen-Wood L, and the English and Romanian Study Team, Institute of Psychiatry. Language development following severe early deprivation. Conference presentation at A fasic Third International Symposium; 1999.

*8. Rutter M, and the English and Roumanian Adoptees (ERA) Study Team. Developmental catch-up and deficit following adoption after severe global early deprivation. J Child Psychol Psychiatry 1998; 39:465–476.

*9. O'Connor T, Rutter M, Beckett C, and the English and Roumanian Adoptees Study Team. The effect of global severe deprivation on cognitive competence: extension and follow-up. Child Dev 2000; 71:376–390.

*10. Lucas A, Morley R, Cole TJ, et al. Breast milk and subsequent intelligence quotient in children born preterm. Lancet 1992; 339:261–264.

11. Brunswick N, McCrory E, Price CJ, et al. Explicit and implicit processing of words and pseudowords by adult developmental dyslexics: a search for Wernicke's Wortschatz? Brain 1999; 122:1901–1917.

12. Fensom L, Bates E, Dale P, et al. Measuring variability in early child language: don't shoot the messenger. Child Dev 2000; 71:323–328.

13. Geschwind N, Galaburda A. Cerebral lateralization: biological mechanisms, associations and pathology: I. A hypothesis and a program for research. Arch Neurol 1985; 42:428–429.

14. Sheridan MD. The developmental progress of infants and young children. 3rd edn. London: HMSO; 1975.

15. Illingworth R. Development of the infant and young child, 9th edn. Edinburgh: Churchill Livingstone; 1987.

16. Milani-Comparetti A, Gidoni EA. Routine developmental examination in normal and retarded children. Dev Med Child Neurol 1967; 9:631–638.

17. Erhardt R. Developmental hand dysfunction: theory, assessment and treatment. San Antonio: The Psychological Corporation; 1994.

18. O'Hare A, Gorzkowska J, Elton R. Development of an instrument to measure manual praxis. Dev Med Child Neurol 1999; 41:597–607.

19. Harris DB. Children's drawings as measures of intellectual maturity. New York: Harcourt, Brace & World; 1963.

20. Vygotsky LS. Thought and language. Cambridge, MA: Harvard University Press; 1986.

21. Bruner J. Child's talk: learning to use language. New York: WW Norton; 1983.

22. Mundy P. Joint attention and social–emotional approach behavior in children with autism. Dev Psychopathol 1995; 7:63–82.

23. Bates E, Dale P, Thal D. Individual differences and their implications for theories of language development. In: Fletcher P, MacWhinney B, eds. The handbook of child language. Oxford: Blackwell; 1995.

24. Fenson L, Dale PS, Resnick JS, et al. MacArthur's communicative development inventories. San Diego: Singular Publishing; 1993.

25. Volterra V, Erting CJ, eds. From gesture to language in hearing and deaf children. Berlin: Springer; 1990.

26. Crystal D. Listen to your child. Middlesex: Penguin Books; 1986.

27. Astington JW, Jenkins JM. Theory of mind development and social understanding. In: Dunn J, ed. Connections between emotions and understanding in development. J Cognit Emot Special Isssue. 1995.151–167.

28. Wainryb C, Shaw L, Maianu C. Tolerance and intolerance: children's and adolescents' judgments of dissenting beliefs, speech, persons and conduct. Child Dev 1998; 69:1541–1555.

29. Stanley O, Dolby S. Learning in pre-school children with neurological disability. Arch Dis Child 1999; 80:481–484.

30. Wimmer H, Perner J. Beliefs about beliefs: representation and constraining function of wrong beliefs in young children's understanding of deception. Cognition 1983; 13:103–128.

31. Chaplais JD, Macfarlane A. A review of 404 late walkers. Arch Dis Child 1984; 59:512–516.

32. Hall DMB. Health for all children. The Report of the Joint Working Party on Child Health Surveillance. 3rd edn. Oxford: Oxford University Press; 1996.

33. Law J, Boyle J, Harris F, et al. The feasibility of universal screening for primary language delay: findings from a systematic review. Dev Med Child Neurol 2000; 42:190–200.

34. Law J, Boyle J, Harris F, et al. Screening for primary language delay: a systematic review of the literature. Health Technol Assess 1998; 2:1–184.

35. Wilson J, Jungner G. Principles and practice of screening for disease. Public Health Papers No. 34. Geneva: WHO; 1968.

36. Cochrane A, Holland W. Validation of screening procedures. Br Med Bull 1969; 27:3–8.

37. Davis A, Bamford J, Wilson I. A critical review of the role of neonatal hearing screening in the detection of congenital hearing impairment. Health Technol Assess 1997; 1:(10):i–iv.1–176.

38. American Academy of Pediatrics. Committee on Children with Disabilities. Screening infants and young children for developmental disabilities. Pediatrics 1994; 93:863–865.

39. National Research Council. Educating children with autism. Committee on Educational Interventions for Children with Autism. Division of Behavioral and Social Sciences and Education. Washington: National Academy Press; 2001.

40. Baird G, Charman T, Baron-Cohen S, et al. A screening instrument for autism at 18 months of age: a six-year follow-up study. J Am Acad Child Adolesc Psychiatry 2000; 39:694–702.

41. Baird G, Charman T, Cox A, et al. Screening and surveillance for autism and pervasive developmental disorders. Arch Dis Child 2001; 84:468–475.

42. Glascoe F. A method for deciding how to respond to parents' concerns about development and behavior. Ambul Child Health 1999; 5:197–208.

43. Glascoe FP. The value of parents' concerns to detect and address developmental and behavioral problems. J Pediatr Child Health 1999; 35:1–8.

44. Belsky J, Melhuish E, Barnes J, et al. Effects of SureStart local programmes on children and families, early findings from a quasi-experimental cross sectional study. BMJ 2006; 332 (7556):1476.

45. Blair M, Hall D. From Health Surveillance to health promotion: the changing focus in preventive children's services. Arch Dis Child 2006; 91: 730–735.

46. British Association for Community Child Health. Child Development and Disability group of the RCOCH. Standards for child development services. A guide for commissioners and providers. London: Royal College of Paediatrics and Child Health; 2001.

47. Lord C, Rutter M, Le Couteur A. Autism diagnostic interview – revised. J Autism Dev Disord 1994; 24:659–686.

48. Blair E, Stanley F. Aetiological pathways to spastic cerebral palsy. Pediatr Perinat Epidemiol 1993; 7:302–317.

49. Gesell A. The first five years of life. London: Methuen; 1950.

50. Lord C, Risi A, DiLavore P, et al. The autism diagnostic observation schedule – generic. Los Angeles: The Western Psychological Corporation; 1999.

51. Wiart L, Darrah J. Review of four tests of gross motor development. Dev Med Child Neurol 2001; 43:279–285.

52. O'Brien G, Pearson J, Berney T, et al. Measuring behavior in developmental disability: review of existing schedules. Dev Med Child Neurol 2001; 43:(suppl):1–72.

53. Robson P. Shuffling, hitching, scooting or sliding: some observations in 30 otherwise normal children. Dev Med Child Neurol 1970; 12:608–617.

54. Robson P. Prewalking locomotor movements and their use in predicting standing and walking. Child Care Health Dev 1984; 10:317–330.

55. Milani-Comparetti A, Gidoni EA. Pattern analysis of motor development and its disorders. Dev Med Child Neurol 1967; 9:625–630.

56. Sonksen P, Petrie A, Drew K. Promotion of visual development of severely visually impaired babies: evaluation of a developmentally based program. Dev Med Child Neurol 1991; 33:320–335.

57. Sonksen PM, Dale N. Visual impairment in infancy: impact on neurodevelopmental and neurobiological processes. Dev Med Child Neurol 2002; 44:782–791.

58. Sonksen PM. The assessment of vision in the preschool child. Arch Dis Child 1993; 68:513–516.

59. Salt A, Sonksen P, Wade A, et al. The maturation of linear acuity and compliance with the Sonksen–Silver acuity system in young children. Dev Med Child Neurol 1995; 3:505–514.

60. Bailey IL, Lovie JE. New design principles for visual acuity letter charts. Am J Optom Physiol Opt 1976; 53:740–745.

61. Sheridan MD. The clinical assessment of visual competence in babies and young children. In: Smith V, Kean J, eds. Visual handicap in children. London: Heinemann; 1979.

62. Salt A, Wade A, Proffitt R, et al. The Sonksen logMAR Test of visual acuity: I. Developmental compliance and reliability. Submitted.

63. Sonksen PM, Wade A, Proffitt R, et al. The Sonksen logMAR Test of visual acuity: II Age norms from 2.9 to 8 years. Submitted.

64. Kay Picture Test. PO Box 156, Coventry CV8 3LJ. 1983.

65. Jones D, Westall C, Averbeck K, et al. Visual acuity assessment: a comparison of two tests for measuring children's vision. Ophthalmic Physiol Opt 2003; 23:541–546.

66. Teller DY, McDonald MA, Preston K, et al. Assessment of visual acuity in children: the acuity card procedure. Dev Med Child Neurol 1986; 28:779–789.

67. Mackie RT, McCulloch DL. Assessment of visual acuity in multiply handicapped children. Br J Ophthalmol 1995; 79:290–296.

68. Sonksen PM, Macrae AJ. Vision for colored pictures at different acuities. Dev Med Child Neurol 1987; 29:337–347.

69. Russell-Eggitt I, Harris CM, Kriss A. Delayed visual maturation: an update. Dev Med Child Neurol 1998; 40:130–136.

70. Dutton GN. The Edridge Green Lecture. Cognitive vision, its disorders and differential diagnosis in adults and children: knowing where and what things are. Eye 2003; 17:289–304.

71. Fortnum HM, Summerfield AQ, Marshall DH, et al. Prevalence of permanent childhood hearing impairment in the United Kingdom and implications for universal neonatal screening: questionnaire based ascertainment study. BMJ 2001; 323:536–539.

72. Wells G. Language development in the preschool years. Cambridge: Cambridge University Press; 1985.

73. Willcutt EG, Pennington BF, Olson RK, et al. Neuropsychological analyses of comorbidity between reading disability and attention deficit hyperactivity disorder: in search of the common deficit. Dev Neuropsychol 2005; 27:35–78.

74. Waber DP, Forbes PW, Wolff PH, et al. Neurodevelopmental characteristics of children with learning impairments classified according to the double-deficit hypothesis. J Learn Disabil 2004; 37:451–461.

75. Lorber J, Priestley BL. Children with large heads: a practical approach to diagnosis in 557 children, with special reference to 109 children with megalencephaly. Dev Med Child Neurol 1981; 23:494–504.

76. Code of Practice Guidelines in the UK. Special educational needs, code of practice. Department of Education and Skills 581/2001. Online. Available at: http://www.dfes.gov.uk

77. Baird G, McConachie H, Scrutton D. Parents' perceptions of disclosure of the diagnosis of cerebral palsy. Arch Dis Child 2000; 83:475–480.

78. NHS Executive Guide to Good Practice: Child Health in the Community. 1996.

79. www.rightfromthestart.org.uk

80. Dorling J, Salt A. Assessing developmental delay; evidenced based case report. Br Med J 2001; 323:148–150.

81. Whitehurst GJ, Fischel JE. Early developmental language delay: what, if anything, should the clinician do about it? J Child Psychol Psychiatry 1994; 35:613–648.

82. Stothard S, Snowling M, Bishop D, et al. Language impaired preschoolers: a follow-up to adolescence. J Speech Lang Hear Res 1998; 41:407–418.

83. Clegg J, Hollis C, Mawhood L, et al. Developmental language disorders – a follow-up in later adult life. Cognitive, language and psychosocial outcomes. J Child Psychol Psychiatry 2005; 46:128–149.

84. Together From The Start – Practical guidance for professionals working with disabled children (birth to third birthday) and their families. May 2003. Reference number: LEA/0067/2003. Department for Education and Skills. London: HMSO.

85. Every Child Matters. Together from the Start. London: HMSO Online. Available at: http://www.dh.gov.uk/en/Publicationsandstatistics/Publications/PublicationsPolicyAndGuidance/DH_4007526.

86. McConachie H, Salt AT, McLachlan A, et al. How do child development teams work? Findings of a UK national survey. Child Care Health Dev 1999; 25:157–168.

87. King S, Teplicky R, King G, et al. Family-centered service for children with cerebral palsy and their families: a review of the literature. Semin Pediatr Neurol 2004; 11:78–86.

88. King GA, Rosenbaum PL, King SM. Evaluating family-centred service using a measure of parents' perceptions. Child Care Health Dev 1997; 23:47–62.

89. Lloyd-Evans A. Standards for child development services. Produced for the British Association of Community Child Health. London: Royal College of Paediatrics and Child Health; 2001.

90. Greco V, Sloper P, Webb R, et al. An exploration of different models of multi-agency partnerships in key worker services for disabled children: effectiveness and costs. Department for Education and Skills Research Report 656. London: HMSO; 2005.

91. Greco V, Sloper P, Barton K. Care co-ordination and key worker services for disabled children in the UK (348KB PDF). Research Works, 2004–1. York: Social Policy Research Unit, University of York; 2004.

92. Milner J, Bungay C, Jellinek D, et al. Needs of disabled children and their families. Arch Dis Child 1996; 75:399–404.

93. Baird G, Simonoff E, Pickles A, et al. Prevalence of disorders of the autism spectrum in a population cohort of children in South Thames: the Special Needs and Autism Project (SNAP). Lancet 2006; 368:(9531):210–215.

8

History, examination, basic investigations and procedures

Julie-Clare Becher, Ian Laing

INTRODUCTION

Despite the development of sophisticated laboratory and imaging techniques, the foundation of sound clinical practice continues to be history taking and clinical examination.[1] The aims of the consultation can be measured by the ability to establish the relevant facts of the history, elicit the findings from clinical examination, formulate a diagnosis or diagnoses and plan ongoing investigations and management. It is also important to establish and maintain a partnership between the family and the medical profession, measured in trust, motivation and empowerment. Such a partnership is engendered by good communication, provision of information and credibility.

The pediatric history and examination also serve as a record of information for future health surveillance or clinical governance. It has an important role to promote health and prevent disease and to diagnose secondary illness (Table 8.1).

Table 8.1   Purpose of the pediatric consultation

Diagnosis of primary disease
Establishment of an effective partnership with the family
Record of health and development
Diagnosis of secondary or concurrent illness
Information for health systems to use as audit
Health promotion and disease awareness

Of these functions, the opportunity for health promotion and disease prevention is most overlooked by health professionals. Guidance can be provided on a variety of health and lifestyle issues such as nutrition, dental health, drug abuse, injury prevention, exercise and contraceptive counselling. Educational fragments can be provided during the examination to help enable parents to recognize health and disease.

Pediatric history taking and examination is an art that requires thoughtfulness, patience, and versatility. Through practice it should become smooth and spontaneous. A skilled interviewer will pick up on subtleties and explore these clues. The pediatric history presents different challenges from the consultation in adults.

1. Childhood is characterized by considerable physical, cognitive and psychosocial growth and development.
2. The presentation of disease in children may differ; many symptoms and signs are nonspecific.
3. The history is usually taken from a third person.
4. Young children have limited verbal skills and comprehension.
5. Children are often uncooperative and unpredictable.

AGE-APPROPRIATE CONSULTATION AND COMMUNICATION SKILLS

The specialty of pediatrics spans around 16 years and unless specializing as an adolescent pediatrician or neonatologist, a doctor must learn an array of interview and examination techniques to allow him versatility in his interaction with children. A child has autonomy and a separate identity from that of his parents and respect for this is fundamental to trust and communication even in the smallest child. A key right in the United Nations Convention on the Rights of the Child is a child's right to express views in all matters that affect them, and for due weight to be given to their views.[2] Health care professionals have an important role in sharing information with children and listening to their needs, empowering them to make confident decisions with their parents about treatment. Support of parents, who may express different needs and desires from those of their child, is also crucial in this process.

The age of the child will determine the nature and presentation of the condition, how the interview is conducted and the subsequent management of the condition. Remember that the younger the child the less specific the symptoms will be. The age of the child will also influence how he or she understands and responds to illness and its treatment. Provision of information should always be appropriate to the developmental age of the child. Children can be divided by age groups:

Neonates	First 28 days of life
Infants	First year
Preschool children	1–4 years
School children	5–16 years
Adolescents	13–16 years

Establishing rapport and gaining the parent's trust facilitates the relationship with the child. First impressions are important. Your attitude, demeanor and dress will influence the doctor–parent/patient relationship from the outset and it is important to be neat, clean and polite. On the other hand, take time to note the attitude, demeanor and dress of your patient. These nonverbal clues can be very valuable and often will add information to the history.

Ensure that the consultation will be quiet and private. This may be difficult in the hospital setting where medical students and nursing staff may be present. Consider the patient's dignity and privacy in all circumstances. Always introduce yourself and any other staff present. Ensure your hands and nails are clean and that you wash your hands before and after examining the child. Avoid having a desk between you and the family. Make eye contact and avoid scribbling in notes or typing on a keyboard while you or the parent is talking.

TIPS FOR COMMUNICATING WITH CHILDREN

- Make the area safe and welcoming.
- Be friendly and smile.
- Be confident but gentle; warm hands and equipment help!
- Get down to their eye level and call them by their name.
- Distract, captivate and reward.
- Offer praise for cooperation.
- Talk about popular characters such as Thomas the Tank Engine, Postman Pat.
- Let them play with any equipment, if it is safe to do so.
- Mock examinations may allay fear, e.g. auscultating a teddy.
- Address questions to the child when appropriate and listen to all verbal offerings.
- Use language that they will understand.
- Older children appreciate being part of the discussion about what is wrong and how to make it better.
- Avoid the surprise factor – always explain what you are going to do in advance, but avoid *asking* young children to cooperate, they will often refuse! It may be better to tell them what is required of them.
- Have a small space or area with a chair and some toys or books.
- Be opportunistic, abandon structured examination techniques, and do what you can when you can.
- Leave unpleasant procedures to the end.
- Be sensitive to their modesty; let parents undress their child.

Infants and very young children will often be held on their parent's lap. No attempt should be made to remove them from that place of safety unless examination is required that necessitates it. In such a case the parent should place the child on the bed but remain beside them. Older pre-school children can be examined while at play with the parent nearby.

Children of an older age appreciate being asked about their health and concerns and they should be involved in any questioning, discussion of diagnosis, and plan of management. Some may be shy about answering questions but should be encouraged to take part in the process.

Adolescents may prefer to be interviewed without their parents and this should be respected. They should be aware that the content of the consultation will remain confidential. If information is required from their parent this should be made clear. Girls should be examined by a male doctor in the presence of their mother or a chaperone.

Remember that mothers are excellent observers of their own children and they will often surprise with their intuition. They will often have their own ideas as to what is the matter. Remember to get a mother to define the language she uses: 'constipation' to her may be passing a single hard stool, 'hyperactive' to one mother may be another's normal boisterous toddler.

CULTURAL AND RELIGIOUS CONSIDERATIONS

The cultural aspects of history taking and examination are become increasingly important. Where previously families lived in large supportive communities, the family of modern society is a small unit of parents and their children, often with little input or contact from extended family. Furthermore, increasing rates of marital breakdown mean that many children are now brought up by a single parent or care is shared by parents who live apart. In the UK, one quarter of children are brought up in lone-parent households.[3] Many children live between two homes. Owing to changes in working patterns, children are more likely to attend childcare facilities than previously. Social isolation with little contact from neighbors or relatives is common. Social inequalities in health persist even in resource rich countries, where child poverty is not unusual.

Classical pediatric morbidities such as infectious diseases and infant mortality have given way to the modern morbidities of learning disabilities, family dysfunction and emotional disorders. One in ten British children have a clinically diagnosed mental health disorder, including conduct, emotional and hyperkinetic disorders.[4] As many children respond to stress with a variety of somatic, psychological and behavioral strategies, today's pediatrician must have an appreciation of the interplay of family dynamics and social stresses on health.

The world has become smaller as travel and migration have increased. Children come from more diverse ethnic, religious and multicultural backgrounds than ever before and will present with unfamiliar medical and social problems as well as traditional conditions. To succeed in the role of pediatrician, an understanding of the complexities of such a culturally diverse society must be learned.

In the UK, around 8% of our society is from ethnic minorities, many having been born in this country. Visitors from the continent and immigrants from further afield are common and many will experience the new culture as unsympathetic and cold. Religious and cultural differences may influence the approach to illness and management. Expression of pain and grief vary considerably across cultures. Beliefs about death and what happens after death may be very different to one's own philosophy and this should be understood and accepted. Be sensitive of cultural differences to hand-shaking, hand gestures and eye contact. There may be very diverse approaches to infant feeding among different ethnic groups. Not only may racial differences influence a patient's approach to disease but race-specific diseases also need to be considered in the diagnosis (Table 8.2). Similarly there are ethnic variations in birthweight, growth and in neurodevelopment with black children frequently having more advanced motor skills than other racial groups. Screening and immunization requirements may also differ.

There may be considerable communication difficulties in the face of limited English.

Where a parent does not speak your language or is deaf or has communication difficulties, it is important to establish optimal communication. This may mean finding an interpreter, someone who can sign or a friend or relative who is used to communicating with this individual. In some cultures female emancipation lags behind that of Western society and a woman may commonly depend on her husband or male family member to translate for her. Remember that in order to protect her they may decide to hold back important details from her. Always document the name of the translator and their relationship to the parent.

The traditional doctor–patient relationship is now regarded as overly paternalistic and inhibiting. Most parents now want to take an active part in decisions about their child's health. Many will have researched what they believe is the problem before the consultation. The explosion of the World Wide Web has allowed people open access to a wide range of information. Media coverage of many health matters means that people are more knowledgeable about their health and their rights as a patient. Increasing numbers of parents seek alternative or complementary therapies for their child seeing such approaches as 'kinder', 'less toxic' and more holistic. It is acknowledged that few such parents will discuss with their doctor their use of such therapies.[5]

CONFIDENTIALITY

Doctors have a duty of confidentiality to all patients including children. Health professionals must decide for themselves when they feel a child shows sufficient maturity to take responsibilities for decisions regarding themselves ('competency'). Details of the child's health can only be shared with individuals who are involved in that child's care. Disclosure to other individuals such as researchers, insurance companies and lawyers requires fully informed, written consent. It is only justified to disclose information without consent if it is thought a child may suffer through nondisclosure. In such cases the parent should be informed of the pending disclosure prior to this decision. The confidentiality of older 'competent' children, incurs the same respect. Adolescents often underutilize health care resources because of concern about confidentiality yet effective care at this age can help to preserve good health, development and future opportunities. Sensitive issues such as substance abuse and sexually transmitted diseases are more easily discussed with parents absent. It may be important to encourage the young person to involve their parents if it is in their best interests to do so. They must also be aware of circumstances that may require disclosure of confidential information, such as a life-threatening emergency. The General Medical Council has produced Standards of Practice on Patient Confidentiality, and the American Academy of Pediatrics has a policy statement on Confidentiality in Adolescent Health Care, both available on respective web sites (*www.gmc-uk.org* and *www.aap.org*).

PRIVACY AND CHAPERONES

Consideration of privacy at all ages is important. Always explain to a child that you are going to look at them and touch them and ask permission from all but the smallest of children for examination. Many children find even a cursory examination scary, especially with the appearance of stethoscopes and other equipment and it is important to gain their trust during the interview.

If any part of the exam will be painful or uncomfortable, this should be explained beforehand. The doctor must be sensitive to the patient's feelings about examination of the genital, breast or anal area and remember that even young children may feel embarrassed about undressing in front of a stranger. It is seldom necessary to completely undress children older than 1 year. Selective undressing of the upper or lower half of the body as examination proceeds is a more sensitive approach. If the mother is not present it may be appropriate to ask for a chaperone to be present during the examination. A chaperone protects the interests of both the patient and the pediatrician but their presence may be awkward if the parent or patient has requested confidentiality.

DOCUMENTATION

Documentation of the consultation, the diagnosis and plan of management make up a written record of the patient's medical condition to be shared by all who are responsible for the care of the patient. Notes therefore must be legible, accurate and clearly dated and signed. Under the Freedom of Information Act 2000,[6] parents are allowed free access to their child's notes and as such the record should be free of disparaging or judgmental remarks and hearsay. The legislation also gives parents the right to check for any errors in the record and insist that amendments be made if required. Similarly the notes are a legal record and may be used subsequently in a court of law. Avoid abbreviations unless they are in common usage and unambiguous. The extent of rashes, injuries and tenderness may be best documented in a diagram.

In the UK medical records belong to the NHS Department of Health and in children they are kept for a minimum of 25 years.

Table 8.2 Diseases commoner to particular ethnic groups

Ethnic groups	Diseases
African	Sickle cell disease, glucose-6-phosphate dehydrogenase deficiency, tuberculosis, HIV
Amish	Ellis–van Creveld syndrome
Ashkenazi Jews	Gaucher disease, Tay–Sachs disease, breast and ovarian cancers, other autosomal recessive diseases
Asian Indians	Tuberculosis, autosomal recessive diseases
Chinese	Nasopharyngeal carcinoma, glucose-6-phosphate dehydrogenase deficiency
Hopi Indians	Oculocutaneous albinism
Mediterranean	Thalassemia, glucose-6-phosphate dehydrogenase deficiency
Yupik Eskimos	Congenital adrenal hyperplasia

Most patient records are shared by members of the multidisciplinary team, facilitating communication, avoiding duplication and encouraging a shared approach to patient care. Parent-held records are used in the UK until the age of 5 years, as a method of sharing communication between health professionals and parents. These also record developmental milestones and provide parents with substantial health advice.

Structured proformas for history taking and examination are used in some hospital settings where there is high patient volume and need for repeated screening procedures. Although these aids may facilitate rapid and thorough information gathering, there is a risk of careless ticking of boxes and under-documentation of free text that may compromise an objective and thoughtful approach to the history-taking.

CLINICAL HISTORY

Before taking the history, the clinician should ensure that they read any appropriate referral letters and look through any available records. The history should be recorded clearly in the patient's notes with the date and time of consultation. The signature and printed name of the clinician should follow this record. Although history and examination are usually recorded freehand, many hospitals use proformas for admissions or clinic attendances to ensure optimal information is recorded. Recent introduction of computerized patient records have allowed more readable records and have many advantages such as easy retrieval of standardized information, but the process of entering information on a keyboard may interfere with the interview ambience. An open style of questioning invites the parent to talk whereas closed questions seek specific information that may add clarification to the history. As direct questioning allows the parent little scope for qualification, care must be taken that this type of questioning does not result in a biased response. A combination of both styles will be used during the history taking. Listen without interruption to the parents' concerns and encourage them to talk through looking interested and making encouraging comments. Direct your questioning to the child if he is old enough.

Throughout the clinical history, the examination is already taking place through careful observation of the child, his play and his interaction with family members. A quick evaluation of his level of wellness will determine the need for immediate resuscitation. Although most medical students learn to take a history and examination through a structured approach, this is not always possible or necessary in children, to whom a problem-based approach is more appropriate, focussing on the relevant aspects of the history (Table 8.3).

PRESENTING COMPLAINT

Document the child's name, age, sex and date of birth.

Find out the reason for presentation, 'the problem'. The complaint will direct a line of questioning specific to that symptom, in order to amplify and clarify the problem (Table 8.4). Ask the parents to describe the complaint, in their own words and at their own pace. Find out how long it has been present and how it started. Was there a precipitating factor? Does anything make it better? Does anything make it worse? What made them come to a doctor? What do they think the problem is? When a full picture of the presenting complaint has been obtained, the doctor will have a likely or differential diagnosis on which to direct the rest of the history taking and examination. A full systems review is not usually necessary and a selective approach may be more appropriate.

PAST MEDICAL HISTORY

Obtain details of the child's birth and any antenatal or postnatal complications. Birthweight and gestation may be relevant. In children under the age of 2 who were born prematurely, chronological age in relation to gestation should be recorded.

Ask about general health and any chronic illnesses. Ask about any injuries or accidents. Find out whether there have been any previous presentations to the family doctor, any hospital admissions or attendance at specialist clinics. Ask about previous infectious diseases such as chicken pox, measles, pertussis or mumps and recent exposure to such diseases.

FEEDING AND GROWTH

Find out what the child's general appetite is like and what kind of diet they have. Many parents who think their child has a balanced diet are unaware of what that means. In infants, ensure milk intake is adequate. In breast-fed infants, know the signs of a good milk supply and intake. In formula-fed infants, ensure parents know how to make up the feed correctly. Find out whether there are any difficulties with feeding such as choking or vomiting after a feed. Ask about bowel habit and in particular any change in bowel habit.

If there are concerns about a child's growth, ask to see any previous records the parents may have for comparison. Growth is detailed in Chapter 15.

DEVELOPMENTAL HISTORY

Knowledge of the normal developmental milestones is important if a delay or arrest of development is suspected. Normal development is detailed in Chapter 7. Ask the age at which of the major milestones (smiling, sitting alone, walking, talking, toilet-training) were achieved. Remember however that recall may be poor and unreliable.[7] Previous examination notes or the child health surveillance record may be useful. All areas of development should be covered including gross and fine motor development, speech and language, cognitive development, hearing and vision. Ask whether there are any developmental concerns.

SOCIAL, SCHOOL AND FAMILY HISTORY

The social history is a chronicle of human interactions and describes the relationship of the child with his family, environment and school. The child should not be seen in isolation from his or her family and extended social environment. Illness in the child can cause anxiety or depression, and may impact on family dynamics or ability to attend or function optimally at school. In children, worries about unfavorable home or school circumstances can translate into psychosomatic symptoms (Table 8.5). Importantly some problems present due to a change in the family's ability to cope: examples include mental health problems, physical illness or changes in social circumstances.

Take details about the other members of the family and the child's relationship to them. Find out if the parents are living together and if not, whether the patient has contact with the absent parent. Ask the occupation of the parents. Note the ages of parents and siblings and the presence of any current illness or inherited conditions. Construction of a family tree (a genogram) may be helpful and easily interpreted when a stan-

Table 8.3 Taking a pediatric history

Name, age, sex, date of birth
Presenting complaint: what symptoms, when and for how long, precipitating and relieving factors, treatment already given/advice already sought
Past medical history: perinatal (pregnancy, birth and neonatal problems), accidents, operations, surgery, hospital visits, infectious diseases and contacts
Feeding and growth: appetite, diet, growth
Developmental history: gross and fine motor, speech and language, cognitive, hearing, vision
Social, school and family: parents, carers, siblings, family history of disease, housing, school progress, friends, hobbies, sleeping pattern, foreign travel
Drug history: dosages, frequency, allergies
Immunizations
Summary: 'Is there anything else you would like to tell me?'

Table 8.4 Clinical history points and relevant amplification

System	Symptom	Amplification
General	Pyrexia and night sweats	Duration, method of ascertaining temperature, rigors, sheet changing
	Weight loss	Amount, method of weighing, duration, other symptoms
	Rashes	Site, size, number of lesions, color, nature (petechiae, purpura, macules, papules, pustules, vesicles, bullae, ulcers), associated pain or pruritus
	Cyanosis	Peripheral or central, intermittent or persistent, association with environmental temperature
	Pain	Onset, nature, duration, severity, precipitating factors, relieving factors, associated symptoms, treatment sought
Respiratory	Discharge from nose, eyes or ears	Nature and duration
	Sore throat or earache	Localization, associated pyrexia or other respiratory symptoms
	Cough	Character, duration, exacerbating factors, sleep disturbance, association with pain, whoop, vomiting, other respiratory symptoms, nature of sputum
	Stridor	Associated color change or apnea
	Wheeze	Precipitating or exacerbating factors, diurnal variation, home peak flow testing
	Snoring	Change in cry or voice, mouth breathing
	Dyspnea	At rest or with exercise, intermittent or persistent, nocturnal or diurnal, association with cough, cyanosis or breath-holding
	Apnea	Duration, association with infection or airway obstruction
Cardiovascular	Breathlessness	At rest, or exertion or with feeding
	Tiredness and lethargy	Exercise tolerance, interest in play
	Slow feeding	Associated breathlessness
	Poor weight gain	Dietary intake
	Pallor or cyanosis	Intermittent or persistent, associated with crying or straining
Gastrointestinal	Appetite and feed tolerance need for special diet	Temporary or persistent impairment, food faddism, parental attitudes towards diet, vitamin or other supplementation
	Dysphagia	Often functional food refusal rather than organic, in organic dysphagia food is swallowed but soon regurgitated
	Thirst	Assess total daily intake of fluid and output of urine
	Vomiting	Amount, frequency, association with feeds, effortless or projectile, bilious or bloodstained, association with pain or impairment of consciousness
	Constipation	Consistency, frequency, pain on defecation
	Diarrhea	Nature of stool, consistency, frequency, presence of blood
	Abdominal pain	Site, nature, timing, duration, intermittent or constant, aggravation by breathing or movement, relationship of feeds, bowel movements or micturition, association with other gastrointestinal symptoms, sore throat, cough or purpura
	Jaundice	Onset, duration, nature of stool and urine, associated vomiting
Genitourinary	Incontinence or bed-wetting	Day or night, deterioration from before or regression in development, associated urinary symptoms, parental reaction, stress or bullying, treatment sought or tried
	Increased urinary frequency	Recent change in pattern, urine volume
	Dysuria	Pain, burning or cry related to micturition
	Change in odor or appearance of urine	Associated urinary symptoms, hematuria
Neurodevelopmental	Headaches	Site, manner of onset, severity, associated symptoms, aura
	Visual disturbances	Fixation and following, myopia or hypermetropia, color blindness, colliding with objects, associated symptoms
	Speech	Delay in onset or regression, nature, difficult comprehension or expression
	Hearing	Unresponsiveness or inattentiveness, functional or organic, family history
	Fits, faints, floppiness	Time, duration, frequency, tonic and clonic components, state of consciousness, known triggers, associated color change, oculogyrus, choking or incontinence, injury sustained
	Abnormalities in posture, gait or coordination	Deterioration from before or regression in development, falling and injury
	Involuntary movement	Nature, aggravating factors, injury suffered as a result
	Changes in mood, activity or behavior	Performance in normal play and household activities, interest in surroundings and excursions, tiring easily
	School performance	Normal or special school, extra support, bullying

Table 8.5 Psychosomatic manifestations of stress

Somatic	Psychological
Headache	School refusal/truancy
Blurred or tunnel vision	Conduct disorders
Blackouts	Anorexia nervosa/bulimia
Tics	Sleep disorders, e.g. sleep-walking
Abdominal pain or infantile	Attention deficit/hyperactivity disorder
colic	Anxiety and depression
Nausea and vomiting	Self-harm
Constipation	Suicide/parasuicide
Enuresis/encopresis	
Poor appetite	
Weight loss	
Cough	
Eczema	
Other pain, e.g. back, neck, throat	

Table 8.6 External factors that may impact on a child's health

Marital discord or breakdown
Parental illness or disability, including psychiatric illness
Bereavement stress
Parental absence
Unemployment
Poverty
Domestic violence
Physical, mental, emotional or sexual abuse
Parental substance abuse
Moving house
Immigration
New baby
Bullying
School stress: moving school, exams, learning difficulty

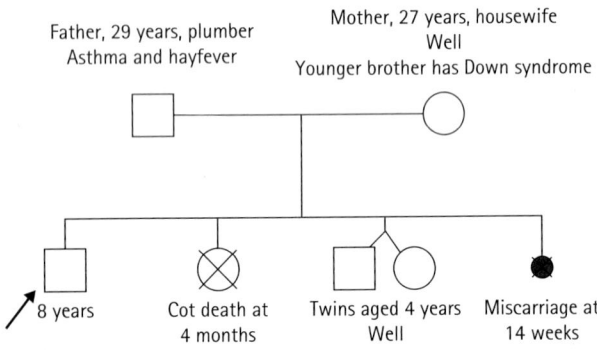

Legend:
• Squares indicate males and circles female
• The index case is marked with an arrow
• The birth order should be set out from left to right
• A crossed out symbol indicates a death
• Spouses are connected with lines, separations and divorces indicated by slash lines running through the lines
• Birth, marriage, divorce, or death dates may be indicated by the initial and date (e.g. b.89)

Fig. 8.1 Example of a genogram.

Table 8.7 Current immunization schedule for children living in the UK[11]

Age at immunization	Diseases protected against
2 months	Diphtheria, tetanus, pertussis, polio and *Haemophilus influenza* type B Pneumococcus
3 months	Diphtheria, tetanus, pertussis, polio and *Haemophilus influenza* type B Meningitis C
4 months	Diphtheria, tetanus, pertussis, polio and *Haemophilus influenza* type B Meningitis C Pneumococcus
Around 12 months	*Haemophilus influenza* type B and meningitis C
Around 13 months	Measles, mumps and rubella
3 years 4 months– 5 years	Diphtheria, tetanus, pertussis, polio Measles, mumps and rubella
13–18 years	Diphtheria, tetanus and polio

dardized version is used (Fig. 8.1).[8] It may be relevant to find out whether the parents are consanguineous. Find out what impact the child's illness may have had on the family. Ask who looks after the child normally.

Check that the housing is adequate and whether there are any smokers and/or pets in the household.

Ask the name of the school and the class teacher. Ask whether the child is performing at his expected level and about school absences. It may be relevant to seek permission from the parents to obtain information from the class teacher about educational progress or behavioral difficulties.

Find out whether there have been any significant events in the child's life recently (Table 8.6). Ask about friends and whether the child attends any clubs or has any hobbies. Ascertain that the child gets adequate exercise through the week. Ask about sleep routine and behavior. A history of recent foreign travel may be relevant.

It may be appropriate in an adolescent patient to ask about lifestyle issues such as sexual history, smoking and use of recreational drugs. Remember that most will prefer that their parents are not present. Over 25% of adolescents will have had sexual intercourse before their 16th birthday. According to the 2000/2001 General Household Survey, 23% of British adolescents aged 11–15 admitted to having had an alcoholic drink in the previous week and such young people have doubled their average intake in the last decade.[9] As many as 15% of British children aged 11–15 years will have used illicit drugs in the last year and around 10% will smoke cigarettes regularly.[10]

DRUG HISTORY

Ask whether the child has been prescribed any medications or supplements and check that the child has been taking them as prescribed. Drug dosages and frequency of administration should be noted. Ascertain whether there are have been any reactions to medications that may have caused a rash, diarrhea or anaphylaxis. Ask about nondrug allergies.

IMMUNIZATIONS

Know the current immunization schedule (Table 8.7)[11] and ascertain that the child is immunized fully to date. There may have been additional immunizations such as BCG or hepatitis B, particularly at birth.

SUMMARY

Before examining the child, summarize the information you have received from the parent to check it is correct and ask whether there are any other concerns.

PHYSICAL EXAMINATION

Examination begins at the moment the child and family enter the room. Careful observation often reveals more than hands-on examination, as localizing signs are often absent in children.

There is no single examination technique that is appropriate to all ages and situations. Doctors should develop their own style, inclusive of patience and empathy. It is usually not appropriate to examine each individual system in all children and the doctor should be guided by the clinical history and his initial observations. However for the purpose of this chapter, individual systems will be detailed. Tables 8.8 and 8.9 provide possible interpretations for some common physical signs. Landmarks for a child's chest are shown in Figure 8.2.

GENERAL ASSESSMENT

- Inspect the child and observe whether the child is well or ill and whether he is in pain or comfortable.

- Observe behavior, demeanor and the interaction of the child with other family members. Is the child well cared for?
- Observe for signs of hydration and state of alertness.
- Look for signs that the child is well-nourished and appropriately grown for age.

GROWTH

Growth parameters should be plotted on centile charts appropriate for the sex and age of the child. Use the most up-to-date charts available that will be most representative of the current population. In the UK, these are the UK90 growth charts, constructed from cross-sectional measurements of seven UK cohorts measured in 1990.[12,13] There are

Table 8.8 Common physical signs and their possible causes

System	Sign	Possible causes
Skin	Albinism	Inherited, Chediak–Higashi syndrome
	Alopecia	Stress, protein deficiency, iron or zinc deficiency, hypopituitarism, rapid weight loss, SLE, hypothyroidism, thyrotoxicosis, diabetes mellitus, renal failure, drugs
	Bruising	Hemophilia, non-accidental injury, leukemia, ITP, liver failure, scurvy, Cushing syndrome, drugs
	Butterfly rash	SLE, photodermatitis
	Café-au-lait spots	Neurofibromatosis, tuberous sclerosis
	Cyanosis	Congenital cyanotic heart disease, persistent pulmonary hypertension, cardiovascular collapse, respiratory failure
	Depigmentation	Pityriasis versicolor or alba, vitiligo, postinflammatory, hypopituitarism, leprosy
	Dermographism	Allergy or hypersensitivity
	Herald patch	Pityriasis rosea, drugs
	Hirsutism	Congenital adrenal hyperplasia, pituitary–gonadal tumors, hypothyroidism, steroid therapy, Albright syndrome, mucopolysaccharidoses
	Lymphadenopathy	Infection, chronic inflammation, lymphoma, metastases
	Petechiae/purpura	Meningococcal septicemia, ITP, vasculitis, leukemia, DIC, Henoch–Schönlein purpura, Waterhouse–Friderichsen syndrome, Cushing syndrome, congenital infection, neonatal alloimmune thrombocytopenia, hemorrhagic disease of the newborn, infective endocarditis, trauma, drugs
	Scaly rash	Seborrheic dermatitis, pityriasis rosea, psoriasis
	Spider nevi/telangiectasia	Liver cirrhosis, thyrotoxicosis, systemic sclerosis, hepatitis, ataxia telangiectasia
	Striae	Cushing syndrome or disease
	Subcutaneous nodules	Neurofibromatosis, tuberous sclerosis, rheumatic fever, sarcoid
	Target lesions	Erythema multiforme, Stevens–Johnson syndrome
	Tissue crepitations	Subcutaneous emphysema
	Vesicles	Herpes zoster, herpes simplex, impetigo, contact dermatitis, pemphigus, pemphigoid, incontinentia pigmenti, epidermolysis bullosa, burns, drugs
	White forelock	Waardenburg syndrome
	Xanthoma	Hyperlipidemia, diabetes, cholestasis
	Xeroderma	Ichthyosis, hypothyroidism, seborrheic dermatitis, eczema, psoriasis
Head	Microcephaly	Congenital infection, chromosomal abnormality, perinatal asphyxia
	Macrocephaly	Hydrocephalus, achondroplasia, gigantism, mucopolysaccharidoses, familial megalencephaly
	Acrocephaly	Apert and Crouzon syndromes
	Brachycephaly	Positional, Down syndrome
	Dolichocephaly	Ex-preterm infant
	Plagiocephaly	Positional, coronal suture craniosynostosis
	Scaphocephaly	Sagittal suture craniosynostosis
	Prominent occiput	Edward syndrome, Beckwith–Wiedemann syndrome
	Frontal bossing	Rickets, chondrodysplasia, storage diseases
	Craniotabes	Rickets, prematurity
	Scalp defects	Patau syndrome
	Bulging fontanelle	Raised intracranial pressure, meningitis
	Sunken fontanelle	Dehydration
	Delayed fontanelle closure	Rickets, hypothyroidism, hydrocephalus, chondrodysplasias and chondrodysgeneses, other chromosomal abnormality
Face and neck	Moon face	Cushing syndrome or disease, Prader–Willi syndrome
	Triangular face	Russell–Silver syndrome, osteogenesis imperfecta, Turner syndrome
	Coarse face	Hypothyroidism, mucopolysaccharidoses
	Micrognathia	Familial, Pierre-Robin sequence, other chromosomal abnormalities

(Continued)

Table 8.8   Common physical signs and their possible causes—cont'd

System	Sign	Possible causes
	Torticollis	Sternomastoid tumor, corpus striatum or labyrinthine disease, 11th cranial nerve palsy
	Neck webbing	Turner syndrome, Noonan syndrome
	Saddle nose	Down syndrome, chondrodysplasias, fetal teratogenicity
Eyes	Aniridia	Aniridia–Wilms tumor association
	Blue sclera	Osteogenesis imperfecta
	Buphthalmos	Congenital glaucoma
	Cataract	Congenital infection, Down syndrome, galactosemia, Alport syndrome, diabetes mellitus, malnutrition, trauma, ocular tumors, retrolental fibroplasia
	Chorioretinitis	Congenital cytomegalovirus infection
	Choroidal tubercles	Tuberous sclerosis
	Coloboma of eyelid	Treacher–Collins and Goldenhar syndromes
	Coloboma of iris	Idiopathic, CHARGE syndrome, Patau syndrome
	Corneal clouding	Hurler syndrome, other mucopolysaccharidoses
	Enophthalmos	Dehydration, malnutrition, Horner syndrome
	Exophthalmos	Thyrotoxicosis, cerebral, optic or orbital tumor, neurofibromatosis, malignant hypertension, Apert and Crouzon syndromes, Cushing disease
	Epicanthic folds	Down syndrome, other chromosomal abnormalities
	Hypertelorism	Various chromosomal abnormalities
	Hypotelorism	Holoprosencephaly syndrome, Patau syndrome
	Lens dislocation	Marfan syndrome, homocystinuria
	Lid retraction	Thyrotoxicosis
	Miosis	Bright light, convergence, narcotics, sympathetic nerve paralysis, Horner syndrome, drugs
	Mydriasis	Darkness, thyrotoxicosis, anxiety, iritis, inflammatory adhesions, coma, drugs
	Nystagmus	Normal in some infants and with watching moving object, labyrinthine and vestibular disease, brainstem lesions, central vision loss, septo-optic dysplasia, Friedreich's ataxia
	Optic atrophy	Glaucoma, retinal ischemia, optic neuritis, retinitis pigmentosa
	Papilledema	Raised intracranial pressure, optic neuritis, hypertension
	Periorbital edema	Nephrotic syndrome
	Ptosis	Bell's palsy, Horner syndrome, myasthenia gravis, 3rd cranial nerve palsy, congenital
	Raccoon sign	Basal skull fracture
	Retinal hemorrhages	Non-accidental injury, trauma, leukemia, hypertension, bacterial endocarditis, bleeding diathesis
	Retinal pigmentation	Congenital infection, mucopolysaccharidoses, Laurence–Moon–Biedl syndrome
	Strabismus	Intermittent normal in neonates, fixed due to birth trauma, raised intracranial pressure, 3rd, 4th or 6th cranial nerve palsy, severe miosis, chromosomal abnormality
	Sunsetting	Hydrocephalus
	Xanthelasma	Hyperlipidemia, cholestasis
Ears	Low-set ears	Branchial developmental abnormalities, various chromosomal abnormalities
	Malformed auricles	Various chromosomal abnormalities
	Deafness	Familial, congenital infection, postmeningitis, branchial developmental abnormalities, other metabolic and chromosomal abnormalities
	Pre-auricular tags or pits	Beckwith–Wiedemann syndrome, Treacher–Collins syndrome, may be associated with deafness
	Earlobe crease	Beckwith–Wiedemann syndrome
Mouth	Xerostomia	Anxiety, pyrexia, dehydration, diabetes mellitus and insipidus, cystic fibrosis, drugs
	Risus sardonicus	Tetanus
	Stomatitis	Iron deficiency, herpes simplex, Stevens–Johnson syndrome, Kawasaki disease
	Cleft lip/palate	Idiopathic, Pierre Robin syndrome, Patau syndrome, fetal teratogenicity
	Smooth philtrum	Fetal alcohol syndrome
	Blue gums	Lead poisoning
	Gum hypertrophy	Chronic phenytoin administration
	Glossoptosis	Down syndrome
	Macroglossia	Hypothyroidism, Beckwith–Wiedemann syndrome, mucopolysaccharidoses, other storage diseases
	Strawberry tongue	Scarlet fever, vitamin B deficiency
	White tongue	Milk, thrush, leukoplakia
	Anodontia/hypodontia	Osteochondrodysplasias, ectodermal dysplasia, Down syndrome
	Enamel hypoplasia	Tuberous sclerosis, Williams syndrome, Prader–Willi syndrome
Cardiovascular	Tachycardia	Exercise, pain, hypovolemia, infection, thyrotoxicosis, cardiac failure, anaphylaxis, pheochromocytoma, drugs
	Bradycardia	Hypothyroidism, heart block, raised intracranial pressure, hypothermia, cardiac failure, drugs
	Hypertension	Anxiety, renal disease, pheochromocytoma, aortic coarctation, raised intracranial pressure, Conn and Cushing syndromes, SLE, drugs
	Hypotension	Cardiac failure, hypovolemia, cardiogenic or septic shock, anaphylaxis, Addison's disease, electrolyte imbalance, hypothyroidism, drugs

(Continued)

Table 8.8   Common physical signs and their possible causes—cont'd

System	Sign	Possible causes
	Atrial fibrillation	Wolff–Parkinson–White syndrome, thyrotoxicosis, rheumatic valve disease, carditis
	Bounding pulse	Pyrexia, thyrotoxicosis, anemia, hypercarbia
	Collapsing pulse	Aortic regurgitation, PDA, VSD, heart block, thyrotoxicosis, hyperdynamic circulation
	Plateau pulse	Aortic stenosis, aortic coarctation
	Pulsus paradoxus	Severe asthma, pericardial effusion or tamponade, constrictive pericarditis
	Gallop rhythm	Left ventricular failure, cardiac dilatation, constrictive pericarditis
	Systolic murmur	Physiological, VSD, PDA, ASD, pulmonary stenosis, aortic coarctation, aortic stenosis, hyperdynamic circulation, mitral regurgitation, tricuspid regurgitation, cardiomyopathy
	Diastolic murmur	Venous hum, PDA, large VSD, mitral stenosis, aortic regurgitation, pulmonary regurgitation, tricuspid stenosis
	Thrill	Palpable murmur
	Pericardial rub	Pericarditis, rheumatic fever, pleurisy, pneumonia
	Bruits	Artery stenosis, arteriovenous malformation
	Thrust/heave	Apical – left ventricular hypertrophy, lower left sternal edge – right ventricular hypertrophy
Respiratory	Barrel chest	Emphysema, asthma
	Pectus carinatum	Asthma, rickets, chromosomal or metabolic abnormalities
	Pectus excavatum	Asthma, rickets, chromosomal or metabolic abnormalities
	Thoracic rosary	Rickets
	Barking cough	Croup
	Hemoptysis	Airway trauma, foreign body inhalation, infection, malignancy, arteriovenous malformation, bleeding diathesis
	Stridor	Croup, epiglottitis, laryngitis, laryngomalacia, infectious mononucleosis, diphtheria, subglottic hemangioma or cyst
	Wheeze	Asthma, bronchitis
	Bronchial breathing	Normal in young children, pneumonia
	Coarse crepitations	Bronchiolitis, bronchiectasis
	Fine crepitations	Pulmonary edema, atelectasis, pneumonia
	Pleural rub	Pleurisy, pneumonia, pulmonary thrombosis
	Hyperventilation	Anxiety, pain, pyrexia, metabolic acidosis, infection, hypoxia, drugs, Rett syndrome
	Hypoventilation	Raised intracranial pressure, drugs, lung disease
Gastrointestinal	Abdominal distension	Intestinal obstruction, ileus, peritonitis, ascites, masses, pregnancy, organomegaly
	Scaphoid abdomen	Congenital diaphragmatic hernia
	Abdominal mass	Organomegaly, tumor, fluid, hernia, cyst, abscess, pregnancy
	Hernias	Ex-preterm infant, hypothyroidism, Beckwith–Wiedemann syndrome, mucopolysaccharidoses
	Omphalocele	Idiopathic, Beckwith–Wiedemann syndrome, Patau syndrome, Edward syndrome
	Hepatomegaly	Congestive cardiac failure, any cause of infectious hepatitis, metabolic or liver storage disease, malignancy
	Splenomegaly	Infectious mononucleosis, infective endocarditis, portal hypertension, leukemia, lymphoma, hemolytic anemia, malaria
	Abdominal rigidity	Peritonitis
	Rebound tenderness	Peritonitis
	Visible peristalsis	Pyloric stenosis, acute intestinal obstruction
	Shifting dullness	Ascites
	Fluid thrill	Ascites
	Borborygmi	Intestinal obstruction, toxic enteritis
	Pale stool	Pancreatic insufficiency, bile duct obstruction
	Melena	Upper intestinal bleeding, iron therapy
	Green stool	Intestinal hurry, starvation
	Anal defects	VATER association, caudal regression sequence
Nervous	Hypertonia	Upper motor neurone lesions, extrapyramidal lesions, asphyxia, kernicterus, raised intracranial pressure, meningitis, cerebral palsy
	Hypotonia	Lower motor neurone lesions, prematurity, cerebellar lesions, myopathies, metabolic and chromosomal abnormalities
	Clasp-knife rigidity	Upper motor neurone lesion
	Cog-wheel rigidity	Extrapyramidal lesions, cerebral palsy
	Neck stiffness	Meningeal irritation
	Opisthotonus	Meningitis, cerebellar lesions, tetanus
	Myoclonus	Upper motor neurone lesions
	Brisk tendon reflexes	Upper motor neurone lesions, thyrotoxicosis, anxiety, tetanus
	Diminished tendon reflexes	Peripheral neuropathies, hypothyroidism, syringomyelia, lower motor neurone lesions
	Muscle fasciculation	Lower motor neurone lesions, muscular dystrophies, hypocalcemia, thyrotoxicosis, depolarizing drugs

(Continued)

Table 8.8 Common physical signs and their possible causes—cont'd

System	Sign	Possible causes
	Athetosis	Kernicterus, juvenile Huntington's chorea, Wilson's disease, Lesch–Nyhan syndrome, basal ganglia or extrapyramidal lesions, drugs
	Chorea	Ataxia-telangiectasia, Angelman syndrome, Cockayne syndrome, cerebellar or brainstem lesions, drugs (including alcohol and antiepileptics), vestibular neuronitis
	Intention tremor	Cerebellar or brainstem lesions, Friedreich's ataxia, mercury poisoning
	Postural tremor	Anxiety, thyrotoxicosis, alcohol, Wilson's disease, cerebellar lesions, drugs
	Dysdiadochokinesia	Cerebellar lesions
	Asterixis	Encephalopathy, liver failure, metabolic disease
	Meningomyelocele	Maternal folate deficiency, fetal teratogenicity, chromosomal abnormality
	Encephalocele	Meckel–Gruber syndrome
Locomotor	Scoliosis	Congenital vertebral anomaly, developmental abnormality, disc prolapse, Marfan syndrome, Coffin–Lowry syndrome
	Buffalo hump	Cushing disease, steroid therapy
	Short limbs	Chondrodysplasias, osteogenesis imperfecta, fetal varicella syndrome
	Cubitus valgus	Turner syndrome
	Fixed flexion deformities	Arthrogryposis multiplex congenita usually due to oligohydramnios sequence
	Joint erythema	Septic arthritis, inflammatory arthropathy, rheumatic fever
	Joint hypermobility	Familial, enthesopathy, Marfan syndrome, Ehlers–Danlos syndrome, acromegaly
	Myotonia	Myotonic dystrophy, hyperkalemia
	Muscular atrophy	Lower motor neurone lesions, muscular dystrophies, prolonged immobilization
	Muscular hypertrophy	Duchenne's muscular dystrophy
Hands and feet	Finger or toe clubbing	Chronic cardiac, respiratory or gastrointestinal disease, congenital cyanotic heart disease, tumors, suppurative disease
	Koilonychia	Iron deficiency anemia
	Nail pitting	Eczema, psoriasis, chronic paronychia, alopecia areata
	Thickened nail	Psoriasis, chronic paronychia or fungal infection, lichen planus
	Onycholysis	Trauma, fungal infections, eczema, psoriasis, diabetes, drugs
	Splinter hemorrhages	Infective endocarditis, blood dyscrasias, eczema, psoriasis, trauma
	Arachnodactyly	Marfan syndrome
	Brachydactyly	Down syndrome, Ellis van Creveld syndrome
	Camptodactyly	Edward syndrome
	Clinodactyly	Down syndrome, other chromosomal abnormalities
	Polydactyly	Familial, Patau syndrome, other chromosomal abnormalities
	Syndactyly	Acrocephaly–syndactyly syndrome, various chromosomal abnormalities
	Thumb hypoplasia	Thrombocytopenia-absent radius syndrome, Fanconi anemia, Holt–Oram syndrome
	Single transverse palmar crease	Normal, chromosomal abnormality
	Wrist drop	Radial nerve lesion, peripheral neuropathy, muscular dystrophy
	Talipes equinovarus	Positional, oligohydramnios sequence, muscular dystrophy, chromosomal abnormality
	Pes cavus	Familial, Friedreich's ataxia, spina bifida, sacral dermoid
	Pes planus	Physiological lax ligaments, tarsal coalition, cerebral palsy, polio
	Peripheral edema	Cardiac failure, venous thrombosis, hypoproteinemia, nephrotic syndrome, renal failure, prolonged immobilization
	Carpopedal spasm	Hypocalcemia
Reproductive	Gynecomastia	Puberty, obesity, thyrotoxicosis, pituitary–adrenal–gonadal disease, liver disease, drugs
	Galactorrhea	Normal in some newborns, pituitary–adrenal tumors, hormonal therapy, thyroid disease, pregnancy and nursing
	Ambiguous genitalia	Congenital adrenal hyperplasia, hermaphroditism, Prader–Willi syndrome, other chromosomal abnormality
	Cryptorchidism	Delayed testicular descent, causes of ambiguous genitalia
	Testicular mass	Hydrocele, hernia, tumor, orchitis

ASD, atrial septal defect; CHARGE (syndrome), ocular coloboma, heart defects, atretic choanae, retarded growth or development, genital hypoplasia, and ear anomalies; DIC, disseminated intravascular coagulopathy; ITP, idiopathic thrombocytopenic purpura; PDA, patent ductus arteriosus; SLE, systemic lupus erythematosus; VATER, vertebral defects, imperforate anus, tracheo esophageal fistula, and radial and renal dysplasia; VSD, ventricular septal defect.

Table 8.9 Eponymous signs

Eponymous sign	Sign description	Possible causes
Austin Flint murmur	Murmur at apex, onset with third heart sound and loudest at mid-diastole	Aortic regurgitation
Argyll Robertson pupil	Small unequal pupils that react to convergence but not to light	Neurosyphilis, diabetes
Battle's sign	Retromastoid bruising behind ears	Petrous bone fracture
Beau's ridges	Transverse ridging of nail plate	Hypoalbuminemia, steroid therapy, cytotoxics, severe illness
Brushfield spots	Focal areas of iris stromal hyperplasia giving appearance of white spots	Down syndrome
Charcot joint	Severely disorganized, arthritic joint that is pain-free	Tabes dorsalis, diabetic neuropathy, leprosy, myelomeningocele
Cheyne–Stokes respiration	Respirations that decrease in frequency, then stop temporarily before restarting and building up again	Damage to cerebral respiratory center terminal stage
Corrigan's sign	Vigorous pulsation of major head and neck arteries causing head or ears to move	Aortic regurgitation, PDA, VSD
Cullen's sign	Spontaneous umbilical bruising	Hemoperitoneum
Dance's sign	Right iliac fossa depression in distressed infant	Intussusception
Epstein's pearls	Epithelial inclusions along midline of hard palate	Normal in neonates
Erb's palsy	Arm held adducted and internally rotated, extended at elbow, with forearm and palm pronated	C5/6/7 damage
Gottron's sign	Scaly patches over dorsal finger joints, with subungual erythema and cuticular telangiectasia	Polymyositis, dermatomyositis
Graham Steel murmur	Soft, high-pitched murmur in second left intercostal space in early diastole	Pulmonary regurgitation from pulmonary hypertension
Harrison's sulcus	Chest deformity with subcostal groove along attachment of diaphragm	Chronic asthma, rickets
Henoch–Schönlein purpura	Extensive purpuric and ecchymotic lesions on extensor surfaces of limbs	Idiopathic, post-streptococcal, drug-induced
Hoffmann's reflex	Foot dorsiflexion causes calf muscle pain	Calf thrombophlebitis or cellulitis
Jacobsen–Holdsnedt phenomenon	Mediastinum displaced away from affected side during expiration on X-ray	Unilateral obstructive emphysema, e.g. foreign body inhalation
Janeway lesion	Small purplish nodules on palms or soles	Infective endocarditis
Kayser-Fleischer ring	Green–brown ring at outer edge of cornea	Wilson's disease
Kehr's sign	Left shoulder tip pain with acute abdomen	Splenic rupture
Koplik spots	Gray spots in the mucous membranes of the mouth	Measles
Kussmaul breathing	Deep sighing respirations	Diabetic ketoacidosis, uremia, other metabolic acidosis, neurogenic hyperpnea
Murphy's sign	Pain and interruption of inhalation during palpation of right upper abdominal quadrant	Cholecystitis

PDA, patent ductus arteriosus; VSD, ventricular septal defect.

separate charts available for children with Down syndrome, Turner syndrome and sickle cell disease. Growth standards of exclusively breast-fed babies have also recently been published by the World Health Organization.[14] A single measurement of weight or height is rarely helpful. Compare current growth parameters with any previously recorded. Assess whether the growth velocity has been satisfactory.

In infants, weight should ideally be measured in electronic scales with the baby completely undressed. Older children should stand on scales and should have their shoes and outdoor clothing off. The method by which parent and child are weighed together and the parent's weight is then subtracted to get the child's weight is not reliable. Weight should be measured and recorded in kilograms.

In newborn babies, weight loss of up to 12 per cent is normal in the first 5 days of life, but birth weight should be regained by 10 days of age. Thereafter weight gain is approximately 200 g/week with birth weight doubled by 5 months and tripled by 1 year. In children, the expected weight in kg can be estimated by the formula: $2 \times$ (age in years + 4). However constitutional and ethnic variations in weight should be appreciated.

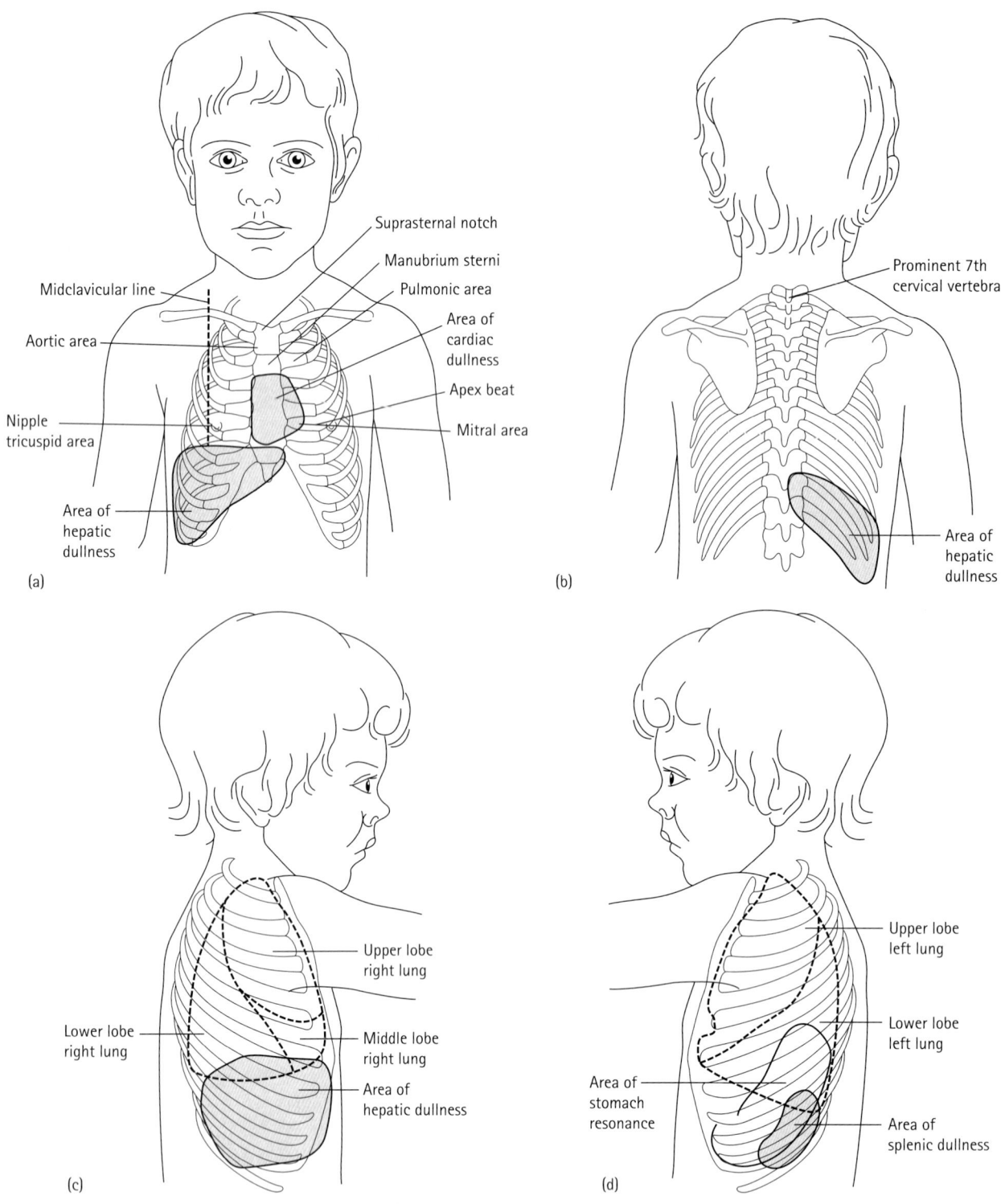

Fig. 8.2 Landmarks in a child's chest: (a) anterior, (b) posterior, (c) right lateral, (d) left lateral.

Crown–heel length is measured in infants lying supine and fully extended on a stadiometer. It should be recognized that this method of measurement is relatively inaccurate due to variation in the 'stretchiness' of a child due to stress, well-being and the time of day, with children similar to adults in being 1 cm taller on average in the morning. In children older than 1 year of age and who are able to stand, standing height should be measured with shoes off on a measuring wall ruler. Height should be measured and recorded in centimeters. At birth length is approximately 50 cm, increasing to 75 cm at 1 year of age and 100 cm by 4 years. An infant grows on average 14–16 cm/year, a pubertal child 7–12 cm/year and in the mid-childhood years, growth is around 4–6 cm/year. Height velocity charts may be useful in plotting speed of growth around puberty. Remember that body proportions change with age (Fig. 8.3).

Body mass index (BMI) or weight in relation to stature (weight[kg]/height^2[m^2]) may be a more useful measurement of body fat mass in children over 2 years.[15] Both the UK government and the American Academy of Pediatrics have recently advocated the routine monitoring

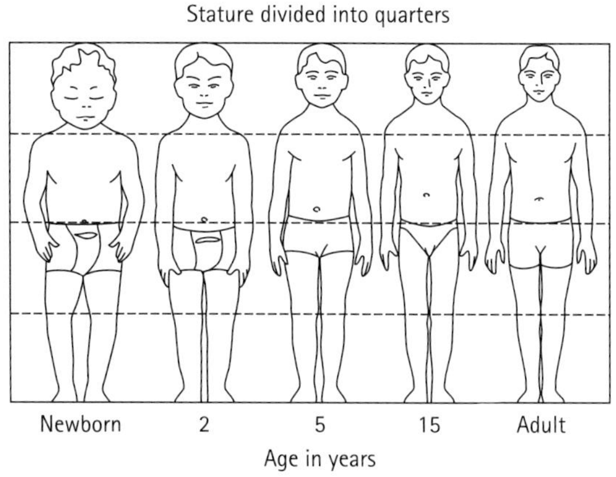

Stature divided into quarters

Newborn   2   5   15   Adult

Age in years

Fig. 8.3 Body proportions at different ages.

of BMI in schoolchildren to identify those who are, or who are at risk of, becoming obese (BMI >97th centile for age).[16,17]

Occipitofrontal circumference (OFC) is the largest circumference around the forehead and occiput. It should be measured with a disposable nonstretch tape and is measured in centimeters to the nearest millimeter. Measure it three times, and then record the largest measurement. The OFC in a term baby is approximately 35 cm, and should enlarge by 12 cm in the first 12 months of life and a further 2 cm by the second year. The subsequent annual increase is 0.5 cm from 2 to 7 years and 0.3 cm from 8 to 12 years. Centile charts are available through childhood and adulthood.

Other signs of adequacy of nutrition should be sought. Children who are failing to thrive will have loose skin folds with a lack of subcutaneous fat. Nutritional deficiencies may manifest as angular stomatitis, glossitis, skin rashes, anemia, bleeding gums, bruises or bowing of the legs. Dissociation between growth parameters may indicate underlying disease such as hypothyroidism, malnutrition, obesity or Marfan syndrome.

TEMPERATURE

Temperature can be measured at various sites (rectal, sublingual, axillary or tympanic) and with a variety of different devices (mercury thermometer, digital thermometer, tympanic infrared thermometer or color-change chemical thermometer). Rectal, sublingual and tympanic temperatures correlate with core temperature better than axillary temperature.[18–20] Axillary temperatures are accurate in neonates and are representative of sublingual or rectal temperatures, detecting pyrexia with a sensitivity of 98%.[21,22] However in older infants and children, axillary temperatures perform less well and detect pyrexia with sensitivity of only 47%.[22] One degree Celsius should be added to the axillary temperature for any child older than 1 month of age.[21] Forehead liquid crystal strips are even less accurate than axillary temperature.[21]

Tympanic membrane thermometry is a newer development that has been evaluated for use in infants, including well preterm infants.[23] Temperature should be measured in degrees Celsius. The normal core temperature should be 36.5–37.5°C.

EXAMINATION OF INDIVIDUAL SYSTEMS

MORPHOLOGY

Examine the head, face, neck, eyes, ears, mouth, hands and feet for signs of abnormal morphology (Table 8.8). Different head shapes are shown in Figure 8.4. Examine the ears for position, size and shape. A normally positioned ear should have its upper third above a horizontal line at eye level, with the helix joining the skull at a horizontal plane through both inner canthi. The presence of low-set ears may be supportive of a chromosomal anomaly, particularly when associated with other dysmorphology. The distance between the eyes can be measured in terms of innercanthal, midpupillary or outer-canthal measurements. Normograms for these and for ear length are available in textbooks of morphology.[24]

SKIN, MUCOUS MEMBRANES AND LYMPH NODES

Examine the skin for rashes, bruises, skin integrity and birthmarks. Common lesions are detailed in Table 8.8. Lesions can be documented in a diagram or by photographs where necessary.

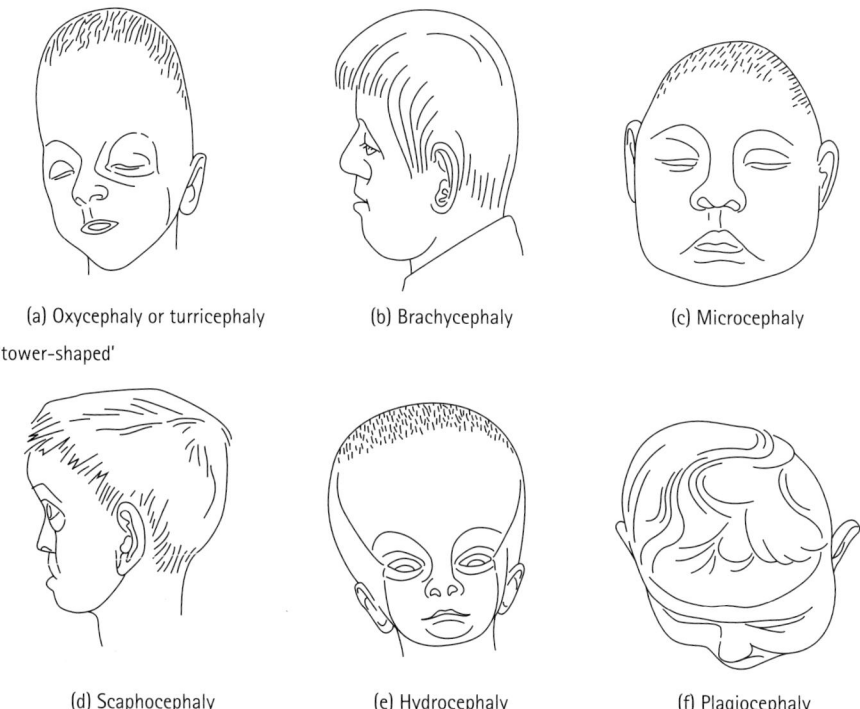

Fig. 8.4 Head shapes.

(a) Oxycephaly or turricephaly
'tower-shaped'

(b) Brachycephaly

(c) Microcephaly

(d) Scaphocephaly
'boat-shaped'

(e) Hydrocephaly

(f) Plagiocephaly

Rashes should be described in terms of color, distribution, size, nature (macules, papules, vesicles, pustules), ability to blanch under pressure, and whether it is itchy or not. Look for the presence of atopic dermatitis characterized by pruritic, erythematous papules and vesicles with serous discharge and signs of skin trauma from scratching. Seborrheic dermatitis (cradle cap) on the other hand is not itchy and the salmon-colored greasy scales characteristically affect the scalp but also commonly the face, neck, groin and axillae.

There may be jaundice or excessive pallor. Hypercarotenemia may be seen in infants who consume large amounts of carrot and squash, and can be distinguished from jaundice by the absence of orange–yellow discoloration of the sclerae. Assess the mucous membranes for central cyanosis and signs of hydration. Observe in the mouth for gum disease and dental caries.

Examine for lymphadenopathy in the neck, groin and axilla. Multiple, palpable, nontender and generally small, shotty nodes are common in children following upper respiratory infection. The size, number, and consistency of palpable lymph nodes should be documented as well as any associated erythema and tenderness. Remember to check the surrounding area for presence of any infection or inflammation that may have resulted in lymphadenopathy.

CARDIOVASCULAR SYSTEM

Inspection

Examine the hands for:
- palmar erythema;
- cyanosis;
- finger clubbing – in cyanotic heart disease usually only after 6 months of age;
- nail bed hemorrhages – rare, seen in infective endocarditis.

Examine the face for:
- dysmorphic features – heart disease is more common in children with other congenital abnormalities or syndromes;
- central cyanosis or pallor;
- sweating.

Examine the precordium for:
- signs of respiratory distress;
- scars – usually a sternotomy scar or a left thoracotomy but be aware that modern advances in laparoscopic surgery may result in lack of traditionally recognized scars;
- a hyperdynamic precordium from a ventricular impulse;
- count the respiratory rate and look for signs of respiratory distress;
- check the oxygen saturations using a pulse oximeter;
- assess general level of nutrition and ease of activity.

Palpation

Feel whether the child is warm and well-perfused. There may be prolongation of the capillary refill time. This may be an indicator of shock if it is very prolonged, but as a sign it has notoriously poor inter-rater agreement.[25]

Examine the pulse. In infants measure the brachial pulse; in older children measure the radial pulse. Remember that the pulse rate will vary with temperature, activity and stress.

Rate (Table 8.10)
Rhythm

Sinus arrhythmia, where the rhythm and volume of the pulse varies with respiration, is common in children.

Volume

Volume is small in circulatory collapse and aortic stenosis and increased in high-output states such as anemia, patent ductus arteriosus and fever. Following a Blalock–Taussig shunt procedure volume may be decreased or absent.

The jugular venous pressure is often difficult to assess in younger children but prominent pulsation may be seen in tricuspid regurgitation and cannon waves in heart block.

Palpate the femoral pulses. Absent or reduced femoral pulses are suggestive of coarctation of the aorta as is radiofemoral delay, which may be difficult to appreciate in faster heart rates.

Palpate the precordium for the position of the apex beat, usually located in the 4th or 5th intercostal space in the midclavicular line. Note any parasternal heave from a ventricular impulse or a thrill from a palpable murmur. Feeling in the suprasternal notch for a thrill can be uncomfortable for children and should only be checked if aortic stenosis is suspected.

Palpate the abdomen for an enlarged liver and spleen. Assess any lower limb edema. Both hepatosplenomegaly and limb edema are late signs of heart failure.

Auscultation

Auscultate at the apex to identify the heart sounds. The first sound tends to be single and the second sound split with variation during respiration, splitting increasing with inspiration. A third heart sound at the apex is common in infants and younger children. Listen for the murmurs in the positions shown in Figure 8.5 with the bell and then diaphragm of the stethoscope.

Assess and describe any murmur.

Timing   – systolic, diastolic, continuous
Phase   – early, mid, late
Duration   – short, pansystolic
Loudness   – Grades 1–2– very soft
                           Grade 2   – soft
                           Grade 3   – easy to hear, no thrill
                           Grade 4–6 – loud with a thrill
                           Grade 5   – heard with a stethoscope held off the chest
                           Grade 6   – heard without stethoscope
Site of maximal intensity
Radiation   – examples: to neck in aortic stenosis
                     to back in aortic coarctation/ pulmonary stenosis
                     to right axilla in atrial septal defect

Innocent murmurs are common in children and are characterized by being soft, short, midsystolic, localized, and varying with position and respiration. They are commonest at the lower left sternal edge. They are usually musical or vibratory, do not conduct and are not associated with other signs of heart disease. A venous hum is caused by blood flow in the great veins and is heard as a low-pitched machinery-type murmur in the upper right side of the chest that varies with position, becoming louder when sitting up. It may be eliminated by gentle pressure on the neck. Characteristics of a significant murmur are shown

Table 8.10 Normal ranges or values for physiological variables across different ages

Sign	Preterm neonate	Term neonate	Up to 1 year	1–5 years	10 years
Heart rate (beats per min)	120–160	100–140	80–120	70–100	60–80
Blood pressure (mmHg)					
Systolic	*Mean* BP at least numerically		80	85	95
Diastolic	equivalent to gestational age		50	55	60
Respiratory rate (breaths per min)	40–60	30–50	20–40	20–30	15–20

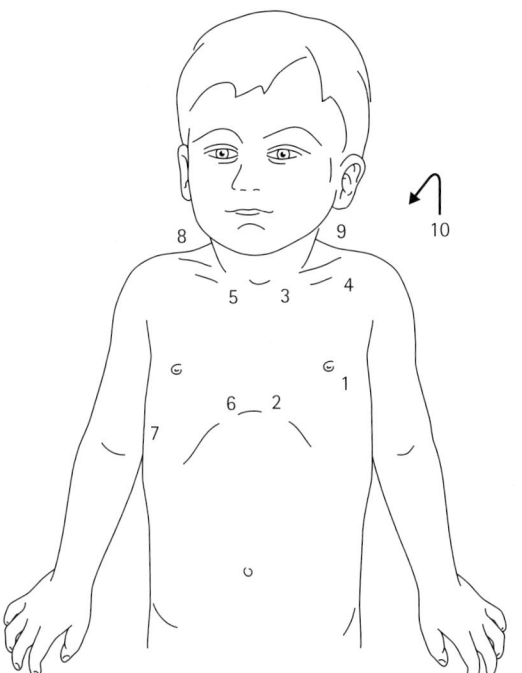

Fig. 8.5 Auscultation positions. 1, apex; 2, left lower sternal edge; 3, left upper sternal edge; 4, left infraclavicular; 5, right upper sternal edge; 6, right lower sternal edge; 7, right midaxillary line; 8, right side of neck; 9, left side of neck; 10, posteriorly. (From Laing & McIntosh[42] with permission of Baillière Tindall).

Table 8.11 Characteristics of a significant murmur

Pansystolic or diastolic
Heard best at the upper left sternal edge
Harsh quality
Abnormal 2nd heart sound
Early or mid-systolic click

in Table 8.11.[26] Murmurs with a thrill and those that are diastolic are always significant. All significant murmurs should be referred to a pediatric cardiologist.

Measure the blood pressure

Practice in pediatric blood pressure measurement has been found to vary widely in the UK with further variation in what are regarded as acceptable limits for normal blood pressure.[27,28] Further difficulties arise due to discrepancies in measurements between devices.

The gold standard for blood pressure measurement is invasive continuous intra-arterial waveform monitoring. This method allows trend evaluation of the blood pressure as well as observation of the waveform, and may indicate pathology. Non-invasive methods include the manual auscultatory method and also automatic oscillometric and Doppler methods. Although non-invasive oscillometric measurements have been found to be reliable in healthy settled neonates,[29] they may be less reliable in critically ill infants.[30] Pulse oximetry waveform systolic blood pressure measurement is a newer development that has been found to be more accurate than oscillometric devices in both postoperative children and sick neonates,[31,32] This method may be particularly useful in patients on transport.[33]

In neonates, the mean blood pressure should be at least numerically equivalent to the infant's gestational age in weeks.[34,35] A guide to normal blood pressure values in older children is given in Table 8.10. A rough guide to remembering expected blood pressure values in children is:

Systolic BP = 100 mmHg at 6 years. After 6, BP rises by around 2.5 mmHg a year
Diastolic BP = 60 + age in years

Blood pressure measurements should be considered with respect to the child's size and gender as well as age and pediatric normograms are available.[36–38] Although there are limitations to using an absolute cut off in children, hypertension is generally defined as an average systolic and/or diastolic blood pressure ≥95th percentile for age and sex with resting measurements obtained on at least three different occasions.[38]

Technique for manual auscultatory method (korotkoff's method[39])

Explain the procedure to the child before you start. The child should be relaxed, as pressures recorded during crying or struggling are unreliable. The child should be sitting with the right arm exposed and resting on a surface at the level of the heart.

Select the largest cuff that will fit the child's arm comfortably. The cuff should encircle the arm and cover around 75% of the distance between the shoulder tip and elbow. A cuff that is too small will give artificially high readings. Doppler, oscillometric and ultrasonic machines will measure the blood pressure automatically. The cuff should be inflated to around 20 mmHg above the point at which the radial pulse disappears. The cuff should be deflated slowly at a rate of about 3 mmHg/s while light auscultation of the brachial artery is performed. The systolic blood pressure is measured as the pressure at which the pulse is first heard. Continue deflation until the sounds become muffled or disappear; this is the diastolic blood pressure. The blood pressure should be measured and recorded in millimeters of mercury (mmHg).

RESPIRATORY SYSTEM

Inspection

Observe and listen for signs of respiratory disease:
- measure respiratory rate (Table 8.10) and observe the pattern of breathing;
- cyanosis (measure SaO_2 with a pulse oximeter, if necessary);
- inspiratory stridor;
- expiratory wheeze;
- grunting;
- nasal flaring;
- cough – may be barking in croup, or moist and wheezy in bronchiolitis;
- tracheal tug;
- use of accessory muscles: intercostal and sternocleidomastoid;
- retractions: subcostal, intercostal, supraclavicular, suprasternal (tracheal tug) or sternal;
- ease of speech and feeding;
- nasal discharge, snuffliness, upper airway secretions;
- posture and level of activity;
- finger clubbing – seen in chronic suppurative conditions such as cystic fibrosis;
- examine any sputum.

Look at the chest for scars, asymmetry and shape. The chest may be barrel-shaped in asthma and a Harrison's sulcus from diaphragmatic tug may be present in poorly controlled asthma and chronic lung disease of prematurity.

Observe for paradoxical respirations with sternal recession and abdominal distension during inspiration and the reverse during expiration. A degree of abdominal breathing is common in infants but excessive use of the abdominal muscles may indicate respiratory distress.

Children over the age of 5 may be able to generate a peak expiratory flow rate. This measurement is commonly used to assess the severity of asthma and response to treatment. It is measured in L/min and can be compared against normal values for height and sex.

Palpation

Examining the position of the trachea in the suprasternal notch may cause discomfort to some children and is rarely useful.

Assess chest expansion. With thumbs meeting over the sternum and the hands placed gently around the chest, ask the child to take a deep breath. In normal school-aged children, the thumbs should move apart about 3–5 cm.

Percussion is rarely performed in the infant as it can make the child cry and obscures other signs. In older children, explain what you are going to do prior to percussion. Percuss anteriorly and posteriorly, appreciating any dullness suggestive of effusion or consolidation, and hyper-resonance suggestive of a pneumothorax. Always make symmetrical comparisons.

Palpate the abdomen for downward displacement of the liver.

Auscultation

Use the diaphragm of the stethoscope. Listen anteriorly, posteriorly and in the axillae. Assess equality of air entry bilaterally. Listen to the quality of the breath sounds, which may be harsh, high pitched or bronchial. Harsh breath sounds from the upper airways are easily transmitted to the upper chest in young children. Bronchial breath sounds are higher-pitched than vesicular breath sounds and both inspiration and expiration are equal in length. Listen for any added sounds such as crackles (crepitations), wheeze or pleural rub. Crackles are discontinuous moist sounds from the opening and closing of the bronchioles. Wheeze is the high-pitched expiratory sound from distal airway obstruction. Remember that in infants significant lung disease may be present in the absence of signs on auscultation.[40]

GASTROINTESTINAL SYSTEM

The child should lie supine. In small infants, examination may take place with the child lying in the parent's arms.

Inspection

Assess nutritional status. Look at the eyes for jaundice and anemia. Check for finger clubbing, which may be present in chronic inflammatory bowel disease. Look in the mouth for angular stomatitis, glossitis and mucosal ulceration or bleeding.

Look at the abdomen for distension, visible bowel loops or masses and scars. If there is any swelling, note the site and size of this. Generalized distension may occur with fat, fluid, feces or flatus. Distinguish true distension from the normal protuberant 'pot belly' seen in pre-school children. There may be swelling in the flanks if there is ascites. Gross ascites may lead to eversion of the umbilicus. Localized swellings may be due to enlarged organs, a distended bowel loop, intra-abdominal masses or herniae. Umbilical herniae are common in the infant and usually resolve by 18 months of age. In intestinal obstruction, peristalsis may be visible. It may be relevant to examine the stool and urine.

Palpation

Ensure the child is comfortable and relaxed. Ask about any tenderness. Warm your hands. Palpation often provokes giggling in tickly children. Distract the child by asking him questions about school or a favorite toy. Using the child's hand to palpate may help. If the child is unable to settle, bending the child's knees will relax the stomach muscles. In a crying baby, palpate during inspiration or later during sleep. Gently palpate in all four quadrants to assess tenderness and guarding, observing the child's face for signs of pain throughout. Assess any organomegaly, masses and tenderness (Fig. 8.6).

Liver

The liver is normally felt 1–2 cm below the costal margin in the mid-clavicular line in children up to the age of 3 years. In pathological conditions it enlarges towards the right iliac fossa and will move with respiration. Palpate from the right iliac fossa, using the tips of the fingers or the side of the index finger. Remember that in respiratory disease the liver may be pushed down by a flattened diaphragm, giving

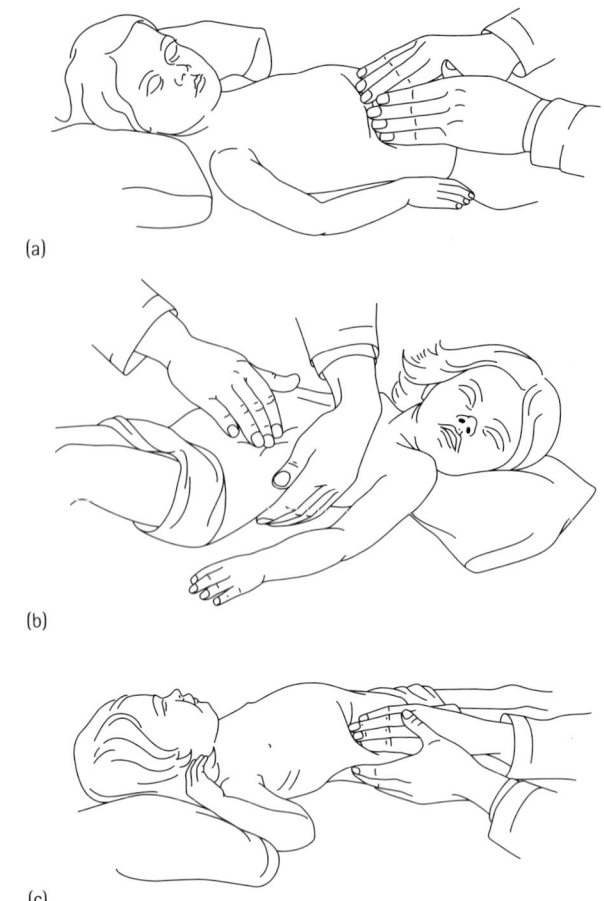

(a)

(b)

(c)

Fig. 8.6   Palpation: (a) liver, (b) spleen, (c) kidney.

the impression of hepatomegaly. Therefore always percuss the upper edge of the liver and measure the full size in centimeters with a tape measure.

Spleen

A spleen is sometimes palpable under the costal margin in normal young children – usually after a minor viral infection. The spleen enlarges towards the right from the left costal margin, although in small infants, extension towards the left iliac fossa is more usual. Laying the child slightly on the right side may allow easier palpation of this organ. Features that distinguish an enlarged spleen from the left kidney are the presence of a notch, inability to feel above it, dullness to percussion and that it is not ballotable. Measure the extent below the costal margin in centimeters with a tape measure.

Kidneys and bladder

Although a kidney may be felt in the newborn infant, it should not be palpable in older infants and children. An enlarged kidney may be felt on deep palpation with one hand but a bimanual approach is easier, with one hand underneath the child and one on the abdomen. Kidneys move on respiration, have a smooth outline and can be accessed from the area above them. Feel for tenderness in the flanks posteriorly. A full bladder may be palpable.

Other

If ascites is suspected, check for a fluid thrill and percuss for shifting dullness. Percuss the child's abdomen to outline areas of dullness and tympany. Ask the child to roll onto his side and after 1 min, percuss again, noting any shift in the area of dullness, which may suggest ascites. Assess the size, shape and characteristics of any masses. Check in the groins for swellings suggestive of a hernia, lymph nodes or gonads. Inguinal herniae, in contrast to an umbilical hernia, are always pathological and require referral to the surgeons. The anus should be inspected where guided by the clinical history. Rectal examination is seldom necessary and is discussed later.

Auscultation

Bowel sounds may be hyperactive in intestinal obstruction and acute infective diarrhea or absent in peritonitis or ileus.

GENITOURINARY SYSTEM

If the genitals require examination, ensure that a parent or chaperone is present and that this is recorded in the notes. If sexual abuse is suspected the child should be assessed by a child protection specialist.

Boys

Examine the penis for size and ensure that the urethral meatus is at the tip. In hypospadias the meatus is on the ventral surface of the penis (head, shaft or perineum) and in epispadias, it is positioned on the dorsum. Although a phimosis is common in infancy, by 4 years of age the foreskin can be retracted in most uncircumcised males. Examine the scrotum. Ensure both testes are palpable. If a testis is unable to be felt, determine whether it is truly undescended or simply retractile by asking the child to squat. This will abolish the cremasteric reflex and a retractile testis will be felt. It may be relevant to measure the size of the testes, in which case, use an orchidometer. Feel for other scrotal masses and if found, transilluminate the swelling with a pen torch. Fluid will transilluminate and the commonest cause is a hydrocele. An inguinal hernia is another common scrotal mass and will not transilluminate. Inguinal herniae require surgical referral, particularly if irreducible, in which case it should be treated as an emergency.

Girls

Look for the size of the clitoris and the labia, the position of the vagina and the presence of any vaginal discharge. The differentiation of notches and clefts in the hymen may be important in suspected child sexual abuse.[41]

SEXUAL MATURATION

The age at development of the secondary sexual characteristics varies greatly. On average, the onset of puberty is 1–2 years earlier in girls than boys. Breast and pubic hair development may begin as early as 8 years whereas testicular development in boys starts at around 9–10 years. The adolescent growth spurt occurs around 12 years in girls and 14 years in boys.

In girls, growth of pubic hair and breast development are assigned a sexual maturity rating as established by Tanner in 1962 (Fig. 8.7).[42] In boys, a similar rating is used to document the growth of pubic hair and the development of the penis, testes and scrotum (Fig. 8.7).[42]

RETICULOENDOTHELIAL SYSTEM

Symptoms and signs of dysfunction of the reticuloendothelial system are typically nonspecific and although examination is important in guiding investigations, the diagnosis is usually made on examination of blood count and film, and sometimes the bone marrow.

Inspection

Look for evidence of weight loss and general indices of nutrition. The child may be lethargic or listless. Look for pallor, jaundice, bruises, mucosal bleeding, petechiae and skin rashes. There may be angular stomatitis and glossitis on examination of the mouth. Take the child's temperature and inspect for signs of infection, remembering to look for candida. Look for evidence of marrow hyperplasia with overgrowth of the frontal and maxillary bones. Examine the gums

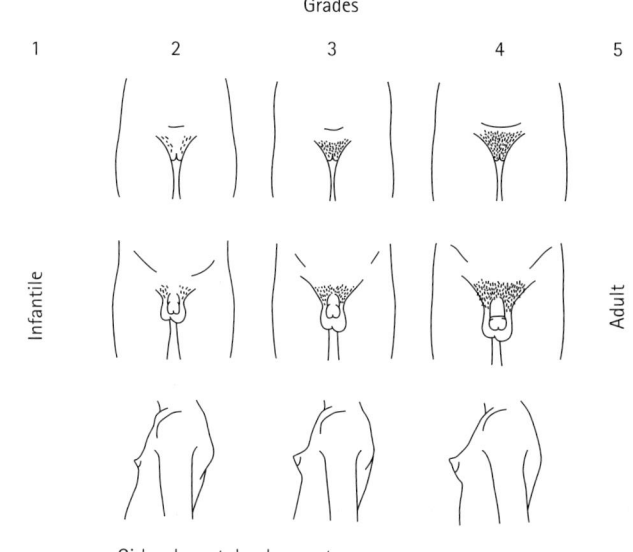

Girls – breast development:
Stage 1: as in early childhood
Stage 2: breast bud
Stage 3: breast and areola enlarging
Stage 4: areola and papilla form a secondary mound distinct from enlarging breast
Stage 5: mature

Boys – genital development:
Stage 1: testes, scrotum and penis as in early childhood
Stage 2: some enlargement of testes and scrotum
Stage 3: early lengthening of penis
Stage 4: enlarged penis in length and breadth, with glans development
Stage 5: adult genitalia

Girls and boys – pubic hair:
Stage 1: no pubic hair
Stage 2: sparse growth of pubic hair on each side of penile root or on labia
Stage 3: darker coarse hair meeting on symphysis
Stage 4: adult hair, no spread to medial surface of thighs
Stage 5: adult in quantity and type with spread to medial surface of thighs

Fig. 8.7 Pubertal development grading. (From Laing & McIntosh[42] with permission of Baillière Tindall)

for hypertrophy. Observe for breathlessness or other signs of respiratory distress.

Look at the abdomen for any distension, dilated superficial veins and scars suggestive of a splenectomy.

Palpation

Palpate for enlarged lymph nodes in the neck, axillae and groin. Palpate the abdomen for enlargement of the liver and spleen.

Auscultation

Listen to the heart sounds, noting any tachycardia and the presence of a flow murmur, which may be present in anemia.

NERVOUS SYSTEM

Although in older children a full detailed neurological examination can be carried out as in adults (Table 8.12), observation and clinical history will allow a reasonable assessment of neurological function in smaller children. Some useful neurological tests are listed in Table 8.13 Neurodevelopmental examination is detailed in Chapter 7.

Table 8.12 Schema for neurological examination in children

Assessment of level of consciousness and mental state
Inspection – size and shape of head, dysmorphic features, neurocutaneous lesions
Meningeal signs – if prompted by symptoms
Motor system – tone, power, reflexes
Sensation – if prompted by symptoms
Cerebellar function – gait, balance and coordination
Cranial nerves

Inspection

Assess the level of consciousness and mental state. Observe the child's posture for asymmetry, unusual posture of limbs (such as scissoring of the legs, hemiplegia or windswept posture) and involuntary movements. Look for any neurocutaneous stigmata such as café-au-lait spots, shagreen patches, depigmented macules and facial capillary hemangiomas. Examine the child's head for size, shape and any unusual facial features. Observe any muscular fasciculation, particularly in the tongue.

Watch the child move around, looking for paucity or weakness of movement, balance and general tone.

In babies, feel the fontanelles and the cranial sutures, noting whether they are open or closed. The anterior fontanelle measures approximately 0.5–2.5 cm in diameter at birth, although the size may vary considerably depending on the degree of molding. It should close by 18 months. The posterior fontanelle measures around 0.5 cm across and closes shortly after birth. The cranial sutures may be overriding at birth due to molding in the birth canal. Feel the sutures for premature fusion (craniosynostosis) or separation, which may indicate hydrocephalus or raised intracranial pressure. If an arteriovenous malformation is suspected, auscultation over the skull may yield cranial bruits.

Meningism

The classical signs of meningism (neck stiffness, photophobia and in infants, a bulging fontanelle) develop relatively late in the course of

Table 8.13 Neurological and locomotor tests

Test name	Test description	Possible causes
Babinski's sign	Stroking lateral plantar surface from heel to toes causes extension of great toe	Normal in infants, upper motor neurone lesions
Barlow's test	With one hand stabilizing pelvis, the other hand abducts infant's hip. Pressure is then applied backwards and outwards with the thumb on the inner upper thigh while abducting same hip in an attempt to dislocate an unstable hip	Unstable hip
Bragaard test	Dorsiflexion of foot following straight leg raising causes pain in leg and lumbar region	Sciatic nerve root impingement
Brudzinski's sign	Flexing head causes legs to be drawn up	Meningeal irritation
Chvostek's sign	Tapping facial nerve lightly causes contraction of ipsilateral facial muscles	Hypocalcemia
Gower's maneuver	Child getting up from floor by walking hands up legs	Duchenne muscular dystrophy
Kernig's sign	With hip flexed, any attempt to straighten knee results in hamstring or lumbar spasm	Meningeal irritation
Lachman's test	With knee almost fully extended, tibia can be moved forward on femoral condyle	Anterior cruciate ligament laxity or rupture
McMurray test	Flex hip and knee to 90 degrees. Grasp heel with one hand and steady knee with other. Slowly extend knee using heel movement, while palpating joint line. Do with tibia in external and internal rotation. A clunk indicates displaced cartilage	Cartilage displacement in knee
Moro reflex	See Table 8.16	
Ortolani's test	With one hand stabilizing pelvis, abduct hip and press forward with middle finger on greater trochanter. A dislocated hip can be felt to slip forward into joint again with a 'clunk'	Congenital dislocation of the hip
Romberg's sign	Closing eyes while standing with feet together causes severe swaying or falling over	Proprioceptive or vestibular deficit, posterior column lesion, intoxication
Simmond's test	With patient lying prone, squeezing calf results in absence of plantar flexion of foot	Ruptured Achilles tendon
Thomas test	With patient supine, place one hand between lumbar spine and couch. Flex normal hip to limit to straighten lumbar spine. Opposite leg will rise off couch if fixed flexion deformity present	Flexion deformity of hip
Trendelenburg's test	While standing, pelvis tilts down towards side on which leg is lifted. Opposite side is impaired	Congenital dislocation of the hip, muscular dystrophy
Trousseau's sign	Circumferential pressure of limb causes carpopedal spasm	Hypocalcemia, alkalosis, Bartter syndrome

meningitis. Early symptoms of bacterial meningitis include leg pains, cold peripheries and skin mottling.[43] There may be a history of poor feeding, vomiting and irritability. If the history is suspicious of meningitis, look for neck stiffness. However, this is an unreliable sign in children and can also be present in tonsillitis or in a generalized flu-like illness. A child who has true neck stiffness will not move his neck actively and may even lie in an extended position. Ask him to touch his chin to his chest and each shoulder, and then ask him to look up above. Gently flex the neck while watching the child's face for signs of pain and feeling for resistance. With the child lying supine, flex the child's leg at the hip and knee. Straighten the leg at the knee, observing for neck pain and resistance to extension (Kernig's test).

Ask about photophobia and observe the child's response in a well-lit room and to a bright light shone in the eyes. In infants, assess the tension of the anterior fontanelle remembering that crying and struggling babies will have a bulging tense fontanelle too.

Tone

Tone is defined as the resistance to passive movement felt across a joint and should always be assessed with the head in the midline. Observe the posture. A child with generalized hypotonia will lie in a frog-like posture and will 'slip through your hands' when holding him upright. Hypertonic children may lie in a hyperextended position, with arching of the neck and fisting of the hands. Truncal tone can be assessed on pulling to sit or holding prone in the younger child and in the ability to sit in older children. Assess tone in the limbs, checking for spasticity and clonus or untoward floppiness. This is best assessed in children while they are distracted with another activity. Increased tone in the lower limbs may result in scissoring of the legs when a child is held upright. In children who are walking, heels should touch the ground. Increased tone may lead to joint contractures whereas floppiness may result in hypermobile joints or even dislocations.

Power

Power is the measure of strength of muscle groups and can be graded as follows:

Grade
0 – no movement
1 – minimal movements present
2 – movements but not against gravity
3 – voluntary antigravity movements
4 – movements against resistance
5 – normal strength

The symmetry of active movements should be noted. Assess muscle bulk. Pseudohypertrophy is the fatty infiltration of weak muscles seen in Duchenne muscular dystrophy.

In children who are not yet walking, a useful test of gross motor function is the 180-degree test:
- With the baby lying supine, observe anti-gravity movements and whether he can roll from supine to prone.
- Pull the baby by the hands to the sitting position, assessing head lag.
- Does the baby sit unsupported? What head control does the baby have? Are there protective righting reflexes, present from 5–6 months? The baby puts one arm out to right himself when gently pushed over to one side.
- With hands under the axillae, stand the baby on a flat surface. Does he weight bear?
- Lift the baby upright, assessing tone and posture of the legs.
- Watch for the protective parachute reflex, present from around 6–9 months, as you lay the baby prone. The baby will extend his arms to protect himself.
- With the baby prone, observe head lifting and whether the baby is able to support himself on flexed or extended arms and lift his chest off the bed.
- Observe rolling from prone to supine.

In children who are walking, assess gross motor function in a range of activities including running, jumping, hopping, squatting and climbing steps. Fine-motor power can be assessed as in adults.

Deep tendon reflexes

Examination of the deep reflexes includes biceps, triceps, pronator, knee and ankle. In small infants, percussion of the reflexes can be done using a brisk tap with the fingertips; in older children a tendon hammer should be used. Explain to the child before you start the examination what it entails as some children find it alarming. A few beats of clonus in the ankle reflex are normal in small infants but in conditions with increased tone, clonus is exaggerated and sustained.

Sensation

Formal assessment of sensation is laborious and difficult to carry out in infants and in small children who lack cooperation. It is not part of the routine examination. In younger children, stroking or tickling may result in withdrawal of the limb and may be a useful screening tool. If suspicious symptoms are present, formally assess sensation in all dermatomes (Fig. 8.8). Explain the procedure clearly to the child and

Fig. 8.8 Cutaneous nerve segments. **(From Geigy[112] with permission).**

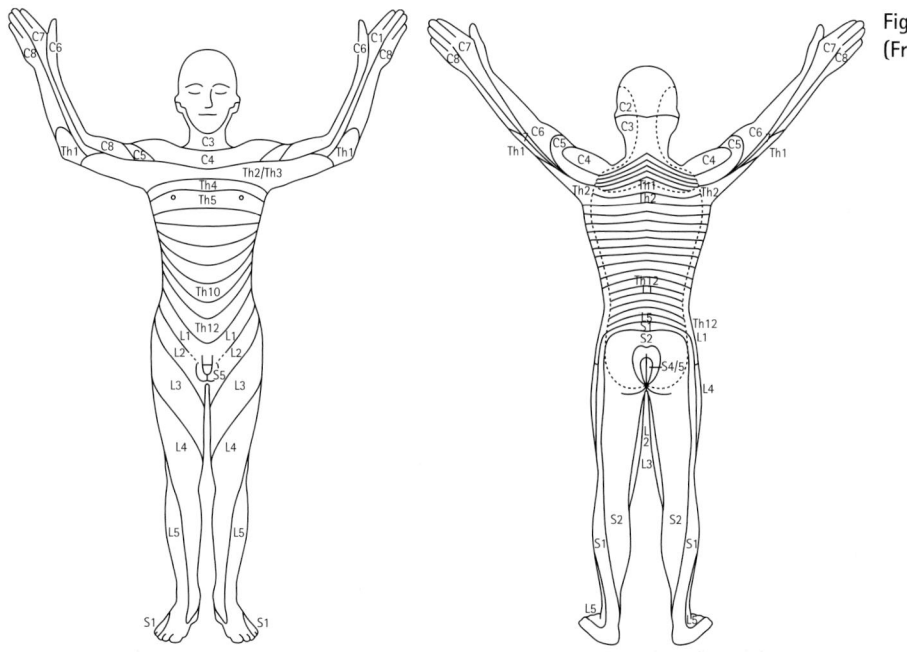

let him know what response is expected of him. Demonstrate the test with the child's eyes open initially. The child should subsequently have his eyes shut. Assess the child's responses to light and deep touch, pain, temperature, vibration and proprioception.

Cerebellar function

Formal assessment of cerebellar function requires cooperation and is not recommended in infants and younger children. Older children may enjoy the different tasks:

1. Assess the child walking for broad-based features.
2. Listen to the child's speech – slow, slurred speech is characteristic of cerebellar disease.
3. Observe tongue movements – small spastic tongue is classical of cerebellar pathology.
4. Assess balance with one-legged standing, heel–toe test and the Romberg test. The Romberg test involves getting the child to stand with the eyes shut while gently pushing his shoulders from side to side to push him off balance. Explain before the test what it entails and reassure any worried child that you will catch him if he falls.
5. Stand the child with eyes shut and arms outstretched in front, palms facing downward. Push the wrist quickly downward and observe the returning movement. In cerebellar disorders the hand may shoot up past its original position.
6. Examine the eye movements for nystagmus. In cerebellar disease, the nystagmus is typically of large amplitude and low frequency.

7. Heel–shin coordination test – repetitive sliding of the heel of one foot up and down the shin of the other leg. Watch for inaccuracy of placement and 'wobbliness'.
8. Finger–nose test. Get the child to touch your finger then touch his nose repetitively while you move your finger into random positions within his reach. Watch for past-pointing, where the child's finger overshoots the target, and tremulous intent, where attempt at accuracy of the action is associated with increased tremor.
9. Fine motor movements of the fingers – 'playing the piano' and quick repetitive opposition of thumb with each finger.
10. Test for dysdiadochokinesis – ask the child to clap one hand repetitively with the alternating palm and dorsum of the other hand.

Cranial nerves

Testing of the cranial nerves in children requires practice, patience and ingenuity. Much information can be gathered from watching a child's facial expression and eye movements, observing him eating and listening to him talking. Most children will be only too delighted to stick their tongue out at you! Parental concerns about hearing and vision should be taken seriously and usually warrant specialist referral. Smell and taste are not tested routinely in children.

Detailed assessment of the cranial nerves can be performed in older, cooperative children (Table 8.14). Ophthalmoscopy is described in detail in Chapter 31.

Table 8.14 Testing of cranial nerves

	Cranial nerve	Test for integrity
I	Olfactory nerve	Before testing, check each nostril is patent. Test the sense of smell in each nostril, by occluding one at a time. Present common odors such as coffee, chocolate, soap and orange peel
II	Ophthalmic nerve	Test the visual fields, and visual acuity (with glasses on if normally worn) with a Snellen or Logmar chart in school-age children. Charts that use shapes instead of letters are available for younger children. Examine the fundi
III IV VI	Oculomotor nerve Trochlear nerve Abducent nerve	Test the eye movements, looking for nystagmus, squint, head tilting and dysconjugate movements. Ask if he has double or blurred vision during the examination. Examine the pupils for shape and symmetry. Test the direct and consensual papillary reflexes to light and the accommodation reflex
V	Trigeminal nerve	With the child's eyes closed, test facial sensation in ophthalmic, maxillary and mandibular areas with a piece of cotton wool or your fingers. Test sensation over the anterior part of the tongue with an orange stick. The corneal reflex can be unpleasant to test. Touch a piece of damp cotton wool to the lower lateral quadrant of the eye while the child is looking upwards. Check for blinking. Ask the child to bite down hard and test the bulk of the masseter muscle. Test for a jaw jerk by gently tapping the chin with a tendon hammer while the mouth is loosely open
VII	Facial nerve	Test the muscles of facial expression by asking the child to look angry, happy, surprised and to show his teeth. Ask him to pretend to blow up a balloon. Look for asymmetry and feel for weakness. Test common tastes such as sugar, salt, lemon juice on the anterior part of the tongue
VIII	Vestibulocochlear nerve	Test the hearing and balance. Hearing can be tested crudely by distraction testing
IX X	Glossopharyngeal nerve Vagus nerve	Test common tastes such as sugar, salt, lemon juice on the posterior part of the tongue. Testing pharyngeal sensation is unpleasant and should be reserved for those children with swallowing difficulties. Use an orange stick and gently test sensation on both sides. Ask the child to say the sounds 'aah', 'c' and 'g' and watch the movement of the palate. Test the gag reflex if there are swallowing difficulties
XI	Accessory nerve	Inspect and palpate the sternocleidomastoid and trapezius muscles for bulk. Holding the chin on one side, ask the child to turn the head to that side against resistance thus testing the power of the sternocleidomastoid muscle on the opposite side. Test the power of the trapezius muscle by asking the child to shrug his shoulders as you exert downward pressure
XII	Hypoglossal nerve	Ask the child to stick out his tongue and waggle it from side to side. Look for deviation and fasciculation. Ask him to push his tongue against the inside of each cheek, while you assess power from the outside

LOCOMOTOR SYSTEM

Inspection

Watch the child as he moves around. In infants observe how he reaches for objects and crawls or bottom-shuffles. In older children observe the gait while walking, running, jumping, hopping and climbing stairs. Observe any unusual positioning, guarding and swelling. Look for erythema or any contractures around a joint. Look at the soles of the child's shoes for asymmetry of tread and scuffing.

Palpation

Ascertain any tenderness before you start and watch the child's face throughout the examination. Remember that pain may be referred, such as hip pathology presenting as pain in the knee. Examine the upper and lower limbs and then the joints for swelling, tenderness, heat, crepitus and range of movement. Find out the extent of voluntary active movement before manipulating a joint passively.

Examine the spine for sacral sinuses, nevi, swellings and tufts of hair. Check the spine for scoliosis, kyphosis and lordosis with the child standing erect initially. True scoliosis can be demonstrated if an apparent hemithoracic convexity persists on bending over forwards. Some useful locomotor tests are detailed in Table 8.13. Measurement of limb lengths may be relevant and normograms are available in textbooks of morphology.[24]

INVASIVE EXAMINATIONS

Invasive examinations are not part of the routine examination and should be performed only when guided by relevant information in the clinical history. Such examinations usually cause distress or discomfort and should be performed at the end of the examination.

EXAMINATION OF AUDITORY CANAL

The ears are best examined in younger children with the child held sideways in the parent's lap. The parent should be shown how to hold the head to prevent trauma if the child wriggles (Fig. 8.9).[42] Use an appropriately sized attachment of the otoscope. Hold the pinna with one hand and insert the otoscope into the external ear canal. Note the integrity and color of eardrum and any discharge.

EXAMINATION OF OROPHARYNX

If unable to cooperate, the child should be positioned on the parent's lap facing the examiner with the parent's hand firmly on the forehead to prevent the child lunging forward (Fig. 8.10).[42] Using a light source and a tongue depressor inspect the tonsils and pharynx. The size of the tonsils in children may be considerable and usually is of no clinical significance. Note any erythema, ulceration, exudates or palatal petechiae. Candidal infection of the oropharynx leads to white adherent mucosal plaques. The mucosa will bleed if the plaque is scraped off in contrast to milk residue, which is also common in babies. It is useful to be prepared and take a swab for microbiological investigation if warranted, rather than repeat the procedure. Use this opportunity to inspect the condition of the gums and the teeth for caries. Although this examination is a usual procedure in suspected upper respiratory infection, beware of the toxic, febrile child with drooling and stridor. This child may have acute epiglottitis and inspection of the pharynx in this way may precipitate acute respiratory obstruction.

RECTAL EXAMINATION

This may be necessary to assess fecal impaction and check for anal fissures or trauma. It may also be required when child sexual abuse has been suggested, when it should be performed by a child protection specialist. Its usefulness in assessing pain in acute appendicitis is debatable.[44] Explain to the child what you are about to do. Ask the child to lie on his side with his legs drawn up to his chest. Note the appearance of the anus and the

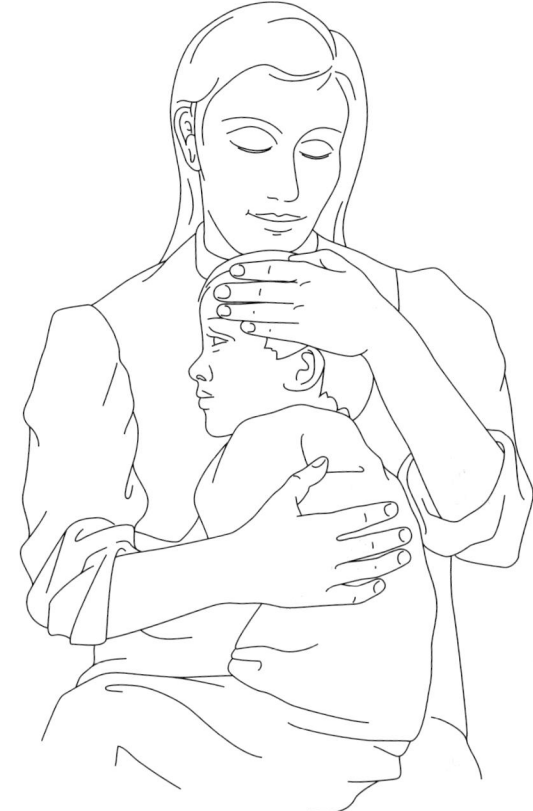

Fig. 8.9 Method of holding a child for otoscopy. (From Laing & McIntosh[42] with permission of Baillière Tindall)

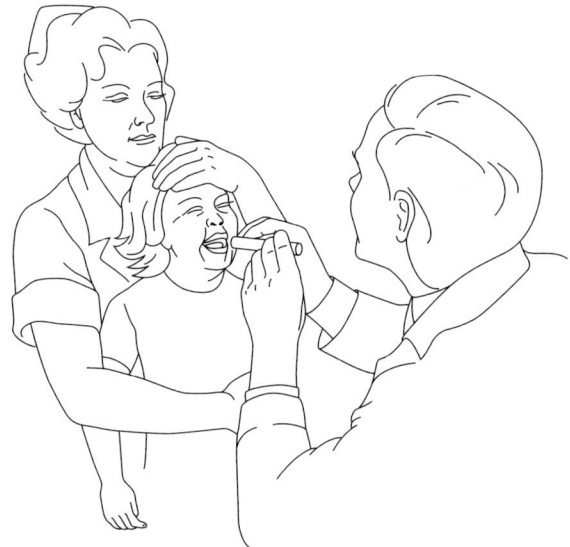

Fig. 8.10 Examining the oropharynx in an uncooperative child. (From Laing & McIntosh[42] with permission of Baillière Tindall)

presence of any threadworms, excoriation or bleeding. On spreading the buttocks apart, a fissure may be seen, commonly at 6 and 12 o'clock positions. Use lots of lubricant on a gloved little finger. The anal tone may be increased in anal stenosis or decreased (patulous) in spinal cord lesions. The specificity of the reflex anal dilatation test for recurrent anal abuse has been questioned.[41] Appreciate any tenderness and feel for any masses. Examine the appearance of rectal contents on withdrawal of your finger.

VAGINAL EXAMINATION

Vaginal examination may be necessary in cases of suspected child abuse and in this case should be performed by a clinician skilled in this procedure. Small children may have vaginal discharge secondary to a self-inserted foreign body. This generally requires exploration under sedation.

SUMMARY

Summarize the key problems and the list of differential diagnoses. Decide whether any investigations are required to firm up the diagnosis. Formulate a management plan, which may be a period of observation or a therapeutic intervention. Decide on a date for review if necessary and/or whether referral to other specialties is required.

Provide verbal information for the family and include the child where appropriate in the discussion. Support the information by written information, in the form of a note or entry in the parent-held records, a published pamphlet or sending a copy of the clinic letter. Some conditions are best explained with diagrams. Although the Internet is a rich source of information, it may be wise to explain the limitations of this resource.

The likely outcome should be made clear but parents should also know what to do or who to contact if things do not progress as expected. Parents should be clear about arrangements to be seen again. It is often useful to ask parents to recount the information they have been given to ascertain they have understood the plan of action. Ensure your findings are documented accurately and that your notes are dated and signed.

THE NEWBORN

History and examination of the newborn is a well-established element of routine screening in many countries and takes place usually within the first 3 days of birth. In the UK it is a standard part of child health surveillance.[45] There is no evidence supporting the most optimal time for the examination but traditionally it has been postponed until after the first 24 h of life so that the murmur of a patent ductus arteriosus has disappeared and the infant has had some time to establish feeding. It is recommended in the UK that each infant should be examined before 72 h of age.[46] There is no evidence to support a second neonatal examination,[47] but in the UK this examination is repeated in the primary care setting at around 6 weeks of age.

The purpose of the newborn examination is to identify congenital abnormalities, exclude disease where possible, and establish a baseline for future comparison in that child (Table 8.15). As well as reassuring the majority of parents that their child appears healthy, it also provides an opportunity for health promotion. Recording of information also serves a wider purpose of informing on population health by providing data on weight and head circumference.

Congenital anomalies are present in 9% of newborns,[48] but many may be difficult to identify at this early stage or may be missed by inexperienced staff. The newborn examination therefore has important limitations. Many conditions are asymptomatic in the first days or weeks of life and signs and symptoms evolve over time. Some conditions such as hypoplastic left heart and metabolic conditions will evolve over the first days of life, others such as ventricular septal defect only become apparent at a few days or weeks when pulmonary vascular resistance drops and the murmur of a left-to-right shunt becomes audible. Infants with antenatally occurring brain damage may appear neurologically normal at birth and take many months to show signs of spasticity and neurodevelopmental delay. It is important to remember, therefore, that the findings of the newborn examination are specific to that particular point in time.

As well as looking for congenital anomalies, the doctor should ascertain that the baby is well, feeding adequately and behaving appropriately. The pediatrician should have a working knowledge of the effects of the intrauterine environment on the fetus, the physiological changes that occur during and after birth, and an understanding of feeding behavior. Although 'baby checks' are usually carried out by a relatively inexperienced member of pediatric staff, it is important that this doctor has an appreciation of the wide spectrum of normality in the newborn as well as a familiarity with the common pathologies. The junior pediatrician must have ready access to senior advice.

Many women are emotionally labile in the postpartum period. Some mothers may have undergone difficult and traumatic labors; others will never have handled a baby before. Most will have had little sleep in the preceding days or weeks. Remember that even minor problems such as an innocent murmur, jaundice or positional talipes can provoke intense anxiety in the parents and should be discussed sensitively and patiently. Never be judgmental or patronizing.

The newborn examination is also an important opportunity to discuss with the mother any concerns about her baby and his feeding as well as offering reassurance that the examination has not detected anything abnormal. Health promotion such as advice about breast-feeding, immunizations and prevention of cot death can be offered at this time. In addition, parents may seek advice on getting their baby to sleep, what to do when their baby is crying and how to manage sibling rivalry. Written information on these subjects may be available in hand-held records or in leaflet form but the doctor should be prepared to discuss these topics and offer sensible advice. Time taken to provide parents with such health care information may enhance parental satisfaction with the newborn examination.[49]

NEONATAL HISTORY

As with the pediatric history and examination, all information should be recorded accurately and legibly, and signed and dated by the clinician. It is always good practice to check through maternal notes beforehand as parents may fail to disclose important information or realize its relevance.

Introduce yourself and ask the names of the people present and their relationship to the baby. Observe the maternal interaction with her baby. The following important details of the history should be ascertained from the patient records and the mother.

MATERNAL HISTORY

- Maternal age
- General health and pre-existing medical or psychiatric conditions
- Previous obstetric history including miscarriages and fetal losses
- Inherited conditions, including those on her partner's side, particularly developmental dysplasia of the hip and congenital heart disease
- Social circumstances, including occupation, home support and when she hopes to go home.

PREGNANCY HISTORY

- Maternal health during pregnancy – pregnancy-induced hypertension, diabetes, thyroid disease etc.;
- Antenatal concerns about the fetus – poor growth, abnormal serum screening, results of amniocentesis or chorionic villous sampling, excessive or inadequate amounts of liquor and antenatally diagnosed anomalies;
- Antenatal incidents – infections, hemorrhage, trauma and episodes of reduced fetal movements;
- Smoking, alcohol and use of recreational drugs during pregnancy should be sensitively discussed;
- Prescribed medications.

Table 8.15   Role of the newborn examination

To detect congenital anomaly
To exclude disease
To record baseline information for future health surveillance
To reassure parents
To provide health education through anticipatory guidance and supporting parenting skills
To inform population statistics

LABOR AND DELIVERY

- Onset of labor – spontaneous, induced or no labor
- Duration of rupture of membranes
- Mode of delivery
- Medications during labor, including spinal anesthetics and antibiotics
- Presentation of the baby
- Problems during labor – meconium, failure to progress, fetal distress, bleeding, pyrexia
- Condition of the baby at delivery and need for resuscitation.

INFANT HISTORY

- Gender
- Gestation
- Birth weight
- Current parental concerns
- Feeding history.

Although the management and assessment of breast-feeding has traditionally been the role of midwifery staff, it is important that the pediatrician is also able to assess the adequacy of lactation:

- Is the baby waking for feeds regularly without stimulation? A newborn infant typically wants to breast-feed 8–10 times a day in the first few days of life.
- Is the baby rooting and attaching well to the breast? The mouth should be wide-open, with the lower lip rolled down, the chin pressed into the breast and the nose free. The mother should not feel pain if the baby is optimally attached.
- Is the sucking rhythmic and sustained? At the beginning of a feed the baby takes short shallow sucks followed by long deep sucks and audible swallowing.
- Is the baby passing adequate amounts of stool and urine? Most babies will pass meconium (green–black) for the first 2 d of life with changing stool (yellow–brown) appearing by days 3–4. The first stool should be passed within 48 h and urine within 24 h.
- Is weight loss excessive? Most babies lose weight following birth but the majority has regained their birthweight by around 10 d. If a breast-fed infant has a weight loss of greater than 10–12%, consideration should be given to excluding hypernatremic dehydration secondary to lactation insufficiency.[50]

NEONATAL EXAMINATION

As with the pediatric examinations, this should be carried out where possible with the parents present, in a well-lit, warm and quiet room, where privacy can be respected and interaction between the mother and baby can be observed. It is advisable to examine the baby between feeds and for the examination to be guided by the infant's clinical condition.

It is essential that good hand hygiene is observed at all times and that any equipment is cleaned before and after examination. Although all organ systems must be examined fully, the newborn examination is often opportunistic as babies become cold quickly when undressed and fretful when disturbed. Uncomfortable procedures such as examination of the hips or elicitation of the Moro reflex should be deferred to the end of the examination. Through time and practice each pediatrician will develop their own system for examination, which should be thorough and accurate. A top-to-toe assessment, rather than a system-orientated approach, is useful. Speaking soothingly to the infant may help to calm him and the mother.

Inspection

The baby should be observed lying supine for general assessment before touching or undressing. Observe the following points:

- General wellness – does the baby look well?
- Level of alertness – the rousability, consolability and nature of the baby's cry should be noted.
- Nutrition – the weight and head circumference (OFC) of the baby should be plotted on a growth chart appropriate for gender and race. In term infants the weight should be 2.9–4.1 kg and the OFC should measure 33–37 cm. An assessment of skin folds and fat stores can be made through examination. An assessment of gestational age can be made if there is doubt as to the infant's maturity (see Chaplter 12).
- Posture and movement – a normal full-term baby should lie in a flexed position and make many random gross movements of his limbs, trunk and head. The presence of asymmetry should be noted. Jitteriness is common and is seen in almost half of all babies in the first few days.
- Color – jaundice, cyanosis, plethora, pallor, meconium staining.
- Work of breathing – respiratory rate, nasal flaring, tracheal tug, tachypnea, grunting.
- Observe the facies for any dysmorphic features.

Skin

Observe the skin color:

- Plethora may be due to vasodilatation or an increase in circulating red blood cells.
- Pallor may be due to anemia or vasoconstriction.
- Jaundice is common, affecting 30% of newborns between 2 and 4 d of age. It is always an abnormal finding in the first 24 h of life and should prompt investigation for hemolytic disease of the newborn.
- Acrocyanosis where the baby has blue peripheries but is centrally pink is normal in the first 2 weeks of life.
- Central cyanosis is best assessed on the tongue and if present, requires urgent investigation. Cyanosis can be difficult to assess in very pale babies or in those with racial pigmentation. Plethoric babies or those with facial congestion or bruising often appear cyanosed even when well oxygenated. If in doubt carry out pulse oximetry.
- Meconium staining of the skin is often a feature in post-mature infants who have passed meconium in utero some days before delivery. It is most commonly seen around the nails and umbilical cord.
- A harlequin color change is an uncommon episodic but usually benign manifestation of vasomotor instability in the newborn period. When the baby is lying on his side the dependent part appears red but the nondependent part is pale. It is commonest in the low-birthweight infant and may be associated with systemic infection in the unwell infant.

Birthmarks should be noted. Capillary hemangiomas over the eyelids, glabella and nape of neck ('stork marks') are common and fade quickly with time. Cavernous hemangiomas are usually not present at birth but develop over the early weeks and months and typically involute completely by school age. Although often alarming in size and swelling, they require no treatment unless excessively large, when they can be associated with platelet consumption and heart failure, or unless interfering with vision or obstructing the airway. A capillary nevus or port-wine stain, however, is permanent and when located in the distribution of the trigeminal nerve, is often associated with an underlying vascular malformation in the meninges that can interfere with brain development and cause seizures (Sturge-Weber syndrome). Mongolian blue spots are areas of bluish pigmentation, usually over the lower spine and buttocks that are present usually but not invariably in non-Caucasian infants. These also fade over the first year.

The skin in post-mature babies may appear dry and cracked, especially on the feet. This resolves over the ensuing days without treatment. More rarely ichthyosis may be indicative of a more chronic skin condition.

Erythema toxicum is a common benign eruption in full-term babies. Typically the lesion is a red macule with a pale yellow papule in the center. It is occasionally vesicular. The rash is widespread and typically waxes and wanes over the first 2 weeks of life. Although not performed as a diagnostic test, skin scrapings reveal eosinophils. It should be distinguished from staphylococcal infection, which requires antimicrobial treatment. Such infection usually results in a more localized distribution of frankly erythematous pustules.

Milia are tiny white blocked sebaceous glands on the nose and forehead that resolve over a few weeks.

Subcutaneous fat necrosis secondary to local trauma during labor and delivery presents as hard lumps under the skin that initially may be red and painful. These subside with time but there may be residual palpable calcification. Document any bruising or other signs of trauma.

Engorgement of the mammary tissue secondary to placental transfer of maternal hormones may be present in both boys and girls. Rarely neonatal mastitis due to bacterial infection may cause erythema and swelling of the mammary tissue.

Palpable lymph nodes are found in around one third of normal newborn infants and are usually of no clinical significance. They often persist into later infancy.[51]

Head and neck

Note the shape of the head according to Figure 8.4. Examine the size of the anterior fontanelle, which may vary between 1 and 5 cm across. Normal tension should be noted. Bulging of the fontanelle in a baby who is calm and settled warrants investigation. Palpate the posterior fontanelle, which should be open and usually smaller than the tip of your finger. Palpate the sutures, which in the newborn are commonly overlapping (moulding). Premature fusion (craniosynostosis) or excessive separation of the sutures should be investigated.

Note any signs of trauma from delivery such as scalp lacerations from electrodes, or bruising from forceps or vacuum extraction. A cephalhematoma is a subperiosteal hemorrhage confined within the margins of the skull sutures. Occasionally it may be bilateral. A caput succedaneum is a soft boggy swelling, usually over the vertex, which represents diffuse edema secondary to pressure during birth. Rarely this is associated with a rapidly enlarging hematoma under the aponeurosis causing a subgaleal hemorrhage. This should be taken seriously as it is life threatening. Facial congestion or petechial hemorrhages in the distribution of the superior vena cava are common and resolve spontaneously.

An encephalocoele occurs in the midline usually in the occipital region and contains meninges with or without brain tissue. Rarely it may be located anteriorly.

Cutis aplasia is a congenital absence of an area of scalp that may be isolated or have syndromic associations. It is often oval shaped and occurs in the midline at the vertex. It is usually associated with a halo of alopecia.

Examine the neck for presence of developmental anomalies such as branchial fistulae and sinuses. These may occur bilaterally in the newborn and the external opening, which may secrete mucous, usually found in the lower third of the neck anterior to the sternocleidomastoid muscle. Palpate at the back for an extra fold of nuchal skin, which is characteristically seen in Down syndrome, and look for webbing of the neck, which may suggest Turner syndrome. Palpate for any swellings such as the soft fluctuant swelling of a cystic hygroma or the firm restrictive 'tumor' caused by hemorrhagic fibrosis in the sternocleidomastoid muscle. This sternomastoid 'tumor' may result in torticollis of the neck to the affected side. The clavicles should be palpated for fractures.

Ears

Examine for shape and position. Folded ears are common and result from in utero positioning. These are usually only temporarily deformed. Where there is true underdevelopment of the helix and antihelix ('bat ear'), successful correction of the deformity with splinting may avoid surgery. Low-set ears are found in a number of syndromes and chromosomal anomalies. Look for pre-auricular tags or pits. If isolated, they are usually only of cosmetic significance but warrant assessment of hearing. They may occasionally be associated with abnormalities of the genitourinary tract in infants who have coexistent anomalies.

Eyes

Note the size and shape of the eyes. Note any slanting of the palpebral fissures, epicanthic folds, colobomata (keyhole-shaped pupil secondary to a defect of the iris, associated with other congenital anomalies) and Brushfield spots (white flecks on the iris characteristic of Down syndrome).

Subconjunctival hemorrhages are common following delivery but the cornea should be otherwise clear or icteric in the presence of hyperbilirubinemia. Discharge from the eyes and the presence of conjunctivitis should be noted. Impaired lacrimal drainage is common in the newborn period and may cause 'sticky eyes'. Copious purulent discharge and erythema of the surrounding eyelids requires microbiological investigation and treatment as it may be due to the gonococcus in the first few days or Chlamydia a little later.

The red reflex is a reflection of light from the retina when an ophthalmoscope is shone through the iris. Puffiness of the eyelids may make this examination difficult in the first couple of days of life. Absence of the red reflex suggests a cataract, corneal opacity or rarely a retinoblastoma and always warrants further investigation. Although congenital cataracts are present in around 3/10 000 live births, routine newborn examination only detects around 35% of these.[52] Infants of nonCaucasian origin may have retinal pigmentation that alters the appearance of the classical red reflex. Isolated retinal hemorrhages are common after birth and are of no significance.

Nose

Both nostrils should be patent and this can be ascertained by occluding each nostril separately with a finger whilst the mouth is closed. 'Snuffliness' is relatively common due to congestion of small nasal passages and should clear over the first couple of days. Excessive sneezing may indicate drug withdrawal.

Mouth

Observe any asymmetry of the mouth and nasolabial folds suggestive of facial nerve palsy. Note any micrognathia, if present. A cleft lip may be unilateral, bilateral or midline. Assessment of the mouth includes both digital examination and visual inspection of both the soft and hard palate to exclude both submucosal and overt clefts. Palatal clefts may be unilateral, bilateral or midline and may involve the alveolus. A high-arched palate may be present as part of a syndrome such as Pierre Robin syndrome or cranial deformities.

Cyst-like thickenings of the oral epithelium are called 'Epstein's pearls' and may be found on the gums. They are usually but not always in the midline and are of no clinical significance. Congenital teeth are rare but represent the first deciduous teeth and should not be removed unless loose. A bluish swelling on the floor of the mouth is likely to be a mucous retention cyst (ranula) originating from the sublingual or submandibular salivary ducts and requires no treatment. White deposits on the tongue and buccal mucosa may be secondary to milk deposits or from *Candida albicans* infection. Milk deposits are easily scraped away but *Candida* is adherent and tends to bleed on scraping.

The presence of a sublingual frenulum is common but true tongue-tie, where the frenulum is short and restrictive, is rare and may result in feeding difficulties if present.

Hands and feet

Check for a full complement of fingers and toes and for normal palmar creases. Although a single palmar crease is present in 4% of the Caucasian population, it may be associated with chromosomal abnormalities. Ensure there is no syndactyly (joined digits) or polydactyly (extra digits). Polydactyly may be pre-axial (on the radial side) or postaxial (on the ulnar side). Both fused and extra digits are commonly familial but may be associated with dysmorphic syndromes. Rocker-bottom feet may be found in Edwards syndrome (trisomy 18) and other syndromes. Puffiness of the hands and feet ('lymphedema') with hypoplastic nails is seen in Turner syndrome.

RESPIRATORY EXAMINATION

Assess the respiratory rate before handling the infant (Table 8.10). The pattern of respiration in the newborn infant is often irregular with alternating short pauses and relative tachypnoea (periodic breathing). Observe for signs of respiratory distress including subcostal and sternal retractions. Listen for grunting (an expiratory sound and a nonspecific sign of respiratory distress) or stridor (an inspiratory sound indicating a congenital laryngeal problem such as laryngomalacia, tracheal stenosis, webs or cleft, or rarely compression of the larynx by a vascular ring).

Observe any chest deformity. Percussion is never helpful and may distress the baby. Auscultation rarely yields extra information in the absence of respiratory symptoms. Auscultate the chest with the diaphragm of the stethoscope, anteriorly, laterally and posteriorly for symmetry of breath sounds. Crepitations may be present in the hours following birth due to retained lung liquid but should rapidly clear.

CARDIOVASCULAR EXAMINATION

Congenital heart defects affect 7–8 per 1000 live-born infants and account for 3% of all infant deaths and 46% of deaths due to congenital malformations. Early detection can improve the outcome of congenital heart defects,[53] but many infants with significant cardiac defects have normal cardiovascular examinations in the first week of life.[54] Moreover, while the newborn examination identifies around 45% of congenital cardiac disease; one third of affected infants will present with symptoms or noncardiac abnormalities before this examination.[55]

Observe the color of the baby for cyanosis, which may be difficult to see under normal lighting conditions. If in doubt measure the oxygen saturation with a pulse oximeter. Assess perfusion, remembering that it is normal for the hands and feet of a newborn baby to be cold and appear blue (acrocyanosis). Remember that cardiac disease, particularly cardiac failure, may cause tachypnea.

Palpate the precordium for the apex beat, which should be present in the fourth intercostal space around the mid-clavicular line. A parasternal heave and thrill is best felt by the palm of the hand and not the fingers. A heave may lift your hand, and a thrill may be palpable as a vibration.

Auscultate the chest. Measure the heart rate (Table 8.10). Remember that the heart rate varies in response to physical activity and level of alertness. In a newborn baby it may vary between 80 bpm in deep sleep and 160 bpm when crying and active. Listen for heart sounds and murmurs in the suggested positions shown in Figure 8.5.[42] Use both the bell (for low-pitched sounds) at the apex and the diaphragm (for high-pitched sounds) in all positions. Describe the quality and any splitting of the heart sounds as well as any additional heart sounds or murmurs. The second sound is often loud and single shortly after birth but splitting can be detected by around 48 h in most infants. Around 60% of newborn infants will have murmurs in the first few hours of life but many are transient and not related to cardiac pathology. Around 20–54% of murmurs will have structural cardiac disease on echocardiography but many are small ventricular septal defects that close spontaneously in the first few months of infancy.[54,56,57] Innocent murmurs are characterized by a normal clinical examination, normal pulses, soft 1–2/6 systolic murmur heard at the left sternal edge and normal heart sounds with no clicks.[58]

Gently extend the hips and palpate the femoral pulses in each inguinal crease over the femoral triangle with the thumbs. Remember that this may upset a baby and should be left until the end. In restrictive left output conditions such as aortic coarctation or valvular stenosis, femoral pulses may be reduced in volume or difficult to feel. If so, it is mandatory to perform a four-limb blood pressure and refer urgently to a cardiologist. Remember a baby with coarctation may have normal femoral pulses in the first few days due to the presence of a patent ductus arteriosus.

The abdomen should be palpated and the size of the liver measured in the midclavicular line.

Non-invasive measuring of the blood pressure is difficult and often inaccurate in healthy newborn infants. It is seldom part of the routine examination. In sick newborns, intra-arterial blood pressure can be measured accurately.

ABDOMINAL EXAMINATION

The abdomen should be inspected for distension. Mild distension due to recent feeding or swallowed air from crying is not unusual. Owing to lax abdominal musculature, visible bowel loops and diastasis of the rectus sheath are common features. The xiphisternum at the caudal end of the sternum is often clearly visible.

The cord should be inspected to ensure it is clean with no surrounding erythema. The cord separates at around 10 d of age but may still be adherent until 14 d. The three umbilical vessels (one vein and two arteries) may be seen shortly after birth. An isolated single umbilical artery is associated with a marginal increase in the incidence of renal anomalies. However these are almost universally mild and self-limiting, and imaging investigations should only be pursued in the face of other congenital anomalies.[59] An umbilical hernia is common and of little clinical significance. It should be distinguished from an omphalocele, where there is herniation of the abdominal contents through the umbilicus within a sac of peritoneum, and gastroschisis, where an anterior abdominal defect usually to the right of the umbilicus allows protrusion of the gut and intra-abdominal contents. A flare of erythema around the cord may indicate infection (omphalitis).

Superficial and then deep palpation of the abdomen with warmed hands may reveal the presence of masses such as enlarged liver or spleen. If the baby has just fed, be careful not to provoke vomiting. A liver edge up to 2 cm below the costal margin is a normal finding in this age group.

The spleen is not often palpable but in some infants with lax abdominal muscles it may be felt under the ribcage. The spleen of the newborn expands down the left flank rather than towards the right (Fig. 8.11).[42]

The kidneys are often palpable and are best examined using a finger and thumb encircling the flank (Fig. 8.11).[42]

The anus should be patent and not positioned anteriorly. Any nappy dermatitis should be noted. Stool should be inspected if available. Rectal examination is not a part of the routine examination. If clinically indicated it should be carried out by the examiner's well-lubricated fifth finger.

GENITALIA
Boys
Examine the penis for shape and size. It is common for babies to have a degree of phimosis and attempts should not be made to retract the foreskin at this age.

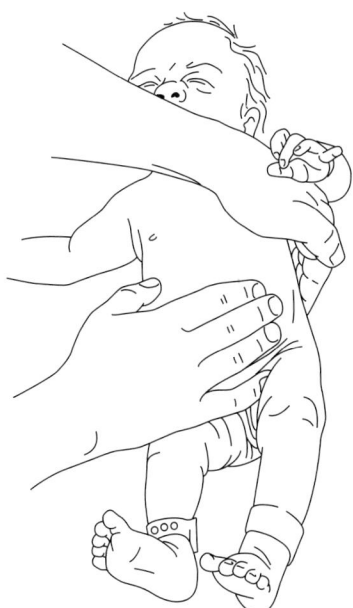

Fig. 8.11 Palpation of the infant spleen/kidney. (From Laing & McIntosh[42] with permission of Baillière Tindall)

The position of the urethral meatus should be noted and should be at the tip of the penis. In hypospadias the meatus is positioned on the ventral surface of the penis. It may be associated with a tethering of the foreskin known as 'chordee'. In epispadias, the urinary outlet is situated on the dorsum of the penis. Abnormal meatal position usually requires surgery and parents should be cautioned not to arrange circumcision, as the foreskin may be required during reconstruction. Ask about or if possible, observe the urinary stream. A poor stream may warrant further investigation for meatal stenosis or posterior urethral valves.

Examine the scrotum and testes. The scrotum should be inspected for evidence of pigmentation. Although common in infants of darker skin color, consideration should always be given to the diagnosis of congenital adrenal hyperplasia. Both testes should be palpable in the scrotum or high in the scrotum outside the inguinal canal. Some testes will be retractile and move from the scrotum to the inguinal canal on stimulation. These can be gently milked along the inguinal canal to the scrotum. The right testis descends later than the left. A unilateral undescended testis is present in 5% of male infants and should descend by around 3 months of age. Bilateral undescended testes warrant further investigation. Testicular torsion, suggested by bluish black discoloration of the scrotum with a hard tender testis, requires urgent surgical attention. A hydrocele may be present after birth. Containing fluid, a hydrocele will transilluminate and may extend superiorly, communicating with the abdominal cavity. It usually resolves over the coming months. Indirect inguinal hernias are also common and warrant surgical referral, particularly where irreducible, when urgent surgical repair is required.

Girls

The labia majora and minora should be separate and not fused. In term infants, the labia minora should be covered by the labia majora and should meet at the anterior aspect of the clitoris. In preterm infants, the labia majora may be underdeveloped and retracted laterally, causing the labia minora to appear more prominent. Labial swellings may indicate the presence of testes. Clitoral enlargement or pigmentation is suggestive of congenital adrenal hyperplasia. Vaginal tags are small remnants of mucosal tissue protruding from the posterior end of the vagina. These are of no clinical significance and regress over the ensuing months. A white mucoid discharge is normal. It is common at the end of the first week of life for a small amount of blood to be passed in response to the withdrawal of maternal hormonal influence (pseudomenses).

NEUROLOGICAL ASSESSMENT

The nervous system of the newborn is in a rapid state of development and any examination must allow not only for any pathological variations but also for the state of maturity of the infant.

Listen to the quality of the cry and assess the consolability of the infant. The infant's behavioral state should be noted.

The posture of a term infant should be flexed and symmetrical, with the knees tucked under the pelvis when prone. A frog-legged posture with abduction of the hips suggests generalized hypotonia. Abnormal posturing of the feet and hands should be noted, e.g. fisting, thumb adduction, big toe extension. Nerve palsies caused by a traction injury during birth may affect the upper roots of the brachial plexus (C5, C6) leading to an Erb's palsy with internal rotation and adduction of the arm with the hand held in a 'waiter's tip' position. Less commonly, the lower roots (C8, T1) are damaged, resulting in a Klumpke's palsy. This affects innervation of the small muscles of the hand and causes weakness of the wrist and finger flexors. A facial nerve palsy may present with asymmetry of the facies, particularly when crying, failure of eyelid closure and difficulty in feeding. Feeding support and lubrication of the eye may be required while the palsy resolves. Most palsies resolve over the ensuing weeks.

All assessments of tone must be performed with the head in the midline so as to avoid elicitation of the asymmetric tonic neck reflex (Fig. 8.12).[42] Tone may vary with the level of alertness and with relation to

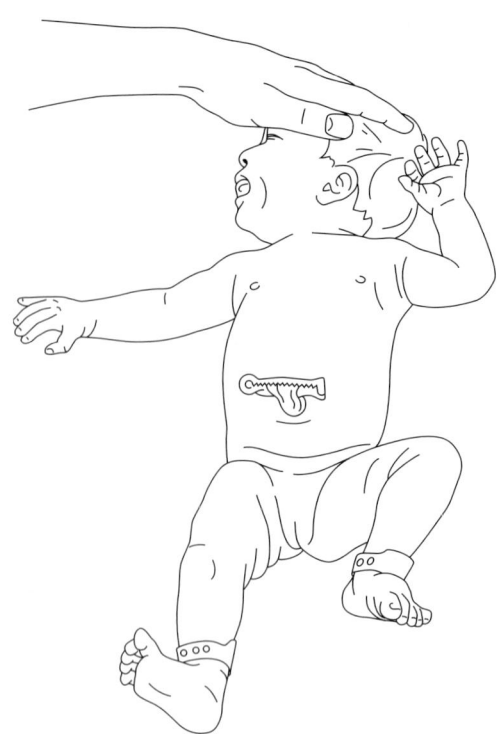

Fig. 8.12 Tonic neck reflex. (From Laing & McIntosh[42] with permission of Baillière Tindall)

feeds. Small-for-gestational-age infants may be relatively hypertonic and hyperalert at birth. Recoil of the limbs may give information about tone. Head lag on arm traction in the pull-to-sit maneuver should be assessed. On sitting supported, the baby should have a curved back and intermittently raise his head. When held prone, some flexion of the limbs against gravity should be present, the head is lifted intermittently in line with the body and truncal tone should be evident. Infants with Down syndrome are almost universally hypotonic. Back and neck arching (opisthotonus), limb extension and stiffness may be features of an intracranial pathology such as meningitis, asphyxia, hemorrhage or kernicterus.

General quality and quantity of spontaneous movements should be observed. The baby should exhibit frequent generalized fluent and alternating movements when awake. Antigravity movements of all limbs should be present, as should strong resistance to passive movement. Intermittent lifting of the head when prone is normal. Around a half of all newborn babies exhibit jitteriness[60] but if this is excessive, it may indicate drug withdrawal, metabolic disturbance or intracranial pathology.

Although not performed routinely, deep tendon reflexes of the knee, ankle and biceps can be elicited in the newborn infant and may be warranted in the face of other neurological abnormality (Table 8.16). These can be performed with a sharp tap of the middle finger or a small patella hammer. The presence of clonus should be noted. Although muscular fasciculation is rare in the newborn infant, it may be visible in the tongue in the presence of anterior horn cell disease.

Sensory examination is limited to withdrawal from tactile stimuli. Painful stimuli should not routinely be inflicted on the normal newborn infant. Vision can be assessed crudely. A baby should open his eyes in a darkened room and screw up his eyes when exposed to bright light. In the first week of life a newborn baby will fix on a human face or red ball at a distance of around 15–25 cm and can follow it horizontally and vertically over a short arc. An intermittent divergent or convergent squint is common in the full-term infant. Roving eye movements, persistent nystagmus and the sun-setting sign are always abnormal. A crude assessment of hearing is the observation that a baby will startle at a loud noise and may be consoled by a quiet calming voice. Universal newborn hearing screening, by elicitation of auditory brainstem-evoked responses or evoked otoacoustic emissions, has recently been introduced across the UK.

Table 8.16   Neonatal reflexes

Primitive reflexes Cranial nerve reflexes (relevant cranial nerves)	How elicited	Time of appearance	Usual time of disappearance of those reflexes that are time limited	Possible significance if abnormal
Sucking (IX, X, XII)	On feeding	Birth	When voluntary control of feeding achieved at 6–9 months	General neurological depression, hypotonia, immaturity or bulbar palsy
Swallowing (IX, X, XII)	On feeding	Birth	When voluntary control of feeding achieved at 6–9 months	General neurological depression, hypotonia, immaturity or bulbar palsy
Rooting (V)	On light contact with infant's cheek the infant turns towards the point of contact	Birth	9 months	General neurological depression, hypotonia, immaturity or bulbar palsy
Glabella (V, VII)	A sharp tap on the glabella produces momentary tight closure of the eyes	Birth	Variable persistence	Apathy or facial palsy if absent; accentuated in hyperexcitability
Head turn to light (II)	With infant supine light from a diffuse source is allowed to fall on one side and then on the other side of the infant's face and he turns his head to the light (the infant must be in a quiet relaxed state)	Several weeks	–	General neurological depression, hypotonia, ?impaired vision
Pupillary (II, also III and V)	Shade one eye with the hand for a moment or two and then withdraw it	Birth	–	General neurological depression, ?impaired vision
Optic blink (II)	Shine a bright light suddenly at the eyes	Birth	–	General neurological depression, ?impaired vision
Doll's eye (III, IV, VI)	Turn head slowly to right or left watching position of eyes (normally eyes do not move with head)	Birth	2 weeks	Ophthalmic muscle palsies (ophthalmoplegia)
Acoustic blink (VIII)	Clap the hands about 30 cm from the infant's head. Avoid producing an air stream across the face. Rapid habituation – no response to test – normally achieved	After a few days	–	?Impaired hearing
Labyrinthine (rotation) (VIII, also III, IV, VII)	(a) Hold baby upright with examiner's hands under infant's arms. Spin round so that baby turns with examiner, first one direction then the other (the head should turn towards direction in which baby is being turned)	Birth	–	Disturbed vestibular function or ophthalmoplegia
	(b) Baby similarly held but head held firmly by examiner's forefinger and middle finger which, on each side, are extended upwards against the side of the baby's head. Similar rotation (the baby's eyes should turn towards the turning direction)			Disturbed vestibular function or ophthalmoplegia
Gag (IX, X, XII)	Touch posterior pharynx, e.g. with spatula	Birth	–	General neurological depression or bulbar palsy
Cough (IX, X, XII)	Generated spontaneously on irritation of the respiratory passages	Weak for several weeks after birth	–	General neurological depression

(Continued)

Table 8.16   Neonatal reflexes—cont'd

Primitive reflexes Cranial nerve reflexes (relevant cranial nerves)	How elicited	Time of appearance	Usual time of disappearance of those reflexes that are time limited	Possible significance if abnormal
Cutaneous reflexes Palmar/foot grasp	Place the examiner's forefinger in the palm/sole of the infant's hand/foot, which then closes round the examiner's finger, maintaining a grip	Birth	2–3 months (palmar), 7–8 months (foot)	General neurological depression, hypotonia: hemisyndromes, Erb palsy or clavicular fracture. May persist beyond normal time in spastic cerebral palsy
Abdominal	Stroke a pin or thumbnail from the side to the center of the abdomen (a response is only possible if muscles are fully relaxed)	7 d	–	Absence does not necessarily imply abnormality
Anal	Contraction of the external anal sphincter when the skin round it is stroked with a pin	Birth	–	Damage to sacral cord (e.g. spina bifida)
Cremaster	Stroking the medial side of the thigh with a pin or thumbnail results in pulling up of the testes	10 d	–	Absent in spinal cord lesion
Withdrawal	On pricking the sole of the foot with a pin there is rapid flexion of the hip, knee and foot	Birth	–	Hemisyndromes; absent or weak in spina bifida and after breech delivery with extended legs
Plantar (Babinski)	Stroking the foot along the lateral side with pin or thumbnail produces dorsal flexion of the big toe and spreading of the other toes in infancy (and plantar flexion of the other toes in older children who are walking). Do not mistake a grasp reflex of the foot for a flexor plantar response	Birth	–	Defects of lower spinal cord, hemisyndromes
Extensor reflexes Asymmetrical tonic neck	With baby in supine position rotate the head to one side. This produces increased tone in, and partial extension of, the arm and leg on the side to which the head is rotated, and there may be flexion of the arm and leg on the contralateral side	1 month	3–5 months	Medullary or spinal cord damage. Readily elicited in immature infant. May persist beyond normal time in cerebral palsy
Crossed extensor reflex	Passively extend one lower limb pressing the knee down, and with a pin stimulate the sole of the foot of this fixated leg. Flexion and slight abduction of the unstimulated lower limb normally occurs	A few days after birth	1 month	Absent in lesions of spinal cord and weak in peripheral nerve damage
Trunk incurvation (Galant)	Stroke a pin or thumbnail along the paravertebral line about 3 cm from the midline from the shoulder to the buttock (the back should curve with the concavity to the stimulated side)	5–6 d	7–8 d	Hemisyndromes; spinal cord damage – with indication of segmental level
Perez	Elicited as for Galant but by stroking over central vertebral spines (the infant arches backwards, the buttocks rise and the anus dilates)	5–6 d	–	As for trunk incurvation reflex
Moro	Hold baby in supine position with shoulders and back supported on left hand and arm of the examiner and head (occiput) on the right hand. Allow the head to fall back suddenly (catching it again with the right hand after it has fallen a short distance) while the rest of the body remains supported. The arms rapidly abduct and come together again with an embracing movement and the legs flex	Birth	2–3 months	General neurological depression, hypotonia. Prolongation of tonic phase of response in immaturity. Hemisyndromes, fractured clavicle or humerus. May persist beyond normal time in cerebral palsy

(Continued)

Table 8.16   Neonatal reflexes—cont'd

Primitive reflexes Cranial nerve reflexes (relevant cranial nerves)	How elicited	Time of appearance	Usual time of disappearance of those reflexes that are time limited	Possible significance if abnormal
Hand opening	Stroke the dorsum of the hand	Birth	2–3 months	General neurological depression; hemisyndrome
Progression Walking/stepping	Hold infant in standing position and place foot on a flat surface. The leg extends to take the infant's weight (supporting reaction), the opposite leg flexes then extends, and as it takes weight the original leg flexes	4 d	2 months	General neurological depression, hypotonia: paresis of lower limbs
Placing	With the baby held upright between the hands of the examiner the dorsal part of the foot is brought lightly in contact with the edge of the table. Normally the baby flexes knee and hip and places foot on the table	4 d	5–9 months	General neurological depression, hypotonia: paresis of lower limbs
Crawling	Infant prone. Crawling movements may occur spontaneously but can be reinforced by the examiner pressing his thumb gently into the sole of the infant's foot (the crawling reflex is more easily elicited in the immature infant than the walking reflex)	4 d	4 months	General neurological depression, hypotonia; paresis of lower limbs
Tendon reflexes Jaw jerk	Sharp tap on the examiner's index finger placed on patient's chin below the lip	2 d	–	Absent in brainstem lesions or 5th cranial nerve damage; exaggerated in hyperexcitability, e.g. hypocalcemia
Biceps	A tap on the examiner's finger placed on the biceps muscle causes contraction of the muscle	2 d	–	Absent in general neurological depression and hypotonia; exaggerated in hyperexcitability
Knee jerk	A tap on the patellar tendon with the knee in the flexed position produces quadriceps contraction	2 d	–	Absent in general neurological depression and hypotonia; exaggerated in hyperexcitability
Ankle	With infant prone, knee slightly flexed and the fore part of the foot held lightly in the examiner's hand a tap over the tendo Achillis produces plantar flexion of the foot (response better felt than seen)	Birth	–	Absent in general neurological depression and hypotonia; exaggerated in hyperexcitability
Ankle clonus	Rapid dorsiflexion of the foot with the examiner's hand on the distal part of the sole produces a succession of rapid contractions of the calf muscle (only briefly sustained in a normal infant)	Birth	–	Absent in general neurological depression and hypotonia; exaggerated in hyperexcitability

Primitive reflexes

The primitive reflexes are detailed in Table 8.16. The value of examination of the primitive reflexes lies in their asymmetry, absence or persistence in certain pathological conditions. Although it is not necessary to conduct the full battery of the reflexes at each newborn examination, it is important to have a working knowledge of the characteristics of each in case of suspected abnormality during examination. Generally, the feeding reflexes (root and suck responses), Moro, palmar and plantar and vestibular reflexes should be assessed at each examination.

Spine and locomotor system

The spine should be inspected with the infant prone, checking that it is straight with no curvature. Examine for evidence of a midline defect such as a meningomyelocele or signs of spina bifida occulta, e.g. midline swelling, dimples, nevi and tufts of hair. Sacral dimples are usually blind-ending pits at the base of the spine that are rarely of significance.[61] A sacral sinus, in persistent communication with the spinal cord, is usually lateral to the midline above S2 and warrants further investigation as it carries a risk of meningitis and may overlie spinal defects.

The limbs should move spontaneously and against gravity. Muscle mass should be appropriate for gestation. Owing to the restriction of movement in utero both the elbows and the knees may have a 30-degree limitation of extension that corrects over the first week. If there is a history of difficult delivery or shoulder dystocia, there may be reduced movement of the arm or callus formation over the clavicle at a few days of age. Babies who were in extended breech position in utero may have fully extended knees for some days after birth.

Examine the hips for developmental dysplasia (DDH). Incidence of this condition varies depending on the screening and classification methods used[62] and is probably around 1.2/1000 live births in the UK. The issues of screening and treatment of DDH are complex and have been reviewed in detail on behalf of the American Academy of Pediatrics.[63] Lay the baby supine on a firm surface (Fig. 8.13).[42] Keep the baby calm and relaxed if possible. If the baby is active or distressed, there will be muscular contraction around the hip that will limit examination. Look at the thighs for symmetry of the creases. Examine each hip separately. Hold the knee and hip flexed and adducted with the middle finger on the greater trochanter and the thumb on the medial aspect of the thigh. Stabilize the pelvis with your other hand. Exert gentle downward and lateral pressure. A clunk may be heard as the hip dislocates out of the acetabulum (Barlow maneuver). The dislocation may reduce spontaneously with relief of downward pressure but may also be reduced with the Ortolani maneuver. In this maneuver, the greater trochanter of the already dislocated hip is relocated into the acetabulum with forward pressure of the middle finger while the hips are being abducted. Established dislocation may also present with limitation of hip abduction. Ligamentous clicks related to the presence of maternal hormones are common and must be distinguished from true instability. Ultrasound screening of the hips is available in some centers but evidence is as yet lacking for its use in universal screening of the newborn.[64]

Examination of the feet for talipes (equinovarus, plantar flexion with medial rotation or calcaneovalgus, lateral rotation of the foot) should be performed. Most cases of talipes are postural deformities only and will resolve with or without gentle manipulation. Talipes may be a result of in utero 'squashing' and can be associated with positional scoliosis, plagiocephaly, 'bat ear' and developmental hip dysplasia.[65] In some cases

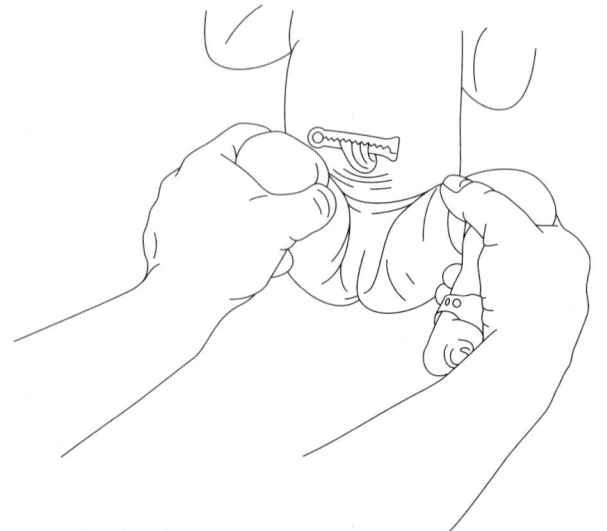

Fig. 8.13 Hip examination. (From Laing & McIntosh[42] with permission of Baillière Tindall)

the deformity cannot be corrected with manipulation and will require orthopedic assessment.

SUMMARY

The quality of information obtained from the newborn examination depends on the skill and diligence of the examiner. This takes practice and patience to achieve. All information should be recorded clearly at the end of the examination and any abnormal findings reported in a simple and sensitive manner to the parents, with supportive written information where possible. A clear plan for follow-up, treatment or specialist referral should be documented and implemented.

GENERAL PRINCIPLES OF COMMON INVESTIGATIONS

INTRODUCTION

Modern medicine has become dominated by the introduction of ever-more sophisticated and expensive tests. Although these may be vital in securing a diagnosis, their sensible use and safe interpretation are crucially dependent on good basic clinical skills. After reaching a hypothesis suggested by careful history taking and thorough examination, the clinician must decide whether laboratory tests or imaging will help in confirming the diagnosis suggested by the signs and symptoms. The decision to order such tests will be influenced in part by the probability and utility of the possible outcomes of the test, which may be invasive or costly.

The probability of the test is the likelihood it will be positive or negative in that particular patient or situation and is usually based on strong clinical research studies. All diagnostic tests can produce false negatives and false positives. The accuracy of a test to diagnose a particular condition can be expressed in terms of its sensitivity and specificity. Sensitivity is the percentage of the test population who has the index condition and are test positive. A very sensitive test will detect most people with the disease but may produce abnormal findings in healthy individuals (false positives). Specificity is defined as the percentage of the test population who are healthy and who test negative. A very specific test may miss the diagnosis in affected patients (false negatives) but is likely to be very accurate when the test is positive.

The utility of a test refers to the worth or value of the outcome and can be objective (measured in monetary terms or expected years of life) or subjective (stated in relation to the anticipated value to the patient or society). Other factors influencing the ordering of investigations will be the availability of the necessary technology and the expertise required to perform and/or interpret the test.

Tests may be reported in terms of qualitative (e.g. yes or no, blood groups) or quantitative results. Quantitative test results are usually referenced against a range produced from results of the same test in the normal healthy population. Such results usually fall within a normal distribution and the normal range represent two SDs either side of the mean, that is, 95% of the population. A healthy member of the normal population will have a 5% chance of a test result that falls outwith this reference range (false positive). Disease populations also have a distribution of test results and sometimes these may overlap with one or other extreme of the normal healthy population (false negative). The larger the difference between the test result and the limits of the normal population, the greater the chance that the test will be truly positive. Indiscriminate testing should be avoided as an increased number of tests will result in more likelihood of a false-positive result being generated. Be guided instead by clinical acumen. A constellation of positive signs and symptoms will increase the prior probability that a chosen test will be abnormal. Therefore the value of a test is determined by the prevalence of the condition in the test population (Baye's theorem). Bayesian analysis dictates that the value of a test is at its best when there is an intermediate pre-test probability of a disease. Although clinicians seldom have such exact statistics available they must be aware of the importance of the integration of clinical information with diagnostic tests.

Samples for investigations should be collected appropriately and responsibly to ensure that test results are an accurate representation of that specific patient. Children particularly will have limited understanding or tolerance of clinician error if a sample has to be repeated.

HOW TO MINIMIZE SPURIOUS RESULTS

- Use the correct container.
- Fill it with the recommended volume.
- Do not shake samples, just mix.
- Label the container with the correct patient details.
- Avoid unnecessary delays in reaching the laboratory.

The following section outlines some of the more common investigations of blood, cerebrospinal fluid and urine; more specialized tests and implications of abnormal results will be discussed in detail in the relevant chapters. All reference ranges are given in Appendix.

Blood

Full blood count and film

Normal blood count values are given in Appendix.

The full blood count and film provide information about:

- red blood cells (number, size, volume, hematocrit, hemoglobin, Hb concentration, morphology);
- white blood cells (number, type, morphology);
- platelets (number and morphology).

Results depend not only on the quality of sampling, as small clots within the sample can affect all parameters, but also on the site of sampling: compared to venous blood, capillary samples tend to overestimate hemoglobin levels, hematocrit and white cell counts, and underestimate platelet counts.[66]

Red blood cells

1. Hemoglobin (Hb): the normal Hb concentration varies through childhood, reaching adult values by 12 years of age. A newborn infant has an Hb concentration of between 150 and 240 g/L. This higher concentration may be caused by the high circulating red cell volume necessary in the relatively hypoxic conditions in the womb. The Hb drops to a nadir of 90–130 g/L after delivery at around 8–12 weeks and gradually increases over the first year of life. The subsequent Hb range in childhood is between 110 and 150 g/L. A similar trend is seen in hematocrit and mean cell volume (see Appendix).

2. The hematocrit (Hct) or packed cell volume (PCV) is a measure of the blood volume occupied by red blood cells. In most laboratories the Hct will be calculated by an automated analyzer. Manually measured hematocrits may still be performed in some centers. As this latter method uses centrifuge to separate the blood into layers of plasma, red cells and white cell/platelets, the hematocrit will always be slightly higher than automated hematocrits, as the degree to which the blood can be separated is limited.
   - In the newborn, a high Hct (a venous Hct > 65%) exists in conditions where there is an excess of red cells secondary to endogenous production (intrauterine growth restriction, infant of a diabetic mother, chromosomal disorders) or to exogenous transfusion (excessive blood transfusion, twin–twin transfusion syndrome, delayed cord clamping).
   - In older children, polycythemia is seen in dehydration, cyanotic heart disease, chronic hypoxia, following renal transplant and in association with some rare tumors (pheochromocytoma, cerebellar hemangioblastoma). Polycythemia vera (primary polycythemia) is very rare in children.
   - A low Hct may be due to dilution, blood loss, increased destruction or decreased production of red cells.

3. The 'mean cell volume' (MCV) is the average volume of the cells, measured in femtoliters (fl). Apart from in early infancy, where the size of the red blood cells is larger (90–125 fl), the mean cell volume in childhood is around 75–90 fl. Anemia may be classified as microcytic or macrocytic depending on this value.
   - Anemia with a low MCV suggests failure of Hb synthesis, commonly secondary to iron deficiency anemia but may also be due to chronic disease or hemolysis. Measurement of serum iron, transferrin and ferritin may help to distinguish between these causes.
   - Anemia with a high MCV suggests failure of DNA synthesis and is seen in conditions resulting in B_{12} or folate deficiency.

White blood cell count

The total white cell count (WCC) is a summation of the various white cell subgroups including neutrophils, lymphocytes, basophils, eosinophils and monocytes. It is measured in the number of cells per liter. Neutrophils and lymphocytes make up around 90–95% of the total white cell count but the relative proportion of each of these subgroups varies throughout childhood. The WCC is high at birth, with a predominance of neutrophils, and falls to normal values of $6–15 \times 10^9$/L in the subsequent days. Lymphocytes decrease during the first few days of life and then increase until the second week. Thereafter the lymphocyte is the predominant white cell, making up 60% of the total white cell population until mid-childhood, when the neutrophil is predominant. An excessive increase of any of the white cell subgroups may indicate a hematological malignancy:

- A raised neutrophil count is indicative of bacterial infection and is rarely secondary to stress or leukemia. Steroids may also increase circulating neutrophils.
- Neutropenia is commonly seen in viral infections, but may also be seen in severe sepsis, cyclical neutropenia and bone marrow suppression. In the newborn period it is observed in infants with severe intrauterine growth restriction and in growing premature infants.
- A lymphocytosis may be seen in viral infections, pertussis and leukemias.
- Eosinophils are typically raised in allergic conditions and parasitic infections.
- An increase in monocytes is seen in chronic inflammation and in granulomatous diseases.

Platelet count

Platelets are measured as the number per liter. The platelet count is constant throughout life at around $150–450 \times 10^9$/L.

- Thrombocytosis (platelet count $> 450 \times 10^9$/L) is a feature of infection, hemorrhage, Kawasaki disease, malignancy (lymphoma, neuroblastoma, acute megakaryocytic leukemia), anemia (iron/vitamin E deficiency) and also occurs post-splenectomy.
- Thrombocythemia is a sustained platelet elevation over 800×10^9/L. The principal stimulation of platelet production, thrombopoietin, is raised in inflammatory disorders as part of the acute phase reaction, and thrombocythemia is a common feature of such conditions. Essential or primary thrombocythemia is very rare in children.
- Thrombocytopenia is defined as a platelet count of less than 100×10^9/L. The commonest cause is a clot in the sample or poor sampling technique. Always repeat the sample before treatment if the result is unexpected. Any patient with a confirmed thrombocytopenia should have a coagulation profile measured. Thrombocytopenia may be due to blood loss, increased destruction (infection, disseminated intravascular coagulation, immune thrombocytopenia), decreased production (infection, congenital platelet disorders, asphyxia, drugs or marrow infiltration) or sequestration (hypersplenism). In the infant with intrauterine growth restriction, thrombocytopenia may occur secondary to decreased production (lineage steal[67]) or increased platelet consumption (placental vascular disease[68]).

Blood film

Microscopic examination of a film will inform about cell morphology and may reveal:

- abnormal cell forms such as Howell-Jolly bodies (damaged or absent spleen);
- sickle cells (HbS hemoglobinopathy);
- spherocytes (autoimmune hemolytic anemia, hereditary spherocytosis, sepsis);
- Heinz bodies (enzyme deficiencies);
- target cells (iron deficiency, hemoglobinopathies, post splenectomy)
- schistocytes and fragments (burns, prosthetic heart valves, disseminated intravascular coagulation (DIC), microangiopathy) coarse basophilic stippling of red cells (lead poisoning);
- reticulocytes (immature red blood cells seen in response to hemorrhage or hemolysis).

Occasionally films will be stained specifically to look for parasites such as malaria and microfilaria.

Coagulation screen

The clotting cascade and abnormalities thereof are described in detail in Chapter 23. Reference values for newborn infants and older children are given in Chapter 39, Appendices. Attention to optimal sampling is important, as activation of clotting during traumatic or lengthy sampling is common and samples taken from indwelling lines are frequently contaminated with heparin. A routine coagulation screen consists of measurements of the prothrombin time (PT), activated partial thromboplastin time (APTT), fibrinogen and fibrin degradation products (FDPs) or D-dimers. An abnormal coagulation screen may prompt further tests such as the thrombin time, bleeding time and levels of specific factors. Both the PT and APTT are compared against simultaneous control samples using the same methodology. The PT and PTT remain normal until factor levels drop to about 25–40% depending on the reagents used.[69] The PT and PTT measure the time to fibrin clot formation and as such, neither test will detect even severe deficiency of factor XIII, which is responsible for covalent cross-linking of the fibrin mesh.

Prothrombin time. The PT

- measures the generation of thrombin after the addition of tissue factor in vitro;
- tests the integrity of the extrinsic and common pathways (factors I, II, V, VII, X);
- may also be used to monitor warfarin therapy and assess liver damage.

Activated partial thromboplastin time. The APTT

- measures the generation of thrombin after the addition of contact-activating factor (e.g. kaolin, silica);
- tests the integrity of the intrinsic and common pathways (factors I, II, V, VIII, IX, X, XI, XII);
- can be used to monitor treatment effects of heparin.

In prolongation of the APTT, a 'mix' is often performed to distinguish between the presence of an 'inhibitor' (such as heparin or other anticoagulant) and a factor deficiency. The patient's plasma is mixed 50:50 with normal plasma. If the abnormality of APTT does not disappear, the patient's plasma is likely to contain an inhibitor. If the mix results in at least partial correction of the APTT, a factor deficiency is more likely.

Fibrinogen. Fibrinogen (Factor I) is a protein synthesized in the liver and normally has a concentration between 1.5 and 4.0 g/L. Low levels are seen in liver disease, in disseminated intravascular coagulation and in preterm infants. As fibrinogen is required in the final stage of coagulation, in converting thrombin (IIa) to fibrin (Ia), a low fibrinogen (0.6–0.8 g/L) will also result in prolonged PT and APTT.

Fibrin degradation products (FDPs) or D-Dimers. Both types of fragments result from the breakdown of a cross-linked fibrin mesh by plasmin and are increased in DIC and in the presence of large thromboses. An abnormal coagulation screen may be due to:

1. poor sampling;
2. decreased or abnormal factor production:
   - vitamin K deficiency, malabsorption, liver disease, warfarin;
   - hemophilias A, B and von Willebrand disease.
3. antagonism – heparin, lupus anticoagulant;
4. consumption or blood loss – DIC (including hemolytic uremic syndrome), sepsis, large thrombosis or hemorrhage.

Blood cultures

Blood cultures should always be taken as a sterile procedure to minimize contamination with skin commensals. In the newborn, the optimal specimen volume is around 1 ml, as lower volumes may be inadequate to detect low colony–count sepsis.[70] In extremely low-birth-weight infants however, consideration must be given to whether improved blood culture yield justifies the risk of a relatively large blood sample. In older children, 2–10 ml blood is desirable, although it is always worth culturing smaller volumes because high levels of bacteremia (>1000 CFU/ml of blood) are found in some infants. In blood-borne infections, there is seeding of bacteria at a fairly constant rate. In other infections, transient seeding of organisms from a focus of infection, such as an abscess, is followed around 45 min later with pyrexia. Organisms grown from blood that has been sampled from intravascular catheters may represent commensals instead of true line infection.

Blood should be collected into a bottle with specific media for growing aerobic and non-aerobic organisms. The bottle is then incubated for 48 h. In modern systems, colorimetric carbon dioxide sensors measure microbial growth and an alarm is activated. The sample can then be Gram stained, cultured on appropriate bacteria medium and sensitivity to various antibiotics is assessed. Some bacteria such as *Mycobacteria* require specialist and prolonged culture.

Urea, electrolytes and creatinine

Fluid and electrolyte disturbances are detailed in Chapter 17. Assessment of urea and electrolytes should be made in association with other parameters of hydration and renal function including clinical signs of hydration, blood pressure, measures of end-organ perfusion (level of consciousness, temperature, urinary output, assessment of skin perfusion), weight and acid-base status. Supplementary information from paired urinary and plasma osmolality, urinalysis and urinary electrolytes may be useful. It is important to have an appreciation of the age-dependent variations in body water distribution and renal function.

Sodium

Sodium is predominantly an extracellular cation. The plasma sodium is a measure of body water as well as intravascular sodium, particularly in the newborn infant, where plasma sodium is a proxy of hydration. Sodium diffuses freely between the body compartments but the activity of the Na^+/K^+ ATPase transport mechanism means that it remains mainly in the extracellular compartment. The regulation of plasma sodium is closely related to water, which is regulated by antidiuretic hormone acting on the renal collecting ducts. Control over absorption and excretion of sodium is primarily by the renin-angiotensin system prompted by changes in perfusion pressure at the renal juxtaglomerular apparatus. Plasma sodium values are influenced by poor sampling technique: hemolyzed samples will have artificially low sodium.

Hyponatremia (Na < 135 mmol/L) may be due to:

- decreased total body sodium (congenital adrenal hyperplasia, diarrhea, vomiting);
- normal total body sodium and increased body water (syndrome of inappropriate antidiuretic hormone, water intoxication, excessive hypotonic infusions, acute renal failure);
- increased total body sodium and greater retention of water (cardiac failure, nephrotic syndrome, cirrhosis).

It may be difficult to determine which of these causes is responsible and the child will need careful clinical assessment with weighing, acid-base balance, paired urine and plasma electrolytes and osmolality (Table 8.17).

Hypernatremia (Na >150 mmol/L) may be due to:

- sodium loss with greater loss of water (dehydration due to vomiting, diarrhea);

Table 8.17   Additional tests in the investigation of hyponatremia

	Renal failure	Adrenocortical failure	Inappropriate ADH	Hemodilution	RTA
Serum K (mmol/L)	> 5.5	> 5.5	<4	<4	<4
Urine osmolality (mosm/L)	–	–	high	low	low
Blood osmolality (mosm/L)	–	–	low	low	n
Urine/blood osmolality	< 1.1	> 1.1	>2	<1.1	–
Urine Na (mmol/L)	> 20	> 20	n or ↑	n or ↓	↑
Urine Na/K	> 1.5	> 1.5	n	n	n
Blood pH	–	–	–	–	< 7.2
Urine pH	–	–	–	–	> 5.6

RTA, renal tubular acidosis; ADH, antidiuretic hormone.

- normal total body sodium with water loss (fever, radiant heaters, diabetes insipidus, poor breast-feeding);
- increased total body sodium (hyperosmolar feeds, excessive sodium supplementation).

Potassium

Potassium is also freely diffusible across cell membranes but the active transport mechanism means that it is predominantly an intracellular cation. Plasma potassium may not reflect total body levels, as there may be considerable flux between the body compartments. For example, insulin and alkalosis may result in low plasma potassium due to an intracellular influx, whereas the reverse is seen in acidosis and drugs such as digoxin and beta-blockers. Despite its mainly intracellular presence, small changes in plasma potassium concentration can have major changes in membrane excitability. Renal excretion of potassium is dependent on renal tubular function, urine flow rate and aldosterone.

Hypokalemia (K^+ < 3.5 mmol/L) occurs with:

- persistent vomiting, diarrhea, or alkalosis;
- diabetic ketoacidosis;
- rarely due to diuretic therapy, renal tubular defects and endocrine disturbances such as Cushing disease and hyperaldosteronism.

Hyperkalemia (K^+ >6.5 mmol/L) may be factitious due to in vitro hemolysis. True hyperkalemia where there is elevation of total body potassium occurs:

- in renal failure (decreased excretion);
- following increased load (crush injuries, hemolysis, gastrointestinal hemorrhage or tumor lysis syndrome);
- occasional causes include massive hemolysis, congenital adrenal hyperplasia and drugs such as spironolactone, and angiotensin-converting inhibitors.

Urea

Urea is a nontoxic substance made by the liver as a means of clearing ammonia from protein metabolism. Urea is filtered by the glomerulus. If the glomerular filtrate is flowing slowly through the proximal tubule, urea tends to be passively reabsorbed and returns to the bloodstream. By itself it is a poor marker of renal excretory function.

Uremia may be due to:

- increased protein catabolism from high protein diets, severe physiological stress or gastrointestinal bleeding;
- impaired kidney function: pre-renal (underperfusion of the kidney), renal (intrinsic renal tubular or glomerular pathology), or post-renal (obstruction to urinary flow);
- contraction of the extracellular compartment in dehydration.

Laboratory differentiation of these causes is detailed in Chapter 17. A decreased plasma urea is seen in:

- low protein states (e.g. starvation, malabsorption);
- severe liver disease;
- overhydration.

Creatinine

Creatinine is the most commonly used way of assessing the excretory function of the kidneys. This breakdown product of creatine and phosphocreatinine is released from skeletal muscle at a steady rate. Serum creatinine correlates with the percentage of skeletal muscle mass and as such may be higher in boys than girls. Creatinine is filtered freely by the glomerulus, and a small amount is also secreted into the glomerular filtrate by the proximal tubule. However due to this tubular secretion, creatinine will overestimate glomerular filtration rate (GFR) at low filtration rates and as such elevated serum creatinine alone is an insensitive index of decreased GFR. More accurate estimations of renal function in children can be derived from various formulae that use height, creatinine and a constant to calculate the GFR.[71,72]

In children, increased creatinine is seen commonly in:

- impaired kidney function;
- massive tissue trauma, e.g. crush injuries and burns.

Ingestion of cooked meat and vigorous exercise may cause a temporary increase in creatinine.

Glucose

The normal range of blood glucose concentration is lower in the newborn compared to the child. The newborn infant undergoes a process of extrauterine adaptation during which the brain relies on ketones and lactate for fuel while glycogenolysis and gluconeogenesis are switched on. As such newborn infants appear to tolerate lower levels of hypoglycemia than older children. The exception may be those infants whose ketogenic potential may be impaired due to growth restriction or prematurity, or where ketogenesis is switched off due to hyperinsulinism. Although controversy exists as to the definition of neonatal hypoglycemia that requires treatment ('operational threshold'), it has been shown that at levels below 2.6 mmol/L, acute alteration of cerebral physiology may occur.[73] However, many healthy full-term infants appear clinically asymptomatic when hypoglycemic. There is little information about the long-term sequelae of transient neonatal hypoglycemia to dictate acute management. Clinicians should be guided by the infant's clinical status and the potential of a particular child to generate alternative brain fuels.[74] In the older child, blood glucose concentrations between 4.5 and 6 mmol/L indicate good glucose homeostasis.

Plasma or serum is the preferred sample for laboratory measurement whereas whole-blood methods are used in point-of-care testing. However whole-blood samples may be affected by hematocrit or skin-cleansing agents, and are generally 10–18% lower than plasma samples.[75]

Hypoglycemia is seen in:

- hyperinsulinism (exogenous insulin, islet cell adenomas or hyperplasia, oral hypoglycemic agents, infant of a diabetic mother);
- decreased glucose production (inherited metabolic conditions);
- decreased fuels and fuel stores (fasting, malnutrition, malabsorption, small-for-gestational age infants);

Table 8.18   Normal blood gas values in children (see Chapter 12 for newborn values)

	pH	pCO_2 (kPa)	pO_2 (kPa)	Base excess (mmol/l)	HCO_3^- (mmol/l)
Arterial blood	7.38–7.45	4.5–6.3	11.3–14.0	+2.5 to –2.5	23–27
Venous blood	7.35–7.40	6.0–7.6	Variable	+2.5 to –2.5	24–29

- inadequate counter-regulatory hormones (growth hormone or cortisol deficiency);
- increased fuel demand (fever, exercise).

Hyperglycemia (> 7 mmol/L after a 4-hour fast) is seen:
- commonly in children with diabetes mellitus;
- in high-stress conditions, e.g. in sepsis and following cardiovascular collapse;
- in the extreme preterm infant receiving i.v. nutrition (hyperglycemia may be due to decreased insulin production and impairment of end-organ sensitivity).

Blood gas analysis

Acid-base balance in the newborn is discussed in Chapter 12 and in older children in Chapter 17. Normal values in well children are shown in Table 8.18. Blood gas analyses are usually performed on arterial or capillary samples.

Hydrogen ion concentration is precisely regulated by three systems that act to prevent excessive changes in pH:

1. the chemical acid–base buffer systems of the body fluid that combine with acid or base. The bicarbonate buffer system is the most important, but others include the phosphate and the protein (important intracellularly) buffer systems;
2. the respiratory center that regulates removal of CO_2, and therefore H_2CO_3;
3. the kidneys, which can excrete acid or alkaline urine.

Low pH values indicate acidosis, and high values, alkalosis. Both these extremes may have respiratory or metabolic causes (Table 8.19). pCO_2 and pO_2 values indicate the success of gas exchange at the alveolar–capillary interface. The metabolic component (the base excess or bicarbonate level) is calculated by allowing for the effect of pCO_2 on the pH, i.e. any change unexplained by the pCO_2 indicates a metabolic abnormality.

Metabolic acid is any acid in the body except carbonic acid. Such acids are not respirable and need to be neutralized, metabolized or excreted via the kidney. The base excess (BE) refers to the amount of acid required to return the blood pH to normal (pH 7.38–7.45) and is measured in mmol/L. The relationship between bicarbonate and metabolic acidosis is not consistent or linear and therefore the base excess is considered the best measure of the metabolic disturbance.

Metabolic acidosis may be due to loss of base or gain of acid. Calculation of the anion gap may help to differentiate the two. The anion gap represents the difference between serum anions and cations and is calculated by the following equation:

$$\text{Anion gap} = (Na^{++}\ K^+)^- (Cl^-\ \text{and}\ HCO_3^-)$$

The difference is usually 12 mmol/L (range 8–16 mmol/L). In metabolic acidosis secondary to bicarbonate loss, the anion gap will be normal as Cl^- rises proportionally. An acidosis secondary to accumulation of an anion such as lactic acid will have an increased anion gap (Table 8.19).

Table 8.19   Causes of acid–base disturbance

	Acidosis (pH <7.35)	Alkalosis (pH >7.45)
Respiratory	pCO_2 > 6.5 kPa Respiratory failure – severe asthma – pneumothorax – blocked airway – pulmonary edema – poor respiratory drive	pCO_2 < 4.5 kPa Hyperventilation – hysteria, excessive crying – iatrogenic – early salicylate poisoning – brainstem dysfunction Hyperammonemia
Metabolic	BE < –4 mmol/L Increased anion gap Lactic acidosis – hypoxia – prolonged exercise – poor tissue perfusion due to sepsis, hypovolemia, anaphylaxis – primary lactic acidosis, defects of gluconeogenesis, fatty acid oxidation Ketoacidosis – diabetes mellitus – organic and branched chain amino acidemias Impaired renal handling of H^+ – renal failure – renal tubular acidosis type 1 Ingestion of excess salicylate, ethanol, methanol, ethylene glycol Normal anion gap Loss of bicarbonate – diarrhea – renal tubular acidosis type 2 – intestinal fistulae	BE > + 4 mmol/L Loss of acid (e.g. H^+, K^+) – pyloric stenosis – recurrent vomiting – diuretic therapy Gain of bicarbonate – secondary to over-replacement in metabolic acidosis

Cerebrospinal fluid

As sampling of the cerebrospinal fluid (CSF) is an invasive procedure with risks of infection and cardiorespiratory compromise, it is essential that consideration is given to the extent of investigations required to confirm the suspected diagnosis, so that repeat punctures are not required. Prior liaison with microbiologists and biochemists may be advisable if unusual conditions are suspected. Traumatic taps are common, affecting at least 15–20% of all pediatric lumbar punctures and can make interpretation of findings difficult.[76] Trauma may be caused to the lumbar veins by introducing the needle too far during the procedure. Having an experienced assistant to hold the child as well as a skilled clinician performing the procedure may optimize the chances of obtaining noncontaminated CSF.

Color

The color of normal CSF is clear. Yellow discoloration (xanthochromia) is seen in the presence of old hemorrhage and in hyperbilirubinemia. Blood from a traumatic puncture may contaminate the initial drops of CSF, or uniformly blood-stained CSF may be due to intracranial hemorrhage. The color may be hazy, turbid or frankly purulent in meningitis.

Glucose

The CSF glucose level should be at least 60% of the simultaneous blood glucose level. If it is lower, this indicates that glucose is being utilized by constituents within the CSF such as bacteria, or white and red cells. It is characteristically very low in tuberculous meningitis and often normal in viral meningitis. Normal glucose levels do not rule out infection, because up to 50% of patients who have bacterial meningitis will have normal CSF glucose levels.

Protein

Protein in the CSF is dependent on age (it may be as high as 2500–3000 mg/L in the newborn), the presence of blood (intracranial hemorrhage, traumatic tap) or other cells (white cells, bacteria, liquefying brain tissue). Normal childhood values are around 150–450 mg/L after infancy.

Microscopy

Microscopic examination of the CSF will ascertain the number of white cells and red cells in the sample of CSF and whether there are any organisms present. It is important to remember however that the CSF may be normal in early infection. Do not try and distinguish bacterial and viral meningitis on the basis of clinical or preliminary CSF findings. If CSF findings are suggestive of viral meningitis, treat with antibiotics until it is proven 'culture-negative'.

White cells should be less than 5/mm³ but in the full-term newborn on the first day of life, values of up to 30/mm³ may be normal. Preterm infants may have white cell counts in excess of 30/mm³. An excess of white cells is suggestive of infection. Cytospin and subsequent staining may give information as to the subgroup of white cell present. Although neutrophils predominate in bacterial meningitis, lymphocytes may be the predominant cell in the newborn period, and in partially treated meningitis or Listeria monocytogenes meningitis.

Increased numbers of red and white cells are commonly seen in a traumatic tap and following intracranial hemorrhage. As many as 20% of pediatric lumbar punctures may be traumatic. As such it is conventional to correct the number of white cells depending on the number of red cells seen: 1 white cell allowed for every 500 red cells in the CSF.[77] The accuracy of this method is disputed however, as the ratio may vary depending on the peripheral white cell count. Taking this into consideration, some assume that the ratio of white blood cells to red blood cells in the peripheral blood remains constant when peripheral blood is introduced into the subarachnoid space. Therefore, the expected or predicted CSF white cells can be calculated on the basis of the peripheral blood count and the CSF red cells. This predicted white cell value can then be subtracted from the actual or observed CSF WBC. A true increase in CSF

white cells exists when the observed CSF white cell count is greater than the predicted count. Debate exists as to whether or not this is any more reliable as a predictor of the presence or absence of infection. In fact some have found a reduction in the observed white cell count compared to the predicted, and have postulated that white cells may adhere to the meninges or may undergo lysis on transport.[78]

Morphology and Gram staining characteristics will give a clue as to the nature of any organism, but the Gram stain can be affected by laboratory techniques and expertise, as well as bacteria load. The CSF Gram stain has a sensitivity of between 60% and 92% in children not treated previously with antibiotics.[79,80] Cytospin may increase the ability to detect bacteria, especially in partially treated or very early meningitis, when numbers of bacteria may be low. Culture of the organism is required for definitive diagnosis but antibiotic treatment prior to lumbar puncture can decrease the sensitivity. The common central nervous system pathogens are Group B Streptococcus (Gram-positive coccus), Streptococcus pneumoniae (Gram-positive coccus), Neisseria meningitides (Gram-negative diplococcus), Haemophilus influenzae (Gram-negative bacillus), Escherichia coli (Gram-negative bacillus) and Listeria monocytogenes (Gram-positive bacillus).

The polymerase chain reaction (PCR) has superseded latex agglutination techniques in the diagnosis of meningitis. PCR is fast, has high sensitivity and specificity for many central nervous system infections, and requires only small volumes of CSF. PCR has been especially useful in the diagnosis of viral meningitis, where it has a very high sensitivity for herpes simplex virus type 1, Epstein Barr virus, cytomegalovirus, varicella zoster virus and enterovirus.[81,82] In bacterial meningitis, PCR is in common usage for diagnosis of N. meningitides, H. influenzae, Streptococci, Listeria and E. coli,[83,84] particularly when antibiotics have been started prior to lumbar puncture.

Urine

Urine for culture should be collected by an optimal method:
- Clean catch and mid-stream specimens and suprapubic aspiration of urine are the methods least likely to be contaminated by organisms from the perineum.
- The bag method is highly prone to contamination and the bag is uncomfortable to remove. It should therefore never be used for culture and only for collection of urine for metabolic analysis, output measurements or for estimation of electrolytes.
- Urine for microscopy must be refrigerated. If it cannot be examined promptly; delays of more than 2 h between collection and examination often cause unreliable results.

Microscopy

Microscopy of urine yields important information as to the presence of cells, casts, crystals and micro-organisms.

Leucocytes

Counts of fewer than 3 white cells/mm³ of uncentrifuged urine or 5 white cells/high power field of centrifuged urine are normal. Usually, the cells are granulocytes. Higher numbers (pyuria) may be present in urinary tract infection but are also common in any pyrexial illness and in the presence of renal calculi. In 30% of urinary tract infections, there are no or only a few white blood cells in the urine. Most of these are in children with recurrent infections.

Red cells

Normal values are fewer than 3 red cells/mm³ of uncentrifuged urine or 2 red cells/high power field of centrifuged urine. As well as identifying red cells, microscopy may also reveal red cell casts and dysmorphic red cells that have odd shapes because of their passage through an abnormal glomerulus. Such odd-shaped erythrocytes suggest glomerular disease. Hematuria may be microscopic only or macroscopic, and may originate from anywhere in the renal tract. Glomerular and tubular causes are often associated with significant proteinuria, whereas infection, tumors and calculi are less so. Exercise-induced hematuria is relatively common, benign and self-limiting. Red cells may also be found following bladder procedures.

Epithelial cells

Epithelial cells originating from the renal tubule are usually present in the urine in small numbers. However, in nephrotic syndrome and in conditions leading to tubular degeneration, they are seen in greater quantity and typically contain oval fat bodies.

Casts

Casts in the urinary sediment may help to localize disease to a specific location in the genitourinary tract. Urinary casts are formed only in the distal convoluted tubule or the collecting duct during periods of urinary concentration or stasis or when the urinary pH is very low. The proximal convoluted tubule and loop of Henle are not locations for cast formation. The predominant cellular elements determine the type of cast:

- Hyaline casts are composed primarily of a mucoprotein (Tamm-Horsfall protein) secreted by tubule cells. It is found in pyelonephritis and chronic renal disease, but may be a normal finding, especially in pyrexial illnesses or following exercise;
- Red blood cell casts – indicative of glomerulonephritis or severe tubular damage. May be present following strenuous activity or renal trauma;
- White blood cell casts are most typical for acute pyelonephritis, but they may also be present with glomerulonephritis. Their presence indicates renal inflammation because such casts will not form outside the kidney;
- Granular casts – seen in acute and chronic renal failure;
- Epithelial casts – suggest tubular damage and are found in acute tubular necrosis, interstitial nephritis and nephritic syndrome;
- Fatty casts – lipid-laden renal tubule casts found in nephritic syndrome.

Crystals

Occasional crystals of triple phosphate, uric acid or calcium oxalate are common and usually of no significance. However they may be present in larger amounts in hyperuricemia, cystinuria or in *Proteus* infection. More unusually, crystals such as cystine (in urine of neonates with congenital cystinuria), tyrosine (congenital tyrosinosis) or leucine (maple syrup urine disease) may be seen. All of these rare forms may be observed in the urine of children with severe liver disease.

Bacteria

Bacteria are not an unusual finding in urine because of the large number of commensals around the urethral meatus in both boys and girls. Bacteria in urine specimens will also rapidly multiply in room temperature. Gram stain of uncentrifuged urine has a sensitivity of 93% and specificity of 95% for urinary tract infection on a recent meta-analysis:[85]

- The presence of any organism from a suprapubic aspirate should be considered significant.
- Culture of urine should follow microscopy of urine.
- Generally, more than 100 000/ml of one organism is defined as significant bacteriuria.
- Mixed organisms are suggestive of contamination.

Urinalysis

Urinalysis is performed by a variety of bedside testing methods. Dipsticks will test a sample of urine for specific gravity, pH, glucose, blood, protein, ketones, leukocyte esterase and nitrites. Dipstick testing is notorious for false negatives and false positives in the presence of specific medications and various urinary characteristics.[86]

Specific gravity

Specific gravity (SG) is the ratio of the weight of a volume of urine to a similar volume of water. Because of their weight, glucose and protein can affect the SG. The SG of urine is a proxy for its osmolality and should be between 1005 and 1030. As well as reflecting the hydration of the patient, it is also a measure of the concentrating ability of the kidneys. Dipsticks estimate SG poorly and more accurate estimation requires visualization of urine on a refractometer.

Lower SG values indicate dilute urine and may be due to:

- high fluid intake;
- diabetes insipidus;
- diuretics;
- impaired renal function.

High SG values indicate concentrated urine and are found in:

- dehydration;
- syndrome of inappropriate secretion of antidiuretic hormone;
- glycosuria.

Urinary pH

The normal pH of urine is 4.6–8.0 depending on diet and acid-base status. Acidification takes place in the renal tubule and the collecting ducts.

Alkaline urine (pH > 8) is found in:

- *Proteus* or *Pseudomonas* urinary tract infections;
- respiratory alkalosis;
- renal tubular acidosis (RTA);
- normokalemic metabolic acidosis.

Acidic urine (pH < 4.6) is found in:

- other urinary tract infections;
- respiratory and metabolic acidosis (not RTA).

Glycosuria

Plasma glucose is filtered in the glomerulus but almost all of it is reabsorbed in the proximal convoluted tubule, such that less than 0.1% of glucose normally filtered by the glomerulus appears in urine (<130 mg/24 h). Glycosuria is found when the filtered glucose is in excess of the reabsorptive capabilities of the tubule:

- in hyperglycemia (commonly diabetes mellitus);
- in the premature infant who typically has a low renal threshold for glucose;
- in Fanconi's syndrome where there is proximal tubule dysfunction.

Dipsticks employing the glucose oxidase reaction for screening (Clinistix) are specific for glucose but can miss other reducing sugars such as galactose, lactose, pentose and fructose. These sugars are best detected with the Clinitest (a modified Benedict's copper reduction test) but positive results may also be obtained in the presence of glucuronates, cephalosporins and vitamin C. In the case of a positive result, chromatography will confirm the presence and type of sugar.

Hematuria

A positive dipstick for blood may indicate hematuria, myoglobinuria or hemoglobinuria. Microscopy is required to distinguish hematuria from other conditions.

Proteinuria

Only low-molecular-weight plasma proteins are filtered at the glomerulus and most are reabsorbed by the renal tubule. However, a small amount of filtered plasma protein and protein secreted by the distal tubule (Tamm-Horsfall protein) can be found in normal urine. Dipsticks are impregnated with tetrabromophenol blue, which changes color according to the amount of protein present in the urine. This reagent is sensitive to albumin but may not detect low concentrations of gamma globulins and Bence Jones proteins, which require other diagnostic methods. Alkaline and highly concentrated urines may result in false positives whereas acidic, dilute urines may prove to be falsely negative.

Normal total protein excretion does not usually exceed 4 mg/h/m^2 in the child in any single specimen. More than 150 mg/d is defined as 'proteinuria'. Proteinuria more than 40 mg/h/m^2 is severe and known as 'nephrotic syndrome'. The majority of patients with proteinuria on dipstick testing will not have significant renal disease.

Proteinuria may result from:

- increased glomerular permeability (glomerulonephritis, congenital nephrosis);
- impaired tubular reabsorption (Fanconi syndrome, acute tubular necrosis, interstitial nephritis);
- orthostatic or postural proteinuria – a benign condition that results from prolonged periods of standing; it is confirmed by obtaining a negative urinalysis result after 8 h in supine position;
- transient proteinuria may be found in pyrexial illness and following vigorous exercise;
- dipstick tests for trace amounts of protein yield positive results at concentrations of 5–10 mg/100 ml – lower than the threshold for clinically significant proteinuria. A result of 1+ corresponds to approximately 30 mg of protein per 100 ml and is considered positive; 2+ corresponds to 100 mg/100 ml, 3+ to 300 mg/100 ml, and 4+ to 1000 mg/100 ml.

Although dipsticks are sensitive in detecting proteinuria, accurate measurement requires a 24-hour urine collection. In small children this may not be practicable and a random single sample estimation of urinary protein/creatinine ratio may give useful information more easily.[87]

Ketones

Acetone, acetoacetic acid and beta-hydroxybutyric acid resulting from either diabetic ketosis or other forms of calorie deprivation (starvation), are easily detected with dipsticks containing sodium nitroprusside.

Leukocyte esterase and nitrites

Leukocyte esterase (LE) is an enzyme produced by neutrophils and a positive test indicates pyuria. Pyuria occurs in a variety of conditions including infection, inflammation, pyrexial illness and malignancy. Nitrites are formed in the urine from the conversion of nitrates by bacteria. A positive result indicates bacteria present in amounts of 10^4/ml or greater but a negative result does not rule out infection. Negative results are common in infants where frequent voiding may preclude bacterial nitrate reduction and in infections with non-nitrate-reducing organisms. A recent meta-analysis of pediatric articles concluded that LE and nitrites in combination have a sensitivity of 88% and specificity of 96% in the detection of urinary tract infection, and perform nearly as well as Gram staining of urine.[85]

PRINCIPLES AND PRACTICALITIES OF DIAGNOSTIC IMAGING

Imaging of the pediatric patient is performed to detect congenital abnormality, diagnose disease or injury, assess response to treatment and locate the position of foreign bodies such as surgically placed lines. Although more sophisticated modalities such as magnetic resonance and radioisotope imaging have revolutionized the specialty, the mainstay of pediatric radiology continues to be conventional X-ray imaging and ultrasonography. This section details the principles of the various imaging techniques; the application of these techniques to the various body systems is discussed in the relevant chapters of this textbook.

RADIATION PROTECTION

The scientific measurement of radiation dose (the 'effective dose') is the millisievert (mSv). Because the body tissues have differential sensitivity to radiation exposure, particularly in childhood, the actual dose to different tissues and organs varies. The stated 'effective dose' is an average value of effect on the entire body. Background exposure from natural environmental sources is around 2–3 mSv/year but varies depending on location.

Children are particularly sensitive to radiation, with specific risks to the thyroid gland, breast tissue, bone marrow and gonads. This means that a similar radiation dose per gram of tissue has a greater potential for developing fatal cancer.[88] Furthermore, children have a longer lifespan in which to manifest radiation-related cancer. Radiation for older adults and the elderly does not carry the same cancer risk, as many radiation-induced cancers will not become evident for many decades. Consequently children are recognized as being twice as likely to develop late manifestations of detrimental radiation effects than adults for the same effective dose.[89] Table 8.20 shows the effective dose of an X-ray examination in childhood and the lifetime risk of fatal cancer secondary to that examination.[90] In the Ionizing Radiation (Medical Exposure) Regulations,[91] children are recognized therefore, as warranting special consideration.

The aim of a good pediatric radiology department is to have agreed protocols and diagnostic pathways, standardized techniques, comparable diagnostic image quality and dose within the published reference ranges. Minimization of dose can be achieved in four key areas:

1. justification: benefit must outweigh harm;
2. optimization: adequate diagnostic quality at the lowest achievable dose;
3. evaluation: availability of quality criteria references for a diagnostic image;
4. radiation protection:
   - equipment and techniques should comply with national regulations;
   - doses should be recorded for each patient and should comply with standard diagnostic reference levels.[92–94]

CONSIDERATIONS FOR A PEDIATRIC RADIOLOGY DEPARTMENT

The correct and optimal use of imaging depends on close teamwork between the clinician and the radiologist. This applies not only to the planning of initial investigations but also to prompt feedback about results and whether secondary investigations are required. Investigation should proceed along recognized flow channels, beginning with the least invasive procedure. Many hospitals have interdepartmental meetings that promote education and collaboration.

Gaining a child's trust and cooperation is essential for optimizing image quality, thereby reducing radiation exposure and investigation times. It is highly desirable that radiology staff have training in communicating with and managing children. Clear and simple explanations of the planned procedure should be available to the parent and, where appropriate, to the child prior to the examination. The department should be friendly and clean, with books or toys available in the waiting area. Waiting times should be minimized. Praise for the child's cooperation is important and reward in the form of stickers or certificates can be useful. Simple and safe restraints and supports should be on hand for immobilization of particular body areas. A variety of sizes of shields for gonad protection should be available. A chest X-ray should never include ovaries and an abdominal X-ray should never include testes.

Policies for safe sedation and anesthesia should be in place and undergo regular review. The IRR99 advises a quality assurance program in each department to ensure optimal diagnostic images are produced at the lowest possible exposure to the child.[95]

Table 8.20 Lifetime risk of developing a fatal cancer following X-ray exposure in childhood[90]

Examination	Effective dose (mSv)	Lifetime risk of fatal cancer
Chest	0.01	1/million
Spine	0.07	1/150 000
Abdomen	0.1	1/100 000
Micturating cystourethrogram	1.0	1/10 000
CT head	2	1/5000
CT body	10	1/1000

CONVENTIONAL X-RAYS

X-rays are high-frequency electromagnetic waves that are radiated through a patient. The emergent X-ray beam excites a fluorescent screen that produces light exposure on the photographic film. The image produced by X-ray depends on the density of the tissues through which the radiation passes. These are normally bone, soft tissue, air and fat. The different body tissues absorb the X-ray variably, with bone and calcified structures absorbing most radiation and air absorbing least. The absorption differences between tissues can be enhanced by the administration of contrast such as barium, or iodine in a water-soluble form.

Barium is a safe, dense and inert medium and is used exclusively in gastrointestinal studies. When supplemented with bicarbonate, the resultant barium/air interface will detail mucosal irregularities such as ulceration and polyps. Non-ionic water-soluble contrasts are now used routinely for i.v., intra-arterial and intrathecal examinations. Owing to a relatively low osmolality, non-ionic contrast media are ideal for investigation of gastrointestinal pathology such as gastro-esophageal reflux and aspiration, tracheo-esophageal fistula and bowel obstruction. Although low osmolar non-ionic contrast is regarded as safer than other media, any use of contrast poses risks over and above that of the plain X-ray, due to potential allergic and nephrotoxic effects.[96]

X-rays are typically the primary imaging modality for investigation of suspected fractures, chest pathology and bowel obstruction or perforation. X-rays may also be performed to monitor response to therapy such as healing of a fracture, drainage of a pleural effusion or antimicrobial treatment of pneumonia. They are regularly used to locate the position of endotracheal, feeding tubes and indwelling vascular catheters. Because most X-rays are performed by radiographer, a clinician will commonly see the film before a radiologist is able to report it. As such, clinicians must be able, not only to assess any abnormality, but also to have an appreciation of the normal radiological appearances and the quality of the film. A standard approach is shown below.

Standard approach to assessing an X-ray

1. Use good viewing conditions, i.e. a light box in a darkened room.
2. Check that the child's name, date of birth and date of examination are correct.
3. Note the orientation of the X-ray, e.g. anterior–posterior film, posterior–anterior film, lateral, sagittal, coronal, transverse etc. and check which sides are marked 'left' and 'right'.
4. Assess the quality of the X-ray:
   - is the child in an optimal position or was the film taken with the child rotated laterally, or in a scoliotic or lordotic position? Rotation in an infant's chest X-ray can be assessed by comparing symmetry of the anterior ends of the ribs; in an older child compare the symmetry of the medial ends of the clavicles;
   - has the area of interest been fully imaged, e.g. in a chest X-ray, are the apices and costophrenic angles of the lungs shown?;
   - is the X-ray adequately penetrated? In a chest X-ray, the vertebral bodies should be visible through the heart shadow;
   - in a chest X-ray, was the X-ray taken during inspiration? If so, there should be eight ribs visible above the hemidiaphragm;
   - are there artefacts from overlying or underlying equipment or clothing that obstruct the view of the area of interest?
5. Comment on any foreign bodies such as indwelling lines, endotracheal or nasogastric tubes. Foreign bodies may be in front of the child, inside the child or behind the child;
6. Describe any abnormalities of:
   - the soft tissues: localized or generalized swelling, calcification, foreign bodies, trauma;
   - the bones: density, deformity, fracture, inflammatory change;
   - the organs: detailed in individual chapters.
7. Summarize the positive findings.

Fluoroscopy is a technique by which dynamic X-rays are recorded and viewed in real-time. The X-ray beam is projected through a patient to a fluoroscopic screen and this image is coupled to an intensifier and video camera, allowing images to be viewed instantaneously. It is particularly useful in barium studies, urography and during interventional procedures.

ULTRASOUND

Ultrasonography (USS) is an established non-ionizing bedside tool that has become the first-line imaging modality in many conditions in children. A transducer sends high-frequency (between 3 and 12 MHz) sound waves through a tissue. A coupling gel is used to enhance transmission by improving contact between the transducer and the skin. The sound wave is partially reflected from the interface between different tissues and returns to the transducer as an echo. These echoes are converted into electrical pulses that are processed and transformed into a digital image. High-frequency sound waves have a short wavelength, and such images have a high resolution. However, the attenuation of the sound wave is increased at higher frequencies, so in order to have better penetration of deeper tissues, a lower frequency (3–5 MHz) may be used.

USS is portable and easy to use, and patients rarely require sedation. It has disadvantages in being dependent on the technology of the system and the knowledge and skills of the operator. Sound waves pass poorly through bone so examination of the brain is limited to infancy. Reflection of sound waves by gas can make examination of the chest and abdomen difficult. Although no known risks have been recorded in vivo, ultrasound is a form of energy and there remains concern about its safety, especially at higher power levels that can cause significant heating in tissues. Consideration should be given to keeping acoustic power, pulse amplitude and examination time to a minimum. The greatest risk of USS is sometimes considered to be erroneous diagnosis in the hands of unskilled operators.

Although used therapeutically in adults in lithotripsy, phacoemulsification and thrombolysis, the uses of USS in pediatrics are diagnostic and for image guidance in interventional radiology. Newer developments in USS technology have allowed three-dimensional (3D) and more recently, four-dimensional (real-time 3D) imaging. These tools offer more accurate assessment of fetal morphology, in particular the face, heart and extremities.[97]

Echocardiography is used widely for the detection of abnormalities of the heart and surrounding vessels. M-mode (1D) and 2D echocardiography inform anatomy and movement of the heart muscle and valves, while Doppler ultrasound gives information of blood flow direction and velocity. The information retrieved by Doppler can be portrayed as a spectral graph of frequency or velocity versus time, or as an image using color Doppler (directional Doppler). Color Doppler processes frequency shift and phase information, allowing blood cells to be coded in color depending on their direction and speed. Conventionally, red shows blood flow towards the transducer, blue indicates flow in the opposite direction and a red–blue mosaic indicates turbulence of blood flow. The color image, superimposed on the grayscale background of the 2D image has revolutionized the diagnosis of congenital heart disease. Doppler may also be used to measure flow and hemodynamic disturbances elsewhere in the circulation, namely in and around aneurysms, thromboses and stenoses. Altered blood flow in the brain secondary to increased intracranial pressure or impaired cerebral autoregulation is manifest as a change in the resistance or pulsatility index, as measured by Doppler USS.[98,99]

Contrast-enhanced USS with injected microbubbles of air improves ultrasound signal backscatter and is used in both echocardiography and urography.

COMPUTERIZED TOMOGRAPHY

This technique was introduced into clinical practice in 1972 and offers high-quality cross-sectional views of the body. A large series of 2D images is taken around a single axis of rotation and these are processed by digital geometry to generate a 3D image of internal anatomy. Various structures can be delineated based on their ability to block the X-ray beam. Tissues that most attenuate the beam appear white (bones), and tissues that cause less attenuation appear darker (air-filled lungs, fat). Although historically images were generated in an axial plane, modern scanners have allowed the data to be reformatted in alternative planes and even in 3D forms.

Major advances in CT systems, computer technology and reconstruction algorithms have resulted in a dramatic reduction in the acquisition speed such that a modern scanner can reconstruct a 1000-image study in less than 30 s. Spiral or helical techniques have reduced movement artefacts, particularly those related to breathing and gastrointestinal motility. Such systems have reduced the need for sedation and anesthesia in children.[100] The shorter imaging times makes it easier for children to lie still and hold their breath during critical parts of the examination.

Compared to conventional X-rays, CT improves low contrast resolution of soft tissues and can distinguish tissues that differ in density by less than 1%. However this high resolution is at the expense of a highly absorbed radiation dose (Table 8.20).[90] European guidelines advise on quality criteria for a CT examination that will provide the required clinical information in its optimal form, with minimum dose to the patient.[101]

CT is particularly useful in the diagnosis of bony abnormalities, particularly craniofacial injuries, in the imaging of the chest parenchyma and in acute abdominal trauma. CT also detects blood and calcification easily. Compared to MRI however, soft tissue contrast is relatively low and this can be a problem in the brain, where the differences between white and grey matter are small. Contrast will enhance tissue differentiation and is particularly useful in the evaluation of tumors and lymphadenopathy, although MRI remains a more sensitive tool.

MAGNETIC RESONANCE IMAGING

This technique depends on the ability of nuclei within a tissue to resonate under certain conditions in the presence of a magnetic field. The nuclei first align themselves in a parallel or anti-parallel direction in response to a strong magnetic field. The tissue is then briefly exposed to pulses of electromagnetic energy (radiofrequency [RF] pulses), which causes some of the nuclei to assume a temporary high-energy state. As the high-energy nuclei relax and realign, they emit energy at rates that are recorded to provide information about their environment.

Generally, image contrast is created by using a selection of image acquisition parameters that weights signal according to the different phases in the relaxation processes that establish equilibrium following the RF pulses (T1, T2 or T2*). In the brain, T1 weighting causes axons (white matter) to appear white, congregations of neurons to appear gray, and cerebrospinal fluid to appear dark. The contrast of white matter, gray matter and cerebrospinal fluid is reversed using T2 or T2* imaging.

Different strengths of magnet are available. The low-strength magnets (0.18–0.23 T) are usually of an open configuration and as such are less claustrophobic. Mid-strength magnets of up to 2 T are of a tunnel configuration and are noisier and more expensive. The high-strength systems have the advantage of faster image acquisition and better resolution.

The time for data acquisition by MRI is relatively long, with several periods of acquisition lasting up to 10 min each. This may be difficult for the young or poorly cooperative child and sedation or even anesthesia may be necessary.

MRI is now used in fetal imaging in the delineation of congenital anomaly and acquired damage.[102] It has been important in the identification and classification of many congenital brain abnormalities[103] and in the documentation of the development of the premature brain.[104] It has been evaluated as an alternative to postmortem, where it performs relatively poorly but may be useful where consent has not been granted for pathological examination.[105]

Diffusion-weighted imaging (DWI) measures diffusion of water molecules within a tissue and can demonstrate impairment of this diffusivity, particularly within the brain, where DWI has high sensitivity for detecting infarction within minutes of occurrence. In the newborn, abnormal signaling in the brain on DWI predicts outcome following hypoxia-ischemia.[106]

Diffusion tensor imaging (DTI) makes use of the assumption that water molecules within a tissue do not exhibit Brownian motion but instead move in a particular direction, e.g. along an axon with the nervous system. DTI has been pioneering in producing maps of fiber directions within the brain to examine connectivity.[107]

MR spectroscopy allows study of the biochemistry of the brain by providing information about the relative concentrations of certain metabolites in specific areas of the brain. Contrasts with specific magnetic properties (such as gadolinium) may be required to delineate areas of interest.

The advantage of MRI technology is that, as far as we know today, it is harmless to the patient, using non-ionizing radiation that is in the radiofrequency range. While a CT scan may have good spatial resolution (i.e. the ability to differentiate two structures that are a small distance apart), MRI has better contrast resolution (i.e. the ability to distinguish between two structures that are similar but not identical) and provides excellent soft tissue differentiation apart from in the chest, where CT remains superior. MRI is poorer in depicting bone or blood compared to other imaging modalities.

The presence of pacemakers and other metallic implants is a contraindication to MRI as they may cause arrhythmias, trauma due to movement of the object, thermal injury from induction heating or failure of the implanted device. Owing to the construction of many scanners, children may feel claustrophobic during the examination. In addition, the loud noise and vibration resulting from rapidly alternating magnetic gradients interacting with the main magnetic field can be highly disturbing. Children may be distracted from the excessive noise by listening to music or a story through earphones but some still find it distressing that they are unable to hear their nearby parents.

NUCLEAR MEDICINE

Nuclear medicine uses radioactive isotopes for the diagnosis and treatment of patients. Where conventional radiology provides information mostly on structure, nuclear medicine provides complementary data on function.

The most commonly used radionuclide is ^{99m}Tc but ^{123}I, ^{131}I, ^{133}Xe and ^{81m}Kr are occasionally used. The dose of radionuclide is calculated from the weight and surface-area of the child. The radiation dose is usually less than that received through equivalent X-rays. Radionuclides are absorbed by healthy tissue at a rate different from tissue undergoing a disease process. The tissue, having absorbed the radionuclide, emits gamma radiation that is detected by a camera. A deviation in normal rates of absorption may be an indication of abnormal metabolic activity.

The use of nuclear medicine in pediatrics is primarily diagnostic:

- detection of congenital abnormalities such as Meckel's diverticulum, lung anomalies, biliary atresia;
- diagnosis of inflammation/infection – white cell scans;
- assessment of swallowing and gastro-esophageal reflux;
- assessment of differential renal function and vesico-ureteric reflux;
- assessment of pulmonary perfusion;
- investigation of bony pathology – tumors, infection, trauma, avascular necrosis.

Nuclear medicine is a common therapeutic option in adults, utilized in the treatment of thyroid disease, neural crest tumors and the palliation of metastatic bone pain. In children monoclonal antibodies such as metaiodobenzylguanidine (MIBG) have been labeled with large doses of ^{131}I and successfully used in the treatment of neuroblastoma.[108]

SINGLE-PHOTON EMISSION COMPUTERIZED TOMOGRAPHY (SPECT)

Single-photon emission computerized tomography (SPECT) is an allied nuclear medicine blood flow technique where a gamma camera rotates around the body at the time of examination, collecting data from all angles. A series of axial images of the internal anatomy is generated, which allow more precise localization of activity. SPECT can be used to observe biochemical and physiological processes, as well as the size and volume of structures. The main use of SPECT in children has been in the identification of epileptogenic foci in the brain prior to neurosurgical removal[109] and in the diagnosis and monitoring of areas of abnormal bone metabolism such as spondylolysis[110] and tumors.

INTERVENTIONAL RADIOLOGY

The field of interventional radiology is expanding rapidly with radiologists now performing many procedures that were previously the responsibility of surgeons. In children because of their small size and sensitivity to radiation, ultrasound rather than CT is the usual choice for image guidance. Commonly performed procedures include vascular and enteric access, biopsy (liver, kidney, tumor), aspiration and drainage (abscess, effusion), stenting procedures (esophageal, ureteric, biliary), angiography, nephrostomy and sclerotherapy of lymphatic or vascular malformations. Many children will require sedation or anesthesia during the intervention but in general such procedures are easier than in adults, even accounting for difficulties in vascular access. Image-guided central venous access has the advantages of a very high success rate, the ability to access innovative vessels (collaterals or recanalization of occluded veins), optimization of tip position and the opportunity to combine it with other image-guided procedures such as biopsy.

GENERAL PRINCIPLES OF COMMON PRACTICAL PROCEDURES

INTRODUCTION

The process of obtaining informed consent, specific for various tests and procedures has become arguably more important with the public's wish and expectation that they should be involved in medical decisions. In requesting consent for a test or procedure from a child, parents or other health professionals, it is important to know what is involved in that procedure. Parental understanding will allow the child to be better prepared and will ensure optimum benefit is provided to the patient from each procedure. Even relatively simple medical words and phrases are difficult for most parents and children to understand, and innocent words can sound extremely frightening (murmur, tumor, anesthetic, etc.) Children and parents may be reluctant to ask for a 'translation' when the explanation is theoretically in their own language. Help them by considering the words you will use, in what context and how they might be misinterpreted. If you are explaining procedures to someone in whom your language is not his mother tongue, use a translator (do not rely on relatives if this is an important procedure or one that carries significant risk). In general:

1. Know how to explain procedures to parents and children. Do not explain a procedure if you are not fully aware of what will be involved: go and find out about it. Consider:
   - Why is the procedure necessary?
   - When and where will it take place?
   - What grade of staff will be performing it?
   - What problems might be encountered and what risks are possible?
   - Ensure that you are able to explain the balance of risk versus benefit of the procedure *in that child.*
2. Local variation in procedures will be present. Try and find out how the procedures vary and give up-to-date information.
3. Be able to appreciate the hazards associated with procedures for both patients and staff, and therefore how to avoid them.
4. Do not perform procedures for which you are not adequately trained. In this section common procedures are explained and their benefits, risks and hazards discussed. There will be local variation in how procedures are performed, so find out how these differ in your locality. This will be important from the perspective of clinical governance.

PREPARING PATIENTS FOR PROCEDURES

Informed consent

Consent should usually be obtained by the person doing the procedure or at least by someone who is capable of doing it. Issues with regard to consent are dealt in Chapter 10. Remember that issues of consent apply to both parents and children.

Talking to children about procedures[111]

Misconceptions exist that delaying or not explaining procedures to children protects them from pain and fear. Such mistaken beliefs often arise because staff and/or parents fail to appreciate the level of understanding of the child or because they have little ability to adapt their communication to language that the child will understand. If parents do not wish to have a procedure explained to their young child, then those wishes should generally be respected, though parents should understand the procedure and not try to protect themselves by not telling the child. The parents should be made aware of the consequences of not discussing an important procedure with their child. Even if parents are present during a procedure, the child should be the focus of explanation. Do not ignore the child hoping they will pick up information given to the parents.

When talking to a child, introduce yourself and take account of the cognitive level of the child and his language. Don't patronize, and consider throughout the consultation whether you retain his interest and understanding. In your introduction, recognize (as the child will) your authority as an adult, but be respectful of the child's status. Give a clear introduction to the topic or plan to be discussed and be careful not to make promises you will not be able to keep (e.g. confidentiality etc.) Communicate on the same physical level, and begin the conversation with a nonthreatening topic. Warn the child the main topic to be discussed is a serious one, and enquire as to what the child understands about that topic already. Always give adequate time for the child to respond or ask questions and listen carefully to his response, but do not pressurize the child into giving a response. Do not attempt to anticipate his answers. Go at the child's pace and check the child has understood. Any explanation should be a clear and simple, optimistic (but realistic) narrative of the events. There is a tendency to overestimate what information has been conveyed and how much has been understood, and a tendency to underestimate what the child has acquired from other sources.

The child will often give clues as to when he feels the conversation is over. If the procedure is complex, then it is often not possible to cover everything at one meeting and a further time can be arranged. End by summarizing what has been discussed, including the child's viewpoints; offer a plan. Explain that you are available to discuss the procedure and how the child and parents can contact you.

Use of play specialists

Play specialists are a well-trained and respected part of the pediatric team in any hospital. They have knowledge of infant and childcare, nursing and teaching. They may be able to advise doctors and nurses of a particular child's needs. The play specialist is able to introduce different types of play and activities to individual children based on their age and development. Children use play as a medium to express feelings. Familiar play helps children to normalize a clinical environment, with reduction in their anxiety and stress.

Hospital play specialists have a significant role in preparing children for procedures during their stay in hospital. Preparation can be achieved by use of photo books and role playing. Children can also be given the opportunity to touch and play with medical equipment in a safe and controlled environment, i.e. syringe painting, dolls fitted with cannulae, nasogastric tubes etc. As a familiar face to the children, play specialists can have a significant effect in relaxing them during procedures by using distraction methods.

Procedural pain

The management of pain during procedures is described in detail in Chapter 38.

The management of procedural pain in children should be by the simplest effective technique, multimodal, pre-emptive where possible, and frequently reassessed and titrated to the child's needs.

Pre-emptive pain control helps to minimize fear and anxiety associated with the procedure, reduces the stress response, prevents the 'wind up' phenomenon of central nervous system sensitization to noxious stimuli and tissue release of pain mediators. Pain prevention should be tailored to the individual child's needs using a combination of nondrug techniques, local anesthetic, simple analgesics and opioids, and sedation where appropriate. By using a multimodal approach the required doses of stronger agents can be reduced and in turn this reduces the incidence of adverse effects. Management of pain requires regular pain assessment and this must be linked to appropriate action.

Nonspecialist practical procedures

Clinical governance dictates that procedures should only be carried out by those who have had fully supervised training. The descriptions provided here are insufficient to enable you to perform these tasks, but they should provide enough information for you to be familiar with what is involved so that you can describe them adequately to parents and patients. Techniques for more specialist procedures are discussed in the relevant chapters.

Title. Peripheral venous sampling

Procedure. The most common form of blood sampling takes blood from a peripheral vein. In children, the veins in the arm (brachial) and back of the hand are most frequently used.

Complications. Localized hematoma (bruise) may occur, which will disappear in a few days. Tourniquets will produce elevation of plasma calcium estimation.

Hazards. In children, separate needle and syringe are still used more frequently than closed needle systems. These are more hazardous to users and patients in terms of needle stick injury. Needles with the hub broken off should not be used under any circumstances. Neonatal venepuncture needles are now available. Gloves should be worn during all blood-taking procedures.

Title. Peripheral capillary sampling

Procedure. This method of blood sampling is satisfactory for assessing arterialized carbon dioxide and pH in the peripheral blood. It can also be used for complete blood counts and glucose estimation. In the neonate the side of the heel is used and in older infants and children the finger tip. The procedure is quick and although some centers use an anesthetic cream for such intervention, this may cause blood vessel constriction that can reduce the amount of sample. A spring-loaded lancet reduces damage to skin and is least painful. A capillary tube collects the sample from the skin, which is sometimes smeared with Vaseline to help localize the blood. The area is compressed with cotton wool following the procedure to stop bleeding.

Complications. Biochemical tests on capillary samples may have errors, especially elevation of potassium and calcium measurements. In neonates, very deep stabs on the heel have been rarely associated with osteomyelitis.

Hazards. Automated spring-loaded lancets need to be disposed of in a similar way to other 'sharps'. Blood sampling should be performed wearing gloves.

Title. Peripheral arterial sampling

Procedure. This is required for measurement of arterial oxygen, and also carbon dioxide and pH. Transcutaneous oxygen and saturation monitoring has reduced the need for frequent arterial sampling to estimate arterial oxygen. The most common site for an arterial sample is the radial artery but the posterior tibial artery is sometimes used in the neonate. Other arteries can be used as long as an adequate alternative arterial supply can be demonstrated to that area of tissue. Fixed sampling syringes are now in common use and contain heparin to stop the sample clotting. Arterial sampling can be painful (use local anesthetic cream, or subcutaneous local anesthetic injection without adrenaline). The pulse is identified and the needle inserted at a 45-degree angle. Pressure will need to be applied to the site for up to 5 min after removal of the needle before bleeding stops.

Complications. Hematoma frequently forms during arterial sampling, either because of insufficient pressure applied to the overlying skin once the needle is withdrawn, or because the needle pierces the artery at an oblique angle, limiting blood drawn but damaging the vessel wall. Occasionally, arterial spasm can severely limit arterial supply to the limb peripheral to the sampling site: this should correct over a few minutes, though occasionally an arterial vasodilator, such as topical nitroglycerin ointment may have to be applied.

Hazards. Sharps need to be disposed of appropriately. Gloves should be worn, and because of the possible spray of arterial blood users may wish to use protective eyewear.

Title. Peripheral venous access

Procedure. A peripheral venous cannula is frequently placed in children. In neonates, veins may easily be seen but may be too small to cannulate; in toddlers veins may be difficult to see because of subcutaneous fat. At all ages, knowledge of the distribution of large subcutaneous veins is valuable. Local anesthetic cream should be used where possible. A tourniquet may be applied to help fill veins, though it is often helpful to have a second person to apply a tourniquet with their hand (ensuring that little wriggles don't ruin your attempts to site the cannula). Parents should be warned that this technique is difficult and even in experienced hands several attempts may be required. In very young children with poor venous access, a scalp vein may be the most sensible option, though many parents may find it particularly distressing because hair in the region has to be shaved to enable fixation. Peripheral venous cannulation represents a standard technique to most doctors, yet is associated with significant stress to many parents. Children may need securing to ensure a quick and relatively painless procedure. The cannula should be secured effectively to ensure the child does not remove it as soon as it is in place.

Complications. Hematoma formation is common. Occasionally, particularly when using scalp veins, an artery may be mistaken for a vein during cannulation. Any pulsatility of flow during cannulation is arterial and the cannula should be withdrawn (using 5 min of pressure) immediately.

Hazards. Sharps must to be disposed of appropriately. Gloves should be worn.

Title. Peripheral venous cutdown access

Procedure. This procedure is used when no veins can be identified for percutaneous cannulation. Children needing this procedure are commonly in extremis, but every attempt should be made to ensure adequate explanation and pain relief. The sterile procedure usually cannulates the long saphenous vein just above the ankle, by making an incision in the skin and dissecting back the tissues until the vein is identified. A small slit in the vein then allows the cannula to be inserted. The catheter is sutured in place.

Complications. Bleeding at the site may occur when circulation is re-established if sutures are not secure enough.

Hazards. This is a sterile surgical procedure with full protection against blood biohazard.

Title. Intraosseous needle insertion

Procedure. This is an emergency procedure used when no veins can be identified for peripheral cannulation. In a shocked child with hypotension, this procedure should be performed after no more than two quick attempts at peripheral cannulation. The tibia is the most common site for insertion, though the femoral head and other sites are possible. The child is frequently in extremis and pain relief may not be possible without access in an unstable child. The position of insertion is just below the tibial tuberosity on the anteromedial aspect of the tibia. The needle is screwed steadily into bone until the outer cortex is felt to give way. The bone marrow that can be aspirated can be sent for blood glucose and electrolyte concentration, in addition to blood culture. All i.v. preparations can be given via intraosseous needle. Though the needle is fairly secure within the bone, it should be attached with tapes. When circulation is re-established, i.v. access should be obtained and the intraosseous needle withdrawn.

Complications. Leak of instilled fluid into the skin around the site of the needle may occur if the needle is not properly sited. The needle can occasionally exit the bone on the opposite side and this should be checked for before fluid is instilled.

Hazards. When dropped, intraosseous needles tend to fall on the handle exposing the needle upright: great care is needed to alert others in the vicinity if the needle is dropped. Sharps need to be disposed of appropriately. Gloves should be worn.

Title. Peripheral arterial access

Procedure. This is only needed if a child requires intensive care. In older children the radial or femoral arteries are typically cannulated. In neonates the radial and posterior tibial are most commonly used. As far as parents are concerned, the procedure is similar to peripheral venous cannulation. In practice, arterial cannulation is more difficult, particularly as the arterial pulse can sometimes be difficult to localize precisely, and the elastic wall of the artery and arterial spasm may impede cannulation. In small infants, a cold light transilluminator may help to locate the radial or posterior tibial artery. The small risk of peripheral ischemia following insertion of an arterial catheter should be balanced against the benefit of continuous arterial access (and the availability of continuous direct arterial blood pressure). Local anesthetic should be used for insertion. The artery can be cannulated in a similar way to venous cannulation. Some prefer to transfix the artery with the cannula needle, withdrawing slowly until the end of the needle is within the artery, shown by a flashback into the hub of the cannula. The cannula, once in place, needs careful and continued observation for signs of peripheral ischemia and localized hematoma or leak. Arterial spasm and peripheral ischemia are discussed in the section on arterial sampling (see earlier).

Complications. Peripheral ischemia; blood loss from puncture site or misconnected blood pressure monitoring circuit.

Hazards. Sharps need to be disposed of appropriately. Gloves should be worn. Arterial lines should be labeled clearly so that i.v. drugs are not infused inadvertently.

Title. Lumbar puncture

Procedure. A lumbar puncture enables access to the cerebrospinal fluid (CSF) surrounding the spinal cord. It is performed safely in the majority of children, however caution is needed if there is a question of raised intracranial pressure (i.e. meningism, headache, vomiting). In children younger than 1 year of age with a soft patent anterior fontanelle the procedure is considered safe. In children without a patent anterior fontanelle, it is not possible to reliably identify raised intracranial pressure by fundoscopy alone and so a cranial CT may be required, or, if the index of suspicion of meningitis is high, then i.v. antibiotics can be started and a lumbar puncture performed at a later time. Children with coagulopathy or respiratory instability are also at risk from the procedure. Children and infants usually lie on their left side for the procedure, with oxygen saturation and heart rate monitoring. Occasionally an upright flexed sitting position may be used. Local anesthetic cream should be used if time allows, but in suspected meningitis, risks of delaying antibiotic administration outweigh the benefits of analgesia. Complete aseptic technique should be used, including gown and sterile gloves. The key to success is having the back well flexed and perfectly perpendicular to the edge of the bed. An assistant who will maintain the position when the needle enters the back is very important. The needle is placed in the lower back, between L3 and L4 (the space directly below the superior iliac crest when the child is lying on his side). Pressure estimation with a manometer may be warranted prior to removal of approximately 2 ml of CSF for biochemical and microbiological examination. Two or three attempts may be required to find the spinal fluid space, particularly if the child is active. Following removal of enough fluid, the central portion of the needle is replaced and the needle withdrawn; a sealant spray or liquid is quickly applied to close the puncture hole and a dressing or sticking plaster is placed over the site.

Complications. Occasionally a blood vessel close to the spine may be hit by the needle and the sample will be heavily blood stained; these samples should still be sent for culture. If this occurs then a further attempt one intervertebral space higher may be attempted. Headache is a common side effect following lumbar puncture, and should settle with simple pain relief over 48 h. Occasionally continued seepage of CSF may require firm pressure with a sterile dressing until leakage stops. In children with raised intracranial pressure a lumbar puncture may result in 'coning', where the base of the brain is pushed down into the base of the skull, depressing the respiratory center and other autonomic control centers; this is a neurological emergency requiring urgent intensive care support. Prior scanning by CT or MRI may detect increased pressure and advise against lumbar puncture.

Hazards. Sharps are used and should be disposed of appropriately. CSF should be considered an infected biohazard.

Title. Clean-catch urine sampling

Procedure. This is performed in children suspected of having a urinary tract infection (bag urine collection is frequently contaminated, and the result sets off a whole series of unnecessary investigations). The child should be well hydrated and be sat on a parent's knee with no nappy (diaper). The genitals should be cleaned with sterile water (not disinfectant) and left to dry. The hands of the person collecting the sample should be washed prior to collection. A small sterile container should be held ready, waiting for the child to pass urine and a sample (approximately mid-stream), obtained as soon as the event occurs. Good observation and rapid reflexes are required, as the opportunity may not arise again for many more hours.

Complications. None

Hazards. Hands should be thoroughly washed after sample collection as they may be contaminated with bodily fluids.

Title. Suprapubic urine sampling

Procedure. This technique enables a rapid and clean sample of urine to be obtained. It is particularly useful if children are unwell with a suspected urinary tract infection and antibiotics need to be started. The bladder is an abdominal organ in the baby but becomes more and more pelvic as the infant grows. As such, the procedure is most easily performed in children younger than 18 months of age. The child needs to be lying supine with legs kept still. Local anesthetic cream should be used for analgesia. The bladder should be palpated (or percussed), or alternatively can be identified on ultrasound: in an emergency the bladder can be sampled without these, but may contain no urine (a 'dry' tap). The suprapubic area should be cleaned with antiseptic fluid and then a small needle attached to a syringe is inserted perpendicular to the skin in the midline just above the symphysis pubis in the infant: in the older child the needle may need to be directed more into the pelvis. Urine is withdrawn into the syringe and the needle removed. Pressure need only be applied to the area for a short time and then the area left without dressing if there is no bleeding.

Complications. 'Dry' tap: knowledge of when the infant/child last passed urine and good clinical practice should minimize the number of these. Ultrasound may confirm the presence of urine in the bladder. Hematuria may be noted for a short period after the procedure. The child may void during skin preparation; have a container ready to catch the stream. Occasionally adjacent bowel can be punctured; this typically does not cause a problem as the hole created is small and self-healing.

Hazards. Care should be taken as the child may move during the procedure if not correctly nursed, causing needlestick injury. Sharps should be disposed of carefully.

REFERENCES (*Level 1 Evidence)

1. Miall LS, Davies H. An analysis of paediatric diagnostic decision-making: how should students be taught? Med Educ 1992; 26:317–320.
2. United Nations. Convention on the Rights of the Child. Article 12. Geneva; 1989.

3. Department of Health. http://www.statistics.gov.uk/focuson/families Last accessed 12th November 2006.
*4. Office of National Statistics for the Department of Health and the Scottish Executive. Survey of the mental health of children and young people in Great Britain. 2005.

5. Kemper KJ. Complementary and alternative medicine for children: does it work? Arch Dis Child 2001; 84:6–9.
6. Freedom of Information Act. 2000.
7. Majnemer A, Rosenblatt B. Reliability of parental recall of developmental milestones. Pediatr Neurol 1994; 10:304–308.

8. Jolly W, Froom J, Rosen MG. The genogram. J Fam Pract 1980; 10:251–255.

9. General Household Survey 2000/1. http://www.statistics.gov.uk/CCI/nugget.asp?ID=1328&Pos=4&ColRank=2&Rank=800 Last accessed 12th November 2006.

10. General Household Survey 2000/1. http://www.statistics.gov.uk/cci/nugget.asp?id=719 Last accessed 14th August 2006.

11. Department of Health. www.immunisation.nhs.uk Last accessed 12th November 2006.

*12. Preece MA, Freeman JV, Cole TJ. Sex differences in weight in infancy. Published centile charts for weights have been updated. Br Med J 1996; 313:1486.

*13. Freeman JV, Cole TJ, Chinn S, et al. Cross sectional stature and weight reference curves for the UK, 1990. Arch Dis Child 1995; 73:17–24.

*14. WHO Child Growth Standards based on length/height, weight and age. Acta Paediatr Suppl 2006; 450:76–85.

15. Hall DM, Cole TJ. What use is the BMI? Arch Dis Child 2006; 91:283–286.

*16. House of Commons: Health Committee. Obesity: third report of session 2003–04. Vol. 1. London: The Stationery Office; 2004.

*17. Krebs NF, Jacobson MS. Prevention of pediatric overweight and obesity. Pediatrics 2003; 112:424–430.

*18. Schmitz T, Bair N, Falk M, et al. A comparison of five methods of temperature measurement in febrile intensive care patients. Am J Crit Care 1995; 4:286–292.

*19. Robinson JL, Seal RF, Spady DW, et al. Comparison of esophageal, rectal, axillary, bladder, tympanic, and pulmonary artery temperatures in children. J Pediatr 1998; 133:553–556.

*20. Erickson RS, Woo TM. Accuracy of infrared ear thermometry and traditional temperature methods in young children. Heart Lung 1994; 23:181–195.

21. Shann F, Mackenzie A. Comparison of rectal, axillary, and forehead temperatures. Arch Pediatr Adolesc Med 1996; 150:74–78.

22. Osinusi K, Njinyam MN. Comparison of body temperatures taken at different sites and the reliability of axillary temperature in screening for fever. Afr J Med Med Sci 1997; 26:163–166.

23. Hicks MA. A comparison of the tympanic and axillary temperatures of the preterm and term infant. J Perinatol 1996; 16:261–267.

24. Jones KL. Smith's Recognizable patterns of human malformation. 6th edn. Philadelphia: Elsevier Saunders; 2006.

25. Carcillo JA, Fields AI. Clinical practice parameters for hemodynamic support of pediatric and neonatal patients in septic shock. Crit Care Med 2002; 30: 1365–1378.

26. McCrindle BW, Shaffer KM, et al. Cardinal clinical signs in the differentiation of heart murmurs in children. Arch Pediatr Adolesc Med 1996; 150: 169–174.

27. Lip GY, Beevers M, Beevers DG, et al. The measurement of blood pressure and the detection of hypertension in children and adolescents. J Hum Hypertens 2001; 15:419–423.

28. Goonasekera CD, Dillon MJ. Measurement and interpretation of blood pressure. Arch Dis Child 2000; 82:261–265.

29. Sarici SU, Alpay F, Okutan V, et al. Is a standard protocol necessary for oscillometric blood pressure measurement in term newborns? Biol Neonate 2000; 77:212–216.

30. Gevers M, van Genderingen HR, Lafeber HN, et al. Accuracy of oscillometric blood pressure measurement in critically ill neonates with reference to the arterial pressure wave shape. Intensive Care Med 1996; 22:242–248.

31. Movius AJ, Bratton SL, Sorensen GK. Use of pulse oximetry for blood pressure measurement after cardiac surgery. Arch Dis Child 1998; 78:457–460.

32. Langbaum M, Eyal FG. A practical and reliable method of measuring blood pressure in the neonate by pulse oximetry. J Pediatr 1994; 125:591–595.

33. Gilmore B, Hardwick W, Noland J, et al. Determination of systolic blood pressure via pulse oximeter in transported pediatric patients. Pediatr Emerg Care 1999; 15:183–186.

*34. Cunningham S, Symon AG, Elton RA, et al. Intra-arterial blood pressure reference ranges, death and morbidity in very low birthweight infants during the first seven days of life. Early Hum Dev 1999; 56:151–165.

35. Engle WD, Rosenfeld CR. Neutropenia in high-risk neonates. J Pediatr 1984; 105:982–986.

*36. de Swiet M, Fayers P, Shinebourne EA. Blood pressure in first 10 years of life: the Brompton study. Br Med J 1992; 304:23–26.

*37. de Man SA, Andre JL, Bachmann H, et al. Blood pressure in childhood: pooled findings of six European studies. J Hypertens 1991; 9:109–114.

*38. Report of the Second Task Force on Blood Pressure Control in Children–1987. Task Force on Blood Pressure Control in Children. National Heart, Lung, and Blood Institute, Bethesda, Maryland. Pediatrics 1987; 79:1–25.

39. Korotkoff N. To the question of methods of determining the blood pressure (from the clinic of Professor SP Federov) [Russian]. Reports of the Imperial Military Academy 1905; 11:365–367.

40. Margolis P, Gadomski A. The rational clinical examination. Does this infant have pneumonia?. JAMA 1998; 279:308–313.

41. RCPCH. CSA Guideline. Royal College of Paediatrics and Child Health – The Evidence Base for the Physical Signs of Child Sexual Abuse 2007.

42. Laing IA, McIntosh N. Paediatric history and examination. London: Baillière Tindall; 1994.

43. Thompson MJ, Ninis N, Perera R, et al. Clinical recognition of meningococcal disease in children and adolescents. Lancet 2006; 367:397–403.

44. Dixon JM, Elton RA, Rainey JB, et al. Rectal examination in patients with pain in the right lower quadrant of the abdomen. Br Med J 1991; 302:386–388.

45. Hall E. Health for all children. 4th edn. Oxford: Oxford University Press; 2003.

46. www.nice.org.uk/CG037 Last accessed 12th August, 2006.

*47. Glazener CM, Ramsay CR, Campbell MK, et al. Neonatal examination and screening trial (NEST): a randomised, controlled, switchback trial of alternative policies for low risk infants. Br Med J 1999; 318:627–631.

*48. Congenital Anomaly Statistics. HMSO; 2005.

49. Wolke D, Dave S, Hayes J, et al. Routine examination of the newborn and maternal satisfaction: a randomised controlled trial. Arch Dis Child Fetal Neonatal Ed 2002; 86:F155–F160.

50. Laing IA, Wong CM. Hypernatraemia in the first few days: is the incidence rising? Arch Dis Child Fetal Neonatal Ed 2002; 87:F158–F162.

51. Bamji M, Stone RK, Kaul A, et al. Palpable lymph nodes in healthy newborns and infants. Pediatrics 1986; 78:573–575.

52. Rahi JS, Dezateux C. National cross sectional study of detection of congenital and infantile cataract in the United Kingdom: role of childhood screening and surveillance. The British Congenital Cataract Interest Group. Br Med J 1999; 318:362–365.

53. Knowles R, Griebsch I, Dezateux C, et al. Newborn screening for congenital heart defects: a systematic review and cost-effectiveness analysis. Health Technol Assess 2005; 9:1–168.

54. Ainsworth S, Wyllie JP, Wren C. Prevalence and clinical significance of cardiac murmurs in neonates. Arch Dis Child Fetal Neonatal Ed 1999; 80:F43–F45.

55. Wren C, Richmond S, Donaldson L. Presentation of congenital heart disease in infancy: implications for routine examination. Arch Dis Child Fetal Neonatal Ed 1999; 80:F49–F53.

56. Patton C, Hey E. How effectively can clinical examination pick up congenital heart disease at birth? Arch Dis Child Fetal Neonatal Ed 2006; 91:F263–F267.

57. Farrer KF, Rennie JM. Neonatal murmurs: are senior house officers good enough? Arch Dis Child Fetal Neonatal Ed 2003; 88:F147–F151.

58. Arlettaz R, Archer N, Wilkinson AR. Natural history of innocent heart murmurs in newborn babies: controlled echocardiographic study. Arch Dis Child Fetal Neonatal Ed 1998; 78:F166–F170.

*59. Thummala MR, Raju TN, Langenberg P. Isolated single umbilical artery anomaly and the risk for congenital malformations: a meta-analysis. J Pediatr Surg 1998; 33:580–585.

60. Parker S, Zuckerman B, Bauchner H, et al. Jitteriness in full-term neonates: prevalence and correlates. Pediatrics 1990; 85:17–23.

61. Gibson PJ, Britton J, Hall DM, et al. Lumbosacral skin markers and identification of occult spinal dysraphism in neonates. Acta Paediatr 1995; 84: 208–209.

62. Bialik V, Bialik GM, Blazer S, et al. Developmental dysplasia of the hip: a new approach to incidence. Pediatrics 1999; 103:93–99.

*63. Clinical practice guideline: early detection of developmental dysplasia of the hip. Committee on Quality Improvement, Subcommittee on Developmental Dysplasia of the Hip. American Academy of Pediatrics. Pediatrics 2000; 105:896–905.

*64. Woolacott NF, Puhan MA, Steurer J, et al. Ultrasonography in screening for developmental dysplasia of the hip in newborns: systematic review. Br Med J 2005; 330:1413.

65. Philippi H, Faldum A, Jung T, et al. Patterns of postural asymmetry in infants: a standardized video-based analysis. Eur J Pediatr 2006; 165: 158–164.

66. Kayiran SM, Ozbek N, Turan M, et al. Significant differences between capillary and venous complete blood counts in the neonatal period. Clin Lab Haematol 2003; 25:9–16.

67. Meberg A, Jakobsen E, Halvorsen K. Humoral regulation of erythropoiesis and thrombopoiesis in appropriate and small for gestational age infants. Acta Paediatr Scand 1982; 71:769–773.

68. Trudinger B, Song JZ, Wu ZH, et al. Placental insufficiency is characterized by platelet activation in the fetus. Obstet Gynecol 2003; 101:975–981.

69. Santoro SA, Eby CS. Laboratory evaluation of hemostatic disorders. In: Hoffman R, Benz EJ, Shattil SJ (eds) Hematology. Basic principles and practice. Philadelphia PA: Churchill Livingstone; 2000.

70. Schelonka RL, Chai MK, Yoder BA, et al. Volume of blood required to detect common neonatal pathogens. J Pediatr 1996; 129:275–278.

*71. Schwartz GJ, Haycock GB, Edelmann CM Jr, et al. A simple estimate of glomerular filtration rate in children derived from body length and plasma creatinine. Pediatrics 1976; 58:259–263.

*72. Counahan R, Chantler C, Ghazali S, et al. Estimation of glomerular filtration rate from plasma creatinine concentration in children. Arch Dis Child 1976; 51:875–878.

73. Koh TH, Aynsley-Green A, Tarbit M, et al. Neural dysfunction during hypoglycaemia. Arch Dis Child 1988; 63:1353–1358.

74. Deshpande S, Ward PM. The investigation and management of neonatal hypoglycaemia. Semin Fetal Neonatal Med 2005; 10:351–361.

75. Burrin JM, Alberti KG. What is blood glucose: can it be measured? Diabet Med 1990; 7:199–206.

76. Yogev R. Meningitis. In: Jenson B, Baltimore RS, eds. Pediatric infectious diseases. Philadelphia, PA: WB Saunders; 2002.630–650.

77. Fuchs S. Neurologic disorders. In: Barkin R, ed. Pediatric emergency medicine. St Louis, MO: Mosby; 1997.972–1024.

78. Mazor SS, McNulty JE, Roosevelt GE. Interpretation of traumatic lumbar punctures: who can go home? Pediatrics 2003; 111:525–528.

*79. Marton KI, Gean AD. The spinal tap: a new look at an old test. Ann Intern Med 1986; 104:840–848.

*80. Hristeva L, Bowler I, Booy R, et al. Value of cerebrospinal fluid examination in the diagnosis of meningitis in the newborn. Arch Dis Child 1993; 69:514–517.

81. Read SJ, Mitchell JL, Fink CG. LightCycler multiplex PCR for the laboratory diagnosis of common viral infections of the central nervous system. J Clin Microbiol 2001; 39:3056–3059.

82. Espy MJ, Uhl JR, Sloan LM, et al. Real-time PCR in clinical microbiology: applications for routine laboratory testing. Clin Microbiol Rev 2006; 19:165–256.

*83. Backman A, Lantz P, Radstrom P, et al. Evaluation of an extended diagnostic PCR assay for detection and verification of the common causes of bacterial meningitis in CSF and other biological samples. Mol Cell Probes 1999; 13:49–60.

*84. Tzanakaki G, Tsopanomichalou M, Kesanopoulos K, et al. Simultaneous single-tube PCR assay for the detection of Neisseria meningitidis, Haemophilus influenzae type b and Streptococcus pneumoniae. Clin Microbiol Infect 2005; 11:386–390.

*85. Gorelick MH, Shaw KN. Screening tests for urinary tract infection in children: A meta-analysis. Pediatrics 1999; 104:e54.

86. Simerville JA, Maxted WC, Pahira JJ. Urinalysis: a comprehensive review. Am Fam Physician 2005; 71:1153–1162.

*87. Abitbol C, Zilleruelo G, Freundlich M, et al. Quantitation of proteinuria with urinary protein/creatinine ratios and random testing with dipsticks in nephrotic children. J Pediatr 1990; 116:243–247.

88. Brenner DJ. Estimating cancer risks from pediatric CT: going from the qualitative to the quantitative. Pediatr Radiol 2002; 32:228–233.

89. Cox R, MacGibbon BH. Estimates of late radiation risks to the UK population. Documents of the NRPB. 1993;4.

90. Cook JV. Radiation protection and quality assurance in paediatric radiology. Imaging 2001; 13: 229–238.

*91. Department of Health. Ionising Radiation (Medical Exposure) Regulations (Statutory Instrument 2000 No. 1059). London: HMSO; 2000.

*92. European guidelines on quality criteria for diagnostic radiographic images in paediatrics, EUR 16261 EN. London: HMSO; 1996.

*93. Guidelines on patient dose to promote the optimisation of protection from diagnostic medical exposures. Documents of the NRPB. 1999;10.

*94. Hart D, Wall BF, Shrimpton PC, et al. Reference doses and patient size in paediatric radiology, R318. Chitton, UK: NRPB; 2000.

*95. The Ionising Radiations Regulations 1999. Statutory Instrument 1999 No. 3232. London: HMSO; 1999.

96. Stacul F. Current iodinated contrast media. Eur Radiol 2001; 11:690–697.

97. Avni FE, Cos T, Cassart M, et al. Evolution of fetal ultrasonography. Eur Radiol 2006;

98. Quinn MW, Ando Y, Levene MI. Cerebral arterial and venous flow-velocity measurements in post-haemorrhagic ventricular dilatation and hydrocephalus. Dev Med Child Neurol 1992; 34: 863–869.

99. Levene MI, Fenton AC, Evans DH, et al. Severe birth asphyxia and abnormal cerebral blood-flow velocity. Dev Med Child Neurol 1989; 31:427–434.

100. Pappas JN, Donnelly LF, Frush DP. Reduced frequency of sedation of young children with multisection helical CT. Radiology 2000; 215:897–899.

*101. European Guidelines on Quality Criteria for Computed Tomography. EUR 1999; 16262:

102. Hubbard AM. Ultrafast fetal MRI and prenatal diagnosis. Semin Pediatr Surg 2003; 12:143–153.

103. Barkovich AJ, Kuzniecky RI, Jackson GD, et al. A developmental and genetic classification for malformations of cortical development. Neurology 2005; 65:1873–1887.

104. Childs AM, Ramenghi LA, Cornette L, et al. Cerebral maturation in premature infants: quantitative assessment using MR imaging. AJNR Am J Neuroradiol 2001; 22:1577–1582.

105. Griffiths PD, Paley MN, Whitby EH. Postmortem MRI as an adjunct to fetal or neonatal autopsy. Lancet 2005; 365:1271–1273.

106. Hunt RW, Neil JJ, Coleman LT, et al. Apparent diffusion coefficient in the posterior limb of the internal capsule predicts outcome after perinatal asphyxia. Pediatrics 2004; 114:999–1003.

107. Mukherjee P, McKinstry RC. Diffusion tensor imaging and tractography of human brain development. Neuroimaging Clin N Am 2006; 16: 19–43, vii.

*108. Matthay KK, Tan JC, Villablanca JG, et al. Phase I dose escalation of iodine-131-metaiodobenzylguanidine with myeloablative chemotherapy and autologous stem-cell transplantation in refractory neuroblastoma: a new approaches to Neuroblastoma Therapy Consortium Study. J Clin Oncol 2006; 24:500–506.

109. Kaminska A, Chiron C, Ville D, et al. Ictal SPECT in children with epilepsy: comparison with intracranial EEG and relation to postsurgical outcome. Brain 2003; 126:248–260.

110. Logroscino G, Mazza O, Aulisa G, et al. Spondylolysis and spondylolisthesis in the pediatric and adolescent population. Childs Nerv Syst 2001; 17:644–655.

111. Alderson P, Montgomery J. Health care choices: Making decisions with children: Summary of conclusions. Bulletin of Medical Ethics 1996; 117:8–11.

112. Geigy JR. Folia Medica scientific table. 1000. In: Diem K, Lentner C, eds. Documenta Geigy Scientific Tables. Basel, Switzerland: Ciba-Geigy; 1975.

9

Pediatric prescribing

George Rylance

INTRODUCTION

Prescribing for children encompasses a number of knowledge-based skills and practical considerations. These include knowledge and understanding of inter- and intraindividual variation relating to age, body composition, differential maturation of body organs, and state of health.

Pharmacokinetics is the mathematical expression of the drug handling processes of absorption, distribution, metabolism and excretion which determine a medicine's disposition in the body. Pharmacodynamics describes what the medicine does to the body and therefore the processes linking the concentration of a drug in a body fluid with pharmacological effect. This is essentially the interaction of a drug with a receptor at the site of action.

DRUG HANDLING PROCESSES

Unless they are administered directly into the vascular system, all medicines need to be absorbed. Most will depend on absorption from the gastrointestinal tract.

GASTROINTESTINAL ABSORPTION

The rate and extent of gastrointestinal absorption is affected by gut pH and flora, gastric contents and emptying time, gut motility and absorptive surfaces. All vary somewhat according to age and with certain disease processes. After the neonatal period, there are a few differences with age and gastrointestinal absorption of medicines is usually predictable in rate and extent. The unpredictability of the newborn period relates to reduced gastric acid secretion, reduced gastric emptying time, and reduced intestinal motility and biliary function. The oral route is preferred for drug administration generally.

OTHER ROUTES OF DRUG ABSORPTION

Absorption from **muscle** is unpredictable. Drugs which are not water soluble tend to precipitate with resultant delayed or decreased absorption. The rate and extent is also compromised by poor perfusion in serious illness.

Absorption through **skin** is more important with regard to toxicity than benefit. Preterm skin represents much less of a barrier than that of a full-term baby and hexachlorophene, aniline dye, and steroid toxicity have been reported. However, the same characteristics afford a potential for drug delivery via topical creams and patch formulations although these are limited in application.

DISTRIBUTION

The composition of body water compartments, protein binding, regional blood flow and membrane permeability are important determinants of drug distribution in the body. The relatively large total and extracellular body water compartments in the newborn and infancy period largely account for the greater drug distribution volumes in young children.

Drug distribution is also affected by the extent and characteristics of protein binding. The lower protein binding for drugs in particular in the newborn and infant probably relates to the amount of albumin available, different affinity, and competitive displacement by endogenous substances (e.g. bilirubin; free fatty acids). The greater free fraction at this age contributes to a larger distribution volume and increase in clearance. Although albumin is the major drug-binding protein, lipoproteins and alpha-1 acid glycoprotein are important and their concentration is influenced by age, nutrition and disease processes.

METABOLISM

Removal of a drug from the body occurs as soon as it is absorbed. The process of removal for many drugs includes biotransformation into more water-soluble compounds so facilitating elimination through the kidney or in bile. For most drugs, this process makes them less active or completely inactive although some 'parent' drugs are converted from active to other active compounds (theophylline to caffeine and morphine to morphine-6-glucuronide) and in some cases to more active compounds (carbamazepine to its 10′11 epoxide metabolite).

Most biotransformation processes occur in the liver although some occur in the intestine. There are two phases of metabolism, both occurring mainly within the hepatocyte. Phase I reactions are enzymatic and involve oxidation, reduction, hydroxylation or hydrolysis; Phase II reactions are mainly those of conjugation with glucuronide, sulfate or glycine.

The cytochrome P450 mixed function oxidase system is the most important biotransformation system incorporating many enzymes and isoenzymes. In general, these enzyme systems are immature at birth and particularly so in premature newborns. There is therefore relatively slow clearance of most metabolized drugs in the first 2 or 3 months of life. Between 2 and 6 months, clearance is more rapid than in adults and even more so for most drugs from 6 months to 2 years. From 2 to 12 years, somewhat faster clearance rates than in adults are maintained but after 12 years, adult values are the norm (Table 9.1).

159

Table 9.1 Approximate elimination half-life (t½) and total clearance (Cl) for drugs in children relative to adult values for different elimination pathways (from published literature database)

		Preterm newborn	Full-term newborn	1 week– 2 months	2 months– 6 months	6 months– 2 years	2 years– 12 years	12 years– 18 years
All drugs	t½	3.8	1.85	1.8	1.1	0.75	0.95	1.05
All drugs	Cl	0.5	0.7	0.75	1.2	1.7	1.35	1.0
Renally cleared drugs	t½	2.7	2.6	1.1	0.75	0.6	1.1	–
Metabolized drugs Cytochrome P450 Isoenzyme 1A2 (caffeine, theophylline)	t½	–	9.1	4.0	1.2	0.6	0.6	–
Metabolized drugs Cytochrome P450 Isoenzyme 3A	t½	5.1	1.9	1.75	0.35	0.5	0.75	0.75
Metabolized drugs Cytochrome P450 All isoenzymes	t½	4.4	1.75	3.5	1.25	0.6	0.75	0.95
Phase II glucuronidation drugs	t½	4.2	2.8	2.1	0.9	1.15	1.3	1.5

EXCRETION

Glomerular filtration of drugs depends on renal blood flow, protein binding and the functionality of the glomeruli. The relatively low glomerular filtration rates in premature and full-term newborns result in the half-lives of renal cleared drugs being approximately two to three times longer than those in adults, and this difference is maintained up to 1–2 weeks age. Thereafter, rates are similar in infants and adults up to 2 months. Half-lives are subsequently faster until about 2–3 years.

PHARMACOKINETICS

Pharmacokinetics refers to the mathematical expressions of drug changes in the body. **Bioavailability** describes the fraction (percentage) of drug reaching the systemic circulation of that presented to the body. For intravenously administered drugs, this is considered to be 1 (100%). For other routes of administration, values are usually somewhat less than 100% and this amount (and the rate of absorption) depends on a number of physicochemical properties of the drugs and other factors related to the patient. Reduced blood flow to the gut in intestinal and systemic illness tends to slow the rate and extent of absorption but food in the gut only tends to delay absorption.

Volume of distribution describes an apparent hypothetical volume within which a drug is distributed. It tends to be larger in babies, infants and young children than in adults. The relationship between dose (bioavailable dose = FD), volume of distribution (aV_d), and concentration (c) is given by the equation:

$$c = FD/aV_d \qquad \text{Equation 1}$$

In simplistic terms, it is like achieving a pink volume of liquid (c) when an amount of red dye (D) is put into a bucket of water (aV_d). In clinical terms, it determines what loading dose, either initially ($c \times aV_d$) or during maintenance therapy ((desired – measured concentration) $\times aV_d$) is required, e.g. to stop fitting using phenytoin.

The (**elimination**) **half-life (t1/2)** describes the time it takes for a drug concentration in any body fluid to reduce by half. It most frequently refers to blood. Mathematically its value is given by dividing 0.693 by the slope of the terminal portion of the log concentration–time 'curve' or elimination rate constant (k_e):

$$\mathbf{t1/2} = 0.693/k_e.$$

Clearance is the volume from which drug is removed per unit time. The concept of renal clearance is well understood. Drug clearance usually refers to total body clearance (Cl) and is the product of apparent volume of distribution and the elimination rate constant:

$$Cl = K_e \cdot aV_d \text{ or } Cl = (0.693/t1/2) \cdot aV_d.$$

PRESCRIBING PRINCIPLES

Choice of drugs depends on a number of factors. Of course, the benefit–risk assessment has to be positive, and the drug delivery needs to be practically feasible. This will depend on an assessment of handling, kinetics and formulation availability. For antibiotics the choice is further determined by the likely or known causal organism, the minimum inhibiting concentration (MIC), and the ability to reach the site of action.

In considering the **administration route** for most drugs, the oral route is preferred but is inappropriate if there is significant vomiting and when gut perfusion is compromised by systemic illness. Gut pathology and immaturity (first week or two of life) are significant and important considerations. The intramuscular route only serves the purpose of 'one-off' administration because of pain and unpredictable bioavailability. The skin route is more of a toxicity consideration but some benefit is afforded in the newborn and for a small but increasing number of drugs available as patches. Inhalation of antibiotics in cystic fibrosis, and steroid and/or beta-2 agonists in asthma are established examples for this route. The rectal route is more unpredictable than the oral route but affords possibilities in vomiting, 'nil by mouth', and upper gut pathologies. Rectal administration is well established in some acute situations (benzodiazepines in continuing fits) and in situations where skilled personnel are not available, e.g. home use of diazepam, paracetamol and antiemetics. More recent use of intranasal or buccal delivery has proved efficacious for midazolam as sedation and in stopping fits.

Some drugs are not stable when administrated orally but most drugs are and therefore should be given by this route. Liquids are most rapidly absorbed giving shorter times to peak concentrations. Tablets that require disintegration and dissolution are more slowly absorbed as a result. **Choice of formulation** is also important because of variation in palatability.

Dose determination is especially difficult given the wide inter- and intraindividual variability of pharmacokinetic parameters with age. Pharmacodynamic and receptor variability are less well worked out but are likely to be of similar or even greater importance. For drugs where there is only a small difference between appropriately effective and toxic concentrations (drugs with low or narrow **therapeutic indices**), individualization of dosage is even more important.

If there is a clear endpoint of efficacy (e.g. blood pressure lowering; stopping fits) and if there is a wide therapeutic index, titration with increasing doses is appropriate. For some problems and drugs, plasma concentration therapeutic ranges are established and doses are then determined by the target concentration. Pharmacokinetic knowledge determines dosage in these situations. For example, and using the rearranged Equation 1, the required single dose is the product of target concentration and apparent volume of distribution. For phenytoin use in a child who continues to convulse, the equation for an infant of 3 months could be:

$$\text{i.v. dose (mg/kg)} = aV_d(0.75\,\text{L/kg}) \times \text{desired concentration}$$
$$(20\,\text{mg/L}) = 15\,\text{mg/kg}.$$

The repeated doses that are necessary are determined by a drug's clearance; the frequency of dosing by its half-life (for drugs for which there is a relationship between concentration in blood and clinical effect). The dose is given by:

$$\text{Dose} = \text{concentration (mg/L)} \times \text{clearance (L.kg.h}^{-1}) \times \text{dose interval (h)}.$$

The **frequency of dosing** will not result in wide fluctuation between doses if the dose interval approximates the half-life.

Many of these considerations relate to knowledge about the kinetics of the drug, and the recommended dose regimens in prescriber reference sources are based on these and other factors where such knowledge exists.

Therapeutic drug monitoring whereby drug concentrations are measured to determine dose regimens is not practically useful for drugs (the majority) which have clearly defined and easily measured clinical effects or endpoints. For the remainder, drug level monitoring is potentially useful but established therapeutic ranges are available for only a few. Phenytoin and gentamicin are the best known examples. Concentration monitoring is especially useful in potential drug–drug interaction scenarios, where the therapeutic index is narrow, and in situations of therapeutic failure or potential noncompliance.

Practical conditions for measurement include: 'steady state' concentrations (at least five elimination half-lives should have elapsed since starting therapy in chronic situations); time of likely peak concentration; whether measurement is primarily for efficacy or toxicity (peak or trough [pre dose] concentrations may be more related to one or the other).

Length of treatment is determined by published data related to the condition treated and individual patient response. **Compliance** with therapy in chronic situations may frequently be no more than 50% of that prescribed or intended. Its relevance in the assessment of therapeutic failure should not be underestimated.

DRUG INTERACTIONS

Drugs primarily interact with food and other drugs. However, for most drugs, food is not of major clinical significance.

Interactions with other drugs – the effects of one drug changed by another – are important if they lead to toxicity or reduced efficacy. Drug absorption interactions are relatively unimportant. However, other pharmacokinetic interactions based on protein binding or drug clearance are potentially of much greater clinical relevance. Drugs which are more than 90% protein bound and with relatively low volumes of distribution are those for which interactions should be considered although changes arising from displacement of one drug from protein binding sites by another and so increasing the amount of 'free drug' are rarely of clinical importance because of the transient nature of this effect.

Drugs which influence the metabolism of others by inhibiting or inducing the mixed function oxidase system are frequently of clinical concern. Rifampicin, carbamazepine, phenytoin and phenobarbital are examples of enzyme-inducing drugs which lower the concentration of some other drugs. Cimetidine, erythromycin and sodium valproate are enzyme-inhibiting drugs which increase the concentrations of those other drugs dependent on similar mechanisms for clearance.

DRUGS IN BREAST MILK

The context of consideration should always be 'which drugs should not be used or deserve special consideration in breast-feeding mothers?' rather than 'should mothers be allowed to breast-feed when taking these drugs?' Few drugs require particular consideration. These are listed with effects and special considerations in Table 9.2. In general, the following considerations are relevant:

- Is a drug really necessary? If it is, a discussion between the pediatrician and mother's doctor is necessary.
- If a drug is needed, choose one which is the safer of alternatives, e.g. warfarin rather than phenindione; paracetamol rather than aspirin.
- Consider the benefit of measuring the drug concentration in the baby.
- Drug exposure may be reduced by taking medication just before a baby's long sleep, or just after breast-feeding.

UNLICENSED MEDICINES AND USE OF LICENSED MEDICINES FOR UNLICENSED APPLICATIONS

More than 30% of medicines used in hospital practice are either unlicensed, or are used outwith the license indications. The Joint Standing Committee on Medicines of the Royal College of Paediatric and Child Health and the Neonatal and Paediatrics Pharmacists Group has recognized the need for those who prescribe for children to prescribe unlicensed medicines, or use medicines 'off label' and has provided the following information and guidance:

- Those who prescribe for a child should choose the medicine which offers the best prospect for the child, with due regard to cost.
- The informed use of licensed medicines for unlicensed applications and unlicensed medicines is necessary in pediatric practice.
- Health professionals should have ready access to sound information on any medicine they prescribe, dispense or administer, and its availability.
- In general, it is not necessary to obtain explicit consent of parents, carers or child patients to prescribe or administer licensed medicines for unlicensed applications, or to prescribe unlicensed medicines.
- *Those with administrative responsibilities* should support therapeutic practices that are advocated by a respectable, responsible body of professional opinion.

WHAT PARENTS AND CHILDREN NEED TO KNOW ABOUT MEDICINES

The prescriber needs to recognize the need for information provision and the following is an appropriate and basic check list:

- Medicine generic/brand name;
- How the medicine is expected to help. What results are expected? How long it takes to start working;
- How much to take at one time and how often;
- For how long the medicine will need to be taken;
- When to take the medicine. Before or after meals? At bed time? At special times?;
- How to take the medicine. Can it be diluted? With juices? With food?;
- Other medicine, foods, drinks which shouldn't be taken with the medicine;
- What restriction on activities is necessary?;
- Possible side-effects. When might they occur? Can they be reduced? Will they go away by themselves?;

Table 9.2   Drugs and breast milk

Problem area	Drug	Effect
Cytotoxics	Cyclophosphamide Ciclosporin Doxorubicin Methotrexate	Possible immunosuppression; unknown effect on growth or association with carcinogenesis
Abuse/social	Amfetamine Cocaine Heroin Phencyclidine	Irritability, poor sleeping Irritability; vomiting; seizures Tremors; restlessness; poor feeding Potent hallucinogen
Radiopharmaceuticals (cessation of breastfeeding according to time of effect)	Copper 64 (^{64}Cu) Gallium 67 (^{67}Ga) Iodine 123 (^{123}I) Iodine 125 (^{125}I) Iodine 131 (^{131}I) Technetium 99m (^{99m}Tc)	Radioactive 50 h (3 d) Radioactive 2 weeks (2 weeks) Radioactive 30 h (2 d) Radioactive 12 d (2 weeks) Radioactive 2–14 d (2 weeks) Radioactive 15 h–3 d (3 d)
Other drugs to be cautious about	Atenolol Clemastine Ergotamine Lithium Phenindione	Cyanosis; bradycardia Drowsiness; irritability; high-pitched cry (1 case) Vomiting; diarrhea; fits Half therapeutic concentration Increased prothrombin time and partial prothrombin time

- When to seek help if problems occur;
- What to do and how long to wait if things don't get better;
- How to keep the medicine safely and in what storage provision;
- Expiry date;
- How to renew the medicine by prescription.

FURTHER READING

1.   American Academy of Pediatrics Committee on Drugs. Transfer of drugs and other chemicals into human milk. Pediatrics 2001; 108:776–789.

2.   Drug Information for the Health Care Professional 2002, 22nd edn. United States Pharmacopeia Micromedex. Thomson Healthcare.

3.   Ginsberg G, Hattis D, Sonawane B, et al. Evaluation of child/adult pharmacokinetic differences from a database derived from the therapeutic drug literature. Toxicol Sci 2002; 66:185–200.

4.   Medicines for Children. Royal College of Paediatrics and Child Health and Neonatal and Paediatric Pharmacists Group. London: RCPCH; 1999.

10

Ethics

Ben Stenson, Sheila McLean

INTRODUCTION

Everyone involved in the care of children has a duty of care that requires them to promote the best interests of the child. Decisions or recommendations made on behalf of children, as well as being medically appropriate, must be consistent with both ethics and law. To the fullest extent possible they should be joint decisions involving all of those with a legitimate role in the partnership of care and they must respect the human rights of everyone whose lives may be affected by them. In most everyday clinical situations the options available are relatively straightforward, the communication is harmonious and everyone involved agrees on the appropriate course of action. However, when situations are more complex major difficulties can arise.

The actions of health professionals are subject to external scrutiny more than ever before. Highly publicized enquiries into standards of practice in relation to postmortem examinations, organ retention, research conduct and children's cardiac surgery (see Appendix) have tested the trust of the public in the medical profession. Doctors need to become comfortable with the fact that their recommendations may be questioned rather than accepted uncritically, both at the time they are made and in retrospect once the outcome of a clinical situation is known. Practicing medicine under these circumstances requires familiarity with ethical reasoning, legal issues and the professional standards of behavior expected by regulatory bodies as well as with technical medical information. The aim of this chapter is to provide basic guidance in these matters. The same broad principles governing conduct apply wherever medicine is practiced but legal matters vary significantly by jurisdiction. The legal issues discussed here represent the position in UK jurisdictions. Guidance on professional matters can be found on the General Medical Council website (see Appendix).

CHILDREN'S RIGHTS

The UN Convention on the Rights of the Child[1] was endorsed by the UK Government in 1991. Although it influenced subsequent legislation, it was not directly translated into law, unlike the European Convention on Human Rights,[2] which became fully incorporated into UK law in October 2000 following the enactment of the Human Rights Act 1998.[3] The impact of this legislation on medical professionals is that their decisions will be tested against human rights norms and jurisprudence, as well as professional considerations. Up-to-date information about developments in the application of this new legislation can be obtained from the British Medical Association website (see Appendix). The rights of one individual can often conflict with the rights of another and determining which right carries most importance in a given situation can be difficult. Clinicians are encouraged to seek legal advice if they are in doubt in these matters.

As far as health issues are concerned, the main rights that are likely to affect medical practice are the right to life (article 2 of the Convention), the right not to be subjected to inhuman or degrading treatment (article 3), and the right to private and family life (article 8). Some other rights may be relevant, including the right to marry and found a family (article 12), which may affect fertility questions and the right not to be subjected to discrimination (article 14). The precise effect of these rights in the health context is not yet settled, but human rights arguments have already been taken into account in a number of important cases involving treatment decisions. At this stage, however, it must be pointed out that the human rights guaranteed in the Convention are not absolute (with the exception of article 3). Individual states benefit from what is called a 'margin of appreciation', which allows them to interpret the rights in a way that suits their own social and cultural principles.

CHILDREN AND CAPACITY – COMMUNICATION AND CONSENT

Honest, open communication is an essential foundation of ethical practice. Many differences of opinion originate from misunderstandings or inadequate information. The input of time required for optimal communication is substantial but the investment is usually repaid in the form of greater trust and confidence on the part of patients and parents. Communication is a two-way process and, where possible, should involve substantial listening as well as talking. When information has been shared and decisions or recommendations have been made openly there are greater grounds for confidence in their validity. However, there are issues associated with communicating with children that need to be specifically addressed, and these will vary with the age of the child.

THE VERY YOUNG CHILD

It is self-evident that very young children are not able to receive information, nor to express an opinion about proposed medical treatment. In this situation, parents have both the right and the responsibility to make decisions on behalf of their child, but they must act in the child's best interests (this will be considered in more depth later). For the moment, it is worth noting that parents, if they are to meet this standard, need access to accurate and clear medical information. Additionally, where there is a clear medical recommendation it should be made. Parents will generally wish to be guided by expert clinical recommendations, although they may not always agree with them. In some cases, it may be appropriate to offer to arrange for a second opinion, and of course interpreters can assist in overcoming language barriers. Discussion with the family's religious adviser may give an insight into the background to specific moral standpoints, although this should only be done with the consent of the family so as to avoid problems with confidentiality. There is an ongoing need to re-visit information and decisions with families to maintain confidence and to ensure the continued validity of the consent.

THE OLDER CHILD

Although the age of majority (the time at which a child becomes an adult) is set by law,[4,5] children become more mature as they age, and it is clear that children under the age of majority may have legal authority to make their own medical decisions. Great care should be taken in assessing whether or not a young person is sufficiently mature when they express an opinion about their treatment, but it should not simply be assumed that a child is not competent merely because they reject the medical recommendation.

A valid consent may, therefore, be given by a child under the age of 16, provided that the nature and implications of the treatment can be understood. Whether or not a child has the capacity to consent depends, then, on the maturity of the individual and on the complexity of the issues that have to be decided. A comparatively young child may be able to give consent to an uncomplicated procedure with no long-term implications for health (minor surgery, for example, or the administration of an antibiotic to combat an infection) whereas it will clearly require considerably greater understanding to consent to procedures involving greater risk. The law does not, and cannot, set out precise criteria for determining capacity: this will entail an assessment of the facts of each case. Once a child is deemed competent to consent to treatment (and this is a decision generally left to the attending doctors) it is not necessary to have parental consent as well. Only a single valid consent is required to enable treatment to proceed legally. The child should be encouraged to involve the parents, but this choice belongs to the competent child. A parental refusal of consent cannot override the consent of a competent child.

Once the child is seen to be capable of acting autonomously, there is no need for a proxy decision maker. Although it may seem logical from this position that a child who is competent to consent to medical treatment should also be competent to refuse it, courts have deemed young people who refuse medical treatment where a parent has consented not to be competent and have allowed treatment to proceed against the wishes of the child. In the English case of *Re W*,[6] a 16-year-old girl refused treatment for anorexia nervosa in spite of the grave threat that the illness posed to her health. Although she was legally entitled to consent to treatment, the court ruled that this did not imply a correlative authority to refuse it, and that parental consent in such circumstances would override the child's opposition until such time as the child reaches the age of majority (18 years in England and Wales). This means that provided that parental consent is obtained, treatment in the best interests of the child may be imposed even if the child satisfies legal criteria of competence. This is justified on the grounds that there is a difference between consent to treatment and its refusal; the latter requires greater maturity and understanding than the former. Ultimately, the need to preserve life may override other considerations. However in Scotland, where a young person acquires full decision-making capacity at 16 years of age, the courts would have no right to interfere with their decision, and arguably Scots law gives more rights to children under the age of 16 than does the law in England and Wales.[7]

Although children may be permitted to consent to treatment under the age of majority, this too may be ignored in the face of more important considerations. In *Re M*,[8] for example, the court authorized a heart transplant operation in the case of a 15-year-old girl who expressed strong objections to further treatment. This was done on the explicit grounds that the need to preserve her life outweighed the risks entailed and in the face of the possibility that she might in the future resent her wishes being ignored. A Human Rights Act challenge to this position is conceivable. Both article 3 and article 8 of the Convention provide some protection for the realm of private decision-making. It could be argued that subjecting a competent child to a strongly resisted procedure constitutes inhumane treatment, although this would have to be balanced against parental rights under article 8 to make decisions relating to family life. It is unlikely, though, that a court would allow a child to embark on a life-threatening course of action (even with parental approval). The law is prepared to be paternalistic in relation to the decisions that children make. Certainly autonomy may be encouraged, but courts have sometimes regarded it as a negation of the principle of respect for autonomy to allow choices that would prevent the development of the full autonomy that usually comes with adulthood.

However, maximizing children's autonomy is a worthwhile goal, and will depend in part on the quality of the communication with the child. Communication should always be truthful and realistic. Information about risks and benefits should reflect local experience as well as the outcomes described in the medical literature. In cases of possible medical error patients and parents should be informed and this should be documented. It may occasionally be justifiable to withhold information but only if disclosing it would cause serious harm to the patient or another person. The General Medical Council publication *Good Medical Practice* outlines professional standards on which continuing medical registration is dependent.[9] 'If a patient under your care has suffered harm, through misadventure or for any other reason, you should act immediately to put matters right, if that is possible. You must explain fully and promptly to the patient what has happened and the likely long- and short-term effects. When appropriate you should offer an apology.... In the case of children the situation should be explained honestly to those with parental responsibility and to the child, if the child has sufficient maturity to understand the issues.'

Sometimes parents and professionals may feel that giving a child full details is not in their best interests, but this should be the exception rather than the rule.

BEST INTERESTS OF CHILDREN

At the center of issues relating to the care of children is the requirement to safeguard the best interests of the child. A person's best interests are not definable in simple terms of physical health. A complex interaction of physical, emotional and social factors is involved. The health gains of a procedure alone may not, therefore, be sufficient to determine a clear best interest. If the child does not wish to be treated or investigated it may not be justifiable to do so. The negative impact on the child – and on relationships with the child – of performing a procedure against their wishes may outweigh any health benefit obtainable. On the other hand, while adults are free to make choices that to others might seem unwise and to take actions that place themselves at risk of harm, children who are in the process of developing competence or capacity as decision makers do not enjoy the same degree of autonomy. Until they become competent, others have rights and responsibilities to decide on their best interests for them. When a child's best interests are judged by a proxy decision maker it is, however, important to separate the interests of the child from those of the decision maker.

There are many reasons why caregivers and parents or young people may evaluate best interests differently. Health care professionals tend to be enthusiasts for positive action in response to health problems. They are strongly motivated to improve outcomes and tend to believe that scientific advances will help them to do so. If treatments are not working there is a natural urge to look for alternatives and a reluctance to accept failure. This so-called technological imperative[10] could lead a clinician to favor using treatments that a patient, or a different clinician, might not wish to agree to. The converse is also true. Experienced clinicians can sometimes be more pessimistic than parents or young people about what the future might hold.[11] It is important for clinicians to analyze whether their personal beliefs may affect the advice or treatment that they offer patients and to be open about this in order that patients can see another professional if they wish.

The values and experiences of parents and young people are also highly variable. Where the child is very young, and cannot express an opinion, parents may seek to impose their own views on the child. For example, people with particular religious beliefs may wish to reject certain treatments for their child (such as blood transfusion) that doctors believe to be vital – even life-saving. From the parents' point of view, the child's best interests are served by following their religious tenets; for doctors, their best interests are more likely to be concerned with continuing to live. Where such disputes arise, clinicians should seek legal advice and this may ultimately mean that the decision for the child is made by a court of law. This decision may not agree with the parents' views, of course, but the right of parents to be involved in their child's treatment decisions was recently reinforced by the European Court of Human Rights in the case of *Glass v United Kingdom*.[12] This case involved a serious (and ultimately violent) dispute between a family and the doctors caring for their son. Although it is authority for the right of parent(s) to be involved in the treatment plan for incompetent children, it should be treated with some caution. The legal finding against the health care professionals concerned was made directly because there were options for resolution – that is seeking a declaration from the High Court – that they had not taken. In that sense, it is of limited relevance, but it is an important case in establishing both the need to negotiate with families (and where this proves unsuccessful, to seek legal authority) and in its reinforcement of the family's rights in decision-making for incompetent children.

In the case of older children, it is important that their views are heard and, where appropriate, accommodated. We have already seen that decisions to reject recommended treatment can be overcome by the court or by the parents in England and Wales (even after the young person has reached the age of 16). In Scotland the position is different. At 16, a child becomes an adult for these purposes and his/her decisions cannot be interfered with by parents. In addition, the right of children under the age of 16 to make their own decisions (if they are sufficiently mature) about medical treatment is clear, and it has long been assumed that this includes the right to refuse treatment. The terms of s. 2(4) of the Age of Legal Capacity (Scotland) Act 1991[5] establish that a child under the age of 16 in Scotland can indeed make his or her own decisions if sufficiently mature. That this might include the right to refuse treatment seems to be clarified by the case of *Re Houston*.[13] In this case, a young man who suffered from mental illness was deemed competent to refuse medical treatment. It should be noted, however, that *Houston* is the only case that has been considered in Scotland on this ground, and it is a decision of one of the lower courts. It would not, therefore, be binding in a more senior court. The legislation does not specifically mention refusal, but it does seem clearly to give decision-making authority to competent people under the age of 16. What is important to bear in mind is that, in the case of older children, it is not their chronological age that necessarily is of importance; rather it is their understanding and maturity.

WITHHOLDING/WITHDRAWING TREATMENT

It is clear from the medical literature that it is common practice for life-prolonging treatment to be withdrawn. Discussions with parents about limitation and possible withdrawal of treatment may occur in up to 70% of deaths in UK neonatal units[14] and between 43% and 72% of deaths in pediatric intensive care units.[15] Since many of the issues raised by life-and-death dilemmas are ethical/legal and not medical, some commentators, notably philosophers and lawyers, believe that doctors and parents are not competent to make such decisions on their own and that the law should dictate this process. However, not every decision needs to be made by a court, and indeed it would be impossible for medicine to function if doctors were constantly required to seek legal endorsement of their clinical decisions. At the same time, the protection of human life is a matter of central concern for the law, and therefore any medical and parental decisions must be made against a background of certain legal limits as to what is permissible. Within these limits, there remains considerable room for nuanced and sensitive decisions to be made by those most intimately involved in the life of the child and his or her medical care. When this process fails, however, courts will likely become involved as the ultimate arbiter of the child's best interests.

The starting point of any discussion of this issue is the stark proposition that any deliberate act intended to bring life to an end normally amounts to the crime of murder. This is the case even if the person carrying out the act acted with the motive of ending the victim's suffering (assisted suicide or euthanasia). Although there have not been many convictions of doctors in the UK for killing their patients with this motive in mind, this is more because of the difficulty of getting juries to convict in such cases than of any ambiguity in the law. A recent attempt to change the law in the UK has been put on hold, and seems unlikely to succeed. Euthanasia is legal under some circumstances in the Netherlands, Belgium and the Northern Territory of Australia, where the State law was overruled by Federal legislation. Physician-assisted suicide is also explicitly permitted in the US state of Oregon, and is widely tolerated in Switzerland. The legal prohibition of assisted dying within the UK does not, however, prevent the appropriate and medically indicated use of pain-killing drugs that will have the incidental effect of shortening the life of the patient. This is justified by the doctrine of double-effect, which holds that pursuing a legitimate goal (in this case, pain relief) is justified even if this will have the inevitable effect of causing an undesirable event (the death of the patient). The fact that death is foreseen is not, in terms of this doctrine, the same as it being intended, although in other areas of law this description of the event has been challenged. For example, it was said in the case of *R v Woollin*[16] that where an outcome was foreseen as inevitable it must also be regarded as intentional. In other words, in the medical context, if a significant increase in analgesia predictably results in death, then the doctrine of double-effect may not be sufficient to avoid criminal charges.

Assisted dying is one thing, but the withdrawal or denial of treatment is regarded as quite different. It has long been accepted that it is lawful to withdraw life-prolonging treatment if it is no longer in a person's best interests and that it is lawful to withhold treatment for the same reason. This has been established in a series of cases in which the courts have considered the circumstances in which it is proper to withdraw support for infants and young children for whom the prognosis is bleak. In most of these cases the courts have recognized that where a child's suffering would be intense and where no reasonable quality of life could be achieved, then it is futile to continue with treatment. An example of such a decision is *A National Health Service Trust v. D*[17], in which the child in question had been born with chronic and worsening lung disease and suffered in addition from heart failure, hepatic and renal dysfunction as well as severe developmental delay. There was a difference of opinion in this case between the parental and medical views as to whether resuscitation should be attempted in future; the court endorsed the medical conclusion of futility. In reaching its conclusion, the court addressed arguments based on European Convention rights. In particular, the court said that the decision not to resuscitate was compatible with article 2 of the Convention (the right to life). It also expressed the view that such a course of action was in accordance with article 3, which requires that a person should not be subjected to inhuman or degrading treatment; undue prolongation of life through excessively zealous treatment could infringe the right to die with dignity. This decision is significant, in that it demonstrates that human rights provisions will not be interpreted in such a way as to oblige doctors to provide treatment in those circumstances where their clinical and indeed human judgment suggest otherwise.

The practice of withholding or withdrawing life-prolonging treatment is acknowledged and endorsed by the British Medical Association[18] and by the Royal College of Paediatrics and Child Health.[19] There is presently no legal requirement for the involvement of the courts in medical decisions of this nature, unless, as we have seen, there is a dispute that cannot otherwise be resolved. It is desirable, however, that decisions of such gravity, made on behalf of dependent individuals, are not taken by a single person but reflect the views of a body of people with an intimate involvement in the situation. This can provide a safeguard against the possibility that a decision could be overly influenced by the polarized views or values of one person. Openness should promote better decision-making. Clear documentation of the issues being addressed, the individuals involved and their viewpoints is an important part of this. Nor should decisions of this nature be rushed. In emergencies where the appropriate course of action is unclear and a plan has not been documented, trainee doctors should administer life-sustaining treatment until a senior and more experienced doctor arrives. With these safeguards in place it is reassuringly uncommon for parents to think later that the wrong decision was made.[20] It is not essential for there to be unanimity of views on the part of the medical team. There should be substantial consensus and the weight attributed to individual dissent will depend on the experience and knowledge of the person expressing it.

Withdrawal of life-prolonging treatment does not imply withdrawal of care. Care that is directed at maintaining the comfort and dignity of the patient (palliative care) is always required. The clinical team should continue to consider the child's physical, emotional and spiritual needs. Food and fluid should usually be offered (but not forced) on a regular basis. The role of assisted feeding by nasogastric tube or gastrostomy can be a source of difficulty. There is a spread of opinion as to what circumstances determine whether this is a life-prolonging medical treatment, a comfort measure or a basic necessity. In some circumstances such as the persistent vegetative state it may be seen to be in a person's best interests for feeding or i.v. fluids to be withdrawn. It is important to consider whether these measures are benefiting the patient. These issues must be handled sensitively, taking into account the views of the family and the staff.

Where consideration is being given to withdrawal of treatment there may be a number of treatments in use, such as mechanical ventilation, antibiotics, analgesics or sedatives and paralyzing agents. It is not appropriate to wait for the effect of the medications to wear off before withdrawing the ventilation. This would effectively amount to giving one futile treatment because you were already giving another. Analgesics should be continued after the withdrawal of ventilation. The primary intention of administering analgesics is to control pain and distress, and this has a clear benefit to the patient. A side effect of opioids may be that they suppress breathing and could shorten life; however this is not the purpose for which they are being administered. Subject to the caveat discussed earlier, the principle of double-effect is recognized and accepted in law.[21] The situation is a little more finely balanced in the case of paralyzing agents. If ventilation is withdrawn in a paralyzed patient, death will certainly follow shortly afterwards. These agents are generally being given to facilitate ventilation in a critically ill patient with severe cardio-pulmonary failure. Under these circumstances death is inevitable after withdrawal of ventilation whether paralyzing agents are being used or not. Paralyzing agents may therefore reasonably be continued up to the point that ventilation is withdrawn but should not be administered after extubation. In the absence of cardiopulmonary failure, paralyzing agents are unlikely to be in clinical use and should not be given to patients who are not going to be ventilated.

The Ethics Advisory Committee of the Royal College of Paediatrics and Child Health published guidance for professionals about withdrawing or withholding life-sustaining treatment from children.[19] This is available online (http://www.rcpch.ac.uk/publications/recent_publications/Witholding.pdf). The guidance highlights a number of axioms on which ethical decision-making about the withholding or withdrawal of life-prolonging treatment may be based:

1. There is no significant ethical difference between withdrawing (stopping) and withholding treatments, given the same ethical objective.
2. Optimal ethical decision-making concerning children requires open and timely communication between members of the health care team and the child and family, respecting their values and beliefs and the fundamental principles of ethics and human rights.
3. Parents may ethically and legally decide on behalf of children who are unable, for whatever reason, to express preferences, unless they are clearly acting against the child's best interest or are unable, unwilling or persistently unavailable to make such decisions on behalf of their child.
4. The wishes of a child who has obtained sufficient understanding and experience in the evaluation of treatment options should be given substantial consideration in the decision-making process.
5. The antecedent wishes and preferences of the child, if known, should also carry considerable weight given that conditions at the time for action match those envisaged in advance.
6. In general, resolution of disagreement should be by discussion, consultation and consensus.
7. The duty of care is not an absolute duty to preserve life by all means. There is no obligation to provide life-sustaining treatment if: (1) its use is inconsistent with the aims and objectives of an appropriate treatment plan or (2) if the benefits of that treatment no longer outweigh the burden to the patient.
8. It is ethical to withdraw life-sustaining treatment if refused by a competent child, or from children who are unable to express wishes and preference when the health care team and parent/carers agree that such treatment is not in the child's best interests.
9. A redirection of management from life-sustaining treatment to palliation represents a change in beneficial aims and objectives and does not constitute a withdrawal of care.
10. The range of life-sustaining treatments is wide and will vary with the individual circumstances of the patient. It is never permissible to withdraw procedures designed to alleviate pain or promote comfort.
11. There is a distinction to be drawn between treatment of the dying patient and euthanasia. When a dying patient is receiving palliative care, the underlying cause of death is the disease process. In euthanasia, the intended action is to cause death.
12. It follows that use of medication and other treatments that may incidentally hasten death may be justified if their primary aim is to relieve suffering. The Ethics Advisory Committee of the Royal College of Paediatrics and Child Health does not support the concept of euthanasia.
13. Legal intervention should be considered when disputes between the health care team, the child, parents and carers cannot be resolved by attempts to achieve consensus.

The guidance document outlines five situations where it may be ethical and legal to consider withholding or withdrawal of life-sustaining medical treatment from children:

1. **The Brain-dead Child.** In the older child where criteria of brainstem death are agreed by two practitioners in the usual way it may still be technically feasible to provide basic cardio-respiratory support by means of ventilation and intensive care. It is agreed within the profession that treatment under such circumstances is futile and the withdrawal of current medical treatment is appropriate.
2. **The Permanent Vegetative State.** The child who develops a permanent vegetative state following insults, such as trauma or hypoxia, is reliant on others for all care and does not react or relate to the outside world. It may be appropriate to withdraw or withhold life-sustaining treatment in these circumstances. In England and Wales, withdrawing such treatment requires the authority of the courts.[22] In Scotland, no such permission is demanded, although the Lord Advocate has indicated that only in those cases where it has been obtained will there be a guarantee of no prosecution.

3. **The No Chance Situation.** The child has such severe disease that life-sustaining treatment simply delays death without significant alleviation of suffering. Treatment to sustain life in this case is inappropriate.

4. **The 'No Purpose' Situation.** Although the patient may be able to survive with treatment, the degree of physical or mental impairment will be so great that it is unreasonable to expect them to bear it.

5. **'The Unbearable Situation'.** The child and/or family feel that in the face of progressive and irreversible illness further treatment is more than can be borne. They wish to have a particular treatment withdrawn or to refuse further treatment irrespective of the medical opinion that it may be of some benefit.

The document concludes that:

'In situations that do not fit with these five categories, or where there is uncertainty about the degree of future impairment or disagreement, the child's life should always be safeguarded in the best way possible by *all* in the health care team, until these issues are resolved.'

Decisions about withdrawing or withholding life-prolonging treatment are likely to be based on probabilities rather than on certainties. Parents need to be prepared for what might follow. Death may take minutes or hours or may not occur at all. Protracted deaths are particularly stressful for parents and may cause them to doubt the wisdom of the decision. There is a danger that withdrawing or withholding treatment in a child who goes on to survive may mean that the eventual outcome is worse than would otherwise have been the case. Unexpected survivors need ongoing support, evaluation and respect.

Disputes about where the balance between the views of doctors and parents should lie are at their most acute when the outcome of following one or the other would result in the death of a child. Again, in these cases, it is wise to seek legal advice and the ultimate decision may become that of the courts.

Several UK cases have involved this situation. In *Re C (a minor)*,[23] a decision of the Family Division of the High Court of England and Wales, there was a difference of opinion between the parents and the doctors of a 16-month-old child suffering from spinal muscular atrophy. The medical view was that further ventilation in the event of a collapse was futile, a view that was not shared by the parents who, for religious reasons, believed that everything possible should be done to save human life. The court declined to endorse the parental view. In *R v. Cambridge District Health Authority, ex parte B*,[24] the father of a child requiring treatment with a limited chance of success challenged the decision of the area health authority that this treatment was not justified. This was unsuccessful, the Court of Appeal accepting that decisions have to be made about the allocation of resources and that parents could not upset such hard decisions, provided that they were reasonably reached by those making them.

Parental wishes were at the center of two further life-or-death cases: *Re T (a minor) (wardship: medical treatment)*[25] and, more recently, *Re A (children)*.[26] In *Re T* a parental decision to refuse a liver transplant for a child suffering from biliary atresia was upheld, even although medical opinion was that this could add several years to the child's life. This was an exceptional case and in *Re A (children)*, the highly publicized conjoined twins case, parental opposition to surgery to separate the children was overruled.

More recently two further cases have highlighted the complexities of these decisions. In the case of Charlotte Wyatt, who was born with multiple life-threatening pathologies, the views of the clinicians caring for her were that she would be best served by being allowed to die. In their view, aggressive treatment was not appropriate; indeed, it was essentially futile. Her parents, however, wanted treatment to continue and were determined that she should receive every assistance to live. In the event, Charlotte lived for many months longer than her doctors would have predicted, although it is impossible to judge objectively the quality of her life.

In October 2004, the High Court in England declared that Charlotte's best interests, in the event that she suffered from an infection which led, or might lead, to a collapsed lung, would be served by providing 'all suitable medical care including antibiotics'.[27] Should, however, she require intubation and/or ventilation, it would be lawful for her doctors to decide not to provide this treatment. Her doctors could also lawfully decide that it was appropriate to administer continuous positive airway pressure (CPAP), but if she were 'visibly distressed' by this, it would also be lawful to withdraw it. Finally, it would be lawful for her doctors to use symptomatic relief to make her more comfortable, even if that might depress her efforts to breathe (double-effect). In December 2004, the judge made three further declarations, and the case was heard again in January 2005, when the court instructed that further experts should be engaged to discover whether or not Charlotte's condition was improving, as her parents insisted it was. Later in 2005, in the High Court, the judge lifted an order saying that doctors would not be acting unlawfully if they decided not to give Charlotte artificial ventilation in a life-threatening situation, and indicated that her parents should reach agreement with the doctors about their daughter's treatment if a crisis arose. However, in February 2006, Charlotte's condition had worsened, and in his latest ruling Mr Justice Hedley said that Charlotte's deterioration meant that circumstances had changed. She had developed a cough, probably caused by a viral infection, and was having difficulty breathing. Mr Justice Hedley therefore agreed that doctors could lawfully decide not to resuscitate her if they feel it would not be in her best interests to do so.

The second case is referred to as *Re MB*.[28] In this case, the child was found to have a degenerative, inherited condition that would ultimately require him to be artificially ventilated before his inevitable death. The parents wished all treatment – including artificial ventilation – to be used; the clinicians, on the other hand, believed that the child's best interests would not be served by imposing painful, distressing and ultimately futile treatment. The court acknowledged that the views of each were important, but that its task was objectively to establish the best interests of the child. In the event, the judge declared that it was in the child's best interests for current treatment (including continuous pressure ventilation) to be continued. However, should interventions such as cardiopulmonary resuscitation (CPR) or the i.v. administration of antibiotics be required, it would be in his best interests to withhold them. However, if parents and doctors are in agreement that treatment should be continued, then the Law will not need to be involved. Should parents wish no treatment to be given and the doctors disagree, again they should seek legal advice. In one such case, the court allowed parents to refuse treatment even although the doctors believed that it would be life-saving, showing just how complex this situation can be.[29]

PARENTAL RESPONSIBILITY

Broadly the obligations of parents are to care for the child and to raise him or her to moral physical and emotional health. This is the fundamental task of parenthood and the only justification for the authority that it confers. This is enshrined in The Children Act 1989,[30] which applies in England and Wales, and the Children (Scotland) Act 1995,[31] which is the equivalent Scottish legislation. Having said that, parental decisions that are not in the best interests of their children can be overridden by the courts, as has been reported. However, given that parents have the primary rights and responsibilities in respect of their children under these Acts, it is important to discover who actually has parental rights, bearing in mind that in an emergency, where treatment is necessary to prevent serious deterioration in a child's condition or to save its life, treatment can proceed without consent.

Who is a parent?

The biological parents are the legal parents unless a child has been adopted; however biological parenthood does not necessarily confer parental responsibility under the Acts (except where parental rights have been acquired following a surrogacy arrangement in terms of s.30 of the Human Fertilisation and Embryology Act 1990.[32] The mother has parental responsibility, and so does the father, provided that he was married to the mother at the time of the conception or the birth, or if he marries her after the birth. Once a parent has obtained parental responsibility, it is not lost in the event of divorce. It is possible that the Human Rights Act could be used by unmarried fathers to establish their parental responsibility on the basis of their right to enjoy family life if the mother of the child is not permitting them involvement, but the outcome of any such challenge is unclear.

Of course, a parent is not always available. The person who has care of the child under these circumstances (e.g. a grandparent or carer) has a responsibility under the Children Act to do 'what is reasonable in all the circumstances of the case for the purposes of safeguarding or promoting the child's welfare. This could in theory include giving consent to medical treatment, but carers should not give consent if they know that the parent is likely to object.

In England, Wales and Northern Ireland if the parents are not married, the father can gain parental responsibility by entering into a parental responsibility agreement with the mother and registering it in the Principal Registry of the Family Division of the High Court. A father can also be granted parental responsibility by a court. Adoptive parents have parental responsibility. The courts can grant parental responsibility to others such as a guardian or a local authority where the child is made the subject of a care order or a residence order. The parental responsibility that accompanies these orders lasts for the duration of the order. The court itself can also give consent to treatment on behalf of a child and can make specific issue orders or prohibited steps orders limiting parental responsibility in specified circumstances. The High Court can make the child a ward of court, which requires all important decisions about the welfare of the child to be referred to the Court. In an emergency the High Court is available at all hours and, if appropriate, a duty judge can be obtained through the security officer at the Royal Courts of Justice. The judge may deal with the issue by telephone or in person. A medical adviser should be available to speak to the judge in such circumstances.

In Scotland, unmarried fathers can gain parental responsibility through a voluntary parental responsibility agreement with the mother, registered in the Books of Council and Session. Fathers can also apply to the Sheriff Court or the Court of Session for an order granting them parental responsibilities and rights. Adults can gain parental responsibility by being appointed as guardians or on the order of a court. The Court of Session can give consent on behalf of a child who is not competent but, as we have seen, probably cannot override the refusal of a competent young person, although this has not been tested. As in the rest of the UK, the courts are available at all hours, if necessary, and can respond promptly. Both the Sheriff Court and the Court of Session can make decisions about medical issues. Contact should be made with the local Sheriff Court or with the Keepers office and if appropriate a Sheriff or Judge Depute will be contacted. As before, a medical advisor should be available via telephone or in person to answer any questions. The court can make specific issue orders or prohibited steps orders. One further arena for welfare-based decisions is the Children's Hearing System. If someone believes that a child requires compulsory measures of supervision, an official called a 'Reporter' will investigate and decide whether a ground for referral to a children's hearing is established, e.g. that the child is likely to suffer serious impairment in his health or development due to a lack of parental care. If such a ground is established a hearing is arranged. If the young person and the parents accept the ground for referral the hearing can then decide on the case and issue an appropriate order. If the ground is not accepted then the case must be determined by a Sheriff Court. If the Sheriff decides that the ground is valid the case is returned to the Children's Hearing, which can make supervision decisions; otherwise it is dismissed.

Under the Adoption and Children Act (2002)[33] in England and Wales and the Family Law Scotland Act 2006,[34] unmarried fathers now automatically gain parental responsibility if they are named as the father on the birth certificate.

CONFIDENTIALITY

Adults should be able to assume that health care professionals dealing with personal information about them will maintain confidentiality.

Confidentiality may be broken but only when consent (express or implicit) is given for disclosure or where it becomes necessary to breach confidence to protect others from a risk of serious harm. When children have been deemed competent their right to confidentiality must be respected, as long as this is judged to be in their best interests. (This was established legally in the case of *Gillick v. West Norfolk and Wisbech Area Health Authority*.[35]) When serious issues are being considered, the competent child should be encouraged to involve their parents but the choice belongs to the competent child. Less mature children may also wish for matters to remain confidential. They too should be encouraged to share information with their parents voluntarily and their confidence should not be broken lightly. If the information involves serious matters relating to the health or well-being of the incompetent child, the health care professional will have to disclose the information but they should not do so without informing the child of their intention and explaining their reasons for disclosing the information. In cases of abuse or neglect there is a responsibility to disclose information to the social services to protect the child from possible harm. It may be justifiable not to inform the child of your intention to disclose this information but only if doing so would introduce a serious risk to their health and well-being.

Medical records are confidential, which means that parents may not see the medical records of their competent child without their permission. Children have a right of access to their own records under the Access to Health Records Act 1990[36] provided that the child is capable of understanding the nature of his or her application for access (s. 4 of the Act). This right of access to the record may also be exercised by the parent or guardian on behalf of the child. As in the case of an application by an adult to see medical records, information can be withheld when the person holding the record believes that disclosing it will cause serious harm to the patient or another person.

Where personal health information potentially attributable to an individual is published or presented, consent should be sought for the disclosure, although under section 60 of the Health and Social Care Act 2001[37] the nonconsensual use of identifiable patient information for the purposes of research and the improvement of treatment services may be authorized in certain circumstances. In the normal case, consent for the use of identifiable patient information should specify the ways in which the information will be disclosed. When such information is disclosed for research purposes to others who are not directly involved in the care of the patient, consent should also be sought. Anonymized information is not protected in the same way, and considerable benefit is obtained from clinical improvement activity and research work in which clinicians analyze their patient information databases and the anonymized databases of others. Such work would become impracticable if individual patient consent was required and there would be a potential for considerable loss of health benefit to patients.

Since the Caldicott Report,[38] within the UK each health care organization must appoint a Caldicott Guardian. This is usually a senior health professional responsible for safeguarding the confidentiality of patient information.

DUTY OF CARE OF THE HEALTH PROFESSIONAL

The clinician has an ethical and legal duty of care to protect the life and health of his or her patients. Treatment decisions should be consistent with the basic ethical principles of beneficence and nonmaleficence, which require that the benefits must outweigh the burdens. In the UK, doctors alone have the right to decide whether a treatment is medically appropriate and patients have no right to insist on treatment from a doctor if that doctor does not consider it to be in their best interests. Similarly, parents have no right to obtain such treatments for their children. The courts cannot oblige doctors to undertake any specific medical intervention, even if parents wish to insist on it – although courts may agree with parents that treatment is appropriate, as we have already seen.

If the clinician is being pressed to administer a treatment deemed inappropriate, all efforts should be made to resolve the situation through further discussion. If these efforts do not succeed, the clinician should go to reasonable lengths to find an alternative clinician for the family, although if good decision-making practices have been followed there may not be one easily identifiable. If these measures do not succeed and the clinician has the support of his colleagues then he cannot be forced to treat. However, the parents should be informed of their right to obtain judicial review if they wish. Following the *Glass* judgement,[12] it is clear that parents have this right. However, it would be for the parents in this situation, rather than the doctors, to initiate any such action as the doctor's actions are regarded as appropriate professionally. If the medical reasoning has been sound and the clinician's colleagues support him then there is a strong prospect that the decision not to treat will be upheld. If a doctor refuses to give a treatment then this decision may later be challenged legally on the grounds that it amounts to a failure to discharge the duty of care owed to the patient. If there has been such a failure, then this may amount to negligence, the presence of which is determined by applying the test of whether the doctor has acted in accordance with the practice accepted by a responsible body of medical practitioners skilled in that particular art, and that his decision was logical. In other words, a specialist must practice with the ordinary skill of his speciality.[39,40]

Doctors have no legal authority to institute treatment in the absence of consent but they have a duty of care and an ethical responsibility to institute emergency treatment deemed to be in the child's best interests. If there is doubt as to the best interests in an emergency, then this same duty should compel them to act on the presumption that the child would want to be saved, at least until there has been time for further consideration. Under these circumstances, if the action satisfied the legal test described earlier, it is highly likely (even if not absolutely certain) that the courts would support it.

If the patient or parents refuse consent to important but nonurgent treatment, attempts should again be made to resolve the dispute through further communication. A second opinion, particularly from an acknowledged expert, may help. If these measures do not succeed and the clinician has support for his position from his colleagues, judicial resolution should be sought. Again the sharing of the information with colleagues and presence of their support will increase the chances that the court will endorse the doctor, but if the decision-making process has lacked balance then the court will rightly support the alternative position. One viewpoint is that seeking a judicial resolution might take the pressure off the relationship between the family and the clinician. In reality it probably just relocates the conflict from the consulting room to the courtroom without substantially changing the individuals involved, the balance of power or the nature of the conflict.[41]

GENETIC TESTING

Recent progress in elucidating the genetic basis of disease has been beyond all expectation and continued progress is likely. This carries great potential to improve health through new approaches to the diagnosis, treatment and prevention of illness. Further progress must be made before gene therapy becomes widespread but diagnosis and screening are already widely established. This gives rise to a number of ethical issues.[42] Rare and serious diseases that affect the health of children can be detected and this has obvious potential benefit to children. The new science also offers increasing capacity to detect predisposition to illnesses or even behavioral traits that may affect individuals only in adulthood. The results of such tests may have marked adverse effects on a child and on their future potential. As well as the person being tested, genetic tests also affect many others who are related to them. They may influence parental reproductive decisions. They may cast doubt on parenthood. They may raise similar issues for siblings. False-positive and false-negative results can cause considerable anxiety. Genetic tests should therefore only be used with caution, informed consent and adequate counseling. In general, tests on children should only be performed when a direct benefit to the child is anticipated during childhood. If the test will give information that will not have great relevance to the child

until adulthood, then it should be deferred until the child is competent to decide for him- or herself whether or not to agree to testing. This cautious approach to the genetic testing of children has been endorsed in the UK by the Government's Advisory Committee on Genetic Testing and by its successor body, the Human Genetics Commission (see Appendix).

Consent to genetic testing raises questions that have yet to be firmly settled. In the case of routine nongenetic tests carried out in a clinical context, all that is required is that there should be consent to the necessary medical procedures (by the competent child or by the parent or guardian). It is not necessary to explain the implications of every biochemical test, for example, that will be carried out on a sample. Where, however, the test has particular significance (such as a human immunodeficiency virus [HIV] test), the person giving consent should know the nature of the test being proposed. Genetic tests have special features that should be explained in general terms to the patient. In particular, genetic tests may have implications for other family members, and if this is the case then this should be discussed with the parent (and with the child, if the child is sufficiently mature to understand what is entailed by the information). Further questions are raised by multiplex testing, which may involve testing for a number of different genetic characteristics through devices capable of detecting numerous DNA sequences. It may be unrealistic to expect a full explanation to be given of everything that such a test may do, and for this reason consent should be valid if it is explained to the patient that a number of genetic characteristics may be revealed by the test and that this information may be retained on the record. Obviously this must be done sensitively, as nothing will be gained by giving complicated explanations that may serve only to alarm the patient unnecessarily. In respect of consent to testing, all that the law requires is that the doctor should give the patient that amount of information that is reasonable in the circumstances. A sound sense of current professional consensus on these issues is probably as good a guide as any as to how the matter should be approached.

Paternity testing may be requested by parents. This should not be performed without the involvement of both parents unless authorized by a court. Courts usually determine that testing is in the interests of the child. The child and family may need a lot of support and counseling. Guidelines on this subject are now available (see Appendix).

RESEARCH

There is no doubt that medical research can be in the best interests of children. Without it, medicine would be unable to progress, ineffective treatments would not be discarded, effective new treatments not introduced, and dangerous ones not identified. Carrying on in ignorance where properly conducted research could determine the optimal path is unethical. However, while research may benefit society it can sometimes be of little benefit to the individual under study. This may be irrelevant in the case of competent adults, who can consent to participate in ethical research even if it is of no therapeutic benefit to them. The involvement of children in research is more problematic. Research that is of potential therapeutic benefit to the child is acceptable, and can be consented to by the parent on behalf of the child. Nontherapeutic research, however, is of no benefit to the child, unless, possibly, the child has a sibling or other close relative who suffers from the condition that is the subject of research. In such a case, it is possible to argue that the child benefits from helping to advance knowledge of a condition that affects him or her through the family link. There are other ways in which participation might be in the best interests of the child. Patients enrolled in studies tend to experience some improvement in their clinical outcomes when compared with similar patients who are not being studied.[43] This inclusion benefit may relate to the closer supervision necessary to perform successful research. Where there is no such justification, then it must be asked whether it is either ethical or legal to involve children in nontherapeutic research.

One further constraint on the involvement of children in research relates to the question of risk. There is widespread agreement that it is ethical to use children in medical research provided that the research in question involves a negligible risk of harm to the child. There is a range of views as to how this risk is to be assessed. The legal position on this issue is more complex. It has been suggested in the past that the Law prevented participation by children even in nonrisky research on the grounds that parental consent, which would be needed, cannot be given in respect of anything that is not in the best interests of the child. On this view it would be impossible, then, for a parent ever to agree to something from which the child would not benefit. However, the view has also emerged that a parent may consent to that which does not actually threaten the child's interests. This would mean that nontherapeutic research on children is permissible, with parental consent, as long as the risk is negligible. It is not yet settled whether this latter view would be taken by the Law, particularly given the best interests requirement that predominates judicial decision-making in this area.

It should be stressed that if the child is old enough to have views on involvement, these views should be taken into account (even if the child does not have the capacity to consent in general). If a research procedure involves discomfort, and the child objects, then it would be unethical to continue with the procedure. From the legal point of view it would clearly not be in the child's best interests to proceed with unwelcome procedures.

In 2000, The Ethics Advisory Committee of the Royal College of Paediatrics and Child Health published guidelines for the ethical conduct of medical research involving children.[44] Six principles were outlined:

1. Research involving children is important for the benefit of all children and should be supported, encouraged and conducted in an ethical manner.
2. Children are not small adults; they have an additional, unique set of interests.
3. Research should only be done on children if comparable research on adults could not answer the same question.
4. A research procedure that is not intended directly to benefit the child subject is not necessarily either unethical or illegal.
5. All proposals involving medical research on children should be submitted to a research ethics committee.
6. Legally valid consent should be obtained from the child, parent or guardian as appropriate. When parental consent is obtained, the agreement of school-age children who take part in research should also be requested by researchers.

In 2005, the Additional Protocol to the Convention on Human Rights and Biomedicine, Concerning Biomedical Research (Council of Europe)[45] also considered research on incompetent people, and proposed the following guidelines:

ARTICLE 15 – PROTECTION OF PERSONS NOT ABLE TO CONSENT TO RESEARCH

1. Research on a person without the capacity to consent to research may be undertaken only if all the following specific conditions are met:
   i. the results of the research have the potential to produce real and direct benefit to his or her health;
   ii. research of comparable effectiveness cannot be carried out on individuals capable of giving consent;
   iii. the person undergoing research has been informed of his or her rights and the safeguards prescribed by law for his or her protection, unless this person is not in a state to receive the information;
   iv. the necessary authorization has been given specifically and in writing by the legal representative or an authority, person or body provided for by law, and after having received the information required by article 16, taking into account the person's previously expressed wishes or objections. An adult not able to consent shall as far as possible take part in the authorization procedure. The opinion of a minor shall be taken

into consideration as an increasingly determining factor in proportion to age and degree of maturity;
   v. the person concerned does not object.
2. Exceptionally and under the protective conditions prescribed by law, where the research has not the potential to produce results of direct benefit to the health of the person concerned, such research may be authorized subject to the conditions laid down in paragraph 1, subparagraphs ii, iii, iv, and v above, and to the following additional conditions:
   i. the research has the aim of contributing, through significant improvement in the scientific understanding of the individual's condition, disease or disorder, to the ultimate attainment of results capable of conferring benefit to the person concerned or to other persons in the same age category or afflicted with the same disease or disorder or having the same condition;
   ii. the research entails only minimal risk and minimal burden for the individual concerned; and any consideration of additional potential benefits of the research shall not be used to justify an increased level of risk or burden.
3. Objection to participation, refusal to give authorization or the withdrawal of authorization to participate in research shall not lead to any form of discrimination against the person concerned, in particular regarding the right to medical care.

The UK has not yet ratified this Convention, but it is likely that these guidelines will be seen as persuasive, and they should certainly be taken into account in the interests of best practice.

The same basic principles apply when consent is obtained for research studies as when consent is obtained for treatment or examination. The person must be given adequate information to enable them to understand the nature and purpose of the research and weigh up its risks and benefits, otherwise it will be invalid. However, consent can be difficult to achieve when the individual is already heavily burdened with complex information,[46] and even when people have given written consent they do not always remember that they did so.[47] Recollection of the information that they were given is often poor and their understanding of what they consented to may be incorrect.[48] For these reasons researchers should regard the process of seeking consent as ongoing throughout the duration of their involvement with any patient. They should maintain the child's and the parents' awareness that they are enrolled in a study, explaining any procedures, tests or treatments that are being used and making clear whether they are part of standard care or are being performed specifically for the purposes of the study.

Wherever possible, a reasonable amount of time should be allowed between informing a family about a research study and obtaining consent. This can be impracticable in some studies where interventions are performed under pressure of time, e.g. in the immediate newborn period. The child and family should be aware that they are free to withdraw from a study at any time without penalty. Important details about the study should be given in the form of a printed information sheet that the patient can keep, as well as being communicated verbally. Financial rewards should not be offered to families other than reasonable expenses. Pressure should not be exerted. If the child and family wish to know the final results of the research then these should be made available to them as soon as is practicable. There may be considerable delay in this if long-term follow-up requires blinding to be maintained.

Poorly designed research is unethical research. Peer review and statistical advice should be sought during study design. Often the results of studies can be disappointing, with no positive finding. It is still important to attempt to publish these studies to avoid others repeating the work and burdening future participants unnecessarily. Failure to publish negative results is an important source of bias in the literature. This has been made difficult by the competition for publication in a limited amount of journal space. With advances in technology this should lessen as electronic publishing will provide the space for studies that cannot compete successfully for mainstream scientific journal exposure.

A great deal of research is commercially sponsored.[49] As well as potentially affecting the outcomes of future patients, the results of such studies are economically important to individuals or companies. Clinicians entering into agreements to organize such studies should not do so if they are not given a say in the study design, access to the full data and freedom to publish the data, even if the results are not flattering to the product in question. At the time of submission for publication, authors should disclose all financial interests between themselves and others that might influence their work.

MENTAL HEALTH CARE

When treating people for mental illness the same ethical principles apply as when treating others. The Mental Health Acts[50,51] describe statutory powers that allow patients to be detained in hospital and treated for mental illness in the interests of their own health. There is no specific statutory authority to treat physical disorders of those receiving treatment under the Mental Health Acts. Psychiatric treatment can proceed without consent where a patient has been compulsorily admitted under the relevant Act. Children or young people who have been detained under the Mental Health Acts have the right to a hearing either before a tribunal or, in Scotland, the Sheriff Court. The tribunal, or court, may order the discharge of a detained patient if the patient is found not to have a mental disorder of a nature or degree justifying detention in hospital. Alternatively, even if a disorder is present, discharge may be ordered if the detention is not justified in the interests of the patient's health or safety, or in order to protect others.

A ROLE FOR ETHICS COMMITTEES?

Given the uncertainty faced by many caregivers in complex ethical and legal situations, some consider that there may be a role for institutional ethics committees to provide advice, education and support.[52] Doctors and nurses do not express widespread support for a decision-making role for such committees[53] and neither do parents.[54] In the UK, any medical decision made would remain the legal and professional responsibility of the doctor concerned. More work is required to establish the value of these committees. There is however, a clear need for better education of health care staff in the ethical and legal matters.[53] Further information about existing committees can be obtained from the UK Clinical Ethics Network website (http://www.ethics-network.org.uk).

CONCLUSION

Treating children is a particularly complex area of the medical enterprise. Care should be taken to identify the child's best interests, to communicate carefully with the child (where possible) and the parents, and – where the child is sufficiently mature – serious and appropriate weight should be given to their views. The legal trend is increasingly to prioritize and respect autonomy, but children's autonomy and their best interests may sometimes appear to conflict. Resolving this tension requires careful and sensitive communication. In the event that no agreement can be reached, it may be necessary to seek legal advice, and even to involve the courts.

APPENDIX – INFORMATION RESOURCES

ETHICAL AND LEGAL ISSUES

Consent, Rights and Choices in Health Care for Children and Young People. London: BMJ Books; 2001. This book gives an excellent detailed overview of many of the issues discussed in this chapter.

Mason and McCall Smith's Law and Medical Ethics, 7th edn. Oxford University Press; 2006. This is an outstanding textbook on the whole area of medical law and ethics.

ROYAL LIVERPOOL CHILDREN'S INQUIRY

The Royal Liverpool Children's Inquiry Report (The Redfern Report) London: The Stationery Office; 2001. http://www.rlcinquiry.org.uk/

NORTH STAFFS INQUIRY

Report of a review of the research framework in North Staffordshire Hospital NHS Trust (Griffiths report). This can be found on the Department of Health Website, policy and guidance section http://www.dh.gov.uk/PolicyAndGuidance/fs/en *See also*: Hey E, Fleming P, Sibert B Learning from the sad, sorry saga at Stoke. Arch Dis Child 2002; 86:1–3.

BRISTOL INQUIRY

Public Inquiry into Children's Heart Surgery at the Bristol Royal Infirmary 1984–1995. In: Learning from Bristol. London: Stationery Office; 2001. (Cmnd 5207.) http://www.bristol-inquiry.org.uk/

SCOTLAND

Report of the Independent Review Group on Retention of Organs at Post-Mortem, Edinburgh: Stationery Office; 2001

GENERAL MEDICAL COUNCIL

Standards of practice on which ongoing professional registration within the United Kingdom depend are outlined on the General Medical Council web-site at http://www.gmc-uk.org. This site covers a broad range of issues including, duties of a doctor, good medical practice, medical research guidance, withholding and withdrawing treatment, confidentiality, consent, and guidance for doctors asked to circumcise male infants.

BRITISH MEDICAL ASSOCIATION

Up-to-date information about the impact of the European Convention on Human Rights on medical practice within the UK can be obtained from the BMA web-site at http://www.bma.org.uk.

HUMAN GENETICS COMMISSION

http://www.hgc.gov.uk/Client/library.asp Includes: 'Whose hands on your genes?' (November 2000) – A consultation document on the uses of human genetic information, followed by a report on this subject (May 2002).

PATERNITY TESTING

Code of Practice and Guidance on Genetic Paternity Testing Services (Department of Health Guidance Document). This can be found on the Department of Health policy and guidance section http://www.dh.gov.uk/PolicyAndGuidance/fs/en website.

PUBLICATION ETHICS

Guidelines on good publication practice have been published by the Committee on Publication Ethics. Http://www.publicationethics.org.uk.

REFERENCES

1. UN Convention on the Rights of the Child 1989 available at http://www.unicef.org/crc.

2. European Convention on Human Rights 1950 available at http://www.hri.org/docs/ECHR50.html.

3. Human Rights Act 1998.

4. Family Law Reform Act, 1969.

5. Age of Legal Capacity (Scotland) Act 1991.

6. Re W. (a minor) (medical treatment) [1992] 4 All ER 627.

7. Elliston S. If you know what's good for you. In: McLean SAM, ed. Contemporary issues in law, medicine and ethics. Aldershot: Dartmouth; 1996.

8. Re M (child: refusal of medical treatment) [2000] 52 BMLR 124.

9. General Medical Council. Good medical practice. London: GMC; 1998.

10. Guillemin JH, Holmstrom LL. Mixed blessings: Intensive care for newborns. New York: Oxford University Press; 1986.

11. Streiner DL, Saigal S, Burrows E, et al. Attitudes of parents and health care professionals toward active treatment of extremely premature infants. Pediatrics 2001; 108:152–157.

12. Glass v United Kingdom [2004] BMLR 120.

13. Re Houston (applicant) [1996] 32 BMLR 93.

14. McHaffie HS et al. Crucial decisions at the beginning of life. Radcliffe Medical Press; 2001 Abingdon, Oxon, OX14 IAA.

15. McCallum DE, Byrne P, Bruera E. How children die in hospital. J Pain Symptom Management 2000; 20:417–423.

16. R v Woollin [1999] 1 AC 82.

17. A National Health Service Trust v. D. [2000] 55 BMLR 19.

18. British Medical Association. withholding and withdrawing life prolonging medical treatment. 3rd Edition 2007 Blackwell BMJ Books, Oxon.

19. Royal College of Paediatrics and Child Health, Ethics Advisory Committee 2004. Witholding or withdrawing life sustaining treatment in children. A framework for practice. 2nd edn. London: Royal College of Paediatrics and Child Health.

20. McHaffie HE, Lyon AJ, Hume R. Deciding on treatment limitation for neonates: the parents' perspective. Eur J Pediatr 2001; 160:339–344.

21. R v Adams [1957] Crim LR ;365.

22. Airedale NHS Trust v Bland [1993] 1 All ER 821.

23. Re C (a minor) [1997] 40 BMLR 31.

24. R v Cambridge District Health Authority, ex parte B [1995] 25 BMLR 5.

25. Re T (a minor) (wardship: medical treatment) [1996] 35 BMLR 63.

26. Re A (children) (conjoined twins: surgical separation) [2000] 4 All ER 961.

27. Wyatt (a child) (medical treatment: parents' consent) [2004] Fam Law 866.

28. Re MB [2006] EWHC 507 (Fam).

29. Re T. (a minor) (wardship: medical treatment) [1989] 2 All ER 782.

30. Children Act 1989.

31. Children (Scotland) Act 1995.

32. Human Fertilisation and Embryology Act 1990.

33. Adoption and Children Act (2002).

34. Family Law Scotland Act 2006.

35. Gillick v. West Norfolk and Wisbech Area Health Authority [1996] 3 All ER 402.

36. Access to Health Records Act 1990.

37. Health and Social Care Act 2001.

38. Report on the review of patient-identifiable information. The Caldicott Committee. Department of Health; December 1997.

39. Bolam v Friern Hospital Management Committee [1957] 2 All ER 118.

40. Bolitho v. Hackney Health Authority [1998] AC 232.

41. Stenson B, McIntosh N. The rights and duties of parents in the neonatal unit: the limits of informed consent. Semin Neonatol 1998; 3:291–296.

42. American Academy of Pediatrics, Committee on Bioethics 2001 Ethical issues with genetic testing in pediatrics. Pediatrics; 107:1451–1455.

43. Lantos JD. The 'Inclusion benefit' in clinical trials. J Pediatr 1999; 134:130–131.

44. McIntosh N, Bates P, Brykczynska G, et al. Guidelines for the ethical conduct of medical research involving children. Royal College of Paediatrics, Child Health: Ethics Advisory Committee. Arch Dis Child 2000; 82:177–182.

45. Additional Protocol to the Convention on Human Rights and Biomedicine, Concerning Biomedical Research 2005, available at http://conventions.coe.int/Treaty/en/Treaties/Html/195.htm

46. Anonymous. Your baby is in a trial. (Editorial). Lancet 1995; 345:805–806.

47. Stenson BJ, Becher JC, McIntosh N. Neonatal research: the parents' perspective. Arch Dis Child Fetal Neonatal Ed 2004; 89:F321–F323.

48. Snowdon C, Garcia J, Elbourne D. Making sense of randomisation: responses of parents of critically ill babies to random allocation of treatment in a clinical trial. Soc Sci Med 1997; 45:1337–1355.

49. Davidoff F, et al. Sponsorship, authorship and accountability. The Lancet 2001; 358:854–856.

50. Mental Health Act 1983.

51. Mental Health (Scotland) Act 1984.

52. Larcher VF, Lak B, McCarthy J. Paediatrics at the cutting edge; do we need clinical ethics committees? J Med Ethics 1997; 23:245–249.

53. McHaffie HE, Fowlie PW. Life and death decisions. Doctors and nurses reflect on neonatal practice. Hale: Hochland and Hochland; 1996.

54. Lee SK, Penner PL, Cox M Comparison of the attitudes of health care professionals and parents toward active treatment of very low birth weight infants. Pediatrics 1991; 88:110–114.

Section 2
Perinatal/neonatal medicine

11

Fetal medicine

Stephen C Robson, Steven Sturgiss

PRENATAL SCREENING AND DIAGNOSIS OF CONGENITAL ABNORMALITIES

Congenital abnormalities occur in 3–4% of newborn infants and are responsible for between 10 and 15% of perinatal deaths and 30–40% of postneonatal deaths.[1] Even if not lethal, many congenital abnormalities cause significant long-term morbidity. The benefits of prenatal diagnosis include enhanced parental and neonatal preparedness and optimization of delivery. For those anomalies likely to be associated with death and/or significant disability, parents can be offered pregnancy termination. Antenatal screening for trisomy 21 receives much attention, but structural malformations account for 63% of therapeutic pregnancy terminations for fetal abnormalities.[2]

MATERNAL SERUM SCREENING

Maternal serum screening (MSS) for trisomy 21 is carried out with a combination of maternal age and biochemical analytes. Measurements of alpha-fetoprotein (AFP) and human chorionic gonadotrophin (hCG) in the second trimester constitute the double test; the addition of unconjugated estriol (μE3), or μE3 and inhibin A make the triple and quadruple tests, respectively. The detection rates for trisomy 21 with the double (60%), triple (68%) and quadruple tests (79%) are all substantially greater than using maternal age alone. These test characteristics are based on a false-positive rate (FPR) of 5% and a threshold for offering invasive testing of 1 in 200–250.

More recently, pregnancy-associated plasma protein-A (PAPP-A) and hCG have been used as first trimester serum markers, with a detection rate of 63%. Combined first and second trimester serum screening (the serum integrated test) has been reported to give detection rates of about 85% with a false-positive rate of 2.7%.[3]

ULTRASOUND

FIRST TRIMESTER
Structural anomalies
First trimester anatomy screening identifies 32–65% of major structural abnormalities in low-risk populations, and 57–74% in high-risk cases. The anomalies that have been detected in the first trimester include anencephaly, holoprosencephaly, cystic hygroma, multicystic kidneys, megacystis and anterior abdominal wall defects.

Nuchal translucency
Screening with nuchal translucency (NT), measured as the maximum thickness of the subcutaneous tissue overlying the cervical spine at 11–14 weeks, identifies 74–82% of fetuses with trisomy 21 for a FPR of 5%. NT also acts as a marker for other trisomies (18, 13), sex chromosome abnormalities, syndromic disorders and structural abnormalities including cardiac defects (Table 11.1); in one large study 56% of the major cardiac anomalies occurred in fetuses with a NT above the 95th centile at 10–14 weeks' gestation.[4] Others have demonstrated that the prevalence of major cardiac defects in euploid fetuses with NT > 3.5 mm is 5–6%. However, the sensitivity of NT screening for cardiac abnormalities is low (15%). The overall chance of delivering a healthy infant declines with increasing NT; 86% at 3.5–4.4 mm, 77% at 4.5–5.4 mm, 67% at 5.5–6.4 mm, and less than 31% for an NT > 6.5 mm.[5]

Other first-trimester ultrasonographic markers for T21 include absence of the nasal bone, increased impedance to flow in the ductus venosus and tricuspid regurgitation. The incorporation of one or more of these markers into a screening program for T21 increases the first trimester detection rate to about 92–94%, for a FPR of about 2–3%.

Strategies incorporating first trimester ultrasonography have the additional benefits of providing parents with early reassurance and **175**

Table 11.1 Anomalies associated with nuchal translucency in euploid fetuses

Cardiac	Other structural
Tetralogy of Fallot	Diaphragmatic hernia
Hypoplastic left heart	Pentalogy of Cantrell
Transposition of the great arteries	Exomphalos
Coarctation of the aorta	Body stalk anomaly
Aortic stenosis or atresia	Caudal regression
Ventricular and atrioventricular septal defects	Achondrogenesis
Other complex cardiac defects	

Genetic syndrome	Other conditions
Mucopolysaccharidosis type VII	Homozygous alpha-thalassemia
Zellweger	Twin–twin transfusion syndrome
Spinal muscular atrophy	Parvovirus infection
Noonan	
Robinow	
Cleidocranial dysplasia	
Jarcho–Levin	

Table 11.2 Sensitivities of routine ultrasonography for the detection of anomalies in organ systems

	Total n	(%)	
Central nervous system			
Anencephaly	29/29	(100)	
Spina bifida	18/22	(82)	
Hydrocephaly	8/20	(40)	
Holoprosencephaly	3/5	(60)	
Other	9/13	(69)	
Total	*67/89*	*(75)*	
Cardiovascular system			
Septal defects	4/54	(7)	
Transposition	0/9	(0)	
Other complex heart	18/78	(23)	
Total	*22/141*	*(16)*	
Urinary tract			
Obstructive uropathy	164/171	(96)	
Renal agenesis	10/11	(91)	
Renal dysplasia	13/24	(54)	
Other	7/9	(78)	
Total	*194/215*	*(90)*	
Thoracic abnormalities			
CCAM	6/6	(100)	
Diaphragmatic hernia	8/13		(62)
Pleural effusion	1/3		(33)
Other	2/5		(40)
Total	*17/27*		*(63)*
Abdominal/gastrointestinal			
Exomphalos	9/9	(100)	
Gastroschisis	6/6	(100)	
Small bowel obstruction	2/5		(40)
Esophageal atresia	2/11		(18)
Other	2/25		(8)
Total	*21/56*		*(38)*

Summary data from five studies of routine ultrasonography in low risk populations.[7-11]
CCAM, congenital cystic adenomatoid malformations.

the early detection of nonviable and multiple pregnancies. It is perceived that termination of pregnancy in the first, as compared to the second trimester, is safer and less likely to result in psychological sequelae. Termination prior to 15 weeks of pregnancy can be carried out by suction aspiration, obviating the need for a medical procedure involving vaginal expulsion of the conceptus. However, recent evidence suggests that the emotional responses to termination for an abnormal fetus are independent of the gestational age and method of termination.[6] Other potential problems with early pregnancy screening include the narrow time interval for screening and diagnosis, the higher loss rate of chorionic villus sampling compared with amniocentesis, lack of pathological confirmation of diagnosis, and the high spontaneous loss rate in abnormal pregnancies (particularly trisomies and cystic hygroma).

SECOND TRIMESTER
Structural anomalies
Ultrasound screening between 18 and 20 weeks of pregnancy identifies 61–85% of fetal anomalies in low-risk populations.[7-11] The sensitivities for individual anomalies are shown in Table 11.2. Although one large trial[12] reported very poor detection rates (17%), subsequent analysis indicated that the low sensitivities were due in part to poor sonographer training. A recent meta-analysis of eight studies showed that, when compared with selective examination, routine second trimester screening is associated with earlier diagnosis of twin pregnancy and a reduced incidence of induction of labor for post-term pregnancy,[13] but no apparent benefit in terms of perinatal mortality. It is likely that this result is explained by the rarity of perinatal deaths (10 per 1000), variable detection rates, and some parents opting to continue their pregnancy even when a lethal anomaly is diagnosed.

Markers of chromosomal anomalies
Many aneuploid fetuses exhibit major structural anomalies and/or minor findings of little or no functional significance (soft markers). For each soft marker, a likelihood ratio for aneuploidy is calculated from the ratio of the frequencies in affected and normal fetuses. Likelihood ratios (LRs) for potential ultrasound markers associated with trisomy 21 are shown in Table 11.3. Maternal age is used for the prior risk, and the risk factors applied sequentially when more than one is present. A normal scan without anomalies or soft markers reduces the risk for trisomy 21 by about 40–45% (i.e. LR 0.6).

COMBINED SERUM AND ULTRASOUND SCREENING

COMBINED TEST
Screening with a composite-adjusted risk derived from measurement of NT and maternal serum PAPP-A and hCG in the first trimester is known as the *combined test*. The detection rate for trisomy 21 is increased to about 85–89% for the same FPR of 5%. This test retains the perceived benefits of first trimester ultrasonography and early diagnosis.

Table 11.3 Ultrasound markers for trisomy 21

Sonographic feature	Likelihood ratio for trisomy 21
Nuchal fold 6+ mm	10.0
Echogenic bowel	5.5
Short femur	2.5
Mild pyelectasis	1.5
Choroid plexus cyst	1.5
Sandal gap	1.5

INTEGRATED TEST

The combination of multiple first and second trimester ultrasonographic and serum markers for trisomy 21 is known as the *integrated test*. Typically, this involves a composite adjusted risk based on first trimester NT, as well as first and second trimester serum screening. The multiplicity of markers involved in this form of screening is associated with test characteristics that are better than with any other form of screening; the detection rate for trisomy 21 is 95% for a FPR of 5%. Alternatively, FPRs can be reduced to < 1% while maintaining sensitivity at ~85%.[3]

This screening strategy is referred to as *non-disclosure sequential screening*, and involves withholding results from women until the second trimester serum markers have been measured. There are, however, concerns that pregnant women and clinical staff might find the non-disclosure of high-risk first trimester results to be unacceptable, and a breach of patient autonomy by the denial of the perceived benefits of first-trimester screening.

CONTINGENT SCREENING

These concerns about non-disclosure screening have led to the development of an alterative form of sequential screening, in which a first trimester test is used to triage the screened population into three groups: one group (high-risk screen positive) that is immediately offered a diagnostic test, a second group (screen negative) that receives no further screening, and a third group (intermediate risk) in which the first trimester results are reused in the second trimester as part of a subsequent integrated test. Theoretical modeling suggests that first-trimester completion is achievable in about 75% of women for a 30% early detection rate and a 55% second trimester detected rate (net 85%) with a false-positive rate only 0.1% above that achievable by the Integrated test.[14]

Contingent screening retains the perceived benefits for a substantial proportion of screened women, but there are concerns about the complexity of the test, and whether or not the real-life performance characteristics will match those demonstrated in modeled scenarios.

SAFETY OF ULTRASOUND

Ultrasound induces the thermal effects and gas bubble formation (cavitation). There is no evidence of teratogenesis in humans despite the widespread use of prenatal ultrasound for more than 20 years. Newnham et al[15] reported that mothers exposed to five or more third-trimester ultrasound examinations delivered babies weighing about 25 g less than controls. These results have not been confirmed in other studies. Case–control or randomized, controlled studies have shown small but significant increases in speech problems, dyslexia, abnormal grasp, and non-right handedness.[13] However, there is little consistency between these studies, which are all prone to methodological problems including errors due to chance in multiple hypothesis testing.

MANAGEMENT OF PRENATALLY DETECTED STRUCTURAL ANOMALIES

PRINCIPLES OF MANAGEMENT

The prenatal diagnosis of a fetal malformation should prompt referral to a clinician with expertise in the antenatal management of such conditions. Regional fetal medicine centers have been established with core teams of experts specialized in ultrasonography, invasive assessment and intrauterine therapy. The initial management includes a detailed characterization of the malformation, as well as a thorough search for associated anomalies. Many structural anomalies are associated with an increased risk of chromosome abnormalities, and the management will usually include the offer of prenatal karyotyping. Parents are provided with considerate, empathetic and knowledgeable counseling based, wherever possible, on relevant prenatal literature. The prognosis

for lesions diagnosed during pregnancy is often very different from those diagnosed after delivery. A single clinician leads and coordinates this process, which often includes colleagues in genetics, neonatology and neonatal surgery. Decisions regarding further testing, surveillance during pregnancy, and the time and place of delivery are individualized according to the underlying problem.

Termination of pregnancy (TOP) in the UK is allowable at any gestation if there is a substantial risk of serious handicap. The interpretation of risk and handicap, and by implication the decision to offer termination of pregnancy, is presently at the discretion of the clinician(s) involved with the case. The Royal College of Obstetricians and Gynaecologists has issued guidelines recommending fetocide for TOPs after 22 weeks' gestation.[16]

CENTRAL NERVOUS SYSTEM

Ventriculomegaly

Ventriculomegaly (ventricular width ≥10 mm) describes dilatation of the lateral ventricles whereas hydrocephalus refers to a pathological increase in intracranial cerebrospinal fluid, which is usually associated with increased intracranial pressure and enlargement of the fetal head. Ventriculomegaly occurs in 0.05–0.3% of all pregnancies.

The causes of ventriculomegaly include constitutional increase in size, obstruction to the flow of fluid through the ventricular system, other central nervous system (CNS) anomalies (e.g. neural tube defects, hemorrhage, or migration defects), infection (cytomegalovirus, toxoplasmosis, adenovirus), genetic disorders and karyotype abnormalities (trisomies 21, 18 and 13, as well as triploidy and translocations). Associated anomalies are found in 70% of cases. Additional investigations should include fetal echocardiography, an infection screen, and the offer of invasive testing to determine the fetal karyotype. Consideration should be given to magnetic resonance imaging (MRI), which at gestations beyond 23 weeks has been claimed to provide additional information – particularly in the evaluation of the posterior fossa, midline structures (corpus callosum) and cortex. Examples of alterations to the diagnosis after MRI in cases with apparently nonspecific hydrocephalus include aqueductal stenosis, agenesis of the corpus callosum, migrational abnormalities, or late presenting Chiari II malformations.[17,18] There is uncertainty about the amount of useful additional information from MRI following ultrasonography by experienced specialists.

In general, the prognosis for fetuses with ventriculomegaly and other abnormalities is very poor. However, quantification of individual risk for adverse outcome when the underlying diagnosis is unclear can be difficult. The management and prognosis for fetuses with isolated ventriculomegaly are influenced by the severity of the ventricular dilatation.

Mild/moderate ventriculomegaly

Ventricular widths between 10 and 15 mm are often subdivided into mild (ventricular width 10–12 mm) and moderate (12.1–14.9 mm) ventriculomegaly. About 2–3% of fetuses with apparently isolated mild/moderate ventriculomegaly will have a karyotype abnormality. If all investigations are normal, about 93–97% of surviving fetuses with mild ventriculomegaly will have a normal outcome,[19] but the chance of a normal outcome with moderate ventricular dilatation decreases to about 75–80%. It has been reported that neonatal survival to 2 years of age in fetuses with the antenatal diagnosis of moderate ventriculomegaly is about 80%.[20] Serial scans are undertaken throughout pregnancy to monitor the ventricular size. Resolution of the ventriculomegaly occurs in about one third of cases and increases the chance of a normal outcome.

Severe ventriculomegaly

For severe ventriculomegaly (ventricular width ≥15 mm), the incidence of chromosome abnormalities is ~ 10%. With apparently isolated severe ventriculomegaly the neonatal/infant mortality rate is ~ 50%, with about 50% of surviving infants exhibiting abnormal neurodevelopment.[21] Where severity has been reported, about 20% were mildly affected and 80% moderate to severe. Postnatal ventriculoperitoneal shunting is required in 60% of cases. For parents continuing their pregnancy, serial scans should be undertaken to monitor ventricular size. In cases with rapidly progressive disease and/or hydrocephalus, delivery should be considered as soon as fetal maturity can reasonably be assumed. There is no benefit from routine Cesarean section, but the macrocephaly can be severe enough to preclude vaginal delivery. In utero ventriculoperitoneal shunting does not improve outcome, and frequently results in intracranial hemorrhage with in utero demise. Cephalocentesis may be justified to avoid traumatic delivery but also has a very high mortality rate.

Spina bifida

The incidence of neural tube defects in the UK has declined from 5.5 to 1.0 in 1000 over the last 20 years. Part of this reduction might be due to periconceptual folate supplementation, which reduces the incidence of neural tube defects by 75%.[22] The ultrasound features include widening of the spinal posterior ossification centers (dysraphism), a sacular protrusion and/or a defect in the overlying skin. Virtually all cases of myelomeningocele manifest cranial features including microcephaly, scalloping of the frontal bones (lemon sign), ventriculomegaly, obliteration of the cisterna magna and/or an absent or abnormally shaped cerebellum (banana sign) as a consequence of the Arnold–Chiari malformation. Associated anomalies occur in most other systems, but the commonest are urogenital anomalies (9%) including renal agenesis, horseshoe kidneys and ureteral duplications. Karyotype abnormalities, mainly trisomy 18, occur in 2% of apparently isolated cases.

There is a wide spectrum of outcomes for newborns with spina bifida – with the upper level of the lesion being the greatest determinant of eventual neurologic function. Infants with the prenatal diagnosis of a thoracic lesion are rarely ambulatory, whereas 90–100% of infants with a sacral or lower lumbar (L5) defect are ambulatory most of the time.[23] Mid-lumbar lesions are associated with ambulation in about 50% of cases.

The majority (60–70%) of infants with spina bifida will have a normal IQ, and even more (about 85%) will attend high school and/or college. Intellectual restriction in children with spina bifida is usually associated with complications of shunt placement, but recent data indicates that shunt placement is carried out less frequently than previously. About 70% of infants with sacral lesions require a shunt, with rates rising to about 90% with a lumbar, and 100% with thoracic lesions.

Continence problems are common, but about 75–85% of patients with spina bifida will achieve social continence using techniques such as clean intermittent catheterization.

There is concern that the counseling of parents following the diagnosis of spina bifida has been unduly pessimistic.[24] It is certainly true that some children will experience devastating sequelae, but many more will go on to have normal intelligence, reasonable ambulation and social continence.

Agenesis of the corpus callosum

Agenesis of the corpus callosum (ACC) is found in 1 in 19 000 unselected autopsies and 2.3% of children with mental retardation. The corpus callosum can be identified with coronal ultrasound views after 20 weeks' gestation. However, these views are not part of the standard ultrasound scan, and it is likely that many cases are unrecognized. In low-risk cases, the diagnosis will only be made through identification of associated anatomic alterations including mild ventriculomegaly, absence of the cavum septum pellucidum, and enlargement or upward displacement of the third ventricle.

In total, 80% of cases are associated with other anomalies including hydrocephalus, Dandy-Walker syndrome, neuronal migration disorders and aneuploidy (trisomies 13 and 18). Normal outcome occurs in 85% of cases with apparently isolated ACC and in 13% of cases with additional scan abnormalities.[25]

Holoprosencephaly

Holoprosencephaly is characterized by failed septation of the midline forebrain structures, and is frequently accompanied by midfacial abnormalities. The forebrain abnormalities are subdivided into lobar, semilobar, and alobar types according to increasing degree of failed septation. Population-based studies suggest a prevalence of 1.1 to 1.2 cases per 10 000 pregnancies.[26] Associated syndromic (including Smith–Lemli–Opitz, Hall–Pallister, pseudotrisomy 13, and Meckel) and structural anomalies are common. Trisomy 13, the most commonly identified cause, and other chromosomal abnormalities (trisomy 18 and rearrangements or deletions) account for nearly 50% of cases.

The prognosis is very poor; overall, about 70% of affected infants die within 1 year, and all diagnosed infants exhibit developmental delay, which is often severe. It is possible that individuals with subtle forms of undiagnosed lobar holoprosencephaly exist with little or no neurological abnormality. Even when a case of holoprosencephaly appears to be sporadic, the recurrence risk (13–14%) remains higher than with other major malformations. The high incidence of syndromic and subtle familial cases and the high recurrence rates emphasize the importance of full investigation and detailed postnatal counseling.

Dandy–Walker malformation

Dandy–Walker malformation (DWM) describes agenesis or hypoplasia of the cerebellar vermis with communication between the fourth ventricle and the cisterna magna. Chromosome abnormalities are present in 15–45% of cases and around 45% have other CNS anomalies, including holoprosencephaly, ventriculomegaly and neuronal migration defects. Non CNS structural and syndromic anomalies are present in two thirds of cases. Prenatal series report a 40% risk of fetal or neonatal death and almost all reported survivors are symptomatic with developmental/motor delay, seizures and spasticity. It is possible that isolated DWM is associated with a lower risk of neurodevelopmental problems, but very few genuinely isolated cases have been reported.

URINARY TRACT

Hydronephrosis

Renal pelvic dilatation (RPD) is usually defined as an anteroposterior diameter of the renal pelvis of ≥ 5.0 mm in the second trimester and/or ≥ 7.0 mm in the third trimester. It affects 1% of pregnancies and is commoner in male fetuses. Using a threshold of 4 mm at 20 weeks of pregnancy increases the sensitivity for detecting significant nephrouropathy from 53% to 76% but increases the false-positive rate. Antenatal RPD can be a variant of normal or can be secondary to urinary tract pathology (pelviureteric junction obstruction [PUJO], vesicoureteric reflux [VUR], vesicoureteric junction obstruction, posterior urethral valves and obstruction in a duplex system).[27] Bladder and/or ureteric dilatation suggest the presence of lower urinary tract uropathy, but their absence does not exclude this possibility. The presence of caliectasis and parenchymal thinning is associated with an increased likelihood of obstruction.

Mild/moderate renal pelvic dilatation

Mild second trimester RPD (5–10 mm) resolves during pregnancy in 66–80% of cases.[27] Significant nephrouropathies are more likely if RPD persists in the third trimester (40%) than if it resolves (12%)[28] and therefore a follow-up scan should be performed at 32 weeks' gestation. Progression from mild to severe (≥ 15 mm) dilatation is uncommon (< 5% of cases). Most cases of pathology have a third trimester RPD ≥ 10 mm (sensitivity 80%, specificity 93%) with the exception of VUR, which occurs in 10–15% of cases even with mild RPD. Where RPD persists at 32 weeks, an ultrasound scan should be performed 3–7 d after delivery unless prenatal ultrasound findings suggest lower urinary tract obstruction where an earlier scan (24–48 h) is indicated.[27] Many units recommend antibiotic prophylaxis, as well as investigation for VUR for those babies with prenatal RPD because postnatal ultrasound is an unreliable modality for the detection of VUR. However reflux associated with mild RPD is usually low grade, found more often in males and has a high probability of resolving spontaneously. Increasingly the weight of published evidence suggests that routine micturating cystourethrography is no longer justified.[27] Few (< 3%) fetuses with fetal RPD < 15 mm will ultimately require surgery.[27]

Severe Renal Pelvic Dilation (RDP)

Almost all fetuses with severe RPD (> 15 mm) will have significant renal pathology, most commonly PUJO. There is a relationship between severity of prenatal RPD and differential function in the obstructed kidney as assessed by MAG3 isotope renography. The requirement for pyeloplasty (based on differential function) increases with the extent of fetal RPD; 7% at 15–20 mm, 29% at 20–30 mm, 65% at 30–50 mm and 100% at > 50 mm.[27] The overall prognosis for fetuses with isolated unilateral dilatation is usually excellent. A more cautious approach needs to be taken with bilateral disease. Reduction or absence of amniotic fluid suggests severe renal dysfunction and a very poor prognosis. Serial scans should be undertaken to assess the degree of dilatation and amniotic fluid volume. Progressive dilatation and/or diminution of amniotic fluid volume near term (37 weeks) are indications for delivery.

Renal agenesis

Unilateral renal agenesis occurs in 1 in 1000 pregnancies, and bilateral renal agenesis 1 in 4000. Bilateral renal agenesis is always associated with severe oligohydramnios from about 15 weeks' gestation. Earlier in pregnancy, a large proportion of the amniotic fluid originates from the fetal membranes. The differential diagnosis of severe oligohydramnios includes other causes of impaired urine production (bilateral multicystic kidney disease, urinary tract obstruction), fetal growth restriction and amniorrhexis. The sonographic demonstration of kidneys and bladder is very difficult in the absence of amniotic fluid. Transvaginal and color Doppler sonography may help but a definitive diagnosis often requires amnioinfusion and occasionally infusion of fluid into the fetal abdomen.

Low urinary tract obstruction

Posterior urethral valves (PUVs) are the most common cause of severe lower urinary tract obstructive uropathy, occurring in 1 in 5000–8000 male fetuses. Ultrasonographic appearances include a dilated thick-walled bladder, a dilated posterior urethra, and oligohydramnios. The obstruction is classified as complete when there is anhydramnios, or incomplete when the amniotic fluid volume is normal or slightly reduced. The most important differential diagnosis is severe bilateral VUR producing the megacystis–megaureter association. However, with reflux, the bladder is often thin-walled and the liquor volume is normal. Urethral atresia can also lead to severe bladder dilatation and has a worse prognosis because of the associated cloacal anomalies. Associated abnormalities are seen in 43% of fetuses and include cardiac anomalies, bowel rotation, imperforate anus and vesicorectal fistula. Karyotype abnormalities occur in up to 8% of cases.

The prognosis for PUV is dependent on the degree of obstruction and the extent of renal dysplasia.

Complete obstruction

Complete obstruction is associated with anhydramnios and a very poor prognosis as a consequence of renal dysplasia and pulmonary hypoplasia. Decompression of the dilated bladder with a vesicoamniotic shunt can increase amniotic fluid volume and protect the fetus from pulmonary hypoplasia. Shunt placement is only worthwhile in fetuses with satisfactory residual renal function, as assessed with ultrasonography and measurement of urinary electrolytes after vesicocentesis. Kidneys with bilateral cystic change will always be severely dysplastic. Normal ranges have been established for fetal urinary sodium, calcium, phosphate, osmolality and beta 2-microglobulin. In borderline cases, analysis of fresh urine from a repeat vesicocentesis after 2–3 d can provide more definitive results. With appropriate case selection, survival rates of 67% have been reported after vesicoamniotic shunt procedures.[29] A recent systematic review and meta-analysis concluded that bladder shunting improves perinatal survival in fetuses with lower urinary tract obstruction, particularly those with poor predicted prognoses.[30] The quality of evidence leading to this conclusion was, however, noted to be poor. The complications of shunt placement include chorioamnionitis, anterior abdominal wall defects, and fetal demise; the overall procedure-related fetal loss rate is about 5%. Even when the shunt works satisfactorily, many fetuses develop renal dysplasia requiring renal support within the first year of life. A multi-centre randomized controlled trial comparing intra-uterine vesico-amniotic shunting vs. not shunting in the treatment of congenital bladder outflow obstruction is currently underway.

Incomplete obstruction

Fetuses with no or mild oligohydramnios throughout pregnancy are protected from pulmonary hypoplasia and are very likely to survive. Some degree of renal dysplasia is common, but the severity is highly variable and difficult to predict. Vesicocentesis might be indicated in those fetuses with borderline amniotic fluid volume. Management during pregnancy should include serial scans to monitor amniotic fluid volume and renal appearances.

Cystic kidney disease

Multicystic renal dysplasia is the commonest form of cystic kidney disease diagnosed in utero. Bilateral disease occurs in 23% of cases, and is characterized by paraspinal cystic masses, a nonvisible bladder, and severe oligohydramnios. Pulmonary hypoplasia is invariable resulting in neonatal death. The prognosis for unilateral disease is dependent on the presence of contralateral renal anomalies, which occur in up to 39% of cases and include renal agenesis, renal hypoplasia, pelviureteric junction obstruction and VUR. Reflux occurs in 15% of cases, but is not always apparent prenatally. If the contralateral kidney appears normal, and there are no apparent systemic anomalies, the prognosis is excellent. A further ultrasound scan should be carried out in the third trimester of pregnancy to monitor the size of the diseased kidney. Postnatal investigations should include a renal scan and a micturating cystourethrogram with antibiotic cover.

Autosomal recessive and dominant renal cystic disease are usually only diagnosed in cases with a family history. The management is individualized according to the underlying pathology and degree of in utero renal dysfunction as assessed from amniotic fluid volume. Specialist neonatal nephrologic advice is required.

ABDOMINAL WALL

Exomphalos

Exomphalos is an incomplete return of the abdominal contents into the abdominal cavity, which is complete by 11–12 weeks' gestation. The incidence is 1–3 per 1000 pregnancies. The lesion is highly variable in size and appears as an anterior extrusion of abdominal contents contained within a sac, which occasionally ruptures. The umbilical vein will be seen coursing through the sac, in contrast to a gastroschisis, where the cord insertion is intact. Other abnormalities are common. Cardiac malformations are seen in up to 50%, limb abnormalities in 30%, and karyotype abnormalities in 28–36%, mainly trisomy 18. The smaller umbilical hernias, and lesions diagnosed early in pregnancy (<15 weeks) are associated with even higher rates of aneuploidy. Associated genetic anomalies include the Beckwith–Wiedemann and de Lange syndromes.

Survival rates for isolated lesions are in excess of 90%, but some babies will require staged repairs and need to be in hospital for many weeks. Larger lesions are associated with reduced survival rates (~ 75%), as is the presence of additional abnormalities. Periodic ultrasound surveillance should be undertaken, but the incidence of complications such as bowel constriction is low. There is no merit in routine Cesarean section, but this might be justified for the very extensive lesions where the fetal liver is completely extruded.

Gastroschisis

A gastroschisis is a herniation of the intra-abdominal contents through a defect in the abdominal wall, usually just to the right of the cord insertion. The ultrasonographic features include free loops of bowel floating in the amniotic fluid, associated with an intact cord insertion. Gastroschisis is not usually associated with other anomalies, but some studies have reported cardiac anomalies in up to 5% of cases. About

50% of fetuses will be small for gestational age (SGA), and there is an increased risk of hypoxic intrauterine death. Intestinal atresias or stenosis secondary to intestinal ischemia are reported in up to 30% of cases. Survival rates for isolated cases without liver herniation approach 95%. Management should include periodic surveillance during pregnancy to establish fetal size, growth, placental function and bowel status. Bowel luminal diameters of 11–17 mm have been associated with an increased incidence of bowel complications at surgery. Delivery should be in a unit with neonatal surgical facilities. There is no merit in routine Cesarean section.

THORAX
Diaphragmatic hernia

Left-sided congenital diaphragmatic hernia (CDH) is usually suspected when the fetal heart is displaced to the right side of the chest, and/or the stomach is seen in the thoracic cavity. If neither of these signs is evident, the diagnosis is often missed. The prenatal diagnosis of a right-sided CDH is especially difficult; the echogenicity patterns of the fetal lung, liver and small intestine are very similar. About 60% of CDHs evade prenatal diagnosis. Associated anomalies occur in 30% of cases, and include abnormalities of the cardiovascular, genitourinary, musculoskeletal, and central nervous systems, as well as aneuploidy (mainly trisomy 18) in 10–15% of cases. Reported survival rates for isolated lesions diagnosed in utero are 50–60% but this falls to 10% when there are coexistent anomalies. The prognosis is dependent on contralateral lung development, but ultrasound assessment of lung size and growth is imprecise. Early diagnosis, the presence of liver in the chest, hydramnios and hydrops are associated with a worse outcome. The ratio of fetal lung area to head circumference ratio (LHR) measured with ultrasonography at 22–28 weeks appears to be predictive of survival, but only in fetuses without intrathoracic herniation of the liver – ranging from 58% with a LHR < 1.0, to 89% with a LHR > 1.6.[31]

Management should include fetal echocardiography and ultrasound scans every 2 weeks during the third trimester to look for hydramnios and hydrops. Delivery should be in a unit with specialist neonatal and pediatric surgical facilities. There is no contraindication to vaginal delivery. The extent to which outcome can be improved with prenatal surgery remains to be determined.

Cystic adenomatoid malformation

Congenital cystic adenomatoid malformations (CCAMs) are classified on the basis of ultrasound appearances as macrocystic (type 1), mixed (type 2) or microcystic (type 3). Microcystic lesions appear predominantly echogenic, whereas macrocystic lesions contain one or more unilocular cysts. The differential diagnosis includes CDH, pulmonary sequestration, and bronchial atresia. In difficult cases, intrathoracic instillation of fluid helps differentiate a CDH. Doppler color flow imaging may visualize a direct vascular connection to the aorta in sequestration. Associated anomalies are rare but hydrops can occur as a result of distortion of the thoracic great arteries/veins, or myocardial dysfunction.

The prognosis for a CCAM in the absence of hydrops is very favorable. In about 20–30% of cases, there is partial or apparently complete resolution of the lesion in utero. Ultrasound scans should be performed every 4 weeks to exclude hydrops, but this rarely develops if it is not present at diagnosis. The place of delivery can be decided according to the size of the lesion. The prognosis for fetuses with hydrops is much less favorable. However, even when hydrops is present in early pregnancy, serial scans have documented apparent shrinkage and resolution of the lesion with disappearance of the hydrops.

GASTROINTESTINAL ABNORMALITIES
Duodenal atresia

Duodenal atresia affects 1 in 5000 pregnancies. The typical ultrasonographic appearances include a 'double-bubble', with the stomach and dilated duodenum forming similarly sized and connected fluid-filled structures, and hydramnios, which can predispose to premature labor. The diagnosis is not usually evident before the end of the second trimester. Associated anomalies include vertebral defects, imperforate anus, tracheoesophageal fistula with esophageal atresia, and radial and renal dysplasia (complex) (VATER) association and trisomy 21, which is present in 30% of cases. The prognosis for fetuses with isolated duodenal atresia is very good. Regular ultrasound surveillance should be carried out to monitor amniotic fluid volume. Hydramnios can be severe and warrant amnioreduction.

Other bowel obstruction

The appearance of multiple fluid-filled bowel loops suggests small bowel obstruction. Precise localization of the obstruction is not possible, but the greater the number of dilated bowel loops and the greater the dilatation, the more distal the atresia. Conversely the greater the volume of amniotic fluid, the more proximal the obstruction. Associated anomalies external to the gut are uncommon. The prognosis is usually excellent, but the outlook needs to be more guarded when multiple atresias are suspected. Serial ultrasound scans are performed to monitor amniotic fluid volume. Amnioreduction is occasionally required.

Meconium ileus

Meconium ileus should be suspected when the bowel is dilated and hyperechogenic. Virtually all cases are due to cystic fibrosis, which can usually be confirmed with parental and fetal genotyping. About 98% of the cystic fibrosis gene mutations have been characterized and can be identified with DNA studies. The immediate prognosis for meconium ileus is good, but the longer term prognosis is determined by the underlying condition.

CARDIAC ABNORMALITIES

Congenital heart disease occurs in 0.4–1.0% of live births and accounts for 35% of infant deaths secondary to congenital disease. Screening using the four-chamber view of the fetal heart will detect about 20% of cardiac abnormalities. Sensitivity is increased by incorporating views of the arterial connections. Chromosomal anomalies have been reported in up to 30% of fetuses with prenatally detected heart disease; trisomy 18 is detected as frequently as trisomy 21, with Turner syndrome the next most common. Karyotype analysis should include a search for microdeletions localized to the long arm of chromosome 22 (22q11), which result in DiGeorge syndrome.

A detailed discussion about the diagnosis and management of the individual cardiac abnormalities amenable to prenatal diagnosis is outwith the scope of this chapter. Interested readers are referred to Allan et al.[32] The prognosis for malformations detected with prenatal ultrasonography is usually worse than for those first seen after delivery. Counseling should be undertaken by clinicians specializing in the field of prenatal echocardiography.

SKELETAL DYSPLASIAS

The commonest lethal skeletal dysplasia seen prenatally is thanatophoric dysplasia with an incidence of 1 in 10 000 births. Other lethal dysplasias include achondrogenesis (1 in 40 000 births) and osteogenesis imperfecta (1 in 55 000). The prenatal diagnosis of skeletal dysplasias is complex and beyond the scope of this chapter. Interested readers are referred to Griffin.[33] Frequently the precise diagnosis is not made until after delivery or autopsy. The lethal anomalies can usually be identified by either severe micromelia (long bone lengths > 4 SDs below the mean for gestation), narrow chest dimensions, or associated anomalies.

INVASIVE PROCEDURES AND FETAL SURGERY

The commonest indication for invasive testing is to establish the fetal karyotype in situations of high risk such as advanced maternal age, abnormal MSS or the ultrasonographic visualization of anomalies or soft markers. The number of monogenic disorders amenable to prenatal diagnosis by polymerase chain reaction (PCR) analysis of DNA is increasing rapidly, and has virtually replaced diagnosis by enzyme assay. Other indications include suspected fetal infection and alloimmunization.

All invasive procedures should be performed with real-time ultrasound guidance by appropriately trained and experienced operators. The Royal College of Obstetricians and Gynaecologists has recently issued guidelines suggesting that operators should undertake a minimum of 30 amniocenteses a year in order to maintain skills.[34]

AMNIOCENTESIS

Amniocentesis can be carried out from 15 weeks' gestation onwards. Early (11–14 weeks) amniocentesis is more hazardous than either chorionic villus sampling (CVS) or second trimester amniocentesis.[35] The cells in the amniotic fluid are mostly in interphase, and are prepared for metaphase analysis by culture in flasks for 2–3 weeks. More rapid culture on cover slips reduces reporting time to 7–10 days, but is more costly. Rapid detection of trisomy 21 and other trisomies is possible with quantitative PCR, but the information provided is probe specific.

The only randomized, controlled study of pregnancy outcomes following amniocentesis reported a procedure-related loss rate before viability of 1%.[36] Procedure-related losses occur up to 6 weeks after the test, but the maximal risk appears to be within 1–2 weeks. Experienced operators have lower complication rates; those undertaking < 50 procedures in 3 years had a single pass success rate of 82% compared with 93% for those carrying out > 50 procedures.[37] It is likely that the majority of losses occur as a result of infection.

CHORIONIC VILLUS SAMPLING

CVS in the first trimester of pregnancy can be performed transabdominally or transcervically using biopsy forceps or aspiration. Direct chromosome preparations from the cytotrophoblast provide provisional information about the fetal karyotype within 48 h. Rapid culture of the mesenchymal core allows full cytogenetic analysis using G-banding and also obviates diagnostic errors due to mosaicism in the fetus and/or placenta (see later). Chorionic villi are also an excellent source of DNA, supplying sufficient amounts for most molecular genetic techniques without prior culture. It is recommended that CVS is performed after 10 weeks of pregnancy when there is no increased risk of severe limb deficiencies and the hypoglossia/hypodactyly syndrome. Transabdominal placental sampling can also be performed in the second and third trimesters, but is more prone to failure as a result of reduced mitotic activity of the cytotrophoblast.

Meta-analysis of three randomized trials[38] showed pregnancy loss rates before viability to be significantly greater following first trimester CVS compared to midtrimester amniocentesis (odds ratio [OR] 1.37, 95% confidence interval [CI] 1.18–1.60.) However, a large number of the CVS procedures were carried out using a transcervical approach, which is associated with a higher incidence of procedure-related miscarriage.

Diagnostic errors can occur due to confined placental mosaicism (CPM), where aneuploid cells (mosaic and rarely nonmosaic) occur in the placenta but not in the fetus. In one large series, mosaicism was present in 30 (1.2%) of 2483 CVS cases.[39] Confined placental mosaicism within the cytotrophoblast will be apparent in the direct preparation, but not the longer term mesoderm culture. For those cases where the long-term culture confirms the mosaicism, or shows mosaicism not found on direct analysis, further investigation is warranted with either detailed ultrasonography, amniocentesis, fetal blood sample or skin biopsy. The input of genetics experts is essential to the management of couples in this very difficult situation.

FETAL BLOOD SAMPLING BEFORE LABOR

Fetal blood can be obtained from the umbilical vein, the intrahepatic vein, or the heart from about 18 weeks' gestation onwards. The main indications for fetal blood sampling are urgent fetal karyotyping after 18 weeks and measurement of hematologic parameters in fetuses at risk of alloimmune anemia or thrombocytopenia. Other indications include suspected fetal infection, later pregnancy DNA analysis, and investigation of mosaic results from either amniocentesis or CVS.

The post-procedure pregnancy loss rate following fetal blood sampling is about 1%. Loss rates are related to the indication for sampling; in one study loss rate was 1.5% for prenatal diagnostic procedures, 14% for fetuses with suspected placental dysfunction and 25% for fetuses with fetal hydrops.[40]

OTHER TISSUE BIOPSIES

Fetal skin biopsies are performed for suspected dermatological disorders such as harlequin ichthyosis or congenital bullous epidermolysis. Skin biopsies are also potentially useful in the investigation of fetuses with a suspected mosaic karyotype. Fetal liver and muscle biopsies have also been reported, but there are few indications.

FETAL SURGERY

Despite many advances in prenatal diagnosis, the fetus remains inaccessible. Established in utero therapeutic procedures include transabdominal intravascular transfusion of red cells or platelets, as well as placement of pleuroamniotic and vesicoamniotic shunts. The transplacental route is used for the delivery of antiarrhythmic agents for the treatment of complex cardiac arrhythmias.

The desire to perform more complex surgical treatments led to the development of open fetal surgery for conditions such as CDH, sacrococcygeal teratoma, CCAM of the lungs and obstructive uropathies. In severe form these conditions have a very poor prognosis due in part to progressive organ damage throughout the second trimester. In open surgery, the fetus is partially extracted, undergoes surgery, and is then returned to the amniotic cavity. Success rates have been severely limited by the high incidence of preterm labor, premature rupture of membranes and placental abruption. The median interval between surgery and delivery is 4 weeks with a median gestational age at delivery of only 25 weeks.

Endoscopic fetal surgery is less traumatic to the uterus and membranes, and is associated with fewer complications. In a series of 15 fetal endoscopic tracheal occlusion (FETO) procedures for severe CDH, only two mothers (13%) delivered within 2 weeks of surgery.[41] Prenatal tracheal occlusion obstructs the normal egress of lung fluid, increases transpulmonary pressure, leading to enhanced lung growth. The ability to predict outcome by measurement of the lung:head ratio (LHR) in fetuses with severe CDH has been used to select cases more likely to benefit from FETO; in a recent series, neonatal survival following FETO when the LHR was < 1.0 was 57%, as compared with 11% with an expectant approach.[42]

Other possible indications for endoscopic fetal surgery include amniotic bands and obstructive uropathies. Fetal surgery is an intriguing future development, but rigorous assessment is required before these techniques become more widely available.

ASSESSMENT OF FETAL SIZE AND WELL-BEING

DEFINITIONS

Perinatal mortality and morbidity are linked not only to gestational age but also to fetal growth. Screening previously focused on the detection of the small fetus but obstetricians now appreciate the differences between size and growth. Size is an endpoint, typically weight at birth, whereas growth is the process by which this endpoint is reached. Size is determined by a combination of local factors in tissues and organs, together with systemic nutritional and endocrine factors. Genetic influences, which are the primary determinant of fetal size, probably act primarily at the local level.

'Small for gestational age' refers to a fetus that is below a specific weight or anthropometric threshold. The commonly used thresholds for clinical and ultrasonic measurements are the 10th and 5th centiles. Approximately 40% of SGA infants are growth restricted as assessed by morphometric measures of wasting (ponderal index, midarm to head circumference [MAC:HC] ratio, skinfold thickness). These fetuses have failed to achieve their genetically programmed growth potential usually because of placental dysfunction and/or maternal disease. The remainder of SGA infants are thought to be constitutionally small.

SGA fetuses are at greater risk of stillbirth, acidemia at birth, low Apgar scores, neonatal complications, neurodevelopmental impairment as well as non-insulin-dependent diabetes and hypertension in later life. They are therefore the single largest group of fetuses tested for wellbeing. The reason that studies of SGA infants have shown poor perinatal outcome is likely to be due to the high incidence of true fetal growth restriction (FGR) in this group. Morbidity is much commoner in SGA infants with evidence of wasting and there is little evidence that small infants who reach term without evidence of growth restriction are at increased perinatal risk.[43]

ETIOLOGY OF FETAL GROWTH RESTRICTION (FGR)

The etiology of FGR is diverse but can be broadly classified according to the site of the primary pathology (Fig. 11.1). Some factors (e.g. maternal smoking) may affect fetal growth through several mechanisms. Genetic alterations associated with FGR can be divided into chromosomal anomalies, CPM and syndromes. Overall 4–7% of SGA fetuses will be aneuploid, the commonest abnormalities being triploidy and trisomies 13, 18 and 21. In CPM two or more cell lines with different karyotypes are present, both being derived from the same zygote. Cytogenetic abnormalities restricted to the placenta that have been associated with FGR include trisomy 16, trisomy 22 and trisomy 9. Growth restriction is also part of the phenotype of a large number of syndromes, some of which involve a primary disturbance of bone growth (e.g. osteogenesis imperfecta) and others associated with generalized (proportionate) reduction in body growth (e.g. Silver–Russell syndrome).

Congenital viral infection probably accounts for up to 5% of FGR. A causal relationship is clear for cytomegalovirus and rubella virus but probably also exists for varicella-zoster and human immunodeficiency viruses.

Abnormalities of uteroplacental perfusion and stem artery structure underlie a significant proportion of preterm FGR. Failure of extravillous trophoblast invasion and spiral artery transformation, leading to placental ischemia, is generally associated with maternal pre-eclampsia. However identical changes can be seen in the myometrial spiral arteries of 60–80% of growth-restricted fetuses born to women without hypertension.

SCREENING AND DIAGNOSIS OF SGA/FGR
Clinical assessment
Methods of detecting SGA fetuses include antenatal clinical examination, measurement of symphysis-fundal height (SFH), fetal anthropometry and ultrasound estimated fetal weight (EFW). All measurements require an accurate estimation of gestational age based on fetal crown–rump length prior to 13 weeks' gestation or fetal head circumference between 16 and 24 weeks' gestation (95% prediction interval ± 5 d).

Abdominal palpation remains a routine part of obstetric examination, despite the fact that the sensitivity for detection of a SGA infant is only 20–30% and the positive predictive value (PPV) no greater than 40%. Measurement of SFH is an alternative but a systematic review, which identified only one controlled trial which showed that SFH measurement did not improve perinatal outcome.[44] Serial SFH measurements may improve sensitivity and specificity as may the use of customized SFH charts. The customized antenatal growth chart displays computer generated curves for fetal weight and SFH, adjusted for physiological variables (maternal height, weight at booking, parity and ethnic group). One controlled trial has shown that use of customized charts improved detection rate of SGA infants (48% versus 29%, OR 2.2 [95% CI 1.1–4.5]) and reduced the number of women admitted (OR 0.6, 95% CI 0.4–0.7).[45] SFH should be measured at each antenatal assessment after 24 weeks of pregnancy. Ultrasound assessment is indicated if the SFH falls below the 10th centile.

Ultrasound anthropometry
A large number of ultrasonic anthropometric measurements have been used to predict fetal size but abdominal circumference (AC) and EFW are the most accurate.[46] Fetal AC is measured at the level of the hepatic vein. Fetal weight can be calculated from a variety of formulae incorporating routine ultrasonic anthropometric measurements (AC, BPD, HC and femur length [FL]). Systematic review suggests that an AC < 10th centile has the highest sensitivity, predicting 84% of SGA infants in high-risk women with an overall OR of 18 (95% CI < 10–34).[46] Reported sensitivities for EFW < 10th centile are lower and more variable (33–89%) although the overall OR is higher (39 [95% CI 29–52]). FPRs are comparable (20–25%) but can be reduced by the use of customized

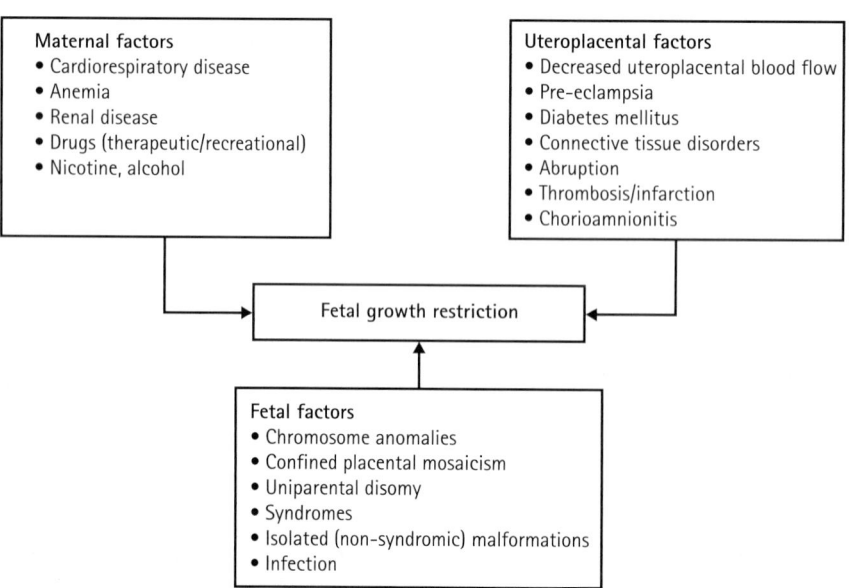

Fig. 11.1   Etiology of fetal growth restriction according to site of primary pathology.

ultrasound charts which adjust for physiological variables; in one study 27.5% of cases classified as SGA using an unadjusted EFW < 10th centile were reclassified as appropriate for gestational age (AGA) using the customized cut-off.[47] Fetuses identified as small by customized charts are more likely to suffer adverse perinatal outcome; the OR for stillbirth was 6.1 (95% CI 5.0–7.5) for fetuses classified as SGA by customized charts but AGA by population charts compared with 1.2 (CI 0.8, 1.9) for those classified as SGA by population charts but normal by customized charts.[48] Fetal anthropometric ratios (e.g. HC:AC and FL:AC) are less predictive of SGA than AC or EFW and there is no evidence that disproportion adds to the prognostic significance over and above the severity of growth restriction.

Despite the evidence that ultrasound anthropometry is effective at detecting small fetuses, there is no evidence that routine late pregnancy ultrasound in low-risk or unselected women confers benefit to mother or baby; systematic review of seven randomized trials (25 000 women) suggests that, while screened women are less likely to deliver post-term (OR 0.69 [95% CI 0.58–0.81]), perinatal mortality is no different (OR 1.12 [95% CI 0.75–1.68]).[49] Most of these studies investigated the value of a one-off measurement of size rather than the trend (reflecting growth) and none included umbilical artery Doppler (see later).

Reference charts of AC and EFW, derived from longitudinally collected measurements, can be used to assess fetal growth. Several studies have confirmed that serial measurements of AC and EFW are superior to single estimates in the prediction of wasting at birth and perinatal morbidity; a change in EFW SD (z) score of ≥ -1.5 detects 80% of babies with an abnormal MAC:HC ratio (OR 14.6 [95% CI 2.8–76.5]) and 54% of babies with suboptimal neonatal outcome (OR 3.6 [95% CI 1.3–9.5]).[50] Where growth restriction is suspected, measurements of size should be performed every 2 weeks as shorter intervals increase the FPR.

Uterine artery doppler

Because of the association between abnormal placentation and FGR, there has been considerable interest in the ability of uterine artery Doppler to predict FGR. Uterine arteries can be readily identified transabdominally with color flow Doppler and reproducible waveforms obtained by pulsed Doppler. A positive test (defined as an abnormal waveform ratio and/or a diastolic notch) between 20 and 24 weeks predicts pre-eclampsia, FGR and perinatal death in low- and high-risk populations. A recent systematic review of 74 studies found a sensitivity and specificity for predicting FGR in a low-risk population of 33% (95% CI 26–40) and 91% (95% CI 87–94). Sensitivity increased to 69% (95% CI 54–83) in a high-risk population while specificity fell (69% [95% CI 46–90]).[51] More importantly the test is more predictive of FGR necessitating delivery before 34 weeks' gestation (LRs > 5). In one screening study, 14% of fetuses where the mother had an abnormal uterine artery waveform (pulsatility index > 95th centile) developed FGR (fetal AC < 5th centile) and, of this group, 40% required delivery < 34 weeks.[52]

There is also accumulating evidence that several of the analytes used in maternal serum screening for Down syndrome (e.g. PAPP-A, hCG, AFP and uE3) can also be used to screen for FGR, pre-eclampsia and adverse perinatal outcome. Thus in the future it may be possible to offer multiparameter screening for 'poor placentation' between 12 and 24 weeks.

ASSESSMENT OF FETAL WELL-BEING
Principles

Fetal death from hypoxic ischemia may occur acutely, as a result of a sudden insult (e.g. cord accident or placental abruption), or may be the result of chronic placental dysfunction. In the latter case, FGR (but not necessarily SGA) is invariably present. Current understanding of the adaptive responses and consequences of progressive fetal hypoxemia is primarily derived from animal studies but antenatal fetal blood sampling has provided important insights into human FGR. In the face of progressive hypoxemia (fetal pO_2 > 2 SDs below mean for gestation) the fetus makes a number of circulatory and metabolic adaptations to optimize the available oxygen and nutrient supply. With progressive placental insufficiency the fetus becomes acidemic (pH > 2 SDs below mean for gestation) and ultimately suffers end-organ damage prior to death. Up to 40% of severely growth restricted fetuses (AC > 2 SDs below the mean for gestation) are acidemic. This is an important outcome as there is evidence that chronic fetal acidemia is associated with reduced neurodevelopmental outcome as assessed by Griffiths neurodevelopmental quotient at a mean age of 29 (range 12–52) months.[52]

A number of biophysical tests are available to assess fetal well-being. These include fetal Doppler arterial and venous flow velocity waveforms, cardiotocography (CTG), amniotic fluid volume (AFV) and the biophysical profile score (BPS). For many of these tests the relationship between test result and antenatal hypoxemia/acidemia has been defined, thereby obviating the need for fetal blood sampling, which carries a significant risk in FGR. In this context a normal test result implies the absence of acidemia and therefore fetal well-being. As the only effective intervention available to the obstetrician is delivery, the presence of fetal well-being justifies expectant management, at least prior to term, unless there is coexistent maternal disease necessitating delivery. When the test is abnormal, the likelihood of acidemia and the risk of end-organ damage/death with further expectant management have to be balanced against the risks of premature delivery.

Umbilical artery doppler

Reproducible Doppler velocity waveforms can be obtained from the umbilical artery (UA) using pulsed Doppler. A variety of descriptive indices have been used to characterize the waveform including pulsatility index (PI), resistance index and systolic:diastolic ratio. Mean PI declines during pregnancy with the 95th centile value falling from around 2.0 at 20 weeks to 1.4 at term. Waveform indices are independent of the angle of ultrasound insonation and reflect downstream blood flow resistance. With progressive placental damage and vascular occlusion, PI increases and in some cases this may progress to absent or even reversed end-diastolic velocities (A/R EDV). Between 40% and 45% of fetuses with an elevated PI (but EDV present) are hypoxemic and 20–30% are acidemic. In contrast 80–90% of fetuses with AEDV are hypoxemic and 45–80% are acidemic. Loss of EDV is a key finding, which has a profound impact on outcome and management. Overall perinatal mortality in this group is around 40%,[53] justifying delivery on this finding alone after 32 weeks' gestation and possibly earlier.

Systematic review of randomized trials in high-risk pregnancies (mainly in association with hypertensive disorders and FGR) has indicated that management based on UA Doppler significantly improves important obstetric outcomes, including fewer admissions (OR 0.56 [95% CI 0.42–0.72]) and fewer labor inductions (OR 0.83 [95% CI 0.74–0.93]).[54] There was also a trend to reducing perinatal mortality (OR 0.71 [95% CI 0.50–1.01]). There is also evidence that UA Doppler is superior to CTG and the BPS in predicting outcome in SGA fetuses and that it reduces use of resources.[55] Thus UA Doppler should be the primary mode of fetal monitoring in the high-risk fetus. Screening low-risk fetuses by UA Doppler however does not reduce perinatal mortality or morbidity and is not recommended.

Fetuses with a normal UA Doppler and normal anatomy can be managed as a 'normal small fetus'; in this group twice-weekly monitoring results in earlier deliveries and more inductions of labor than fortnightly monitoring without any difference in neonatal morbidity.[56] Thus, in the absence of maternal hypertension, provided UA Doppler and fetal growth remain normal fortnightly surveillance can be maintained until delivery. Fetuses with abnormal UA Doppler, especially those with A/R EDV, require more intensive surveillance. The average interval between loss of EDV in the UA and the development of a terminal CTG is 7 d, although the range is wide (1 d to more than 4 weeks). Gestational age > 30 weeks, the presence of maternal hypertension and Doppler venous abnormalities are associated with a reduced interval. The optimal monitoring strategy in this group is unclear and may involve targeted fetal

Doppler (arterial and venous), BPS or both. Quality randomized trials are urgently needed in this area.

Fetal arterial and venous doppler

Redistribution of cardiac output to the cerebral circulation is one of the earliest signs of hypoxemia. This is reflected by an increase in the umbilical artery:middle cerebral artery (MCA) PI ratio to greater than 1 (~95th centile) or a decrease in the middle cerebral artery PI. Despite being a sensitive indicator of hypoxemia, there is no evidence that MCA Doppler is a better predictor of adverse outcome than UA Doppler. However the absence of cranial redistribution may provide better negative prediction in the preterm fetus; when gestational age at first Doppler was less than 32 weeks, the MCA PI had a sensitivity of 95.5% and a negative predictive value of 97.7% (negative LR 0.10) for major adverse outcome (death, neurological complications and necrotizing enterocolitis).[57] Compared to fetuses without cranial redistribution, those with cerebral sparing appear to have no long-term adverse neurodevelopmental effects although larger follow-up studies are needed.

Fetal venous Doppler abnormalities generally follow loss of EDV in the UA and are thought to reflect ventricular function and, to a lesser extent, cardiac afterload. Waveforms from the ductus venosus (DV) show a systolic and a diastolic peak followed by a trough ('a' wave) related to atrial contraction. With increasing hypoxemia, the 'a' wave decreases and then reverses and pulsations may be evident in the umbilical vein (UV); 90% of fetuses with these findings are acidemic and they have the highest sensitivity for perinatal death and serious morbidity.[58] In fetuses with loss or reversal of EDV in the UA, abnormal DV Doppler waveforms and gestational age at delivery show the strongest association with perinatal death.[59] Perinatal mortality in this group is increased by 20–25% in the presence of abnormal DV waveforms.[58,59] Hence many authorities regard reversal of the DV 'a' wave and/or UV pulsations as indications for delivery irrespective of biophysical parameters. As myocardial function worsens, tricuspid valve regurgitation may appear and there may be a loss of brain sparing with normalization of the MCA PI. These are pre-terminal events and fetal death is likely within 48 h.

Biophysical profile scoring (BPS)

The BPS incorporates CTG, AFV and three dynamic ultrasound variables (fetal movement, fetal breathing and fetal tone). Each component is scored 0 (abnormal) or 2 (normal). A total score of 8 or 10 is normal and excludes acidemia.[60] Perinatal mortality within 7 d of a normal BPS is ≤ 1 per 1000 and no test has a lower false-negative rate. Scores of 4 or less are regarded as abnormal; > 90% of fetuses will be acidemic and 50% will have an umbilical vein pH < 7.25. Adverse outcome increases with declining score: perinatal mortality increases from 12.5% with a score of 4 to 100% with a score of 0 without intervention (and 43% despite intervention), while the rate of cerebral palsy increases from ~2 to 25% respectively.[60] A score of 6 is equivocal necessitating repeat testing, usually within 12–24 h. Systematic review of four poor-quality studies (fewer than 3000 subjects) indicates that BPS does not improve perinatal outcome but insufficient data are available to assess the true value of the test.[61] Given the absence of benefit from randomized trials and that the BPS is a time-consuming test, it is not recommended for primary surveillance in high-risk fetuses. However, based on the results of observational studies, BPS may have a role in monitoring preterm fetuses with A/R EDF in the UA when a normal score allows continued expectant management. In the authors' large series of 137 fetuses with growth restriction and A/R EDF monitored with daily BPS, in utero demise in actively managed cases (i.e. where delivery in the fetal interests was offered) was 4%.[62]

CTG and AFV have been used in isolation as tests of fetal well-being although there is little evidence to support this. The CTG records autonomic reflexes superimposed on intrinsic cardiac activity. In addition to the baseline fetal heart rate (FHR) and variability, the CTG records periodic changes (accelerations and decelerations). Two 15 b.p.m. accelerations lasting ≥ 15 s in a 20-minute period are regarded as reassuring. Preterm accelerations are less marked. Unlike the BPS where only 0.7% of tests are abnormal (score ≤ 4) and 1.7% are equivocal, up to 15% of CTGs will be nonreassuring. This proportion increases as gestation declines. A nonreassuring CTG is a poor predictor of perinatal death within 7 d (< 10%). The features most predictive of acidemia are reduced FHR variability (< 5 b.p.m.) and decelerations (positive predictive value 65% and 75%, respectively). When both are present (so-called 'terminal' CTG), the overall mortality rate is around 45%. Use of CTG in high-risk pregnancies is not associated with better perinatal outcome; in fact systematic review of four randomized trials showed a trend towards increasing perinatal mortality in the CTG group (OR 2.85, 95% CI 0.99–7.12).[63] Computerized analysis of the CTG provides a more objective measure of FHR variability; several parameters have been studied but the short-term variability (STV) appears to be the most useful; around 60% of fetuses with a STV < 3.5 ms are acidemic. Computer systems have been shown to be more accurate predictors of umbilical acidemia than clinical experts but it is unclear whether use of this technology (as opposed to visual analysis) improves perinatal outcome.

There are many definitions for reduced AFV but the two most widely accepted are a maximum vertical pocket < 2 cm or a four-quadrant amniotic fluid index (AFI) < 5 cm. Both correlate very poorly with actual AFV and neither accurately predicts perinatal outcome. Systematic review of 18 studies indicated that an AFI < 5 cm was associated with an increased risk of Cesarean section for fetal distress (relative risk [RR] 2.2, 95% CI 1.5–3.4) and Apgar score < 7 at 5 min (RR 5.2, 95% CI 2.4–11.3),[64] but not with neonatal acidosis. Large observational studies have shown an association between reduced AFV and perinatal mortality but the predictive value is poor (< 10%). There is little evidence to support intervention with isolated oligohydramnios when the UA Doppler is normal.

The sequence and timing of circulatory changes in FGR with progressive hypoxemia/acidemia have been determined and are summarized in Figure 11.2. In a serial study of preterm growth-restricted fetuses, 73% showed this pattern of Doppler deterioration prior to emergency delivery (median gestation of 30 weeks) for a BPS of ≤ 6.[65] In the majority, Doppler deterioration was confined to the week prior to delivery, was most marked for the UA and DV and was complete 24 h before BPS decline. The decline in BPS typically involved cessation of breathing movements 2–3 d before delivery, followed by a decline in AFV and then a loss of fetal movement and tone on the day of delivery.

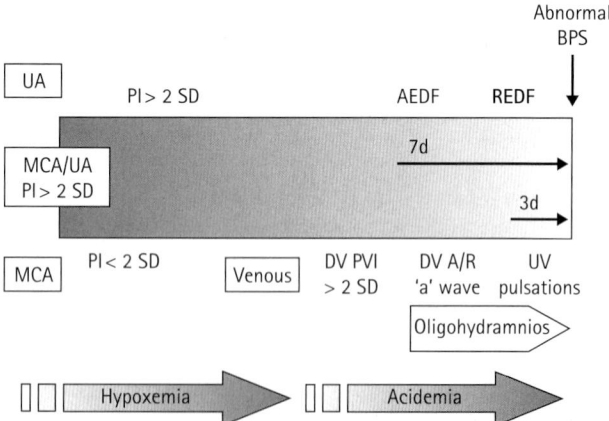

Fig. 11.2 The sequence and timing of Doppler changes in FGR with progressive hypoxemia/acidemia. Doppler changes are usually (but not invariably) preceded by a decline in fetal growth (as assessed by serial changes in abdominal circumference or weight). AEDF, absent end diastolic frequencies; BPS biophysical profile score; d, days; DV A/R, ductus venosus absent/reversed; MCA, middle cerebral artery; PI, pulsatility index; PVI, peak velocity index; REDF, reversed end diastolic frequencies; SD, standard deviation; UA, umbilical artery; UV, umbilical vein.

Table 11.4 Indications for ultrasound to assess fetal size and well-being

Maternal medical history	Current pregnancy history
Hypertension	SFH < 10th centile
Antiphospholipid syndrome	Pregnancy-induced hypertension
Sickle cell disease	Antepartum hemorrhage
Renal disease	Oligohydramnios
Cardiopulmonary disease	Post-term
Insulin-dependent diabetes	Abnormal uterine artery Doppler waveforms
mellitus	Elevated maternal AFP

Previous obstetric history
Stillbirth
Pre-eclampsia
SGA infant
Cesarean section for fetal distress
Placental abruption

AFP, alpha-fetoprotein; SFH, symphysis–fundus height; SGA, small for gestational age.

Organization of screening

Women with risk factors for FGR and fetal acidemia/perinatal mortality (Table 11.4) should have ultrasound screening for fetal size and well-being by AC and UA Doppler. The timing and frequency of assessment should be determined by the degree of risk and the outcome of uterine artery Doppler screening at 20–24 weeks of pregnancy. In those with a normal uterine artery Doppler, a single screen at 32–34 weeks may be appropriate but where risk is high (e.g. previous stillbirth associated with FGR, abnormal uterine artery Doppler), 2-weekly surveillance from 26 weeks is justified.

The authors' current management guidelines following the initial AC and UA Doppler are shown in Figure 11.3. Where the mother does not have pre-eclampsia and the UA Doppler is normal UA Doppler testing is repeated weekly. This is increased to twice weekly if the UA PI becomes abnormal (but with EDF present). Once there are A/R EDF in the UA this is regarded as an indication for daily BPS and DV Doppler studies and an indication for delivery, irrespective of the results of other monitoring tests, after 32 weeks' gestation. Deterioration of the DV Doppler, with reversal of the 'a' wave, usually heralds a decline in the BPS. Unless parents have made an informed decision not to intervene due to the expected poor prognosis (< 500 g and < 28 weeks' gestation) the authors would deliver when the BPS or DV Doppler became abnormal between 28 and 32 weeks' gestation. Based on the authors' previous experience,[62] the BPS alone is still used to time delivery < 27 weeks. However the benefit of using the BPS rather than abnormalities in the DV waveform to time delivery have not been studied. In this group, the authors routinely offer Cesarean section as in excess of 75% will develop fetal distress if exposed to labor.

Conclusion

All SGA fetuses should be monitored with UA Doppler. Several studies have demonstrated that fetuses not identified as SGA have a higher rate of adverse fetal outcome (OR 4.1 [95% CI 2.5–6.8]) than those identified as SGA and monitored with UA Doppler.[66] Widespread use of UA Doppler is also likely, at least in part, to account for the proportionally larger reductions in perinatal mortality and cerebral palsy in very low birth weight (VLBW) growth-restricted infants compared with VLBW infants overall seen over the last 20 years: 67% [95% CI 51–80] in 1983–1987 versus 5% [95% CI 2–13] in 1998–2002 compared to 54% [95% CI 44–64] in 1983–1987 versus 20% [95% CI 15–25] in 1998–2002, respectively.[67]

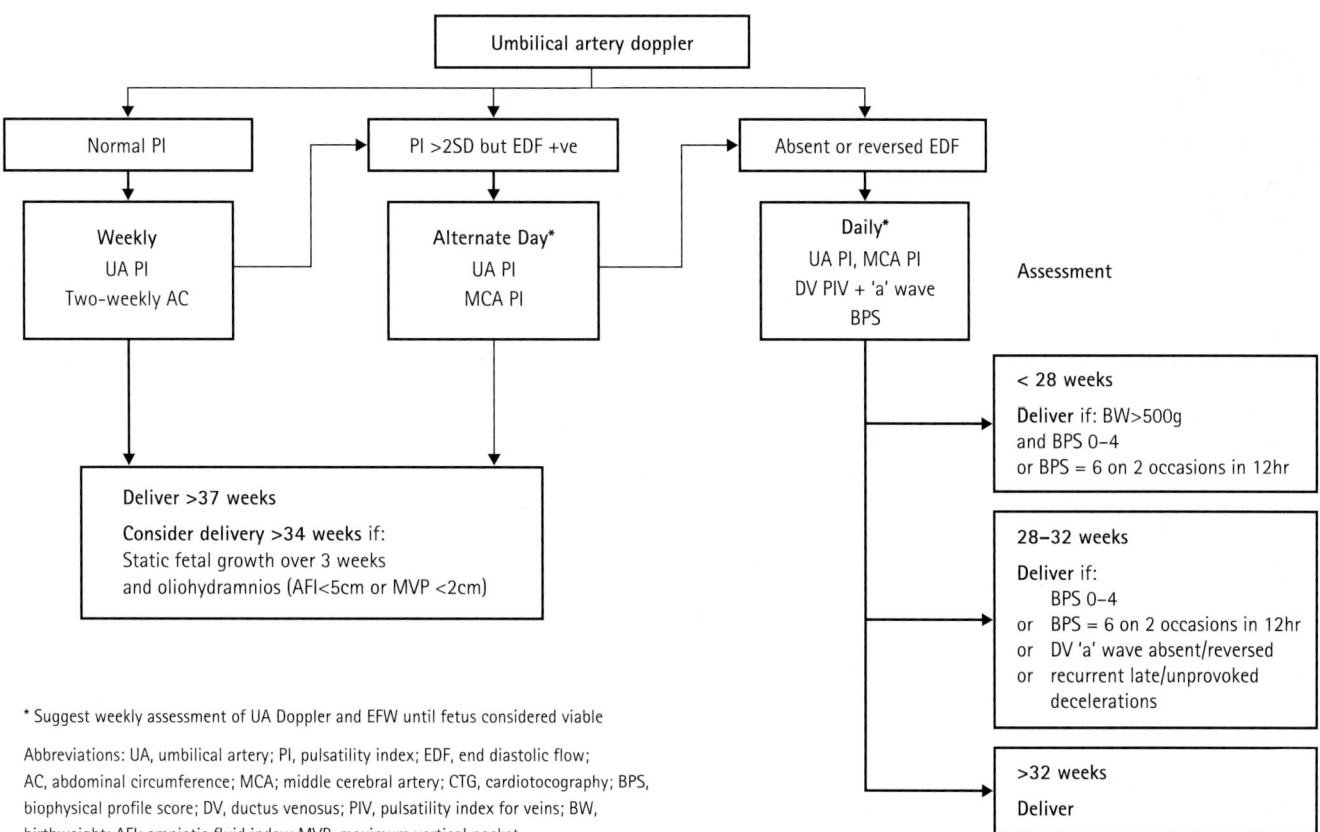

* Suggest weekly assessment of UA Doppler and EFW until fetus considered viable

Abbreviations: UA, umbilical artery; PI, pulsatility index; EDF, end diastolic flow; AC, abdominal circumference; MCA; middle cerebral artery; CTG, cardiotocography; BPS, biophysical profile score; DV, ductus venosus; PIV, pulsatility index for veins; BW, birthweight; AFI; amniotic fluid index; MVP, maximum vertical pocket

Fig. 11.3 Guidelines for management of high-risk fetuses based on ultrasound morphometry and umbilical artery (UA) Doppler. We base the decision to deliver fetuses with absent or reversed end diastolic frequencies (A/R EDF) prior to 34 weeks on the biophysical profile scoring (BPS). Randomized trials are needed to determine if this is a better strategy than using Doppler alone. AC/EFW, abdominal circumference/estimated fetal weight; AF, amniotic fluid; CTG, cardiotocography; DV, ductus venosus; EDF, end diastolic frequencies; SD standard deviation; UV, umbilical vein.

MULTIPLE PREGNANCIES

TWINS

Perinatal complications

Perinatal mortality in twins is about five times greater than in singletons. The majority of adverse outcomes occur as a result of either preterm delivery, which occurs in 30–50% of twin pregnancies, or FGR. The predominant prenatal prognostic factor for twins is chorionicity. Relative to dichorionic twins, monochorionic twins are at greater risk of fetal loss at 10–24 weeks' gestation (12.2% versus 18.0%), perinatal mortality (2.8% versus 1.6%), preterm delivery < 32 weeks (9.2% versus 5.5%) and birth weight < 5th centile in both twins (7.5% versus 1.7%).[68] The marked increase in the number of second trimester losses is a consequence of the fetoplacental vascular anastamoses that are present in more than 98% of monochorionic pregnancies. Hemodynamic imbalance between the two circulations is responsible for acute and chronic transfusion syndromes.

Prenatal ultrasonography in twins

Prenatal ultrasonographic assessment of fetal sex and placental/membrane morphology is highly accurate in predicting chorionicity. The lambda sign, an echogenic chorionic tissue projection into the base of the intertwin membrane, is evident in all dichorionic pregnancies at 10–14 weeks' gestation but disappears by the 20th week in about 7% of dichorionic pregnancies with fused placenta. Monochorionic twins should be scanned every 2 weeks to look for evidence of transfusion pathology. Dichorionic twins with normal biometry, umbilical Doppler values and amniotic fluid levels should be scanned every 4–6 weeks from 24 weeks onwards to monitor growth and well-being.

Discordant size and growth

A 20–25% discordance in size between twins is associated with an increased incidence of adverse pregnancy outcomes. The differential diagnosis includes constitutional size difference, uteroplacental dysfunction, and fetal abnormalities as well as twin–twin transfusion syndrome (TTTS) in monochorionic twins. Detailed ultrasonography including Doppler analysis of the umbilical, fetal and uteroplacental circulations will usually determine the etiology. The assessment of fetal well-being is based on the same principles as for singletons, but decisions regarding premature delivery need to consider the outcome of the healthy twin.

Twin–twin transfusion syndrome

The TTTS occurs in about 10–15% of monochorionic twins and accounts for 17% of perinatal deaths. The syndrome develops when there is unbalanced shunting of blood from one twin (the donor) to the other (the recipient) through arteriovenous anastomoses in the placenta. The donor twin progressively becomes anemic, growth restricted, and oliguric. The resulting oligohydramnios can be so severe that the donor becomes shrouded in the amniotic membrane ('stuck twin'). The recipient becomes plethoric, polyuric, and can eventually develop cardiomegaly and cardiac failure manifest as hydrops. The polyuria leads to hydramnios, which predisposes to miscarriage and/or extreme prematurity. The wide spectrum of severities is incorporated into a sonographic staging classification, as first proposed by Quintero et al:[69]

Stage I: The bladder of the donor twin is still visible, and Doppler studies are still normal.

Stage II: The bladder of the donor twin is not visible (during the length of the examination, usually 1 h), but Doppler studies are not critically abnormal.

Stage III: Doppler studies are critically abnormal in either twin and are characterized as absent or reverse end-diastolic velocity in the umbilical artery, reverse flow in the ductus venosus, or pulsatile umbilical venous flow.

Stage IV: Ascites, pericardial or pleural effusion, scalp edema, or overt hydrops are present.

Stage V: One or both twins are dead.

Mortality rates for severe (grade II+) untreated TTTS at < 22 weeks approach 95%. Therapeutic options include serial amnioreduction, endoscopic laser coagulation of placental vascular anastamoses, and selective termination of one fetus with bipolar cord diathermy.

Serial amnioreduction

Therapeutic amniocentesis reduces the amniotic fluid volume and/or pressure, thereby reducing the risk of preterm birth and amniorrhexis. The procedure sometimes results in reappearance of fluid in the donor sac. This might reflect alterations in the hemodynamic characteristics of the shunt caused by a reduction in hydrostatic pressure.

Endoscopic laser coagulation of placental vascular anastomoses

Endoscopic laser coagulation obliterates the communicating placental vessels between the twins. A combination of ultrasonography and direct vision are used to examine systematically the chorionic plate along the whole length of the intertwin membrane and identify the crossing vessels. The main advantage of this treatment is that the potential for further intertwin vascular shunting is substantially reduced, thereby removing the need for repeated interventions, and theoretically improving the health of surviving twins by reducing cardiovascular instability.

Comparison of outcomes following endoscopic laser coagulation or amnioreduction

Data from a recent multicentre randomized, controlled trial indicated that endoscopic laser coagulation for all grades of TTTS – as compared with amnioreduction – was associated with a higher likelihood of one or both twins surviving to 28 d of age (76% vs. 56%) or 6 months.[70] Analysis of data from a large comparative case series confirmed better outcomes following endoscopic laser surgery in pregnancies complicated by stage III/IV TTTS, but the outcomes for stage I/II disease were similar after both forms of treatment.[71]

Detailed long-term follow-up of babies surviving laser surgery for severe TTTS has revealed that up to 11% will experience minor neurologic disability, and a further 11% will develop major neurologic morbidity.

Selective feticide

The spontaneous death of one twin is often associated with either loss of the sib, or resolution of the hydramnios. Selective feticide of one twin with a mechanical procedure, such as umbilical cord ligation, has been reported with good short-term results. However, there is concern regarding the potential for acute transfer of blood into the placenta of the demised twin.

Single fetal demise

Single fetal death occurs in 0.5–6.8% of twin pregnancies. The earlier twins are diagnosed, the more likely one twin is to demise. The three major factors affecting outcome are the gestational age at death, the cause of death and the chorionicity of the twins. With dichorionic twins, provided the cause of death is intrinsic to the dead twin, complications are unusual. However, the death of a monochorionic twin may be followed by cerebral infarction in the surviving co-twin, as well as renal, hepatic and cutaneous damage. In 13 studies, single fetal death was associated with serious morbidity in 24% of 119 surviving monochorionic children.[72] It is likely that the cause of the neurological damage is acute exsanguination of the surviving twin into the circulation of the dead twin through placental vascular anastomoses.

The optimal management of single fetal death ≥ 36 weeks' gestation is elective delivery. For dichorionic twins remote from term, an expectant approach leads to enhanced maturity and an increased chance of survival. For the survivors of monochorionic single fetal deaths, there is debate as to whether the optimal management is delivery or expectant.

However, delivery is unlikely to improve outcome if the reason for neurological injury is acute hypoperfusion immediately after the demise of the sibling. Thus a conservative approach is usually adopted with serial ultrasound follow-up (and/or MRI) to look for ventriculomegaly, porencephaly, and microcephaly.

Fetal anomalies

Fetal anomalies are more common in twin pregnancies, particularly monozygous twins, compared to singletons (OR 1.25, 95% CI 1.21–1.28).[73] Even in monozygous twins it is more common for twins to be discordant for anomalies. When ultrasound or genetic studies demonstrate that twins are discordant for a major anomaly, parents are faced with a choice between continuation, TOP, or selective feticide. The risks of selective feticide are dependent on gestation and chorionicity. In dichorionic twins, selective feticide with intracardiac injection of potassium chloride is associated with miscarriage rates varying between 5% at 11–12 weeks and 9% at 16–20 weeks' gestation. The chance of co-twin demise is much reduced if the procedure is carried out during the third trimester after fetal maturity is established, but parents find this option emotionally more difficult.

Selective feticide in monochorionic twins is problematic. Potassium chloride injected into the heart of the abnormal twin might enter the circulation of the normal twin through placental vascular connections. Recent experience with this technique appears to be encouraging; with co-twin survival rates of about 80–85%, and very low rates of immediate neonatal morbidity. However, further investigation is required before definitive conclusions can be drawn regarding the safety of this procedure.

Monoamniotic twins

About 1% of monozygous twins are monoamniotic. Mortality rates (10–40%) are greater than for all other forms of twins due to the increased incidence of fetal anomalies, cord entanglement, prematurity and trauma during labor. Stillbirths at > 24 weeks are unusual in women admitted to hospital for daily fetal monitoring, but there is no consensus about the optimal technique for monitoring these very high-risk pregnancies. Prophylactic early delivery is usually recommended at about 32–34 weeks' gestation by Cesarean section.

HIGHER ORDER MULTIPLES

The natural incidence of triplets is 1 in 8000 pregnancies. With assisted reproductive techniques, the incidence has increased to between 1 in 850–2000. The mean gestation at delivery is 33 weeks with a mean birth weight of 1800 g. Preterm delivery at less than 28 weeks' gestation occurs in 7% of cases, and at less than 32 weeks in 28%. Perinatal mortality rates vary from 48 to 151 per 1000 pregnancies. Cerebral palsy occurs in about 3% of long-term survivors. For quadruplets, perinatal mortality rates are between 67 and 104 per 1000, with cerebral palsy occurring in 10% of survivors. The outcomes for higher order multiple pregnancies are even worse.

Multifetal pregnancy reduction (MFPR)

Although advances in prenatal and neonatal care have resulted in significant improvement in perinatal mortality for higher order multiple pregnancies, there remains concern about long-term morbidity for both the offspring and the family. One option is MFPR, which is usually performed by intrathoracic injection of potassium chloride. Success rates of 100% are typical.

The majority of pregnancies are reduced to twins. This leaves 'margin for error' if there is a problem with a remaining fetus. The frequency of complications, mainly miscarriage or preterm delivery, is a function of the starting number of fetuses (Table 11.5).[74] The outcome for pregnancies reduced to twins is comparable to nonreduced twins. There is general agreement that gestation at delivery (and birth weight) are improved following triplet reduction to twins, but it might be that pregnancy loss rates in centers without a substantial experience of MFPR are greater than those generally reported in the literature. There are no doubts that outcomes are improved following MFPR for quadruplets and higher order multiple pregnancies.

ALLOIMMUNIZATION

RED CELL ANTIBODIES

When maternal antibodies to antigens on fetal red cells cross the placenta they can result in hemolysis. The risk of hemolytic disease of the newborn (HDN) requiring treatment is dependent on the red cell antigen (Table 11.6). Transplacental fetomaternal hemorrhage (FMH) is the most common cause of alloimmunization. Heterologous blood transfusion is the second, but is the most common cause of sensitization to the uncommon antigens. Of the five major antigenic loci determining rhesus (Rh) status (C, D, E, c, e), D is the most immunogenic, followed by c. Approximately 85% of the Caucasian population are RhD positive, 45% being homozygous for the D antigen. Routine screening for red cell antibodies is undertaken at booking and around 30 weeks of pregnancy. Alloimmunization is now sufficiently uncommon that all cases at risk of significant hemolysis should be managed by, or in collaboration with, a regional center.

Anti-D prophylaxis

Anti-D immunoglobulin (Ig) should be given to all nonsensitized RhD-negative women within 72 h of the delivery of a RhD-positive infant. A dose of 100 μg (500 iu) is capable of suppressing immunization by 4–5 ml RhD-positive cells. A Kleihauer test is routinely undertaken to detect larger FMH requiring additional anti-D Ig. Prophylaxis is also given after potentially sensitizing events during pregnancy (e.g. antepartum hemorrhage, invasive prenatal diagnosis) and after therapeutic TOP, ectopic pregnancy, and uterine evacuation of a spontaneous or incomplete abortion. Between 1 and 1.5% RhD-negative women develop anti-D antibodies during a first or subsequent pregnancy due to 'silent' FMH. Evidence from several studies indicates prophylactic anti-D during pregnancy in the early third

Table 11.5 Multifetal pregnancy reduction: pregnancy losses or deliveries as a function of starting number (S) before reduction

		Losses			Deliveries		
		< 24 weeks	25–28 weeks	29–32 weeks	33–36 weeks	37+ weeks	
	N	n (%)	n (%)	n (%)	n (%)	n (%)	Mean GA
S 6+	96	22 (22.9)	11 (11.5)	11 (11.5)	33 (34.4)	19 (19.8)	33.6
S 5	170	29 (17.1)	9 (5.3)	21 (12.4)	55 (32.4)	56 (32.9)	34.5
S 4	653	90 (13.0)	32 (4.9)	68 (10.4)	221 (33.8)	242 (37.1)	35.0
S 3	759	58 (7.6)	25 (3.3)	57 (7.5)	263 (34.7)	356 (46.9)	35.5
S 2	111	10 (9.0)	4 (3.6)	4 (3.6)	12 (10.8)	81 (73.0)	35.6

Collaborative data from 1789 patients having multifetal pregnancy reduction to twins, or singletons when reducing from twins.[74] GA, gestational age.

Table 11.6   Red cell antigens causing hemolytic disease of the newborn (HDN)

Can cause severe HDN and intrauterine death	Severe HDN uncommon
Rhesus – D, c, e, C, E	Kidd – JK^a
Kell	Duffy – Fy^a
	Kp$^{a or b}$
	k
	S

Severe HDN rare	Never cause HDN
Fy^b	Le$^{a or b}$
Jk^b	p
Lu^a	
Hutch	
M,	
N,	
S,	
U	

trimester reduces this to 0.2% or less and antenatal prophylaxis is now recommended.

Management of women with anti-D

Once anti-D antibodies are detected the father's RhD type should be determined. Significant hemolysis does not occur with anti-D concentrations ≤ 4 iu/ml and there is no need for intervention. Antibody testing should be repeated monthly to 28 weeks and fortnightly thereafter. Above 4 iu/ml there is a risk of anemia but this is not accurately predicted by anti-D concentration; between 4 and 15 iu/ml mild to moderate anemia, requiring postnatal transfusion, may occur but severe anemia (hemoglobin < 7 g/dl) is uncommon. Above 15 iu/ml, and particularly in the presence of rapidly rising levels, the risk of severe anemia has been reported to be as high as 50%. Where there is a risk of significant hemolysis and the partner is heterozygous for the RhD antigen, the fetal RhD genotype can be predicted using real-time PCR on cell-free fetal DNA within the maternal circulation.

In women with anti-D > 4 iu/ml and an RhD-positive fetus, the risk of fetal anemia is assessed by ultrasonographic measurement of cerebral peak systolic blood flow; the sensitivity of an increased peak velocity of systolic blood flow for severe fetal anemia is ~100% with a FPR of 12% (positive LR 8.5, 95% CI 4.7–15.6, negative LR 0.02, 95% CI 0.00–0.25).[75] This increase in peak velocity is likely to be a result of increased cardiac output and/or reduced blood viscosity.

The management of increased peak systolic velocity (i.e. > 1.5 Multiples of the Median [MoMs]) at gestations < 33 weeks is cordocentesis to measure the fetal hematocrit (or hemoglobin). The risk of increased sensitization, especially with transplacental passage of the needle, and fetal death suggests that fetal blood sampling should be reserved for fetuses perceived to be at highest risk. Intravascular transfusions are begun when the fetal hematocrit declines below > 30% (less than the 2.5th centile after 20 weeks). The timing of subsequent blood sampling in fetuses with a hematocrit > 30% is determined by the strength of the positive direct antiglobulin test and the fetal reticulocyte count. Compatible (RhD negative), fresh, leukocyte depleted blood, resuspended in saline to a hematocrit of ~70–75%, is transfused into either the umbilical vein (at the placental cord insertion) or the intrahepatic vein. The volume of blood required to attain the desired hematocrit (typically 40–50%) can be estimated from the initial fetal and donor hematocrits together with the estimated fetoplacental blood volume. The second

transfusion is arbitrarily undertaken 2 weeks after the first, or at a time when the peak systolic velocities increase beyond the treatment threshold. The timing of subsequent transfusions is then determined from the fall in hematocrit, which becomes more consistent over time (typically ~1%/d) as fetal erythropoiesis is suppressed and only donor blood is circulating. Intraperitoneal transfusion is less effective and associated with a greater risk of fetal death compared with intravascular transfusion. Furthermore combining intraperitoneal and intravascular transfusion confers no advantage. The aim with fetal transfusion is to reach a gestational age of at least 36 weeks before delivery.

Mortality rate per intravascular transfusion is ~ 3%, with higher rates reported when transfusion is required prior to 20 weeks' gestation and in hydropic fetuses. Overall 84% of fetuses (94% without hydrops and 74% with hydrops) requiring in utero transfusion will survive[76] with < 10% suffering developmental problems.[77] Postnatal exchange transfusion is rarely necessary when there have been at least two antenatal transfusions. Top-up transfusions are frequently necessary because of late anemia prior to resumption of normal erythropoiesis.

Management of women with other alloantibodies

Anti-c antibodies can be quantitated accurately and management of women with anti-c levels > 4 iu/ml follows similar guidelines to anti-D, including fetal genotyping from maternal blood. Antibody levels for other red cell antibodies are measured by indirect antiglobulin test. The reciprocal of the highest dilution of serum that causes agglutination is the titer. Severe hemolysis rarely, if ever, occurs with titers ≤ 1 in 32 with the exception of anti-Kell, where severe anemia has been reported with titers as low as 1:2. In Kell disease the main cause of fetal anemia is erythroid suppression rather than hemolysis. Determination of the partner's Kell status is vital as only 9% will be Kell positive, with virtually all being heterozygous. Thus very few fetuses of women with anti-Kell are actually at risk.

PLATELET ANTIBODIES

In alloimmune thrombocytopenia (AIT), maternal antiplatelet antibodies to a paternally derived platelet antigen, usually PLA1, cross the placenta and destroy fetal platelets. Neonatal AIT occurs in 1 in 2000–5000 births with intracranial hemorrhage (ICH) in 15–20% of cases. Between 30% and 50% of ICH occurs in utero, usually after 30 weeks' gestation. The mother is healthy and her first child is affected in 50% of cases. Recurrence rates are very high (> 85%). Management is controversial, but often based on stratification by the history of previous siblings.

Women with a history of an infant with an ICH during pregnancy are usually treated with i.v. immunoglobulin (1 g/kg/week) from about 12 weeks, followed by fetal blood sampling at 22–24 weeks.[78] If severe thrombocytopenia (platelet count < 30 × 10⁹/L) is confirmed the dose of i.v. immunoglobulin can be doubled, or prednisone can be added to the therapy. Because the response is not consistent, repeat fetal blood sampling 2–4 weeks later is necessary. A falling platelet count, particularly to < 20 × 10⁹/L, is an indication for platelet transfusion. Transfusion raises the platelet count for only a few days and therefore needs to be repeated weekly. Platelet transfusions are more likely to be complicated by fetal bradycardia and death than red cell transfusions and therefore delivery around 34 weeks, usually by Cesarean section, is appropriate. Where the initial platelet count is > 50 × 10⁹/L it is reasonable to repeat blood sampling 4–6 weeks later.

Women with no prior history of a fetus with an antenatal ICH are often treated with IVIG from about 20 weeks, followed by fetal blood sampling close to 32 weeks. The management thereafter is determined by the platelet count, as described earlier.

REFERENCES (* Level 1 evidence)

1. Northern Regional Maternity Survey Office Annual Report 1995. Newcastle-upon-Tyne: Survey Office; 1997.

2. Boyd PA, Chamberlain P, Hicks NR. 6-year experience of prenatal diagnosis in an unselected population in Oxford, UK. Lancet 1998; 352:1567–1569.

3. Wald NJ, Rodeck C, Hackshaw AK, et al. First and second trimester antenatal screening for Down's syndrome: the results of the serum, urine and ultrasound screening study (SURUSS). Health Technol Assess 2003; 7:1–88.

4. Hyett JA, Moscoso G, Nicolaides KH. First trimester nuchal translucency and cardiac septal defects in fetuses with trisomy 21. Am J Obstet Gynecol 1995; 172:1411–1413.

5. Souka AP, Krampl E, Bakalis S, et al. Outcome of pregnancy in chromosomally normal fetuses with increased nuchal translucency in the first trimester. Ultrasound Obstet Gynecol 2001; 18:9–17.

6. Statham H, Solomou W, Chitty L. Prenatal diagnosis of fetal abnormality: psychological effects on women in low-risk pregnancies. Best Pract Res Clin Obstet Gynaecol 2000; 14:731–747.

7. Chitty LS, Hunt GH, Moore J, et al. Effectiveness of routine ultrasonography in detecting fetal abnormalities in a low risk population. BMJ 1991; 303:165–169.

8. Shirley IM, Bottomley F, Robinson VP. Routine radiographer screening for fetal abnormalities in an unselected low risk population. Br J Radiol 1992; 65:564–569.

9. Luck CA. Value of routine ultrasound scanning at 19 weeks: a four year study of 8849 deliveries. BMJ 1992; 304:1474–1478.

10. Bernaschek G, Stuempflen I, Deutinger J. The value of sonographic diagnosis of fetal malformations: different results between indication-based and screening-based investigations. Prenat Diagn 1994; 14:807–812.

*11. Crane JP, LeFevre ML, Winborn RC, et al. A randomized trial of prenatal ultrasonographic screening: Impact on the detection, management and outcome of anomalous fetuses. Am J Obstet Gynecol 1994; 171:392–399.

*12. Ewigman BG, Crane JP, Frigoletto FD, et al. Effect of prenatal ultrasound screening on perinatal outcome. N Engl J Med 1993; 329:821–827.

*13. Neilson JP. Ultrasound for fetal assessment in early pregnancy (Cochrane Review). In: The Cochrane Library, Issue 4. Oxford: Update Software; 2001.

14. Wright D, Bradbury I, Benn P, et al. Contingent screening for Down syndrome is an efficient alternative to non-disclosure sequential screening. Prenat Diagn 2004; 24:762–766.

*15. Newnham JP, Evans SF, Michael CA, et al. Effects of frequent ultrasound during pregnancy: a randomised controlled trial. Lancet 1993; 342: 887–891.

16. Royal College of Obstetricians and Gynaecologists. Termination of pregnancy for fetal abnormality. London: RCOG; 1996.

17. Malinger G, Ben-Sira L, Lev D. Fetal brain imaging: a comparison between magnetic resonance imaging and dedicated neurosonography. Ultrasound Obstet Gynecol 2004; 23:333–340.

18. Twickler DM, Magee KP, Caire J, et al. Second-opinion magnetic resonance imaging for suspected fetal central nervous system abnormalities. Am J Obstet Gynecol 2003; 188:492–496.

19. Vergani P, Locatelli A, Strobelt N, et al. Clinical outcome of mild fetal ventriculomegaly. Am J Obstet Gynecol 1998; 178:218–222.

20. Gaglioti P, Danelon D, Bontempo S, et al. Fetal cerebral ventriculomegaly: outcome in 176 cases. Ultrasound Obstet Gynecol 2005; 25:372–377.

21. Sparey C, Robson S. Fetal cerebral ventriculomegaly. Fetal Mat Med Rev 1998; 10:163–179.

*22. Lumley J, Watson L, Watson M, et al. Periconceptional supplementation with folate and/or multivitamins for preventing neural tube defects. [Systematic Review] Cochrane Pregnancy and Childbirth Group Cochrane Database of Systematic Reviews . Issue 4, 2001.

23. Biggio JR, Owen J, Wenstrom KD, et al. Can prenatal ultrasound findings predict ambulatory status in fetuses with open spina bifida? Am J Obstet Gynecol 2001; 185:1016–1020.

24. Bruner JP, Tulipan N. Tell the truth about spina bifida. Ultrasound Obstet Gynecol 2004; 24:595–596.

25. Gupta JK, Lilford RJ. Assessment and management of fetal agenesis of the corpus callosum. Prenat Diagn 1995; 15:301–312.

26. Bullen PJ, Rankin JM, Robson SC. Investigation of the epidemiology and prenatal diagnosis of holoprosencephaly in the North of England. Am J Obstet Gynecol 2001; 184:1256–1262.

27. Thomas DFM. Fetal urology and prenatal diagnosis: current themes. Fetal Mat Med Rev 2004; 15:343–364.

28. Ismaili K, Hall M, Donner C, et al. Results of systematic screening for minor degrees of fetal renal pelvis dilatation in an unselected population. Am J Obstet Gynecol 2003; 188:242–246.

29. Johnson M, Bukowski TP, Reitleman C, et al. In utero surgical treatment of fetal obstructive uropathy: a new comprehensive approach to identify appropriate candidates for vesico-amniotic shunt therapy. Am J Obstet Gynecol 1994; 170:1770–1779.

30. Clark TJ, Martin WL, Divakaran TG, et al. Prenatal bladder drainage in the management of fetal lower urinary tract obstruction: a systematic review and meta-analysis. Obstet Gynecol 2003; 102:367–382.

31. Jani J, Keller RL, Benachi A, et al. Prenatal prediction of survival in isolated left-sided diaphragmatic hernia. Ultrasound Obstet Gynecol 2006; 27: 18–22.

32. Allan L, Hornberger L, Sharland G. Textbook of fetal cardiology. London: Greenwich Medical Media; 2000.

33. Griffin DR. Skeletal abnormalities. In: James DK, Steer PJ, Weiner CP, et al, eds. High risk pregnancy. London: WB Saunders; 1999; 465–488.

34. Royal College of Obstetricians and Gynaecologists. Amniocentesis. Clinical Guideline No. 8. London: RCOG; 2001.

*35. Canadian Early and Mid Trimester Amniocentesis Trial Group. Randomized trial to assess safety and fetal outcome of early and midtrimester amniocentesis. Lancet 1998; 351:243–249.

*36. Tabor A, Philip J, Madsen M, et al. Randomised controlled trial of genetic amniocentesis in 4606 low-risk women. Lancet 1986; i:1287–1293.

37. Silver RK, Russell TK, Kambich MP, et al. Midtrimester amniocentesis. Influence of operator caseload on sampling efficiency. J Reprod Med 1998; 43:191–195.

*38. Alfirevic Z, Gosden CM, Neilson JP. Chorion villus sampling versus amniocentesis for prenatal diagnosis. [Systematic Review] Cochrane Pregnancy and Childbirth Group Cochrane Database of Systematic Reviews 2001; Issue 4.

39. Kalousek DK, Vekemans M. Confined placental mosaicism. J Med Genet 1996; 33:529–533.

40. Maxwell D, Johnson P, Hurley P, et al. Fetal blood sampling and pregnancy loss in relation to indication. Br J Obstet Gynaecol 1991; 98:892–897.

41. Flake AW, Crombleholme TM, Johnson MP, et al. Treatment of severe congenital diaphragmatic hernia by fetal tracheal occlusion: clinical experience with 15 cases. Am J Obstet Gynecol 2000; 183:1059–1066.

42. Jani JC, Nicolaides KH, Gratacos E, et al. Fetal lung-to-head ratio in the prediction of survival in severe left-sided diaphragmatic hernia treated by fetal endoscopic tracheal occlusion (FETO). Am J Obstet Gynecol 2006; 195:1646–50.

*43. Soothill PW, Bobrow CS, Holmes R. Small for gestational age is not a diagnosis. Ultrasound Obstet Gynecol 1999; 13:225–228.

*44. Neilson JP. Symphysis-fundal height measurement in pregnancy. Cochrane Database Syst Rev 2000; CD000944.

45. Gardosi J, Francis A. Controlled trial of fundal height measurement plotted on customised growth charts. Br J Obstet Gynaecol 1999; 106:309–317.

46. Chang TC, Robson SC, Boys RJ, et al. Prediction of the small for gestational age infant: which ultrasonic measurement is best? Obstet Gynecol 1992; 80:1030–1038.

47. Mongelli M, Gardosi J. Reduction of false-positive diagnosis of fetal growth restriction by application of customized fetal growth standards. Obstet Gynecol 1996; 88:844–848.

48. Clausson B, Gardosi J, Francis A, et al. Perinatal outcome in SGA births defined by customised versus population-based birthweight standards. Br J Obstet Gynaecol 2001; 108:830–834.

*49. Bricker L, Neilson JP. Routine ultrasound in late pregnancy (after 24 weeks' gestation). [Systematic Review] Cochrane Pregnancy and Childbirth Group. Cochrane Database of Systematic Reviews 2007; 1.

50. Robson SC, Chang TC. Measurement of human fetal growth. In: Hanson MA, Spencer JAD, Rodeck CH, eds. Fetus and neonate physiology and clinical applications, vol. 3 (Growth). Cambridge: Cambridge University Press; 1995; 297–325.

51. Cnossen JS, Morris K, ter Riet G, et al. Uterine artery Doppler to predict preeclampsia and fetal growth restriction: a systematic review and bivariate meta-analysis. (submitted for publication).

52. Soothill PW, Ajayi RA, Campbell S, et al. Relationship between fetal acidemia at cordocentesis and subsequent neurodevelopment. Ultrasound Obstet Gynecol 1992; 2:80–83.

53. Karsdorp VHM, van Vugt JM, van Geijn HP, et al. Clinical significance of absent or reversed end-diastolic velocity waveforms in umbilical artery. Lancet 1994; 344:1664–1668.

*54. Neilson JP, Alfirevic Z. Doppler ultrasound for fetal assessment in high risk pregnancies. [Systematic Review] Cochrane Pregnancy and Childbirth Group. Cochrane Database of Systematic Reviews. 2007; 1.

55. Soothill PW, Ajayi RA, Campbell S, et al. Prediction of morbidity in small and normally grown fetuses by fetal heart rate variability, biophysical profile and umbilical artery Doppler studies. Br J Obstet Gynaecol 1993; 100:742–745.

*56. McCowan LM, Harding JE, Roberts AB, et al. A pilot randomized trial of two regimes of fetal surveillance for small-for-gestational age fetuses with normal results of umbilical artery Doppler velocimetry. Am J Obstet Gynecol 2000; 182:81–86.

57. Fong KW, Ohlsson A, Hannah ME, et al. Prediction of perinatal outcome in fetuses suspected to have intrauterine growth restriction: Doppler US study of fetal, cerebral, renal and umbilical arteries. Radiology 1999; 213:681–689.

58. Baschat AA. Doppler application in the delivery timing of the preterm growth-restricted fetus: another step in the right direction. Ultrasound Obstet Gynecol 2004; 23:111–118.

59. Schwarze A, Gembruch U, Krapp M, et al. Qualitative venous Doppler flow waveform analysis in preterm intrauterine growth-restricted fetuses with ARED flow in the umbilical artery – correlation with short-term outcome. Ultrasound Obstet Gynecol 2005; 25:573–579.

60. Manning FA. Fetal biophysical profile: a critical appraisal. Fetal Mat Med Rev 1997; 9:103–123.

*61. Alfirevic Z, Neilson JP. Biophysical profile for fetal assessment in high risk pregnancies. [Systematic

Review] Cochrane Pregnancy and Childbirth Group Cochrane Database of Systematic Reviews. 2001; Issue 3.

62. Hornbuckle J, Sturgiss SN, Robson SC. Management of fetuses with absent and reversed end Diastolic frequencies (AREDF) of the umbilical artery: outcome of a policy of daily biophysical profile (BPP). J Obstet Gynecol 2003; 23:(Suppl 1):S35.

*63. Pattison N, McCowan L. Cardiotocography for antepartum fetal assessment. [Systematic Review] Cochrane Pregnancy and Childbirth Group Cochrane Database of Systematic Reviews 2001; Issue 3.

*64. Chauhan SP, Sanderson M, Hendrix NW, et al. Perinatal outcome and amniotic fluid index in the antepartum and intrapartum periods: a meta-analysis. Am J Obstet Gynecol 1999; 181:1473–1478.

65. Baschat AA, Gembruch U, Harman CR. The sequence of changes in Doppler and biophysical parameters as severe fetal growth restriction worsens. Ultrasound Obstet Gynecol 2001; 18:571–577.

66. Lindqvist PG, Molin J. Does antenatal identification of small-for-gestational age fetuses significantly improve their outcome. Ultrasound Obstet Gynecol 2005; 25:258–264.

67. Spinillo A, Gardella B, Preti E, et al. Rates of neonatal death and cerebral palsy associated with fetal growth restriction among very low birthweight infants. A temporal analysis. BJOG 2006; 113:775–780.

68. Sebire NJ, Snijders RJ, Hughes K, et al. The hidden mortality of monochorionic twin pregnancies. Br J Obstet Gynaecol 1997; 104:1203–1207.

69. Quintero R, Morales W, Allen M, et al. Staging of twin–twin transfusion syndrome. J Perinatol 1999; 9:550–555.

70. Senat M, Deprest J, Boulvain MD, et al. Endoscopic Laser surgery versus serial amnioreduction for severe twin-to-twin transfusion syndrome. N Engl J Med 2004; 351:136–144.

71. Quintero RA, Dickinson JE, Morales WJ, et al. Stage-based treatment of twin–twin transfusion syndrome. Am J Obstet Gynecol 2003; 188:1333–1340.

72. Van Heteren CF, Nijhuis JG, Semmekrot BA, et al. Risk for surviving twin after fetal death of co-twin in twin–win transfusion syndrome. Obstet Gynecol 1998; 92:215–219.

73. Mastroiacovo P, Castilla EE, Arpino C, et al. Congenital malformations in twins: an international study. Am J Med Genet 1999; 83:117–124.

74. Evans MI, Dommergues M, Wapner RJ. International collaborative experience of 1789 patients having multifetal pregnancy reduction: a plateauing of risks and outcomes. J Soc Gynecol Invest 1996; 3:23–26.

75. Mari G, Deter RL, Carpenter RL, et al. Non-invasive diagnosis by Doppler ultrasonography of fetal anaemia due to maternal red-cell alloimmunization. New Engl J Med 2000; 342:9–14.

76. Schumacher B, Moise KJ. Fetal transfusion for red blood cell alloimmunization in pregnancy. Obstet Gynecol 1996; 88:137–150.

77. Doyle LW, Kelly EA, Rickards AL, et al. Sensorineural outcome at 2 years for survivors of erythroblastosis treated with fetal intravascular transfusion. Obstet Gynecol 1993; 81:931–935.

78. Berkowitz RL, Bussel JB, McFarland JG. Alloimmune thrombocytopenia: State of the art 2006. Am J Obstet Gynecol 2006; 195:907–913.

12

The newborn

Neil McIntosh, Ben Stenson

INTRODUCTION

DEFINITIONS – WORLD HEALTH ORGANIZATION (WHO)

GESTATION (INDEPENDENT OF BIRTH WEIGHT)

1. Preterm = less than 37 completed weeks of gestation (258 days).
2. Full-term = between 37 weeks and 42 completed weeks of gestation (259–293 days).
3. Post-term or postmature = more than 42 completed weeks (294 days).

Dates are taken from the first day of the last menstrual period. Conception is presumed to be approximately 2 weeks after this date. Ultrasound dates are based on conception and have to be altered to fit with the dates estimated from the last menstrual period.

BIRTH WEIGHT (INDEPENDENT OF GESTATION)

1. Low birth weight = less than 2500 g.
2. Very low birth weight = less than 1500 g (accepted by convention).
3. Extremely low birth weight (USA – very, very low birth weight) = less than 1000 g (accepted by convention).
4. Impossibly or incredibly low birth weight = (less than 750 g).

SIZE FOR GESTATION (Fig. 12.1)

1. Small for gestation (SGA) = less than 10th centile in weight expected for gestation (small for dates).

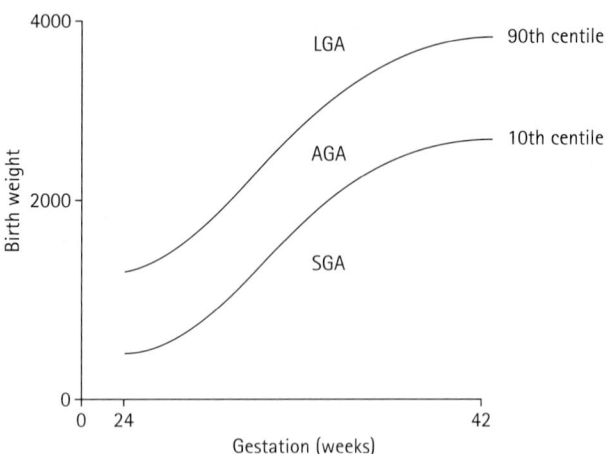

Fig. 12.1 Size for gestation based on population centiles for birth weight with gestation: LGA, large for gestational age; AGA, appropriate for gestational age; SGA, small for gestational age (less than the 10th centile expected weight for gestation).

2. Appropriate for gestation (AGA) = between 10th and 90th centiles of weight expected for gestation.
3. Large for gestation (LGA) = more than 90th centile in weight expected for gestation.

NB: The expected weight centiles will vary with the population. The terms immature, premature and dysmature should no longer be used.

AGE

In utero
1. Less than 1 week = fertilized egg to the formation of the blastocyst.
2. 1–12 weeks = embryo.
3. 12 weeks – delivery = fetus.
4. 24 weeks or more = current period of 'legal' viability in the UK.

In the UK it is uncommon to terminate a pregnancy after 20 weeks of gestation, though it is legal through to term for major fetal anomaly or maternal life-threatening problem (Human Embryo and Fertilisation Act 1990[1].)

Abortion is the expulsion of the dead fetus prior to 24 weeks' gestation (168 days). A dead fetus expelled after this time is a **stillbirth**. Note that a liveborn baby is a baby of *any gestation* that has signs of life (e.g. only a heart beat) at delivery. Many miscarriages before 20 weeks' gestation will show signs of life.

The neonate
1. Perinatal period = the period from 24 weeks' gestation or the time of the live birth if less than 24 weeks' gestation, to 7 days of postnatal age.
2. Early neonatal period = the first 7 days of life of a liveborn infant of *any* gestation.
3. Late neonatal period = 8–28 days after birth.
4. Neonatal period = the first 28 days of life of a liveborn infant of *any* gestation.
5. Infancy = the first year of life.

MORTALITY RATES
1. Stillbirth rate = number of stillbirths per 1000 total births.
2. Perinatal mortality rate (PMR) = number of stillbirths + early (up to 7 days) neonatal deaths per 1000 total births.
3. Neonatal mortality rate (NNMR) = number of deaths in the first 28 days per 1000 live births.
4. Infant mortality rate (IMR) = number of deaths in the first 365 days per 1000 live births.

Maternity units should collect the figures for PMR, NNMR and also neonatal deaths before discharge from hospital. Reduction of NNMR simply by postponing the deaths out of the neonatal period is not the ideal of neonatal care. Bronchopulmonary dysplasia, infection and necrotizing enterocolitis are the current problems that lead to late deaths after 28 days. The 'corrected' WHO neonatal mortality rate is the number of deaths in the first 28 days of life (birth weight greater than 1000 g) per 1000 live births.

THE ECONOMICS OF NEWBORN CARE

INTRODUCTION

The increasing incidence and improved survival chances of infants of low birth weight and low gestational age, as well as the diffusion of new technologies for mature infants, have increased the demand for specialist neonatal care in many industrialized countries.[2] This has generated considerable debate about the correct level of funding for neonatal care. Economic evaluation provides a framework for assessing the costs and benefits of neonatal care, and for identifying the combination of human and material inputs that maximize health benefits or other measures of social welfare. This section outlines the methods of economic evaluation of health care and, in the process, describes the key economic issues raised by studies of neonatal care.

STUDY DESIGN

Economic evaluations of neonatal interventions can be conducted on the basis of observational evidence, such as before-and-after studies, case-control studies or ad hoc syntheses of evidence from several sources. However, health economists tend to consider prospective economic evaluations conducted alongside randomized controlled trials as possessing the highest internal validity.[3] A number of trial-based economic evaluations of neonatal interventions has been reported in the literature in recent years, including studies of ultrasonography in the diagnosis and management of developmental hip dysplasia,[4] neonatal extracorporeal membrane oxygenation (ECMO)[5] and indomethacin prophylaxis for patent ductus arteriosus.[6] The randomized controlled trial is considered to act as the primary vehicle for collecting unbiased information on both the costs and consequences of the interventions being evaluated and a means of simulating real world conditions. However, there are many circumstances in which the use of a single randomized controlled trial as a vehicle for economic analysis of a neonatal intervention will provide an inadequate and partial basis for decision making. For example, the sample size of the trial may be inadequate for true differences in outcomes between the experimental and control groups to be recognizable with statistical methods. If this is the case, then the clinical effectiveness estimate might have to be derived from meta-analyses or overviews of the relevant controlled trials in the area, or the cost estimates might have to be derived from several studies.[7] In addition, many randomized controlled trials of neonatal interventions focus upon intermediate outcomes rather than the long term outcomes that might be of interest. For example, a number of trials have shown that giving preterm infants systemic corticosteroids in the first few days of postnatal life improves short term respiratory outcomes, such as reducing oxygen dependency, but also appears to increase the rate of adverse neurological outcomes over the longer term.[8] There are many circumstances, therefore, in which decision-analytic modelling techniques have to be used to extrapolate the relevant data beyond the time horizon of the randomized controlled trial in order to reflect long term outcomes.

FORM OF ECONOMIC EVALUATION

Four broad forms of economic evaluation have been reported in the literature.[3] *Cost-minimization analysis* is the simplest form of economic evaluation and establishes the least costly method of achieving given outcomes. It is only appropriate if all outcomes are known or found to be identical. Birnie et al[9] performed a cost-minimization analysis of domiciliary antenatal fetal monitoring in high-risk pregnancies. The investigators found that, compared with in-hospital monitoring, domiciliary monitoring is safe (when measured in terms of a range of neonatal outcomes) and reduces health service costs by one half.

Cost-effectiveness analysis compares the costs of health interventions to their consequences where the consequences are measured in natural or physical units. Cost-effectiveness analysis can only be used to compare interventions that produce the same kinds of consequences. It cannot be used to compare an economic evaluation whose primary outcome is cases of necrotizing enterocolitis avoided with an economic evaluation whose primary outcome is days of oxygen dependency avoided. To make these broader comparisons, a common 'currency' for measuring consequences is needed. The common currency is achieved in two distinctly different ways, one leading to *cost-utility analysis* and the other leading to *cost-benefit analysis*. In both cases, by placing a value on the consequences of interventions, either through preference weighting or value weighting, the methods can address questions of allocative efficiency, i.e. the efficient allocation of scarce resources across different areas of neonatal care.

In *cost-utility analysis*, the consequences of health interventions are measured in quality-adjusted life years (QALYs), which attempt to capture the health gains derived from health interventions in a single metric that combines life years gained and enhancement of health-related quality of life.[10] The QALY displays cardinal properties, such that four years of a child's life in a health state judged to be halfway between death and full health would be considered equivalent to two years in full health. The advantage of the QALY metric is that it allows neonatal interventions with diverse consequences to be compared. QALYs have been estimated for a number of neonatal interventions, including predischarge monitoring for apnea of prematurity,[11] neonatal surgery and subsequent treatment for congenital diaphragmatic hernia,[12] neonatal surgery and subsequent treatment for congenital anorectal malformations,[13] alternative models of neonatal intensive care,[14,15] and prophylactic indometacin in very low birth weight infants.[16]

In *cost-benefit analysis*, the consequences of health interventions are measured and valued in monetary units, most commonly by asking relevant individuals how much they would be willing to pay to obtain the consequences. This is most frequently done using the willingness to pay approach. Hence, for a new neonatal screening program, the analyst could describe to potential parents how many life years the program could be expected to add and what the health of the child would be during those years, and then ask them how much they would be willing to pay to obtain those health benefits. In cost-benefit analysis, both the costs and consequences of an intervention are valued in the same units, monetary units, and thus cost-benefit analysis is the only technique that can determine in and of itself that an intervention is worth delivering in economic terms (benefits exceed the costs, thus generating positive net benefit).

PERSPECTIVES FOR ECONOMIC EVALUATION

Economic evaluations can be undertaken from a number of different perspectives or viewpoints. The broadest, most comprehensive perspective is the societal perspective in which all costs are counted regardless of who incurs the costs. In neonatal care, a societal perspective is often relevant. Low birth weight babies, for example, may require support from social service departments upon their discharge from hospital. The parents of sick neonates may have to forego other productive activities (paid or unpaid work) in order to spend time with them; their transport costs to and from the neonatal unit may be considerable, and care for other children may have to be arranged.[17] Other perspectives can also be adopted in studies, such as the perspective of a particular agency, the entire health care system or the perspective of the family. Recently, the National Institute for Health and Clinical Excellence (NICE) in England and Wales recommended that the most relevant costs for economic evaluation are those incurred by the National Health Service and personal social service providers.[18] Alternative perspectives are often useful as

a means of predicting who will favor a new program and who will not, and thus to help an appropriate implementation strategy.

DISCOUNTING IN ECONOMIC EVALUATION

Health care interventions often generate streams of costs and consequences that occur over time and into the future. For example, an effective treatment for preterm infants may reduce the number of hospital admissions during childhood and reduce the pool of disabled children that need to be cared for by society. Analysts are not only concerned about the costs and consequences of the intervention during the neonatal period, but also those costs and consequences that occur throughout childhood and beyond. By discounting, all costs and consequences that occur in future years are reduced by a discount factor to their equivalent present values. The discounted amounts, the equivalent present values, are totalled and then all programs can be fairly compared on the basis of their present values. The discount rates applied within economic evaluations of neonatal interventions have varied markedly across jurisdictions and over time. Recently, NICE has recommended that economic evaluations conducted in England and Wales should discount costs and, more controversially, health consequences, at an annual rate of 3.5%.[18] The effect of discounting health consequences as well as costs is that many neonatal screening programs will appear to be penalized as their benefits are often felt over the longer term. When the results are potentially sensitive to the discount rate used, then sensitivity analyses that vary the discount rate between 0% and 6% are recommended in order to assess the impact on the final results.[18]

COMPONENTS OF ECONOMIC EVALUATION

It is useful to view the various costs and consequences of neonatal programs as building blocks, which can be assembled in an economic evaluation in different ways.

Costs

The costs of neonatal programs can be calculated using a number of different approaches. The most common alternative approaches are based on cost accounting methods, either using detailed information about resources used by individual patients (the 'bottom up' approach), or by allocation of total costs by unit workload (the 'top down' approach). Many studies, particularly those conducted in countries, such as the United States, where there is a comprehensive system of billing and fee-for-service payment of providers, cite charges for neonatal care rather than costs. However, it is worth noting that health care charges may include elements arising from corporate financial decisions and may therefore be poor proxies for the costs of providing neonatal care. If the study adopts a societal perspective, the impact of the neonatal program on other sectors of the economy and on families and carers should also be considered. Estimation of these broader costs may use a number of methods including time and motion studies, diary methods, work sampling, interviews with key caregivers, case note analysis and patient activity databases.[19]

Consequences

The consequences of neonatal programs can be described in terms of either: (1) resources saved, or (2) health effects.

Resources saved

Neonatal programs can save resources for the health sector, for other sectors of the economy and for patients and informal carers. For example, an effective intervention for preterm birth might avoid hospital readmissions, the consumption of special education services, and the time taken off work by parents to care for a disabled child. The methods for measuring these resource savings are identical to those outlined in the section on costs. These resource savings are simply the costs that would have been incurred if the program had not been provided. Indeed, all assessments of costs and consequences within an economic evaluation framework are comparative to an alternative.

Health effects

In addition to potential resource savings, neonatal interventions will hopefully also directly impact upon the health of the child. These health effects can be measured in natural or physical units (for example, cases of necrotizing enterocolitis avoided) that can then be incorporated into a cost-effectiveness analysis. Alternatively, they can be measured in terms of health state preferences in the construction of QALYs for incorporation into a cost-utility analysis, or in willingness to pay terms for incorporation into a cost-benefit analysis.

QALYs. For cost-utility analysis, the quantity and health-related quality of life effects of a neonatal intervention are combined into a composite metric, the QALY. The life years gained component of the QALY metric is relatively uncontroversial. It is ideally calculated through clinical trials of the intervention being evaluated, incorporating long term follow-up of patients and controls. In contrast to the life years gained component of the QALY metric, estimation of the *health-related quality of life* component has generated great interest amongst health economists. Several scaling techniques have been developed with the view to estimating these weights, the most prominent of which are the rating scale, the standard gamble approach and the time trade-off approach. The scaling techniques vary in their strength of foundation in economic theory and health economists are still debating their relative merits.[20]

An alternative approach to measuring the health-related quality of life weight of a health state is provided by multi-attribute utility measures, which are generic health-related quality of life instruments with pre-existing preference weights which can be attached to each permutation of responses. The available multi-attribute utility measures include the EQ-5D[21] and the Health Utilities Index (HUI).[22] Oostenbrink et al[23] compared the EQ-5D with the Mark 3 version of the HUI to value the health states associated with childhood bacterial meningitis. A panel of 28 pediatricians classified seven health state descriptions which included deafness, epilepsy, mental retardation and paresis. They found that HUI Mark 3 preference values were substantially lower than the EQ-5D values for all health state descriptions, although the ranking of the health states was the same. Greatest differences were found in states associated with deafness and mental retardation. This reflects the fact that the EQ-5D does not include dimensions for cognition or sensation, so these aspects of health-related quality of life are only covered by their effects on functional domains such as 'usual activities' or 'anxiety/discomfort'. It should be noted that there are a number of methodological problems that have constrained the application of all multi-attribute utility measures in the neonatal context.[24] Most notably, the measures tend to incorporate a core set of health attributes that reflect human experiences as a whole and ignore attributes that might be considered relevant in the neonatal context, such as health care needs and gross motor mobility. In addition, there is a great deal of uncertainty concerning the appropriate respondents for the preference elicitation tasks.[24]

Willingness to pay. An alternative approach to valuing health effects is the willingness to pay approach for incorporation into cost-benefit analysis. The willingness to pay approach is considered to provide values that reflect individuals' strength of preference for health interventions.[3] Willingness to pay questions can be classified in either open-ended or closed-ended form; the latter offers respondents an opportunity to accept or reject a series of price levels for the intervention being valued. Population values may be obtained using a variety of survey techniques, including face-to-face interviews, telephone interviews and postal surveys. As with the various QALY-based approaches, a particular methodological concern when applying the willingness to pay approach in the neonatal context is identifying the appropriate respondent for the task. Valuations might be obtained from clinicians, parents or the general public. The primary justification for using clinicians is that they are knowledgeable about neonatal care and its sequelae and may be more accessible than some patient groups and their families. The primary justification for selecting a sample of parents is that the parents might be considered the final arbiter of the child's best interests, particularly after the child has been discharged from the neonatal unit; parents might have the greatest sense of what the child himself might perceive as

a worthwhile existence, and what the child might view as intolerable. The rationale for measuring the preferences of the general public is related to policy decision-making, i.e. the consideration that decisions pertinent to public policy should be based on public opinion.

COMPARATIVE ANALYSIS OF COSTS AND CONSEQUENCES

Economic evaluation synthesizes evidence on costs and consequences within an explicit framework, enabling decision-makers to assess whether a neonatal intervention offers good 'value for money'. Data on either costs or consequences, when viewed in isolation, do not provide decision-makers with the information required for value for money assessments.

In cost-minimization analysis, the decision rule for decision-makers is straightforward. If health effects are equivalent, then the cheaper neonatal intervention is preferable. Similarly, in cost-benefit analysis, the decision rule for decision-makers is straightforward. If the monetary valuation of the consequences of a neonatal intervention exceeds the net costs of the intervention, then the intervention should be provided since there is a net gain to society. In cost-effectiveness analysis and cost-utility analysis, however, the decision rule becomes rather more complex, since costs and health effects are expressed in different metrics. In analytical terms, there is a number of possible scenarios that can be summarized in a 'cost-effectiveness plane' (Fig. 12.2). The same scenarios apply whether the health effects are measured in natural or physical units, such as life years gained, for the purposes of cost-effectiveness analysis, or in QALYs for the purposes of cost-utility analysis.

In the cost-effectiveness plane, the difference in health effects between a neonatal intervention and its comparator is plotted along the horizontal axis, whilst the difference in cost between a neonatal intervention and its comparator is plotted on the vertical axis. In the south-east (SE) and north-west (NW) quadrants of the cost-effectiveness plane, one intervention is clearly more effective and less costly than the other and, therefore, this intervention would be a clear winner in cost-effectiveness or cost-utility terms. In the south-west (SW) and north-east (NE) quadrants, however, one intervention is both more effective and more costly, and decision-makers need to assess whether the additional costs are worth the greater effectiveness. Currently, there is very little explicit guidance on what decision-makers are willing to pay for health gains generated by new neonatal technologies. There is some evidence to suggest that NICE holds a willingness to pay threshold of approximately £30 000 for an additional QALY in the general population.[25] However, it is conceivable that members of the general population attach greater weight to health gains made by children, particularly compromised infants, and that decision-makers should weight their decisions in favor of these particular groups.

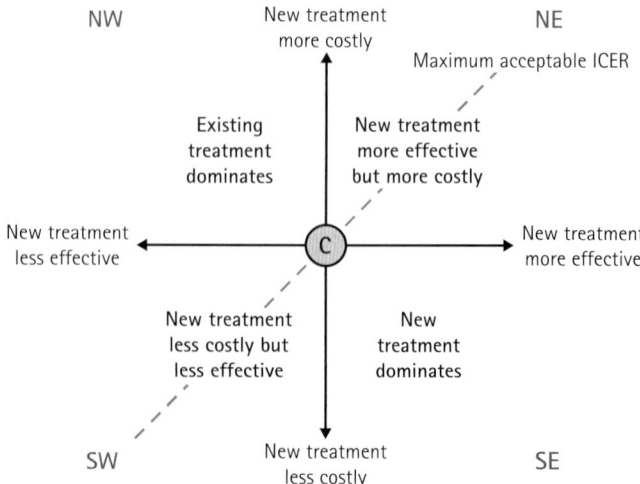

Fig. 12.2 The cost-effectiveness plane. ICER, incremental cost effectiveness ratio.

CONCLUSIONS

Economic evaluation provides a means of allocating finite health care resources in an efficient manner. It can inform decision-making processes at many levels, from national decision-making bodies, such as NICE, to decisions by local health care providers. However, it is important to mention some of the limitations of the approach. Although health economists agree about the objectives of economic evaluation, they disagree about a number of methodological issues. For example, some health economists argue that cost-benefit analysis is the optimal form of economic evaluation because of its foundation on welfare economic theory, whilst others promote cost-utility analysis because of its broader acceptance by the research community. Some health economists argue that economic evaluation of health interventions should be limited to a health service perspective, whilst others promote a broader societal perspective. There is also a number of methodological concerns that are unique to economic evaluation of neonatal care, such as the methods for summarizing the consequences of interventions that have a direct impact upon the health of two individuals, the mother and her infant, in a single estimate of cost-effectiveness.[26] Even without these methodological concerns, economic evaluation should not be viewed as a panacea for decision-makers, but rather as an additional strand of evidence that can facilitate evidence-based decision-making.

THE NORMAL FETAL–NEONATAL TRANSITION

The most vital change immediately after birth is for the lungs to expand to take in air. If lung expansion fails, death will occur quite rapidly and shortly after the umbilical cord is clamped. Almost as important as lung expansion is the change from the fetal type circulation, with the cardiac output bypassing the lungs, to the postnatal pattern where the cardiac output from the right side of the heart will perfuse the lungs and be oxygenated (Fig. 12.3). Less urgent changes in the other organ systems must take place over the next days and weeks in order to ensure a viable postnatal existence.

THE LUNGS (Fig. 12.4)

The lungs of the fetus in utero are filled with a unique fluid which near term is being produced at a rate of about 3 ml/kg/h. Clearance of this fluid is crucial for successful air breathing and begins during labor. Each uterine contraction has been shown to generate surges of fetal catecholamines which reduce the rate of lung liquid secretion and, as labor progresses, lead to active resorption. Elective delivery of the baby before labor will lead to babies being born with wet lungs which result in transient tachypnea of the newborn (p. 250). Additional lung fluid is dispersed during the second stage of labor by a compression force of up to 160 cm of water and the elastic recoil from this vaginal squeeze may draw up to

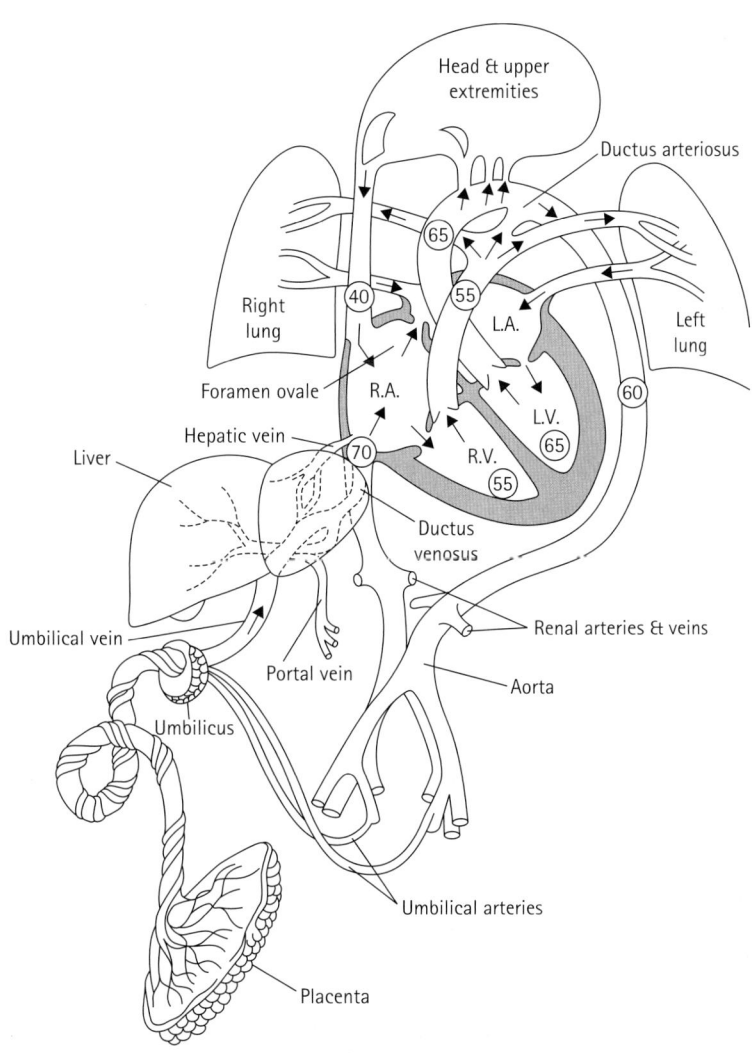

Fig. 12.3   Fetal circulation. The circled figures indicate oxygen saturation at various points, e.g. blood 70% saturated at point where inferior vena cava enters right atrium. L.A., left atrium; L.V., left ventricle; R.A., right atrium; R.V., right ventricle.

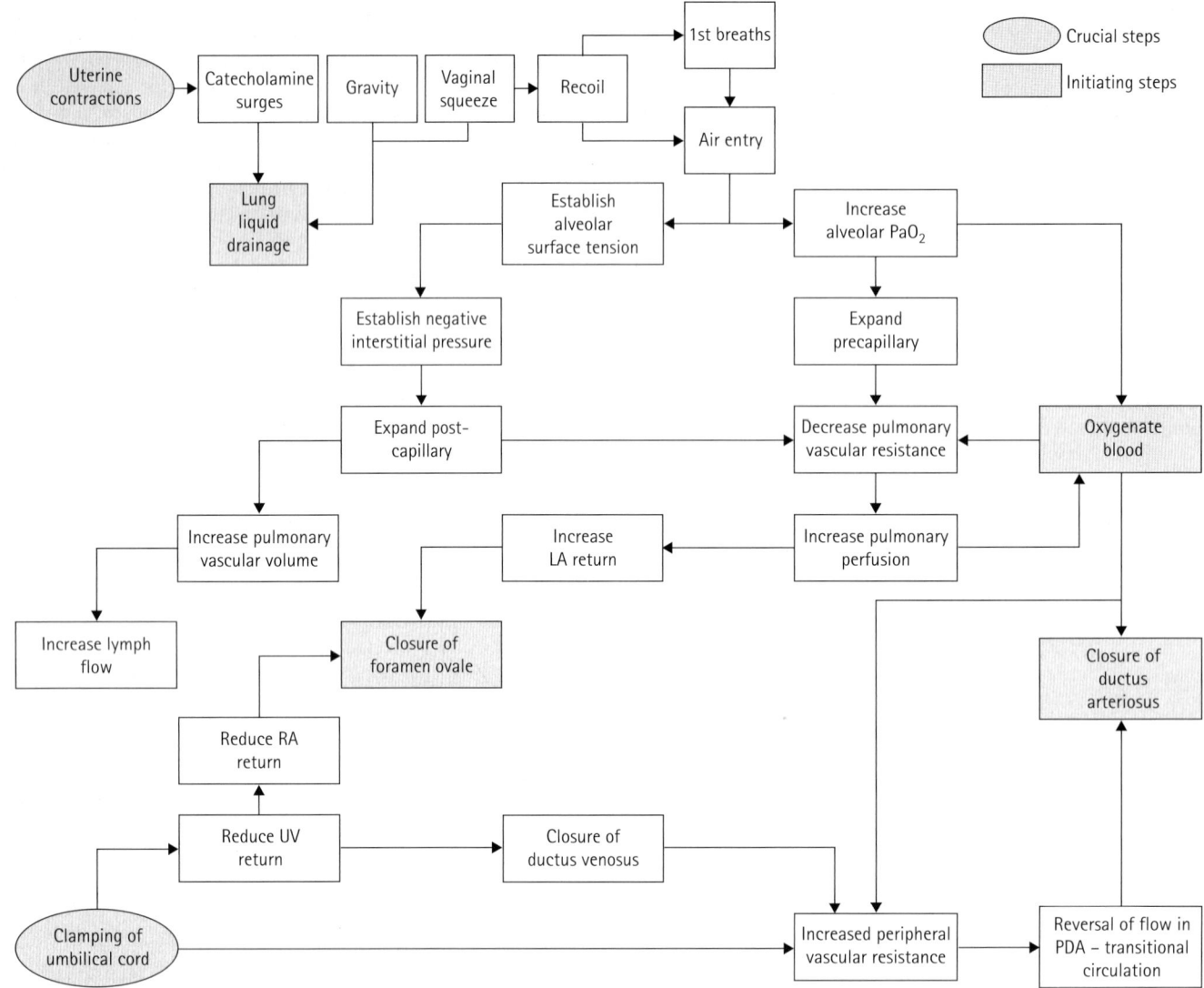

Fig. 12.4 The steps involved in lung expansion and the change in circulation after birth. LA, left atrium; PDA, persistent ductus arteriosus; UV, umbilical vein.

50 ml of air into the chest. Where a mother delivers her infant from a squatting position, further fluid drains by gravity in the vertex delivery. Cesarean section can reduce the effectiveness of all these mechanisms to give an increased incidence of respiratory problems from wet lungs, but even the normal vaginally delivered infant will have a quantity of fluid in his lungs at the moment of birth.

The first gasps or cries of the baby achieve a transthoracic pressure of 70–90 cm of water and a tidal wave of air passes into the upper respiratory passages and larynx. This air initiates Head's paradoxical reflex which potentiates the first gasp. The Valsalva maneuver achieved by the infant crying against a partially closed glottis pushes further fluid from the airway through to the lymphatics. The first breath may generate a pressure as high as 70–120 cm water and may achieve a volume of 80 ml of air in the lungs. The gasps occurring immediately after birth are crucial for the success of air breathing. It is not clear which of the many stimuli that occur after birth are most important in initiating breathing. It may be the deluge of sensory information as the baby delivers – tactile (midwife's hands), thermal (air temperature in the delivery room and evaporation of liquor from the skin), noise, position, light, gravity, pain, etc. It is likely that chemoreceptor input caused by hypoxia and hypercarbia in the last moments before delivery (physiological asphyxia) are also important; however, severe hypoxia and acidemia may depress the respiratory center.

There are two major reasons for the failure of the lungs to expand at birth:
1. The lungs may be unable, physically, to expand, either because they have failed to develop properly in utero (e.g. Potter syndrome, prolonged liquor leakage, diaphragmatic hernia) or because the airway is obstructed (congenital laryngeal web, acquired meconium aspiration).
2. The brain may fail to initiate the expansion of the lungs (e.g. extreme immaturity, oversedation with obstetric prescribed narcotics or brain damage occurring during either the pregnancy or the delivery).

Effective means of resuscitation at birth are crucial in these situations (p. 207) and in resource rich countries should be available to all infants born.

HEART AND CARDIOVASCULAR SYSTEM

The left and right ventricles of the fetus both receive blood returning from the body (cf. after birth). Partly oxygenated blood [$PaO_2 = 3.7$–4.7 kPa (25–35 mmHg)] returning from the placenta via the ductus venosus and inferior vena cava is returned to the right atrium but is deflected by the 'valve' of the inferior vena cava through the patent foramen ovale into the left atrium. In utero only 5–10% of the cardiac output goes to and returns from the lungs; therefore the blood passing from the left atrium to the left ventricle is largely the oxygenated supply from the placenta. Left ventricular contraction powers blood to the aortic arch with its major vessels; thus the coronary and carotid arteries of the fetus, the priority areas, receive blood with the best possible oxygen content. Blood returning from the coronary sinus and the superior vena cava to the right atrium passes to the right ventricle and the pulmonary trunk. The high pulmonary vascular resistance of the fetus and the presence of the patent ductus arteriosus ensure that the right ventricular output predominantly (90%) supplies the descending and abdominal aorta and the viscera. Fifty percent of the abdominal flow goes via the two umbilical arteries to the placental bed where exchange of blood gases and other nutritional and excretory substances occurs (Fig. 12.4). The distribution of blood flow in utero is primarily dependent on the high vascular resistance of the unexpanded fetal lung and the low vascular resistance of the placenta. Fetal pulmonary arterioles have a thick medial muscle layer. The low fetal PaO_2 is thought to keep the vessels constricted. With the first gasps there is a rapid rise in the oxygen tension within the alveoli, and the arteriolar musculature relaxes and pulmonary perfusion occurs. The sudden increase in pulmonary venous return of well-oxygenated blood to the left atrium functionally closes the foramen ovale within minutes or hours of birth and this now well-oxygenated blood [PaO_2 greater than 7 kPa (50 mmHg)] is ejected up the aortic arch from the left ventricle. The closure of the ductus arteriosus is thought to be a result of the increased oxygen content. The ductal muscle in utero is maintained in a relaxed state by the combination of the relative hypoxia and the presence of high circulating levels of prostaglandins produced by the placenta.

The clamping of the umbilical cord raises the systemic vascular resistance and, as a consequence, blood may pass in the reverse direction through the patent ductus. This 'transitional circulation' may revert back to the fetal situation (right to left) if satisfactory oxygenation is not achieved (persistent pulmonary hypertension of the newborn, p. 268). Functional closure of the ductus usually takes place within the first 24 h (and usually much earlier) after birth, but before this a systolic murmur may be present at the base of the heart from transient left to right ductal flow. After birth the pulmonary artery pressure falls from about 3.3–5.3 kPa (25–40 mmHg) on the first day to 2 kPa (15 mmHg) after 6 weeks. During this time there is a rise in the systemic blood pressure from 45–55 mmHg (6–7.3 kPa) to approximately 70 mmHg (9.3 kPa).

BRAIN AND CENTRAL NERVOUS SYSTEM

The brain and central nervous system develop steadily through fetal life, infancy and childhood. There are no dramatic changes that occur with or because of birth itself although sensory experience following birth is obviously different. At birth the cerebellum is more maturely developed than the cerebrum. Neuronal development and dendritic connections are more evident and myelination is already occurring from the oligodendroglia. Cerebral myelination and dendritic connections are predominantly postnatal events.

Brainstem and higher reflexes develop in late fetal life in an orderly fashion and can be used to estimate gestation. Interruption at any stage will cause damage. The seriousness of ensuing problems will depend on the maturity of the brain at the time the damage occurs.

Some recognition patterns seem innate in the newborn. Immediately after birth many newborns will follow a simple stylized face through 180 degrees, though if the features are scrambled this will not occur. Other experiments show rapid learning ability; for example by the fifth day of life the breast-fed infant will be able to detect his own mother by his sense of smell.

THE GUT AND DIGESTION

Swallowing is well developed by the fourth month of in utero life. The inability to swallow in utero leads to hydramnios. Sucking develops rapidly after birth; usually the baby increases the number of sucks in a burst from 5–6 on the first day to 30 or more by day 3. Babies born at 28 weeks' gestation may also suck but the effective coordination of sucking, swallowing and breathing does not occur until 34–35 weeks' gestation. The importance of sucking and swallowing after birth is obvious but these have to be matched by the ability of the rest of the gastrointestinal tract to digest and absorb the food. Intestinal motor activity and the migrating motor complex are developed by 34 weeks' gestation but it is possible that feeding facilitates this development in a baby born earlier.[27] Radiological investigation will show that air usually passes to the large bowel by 2 h of postnatal age, even in the very preterm infant. Most of the intestinal enzymes are present at birth but their full activity and that of the various gastrointestinal hormones are further induced by feeding. Breast milk is undoubtedly and not surprisingly better tolerated than other food and no additional nutritional supplements are required for at least 4–5 months of life in the full-term infant.

Meconium should be passed within 24 h of birth (95%). Should the baby fail to pass meconium, medical staff should be notified as an intestinal atresia, Hirschsprung disease or meconium ileus may be the cause.

THE KIDNEYS AND RENAL FUNCTION

Dynamic measurements of bladder volume by ultrasound show that the fetus at full term will be producing 7 ml of urine/kg/h; thus glomerular filtration from the full complement of nephrons (present by 35 weeks' gestation) is considerable. Fine control of water balance in utero has been the concern of the placenta, and after birth both glomerular and tubular immaturity mean that fluid and electrolyte insults on the newborn are poorly tolerated. The glomerular filtration rate (GFR) of the term infant is only 10 ml/min/m^2, increasing to 15 ml/min/m^2 by the end of the first week. Renal blood flow is low at birth and the juxtaglomerular nephrons are preferentially perfused. Sodium resorption is well developed in the full-term infant (though not in the preterm) as the tubules are comparatively mature and the circulating aldosterone levels are high. The maximum urine osmolality is relatively low, not because of the baby's inability to secrete the antidiuretic hormone, arginine vasopressin (AVP), from the posterior pituitary but because the low solute and nitrogen content of breast milk result in a low solute concentration in the interstitial compartment of the medulla. Increasing the protein intake of the infant increases the maximum urine osmolality that is possible.

The renal bicarbonate threshold is low and there may be limited hydrogen ion excretion due to reduced phosphate availability. Both of these may lead to acidosis. The tubular cells are also less able to produce ammonia. This is more marked in preterm infants, particularly with high protein and acid loads, and leads to the late metabolic acidosis of prematurity.

The breast-fed infant receives low solute food with adequate nitrogen and calories: there is little stress on the kidneys. Unmodified cows' milk or solids contain too much solute and nitrogen and can rapidly lead to metabolic difficulties such as cows' milk tetany (p. 373) and hypernatremia (p. 220).

Congenital abnormalities of the kidney and renal excretory systems lead to metabolic upset developing over the first days or weeks of life depending on their severity. The common coexistence of pulmonary hypoplasia with complete renal agenesis (Potter syndrome) ensures this abnormality presents as an acute respiratory difficulty, usually with rapid death.

LIVER FUNCTION

Immaturity of liver function leads to jaundice (p. 279) and also to the newborn's inability to tolerate drugs which are usually excreted via the biliary tree. The 'gray baby' syndrome is due to increased free and conjugated chloramphenicol levels in the serum leading to vomiting, poor sucking, respiratory distress, abdominal distention, diarrhea and eventually collapse. Liver immaturity may be a factor in the development of hemorrhagic disease of the newborn (p. 295) though damage to the liver from hypoxia and an inadequate supply of vitamin K are likely to be more important components.

BLOOD

The fetal hemoglobin predominant in the full-term newborn (80%) is ideal for oxygen uptake across the placenta at the low oxygen tensions that are present in utero. After birth this fetal hemoglobin is less able to unload oxygen at the tissues. Red cell 2,3-diphosphoglycerate levels increase rapidly in the newborn period to improve oxygen delivery and release, and the oxygen dissociation curve shows a shift to the right.

The blood volume of the newborn depends on the age at which the umbilical cord is clamped. Clamping within the first 15 s after delivery leads to a blood volume of around 75 ml/kg but delayed clamping increases this, the contracting uterus expelling blood from the sinuses of the placenta to the baby (Fig. 12.5). If the cord is not clamped for 3 min after delivery, the blood volume may be 95–100 ml/kg. In the term baby this is associated with a higher incidence of respiratory problems and jaundice but in the preterm infant, where the hemoglobin and red cell volume at birth tend to be lower, a 30 s delay in cord clamping with the newborn infant lower than the placenta may reduce the respiratory problems and the subsequent requirement for top-up blood transfusions.

ENDOCRINE SYSTEM

Numerous hormonal changes take place during labor and immediately after birth which allow the infant to adjust to the change in the environment and the loss of the placental supply of nutrients and minerals. There is a rapid surge in thyroid hormones, thought to be a response to cold exposure. Cortisol and ACTH rise with labor and peak a few hours after delivery in response to stress. Intact pituitary, thyroid, parathyroid, adrenal and pancreatic functions are required to maintain glucose, calcium and electrolyte homeostasis. Babies with disorders of pituitary function may present with hypoglycemia or prolonged jaundice, and this may be associated with midline structural abnormalities of the brain (septo-optic dysplasia). Inborn errors of

adrenocortical steroid synthesis (congenital adrenal hyperplasia) can present with ambiguous genitalia and/or salt loss.

THE IMMUNE RESPONSE AND INFECTION

Once delivered from the protected environment of the uterus, the baby is subjected to many potentially infectious agents. IgG transferred actively across the placenta in the last trimester of pregnancy will last for only a short time (up to 6 months). During this time the infant must develop his own antibodies. Although both B and T cells are potentially functional in utero the virginal experience (in relation to foreign antigen) in the uterus leads to a gap of cell-mediated immunity in the neonatal period. It is sensible for people overtly suffering with viral or bacterial infections not to be intimately involved with the management of newborn infants. Exposure to a pathogen leads to a response at a rate similar in the baby to that seen in older age groups. Absence of either B or T cell functions after birth leads to severe infections and if the diagnosis is not considered, the infant may die (Ch. 27).

ROUTINE CARE OF THE FULL-TERM INFANT

EXAMINATION OF THE NEONATE

It is standard practice in the UK and many other countries for all newborn babies to have a formal clinical examination in the first few days of life. This is often referred to as the routine newborn examination and it can be defined as the detailed professional examination in the first few days of life of a baby who, at the start of the examination, is thought to be well and without significant problems. Examination of a baby to whom attention has been drawn, for example because of cyanosis, feeding problems, apneic episodes or an obvious congenital anomaly, is not a routine newborn examination.[29] In the UK, where most births take place in maternity units rather than the mother's home, this examination usually takes place before the family returns home.

The aims of the routine newborn examination are as follows:
- To ascertain the family's concerns and to provide the chance to discuss them.
- To consider the baby in the light of the mother's medical history, the family's medical history and any relevant concerns raised during the course of the pregnancy and delivery.
- To note birth weight and a baseline measurement of head circumference.
- To verify that the baby is appropriately nourished, is feeding acceptably and has passed urine and meconium.
- To appreciate the presence of clinical signs (e.g. cyanosis, respiratory distress, or inappropriate drowsiness) which identify the occasional baby who is clearly unwell.
- To perform a systematic examination of the baby with the aim of detecting variations of normal which may only need explanation (e.g. 'stork marks'); or which may need investigation (e.g. jaundice); or which require referral for treatment (e.g. posterior palatal cleft).[30]
- To examine the baby for specific target conditions, in particular congenital cataracts, congenital heart disease, developmental dysplasia of the hip, and cryptorchidism.[31]
- To ensure that the findings of the examination, and any plans for follow-up or treatment, are appropriately recorded and effectively communicated to the parents and to those involved in providing future health care to the family.

The mother's handling of her baby while the history is taken and her behavior during the examination may alert the doctor to problems in the developing relationship between mother and baby.

EFFECTIVENESS OF THE ROUTINE NEWBORN EXAMINATION

Many of the aims of the routine newborn examination fit within the definition of screening. The criteria for appraising screening programs were set out by Wilson & Jungner[32] and enlarged upon by Cochrane & Holland.[33]

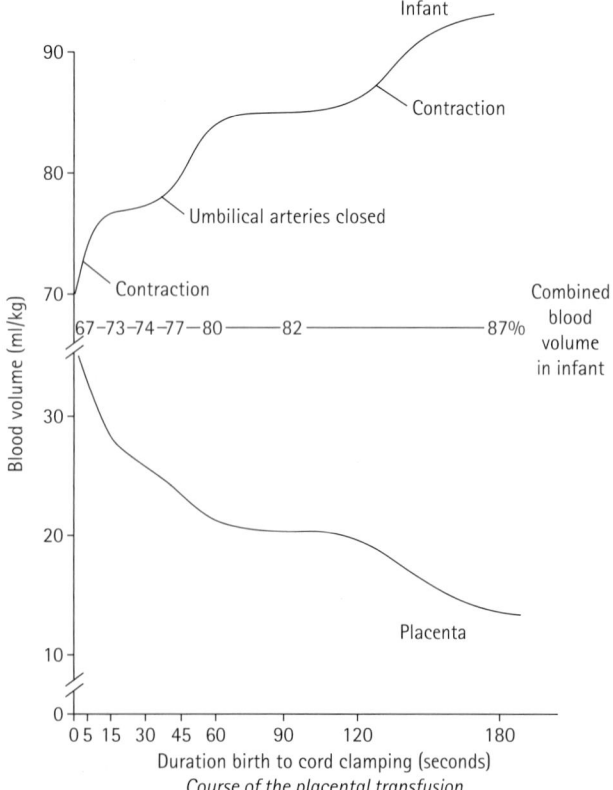

Fig. 12.5 Variation in infant's blood volume with time of clamping of the umbilical cord. (From Smith and Nelson 1976[28] with permission.)

If applied to the routine newborn examination these would essentially demand that the examination detect significant malformations reliably and accurately; that these conditions would, if left undetected, result in a worse outcome for the baby; that they are treatable; and that the mode of examination is acceptable to the parents. These criteria have been further developed in the UK by the National Screening Committee.[34] This body defines screening as 'the systematic application of a test or inquiry, to identify individuals at sufficient risk of a specific disorder to warrant further investigation or direct preventive action, amongst persons who have not sought medical attention on account of symptoms of that disorder'.

In these days of increasing patient expectations it is important not to exaggerate the effectiveness of the routine newborn examination. When evaluated as a screening test for the four target conditions mentioned below, the routine newborn examination does not perform well. Some justification for including these conditions in the newborn examination and some idea of the performance of the examination in the detection of affected children can be found in the next few paragraphs.

CONGENITAL CATARACT

Congenital cataract occurs in 2–3 babies per 10 000 births in the UK and is well recognized as a preventable cause of blindness.[35] All babies should have their eyes examined and the presence of a red reflex confirmed as part of the routine newborn examination. If no red reflex is seen then urgent referral for ophthalmological examination is justified. Early surgical removal of dense opacities together with refractive correction produces the best results in terms of visual acuity.[36] Most ophthalmologists would wish to remove cataracts well before 8 weeks because studies show that delay beyond this age results in a measurable reduction in the quality of vision when compared with earlier correction.[37] A recent UK study showed that only 35% of infant cataracts were detected at routine newborn examination.[38]

CONGENITAL CARDIAC MALFORMATION

Unrecognized cardiac malformation carries a serious risk of avoidable mortality, morbidity and handicap[39] but detecting such malformations in the newborn period is difficult for a number of reasons.[40] The prevalence is low (~ 6 per 1000 births) and most babies show no signs or symptoms in the newborn period.[41] Murmurs can be heard in about 1–2% of babies undergoing routine newborn examination but less than half of these indicate cardiac malformation.[42] Conversely, less than half the babies with such malformations have a murmur in the newborn period.[29] Finally the most dangerous diagnoses (systemic ventricle outflow tract obstructions) have a combined prevalence of only 1:1500[41] and usually become symptomatic only after they are already established on a rapidly deteriorating course which can lead to death in a matter of hours.[43] It is thus perhaps not surprising that the routine newborn examination only detects about 45% of congenital cardiac malformations and that serious conditions are no more likely to be detected than less serious ones.[29]

DEVELOPMENTAL DYSPLASIA OF THE HIP

Developmental dysplasia of the hip (DDH) resulting in dislocation at about 1 year of age could be expected to occur in about 1 per 1000 live births in the UK in the absence of screening.[44] Even though universal screening was introduced in this country in 1969,[45] a national review 30 years later suggests that the number of children receiving surgery for this condition has not been reduced.[46] Results from South Australia appear more successful, though this is exaggerated by their presumption that all positive neonatal findings represented true cases.[47]

However, screening for this condition aims to achieve good hip structure and function, not merely to avoid surgery. No study has yet looked at the quality of hips in surgically treated screened and unscreened cases. In the past, departments with a special interest in this condition have been estimated to detect a little over 60% of cases at a 'cost' of splinting 10 or more false positives for every true case.[44] The

number of cases unnecessarily treated may be able to be safely reduced if ultrasound examination is included in the assessment of possible cases. Primary screening with ultrasound is unlikely to be helpful.[48] Complications can result from nonsurgical treatment.[49] An extensive review of the literature and various detection strategies are outlined in a clinical practice guideline recently issued by the American Academy of Pediatrics and its technical report.[50,51]

CRYPTORCHIDISM

About 2% of term male babies have one or both testes undescended but most of these will descend in the first few months of life, probably as a result of the postnatal testosterone surge.[52] Many of those that have not descended by the age of 4 months will probably not descend until puberty when human chorionic gonadotrophin and testosterone levels increase once again. Most surgeons regard boys as cryptorchid if one or both testes are not descended at 1 year of age. In the cohort studied by Scorer & Farrington in the 1950s this definition applied to 0.8%.[52]

While it is reasonably clear that cryptorchidism is associated with both reduced fertility[53] and an increased risk of testicular malignancy[54] it is less clear that either of these risks is reduced by orchidopexy.[55] However, histological changes occur in testes not brought down in the first 2 years of life which are not apparent in those brought down earlier.[56]

WHO PERFORMS THE ROUTINE NEWBORN EXAMINATION

In the UK at the present time most routine newborn examinations are performed by junior medical staff attached to a pediatric department for a period lasting perhaps 6 months. Training to perform such examinations is not standardized and supervision is variable. Recent data have shown that when neonatal nurse practitioners are responsible for performing these examinations the results are possibly improved.[57] This may be due to two factors: first, nurse practitioners receive specific training before taking on this responsibility; second, nurse practitioners are likely to remain in post for considerably longer, and thus are likely to gather considerably more experience of the examination than the average pediatric senior house officer.

A detailed description of a suitable approach to neonatal history taking and examination is given in Chapter 8.

LABOR WARD ROUTINES

AIRWAY

Around 95% of term infants establish spontaneous respiration by one minute of age and rapidly become vigorous and pink. Suctioning these infants after delivery is unnecessary and may provoke bradycardia and apnea. If there was meconium staining of the liquor, prophylactic suctioning of the airway of the emerging baby at the maternal perineum before the delivery of the shoulders is of no benefit.[58] Airway suctioning after delivery of vigorous infants also carries no advantage.[59] A significant proportion of the infants who end up needing extensive resuscitation after birth cannot be predicted in advance of delivery. Although the empirical risk of this is small, this is one of the reasons that justify a recommendation that all infants should be delivered in hospital. Although they are clinically pink and healthy, term infants without breathing difficulties still have oxygen saturations in the low 80s at the time of the 5 minute Apgar score.[60] There is no evidence that they benefit from oxygen supplementation.

THERMAL STABILITY

Newborn infants lose heat rapidly, particularly if they have low birth weight. They should be dried with a warm towel as soon as possible after birth. This only takes seconds and should not prevent close contact between the baby and the mother from being established promptly. The delivery room should be kept warm and draught free. Routinely bathing infants in the delivery room is not beneficial and places them at risk of hypothermia.

CORD CARE

The cord should be clamped with a disposable clamp or tied twice with a cord ligature to prevent accidental hemorrhage. The optimal timing of cord clamping and the preferred position of the infant in relation to the mother prior to cord clamping remain uncertain.[61,62] Delayed clamping of the cord in preterm infants increases blood volume and may be advantageous. In term infants the increased blood volume may decrease the risk of later anemia but this must be balanced against the risk of occasional polycythemia and volume overload.

SUCKLING

With a minimum of delay, the infant should be given to the mother. Skin to skin contact between the baby and mother will help keep the baby warm and encourage early suckling, which promotes successful breast-feeding.

APGAR SCORES

The condition of the infant should be continually assessed during the first minutes of life. A policy of assigning Apgar scores at 1 and 5 minutes of age helps to ensure that assessment takes place (p. 204).

OTHER ISSUES

Mistaken identity must be prevented. Someone who was present at the birth should stay with the baby at all times until two identity labels have been securely fastened to the baby, particularly if the baby is removed from the birthing room for resuscitation. At some point, the baby should be weighed, vitamin K should be given (p. 295) and the baby should be inspected for congenital malformations, dysmorphic features and signs of illness.

POSTNATAL WARD ROUTINES

Unless they are unwell, babies should generally remain with their mother rather than be admitted to a separate nursery. A further assessment of the general well-being and temperature of the infant should be made at the time of admission to the postnatal ward.

Long postnatal ward stays in healthy mothers and infants used to be the norm but discharge home soon after birth is now increasingly common. This means that an increasing proportion of the problems which occur during neonatal adaptation now develop after discharge and require re-admission to hospital.[63] High levels of support for mothers and infants in the community are required to prevent occasional serious morbidity. Hypernatremic dehydration due to inadequate milk intake in breast-fed infants is common[64] and kernicterus has reappeared.[65]

At some point in the newborn period the infant should be thoroughly examined by someone competent in neonatal hip examination, auscultation and ophthalmoscopy (p. 135). Once milk feeds are established, a capillary blood sample is collected onto filter paper (the Guthrie test). This is used for screening for hypothyroidism and phenylketonuria. A sample is also archived. A formidable array of tests is now possible on these samples and many new screening tests are proposed but not yet offered universally. Archived blood spots have also been used for population-based research and anonymous screening.

VITAL FUNCTIONS

Most infants (95%) are observed to pass urine during the first 24 hours after birth. Those who do not probably did so at the time of delivery. By 48 hours 99% of infants have micturated and failure to do so should prompt further assessment. Meconium is also passed soon after birth by most infants. Failure to do so by 24 hours may indicate an underlying cause such as Hirschsprung disease or meconium ileus and further investigation may be required if there is clinical suspicion. Infants should be kept under review until normal meconium passage has been documented.

After 2–3 days of milk feeding the dark green meconium (bile stained intestinal secretions, intestinal debris and cells) becomes mixed with milk stool and after a further 2–3 days yellow milk stools are present. Delay in the development of changed stools in a breast-fed infant should prompt assessment of the adequacy of the milk intake. There is wide variation between healthy infants in the frequency of passage of stool in the first weeks. Breast-fed infants tend to pass loose yellow stools that may be mistaken for diarrhea, many times per day. The stool frequency of formula-fed infants tends to be lower and the consistency more solid.

Most babies lose weight in the days after birth. A 10% weight loss in the first 4 days is common as excess extracellular fluid is excreted. Thereafter, provided that the milk intake is adequate, a steady pattern of weight gain of approximately 25 g/day is observed. The weight gain may be established more slowly in breast-fed infants and this can undermine maternal confidence in breast-feeding. A very small number of breast-fed infants do not establish an adequate milk intake, continue to lose weight and develop hypernatremic dehydration which can be life threatening.[64] They are often felt to have been feeding satisfactorily although clues to an inadequate intake may have been present such as delay in developing changed stool. One approach to preventing this problem is to weigh all breast-fed infants at the time of the Guthrie test with the aim of identifying excess weight loss before illness develops.

Vomiting is common in the healthy newborn but may be a sign of abnormality. Occasional mucus or milk vomits are acceptable. Bilious or blood-stained vomits require prompt investigation (p. 273). The commonest explanation for blood-stained vomits in the newborn period is maternal blood swallowed, either during delivery or when feeding from a cracked nipple.

The umbilical stump remains a potential portal for infection until it has healed. It is important to keep the area clean as the stump necroses and separates. Some advocate the regular application of surgical spirit, chlorhexidine powder or antiseptic dyes to the umbilical stump. Trials of these practices in resource rich countries do not demonstrate them to be advantageous.[66] Periumbilical erythema indicates infection and requires prompt medical review.

Mothers may require support and education in the basics of baby care, including feeding, feed preparation, bathing and temperature control. If the environmental temperature is warm enough for the mother to be clothed only in a nightdress then the baby should be warm enough in a babygrow under two blankets. Overheating is probably as common as hypothermia in term infants. Both may be dangerous. Epidemiological data demonstrate that the incidence of sudden infant death syndrome is lower when infants sleep supine rather than prone.

GENITALIA

Routine circumcision is a nonmedical ritual that should not be imposed on infants of either sex.

FEEDING THE FULL-TERM NEWBORN

Newborn infants make a rapid change from the parenterally nourished in utero environment to the outside world where their nutritional needs are normally met by enteral nutrition alone. A small minority of infants encounter problems when trying to make that change. This may be because of impaired metabolic adaptation shortly after birth or because they are unwell in some way, e.g. with sepsis. Some infants with structural gastrointestinal abnormalities may be unable to tolerate enteral feeds but for the vast majority of infants milk feeding is established soon after birth. Despite extensive research, there are few adequately conducted or controlled trials of feeding in full-term infants. What good evidence there is, however, continues to demonstrate major short and long term benefits for breast milk.

BREAST MILK

Evolution has designed breast milk to satisfy the needs of newborn infants. Despite rising prolactin levels during pregnancy, lactogenesis is inhibited by the concomitant high levels of progesterone. A further rise in prolactin, and withdrawal of other circulating hormones (progesterone, estrogen and placental lactogen) leads to milk production. Early skin-to-skin contact involves placing the newborn infant on the mother's bare chest and helps to release maternal oxytocin.[67] Oxytocin causes uterine contraction (and so reduces the risk of maternal post-partum hemorrhage), raises maternal skin temperature and decreases maternal anxiety. Systematic review has shown a significant benefit of skin-to-skin on breast-feeding at 1–3 months post birth [odds ratio (OR) 2.15] and breast-feeding duration.[67]

Nipple stimulation helps release further prolactin, and oxytocin leads to contraction of the myoepithelial cells surrounding the lactiferous sinuses resulting in milk ejection (the 'let down' reflex). Initially small amounts of colostrum are produced – this is high in protein and immunoglobulins, and contains a variety of hormonal factors and cells. Transitional milk produced after the first few days also contains higher concentrations of fat and lactose. Towards the end of the second week, 'mature' milk is produced. This continues to contain a bewildering array of substances: enzymes, growth factors, cytokines and prostaglandins.

After the first 2–3 days, further suckling results in milk production and many mothers will experience full and possibly tender breasts. Regular feeding and emptying of the breast results in continued milk production. The composition of milk changes during a feed (hind milk is much higher in fat) so successful breast-feeding involves emptying one breast before moving to the other. Cesarean section (compared to normal vaginal delivery) results in lower volumes of milk production over the first few postnatal days. Maternal opioid analgesia also seems to impair breast-feeding initiation.

SUPPORTING BREAST-FEEDING

Hospital routines and environments are not necessarily conducive to breast-feeding. Wards are often busy and noisy, and may not provide adequate privacy. Sleep and rest (for both mother and baby) may be compromised. Education is effective at increasing breast-feeding initiation rates.[68] Many mothers benefit from support from established breast-feeding support staff. UNICEF has developed 'The 10 steps to successful breastfeeding' – evidenced-based standards that maternity providers can use to examine their own practice.[69] These state that every facility providing maternity services and care for newborn infants should:

1. Have a written breast-feeding policy that is routinely communicated to all health care staff.
2. Train all health care staff in skills necessary to implement this policy.
3. Inform all pregnant women about the benefits and management of breast-feeding.
4. Help mothers initiate breast-feeding within half an hour of birth.
5. Show mothers how to breast-feed, and how to maintain lactation even if they should be separated from their infants.
6. Give newborn infants no food or drink other than breast milk, unless medically indicated.
7. Practice rooming-in – that is, allow mothers and infants to remain together – 24 hours a day.
8. Encourage breast-feeding on demand.
9. Give no artificial teats or pacifiers (also called dummies or soothers) to breast-feeding infants.
10. Foster the establishment of breast-feeding support groups and refer mothers to them on discharge from the hospital or clinic.

Units that can meet these standards can be accredited with the 'Baby Friendly Initiative' (BFI) award.[70] Recent surveys (2005) have shown improvements with breast-feeding initiation rates in the UK currently at 76%.[71] Unfortunately, a rapid fall off in breast-feeding prevalence still seems common with less than half of all babies being breast-fed at 4 weeks' postnatal age.

Over the first 1–2 postnatal days some babies will only feed 3–4 times a day but this rapidly increases and most will be feeding every 2–3 hours by the end of the first week. This often settles to 3–4 hourly in the second postnatal week. Antenatal and postnatal education needs to alert mothers to this so they are prepared. Frequent feeding by breast-fed infants may be misinterpreted. Mothers who cease breast-feeding often express the concern that their baby was 'not satisfied'.

Early growth differs little between those fed breast or formula milk. Observational studies suggested that weight gain later on in the first year of life may be less in those breast-fed, although whether this is due to unmeasured confounding or a biologic effect of formula feeding remains unclear.[72] Body composition also differs – breast-fed babies tend to have a lower fat mass.

Failure of breast-feeding still occurs in the first few days. Improved education and support in the antenatal and postnatal period will reduce this, but support following hospital discharge still seems to be lacking. Early discharge may exacerbate the problem. Affected babies have often lost > 10–12% of their birth weight, and may be jaundiced and hypernatremic. Coexisting morbidity (e.g. infections) requires consideration. Most can be managed with enteral rehydration (with breast or formula milk). Intravenous rehydration is complicated and potentially more dangerous and should be reserved for those unable to tolerate enteral feeds and/or those with very high sodium levels.

BREAST MILK SUBSTITUTES

Formula milks based on cows' milk have been used for decades in place of breast milk. The macronutrient composition is designed to mimic that of breast milk (~ 65 kcal/100 ml and 1.3–1.5 g protein/100 ml) and requires that the relatively high levels of protein, sodium and phosphate in cows' milk are reduced. Modification of the protein and albumin is necessary, fat blend is altered, and iron and a range of vitamins and other micronutrients are added or modified. There are no good data to support the addition of long chain polyunsaturated fatty acids[73] or other substances (such as nucleotides) in term formulas. Most of these are probably safe but few have been subject to adequate controlled study.

In resource rich countries the risks of preparation using contaminated water or inadequate washing or sterilization of bottles are small. In countries where clean water is not available and where perinatal education may be lacking, formula feeding is associated with higher rates of serious infections and death. Promotion of breast-feeding remains one of the most cost-effective health interventions available. However, there will always be a need to produce and prepare safe formula milk where breast-feeding is not possible or recommended (e.g. maternal HIV positivity in resource rich countries, rare metabolic problems such as galactosemia or maternal cytotoxic therapy). These babies' parents also deserve appropriate education and support. This should emphasize the importance of hygiene and sterile water (boiled water that has cooled) and the avoidance of adding extra scoops to promote more rapid weight gain. Formula-fed babies generally feed less often than breast-fed infants.

BREAST VERSUS BOTTLE FEEDING

Level 1 evidence from prospective trials directly comparing breast and formula milk is generally lacking as such trials may be considered unethical, but studies in preterm infants have been undertaken and provide compelling evidence of advantage. Epidemiological studies suggest a decrease in the incidence of sudden unexpected death in infancy.[74] The Promotion of Breastfeeding Intervention Trial (PROBIT), conducted in Belarus in over 17 000 mother – infant pairs, compared infant outcomes between those born in UNICEF BFI modeled hospitals (intervention) or standard practice.[75] Significant increases in breast-feeding rates occurred in BFI hospitals and were paralleled by reduced risks of gastrointestinal infections and atopic eczema.

There is also increasing evidence of long term advantage for breast milk. Blood pressure in childhood and adolescence is typically 4–6 mmHg lower, plasma lipid profiles are more 'beneficial', and obesity is reduced (typical OR ~0.75).[76] There seems to be significant cognitive advantage of breast milk with adjusted benefits of 2–3 IQ points for term infants and possibly 5–6 IQ points for preterm infants. Data on the risks for later development of diabetes, celiac disease, inflammatory bowel disease and neoplasia suggest breast milk benefit but remain uncertain.[76]

THE HIGH RISK NEWBORN

BIRTH TRAUMA

A birth injury is a potentially avoidable mechanical injury occurring during labor or delivery (thus excluding damage from amniocentesis or intrauterine transfusion). Asphyxia and injury may occur together as the identification of a fetus in suboptimal condition inevitably leads to a rushed delivery. Even competent obstetric intervention in this situation may lead to injury but it is often possible that more serious damage such as severe asphyxia or death may have been prevented. Improvements in antenatal care and obstetric practice have reduced the incidence of birth trauma but where obstetric provision is poor, injuries are both common and severe. In resource rich countries, possibly because of the low incidence, obstetric anxiety and guilt may be an inevitable sequel to each case. It is important that information is given to the parents immediately problems are identified in order to avoid misunderstandings and recrimination. Sensitive counseling is a most important aspect of management. Estimates of incidence are meaningless as the frequency varies with the quality of obstetric practice but the more difficult or prolonged the labor and delivery, the more likely it is that trauma will occur. Conditions predisposing to injury are listed in Table 12.1.

SOFT TISSUE INJURIES

Abrasions and *blisters* from forceps or vacuum deliveries, *punctures* from scalp electrodes or blood samples and *incisions* from hurried Cesarean sections lead to potential infection sites. *Bruises* from trauma may be severe in preterm deliveries and extensive into the buttocks following breech deliveries leading later to jaundice and anemia and occasionally disseminated intravascular coagulation. Vitamin K should be given and phototherapy considered early. The *sternomastoid tumor* is originally a hemorrhage. Do *not* call it a tumor in front of parents. It may require passive physiotherapy. *Petechiae* are common over the head and neck following shoulder dystocia, face presentation or a nuchal cord. *Subconjunctival hemorrhages* are common in spontaneous deliveries (the mother may be worried about the baby's vision – reassure). *Subcutaneous fat necrosis* may be from obvious pressure from forceps or mother's pelvis, the thickened rubbery skin sometimes softening with resolution. This necrosis may occur over the back of head, cheek, outside of upper arm or greater trochanter of the femur. No treatment is required. *Fractures* (Table 12.2), deformity or pseudoparalysis may be observed and crepitations or later callus may be palpable. Pain relief is important.

INTRA–ABDOMINAL INJURIES

Hepatosplenomegaly (e.g. rhesus hemolytic disease), coagulation disorders and hypoxia, breech deliveries and cardiac massage all predispose to *subcapsular hematomas of the liver and spleen*. Anemia, pallor, tachycardia and tachypnea may be the presenting features or rupture may occur (immediately or days later) to give hypovolemic shock and death. *Adrenal hemorrhages* may follow severe infection, severe asphyxia

or coagulation disorder. Hypovolemic shock with a flank mass and overlying skin discoloration may be evident. Adrenal failure may require treatment (p. 487) and later calcification may occur. All hemorrhages predispose to jaundice. Ultrasound assists in diagnosis.

EXTRACRANIAL INJURIES

The *caput succedaneum* (present at birth) is a serosanguineous subcutaneous effusion over the presenting part in a vaginal delivery. It crosses the suture lines and disappears rapidly. *Subaponeurotic hemorrhages* are rare. They may follow vacuum deliveries or less commonly other instrumental deliveries. The hemorrhage is between the scalp aponeurosis and the periosteum and if it is massive it may present with hypovolemic shock and be fatal. Vitamin K (1 mg) intramuscularly should be given to all vacuum deliveries. Once diagnosed, full clotting tests should be performed and 10 ml/kg of fresh frozen plasma should be given followed by cross-matched blood. Later there may be jaundice and anemia. The *chignon* is usual from a vacuum delivery and requires no treatment. A *cephalhematoma* may follow an instrumental or less commonly a spontaneous delivery. This subperiosteal hematoma is limited by each cranial bone and is probably always associated with a hairline fracture. There is no scalp discoloration and it appears *after* birth. Jaundice may develop and phototherapy may be required. The hematoma usually resolves over 2–8 weeks with hardening of the edge and at this stage may mimic a depressed fracture. Thickening of the diploë on skull X-ray may be apparent for years. The commonest site is parietal (sometimes bilateral) followed by frontal and then occipital. No treatment is required. Do *not* drain as this potentially allows infection into the hematoma.

INTRACRANIAL INJURIES

Asphyxia and intracranial birth injury show similar clinical features and frequently coexist. Prenatal asphyxia or congenital abnormality may have initiated an instrumental delivery so it may be impossible to attribute abnormal features neonatally or later neurodevelopmental problems to one cause rather than the other. It is also possible that prenatal asphyxia may make a baby more vulnerable to birth injury by causing a high venous pressure, acidosis or disordered coagulation.

Intraventricular hemorrhage (p. 307)

This hemorrhage usually found in preterm infants is not now thought to be related to birth injury. In the asphyxiated full-term infant the choroid plexus may bleed into the ventricle.

COMPRESSION HEAD INJURIES

Cephalopelvic disproportion and instrumental delivery will predispose to intracranial injury. In many cases there will be obvious extracranial injury. Hypoxic–ischemic encephalopathy and cerebral edema (p. 205) may contribute to the clinical signs. If intracranial hemorrhage is massive, resuscitation may prove impossible or when initially successful the infant may survive only a few hours with generalized hypotonia progressing later to rigidity with convulsions and deep gasping respirations. Supratentorial bleeds lead to a tense fontanelle but posterior fossa bleeds do not. Head retraction may be marked, retinal hemorrhages may occur rapidly and the infant may have a high-pitched cry or may moan continuously. If unconscious the infant may make no sound.

Less severe hemorrhage leads to apathetic periods interspersed with periods of extreme irritability. The hemisyndrome may be evident with eyes and head turned to one side and paucity of movement on the other. Up to 50% of such infants convulse and tonic fits have a worse prognosis.

Subarachnoid hemorrhage

This may occur in preterm and term infants following perinatal hypoxia. The baby may be pale and irritable with a high-pitched cry, neck retraction and sometimes a full fontanelle. Diagnosis is difficult by ultrasound but the presumptive diagnosis by lumbar puncture may be confirmed by CT or MRI scan.

Table 12.1 Conditions predisposing to birth injury

Poor maternal health	Cephalopelvic disproportion
Maternal age (very young and old)	Hydrocephalus
Grand multiparity	Macrosomia
Twins (particularly the second)	Dystocia
Prematurity/low birth weight	Contracted pelvis
Malpresentation	Instrumental delivery

Table 12.2 Fractures

	Specific cause	Potential problem	Treatment	Comment
Skull				
Linear	1. Forceps pressure 2. Pubic pressure 3. Sacral pressure 4. Ischial spine pressure	Usually none, rarely subdural or extradural hemorrhage		
Depressed	Forceps	Underlying brain injury	1. If asymptomatic, none 2. If symptomatic, elevate	Prevent sustained cortical pressure
Occipital subluxation	Traction on spine in breech deliveries with head fixed in the pelvis	Rupture of underlying venous sinus		Usually fatal from subdural hemorrhage or tentorial tear
Clavicle (common)	1. Breech – extended arms 2. Difficult shoulder in vertex delivery	Associated brachial plexus injury	1. None – or if pain: treat pain 2. Bandage arm to chest with pad in axilla for 10 days	Prognosis excellent
Humerus	Breech – bringing down a displaced arm	Nerve damage	As for clavicle	Prognosis excellent
Femur	Extended breech	Sciatic nerve damage	1. Immobilize leg onto abdomen for 2–4 weeks (the in utero position) 2. Gallows traction	Position unimportant, molding will repair
Epiphyseal separation		Callus interferes with joint mobility and bone growth		1. On the upper femur, pain on external rotation 2. Outlook good
Nose	Dislocation of nasal cartilage	Difficulty feeding	1. Insert oral airway 2. Straighten surgically	Nares asymmetrical and nose flat

Subdural hemorrhage (hematoma)

Tears of the tentorium cerebelli or less often the falx cerebri are rare nowadays. If the hemorrhage is not rapidly fatal and if it is supratentorial, localization leads to hematoma. Signs of cerebral irritation settle after 48–72 h but later in the first week the head circumference begins to increase fast and there is clinical deterioration. Vomiting is common. Diagnosis is by CT or MRI scan and treatment by subdural taps at the lateral edge of the anterior fontanelle. Ultrasound may show midline shift but it is frequently difficult to see the subdural region to visualize the hemorrhage itself.

Management of intracranial injury

Any baby suspected of having an intracranial injury should be closely observed in an incubator with monitoring of PaO_2 and $PaCO_2$. Temperature, blood pressure, fluid balance, and metabolic problems of blood sugar, calcium and coagulation should be corrected.

The use of anticonvulsants may be required for convulsions (p. 304). Careful fluid balance is needed and it is wise to restrict intake initially to intravenous 10% dextrose at 50 ml/kg/24 h (to reduce edema secondary to inappropriate vasopressin secretion). Manual expression of the bladder may be needed. Treatment may be required for cerebral edema (p. 206).

PERIPHERAL NERVE INJURIES

Sixth nerve palsy seen for a few days after birth is probably associated with cerebral edema and trapping of the nerve on the tentorium. *Facial nerve damage (VII)* is usually peripheral from forceps pressure or from pressure on the maternal pelvis (spontaneous deliveries). No facial movement or forehead movement is seen when the infant cries. The corner of the mouth droops with dribbling at feeds and the eye fails to close (this requires protection). Recovery usually occurs over weeks but if after months there has been no recovery surgical neuroplasty should be considered. Rarely a central nuclear agenesis leads, if one sided, to paralysis of the lower half of the face.

Neck retraction in breech deliveries or shoulder dystocia damages the upper brachial plexus roots to give *Erb palsy (C5, C6)* or *phrenic palsy (C3, C4, C5)*. The arm is limp with forearm pronated and wrist flexed (waiter's tip position) from paralysis of deltoid, biceps, brachioradialis and long wrist extensors. Finger movements and therefore grasp reflex are normal. The biceps and Moro reflexes are absent on the affected side. Initial splinting of the arm to the side of the head probably makes little difference to the rate of recovery which is usually within 3 weeks (if severe it may take up to 2 years). If severe, and little recovery is detected after 3 weeks, a neurological service should be involved in management. Phrenic involvement presents as acute cyanosis and irregular labored breathing. There are reduced breath sounds and an absent abdominal bulge on inspiration because of paradoxical diaphragmatic movement. Diagnosis is by ultrasound or fluoroscopy. Treatment is with oxygen and intravenous fluids and then the gradual introduction of enteral feeds. If there is no improvement in 2 months (on ultrasound), diaphragmatic plication is indicated to prevent recurrent infection and bronchiectasis. *Klumpke palsy (C8, T1)* may occur with a breech delivery when the arms are extended up beside the head and the lower roots are stretched. The hand and forearm are paralyzed and there may be an ipsilateral Horner syndrome. Edema and hemorrhage cause temporary problems but avulsion may lead to permanent disability so a neurological service should be involved soon after birth. Traditional treatment, strapping the upper limb to the trunk, probably makes little difference to the rate of recovery. *Radial nerve* damage is temporary and leads to wrist drop. It may be due to fat necrosis involving the nerve but frequently no predisposing factor can be found. Treat with a cock up splint.

In general peripheral nerve injuries need gentle passive exercise of the limb several times a day with splinting to avoid contractures. If paralysis continues for more than 3 months, recovery is unlikely. Neuroplasty and tendon transplant have usually been considered at 3–4 years of age but there has been a recent move in brachial plexus injuries to explore and attempt repair much earlier if there has been no improvement by a few months of age.

SPINAL CORD INJURIES

The lower cervical or upper thoracic cord may be bruised or rarely transected by forceful longitudinal or lateral traction on the spine. Subluxation or fractures of the vertebrae may occur with breech deliveries where the head is hyperextended or in a vertex delivery with shoulder dystocia. Coincident brachial plexus injury is common. The infant may be normal at birth or shocked but paralysis with flaccidity below the lesion quickly occurs with accompanying constipation and urinary retention. Intercostal paralysis leads to respiratory recession (Fig. 12.6). Spinal reflex activity returns after a short time. The initial flaccidity and immobility are replaced after several weeks by rigid flexion at hip, knee and ankle with increased tone and spasms. Absent sensation and automatic bladder function necessitate treatment similar to that of the baby with a meningomyelocele (p. 832). Diagnosis may be confined by MRI or myelography. There is no reparative treatment but multidisciplinary involvement inclusive of physiotherapy may prevent or reduce contractural difficulties in the future.

PERINATAL ASPHYXIA

When related to pathophysiological processes, asphyxia is the combination of both a lack of oxygen (hypoxia) and perfusion (ischemia) to an organ. In current clinical usage there remains variability in both the meaning and interpretation of the term 'birth asphyxia'. Hence when determining the incidence, etiology and outcome of birth asphyxia there is wide variation. Many have suggested that this term should no longer be used.[77] Undoubtedly hypoxia–ischemia (HI) can lead to severe brain injury but a major concern regarding the term is in those children who develop long term neurodisability such as cerebral palsy. In these children there is often a false assumption that they were 'injured' during the events of labor and delivery with the result that obstetricians and midwives are targeted as the person responsible for those neurologic injuries.[78] In resource rich countries two of every 1000 liveborn children develop cerebral palsy (CP). Evidence suggests that 70–80% of these CP cases are due to prenatal factors and that birth asphyxia plays a relatively minor role (< 10%).[79]

However, of the approximately 130 million births worldwide each year, four million infants will suffer from birth asphyxia; of these, one million will die and a similar number will develop serious long term neurological sequelae. Ninety-eight percent of these neonatal deaths take place in resource limited countries. This leads to a neonatal mortality rate of about 4–5 per 1000 in resource rich countries and nearly 10 times this in resource limited countries.[80,81] Although restricted antenatal and peripartum care are important contributors to the high rates in resource limited countries, birth asphyxia remains a problem in resource rich countries with little reported improvement over the last two decades, and factors such as hospital shift work and night time working arrangements appear to contribute to higher risk periods for the occurrence of birth asphyxia in resource limited countries.[82]

The World Health Organization definition of birth asphyxia in the International Classification of Diseases (ICD-10) is based on the Apgar scoring system (see Table 12.3). Apgar scores are a method of describing the condition of an infant at birth, originally described by Virginia Apgar.[83] Using these markers of heart rate, respiratory effort, tone, reflex activity and color, a score is established at 1 min then at 5 min intervals as necessary (maximum score 10). The ICD-10 definition of asphyxia is dependent on the Apgar score at 1 min of age. An Apgar score at 1 min of 0–3 defines severe birth asphyxia and an Apgar score of 4–7 defines moderate asphyxia. There is much debate as to whether this definition is of clinical use. Specifically, regarding prognosis, Apgar scores in individual cases do not appear to correlate well with outcome and hence are frequently interpreted incorrectly from a view of long term prognosis.[84] Despite the controversy, this definition of severe birth asphyxia (Apgar < 3) appears useful in identifying a high risk group requiring further observation of their neurological condition[85,86] with an understanding that it overestimates eight-fold the scale of the problem. Table 12.4 summarizes the proportion of infants that either die or develop cerebral palsy with different Apgars at different time points immediately after birth.[87]

Newer terms include 'birth depression', which is a descriptive term to indicate a newborn with poor Apgars but without passing judgment on etiology. The use of the word 'perinatal' rather than 'birth' supports the pathological processes that may begin many hours before birth and

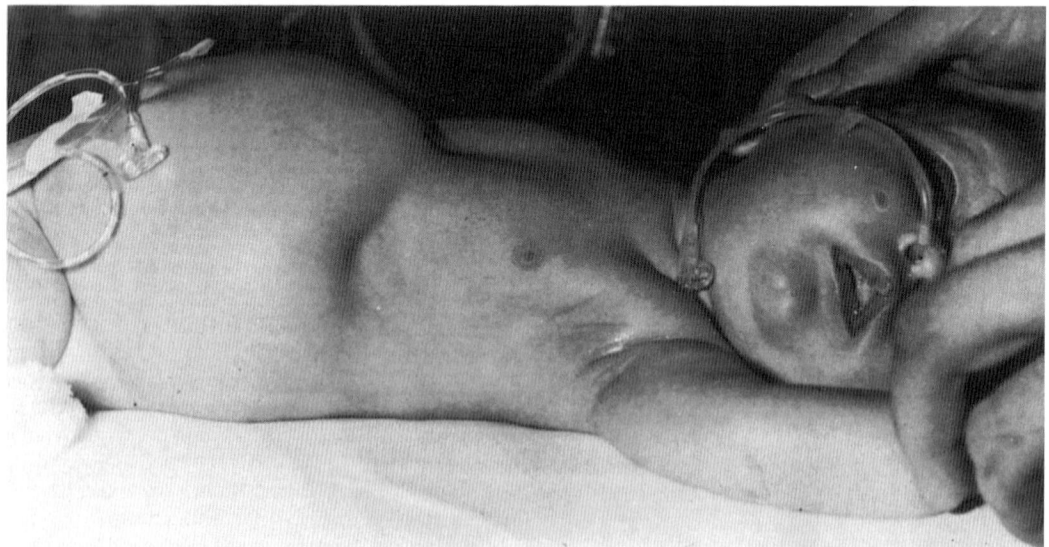

Fig. 12.6 Thoracic indrawing in newborn infant with broken neck.

Table 12.3 The Apgar score

Sign	0	1	2
Heart rate	Absent	< 100/min	> 100/min
Respiratory effort	Absent	Weak cry	Strong cry
Muscle tone	Limp	Some flexion	Good flexion
Reflex irritability on suctioning pharynx	No response	Some movement	Cry
Color	Pale	Centrally pink, peripherally blue	Pink all over

Table 12.4   Risk of death or cerebral palsy (CP) in infants > 2500 g with Apgar scores of 0–3 at varying times from birth (data from Nelson & Ellenberg[87])

Age (min)	Death in first year (%)	CP > 2500 g (%)
1	3	0.7
5	8	0.7
10	18	5
15	48	9
20	59	57

continue for many hours afterwards. There are numerous causes, and the clinical manifestations vary. Infants who experience mild asphyxia may show no neurological injury. However, severe asphyxia may be fatal in utero, or immediately after birth, with survivors showing extensive neurological sequelae, with or without cognitive deficits.

ETIOLOGY OF PERINATAL ASPHYXIA

The fetoplacental unit seems well prepared to deal with transient episodes of hypoxia–ischemia. During contractions of the uterus, placental gas exchange is commonly interrupted and there are mechanisms that protect the fetus during these episodes. These mechanisms include increased extraction of oxygen from the blood,[88] redistribution of the fetal blood supply to the brain and heart at the expense of the gastrointestinal tract, kidneys and muscle, etc. The neonatal brain also appears to be able to utilize other substrates instead of glucose (such as lactate and ketones).[89] On top of this usual process other stresses may occur and these stresses may be acute or chronic or acute on chronic. Examples of these stresses include altered placental gas exchange such as may occur in placental insufficiency or abruption, interruption to the umbilical circulation (cord prolapse or cord compression), reduced maternal placental perfusion (such as may occur with maternal hypo/hypertension), impaired maternal oxygenation, or in the newborn infant the failure to establish adequate circulation after birth.

ASSESSMENT OF FETAL WELL-BEING (see Ch. 12)

Many different assessments attempt to predict fetal well-being. These include observing for the passage of meconium, electronic fetal heart rate monitoring via a cardiotocograph (CTG) and the assessment of fetal acid–base balance. Umbilical cord blood gas and pH values should always be obtained in the high risk delivery and whenever newborn depression occurs. The most useful umbilical cord blood parameter is arterial pH. It is more representative of the fetal metabolic condition because arterial acidemia may occur with a normal venous pH. In general, the lower range for normal arterial pH extends down to 7.10 and that for venous pH to 7.20. It is the gold standard assessment of uteroplacental function and fetal oxygenation/acid–base status at birth.[90] The CTG parameters associated with asphyxia include abnormal fetal heart rate variability, repeated late decelerations, repeated variable decelerations, occasional late or variable decelerations and also a lack of accelerations.[91] However, these associations are not helpful in individual cases as they have poor correlation with longer term outcome in newborn infants. Nonreassuring fetal heart rate patterns, prolonged labor, meconium-stained fluid, a low 1 min Apgar score, and mild to moderate acidemia have no predictive value for long term neurological injury without signs of encephalopathy and seizures.[92] It is therefore essential that the entire pregnancy, labor, delivery and the period well beyond birth are examined to understand fully the pathophysiological mechanisms that are responsible for any particular infant's brain injuries, and their long term impact on the child.[78] It is extremely important when faced with a newborn infant with low Apgars to immediately provide proper resuscitation and ongoing support whilst allowing time for further evaluation.[92]

EXTENT OF INJURY FOLLOWING PERINATAL ASPHYXIA

After a severe hypoxic–ischemic insult, multiorgan system failure is common including neurological, hepatic, cardiac, pulmonary and renal systems.[93,94] However, apart from brain injury there appears to be no relationship between individual or combinations of organs involved and long term outcomes.[95] Ultimately, if the HI insult is overwhelming then death may occur.

HYPOXIC–ISCHEMIC ENCEPHALOPATHY (HIE)

When the brain is affected by an HI insult there may be both short and long term sequelae. Infants show a sequence of often transient encephalopathic behavior, often lasting for many days, and this is dependent on the severity and duration of the asphyxial event. In the acute setting, the clinical features that result from an HI insult in the term newborn brain reflect an evolving process characterized by an initial primary injury followed by a secondary phase of brain damage lasting several hours or even days after the insult.[96] Experimental studies have shown that a severe HI insult results in an evolving process of adverse biochemical events that include increased levels of neurotransmitters, excessive production of free radicals, increased intracellular calcium and stimulation of inflammatory mediators that initiate apoptotic cell death.[97,98] HIE is the clinical marker of cerebral tissue that has suffered severe damage and may result in perinatal mortality or permanent neurodevelopmental disability. Between 2 and 6 infants per 1000 live births develop HIE[99] which cannot be reliably diagnosed in premature babies. Grading systems define the degree of encephalopathy in term babies[100,101] (Table 12.5). Mild HIE usually recovers completely within 48–72 h and moderate HIE often continues to show significant acute neurological signs for 7–10 days. However, babies with severe HIE may remain persistently neurologically abnormal although the signs of acute encephalopathy often improve prior to discharge home. In the longer term approximately 25% of infants with moderate HIE will develop cerebral palsy, whilst historically the majority of infants with severe encephalopathy either die or survive with multiple disabilities.[102] It is important to note that asphyxia is not the only cause of neonatal encephalopathy[103] and as well as looking for supportive evidence of perinatal HI, such as signs of fetal distress, acidosis and poor Apgars, the alternative causes listed in Table 12.6 should be considered.[104]

MANAGING PERINATAL ASPHYXIA

In the antenatal period the reliability of continuous heart rate monitoring of the fetus during labor as well as validity of certain heart rate changes for the detection of developing hypoxia is a matter of ongoing dispute. In the presence of clearly pathological heart rate patterns hypoxic damage may already have occurred. Suspicious or 'nonreassuring' heart rate alterations are frequent and only in a small percentage is there a real threat to the fetus in the form of severe hypoxia. Up until now there is no proof that a combination of continuous fetal heart rate monitoring with additional tests can prevent hypoxic damage to the fetus. However, despite the high false positive rate, continuous intrapartum electronic fetal monitoring is recommended for pregnancies where there is an increased risk of perinatal death, cerebral palsy or neonatal encephalopathy. Fetal scalp blood sampling is recommended in association with electronic fetal monitoring patterns that are uninterpretable or nonreassuring, such as sustained minimal or absent variability, uncorrectable

Table 12.5   The major clinical features for grading the severity of hypoxic–ischemic encephalopathy

Mild	Moderate	Severe
Irritability	Lethargy	Coma
Hyper-alert	Seizures	Prolonged seizures
Normal tone	Differential tone (legs > arms) (neck extensors > flexors)	Severe hypotonia
Weak suck	Poor suck, requires tube feeds	No sucking reflex
Sympathetic dominance	Parasympathetic dominance	Coma, requires respiratory support

Table 12.6 Differential diagnosis for hypoxic–ischemic encephalopathy

Infective	Meningitis (bacterial or viral) Encephalitis (herpes simplex)
Traumatic brain lesion	e.g. Subdural hemorrhage
Vascular	Neonatal stroke Shock secondary to acute blood loss (antepartum/intrapartum)
Metabolic	Hypoglycemia Hypo/hypernatremia Bilirubin encephalopathy
Inborn error of metabolism	Urea cycle defects Pyridoxine dependency Lactate acidemias Amino acidemias (e.g. NKH) Organic acidemias
Congenital brain malformation	e.g. Neuronal migration disorder
Neuromuscular disorder	e.g. Spinal muscular atrophy
Maternal drug exposure	Acute or chronic

Table 12.7 Identification of infants at highest risk of evolving brain injury

Criteria A – One of the following must be present
Apgar score of ≤5 at 10 min of age
Continued need for resuscitation (including mask ventilation) at 10 min after birth
Acidosis within 60 min of birth [defined as any pH < 7 in umbilical cord or infant blood (arterial or capillary)]
Base deficit ≥ 16 mmol/L in umbilical cord or any sample (arterial, venous or capillary) within 60 min of birth

Criteria B – Abnormal neurological status
Infants that meet criteria A should then be assessed to determine whether they are affected neurologically
Altered state of consciousness (reduced or absent response to stimulation) *and*
Abnormal tone (hypotonia or flaccidity) *and*
Abnormal primitive reflexes (weak or absent suck/Moro)
Or seizures in isolation

Criteria C – Neurophysiological abnormality
Abnormal EEG or amplitude integrated EEG

late decelerations, increasing fetal tachycardia and abnormal fetal heart rate characteristics on auscultation. Recent advances such as fetal pulse oximetry, ST waveform analysis and near infrared spectroscopy as adjuncts to electronic fetal medicine are not recommended as standard care at present.[105]

In the perinatal period, staff training improves outcome. The introduction of obstetric emergencies training courses has been shown to lead to a significant reduction in both low 5 min Apgar scores and the incidence of hypoxic–ischemic encephalopathy,[106] and a significant improvement in neonatal Apgar scores has also been shown with neonatal resuscitation training.[107]

In the postnatal period, the current treatment approach to a term (or near term) infant at risk of progression to neonatal encephalopathy after intrapartum hypoxia–ischemia is fourfold: resuscitation, identification, supportive and neuroprotective strategies. Effective resuscitation is the main priority in the infant born with poor Apgars. Recent evidence regarding the resuscitation of infants with poor Apgars (1 min Apgar < 4) in either ambient air versus pure oxygen suggests that although mortality rates are similar, those infants resuscitated in air recover faster than those resuscitated in oxygen.[108] Once the infant has been resuscitated then early identification of the infant at highest risk for evolving brain injury is necessary. This identification is based on the criteria of a sentinel event during labor, prolonged depression at birth with the need for resuscitation, evidence of severe fetal acidemia based on a cord umbilical arterial pH less than 7 and/or a base deficit more than −16 < mmol/L. The entry requirement to the majority of large randomized studies of neuroprotective strategies is stepwise through criteria A to C as summarized in Table 12.7.

The assessment of amplitude integrated EEG (aEEG) using a cerebral function monitor (CFM) in the identification of at risk infants is based on studies of infants between 3 and 6 h of age after HI and has been shown to be highly sensitive and specific in determining which of these children are most at risk of death or disability.[109–111] Infants meeting criteria A, B and C have a 70% chance of mortality or long term severe neurodisability. Based on animal experiments, the therapeutic window for neonates with signs of perinatal hypoxia–ischaemia is probably less than 6 h, and early selection of patients is of utmost importance. At present, neurophysiological methods such as (amplitude integrated) EEG and evoked potentials have the best predictive value.[112]

It is important that supportive therapy is instituted to maintain adequate ventilation; in particular severe hyperoxemia and severe hypocapnia are associated with adverse outcome in infants with post-asphyxial HIE. During the first hours of life, oxygen supplementation and ventilation should be rigorously controlled.[113] Mean arterial blood pressure should be kept within the perinatal range so as to avoid fluctuations in cerebral perfusion. Glucose should be kept in the normal range to avoid hypoglycemia, and seizures should be treated. Animal studies have also suggested that preventing spontaneous hyperthermia after HI in the newborn is neuroprotective.[114]

There is insufficient evidence from randomized controlled trials to determine whether the infusion of sodium bicarbonate reduces mortality and morbidity[115] or that fluid restriction is beneficial[116] or that prophylactic use of anticonvulsants confers benefit other than in the treatment of prolonged or frequent clinical seizures.[117]

Until recently there has been no neuroprotective treatment available for infants with HIE. Induced systemic hypothermia is currently the only strategy that has been evaluated in large, multicenter randomized studies. The results of studies in human infants suggest that not only is cooling safe (when used in a tightly controlled fashion within a clinical trial) but that it also appears to confer a beneficial effect. One large study used a cooling cap device to induce selective head cooling whilst lowering rectal temperature to 34.5°C; another large study induced total body hypothermia using a cooling blanket system reducing core temperature to 33.5°C. The majority of clinical cooling studies in infants induced hypothermia for a period of 72 h. No significant side-effects were noted with this degree of cooling. The combined data from these studies indicate that hypothermia is associated with a reduction in the incidence of death and/or severe disability at 18 months follow-up, with the most significant effect observed in infants who at the start of therapy presented with moderate encephalopathy and/or did not exhibit seizures.[118–120] However, there remain many unanswered questions about this type of treatment (such as the long term effects of hypothermia) and the fact that only a subgroup of babies seems to benefit. There are also no data on optimal duration, degree of cooling, best method, or whether the methods and degree of cooling should be adapted to the type or timing of brain injury. Therefore many people still feel that further data are needed before health care policies can be changed to make cooling the standard of care for all babies with suspected birth asphyxia.

For clinicians practicing in the UK the results of a large multicenter study of total body cooling to 33.5°C are still awaited.[121] Until the results of this study become available, clinicians involved in the study have permission to induce hypothermia in infants with HIE (using both the study protocol and eligibility criteria from the trial – see Table 12.7). Data from patients cooled in this way are collected as part of a national register. A similar system has been used in the USA for clinicians pending longer term safety data.

PROGNOSIS AFTER HIE

Early indicators of prognosis are invaluable in the clinical setting and especially when discussing issues with parents. As previously mentioned, aEEG in the first 3–6 h can be used to predict future outcome. Early EEG is an excellent prognostic indicator for a favorable outcome if normal within the first 8 h of life and for a poor outcome if the background activity continues to be low or grossly abnormal beyond 8–12 h of life. However, an inactive or very depressed EEG within the first 8 h of life can be associated with good outcome if the EEG activity recovers within 12 h.[122,123] The highest recorded lactate level in the first hour of life and serial measurements of lactate (to determine how quickly the levels fall) are important predictors of moderate to severe HIE.[124] Plasma nonprotein bound iron is also a good early predictive marker of neurodevelopmental outcome, with 100% sensitivity and 100% specificity for good neurodevelopmental outcome at 0–1.16 micromol/L, and for poor neurodevelopmental outcome at values > 15.2 micromol/L.[125] At 24 h of age neurological assessment using a Sarnat assessment score as well as ultrasound Doppler assessment of resistance index of blood flow in the anterior cerebral artery also add valuable information about prognosis in the individual patient.[100,126] Imaging of the brain with an MRI scan in the first week of life also provides further information to determine prognosis. Abnormal signal intensity in the posterior limb of the internal capsule (PLIC) is an accurate predictor of neurodevelopmental outcome in term infants suffering HIE.[127] The apparent diffusion coefficient (ADC) value in the PLIC is also an indicator of ischemic injury.[128] It is of interest that the distribution of injury appears to be different in those infants that have undergone hypothermia. The hypothermia group appear to have had less cortical gray matter signal abnormality on MRI which may indicate differing regional benefit from systemic hypothermia.[129]

THE IMPORTANCE OF AUTOPSY

It is a sad fact that many infants die of overwhelming HI injury. In those cases it is essential that a postmortem is offered to the parents. HIE is a symptom rather than a final clinical diagnosis. A full autopsy is required to fully explore the reasons for fatal neonatal HIE and it may also provide information that is important medicolegally. One study reported that significant new information was added to the clinical diagnoses in over 60% of cases after autopsy.[130] Detailed autopsy examination should include the search for infection. The placenta should be examined for the presence of thrombosis and infarction. Careful autopsy of the neck and paravertebral tissues, spinal cord, brainstem and nerve roots is important where trauma is suspected. Metabolic disease, including peroxisomal disorders, nonketotic hyperglycinemia, lipid and glycogen storage disorders and mitochondrial diseases may cause profound hypotonia and respiratory failure at birth or shortly afterwards.[131]

RESUSCITATION IN THE NEWBORN

In Western countries relatively few mature newborn infants require active resuscitation at birth. In Sweden, just 1% of babies weighing over 2.5 kg required artificial ventilation, but significantly 20% of these were unexpected in babies with no obvious risk factors.[132] In the UK, a comparison between two large obstetric units found that there was a five-fold variation in the proportion of newborn infants who required intubation; 2% versus 10%. In resource limited countries it is estimated that 1 million babies a year die of asphyxia and that lack of simple airway interventions is a significant factor in many of these deaths. The more preterm the delivery, the more likely it will be that the baby needs active resuscitation.

The physiology of fetal hypoxia leading to the need for resuscitation at birth is well understood and has been known for many years. In recent years, a number of national and multidisciplinary groups have described optimal practice for neonatal resuscitation based on the best available scientific evidence.[133–135] Although there are some differences in detail between these recommendations, these are relatively minor. Current British recommendations are outlined in this section.

THE PHYSIOLOGICAL RESPONSE TO HYPOXIA

Our understanding of the newborn's response to hypoxia is based on neonatal animal experiments published in the 1960s[136,137] and is summarized in Figure 12.7. At the onset of hypoxia there is a period of small-volume but rapid breaths lasting for several minutes followed by a period of primary apnea. Prior to primary apnea the heart rate and blood pressure are maintained. Once apnea occurs the heart rate falls, but with increasing stroke volume a good cardiac output is maintained with continued perfusion of the vital organs. At this stage the baby looks cyanosed.

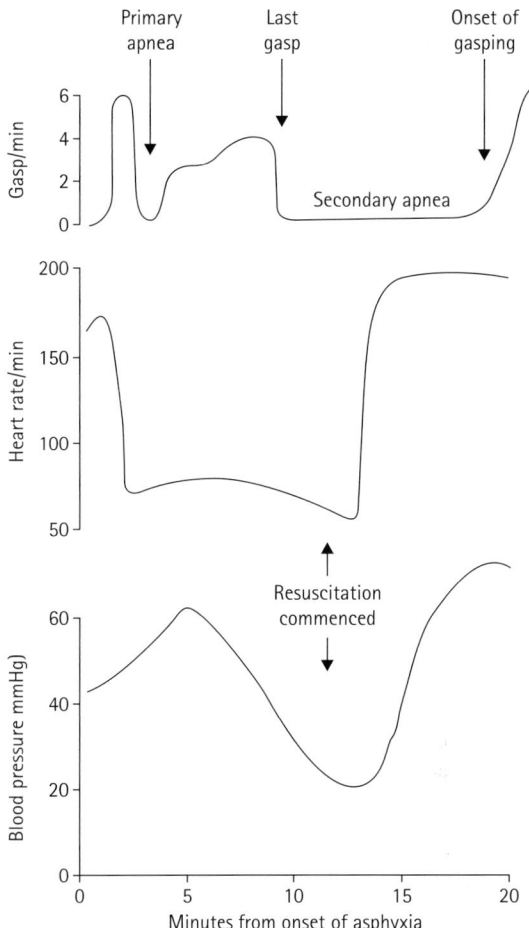

Fig. 12.7   The effects of asphyxia on a newborn animal showing primary and secondary apnea. (Redrawn from Dawes 1968[137] with permission of Blackwell Scientific Publications.)

If hypoxia continues then after a period of primary apnea lasting up to 5 minutes, spontaneous gasping occurs (10–15 per minute) and this lasts for a further period of 5–6 minutes before a second period of apnea develops. This is referred to as terminal apnea and if nothing is done to resuscitate the animal at this time death will occur within another 10 minutes. During the period of primary apnea and subsequent gasping, blood pressure and heart rate are maintained, but with increasing metabolic acidemia. Cardiovascular deterioration commences with the onset of terminal apnea.

These timings are based on rhesus monkey studies but are likely to reflect the human situation although the timing of the sequence of events may be a little shorter than in monkeys.

THE PRINCIPLES OF NEONATAL RESUSCITATION

All babies must be born in an environment where they have rapid access to expert resuscitation skills. In home births there must be two attendants, one of which will be responsible for resuscitating the baby (if necessary) and who has appropriate training and knowledge of the equipment, which should be in full working order. Most babies will require no active resuscitation other than gentle stimulation, but others are slow to adapt to their extrauterine environment and some active steps will need to be taken by caregivers. The vigor of the response will depend on the stage of the baby's reaction to the hypoxic event. The baby who is not breathing may start to breathe spontaneously if in the stage of primary apnea but will not if in secondary apnea. Whether the baby is in primary or secondary apnea may be difficult to determine clinically. Consequently, the attendant must undertake a measured response and be prepared to escalate resuscitative measures if the initial response is inadequate.

Table 12.8   Indications for calling a pediatrician to be present at a delivery

Prematurity
  Gestation <36 weeks
Fetal distress
  Thick meconium staining
  Severely abnormal CTG
  Fetal scalp acidosis (pH <7.2)
Operative delivery
  Any delivery under general anesthesia
  Mid-cavity or rotational forceps
Multiple pregnancy
Significant antepartum hemorrhage
Fetal disease
  Known major congenital abnormality
  Rhesus disease

CTG, Cardiotocograph.

Many, but by no means all, infants who are born in a depressed state can be anticipated. Table 12.8 lists the indications for calling a pediatrician or other person competent to resuscitate the newborn infant.

PREPARATION PRIOR TO DELIVERY

The pediatrician called for a high risk delivery should spend some time prior to delivery acquainting himself with the mother's medical and antenatal history. It is important to check all the equipment that may be required prior to delivery and not rely on the fact that this should have been done by others.

Resuscitation trolley

A stop clock permanently fixed to the trolley is started at delivery, giving the operator a reference point for the duration of resuscitation. An integral overhead heater should be of fixed height above the infant with a dial to give variable temperature settings.

Medical gases

It is most important that both air and oxygen are readily available, together with appropriate reduction valves so that a variable and measurable flow of gas can be given to the infant. As well as controlling the flow of gas, a blow-off valve must be fitted so that the baby's lungs are not overdistended by unacceptably high pressures.

Suction

The presence of suction apparatus on the resuscitation trolley is essential. This must also be fitted with an accurate valve device with a display of negative pressure as too high a suction pressure may damage the infant's respiratory tract. Mouth suction must not be used. A number of suction catheters of different sizes (FG 4, 6 and 8) must also be at hand with appropriate connectors to attach to the suction device.

Bag and mask

Bag and mask resuscitation equipment is essential in every hospital where babies are delivered or cared for and all staff must be familiar with their effective use. The method for appropriate bag and mask ventilation is described below. A number of different bags exist, the best being the Laerdal type. These are fitted with a blow-off valve which can be adjusted to give a maximum inflation pressure. Tubing can be fitted to these devices so that the baby can be ventilated with additional oxygen. As well as the bag, a tight-fitting deformable silastic Laerdal face mask is essential. These should be of variable sizes to fit the faces of the smallest and the biggest babies likely to be encountered. The technique is described below.

Intubation equipment

Two laryngoscopes should be available with fresh batteries and these should be checked prior to delivery of the baby. A selection of endotracheal tubes should be present varying in size from 2.5 to 4.0 mm. The correct connector must also be available together with a malleable metal introducer. Reliable means of securing the tube to the baby's face should also be available and the assisting nurse must be skilled in the fixation of the tube. A stethoscope should be worn by the resuscitator prior to delivery of the baby.

A SCHEME FOR RESUSCITATION

All staff responsible for neonatal resuscitation must have received appropriate training and regular retraining to maintain appropriate skills. In Britain the Resuscitation Council (UK) has developed the Newborn Life Support course, which is now widely available. The following are currently recommended by this course[133] and summarized in Figure 12.8.

The need for resuscitation must be carefully assessed and an incremental approach is required depending on the condition of the baby and the response to initial measures. The six steps in this approach are as follows:
1. Conserve heat: dry and cover the baby.
2. Assess the need for resuscitation.
3. Airway: check and stabilize.
4. Breathing: bag and mask inflation.
5. Circulation: start chest compressions.
6. Drugs if required.

Assess

Whilst drying the baby observe its responses. Watch the baby's color, respiratory efforts, heart rate and tone. Most babies will rapidly adapt to birth with improving color, increasing heart rate with the development of spontaneous breathing or crying activity. If the baby has a heart rate >100 bpm and has reasonable tone, it is reasonable to wait for up to 3 minutes for the baby to breathe spontaneously. If this is the case then nothing more needs to be done once the baby is breathing and pink; it can then be given to the mother. In premature babies great care must be taken to avoid hypothermia (see below).

Airway

The airway must be clear for breathing to occur. The commonest cause of an impaired airway is positional: the baby lies with his head flexed causing the tongue to fall back and obstruct the pharynx. The baby's head must be put into the neutral position with the jaw drawn forward (jaw thrust maneuver – Fig. 12.9). Do not overextend the neck.

Sometimes the airway must be cleared, particularly if meconium is present (see below). This is best done by visualizing the oropharynx with a laryngoscope and giving gentle suction. Do not blindly use a suction catheter to suck out the mouth as stimulation of the posterior pharynx and larynx may induce vagal stimulation with apnea and bradycardia.

Rarely the baby may have an anatomical abnormality of the face, jaw or palate and an oropharyngeal airway (Guedel) of the appropriate size should be available to insert into the baby's mouth with its tip beyond the back of the tongue.

Inflation breaths

If the baby fails to breathe 30–60 s after an airway has been established then the lungs must be inflated with gas. This is done by giving 5 long inflation breaths each lasting 2–3 s with an opening pressure of $30 \, cmH_2O$ in term babies (less in preterm infants). This is performed with an appropriately sized soft, tight-fitting face mask which makes a good seal around the baby's mouth and nose. The lungs are expanded by a self-inflating bag (Fig. 12.10). An alternative is a T-piece attached to the mask and pressurized gas directed into the baby's lungs by occluding the T-piece with a finger for the requisite period of 2–3 s. The pressurized gas must blow off at a predetermined level (usually $30 \, cmH_2O$), often by an underwater seal.

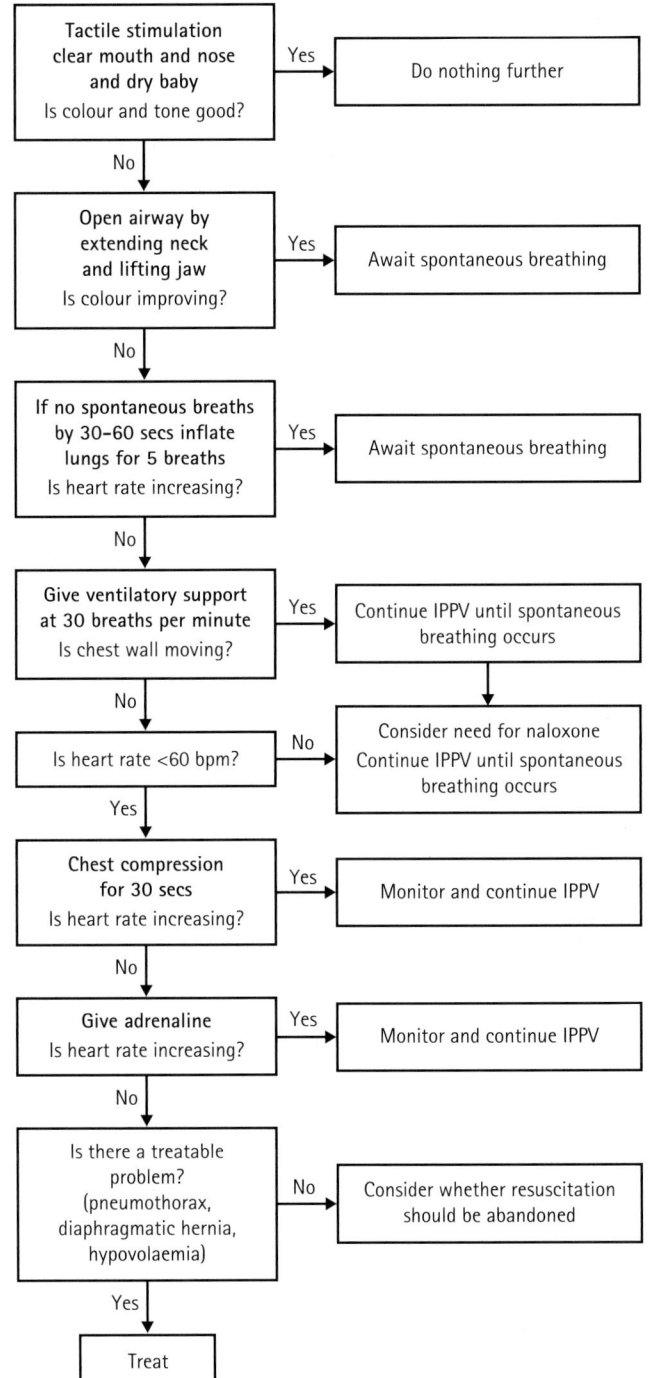

```
┌─────────────────────┐
│ Tactile stimulation │  Yes  ┌──────────────────────┐
│ clear mouth and nose│──────▶│  Do nothing further  │
│    and dry baby     │       └──────────────────────┘
│ Is colour and tone  │
│       good?         │
└─────────────────────┘
          │ No
          ▼
┌─────────────────────┐
│   Open airway by    │  Yes  ┌──────────────────────────┐
│   extending neck    │──────▶│ Await spontaneous breathing│
│   and lifting jaw   │       └──────────────────────────┘
│ Is colour improving?│
└─────────────────────┘
          │ No
          ▼
┌─────────────────────┐
│If no spontaneous    │  Yes  ┌──────────────────────────┐
│breaths by 30–60 secs│──────▶│ Await spontaneous breathing│
│inflate lungs for 5  │       └──────────────────────────┘
│breaths              │
│Is heart rate        │
│increasing?          │
└─────────────────────┘
          │ No
          ▼
┌─────────────────────┐
│ Give ventilatory    │  Yes  ┌──────────────────────────┐
│ support at 30       │──────▶│ Continue IPPV until      │
│ breaths per minute  │       │ spontaneous breathing    │
│ Is chest wall       │       │ occurs                   │
│ moving?             │       └──────────────────────────┘
└─────────────────────┘
          │ No
          ▼
┌─────────────────────┐  No   ┌──────────────────────────┐
│ Is heart rate       │──────▶│ Consider need for naloxone│
│ <60 bpm?            │       │ Continue IPPV until      │
└─────────────────────┘       │ spontaneous breathing    │
          │ Yes               │ occurs                   │
          ▼                   └──────────────────────────┘
┌─────────────────────┐
│ Chest compression   │  Yes  ┌──────────────────────────┐
│ for 30 secs         │──────▶│ Monitor and continue IPPV│
│ Is heart rate       │       └──────────────────────────┘
│ increasing?         │
└─────────────────────┘
          │ No
          ▼
┌─────────────────────┐  Yes  ┌──────────────────────────┐
│ Give adrenaline     │──────▶│ Monitor and continue IPPV│
│ Is heart rate       │       └──────────────────────────┘
│ increasing?         │
└─────────────────────┘
          │ No
          ▼
┌─────────────────────┐
│ Is there a treatable│  No   ┌──────────────────────────┐
│ problem?            │──────▶│ Consider whether         │
│ (pneumothorax,      │       │ resuscitation should be  │
│ diaphragmatic       │       │ abandoned                │
│ hernia,             │       └──────────────────────────┘
│ hypovolaemia)       │
└─────────────────────┘
          │ Yes
          ▼
┌─────────────────────┐
│       Treat         │
└─────────────────────┘
```

Fig. 12.8   Summary of approach to neonatal resuscitation.

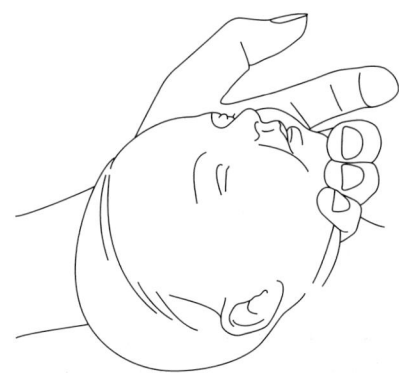

Fig. 12.9   Slight head extension with chin support to open airway.

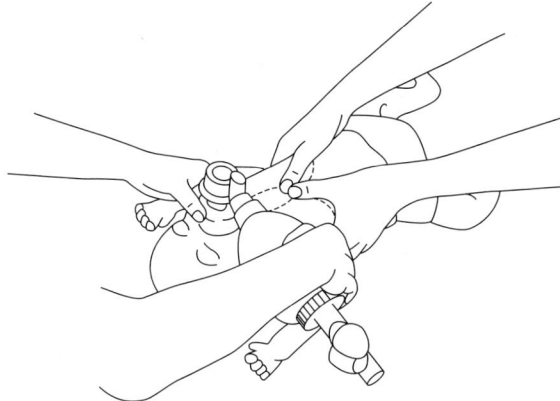

Fig. 12.10   Cardiorespiratory resuscitation. One operator inflates the baby's lungs with the bag and mask. The head is slightly extended and the chin pulled forward. The other operator gives external cardiac massage with hands encircling the chest. (From Levene et al 1987 with permission of Blackwell Scientific Publications.)

After 5 breaths observe its effect. There should be an increase in heart rate; if there is not, the lungs are not being appropriately inflated. Immediately check that the chest is moving with inflation breaths. If it does not, then the airway is probably not clear. Readjust the baby's position and check the seal of the mask on the baby's face. Repeat 5 breaths and if there is still no chest movement consider the following:

- Does the baby need more jaw thrust?
- Does he need longer inflation breaths?
- Is there an obstruction in the oropharynx (consider laryngoscopy and suction)?
- Does the baby need a Guedel airway?

Once the lungs are inflated, continue shorter breaths at 30 per min until the baby establishes spontaneous respiration. In most babies bag and mask ventilation is all that is required. Intubation may be necessary if bag and mask resuscitation fails, during prolonged resuscitation, where copious tracheal suction is required or if surfactant administration is anticipated. A recent study has suggested that use of a laryngeal mask airway is as effective and rapid as intubation in achieving a secure airway.[138]

Circulation

With appropriate inflation breaths the baby's heart rate should improve and the baby will become pink. If the chest is inflating well and the heart rate remains slow (< 60 bpm) circulatory support is required. This requires two people: one to maintain ventilation and the other to give chest compressions. With the fingers over the baby's spine, the resuscitator's thumbs are placed on the sternum just below the internipple line and the lower third of the sternum is compressed by one third of the depth of the chest (Fig. 12.10). The ratio of compressions to breaths is 3:1 to achieve 90 compressions and 30 breaths per min.

Drugs

In most cases the baby recovers rapidly with appropriate ventilation and chest compression, but sometimes further resuscitation with drugs is required. It is essential to first establish an effective route by which the drugs can be given. The most rapid way is to insert a sterile catheter into the umbilical vein into the inferior vena cava. A rough guide to achieve this is to insert the radio-opaque cannula the distance from the umbilicus to the internipple line. The sequence of drug administration depends on the baby's response and is hierarchical as follows:

- Sodium bicarbonate, 2–4 ml/kg of 4.2% solution. It is not necessary to correct a metabolic acidosis but merely to improve the intracardiac pH. Although sodium bicarbonate is widely used, a recent randomized controlled trial showed no benefit in terms of survival or neurological complications in a group of asphyxiated newborn infants still requiring intubation 5 min after birth.[139]

- Adrenaline (epinephrine) 0.1 ml/kg of 1:10 000 dilution. Do not use more concentrated solutions. This should only be given after sodium bicarbonate as cardiac receptors are less sensitive in the presence of severe acidosis. Up to three repeated doses may be given if there is no response. An alternative route of administration is via the endotracheal tube but other drugs must not be given through the tube and it is preferred to give all the drugs via the umbilical venous catheter.
- 10% Dextrose at 2.5 ml/kg.
- Volume infusion with 0.9% saline 10 ml/kg.
- Naloxone is only indicated when the baby appears to have respiratory depression as a result of maternal opiate administration within 3 h prior to delivery. Small doses of naloxone (40 mcg ampoule of 'neonatal' Narcan) provide only transient antagonism of respiratory depression and a full dose (200 mcg) intramuscularly should be given if naloxone is indicated. Intramuscular use is preferred to intravenous except if the baby is shocked with poor tissue perfusion. Never use naloxone without suspicion of neonatal opiate depression. Do not give naloxone to the baby of an opiate dependent mother as this may cause acute and severe withdrawal symptoms in the baby.

There is no evidence that calcium infusion is of any benefit in cardiac resuscitation.

CONTROVERSIES IN NEONATAL RESUSCITATION

Volume expansion

Administration of 10 ml/kg 0.9% saline in babies with circulatory failure is recommended. Care should be taken if large volume administration is given (> 40 ml/kg) as this may exacerbate metabolic acidosis due to hyperchloremia.[140] Hypovolemia at delivery may arise as a result of prenatal bleeding, premature clamping of the cord, when the baby is held above the mother prior to cord clamping or with a nuchal cord and failure of adequate blood flow to the fetus from the placenta. If the baby is shocked at birth and is thought to have recently sustained a significant hemorrhage then he should be given an infusion of group O rhesus negative blood immediately.

There remains considerable controversy about the role of albumin in treating hypovolemia. There is no evidence that giving human albumin improves survival when compared to giving saline.[141] An isotonic crystalloid solution such as normal saline is recommended in both the British and American Neonatal Resuscitation guidelines.

Resuscitation in room air or 100% oxygen

In 1999 the International Liaison Committee on Resuscitation recommended that resuscitation of the newborn should be performed with 100% oxygen,[142] but there has been concern about the potential adverse effects of high oxygen concentrations and in particular increasing the work of breathing in newborn infants and the generation of excess free radicals with adverse effect to the eyes, lungs and brain. High concentrations of oxygen have also been shown to reduce cerebral blood flow. A recent Cochrane review[143] identified five studies where babies were randomized at resuscitation to receive either 100% oxygen or room air. Those babies given air had significantly better Apgar scores[144,145] and time to first breath was longer in the 100% oxygen group.[145,146] It is suggested that the effects of 100% oxygen may be more adverse in preterm infants than at term.[147] Pooled analysis of four trials where mortality was reported showed a significant reduction in mortality rate in the room air compared with the 100% oxygen resuscitated group. In one trial where follow-up data on survivors at 18–24 months was described there were no significant differences in the rates of adverse neurodevelopmental outcome. The conclusion of this Cochrane review was that there were insufficient data to support the routine policy of resuscitation with room air. Until this controversy has been fully resolved the most appropriate recommendation is to use a blender on the resuscitation trolley so that 30–40% oxygen is used initially and modified according to the baby's oxygen saturation.[148]

Meconium stained liquor

In the presence of severe prenatal hypoxia, fetal gasping may cause aspiration of meconium deep into the bronchial tree. Approximately 15% of babies are born with meconium staining of the liquor and in approximately 5% meconium aspiration syndrome (MAS) occurs. In the US 25–60% of infants with MAS require mechanical ventilation.[149,150] Strategies to reduce the risk of MAS such as amnioinfusion (injection of fluid into the amniotic cavity intended to dilute the meconium prior to delivery) have been evaluated in a Cochrane review.[151] This showed that amnioinfusion significantly reduced the incidence of meconium aspirate. More recently a large international multicenter study[152] enrolling almost 2000 women showed no reduction in the rate of moderate or severe meconium aspiration syndrome and the authors concluded that meconium staining of the amniotic fluid is not an indication for amnioinfusion for women in labor.

Suctioning of the oro- and nasopharynx after birth of the head and before delivery of the baby's trunk has also been suggested to be effective,[153] but others have not shown a similar beneficial effect (see Wiswell 2001[154] for review) and this technique remains of unproven benefit. A further strategy is endotracheal intubation at birth for babies born through thick meconium stained liquor so that effective suctioning of the airways can be undertaken. This has been evaluated within the context of a Cochrane review.[155] Four randomized controlled trials of intubation at birth in vigorous term infants born through meconium stained liquor were identified. There was no evidence that routine intubation with lavage in vigorous term meconium stained babies reduced the incidence of significant lung disease. Chest compression immediately after birth to avoid aspiration of meconium is dangerous and should not be performed.

The US recommendations for resuscitation of a baby born through meconium stained liquor are initially thorough suctioning of the mouth, nose and pharynx with either a bulb syringe or 12–14F suction catheter as soon as the head is delivered and before the body emerges. After delivery, if the baby is in a *depressed* state (slow to establish regular breathing, reduced tone, or heart rate < 100 bpm) then immediate direct laryngoscopy should be performed with intubation/suctioning of any residual meconium from the trachea under direct vision. Saline lavage is not recommended. Delay gastric suctioning of meconium until initial resuscitation is complete. If the baby is vigorous, intratracheal suctioning is not recommended. This technique has not been subject to meta-analysis.

Hypothermia

There is accumulating evidence that controlled hypothermia to 35 °C for 72 hours may significantly reduce the adverse outcome (death and disability) in term babies born with severe birth asphyxia. Wyatt JS, Gluckman PD, Lin PY, et al. Determinants of outcomes after head cooling for neonatae encephalophaty. Pediatrics 2007;119:912–21. This is the subject of ongoing research (TOBY TRIAL). It is, however, not appropriate to inadvertently allow a baby to become cold during resuscitation and it is particularly disadvantageous in preterm infants, in whom it has been shown to increase mortality. Conversely, inadvertent hyperthermia must be avoided during resuscitation and this may occur as a result of an overhead warmer. This may cause an exacerbation of cerebral injury.

Various methods have been evaluated to maintain body temperature in prematurely born infants whilst in the delivery room. One method uses a barrier to prevent heat loss: four studies have evaluated either wrapping the baby from the neck down in a plastic sheet or placing the baby in a warmed plastic bag secured at the baby's neck. A Cochrane systematic review of these randomized controlled trials showed that this method significantly reduced heat loss in premature babies below 32 weeks[156] and was particularly effective in babies below 28 weeks of gestation. These studies did not show that there was a significant reduction in duration of hospital admission, major brain injury or duration of oxygen therapy. Another study of reducing heat loss by a tightly fitting hat showed that this method of reducing heat loss was ineffective.

Early versus delayed umbilical cord clamping

Controversy exists concerning the timing of clamping of the umbilical cord following birth. Delayed clamping allows blood to be transferred from the placenta to the baby until pulsation of the cord ceases. It has been suggested that this may result in a lower incidence of respiratory distress and the need for fewer blood transfusions. Early clamping will allow the baby to be more rapidly resuscitated and in theory prevent hypothermia, polycythemia and hyperbilirubinemia in premature infants. Seven randomized controlled trials have been conducted to compare early clamping (less than 30 s) with delayed cord clamping (30–120 s) and these studies have been evaluated in a Cochrane review.[157] Delayed clamping was associated with a reduced number of blood transfusions, less hypotension and fewer intraventricular hemorrhages compared with a group who had early clamping. The current evidence supports the recommendation that delayed clamping is of benefit in prematurely born infants.

WHEN TO STOP RESUSCITATION

All babies should be considered for active resuscitation unless they are macerated or show an obvious lethal congenital malformation. The prognosis for very immature babies of 23 weeks' gestation and below is extremely poor[158,159] and it is important to discuss with the parents prior to the delivery in light of the poor prognosis whether it is appropriate to offer vigorous resuscitation. The parents should be encouraged to consider whether they wish their baby to receive resuscitation at birth and their views should be respected. If the baby is vigorous at birth it may be appropriate to resuscitate fully and transfer the baby to the neonatal unit where with time a more considered decision can be made about the continuation of intensive care.

In mature infants failure to achieve a spontaneous cardiac output after 10 min of vigorous resuscitation indicates a very poor prognosis and resuscitation should be abandoned. A more difficult situation is when the baby has a reasonable cardiac output but fails to breathe. Other causes of respiratory failure must first be considered such as maternal drug effect and neuromuscular disorders. If the baby is not breathing by 40 min and particularly if he remains extremely depressed with severe hypotonia, then further active resuscitation should be considered to be inappropriate. The most senior doctor available should make this decision. If there is any doubt it is best to take the baby to the neonatal intensive care unit until such time as a full assessment can be made. It is much easier for the parents to mourn the loss of their baby if they are convinced that full resuscitation

was attempted and they will come to terms with it better if they have time to understand the severe problems that are present. Parents should be encouraged to hold their baby when resuscitative efforts are abandoned.

THE SMALL FOR GESTATIONAL AGE INFANT (Fig. 12.11)

The World Health Organization in 1950 defined a baby as small for gestational age (SGA) when it was below the 10th weight centile for gestation. At that time perinatal mortality of this group even in the Western world was very high. Obstetric deaths due to placental failure in utero and acute intrapartum asphyxia were relatively common. Neonatal problems such as pulmonary hemorrhage and hypoglycemia were inadequately treated and the mortality and morbidity from congenital rubella was more common (immunization schedules were not introduced until 1966 in the UK). Times have now changed but the definition has not. With modern antenatal and intrapartum care it is unusual for the pediatrician to be confronted by an unexpectedly small baby. Intrauterine and peripartum asphyxia and death are rarities. Rubella embryopathy is much less common and ultrasound policies for infants early diagnosed as small may allow termination of pregnancy for a lethal congenital abnormality. Better feeding policies postnatally have made all but the smallest of light for dates babies (SGA) manageable with care on the postnatal wards. It is unlikely that the baby more than 1800 g birth weight will need to be transferred to the neonatal unit if delivery care and care on the postnatal wards are appropriate.

ETIOLOGY
Maternal causes

These consist of in utero starvation and placental insufficiency [essential hypertension, pregnancy associated hypertension (PET), chronic renal disease, long-standing diabetes, heart disease in pregnancy, multiple pregnancy, poor socioeconomic circumstances with severe malnutrition, excess smoking, excess alcohol, living at high altitude]. Classically, placental insufficiency leads to asymmetric growth retardation, the weight being more affected than the length or particularly the

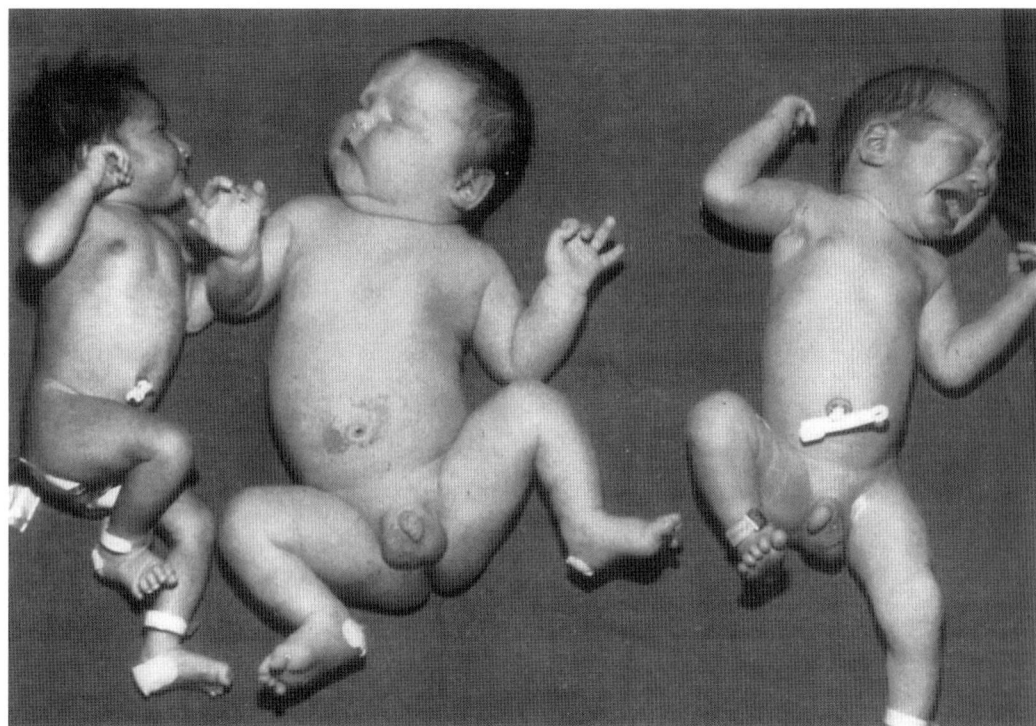

Fig. 12.11 Size with gestation. The baby on the left at 1.7 kg and 39 weeks is small for gestational age. The baby on the right is 1.9 kg and 34 weeks' gestation and is both appropriate for gestation and preterm. The center baby at 4.4 kg and 39 weeks' gestation is large for gestational age.

head circumference. The obstetrician may identify this problem in utero, ultrasound showing a small abdominal and thoracic circumference and a relatively spared head circumference. Small mothers and elderly primigravidae tend to have smaller than average babies.

Fetal causes

These include congenital abnormality (chromosomal and many syndromes, e.g. Potter) and congenital infection (rubella, toxoplasmosis, cytomegalovirus, herpes simplex and syphilis) as well as early fetal toxins such as alcohol, phenytoin and warfarin. Such infants usually display symmetrical growth retardation, the head size being as retarded as the weight and length.

PROBLEMS OF THE SGA BABY

Hypoglycemia

A large proportion of SGA babies develop hypoglycemia, which may be present before birth. The etiology after birth is complex.

1. Reduced glycogen deposits (in liver, muscle and heart).
2. The brain and heart (but not the liver, spleen, thymus and adrenals) are large in proportion to the rest of the body and have high energy substrate demands.
3. A reduced catecholamine response to a falling blood sugar suggests that the adrenal medulla is failing with consequent reduced glycogenolysis.
4. Rapid glucose disappearance may in some cases be due to high insulin levels. However many infants show a reduced insulin response to a glucose load which suggests either a defect in peripheral glucose utilization or reduced insulin sensitivity.
5. Defective lipolysis is suggested by reduced levels of beta-hydroxybutyrate and lack of the normal inverse relationship between free fatty acids and blood sugar.
6. Hepatic gluconeogenesis is reduced. Frequently there are elevated levels of alanine, lactate and pyruvate and an alanine load does not provoke an appropriate increase in blood sugar. There may be a delay in the postnatal development of hepatic gluconeogenic enzymes.

Hypoglycemia may lead to neuroglycopenia. Clinical signs of apnea and convulsions do not occur until a blood sugar of less than 1 mmol/L has been present for several hours, probably because alternative substrates are available (glycerol, lactate, beta-hydroxybutyrate, acetoacetate). Nevertheless, Koh et al[160] have shown that auditory evoked potentials are compromised at much higher blood sugar levels so it is important to be obsessional in blood sugar management in these small infants.

Practically, in all except the very small for gestational age (less than 3rd centile), management can and should be on the postnatal ward.

Breast-feeding mothers are encouraged to breast-feed 3-hourly, and prefeed dextrostix or BM stix are done after 6 h for 48 h. If hypoglycemia less than 2.6 mmol/L is detected, 8 ml/kg of formula are given after each breast-feed on day 1 and 12 ml/kg after each feed on day 2, if necessary by nasogastric tube. After 48 h, if there has been no hypoglycemia the bottle feeds after the breast can be withdrawn gradually as the mother's milk comes in.

Bottle-fed babies should be given 90, 120, 150 ml/kg/day respectively on each of the first 3 days of life. Prefeed dextrostix or BM stix should be done at 6, 9, 12, 18, 24, 30, 36 and 48 h. If the blood sugar is low, <2.6 mmol/L, or the baby is asymptomatic add 2 ml/kg/feed of 50% dextrose. If the dextrostix is still low or the baby is vomiting or the hypoglycemia is symptomatic a drip of at least 90 ml/kg/24 h of 10% dextrose is required.

Hypoglycemia is unlikely to be problematic after 48 h of age if it has not been so beforehand.

A baby both small for gestational age and less than 1800 g should probably be admitted to the neonatal unit for observation and treatment.

Infants with transient diabetes mellitus are usually small for gestational age.

Hypothermia

SGA infants may be born with a temperature above mother's as the inefficient placenta will not exchange heat. The scraggy baby with large surface area:body weight ratio may cool fast after delivery if appropriate steps are not taken to prevent this (p. 221).

Polycythemia

The high altitude effect associated with poor placental oxygen transfer leads to increased packed cell volume, red cell mass and high erythropoietin levels. This may lead to viscosity problems. Sheer stresses may reduce the platelet count and on rare occasions liberated platelet thromboplastins may set off disseminated intravascular coagulation (DIC). It is appropriate if the baby looks plethoric to do a venous packed cell volume (PCV) and also platelet count and clotting tests. Treatment with partial exchange transfusion may be required on occasions and vitamin K should be given (p. 295).

Neutropenia and thrombocytopenia

Severely SGA infants, particularly those less than 1000 g birth weight, may show neutropenia and thrombocytopenia.[161] Platelets may be reduced in number partly by the mechanisms mentioned above but it may be that the marrow in utero is more committed to manufacture of red cell series (high normoblasts) because of hypoxia and there is a temporary reduction in the ability to produce other cells after birth.

Hypocalcemia

This is less commonly seen now that babies are delivered in good condition by the obstetric team. It was probably related to perinatal asphyxia but the pathophysiology is not clear.

Infection

With modern management it is rare for SGA infants to develop a postnatal infection unless they are in addition very preterm.

Congenital abnormality

Three to six percent of SGA babies have congenital abnormalities; these are usually obvious and lethal such as the chromosome abnormalities, Potter syndrome and the baby with disseminated congenital infection.

Meconium aspiration

This is rare with modern obstetric management.

Pulmonary hemorrhage

This was probably related to intrapartum asphyxia and polycythemia. Modern obstetric and pediatric practice should identify and rectify these problems before hemorrhage results.

Other humoral and metabolic abnormalities

High ammonia, urea and uric acid levels after birth may reflect the reduced calorie reserve of these infants or a protein catabolic state. High circulating cortisol, corticosterone and growth hormone levels have also been demonstrated at birth.

CLINICAL FEATURES OF SGA BABIES

A minority of infants will have obvious congenital abnormalities, chromosome defects or intrauterine infection. Most infants will be scraggy individuals with wasting, particularly of the thighs. The fingernails are mature and long and cracks and desquamation of the skin begin rapidly after birth. The infant is usually active and vigorous and apparently anxious lest his starved state in utero may continue after birth. Sucking is usually strong and the weight loss after birth is less than for an appropriately sized baby.

MANAGEMENT

Early obstetric diagnosis should be followed by a planned delivery in the presence of pediatric staff capable of skilled resuscitation. Labor and birth are asphyxial stresses so labor should be carefully monitored. The baby may be hypoglycemic at birth so a dextrostix should be performed immediately. If there are no signs of anomaly or infection the major pediatric concerns are to prevent hypothermia and hypoglycemia – hopefully on the normal postnatal ward.

OUTCOME

Babies with asymmetric growth retardation usually catch up to within the normal centiles after birth whereas many symmetrically growth retarded infants do not. Unless they suffer symptomatic hypoglycemia, they will in all probability develop with a normal DQ and later IQ. Babies that are SGA because of syndromes, chromosome abnormalities and intrauterine infections will have a high neonatal mortality and later morbidity.

THE LARGE FOR GESTATIONAL AGE INFANT (Fig. 12.11)

By definition heavier than the 90th weight centile for gestation.

ETIOLOGY

1. Constitutionally large baby from heavy large mother.
2. Maternal diabetes or prediabetes – the infant of the diabetic mother (IDM) or the infant of the gestational diabetic mother (IGDM).
3. Severe erythroblastosis.
4. Other causes of hydrops fetalis and ascites.
5. Transposition of the great arteries (sometimes).
6. Syndromes:
   a. Beckwith–Wiedemann (BW) syndrome (p. 337)
   b. Sotos syndrome
   c. Marshall syndrome
   d. Weaver syndrome.

PROBLEMS OF LARGE FOR GESTATIONAL AGE (LGA) BABIES

Birth asphyxia and trauma

Shoulder dystocia may delay delivery leading to low Apgars, acidosis, meconium aspiration and hypoxic–ischemic encephalopathy and the consequent interventions may lead to fractured clavicle or long bones, brachial plexus injury (Erb or phrenic palsy), subdural or cephalhematoma and skin bruising (later resulting in jaundice).

Hypoglycemia

The IDM, IGDM, baby with erythroblastosis and BW syndrome baby all have hyperinsulinism leading to reactive hypoglycemia after birth.

Polycythemia

Unusual.

Apparent large postnatal weight loss

A 5 kg baby may naturally lose more than 0.5 kg in weight over a few days (10% body weight being 500 g) even if supplied with adequate milk.

CARE OF THE PRETERM INFANT

DEVELOPMENTAL CARE

INTRODUCTION

Changes in neonatal care over the last 25 years have had a significant impact on infant mortality and morbidity. The increasing survival of low birth weight infants and especially those born at the limits of viability has created new challenges; in particular how best to reduce the increasing incidence of developmental delay, neurosensory impairment and cerebral palsy that accompanies extreme prematurity.[162,163] These infants, with their rapidly developing and extremely vulnerable brains, spend many weeks in an environment that is in stark contrast to that of the protective uterus. Whilst it is accepted that fetal development and experience might not be an appropriate model for determining newborn care, animal studies provide evidence that positive and negative early experiences can alter the structure and function of the developing brain.[164]

The theoretical framework underpinning the 'developmentally supportive' model of care is that the neonatal intensive care unit (NICU) environment and activities associated with medical and nursing interventions are developmentally unexpected and therefore are likely to be stressful for both infant and parent. Decreasing this stress enables greater physiological and behavioral stability, better attainment of developmental skills and more positive engagement with the caregiver.[165] The provision of developmental care interventions is based on recognizing stress and stability cues in the infant (and parent), using them to positively modify environmental stimuli, care activities, and human interactions.

FETAL SENSORY RESPONSES

From conception to birth, fetal development and maturation is continuously influenced by the varied sensory experiences within the uterus. The neurosensory system develops in an orderly and predictive manner so that by 28 weeks' gestation the neural pathways for tactile, vestibular and chemosensory perception are well established and functional: contralateral movement to touch,[166] sucking,[167] altered swallow pattern to changes in amniotic fluid composition,[166] tachycardia and excessive movement with vibroacoustic stimulation[168,169] are seen. At this gestation the auditory and visual pathways are still establishing but the fetus responds physiologically and behaviorally to stimulation and is able to recognize the maternal voice.[170–172]

NICU ENVIRONMENT

In the mid 1970s Cornell and Gottfried[173] summarized the literature on sensory stimulation of premature infants and concluded that the NICU environment was not lacking in stimulation but rather it was inconsistent and inappropriate to the needs of the newborn. Neonatal units are frequently places of extreme stimulation because they present experiences which are not the norm for the developing infant:

- Cutaneous stimulation commonly takes the form of medical/nursing procedures with little opportunity for gentle and comforting care.
- Movement is often prohibited and restricted by the use of equipment and/or bedding.
- Alcohol or other antiseptic solutions are frequently presented to infants and positive taste experiences are seldom reinforced unless the infant is receiving oral feeds.
- Sound is created by staff/parent activities and conversation, use of routine equipment and alarm mechanisms; the reported range of sound within the NICU is between 53 and 90 dB with bursts of excessive loudness over 90 dB with no attenuation of higher frequencies.
- Lighting levels depend upon postmenstrual age (reflecting maturity), illness acuity, number and location of exposed windows, incubator/cot position within the unit and seasonal changes. Exposure can be between 24 and 150 foot-candles; this might be continuous lighting, intermittent for procedures and/or treatment (phototherapy = 300–400 foot-candles) or natural daylight (1000 foot-candles).

Stimulation from the NICU environment has a physiological and functional impact on the infant. Whilst some changes in state are considered to be normal arousal responses others are considered to be stress signals.

Caregiving activities

Prematurely born infants respond to touch differently than term infants; they show an increased sensitivity in both flexion withdrawal and general body movements.[174] This increased sensitization may account for the stress responses seen in relation to routine caregiving[175–177] and oral feeding.[167] Whilst individually these disruptions may be short lasting, they may endure throughout the first year of life and can lead to complications in adulthood.[178–180]

Minimal handling and clustering of care procedures has become the norm so that the infant has prolonged rest periods between disturbances. However these practices appear to stress the infant[181] and increase the infant's sensitivity to painful interventions.[182,183] The available literature suggests it would be prudent to reduce the frequency of handling episodes and perhaps more importantly to reconsider the number of interventions clustered together at any one time.

When a procedure or investigation has been completed, the infant is positioned to promote physiological stability and secure fixation of equipment. Traditional positioning strategies, for example the use of flat unyielding surfaces and prolonged lying in either supine or prone position, may have long-lasting effects on the infant and child. Whilst quality of movement and subsequent performance is strongly correlated with degrees of neurological abnormality,[184] preterm infants who have little or no cerebral abnormality on ultrasound scanning exhibit dysfunction in movement and postural control as they grow older.[185] It is suggested these abnormalities stem from early experiences of being less mobile with less opportunity to 'learn' from the different positions.[186] 'Supportive positioning' attempts to override these limitations by incorporating techniques and aids that promote physiological stability whilst encouraging a balance between flexion and extension and facilitating self-regulatory behavior.[187] Use of these strategies results in significantly fewer stress responses as denoted by a lower heart rate, improved oxygenation, less crying and fewer sleep state changes.[188,189] Other handling techniques that seem to have benefit are comforting touch and massage and skin-to-skin care.[190] In the systematic review by Vickers[191] gentle still touch showed no negative effects on infants but did reduce motor activity and behavioral distress. Studies on massage showed that the intervention brought about physiological stability in more mature infants but induced hypoxia and tachypnea in the immature infant. Studies on skin-to-skin care (as reported by Harrison[190]) indicate that there are physiological and behavioral advantages for the infant if held in the 'kangaroo position'. The systematic review by Conde-Agudelo[192] concludes that although kangaroo mother care appears to reduce severe infant morbidity without any serious deleterious effect reported, there is still insufficient evidence to recommend its routine use in LBW infants.

This work highlights the fragility of premature infants to non-noxious stimuli and should remind the caregiver to consider frequency and timing of interventions.[176]

Environmental effects

Two features of the environment that have been examined extensively are sound and light. In the NICU the infant is exposed to chaotic and variable levels of sound originating from a multitude of sources. In terms of perceived loudness, for each increase of 6 dB, the perceived loudness doubles. Even when the unit is thought to be quiet (35 dB), the level perceived by the infant might exceed 60 dB.[193] Morris et al[194] reviewed the literature about the effects of sound on the newborn. The authors describe physiological and behavioral responses of infants to mild to high range (55–100 dB) stimuli. When presented with sound stimuli, infants increase their heart rates whilst respiration effects are more variable and associated with maturity, age and previous exposure. Low frequency stimulation is also noted to increase blood pressure and produce fluctuations in intracranial pressure and oxygenation. Unlike the term infant, the premature infant does not readily habituate to the stimulus but is continuously aroused by it. Whilst respiratory pattern appears to be more related to sleep wake state than acoustic stimulation, acoustic stimulation can affect sleep state and thus adversely influence respiratory pattern and oxygenation.[195] The literature to date focuses on immediate and medium term deleterious effects of sound in the infant but little is known about the optimal sound level for stability.[194,196] Slevin[197] showed that introducing a quiet period altered ambient noise levels and staff behavior considerably but these changes had little effect on the infant's heart and respiratory rate and oxygenation. Rather the impact was seen by an increase in restfulness. Supplemental sound interventions appear promising for the stable infant greater than 28 weeks' postmenstrual age. In a meta-analysis on music therapy for premature infants, Standley[198] concludes that 'Music alone or combined with the human voice would seem to be a valuable resource for enhancing developmental goals in the NICU, functioning to reduce stress, to provide developmental stimulation during a critical period of growth, to promote bonding with parents, or to facilitate neurological, communication, and social development'.[198]

Concern has also been raised as to whether, in the absence of impairment of functional hearing, there is some alteration in the recognition and integration of sound. The high levels of continuous sound or 'white noise' and lack of rhythm mask the infant's ability to make associations between source and sound; it has been postulated that this may account for the difficulties which preterm infants experience with concept learning and recognition.[199] Apart from these physiological and behavioral responses, prematurely born infants also show more hearing related disorders than term infants (approximately 13% of premature infants experience significant hearing loss compared to 2% of term infants). However there is little to suggest a cause and effect response between the NICU sound environment and the impairment.

At term the visual system is functionally relatively immature. Given this and the typical lighting of the NICU, concern has been expressed about the impact that light levels and lighting pattern might have on the visual system of the developing infant.[200] In the healthy preterm infant visual maturation proceeds in the expected fashion irrespective of the exposure of the infant to light. However, between 1% and 3% of the preterm population have visual impairments which are associated with birth weight, cerebral hypoxia/hyperoxia, intraventricular hemorrhage and lung function.[201] Studies have generally focused on light exposure and the effect of illumination on the incidence of retinopathy, physiological stability and the development of circadian rhythm.

There is no evidence to suggest that continuous bright or variable lighting affects the incidence of retinopathy.[202] It does however affect physiological stability and circadian rhythm development. High lighting level is implicated in disturbing sleep and producing stress-like responses in the infant: variable heart rate pattern, increased respiratory rate and activity and a reduction in oxygenation.[203–205] Cycled levels of lighting appear to have the greatest impact on infant well-being. When compared to continuous high or dim lighting, cycled lighting promotes physiological stability, improved growth, increased sleep time and earlier entrainment of circadian rhythms.[200,204–207]

Newborn infants have acute chemosensory perception. When presented with various olfactory stimuli preterm infants respond with facial movements and changes in heart and respiratory rate and cerebral oxygenation.[208–211] These alterations equate with stress signals and are seen more often in infants presented with noxious compared to pleasant or control odors. Schaal[208] describes several studies where the maternal odor or that of breast milk elicits a calming effect on full-term infants and higher non-nutritive sucking episodes when compared with formula milk or neutral odors in preterm infants.

A recent systematic review of non-nutritive sucking found that the activity was associated with decreased length of stay for infants on the NICU and was beneficial in promoting the transition of infants from gastric to oral feeding.[212] Furthermore it is found to be effective in decreasing the effect of a painful intervention (eye examination). The magnitude of the effect was greater when non-nutritive sucking was combined with the administration of sucrose.[213] Although odors and non-nutritive sucking can help relieve stress, Schaal[208] cautions that care should be taken not to produce negative conditioning which might interfere with the infant's developing social relationship.

CONCLUSION

This review has considered the effects of single interventions on the reduction of infant stress and promotion of infant stability. Multimodal stimulation, specific developmental care assessment programs and parent support have not been taken into account. When proposing interventions to reduce stress and promote stability, it should be noted that it is unlikely that any one intervention has a single mode of action. For example, modifying the environment to promote auditory recognition may positively impact on the development of visual and motor systems and collectively or individually these may affect the developing parent – infant relationship.

SPECIAL CARE – FLUID BALANCE

During fetal life, the placenta maintains biochemical homeostasis even in the absence of fetal renal function. Immediately following birth, however, the kidney becomes essential for chemical and fluid balance. The preterm infant is particularly vulnerable, and dehydration and hyponatremia are the commonest problems.[214]

BODY WATER CONTENT AND DISTRIBUTION
Changes in body fluid related to delivery

Plasma sodium concentration in the newborn correlates closely with maternal plasma sodium concentration at delivery.[215] Crystalloid fluids administered to laboring mothers equilibrate across the placenta and increase fetal extracellular fluid (ECF) volume. Subsequently, at delivery, stress hormones, including glucocorticoids, aldosterone, antidiuretic hormone and angiotensin[216] are elevated in the newborn and may contribute to salt and/or water retention.

Postnatal changes

The ratio of ECF to intracellular fluid (ICF) decreases in the immediate postnatal period owing to water loss from the ECF space. A postnatal weight loss of 5–8% of birth weight is common in term infants, the nadir occurring around the fifth day with birth weight usually regained by the tenth day. An even greater percentage weight loss of 12–21% may occur in premature infants.[217] Whilst some of this weight loss is meconium, vernix and the umbilical stump, most is water derived from the ECF space.

ECF comprises interstitial fluid and circulating blood and most of the early postnatal weight loss is due to a reduction in interstitial fluid volume since plasma volume is well maintained over the first week of postnatal life. The interstitial fluid lost from the body as urine is virtually isotonic,[218] and the negative sodium and water balance and weight loss which result from this appear to be obligatory as these are not prevented by administration of water, sodium or both.[219]

WATER BALANCE

To maintain a stable water balance:
- Water intake
- = water for growth
- + insensible losses (respiratory losses + transepidermal losses)
- + sensible losses (sweat + urine + fecal losses).

Pre-existing deficits or overload must also be corrected to achieve fluid balance.

Water for growth

Approximately 75% of increase in weight in utero is water. If the intrauterine growth velocity of approximately 16 g/kg/24 h[220] is to be sustained in infants born preterm, 12 ml/kg/24 h of water intake will be diverted towards growth, mostly into the ICF space. However, if the infant is not being fed enterally or parenterally, this consideration of water for growth is irrelevant as intravenous crystalloid solutions contain no nitrogen for anabolism.

Respiratory water losses

Inspired air is humidified and warmed by the respiratory tract so that expired air leaves the nose and mouth almost fully saturated at a temperature of 35–36 °C. The amount of water lost from the respiratory tract is inversely proportional to the humidity of the inspired air – highest when the inspired air is dry and non-existent when it is fully saturated. Such water loss will also depend on the minute volume, the product of tidal volume and respiratory rate – around 7 ml/kg/24 h at an ambient humidity of 50% in term infants[221] and similar in preterm infants in the absence of respiratory disease. The management of the fluid balance of the very immature infant is, therefore, simplified if a high humidity (> 90%) is provided within the incubator or ventilator circuit.

Transepidermal water loss

Transepidermal water loss (TEWL) is the passive diffusion of water through the epidermis and is dependent on the ambient humidity and temperature. TEWL is lower in the full-term newborn (6–10 ml/kg/24 h) than in the child or adult. Values are much higher in preterm infants in the days after birth, especially before 30 weeks' gestation, as a result of their poorly developed keratinized layer of epidermis. As the stratum corneum rapidly matures in the first 2 weeks of life, TEWL falls towards term values.[222] The relationship between TEWL and ambient relative humidity is such that TEWL is much higher if the surrounding air is dry and is abolished when it is fully saturated. TEWL is also increased by phototherapy and radiant heat. As infants nursed naked on radiant heaters can lose 200–300 ml/kg/day as TEWL, the management of the fluid balance of very immature infants is simplified if a high ambient humidity is routinely provided within the incubator for infants less than 30 weeks' gestation or less than 1000 g in the first week (Grade D, Level 5).[223] Humidification close to 100% can be achieved if incubator ports are kept closed, reducing TEWL by 50% in infants 24–27 weeks' gestation.

Respiratory and transepidermal water loss together make up insensible water loss. This, measured as insensible weight loss, is around 15 ml/kg/24 h for a term infant. Values in preterm infants are higher (especially in the very immature infant in the early neonatal period, because TEWL is so high), ranging from 15 to 120 ml/kg/24 h, and depend on gestational age, postnatal age and ambient conditions.[224] Insensible water loss is best derived by adding 7 ml/kg/24 h (respiratory water loss) to the values of TEWL shown in Table 12.9.[222]

Sweating

The ability to sweat is impaired in the term newborn compared with children or adults. If heat stress is sufficient to raise the body temperature above 37.5 °C, evaporative water loss increases by a factor of two to four – an increase from 15 to 30–60 ml/kg/24 h. Before 30 weeks' gestation, sweating is absent in the first 2 weeks and can be ignored in fluid balance consideration. From 30 weeks to 36 weeks' gestation, sweating does not appear until a few days after birth and is limited compared with that of a term infant.

Fecal water loss

Fecal water losses are usually around 5–10 ml/kg/24 h. However, such losses can be excessive and may lead to profound fluid imbalance in infants with diarrhea or an enterostomy. As infants with high

Table 12.9 Average values of transepidermal water loss (in ml/kg/24 h) at an ambient relative humidity of 50%. There is wide individual variation in the higher values. Data from Hammarlund et al[222]

Gestation (weeks)	Postnatal age (days)						
	1	3	5	7	14	21	28
25–27	110	71	51	43	32	28	24
28–30	39	32	27	24	18	15	15
31–36	11	12	12	12	9	8	7
37–41	6	6	6	6	6	6	7

fecal losses increase renal reabsorption of water and sodium, tracking of renal sodium excretion can be useful as a low urinary sodium may precede other signs of dehydration.

Urinary losses

During early postnatal life, the kidney of even a full-term infant has a limited capacity to produce concentrated urine and fractional sodium excretion is usually high. In the immediate period after birth, urine production falls and the urine becomes more concentrated. Failure to pass urine postnatally is not clinically significant until 24 h have elapsed (7% of neonates do not void in the first 24 h),[225] unless there are other pointers to a urogenital abnormality. This oliguric period may be due to the high levels of antidiuretic hormone in the newborn following birth as there is no evidence of a fall in glomerular filtration rate (GFR). Indeed, over the first week of postnatal life, both GFR[226] and blood pressure increase in term and premature infants and the initial period of oliguria and relatively concentrated urine is followed by a diuresis of isotonic, or even hypotonic, urine[227] and contraction of the ECF volume. Overall, in the VLBW infant, GFR varies from 0.4 to 1.0 ml/min/kg with a mean of 0.7 ml/min/kg at 26 weeks' gestation and 0.84 ml/min/kg at 33 weeks.[226] Given the reported maximum concentrating capacity of 800 mOsm/kg of urine (Table 12.10), compared to 1200 mOsm/kg of urine for an adult, and average renal solute load, fluid intake should be such as to maintain a minimum urine output of 1 ml/kg/h.

WATER REQUIREMENTS

The aims of fluid management are to maintain satisfactory volumes of total body water (TBW), ICF and ECF, normal tissue perfusion, a normal blood pressure and a normal plasma sodium concentration. Changes in plasma sodium during the first week of life are usually due to changes in water balance rather than sodium balance.[219] In the first week of preterm life, hypernatremia is commonly secondary to inadequate fluid replacement in the face of excessive insensible losses and hyponatremia is usually due to excessive intravenous fluids.

Four randomized controlled trials were included in a Cochrane review of liberal water intake (the standard or control group) versus a restricted water intake[227] (Grade A level 1a). In the von Stockhausen study[228] (n = 56, 'most of whom were premature' – published in German), the prescribed water intake was given only during the first 3 days of life; in the Lorenz study[229] (n = 88, 750–1500 g), only during the first 5 days; in the Tammela study[230] (n = 100, <1751 g), between 24 h and 28 days; in the Bell study[231] (n = 170, 751–2000 g), before 72 h up to 30 days (Table 12.11).[228–231]

A significantly greater postnatal weight loss occurred in the restricted water intake groups. There was no difference in intracranial hemorrhage, and the trend towards less bronchopulmonary dysplasia in the restricted water intake groups was not statistically significant. The risks of persistent ductus arteriosus, necrotizing enterocolitis and death (Table 12.12) were statistically significantly lower with restricted water intake in the overall analysis.

The interpretation of the overall analysis was heavily influenced by the Bell study since this contained most participants. This study also continued the restriction for the longest duration. Moreover, all the infants were enrolled at least a decade ago and only limited numbers of ELBW infants were included and there would be few units in the UK now using fluid regimens in early postnatal life as liberal as those in these trials. These studies did not control for sodium intake and it is not clear

Table 12.10   Normal renal function in newborn infants in the first week of life

Glomerular filtration rate	0.35–0.85 ml/kg/min
Urine flow rate	1.0–3.0 ml/kg/h
Urine osmolality	45–800 mOsm/kg

Table 12.11   Fluid regimens

	Restricted water intake (ml/kg/day)	Liberal water intake (ml/kg/day)
Von Stockhausen[228]	60	150
Lorenz[229]		
Day 1	65–70	80
Increasing gradually to day 5	80	140
Tammela[230]		
Day 1	50	80
Day 2	60	100
Day 3	70	120
Day 4	80	150
Day 5	90	150
Day 6	100	150
Day 7	120	150
Thereafter	150	200
Bell[231]	Mean 122 ml/kg/day throughout study period	Mean 169 ml/kg/day throughout study period

how many infants were exposed to antenatal steroids or postnatal surfactant. Furthermore, the analysis included five infants in the Tammela study who died on the first day of life. It could be argued these were too early to be influenced by the fluid regimen. If these five, who were all in the liberal fluid group, were excluded from analysis, restriction of water intake would no longer significantly affect the risk of death. This Cochrane review[227] does not include the study by Kavvadia et al[225] (n = 168, 486–1500 g), described below, which may ultimately influence the overall analysis of the systematic review. Future work required in this regard is outlined in Table 12.13.

GESTATIONAL AGE AND POSTNATAL AGE

Fluid requirements depend on gestational age. The premature infant has a greater surface area to volume ratio, a thinner epidermis and more limited renal water conservation than a term infant. The premature infant is also more likely to require ventilation and phototherapy, and be nursed under a radiant heater. Fluid requirements also vary with postnatal age, increasing during the first week of life to cope with the transition from oliguria to diuresis and reaching a plateau as water balance is restored and birth weight is regained. Fluid requirements do not fall again until after the first 6 months of life.

If the infant is fed enterally, all or part of the water requirement is delivered in breast or formula milk. If the infant is not fed, all the water must be administered intravenously. This may be incorporated into a total parenteral nutrition regimen (providing other essentials such as nitrogen) or as 10% dextrose solution on the first day and 10% dextrose/0.18% saline thereafter (see section on sodium balance).

Water requirements for well infants may be given according to Table 12.14 and, provided there is no water retention due to inappropriate secretion of antidiuretic hormone (ADH) or excessive water loss due to transepidermal evaporation, plasma sodium concentration generally remains within the normal range as urinary losses are initially isotonic. However, greater caution is advisable in sick and ELBW infants for whom more cautious daily increments should be guided by changes in daily body weight, hyper- or hyponatremia and calculated and insensible losses. Thus, fluid administration must be adjusted in light of continuing assessment of fluid balance and the presence of the conditions in Table 12.15.

CRYSTALLOID VERSUS COLLOID

Colloid is not routinely given to newborn infants as part of their fluid balance management. Historically, colloid was used in an attempt to

Table 12.12 Risks of persistent ductus arteriosus, necrotizing enterocolitis (NEC) and death on low compared to high fluid intake regimen

	Typical RR (95% CI)	Typical RD (95% CI)	Number needed to treat to prevent one case (95% CI)
Persistent ductus arteriosus	0.40 (0.26, 0.63)	−0.19 (−0.27, −0.11)	5.3 (3.7, 9.1)
NEC	0.30 (0.13, 0.71)	−0.08 (−0.14, −0.03)	11.9 (7.2, 33.3)
Death	0.52 (0.28, 0.96)	−0.06 (−0.12, −0.01)	15.9 (8.4, 167)

Table 12.13 Future work required

- ELBW infants
- Critical period over which water intake must be controlled
- A larger study to determine whether mortality really is reduced
- New trials with the previous 'restricted' regimens as the control arm and even greater restriction during the early postnatal period as the intervention arm, provided infants are nursed in incubators rather than under radiant warmers

ELBW, extremely low birth weight.

Table 12.14 Daily fluid requirements for well infants (ml/kg/24 h)

	Day 1	Day 2	Day 3	Day 4	Day 5
Premature infants	60	90	120	120–150	120–150
Term infants	40	60	80	110	120–150

Table 12.15 Fluid intake alterations

Conditions in which fluid restriction should be considered
  ELBW infants nursed in 100% humidification with humidified respiratory gases
  Persistent ductus arteriosus, especially if indometacin given
  Hypoxic–ischemic encephalopathy
  Severe respiratory distress
  Oliguric renal failure
  Inappropriate release of ADH

Conditions in which fluid requirements are increased
  Excessive insensible water loss
  Use of a radiant warmer
  Phototherapy
  Vomiting
  Diarrhea
  Polyuria (e.g. due to glycosuria or following relief of obstructive uropathy)

ADH, antidiuretic hormone; ELBW, extremely low birth weight.

treat reduced tissue perfusion and hypotension but these are better managed with dopamine (Grade A, Level 1a).[232] Whether colloid administration may actually increase mortality in resuscitation and intensive care settings[233] is controversial and caution is necessary in interpreting studies involving heterogeneous indications and patient groups. The possible role of colloid in the genesis of chronic lung disease (CLD) is discussed below.

ASSESSMENT OF WATER BALANCE

Water and sodium constitute the major solvent and solute of the ECF and water balance cannot be assessed independently of that of sodium. Most clinical and laboratory observations give information about the ECF volume rather than ICF volume.

Clinical examination

Heart rate, systemic arterial blood pressure, central venous pressure and skin–core temperature gradient are all variables which are related to intravascular volume and cardiac output. However, these signs are crude monitors of fluid balance, and tachycardia, hypotension and poor perfusion are features of decompensation following significant hypovolemia. Moreover, many factors other than fluid balance modulate cardiovascular responses.

Classic signs of decreased interstitial fluid volume are sunken eyes, a depressed fontanelle and reduced skin turgor but only semiquantitative interpretation is possible and this is much more difficult in premature infants in whom these skin changes may be less apparent. Furthermore, edema is not a reliable sign of fluid overload in the premature infant.[234]

Fluid balance charts

If obsessionally maintained, these are a helpful guide to monitoring fluid balance. Obviously, interpretation of the cumulative arithmetic balance must include possible insensible losses and may be very misleading if these are overlooked. The omission of volumes administered to flush vascular cannulae and as drug vehicles, as well as the omission of the blood volumes sampled (injudicious sampling may cause significant cumulative losses leading to anemia[235] and even hypovolemia), are important sources of error in calculated fluid balance.

Body weight

This is the best cot-side guide to TBW. Where fluid balance is important, the infant should be weighed daily, on the same scales and at the same time, particularly in relation to feeds. Serial body weights are of great value in distinguishing hyponatremia due to water overload from that due to sodium depletion. However, a stable or increasing body weight must be interpreted alongside the infant's evolving clinical condition as it may be falsely reassuring under circumstances in which TBW and intravascular volume do not move in parallel, e.g. concealed losses from the intravascular compartment into the so-called 'third space' in peritonitis and ileus, in hydrops and in congestive cardiac failure.

Urine flow rates

Estimation of urinary fluid loss is helpful in the fluid management of the preterm infant as are urine chemistry (see below), urine pH, glucose testing, specific gravity and osmolality (Fig. 12.12).[236] A urine specific gravity of between 1.005 and 1.012 is desirable as the newborn kidney is not then at the limits of its concentrating or diluting capacity. Specific gravity and osmolality are unreliable in the presence of glycosuria or significant proteinuria. The normal range for urine flow rates is given in Table 12.10. Although catheterization is best avoided wherever possible, urine output must be assessed in all infants when fluid balance is considered critical, particularly if there is evidence of renal disease. Bag collections may be reliable in male infants but the adhesive used may damage the skin of a very immature infant. Alternatively, the infant may be nursed on a plastic sheet and the urine collected with a syringe. Nursing infants on cotton wool or absorbent, plastic coated nappies which are weighed before and after micturition also have roles but may overestimate fluid loss in high incubator humidity.

Urine and plasma biochemistry

Plasma creatinine concentration is of limited value as an index of glomerular filtration in the newborn because:

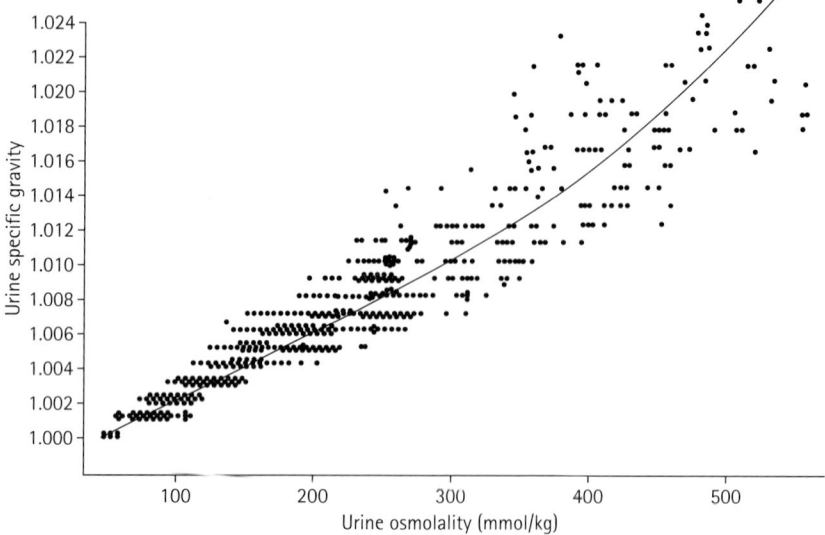

Fig. 12.12   Comparison of urinary specific gravity and urinary osmolality in 1000 urine samples. Third order regression line is shown: r = 0.97. (From Jones et al 1976[236] with permission.)

1. Initially the neonatal concentration mirrors the maternal concentration before birth.
2. Non-creatinine chromogens may interfere with measurement.
3. The reference range is wide.[226,237]

Similarly, the interpretation of urinary electrolytes is also difficult as the ranges encountered are so wide (Table 12.16).[238-240] Interpretation should always be made in the light of simultaneous plasma electrolytes and a clinical assessment. As fractional sodium excretion declines with increasing gestation and increasing postnatal age, fluid intake is best adjusted to maintain a normal plasma sodium concentration rather than relying on urinary measurements. Moreover, a high fractional sodium excretion may reflect excessive sodium supplements once these have been initiated.

Despite these caveats, urinary chemistry may be of value in distinguishing oliguria due to hypovolemia (guiding an increase in fluid administration) from established renal failure, when fluid intake should be restricted. As another cause of oliguria is inappropriate ADH secretion, urinary electrolytes and osmolality are necessary for the definitive diagnosis before initiating fluid restriction. Although in VLBW infants, random urine creatinine concentration is related to instantaneous urine flow rate by the formula: urine flow rate (ml/kg/24 h) = 90/urine creatinine concentration (μmol/L), the 95% confidence limits are wide.[237]

Plasma albumin and colloid osmotic pressure

Albumin concentration accounts for 70% of colloid osmotic pressures (COP). The two measurements are closely correlated in the premature newborn and both increase postnatally, in a similar fashion to the increase in fetal albumin concentration in utero. However, low albumin concentrations

Table 12.16   Normal reference values for urinary excretion

Term infants	Mean	SD
Sodium*	1.63	(0.78) mmol/kg/24 h
Potassium*	0.68	(0.31) mmol/kg/24 h
Creatinine[†]	0.45	(0.23) mmol/24 h
Preterm infants	Median	Range
Sodium[§]	2.23	(0.18–4.12) mmol/kg/24 h
Potassium[§]	0.75	(0.06–3.50) mmol/kg/24 h
Creatinine	0.06	(0.03–0.36) mmol/kg/24 h

* Full term, appropriate weight, breast-fed babies during the first and second weeks of life.[238]
[†] Normal full term infants during the first month of life.[239]
[§] Male infants, 24–36 weeks' gestation, during the first week of life
(Stephenson & Broughton Pipkin, unpublished observations.)

correlate poorly with clinical edema[234] and, although high albumin concentrations may reflect reduction in plasma volume ('hemoconcentration'), this relationship has not been demonstrated directly.

Packed cell volume

Packed cell volume (PCV) falls with decreasing gestation and increasing postnatal age, but with great variability between individuals, so that single measurements are a poor guide to fluid balance. However, if serial measurements of PCV (a simple and reproducible task) show a rising trend in a sick infant, in whom erythropoiesis is usually depressed, then fluid intake is probably insufficient. Falling levels of PCV may be due to blood loss, red cell destruction or hemodilution and are, therefore, difficult to interpret.

POSSIBLE CLINICAL CONSEQUENCES OF WATER OVERLOAD AND DEFICIENCY

Poor control of water balance leads to both volume and osmolar changes within body fluid compartments. Overload of water and sodium, which if it is isotonic expands only the ECF, has been implicated in the pathogenesis of a number of neonatal disorders. The consequences of pure water overload and deficiency are discussed under the headings hyponatremia and hypernatremia.

Respiratory distress syndrome (RDS) and chronic lung disease (CLD)

In infants with RDS, the oliguric phase following birth persists for longer and there is correlation between the degree of oliguria and the minimum PaO_2.[241] There is also correlation between the duration of oliguria, the duration of oxygen therapy and the risk of bronchopulmonary dysplasia (BPD). Pharmacological muscle relaxation, at least with pancuronium, exacerbates this fluid retention with peripheral edema and weight gain[242] and special attention should be paid to fluid balance and brevity of the period of muscle relaxation. Colloid administration appears to adversely affect short term measures of lung function in the perinatal period.[243]

The orthodox view is that the onset of the diuretic phase precedes improvement in respiratory function but this has been questioned.[244,245] High levels of ADH[241] and angiotensin II have been reported in RDS, which would contribute to salt and water retention, and increased levels of atrial natriuretic peptide (ANP)[246] which would antagonize these hormones have been reported during the diuretic phase of RDS.[247] The use of diuretics in the treatment of acute RDS and CLD has given differing results (see also Energy, fluid and electrolyte requirements, Chronic lung disease).

The role of fluid intake between the first and seventh postnatal days (Table 12.17) in CLD has been studied in a trial in which 168 VLBW

Table 12.17 Prescribed fluid regimens

	Documented mean restricted fluid intake (crystalloid + colloid) (ml/kg/day)	Documented mean standard fluid intake (crystalloid + colloid) (ml/kg/day)
Day 1	66	86
Day 2	79	93
Day 3	84	114
Day 4	103	124
Day 5	121	142
Day 6	136	148
Day 7	146	159

ventilated infants, at high risk of CLD and routinely exposed to antenatal steroids and postnatal surfactant,[225] were randomized to liberal or restricted water intakes. Actual intakes initially exceeded the recommended regimen by up to 26 ml/kg/day, although variances from the trial protocol became smaller after the first 48 h of life.

There were no significant differences in the two primary outcome measures, the proportions developing chronic lung disease or surviving without chronic lung disease. There were no differences in the secondary outcomes of persistent ductus arteriosus, intracranial hemorrhage, NEC and death. Significantly fewer infants who received the restricted regimen received postnatal steroids after the first week (19% versus 43%), prescribed for infants fully ventilator dependent beyond 7 days or in 40% O_2 after 3 weeks, although it is unclear whether this was enforced by trial protocol or left to the clinicians' discretion. However, since the duration of ventilation (median 7 days in both) and O_2 dependency (median 40 days in the restricted group and 38 in the standard group) was similar, it is difficult to explain the difference in steroid therapy except to note that the trial was not blinded. In a post hoc analysis, volume of colloid infused was associated with duration of oxygen dependency. However, this was not a randomized intervention and colloid may well have been administered to sicker infants.

Persistent ductus arteriosus (PDA)

PDA is extremely common in premature infants and this has been associated with high fluid intake.[231] The persistence of the duct may be partly due to failure of the usual postnatal contraction in ECF and this, in turn, may be responsible for the elevated levels of ANP found with persistent ductus arteriosus.[248,249] Moreover, prostaglandin E_2, which is the most potent dilator of the duct,[250] is also involved in regulation of sodium balance, causing natriuresis. Elevated levels of PGE_2 may, therefore, be provoked by salt and water retention.

There has been no systematic trial of the place of fluid restriction in the treatment (as opposed to prevention) of PDA and, as in cardiac failure, given the importance of adequate calorific intake it may be more rational to restrict sodium and maintain fluid intake, using diuretics to reduce fluid overload if necessary. Diuretics can also be used with indometacin in the treatment of PDA since PGE_2 synthesis is inhibited by indometacin and fluid retention may result (see p. 267) although caution is important in the face of fluid depletion.[251]

In a number of other conditions, such as cardiac failure, renal failure or ascites, salt and water overload occurs as a *consequence* of organ dysfunction rather than as an etiological factor.

SPECIAL CARE – SODIUM AND POTASSIUM

BODY SODIUM CONTENT AND DISTRIBUTION

Sodium is the major extracellular cation. As the percentage of body weight which is ECF falls during fetal life, so the sodium content in the fetus falls from 94 mmol/kg at 25 weeks' gestation to 74 mmol/kg at term. However, with the continued increase in absolute fetal weight, there is a daily accretion of sodium in utero of about 1 mmol/kg/24 h.

Following birth, as there is isotonic contraction of the ECF, there is an inevitable loss of sodium during the first week which averages 14 (range 6–22) mmol/kg. This loss cannot be prevented but may be excessive if sodium intake is inadequate.[252] Negative sodium balance is maximal on day 4 and becomes positive by day 6 or 7,[253] provided sodium intake is maintained at 6–8 mmol/kg/24 h.

REGULATION OF SODIUM HOMEOSTASIS

The control of sodium and water balance is regulated by a number of homeostatic mechanisms to maintain a normal plasma sodium concentration (132–142 mmol/L) and normal circulating volume. Moreover, conservation of sodium throughout childhood is essential for growth. The regulating mechanisms are:

1. sodium and water intake under the influence of thirst;
2. glomerular filtration rate which determines the amount of sodium and water delivered to the renal tubules;
3. reabsorption of sodium and water by the renal tubules and collecting ducts.

The healthy term infant can respond to thirst by demand feeding but infants of less than 34 weeks' gestation have little control over intake (as solutes are delivered not sought). Moreover, as the rise in GFR over the first week outstrips the more gradual improvement in renal tubular sodium reabsorption, transient glomerulotubular imbalance develops and a high fractional sodium excretion results. Sodium sensors in the macula densa are stimulated by this high delivery of sodium to the distal tubule, as shown by correlation between urinary sodium and plasma renin even in very premature infants.[254] However, the immature nephron appears to be unresponsive to the high circulating concentrations of angiotensin II and aldosterone generated by this system. ANP levels are high in the immediate newborn period[255] and ANP inhibits the sodium-retaining actions of both angiotensin and aldosterone.[256]

This initial sodium-losing state continues until the end of the first week following which positive sodium balance ensues to ensure growth. Maturation of the aldosterone-dependent distal tubular reabsorption, which is gestation dependent but accelerated by birth, appears to be responsible for the transition to net sodium gain, since proximal tubular reabsorption is unchanged.

During the initial period of glomerulotubular imbalance, urine flow rates do not increase significantly[257] although GFR is increasing. This suggests that the collecting ducts are sensitive to ADH, the levels of which are high in the immediate newborn period.[253] The feedback control of ADH secretion is operative from 26 weeks' gestation (although inappropriate secretion of ADH also occurs commonly in this group[253]) and, as a result, plasma osmolality is normally maintained within a narrow range of 282–298 mOsm/kg despite variable water intake.

SODIUM BALANCE

To maintain a stable plasma sodium concentration and allow growth:

Required sodium intake

= sodium for growth (mostly increase in ECF)

+ sodium lost [in urine + in sweat (after 36 weeks' gestation) + in feces].

Sodium for growth is roughly 1–2 mmol per week over the first year of life and fecal sodium losses are trivial (0.23 mmol/kg/24 h) in the absence of diarrhea. In a healthy term infant, urinary sodium losses (1–2 mmol/kg/24 h) far exceed other losses and in VLBW infants urinary sodium losses up to 20 mmol/kg/24 h occur.[258]

As urinary sodium losses account for the greatest sodium losses in the newborn period, but there is initial oliguria after birth, no sodium intake is required for the first 24 h of postnatal life. During the succeeding week, 4–8 mmol/kg/24 h is usually adequate. Thereafter, term infants may require as little as 1 mmol/kg/24 h, whereas immature infants may require 8–12 mmol/kg/24 h if 'late' hyponatremia is to be avoided (see below). The needs of a term infant are ideally supplied by human breast milk which, with a nominal intake of 150 ml/kg/24 h, provides 4 mmol/kg/24 h on day 3 but only 1.2 mmol/kg/24 h after a month, the sodium concentration of breast milk naturally falling with time. Preterm human milk alone can rarely keep pace with the obligate renal losses in preterm infants of < 2 kg. The addition of breast milk fortifiers or preterm formula milk (if human breast milk cannot be provided) provides a sodium content 14–26 mmol/L. Nevertheless, additional sodium supplements may also be required if the plasma sodium concentration is to be maintained. When enteral fluids are contraindicated and parenteral fluids are given, sodium homeostasis can be achieved by supplying sodium alongside nitrogen-containing parenteral nutrition or by giving 10% dextrose on day 1 and 10% dextrose and 0.18% saline (30 mmol/L NaCl). Thereafter the rates for well infants in Table 12.14 deliver 4.5 mmol/kg/24 h of sodium by day 5 if 150 ml/kg/24 h 10% dextrose/0.18% saline is administered.

Changes in plasma sodium concentration during the first week of life are more often due to changes in water balance than sodium balance[253] so the volumes of water may need to be adjusted on the basis of frequent plasma sodium estimations.

HYPONATREMIA

The causes of hyponatremia (plasma sodium < 130 mmol/L) are listed in Table 12.18. Water overload is the major cause during the first week of life but, thereafter, sodium depletion becomes more important. Under conditions of sodium depletion, initially the kidney loses water to maintain a normal plasma osmolality but eventually the need to conserve plasma volume becomes the overriding stimulus, there is *appropriate* release of ADH and hyponatremia occurs.

The clinical features of hyponatremia have three origins:

1. Hypotonia, lethargy and convulsions due to the hyponatremia, irrespective of the cause. These symptoms are not usually seen until plasma sodium falls below 125 mmol/L and are partly related to the acuteness of the fall.
2. Inappropriate weight gain with iatrogenic water overload in early postnatal life or weight loss with sodium depletion in later postnatal life.
3. Features associated with the underlying disease.

The underlying cause should be treated but, in the interim, symptomatic treatment may be necessary to achieve a safe plasma sodium concentration. It is critical that a definitive diagnosis is made as the appropriate treatment may be either fluid restriction or sodium supplementation.

Table 12.18   Causes of hyponatremia in the newborn

A. Water overload
1. Maternal water overload prior to birth
2. Iatrogenic water overload following birth
3. Decreased free water clearance in a sick preterm infant
4. Inappropriate release of antidiuretic hormone
   Cerebral disease (birth asphyxia, meningitis)
   Respiratory disease (pneumonia, pneumothorax)

B. Sodium depletion
   This is usually accompanied by a lesser degree of water depletion
1. Excessive gastrointestinal losses (vomiting, diarrhea, nasogastric aspirate, enterostomy loss)
2. Excessive removal (repeated drainage of ascites, pleural fluid or CSF)
3. Excessive renal losses
   a. Primary renal tubular problems
      (i) 'late' hyponatremia of prematurity
      (ii) following relief of obstructive uropathy
      (iii) Fanconi syndrome
      (iv) Bartter syndrome
   b. Hypoadrenalism
      (i) congenital adrenal hyperplasia
      (ii) congenital adrenal hypoplasia
      (iii) hypoaldosteronism
      (iv) pseudohypoaldosteronism

If there is water overload, renal failure or hyponatremia following indometacin treatment, fluids should be restricted rather than more sodium given.

If there is a sodium deficit, the number of millimoles required is given by the formula:

$$(135 - \text{plasma sodium concentration}) \times \text{body weight(kg)} \times 2/3$$

This should be replaced slowly over 24 h by giving sodium intravenously [adding appropriate amounts of 30% NaCl (5 mmol/ml) to intravenous fluids].

In a symptomatic infant (irritable, apneic or convulsing), or in an infant with a genuine plasma sodium < 120 mmol/L, resuscitation should be initiated with a slow bolus of 15 ml/kg 0.9% saline (150 mmol/L).

In premature infants, a high incidence of 'late' hyponatremia is well recognized and, in contrast to the first postnatal week, this is frequently due to total body sodium depletion (accompanied to a lesser extent by water depletion) with poor weight gain or even weight loss. The sodium depletion is due to prolongation of the period of obligate renal sodium loss, possibly due to a delay in endocrine maturation, so that plasma sodium concentration is dependent on sodium intake which must be increased accordingly. This may be provided within parenteral nutrition or supplementation of enteral feeds using 30% NaCl (5 mmol/ml).

HYPERNATREMIA

Hypernatremia is almost invariably the result of water depletion (Table 12.19) and is associated with weight loss, failure to thrive or irritability. Hypertonicity and convulsions may occur when plasma sodium exceeds 150 mmol/L. A 'doughy' quality of the skin and a paradoxically full fontanelle may also suggest hypernatremic dehydration. The osmotic gradient favors maintenance of the ECF at the expense of the ICF and the diagnosis may be delayed as signs of hypovolemia and decreased skin turgor occur late. As hypernatremia may occur where restrictive fluid administration regimens in ELBW infants underestimate their excess fluid losses, daily body weights and twice daily plasma sodium measurements are a helpful guide to fluid management.

Treatment is difficult as persistence of hypernatremia is associated with cerebral hemorrhage and renal vein thrombosis in the newborn but overaggressive correction may cause cerebral edema as water enters cells down the osmotic gradient. A solution of 0.9% saline should be used initially and the deficit should be corrected slowly over 48 h.

BODY POTASSIUM CONTENT AND DISTRIBUTION

Potassium is the major intracellular cation. Although fetal growth is accompanied by a more than commensurate increase in total body potassium (as the ICF fraction of TBW increases), the potassium concentration in blood throughout life is virtually unchanged from 15 weeks' gestation.[259] Plasma potassium concentration is a major determinant of the cell membrane potential and if significant changes do occur, they must be corrected. As the vast majority of body potassium is intracellular, significant body depletion of potassium may occur for only a modest reduction in measured extracellular

Table 12.19   Causes of hypernatremia in the newborn

A. Water depletion
1. Inadequate intake
2. Excessive transepidermal water loss
3. Excessive renal losses
   a. Glycosuria
   b. Diabetes insipidus

B. Sodium overload
   Isolated sodium overload is rare as water is usually retained with sodium. It is caused by the administration of hypertonic solutions, such as sodium bicarbonate

potassium concentrations below a laboratory reference range. Similarly, as only 2% of total body potassium is found in ECF, large changes may occur in total body potassium without significantly altering plasma potassium concentration. In ventilated premature infants, a negative potassium balance of 10% of total body potassium occurs over the first 4 postnatal days, but hypokalemia (measured as ECF potassium concentration) is a rare problem. Subsequently, provided potassium-containing fluids are provided, positive potassium balance is restored and net potassium accumulation then continues at an average of 1 mmol/24h over the first year of life (approximately 0.3 mmol/kg/24h initially and 0.05 mmol/kg/24h at 1 year).

POTASSIUM BALANCE

Required potassium intake = potassium for growth
+ potassium lost (in urine + from GI tract).

As with sodium balance, urinary losses far exceed other losses, particularly during early newborn life. As the newborn's prostaglandin E_2 levels decline, the distal tubule becomes more aldosterone responsive (leading to reabsorption of sodium from the tubular lumen in exchange for excretion of potassium) so that the urinary potassium to sodium ratio increases with postconceptional age. Urinary potassium excretion in VLBW infants is 1–5 mmol/kg/24h.[258,260] Gastrointestinal losses are normally less than 0.5 mmol/kg/24h but very significant cumulative losses of potassium can occur if gastric contents are aspirated and not replaced, in fluid lost from enterostomies and in ileus.

For most infants in the newborn period, daily potassium intake of 3 mmol/kg/24h is usually adequate. Human breast milk provides 2.25 mmol/kg/24h (assuming 150 ml/kg/24h intake). The sodium: potassium ratio in mature human breast milk is about one, the same as the ratio in the urine of healthy term infants.[258]

HYPOKALEMIA

Symptoms of hypokalemia rarely occur until the plasma potassium concentration is more than 0.5 mmol/L below the lower limit of the normal range (3.0–6.6 mmol/L up to 1 month of age) with a concomitant increase in plasma bicarbonate being common. As the clinical features of weakness, hypotonia, hyporeflexia and lethargy are extremely difficult to recognize in the newborn, plasma potassium should be measured frequently in sick infants. Such infants should receive continuous cardiac monitoring (ECG features of hypokalemia are small T waves, depression of the ST sequence, and the appearance of U waves) because cardiac arrhythmias may occur. Loop diuretics and aminophylline[261] predispose to hypokalemia in the newborn and hypokalemia sensitizes the heart to digoxin.

Causes of hypokalemia are listed in Table 12.20. Treatment is by oral or intravenous (5 ml of 20% solution contains 1g or 13 mmol) potassium chloride administration, depending on the infant's condition and the severity of the hypokalemia, and by reversal of the underlying cause if possible. Intravenous potassium supplements should not exceed a con-

centration of 40 mmol/L. ECG monitoring is mandatory, infusion through a central venous catheter is preferable (provided the tip is not in the right atrium), and potassium added to fluid in plastic containers must be well mixed to prevent adherence. Potassium should not be added to blood products as it may cause red cell lysis. Oral potassium supplements should be avoided in gastrointestinal disorders because they may cause vomiting, ulceration and stricture. Diuretics should be stopped if possible or the potassium-sparing aldosterone antagonist, spironolactone, added.

HYPERKALEMIA

The causes of hyperkalemia are listed in Table 12.21. Plasma potassium concentrations above the 'normal' range occur in 3.5% of infants under 1500 g, particularly sicker infants less than 28 weeks.[258,262] Acute rises in plasma potassium can occur with intravenous administration but, apart from this, hyperkalemia due to excessive intake is rare because the kidney has a large reserve for potassium excretion. Hyperkalemia is more commonly due to a failure of excretion by the distal tubule, and this is supported by the finding of impaired renal function in 50% of cases of hyperkalemia in VLBW infants.[262] Altered Na^+, K^+-ATPase cation pump function may contribute to this non-oliguric hyperkalemia of the preterm neonate.[263] Preterm infants have lower erythrocyte intracellular sodium concentrations and higher intracellular potassium concentrations suggesting Na^+, K^+-ATPase enzyme activity is increased.[264]

As with hypokalemia, there may be apathy, weakness, hypotonia and hyporeflexia and also ileus. The ECG shows tall peaked T waves and arrhythmias occur in 60% of premature infants with serum potassium above 7.5 mmol/L, the commonest being supraventricular tachycardia.[262] Hyperkalemia > 7.5 mmol/L (or 6.5–7.5 mmol/L if there are associated ECG abnormalities) requires urgent treatment to redistribute potassium into cells as measures to improve renal excretion are too slow. Although Grade A evidence is lacking in the newborn, salbutamol has been shown to be an effective short term measure for the emergency management of hyperkalemia in older children[265] and adults and has the potential to have fewer short term side-effects than insulin/dextrose.[266] The myocardium is stabilized by intravenous calcium whilst the other measures in Table 12.22 take effect.

SPECIAL CARE – THERMOREGULATION

Soranus of Ephesus (98–131AD), in his treatise *On Diseases of Women*, clearly understood the importance of keeping newborn infants warm. In late 19th century Paris, Tarnier and Budin reduced by half the mortality of infants under 2000 g birth weight by nursing them in a warming chamber they designed from an incubator used for rearing poultry.[267] In a series of randomized controlled trials in the 1950s, William Silverman showed that keeping babies warm resulted in a 25% absolute reduction in mortality in all birth weight groups, including those under 1000 g.[268–270] Despite these studies, recent data show that newborn babies still get cold and hypothermia, especially in the preterm infant, remains associated with increased mortality.[271–274]

Table 12.20 Causes of hypokalemia in the newborn

Gastrointestinal losses
Vomiting or excessive nasogastric aspirate
Diarrhea
Enterostomy losses
Ileus
Renal losses
Bartter syndrome
Fanconi syndrome
Following relief of obstructive uropathy
Diuretic therapy
Alkalosis from any cause
Inadequate intake
Inadequate enteral or intravenous supplements

Table 12.21 Causes of hyperkalemia in the newborn

Erroneous
Sample hemolysis
Sample contamination with EDTA
Excessive intake/production
Iatrogenic supplementation of i.v. fluids or parenteral nutrition
Excessive hemolysis (e.g. accompanying intraventricular hemorrhage in VLBW infant)
Inadequate excretion
Acute renal failure
Hypoadrenalism (especially congenital adrenal hyperplasia and hypoplasia)
Hypoaldosteronism

Table 12.22   Management of hyperkalemia in the newborn

1. Discontinue all potassium administration, potassium-conserving diuretics and potentially nephrotoxic drugs. Correct prerenal failure due to hypovolemia, treat sepsis (avoiding potassium-containing penicillin salts) and optimize nutrition to minimize catabolism. Monitor ECG continuously
2. Intravenous salbutamol 4 mcg/kg over 5 min – can repeat if necessary
3. Intravenous 10% calcium gluconate 0.5 ml/kg over 5 min
4. Intravenous 4.2% sodium bicarbonate 4 ml/kg over 5 min
   This should be given via a different vein or after flush to prevent precipitation
5. A glucose + insulin infusion (less safe than salbutamol)
   Give 1 g/kg glucose + insulin 0.1 unit/kg infusion over 2 h, mixed in the same syringe, measuring venous blood sugar and plasma potassium concentrations hourly. Consider dialysis
6. Calcium resonium enema 0.5 g/kg, retained for at least 30 min. This can be repeated 8-hourly

Children and adults maintain a constant deep body temperature over a wide range of ambient thermal conditions (they are homeothermic). This is achieved by physiological and behavioral responses that control the rate at which heat is produced or lost. The newborn infant is also homeothermic but control of body temperature can only be achieved over a narrower range of ambient conditions. The preterm infant has even greater difficulty and the most immature infants behave at times as if they are poikilothermic – their body temperature tending to drift up or down with the ambient temperature. The aim in neonatal care is to provide a thermal environment which keeps body temperature in the normal range and which does not stress the infant to produce or lose large amounts of heat.

HEAT BALANCE
Heat production
Heat is produced as a by-product of cell metabolism. The basal metabolic rate is the lowest obligatory rate of heat production which occurs when an individual is starved, quiet and resting. In the newborn this is usually taken as the minimal rate of oxygen consumption in an infant who is lying still and asleep, at least 1 h after a feed in a neutral thermal environment. Values depend on gestation and postnatal age.

Heat loss
Convection
Heat is lost from the skin surface to the surrounding air by convection. Loss is high if there is rapid movement of cold air over the exposed skin. A naked baby in a cold drafty room has a high convective heat loss.

Radiation
Heat is lost from the skin to the nearest surface facing the baby. Radiative heat loss varies with the temperature of that surface and its distance from the skin, but is independent of the temperature of the intervening air. A naked infant can radiate large amounts of heat to the cool walls of an incubator even if the air is warm. An overhead warmer provides heat by radiation.

Evaporation
Heat is lost as water evaporates from the surface of the skin (560 cal/ml of water). A newly born infant wet with amniotic fluid loses heat as the skin dries. Evaporative heat loss is low in mature infants unless they are sweating in response to heat stress. Losses are high in preterm infants who have a high transepidermal water loss (TEWL) due to passive diffusion of water through the thin, poorly keratinized immature epidermis. TEWL is related to both gestational and postnatal age.[275–277]

Conduction
Newborn infants are not usually in direct contact with a structure of high thermal capacity, so conductive losses are small. Heat can be gained by conduction if the baby is lying on a heated gel- or water-filled mattress.

Heat production must be balanced by that lost from convection, radiation, evaporation and conduction. The more immature the infant, the greater the difficulty in temperature control. Heat loss is related to surface area which is relatively high in the smaller babies. There is poor insulation due to lack of subcutaneous tissue, and the poorly developed stratum corneum results in high TEWL and evaporative heat loss. The ability to conserve heat by vasoconstriction is limited and heat production, which is related to mass, is low. This poor response to relatively high heat losses means that hypothermia is a common problem in the immature baby.

RESPONSE TO THERMAL STRESS
The thermoneutral environment is a range of environmental temperature over which an infant has a minimum rate of heat production and is not sweating. Within this range, small adjustments to thermal control can be made by alterations in posture, activity and skin blood flow with deep body temperature remaining constant.[278] The thermoneutral range is wide if the infant is mature and well insulated by clothes and bedding, but narrow in the small and naked baby. As environmental temperature falls below the lower end of the thermoneutral range, metabolic heat production increases. This is mainly the result of oxidation of brown adipose tissue which is distributed in the neck, between the scapulae and along the aorta. The metabolism of brown fat to produce heat is controlled by catecholamine release (nonshivering thermogenesis). A term newborn infant can double his resting heat production in this way without any increase in activity.[279] As environmental temperature continues to decline, heat production reaches a maximum and below this point the body temperature falls. If environmental temperature rises above the upper end of the thermoneutral range, sweating occurs until a point is reached when the heat lost by sweating is insufficient and body temperature starts to rise.

In all infants heat production is delayed during adaptation to extrauterine life, especially if there is asphyxia, hypoxia or maternal sedative administration. Heat production per unit area is lower in preterm infants, particularly below 28 weeks' gestation, and the immature infant has a more prolonged impairment of nonshivering thermogenesis.

Sweating occurs from birth in infants above 36 weeks' gestation but is delayed by 2–3 weeks in the most immature infants.[280] This is a result of neurological rather than glandular immaturity. Sweating is a relatively poor defense against overheating in the newborn because the production of sweat per unit area of skin is low compared with a child or adult. The term newborn can alter skin blood flow effectively, and hence the amount of heat lost by convection and radiation, but this is impaired in the very immature infant. Change of posture to increase or decrease the surface area available for heat loss by convection and radiation is important in thermoregulation. It occurs in the healthy term infant and to some extent in the preterm infant but not in the presence of illness.

BODY TEMPERATURE AND ITS MEASUREMENT
Measurement of body temperature is the only practical way of assessing the thermal environment in day-to-day care. It is crude because it tells us nothing about the amount of energy the baby may be using to maintain its body temperature. An infant can be exposed to very significant thermal stress and still maintain a normal deep body temperature. The corollary of this is that just because a baby has a normal deep body temperature does not necessarily mean that it is in a neutral thermal environment.

Deep body temperature varies depending on the metabolic rate of the tissue, with the brain having the highest temperature. Esophageal temperature, measuring the temperature of the blood in the great veins close to the heart, is often used to represent deep body temperature but this is not used in routine care. Tympanic temperature closely correlates with brain temperature but is impractical in the newborn. In clinical practice we need an easily measured temperature that is at least close to, and follows changes in, deep body temperature.

Rectal temperature should no longer be used in infants and children as there is a significant risk of damage to the mucosa. Temperature in the rectum is an unreliable measure as it is affected by the depth of insertion of the thermometer, whether the baby has just passed a stool and by the temperature of the blood returning from the lower limbs. It is very difficult to retain rectal probes in the same position to allow continuous monitoring of temperature.

Axillary temperature is a reasonable guide to deep body temperature. The bulb of the thermometer should be held in the roof of the axilla with the infant's arm pressed against the side of the chest until a stable reading is obtained, usually by 3 min. The normal range is 36.3–37.0 °C.

Skin temperature reflects tissue insulation and environmental conditions as well as deep body temperature. In the preterm baby, the temperature of the skin over the liver can be used to monitor trends in deep body temperature. If the infant lies on a temperature probe which is insulated on the outside, the skin under the probe cannot lose heat and so equilibrates with the deep body temperature. This is the zero heat flux temperature and is a practical method for continuous monitoring of a central temperature.[281]

A single temperature, measured intermittently, gives limited information on the thermal state of the baby. Particularly in the sick or unstable baby, more information can be obtained from the continuous measurement and display of a central (abdominal, axillary or zero heat flux) and a peripheral (foot) temperature. Changes in peripheral temperature can detect cold stress before the central temperature falls. The preterm baby who appears to be comfortable in its environment will have a central temperature, measured from a skin probe, of 36.8–37.3 °C and a central–peripheral temperature difference of 0.5–1 °C. An increasing central–peripheral temperature difference, particularly above 2 °C, is commonly due to cold stress and occurs before any fall in central temperature. Hypovolemic babies will vasoconstrict their peripheral circulation in an attempt to maintain blood pressure. This results in a rise in central–peripheral temperature difference but, in such cases, there are other signs of hypovolemia such as a rising heart rate and falling blood pressure.[282] A high central temperature, particularly if unstable, along with a wide central–peripheral gap is seen in septic babies.[283]

MANAGEMENT OF THE THERMAL ENVIRONMENT
At delivery
The newborn baby loses heat by convection and radiation, but evaporation of amniotic fluid from the skin is the greatest source of heat loss. Delivery rooms should be warm, with a minimum temperature of 25 °C. The term newborn infant should be dried at delivery, wrapped in a warm dry blanket and given to the mother. Skin to skin contact with the mother is an effective way of maintaining body warmth but it is important to cover the baby to prevent heat loss from exposed skin on the back. Exposure for weighing, cord care and fixing of name bands should be minimized and bathing avoided.

In the preterm infant low temperature on admission to the neonatal unit has been associated with increased mortality and morbidity. Evaporation, the major source of heat loss, can be significantly reduced using occlusive dressings.[284] Clean plastic bags are easier to use and prevent hypothermia immediately after delivery.[285,286] The baby can be slid into the bag, up to the neck, whilst still wet. The head is covered with a hat. No blankets are used, allowing radiant heat to warm the infant through the bag. Clinical inspection and auscultation during resuscitation can be done through the bag and if vascular access is needed a small hole can be cut in the plastic over the vessel to be cannulated. The infant can be transported while still in the bag, which is only removed once the baby is in a humidified environment.

Nursing
The healthy term newborn will maintain a normal temperature if nursed fully dressed in a cot in a warm room. Most healthy preterm babies can be managed in the same way, although comparative data between open cot and incubator care are limited.[287] Some very small infants may need to be nursed clothed in an incubator to provide a sufficiently warm ambient temperature.
- Over 2 kg: nurse clothed, with bedding in a cot, in a room temperature of about 24 °C.
- 1.5–2 kg: nurse clothed with a hat and bedding in a cot, in a room temperature of about 26 °C.
- Below 1.5 kg: nurse clothed with a hat, in an incubator temperature of 30–32 °C.

Heated cot
A water-filled mattress, heated to a set temperature between 35 and 38 °C, can be used to provide conductive heat to a preterm infant nursed in a cot. This can be as effective as an incubator for keeping small babies warm, resulting in similar rates of resting metabolism and growth.[288,289] It is cheap, simple and does not depend on a constant unbroken supply of electricity (because of its stored heat), so that it is particularly useful in resource limited countries. It is only of use if the infants are healthy and do not need to be nursed naked for observation and access. It has been effectively used as a method of rewarming cold preterm infants.[290] Gel-filled heated mattresses are also available but are more expensive.

Incubator
The incubator provides a warm environment suitable for nursing small or sick infants, particularly if they need to be naked for observation and access. Air within the canopy is warmed by a heater and circulated by a fan. The heater output can be controlled in two ways. In air mode the incubator air temperature is set to a point between 30 and 37 °C and the heater is thermostatically controlled to reach and maintain this temperature. In servo mode a thermister probe is taped to the infant's abdominal skin and the desired skin temperature is set – the heater output varies to provide an air temperature which maintains the set skin temperature. In practice, air mode control is simpler to use, safer and results in a very constant ambient air temperature regardless of the condition of the infant and the amount of care being received. Servo control results in wide fluctuations in air temperature, particularly during handling, and in the preterm baby this has been associated with an increase in apnea and possibly a poorer outcome.[291,292] The probe can become detached or wet, and the infant's own attempts at thermoregulation are overridden so that a fever may be disguised.

Suggested air temperature (Table 12.23)[278,293] and skin temperature settings (Table 12.24)[294] for the two modes of control are shown.

Table 12.23 Average incubator air temperatures needed to provide a suitable environment for naked, healthy infants (from Rutter[294])

Birth weight (kg)	37° C	36° C	35° C	34° C	33° C	32° C
Less than 1.0	For 1 day	After 1 day	After 2 weeks	After 3 weeks	After 4 weeks	After 6 weeks
1.0–1.49			For 10 days	After 10 days	After 3 weeks	After 5 weeks
1.5–1.99				For 10 days	After 10 days	After 4 weeks
2.0–2.5				For 2 days	After 2 days	After 3 weeks
More than 2.5					For 2 days	After 2 days

Table 12.24 Suggested abdominal skin temperature settings for infants nursed in servo mode incubators or under radiant warmers (from Rutter[294])

Weight (kg)	Abdominal skin temperature (°C)
Less than 1.0	36.9
1.0–1.49	36.7
1.5–1.99	36.5
2.0–2.5	36.3
More than 2.5	36.0

These are a guide only and there will be variation in individual requirements. In particular, dressed babies will need lower incubator temperatures. Monitoring of body temperature is essential to allow appropriate changes in environmental settings.

The naked infant will lose heat by radiation to the cooler walls of the incubator. This can be reduced by raising the temperature of the nursery, and therefore of the incubator wall, raising the incubator air temperature, using a radiant heat shield within the incubator which warms to the air temperature and shields the infant from the canopy, or by using a double-walled incubator.

In infants below 30 weeks' gestation, especially if weighing less than 1 kg, evaporative water and heat loss is high during the first days of life and may exceed the infant's own heat production. Raising the humidity of the air around the body will reduce evaporative losses so that a normal body temperature can be achieved and fluid losses minimized. Beyond 1 week of age the immature infant's skin has matured to such an extent that evaporative water and heat losses are less important and added humidity is rarely required.[295] Incubators using a sealed system do not need to be run dry for part of the day and there does not appear to be any increased risk of infection when humidity is used. Evaporative heat losses can also be reduced by covering the baby with a plastic sheet. This reduces visibility and when removed to handle the baby there are high evaporative losses. The use of semipermeable non-adhesive skin dressings lowers TEWL and reduces the number of bacteria in the covered skin. Emollients have also been used to cover the skin and reduce fluid loss. They are safe and reduce excessive drying, skin cracking and fissuring. However the effect of these products wears off after about 3 h, necessitating repeated application.

There are few data available to help in deciding the optimum time to make the transition from incubator to cot.[296] Traditionally this is usually based on weight, with most babies able to maintain their temperature in a cot, and continue to gain weight, when they are between 1700 and 1800 g.

Radiant warmer

The infant lies naked on a platform with a radiant heat source above. The output of the heater is controlled by a temperature sensor in contact with the infant's skin, set to the desired temperature. The sensor should be taped to the abdomen or chest rather than a limb and must be shielded from the heat source. The normal range of abdominal skin temperature under neutral thermal conditions for infants of different size is shown in Table 12.24.

Heat losses by convection and radiation are high when radiant warmers are used. Evaporative water loss is also very high, a mean of about 23 ml/kg/day,[297] due to the low relative humidity in the surrounding air. These losses are all balanced by a large radiant heat gain from the heater. Wide fluctuations in heater output occur, producing a very uneven, asymmetrical thermal environment compared with an incubator. In the more immature infants, evaporative water loss may lead to hypernatremia and dehydration. The wide fluctuations in thermal environment and high evaporative water losses can be reduced by placing a small clear plastic canopy over the infant – radiant heat can still reach the infant but heat losses by convection, radiation and evaporation are greatly reduced.

Overheating can occur and regular measurement of the infant's body temperature by an independent method is essential. It is important to be sure that the skin temperature probe is securely attached to the baby. If the heater is switched off, moved to one side or if something is interposed between the infant and the heat source, the infant's heat losses are very great and rapid cooling occurs. The advantage of radiant warmers is that they allow access to the infant for practical procedures whilst keeping the infant warm.

Babies nursed with similar skin temperatures have a higher basal metabolic rate when managed under radiant heaters compared with incubators. However, no study has shown any significant difference in outcome for babies nursed using either device.[297]

Transport

The newborn, and in particular the preterm infant, is at high risk of cold stress during transport. High radiant heat losses, especially in cold weather, can be reduced by covering the incubator and using blankets around the baby. Evaporative heat loss can be reduced by putting the baby in a plastic bag. If ventilator gases are not heated and humidified there will be high evaporative heat losses from the respiratory tract. Heated gel mattresses that can be used during transport are available, with the baby gaining heat by conduction. All units transporting babies should collect data on temperature control during transfer and use this to audit the efficacy of the transport process.

Surgery

There is a major risk of cold stress during surgery. The baby is starved and anesthetized, reducing the normal metabolic response to cold. The operating theater is often cool and the baby may have had to travel some distance from the nursery. Exposure of the skin and moist organs increases heat loss significantly. Heat losses can be minimized by increasing the environmental temperature to 28–30 °C, exposing only the minimum area during surgery and adding a supplementary heat source such as an electric heating pad or radiant heater.

DISORDERS OF BODY TEMPERATURE IN THE NEWBORN

A low body temperature (below 36°C)

Mild hypothermia (central temperature 34–36 °C) is not uncommon. In hospital it is most often seen following resuscitation or when infants are exposed to a cool delivery room or theater. This is easily preventable by paying careful attention to keeping infants warm after delivery. Moderate (30–34 °C) or severe (below 30 °C) hypothermia due to cold exposure occurs most often when infants are born outside hospital, either unexpectedly or after a concealed delivery – if the infant is small, born into a toilet, abandoned, or inadvertently exposed to cold, severe hypothermia may result.

Accidental hypothermia also occurs later in the newborn period or early infancy because of inadvertent cold exposure due to inadequate clothing or cold thermal environments. Infants with bacterial sepsis or with respiratory syncytial virus (RSV) infection are prone to mild hypothermia – so too are infants in severe heart failure or with marked cyanosis. Malnutrition predisposes to hypothermia because of poor tissue insulation and an impaired metabolic response to cold. Hypothyroidism also results in an impaired metabolic response to cold. Drugs given to the mother which cross the placenta have a similar effect on the newborn infant, particularly the long-acting sedatives such as diazepam. Intentional hypothermia is used as an adjunct to cardiopulmonary bypass, the body temperature being lowered to about 28 °C by surface cooling with ice to reduce the metabolic demands of the brain. The infants tolerate this brief, acute severe hypothermia well. Whole body or local head cooling appears to be effective in reducing brain damage in asphyxiated animals and trials have shown potential benefit in newborn infants following birth asphyxia.[298,299]

Hypothermic infants develop symptoms when their deep body temperature falls below 34 °C. They become lethargic, feed poorly and have a weak cry and reduced movements. If exposure to cold has been persistent there may be peripheral edema, sclerema and marked facial erythema in the presence of a strikingly cold skin – these are the features of neonatal cold injury. In very severe hypothermia there is profound bradycardia with slow, shallow respiration and the infant may appear to be dead.

There are anecdotal reports of such infants being left for dead yet eventually making a full recovery. The diagnosis of hypothermia is made by recording a low rectal temperature – it is important that a low reading thermometer is used, not the standard clinical thermometer with a minimum reading of 35°C.

The treatment of accidental hypothermia is rewarming. If there is an underlying cause, this obviously also needs to be treated. There is limited information about the correct rate for rewarming cold infants but in cases of mild hypothermia this can take place rapidly. In moderate or severe cases there is concern that rapid rewarming of the infant's surface causes peripheral vasodilation, diversion of blood from the core and therefore hypotension. There is no evidence for the routine use of plasma expanders in these cases. Following acute accidental hypothermia it appears to be safe to restore deep body temperature to normal over a few hours. This can be achieved using a radiant warmer, an incubator or a heated cot.[290]

Hypoglycemia may occur during rewarming and should be anticipated and prevented with an intravenous infusion of 10% dextrose. Care should be taken in interpreting blood gas results – a metabolic acidosis at 37°C is less severe at 30°C and should not be overenthusiastically treated. Abdominal distention is common as a result of ileus and feeding should not be started until a normal body temperature is achieved. NEC and hemorrhagic pulmonary edema have been described. The reported mortality rate in severe hypothermia is 25–50% but this includes infants with overwhelming sepsis or congenital abnormalities that predisposed them to cold. Most survivors develop normally.

A high body temperature (above 38°C)

An infant with a high body temperature may be either febrile or overheated. A febrile infant has a high set point temperature and behaves as if cold. He makes physiological and behavioral responses which reduce heat loss, increase heat production and therefore raise body temperature. Although he has a raised central temperature, his central–peripheral temperature difference will be high (above 2°C). An overheated infant makes physiological and behavioral responses in an effort to increase heat loss and therefore lower body temperature. In this case the central temperature will be high but the central–peripheral temperature gap will be small (below 1°C). Overheated infants simply need a cooler environment, not a series of painful investigations to find an infective cause for the 'fever'. In a large study of term infants with a high body temperature, 90% were found to be overheated and only 10% had infection.

The newborn infant may develop a raised body temperature in the presence of infection but this is usually not marked. It is not known why serious infection in a newborn seems to elicit such a mild febrile response when mild infection in a toddler is often associated with a very high body temperature. Infection is not the only cause of a raised set point temperature in the newborn; it is also caused by a severe cerebral abnormality, either congenital (holoprosencephaly, hydranencephaly, encephalocele) or acquired (birth asphyxia). Such infants have hypothalamic dysfunction leading to poor temperature control.

Overheating is less common than accidental hypothermia in the newborn. Mild degrees occur when active, large infants are overwrapped and left in a warm room, or when small infants are overheated by an incubator or radiant warmer. Severe overheating occurs when there is electrical or mechanical failure of a warming device, or when an incubator is exposed to direct sunlight (this turns it into a greenhouse). It can also occur if infants are left in closed cars exposed to direct sunlight.

Mild overheating has been suggested as a predisposing factor in apnea of prematurity but otherwise seems not to be dangerous. Severe overheating leading to hyperpyrexia (rectal temperature above 41°C) has caused sudden death in the newborn without prior symptoms.

SPECIAL CARE – ENTERAL NUTRITION

Preterm babies have very little stored energy and urgently need adequate nutrition in order to survive beyond a few days. Subsequently, good nutrition is essential to promote the rapid growth which characterizes this period of life, and is important for long term outcome.[300] Nutrients can be provided parenterally or enterally but the aim in all infants is to use full enteral feeding as soon as it is safe. This section reviews the balance of benefits and risks of enteral feeding and recommends suitable intakes, aimed at promoting growth and avoiding deficiencies.

DEVELOPMENT OF GUT FUNCTION

The motility, digestive and absorptive functions of the gut develop in utero. Gut development continues postnatally and enteral feeding influences this. An understanding of gut development is essential to the discussion of benefits and risks of enteral feeding.

Sucking, swallowing, gastric emptying and small gut peristalsis are inefficient in the preterm baby.[301] The fetus begins to swallow at 16 weeks but in babies born before 34 weeks' gestation feeding behavior is characterized by short bursts of sucking, a small intake of milk, uncoordinated swallowing, and nonpropagative, disorganized esophageal motor activity.[302] Lower esophageal sphincter pressure is low,[303] predisposing to gastroesophageal reflux. Gastric emptying time is prolonged to about twice that of the term infant, and is even longer in the presence of illness or when feeds are of high energy density, fat or carbohydrate content.[301] In the fetus small intestinal transit is seen from 30 weeks, but the normal pattern of migrating motor complexes and peristalsis is not observed until a few weeks later. The coincidence of nutritive sucking, swallowing and gut motor activity at about 34 weeks is a good example of developmental coordination.

Gastric acid production is present by 24 weeks' gestation. Pepsin production is low, but this does not appear to inhibit utilization of dietary protein and may enhance the passage of intact IgG and IgA into the small bowel. Pancreatic enzyme secretion is reduced in the term infant, and in the preterm infant levels of trypsin, lipase, amylase and bicarbonate secretion are further reduced.[304] In the preterm baby, studies using test meals have demonstrated inadequate intraluminal digestion of fat, protein and carbohydrate, but clinical malabsorption is rare. Fat absorption, for example, limited by low pancreatic lipase and low intraluminal bile salt concentration, may be improved by the high contribution of lingual and gastric lipase and bile salt dependent lipase in breast milk. Alpha-glucosidase (sucrase, maltase and isomaltase) activities are about 70–80% of normal at 32 weeks' gestation.[305] Lactase is at 25% of adult levels at 26 weeks and increases markedly towards term.[306]

Intestinal permeability is increased in the preterm baby and results in increased macromolecular transport across the epithelium.[307] This may be relevant to the development of NEC by allowing bacteria and their antigens to penetrate the gut wall.

INTRODUCTION OF ENTERAL FEEDS

Healthy preterm babies should be fed within 1 or 2 h of birth, in order to prevent hypoglycemia and to maintain hydration. Deciding when to feed enterally in intensive care is a more contentious matter and practice varies widely.[308] Most would not attempt enteral feeding in ill preterm infants, unstable on intensive care. In the preterm infant who is stable on intensive care and receiving ventilatory assistance, should milk feeds be given? The main arguments for not feeding are the fear of milk aspiration, respiratory embarrassment through gastric distention, and NEC (see Complications of feeding). With a cautious approach, however, many neonatal units successfully milk feed babies on ventilators. Milk feeds should be stopped for a period following extubation, to allow recovery of laryngeal protective reflexes.

The growth-restricted infant also merits particular care. In intrauterine growth restriction (IUGR) with abnormal fetal Doppler studies, fetal gut perfusion is reduced, predisposing the infant to NEC.[309] A large European study of women whose pregnancies were complicated by hypertension or IUGR showed no significant increase in NEC in infants with a history of abnormal fetal Doppler studies, however IUGR was present in less than 50% of the cases.[310] A meta-analysis of 14 studies compared the incidence of NEC in infants who had exhibited absent or reversed end-diastolic flow on fetal Doppler, compared to those with normal flow. Affected babies showed a significant increase in NEC with OR 2.13 (95% CI 1.49–3.03).[311] In infants with IUGR, notably those with the triad of IUGR, abnormal fetal Doppler studies and fetal echogenic gut, difficulty with enteral feeds is common.[312] It is common practice to delay introduction of milk feeds in these infants[313] although there is no clear evidence that this is of benefit. Parenteral nutrition accompanied by a period of trophic feeding (see below) and a gradual increase in enteral feed volumes seems a pragmatic approach while awaiting further research evidence.

TROPHIC FEEDING (TF)

TF is also known as minimal enteral feeding, hypocaloric feeding and gut priming. It is an important advance in the use of enteral feeding, entailing the administration of small, nutritionally inconsequential amounts of milk in order to confer the benefit of milk feeds on the infant receiving parenteral nutrition.[314]

Physiology

Absence of enteral feeding is associated with reduced gastrointestinal growth and maturation. Gastric, intestinal and pancreatic weight and DNA content is reduced if milk is withheld, changes that occur in the first days of enteral starvation.[315,316] Bile flow is reduced and this may underlie the high incidence of conjugated hyperbilirubinemia in infants on parenteral nutrition.

The administration of TF has major advantages in inducing maturation of gastrointestinal motor function,[317] an effect which is not seen if water is given. This translates to more rapid whole gut transit time in infants receiving TF.[318,319] Milk tolerance is improved with a reduction of 4 days in time to reach full feeds.[314,320] Gastric emptying is not altered in infants who have received TF (Fig. 12.13).[318]

TF induces surges in gut hormones[321] including motilin and enteroglucagon which are known to be trophic and promote normal motility. In animals, enteral feeds enhance digestive capacity, with increase in gastric lipase, intestinal lactase activity, and pancreatic responsiveness to glucose. TF has also been shown to induce lactase activity measured in duodenal aspirate,[322] which was subsequently found to relate to improved milk tolerance.[323] Chymotrypsin activity is not altered by TF.[322]

Clinical trials

A Cochrane review of TF compared to no feeds, including 617 infants in nine trials, showed a mean reduction in days to full feeding of 2.6 days (95% CI −4.12, −0.99), and showed no difference in NEC (RR 1.16, 95% CI 0.75, 1.79).[324] Comparison of TF with advancing feeds in 141 infants resulted in longer time to achieve full feeds, with a mean weighted difference of 13.4 days, but a lower incidence of NEC (RR 0.14, 95% CI 0.02, 1.07). The feeding regimen used was not typical of UK practice.

TF appears to confer a reduction in time to full enteral feeds, improved milk tolerance, shorter hospital stay, more rapid full nipple feeding and accelerated growth in the first 6 weeks.[314] Avoidance of cholestatic jaundice has not been explored by studies with sufficient power. One trial showed a large reduction in culture positive sepsis with parallel decrease in days with elevated C-reactive protein in the infants who received TF.[320] An associated reduction in upper gut colonization with coagulase negative staphylococci may, in part, explain this observation.

None of the 10 randomized controlled trials examining TF has demonstrated any adverse effects.[314] There is no evidence to suggest an increase in respiratory problems.

NUTRITIONAL REQUIREMENTS OF THE PRETERM INFANT

Table 12.25 compares body composition of infants of 26 weeks' gestation and term. Fetal and infant metabolic demands differ, and nutrient requirements based on prenatal growth may not be appropriate for the preterm baby. Current consensus, however, is that the fetal growth curve seems a reasonable 'gold standard', and a growth rate falling far below it should be regarded as a risk factor for poor long term outcome.[325,326] Composition of growth varies during late fetal life. For example, in the term infant, during the first weeks after birth over 40% of weight gain is fat and about 12% protein, whereas in late fetal life only 15–20% of the weight gain is fat, and protein accretion rates are higher. It is also extremely hard in the preterm infant to achieve fetal accretion rates of calcium (3 mmol/kg/day) and phosphate (2 mmol/kg/day).

The nutritional requirements of the preterm baby for the major nutrients, electrolytes, minerals, vitamins and trace elements remain uncertain. European consensus was reached by ESPGAN in 1987[327] and a trans-Atlantic agreement reached in 1993.[325] The latter has recently been revised and gives the most up-to-date evidence base for intake of individual nutrients as well as different fortifiers and formulae.[328] Aiming for a growth rate of 15–18 g/kg/day, the requirements of the preterm baby for the major nutrients (Table 12.26) and electrolytes, minerals, vitamins and trace elements (Table 12.27) are shown.

THE CHOICE OF MILK FOR THE PRETERM INFANT

The chosen milk should meet nutritional requirements, be well tolerated, digested and absorbed and minimize risk of adverse effects,

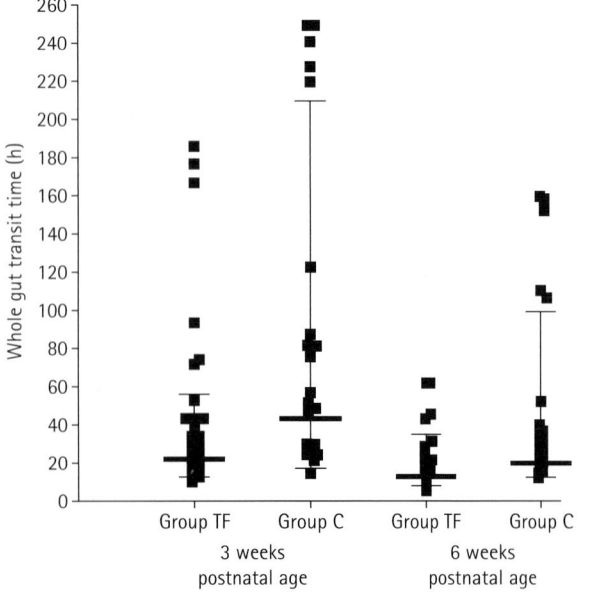

Fig. 12.13 Individual whole gut transit time at 3 and 6 weeks of postnatal age. Broad horizontal bars represent median; narrow horizontal bars interquartile ranges: p < 0.05 at 3 and 6 weeks.

Table 12.25 Some aspects of body size and composition at 26 weeks gestation and at term

	26 weeks	40 weeks
Weight	850 g	3500 g
Length	34 cm	51 cm
Brain weight	260 g	490 g
Body water	730 ml	2400 ml
Body sodium	70 mmol	280 mmol
Total nitrogen	10 g	60 g
Fat	6 g	540 g
Calcium	6 g	35 g
Phosphate	3 g	18 g

Table 12.26 Requirements of the preterm baby for the major nutrients

Calories	130 kcal/kg/day
Water	150–180 ml/kg/day
Carbohydrate	16 g/kg/day
Fat	7 g/kg/day
Protein	3.5 g/kg/day

Table 12.27 Requirements of the preterm baby for electrolytes, minerals, trace elements and major vitamins

Sodium	2.5–5 mmol/kg/day
Potassium	2.5–3.5 mmol/kg/day
Chloride	2.5–3.5 mmol/kg/day
Calcium	2–3 mmol/kg/day
Phosphate	2–3 mmol/kg/day
Magnesium	0.5 mmol/kg/day
Iron	2 mg/kg/day
Copper	120 µg/kg/day
Zinc	1000 µg/kg/day
Vitamin A	1000 IU/day
Vitamin D	400 IU/day
Vitamin C	30 mg/day
Vitamin E	8 mg/day
Vitamin B_{12}	0.3 µg/day
Folic acid	50 µg/day

notably NEC. The choice of milk also has effects upon neurodevelopmental outcome and intelligence, with breast milk conferring significant advantage.[329] All mothers of preterm infants should thus be encouraged to express their milk, which is the feed of choice. As will be described below, human milk fulfills all requirements listed above, apart from meeting nutritional requirements, and for some nutrients supplements will be required.[330]

Human milk

In the preterm infant human milk is better tolerated and full enteral feeding is achieved more rapidly than with formula,[331] gastric emptying is quicker[332] and stool frequency greater.

The advantages of human milk are now well established: considerable reduction in risk of NEC;[333] protection against gastrointestinal and respiratory tract infection in the first years of life;[334] reduction in atopic symptoms in infants with a family history of atopy;[335] and, most importantly, its association with optimal neurodevelopmental and intellectual outcome.[300,329] The semi-essential long chain polyunsaturated fatty acids contained in breast milk are structurally important in the central nervous system and may underlie this advantage of breast milk.[336] Breast milk may also protect against adult disease such as diabetes mellitus and Crohn's disease and confer protection against cardiovascular disease through nutritional programming, whereby early nutritional experience exerts a later effect upon health, independent of other influential factors during life.[337–339] Human milk also contains growth factors, IgA and immunoprotective factors.

There are two main problems with human milk: it is not always available, and its energy, protein, calcium, phosphate and sodium content do not meet theoretical nutrient requirements despite optimal absorption of breast milk.

Breast milk varies in composition and is particularly affected by gestation, postnatal age and method of collection. The mothers of term and preterm infants produce milk which is different in important respects during the first 2–3 weeks after birth. Preterm milk has about a three times higher concentration of sodium, protein and IgA, and a lower water content producing a general increase in the concentration of most constituents, but not calcium or phosphate. Method of collection is important, and drip milk is of lower energy content than expressed milk (Table 12.28). Banked donor milk from term mothers produces less good weight gain than either expressed preterm milk or preterm formula. Breast milk can be given in larger volumes than formula milk at around 180–200 ml/kg/day.

If donated milk is used, great care must be taken to prevent transmission of HIV[340] and hepatitis B and C, through screening of donors and pasteurization. Records are kept on all donors and recipients. This disincentive to the use of donor milk led to a reduction of milk banking, but several banks still exist and their role is currently being evaluated.[341]

Breast milk fortification

Fortification of breast milk is now used in most neonatal units in the UK.[308] Breast milk fortifiers are powders added to breast milk to increase energy, protein, carbohydrate, sodium, calcium and phosphate contents of the milk (Table 12.29). Most studies have found acceptable

Table 12.28 Composition of milks

Per 100 ml	Colostrum	Mature breast milk	Drip breast milk (foremilk)	Unmodified cows' milk	*Whey based	Casein based
Energy (kcal)	67	70	45	65	67	67
Protein (g)	2.3	1.34	1.0	3.2	1.5	1.6
Fat (g)	2.95	4.2	2.2	3.8	3.6	3.6
Carbohydrate (g)	5.7	7.1	6.5	4.7	7.2	7.0
Sodium (mg)	50	19		77	23	22
Calcium (mg)	48	27		137	66	56
Phosphorus (mg)	16	14		91	42	44
Iron (µg)	100	50		45	700	800
Vitamin A (µg)	161	60		23	60	75
Vitamin C (µg)	7.2	5.2		1.1	8.0	9.0
Vitamin D (µg)	0.04	0.1		0.02	1.0	1.1
Vitamin E (mg)	1.5	0.24		0.06	0.6	0.74
Vitamin B_6 (mg)	–	0.018		0.05	0.04	0.06

Table 12.29 Nutrient change in 100 ml breast milk after fortification

Nutrient	Energy (kcal)	Protein (g)	Carbohydrate (g)	Fat (g)	Sodium (mmol)	Calcium (mmol)	Phosphorus (mmol)
Increase	10–14	0.6–1.0	2.0–2.4	Small	0.3–0.9	1.0–2.2	0.7–1.2

tolerance of feeds and gastric emptying during introduction of forti-fied milk feeds.[342,343] Two studies however have shown less good feed tol-erance and one a trend towards increased risk of NEC.[344]

Growth and mineral accretion is improved with fortification[345] although the impact on long term outcome is not clear. At 18 months, infants given fortifier show no neurodevelopmental advantage over those whose milk was not fortified.[344] A recent trial exploring protein content of fortifier has shown improved growth and increase in head circumference with a higher protein content.[346]

The optimal use of breast milk fortifier and its ideal composition is not fully established. In most centers fortifier is only used after full feed-ing with breast milk is achieved, and either growth failure is observed, or protein indices such as blood urea/nitrogen or serum albumin lev-els are low. This strategy avoids fortification during the introduction of feeds when the infant's mother is producing milk with a naturally high nutrient content.

Preterm formula milks

Preterm formulae are based upon human milk. The principal differ-ences are: more protein (approx. 1.8–2.5 g/100 ml); more energy (approx. 75–90 kcal/100 ml); higher sodium, calcium and phospho-rus content; and the addition of iron and vitamins, especially D, E and the B complex. Some lactose is replaced with glucose or its polymers, and a small proportion of fat may be given as medium chain triglycer-ide to improve fat absorption. The addition of long chain polyunsatu-rates (see above), similar to those found in breast milk, has been shown to produce more rapid maturation of the visual pathway and may con-fer neurodevelopmental advantage.[336] Purified sources of these fats are now added to formula milk. Preterm formulae work well, growth rates are good, nutritional deficiencies are rare, and medium term growth and development outcome almost matches that seen with breast milk.[300]

Other milks

Term formula is not adequate for the preterm infant.[347] Preterm formula is given until an infant weighs 2.0–2.5 kg. Most, who are not breast-fed, then go on to a whey-dominant term formula. Many preterm infants remain underweight at term, and better weight gain may be seen after discharge home if a formula of composition between preterm and term formula is given.[328,348] Infants may compensate by taking a larger volume of formula, but male infants have increased linear growth and head cir-cumference if fed a nutrient enriched formula for 6 months post term.[349] A number of preterm post-discharge formulae are now available. At no time during the first year of life is unprocessed cows' milk a suitable food for the preterm baby.

Special milks are occasionally required to treat cows' milk protein or lactose intolerance and inborn errors of metabolism. This should be done in collaboration with a pediatric dietitian. Soya milks are not designed to meet the needs of preterm infants, are potentially aller-genic and have levels of phytoestrogens which may be harmful. They are not recommended for infants under one year (Department of Health January 2004).

FEEDING IN PRACTICE

No-one is in a better position to make individual decisions about feed-ing than the experienced neonatal nurse caring for an infant. Feeding policy and each infant's nutrition should be managed jointly by nurs-ing and medical staff, while empowering the neonatal nurse to make feeding management decisions when necessary.

Enteral feeding should be introduced gradually and increased with care. Tolerance should be assessed and, whenever possible, infants should be weighed and measured regularly. It is reasonable to begin with 0.5–1 ml/kg/h in a baby of less than 30 weeks' gestation, increas-ing by 0.5–1 ml/kg every 6–12 h. In more mature babies, larger start-ing volumes and a faster rate of progress may be indicated. In a healthy baby, enteral feeds may be given at 75 ml/kg on day 1, 90 ml/kg on day

2, 120 ml/kg on day 3, 135 ml/kg on day 4 and 150 ml/kg on day 5, with subsequent increases up to a maximum of 180 ml/kg/day accord-ing to tolerance and growth rate. Preterm formula is usually given at 160 ml/kg/day and fortified breast milk at 160–180 ml/kg/day.

Full nipple feeding from breast or bottle depends upon maturity and health. In most it is achieved at a postmenstrual age of 34–37 weeks.

Avoidance of NEC

Trials of strategies aimed at preventing NEC are inherently difficult. The condition is unpredictable with variation in incidence that demands very large studies to obtain adequate power. There is some evidence for the following in order to avoid NEC during enteral feeding:

Use of breast milk was protective in a large multicenter trial of 926 infants randomized to donor breast milk or formula as sole diet or sup-plement to mother's own milk with an odds ratio of 10.6.[333] Avoidance of hyperosmolar feeds[350] and rapid, incautious increase in feed volume[351] has also shown some benefit. Delaying introduction of milk in infants with IUGR is common practice and is currently being evaluated in the 'ADEPT' trial, comparing introduction of a graded feeding schedule on either day 2 or day 6 after birth in IUGR infants with abnormal fetal Doppler blood flow.[352]

Control of infection in epidemic NEC has been evaluated in a num-ber of trials. A systematic review in the Cochrane Library demonstrated a statistically significant reduction in NEC with use of prophylactic oral antibiotics, but also an increase in colonization with resistant bacteria and concluded there was insufficient evidence to recommend this prac-tice.[353] Manipulation of enteric organisms by inclusion of either prebiotics (oligosaccharides which promote colonization with benign bifidobact-eria), or probiotics (actual organisms of the genera lactobacilli and bifido-bacilli) in preterm infants' diets shows some promise as a method by which healthy gut colonization may be achieved and risk of NEC may be reduced.[354,355] Continuous or intermittent feeds have also been consid-ered. A systematic review included six trials and showed a trend towards improved tolerance with bolus feeds, but faster weight gain in infants under 1000 g with continuous feeds. There was no difference in NEC and insufficient evidence to make clear recommendations.[356]

Feeding tube placement

Meta-analyses of trials of tube placement have shown a 15% (95% CI 5–23) increase in mortality in association with transpyloric feeding compared with gastric feeding.[357] Transpyloric feeding can no longer be recommended.

The choice between nasal and oral tube passage is more a mat-ter of esthetics than of clinical importance. Nasal tubes are easier to fix but may increase resistance to air flow through the nose and increase the work of breathing. Most commonly fine bore nasogas-tric tubes are used.

Non-nutritive sucking (use of a dummy during gastric tube feeds) has no effect upon gastric emptying or nutrient absorption, but meta-analysis shows a mean reduction of hospital stay of 6 days (95% CI 2–10).[357]

Weaning from tube to breast or bottle feeds is usually a gradual pro-cess and most experienced neonatal nurses say that if rushed, it will take longer. There may be parental pressure to accomplish the task as soon as possible as the time for discharge approaches. Special soft teats are available for preterm babies and do seem to have some advantages over conventional teats.

NUTRITIONAL SUPPLEMENTS
Protein and energy

There is no need to routinely supplement fortified breast milk or pre-term formula. Occasionally an energy supplement (glucose polymers or a mixture of glucose polymers and fat) is needed when larger feed vol-umes are not possible (e.g. heart failure). These supplements are usually well tolerated when added to milk at a rate up to 5 g/100 ml. Energy:pro-tein ratio should not exceed 100 kcal/2 g of protein. Special high energy formulae are also available.

Vitamins

Preterm infants are denied some of the placental transfer of fat soluble vitamins which occurs in the third trimester and although breast milk will provide adequate amounts of most vitamins, it contains little vitamin D or vitamin K. Infants born below 34 weeks and more mature infants with perinatal complications should have supplements for the first 1–2 years of life. Preterm formulae and breast milk fortifiers contain additional vitamins. All preterm infants should receive vitamin K (phytomenadione 0.4 mg/kg) at birth for prevention of hemorrhagic disease of the newborn and in most this is given parenterally (p. 295). Extra vitamin K should be given i.m. if the preterm baby needs to undergo surgery or has clinical liver disease or severe diarrheal illness during the first 4 months of life. A daily intake of vitamin D of 400 IU (10 mcg) will prevent deficiency.

Multivitamin preparations used for breast- and term formula-fed infants usually contain vitamins A, C, and D, B_1, B_2, nicotinamide and pyridoxine.[358]

Sodium

The preterm infant requires 2.5–5 mmol/kg/day of sodium, usually as chloride. When intake is poor, urinary excretion may well exceed intake, leading to poor growth and hyponatremia. Routine supplementation of fortified breast milk or preterm formula is not necessary. Initially after birth, preterm milk may contain 20 mmol/L of sodium but this falls over 2–3 weeks to levels seen in mature human milk, at about 7 mmol/L. This is one reason, as suggested above, to fortify breast milk only when lactation is established. If feeding with unfortified breast milk, a sodium supplement should be considered. Certainly, if a preterm baby is not growing well, it is always worth checking the serum and urinary sodium concentrations, as the response to an additional 2–4 mmol/kg/day of sodium (as chloride) can be dramatic. Serum concentrations should be monitored during therapy.

Calcium and phosphorus

Metabolic bone disease of prematurity (previously, osteopenia of prematurity or neonatal rickets) is largely due to substrate deficiency which is the almost inevitable consequence of preterm delivery. In fetal life, active transport across the placenta during the final trimester results in fetal accretion rates which cannot be matched by enteral or parenteral supplementation after birth because when sufficient calcium and phosphate is added to feeds, precipitation of insoluble salts occurs. It is, however, known that addition of calcium and phosphate to enteral feeds will result in improved bone mineral density and lower levels of alkaline phosphatase.[357,359]

Addition of calcium and phosphate to preterm formulae or fortified breast milk is usually unnecessary. If unsupplemented breast milk is used, a supplement of phosphorus (as buffered sodium phosphate 1–2 mmol/kg/day) is recommended. Serum chemistry and alkaline phosphatase should be monitored. Adequate provision of substrate should prevent fractures although special care should be taken in infants exposed to systemic steroids or long term diuretics.

Iron

Iron absorption from human milk is very efficient, but its iron content is low. The iron accretion rates of the third trimester cannot be achieved in human milk fed preterm infants. Fortification and preterm formulae provide additional iron but this may be inadequate and most preterm infants are supplemented with 2 mg/kg/day of iron from 6–8 weeks of age until about 6 months corrected age.

COMPLICATIONS OF FEEDING
Milk aspiration

Regurgitation of milk into the esophagus, as shown by esophageal pH monitoring, is common among preterm babies[360] but significant aspiration is uncommon in infants receiving milk feeds during intensive care. The extent to which milk aspiration contributes to chronic lung disease

or recurrent apneic attacks remains uncertain, but in the infant who has atypical disease with unexplained deterioration or failure to respond to standard therapy, gastroesophageal reflux and aspiration should be considered. Prone positioning, thickening agents and smaller, more frequent feeds may help. Xanthines may be withdrawn. A number of trials have investigated the role of low dose oral erythromycin as a pro-kinetic agent, either prophylactic or as rescue treatment. While some report success, a systematic review found too many differences in trial design to perform a meta-analysis and concluded this treatment could not yet be widely recommended.[361]

Respiratory embarrassment resulting from gastric distention

When the lungs are normal, tube feeding has little or no effect on lung function, but when the lungs are abnormal a tube feed of only 5 ml of milk has been shown to produce a small reduction in arterial PO_2 for about 30 min. During suckling, a fall in arterial PO_2 and a small rise in arterial PCO_2 has been shown in preterm infants. It is important to be aware of this effect in babies recovering from respiratory distress syndrome (RDS) and those with bronchopulmonary dysplasia.

Food intolerance

Intolerance of cows' milk protein seems uncommon among preterm babies, perhaps reflecting the relative unresponsiveness of their immune system. It may present as colitis with fresh bleeding per rectum. Lactose intolerance is more common, especially after NEC or gut surgery. Treatment by exclusion diet is appropriate as long as the substitute food is carefully chosen with the nutritional needs of the preterm baby in mind. The advice of the pediatric dietitian is most helpful.

NUTRITIONAL ASSESSMENT

The final validation of any nutritional regimen is satisfactory growth and prevention of deficiency states. Careful and frequent assessments of the growth of the preterm baby should be made. Weight, length and occipitofrontal circumference are measured at least weekly and related to centile charts. In addition to the routine measurements, reference data are available for skinfold thickness, mid-upper arm circumference (MUAC) and MUAC:head circumference ratio which can be used as indicators of fat deposition and lean body mass.

Hematological and biochemical assessments should be undertaken regularly to look for signs of nutritional deficiency such as: anemia due to iron deficiency; raised alkaline phosphatase and low serum phosphate related to metabolic bone disease; hypoalbuminemia suggesting absolute or relative protein deficiency; hyponatremia; hypocalcemia; metabolic acidosis due to excessive protein intake, etc.

Finally, growth monitoring and dietary advice are an important part of follow-up for the VLBW infant after discharge, and throughout the first year.

INTENSIVE CARE OF THE NEWBORN

ORGANIZATION OF NEONATAL INTENSIVE CARE SERVICES

It is now accepted that 1.0–1.9 neonatal intensive care cots are required per 1000 deliveries.[362] Each unit providing for anything other than anticipated normal deliveries should have special care back-up facilities. Providing neonatal intensive care requires highly trained medical and nursing staff and complex equipment. Continuous back-up maintenance and service support is required. Without such expertise and support outcomes are likely to be compromised and consequently such care should only be carried out in recognized centers.[362] There is evidence that outcomes are improved when intensive care is centralized but this has not been observed universally.[363] Neonatal patient outcomes are worse when nursing care is not delivered by specially qualified neonatal nurses[364] and when unit workloads are close to maximum capacity according to available nurse staffing.[365]

HIERARCHY OF CARE

Every hospital concerned with the delivery of babies should *at all times* provide expertise for the resuscitation of the newborn (basic neonatal life support) – this can be by trained medical or nursing staff and it is the training of these staff that is critical rather than their job title. In addition, all district hospital maternity services should have a neonatal unit that can provide special care. This care can be given by midwives under the supervision of staff trained in neonatal care but the skill mix must be adequate. There should be staff capable of providing advanced neonatal life support and ongoing medical input on site at all times. These can be doctors or advanced neonatal nurse practitioners (ANNP).[366] The British Association of Perinatal Medicine has published a guidance document to assist those planning new neonatal units.[367]

The special care unit (level 1 care – USA) must be capable of providing safe temperature control, oxygen therapy, intravenous access and therapy, and treatment for hypoglycemia, hypocalcemia, hyperbilirubinemia and infection. Though not intended to carry out ongoing intensive care, the special care unit must still provide expertise for the safe resuscitation and stabilization of the unexpected critically ill child prior to transport.

The subregional center (level 2 – USA) will usually be sited in a larger hospital and will be able to offer short term neonatal intensive care to its own deliveries. Infants likely to require long periods of intensive care (e.g. the ELBW infant or infant requiring surgical treatment) would reasonably be diverted to the perinatal intensive care unit (ICU) which when busy could itself refer back shorter term problems and high dependency cases.

Each region should have one or more perinatal ICUs (level 3 – USA) (Table 12.30) dealing with the very high risk mother and infant. These centers provide care for all the most difficult medical problems of the region but also are intimately concerned with the improvement of standards in the region by specialist education and research. Some of these centers will also provide neonatal surgical care. In the UK, extracorporeal membrane oxygenation (ECMO) is provided supraregionally at four centers (level 4).

CATEGORIES OF NEONATAL CARE

The British Association of Perinatal Medicine revised the definitions of categories of care for babies in 2001[362] and recommended that babies categorized as intensive care should receive 1:1 care from a qualified neonatal nurse. High dependency care babies should have at least one nurse for every two babies, and special care babies at least one nurse for every four babies. The most dependent intensive care babies will require more than one nurse.

TRANSPORT OF SICK OR HIGH RISK NEONATES

Introduction

With different hospitals capable of providing different levels of care and the evolution of networks it is inevitable that a significant number of infants will require transfer to another center for care that is not available where the infant was originally destined to deliver. If the issue can be anticipated before delivery, e.g. in the case of antenatally diagnosed problems or planned surgical deliveries of pregnancies with complications arising before term, then transfer of the mother with the infant in utero is generally the preferred option. Even if this is optimized, a large number of postnatal transports will be required for acute care and to return convalescing infants to their referring unit. In Scotland there are around 50 000 total births per annum and this gives rise to approximately 1300 neonatal transfers per year, of which around 30% are emergencies.

Table 12.30 The perinatal intensive care unit (ICU) (at least one in every health region)

Facilities
1. Obstetric ICU facilities/fetal medicine service
2. Neonatal ICU facilities
   a. Minimum medical provision
      Resident junior doctor or ANNP always on duty
      Resident Specialist Registrar or highly experienced ANNP always on duty
      Consultant Neonatologist always on call
   b. Nursing provision
      One qualified neonatal nurse per intensive care baby per shift*
   c. 24 h back-up provisions
      Radiology service to the unit
      Biochemistry with blood gases and electrolytes
      Hematology service for diagnosis and transfusion
      Microbiological service
      Medical physics and electronics
   d. Specialist facilities: surgery, cardiology, audiology, ophthalmology, pharmacy and physiotherapy

Responsibilities
1. Provision of medical neonatal intensive care
2. Provision of surgical neonatal intensive care
3. Administrative liaison within the region
4. Neonatal education for the region
   a. Ward rounds and seminars for nursing and medical visitors to the ICU
   b. Medical and nursing outreach by staff to the district and subregional centers
5. Regional audit
6. Training base for medical and neonatal nursing staff
7. Research
   Epidemiological, applied, basic

---

* Although recommended and ideal, the provision of one neonatal intensive care trained nurse per intensive care baby per shift is not available anywhere in the UK at this stage. One is forced back to stipulating that there be adequate overall numbers of trained nurses and a reasonable skill mix of trainers to trainees. This in fact means that most units are unable to take all the sick infants that they are asked to because of insufficient nursing staff.

Neonatal transport is best delivered by a dedicated transport service and this is now generally organized on a regional or network basis. This enables the provision of trained staff with appropriate equipment whenever needed, without compromising the core staffing of any individual unit. Despatching a transport team and traveling to the referring unit takes time and this means that support cannot be immediate; referring units must be capable of providing whatever initial resuscitation and stabilization is required. Training in these matters may be required as part of the overall risk management of a network and transport service. Individual units need an agreed policy on which categories of infants should be transferred and to which units the babies would usually travel. It should be clearly defined who is responsible for identifying an appropriate cot and who is the senior clinician responsible for the infant before, during and after the transfer. Good communication between senior clinicians is essential. Transport may be by road, helicopter, fixed wing aircraft or a combination of these.

Equipment

Transport equipment should enable the provision of full neonatal intensive care during the journey. Regulations cover the specification of the equipment to ensure that it is fit for purpose and is light enough to be moved by transport staff without compromising health and safety. A transport trolley incorporating portable incubator, ventilator, gas supply, monitor, infusion pumps and battery power is usually used. Systems have been designed to enable this to be fixed securely in the ambulance

Table 12.31 Indicators for antenatal (in utero) transfer

1. Obstetric assessment of the high risk fetus where urgent delivery is likely (e.g. IUGR, fetal cardiac rhythm disorder)
2. The severely ill mother (e.g. with pregnancy-associated hypertension) at an early stage of pregnancy with a potentially viable fetus
3. Early preterm labor where the referring hospital has inadequate facilities
4. Hemolytic disease with a severely affected fetus
5. Fetal malformation needing postnatal surgery
6. Prolonged and preterm rupture of the fetal membranes with resulting oligohydramnios
7. Any other situation where advanced neonatal resuscitation is anticipated

and inside dedicated transport aircraft. There is no longer a justification for attempting transport on an ad hoc basis without such equipment. The transport staff will also carry equipment bags with a full range of resuscitation and stabilization equipment, as well as any drugs that might be required. Presently available transport systems do not enable the provision of high frequency oscillatory ventilation and infants on this treatment need to be stabilized on conventional ventilation before transfer. The provision of a fully equipped and trained service means that the transport team can spend whatever time is necessary in the referring unit to secure the stability of the patient before transport so that the actual transport of the baby can be as unhurried as possible. This minimizes the need for the use of blue lights and hazardous driving.

Antenatal (in utero) transfer (Table 12.31)

With few exceptions the best portable incubator for the high risk problem is the uterus, with delivery of the infant where support and expertise are readily available. Such transfers should be with agreement between district and central obstetric consultants and should also involve the neonatal staff of the ICU. Mothers in advanced stages of preterm labor may need delivery peripherally to avoid the danger of a delivery in the ambulance. The mother with severe pregnancy-associated hypertension or antepartum hemorrhage should be stable before transfer and an obstetric doctor should accompany her. Systems for transferring mothers are not yet as well developed as those for transporting infants.

PRACTICAL PARENTERAL NUTRITION

All units providing neonatal intensive and high dependency care must be able to provide optimal parenteral nutrition for sick, full-term and preterm infants. All regimens should provide complete nutrition in terms of macronutrients (protein, carbohydrate and fat) and micronutrients, with minimal adverse nutritional or other consequences. Energy and nutrient stores are mainly laid down in the third trimester of pregnancy, so parenteral nutrition of the preterm infant must supply energy and nutrients not only to meet basic needs, but also to promote growth, which occurs at a rate of 15 g/kg/d or 1.5% of body weight at this stage.[368] About 15 years ago, it was stated that there was a dearth of well-designed studies of parenteral nutrition use in the newborn,[369] and despite the advent of evidence-based medicine and the Cochrane Collaboration, there remain few high quality systematic reviews with homogeneous studies, and low numbers of randomized controlled trials of parenteral nutrition of the newborn without major methodological flaws. This is exemplified by the joint ESPGHAN/ESPEN guidelines on pediatric parenteral nutrition,[370] which by necessity are based mainly on adult data and expert opinion due to the scarcity of good pediatric trials.

INDICATIONS IN THE NEONATAL UNIT

Parenteral nutrition may provide all the nutritional requirements of the infant (total parenteral nutrition, TPN) or may more usually be supplemented by some enteral nutrition (partial parenteral nutrition, PPN). Low volume or 'minimal' enteral feeding should be started in all sick newborn infants.[371]

There are three major indications for parenteral nutrition in the neonatal unit:

1. surgical lesions such as omphalocele or gastroschisis, or following extensive bowel resection (PPN if possible, or TPN);
2. the medical (and surgical) treatment of necrotizing enterocolitis (NEC) (usually TPN);
3. in immature and usually very premature infants where enteral feeds cannot be fully established, due to gastrointestinal immaturity (PPN).

NUTRITIONAL REQUIREMENTS DURING PARENTERAL NUTRITION

Fluid and sodium

After birth, loss of interstitial fluid causes contraction of the extracellular compartment, and the resulting loss of sodium and water accounts in part for the early postnatal weight loss seen in all babies.[368] After this, growth can only be supported by a positive sodium balance. Some preterm babies have renal salt wasting, and thus very high sodium needs. Fluid needs vary depending upon maturity, postnatal age and environment, and may be huge in very immature infants; cohort and case control studies have suggested that excessive fluid intake in early life is associated with worse outcome in preterm infants in terms of chronic lung disease and NEC.

Energy

It has been suggested that a parenteral energy intake of 90 kcal/kg/d with adequate nitrogen intake will support weight gain in preterm infants equivalent to the intrauterine rate.[369] The energy needs of the very preterm or ventilator dependent baby are likely to be higher.[372] Chronic energy imbalance is common in very preterm babies, particularly those with chronic lung disease, and there is often a major problem in the shortfall between prescribed and actual energy intakes.[373] Multiple reasons contribute to this shortfall, such as the need for fluid restriction, intolerance of standard dextrose infusions, withholding parenteral lipid due to concerns about clinical status, delay in commencing and advancing enteral feeds, and technical problems such as delay in re-establishing venous access. Only determined efforts to monitor and negate this shortfall in energy intake will help prevent the growth problems that are very common at hospital discharge of very preterm infants.[374]

Protein

Although milks provide between 2 and 4 g/kg/d of protein, most preterm infants receive only 2.5 g/kg/day of parenteral amino acids, and few randomized controlled studies have assessed higher intakes.[374] During evolution, the animal kingdom lost the enzyme capacity to synthesize nine amino acids and therefore were dependent upon supply from exogenous sources for these *essential* amino acids; the remainder were termed *non-essential*. A more accurate terminology has been created,[375] which now divides amino acids into *indispensable* (equivalent to essential), *conditionally indispensable* (whose rates of biosynthesis may be inadequate, particularly during certain pathophysiological or metabolic states), and *dispensable* (no dietary need for preformed amino acids, but do contribute to nonspecific nitrogen pool). The original parenteral amino acid solutions were protein hydrolysates, and were replaced by crystalline amino acid solutions, which were then specifically refined for use in children; problems such as hyperammonemia, metabolic acidosis and hyperphenylalaninemia were associated with the use of these in newborn infants. The latest amino acid preparations for neonatal TPN contain amino acids felt to be conditionally indispensable for the newborn. They have low phenylalanine contents, are carbohydrate and electrolyte free and are based upon the amino acid profile of either human breast milk or cord blood.[376]

Fat

The absence of an intravenous lipid emulsion in early parenteral nutrition regimens led to a syndrome of essential fatty acid deficiency with inadequate growth and a scaly dermatitis. In the UK and Europe lipid solutions can be obtained as 10% or 20% concentrations; randomized controlled trials have demonstrated the superiority of use of 20% emulsions.[377] These solutions are usually based on soya oil, although olive oil based solutions and solutions containing medium chain triglycerides are available; few studies have compared different types of solutions. Preterm infants can tolerate incremental increases up to 3.5–4.0 g/kg/day of parenteral lipid without side-effects.[374] Concerns about undernutrition in the sick preterm infant have led to the use of parenteral lipid solutions soon after the commencement of parenteral nutrition. A Cochrane review[378] of five RCTs containing 397 preterm infants found no statistically significant effects on either benefits or adverse outcomes of early introduction of lipids, defined as before day 6 of life.

Carbohydrate

Term newborns have a significantly higher glucose requirement than older children, and preterm infants have the highest needs of all. It is usual to start with a 10% dextrose solution at approximately 6 g/kg/d (4 mg/kg/min), and to increase this incrementally if there is no hyperglycemia. Continuous insulin infusions have been used as an effective treatment of hyperglycemia in preterm infants.[374]

Vitamins and minerals

In the past the vitamin and mineral requirements of preterm infants have often been poorly met with parenteral feeding; a typical parenteral prescription that meets these needs is shown in Table 12.32 using the Scottish standard neonatal bag.

Other additives

Heparin increases the clearance of lipid from the circulation; there is a belief, not backed up by any evidence, that addition of 1 IU/ml to parenteral nutrition solutions preserves i.v. line patency and promotes lipolysis. Preterm infants have low concentrations of carnitine, required for oxidation of long chain fatty acids; a Cochrane review evaluated the many studies of supplemental carnitine in parenterally fed newborns, and concluded that there was no evidence to support its use.[379]

Table 12.32 A typical parenteral nutrition prescription using the standard Scottish neonatal bag for a 20-day-old infant of 1500 g with necrotizing enterocolitis (150 ml/kg/d). Note further additions of electrolytes may be added to the bag. (Courtesy of David Hoole, Senior Pharmacist, Royal Hospital for Sick Children, Edinburgh.)

Aqueous bag		Lipid bag	
Vaminolact[+]	68 ml	Intralipid 20%[+]	26 ml (3.5 g/kg/d)
Glucose 20% w/v	96 ml	Vitlipid Infant[+]	6 ml (4 ml/kg/d)
Solvito[+]	1.5 ml (1 ml/kg/d)		
Potassium chloride 15%	0.95 ml		
Sodium glycerophosphate 21.6%	1.9 ml		
Magnesium sulfate 2 mmol/ml	0.13 ml		
Peditrace[+]	1.5 ml (1 ml/kg/d)		
Calcium gluconate 10% w/v	8.5 ml		
Water for injections	15 ml		
Total	193 ml		32 ml

The final solution has the following composition:

Amino acids	4.8 g (3.2 g/kg/d)
Retinol	414 µg (276 µg/kg/d)
Nitrogen	0.64 g (0.43 g/kg/d)
Ergocalciferol	6 µg (4 µg/kg/d)
Carbohydrate	19.1 g (12.7 g/kg/d)
Tocopherol	3.84 mg (2.56 mg/kg/d)
Sodium	3.8 mmol (2.5 mmol/kg/d)
Phytomenadione	120 µg (80 µg/kg/d)
Potassium	1.9 mmol (1.3 mmol/kg/d)
Lipid	5.2 g (3.5 g/kg/d)
Calcium	1.9 mmol (1.3 mmol/kg/d)
Phosphate	1.9 mmol (1.3 mmol/kg/d)
Magnesium	0.26 mmol (0.17 mmol/kg/d)
Vitamin B$_1$	0.38 mg (0.25 mg/kg/d)
Vitamin B$_2$	0.54 mg (0.36 mg/kg/d)
Nicotinamide	6.0 mg (4.0 mg/kg/d)
Pantothenic acid	2.25 mg (1.5 mg/kg/d)
Biotin	9.0 µg (6.0 µg/kg/d)
Folic acid	60 µg (40 µg/kg/d)
Vitamin B$_6$	0.6 mg (0.4 mg/kg/d)
Vitamin B$_{12}$	0.75 µg (0.5 µg/kg/d)
Vitamin C	15 mg (10 mg/kg/d)
Copper	0.47 µmol (0.31 µmol/kg/d)
Zinc	5.7 µmol (3.8 µmol/kg/d)
Manganese	0.027 µmol (0.018 µmol/kg/d)
Selenium	0.038 µmol (0.025 µmol/kg/d)
Fluoride	4.5 µmol (3.0 µmol/kg/d)
Iodide	0.012 µmol (0.008 µmol/kg/d)

[+] Fresenius Kabi, UK.

Other additives have been given to parenteral nutrition in the newborn to try to either improve clinical outcome or prevent adverse outcomes. Cysteine, cystine or N-acetyl cysteine supplementation has been parenterally fed to neonates. L-cysteine is a conditionally indispensable amino acid for neonates, and is a precursor of the antioxidant glutathione. A Cochrane review of six RCTs of mainly preterm infants, of which five were short term studies, concluded that the available evidence does not support the routine use of these substances.[380] There has long been an interest in glutamine supplementation to prevent morbidity and mortality in preterm infants. In a Cochrane review[381] of glutamine supplementation in preterm infants, six RCTs were identified, of which two (involving 1468 infants) were of parenteral glutamine administration. There was no evidence that the routine use of glutamine supplementation altered mortality or other important clinical outcomes for very low birth weight infants. Arginine can act as a substrate for the production of nitric oxide in the tissues and arginine supplementation may help in preventing NEC – decreased concentration of nitric oxide is proposed as one of the possible cellular mechanisms for NEC. A Cochrane review[382] of arginine supplementation to parenteral nutrition to prevent NEC in preterm infants identified only one RCT, involving 152 infants, and concluded that this was insufficient evidence and that a large multicenter RCT was required.

TECHNIQUE OF PREPARATION, ADMINISTRATION AND MONITORING

As for all nutritional support, involvement of a multidisciplinary nutrition support team (NST) will optimize parenteral feeding and reduce complications (Table 12.33).[383] Nutrition support teams have long been used in pediatric hospitals on the basis that they improve nutritional management of sick children. This includes screening for nutritional risk, identification of patients requiring nutritional support, and the provision of adequate nutritional management, education and training of hospital staff. This is provided by a multidisciplinary team with expertise in all aspects of clinical nutrition care.[383] The use of neonatal NSTs has been slow to develop, with many major neonatal units still not having a specialist dietitian with a neonatal interest, let alone a nutrition support nurse. A common practice in the United Kingdom is that parenteral nutrition is provided using a standard neonatal infusion bag (see Table 12.32). There are concerns that this does not meet the currently recommended nutrient guidelines,[370] so increasing risk of undernutrition with prolonged use.

Once it appears that an infant will require prolonged parenteral nutrition (beyond the corrected age of term), is having complications related to parenteral nutrition, or seems to have irreversible intestinal failure, it is transferred to a pediatric teaching hospital with a pediatric nutrition support team, a pediatric gastroenterology and nutrition department, a pediatric surgical department, and a defined pediatric pharmacy, all with appropriate expertise. In Table 12.34, a typical parenteral prescription that meets the currently recommended nutrient guidelines[370] is shown for the same infant as Table 12.32, in this case using the Royal Hospital for Sick Children, Edinburgh, standard

Table 12.33 Complications of parenteral nutrition

1. Catheter related
   a. Sepsis – bacterial or fungal
   b. Thrombosis/obstruction
   c. Hemorrhage
   d. Extravasation of fluid from peripheral lines
   e. Catheter displacement, breakage or removal
2. Metabolic related
   a. Cholestasis – often reversible, and reduced by minimal enteral feeding
   b. Fat embolism, lipid overload – rare
   c. Hyperglycemia and glycosuria
   d. Hyperammonemia and acidosis – rare

0–2-year-old infant infusion bag. This standard bag has met the needs of more than 95% of all 0–2-year-olds, including neonates with prolonged intestinal failure, in the last 2 years. The exceptions have been severely ill infants in intensive care with major fluid restriction and multiple infusions of medications.

Prescription of TPN is often aided by the use of computer programs, although nutritional regimens may be individualized depending on the degree of prematurity, postnatal age, concurrent illness, enteral feed tolerance, and presence of undernutrition requiring catch-up growth.[368] Whether the final solution is infused by central or by peripheral vein, it should be made up by pharmacy under laminar flow conditions to prevent contamination. It should be run through from the bag to the giving set delivery point so that all that is required on the neonatal unit is the linking of the sterile connection of the set to the intravenous line on the baby. The lipid should join the main set by a Y-connector just prior to this connection. Covering the bags with colored polyethylene will reduce the photodegradation of vitamins. In many units, it is practice to use in-line filters for intravenous solutions. A Cochrane review of three randomized controlled trials of 262 infants found insufficient data to determine any benefit to their use.[384]

Since Wilmore & Dudrick's original description in 1968,[385] central lines have frequently been used to give parenteral nutrition. This is because access to the circulation can be very difficult in infants, particularly if prolonged parenteral nutrition is required. Peripheral venous cannulae have a limited life span and are associated with infiltration of the infusate and skin sloughs.[369] Frequent occlusion will result in increased handling of the baby and interruption of nutrient supply. Central access is usually provided by noncuffed silicone catheters that are inserted percutaneously and threaded to a central position. Due to concerns about pericardial effusions, these are usually placed close to, but not in, the right atrium. In most units, parenteral nutrition is given initially by peripheral cannulas, with a change to percutaneous central venous catheters if it appears that the child will need more than a few days of nutrition. In a Cochrane review of three randomized controlled trials of 262 infants, there was a suggestion that use of percutaneously replaced central venous catheters improved nutrient intake, with no evidence of increased adverse events.[386] If longer term parenteral nutrition is required, at some stage a surgically placed central venous catheter with a tunneled subcutaneous portion (such as a Hickman catheter) will be needed. It is important to liaise with both a pediatric surgeon interested and experienced in vascular access and a pediatric gastroenterology and nutrition team if a preterm infant is thought to require prolonged parenteral nutrition but is not yet well enough to be transferred to a pediatric unit. Many infants run into problems out of hours with vascular access, and end up having lines placed in external jugular veins or femoral veins. For children with prolonged intestinal failure, emergency line placement in these sites may be associated with thrombosis and loss of central venous access, potentially in all four major central venous quadrants (upper right, upper left, lower right and lower left), a situation which either requires novel methods of vascular access or will push a child towards an assessment for small intestinal transplantation.

Monitoring of growth and biochemical and metabolic tolerance of parenteral nutrition is mandatory. A few infants, for example those with intestinal failure due to short gut syndrome (see later), will require prolonged parenteral feeding in hospital or at home, and early liaison with pediatric gastroenterologists is advised.

BLOOD GASES AND RESPIRATORY SUPPORT

Optimal respiratory support requires meticulous attention to blood gases, equipment settings, blood pressure and infant behavior. Maintenance of appropriate gas exchange with minimal complications requires knowledge of:
1. lung mechanics;
2. mechanisms of lung injury;
3. the principles of gas exchange;
4. appropriate blood gas values;
5. measurement of blood gases.

Table 12.34 A typical parenteral nutrition prescription using the standard RHSC Edinburgh (0–2 years) TPN bag for a 20-day-old infant of 1500 g with necrotizing enterocolitis (max nutrition supplied on 135 ml/kg/d). Note further additions of electrolytes may be added to the bag. (Courtesy of David Hoole, Senior Pharmacist, Royal Hospital for Sick Children, Edinburgh.)

Aqueous bag		Lipid bag	
Vaminolact[†]	90 ml	Intralipid 20%[†]	26 ml (3.5 g/kg/d)
Glucose 50% w/v	54 ml	Vitlipid Infant[†]	6 ml (4 ml/kg/d)
Solvito[†]	1.5 ml (1 ml/kg/d)		
Sodium glycerophosphate 21.6%	1.3 ml		
Magnesium sulfate 2 mmol/ml	0.17 ml		
Peditrace[†]	1.5 ml (1 ml/kg/d)		
Calcium chloride 1 mmol/ml	1.4 ml		
Sodium chloride 30%	0.77 ml		
Water for injections	21 ml		
Total	172 ml		32 ml

The final solution has the following composition:

Amino acids	6.3 g (4.2 g/kg/d)
Retinol	414 µg (276 µg/kg/d)
Nitrogen	0.84 g (0.56 g/kg/d)
Ergocalciferol	6 µg (4 µg/kg/d)
Carbohydrate	27 g (18 g/kg/d)
Tocopherol	3.84 mg (2.56 mg/kg/d)
Sodium	6.5 mmol (4.3 mmol/kg/d)
Phytomenadione	120 µg (80 µg/kg/d)
Potassium	3.7 mmol (2.5 mmol/kg/d)
Lipid	5.2 g (3.5 g/kg/d)
Calcium	1.4 mmol (0.9 mmol/kg/d)
Phosphate	1.3 mmol (0.86 mmol/kg/d)
Magnesium	0.34 mmol (0.23 mmol/kg/d)
Vitamin B_1	0.38 mg (0.25 mg/kg/d)
Vitamin B_2	0.54 mg (0.36 mg/kg/d)
Nicotinamide	6.0 mg (4.0 mg/kg/d)
Pantothenic acid	2.25 mg (1.5 mg/kg/d)
Biotin	9.0 µg (6.0 µg/kg/d)
Folic acid	60 µg (40 µg/kg/d)
Vitamin B_6	0.6 mg (0.4 mg/kg/d)
Vitamin B_{12}	0.75 µg (0.5 µg/kg/d)
Vitamin C	15 mg (10 mg/kg/d)
Copper	0.47 µmol (0.31 µmol/kg/d)
Zinc	5.7 µmol (3.8 µmol/kg/d)
Manganese	0.027 µmol (0.018 µmol/kg/d)
Selenium	0.038 µmol (0.025 µmol/kg/d)
Fluoride	4.5 µmol (3.0 µmol/kg/d)
Iodide	0.012 µmol (0.008 µmol/kg/d)

[†] Fresenius Kabi, UK.

LUNG MECHANICS

To inflate the lungs, work must be done against their elastic recoil and resistance. Even with adequate surfactant most of this recoil is attributable to surface tension. Lung compliance is the change in lung volume per unit change in pressure. This is proportional to the number of recruited alveoli and is therefore determined by the size of the lungs but is reduced by atelectasis or consolidation and improves as these improve. Resistance reflects airway caliber and increases with airway narrowing.

The pressure–volume curve of the lungs

When lungs are inflated from complete atelectasis, large pressure changes are required to begin opening the alveoli. Once opened, they inflate easily and smaller changes in pressure achieve large changes in volume. As the alveoli become overdistended, further pressure changes add little volume. During deflation the alveoli do not collapse completely. Surfactant enables lung volume to remain higher per unit pressure than during inflation. Around 30 ml/kg body weight of gas remains in the lungs at end-expiration. This functional residual capacity (FRC)

enables gas exchange to continue during expiration. Surfactant deficiency impairs deflation stability causing alveolar collapse, reduced FRC and impaired gas exchange. Once the alveoli collapse, high pressures are required to re-recruit them.

The time required to inflate or deflate the lungs depends on the tidal volume, the pressure applied and the resistance to flow. If resistance is high, as in chronic lung disease or endotracheal tube obstruction, the same volume takes longer to exchange. Where compliance is low, as in RDS, the recoil pressure is high and the lungs empty rapidly.

MECHANISMS OF LUNG INJURY

The same mechanisms of lung injury operate in all age groups.[387,388] High volume injury (volutrauma) occurs when the airspaces are inflated to excess end-inspiratory volume. Low volume injury (atelectrauma) occurs when the lungs are allowed recurrently to collapse at end-expiration and are re-inflated with each breath. Both mechanisms cause epithelial disruption and alveolar capillary leak. This causes accumulation within the airspaces of proteinaceous material which inhibits surfactant function and adds further to the cycle. Injury may begin within minutes and is accompanied by inflammation, the persistence of which has been implicated in the pathogenesis of chronic lung disease.[389]

Respiratory support techniques should aim to maintain optimal alveolar recruitment and limit excess tidal volume. This is associated with lower mortality and more rapid resolution of pulmonary inflammation in adults.[390,391] There are no published trials examining this approach in neonates. A healthy, term infant breathes with a tidal volume of around 7–9 ml/kg.[392] In the presence of lung disease there may be less fully functional alveoli than normal. Ventilator tidal volumes of around 4–7 ml/kg may be more appropriate if focal overinflation is to be minimized.

Oxygen in high concentration generates free radicals. The preterm infant has poorly developed antioxidant lung defenses and may be at greater risk of oxygen toxicity. Failure to maintain adequate end-expiratory lung volume causes hypoxia and results in greater exposure to supplemental oxygen.

PRINCIPLES OF GAS EXCHANGE

If ventilation and perfusion are well matched, gas tensions in the blood equilibrate with those in the airspaces. Mechanisms of ventilation/perfusion mismatching and impaired gas exchange are illustrated in Figure 12.14.

Oxygenation

When alveoli collapse or are filled with blood, edema or exudate, blood perfusing them traverses the lungs without exchanging gas (right to left shunt). If the pulmonary vascular resistance is elevated, extrapulmonary right to left shunt can take place through the foramen ovale and ductus arteriosus. This occurs in association with acidosis, hypoxia, hypercarbia, lung disease or persistent pulmonary hypertension of the newborn and is worsened by low systemic blood pressure. High ventilator pressures may also compromise pulmonary blood flow. If cardiac output is low, the blood perfusing the alveoli has lower oxygen tension and higher carbon dioxide tension than normal and equilibration with alveolar gas may be incomplete. If blood volume is low the increased rate of recirculation may reduce the time available for equilibration. Inadequate alveolar ventilation results in lower alveolar oxygen tension and hypoxia.

Mild degrees of shunt can be compensated for by increasing the inspired oxygen concentration. If the shunt is more substantial, increased inspired oxygen is ineffective. The vast majority of the oxygen carried in blood is bound to hemoglobin. Relatively little can dissolve in the plasma. Once hemoglobin is fully saturated, further large increases in oxygen tension (PO_2) generate small increases in total blood oxygen content as they only reflect increased dissolved oxygen in plasma. When fully saturated blood from alveoli with good ventilation/perfusion matching is mixed with large amounts of desaturated shunt blood, the mixture cannot be fully saturated. Severely compromised oxygenation can only be improved by decreasing the degree of shunt. This requires recruitment of unventilated alveoli or improvement of pulmonary perfusion. By improving pulmonary perfusion, correction of hypotension may improve gas exchange without alteration of the ventilator settings.

Carbon dioxide elimination

Carbon dioxide is more soluble in plasma than oxygen and its pulmonary diffusion capacity is greater. The relationship between blood carbon dioxide content and arterial carbon dioxide tension ($PaCO_2$) is linear. Carbon dioxide elimination is proportional to total alveolar ventilation. This can be expressed as minute ventilation (tidal volume times respiratory rate). In respiratory failure or where there is right to left shunting, the carbon dioxide tension of blood returning from alveoli with good ventilation/perfusion matching can be lowered by increased alveolar ventilation. This can compensate for the elevated carbon dioxide of shunt blood and normalize $PaCO_2$. Minute ventilation may be inadequate with poor respiratory drive, airway obstruction, widespread atelectasis or increased respiratory dead space.

MEASUREMENT OF BLOOD GASES

All neonatal units should have immediate 24 h access to a blood gas analyzer. Blood samples are usually obtained from an umbilical arterial catheter, or by indwelling catheter or needle puncture from the radial or posterior tibial arteries after assessing the collateral circulation. Use of end arteries (temporal, brachial or femoral) is less desirable because of the risk of irreversible ischemia.

Measurements of PO_2 in capillary or venous blood underestimate arterial oxygen tension (PaO_2) and cannot be relied on. Capillary blood obtained by heel prick provides an acceptable estimate of arterial PCO_2, pH and base excess, but warming the heel to 40 °C does not significantly improve accuracy of PO_2.[393]

Continuous monitoring of blood gas tensions or oxygen saturation is an important supplement to, but not a substitute for, intermittent sampling. Continuous measurements can be made by an indwelling device in the umbilical artery.[394] Transcutaneous monitors generate local hyperemia by gently heating the skin. Diffusion of gases through the skin then permits measurement of gas tensions and both PO_2 and PCO_2 can be measured. This technique is unreliable when the skin is poorly perfused or compressed and becomes less reliable as the skin thickens with age. In very immature infants, repeated reattachment of the electrode can damage the skin. Pulse oximetry is easier and less invasive but gives less information. A probe transilluminates a body part and measures the light absorption characteristics of oxygenated hemoglobin. Pulse oximeters can be used at all gestations, require no calibration and are not affected by changes in skin thickness or perfusion. The technique is very prone to movement artefact, although new signal processing techniques can reduce this problem.[395] In the steep portion of the oxygen–hemoglobin dissociation curve, small changes in PO_2 cause large changes in O_2 saturation, so in this range the pulse oximeter reflects hypoxia and oxygen availability to tissues better than $tcPO_2$ measurements. In the flat portion of the oxygen–hemoglobin dissociation curve large changes in PO_2 cause small changes in O_2 saturation, so hyperoxia cannot safely be excluded when $tcSaO_2$ is 95–100% and $tcPO_2$ monitoring is more reliable.

RECOMMENDED BLOOD GAS VALUES

Present recommendations are based on physiological reasoning and clinical observations. There is a need for prospective trials which compare the outcomes of infants with different target blood gas values as the interventions introduced to normalize blood gases may be harmful.

Oxygenation (PaO_2, $tcPO_2$ and $tcSaO_2$)

Values for $tcPO_2$ and $tcSaO_2$ in the first weeks of life from healthy term and preterm infants[396,397] are shown in Table 12.35. In preterm infants hyperoxia is associated with increased risk of chronic lung disease, retinopathy of prematurity[398] and periventricular leukomalacia.[399] Even modest variations in oxygen administration policy may be associated with significant changes in risk of adverse outcome.[400] There is considerable variation in policy between units.[401] Randomized controlled trials are under way in the USA, Australia and New Zealand and the United Kingdom comparing different target ranges for oxygen saturation. At all

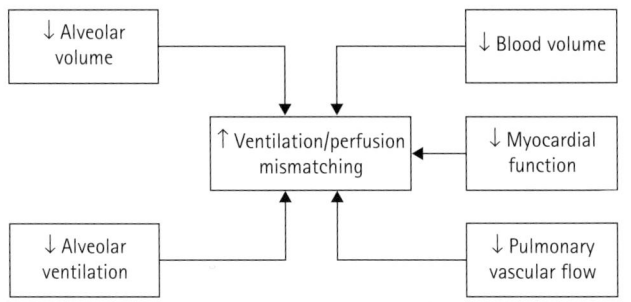

Fig. 12.14 Mechanisms leading to ventilation/perfusion mismatching.

Table 12.35 Normal range of tcPO₂ and tcSaO₂ in healthy infants in air* (adapted from Mok et al 1986,[396] 1988[397])

	Awake	Quiet sleep	Active sleep
Term infants (n = 55)			
tcPO₂ (kPa†)			
Postnatal age			
< 1 week	8.5–13.0	7.8–12.1	6.7–12.8
6 weeks	9.1–12.2	7.1–12.3	7.1–12.4
tcSaO₂ (%)			
Postnatal age			
< 1 week	91.8–100	87.4–98.3	86.1–98.4
6 weeks	95.0–99.0	89.4–98.1	87.5–98.5
Preterm infants (n = 28)			
tcPO₂ (kPa†)			
Postconceptional age			
29–34 weeks	4.7–11.0	6.4–11.7	4.7–11.1
36–38 weeks	6.8–12.5	7.0–12.9	6.7–12.0
tcSaO₂ (%)			
Postconceptional age			
29–34 weeks	86.6–96.3	86.0–96.1	86.6–96.5
35–38 weeks	86.8–96.8	87.6–97.9	88.6–96.8

* No infant appeared cyanosed or had signs of respiratory distress during any of the studies.
† To convert oxygen tension in kPa to mmHg, multiply by 7.5.

gestations prolonged severe hypoxia causes organ damage. Until new data become available, a reasonable policy for preterm infants receiving respiratory support is to aim for PaO₂ or tcPO₂ between 6.7 and 10.7 kPa (50–80 mmHg) or tcSaO₂ between 86 and 94%.

Carbon dioxide tension

Hypercapnia produces pulmonary vasoconstriction, but cerebral vasodilatation. In a prospective study of 200 very low birth weight infants, PaCO₂ > 7 kPa (52.5 mmHg) was associated with both periventricular hemorrhage and periventricular leukomalacia.[402] Severe hypocapnia causes a profound reduction in cerebral blood flow, and has been associated with periventricular leukomalacia, intracerebral hemorrhage and cerebral palsy.[399,403–405]

Broad consensus in current practice is to keep PaCO₂ between 4.7 and 8 kPa (35–60 mmHg).[406] However in severe respiratory failure some authors *routinely* keep PaCO₂ between 6.7 and 8 kPa (50–60 mmHg) or higher, provided arterial pH remains above 7.25. By allowing lower ventilator pressures to be used, it is suggested, may increase the number of infants surviving without chronic lung disease.[407–410] Whether allowing higher values of PaCO₂ may also increase the risk of cerebral insult and handicap in preterm infants is uncertain. Data from prospective trials in newborn infants are limited and inconclusive at present.[411] In the meantime a reasonable compromise is to aim for PaCO₂ between 5.3 and 7.0 kPa (40–52.5 mmHg) in preterm infants below 33 weeks' gestation during the first 3 days of life. In term infants or older preterm infants, higher levels of PaCO₂ are probably acceptable in order to limit ventilator pressures, provided acidosis is avoided. Iatrogenic hypocapnia should be avoided.

pH

Acidosis causes cerebral vasodilatation and alkalosis cerebral vasoconstriction. Acidosis may also promote pulmonary vasoconstriction and right to left shunting. In preterm infants, pH < 7.20 has been associated with periventricular hemorrhage[412] and pH < 7.1 with periventricular leukomalacia.[402] In very low birth weight infants pH < 7.20 has been associated with retinopathy of prematurity.[398] Acidosis may be due to tissue hypoxia, respiratory failure, excess acid load, renal dysfunction or inborn error of metabolism. It is unlikely that a pH value will have

the same implications whatever its origins. Simultaneous measurements of plasma lactate may give additional information. Interventions aimed at altering pH should reflect the likely underlying explanation. On present information, a reasonable policy for infants receiving respiratory support is to keep pH between 7.20 and 7.45.

RESPIRATORY SUPPORT

Reducing the need for respiratory support by antenatal steroids or methylxanthines

Treating mothers at risk of preterm delivery with antenatal steroids reduces infants' risks of RDS, death and brain damage by around 50%[413] and should be a standard of care. In women at less than 32 weeks' gestation who remain undelivered but still at risk of preterm birth 7 days after treatment, repeating the steroids weekly reduces the severity of neonatal lung disease but does not alter the risk of air leak, chronic lung disease, major cerebral ultrasound scan abnormality or death.[414] Long term follow-up data are required to determine the full balance of risks and benefits of this approach.

Trials demonstrate that methylxanthines such as caffeine and theophylline reduce the occurrence of apnea of prematurity and decrease the need for ventilation.[415,416] This is associated with lower risk of bronchopulmonary dysplasia.[417] Long term follow-up data are awaited to determine whether there are any other health benefits or risks.

Continuous positive airway pressure

Continuous positive airway pressure (CPAP) helps to establish and maintain alveolar recruitment. This protects against low volume lung injury, improves gas exchange and reduces work of breathing. CPAP may also maintain the patency of the upper airways and reduce the frequency of apnea. Use of nasal CPAP in preterm infants after extubation is associated with a lower risk of extubation failure.[418] CPAP can be generated by placing the outlet tubing of a gas source under water (bubble CPAP), by a mechanical ventilator, or by a flow generated method (Infant flow™ driver or Benveniste valve). None is proven to be clearly superior in clinical trials. Epidemiological data suggest that chronic lung disease may be observed less frequently when CPAP is preferred to mechanical ventilation in preterm infants[419] but so far trials have not confirmed this.[420,421] Two current randomized controlled trials (the COIN trial and the SUPPORT trial) may help to answer this question.

When nasal CPAP is delivered using a mechanical ventilator, nasal intermittent positive pressure ventilation can be delivered and this can be synchronized to the infant's breathing pattern. This has been called 'non-invasive ventilation'. Similar support can be delivered using a device that can generate bi-level CPAP. Three small trials comparing synchronized nasal intermittent positive pressure ventilation (SNIPPV) with conventional CPAP in infants post extubation suggest that SNIPPV may reduce the risk of extubation failure.[422]

Nasal CPAP can be combined with surfactant administration to treat RDS.[423,424] Infants with worsening respiratory failure are sedated, intubated, surfactant is administered and the infants are extubated and returned to CPAP. This may reduce the number of infants that require ventilation but it has not been demonstrated to be superior to elective intubation soon after birth for prophylactic surfactant treatment.

Indications for respiratory support by endotracheal tube

No consensus exists as to when to start intermittent positive pressure ventilation by endotracheal tube. Some start it electively at birth in the smallest infants, others use it as rescue therapy in infants failing on CPAP. Prolonged apnea, or progressive respiratory failure are the principal indications. Intubation can be hazardous. An endotracheal tube prevents laryngeal closure which removes the infant's capacity to maintain lung volume by grunting. Adequate positive end-expiratory pressure (PEEP) is required to prevent atelectasis. By narrowing the airway the resistive work of breathing is increased. The extra work is done by the ventilator except at low ventilator settings. Other complications include blockage or malplacement of the tube, airway injury, impaired muco-ciliary clearance, infection and aspiration, which all may contribute to chronic lung disease.

CONTROLLING GAS EXCHANGE BY MECHANICAL VENTILATION

Despite variations in the type and severity of neonatal respiratory disorders, alterations in ventilator settings often have predictable effects on oxygenation and $PaCO_2$. These are summarized in Tables 12.36 and 12.37.

Mean airway pressure and oxygenation

Herman & Reynolds[425] showed in infants with severe hyaline membrane disease a linear relationship between mean airway pressure and oxygenation, expressed as A-aDO$_2$ (Fig. 12.15). Improved oxygenation was mainly attributed to improved alveolar inflation with reduced intrapulmonary right to left shunt. Increases in (1) peak pressure, (2) inspiratory:expiratory ratio and (3) positive end expiratory pressure were thought to (a) expand collapsed lung units, (b) hold them open longer and (c) prevent their collapse during expiration. With stiff lungs in severe disease, high mean airway pressures had no effect on cardiac output or arterial blood pressure. Stewart et al[426] achieved greater increases in oxygenation per

Table 12.36 Ventilator settings and gas exchange: methods of increasing oxygenation

Maneuver	Probable underlying mechanisms
1. ↑ FiO_2	a. ↑Saturation of alveolar capillary blood b. Relieving hypoxia can decrease pulmonary vascular resistance, reducing extrapulmonary right to left shunt through fetal channels
2. Adding CPAP	Maintains lung volume in spontaneously breathing infants with reduced lung compliance
3. ↑ PIP	These three maneuvers increase MAP, hence lung volume and oxygenation
4. ↑ PEEP	The stiffer the lungs, the greater the MAP needed for optimum lung expansion
5. ↑ I:E ratio	NB: In mild or improving disease, excessive MAP may cause hypoxia by obstructing the pulmonary circulation (causing right to left shunt) and it may also decrease cardiac output
6. Achieving synchronous ventilation	a. Maximizes efficiency of baby's contribution to gas exchange b. ? Minimizes compression of pulmonary circulation during ventilator inflation and consequently reduces right to left shunting
7. Correcting hypovolemia and hypotension	If there is evidence of hypovolemia hypotension (systemic hypotension ± peripheral vasoconstriction), correcting it with an infusion of blood, plasma or an inotrope may reduce extrapulmonary right to left shunt, improving pulmonary perfusion and oxygenation without a change in ventilator settings
8. Exogenous surfactant	Increases alveolar recruitment and improves deflation stability by decreasing surface tension

CPAP, Continuous Positive Airway Pressure; I:E Ratio, Inspiratory:Expiratory Ratio; Mean Airway Pressure, MAP; PEEP, Positive end-Expiratory Pressure; PIP, Peak Inspiratory Pressure.

Table 12.37 Ventilator settings and gas exchange: methods of decreasing $PaCO_2$

Maneuver	Probable underlying mechanisms
1. Reduce excess CPAP	In a spontaneously breathing baby, excess CPAP a. Decreases compliance and tidal volume b. Obstructs the pulmonary circulation c. Increases the work of breathing
2. ↑ Ventilator rate	Increases minute volume
3. ↑ PIP	Increases tidal volume and therefore minute volume
4. ↓ PEEP	

In severe disease, with stiff lungs:

5. ↑ Inspiratory time	If expansion of the chest wall is poor and $PaCO_2$ is elevated, increasing the inspiratory time may improve alveolar ventilation and decrease $PaCO_2$. *Increasing the expiratory time may have the opposite effect*

In mild or improving disease, with compliant lungs:

6. ↑ Expiratory time	Compliant lungs need longer to deflate. If expiratory time is too short, inadvertent PEEP is produced and alveolar ventilation is decreased. Inadvertent PEEP can be reduced by increasing expiratory time

CPAP, continuous positive airway pressure; PEEP, positive end-expiratory pressure; PIP, peak inspiratory pressure.

unit increase in mean airway pressure by raising positive end expiratory pressure (PEEP) than by adjusting inspiratory:expiratory ratio or peak inspiratory pressure (PIP). With earlier intervention and less severe lung disease shorter inspiratory times and faster rates were associated with improved outcomes.[427,428] High airway pressures are now seldom required. In mild disease, excess airway pressures may cause lung injury and impair gas exchange by compromising the pulmonary and systemic circulation. If oxygenation is good with low FiO_2, high PEEP and long inspiratory times are inappropriate. However, extremely short inspiratory times may compromise lung inflation. Field et al[429] found a significant fall in tidal volume at inspiration times under 0.3 s.

Minute ventilation, carbon dioxide exchange and inadvertent PEEP

Herman and Reynolds[425] showed that $PaCO_2$ (a) falls with increasing ventilator rate (increased minute volume), and (b) rises with increases

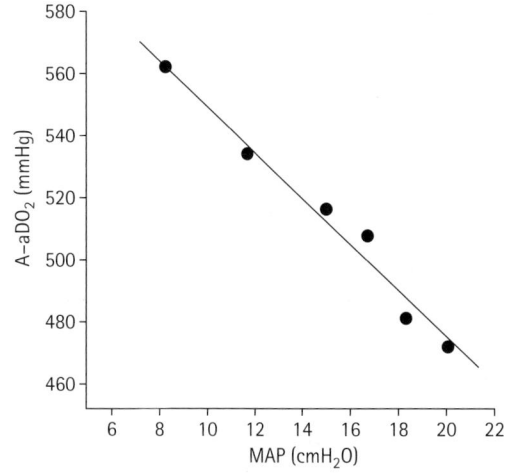

Fig. 12.15 Inverse relationship between mean airway pressure (MAP) and A-aDO$_2$ in severe hyaline membrane disease, indicating that MAP is directly proportional to oxygenation. (From Herman & Reynolds 1973[425] with permission.)

in PEEP (i.e. decreased minute volume). Bartholomew et al[430] showed that the average effect on tidal volume of a 1 cmH$_2$O change in PEEP was comparable to that of a 2 cmH$_2$O change in PIP in infants with hyaline membrane disease. This probably reflects the sigmoid shape of the pressure–volume curve.

Inadvertent PEEP occurs when the expiration time is too short to allow adequate deflation before the next inflation is imposed.[431] The gas trapped in the lungs increases the respiratory dead space and may compress the pulmonary circulation, impairing gas exchange. The intrapulmonary pressure does not fall as far as the PEEP set on the ventilator. Inadvertent PEEP may be dangerous[432] and is most likely when compliance is improving and airway resistance is elevated, as in chronic lung disease. Reducing the ventilator rate by lengthening expiration time may improve gas exchange under these circumstances by allowing more complete expiration.

HUMIDIFICATION

Bypassing the upper airway with an endotracheal tube makes the baby dependent on external humidification. Inadequate humidity slows mucociliary clearance causing viscid secretions and may predispose to pneumothorax and chronic lung disease.[433] The presence of condensate in the ventilator tubing indicates that relative humidity is close to 100% but unless the gas temperature is above 30.5 °C the absolute humidity will be inadequate. Inspired gas temperature or humidity may vary considerably[434,435] and should be measured continuously, close to the patient's airway. Excess humidification may cause fluid overload, increased respiratory system resistance and surfactant dysfunction.

ENDOTRACHEAL LAVAGE, SUCTION AND PHYSIOTHERAPY

Clearance of secretions by intermittent endotracheal tube lavage and suction reduces respiratory system resistance[436] and may prevent tube blockage. However, endotracheal suction is associated with hypoxia, bradycardia, increased blood pressure[437] and altered cerebral hemodynamics[438] and should be used in a measured way, particularly in the first 48 h of life when secretions are scant.

ADDITIONAL TECHNIQUES

The latest neonatal ventilators offer a wide range of new ventilation modes. These utilize the capacity to monitor the interaction between the baby and the ventilator and to measure flow and volume at the airway. The situation is made confusing by the lack of a standard terminology.

Synchronous ventilation modes

If the ventilator rate is set slightly faster than the spontaneous respiratory rate, many babies begin to breathe synchronously with the ventilator and show improved gas exchange.[439] Breath-sensing technology now eliminates the need for this entrainment. Modern ventilators can detect the onset of spontaneous inspiration quickly enough for a ventilator breath to be delivered in synchrony. To prevent the inflation continuing after the onset of spontaneous expiration, short inspiratory times are required. Inspiratory efforts can be measured directly at the patient airway or sensed by changes in the ventilator circuit pressure or flow, thoracic impedance, or pressure changes in a Graseby capsule attached to the abdomen. Increased trigger sensitivity allows smaller respiratory efforts to be sensed but also promotes accidental triggering (autocycling) by other signals such as air leak around the endotracheal tube or water in the ventilator circuit. Autocycling is common[440] and may cause hypocapnia in triggered modes where the ventilator rate is unrestricted.

Synchronized intermittent mandatory ventilation mode (SIMV) leaves the clinician in control of ventilator rate, inspiratory time and pressures. The ventilator divides the minute into equal blocks of time determined by the set rate. In the first part of each time block (trigger window) the ventilator can sense an inspiratory effort and deliver a trig-

gered breath. If no breath is sensed, a mandatory breath is delivered. There is then a brief refractory phase. Weaning is accomplished as the clinician chooses. The need for a preset inspiratory time and a refractory period in each time block limits effective SIMV to slower respiratory rates because the trigger window is narrow at higher rates.

In patient triggered ventilation mode (PTV), all inspiratory efforts made by the infant of greater than trigger threshold are rewarded by a ventilator breath. The infant determines the ventilator rate and the clinician the inspiratory time and pressures. A mandatory back-up rate is delivered in the event of apnea or failure to trigger. Weaning is accomplished by decreasing the pressures. Assist control is another term for PTV.

In comparison with unsynchronized ventilation, tidal volume and gas exchange were superior on SIMV.[441,442] A meta-analysis of trials of both PTV and SIMV in comparison with conventional IMV suggests that synchronized modes may be associated with more rapid weaning from ventilation but not with altered clinical outcomes.[428]

Pressure support ventilation is a further adaptation of PTV where changes in flow at the airway are used to initiate and terminate inspiration, leaving the infant in control of everything except pressure. Further adaptations now permit delivered volume to be adjusted breath by breath in relation to measurements of tidal volume. This volume controlled approach can be applied in association with the other modes of ventilation. The value of these newer modes is presently unclear. Volume guarantee ventilation has been associated with less hypocarbia[443] and less lung inflammation[444] but so far trials powered to examine clinical outcomes have not been performed.

Paralysis

Greenough et al[445] demonstrated in randomized trials that ventilated infants breathing asynchronously sustain fewer pneumothoraces if paralyzed with pancuronium. Shaw et al[446] found that routine paralysis of all ventilated infants was not more effective than selective treatment of those breathing asynchronously. Prolonged neuromuscular blockade is associated with decreased lung compliance[447] and edema. When pancuronium is administered rapid hypoxia can develop if ventilation is inadequate. With milder lung disease and gentle ventilation, paralysis is seldom required.

High frequency ventilation

High frequency ventilation describes any technique using ventilator rates of 60/min or more. It can be divided into three major types: high frequency positive pressure ventilation (HFPPV 60–150/min – see ref 427 and previous discussion on synchronous ventilation); high frequency oscillatory ventilation (HFOV 180–3000/min); and high frequency jet ventilation (HFJV 200–600/min).

High frequency oscillatory ventilation

HFOV eliminates the large changes in lung volume generated with conventional ventilation. A continuous distending pressure is applied to establish and maintain alveolar recruitment. As with conventional ventilation, oxygenation is determined by the mean airway pressure. The FiO$_2$ becomes low once alveolar recruitment is established.[448] In addition, the ventilator produces oscillations in pressure, above and below the mean airway pressure, at around 10 Hz (3–50 Hz). These oscillations have little effect on the mean airway pressure but cause small volumes of gas to move in and out of the lungs. The tidal volume (typically around 2 ml/kg) is determined by the amplitude of the oscillations and is much lower than with conventional ventilation. Carbon dioxide elimination on HFOV is proportional to tidal volume squared.[449] Because of the high frequency employed, there is only time for around 10% of the pressure oscillation in the ventilator circuit to reach the airspaces. Increasing the frequency reduces the tidal volume.[450] Carbon dioxide elimination is optimal at around 10 Hz.[451] By maintaining alveolar recruitment and avoiding overinflation, both low volume (atelectrauma) and high volume (volutrauma) lung injury may be avoided.

The indications for HFOV are unclear. Some infants with severe lung disease appear to be easier to stabilize on HFOV than conventional ventilation. A meta-analysis of trials of elective early HFOV versus conventional ventilation shows no advantage to routine early HFOV.[452] In an uncontrolled prospective study, 21 out of 46 term or near term infants with severe respiratory failure who were referred for extracorporeal membrane oxygenation (ECMO) were successfully managed with HFOV without an increase in mortality or morbidity.[453] No clear advantage was demonstrated in a small randomized controlled trial[454] although some infants failing on conventional ventilation could be successfully managed with HFOV. In a randomized controlled trial of rescue HFOV in preterm infants with severe respiratory distress syndrome, HFOV was associated with reduced risk of new air leak but increased risk of intraventricular hemorrhage and no effect on mortality or chronic lung disease.[455]

High frequency jet ventilation

The principles of ventilation strategy with HFJV are similar to those with HFOV.[456] With this technique high frequency positive pressure pulses of gas are introduced into the endotracheal tube through a cannula within its lumen. These pulses entrain additional gas through the endotracheal tube. Expiration is passive and is promoted by the use of low I:E ratios. Rate, peak pressure and inspiratory time are controlled and tidal volume and mean airway pressure are dependent on them. The optimum frequency for carbon dioxide elimination tends to be lower than with HFOV. HFJV has been associated with improved gas exchange in RDS.[457] A meta-analysis of three small trials of elective high frequency jet ventilation for RDS suggests that HFJV may be associated with a decreased risk of chronic lung disease at 36 weeks' gestation but too few infants have been studied to recommend this for routine practice.[458]

Extracorporeal membranous oxygenation

This technique uses an artificial membrane oxygenator to achieve gas exchange outside the body. It is used where there is severe reversible respiratory failure such as in persistent pulmonary hypertension of the newborn, severe lung disease or diaphragmatic hernia. The rarity of such sick infants and the complexity of the treatment mean that it is only available in a few centers and infants must be transferred for treatment. Among 190 infants in severe respiratory failure, the risk of death or disability at 1 year was reduced by 50% among those randomly allocated to be transferred to an ECMO facility versus those who remained in their local center.[459] Exactly which infants should be referred for ECMO is unclear because nitric oxide, HFOV and surfactant treatment for term respiratory failure reduce the need for ECMO but were not in widespread use when the UK ECMO study began. It is essential not to allow infants to die of potentially reversible respiratory failure without reaching an ECMO center. Sick infants should be discussed with an ECMO specialist early in their illness.

Pulmonary vasodilators

Pulmonary vasodilators may improve oxygenation where there is right to left shunt secondary to increased pulmonary vascular resistance. They have not been shown to reduce mortality. The most promising agent is nitric oxide. Others include sildenafil, prostacyclin (PGI$_2$), glyceryl trinitrate, nitroprusside, magnesium and tolazoline. Systemically administered vasodilators may cause hypotension.

Nitric oxide

Vascular smooth muscle relaxation is induced by nitric oxide.[460] Inhaled nitric oxide is inactivated by combining with hemoglobin to form methemoglobin, which largely confines its effects to the lungs. Nitric oxide reacts with oxygen to form nitrogen dioxide, nitric and nitrous acid, raising issues of toxicity. US safety regulations recommend that nitrogen dioxide exposure should not exceed 5 ppm in an 8 h period. Miller et al[461] found that in an infant ventilator circuit, nitric oxide concentrations greater than 80 ppm resulted in nitrogen dioxide levels greater than 5 ppm in the presence of 90% oxygen. Nitric oxide concentrations of less than 70 ppm did not result in excess nitrogen dioxide. A meta-analysis of randomized trials of nitric oxide in term or near term infants with respiratory failure suggests that around 50% of infants show improved oxygenation and this is associated with a significant reduction

in the number of infants who require ECMO.[462] A reasonable starting dose is 20 ppm. Trials in preterm infants with respiratory failure have not demonstrated benefit from nitric oxide.[463] When nitric oxide is discontinued, a rebound worsening of oxygenation is frequently observed whether or not the infant responded to treatment.[464] This is minimized if the nitric oxide is weaned down to 1 ppm before it is discontinued. Methemoglobin levels and NO$_2$ levels should be monitored. Because nitric oxide may inhibit platelet adhesion, caution is warranted in the presence of hemorrhage or thrombocytopenia.

Hyperventilation

Hyperventilation to unphysiological levels of pH > 7.6 can reverse extrapulmonary right to left shunt in severe pulmonary hypertension.[408,465] A similar effect is achieved through infusion of alkali to high pH.[466] However, since both maneuvers may cause cerebral ischemia their use is not recommended. They should not be preferred to nitric oxide treatment or transfer to an ECMO center.

NEURODEVELOPMENTAL OUTCOME

Survival with good health into childhood and beyond is the true measure of success of perinatal care. Severe neurodevelopmental disability remains the worst adverse long term outcome associated with prematurity. The types of neurological disability seen amongst preterm survivors include spastic diplegia, spastic hemiplegia and quadriplegia with and without intellectual impairment. Other problems include blindness, deafness and severe epilepsy. Minor motor problems, specific learning disorders and attention deficits are commonly recognized amongst school-age survivors.

The median prevalence of cerebral palsy in a meta-analysis of 111 studies reporting outcome of VLBW survivors was 7.7%.[467] The median prevalence of any disability in VLBW survivors was high at 25% with a positive correlation between the reported incidence of disability and length of follow-up. Time trends showed that the prevalence of cerebral palsy increased in the VLBW population in the 1980s but data from cerebral palsy registries have shown a recent welcome decline in the prevalence, with severe motor disability being found in around 12 per 1000 VLBW survivors.[468] The risk of cerebral palsy was strongly related to gestational age in this Oxford study, with a 40-fold higher incidence amongst babies born at less than 28 weeks of gestation when compared to those at term (Fig. 12.16). Whilst increasing survival means that there has been a net gain of normal survivors amongst the VLBW group over time, there is still no room for complacency.

EVALUATING THE OUTCOME STUDIES

The vast literature reporting the outcome of preterm babies can be a minefield for the unwary reader. The results of outcome studies show a huge variation and there has been little improvement in methodology over time. A recent evaluation confirmed that there can be considerable selection bias.[469] Recently a collaboration between cerebral palsy registers has been set up in Europe and work has begun on harmonization of definitions; in future the very large population base of this collaboration should lead to extremely valuable information on trends in the subtypes of cerebral palsy.[470]

Population

Most reports of preterm morbidity are hospital based making it difficult to compare results as referral practices vary widely between units. Birth weight cut-offs are extensively used, perhaps the most frequent being the reporting of the outcome for babies less than 1500 g. Small for dates infants of around 30 weeks' gestation are over-represented in these reports. The ideal study would report results from an entire geographical region and contain information about the outcome of all pregnancies ending between 22 and 32 weeks' gestation. The EPICURE study comes closest to this, and has provided data on the outcome of all pregnancies ending between 20 and 25 weeks of gestation in the UK in 1995; EPICure

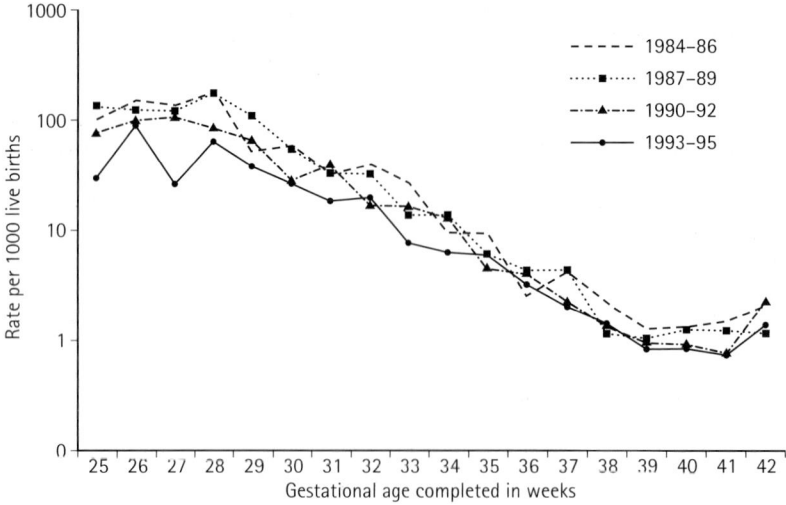

Fig. 12.16   Cerebral palsy rate per 1000 live births by completed week of gestation. (Adapted from Surman et al 2003[468] with permission.)

II is currently recruiting cases and the 10-year outcome of EPICure I will soon be available.[471] Recent reports remind us that babies of 32–36 weeks' gestation are also at increased risk of death and disability, and the population is larger than that of babies born at 23–25 weeks.[472,473]

Treatment of multiples

As many as a quarter of most preterm cohorts are one of a multiple delivery, and this trend seems set to continue. Some outcome studies exclude multiples, and many do not differentiate between singleton and multiple deliveries making specific counseling difficult. Although some researchers say that the outlook is not different for preterm twins compared to singletons there is considerable evidence that twinning is associated with an increased risk of cerebral palsy, and that the proportion of cerebral palsy accounted for by multiple births has increased.[468] This is particularly important when there is intrauterine death of a co-twin, where the risk of significant handicap may be as great as 1 in 10.[474]

Reason for prematurity

As more data accrue, it becomes possible to analyze outcome by etiology of prematurity. There are differences between the outcomes of babies born because of maternal pre-eclampsia (about 12% of preterm deliveries), prolonged rupture of membranes (22%), placental abruption (4%), IUGR (4%), idiopathic preterm labor (40%) or multiple pregnancy (20%). Chorioamnionitis carries a particularly high risk of subsequent periventricular leukomalacia and spastic diplegia.[475] The obstetric team's perception of the chance of survival has also been shown to influence outcome.

Missing cases

Tracing the movements of babies is never easy. Frequent changes of surname and address are common and some leave the country of their birth altogether. Work from the Northern region of the UK continues to show that the last few babies remaining to be found in a follow-up study contain a disproportionate number of handicapped infants.[476] The reasons for the discrepancy include the fact that the parents of the handicapped infants are already busy with hospital attendances or that they do not wish to confront the adverse outcome. Studies reporting less than 95% follow-up are likely to be underestimating handicap and an ideal study would have 100% ascertainment.

Duration and timing of follow-up

The diagnosis of cerebral palsy cannot be made with any degree of confidence before 2 years, and may not be stable until 5 years or more. Late deaths will alter the denominator if the handicap rates are to be reported for survivors rather than for live births, another potential source of difficulty when trying to compare studies. Some report neo-

natal survival, some survival to discharge, and some survival to the time of late follow-up. There is a tendency to use cranial ultrasound results as a proxy for the more expensive and time-consuming neurodevelopmental assessments; this will underestimate the number of cases and is becoming less accurate as the incidence of large hemorrhages and 'periventricular leukomalacia' continues to reduce because periventricular leukomalacia is not reliably detected with ultrasound.

Definition of disability

This is perhaps the most variable of the many problems with the outcome studies. The WHO international classification of impairment, disabilities and handicap contains useful definitions which are listed in Table 12.38. Usually major handicap includes cerebral palsy, severe developmental delay (more than two or three standard deviations below the mean on the particular test used), blindness and deafness. There are differences of opinion regarding inclusion of conditions such as epilepsy and shunted hydrocephalus. The latter can cause impairment without disability, as can a mild hemiplegia. Types of cerebral palsy include spastic, ataxic, dyskinetic (athetoid and dystonic) and hypotonic and can involve a single limb through to quadriplegia. Few groups have enough subjects to allow analysis of outcome according to type of cerebral palsy: there are probably different associated antecedent variables for spastic diplegia, hemiplegia, athetosis and quadriplegia. Important associations may be missed by 'lumping' adverse outcome in small studies.

Table 12.38   WHO definitions of impairment, disability and handicap

Impairment
Any loss or abnormality of psychological, physiological or anatomical structure or function: in principle impairments represent disturbances at organ level

Disability
Any restriction or lack (resulting from an impairment) of ability to perform an activity in the manner or within the range considered normal for a human being. A disability thus reflects the consequence of an impairment in terms of functional performance and activity by an individual

Handicap
A disadvantage for a given individual resulting from an impairment or disability that limits or prevents the fulfillment of a role that is normal (depending on age, sex and social and cultural factors). Handicap thus reflects interaction with the surroundings and is a difficult outcome to use for comparison as it depends on attitudes within the family and society to disability

Minor disability, clumsiness, language disorder, school failure and behavior disorder are even more difficult to define and the wide range in the reported incidence between studies reflects this.

Diagnosis of disability

The tests used to diagnose disability should be reproducible and have been previously evaluated in an appropriate population in order to minimize problems such as intraobserver variability. At present there is a large number of tests applied at different ages by people of varying levels of experience and this can severely bias results. Well validated in this respect are the Bayley and Griffiths scales of infant development, and the Amiel-Tison method of neurological examination.

Control groups

In a cohort descriptive follow-up study of all children below a certain weight there can be no control group. Consideration needs to be given to the inclusion of control subjects such as term infants, particularly in view of the known effects of socioeconomic deprivation on the incidence of prematurity. As studies of preterm outcome begin to report school performance, variables such as birth order and social class will become relatively more important factors than they are in the current descriptions of the prevalence of major handicap.

OUTCOME RELATED TO BIRTH WEIGHT, SEX, GESTATIONAL AGE AND OTHER FACTORS

That the incidence of handicap increases with decreasing birth weight and gestational age was shown as early as 1956. Most large regional studies reporting the outcome of VLBW babies born during the last 50 years record serious disability in less than 10% of the survivors, increasing to 13–25% of affected children when moderate disability is included. The interaction of birth weight and gestational age on survival and disability can be studied by those who have access to large datasets. One approach is to calculate the birth weight ratio, which is the actual birth weight divided by the mean birth weight for the same gestational age.[477] A birth weight ratio of 0.8 corresponds to the 10th centile. This is a statistically useful tool because the number generated is a normally distributed continuous variable. Morley and her colleagues[477] were unable to show any association between birth weight ratio and neurodevelopmental outcome at 18 months, but others have reported a higher mortality and morbidity for very preterm growth retarded infants.[478,479] In the longer term, most follow-up studies describe worse cognitive outcome for preterm SGA infants when compared with appropriate for gestational age controls.[480]

Male sex has been associated with a doubling of the risk of death and/or handicap in almost every study which has included sex as a factor in logistic regression analysis. Some studies suggest an increased chance of survival amongst black preterm babies, whereas others show the opposite.[481]

Outcome related to gestational age

Survival at 22 weeks' gestation remains very rare, but at 23 weeks the chance of survival has improved considerably over the last decade, providing the fetus is well grown and weighs more than 500 g. For the small number of babies born preterm and with birth weight less than 500 g the outcome remains dismal, probably reflecting the combined effects of prematurity and severe intrauterine growth failure. For appropriately grown babies of 23 weeks' gestation many centers around the world are now reporting 50% survival, improving to 70% at 24 weeks and 80% at 25 weeks.[482] These data are in contrast to the more gloomy outlook revealed in the 1995 EPICURE study, which considered the population of the UK rather than single center outcomes,[471] and a wide range of outcome at 23, 24 and 25 weeks was reported in a careful review of outcome studies reporting births in the 1990s.[483] A comparison between EPICURE, data from UCLH, and that from Minneapolis[482] is shown in Figure 12.17. After 28 weeks' gestation survival is now regularly reported as above 90%.

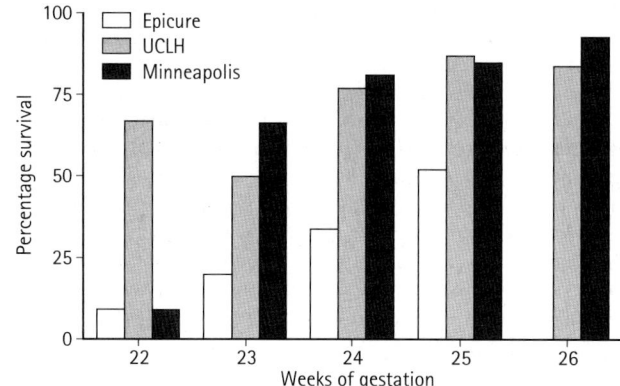

Fig. 12.17 Survival rates (percentage) for each week of gestation between 22 and 26 weeks. Data adapted from EPICURE, UCLH, and Minneapolis.[471,482]

The major neonatal complications which influence later development remain preterm brain injury (intraventricular hemorrhage or periventricular leukomalacia), chronic lung disease, necrotizing enterocolitis and sepsis. Chronic lung disease continues to occur in a significant proportion of VLBW infants and is associated with long hospital stays, poor weight gain and episodes of infection; all of these probably affect neurodevelopment. NEC that requires surgery doubles the risk of an adverse neurodevelopmental outcome.[484]

The rates of disability, and cerebral palsy in particular, increase with decreasing gestational age (Fig. 12.16). Precise estimates of neurodevelopmental outcome at 23–26 weeks are still hard to find and vary widely, but 34% of the Minneapolis cohort born at 23 weeks had severe disability at follow-up, with 52% normal at a mean age of about 4 years, and this fits fairly well with many of the studies summarized by Hack & Fanaroff.[482,483] Four years is too young to assess school performance or attention deficit hyperactivity disorder (see below). At 24–26 weeks the percentage of children who survive with severe neurodisability is around 20%, with a similar percentage affected by minor disability. Many disabled ex-preterm children continue to have multiple impairments, and Maureen Hack pointed out that her meta-analysis gave strikingly similar results to that performed by Rennie in 1996.[485]

SENSORY HANDICAP

In addition to the high cerebral palsy rate in VLBW infant survivors there are a significant number of visually impaired children, often as a consequence of retinopathy of prematurity. About 3% are blind, and many more have severe myopia: about a quarter of the children in most cohorts need prescription glasses. Deafness afflicts slightly fewer children but is still a problem in about 1–2%. Early diagnosis by screening can help limit the handicap resulting from this latter disability. Long term follow-up studies in the state of Victoria have been in place since the early 1980s, and the most recent cohort had far fewer blind children (1%) than earlier cohorts.[486]

MINOR HANDICAPS AND SCHOOL FAILURE

Follow-up to school age and beyond has been reported for several cohorts of ex-preterm children. More of the children are left-handed, which has been suggested as a possible risk factor for a later risk of schizophrenia. More are hyperactive with a short attention span and require special help at school.[487] The meta-analysis of Aylward showed a mean reduction of six points in IQ when disabled survivors were excluded[488] and more recent studies continue to show a downwards shift of similar magnitude.[489] There is a considerable overlap between behavioral disorders, neurodevelopmental abnormalities and school problems – 'clumsiness' may be a marker for this type of dysfunction, which remains very common.[490] More (14%) Finnish LBW children born in 1966 than controls

(6%) were educationally subnormal at the age of 14, but when the disabled survivors were excluded similar numbers succeeded in higher education.[491] The Bavarian follow-up study showed that ex-preterm children had significant problems with sequential and simultaneous information processing and language.[492] These problems are not limited to those with obvious white matter disease of prematurity, and MRI cohort studies are revealing abnormalities in brain volume, gyral folding and subtle white matter damage which may be important (see below). 'Executive function' is a term used to describe the end result of a series of processes involving goal setting, planning, problem solving, attention and concentration on tasks; this ability is often impaired in ex-preterm children.[493] Nevertheless, many young adults who were born very preterm rate their own quality of life as high.[494]

OUTCOME RELATED TO NEUROIMAGING APPEARANCES

Cohort screening of asymptomatic VLBW infants with cranial ultrasound continues to show a high incidence of lesions involving the periventricular zone. Damage to premyelin cells abundant in this region provides a convenient explanation for the high prevalence of cerebral palsy. Cysts in the parenchyma and cerebral atrophy indicate loss of white matter and are the strongest predictors yet found for cerebral palsy. Delayed myelination has been confirmed with later MRI studies, suggesting that the cysts are markers of even more diffuse injury to oligodendroglia. Ultrasound is a poor predictor of periventricular leukomalacia diagnosed later with MRI, detecting only about 30% of cases. Most studies are in remarkable agreement about the outcome of cystic change, showing a five-fold increase in the risk of cerebral palsy following ultrasound diagnosis of any parenchymal lesion, and a 15-fold increase in the presence of bilateral occipital periventricular leukomalacia. Accumulated experience is still relatively meager, however, and the predictions have wide confidence intervals due to the small numbers of cases. Visual handicap can be accurately predicted from ultrasound abnormalities. A normal scan is not therefore a guarantee of a normal outcome, although the chances are about 90%.[495] The risk may be higher in the group weighing less than 1 kg.[496]

Germinal matrix hemorrhage, subependymal hemorrhage

There is consistent agreement that the appearance of increased echodensity in the region of the germinal matrix capillary bed carries no increased risk of adverse outcome. This is probably also true for intraventricular hemorrhage which is not associated with ventricular enlargement. Again, more recent studies suggest that for the highest risk subgroup of extremely low birth weight infants, even this lowest grade of intracranial hemorrhage does carry an increased risk of adverse outcome.[497] The mechanism of this effect remains to be elucidated; isolated intraventricular hemorrhage is not associated with impaired myelination in MRI studies,[498] but bleeding into the germinal matrix may damage the subplate neurons with a consequent reduction in the population of the cortex.[499]

Ventricular dilation and progressive hydrocephalus

The natural history of ventriculomegaly secondary to the presence of blood in the ventricular cavity in VLBW infants is that about 50% will progress to require a ventriculoperitoneal (VP) shunt insertion and the remainder will arrest or regress. Attempts at preventing the progression by early cerebrospinal fluid (CSF) drainage have proved unsuccessful. Many of these infants have associated parenchymal lesions of the brain making the assessment of risk due to persistent dilation alone very difficult. Nevertheless, the prognosis of shunted hydrocephalus in the preterm infant with post-hemorrhagic hydrocephalus remains concerning, with 75% of those enrolled in the ventriculomegaly trial ending up with cerebral palsy.[500] More recent studies claim better results, and some are of the view that the criteria for treatment in the ventriculomegaly trial were set too high.[501] Even nonprogressive ventriculomegaly probably reflects significant white matter damage, and carries a substantial risk of cognitive delay.

Noncavitating transient parenchymal echodensity, and the MRI finding of DEHSI

The incidence with which a 'flare' or 'blush' is seen in the parenchyma surrounding the ventricle varies widely with the observer and the frequency of ultrasound scanning, and the importance of transient 'flare' seen with ultrasound remains uncertain. Now that several centers have imaged cohorts of preterm babies with MRI, it has become obvious that subtle white matter deficits are common. Diffuse excessive high signal intensity (DEHSI) is found in up to 70% of VLBWI imaged with MRI at term.[502] Increasing severity of periventricular white matter signal intensity at term is associated with poorer performance on the Bayley scales, as well as with an increased risk of cognitive and motor impairment.

Persistent parenchymal echodensities and porencephalic cysts

A single large echodense area in the parenchyma of the brain may be the end result of one or several pathological events including venous infarction, secondary hemorrhage into an ischemic area or a primary hemorrhagic event due to transmission of a hypertensive peak or release of vasoactive substances.

Large parenchymal lesions often cavitate to form porencephalic cysts: these are associated with a risk of hemiplegia rather than spastic diplegia; the risk is high and further information can be obtained by imaging the posterior limb of the internal capsule with MRI.

Periventricular leukomalacia

There is no doubt that cystic periventricular leukomalacia is the most powerful predictor of cerebral palsy amongst the neonatal cranial ultrasound lesions so far described.[503] In many cohort follow-up studies almost all the cases of cerebral palsy had bilateral occipital leukomalacia in the neonatal period. Single cysts and cysts confined to the frontal region have a better outcome than multiple bilateral occipital cysts, where the outlook is universally dismal.

NEONATAL DEATH

Although neonatal deaths have become uncommon, they are still frequent enough both on the labor ward and on the neonatal unit for consideration of best management to be important. Neonatal intensive care units have developed to rescue preterm and sick infants but there is still a steady trickle of deaths in a neonatal unit from congenital abnormality and the problems of extreme prematurity. With all formal nursing and medical training geared to rescue, the death of the patient is often regarded as failure. As an occasional occurrence, a neonatal death may be rapidly 'set aside', but in a referral unit the frequency and regularity of such events cannot be easily avoided. The emotional load of guilt and depression that arises with frequent deaths almost certainly plays a part in the high turnover of nursing staff and the incidence of 'burnout' in physicians. In the arena of neonatal intensive care, perinatal mortality meetings and more universally perinatal mortality statistics highlight the unsatisfactory nature of death, yet many will be inevitable.

PARENTAL GRIEF

The grief of the parents after a neonatal death seems independent of the size of the offspring. Such grief is present even when the infant is nonviable or lives for only a very short time and there is an identical reaction after a stillbirth. The failure of a mother to come to terms with a perinatal death can lead to emotional problems. Over 30% of mothers in a study by Cullberg[504] had overt psychiatric problems in the 2 years after such an event. It was the recognition that psychiatric sequelae could be considerably reduced by parents touching their infants before and after death that led to an acknowledgment that the management of death is as important as the rescue of life. This has recently been questioned.

THE DEATH

The death of a baby in the neonatal unit is an undignified event for the baby and the family, especially when 'rescue therapy' is given until the last moment. It is difficult for the parents to express their true emotions in the intensive care unit where staff are busy with other critically ill patients. It is difficult for staff to cope on the one hand with the rescue care for some patients and still provide sensitivity for grieving parents in the same nursery. It is particularly difficult for parents of other babies in a unit with an open visiting policy. The emphasis in neonatal death must be changed from a medical failure, which must be rapidly forgotten, to an event, tragic indeed, but in which the parents are if at all possible closely involved. Deaths in a neonatal unit should occur, if possible, with the parents present and life support can often be withdrawn with the baby in the mother's or father's arms. Thus in many instances the time of death is itself organized for the benefit of the parents. Death then becomes a reality and with this involvement parents may feel, in retrospect, that they have done their best for their infants by allowing death to occur in a dignified way in the presence of love and company. In an attempt to dissociate death from the urgency of the intensive care unit it is helpful to set aside a room for the parents in the unit which can be used for terminal care. This room may be less clinical than the main nurseries with wallpaper, curtains, a rug and easy chairs. Full supportive care can still be given but in this setting the parents will be more able to provide hospice type care for their infant's last hours or sometimes days and will more easily be able to come to terms with the impending death. The availability of a special room allows extended families to be involved in culturally important ritual. During the terminal period a senior member of the nursing and medical staff should be available to provide continuity and it must be made clear to the parents that someone will always be present unless they wish otherwise. The cultural and religious background of the families must be acknowledged so that a flexible and individual approach can be developed. Discussions early on with the parents should elaborate their religious beliefs and standpoints and outside support from a priest, mullah, rabbi, etc., should be encouraged if appropriate. The introduction of this support at an early stage in a critically ill infant is important as it allows more constructive relationships to develop than when the meeting is for the baptism of a terminally ill infant. In Christian families hospital chaplains and social workers can be actively involved with the family from an early stage. The presence of young siblings can enrich the feeling of family togetherness at this time of grief and is unlikely to damage the siblings.[505] Ritual is important. If an emergency baptism is required this should be memorable with a proper silver christening bowl to facilitate baptism with meaning and dignity. It is important to *suggest* to parents that they might like to hold or groom their dead infant. This may be met with agitation and a certain degree of horror, particularly by European parents, but after a short time many mothers will request such involvement. In some instances parents have left the hospital to obtain their own baby clothes in which to dress their infant in the laying out process. Photographs of the infant will usually have been taken during life but if the life span has been short it is suggested that pictures of the dead infant are taken, often in the parents' arms. Frequently the baby can be specially clothed to enable a better photograph for remembrance to be taken than the ones in life, which have had evidence of intensive care support. The neonatal unit can provide the parents with a bereavement folder which combines advice and information (to help them at this time) with mementos of their baby (lock of hair, name band, hand and foot prints, etc.).

THE IMMEDIATE AFTERMATH OF DEATH[506]

Their baby's death is an intensely private and personal experience for all parents. Many will wish to follow the customs of their own culture or the rites of their own particular religion and these wishes should be respected. It is important that no assumptions are made. It may be helpful to ask parents as sensitively and gently as possible to explain their needs. If language problems make this or any other discussion with parents difficult every effort should be made to find an appropriate and skilled interpreter. Parents who have a specific religious commitment may want to make contact with their minister, priest or other religious leader and he or she will advise them about their baby's funeral as well as provide support and help. Some parents who do not hold any particular religious belief will still find comfort with a simple ceremony in the hospital, perhaps in the hospital chapel with their families and the nursing and medical staff involved in the care of their infant taking part. This may be suggested, bearing in mind that it is not appropriate for all parents. Parents will inevitably be bewildered by a neonatal death. It may be their first experience of losing a close relative and sensitivity is required by staff at all stages.

AUTOPSY IN THE UK

The parents themselves may request an autopsy. If they make such a request it should always be fulfilled. The autopsy may be necessary because the cause of death is unclear. In this case a coroner (or in Scotland, a procurator fiscal) will be involved because the medical practitioner is unable to issue a death certificate of the medical cause of death. In this event it is not open to the parents to withhold their consent but parents can withhold their authorization if the medical practitioner is prepared to put a cause of death on the death certificate. I believe that all babies should have an autopsy independent of whether the cause of death is apparently known. I believe this because:

1. Even today and with modern imaging techniques, in a significant proportion of autopsies further information is discovered which has a direct bearing on the counseling of the parents for the future.[507]
2. It is important for the medical staff to know that their diagnosis has been accurate and that their management has not caused pathology. It is only in this way that medical science can progress.
3. At some stage in the future it is not uncommon that parents will have anxieties that something went undiscovered in their baby and that this led to the death. The autopsy is often a more objective measure of cause of death.
4. Retained tissue as organ blocks may be helpful at a future date to make a specific genetic diagnosis.

Where the parents' authorization is necessary, it is highly desirable that they can give this freely. An honest and unhurried approach to parents by consultant or senior resident (not a junior staff member), explaining the reasons for an autopsy and what it involves, will help them to reach a decision. Parents will also feel more comfortable if the request is made as a normal rather than an exceptional procedure. Although the consent of only one parent is required by law, it is advisable that whenever possible parents should be asked to sign the consent form together. It will help parents to make their decision if they are given clear information about the following:

1. Why it is thought an autopsy is necessary and why their authorization is being sought. Although many parents wish to be given the reason for their baby's death, many also find the thought of an autopsy distressing. It is important that they can feel their baby is still theirs and is not becoming a hospital specimen.
2. The possible outcome of the examination. While it should be explained that an autopsy can provide a definite cause of death, parents should also be warned that an indecisive result is possible.
3. Where, when and by whom the autopsy will be performed. Parents are also likely to want information and reassurance about the whereabouts of and their access to their baby and, if the autopsy is to be performed at another hospital, the body should not be removed to that hospital until the day of the autopsy and should be returned as quickly as possible after the examination.
4. When, to whom and how the results of the autopsy will be made available. If you are not prepared to give the full information to the parents you should not be doing an autopsy.

Most parents feel anxious about authorizing an autopsy and need reassurance. A particular fear is the damage which will be done to their baby. With good practice by the pathologist (who can be introduced to the parents), it is possible for the baby to be restored and carefully dressed so as to be acceptable for the parents to see again before the funeral. If the parents are to hold their infant following the autopsy, they should be warned that he or she will be lightweight as in most cases the brain will be removed for later processing. It may also be suggested that the parents might like to provide clothes including a bonnet for the baby to be dressed in after the autopsy or the parents may prefer a funeral director to prepare the baby for them.

The results of an autopsy are anxiously awaited by most parents and there should be a minimum of delay in providing parents not only with the results but also with the opportunity to discuss them fully. The full autopsy report should be sent to the parents with an appointment shortly after so that they can bring it and discuss it fully with the pediatrician involved. In this way they have both written information and the access to a pediatrician to discuss all the implications. If necessary the results can be discussed also with an obstetrician. If an autopsy shows the baby's death to be the result of a genetic disorder, parents should be offered the opportunity for later genetic counseling.

CERTIFICATION AND REGISTRATION PROCEDURES IN THE UK

When a baby is born alive and subsequently dies, irrespective of the gestation or the duration of life, the medical practitioner who attended the baby is required by law to issue a medical certificate giving the cause of death. This certificate is required to enable the death to be registered. If the cause of death is not immediately apparent the medical practitioner may have to report the death to the coroner (or in Scotland, a procurator fiscal). The law requires that all births and deaths be notified to the registrar of births and deaths. It is best if parents can deal with the registration themselves and *both together* and this is necessary where the couple are unmarried and wish both parents' names entered on the certificate. The medical practitioner who attended the baby during his or her last illness will issue a medical certificate giving the cause of death. This certificate must be produced to the registrar of births and deaths within 5 days of the baby's death (8 days in Scotland). The registrar will issue a green certificate after registration (the certificate for disposal) to permit burial or cremation. This certificate is required before the funeral can take place. It is free of charge. The registrar will also issue, on request, a copy of a certified entry (a death certificate) for a small fee. It is helpful if parents are told in advance that this certificate is available since to many parents it is a valuable memento of their baby. Parents should be told in advance when registering a baby's death that the registrar can enter the baby's forename as well as the surname if they so wish. This may be particularly important for those parents whose baby died soon after birth, as they can then give some thought to the naming of the child before registering the death.

'Death grants' have now been abolished in the UK, but parents can apply to the Department of Social Security for a grant or loan to cover the funeral expenses. In Scotland, the health board will meet the funeral costs for stillborn babies and terminations.

THE FUNERAL IN THE UK

Ceremonies can take many different forms and may be religious or non-religious. The certificate of disposal (Form 14) issued after registration is needed by the undertaker before a cremation can take place but is not needed for a burial. It should be handed to the funeral director or, if the parents have asked the hospital to take responsibility for the funeral, to the hospital. The funeral director involved will complete all necessary documentation according to the kind of funeral requested. It is also the parents' choice whether their baby is buried or cremated. The cremation of a baby leaves no remains whatsoever (ashes) and the parents should be aware of this. A baby cannot be cremated without the parents' formal consent. If the funeral is privately arranged the funeral director will organize all steps in conjunction with the parents. If on the other hand the parents wish for a hospital contract funeral, they must be aware that there may be some emotional risks in accepting this option. If there is any anxiety about this the parents can always contact the British Institute of Funeral Directors or the Stillbirth and Neonatal Death Society (SANDS).

GRAVES, MEMORIALS AND REMEMBRANCE

Depending on the funeral that the parents opt for, the baby may be buried with other babies in a common grave though this practice is becoming less common. Many parents find it comforting to know that their baby is buried with other babies but for others this is distressing and sometimes it takes a while before the grave is full (usually no more than 10 babies should be buried in one grave). Most parents accept a multiple grave so long as they are told about it in advance and do not find out about it when it is too late to consider alternatives. The common grave should be located in a special children's area of a cemetery with a general memorial stone. Parents should be warned that unless they purchase exclusive right to burial, they do not have the right to erect any kind of memorial of their own. If the parents buy exclusive right of burial they can mark their baby's grave with a memorial provided that it complies with local regulations. All crematoria and some cemeteries have a book of remembrance for individual entries. Many specialist neonatal units also have a book of remembrance for infants dying in their units. This book may be located on the neonatal unit or in the hospital chapel. A full page can be allocated to each baby with a personal inscription designed by the parents. This can be made in copperplate writing. The parents can then see the book at any time by arrangement with the hospital chaplain or neonatal unit staff.

LATE BEREAVEMENT COUNSELING AND SUPPORT

It is now accepted that the aftercare of the parents and siblings is important for subsequent emotional well-being. The parents should be seen several times after the death of their infant. On the first occasion, usually on the day of death, sympathy is shown for the parents' situation. Explanation about the cause of death is often inappropriate at this stage and intrudes into the grief. Over the next few days, necessary formalities have to be completed and this can be a bewildering time. The parents need to be seen on the day after the death to explain what has to be done. If the mother is mobile (that is, not just postoperative after a Cesarean section) it is appropriate to encourage both parents to complete the formalities together rather than the man take on an organizational role. A social worker or member of the clergy may help in shepherding them through these routines. It is also at this second interview that permission is asked by a senior pediatrician for the autopsy. The final task on this second visit is to guide the parents through a few of the reactions and emotions that they will suffer in the ensuing period. At between 1 and 2 weeks after the death the parents are seen a third time. They will have received a copy of the morbid anatomy findings of the autopsy and this interview will explain the findings (the histology will return later and necessitate a further visit). If possible, the senior nurse who has been involved in the terminal events will also be present. It is important not to see the parents in the neonatal unit or in the middle of the busy outpatient session where other babies and infants intrude too easily into their consciousness. The distress and anxieties of the ensuing weeks are again raised and suggestions are made as to how best to deal with them. A final optional appointment is given for about 3 months at which outstanding questions may be clarified and at which pathological grief, if present, should be evident. At all stages hospital social workers and chaplains should be informed (not necessarily to be active) of what is proceeding and the GP should have a full letter with regard to each interview. Genetic counseling should be arranged for the future if this is appropriate from the results of the autopsy.

VOLUNTARY SUPPORT ORGANIZATIONS

The Stillbirth and Neonatal Death Society (SANDS), 28 Portland Place, London W1B 1LY. SANDS national helpline: 020 7436 5881.
The British Institute of Funeral Directors, 41 Bridge Street, Tranent, East Lothian, EH33 1AH.

BOOKLETS

Support For You When Your Baby Dies. Outlines the support offered by SANDS to bereaved parents and those caring for them.
Saying Goodbye to Your Baby (1999) by Priscilla Alderson. Available from SANDS and the National Childbirth Trust, 9 Queensborough Terrace, London W2 3TB.
Miscarriage, Stillbirth and Neonatal Death: Guidelines for Professionals. Available from SANDS.

STAFF SUPPORT

With the realization that the support and understanding of health professionals can play a vital role in the eventual recovery of the parents, there has also come the realization that this involvement can itself cause emotional stress and tension in the staff. After a death it is important not only to analyze in detail traditional physiological and pathological events but also to consider the stress aspects for the parents and the nursing and medical staff. Some units may feel it is important to involve formal psychiatric help in this process but regular discussion on a less formal basis (and at particular times of need) can be more important (our regular involvement of chaplaincy staff with parents in a neonatal unit pays dividends for the staff themselves at 'crisis times'). In this way we hope that the people involved in a neonatal death and who will inevitably be under considerable stress will not reach the point of physical and emotional exhaustion.

PROBLEMS OF THE NEWBORN

PULMONARY DISORDERS AND APNEA

LUNG EMBRYOLOGY

Viability of the preterm baby is limited by lung development. The airways begin as an outpouching from the primitive gut at 24 days. By 26 days two primary branches, which will form the major bronchi, can be discerned. This is called the *embryonic phase* and it ends about the 6th week. The *pseudoglandular phase*, from the 7th to 16th week, consists of branching of the endodermal tube into surrounding mesenchyme. By 10 weeks cartilage is deposited in the bronchi and by 16 weeks formation of new bronchi is almost complete. The *canalicular phase*, from 16 to 26 weeks, comprises canalization of the airways, increased capillary growth and differentiation of type I pneumocytes (needed for gas exchange) from type II pneumocytes which produce surfactant. The terminal *saccular phase* begins from 24 to 26 weeks and continues until term. Terminal air sacs or alveoli appear as outpouchings of the bronchioles after 26 weeks and increase in number to form multiple pouches of a common chamber called the alveolar duct. From 26 weeks the capillary network, which arises at about 20 weeks from vascular structures in the mesenchyme, proliferates close to the developing airway to constitute the *alveolar phase* which continues postnatally for about 2 years. There is a continuum between antenatal and postnatal lung development. Normal alveolarization proceeds rapidly to achieve alveolar numbers that are between 20 and 50% of the adult number of 300×10^6 by 40 weeks' gestation. Normal lung development can be disrupted by antenatal events which lead to preterm birth. Before 24–26 weeks gas exchange must take place across terminal bronchioles into the developing capillary network.

Lung growth

Growth factors have a major role in lung growth and development. Mechanical and humoral factors also influence growth of the fetal lung. Lung growth requires distention of the fluid-filled lung, with tracheal fluid acting as an internal template or splint. Absence of lung fluid at appropriate pressure leads to pulmonary hypoplasia. Lung hypoplasia may be caused by oligohydramnios from renal agenesis, bladder neck obstruction or rupture of the membranes before 20 weeks. These lungs are structurally immature with persistent cuboidal epithelium and lack of elastic tissue. They are also biochemically immature, containing low levels of phospholipids. Lung growth is also regulated by external forces, which include the phasic negative pressure of fetal breathing and the tonic negative pressure of diaphragmatic tone. Hypoplastic lungs may also result from absence of fetal breathing movements in babies with central nervous system anomalies, congenital muscle disorders or absent diaphragm. These lungs, although small, appear to be appropriately developed and have normal content of phospholipids. Pulmonary hypoplasia may also be caused by thoracic space-occupying lesions such as diaphragmatic hernia, lung cysts, or pleural effusions which may be associated with severe fetal hydrops.

Lung maturation

After birth alveolar stability is dependent upon release of pulmonary surfactant. Synthesis and release of surfactant rely mainly on humoral control mechanisms. Alveolar type II cells, which synthesize surfactant, have microvilli on the luminal surface and contain lamellar bodies. They constitute 16% of alveolar cells but only 7% of the alveolar surface area and can differentiate to form the larger, thinner type I cell which covers the remaining 93% of the alveolar surface. The lamellar bodies (storage sites for surfactant) are first recognized at about 22 weeks. They contain about 80% phosphatidylcholine, mostly dipalmitoylphosphatidylcholine (DPPC) but also unsaturated phosphatidylglycerol (PG). PG is used as a marker of lung maturity and levels rise as phosphatidylinositol levels decrease towards term. Lamellar bodies also contain surfactant proteins A, B and C (SP-A, B, C). A fourth surfactant apoprotein, SP-D, is not stored in the lamellar bodies and is secreted separately. SP-A and SP-D have major roles in host defense of the lung whereas SP-B and SP-C have surface active properties, helping to spread and recycle surfactant. Mature SP-B increases in amniotic fluid in late gestation and SP-A is the last surfactant protein to appear in amniotic fluid.

Mechanisms controlling lung maturation

Glucocorticoids. These induce both structural and biochemical changes in alveolar type II and type I cells. They act on lung fibroblasts to produce fibroblast pneumocyte factor (FPF) which in turn stimulates surfactant synthesis by alveolar type II cells. Glucocorticoids also increase the numbers of lamellar bodies, the rate of choline incorporation into phosphatidylcholine, the amount of DPPC in tracheal fluid and the lung content of SP-A. Induction of FPF is relatively slow, which may account for the delayed clinical effect of maternal glucocorticoid (betamethasone) treatment.
Thyroid hormones. Thyroid hormones increase synthesis of surfactant lipids in type II cells, probably by making the cells more responsive to FPF. They act earlier in the phospholipid biosynthetic pathway and are synergistic when used with glucocorticoids in animal studies. Synthetic analogues of T_3 and thyrotropin releasing hormone (TRH) cross the placenta but clinical trials have shown poorer outcomes when mothers have been given combination treatment of TRH plus glucocorticoid.[508,509]
Insulin. Hyperinsulinemia is associated with reduced surfactant production. In pregnancies complicated by inadequately controlled maternal diabetes, fetal hyperinsulinemia is associated with an increased risk of neonatal RDS.
Catecholamines. Epinephrine, but not norepinephrine, decreases tracheal fluid secretion and increases surfactant release. The concentration of beta-adrenergic receptors in lung increases at term and in response to glucocorticoids. Beta-adrenergic agents delay preterm labor; if used in association with betamethasone, they have a synergistic effect in preventing RDS.
Other hormones and agents. Prolactin levels are lower in babies with RDS. Estrogen, testosterone, epidermal growth factor, prostaglandins, cholinergic agonists and leukotrienes have all been postulated as having roles in fetal lung development.

Role of surfactant and fetal lung fluid

Fetal lungs are filled with liquid secreted by the epithelium of potential airspaces. Before birth absorption across the epithelium is initiated by increased circulating catecholamines associated with labor contractions. Air-filled lungs after birth retain a thin fluid layer in the alveoli. Pulmonary surfactant forms an insoluble film at the alveolar air–liquid interface, lowering surface tension and improving alveolar stability during expiration. Surfactant allows very low transpulmonary pressures to be used during normal respiration and also has a role in host defense mechanisms of the lung mainly through the actions of SP-A and SP-D.

Surfactant secretion is stimulated by lung inflation. When surfactant is released the contents of lamellar bodies are extruded into the alveoli as tubular myelin, which is formed into the surfactant monolayer by actions of surfactant proteins SP-B and SP-C. SP-B also regulates surfactant protein metabolism and enhances uptake of phospholipids by type II cells in vitro. SP-A and SP-D have a role in the feedback control of surfactant secretion. The surface film needs to be constantly replenished from freshly secreted surfactant and recycling occurs within type II cells. As much as 85–90% of surfactant is recycled. Clearance of surfactant is rapid and may be increased in the newborn period or after hyperventilation. Specific proteins may regulate clearance of surfactant back to type II cells and small amounts are also phagocytosed by alveolar macrophages and cleared up the airways.

Further reading

Warburton D, Schwarz M, Tefft D, et al. The molecular basis of lung morphogenesis. Mech Dev 2000; 92:55–81. (Review article with 258 references)

Cardoso WV. Transcription factors and pattern formation in the developing lung. Am J Physiol 1995; 269:L429–442. (Review article with 185 references)

Bolt RJ, van Weissenbruch MM, Lafebre HN, et al. Glucocorticoids and lung development in the fetus and preterm infant. Pediatr Pulmonol 2001; 32:76–91. (Review article with 256 references)

Jobe AH, Ikegami M. Lung development and function in preterm infants in the surfactant era. Annu Rev Physiol 2000; 62: 825–846. (Review article with 98 references)

RESPIRATORY DISTRESS SYNDROME (HYALINE MEMBRANE DISEASE)

RDS is a condition of pulmonary insufficiency commencing at, or shortly after birth and increasing in severity over the first 2 days of life. If RDS is left untreated death can occur from progressive hypoxia and respiratory failure. In survivors resolution begins between 2 and 4 days. It is due to a lack of alveolar surfactant along with structural immaturity of the lung and is mainly confined to preterm babies, with incidence increasing as gestation decreases.[510] RDS is also known as hyaline membrane disease because of histological features at autopsy. Incidence is 2–3% of all births but it is important as it is responsible for the deaths of many preterm infants throughout the world each year. There is evidence that increased use of prenatal glucocorticoid treatment and perhaps prophylactic surfactant therapy have led to a reduction in both the incidence and severity of RDS (Table 12.39).[511] Apart from prematurity, other factors are known to affect the incidence of RDS (Table 12.40).

Table 12.39 Risk of RDS by gestational age groups

Gestation (weeks)	Risk of RDS (%)
<27	41.5
27–28	54.0
29–30	44.6
31–32	37.2
33–34	12.0
35–36	2.0
37–42	0.1

After Rubaltelli et al.[511]

Table 12.40 Factors affecting the incidence of RDS

Decrease	Increase
Intrauterine growth retardation	Asphyxia
Prolonged rupture of membranes	Severe rhesus disease
Maternal steroid therapy	Maternal diabetes
Maternal smoking	Maternal hypertension
Sickle cell disease	Antepartum hemorrhage
Heroin	Elective Cesarean section
Alcohol	Second twin
Black infants	Family history
Girls	Boys

Pathogenesis and natural course of RDS

Deficiency of surfactant leads to alveolar collapse, reduced lung volume, decreased lung compliance and ventilation–perfusion abnormalities. Right to left shunting of up to 70% or more occurs through collapsed lung (intrapulmonary) or across the ductus arteriosus and the foramen ovale (extrapulmonary) if pulmonary hypertension is severe. Persistent hypoxemia ($<4\,kPa$) causes metabolic acidosis and respiratory acidosis will also be present because of alveolar hypoventilation. This further reduces surfactant production and affects pulmonary vascular resistance, myocardial contractility, cardiac output and arterial blood pressure. Perfusion of the kidneys, gastrointestinal tract, muscles and skin is reduced leading to edema and electrolyte disorders.

Surfactant deficiency in RDS is primary and due to immaturity; the normal pool size of 100 mg of phospholipids/kg at term is reduced to $<5\,mg/kg$ in babies with severe RDS. In some babies there is sufficient surfactant at birth to sustain normal respiration but this is gradually used up so that a milder form of RDS can present some hours after birth. Surfactant may also be inactivated by plasma proteins leaking into the alveoli and this form of ARDS may be seen in infants born to mothers with severe pregnancy-induced hypertension. Usually after 2–3 days endogenous surfactant production begins and is followed by clinical recovery. Surfactant replacement will hasten recovery and does not delay the onset of endogenous surfactant production.

Pathology

Macroscopically the lungs appear collapsed and liver-like and sink in water. Microscopic examination shows generalized collapse of alveoli with eosinophilic membranes in infants surviving more than a few hours. The membranes begin to break up by the third day and are removed by macrophages. Sometimes there is frank pulmonary hemorrhage and interstitial emphysema. The muscle layer of the walls of pulmonary arterioles is thickened and pulmonary lymphatics are dilated. Surfactant treatment may modify the pathological features of RDS reducing epithelial necrosis, interstitial emphysema and pulmonary interstitial hemorrhage.

Clinical features

The disease has a wide spectrum of severity from mild respiratory distress lasting 2 or 3 days to a rapidly fatal illness causing death within a few hours. The early clinical signs are shown in Table 12.41. Each of these clinical signs may be explained by disturbed lung function. Increased respiratory rate is caused by the demand of increased alveolar ventilation and is related to blood gas changes of hypercarbia and hypoxemia. Later slow or decreasing respiratory rate which may progress to apnea

Table 12.41 Early clinical signs of RDS

Tachypnea (>60/min)
Expiratory grunting
Sternal and intercostal recession
Cyanosis in room air
Delayed onset of respiration in very immature babies

may be related to diaphragmatic muscle fatigue. The sternal and inter-costal recession or retractions are due to reduced lung compliance as a result of surfactant deficiency. Expiratory grunting results from expiration against a partially closed glottis in an attempt to prevent alveolar collapse but may be absent in the very immature or seriously ill baby. Cyanosis is due to decreased arterial oxygen tension caused by right to left interatrial and ductus shunts and to increasing intrapulmonary shunting after the first 12 h of life due to perfusion of collapsed or poorly ventilated parts of the lungs.

In severe disease, immature babies or those with asphyxia, positive pressure ventilation may be needed from birth. In more mature babies grunting and retractions are prominent and cyanosis may be apparent from soon after birth. Oxygen concentrations of greater than 60% are often needed to abolish cyanosis, and respiratory failure with hypercarbia and acidosis frequently supervenes, so that mechanical ventilation becomes necessary. Clinical signs outside the respiratory system also occur (Table 12.42).

The classic signs of RDS have become outdated for two reasons. First, most of the babies cared for in neonatal units are very immature and they often present with apnea at birth; second, prophylactic surfactant treatment is widely practiced for these babies and significantly modifies the clinical course and chest radiographic appearances.

Investigations

These are needed to confirm the diagnosis and exclude disorders in the list of differential diagnoses (Table 12.43). The chest radiograph is the best way to confirm the diagnosis but there are two caveats: first, congenital pneumonia can have a similar picture often coexisting with RDS and, second, surfactant treatment rapidly improves the chest radiographic appearances and with prophylactic therapy this often happens before radiographs are taken.

Classic radiographic signs are a diffuse reticulogranular pattern of mottling of the lung fields, described as a 'ground glass' appearance with superimposed 'air bronchograms' due to air in the major bronchi being highlighted against the opacified lung (Fig. 12.18). With increasing severity the opacification increases and becomes confluent so that the heart borders are obscured. The radiological appearances may be atypical with asymmetry when changes are more pronounced on the right side or are confined to the lower lobes. Uneven distribution of

Table 12.42 Nonrespiratory clinical signs in severe RDS

Hypotonia	Jaundice
Decreased movements	Hypothermia
Edema	Abdominal distention
Loss of heart rate variability	Decreased urinary output

Table 12.43 Differential diagnosis of RDS

Congenital pneumonia
Aspiration pneumonia
Meconium aspiration syndrome
Air leak – pneumothorax, pulmonary interstitial emphysema and pneumomediastinum
Transient tachypnea of the newborn
Lobar emphysema
Pulmonary hypoplasia
Diaphragmatic hernia
Heart failure
Persistent pulmonary hypertension
Asphyxia and raised intracranial pressure
Metabolic acidosis/inborn errors of metabolism
Congenital neuromuscular disorders
Anemia, hypovolemia and polycythemia

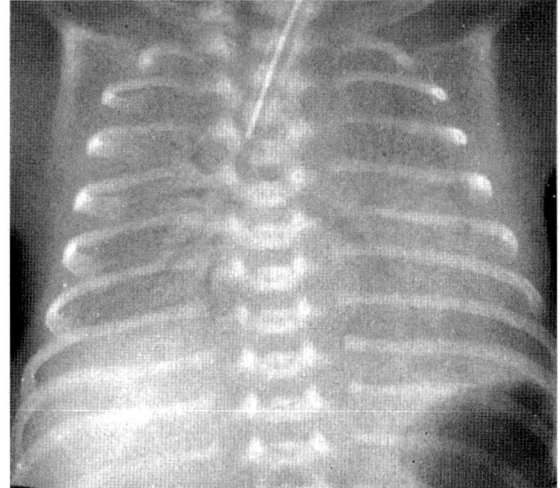

Fig. 12.18 Radiograph of severe RDS with widespread reticulogranular mottling and air bronchograms amounting to grade IV disease.

reticulogranularity on chest radiograph may be due to underlying pneumonia or maldistribution following surfactant treatment.

Other investigations may be biochemical, hematological or microbiological. Serial analyses of pH and arterial blood gases are essential for clinical management. Continuous measurements of oxygen and carbon dioxide tensions may be made transcutaneously, and oxygen saturation can be assessed non-invasively by pulse oximetry but this has a major disadvantage of failing to exclude hyperoxia. These measurements are necessary to follow the clinical course of a baby with RDS and to detect early signs of deteriorating respiratory function allowing effective interventions such as surfactant therapy, CPAP or assisted ventilation. Hematological and microbiological investigations are needed to exclude underlying infection especially that due to group B streptococcus (GBS).

Natural history

The clinical course of classic RDS is that of increasing severity during the first 24–48 h, followed by a period of stability lasting another 48 h before improvement occurs. Severity of the disease may be expressed in terms of oxygen requirements and need for assisted ventilation. In the 24 h prior to recovery a diuresis usually occurs. The widespread introduction of prophylactic surfactant therapy has meant that this natural history is unfamiliar to today's resident pediatricians although the occasional more mature infant with RDS may be encountered.

Prevention

Antenatal glucocorticoid administration reduces the incidence and severity of RDS provided 48 h of treatment is possible. Improved survival and reduced risk of complications such as pneumothorax, intraventricular hemorrhage (IVH) and persistent ductus arteriosus (PDA) but not bronchopulmonary dysplasia (BPD) have also been demonstrated.[512] RDS may also be prevented or at least ameliorated if care is taken to prevent hypoxemia, acidosis and hypothermia in preterm babies. Gentle resuscitation at birth with early expansion of the alveoli or terminal airways in the very preterm baby, especially those of less than 30 weeks' gestation, is very important. This may be facilitated by giving prophylactic surfactant or early use of CPAP.

Later surfactant replacement will also modify the course of RDS and in general the earlier it is given the greater the benefit.[513] Babies who might benefit most from prophylactic treatment at birth are those of less than 30 weeks' gestation, those needing endotracheal intubation for resuscitation or those who were not treated with prenatal corticosteroids.

Treatment

The objectives of treatment are to maintain normal blood gases, pH, biochemistry and physiology (blood pressure, temperature and renal function) and in addition to avoid complications of both the disease and the treatments. Surfactant replacement therapy is an effective way of accomplishing these objectives. There are two basic types of surfactant, synthetic and natural, and both have been shown to improve survival by about 40% and reduce the risk of pneumothorax by 30–70% in babies with RDS.[514–516] Natural surfactants containing the proteins SP-B and SP-C are more effective than the protein-free synthetic surfactants[517] with improved survival and a reduced risk of pneumothorax. There are many natural surfactant preparations, prepared from animal lungs – Survanta™ (bovine), Alveofact™ and Infasurf™ (calf) and Curosurf™ (porcine)–and there may be subtle differences between them in terms of efficacy.[518] The optimal dose of surfactant is from 100 mg/kg to 200 mg/kg and repeated doses may be needed for babies who show relapse.[519] Natural surfactants may be given to babies with moderate to severe RDS as soon after birth as possible or used prophylactically for very immature infants. Newer synthetic surfactants with SP-B analogues will soon be available but to date there are insufficient data on safety and efficacy to recommend them in place of natural surfactants.

Maintenance of temperature
Occlusive wrapping in a polythene bag at birth helps to maintain temperature during resuscitation.[520] Preterm infants should be nursed in incubators or under radiant warmers. In order to maintain adequate temperature in very preterm infants incubators need high humidity and double walls (see p. 223).

Maintenance of normoxemia
The aim is to achieve satisfactory oxygenation. For more mature babies (> 30 weeks) with spontaneous respiration, humidified oxygen may be administered directly into the incubator. For very immature infants (< 30 weeks) or when respiratory failure supervenes, some form of assisted ventilation may be necessary (see below). Excessive handling should be avoided as this causes hypoxemia and leads to deterioration. Monitoring of oxygenation is essential as too little oxygen will cause hypoxemia and metabolic acidosis and too much oxygen has been associated with the development of retinopathy of prematurity and BPD. Studies are currently underway to determine optimal oxygen saturation targeting using pulse oximetry. An initial right radial artery blood sample is helpful. An arterial catheter should be inserted in babies needing greater than 40% oxygen after the first hour (or greater than 30% oxygen in babies of less than 1200 g birth weight). Continuous methods of assessing oxygenation such as intravascular electrodes, transcutaneous monitors and pulse oximeters do not remove the need for intermittent arterial blood sampling to check calibration and measure pH, arterial carbon dioxide tension and base deficit. Oxygen delivery is affected by arterial oxygen tension, oxygen-carrying capacity, oxygen affinity, peripheral blood flow, temperature and pH. Fetal Hb allows more oxygen to be carried in the blood at any oxygen tension (greater affinity) but less oxygen will be released to the tissues. Transfusions of adult blood may improve tissue oxygen delivery.

Correction of acid–base abnormalities
Respiratory acidosis due to raised arterial carbon dioxide tension is common in severe RDS. Hypercarbia can only be treated adequately by improving ventilation. Metabolic acidosis may arise from hypoxemia, hypotension, infection, renal failure, PDA or IVH. Treatment of the underlying cause, for example by increasing oxygen concentrations, giving blood or treating the PDA, may be more appropriate than infusion of sodium bicarbonate. The aim should be to keep the pH above 7.25. If the base deficit becomes greater than 10 mmol/L then sodium bicarbonate should be considered. The dose may be calculated as follows:

$$\text{dose (mmol)} = \text{base deficit (mmol/L)} \times \text{weight(kg)} \times 0.3$$

Molar sodium bicarbonate 8.4% (1 mmol/mL) is the most frequently used alkali in clinical practice but it is hyperosmolar and rapid infusions have been associated with the development of IVH. Severe tissue injury

may result from extravasation. It also has a high sodium content and will raise $PaCO_2$ unless ventilation is adequate. Sodium bicarbonate should be diluted and given slowly (not faster than 1 mmol/min) by peripheral venous infusion. Serum sodium levels should be monitored regularly.

Energy, fluid and electrolyte requirements
The preterm baby with RDS has reduced stores of carbohydrate (as glycogen), fat and protein (as skeletal muscle), and also has increased metabolic requirements from extra work of breathing. Providing adequate exogenous sources of energy as parenteral nutrition for these sick babies is technically difficult. Most babies should be started on intravenous fluids of 70–80 ml/kg/d[521] while kept in > 80% humidity in an incubator. Indeed, 60 ml/kg/d may be better than 80 ml/kg/d in babies > 32 weeks' gestation. Sodium intake should be restricted over the first few days of life and initiated after onset of diuresis with careful monitoring of fluid balance and electrolyte levels. Fluid requirements may be monitored by looking at plasma sodium, urine output and specific gravity, osmolality and by regular weighing. Excessive fluid intake is associated with increased risk of PDA, NEC and BPD.

Oliguria in severe RDS is common for the first 48 h due to effects of asphyxia, hypotension and possibly inappropriate ADH secretion. Care must be taken to avoid fluid and electrolyte overload. Subsequently, when diuresis occurs, the large urinary losses mean that extra fluid, sodium and potassium intake will be necessary to prevent hyponatremia or hypokalemia (see p. 220).

There should be early introduction of protein, calories and lipids in parenteral nutrition (PN).[522] Early use of PN improves survival by 40% in infants of 28–30 weeks with RDS.[523] Once the baby shows signs of recovery, extra energy should be provided in the form of enteral milk feeds started very gradually to reduce the risk of NEC.[524]

Assisted ventilation
CPAP. Continuous positive airways pressure (CPAP) is a distending pressure which prevents alveolar collapse during expiration and thus improves oxygenation. CPAP is often used as a substitute for mechanical ventilation to provide respiratory support for babies with RDS.[525] The indications for using CPAP in RDS are not absolute and may depend upon maturity of the baby (Table 12.44). Babies with mild RDS can often be managed on CPAP without needing surfactant treatment. In babies who do require surfactant, mechanical ventilation can also be avoided by the 'INSURE' technique (INtubate – SURfactant – Extubate to CPAP).[526] There are various methods of applying CPAP, but today nasal prongs using a ventilator circuit or a flow driver are generally used. There is no evidence to date of any differences in long term outcomes among various devices used to provide nasal CPAP, however studies have shown that short binasal prongs are better than a single prong at reducing the need for re-intubation.[527] Recently devices such as the infant flow driver have been developed with the technology to provide a background of synchronized nasal ventilation (NIPPV). This can reduce extubation failure rates but it is not yet clear if there are any long term advantages.[528]
Mechanical ventilation. Mechanical ventilation (MV) is used to treat respiratory failure or intractable apnea (Table 12.45). For babies less than 30 weeks' gestation, $PaCO_2$ of > 8 kPa is usually accepted as an indication for MV. The aim of MV is to provide acceptable blood gases whilst minimizing lung injury, hemodynamic impairment or other adverse events. The strategy for minimizing lung injury is to optimize

Table 12.44 Indications for CPAP in RDS

1. Early treatment of infants < 30 weeks if good spontaneous respiratory effort
2. After surfactant treatment in infants > 27 weeks
3. For infants > 30 weeks and oxygen need > 30% to keep PaO_2 > 8 kPa (60 mmHg)
4. Recurrent apneic attacks
5. Weaning from IPPV and after extubation

Table 12.45 Indications for IPPV in RDS

1. Failure to establish respiration at birth
2. To administer surfactant at birth in infants <27 weeks
3. To administer surfactant in infants >27 weeks and <32 weeks when they need >30% oxygen
4. In infants >32 weeks when respiratory failure develops
   pH <7.20
   $PaCO_2$ >9 kPa (68 mmHg)
   PaO_2 <7 kPa (53 mmHg) in 60% oxygen
5. Intractable apneic attacks not responding to other measures

Table 12.46 Complications of RDS

1. Persistent ductus arteriosus
2. Intraventricular hemorrhage
3. Pulmonary
   a. Air leaks
      Pneumothorax
      Pneumomediastinum
      Pulmonary interstitial emphysema
      Pneumopericardium
      Pneumoperitoneum
      Air embolism
      Subcutaneous emphysema
   b. Chronic lung disease
   c. Pneumonia
      Aspiration
      Bacterial
4. Complications of mechanical ventilation (see above)
5. Long term neurological sequelae

lung volume with avoidance of excessive tidal volumes and atelectasis.[529] MV can be provided as intermittent positive pressure ventilation (IPPV) or high frequency oscillatory ventilation (HFOV).[530] HFOV may result in less lung injury thereby reducing BPD,[531] however the quality of the intensive care team may determine outcome to a greater degree than the type of ventilator used, and with the introduction of low tidal volume MV the benefits of HFOV over IPPV in lowering incidence of BPD have probably diminished.

A neonatal version of time-cycled, pressure-limited ventilation is provided by many manufacturers in several modalities such as: IPPV, intermittent mandatory ventilation (IMV), synchronized intermittent mandatory ventilation (SIMV), assist control (AC) or synchronized IPPV (SIPPV), pressure support ventilation (PSV) or volume guarantee (VG). VG combines the advantages of pressure-limited, time-cycled, continuous-flow ventilation with those of volume-controlled ventilation by autoregulating peak pressures within preset limits to achieve tidal volumes set by the user.

IPPV is performed through an endotracheal tube inserted through either the nose or mouth into the trachea. The initial ventilator settings employed will depend upon the maturity of the baby and the severity of the lung disease. For the baby < 30 weeks' gestation with severe lung disease, the aim of IPPV should be to expand the lungs as early as possible with the lowest peak airway pressure possible. Peak airway pressures of 15–25 cmH₂O are often needed initially, with PEEP (positive end-expiratory pressure) of 3–5 cmH₂O and ventilator rate of 40–60/min with a relatively short inspiratory time of 0.3–0.4 s.[532] Mechanical ventilation of the more mature baby with severe RDS may need higher peak airway pressures and lower rates. Sometimes muscle relaxants and sedation with morphine or fentanyl are needed to prevent these babies 'fighting' the ventilator which will increase the risk of pneumothorax.

If gas exchange remains impaired in a ventilated infant after surfactant treatment, oxygenation may be improved by increased mean airway pressure (MAP) or use of HFOV. Muscle relaxation with pancuronium (0.03 mg/kg) or vecuronium (0.05 mg/kg/h by infusion after a loading dose of 0.1 mg/kg) may be required. A further dose of surfactant may be required. Inhaled nitric oxide does not benefit preterm babies with acute RDS.[533] As the baby's condition improves the ventilator settings can be reduced. Peak inspiratory pressure should be lowered first, along with inspired oxygen concentration. Later, ventilator rates can be lowered keeping inspiratory time constant at about 0.4 s. Following surfactant treatment ventilator settings can usually be reduced quite rapidly. Patient triggered ventilation (PTV) can shorten the duration of mechanical ventilation during the weaning process in preterm babies, however there is no evidence of any long term benefit in terms of survival or reduction in BPD.[534] Methylxanthines such as caffeine are used as respiratory stimulants to promote successful weaning.[535] Extubation may be successful from MAP of 6–7 cmH₂O on conventional ventilation and from 8–9 cmH₂O on HFOV, even in very preterm babies. After extubation nasal CPAP reduces the need for re-intubation.[536]

Complications of RDS (Table 12.46)
Persistent ductus arteriosus (PDA)
The ductus arteriosus is likely to remain open in babies with severe RDS for a number of reasons: prematurity with poorly developed ductus musculature, reduced arterial oxygen tensions and inadequate metabolism of prosta-

glandins in the lungs.[537] Fluid overload and surfactant replacement may also increase the risk of PDA. The management is discussed on page 267.

Intraventricular hemorrhage (IVH) (p. 307)
IVH can cause acute deterioration in infants with RDS and may be predisposed to by other causes of collapse such as pneumothorax.[538] Maintenance of physiological stability and prevention of air leak by manipulation of ventilator settings or surfactant replacement has reduced the incidence of IVH in recent years.[539]

Pulmonary air leaks (p. 253)
The incidence of these depends upon the severity of RDS and the need for assisted ventilation. For babies with RDS not needing assisted ventilation the incidence is 5–10%. In the decades of the 1970s and 1980s, if CPAP was needed the incidence was about 10–15% and with IPPV 10–30%.[540] Since that time surfactant replacement,[513–515] together with better ventilators,[541] have reduced the incidence of pneumothorax to less than 5%, which means that many residents have not had much experience in insertion of chest drains.

Bronchopulmonary dysplasia (p. 259)
This condition was not described until after the introduction of mechanical ventilation to treat RDS.[542] Positive pressure mechanical ventilation along with oxygen toxicity and chorioamnionitis have a significant role in pathogenesis. About 20% of babies needing MV for RDS will develop this complication[543] but infants with mild or no RDS can also develop BPD, particularly in the presence of chorioamnionitis.[544]

Pneumonia (p. 250)
Pneumonia may coexist with RDS or be secondary associated with the presence of an endotracheal tube. Cultures of tracheal aspirates are of limited use in diagnosis of secondary infection but may guide the choice of antibiotics should the infant deteriorate. The presence of both pus cells and organisms in tracheal aspirates, development of patchy opacity on chest radiograph and general deterioration with elevated serum inflammatory markers along with positive blood cultures help to make the diagnosis.[545] Appropriate antibiotic treatment is then necessary. Aspiration pneumonia may also be common and may cause acute deterioration. In one study it occurred in up to 80% of mechanically ventilated neonates.[546] The chest radiograph may show areas of collapse and consolidation, especially in the right upper or right lower lobes. Antibiotic therapy and gentle chest physiotherapy may be helpful.

Long term neurological sequelae (p. 239)
There is recent evidence that modern neonatal intensive care has not only reduced neonatal mortality very considerably, but has also improved the

quality of survival. A major contributing factor is the improved understanding of the pathogenesis of RDS as well as improved methods of prevention and treatment. For babies of > 30 weeks' gestation, ventilatory techniques are now well standardized and technical difficulties are minimal. Babies in whom RDS is the primary indication for mechanical ventilation are unlikely to develop permanent brain injury unless there is severe asphyxia or extensive IVH. The introduction of surfactant therapy after 1988 was largely responsible for the sharp reduction in the RDS-specific infant mortality rate from 2 per 1000 births in 1970 to 0.4 per 1000 in 1995.[547]

TRANSIENT TACHYPNEA OF THE NEWBORN

First described in 1966,[548] transient tachypnea of the newborn occurs in both term and preterm babies, affecting about 1% of all births.[511] The risk is increased after Cesarean section to about 4% but the timing of elective Cesarean section is important, with the risk markedly decreasing between 37 and 40 weeks' gestation.[549]

Etiology and pathogenesis

Transient tachypnea of the newborn (TTN) has been attributed to delayed resorption of fetal lung fluid, and predisposing factors include elective Cesarean section, perinatal asphyxia, excessive maternal analgesia, maternal diabetes, hypothermia and male gender. Many of these factors are associated with increased production or decreased resorption of lung fluid.[550] Catecholamine levels after elective Cesarean section are lower than those following vaginal delivery with the result that fetal lung fluid production continues after birth. Mild left ventricular dysfunction is also found in echocardiographic studies of babies with TTN.[551] More severe TTN may present clinically as persistent pulmonary hypertension.[552]

Clinical presentation

Most affected babies are either term or near term infants; there is a male preponderance of 3:1. Tachypnea is apparent from about 1 h after birth, with respiratory rates of up to 120/min. Subcostal recession, grunting and cyanosis may be present but are not prominent features. Affected babies have barrel chests with increased anteroposterior diameter. Babies with a picture of persistent fetal circulation are uncommon, but present with marked cyanosis and often need mechanical ventilation.

Diagnosis

The chest radiograph shows hyperinflated lung fields, perihilar opacities, increased vascular markings, fluid in the transverse fissure and small pleural effusions (Fig. 12.19). Two important differential diag-

noses should be considered in atypical infants. Early onset group B streptococcal (GBS) sepsis can mimic TTN initially but if unrecognized and untreated will be fatal. Blood culture, full blood picture and measurement of inflammatory markers will help to make this diagnosis. Some forms of congenital heart disease, for example anomalous pulmonary venous drainage, can also mimic TTN. Chest radiograph and echocardiography are helpful if a cardiac anomaly is suspected.

Management

Oxygen is often needed for 2 or 3 days but respiratory failure is uncommon unless a pulmonary air leak or pulmonary hypertension occurs. Pulse oximetry is used to monitor the oxygen needs. Only rarely are oxygen concentrations above 40% necessary. Penicillin should be given until GBS sepsis has been excluded. Diuretics do not alter the clinical course of TTN.[553]

Outcome

Most infants recover within 2–3 days. A few develop pneumothoraces and a few may need mechanical ventilation. The mortality rate should approach zero and survivors should have normal neurodevelopment. Recent studies have reported an association between TTN and the subsequent development of childhood asthma.[554]

PNEUMONIA

Pneumonia is probably the most common serious infection of the newborn. It may be either congenital or acquired, although intrapartum infection can occur and may not fit easily into either category (Table 12.47).

Incidence

Preterm babies are more at risk for at least three reasons. First, chorioamnionitis is a common stimulus for preterm labor;[555] second, preterm babies have problems with host defense mechanisms; third, they are more likely to need intensive care and thus be exposed to risks of acquired infections. Early onset pneumonia has been estimated to occur in 1.79 per 1000 live births.[556] Pneumonia complicates endotracheal intubation for mechanical ventilation of very low birth weight babies in about 30% of cases.[557]

Pathogenesis

Pneumonia acquired congenitally or intrapartum usually presents within the first 4–6 h of life. Nosocomial infections are of later onset although colonization with organisms acquired during birth can lead to subsequent infection occurring after 7 days. This may occur in late onset GBS infections.

Transplacentally acquired pneumonia may be due to viruses (CMV, coxsackie, herpes simplex and rubella), bacteria (*Listeria monocytogenes*, coliforms, pneumococci and streptococci) or toxoplasmosis. The ascending route of infection is most important in early onset infection and organisms found in the maternal genital tract and in the baby's lungs are very similar. Prolonged rupture of the membranes, maternal GBS colonization and prematurity significantly increase risk of ascending infection with chorioamnionitis and pneumonia.[558] Ascending infection can also occur through intact membranes and cause illness or perinatal death.[559] Organisms involved in ascending infection are coliforms, streptococci, *Haemophilus influenzae*, pneumococci, staphylococci and herpes simplex virus.

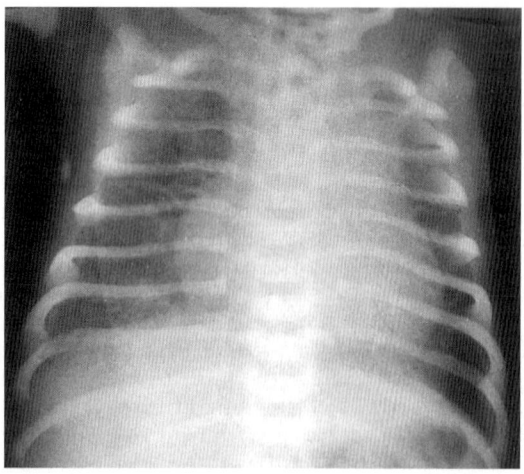

Fig. 12.19 Radiograph of TTN with overinflated lungs, fluid in the right costophrenic angle and horizontal fissure. The skinfold line seen at the right base may be mistaken for a pneumothorax.

Table 12.47 Pathogenesis of neonatal pneumonia

Congenital (transplacental acquisition)
Intrapartum
    a. Ascending infection and chorioamnionitis
    b. Aspiration of infected secretions at delivery
Acquired
    Nosocomial – often during mechanical ventilation or late infection
    after colonization at birth

Intrapartum aspiration of infected secretions can cause infection with *L. monocytogenes*, streptococci, herpes simplex and varicella. Nosocomial or environmentally acquired infection can be transmitted by hospital staff, usually from poor handwashing. Organisms involved are usually staphylococci, streptococci and RSV. Sometimes infection is acquired from nursery equipment and the organisms involved are pseudomonas, serratia, klebsiella and listeria. Late onset infection may also be due to delayed invasion of organisms acquired at birth. This typically occurs with certain serotypes of streptococci and listeria and is probably not preventable by prophylactic antibiotic use.

Early onset pneumonia
Clinical features
Intrapartum stillbirth may occur, although often the baby is born alive but appears septicemic and needs resuscitation. The onset of respiratory signs may be more gradual with a clinical picture very similar to that of RDS (Table 12.41). Helpful distinguishing features include temperature instability, hypotension, apneic spells and acidosis. Sometimes a skin rash or hepatosplenomegaly (listeriosis) will be present or the baby may be malodorous (coliforms or bacteroides). The severity of respiratory distress is variable and some babies may have profound shock and metabolic upsets with right to left shunting and a clinical course resembling severe persistent fetal circulation whereas others have respiratory signs such as tachypnea.

A chest radiograph is necessary to exclude other causes of respiratory distress. With transplacentally acquired infection there are diffuse, interstitial opacities giving a ground glass, reticular pattern which may be indistinguishable from RDS or there may be extensive consolidation (Fig. 12.20). With ascending infection there may be alveolar involvement which produces bilateral coarse opacities which are much less uniform (Fig. 12.21). Air bronchograms may also be seen, especially if the opacities become confluent.

Pneumonia acquired following aspiration is usually less evenly distributed on chest radiograph and may show as segmental or lobar collapse (Fig. 12.22).

Diagnosis
Clinical diagnosis is confirmed by culturing organisms from tracheal fluid or blood along with typical changes on chest radiograph. There is not time to wait for culture results before starting treatment, and hematological (white cell and platelet counts) and biochemical (C-reactive protein) tests are not sensitive enough to be relied upon if negative. If in doubt, it is best to start antibiotics after cultures have

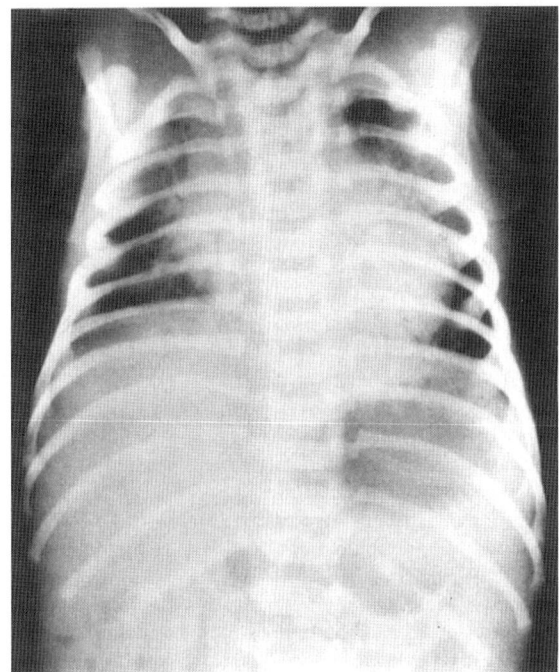

Fig. 12.21 Radiograph of intrauterine pneumonia from ascending infection showing patchy bronchopneumonic consolidation.

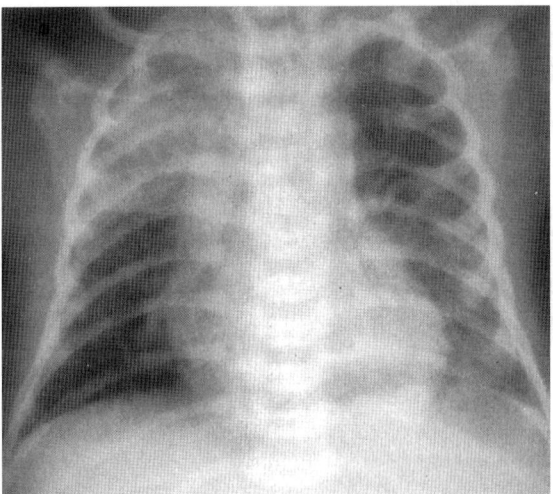

Fig. 12.22 Chest radiograph showing aspiration pneumonia with collapse and consolidation in right upper lobe.

been taken. If tracheal aspirate can be obtained and examined within 8 h of birth there is a good correlation between organisms seen and those subsequently cultured.

Differential diagnosis
This includes RDS, TTN and meconium aspiration syndrome in addition to causes of severe asphyxia at birth including pulmonary hypoplasia. Often these conditions coexist and all babies with respiratory distress should be assumed to have GBS infection until proven otherwise. Severe pneumonia may also be difficult to distinguish from cyanotic heart disease and persistent fetal circulation.

Management
Prevention. Early onset GBS infection can be predicted from maternal risk factors such as prolonged rupture of the membranes, colonization of the genital tract, spontaneous preterm labor and maternal pyrexia in labor. In women with these risk factors who are colonized with GBS and who are treated with

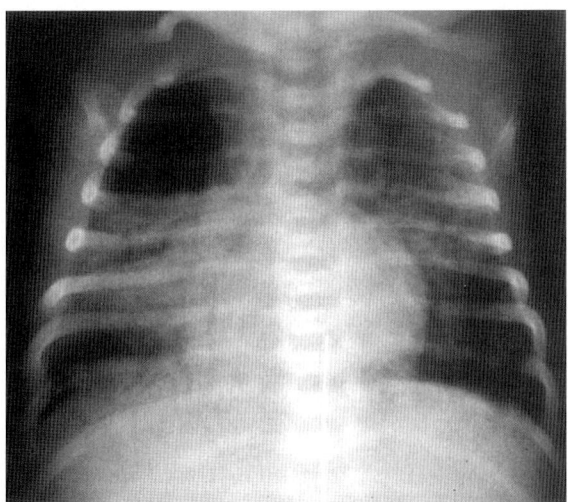

Fig. 12.20 Radiograph of congenital listeriosis showing extensive consolidation in both midzones but more marked on the right. An arterial catheter is seen with its tip at T7 and T8.

intravenous penicillin in large doses during labor there is a significant reduction in neonatal infection.[560] Penicillin may also be effective in pregnancies complicated by infection with listeria, haemophilus and pneumococci but other Gram negative organisms and anaerobes will not usually be sensitive. A combination of ampicillin and metronidazole improves the spectrum of cover in these high risk cases. Maternal erythromycin improves neonatal outcome when there is preterm prelabor rupture of the membranes.[561]

Treatment. Babies born to mothers with the risk factors mentioned above should have cultures taken and be given antibiotic prophylaxis. There is no evidence that routine penicillin prophylaxis for all preterm babies is effective and this approach might increase risk of Gram negative infections. Routine monitoring of respiratory rate for 24 h on the postnatal ward is effective in shortening the time to diagnosis and treatment of the occasional late-presenting case.[562]

For symptomatic infants with respiratory distress, penicillin therapy should be started after appropriate cultures have been taken; the antibiotic can be stopped after 48 h if cultures are negative and the baby's condition improved or a clear diagnosis of non-infective illness has been made. If infection is strongly suspected, cultures become positive or the infant deteriorates, an aminoglycoside such as gentamicin should be added to the antibiotic regimen.

Treatment of the ill baby requires good resuscitation, stabilization and respiratory support, in addition to antibiotics given after cultures have been taken. Blood or plasma transfusion, inotropic drugs and correction of acidosis are all important. Penicillin or ampicillin and gentamicin or amikacin in combination provide the best cover for early onset pneumonia. Cefotaxime has also been advocated because of increased Gram negative cover and better penetration into lung tissue, although with cephalosporins there is an associated increased risk of fungal sepsis.[563]

Surfactant treatment may be helpful to treat respiratory failure from surfactant inactivation in streptococcal pneumonia but it is less effective than in infants with RDS.[564] The role of intravenous immunoglobulin therapy in neonatal pneumonia remains to be determined.[565]

Late onset pneumonia

This may be associated with mechanical ventilation, aspiration or bacteremia or occur secondary to late invasion with an organism acquired during birth, e.g. GBS or *L. monocytogenes*. Occasionally unusual organisms such as chlamydia, candida, CMV, herpes simplex, RSV or mycoplasma are implicated although staphylococci and coliforms are much more commonly found.

Clinical features

Late onset pneumonia occurs after 24 h and presents with signs of respiratory distress although preterm babies may develop apnea. There may be systemic signs with pyrexia in term and hypothermia in preterm babies. Bacteremia and meningitis may coexist.

A chest radiograph is necessary for diagnosis, and culture of blood, tracheal aspirate and CSF should be performed. The differential diagnosis includes PDA and heart failure, aspiration pneumonia, early chronic lung disease or an inborn error of metabolism.

Management

General supportive measures, antibiotics and perhaps gentle chest physiotherapy form the basis of management. Antibiotic selection must cover staphylococci and Gram negative organisms and, if meningitis is suspected, be capable of penetrating the CSF. A combination of flucloxacillin and amikacin or one of the third generation cephalosporins, e.g. cefotaxime, is usually satisfactory. For pseudomonas infections ceftazidime is used and some staphylococcal infections respond only to vancomycin or teicoplanin.

Outcome

Early onset pneumonia has a high mortality of about 50%, especially when due to GBS which often affects very immature babies who have septicemia with pneumonia. Late onset pneumonia has a mortality rate of less than 15% despite its association with bacteremia and meningitis.

MECONIUM ASPIRATION SYNDROME

This is a serious and potentially preventable condition occurring usually in term and post-term babies.

Incidence

Meconium staining of the amniotic fluid is found in about 9% of deliveries at term, however in resource rich countries the incidence of meconium aspiration requiring intubation and mechanical ventilation is low (0.43 per 1000 births).[566] The incidence may be falling because of increased induction of labor in prolonged pregnancy beyond 41 weeks and better monitoring for signs of fetal distress in labor.[567]

Etiology and pathogenesis

In the term or post-term infant asphyxia prior to birth stimulates intestinal peristalsis and relaxation of the anal sphincter. Meconium passage is most likely to occur in the post-term baby, the term baby after asphyxia or the baby with IUGR. It rarely happens in the preterm baby of < 34 weeks' gestation and if it does one should consider an alternative cause such as congenital infection, especially that due to listeriosis[568] or GBS. Once meconium reaches the major airways, respiration after birth ensures distal migration into the smaller airways. This may lead to obstruction with air trapping and atelectasis with pneumothorax occurring in 5–10% of cases.[566]

Other factors producing lung disease are chemical pneumonitis and secondary bacterial infection. Progression to persistent pulmonary hypertension occurs in about 20% of cases, particularly those with asphyxial insult or pneumothoraces.[569]

Clinical features

Affected babies are usually post-term or growth retarded. There may be meconium staining of the skin, umbilical cord and nails. The baby may present with respiratory distress from birth but respiratory signs may gradually develop over 12 h with tachypnea, cyanosis, indrawing and a hyperinflated chest. There may be profound hypoxemia although hypercarbia is less common. Metabolic acidosis and hypoglycemia are common and postasphyxial signs may be found in the central nervous system, kidneys and heart.

Diagnosis

Diagnosis is made on the basis of meconium-stained amniotic fluid, presence of meconium in the trachea and radiological changes. On chest radiograph there is overinflation of the lungs with widespread coarse, fluffy opacities (Fig. 12.23). Sometimes the appearances are confined to

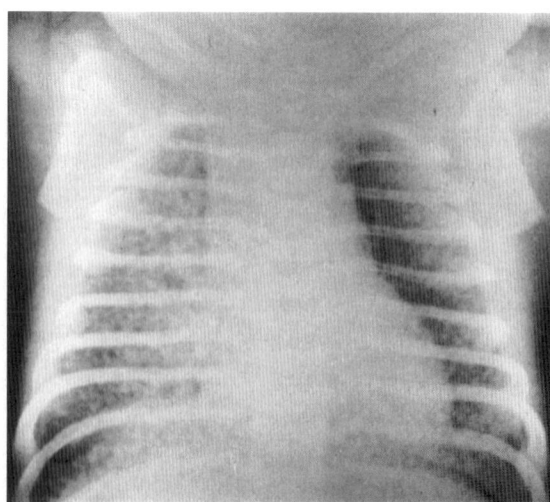

Fig. 12.23 Radiograph of meconium aspiration syndrome with overinflated lungs, depressed diaphragm and coarse modular opacities alternating with areas of focal overinflation.

the right lung or right upper lobe. Pneumothorax, pneumomediastinum and cardiomegaly may be present. Radiological clearing is usually slow over 10 days but in some babies the meconium disappears within 2–3 days possibly by ciliary action, phagocytosis or enzymatic lysis.

Management

This comprises prevention by intervention in pregnancy, labor or at birth and the treatment of established aspiration.

Prevention

Meconium aspiration syndrome should be largely preventable by careful antenatal monitoring, rapid delivery for fetal distress and rapid resuscitation with tracheal suctioning at birth if indicated. A pediatrician skilled at neonatal resuscitation should attend all deliveries complicated by meconium staining of the amniotic fluid. Suctioning of the mouth and nose after delivery of the head but before delivery of the shoulders was previously advocated, however a large randomized trial showed that this technique had no impact on the incidence of meconium aspiration.[570] Meconium aspiration often occurs before birth. Intubation of all meconium-stained babies and careful tracheal toilet has been advocated to prevent aspiration, however randomized trials have shown no benefit of routine endotracheal intubation in babies who are vigorous at birth.[571] Intubation should be reserved for babies with signs of respiratory depression and asphyxia. Tracheal aspiration using a wide bore suction catheter or an endotracheal tube adapter should be repeated until the trachea is cleared. Saline washouts should be avoided as this may liquefy the meconium allowing it to pass distally. Positive pressure ventilation should be postponed if possible until tracheal aspiration has been completed.

Treatment

All babies with meconium below the vocal cords should be admitted to the neonatal unit for observation and further management. All symptomatic babies should have a chest radiograph performed and oxygen supplementation as indicated by blood gas analyses and pulse oximetry. Babies with mild disease may need only humidified oxygen in a headbox. Gentle chest physiotherapy and postural drainage may be helpful. Broad spectrum antibiotics should be given to treat any coexistent pneumonia or congenital sepsis. There is no benefit from hydrocortisone and it may even delay recovery. Surfactant bolus treatment may hasten recovery but larger (150 mg/kg) and more frequent (6-hourly) doses are required,[572] presumably to overcome inactivation of surfactant by meconium. Dilute surfactant lavage may also help to remove particulate material from the airways[573] but this cannot be recommended as a routine treatment.

Severely asphyxiated babies with meconium aspiration often have multisystem involvement and require careful management. Mechanical ventilation may be indicated to treat respiratory failure and severe hypoxemia. Rapid ventilator rates with low PEEP are advised because of risk of pneumothorax and cardiovascular side-effects. Muscle relaxation or sedation with morphine or fentanyl is often necessary. If hypoxemia due to right to left shunting persists the PEEP may be increased up to $6 \, cmH_2O$ or higher and use of inhaled nitric oxide might reduce ventilation–perfusion mismatching and obviate the need for ECMO.

Outcome

Infants with mild disease who do not require assisted ventilation recover within a few days. Recent reports suggest mortality rates of about 2.5%.[566] Both mortality and long term neurodevelopmental sequelae are related to the severity of the underlying perinatal asphyxia. There is an increased risk of asthma among survivors of meconium aspiration syndrome compared with the general childhood population.[574]

OTHER ASPIRATION PNEUMONIAS

Aspiration may occur before, during or after birth. Apart from meconium the substances aspirated may be amniotic fluid, blood, secretions or milk.

Incidence

This is unknown but early contrast radiography studies showed that 10–15% of newborn babies aspirate fluid into their lungs during the first few days after birth. The incidence of milk aspiration in preterm babies probably has substantially decreased with introduction of more cautious feeding regimens for preterm babies. Ventilated preterm babies probably aspirate secretions quite frequently; one study suggested that this occurred in as many as 80% of such babies.[546]

Etiology

Aspiration can occur before birth and amniotic debris including squamous cells has been found in lungs of stillborn babies. Aspiration of small amounts of fetal and maternal blood does not appear to cause major problems and they are rapidly removed from the lungs. If purulent secretions are aspirated during birth there is increased risk of subsequent bacterial pneumonia. Aspiration of milk may occur in the very preterm infant, those with swallowing disorders, and those with esophageal atresia and tracheoesophageal fistula. Before 34 weeks, sucking and swallowing are uncoordinated and most babies need gastric tube feeds. Aspiration of liquids may cause apnea as part of a protective laryngeal reflex.

Clinical features

Aspiration before or during birth may cause signs of asphyxia and immediate respiratory distress in the same way as meconium aspiration syndrome. Aspiration after birth presents with apneic or cyanotic attacks and there may be choking or signs of airway obstruction. After such an episode there may be tachypnea and indrawing.

Apart from immaturity, babies at risk of aspiration are those who have suffered asphyxia or those with neuromuscular disorders such as congenital myotonic dystrophy. If there are recurrent episodes of aspiration, an underlying disorder such as H-type tracheoesophageal fistula or posterior laryngeal cleft should be excluded. In supine infants aspiration is most likely to occur into the right upper lobe and crepitations may be heard there. Occasionally there may be complete collapse of a lobe with mediastinal shift.

Diagnosis

The chest radiograph may be clear or show localized or diffuse opacities and areas of atelectasis. These changes are most frequently seen in the right upper lobe (Fig. 12.22). Tracheal aspirate may show fat-laden macrophages in babies who have aspirated milk. If gastroesophageal reflux is suspected a contrast swallow may be necessary. Esophageal pH studies are of limited value in the newborn period.[575] Videofluoroscopy may demonstrate aspiration of secretions or milk even in the absence of reflux.[576]

Management

Direct laryngoscopy and careful suction of the airways should be performed to resuscitate babies who have aspirated. Supportive care includes oxygen to correct hypoxemia, intravenous fluids and the treatment of acidosis. Broad spectrum antibiotics should be given if the aspiration is large or the secretions aspirated appear to be infected. Careful nursing is important; gastric emptying is most rapid with the baby lying either prone or on the right side.

PULMONARY AIR LEAKS

These comprise pneumothorax, pulmonary interstitial emphysema, pneumomediastinum, pneumopericardium, pneumoperitoneum, subcutaneous emphysema and air embolism.

Etiology and pathogenesis

Alveolar rupture occurs more commonly in the neonate than at any other time of life. It is more likely to occur in states of hyperinflation of the chest and risk is increased because of lack of pores of Kohn which are communications between alveoli.

Air leak occurs at the base of a group of alveoli and tracks into the perivascular sheath at the center of the pulmonary lobule. Air later tracks along the bronchovascular spaces to the hilum where it dissects into the mediastinum and pleural space. Air may also form subpleural blebs which can later rupture to cause a pneumothorax. Extension of air into subcutaneous tissues of the neck will cause surgical emphysema, and down along perivascular or periesophageal tissue sheaths to form a pneumoperitoneum. A pneumothorax may result from high transpulmonary pressures generated by the first breath but it more usually arises later because of some underlying lung pathology such as RDS, aspiration syndromes or pulmonary hypoplasia with associated need for positive pressure ventilation. Traumatic pneumothorax may occur from perforation of the lung by a suction catheter or a chest drain. Although the more mature lung ruptures at lower transpulmonary pressures than the immature lung, pneumothorax is more common in the preterm baby who is more likely to have respiratory distress.

Pneumothorax

This is accumulation of air within the pleural cavity and usually occurs following a pneumomediastinum, although the latter may not be obvious clinically or radiologically.

Incidence

About 1% of term babies have an asymptomatic pneumothorax. Symptomatic pneumothorax is less common occurring in about 1 in 1000 live births. Prior to surfactant therapy mild RDS had an incidence of pneumothorax of about 5% increasing to 10–20% with continuous positive airway pressure and to 20–40% with positive pressure ventilation. However, since introduction of surfactant therapy the incidence of pneumothorax has fallen to about 5% overall. Up to 10% of babies with meconium aspiration syndrome develop pneumothoraces.[566]

Clinical presentation

Most babies with spontaneously occurring pneumothoraces who have no underlying lung pathology have minimal signs of respiratory distress and the pneumothorax is seen as an incidental finding on a chest radiograph taken for another reason. Most significant pneumothoraces occur in babies with underlying pulmonary disease and the diagnosis should be suspected in any such baby whose condition suddenly deteriorates. If the baby is breathing spontaneously, tachypnea, grunting and cyanosis are often the presenting signs. In a unilateral pneumothorax there may be shift of the mediastinum (apex beat) away from the side of the pneumothorax and breath sounds may be reduced on the affected side. The affected hemithorax or the abdomen may appear distended because of increased tension within the pleural space. There may be hyperresonance to percussion on the affected side and hypotension may occur because of venous compression and reduced cardiac output. With a small pneumothorax there may be an increase in cardiac output, heart rate and blood pressure so that continuous monitoring of blood pressure can help make the diagnosis.[577]

In about 10% of cases pneumothoraces will be bilateral and this causes a major hemodynamic upset which for the very preterm baby may prove fatal.[578] In survivors there is an increased likelihood of IVH and adverse neurodevelopmental outcome.[579]

Diagnosis

The chest radiograph confirms the diagnosis. Anteroposterior (AP) (Fig. 12.24) and lateral views should be taken.[580] The lateral will show air in the anterior mediastinum and the thymus may be lifted up, which may also be evident on the AP film (Fig. 12.25). If the pneumothorax is extensive there will be collapse of the lung and mediastinal shift away from the affected side (Fig. 12.24). For the baby who deteriorates suddenly, there may not be time to wait for a chest radiograph, and two alternative methods of confirming the diagnosis of pneumothorax can be used. For the baby in extremis diagnostic pleural aspiration using a needle, syringe and three-way tap can be performed without delay. The second or third intercostal space in the mid-clavicular line should be used for this procedure

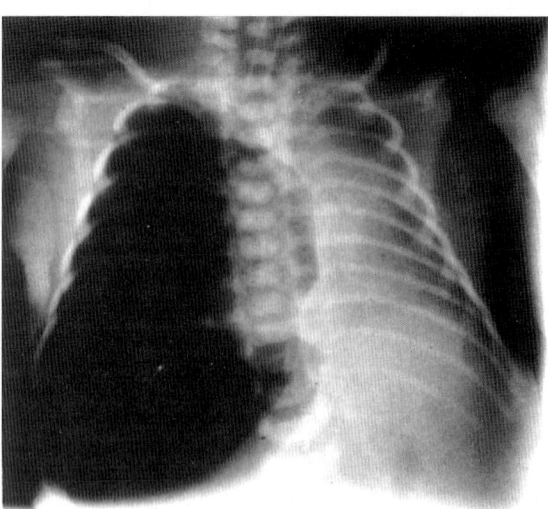

Fig. 12.24 Radiograph of a right tension pneumothorax with depression of the diaphragm and shift of the mediastinum to the left. There is also mediastinal herniation.

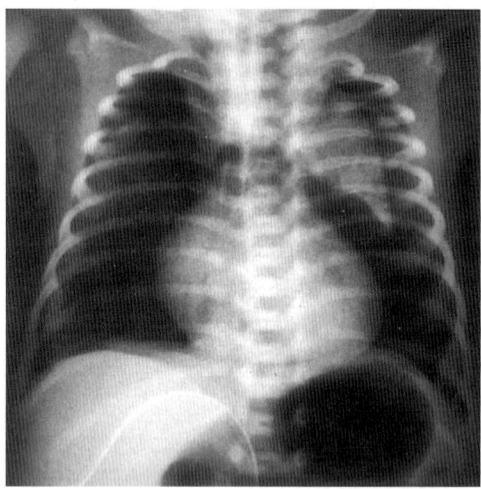

Fig. 12.25 Radiograph showing bilateral pneumothoraces and a large pneumomediastinum with elevation of the lobes of the thymus clear of the cardiac shadow (the sail sign). The endotracheal tube is shown with its tip in the right mainstem bronchus.

which is both diagnostic and therapeutic. Transillumination of the chest with a fiberoptic bright light can be used to rapidly diagnose large pneumothoraces in less severely ill babies. This technique is less useful for diagnosing small pneumothoraces or those occurring in term babies.

Treatment

No treatment is necessary if the infant is asymptomatic. Increasing inspired oxygen levels has been shown to speed the resolution of pneumothoraces in animal studies,[581] but the benefits of this versus the risks of hyperoxia have not been evaluated in human newborns. The only satisfactory treatment of a tension pneumothorax is drainage, usually by insertion of a pleural catheter connected to a nonreturn valve such as an underwater seal drain. The catheter should be large bore and placed in the anterior mediastinal space with care to avoid perforation of the lung. Local anesthetic should be used before making a small skin incision and careful dissection of the intercostal muscle. Use of an artery forceps will prevent overpenetration of the trocar into the chest. Continuous suction of 10–20 cmH$_2$O may occasionally be needed to prevent reaccumulation of the pneumothorax. Simple needle aspiration may be successful and avoid the need for insertion of a chest drain, especially when the pneumothorax is not under great tension.

Careful fluid balance should be observed as increased vasopressin secretion, leading to fluid retention, may occur after a pneumothorax although this is not common.[582] Fibrin glue pleurodesis has been used to treat persistent pneumothorax.[583]

Prevention

Timely use of prophylactic and rescue natural surfactant results in dramatic reduction in the incidence of pneumothorax.[513–517] Air leaks may also be reduced by muscle relaxation for babies with asynchronous breathing on mechanical ventilation,[584] however there are concerns about using paralysis over prolonged periods.[585] Faster mechanical ventilator rates with short inspiratory time are protective.[532] Modern ventilation methods with targeted tidal volumes also reduce rates of pneumothoraces.[541]

Prognosis

Pneumothorax is associated with increased morbidity and mortality depending upon the nature of the underlying lung disease and gestational age of the baby. Both mortality rate and IVH rate are approximately doubled following pneumothorax.

Pulmonary interstitial emphysema

This is the presence of air in the interstitium or perivascular tissues of the lung and it is probably a prerequisite of all other forms of air leak.

Incidence

The true incidence of pulmonary interstitial emphysema (PIE) is uncertain but it has been described in about 10% of neonatal autopsies. The incidence in control groups of the randomized surfactant trials varied from 25 to 50%. With introduction of surfactant therapy, widespread use of CPAP and more gentle forms of assisted ventilation the incidence of PIE is now much lower than this.

Pathogenesis

After alveolar rupture, air escapes into the pulmonary interstitium to form regular air-filled cysts varying from 0.1 to 1.0 cm in diameter. These are localized to the interlobular septa and extend radially from the hila of each lung to form a diffuse or a localized pattern. Lung function is impaired by compression of normal lung tissue, decreased compliance and obstruction of pulmonary blood flow. PIE is associated with raised leukocyte elastase levels in tracheal aspirates suggesting that intrauterine infection or prior lung injury may predispose.[586]

Clinical presentation

When PIE is localized it may be asymptomatic or the baby may gradually deteriorate. If it becomes diffuse there is progressive hypoxemia and ventilation–perfusion imbalance necessitating an increase in ventilator settings. There is usually decreased chest wall movement with hyperinflation of the chest and muffling of the heart sounds.

Diagnosis

Chest radiograph may show areas of translucency and collapse scattered throughout the lung fields rather like a snowstorm, also described as 'lacy lungs' (Fig. 12.26). If the changes are localized to one lung there may be marked overinflation and shift of the mediastinum as in a tension pneumothorax. Pseudocysts may form within the pulmonary parenchyma beneath the visceral pleura or along fissure lines.

Treatment

For diffuse PIE, fast rate mechanical ventilation using low pressures has been advocated. Permissive hypercapnia is used to minimize ventilator pressures, and maintaining pH levels above 7.20 is acceptable. More aggressive treatment has been used to manage severe unilateral forms of PIE and includes selective intubation of the normal lung to allow the emphysematous lung to collapse,[587] selective bronchial obstruction of the affected side, artificial creation of a pneumothorax by probing[588] or percutaneous drainage of large pneumatoceles.[589] HFOV has been advocated as a method of treating PIE[590] but there have been no randomized trials.

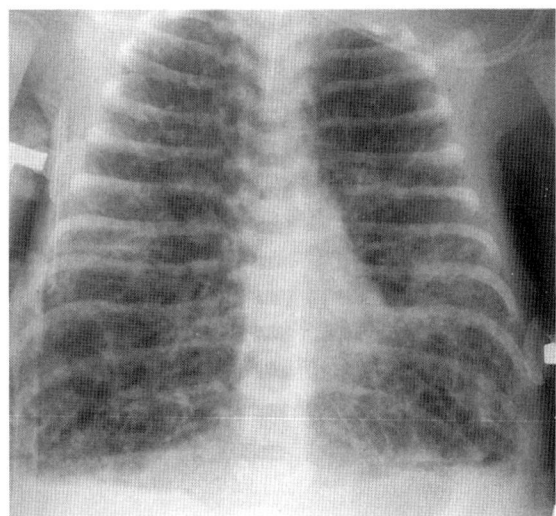

Fig. 12.26 Radiograph showing bilateral diffuse pulmonary interstitial emphysema with marked overinflation of the chest, lowered diaphragm and narrowed heart shadow.

Prognosis

Severe diffuse PIE occurring soon after birth has a very high mortality rate. For babies weighing less than 1000 g, the mortality of 67% is more than twice that of babies without PIE.[591] Complications such as pneumothorax and IVH are common and affected babies need prolonged ventilator support with most survivors developing BPD.

Pneumomediastinum

Incidence

Pneumomediastinum probably occurs prior to all cases of pneumothorax but it often goes unrecognized.

Clinical presentation

Pneumomediastinum may occur with other air leaks or in isolation, when it is asymptomatic in over 90% of cases, being noticed incidentally on a routine chest radiograph. If there are symptoms the baby may have tachypnea, cyanosis and an overinflated chest which is hyper-resonant to percussion. Occasionally a large pneumomediastinum causes severe symptoms by compressing the heart and lungs.

Diagnosis

This is confirmed by chest radiograph. The lateral view is most helpful to demonstrate air lying anteriorly. The thymus may be lifted off the mediastinum in the anteroposterior view giving rise to the 'sail sign' or 'spinnaker sign' (Fig. 12.25).

Treatment

In pneumomediastinum the air is loculated so that drainage is impracticable. The rate of absorption can be accelerated by breathing higher oxygen concentrations, but this should rarely be needed and only used in term babies.

Pneumopericardium

This occurs in about 1.6% of babies with RDS.[578]

Clinical presentation

Pneumopericardium is occasionally asymptomatic but more usually presents with pallor, shock and hypotension due to cardiac tamponade. In most cases it is associated with other forms of air leak.

Diagnosis

Chest radiograph shows a complete ring of air around the heart. The transverse diameter of the heart is reduced if tamponade is present and substernal transillumination may be used to make a rapid diagnosis in the baby who suddenly deteriorates during mechanical ventilation.

Treatment

The only effective treatment for pneumopericardium with tamponade is immediate drainage of air from the pericardial sac using a needle and syringe directed anteriorly and superiorly from below the xiphisternum. Recurrence of tamponade is common and permanent drainage is often needed.

Prognosis

The mortality is high despite early drainage with more than half of affected babies dying.

Pneumoperitoneum

Air in the peritoneal cavity may result from a pulmonary air leak or a ruptured abdominal viscus.

Incidence

Incidence of pneumoperitoneum as a complication of mechanical ventilation is about 2%.[578]

Clinical presentation

Pneumoperitoneum may be asymptomatic or present as abdominal distention. There are usually other signs of air leak (Fig. 12.27).

Treatment

Aspiration is only necessary if abdominal distention is severe enough to compromise ventilation.

Subcutaneous emphysema

This is rare in the neonate and when it does occur it is usually associated with pneumomediastinum. Air from the superior mediastinum passes along the perivascular fascia to the subclavicular area before spreading subcutaneously. Apart from swelling and a typically crackling feel to the affected skin there are few other signs and the air usually absorbs in a few days.

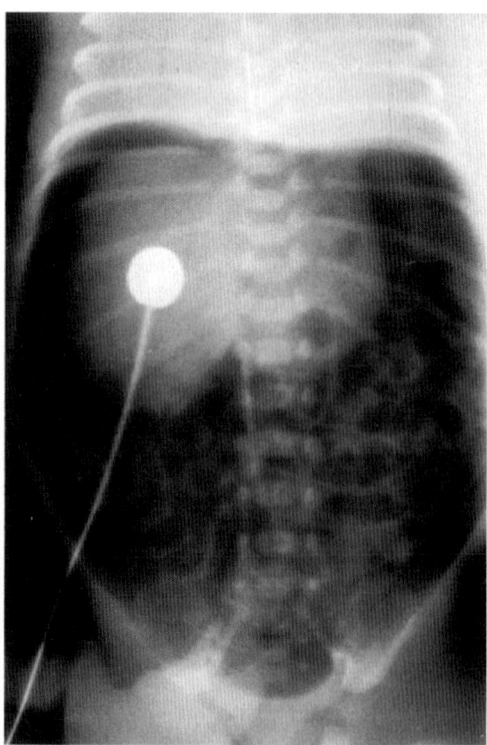

Fig. 12.27 Radiograph showing a large pneumoperitoneum with the liver clearly outlined by the air in the peritoneal cavity. The lungs appear collapsed and airless.

Air embolism (pneumatosis arterialis)

This is an uncommon and almost universally fatal condition which may present as air being withdrawn from an umbilical arterial catheter in an infant who has collapsed.[592] Air embolism results from rupture of pulmonary veins associated with raised intra-alveolar pressure during mechanical ventilation of very preterm babies. Affected babies have other forms of air leak and deteriorate acutely with pallor, bradycardia and hypotension. Chest and abdominal radiographs show gas shadows in the heart chambers and major arteries. There is no effective treatment and massive air embolism is usually fatal. The introduction of surfactant therapy and gentler forms of assisted ventilation has greatly reduced the risk of this serious condition.

PULMONARY HEMORRHAGE

Sometimes called massive pulmonary hemorrhage, this poorly understood condition has a sudden onset and a high mortality.

Incidence

Isolated pulmonary hemorrhage is a rare condition occurring in approximately 1/1000 live births. Between 2 and 5% of babies with RDS develop pulmonary hemorrhage.[593]

Etiology and pathogenesis

Pulmonary hemorrhage can occur in SGA babies with no underlying lung disease but more usually there has been a history of severe perinatal asphyxia, hypothermia, rhesus isoimmunization, pneumonia, hypoglycemia, coagulation disorder or fluid overload, particularly when a PDA is present.[594] Pulmonary hemorrhage is probably a form of hemorrhagic pulmonary edema as the hemorrhagic fluid usually has an hematocrit of less than 10%. Pulmonary hemorrhage may be secondary to aspiration, hypoproteinemia and lung tissue damage from pneumonia, RDS, oxygen toxicity or mechanical ventilation. There is an association with surfactant treatment, especially in the very immature infant treated with synthetic surfactant.[593,595]

Clinical presentation

The onset is frequently between the second and fourth day after birth when an infant with improving respiratory distress suddenly deteriorates with shock, cyanosis, bradycardia and apnea. Pink or red frothy fluid is aspirated from the mouth and lungs and urgent resuscitation is needed to prevent death. In ventilated babies, blood-stained fluid appears in the endotracheal tube during suctioning. Auscultation reveals widespread crepitations.

Diagnosis

Chest radiograph shows large areas of consolidation with diffuse opacification. In massive pulmonary hemorrhage the lungs may appear completely white and there may be cardiomegaly. Sometimes the diagnosis is only confirmed at autopsy when widespread intra-alveolar and interstitial hemorrhage is found.[596]

Treatment

Immediate resuscitation of the collapsed baby is important with endotracheal intubation for mechanical ventilation and cautious volume expansion with blood or plasma. High PEEP may help to reduce bleeding by tamponade, and a diuretic such as furosemide may reduce pulmonary edema. If the ductus arteriosus is widely patent indometacin or ibuprofen should be administered intravenously. Correction of acidosis and underlying coagulation disorder is beneficial and antibiotics should be given if infection is suspected. Repeated doses of surfactant may be beneficial.[597]

Prognosis

Until recently massive pulmonary hemorrhage was invariably fatal but prompt use of mechanical ventilation with PEEP has improved the outlook. Pulmonary hemorrhage is associated with a four-fold increased risk of CLD, seven-fold risk of death and three-fold risk of major IVH.[598] In survivors there is no apparent increase in long term morbidity at 2 year follow-up.

Prevention

Prevention is most important because of the poor outlook once major pulmonary hemorrhage has occurred. Asphyxia, hypothermia, hypoglycemia and acidosis should be avoided in SGA babies. Coagulation defects should be corrected early and large PDAs should be treated with indometacin or ibuprofen.

DEVELOPMENTAL ANOMALIES OF THE LUNG
Pulmonary hypoplasia

In this condition, which is frequently bilateral, the lungs are smaller than normal. Unilateral hypoplasia may be primary but is more often associated with other congenital malformations such as diaphragmatic hernia.

Incidence

Pulmonary hypoplasia is found in 15–20% of early neonatal deaths and is now the commonest single abnormality at autopsy.[599] Milder cases survive and are probably underdiagnosed.

Etiology and pathogenesis

Pulmonary hypoplasia occurs as a primary lesion in about 10% of cases but is most often associated with other malformations that restrict lung growth (Table 12.48). Pulmonary hypoplasia, as a result of oligohydramnios, is caused by the combined effects of reduced lung fluid volume and impaired fetal breathing movements.

Clinical presentation

Diagnosis may be suspected prenatally if there has been prolonged rupture of the membranes, especially if this occurs before 24 weeks or an ultrasound scan has demonstrated congenital diaphragmatic hernia or a chondrodystrophy. Babies with pulmonary hypoplasia may present at birth with signs of asphyxia and difficulties in resuscitation. Some have Potter syndrome and do not survive; pneumothoraces readily develop during resuscitation. With less severe degrees of hypoplasia the presentation is less acute with mild but prolonged respiratory distress and oxygen dependency. Congenital diaphragmatic hernia must be excluded by chest radiograph (Fig. 12.28). Such a hernia is usually left-sided, in 80% of cases occurring through the foramen of Bochdalek and there is displacement of the mediastinum to the right by stomach and bowel. About 25% of cases have associated congenital heart lesions which increase mortality.

Diagnosis

In life it is difficult to confirm the diagnosis unless an associated abnormality such as Potter syndrome, diaphragmatic hernia, Jeune syndrome or prolonged oligohydramnios is present. Sometimes chest radiograph shows small lungs with a bell-shaped thorax. At autopsy lung:body weight ratio may be helpful and ratios of <0.012 for babies over 28 weeks' gestation and <0.015 for lower gestations are used to define pulmonary hypoplasia.[600] Strict confirmation of the diagnosis requires more sophisticated autopsy analysis such as radial alveolar counts or DNA estimation.[601]

Table 12.48 Pathogenesis of pulmonary hypoplasia

1. Oligohydramnios: renal agenesis, urinary tract obstruction, prolonged rupture of the membranes
2. Lung compression: diaphragmatic hernia, lung cysts, pleural effusions, erythroblastosis, chondrodystrophies
3. Absent fetal breathing movements: anencephaly, neuromuscular disorders

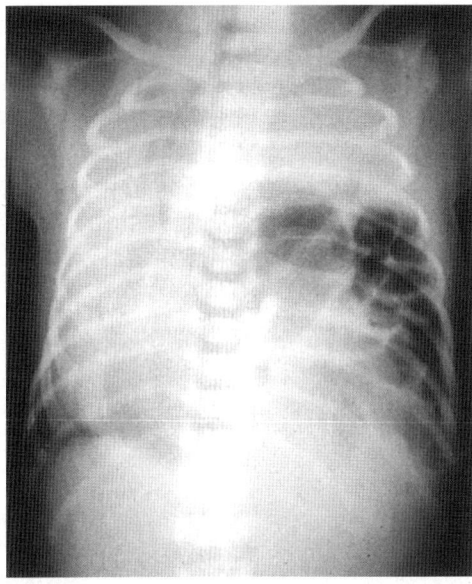

Fig. 12.28 Radiograph of a large left-sided diaphragmatic hernia with mediastinal shift to the right. Air in the stomach and intestine is due to resuscitation with bag and mask.

Management

Outlook depends upon severity of respiratory signs and the associated congenital anomalies. Severe pulmonary hypoplasia occurring with oligohydramnios is usually fatal but on occasions mechanical ventilation with high pressures has been successful in 'opening up' the lungs.[602] Surfactant replacement therapy is often used for associated RDS but it is not clear if it makes any difference.[603] Inhaled nitric oxide has been shown to improve oxygenation but more studies are needed.[604] Babies with diaphragmatic hernia need surgical correction, but even with this, severe unilateral pulmonary hypoplasia can be associated with marked pulmonary hypertension which does not respond to mechanical ventilation or vasodilators such as inhaled nitric oxide. ECMO is less effective in treating congenital diaphragmatic hernia than other causes of respiratory failure in term infants.[605] For babies who survive the neonatal period, lung growth occurs and their prognosis improves.

Congenital lobar emphysema

In this uncommon condition overinflation of one or more lobes occurs secondary to bronchial obstruction or deficiency of bronchial cartilage. The left upper lobe and the right middle lobe are most commonly affected and babies present with signs of respiratory distress and occasionally wheezing. Boys are affected twice as commonly as girls. Chest radiograph may initially show lobar opacification due to fluid trapped beyond the obstruction but later the affected lobe becomes overdistended and there may be shift of the mediastinum (Fig. 12.29). Diagnosis can also be confirmed by CT scan and lung scintigraphy showing reduced perfusion in the affected lobe. If symptoms are slight, conservative management is preferred.[606] For babies with persistent respiratory failure, surgical excision of the affected lobe is necessary. In about 30% of affected babies there is an associated congenital heart defect.

Cystic adenomatoid malformation

This is a rare form of congenital cystic disease of the lung which has three pathological types[607] (Table 12.49). The middle or upper lobes are usually affected and the condition is unilateral. At worst polyhydramnios and hydrops can occur in utero. About 25% of babies present with respiratory distress soon after birth, the remainder are asymptomatic.[608] Antenatal diagnosis by ultrasound is common and in some cases the lesion seems to regress before birth. Chest radiograph shows cystic overdistention of the affected lung in about 75% of asymptomatic cases.

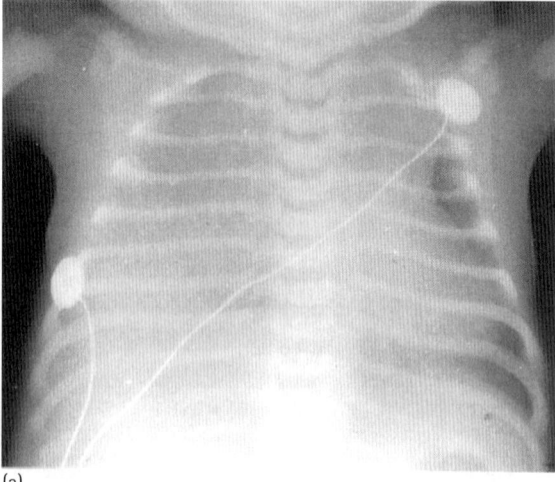

(a)

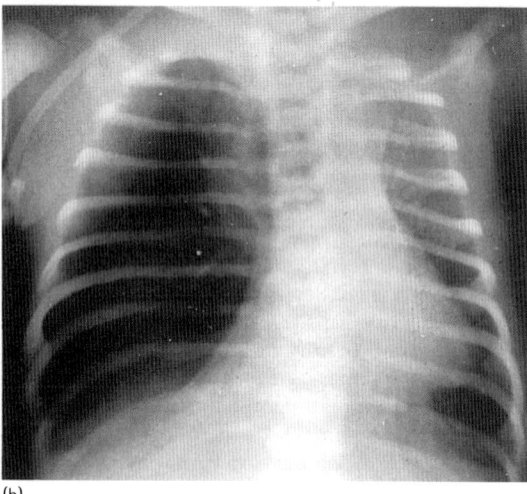

(b)

Fig. 12.29 (a) Congenital lobar emphysema showing retained lung fluid on the right as a result of bronchial obstruction, and displacement of the heart shadow to the left. (b) After 24 h with clearance of the lung fluid the right lung shows gross overinflation and the mediastinal displacement is more clearly demonstrated.

Table 12.49 Types of cystic adenomatoid malformation (CAM)

Type	Frequency (%)	Features
I	70	Multiple large cysts which mimic type III lobar emphysema
II	20	Medium sized cysts (12 mm in diameter)
III	10	Small cysts evenly distributed in a bulky lung

However, when ultrasound findings return to normal and neonatal chest radiograph is normal many congenital pulmonary lesions are still demonstrable on CT scanning so careful follow-up is still indicated.[609] Early surgical excision is required for symptomatic cases and should also be considered for asymptomatic antenatally diagnosed lesions, because of risks of later infection and the possibility of malignant transformation, although this can be deferred for some time after birth.[610]

Other lung cysts

Neurenteric cysts present as a mediastinal mass on chest radiograph in association with vertebral anomalies. Gastrogenic cysts, containing gastric mucosa, may ulcerate and cause hemoptysis. Duplication cysts of the duodenum may extend through the diaphragm and, if associated with a vertebral anomaly, can cause meningitis.

Bronchogenic cysts

These may present as episodes of wheezing or stridor. They are found near the carina but may be radiolucent on chest radiograph. If bronchial obstruction occurs there may be retained lung fluid giving rise to confluent opacity of one lung or lobe on radiography. Antenatal diagnosis by ultrasound scan is possible.

Sequestration of the lung

This is a mass of embryonic lung tissue that does not communicate with the bronchial tree and has a systemic rather than a pulmonary arterial supply. It may be intra- or extralobar; in the latter communication with foregut and other congenital anomalies including congenital heart disease are common. Males are more commonly affected and in about three quarters of cases the sequestration is left-sided. Ultrasound can be used to make the diagnosis prenatally and hydrops fetalis may occasionally occur. Extralobar lesions are more likely to be symptomatic but abnormality on chest radiograph is the commonest presentation. A triangular density at the left lung base extending to the mediastinum gives rise to the 'scimitar sign'. Bronchoscopy, radionuclide scanning or aortography may be needed to confirm the diagnosis. In 65% of cases there are associated anomalies.[611] Surgery for intralobar sequestrations prevents repeated respiratory infections and may also be needed for extralobar lesions that are symptomatic.[612]

Chylothorax

This is a form of pleural effusion in which chyle or lymphatic fluid appears in the pleural cavity. It is typically unilateral with 60% being right-sided and may be congenital or acquired, both being more common in males. In congenital or spontaneous chylothorax there is usually an anomaly of lymphatic drainage and chylous ascites and lymphedema are associated. Acquired chylothorax may follow birth trauma or thoracotomy. About half of affected babies present with respiratory distress soon after birth and a further one quarter have symptoms by the end of the first week. Breath sounds are reduced on the affected side and there is mediastinal shift away from this side. Chest radiography shows diffuse opacity with depressed diaphragm and mediastinal shift. A pleural tap will show clear yellow fluid soon after birth and only after feeding does the effusion appear chylous. The fluid is sterile and contains large numbers of lymphocytes and fat globules. Treatment is initially by needle thoracocentesis, although if several taps are needed a chest drain is better.[613] Occasionally prolonged drainage is required but there is a risk of protein and lymphocyte depletion. If reaccumulation becomes a problem, use of a milk formula containing medium chain triglycerides reduces production of chyle. Occasionally it is necessary to discontinue oral feeds and use total parenteral nutrition. Recently somatostatin analogues have successfully treated persistent chylous effusions.[614]

Pleural effusion can also occur in cases of hydrops fetalis, Turner syndrome, pneumonia and congestive heart failure.

Pulmonary lymphangiectasis

In this rare condition there is bilateral cystic dilation of pulmonary lymphatics with obstruction of lymph drainage. Three types have been described: a primary isolated developmental defect accounting for 70% of cases; a generalized type which presents with widespread edema, malabsorption, hemihypertrophy and other anomalies; and a type associated with congenital heart disease and obstruction of pulmonary venous return (total anomalous pulmonary venous drainage, closure of atrial septum in hypoplastic left heart syndrome or pulmonary vein atresia).

Babies with primary lymphangiectasis are often born at term and have progressive respiratory distress which until recently was uniformly fatal.[615] Clinical and radiological features mimic RDS so that there is underdiagnosis of this condition. Chest radiograph may show reticulogranular mottling with hyperaeration, and dilated lymphatics may sometimes be seen. Confirmation of the diagnosis is by lung biopsy or at autopsy.

Choanal atresia

Obstruction to the nasal airway may be unilateral or bilateral, membranous or bony. Incidence is about 0.3 per 1000 births with girls affected twice as commonly as boys. About two thirds of cases are unilateral and in about half there are associated anomalies such as coloboma, heart defects, micrognathia and tracheoesophageal fistula. If the obstruction is bilateral, babies often present with great distress at birth, although when crying they may remain pink. Babies with unilateral choanal atresia may be asymptomatic or present later with a purulent nasal discharge. Diagnosis may be confirmed by attempting to pass a fine feeding tube or suction catheter, instilling saline into the nostril, or nasal tympanometry.[616] The infant with bilateral choanal atresia needs an oral airway or oral endotracheal intubation followed by a surgical procedure. A transnasal or transpalatal approach may be used to open the posterior choanae and patency is maintained by inserting silastic tubes for up to 2 months. Operative correction of unilateral choanal atresia may be postponed until the child is several years old.

Laryngomalacia

In this condition the larynx appears soft and flexible, associated with an elongated, floppy epiglottis and loose aryepiglottic folds which tend to be drawn over the glottis during inspiration. Also known as congenital laryngeal stridor, it needs to be distinguished from other causes of stridor such as vocal cord paralysis, vascular rings, laryngeal webs and cysts and papillomata. Onset of stridor is usually on the second day but delay of up to 4 months is possible. Usually the stridor persists for less than 1 year. Diagnosis is confirmed by direct laryngoscopy which excludes most other causes of stridor. No specific treatment is required apart from reassurance of the parents although occasionally long term feeding problems and speech difficulties occur.

CHRONIC LUNG DISEASE

BPD remains the major pulmonary complication of preterm delivery. The term BPD was coined in 1967 to describe damage to lungs from high volume mechanical ventilation,[542] with the typical baby being more than 30 weeks' gestation and developing cystic X-ray changes and oxygen requirement beyond 28 days of life. With improved perinatal care the pattern of BPD has changed over the years, with 'new BPD' mainly affecting ELBW babies.[617] The latest definitions divide babies born < 32 weeks' gestation according to severity based on duration of oxygen therapy.[618] Those who require oxygen for < 28 days have no BPD, > 28 days but not beyond 36 weeks' corrected gestation mild BPD, < 30% oxygen at 36 weeks moderate BPD, and > 30% oxygen or on respiratory support severe BPD. This definition correlates well with longer term respiratory and neurological outcomes.[618] Severe BPD is independently predictive of death or neurosensory impairment in the first 18 months of life.[619]

Incidence

Advances in perinatal and neonatal medicine have reduced mortality in ELBW babies resulting in greater numbers of survivors who are at risk of BPD.[620] Incidence increases with decreasing gestation; about 50% of babies < 1000 g and 85% < 700 g are affected.

Etiology and pathogenesis

Rather than BPD being caused by 'ventilator-induced injury' it is now believed that chronic inflammation is important in its pathogenesis.[621] It is common in small preterm babies who, although ventilator dependent for long periods, have not needed high pressures or oxygen concentrations and may occur in infants who did not need assisted ventilation,[622] particularly if there has been chorioamnionitis.[623] Factors associated with development of BPD are listed in Table 12.50. Any of these, particularly in combination, leads to a process of pulmonary inflammation resulting in abnormal lung growth and alveolarization.[621]

Table 12.50 Factors associated with chronic lung disease

Chorioamnionitis
Low gestation
Congenital pneumonia
Mechanical ventilation
Oxygen therapy
Acquired pulmonary infection
Pulmonary interstitial emphysema
Persistent ductus arteriosus
Fluid overload

Pathology

In BPD there is abnormal lung growth and modeling in combination with lung injury leading to scarring and fibrosis. Pathological changes are of arrested lung development with alveolar thickening and enlargement, hypoplasia of alveolar capillary development and decreased lung septation.[617] This pattern occurs in combination with areas of damage shown by septal fibrosis and evidence of hypertensive vascular changes leaving reduced surface area for gas exchange.

Clinical presentation

The usual history is of a preterm baby treated with mechanical ventilation and surfactant for RDS whose condition improves and then deteriorates between 7 and 10 days with increasing oxygen requirements. Mild cases need increased inspired oxygen concentrations for a few weeks but in severe cases there may be progressive respiratory failure with ventilator dependence and later tachypnea, indrawing, wheezing and recurrent apnea with cyanotic spells. Cor pulmonale may develop secondary to pulmonary hypertension, and these babies show hepatomegaly, increased weight gain and edema. Chest radiographs initially show generalized haziness which later can progress to hyperinflation, coarse streaking or at worst cystic changes (Fig. 12.30).

Management

The management priority is prevention by trying to limit pulmonary inflammation. This involves limiting mechanical ventilation and oxygen therapy to the shortest possible time. Management of infection, PDA and fluid balance are also important in trying to prevent BPD. Mechanical ventilation can often be avoided by early surfactant therapy and nasal CPAP,[526] and units with the lowest ventilation rates have the lowest incidence of BPD.[624] Weaning from ventilation may be helped by allowing $PaCO_2$ levels to rise to 7–9 kPa so that peak inspiratory pressures can be lowered. Reduced fluid intake, diuretic therapy and closure of the ductus arteriosus may all assist in weaning. Caffeine has also been shown to

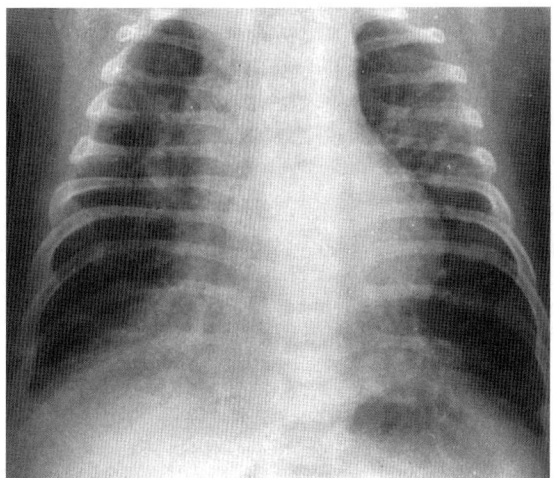

Fig. 12.30 Radiograph of severe CLD (formerly called BPD) with basilar emphysema, coarse stranding and cystic changes.

improve lung function and shorten duration of ventilation with associated reduction in BPD.[535] Dexamethasone reduces BPD in the short term allowing rapid weaning from ventilation[625-627] but there are concerns about both short term complications (hyperglycemia, hypertension and gastrointestinal bleeding and perforation) and long term adverse effects on the central nervous system.[628] Dexamethasone use should be limited to babies who are ventilator-dependent and whose condition is deteriorating. The lowest possible dose should be used for the shortest duration.[629,630] Inhaled steroids may also facilitate extubation but are probably not as effective as dexamethasone in reducing death or later BPD.[631] Adequate supplemental oxygen needs to be given to preterm babies to maintain acceptable oxygen saturation levels of about 88–94%. It is not clear however whether or not to err on the side of higher or lower saturations within this range.[632] Oxygen toxicity contributes to development of BPD and retinopathy of prematurity but hypoxemia increases pulmonary vascular resistance and risk of cor pulmonale with poor growth and development. Intramuscular vitamin A, an antioxidant, has been shown to modestly reduce BPD.[633]

Established BPD is difficult to treat. Adequate nutrition is important and supplemental calories may be given in the form of long chain glucose polymers so that fluid restriction is possible without reducing energy intake. Drugs such as diuretics, inhaled bronchodilators and inhaled steroids may be used to reduce respiratory symptoms but their effects are marginal.[634] Chest infections should be promptly treated with antibiotics. In later infancy RSV infections may cause acute deterioration. Regular intramuscular anti-RSV monoclonal antibody such as palivizumab reduces hospital admission rates[635] although there is still debate over its cost effectiveness.[636]

Prognosis

Many babies with BPD require prolonged oxygen therapy, usually given via nasal cannulae. Home oxygen therapy significantly shortens time in hospital. Mortality in babies with severe BPD is about 25–30%. Surviving babies have frequent lower respiratory tract infections and often require hospital admission with persistent tachypnea, intermittent wheezing and subcostal retractions. Growth and development depend upon severity of lung disease and adverse perinatal events. Growth retardation is present in about one third of survivors and major developmental defects in about 25%.

CHRONIC PULMONARY INFECTION

This may account for a small proportion of cases of neonatal chronic lung disease. Infection with CMV may be congenital or acquired although pneumonitis is uncommon in congenitally infected babies. Interstitial pneumonitis can also occur with congenital toxoplasmosis, rubella, varicella and herpes simplex virus. Acquired infections with enteroviruses, adenovirus, RSV and rhinovirus can cause acute pneumonitis.

Chlamydia may cause a late pneumonitis with tachypnea, cough and chest radiograph showing disproportionately severe infiltrates and hyperinflation. Erythromycin treatment for 14 days is effective. Pneumocystis pneumonia has also been reported in preterm infants and is treated with co-trimoxazole.

SUBGLOTTIC STENOSIS

Subglottic stenosis may be congenital or acquired. Acquired subglottic stenosis is due to prolonged endotracheal intubation and occurs in severe form in about 1% of ventilated babies. Use of endotracheal tubes that are too big, oral rather than nasal intubation and repeated intubations may increase the risk of subglottic stenosis. Presentation is with stridor and respiratory distress after extubation although there may be delayed onset of symptoms for several months with difficulty apparently precipitated by upper respiratory tract infections.

In mild cases treatment with high humidity and supplemental oxygen is sufficient, but use of dexamethasone or inhaled epinephrine has been advocated in more severe cases prior to a trial of extubation.

Sometimes tracheostomy is needed but minor surgery to split the cricoid cartilage anteriorly[637] has been successful as an alternative. Dilatation of the narrowed segment at intervals by an experienced ENT surgeon may be necessary.

CONTROL OF BREATHING

Postnatal control of breathing is complex and involves chemical and nonchemical stimuli and respiratory reflexes. Inspiratory and expiratory centers in the brainstem are influenced by sensors (central and peripheral chemoreceptors) monitoring arterial blood and they maintain normal oxygen tensions and pH despite wide variations in oxygen demand and carbon dioxide production.

Chemical stimuli

Hypoxemia and hypercarbia are the most important chemical stimuli for respiration. Hypoxemia depresses ventilation and blunts the ventilatory response to hypercarbia. For the first week after birth there are three phases of the respiratory response to hypoxemia:

1. initial stimulation of peripheral chemoreceptors causing transient hyperventilation for 1–2 minutes;
2. if hypoxia persists this is followed by central depression with decrease in ventilation;
3. central stimulation by severe hypoxemia causing gasps.

In the preterm baby these responses may persist for up to 6 weeks after birth. Breathing oxygen reduces ventilation by an effect on carotid body chemoreceptors but after several minutes hyperventilation occurs secondary to hypercarbia. This response, mediated by hydrogen ion receptors in the medulla, increases with gestational and also with postnatal age.[638]

Respiratory reflexes

The Head and Hering–Breuer reflexes, arising from lung stretch receptors and mediated through the vagus nerve, are important in modulation of respiratory center output in the newborn. Head's paradoxical reflex, which is present for the first few days after birth, causes an extra inspiratory effort when the upper airways are distended. Its importance is in aeration of the lungs soon after birth. In the Hering–Breuer reflex sustained lung inflation inhibits respiration causing apnea in inspiration. This inflation reflex is stronger in preterm than term babies. The Hering–Breuer deflation reflex comprises an increase in respiratory rate in response to reduced lung volume and may also be important in the preterm baby. There are irritant receptors in the hypopharynx and larynx which, if stimulated by vigorous suctioning or cows' milk, cause apnea.[638]

Apneic attacks

Apnea of prematurity is defined as cessation of breathing for more than 15 s, typically accompanied by desaturation and bradycardia. Periodic breathing is a series of respiratory pauses of about 10 s alternating with periods of hyperventilation of up to 15 s and occurring at least 3 times per min. It is not associated with cyanosis and bradycardia and may be a physiological response in the preterm baby.[639]

Incidence

Apneic attacks occur in most infants < 30 weeks' gestation and in about half of babies of 30–32 weeks decreasing to less than 10% of babies at < 34 weeks. Periodic breathing is also common, occurring in nearly all LBW babies and about one third of term babies.

Etiology and pathogenesis

Many clinical conditions are associated with apnea (Table 12.51). Only after exclusion of those listed from 1 to 6 can a confident diagnosis of apnea of prematurity be made. Immaturity of brainstem respiratory neurons is probably a major underlying factor and apnea may also occur if the medullary centers are immature or depressed by hypoxia. There is no evidence of a temporal relationship between gastroesophageal acid reflux and apneic episodes.[640]

Table 12.51   Clinical conditions associated with apnea

1. Hypoxemia: respiratory distress syndrome, pneumonia, chronic lung disease, recurrent aspiration, airway obstruction
2. Infection: septicemia or bacteremia, meningitis, necrotizing enterocolitis
3. Metabolic disorder: hypoglycemia, hypocalcemia, hypomagnesemia, hypernatremia, hyponatremia, acidosis
4. Central nervous system disorder: seizures, intracranial hemorrhage, drugs and drug withdrawal, kernicterus, cerebral malformation
5. Circulatory disorder: hypotension, congestive heart failure, persistent ductus arteriosus, anemia, polycythemia
6. Temperature instability: hyperthermia, hypothermia
7. Apnea of prematurity: diagnosis by exclusion

Pathophysiology

During a significant apneic attack the preterm baby has bradycardia, peripheral vasoconstriction and a variable alteration of blood pressure which may increase or decrease slightly. The interval between onset of apnea and bradycardia varies between 2 and 30 s. There are three types of apnea based upon polygraphic recordings (Table 12.52).[641] In preterm babies central apnea and mixed apnea occur with about equal frequencies. Use of apnea monitors which detect chest wall movement only will underestimate the incidence of apnea.

Diagnosis

The infant should be examined carefully to look for signs of infection, airway obstruction, seizures or PDA. Laboratory investigations might include full blood picture, blood culture, C-reactive protein (CRP), blood glucose, electrolytes and calcium. Chest radiography, blood gas analysis and pH and examination of cerebrospinal fluid might also be indicated. Only after exclusion of infection, biochemical or drug causes of apnea can an infant be confidently labeled as having apnea of prematurity.

Treatment (Table 12.53)

All preterm babies < 34 weeks' gestation should have continuous monitoring of heart and respiratory rate for several days until apnea has ceased to occur. Pulse oximetry or transcutaneous oxygen monitoring is also desirable in less mature babies. Monitors that respond to chest wall movement (the apnea mattress, pressure sensor pad or pressure-sensitive capsule) will fail to detect obstructive apnea as long as

Table 12.52   Polygraphic classification of type of apnea

1. Central apnea: simultaneous cessation of respiratory effort and airflow at the end of expiration. Probably due to cessation of motor output from the respiratory center in the brainstem
2. Obstructive apnea: cessation of airflow while respiratory effort continues. Seen in babies with the Pierre Robin syndrome for example
3. Mixed apnea: cessation of airflow with continued respiratory effort on some occasions and not on others. Both central and obstructive apneas occur during the same episode

Table 12.53   Management of apnea

1. Immediate resuscitation
2. Exclude underlying cause (Table 12.51)
3. Lower environmental temperature 0.5° C
4. Correct mild hypoxemia and anemia
5. Repeated stimulation
6. Intermittent bag and mask ventilation
7. Continuous positive airway pressure
8. Drug therapy – caffeine, aminophylline, theophylline, doxapram
9. Mechanical ventilation

respiratory movement continues. To detect obstructive or mixed types of apnea, the heart rate and oxygen saturation must also be monitored. Sometimes a simple adjustment of environmental temperature or feed frequency will prevent apneic attacks. During resuscitation, overzealous suctioning must be avoided as this stimulates irritant receptors in the pharynx and perpetuates the apnea and bradycardia. Many apneic attacks are self-resolving and provided bradycardia and hypoxemia do not occur these are probably not harmful.

Repeated stimulation. Stimulation by stroking, gentle rubbing or rocking often prevents or shortens apneic attacks by increasing input to the immature respiratory center by cutaneous, vestibular or proprioceptive pathways.

Intermittent bag and mask ventilation. When peripheral stimulation fails, bag and mask ventilation, using the same oxygen concentration as the baby is breathing, will stimulate spontaneous respiration without increasing the risk of retinopathy of prematurity.

Continuous positive airway pressure (CPAP). CPAP at 4–5 cmH$_2$O reduces apnea by improving oxygenation and increasing functional residual capacity. It may also stabilize the chest wall and eliminate the Hering–Breuer deflation reflex. CPAP decreases incidence of both mixed and obstructive apneas but does not affect central apneas so it might work by helping to relieve upper airway obstruction. Gentle nasal ventilation via CPAP prongs is also helpful in avoiding the need for mechanical ventilation.[528]

Drug therapy. Methylxanthines such as aminophylline, theophylline and caffeine are useful in central as well as obstructive apnea and work by increasing the sensitivity of the respiratory center to hypercarbia, increasing minute ventilation, decreasing hypoxic depression and reducing periodic breathing. Other effects are stimulation of the diaphragm, positive inotropic and chronotropic effects, mild diuresis and increased heat production through utilization of brown fat. Unwelcome effects include decreased cerebral blood flow and some uncertainty about long term outcome.[642] Caffeine has a wider margin of safety than theophylline.[643] Concerns about potential long term adverse effects and the risk: benefit ratio will hopefully be resolved with completion of the CAP follow-up study.[644] Doxapram is a direct respiratory stimulant which has undergone limited study for treatment of neonatal apnea and has the side-effect of jitteriness and raised blood pressure. It appears to have similar efficacy to methylxanthines in the short term but its routine use should be limited because of lack of data on long term safety.[645] Antireflux medications do not reduce the frequency of apnea in preterm infants.[646]

Mechanical ventilation. This is reserved for babies whose apnea is resistant to other measures. Very immature infants and those with bacteremia often need mechanical ventilation and low inflating pressures should be used as lung compliance is usually normal.

Prognosis

In most cases apnea of prematurity resolves at around 34 weeks' corrected gestation and caffeine therapy can be discontinued with continued monitoring for several days afterwards. Recurrent apnea does not appear to have deleterious effects on long term cognitive or neurodevelopmental outcome.[647] There appears to be no relationship between apneic spells in the neonatal period and subsequent sudden infant death syndrome (SIDS). Apnea can recur within 2 months of discharge from hospital if there is a respiratory infection or if general anesthesia is needed for surgery.[648]

NEONATAL CARDIOVASCULAR DISEASE

This section considers normal perinatal cardiovascular changes (Fig. 12.4). Certain situations characteristically associated with the newborn period are then covered in detail. Congenital and acquired cardiac disease is described in detail in Chapter 21.

PERINATAL CARDIOVASCULAR PHYSIOLOGY

Figure 12.3 illustrates fetal circulatory pathways. Labor and delivery trigger a number of cardiovascular events (Fig. 12.4), the occurrence or failure of which have implications for the presentation and management of neonatal cardiovascular disease.

Pulmonary vascular resistance

In healthy term babies the postnatal fall in pulmonary vascular resistance results in a rapid fall in right heart pressures over a few days with adult pulmonary:systemic pressure ratios being established by 2–3 weeks of age. Many factors can inhibit, delay or reverse pulmonary vasodilation in the newborn and these are listed with clinical examples in Table 12.54. The fall in resistance may occur more slowly in certain congenital cardiac abnormalities such as atrioventricular septal defect (AVSD) and large ventricular septal defect (VSD). This delayed fall has implications for the time at which heart murmurs, clinical left to right shunting and heart failure develop. Thus, a small VSD is more likely to produce a murmur in the first few days after birth than a large one and a large VSD rarely causes heart failure in the first few weeks of life. In some congenital heart lesions, pulmonary vascular resistance never falls to normal and pulmonary vascular disease develops without clinical evidence of a large shunt ever having been present. This happens not infrequently in complete AVSD but can also happen with a large VSD, in both cases particularly if the child has Down syndrome. This process is accelerated in the presence of hypoxemia from cardiac or other causes.

Ductus arteriosus

As gestation progresses, ductal smooth muscle becomes less sensitive to dilating circulating prostaglandins and more sensitive to the vasoconstrictor effects of oxygen. At term, increasing arterial oxygen tension causes functional closure of a normal ductus within 2–3 days of birth in virtually all babies. In preterm babies without respiratory distress the time of ductal closure is similar.[649] Babies with structural abnormalities of the cardiovascular system may maintain ductal patency longer than normal before spontaneous closure occurs. There are two groups of congenital heart lesions which are critically dependent on ductal patency for the baby to remain alive (Table 12.55). The first group, those with duct-dependent pulmonary circulation, show appearance of or worsening of cyanosis on ductal closure. The second group consists of those conditions in which the systemic circulation is dependent on the ductus, and collapse with gross heart failure occurs when the ductus closes. An important part of resuscitation in both these groups of infants is the use of prostaglandin E_1 or E_2 to reopen and maintain ductal patency. In addition, babies with transposition without a large VSD will show a marked deterioration in oxygenation when the ductus closes. Persistent ductus arteriosus, either isolated or in association with other cardiac abnormalities, may also be a structural abnormality which will never close. If a normal ductus arteriosus is subject to abnormal conditions, its closure may be delayed. This situation is frequently seen in preterm babies with lung disease and may respond to prostaglandin synthetase inhibitor administration.

Foramen ovale

Increased pulmonary venous return after birth results in closure of the flap-like foramen ovale as left atrial pressure rises. If intra-atrial pressures are abnormal, shunting can occur in either direction through the foramen ovale. Thus left to right shunting may occur in babies with an increase in left atrial pressure (due to left to right shunting through a ductus arteriosus or to obstruction to flow of blood through the left heart) and right to left shunting can occur in persistent pulmonary hypertension or mechanical obstruction to flow through the right heart giving desaturated blood access to the systemic arterial circulation.

Ductus venosus

Blood flow through the ductus venosus falls dramatically when umbilical venous return ceases and functional closure occurs within a few days; however an umbilical venous catheter can sometimes be passed through it into the inferior vena cava and right atrium until at least a week after birth. The clinical relevance of patency of the ductus venosus relates to its usefulness as a route to the heart for central venous pressure monitoring or cardiac catheterization and also to the fact that when it closes, obstruction to pulmonary venous drainage becomes severe in total anomalous pulmonary venous return to the portal vein, causing marked deterioration in cyanosis and respiratory distress.

CARDIOVASCULAR EXAMINATION OF THE NEWBORN

The present history, perinatal and family histories may all give clues to a diagnosis. Routine examination of well babies should include an assessment of the presence or absence of central cyanosis, an evaluation for evidence of heart failure and observations about pulse rate, regularity and character with special reference to the nature of the femoral pulses when compared simultaneously to the right brachial pulse. If the femoral pulses cannot be satisfactorily palpated or are markedly different from right arm pulses, a more thorough cardiovascular assessment including blood pressure measurement in both arms and one leg, ECG and chest X-ray should be performed. Auscultation of the heart should be performed with an attempt to ensure that heart sounds are louder in the left chest than the right. Then attention should be given to whether the second sound is single or fixedly split and then to murmurs. The presence or absence of murmurs is only part of the neonatal cardiovascular examination. Some murmurs are innocent and many severe lesions have unimpressive murmurs or even none.

If cardiac disease is suspected, the precordium, suprasternal notch and subxiphoid region should be palpated for thrills or abnormal impulses, the skull auscultated for bruits, and a more detailed cardiac auscultation for added sounds and full murmur characterization carried out. Reliable blood pressure measurement in newborn infants requires a quiet and relaxed infant and a cuff of appropriate size (a cuff which covers two thirds of the length of the upper arm and in which the bladder either encompasses the entire circumference of the arm or is positioned in such a way as to have the center of the bladder over the brachial artery). Detection of pulse reappearance can be by palpation but a Doppler probe is more sensitive; auscultation is very difficult. Oscillometric devices need to be watched whilst recording to ensure that the infant remains peaceful and are second best to direct invasive

Table 12.54 Situations associated with delay in or reversal of postnatal fall in pulmonary vascular resistance

Factor	Comment
Acidosis, hypoglycemia, hypoxemia, hypercapnia, polycythemia	Wide range of neonatal diseases
High altitude	Mediated via lower oxygen tension
Cardiac disease	See Table 12.64
Respiratory disease	Any cause
Ductal closure in utero	Maternal prostaglandin synthetase inhibitor ingestion
Obstructed middle or upper airway	Any cause

Table 12.55 Duct-dependent congenital heart lesions

Obstruction to flow through right heart
   Pulmonary atresia with intact ventricular septum
   Critical pulmonary stenosis
   Severe tetralogy of Fallot
   Pulmonary atresia with VSD and no aortopulmonary communicating arteries
   Tricuspid atresia (unless with large VSD and without pulmonary stenosis)

Obstruction to flow through left heart
   Aortic atresia
   Critical aortic stenosis
   Hypoplastic left heart syndrome
   Interrupted aortic arch
   Severe coarctation

continuous monitoring of ill infants. The same cuff can be used on the calf with detection of posterior tibial or dorsalis pedis pulses for lower limb systolic pressures. Normal values for systolic pressures in term babies measured non-invasively are given in Table 12.56.[650] Acceptable values in ill preterm babies are different and less clearly defined (Table 12.57).[651,652] Non-invasive pressure up to 20 mmHg systolic higher in the arm than the leg can be normal; discrepancies between arm pressures may give clues as to the site of an aortic arch interruption. Significant coarctation may occasionally be associated with an aberrant right subclavian artery arising distal to the left subclavian, in which case upper to lower limb pulse discrepancy will not exist. Upper limb pressures may be raised in coarctation but in sick infants poor left ventricular function may prevent hypertension.

CARDIOVASCULAR INVESTIGATION OF THE NEWBORN

Chest X-ray

A systematic approach to the chest X-ray allows maximum information to be obtained; the particular points of relevance to cardiovascular diagnosis are listed in Table 12.58. Immediate management of a baby with a cardiac lesion may be greatly influenced by deciding whether lung blood flow is increased (plethoric lung fields, Fig. 12.31) or decreased (oligemic lung fields, Fig. 12.32). Pulmonary venous obstruction produces X-ray appearances often hard to distinguish from respiratory pathology. Clinical conditions associated with each of these abnormalities are given in Table 12.59.

Electrocardiography

This can provide important diagnostic information when significant heart disease is suspected. A detailed consideration of the subject will be found in Chapter 21. It is important to recognize the normal evolution of the ECG in the newborn and to have access to reference information[653] (Table 12.60).

Hyperoxia (nitrogen washout) test

If cyanosis is due to a cardiac cause, high concentrations of inspired oxygen rarely relieve it significantly, although there are exceptions, for example some common mixing conditions. If respiratory disease is the cause there is often relief from increasing inspired oxygen, although this will not be the case in severe respiratory disease and persistent pulmonary hypertension. This is the basis for the hyperoxia test. If a baby is put in 85% or more inspired oxygen for 15–20 min, a right radial arterial blood or right upper trunk transcutaneous oxygen tension should rise to well above 20 kPa. Failure to do so supports a cyanotic cardiac abnormality. Transcutaneous oxygen tension monitors placed on the right upper thorax can give similar information to right radial artery samples but pulse oximetry can be misleading in that elevation of saturation to normal, even to 100%, does not necessarily mean that arterial oxygen tension had risen above 20 kPa. Theoretical fears about precipitating ductal closure mean that the baby should be closely observed during the test; however, the risk of precipitating a problem is extremely small. Marked prematurity is a contraindication because of the possible consequence of retinopathy. Pulse oximetry may have a role in screening for cardiac disease (see below).

Table 12.57 Systemic blood pressure in the neonatal period. Healthy LBW infants (no inotropes, no positive pressure ventilation). Some recordings direct intra-arterial, some oscillometric.[651,652] Reproduced from Rennie JM & Roberton, NRC. Textbook of Neonatology, 3rd edn. Edinburgh: Churchill Livingstone; 1999

Day 1

Birth weight (g)	Number	Systolic range (mmHg)	Diastolic range (mmHg)
501–750	18	50–62	26–36
751–1000	39	48–59	23–36
1001–1250	30	49–61	26–35
1251–1500	45	46–56	23–33
1501–1750	51	46–58	23–33
1751–2000	61	48–61	24–35

Day 1

Gestation (weeks)	Number	Systolic range (mmHg)	Diastolic range (mmHg)
<24	11	48–63	24–39
24–28	55	48–58	22–36
29–32	110	47–59	24–34
>32	68	48–60	24–34

Week 1

Day	Number	Systolic range (mmHg)	Diastolic range (mmHg)
1	183	48–63	25–35
2	121	54–63	30–39
3	117	53–67	31–43
4	85	57–71	32–45
5	76	56–72	33–47
6	59	57–71	32–47
7	48	61–74	34–46

Table 12.58 Chest X-ray: points to look for with reference to the cardiovascular system

Bronchial situs	
Lung fields	Oligemia
	Plethora
	Venous engorgement
	Lung pathology
Heart	Position, apex side
	Size
	Contour
	Aortic arch side
Abdomen	Visceral situs
Skeleton	Abnormalities

Table 12.56 Non-invasive (indirect) arm systolic blood pressures (mmhg) with pulse detected by Doppler probe. All infants 38 weeks' gestation or more (from de Swiet et al[650]). Reproduced from Rennie JM & Roberton NRC. Textbook of Neonatology, 3rd edn. Edinburgh: Churchill Livingstone; 1999

Age (days)	3	4	5	6	7	8–10
Awake						
Mean ± SD	72 ± 6	74 ± 9	77 ± 10	77 ± 10	82 ± 9	88 ± 17
Number of infants	4	71	44	42	9	4
Asleep						
Mean ± SD	68 ± 7	70 ± 8	72 ± 8	72 ± 9	72 ± 9	75 ± 9
Number of infants	72	681	426	322	47	18

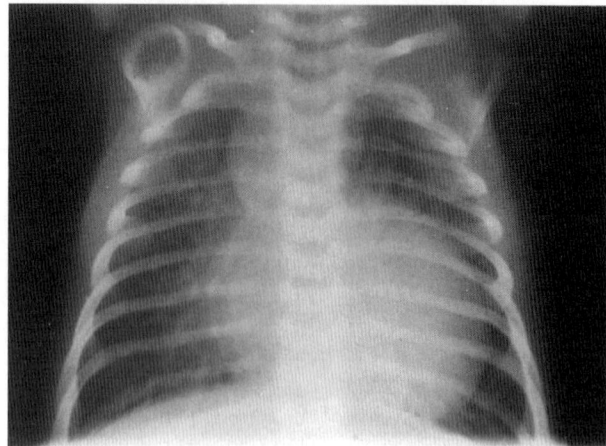

Fig. 12.31 Chest X-ray on cyanotic newborn infant. Lung fields are plethoric (double inlet left ventricle).

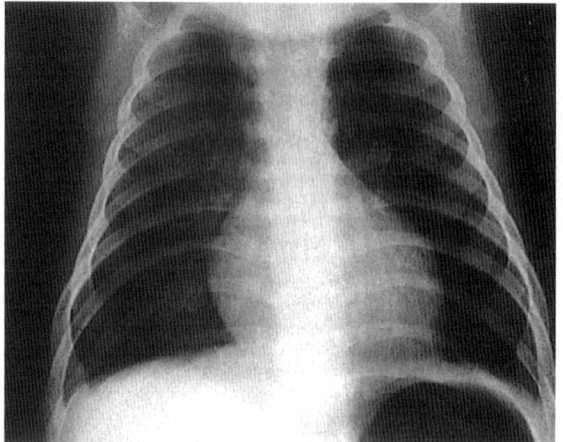

Fig. 12.32 Chest X-ray on cyanotic newborn infant. Lung fields are oligemic (tetralogy of Fallot).

Table 12.59   Lung vascularity on chest X-ray

Oligemia	Tricuspid atresia (unless large VSD)
	Ebstein anomaly
	Pulmonary atresia or critical stenosis
Plethora	Any left to right shunt
	Common mixing without pulmonary stenosis
	Transposition of great arteries
Venous congestion	Obstruction to flow into or through left heart

Echocardiography

Clinical evaluation should always precede echocardiography. Resuscitation and stabilization must always be achieved before transfer to another unit for evaluation. Ultrasound imaging and Doppler assessment allow a precise anatomical and functional diagnosis in the majority of symptomatic neonates with cardiac disease, so that surgery, be it palliative or definitive, is frequently not preceded by cardiac catheterization. The increasing expertise in echocardiography of neonatal pediatricians and the advent of telemedicine are altering transfer patterns of infants with actual or suspected heart lesions.

Cardiac catheterization

Although echocardiography has made neonatal diagnostic cardiac catheterization uncommon, there has been an increase in the number and scope of interventional therapeutic catheterizations in neonates. Good neonatal care is required throughout the procedure. The heart can be approached via umbilical vessels, femoral vessels percutaneously or by cut-down, or rarely by axillary vessel cut-down. The procedure has mortality and morbidity, though these have been greatly reduced by good general neonatal care and by anatomical information obtained from prior echocardiography.

Magnetic resonance imaging and computer assisted tomography

These modalities are increasingly used in specialist congenital cardiac centers.

Table 12.60   Selected ECG measurements in normal pediatric patients

	0–3 days	3–30 days	1–6 months	6–12 months	1–3 years	3–5 years	5–8 years	8–12 years	12–16 years
Heart rate (/min)	90–160	90–180	105–185	110–170	90–150	70–140	65–135	60–130	60–120
PR (ms) lead II	80–160	70–140	70–160	70–160	80–150	80–160	90–160	90–170	90–180
QRS (ms) lead V_s	25–75	25–80	25–80	25–75	30–75	30–75	30–80	30–85	35–90
QRS axis (degrees)	60–195	65–185	10–120	10–100	10–100	10–105	10–135	10–120	10–130
QRS V_1									
Q (mV)	0	0	0	0	0	0	0	0	0
R (mV)	0.5–2.6	0.3–2.3	0.3–2.0	0.2–2.0	0.2–1.8	0.1–1.8	0.1–1.5	0.1–1.2	0.1–1.0
S (mV)	0–2.3	0–1.5	0–1.5	0–1.8	0.1–2.1	0.2–2.1	0.3–2.4	0.3–2.5	0.3–2.2
QRS V_6									
Q (mV)	0–0.2	0–0.3	0–0.25	0–0.3	0–0.3	0.02–0.35	0.02–0.45	0.01–0.3	0–0.3
R (mV)	0–1.1	0.1–1.3	0.5–2.2	0.5–2.3	0.6–2.3	0.8–2.5	0.8–2.6	0.9–2.5	0.7–2.4
S (mV)	0–1.0	0–1.0	0–1.0	0–0.8	0–0.6	0–0.5	0–0.4	0–0.4	0–0.4
TV_1 (mV)	−0.4→0.4	−0.5→0.1	−0.6→0.1	−0.6→0.1	−0.6→0.1	−0.6→0	−0.5→0.2	−0.4→0.3	−0.4→0.3

Reproduced from Emmanouilides et al 1995, as adapted from Davignon A, Rautaharju P, Barselle E, Soumis F, Megelas M. Normal ECG standards for infants and children. Pediatric Cardiology 1979/80; 1:123–124
Values reported as 2–98% (approximate).

PATTERNS OF CARDIOVASCULAR DISEASE IN THE NEWBORN

Congenital disease accounts for most cardiac disease in the newborn but acquired disease can occur as a result of birth asphyxia, viral infections and other severe postnatal illnesses. Congenital heart disease presents in the newborn period in approximately 4 per 1000 live births. Congenital heart disease may be structural or functional, the latter group including conduction disturbances, dysrhythmias and heart muscle disease.

PRESENTATION AND MANAGEMENT OF CARDIOVASCULAR DISEASE IN THE NEWBORN

Fetal diagnosis[654]

Detailed fetal echocardiography may show cardiac abnormalities from 13 weeks' gestation onwards. Investigation is performed when a factor increasing the risk of heart disease is identified such as:

- increased nuchal translucency with normal karyotype;
- monochorionic twins;
- abnormal heart suspected at general anomaly scan;
- chromosomal or noncardiac abnormality detected in fetus;
- parental congenital heart disease;
- maternal diabetes;
- parental illness with fetal cardiac implications (e.g. autosomal dominant condition with cardiac aspects, maternal collagen vascular disease).

Detailed fetal echocardiography of all pregnancies is too resource consuming to be practiced in many places, especially as evidence for improved postnatal outcomes after prenatal cardiac diagnosis is conflicting.[655–658] When a baby is born in whom a fetal diagnosis has been made, this must be confirmed by postnatal echocardiography. A normal fetal cardiac scan should not prevent postnatal echocardiography being performed if clinical features point to the possibility of cardiac disease in the newborn.

Cyanosis

Recognition of central cyanosis in a newborn infant is not always easy. Factors that complicate the assessment include a high hematocrit, traumatic petechiae on the face, racial pigmentation and acrocyanosis. A plethoric newborn infant may be normally saturated but still have enough deoxygenated Hb to look centrally cyanosed. Occasionally non-invasive monitoring or even blood gas sampling will be needed for confirmation. Some 'cyanotic' congenital heart disease may not produce recognizable cyanosis in a newborn baby (unobstructed total anomalous pulmonary venous drainage, double inlet and double outlet ventricles with high lung blood flow and good mixing, and tetralogy of Fallot in which right ventricular outflow obstruction progresses through infancy and is often only mild in the newborn period). Once central cyanosis is identified the immediate priority is to assess that airway and respiration are adequate, regardless of suspected cause. Detailed review of history and a complete physical examination are then important. Features of the different groups of causes and management pathways for a suspected cardiac cause are given in Tables 12.61 and 12.62, respectively. In an ill infant with cyanosis from cardiac disease, the most important specific management issue is whether or not ductal patency needs to be secured with prostaglandin; if in doubt, a trial of the drug is appropriate. Prostaglandin E_1 or E_2 may be given intravenously; prostaglandin E_2 may be given orally or nasogastrically, hourly in the first instance. Doses are given in Table 12.63.

Oxygenation is improved by prostaglandin in conditions with obstructed right heart flow (oligemic lungs on X-ray) and in many cases of transposition of the great arteries. Short term side-effects of prostaglandin include pyrexia, apnea, jitteriness, convulsions, flushing and diarrhea. These often improve with dosage reduction without loss of therapeutic effect. The drug should be stopped if no benefit is seen after 1–2 h. Persistent pulmonary hypertension in the newborn (PPHN, see below) can at times be difficult to distinguish from cardiac disease even with echocardiography and the two may coexist (Table 12.64).

Table 12.61 Clinical features and investigations which help rapid differentiation of causes for central cyanosis

Causes of cyanosis	Clinical features	Investigations
Respiratory	Marked respiratory distress (unless PPHN in addition) Color improves in oxygen usually	Abnormal lung fields on X-ray Hypercapnia Hyperoxia test (pass)
Cardiac	May have other cardiac signs May have little or no respiratory distress	X-ray may help, lung pathology absent Normo- or hypocapnia Hyperoxia test (fail) ECG abnormal
Neurological (respiratory depression)	Slow respiration Color improves on stimulation and in oxygen. May have other neurological or syndrome features	X-ray normal Hypercapnia Hyperoxia test (pass)
Hematological (methemoglobinemia)	Black mucous membranes, not typical cyanosis, usually very well	Blood gas normal Hyperoxia test (pass)

In all groups history may provide valuable clues.
PPHN, persistent pulmonary hypertension in the newborn.

Table 12.62 Management approach to cyanosis due to a suspected cardiac cause

1.	General measures	Temperature control, avoid hypoglycemia, ensure ventilation adequate
2.	Arterial blood gas	Treat respiratory acidosis Treat metabolic acidosis Ventilate if necessary (hypoxemia alone not indication to ventilate) Consider value of hyperoxia test
3.	Chest X-ray	Diagnostic clues may be present Management Oligemia – trial of prostaglandin Plethora – trial of prostaglandin if very hypoxemic or metabolic acidosis
4.	ECG	May help with specific diagnosis
5.	Drugs	Prostaglandin (see above) Alkali Diuretics if heart failure/pulmonary congestion Antibiotics if significant risk of serious infection
6.	Echocardiography	Precise diagnosis often possible (transfer if necessary when stable)

Heart failure

Features of heart failure include respiratory distress, sweating, hepatomegaly and in severe cases (particularly where failure has been present antenatally) ascites, generalized edema, pleural and pericardial effusions. Tachycardia, gallop rhythm and clinical features of the cause should also be looked for. Structural heart disease (particularly severe left ventricular outflow obstruction), rhythm disturbances, myocardial diseases (cardiomyopathy of any sort, myocarditis and myocardial ischemia or infarction) and noncardiac diseases may all cause heart failure.

Table 12.63 Drug dosage table

Drug	Route	Dose	Frequency
Prostaglandin			
E_1	i.v.	0.005–0.1 µg/kg/min	–
E_2	i.v.	0.005–0.05 µg/kg/min	–
E_2	Nasogastric	25 µg/kg/h	Hourly initially
Indometacin	i.v.	0.2 mg/kg over 30 min	8- to 12-hourly × 3
Tolazoline	i.v.	0.5 mg/kg over 5 min then 0.5 mg/kg/h	–
Prostacyclin	i.v.	2–20 ng/kg/min	–
Dopamine	i.v.	2–20 µg/kg/min	–
Dobutamine	i.v.	2–20 µg/kg/min	–
Captopril	Oral/ nasogastric	0.1–0.5 mg/kg/dose	8-hourly
		Start with lowest dose	

Table 12.64 Structural cardiac lesions which may be associated with persistent pulmonary hypertension in the newborn infant

Pulmonary venous hypertension	Pulmonary vein stenosis Obstructed total anomalous pulmonary venous drainage Absent left atrioventricular connection with restrictive foramen ovale Left ventricular dysfunction (any cause) Left ventricular outflow obstruction (any cause)
Left to right shunts independent of pulmonary vascular resistance	Atrioventricular septal defect Cerebral arteriovenous malformation Coronary arteriovenous fistula
Severe tricuspid regurgitation	Ebstein anomaly

Intracerebral and more rarely other arteriovenous malformations, generalized viral and bacterial infections, noncardiac hypoxemia, severe anemia, marked polycythemia and excessive fluid administration may all precipitate cardiac decompensation.

Cyanosis and heart failure

Cyanosis is a feature only of very severe heart failure, and heart failure does not develop in many conditions which cause severe cyanosis. Thus, if both cyanosis and heart failure are present, this may be a useful diagnostic aid (Table 12.65).

Collapse

This may be a feature of duct-dependent systemic circulation (Table 12.55). Such lesions are also characterized by respiratory distress, massive hepatomegaly, cardiomegaly with congested lung fields on X-ray, right ventricular dominance on ECG and metabolic acidosis. Differential diagnosis includes septicemia and metabolic disorders but if any doubt exists, resuscitation should include prostaglandin, which will almost invariably produce rapid improvement if the diagnosis is cardiac.

Arrhythmia

Tachyarrhythmias may produce collapse, although supraventricular tachycardia (SVT) may produce either no symptoms or heart failure. Ventricular tachycardia may be life threatening or asymptomatic with a benign natural history and eventual spontaneous resolution. It is an indication for urgent cardiological referral. Complete heart block may be well tolerated, especially if the ventricular rate is above 55/min and rises on activity. Although Stokes–Adams attacks may

Table 12.65 Structural cardiac lesions characteristically showing both heart failure and arterial desaturation in the newborn period. Such lesions with pulmonary stenosis in addition are unlikely to have heart failure

Transposition	(i) with large VSD and PDA
	(ii) with coarctation
Truncus arteriosus	
Tricuspid atresia	(i) with large VSD
	(ii) with TGA and coarctation
Double inlet ventricle	
Total anomalous pulmonary venous drainage with obstructed pulmonary veins	
Hypoplastic left heart syndrome	
Cerebral arteriovenous malformation (vein of Galen aneurysm)	

PDA, persistent ductus arteriosus; TGA, transposition of the great arteries; VSD, ventricular septal defect.

occur, cardiac failure is the more usual problem in the neonate with complete heart block and both are indications for pacemaker insertion, as is a heart rate below 50/min even in the absence of symptoms. Chronotropic drugs rarely have much effect on ventricular rate. The association of rhythm disturbances with structural heart disease must be remembered and the majority of babies with complete heart block without structural heart disease have mothers with serological evidence with or without clinical features of lupus erythematosus or other collagen vascular diseases.[659,660] Supraventricular ectopics (SVEs) are common in normal fetuses and newborns; they are not always conducted to the ventricles (blocked SVEs) in which case they result in a slow and or irregular pulse. In the absence of other cardiovascular signs or ECG abnormalities SVEs do not point to the presence of structural heart disease and resolve within 3 months of birth. There would appear to be an increased risk of SVT in infants with SVEs although clear information on the incidence is not available. Ventricular ectopics (VEs) are found in more than 30% of normal newborn infants and usually resolve rapidly. However if they are a sign of structural heart disease, heart muscle disease or a congenital long QT syndrome there is a risk of serious ventricular dysrhythmias. A variety of acute metabolic disturbances can precipitate rhythm disturbances but do not require detailed cardiac investigation if rhythm and ECG return to normal when plasma biochemistry is corrected.

Cardiac murmur

Murmurs are often heard at routine examination of newborn infants. Other features of cardiac disease must be sought by thorough cardiovascular examination as the presence of a murmur is associated with cardiac disease in up to 50%.[661] Asymptomatic murmurs with no other abnormal features may be innocent and have been found in up to 2% of term infants in the first few days after birth;[662] Table 12.66 lists the characteristics of innocent neonatal murmurs. Trained staff are efficient at identifying murmurs indicative of important structural heart disease without investigation by ECG and chest X-ray.[663,664] It is possible that adding foot pulse oximetry or right arm and foot oximetry to clinical screening examination might further improve the pick up rate of heart (and respiratory) lesions if babies with a reading from the foot of less than 95% are reassessed.[665] However, the widespread use of this technique has yet to be evaluated.[666] Some cardiac abnormalities can be associated with asymptomatic murmurs without any other physical signs and with normal ECG and chest X-ray. Tricuspid regurgitation and VSD may produce similar pansystolic murmurs at the lower left sternal edge. Tricuspid regurgitation producing a murmur in an otherwise well baby is of no long term significance; a VSD heard in the early neonatal period may never cause symptoms and has a high chance of spontaneous resolution.[667] Aortic and pulmonary valve stenosis (including tetralogy

Table 12.66 Features of innocent neonatal murmurs: in all groups the remainder of the examination is normal

Source/type	Features of murmur	Other points
Pulmonary arteries	Bilateral, base of heart, also over scapulae and lateral chest High pitched mid-systolic	Gone by 6 months
Ductus arteriosus	Pulmonary area rarely diastolic	Gone by 2–3 days
Tricuspid regurgitation	Same as VSD, heard day 1	May be perinatal asphyxia Goes in a few days–weeks
Still's innocent	Vibratory	Rarely heard in newborn
murmur	Mid-systolic Between LLSE and apex	May last years

LLSE, lower left sternal edge.

of Fallot) will produce a murmur at birth; evaluation including ECG, chest X-ray and if possible echocardiography is necessary before allowing a baby home if significant outflow tract obstruction is suggested by a loud murmur at the base. The normal murmur from pulmonary artery branches in the newborn is not as loud or as harsh as that from semilunar valve stenosis and radiates laterally.

Hypertension

Neonatal hypertension is usually only identified in infants with other cardiovascular signs or in those known to be at increased risk such as those with chronic lung disease or cocaine-using mothers. Treatment of neonatal hypertension is only occasionally necessary, but attention to the underlying cause is always appropriate (Table 12.67).

Association with other abnormalities

Many syndromes include cardiac abnormalities;[668] in some the cardiac malformation may be a major determinant of length or quality of life. Any infant with a congenital abnormality should at very least have a full physical examination of the cardiovascular system so as to detect abnormalities which may influence management and allow comprehensive counseling of families.

Table 12.67 Causes of hypertension in the newborn

Renal	Renal vein thrombosis
	Renal arterial emboli/thrombosis
	Dysplastic renal disease
	Polycystic renal disease
	Urinary tract obstruction
	Renal infection
	Renal failure (any cause)
Cardiovascular	Coarctation
Endocrine	Congenital adrenal hyperplasia
	Hyperaldosteronism
	Hyperthyroidism
	Pheochromocytoma
	Neuroblastoma
Respiratory disease	Bronchopulmonary dysplasia (mechanism unknown)
Neurological disease	Raised intracranial pressure (any cause)
Drugs	Corticosteroids
	Methylxanthines
	Phenylephrine (in eyedrops)

CARDIOVASCULAR ASPECTS OF NEONATAL DISEASES
Respiratory distress syndrome
Persistent ductus arteriosus (PDA)

Patency of the ductus arteriosus is associated with worse RDS, and delayed closure of the ductus can result in the need for continuing ventilation, but clear evidence of reduced long term morbidity or mortality from prophylactic or therapeutic intervention is not available.[669] Antenatal prostaglandin synthetase inhibitor administration predisposes to postnatal delayed closure of the ductus and makes the ductus less responsive to indometacin.[670] The efficacy of antenatal steroid administration in reducing incidence and severity of RDS may in part be due to increasing ductal sensitivity to postnatal constricting influences. Cautious fluid regimens in babies with RDS are associated with a lower incidence of PDA. Etamsylate[671] given to reduce intracerebral hemorrhage has been found to be associated with a lower incidence of PDA. Prophylactic duct closure with indometacin reduces but does not abolish the occurrence of later symptoms;[672] similar effects are described for ibuprofen.[673] The failure to demonstrate better outcomes following prophylactic use of indometacin[674,675] or ibuprofen[676] indicates the need for caution but long term outcome information following treatment only of babies at increased risk of symptomatic PDA is not available.

Prediction in the first 3 days of life of high risk of future symptomatic PDA is possible if a duct more than 1.5 mm in diameter is seen on color flow Doppler[677] or if low velocity continuous left to right shunting is demonstrated by pulsed wave Doppler.[678] The typical clinical features of PDA may be hard to detect in a baby with respiratory disease and PDA may cause no murmur or more usually just a systolic one. Other features of PDA in the context of the preterm include apnea, hypotension, heart failure, NEC and metabolic acidosis. When ventilator requirements are increasing after apparently passing the peak of RDS and a continuous murmur is present, the diagnosis is easy; when features are less obvious, the possibility of left to right shunting through a PDA must be remembered. The ECG is not helpful and chest X-ray is often noncontributory. If there is clinical doubt, echocardiography imaging, M mode[679] and Doppler examination are required[680] looking for the features mentioned above and also for mean and diastolic velocities in the left pulmonary artery.[681]

Symptomatic PDA should be vigorously treated with fluid restriction, correction of anemia and cautious use of diuretics, which may derange electrolytes. If these measures do not rapidly control the situation, indometacin has long been known to be effective in closing the ductus in approximately 70% of premature infants.[682] Intravenous indometacin (0.2 mg/kg) for 3 doses 8–24 h apart should be used; an infusion over at least 30 min is preferable to a bolus injection because of effects on blood pressure and cerebral circulation[683] although even slow infusions reduce cerebral oxygen delivery.[684] Less than three doses may be used if the Doppler velocity across the ductus can be shown to evolve to a closing pattern after the initial dose.[685] It is possible that ibuprofen may be less active on the cerebral circulation and just as effective at closing the ductus[686,687] although pulmonary hypertension and chronic lung disease may be more common than after indometacin use, therefore at present it has no clear advantage over indometacin.[688] Fluid retention and elevation of creatinine are temporary adverse effects of indometacin; thrombocytopenia is usually considered a contraindication to its use, as are renal failure and NEC. A repeat course may be used if the beneficial effect is transient although an asymptomatic murmur which reappears after natural or pharmacological ductal closure is more likely to be arising from the pulmonary artery branches than from the ductus.[689] A 5-day course of indometacin[690] or a 6-day low dose course[691] is effective at closing the ductus with a lower relapse rate. Biochemical evidence of renal dysfunction is less on the low dose regimen. The effect on cerebral hemodynamics of prolonged indometacin treatment has not been studied. Two unsuccessful short courses, unacceptable side-effects or a definite contraindication mean that surgical ligation or clipping of the ductus should be carried out. This can be done in the neonatal nursery with low mortality and morbidity. Transcatheter[692] and thoracoscopic[693] closure of the ductus is now reported in babies under

2000 g but not in those under 1000 g. Whether or not echocardiography is regarded as mandatory before using prostaglandin synthetase inhibitor drugs, it certainly is before surgical ligation to confirm the diagnosis and to rule out structural congenital heart disease and systemic to pulmonary collateral arteries which can be found in preterm infants[694] and which cause a continuous murmur.

Persistent pulmonary hypertension of the newborn (PPHN)

Pulmonary hypertension may complicate a variety of neonatal respiratory illnesses (Table 12.54). Diagnosis is helped by recognizing risk factors and by excluding structural heart disease. Lower saturations in the feet than the right hand are characteristic if the ductus arteriosus is open (this is also a feature of structural heart lesions with obstruction of the aortic arch).

Management in general consists of treating predisposing and aggravating factors aggressively, ensuring adequate alveolar recruitment and systemic blood pressure and normalizing acid–base balance. Consideration should then be given to the use of vasodilators. Oxygen and inhaled nitric oxide[695] are the only specific pulmonary vasodilators. The optimum dosage of nitric oxide is unclear but may be 20 parts per million (ppm)[696] and there may be disadvantages to initiating therapy at a lower dose.[697] There are benefits in tailoring ventilatory modes to the individual patient which may be additive to the effects of nitric oxide.[698] Plasma expansion and inotropes may both be needed. ECMO is effective in PPHN but exact indications for its use are unclear, as newer treatment protocols are more effective than those used when ECMO was first introduced. Intravenous magnesium sulfate, prostacyclin and tolazoline may be effective and the latter drug has also been used by inhalation. These treatments have not been extensively evaluated in randomized controlled trials. All infused drugs will lower systemic as well as pulmonary vascular resistance, so blood pressure must be invasively and continuously monitored when they are used. Modest hyperventilation to a carbon dioxide tension of 3–4 kPa or administration of alkali lower pulmonary vascular resistance but have adverse effects on cerebral perfusion and are seldom used.

Asphyxia

Persistent pulmonary hypertension

This may also be a feature of perinatal asphyxia, with or without meconium aspiration pneumonitis (see above).

Myocardial ischemia and infarction

Electrocardiographic[699] and pathological[700] studies indicate that myocardial ischemia is common in neonates stressed by asphyxia. Even in mild cases there may be the murmur of tricuspid regurgitation which may be associated with ischemic ECG changes. In severely asphyxiated infants, hypotension from myocardial dysfunction may need inotrope support, and any type of arrhythmia can occur. Discrete areas of myocardial infarction can occur secondary to thromboembolic phenomena pre- or postnatally; this is rare but has a high mortality.[701]

Infection

Generalized and pulmonary bacterial and viral infections in the newborn may predispose to PPHN. Myocarditis is a feature of disseminated viral infections, and heart failure, shock and arrhythmias may result. Shock may also be caused by peripheral vasodilation and capillary leakage in severe bacterial sepsis. Endocarditis is increasingly being recognized in already sick newborn infants.[702] Clinical features are nonspecific. There is rarely underlying structural heart disease. The diagnosis is suggested by multiple septic lesions appearing over time or recurrent bacteremia or fungemia, particularly in the presence of intravenous long lines. Ultrasound scanning can make, but not exclude, the diagnosis. Masses within the heart chambers or in great vessels can be vegetations in association with infection, non-infected thrombus (usually related to presence of an indwelling catheter at that site at some time) or tumors. Prolonged appropriate multiple antimicrobial therapy is indicated for endocarditis.

Metabolic diseases

There are many inborn errors of metabolism and storage diseases which may be associated with cardiomyopathy. Hypertrophic cardiomyopathy seen in the newborn infants of diabetic mothers is worth specific mention because although it is frequently asymptomatic it may cause severe heart failure with gross cardiomegaly and ECG changes. The possibility of cardiac dysfunction in the respiratory problems encountered in infants of diabetic mothers needs careful individual assessment, as in some it will be a major contributory factor. This cardiomyopathy is self-limiting, resolving completely in 6–12 months.[703] Inotropes and vasodilators should be avoided in this condition because they may aggravate left ventricular outflow obstruction. Dilated cardiomyopathy may present symptomatically in the newborn period and a vigorous search for familial, infective and metabolic causes is indicated.

GENERAL MANAGEMENT OF NEONATAL HEART DISEASE

All the principles for care of the newborn infant apply to the baby with definite or suspected cardiac disease. These principles should not be neglected because of a desire to get the correct diagnosis or to transfer the infant elsewhere.

Ductal manipulation

The major resuscitative decision with respect specifically to heart disease is whether or not to use prostaglandin. In an unwell baby with poor systemic perfusion the possibility of critical left heart obstruction must always be borne in mind and unless it can be confidently excluded a trial of prostaglandin is appropriate. A cyanosed infant who is well does not need prostaglandin urgently but if there is metabolic acidosis or respiratory distress for which no primary respiratory cause is apparent prostaglandin should be commenced. Pharmacological duct closure with indometacin is never as urgent and if any doubt exists about the diagnosis, echocardiography is essential, as indeed it is before surgical intervention.

Heart failure

Fluid restriction in the short term, optimal oxygenation and the treatment of anemia are important. Digoxin use is time honored but controversial in the treatment of heart failure when associated with left to right shunt. Diuretics, usually furosemide with or without a potassium sparing diuretic, are particularly effective in relieving symptoms. Vasodilators in neonatal heart failure are relatively untried, although angiotensin-converting enzyme inhibitors are widely used in infants.[704,705] Aggressive drug therapy for heart failure is appropriate in order to allow adequate nutrition.

Hypotension/low output states

There is no single objective method of assessing clinically the adequacy of the circulation in a newborn infant. Decisions to provide circulatory support are not based on any one parameter alone. Normal ranges for blood pressure can be derived from healthy infants but they do not determine what is an adequate or beneficial blood pressure and there are no randomized trials assessing the outcomes of sick infants treated with different target ranges for blood pressure.

Clinical assessment of end organ perfusion is more important than aiming at a particular blood pressure.[706] If the urine output is good, there is no metabolic acidosis and there is good peripheral perfusion, the circulation is likely to be adequate whatever the blood pressure. However, preterm infants with higher blood pressure tend to have better clinical outcomes than those with lower blood pressure and, perhaps because it is easily measured, treatment decisions are strongly influenced by blood pressure measurements.

The broad consensus is that if the mean arterial blood pressure is around the gestational age in weeks then it is likely to be adequate;[707] ensuring optimal circulating volume should precede or accompany inotrope support.[708] However, in the majority of cases hypovolemia is unlikely to be the explanation and repeated boluses of colloid for hypotension in preterm infants may be harmful. Early intervention with dopamine or dobutamine[709,710] should be considered. Echocardiography is helpful if doubt about the need for inotrope support exists and central venous pressure measurements may help.

A small number of infants remain hypotensive despite maximal inotropic support and volume replacement. Some of these infants respond well to small doses of hydrocortisone. It is not clear to what extent newborn infants can increase cardiac output by increasing myocardial contractility rather than heart rate. Bradycardia, be it sinus or due to atrioventricular block, resulting in circulatory compromise should be treated by identifying and removing the cause, aided if necessary by drugs such as atropine and isoprenaline or by pacing. Primary tachyarrhythmias such as atrial flutter and atrioventricular re-entry tachycardia (see Ch. 21) can be hard to distinguish from reactive sinus tachycardia but must be recognized and treated if compromising cardiac output. The rare cases of cardiac tamponade from pericardial fluid or air require drainage.

Arrhythmias

Management of these in newborn babies is governed by the same principles as throughout infancy and is discussed in Chapter 21.

Drug therapy

Recommended drugs and dosages for the treatment of neonatal cardiovascular disease are given in Table 12.63.

Interventional cardiac catheterization

Rashkind balloon atrial septostomy still forms part of the emergency management of a number of conditions, particularly transposition of the great arteries (TGA). If diagnostic catheterization is not needed, a balloon atrial septostomy can be performed by an experienced operator under ultrasound control in the neonatal nursery. Balloon valvuloplasty is used in some centers for both critical aortic and critical pulmonary valve stenosis.[711] Balloon dilatation of neonatal coarctation is generally not as effective as surgery. The role of ductal stenting in duct-dependent lesions is being explored.[712] Transcatheter ductal closure is not yet feasible in babies under about 1500 g.[692]

Surgery

Cardiac surgery in the newborn can be palliative or corrective, closed or open. Surgical treatment for particular conditions is discussed in Chapter 21 and it must be remembered that local practices vary a great deal. In general there is a trend towards performing corrective open procedures at increasingly younger ages. Whatever approach is taken, results are better when infants come to operation well resuscitated and stable.

STRUCTURAL HEART DISEASE IN THE PRETERM INFANT

Respiratory pathology and infective processes are so common in the preterm infant that cardiac disease can be forgotten or masked. It is extremely important to bear in mind the possibility of structural and functional cardiac disease as the cause of or a contributory factor to symptoms and signs in the premature infant. In many cases pharmacological or surgical management is possible with ultimate good outcome. Preterm babies may go into heart failure at an earlier postnatal age with a given condition, such as VSD, than a term baby for reasons that are not entirely clear.

CARDIOVASCULAR ASPECTS OF CHRONIC PULMONARY DISEASE IN THE NEWBORN

The role of PDA in prolonging acute respiratory failure in RDS has been discussed above. Chronic lung disease will make clinical features of a left to right shunt of any sort very hard to recognize but treatment of the cardiac abnormality may help the respiratory condition. Chronic respiratory failure may cause right heart failure; it is important to avoid hypoxemia in such infants and to treat intercurrent infections and secretion retention vigorously.

GASTROINTESTINAL PROBLEMS AND JAUNDICE OF THE NEONATE

EMBRYOLOGY AND MALFORMATIONS

The gut is derived from the embryonic yolk sac which differentiates in early life into the fore-, mid- and hindgut. The foregut gives rise to the pharynx, thyroid, thymus, parathyroid glands, respiratory tract, esophagus, stomach, upper duodenum, liver and pancreas. The midgut gives rise to the lower half of the duodenum, small intestine and large intestine as far as the distal third of the transverse colon. The rest of the large bowel arises from the hindgut. Agenesis of a complete segment is rare; rather, constriction (atresia) of a small portion is more common and can occur at any level because normal development includes luminal obliteration by mucosal growth, followed by recanalization.[713] Atresia is more common at sites where the development of the gut is complex, like the respiratory diverticulum of the foregut (see below).

Between 4 and 6 weeks of fetal life the cranial portion of the foregut differentiates into a complicated branchial arch system which is transitory and obliterated by 7 weeks. Failure of obliteration may result in a persistent sinus, fistula or epithelial lined cyst (e.g. neurenteric cyst). The partitioning of the foregut into the pharynx and trachea may also be incomplete and various types of tracheoesophageal fistula with or without esophageal atresia will result. Abnormal development of the lower end of the foregut may result in a diaphragmatic hernia whilst failure of esophageal differentiation causes achalasia of the cardia or more rarely an esophageal web.

The stomach is relatively immune to embryological malformation. However, the terminal portion of the foregut and cranial end of the midgut undergo major growth in length with consequent herniation from the umbilical cavity (Fig. 12.33).[714] As it returns to the abdomen there is a complex counterclockwise rotation (ultimately 270 degrees) resulting in the fixation of the cecum in the right iliac fossa and the passage of the transverse colon and mesentery over the second and third parts of the duodenum. The first possible failure is that of the endoderm of the yolk sac to separate from the notochord during the third week which

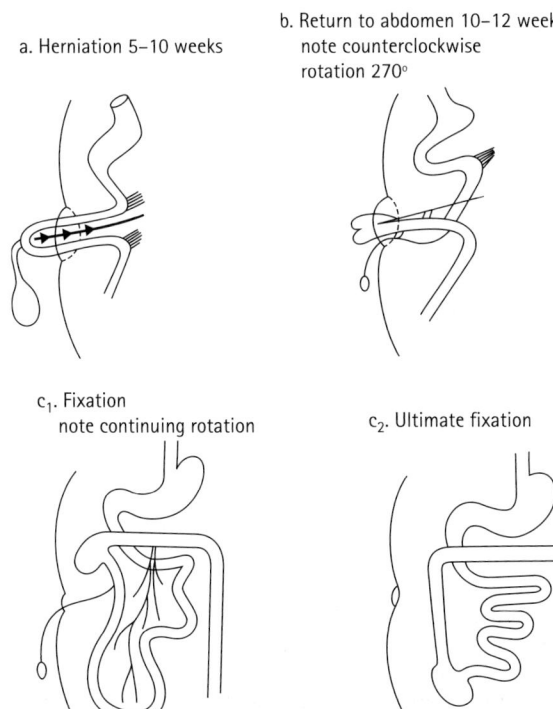

a. Herniation 5–10 weeks

b. Return to abdomen 10–12 weeks note counterclockwise rotation 270°

c₁. Fixation note continuing rotation

c₂. Ultimate fixation

Fig. 12.33 The course of events leading to fixation and final position of the gut within the abdomen. (From Lebenthal et al 1988[714])

results in a variety of reduplications of the intestine. Incomplete failure of the vitellointestinal duct to regress in the fifth week results in a Meckel's diverticulum and complete failure results in an umbilical fistula. Finally failure in herniation return and fixation of the intestine between the fifth and twelfth weeks may cause major defects such as exomphalos and malrotation.

The cloaca is divided by a membrane at 6 weeks into the sagittally oriented rectum posteriorly and the urogenital sinus. Anomalies in rectal differentiation cause a variety of defects ranging from imperforate anus and rectovaginal fistulae to sacral sinus formation. Because rectal differentiation is contemporaneous with that of esophageal differentiation, defects in both structures are often found in the same patient.

The liver is derived from an outpouching of the ventral portion of the duodenum at 4 weeks and defects in its development are rare (Fig. 12.34).[714] Defects in the development of the biliary tree from the cystic duct are more common with either cystic dilation (choledochal cyst) or failure of canalization (biliary atresia) being the commonest disorders. Defects in pancreatic development are also rare but because the final gland is produced by the fusion of a dorsal pancreas from an outpouching of the duodenum just cranial to the hepatic diverticulum and a ventral pancreas from an outpouching in the caudal angle between the gut and hepatic diverticulum (Fig. 12.34) failure of this fusion process may result in an anular pancreas. Cellular differentiation of all the organs of the gut occurs early and is complete in most cases by the end of the first trimester. Intestinal epithelial cells of the first trimester human fetus resemble immature crypt cells of the adult intestine. Morphogenesis of the intestinal epithelium (including differentiation of crypts and villi as well as the intracellular organelles) is completed by about 22 weeks' gestation. Thus, the anatomical development of the gut is complete by the birth of even the 24-week infant and the limiting factor in feeding is the maturation of functional activity.

ONTOGENY OF GUT FUNCTION
Carbohydrate absorption
The absorption of carbohydrates seems to pose no problem even for premature neonates. Human milk and most formula milks usually contain only lactose, thus pancreatic digestion is relatively unimportant and the low levels of amylase detected in the duodenal juice of premature and term infants do not matter. More modified milks contain such elements as corn syrup, amylose or maltodextrins in order to reduce their osmolality; however, glucoamylase and sucrase-isomaltase activity should be adequate for their digestion. The disaccharidases develop in close association with the enterocyte itself and disaccharidase activity first appears with the villus formation. Lactase, however, develops later in comparison with sucrase-isomaltase activity (8–10 months' gestation) but lactose intolerance is very rarely seen in the very low birth weight infant, presumably because of enzyme induction.

Intestinal absorption of nutrients and electrolytes is dependent on the development of appropriate cellular active transport processes.

Studies of everted fetal intestinal sacs have shown that cotransport of glucose/galactose by the sodium-glucose linked transporter (SGLT1) is present as early as 10 weeks and there is a three-fold increase in the uptake by 18 weeks. Studies of glucose-evoked potential difference across the duodenum in neonates have confirmed the presence of active glucose transfer in premature neonates, although the number of monosaccharide transporters is reduced in the premature compared with the term infant. Thus carbohydrate digestion/absorption is adequate in the premature infant.

Protein absorption
Protein digestion is initiated in the stomach and gastric peptic activity increases rapidly after birth (from 2 to 50% adult reference levels by 2 months in term infants). Gastric acid secretion (which is necessary for full peptic activity, the optimal pH for pepsin being 4–5) does not occur at maximal activity in the preterm infant for about 1 month. It is, however, rapidly buffered by milk because of the overall decreased secretory mass in these infants.

Although tryptic activity is low at birth, pancreatic enzyme induction results in high levels by the first week of life in term/preterm infants. Brush border oligopeptidase activity is similar to that found in adults by the early part of the second trimester and protein digestion appears adequate. Active absorption of L-alanine and L-leucine has also been demonstrated in everted sacs from both 10- and 18-week fetuses. Peptides as well as amino acids can be absorbed by the enterocyte which further enhances the efficiency of protein absorption.

Fat absorption
Lipid digestion is more complex and requires more adaptive mechanisms to ensure maximal absorption of this major source of energy by preterm infants. Four major lipases exist:
1. lingual lipase – this is often bypassed by nasogastric tubes although nonnutritive sucking may increase the contribution of this enzyme;
2. gastric lipase (first demonstrated as having a role in the gastric aspirates of infants with esophageal atresia);
3. pancreatic lipase (this shows rapid substrate induction);
4. bile salt-stimulated lipase (present in high quantities in human milk, irrespective of prematurity and milk volume).

Together, these contribute more than sufficient lipolytic activity even in the preterm infant. Unfortunately, bile salt production in such infants barely reaches the critical micellar concentration and this becomes the rate-limiting factor in fat digestion. However, the palmitic acid of human milk fat is predominantly esterified at the triglyceride 2 position which matches the stereospecificity of pancreatic lipase reducing the need for bile salts. Milk manufacturers tend to compensate for the inefficient fat absorption of their milks by supplementing them with medium chain triglycerides (at the expense of increasing osmolality). The products of fat digestion are absorbed, resynthesized as triglycerides and secreted into the lymphatic system as chylomicrons. Medium chain triglycerides (8–10 carbon chain length) are absorbed without bile salts, and pass to the liver in the portal system.

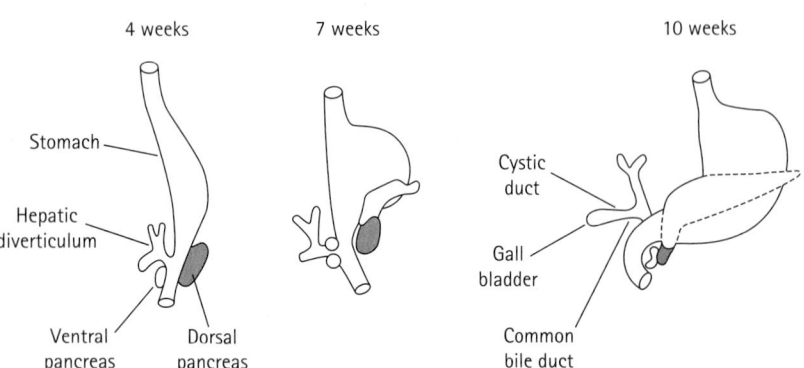

Fig. 12.34 The development of the liver/pancreas from an outpouching of the ventral portion of the duodenum. (From Lebenthal et al 1988[714])

4 weeks   7 weeks   10 weeks

Stomach

Hepatic diverticulum

Cystic duct

Gall bladder

Ventral pancreas   Dorsal pancreas   Common bile duct

Salt and water absorption

Salt and water absorption by the enterocyte is present in the early stages of cellular differentiation. It has been shown that adenylate cyclase and Na/K ATPase activities, both closely related to the electrolyte transport processes, develop concomitantly with the brush border translocation mechanisms. Equilibrium dialysis studies of colonic transport mechanisms in the premature infant have demonstrated that the sodium chloride exchange mechanisms are highly active (presumably under the influence of the high levels of aldosterone seen in these infants). Basic transport processes clearly function in early life.

Intestinal motility

The limiting factor in feeding premature infants is intestinal motility, the ontogeny of which lags behind digestion and absorption. The ability to suck is not present until about 34 weeks' gestation (although it can occur earlier) but this can be bypassed by tube feeding. Gastric emptying, although poor at birth, is fully functional by 24 h postnatally. It is controlled by duodenal receptors in similar fashion in both premature and mature infants by nutrient density and specific constituents of the meal and is inhibited by pathological processes (e.g. RDS and asphyxia). Small intestinal motor activity is divided into fasting and postprandial motor patterns. The fasting migrating motor complex does not fully develop until about 34 weeks' gestation (in association with the onset of sucking).[715] Postprandial activity does not occur until later and seems to be a learned phenomenon increasing with the increasing nutritional density of the feeds. Before 34 weeks a highly propulsive activity, the fetal motor complex, is seen which allows the intestine to function and feeding to be effective. Before 26 weeks, only small nonpropagated contractions are seen and so enteral feeds may not be tolerated initially. More mature motor function may be induced by feeding, allowing many infants of lower gestation to tolerate enteral feeding. The development of colonic motility has not been studied but appears to be adequate although regular glycerin suppositories may be needed initially. It is also clear that the gut motor function is critically dependent upon the well-being of the infant. Thus, sick infants will show delayed maturation (or regression) of gut motor activity and it is this which causes the functional ileus seen in such infants. More rarely disorders of the nervous system of the gut may present with a true pseudo-obstruction and disordered distal migration of the myenteric nerves can give rise to aganglionic segments as in Hirschsprung disease.

Postnatal development

There are three elements of postnatal development of the gastrointestinal tract that are of fundamental importance in the consideration of neonatal and later childhood intestinal disease.[716] First is the huge capacity for postnatal growth of small and large intestine. The small intestine increases in length from 4 mm at 4 weeks' gestation to 250–300 cm at term, and the colon is 30–40 cm at term. The postnatal growth of the intestine is at least ten-fold, with the small intestine reaching 4–6 m, and the colon 1.5–2.0 m.[717] Second, there is increasing evidence that postnatal modelling events, either as part of normal growth or as a response to injury or inflammation, may proceed under very similar regulation to embryonic development.[716] This will soon be the source of therapeutic development. Last is the central role of the intestinal immune system – the intestine is the largest immune organ in the body. Very recent environmental and cultural changes in human life have resulted in changes in tolerance to dietary antigens and the enteric flora, and may be the cause of the rapid rise in inflammatory bowel diseases and atopic diseases.[716]

PROBLEMS

The common problems of feeding intolerance, feeding difficulties, vomiting, diarrhea, constipation and gastrointestinal bleeding in the neonatal period will be considered, and then the specific problems of necrotizing enterocolitis (NEC) and intestinal failure, principally due to short bowel syndrome.

Feeding intolerance (Table 12.68)

This is a common problem in the neonatal nursery, becoming manifest as increasingly large aspirates and failure to tolerate milk in the

Table 12.68 Feeding disorders

Etiology	Investigations
a. 'Feeding intolerance'	
Prematurity	History and examination
Ileus	Nursing observation
Sepsis	Abdominal distention
Major clinical deterioration	Septic screen
Necrotizing enterocolitis	Distention – abdominal wall crepitus, tenderness
	Abdominal X-ray
	Proctoscopy
Asphyxia	
Drugs	
All causes of vomiting	
b. 'Feeding difficulties'	
Maternal factors	History and examination
Poor milk supply	Nursing observation
Cracked nipples/breast abscess	
Tension/anxiety	
Poor ability to suck	
Tachypnea/RDS	
Anatomical abnormality	
Micrognathia	
Macroglossia	
Cleft palate	
Asphyxia	
Bulbar/suprabulbar palsy	Jaw jerk positive
Moebius syndrome	
Myopathies	Absent reflexes
	Electromyogram nerve conduction studies
Familial dysautonomia	Jewish race
	Histamine prick test
	Pupillary response to metacholine

tube-fed infant. Care must be taken to check for blood or bile in the aspirate. The former suggests a gastritis and the latter functional or surgical obstruction. Prematurity is the usual cause for failure to tolerate feeds although most infants after the age of 28 weeks will tolerate continuous tube feeds which are started gradually at 1 ml/h and increased, as tolerated, to full requirements over the course of the first week. In their Cochrane review of ten randomized trials, Premji & Chessell[718] concluded that the evidence to date could not reliably discern between the clinical benefits and risks of continuous versus intermittent milk feeding of preterm infants. A further Cochrane review concluded that the ideal rate of advancement of feeds for preterm infants remains unclear.[719] Hourly intermittent bolus feeds are then introduced and by about 34 weeks' gestation, with the onset of suckling, the infant will tolerate 3- to 4-hourly feeds and is ready for the introduction of orogastric feeding. Attempts to introduce these steps too quickly will result in an increase in the volume of stomach contents aspirated before the next feed (or hourly if continuously fed). Continuous feeds should be continued in infants with short bowel syndrome or other causes of intestinal failure, together with very slow advancements and ongoing parenteral nutrition. Experienced nurses are normally able to distinguish any increase in aspirate due to overly aggressive feeding changes from that occurring unexpectedly and indicating pathology in the gastrointestinal tract. A Cochrane review of 15 randomized trials concluded that non-nutritive sucking by preterm infants aided the transition to bottle feedings and gave better bottle-feeding performance.[720] Most of the causes of vomiting in the neonatal period could present in this manner but most commonly such an increase in aspirate heralds the onset of ileus secondary to sepsis, a major deterioration in the child's general condition or NEC. Asphyxia may be complicated by gastric stasis and is the commonest organic cause of poor feeding postnatally in the term infant. Failure to start oral feeding for more than 1 week indicates a poor prognosis. Drugs used postnatally, especially phenobarbitone and diazepam, can delay gastric emptying and enteral feeding may not be possible in the ventilated and paralyzed infant. Other drugs have been assessed in randomized trials for improvement of motility in preterm infants with feeding intolerance, but some, such as erythromycin,[721] do not have current evidence to support such use, and others, such as cisapride,[722] have been withdrawn from use due to side-effects.

Feeding difficulties (Table 12.68)

It may be difficult to establish feeding even in the term infant. Breast problems such as cracked nipples or a breast abscess may prevent breast-feeding, the gold standard route of feeding for both preterm and term infants, but the baby will quickly accept bottle-feeding. Maternal anxiety, however, may prevent the establishment of breast-feeding and can also lead to clumsy or inappropriate methods of bottle-feeding (resulting usually in overfeeding and vomiting but occasionally in inadequate feeding and failure to thrive). A recent Cochrane review evaluated 34 eligible randomized controlled trials containing nearly 30000 mother–infant pairs, and concluded that there was clear evidence that professional support and lay support could prolong duration of breast-feeding and promote exclusive breast-feeding respectively.[723]

Disorders of sucking and swallowing can occur. Anatomical abnormalities such as micrognathia, macroglossia and cleft palate often result in poor sucking and slow feeding. Neurological conditions other than asphyxia tend to present with uncoordinated sucking and swallowing causing oral or nasal regurgitation, sometimes accompanied by the signs of a suprabulbar palsy with tongue thrust and a positive jaw jerk. The rare congenital Moebius syndrome with bilateral facial palsy (and other cranial nerve palsies) due to congenital agenesis of the cranial nerves also results in a poor suck and uncoordinated swallowing. Unilateral nerve lesions do not usually cause problems and where present should be distinguished from myopathies such as mitochondrial myopathy which may cause dysphagia in the neonatal period. The Riley–Day syndrome (familial dysautonomia) may also present in the neonatal period with disorders of swallowing but usually dysphagia occurs later in childhood. Where there is excessive drooling of saliva in association with swallowing difficulties a tracheoesophageal fistula should be considered although the usual clinical picture (coughing, excessive saliva, cyanotic and apneic spells) is quite distinctive and is rapidly diagnosed within a few hours of birth by a plain X-ray with a nasogastric tube inserted.

Vomiting

Vomiting is common in newborn infants. Assessment should always include the overall clinical condition and other symptoms and signs, as well as the volume, frequency and contents of the vomitus (causes and investigations in Table 12.69).

Posseting

Posseting (the regurgitation of small amounts of milk after feeds) is common in the neonatal period and is easily distinguished from pathological vomiting by experienced mothers and midwives. Regurgitation and vomiting both indicate underlying disorders in the newborn period (vomiting is a more serious problem). Rumination is a rare disorder, possibly familial. The baby regurgitates small amounts of food into the mouth which is then chewed with apparent self-gratification. It usually presents after the neonatal period.

Feeding disorders

Feeding disorders are the commonest cause of vomiting in the first month of life after leaving hospital. Greedy babies swallow air. This leads to excessive posseting or vomiting and can usually be recognized by experienced health visitors. Overfeeding or the improper preparation of the bottles is more difficult to spot and commonly presents as vomiting to casualty departments. A careful history of type, amount and constitution of feed is vital in every case of vomiting. With correction of mother's mistakes

Table 12.69 Vomiting

Etiology	Investigations
Feeding disorders	
Overfeeding	Feeding history and observation
Air swallowing	
Maternal stress	Family history
Esophageal disorders	
Tracheoesophageal fistula/frothy vomit day 1	CXR/AXR with large nasogastric tube
Hiatus hernia	Barium swallow/pH study
Gastric disorders	
(Gastritis)	
Maternal debris	Stomach washout
Blood – hemorrhagic disease of the newborn	Clotting screen
Maternal stress illness	History
Pyloric stenosis	Test feed
	Ultrasound/barium meal
Small intestinal disorders	
Congenital	
Duodenal atresia	AXR
Extrinsic duodenal obstruction	AXR
Malrotation	AXR
Volvulus	AXR
Meconium ileus	AXR (calcification)
Intestinal duplication	AXR
Acquired	
Pseudo-obstruction/sepsis	Full blood count, septic screen
NEC	AXR – free or intramural gas
Proctocolitis	Stool cultures
Food allergy	Dietary manipulation
Incarceration/strangulation	Inspection
Inguinal herniae	AXR
Extraintestinal disorders	
Intracranial lesions	
Asphyxia, meningitis	
Intracranial hemorrhage	
Hydrocephalus/SOL	
Renal disorders	
Urinary tract infection	MSU/bag urine
Obstructive uropathy	Renal ultrasound
Metabolic disorders	
Galactosemia	Urine sugar
Hyperammonemias	Urine amino acids
Phenylketonuria	Urine amino acids
Organic acidemias	pH urine
Congenital adrenal hyperplasia	Electrolytes
Drugs	Theophylline

AXR, abdominal X-ray; CXR, chest X-ray; MSU, mid stream urine; NEC, necrotizing enterocolitis; SOL, space-occupying lesion.

the symptoms rapidly resolve. However, maternal anxiety or depression is often a coexistent factor in such cases and contributes to the fussy eating and vomiting in these babies. Evidence of affective disorder or postnatal depression in the mother should be sought during history taking and a full family history often reveals predictable stressors such as death of a sibling or other close relative, or a previous stillbirth or neonatal death.

Organic causes of vomiting

Vomiting in the first week of life. Vomiting at this time may be due to difficulties in establishing appropriate feeding. However, more specific organic causes must be excluded by appropriate means. All causes of vomiting (Table 12.69) may present at any time, but in this early period, consideration of the vomitus and baby together with an abdominal X ray can narrow the differential diagnosis. For example:

1. Vomitus
   - Frothy
     - tracheoesophageal fistula
   - Blood
     - maternal – swallowed
     - hemorrhagic disease
     - gastric erosions/stress ulcers
   - Bile
     - intestinal obstruction
     - intestinal perforation/peritonitis
     - intestinal pseudo-obstruction
   - Milk only
     - feeding disorder
     - gastroesophageal reflux
     - food allergy
2. Baby well: abdomen normal
   - AXR – fluid level
     - duodenal/intestinal atresia
     - meconium ileus
     - large bowel obstruction/Hirschsprung disease
   - AXR – no fluid levels
     - gastroesophageal reflux
     - milk allergy
3. Baby sick
   - Abdomen normal: AXR – ± fluid levels + watery diarrhea
     - sepsis/UTI
     - increased intracranial pressure/meningitis
     - renal tract disorders
     - metabolic disorders
   - Abdomen distended/tender: AXR – fluid levels (watery or bloody diarrhea)
     - necrotizing enterocolitis
     - obstruction/perforation
     - volvulus
     - intussusception.

The commonest cause for vomiting in the first 2 days of life is neonatal gastritis due to irritation from swallowed liquor and debris from the birth canal. One or two stomach washouts will identify the debris (and the altered maternal blood) and cure the problem. The baby remains well throughout. If the baby is sick, other signs are present or the vomiting persists, then fuller investigations are required. Clearly a septic screen comprising full blood count (FBC), clotting studies, blood cultures, mid stream specimen of urine (MSSU) and possibly lumbar puncture (LP)] is indicated in a baby who is unwell, and all vomiting babies need urea and electrolytes checked. Hematemesis may require transfusion and treatment with vitamin K or fresh frozen plasma (FFP) as indicated. Stress ulceration is rare but usually settles with i.v. ranitidine or omeprazole.

Bile-stained vomiting is a more sinister sign and usually indicates NEC, obstruction or some other surgical condition. Request for a surgical opinion should always be considered. The higher the obstruction, the earlier the presentation; thus duodenal atresia, jejunal atresia, malrotation and volvulus and high duplications all present in the first 2 days of life with marked vomiting and intolerance of feeds. Low obstructions due to Hirschsprung disease, milk plug functional obstruction and anal atresia may present more insidiously with a period of constipation before vomiting starts towards the end of the first week. Meconium ileus due to cystic fibrosis presents at any time in the first week (usually in the first few days). Acquired obstruction obviously tends to present later but one should always examine the abdomen carefully for signs of strangulated herniae and intussusception and the presence of anal atresia. These conditions are discussed in more detail in Chapter 37.

The abdominal X-ray is pivotal in making the initial diagnosis. Fluid levels indicate both the obstruction and the level of obstruction. Duodenal atresia causes a classic double bubble whilst high obstructions reveal small bowel fluid levels with no gas in the rectum. Colonic disorders may have many fluid levels but often require contrast enemas to distinguish between long segment Hirschsprung disease, meconium ileus of cystic fibrosis (although abdominal calcification may be seen following intra-uterine perforation) and the even more rare true pseudo-obstruction (visceral myopathy or neuropathy). Free abdominal gas indicates an intestinal perforation that is usually due to NEC but occasionally spontaneous or associated with an atretic segment. Volvulus secondary to malrotation is dramatic with large dilated loops (the American football sign) or may be inferred from the abnormal distribution of the bowel gas in malrotation (although this usually requires upper gut contrast studies for accurate delineation). When fluid levels are less marked and the infant is sick or jaundiced, ileus due to sepsis is likely.

Surgical disorders when identified will require prompt transfer to a unit specializing in neonatal surgery. An intravenous infusion of 10% dextrose should be started and the infant kept warm in the incubator. The stomach should be aspirated hourly and the aspirate replaced as normal saline intravenously. If the infant is shocked, resuscitation with 10–20ml/kg of fluid is required. If the infant is sick, parenteral antibiotics must be started whilst awaiting the result of the septic screen. In cases of tracheoesophageal fistula, a large bore double lumen tube (Replogle tube) is passed into the proximal pouch. Air is passed into one lumen and aspirated with any secretions from the other. Continuous drainage in this way prevents apnea and aspiration episodes. The infant is nursed prone with a slight head tilt.

General disorders. Nongastrointestinal causes for vomiting must always be borne in mind. Sepsis will cause an ileus, as already described. Urinary tract infection without bacteremia, however, has long been recognized to present with gastrointestinal symptoms, most commonly with vomiting. Obstructive renal disease may also present in this way in the absence of infection. Urine culture and microscopy must always be performed. Plasma urea and electrolytes are also important to identify acidosis (renal and metabolic disease) and alkalosis (pyloric stenosis occasionally presents early in the neonatal period). Intracerebral asphyxial insults may cause vomiting acutely due to raised intracranial pressure, and meningitis may present as vomiting at any age. Other cerebral causes of vomiting such as hydrocephalus, space-occupying lesions and the diencephalic syndrome rarely present in this fashion in the neonatal period. Metabolic disorders are a cause of vomiting in the neonatal period and should always be considered if metabolic acidosis (and/or hypoglycemia) is present, or if a baby appears septic but has a metabolic alkalosis (urea cycle disorders). Galactosemia may present as early as the first day and the urine must always be tested for reducing substances. Usually the infants with metabolic disorders start vomiting after milk feeding has been established and they have been exposed to a reasonable protein load (e.g. the hyperammonemias, disorders of amino acid metabolism and the nonketotic hypoglycemias). The presence of constipation with vomiting in a dysmorphic infant may suggest the presence of idiopathic hypercalcemia; vomiting with dehydration and electrolyte disturbance (sometimes with diarrhea) may be due to congenital adrenal hyperplasia. The organic acidemias must be excluded by specific assays (dicarboxylic aciduria) on acute phase urines collected when the patient is symptomatic and, where possible, acidotic. After the first week of life acquired metabolic disorders such as diabetic ketoacidosis and Munchausen syndrome by proxy may rarely have to be considered.

Persisting vomiting/vomiting after the first week of life. Babies presenting after the first week of life tend to have acquired problems although lower intestinal obstructions, malrotation and, in the very low birth weight baby, NEC, may present later. Vomiting is one of the commonest presentations to a pediatric unit and consideration of the baby's clinical state again allows a fairly rapid differentiation of causes:

- Baby well: abdomen normal
  - posseting
  - feeding disorder
  - gastroesophageal reflux
  - gastrointestinal food allergy
  - pyloric stenosis
  - urinary tract infection

- Baby unwell: abdomen distended
  - late obstruction
  - peritonitis/appendicitis
  - intussusception
  - NEC.

Persistent vomiting even in a relatively well baby, and especially if accompanied by poor growth, may indicate a more serious underlying disorder. If investigations are normal, a feeding disorder is excluded and the vomiting still persists then the differential diagnosis usually rests between a dietary food intolerance and gastroesophageal reflux.

Gastroesophageal reflux (GOR). GOR may present with vomiting in the first month of life. It must be remembered that GOR is a physiological condition, associated with transient relaxation of the lower esophageal sphincter, and should only be investigated and treated if there is GOR-associated disease present (GORD) – esophagitis, strictures, chronic aspiration, failure to thrive. In the term baby, GORD can be investigated with upper gastrointestinal endoscopy, pH meter or radiolabeled milk scan, although many would use an empirical trial of treatment first. The role of contrast studies is not for diagnosis but rather to rule out anatomical lesions (malrotation) or esophageal strictures. Infants at risk of GORD include those with repaired esophageal atresia, those with bronchopulmonary dysplasia, and those with severe neurodevelopmental problems. Infants with severe neurodevelopmental problems develop a generalized gastrointestinal dysmotility, manifest by GOR and duodenogastric reflux, leading to bilious vomiting, and may be intractable. In the premature infant recurrent consolidation due to aspiration from GOR may lead to a disorder indistinguishable from bronchopulmonary dysplasia. GOR may also be a major cause of apneic spells resistant to methylxanthine therapy. Esophageal pH studies may confirm this, although they undoubtedly underestimate postprandial reflux in the preterm baby where the decreased acid production of the stomach is readily buffered for prolonged periods by the milk feed. Sometimes it is more practical to again treat such infants empirically. Treatment includes pharmacological, surgical and nonpharmacological, nonsurgical options such as positioning and feed thickeners. The role of the last group of measures has recently been systematically reviewed, and it was concluded that commonly used conservative measures do not have any proven efficacy in GORD in infancy.[724] Positioning at 60 degree elevation in seats was found to increase reflux compared to prone positioning, and thickened formulas reduced vomiting but not reflux.[724] The supine position is currently recommended for infants due to reduced risk of SIDS. There are no high quality randomized trials of drug or surgical therapy confined to infancy with GOR as a primary outcome, so systematic review is currently unhelpful. Antacids and alginates, prokinetic agents such as domperidone, antisecretory agents such as ranitidine, and proton pump inhibitors such as omeprazole are all used in the treatment of GORD in infancy, although few are licensed for this. Fundoplication, increasingly by the laparoscopic route, is reserved for persisting and severe GORD. Severe gastrointestinal dysmotility may require nasojejunal or transgastric jejunal feeding, with gastric (nasogastric or gastrostomy tube or gastric port) access for aspiration, drainage and medication administration.

Gastrointestinal food allergy. Food allergy is becoming increasingly common in children and may present in the first weeks of life, even in solely breast-fed babies.[725] Sensitization can occur due to minute doses of antigens (usually glycoproteins) passing into breast milk. Symptoms such as vomiting follow food ingestion, due to an abnormal immunologically mediated reaction within the gastrointestinal tract. These reactions can be type I immediate hypersensitivity, which will present with vomiting, or type IV delayed hypersensitivity, which presents with poor growth, diarrhea and rectal bleeding. For acute allergy, careful history will reveal the ingestion of an allergen, such as cows' milk protein, followed by vomiting, and occasionally pallor, diarrhea and rarely acute anaphylaxis. There is often a family history of atopy and atopic eczema may be present. The best investigation is exclusion, causing relief of symptoms, and challenge, which may need to be in a controlled environment. The presence of specific IgE antibodies and positive skin-prick tests are not valuable for delayed reactions. Treatment is elimination of cows' milk, usually by substitution with an extensively hydrolyzed protein feed or amino acid based feed (Neocate, SHS, Liverpool).

Neonatal diarrhea (Table 12.70)

Diarrhea is a relatively uncommon symptom in the neonatal period although most breast-fed children will have loose yellow seedy stools. Mothers and midwives are very clear when the stools are pathological, usually because they are watery with little or no solid matter, are increased in frequency or contain blood and mucus. The commonest cause of loose stools is phototherapy but this causes no harm as long as the fluids are increased appropriately. Loose stools may occur with nasojejunal tube feeding. The commonest serious causes of diarrhea are gastroenteritis and NEC and the latter should always be considered in infants with diarrhea. Usually, however, the characteristic bloody/mucusy stool together with the abdominal distension and X-ray signs give the diagnosis.

Outbreaks of viral gastroenteritis are not unknown in the neonatal unit and the infants respond to the normal management of such infections. Stools should be sent for cultures and electron microscopy for viruses. A full infection screen should be performed to exclude systemic causes of diarrhea. Diarrhea always causes loss of water and electrolytes, and dehydration can rapidly occur; the newborn are more susceptible

Table 12.70 Neonatal diarrhea

Etiology	Investigations
Iatrogenic	
Phototherapy	
Nasojejunal tube feeding	
Narcotic withdrawal	Drug history – maternal, neonatal
Infective	
Gastroenteritis	
Viral	Stool electron microscopy
Bacterial	Culture
Systemic infection	Infection screen
Surgical	
Necrotizing enterocolitis	Abdominal X-ray
Appendicitis	
Hirschsprung disease	Rectal examination, biopsy
Congenital enteropathy	
Lactase deficiency	Stool sugars – Clinitest, chromatography
Sucrase-isomaltase deficiency	Biopsy
Glucose-galactose malabsorption	
Congenital Na/H exchange deficiency	
Congenital chloridorrhea	Stool electrolytes/osmolality
Congenital microvillus atrophy	
Tufting enteropathy	
Abetalipoproteinemia	Fasting cholesterol/lipids + biopsy
Acrodermatitis enteropathica	Plasma zinc
Acquired enteropathy	
Food allergy	Family history, eosinophilia on biopsy
Immunodeficiency (SCID)	Immunoglobulins, lymphopenia
Metabolic disorders	
Congenital adrenal hyperplasia	Electrolytes
Dicarboxylic aciduria	Venous pH, urine organic acids
Drugs	
Antibiotics	
Prostaglandins	
Theophylline	
Pancreatic insufficiency	
Cystic fibrosis	
Shwachman–Diamond syndrome	

SCID, severe combined immunodeficiency.

to this, due to gut immaturity. The baby should be rehydrated with oral rehydration therapy (ORT) by oral or nasogastric tube, or intravenous fluids as necessary. Once replacement of deficit has occurred, reinstitution of feeds should occur, with maintenance fluids and ongoing losses replaced with ORT or i.v. fluids. Complications of diarrhea include electrolyte disturbance with acidosis, nosocomial spread of the disease (the infants should be isolated), secondary lactose intolerance (check for stool pH and reducing sugars), and secondary cows' milk protein intolerance.

Other causes of diarrhea are all rare, and may present as intractable or protracted diarrhea, defined as watery diarrhea for more than 2 weeks. It is often associated with malabsorption and undernutrition. Many of these infants eventually will be found to have a specific diagnosis,[726] but a group remains in which no primary cause can be determined. Congenital disorders of the enterocyte usually cause loose stools in the neonatal period although they may present later with intractable diarrhea since the pathological nature of the stools is not always appreciated initially. An antenatal ultrasound may have shown distended fluid-filled bowel loops. Food allergy, particularly the delayed type, may present as diarrhea. The more specific entity of cows' milk colitis, however, presents with bloody diarrhea and must be differentiated from NEC and other conditions (intussusception, Meckel's diverticulitis and volvulus). Diagnosis rests on the resolution of the symptoms after appropriate substitution of the feed. Where the infant's size and condition permit, a rectal biopsy may show eosinophils in the inflammatory infiltrate. Autoimmune enteropathy and immunodeficiency, especially severe combined immunodeficiency (SCID) and IPEX syndrome (immune dysregulation, polyendocrinopathy, enteropathy and X-linkage), may present with diarrhea and even a protein-losing enteropathy in the neonatal period. Lymphopenia on the blood film and other coexistent signs of infection (such as an interstitial pneumonia on chest X-ray) should alert one to this diagnosis. Similarly, abnormalities of the urea and electrolytes or acidosis should suggest the possibility of a metabolic disorder and one should always inquire jointly of the mother's and baby's drug history. Intractable or protracted diarrhea of infancy may helpfully be divided into those entities having normal villous–crypt axis (transport defects, acrodermatitis enteropathica, enzyme deficiency) and those with villous atrophy (congenital enterocyte disorders, autoimmune enteropathy, IPEX syndrome, allergic enteropathy and infectious and postinfectious enteropathies).[726]

Nutritional management remains the cornerstone of treatment of intractable diarrhea, and the majority require parenteral nutrition, with very careful and slow introduction of enteral feeds.[726] In many cases, home parenteral nutrition or intestinal transplantation are the only long term therapeutic options.

Neonatal constipation (Table 12.71)

The failure to pass meconium in the first 24 h in a term baby is a significant symptom and should prompt a search for the underlying cause. In a preterm baby, however, failure to open the bowels is not uncommon and many neonatal units use glycerin suppositories (chips) from day 1 to encourage bowel actions and facilitate tolerance of enteral feeds. After prematurity, the most common organic cause of constipation in the first weeks of life is Hirschsprung disease and this must be excluded by rectal examination followed by suction biopsy in all term infants when constipation follows on failure to pass meconium within the first 48 h. Hirschsprung disease has an incidence of 1 in 5000 live births, and has complex inheritance; multiple genes have been found to be involved.[727] Neonatal constipation should always be taken seriously; failure to open the bowels at least every other day is outside the range of normality. Clinical findings and simple investigations as outlined in Table 12.71 should allow one to identify most organic causes.

The management of simple constipation in the neonatal period is similar to that at an older age. Correction of a feeding disorder and provision of an adequate amount of extra water to slake thirst (especially in hot weather) will correct most cases. If this proves insufficient, intermittent suppositories are occasionally successful but more usually infants will need a stool softener (lactulose 2.5 ml b.d.) for a period of time to regularize the bowel habit. Impaction, if present, must be relieved before a regular bowel habit is restored.

Table 12.71 Neonatal constipation

Etiology	Investigation
1. Ileus	
Prematurity	Abdominal X-ray
Major insult – sepsis	Abdominal X-ray
Asphyxia	Abdominal X-ray
2. Pseudo-obstruction	
Neuropathy	Abdominal X-ray, barium meal and follow through
Myopathy	Rectal biopsy
3. Meconium plug	
4. Low bowel obstruction	
Meconium ileus/cystic fibrosis	Immunoreactive trypsin
Hirschsprung disease	Rectal examination, barium enema
Colonic atresia	
5. Anorectal anomalies	
Imperforate anus – anal atresia, anorectal atresia	Rectal examination
Rectal atresia	
Anal stenosis/stricture	
Rectal stenosis/stricture	
6. Metabolic disorder	
Hypothyroidism	Thyroxine, thyroid stimulating hormone
Hypercalcemia	Calcium
Salt- and water-losing states	Urea and electrolytes
Renal tubular acidosis	Urine pH
7. Overfeeding	

Gastrointestinal bleeding

Gastrointestinal bleeding in the newborn is a potentially serious problem.[728,729] It can present in four ways – hematemesis, hematochezia (bright red blood passed per rectum), melena or occult bleeding. The initial assessment should rapidly address the need for resuscitation, and whether bleeding is ongoing. Recognition of shock should not rely on hypotension, a late and ominous finding in infancy. Differentiation of upper from lower gastrointestinal bleeding will guide the order of investigations and the therapy. Hematemesis is a clear guide of upper bleeding, melena suggests a source far from the rectum, and hematochezia can occur with small intestinal or colonic bleeding. Diagnostic techniques include upper and lower gastrointestinal endoscopy using neonatal endoscopes, scintigraphy (Meckel's scan), ultrasonography, other imaging, and rarely laparoscopy or laparotomy.

Swallowed maternal blood explains many cases of bleeding in the newborn.[728,729] Small amounts of fresh blood or coffee-ground material in vomitus is not rare, and if self-limiting the prognosis is good. The common sources of upper gastrointestinal bleeding in the newborn are nasopharyngeal bleeding, swallowed maternal blood, esophagitis, gastritis and stress ulcer; rarer causes include vitamin K deficiency, bleeding disorders, duplication cyst, trauma from tubes, food allergy and vascular malformations. The common sources of lower gastrointestinal bleeding in the newborn are anal fissure, enteritis, intussusception, NEC, food allergy and an upper source; rarer causes include vitamin K deficiency, bleeding disorders, pseudomembranous colitis, duplication cyst, Meckel's diverticulum, Hirschsprung's enterocolitis, ischemia and vascular malformations. Treatment of all moderate and severe cases includes assessment, resuscitation, appropriate venous access, consultation with a pediatric surgeon, then identification and treatment of the cause.

Necrotizing enterocolitis

Necrotizing enterocolitis (NEC) is a much feared condition in every neonatal unit, and has a much higher incidence in the very low birth weight infant, with an incidence of 2–5% in the UK, where a survey by the British Paediatric Surveillance Unit to the end of 1994 reported over 300 new cases, with a total mortality of 22%.[730] In the USA, NEC is reported to occur in 4–13% of VLBW infants.[731] In high risk groups, such as those of birth weight < 1 kg, up to 25% of survivors experience long term adverse sequelae.[732] The etiology is unknown but is likely to be multifactorial with superinfection by gas-forming bacteria and failure of the mucosal barrier in the immature gut playing important roles. Other contributing elements include inadequate oxygen transport to the gut mucosa and substrate in the form of enteral feeds.[733] Precipitating factors include hyperosmolar feeds, perinatal asphyxia, polycythemia and umbilical vessel catheterization. A clear association has emerged between the presence of reversed end-diastolic flow in the umbilical artery in utero in the severely growth retarded infant and the development of NEC in the first weeks of life.

The prevention of NEC in the neonatal unit has been addressed in eight Cochrane reviews.[718,719,734–739] None of those concerning feeding strategies[718,719,734,735] contains enough high quality randomized trials of sufficient power to demonstrate superiority of one feeding regimen over another. Similarly, a review found only one small randomized trial of arginine supplementation to parenteral feeds to prevent NEC, with insufficient power to support this action.[736] Three randomized trials (involving 2095 newborn) of oral immunoglobulin usage were reviewed by Foster & Cole,[737] who concluded that the evidence did not currently support this strategy. Five eligible randomized trials (involving 456 infants) of enteral antibiotic prophylaxis were reviewed by Bury & Tudehope,[738] who concluded that a larger single randomized trial was needed to assess benefit and harm. A review of three randomized trials suggested restricted fluid intake for preterm infants could prevent NEC, although

one was of low methodological quality.[739] Bell[733] has reviewed other proposed strategies for the prevention of NEC, including significant risk reduction by the use of antenatal corticosteroids[740] and feeding with breast milk.[741] Schanler[742] has recently summarized three randomized trials of probiotic usage in more than 1100 preterm infants to prevent NEC, and also showed a significant risk reduction but some unanswered questions.

The disease presents with increasing aspirates (usually bile-stained) or vomiting (usually bilious but occasionally blood-stained). Diarrhea follows (or occasionally precedes) the failure to tolerate feeds and may be watery or contain mucus and visible blood and pus. The baby is often unwell, lethargic and having apneic episodes. Examination reveals a tense distended tender abdomen which is quiet (or silent if perforation has taken place). Tenderness and/or guarding suggest peritonitis has supervened and in the later stages there may be edema and inflammation of the abdominal wall (producing a 'peau d'orange' appearance in the skin) or an underlying abdominal mass. Blood cultures are positive in 18–60% of cases and septic or hypovolemic shock may be a complication and the infant may collapse and die. Diagnosis is classically made on the plain abdominal X-ray. This initially shows separation of the bowel loops due to ascites with fluid levels. Then the periluminal tramlines indicating intramural gas appear (Fig. 12.35a) especially in the cecum, ascending and descending colon and sigmoid. Later signs include gas in the portal tree (Fig. 12.35b) and gas under the diaphragm following perforation. In the early stages the diagnosis may also be suggested by the presence of a proctocolitis using an auroscope as a proctoscope.

A pancolitis is usually found at postmortem. The histology reveals a characteristic hemorrhagic inflammatory infiltration. The differential diagnoses include generalized sepsis, meconium ileus, malrotation

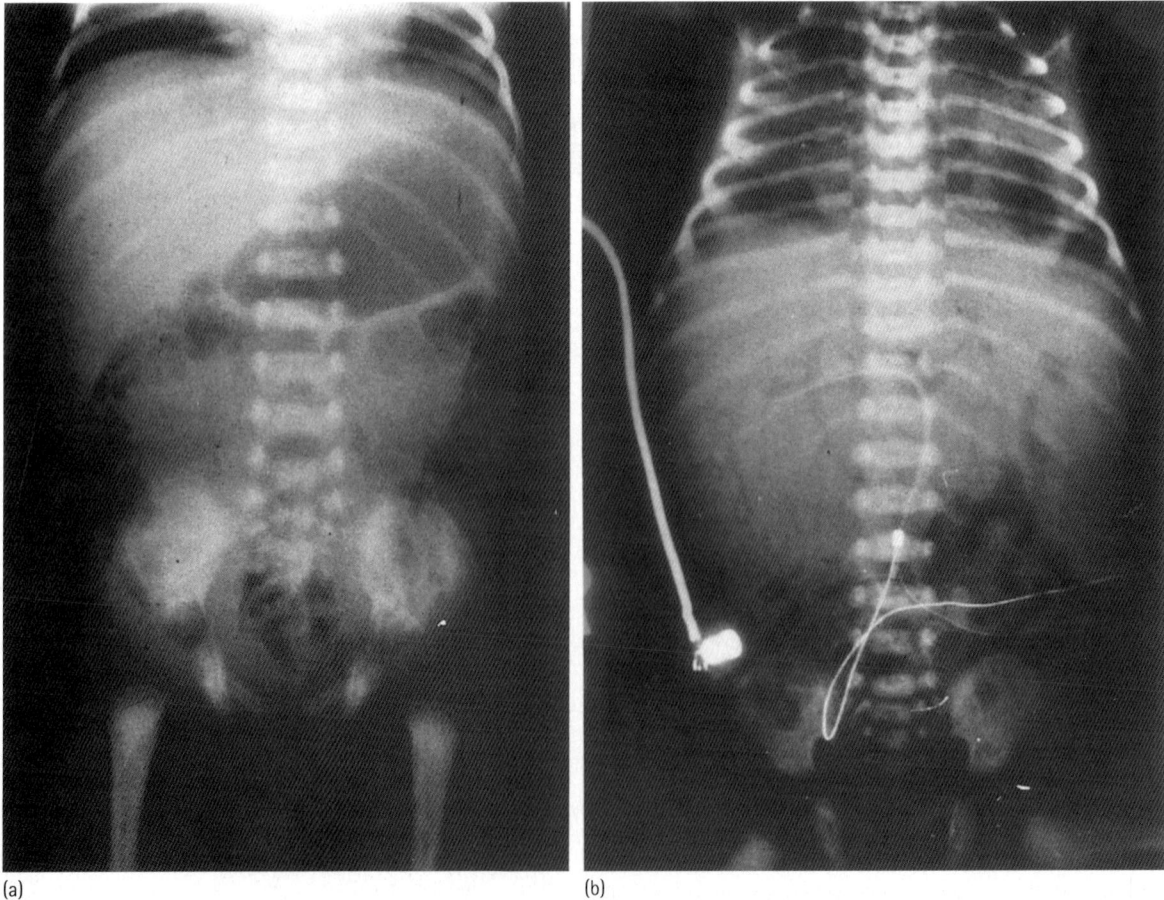

(a)   (b)

Fig. 12.35 (a) Necrotizing enterocolitis. Double lumen to the colon can be seen clearly at the hepatic flexure and triple lumen in the descending colon – both effects caused by intramural gas. (b) Gas tracts ramifying throughout the liver in portal vessels and periportal tissue. Arterial catheter is adequately sited. The venous catheter passes into the right hepatic vein.

Table 12.72 Cause of abdominal distention

1. Intestinal obstruction
2. Ileus and intestinal pseudo-obstruction
3. Intestinal perforation
   - Congenital/spontaneous
   - Acquired
4. Ascites
   - Congestive cardiac failure/hydrops fetalis
   - Peritonitis/necrotizing enterocolitis
   - Hypoalbuminemia/nephrotic syndrome
   - Urinary/ruptured urinary tract with urethral valves
   - Biliary/spontaneous rupture of bile duct
   - Chylous/disordered lymphatic drainage
5. Mass
   - Hydronephrosis
   - Congenital malignancy, Wilms'/neuroblastoma
   - Reduplication
   - Ovarian

and volvulus, hemorrhagic disease of the newborn, cows' milk colitis and intussusception and the even rarer neonatal appendicitis. The other causes of abdominal distention (Table 12.72) must also be considered, especially spontaneous perforation of the gut and other causes of ascites.

Management is initially medical and conservative.[743] Oral feeds should be stopped and the stomach placed on free drainage. A septic screen is performed and it is customary to give broad spectrum intravenous antibiotics. Blood counts, clotting screen, urea and electrolytes and albumen are checked and appropriate supportive management given as indicated. Intravenous feeding through a central line should be instituted for 10 days and the bowel rested. Afterwards feeds should be introduced slowly. Expressed breast milk or a preterm formula is used, although a protein hydrolysate may be needed as lactose and cows' milk protein intolerance are often seen in the recovery phase in these infants. Surgery is required for the acute complications of perforation, ongoing necrosis, progressive shock and bleeding, or if there is failure to improve with medical therapy. Later complications (stricture formations with subacute small bowel obstruction, blind loop syndrome and rectal bleeding) may also require surgery, as may a recurrence which occurs in 10% of patients. Short bowel syndrome (see below) may occur.

Neonatal intestinal failure

Intestinal failure is defined as a reduction of functional gut mass below that needed to allow sufficient digestion and absorption of fluids and nutrients for growth in infants and children.[744] In neonatal practice, this will be severe congenital or early onset disorders needing protracted or indefinite parenteral nutrition. Intestinal failure is usually divided into three groups:[744,745] an anatomical reduction giving short bowel syndrome (SBS), neuromuscular disease of the gastrointestinal tract such as chronic intestinal pseudo-obstruction syndrome (myopathy or neuropathy) or long segment Hirschsprung syndrome, and lastly the congenital enterocyte disorder such as microvillous inclusion disease and intestinal epithelial dysplasia. Short bowel syndrome is by far the predominant cause of neonatal intestinal failure and is therefore considered in more detail below. The small intestine is only 115 cm length at 27 weeks and is 250 cm at term. There is maximal growth in the first year of life and adults have a mean of 6.2 m. The capacity for small intestinal growth is highest in preterm infants. There is regional gut function, with the stomach acting as a reservoir, then the jejunum has most nutrient absorption but is very porous for water and electrolytes. The ileum is involved mainly in fluid and electrolyte absorption, with less general absorption of nutrients except for specific absorption of vitamin B_{12} and bile acids. The ileocecal valve acts as a barrier to colonic bacteria and in the colon there is absorption of sodium, water and some carbohydrate and fat.

The early management of intestinal failure in the neonatal unit is vital. This includes:

- careful charting of input and output;
- use of a stoma bag to measure effluent if applicable;
- replacement of stoma losses in terms of fluid and electrolytes;
- meticulous checking of growth, recording of growth and consultation of the results;
- checking of urinary sodium levels, even when serum levels are normal;
- a very slow increase in enteral feeds, be it expressed breast milk, protein hydrolysate or elemental feed;
- use of continuous enteral feeding via a pump;
- treatment of gastric hyperacidity with H_2 receptor agonists or proton pump inhibitors.

Short bowel syndrome is defined functionally, rather than anatomically; it exists where there is malabsorption in the presence of a shortened small intestine. Intestinal adaptation begins with gut resection and there is epithelial hyperplasia to increase surface area and later muscular hypertrophy. This will result in improved digestive and absorptive function, and the ileum has the best adaptive capacity. This process will not occur without enteral nutrition. The consequences of a major loss of small bowel include malabsorption of nutrients, vitamins and minerals, gastric acid hypersecretion, functional pancreatic insufficiency, water and electrolyte losses, hyperoxaluria, biliary lithiasis, liver disease and bone disease. The relative degree of jejunal, ileal and colonic loss in this syndrome determines the pathophysiological effects and thus the management. By far the commonest cause of short bowel syndrome is NEC, but many other prenatal (vascular accidents, atresias, volvulus, abdominal wall defects) and postnatal (volvulus, thrombosis) etiologies exist.

The development and refinement of parenteral nutrition, techniques and equipment for prolonged central venous access, new enteral formula development and the back-up of intestinal and/or liver transplantation have changed this disorder from one that was fatal 30 years ago to one where infants may have a prolonged life span into adult life.[745] Management of short bowel syndrome is a gradually changing multistage process.[744,745] There has to be institution of appropriate parenteral nutrition and restoration of fluid and electrolyte balance. When the infant is stabilized, enteral feeding should be initiated. The aim is to increase enteral feeds within the limits of tolerance until weaned from TPN. If parenteral nutrition will be prolonged, management at home should be considered, with appropriate training and support. Once a child has adapted, parenteral nutrition should be stopped and the child maintained on a combination of oral and/or enteral tube feeding. The child will continue to need to be monitored for growth and complications. Given that it is a relatively rare and highly complex problem, assessment and management must involve tertiary center pediatric gastroenterologists and pediatric surgeons.

There are few randomized trials of components of management of short bowel syndrome. Other medical management includes treating hypergastrinemia, cycling TPN, and treatment of small bowel bacterial overgrowth. Surgical management includes stricturoplasties, tapering procedures and consideration of small bowel and/or liver transplant if vascular access or chronic liver disease become problematic. Complications include macro- and micro-nutrient deficiency, intestinal failure-associated liver disease,[746] central venous catheter thrombosis and infection, and small bowel bacterial overgrowth. Prognosis depends upon presence of the ileocecal valve, length and quality of remaining bowel, number of anastomoses, and small bowel bacterial overgrowth. Intestinal failure and short bowel syndrome are discussed further in Chapter 19.

BILIRUBIN METABOLISM[747,748]

Bilirubin is one of the end products of heme catabolism and in normal circumstances has to be processed by the liver for its excretion. In early neonatal life there is a much greater production of bilirubin.

The hemoglobin mass at birth is high (and further increased by such factors as delayed clamping of the cord) and contains approximately 80% fetal hemoglobin. This is replaced within 4 months by adult hemoglobin. This obligatory red cell turnover is the major factor in the excess bilirubin production (each 1 g Hb produces 600 µmol of bilirubin). To this must be added the bilirubin produced by bruising, cephalhematoma and shunt bilirubin (bilirubin produced by heme pigments in the reticuloendothelial system that are never incorporated into hemoglobin: approximately 20% of the total bilirubin production).

Heme is metabolized to biliverdin by heme oxygenase (Fig. 12.36)[749] which is found in the liver, spleen and macrophages and whose activity is increased many-fold in the face of such an increased substrate load. The biliverdin is rapidly reduced to bilirubin by biliverdin reductase using NADPH as a proton donor. The end product, bilirubin XIIa, is insoluble because of the hydrogen bonding between the two pyrrole rings (a process facilitated by the ionization of the molecule that occurs below pH 7.4) (Fig. 12.37).[750] The insoluble bilirubin is tightly bound to albumin (binding capacity 0.5–1.0 mmol bilirubin per mol albumin). At a bilirubin concentration of 340 mmol/L the molar ratio exceeds 1:1 and dissociation of the bilirubin occurs readily. Because of its fat solubility (increased at low pH) this bilirubin is readily deposited in the tissues.

Bilirubin is transported through the hepatocyte membrane by a carrier-mediated process and is then carried to the endoplasmic reticulum after binding to cytosolic glutathione-S-transferases (ligandins). These also have low concentrations at birth but increase to adult levels by 5–10 days of age. In the endoplasmic reticulum the bilirubin is conjugated with a uridine moiety to bilirubin monoglucuronide by the enzyme glucuronyltransferase, properly termed UGT1A1, which is essential for efficient biliary excretion of bilirubin. UGT1A1 also has a low activity at birth but following induction by the high bilirubin load, adult levels are reached by 14 days of age irrespective of gestation (a birth-related event). The activity of this enzyme can be induced by phenobarbitone or other microsomal enzyme-inducing drugs. The bilirubin monoglucuronide is further converted to bilirubin diglucuronide by UGT1A1 and then transported across the canalicular membrane by an energy-dependent carrier-mediated system, using various export pumps, including MRPR2, MDR3 and the bile salt export pump.[748] Conjugated bilirubin is excreted into the duodenum. Degradation by intestinal bacteria produces urobilinogen, most of which is reabsorbed from the intestine and undergoes enterohepatic recirculation. A minor fraction is excreted in the urine. The oxidation product urobilin/stercobilin contributes color to normal urine and stools.

The excretory mechanisms described above result in a high concentration of bilirubin in the bile. In the adult this consists mostly of bilirubin IXa, a pigment which cannot be excreted without conjugation which alters its involuted hydrogen-bonded conformation. However, the other bilirubin isomers can be excreted directly in the bile since they are naturally water soluble. The major photochemical effect of phototherapy makes use of this fact. Under blue light (420–480 nm) bilirubin IXa is converted by photoisomerization to Z-lumirubin (Fig. 12.38).[751] There is a 180 degree rotation of a terminal pyrrole which prohibits intramolecular hydrogen bonding, thus disrupting the tertiary structure of the bilirubin IXa isomer, and exposes the carboxyl radical, thus creating a polar water-soluble pigment which can be excreted in the bile.

The newborn infant is unable to cope with the normal bilirubin load and thus a degree of jaundice is to be expected. This is recognized by the term physiological jaundice of the newborn. Postnatally there is a rapid rise in the bilirubin due to a combination of high bilirubin load and decreased hepatic excretion. Following the initial rise there is a slow fall due to the slow development of hepatic carrier proteins (induction of ribosomal enzyme complexes). The maximum allowable level of physiological jaundice is not clear. A level as low as 210 µmol/L by the third day of life has been claimed to indicate the need for further investigation but, in practice, most clinicians probably would not investigate the cause of jaundice unless the patient required phototherapy or other clinical features were present, the most important of which is the postnatal age of patient.

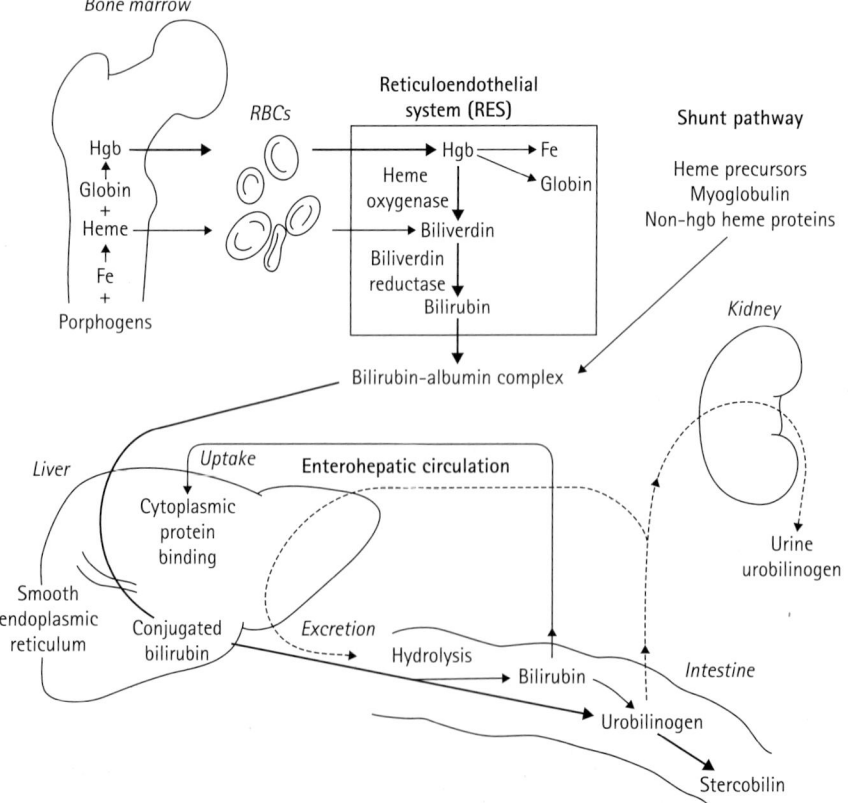

Fig. 12.36   The pathway of bilirubin production, transport and metabolism. (From Garcia 1972,[749] reprinted with permission.)

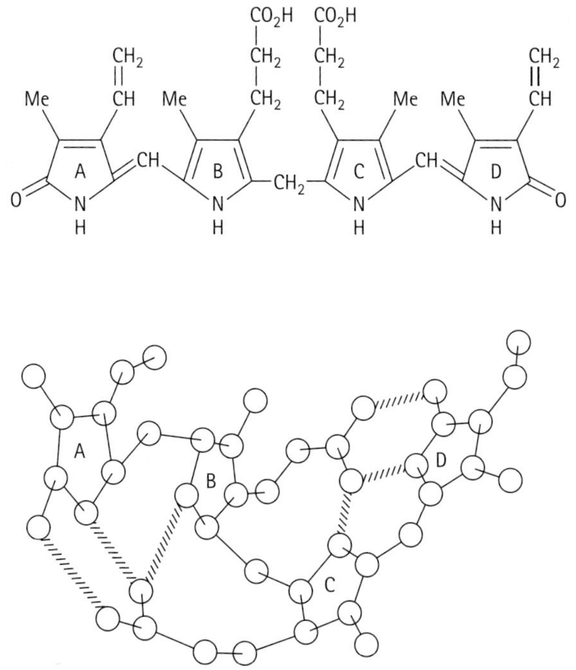

Fig. 12.37 Primary structure of bilirubin above, and below tertiary structure with hydrogen bonds shown as shaded lines. This folded structure serves to mask the polar carboxyl residues and renders the bilirubin molecule water insoluble/fat soluble. (From Schmidt 1978[750].)

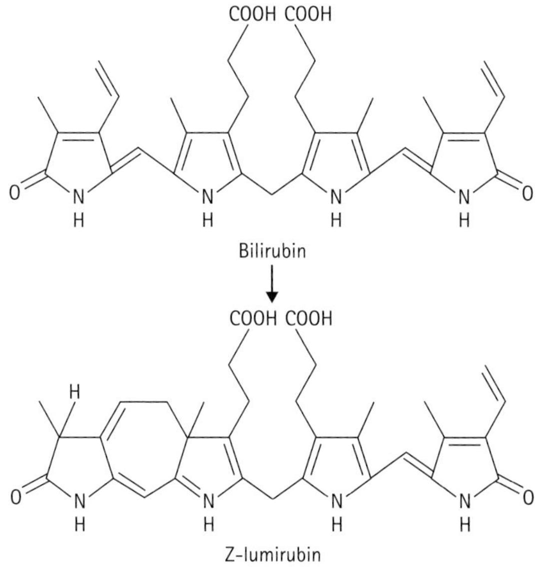

Bilirubin

Z-lumirubin

Fig. 12.38 Photoisomerization by light converts the stable isomer of bilirubin to the thermodynamically unstable Z-lumirubin (From McDonagh et al 1982[751].)

NEONATAL JAUNDICE (Table 12.73)

Early jaundice (< 10 days)

First 24 hours (hemolytic disease of the newborn, HDN)

This is by far the most dangerous form of jaundice in the newborn as the bilirubin levels can rise rapidly into the toxic range. The most common cause is rhesus hemolytic disease although with current obstetric management it is now rare in resource rich countries. Sensitization of the mother (usually by small fetomaternal transfusions in previous pregnancies and particularly deliveries) will result in the production of anti-D IgM and IgG. The latter is responsible for rhesus disease in the

Table 12.73 Neonatal jaundice

Mechanism	Cause	Investigation
1. Early jaundice (< 10 days)		
a. *First 24 h*		
Immune hemolysis	Rhesus disease	Direct Coombs' test
	ABO incompatibility	Maternal/infant
	Rare blood group antibodies	blood group
Non-immune hemolysis	Glucose-6-phosphate dehydrogenase (G6PD) deficiency	Family history G6PD assay
	Pyruvate kinase (PK) deficiency	PK assay
	Congenital spherocytosis	Blood film
		Full blood count
Sepsis		Septic screen
b. *After 24 h*		
Physiological jaundice	Prematurity	
	Hypoglycemia	
	Hypoxia	
	Dehydration intestinal stasis	
Excess bilirubin production	Bruising	
	Cephalohematoma	
	Disseminated intravascular coagulation	
	Intraventricular hemorrhage	
	Polycythemia	Full blood count
	Ingestion maternal blood (Melena)	
Infection	Sepsis	Septic screen
	Intrauterine infection	IgM, torch screen
Congenital nonhemolytic hyperbilirubinemia	Crigler–Najjar syndrome Gilbert syndrome	
Metabolic	Galactosemia	Urine-reducing substances
Congenital hemolytic anemia		
2. Prolonged jaundice (> 10 days)		
a. *Prolonged unconjugated hyperbilirubinemia*		
Breast milk	Breast milk jaundice	Trial of formula milk
	Inhibitor of glucuronyl transferase	
Sepsis	New/persisting	Full blood count, septic screen
Metabolic	Hypothyroidism	Thyroxine, TSH
	Aminoacidemias	Plasma/urine amino acids
	Galactosemia	Urine-reducing substances
	Fructosemia	Liver function tests
	Cystic fibrosis	Immunoreactive trypsin
Increased enterohepatic circulation	Intestinal obstruction	Abdominal X-ray
	Pyloric stenosis	
	Atresia	
	Hirschsprung disease	
	Meconium ileus	
	Meconium plug	
	Pseudo-obstruction	
	Fasting	
	Underfeeding	
	Drugs	

(Continued)

Table 12.73 Neonatal jaundice—cont'd

Mechanism	Cause	Investigation
Persisting hemolysis	Rhesus incompatibility (inspissated bile syndrome)	
	Hemoglobinopathy	
	G6PD deficiency, PK deficiency	
	Vitamin E deficiency	
Congenital nonhemolytic hyperbilirubinemia	Crigler–Najjar syndrome	
	Gilbert syndrome	
Decreased hepatic uptake	Persisting shunt through ductus venosus	
b. *Prolonged conjugated hyperbilirubinemia*		
Intrahepatic cholestasis		
Infections		
Acquired	Septicemia/bacteremia	Septic screen, chest X-ray
	Urinary tract infection	MSU
	Listeriosis	
	Tuberculosis	
Congenital	Syphilis	
	Malaria	
	Toxoplasmosis	Torch screen
	Hepatitis B, C	Hepatitis B antigen, DNA
		Hepatitis A IgM, HCV RNA
	Epstein–Barr virus	Viral titers
	Rubella	Viral titers
	Coxsackie B, A9	Viral titers
	Cytomegalovirus	Viral titers
	Varicella-zoster	Viral titers
	Herpes simplex	Viral titers
	ECHO virus, adenovirus	Viral titers
	HIV infection	Maternal HIV titers
	Parvovirus B19	
Metabolic disorders	Alpha1-antitrypsin deficiency	Alpha1-antitrypsin
	Cystic fibrosis	Immunoreactive trypsin
		Sweat test
	Galactosemia	Urine-reducing substances
	Fructosemia	WBC enzyme assay
	Tyrosinemia	Plasma/urine amino acids
	GM1 gangliosidosis	Storage vacuoles Lymphocytes
	Gaucher syndrome	WBC enzyme assays
	Niemann–Pick disease	Urine oligosaccharides
	Mucopolysaccharidosis	Urine mucopolysac-charides
	Sialosis	
	Wolman disease	
	Zellweger syndrome	Serum catalase/VLC fatty acids
	Dubin–Johnson syndrome	
	Rotor syndrome	
	Glutaric aciduria Type II	Urine organic acids
	Bile acid synthesis disorders	

Table 12.73 cont'd

Mechanism	Cause	Investigation
Endocrine	Hypothyroidism	Thyroxine, TSH
	Hypoadrenalism	Urea and electrolytes, 17-OH-progesterone, cortisol, aldosterone
	Hypopituitarism	ACTH
	Diabetes insipidus	Plasma/urine osmolality
	Hypoparathyroidism	
Vascular	Veno-occlusive disease	Ultrasound liver
	Poor perfusion syndromes	
	Budd–Chiari syndrome	
	Hemangioendothelioma	
	Lymphatic defects, familial cholestasis with lymphedema	
Miscellaneous	Infantile polycystic disease	Ultrasound kidney and liver
	Toxins	
	Parenteral nutrition	
	Drugs	
	Halothane	
	Chromosomal disorders – trisomies 21, 18, 13	Chromosomes
	Biliary duct paucity (Alagille syndrome, non-syndromic)	
	Progressive familial intrahepatic cholestasis (Byler syndrome)	
	Posthemolytic hepatic dysfunction	
	Neonatal lupus	
Idiopathic neonatal hepatitis		
Extrahepatic cholestasis	Extrahepatic biliary atresia	
	Choledochal cyst	Ultrasound liver
	Bile duct stenosis	
	Spontaneous perforation of bile duct	Abdominal X-ray, ascites
	Gallstones	
	Ascending cholangitis	

ACTH, adrenocorticotropic hormone; HCV, hepatitis C virus; MSU, mid stream urine; PK, pyruvic kinase; TSH, thyroid stimulating hormone; VLC fatty acids, very long chain fatty acids; WBC, white blood cells.

neonate which is characterized by a (often highly) positive Coombs' test and extravascular hemolysis in the spleen. ABO incompatibility, now the most common cause for HDN (mother usually blood group O, infant blood group A or B) in the UK, occurs in 15% of pregnancies. It is particularly common in those of African origin. Again the IgG antibody is the important hemolysin but in this case the Coombs' test is often negative (possibly due to the decreased number of A and B sites on the fetal erythrocyte). Laboratory investigation is notoriously unreliable at predicting infants at risk from ABO hemolytic disease but microspherocytosis on the blood film is a useful diagnostic pointer to the condition. Red blood cell destruction occurs primarily by extravascular mechanisms and is more rapid in ABO incompatibility with the antibody disappearing within 2–3 days. Occasionally minor blood group antibodies (anti-Kell, anti-Duffy) cause hemolytic disease and these are usually Coombs' positive.

Hemolysis also occurs in the absence of blood group incompatibility. Sepsis is said to cause jaundice at this age and should always be excluded. In fact, it rarely turns out to be responsible for such early jaundice but congenital infections, e.g. rubella, syphilis and toxoplasmosis, can present this way. The most common non-immunological cause of hemolytic jaundice within 24 h is congenital hemolytic anemia due to a red cell metabolic defect [e.g. glucose-6-phosphate dehydrogenase (G6PD) deficiency or pyruvic kinase (PK) deficiency] or structural defect (congenital spherocytosis, elliptocytosis and pyknocytosis). In these cases there is often a family history. G6PD deficiency occurs more commonly in patients of Mediterranean, African or Oriental origin. Appropriate hematological investigations and enzyme assays usually provide a rapid diagnosis.

After 24 hours

Sixty-five percent of normal neonates exhibit clinical jaundice (85 μmol/L or 5 mg/dL). In most patients excessive jaundice at this stage is due to exacerbation of the normal physiological jaundice of the newborn. The 95th percentile for term infants is 190 μmol/L (11.5 mg/dl) for bottle-fed and 240 μmol/L (14.5 mg/dl) for breast-fed infants. The more premature the infant the more immature the liver although this may be balanced by decreased bilirubin production since exchange transfusion is rarely required despite the almost obligatory use of phototherapy in infants of less than 30 weeks' gestation. Excessive production of bilirubin from severe bruising or cephalhematomata, polycythemia or ingestion of maternal blood commonly causes jaundice in this period.

The most important cause to consider is acquired bacterial infection or rarely congenitally transmitted infections (CMV, rubella, toxoplasmosis, syphilis). Direct involvement of the liver by the infective process is one reason for the jaundice, as is increased bilirubin breakdown with disseminated intravascular coagulation. However, it is likely that the nature of the hyperbilirubinemia is multifactorial.

Inadequate calorie intake and decreased glucose production will lead to a reduction in glycogen and energy available for the production and conversion of the uridine diphosphoglucuronic acid required for the conjugation of the bilirubin glucuronyltransferase. Acidosis may increase bilirubin levels but, more importantly, increases bilirubin toxicity due to the alteration of the equilibrium between free bilirubin and its acid salt, thus decreasing the maximum tolerable level of bilirubin. Dehydration probably increases the bilirubin levels by prolonging gut transit and therefore increasing the enterohepatic circulation. In such conditions as failure to pass meconium, pyloric stenosis and cystic fibrosis with meconium ileus, there will be an increase in the hydrolysis of the conjugated bilirubin by the alkaline duodenal juices and the mucosal beta-glucuronidases of the small intestine, thus increasing the bilirubin returned to the blood via the enterohepatic circulation.

In most cases of neonatal jaundice, the bilirubin levels will fall below the phototherapy range before the end of the second week of life. However, in the premature infant phototherapy may be required for longer. One group of patients that presents with severe early neonatal jaundice that continues beyond the first 10 days (and may also present later) are the rare patients with congenital nonhemolytic hyperbilirubinemias. The most important of these, Crigler–Najjar syndrome, presents as two variants:

1. the autosomal recessive type I with absence of uridine diphosphoglucuronyltransferase (UDPGT) in the liver, characterized by persistent severe unconjugated hyperbilirubinemia;
2. the autosomal dominant type II with defective rather than absent UDPGT activity in which the bilirubin levels are lower (< 340 μmol/L).

This latter variant (known also as Arias syndrome) may present much later in life and for this reason is said to merge diagnostically into the commonest of the unconjugated hyperbilirubinemias, Gilbert syndrome, which is more common in men and usually presents after puberty. The other familial conjugated hyperbilirubinemias (Dubin–Johnson and Rotor syndrome) hardly ever present at birth.

Management of early jaundice

Investigation and treatment of cause. It is important that the etiology of the hyperbilirubinemia should be established. A careful obstetric and family history (e.g. spherocytosis) is important. A full blood count, direct Coombs' test, grouping of mother and baby and testing the urine for reducing substances are the usual minimum of investigations required. If infection is suspected a septic and TORCH (congenital infection) screen can be added. Where the hemolysis remains unexplained further hematological investigation (e.g. enzyme assays for G6PD deficiency and PK deficiency) will be needed. In most cases no treatment for the cause of the hemolysis will be available though it behoves the pediatrician to ensure that the mother is given anti-D globulin where indicated. Advice on drugs to be avoided in the future must be made available to the patients with G6PD deficiency. Infection should be treated as indicated.

Treatment of jaundice. *Phototherapy.* The aim of therapy is to keep the level of bilirubin below the toxic level. Phototherapy must be started early enough to prevent the expected rise in bilirubin but not at a level which causes unnecessary work for the nursing staff and, more importantly, an unnecessary separation of mother and baby. Most units have their own chart for plotting bilirubin levels and action lines to indicate the levels at which phototherapy (and exchange transfusion) are indicated. Where a rapidly rising bilirubin is expected such as hemolytic disease and jaundice at less than 24 h, phototherapy should be started straight away and the sequential bilirubin results should be graphed. At a later stage the need for phototherapy is more debatable. As a general rule the more premature the infant the lower the levels of bilirubin that are tolerated and thus a good guiding figure is that phototherapy is indicated when the bilirubin rises above a level given by the formula: birth weight in kg × 100. In term babies, phototherapy should be given when the bilirubin rises above 300 μmol/L.

There are many potential complications to phototherapy:

1. Equipment failure/design drawbacks: the lamps must produce radiation in the blue range of 450–460 nm with a minimum irradiance of flux of 4 μW/m²/nm. The new generation of phototherapy units is much more efficient than the old (although the blue light is off-putting for the parents). It seems prudent to protect the eyes since changes of premature aging have been induced by phototherapy in newborn monkeys but no detrimental effect is recorded in the human infant.
2. Dehydration: this is by far the most important complication and is the result of increased insensible water loss through the skin and increased stool water content. Increasing the fluid intake of infants under phototherapy by 15 ml/kg/day will correct this.
3. Loose stools: Z-lumirubin excreted in the bile is a highly polar, nonphysiological substance which has a direct secretory effect on intestinal mucosa leading, inevitably, to loose stools. These are not troublesome and frank diarrhea never results. The increased fluid intake is the only therapeutic manipulation required. (Lactose intolerance, however, may also occur.)
4. Parental anxiety: the separation of mother and baby and the terrible color given to the infant by the effective blue lamps are naturally upsetting to parents and a sympathetic explanation of what is happening is mandatory. The best way of minimizing this anxiety is to pay scrupulous attention to the need for phototherapy and to minimize the duration of such therapy.
5. Other effects have been noted experimentally (copper retention, abnormal porphyrin metabolism and damage to DNA in cell cultures) but they do not seem relevant in clinical practice. Bronzing or discoloration of the skin can also occur when phototherapy is used in patients with a cholestatic element to their jaundice.

Exchange transfusion. The exchange transfusion of blood via an umbilical artery or vein is the most efficient way of removing bilirubin (and other noxious substances). It is employed when bilirubin levels reach the toxic range determined both by the gestational age and the clinical state of the baby. Sicker babies with their attendant metabolic derangements such as acidosis are transfused at lower levels. Acceptable criteria for exchange transfusion would be a serum bilirubin of 340 μmol/L (term babies), 300 μmol/L (infants < 2500 g), 250 μmol/L (infants <1500 g) and 170 μmol/L (infants < 1000 g). In practice, however, most exchange transfusions in the smaller infants (<1500 g) are performed for reasons other than jaundice (usually a septic child in extremis or for disseminated intravascular coagulation). Most physicians would not immediately exchange an asymptomatic term baby even with severe physiological jaundice greater than 340 μmol/L assuming there was a fairly prompt response to phototherapy (usually given with double lamps in such situations). The commonest indication for exchange transfusion is a rapidly rising bilirubin in the first 24 h of life in babies with hemolytic disease of the newborn (p. 288). The technique is described on page 288. The complications are listed in Table 12.74 together with suitable avoiding action.

Other methods. Attention to clinical detail (for example the correction of acidosis, treatment of infection and maintenance of hemodynamic stability) is valuable. In the small premature infant judicious use of 20% albumen (4–5 ml/kg) will buy time under phototherapy and often obviate the need for a formal exchange transfusion. In the rarer congenital nonhemolytic disorders (Crigler–Najjar type II and Rotor syndrome) hepatic enzyme inducers such as phenobarbitone (1–8 mg/kg/24 h) are used in addition to prolonged daily phototherapy to control the bilirubin levels.

Prolonged jaundice

Any jaundice beyond 10 days in a term infant is pathological but preterm infants (especially very low birth weight infants) often have jaundice that persists beyond this time for which no cause is found. It is probably wise, however, to investigate all these patients in the same way so that rarer conditions presenting in premature infants are not missed. The basic investigation is the estimation of the percentage of conjugated bilirubin; the majority of patients will have an unconjugated hyperbilirubinemia (conjugated bilirubin <25% of total). Conjugated hyperbilirubinemia (>25% of total) is an indication of intra- or extrahepatic cholestasis and is accompanied by bilirubinuria and dark urine (conjugated bilirubin >25 μmol/L). Early diagnosis, supportive care and specific therapy is mandatory.[752]

Prolonged unconjugated hyperbilirubinemia

Breast milk jaundice. The usual cause of such prolonged jaundice is breast milk jaundice but to diagnose this without estimating the percentage of conjugated bilirubin would be negligent. The bilirubin is usually less than 200 μmol/L, but can rise to values up to 400 μmol/L (usually less than 20% conjugated); the patient, however, is well and no treatment is necessary.[753,754] The jaundice usually settles by about 6 weeks although it may occasionally continue up to 4 months. Discontinuation of breast-feeding leads to a rapid fall in the bilirubin. The etiology of this condition long remained obscure and was thought to be due to various constituents of the milk. Breast milk consists of milk constituents which are parceled in maternal breast milk membrane prior to their secretion from the acini of the gland. This membrane is a protein structure and has a functional activity in its own right, e.g. enzymatic (breast milk lipase) and transport (membrane-bound iron). Both of these greatly increase the nutritional efficiency of milk. In patients with breast milk jaundice a beta-glucuronidase has been shown to be present in mother's milk and in the infant's feces (the activity in the stool disappearing with the cessation of breast-feeding coincident with a fall in unconjugated hyperbilirubinemia). It seems likely, therefore, that breast milk jaundice is due to the breast milk beta-glucuronidase causing deconjugation of the bilirubin diglucuronide and intestinal absorption of the fat-soluble bilirubin through the intestinal mucosa, increasing the enterohepatic circulation of bilirubin (Fig. 12.36) and thus increasing the level of unconjugated bilirubin in the blood.[749] It is relevant at this point to contrast this with the mechanism seen in the very rare Lucy Driscoll syndrome in which there is a definite inhibitor of bilirubin glucuronide in mother's milk (recoverable in the infant's serum) and which results in the development of jaundice in all of the mother's offspring (despite her apparent good health). This entity may present in the first few days of life and is occasionally severe enough to require exchange transfusion.

Hypothyroidism. It is mandatory to exclude hypothyroidism as a cause of persistent unconjugated hyperbilirubinemia although in countries with a neonatal screening program for hypothyroidism this is hardly ever a presenting symptom.

Intestinal stasis. The second most common cause now for persistent unconjugated jaundice is an increased enterohepatic circulation of bilirubin. In the normal situation 25% of the conjugated bilirubin reaching the duodenum is deconjugated and reabsorbed. This may be increased in situations of stasis where the alkaline intestinal juices and the mucosal bilirubin diglucuronidases (together with bacterial organisms in conditions of overgrowth) have longer to act on this substrate. Thus surgical conditions such as Hirschsprung disease, intestinal atresia, pyloric stenosis and the meconium ileus of cystic fibrosis are often complicated by jaundice. Cystic fibrosis may also cause unconjugated jaundice due to hepatic involvement, and such involvement may explain why other conditions can present in this fashion (i.e. sepsis, galactosemia and fructosemia).

Hemolytic causes. Finally, the hemolytic anemias, especially rhesus hemolytic disease and more consistently the rare hemolytic congenital hyperbilirubinemias, will be a cause of prolonged unconjugated jaundice. The management of all such jaundice is the identification and treatment of the underlying disorder as indicated in Table 12.73.

Prolonged conjugated hyperbilirubinemia

This discussion will center on the presentation of the child with prolonged conjugated jaundice to the general pediatrician. The more complicated perspective of the specialist referral center will be dealt with in the section on liver disease (Ch. 19). The main aim of the general pediatrician is to recognize that a cholestatic syndrome is present. The signs listed in Table 12.75 should alert the physician to the presence of such a syndrome. Whilst jaundice is the usual presenting symptom, other complications, especially bruising and other evidence of defective hemostasis, hypoalbuminemia or hypoglycemia may also be presenting features. (One should never diagnose hemorrhagic disease of the newborn, especially in a jaundiced child, without checking the liver function tests and percentage conjugated bilirubin.) Clues that suggest an underlying disorder are shown in Table 12.75.

The management of prolonged cholestatic jaundice is aimed at identifying conditions requiring immediate treatment and supportive therapy and then distinguishing between intra- and extrahepatic cholestasis. Blood cultures and a septic screen together with a screen

Table 12.74 Complications of exchange transfusion

Infection	Sepsis	Strict aseptic technique Fresh blood
	CMV	Appropriate screening donors
	Hepatitis	
Hypothermia		Warm blood/baby
Cardiovascular instability	Transient hypovolemia	Small aliquots (10–20 ml)
	Hypervolemia	Meticulous recording of exchanges
	Cardiac dysrhythmia	Cardiac monitoring
Electrolyte disorders	Hyperkalemia	Monitor electrolytes and blood sugar before and after exchange
	Hypoglycemia	
	Hypocalcemia	Check citrate concentration of donor blood
	Acidosis	
Complications of catheter	Embolic	Minimize duration of catheterization
	Hemorrhage (late portal vein thrombosis)	
Inadequate exchange		Use 170–200 ml/kg over 100 min for full exchange

Table 12.75 Clinical features that alert one to the presence of conjugated hyperbilirubinemia

a. *Evidence of hepatic disease*

Jaundice	Urine – Yellow, not colorless from birth. Dark later with bilirubin⁺⁺ on Stick test
	Stools – Pale yellow to white (may be green)
Hepatomegaly	
Pruritus	
Splenomegaly, ascites, edema	
Evidence of bleeding tendency	–Bruising
	Bleeding
Failure to thrive	
Investigations –	Increased bilirubin, conjugated bilirubin >80%
	Increased alanine aminotransferase
	Increased aspartate transaminase
	Increased γ-glutamyltransferase
	Increased α-fetoprotein
	Prolonged prothrombin time
	Low albumin
	Low blood sugar

b. *Features of underlying etiology*

Maternal history, skin lesions	– Congenital infections
Purpura, choroidoretinitis	– Congenital infections
Cataracts	Galactosemia (urine positive for reducing substances)
	Lowe syndrome (aminoaciduria)
Multiple congenital	– Trisomy 13, 18, 21 abnormalities
Ascites, bile-stained hernia	– Spontaneous perforation of bile ducts
Cystic mass below the liver	– Choledochal cyst
Situs inversus, midline, liver	– Extrahepatic biliary atresia
Malposition of the viscera	– Biliary hypoplasia
Systolic murmur, dysmorphic facies	
Cutaneous hemangioma	– Hepatic/biliary hemangiomata
Marked splenomegaly	– Lysosomal storage disorder
Hypoglycemia	– Pituitary deficiency

c. *Features indicating the nature of the cholestasis*

Incomplete stool pallor	– Intrahepatic cholestasis plus low birth weight, moderate hepatomegaly
Complete stool pallor:	– Intrahepatic cholestasis
<10 days transient	
>10 days permanent	– Extrahepatic cholestasis
	Plus normal birth weight, firm hard hepatomegaly

for intrauterine infections (TORCH, VDRL) should be sent in all infants. Parenteral antibiotics should be started if the infant appears unwell. Urine should be tested for reducing substances and sent for sugar chromatography to exclude galactosemia and fructosemia. It is also sensible to exclude galactose and fructose from the diet until the results of this are known. It should be remembered that all infants less than 2 weeks of age (and babies with renal tubular disorders, e.g. Lowe syndrome) can have reducing substances in the urine. Furthermore, infants with liver disease can both have sugar in the urine and present with septicemia. Initial investigations should include urine for amino acid chromatography to identify particularly tyrosinemia, and blood for alpha1-antitrypsin phenotyping and serum immunoreactive trypsin (if available), or fecal elastase. Endocrinological disorders and other rare metabolic disorders should be considered and investigated as seems appropriate to the infant. Liver function tests are not discriminatory but serum alpha-fetoprotein is particularly raised in tyrosinemia. A hemorrhagic diathesis should be

treated with vitamin K (1 mg i.v.) and fresh frozen plasma if bleeding continues. Other supportive measures for liver failure may be needed.

The next step is to distinguish between intra- and extrahepatic cholestasis. The color of the stool is a useful guide (Table 12.75). Incomplete stool pallor together with evidence of intrauterine growth retardation suggests a prenatal hepatitis causing intrahepatic cholestasis. Complete stool pallor lasting longer than 2 weeks, especially if accompanied by a large hard liver or a conjugated bilirubin level of >80%, suggests extrahepatic biliary obstruction and referral to a specialist to exclude biliary atresia is required without delay. Where the diagnosis is less clear cut or delay in referral is experienced, a hepatobiliary ultrasound (to exclude a choledochal cyst) or technetium-99 m HIDA cholescintigraphy (to demonstrate hepatic uptake and functional bile flow) may all be considered. The gold standard for the diagnosis of intra- and extrahepatic cholestasis remains, however, the percutaneous liver biopsy (see Table 12.75). This will also provide for the differentiation between neonatal hepatitis syndrome and bile duct paucity. Paucity of the bile ducts may be further differentiated into syndromic (Alagille syndrome – characteristic facies, butterfly wing vertebra, peripheral pulmonary artery stenosis and retinopathy) and nonsyndromic. Neonatal hepatitis is the end result of many hepatic insults. In some cases, however, no cause can be found and the final diagnosis is idiopathic neonatal hepatitis. These entities are discussed further in Chapter 19.

Management of neonatal liver disease is supportive and, where possible, definitive.[753] Nutritional support aims to provide sufficient energy and nutrients to combat maldigestion and malabsorption, and specialized formulas are used. Fat soluble vitamin supplementation is required for all cholestatic infants. Management is discussed further in Chapter 19.

HEMATOLOGICAL PROBLEMS OF THE NEWBORN

DEVELOPMENTAL HEMOPOIESIS
Hemopoietic stem cells and hemopoiesis

Hemopoiesis is the process which generates life-long production of cells of all the hemopoietic lineages. The principal lineages and current views of the organization of hemopoiesis are shown in Figure 12.39. The most primitive cells are the pluripotent hemopoietic stem cells. These stem cells are characterized by their astonishing capacity to choose between one of two destinies depending on the genes they express: they either undergo self-renewal (i.e. they maintain exactly the same pluripotent characteristics after cell division) or alternatively they differentiate. At an early stage in this process of differentiation stem cells commit themselves, via a distinct pattern of gene expression, to producing cells of the lymphoid lineage (lymphoid stem cells) or nonlymphoid lineage (myeloid stem cells).

Myeloid stem cells are able to further differentiate into hemopoietic progenitor cells of all the remaining lineages (erythroid, megakaryocyte, eosinophil, granulocyte, monocyte and basophil) as shown in Figure 12.39. By coordinated expression of many genes in response to a range of stimuli, including hemopoietic growth factors, these cells develop into mature peripheral blood cells. The process of hemopoiesis outlined here is broadly similar in adults, children, neonates, the fetus and the embryo. However, there are differences in the regulation of this process and its cellular components during development which contribute to the nature and management of the neonatal hematological problems described in this section.

Sites of hemopoiesis

While virtually all hemopoiesis in children and adults takes place in the marrow, the principal sites of hemopoietic activity change during development. The first signs of hemopoiesis in humans occur in the third week of gestation in the yolk sac; by 5 weeks' gestation the majority of hemopoietic stem cells arise from the embryonic dorsal aorta in the aorto-gonad-mesonephros (AGM) region.[755] Soon afterwards these hemopoietic stem cells migrate to the liver. By the eleventh week,

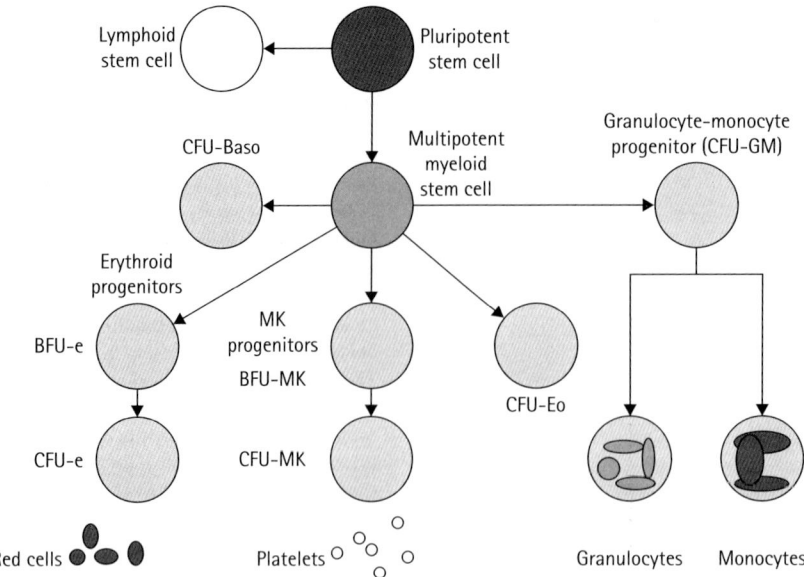

Fig. 12.39 Hemopoiesis: a schematic outline. BFU-e, burst-forming unit erythrocyte; BFU-MK, burst-forming unit megakaryocyte; CFU-baso, colony-forming unit basophil; CFU-e, colony-forming unit erythrocyte; CFU-Eo, colony-forming unit eosinophil; CFU-MK, colony-forming unit megakaryocyte; MK, megakaryocyte.

hemopoiesis begins in the bone marrow although the fetal liver remains the principal site of hemopoiesis until the end of the third trimester.

Erythropoiesis

A number of characteristics of erythropoiesis in the newborn are relevant to our understanding of the normal changes in hemoglobin (Hb) during this period and to identifying significant abnormalities of erythropoiesis in neonates.

(i) Erythropoiesis is switched off at birth

Production of new red blood cells and the rate of Hb synthesis fall dramatically after birth and remain low for the first 2 weeks of life. The exact mechanisms for these changes are unknown but probably reflect the sudden increase in tissue oxygenation at birth and downregulation of erythropoietin production. Although erythropoiesis begins to increase after the first 2 weeks, this starts at the erythroid progenitor stage of differentiation and the rise in Hb is not apparent until many weeks later and reaches a maximum only by 3 months of age when a healthy infant should be able to produce up to 2 ml packed red cells/day. Studies in preterm neonates have suggested that over the first 2 months of life the maximal rate of red cell production is ≤ 1 ml/day since preterm babies receiving erythropoietin are unable to maintain their Hb if > 1 ml of blood/day is venesected for diagnostic purposes.

(ii) Neonatal red cells have a reduced life span

Calculated actuarial red cell life spans for preterm infants are 35–50 days compared to 60–70 days for term infants and 120 days for healthy adults.[756] The reasons are unclear and are likely to mainly reflect changes in the red cell membrane.

(iii) Neonatal red cell membranes and intracellular metabolism are different from adult red cells

Differences in the red cell membranes of neonates include: increased resistance to osmotic lysis, increased mechanical fragility, increased total lipid content and an altered lipid profile, increased insulin-binding sites and reduced expression of blood group antigens such as A, B and I. There are also numerous differences in metabolism between neonatal and adult red blood cells both in the glycolytic and pentose phosphate pathways which lead to an increased susceptibility to oxidant-induced injury, although the clinical implications of these differences remain unclear.

(iv) The principal hemoglobin at birth is hemoglobin F

Knowledge of the normal evolution of embryonic, fetal and 'adult' Hbs during development is essential to our understanding of hemoglobinopathies and how they present in neonates. The first globin chain produced is epsilon globin, followed almost immediately by alpha- and gamma-globin chain production. HbF (alpha2gamma2) is therefore produced from very early in gestation (4–5 weeks) and is the predominant Hb until after birth. Adult Hb (Hb A: alpha2beta2) is also produced from an early stage (6–8 weeks' gestation) but remains at low levels (10–15%) until 30–32 weeks. After this time the rate of HbA production increases at the same time as HbF production falls, resulting in an average HbF level at birth of 70–80%, HbA of 25–30%, small amounts of HbA2 and sometimes a trace of Hb Barts (beta4) (Table 12.76).

After birth and over the first year of life HbF falls in healthy term and preterm babies (to 2% at age 12 months) with a corresponding increase in HbA. In term babies there is little change in HbF in the first 15 days after birth but it declines steeply thereafter as neonatal erythropoiesis starts. In preterm babies who are not transfused, HbF may remain at the same level for the first 6 weeks of life before HbA production starts to increase. It is this delay in HbA production which can make the diagnosis of beta-globin disorders difficult in the neonatal period. By contrast, the fact that alpha-globin chains are absolutely essential for the production of both HbF and HbA, means that alpha-thalassemia major causes severe anemia from early in fetal life.

Table 12.76 Composition of embryonic, fetal and adult Hbs

Hb	Globin chains		
	Chromosome 16 α-gene cluster	Chromosome 11 β-gene cluster	Gestation
Embryonic			
Hb Gower 1	ξ2	ε2	From 3 to 4 weeks
Hb Gower 2	α2	ε2	
Hb Portland	ε2	γ2	From 4 weeks
Fetal			
HbF	α2	γ2	From 4 weeks
Adult			
Hb A	α2	β2	From 6 to 8 weeks
HbA2	α2	ε2	From 30 weeks

(v) Regulation of erythropoiesis in the fetus and newborn: role of erythropoietin

The principal cytokine regulating erythropoiesis in the fetus and newborn is erythropoietin. Since erythropoietin does not cross the placenta, erythropoietin-mediated regulation of fetal erythropoiesis is predominantly under fetal control. The only known stimulus to erythropoietin production under physiological conditions is hypoxia with or without anemia. This explains the high erythropoietin levels in fetuses of mothers with diabetes or hypertension or those with IUGR or cyanotic congenital heart disease where the fetus and newborn are polycythemic rather than anemic; erythropoietin is also increased in fetal anemia of any cause including hemolytic disease of the newborn.[757]

Platelet production in the fetus and neonate

Platelets first appear in the fetal circulation at 5–6 weeks' postconceptional age. During the second trimester the platelet count rises to $175–250 \times 10^9/L$.[758] The principal cytokine regulating platelet production is thrombopoietin. Thrombopoietin stimulates megakaryocyte progenitors and mature megakaryocytes. In neonatal thrombocytopenia thrombopoietin levels rise when the platelet count and/or circulating megakaryocyte progenitors are low (e.g. early onset thrombocytopenia associated with maternal PET and/or IUGR) while thrombopoietin levels remain low where thrombocytopenia is secondary to increased platelet destruction (e.g. idiopathic thrombocytopenic purpura; ITP). Although thrombopoietin is detectable in all healthy neonates, the ability to upregulate thrombopoietin is reduced in the fetus and newborn which limits their capacity to increase platelet production at times of need, e.g. during neonatal sepsis.[759]

Neutrophil production (granulopoiesis) in the fetus and neonate

There are few circulating neutrophils in first trimester blood (around 1% of circulating nucleated cells). The number of granulocytes in fetal blood remains low ($0.1–0.2 \times 10^9/L$) throughout the second trimester gradually rising to over $2 \times 10^9/L$ by term, with slightly lower numbers in preterm neonates (Table 12.77). The principal difference between granulopoiesis in the newborn and later in infancy is the diminished size of the neutrophil storage pool, particularly in preterm infants and most markedly so in those with IUGR or exposure to maternal hypertension. (The neutrophil storage pool reflects the available reserve of neutrophils which the fetus or neonate can mobilize in response to infection.) This may explain the frequency of bacterial infection in such infants. In healthy term and preterm neonates the ratio of immature band forms to mature neutrophils is normal. This has led to widespread use of 'I/T' (immature/total) ratios as an indicator of neonatal sepsis. However, there are several important limitations to their value. In particular,

preterm infants born to mothers with chorioamnionitis frequently have markedly increased numbers of all types of immature granulocytic cells on their blood film including metamyelocytes, myelocytes, promyelocytes and blast cells; this appearance in the first few days of life is not usually indicative of sepsis, instead reflecting the normal hematological response of a neonate to preterm delivery. The most useful diagnostic clue to the coincident presence of sepsis is a marked peak in the numbers of band forms compared to other granulocytic cells.[760] The regulation of granulopoiesis is not fully understood. Various cytokines, such as granulocyte colony-stimulating factor (G-CSF) and granulocyte–macrophage colony-stimulating factor (GM-CSF), stimulate granulocyte production in vitro and in vivo but their exact physiological role is unclear.[760]

Other leukocytes

All types of leukocyte found in adult blood are also seen in the fetus and the newborn. Monocytes circulate from 4–5 weeks' gestation and eosinophils and basophils from 14–16 weeks' gestation, each cell type being present in low numbers and increasing slowly to the normal values at term (Table 12.77). There are few studies of lymphopoiesis in the human fetus. There appears to be no lymphopoiesis in the yolk sac, but both T lymphocytes and B lymphocytes are found in small numbers in the fetal liver by 8 weeks' gestation. Shortly thereafter T lymphocytes are detectable in fetal blood and thymus, with marrow T lymphocyte production established during the second trimester. By term T lymphocytes form 40–45% of circulating mononuclear cells with a CD4:CD8 ratio of around 5.0, slightly higher than in adult blood (3.1:1). B lymphocytes are found in fetal blood and bone marrow from around 12 weeks' gestation and constitute 4–5% of circulating mononuclear cells by term.[761]

HEMATOLOGICAL VALUES AT BIRTH

Practical issues: establishing normal values and identifying artefacts

One of the most important aspects of neonatal hematology is knowledge of what is normal in the neonatal period and the factors that impact upon the importance of a laboratory result. These include:

1. *Site of sampling*: capillary or skin puncture samples yield higher Hb levels (2–4 g/dl higher) and hematocrits (up to 20% higher) than venous or arterial samples collected simultaneously.[762]
2. *Quality of the blood sample*: common problems include clotted or partially clotted samples particularly when the baby is polycythemic; and poorly preserved white cell morphology due to excess ethylenediaminetetraacetic acid (EDTA) if there is delay in samples reaching the laboratory or a high blood:anticoagulant ratio.
3. *Gestational age-related changes in hematological values*: while there are no significant differences in Hb, hematocrit, white blood cell (WBC) count or platelet count with gestational age from 24 weeks to term, the normal mean cell volume (MCV) is higher in preterm infants (Tables 12.77 and 12.78); the number of reticulocytes is twice as high in preterm compared to term infants (6% at 24–25 weeks versus 3.2% at term); and the numbers of circulating nucleated red cells in healthy preterm infants are around twice as high ($\leq 20 \times 10^9/L$) as in term babies.
4. *Postnatal changes in hematological values*: the marked changes after birth in almost all hematological parameters over the first few weeks of life make it essential to know the postnatal age of a baby to make a sensible interpretation of the hematological results.
5. *Effect of timing of cord clamping and other aspects of delivery on hematological values in the newborn*: Since the placental blood vessels in a term baby contain 50–200 ml of blood, delaying clamping of the cord and holding the baby below the level of the placenta to allow emptying of this blood into the baby's circulation can increase the blood volume by 50–60% with a consequent increase in Hb (to > 19 g/dl versus 15–16 g/dl with early clamping of the cord); similar differences are seen in preterm babies.[764]

Table 12.77   Representative normal hematological values at birth and over the first 2 months of life in term babies

	Birth	2 weeks	2 months
Hb (g/dl)	14.9–23.7	13.4–19.8	9.4–13
Hematocrit	0.47–0.75	0.41–0.65	0.28–0.42
Mean cell volume (fl)	100–125	88–110	77–98
Reticulocytes ($\times 10^9/L$)	110–450	10–85	35–200
White blood cells ($\times 10^9/L$)	10–26	6–21	5–15
Neutrophils ($\times 10^9/L$)	2.7–14.4	1.5–5.4	0.7–4.8
Monocytes ($\times 10^9/L$)	0–1.9	0.1–1.7	0.4–1.2
Lymphocytes ($\times 10^9/L$)	2.0–7.3	2.8–9.1	3.3–10.3
Eosinophils ($\times 10^9/L$)	0–0.85	0–0.85	0.05–0.9
Basophils ($\times 10^9/L$)	0–0.1	0–0.1	0.02–0.13
Nucleated red blood cells ($\times 10^9/L$)	<5	<0.1	<0.1
Platelets ($\times 10^9/L$)	150–450	150–450	150–450

These data are obtained from a number of sources and have been chosen to represent data most useful for interpreting the significance of hematological results.

Table 12.78 Representative normal hematological values at birth in preterm babies

	24–25 weeks	26–27 weeks	28–29 weeks	30–31 weeks
Hb (g/dl)	19.4 ± 1.5	19.0 ± 2.5	19.3 ± 1.8	19.1 ± 2.1
Hematocrit	0.63 ± 0.04	0.62 ± 0.08	0.60 ± 0.07	60 ± 0.08
Mean cell volume (fl)	135 ± 0.02	132 ± 14.4	131 ± 13.5	127 ± 12.7
Reticulocytes ($\times 10^9$/L)	279 ± 23	454 ± 15	347 ± 12	278 ± 10
Platelets ($\times 10^9$/L)	150–450	150–450	150–450	150–450

Data adapted from Brugnara & Platt 2003.[763]

Normal values for red blood cells and blood volume

Normal values at birth for Hb, hematocrit and MCV are shown in Tables 12.77 and 12.78 for term and preterm babies respectively. In term babies the Hb, hematocrit and red cell indices fall slowly over the first few weeks reaching a mean Hb of 13–14 g/dl at 4 weeks of age and 9.5–11 g/dl at 7–9 weeks of age. For preterm infants changes in the first few weeks of life are often difficult to interpret because of their variable clinical course and transfusion requirements. However, studies of well preterm infants carried out in the 1970s show a more rapid and steeper fall in Hb reaching a mean of 6.5–9 g/dl at 4–8 weeks' postnatal age.[763] The reticulocyte count and numbers of nucleated red cells also fall rapidly after birth as erythropoiesis is suppressed. The reticulocyte count starts to increase in term babies at 7–8 weeks of age and in preterm babies at 6–8 weeks of age.

Normal blood volume at birth varies with gestational age as well as the timing of the clamping of the cord. In healthy term infants average blood volume is around 80 ml/kg. The blood volume is higher in preterm infants with an average of 106 ml/kg. Term and preterm babies have adequate stores of iron, folic acid and vitamin B$_{12}$ at birth. However, stores of both iron and folic acid are lower in preterm infants and are depleted more quickly, leading to deficiency after 2–4 months if the recommended daily intakes are not maintained (see p. 227 and Ch. 16). In general, even term neonates with a normal Hb at birth will have depleted their iron stores by the time they have doubled their birth weight.

Normal values for white cells

The neutrophil and monocyte count vary over the first few days of life even in healthy babies. For the first 12 h they increase then fall to a nadir at 4 days of age. Normal values for neutrophils at birth are also affected by other factors including antenatal history, perinatal history, ethnic origin, site of blood sampling and whether or not the baby has been crying. The neutrophil count is higher in capillary samples and after vigorous crying; it is lower in neonates with IUGR, those born to mothers with hypertension or diabetes and in neonates of African origin.[757,760] Some cell types not found in healthy adults are seen in healthy preterm babies – these include blast cells, other early myeloid cells, nucleated red cells and even occasional megakaryocytes.

Normal platelet count and platelet function

Blood platelet counts at birth in term and preterm neonates are within the normal adult range.[765] Many studies have found impaired function of neonatal platelets in vitro in term and preterm infants; the most consistent abnormalities are reduced aggregation in response to epinephrine (adrenaline), ADP and thrombin. However, these abnormalities do not appear to be of major clinical significance: there is no increased bleeding tendency in neonates with normal platelet counts and coagulation parameters and the bleeding time tested with adult and neonatal devices is normal in term and preterm infants (≤ 135 s).

RED CELL DISORDERS

Anemia

Anemia is the commonest hematological abnormality in the newborn. The cause is often multifactorial. Nevertheless a logical approach and appropriate use of straightforward investigations, as outlined below and summarized in figure 12.40, reveal the cause in most babies. The general management of neonatal anemia, including red cell transfusion, is outlined on page 290.

Definition. Anemia is defined as an Hb concentration below the normal range for a population of age- and sex-matched individuals. Normal values for term and preterm infants at birth are shown in Tables 12.77 and 12.78; from this it can be seen that, regardless of gestation, any neonate with a Hb of < 14 g/dl at birth on a properly taken blood sample would be considered anemic.

Physiological impact of anemia in the neonate

Anemia is one of the main factors, together with cardiopulmonary function and the position of the Hb–oxygen dissociation curve, which influences tissue oxygenation. The clinical significance of anemia in the newborn does not therefore depend solely upon the Hb concentration. The two most important factors determining the position of the Hb–oxygen dissociation curve are the HbF and 2,3-DPG concentrations within the red blood cells: a high HbF and low 2,3-DPG both cause the curve to be shifted to the left, i.e. the affinity of Hb for oxygen is increased so less oxygen is released to the tissues. This is the situation just after birth and will be more marked in preterm babies with higher HbF concentrations. Over the first few months of life 2,3-DPG levels rise and HbF levels fall so the Hb–oxygen dissociation curve gradually shifts to the right, i.e. the oxygen affinity of Hb falls and oxygen delivery to the tissues increases. This increase in oxygen delivery ameliorates the effects of the falling Hb over the first months of life.

Pathogenesis and causes of neonatal anemia

Anemia in the neonatal period has distinct physiological features compared to older children and a distinct pathogenesis. Interpretation of diagnostic investigations has to be made on a background of changes in the red cell membrane, red cell enzymes and Hb production which vary with gestational and postnatal age. Furthermore, anemia in the neonate may be attributable to pregnancy-related or pre-existing disorders in the mother. Anemia results from one or more of the following mechanisms:

1. inappropriately reduced red cell production (see below);
2. increased red cell destruction/reduced red cell life span (p. 288);
3. blood loss (p. 289);
4. a combination of these mechanisms (anemia of prematurity, p. 290).

Using this approach the principal causes of anemia in the term and preterm neonate are shown in Table 12.79 and a diagnostic approach to identifying these causes is shown in Figure 12.40.

Anemia due to reduced red cell production

The main diagnostic clues are a combination of a low reticulocyte count ($< 20 \times 10^9$/L) together with a negative direct antiglobulin test (Coombs' test). The most important causes are red cell aplasia due to parvovirus B19 and Diamond–Blackfan anemia (DBA). Reduced red cell production may also be due to abnormal red cell development, usually congenital dyserythropoietic anemia (CDA) or part of a global failure of hemopoiesis, e.g. in CMV infection, Pearson syndrome or congenital leukemias (see p. 292).

Anemia due to parvovirus B19 and other congenital infections

Parvovirus B19 causes selective red cell aplasia when maternal infection occurs during the first or second trimester. The anemia and reticulocytopenia are severe and may present as hydrops fetalis; the leukocyte and platelet count are usually, but not always, normal.[766] The diagnosis of fetal/neonatal parvovirus B19 may be very difficult to make and should

Table 12.79 Causes of neonatal anemia

A. Impaired red cell production
- Congenital infection, e.g. CMV, rubella
- Diamond–Blackfan anemia
- Pearson syndrome
- Congenital dyserythropoietic anemia
- Transient erythroblastopenia of childhood (rare in neonates)
- Congenital leukemia

B. Increased red cell destruction (hemolysis)
- Alloimmune: hemolytic disease of the newborn (Rh, ABO, Kell, other)
- Autoimmune, e.g. maternal autoimmune hemolysis
- Infection, e.g. bacterial, syphilis, malaria, CMV, toxoplasma, herpes simplex
- Red cell membrane disorders, e.g. hereditary spherocytosis
- Infantile pyknocytosis
- Red cell enzyme deficiencies, e.g. pyruvate kinase deficiency
- Some hemoglobinopathies, e.g. alpha-thalassemia major, HbH disease
- Macro/microangiopathy, e.g. cavernous hemangioma, DIC
- Galactosemia

C. Blood loss
- Occult hemorrhage before birth, e.g. twin-to-twin, fetomaternal
- Internal hemorrhage, e.g. intracranial, cephalhematoma
- Iatrogenic: due to frequent blood sampling

D. Anemia of prematurity:
- Impaired red cell production plus reduced red cell life span

CMV, cytomegalovirus; DIC, disseminated intravascular coagulation.

Table 12.80 Hematological causes of hydrops fetalis

A. Reduced red cell production
   Parvovirus B19
   Diamond–Blackfan anemia
   Congenital dyserythropoietic anemia
   Congenital leukemia

B. Increased red cell destruction (hemolysis)
   Pyruvate kinase deficiency
   Alpha-thalassemia major
   Hemolytic disease of the newborn – Rhesus, Kell, ABO (rare)

C. Blood loss
   Twin-to-twin transfusion
   Fetomaternal hemorrhage

be considered in every 'unexplained' case of fetal hydrops (Table 12.80) or neonatal red cell aplasia.[767] Other infections which cause anemia due to reduced red cell production include: CMV, toxoplasmosis, congenital syphilis, rubella and herpes simplex; in these cases the reticulocytopenia is less marked or absent and the blood film often shows abnormal 'viral' lymphocytes, thrombocytopenia and/or neutropenia.

Management. Antenatally diagnosed parvovirus with early hydrops can be treated with intrauterine transfusions. Neonates with red cell aplasia secondary to parvovirus B19 should be treated with red cell transfusion; those who fail to recover should be given intravenous immunoglobulin (IVIG) to help eradicate persistent viral infection.[766]

Congenital red cell aplasia, including Diamond–Blackfan anemia

The principal cause of congenital red cell aplasia is DBA. The incidence is 5–7 cases/million live births. Most cases present at 2–3 months of age when transfusion-dependent anemia becomes apparent. Around 25% of cases present at birth and rare cases present in utero in the second trimester with anemia and/or hydrops. Around 50% of patients also have a distinct facial appearance and/or short stature, thumb abnormalities, genitourinary and cardiac abnormalities. Mutations of the RPS19 gene

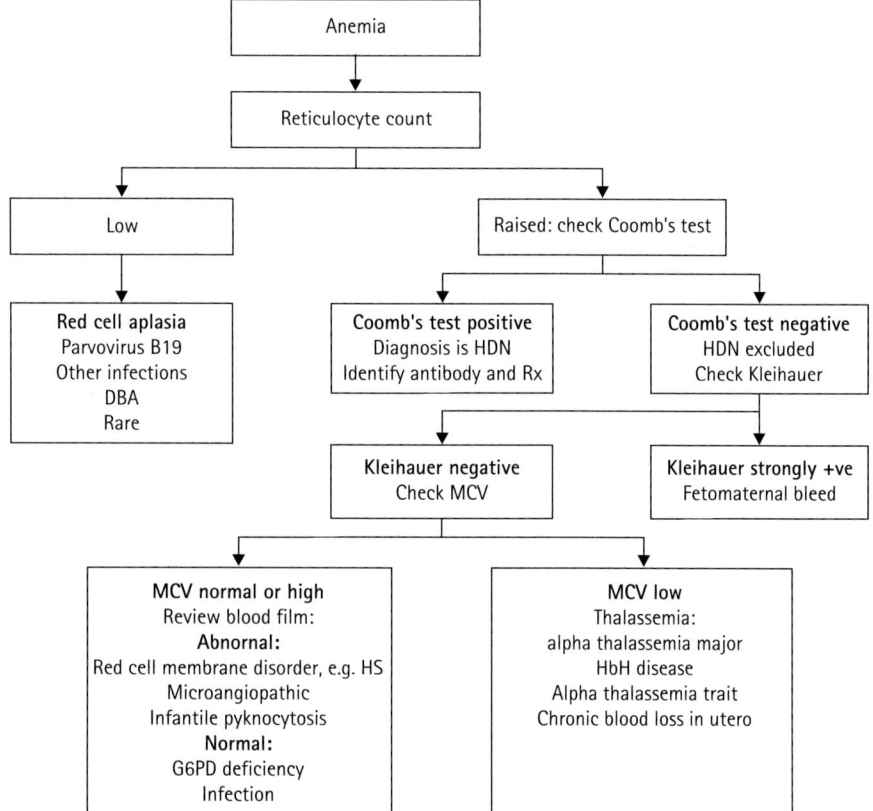

Fig. 12.40 Diagnostic approach to neonatal anemia. G6PD; glucose-6-phosphate dehydrogenase; DBA, Diamond–Blackfan anemia; HDN, hemolytic disease of the newborn; HS, hereditary spherocytosis; MCV, mean cell volume.

are found in 25% of cases of DBA; this causes a defect in ribosome biogenesis. The genetic basis of DBA in the remaining families is currently unknown although the majority of cases are familial and at least two other genetic loci have been identified.[768] Red cell adenosine deaminase activity (measured pre-transfusion) is elevated in some patients and family members and may help diagnosis in patients without an RPS19 mutation.

Other inherited/congenital disorders which may present with anemia due to reduced red cell production include CDA and Pearson syndrome. Most types of CDA present in childhood but a significant number do present with transfusion-dependent anemia in the neonatal period. Most affected babies are normally grown with no dysmorphic features, have a normocytic anemia with normal white cells and platelets but a low reticulocyte count. The genetic basis is unknown but most cases are autosomal recessive. Pearson syndrome, which is caused by mutations in mitochondrial DNA, presents in neonates who are SGA and thrive poorly in the first few weeks of life due to anemia and exocrine pancreatic dysfunction. The anemia is normocytic and associated thrombocytopenia and neutropenia are common; abnormal leukocyte vacuolation may be seen in the peripheral blood and highly characteristic vacuolation of early erythroid cells on the marrow aspirate should prompt blood to be sent for mitochondrial DNA analysis to establish the diagnosis. The other inherited bone marrow failure syndromes, e.g. Fanconi anemia, rarely present at birth.

Management. Management of these disorders is discussed in detail in Chapter 23. In the neonatal period the main issues are making the diagnosis and judicious use of red cell transfusion (see p. 290). Steroids are rarely used for DBA in the neonatal period as they are only indicated in transfusion-dependent children and have significant side-effects in this age group.

Anemia due to increased red cell destruction/reduced red cell life span (hemolytic anemia)

Recognition of neonatal anemia due to hemolysis is clinically extremely important even if the anemia is mild and apparently trivial. This is because transient or mild hemolysis in the neonatal period may be the first sign of an underlying problem with more serious manifestations later on in childhood (e.g. red cell enzymopathies or hemoglobinopathies) or problems which might affect future siblings (e.g. alloimmune anemia due to maternal red cell antibodies).

The principal diagnostic clues suggesting hemolysis are: increased numbers of reticulocytes, unconjugated hyperbilirubinemia, a positive Coombs' test (if immune) and characteristic changes in the morphology of the red cells on a blood film (e.g. hereditary spherocytosis). The main types of neonatal hemolytic anemia are listed in Table 12.79. It is usually straightforward to distinguish the cause. The first step should be a Coombs' test, which will be positive only in the presence of immune hemolytic anemia.

Immune hemolytic anemias including hemolytic disease of the newborn (HDN)

By far the most common cause of Coombs'-positive hemolysis is hemolytic disease of the newborn (HDN) due to transplacental passage of maternal IgG alloantibodies to red cell antigens. Maternal autoimmune hemolytic anemia occasionally causes a positive Coombs' test in the neonate; however, both hemolysis and anemia in the baby are extremely rare.

Alloantibodies which can cause HDN include anti-D, anti-c, anti-E, anti-Kell, anti-Kidd (J^k), anti-Duffy (F^y) and antibodies of the MNS blood group system, including anti-U. Anti-D remains the most frequent alloantibody to cause significant hemolytic anemia; it affects 1 in 1200 pregnancies and still results in around 50 deaths per year in the UK.[769] Anti-Kell antibodies also cause severe fetal and neonatal anemia since they inhibit erythropoiesis as well as producing hemolysis. Although ABO incompatibility between mother and fetus is present in approximately 25% of pregnancies, hemolysis is relatively uncommon. This is because the majority of naturally occurring anti A and B antibodies are

of the IgM subclass that do not cross the placenta. In addition, neonatal red cell A and B antigens are not fully glycosylated and are therefore weakly antigenic at birth; there is also widespread expression of A and B antigens on other cells throughout the body thereby 'mopping up' any antibody that crosses the placenta. Nevertheless ABO HDN occurs around 1 in 150 births. It affects neonates born to women of blood group O and is confined to the 1% of such women with high titer IgG antibodies. Hemolysis due to anti-A is more common than anti-B. The main clinical feature is hyperbilirubinemia which may be severe. Anemia is usually mild or absent and where there is significant anemia it is usually associated with anti-B antibodies. HDN is a rare cause of 'blueberry muffin' baby.

Management of HDN due to Rh or Kell alloantibodies. The antenatal diagnosis and management of pregnancies affected by red cell alloimmunization are discussed in Chapter 11. Close cooperation between obstetric, pediatric and hematology teams is essential for good management.[769] All neonates at risk of HDN should have cord blood taken for Hb, bilirubin and a Coombs' test and should remain in hospital until hyperbilirubinemia and/or anemia have been properly managed. Phototherapy should be given to all Rhesus-alloimmunized infants from birth as the bilirubin can rise steeply after birth and this expectant approach will prevent the need for exchange transfusion in some infants.

Exchange transfusion is required for:
1. severe anemia (Hb < 10 g/dl at birth) or;
2. severe and/or rapidly increasing hyperbilirubinemia as indicated by standard graphs.

Blood for exchange transfusion should be Group O, Rh D-identical with the neonate, Kell-negative and < 5 days old. Current recommendations state that the blood should be CMV-negative but universal leukocyte depletion in the UK means that CMV-untested blood is likely to be of equivalent safety to CMV-negative blood even in the newborn.[770] The blood should be irradiated *if* the baby has received intrauterine transfusion; irradiation of blood for exchange is not essential otherwise but may be carried out in some centers if it can be performed without delay. Packed red blood cells are suitable for neonatal exchange transfusion provided they have a hematocrit of <0.6. The technique for exchange transfusion is described on page 98. There is some evidence that IVIG may be helpful in preventing exchange transfusion in neonates with immune hemolytic anemia. It is postulated that this exogenous source of antibodies might block destruction of antibody-coated red cells in the reticuloendothelial system. A recent Cochrane review concludes that studies so far are of limited applicability and high quality large studies are needed.[771] 'Late' anemia is seen in some babies with milder hemolytic disease who do not require exchange transfusion and in babies who have had earlier exchange transfusion. This presents at a few weeks of age and is due to ongoing hemolysis and postnatal suppression of erythropoiesis. Such babies may require 'top-up' transfusion (see p. 290) but irradiated blood must be used for infants who have previously received intrauterine transfusion to prevent the risk of transfusion-associated graft versus host disease.

Non-immune hemolytic anemia presenting in neonates

Causes of non-immune hemolysis in neonates are shown in Table 12.79. The main diagnoses to consider are:
- red cell membrane disorders;
- red cell enzymopathies;
- hemoglobinopathies.

A number of congenital and primary infections can also cause hemolytic anemia in the neonatal period including CMV, toxoplasmosis, congenital syphilis, rubella, herpes simplex and, rarely, malaria (see also Ch. 28).

Red cell membrane disorders. Red cell membrane disorders can usually be identified by the characteristic shape of red cells on a blood film. Hereditary spherocytosis (HS) occurs in 1 in 5000 births. HS is autosomal dominant but around 25% of cases are sporadic due to new mutations; it is genetically heterogeneous – mutations in spectrin, ankyrin, protein 4.1 and protein 3 have all been reported. The usual presentation of HS in neonates is unconjugated hyperbilirubinemia. Most affected neonates are not anemic at birth but may become anemic during the first month of life due to increased splenic function and the physiological shutdown of erythropoiesis at birth.[772] The blood film in HS shows moderate numbers of spherocytes; the appearance is identical to that of ABO HDN but the two disorders are distinguishable by the negative Coombs' in HS. Recent guidelines for the diagnosis and management of HS have been published.[773] Hereditary elliptocytosis is a more complex disorder caused by mutations in the genes for spectrin, ankyrin or Band 4.1. In the common, autosomal dominant form, heterozygotes have no clinical manifestations (i.e. no anemia and no jaundice) apart from elliptocytes on the blood film. More important clinically are neonates who have more than one mutation in a red cell membrane protein (they may be homozygous or compound heterozygotes) as they present with the disease hereditary pyropoikilocytosis (HPP). In HPP hemolytic anemia is severe in the neonatal period and many infants require transfusion. The diagnosis of HPP should be easily made by examining blood films from the baby and both parents; a useful diagnostic clue is the low MCV at birth (< 70 fl).

Management. Babies with chronic hemolysis secondary to red cell membrane abnormalities should be given folic acid (i.e. all affected babies except hereditary elliptocytosis heterozygotes who have no significant hemolysis). Red cell transfusion may be required in the neonatal period and, especially in HPP, sometimes indefinitely until the child is old enough to undergo splenectomy. It is important to carry out definitive diagnostic investigations on pretransfusion blood samples to minimize diagnostic confusion due to transfused cells.

Red cell enzymopathies. Red cell enzymopathies present in neonates with unconjugated bilirubinemia with or without anemia and, unlike the membrane disorders, usually do not have characteristic changes on the blood film. The most common is G6PD deficiency, which has a high prevalence in individuals from central Africa (20%) and the Mediterranean (10%). G6PD deficiency, which is X-linked, predominantly affects boys although female carriers may have milder symptoms. In neonatal G6PD deficiency jaundice usually presents within the first few days of life and is often severe; anemia is uncommon and the blood film is usually completely normal and so the diagnosis must be made by assaying G6PD on a peripheral blood sample. This predominance of jaundice over hemolysis probably results from hepatic dysfunction caused by G6PD deficiency in the liver.[774] In addition there is an association between the degree of hyperbilirubinemia and co-inheritance of Gilbert syndrome due to a polymorphism in the promoter of the gene uridine diphosphate glucuronyltransferase (UGT1A). The second most common red cell enzymopathy in neonates, pyruvate kinase deficiency, is more heterogeneous varying from anemia severe enough to cause hydrops fetalis to a mild unconjugated hyperbilirubinemia; the blood film is sometimes distinctive but often shows nonspecific changes of nonspherocytic hemolysis.[775] Neonatal hemolytic anemia may be the only presenting feature of triosephosphate isomerase deficiency, the devastating neurological features of this disorder only becoming apparent 6–12 months later. Persistent hemolysis should therefore always be investigated.

Management. The most important management issues in these disorders are making the diagnosis and issuing parents of babies with G6PD deficiency with the appropriate information about which medicines, chemicals and foods may precipitate hemolysis (Table 12.81). If transfusion is required, conventional guidelines for neonatal transfusion can be followed. Folic acid supplements are not required in most cases of G6PD deficiency but are necessary in any baby with chronic hemolysis, e.g. pyruvate kinase deficiency.

Hemoglobinopathies. Hemoglobinopathies, with the exception of alpha-thalassemia major, do not usually present in the neonatal period. Alpha-thalassemia major (all four alpha-globin genes deleted) occurs predominantly in families of south-east Asian origin and presents with mid-trimester fetal anemia or hydrops fetalis, which is fatal within hours of delivery. The only long term survivors of alpha-thalassemia major received intrauterine transfusions. The diagnosis is made by Hb electrophoresis or high performance liquid chromatography (HPLC; which

Table 12.81 Drugs and chemicals associated with hemolysis in patients who are G6PD deficient

A. Antimalarials
Primaquine
Pamaquine
(Quinine)*
(Chloroquine)*
B. Antibiotics
Nitrofurantoin
Sulfones, e.g. dapsone
Sulfonamides,** e.g. sulfamethoxazole (Septrin)
Quinolones, e.g. nalidixic acid, ciprofloxacin
(Chloramphenicol)†
C. Analgesics
Aspirin (in high doses)
Phenacetin
D. Chemicals
Naphthalene (mothballs)
Divicine (broad beans)
Methylene blue

*Acceptable in acute malaria.
**Some sulfonamides do not cause hemolysis in most G6PD deficient patients, e.g. sulfadiazine.
†To be avoided in some types of G6PD deficiency (can be taken by patients with the common, African A- form of G6PD deficiency).

shows mainly Hb Barts); the blood film shows hypochromic, microcytic red cells with circulating nucleated red cells. Symptoms and signs of the major beta-globin hemoglobinopathies (sickle cell disease and beta-thalassemia major) are rare in neonates although modern techniques (e.g. HPLC, isoelectric focusing) allow the diagnosis to be made on neonatal blood samples where family studies indicate that both parents are carriers. Many countries and regions with a high prevalence of hemoglobinopathies, including the UK, have neonatal screening programs to facilitate early diagnosis which is particularly important in sickle cell disease in order to start penicillin prophylaxis as soon as possible.

Management. Transfusion for hemoglobinopathies is rarely required in the neonatal period. It is important to carry out diagnostic investigations on pretransfusion samples and analysis of parental samples is also essential. Folic acid should be given, until transfusion dependence occurs, as all patients have chronic hemolysis and penicillin prophylaxis should be commenced in babies with all forms of sickle cell disease.

Anemia due to blood loss

Anemia due to blood loss may occur during fetal life, at the time of delivery or postnatally (Table 12.79). In neonatal inpatients the most common cause of anemia is blood loss secondary to iatrogenic blood letting.

Blood loss prior to birth, including twin-to-twin transfusion

This usually follows twin-to-twin transfusion, feto-maternal transfusion or trauma but may be spontaneous. The degree of anemia is variable and the clinical presentation depends on the amount and rate of blood loss. The most useful diagnostic tests are a blood film and a Kleihauer test on maternal blood to quantitate the number of HbF-containing fetal red blood cells in the maternal circulation. Where there is chronic blood loss the baby is often well but may present with cardiac failure; the blood film is hypochromic/microcytic. Where the baby has bled acutely just prior to delivery, it will have signs of circulatory shock and the maternal Kleihauer will show a large feto-maternal bleed; in this situation the Hb may be normal at delivery but fall rapidly as hemodilution occurs and the blood film is normochromic/normocytic with large numbers of nucleated red cells. Twin-to-twin transfusion occurs only in monochorionic twins with monochorial placentas. In this situation fetal–fetal transfusion may occur in up to one third of cases producing a discordance in birth weight and Hb (> 5 g/dl). Diagnosis is usually made antenatally by detection of markedly different amniotic fluid volumes between the twins in the second trimester.

Blood loss at or after delivery

This is usually due to obstetric complications, such as placenta previa, placental abruption or incision of the placenta during Cesarean section. Such babies are often extremely unwell with circulatory shock, anemia worsening rapidly after birth, large numbers of circulating nucleated red cells and disseminated intravascular coagulation. Similar hematological changes occur after massive internal bleeding in the baby, e.g. subarachnoid or retroperitoneal bleeding, and may be particularly severe where there is damage to the liver. While most cases of internal bleeding will be associated with traumatic delivery, it is important to search for any underlying bleeding disorder in such babies (see p. 293).

Anemia of prematurity

The normal fall in Hb after birth is greater in preterm compared to term neonates and has been termed 'physiological anemia of prematurity' since it does not appear to be associated with any abnormalities in the baby. The pathogenesis is not fully elucidated but contributory factors include:

- reduced red cell life span;
- inappropriately low erythropoietin;
- nutritional deficiency (iron and folic acid);
- rapid growth rate.

The nadir of Hb in a well term infant is as low as 9.4–11 g/dl at 8–12 weeks of age (Table 12.77); for a preterm infant the nadir in Hb occurs earlier (4–8 weeks of age) and is lower (6.5–9 g/dl). The diagnosis is usually straightforward – a well preterm baby has a slowly falling Hb with a completely unremarkable blood film showing normochromic/normocytic red cells, slightly low reticulocytes (20 × 10⁹/L) and no nucleated red cells.

Management. This is discussed in detail below. The most important aspects are minimizing the severity of anemia and judicious use of red cell transfusion. Erythropoietin may have a role in some babies (see below).

A simple diagnostic approach to neonatal anemia

Red cell disorders associated with anemia present in three main ways: with a low Hb (anemia), with jaundice and with hydrops. A diagnostic algorithm to help in identifying the cause of neonatal anemia and the most useful investigations is shown in Figure 12.40. Hematological causes of neonatal jaundice and of hydrops are shown in Tables 12.80 and 12.82.

Management of neonatal anemia

There are two facets to management:
1. identifying the underlying cause of the anemia where possible; and
2. deciding whether or not to transfuse.

A brief summary of the indications for red cell transfusion is outlined (Table 12.83). Management of neonatal anemia associated with specific hematological disorders is discussed in the relevant sections (Ch. 23). With increasing recognition of potential transfusion hazards, prevention of neonatal anemia has become extremely important.

Red cell transfusion for neonatal anemia

The threshold levels of anemia which should trigger red cell transfusion in neonates remain controversial. There are several useful reviews and guidelines produced by professional bodies; almost none are evidence based. Nevertheless, compliance with transfusion guidelines reduces transfusion requirements and donor exposure.[776,777] A pragmatic approach is to use the published guidelines to produce local, consensus-based neonatal transfusion protocols which can be enforced and monitored to maintain a consistent and sensible transfusion policy for all neonates (Table 12.83). The red cells used should be packed

Table 12.82 Hematological causes of neonatal jaundice

A. Red cell membrane disorders
   Hereditary spherocytosis
   Hereditary pyropoikilocytosis
   Other: e.g. homozygous hereditary elliptocytosis
B. Red cell enzymopathies
   G6PD deficiency
   Pyruvate kinase deficiency
   Other: e.g. glucose phosphate isomerase deficiency
C. Hemoglobinopathies
   Alpha-thalassemias
   Gamma-thalassemias
   Other: sickle cell syndromes (occasionally)
D. Immune
   Hemolytic disease of the newborn
   Maternal autoimmune hemolytic anemia
   Drug induced
E. Infection
   Bacterial
   Viral, e.g. CMV, rubella, herpes simplex
   Protozoal, e.g. toxoplasma, malaria, syphilis

Table 12.83 Indications for 'top up' red cell transfusion in preterm infants: based on a summary of national consensus-based guidelines

1. Severe pulmonary disease (babies on mechanical ventilation) Hb < 13 g/dl
2. Acute blood loss with shock
3. Stable newborn with clinical signs of anemia (e.g. tachycardia, poor weight gain) Hb 8–10.5 g/dl (threshold varies in different national guidelines)
4. Stable newborn without signs of anemia Hb < 7 g/dl

These guidelines can be used as the basis to produce more specific local neonatal transfusion protocols which may specify different thresholds for transfusion depending upon other important clinical variables, e.g. the postnatal age of the infant, the FiO₂, whether the baby is on CPAP, whether there are associated major complications, e.g. septic shock, NEC, planned surgery.

cells (hematocrit 0.5–0.7) which are ABO and Rh D-compatible with the mother and the baby and which are < 35 days old. Specially prepared satellite packs should be used wherever possible to allow multiple-transfused neonates to receive blood from the same donor.

Prevention of neonatal anemia, including the role of erythropoietin and hematinics

Approaches to preventing or minimizing neonatal anemia include:
1. limiting iatrogenic blood loss by appropriate use of blood tests;
2. iron and folate supplementation for all preterm infants;
   - iron 3 mg/kg/day from 4–6 weeks of age (a pragmatic approach is to give 1 ml of sodium iron edetate – 'Sytron' – once daily)
   - folic acid 15 mcg daily or 500 mcg once weekly;
3. judicious use of erythropoietin.

There have been many controlled trials of erythropoietin for prevention of neonatal anemia. The subject has been extensively reviewed[778,779] and is only briefly summarized here. Erythropoietin is able to reduce red cell transfusion requirements in preterm infants. However, in most studies only the relatively well infants with low transfusion requirements benefit from this as, even in high doses, the erythropoietin-mediated increase in red cell production is unable to increase sufficiently to cope with the need for frequent phlebotomy and multiple transfusions in sick preterm infants. The use of erythropoietin in the first week of life has been associated with an increase in retinopathy of prematurity and therefore is not currently recommended.[779] Erythropoietin has a useful role where red cell transfusions cannot be used (e.g. preterm babies of Jehovah's witnesses). Hb does not start to rise until about 10–14 days after erythropoietin has been commenced and iron supplements should be started as soon as possible to prevent the rapid development of iron deficiency in erythropoietin-treated infants.

Polycythemia

For both term and preterm infants polycythemia can be defined as a central venous hematocrit of >0.65; above this level there is an exponential rise in blood viscosity. Clinical manifestations include lethargy, hypotonia, hyperbilirubinemia and hypoglycemia. Polycythemia may also be a contributory factor in neonatal seizures, stroke, renal vein thrombosis and NEC. Causes of polycythemia include:

- IUGR;
- maternal hypertension;
- maternal diabetes;
- endocrine disorders: thyrotoxicosis, congenital adrenal hyperplasia;
- chromosomal disorders – trisomy 21, 18 or 13;
- twin-to-twin transfusion;
- delayed clamping of the cord.

Treatment of neonatal polycythemia is controversial. A recent meta-analysis suggested no proven benefit of partial exchange transfusion in terms of long term neurological outcome or early neurobehavioral assessment although there may be an earlier improvement in symptoms. There is also a suggestion of increased risk of gastrointestinal symptoms, in particular NEC, in exchanged neonates.[780] If partial exchange transfusion is felt to be necessary then a crystalloid solution such as normal saline should be used.[781] The aim of exchange transfusion is to reduce the hematocrit to 0.55. The formula for calculating the volume to be exchanged in ml is:

$$\frac{\text{Blood volume} \times \text{Observed PCV} - \text{Desired PCV}}{\text{Observed PCV}}$$

Controlled studies show no evidence to support the use of fresh frozen plasma or albumin for this procedure, both of which carry the risk of transfusion-transmitted infection.[781]

WHITE CELL DISORDERS
Neutropenia
Definition and causes of neonatal neutropenia

Neutropenia is fairly common in preterm neonates but is uncommon in term infants. Since normal values are dependent on age and gestational age, a pragmatic approach is to consider a neutrophil count at birth of $<2 \times 10^9$/L as abnormal and worth monitoring and a neutrophil count during the first month of life of $<0.7 \times 10^9$/L as significant enough to merit further investigation. Causes of neonatal neutropenia are shown in Table 12.84. In preterm neonates the commonest cause is neutropenia in association with IUGR and/or maternal hypertension. The second most frequent cause in preterm infants, and the most common cause in term infants, is neutropenia secondary to bacterial or viral infection.

Immune neutropenias

Although uncommon, immune neutropenia may be severe in the newborn. Both autoimmune and alloimmune neutropenia occur. Autoimmune neutropenia is secondary to maternal autoimmune disease [e.g. systemic lupus erythematosus (SLE)] and is self-limiting. Alloimmune neutropenia occurs where fetal neutrophils express paternally derived neutrophil-specific antigens not present on maternal neutrophils and against which the mother produces IgG neutrophil alloantibodies. The causative antibodies are usually anti-NA1 or anti-NA2. It is said to occur in 3% of all deliveries but it seems likely that most cases are so mild they do not present to medical attention. The more severe cases present in the first few days of life with fever and infections of the respiratory tract, urinary tract and skin, particularly due to *Staphylococcus aureus*. The neutropenia is self-limiting, usually resolving within 1–2 months, and the mainstay of treatment is antibiotics.

Table 12.84 Causes of neonatal neutropenia

1. Immune
   Alloimmune
   Autoimmune
2. Infection
   Acute, perinatal bacterial infection, e.g. group B streptococcus
   Congenital infections, e.g. CMV
   Postnatal bacterial infections
   Postnatal viral infections, e.g. CMV
3. Necrotizing enterocolitis
4. Placental insufficiency
   Maternal hypertension
   Intrauterine growth restriction
   Maternal diabetes
5. Genetic
   Trisomies: 21, 13 and 18
   Kostmann syndrome
   Shwachman syndrome
   Pearson syndrome
   Reticular dysgenesis
   Metabolic disorders, e.g. hyperglycinemia; isovaleric, propionic and methylmalonic acidemia
6. Marrow replacement
   Congenital leukemia

Non-immune neutropenias

The commonest non-immune cause in preterm infants is neutropenia secondary to IUGR and/or maternal hypertension; it may also occur in infants of diabetic mothers. The exact pathogenesis is unknown. Neutrophil production secondary to reduced numbers of neutrophil progenitors (CFU-GM) is found and most affected neonates have associated thrombocytopenia and increased erythropoiesis (polycythemia and/or increased circulating nucleated red cells).[757] The hematological abnormalities appear secondary to fetal tissue hypoxia. Increased erythropoietin is likely to play a role, perhaps by enhancing erythropoiesis at the expense of neutrophil and platelet production. Neutropenia secondary to IUGR/maternal hypertension reaches its nadir on day 2/3 of life and recovers spontaneously by day 7–10. The severity is directly related to the severity of the IUGR/maternal hypertension. Attempts have been made to prevent or ameliorate sepsis in neutropenic infants by the use of growth factors (recombinant G-CSF or GM-CSF) either therapeutically or prophylactically, or by direct infusion of donor granulocytes. Despite a number of small double-blind placebo-controlled trials none of these approaches has currently been shown to be of clinical benefit.[782,783]

Other non-immune causes of neutropenia are listed in Table 12.84. The most important is neutropenia secondary to infection. Any bacterial infections cause acute neutropenia – where this is short lived (6–12 h) it is a normal response, but neutropenia lasting >12 h in the setting of acute bacterial infection is a poor prognostic sign. Examination of the blood film is often helpful in differentiating neutropenia secondary to infection from that due to viral infection or IUGR. The classic signs of acute bacterial infection are the presence of an increased percentage of band neutrophils and toxic granulation of immature and mature neutrophils followed after 1–2 days by a mature neutrophilia and after 3–5 days by eosinophilia. By contrast, there is no increase in band cells or toxic granulation in viral infections; instead atypical 'viral' lymphocytes are seen. Rare causes of neonatal neutropenia include Kostmann disease and bone marrow failure syndromes. These should be sought where the neutropenia is prolonged, there is a relevant family history, there is consanguinity or if the baby has typical dysmorphic features.

Hemopoietic stem cell disorders including leukemias and myeloproliferative disorders

Congenital leukemias

Congenital leukemia is rare but the diagnosis is usually straightforward. The most common types are acute monoblastic leukemia and acute megakaryoblastic leukemia; around 25% of cases occur in babies with Down syndrome (see Ch. 14). Both have similar presentations but can be differentiated by cytogenetic and immunophenotypic studies on bone marrow and blood leukemia cells. The usual presentation is with clinical signs of anemia and skin lesions caused by focal infiltration by leukemic cells. Congenital leukemia may present as a 'blueberry muffin' baby or hydrops fetalis. The prognosis in infants without Down syndrome is extremely poor; few are cured by chemotherapy and bone marrow transplantation may be the best option.[784]

Hematological abnormalities in neonates with Down syndrome and other trisomies

Hematological abnormalities are more common in neonates with chromosomal disorders, including Down syndrome, trisomy 13 and trisomy 18, all of which may be associated with pancytopenia. Most babies with Down syndrome have a normal blood count; the remaining 10% have one of three hematological presentations:

1. acute leukemia (see p. 334);
2. transient abnormal myelopoiesis (TAM);
3. mild pancytopenia with subtle myelodysplastic changes.

TAM presents with leukocytosis and an abnormal blood film with circulating blast cells. In most cases no treatment is required and TAM almost always resolves by the age of 2–3 months.[785] In some cases affected infants may present with severe hepatic or pulmonary impairment due to fibrosis or infiltration with hemopoietic cells. These babies may respond to low dose cytarabine chemotherapy. The majority of cases of TAM spontaneously resolve but 20–30% of babies go on to develop acute megakaryoblastic leukemia (AMKL) within the first four years of life. This disease is of considerable scientific interest as virtually 100% of affected babies with TAM and AMKL harbor mutations in the X-linked hemopoietic transcription factor GATA-1. This, alongside the tight association between trisomy 21 and TAM/AMKL, makes it an excellent biological model with which to try to understand the stepwise acquisition of molecular and cellular abnormalities underlying the development of leukemia in all children.[786] Large national prospective studies are under way to try to acquire knowledge of the natural history of hemopoietic abnormalities in Down syndrome and evaluate markers that may predict which children are likely to develop leukemia in later infancy/childhood.

Abnormal leukocytes in neonatal systemic disease

The blood film often provides clues to other underlying disorders in the newborn. As well as classic features of acute bacterial and viral infections (see p. 322), characteristic changes can be seen in fungal infection where vacuolation of the neutrophils and monocytes may be prominent and fungi may be seen within the phagocytic cells. In NEC, neutrophil and monocyte vacuolation is also common. A number of metabolic and storage disorders produce changes in the appearance of leukocytes which can be seen on carefully examined blood films:

- leukocyte vacuolation in Pearson syndrome;
- giant neutrophil granules in Chediak–Higashi syndrome;
- Alder Reilly leukocyte granules in Hunter syndrome, Hurler syndrome and Sanfilippo syndrome;
- lymphocyte vacuolation in Wolman disease, alpha-mannosidosis, sialidosis and Sanfilippo syndrome.

HEMOSTASIS AND THROMBOSIS

Normal hemostasis

Hemostasis involves a complex balance between activators and inhibitors of the coagulation cascade and a system to break down and limit clot size (fibrinolysis).[787] There are five main components: blood vessels, platelets, coagulation factors, coagulation inhibitors and fibrinolysis.

Blood vessels

Local damage to the vasculature leads to release of tissue factor and exposure of procoagulants in the subendothelium including collagen and von Willebrand factor (vWF). This results in platelet adhesion followed by coagulation. Key inhibitors of coagulation are also present on the endothelial surface including antithrombin, protein C and protein S. Hence endothelium is responsible for directing coagulation to the site of injury and then limiting the extent of thrombus formation via inhibitors.

Platelets

Platelets aggregate at sites of injury and are vital for primary hemostasis. They also provide a phospholipid surface essential for the coagulation cascade. Both quantitative and qualitative defects can lead to bleeding disorders.

Coagulation factors

Traditional versions of the coagulation cascade based on in vitro clotting tests delineated intrinsic and extrinsic pathways and sequential activation of coagulation factors. It has become clear that the process in vivo is quite different and a new pathway has been proposed (Fig. 12.41). Clotting factors generally exist as inactive precursors and require activation to take part in coagulation. The key initiating event is exposure of tissue factor in response to endothelial damage. Tissue factor activates factor VII to form a complex, TF – VIIa, which cleaves factor X to its active form Xa. Xa can convert prothrombin to thrombin with low efficiency but this generation of small amounts of thrombin then activates feedback loops to increase coagulation factor activation. Factor VIII (activated by thrombin) and factor IX (activated by TF – VIIa and factor XI) form a complex VIIIa – IXa known as tenase. Tenase generates activated factor X with great efficiency. Thrombin also activates factor V, and a Xa – Va complex is formed which cleaves prothrombin to form thrombin. Thrombin generation leads to conversion of fibrinogen to fibrin with subsequent crosslinking by factor XIII.

Inhibitors of coagulation

Upon localized initiation of clotting, spread throughout the vasculature is prevented by inhibitors. Protein C is activated by thrombin. Once

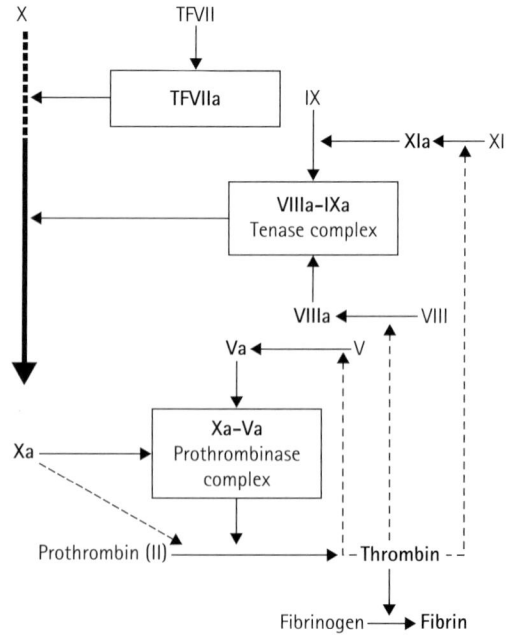

Fig. 12.41 Coagulation cascade. Thick dashed arrows indicate low efficiency pathways. Thin dashed arrows indicate feedback activation loops. Boxes indicate complexes on phospholipid surface.

activated, protein C forms a complex with protein S which increases its activity 10-fold. The activated protein C complex (APC) cleaves and inactivates factors V and VIII. A mutation in factor V (factor V Leiden) at the cleavage site, preventing factor V inactivation by APC, is associated with thrombophilia. Antithrombin and heparin cofactor II are both potent direct inhibitors of thrombin; levels of these proteins are low at birth but rarely cause thrombosis.[788]

Fibrinolysis

Fibrinolysis limits fibrin deposition at the site of injury. The key enzyme is plasmin. This is produced by the action of tissue plasminogen activator whose activity is catalyzed by fibrin itself. Fibrin breakdown is accompanied by the production of degradation products (FDPs) and D-dimers.

Coagulation in the fetus and newborn

Coagulation proteins are synthesized from the fifth week of gestation onwards and do not cross the placenta.[788] Levels gradually rise towards birth but many do not attain adult values during the neonatal period. Birth may cause activation of coagulation, hence levels in preterm infants may be significantly higher than those found in fetuses of the same gestational age. Normal values vary with gestational and postnatal age (Table 12.85).[789–791]

Diagnostic approach to bleeding in neonates
Clinical presentation of bleeding disorders

Neonates exhibit patterns of bleeding distinct from those in older children. Bleeding from the umbilical cord stump, venepuncture sites, cephalhematomas after vacuum extraction, intracranial and pulmonary hemorrhage can occur. Bleeding post circumcision is a relatively common presentation of hemophilia in the neonate, but hemarthroses are extremely rare. The most likely cause of bleeding in neonates depends on gestational age and whether the child is clinically well or unwell. A thorough clinical assessment is essential and should include sites and severity of bleeding, predisposing factors, drug history (infant and maternal) including vitamin K and a family history of possible coagulation disorders.

Screening tests for bleeding disorders

Initial screening tests should comprise:
1. *prothrombin time* (PT) – measures activity of factors II, V, VII and X;
2. *activated partial thromboplastin time* (APTT) – measures factors II, V, VIII, IX, X, XI and XII;
3. *thrombin time* (TT) – prolonged by quantitative and qualitative disorders of fibrinogen, the presence of inhibitory factors such as fibrin/FDPs and the presence of heparin;
4. fibrinogen level;
5. platelet count.

Table 12.85 Reference values for (a) healthy full-term infants and (b) preterm infants during the neonatal period

a) Full-term infants

Coagulation tests	Full-term Day 1 Mean (95% limits)	Full-term Day 5 Mean (95% limits)	Full-term Day 30 Mean (95% limits)
PT (s)	13.0 (10.1–15.9)	12.4 (10.0–15.3)	11.8 (10.0–14.3)
APTT (s)	42.9 (31.3–54.5)	42.6 (25.4–59.8)	40.4 (32.0–55.2)
TT (s)	23.5 (19.0–28.3)	23.1 (18.0–29.2)	24.3 (19.4–29.2)
Fibrinogen (g/L)	2.83 (1.67–3.99)	3.12 (1.62–4.62)	2.70 (1.62–3.78)
Factor V (u/ml)	0.72 (0.34–1.08)	0.95 (0.45–1.45)	0.98 (0.62–1.34)
Factor VII (u/ml)	0.66 (0.28–1.04)	0.89 (0.35–1.43)	0.90 (0.42–1.38)
Factor VIII (u/ml)	1.00 (0.50–1.78)	0.88 (0.50–1.54)	0.91 (0.50–1.57)
Factor IX (u/ml)	0.53 (0.15–0.91)	0.53 (0.15–0.91)	0.51 (0.21–0.81)
Factor X (u/ml)	0.40 (0.12–0.68)	0.49 (0.19–0.79)	0.59 (0.31–0.87)
Factor XI (u/ml)	0.38 (0.10–0.66)	0.55 (0.23–0.87)	0.53 (0.27–0.79)
Factor XII (u/ml)	0.53 (0.13–0.93)	0.47 (0.11–0.83)	0.49 (0.17–0.81)
Factor XIIIa (u/ml)	0.79 (0.27–1.31)	0.94 (0.44–1.44)	0.93 (0.39–1.47)
vWF (u/ml)	1.53 (0.50–2.87)	1.40 (0.50–2.54)	1.28 (0.50–2.46)
Antithrombin (U/ml)	0.63 (0.39–0.87)	0.67 (0.41–0.93)	0.78 (0.48–1.08)
Protein C (U/ml)	0.35 (0.17–0.53)	0.42 (0.20–0.64)	0.43 (0.21–0.65)
Protein S (U/ml)	0.36 (0.12–0.60)	0.50 (0.22–0.78)	0.63 (0.33–0.93)

b) Preterm infants

Coagulation tests	Premature 30–36 weeks Day 1 Mean (95% limits)	Premature 30–36 weeks Day 5 Mean (95% limits)	Premature 30–36 weeks Day 30 Mean (95% limits)	Premature 30–36 weeks Day 90 Mean (95% limits)	Premature 24–29 weeks Day 1 Mean (95% limits)
PT (s)	13.0 (10.6–16.2)	12.5 (10.0–15.3)	11.8 (10.0–13.6)	12.3 (10.0–14.6)	14.5 (11.7–21.6)
APTT (s)	53.6 (27.5–79.4)	50.5 (26.9–74.1)	44.7 (26.9–62.5)	39.5 (28.3–50.7)	69.5 (40.6–101)
TT (s)	24.8 (19.2–30.4)	24.1 (18.8–29.4)	24.4 (18.8–29.9)	25.1 (19.4–30.8)	
Fibrinogen (g/L)	2.43 (1.50–3.73)	2.80 (1.60–4.18)	2.54 (1.50–4.14)	2.46 (1.50–3.52)	1.35 (0.62–4.21)
Factor V (u/ml)	0.88 (0.41–1.44)	1.00 (0.46–1.54)	1.02 (0.48–1.56)	0.99 (0.59–1.39)	
Factor VII (u/ml)	0.67 (0.21–1.13)	0.84 (0.30–1.38)	0.83 (0.21–1.45)	0.87 (0.31–1.43)	
Factor VIII (u/ml)	1.11 (0.50–2.13)	1.15 (0.53–2.05)	1.11 (0.50–1.99)	1.06 (0.58–1.88)	
Factor IX (u/ml)	0.35 (0.19–0.65)	0.42 (0.14–0.74)	0.44 (0.13–0.80)	0.59 (0.25–0.93)	
Factor X (u/ml)	0.41 (0.11–0.71)	0.51 (0.19–0.83)	0.56 (0.20–0.92)	0.67 (0.35–0.99)	
Factor XI (u/ml)	0.30 (0.08–0.52)	0.41 (0.13–0.69)	0.43 (0.15–0.71)	0.59 (0.25–0.93)	
Factor XII (u/ml)	0.38 (0.10–0.66)	0.39 (0.09–0.69)	0.43 (0.11–0.75)	0.61 (0.15–1.07)	
Factor XIIIa (u/ml)	0.70 (0.32–1.08)	1.01 (0.57–1.45)	0.99 (0.51–1.47)	1.13 (0.71–1.55)	
vWF (u/ml)	1.36 (0.78–2.10)	1.33 (0.72–2.19)	1.36 (0.66–2.16)	1.12 (0.75–1.84)	
Antithrombin (U/ml)	0.38 (0.14–0.62)	0.56 (0.30–0.82)	0.59 (0.37–0.81)	0.83 (0.45–1.21)	
Protein C (U/ml)	0.28 (0.12–0.44)	0.31 (0.11–0.51)	0.37 (0.15–0.59)	0.45 (0.23–0.67)	
Protein S (U/ml)	0.26 (0.14–0.38)	0.37 (0.13–0.61)	0.56 (0.22–0.90)	0.76 (0.40–1.12)	

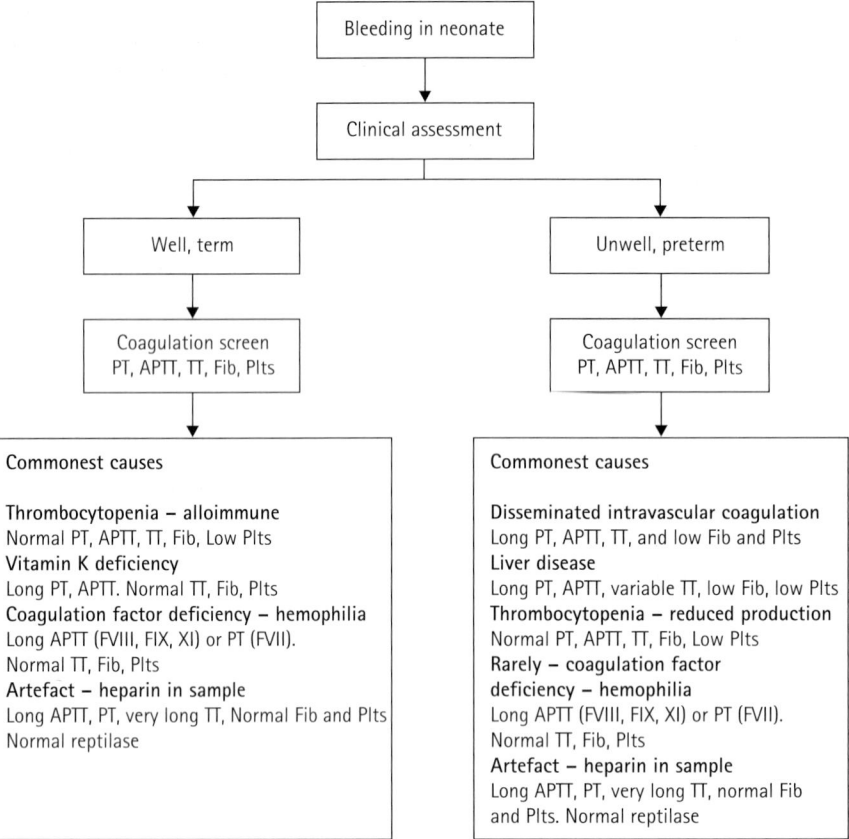

Fig. 12.42 Diagnostic algorithm for bleeding in neonates. APTT, activated partial thromboplastin time; Fib, fibrinogen; Plts, platelets; PT, prothrombin time; TT, thrombin time.

Results of these tests along with clinical history can guide subsequent investigation. Bleeding times are generally unhelpful. A diagnostic algorithm is shown in Figure 12.42.

Interpretation of laboratory coagulation tests

Coagulation testing in neonates is often difficult. Since testing is done on plasma, the high hematocrit in many neonates means the blood volumes required for testing are relatively large even when using specially adapted microtechniques. Activation of coagulation during sampling is common when venepuncture is difficult and invalidates results. Samples from indwelling lines are frequently heparin contaminated. Laboratories may use various tests to distinguish the presence of heparin in a sample including measuring the degree of correction of the thrombin time with protamine or normal patient plasma. A *reptilase time* (so named because snake venom is used in the test) can also be very helpful; it assesses the same components as a TT but is unaffected by heparin. In coagulation factor assays, the lower limit of the normal range in neonates often overlaps with those seen in deficiency states (especially seen with factor II, factor X and factor XI). In such circumstances demonstrating heterozygote levels of factor activity in parents is useful.

Inherited coagulation disorders

Inherited coagulation disorders are rare but often present in the neonatal period so a high index of suspicion is needed. The commonest are the X-linked disorders factor VIII (hemophilia A) and factor IX (hemophilia B) with a frequency of 1 in 10 000 and 1 in 60 000 male births respectively. Most other factor deficiencies are autosomal recessive. All produce prolongation of coagulation screening tests with the exception of factor XIII deficiency and, rarely, von Willebrand disease (vWD). Therefore a normal coagulation screen in a child with unexplained bleeding does not exclude all inherited coagulation disorders and further specialized tests may be needed.

This section addresses neonatal aspects of inherited coagulation abnormalities. A comprehensive discussion of these conditions is provided elsewhere (Ch. 23).

Factor VIII deficiency

Clinical presentation. This may be diagnosed or suspected antenatally in families with a history of hemophilia. One third of cases represent new mutations and are therefore unsuspected at birth. They may present with intracranial hemorrhage, subgaleal or cephalhematomas, bleeding post circumcision or from venous or arterial puncture sites. The hemorrhage may be life threatening. Prolonged bleeding from the umbilical cord is less common. Large bruises may occur and the diagnosis may be made during investigations of possible non-accidental injury.

Diagnosis. Coagulation tests show a very prolonged APTT with normal PT, TT, platelets and fibrinogen. The definitive diagnosis is made by measurement of factor VIII clotting activity which is < 50%; all other factors, including vWF antigen, are normal. Disease severity is classified according to factor VIII activity with levels < 1% indicative of severe disease.

Management. Adequate family support is vital and early liaison with a hemophilia center is essential. Treatment should be with recombinant factor VIII concentrate for bleeding episodes. The best mode of delivery is controversial; there is no evidence that elective Cesarean section eliminates bleeding; spontaneous vaginal delivery is acceptable but vacuum extraction should be avoided due to the high rate of subgaleal bleeds and cephalhematomas. There is debate as to whether known hemophiliac newborns should be given prophylactic factor VIII following delivery to reduce the risk of intracranial bleeding, currently estimated to have an incidence of around 3–5%. Large prospective cohort studies are needed.[792] Known or suspected hemophiliac newborns should always have a cord blood sample taken for a coagulation screen and factor VIII level as this avoids possible iatrogenic bruising or bleeding secondary to difficult venepuncture in the first few days of life. Vitamin K should be given at birth but the intramuscular route avoided because of hematoma formation.

Factor IX deficiency

This has an identical clinical phenotype to factor VIII deficiency and can only be distinguished by specific factor assays. Unlike factor VIII, factor IX is vitamin K dependent and hence its activity also falls in liver disease and vitamin K deficiency. However there is seldom diagnostic confusion as the latter diseases produce prolongation of other screening tests and characteristic clinical features. Treatment of bleeding is with recombinant factor IX concentrate.

von Willebrand disease

This is a complex group of conditions caused by quantitative or qualitative defects in vWF. Neonatal presentation is rare as levels of vWF are elevated at birth.[788] However, one of the most severe forms, type 3 vWD, may present in the neonatal period. In this case factor VIII levels are very low, vWF is virtually absent and the patient presents in a similar way to hemophilia A. Clues to the diagnosis are the absence of X-linked inheritance and poor response to factor VIII concentrates. Quantification of vWF makes the diagnosis. Treatment of bleeding is with a viricidally treated intermediate purity factor VIII concentrate containing the high molecular weight multimers of vWF. Desmopressin (DDAVP) can be used in older children with mild to moderate vWD but should be avoided in neonates and younger children due to the risk of hyponatremic convulsions.

Factor XIII deficiency

Factor XIII deficiency presents with umbilical stump bleeding and/or intracranial hemorrhage. Routine coagulation screens are normal. Diagnosis is made by measuring clot lysis in 5 M urea solution; molecular tests for the common mutations are also available. Treatment is with factor XIII concentrate.

Other rarer inherited coagulation factor deficiencies

These can present in the neonatal period with bleeding or unexplained prolongation of coagulation tests. The majority are autosomal recessive. Factor XI deficiency can produce hemophiliac-type bleeding and is commoner in Ashkenazi Jews. Factor VII deficiency can produce a very severe bleeding disorder with a high incidence of intracranial hemorrhage. Recombinant factor VII concentrate can be used but is expensive and has a very short half-life. Factor XII deficiency produces a markedly prolonged APTT but no clinically apparent bleeding disorder. Dysfibrinogenemias are rare and can produce both hemorrhage and thrombosis.[793]

Acquired disorders of coagulation

Vitamin k deficiency (hemorrhagic disease of the newborn)

Vitamin K is essential for the production of active forms of factors II, VII, IX, X and protein C and S. Placental transfer of vitamin K occurs but is insufficient to build up adequate stores in the neonate and without supplementation levels fall during the first few days of life. Untreated vitamin K deficiency can lead to hemorrhagic disease of the newborn. It can be classified according to age of onset into classic, early and late.

Classic. This presents at 2–7 days old, generally in breast-fed term healthy infants. The incidence in babies not receiving supplementation is 0.4–1.7/100 births. Causes include: low vitamin K content in breast milk (< 5 mcg/L compared to 50–60 mcg/L in formula milk), poor oral intake and a sterile gut. It can be prevented by vitamin K supplementation at birth.

Early. This presents within the first 24–48 h and is associated with severe vitamin K deficiency in utero. The usual cause is maternal medication that interferes with vitamin K, e.g. anticonvulsants (phenobarbital, phenytoin), antituberculous therapy and oral anticoagulants. It cannot be prevented by vitamin K supplementation at birth.

Late. This occurs from 2 weeks to 6 months of age. It is usually associated with disorders that reduce vitamin K absorption, e.g. alpha1-antitrypsin deficiency, biliary atresia, liver disease and malabsorptive states. Breast-fed babies are also at risk. It is prevented by a single intramuscular dose or repeated oral doses of vitamin K. Prolonged vitamin K supplementation should be given to all babies with chronic liver disease or other risk factors.

Bleeding manifestations include gastrointestinal, cutaneous and intracranial bleeding. Gastrointestinal bleeding in newborns can be differentiated from melena secondary to swallowed maternal blood by the Apt test which distinguishes fetal from adult hemoglobin, although this test is no longer widely available. Isolated prolongation of the PT is the earliest laboratory sign of vitamin K deficiency, followed by prolongation of the APTT. Low levels of vitamin K dependent factors are seen, and inactive forms (proteins induced by vitamin K absence; PIVKAs) can be measured. Treatment is with 1 mg vitamin K subcutaneously or intravenously (not i.m. due to risk of hematoma) which will usually correct the coagulopathy within a few hours; fresh frozen plasma (FFP) at a dose of 10–15 ml/kg may be given for active bleeding prior to vitamin K taking effect. In the presence of life-threatening bleeding, prothrombin complex concentrate may be more effective in restoring adequate clotting factor levels but there are few data in neonates.[793]

Vitamin K supplementation at birth. Vitamin K supplementation prevents classic and late vitamin K deficiency bleeding. Controversy surrounds the best mode of administration. Studies by Golding et al[794] suggested a link between intramuscular vitamin K at birth and later childhood malignancies. These studies have been criticized on methodological grounds. No link between oral vitamin K and malignancy has been reported but disadvantages of oral vitamin K include unnoticed regurgitation, unpredictable absorption and the need for repeated dosing. In one study there were no cases of vitamin K deficiency bleeding in 320 000 infants given 1 mg i.m. vitamin K at birth, but 32 cases of late disease in 1 200 000 infants given 1 mg orally at birth, 1 week and 1 month of age.[795] A systematic review[796] concludes that:

1. intramuscular vitamin K has been proven to prevent classic disease;
2. oral vitamin K has been proven to improve biochemical parameters of vitamin K deficiency in the first week of life;
3. the efficacy of oral supplementation in preventing late disease is unproven.

Disseminated intravascular coagulation (DIC)

The pathophysiology of DIC is complex but involves widespread uncontrolled activation of the coagulation cascade with subsequent consumption of clotting factors and a combination of thrombotic and hemorrhagic manifestations. The initial trigger is usually the release of tissue factor and cytokines from damaged endothelium or monocytes. A number of neonatal disorders resulting in severe hypoxia and/or acidosis can precipitate DIC including peripartum hemorrhage, severe birth asphyxia, meconium aspiration and sepsis. Clinically DIC is seen in sick neonates and presents with generalized bleeding. The PT, APTT and TT are prolonged; platelets and fibrinogen are low. Although D-dimers are of some use in monitoring DIC they should be interpreted with caution as they are not specific and can be found in healthy neonates with no evidence of coagulopathy.[793] The mainstay of management is treatment of the underlying cause. In the presence of uncontrolled bleeding, platelet infusion and FFP or cryoprecipitate may be needed. Platelets should be maintained above 50×10^9/L and fibrinogen > 1 g/L.

Other acquired coagulation disorders

Serious liver disease can cause a severe coagulopathy compounded by hepatocyte immaturity, vitamin K deficiency and DIC. Platelets may be low due to impaired production, increased consumption and splenic sequestration. Coagulopathy can be seen with metabolic defects such as hyperammonemia. Extracorporeal membrane oxygenation often causes coagulation and platelet disturbances due to consumption of clotting factors and platelets and heparinization. Consumptive coagulopathy with thrombocytopenia can be seen with giant hemangioendotheliomas (Kasabach–Merritt syndrome).

Neonatal thrombocytopenia

Incidence of neonatal thrombocytopenia

Thrombocytopenia (platelets $< 150 \times 10^9$/L) is relatively common in neonates, occurring in 1–5% of all newborns, in 22–35% of neonates admitted to NICUs and in up to 50% of neonates who are preterm and sick.[797] Severe thrombocytopenia (platelets $< 50 \times 10^9$/L) occurs in 0.2% of neonates.

Causes and natural history of neonatal thrombocytopenia

Neonatal thrombocytopenia usually presents in one of two patterns: early (within 72 h of birth) and late (after 72 h of life). Early thrombocytopenia is more common; the principal causes are shown in Table 12.86. The most frequent cause of early thrombocytopenia in preterm infants is 'placental insufficiency'; this is self-limiting, usually within 10 days, and is rarely severe except in neonates with profound IUGR. It is caused by reduced platelet production. The most important cause of early neonatal thrombocytopenia from a clinical viewpoint is neonatal alloimmune thrombocytopenia (NAITP) (see below). The most common and clinically important causes of late thrombocytopenia are sepsis and NEC.[797]

Neonatal alloimmune and autoimmune thrombocytopenia (NAITP)

NAITP is the platelet equivalent of hemolytic disease of the newborn. Fetal and neonatal thrombocytopenia result from transplacental passage of maternal platelet-specific antibodies; in 80% of cases these are anti-HPA-1a antibodies and in 10–15% anti-HPA-5b. Although NAITP is uncommon, affecting 1:1000 pregnancies, it is frequently severe and occurs in the first pregnancy in almost 50% of cases. Intracranial hemorrhage occurs in 10% of cases with long term neurodevelopmental sequelae in 20% of survivors. Diagnosis is made by demonstrating platelet antigen incompatibility between mother and baby. Therapy for NAITP remains controversial (reviewed in Ouwehand et al[798]). Antenatal management may include fetal blood sampling, fetal transfusion with HPA-compatible platelets and/or maternal IVIG therapy; each approach has evidence to support it. All severely affected babies should receive HPA-compatible platelets until a stable platelet count $> 50 \times 10^9$/L is achieved.

Neonatal autoimmune thrombocytopenia occurs secondary to transplacental passage of maternal platelet autoantibodies, usually maternal ITP. Thrombocytopenia affects the infants of 10% of affected mothers;

Table 12.86   Causes of neonatal thrombocytopenia

Early (<72 h)	Placental insufficiency (PET, IUGR, diabetes)
	NAITP
	Birth asphyxia
	Perinatal infection (group B strep, *Escherichia coli*, *Listeria*)
	Congenital infection (CMV, toxoplasmosis, rubella)
	Maternal autoimmune (ITP, SLE)
	Severe rhesus HDN
	Thrombosis (renal vein, aortic)
	Aneuploidy (trisomy – 21, 18, 13)
	Congenital/inherited (TAR, Wiskott–Aldrich)
Late (>72 h)	Late-onset sepsis and NEC
	Congenital infection (CMV, toxoplasmosis, rubella)
	Maternal autoimmune (ITP, SLE)
	Congenital/inherited (TAR, Wiskott–Aldrich)

CMV, cytomegalovirus; HDN, hemolytic disease of the newborn; ITP, idiopathic thrombocytopenic purpura; IUGR, intrauterine growth restriction; NAITP, neonatal alloimmune thrombocytopenia; NEC, necrotizing enterocolitis; PET, pre-eclampsia; SLE, systemic lupus erythematosus; strep, streptococcus; TAR, thrombocytopenia with absent radii.

thrombocytopenia is usually mild and intracranial hemorrhage occurs in 1% or less. In affected babies with severe thrombocytopenia treatment with IVIG is usually effective.

Management of neonatal thrombocytopenia

The antenatal management of immune thrombocytopenias is described in chapter 11. For other forms of neonatal thrombocytopenia therapy mainly depends upon the appropriate use of platelet transfusion. Evidence-based guidelines for neonatal platelet transfusion therapy are yet to be defined; consensus guidelines are available, most of which recommend platelet transfusion for sick neonates where the platelet count is $< 50 \times 10^9$/L; for stable, relatively well preterm and term infants platelet counts of $30-50 \times 10^9$/L do not appear to be associated with an increased risk of hemorrhage; this approach conforms to the current UK guidelines.[777]

Thrombosis in neonates

Neonates and infants have the highest rate of thrombotic problems within the pediatric population. Most thromboses occur in sick or preterm neonates and are due to acquired risk factors, especially the presence of an indwelling central line. Inherited deficiencies of coagulation inhibitors can lead to dramatic thrombosis in otherwise healthy neonates.

Inherited thrombotic disorders

Protein C deficiency. Homozygous or compound heterozygous protein C deficiency usually presents within the first few days of life with purpura fulminans. This is characterized by a rapidly progressive hemorrhagic necrosis of the skin accompanied by dermal vessel thrombosis which is most pronounced in the extremities. Babies may also show evidence of intrauterine thrombosis with cerebral and ophthalmic damage at birth. Occasionally isolated vessel thrombosis may occur. Diagnosis is made by the characteristic clinical picture in conjunction with very low levels of protein C in the patient and heterozygote levels in the parents. Treatment is with FFP or protein C concentrate. Oral anticoagulation is used in the medium to long term to prevent recurrence but its introduction must be covered by infusion of a source of protein C and very careful monitoring is needed to prevent subtherapeutic levels which are associated with recurrence of thrombosis.

Protein S deficiency. This presents in a similar way to protein C deficiency. Treatment is with FFP.

Antithrombin deficiency. This is very rare in the homozygous state. Myocardial infarction, aortic thrombosis and cerebral thrombosis have all been reported in neonates. Antithrombin concentrate is commercially available.

The role of thrombophilia screening in neonatal thrombosis. Homozygous protein C, S and antithrombin deficiency are the only inherited thrombophilic mutations shown to directly cause neonatal thrombotic problems. Many studies have documented the presence of other thrombophilic mutations such as factor V Leiden and the prothrombin 202010A promoter mutation in neonatal thrombotic disease, both venous and arterial, but whether these mutations are causative and the role they play in the natural history of these disorders is uncertain. In order to justify testing for these defects it must be shown that the result influences treatment or prognosis. At present there is insufficient evidence to support routine testing but ongoing international registries of pediatric thrombosis are currently collecting data and the position may become clearer in the future.[793]

Acquired thrombotic problems

Risk factors for thrombosis include the presence of a vessel catheter, shock syndromes (septic, hypoxemic or hypovolemic) and, rarely, the presence of maternal lupus anticoagulant.

Catheter-related thrombosis. This is the commonest cause of neonatal thrombosis, being responsible for > 80% of venous and > 90% arterial thrombosis. Symptomatic thrombosis occurs in 1% of neonates with indwelling vascular catheters, but postmortem studies suggest rates of asymptomatic thrombosis up to 20–30%. Arterial thrombosis can lead to peripheral gangrene and renal hypertension. Venous thrombosis can cause portal hypertension and varices. Neonatal thrombosis is increasingly recognized as a risk factor for post-thrombotic syndrome, often presenting much later in childhood with skin changes, chronic edema and limb pain or dysfunction.[799] The gold standard for diagnosis of venous thrombosis is contrast angiography, although Doppler ultrasound or magnetic resonance angiography may also be useful. Injection of contrast down a catheter lumen (lineogram) may miss significant thrombosis. The optimal treatment in the neonatal setting is controversial and large randomized trials are urgently needed.[800] Because of differences between the neonatal coagulation system and those of older children and adults extrapolation of guidelines from older age groups to neonates is difficult. In general treatment depends on the severity and extent of thrombosis. The first step is prompt removal of the catheter. If signs progress or have not resolved by 24 h, heparin is the drug of choice but requires a dosing regimen adapted for neonates. Duration of therapy is generally shorter than for older children with 10–14 days of initial treatment followed by re-imaging and discontinuation unless there is new or extending thrombus at this time.[793] Local or systemic thrombolysis with tissue plasminogen activator (tPA) can be considered where there is associated organ dysfunction or limb viability is threatened but can cause high rates of bleeding including intracranial hemorrhage and needs specialist advice and monitoring. Prevention of thrombosis is paramount, e.g. correct catheter positioning, prompt removal once unnecessary. Prophylactic low dose heparin prolongs catheter patency but its role in preventing thrombosis is unproven.[801]

Non-catheter-related thrombosis. The commonest non-catheter-related thrombosis is renal vein thrombosis. Nearly 80% present in the neonatal period and thrombosis may occur in utero. One quarter are bilateral. Presentation is with a flank mass, hematuria, proteinuria, thrombocytopenia and reduced function of the involved kidney. Predisposing factors include reduced renal blood flow, increased viscosity, hyperosmolar states and hypercoagulability; therefore risk factors are sepsis, maternal diabetes, polycythemia, dehydration and prothrombotic mutations. Treatment is supportive. Heparin and thrombolysis are reserved for extensive bilateral cases. Long term outlook is variable.

Neonatal stroke. Neonatal stroke is rare. Causes include bacterial meningitis, hypoxic–ischemic damage and birth trauma. Many cases are idiopathic. Some studies show an increased prevalence of thrombophilia in affected neonates, particularly factor V Leiden.[802] Maternal or neonatal anticardiolipin antibodies have also been linked to neonatal stroke; these are often transient and their causal role is not yet established. This is a rapidly evolving field. It is likely that thrombophilia plays a role in neonatal stroke but additional risk factors are probably also needed.

NEONATAL NEUROLOGY

NEUROLOGICAL ASSESSMENT

Introduction

Clinical examination of the neonatal nervous system is, of necessity, dominated by assessment of motor function. Over time the emphasis has shifted from examination of primitive reflexes to the assessment of the newborn's spontaneous behavior and the way that the baby interacts with adults and deals with stimuli. The following description is based on the work of many pioneers such as Saint-Anne Dargassies,[803] Amiel-Tison & Grenier,[804] Prechtl and his colleagues,[805–808] Brazelton[809,810] and Dubowitz and her colleagues.[811,812]

State

Normal babies show different states of alertness (Table 12.87).[805,809] The fetus exhibits similar states, apart from crying. Babies born before 36 weeks' gestation spend a great deal of time asleep and fall asleep easily when awakened. Preterm sleep states are less easily characterized than at term. Term babies spend about 50 min of each hour asleep, 50% of the time in quiet sleep. Babies who are continually in one state may be abnormal. One example is the baby who is 'hyperalert' due to withdrawal

Table 12.87 Normal neonatal states of Prechtl and Brazelton

Prechtl & Bientema[805]	
State 1	Eyes closed, regular respiration, no movements
State 2	Eyes closed, irregular respiration, no movements
State 3	Eyes open, no gross movements
State 4	Eyes open, gross movements, no crying
State 5	Crying
Brazelton[809]	
State 1	Deep sleep, regular breathing, no movements
State 2	Light sleep, irregular respiration, rapid eye movements, eyes closed
State 3	Drowsy, eyes open or closed, some activity – smooth
State 4	Alert, minimal motor activity
State 5	Eyes open, considerable motor activity
State 6	Crying

symptoms after maternal drug abuse, who spends little time asleep and more time crying than is usual. Inability to rouse a baby from sleep is pathological and a baby who is persistently in state 1 is in a coma.

Crying and consolability

During an examination most babies will cry but are consolable. Soundless or hoarse crying can result from a congenital abnormality such as vocal cord palsy, or from an acquired problem such as trauma from intubation or damage to the recurrent laryngeal nerve during thoracic surgery. High pitched or excessive crying can indicate cerebral irritability due to neonatal encephalopathy. Asymmetrical crying facies is usually due to agenesis or hypoplasia of the depressor anguli oris muscle and needs to be differentiated from facial palsy. Asymmetrical crying facies can be a marker of congenital heart disease although it is usually an isolated malformation.

Posture, spontaneous movement and tone

Normal muscle offers a resistance to stretch felt by the examiner as tone. Tone increases with gestational age and is high in term babies. Term babies lie with their limbs flexed and adducted, unlike preterm babies who adopt an extended posture (Fig. 12.43). Asymmetrical tone does not always indicate asymmetrical pathology in the newborn period.

A term newborn makes smooth, spontaneous symmetrical limb movements which stop when the baby's attention is diverted.[808] Finger movements are elegant and varied, involving the thumb which can be abducted away from the palm by term.[808] In general, the movements of the newborn have a writhing quality, which changes to fidgety after 6–9 weeks of age. Fidgety movements persist until around 6 months of age, when intentional and anti-gravity movements start to dominate. The repertoire of movement is varied and not stereotyped. A persistently adducted thumb (cortical thumb) is abnormal, and brain damaged babies often have fisted hands and a paucity of fine finger movements.

Jitteriness

The normal term newborn is in a state of hypertonicity, with brisk reflexes tending to clonus. This 'transient spasticity' gradually relaxes over the first 8–10 months in a caudocephalad direction. The high tone can lead to the clinical sign of jittering. Jittering is a high frequency, generalized, symmetrical tremor of the limbs which is stilled by flexion or by inducing the baby to suck on a finger. Jittering is common in the first 2 or 3 days in term babies but if it is excessive or persistent deserves investigation. Repetitive chewing movements or tongue thrusting are not part of jitteriness and imply seizures. Jitteriness is stimulus-sensitive whereas seizures are not and in seizures the movements have a fast and slow component whereas in jittering the tremor is symmetrical.

Limb tone and power

Before passive movements are used to assess tone it may be possible to observe spontaneous movements of the limbs against gravity. Failure to

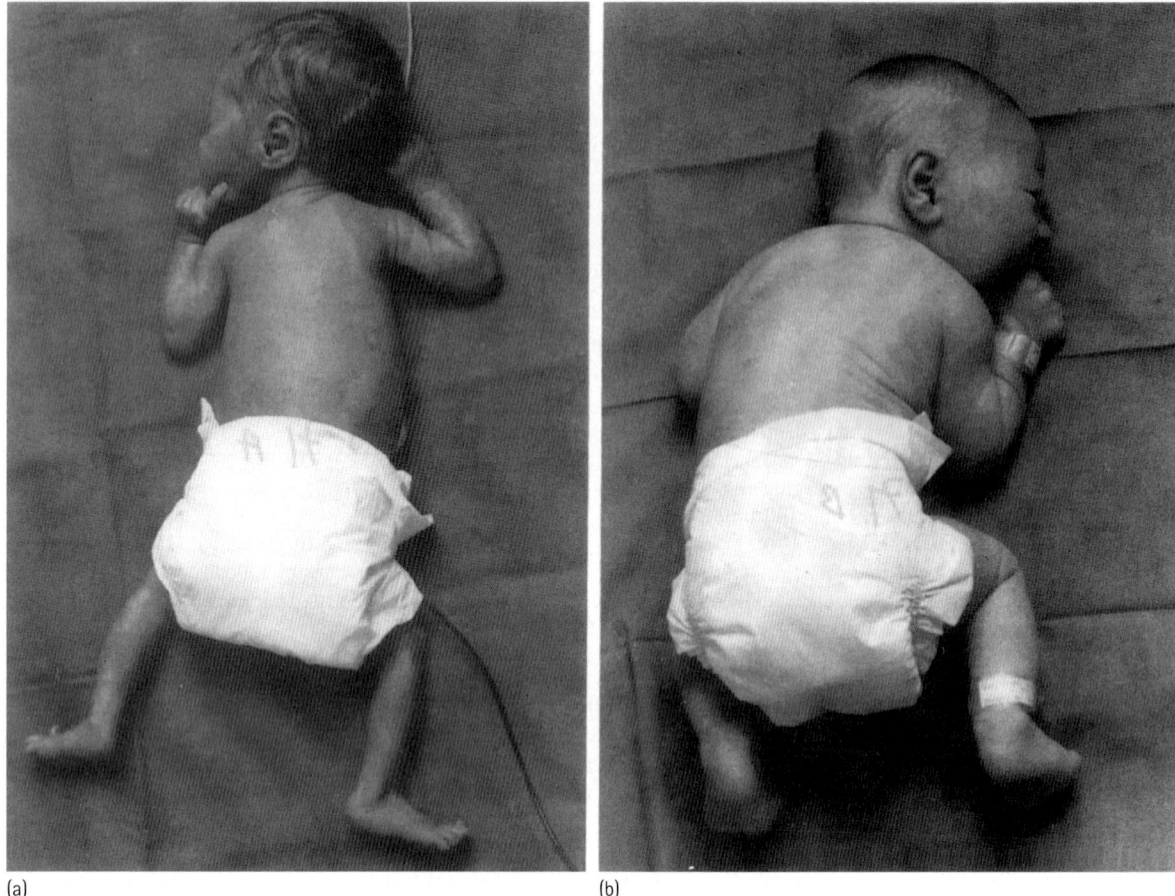

Fig. 12.43   Comparison between low tone in preterm baby (normal) (left) and the high flexor tone of a healthy term baby (right).

move part or whole of a limb may be due to pain or paralysis. Limb tone is influenced by the tonic neck reflex in newborns which means it is important to have the head in the midline before beginning to elicit the response to passive movements. Passive movements involve gentle flexion of the upper and lower limbs, then rapid extension and observation of recoil.

Trunk and neck tone and power

Normal term babies have sufficient power in their neck muscles to lift their heads slightly when prone or supine. Preterm babies can manage to turn their heads from side to side but have much less power with complete head lag when pulled to sit. In order to judge tone in the neck and trunk, babies should be pulled to sit by holding them at the shoulders and then allowing them to fall back again. If the head is unsupported it will gradually fall forwards or backwards: normal term babies will be able to raise their heads to the vertical again from either direction. There is balance between the neck flexors and extensors during pull-to-sit and back-to-lying maneuvers at term so that the head is held in line with the body during both phases. Immature babies usually have better control in back-to-lying. To assess truncal tone, lie the child on his back and try to push his bottom towards his head using his thighs (Fig. 12.44).[813] With the baby lying on his side, hold the lumbar region and pull both legs backwards with the other hand grasping the ankles. Trunk flexion should always exceed extension. Arching of the trunk is abnormal; backwards arching of the whole back and neck is called opisthotonos. Opisthotonos is an important sign of neurological abnormality in the newborn.

Reflexes

Tendon and Babinski reflexes

Eliciting tendon reflexes is of less value in the newborn period than later in childhood. Knee and biceps jerks can usually be obtained.

Reflexes at term are very brisk due to the high tone, and a few beats of clonus at the ankle are usual. The plantar reflex of Babinski is always extensor and is best omitted as the stimulus often results in a withdrawal response.

Primary neonatal reflexes

Whilst the multiplicity of these responses and the timing of their appearance and disappearance is fascinating it is only necessary to have a working knowledge of a few. The reflexes have parallels in animals: the Moro reflex enables young primates to hold on to their mothers. Primitive reflexes normally habituate after repeated performance: this 'conditioning' is apparent even in fetal life. Persistence of neonatal reflexes can considerably inhibit normal movement in children with cerebral palsy.

Moro

This reflex is elicited by allowing the previously supported head of a baby to fall backwards slightly, whereupon the baby extends and adducts both upper limbs, opening the hands (Fig. 12.45). Babies of greater than 33 weeks' gestation subsequently abduct their arms. The Moro response is present from 28 weeks of gestation and usually disappears by 4 months. Persistence beyond 6 months is always abnormal.

Asymmetric tonic neck reflex

Starting with the baby supine and the head in the midline the head is slowly turned to one side. This results in increased extensor tone in the arm on the side to which the head is turned and increased flexor tone in the arm on the opposite side (fencing posture). A persistent asymmetric tonic neck reflex can dominate the movement patterns of children with cerebral palsy for many months, even years.

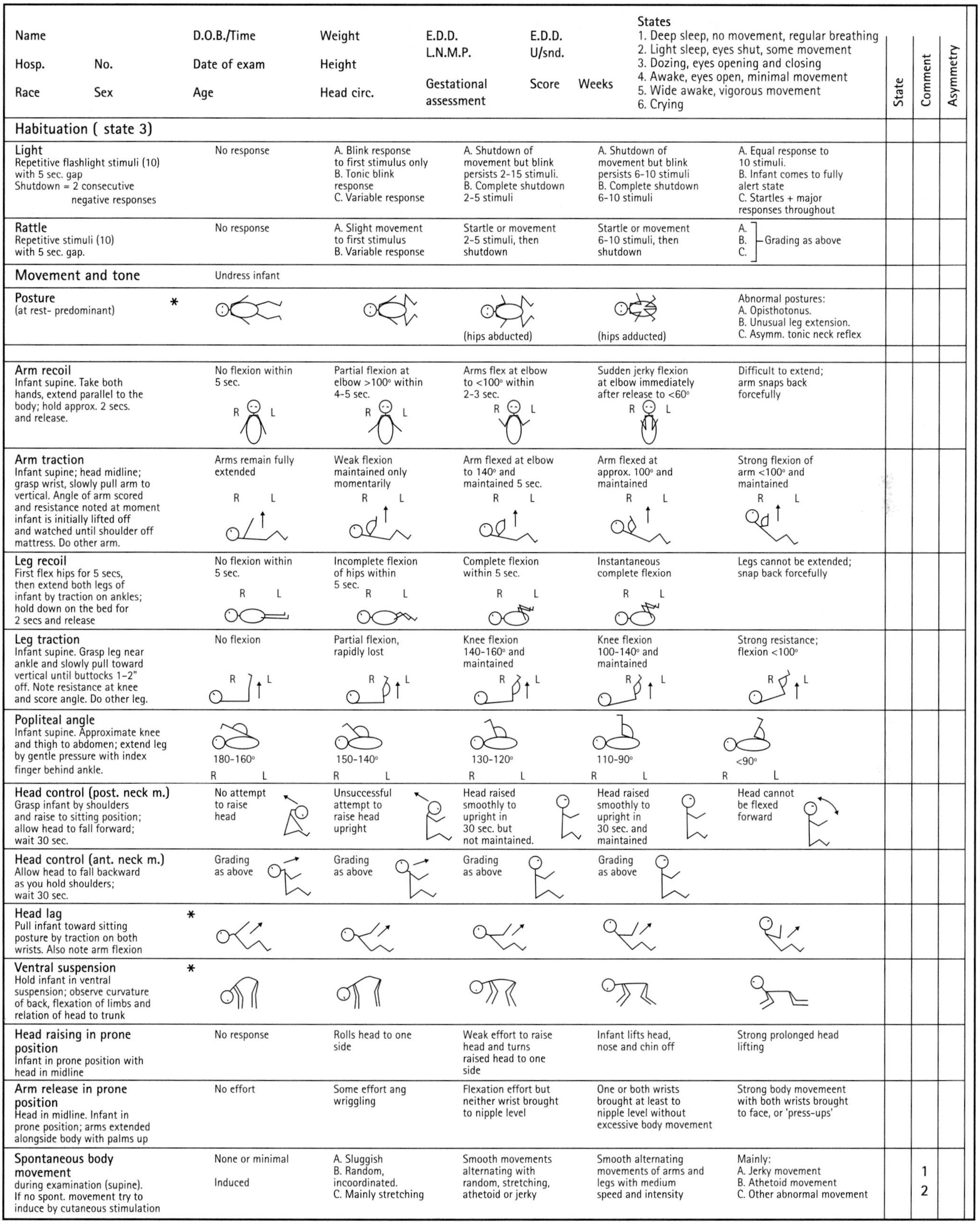

Name	D.O.B./Time	Weight	E.D.D. L.N.M.P.	E.D.D. U/snd.	States 1. Deep sleep, no movement, regular breathing	State	Comment	Asymmetry
Hosp. No.	Date of exam	Height			2. Light sleep, eyes shut, some movement 3. Dozing, eyes opening and closing			
Race Sex	Age	Head circ.	Gestational assessment	Score Weeks	4. Awake, eyes open, minimal movement 5. Wide awake, vigorous movement 6. Crying			

Habituation (state 3)

Light Repetitive flashlight stimuli (10) with 5 sec. gap Shutdown = 2 consecutive negative responses	No response	A. Blink response to first stimulus only B. Tonic blink response C. Variable response	A. Shutdown of movement but blink persists 2-15 stimuli. B. Complete shutdown 2-5 stimuli	A. Shutdown of movement but blink persists 6-10 stimuli. B. Complete shutdown 6-10 stimuli	A. Equal response to 10 stimuli. B. Infant comes to fully alert state C. Startles + major responses throughout			
Rattle Repetitive stimuli (10) with 5 sec. gap.	No response	A. Slight movement to first stimulus B. Variable response	Startle or movement 2-5 stimuli, then shutdown	Startle or movement 6-10 stimuli, then shutdown	A. B. ⎱Grading as above C.			

Movement and tone   Undress infant

Posture (at rest- predominant) *			(hips abducted)	(hips adducted)	Abnormal postures: A. Opisthotonus. B. Unusual leg extension. C. Asymm. tonic neck reflex			
Arm recoil Infant supine. Take both hands, extend parallel to the body; hold approx. 2 secs. and release.	No flexion within 5 sec. R L	Partial flexion at elbow >100° within 4-5 sec. R L	Arms flex at elbow to <100° within 2-3 sec. R L	Sudden jerky flexion at elbow immediately after release to <60° R L	Difficult to extend; arm snaps back forcefully			
Arm traction Infant supine; head midline; grasp wrist, slowly pull arm to vertical. Angle of arm scored and resistance noted at moment infant is initially lifted off and watched until shoulder off mattress. Do other arm.	Arms remain fully extended R L	Weak flexion maintained only momentarily R L	Arm flexed at elbow to 140° and maintained 5 sec. R L	Arm flexed at approx. 100° and maintained R L	Strong flexion of arm <100° and maintained R L			
Leg recoil First flex hips for 5 secs, then extend both legs of infant by traction on ankles; hold down on the bed for 2 secs and release	No flexion within 5 sec. R L	Incomplete flexion of hips within 5 sec. R L	Complete flexion within 5 sec. R L	Instantaneous complete flexion R L	Legs cannot be extended; snap back forcefully			
Leg traction Infant supine. Grasp leg near ankle and slowly pull toward vertical until buttocks 1-2" off. Note resistance at knee and score angle. Do other leg.	No flexion R L	Partial flexion, rapidly lost R L	Knee flexion 140-160° and maintained R L	Knee flexion 100-140° and maintained R L	Strong resistance; flexion <100° R L			
Popliteal angle Infant supine. Approximate knee and thigh to abdomen; extend leg by gentle pressure with index finger behind ankle.	180-160° R L	150-140° R L	130-120° R L	110-90° R L	<90° R L			
Head control (post. neck m.) Grasp infant by shoulders and raise to sitting position; allow head to fall forward; wait 30 sec.	No attempt to raise head	Unsuccessful attempt to raise head upright	Head raised smoothly to upright in 30 sec. but not maintained.	Head raised smoothly to upright in 30 sec. and maintained	Head cannot be flexed forward			
Head control (ant. neck m.) Allow head to fall backward as you hold shoulders; wait 30 sec.	Grading as above	Grading as above	Grading as above	Grading as above				
Head lag Pull infant toward sitting posture by traction on both wrists. Also note arm flexion *								
Ventral suspension Hold infant in ventral suspension; observe curvature of back, flexation of limbs and relation of head to trunk *								
Head raising in prone position Infant in prone position with head in midline	No response	Rolls head to one side	Weak effort to raise head and turns raised head to one side	Infant lifts head, nose and chin off	Strong prolonged head lifting			
Arm release in prone position Head in midline. Infant in prone position; arms extended alongside body with palms up	No effort	Some effort ang wriggling	Flexation effort but neither wrist brought to nipple level	One or both wrists brought at least to nipple level without excessive body movement	Strong body movement with both wrists brought to face, or 'press-ups'			
Spontaneous body movement during examination (supine). If no spont. movement try to induce by cutaneous stimulation	None or minimal Induced	A. Sluggish B. Random, incoordinated. C. Mainly stretching	Smooth movements alternating with random, stretching, athetoid or jerky	Smooth alternating movements of arms and legs with medium speed and intensity	Mainly: A. Jerky movement B. Athetoid movement C. Other abnormal movement		1 2	

Fig. 12.44 The Dubowitz score. (From Dubowitz & Dubowitz 1981,[811] courtesy of Spastics International Publishers Ltd.)

(Continued)

Placing and stepping

By stimulating the dorsum of the foot, usually by bringing it into contact with the edge of the couch, a mature baby can be induced to 'step' over the edge. With the feet in contact with a solid surface the baby will 'walk'.

Rooting, sucking and swallowing

Stroking the upper lip of a baby of 28 weeks' gestation and above results in the baby 'searching for the nipple' and tests the sensation in the distribution of the 5th cranial nerve. Sucking involves the motor activity of cranial nerves V, VII, XII; swallowing involves IX and X. The sensory input for the sucking reflex

Tremors — Mark: Fast (>6/sec.) or Slow (<6/sec.)	No tremor	Tremors only in state 5-6	Tremors only in sleep or after Moro and startles	Some tremors in state 4	Tremulousness in all states		
Startles	No startles	Startles to sudden noise. Moro, bang on table only	Occasional spontaneous startle	2-5 spontaneous startles	6+ spontaneous startles		
Abnormal movement or posture	No abnormal movement	A. Hands clenched but open intermittently. B. Hands do not open with Moro	A. Some mouthing movement. B. Intermittent adducted thumb	A. Persistently adducted thumb. B. Hands clenched all the time	A. Continuous mouthing movement B. Convulsive movements		
Reflexes							
Tendon reflexes Biceps jerk Knee jerk Ankle jerk	Absent		Present	Exaggerated	Clonus		
Palmar grasp Head in midline. Put index finger from ulnar side into hand and gently press palmar surface. Never touch dorsal side of hand	Absent	Short, weak flexion	Medium strength and sustained flexion for several secs.	Strong flexion; contraction spreads to forearm	Very strong grasp. Infant easily lifts off couch		
Rooting Infant supine; head midline. Touch each corner of the mouth in turn (stroke laterally)	No response	A. Partial weak head turn but no mouth opening B. Mouth opening, no head turn	Mouth opening on stimulated side with partial head turning	Full head turning, with or without mouth opening	Mouth opening with very jerky head turning		
Sucking Infant supine; place index finger (pad toward palate) in infant's mouth; judge power of sucking movement after 5 sec.	No attempt	Weak sucking movement: A. Regular B. Irregular	Strong sucking movement, poor stripping A. Regular B. Irregular	Strong regular sucking movement with continuing sequence of 5 movements. Good stripping	Clenching but no regular sucking		
Walking (state 4, 5) Hold infant upright, feet touching bed, neck held straight with fingers	Absent		Some effort but not continuous with both legs	At least 2 steps with both legs	A. Stork posture; no movement. B. Automatic walking		
Moro One hand supports infant's head in midline, the other the back. Raise infant to 45° and when infant is relaxed let his head fall through 10°. Note if jerky. Repeat 3 times	No response, or opening of hands only	Full abduction at the shoulder and extension of the arm 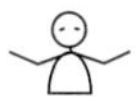	Full abduction but only delayed or partial adduction 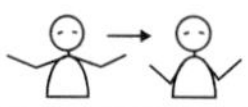	Partial abduction at shoulder and extension of arms followed by smooth adduction 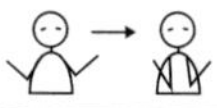 A. Abd>Add B. Abd=Add C. Abd<Add	A. No abduction or adduction; extension only B. Marked adduction only 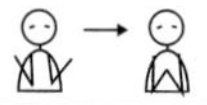	J	S
Neurobehavioural items							
Eye appearances	Sunset sign Nerve paisy	Transient nystagmus. Strabismus. Some roving eye movement	Does not open eyes	Normal conjugate eye movement	A. Persistent nystagmus B. Frequent roving movement C. Frequent rapid blinks		
Auditory orientation (state 3, 4) To rattle. (Note presence of startle)	A. No reaction B. Auditory startle but no true orientation	Brightens and stills; may turn toward stimuli with eyes closed	Alerting and shifting of eyes; head may or may not turn to source	Alerting; prolonged head turns to stimulus; search with eyes	Turning and alerting to stimulus each time on both sides	S	
Visual orientation (state 4) To red woollen ball	Does not focus or follow stimulus	Stills; focuses on stimulus; may follow 30° jerkily; does not find stimulus again spontaneously	Follows 30-60° horizontally; may lose stimulus but finds it again. Brief vertical glance	Follows with eyes and head horizontally and to some extent vertically, with frowning	Sustained fixation; follows vertically, horizontally, and in circle		
Alertness (state 4)	Inattentive; rarely or never responds to direct stimulation	When alert, periods rather brief; rather variable response to orientation	When alert, alertness moderately sustained; may use stimulus to come to alert state	Sustained alertness; orientation frequent, reliable to visual but not auditory stimuli	Continuous alertness, which does not seem to tire, to both auditory and visual stimuli		
Defensive reaction A cloth or hand is placed over the infants face to partially occlude the nasal airway	No response	A. General quietening B. Non-specific activity with long latency	Rooting; lateral neck turning; possibly neck stretching.	Swipes with arm	Swipes with arm with rather violent body movement		
Peak of excitement	Low level arousal to all stimuli; never > state 3	Infant reaches state 4-5 briefly but predominantly in lower states	Infant predominantly state 4 or 5; may reach state 6 after stimulation but returns spontaneously to lower state	Infant reaches state 6 but can be consoled relatively easy	A. Mainly state 6. Difficult to console, if at all B. Mainly state 4-5 but if reaches state 6 cannot be consoled		
Irritability (states 3,4,5) Aversive stimuli: Uncover Ventral susp. Undress Moro Pull to sit Walking reflex Prone	No irritable crying to any of the stimuli	Cries to 1-2 stimuli	Cries to 3-4 stimuli	Cries to 5-6 stimuli	Cries to all stimuli		
Consolability (state 6)	Never above state 5 during examination, therefore not needed	Consoling not needed, Consoles spontaneously	Consoled by talking, hand on belly or wrapping up	Consoled by picking up and holding; may need finger in mouth	Not consolable		
Cry	No cry at all	Only wimpering cry	Cries to stimuli but normal pitch	Lusty cry to offensive stimuli; normal pitch	High pitched cry, often continuous		

Notes   * If asymmetrical or atypical, draw in on nearest figure
         Record any abnormal signs (e.g. facial palsy, contractures, etc.)

Fig. 12.44 Continued

comes from the hard palate, not the tongue or cheek. Coordination between sucking and swallowing exists from 28 weeks' gestation but the strength to sustain it and to synchronize breathing is only adequate after 32–34 weeks' gestation. Sucking gradually builds up from bursts of three at a time to eight or more, with a reduction in the interburst interval. If sucking is absent, test the gag reflex by gently stroking the soft palate with a cotton bud.

Palmar and plantar

The palmar reflex results from stroking the palmar surface of the hand, eliciting a grasp that is often strong enough to lift the baby from the crib. It is present from 26 weeks' gestation and persists up to 4 months. Stroking the ball of the foot results in curling of the toes in a similar manner to the palmar response.

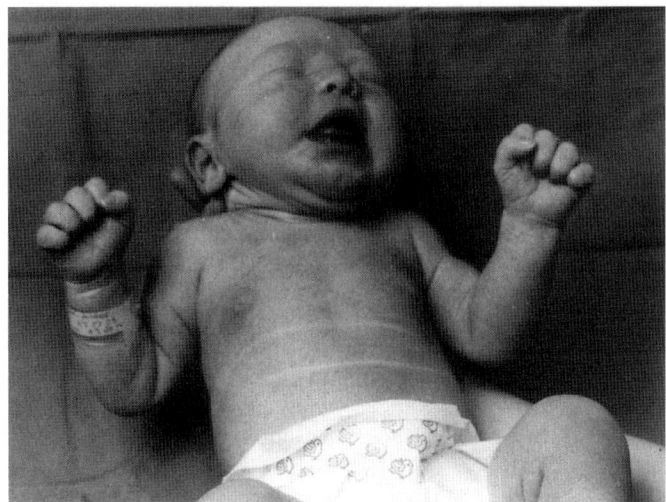

Fig. 12.45 The fully developed Moro reflex, abduction phase.

Special senses
Examination of the eyes and vision
Babies can usually be induced to open their eyes by holding them face to face and spinning them round, or they often open their eyes when sucking. The eyes are in alignment, although a slightly dysconjugate horizontal position is not abnormal in the first 6 weeks. Vertical or skew deviation is always abnormal and has been seen in association with periventricular hemorrhage. Sunsetting should be noted although it is not as reliable a sign of raised intracranial pressure as later in childhood. The 'doll's eye' maneuver induced by rotating the head from side to side results in reflex deviation of the eyes to the opposite side. It is normally present even in preterm babies, and absence of this reflex indicates severe brainstem damage. Pupil reactions to light are present after 30 weeks' gestation. Visual fixation of a suitable target such as a red woolly ball or a target of broad concentric rings is present from 32 weeks' gestation, and by 34 weeks babies track briefly. By term, babies can reliably fix and track an object held 20–30 cm away from the face, and persistent failure to follow a suitable object should give rise to concern. Blinking in response to a bright light is a subcortical response and has been recorded in anencephalic and holoprosencephalic babies. Tracking in infancy is not a guarantee of later intact visual function and may be subcortically mediated.[814] Optokinetic nystagmus is present from 36 weeks and preferential looking towards gratings of varying thickness can be used to assess acuity. Visual cortical function is achieved by 6 weeks.[815] Visual evoked potentials are discussed below, in the investigation section.

Hearing
Babies from 28 weeks' gestation onwards can be shown to respond to noise, usually by turning the head or increased body movements. For electrophysiological methods of assessing the auditory pathway, see investigation section below.

Smell
There is no doubt that babies, including preterm babies, can detect smells. Babies of all gestations have been found to respond to odors such as peppermint, or breast pads soaked in their own mother's breast milk.

Sensory testing
Withdrawal
Babies respond to pinprick stimuli with gross body movements or grimacing and there is no doubt that even very preterm babies feel pain. The classic withdrawal response of flexion of the lower limb and extension of the opposite leg in response to pricking the sole of the foot requires motor integrity also, and habituates easily.

Occipitofrontal head circumference and fontanelles
Examination is not complete without measuring and charting the occipitofrontal circumference and noting the presence and tension of the fontanelles. An extremely large anterior fontanelle can indicate hypothyroidism; a non-existent fontanelle can mean craniosynostosis. Useful information can be obtained by palpation of the sutures which can be widely spaced (diastasis) or overlapping. During the first 3 months of life the head grows at least 0.5 cm a week, and insufficient head growth is an ominous sign.

INVESTIGATION OF THE NEWBORN NERVOUS SYSTEM
Imaging
Ultrasound is the imaging procedure of first choice in the newborn. The method is relatively cheap, portable and safe, enabling repeated examinations. Intracranial hemorrhage can be identified fairly reliably. The cystic lesions of periventricular leukomalacia can be imaged down to a resolution of 1–2 mm, although ultrasound detects only about a third of cases of periventricular leukomalacia when compared to MRI. Ultrasound is insensitive for the detection of lesions of the extracerebral space and in the posterior fossa. Several atlases of cranial ultrasound pictures exist.[816]

MRI provides exquisite anatomical information but requires careful supervision and attention to detail particularly when it involves babies requiring artificial ventilation, in order to ensure that all ferrous metal components are excluded for safety. MRI is the method of choice for imaging the neonatal brain and avoids the radiation exposure of CT. CT should be reserved for emergencies and occasions when there is concern about intracranial bleeding. For those who wish to learn more about MRI the books by Rutherford[817] and Barkovich[818] are useful resources.

Examination of CSF
Lumbar puncture is often easier with the baby sitting up in the newborn period, and this position results in a more stable oxygen level. The spinal cord of the newborn extends to L3 so that the L3/L4 space is the best one to choose. A blood sample for plasma glucose estimation should be collected before performing the lumbar puncture as the stress response raises the blood sugar level. The CSF glucose value is usually 70–80% of the plasma glucose and should be at least 50% of it. A proper styleted lumbar puncture needle should be used as there have been cases of epidermoid tumors resulting from the implantation of a tiny core of skin during neonatal lumbar puncture with an unstyleted needle. In the neonatal period CSF may be xanthochromic because of jaundice or old intraventricular hemorrhage. The cell count is higher than later in childhood. In preterm neonates the red and white cell counts can each be up to 30/mm³ (Table 12.88). A study with careful documentation showed that the mean value was 7 white cells/mm³ with two standard deviations from the mean being 21.[820] Martin-Ancel suggested that the upper limit of normal at term is 5 white cells/mm³ although these workers found that counts of up to 30 occurred in babies without evidence of CNS infection.[821] There is some consensus emerging that the upper limit of normal white cell count in the CSF of a term baby should be set at 21 white cells/mm³, and a recent study found that this led to a sensitivity of 79% and a specificity of 81% for the diagnosis of meningitis, although 12% of the cases would still have been missed; choosing 1 as the upper limit was over-sensitive.[819]

In general the Gram stain will reveal organisms when the CSF white cell count is high in a baby who has not been treated with antibiotics; when no organisms are seen it is important to think of viral meningitis and to start treatment with aciclovir. Red cell counts of more than 1000/mm³ make the interpretation of CSF results impossible: applying correction factors using the ratio of white cells to red cells has been shown to be inaccurate. The only course of action is to repeat the lumbar puncture after 12 h.

Estimation of intracranial pressure (ICP)
ICP usually refers to pressure within the CSF space, and when subtracted from the arterial pressure gives the cerebral perfusion pressure. Rising

Table 12.88   Normal values for csf in neonates

Type of baby	Red cell count (per cubic mm)	White cell count (per cubic mm)	Protein (g/L) (mmol/L)	Glucose
Preterm <7 days	~30	9 (0–30)	1 (0.5–2.9)	3 (1.5–5.5)
Preterm >7 days	~30	12 (2–50)	0.9 (0.5–2.6)	3 (1.5–5.5)
Term <7 days	<10	5 (0–21)*	0.6 (0.3–2.5)	3 (1.5–5.5)
Term >7 days	<10	3 (0–10)	0.5 (0.2–0.8)	3 (1.5–5.5)

*See text; more than 21 white cells/mm³ has a sensitivity of 79% and a specificity of 81% for the diagnosis of meningitis in the newborn, but on occasion babies can have a positive CSF culture with white cell counts lower than this.[819]

ICP results in a reduction in cerebral perfusion unless the usual reflex elevation in systemic blood pressure occurs (the Cushing response). The Cushing response may be inadequate in the newborn.[822]

Normal value of ICP in the newborn
Measured directly with pressure transducers at lumbar puncture the pressure is 0–5.5 mmHg.

Electroencephalography
Conventional multichannel EEG recordings are difficult to obtain in newborn babies but provide the most complete information. The montage of electrodes is hard to apply and maintain and many babies requiring investigation are in ICUs which are electrically noisy. Continuous monitoring is possible with several types of cerebral function monitor (CFM) which display amplitude integrated and compressed EEG (aEEG) at the cot side. Modern digital technology now allows multichannel EEG recordings to be made and stored at the cotside, with simultaneous video and physiological monitoring. Cotside aEEG is increasingly used as a tool with which to support the diagnosis of encephalopathy and/or seizures, and to assist with prognosis although at least one formal EEG is recommended. Guidance on the interpretation of aEEG patterns is available.[823]

Maturation of EEG
The EEG of very preterm babies is markedly discontinuous (Fig. 12.46) with a pattern of high voltage slow activity with suppressed EEG activity termed 'trace alternant'. This pattern can still be seen during normal sleep in mature babies, but with increasing gestation there is a reduction in amount and duration of trace alternant activity. There is also a pattern, called 'delta brush', of fast waves superimposed on delta waves which can be misinterpreted as convulsive activity. A persisting severe abnormality of the background EEG activity predicts later adverse outcome in both preterm and term babies.[824–826]

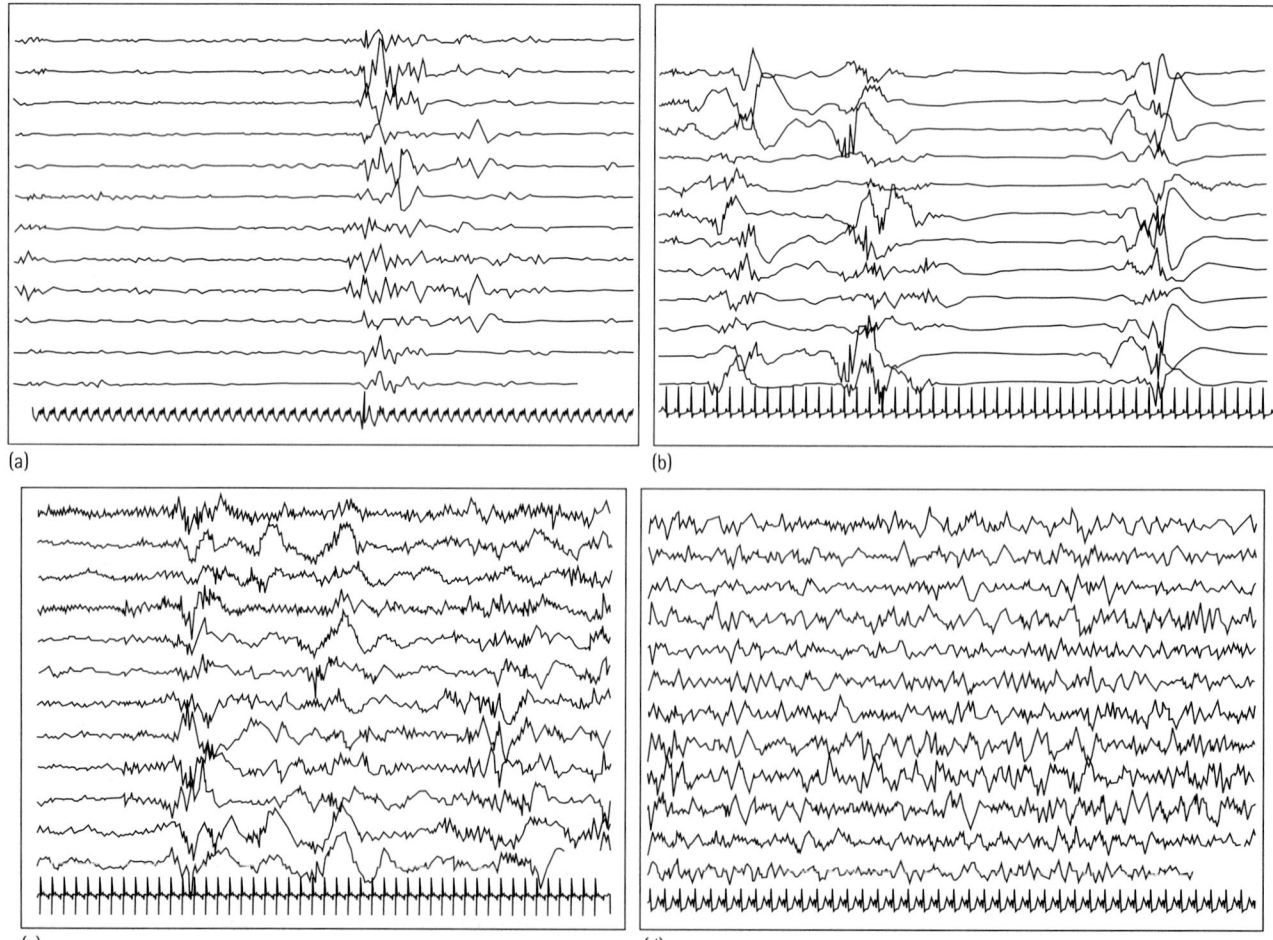

(a)   (b)   (c)   (d)

Fig. 12.46   Maturation of the normal EEG in preterm babies: (a) 25 weeks; (b) 29 weeks; (c) 35 weeks; (d) 40 weeks.

Investigation of the visual pathway

Visual evoked potentials (VEP) are produced within the occipital cortex as a result of repeatedly applying an appropriate visual stimulus so that the minute electrical response to it, which will be identical each time, can be extracted from the random background electrical noise (EEG) by computerized averaging. Stroboscopic or flashing red lights are used which can penetrate closed eyelids. The electrical response 'matures' with advancing gestation and can be detected from 25 weeks. Study of VEPs has been found to be of value in predicting outcome after birth asphyxia[827] and is a sensitive test for the integrity of the visual pathway. Absent VEPs predicted cortical blindness in preterm babies with extensive cystic leukomalacia.[828]

Investigation of the auditory pathway

Neural pathways for hearing are established and can be tested within hours of birth. The fetus responds to low frequency sounds applied to the maternal abdomen from 19 weeks of gestation, with a gradual increase in the range of frequency response and sensitivity.[829] Young children who are fitted with hearing aids early have an excellent chance of developing normal speech, but the current average age for the acquisition of hearing aids is often almost 2 years. Universal neonatal hearing screening was established in all regions of England and in Scotland by the end of 2005, and so far the yield of babies diagnosed with bilateral permanent deafness is around 1 per 1000. This program replaced the previous 8 month health visitor 'distraction' test, which had proved unsatisfactory and has been phased out. The new program identifies cases far earlier than before, with a median age of 10 weeks. Newborn hearing screening is carried out with automated auditory evoked potentials or by the study of automated oto-acoustic emissions; the auditory response cradle proved unreliable and is not used for the national screening program (www.library.nhs.uk/screening).

CONVULSIONS IN THE NEWBORN
Diagnosis and incidence

Convulsions are more frequent on the first day of life than at any other time, although the diagnosis is easily missed because their manifestations can be extremely subtle.[830] Subtle seizures are the most common type, occurring in 75% of the cases described by Scher et al[831] (Table 12.89). Repetitive lip smacking, cycling or swimming movements, deviation of the eyes and apnea can all be epileptic in origin but are sometimes difficult to distinguish from normal movements or jittering.

Continuous monitoring has shown that electrical seizures occur more frequently in the newborn than clinically suspected seizures, and conversely that stereotyped repetitive activity which looks like a seizure is not always associated with EEG change.[833,834] This phenomenon of electroclinical dissociation is more prevalent in the neonatal period than later in life. Recognition of seizure activity may be particularly important in babies who are paralyzed as prolonged seizures (> 30 min in animals) are accompanied by an increase in cerebral metabolic rate which outstrips the available energy supply and leads to cerebral damage. Changes in cerebral energy metabolites and cerebral blood flow velocity have been seen even in the brief seizures characteristic of the human neonate.[835]

The incidence of seizures in term babies is reported at between 1.6 and 14 per 1000 deliveries. Higher incidences were reported prior to the introduction of low-phosphate milks, and half the babies in early series were hypocalcemic. More recent series give an estimate of around 5 per 1000; in most series a quarter of the cases are amongst babies of less than 30 weeks' gestation and a half are less than 37 weeks.[836] The incidence of clinically diagnosed seizures in VLBW babies varies from 50 to 130 per 1000.[837,838]

Etiology
Intracranial injury

The majority of cases of seizures in term babies are associated with hypoxic–ischemic encephalopathy (HIE) (Table 12.90).[830,839–842,844] Newer imaging methods have revealed focal cerebral artery infarction (stroke) to be more common than previously suspected, with the left middle cerebral artery the most commonly affected.[845,846] A thrombophilia screen (looking for inherited disorders such as factor V Leiden) should be carried out in cases of neonatal stroke. Intracranial hemorrhage is the commonest cause of seizure in the preterm neonate.

Maternal drug withdrawal

Methadone withdrawal is more likely to produce seizures than heroin, but modern treatment for neonatal abstinence syndrome is aimed at preventing seizure, which has now become rare. Withdrawal from maternal selective serotonin reuptake inhibitors (SSRIs) such as paroxetine is probably increasing as a cause of neonatal seizure.

Metabolic causes

The metabolic causes of hypocalcemia, hypoglycemia, hyponatremia and hypomagnesemia now account for less than 10% of cases of neonatal seizure but remain important because they are readily treatable. Hypomagnesemia coexists with hypocalcemia about half the time, and recognition is important because administration of calcium can cause the serum magnesium to drop further. Pyridoxine dependency can be a difficult diagnosis to make; the disorder is autosomal recessive and the fits are intractable until an infusion of 100 mg pyridoxine is given, ideally under EEG monitoring. The response may take up to half an hour. Pyridoxine is necessary for the manufacture of gamma-aminobutyric acid, which is the major inhibitory neurotransmitter, and hence in the familial form of the disease replacement needs to be life-long. Temporary deficiency has also arisen following vomiting and incorrectly designed formula baby milks. Inborn errors of metabolism such as nonketotic hyperglycinemia can cause seizure and these should be suspected if the onset is late and related to milk feeds. Preterm babies can develop transient hyperammonemia and hyperlactemia causing seizures. 'Fifth day fits' were commonly reported in the 1970s and 1980s, but this condition is now rarely diagnosed.

Infection

Infection accounts for about 8% of cases of neonatal seizure and evidence of bacterial or viral infection should always be sought, including congenital infections such as CMV.

Inherited and congenital disorders

Benign familial convulsions are dominantly inherited and occur in the first 3 weeks of life. The fits can be very frequent but they are usually brief and the prognosis is excellent. The diagnosis rests on excluding other causes and the presence of a positive family history. The chromosomal defect has recently been mapped to the long arm of chromosome 20. Benign neonatal sleep myoclonus may give rise to dramatic manifestations in otherwise entirely healthy newborns who have an excellent prognosis.

Sometimes neonatal seizures are the first manifestation of a congenital neurological disorder and these are more likely if the fits are intractable. The condition called 'early infantile epileptic encephalopathy'

Table 12.89 Types of seizure in the newborn (adapted from Volpe[832])

Type	Clinical manifestation
Subtle	Eye signs – eyelid fluttering, eye deviation, fixed open stare, blinking Apnea Cycling, boxing, stepping, swimming movements of limbs Mouthing, chewing, lip smacking, smiling
Tonic	Stiffening. Decerebrate posturing
Clonic	Repetitive jerking, distinct from jittering Can be focal or multifocal
Myoclonic	Rapid single repetitive contraction of muscle groups Sleep myoclonus is benign.

Table 12.90   Causes of neonatal convulsions

	1	2	3	4	5*	6†	7
Number of cases in report	–	–	71	131	100	40	100
Hypoxic–ischemic encephalopathy	53%	16%	49%	30%	49%	37%	32%
Intracranial hemorrhage	17%	–	14%	–	7%	12%	16%
Cerebral infarction (stroke)	–	–	–	–	12%	17%	7%
Meningitis	8%	3%	2%	7%	5%	5%	14%
Maternal drug withdrawal	–	–	4%	–	–	–	–
Hypoglycemia	3%	2%	0.1%	5%	3%	–	2%
Hypocalcemia, hypomagnesemia	–	–	–	22%	–	–	4%
Rapidly changing serum sodium	–	–	–	–	–	–	–
Congenitally abnormal brain	–	8%	–	4%	3%	17%	3%
Fifth day fits	–	52%	–	–	–	–	–
Benign familial neonatal seizures	–	–	–	–	–	–	1%
Benign neonatal sleep myoclonus	–	–	–	–	–	–	1%
Pyridoxine dependent seizures	–	–	–	–	–	–	–
Hypertensive encephalopathy	–	–	1.4%	–	–	–	–
Kernicterus	–	–	–	–	1%	–	–
Inborn errors of metabolism	–	–	–	–	3%	–	3%

*This series included >31 week gestation infants only.
†This series was limited to cases presenting in the first 48 hours of life.
Blanks occur where no cases were recorded in a particular study.
Data in column 1 are from Levene & Trounce,[839] column 2 from Goldberg,[840] column 3 from Andre et al,[841] column 4 from Bergman et al,[842] column 5 from Estan & Hope,[843] column 6 from Lien et al,[844] column 7 from Mizrahi & Kellaway.[830]

presents as severe tonic spasms and many of these babies have cerebral malformations. Cases of Aicardi syndrome (female children with infantile spasms, agenesis of the corpus callosum and a characteristic EEG) would also fall into this group. The phakomatoses occasionally present in the neonatal period, and syndromes such as Zellweger or Smith–Lemli–Opitz can cause neonatal seizures.

Investigations of seizures

These follow from the possible causes listed above. Information regarding the pregnancy, labor and delivery is vital. Essential laboratory investigations include estimation of calcium, magnesium, glucose, acid–base balance and sodium in the blood together with a full infection screen including a lumbar puncture, specimens for virology and a congenital infection screen. A cranial ultrasound scan should be included as a first line investigation. If the cause is not revealed, second line investigations include MRI, samples to look for maternal 'street' drugs, urinary and blood amino acid estimation, chromosomal analysis, blood ammonia, measurement of organic acids and consideration of a trial of pyridoxine. The value of an EEG examination has already been discussed. Information about the background interictal EEG is useful in prognosis, particularly if the EEG is made at 12–48 hours of age.[826,847]

Treatment
General guidelines

Treatment is best given intravenously as intramuscular absorption is erratic and the neonate has little muscle mass. Facilities to site and maintain intravenous lines and to institute artificial ventilation are necessary, as many of the available drugs depress respiration and ventilation can become inadequate due to frequent convulsions. The high total body water of the neonate means a large volume of distribution hence the loading doses are relatively large. Most of the antiepileptic drugs (AEDs) are protein bound and can interact with other drugs and bilirubin. Many AEDs act by enhancing the inhibition of the gamma amino butyric acid (GABA) receptors, particularly the chloride permeable $GABA_A$ receptors. The neonatal neurone has a high chloride content and consequently the developing brain has a different response to GABA compared to the adult brain; in other words GABA becomes excitatory rather than inhibitory. Recently, it has been discovered that the neonatal brain continues to express a $Na^+K^+2Cl^-$ (NKCCl) cotransporter after birth, explaining the high intracellular chloride levels which

have been observed at this time.[848] This provides an elegant explanation for the observation that standard AEDs do not work well in newborn babies and leads to the intriguing possibility that drugs which act on the NKCCl transporter would work better. Recently, there has been the exciting observation that bumetanide, which is widely used as a diuretic and has a good safety profile, suppresses seizures in rat pups, and anecdotal case reports are likely to follow. In the meantime, the best current advice is to use phenobarbital in an adequate dose with an early blood level, and to follow with intravenous phenytoin if seizures are not controlled.[849,850] Midazolam is a popular third line antiepileptic drug and has a good safety profile, albeit evidence for effect on electrographically determined seizures in the newborn is lacking.[851] Thiopental coma did not improve the outcome in a controlled clinical trial[852] and in resistant cases lidocaine may be the best alternative, although it accumulates and should not be continued for more than 48 hours.[853]

Phenobarbital

It is reasonable to give 30 mg/kg of phenobarbital as a loading dose to a baby who is already ventilated, otherwise use 15 mg/kg. Gilman et al achieved seizure control with phenobarbital alone in 77% of cases using a rapid sequential method in which they gave 15–20 mg/kg initially then further doses of 5–10 mg/kg every 30 min up to a maximum of 40 mg/kg and serum level of over 40 mg/L.[854] The half-life of phenobarbital is very long and there have been concerns about toxic effects on the developing brain, including apoptosis.

Sodium valproate

Hepatotoxic effects, hyperammonemia and hyperglycinemia may limit the use of this drug in the newborn. Valproate proved effective in six intractable cases of neonatal seizure.[855]

Duration of treatment

Concern about the effects of anticonvulsant treatment on the developing brain means that most neonatologists would only discharge a baby on maintenance phenobarbital if the neurological examination was abnormal, discontinuing treatment before discharge in those who were neurologically normal. As many as 56% of babies developed subsequent epilepsy in one series[856] although 30% is probably a more realistic figure.[830,831] For babies who are discharged on anticonvulsants consider discontinuation of treatment if the baby is seizure-free at 9 months.

Prognosis

This is related to the cause of the seizures. Following hypoxic–ischemic encephalopathy at term about 25% of those who fit will have sequelae. Many surviving preterm babies who suffered seizures have a disability, and a more precise prognosis in this group can be obtained by considering the findings on MRI. The prognosis after hypocalcemic seizure and in familial neonatal seizure is excellent. Symptomatic hypoglycemia and meningitis have a 50% chance of sequelae in the survivors. A normal background interictal EEG at term is a good prognostic factor. The value of a normal neurological examination at discharge in providing early reassurance should not be underestimated either; in one series 11 of 14 babies with seizures who were normal at 4 years were assessed as normal at this stage. However, this apparently normal group of Oxford children then had problems with spelling and memory in adolescence.[857]

INFECTION OF THE NERVOUS SYSTEM IN THE NEWBORN

Neonatal meningitis

Incidence and cause

Meningitis is more common during the first month of life than at any other time: the incidence has been estimated as 0.25–0.5 per 1000 in normal weight babies and 1–2 per 1000 in those below 2.5 kg at birth. Gram negative organisms are more often implicated than later in childhood. The commonest causative organisms are *Escherichia coli* and group B streptococcus (GBS). The incidence of GBS meningitis has fallen in Australia and New Zealand since the widespread introduction of GBS screening and intrapartum antibiotic prophylaxis.[858] There are no plans to introduce GBS screening in the UK. *Listeria monocytogenes* neonatal meningitis has become very rare in the UK since the Government issued advice to pregnant women about avoiding soft cheese and cook-chill food in the late 1980s. A wide variety of different organisms have been reported, particularly in the LBW baby. Staphylococci have a predilection for ventriculoperitoneal shunts. Table 12.91 lists 10 important causative bacteria.

Clinical signs and diagnosis

The diagnosis can be difficult and if infection is considered as a cause for a baby's symptoms then a lumbar puncture must be performed. Examples of babies who should have LP performed include those who are shocked or who present later with subtle signs such as apnea or lethargy. Seizures are an indication for LP, and the investigation should be part of a septic screen done for prolonged rupture of membranes. Babies developing hydrocephalus deserve to have at least one LP even if the etiology is thought to be posthemorrhagic hydrocephalus, as ventriculomegaly can result from low grade staphylococcal infection. Cerebral ultrasound scans may reveal intraventricular strands. The yield of positive CSF cultures is relatively low, around 1% in most series, but the observation that the organism will not always be grown from the blood culture remains true, and there is still no substitute for lumbar puncture as part of a septic screen in a symptomatic baby.[819] As previously discussed, the definition of what constitutes a normal neonatal CSF remains elusive but in a 'clean' tap at term more than 21 white cells/mm³, and certainly more than 30 are suspicious. If a high number of white cells are found but no organisms are seen on Gram staining in a baby not previously treated with antibiotics, then think of viral meningitis and start aciclovir pending further results including polymerase chain reaction (PCR) for herpes simplex.

Treatment

Antibiotics alone do not treat meningitis, and the importance of supportive treatment must not be underestimated. Babies are often shocked, requiring measures such as artificial ventilation, inotropic support, frequent monitoring of their acid–base state, careful fluid balance and maintenance of nutrition. There is no convincing evidence that adjunctive therapy such as steroid or immunoglobulin administration, exchange transfusion or monoclonal antibody treatment helps in neonatal meningitis.

Most treatment is started without knowledge of the infecting organism. Third generation cephalosporins offer excellent penetration into CSF with wide spectrum of activity including Gram negative organisms. Of those available, cefotaxime is probably the best choice and the outcome of neonatal meningitis has improved since the introduction of third generation cephalosporins. Before the organism is identified a broad spectrum of coverage with good CSF penetration can be achieved with cefotaxime, penicillin and gentamicin. The combination of ampicillin and an aminoglycoside is still chosen by some authorities. Vancomycin should be considered in preterm babies at high risk of *Staphylococcus epidermidis* infection. Antibiotics should be continued for 2–3 weeks, longer with Gram negative infections than for GBS. Recent advice to stop antibiotic treatment 2–3 days after the C-reactive protein returns to normal seems sensible. A repeat lumbar puncture should be carried out if there is a failure of clinical response and/or a failure of the laboratory indices of infection to return to normal. An intraventricular tap may be required if the ventricles are seen to enlarge on serial ultrasound scans, and intraventricular therapy should be considered via a surgically implanted reservoir in this situation.

Prognosis

The mortality of neonatal meningitis has fallen since the introduction of neonatal intensive care and the use of cephalosporins. In England and Wales, the mortality has fallen from 29% in 1985 to 10% in 1996–97.[859] The 1985–87 cohort have been followed up, and neurodevelopmental sequelae continue to be a problem in the survivors, with only 63% reported to have an entirely normal outcome. Deafness is the most common disability, and 10% had a severe disability (usually cerebral palsy).

Viral and protozoal infections

These may be acquired in utero or postnatally and can cause severe neurological impairment. The acronym TORCH has been used to summarize the infections *Toxoplasma*, rubella, CMV and herpes, to which should be added human immunodeficiency virus and varicella zoster.

Rubella

Rubella infection in the first 16 weeks of pregnancy can result in a severely damaged baby with cataracts, sensorineural deafness, congenital heart disease, microcephaly, hepatosplenomegaly and thrombocytopenia. The condition is preventable by achieving high immunization coverage.

CMV

CMV can present in a dramatic form with jaundice and petechiae, the 'blueberry muffin' baby. Most babies who are symptomatic at birth will be handicapped. Only 1% of babies born with congenital CMV infection are symptomatic, however, most babies being clinically unaffected by the infection. Perhaps 6% have significant hearing loss at follow-up.[860]

Table 12.91 Bacterial causes of neonatal meningitis

Organism	Incidence
Escherichia coli	34%
Group B streptococci	30%
Other Gram negative bacilli	8%
Listeria monocytogenes	6%
Staphylococci	4.5%
Other streptococci	4%
Pneumococcus	3%
Pseudomonas	3%
Haemophilus	2%
Meningococcus	2%

Varicella zoster

Varicella zoster can result in severe damage with cicatricial skin scarring, cataracts and seizures. Sequelae are more likely following infection in the first trimester, when the risk was 1/11 in one study.[861] Transmission later in pregnancy can result in zoster or chickenpox in the newborn. If the maternal infection occurs within −5 to +5 days of delivery, the fetus will be unprotected by maternal antibody and should be treated with aciclovir and zoster immune globulin.

Herpes simplex virus

Herpes simplex virus can result in severe illness in newborns, and there is not always a clear history of a primary maternal genital infection because the lesions can be hidden on the cervix. There is a high incidence of meningitis and encephalitis. The infection should be treated with aciclovir. Herpes can be difficult to diagnose but the virus can be identified on electron microscopy, or a search for viral DNA can be made with a specific PCR test.

Human immunodeficiency virus

This retrovirus can cause meningitis and encephalopathy. Vertical transmission occurs in 13–45% of cases, a risk which can be reduced by zidovudine and by Cesarean section delivery. Neurological manifestations of HIV include encephalopathy and microcephaly.

Toxoplasma gondii

This protozoan can cause neurological sequelae when acquired in uterine life and the diagnosis is important because the condition is treatable. The organism is mainly acquired from cat litter or consumption of undercooked meat, and the infection may produce only mild symptoms in the mother. Birth prevalence is about 0.5 per 1000 in the UK. The classic triad of hydrocephalus, chorioretinitis and intracranial calcification is extremely rare, with only four such cases reported in the UK between 1975 and 1980. Specific IgM antibody can be demonstrated in the baby who should be treated with pyrimethamine + sulfadiazine followed by spiramycin. The prognosis of symptomatic congenital toxoplasmosis is poor, with 50% suffering impaired vision and 85% mental retardation.

Spirochetal and fungal infections

The incidence of congenital syphilis is rising commensurate with the rise in the use of crack cocaine. All babies suspected of having congenital syphilis should receive penicillin, and this is also the drug of choice for neonatal Lyme disease. Fungal meningitis and abscess formation is mainly a problem of the VLBW baby requiring intensive care, in whom the morbidity from this complication is high.

DEVELOPMENTAL ABNORMALITIES

See Chapter 22 for further information about these conditions.

METABOLIC AND ENDOCRINE DISORDERS
Introduction

Whilst adequate energy is essential to sustain adequate growth of the brain, nutrients also need to be in the appropriate concentrations and supported by the correct hormonal milieu. Inborn errors of metabolism can alter the relative concentrations of amino acids and many of these conditions present in the newborn period with neurological symptoms. High ammonia levels are toxic to the nervous system so that disorders of the urea cycle also present with severe derangement of neurological function. Lack of thyroid hormone causes failure of neurological maturation which rapidly results in permanent damage; the prevention of cretinism by early identification of such individuals with screening and replacement therapy has been a significant advance. Preterm babies have low thyroxine in early postnatal life and studies have suggested a correlation between low levels of thyroid hormones and adverse neurodevelopmental outcome although replacement therapy has not proved a success.

Urea cycle defects

Hyperammonemia may present with severe neurological disturbance in the newborn period. Recognition is important because many of the conditions are inherited and the babies often succumb without the correct diagnosis being made. There may be lethargy, vomiting and convulsions. Plasma ammonia concentrations above 200 mg/L are toxic and can result from liver failure, enzyme defects of the urea cycle or other disorders of amino acid metabolism such as propionic acidemia and lysine intolerance. Further investigation consists of enzyme assay using leukocytes or liver cells.

Hyperbilirubinemia

Unconjugated bilirubin is lipid soluble and hence able to cross the blood–brain barrier. The classic neurological syndrome of acute bilirubin encephalopathy, presenting with opisthotonic posturing and fits, is rare but has re-emerged in recent years. Babies who are most at risk are those who are near term and those discharged early. Acute bilirubin encephalopathy carries a high risk of permanent damage due to kernicterus, with athetoid cerebral palsy and deafness. Kernicterus can now be imaged with MRI, and there are characteristic changes in the globi pallidi.

Hypoglycemia

Prolonged low glucose levels damage the newborn nervous system which is unable to utilize alternative energy sources. There has been much debate regarding the degree and duration of hypoglycemia required to be responsible for permanent brain damage. That damage can result from a prolonged period of symptomatic hypoglycemia at term is not in doubt, however. The evidence that asymptomatic hypoglycemia can cause permanent sequelae is not convincing. In preterm babies, there has been a suggestion that persisting glucose levels below 2.6 mmol/L were associated with a reduction in Bayley motor and mental development scores at 18 months. However, much more evidence is needed before definite guidelines can be formulated regarding moderate or asymptomatic hypoglycemia.

NEONATAL CEREBRAL INJURY

Perinatal stress such as hypotension or trauma can result in cerebral injury, and intracranial and extracranial hemorrhage remain a problem although the incidence has declined considerably. There are a number of important potential causes of intracranial hemorrhage at term (including inherited or acquired coagulopathy), listed in Table 12.92. The preterm brain is especially vulnerable to postnatal damage from hemorrhage because of the presence of residual germinal matrix tissue, the extent of which can be appreciated with MRI. Neonatal brain injury is best considered as a spectrum with the end result depending on the type and degree of insult, the gestational age of the baby and any underlying factors. The problem is an important one because there is a relationship with later handicap.

Table 12.92   Causes of intracranial hemorrhage at term

Choroid plexus hemorrhage, often secondary to straight sinus thrombosis
Hemorrhage into residual germinal matrix tissue
Hemorrhagic cerebral venous infarction
    Thalamic – venous thrombosis into the straight sinus
    Parasagittal – venous thrombosis into the parasagittal sinus
Temporal lobe – venous thrombosis of the vein of Labbe, the transverse sinus, the sigmoid sinus
Hemorrhagic cerebral arterial infarction
    'Stroke' of the middle cerebral or other arterial territory
Primary 'lobar' cerebral hemorrhage
    Cause unknown
    Bleeding diathesis; NAITP, inherited or acquired coagulopathy, vitamin K deficiency

NAITP, neonatal alloimmune thrombocytopenia.

Subgaleal (subaponeurotic) hemorrhage

The space between the scalp and the subaponeurotic layer outside the skull is a potentially large one, and significant blood loss can occur at around the time of birth (Fig. 12.47). There is a very strong association between subgaleal hematoma and ventouse delivery. Babies can become shocked very quickly after birth as a result of the massive blood loss, and the mortality of the condition remains high, around 20% in many series. The diagnosis rests on a high index of suspicion, and the demonstration of a fluctuant boggy swelling in the scalp which crosses suture lines.

Subarachnoid hemorrhage

A small amount of subarachnoid blood is quite common after normal delivery, and as ever with bleeding disorders in the neonatal period it is important to exclude vitamin K deficiency bleeding. The outcome is generally good, but the presence of subarachnoid blood can cause seizures.

Subdural hemorrhage

The incidence of this complication has fallen with more careful obstetric practice, although a small subdural collection is surprisingly common even after a normal delivery. The hematoma is thought to result from tearing of the bridging veins. Tears of the dura can lead to posterior fossa collections resulting in brainstem compression and coning. Ultrasound is not good at detecting subdural hemorrhage, and suspicion of the diagnosis is an indication for an urgent CT scan; a neurosurgical opinion is important as drainage may be required.

Thalamic hemorrhage

This type of intracranial bleeding may be primary or secondary to extension from germinal matrix bleeding; sinus thrombosis is thought to be an important contributory factor, and venous infarction is thought to be the origin of many types of intracranial hemorrhage at term (Table 12.92). Term babies with primary thalamic bleeding can present at about 10 days of age with eye signs (deviation and sunsetting) and fits.

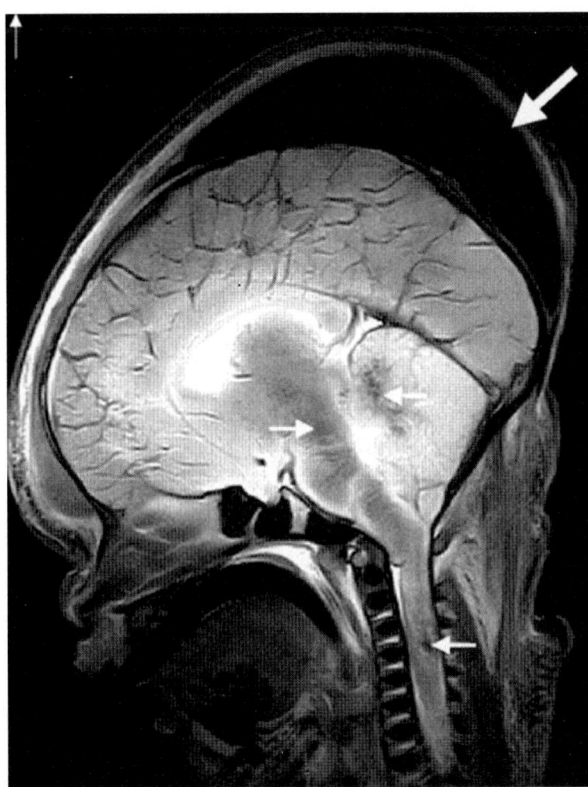

Fig. 12.47 MRI showing a massive subgaleal collection associated with hypoxic–ischemic damage. (From Cheong et al[862] with permission.)

Periventricular hemorrhage (PVH)

The preterm brain contains the germinal matrix, which contains actively dividing neuroblasts and glioblasts. The blood supply is via a capillary bed supplied by Heubner's artery, which is a branch of the anterior cerebral artery. The region of the germinal matrix situated at the head of the caudate nucleus is prone to bleeding, and this is the most common form of intracranial hemorrhage in preterm babies, although the germinal matrix is extensive and bleeding can occur at any site. The incidence of intracranial hemorrhage diagnosed with ultrasound in VLBW babies has reduced from around 40% to 15–20% since the widespread introduction of antenatal steroids and postnatal surfactant.[863,864] Rates as low as 13% have been reported from some centers, although one Canadian study found a wide range of incidence.[865]

The term PVH is often used as a generic one, encompassing several different types of hemorrhage in preterm babies. The mildest form is germinal matrix or subependymal bleeding alone. This is often abbreviated to GMH or SEH and is equivalent to grade 1 PVH in the classification of Papile et al.[866] Bleeding into the ventricular system, or intraventricular hemorrhage (IVH) was classified by Levene & de Crespigny[867] in 1983 as grade 2 PVH, but was subdivided by Papile into grade 2 when the ventricle was not distended and grade 3 when it was. Bleeding into the parenchyma of the brain (ParH) was classified by Levene as grade 3 PVH and by Papile as grade 4. A parenchymal hemorrhagic lesion is illustrated with the ultrasound scan appearance in Figure 12.48. Few now believe that parenchymal hemorrhage represents direct extension of intraventricular bleeding, and it is now clear that all echodense lesions diagnosed with ultrasound are not hemorrhagic in nature. As a result the older classification systems are no longer appropriate.

Repeated ultrasound scanning of cohorts of VLBW babies has revealed that the incidence and degree of hemorrhage relate to the birth weight and gestational age. The complication develops in early postnatal life, with the majority of lesions present 24h after birth. There are several risk factors. These include:

- gestational age;
- birth weight;
- RDS;
- artificial ventilation;
- hypercarbia;
- pneumothorax.

Less conclusive evidence exists for variables such as the mode and place of delivery, use of beta-sympathomimetics during labor, presence of coagulopathy, acidosis, bicarbonate administration, low blood pressure, fluctuating cerebral blood flow velocity and the administration of vasodilators such as tolazoline. The main problem is in distinguishing antecedent from associate. The best unifying hypothesis is that GMH-IVH results from a disturbance of cerebral blood flow in babies who are poor at cerebral autoregulation, and in whom there is often a bleeding tendency.

Periventricular leukomalacia

Periventricular leukomalacia (PVL) was first recognized by pathologists. The 'white spots' appear at the boundary zone of the cerebral circulation in the immature brain and it seems likely that a period of low cerebral blood flow is often exacerbated by flow–metabolism uncoupling. Small cysts can be diagnosed during life with ultrasound (Fig. 12.49), but many cases of PVL are 'ultrasound negative' and are only diagnosed later on because of disability or MRI. Cysts can be imaged in between 8 and 17% of babies less than 1500g. Some series include parenchymal echodense lesions persisting for more than 2 weeks but not evolving into cysts, and report a higher incidence of 25%.[868] There can be some difficulty in distinguishing this type of 'flare' from the normal peritrigonal 'blush' described by Di Pietro et al,[869] which is normal. It is very important to describe the ultrasound appearances in detail; an echodense lesion in a 1-day-old preterm baby is not at all the same entity as the pathological identification of cystic change in the white matter. Paneth et al[870] found white matter damage at postmortem in preterm babies with cerebral echodensity during life, but in very few were the lesions typical of classic periventricular leukomalacia. In many babies the white matter damage, with liquefactive necrosis and perivascular hemorrhage, was not restricted to the periventricular

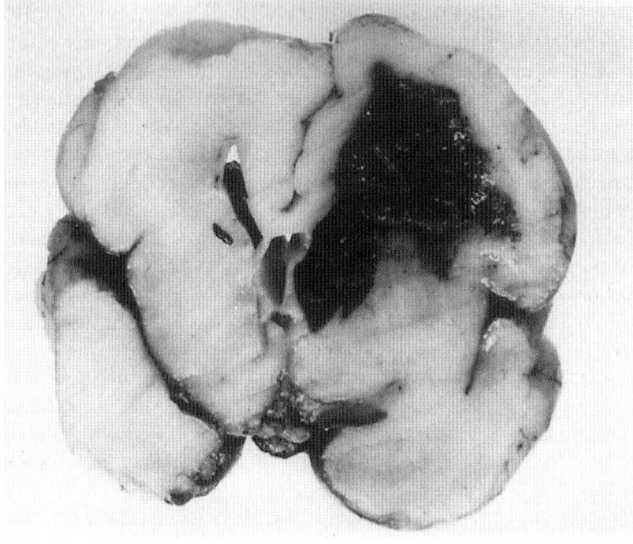

(a)

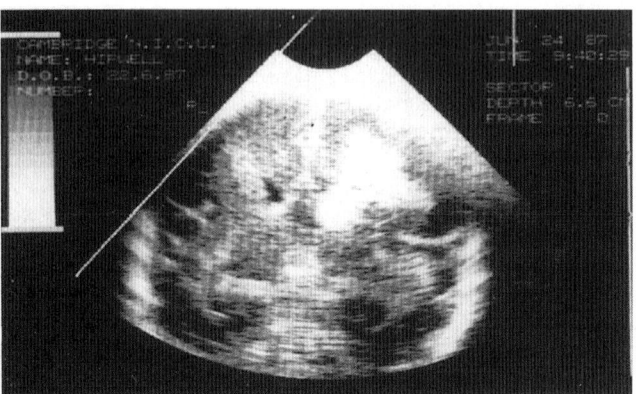

(b)

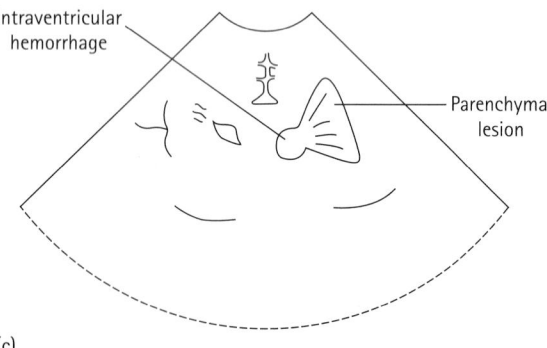

(c)

Fig. 12.48 Periventricular hemorrhage, (a) at postmortem and (b) imaged with ultrasound in life, (c) with diagrammatic representation.

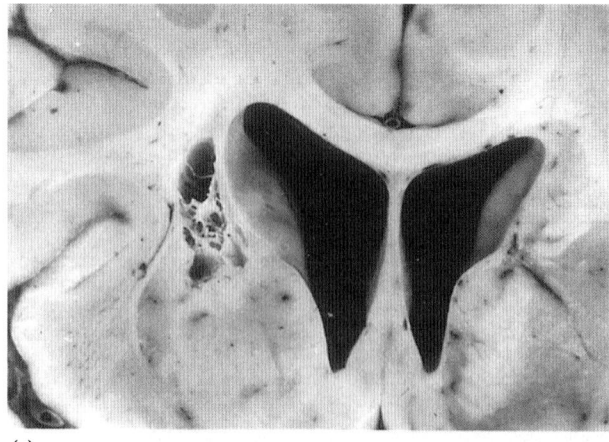

(a)

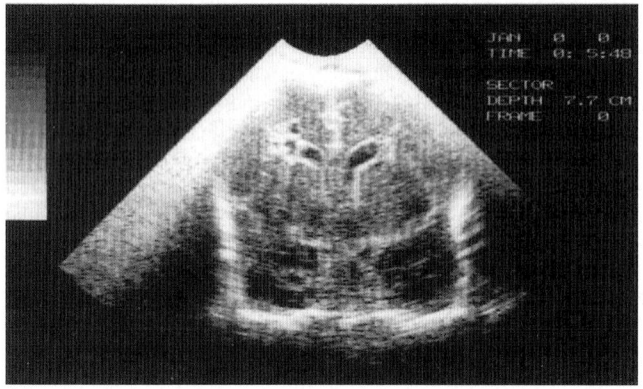

(b)

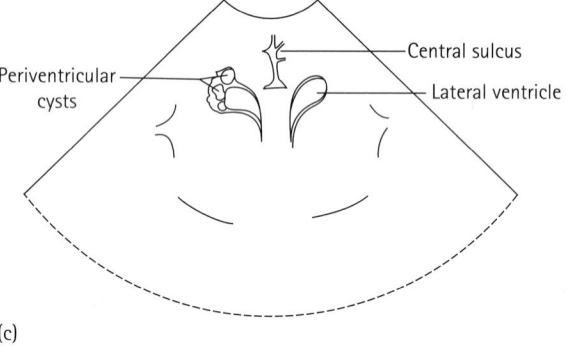

(c)

Fig. 12.49 Periventricular leukomalacia (a) at postmortem and (b) imaged with ultrasound in life, (c) with diagrammatic representation.

region. Cysts disappear after a few months and are replaced by a thinning of the myelin layer. MRI confirms reduction in myelin content of the brain in babies with PVL, and shows that white matter damage is far more common than is suspected with ultrasound imaging alone.[871] The significance of the MRI finding of diffuse excessive high signal intensity (DEHSI) in the white matter has yet to be defined; DEHSI is very common in ex-preterm babies on MRI scans made at term corrected age.

No agreement has yet been reached on the precise definition of the ultrasound appearances of a 'flare' but follow-up suggests that a persistent flare is predictive of outcome and hence represents genuine white matter injury. Early echodense lesions appear 24–48 h after an insult and are often followed in 2–4 weeks by appearance of cystic change. Studies are still emerging regarding the antecedents: antepartum hemorrhage, asphyxia, hypocarbia, and cytokine damage associated

with chorioamnionitis and surgery (particularly for NEC) all appear to be important antecedent factors. The outlook for the survivors with bilateral occipital cystic PVL remains poor, although babies with small cysts confined to the frontal cortex can do well.

Intracerebellar hemorrhage

Cerebellar bleeding can occur as an extension from intraventricular or subarachnoid bleeding or as an isolated clinically silent event in premature babies, and is increasingly recognized as a complication of prematurity.[872] It has been described in association with tight bands around the head. Management is usually conservative and a good outcome has been described at term although preterm babies fare less well.

HYDROCEPHALUS AND VENTRICULOMEGALY

For more information on these conditions see Chapter 22. The following discussion is limited to preterm posthemorrhagic hydrocephalus and the outcome after an in utero diagnosis of ventriculomegaly.

Etiology

Important causes to consider in the newborn period include:

1. cerebral malformations – Arnold–Chiari malformation, Dandy–Walker cysts, aqueduct stenosis, arachnoid cysts causing obstruction to CSF flow;
2. craniosynostosis, e.g. Apert syndrome;
3. obstruction by a mass – vein of Galen aneurysm, tumors;
4. posthemorrhagic hydrocephalus, particularly in preterm babies;
5. postmeningitic hydrocephalus;
6. X-linked congenital hydrocephalus.

Posthemorrhagic hydrocephalus in preterm babies

This is the most frequent cause of acquired hydrocephalus arising in the neonatal period, and usually occurs secondary to periventricular hemorrhage. The natural history of ventricular dilation secondary to PVH is that at least half the cases will not progress to require shunting, an important consideration when assessing uncontrolled studies claiming effective 'cures'.[873]

Treatment

There is no place for compressive head wrapping, glycerol or isosorbide in the treatment of hydrocephalus in babies. The definitive treatment is surgical placement of a ventriculoperitoneal shunt and this will be required in most cases of congenital hydrocephalus. The difficult management decisions usually occur in preterm babies with posthemorrhagic dilation, as in some the ventriculomegaly will arrest, and some are too ill to undergo surgery. Suggestions that shunt placement could be avoided by early intervention with CSF drainage have not been borne out; trials of 'washing out' fibrinogen with CSF irrigation are under way. Acetazolamide and spironolactone were not of any benefit in a randomized controlled trial.[874] Management of this condition should therefore include a single diagnostic lumbar puncture in order to establish the intracranial pressure, whether the ventriculomegaly is of the communicating type and to exclude infection, and then a wait-and-see policy should be adopted with intervention planned if the head growth is more than twice the usual rate or the baby develops symptoms of raised intracranial pressure.

Ventriculoperitoneal shunts

These can be inserted in babies as small as 1500 g. There is a high complication rate in such babies, 30% in some series, with frequent episodes of blockage. Many surgeons like to wait until the CSF protein is below 1.5 g/L before insertion, particularly in posthemorrhagic hydrocephalus when blood in the CSF makes it viscous. Ventriculoatrial shunting is no longer the method of choice, as the complications specific to this route were serious and included shunt nephritis, systemic sepsis and pulmonary hypertension.

Prenatally diagnosed ventriculomegaly

Pediatricians are increasingly asked for help in counseling parents whose fetus has enlarged ventricles diagnosed on an antenatal ultrasound scan. Ventriculomegaly is the most commonly detected abnormality of the fetal brain, occurring in about 1–2 per 1000 of all fetuses. The usual basis of diagnosis is a lateral ventricular width, measured in a true transverse axial plane across the most posterior portion of choroid plexus in a fetus of more than 14 weeks, of more than 10 mm. A distinction is usually made between 'borderline' ventriculomegaly (10–12 mm), 'mild' ventriculomegaly (12–15 mm), and 'severe' ventriculomegaly (>15 mm). Many of the fetuses will be found to have other abnormalities, and a specific search should be made for intrauterine infection, chromosomal abnormality and spina bifida. Even in the best hands some important associated cerebral malformations (notably agenesis of the corpus callosum) can be missed antenatally. The outlook for the group with ventriculomegaly and another abnormality in the CNS is generally poor, and many couples choose termination of pregnancy after counseling, particularly if the diagnosis is made early

enough. Of those diagnosed later, the differentiation between progressive and nonprogressive enlargement needs to be made. If the hydrocephalus is progressive and the pregnancy past 32 weeks' gestation then early delivery and postnatal treatment may be considered. Fetuses with isolated borderline ventriculomegaly (10–12 mm) which does not progress have a good prognosis, about 90% being normal at follow-up although there is a risk of developmental delay.[875,876] Those with a persisting ventriculomegaly above 15 mm do badly.

Prognosis

This depends on the underlying condition, and is worse for posthemorrhagic hydrocephalus than the congenital syndromes. Surgery has radically improved the outlook for some children with hydrocephalus, who can now expect to survive and attend normal school. Overall about 86% now survive and two thirds will have normal intelligence. For preterm babies the prognosis relates to the severity of the associated periventricular hemorrhage and the presence of fits in the neonatal period.

RENAL DISEASE IN THE NEONATE

DEVELOPMENT OF THE RENAL TRACT

The human embryo develops three sets of 'kidneys': the pronephros and the mesonephros which predominantly involute, and the metanephros which is the precursor of the functional kidney (Fig. 12.50). The metanephros can be identified from about 6 weeks post fertilization. It consists of the ureteric bud, which is a branch of the caudal mesonephric duct, and the metanephric mesenchyme, which is a concentration of intermediate mesoderm. The ureteric bud develops to form the collecting ducts, renal pelvis, ureter and bladder trigone. The metanephric mesenchyme forms the functional nephron.

The ureteric bud branches and a condensation of metanephric mesenchyme forms at the tip of each branch. Each condensation develops a

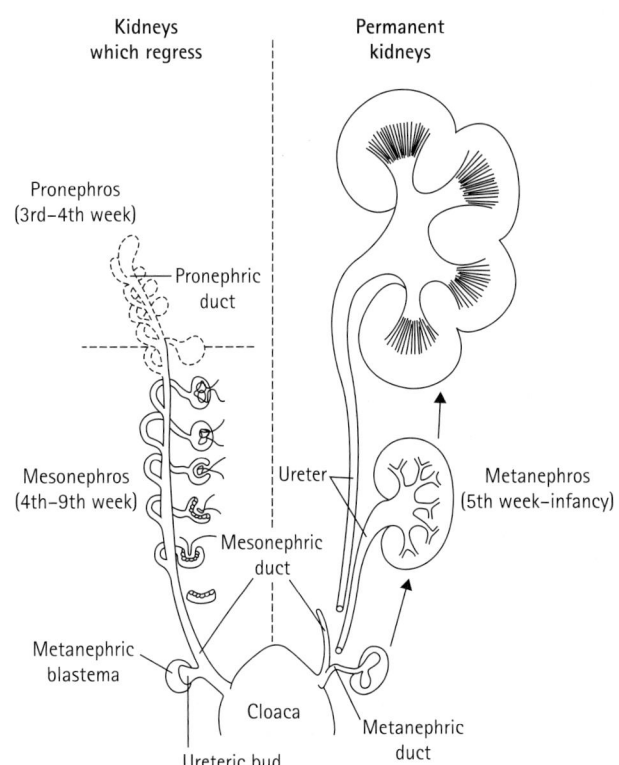

Fig. 12.50 Development of the three paired kidneys in utero. The pronephros and the mesonephros are shown on the left. On the right the development of the metanephros. (From Evan & Larsson 1992[877] with permission.)

lumen, which elongates to form a tubule and develops into primitive glomerular and proximal tubular epithelia (S-shaped body). Nephrogenesis continues with the distal end of the S-shaped body fusing with the neighboring ureteric bud to form a new layer of nephrons. Nephrogenesis continues up to 34–36 weeks' gestation after which no new nephrons are formed. Further expansion in nephron mass is achieved by increased tubular length and glomerular size.

DEVELOPMENT OF RENAL FUNCTION

Fetal urine production begins between 6 and 10 weeks of gestational age and is initially an ultrafiltrate of plasma. The glomerular filtration rate (GFR) increases with gestational age and is higher in the fetus than in an age matched premature infant. Fetal homeostasis is maintained by the placenta. Postnatally GFR continues to increase until 2 years when it becomes equivalent to that of an adult when corrected for surface area (Table 12.93).[878] The relatively low neonatal GFR is both efficient and sufficient given the increased energy requirements that would be needed to deliver an increased GFR, the biochemical compatibility of breast milk and the effects of neonatal growth. However, the relatively low neonatal GFR must be considered when administering drugs that require renal excretion.

Fetal urine production rises from 4.5 ml/kg/h at 20 weeks to 6 ml/kg/h at 32 weeks and 8 ml/kg/h at 39 weeks and is the predominant contributor to amniotic fluid. The urinary excretion of sodium decreases progressively during fetal development from 120 mmol/L of amniotic fluid at 20 weeks to 50 mmol/L at term. It remains higher than that of an age matched neonate and increases sharply following birth. Infants born after 33 weeks' gestation are able to decrease their fractional excretion of sodium to less than 1% within 24 hours of delivery. Most premature infants lack this ability and continue to excrete an excessive amount of urinary sodium and are at risk of intravascular volume depletion and hyponatremia. The ability to conserve water is also impaired in the newborn because the osmotic threshold for ADH release is higher, the loops of Henle are shorter, the counter-current multiplier system is inefficient and there is a relative paucity of urea.

ABNORMALITIES OF THE RENAL TRACT

Congenital anomalies of the urinary tract comprise up to 17% of antenatally diagnosed abnormalities[879] and are classified according to the anatomical area affected or the morphological appearance noted. The complexity of renal development and the interactions between mesenchyme and ureteric bud increase the propensity for abnormal development, as defects in one will often affect the associated development of the other. Advances in the understanding of the molecular and genetic mechanisms of abnormal urinary tract development have demonstrated gene defects associated with specific morphological abnormalities and the potential molecular pathogenesis of these defects. Classification of morphological abnormalities is therefore possible based upon either a descriptive or a molecular/genetic basis and will be discussed further in Chapter 18. Such abnormalities however have a major impact on the prevalence of end-stage renal failure in all age groups.

Renal agenesis is reported unilaterally in about 1 in 1400 infants, although precise figures are uncertain because many patients are

asymptomatic.[880] It may arise because of failure of the ureteric bud to develop, failure of the ureteric bud to contact the metanephric blastema, or failure of the bud and the metanephric blastema to interact and induce nephrogenesis. Bilateral renal agenesis is reported in 1 in 4000 births, with a male to female ratio of 2.5 to 1.[880] Bilateral renal agenesis is associated with oligohydramnios, Potter's sequence and fetal or perinatal death. Unilateral renal agenesis is generally asymptomatic, but abnormalities in the contralateral kidney have been reported[881] and it is often associated with abnormalities of other organs. The risk of recurrence can be determined in syndromic cases or if the mode of inheritance is known. The recurrence risk is 3% if there are no renal abnormalities in first degree relatives.[882] One study reported associated urogenital abnormalities in 9% and unilateral renal agenesis in 4.5% of first degree relatives of infants with bilateral renal agenesis.[883]

Misplacement of the ureteric bud on the mesonephric duct may lead to abnormal nephrogenesis and renal dysplasia. This is characterized histologically by the presence of primitive ducts and foci of metaplastic cartilage with or without cyst formation.[884] The association of reflux with renal dysplasia may occur as a result of the ureteric bud arising below the normal position. This then presents at the urogenital sinus earlier in gestation and migrates further laterally presenting a larger ureteric orifice which is consequently more prone to reflux.[885] As with renal agenesis, renal dysplasia may be found as a component of several differing syndromes with considerable clinical variation.

Multicystic dysplasia is characterized by the presence of multiple, noncommunicating and nonfunctioning renal cysts varying in size from a few millimeters to several centimeters. It is unilateral in 76% and bilateral in the remainder[886] with a reported incidence of 1 in 3–4000 and 1 in 10 000 live births respectively.[887] It is the commonest cause of an abdominal mass in the newborn. Consistent evidence demonstrates that the perceived risk of hypertension or malignancy is unfounded[888–890] and that serial ultrasounds to ensure regression are all that is required.

Cystic disease of the kidneys may occur in isolation or in association with recognized syndromes. Isolated renal cystic disease in the absence of urinary tract obstruction may be identified antenatally as large hyperechoic kidneys on ultrasound. The presence of oligohydramnios is a poor prognostic sign and is frequently associated with neonatal death from pulmonary hypoplasia. Autosomal recessive polycystic kidney disease (ARPKD) is sometimes referred to as infantile polycystic kidney disease. This is a misnomer because the adult form (autosomal dominant, ADPKD) may also present in infancy. ARPKD is an uncommon disorder occurring in 1 in 40 000 births,[890] the gene for which is mapped to chromosome 6.[891] It is characterized histologically by bilateral renal enlargement with numerous microscopic corticomedullary cysts. Associated liver changes including bile duct proliferation with portal fibrosis are invariably present. The prognosis of this condition is dependent on the severity of renal disease in the perinatal period with the most severely affected dying within the first year of life. ADPKD has a gene frequency of 1 in 1000[892] and has multiple gene loci, the commonest of which is on the short arm of chromosome 16.[892] The clinical course for ADPKD is generally more benign. However, cases that are detected antenatally have a similar prognosis to infants with antenatally detected ARPKD, with mortality approaching 50% in the first year of life.[893]

Failure of the kidney to ascend from the pelvis is the commonest form of renal ectopia. It has an incidence of 1 in 1200 in postmortem studies.[894] The ectopic kidney derives its blood supply from an anomalous source in the aorta or the pelvic vessels. Fusion of ectopic kidneys may occur in the midline, producing a discoid or 'pancake' kidney or following migration of the ectopic kidney to the contralateral side where fusion occurs with the normal kidney on that side. Fusion of kidneys also occurs to form a horseshoe kidney with an incidence of 1 in 400, where both kidneys are fused at the lower poles. Horseshoe kidneys are found at the level of the lumbar vertebrae as ascent is limited by the presence of the aortic bifurcation and the inferior mesenteric artery. As with ectopic kidneys, horseshoe kidneys are frequently asymptomatic but complications from a malrotated pelvis or ureter may result in

Table 12.93 Increase in relative glomerular filtration rate in infancy. Values expressed as mean (± 2 SD)

Age	ml/min	ml/kg	ml/min/1.73 m²
1 week	3.75 (2.5–5)	1.2 (0.8–1.6)	30 (20–40)
1 month	6 (4–8)	1.5 (1–2)	50 (30–70)
3 months	10.5 (7–14)	1.89 (1.2–2.4)	60 (40–80)
6 months	18.5 (12.5–25)	2.4 (1.6–3.2)	80 (60–100)
1 year	30 (20–40)	2 (2–4)	100 (75–125)
2 years	45 (30–60)	3.3 (2.2–4.4)	120 (90–150)

infection, ureteric obstruction or nephrolithiasis. Additionally there is an increased risk of neoplasia in horseshoe kidneys, most commonly Wilms' tumor.[895]

Abnormalities in ureteric development are the commonest abnormalities of the renal tract with duplex systems reported in up to 4% of the population.[896] This arises when two ureteric buds occur on one side and induce nephrogenesis in an upper and lower renal moiety, resulting in drainage through either a common or two separate ureters. The lower ureter migrates laterally, crossing the upper ureter, and is more prone to vesicoureteric reflux. The upper ureter is more prone to ectopic insertion and ureterocele development. These abnormalities are frequently asymptomatic.

Obstruction of the ureter due to stenosis at the pelviureteric junction or the vesicoureteric junction or due to external compression may result in hydronephrosis. Fetal ureteric obstruction may lead to renal dysplasia,[897] depending on the duration and the degree of ureteric obstruction. The investigation and postnatal management of these conditions will be discussed later. Bladder outflow obstruction is more common in males. It may be due to posterior urethral valves. Less commonly it is a feature of prune belly syndrome. This may be a consequence of transient fetal urethral obstruction and features include oligohydramnios, pulmonary hypoplasia, Potter's facies, a deficiency in the abdominal wall musculature, cryptorchidism, megacystis, megaureter and variable progression to renal failure. The role of fetal interventional surgery for bladder outflow obstruction is unclear. Benefits in pulmonary growth may occur following the insertion of a vesico-amniotic shunt in the presence of oligohydramnios, however the impact on postnatal renal function has been disappointing.[898,899]

ASSESSMENT AND INVESTIGATION OF THE NEONATE WITH RENAL DISEASE

Careful history taking is important. An infant with autosomal dominant polycystic kidney disease may have asymptomatic parents but affected members of the extended family. Specific gene defects are recognized for many syndromic conditions, offering the possibility of pre-implantation or antenatal gene testing. In several conditions more than one gene defect exists, requiring linkage analysis to determine the presence of the condition in the fetus. A useful summary published by Rizk & Chapman outlines the genetic and clinical features of cystic and inherited conditions.[900]

Details of the pregnancy are also important. Oligohydramnios may indicate renal agenesis or dysplasia. Polyhydramnios occurs in association with fetal polyuric states such as nephrogenic diabetes insipidus or Bartter syndrome. The placenta may be enlarged (> 25% of birth weight) in autosomal recessive congenital nephrotic syndrome (Finnish type), which is also associated with an elevated maternal alpha-fetoprotein. The presence of a single umbilical artery may be associated with abnormalities of the renal tract. Thummula et al[901] performed a meta-analysis of 37 studies. Single umbilical artery was noted in 0.55% of live-born fetuses and was associated with a congenital abnormality rate of 27%, including abnormalities of the renal tract in 16%. More than half of the abnormalities were minor or self-limiting and isolated single umbilical artery in an asymptomatic infant was not considered to be an indication for detailed urological investigation.

The use of antenatal ultrasound to detect fetal anomalies is now routine in many areas and has a created a previously unknown patient population. The finding of a renal abnormality on antenatal ultrasound should be treated with caution in all but the most severe cases as studies have shown that the majority of abnormalities detected are of hydronephrosis and are minor or self-limiting.[902] Parents should be reassured of this during the pregnancy. The identification and investigation of infants with antenatal hydronephrosis is not standardized and is determined by local protocols. Measurement thresholds for renal pelvis dilatation considered to be consistent with a degree of hydronephrosis increase with advancing gestation from > 6 mm at 20 weeks to > 8 mm at 20–30 weeks and > 10 mm at over 30 weeks.[903–905] These measurements should not be viewed in isolation. Infundibular or

Table 12.94 Etiology of hydronephrosis detected antenatally[913]

Transient/physiological	63%
Pelviureteric junction obstruction	11%
Vesicoureteric reflux	9%
Megaureter	4%
Multicystic dysplastic kidney	2%
Ureterocele	2%
Posterior urethral valves	1%

calyceal dilatation is never a normal variant.[906] Ureteric dilatation, parenchymal thinning or abnormalities of the urinary bladder increase the likelihood of postnatal pathology. The definition of significant renal pelvic dilatation varies, with most studies accepting 10 mm as a threshold.[907–911] The etiology of hydronephrosis is consistent across studies[912,913] and is shown in Table 12.94. The current guidelines for the management of antenatally diagnosed renal pelvis dilatation adopted by the Scottish Paediatric Renal Group are shown in Figure 12.51. It is accepted that minor degrees of vesicoureteric reflux may be missed by the omission of a micturating cystourethrogram in some infants, however the clinical significance of this is felt to be minimal.

PHYSICAL EXAMINATION

Renal disease in the neonatal period may present with nonspecific features such as poor feeding, weight loss, irritability, fever, jaundice or diarrhea. The possibility of associated renal abnormalities is increased in the presence of other congenital abnormalities or syndromes.

Inspection of the infant may reveal features consistent with oligohydramnios such as the classic Potter's facies or orthopedic anomalies, including talipes equinovarus. Urinary tract pathology should be anticipated when neural tube defects are identified. Examination of the external genitalia and visualization of the urinary stream are particularly important in the male infant as dribbling or a hesitant stream may be associated with posterior urethral valves. Approximately 30% of neonates void during or immediately after delivery, 92% within 24 h and 99% within 48 h. Failure to do so requires clinical assessment to exclude dehydration or bladder outlet obstruction. Ultrasonically confirmed bladder distention requires catheter drainage either per urethra or, in some units, suprapubically if there is a suspicion of a posterior urethral valve.

Most abdominal masses that are palpable in the newborn period are renal in origin.[914] Normal kidneys may be readily palpated with bi-manual examination. Ascites is rarely renal in origin. It may occur in association with generalized edema from fluid overload secondary to renal failure, or in association with hypoalbuminemia secondary to fetal hydrops or congenital nephrotic syndrome.

INVESTIGATION – URINALYSIS

Frank hematuria is far less common than microscopic hematuria in the neonatal period. Possible etiologies are highlighted in Table 12.95. The association of an abdominal mass, hematuria and thrombocytopenia in a sick neonate raises the possibility of renal vein thrombosis. Doppler ultrasound should be used to ascertain the extent of the thrombosis of the renal vein and any extension into the inferior vena cava or into the contralateral renal vein. Renal vein thrombosis occurs in association with perinatal asphyxia and umbilical venous catheterization. The possibility of an inherited thrombophilia should be assessed by investigation of the child and the parents. Abnormalities have been reported in approximately 40% of cases.[915,916] There are no published data relating to the use of prophylactic anticoagulant therapy in this population. Bilateral renal vein thrombosis or extending caval thrombosis are cited as relative indications for the commencement of anticoagulant or less commonly thrombolytic therapy.[915–917] Intravenous unfractionated heparin, 20–25 u/h aiming for an activated partial prothrombin time of 1.5–2.5, has been used. Low molecular weight heparin at a dose

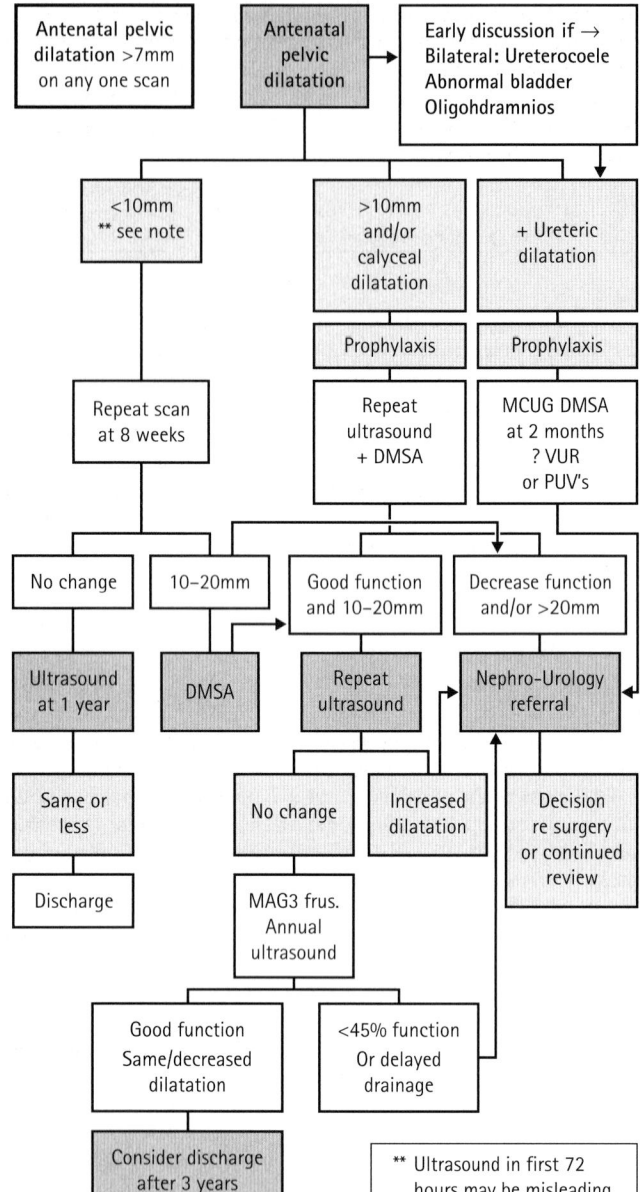

Fig. 12.51   Current guidelines for the management of antenatally diagnosed renal pelvis dilatation adopted by the Scottish Paediatric Surgical Group (with permission). * Ultrasound in the first 72 h may be misleading. DMSA, dimercaptosuccinic acid; MCUG, micturating cystourethrogram; PUV, posterior urethral valves; MAG3 frus., MAG3 scan.

of 150 u/kg twice daily administered subcutaneously, aiming for an anti-factor Xa level of 0.5–0.9 IU/ml, has also been described. The outcome of renal vein thrombosis is generally good with a reported incidence of end-stage renal failure of less than 10%, and hypertension in up to 25%. However, significant degrees of renal damage are consistently reported[915,916,918] with recent evidence suggesting that a renal length over 6 cm is always associated with long term renal dysfunction.[915]

Hypercalciuria may lead to nephrocalcinosis, which is reported in up to two thirds of very low birth weight neonates and is associated with tubular and glomerular dysfunction. Recent studies however suggest that in the majority of cases nephrocalcinosis resolves with no evidence of residual renal dysfunction.[919]

Proteinuria in the neonatal period is physiological[920] and is higher in the preterm than the term infant. Proteinuria exceeding 10 mg/m^2/h after 5 days of age requires further investigation; possible etiologies are listed in Table 12.96.

Table 12.95   Causes of hematuria in the neonatal period

Coagulation disorders
Vascular disorders
    Acute tubular necrosis
    Corticomedullary necrosis
    Renal vascular thrombosis
    Adrenal hemorrhage
Cystic disease
    Cystic dysplasia
    Multicystic dysplastic kidney
    ARPKD/ADPKD
Neoplasia
    Wilms' tumor
    Mesoblastic nephroma
    Angioma
Infection
Trauma
Obstruction
Interstitial nephritis

Table 12.96   Etiology of proteinuria in the neonate

Physiological
Renal vascular thrombosis
Cortical necrosis
Congenital nephrosis
    Finnish type
    Denys–Drash
    Nail–patella syndrome
Infection
    Urosepsis
    Syphilis
    Toxoplasmosis
    Cytomegalovirus
Nephrotoxic agents – including drug therapy

INVESTIGATION – BLOOD BIOCHEMISTRY

Following birth the plasma creatinine reflects the maternal creatinine and is elevated, particularly in preterm infants. Levels fall by the end of the first week. However, this fall may take several weeks in preterm infants due to tubular reabsorption of creatinine and a lower GFR. Urea concentration is affected by many variables including protein intake, hydration status and metabolic state and as such is unreliable in assessing renal function.

Urinary sodium excretion is greater in preterm infants as a consequence of relative aldosterone resistance and this can mean that sodium supplementation is necessary. Bicarbonate loss is also greater in preterm infants, causing them to exist in a more acidotic state. However the excretion of an acid load is not impaired, allowing the preterm infant to thrive.

INVESTIGATION – IMAGING

Ultrasound examination of the fetal and neonatal urinary tract has been discussed earlier in relation to the investigation of antenatally observed hydronephrosis. The relatively low volume of urine produced by neonates in the first 48 h post partum may mask hydronephrosis persisting postnatally and for this reason delaying the initial postnatal ultrasound scan beyond this period has been advocated. This should not occur for cases of moderate to severe antenatally detected hydronephrosis (renal pelvis diameter > 15 mm) who require imaging within the first 48 h post partum. The use of nuclear scintigraphy in the assessment of the neonatal renal tract is well established with dynamic isotopes such as ^{99m}Tc-labeled diethylenetriaminepentaacetate (DTPA) and mercaptoacetyltriglycine (MAG-3) providing data on renal perfusion. As they are dynamic isotopes they also provide data on renal excretion, particularly in cases of suspected pelviureteric junction obstruction. However they are of limited benefit in assessing obstruction in the lower ureter at the vesicoureteric junction, which remains one of the few indications for the use of an intravenous pyelogram in the investigation of the neonatal renal tract other than prior to surgical intervention in cases of established obstruction. Assessment of differential renal function may be undertaken using these isotopes. ^{99m}Tc-labeled diethylmercaptosuccinic acid (DMSA) is more sensitive and provides data on renal scarring. Because DMSA does not adhere well to immature tubular epithelium, unreliable results may be obtained in preterm infants, and in our institution DMSA imaging is not undertaken prior to 3 months of age.

Micturating cystourethrogram (MCUG) is mandatory for the assessment of infants with neonatal urosepsis with particular attention in males to the possibility of a posterior urethral valve. The role of the MCUG in the investigation of minimal antenatal hydronephrosis or in the investigation of a neonate in whom the sibling has reflux nephropathy is less clear. Recent evidence suggests that investigation in this cohort is seldom required and that ultrasound is a suitable alternative to MCUG.[921]

CLINICAL CONDITIONS AFFECTING THE NEONATE
Acute renal failure
Acute renal failure is a frequent occurrence in the neonatal intensive care setting, with up to a quarter of neonates presenting to intensive care showing evidence of renal failure.[922] The diagnosis of acute renal failure is dependent on repeated measurements of the plasma creatinine, as variations in gestation and maternal creatinine in combination with the normal postpartum diuresis make estimation of GFR from a single plasma creatinine measurement very difficult. A rise in plasma creatinine or indeed a failure to observe the physiological decline in creatinine post partum both indicate renal functional impairment. Preterm infants may have a transient period of oliguria ($< 300\,ml/m^2/d$). The main cause of oliguria in the neonatal period is inadequate renal perfusion (pre-renal failure) as a consequence of hypotension, hypovolemia, hypoxia and acidosis. Early correction of impaired renal perfusion with volume expansion or pressor support may prevent progression to established renal failure. In the absence of pre-renal failure the most common cause is intrinsic renal disease. Ultrasound examination should be used to exclude congenital uropathy.

The general principles of management of acute renal failure are discussed in Chapter 18. There are some additional considerations in the management of neonatal acute renal failure. The relatively high surface area to weight ratio of the neonate results in increased insensible fluid losses. These are around 0.5–1 ml/kg/h in term infants, but due to higher transepithelial fluid losses they may be as high as 3 ml/kg/h in preterm infants.[923] Renal replacement therapy using peritoneal dialysis can be undertaken successfully in neonates with acute renal failure.[924] Improvements in vascular access and the use of pumped extracorporeal circuits have also made continuous renal replacement therapies a viable alternative, not withstanding the attendant risks of vascular access and systemic anticoagulation. The outcome of non-oliguric renal failure is excellent[925] as it is almost exclusively a secondary event that responds to treatment of the initial cause.[926] However, oligo-anuric renal failure has a reported mortality of up to 78%.[925]

Chronic renal failure
Chronic renal failure may develop in infants who fail to recover from acute renal failure and in infants with congenital renal abnormalities. Imaging of the renal tract will generally define the underlying etiology. In rare cases a renal biopsy may be required. The general principles of management of chronic renal failure are discussed in Chapter 18 . In the

neonatal period particularly close attention to fluid balance and nutritional intake is required as many of these infants are polyuric, requiring over 200 ml/kg/day, and consequently require the input from specialist dietetic staff and frequent checks of body weight. Whilst chronic hemodialysis is feasible in smaller infants,[927] the renal replacement modality of choice is peritoneal dialysis. The impact on the family of having a baby with complex medical needs is profound and the services of the multidisciplinary team should be made available, including that of an appropriately trained psychologist.

Hypertension
Hypertension is uncommon in the neonatal period and occurs most commonly in the intensive care setting.[928] As in older children, hypertension in the neonate is defined as a blood pressure greater than the 95th percentile for age, gender and weight.[929] Blood pressure measurement in sick neonates in intensive care is generally achieved by direct arterial measurement through the umbilical artery. Automated oscillometric blood pressure recording is also frequently used, although care must be taken in using the appropriate cuff size to avoid serious inaccuracies. The main causes of hypertension in the neonate are listed in Table 12.97. It is most commonly observed in sick infants where the etiology is multifactorial and the hypertension generally resolves with clinical improvement. Persisting hypertension is most commonly a consequence of renovascular or renal parenchymal disease. Determining the etiology of hypertension in the neonate can generally be achieved through a careful history and physical examination. Investigations other than renal tract imaging are rarely required. Treatment of the sick hypertensive neonate is best achieved using an intravenous agent, which allows immediate dose titration according to response. In neonates with blood pressure controlled with intravenous agents or those with mild hypertension, oral therapy should be commenced that is relevant to the etiology of the hypertension, e.g. in the presence of chronic lung disease and steroid usage, diuretic therapy would be the initial treatment of choice. The choice of antihypertensives is frequently dictated by local expertise and is reviewed in detail by Flynn.[929]

Urinary tract infection
Urinary tract infection (UTI) in the neonatal period is more common in males and is significantly associated with abnormalities of the renal

Table 12.97   Etiology of hypertension in the neonate

Renal
Polycystic kidney disease
Renal dysplasia
Obstructive uropathy
Renal failure
Vascular
Renal artery stenosis
Aortic coarctation
Mid-aortic syndrome
Tumor
Neuroblastoma
Mesoblastoma
Pheochromocytoma
Endocrine
Adrenal hyperplasia
Cushing syndrome
Thyrotoxicosis
Central nervous system
Raised intracranial pressure
Meningitis
Seizures
Miscellaneous
Neonatal abstinence syndrome
Idiopathic

tract.[930,931] The clinical features of a neonate with UTI are nonspecific and include vomiting, weight loss, poor feeding, fever, diarrhea and jaundice, and therefore a high index of suspicion is required. Treatment should be initiated without delay following specimen collection and should be administered intravenously in the first instance. The choice of antibiotic is likely to be determined by local preference with the majority of organisms responding to the standard neonatal sepsis protocol. Following treatment, prophylactic antibiotic therapy is advised at least until the completion of radiological investigation, the protocol for which is discussed further in Chapter 18.

EYE PROBLEMS IN THE NEWBORN

A normal visual input is important for a child's development. This section will be concerned with the developing visual system, and the various problems which may befall it in the neonatal period.

THE DEVELOPING VISUAL SYSTEM
Ocular growth
The ocular growth of the extremely preterm infant is particularly active, the retinal surface area doubling between 24 weeks' gestation and term. By term the infant's eye is at a relatively advanced stage of development: it increases only three times in volume to reach adult size, compared to the rest of the body which increases 20 times. In the first 2 years the surface area increases by a further 50%. Most of the postnatal growth of the eye takes place in its posterior segment, particularly in the peripheral regions of the retina. There is little growth in either the retina around the macula[932] or the anterior segment of the eye[933] so the line of sight is relatively unperturbed during development. The length of the globe does not reach its adult value of approximately 24 mm until the second decade.

Cornea
The normal cornea is hazy until about 27 weeks' gestation. Slight haze in preterm and term infants is not rare depending on the degree of immaturity. It clears rapidly. A cloudy cornea may be caused by infantile glaucoma (see below and Fig. 12.52), a corneal dystrophy, malformation of the anterior segment, and rarely, in congenital rubella, by keratitis.

Lens
Subtle lens opacities are quite common in preterm neonates. These are in the form of vacuoles and are best seen using the direct ophthalmoscope. They are transient, of no long term significance and their etiology is unknown. Congenital cataract is considered elsewhere (Ch. 31).

Vascular development
Transient vascular systems. In fetal life the eye has two transient vascular systems. The hyaloid vascular complex, which fills the vitreous cavity and extends forwards, also contributes to the second system, the tunica vasculosa lentis, a vascular structure which surrounds the lens. The hyaloid artery disappears by 28 weeks' gestational age while the tunica vasculosa lentis regresses between 28 and 34 weeks' gestational age. As the latter can readily be visualized by direct ophthalmoscopy the degree of regression can be used as a crude estimate of gestational age. Failure of regression can be an important sign of severe retinopathy of prematurity.
Retinal vasculature. The retina is avascular until the fourth month of gestation, relying entirely on the underlying choroidal circulation for its nutrients. From this time the mesenchymal precursors of the retinal vessels grow out from the optic disc and reach the periphery of the nasal retina around 32 weeks' gestational age, whilst in the temporal retina, which is the last area to be vascularized, this process is not complete until around term. The stimulus for vessel growth is tissue hypoxia mediated through retinal astrocytes and Muller cells, which secrete vascular endothelial growth factor (VEGF). VEGF is a vascular survival factor and, in synergy with IGF-1, is vital to the formation and maintenance of a normal mature retinal circulation.[934]

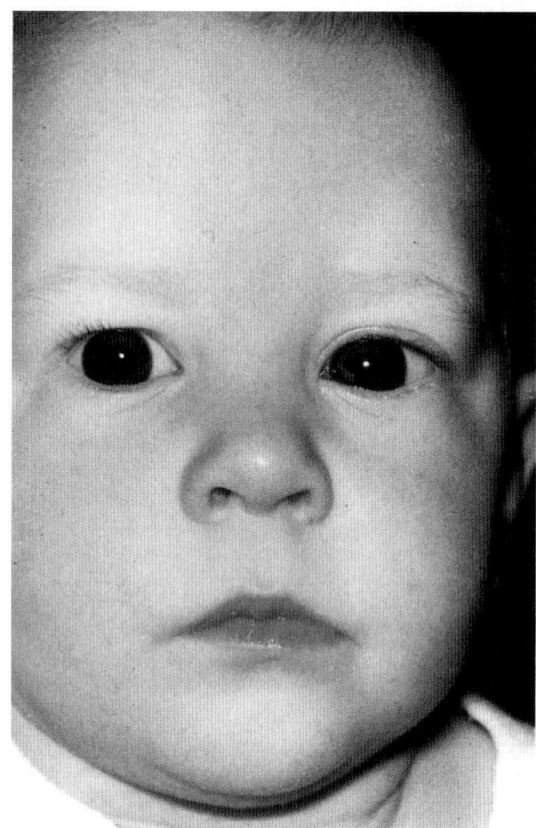

Fig. 12.52   Congenital glaucoma in the left eye. This eye is larger than its fellow, and the cornea is also slightly hazy (dulled corneal light reflex).

Visual pathway development
The retina has its full complement of cells by 24 weeks' gestational age, but retinal maturational changes continue, particularly in the fovea, for another 4 years or so. Myelination between the globe and the lateral geniculate nucleus starts at about 24 weeks' gestational age and is complete by 2 years. In the posterior visual pathway dendrite formation and synaptogenesis both lead to an increase in volume of the lateral geniculate nucleus and the visual cortex over the first 6 or so months of postnatal life, while myelination continues for at least a decade.

Ocular growth, the maturational changes within the eye, and the posterior sections of the visual system are all dovetailed so that they proceed at a predetermined and relatively unimpeded rate to reach a successful functional outcome. That this occurs relatively unimpeded is quite remarkable for the baby born before term, who is reared in an environment that is relatively hostile compared to the womb.[935]

OPHTHALMIA NEONATORUM

Defined as conjunctivitis developing within the first 4 weeks after birth of life (Fig. 12.53), ophthalmia neonatorum is a notifiable condition as in the past it was one of the most important causes of childhood visual disability. Fortunately, in most countries, the situation has now changed, but even today permanent ocular damage can result and treatment must be appropriate and prompt. Although the clinical features of the various types of ophthalmia neonatorum are suggestive of a particular diagnosis they are not sufficiently characteristic to make a definitive diagnosis. A large number of organisms have been implicated and in order of frequency these are *Chlamydia trachomatis*, *Staphylococcus* sp., *Neisseria gonorrhoeae*, *Streptococcus* sp., *Haemophilus* sp., *E. coli*, and less frequently a number of other organisms including *Pseudomonas aeruginosa* and the herpes simplex virus.

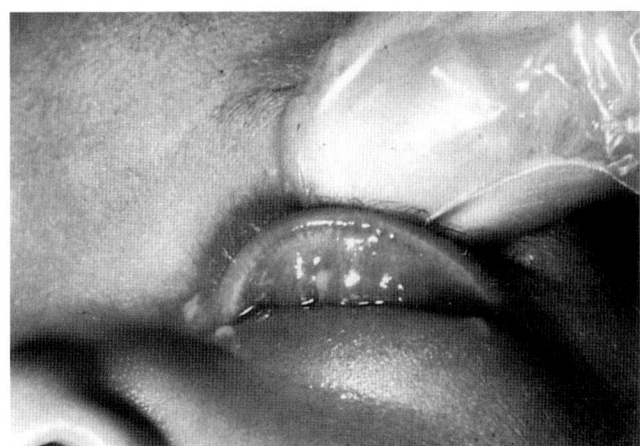

Fig. 12.53 Ophthalmia neonatorum.

Chlamydia trachomatis

This is the commonest cause of ophthalmia neonatorum (developing in 10–50% of those infants exposed) and although the clinical picture may be mild, subclinical infections are not unusual. About 70% babies with chlamydial infection are culture positive in the nasopharynx and pneumonia can develop.[936] The incubation period is usually 5–14 days with a peak incidence in the second week after birth. The condition can be unilateral or bilateral and may range from a mild erythematous response to a severe pseudomembranous conjunctivitis (streptococci are another cause of a pseudomembranous reaction). Only in the most severe infection is the discharge copious and purulent. Even mild disease can cause corneal scarring (pannus), but the risk of this complication is lessened by prompt treatment.[936,937]

Neisseria gonorrhoeae

This infection is acquired during passage down the birth canal of the mother who has either untreated or partially treated gonorrhea. Worldwide it is estimated that there were over 62 million new cases in 1999.[938] The incubation period is usually 2–5 days but conjunctivitis may present up to 3 weeks after delivery. Characteristically the gonococcus causes a marked inflammatory reaction with lid and conjunctival edema, and a copious purulent, greenish, sometimes blood-stained discharge held under pressure by the swollen eyelids. Disseminated infection can occur. This organism is particularly virulent as it alone can penetrate the intact cornea to cause blindness.

Herpes simplex virus

When ophthalmia neonatorum is caused by this virus it is usually as part of a generalized infection. In addition to the conjunctivitis, corneal clouding and dendritic ulceration occur. In contrast to herpes simplex infections developing at other times of life, neonatal herpes has a propensity to affect both eyes, and to differentiate it from other causes of ophthalmia neonatorum there may be vesicular formation of the eyelid skin and corneal involvement.

Other organisms

These do not individually give rise to distinctive clinical features, although in general a purulent discharge indicates bacterial origin or secondary involvement.

Diagnosis and treatment

As the clinical features are at best suggestive but not pathognomonic, accurate diagnosis rests with laboratory tests. Culture media (blood and chocolate agar) should be inoculated immediately as *N. gonorrhoeae* cannot resist drying. Swabs from the conjunctivae must be taken before any topical or systemic antibiotic is administered. A further tissue specimen which must contain epithelial cells is applied directly to microscope slides and stained by Gram and Giemsa stains, looking in

the latter for the intracytoplasmic inclusions of *Chlamydia*, and multinucleated giant cells and intranuclear inclusions of herpes simplex. Direct enzyme immunoassay or immunofluorescent antibody assay of conjunctival discharge has high specificity and sensitivity for *Chlamydia*. Impression cytology of conjunctival cells is a rapid technique for diagnosing *Chlamydia*.[936]

In several countries, and many of the states in the USA, but not the UK, prophylaxis is routine and sometimes is mandatory, using 1% silver nitrate, 1% tetracycline ointment, or 0.5% erythromycin ointment. Neither silver nitrate nor erythromycin is protective against *Chlamydia*. Povidone–iodine 2.5% is more effective than all other prophylactic agents, is simple and cheap to prepare and yet, for reasons not readily apparent, is not used routinely.[939,940] Whichever preparation is used it is applied once to both eyes soon after birth. Silver nitrate is ineffective against established infection. Silver nitrate causes a chemical conjunctivitis which resolves after one or two days. All cases of ophthalmia neonatorum should be managed as though they are contagious and in many cases there will be infection by multiple organisms. Thus, gonococcal infection is frequently accompanied by chlamydial infection and infants need to be investigated appropriately; many will need to be treated for both conditions. It is also important to appreciate that both gonococcal and chlamydial infections may have a systemic component and treating the eye alone is not enough. Treatment must be started immediately, guided by clinical findings and the results of the histological stains. The first line of treatment for gonococcal infections is ceftriaxone administered by intramuscular or intravenous routes (25–50 mg/kg) as a single dose, although multiple doses may be preferred by some pediatricians.[938] Resistance to ceftriaxone has not been reported. For chlamydial infection oral erythromycin for 2 weeks remains the treatment of choice; as efficacy of treatment is 80%, a second course may be required.[936,937] For both gonococcal and chlamydial infections once systemic treatment has commenced topical antibiotics are not necessary, although it is important that the conjunctival discharge is washed away frequently by saline irrigation. In other words, treat the baby and the eye is naturally covered by this; the reverse is not true.

BIRTH TRAUMA
Eyelids and orbit

Ecchymosis of the eyelids is common but is of no long term consequence. Orbital hemorrhage causing proptosis occurs occasionally and is usually the consequence of a prolonged and difficult labor.

Ocular hemorrhages

Hemorrhages into various ocular tissues are frequent with all types of delivery. Conjunctival hemorrhages resolve rapidly and without sequelae. It is not uncommon for the iris blood vessels to be markedly engorged following birth, and on occasion bleeding into the anterior chamber occurs causing a hyphema which also settles spontaneously.

The retina is the most frequent site of hemorrhage following birth. In decreasing frequency they may result from delivery by vacuum extraction, vaginal and forceps delivery, and least often following Cesarean section.[941] Frequently but not invariably bilateral, most retinal hemorrhages resolve spontaneously without trace over the ensuing days and weeks. If the hemorrhage is large and has a preretinal or vitreous extension this process may take up to 2–3 months, but even so it does not result in adverse sequelae. Neonatal retinal hemorrhages do not cause amblyopia. Sometimes it can be difficult to differentiate between retinal hemorrhages due to the birth process and a later acquired non-accidental injury. The distinction, which can be extremely difficult, rests on the history and whether the features of the hemorrhage are compatible with the history.

Cornea

The cornea may be damaged by forceps injury. This is usually unilateral and causes a cloudy cornea. The first priority is to distinguish corneal cloudiness due to injury from infantile glaucoma (Fig. 12.54) which requires prompt treatment. Although in glaucoma the corneas

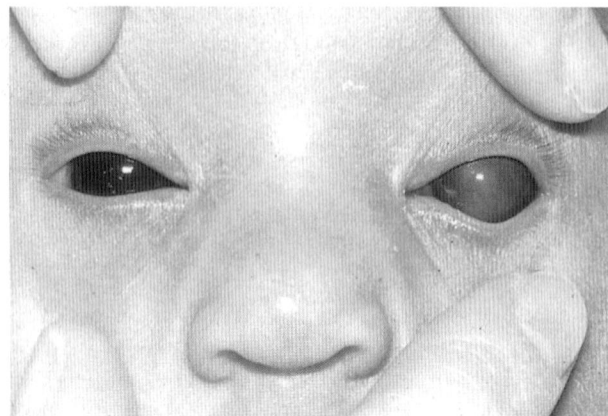

Fig. 12.54 Left cloudy cornea due to malformation of the anterior segment, the so-called anterior cleavage syndrome.

are characteristically enlarged, in the neonatal period this may be yet to develop and it is essential therefore to measure the intraocular pressure. Clouding following forceps trauma clears over a few weeks, but in the long term astigmatism, amblyopia and strabismus are likely sequelae.

Cranial nerve palsies

Palsy of one of the ocular motor nerves is not rare and has in the past often been attributed to birth trauma – almost certainly incorrectly.

RETINOPATHY OF PREMATURITY

Retinopathy of prematurity (ROP) is a potentially blinding disorder affecting infants born prematurely. Described first in the 1940s, there was an epidemic of retrolental fibroplasia (RLF), as it was then known. This was brought to an end in the early 1950s by the discovery that the high concentrations of oxygen being given at that time were important in its etiology. Concomitant with the increased survival of the extremely immature neonate over the past few decades, the incidence of ROP has again risen.

Pathogenesis

ROP is a condition of the immature retinal vasculature and does not develop after the retina is fully vascularized. Retinopathy develops at the junction of the vascularized and yet to be vascularized retina. There are three theories of ROP pathogenesis. According to the first, classic theory,[942,943] the retinal vessels constrict and their endothelial cells are damaged due to raised (i.e. above normal for the fetus) PaO_2 levels. This leads to the production of angiogenic factors and subsequent vasoproliferation. The second theory[944] also postulates the production of angiogenic factors but proposes that this is not induced by vasoconstriction but by direct oxidative insult to the mesenchymal precursors (spindle cells), which then synthesize and secrete angiogenic factors generating the retinal vasoproliferative response.

Both theories invoke an oxidative insult, which might be due to a direct cytotoxic action of oxygen itself,[942] indirectly due to ischemia consequent upon the vasoconstriction,[943] or indirectly by oxygen-generated free radicals.[944] The most recent and third theory invokes growth factors and apoptosis.[945,946] The maintenance of the retinal vascular tree depends on a continuous supply of the survival factor VEGF acting in synergy with IGF-1.[934] Hyperoxia downregulates VEGF so halting retinovascular development and inducing endothelial apoptosis and excessive capillary regression. The resultant retinal ischemia generates an upregulation of VEGF, which in turn induces angiogenesis and the vasoproliferative response known as ROP.[946]

All theories concur that oxygen is implicated directly or indirectly in the initiation of ROP. However, once ROP has developed the retina is rendered ischemic and it is this ischemia which contributes to the vasoproliferative response of severe disease. Oxygen-dependent VEGF is implicated in all

stages of ROP development, and oxygen-independent IGF-1 permits VEGF to function maximally.[934] A trial to reduce the severity of the retinal ischemia associated with severe ROP by oxygen administration was unsuccessful.[947]

Risk factors

Clinicians have tended to regard severe ROP as an inevitable, albeit unpredictable, occasional consequence of extreme prematurity. However, recent advances in our understanding allow us to challenge this complacency. By far the most powerful ROP risk factor is the degree of immaturity. However, many other risk factors have been implicated, of which the best known is supplemental oxygen administration. Interest in the role of oxygen in its pathogenesis has reawakened[948] with the finding that oxygen administration in the first few weeks of life is a risk factor for ROP incidence and severity. Fluctuations, even within the normal range, can increase the risk of severe ROP, and PaO_2 monitoring – being intermittent – may mask important variations.[949] These findings have major implications for neonatal care. Nevertheless, it has not been possible to define a concentration or duration of oxygen which is, or is not, associated with ROP. The current consensus is that hyperoxia is important in ROP initiation and the challenge for the future is to determine the safe lower oxygen limit so that severe ROP does not develop and there is no increase in neurodisability.[948,950] Hypoxia on the other hand may increase the severity of established ROP, which is known to be ischemic. Other possible risk factors include: ethnic origin, multiple birth, intrauterine growth retardation, blood transfusions, apneic episodes, hypercarbia, low pH, intraventricular hemorrhage and periventricular leukomalacia. A randomized controlled trial showed that early exposure to light is not a factor in ROP development.[951,952]

Classification

The International Classification of Retinopathy of Prematurity was revised in 2005.[953] The major features of the revised classification are the introduction of the concept of a more virulent form of retinopathy [aggressive posterior ROP (AP-ROP)] and the description of an intermediate level of plus disease (preplus).

Acute phase ROP (Fig. 12.55)

This is described by four parameters: severity by stage (1–5 and AP-ROP), location by zone (1–3), extent [clock hours of the retinal circumference (Fig. 12.56)], and the presence of 'preplus' or 'plus' disease (Fig. 12.57).

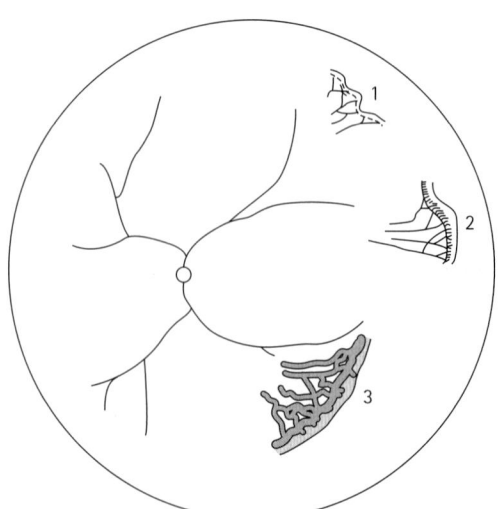

Fig. 12.55 Acute ROP: the first three stages of acute ROP presented for diagrammatic purposes on one retina. Each is shown as a short segment, but can extend over 360 degrees. Stage 1, demarcation line; stage 2, ridge; and stage 3, ridge with extraretinal fibrovascular proliferation. Note abnormal peripheral vascular arborization in all stages, but in stage 3 the vessels are engorged and the lesion is more posteriorly located. Note also that the retina is not fully vascularized.

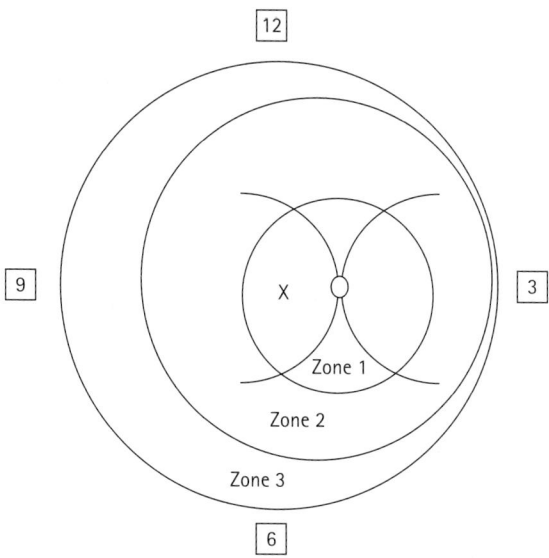

Fig. 12.56 Acute ROP: diagram of the retinal zones. Acute ROP develops at the advancing edge of the growing retinal blood vessels and ROP commencing in zone 1 has a marked propensity to become severe. Numbers on the periphery denote the hours of the clock which are used to describe extent.

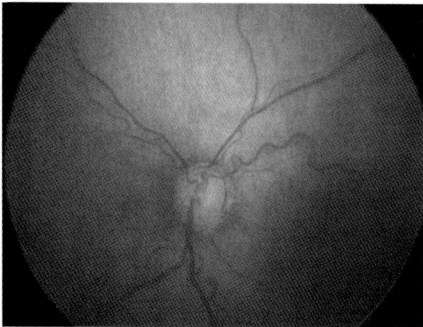

Fig. 12.57 Plus disease – retinal venous congestion and arteriolar tortuosity. Plus disease is the major indication that treatment is indicated.

Severity:

Stage 1 – demarcation line, lying within the plane of the retina at the junction of the vascularized and avascular retina. The demarcation line is the accumulation of the mesenchymal precursors of the retinal vessels.

Stage 2 – ridge; the demarcation line extends out of the plane of the retina (Fig. 12.58).

Stage 3 – ridge with extraretinal fibrovascular proliferation. This is the stage of frank neovascularization, i.e. definitive new vessels are formed (Fig. 12.59).

Stage 4 – subtotal retinal detachment.

Stage 5 – total retinal detachment.

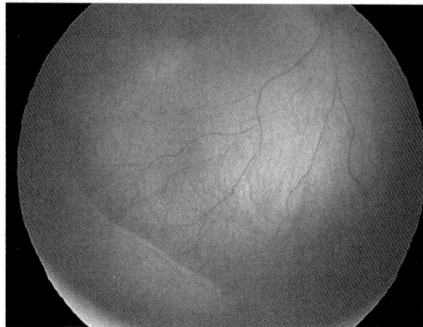

Fig. 12.58 Stage 1 and 2 acute ROP. With a prominent ridge this is mostly stage 2, but to the left of the figure the ridge flattens to become stage 1.

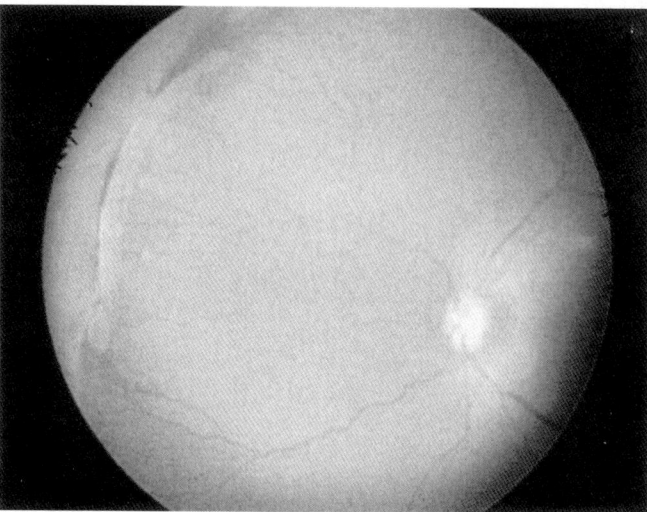

Fig. 12.59 Stage 3 ROP – ridge with fibrovascular proliferation. Hemorrhage disconnects a portion of the ROP lesion from the ridge.

Aggressive posterior retinopathy of prematurity (AP-ROP). Located in zone 1 or posterior zone 2, this form of ROP is uncommon, but untreated it rapidly progresses to stage 5. It is characterized by its posterior location, the prominence of plus disease and the deceptively featureless nature of the retinopathy.

Location. Retinal blood vessels grow centrifugally from the optic disc at the centre of zone 1 to zone 3. ROP in zone 1 is far more likely to become severe, and even if treated there is a far greater likelihood of a poor outcome than ROP in zone 3.[954]

Extent. The extent of ROP around the circumference is described in clock hours and this is one of the parameters used to indicate treatment.

'Preplus' and 'plus' disease. Important signs of ROP severity, in order of severity, include: congestion and tortuosity of the retinal vessel at the posterior pole, congestion of the iris vessels so that the pupil does not dilate readily with mydriatics (pupil rigidity), and vitreous haze. In practice, the critical signs are venous congestion and arteriolar tortuosity at the posterior pole as these signs drive treatment. Plus disease is defined as vascular abnormalities in at least two retinal quadrants close to the optic disc. Because plus cannot be sensibly quantified, the revised classification introduced the concept of preplus which describes rather loosely retinal vessels that are not normal but do not (yet) meet the criteria for plus.

Regressed ROP

Not all ROP undergoes complete resolution. Signs in the fundus which signify previous acute ROP are described according to their location, posterior or peripheral, and according to the structures involved, thus:

Vascular – tortuosity, abnormal branching and arcades, and the straightening ('dragging') of the vessels around the disc (Fig. 12.60).

Retinal – pigmentation, folding, stretching, detachment and vitreoretinal membranes.

Incidence

The incidence and severity of acute ROP rises with decreasing birth weight and gestational age. Quoted figures vary widely, probably due more to examination technique and frequency than neonatal factors. About 30–60% of babies weighing less than 1500 g develop some ROP. Severe disease is virtually confined to those infants < 1500 g birth weight and affects about 6% infants < 1250 g birth weight.[955]

Natural history

As the temporal retina is the last area to be vascularized, most acute ROP develops in that region, although in extremely immature babies it often starts in the nasal retina. The age at onset of acute ROP is governed by the postmenstrual age (PMA) of the baby rather than neonatal

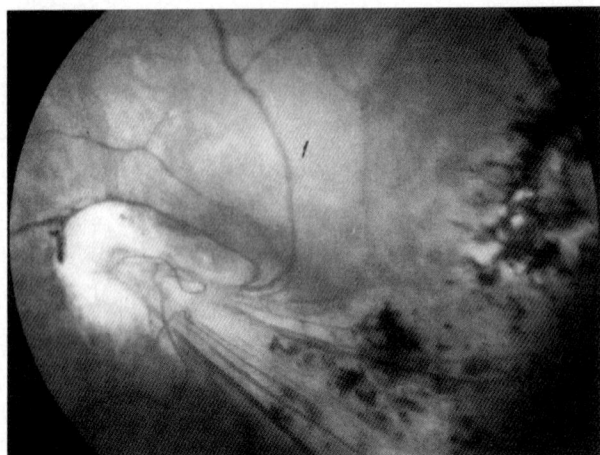

Fig. 12.60   Signs of regressed ROP. Retinal fold extending from the 'dragged' optic disc. Peripheral pigmentation corresponds to the site of the acute lesion. (Reproduced with permission, Editor of the Practitioner.)

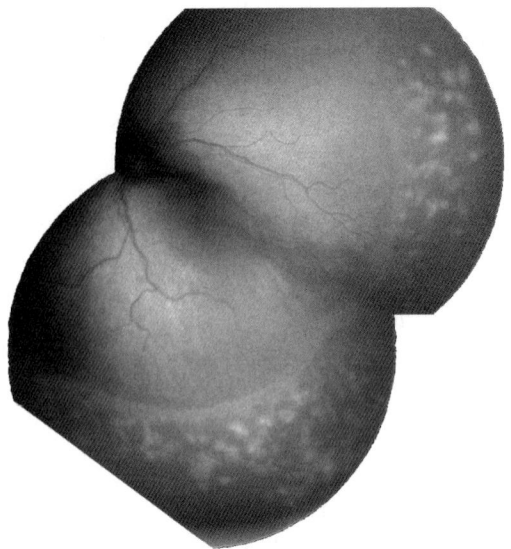

Fig. 12.61   Laser treatment for acute ROP. Laser has been applied to the avascular retina anterior to the ROP lesion.

events. Thus contrary to expectation, ROP develops later postnatally in the smaller, very immature baby who is ill, compared to his larger, usually fitter more mature counterpart. Retinopathy of prematurity exceptionally requires treatment around 31 weeks' PMA, and never after complete retinal vascularization. The average age for treatment at 'threshold' is 37 weeks' PMA while that for 'prethreshold type 1' is 35 weeks' PMA (see below).[956,957]

Treatment

Treatment is not required for mild ROP as this spontaneously resolves, while the outcome for stages 4 and 5 is so dismal that intervention cannot be justified. For many years, the indication for intervention was 'threshold' ROP, at which stage the untreated risk of blindness is 50%.[958] 'Threshold' is defined as stage 3 ROP in zone 1 and 2 which extends over 5 or more continuous, or 8 or more cumulative, clock hours of the retinal circumference in the presence of 'plus' disease. The subsequent Early Treatment for Retinopathy of Prematurity (ETROP) Randomized Trial[957] reported benefit of treatment at an earlier stage and resulted in a revision of the recommendations for treatment to 'prethreshold type 1', defined as:

1. zone 1, any stage of ROP with plus disease;
2. zone 1, stage 3 with or without plus disease; or
3. zone 2, stage 2 or 3 with plus disease.

Note that the revised treatment criteria include what was known as threshold but also include treating some eyes at an earlier stage known as prethreshold. Critically, the decision to treat has shifted from a complex assessment of the entire retina to the diagnosis of plus which is centered on the optic disc. Practically, the mean age for achieving the former is 37 weeks' and for the latter 35 weeks' PMA. It is important to emphasize that the time available for treatment once 'threshold' ROP has been reached is short, and ideally treatment should normally be undertaken within 48 h.

Cryotherapy and laser

In 1988 the US-based Multicenter Trial of Cryotherapy for ROP demonstrated that cryotherapy reduced the unfavorable outcome of 'threshold' stage 3 ROP by about 50%[958] and this was maintained 10 years on.[959] However, 45% of children treated at threshold had a visual acuity of 6/60 or worse and this led to the early treatment (ETROP) study which reported a further improvement in outcome to treatment at prethreshold compared to conventional treatment (at threshold).[957]

Over the past decade, laser delivered through an indirect ophthalmoscope has largely supplanted cryotherapy as the treatment for severe ROP. Either cryotherapy or laser is applied to the peripheral retina anterior to the ridge (Fig. 12.61) over the full circumference of the globe. The

procedure can be performed either under general anesthesia or sedation. While not all eyes respond to treatment, with early treatment at prethreshold both structural and functional outcomes are improved.[960]

ROP screening

Screening is recommended for ROP that requires treatment.[955,961,962] UK guidelines specify that all babies of birth weight <1501<g and/or <32 weeks' gestational age are screened. Examinations for babies born before 27 weeks' gestational age should commence at 30–31 weeks' PMA, while for babies born at 27 weeks or over examinations should begin at 4–5 weeks postnatally. Examinations should be undertaken at least every 2 weeks (more frequently for babies with or at high risk of imminent severe disease) and continue until retinal vascularization is well into zone 3. As a rule the screening program should not cease before 37 weeks' PMA.[957,961]

Treatment for end-stage disease

Not all ROP responds to treatment, and retinal detachment surgery and vitrectomy have been used for end-stage ROP. Vitrectomy is technically well within the scope of many surgeons but to date the visual results have been so poor that it is not recommended. Acute glaucoma sometimes develops in advanced disease. Removal of the lens may be helpful although this carries a risk of globe shrinkage.

Differential diagnosis

For the preterm neonate this question hardly ever arises but there are a number of conditions that simulate ROP which may present in the full-term baby or in later life. These include autosomal dominant familial exudative vitreoretinopathy, Norrie disease, fetal ischemia (porencephaly, anencephaly), and Coats disease. The distinction may be impossible on ophthalmological criteria alone, and the family history and systemic aspects must be taken into account.

OPHTHALMIC SEQUELAE OF PRETERM BIRTH
Sequelae of ROP

Spontaneous and complete regression is the rule for mild ROP (stages 1 and 2) so that long term outcome is not significantly different from children born preterm who never developed ROP.[963] The single exception to this statement is strabismus, which is related to both ROP presence and stage. Severe ROP, even after treatment, generates sequelae which include refractive errors (myopia, astigmatism), strabismus, and visual acuity deficits ranging from the very mild to complete blindness. All stages 4 and 5 have a dismal visual outcome. The eye after severe ROP is relatively unstable and a serious late complication of ROP is retinal detachment, which can develop at any age, even in adulthood.[959]

Sequelae of prematurity

Visual development proceeds according to postmenstrual age rather than postnatal age and failure to appreciate this can result in unnecessary concern about visual functions in early infancy. Infants and children who were born prematurely, even after ROP has been accounted for, are more prone to suffer a range of visual pathway defects.[963–968] In reality the effects of ROP and neurological insults cannot be differentiated as the proportional effect of neurological damage suffered in the perinatal period compared to that due to prematurity per se is unknown. Neurological insults can vary in location and severity and not surprisingly result in a range of neuro-ophthalmic defects including reduced vision, eye movement disorders, refractive errors and optic atrophy. The causes of reduced vision depend on the nature of the insult, and the severity of the deficit can range from minimal to severe (cortical visual impairment).[969,970] Eye movement disorders include strabismus, gaze and saccadic palsies, and nystagmus. These are commonly associated with neurological insult; indeed the last three mentioned are almost certainly its direct consequence. The incidence of squint ranges from 11% to over 30%[963,971] and is particularly high in those with neurological damage such as cystic periventricular leukomalacia, especially if the lesion is posteriorly located. Myopia can be due to ROP,[972] but even in the absence of ROP the ex-preterm child and teenager is more likely to be myopic than his ex-full-term counterpart.[963,973]

ROUTINE NEONATAL EYE EXAMINATION

Every baby should have an eye examination in the very early neonatal period before discharge from hospital or equivalent.[974] The following aspects need to be included and although the list looks formidable at first glance each examination need not take more than a minute or so. The neonatal eye examination while seemingly simple is not that easy to perform (puffy eyelids, etc.) and only 50% of congenital cataracts are diagnosed by 10 weeks of age, while 30% remain unidentified until after the first year.[975]

Look for conditions affecting both eyes, but be especially suspicious of asymmetry between the eyes.

Signs of significant birth trauma

These have already been covered, and the word significant is included so that the pediatric resident performing this examination does not feel obliged to dilate pupils in order to look for retinal hemorrhage. Using the direct ophthalmoscope as torchlight, the anterior segment of the eye can be examined for corneal cloudiness, hyphema, etc.

Ocular malformation

With the ophthalmoscope the following are examined:
- *Lids* – ptosis, hemangioma, dermoids.
- *Globe size*
  - microphthalmos
  - macrophthalmos, most important as this could be infantile glaucoma, but in the neonatal period the eyes may still be of normal size.
- *Conjunctiva* – injection or dermoid.
- *Cornea* – cloudiness, consider infantile glaucoma (Fig. 12.52). Opacities may be part of a malformation (Fig. 12.54).
- *Iris* – coloboma.

Leukocoria (white pupil)

This is an important clinical sign which may signify a condition that is potentially lethal or may have severe consequences for vision. The red reflex is looked for by viewing the undilated pupil through a direct ophthalmoscope which is held at 33 cm from the eye. The absence of a red reflex must always be taken seriously and it requires *urgent* specialist referral. The red reflex can be difficult to visualize in the darkly pigmented baby, so take extra care under these circumstances.

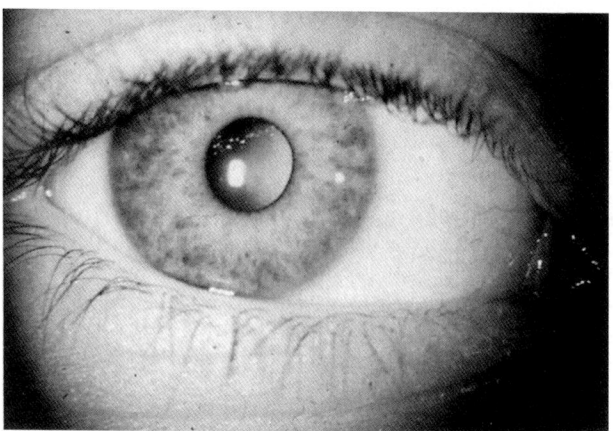

Fig. 12.62 Leukocoria, a frequent presenting sign of retinoblastoma and cataract.

Causes of leukocoria (Fig. 12.62) include cataract, tumors (retinoblastoma), malformations (persistent hyperplastic primary vitreous, coloboma, retinal dysplasia as in Norrie disease and lissencephaly), myelinated nerve fibers, and inflammations (endophthalmitis). Conditions such as end-stage ROP, Coats disease and toxocariasis also can give a white pupil but always after the neonatal period.

Ophthalmic family history

It is important to examine the eyes if there is a family history of a serious ophthalmic problem. In some conditions, for example dominantly inherited retinitis pigmentosa, the eyes at this time will be normal and it is not possible to determine whether or not the baby will be affected later. Certain fears can only be eliminated by a detailed examination and the diplomatic effect of this early examination is considerable and provides a good start to any subsequent involvement. A positive family history of infantile glaucoma and retinoblastoma even in the presence of a *normal* neonatal eye examination requires urgent referral and continued ophthalmological review.

INFECTION AND IMMUNITY IN THE NEWBORN

EPIDEMIOLOGY

Neonatal infections are estimated to cause 1.6 million deaths per year, accounting for 40% of all neonatal deaths in resource limited countries (reviewed in ref 976). The incidence of neonatal sepsis is uncertain, in part because definitions vary (bacteremia only, ± focal sepsis, ± clinical sepsis), as do definitions of its timing of onset [early onset (EO) sepsis is variably defined as < 48 hours, < 72 hours, < 5 days or < 7 days of age]. Postmortem examinations suggest that under-reporting is common.[977]

In resource limited countries, rates of bacteremia range from 1.7 to 33 and rates of clinical sepsis from 6.5 to 38 per 1000 live births. Such bacteremia rates are 3–20-fold higher than those of resource rich countries.[976] For example, Isaacs et al report an EO sepsis rate (< 48 hours of age) of 1.4/1000 live births from Australasian neonatal units,[978] Haque et al report rates of 1.6/1000 (< 72 hours of age) and 8.4/1000 (total) from a single UK unit[979] and Escobar et al report a rate of 1.2/1000 (total) for infants ≥ 2000 g from six US neonatal units.[980] Few population based UK data are available but a national (UK and Ireland) surveillance study in 2000–2001 identified 568 cases of group B streptoccocal (GBS) sepsis in the first 3 months of life (total incidence 0.72/1000), of which 0.48/1000 were EO (< 7 days of age),[981] and another national study estimated the incidence of fungal sepsis in VLBW UK infants at 10/1000 live births.[982]

The incidence of sepsis is higher among babies of low birth weight. Blood culture-proven EO sepsis (< 72 hours of life) was 15/1000 in very low birth weight infants (< 1500 g) in the US National Institute of Child Health and Human Development (NICHHD) Neonatal Research

Network with a late onset sepsis incidence of 210/1000.[983,984] The mortality is also higher in the VLBW population: 37% for EO and 18% for late onset sepsis.[983,984] The mortality from fungal sepsis in UK VLBW infants is 41%.[982]

One reason for uncertainty regarding the total burden of neonatal infection is that although sepsis may be diagnosed clinically, on the basis of clinical or laboratory markers, conventional blood or other sterile site cultures may be negative. Overall incidence estimates based only on culture positive infection may therefore underestimate the true burden of infection. Various factors may decrease the yield of blood cultures in the presence of true infection. This is particularly so in the case of pneumonia where bacteremia may be infrequent.[985] Antibiotics administered to mothers during labor may suppress the growth of bacteria in neonatal cultures and cultures may not be taken prior to the administration of antibiotics to the neonate. It is also possible that the volume of blood obtained from some neonates may be insufficient to grow the organism.[986] Using a definition of 'probable' GBS sepsis, for example, defined by positive surface swab cultures in the presence of clinical sepsis with no other explanation, several UK studies have suggested the incidence of GBS disease to be 1–3-fold higher than that defined by positive sterile site cultures alone.[987–989] Similarly, a US study estimated the incidence of culture proven infection to be 1.2/1000 live births and the additional incidence of clinical infection to be 2.2/1000.[980]

Neonatal infection is associated with significant morbidity. Approximately half of those with neonatal meningitis have long term neurodevelopmental problems at 5 year follow-up.[990] In a cohort of extremely low birth weight infants those who had neonatal infections were more likely to have cerebral palsy and a range of adverse neurodevelopmental sequelae. This was seen in those with sepsis alone, those with meningitis and, significantly, those with culture negative (clinical) sepsis as well.[991]

The most frequent organisms associated with neonatal infection are shown in Table 12.98.

Gram positive bacteria are the most frequent pathogens because of the increasing importance of coagulase negative staphylococci (CONS). They are particularly associated with low birth weight, use of intravascular catheters, late onset sepsis and nosocomial transmission. It can be difficult to differentiate contamination of blood cultures by CONS from true infection. CONS infection is associated with a low mortality.[993] Group B streptococcus, however, remains the most frequent cause of EO sepsis. Gram negative bacteria, especially those associated with multiple antibiotic resistance, are an important cause of infection and are increasingly associated with outbreaks in neonatal units. Fungal infections, most commonly *Candida albicans*, are an infrequent cause of neonatal sepsis and the incidence of invasive fungal infection in VLBW infants in the UK appears to be lower than that reported in studies from tertiary centers in North America and elsewhere. The mortality associated with fungal

Table 12.98 Organisms associated with early and late onset neonatal sepsis

	Organism
Early onset sepsis (0–6 days)	Group B streptococcus
	Escherichia coli
	Other Gram negative organisms, e.g. *Pseudomonas* sp., *Klebsiella* sp., *Haemophilus influenzae*
	Listeria monocytogenes
Late onset sepsis (7–90 days)	*Staphylococcus epidermidis* (and other coagulase negative staphylococci)
	Escherichia coli
	Other Gram negative organisms, e.g. *Serratia* sp., *Enterobacter* sp., *Citrobacter* sp.
	Staphylococcus aureus (including MRSA[992])
	Group B streptococcus
	Candida albicans (*Candida parapsilosis*)

infections is, however, considerable.[982] A UK-based analysis of neonatal deaths arising from maternal infection (defined as neonatal symptoms present in the first 48 hours of life) for the years 1981–1996 suggested that the top three identifiable bacteria were GBS (33%), *E.coli* (15%) and *Listeria monocytogenes* (6%).[994] A similar order of bacteria is responsible for neonatal meningitis in the UK with surprisingly little change between the 1980s and the 1990s.[995,996] Group B streptococcus remains the leading pathogen (39% of cases in 1985–7 and 48% in 1996–7), followed by *E. coli* (26% and 18%), other Gram negative rods (12% and 8%), *Streptococcus pneumoniae* (6% both periods) and *Listeria monocytogenes* (7% and 5%). The overall incidence of neonatal bacterial meningitis also has not changed: 0.22 cases/1000 live births (1985–7) versus 0.21 cases/1000 (1996–7). A Canadian review of 101 cases of neonatal meningitis (1979–1998) determined that 50% were due to GBS, 25% *E. coli*, 8% other Gram negative rods, 6% *Listeria monocytogenes*, and 3% nontypeable *Haemophilus influenzae*.[997] Other studies have noted an increase in meningitis due to *Enterobacter* sp. and *Serratia marcescens*; the majority of these Gram negative organisms were isolated from premature infants with late onset meningitis.[998,999] In resource limited countries, GBS meningitis appears to be much less frequent,[1000] although this is not universal.[1001,1002] Gram negative enteric organisms appear to account for the majority of early onset and *Streptococcus pneumoniae* for late onset meningitis in resource limited countries.[1000]

PATHOGENESIS AND RISK FACTORS FOR NEONATAL INFECTION

Neonatal infection may be acquired in utero (congenital infection), during delivery (from the maternal genital or gastrointestinal tracts), while in the neonatal unit or from the home or community after discharge. The mother's race, age, socioeconomic status, and her susceptibility to certain pathogens (e.g. rubella, CMV) may increase the risk of transmission of microorganisms through the placenta to cause congenital infection. Maternal infection may be symptomatic or asymptomatic and signs of congenital infection in the baby may not appear for weeks, months or even years after birth. One of the main reasons for dividing neonatal bacterial infections into early onset and late onset is that this will often reflect the source of the infection. EO infections are usually caused by organisms which colonize the genital and gastrointestinal tracts of healthy women and transmission occurs just prior to or during delivery. Symptoms and signs will often manifest during the first week of life. Examples include group B streptococcus and *E. coli*. Prematurity, prolonged rupture of membranes (PROM), chorioamnionitis, maternal fever during labor and maternal urinary tract infection are all associated with an increased risk of early onset infection. In one US study an obstetric risk factor (preterm delivery, intrapartum fever or PROM > 18 h) was present in 49% of EO GBS and 79% of EO sepsis due to other bacteria[1003] and in a UK case control study, the odds ratios for EO GBS were 25.8 for PROM, 11 for rupture of membranes before labor onset, 10.4 for prematurity and 10 for intrapartum fever.[1004]

The source of late onset infection may also be the maternal genital tract, but more frequently infection will be derived from the environment or from other humans. Examples include the hands of health care workers (or parents and siblings), contaminated equipment, contaminated breast or formula milk feeds, blood transfusions or droplets from the upper respiratory tract of infected adults or children. The clear evidence that improvements in hand hygiene policies and rational antibiotic prescribing can reduce infant colonization and late onset infection rates demonstrates the importance of these particular environmental factors.[1005,1006]

The most important overall risk factor for neonatal bacterial infection, both early and late onset, is prematurity/low birth weight; such infants have a 3–10-fold greater risk of sepsis and/or meningitis than term infants. Yet the relationship between infection and preterm delivery is a complex one. There is increasing evidence that preterm delivery may itself reflect an excessive and inappropriate maternal response to infection or inflammation. For example, approximately 60% of mothers delivering extremely preterm (< 28 weeks' gestation) have histological evidence of chorioamnionitis.[1007]

HOST DEFENSES

At birth the fetus passes from the sterile intrauterine environment through a birth canal that is colonized with potentially lethal bacteria to an extrauterine coexistence with microorganisms.

Host defense against invading microbial pathogens relies on the immune system (innate and adaptive), although the first barrier to infection is actually the mucosae (i.e. skin and mucous membranes). This barrier is frequently breached by medical procedures, e.g. cutting the umbilical cord, endotracheal intubation and breaking the skin to insert intravascular catheters, etc. It is an even more fragile barrier in preterm infants.

Innate immune system

Once a bacterium enters the body the innate immune system is encountered. This consists of the complement system and the phagocytes and antigen presenting cells (macrophages, monocytes, dendritic cells, polymorphonuclear granulocytes). Additional protection may also be derived from the presence of maternal antibody (see below). A number of events occur in parallel. Bacteria are recognized nonspecifically via complement receptors that then interact with opsonizing serum components such as antibodies. At the same time, phagocytes sample pathogen-associated molecular patterns (PAMPs). PAMPs are evolutionarily conserved among microorganisms (including bacteria, fungi, protozoa and viruses) but absent from eukaryotic cells. Sensing of PAMPs occurs through pattern recognition receptors present on the cell surface or within the cell such as Toll-like receptors (TLR). TLRs carry individual specificity for a certain range of PAMPs; for example, TLR 4 is the receptor for the lipopolysaccharide of Gram negative bacteria. TLRs are pivotal in both recognition and then in transduction of recognition signals across the host cell membrane. Recognition signals then trigger expression of genes, the products of which include inflammatory cytokines (e.g. TNF-alpha, IL-6, IL-12) and co-stimulatory molecules which control innate immune responses [e.g. recruitment of further polymorphonuclear leukocytes (PMNs)] as well as the development of antigen-specific acquired immunity (for a comprehensive review of TLRs see ref 1008).

The complement system also has a major role in the defense against bacterial, viral and fungal infections. The classic pathway is activated mainly by antigen–antibody complexes or aggregated immunoglobulins. The alternative (properdin) pathway is activated by endotoxins or complex polysaccharides. There is no transfer of complement from mother to fetus. Although complement synthesis begins early in the first trimester, term infants have slightly diminished classic and significantly diminished alternative pathway levels. C3, C4 and C5 are the most important functional components of the system and are approximately 50% of adult levels in term infants. Much lower levels are seen in preterm infants, leading to markedly reduced opsonizing capacity. The receptor for C3b0001 on neonatal PMNs is also decreased, leading to depressed cell adherence, phagocytosis, mobility and activation of adhesion reactions.

Phagocytosis of microbes by dendritic cells and macrophages triggers both degradation of pathogens and subsequent presentation of pathogen-derived peptide antigen, both to TLR (as above) as well as to naive T cells. This in turn stimulates antigen-specific acquired immunity (see below).

Neonatal sepsis is a highly inflammatory process that culminates in septic shock and multiorgan failure. In newborn infants excessive cytokine concentrations can be measured in the serum, and neonatal phagocytes and monocytes can form large amounts of the cytokines TNF, IL-1, IL-6 and IL-8 in response to infection.[1009,1010] The ability to produce proinflammatory cytokines is an initially protective physiological response to microorganisms. However, an immature regulatory response both in production of and response to anti-inflammatory cytokines is reported in both term and preterm infants.[1011] This may predispose preterm infants to the harmful effects of proinflammatory cytokines including severe organ sequelae during infection.

In contrast to the preserved proinflammatory capacity of neonatal phagocytes, there do appear to be deficiencies in the other key mechanisms required for bacterial elimination: chemotaxis, phagocytosis and intracellular and extracellular bacterial killing. For example, chemotaxis of neonatal polymorphonuclear granulocytes is impaired as a consequence of decreased membrane deformability. Neonatal granulocytes also migrate at reduced speed compared with adult granulocytes. Phagocytosis is further hampered by low serum concentrations of opsonizing complement factors and immunoglobulins, especially so in preterm infants. In order to kill bacteria, toxic oxygen products (superoxide, hydroxyl radicals and hydrogen peroxide) need to be generated. The cationic proteins, lactoferrin and a lysosomal enzyme (myeloperoxidase) interact with hydrogen peroxide to form hypochlorite ions, which are bactericidal. Intracellular oxidative killing is, however, depressed in newborn phagocytes. All these essential functions are depressed further when an infant is stressed by infection. (For a review see ref 1012.)

Adaptive immune system

B and T lymphocytes use antigen receptors such as immunoglobulins and T cell receptors to recognize microorganisms. Although antigen-specific IgG can be produced early, even in utero, the response in infants is both qualitatively and quantitatively different to that of older children and adults. A gradual maturation of antibody responses is seen over the first 2 years of life and this is reflected in the increasing capacity to mount antibody responses to vaccines. Secretory IgA is present in large amounts in colostrum and breast milk and has a role in preventing mucosal infections but the most important compensation for this immunoglobulin deficiency is the presence of maternal antibody. Maternofetal transport of IgG commences around the 17th gestational week, is at equilibrium around the 33rd week and reaches up to 2-fold higher values in the neonate at term. Fetal levels of IgG at 17–22 weeks' gestation are therefore only 5–10% of maternal levels. This is one major explanation for the increased susceptibility to infection of preterm infants. There are also differences in the four IgG subclasses with preferential transfer of IgG1.[1013] An example of the importance of immunoglobulin is the association between bacterium-specific IgG and susceptibility to infection; infants who lack specific antibody to GBS polysaccharide capsule are more likely to develop invasive GBS disease than those with adequate levels.[1014]

Adult-like antigen-specific T cell responses can be achieved earlier than B cell responses. For example, BCG immunization at birth elicits comparatively stronger IFN-gamma (i.e. T cell) than IL-5 (i.e. B cell) responses that are similar to adult responses.[1015] However, early life T cell responses, like B cell responses, are also subject to immune maturation. For example, stronger purified protein derivative (PPD) responses are seen when BCG vaccination is delayed from birth to 2–6 months of age.[1016] Immaturity of antigen-presenting cells is considered a critical determinant of early infant T cell responses: the response of neonatal dendritic cells to in vitro activation by TLR ligands is incomplete and results in limited IL-12 responses as compared to adult responses.[1017] T cell responses, however, are largely unaffected by the presence of maternal antibody.[1018]

Many aspects of the infant's immune system immaturity will be more pronounced in preterm infants. Even at 8 weeks of age preterm infants have lower absolute counts of lymphocytes, T cells, B cells, and T helper cells and a lower CD4:CD8 ratio than term infants. By the age of 7 months B cell numbers in the preterm group have reached term equivalent, but the reduced absolute lymphocyte count, total T cell count, and T helper count persist.[1019] The range of antigens recognized by preterm B cells may also be limited when compared to term infants because intense development of the B cell receptor repertoire occurs during the third trimester of pregnancy. However, there is intriguing evidence that premature exposure to antigens can accelerate this development. The significance of this is that infants born at 28 weeks' gestation may actually have a more diverse antibody repertoire by the time they reach 'term' than infants who are born at term.[1020,1021]

Another consideration in the immune response of preterm infants is the possible impact of iatrogenic factors. Disruption of the mucosal barrier by medical procedures is mentioned earlier. Additionally, preterm infants may be exposed to corticosteroids, antenatally and/or postnatally, and may receive blood and immunoglobulin transfusions during their neonatal stay. It is conceivable that any of these might impair the immune responses of preterm infants. There is suggestive evidence that steroids administered for chronic lung disease, for example, may suppress antibody responses to diphtheria/tetanus/pertussis (DTP) and Hib vaccines[1022,1023] and in a US study of VLBW infants, those who received a 14 day course of dexamethasone were more likely to develop a bloodstream or cerebrospinal fluid infection than those who received placebo.[1024]

Administration of antenatal steroids does not seem to reduce the responses to meningococcal C conjugate vaccine.[1025] There are no data on the impact of blood transfusions or immunoglobulin infusions on the development of antibody responses of premature infants.

SEPSIS SYNDROME

As a result of their breakdown by the host inflammatory response, Gram positive bacteria release peptidoglycans and Gram negative bacteria release lipopolysaccharide-A (LPS-A) or endotoxin. These substances can lead to the release of inflammatory mediators as described above. They can also activate the complement, coagulation and fibrinolytic cascades leading to the formation of vasoactive and proinflammatory agents. The net effect is the initiation of a cascade of events that leads to the sepsis syndrome, septic shock, multiple organ failure and death (Fig. 12.63).

Clinical manifestations

Neonatal infections are caused by a number of organisms (Table 12.98) and can present in many different ways. As described earlier, it is useful to classify them as early onset (EO) and late onset (LO). The advantage of such a classification is that it helps in determining the most probable organism and mode of transmission and thus guides empiric treatment. Whilst most clinicians use this general classification there is no consensus as to the precise definition. Some define EO as infection occurring between birth and 48 hours, 72 hours, 5 days or up to 7 days of life. LO infection occurs up until 3 months of life. EO infection is generally caused by organisms acquired from the mother at or during birth (vertical transmission) whilst LO infection is more likely to be caused by organisms from the environment (nosocomial or community sources).

Maternal chorioamnionitis (e.g. abdominal pain, fever, discharge), PROM and urinary tract infection may provide important clues to early diagnosis of sepsis in the newborn. Signs and symptoms of sepsis in the newborn are often nonspecific (Table 12.99) and may evolve over time. Sepsis may be fulminant, leading to death in several hours from multiorgan failure, or may be more protracted. The most frequent indicators are lethargy, poor feeding, abdominal distention, prolonged capillary filling time, glucose intolerance and unexplained persistent acidosis. Physical examination may not be very helpful but particular note should be made of the baby's responsiveness and the respiratory and heart rates.

Laboratory investigations

There is no single reliable test for neonatal sepsis. Ultimate proof rests on recovering an infecting organism from a normally sterile body fluid, e.g. blood, CSF, urine or aspirate from an infected lesion or tissue. Even though culture remains the gold standard it is recognized, as described earlier, that clinical sepsis may be evident even in the absence of positive sterile site cultures. The list of tests which may suggest infection is large (Table 12.100).

Table 12.99 Most frequent signs and symptoms in neonatal sepsis

Symptoms	Signs
Lethargy	Temperature instability
Poor feeding	Prolonged capillary filling time (hypotension)
Apnea	'Does not look well'
Respiratory distress	Widening toe–core temperature difference
Pallor	Hepatomegaly
Mottling	Splenomegaly
Cyanosis	Full fontanelle
Abdominal distention	Abnormal neurological reflexes
Vomiting/increasing gastric residue	Glucose intolerance
	a. Hyper/hypoglycemia
Jaundice	b. Glucosuria
Petechiae, purpura, bleeding from prick sites	Persistent acidosis
Irritability	Painful bones/joints
Seizures	Sclerema

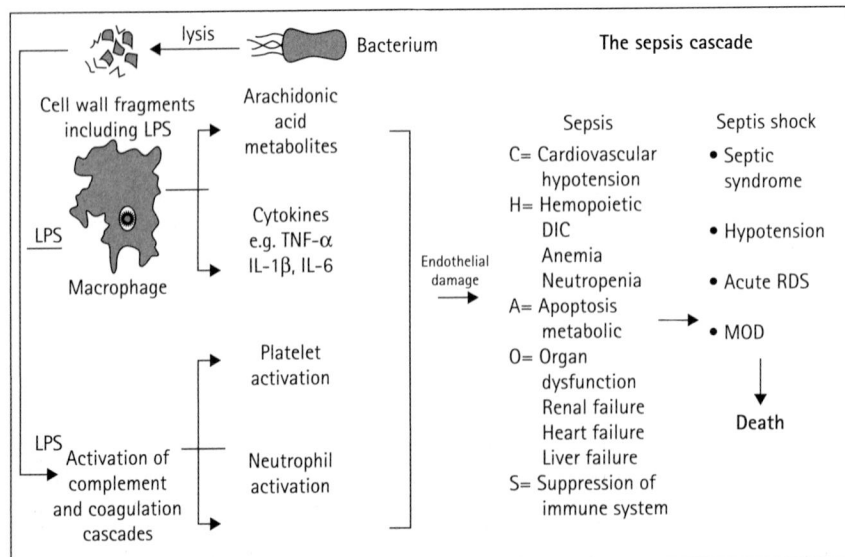

Fig. 12.63 The 'sepsis cascade': DIC, disseminated intravascular coagulation; IL, interleukin; LPS, lipolysaccharide; MOD, multiple organ dysfunction; RDS, respiratory distress syndrome; TNF, tumor necrosis factor. (Modified from Endotoxin and Septic shock – the Antibiotic connection 1994.) (Published with permission and courtesy of Dr S K Jackson and Bayer plc UK from their publication.)

Table 12.100 Accuracy of diagnostic tests or combinations of tests for early onset neonatal sepsis (from Mishra et al,[1026] with permission)

Test	Sensitivity (%)	Specificity (%)	Positive predictive value (%)	Negative predictive value (%)
CRP	60–82	93–96	95–100	75–87
CRP, FBC, gastric aspirate	97	61	53	98
Procalcitonin	82–100	87–100	86–98	93–100
CD11b	96–100	81–100	22–100	100
CD64	64–97	72–96	64–88	84–98
CD64, IL-6 or CRP	81–97	71–87	63–74	86–98
GCSF ≥ 200 pg/ml	95	73	40	99
Umbilical cord IL-6	87–90	93	93	93–100
IL-6	67–89	89–96	84–95	77–91
IL-6 and/or CRP	93	88–96	86–95	95
IL-8	80–91	76–100	70–74	91–95
IL-8 and/or CRP	80	87	68	93
PCR for genomic DNA in blood culture	100	100	100	100

CRP, C-reactive protein; FBC, full blood count; GCSF, granulocyte colony-stimulating factor; IL-6, interleukin 6; IL-8, interleukin 8; PCR, polymerase chain reaction.

Microbiological tests

Blood culture. Blood cultures remain the mainstay for investigation of neonatal sepsis although results are not immediately available. In one prospective study virtually all cultures growing clinically significant Gram positive and Gram negative organisms were positive by 24–36 h of incubation. Cultures growing *Staphylococcus epidermidis* were virtually all positive after 36–48 h and 88% of cultures growing yeasts were positive by 48 h.[1027] The yield of blood cultures may depend on such things as skin disinfection technique, sample volume and the number of cultures taken as well as technical factors: the dilution of blood to culture medium and the blood culture system used (reviewed in ref 1028).

CSF culture. Examination of cerebrospinal fluid (CSF) via lumbar puncture (LP) is the only way to confirm meningitis because clinical signs are nonspecific and unreliable and blood cultures may be negative in 15–55% cases.[1029–1031] An LP should be done in all neonates with suspected meningitis, with suspected or proven late onset sepsis and should be considered in all neonates in whom sepsis is a possibility. The role of LP in neonates who are healthy appearing but have maternal risk factors for sepsis is more controversial; the yield of the LP in these patients is likely to be low.

It is generally believed that the interpretation of CSF tests in the newborn differs from that in older children. Previous studies have suggested average white cell counts of between 3 and 11/mm³ with an upper limit of 42 white cells/mm³ to be normal, but it is not clear how 'normal' these infants actually were.[1032] A recent small study of healthy term infants suggested that an upper limit of 5 white cells was more appropriate.[1032] The cell counts in preterm infants are likely to be higher.

Urine culture. Uncontaminated urine is difficult to obtain. The best method is suprapubic aspiration. Infection should be considered present if there are more than 10 leukocytes/mm³ in uncentrifuged well-shaken urine or when more than 10⁵ colony-forming units (CFU) of bacteria/ml of urine are cultured. However, the latter figure is a cut-off derived from mid stream or clean catch specimens where specimen contamination from anterior urethral or perineal skin organisms may occur. Thus, where urine is collected by catheterization or suprapubic aspiration, lesser growths of organisms may indicate infection. The yield from urine collections when done as a screen for early onset infection is lower than when it is done as a screen for late onset infection.[1033,1034] Urine culture may also be useful for detecting systemic fungal infections.

Superficial and other cultures. Routine cultures from the umbilicus, skin, nose, rectum, pharynx, etc., demonstrate colonization rather than invasive disease and are not generally helpful.[1035] There may be a role for such screening in the context of an outbreak investigation. Positive cultures from other normally sterile sites such as joint fluid will reflect true infection. Positive cultures from tracheal or lower respiratory tract specimens may be useful, especially in the context of a new pneumonia, but otherwise may simply reflect colonization and are common in ventilated preterm infants.[1036]

Hematological tests

Neutrophil counts are more valuable than total white cell counts. The early 'band' (metamyelocyte and myelocyte) count and its ratio with total neutrophils (I:T ratio) is more important. An I:T ratio greater than 0.2 suggests infection but still has a poor positive predictive value. Other characteristics seen in adults, e.g. toxic granulation, vacuolation, Dohle bodies and decreased leukocyte alkaline phosphatase activity, are not reliable in neonatal sepsis. There may be a coagulopathy but this is not specific. A platelet count less than 150×10^9/L is suggestive of sepsis but may also be caused by other conditions.

Serological tests

Antibody tests are generally used for diagnosing congenital infections, especially those encompassed by the TORCH acronym: toxoplasmosis, other (such as HIV and syphilis), rubella, cytomegalovirus and herpes simplex virus. Over time many of these are being supplanted by PCR amplification of specific pathogen-related nucleic acid.

Serological assays are dependent on the host response to infection. Recent infection is recognized by a 4-fold or greater rise in titer when acute and convalescent sera are run in the same assay at the same time. The presence of specific IgM is evidence of recent infection and the presence of pathogen-specific IgM in the infant is particularly useful as this will represent the infant's antibody response, as opposed to IgG, which may reflect transplacental transfer of maternal IgG. However, the sensitivity of this test is variable and especially so in the older infant in whom a congenital infection is being retrospectively considered. Similarly, maternal pathogen-specific IgM may be useful although it can persist for long periods of time and thus may reflect prenatal rather than antenatal infection.[1037] The particular assays used are important.[1038] An alternative means of diagnosing antenatal infection is to compare the pathogen-specific IgG titers between early/pre pregnancy and those of late pregnancy, assuming such samples are available. IgG avidity is also used in an attempt to differentiate recent primary infection (low avidity) from recurrent or past infection (high avidity).[1039]

Other diagnostic tests

There is a great need for a reliable diagnostic test (or combination of tests) for the early diagnosis of neonatal infection. There is considerable antibiotic use on neonatal units because of concern about infection; however, most babies who receive antibiotics will not actually have a bacterial infection. The ideal early diagnostic test for neonatal infection would have 100% sensitivity (all babies with the infection have a positive test) and 100% specificity (all babies without the infection have a negative test). This is unlikely to be achieved as many tests are assessed on a continuous scale where there is overlap between infected and non-infected babies. However, cut-offs can be set at which most infections are detected and most non-infections are defined correctly. In the case of neonatal sepsis a test with higher sensitivity, i.e. 100%, is probably required because of the implications of missing and not treating a true infection. A large number of tests have been studied although the methodological quality of studies is variable, e.g. often small sample sizes are used. These are summarized in Table 12.100, which is taken from a useful review in this area.[1026] Markers of infection that have been studied include acute phase reactants (such as CRP and procalcitonin), cell surface markers (such as neutrophil CD11 and CD64), granulocyte colony-stimulating factor concentrations, cytokines (such as IL6 and IL8) and nucleic acid amplification techniques (PCR).

Management

Prompt, effective therapy is important as babies with infection may deteriorate rapidly. Supportive care, antimicrobial therapy and host defense modulation are all important. As highlighted in Figure 12.63, the cascade of sepsis, cytokine and inflammatory cell interaction at the endothelial level leads to CHAOS (cardiovascular instability, hematological abnormalities, increased apoptosis, organ dysfunction and suppression of immunity). Efforts should be made to correct this chaos.

Septic babies may rapidly lose fluid into the extravascular space (third spacing). Meticulous attention to fluid balance and blood pressure is required to maintain tissue perfusion. Increased fluids may be necessary as may blood transfusion to maintain an adequate hematocrit. Inotropic support should be started sooner rather than later because systemic hypotension can result in end organ damage, e.g. renal and cerebral. Acid–base balance should be maintained. It is important to maintain tissue oxygenation and nutrition by providing adequate oxygen and calories. Frequently, clinicians stop feeding babies with sepsis although there is no evidence that feeding is harmful in babies with sepsis without intestinal pathology. Calories should be provided parenterally if enteral feeding is not possible. Maintaining tight glycemic control may be important.[1040,1041] Single or multiorgan failure in sepsis is not uncommon and this should be managed accordingly.

Antimicrobial therapy

Because neonatal pharmacokinetics differs from that in later life, most antimicrobial drugs require modification of dose, dose intervals and duration in the newborn. Slower metabolism and delayed excretion of many drugs in the newborn may prolong their half-life, particularly in the very premature. Other factors include the larger volume of extracellular fluid, the amount of serum protein available for binding and drug competition with bilirubin at protein binding sites. For detailed information about individual antimicrobials the reader should refer to a specialized text.

The specific agent(s) chosen to treat infection are determined by knowledge of local pathogens and their susceptibilities, the nature of the illness and the unit policy. Since initial empirical treatment in suspected sepsis cannot cover all possible pathogens, value judgments have to be made. Use of the narrowest spectrum antibiotics possible is encouraged. Routine use of cephalosporins as first line therapy is discouraged due to the emergence of resistant pathogens[1042] and routine empiric use of vancomycin for late onset sepsis is also discouraged as it is unnecessary and may also promote resistance.[1043] Third generation cephalosporins are particularly useful in the treatment of meningitis due to their antimicrobial spectrum and penetration into the CSF.[1044]

Most antibiotics should be administered intravenously. Intramuscular injections are painful and should be avoided. Absorption after oral therapy in the newborn is erratic and cannot be relied upon. For some antibiotics drug levels must be carefully monitored.

There is no consensus on the duration of therapy. If the baby is well, antibiotics should be stopped as soon as negative culture results are available. If the cultures are positive then at least 7 days of treatment is traditional, and if the clinical suspicion of sepsis is high in the face of negative cultures, at least 5 days of treatment is often recommended. Earlier discontinuation of antibiotic treatment may be possible in selected infants.[1045] One exception is pneumonia where blood cultures are often negative.[985]

There are no controlled clinical trials to guide the recommended duration of antibiotic therapy for neonatal meningitis. Historically, therapy has been continued for 2–3 weeks after sterilization of CSF cultures. This equates to a minimum of 14 days for GBS and *Listeria monocytogenes* meningitis and 21 days for Gram negative meningitis.[1044] Osteomyelitis should be treated for at least 4–6 weeks.

Adjunctive therapies

As outlined above, the relative immunodeficiency of the newborn infant, which is exaggerated in premature and sick neonates, includes quantitative and qualitative deficits in phagocytes, complement components, cytokines and immunoglobulins. Therapies that modulate or augment these host defenses may attenuate the virulence of neonatal infections. Unfortunately, the evidence for the clinical efficacy of many such therapies is currently lacking.

Fresh frozen plasma (FFP)

There is no evidence to support the routine use of FFP in sepsis.

White cell transfusion

Neonates, especially preterm neonates, have an immaturity of granulopoiesis and a limited capacity for progenitor cell proliferation. Neutropenia is a frequent finding in septic neonates and is a risk factor for death. Transfusion of granulocytes to septic neutropenic neonates may therefore reduce mortality and morbidity. However, a Cochrane review concluded that there is inconclusive evidence from randomized controlled trials to support or refute the routine use of granulocyte transfusions in neonates with sepsis and neutropenia. When granulocyte transfusion was compared with placebo or no transfusion, there was no significant difference in all-cause mortality [typical RR 0.89 (95% CI 0.43, 1.86)].[1046]

Exchange transfusion

There is no evidence to support the routine use of exchange transfusion in sepsis.

Pentoxifylline

This methylxanthine derivative inhibits TNF-alpha production, preserves microvascular blood flow, inhibits neutrophil deformability and increases the respiratory burst. Two randomized controlled trials of 140 preterm infants showed an 86% reduction in mortality. The conclusion of a Cochrane review was that given the relatively small numbers of infants and considerable methodological weaknesses, larger studies are required before this therapy can be recommended.[1047]

G-CSF and GM-CSF

In studies involving newborn babies G-CSF and GM-CSF have been shown to increase neutrophils and granulocyte counts and enhance their functional activity. Studies have been performed using these agents as prophylaxis against sepsis as well as for treatment during sepsis. A Cochrane review analyzed seven treatment studies which included 257 infants with suspected systemic bacterial infection and three prophylaxis studies comprising 359 neonates. From the treatment studies there was no evidence that the addition of G-CSF or GM-CSF to antibiotic therapy reduced immediate all-cause mortality. No significant survival advantage was seen at 14 days from the start of therapy [typical RR 0.71 (95% CI 0.38, 1.33)]. However all seven of the treatment studies were small, the largest recruiting only 60 infants. The subgroup analysis of 97 infants from three treatment studies who, in addition to systemic infection, had clinically significant neutropenia ($< 1.7 \times 10^9$/L) at trial entry, did show a significant reduction in mortality by day 14 [RR 0.34 (95% CI 0.12, 0.92); NNT 6 (95% CI 3–33)]. Prophylaxis studies have not demonstrated a significant reduction in mortality in neonates receiving GM-CSF [RR 0.59 (95% CI 0.24, 1.44)]. The identification of sepsis as the primary outcome of prophylaxis studies has been hampered by inadequately stringent definitions of systemic infection. The authors' conclusions were that there is currently insufficient evidence to support the introduction of either G-CSF or GM-CSF into neonatal practice, either as treatment of established systemic infection to reduce resulting mortality, or as prophylaxis to prevent systemic infection in high risk neonates. No toxicity was reported in any study included in this review. The limited data suggest that G-CSF treatment may reduce mortality when systemic infection is accompanied by severe neutropenia and should be investigated further.[1048]

IVIG

Administration of intravenous immunoglobulin provides IgG that can bind to cell surface receptors, provide opsonic activity, activate complement, promote antibody dependent cytotoxicity, and improve neutrophilic chemoluminescence. Intravenous immunoglobulin thus has the potential of preventing or altering the course of neonatal infections. A Cochrane systematic review assessed the effectiveness and safety of intravenous immunoglobulin (IVIG) administration (compared to placebo or no intervention) to preterm (< 37 weeks' gestational age at birth) and/or low birth weight (LBW) (< 2500 g BW) infants in preventing nosocomial infections. When all 19 eligible studies were combined there was a statistically significant reduction in sepsis (p = 0.02), RR [0.85 (95% CI 0.74, 0.98)], NNT 33. A statistically significant reduction was found for any serious infection, one or more episodes, when all studies were combined [RR 0.82 (95% CI 0.74, 0.92); NNT 25 (95% CI, 16.7, 50)]. There were no statistically significant differences for mortality from all causes, mortality from infection, incidence of necrotizing enterocolitis, bronchopulmonary dysplasia or intraventricular hemorrhage or length of hospital stay. No major adverse effects of IVIG were reported in any of the studies. The absence of significant impact on these other outcomes, especially mortality, leads the reviewers to conclude that any benefit was marginal.[1049]

In a review of trials of immunoglobulin use in treatment of proven or probable sepsis, six studies (n = 318) reported on the outcome of mortality for randomized patients with clinically suspected infection. The results showed a reduction in mortality following IVIG treatment [typical RR 0.63 (95% CI; 0.40, 1.00)]. Treatment with IVIG (seven trials, n = 262) in cases of subsequently proven infection did result in a statistically significant reduction in mortality [typical RR 0.55 (95% CI; 0.31, 0.98)]. The authors concluded that there is insufficient evidence to support the routine administration of IVIG to prevent mortality in infants with suspected or subsequently proved neonatal infection. Further studies were encouraged.[1050] A large international study is in progress (www.npeu.ox.ac.uk).

Corticosteroids

In the light of the benefits reported with dexamethasone treatment in childhood meningitis, corticosteroids were an obvious consideration for the management of neonatal meningitis. In a study from Jordan, 52 cases of neonatal meningitis (84% Gram negative) in full-term neonates were alternately assigned to dexamethasone treatment (0.15 mg/kg every 6 h for 4 d).[1051] The mortality (22% dexamethasone vs. 28% controls) and the morbidity at 2 years (30 vs. 39%) were not significantly different and it was concluded that adjunctive dexamethasone therapy does not have a role in neonatal meningitis.

Prevention

The source of infection in late onset cases may be nosocomial or community spread. It follows that any steps taken to prevent the spread of organisms in a neonatal unit may reduce the likelihood of late onset infection. Judicious antibiotic use including the use of narrow spectrum antibiotics, stopping antibiotics when cultures are negative and not using antibiotics to treat colonization or as prophylaxis,[1006,1052] as well as enforcement of hand hygiene policies,[1053] are obvious prevention strategies for neonates remaining in the hospital. Breast-feeding appears to be protective against nosocomial infection in general, although its main benefit seems to be in preventing infections due to *Staphylococcus epidermidis*.[1054–1056]

SPECIFIC NEONATAL INFECTIONS
Group B streptococcal infection
Epidemiology

In Europe, Australasia and North America, GBS is the commonest Gram positive bacterium causing neonatal septicemia. Early onset (EO) GBS disease may be defined as infection presenting in the first 6 days of life (though some use the first 2, 3 or 5 days as the cut-off) and accounts for approximately 60–70% of all GBS disease in the first 3 months of life. Of the 9 serotypes that exist, types III, Ia, II and V are responsible for most EO disease.[1057,1058] Maternal carriage of GBS in the gastrointestinal and/or genital tracts is a prerequisite for EO disease, vertical transmission occurring prior to or during birth. An estimated 20–30% of pregnant women are GBS colonized,[1059,1060] 50% of babies become colonized perinatally and 1% become infected. Late onset (LO) disease appears to have a different pathophysiology. It is predominantly caused by serotype III and is acquired perinatally, nosocomially or from community sources.[981,1057]

Incidence measured by multistate, population-based, active surveillance in 1990 in the USA identified an early onset disease rate of 1.4 per 1000 live births, with a lower rate of 0.4 per 1000 births recorded for late onset infections occurring in infants between 7 and 90 days of age.[1061] This equated to 7600 cases and 310 deaths per year. Both early and late onset GBS disease occurred at significantly higher rates among African American newborns compared with whites, as well as among low birth weight or preterm infants.[1061,1062] In the UK, a study carried out between 1977 and 1978 involving 25 centers in England and one in Scotland observed an incidence of invasive GBS disease in infants < 2 months of age of 0.3 cases per 1000 live births. Through the late 1990s studies from different centers in England reported incidence figures ranging from 0.6 to 1.2 cases per 1000 live births. In 2000–2001, national surveillance was enhanced and cases of invasive GBS disease (culture positive) in infants < 90 days of age were identified through active surveillance involving pediatricians, microbiologists and parents. A total of 568 cases were identified: an incidence of 0.72/1000 live births (95% confidence interval 0.66–0.78), 0.47/1000 (0.42–0.52) for early onset disease and 0.25/1000 (0.21–0.28) for late onset disease.[981] Regional variation was marked; the incidence in Scotland, for example, was 0.42 per 1000 while it was 0.9 per 1000 live births in Northern Ireland. As indicated earlier, the true burden of GBS sepsis (if culture negative cases are included) may indeed be higher.

GBS disease is associated with significant morbidity and mortality. GBS meningitis leaves half those infected with long term neurodevelopmental effects at 5 year follow-up.[990] Neurodevelopmental impairment may also be associated with clinical (i.e. culture negative) neonatal sepsis.[991] Case fatality rates for GBS disease are estimated at between 9% in Oxford (1990–6) and 15% in London (1990–9),[1063] with a UK national figure of 10% (2000–1).[981] In the USA between 1993 and 1998 the case fatality rates for EO and LO disease were 4.7% and 2.8% respectively. GBS is also a well recognized cause of stillbirth, but in the absence of clear case definitions and with variable autopsy rates, this burden is more difficult to quantify.

Risk factors include exposure to a heavy inoculum of GBS and to a strain with a high potential for invasiveness, preterm delivery, maternal chorioamnionitis, rupture of membranes more than 18 h prior to delivery, intrapartum pyrexia, GBS bacteriuria during the current pregnancy and a previous baby with GBS infection. There is a clear correlation between neonatal disease and low levels of maternal antibody to the capsular polysaccharide of the colonizing strain of GBS at the time of delivery.[1014]

Clinical features

Signs of EO sepsis may mimic those of RDS, birth asphyxia or cyanotic congenital heart disease. Disease occurs rapidly, being evident at birth or within 12 h in over 90% of cases, and presenting with overwhelming sepsis (60%) or pneumonia (25%).[981] Up to 50% of LO cases present with meningitis but focal infections such as cellulitis, abscesses, arthritis, osteomyelitis, ethmoiditis, fasciitis and conjunctivitis may also occur.

Cultures are diagnostic; rapid diagnosis is possible using antigen detection assays but these may be unreliable.

Treatment

The combination of a penicillin and an aminoglycoside has been the mainstay of GBS treatment for decades. The rationale for this choice is that in vitro and animal studies suggest improved outcome with the combination over a penicillin given alone.[1064] Cefotaxime is an alternative but broad spectrum. Ceftriaxone could be substituted for cefotaxime for once a day administration, but there is substantially less experience with this drug in neonates, some uncertainty because of its ability to displace bilirubin from plasma protein, and cases of associated cholestasis and gallbladder hydrops have been reported. Once clinical improvement has been documented and the CSF has been sterilized, there is probably no indication for continuing an aminoglycoside. Penicillin alone can be used to complete therapy. Treatment is usually given for 7–10 days. For GBS meningitis it is recommended to use high doses of penicillin for a minimum of 14 days.

Prevention

Clinical trials during the 1980s assessed the use of antibiotics to reduce transmission from the pregnant woman to her fetus or newborn. Antenatal antibiotics failed to eliminate vaginal colonization, consistent with a persistent gastrointestinal reservoir and/or reinfection from a sexual partner. Postnatal penicillin seemed to reduce the occurrence of infections that were not very early in onset but had no effect on group B streptococcal disease in the low birth weight population where disease occurrence and severity was greatest.[1065] Antimicrobials administered after onset of labor or rupture of the membranes were consistently effective in reducing transmission of infection and, where measured, also reduced early onset disease. A systematic review in 2000, which included five studies, concluded that intrapartum antibiotic prophylaxis (IAP) reduced the colonization rate of newborns [odds ratio (OR) 0.1, 95% confidence limits 0.07–0.14] and reduced the incidence of EO GBS (OR 0.17, 0.07–0.39). The reduction in mortality did not reach statistical significance (OR 0.12; 0.01–2.0), probably reflecting the relatively small sample size of these studies.[1066] The main issue is how to target IAP appropriately. Two strategies emerged, based on clinical risk factors or based on swab-based screening.

Clinical risk-based strategy for GBS prevention. The risk-based strategy was based on multiple studies indicating that certain clinical risk factors were overly represented in mothers of infants who went on to develop EO GBS disease. With this strategy prenatal screening cultures are not obtained and IAP is directed to any woman with prolonged membrane rupture, gestation < 37 weeks, or intrapartum fever. Additionally, IAP is given to women with antenatal GBS bacteriuria (a marker of heavy colonization and a risk factor for EO GBS disease) and to those who had experienced a previous delivery of a neonate with group B streptococcal disease.

Swab-based strategy for GBS prevention. With a swab screening-based strategy cultures are obtained by swab of both lower vagina and rectum at 35–37 weeks' gestation. Swabbing of both sites significantly increases the yield over one site.[1067] Specimens are then processed with selective broth media containing either nalidixic acid and gentamicin or nalidixic acid and colistin. This is to prevent the overgrowth of other commensal bacteria and again results in a significant increase in GBS isolation over use of nonselective media.[1067] After onset of labor or rupture of membranes, IAP is then given to women who are identified as GBS carriers. If no culture result is available, intrapartum prophylaxis is only given to those women who develop intrapartum fever, threatened preterm delivery (< 37 weeks), or membrane rupture over 18 h. As with the risk-based strategy, IAP is also given to women with antenatal GBS bacteriuria and to those who have experienced a previous delivery of a neonate with group B streptococcal disease.

In the USA, application of either of these prevention strategies was associated with a reduction in the occurrence of GBS disease. Early onset disease fell from 1.7 to 0.5 cases per 1000 live births between 1993 and 1998, while late onset disease was stable.[1068] Death certificate analysis also documented a steeper decline in early sepsis deaths temporally associated with prevention implementation, without similarly steep declines in other causes of deaths including late sepsis deaths.[1069] A retrospective cohort study was conducted among a birth cohort of more than 600 000, and including 312 early onset GBS cases, to assess the relative effectiveness of the two strategies. Adjusting for confounders, women who were screened for GBS prenatally had more than 50% less risk of delivering a baby with GBS disease than did those exposed to the risk-based strategy (relative risk for EO disease following screening-based versus risk-based IAP 0.46; 95% confidence limits 0.36–0.60).[1070]

In the UK the background rate of culture proven GBS diseases appears lower than that of the USA and the cost effectiveness arguments may be different. Concerns persist about unintended consequences of widespread IAP use such as antibiotic resistance and drug side-effects. National UK guidelines for GBS prevention recommend targeting IAP to mothers based on clinical risk factors (www.rcog.org.uk).

An important issue, about which there are few data to guide practice, is the assessment and management of the baby born to a mother who has received IAP. If the mother receives appropriate antibiotics at least 2 h before delivery and the baby is well and not born prematurely, no further intervention is required. However, if the baby is born prematurely or appears unwell then consideration should be given to performing a full sepsis screen and starting the baby on antibiotics until culture results are available.

Listeriosis

L. monocytogenes is a Gram positive bacillus which causes EO and LO sepsis and meningitis. EO infection is frequently associated with signs of maternal infection and clinical presentation, as with GBS, may be with pneumonia or sepsis. Maternal infection may also result in abortion, stillbirth or preterm delivery. LO sepsis is more likely to present with meningitis. Microabscesses, skin granulomas, hepatosplenomegaly and passage of meconium by preterm infants should arouse the suspicion of *L. monocytogenes* infection.

Diagnosis is based on culture.

Listeria monocytogenes is not susceptible to cephalosporins. Ampicillin is the mainstay of therapy. The combination of ampicillin and gentamicin is synergistic in vitro and provides more rapid bacterial clearance in animal models of infection. Thus this combination is favored for initial therapy, with cessation of the aminoglycoside when the patient has improved clinically. The duration of therapy is 14 days for sepsis and at least 14 days for meningitis.

Neonatal meningitis (see also p. 305)
Incidence

The age at presentation with meningitis will suggest both the probable organisms and their likely mode of acquisition. EO infection, particularly in the first two days of life, reflects vertical transmission while LO infection suggests nosocomial or community acquisition. EO meningitis is more likely to be due to GBS, *Escherichia coli* and *Listeria monocytogenes* while LO meningitis may be caused by other Gram negative organisms as well as staphylococcal species. In the majority of cases a bacteremia permits the organism to traverse the blood–brain barrier (BBB). The risk appears to correlate with the magnitude of bacteremia. It is estimated that meningitis complicates 20% of early onset and 10% of late onset sepsis.[1071] Direct infection of the central nervous system via a myelomeningocele, congenital dermal sinus, infected cephalhematoma, osteomyelitis of the skull or otitis media may also occur. The BBB separates vascular and CNS compartments and is composed of brain microvascular endothelium with tight junctions. Penetration of the BBB may occur via the paracellular route, as a result of damage and disruption, via macrophages/monocytes and via the transcellular route. The latter appears to predominate for most bacteria. Generalized inflammation, brain swelling and vasculitis along with cortical thrombophlebitis may cause brain damage. Thrombosis and infarction may occur. At autopsy, subarachnoid inflammatory exudate is more prominent at the base of the brain than over the cortex. Damage to the choroid plexus and ventriculitis may lead to encephalopathy and blockage of the foramina and aqueduct resulting in hydrocephalus.

Comparison of data from two studies of neonatal meningitis conducted in England and Wales between 1985–7 and 1996–7 suggests that the bacteria responsible for meningitis have changed very little over this decade.[995,996] Group B streptococcus remains the leading pathogen, followed by E. coli, other Gram negative rods, Streptococcus pneumoniae and Listeria monocytogenes. The overall incidence of neonatal bacterial meningitis also has not changed: 0.22 cases/1000 live births (1985–7) versus 0.21 cases/1000 (1996–7). Under-reporting is probably common.

These data are consistent with other UK studies[1072] as well as with data from other industrialized countries.[1071,1073,1074] In developing countries, Gram negative enteric organisms appear to account for the majority of early onset and Streptococcus pneumoniae for late onset meningitis.[1000]

Aseptic or viral meningitis is uncommon in the newborn, though adenovirus and enteroviruses have been implicated. Herpes simplex virus is a rare but important cause of meningoencephalitis and aciclovir therapy must be started promptly if the outcome is to be favorable. This pathogen should be considered in all cases of meningitis where the initial Gram stain is negative for bacteria.

Mortality and morbidity

A reduction in mortality between the 1980s and the 1990s is evident from the two England and Wales studies (from 25% to 10%). A case control study from the 1985–7 national neonatal meningitis cohort has determined the neurodevelopmental outcome at 5 years of age.[990] Surprisingly it showed there to be very little difference between GBS and E. coli regarding disability at 5 years of age (~50% each) but a dismal outcome following meningitis due to other Gram negative organisms (78% with disability at 5 years of age). In another study, the neurodevelopmental outcome of VLBW infants with meningitis at 20 months' corrected age revealed a similar figure; 51% had impairment.[997] Comparison with data from older studies[1073–1075] suggests that despite declines in mortality, morbidity has not changed significantly between the 1970s and 1990s.

Clinical manifestations

Any of the clinical signs and symptoms listed in Table 12.99 may be present in meningitis. Temperature instability, lethargy, feed intolerance, recurrent apnea and bradycardia, sugar intolerance and unexplained hyponatremia are more frequent in VLBW babies. Bulging or full fontanelle and neck stiffness are late manifestations and occur in only 28% and 15% of cases, respectively.[1076]

Diagnosis

Examination of CSF via LP is the only way to confirm meningitis. See the discussion under microbiological tests, above.

There are few contraindications to performing a LP. Cardiorespiratory compromise during the procedure can be minimized using a modified left lateral position (hip flexion at 90 degrees without flexion or extension of the neck).[1077] In an unstable neonate the procedure can be deferred until stabilization is achieved.

Management

Antibiotic therapy. Appropriate antibiotic therapy is a critical aspect of management. Antibiotic choice is empirical, based on age at onset, likely pathogens and antibiotic susceptibility patterns, with a focus on GBS, E. coli, other Gram negative organisms and Listeria monocytogenes. A reasonable regimen therefore is a combination of ampicillin, gentamicin and cefotaxime.[1044] Antibiotics are then modified according to culture and antibiotic susceptibility results. Empirical choice in an individual neonatal unit must also consider data regarding pathogens and their susceptibility within that unit. The goal of antibiotic therapy is to achieve sterilization of CSF. Delayed CSF sterilization is a particular feature of Gram negative meningitis and may in part account for its higher

mortality compared with GBS. CSF sterilization is dependent on achieving bactericidal antibiotic concentrations within the CSF. This will be influenced by the dose of antibiotic that can be administered safely, the penetration of the antibiotic into the CSF and the minimum bactericidal concentration (MBC) of the infecting organism. For example, the aminoglycosides have relatively good CSF penetration but the concentrations achieved at standard doses may only be minimally above the MBC of Gram negative organisms. A low margin of error between therapeutic and toxic concentrations means that aminoglycoside doses cannot be safely increased to compensate. In contrast, although the CSF penetration of third generation cephalosporins may be modest, the CSF concentrations usually achieved are many-fold higher than the minimum bactericidal concentrations for Gram negative bacteria, and cephalosporin dosage is not limited by toxicity.[1078]

The antibiotic considerations for GBS and Listeria meningitis are discussed above. The treatment of Gram negative meningitis (e.g. E. coli, Klebsiella, Enterobacter, Citrobacter, Salmonella, Proteus, Pseudomonas and Serratia) has traditionally been with a combination of ampicillin and an aminoglycoside. However, these Gram negatives frequently are resistant to ampicillin, CSF aminoglycoside concentrations often are minimally above their minimum inhibitory concentrations, CSF cultures remain positive longer than with GBS meningitis, and morbidity and mortality from Gram negative meningitis remain high. This led to consideration of intrathecal and intraventricular administration of antibiotics such as gentamicin, but trials have demonstrated these to be unhelpful strategies.[1079,1080] No further trials have been performed. While certain infants with obstructive ventriculitis complicating Gram negative meningitis may require administration of intraventricular aminoglycoside to assist in sterilization of the CSF, this therapy is not recommended routinely. Cefotaxime (or ceftazidime in the case of P. aeruginosa) is recommended for therapy in suspected neonatal Gram negative meningitis in combination with an aminoglycoside, usually gentamicin. Once susceptibility is documented, the combination is continued for at least 14 days after CSF cultures have sterilized. Thereafter cefotaxime alone is used to complete a minimum total therapy of 21 days. Meropenem has not been sufficiently studied for safety and efficacy in neonates, and is not recommended unless an extended spectrum beta lactamase-producing organism is identified. In this circumstance, meropenem in combination with an aminoglycoside should be administered for the entire course of therapy.

Coagulase negative staphylococci (CONS) rarely invade the CSF except as a complication of bacteremia accompanying intraventricular hemorrhage in VLBW neonates, in the presence of a foreign body, i.e. a ventriculoperitoneal shunt, or after contamination following neurosurgery or direct entry into the ventricular space, i.e. following ventricular fluid aspiration. Such infections are late onset. Most CONS are resistant to penicillin and flucloxacillin, necessitating the use of vancomycin for proven CONS central nervous system infection.

Repeat lumbar punctures. A repeat lumbar puncture 24–48 h into antibiotic therapy should be considered in cases of Gram negative meningitis in order to document CSF sterilization. Persistence of infection may indicate a focus, such as obstructive ventriculitis, subdural empyema or multiple small vessel thrombi. Infants with positive CSF cultures after initiation of appropriate therapy are at risk of these complications as well as a poor outcome. In this situation immediate diagnostic imaging is recommended. The choice and dosage of antibiotics also should be reviewed and (rarely) intraventricular administration considered. Delayed CSF sterilization and/or abnormalities found on neuroimaging may be an indication for prolonging the total course of therapy (see below).

With regard to LP at the end of treatment, Schaad et al reviewed 27 cases of recrudescence and relapse following bacterial meningitis in childhood (including 9 neonates). In the majority recrudescence/relapse could be explained by inadequate dosage of antibiotics, inadequate length of course or persistent infection in meningeal or parameningeal sites, e.g. subdural empyema, brain abscess or ventriculitis. They concluded that an LP at the end of therapy was unnecessary if the clinical response was otherwise uneventful as they found that normal CSF findings may not exclude a relapse and abnormal CSF findings may not be predictive of relapse.[1081] However, in neonates where abnormal neurological findings persist, especially focal deficits, or where CSF cultures are positive for more than 48–72 h into therapy, prolonging therapy may assist in preventing a relapse of infection. Examination of the CSF as well as neuroimaging in these circumstances may assist in determining an optimal duration of antibiotic therapy.

Intensive care support. The appropriate and early use of supportive care including fluid management, inotropes, anticonvulsants and ventilation appears to be a critical part of neonatal meningitis management. There are no clinical trials, however, which address this.

Imaging. Neuroimaging is recommended to detect the complications of meningitis. Complications should be suspected when the clinical course is characterized by shock, respiratory failure, focal neurological deficits, a positive CSF culture after 48–72 h of appropriate antibiotic therapy or by infection with certain organisms. *Citrobacter koseri* and *Enterobacter sakazakii* meningitis, for example, are frequently associated with the development of brain abscesses, even in infants who have a benign clinical course.[1082,1083] The most useful and non-invasive method early in the course is ultrasonography, which will provide information regarding ventricular size and the presence of hemorrhage. Computerized tomography will be useful in detecting cerebral abscesses and later in the treatment course in identifying areas of encephalomalacia that may dictate prolonged therapy.

NOSOCOMIAL INFECTIONS

Nosocomial infections are an important problem in VLBW infants, associated with a number of complications and a risk factor for death and for prolonged hospital stay. Nosocomial means hospital acquired and the majority of late onset infections are likely to be nosocomial in origin. In their most recent surveillance data, the National Institute of Child Health and Human Development Neonatal Research Network included 6215 infants who survived beyond 3 days and 1313 (21%) had one or more episodes of blood culture-proven late onset sepsis.[984] The vast majority (70%) were caused by Gram positive organisms, with CONS accounting for 48% of infections. Other Gram positive organisms included *Staphylococcus aureus*, *Enterococcus* and GBS. The most frequent Gram negative agents were *E. coli*, *Klebsiella*, *Pseudomonas* and *Enterobacter* species. Rate of infection was inversely related to birth weight and gestational age. Complications of prematurity associated with an increased rate of late onset sepsis included patent ductus arteriosus, prolonged ventilation, prolonged intravascular access, bronchopulmonary dysplasia and necrotizing enterocolitis. Infants who developed late onset sepsis had a significantly prolonged hospital stay (mean length of stay: 79 vs. 60 days). They were significantly more likely to die than those who were uninfected (18% vs. 7%), especially if they were infected with Gram negative organisms (36%) or fungi (32%). The mortality associated with CONS infection is probably very low.[993] In the Stoll multicenter analysis, there was considerable center-to-center variability in the incidence of late onset sepsis, with rates ranging from 10.6% to 31.7% of VLBW infants.[984] This may reflect different infection control practices in different centers.

Coagulase-negative staphylococci (CONS)

Most infants are colonized with *Staphylococcus* by the fifth day of life. Although they may sometimes be culture contaminants there is clear evidence that CONS are also pathogens. They are often associated with the use of vascular catheters. In contrast to *S. aureus* they produce a limited range of virulence factors but it is the ability of CONS to form an adherent multilayered biofilm on polymer surfaces which is considered their main virulence determinant. There are numerous species of CONS but the majority of infections are due to *Staphylococcus epidermidis*.

Clinical features

Presentation is usually subtle rather than acute. Episodes of apnea or bradycardia, low grade acidosis, pyrexia and increased oxygen

Table 12.101 Incidence of catheter related coagulase negative staphylococcal infection by duration of catheter insertion[1085]

Duration of insertion	Incidence (%)
0–7 days	5
8–14 days	15
15–21 days	41
22 days or more	58

requirements may be observed. The usual site of infection is a catheter or other intravascular device. The main risk factors for catheter related sepsis are catheter hub colonization, exit site colonization, duration of total parenteral nutrition, ELBW (<1000 g) at the time of catheter insertion and postnatal age (>1 week) at the time of insertion.[1084] Rates of sepsis are related to duration of catheter insertion (Table 12.101).[1085]

Treatment

Intravascular catheters should be removed if at all possible. Where CONS are isolated from blood cultures, consideration should first be given to their significance. Isolation from two or more blood cultures, a pure growth (vs. mixed growth), growth of organism within 48 h and accompanying clinical signs of sepsis all lend support to the significance of a positive culture. Although a proportion of strains may retain susceptibility to flucloxacillin, most will require therapy with vancomycin. Monitoring of serum concentrations is advised. There is no consensus about duration of antibiotic therapy. Antibiotics should be stopped if the baby is clinically well, has a normal white cell count and a CRP level of <10 mg/dl.

Staphylococcus aureus

S. aureus infections are an increasing problem in neonatal units. Rates of infection have risen over the last decade in all age groups, including neonates, and the proportion of isolates that are meticillin resistant (MRSA) is increasing. In England and Wales in 2001, for example, 13% of all strains in the neonatal period were MRSA as compared with 0–3% between 1990 and 1994.[992] In the USA in particular, community acquisition of MRSA in babies after discharge from hospital is also increasing.[1086] In terms of clinical presentation, MRSA appears to be more likely to present with skin sepsis than meticillin sensitive *S. aureus* (MSSA), although it may also be associated with bacteremia and bone and joint infections as with MSSA.[1086,1087] In one study, babies with MRSA were more likely to be born more prematurely than those with MSSA and the mortality was also higher.[1087]

Treatment

For local umbilical cord infections, cleaning with alcohol or with chlorhexidine solution may be enough. Systemic infection is best treated with an antistaphylococcal penicillin such as flucloxacillin. MRSA will require vancomycin.

Pneumonia (p. 250)

In a review of autopsies performed on 111 ELBW infants between 1990 and 1993, the major cause of death was found to be infection of the amniotic fluid leading to pneumonia.[977] Neonatal pneumonia may be acquired in utero (congenital), during birth or nosocomially. Congenital pneumonia may be caused by TORCH group organisms, or be secondary to chorioamnionitis associated with bacteria such as GBS, *E. coli* and *Listeria*. Most infants swallow material during birth but few develop pneumonia. Congenital pneumonia usually presents within the first 24–48 hours of life. Nosocomial pneumonia is a particular problem in ventilated preterm infants. Many of the late onset pathogens described above may be associated with pneumonia and the finding of positive cultures from tracheal or lower respiratory tract specimens may be useful, especially in the context of a new pneumonia, but otherwise may simply reflect colonization.[1036] Respiratory viruses as a cause of pneumonia should also be considered.

C. trachomatis is well recognized as a cause of pneumonia but the role of *U. urealyticum* is less clear. A proposed link with the development of bronchopulmonary dysplasia is also controversial.[1088]

Clinical manifestations

Clinical features include tachypnea, tachycardia, cyanosis and expiratory grunt. Distinction from RDS may be difficult. Symptoms and signs are nonspecific. Babies may show signs of cerebral irritation or be hypotonic and lethargic. They do not feed well and may go into heart failure. *C. trachomatis* infection may produce a staccato cough.

Diagnosis

This is based on history, blood culture, and Gram stain and culture of the tracheal aspirate. Early chest radiographs may be unhelpful but they may be confirmatory if taken 48–72 h after onset of symptoms. Serology may also be helpful.

Treatment

Initial therapy should be with ampicillin/penicillin and an aminoglycoside. Flucloxacillin should be used for *S. aureus* but vancomycin is preferred for *S. epidermidis* and meticillin resistant *Staphylococcus*. Azithromycin or erythromycin is the drug of choice for *Chlamydia* infection. There is no consensus regarding duration of therapy but shorter courses may be as effective as longer courses. In one study, 4 days of antibiotic therapy plus a 24 h period of observation for selected cases of neonatal pneumonia was comparable to 7 days of therapy. However, these infants had also received a single dose of penicillin soon after birth as group B streptococcal sepsis prophylaxis. Additionally, only infants who were asymptomatic after 48 h of antibiotic therapy were included.[1089] In a later study, 4 days was again shown to be adequate and better than 2 days of therapy.[1090] Supportive therapy with oxygen, intravenous fluids, suction and physiotherapy is also required. Drainage of pleural effusion or empyema may be necessary. Overall prognosis is good.

Gastroenteritis

This is uncommon in the newborn but may occur in epidemics. Rotavirus, echovirus and adenovirus infections are the commonest cause. *E. coli*, *Salmonella*, *Shigella*, *Campylobacter* and *Yersinia* are the commonest bacterial agents. There may be vomiting, diarrhea, feed intolerance, dehydration and pyrexia. The mainstay of management is correction of dehydration. Antibiotics should be given if the infection is considered to be invasive.

Necrotizing enterocolitis (NEC) (see also p. 275)

NEC is a major contributor to morbidity and mortality, particularly in small preterm infants. The precise role played by bacteria remains uncertain but NEC has occurred in endemic and epidemic forms suggesting an infectious origin. Most consistent among predisposing factors are low birth weight and prematurity. Others recorded include hypoxia, persistent ductus arteriosus, umbilical catheterization, rapid advancement of feeding (particularly with hyperosmolar milk), Hirschsprung disease, hyperviscosity syndromes and infective diarrhea. Antenatal Doppler studies showing absent/reversed end-diastolic flow in the umbilical artery may also indicate increased risk. In the majority of cases no organism is isolated. Organisms reported in the literature include *E. coli*, *K. pneumoniae*, *Clostridium butyricum*, *Clostridium perfringens*, *Clostridium difficile*, *Salmonella*, *P. mirabilis* and *Ps. aeruginosa*. Viruses such as adeno type 19, coxsackie, corona and enterovirus have also been implicated.

Clinical manifestations

NEC commonly presents in the first 10 days of life in babies weighing less than 1500 g. There is no sex predisposition. Signs include abdominal distention, increasing gastric residue (may become bile stained), absent bowel sounds, vomiting and passage of blood in the stools. X-ray of the abdomen may show bowel wall edema in the early stages followed by pneumatosis intestinalis, perforation and in severe cases gas in the portal tract. Clinical staging using Bell's criteria (stages 1–3) can be useful.

Treatment

Medical management consists of withdrawal of enteral feeds, gastric suction and administration of intravenous fluids and parenteral nutrition. Empirically a combination of ampicillin, an aminoglycoside (gentamicin) and metronidazole is given for 7–10 days. Shorter courses are appropriate where NEC is only suspected (Bell's stage 1). Indications for surgery are debatable and are discussed on page 275. Mortality varies from 15 to 30%.[1091] Stoll and colleagues reported that infants with sepsis and NEC were at high risk of later neurodevelopmental impairment.[991]

Osteomyelitis and septic arthritis

During the first year of life, capillaries perforate the epiphyseal plate providing communication between the joint space and the metaphysis. Thus, septic arthritis and osteomyelitis may often occur together. The source of infection is usually hematogenous but direct trauma during arterial or venous puncture has also been implicated. The commonest organism is *S. aureus*. GBS, *Klebsiella* and *E. coli* are also prominent. In resource limited countries, *Salmonella* is frequent. *S. epidermidis* and *Candida albicans* are emerging as important etiological agents in extremely preterm infants.

Clinical manifestations

Most cases present insidiously. There may be nonspecific symptoms such as poor feeding, lethargy, decreased activity and low grade fever. Mild unexplained acidosis may be a pointer. Local signs include swelling over the affected area or joint, pseudoparalysis of the limb, and irritability on handling the affected body part.

Diagnosis

Diagnosis is based on radiological confirmation although changes are not seen for 10–14 days. Technetium-99 m scan is highly sensitive. Conventional radiographs may miss early lesions. MRI imaging can be helpful. Whole body scanning is advisable as there may be more than one focus of infection. Repeated cultures should be taken.

Treatment

Flucloxacillin and a third generation cephalosporin (cefotaxime) should be started until culture and sensitivity results are available. Therapy should be continued for at least 6 weeks (at least 2–3 weeks intravenously). Orthopedic consultation should always be sought and surgical intervention may become necessary if the response to medical treatment is slow. Mortality is low; however, long term growth impairment may occur if the growth plates are affected.

Urinary tract infection (see also p. 313)

Urinary tract infection occurs in up to 10% of preterm and 1% of term infants. It is more common in males and in infants with kidney or renal tract abnormalities, e.g. obstructive uropathy. It is also seen more frequently in babies whose renal parenchyma may have been damaged, e.g. by asphyxia or dehydration.

The most frequent infecting organism is *E. coli* with *Klebsiella* and other Gram negative bacteria accounting for the rest. In very preterm LBW babies, *C. albicans* is also an important etiological agent.

Clinical manifestations and diagnosis

Clinical signs and symptoms include poor weight gain, jaundice, hepatomegaly and palpable kidneys. There may be generalized septicemia. Diagnosis is confirmed by urine culture (greater than 100 000 CFU/ml) and > 10 white cells/ml in freshly voided or aspirated urine. (See earlier discussion on urine specimens.)

Further investigation with ultrasound, micturating cystourethrogram and isotope scanning (DMSA) is advisable as abnormalities have been detected in up to 45% of cases.

Treatment

Empirical therapy with ampicillin and gentamicin is usually adequate but antibiotics must be changed according to urine culture reports.

There is a recurrence rate of up to 10%, so follow-up is essential. With current therapy, prognosis is excellent where there has been no renal parenchymal damage and there are no congenital abnormalities. If there is evidence of reflux uropathy then antibiotic prophylaxis with trimethoprim should be initiated.

Conjunctivitis (see p. 314)

The incidence of conjunctivitis varies between 7 and 20%. The higher figure comes mainly from premature infants nursed on NICUs.

Clinical manifestations

In a recent US study the most common isolates in neonates with conjunctivitis were CONS, viridans streptococci, *S. aureus* and *H. influenzae*.[1092] Conjunctivitis usually presents within the first week. *Chlamydia* infections usually, but not always, present later. *N. gonorrhoeae* infection is now rare in the UK but if untreated it may lead to corneal ulceration and perforation, iridocyclitis, anterior synechiae and panophthalmitis. *Chlamydia* infection produces a similar clinical picture but only involves the tarsal aspect of the conjunctiva, sparing the cornea.

Diagnosis

This is based on the clinical history, timing, and site of the lesion and on cultures of the discharge. *Chlamydia* infection may be diagnosed by obtaining scrapings from the tarsal conjunctiva and staining with Giemsa stain for intracytoplasmic inclusions.

Treatment

For gonococcus the eye should be cleaned with frequent eye washes of normal saline or water (every 15–30 min at first) followed by instillation of penicillin drops. Penicillin should also be given intravenously for a few days.

For chlamydial infection, 0.5% erythromycin ophthalmic ointment is used with systemic erythromycin therapy for 7–14 days. Chloramphenicol and sulfacetamide ophthalmic preparations may be useful for staphylococcal colonization. The instillation of 1% silver nitrate drops to newborns led to the decline in gonococcal conjunctivitis, but this treatment has generally been abandoned as it leads to significant chemical conjunctivitis.

Otitis media

Examination of the eardrum, particularly in preterm infants, should be a mandatory part of the routine examination of infants with suspected sepsis. The incidence of otitis media in the newborn is 0.6–2.4%. A shorter, widely patent and horizontally placed eustachian tube predisposes to infection. Other factors include chorioamnionitis, asphyxia, prematurity, ventilatory support, cleft palate and Down syndrome. *S. pneumoniae* and *H. influenzae* are the commonest organisms involved. Presentation is nonspecific. Otoscopic examination reveals a dull tympanic membrane which is bulging and has reduced or absent mobility on pneumatic otoscopy. Treatment includes appropriate antibiotics. Outcome is usually favorable but the recurrence rate is high and up to 33% develop chronic otitis media.

Umbilical infection

S. aureus and *E. coli* are the most frequent organisms causing infection of the umbilicus. The incidence is between 0.5 and 2%. Periumbilical erythema is usually the only clinical feature though severe omphalitis has been reported from resource limited countries. Simple cleaning with an antiseptic such as chlorhexidine is sufficient, but for more significant infection broad spectrum systemic antibiotics should be given.

SPECIFIC INFECTIONS

Syphilis

Congenital syphilis is uncommon in resource rich countries; however, there are concerns that this may change. There has been a 255% increase in the diagnosis of syphilis in UK women between 2000 and 2004.[1093] Coupled with this, two recent case series demonstrate that

screening, referral and management of pregnant women with positive serology is poorly done.[1093,1094] Clinicians must therefore not forget congenital syphilis.

T. pallidum is the etiological agent. Transplacental infection rarely occurs before 18 weeks' gestation as the Langhans' layer of the chorion prevents the passage of *Treponema*. Treatment of the mother before the 18th week of gestation will almost always completely protect the fetus. The chances of the fetus remaining uninfected are negligible if the mother is not treated. If the mother has early or latent syphilis the fetus has a 20–70% chance of being infected.

Clinical manifestations

Hematogenous spread in prenatal life determines which fetal organs and tissues are involved. Abortion, stillbirth and hydrops occur in 40% of pregnancies. There may be severe anemia, hepatosplenomegaly or pneumonia soon after birth. One to three weeks later the stigmata of congenital syphilis become evident, e.g. nasal obstruction with serosanguineous discharge, copper-colored maculopapular rash, perianal condylomata, rhagades (fissures at mucocutaneous junctions), loss of hair, exfoliation of the nails, iritis and choroiditis. Poor feeding and fever may be accompanied by jaundice, generalized lymphadenopathy and signs of pancreatitis or hepatitis. Bone lesions are seen in nearly all infants beyond the neonatal period. Most infants born with congenital disease are free of clinical symptoms at the time of birth, and the problem may not appear for more than 2 years.

Diagnosis

This is based on either the visualization of *T. pallidum* by dark ground microscopy or serological tests. The two types of serological tests for syphilis are nontreponemal reaginic tests and treponema-specific tests. Screening nontreponemal tests include the rapid plasma reagin (RPR) test and the Venereal Disease Research Laboratory (VDRL) test. The specific tests measure antibodies specific for *T. pallidum* and include *T. pallidum* immobilization (TPI), fluorescent treponemal antibody absorption (FTA-ABS), and microhemagglutination assay for antibodies to *T. pallidum* (MHA-TP).

Treatment

Infection is suspected with the following: physical or radiographic evidence of active disease; quantitative nontreponemal titer $\geq \times 4$ maternal titer; reactive CSF VDRL test or abnormal CSF cell count and/or protein; positive IgM FTA-ABS; positive dark field microscopy or staining for treponemes in placenta or umbilical cord.

In general, for symptomatic or CNS syphilis a minimum 10-day course of a parenteral penicillin is needed. Procaine penicillin (penicillin G procaine) IM, once daily, 50000 u/kg for 10 days; or iv benzylpenicillin (= penicillin G = crystalline penicillin) 50000 u/kg twice daily for 7 days followed by three times daily for a further 3 days to a total of 10 days. For asymptomatic syphilis a single intramuscular injection of benzathine penicillin G 50–10000 units/kg is recommended by some experts (where available). If maternal treatment was given during the last 4 weeks of pregnancy or the treatment was not with penicillin or treatment was inadequate or status is unknown, the infant should be treated. Penicillin-allergic patients can be given cephalosporins.

Tetanus

This is very unusual in resource rich countries but in some parts of the world neonatal tetanus is responsible for 30–40% of all neonatal deaths. *Clostridium tetani* is a Gram positive anaerobic spore-forming bacillus which produces a toxin, tetanospasmin, that causes muscle spasms and convulsions. The toxin, once fixed to the nervous tissue, cannot be neutralized by antitoxins. Mothers who are immunized protect the fetus through the active transport of antitoxin antibodies across the placenta.

Clinical manifestations

The incubation period is between 3 days and 3 weeks. Most neonatal cases occur between 3 and 10 days after birth. The umbilicus is the main route of entry. The infant usually presents with difficulty in sucking (due to upper lip spasm), excessive irritability and trismus. This is followed very soon by generalized muscle spasms, convulsions, rigidity and fever. There may also be cardiorespiratory difficulties.

Diagnosis

This is usually easy but meningitis, metabolic disorders and ingestion of phenothiazines must be considered in countries where tetanus is unusual.

Treatment

This is based on the provision of an adequate airway and ventilation, neutralization and elimination of toxins, prevention of spasms and convulsions and maintaining hydration and nutrition. Diazepam, either as a bolus (0.1–2 mg) or as a continuous infusion (10–140 mg/kg/d), is useful in reducing muscular spasm. Paraldehyde or barbiturates may also be used. Human tetanus immune globulin should be given if possible as a single dose but equine tetanus antitoxin may also be used. There is evidence that intrathecal administration is superior to intramuscular administration.[1095] Parenteral penicillin 100 000–150 000 IU should be given for at least 10 days. Fluid, electrolytes and nutrition should be maintained. Where facilities are available, mechanical ventilation and neuromuscular blockade have improved the outcome, which remains gloomy in resource limited countries.

Tuberculosis

It is rare to see tuberculosis (TB) during the first month of life. It may be congenitally or postnatally acquired, although the former is very rare. The source of congenital infection will be the placenta or genitourinary lesions with acquisition via the bloodstream or via the inhalation or ingestion of infected amniotic fluid. Acquisition via airborne spread from adults in the environment is the most common route of postnatal infection. Symptoms include poor weight gain, respiratory distress, fever, lethargy, jaundice, lymphadenopathy and hepatosplenomegaly. The diagnosis may be suspected from seeing a primary focus, a miliary pattern or hilar lymphadenopathy on a chest X-ray, or on the basis of maternal history. Placental histology and culture of gastric washings, bronchoalveolar lavage fluid or bone marrow aspiration from the infant may help.

It would appear that the basic principles of TB treatment would apply to neonates as much as to older children with active TB, thus quadruple therapy with rifampicin, isoniazid, ethambutol and pyrazinamide is recommended. In the setting where the mother has active TB but there is no evidence of disease in the infant then the infant should receive isoniazid prophylaxis (INH 10 mg/kg/d) for 3 months, after which a tuberculin test should be done. If this is negative, bacille Calmette–Guérin (BCG) should be given. If the tuberculin test is positive and there is no evidence of active disease, then INH is continued for 6 months. If the mother has active lesions, the infant should be separated from the mother until treatment has commenced.

FUNGAL INFECTIONS
Candidiasis

Up to 33% of pregnant women have vaginal colonization with *Candida* species. Invasive neonatal fungal infection, however, is very uncommon and predominantly seen in low birth weight or preterm infants. In a recent UK surveillance study the incidence of invasive fungal infections in VLBW infants was 10.0 (95% CI 8.0–12.0) cases per 1000 live births. The majority (86%) of the infants were of extremely low birth weight (< 1000 g) and the incidence in this ELBW group was 21.1 (95% CI 16.5–25.7) per 1000 live births.[982] These figures are much lower than those found in other countries, especially the USA. For example in the NICHHD Neonatal Research Network, invasive candidiasis was documented in 7.7% of ELBW infants.[1096] Fungal colonization is an important risk factor for systemic infection. In one US study of VLBW infants, around 27% of infants were colonized (two thirds during the first week of life), one third developed mucocutaneous candidiasis and 8% developed invasive infection.[1097] Colonization is inversely correlated with gestational age at birth, usually occurs in the first 2 weeks of life, and occurs

on the skin and gastrointestinal tract before the respiratory tract.[1098] Other risk factors for fungal infection include antibiotic therapy, intravenous alimentation with fat emulsions and use of postnatal steroids. The commonest fungal pathogens are *C. albicans* and *C. parapsilosis*.

Infection in the newborn may be congenital or late onset and may be local or disseminated. Congenital candidal infections are acquired in the birth canal and usually present within the first 24 h of life as an intense desquamating rash. Pustules and satellite lesions are common, and may be confused with staphylococcal scalded skin syndrome. In late onset mucocutaneous infections, skin lesions appear between the 7th and 10th day as a rash of small papules which coalesces to form cheesy white patches in the mouth, diaper (nappy) area, groin or axillae. Occasionally oral thrush may extend to cause esophagitis.

Clinical signs and symptoms of invasive candidiasis are indistinguishable from bacterial sepsis. Affected infants often develop hyperglycemia and thrombocytopenia. There is a high incidence of renal and central nervous system involvement in systemic candidiasis.[1099] There may be endophthalmitis and the eyes should be examined for white fluffy retinal deposits which can progress to involve the vitreous humor, resulting in blindness. Occasionally *Candida* may cause skin abscesses, osteomyelitis and pneumonia.

Diagnosis

The diagnosis of local disease can be confirmed by microscopy and culture of scrapings from the margins of lesions. Systemic candidiasis is diagnosed by growing fungi from blood, CSF or urine, but cultures may be negative even when multisystem disease is seen at autopsy. Urine microscopy may show yeasts or hyphae. Ultrasound of the kidneys may reveal fungal balls and eye examination may show retinal deposits.

Treatment

Local lesions may be treated by nystatin, 100 000 IU four times a day for 5 days, or with miconazole gel (orally) or cream (for the perineum and buttocks). Nystatin with corticosteroid ointment may be used in severe cases of *Candida* dermatitis.

Systemic candidiasis is best treated by removing all central lines and indwelling catheters and starting the infant on intravenous antifungal agents. Amphotericin B has a long half-life and good penetration into the CSF. The starting dose is between 0.5 mg/kg and 1 mg/kg per day given as an infusion over 4–6 h. Principal adverse effects are nephrotoxicity, marrow suppression and hepatotoxicity. Liposomal amphotericin B is less toxic. The dose of liposomal amphotericin B is 1 mg/kg/d to a maximum of 3–5 mg/kg/d. Treatment should be given for 4–6 weeks. 5-Flucytosine (5-FC) is synergistic with amphotericin and some recommend combined treatment, particularly in the presence of CNS infection. Fluconazole is a broad spectrum antifungal agent that is well absorbed enterally and is a suitable alternative for susceptible *Candida*. Side-effects include hepatotoxicity, skin rashes and thrombocytopenia.

In the recent UK surveillance study, death occurred in 41% of the infected infants before 37 weeks' postconceptional age.[982]

Other fungi

Aspergillus and *Trichophyton* species may cause cutaneous disease. *M. furfur* is responsible for intralipid induced fungemia, since it is a lipophilic fungus that often colonizes skin. Treatment consists of removal of lines, discontinuing lipid infusion and instituting antifungal therapy with any of the above antifungal drugs.

VIRAL INFECTIONS

See Chapter 28.

PARASITIC INFECTIONS
Malaria

Congenital malaria is rare in resource rich countries but increasingly reported among babies born to mothers continually residing in endemic areas. The clinical presentation may be indistinguishable from sepsis; the infant may present with hepatosplenomegaly or jaundice due to hemolysis.

Diagnosis is made on identifying malarial parasites in the blood film. Treatment should be with quinine.

Toxoplasmosis
See Chapter 28.

NEONATAL NEOPLASIA

Of those rare tumors that present at birth or in the neonatal period less than half will be malignant. It is important to know the natural history as even huge tumor masses or apparently disseminated disease may regress completely and spontaneously. As survival from childhood cancer has improved, death certificate data have become progressively less accurate as an indicator of frequency. Estimates of incidence vary because most reports are referral center rather than population based and some exclude benign tumors. In the USA the best estimate of different malignancies is based on an analysis of 10% of the total population over a 3 year period. This suggests an overall incidence of 1 per 27 000 live births (Table 12.102, column 5 for proportions of different tumors). In the UK a prevalence of 1 per 12 500–17 500 has been found but this included benign neoplasia (Table 12.102, column 1). Approximately 1.9% of childhood malignancies will present in the first 28 days of life: 43% of these will present on the first day; 66% by the end of 1 week;[1103] and 0.6% of pediatric malignant deaths will occur during this period. There is some suggestion that the incidence is increasing.[1106]

ETIOLOGY

1. Transplacental metastases of maternal choriocarcinoma, melanoma and leukemia are well described but very rare.
2. Transplacental carcinogenesis. This is definite for the use of maternal stilbestrol which leads to vaginal adenocarcinoma – the latent period is 10–15 years – it has not been reported neonatally.

Transplacental carcinogenesis is also probable for infantile neuroblastoma in the fetal phenytoin syndrome and it is possible for hepatoblastoma when the mother has been taking estrogens in the first trimester.

3. Genetic
   a. Chromosomal
   - Down syndrome 21X3 – acute myelogenous and occasionally acute lymphoblastic leukemia presents neonatally. Leukemoid reactions are comparatively common in the neonatal period; they are difficult to distinguish and 15% will go on to develop leukemia later.
   - Klinefelter syndrome XXY – breast cancer (not reported neonatally), and recent reports of a higher incidence of leukemia.
   - Gonadal dysgenesis 46XY, 45X/46XY, other mosaics – dysgerminomas (not reported neonatally).
   - 13q (retinoblastoma) – may present neonatally. This is the only known inheritable malignancy.
   - Mutations of genes on chromosome 11 (and possibly on other sites) are common in Wilms' tumors.
   - Fanconi anemia – leukemia (not reported neonatally).
   - Bloom syndrome – leukemia (not reported neonatally).
   - Ataxia telangiectasia – lymphoma and gastric carcinoma (not reported neonatally).
   b. Malformation syndromes
   - Aniridia – nephroblastoma (possible neonatally).
   - Hemihypertrophy syndrome – nephroblastoma and hepatoblastoma (not recorded neonatally).
   - Beckwith–Wiedemann syndrome – nephroblastoma and hepatoblastoma (not recorded neonatally).
   - Cryptorchidism – testicular tumors (not recorded neonatally).
   - Other syndromes – chondrosarcoma (not recorded neonatally).
4. Environmental. In 1992 Golding reported an association between intramuscular vitamin K at birth and later (not neonatal) development of cancer.[1107] Many more recent epidemiological and case-control studies have failed to confirm this association.[1108–1100]

Table 12.102 Comparative frequencies of neonatal neoplasms in different series

	Barson[1100] UK (dates variable)[1]	Davis et al[1101] Glasgow, UK (1955–1988)	Broadbent[1102] Oxford, UK (1970–1977)	Campbell et al[1103] Toronto (1922–1982)	Bader & Miller[1104] USA (1969–1971)[2]	Bader & Miller[1104] Deaths, USA (1960–1969)	Fraumeni & Miller[1105] Deaths, USA (1960–1964)
Leukemia	17	Not surveyed	17	8[3]	5	101	44
Teratoma	67	19	16 (malig.)	Not surveyed (regarded benign)	Not surveyed (regarded benign)	11	9
Neuroblastoma	64	7	27	48 (44%)	21	70	27
Soft tissue sarcoma (rhabdo-, leio-, fibro-)	22	8	13	12 (17%)	4	29	12
Wilms' and mesoblastic nephroma	20	9	8	4 (75%)	5	21	9
CNS	17		12	9 (11%)	1	12	7
Hepatoblastoma		3	3	1	0	15	10
Retinoblastoma		4		7 (76%)	0	1	
Others	78[4]	1	5	3 (100%)	3	35	12
Total	285	51	101	102[5] (42%)	39	295	130[6]
Sex incidence	–	–	1:1	1.7:1	–	–	–

[1] Benign and malignant.
[2] Third National Cancer Study (10% US population surveyed); overall incidence neonatal malignancy USA= 130 cases/year.
[3] Long term survival.
[4] Unclear from report.
[5] Represents 1.9% of all childhood malignancy.
[6] Represents 0.6% of childhood deaths from malignancy.

GENERAL MANAGEMENT

The variety of neonatal neoplasia makes it extremely important that all patients are referred to recognized specialist centers with facilities for diagnostic imaging, expert pediatric and molecular pathology, surgery, radiotherapy, chemotherapy and hematology. Tumor markers have an increasingly important role in both diagnosis and monitoring the response to treatment (Table 12.103). Large tumors may be problematic, more from their size interfering with organ function than from tumor load. Surgery can frequently be more conservative than is generally appreciated and may be curative. Back-up with postoperative intensive care is essential. Neonatal tissue (especially brain, bone, lungs, liver and kidneys) is very sensitive to radiotherapy and the anxieties of infection secondary to immune suppression, interference with growth leading to long term musculoskeletal morbidity, or the development of second malignancies means that this therapy should be avoided if possible. Cytotoxic chemotherapy may reduce the infant's effective immune response with in consequence a higher incidence of complications and particularly infection. Chemotherapy can potentially affect a child's subsequent development but small doses will often reduce tumor size very significantly. Centralization of referral also allows more realistic parental and family support.

SPECIFIC DIAGNOSIS AND MANAGEMENT

See Table 12.104.

NEONATAL METABOLIC DISORDERS

HYPOGLYCEMIA

Glucose homeostasis in the fetus and newborn

The fetus receives a constant supply of glucose across the placenta and this largely determines blood glucose concentrations. Fetal metabolism is directed towards synthesis with insulin as the principal anabolic hormone. Hepatic glycogen accumulates during the third trimester and mobilization of this reserve is the principal source of glucose for the first postnatal hours. At delivery, the constant transplacental glucose supply is interrupted, blood glucose falls and the processes of glycogenolysis and gluconeogenesis are activated mainly by catecholamines and cortisol and a concomitant decrease in insulin levels until milk feed intakes increase to levels where this is the main source of glucose precursors.

The maintenance of normoglycemia during the newborn period is dependent on adequate fetal glycogen reserves, effective glycogenolysis and gluconeogenesis, an appropriate balance of insulin:glucagon and an increasing postnatal nutritional intake. Hypoglycemia will result if any of these processes are inadequate.

Neuropathology

Glucose is an essential primary fuel for the brain and cerebral glucose consumption is proportionately high. It seems likely that the term infant brain can utilize ketones, lactate or amino acids as an alternative to glucose. This may explain the vulnerability of infants with nonketotic hypoglycemia to cerebral damage. Neurones and glial cells are susceptible to hypoglycemia, and vulnerable areas are the cerebral cortex, particularly posteriorly in the parieto-occipital region. Less commonly involved are neurones of the hippocampus, caudate nucleus and putamen but any level of the central nervous system may be involved including anterior horn cells of the spinal cord.

Definitions of hypoglycemia

Hypoglycemia was defined as a glucose concentration less than two standard deviations below the mean for a particular population; in the preterm it was defined as < 1.1 mmol/L during the first week of life but in full-term infants the corresponding value was < 1.7 mmol/L for the first 72 h of life and < 2.2 mmol/L after 72 h of age. These criteria imply that preterm infants compared to term are less prone to neurological impairment secondary to hypoglycemia and that resistance to hypoglycemia

is greatest in the immediate postpartum period. A more satisfactory approach is to define hypoglycemia in the context of acute or chronic neurological dysfunction, e.g. moderate hypoglycemia, < 2.6 mmol/L, in preterm infants is associated with reduced mental and motor developmental scores.[1126]

The *symptomatic* response of the neonate to low blood glucose is variable with nonspecific features including pallor, feeding difficulties, hypotonia, tachypnea, abnormal cry, jitteriness, apnea, irritability, coma and convulsions. This lack of symptomatic specificity can make the interpretation of biochemical hypoglycemia difficult such as the intensively cared for infant where comorbidities can cause similar clinical features or where symptomatic responses may be masked with therapeutic muscle paralysis, severe birth asphyxia or extreme prematurity. Hypoglycemia may be intermittent and it is important to check blood glucose at times of vague but suspicious symptoms.

Some otherwise well infants with low blood glucoses are *asymptomatic* suggesting that alternative substrates are available for brain metabolism. Such infants in general have a favorable prognosis. However, acute cerebral dysfunction, as measured by auditory and somatosensory evoked potentials, occurs in the majority of neonates when blood glucose levels fall below 2.6 mmol/L even though 50% of them were still asymptomatic.[1127]

As a consequence of these relationships between blood glucose levels and acute and chronic neurological dysfunction, *blood glucose levels < 2.6 mmol/L are accepted as indicating hypoglycemia* which requires treatment regardless of gestation or postnatal age.

On a practical basis, hypoglycemia can be subclassified into two main groups: *transient* and *persistent* hypoglycemia.[1128]

Transient neonatal hypoglycemia
IUGR

Infants with asymmetric growth retardation are particularly prone to hypoglycemia; the etiology can be multifactorial with metabolic demands of a relatively large brain, depleted glycogen, fat and protein reserves as well as limited gluconeogenic and ketogenic responses which in some are secondary to poorly coordinated counter-regulatory mechanisms.[1129] The presence of prematurity, birth asphyxia or polycythemia can compound the problem.

Enteral feeds should start within an hour of birth. Blood glucose should be monitored frequently, usually hourly, until normoglycemia is attained, when the interval can be extended to 2- then 4-hourly. If normoglycemia cannot be established, then a background intravenous infusion of dextrose is required, starting around 5 mg/kg/min but increasing if necessary the volume per kg and dextrose concentration. Enteral feeds are gradually increased in volume with reciprocal decreases in intravenous dextrose if normoglycemia is maintained. With the discontinuation of intravenous dextrose, the frequency of enteral feeds can be sequentially increased to 2-, 3- and 4-hourly if normoglycemia is established. In a minority of infants where sustaining normoglycemia is problematic and intravenous glucose requirements are high or prolonged, despite established enteral nutrition, concurrent pathology should be considered. Hypoglycemia in growth restricted infants may produce psychomotor delay[1130] and the problems of persistence of hypoglycemia beyond the neonatal period may be underdiagnosed in asymptomatic infants.[1131]

Prematurity

The immaturity of gluconeogenesis, glycogenolysis and limited glycogen and fat reserves make this group vulnerable to hypoglycemia. Early hypoglycemia, within 1 h of delivery, occurs in up to 70% of infants < 30 weeks' gestation before intravenous dextrose infusions are established and thereafter glucose homeostasis can be unstable in sick premature infants. Hypoglycemia is usually transient and correctable with dextrose infusions of 5 mg/kg/min but a higher caloric intake to meet energy demands, either parenterally or enterally, should also be established early. Preterm infants will only partially suppress endogenous glucose production with glucose infusions but also fail to inhibit proteolysis, and early introduction of complete parenteral nutrition (day 1) improves not

Table 12.103   Features of tumors presenting in the neonatal period

Tumor	Presentation	Investigations	Markers	Treatment	Incidence per 100 000 live births in UK	Notes
Teratoma a. Sacrococcygeal b. Head and neck	1. Prenatal US 2. Obvious mass at birth a. On buttocks: may be so large as to obstruct delivery b. On neck: may lead to airway obstruction	CT/MRI	1. Alpha-fetoprotein: raised malignant, normal benign 2. Beta human chorionic gonadotrophin often raised	1. Benign: surgery (remove coccyx or local recurrence common) 2. Malignant: surgery then chemotherapy (etoposide/ bleomycin/ carboplatin) UKCCSG results (Huddart et al[1111]) 3. Significant recurrence rates mandates long term follow-up (using AFP)	0.27	1. At birth 90% benign, 10% malignant (if presents after 2 yr, 90% malignant) 2. 4:1 females:males 3. 20% of those with intra-abdominal extension are malignant (Altman et al[1112]) 4. AFP raised in 70% malignant variety 5. Solid tumors are more likely to have malignant elements 6. Teratomas rarely present as retroperitoneal (abdominal) mass
Leukemia a. Acute myelogenous (nonlymphocytic)	1. Hepatosplenomegaly 2. Petechiae + bruising 3. Skin infiltration (nodules) 4. Respiratory distress (infiltration) 5. Bone pain 6. Meningeal involvement	1. WBC variable, blasts+++, platelets reduced 2. Bone marrow ± biopsy 3. Biopsy skin plaque	1. Enzymes 2. Monoclonal membrane markers 3. Chromosomes (Burmeister & Thiel,[1113] Robinson[1114])	Invariably fatal despite modern chemotherapy ± intrathecal methotrexate	0.29	1. 25% cases are Down syndrome 2. Differential = hemolytic disease, congenital infection, disseminated neuroblastoma 3. Skin lesions may suggest monocytic leukemia 4. Null ALL may rarely present neonatally
b. (Leukemoid reactions)	Down syndrome child with leukemoid blood reaction	1. WBC 2. Marrow		Spontaneous remission, support with platelets, blood, antibiotics, etc.		1. Down syndrome frequent but may be normal karyotype and phenotype 2. Indistinguishable from leukemia but regresses over 1–3 months
Neuroblastoma	1. Abdominal mass 2. SVC obstruction 3. Respiratory obstruction 4. Leukoerythroblastic anemia 5. Bluish subcutaneous nodules 6. Spinal cord compression with pain and paraplegia 7. Horner syndrome from cervical chain involvement	Stage i-confined to structure of origin ii, local unilateral spread iii, bilateral spread iv, remote disease ivs, i or ii with remote disease 1. 24 h catecholamine, VMA–HVA excretion 2. Calcification on X-ray 3. CT/MRI	1. VMA–HVA up in 95% 2. Vasointestinal peptide 3. Neurone specific enolase (Kintzel[1117]) 4. MYCN gene amplification (Schmidt et al[1118])	Stage i – total excision ii – maximal excision + chemotherapy iii – chemotherapy + excision iv – chemotherapy ivs – spontaneous regression usual Chemo usually etoposide and carboplatin	0.45	1. 1:40 neonatal autopsies (Guin et al[1115]) 2. Spontaneous regression common (Bolande[1116]) 3. 60% occur in abdomen or pelvis 4. Prognosis excellent – compare later childhood 5. Accounts for 30–50% neonatal malignancy 6. Mostly stage ivs 7. Associated congenital abnormalities are common (Isaacs[1119])

Tumor	Presentation	Investigations	Markers	Treatment	Incidence per 100 000 live births in UK	Notes
Soft tissue sarcomas Fibro-, spindle cell, leio-, myo-, rhabdomyo-, hemangiopericytomas	1. Mass – particularly in head and neck and extremities	1. Biopsy 2. CT/MRI	Gene markers allow better management and prognostication	1. Excision if possible 2. ± Cytotoxics at reduced dose	0.3	1. If benign soft tissue sarcomas are included the incidence is greater than either leukemia or neuroblastomas 2. Locally aggressive 3. Metastases rare (compare older age groups)
Renal (Bove[1120]) a. Nephroblastoma [Wilms' tumor (WT)]	1. Prenatal US 2. Postnatal abdominal mass 3. Hematuria (rare)	1. US 2. CXR (pulmonary metastases) 3. CT/MRI	1. Increased inactive renin (Johnston et al[1121]) 2. Gene markers (Bown et al[1122])	Stage 1, surgery + vincristine Stage 2, surgery + vincristine + actinomycin (chemo at 50% dose)	0.13	1. A neonatal renal mass is not likely to be malignant 2. True WTs are associated with aniridia, hemihypertrophy, Beckwith syndrome and UG abnormalities 3. Nephroblastomatosis is present in 1:400 autopsies (Machin[1123])
b. Congenital mesoblastic nephroma (more common – Bolande[1124])	1. Prenatal US 2. Postnatal abdominal mass 3. Hematuria (rare)	1. US 2. CXR (pulmonary metastases) 3. CT/MRI	1. Increased inactive renin (Johnston et al[1121]) 2. Gene markers (Bown et al[1122])	Stage 1 – surgery Stage 2 – surgery		1. Commoner than WT and do not metastasize 2. Outlook extremely good
CNS Astrocytomas, teratomas, ependymomas, oligodendrogliomas, craniopharyngiomas, medulloblastomas	1. Prenatal US 2. Hydrocephalus with cephalopelvic disproportion 3. Bulging fontanelle and suture separation 4. Increased ICP with vomiting 5. Convulsions	1. US 2. CT/MRI		1. Surgery 2. Probably not radiotherapy 3. ± Shunt 4. Chemotherapy	0.2	1. High incidence of teratomas 2. Predominantly supratentorial 3. Often large at diagnosis with frequent hemorrhage 4. Prognosis poor 5. Avoid RT until > 2 yr
Hepatoblastoma and hemangioendotheliomas	1. Hepatosplenomegaly 2. ± Respiratory distress 3. ± Gastrointestinal symptoms	1. US 2. CT/MRI	1. Alpha-fetoprotein	1. Surgery 2. ± Preoperative chemotherapy 3. ± low dose RT preop 4. Postop chemotherapy in low dose	0.05	1. A neonatal liver mass is more likely to be a hemangioma or mesenchymal hamartoma and present with cardiac failure or DIC 2. Secondary neuroblastoma or leukemia is commoner than hepatoblastoma in causing hepatomegaly 3. May be associated with hemihypertrophy or Beckwith syndrome

(Continued)

Table 12.103 Features of tumors presenting in the neonatal period—cont'd

Tumor	Presentation	Investigations	Markers	Treatment	Incidence per 100 000 live births in UK	Notes
Retinoblastoma	1. White eye and squint 2. Heterochromia iridis 3. Abdominal mass	1. CT/MRI head and eye 2. CT/MRI – body	1. Operation – enucleation 2. If bilateral – laser photo-coagulation and RT			1. 40–50 new cases per year UK 2. Family history in 10–25%, and this usually bilateral 3. Abnormality of chromosome 13 common 4. Note an orbital mass may be an orbital teratoma
Langerhans' cell histiocytosis (no longer considered a neoplastic process – Chu et al[1125])	1. Skin rash, particularly groins, axillae, neck, and behind the ears. Occasionally trunk. Usually brown–red raised macules which may coalesce or even ulcerate in the skin folds 2. A cradle cap-like skin lesion on the scalp 3. Respiratory distress from infiltration 4. Hepatosplenomegaly 5. Lymphadenopathy 6. Usually little systemic upset	1. Skin biopsy 2. Chest X-ray 3. Skeletal survey for punched out bone lesions 4. Osmolality of urine for diabetes insipidus		1. Spontaneous remission 2. If systemic upset/ progression, steroids ± vincristine or vinblastine ± VP16		1. Proliferation of tissue macrophages. T-suppressor lymphocytes normally control the macrophages

ALL, acute lymphoblastic leukemia; SVC, superior vena cava; VMA, vanillylmandelic acid; HVA, homovanillic acid; UG, urogenital; US, ultrasound; CT, computerized tomography; MRI, magnetic resonance imaging; ICP, intracranial pressure; RT, radiotherapy; DIC, disseminated intravascular coagulation.

only energy–nitrogen balance but reduces the frequency of hypoglycemic episodes.[1132] Hypoglycemia in preterm infants is common and this may impair the early detection of underlying metabolic abnormalities or genetic disorders affecting glucose homeostasis.[1133]

Birth asphyxia

Perinatal stress will deplete glycogen reserves and mitochondrial damage may uncouple oxidative phosphorylation with subsequent anaerobic glycolysis and generation of lactate. Hypoglycemia is usually transient and correctable with an intravenous infusion of dextrose at around 5 mg/kg/min. Hyperglycemia should be avoided as it may exacerbate existing metabolic acidosis and compound the hyperosmolar state. Prematurity, IUGR, adrenal hemorrhage and transient hyperinsulinism are common associations.

Neonatal sepsis

Hypoglycemia and sepsis are commonly associated. Pyrexia may increase the metabolic rate, caloric intake may be decreased and insulin sensitivity may be increased.

Neonatal hypothermia

Hypoglycemia is a common feature and glucose homeostasis should be established as part of the resuscitative measures.

Starvation

Failure to establish adequate enteral intake in full-term infants can result in hypoglycemia and this effect is exaggerated by IUGR, prematurity or birth asphyxia.

Congenital heart disease

Hypoglycemia per se can result in transient cardiomegaly. An association exists between hypoglycemia and acute congestive cardiac failure; the etiology of this may be multifactorial with decreased caloric intake, increased metabolic rate, decreased hepatic perfusion or even focal hepatic necrosis. Hypoglycemia has also been observed in children with severe congenital heart disease without cardiac failure. Management consists of restoration of normoglycemia with intravenous glucose and, in the longer term, adequate caloric intake.

Transient hyperinsulinemia
Infant of diabetic mother

Fetal blood glucose uptake is directly related to maternal blood glucose levels, and fetal hyperglycemia results in hyperplasia of the islets of Langerhans, increased peripheral insulin receptors, a decreased glucagon response to postnatal hypoglycemia and delayed evocation of hepatic gluconeogenic pathways. Meticulous control of maternal diabetes in pregnancy and labor can prevent or reduce the severity and frequency of neonatal hypoglycemia and the incidence of macrosomia, RDS, hyperbilirubinemia, polycythemia and hypocalcemia. The incidence of congenital malformations is higher and includes congenital heart disease, central nervous system abnormalities, vertebral anomalies and the caudal regression syndrome which may present in various forms including sacral agenesis, femoral hypoplasia or sirenomelia. Careful control of maternal diabetes preconceptually and in the early weeks of pregnancy reduces the incidence of malformations.

In the majority of infants, hypoglycemia is transient, <6 h, and asymptomatic. Blood glucose is usually monitored at birth, 1, 2, 4 and 6 h.

Table 12.104 Causes of neonatal hypoglycemia

Transient hypoglycemia	Persistent hypoglycemia
Intrauterine growth retardation	Hyperinsulinism
	Nesidioblastosis
	Insulinoma
Prematurity	Inborn errors of metabolism
	Glycogen storage disease
Birth asphyxia	GSD types I, III, IV
	Galactosemia
Neonatal sepsis	Hepatic gluconeogenic deficiencies
	Fructose-1,6-diphosphatase
Neonatal cold injury	Pyruvate carboxylase
	Phosphoenolpyruvate carboxylase
Starvation	Defects in amino acid metabolism
	Maple syrup urine disease
Congenital heart disease	Methylmalonic acidemia
	HMG-CoA lyase deficiency
Hyperinsulinism	Beckwith–Wiedemann syndrome
Infant of diabetic mother	Propionic acidemia
Erythroblastosis fetalis	Tyrosinemia type I
Maternal drugs	Mitochondrial fatty acid oxidation defects
Maternal glucose infusions	MCAD deficiency
Idiopathic hyperinsulinism	LCAD deficiency
	Electron transport defects
	MAD-S deficiency
	MAD-M deficiency
	RR-MAD deficiency
	Hormonal deficiencies
	Congenital hypopituitarism
	Cortisol deficiency
	Congenital glucagon deficiency

LCAD, long chain acyl-CoA dehydrogenase; MAD-M, mild multiple acyl-CoA dehydrogenase; MAD-S, severe multiple acyl-CoA dehydrogenase; MCAD, medium chain acyl-CoA dehydrogenase; RR-MAD, riboflavin responsive multiple acyl-CoA dehydrogenase.

Enteral feeds are established within the first hour and thereafter 2-hourly until normoglycemia is established. In the minority of infants hypoglycemia may be more prolonged, up to 3 days, and if normoglycemia is not maintained the infants may become symptomatic. In asymptomatic infants who fail to establish normoglycemia with enteral feeds, a single dose of glucagon (0.03–0.1 mg/kg) may prevent recurrence. In the sick infant, or those intolerant of enteral feeds or where hypoglycemia is prolonged, normoglycemia should be maintained by intravenous infusions of dextrose (4–8 mg/kg/min). Symptomatic hypoglycemia requires an initial bolus of intravenous dextrose (0.25–0.5 g/kg) and thereafter a constant intravenous infusion. Enteral feeds are introduced when appropriate with reciprocal reduction in intravenous infusion rates maintaining normoglycemia and avoiding abrupt changes, which can result in reactive hypoglycemia. Rarely, in prolonged hypoglycemia unresponsive to the above measures, hydrocortisone 5 mg/kg 12-hourly has been used.

Erythroblastosis fetalis
An association exists between moderate to severe erythroblastosis fetalis and hypoglycemia secondary to hyperinsulinism. It is estimated that around 20% of infants with cord Hbs < 10 g/dl will have significant hypoglycemia.

Beckwith–Wiedemann syndrome
Affected infants may have exomphalos, macroglossia, visceromegaly, giantism, parallel creases on the ear lobes, hyperinsulinemic hypoglycemia and an increased risk of Wilms' tumor and other malignancies.[1134] All features may not be present and infants with only giantism or exomphalos should have blood glucose levels monitored.

The majority of cases are sporadic with a female predominance but in familial forms possible patterns include autosomal dominant, multifactorial and autosomal dominant sex-dependent inheritance. This multigenic disorder is caused by dysregulation of the expression of imprinted genes in the 11p15 chromosomal region with close associations to insulin-like growth factor (IGF)-2 and tumor suppressor genes[1135] and genes implicated in regulation of insulin release.[1136]

Hypoglycemia is usually transient but may be prolonged and severe and occasionally persists into adulthood. Symptomatic hypoglycemia is estimated to occur in around 50% of individuals and may contribute to the mental deficiency recognized as part of this syndrome. The management of persistent hyperinsulinemia is discussed below.

Maternal drugs
Neonatal hyperinsulinemic hypoglycemia has been reported after maternal administration of chlorpropamide. Thiazide diuretics probably stimulate beta-cell function. Beta-mimetics stimulate insulin production and also reduce fetal hepatic glycogen deposition. Maternal valproate has been associated with infant hypoglycemia and features of withdrawal.
Intrapartum glucose infusion. Fetal insulin secretion can be induced by intrapartum maternal glucose infusions. The incidence of resultant neonatal hypoglycemia is related to maternal blood glucose levels particularly when above 6.6 mmol/L or when maternal glucose infusions are greater than 20 g/h.

Idiopathic transient neonatal hyperinsulinism
The etiology of hypoglycemia in growth retarded infants is multifactorial but in some infants where normoglycemia is not established by 72 h, in spite of adequate nutrition, the possibility of hyperinsulinism should be considered and investigated. This syndrome also occurs in full-term, appropriate for gestational age infants after normal pregnancies and deliveries, without maternal diabetes or drug ingestion. The resolution of transient hyperinsulinemia may take days, weeks or in some instances months, and on occasions diazoxide is required to control hypoglycemia. The etiology of transient hyperinsulinism is unknown; it is regarded as a temporary imbalance in the regulatory development of insulin secretion.

Persistent hypoglycemia
Persistent hyperinsulinemia
Recurrent or persistent hyperinsulinemia is the commonest cause of prolonged severe hypoglycemia during the first year of life. The majority of cases present with early neonatal hypoglycemia and are recognized causes of neonatal death and sudden infant death. Most are caused by loss of function of the beta-cell K_{ATP} channel function and causative mutations are found in related genes on chromosome 11 (11p15.1) with both autosomal recessive and dominant inheritance.[1137] Dominantly inherited activating mutations in the glutamate dehydrogenase (GLUD1) gene are associated with hyperammonaemia.[1138] There are mutations in the genes for glucokinase, L-3-hydroxyacyl-CoA dehydrogenase and carbohydrate-deficient glycoprotein syndrome type 1b.[1137] However, no genetic etiology has yet been determined for as many as 50% of the cases. In the neonatal group, the underlying pathology is usually diffuse hyperplasia of the endocrine pancreas whereas in older children solitary islet cell adenomas predominate. However, congenital islet cell adenomas are described in neonates and hyperinsulinemic hypoglycemia, whilst the features of diffuse hyperplasia have also been described in adults. Histological features vary widely. In most instances there is an increase in pancreatic beta-cells, either organized in groups or as individuals. Somatostatin cells are usually decreased.

Diagnosis of hyperinsulinism
Normoglycemia, > 2.6 mmol/L, may only be attained in infants with hyperinsulinism with increased glucose infusion rates (> 8 mg glucose/kg/min and in individual cases sometimes > 20 mg glucose/kg/min).

Insulin secretion is inappropriately high in comparison to simultaneously measured blood glucose. Insulin prevents ketogenesis by inhibiting lipolysis and in hyperinsulinism there is no increase in blood ketones. Insulin increases hepatic glycogen reserves and liver size may increase due to glycogen deposition. The measurement of blood ammonia is essential to exclude hyperammonemic hyperinsulinemia.[1138]

Management

Immediate management is to attain normoglycemia by intravenous infusion of dextrose, which may require rates > 15 mg/kg/min, and the establishment of a normal feed volume in content and volume for age. Hypostop and/or glucagon may be useful as a temporary measure, e.g. resiting intravenous sites. Diazoxide inhibits insulin release, acting as a specific K_{ATP} channel opener, and hence the therapeutic effects are variable and unpredictable, some infants showing initial benefit with a subsequent return to hypoglycemia. Diazoxide in oral dosage up to 5–20 mg/kg/day orally 8-hourly is usually combined with chlorothiazide 7–10 mg/kg/day in two divided doses, which potentiates its effects and reduces the associated water retention. Both these agents activate potassium channels by different mechanisms, the diuretic also being given concurrently for its ability to overcome the fluid-retaining effects of diazoxide. Other complications of diazoxide therapy include edema, nonketotic hyperosmolar coma, blood dyscrasias and generalized hypertrichosis. Nifedipine 0.25–2.5 mg/kg/day may be of value as an adjuvant therapy but the precise role of calcium channel blockers has not been defined. The advantages of the above treatments are that they can be given orally and second line drugs require intravenous or subcutaneous infusions. Glucagon infusions at rates between 5 and 10 mcg/kg/h in isolation, or at 1.0 mcg/kg/h combined with the synthetic somatostatin analogue octreotide 10 mcg/kg/h may be useful. Surgery may have to be considered in infants where hypoglycemia is still a significant problem despite adequate medical treatment. There is no diagnostic metabolic or endocrine test to distinguish a diffuse pancreatic disorder from an adenoma in a newborn or infant. In older children, distinguishing an adenoma from diffuse hyperplasia is now potentially possible using percutaneous transhepatic pancreatic venous sampling for insulin, glucose and C-peptide to identify 'hot spots' of insulin hypersecretion. Where no tumor is localized pre- or perioperatively, subtotal or total pancreatectomy may have to be considered, balancing the detrimental effects of hypoglycemia against postpancreatectomy diabetes. The management recommended above is consistent with the consensus view of the European Network for Research into Hyperinsulinism.[1137,1139]

Inborn errors of metabolism

Glycogen storage disease

Type I glycogen storage disease, glucose-6-phosphatase deficiency and associated transporter defects, may present in its severest form in the neonatal period with hepatomegaly, profound hypoglycemia and lactic acidosis.[1140]

Hepatic gluconeogenic enzyme deficiencies

Fructose-1,6-diphosphatase (p. 344) deficiency causes fasting hypoglycemia, lactic acidosis, ketosis, hyperuricemia and hyperlipidemia and hepatomegaly.

Phosphoenolpyruvate carboxykinase converts oxaloacetic acid to phosphoenolpyruvate. Defects of the enzyme restrict the utilization of lactate and gluconeogenic amino acids and this results in hypoglycemia, lactic acidosis and hyperalaninemia.

Pyruvate carboxylase converts pyruvate to oxaloacetic acid and deficiency limits gluconeogenesis from lactate and alanine. Hypoglycemia may not be a prominent feature as other gluconeogenic amino acids can enter the tricarboxylic acid cycle and be converted through oxaloacetic acid to glucose.

Galactosemia

Galactosemia commonly presents in the neonatal period with vomiting, diarrhea, failure to thrive, cataracts, hyperbilirubinemia and hypoglycemia.

Defects in amino acid metabolism

Maple syrup urine disease (p. 344) in neonates may present with vomiting, failure to thrive, a characteristic odor and hypoglycemia with a rapid progression to severe neurological symptoms.

3-hydroxy-3-methylglutaryl-CoA lyase deficiency (HMG-CoA lyase deficiency) has features of hypoglycemia, hyperammonemia and metabolic acidosis without ketonuria. Initial presentation may be in infancy, early childhood or the neonatal period.

Methylmalonic acidemia and propionic acidemia can present in the neonatal period with hypoglycemia and ketoacidosis.

Mitochondrial defects of fatty acid oxidation

Medium chain or general acyl-coa dehydrogenase (MCAD) deficiency (p. 337). This is the commonest of the inborn errors of mitochondrial fatty acid catabolism and crises are commonly precipitated by infectious episodes with fever, diarrhea, vomiting, poor feeding, lethargy and coma. Hepatomegaly is inconsistently present secondary to fatty infiltration. Hypoglycemia is always present. Plasma ammonia may be normal or slightly elevated. Ketonuria is classically absent or inappropriately low. MCAD deficiency has been reported as a cause of sudden and unexpected death in infants. The diagnosis of MCAD deficiency can be made by DNA molecular analysis (90% have a common allelic variant) and/or plasma acylcarnitines. The severity of clinical symptoms can be prevented by frequent meals, additional carbohydrate intake during stress and supplements of carnitine if required.

Long chain acyl-CoA dehydrogenase (LCAD) deficiency (p. 337). Attacks of hypoglycemia and hypotonia occur with hepatocardiomegaly during episodes of exacerbation. In a few infants a sensorimotor neuropathy or pigmentary retinopathy has been described. LCAD deficiency may initially present in the newborn infant.[1141]

Hormone deficiencies

Congenital hypopituitarism. Infants are usually at term, normally grown and without other central nervous system defects but there may be a conjugated or unconjugated hyperbilirubinemia. In affected males external genitalia may be small with micropenis. A few infants have associated midline defects including cleft lip and palate or septo-optic dysplasia. Pituitary hormone deficiencies may be partial or complete and are usually multiple. Cortisol and thyroid replacement may be required from the newborn period.

Cortisol deficiency states. Hypoglycemia may be seen in congenital adrenal hyperplasia, bilateral adrenal hemorrhage and congenital adrenal hypoplasia.

Congenital glucagon deficiency. Two cases have been reported and hypoglycemia described in both.

Investigation of hypoglycemia

The majority of infants will have transient hypoglycemia associated with a clinical risk factor (Table 12.104) and do not require extensive investigation. If hypoglycemia persists or is recurrent the infant should be investigated. The priority of investigations may be determined by clinical features or a family history of inborn errors of metabolism or sudden infant death syndrome.

Hypoglycemia should always be confirmed by formal laboratory analysis using a glucose oxidase method. Glucose requirements of the infant should be calculated in mg/kg/min.

Investigations include a full blood count to exclude polycythemia, a blood gas to determine the presence of a metabolic acidosis and plasma electrolytes, essential if adrenal dysfunction is suspected.

Plasma should be collected at the time of hypoglycemia for insulin, C-peptide, ketone bodies (usually beta-hydroxybutyrate), amino acids, lactate, growth hormone, cortisol and ACTH levels. Prior discussion with the investigating laboratory is essential.

Urine should be collected at around the time of hypoglycemia and screened for pH, reducing compounds (Clinitest), ketones and keto acid with 2,4-dinitrophenylhydrazine and for the variety of compounds that react with ferric chloride. Urine should also be analyzed for amino acid and organic acids.

Acylcarnitine profiles using tandem mass spectrometry on dried blood spots are increasingly being used as a diagnostic tool for disorders of intermediate metabolism. Complete characterization of a metabolic defect may require provocation or loading tests or enzyme studies on fibroblasts, leukocytes or tissue biopsies or analysis of DNA.

HYPERGLYCEMIA

Hyperglycemia in the newborn is defined as blood glucose > 7 mmol/L after a 4 h fast and this value may be used in the diagnosis and subsequent management of the rare phenomenon of transient neonatal diabetes mellitus.

Hyperglycemia in preterm infants

Hyperglycemia is commonly seen in nonfasting preterm infants where blood glucose concentrations > 10 mmol/L are not uncommon, may occasionally exceed 20 mmol/L and are most frequently associated with either dextrose infusions or parenteral nutrition. The pathogenesis of this hyperglycemia is uncertain and may include failure to suppress endogenous glucose production, an attenuated insulin release or a decrease in end-organ sensitivity to insulin.[1142] Some regimens for parenteral nutrition include insulin to control not only the hyperglycemia but to improve anabolism and activate lipid clearance.

The adverse effects of hyperglycemia include osmotic diuresis and dehydration, an increase in plasma osmolality and generation of a metabolic acidosis through lactate production.

Blood glucose values that constitute hyperglycemia in preterm infants are not well defined. Most consider it desirable to maintain blood glucose < 10 mmol/L, either by decreasing the amount of dextrose infused or prescribing insulin 0.05–0.1 IU/kg/h. Whether to control moderate hyperglycemia, 5–10 mmol/L, depends on clinical circumstances. Renal glucose thresholds can be as low as 5 mmol/L in extremely preterm infants and a glucose-induced osmotic diuresis might be an indication to treat with insulin.

Hyperglycemia is also associated with infection, intracranial hemorrhage, severe RDS, NEC, or pain. Aminophylline and dexamethasone may exacerbate hyperglycemic tendencies.

Hyperglycemia in full-term infants

Early postnatal hyperglycemia has been described in association with compensatory responses to birth asphyxia probably involving rapid mobilization of hepatic glycogen by a combination of glucagon and epinephrine secretion and suppression of insulin release. Early hypoglycemia is much more common in this group although late hyperglycemia and instability of glucose homeostasis is seen in severely birth asphyxiated infants who often have associated hepatic damage.

Transient diabetes mellitus

The onset of permanent diabetes mellitus is rare in infants less than 6 months of age. A transient form of diabetes mellitus may present as early as the first postnatal day or as late as 6 weeks of age. The infants are usually small for gestational age and present, in spite of adequate nutrition, as failure to thrive with wasting and dehydration but with a characteristic 'alert appearance'. Blood glucose levels are variable and may be as low as 13 mmol/L or as high as 110 mmol/L. Glycosuria leads to dehydration, which may be rapid in onset and severe. Ketonuria is absent or minimal, in contrast to later onset permanent diabetes mellitus. Insulin levels are inappropriately low for blood glucose concentrations. Management consists of correction of the dehydration and insulin to achieve normoglycemia. A few infants can be managed without continuation of insulin but the majority require regular insulin in dosage varying from 1 to 3 IU/kg/day for periods as short as 14 days or as long as 18 months. These infants are extremely insulin sensitive. After initial correction of dehydration and establishment of enteral feeds

they can usually be managed on a once or twice daily insulin regimen. In the majority, the dose of insulin can be tapered slowly before completely stopping.

In most instances, the condition is sporadic in occurrence although familial cases are reported with a few infants born to diabetic mothers. The etiology of transient diabetes mellitus is thought to be a temporary delay in maturation of beta-cell function and control. A few infants have been reported where there was an initial period of hypoglycemia, but within 3–14 days this gave way to hyperglycemia and transient diabetes mellitus. Permanent diabetes mellitus or later recurrence has been reported in a few individuals.

Leprechaunism. A constellation of mutations in the insulin receptor gene gives rise to this syndrome of IUGR with minor dysmorphic features and characterized by insulin resistance, elevated plasma insulin levels and glucose intolerance. Infants usually die in the first year of life.

DISORDERS OF CALCIUM AND MAGNESIUM METABOLISM

Normal fetal and neonatal calcium homeostasis

In utero, there is an active movement of calcium from mother to fetus such that by term fetal blood levels are approximately 10% higher than maternal values. This relatively hypercalcemic state suppresses fetal parathormone secretion and stimulates calcitonin release, conditions which favor fetal mineral deposition. After birth, the infant parathyroid remains suppressed and this transient hypoparathyroid state results in a fall in plasma calcium. In the normal term infant, the plasma calcium decreases during the first 24–72 h after birth, reaching values as low as 1.75–2.0 mmol/L. This state of relative hypocalcemia stimulates parathormone release and suppresses calcitonin secretion. Calcium levels gradually increase to within the normal range for infants by 4–5 postnatal days. This transition in calcium metabolism is usually without clinical features but symptomatic hypocalcemia develops if these mechanisms are delayed or exaggerated.

Hypocalcemia

Mild functional asymptomatic hypocalcemia occurs normally within the first few days of life but levels which constitute biochemical hypocalcemia can be defined as a corrected plasma calcium < 1.75 mmol/L or an ionized calcium < 0.625 mmol/L. Such infants are at risk of symptomatic hypocalcemia. The ionized state is the metabolically active form but dynamic equilibrium and interchange occurs between calcium in the various plasma fractions. Approximately 80% of protein-bound calcium is attached to albumin and the remaining 20% to globulin: binding to albumin is pH sensitive and acidosis results in an increased ionized calcium and alkalosis a decrease in ionized calcium. Clinical assessment of ionized calcium can be made by electrocardiographic observations of the corrected QT interval (QTc interval). It is prolonged >0.19 s in full-term infants and >0.20 s in preterm infants who have a low ionized calcium value.

There are a number of clinical conditions where hypocalcemia is the presenting feature (Table 12.105) but the commonest of these is early neonatal hypocalcemia.

Early neonatal hypocalcemia

The onset of early neonatal hypocalcemia is typically in the first few days of life and most often between 24 and 48 h. At greatest risk are LBW infants, both premature and growth retarded, birth asphyxiated infants and the infant of the diabetic mother.

Pathogenesis. The etiology of early neonatal hypocalcemia is usually multifactorial. Most symptomatic infants will have had suboptimal postnatal calcium intake. The postnatal rise in parathormone may be delayed in preterm infants, and indeed most infants with early neonatal hypocalcemia have low or undetectable levels of immunoreactive parathormone. Calcitonin levels are normally elevated in the early newborn period but exaggerated concentrations have been documented in premature as well

Table 12.105   Causes of neonatal hypocalcemia

Neonatal hypocalcemia
    Early
    Late (neonatal tetany)

Primary hypoparathyroidism
    Sporadic
    X-linked, autosomal dominant or recessive
    DiGeorge syndrome

Maternal hyperparathyroidism
    Vitamin D deficiency
    Vitamin D dependency
    Rickets/osteopenia of prematurity
    Primary hypomagnesemia

as in asphyxiated hypocalcemic infants. Hyperphosphatemia as a result of hypoxemic tissue damage or excessive catabolism releasing phosphate may lead to hypocalcemia. An intracellular movement of calcium can occur after hypoxic cell injury with depression of plasma calcium levels. Acute respiratory alkalosis can occur in ventilated infants resulting in reduced ionized calcium. Sodium bicarbonate administration or the use of citrated blood in exchange transfusions may create a metabolic alkalosis. Elevated plasma fatty acids generated from intravenous lipid infusions have been reported to lower ionized calcium levels.

Insulin-dependent diabetic mothers tend to have lower plasma magnesium levels throughout pregnancy, and infants have lower cord and 24 h postpartum plasma levels of calcium and parathormone. Chronic maternal hypomagnesemia may cause relative hypoparathyroidism in both mother and fetus. The majority of infants of diabetic mothers are asymptomatic but may show biochemical evidence of hypocalcemia and/or hypomagnesemia. In symptomatic infants with both biochemical abnormalities, the hypocalcemia and hypomagnesemia can be corrected with magnesium treatment.

Clinical features and course.   The symptoms and signs of early neonatal hypocalcemia occur when the calcium falls to < 1.75 mmol/L and can be difficult to differentiate from those of associated pathologies, e.g. HIE or intraventricular hemorrhage, or those of other metabolic abnormalities such as hyponatremia or hypoglycemia.

Management.   Early enteral calcium supplementation has been shown to prevent early neonatal hypocalcemia in preterm infants. Gastrointestinal irritation and increased stool frequency are the only significant side-effects. The vitamin D metabolites 25-hydroxycholecalciferol and 1,25-dihydroxycholecalciferol are also effective in raising plasma calcium levels but are rarely used.

Infants whose only pathology is early neonatal hypocalcemia and who have neurological symptoms should be treated as described for late neonatal hypocalcemia. Calcium gluconate 10% (1 ml/kg) can be given intravenously but cautiously over 10 min with ECG monitoring. Decreases in heart rate require slowing of the intravenous infusion or discontinuation. Maintenance calcium gluconate can be given continuously intravenously or orally (75 mg/kg/day). If peripheral intravenous infusions extravasate they may result in skin slough, tissue necrosis and calcification. The preferred method of maintenance, where there is no central line, is by the enteral route and calcium gluconate 10% 1–2 ml/kg 4- or 6-hourly is usually tolerated.

Late neonatal hypocalcemia (neonatal tetany)

Late neonatal tetany can be regarded as a form of transitory hypoparathyroidism but usually symptomatic hypocalcemia and tetany are only problematic in infants subsequently exposed to high phosphorus intake.

Pathogenesis.   Primary maternal hyperparathyroidism complicating pregnancy is rare but a temporary maternal hyperparathyroid state, secondary to vitamin D deficiency, may be more common. That this type of neonatal hypocalcemia is related to maternal vitamin D

deficiency is supported by nutritional studies and a seasonal incidence in spring and early summer in the northern hemisphere related to low sunshine exposure in the later months of pregnancy, with low levels of 25-hydroxycholecalciferol in both mothers and infants. Enamel hypoplasia is frequently found in affected infants and is indicative of disordered enamel formation during the last trimester of pregnancy.

Occurrence of neonatal tetany in a susceptible population is largely determined by the nature of the milk feed in the newborn period. Cows' milk contains 3–4 times as much phosphorus as human milk. Partially modified cows' milk formulae (particularly tinned evaporated milks), which still had high phosphorus content, were used routinely until the mid 1970s when the incidence of neonatal tetany was as high as 1% of formula-fed infants. With the introduction of feeds with a calcium and phosphorus content approximating to that of human breast milk, neonatal tetany is now rare.

Clinical features.   Late neonatal tetany usually occurs from the second half of the first week up to several weeks, classically in full-term infants born after a normal labor and delivery who are artificially fed. Although affected infants may have appeared a little jittery or tremulous with increasing tactile irritability of muscles, usually they have been otherwise well, feeding normally, responding normally and with a normal cry, before the sudden onset of convulsions.

Fits are usually transitory, lasting for a few seconds and usually focal in nature, and between convulsions the infant is alert. Jitteriness is evident on stimulation, the tendon reflexes are increased and increased muscle tone with extension, in the legs particularly, is usual. Trousseau's sign is seldom positive and Chvostek's sign, which can be elicited freely in the newborn infant, is of little value. Recovery may occur spontaneously, but in others fits may continue for several weeks unless treated.

Diagnosis.   The diagnosis is based on a low serum calcium, < 1.75 mmol/L, and a high serum phosphorus, > 2.6 mmol/L. Occasionally the serum calcium is not markedly lowered and the raised phosphorus level is probably a more important diagnostic criterion. There is usually an associated hypomagnesemia but this is moderate in degree, in the range 0.5–0.6 mmol/L.

The differential diagnosis of neonatal tetany from other types of convulsions usually rests on the absence of an abnormal birth history, the normal behavior of the infant between the attacks, apart from muscular irritability, the absence of other signs which would indicate intracranial birth injury and the presence of normal or increased deep tendon reflexes.

Treatment.   Treatment consists of calcium intravenously or orally, usually in the form of calcium gluconate 10% solution 5 ml/kg/d. Vitamin D has also been used in a dosage of 5000 IU/d orally. Although hypocalcemia is the most obvious biochemical abnormality, the most effective treatment is intramuscular magnesium sulfate (0.2 ml/kg 50% solution per dose), particularly when convulsions are occurring; this can be followed with a further one or two doses at 12-hourly intervals. Intramuscular magnesium controls hypocalcemic tetanic fits more effectively than calcium, and calcium more effectively than phenobarbital.

Prognosis.   The prognosis of neonatal tetany per se is good, most cases making a full recovery without sequelae. Where the hypocalcemia is secondary to an underlying disorder, the prognosis will be of that disorder.

Hypoparathyroidism

Primary hypoparathyroidism is a rare cause of hypocalcemia in the newborn. The diagnosis is confirmed by absent or low parathormone levels in the presence of hyperphosphatemia, hypomagnesemia and low alkaline phosphatase. Sporadic cases occur but most have a genetic basis, usually X-linked recessive, but autosomal recessive and dominant forms have been described.

DiGeorge syndrome is usually sporadic in occurrence and results from an embryological defect of the 4th branchial arch and derivatives of the 3rd and 4th pharyngeal pouches. The pattern of defects includes hypoplasia or absence of the parathyroids, hypoplasia or absence of the thymus and cardiovascular anomalies including aortic and truncal abnormalities with minor facial anomalies. The severity of the congenital heart disease usually determines the early progno-sis. The degree of hypoparathyroidism may be variable and transient forms have been described. The etiology is heterogeneous. Several dif-ferent chromosomal abnormalities have been described but deletions at 22q11.2 are most frequent. Teratogenic causes including retinoic acid and fetal alcohol syndrome are also described. Treatment of hypopara-thyroidism consists of supplementation with vitamin D_2 or its analogs 1alpha-hydroxycholecalciferol or 1,25-dihydroxycholecalciferol.

Maternal hyperparathyroidism

Primary maternal hyperparathyroidism is a rare complication of preg-nancy. Parathyroid adenomas are usually responsible but carcinoma has been described. The maternal diagnosis depends on the demonstra-tion of persistently high plasma calcium, elevated plasma parathormone and low urinary calcium and phosphorus. Complications in pregnancy include hyperemesis gravidarum, weakness, renal calculi, spontane-ous abortion and late fetal death. The most common neonatal compli-cation is hypocalcemic tetany, observed in around 50% of infants born to mothers with untreated disease. The unexpected occurrence of neo-natal tetany may provide the initial clue to the diagnosis of unsuspected maternal hyperparathyroidism. The etiology of neonatal hypocalcemia is thought to reflect prolonged parathyroid suppression from the chronic hypercalcemic state of mother and fetus. However, some infants have normal or elevated parathormone levels and the etiology may be more complex.

The clinical features are those of neonatal tetany. Hypomagnesemia is a frequent occurrence. Most cases of neonatal hypocalcemia second-ary to primary maternal hyperparathyroidism are transient but long term congenital hypoparathyroidism has been described.

Maternal medullary carcinoma of the thyroid

Maternal medullary carcinoma of the thyroid is associated with high calcitonin levels. In the one reported case of this disease, several chil-dren born prior to maternal diagnosis exhibited radiological features of osteopetrosis.

Hypercalcemia

Plasma calcium levels > 2.75 mmol/L (corrected) are generally regarded as constituting hypercalcemia. Clinical manifestations include weak-ness, irritability, hypotonia, poor feeding, weight loss, polyuria, poly-dipsia, constipation and vomiting. The major causes are idiopathic infantile hypercalcemia, hyperparathyroidism, benign familial hyper-calcemia, and vitamin D intoxication, and hypercalcemia associated with inadequate phosphorus intake in extremely immature infants.[1143]

Hypomagnesemia

Plasma magnesium levels in the newborn infant are relatively con-stant through the first week of life (range 0.59–1.15 mmol/L). Hypomagnesemia, < 0.6 mmol/L, does not usually occur during the first few days of life, nor in association with asphyxia, but most commonly occurs towards the end of the first week and later.

Isolated hypomagnesemia can occur as a primary cause of convul-sions but is usually associated with concomitant lowering of the plasma calcium as in late neonatal hypocalcemia. Milk formulae with high phosphorus loads predispose to hypocalcemia and also to hypomagne-semia. Neonatal hypomagnesemia is also associated with maternal mal-absorption, with parathormone deficiency in the infant, with a primary defect of magnesium absorption in the infant (p. 336) or with magne-sium binding by citrate in exchange transfusions.

Treatment of hypomagnesemia is by intramuscular injection of mag-nesium sulfate 50% 0.2 ml/kg dose. This can be repeated for one or two further doses at 12-hourly intervals. If both hypomagnesemia and hypo-calcemia are present, treatment with calcium alone may be ineffective. Improvement may only be achieved after magnesium is prescribed and this often results in the spontaneous rise in serum calcium level. The role of magnesium in relieving the symptoms of hypocalcemia may be due to its capacity to release ionized calcium for effective parathyroid function.

METABOLIC BONE DISEASE IN PRETERM INFANTS

Defective bone mineralization has been recognized in preterm infants for many years but the terminology used to describe this is confusing. The terms *rickets of prematurity* and *osteopenia of prematurity* have been used synonymously. *Osteopenia of prematurity* refers to skeleton hypominer-alization of the preterm infant compared to that resulting from in utero accretion of minerals.[1144] *Rickets of prematurity* implies the presence of radiologically detectable abnormalities, appearances which are histori-cally related to vitamin D deficiency in children, but similar appearances can occur in preterm infants with severe metabolic bone disease. The term osteoporosis has been used to describe radiological rarefaction of bone; where this occurs without obvious rachitic changes it represents a less advanced stage of metabolic bone disease. Substantial deminer-alization, quantified sensitively by means of photon absorptiometry or dual energy radiographic densitometry, can occur before radiological changes are obvious.

Pathogenesis

The etiology of metabolic bone disease in preterm infants is prob-ably multifactorial but a major component is as a consequence of a deficiency of calcium and phosphorus.

The vitamin D status of the infant at birth largely depends on the adequacy or otherwise of maternal vitamin D metabolism. In humans, 25-hydroxycholecalciferol crosses the placenta with a close correla-tion between maternal and cord blood levels both in term and preterm infants.

The preterm infant may not have full expression of hepatic 25-hydroxylation of vitamin D but the majority of studies would sup-port the concept that this ability appears to be achieved very early in postnatal life. Adequate serum levels can be achieved using vitamin D supplements as low as 400–500 IU/day for the first 1–3 months of life. Preterm infants are also capable of 1alpha-hydroxylation of vitamin D, based on serum estimation of 1,25-dihydroxycholecalciferol, which rises sharply during the first week of life when infants are supple-mented with very high vitamin D intakes. On more physiologi-cal dosage regimens of vitamin D, 500 IU/day, lower increments of 1,25-dihydroxycholecalciferol are seen over the first week of life but gradually reach maximal values around 3–4 weeks' postnatal age.

Calcium, unlike phosphorus, is not well absorbed from formula milks. The higher bioavailability in human milk can result in 70% absorption provided that phosphorus and vitamin D contents are adequate. In term milks, the absorption of calcium is in the range of 30–60%, and 80–95% of this absorbed calcium can be retained. Calcium absorption increases with both gestational age and postnatal age. Absolute calcium retention increases with the amount of calcium ingested and with higher calcium intakes can be greater in preterm infants than occurs in utero. The con-centration of calcium in the formula is therefore important, as is the quantity of milk consumed.

Preterm infants absorb phosphorus very efficiently (86–97% of intake) independent of the type of milk or the calcium or phosphorus concentration of that milk. Retention of absorbed phosphorus appears to be directly related to the rates of calcium and nitrogen retention. Calcium and phosphorus absorption are relatively independent. The renal absorption of phosphorus can be almost complete in preterm infants but fractional phosphorus excretion can be increased if phos-phorus is supplied in excess, either in absolute terms or in conditions of relative excess, if calcium is deficient.

The in utero accretion of calcium rises exponentially in the last tri-mester from 114 to 125 mg/kg/day (2.89–3.12 mmol/kg/d) at 26 weeks to 119–151 mg/kg/day (2.97–3.77 mmol/kg/d) at 36 weeks' gestation. Phosphorus accretion over this gestational age range is 60–85 mg/kg/d (1.94–2.74 mmol/kg/d).

The calcium and phosphorus contents of human milk or term for-mulae cannot meet the requirements of the preterm infants if accre-tion of these elements is to continue at intrauterine rates. For example, an extreme preterm infant fed a commercial term formula at 150 ml/kg/d would have a calcium intake of 65 mg/kg/d (1.6 mmol/kg/d) and a phosphorus intake of 40 mg/kg/d (1.6 mmol/kg/d). If the infant typically absorbed 50% of the calcium intake and 90% of the phosphorus intake, then this would give absorbed calcium of only 32 mg/kg/d (0.8 mmol/kg/d) and phosphorus of 36 mg/kg/d (1.2 mmol/kg/d) available for retention. Comparison of these figures with the in utero accretion rates shows how wide the deficits can be between prenatal and postnatal life.

Copper deficiency in preterm infants can easily be confused where the radiological findings are of osteoporosis, flaring of anterior ribs, cupping and flaring of metaphyseal regions of long bones and subperiosteal new bone formation. It is equally possible that deficiencies in other nutrients may contribute to metabolic bone disease in preterm infants.[1145]

Clinical features

The largest number of reports of metabolic bone disease is in extreme preterm infants.[1146] Skeletal mineralization may be compromised by prolonged intravenous nutrition with its inherent limitation of mineral intake as well as concerns about aluminum contamination, fluid restriction resulting in decreased intakes of calcium and phosphorus, prolonged immobility, chronic acidosis, treatment with dexamethasone or furosemide and the use of nonsupplemented human breast milk. Many of these factors are common to infants receiving prolonged intensive care.

In the majority of infants with metabolic bone disease there are no overt findings on clinical examination. Occasionally, clinical features are present in preterm infants with well-established and severe rachitic disease (Fig. 12.64). Metabolic bone disease in preterm infants can be

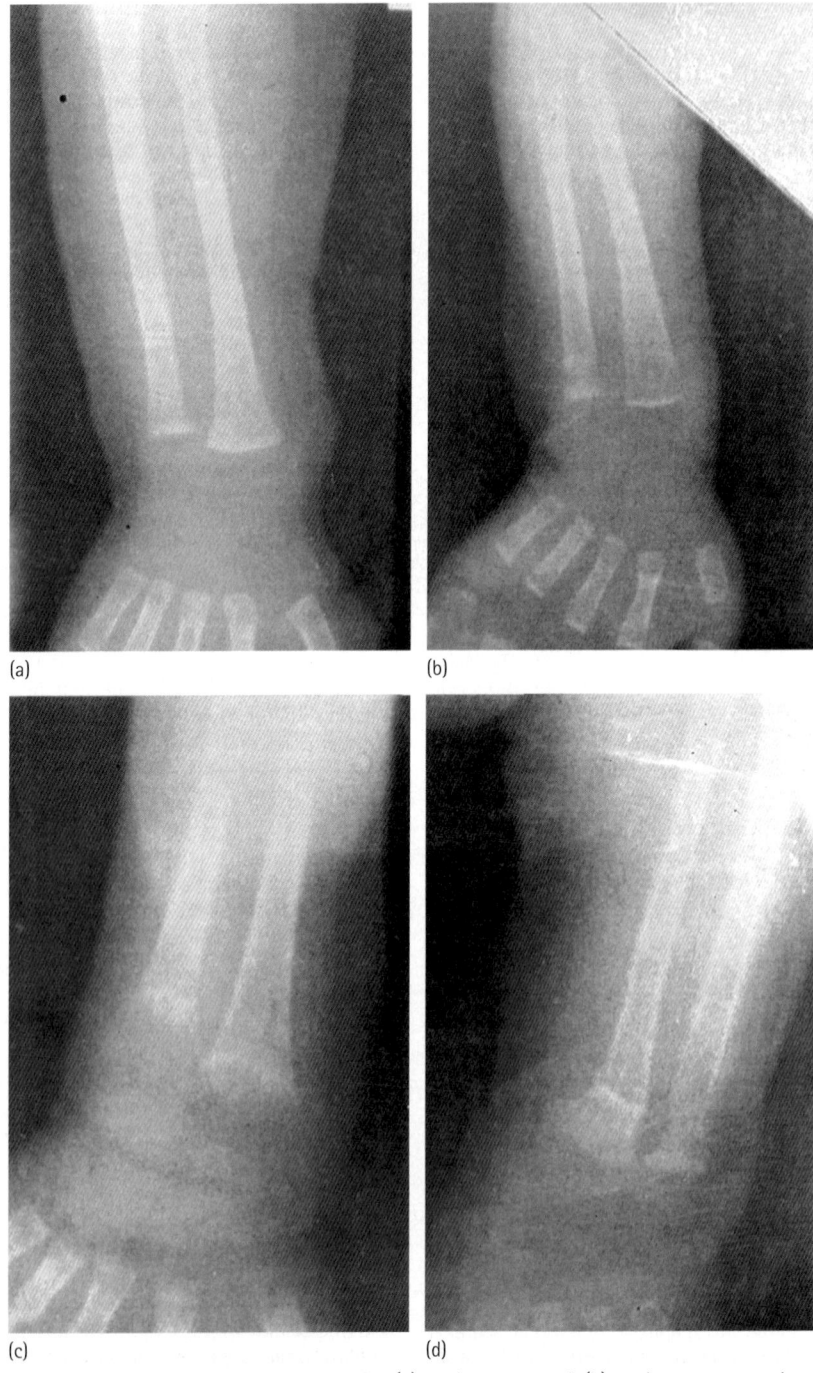

(a)   (b)

(c)   (d)

Fig. 12.64   X-ray grading of changes of rickets of prematurity at the wrist: (a) grade 0 = normal; (b) grade 1 = osteopenia only; (c) grade 2 = cupping and fraying of ulnar metaphysis; (d) grade 3 = spontaneous fracture in association with grade 2 changes. (X-rays by kind permission of Professor N McIntosh.)

associated with impairment of linear growth, spontaneous fractures and chronic respiratory distress.

Investigation and monitoring

Bone mineral content, usually of the forearm, can be measured directly with photon absorptiometry which, when specifically calibrated for small infants, can be precise and accurate.[1147] Bone mineralization is assessed relative to body weight or ulnar length and compared to a gestational age curve which represents in utero mineralization.[1148]

Photon absorptiometry is both sensitive and precise but it is expensive and the equipment bulk makes it impractical for routine use. Dual energy radiographic densitometry overcomes these difficulties.[1149] Radiographic densitometry has the advantage that bone mineral content can be assessed along the length of a bone or comparison easily made between bones. This may be important as bone mineralization is not uniform and wider assessment of the state of mineralization could be a major advantage.

The radiological changes of rickets in preterm infants are cupping and fraying of the metaphyses together with the loss of the provisional zone of calcification (Fig. 12.64). Periosteal reactions and fractures of bone may also occur. Substantial demineralization has to occur before radiological changes become apparent and a dependence solely on radiological methods will seriously underestimate the extent of the spectrum of metabolic bone disease.

In formula-fed infants, plasma calcium and phosphorus values are not good indicators of early metabolic bone disease with plasma calcium only falling significantly in the most severely affected infants with overt radiological rickets and phosphorus values often remaining unchanged. In infants fed human milk, phosphorus depletion is commonly recognized and characterized by hypophosphatemia, hypercalcemia, hypercalciuria, hypophosphaturia and elevated levels of plasma alkaline phosphatase.

Measurement of vitamin D metabolites has limited value in the diagnosis or management of rickets of prematurity.

The use and interpretation of plasma alkaline phosphatase activity as a marker of bone metabolism can be difficult in preterm infants; reference values have been established in cord blood from preterm and term infants and it appears that the bone alkaline phosphatase is the predominant isoenzyme.[1150] The liver isoenzyme is undetectable in preterm and term infant plasma. Plasma fetal intestinal alkaline phosphatase increases dramatically in preterm infants in the postnatal period, peaking at around 2 weeks of age when it may contribute up to 30% of the total activity in plasma. Thereafter peak plasma fetal intestinal alkaline phosphatase activity declines to negligible levels by 6–7 weeks' postnatal age. In preterm infants, total plasma alkaline phosphatase activity in the third trimester decreases with gestational age in infants 5–10 days postnatal age and total alkaline phosphatase has been correlated with the radiological features of rickets and used to monitor the effects of metabolic studies. The wide variability between individual infants makes its usefulness limited on single samples[1151] but sequential measurements from an infant increase its diagnostic value.

In spite of these constraints, the radiological appearances of rickets crudely correlate with total plasma alkaline phosphatase measurements although not with osteopenia or with bone mineral content as measured by photon absorptiometry. Equally high total plasma alkaline phosphatase activity, representing metabolic bone disease in preterm infants, has been related to slower growth rates in the neonatal period and to a significant reduction in attained length at 12 years.[1152] A combination of the criteria serum total alkaline phosphatase activity above 900 IU/L and serum inorganic phosphate concentrations below 1.8 mmol/L yields a sensitivity of 100% at a specificity of 70%. This is probably the best available screening method for low bone mineral density in preterm infants.[1153]

Management

The key to management of this disorder must be prevention, with a sufficient nutritive intake from early postnatal life to allow mineralization to proceed in a manner that avoids clinical and overt radiological rachitic changes. Whether we should go further than this goal and attempt to achieve 'normal' mineralization in all preterm infants using in utero mineral accretion rates is an unresolved question.[1154]

Although vitamin D deficiency is not a major factor in the etiology of metabolic bone disease of preterm infants, it facilitates normal mineralization with intakes of around 500–1000 IU/day. In established metabolic bone disease, modest increases in vitamin D intake, 1000–2000 IU/day, are used for short periods in conjunction with mineral supplementation.

Postnatal retention of calcium and phosphorus can approximate intrauterine accretion in term infants fed formulae with a calcium and phosphorus content similar to that of human milk.[1155] In contrast preterm infants approaching term may have a bone mineral deficit of as much as 30% when compared with full-term infants but have a rapid phase of mineral accretion between 40 and 60 weeks' postconceptional age which reduces perinatal mineralization deficits that might otherwise persist into childhood.[1148] Ziegler[1156] discusses this dilemma and emphasizes that the avoidance of overt bone disease should be the criterion for calcium and phosphorus need, rather than the necessity to achieve fetal accretion rates or in utero rates of mineralization. On this basis the requirement of the preterm infant for calcium and phosphorus is probably greater than the intake from human milk but less than that needed to achieve intrauterine accretion rates. The problem is how much calcium and phosphorus is required to avoid overt bone disease and how this need should be assessed.

A premature infant fed breast milk at 150 ml/kg/d receives an intake of around 55 mg/d (1.3 mmol/d) of calcium and 22 mg/d of phosphorus (0.5 mmol/d) and the postnatal increase in bone mineral content is significantly less than that expected in utero. Supplementation of maternal milk has been attempted with calcium or phosphorus or both, addition of skimmed components of donor human milk, mixing maternal milk with formula containing high concentration of calcium and phosphorus and the use of proprietary powdered fortifiers. Indiscriminate fortification of human milk is to be avoided and reserved for extreme preterm infants where this type of nutrition is the major dietary source. Phosphorus supplements of up to 9 mg/dl (13 mg/100 cal) have been used to maintain the plasma phosphorus greater than 1.5 mmol/dl and avoiding excess urinary calcium losses. Calcium supplements should not be given without a proportionate amount of phosphorus in order to maintain the calcium:phosphorus ratio in the range of 1.4–2.0. Simultaneous additions of calcium and phosphorus salts to milks may result in precipitation. This can be avoided by adding the phosphorus first (usually disodium phosphate) and then calcium (usually calcium gluconate/glubionate).

The American Academy of Pediatrics,[1157] on the basis of estimated fetal requirements, has advised enteral intakes of calcium 185–210 mg/kg/d (4.6–5.2 mmol/kg/d) and phosphorus 123–140 mg/kg/d (4–4.6 mmol/kg/d) for infants between 26 and 31 weeks' gestation. To achieve these intakes, assuming a fluid intake of 150 mg/kg/d, milk formulae would have calcium content of 126–140 mg/dl (3.1–3.5 mmol/dl) and phosphorus 82–93 mg/dl (2.7–3.1 mmol/dl). A more cautious approach has been adopted by the ESPGAN Committee on Nutrition,[1154] representing European opinion, where the recommended calcium content of formulae would be between 56 and 112 mg/dl (1.4–3.8 mmol/dl) with a phosphorus content 40–72 mg/dl (1.3–2.3 mmol/dl). LBW formulae currently available in the UK have calcium contents in the range 70–110 mg/dl (1.7–2.7 mmol/dl) and phosphorus 35–60 mg/dl (1.2–2.0 mmol/dl), compositions not optimal to meet mineral requirements if intrauterine accretion rates are to be attained but levels which should avoid overt bone disease. Excess dietary calcium can cause supermineralization in preterm infants, impede fat absorption as well as that of other minerals and lead to the risk of nephrocalcinosis.

Parenterally fed preterm infants are at particular risk of inadequate supply of calcium and phosphorus.[1158] The solubility and stability of mineral substrate in parenteral solutions depends on a number of factors and precipitation of salts can occur readily, resulting in blocked lines and the potential for microembolization of crystalline particles.

Most parenteral nutrition regimens can routinely achieve intakes of calcium of 1.5 mmol/kg/d and phosphorus 1.0 mmol/kg/d. By prescribing increased amounts of calcium and phosphorus only when fluid and amino acid intakes are appropriate, avoiding prolonged standing times, using the more soluble calcium gluconate rather than the chloride and only adding calcium and phosphorus to already diluted parenteral solutions, precipitation can be avoided and intakes of calcium around 2.0 mmol/kg/d and phosphorus 1.7 mmol/kg/d can be achieved. Further increments may be possible using monobasic potassium phosphate.[1159]

NEONATAL PRESENTATION OF INBORN ERRORS OF METABOLISM

Major advances have been made in the recognition and understanding of many inborn errors of metabolism. Prenatal diagnosis is available for a number of conditions, allowing parents to avoid recurrence of serious disease or early management and treatment to avoid deleterious effects on the developing fetus or neonate. Increasingly successful treatment regimens are being devised but the outcome may depend on the earliest possible recognition and institution of therapy. Only a minority of inborn errors of metabolism are routinely screened for in the newborn and early recognition is often dependent on maintaining a high index of clinical suspicion and a low threshold for sometimes basic and sometimes complex biochemical investigations. This is particularly true where inborn errors can present as acute and serious illness in the newborn period.

The aim of this review is to consider what inborn errors of metabolism can present in the newborn period and their clinical features. Although investigation and management will be discussed, details of individual inborn errors of metabolism are to be found in Chapter 26 and will be cross-referenced, as well as the relevant chapters of The Metabolic and Molecular Bases of Inherited Disease.[1160]

Acute metabolic disorders

A number of metabolic disorders can present with acute overwhelming symptoms in the newborn period, particularly the urea cycle defects, organic acidemias and certain aminoacidopathies (Table 12.106). The majority of these disorders have no detrimental effects on fetal

Table 12.106 Inborn errors of metabolism which may present as acute illness in the newborn period – see also Table 12.104 for metabolic diseases where hypoglycemia is a prominent feature

---

Disorders of amino acid metabolism
Maple syrup urine disease
Phenylketonuria
Tyrosinemia type I
Nonketotic hyperglycinemia
Hyperbeta-alaninemia
Sulfite oxidase deficiency
5,10-Methylene tetrahydrofolate reductase deficiency
Methylmalonic acidemia
Propionic acidemia
Isovaleric acidemia
Beta-methylcrotonylglycinuria
Multiple carboxylase deficiency
Hydroxymethylglutaryl-CoA lyase deficiency
Beta-ketothiolase deficiency
2-Methylacetoacetyl-CoA thiolase deficiency

Urea cycle defects
N-acetylglutamate synthase deficiency
Carbamyl phosphate synthetase deficiency
Ornithine transcarbamylase deficiency
Citrullinemia
Argininosuccinic aciduria
Arginase deficiency

---

development because placental perfusion can correct the disordered metabolic accumulation. As a consequence, the majority of infants are full-term, of normal growth, without dysmorphic features and asymptomatic at birth. An exception to this generalization is where the primary defect is in cerebral metabolism as occurs in nonketotic hyperglycinemia (p. 303). These infants may be born with established brain damage and have clinical features of hypertonia, lethargy, poor feeding and seizures, both grand mal and myoclonic. Other similar conditions include primary lactic acidosis, pyridoxine dependent seizures and primary molybdenum deficiency.

Fetal disorders of fatty acid oxidation can predispose the mother to acute fatty liver of pregnancy and the HELLP syndrome of hemolysis, elevated liver enzymes and low platelet count.[1161]

Many of the disorders are inherited as autosomal recessives and there may be a family history of consanguinity, previous perinatal loss or sudden and unexpected death in infancy. Autopsy findings may have been nonspecific and unrevealing unless specific biochemical investigations were done. A few inborn errors of metabolism have other patterns of inheritance, for example X-linked recessive in ornithine transcarbamylase deficiency.

Clinical features

The initial symptoms are usually nonspecific with lethargy, poor feeding, poor weight gain and vomiting. Diarrhea is less common but occurs in galactosemia (p. 338), and hereditary tyrosinemia (p. 282).

In the case of the infant who is well at birth, the onset of symptoms may be within a few hours of the first milk feed or may be delayed several weeks. The relationship to milk feeds and protein load may be further emphasized when the initial symptoms resolve with a period of intravenous fluids to recur again when milk feeds resume.

Progressive accumulation of intermediate metabolites may have neurotoxic effects and encephalopathic symptoms may accompany the presentation with apnea, periodic respirations, hypotonia, hypertonia, decerebrate rigidity, seizures and coma.

The clinical features ma y mimic the presentation of an acute neonatal infection. Indeed sepsis is a common accompaniment of acute exacerbations of metabolic disease as occurs in maple syrup urine disease (p. 338) galactosemia (p. 338) or the mitochondrial disorders of fatty acid oxidation (p. 338). Certain metabolic disorders may predispose to the risk of infection, for example infants with type I glycogen storage disease.

Clinical examination may be unrevealing. Tachypnea may indicate an underlying metabolic acidosis. Hepatomegaly, if present, classically occurs in the glycogen storage disorders, galactosemia and fructose-1, 6-diphosphatase deficiency (p. 338), but has been described in some infants with urea cycle defects, disorders of mitochondrial fatty acid oxidation and some aminoacidopathies. Cataracts can occur in newborn infants with galactosemia. Dislocated lens, characteristic of homocystinuria and sulfite oxidase deficiency have been described in the first month of life. Abnormal hair fragility can be present in some infants with argininosuccinic aciduria.

The majority of infants with acute metabolic disease do not have congenital anomalies but dysmorphic features are characteristic of some metabolic disorders such as multiple acyl-CoA dehydrogenase deficiency. Ambiguous genitalia occur in association with congenital adrenal hyperplasia.

Abnormal urinary odors may accompany metabolic disorders: phenylketonuria, mousy or musty; maple syrup urine disease, maple syrup or burnt sugar; isovaleric acidemia and glutaric acidemia type II, sweaty feet; beta-methylcrotonylglycinuria, cat urine.

Initial laboratory investigations

Infants suspected of acute metabolic disease require basic investigations not only for clinical management and resuscitation but to begin to determine the nature of the inborn error. Initial investigations should include blood gases, plasma electrolytes, plasma calcium and magnesium, blood glucose and lactate, blood ammonia and a full blood count.

Valuable information can be gained by urine screening tests for pH, glucose (Clinistix), reducing compounds (Clinitest), ketones and keto acids with 2,4-dinitrophenylhydrazine and for the variety of compounds that react with ferric chloride. Urinary creatinine may be useful for standardization of subsequent investigations. These basic investigations should be available in all laboratories and be completed rapidly.

The differential diagnosis and the diseases which may be detected by Clinitest, ferric chloride and 2,4-dinitrophenylhydrazine testing of urine are discussed in Chapter 26.

Metabolic acidosis. This is frequently present in acutely ill infants with galactosemia, gluconeogenic disorders, glycogen storage disease and particularly the organic acidemias (Tables 12.106 and 12.107). Infants with organic acidemias may have a significant anion gap. Secondary lactic acidosis is commonly seen in neonatal medicine secondary to infection, hypoperfusion syndromes, or indeed secondary to other metabolic disorders such as the organic acidemias, urea cycle disorders and fatty acid oxidation defects. Primary lactic acidoses occur in disorders of pyruvate metabolism and mitochondrial respiratory chain disorders.

Hyperammonemia. High blood ammonia is present in the primary enzyme defects of the urea cycle (Table 12.106) and is exacerbated by high protein loads whether from milk or endogenous catabolism. Secondary hyperammonemia is often seen in the defects of mitochondrial fatty acid oxidation and the organic acidemias and in glutamate dehydrogenase associated hyperinsulinemia. Delayed ontogeny of the urea cycle in preterm infants, particularly those receiving high protein loads, may result in severe hyperammonemia. Blood urea may be inappropriately low in the presence of defects of the urea cycle.

Hypoglycemia. This is the predominant feature of the primary defects of carbohydrate metabolism and of mitochondrial fatty acid oxidation but can be present in disorders of amino acid metabolism or organic acidemias. Hypoglycemia is frequently present as part of the acute metabolic derangements in maple syrup urine disease, methylmalonic acidemia, glutaric acidemia type II and hydroxymethylglutaryl-CoA lyase deficiency (Tables 12.106 and 12.107). The list is not exhaustive but illustrates the overlap in presentations and the importance of blood glucose estimations in the investigation, monitoring and treatment of suspected metabolic disease.

Liver transaminases and direct hyperbilirubinemia. Elevated plasma alanine or aspartate aminotransferases are secondary to hepatotoxicity and may be found in galactosemia, type III glycogen storage disease, disorders of mitochondrial fatty acid oxidation and the urea cycle defects (Tables 12.106 and 12.107). Indirect hyperbilirubinemia is a common accompaniment to a wide range of newborn illnesses. A direct hyperbilirubinemia occurs in those diseases that damage the liver, in particular galactosemia, fructose intolerance and tyrosinemia, but is also seen in the later stages of the presentation of urea cycle defects, mitochondrial respiratory chain disorders and alpha1-antitrypsin deficiency.

Thrombocytopenia and neutropenia. These can be features of methylmalonic acidemia, propionic acidemia, isovaleric acidemia and lysinuric protein intolerance. In addition neutropenia has been described in carbamyl phosphate synthetase deficiency and nonketotic hyperglycinemia and glycogen storage disease type Ib. Defective platelet function and bleeding may be a feature of type I glycogen storage disease (Tables 12.106 and 12.107). The presence of neutropenia and/or thrombocytopenia can be indices of sepsis in the newborn infant without an underlying inborn error of metabolism.

Anemia. Anemia can be found in association with methylmalonic aciduria and some of the aminoacidopathies.

Detailed laboratory investigation

If hyperammonemia, unexplained metabolic acidosis or hypoglycemia is present then it must be assumed that the symptoms are secondary to an inborn error of metabolism and the infant thoroughly investigated.[1162] This may require urine and plasma samples to be sent to a specialist laboratory. In general the full range of tests described below may have to be performed, but a priority order of investigations can be made on the basis of clinical features and the results of initial laboratory investigations, e.g. in the case of a vomiting infant with hypoglycemia and a urine positive for reducing substances, urine sugar chromatography will be the first priority to exclude galactosemia. Collaboration and discussion with personnel in a specialist center or laboratory is essential and investigations can be organized for each specific patient. Not all sick newborn infants with metabolic disease need have hypoglycemia, metabolic acidosis or hyperammonemia. For example, infants with nonketotic hyperglycinemia may have severe encephalopathic features but unrevealing initial investigations. Detailed metabolic investigation can be worth pursuing even when initial laboratory results are unsupportive.

Semiquantitative analysis of urinary amino acids can be made relatively rapidly by thin layer or paper chromatography complemented by a complete quantitative amino acid analysis of plasma, CSF or urine. Thin layer chromatography of sugars is semiquantitative but rapid and usually diagnostic. Urinary organic acids may initially be analyzed by gas–liquid chromatography but preferably by gas chromatography–mass spectrometry which can be analyzed from a dried blood spot. Lactate and pyruvate are generally measured in plasma but urinary lactate measurements have been advocated for the differentiation of a primary from a secondary lactic acidosis. Acylcarnitine profiles using tandem mass spectrometry on dried blood spots are increasingly being used as a diagnostic tool.

These investigations may give a definitive diagnosis or one where there is a high index of suspicion of a known inborn error to allow specific treatment to begin. Complete characterization of an inborn error of metabolism may require enzyme studies on fibroblasts, leukocytes or tissue biopsies including DNA analysis.

Acute management of severe metabolic disease

Cardiorespiratory homeostasis and the correction of biochemical abnormalities are the priorities. The extent of resuscitative measures will depend on the clinical state of the infant and often must be instituted before a definitive diagnosis has been established.

Intravenous fluids are given as 10% dextrose solutions; the volume/kg/h will depend on the state of hydration and the presence of renal dysfunction. Hypoglycemia and hypocalcemia should be corrected. Hyperglycemia can potentiate the generation of lactate and should be avoided. This is particularly important for patients with pyruvate dehydrogenase complex defects where a high carbohydrate load can dramatically accentuate the acidosis.

If the infant has a metabolic acidosis with no respiratory acidosis or a compensatory respiratory alkalosis, the metabolic acidosis should be

Table 12.107 Metabolic storage disorders which may be suspected in neonates

Glycogen storage diseases
Type I, glucose-6-phosphatase system deficiencies
Type II, Pompe disease, alpha-1,4-glucosidase deficiency
Type III, debrancher deficiency
Type IV, brancher deficiency

Lipid storage diseases
GM1 gangliosidosis type I
Gaucher disease
Niemann–Pick disease
Wolman disease
Farber disease

Mucolipidoses
Type I, sialidosis
Type II, I-cell disease

Mucopolysaccharidoses
Type VII, beta – glucuronidase deficiency

Glycoprotein storage disease
Fucosidosis

corrected with sodium bicarbonate, initially with boluses to raise the pH to around 7.25 and then maintained if necessary by a slow intravenous infusion. If the infant has a combined respiratory and metabolic acidosis with hypoventilation secondary to cerebral depression, the respiratory component is firstly corrected by ventilatory support and then the metabolic acidosis corrected. Oxygen should be given as required to maintain normal arterial saturation. Muscle paralysis with ventilatory support may have a specific role in severe lactic acidosis reducing the peripheral production. Blood gases and electrolytes should be monitored frequently.

Good tissue perfusion and oxygenation is essential to avoid secondary lactic acidosis. In correction of hypotension it may be more appropriate to use an inotropic agent such as dopamine rather than a high protein load of plasma or blood. As perfusion improves, the metabolic acidosis may worsen as peripheral lactate is brought into the circulation. Convulsive episodes may accentuate anaerobic metabolism and should be treated initially with intravenous phenobarbital.

Vitamins are essential cofactors for some enzymes and in certain conditions where cofactor function is abnormal reduced enzyme activity will result. Prescribing vitamins in doses approximately 10–100 times the daily requirement can increase enzyme activity in some instances. In the situation of the critically ill infant without as yet a specific diagnosis, the empirical use of multivitamins is justified but restricted to biotin (5–10 mg/d) and vitamin B_{12} (1–2 mg). Secondary carnitine deficiency is common in many metabolic disorders, especially fatty acid oxidation defects and organic acidemias, and should be given 100–200 mg/kg/d intravenously by continuous infusion or in divided doses orally.

Protein catabolism can exacerbate most of these disorders and once the infant's condition is stable and the acute metabolic derangements have been corrected, calories can be increased by gradual increments of intravenous 20% dextrose. Hyperglycemia is to be avoided as it may exacerbate metabolic acidosis, and insulin 0.05–0.1 IU/kg can be used to maintain blood glucose < 10 mmol/L. Insulin may also increase anabolism and can be used regularly 4- to 6-hourly. Once the infant is stabilized on this regimen and to maintain anabolism, protein and lipids are introduced either by the enteral or parenteral route. Protein can be commenced at 0.25–0.5 g protein/d and if tolerated increased by the same amount daily to reach 1.5 g/kg/d with an aimed caloric intake of 120 kcal/kg/d.

Specific treatments

Where investigations have led to a definitive diagnosis or where there is a high index of suspicion of an inborn error, specific treatment can be instituted. In urea cycle defects a combination of dietary therapy and the use of drugs to provide alternative pathways for nitrogen excretion can be successful. Arginine functions as an essential amino acid and supplementation will allow excretion of additional nitrogen. Amino acid nitrogen can be excreted as hippuric acid if sodium benzoate is given or as phenylbutylglutamine after administration of phenylbutyrate. The use of medications alone may be sufficient, but dialysis may also be necessary. Hemodialysis and hemodiafiltration are more effective than peritoneal dialysis, and the methods of choice in the initial treatment of urea cycle defects, maple syrup urine disease and the organic acidemias. Exchange transfusion should be reserved for exceptional circumstances.[1163]

Dietary modifications have been particularly successful in phenylketonuria and galactosemia Supplementations of vitamin B_{12} in methylmalonic aciduria, carnitine in organic acidemias, biotin in carboxylase deficiencies and pyridoxine in homocystinuria have been successful in some individuals. Alterations of the ratio of fat:carbohydrate:protein in the diet or the frequency of feeding have been used in the management of type I glycogen storage disease, fructose-1,6-diphosphatase deficiency and the mitochondrial disorders of fatty acid oxidation.

Investigations where death is inevitable

The situation may arise where death is inevitable but the exact definitive diagnosis of an inborn error of metabolism has not been conclusively established. In these circumstances it is important that the fullest information be obtained to advise parents of the risks of recurrence in subsequent pregnancies. An autopsy is vital and should preferably be performed soon after death. The majority of parents, with skilled counseling, will give postmortem permission before the infant dies. At autopsy liver, kidney, skeletal muscle, cardiac muscle and areas of brain thought to be involved should be fixed for light and electron microscopy. Duplicate frozen tissue samples suitable for cryostat sections should be obtained. Skin or pericardial fibroblast cultures should be established. A substantial amount of each tissue should be snap frozen as 0.5 cm³ cubes in liquid nitrogen and stored at −70 °C for subsequent enzyme analysis. Certain disorders, particularly those of membrane associated enzymes where there is a transport function or where the membrane is important for regulatory function or where the enzyme itself is sensitive to freeze-thaw, may best be analyzed on fresh tissue. Specialist advice should be sought. Some parents will agree only to a limited postmortem, for example wedge biopsy or needle biopsy of liver with skin samples for culture from the incision site. In these circumstances all available urine and plasma should be frozen and stored at −70 °C. Blood should be taken into EDTA tubes for subsequent DNA extraction, and a blood spot on a screening card for tandem mass spectrometry.

Suspected metabolic storage disorders

Metabolic storage disorders that may present in the newborn period are shown in Table 12.107 but often symptoms and a diagnosis may be delayed into infancy or childhood depending on the severity of the enzyme deficiency or the rate of expression of pathognomonic features. Infants with glycogen storage disease may have hepatomegaly with or without obvious hypoglycemic symptoms. Pompe disease, type II glycogen storage disease, is not associated with hypoglycemia but infants may have macroglossia, hypotonia, hepatomegaly and cardiomegaly with cardiac failure. In addition to type II glycogen storage disease, cardiac failure and cardiomyopathy may suggest a mitochondrial respiratory chain defect, or a long chain fatty acid oxidation disorder, and Barth syndrome in the presence of neutropenia.[1164]

The clinical features of the mucopolysaccharidoses are rarely fully expressed in the newborn period and a Hurler-like phenotype with coarse facies, macroglossia, limited growth and skeletal abnormalities is more likely to be a lipid or mucolipid storage disorder, particularly GM1 gangliosidosis type I or I-cell disease.

The acute infantile variant of Niemann–Pick disease, Gaucher disease and Wolman disease may present in the newborn period with hepatosplenomegaly, feeding difficulties, vomiting, choking, cyanotic episodes, failure to thrive and disorders of tone. Gastrointestinal symptoms are particularly marked in Wolman disease with diarrhea and abdominal distention in addition to vomiting.

Congenital disorders of glycosylation are rare and involve abnormal glycosylation of certain glycoproteins. The features are variable with cardiomyopathy, pericardial effusions, failure to thrive, abnormal fat distribution and facial dysmorphism.

Metabolic disorders associated with dysmorphic features

Inborn errors of metabolism may be associated with dysmorphic features suggesting that metabolic derangements in utero have disrupted normal fetal ontogeny, for example congenital adrenal hyperplasia in females is associated with ambiguous genitalia.

Peroxisomal disorders

Disorders of peroxisomal biogenesis as well as deficiencies in peroxisomal enzymes may present in the newborn period.[1165]

Zellweger syndrome (cerebrohepatorenal syndrome). This autosomal recessive condition has a number of characteristic clinical features. Craniofacial abnormalities may include a high forehead, flat occiput, wide sutures and fontanelle, absent orbital ridges, micrognathia, redundant neck skinfolds, external ear abnormalities and a high arched palate. The neurological features include hypotonia, poor feeding, nystagmus, hypo- or areflexia, psychomotor retardation and seizures. The brain is abnormal with disordered neuronal migration. Hepatomegaly is characteristic with prolonged jaundice, elevated transaminases and a progression to cirrhosis. The kidneys may show multiple cysts. Ocular abnormalities include cataracts, retinal pigmentation, optic disc pallor and Brushfield spots. Radiologically stippled calcification of the patella or acetabulum may be present. The clinical expression includes milder forms of the disorder.

Neonatal adrenoleukodystrophy. The clinical syndrome and symptoms may be indistinguishable from Zellweger syndrome.[1165] The presence of skeletal stippling or renal cysts at autopsy has not been encountered in neonatal adrenoleukodystrophy.

Infantile Refsum disease. This condition was originally described as an association between elevated plasma phytanic acid in infants with craniofacial dysmorphism, ocular abnormalities, hepatomegaly and psychomotor retardation with peroxisomes absent or deficient.

Rhizomelic chondrodysplasia punctata. This condition is inherited as an autosomal recessive and is characterized by short stature, symmetrical rhizomelia with marked shortening of the humerus and femur and punctate calcification around the epiphysis with coarse irregularity of the metaphyses. Severe psychomotor retardation, hepatomegaly and craniofacial dysmorphism with cataracts and corneal changes complete the clinical picture.[1165]

Hyperpipecolic acidemia. This syndrome is characterized by elevated pipecolic acid in plasma, minor dysmorphic features, optic disc pallor, retinal pigmentation, psychomotor retardation and hepatomegaly with abnormal liver function progressing to cirrhosis. The postmortem findings show adrenal abnormalities, renal cysts, normal neuronal migration in the brain and normal peroxisomes in liver but a disturbance in multiple peroxisomal function.

Zellweger-like phenotype with structurally intact peroxisomes. The biochemical defect in this group is confined to disorders of very long chain fatty acid oxidation or bile salt metabolism but with intact peroxisomes. It includes peroxisomal 3-oxoacyl-CoA thiolase deficiency, peroxisomal acyl-CoA oxidase deficiency and peroxisomal bifunctional enzyme deficiency.

Mitochondrial electron transport chain defects

Multiple acyl-CoA dehydrogenase deficiencies (MAD) or glutaric acidemia type II. MAD deficiency is classified into two variant forms: a severe (MAD-S) neonatal form or glutaric aciduria type II and a mild (MAD-M) variant with later onset.

In the severe neonatal form (MAD-S) two subgroups have been identified: those with congenital abnormalities and those without congenital abnormalities. In MAD-S deficiency with congenital abnormalities, characteristically the infants are born prematurely and may be growth retarded but develop a metabolic acidosis in the first 24 h of life with a characteristic odor of 'sweaty feet'. All patients have died in the first week of life. Neonatal MAD-S deficiency is associated with congenital abnormalities including facial dysmorphism, polycystic kidneys or some form of cystic dysplasia, cerebral abnormalities including disorders of migration, pulmonary hypoplasia, hypospadias and minor abnormalities of nail or palmar creases. At autopsy fatty infiltration of the liver, heart and kidneys is present. In MAD-S deficiency without congenital abnormalities the clinical course is similar with acidosis, hypoglycemia and odor; death occurs rapidly. Both types are a result of deficiencies of electron transport chain flavoprotein or its oxidoreductase. In MAD-M deficiency the clinical presentation is heterogeneous with first symptoms in the neonatal period, childhood or adulthood and characterized by vomiting, acidosis and hypoglycemia.

Riboflavin responsive defects of beta-oxidation or riboflavin responsive multiple acyl-CoA dehydrogenase deficiencies (RR-MAD). Some patients presenting with a Reye-like syndrome or hypoglycemia in the first years of life with defects in beta-oxidation have been shown to be responsive to riboflavin. The biochemical etiology remains to be confirmed but a therapeutic trial with riboflavin should be attempted in all patients presenting with an organic aciduria suggesting an MAD deficiency.

Disorders of cholesterol biosynthesis

Smith–Lemli–Opitz syndrome. Smith–Lemli–Opitz syndrome is a syndrome of mental retardation and multiple congenital malformations. The defect is thought to be in the gene coding for the enzyme 3beta-hydroxysteroid-delta7-reductase with the consequence of reduced conversion of 7-dehydrocholesterol to cholesterol and a reduction in plasma and tissue levels of cholesterol with an increase in 7-dehydrocholesterol. The common dysmorphic features are hypospadias, ambiguous genitalia, syndactyly of the toes, microcephaly, blond hair, anteverted nares, low set ears, palatal abnormalities, micrognathia, congenital heart disease and renal abnormalities. Severe feeding problems are common requiring nasogastric or gastrostomy feeding. Cholesterol supplementation of the diet may increase plasma cholesterol and in some has beneficial effects. Other disorders of cholesterol biosynthesis can result in dysmorphic features but are not as well characterized as Smith–Lemli–Opitz syndrome.[1166]

Miscellaneous conditions with newborn presentations

These include Crigler–Najjar syndrome; cystic fibrosis, alpha1-antitrypsin deficiency; Menkes' kinky hair syndrome, hypophosphatasia; hereditary orotic aciduria; glucose-6-phosphate dehydrogenase deficiency; pyruvate kinase deficiency; pyridoxine dependent convulsions; congenital erythropoietic porphyria; and aminolevulinate dehydratase porphyria (Ch. 26).

REFERENCES (*Level 1 Evidence)

Definitions – World Health Organization (WHO)

1. Human Embryo and Fertilisation Act 1990. London: HMSO; 1990.

The economics of newborn care

2. Macfarlane AJ, Mugford M, et al. Birth counts: statistics of pregnancy and childbirth; 2000. 2, 2nd edn. London: The Stationery Office.
3. Drummond MF, Sculpher MJ, Torrance GW, et al. Methods for the economic evaluation of health care programmes, 3rd edn. Oxford: Oxford University Press; 2005.
4. Gray A, Elbourne D, Dezateux C, et al. Economic evaluation of ultrasonography in the diagnosis and management of developmental hip dysplasia in the United Kingdom and Ireland. J Bone Joint Surg Am 2005; 87:2472–2479.
5. *Petrou S, Bischof M, Bennett C, et al. Cost-effectiveness of neonatal ECMO based on seven year results from the UK Collaborative ECMO Trial. Pediatrics 2006; 117:1640–1649.
6. *Zupancic J, Richardson DK, O'Brien BJ, et al and the Trial of Indomethacin Prophylaxis in Preterms Investigators. Retrospective economic evaluation of a controlled trial of indomethacin prophylaxis for patent ductus arteriosus in premature infants. Early Hum Dev 2006; 82:97–103.
7. Mugford M, Piercy J, Chalmers I. Cost implications of different approaches to the prevention of respiratory distress syndrome. Arch Dis Child 1991; 66:757–764.
8. Brocklehurst P, McGuire W. ABC of preterm birth: Evidence based care. BMJ 2005; 330:36–38.
9. Birnie E, Monincx WM, Zondervan HA, et al. Cost-minimization analysis of domiciliary antenatal fetal monitoring in high-risk pregnancies. Obstet Gynecol 1997; 89:925–929.
10. Torrance GW, Feeny D. Utilities and quality-adjusted life years. Int J Technol Assess Health Care 1989; 5:559–575.
11. Zupancic JA, Richardson DK, O'Brien BJ, et al. Cost-effectiveness analysis of predischarge monitoring for apnea of prematurity. Pediatrics 2003; 111:146–152.
12. Poley MJ, Stolk EA, Tibboel D, et al. The cost-effectiveness of treatment for congenital diaphragmatic hernia. J Pediatr Surg 2002; 37:1245–1252.
13. Poley MJ, Stolk EA, Langemeijer RA, et al. The cost-effectiveness of neonatal surgery and subsequent treatment for congenital anorectal malformations. J Pediatr Surg 2001; 36:1471–1478.
14. Boyle MH, Torrance GW, Sinclair JC, et al. Economic evaluation of neonatal intensive care of very-low-birthweight infants. N Engl J Med 1983; 308:1330–1337.
15. The Victorian Infant Collaborative Study Group. Economic outcome for intensive care of infants of birthweight 500–999 g born in Victoria in the

post surfactant era. J Paediatr Child Health 1997; 33:202–208.

16. Moya MP, Goldberg RN. Cost-effectiveness of prophylactic indomethacin in very-low-birth-weight infants. Ann Pharmacother 2002; 36:218–224.

17. Gennaro S. Leave and employment in families of preterm low birthweight infants. Image J Nurs Sch 1996; 28:193–198.

18. National Institute for Clinical Excellence (NICE). Guide to the methods of technology appraisal. London: NICE; 2004.

19. Broughton PMG, Hogan TC. A new approach to the costing of clinical laboratory tests. Ann Clin Biochem 1981; 18:330–342.

20. Brazier J, Deverill M, Green C, et al. A review of the use of health status measures in economic evaluation. Health Technol Assess 1999; 3:1–164.

21. EuroQol Group. EuroQol – a new facility for the measurement of health-related quality of life. Health Policy 1990; 16:199–208.

22. Torrance GW, Furlong W, Feeny D, et al. Multi-attribute preference functions: Health Utilities Index. PharmacoEcon 1995; 7:503–520.

23. Oostenbrink R, Moll HA, Essink-Bot ML. The EQ-5D and the Health Utilities Index for permanent sequelae after meningitis: A head-to-head comparison. J Clin Epidemiol 2002; 55:791–799.

24. Petrou S. Methodological issues raised by preference-based approaches to measuring the health status of children. Health Econ 2003; 12:697–702.

25. Raftery J. NICE: faster access to modern treatments? Analysis of guidance on health technologies. BMJ 2001; 323:1300–1303.

26. Petrou S, Henderson J. Preference-based approaches to measuring the benefits of perinatal care. Birth 2003; 30:217–226.

The normal fetal–neonatal transition

27. Bisset WM, Watt JB, Rivers JPA, et al. Postprandial motor response of the small intestine to enteral feeding in pre-term infants. Arch Dis Child 1989; 64:1356–1361.

28. Smith CA, Nelson NM. Physiology of the newborn, 4th edn. Springfield; Charles C Thomas; 1976.

Examination of the neonate

29. Wren C, Richmond S, Donaldson L. Presentation of congenital heart disease in infancy: implications for routine examination. Arch Dis Child 1999; 80:F49–F53.

30. Ward-Platt MP. Newborn screening examination (excluding congenital dislocation of the hip). Semin Neonatol 1998; 3:61–66.

31. Hall DMB, ed. Health for all children, 3rd edn. Oxford: Oxford University Press; 1996.

32. Wilson JMG, Jungner G. Principles and practice of screening for disease. Public Health Paper No 34. Geneva: World Health Organization; 1968.

33. Cochrane AL, Holland WW. Validation of screening procedures. Br Med Bull 1971; 27:3–8.

34. National Screening Committee. First report of the national screening committee. Health Departments of the United Kingdom. London: Department of Health; 1998. Also www.open.gov. uk/doh/nsc/nsch.htm.

35. Taylor D, Rice NSC. Congenital cataract, a cause of preventable child blindness. Arch Dis Child 1982; 57:165–167.

36. Taylor D. Congenital cataract: the history, the nature and the practice. Eye 1998; 12:9–36.

37. Rogers GL, Tishler CL, Tsou BH, et al. Visual acuities in infants with congenital cataracts operated on prior to 6 months of age. Arch Ophthalmol 1981; 99:999–1003.

38. Rahi JS, Dezateux C. National cross sectional study of detection of congenital and infantile cataract in the United Kingdom: role of childhood screening and surveillance. BMJ 1999; 318:362–365.

39. Silove ED. Assessment and management of congenital heart disease in the newborn by the district paediatrician. Arch Dis Child 1994; 70: F71–F74.

40. Richmond S, Wren C. Early diagnosis of congenital heart disease. Semin Neonatol 2001; 6:27–35.

41. Wren C, Richmond S, Donaldson L. Temporal variability in birth prevalence of cardiovascular malformations. Heart 2000; 83:414–419.

42. Ainsworth SB, Wyllie JP, Wren C. Prevalence and significance of cardiac murmurs in neonates. Arch Dis Child 1999; 80:F43–F45.

43. Abu-Harb M, Hey E, Wren C. Death in infancy from unrecognised congenital heart disease. Arch Dis Child 1994; 71:3–7.

44. Leck I. Congenital dislocation of the hip. In: Wald N, Leck I, eds. Antenatal and neonatal screening. Oxford: Oxford University Press; 2000.

45. Standing Medical Advisory Committee. Screening for the detection of congenital dislocation of the hip in infants. London: Department of Health and Social Security; 1969.

46. Godward S, Dezateux C. Surgery for congenital dislocation of the hip in the UK as a measure of outcome of screening. Lancet 1998; 351:1149–1152.

47. Chan A, Cundy PJ, Foster BK, et al. Late diagnosis of congenital dislocation of the hip and presence of a screening programme: South Australian population-based study. Lancet 1999; 354:1514–1517.

48. Gardiner HM, Dunn PM. Controlled trial of immediate splinting versus ultrasonographic surveillance in congenitally dislocatable hips. Lancet 1990; 336:1553–1556.

49. Langkamer VG, Clarke NMP, Witherow P. Complications of splintage in congenital dislocation of the hip. Arch Dis Child 1991; 66:1322–1325.

50. Committee on Quality Improvement and Subcommittee on Developmental Dysplasia of the Hip. Clinical practice guideline: early detection of developmental dysplasia of the hip. Pediatrics 2000; 105:896–905.

51. Lehmann HP, Hinton R, Morello P, et al. Developmental dysplasia of the hip practice guideline: technical report. Committee on Quality Improvement, and Subcommittee on Developmental Dysplasia of the Hip. Pediatrics 2000; 105:e57.

52. Scorer CG, Farrington G. Congenital deformities of the testis and epididymis. London: Butterworths; 1971:15–27.

53. Lee PA, O'Leary LA, Songer NJ, et al. Paternity after bilateral cryptorchidism. A controlled study. Arch Pediatr Adolesc Med 1997; 151:260–263.

54. Swerdlow AJ, Higgins CD, Pike MC. Risk of testicular cancer in a cohort of boys with cryptorchidism. BMJ 1997; 314:1507–1511.

55. Colodny AH. Undescended testes – is surgery necessary? N Engl J Med 1986; 314:510–511.

56. Hadziselimovic F. Pathogenesis of cryptorchidism. In: Kogan SJ, Hafez ESE, eds. Pediatric andrology. Vol 7. The Hague: Martinus Nijhoff; 1981.147–162.

57. Lee TWR, Skelton RE, Skene C. Routine neonatal examination: effectiveness of trainee paediatrician compared with advanced neonatal nurse practitioner. Arch Dis Child 2001; 85:F100–F104.

Labor ward routines

58. Vain NE, Szyld EG, Prudent LM, et al. Oropharyngeal and nasopharyngeal suctioning of meconium-stained neonates before delivery of their shoulders: multicentre, randomised controlled trial. Lancet 2004; 364:597–602.

*59. Wiswell TE, Gannon CM, Jacob J, et al. Delivery room management of the apparently vigorous meconium-stained neonate: results of the multicenter, international collaborative trial. Pediatrics 2000; 105:1–7.

60. Lundstrom KE, Pryds O, Greisen G. Oxygen at birth and prolonged cerebral vasoconstriction in preterm infants. Arch Dis Child Fetal Neonatal Ed 1995; 73:F81–F86.

61. Levy T, Blickstein I. Timing of cord clamping revisited. J Perinat Med 2006; 34:293–297.

62. Mercer JS. Current best evidence: a review of the literature on umbilical cord clamping. J Midwifery Womens Health 2001; 46:402–414.

Postnatnal ward routines

63. Danielson B, Castles AG, Damberg CL, et al. Newborn discharge timing and readmissions: California 1992–1995. Pediatrics 2000; 106:31–39.

64. Laing IA, Wong CM. Hypernatraemia in the first few days: is the incidence rising? Arch Dis Child Fetal Neonatal Ed 2002; 87:F158–F162.

65. Manning D, Todd P, Maxwell M. Jane, et al. Prospective surveillance study of severe hyper-bilirubinaemia in the newborn in the United Kingdom and Ireland. Arch Dis Child Fetal Neonatal Ed 2007; 92(5): F342–6.

*66. Zupan J, Garner P, Omari AA. Topical umbilical cord care at birth. Cochrane Database Syst Rev 2004; 3:CD001057.

Feeding the full–term newborn

67. Anderson GC, Moore E, Hepworth J, et al. Early skin-to-skin contact for mothers and their healthy newborn infants. Birth 2003; 30:206–207.

*68. Dyson L, McCormick F, Renfrew MJ. Interventions for promoting the initiation of breastfeeding. Cochrane Database Syst Rev 2005; 2.

69. www.unicef.org.

70. www.babyfriendly.org.uk/home.asp.

71. www.ic.nhs.uk/pubs/breastfeed2005.

72. Kramer MS, Guo T, Platt RW, et al. Breastfeeding and infant growth: biology or bias? Pediatrics 2002; 110:343–347.

*73. Simmer K. Longchain polyunsaturated fatty acid supplementation in infants born at term [Systematic Review]. Cochrane Database Syst Rev 2001; 4:CD000376.

74. Alm B, Wennergren G, Norvenius SG, et al. Breast feeding and the sudden infant death syndrome in Scandinavia, 1992–95. Arch Dis Child 2002; 86:400–402.

*75. Kramer MS, Chalmers B, Hodnett ED, et al. Promotion of Breastfeeding Intervention Trial (PROBIT): a randomized trial in the Republic of Belarus. JAMA 2001; 285:413–420.

76. Fewtrell MS. The long-term benefits of having been breast-fed. Curr Paediatr 2004; 14:97–103.

Perinatal asphyxia

77. ACOG, ACOG Committee Opinion. Number 326. Inappropriate use of the terms fetal distress and birth asphyxia. Obstet Gynecol 2005; 106: 1469–1470.

78. Phelan JP, Martin GI, Korst LM. Birth asphyxia and cerebral palsy. Clin Perinatol 2005; 32:61–76.vi.

79. Jacobsson B, Hagberg G. Antenatal risk factors for cerebral palsy. Best Pract Res Clin Obstet Gynaecol 2004; 18:425–436.

80. Atasay B, Arsan S. Organization of neonatal care services and its importance. J Perinat Med 2003; 31:392–394.

81. Lopez AD, Mathers CD. Measuring the global burden of disease and epidemiological transitions: 2002–2030. Ann Trop Med Parasitol 2006; 100:481–499.

82. Luo ZC, Karlberg J. Timing of birth and infant and early neonatal mortality in Sweden 1973–95: longitudinal birth register study. BMJ 2001; 323:1327–1330.

83. Apgar V. A proposal for a new method of evaluation of the newborn infant. Curr Res Anesth Analg 1953; 32:260–267.

84. AAPCFN. The Apgar score. Pediatrics 2006; 117:1444–1447.

85. Ellis M, Manandhar N, Manandhar DS, et al. An Apgar score of three or less at one minute is not diagnostic of birth asphyxia but is a useful screening test for neonatal encephalopathy. Indian Pediatr 1998; 35:415–421.

86. Asakura H, Ichikawa H, Nakabayashi M, et al. Perinatal risk factors related to neurologic outcomes of term newborns with asphyxia at birth: a prospective study. J Obstet Gynaecol Res 2000; 26:313–324.

87. Nelson KB, Ellenberg JH. Apgar scores as predictors of chronic neurologic disability. Pediatrics 1981; 68:36–44.

88. Bocking AD, White SE, Homan J, et al. Oxygen consumption is maintained in fetal sheep during prolonged hypoxaemia. J Dev Physiol 1992; 17:169–174.

89. Yager JY, Heitjan DF, Towfighi J, et al. Effect of insulin-induced and fasting hypoglycemia on perinatal hypoxic-ischemic brain damage. Pediatr Res 1992; 31:138–142.

90. Thorp JA, Rushing RS. Umbilical cord blood gas analysis. Obstet Gynecol Clin North Am 1999; 26:695–709.

91. Milsom I, Ladfors L, Thiringer K, et al. Influence of maternal, obstetric and fetal risk factors on the prevalence of birth asphyxia at term in a Swedish urban population. Acta Obstet Gynecol Scand 2002; 81:909–917.

92. Leuthner SR, Das UG. Low Apgar scores and the definition of birth asphyxia. Pediatr Clin North Am 2004; 51:737–745.

93. Hankins GD, Koen S, Gei AF, et al. Neonatal organ system injury in acute birth asphyxia sufficient to result in neonatal encephalopathy. Obstet Gynecol 2002; 99:688–691.

94. Trevisanuto D, Lachin M, Zaninotto M, et al. Cardiac troponin I in asphyxiated neonates. Biol Neonate 2006; 89:190–193.

95. Shah P, Riphagen S, Beyene J, et al. Multiorgan dysfunction in infants with post-asphyxial hypoxic-ischaemic encephalopathy. Arch Dis Child Fetal Neonatal Ed 2004; 89:F152–F155.

96. Kirino T. Delayed neuronal death in the gerbil hippocampus following ischemia. Brain Res 1982; 239:57–69.

97. Thoresen M, Satas S, Puka-Sundvall M, et al. Post-hypoxic hypothermia reduces cerebrocortical release of NO and excitotoxins. Neuroreport 1997; 8:3359–3362.

98. Edwards AD, Yue X, Squier MV, et al. Specific inhibition of apoptosis after cerebral hypoxia-ischaemia by moderate post-insult hypothermia. Biochem Biophys Res Commun 1995; 217:1193–1199.

99. WHO. Child health development: health of the newborn. Geneva: World Health Organization; 1991.

100. Sarnat HB, Sarnat MS. Neonatal encephalopathy following fetal distress. A clinical and electroencephalographic study. Arch Neurol 1976; 33:696–705.

101. Levene ML, Kornberg J, Williams TH. The incidence and severity of post-asphyxial encephalopathy in full-term infants. Early Hum Dev 1985; 11:21–26.

102. Yudkin PL, Johnson A, Clover LM, et al. Assessing the contribution of birth asphyxia to cerebral palsy in term singletons. Paediatr Perinat Epidemiol 1995; 9:156–170.

103. Nelson KB, Leviton A. How much of neonatal encephalopathy is due to birth asphyxia? Am J Dis Child 1991; 145:1325–1331.

104. Leonard JV, Morris AA. Diagnosis and early management of inborn errors of metabolism presenting around the time of birth. Acta Paediatr 2006; 95:6–14.

105. Liston R, Crane J, Hamilton E, et al. Fetal health surveillance in labour. J Obstet Gynaecol Can 2002; 24:250–276;quiz 277–280.

106. Draycott T, Sibanda T, Owen L, et al. Does training in obstetric emergencies improve neonatal outcome?. BJOG 2006; 113:177–182.

107. Patel D, Piotrowski ZH, Nelson MR, et al. Effect of a statewide neonatal resuscitation training program on Apgar scores among high-risk neonates in Illinois. Pediatrics 2001; 107:648–655.

108. Saugstad OD, Ramji S, Vento M. Resuscitation of depressed newborn infants with ambient air or pure oxygen: a meta-analysis. Biol Neonate 2005; 87:27–34.

109. Toet MC, Hellstrom-Westas L, Groenendaal F, et al. Amplitude integrated EEG 3 and 6 hours after birth in full term neonates with hypoxic-ischaemic encephalopathy. Arch Dis Child Fetal Neonatal Ed 1999; 81:F19–F23.

110. al Naqeeb N, Edwards AD, Cowan FM, et al. Assessment of neonatal encephalopathy by amplitude-integrated electroencephalography. Pediatrics 1999; 103:1263–1271.

111. Azzopardi D, Guarino I, Brayshaw C, et al. Prediction of neurological outcome after birth asphyxia from early continuous two-channel electroencephalography. Early Hum Dev 1999; 55:113–123.

112. Groenendaal F, de Vries LS. Selection of babies for intervention after birth asphyxia. Semin Neonatol 2000; 5:17–32.

113. Klinger G, Beyene J, Shah P, et al. Do hyperoxaemia and hypocapnia add to the risk of brain injury after intrapartum asphyxia? Arch Dis Child Fetal Neonatal Ed 2005; 90:F49–F52.

114. Yager JY, Armstrong EA, Jaharus C, et al. Preventing hyperthermia decreases brain damage following neonatal hypoxic-ischemic seizures. Brain Res 2004; 1011:48–57.

115. Beveridge CJ, Wilkinson AR. Sodium bicarbonate infusion during resuscitation of infants at birth. Cochrane Database Syst Rev 2006: CD004864.

116. Kecskes Z, Healy G, Jensen A. Fluid restriction for term infants with hypoxic-ischaemic encephalopathy following perinatal asphyxia. Cochrane Database Syst Rev 2005; CD004337.

117. Evans DJ, Levene MI. Anticonvulsants for preventing mortality and morbidity in full term newborns with perinatal asphyxia. Cochrane Database Syst Rev 2001; CD001240.

118. Gluckman PD, Wyatt JS, Azzopardi D, et al. Selective head cooling with mild systemic hypothermia after neonatal encephalopathy: multicentre randomised trial. Lancet 2005; 365:663–670.

119. Eicher DJ, Wagner CL, Katikaneni LP, et al. Moderate hypothermia in neonatal encephalopathy: efficacy outcomes. Pediatr Neurol 2005; 32:11–17.

120. Shankaran S, Laptook AR, Ehrenkranz RA, et al. Whole-body hypothermia for neonates with hypoxic-ischemic encephalopathy. N Engl J Med 2005; 353:1574–1584.

121. http://www.npeu.ox.ac.uk/toby, Whole Body Hypothermia for the Treatment of Perinatal Asphyxial Encephalopathy: The TOBY study.

122. ter Horst HJ, Sommer C, Bergman KA, et al. Prognostic significance of amplitude-integrated EEG during the first 72 hours after birth in severely asphyxiated neonates. Pediatr Res 2004; 55:1026–1033.

123. van Rooij LG, Toet MC, Osredkar D, et al. Recovery of amplitude integrated electroencephalographic background patterns within 24 hours of perinatal asphyxia. Arch Dis Child Fetal Neonatal Ed 2005; 90:F245–F251.

124. Shah S, Tracy M, Smyth J. Postnatal lactate as an early predictor of short-term outcome after intrapartum asphyxia. J Perinatol 2004; 24:16–20.

125. Buonocore G, Perrone S, Longini M, et al. Non protein bound iron as early predictive marker of neonatal brain damage. Brain 2003; 126:1224–1230.

126. Levene MI, Fenton AC, Evans DH, et al. Severe birth asphyxia and abnormal cerebral blood-flow velocity. Dev Med Child Neurol 1989; 31:427–434.

127. Rutherford MA, Pennock JM, Counsell SJ, et al. Abnormal magnetic resonance signal in the internal capsule predicts poor neurodevelopmental outcome in infants with hypoxic-ischemic encephalopathy. Pediatrics 1998; 102:323–328.

128. Hunt RW, Neil JJ, Coleman LT, et al. Apparent diffusion coefficient in the posterior limb of the internal capsule predicts outcome after perinatal asphyxia. Pediatrics 2004; 114:999–1003.

129. Inder TE, Hunt RW, Morley CJ, et al. Randomized trial of systemic hypothermia selectively protects the cortex on MRI in term hypoxic-ischemic encephalopathy. J Pediatr 2004; 145:835–837.

130. Elder DE, Zuccollo JM, Stanley TV. Neonatal death after hypoxic ischaemic encephalopathy: does a postmortem add to the final diagnoses? BJOG 2005; 112:935–940.

131. Squier W, Cowan FM. The value of autopsy in determining the cause of failure to respond to resuscitation at birth. Semin Neonatol 2004; 9:331–345.

Resuscitation in the newborn

132. Palme-Kilander C. Methods of resuscitation in low-Apgar-score newborn infants – a national survey. Acta Paed Scand 1992; 81:739–744.

133. Resuscitation at birth. The newborn life support provider course manual. London: Resuscitation Council; 2001.

134. International Liaison Committee on Resuscitation. The International Liaison Committee on Resuscitation (ILCOR) consensus on science with treatment recommendations for pediatric and neonatal patients: Pediatric basic and advanced life support. Pediatrics 2006; 117:e955–e977.

135. American Heart Association, American Academy of Pediatrics. 2005 American Heart Association (AHA) guidelines for cardiopulmonary resuscitation (CPR) and emergency cardiovascular care (ECC) of pediatric and neonatal patients: Neonatal resuscitation guidelines. Pediatrics 2006; 117:e1029–e1038.

136. Cross KW. Resuscitation of the asphyxiated infant. Br Med Bull 1966; 22:73–78.

137. Dawes GS. Foetal and neonatal physiology. Chicago: Year Book Medical Publishers; 1968.141–159.

138. Esmail N, Saleh M, Ali A. Laryngeal mask airway versus endotracheal intubation for Apgar score improvement in neonatal resuscitation. Egypt J Anesthes 2002; 18:115–121.

*139. Lokesh L, Kumar P, Murki S, et al. A randomised controlled trial of sodium bicarbonate in neonatal resuscitation – effect on immediate outcome. Resuscitation 2004; 60:219–223.

140. Skellet S, Mayer A, Durward A, et al. Chasing the base deficit: hyperchloraemic acidosis following 0.9% saline fluid resuscitation. Arch Dis Child 2000; 83:514–516.

*141. The Albumin Reviewers (Alderson P, Bunn F, Li Wan Po A, et al). Human albumin solution for resuscitation and volume expansion in critically ill patients. Cochrane Database Syst Rev 2004; 4:CD001208.

142. Kattwinkel J, Niermeyer S, Nadkarni V, et al. Resuscitation of the newly born infant: an advisory statement from the Pediatric Working Group of the International Liaison Committee on Resuscitation. Resuscitation 1999; 40:71–88.

*143. Tan A, Schulze A, O'Donnell CPF, et al. Air versus oxygen for resuscitation of infants at birth. Cochrane Database Syst Rev 2005; 2:CD002273.

*144. Ramji S, Ahuja S, Thirupuram S, et al. Resuscitation of asphyxic newborn infants with room air or 100% oxygen. Pediatric Res 1993; 34:809–812.

*145. Saugstad OD, Rootwelt T, Aalen O. Resuscitation of asphyxiated newborn infants with room air or oxygen: an international controlled trial: the Resair 2 study. Pediatrics 1998; 102:el.

*146. Vento M, Asensi M, Sastre J, et al. Resuscitation with room air instead of 100% oxygen prevents oxidative stress in moderately asphyxiated term neonates. Pediatrics 2001; 107:642–647.

147. Saugstad OD. Resuscitation of newborn infants with room air or oxygen. Semin Neonatol 2001; 5:233–239.

148. Milner A. The importance of ventilation to effective resuscitation in the term and preterm infant. Semin Neonatol 2001; 6:219–224.

149. Wiswell TE, Bent RC. Meconium staining and the meconium aspiration syndrome: unresolved issues. Ped Clin North Am 1993; 40:955–981.

*150. Cleary GM, Wiswell TE. Meconium-stained amniotic fluid and the meconium aspiration syndrome. An update. Ped Clin North Am 1998; 45:511–529.

*151. Hofmeyr GJ. Amnioinfusion for meconium-stained liquor in labor. Cochrane Database Syst Rev 2002; 1:CD000014.

*152. Fraser WD, Hofmeyr J, Lede R, et al. Amnioinfusion for the prevention of the meconium aspiration syndrome. N Engl J Med 2005; 353:909–917.

153. Carson B, Losey RW, Bowes WA. Combined obstetric and pediatric approach to prevent meconium aspiration syndrome. Am J Obstet Gynecol 1976; 126:712–717.

154. Wiswell TE. Handling the meconium-stained infant. Semin Neonatol 2001; 6:225–231.

*155. Halliday HL, Sweet D. Endotracheal intubation at birth for preventing morbidity and mortality in vigorous, meconium-stained infants born at term. Cochrane Database Syst Rev 2001; 1:CD000500.

*156. McCall EM, Alderdice FA, Halliday HL, et al. Interventions to prevent hypothermia at birth in preterm and/or low birthweight babies. Cochrane Database Syst Rev 2005; 1:CD004210.

*157. Rabe H, Reynolds G, Diaz-Rossello J. Early versus delayed umbilical cord clamping in preterm infants. Cochrane Database Syst Rev 2004; 4:CD003248.

158. Marlow N, Wolke D, Bracewell MA, et al. Neurologic and developmental disability at six years of age after extremely preterm birth. N Engl J Med 2005; 352:9–19.

159. Levene M. Is intensive care for very immature babies justified? Acta Paediatr 2004; 93:149–152.

The small for gestational age infant

160. Koh TH, Vong SK. Definition of neonatal hypoglycaemia: is there a change? J Paediatr Child Health 1996; 32:302–305.

161. McIntosh N, Kempson C, Tyler RM. Blood counts in extremely low birthweight infants. Arch Dis Child 1988; 63:74–76.

Developmental care

162. Salt A, Redshaw M. Neurodevelopmental follow-up after preterm birth: follow up after 2 years. Early Hum Dev 2006; 82:185–197.

163. Perlman JM. Neurobehavioral deficits in premature graduates of intensive care – potential medical and neonatal environmental risk factors. Pediatrics 2001; 108:1339–1348.

164. Anand KJS, Scalzo FM. Can adverse neonatal experiences alter brain development and subsequent behavior? Biol Neonate 2000; 77:69–82.

165. Als H. A synactive model of neonatal behavioral organization: framework for assessment of neurobehavioral development in the premature infant and for support of infants and parents in the neonatal intensive care environment. Phys Occup Ther Pediatr 1986; 6:3–54.

166. Lecanuet JP, Schaal B. Fetal sensory competencies. Eur J Obstet Gynecol Reprod Biol 1996; 68:1–23.

167. Wolf L, Glass R. Feeding and swallowing disorders in infancy: assessment and management. Arizona Therapy Skill Builders; 1992.

168. D'Elia A, Pighettia M, Vanacoreb F, et al. Vibroacoustic stimulation in normal term human pregnancy. Early Hum Dev 2005; 81:449–453.

169. Tan KH, Smyth R. Fetal vibroacoustic stimulation for facilitation of tests of fetal wellbeing. Cochrane Database Syst Rev 2006; 4.

170. Eswaran H, Lowery CL, Wilson JD, et al. Functional development of the visual system in human fetus using magnetoencephalography. Exp Neurol 2004; 190:S52–S58.

171. Kisilevsky BS, Hains SMJ, Lee K, et al. Effects of experience on fetal voice recognition. Psychol Sci 2003; 14:220–224.

172. Kiuchi M, Nagata N, Ikeno S, et al. The relationship between the response to external light stimulation and behavioral states in the human fetus: how it differs from vibroacoustic stimulation. Early Hum Dev 2000; 58:153–165.

173. Cornell EH, Gottfried AW. Intervention with premature human infants. Child Dev 1976; 47:32–39.

174. Abdulkader HM, Fleetwood-Walker S, McIntosh N. Long term sensitisation of mechanical somatosensory withdrawal responses following preterm birth. Pediatr Res 2005; 58:354.

175. Hellerud BC, Storm H. Skin conductance and behaviour during sensory stimulation of preterm and term infants. Early Hum Dev 2002; 70:35–46.

176. Peters KL. Infant handling in the NICU: does developmental care make a difference? An evaluative review of the literature. J Perinat Neonat Nurs 1999; 13:83–109.

177. Gorski PA, Huntington L, Lewkowicz DJ. Handling preterm infants in hospitals: stimulating controversy about timing of stimulation. Clin Perinatol 1990; 17:103–112.

178. Abdulkader HM, Freer Y, Fleetwood-Walker SM, et al. Bodily progression of motor responses to increasing mechanical force stimulation in the newborn infant and the effect of heel prick. Arch Dis Child 2007; (in Press)

179. Grunau RE, Weinberg J, Whitfield ME. Neonatal procedural pain and preterm infant cortisol response to novelty at 8 months. Pediatrics 2004; 114:e77–e84.

180. King JA, Barkley RA, Barrett S. Attention-deficit hyperactivity disorder and the stress response. Biol Psychiatry 1998; 44:72–74.

181. Mok Q, Bass CA, Ducker DA, et al. Temperature instability during nursing procedures in preterm neonates. Arch Dis Child 1991; 66:783–786.

182. Holsti L, Grunau R, Whifield M, et al. Behavioral responses to pain are heightened after clustered care in preterm infants born between 30 and 32 weeks gestational age. Clin J Pain 2006; 22:757–764.

183. Holsti L, Weinberg J, Whifield MF, et al. Relationships between adrenocorticotropic hormone and cortisol are altered during clustered nursing care in preterm infants born at extremely low gestational age. Early Hum Dev 2006; doi:10.1016/j.earlhumdev.2006.08.005

184. Schmidhauser J, Caflisch J, Rousson V, et al. Impaired motor performance and movement quality in very-low-birthweight children. Dev Med Child Neurol 2006; 48:718–722.

185. Fallang B, Oien I, Hellem E, et al. Quality of reaching and postural control in young preterm infants is related to neuromotor outcome at 6 years. Pediatr Res 2005; 58:347–353.

186. Samsom JF, de Groot L. The influence of postural control on motility and hand function in a group of 'high risk' preterm infants at 1 year of age. Early Hum Dev 2000; 60:101–113.

187. Vaivre-Douret L, Ennouri K, Jrad I, et al. Effect of positioning on the incidence of abnormalities of muscle tone in low-risk, preterm infants. Eur J Paediatr Neurol 2004; 8:21–34.

188. Corff KE, Seiderman R, Venkataraman PS, et al. Facilitative tucking: A non-pharmacologic comfort measure for pain in preterm infants. JOGNN 1995; 24:143–147.

189. Taquino L, Blackburn S. The effects of containment during suctioning and heelstick on physiological and behavioral responses of preterm infants. Neonatal Netw 1994; 13:55.

190. Harrison LL. The use of comforting touch and massage to reduce stress for preterm infants in the neonatal intensive care unit. Newborn and Infant Nursing Reviews 2001; 1:235–241.

191. Vickers A, Ohlsson A, Lacy JB, et al. Massage for promoting growth and development of preterm and/or low birth-weight infants. Cochrane Database Syst Rev 2004; 2.

192. Conde-Agudelo A, Diaz-Rossello JL, Belizan JM. Kangaroo mother care to reduce morbidity and mortality in low birthweight infants. Cochrane Database Syst Rev 2003; 2.

193. Philbin MK. The influence of auditory experience on the behavior of preterm newborns. J Perinatol 2000; 20:S76–S86.

194. Morris B, Philbin MK, Bose C. Physiological effects of sound on the newborn. J Perinatol 2000; 20:S54–S59.

195. Long JG, Philip AGS, Lucey JF. Excessive handling as a cause of hypoxaemia. Pediatrics 1980; 65:203–207.

196. Barreto ED, Morris BH, Philbin MK, et al. Do former preterm infants remember and respond to neonatal intensive care unit noise? Early Hum Dev 2006; 82:(11):703–707.

197. Slevin M, Farrington N, Duffy G, et al. Altering the NICU and measuring infants' responses. Acta Paediatr 2000; 89:501–502.

198. Standley JM. A meta-analysis of the efficacy of music therapy for premature infants. J Pediatr Nurs 2002; 17:107–113.

199. Therien JM, Worwa CT, Mattia FR, et al. Altered pathways for auditory discrimination and recognition memory in preterm infants. Dev Med Child Neurol 2004; 46:816–824.

200. Graven SN. Early neurosensory visual development of the fetus and newborn. Clin Perinatol 2004; 31:199–216.

201. Birch EE, O'Connor AR. Preterm birth and visual development. Semin Neonatol 2001; 6:487–497.

202. Lotas MJ. Effects of light and sound in the neonatal intensive care unit environment on the low-birth-weight infants. NAACOG's Clin Issues Perinat Women's Health Nurs 1992; 3:34–44.

203. Shogan MG, Schumann LL. The effect of environmental lighting on the oxygen saturation of preterm infants in the NICU. Neonatal Netw 1993; 12:7–13.

204. Mann NP, Haddow R, Stokes L, et al. Effect of night and day on preterm infants in a newborn nursery: randomized trial. BMJ 1986; 293:1265–1267.

205. Shiroiwa Y, Kamiya Y, Uchibori S, et al. Activity, cardiac and respiratory responses of blindfold preterm

infants in a neonatal intensive care unit. Early Hum Dev 1986; 14:259–265.

206. Rivkees SA. Emergence and influences of circadian rhythmicity in infants. Clin Perinatol 2004; 31:217–228.

*207. Brandon DH, Holditch-Davis D, Belyea M. Preterm infants born at less than 31 weeks' gestation have improved growth in cycled light compared to continuous near darkness. J Pediatr 2002; 140:192–199.

208. Schaal B, Hummel T, Sousignan R. Olfaction in the fetus and premature infant: functional status and clinical implications. Clin Perinatol 2004; 31:261–285.

209. Bartocci M, Winberg J, Ruggiero C, et al. Activation of olfactory cortex in newborn infants after odour stimulation. Pediatr Res 2000; 48:18–23.

210. Bartocci M, Winberg J, Papendieck G, et al. Cerebral hemodynamic response to unpleasant odors in the preterm newborn measured by near-infrared spectroscopy. Pediatr Res 2001; 50:324–330.

211. Sousignan R, Schaal B, Marlier L. Olfactory alliesthesia in human neonates: Prandial state and stimulus familiarity modulate facial and autonomic responses to milk odors. Psychobiology 1999; 35:3–14.

212. Pinelli J, Symington A. Non-nutritive sucking for promoting physiologic stability and nutrition in preterm infants. Cochrane Database Syst Rev 2005; 4.

213. Boyle EM, Freer Y, Khan-Orakzai Z, et al. Sucrose and non-nutritive sucking for the relief of pain in screening for retinopathy of prematurity: a randomised controlled trial. Arch Dis Child Fetal Neonatal Ed 2006; 91:F166–F168.

Special care – fluid balance

214. Simpson J, Stephenson TJ. Regulation of extracellular fluid volume in neonates. Early Hum Dev 1993; 34:179–190.

215. Tarnow-Mordi W, Shaw JCL, Liu D, et al. Iatrogenic hyponatraemia of the newborn due to maternal fluid overload: a prospective study. Br Med J 1981; 283:639–642.

216. Stephenson TJ, Broughton Pipkin F, Elias-Jones AC. A study of factors influencing plasma renin and renin substrate concentrations in the premature human newborn. Arch Dis Child 1991; 66:1150–1154.

217. Gill A, Yu WYH, Bajuk B, et al. Postnatal growth in infants born before 30 weeks' gestation. Arch Dis Child 1986; 61:549–553.

218. Hamilton CM, Shaw JCL. Changes in sodium and water balance, renal function and aldosterone excretion during the first seven days of life in very low birth weight infants. Pediatr Res 1984; 18:91.

219. Rees L, Shaw JCL, Brook CGD, et al. Hyponatraemia in the first week of life in preterm infants. Part II. Sodium and water balance. Arch Dis Child 1984; 59:423–429.

220. Keen DV, Pearse RG. Birthweight between 14 and 42 weeks' gestation. Diagn Histopathol 1985; 6:89–111.

221. Riesenfeld T, Hammerlund K, Sedin G. Respiratory water loss in fullterm infants on their first day after birth. Acta Paediatr Scand 1987; 76:647–653.

222. Hammarlund K, Sedin G, Stromberg B. Transepidermal water loss in newborn infants. VIII Relations to gestational age and post-natal age in appropriate and small for gestational age infants. Acta Paediatr Scand 1983; 72:721–728.

223. Stephenson TJ, Marlow N, Watkin S, et al. Pocket neonatology. In: Edinburgh: Churchill Livingstone; 2000;426.

224. Costarino A, Baumgart S. Modern fluid and electrolyte management of the critically ill premature infant. Pediatr Clin North Am 1986; 33:153–178.

225. Kavvadia A, Greenough A, Dimitriou G, et al. Randomised trial of fluid restriction in ventilated very low birthweight infants. Arch Dis Child 2000; 83:F91–F96.

226. Wilkins BH. Renal function in sick very low birthweight infants: 1. Glomerular filtration rate. Arch Dis Child 1992; 67:1140–1145.

*227. Bell EF, Acarregui MJ. Restricted versus liberal water intake for preventing morbidity and mortality in preterm infants (Cochrane Review). In: The Cochrane Library, Issue 3, 2001.CD000503. DOI: 10.1002/14651858.CD000503.

228. Von Stockhausen HB, Struve M. Die Auswirkungen einer stark unterschiedlichen parenteralen Flussigkeitszufuhr bei Fruhund Neugeborenen in den ersten drei Lebenstagen. Klin Padiatr 1980; 192:539–546.

229. Lorenz JM, Kleinman LI, Kotagal UR, et al. Water balance in very low-birth-weight infants: relationship to water and sodium intake and effect on outcome. J Pediatr 1982; 101:423–432.

230. Tammela OKT, Koivisto ME. Fluid restriction for preventing bronchopulmonary dysplasia? Reduced fluid intake during the first weeks of life improves the outcome of low birthweight infants. Acta Paediatr 1992; 81:207–212.

231. Bell EF, Warburton D, Stonestreet BS, et al. Effects of fluid administration on the development of symptomatic patent ductus arteriosus and congestive heart failure in premature infants. N Engl J Med 1980; 302:598–604.

*232. Osborn DA, Evans N. Early volume expansion versus inotrope for prevention of morbidity and mortality in very preterm infants (Cochrane Review). In: The Cochrane Library, Issue 2, 2001. Oxford: Update Software.

*233. Schierhout G, Roberts I. Fluid resuscitation with colloid or crystalloid solutions in critically ill patients: a systematic review of randomised trials. Br Med J 1998; 316:961–964.

234. Cartlidge PHT, Rutter N. Serum albumin concentration and oedema in the newborn. Arch Dis Child 1986; 61:657–660.

235. Obladen M, Sachsenweger M, Stahnke M. Blood sampling in very low birth weight infants receiving different levels of intensive care. Eur J Pediatr 1988; 147:399–404.

236. Jones RWA, Rochefort MJ, Baum JD. Increased insensible water loss in newborn infants nursed under radiant warmers. BMJ 1976; 2:1347–1350.

237. Wilkins BH. Renal function in sick very low birthweight infants: 2. Urea and creatinine excretion. Arch Dis Child 1992; 67:1146–1153.

238. Slater JE. Retention of nitrogen and minerals by babies 1 week old. Br J Nutr 1961; 15:83–97.

239. Flood RG, Pinelli RW. Urinary glycocyamine, creatine and creatinine. 1. Their excretion by normal infants and children. Am J Dis Child 1949; 77:740–745.

240. Barlow A, McCance RA. The nitrogen partition in newborn infants' urine. Arch Dis Child 1948; 23:225–230.

241. Tuck S. Fluid and electrolyte balance in the neonate. In: Roberton NRC, ed. Textbook of neonatology. London: Churchill Livingstone; 1986:162–177.

242. Greenough A, Gamsu HR, Greenall F. Investigation of the effects of paralysis by pancuronium on heart rate variability, blood pressure and fluid balance. Acta Paediatr Scand 1989; 78: 829–834.

243. Kavvadia V, Greenough A, Dimitriou G, et al. Comparison of the effect of two fluid input regimes on perinatal lung function in ventilated very low birthweight infants. Eur J Pediatr 1999; 158:917–922.

244. Modi N. Development of renal function. Br Med Bull 1988; 44:936–956.

245. Wilkins BH. Renal function in sick very low birthweight infants: 3. Sodium, potassium and water excretion. Arch Dis Child 1992; 67:1154–1161.

246. Stephenson TJ, Broughton Pipkin F, Hetmanski D, et al. Atrial natriuretic peptide in the preterm newborn. Biol Neonate 1994; 66:22–32.

247. Kojima T, Hirata Y, Fukuda Y, et al. Plasma atrial natriuretic peptide and spontaneous diuresis in sick neonates. Arch Dis Child 1987; 62:667–670.

248. Rascher W, Seyberth HW. Atrial natriuretic peptide and patent ductus arteriosus in preterm infants. Arch Dis Child 1987; 62:1165–1167.

249. Andersson S, Tikkanen I, Pesonen E, et al. Atrial natriuretic peptide in patent ductus arteriosus. Pediatr Res 1987; 21:396–398.

250. Wilkinson AR. Cardiovascular adaptation in the very immature infant. In: Whitelaw A, Cooke RWI, eds. The very immature infant less than 28 weeks' gestation. London: Churchill Livingstone; 1988.

251. Brion LP, Campbell DE. Furosemide for prevention of morbidity in indomethacin-treated infants with patent ductus arteriosus. Cochrane Database Syst Rev 2001; 3:CD001148.

Special care – sodium and potassium

252. Modi N. Sodium intake and preterm babies. Arch Dis Child 1993; 69:87–91.

253. Rees L, Shaw JCL, Brook CGD, et al. Hyponatraemia in the first week of life in preterm infants. Part II. Sodium and water balance. Arch Dis Child 1984; 59:423–429.

254. Broughton Pipkin F, Stephenson TJ. Plasma renin and renin substrate concentrations in the very premature human baby. Early Hum Dev 1989; 19:71.

255. Ito Y, Matsumoto T, Ohbu K, et al. Concentration of human atrial natriuretic peptide in cord blood and the plasma of the newborn. Acta Paediatr Scand 1988; 77:76–78.

256. Stephenson TJ, Broughton Pipkin F. Atrial natriuretic factor: the heart as an endocrine organ. Arch Dis Child 1990; 65:1293–1294.

257. Modi N. Development of renal function. Br Med Bull 1988; 44:936–956.

258. Wilkins BH. Renal function in sick very low birthweight infants: 3. Sodium, potassium and water excretion. Arch Dis Child 1992; 67:1154–1161.

259. Moniz CF, Nicolaides KH, Bamforth FJ, et al. Normal reference ranges for biochemical substances relating to renal, hepatic and bone function in fetal and maternal plasma throughout pregnancy. J Clin Pathol 1985; 38:468.

260. Guignard JP, John EG. Renal function in the tiny premature infant. Clin Perinatol 1986; 13: 377–401.

261. Wilkins B. The renal effects of aminophylline in very low birth weight neonates. Early Hum Dev 1986; 15:184–185.

262. Shortland D, Trounce JCQ, Levene MI. Hyperkalaemia, cardiac arrhythmias and cerebral lesions in high risk neonates. Arch Dis Child 1987; 62:1139–1143.

263. Lorenz M, Kleinman LI, Markarian K. Potassium metabolism in extremely low birth weight infants in the first week of life. J Pediatr 1997; 131:81–86.

264. Vasarhelyi B, Tulassay T, Ver A, et al. Developmental changes in erythrocyte Na+, K+ - ATPase subunit abundance and enzyme activity in neonates. Arch Dis Child 2000; 83:F135–F138.

265. Kemper MJ, Harps E, Hellwege HH, et al. Effective treatment of acute hyperkalaemia in childhood by short-term infusion of salbutamol. Eur J Pediatr 1996; 155:495–497.

266. Mahoney BA, Smith WAD, Lo DS, et al. Emergency interventions for hyperkalaemia. Cochrane Database Syst Rev 2005; 2:CD003235.

Special care – thermoregulation

267.   Cone TE. Perspectives in neonatology. In: Sith GF, Vidyasagar D, eds. Historical review and recent advances in neonatal and perinatal medicine. Mead Johnson Nutritional Division; Evansville, Ind, USA 1983.9–33.

268.   Silverman WA, Blanc WA. Effect of humidity on survival of newly born premature infants. Pediatrics 1957; 20:477–487.

269.   Silverman WA, Fertig JW, Berger AP. The influence of the thermal environment upon survival of newly born preterm infants. Pediatrics 1958; 22:876–885.

270.   Silverman WA, Agate FJ, Fertig JW. A sequential trial of the non-thermal effect of atmospheric humidity on survival of human infants. Pediatrics 1963; 31:710–724.

271.   Hazan J, Maag U, Chessex P. Association between hypothermia and mortality rate of premature infants – revisited. Am J Obstet Gynecol 1991; 164:111–112.

272.   CESDI project 27/28. www.cemach.org. uk/publications/p2728/mainreport.pdf(accessed 01.08.06).

273.   Costeloe K, Hennessy E, Gibson AT, et al, for the EPICure Study Group. The EPICure study: outcomes to discharge from hospital for infants born at the threshold of viability. Pediatrics 2000; 196:659–671.

274.   Lyon AJ, Oxley C. temperature on admission to the neonatal unit – a risk factor or just a reflection of condition at birth? Rhodes: Pediatr Res 2001; 49:200A.

275.   Hammerlund K, Sedin G. Transepidermal water loss in newborn infants. III. Relation to gestational age. Acta Paediatr Scand 1979; 68:795–801.

276.   Hammarlund K, Nilson GE, Oberg PA, et al. Transepidermal water loss in newborn infants. V. Evaporation from the skin and heat exchange during the first hours of life. Acta Paediatr Scand 1980; 69:385–392.

277.   Hammarlund K, Sedin G, Stromberg B. Transepidermal water loss in newborn infants. VIII. Relation to gestational age and postnatal age in appropriate and small for gestational age infants. Acta Paediatr Scand 1983; 72:721–728.

278.   Hey EN. Thermal neutrality. Br Med Bull 1975; 31:69–74.

279.   Hey EN. The relation between environmental temperature and oxygen consumption in the newborn baby. J Physiol 1969; 200:589–603.

280.   Harpin VA, Rutter N. Sweating in preterm babies. J Pediatr 1982; 100:614–618.

281.   Dollberg S, Xi Y, Donnelly MM. A non-invasive alternative to rectal thermometry for continuous measurement of core temperature in the piglet. Pediatr Res 1993; 34:512–517.

282.   Lyon AJ, Pikaar ME, Badger P, et al. Temperature control in infants less than 1000g birthweight in the first 5 days of life. Arch Dis Child 1997; 76:F47–F50.

283.   Messaritakis J, Agnostakis DH, Katerelos C. Rectal-skin temperature difference in septicaemic newborn infants. Arch Dis Child 1990; 65:380–382.

284.   Vohra S, Frent G, Campbell V, et al. Effect of polyethylene occlusive skin wrapping on heat loss in very low birth weight infants at delivery: a randomized trial. J Pediatr 1999; 134:547–551.

285.   Lyon AJ, Stenson B. Cold comfort for babies. Arch Dis Child 2004; 89:F93–F94.

286.   McCall EM, Alderdice FA, Halliday HL, et al. Interventions to prevent hypothermia at birth in preterm and/or low birthweight babies. Cochrane Database Syst Rev 2005; 1:CD004210.pub2.

287.   Gray PH, Flenady V. Cot-nursing versus incubator for preterm infants. Cochrane Database Syst Rev 2001; 2:CD003062.

288.   Sarman I, Tunnell R. Providing warmth for preterm babies by a heated, water filled mattress. Arch Dis Child 1989; 54:29–33.

289.   Greenabate C, Tafari N, Rao MR, et al. Comparison of heated water-filled mattress and space-heated room with infant incubator in providing warmth to low birthweight newborns. Int J Epidemiol 1994; 23:1226–1233.

290.   Sarman I, Can G, Tunell R. Rewarming preterm infants on a heated, water filled mattress. Arch Dis Child 1989; 64:687–692.

291.   Perlstein PH, Edwards NK, Sutherland JM. Apnea in premature infants and incubator air temperature changes. N Engl J Med 1970; 282:461–466.

292.   Perlstein PH, Edwards NK, Atherton HD, et al. Computer assisted newborn intensive care. Pediatrics 1976; 57:494–501.

293.   Sauer PJJ, Dane HJ, Visser HK. New standards for neutral thermal environment of healthy very low birthweight infants in week one of life. Arch Dis Child 1984; 59:18–22.

294.   Rutter N. Temperature control and its disorders. In: Rennie JM, ed. Roberton's Textbook of neonatology, 4th edn. Edinburgh: Churchill Livingstone; 2005.267–279.

295.   Harpin VA, Rutter N. Barrier properties of the newborn infant's skin. J Pediatr 1983; 102:419–425.

296.   New K, Flenady V, Davies MW. Transfer of preterm infants from incubators to open cot at lower versus higher body weight. Cochrane Database Syst Rev 2004; 2:CD004214.

297.   Flenady VJ, Woodgate PG. Radiant warmers versus incubators for regulating body temperature in newborn infants. Cochrane Database Syst Rev 2003; 4:CD000435.

298.   Shankaran S, Laptook AR, Ehrenkranz RA, et al. Whole-body hypothermia for neonates with hypoxic-ischemic encephalopathy. N Engl J Med 2005; 353:1574–1584.

299.   Battin MR, Penrice J, Gunn TR, et al. Treatment of term infants with head cooling and mild systemic hypothermia (35.0 degrees C and 34.5 degrees C) after perinatal asphyxia. Pediatrics 2003; 111:244–251.

Special care – enteral nutrition

*300.   Lucas A, Morley R, Cole TJ, et al. A randomised multicentre study of human milk versus formula and later development in preterm infants. Arch Dis Child Fetal Neonatal Ed 1994; 70:F141–F146.

301.   Kelly EJ, Newell SJ. Gastric ontogeny: clinical implications. Arch Dis Child 1994; 71:F136–F141.

302.   Bisset WM, Watt JB, Rivers JPA, et al. Ontogeny of fasting small intestinal motor activity in the human infant. Gut 1988; 29:483–488.

303.   Newell SJ, Sarkar PK, Durbin GM, et al. Maturation of the lower oesophageal sphincter in the preterm baby. Gut 1986; 29:167–172.

304.   McClean P, Weaver LT. Ontogeny of human pancreatic exocrine function. Arch Dis Child 1993; 68:62–65.

305.   Hamosh M. Digestion in the newborn. Clin Perinatol 1996; 23:191–210.

306.   Schmitz J. Digestive and absorptive function. In: Walker WA, Durie PR, Hamilton JR, et al, eds. Pediatric gastrointestinal disease. Philadephia: BC Decker; 1996.263–279.

307.   Jakobsson I, Lindberg T, Lothe L, et al. Human alpha lactalbumin as a marker of macromolecular absorption. Gut 1986; 27:1029–1034.

308.   McClure RJ, Chatrath MK, Newell SJ. Changing trends in feeding policies for ventilated preterm infants. Acta Paediatr 1996; 85:1123–1125.

309.   Malcolm G, Ellwood D, Devonald K, et al. Absent or reversed end diastolic flow velocity in the umbilical artery and necrotising enterocolitis. Arch Dis Child 1991; 66:805–807.

310.   Karsdrop VHM, Van-Vugt JMG, Van-Geijn HP, et al. Clinical significance of absent or reversed end diastolic velocity waveforms in umbilical artery. Lancet 1994; 344:1664–1668.

311.   Dorling J, Kempley S, Leaf A. Feeding growth restricted preterm infants with abnormal antenatal Doppler results. Arch Dis Child Fetal Neonatal Ed 2005; 90:F359–F363.

312.   Ewer AK, McHugo JM, Chapman S, et al. Fetal echogenic gut: a marker of intrauterine gut ischaemia. Arch Dis Child 1993; 69:510–513.

313.   Newell SJ. Enteral feeding in the micropremie. Clin Perinatol 2000; 27:221–234.

*314.   McClure RJ. Trophic feeding of the preterm infant. Acta Paediatr 2001; 90:(suppl):19–21.

315.   Hughes CA, Dowling RH. Speed of onset of adaptive mucosal hypoplasia and hypofunction in the intestine of parenterally fed rats. Clin Sci (Colch) 1980; 59:317–327.

316.   Goldstein RM, Hebiguchi T, Luk GD, et al. The effects of total parenteral nutrition on gastrointestinal growth and development. J Pediatr Surg 1985; 20:785–791.

317.   Berseth CL, Nordyke C. Enteral nutrients promote postnatal maturation of intestinal motor activity in preterm infants. Am J Physiol 1993; 264:G1046–G1051.

*318.   McClure RJ, Newell SJ. Randomised controlled trial of trophic feeding and gut motility. Arch Dis Child Fetal Neonatal Ed 1999; 80:F54–F58.

*319.   Schanler RJ, Shulman RJ, Lau C, et al. Feeding strategies for premature infants: randomized trial of gastrointestinal priming and tube-feeding method. Pediatrics 1999; 103:434–439.

*320.   McClure RJ, Newell SJ. Randomised controlled trial of clinical outcome following trophic feeding. Arch Dis Child Fetal Neonatal Ed 2000; 82:F29–F33.

321.   Lucas A, Bloom SR, Aynsley Green A. Gut hormones and 'minimal enteral feeding'. Acta Paediatr Scand 1986; 75:719–723.

*322.   McClure RJ, Newell SJ. Randomised controlled study of digestive enzyme activity following trophic feeding. Acta Paediatr 2002; 91:292–296.

*323.   Shulman RJ, Schanler RJ, Lau C, et al. Early feeding, feeding tolerance, and lactase activity in preterm infants. J Pediatr 1998; 133:645–649.

*324.   Tyson JE, Kennedy KA. Trophic feedings for parenterally fed infants. Cochrane Database Syst Rev 2005; 3:CD000504.

325.   Tsang RC, Lucas A, Uauy R, et al. Nutritional needs of the preterm infant: scientific basis and practical guidelines. In: Tsang RC, Lucas A, Uauy R, et al, eds. Baltimore: Williams & Wilkins; 1993.

326.   King C. Growth and outcome. Chapter 8. In: Jones E, King C, eds. Feeding and nutrition in the preterm infant. Edinburgh: Churchill Livingstone; 2005.

327.   ESPGAN. Nutrition and feeding of preterm infants. Acta Paediatr Scand 1987; 336:1–14.

328.   Tsang RC, Uauy R, Koletzko B, et al. Nutrition of the preterm infant: scientific basis and practical guidelines. 2nd edn. Cincinnati, Ohio: Digital Educational Publishing; 2005.

*329.   Lucas A, Morley R, Cole TJ, et al. Breast milk and subsequent intelligence quotient in children born preterm. Lancet 1992; 339:261–264.

330.   King C. Ensuring nutritional adequacy of human-milk-fed preterm babies. Chapter 3. In: Jones E, King C, eds. Feeding and nutrition in the preterm infant. Edinburgh: Churchill Livingstone; 2005.

*331.   Lucas A, Gore SM, Cole TJ, et al. Multicentre trial on feeding low birthweight infants: effects of diet on early growth. Arch Dis Child 1984; 59:722–730.

332.   Ewer AK, Durbin GM, Morgan ME, et al. Gastric emptying in preterm infants. Arch Dis Child 1994; 71:F24–F27.

*333.   Lucas A, Cole TJ. Breast milk and neonatal necrotising enterocolitis. Lancet 1990; 336:1519–1523.

334.   Wilson AC, Forsyth JS, Greene SA, et al. Relation of infant diet to childhood health: seven

year follow up of cohort of children in Dundee infant feeding study. BMJ 1998; 316:21–25.

*335. Lucas A, Brooke OG, Morley R, et al. Early diet of preterm infants and development of allergic or atopic disease: randomised prospective study. BMJ 1990; 300:837–840.

*336. O'Connor DL, Hall R, Adamkin D, et al. Growth and development in preterm infants fed long-chain polyunsaturated fatty acids: a prospective, randomized controlled trial. Pediatrics 2001; 108:359–371.

337. Standing Committee on Nutrition of the British Paediatric Association. Is breast feeding beneficial in the UK?. Arch Dis Child 1994; 71:376–380.

338. Barker DJ. Childhood causes of adult disease. Arch Dis Child 1988; 63:867–869.

*339. Singhal A, Cole TJ, Lucas A. Early nutrition in preterm infants and later blood pressure: two cohorts after randomised trials. Lancet 2001; 357:413–419.

340. Zeigler JB, Cooper DA, Johnson RO, et al. Postnatal transmission of AIDS-associated retrovirus from mother to infant. Lancet 1985; i:896–897.

341. Modi N. Donor breast milk banking. BMJ 2006; 333:1133–1134.

*342. McClure RJ, Newell SJ. Effect of fortifying breast milk on gastric emptying. Arch Dis Child Fetal Neonatal Ed 1996; 74:F60–F62.

343. Ewer AK, Yu VY. Gastric emptying in pre-term infants: the effect of breast milk fortifier. Acta Paediatr 1996; 85:1112–1115.

*344. Lucas A, Fewtrell MS, Morley R, et al. Randomized outcome trial of human milk fortification and developmental outcome in preterm infants. Am J Clin Nutr 1996; 64:142–151.

345. Schanler RJ, Abrams S. Postnatal attainment of intrauterine macromineral accretion rates in low birth weight infants fed fortified human milk. J Pediatr 1995; 126:441–447.

*346. Porcelli P, Schanler R, Greer F, et al. Growth in human milk-fed very low birth weight infants receiving a new human milk fortifier. Ann Nutr Metab 2000; 44:2–10.

*347. Lucas A, Morley R, Cole TJ, et al. Early diet in preterm babies and developmental status at 18 months. Lancet 1990; 335:1477–1481.

*348. Lucas A, Bishop NJ, King FJ, et al. Randomised trial of nutrition for preterm infants after discharge. Arch Dis Child 1992; 67:324–327.

*349. Cooke RJ, Griffin IJ, McCormick K, et al. Feeding preterm infants after hospital discharge: effect of dietary manipulation on nutrient intake and growth. Pediatr Res 1998; 43:355–360.

*350. Book LS, Herbst JJ, Atherton SO, et al. Necrotizing enterocolitis in low birth weight infants fed an elemental formula. J Pediatr 1975; 87:602–605.

*351. McKeown RE, Marsh TD, Amarnath U, et al. Role of delayed feeding and of feeding increments in necrotizing enterocolitis. J Pediatr 1992; 121:764–770.

352. Abnormal Doppler Enteral Prescription Trial (ADEPT). 2001 http://www.npeu.ox.ac.uk/adept

353. Bury RG, Tudehope D. Enteral antibiotics for preventing necrotising enterocolitis in low birthweight or preterm infants. Cochrane Database Syst Rev CD000405.

354. Boehm G, Fanaro S, Jelinek J, et al. Prebiotic concept for infant nutrition. Acta Paediatr Suppl 3003; 441:64–67.

355. Rautava S. Potential uses of probiotics in the neonate. Semin Fetal Neonatal Med 2007; 12:45–53.

*356. Premji S, Chessell L. Continuous nasogastric milk feeding versus intermittent bolus milk feeding for premature infants less than 1500 grams. Cochrane Database Syst Rev 2002; 4:CD001819.

357. Steer PA, Lucas A, Sinclair JC. Feeding the low birthweight infant. In: Sinclair JC, Bracken MB, eds. Effective care of the newborn infant. Oxford: Oxford University Press; 1992.94–140.

358. Leaf A. Vitamins for babies and young children. Arch Dis Child 2007; 92:160–164.

*359. Bishop NJ, King FJ, Lucas A. Increased bone mineral content of preterm infants fed with a nutrient enriched formula after discharge from hospital. Arch Dis Child 1993; 68:573–578.

360. Newell SJ, Booth IW, Morgan ME, et al. Gastro-oesophageal reflux in preterm infants. Arch Dis Child 1989; 64:780–786.

361. Patole S, Rao S, Doherty D. Erythromycin as a prokinetic agent in preterm neonates: a systematic review. Arch Dis Child Fetal Neonatal Ed 2005; 90:F301–F306.

Organization of neonatal intensive care services

362. British Association of Perinatal Medicine. Standards for hospitals providing neonatal intensive and high dependency care (2nd edn) and categories of babies requiring neonatal care. London: BAPM; 2001. Available: http://www.bapm.org/media/documents/publications/hosp_standards.pdf.

363. Marlow N, Gill AB. Establishing neonatal networks: the reality. Arch Dis Child Fetal Neonatal Ed 2007; 92:F137–F142.

364. Hamilton KE StC, Redshaw ME, Tarnow-Mordi W. Nurse staffing in relation to risk-adjusted mortality in neonatal care. Arch Dis Child Fetal Neonatal Ed 2007; 92:F99–F103.

365. Tucker J. UK Neonatal Staffing Study Group. Patient volume, staffing, and workload in relation to risk-adjusted outcomes in a random stratified sample of UK neonatal intensive care units: a prospective evaluation. Lancet 2002; 359:99–107.

366. Hall D, Wilkinson AR. Quality of care by neonatal nurse practitioners: a review of the Ashington experiment. Arch Dis Child Fetal Neonatal Ed 2005; 90:F195–F200.

367. Laing I, Ducker T, Leaf A, et al. Designing a neonatal unit. London: BAPM; 2004. Available: http://www.bapm.org/media/documents/publications/DesigningNNU_May2004b.pdf.

Practical parenteral nutrition

368. Wilson DC. Nutrition of the preterm baby. Br J Obstet Gynaecol 1995; 102:854–860.

369. Heird WC. Parenteral feeding. In: Sinclair JC, Bracken MB, eds. Effective care of the newborn infant. Oxford: Oxford University Press; 1992.141–160.

*370. Koletzko B, Goulet O, Hunt J, et al. Guidelines on paediatric parenteral nutrition of the European Society of Paediatric Gastroenterology, Hepatology and Nutrition (ESPGHAN) and the European Society for Clinical Nutrition and Metabolism (ESPEN), supported by the European Society of Paediatric Research (ESPR). J Pediatr Gastroenterol Nutr 2005; 41:S1–S87.

*371. McClure RJ, Newell SJ. Randomised controlled study of clinical outcome following trophic feeding. Arch Dis Child 2000; 82:F29–F33.

372. Wilson DC, McClure G. Energy requirements in sick preterm babies. Acta Paediatr 1994; 405: (Suppl):60–64.

373. Wilson DC, McClure G, Halliday HL, et al. Nutrition and bronchopulmonary dysplasia. Arch Dis Child 1991; 66:37–38.

*374. Wilson DC, Cairns P, Halliday HL, et al. Randomised controlled trial of an aggressive nutritional regimen in sick very low birthweight infants. Arch Dis Child 1997; 77:F4–F11.

375. Young VR, El-Khoury AE. The notion of nutritional essentiality of amino acids, revisited, with a note on the indispensable amino acid requirement in adults. In: Cynober LA, ed. Amino acid metabolism and therapy in health and nutritional disease. Boca Raton: CRC Press; 1995.191–232.

*376. McIntosh N, Mitchell V. A clinical trial of 2 parenteral nutrition solutions in neonates. Arch Dis Child 1990; 65:612–699.

*377. Cairns PA, Wilson DC, Jenkins J, et al. Tolerance of mixed lipid emulsion in neonates: effect of concentration. Arch Dis Child 1996; 75:F113–F116.

*378. Simmer K, Rao SC. Early introduction of lipids to parenterally fed preterm infants. Cochrane Database Syst Rev 2005; 2:CD005256.

*379. Cairns PA, Stalker DJ. Carnitine supplementation of parenterally fed neonates. Cochrane Database Syst Rev 2000; 4:CD000950.

*380. Soghier LM, Brian LP. Cysteine, cystine or N-acetyl cysteine supplementation in parenterally fed neonates. Cochrane Database Syst Rev 2006; 4:CD004869.

*381. Tubman TRJ, Thompson SW, McGuire W. Glutamine supplementation to prevent morbidity and mortality in preterm Infants. Cochrane Database Syst Rev 2005; 1:CD001457.

*382. Shah P, Shah V. Arginine supplementation for prevention of necrotising enterocolitis in preterm infants. Cochrane Database Syst Rev 2004; 4:CD004339.

383. ESPGHAN Committee on Nutrition. The need for nutrition support teams in paediatric units. Commentary by the ESPGHAN Committee on Nutrition. J Pediatr Gastroenterol Nutr 2005; 41:8–11.

*384. Foster J, Richards R, Showell M. Intravenous in-line filters for preventing morbidity and mortality in neonates. Cochrane Database Syst Rev 2006; 2:CD005248.

385. Wilmore DW, Dudrick SJ. Growth and development of an infant receiving all nutrients exclusively by vein. JAMA 1968; 203:860–868.

*386. Ainsworth SB, Clerihew L, McGuire W. Percutaneous central venous catheters versus peripheral cannulae for delivery of parenteral nutrition in neonates. Cochrane Database Syst Rev 2004; 2:CD004219.

Blood gases and respiratory support

387. Tremblay LN, Slutsky AS, Dreyfuss D, et al. Ventilator-induced lung injury. Mechanisms and correlates. In: Marini JJ, Slutsky AA, eds. Physiological basis of ventilatory support. New York: Marcel Dekker; 1999.

388. Clark RH, Gerstmann DR, Jobe AH, et al. Lung injury in neonates: causes, strategies for prevention, and long term consequences. J Pediatr 2001; 139:478–484.

389. Groneck P, Speer CP. Inflammatory mediators and bronchopulmonary dysplasia. Arch Dis Child Fetal Neonatal Ed 1995; 73:F1–F3.

390. The Acute Respiratory Distress Syndrome Network. Ventilation with lower tidal volumes as compared with traditional tidal volumes for acute lung injury and the acute respiratory distress syndrome. N Engl J Med 2000; 342:1301–1308.

391. Ranieri VM, Suter PM, Tortorella C, et al. Effect of mechanical ventilation on inflammatory mediators in patients with acute respiratory distress syndrome: a randomized controlled trial. JAMA 1999; 282:54–61.

392. American Thoracic Society, European Respiratory Society. Respiratory mechanics in infants. Physiologic evaluation in health and disease. Am Rev Resp Dis 1993; 147:474–496.

393. McLain BI, Evans J, Dear PRF. Comparison of capillary and arterial blood gas measurements in neonates. Arch Dis Child 1989; 63:743–747.

394. Morgan C, Newell SJ, Ducker DA, et al. Continuous neonatal blood gas monitoring using a multiparameter intra-arterial sensor. Arch Dis Child Fetal Neonatal Ed 1999; 80:F93–F98.

395. Bohnhorst B, Peter CS, Poets CF. Pulse oximeters' reliability in detecting hypoxemia and bradycardia: comparison between a conventional and two new generation oximeters. Crit Care Med 2000; 28:1565–1568.

396. Mok JYQ, McLaughlin FJ, Pintar M, et al. Transcutaneous monitoring of oxygenation: what is normal? J Paediatr 1986; 108:365–371.

397. Mok JYQ, Hak H, McLaughlin FJ, et al. Effect of age and state of wakefulness on transcutaneous oxygen values in preterm infants: a longitudinal study. J Pediatr 1988; 113:706–709.

398. Prendiville A, Schulenberg WE. Clinical factors associated with retinopathy of prematurity. Arch Dis Child 1988; 63:522–527.

399. Collins MP, Lorenz JM, Jetton JR, et al. Hypocapnia and other ventilation-related risk factors for cerebral palsy in low birth weight infants. Pediatr Res 2001; 50:712–719.

400. The STOP-ROP Study Group. Supplemental therapeutic oxygen for prethreshold retinopathy of prematurity (STOP-ROP), a randomized, controlled trial. I: primary outcomes. Pediatrics 2000; 105:295–310.

401. Tin W, Milligan DW, Pennefather P, et al. Pulse oximetry, severe retinopathy, and outcome at one year in babies of less than 28 weeks' gestation. Arch Dis Child Fetal Neonatal Ed 2001; 84:F106–F110.

402. Trounce JQ, Shaw DE, Levene MI, et al. Clinical risk factors and periventricular leukomalacia. Arch Dis Child 1988; 63:17–22.

403. Calvert SA, Hoskins EM, Fong KW, et al. Etiological factors associated with the development of periventricular leukomalacia. Acta Paediatr Scand 1987; 76:254–259.

404. Ikonen RS, Janas MO, Koivikko MJ, et al. Hyperbilirubinemia, hypocarbia and periventricular leukomalacia in preterm infants: relationship to cerebral palsy. Acta Paediatr Scand 1992; 81:802–807.

405. Graziani LJ, Spitzer AR, Mitchell DG, et al. Mechanical ventilation in preterm infants: neurosonographic and developmental studies. Pediatrics 1992; 90:515–522.

406. HIFI Study Group. High frequency oscillatory ventilation compared with conventional mechanical ventilation in the treatment of respiratory failure in preterm infants. N Engl J Med 1989; 320: 90–93.

407. Rhodes PG, Graes GR, Patel DM, et al. Minimizing pneumothorax and bronchopulmonary dysplasia in ventilated infants with hyaline membrane disease. J Pediatr 1983; 103:634–637.

408. Wung JT, James S, Kilchevsky E, et al. Management of infants with severe respiratory failure and persistence of the fetal circulation without hyperventilation. Pediatrics 1985; 76:488–494.

409. Avery ME, Tooley WH, Keller JB, et al. Is chronic lung disease preventable? A survey of eight centres. Pediatrics 1987; 79:26–30.

410. Kraybill EN, Runyan D, Bose CL, et al. Risk factors for chronic lung disease in infants with birth weights of 751–1000 grams. J Pediatr 1989; 115:115–120.

411. Woodgate PG, Davies MW. Permissive hypercapnia for the prevention of morbidity and mortality in mechanically ventilated newborn infants. Cochrane Database Syst Rev 2001; 2:CD002061.

412. Skoutelli HN, Dubowitz LMS, Levene MI, et al. Predictors associated with survival and normal neurodevelopmental outcome in infants weighing less than 1001 grams at birth. Dev Med Child Neurol 1985; 27:588–595.

413. Crowley P. Prophylactic corticosteroids for preterm birth. Cochrane Database Syst Rev 2000; 2:CD000065.

414. Crowther CA, Haslam RR, Hiller JE, et al; Australasian Collaborative Trial of Repeat Doses of Steroids (ACTORDS) Study Group. Neonatal respiratory distress syndrome after repeat exposure to antenatal corticosteroids: a randomised controlled trial. Lancet 2006; 367:1913–1919.

415. Henderson-Smart DJ, Steer P. Methylxanthine treatment for apnea in preterm infants. Cochrane Database Syst Rev 2001; 3:CD000140.

416. Henderson-Smart DJ, Davis PG. Prophylactic methylxanthines for extubation in preterm infants. Cochrane Database Syst Rev 2003; 1:CD000139.

417. Schmidt B, Roberts RS, Davis P, et al. Caffeine for Apnea of Prematurity Trial Group. Caffeine therapy for apnea of prematurity. N Engl J Med 2006; 354:2112–2121.

418. Davis PG, Henderson Smart DJ. Nasal continuous positive airways pressure immediately after extubation for preventing morbidity in preterm infants. Cochrane Database Syst Rev 2003; 2:CD000143.

419. Van Marter LJ, Allred EN, Pagano M, et al. Do clinical markers of barotrauma and oxygen toxicity explain interhospital variation in rates of chronic lung disease. Pediatrics 2000; 105:1194–1201.

420. Subramaniam P, Henderson-Smart DJ, Davis PG. Prophylactic nasal continuous positive airways pressure for preventing morbidity and mortality in very preterm infants. Prophylactic nasal continuous positive airways pressure for preventing morbidity and mortality in very preterm infants. Cochrane Database Syst Rev 2005; 3:CD001243.

421. Finer NN, Carlo WA, Duara S, et al. National Institute of Child Health and Human Development Neonatal Research Network. Delivery room continuous positive airway pressure/positive end-expiratory pressure in extremely low birth weight infants: a feasibility trial. Pediatrics 2004; 114:651–657.

422. Davis PG, Lemyre B, de Paoli AG. Nasal intermittent positive pressure ventilation (NIPPV) versus nasal continuous positive airway pressure (NCPAP) for preterm neonates after extubation. Cochrane Database Syst Rev 2001; 3:CD003212.

423. Verder H, Robertson B, Greisen G, et al. Surfactant therapy and nasal continuous positive airway pressure for newborns with respiratory distress syndrome. N Engl J Med 1994; 331:1051–1055.

424. Verder H, Albertsen P, Ebbesen F, et al. Nasal continuous positive airway pressure and early surfactant therapy for respiratory distress syndrome in newborns of less than 30 weeks' gestation. Pediatrics 1999; 103:e24.

425. Herman S, Reynolds EOR. Methods of improving oxygenation in infants mechanically ventilated for severe hyaline membrane disease. Arch Dis Child 1973; 48:612–617.

426. Stewart AR, Finer NN, Peters KL. Effects of alterations of inspiratory and expiratory pressures and inspiratory/expiratory ratios on mean airway pressure, blood gases and intracranial pressure. Pediatrics 1981; 67:474–481.

427. Oxford Region controlled trial of artificial ventilation (OCTAVE) study group. A multicentre randomised controlled trial of high against low frequency positive pressure ventilation. Arch Dis Child 1991; 66:770–775.

428. Greenough A, Milner AD, Dimitriou G. Synchronized mechanical ventilation for respiratory support in newborn infants. Cochrane Database Syst Rev 2004; 18:(4):CD000456.

429. Field D, Milner AD, Hopkin IE. Inspiratory time and tidal volume during intermittent positive pressure ventilation. Arch Dis Child 1985; 60:259–261.

430. Bartholomew KM, Brownlee KG, Snowden S, et al. To PEEP or not to PEEP? Arch Dis Child 1994; 70:F209–F212.

431. Simbruner G. Inadvertent positive end expiratory pressure in mechanically ventilated newborn infants: detection and effect on lung mechanics and gas exchange. J Pediatr 1986; 108:589–595.

432. Stenson BJ, Glover RM, Laing IA, et al. Life threatening inadvertent positive end expiratory pressure. Am J Perinatol 1995; 12:336–338.

433. Tarnow-Mordi WO, Griffiths P, Wilkinson AR. Low inspired gas temperature and respiratory complications in very low birth weight infants. J Paediatr 1989; 114:438–442.

434. Tarnow-Mordi WO, Sutton P, Wilkinson AR. Inadequate humidification of respiratory gases during mechanical ventilation of the newborn. Arch Dis Child 1986; 61:698–700.

435. O'Hagan M, Reid E, Tarnow-Mordi WO. Is neonatal inspired gas humidity accurately controlled by humidifier temperature? Crit Care Med 1991; 19:1370–1373.

436. Prendiville A, Thomson A, Silverman M. Effect of tracheobronchial suction on respiratory resistance in intubated preterm babies. Arch Dis Child 1986; 61:1178–1183.

437. Simbruner G, Coradello H, Fodor M, et al. Effect of tracheal suction on oxygenation, circulation, and lung mechanics in newborn infants. Arch Dis Child 1981; 56:326–330.

438. Perlman JM, Volpe JJ. Suctioning in the preterm infant: effects on cerebral blood flow velocity, intracranial pressure, and arterial blood pressure. Pediatrics 1983; 72:329–334.

439. Greenough A, Greenall F, Gamsu H. Synchronous respiration: which ventilator rate is best? Acta Paediatr Scand 1987; 76:713–718.

440. Bernstein G, Knodel E, Heldt GP. Airway leak size in neonates and autocycling of three flow-triggered ventilators. Crit Care Med 1995; 23:1739–1744.

441. Bernstein G, Heldt GP, Mannino FM. Increased and more consistent tidal volumes during synchronised intermittent mandatory ventilation in newborn infants. Am J Respir Crit Care Med 1994; 150:1444–1448.

442. Cleary JP, Bernstein G, Mannino FL, et al. Improved oxygenation during synchronised intermittent mandatory ventilation in neonates with respiratory distress syndrome: A randomised, crossover study. J Pediatr 1995; 126:407–411.

443. Keszler M, Abubakar K. Volume guarantee: stability of tidal volume and incidence of hypocarbia. Pediatr Pulmonol 2004; 38:240–245.

444. Lista G, Colnaghi M, Castoldi F, et al. Impact of targeted-volume ventilation on lung inflammatory response in preterm infants with respiratory distress syndrome (RDS). Pediatr Pulmonol 2004; 37:510–514.

445. Greenough A, Wood S, Morley CJ, et al. Pancuronium prevents pneumothoraces in ventilated premature babies who actively expire against positive pressure ventilation. Lancet 1984; I:1–3.

446. Shaw NJ, Cooke RWI, Gill AB, et al. Randomised trial of routine versus selective paralysis during ventilation for neonatal respiratory distress syndrome. Arch Dis Child 1993; 69:479–482.

447. Bhutani VK, Abassi S, Sivieri EM. Continuous skeletal muscle paralysis: effect on neonatal pulmonary mechanics. Pediatrics 1988; 81:419–422.

448. Froese AB, Bryan AC. High frequency ventilation. Am Rev Respir Dis 1987; 135:1363–1374.

449. Boynton BR, Hammond MD, Fredburg JJ, et al. Gas exchange in healthy rabbits during high-frequency oscillatory ventilation. J Appl Physiol 1989; 66:1343–1351.

450. Chan V, Greenough A, Milner AD. The effect of frequency and mean airway pressure on volume delivery during high frequency oscillation. Pediatr Pulmonol 1993; 15:183–186.

451. Chan V, Greenough A. The effect of frequency on carbon dioxide levels during high frequency oscillation. J Perinat Med 1994; 22:103–106.

452. Thome UH, Carlo WA, Pohlandt F. Ventilation strategies and outcome in randomised trials of high frequency ventilation. Arch Dis Child Fetal Neonatal Ed 2005; 90:F466–F473.

453. Carter JM, Gerstmann DR, Clark RH, et al. High-frequency oscillatory ventilation and extracorporeal membrane oxygenation for the treatment of acute neonatal respiratory failure. Pediatrics 1990; 85:159–164.

454. Clark RH, Yoder BA, Sell MS. Prospective, randomized comparison of high-frequency oscillation and conventional ventilation in candidates for extracorporeal membrane oxygenation. J Pediatr 1994; 124:447–454.

455. HIFO Study Group. Randomized study of high-frequency oscillatory ventilation in infants with severe respiratory distress syndrome. J Pediatr 1993; 122:609–619.

456. Gerstmann DR, DeLemos RA, Clark RH. High-frequency ventilation: issues of strategy. Clin Perinatol 1991; 18:563–580.

457. Carlo WA, Chatburn RL, Martin RJ. Randomized trial of high frequency jet ventilation in respiratory distress syndrome. J Pediatr 1987; 110:275–282.

458. Bhuta T, Henderson-Smart DJ. Elective high frequency jet ventilation versus conventional ventilation for respiratory distress syndrome in preterm infants. Cochrane Database Syst Rev 2000; 2:CD000328.

459. UK Collaborative ECMO Trial Group. UK collaborative randomised trial of neonatal extracorporeal membrane oxygenation. Lancet 1996; 348:75–82.

460. Ignarro LJ. Biological actions and properties of endothelium derived nitric oxide formed and released from artery and vein. Circ Res 1989; 65:1–21.

461. Miller OI, Celermajer DS, Deanfield JE, et al. Guidelines for the safe administration of inhaled nitric oxide. Arch Dis Child 1994; 70:F47–F49.

462. Finer NN, Barrington KJ. Nitric oxide for respiratory failure in infants born at or near term (Cochrane Review). Cochrane Database Syst Rev 2001; 4:CD000399.

463. Barrington KJ, Finer NN. Inhaled nitric oxide for respiratory failure in preterm infants (Cochrane Review). Cochrane Database Syst Rev 2006; 1:CD000509.

464. Davidson D, Barefield ES, Kattwinkel J, et al. Safety of withdrawing inhaled nitric oxide therapy in persistent pulmonary hypertension of the newborn. Pediatrics 1999; 104:(2 Pt 1):231–236.

465. Dworetz AR, Moya FR, Sabo B, et al. Survival of infants with persistent pulmonary hypertension without extracorporeal membrane oxygenation. Pediatrics 1989; 84:1–6.

466. Schreiber MD, Heymann MA, Soifer SJ. Increased arterial pH, not decreased pACO2, attenuates hypoxia-induced pulmonary vasoconstriction in newborn lambs. Pediatr Res 1986; 20:113–117.

Neurodevelopmental outcome

467. Escobar GB, Littenberg B, Pettiti DB. Outcome among surviving very low birthweight infants: a meta-analysis. Arch Dis Child 1991; 66:204–211.

468. Surman G, Newdick H, Johnson A. Cerebral palsy rates among low-birthweight infants fell in the 1990s. Dev Med Child Neurol 2003; 45:456–462.

469. Evans DJ, Levene MI. Evidence of selection bias in preterm survival studies: a systematic review. Arch Dis Child Fetal Neonatal Ed 2001; 84:F79–F84.

470. Surveillance of Cerebral Palsy in Europe. Surveillance of cerebral palsy in Europe: a collaboration of cerebral palsy registers and surveys. Dev Med Child Neurol 2000; 42:816–824.

471. Wood NS, Marlow N, Costeloe K, et al. Neurologic and developmental disability after extremely preterm birth. N Engl J Med 2000; 343:378–384.

472. Huddy CLJ, Johnson A, Hope PL. Educational and behavioural problems in babies of 32–35 weeks gestation. Arch Dis Child 2001; 85:f23–f28.

473. Kramer MS, Demissie K, Yang H, et al. The contribution of mild and moderate preterm birth to infant mortality. JAMA 2000; 284:843–849.

474. Pharoah POD, Adi Y. Consequences of in-utero death in a twin pregnancy. Lancet 2000; 355:1597–1602.

475. Wu YW, Colford JM. Chorioamnionitis as a risk factor for cerebral palsy. JAMA 2000; 284:1417–1424.

476. Tin W, Fritz S, Wariyar U, et al. Outcome of very preterm birth: children reviewed with ease at 2 years differ from those followed up with difficulty. Arch Dis Child 1998; 79:F83–F87.

477. Morley R, Brooke OG, Cole TJ, et al. Birthweight ratio and outcome in preterm infants. Arch Dis Child 1990; 65:30–34.

478. Kamoji VM, Dorling JS, Manktelow BN, et al. Extremely growth-retarded infants: is there a viability centile?. Pediatrics 2006; 118:758–763.

479. Synnes AR, Ling EW, Whitfield MF, et al. Perinatal outcomes of a large cohort of extremely low gestational age infants (23–28 completed weeks of gestation). J Pediatr 1994; 125:952–960.

480. McCarton CM, Wallace IF, Divon M, et al. Cognitive and neurologic development of the premature, small for gestation age infant through age 6: comparison by birth weight and gestational age. Pediatrics 1996; 98:1167–1178.

481. Bottoms SF, Paul RH, Mercer BM, et al. Obstetric determinants of neonatal survival: Antenatal predictors of neonatal survival and morbidity in extremely low birth weight infants. Am J Obstet Gynecol 1999; 180:665–669.

482. Hoekstra RE, Ferrara B, Couser RJ, et al. Survival and long-term neurodevelopmental outcome of extremely premature infants born at 23 to 26 weeks' gestational age at a tertiary center. Pediatrics 2004; 113:e1–e6.

483. Hack M, Fanaroff A. Outcomes of children of extremely low birthweight and gestational age in the 1990s. Semin Neonatol 2000; 5:89–106.

484. Adams-Chapman I, Stoll BJ. Neonatal infection and long-term neurodevelopmental outcome in the preterm infant. Curr Opin Infect Dis 2006; 19:290–297.

485. Rennie JM. Perinatal management at the lower margin of viability. Arch Dis Child 1996; 74:f214–f218.

486. Doyle LW, Anderson PJ. Improved neurosensory outcome at 8 years of age of extremely low birthweight children born in Victoria over three distinct eras. Arch Dis Child Fetal Neonatal Ed 2005; 90: F484–F488.

487. Bhutta AT, Clevese MA, Casey PH, et al. Cognitive and behavioural outcomes of school-aged children who were born preterm. JAMA 2002; 288:728–737.

488. Aylward GP. Outcome studies of VLBWI: meta-analysis. J Pediatr 1989; 115:515–520.

489. Anderson P, Doyle LW. Neurobehavioral outcomes of school-age children born extremely low birth weight or very preterm in the 1990s. JAMA 2003; 289:3264–3272.

490. Botting N, Powls A, Cooke RWI, et al. Attention deficit hyperactivity disorders and other psychiatric outcomes in very low birthweight children at 12 years. J Child Psychol Psychiatr 1997; 38:931–941.

491. Olsen P, Myrman A, Rantakallio P. Educational capacity of low birthweight children up to age 24. Early Hum Dev 1994; 36:191–203.

492. Skuse D. Survival after being born too soon, but at what cost?. Lancet 1999; 354:354–356.

493. Anderson PJ, Doyle LW. Executive functioning in school-aged children who were born very preterm or with extremely low birthweight in the 1990s. Pediatrics 2004; 114:50–57.

494. Saigal S, Feeny D, Rosenbaum P, et al. Self-perceived health status and health-related quality of life of extremely low birth weight infants at adolescence. JAMA 1996; 276:453–459.

495. Ng PC, Dear PRF. The predictive value of a normal ultrasound scan in the preterm baby – a meta-analysis. Acta Paediatr Scand 1990; 79:286–291.

496. Laptook AR, O'Shea TM, Shankaran S, et al. Adverse neurodevelopmental outcomes among extremely low birth weight infants with a normal head ultrasound: prevalence and antecedents. Pediatrics 2005; 115:673–680.

497. Patra K, Wilson-Costello D, Taylor HG, et al. Grades I–II intraventricular hemorrhage in extremely low birth weight infants: effects on neurodevelopment. J Paediatr 2006; 149:169–173.

498. Inder TE, Warfield SK, Wang H, et al. Abnormal cerebral structure is present at term in premature infants. Pediatrics 2005; 115:286–294.

499. Vasileiadis GT, Gelman N, Han VK, et al. Uncomplicated intraventricular hemorrhage is followed by reduced cortical volume at near-term age. Pediatrics 2004; 114:e367–e372.

500. Ventriculomegaly Trial Group. Randomised trial of early tapping in neonatal posthaemorrhagic periventricular dilatation: results at 30 months. Arch Dis Child 1994; 70:f129–f136.

501. de Vries LS, Liem KD, van Dijk K, et al. Early versus late treatment of posthaemorrhagic ventricular dilatation: results of a retrospective study from five neonatal intensive care units in the Netherlands. Acta Paediatr 2002; 91:212–217.

502. Woodward LJ, Anderson PJ, Austin NC, et al. Neonatal MRI to predict neurodevelopmental outcomes in preterm infants. N Engl J Med 2006; 355:685–694.

503. de Vries LS, van Haastert IL, Rademaker KJ, et al. Ultrasound abnormalities preceding cerebral palsy in high risk preterm infants. J Pediatr 2004; 144:815–820.

Neonatal death

504. Cullberg J. Mental reactions of women to perinatal death. In: Morris N, ed. Psychosomatic medicine in obstetrics and gynaecology. London: 3rd International Congress; 1971.

505. Wilson RE. Parents' support of their other children after a miscarriage or perinatal death. Early Hum Dev 2001; 61:55–65.

506. SANDS. After stillbirth and neonatal death: what happens next. London: Stillbirth and Neonatal Death Society; 1986.

507. Brodlie M, Laing IA, Keeling JW, et al. Autopsies in tertiary referral centre: retrospective study. BMJ 2002; 324:761–763.

Pulmonary disorders and apnea

508. ACTOBAT Study Group. Australian collaborative trial of antenatal thyrotropin releasing hormone (ACTOBAT) for prevention of neonatal respiratory disease. Lancet 1995; 345:877–882.

509. Crowther CA, Hiller JE, Haslam RR, et al. Australian collaborative trial of antenatal thyrotropin releasing hormone: adverse effects at 12 month follow up. Pediatrics 1997; 99:311–317.

510. Taeusch HW, Boncuk-Dayanikli P. Respiratory distress syndrome. In: Yu VYH, ed. Pulmonary problems in the perinatal period and their sequelae. London: Baillière Tindall; 1995.

511. Rubaltelli FF, Bonafe L, Tangucci M, et al and the Italian Group of Neonatal Pneumology. Epidemiology of neonatal acute respiratory disorders. A multicenter study on incidence and fatality rates of neonatal acute respiratory disorders according to gestational age, maternal age, pregnancy complications and type of delivery. Biol Neonate 1998; 74:7–15.

512. Crowley P. Prophylactic corticosteroids for preterm birth. Cochrane Database Syst Rev 2001; 3:CD000065.

513. Soll RF, Morley CJ. Prophylactic versus selective use of surfactant in preventing morbidity and mortality in preterm infants. Cochrane Database Syst Rev 2001; 2:CD000510.

514. Soll RF. Prophylactic natural surfactant extract for preventing morbidity and mortality in preterm infants. Cochrane Database Syst Rev 2001; 3:CD000511.

515. Soll RF. Prophylactic synthetic surfactant for preventing morbidity and mortality in preterm infants. Cochrane Database Syst Rev 2001; 3:CD001079.

516. Soll RF. Synthetic surfactant for respiratory distress syndrome in preterm infants. Cochrane Database Syst Rev 2001; 3:CD001149.

517. Soll RF, Blanco F. Natural surfactant extract versus synthetic surfactant for neonatal respiratory distress syndrome. Cochrane Database Syst Rev 2001; 2:CD000144.

518. Ramanathan R, Rasmussen MR, Gerstmann DR, et al. North American Study Group. A randomized, multicenter masked comparison trial of poractant alfa (Curosurf) versus beractant (Survanta) in the treatment of respiratory distress syndrome in preterm infants. Am J Perinatol 2004; 21:109–119.

519. Soll RF. Multiple versus single dose natural surfactant extract for severe neonatal respiratory distress syndrome. Cochrane Database Syst Rev 2000; 2:CD000141.

520. McCall EM, Alderdice FA, Halliday HL, et al. Interventions to prevent hypothermia at birth in preterm and/or low birthweight babies. Cochrane Database Syst Rev 2005; 25;1:CD004210.

521. Shaffer SG, Weismann DN. Fluid requirements in the preterm infant. Clin Perinatol 1992; 19:233–250.

522. Simmer K, Rao SC. Early introduction of lipids to parenterally-fed preterm infants. Cochrane Database Syst Rev 2005; 2:CD005256.

523. Gunn T, Reaman G, Outerbridge F, et al. Peripheral total parenteral nutrition for premature infants with respiratory distress syndrome: a controlled study. J Pediatr 1978; 92:608–613.

524. Tyson JE, Kennedy KA. Trophic feeding for parenterally fed infants. Cochrane Database Syst Rev 2005; 3:CD000504.

525. Subramaniam P, Henderson-Smart DJ, Davis PG. Prophylactic nasal continuous positive airways pressure for preventing morbidity and mortality in very preterm infants. Cochrane Database Syst Rev 2005; 3:CD001243.

526. Stevens TP, Blennow M, Soll RF. Early surfactant administration with brief ventilation vs selective surfactant and continued mechanical ventilation for preterm infants with or at risk for RDS. Cochrane Database Syst Rev 2002; 2:CD003063.

527. De Paoli AG, Davis PG, Faber B, et al. Devices and pressure sources for administration of nasal continuous positive airway pressure (NCPAP) in preterm neonates. Cochrane Database Syst Rev 2002; 3:CD002977.

528. Lemyre B, Davis PG, De Paoli AG. Nasal intermittent positive pressure ventilation (NIPPV) versus nasal continuous positive airway pressure (NCPAP) for apnea of prematurity. Cochrane Database Syst Rev 2000; 3:CD002272.

529. Attar MA, Donn SM. Mechanisms of ventilator-induced lung injury in premature infants. Semin Neonatol 2002; 7:353–360.

530. Henderson-Smart DJ, Bhuta T, Cools F, et al. Elective high frequency oscillatory ventilation versus conventional ventilation for acute pulmonary dysfunction in preterm infants. Cochrane Database Syst Rev 2003; 1:CD000104.

531. Courtney S, Durand D, Asselin J, et al. Neonatal Ventilation Study Group. High-frequency oscillatory ventilation versus conventional mechanical ventilation for very-low-birth-weight infants. N Engl J Med 2002; 347:643–652.

532. Kamlin CO, Davis PG. Long versus short inspiratory times in neonates receiving mechanical ventilation. Cochrane Database Syst Rev 2004; 4:CD004503.

533. Kinsella JP, Cutter GR, Walsh WF, et al. Early inhaled nitric oxide therapy in premature newborns with respiratory failure. N Engl J Med 2006; 355:354–364.

534. Greenough A, Milner AD, Dimitriou G. Synchronized mechanical ventilation for respiratory support in newborn. Cochrane Database Syst Rev 2004; 4:CD000456.

535. Schmidt B, Roberts RS, Davis P, et al; Caffeine for Apnea of Prematurity Trial Group. Caffeine therapy for apnea of prematurity. N Engl J Med 2006; 354:2112–2121.

536. Davis PG, Henderson-Smart DJ. Nasal continuous positive airways pressure immediately after extubation for preventing morbidity in preterm infants. Cochrane Database Syst Rev 2001; 3:CD000143.

537. Hermes-DeSantis ER, Clyman RI. Patent ductus arteriosus: pathophysiology and management. J Perinatol 2006; 26:Suppl 1:S14–S18.

538. Lipscomb AP, Thorburn RJ, Reynolds EOR, et al. Pneumothorax and cerebral haemorrhage in preterm infants. Lancet 1981; i:414–416.

539. McCord FB, Curstedt T, Halliday HL, et al. Surfactant treatment and incidence of intraventricular haemorrhage in severe respiratory distress syndrome. Arch Dis Child 1988; 63:10–16.

540. Ogata ES, Gregory GA, Kitterman JA, et al. Pneumothorax in the respiratory distress syndrome: incidence and effect on vital signs, blood gases and pH. Pediatrics 1975; 58:177–183.

541. McCallion N, Davis PG, Morley CJ. Volume-targeted versus pressure-limited ventilation in the neonate. Cochrane Database Syst Rev 2005; 3:CD003666.

542. Northway WH, Rosan RC, Porter DY. Pulmonary disease following respirator therapy of hyaline membrane disease. Bronchopulmonary dysplasia. N Engl J Med 1967; 276:357–368.

543. Corcoran JD, Patterson CC, Thomas PS, et al. Reduction in the risk of bronchopulmonary dysplasia from 1980–1990: results of a multivariate logistic regression analysis. Eur J Pediatr 1993; 152:671–681.

544. Sweet DG, Halliday HL. Modeling and remodeling of the lung in neonatal chronic lung disease. Treat Respir Med 2005; 4:347–359.

545. Benitz WE, Han MY, Madan A, et al. Serial serum C-reactive protein levels in the diagnosis of neonatal infection. Pediatrics 1998; 102:E41.

546. Goodwin SR, Graves SA, Haberkern CM. Aspiration in the intubated premature infant. Pediatrics 1985; 75:85–88.

547. Lee K-S, Khoshnood B, Wall SN, et al. Trend in mortality from respiratory distress syndrome in the United States, 1970–1995. J Pediatr 1999; 134:434–440.

548. Avery ME, Gatewood O, Brumley G. Transient tachypnea of newborn. Possible delayed resorption of fluid at birth. Am J Dis Child 1966; 111:380–385.

549. Alderdice F, McCall E, Bailie C, et al. Admission to neonatal intensive care with respiratory morbidity following 'term' elective caesarean section. Ir Med J 2005; 98:170–172.

550. Jain L, Eaton DC. Physiology of fetal lung fluid clearance and the effect of labor. Semin Perinatol 2006; 30:34–43.

551. Halliday HL, McClure G, Reid MMcC. Transient tachypnoea of the newborn: two distinct clinical entities? Arch Dis Child 1981; 56:322–325.

552. Tudehope DI, Smyth MJ. Is 'transient tachypnoea of the newborn' always a benign disease? Report of 6 babies requiring mechanical ventilation. Austr Paediatr J 1979; 15:160–165.

553. Wiswell TE, Rawlings JS, Smith FR, et al. Effect of furosemide on the clinical course of transient tachypnea of the newborn. Pediatrics 1985; 75:908–910.

554. Birnkrant DJ, Picone C, Markowitz W, et al. Association of transient tachypnea of the newborn and childhood asthma. Pediatr Pulmonol 2006; 41:978–984.

555. Newton ER. Preterm labor, preterm premature rupture of membranes, and chorioamnionitis. Clin Perinatol 2005; 32:571–600.

556. Webber S, Wilkinson AR, Lindsell D, et al. Neonatal pneumonia. Arch Dis Child 1990; 65:207–211.

557. Apisarnthanarak A, Holzmann-Pazgal G, Hamvas A, et al. Ventilator-associated pneumonia in extremely preterm neonates in a neonatal intensive care unit: characteristics, risk factors, and outcomes. Pediatrics 2003; 112:1283–1289.

558. Benitz WE, Gould JB, Druzin ML. Risk factors for early-onset group B streptococcal sepsis: estimation of odds ratios by critical literature review. Pediatrics 1999; 103:e77.

559. Naeye RL, Peters EC. Amniotic fluid infections with intact membranes leading to perinatal death: a prospective study. Pediatrics 1978; 61:171–177.

560. Boyer KM, Gotoff SP. Prevention of early-onset neonatal group B streptococcal disease with selective intrapartum chemoprophylaxis. N Engl J Med 1986; 314:1665–1669.

561. Kenyon S, Boulvain M, Neilson J. Antibiotics for preterm rupture of membranes. Cochrane Database Syst Rev 2003; 2:CD001058.

562. Mifsud A, Seal D, Wall R, et al. Reduced neonatal mortality from infection after introduction of respiratory monitoring. BMJ 1988; 296:17–18.

563. Benjamin DK Jr, Stoll BJ, Fanaroff AA, et al. Neonatal candidiasis among extremely low birth weight infants: risk factors, mortality rates, and neurodevelopmental outcomes at 18 to 22 months. Pediatrics 2006; 117:84–92.

564. Herting E, Gefeller O, Land M, et al. Surfactant treatment of neonates with respiratory failure and group B streptococcal infection. Pediatrics 2000; 106:957–964.

565. Ohlsson A, Lacy JB. Intravenous immuno-globulin for suspected or subsequently proven infection in neonates. Cochrane Database Syst Rev 2004; 1:CD001239.

566. Dargaville PA, Copnell B. Australian and New Zealand Neonatal Network. The epidemiology of meconium aspiration syndrome: incidence, risk factors, therapies, and outcome. Pediatrics 2006; 117:1712–1721.

567. Crowley P. Interventions for preventing or improving the outcome of delivery at or beyond term. Cochrane Database Syst Rev 2000; 2:CD000170.

568. Halliday HL, Hirata T. Perinatal listeriosis – a review of twelve patients. Am J Obstet Gynecol 1979; 133:405–410.

569. Hsieh TK, Su BH, Chen AC, et al. Risk factors of meconium aspiration syndrome developing into persistent pulmonary hypertension of newborn. Acta Paediatr Taiwan 2004; 45:203–207.

570. Vain NE, Szyld EG, Prudent LM, et al. Oropharyngeal and nasopharyngeal suctioning of meconium-stained neonates before delivery of their shoulders: multicentre, randomised controlled trial. Lancet 2004; 364:597–602.

571. Halliday HL, Sweet DG. Endotracheal intubation at birth for preventing morbidity and mortality invigorous, meconium-stained infants born at term. Cochrane Database Syst Rev 2001; 1:CD000500.

572. Soll RF, Dargaville P. Surfactant for meconium aspiration syndrome in full term infants. Cochrane Database Syst Rev 2000; 2:CD002054.

573. Wiswell TE, Knight GR, Finer NN, et al. A multicenter, randomized, controlled trial comparing Surfaxin (Lucinactant) lavage with standard care for treatment of meconium aspiration syndrome. Pediatrics 2002; 109:1081–1087.

574. Macfarlane PI, Heaf DP. Pulmonary function in children after neonatal meconium aspiration syndrome. Arch Dis Child 1989; 63:368–372.

575. Mitchell DJ, McClure BG, Tubman TR. Simultaneous monitoring of gastric and oesophageal pH reveals limitations of conventional oesophageal pH monitoring in milk fed infants. Arch Dis Child 2001; 84:273–276.

576. Sheikh S, Allen E, Shell R, et al. Chronic aspiration without gastroesophageal reflux as a cause of chronic respiratory symptoms in neurologically normal infants. Chest 2001; 120:1190–1195.

577. Goldberg RN. Sustained arterial blood pressure elevation associated with small pneumothoraces: early detection via continuous monitoring. Pediatrics 1981; 68:775–777.

578. Madansky DL, Lawson EE, Chernick V, et al. Pneumothorax and other forms of pulmonary air leaks in the newborn. Am Rev Respir Dis 1979; 120:729–737.

579. Laptook AR, O'Shea TM, Shankaran S, et al. NICHD Neonatal Network. Adverse neurodevelopmental outcomes among extremely low birth weight infants with a normal head ultrasound: prevalence and antecedents. Pediatrics 2005; 115: 673–680.

580. Swischuk LE. Two lesser known but useful signs of neonatal pneumothorax. Am J Roentgenol 1976; 127:623–627.

581. England GJ, Hill RC, Timberlake GA, et al. Resolution of experimental pneumothorax in rabbits by graded oxygen therapy. J Trauma 1998; 45:333–334.

582. McIntosh N, Prakesh P, Smith A. Air leaks and vasopressin release. Arch Dis Child 1990; 65:1259–1262.

583. Sarkar S, Hussain N, Herson V. Fibrin glue for persistent pneumothorax in neonates. J Perinatol 2003; 23:82–84.

584. Greenough A, Wood S, Morley CJ, et al. Pancuronium prevents pneumothoraces in ventilated premature babies who actively expire against positive pressure ventilation. Lancet 1984; i:1–3.

585. Cools F, Offringa M. Neuromuscular paralysis for newborn infants receiving mechanical ventilation. Cochrane Database Syst Rev 2005; 2:CD002773.

586. Speer CP, Ruess D, Harms K, et al. Neutrophil elastase and acute pulmonary damage in neonates with severe respiratory distress syndrome. Pediatrics 1993; 91:794–799.

587. Rettwitz-Volk W, Scholosser R, Von Loewenich V. One sided high frequency oscillatory ventilation in the treatment of neonatal unilateral pulmonary emphysema. Acta Paediatr 1993; 82:190–192.

588. Dear PRF, Conway SP. Treatment of severe bilateral interstitial emphysema in a baby by artificial pneumothorax and pneumotomy. Lancet 1984; i:273–277.

589. Fujii AM, Moulton S. Percutaneous catheter evacuation of a pneumatocele in an extremely premature infant with respiratory failure. J Perinatol 2003; 23:516–518.

590. Nelle M, Zilow EP, Linderkamp O. Effects of high-frequency oscillatory ventilation on circulation in neonates with pulmonary interstitial emphysema or RDS. Intensive Care Med 1997; 23:671–676.

591. Hart SM, McNair M, Gamsu HR, et al. Pulmonary interstitial emphysema in very low birthweight infants. Arch Dis Child 1983; 58:612–615.

592. Fenton TR, Bennett S, McIntosh N. Air embolism in ventilated very low birthweight infants. Arch Dis Child 1988; 63:541–543.

593. Raju TNK, Langenberg P. Pulmonary hemorrhage and exogenous surfactant therapy: a meta-analysis. J Pediatr 1993; 123:603–610.

594. Kluckow M, Evans N. Ductal shunting, high pulmonary blood flow, and pulmonary hemorrhage. J Pediatr 2000; 137:68–72.

595. Stevenson DK, Walther F, Long WA and the American Exosurf Neonatal Study Group. 1. Controlled trial of a single dose of synthetic surfactant at birth in premature infants weighing 500–699 grams. J Pediatr 1992; 120:S3–S12.

596. Van Houten J, Long W, Mullet M, et al. Pulmonary hemorrhage in premature infants after treatment with synthetic surfactant: an autopsy evaluation. J Pediatr 1992; 120:S40–S44.

597. Pandit PB, Dunn MS, Colucci EA. Surfactant therapy in neonates with respiratory deterioration due to pulmonary hemorrhage. Pediatrics 1995; 95: 32–36.

598. Pandit PB, O'Brien K, Asztalos E, et al. Outcome following pulmonary haemorrhage in very low birthweight neonates treated with surfactant. Arch Dis Child Fetal Neonatal Ed 1999; 81:F40–F44.

599. Wigglesworth JS, Desai R. Is fetal respiratory function a major determinant of perinatal survival? Lancet 1982; i:264–267.

600. De Paepe ME, Friedman RM, Gundogan F, et al. Postmortem lung weight/body weight standards for term and preterm infants. Pediatr Pulmonol 2005; 40:445–448.

601. Wigglesworth JS, Desai R. Use of DNA estimation for growth assessment in normal and hypoplastic fetal lungs. Arch Dis Child 1981; 56:601–605.

602. McIntosh N. Dry lung syndrome after oligohydramnios. Arch Dis Child 1988; 63:190–193.

603. Tubman TRJ, Halliday HL. Surfactant treatment for respiratory distress following prolonged rupture of membranes. Eur J Pediatr 1990; 149:727–729.

604. Uga N, Ishii T, Kawase Y, et al. Nitric oxide inhalation therapy in very low-birthweight infants with hypoplastic lung due to oligohydramnios. Pediatr Int 2004; 46:10–14.

605. UK Collaborative ECMO Trial Group. UK collaborative randomised trial of neonatal extracorporeal membrane oxygenation. Lancet 1996; 348:75–82.

606. Ozcelik U, Gocmen A, Kiper N, et al. Congenital lobar emphysema: evaluation and long-term followup of thirty cases at a single center. Pediatr Pulmonol 2003; 35:384–391.

607. Stocker JT, Drake RM, Madewell JE. Cystic and congenital lung disease in the newborn. Perspect Pediatr Pathol 1978; 4:93–154.

608. Calvert JK, Boyd PA, Chamberlain PC, et al. Outcome of antenatally suspected congenital cystic adenomatoid malformation of the lung: 10 years' experience 1991–2001. Arch Dis Child Fetal Neonatal Ed 2006; 91:F26–F28.

609. Blau H, Barak A, Karmazyn B, et al. Postnatal management of resolving fetal lung lesions. Pediatrics 2002; 109:105–108.

610. Stanton M, Davenport M. Management of congenital lung lesions. Early Hum Dev 2006; 82:289–295.

611. Stocker JT. Sequestrations of the lung. Semin Diagn Pathol 1986; 3:106–121.

612. Piccione W Jr, Burt ME. Pulmonary sequestration in the neonate. Chest 1990; 97:244–246.

613. Margau R, Amaral JG, Chait PG, et al. Percutaneous thoracic drainage in neonates: catheter drainage versus treatment with aspiration alone. Radiology 2006; 241:223–227.

614. Roehr CC, Jung A, Proquitte H, et al. Somatostatin or octreotide as treatment options for chylothorax in young children: a systematic review. Intensive Care Med 2006; 32:650–657.

615. Dempsey EM, Sant'Anna GM, Williams RL, et al. Congenital pulmonary lymphangiectasia presenting as nonimmune fetal hydrops and severe respiratory distress at birth: not uniformly fatal. Pediatr Pulmonol 2005; 40:270–274.

616. Effat KG. Use of the automatic tympanometer as a screening tool for congenital choanal atresia. J Laryngol Otol 2005; 119:125–128.

617. Jobe AJ. The new BPD: an arrest of lung development. Pediatr Res 1999; 46:641–643.

618. Ehrenkranz RA, Walsh MC, Vohr BR, et al. National Institutes of Child Health and Human Development Neonatal Research Network. Validation of the National Institutes of Health consensus definition of bronchopulmonary dysplasia. Pediatrics 2005; 116:1353–1360.

619. Schmidt B, Asztalos EV, Roberts RS, et al. Trial of Indomethacin Prophylaxis in Preterms (TIPP) Investigators. Impact of bronchopulmonary dysplasia, brain injury, and severe retinopathy on the outcome of extremely low-birth-weight infants at 18 months: results from the trial of indomethacin prophylaxis in preterms. JAMA 2003; 289:1124–1129.

620. Parker RA, Lindstrom DP, Cotton RB. Improved survival accounts for most, but not all, of the increase in bronchopulmonary dysplasia. Pediatrics 1992; 90:663–668.

621. Sweet DG, Halliday HL. Modeling and remodeling of the lung in neonatal chronic lung disease: implications for therapy. Treat Respir Med 2005; 4:347–359.

622. Rojas MA, Gonzalez A, Bancalari E, et al. Changing trends in the epidemiology and pathogenesis of neonatal chronic lung disease. J Pediatr 1995; 126:605–610.

623. Watterberg KL, Demers LM, Scott SM, et al. Chorioamnionitis and early lung inflammation in infants in whom bronchopulmonary dysplasia develops. Pediatrics 1996; 97:210–215.

624. Avery ME, Tooley WH, Keller JB, et al. Is chronic lung disease in low birth weight infants preventable? A survey of eight centers. Pediatrics 1987; 79: 26–30.

625. Halliday HL, Ehrenkranz RA. Early postnatal (< 96 hours) corticosteroids for preventing chronic lung disease in preterm infants. Cochrane Database Syst Rev 2003; 1:CD001146.

626. Halliday HL, Ehrenkranz RA. Moderately early (7–14 days) postnatal corticosteroids for preventing chronic lung disease in preterm infants. Cochrane Database Syst Rev 2003; 1:CD001144.

627. Halliday HL, Ehrenkranz RA. Delayed (> 3 weeks) postnatal corticosteroids for chronic lung disease in preterm infants. Cochrane Database Syst Rev 2003; 1:CD001145.

628. Barrington JK. The adverse neurodevelopmental effects of postnatal steroids in the preterm infant: a systematic review of RCTs. BMC Pediatr 2001; 1:1.Epub 2001 Feb 27.

629. Doyle LW, Davis PG, Morley CJ, et al. DART Study Investigators. Low-dose dexamethasone facilitates extubation among chronically ventilator-dependent infants: a multicenter, international, randomized, controlled trial. Pediatrics 2006; 117:75–83.

630. Grier DG, Halliday HL. Management of bronchopulmonary dysplasia in infants: guidelines for corticosteroid use. Drugs 2005; 65:15–29.

631. Lister P, Iles R, Shaw B, et al. Inhaled steroids for neonatal chronic lung disease. Cochrane Database Syst Rev 2000; 3:CD002311.

632. Askie LM, Henderson-Smart DJ, Irwig L, et al. Oxygen-saturation targets and outcomes in extremely preterm infants. N Engl J Med 2003; 349:959–967.

633. Darlow BA, Graham PJ. Vitamin A supplementation for preventing morbidity and mortality in very low birthweight infants. Cochrane Database Syst Rev 2002; 4:CD000501.

634. Sweet DG, Halliday HL. A risk-benefit assessment of drugs used for neonatal chronic lung disease. Drug Saf 2000; 22:389–404.

635. The IMpact-RSV Study Group. Palivizumab, a humanized respiratory syncytial virus monoclonal antibody, reduces hospitalization from respiratory syncytial virus infection in high-risk infants. Pediatrics 1998; 102:(3 Pt 1):531–537.

636. Embleton ND, Harkensee C, Mckean MC. Palivizumab for preterm infants. Is it worth it?. Arch Dis Child Fetal Neonatal Ed 2005; 90:F286–F289.

637. Michna BA, Krummel TM, Tracy T Jr, et al. Cricoid split for subglottic stenosis in infancy. Ann Thorac Surg 1988; 45:541–543.

638. Martin RJ, Abu-Shaweesh JM. Control of breathing and neonatal apnea. Biol Neonate 2005; 87:288–295.

639. Henderson-Smart DJ. Recurrent apnoea. In: Yu VYH. ed. Pulmonary problems in the prenatal period and their sequelae. London: Baillière Tindall; 1995.

640. Di Fiore JM, Arko M, Whitehouse M, et al. Apnea is not prolonged by acid gastroesophageal reflux in preterm infants. Pediatrics 2005; 116:1059–1063.

641. Milner AD, Boon AW, Saunders RA, et al. Upper airways obstruction and apnoea in preterm babies. Arch Dis Child 1980; 55:22–25.

642. Millar D, Schmidt B. Controversies surrounding xanthine therapy. Semin Neonatol 2004; 9:239–244.

643. Steer PA, Henderson-Smart DJ. Caffeine versus theophylline for apnea in preterm infants. Cochrane Database Syst Rev 2000; 2:CD000273.

644. Schmidt B. Methylxanthine therapy for apnea of prematurity: evaluation of treatment benefits and risks at age 5 years in the international Caffeine for Apnea of Prematurity (CAP) trial. Biol Neonate 2005; 88:208–213.

645. Henderson-Smart D, Steer P. Doxapram treatment for apnea in preterm infants. Cochrane Database Syst Rev 2004; 4:CD000074.

646. Kimball AL, Carlton DP. Gastroesophageal reflux medications in the treatment of apnea in premature infants. J Pediatr 2001; 138:356–360.

647. Koons AH, Mojica N, Jadeja N, et al. Neurodevelopmental outcome of infants with apnea of infancy. Am J Perinatol 1993; 10:208–211.

648. Liu LMP, Cote CJ, Goudsouzian NG, et al. Life-threatening apnea in infants recovering from anesthesia. Anesthesiology 1983; 59:506–510.

Neonatal cardiovascular disease

649. Evans NJ, Archer LNJ. Postnatal circulatory adaptation in healthy term and preterm neonates. Arch Dis Child 1990; 65:24–26.

*650. de Swiet M, Fayers P, Shinebourne EA. Systolic blood pressure in a population of infants in the first year of life: the Brompton study. Pediatrics 1980; 65:1028–1035.

*651. Hegyi T, Carbone MT, Anwar M, et al. Blood pressure ranges in premature infants: 1. The first hours of life. J Pediatr 1994; 124:627–633.

*652. Hegyi T, Anwar M, Carbone MT, et al. Blood pressure ranges in premature infants: 2. The first week of life. Pediatrics 1996; 97:336–342.

*653. Davignon A, Rautaharju P, Barselle E, et al. Normal ECG standards for infants and children. Pediatr Cardiol 1979/80; 1:123–124.

654. Sharland G. Fetal cardiology. Semin Neonatol 2001; 6:3–15.

*655. Allan LD, Apfel HD, Printz BF. Outcome after prenatal diagnosis of the hypoplastic left heart syndrome. Heart 1998; 79:371–374.

656. Kumar RK, Newburger JW. Gauvreau K, et al. Comparison of outcome when hypoplastic left heart syndrome and transposition of the great arteries are diagnosed prenatally versus when diagnosis of these two conditions is made only postnatally. Am J Cardiol 1999; 83:1649–1653.

*657. Tworetzky W, McElhinney DB, Reddy V, et al. Improved surgical outcome after fetal diagnosis of hypoplastic left heart syndrome. Circulation 2001; 103:1269–1273.

*658. Franklin O, Burch M, Manning N, et al. Prenatal diagnosis of coarctation of the aorta improves survival and reduces morbidity. Heart 2002; 87:67–69.

*659. Press J, Uziel Y, Laxer RM, et al. Long-term outcome of mothers of children with complete heart block. Am J Med 1996; 100:328–332.

660. Eronen M, Siren M-K, Ekblad H, et al. Short and long-term outcome of children with congenital complete heart block diagnosed in utero or as a newborn. Pediatrics 2000; 106:86–91.

*661. Ainsworth SB, Wyllie JP, Wren C. Prevalence and clinical significance of cardiac murmurs in neonates. Arch Dis Child 1999; 80:F43–F45.

*662. Arlettaz R, Archer N, Wilkinson AR. Natural history of innocent heart murmurs in newborn babies: controlled echocardiographic study. Arch Dis Child 1998; 78:F166–F170.

663. Farrer KF, Rennie JM. Neonatal murmurs: are senior house officers good enough? Arch Dis Child 2003; 88:F147–F151.

664. Patton C, Hey E. How effectively can clinical examination pick up congenital heart disease at birth? Arch Dis Child 2006; 91:F263–F267.

665. Richmond S, Reay G, Abu Harb M. Routine pulse oximetry in the asymptomatic newborn. Arch Dis Child 2002; 87:F83–F88.

666. Knowles R, Griebsch I, Dezateux C, et al. Newborn screening for congenital heart defects: a systematic review and cost-effectiveness analysis. Health Technol Assess 2005; 9(44):

*667. Roguin N, Du Z-D, Barak M, et al. High prevalence of muscular ventricular septal defect in neonates. J Am Coll Cardiol 1995; 26:1545–1548.

668. Brennan P, Young ID. Congenital heart malformations: aetiology and associations Semin Neonatol 2001; 6:17–25.

*669. Knight DB. The treatment of patent ductus arteriosus in preterm infants. A review and overview of randomised trials. Semin Neonatol 2001; 6:63–73.

670. Norton ME, Merrill J, Cooper BAB, et al. Neonatal complications after the administration of indomethacin for preterm labor. N Engl J Med 1993; 329:1602–1607.

*671. Schulte J, Osborne J, Benson JWT, et al. Developmental outcome of the use of etamsylate for prevention of periventricular haemorrhage in a randomized controlled trial. Arch Dis Child 2005; 90:F31–F35.

*672. Cotton RB, Haywood JL, Fitzgerald GA. Symptomatic patent ductus arteriosus following prophylactic indomethacin. Biol Neonate 1991; 60:273–282.

*673. Varvarigou A, Bardin CL, Chemtob S, et al. Early ibuprofen administration to prevent patent ductus arteriosus in premature newborn infants. JAMA 1996; 275:539–544.

*674. Fowlie PW. Prophylactic indomethacin: systematic review and meta-analysis. Arch Dis Child 1996; 74:F81–F87.

*675. Schmidt B, Davis P, Moddemann D, et al. Long-term effects of indomethacin prophylaxis in extremely low birth weight infants. N Engl J Med 2001; 344:1966–1972.

676. Shah SS, Ohlsson A. Ibuprofen for the prevention of patent ductus arteriosus in preterm and/or low birth weight infants. Cochrane Database Syst Rev 2006; 1:CD004213.

677. Kluckow M, Evans N. Early echocardiographic prediction of symptomatic patent ductus arteriosus in preterm infants undergoing mechanical ventilation. J Pediatr 1995; 127:774–779.

*678. Su B-H, Watanabe T, Shimizu M, et al. Echocardiographic assessment of patent ductus arteriosus shunt flow pattern in premature infants. Arch Dis Child 1997; 77:F36–F40.

679. Iyer P, Evans N. Re-evaluation of the left atrial to aortic root ratio as a marker of patent ductus arteriosus. Arch Dis Child 1994; 70:F112–F117.

680. Evans N. Diagnosis of patent ductus arteriosus in the preterm newborn. Arch Dis Child 1993; 68:58–61.

681. El Hajjar M, Vaksmann G, Rakza T, et al. Severity of the ductal shunt: a comparison of different markers. Arch Dis Child 2005; 90:F419–F422.

*682. Gersony WM, Peakham GJ, Ellison RC, et al. Effects of indomethacin in premature infants with patent ductus arteriosus; results of a national collaborative study. J Pediatr 1983; 102:895–906.

*683. Colditz P, Murphy D, Rolfe P, et al. Effect of infusion rate of indomethacin on cerebrovascular responses in pre term neonates. Arch Dis Child 1989; 64:1–12.

684. Edwards AD, Wyatt JS, Richardson C, et al. Effects of indomethacin on cerebral haemodynamics in very pre term infants. Lancet 1990; 335:1491–1495.

*685. Su BH, Peng C-T, Tsai C-H. Echocardiographic flow pattern of patent ductus arteriosus: a guide to indomethacin treatment in premature infants. Arch Dis Child 1999; 81:F197–F200.

686. Patel K, Marks KA, Roberts I, et al. Ibuprofen treatment of patent ductus arteriosus. Lancet 1995; 346:255.

*687. Van Overmeire B, Follens I, Hartmann S, et al. Treatment of patent ductus arteriosus with ibuprofen. Arch Dis Child 1997; 76:F179–F184.

688. Ohlsson A, Walia R, Shah S. Ibuprofen for the treatment of patent ductus arteriosus in preterm and/or low birth weight infants. Cochrane Database Syst Rev 2005; 4:CD003481.

*689. Arlettaz R, Archer N, Wilkinson AR. Closure of the ductus arteriosus and development of pulmonary branch stenosis in babies less than 32 weeks' gestation. Arch Dis Child 2001; 85:F197–F200.

690. Hammerman C, Aramburo MJ. Prolonged indomethacin therapy for the prevention of recurrences of patent ductus arteriosus. J Pediatr 1990; 117:771–776.

*691. Rennie JM, Cooke RWI. Prolonged low dose indomethacin for persistent ductus arteriosus of prematurity. Arch Dis Child 1991; 66:55–58.

692. Roberts P, Adwani S, Archer N, et al. Catheter closure of the arterial duct in preterm infants. Arch Dis Child 2007; 92: F248–50.

693. Villa E, Folliguet T, Magnano D, et al. Video-assisted thoracoscopic clipping of patent ductus arteriosus: close to the gold standard and minimally invasive competitor of percutaneous techniques. J Cardiovasc Med 2006; 7:210–215.

694. Shaughnessy CD, Reller MD, Rice MJ, et al. Development of systemic to pulmonary collateral arteries in premature infants. J Pediatr 1997; 131:763–765.

*695. Roberts JD, Fineman JR, Morin FC, et al. Inhaled nitric oxide and persistent pulmonary hypertension of the newborn. N Engl J Med 1997; 336:605–610.

*696. Tworetzky W, Bristow J, Moore P, et al. Inhaled nitric oxide in neonates with persistent pulmonary hypertension. Lancet 2001; 357:118–120.

*697. Cornfield DN, Maynard RC, deRegnier RA, et al. Randomized controlled trial of low dose inhaled nitric oxide in the treatment of term and near term infants with respiratory failure and pulmonary hypertension. Pediatrics 1999; 104:1089–1094.

*698. Kinsella JP, Truog WE, Walsh WF, et al. Randomized multicenter trial of inhaled nitric oxide and high frequency oscillatory ventilation in severe, persistent pulmonary hypertension of the newborn. J Pediatr 1997; 131:55–62.

699. Jedeikin R, Primhak A, Shennan AT, et al. Serial electrocardiographic changes in healthy and stressed neonates. Arch Dis Child 1983; 58:605–611.

700. Setzer E, Ermocilla R, Tonkin I, et al. Papillary muscle necrosis in a neonatal autopsy population: incidence and associated clinical manifestations. J Pediatr 1980; 96:289–294.

701. Tillett A, Hartley B, Simpson J. Paradoxical embolism causing fatal myocardial infarction in a newborn infant. Arch Dis Child 2001; 85:F137–F138.

702. Opie GF, Fraser SH, Drew JH, et al. Bacterial endocarditis in neonatal intensive care. J Paediatr Child Health 1999; 35:545–548.

703. Way GL, Woolfe RR, Eshaghpour E, et al. The natural history of hypertrophic cardiomyopathy in infants of diabetic mothers. J Pediatr 1979; 95:1020–1025.

704. Shaw NJ, Wilson N, Dickinson DF. Captopril in heart failure secondary to left to right shunt. Arch Dis Child 1988; 63:360–363.

705. Leversha AM, Wilson NJ, Clarkson PM, et al. Efficiency and dosage of enalapril in congenital and acquired heart disease. Arch Dis Child 1994; 70:35–39.

706. Kluckow M, Evans N. Low systemic blood pressure in the preterm infant. Semin Neonatol 2001; 6:75–84.

707. Joint Working Party of British Association of Perinatal Medicine and the Research Unit of the Royal College of Physicians. Development of audit measures and guidelines for good practice in the management of neonatal respiratory distress syndrome. Arch Dis Child 1992; 67:1221–1227.

708. Keeley SR, Bohn DJ. The use of inotropic and afterload reducing agents in neonates. Clin Perinatol 1988; 15:467–489.

*709. Gill AB, Weindling AM. Randomised controlled trial of plasma protein fraction versus dopamine in hypotensive very low birth weight infants. Arch Dis Child 1993; 69:284–287.

710. Seri I. Circulatory support of the sick preterm infant. Semin Neonatol 2001; 6:85–95.

*711. Hanley FL, Sade RM, Freedom RM, et al. Outcomes in critically ill neonates with pulmonary stenosis and intact ventricular septum: a multi institutional study. J Am Coll Cardiol 1993; 22:183–192.

712. Salmon AP, Keeton BR, Sethia B. Developments in interventional catheterisation and progress in surgery for congenital heart disease: achieving a balance. Br Heart J 1993; 69:479–480.

Gastrointestinal problems and jaundice of the neonate

713. Dyball REJ, Navaratnam V, Tate PA. Basic embryology and the embryological basis of malformation syndromes. In: Rennie JM, Roberton NRC, eds. Textbook of neonatology, 3rd edn. Edinburgh: Churchill Livingstone; 1999:121–132.

714. Lebenthal E, Heitlinger L, Milla PJ. Prenatal and perinatal development of the gastrointestinal tract. In: Milla JP, Muller DPR, eds. Harries Paediatric gastroenterology, 2nd edn. Edinburgh: Churchill Livingstone; 1988.3–29.

715. Bisset WM, Watt JB, Rivers JPA, et al. Ontogeny of fasting small intestinal motor activity in the human infant. Gut 1988; 29:483–488.

716. Walker-Smith J, Murch S, eds. Diseases of the small intestine in childhood, 4th edn. Oxford: Isis Medical Media; 1999:1–10.

717. Weaver LT. Anatomy and embryology. In: Walker WA, Durie PR, Hamilton JR, et al, eds. Pediatric gastrointestinal disease, 2nd edn. St. Louis: Mosby; 1996:9–30.

*718. Premji S, Chessell L. Continuous nasogastric milk feeding versus intermittent bolus milk feeding for premature infants less than 1500 grams. Cochrane Database Syst Rev 2002; 4:CD001819.

*719. Kennedy KA, Tyson JE, Chamnanvanakij S. Rapid versus slow rate of advancement of feedings

for promoting growth and preventing necrotizing enterocolitis in parenterally fed low-birth-weight infants. Cochrane Database Syst Rev 1998; 4:CD001241.

*720. Pinelli J, Symington A. Non-nutritive sucking for promoting physiologic stability and nutrition in preterm infants. Cochrane Database Syst Rev 2005; 4:CD001071.

*721. Ng E, Shah V. Erythromycin for feeding intolerance in preterm infants. Cochrane Database Syst Rev 2001; 2:CD001815.

*722. McClure RJ, Kristensen JH, Grauaug A. Randomised controlled trial of cisapride in preterm infants. Arch Dis Child 1999; 80:F174–F177.

*723. Britton C, McCormick FM, Renfrew MJ, et al. Support for breastfeeding mothers. Cochrane Database Syst Rev 2007; 1:CD001141.

*724. Carroll AE, Garrison MM, Christakis DA. A systematic review of nonpharmacological and nonsurgical therapies for gastroesophageal reflux in infants. Arch Pediatr Adolescent Med 2002; 156:109–113.

725. Walker-Smith J, Murch S, eds. Diseases of the small intestine in childhood, 4th edn. Oxford: Isis Medical Media; 1999.205–234.

726. Sherman PM, Mitchell DJ, Cutz E. Neonatal enteropathies: defining the causes of protracted diarrhea of infancy. J Pediatr Gastroenterol Nutr 2004; 38:16–26.

727. Amiel J, Lyonnet S. Hirschsprung disease, associated syndromes, and genetics: a review. J Med Genet 2001; 38:729–739.

728. Gilger MA. Upper gastrointestinal bleeding. In: Walker WA, Goulet O, Kleinman RE, et al, eds. Pediatric gastrointestinal disease, 4th edn. Hamilton: BC Decker; 2004.258–265.

729. Turck D, Michaud L. Lower gastrointestinal bleeding. In: Walker WA, Goulet O, Kleinman RE, et al, eds. Pediatric gastrointestinal disease, 4th edn. Hamilton: BC Decker; 2004.266–280.

730. British Paediatric Surveillance Unit. Annual Report. London: Royal College of Paediatrics and Child Health; 1997.

731. Lemons J, Bauer CR, Oh W, et al. Very low birth weight outcomes of the National Institute of Child Health and Human Development Neonatal Research Network, January 1995 through December 1996. Pediatrics 107(1). Available at:www.pediatrics.org/cgi/content/full/107/1/e1.

732. Hintz SR, Kendrick DE, Stoll BJ, et al. Neurodevelopmental and growth outcomes of extremely low birth weight infants after necrotizing enterocolitis. Pediatrics 2005; 115:696–703.

733. Bell EF. Preventing necrotizing enterocolitis: What works and how safe? Pediatrics 2005; 115:173–174.

*734. Kennedy KA, Tyson JE, Chamnanvanakij S. Early versus delayed initiation of progressive enteral feedings for parenterally fed low birth weight or preterm infants. Cochrane Database Syst Rev 2000; 1:CD001970.

*735. Tyson JE, Kennedy KA. Trophic feedings for parenterally fed infants. Cochrane Database Syst Rev 2005; 3:CD000504.

*736. Shah P, Shah V. Arginine supplementation for prevention of necrotising enterocolitis in preterm infants. Cochrane Database Syst Rev 2004; 4:CD004339.

*737. Foster J, Cole M. Oral immunoglobulin for preventing necrotizing enterocolitis in preterm and low birth weight infants. Cochrane Database Syst Rev 2004; 1:CD001816.

*738. Bury RG, Tudehope D. Enteral antibiotics for preventing necrotizing enterocolitis in low birth weight or preterm infants. Cochrane Database Syst Rev 2001; 1:CD000405.

*739. Bell EF, Acarregui MJ. Restricted versus liberal water intake for preventing morbidity and mortality

in preterm infants. Cochrane Database Syst Rev 2001; 3:CD000503.

*740. Roberts D, Dalziel S. Antenatal corticosteroids for accelerating fetal lung maturation for women at risk of preterm birth. Cochrane Database Syst Rev 2006; 3:CD004454.

*741. Lucas A, Cole TJ. Breast milk and neonatal necrotising enterocolitis. Lancet 1990; 336:1519–1523.

*742. Schanler RJ. Probiotics and necrotizing enterocolitis in premature infants. Arch Dis Child 2006; 91:F395–F397.

743. Claud EC, Caplan M. Necrotizing enterocolitis. In: Walker WA, Goulet O, Kleinman RE, et al, eds. Pediatric gastrointestinal disease, 4th edn. Hamilton: BC Decker; 2004:873–879.

744. Goulet O, Ruemmele F, Lacaille F, et al. Irreversible intestinal failure. J Pediatr Gastroenterol Nutr 2004; 38:250–269.

745. Gupte GL, Beath SV, Kelly DA, et al. Current issues in the management of intestinal failure. Arch Dis Child 2006; 91:259–264.

746. Kelly DA. Intestinal failure-associated liver disease: what do we know today? Gastroenterology 2006; 130:S70–S77.

747. Weinberg RP. Gastroenterology. I. Bilirubin physiology. In: Roberton NRC, ed. Textbook of neonatology. London: Churchill Livingstone; 1986: 383–393.

748. Wang X, Roy Chowdhury J, Roy Chowdhury N. Bilirubin metabolism: Applied physiology. Curr Paediatr 2006; 16:70–74.

749. Garcia LM. Disorders of bilirubin metabolism. In: Assali NS, ed. Pathophysiology of gestation. Vol III. New York: Academic Press; 1972:457.

750. Schmidt R. Bilirubin metabolism: the state of the art. Gastroenterology 1978; 74:1307–1312.

751. McDonagh AF, Palmer LA, Lightner DA. Phototherapy for neonatal jaundice. J Am Chem Soc 1982; 104:6867.

752. Gourley CR, Arend RA. Beta-glucuronidase and hyperbilirubinaemia in breast fed and formula fed babies. Lancet 1986; i:644–646.

753. Roberts EA. The jaundiced baby. In: Kelly DA, ed. Diseases of the liver and biliary system in children. Oxford: Blackwell Science; 1999:11–45.

754. Gartner IM, Herschel M. Jaundice and breastfeeding. Pediatr Clin North Am 2001; 48: 389–399.

Hematological problems of the newborn

755. Marshall CJ, Thrasher AJ. The embryonic origins of human haematopoiesis. Br J Haematol 2001; 112:838–850.

756. Pearson HA. Life-span of the fetal red blood cell. J Pediatr 1967; 70:166–171.

757. Watts T, Roberts I. Haematological abnormalities in the growth-restricted infant. Semin Neonatol 1999; 4:41–54.

758. Forestier F, Daffos F, Galacteros F, et al. Hematological values of 163 normal fetuses between 18 and 30 weeks of gestation. Pediatr Res 1986; 20:342–346.

759. Watts TL, Murray NA, Roberts IA. Thrombopoietin has a primary role in the regulation of platelet production in preterm babies. Pediatr Res 1999; 46:28–32.

760. Christensen RD, Calhoun DA, Rimsza LM. A practical approach to evaluating and treating neutropenia in the neonatal intensive care unit. Clin Perinatol 2000; 27:577–601.

761. Hann IM. The normal blood picture in neonates. In: Hann IM, Gibson BES, Letsky EA, eds. Fetal and neonatal haematology. London: Bailliere Tindall; 1991.

762. Thurlbeck SM, McIntosh N. Preterm blood counts vary with sampling site. Arch Dis Child 1987; 62:74–75.

763. Brugnara C, Platt OS. The neonatal erythrocyte and its disorders. In: Nathan DG, Orkin SH, Ginsburg D, et al, eds. Nathan and Oski's Haematology of infancy and childhood, 6th edn. Philadelphia: WB Saunders; 2003:19–55.

764. Linderkamp O, Nelle M, Kraus M, et al. The effect of early and late cord-clamping on blood viscosity and other hemorheological parameters in full-term neonates. Acta Paediatr 1992; 81:745–750.

765. Roberts I, Murray NA. Neonatal thrombocytopenia: causes and management. Arch Dis Child Fetal Neonatal Ed 2003; 88:F359–F364.

766. Brown KE. Haematological consequences of parvovirus B19 infection. Baillieres Best Pract Res Clin Haematol 2000; 13:245–259.

767. Lallemand AV, Doco-Fenzy M, Gaillard DA. Investigation of nonimmune hydrops fetalis: multidisciplinary studies are necessary for diagnosis – review of 94 cases. Pediatr Dev Pathol 1999; 2:432–439.

768. Lipton JM. Diamond–Blackfan anemia: New paradigms for a "not so pure" inherited red cell aplasia. Semin Hematol 2006; 43:167–177.

769. Stockman JA. Overview of the state of the art of Rh disease: history, current clinical management, and recent progress. J Pediatr Hematol Oncol 2001; 23:554–562.

770. Williamson LM. Leucocyte depletion of the blood supply – how will patients benefit? Br J Haematol 2000; 110:256–272.

771. Alcock GS, Liley H. Immunoglobulin infusion for isoimmune haemolytic jaundice in neonates. Cochrane Database Syst Rev 2002; 3:CD003313.

772. Delhommeau F, Cynober T, Schischmanoff PO, et al. Natural history of hereditary spherocytosis during the first year of life. Blood 2000; 95:393–397.

773. Bolton-Maggs PH, Stevens RF, Dodd NJ, et al. Guidelines for the diagnosis and management of hereditary spherocytosis. Br J Haematol 2004; 126:455–474.

774. Mehta A, Mason PJ, Vulliamy TJ. Glucose-6-phosphate dehydrogenase deficiency. Baillieres Best Pract Res Clin Haematol 2000; 13:21–38.

775. Zanella A, Fermo E, Bianchi P, et al. Red cell pyruvate kinase deficiency: molecular and clinical aspects. Br J Haematol 2005; 130:11–25.

776. Hume H. Red blood cell transfusions for preterm infants: the role of evidence-based medicine. Semin Perinatol 1997; 21:8–19.

777. Gibson BE, Todd A, Roberts I, et al. Transfusion guidelines for neonates and older children. Br J Haematol 2004; 124:433–453.

*778. Aher S, Ohlsson A. Late erythropoietin for preventing red blood cell transfusion in preterm and/or low birth weight infants. Cochrane Database Syst Rev 2006; 3:CD004868.

*779. Ohlsson A, Aher SM. Early erythropoietin for preventing red blood cell transfusion in preterm and/or low birth weight infants. Cochrane Database Syst Rev 2006; 3:CD004863.

*780. Dempsey EM, Barrington K. Short and long term outcomes following partial exchange transfusion in the polycythaemic newborn: a systematic review. Arch Dis Child Fetal Neonatal Ed 2006; 91: F2–F6.7.

*781. de Waal KA, Baerts W, Offringa M. Systematic review of the optimal fluid for dilutional exchange transfusion in neonatal polycythaemia. Arch Dis Child Fetal Neonatal Ed 2006; 91:F7–F10.

*782. Carr R, Modi N, Dore C. G-CSF and GM-CSF for treating or preventing neonatal infections. Cochrane Database Syst Rev 2003; 3:CD003066.

*783. Mohan P, Brocklehurst P. Granulocyte transfusions for neonates with confirmed or suspected sepsis and neutropaenia. Cochrane Database Syst Rev 2003; 4:CD003956.

784. Bajwa RP, Skinner R, Windebank KP, et al. Chemotherapy and marrow transplantation for congenital leukaemia. Arch Dis Child Fetal Neonatal Ed 2001; 84:F47–F48.

785. Zipursky A. Transient leukaemia – a benign form of leukaemia in newborn infants with trisomy 21. Br J Haematol 2003; 120:930–938.

786. Ahmed M, Sternberg A, Hall G, et al. Natural history of GATA1 mutations in Down syndrome. Blood 2004; 103:2480–2489.

787. Kemball-Cook G, Tuddenham EGD, McVey JH. Normal haemostasis. In: Hoffbrand AV, Catovsky D, Tuddenham EGD, eds. Postgraduate haematology, 5th edn. Oxford: Blackwell Publishing; 2005.

788. Andrew M. The relevance of developmental hemostasis to hemorrhagic disorders of newborns. Semin Perinatol 1997; 21:70–85.

789. Andrew M, Paes B, Milner R, et al. Development of the human coagulation system in the healthy premature infant. Blood 1988; 72:1651–1657.

790. Andrew M, Paes B, Johnston M. Development of the hemostatic system in the neonate and young infant. Am J Pediatr Hematol Oncol 1990; 12:95–104.

791. Seguin JH, Topper WH. Coagulation studies in very low-birthweight infants. Am J Perinatol 1994; 11:27–29.

792. Chalmers EA. Haemophilia and the newborn. Blood Rev 2004; 18:85–92.

793. Williams MD, Chalmers EA, Gibson BE. The investigation and management of neonatal haemostasis and thrombosis. Br J Haematol 2002; 119:295–309.

794. Golding J, Greenwood R, Birmingham K, et al. Childhood cancer, intramuscular vitamin K, and pethidine given during labour. BMJ 1992; 305:341–346.

795. Cornelissen M, von Kries R, Loughnan P, et al. Prevention of vitamin K deficiency bleeding: efficacy of different multiple oral dose schedules of vitamin K. Eur J Pediatr 1997; 156:126–130.

*796. Puckett RM, Offringa M. Prophylactic vitamin K for vitamin K deficiency bleeding in neonates. Cochrane Database Syst Rev 2000; 4:CD002776.

797. Chakravorty S, Murray N, Roberts I. Neonatal thrombocytopenia. Early Hum Dev 2005; 81:35–41.

798. Ouwehand WH, Smith G, Ranasinghe E. Management of severe alloimmune thrombocytopenia in the newborn. Arch Dis Child Fetal Neonatal Ed 2000; 82:F173–F175.

799. Greenway A, Massicotte MP, Monagle P. Neonatal thrombosis and its treatment. Blood Rev 2004; 18:75–84.

800. Manco-Johnson MJ. How I treat venous thrombosis in children. Blood 2006; 107:21–29.

801. Shah P, Shah V. Continuous heparin infusion to prevent thrombosis and catheter occlusion in neonates with peripherally placed percutaneous central venous catheters. Cochrane Database Syst Rev 2005; 3:CD002772.

802. Duran R, Biner B, Demir M, et al. Factor V Leiden mutation and other thrombophilia markers in childhood ischemic stroke. Clin Appl Thromb Hemost 2005; 11:83–88.

Neonatal neurology

803. Saint-Anne Dargassies S. Neurological development in full term and premature neonates. Amsterdam: Elsevier/North Holland/Exerpta Medica; 1977.

804. Amiel-Tison C, Grenier A. Neurological assessment within the first year of life. New York: Oxford University Press; 1986.

805. Prechtl HFR, Bientema D. The neurological examination of the full term newborn infant. Clinics in developmental medicine, No 12. London: SIMP/Heinemann; 1964.

806. Prechtl HFR. The neurological examination of the full term newborn infant, 2nd edn. Clinics in developmental medicine, No 63. London: SIMP/Heinemann; 1977.

807. Prechtl HFR. Qualitative changes of spontaneous movements in fetus and preterm infant as a marker of neurological dysfunction. Early Hum Dev 1990; 23:151–158.

808. Einspieler C, Prechtl HFR, Bos AF, et al. Prechtl's method on the qualitative assessment of general movements in preterm, term and young infants. Clinics in developmental medicine, No 167. Cambridge: Mac Keith Press, Cambridge University Press; 2004.

809. Brazelton TB. Neonatal behavioural assessment scale. Clinics in developmental medicine, No 50. London: SIMP/Heinemann; 1973.

810. Brazelton TB, Nugent JK. Neonatal behavioral assessment scale, 3rd edn. Clinics in Developmental Medicine, No 137. Cambridge: Mac Keith Press, Cambridge University Press; 1995.

811. Dubowitz L, Dubowitz LMS. The neurological assessment of the preterm and full term new born infant. Clinics in developmental medicine, No 79. London: SIMP/Heinemann; 1981.

812. Dubowitz LMS, Dubowitz V, Mercuri E. The neurological assessment of the preterm and full term newborn infant, 2nd edn. Clinics in developmental medicine, No 148. Cambridge: Mac Keith Press, Cambridge University Press; 1999.

813. Amiel-Tison C. Clinical assessment of the infant nervous system. In: Levene MI, Lilford RJ, eds. Fetal and neonatal neurology and neurosurgery, 2nd edn. Edinburgh: Churchill Livingstone; 1995:83–104.

814. Dubowitz LMS, Mushin J, de Vries L, et al. Visual function in the newborn infant: is it cortically mediated? Lancet 1986; i:1139–1140.

815. Braddick O, Wattam-Bell J, Atkinson J. Orientation-specific cortical responses develop in early infancy. Nature 1986; 320:617–619.

816. Rennie JM, Robertson NJ, eds. Neonatal cerebral investigation. Cambridge: Cambridge University Press; 2008.

817. Rutherford M. MRI of the neonatal brain. London: WB Saunders; 2002.

818. Barkovich AJ. Pediatric neuroimaging. 4th edn. Philadelphia: Lippincott Williams & Wilkins; 2005.

819. Garges HP, Moody MA, Cotton CM, et al. Neonatal meningitis: what is the correlation among cerebrospinal fluid cultures, blood cultures, and cerebrospinal fluid parameters? Pediatrics 2006; 117:1094–1110.

820. Ahmed A, Hickey S, Ehrett S, et al. Cerebrospinal fluid values in the term neonate. Pediatr Infect Dis J 1996; 15:298–303.

821. Martin-Ancel A, Garcia-Alix A, Salas S, et al. Cerebrospinal fluid leucocyte counts in healthy neonates. Arch Dis Child 2006; 91:F357–F358.

822. Kaiser AM, Whitelaw AGL. Hypertensive response to increased intracranial pressure in infancy. Arch Dis Child 1988; 63:1461–1465.

823. Hellstrom-Westas L, Rosen I, de Vries LS, et al. Amplitude integrated EEG classification and interpretation in term and preterm infants. NeoReviews 2006; 7:e76–e86.

824. Hellstrom-Westas L, Rosen I, Svenningsen NW. Predictive value of early continuous amplitude integrated EEG recordings on outcome after severe birth asphyxia in full term infants. Arch Dis Child 1995; 72:F34–F38.

825. Eken P, Toet MC, Groenendaal F, et al. Predictive value of early neuroimaging, pulsed Doppler and neurophysiology in full term infants with hypoxic-ischaemic encephalopathy. Arch Dis Child 1995; 73:F75–F80.

826. Holmes GL, Lombroso CT. Prognostic value of background patterns in the neonatal EEG. J Clin Neurophysiol 1993; 10:323–352.

827. Taylor MJ, Murphy WJ, Whyte HE. Prognostic reliability of SEPs and VEPs in asphyxiated newborn infants. Dev Med Child Neurol 1992; 34:507–515.

828. De Vries LS, Connell J, Dubowitz LMS, et al. Neurological, electrophysiological and MRI

abnormalities in infants with extensive cystic leukomalacia. Neuropediatrics 1987; 18:61–66.

829.   Hepper PG, Shahidullah BS. Development of fetal hearing. Arch Dis Child 1994; 71:F81–F87.

830.   Mizrahi EM, Kellaway P. Diagnosis and management of neonatal seizures. New York: Lippincott Raven; 1998.

831.   Scher MS, Aso K, Beggarly ME. Electrographic seizures in preterm and full term neonates: clinical correlates, associated brain lesions and risk for neurologic sequelae. Pediatrics 1993; 91:128–134.

832.   Volpe JJ. Neurology of the newborn, 4th edn. Philadelphia: WB Saunders; 2001:103–133.

833.   Weiner SP, Painter MJ, Geva D, et al. Neonatal seizures: electroclinical dissociation. Pediatr Neurol 1991; 7:363–368.

834.   Boylan GB, Pressler RM, Rennie JM, et al. Outcome of electroclinical, electrographic, and clinical seizures in the newborn infant. Dev Med Child Neurol 1999; 41:819–825.

835.   Boylan GB, Panerai RB, Rennie JM, et al. Cerebral blood flow velocity during neonatal seizures. Arch Dis Child 1999; 80:F105–F110.

836.   Lanska MJ, Lanska DJ, Baumann RJ, et al. A population based study of neonatal seizures in Fayette County, Kentucky. Neurology 1995; 45:724–732.

837.   Van Zeben-Van der Aa DM, Verloove-Vanhorick SP, den Ouden L, et al. Neonatal seizures in very preterm and very low birthweight infants: mortality and handicaps at two years of age in a nationwide cohort. Neuropediatrics 1990; 21:62–65.

838.   Watkins A, Szymonowicz W, Jin X, et al. Significance of seizures in very low birthweight infants. Dev Med Child Neurol 1988; 30:162–169.

839.   Levene MI, Trounce JQ. Neonatal convulsions: towards more precise diagnosis. Arch Dis Child 1986; 61:78–87.

840.   Goldberg JH. Neonatal convulsions – a ten year review. Arch Dis Child 1983; 58:976–978.

841.   Andre M, Matisse M, Vert P, et al. Neonatal seizures – recent aspects. Neuropediatrics 1988; 19:201–207.

842.   Bergman I, Painter MJ, Hirsch RP, et al. Outcome in neonates with convulsions treated in ICU. Ann Neurol 1983; 14:642–657.

843.   Estan J, Hope PL. Unilateral neonatal cerebral infarction in full term infants. Arch Dis Child 1997; 76:F88–F93.

844.   Lien JM, Towers CV, Quilligan EJ, et al. Term early-onset neonatal siezures: obstetric characteristics, etiologic classifications and perinatal care. Obstet Gynaecol 1995; 85:163–169.

845.   Koelfen W, Freund M, Varnholt V. Neonatal stroke involving the middle cerebral artery in term infants: clinical presentation, EEG and imaging studies. Dev Med Child Neurol 1995; 37:203–212.

846.   Nelson K. Stroke in newborn infants. Lancet Neurol 2004; 3:150–158.

847.   Watanabe K, Miyazaki S, Hara K, et al. Behavioural state cycles, background EEGs and prognosis of newborns with perinatal hypoxia. Electroencephalogr Clin Neurophysiol 1980; 49:618–625.

848.   Dzhala VI, Talos DM, Sdrulla DA, et al. NKCC 1 transporter facilitates seizures in the developing brain. Nat Med 2005; 11:1205–1213.

849.   Painter MJ, Scher MS, Stein AD, et al. Phenobarbital compared with phenytoin for the treatment of neonatal seizures. N Engl J Med 1999; 341:485–489.

850.   Rennie JM, Boylan G. Neonatal seizures and their treatment. Curr Opin Neurol 2003; 16:177–181.

851.   Boylan GB, Rennie J, Chorley G, et al. Second line anticonvulsant treatment of neonatal seizures: A video-EEG monitoring study. Neurology 2004; 62:486–488.

852.   Goldberg PN, Moscoso P, Bauer CR. Use of barbiturate therapy in severe perinatal asphyxia. J Pediatr 1986; 109:851–856.

853.   Hellstrom-Westas L, Westergren U, Rosen I, et al. Lidocaine for treatment of severe seizures in newborn infants. Acta Paediatr Scand 1988; 77:79–84.

854.   Gilman JT, Gal P, Duchowny MS, et al. Rapid sequential phenobarbital treatment of neonatal seizures. Pediatrics 1989; 83:674–678.

855.   Gal P, Oles KS, Gilman JT, et al. Valproic acid efficacy, toxicity, and pharmacokinetics in neonates with intractable seizures. Neurology 1988; 38:467–471.

856.   Ledigo A, Clancy RR, Berman PH. Neurologic outcome after electroencephalographically proven neonatal seizures. Pediatrics 1991; 88:583–596.

857.   Temple CM, Dennis J, Carney R, et al. Neonatal seizures: long term outcome and cognitive development among 'normal' survivors. Dev Med Child Neurol 1995; 37:109–118.

858.   May M, Daley AJ, Donath S, et al. Early onset neonatal meningitis in Australia and New Zealand, 1992–2002. Arch Dis Child 2005; 90:F324–F327.

859.   Heath PT, Yusoff NKN, Baker CJ. Neonatal meningitis. Arch Dis Child 2003; 88:F173–F178.

860.   Peckham CS, Johnson C, Aden A, et al. The early acquisition of cytomegalovirus infection. Arch Dis Child 1987; 62:708–785.

861.   Paryani SG, Arvin AM. Intrauterine infection with varicella zoster virus after maternal varicella. N Engl J Med 1986; 314:1542–1546.

862.   Cheong JL, Hagmann C, Rennie JM, et al. Fatal newborn head enlargement: high resolution magnetic resonance imaging at 4.7 T. Arch Dis Child 2006; 91:F202–F203.

863.   Szymonowicz W, Yu VYH, Bajuk B, et al. Neurodevelopmental outcome, periventricular haemorrhage and leukomalacia in infants 1250 g or less at birth. Early Hum Dev 1986; 14:1–7.

864.   Strand C, Laptook AR, Dowling S, et al. Neonatal intracranial haemorrhage: I. Changing pattern in inborn low-birth-weight infants. Early Hum Dev 1990; 23:117–128.

865.   Synnes AR, Chien L-Y, Peliowski A, et al. Variations in intraventricular hemorrhage incidence rates among Canadian neonatal intensive care units. J Pediatr 2001; 138:525–531.

866.   Papile L, Burstein J, Burstein R, et al. Incidence and evolution of subependymal and intraventricular haemorrhage: a study of infants of birth weight less than 1500 g. J Pediatr 1978; 92:529–534.

867.   Levene MI, De Crespigny L ch. Classification of intraventricular haemorrhage. Lancet 1983; i:643.

868.   Trounce JQ, Fagan D, Levene MI. Intraventricular haemorrhage and periventricular leucomalacia: ultrasound and autopsy correlation. Arch Dis Child 1986; 61:1203–1207.

869.   Di Pietro MA, Brody BA, Teele RL. Peritrigonal echogenic 'blush' on cranial sonography: pathologic correlates. Am J Radiol 1986; 146:1067–1072.

870.   Paneth N, Rudelli R, Kazam E, et al. Brain damage in the preterm infant. Clinics in developmental medicine No 131. London: MacKeith Press; 1994.119–137.

871.   Woodward LJ, Anderson PJ, Austin NC, et al. Neonatal magnetic resonance imaging to predict neurodevelopmental outcomes in preterm infants. N Engl J Med 2006; 355:685–694.

872.   Limperopoulos C, Benson CB, Bassan H, et al. Cerebellar haemorrhage in the preterm infant: ultrasonographic findings and risk factors. Pediatrics 2005; 116:717–724.

873.   Whitelaw A, Rivers RPA, Creighton L, et al. Low dose intraventricular fibrinolytic treatment to prevent posthaemorrhagic hydrocephalus. Arch Dis Child 1992; 67:12–14.

874.   Kennedy CR, Ayers S, Campbell MJ, et al. Randomized, controlled trial of acetazolamide and furosemide in posthemorrhagic ventricular dilation in infancy: follow-up at 1 year. Pediatrics 2001; 108:597–607.

875.   Goldstein I, Copel JA, Makhoul IR. Mild cerebral ventriculomegaly in fetuses: characteristics and outcome. Fetal Diagn Ther 2001; 20:281–284.

876.   Gaglioti P, Danelon D, Bontempo S, et al. Fetal cerebral ventriculomegaly: outcome in 176 cases. Ultrasound Obstet Gynecol 2005; 25:372–377.

Renal disease in the neonate

877.   Evan AP, Larsson L. Morphologic development of the nephron. In: Edelmann CM, ed. Pediatric kidney disease. Boston: Little Brown; 1992.20.Fig. 2.1

878.   Haycock G. Perinatal nephrology. In: Gearhart JP, Rink RC, Mouriquand PDE, eds. Pediatric urology. WB Saunders, Phil, USA 2001:14–26.

879.   Stefos T, Plachouras N, Sotiriadis A, et al. Routine obstetrical ultrasound at 18–22 weeks: Our experience on 7,326 fetuses. J Matern Fetal Med 1999; 8:64–69.

880.   Housley HT, Harrison MR. Fetal urinary tract abnormalities. Natural history, pathophysiology and treatment. Urol Clin North Am 1998; 25:63–73.

881.   Cascio S, Paran S, Puri P. Associated urological anomalies in children with unilateral renal agenesis. J Urol 1999; 162:1081–1083.

882.   Van Allen MI. Urinary tract. In: Stevenson RE, Hall JG, Goodman RM, eds. Human malformations and related anomalies. New York: Oxford University Press; 1993;II:501–550.

883.   Roodhooft AM, Birnholz JC, Holmes LB. Familial nature of congenital absence and severe dysgenesis of both kidneys. N Engl J Med 1984; 310:1341–1345.

884.   Fisher C, Smith JF. Renal dysplasia in nephrectomy specimens from adolescents and adults. J Clin Pathol 1975; 28:879–890.

885.   Mackie GG, Stephens FD. Duplex kidneys: a correlation of renal dysplasia with position of the ureteral orifice. J Urol 1975; 11:274–280.

886.   Srivastava T, Garola RE, Hellerstein S. Autosomal dominant inheritance of multicystic dysplastic kidney. Pediatr Nephrol 1999; 13:481–483.

887.   Sanders RC, Hartman DS. The sonographic distinction between neonatal multicystic kidney and hydronephrosis. Radiology 1984; 151:621–625.

888.   Aslam M, Watson AR. Unilateral multicystic dysplastic kidney (MCDK): long term outcomes. Arch Dis Child 2006; 91:820–3.

889.   Narchi H. Risk of hypertension with multicystic kidney disease: a systematic review. Arch Dis Child 2005; 90:921–924.

890.   Narchi H. Risk of Wilm's tumour with multicystic kidney disease: a systematic review. Arch Dis Child 2005; 90:147–149.

891.   Zerres K, Mucher G, Becker J, et al. Prenatal diagnosis of autosomal recessive polycystic kidney disease (ARPKD): molecular genetics, clinical experience, and fetal morphology. Am J Med Genet 1998; 76:137–144.

892.   Gagnadoux MF. Cystic kidney disease. Rev Prat 1997; 15:1536–1540.

893.   MacDermot KD, Saggar-Malik AK, Economides DL, et al. Prenatal diagnosis of autosomal dominant polycystic kidney disease (PKD1) presenting in utero and prognosis for very early onset disease. J Med Genet 1998; 35:13–16.

894.   Daneman A, Alton DJ. Radiographic manifestations of renal anomalies. Radiol Clin North Am 1991; 29:351–363.

895.   Hohenfeller M, Shultz-Lampel D, Lampel A, et al. Tumour in the horse-shoe kidney: clinical implications and review of embryogenesis. J Urol 1992; 147:1098–1102.

896.   Cacciaguerr S, Bagnara V, Arena C, et al. Megacalycosis on duplex upper moiety. Eur J Pediatr Surg 1996; 6:42–44.

897.   Chevalier RC. Pathogenesis of renal injury in obstructive uropathy. Curr Opin Pediatr 2006; 18:153–160.

898. Biard JM, Johnson MP, Carr MC, et al. Long-term outcomes in children treated by prenatal vesicoamniotic shunting for lower urinary tract obstruction. Obstet Gynaecol 2005; 106:503–508.

899. Kitagawa H, Pringle KC, Koike J, et al. Vesicoamniotic shunt for complete urinary tract obstruction is partially effective. J Pediatr Surg 2006; 41:394–402.

900. Rizk D, Chapman AB. Cystic and inherited kidney diseases. Am J Kidney Dis 2003; 42:1305–1317.

901. Thummala MR, Raju TN, Langenberg P. Isolated single umbilical artery anomaly and the risk for congenital malformations: a meta-analysis. J Pediatr Surg 1998; 33:580–585.

902. Lee RS, Cendron M, Kinnamon DD, et al. Antenatal hydronephrosis as a predictor of postnatal outcome: A meta-analysis. Pediatrics 2006; 118: 586–593.

903. Shokeir AA, Nijman RJ. Antenatal hydronephrosis: changing concepts in diagnosis and subsequent management. BJU Int 2000; 85: 987–994.

904. Mandell J, Blyth BR, Peters CA, et al. Structural genitourinary defects detected in utero. Radiology 1991; 178:193–196.

905. Siemens DR, Prouse KA, MacNeilly AE, et al. Antenatal hydronephrosis: thresholds of renal pelvic diameter to predict insignificant postnatal pelviectasis. Tech Urol 1998; 4:198–201.

906. Teele RL, Share JC. Renal screening. In: Ultrasonography in infants and children. Philadelphia: WB Saunders; 1991.137–192.

907. Arger PH, Coleman BG, Mintz MC, et al. Routine fetal genitourinary tract screening. Radiology 1985; 156:485–489.

908. Grignon A, Filion R, Filiatrault D, et al. Urinary tract dilatation in utero: classification and clinical applications. Radiology 1986; 160:645–647.

909. Ransley PG, Dhillon HK, Gordon I, et al. The postnatal management of hydronephrosis diagnosed by prenatal ultrasound. J Urol 1990; 144:584–587.

910. Maizels M, Reisman ME, Flom LS. Grading nephroureteral dilatation detected in the first year of life: correlation with obstruction. J Urol 1992; 148:609–614.

911. Stocks A, Richards D, Frentzen B, et al. Correlation of prenatal pelvic anteroposterior diameter with outcome in infancy. J Urol 1996; 155:1050–1052.

912. Aksu N, Yavascan O, Kangin M, et al. Postnatal management of infants with antenatally detected hydronephrosis. Pediatr Nephrol 2005; 20:1253–1259.

913. Woodward M, Frank D. Postnatal management of antenatal hydronephrosis. BJU Int 2002; 89:149–156.

914. Pinto E, Guignard JP. Renal masses in the neonate. Biol Neonate 1995; 68:175–184.

915. Winyard PJ, Bharucha T, De Bruyn R, et al. Perinatal renal venous thrombosis: presenting renal length predicts outcome. Arch Dis Child Fetal Neonatal Ed 2006; 91:F273–F278.

916. Marks SD, Massicaotte MP, Steele B, et al. Neonatal renal venous thrombosis: clinical outcomes and prevalence of prothombotic disorders. J Pediatr 2005; 146:811–816.

917. Weinschenk N, Pelidis M, Fiascone J. Combination thrombolytic and anticoagulant therapy for bilateral renal vein thrombosis in a premature infant. Am J Perinatol 2001; 18:293–297.

918. Mocan H, Beattie TJ, Murphy AV. Renal vein thrombosis in infancy: long term follow up. Pediatr Nephrol 1991; 5:45–49.

919. Porter E, McKie A, Beattie TJ, et al. Neonatal nephrocalcinosis: long-term follow up. Arch Dis Child Fetal Neonatal Ed 2006; 91:F333–F336.

920. Miltenyi M. Protein excretion in healthy children. Clin Nephrol 1979; 12:216–221.

921. Giel DW, Noe HN, Williams MA. Ultrasound screening of asymptomatic siblings of children with vesicoureteral reflux: a long-term follow-up study. J Urol 2005; 174:1602–1604.

922. Hentschel R, Lodige B, Bulla M. Renal insufficiency in the neonatal period. Clin Nephrol 1996; 46:54–58.

923. Wu PY, Hodgman JE. Insensible water loss in preterm infants: changes with postnatal development and non-ionizing radiant energy. Pediatrics 1974; 54:704–712.

924. Coulthard MG, Vernon B. Managing acute renal failure in very low birthweight infants. Arch Dis Child Fetal Neonatal Ed 1995; 73:F187–F192.

925. Chevalier RL, Campbell F, Brenbridge AN. Prognostic factors in neonatal acute renal failure. Pediatrics 1984; 74:265–272.

926. Moghal NE, Brocklebank JT, Meadow SR. A review of acute renal failure in children: incidence, etiology and outcome. Clin Nephrol 1998; 49:91–95.

927. Al-Hermi BE, Al-Saran, Secker D, et al. Hemodialysis for end-stage renal disease in children weighing less than 10 Kg. Pediatr Nephrol 1999; 13:401–403.

928. Singh HP, Hurley RM, Myers TF. Neonatal hypertension. Incidence and risk factors. Am J Hypertens 1992; 5:51–55.

929. Flynn JT. Neonatal hypertension: diagnosis and management. Pediatr Nephrol 2000; 14:332–341.

930. Zorc JJ, Levine DA, Platt SL, et al. Clinical and demographic factors associated with urinary tract infection in young febrile infants. Pediatrics 2005; 116:644–648.

931. Cleper R, Krause I, Eisenstein B, et al. Prevalence of vesicoureteral reflux in neonatal urinary tract infection. Clin Pediatr 2004; 43:619–625.

Eye problems in the newborn

932. De Silva DJ, Cocker KD, Lau G, et al. Optic disk size and optic disk-to-fovea distance in preterm and full-term infants. Invest Ophthalmol Vis Sci 2006; 47:4683–4686.

933. Fielder AR, Moseley MJ, Ng YK. The immature visual system and preterm birth. In: Hull D, Cooke R, Whitelaw A, eds. The very immature infant Br Med Bulk. 1988;44:1093–1118.

934. Smith LE. IGF-1 and retinopathy of prematurity in the preterm infant. Biol Neonate 2005; 88:237–244.

935. Fielder AR, Moseley MJ. Environmental light and the preterm infant. Semin Perinatol 2000; 24:291–298.

936. Darville T. Chlamydia trachomatis infections in neonates and young children. Semin Pediatr Infect Dis 2005; 16:235–244.

937. Zar HJ. Neonatal chlamydial infections: prevention and treatment. Paediatr Drugs 2005; 7:103–110.

938. Woods CR. Gonococcal infections in neonates and young children. Semin Pediatr Infect Dis 2005; 16:258–270.

*939. Isenberg SJ, Wood LM. A controlled trial of povidone-iodine as prophylaxis against ophthalmia neonatorum. N Engl J Med 1995; 332:562–566.

940. Isenberg SJ, Apt L, Del Signore M, et al. A double application approach to ophthalmia neonatorum prophylaxis. Br J Ophthalmol 2003; 87:1449–1452.

941. Hughes LA, May K, Talbot JF, et al. Incidence, distribution, and duration of birth-related retinal hemorrhages: a prospective study. J AAPOS 2006; 10:102–106.

942. Ashton N. Oxygen and retinal blood vessels. Trans Ophthalmol Soc UK 1980; 100:359–362.

943. Patz A. Retrolental fibroplasia (retinopathy of prematurity). Trans Ophthalmol Soc NZ 1980; 32:49–54.

944. Kretzer FL, Hittner HM. Retinopathy of prematurity: clinical implications of retinal development. Arch Dis Child 1988; 63:1151–1167.

945. Alon T, Hemo I, Itin A, et al. Vascular endothelial growth factor acts as a survival factor for newly formed retinal vessels and has implications for retinopathy of prematurity. Nat Med 1995; 1:1024–1028.

946. Pierce EA, Foley ED, Smith LE. Regulation of vascular endothelial growth factor by oxygen in a model of retinopathny of prematurity. Arch Ophthalmol 1996; 114:1219–1228.

*947. STOP-ROP Multicenter Study Group. Supplemental Therapeutic Oxygen for Prethreshold Retinopathy of Prematurity (STOP-ROP), a randomized, controlled trial. I: Primary outcomes. Pediatrics 2000; 105:295–310.

948. Tin W, Milligan DW, Pennefather P, et al. Pulse oximetry, severe retinopathy, and outcome at one year in babies of less than 28 weeks gestation. Arch Dis Child Fetal Neonatal Ed 2001; 84:F106–F110.

949. Cunningham S, Fleck BW, Elton RA, et al. Transcutaneous oxygen levels in retinopathy of prematurity. Lancet 1995; 346:1464–1465.

950. Tin W, Wariyar U. Giving small babies oxygen: 50 years of uncertainty. Semin Neonatol 2002; 7:361–367.

*951. Reynolds JD, Hardy RJ, Kennedy KA, et al. For the Light Reduction in Retinopathy of Prematurity (LIGHT-ROP) Cooperative Group. Lack of efficacy of light reduction in preventing retinopathy of prematurity. N Engl J Med 1998; 338:1572–1576.

952. Fielder AR, Quinn GE. Retinopathy of prematurity. In: Taylor DSI, Hoyt CS, eds. Pediatric ophthalmology and strabismus, 3rd edn. Elsevier London; 2005.506–530.

953. An International Committee for the Classification of Retinopathy of Prematurity. The International Classification of Retinopathy of Prematurity – Revisited. Arch Ophthalmol 2005; 123:991–999.

954. Kivlin JD, Biglan AW, Gordon RA, et al, for the Cryotherapy for Retinopathy of Prematurity (CRYO-ROP) Cooperative Group. Early retinal vessel development and iris vessel dilatation as factors in retinopathy of prematurity. Arch Ophthalmol 1996; 114:150–154.

955. Fielder AR, Levene MI. Screening for retinopathy of prematurity. Arch Dis Child 1992; 67:860–867.

*956. Palmer EA, Flynn JT, Hardy RJ, et al. The Cryotherapy for Retinopathy of Prematurity Cooperative Group. Incidence and early course of retinopathy of prematurity. Ophthalmology 1991; 98:1628–1640.

957. Early Treatment for Retinopathy of Prematurity Cooperative Group: Revised indications for the treatment of retinopathy of prematurity. Arch Ophthalmol 2003; 121:1684–1696.

958. Cryotherapy for Retinopathy of Prematurity Cooperative Group (CRPCG). Multicenter trial of cryotherapy for retinopathy of prematurity: preliminary results. Arch Ophthalmol 1988; 106: 471–479.

*959. Cryotherapy for Retinopathy of Prematurity Cooperative Group. Multicenter trial of Cryotherapy for retinopathy of prematurity: ophthalmological outcome at 10 years. Arch Ophthalmol 2001; 119:1110–1118.

960. Good WV; Early Treatment for Retinopathy of Prematurity Cooperative Group. The Early Treatment for Retinopathy Of Prematurity Study: structural findings at age 2 years. Br J Ophthalmol 2006; 90:1378–1382.

961. Report of a Joint Working Party of the Royal College of Ophthalmologists and British Association of Perinatal Medicine. Retinopathy of Prematurity: Guidelines for Screening and Treatment. 2007. Royal College of Paediatrics & Child Health, UK.

962. Section on Ophthalmology American Academy of Pediatrics; American Academy of Ophthalmology; American Association for Pediatric Ophthalmology and Strabismus. Screening examination of premature infants for retinopathy of prematurity. Pediatrics 2006; 117:572–576.Erratum in: Pediatrics 2006; 118:1324.

963. O'Connor AR, Stephenson T, Johnson A, et al. Long-term ophthalmic outcome of low birth weight children with and without retinopathy of prematurity. Pediatrics 2002; 109:12–18.

964. Fielder AR, Foreman N, Moseley MJ, et al. Prematurity and visual development. In: Simons K, ed. Early visual development, normal and abnormal. New York: Oxford University Press; 1993.485–504.

965. Crofts BJ, King R, Johnson A. The contribution of low birth weight to severe vision loss in a geographically defined population. Br J Ophthalmol 1998; 82:9–13.

966. Burgess P, Johnson A. Ocular defects in infants of extremely low birthweight and low gestational age. Br J Ophthalmol 1991; 75:84–87.

967. Birch EE, O'Connor AR. Preterm birth and visual development. Semin Neonatol 2001; 6:487–497.

968. Larsson EK, Rydberg AC, Holmstrom GE. A population-based study on the visual outcome in 10-year-old preterm and full-term children. Arch Ophthalmol 2005; 123:825–832.

969. Pike MG, Holmstrom G, de Vries LS, et al. Patterns of visual impairment associated with lesions of the preterm infant brain. Dev Med Child Neurol 1994; 36:849–862.

970. Edmond JC, Foroozan R. Cortical visual impairment in children. Curr Opin Ophthalmol 2006; 17:509–512.

971. Bremmer DL, Palmer EA, Fellows RR, et al. for the Cryotherapy for Retinopathy of Prematurity Cooperative Group. Strabismus in premature infants in the first year of life. Arch Ophthalmol 1998; 116:329–333.

972. Quinn GE, Dobson V, Siatkowski M, et al, for the Cryotherapy for Retinopathy of Prematurity Cooperative Group. Does cryotherapy affect refractive error? Ophthalmology 2001; 108:343–347.

973. Fledelius HC. Pre-term delivery and subsequent ocular development. A 7–10 year follow-up of children screened 1982–84 for ROP. 3) Refraction. Myopia of prematurity. Acta Ophthalmol Scand 1996; 74:297–300.

974. Blair M. The need for and the role of a coordinator in child heath surveillance promotion. Arch Dis Child 2001; 84:1–5.

975. Rahi JS, Dezateux C, for The British Congenital Cataract Interest Group. Measuring and interpreting the incidence of congenital ocular anomalies: lessons from a national study of congenital cataract in the UK. Invest Ophthalmol Vis Sci 2001; 42:1444–1448.

Infection and immunity in the newborn

976. Zaidi AK, Huskins WC, Thaver D, et al. Hospital-acquired neonatal infections in developing countries. Lancet 2005; 365:1175–1188.

977. Barton L, Hodgman JE, Pavlova Z. Causes of death in the extremely low birth weight infant. Pediatrics 1999; 103:446–451.

978. Isaacs D, Royle JA. Intrapartum antibiotics and early onset neonatal sepsis caused by group B Streptococcus and by other organisms in Australia. Australasian Study Group for Neonatal Infections. Pediatr Infect Dis J 1999; 18:524–528.

979. Haque KN, Khan MA, Kerry S, et al. Pattern of culture-proven neonatal sepsis in a district general hospital in the United Kingdom. Infect Control Hosp Epidemiol 2004; 25:759–764.

980. Escobar GJ, Li DK, Armstrong MA, et al. Neonatal sepsis workups in infants >/=2000 grams at birth: A population-based study. Pediatrics 2000; 106:256–263.

981. Heath PT, Balfour G, Weisner AM, et al. Group B streptococcal disease in UK and Irish infants younger than 90 days. Lancet 2004; 363:292–294.

982. Clerihew L, Lamagni TL, Brocklehurst P, et al. Invasive fungal infection in very low birthweight infants: national prospective surveillance study. Arch Dis Child Fetal Neonatal Ed 2006; 91:F188–F192.

983. Stoll BJ, Hansen N, Fanaroff AA, et al. Changes in pathogens causing early-onset sepsis in very-low-birth-weight infants. N Engl J Med 2002; 347:240–247.

984. Stoll BJ, Hansen N, Fanaroff AA, et al. Late-onset sepsis in very low birth weight neonates: the experience of the NICHD Neonatal Research Network. Pediatrics 2002; 110:285–291.

985. Webber S, Wilkinson AR, Lindsell D, et al. Neonatal pneumonia. Arch Dis Child 1990; 65:207–211.

986. Isaacman DJ, Karasic RB, Reynolds EA, et al. Effect of number of blood cultures and volume of blood on detection of bacteremia in children. J Pediatr 1996; 128:190–195.

987. Luck S, Torny M, d'Agapeyeff K, et al. Estimated early-onset group B streptococcal neonatal disease. Lancet 2003; 361:1953–1954.

988. Bedford Russell AR, Breathnach A, Sender P. Confirmed group B streptococcus infection: the tip of the iceberg. Arch Dis Child Fetal Neonatal Ed 2001; 84:F140.

989. Moses LM, Heath PT, Wilkinson AR, et al. Early onset group B streptococcal neonatal infection in Oxford 1985–96. Arch Dis Child Fetal Neonatal Ed 1998; 79:F148–F149.

990. Bedford H, de Louvois J, Halket S, et al. Meningitis in infancy in England and Wales: follow up at age 5 years. BMJ 2001; 323:533–536.

991. Stoll BJ, Hansen NI, Adams-Chapman I, et al. Neurodevelopmental and growth impairment among extremely low-birth-weight infants with neonatal infection. JAMA 2004; 292:2357–2365.

992. Khairulddin N, Bishop L, Lamagni TL, et al. Emergence of methicillin resistant Staphylococcus aureus (MRSA) bacteraemia among children in England and Wales, 1990–2001. Arch Dis Child 2004; 89:378–379.

993. Isaacs D. A ten year, multicentre study of coagulase negative staphylococcal infections in Australasian neonatal units. Arch Dis Child Fetal Neonatal Ed 2003; 88:F89–F93.

994. Embleton ND. Fetal and neonatal death from maternally acquired infection. Paediatr Perinat Epidemiol 2001; 15:54–60.

995. de Louvois J, Blackbourn J, Hurley R, et al. Infantile meningitis in England and Wales: a two year study. Arch Dis Child 1991; 66:603–607.

996. Holt DE, Halket S, de Louvois J, et al. Neonatal meningitis in England and Wales: 10 years on. Arch Dis Child Fetal Neonatal Ed 2001; 84:F85–F89.

997. Doctor BA, Newman N, Minich NM, et al. Clinical outcomes of neonatal meningitis in very-low birth-weight infants. Clin Pediatr (Phila) 2001; 40:473–480.

998. Campbell JR, Diacovo T, Baker CJ. Serratia marcescens meningitis in neonates. Pediatr Infect Dis J 1992; 11:881–886.

999. Hervas JA, Ballesteros F, Alomar A, et al. Increase of Enterobacter in neonatal sepsis: a twenty-two-year study. Pediatr Infect Dis J 2001; 20:134–140.

1000. The WHO Young Infants Study Group. Bacterial etiology of serious infections in young infants in developing countries: results of a multicenter study. Pediatr Infect Dis J 1999; 18:(Suppl):S17–S22.

1001. Nathoo KJ, Pazvakavamba I, Chidede OS, et al. Neonatal meningitis in Harare, Zimbabwe: a 2-year review. Ann Trop Paediatr 1991; 11:11–15.

1002. Nel E. Neonatal meningitis: mortality, cerebrospinal fluid, and microbiological findings. J Trop Pediatr 2000; 46:237–239.

1003. Schuchat A, Zywicki SS, Dinsmoor MJ, et al. Risk factors and opportunities for prevention of early-onset neonatal sepsis: a multicenter case-control study. Pediatrics 2000; 105:21–26.

1004. Oddie S, Embleton ND. Risk factors for early onset neonatal group B streptococcal sepsis: case-control study. BMJ 2002; 325:308.

1005. Ng PC, Wong HL, Lyon DJ, et al. Combined use of alcohol hand rub and gloves reduces the incidence of late onset infection in very low birthweight infants. Arch Dis Child Fetal Neonatal Ed 2004; 89:F336–F340.

1006. de Man P, Verhoeven BA, Verbrugh HA, et al. An antibiotic policy to prevent emergence of resistant bacilli. Lancet 2000; 355:973–978.

1007. Lahra MM, Jeffery HE. A fetal response to chorioamnionitis is associated with early survival after preterm birth. Am J Obstet Gynecol 2004; 190:147–151.

1008. Takeda K, Akira S. Toll-like receptors in innate immunity. Int Immunol 2005; 17:1–14.

1009. Berner R, Welter P, Brandis M. Cytokine expression of cord and adult blood mononuclear cells in response to Streptococcus agalactiae. Pediatr Res 2002; 51:304–309.

1010. Schultz C, Rott C, Temming P, et al. Enhanced interleukin-6 and interleukin-8 synthesis in term and preterm infants. Pediatr Res 2002; 51:317–322.

1011. Schultz C, Temming P, Bucsky P, et al. Immature anti-inflammatory response in neonates. Clin Exp Immunol 2004; 135:130–136.

1012. Kenzel S, Henneke P. The innate immune system and its relevance to neonatal sepsis. Curr Opin Infect Dis 2006; 19:264–270.

1013. Malek A, Sager R, Kuhn P, et al. Evolution of maternofetal transport of immunoglobulins during human pregnancy. Am J Reprod Immunol 1996; 36:248–255.

1014. Baker CJ, Kasper DL. Correlation of maternal antibody deficiency with susceptibility to neonatal group B streptococcal infection. N Engl J Med 1976; 294:753–756.

1015. Marchant A, Goetghebuer T, Ota MO, et al. Newborns develop a Th1-type immune response to Mycobacterium bovis bacillus Calmette–Guerin vaccination. J Immunol 1999; 163:2249–2255.

1016. Sedaghatian MR, Kardouni K. Tuberculin response in preterm infants after BCG vaccination at birth. Arch Dis Child 1993; 69:309–311.

1017. Goriely S, Vincart B, Stordeur P, et al. Deficient IL-12(p35) gene expression by dendritic cells derived from neonatal monocytes. J Immunol 2001; 166:2141–2146.

1018. Gans HA, Maldonado Y, Yasukawa LL, et al. IL-12, IFN-gamma, and T cell proliferation to measles in immunized infants. J Immunol 1999; 162:5569–5575.

1019. Berrington JE, Barge D, Fenton AC, et al. Lymphocyte subsets in term and significantly preterm UK infants in the first year of life analysed by single platform flow cytometry. Clin Exp Immunol 2005; 140:289–292.

1020. Bauer K, Zemlin M, Hummel M, et al. Diversification of Ig heavy chain genes in human preterm neonates prematurely exposed to environmental antigens. J Immunol 2002; 169:1349–1356.

1021. Zemlin M, Bauer K, Hummel M, et al. The diversity of rearranged immunoglobulin heavy chain variable region genes in peripheral blood B cells of preterm infants is restricted by short third complementarity-determining regions but not by limited gene segment usage. Blood 2001; 97:1511–1513.

1022. Robinson MJ, Campbell F, Powell P, et al. Antibody response to accelerated Hib immunisation in preterm infants receiving dexamethasone for chronic lung disease. Arch Dis Child Fetal Neonatal Ed 1999; 80:F69–F71.

1023. Robinson MJ, Heal C, Gardener E, et al. Antibody response to diphtheria-tetanus-pertussis immunization in preterm infants who receive dexamethasone for chronic lung disease. Pediatrics 2004; 113:733–737.

1024. Stoll BJ, Temprosa M, Tyson JE, et al. Dexamethasone therapy increases infection in very low birth weight infants. Pediatrics 1999; 104:e63.

1025. Slack MH, Schapira D, Thwaites RJ, et al. Immune response of premature infants to meningococcal serogroup C and combined diphtheria–tetanus toxoids–acellular pertussis–Haemophilus influenzae type b conjugate vaccines. J Infect Dis 2001; 184:1617–1620.

1026. Mishra UK, Jacobs SE, Doyle LW, et al. Newer approaches to the diagnosis of early onset neonatal sepsis. Arch Dis Child Fetal Neonatal Ed 2006; 91:F208–F212.

1027. Garcia-Prats JA, Cooper TR, Schneider VF, et al. Rapid detection of microorganisms in blood cultures of newborn infants utilizing an automated blood culture system. Pediatrics 2000; 105:523–527.

1028. Buttery JP. Blood cultures in newborns and children: optimising an everyday test. Arch Dis Child Fetal Neonatal Ed 2002; 87:F25–F28.

1029. Wiswell TE, Baumgart S, Gannon CM, et al. No lumbar puncture in the evaluation for early neonatal sepsis: will meningitis be missed? Pediatrics 1995; 95:803–806.

1030. Garges HP, Moody MA, Cotten CM, et al. Neonatal meningitis: what is the correlation among cerebrospinal fluid cultures, blood cultures, and cerebrospinal fluid parameters? Pediatrics 2006; 117:1094–1100.

1031. Visser VE, Hall RT. Lumbar puncture in the evaluation of suspected neonatal sepsis. J Pediatr 1980; 96:1063–1067.

1032. Martin-Ancel A, Garcia-Alix A, Salas S, et al. Cerebrospinal fluid leucocyte counts in healthy neonates. Arch Dis Child Fetal Neonatal Ed 2006; 91:F357–F358.

1033. Tamim MM, Alesseh H, Aziz H. Analysis of the efficacy of urine culture as part of sepsis evaluation in the premature infant. Pediatr Infect Dis J 2003; 22:805–808.

1034. Visser VE, Hall RT. Urine culture in the evaluation of suspected neonatal sepsis. J Pediatr 1979; 94:635–638.

1035. Isaacs D, Wilkinson AR, Moxon ER. Surveillance of colonization and late-onset septicaemia in neonates. J Hosp Infect 1987; 10:114–119.

1036. Cordero L, Ayers LW, Davis K. Neonatal airway colonization with gram-negative bacilli: association with severity of bronchopulmonary dysplasia. Pediatr Infect Dis J 1997; 16:18–23.

1037. Liesenfeld O, Montoya JG, Tathineni NJ, et al. Confirmatory serologic testing for acute toxoplasmosis and rate of induced abortions among women reported to have positive Toxoplasma immunoglobulin M antibody titers. Am J Obstet Gynecol 2001; 184:140–145.

1038. Liesenfeld O, Press C, Montoya JG, et al. False-positive results in immunoglobulin M (IgM) toxoplasma antibody tests and importance of confirmatory testing: the Platelia Toxo IgM test. J Clin Microbiol 1997; 35:174–178.

1039. Lazzarotto T, Varani S, Guerra B, et al. Prenatal indicators of congenital cytomegalovirus infection. J Pediatr 2000; 137:90–95.

1040. Srinivasan V, Spinella PC, Drott HR, et al. Association of timing, duration, and intensity of hyperglycemia with intensive care unit mortality in critically ill children. Pediatr Crit Care Med 2004; 5:329–336.

1041. Alaedeen DI, Walsh MC, Chwals WJ. Total parenteral nutrition-associated hyperglycemia correlates with prolonged mechanical ventilation and hospital stay in septic infants. J Pediatr Surg 2006; 41:239–244;discussion 239–244.

1042. Linkin DR, Fishman NO, Patel JB, et al. Risk factors for extended-spectrum beta-lactamase-producing Enterobacteriaceae in a neonatal intensive care unit. Infect Control Hosp Epidemiol 2004; 25:781–783.

1043. Karlowicz MG, Buescher ES, Surka AE. Fulminant late-onset sepsis in a neonatal intensive care unit, 1988–1997, and the impact of avoiding empiric vancomycin therapy. Pediatrics 2000; 106:1387–1390.

1044. Heath PT, Nik Yusoff NK, Baker CJ. Neonatal meningitis. Arch Dis Child Fetal Neonatal Ed 2003; 88:F173–F178.

1045. Escobar GJ, Zukin T, Usatin MS, et al. Early discontinuation of antibiotic treatment in newborns admitted to rule out sepsis: a decision rule. Pediatr Infect Dis J 1994; 13:860–866.

1046. Mohan P, Brocklehurst P. Granulocyte transfusions for neonates with confirmed or suspected sepsis and neutropaenia. Cochrane Database Syst Rev 2003; 4:CD003956.

1047. Haque K, Mohan P. Pentoxifylline for neonatal sepsis. Cochrane Database Syst Rev 2003; 4:CD004205.

1048. Carr R, Modi N, Dore C. G-CSF and GM-CSF for treating or preventing neonatal infections. Cochrane Database Syst Rev 2003; 3:CD003066.

1049. Ohlsson A, Lacy JB. Intravenous immunoglobulin for preventing infection in preterm and/or low-birth-weight infants. Cochrane Database Syst Rev 2004; 1:CD000361.

1050. Ohlsson A, Lacy JB. Intravenous immunoglobulin for suspected or subsequently proven infection in neonates. Cochrane Database Syst Rev 2004; 1:CD001239.

1051. Daoud AS, Batieha A, Al-Sheyyab M, et al. Lack of effectiveness of dexamethasone in neonatal bacterial meningitis. Eur J Pediatr 1999; 158:230–233.

1052. Isaacs D. Rationing antibiotic use in neonatal units. Arch Dis Child Fetal Neonatal Ed 2000; 82:F1–F2.

1053. Pittet D, Hugonnet S, Harbarth S, et al. Effectiveness of a hospital-wide programme to improve compliance with hand hygiene. Infection Control Programme. Lancet 2000; 356:1307–1312.

1054. Narayanan I, Prakash K, Prabhakar AK, et al. A planned prospective evaluation of the anti-infective property of varying quantities of expressed human milk. Acta Paediatr Scand 1982; 71:441–445.

1055. Hylander MA, Strobino DM, Dhanireddy R. Human milk feedings and infection among very low birth weight infants. Pediatrics 1998; 102:E38.

1056. el-Mohandes AE, Picard MB, Simmens SJ, et al. Use of human milk in the intensive care nursery decreases the incidence of nosocomial sepsis. J Perinatol 1997; 17:130–134.

1057. Weisner AM, Johnson AP, Lamagni TL, et al. Characterization of group B streptococci recovered from infants with invasive disease in England and Wales. Clin Infect Dis 2004; 38:1203–1208.

1058. Zaleznik DF, Rench MA, Hillier S, et al. Invasive disease due to group B Streptococcus in pregnant women and neonates from diverse population groups. Clin Infect Dis 2000; 30:276–281.

1059. Jones N, Oliver K, Jones Y, et al. Carriage of group B streptococcus in pregnant women from Oxford, UK. J Clin Pathol 2006; 59:363–366.

1060. Bergeron MG, Ke D, Menard C, et al. Rapid detection of group B streptococci in pregnant women at delivery. N Engl J Med 2000; 343:175–179.

1061. Zangwill KM, Schuchat A, Wenger JD. Group B streptococcal disease in the United States, 1990: report from a multistate active surveillance system. MMWR CDC Surveill Summ 1992; 41:25–32.

1062. Schuchat A, Oxtoby M, Cochi S, et al. Population-based risk factors for neonatal group B streptococcal disease: results of a cohort study in metropolitan Atlanta. J Infect Dis 1990; 162:672–677.

1063. Mifsud AJ, Efstratiou A, Charlett A, et al. Early-onset neonatal group B streptococcal infection in London: 1990–1999. BJOG 2004; 111:1006–1011.

1064. Bingen E, Lambert-Zechovsky N, Guihaire E, et al. [Optimum choice of antibiotic treatment in neonatal infections due to group B streptococci]. Pathol Biol (Paris) 1986; 34:530–533.

1065. Pyati SP, Pildes RS, Jacobs NM, et al. Penicillin in infants weighing two kilograms or less with early-onset Group B streptococcal disease. N Engl J Med 1983; 308:1383–1389.

1066. Smaill F. Intrapartum antibiotics for group B streptococcal colonisation. Cochrane Database Syst Rev 2000; 2:CD000115.

1067. Toltzis P, Dul MJ, Hoyen C, et al. The effect of antibiotic rotation on colonization with antibiotic-resistant bacilli in a neonatal intensive care unit. Pediatrics 2002; 110:707–711.

1068. Schrag SJ, Zywicki S, Farley MM, et al. Group B streptococcal disease in the era of intrapartum antibiotic prophylaxis. N Engl J Med 2000; 342:15–20.

1069. Lukacs SL, Schoendorf KC, Schuchat A. Trends in sepsis-related neonatal mortality in the United States, 1985–1998. Pediatr Infect Dis J 2004; 23:599–603.

1070. Schrag SJ, Zell ER, Lynfield R, et al. A population-based comparison of strategies to prevent early-onset group B streptococcal disease in neonates. N Engl J Med 2002; 347:233–239.

1071. Isaacs D, Barfield CP, Grimwood K, et al. Systemic bacterial and fungal infections in infants in Australian neonatal units. Australian Study Group for Neonatal Infections. Med J Aust 1995; 162:198–201.

1072. Hristeva L, Booy R, Bowler I, et al. Prospective surveillance of neonatal meningitis. Arch Dis Child 1993; 69:14–18.

1073. Klinger G, Chin CN, Beyene J, et al. Predicting the outcome of neonatal bacterial meningitis. Pediatrics 2000; 106:477–482.

1074. Unhanand M, Mustafa MM, McCracken GH Jr, et al. Gram-negative enteric bacillary meningitis: a twenty-one-year experience. J Pediatr 1993; 122:15–21.

1075. Edwards MS, Rench MA, Haffar AA, et al. Long-term sequelae of group B streptococcal meningitis in infants. J Pediatr 1985; 106:717–722.

1076. Siegel JD. Neonatal sepsis. Semin Perinatol 1985; 9:20–28.

1077. Weisman LE, Merenstein GB, Steenbarger JR. The effect of lumbar puncture position in sick neonates. Am J Dis Child 1983; 137:1077–1079.

1078. Lutsar I, McCracken GH Jr, Friedland IR. Antibiotic pharmacodynamics in cerebrospinal fluid. Clin Infect Dis 1998; 27:1117–1127, quiz 28–29

1079. McCracken GH Jr, Mize SG. A controlled study of intrathecal antibiotic therapy in gram-negative enteric meningitis of infancy. Report of the neonatal meningitis cooperative study group. J Pediatr 1976; 89:66–72.

1080. McCracken GH Jr, Mize SG, Threlkeld N. Intraventricular gentamicin therapy in gram-negative bacillary meningitis of infancy. Report of the Second

Neonatal Meningitis Cooperative Study Group. Lancet 1980; 1:787–791.

1081. Schaad UB, Nelson JD, McCracken GH Jr. Recrudescence and relapse in bacterial meningitis of childhood. Pediatrics 1981; 67:188–195.

1082. Willis J, Robinson JE. Enterobacter sakazakii meningitis in neonates. Pediatr Infect Dis J 1988; 7:196–199.

1083. Graham DR, Band JD. Citrobacter diversus brain abscess and meningitis in neonates. JAMA 1981; 245:1923–1925.

1084. Mahieu LM, De Muynck AO, Ieven MM, et al. Risk factors for central vascular catheter-associated bloodstream infections among patients in a neonatal intensive care unit. J Hosp Infect 2001; 48:108–116.

1085. Gray JE, Richardson DK, McCormick MC, et al. Coagulase-negative staphylococcal bacteremia among very low birth weight infants: relation to admission illness severity, resource use, and outcome. Pediatrics 1995; 95:225–230.

1086. Fortunov RM, Hulten KG, Hammerman WA, et al. Community-acquired Staphylococcus aureus infections in term and near-term previously healthy neonates. Pediatrics 2006; 118:874–881.

1087. Isaacs D, Fraser S, Hogg G, et al. Staphylococcus aureus infections in Australasian neonatal nurseries. Arch Dis Child Fetal Neonatal Ed 2004; 89:F331–F335.

1088. Schelonka RL, Katz B, Waites KB, et al. Critical appraisal of the role of Ureaplasma in the development of bronchopulmonary dysplasia with metaanalytic techniques. Pediatr Infect Dis J 2005; 24:1033–1039.

1089. Engle WD, Jackson GL, Sendelbach D, et al. Neonatal pneumonia: comparison of 4 vs 7 days of antibiotic therapy in term and near-term infants. J Perinatol 2000; 20:421–426.

1090. Engle WD, Jackson GL, Sendelbach DM, et al. Pneumonia in term neonates: laboratory studies and duration of antibiotic therapy. J Perinatol 2003; 23:372–377.

1091. Lin PW, Stoll BJ. Necrotising enterocolitis. Lancet 2006; 368:1271–1283.

1092. Tarabishy AB, Hall GS, Procop GW, et al. Bacterial culture isolates from hospitalized pediatric patients with conjunctivitis. Am J Ophthalmol 2006; 142:678–680.

1093. Simms I, Ward H. Congenital syphilis in the United Kingdom. Sex Transm Infect 2006; 82:1.

1094. Sothinathan U, Hannam S, Fowler A, et al. Detection and follow up of infants at risk of congenital syphilis. Arch Dis Child 2006; 91:620.

1095. Kabura L, Ilibagiza D, Menten J, et al. Intrathecal vs. intramuscular administration of human antitetanus immunoglobulin or equine tetanus antitoxin in the treatment of tetanus: a meta-analysis. Trop Med Int Health 2006; 11:1075–1081.

1096. Cotten CM, McDonald S, Stoll B, et al. The association of third-generation cephalosporin use and invasive candidiasis in extremely low birth-weight infants. Pediatrics 2006; 118:717–722.

1097. Baley JE, Kliegman RM, Boxerbaum B, et al. Fungal colonization in the very low birth weight infant. Pediatrics 1986; 78:225–232.

1098. Kaufman DA, Gurka MJ, Hazen KC, et al. Patterns of fungal colonization in preterm infants weighing less than 1000 grams at birth. Pediatr Infect Dis J 2006; 25:733–737.

1099. Faix RG. Systemic Candida infections in infants in intensive care nurseries: high incidence of central nervous system involvement. J Pediatr 1984; 105:616–622.

Neonatal neoplasia

1100. Barson AJ. Congenital neoplasia: the society's experience. Abstract. Arch Dis Child 1978; 53:436.

1101. Davis CF, Carachi R, Young DG. Neonatal tumours: Glasgow 1955–1986. Arch Dis Child 1988; 63:1075–1078.

1102. Broadbent VA. Malignant disease in the neonate. In: Roberton NRC, ed. Textbook of neonatology. Edinburgh: Churchill Livingstone; 1986.

1103. Campbell AN, Chan HSL, O'Brien A, et al. Malignant tumours in the neonate. Arch Dis Child 1987; 62:19–23.

1104. Bader JL, Miller RW. US cancer incidence and mortality in the 1st year of life. Am J Dis Child 1979; 133:157–159.

1105. Fraumeni JF Jr, Miller RW. Cancer deaths in the newborn. Am J Dis Child 1969; 117:186–189.

1106. Kenney LB, Miller BA, Ries LAG, et al. Increased incidence of cancer in infants in the U.S.: 1980–1990. Cancer 1998; 82:1396–1400.

1107. Golding J, Greenwood R, Birmingham K, et al. Childhood cancer, intramuscular vitamin K, and pethidine given during labour. BMJ 1992; 305:341–346.

1108. McKinney PA, Juszczak E, Findlay E, et al. Case-control study of childhood leukaemia and cancer in Scotland: Findings for neonatal intramuscular vitamin K. BMJ 1998; 316:173–177.

1109. Parker L, Cole M, Craft AW, et al. Neonatal vitamin K administration and childhood cancer in the north of England: Retrospective case-control study. BMJ 1998; 316:189–193.

1110. Frear NT, Roman E, Ansell P, et al, on behalf of the UK Childhood Cancer Study Investigators. Vitamin K and childhood cancer: a report from the UK Childhood Cancer Study. Br J Cancer 2003; 89:1228–1231.

1111. Huddart SN, Mann JR, Robinson K, et al; Children's Cancer Study Group. Sacrococcygeal teratomas: the UK Children's Cancer Study Group's experience. I. Neonatal. Pediatr Surg Int 2003; 19:47–51.

1112. Altman RP, Randolph JG, Lilley JR. Sacrococcygeal teratomata. American Academy of Pediatrics Surgical Section Survey 1973. J Pediatr Surg 1974; 9:389–398.

1113. Burmeister T, Thiel E. Molecular genetics in acute and chronic leukemias. J Cancer Res Clin Oncol 2001; 127:80–90.

1114. Robinson DL. Childhood leukaemia: understanding the significance of chromosomal abnormalities. J Pediatr Oncol Nurs 2000; 18:111–123.

1115. Guin GH, Gilbert EG, Jones B. Incidence of neuroblastoma in infants dying of other causes. Am J Clin Pathol 1969; 51:126–136.

1116. Bolande RP. Benignity of neonatal tumors and concept of cancer repression in early life. Am J Dis Child 1971; 122:12–14.

1117. Kintzel K, Sonntag J, Strauss E, et al. Neuron-specific enolase: reference values in cord blood. Clin Chem Lab Med 1998; 36:245–247.

1118. Schmidt ML, Lukens JN, Seeger RC, et al. Biologic factors determine prognosis in infants with stage IV neuroblastoma: A prospective Children's Cancer Group study. J Clin Oncol 2000; 18:1260–1268.

1119. Isaacs H. Perinatal (congenital and neonatal) neoplasms: a report of 100 cases. Paediatr Pathol 1985; 3:165–216.

1120. Bove KE. Wilms' tumor and related abnormalities in the fetus and newborn. Semin Perinatol 1999; 23:310–318.

1121. Johnston MA, Carachi R, Lindop GB, et al. Inactive renin levels in recurrent nephroblastoma. J Pediatr Surg 1991; 26:613–614.

1122. Bown N, Cotterill SJ, Roberts P, et al. Cytogenetic abnormalities and clinical outcome in Wilms tumor: a study by the U.K. cancer cytogenetics group and the U.K. Children's Cancer Study Group. Med Pediatr Oncol 2002; 38:11–21.

1123. Machin GA. Persistent renal blastoma (nephroblastometosis) as a frequent precursor to Wilms tumour: a pathophysiological and clinical review. Am J Pediatr Haematol Oncol 1980; 2:353–362.

1124. Bolande RP. Congenital and infantile neoplasia of the kidney. Lancet 1974; ii:1497–1499.

1125. Chu AD, D'Angio GJ, Favara B, et al. The Writing Group of the Histiocyte Society. Histiocytosis syndromes in children. Lancet 1987; i:208–209.

Neonatal metabolic disorders

1126. Lucas A, Morley R, Cole TJ. Adverse neurodevelopmental outcome of moderate neonatal hypoglycaemia. BMJ 1988; 297:1304–1308.

1127. Koh THHG, Eyre JA, Tarbit M, et al. Neurophysiological dysfunction in relation to the concentration of glucose in the blood. Early Hum Dev 1988; 17:287.

1128. Aynsley-Green A, Soltesz G. Hypoglycaemia in infancy and childhood. In: Aynsley-Green A, Chambers TL, eds. Current reviews in paediatrics. Edinburgh: Churchill Livingstone; 1985.

1129. Hawdon JM, Ward-Platt MP. Metabolic adaptation in small for gestational age infants. Arch Dis Child 1993; 68:262–268.

1130. Duvanel CB, Fawer C-L, Cotting J, et al. Long-term effects of neonatal hypoglycaemia on brain growth and psychomotor development in small for gestational age preterm infants. J Pediatr 1999; 134:492–498.

1131. Hume R, McGeechan A, Burchell A. Failure to detect preterm infants at risk of hypoglycaemia prior to discharge home. J Pediatr 1999; 134:499–502.

1132. Murdock N, Crighton A, Nelson LM, et al. Low birthweight infants and total parenteral nutrition immediately after birth. II. Randomised study of biochemical tolerance of intravenous glucose, amino acids, and lipid. Arch Dis Child 1995; 73:F8–F12.

1133. Hume R, Burchell A, Williams FLR, et al. Glucose homeostasis in the newborn. Early Hum Dev 2005; 81:95–101.

1134. Elliott M, Bayly R, Cole T, et al. Clinical features and natural history of Beckwith–Wiedemann syndrome: presentation of 74 new cases. Clin Genet 1994; 46:168–174.

1135. Mannens M, Hoovers JM, Redeker E, et al. Parental imprinting of human chromosome region 11p15.3-pter involved in the Beckwith–Wiedemann syndrome and various human neoplasia. Eur J Hum Genet 1994; 2:3–23.

1136. Fournet JC, Mayaud C, de Lonlay P, et al. Unbalanced expression of 11p15 imprinted genes in focal forms of congenital hyperinsulinism – association with a reduction to homozygosity of a mutation in ABCC8 or KCNJ11. Am J Pathol 2001; 158:2177–2184.

1137. Lindley KJ, Dunne MJ. Contemporary strategies in the diagnosis and management of neonatal hyperinsulinaemic hypoglycaemia. Early Hum Dev 2005; 81:161–172.

1138. Stanley CA, Lieu YK, Hsu BYL, et al. Hyperinsulinism and hyperammonemia in infants with regulatory mutations of the glutamate dehydrogenase gene. N Engl J Med 1998; 338:1352–1357.

1139. Shepherd RM, Cosgrove KE, O'Brien RE, et al, on behalf of the EU funded European Network for Research into Hyperinsulinism in Infancy (ENRHI). Hyperinsulinism of infancy: towards an understanding of unregulated insulin release. Arch Dis Child 2000; 82:F87–F97.

1140. Chen Y-T, Burchell A. Glycogen storage diseases. In: Scriver CR, Beaudet AL, Sly WS, et al, eds. The metabolic bases of inherited disease. 7th edn. New York: McGraw Hill; 1995:935–965.

1141. Chalmers RA, English N, Hughes EA, et al. Biochemical studies on cultured skin fibroblasts from a baby with long-chain acyl-CoA of dehydrogenase-deficiency presenting as sudden neonatal death. J Inher Metabol Dis 1987; 10:260–262.

1142. Hawdon JM, Aynsley-Green A, Bartlett K, et al. The role of pancreatic insulin secretion in neonatal glucoregulation. II. Infants with disordered blood glucose homeostasis. Arch Dis Child 1993; 68:280–285.

1143. Lyon AJ, McIntosh N, Wheeler K, et al. Hypercalcaemia in extremely low birthweight infants. Arch Dis Child 1984; 59:1141–1144.

1144. Greer FR. Osteopenia of prematurity. Annu Rev Nutr 1994; 14:169–185.

1145. Giles MM, Laing IA, Elton RA, et al. Magnesium metabolism in preterm infants: effect of calcium, magnesium, postnatal and gestational age. J Pediatr 1990; 117:147–154.

1146. Koo NNI, Gupta JM, Nayanar VV, et al. Skeletal changes in preterm infants. Arch Dis Child 1982; 57:447–452.

1147. Greer FR, MacCormick A. Improved bone mineralisation and growth in premature infants fed fortified own mother's milk. J Pediatr 1988; 112:961–966.

1148. Horsman A, Ryan SW, Congdon PJ, et al. Bone mineral content and body size 65 to 100 weeks postconception in preterm and full term infants. Arch Dis Child 1989; 64:1579–1586.

1149. Lyon AJ, Hawkes DJ, Doran M, et al. Bone mineralisation in preterm infants measured by dual energy radiographic densitometry. Arch Dis Child 1989; 64:919–923.

1150. Crofton PM, Hume R. Alkaline phosphatase isoenzyme in the plasma of preterm and term infants: serial measurements and clinical correlations. Clin Chem 1987; 33:1783–1787.

1151. Nassir DK, Mcintosh N, Lyon A, et al. Ultrasonic diagnosis and monitoring of rickets in immature infants. Br J Radiol 1987; 60:618.

1152. Fewtrell MS, Cole TJ, Bishop NJ, et al. Neonatal factors predicting childhood height in preterm infants: evidence for a persisting effect of early metabolic bone disease? J Pediatr 2000; 137:668–673.

1153. Backstrom MC, Kouri T, Kuusela AI, et al. Bone isoenzyme of serum alkaline phosphatase and serum inorganic phosphate in metabolic bone disease of prematurity. Acta Paediatr 2000; 89:867–873.

1154. ESPGAN Committee of Nutrition. Nutrition and feeding of preterm infants. Acta Paediatr Scand 1987; 336(suppl):9–10.

1155. Giles MM, Fenton MH, Shaw B, et al. Sequential calcium and phosphorus balance studies in preterm infants. J Pediatr 1987; 110:591–598.

1156. Ziegler EE. Nutrient requirements of the preterm infant: an overview. In: Tsang RC, ed. Vitamin and mineral requirements in preterm infants. New York: Marcel Decker; 1985.203–212.

1157. American Academy of Pediatrics. Pediatric nutrition handbook. National Health and Safety performance standards. Oak Grove Village, Illinois: American Academy of Pediatrics; 1985:66–87.

1158. Koo WW. Parenteral nutrition-related bone disease. J Parenter Enteral Nutr 1992; 16: 386–394.

1159. Wong JC, McDougal AR, Tofan M, et al. Doubling calcium and phosphate concentrations in neonatal parenteral nutrition solutions using monobasic potassium phosphate. J Am Coll Nutr 2006; 25:70–77.

1160. Scriver CR, Beaudet al, Valle D, et al, eds. The metabolic and molecular bases of inherited disease, 8th edn. New York: McGraw Hill; 2001.

1161. Matern D, Hart P, Murtha AP, et al. Acute fatty liver of pregnancy associated with short-chain acyl-coenzyme A dehydrogenase deficiency. J Pediatr 2001; 138:585–588.

1162. Burton BK. Inborn errors of metabolism: the clinical diagnosis in early infancy. Pediatrics 1987; 79:359–369.

1163. Chakrapani A, Cleary MA, Wraith JE. Detection of inborn errors of metabolism in the newborn. Arch Dis Child 2001; 84:F205–F210.

1164. Barth P, Wanders RJ, Vreken P. X-linked cardioskeletal myopathy and neutropenia (Barth syndrome-MIM 302060). J Pediatr 2000; 135: 273–276.

1165. Gould SJ, Raymond GV. Valle D. The peroxisome biogenesis disorders. In: Scriver CR, Beaudet al, Valle D, et al eds. The metabolic bases of inherited disease, 8th edn. New York: McGraw Hill; 2001:2287–2324.

1166. Clayton PT. Disorders of cholesterol biosynthesis. Arch Dis Child 1998; 78:185–189.

13

Infant feeding

Anthony F Williams

INTRODUCTION

Promoting, protecting and supporting optimal nutrition is relevant to life-long health and requires not only an understanding of physiological and biochemical facets but an appreciation of the strong social and cultural influences.

BREAST-FEEDING

INCIDENCE OF BREAST-FEEDING

Over the past 15 years the proportion of mothers initiating breast-feeding in the UK has risen (Table 13.1), particularly in areas and social groups with historically low uptake. However the UK is still some way from matching initiation rates typical in Scandinavia and Australasia. Factors that affect the incidence of breast-feeding in the UK are shown in Table 13.2.[1] Social class, educational and geographical gradients are particularly marked. The chosen method of infant feeding is therefore a strong marker of social and educational inequality.

DEFINITION AND PREVALENCE OF 'BREAST-FEEDING'

Because breast-fed babies may receive other fluids and foods it is necessary to define epidemiologically the meaning of 'breast-feeding'. World Health Organization terminology has now been widely adopted (Table 13.3).[2] In the UK the term 'prevalence' has been used in national surveys to describe the proportion partially or exclusively breast-fed at specified ages. A consistent trend has been the rapid decline during the first 6 weeks of life, particularly the first 2. Socially and educationally disadvantaged mothers are more likely to give up. About 80% who stop in the first 2 weeks say that they wanted to breast-feed for longer, the commonest reasons being 'insufficient milk/baby hungry' (44%), 'sore nipples or breasts' (36%) and 'baby would not suck' (20%). As these reflect errors of technique and failure to recognize the normal feeding pattern of the breast-fed baby, better professional education on the management of breast-feeding could help.

CONTRIBUTION OF BREAST-FEEDING TO HEALTH

Infectious and allergic disease

Breast-feeding is crucial to survival in less resource-rich countries: a pooled analysis of data from six countries showed that infants not breast-fed were 2–6 times more likely to die of infections (mainly respiratory and diarrheal disease) in the first 6 months.[3] Risks of not breastfeeding were greatest for those whose mothers were the least educated and for the youngest infants. In Ghana supplementing breast milk with liquids or solids was associated with a fourfold increase in neonatal death; it has been estimated that early establishment of exclusive breast-feeding could reduce neonatal mortality by about one fifth in such circumstances.[4]

The effect size of breast-feeding on maternal and child health in industrialized countries has been harder to confirm: most evidence comes from case–control and cohort studies. Methodological problems include: the variable duration of breast-feeding, imprecise definition of the term 'breast-feeding' (Table 13.3), dependence on recall rather than prospective monitoring of feeding method, confounding by sociocultural factors (Table 13.2), 'ascertainment bias' and inadequate definition of disease outcomes. Although randomized allocation to artificial feeding is clearly unethical, cluster randomization of an intervention increasing the prevalence of breastfeeding, particularly exclusive breastfeeding (the Baby Friendly Initiative, vide infra) has provided level 1 evidence confirming the effect of breastfeeding on child health in an industrialized country setting, Belarus. Infants born in control hospitals were less likely to be breast-fed (either at all or exclusively) and at increased risk of atopic and diarrheal disease, despite a relatively low background prevalence of both.[5]

Breast-feeding and cardiovascular health

Meta-analyses have shown that breast-fed infants in industrialized countries have lower plasma cholesterol in adult life,[6] lower systolic blood pressure[7] and are less obese.[8,9] There are indications that exclusive breast-feeding exerts strongest effects but it has not proved possible to confirm this partly because of imprecise definition (particularly in the largest studies) and partly because of the frequency with which supplementation has been practiced.

Table 13.1   Incidence of mothers initiating breast-feeding in the UK, 1975–2000[53]

	England & Wales	Scotland	Northern Ireland
1975	51	n/a	n/a
1980	67	50	n/a
1985	65	48	n/a
1990	64	50	36
1995	68	55	45
2000	70	77	63
2005	70	54	63

Table 13.2   Factors affecting the incidence of breast-feeding in the UK

Favor breast-feeding
Social class I
Mother educated beyond 18 years of age
Mother over 24 years of age
Live in South-East England
First baby
Breast-fed previous baby

Hinder breast-feeding
Smoking

Breast-feeding and neurological development

Numerous studies have found a statistically significant association between breast-feeding and mental development in infancy and childhood, but potential confounding influences are numerous, e.g. parental alcohol intake, smoking behavior and intelligence. Differences are most marked in preterm infants and in most studies persist after adjustment for confounders.[10] Although attributed to differences in the fat composition of formula and breast milk this is currently unproven.

Breast-feeding and the mother's health

Exclusive breast-feeding assists child spacing by inducing lactational amenorrhea. Globally this may be its most important benefit to maternal health. There is strong evidence that breast-feeding significantly reduces a mother's risk of breast cancer, regardless of menopausal status.[11] Breast-feeding does not adversely influence the mother's bone health.[12] Although some demineralization occurs during lactation there is remineralization on weaning. These events are not preventable by calcium supplementation.[13]

Table 13.3   World Health Organization definitions of 'breast-feeding'[12]

Breast-feeding
Infant has received any breast milk, expressed or from breast

Exclusive breast-feeding
Infant has received only breast milk and no other liquids or solids except vitamin/mineral supplements and medicines

Predominant breast-feeding
Breast milk the predominant source of nourishment but other drinks (e.g. water, herbal drinks, teas, etc.) may have been given

Full breast-feeding
Exclusive or predominant breast-feeding

Complementary feeding
Infant has received breast milk and solid or semi-solid foods

Bottle feeding
Infant has received liquid or semi-solid food from a bottle with a teat

ESTABLISHING AND MAINTAINING BREAST-FEEDING
Breast milk production

Progesterone, prolactin and human placental lactogen induce hyperplasia and hypertrophy of the ducts and acini of the breast during pregnancy. By the second half of pregnancy the breast can secrete small amounts of milk. This preparatory growth period is termed 'lactogenesis stage 1'. At birth the inhibitory influence of maternal progesterone is removed and prolactin released in response to sucking drives milk synthesis. Thus infant demand regulates breast milk supply. Pregnancy is not an essential prerequisite and lactation can be induced to an extent after adoption by infant sucking ('adoptive lactation' or 'relactation').

During the first 3–5 d of life the output of milk increases.[12] This period is termed 'lactogenesis stage 2'. Early milk ('colostrum') is rich in protein, particularly secretory immunoglobulin A. As the output rises protein and electrolyte content falls and carbohydrate and fat content increase. By the fifth day the breasts typically produce more milk than the infant chooses to take. When the breasts were presented in random order (left/right or right/left), 5-day-old babies took significantly less milk from the second breast than the first at a feed, confirming the breasts were not actually 'empty' and the baby chose to leave milk behind.

Other experiments show that the *yield* (or volume obtainable by expressing the breasts over a 24-hour period) usually exceeds the baby's *intake.* In one study it was 7% greater than average intake measured by test weighing and in another an average 'residual volume' of over 100 ml/d (range 0–457 ml/d) could be extracted from the breast in addition to normal intake. Regular pumping increases yield and an increment of 20% has been reported.

It is therefore hard to understand why mothers in the early weeks of life often believe they have 'insufficient milk'. They (and sometimes health professionals) probably fail to recognize differences in the feeding patterns of breast- and bottle-fed babies. Breast-fed babies feed frequently, particularly during the early weeks as production is rapidly increasing; this must not be interpreted as undersupply. The amount of time a baby spends sucking may not reflect the baby's intake as there is very pronounced variation between individual mother–baby pairs.

Breast-feeding management

Important features of breast-feeding management are shown in Table 13.4. Evidence supporting the 'Ten Steps' has been published[14] and supported by a more recent systematic review of interventions increasing duration of breast-feeding.[15] They form the basis for accrediting health care facilities as 'Baby Friendly' (currently 53 accredited maternity

Table 13.4   Steps that help to establish breast-feeding in hospital

Every facility providing maternity services and care for newborn infants should:
1. Have a written breast-feeding policy that is routinely communicated to all health care staff.
2. Train all health care staff in skills necessary to implement this policy.
3. Inform all pregnant women about the benefits and management of breast-feeding.
4. Help mothers initiate breast-feeding as soon as possible after delivery.
5. Show mothers how to breast-feed and how to maintain lactation, even if they should be separated from their infants.
6. Give breast-fed newborn infants no food or drink unless medically indicated.
7. Practice rooming-in – allow mothers and infants to remain together 24 h a day.
8. Encourage breast-feeding on demand.
9. Give no artificial teats or dummies (pacifiers) to breast-feeding infants.
10. Foster the establishment of breast-feeding support groups and refer mothers to them on discharge from the hospital.

Modified from WHO/UNICEF 1989[54]

hospitals and seven primary care facilities in the UK). The effectiveness of the 'Baby Friendly Hospital Initiative' in promoting initiation and maintenance of lactation has been confirmed in a cluster randomized trial performed in Belarus.[5] Babies born in Baby Friendly Hospitals were significantly more likely to be exclusively breast-fed at 3 months and 6 months; similar effects were seen in a randomized study in Brazil.[16] Scottish audit data have also shown that babies born in Baby Friendly Hospitals are more likely to be breast-fed at the end of the first week.[17] It is essential, however, that skilled support for breastfeeding mothers is provided in primary care once the mother has left hospital. There is evidence that *proactive* support is more effective than waiting for the mother to ask for help.[15]

Early feeding, positioning and attachment

Babies should be given an opportunity to breast-feed as soon as possible after birth whilst alert and active. New mothers need to learn that babies do not always cry when hungry, but show signs such as rooting activity. Early feed supervision helps to facilitate correct *positioning* (i.e. baby's body facing mother's body) and *attachment*.

Understanding the mechanics of breast-feeding (Fig. 13.1)[18] helps to ensure correct *attachment* (relationship between baby's mouth and mother's breast). As the baby attaches the nipple and surrounding

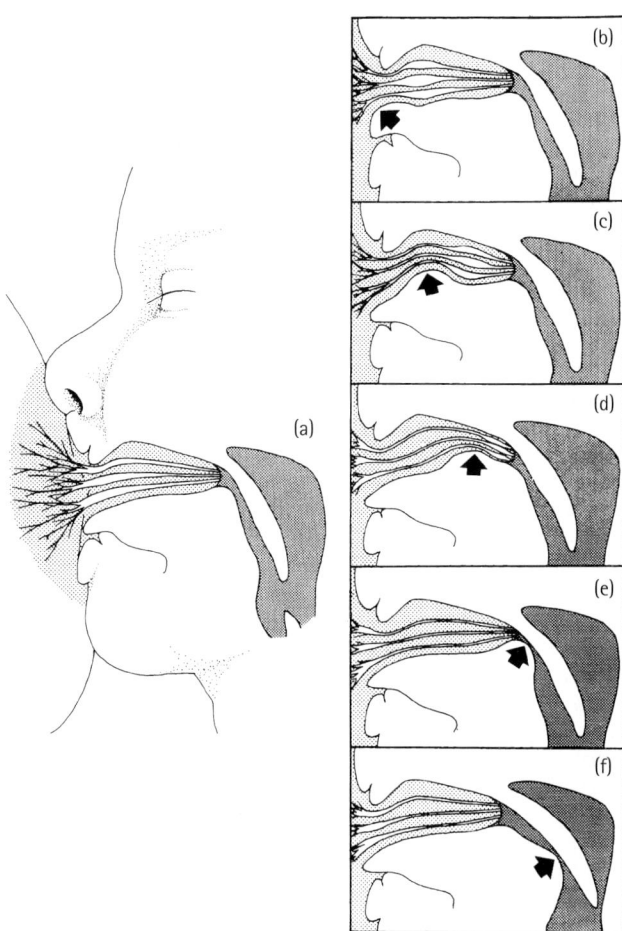

Fig. 13.1 Mechanism of sucking. (From Woolridge 1986[18] with permission) The figure shows a complete 'suck' cycle; the baby is shown in median section. The baby exhibits good feeding technique with the nipple drawn well into the mouth, extending back to the junction of the hard and soft palate (the lactiferous sinuses are depicted within the teat though these cannot be visualized on scans). In ultrasound scans it appears that compression by the tongue, and negative pressure within the mouth, maintain the tongue in close conformation to the nipple and palate. Events are portrayed here rather more loosely to aid clarity.

breast tissue are drawn into the mouth, retained by suction; the nipple is thus elongated to about three times its former length. The lateral margins of the tongue curve upwards to enclose it in a cup formed by tongue and hard palate. Milk is then stripped by a peristaltic wave running anteroposteriorly along the tongue. In this way milk is ejected from the ducts under the positive pressure created by nipple compression; negative pressure retains the nipple in the mouth and draws milk into the stripped ducts. This process is frictionless and the nipple should not be traumatized if the baby attaches correctly.[18] The mechanics of breast- and bottle-feeding are different and many believe babies develop 'nipple confusion' if switched from one to the other (see later).

Incorrect attachment is a common cause of feeding problems.[19] The mother may complain that she has 'insufficient milk' because her baby seems fretful and hungry yet will not suck, or that the nipple is sore, even bleeding. Such symptoms should prompt observation of a feed to check the physical signs of correct attachment, which include:
- baby's chin touching breast;
- baby's lower lip turned out;
- mouth wide open;
- cheeks rounded, not drawn in;
- swallowing seen or heard;
- slow, rhythmical jaw movements with few pauses, not bursts of rapid sucking.

Doubts should prompt expert midwifery assessment of technique rather than resort to ineffective remedies such as creams, sprays or nipple shields. The last may even hinder milk flow. The midwifery skills required are outside the scope of this chapter.

Supplementary feeds

Supplementary feeds of formula or water are unnecessary for healthy, term breast-fed babies. Supplementary water or dextrose feeds are of no value in neonatal jaundice. If anything they *increase* the incidence.[20]

Healthy breast-fed term babies do not require routine blood glucose monitoring. 'Symptomatic' hypoglycemia in a breast-feeding baby should never be attributed to starvation alone; there is likely to be an underlying illness such as infection. Simple supplementary feeding is not therefore the solution.[21]

In some cultures (e.g. south Asian) it is believed that colostrum is detrimental, and 'prelacteal' feeds (e.g. teas, or formula in the UK) are used. It is widely but erroneously believed that this practice has a religious basis; it is contrary, for example, to Islamic teaching and should be discouraged.[22]

Demand feeding

Babies should be allowed to feed until satiated. Limiting sucking time does not reduce the incidence of nipple trauma, which is more likely to be attributable to poor attachment (see earlier). It is impossible to make rules about feed frequency because babies vary greatly. They may feed only a few times in the first 24 h, becoming more active and hungry on the second and third days.

The duration of a breast-feed bears little relationship to the amount consumed. Although a cross-sectional study suggested that, *on average*, 90% of the feed is consumed in the first 4 min, subsequent studies have shown pronounced interindividual variation. It is therefore impossible to formulate a rule applicable to all.

It is not necessary for babies to take both breasts at every feed. Babies can adjust milk intake to allow for variation in fat (i.e. energy) content. Babies extracted more hindmilk, thereby consuming more fat and maintaining a constant total daily energy intake, when mothers offered only one breast at each feed.[23] If the mother curtails feeding at the first breast to offer both routinely, there is a risk that the baby will consume excessive volumes of low-energy foremilk and lactose, producing explosive, watery stools and 'colic'.

Maintaining lactation

Well babies should be with their mothers continuously ('rooming-in'; Table 13.4) in the postnatal period. All breast-feeding mothers should be taught how to express milk by hand, though many prefer to use a pump. If so there is good evidence that pumping both breasts simultaneously (rather than sequentially), coupled with breast massage, increases yield.[24] A mother should express milk at least six times each day if separated from her baby, commencing as soon as possible after the birth. Expressed milk can be given by gavage, bottle or cup, the last being practicable for some babies of 30 weeks' gestation upwards. Cup feeding increases the chances of full breast-feeding at discharge, but may prolong hospital stay.[25]

CONTRAINDICATIONS TO BREAST-FEEDING

There are few absolute contraindications to breast-feeding. Galactosemia is one, and disorders of long-chain fatty acid oxidation another, though with phenylketonuria it is usually possible to continue, supplementing with a low phenylalanine formula according to blood concentrations. Formula supplements may be prescribed in medium chain acyl co-A dehydrogenase deficiency to prevent fasting hypoglycemia during the establishment of lactation. Maternal infections such as hepatitis B and tuberculosis do not contraindicate breast-feeding though the baby should be immunized and treated with appropriate prophylaxis. Maternal hepatitis C infection does not contraindicate breast-feeding.[26]

Human immunodeficiency virus (HIV) infection

In mothers infected antenatally the additional risk of vertical transmission attributable to breast-feeding has been estimated as about 15%, rising to about 30% if the mother is infected whilst breastfeeding. Mothers in the UK known to be HIV antibody positive and those at risk of infection are counseled not to breast-feed. In countries where the risk of malnutrition or infection associated with replacement feeding outweighs the risk of vertical transmission, mothers should be counseled about the risks and benefits, and given specific advice relevant to their circumstances.[27] This may encourage exclusive breastfeeding for the first 6 months with rapid weaning once safe complementary feeding has been established. Breast-feeding support is important as mastitis (including 'subclinical mastitis') significantly increases transmission risk.

Drugs in breast milk

Very few maternal drugs preclude breast-feeding; the decision should be based upon the toxicity of the drug, the quantity that the infant is likely to ingest, and the capacity of the infant to detoxify or excrete. Specific guidance is available from regularly updated texts.[28] The balance of benefit and risk must be considered; highly toxic drugs such as anti-mitotic agents and some retinoids contraindicate breast-feeding even though the amount ingested may be small. The quantity of a drug passed into milk may be measured or estimated from its lipid solubility and pKa. The more ionized the drug at milk pH 7.2 the less likely it is to pass into milk: thus drugs with higher pKa are generally safer. Helpful general guidance is to choose drugs with a shorter half-life and advise that they be taken immediately after a feed: as milk and plasma concentrations are in equilibrium, peak milk concentration will have declined by the next feed.[28]

GROWTH OF BREAST-FED BABIES

Historical growth references such as those of the National Center for Health Statistics (NCHS) and Tanner did not describe accurately the growth of breast-fed infants. In both industrialized and developing countries breast-fed babies grow rapidly in the first 2 months by comparison with those formula-fed, slowing thereafter.[29] Thus charts displayed an apparent slowing of weight velocity, once described as 'growth faltering' of the breast-fed baby and speculatively attributed to energy deficiency.[30] Likewise there was an appearance of rapid early weight gain, which should not be interpreted as 'overfeeding'. These deviations from charts reflected choice of an inappropriate reference population, not suboptimal growth patterns.

The UK 1990 growth reference may better reflect the growth of breast-fed babies, particularly a chart based on the growth of a subset of Cambridge breast-fed babies.[31] A reference based on the growth of healthy babies in six countries born at term to nonsmoking mothers with uncomplicated pregnancies and fed according to World Health Organization recommendations has recently been published.[32] The mean birthweight of this multi-country population was lower than that of babies born in the UK but the charts indicate, as expected, that breast-fed babies are in general heavier in the first 6 months and lighter in the second with respect to the existing UK reference. Differences in length and stature are less marked, but those in weight persist into later childhood.

COMPLEMENTARY FEEDING OF BREAST-FED BABIES

Following systematic review of the evidence, the World Health Organization recently recommended exclusive breast-feeding for the first 6 months of life, with introduction of complementary foods and continued breast-feeding thereafter. By comparison with babies fed exclusively for the first 4 months of life, those exclusively fed for 6 months experienced less diarrheal disease. Maternal postpartum weight loss and duration of lactational amenorrhea were also increased.[33] There have been few randomized studies of the appropriate timing of complementary feeding among breast-fed babies. One in Honduras showed that *total* daily energy intake and growth rate were comparable in early and late-weaned infants, though breast milk intake simply fell in those given solid food intake earlier.[34] There remains a need to examine the effect of energy density of weaning diets on this relationship.

In England the Department of Health recommends exclusive breast-feeding for the first 6 months with introduction of complementary foods and continued breast-feeding thereafter.[35] This is a population recommendation, within which there may be subgroups (such as those of low birth weight) at potential risk of iron or trace mineral deficiency resulting from low stores at birth. As such it is not a rule to be applied inflexibly to all individuals, but guidance. Differences in the social and cultural preferences of mothers mean that complementary foods are introduced for many reasons, for example the need to return to work.

SUPPLEMENTS FOR BREAST-FED BABIES
Vitamin K

Deficiency of vitamin K may result in hemorrhagic disease of the newborn (HDN) (see Chapter 12, Hematologic problems of the newborn). Human milk contains less vitamin K than cows' milk or formula (Tables 13.5 and 13.6) and supplementation from birth has long been recommended. An i.m. injection of vitamin K (1 mg phytomenadione) offers effective prophylaxis but was associated in one study with an increased incidence of childhood malignancy. Although several other studies have not confirmed this association, some parents still prefer oral supplementation. In England the Department of Health recommends that parents are offered this choice, and an information leaflet is available. A preparation licensed for oral administration to healthy term babies (Konakion MM Paediatric, Roche) is now available. It may be given parenterally (i.m./i.v.) to preterm babies or to those with other risk factors (for example instrumental delivery, mother taking anticonvulsants). Some ill babies (for example those with liver disease, malabsorption or on prolonged broad-spectrum antibiotic therapy) require continued supplementation in higher doses. An oral dose (2 mg) given at birth will need to be repeated: the datasheet advises a second 2 mg dose at 4–7 d and further monthly doses during the period of exclusive breast-feeding. Alternative schedules have been recommended but there are no comparative data on safety or efficacy as randomized trials of oral and parenteral dosage have not been performed.[36]

Vitamin D

Young babies meet their vitamin D requirements from stores at birth and sunshine exposure but nutritional rickets is seen in the UK, apparently with increasing frequency. It is associated with late introduction of complementary foods, Asian or black ethnic minority origin, and iron deficiency.[37] A high proportion of young children (between 20 and 35% in a national study of Asian infants and toddlers) have low plasma 25-OH-vitamin D concentrations, particularly during the winter.[38] Preventing rickets requires action before and after birth; a reference nutrient intake (RNI) of 10 mcg/d is set for pregnant and breast-feeding women in the UK, yet very few take a supplement and a high proportion of pregnant women from minority ethnic groups show biochemical evidence of severe deficiency.[39] Breast-fed babies should be given a supplement of 280 iu (7 mcg/d) from 6 months onwards, or from about 2 months in groups at increased risk by virtue of ethnic origins or culture. Other babies should commence vitamin D supplements when no longer receiving fortified infant formula, usually from about 12 months of age. In the USA supplementation with 200 iu/d (5 mcg) vitamin D should start before 2 months of age in all breast-fed babies and in those consuming less than 500 ml formula per day.[40]

Iron

Breast milk contains little iron though bioavailability is high. Birth stores are the principal source in young infants. Thus breast-fed babies do not require iron supplements unless additional risk factors are present, such as low birth weight. There may be adverse effects of iron supplements in babies who do not need them. In one study weight gain was impaired[41] and there are other concerns where malaria is endemic.[42] Moreover iron, copper and zinc compete for absorption, so other trace mineral deficiencies (particularly zinc) might be precipitated.

Water

Breast-fed babies do not need supplementary water: the solute load (vide infra) of breast milk is low enough to permit free water availability even in tropical climates.

INADEQUATE MILK PRODUCTION

Physiological failure of milk supply is rare. Faulty breast-feeding technique usually underlies slow weight gain and expert breastfeeding support is essential. Assessment of the adequacy of breastfeeding should not be made on weight alone. Frequency of feeding, frequency and amount of stools and urine should also be established. A history of early feeding difficulty or nipple pain may be obtained, the baby eventually becoming undemanding. Breast engorgement or mastitis may have occurred, again indicating ineffective drainage. Physical illness in the baby needs to be excluded, particularly if change has been sudden.

Attention to technique and increasing the frequency of feeds, sometimes combined with expression may increase supply. There is no evidence that metoclopramide, domperidone or other galactogogues offer additional benefit.

Test weighing underestimates intake. Electronic scales improve weighing precision but may still undermine the mother's confidence and raise problems of interpretation. Firstly, test weighing must last *at least* 48 h to take account of day-to-day and circadian variation. Secondly, the range of normal is very wide and the baby's milk consumption less than the mother's potential yield; the intake of one group of 3-month-old babies varied from 523–1124 g/d but, on average, a further 100 g could be obtained by expression. Finally, the baby's energy intake cannot be derived from weighed milk intake as the fat content of breast milk varies, tending to be inversely proportional to the volume of milk consumed. Test weighing therefore has little clinical value. Observation of breast-feeding technique (p. 369) and referral to a competent breastfeeding supporter is more likely to help.

BREAST MILK SUBSTITUTES

If a mother cannot breastfeed, or chooses not to, a replacement feed is required. The term 'breast milk substitute' describes 'any food marketed or otherwise represented as a partial or total replacement for breast milk, whether or not suitable for the purpose.' 'Infant formula' is a breast milk substitute formulated in accordance with Codex Alimentarius standards and the replacement feed of choice where feasible. In Europe 'infant formula' is legally defined as 'a product that by itself meets the nutritional requirements of normal healthy infants in the first 6 months of life'. Its composition is determined by European and UK legislation. 'Follow-on formula' is intended for normal healthy infants over 6 months of age as 'the principal liquid element in a progressively diversified diet'. It is not legally required to meet by itself the infant's nutritional needs.

Unmodified milks from cows, sheep, goats and other animals are unsuitable for infants. Amongst other things they generate a high *renal solute load*, have inappropriate calcium:phosphorus ratios, and are low in iron and other micronutrients. Historically the composition of human milk has guided the nutrient content of infant formula, except where significant differences in bioavailability exist (e.g. iron and protein [see later]). More recently it has been proposed that innovations should also strive to approximate health outcomes characteristic of the healthy breast-fed infant. This reflects appreciation of the superiority of human milk and its molecular complexity, and the development of novel processes (such as recombinant DNA technology) to manufacture human milk constituents. Adequately controlled studies must document both the efficacy and safety of such developments.[43]

COMPOSITION OF HUMAN MILK

The composition of expressed human milk has been extensively studied. Table 13.5 shows the composition of mature human milk expressed by UK mothers.[44] It is worth noting briefly some factors that affect milk composition and important qualitative nutritional differences between human milk and formula.

Table 13.5 Composition of mature human milk

Total nitrogen	2.1 g/L
Protein	10.7 g/L
Casein	41% of total protein
α-lactalbumin	28% of total protein
Lactoferrin	14% of total protein
Serum albumin	2% of total protein
Lysozyme	1% of total protein
Secretory IgA	14% of total protein
Nonprotein nitrogen	0.4 g/L
Fat	42 g/L
Cholesterol	0.42 mmol/L
Carbohydrate	74 g/L
Total energy	700 kcal/L
Sodium (23)	6.5 mmol/L
Potassium (39)	15.4 mmol/L
Calcium (40)	8.8 mmol/L
Magnesium (24)	1.2 mmol/L
Phosphorus (31)	4.8 mmol/L
Chloride (35)	12.3 mmol/L
Iron (56)	13.6 μmol/L
Copper (64)	6 μmol/L
Zinc (65)	45 μmol/L
Vitamin A (retinol)	600 μg/L
Vitamin D	0.1 μg/L
Vitamin E	3500 μg/L
Vitamin K	15 μg/L
Thiamin (B$_1$)	160 μg/L
Riboflavin (B$_2$)	310 μg/L
Nicotinic acid	2300 μg/L
Pyridoxine (B$_6$)	59 μg/L
Vitamin B$_{12}$	0.1 μg/L
Folic acid	52 μg/L
Pantothenic acid	2600 μg/L
Biotin	7.6 μg/L
Vitamin C	38 mg/L

After DHSS 1977.[55] Atomic weights of minerals in parentheses.

Factors affecting milk composition

Gestation of baby

The milk of mothers delivering prematurely tends to be higher in protein and sodium content but lower in lactose. Differences can be partly explained by reduced milk output, but serum leakage due to immaturity of mammary epithelial integrity might also be relevant.

Maternal diet and nutritional state

The effect of energy intake on the output and macronutrient content of breast milk has been overstated. Milk production is relatively unaffected by maternal body mass index (BMI). The fat content does, however, reflect qualitatively the amount and type of fat the mother consumes in her diet and her body stores.

Stage of lactation

Stage of lactation affects all milk constituents. Early milk is arbitrarily classified as *colostrum* (0–5 d) or *transitional* milk (5–10 d). Thereafter it is termed *mature*. Protein concentration changes greatly in the early stages. The immunoglobulin content of colostrum falls about 50-fold in the first week but total output of immunoglobulin A changes little because the milk output increases. Sodium concentration similarly falls in early lactation as the lactose concentration rises. Amongst the micronutrients, iron and copper concentrations fall slowly during lactation but zinc drops about 10-fold over a year. The changes in protein, lactose and sodium content reverse at weaning so that colostrum, weaning milk and 'preterm milk' show similarity in composition.

Changes within a feed

Fat concentration changes most, more than doubling during a feed. This may be a simple physical effect as it can to an extent be mimicked by squeezing milk from a sponge.

Time of day

Fat concentration shows most change and is related to the interval since the last feed: the longer it is, the lower the foremilk fat. Variation in nursing patterns affects circadian changes in fat concentration for this reason.

Protein and nonprotein nitrogen

Estimates of human milk protein concentration vary between 0.8 and 1.3 g/d for methodological reasons. The *crude protein* content is total nitrogen (g) × 6.38. It is higher than the true figure as 25% of total nitrogen is *nonprotein nitrogen*. Some of this, including urea, is incorporated into body protein together with the principal nutritional proteins, alpha-lactalbumin and casein. Many milk proteins (e.g. secretory immunoglobulin A, lactoferrin) have important functions other than nutrient provision; they can be recovered from the stool though digestibility increases with age. The differing digestibility of human and cows' milk proteins partly explains why the crude protein content of infant formula does not equate with that of human milk.

A further reason is the difference in *protein quality*, i.e. the relative match between the amino acid content of dietary protein and the requirement for growth and metabolism. Protein quality can be expressed numerically either by essential 'amino acid score' or 'net protein utilization', the proportion of ingested protein that is retained. Human milk is used as a reference protein in both cases, e.g. by regulation an infant formula must be based on soya or cows' milk protein. The latter has broadly two classes: whey (or acid-soluble) proteins and caseins (acid-precipitable curd). As whey and casein differ in amino acid composition the quality of cows' milk protein can be manipulated by changing the whey:casein ratio from 20:80 to 60:40. Such formulae are known as *whey dominant*. The claim that casein dominant formula 'satisfies hungry babies' has no justification, though UK babies commonly change to it within the first 6 weeks.[1]

The plasma amino acid concentrations of babies fed formulas containing 1.25 or 1.3 g/100 ml cows' milk protein as opposed to the usual 1.5–2.0 g/dl (Table 13.6) more closely approximate those of breast-fed babies. The whey:casein ratio also has less effect at these intakes. Thus the protein content of current formulae might be higher than necessary. It is possible that the higher protein intake of formula-fed babies explains the differences in growth and body composition observed during infancy. However breast-fed babies also self-regulate energy intake at lower levels, and have lower levels of energy expenditure.

Fat

Breast milk contains long- (LCT) and medium-chain triglycerides (MCT). In recent years it has been speculated that provision of the polyunsaturated fatty acid (PUFA) precursors linoleic (C_{18}–2ω6) and linolenic acid (C_{18}–3ω3) in formula is insufficient to meet the demands of the growing nervous system for the long-chain polyunsaturated fatty acid (LCPUFA) docosohexaenoic acid (C_{22}–6ω3) but there is no conclusive evidence that the addition of LCPUFAs to formula is of significant short- or long-term health benefit for term infants.[45]

Iron

Cows' milk contains less iron than human milk and, furthermore, cows' milk iron is less bioavailable. Formulae are therefore enriched with iron salts. Formulae sold in the USA vary widely in iron content; so-called 'regular' formula contains 1 mg/L iron whereas 'iron-fortified' formulae contain > 10 mg/L. A US randomized trial showed superior iron status and psychomotor development among infants fed 'iron-fortified' formula.[46] Formulas sold in the UK contain 5–7 mg/L iron and it is not possible to extrapolate the results of the US study to UK practice. If the mother is not breast-feeding, continued use of infant formula to at least 12 months of age is important in building iron stores and preventing iron deficiency in the toddler years. 'Follow-on' formulas offer no advantage over infant formulas in this respect, though either is preferable to cows' milk.

MANUFACTURE OF INFANT FORMULA

Manufacture of infant formula in simple terms changes the composition of cows' milk (Table 13.6) as follows:

1. The protein and electrolyte content of cows' milk (see 'solute load' later) are reduced.
2. The whey:casein blend may be altered to improve protein quality and digestibility.
3. The calcium and phosphorus content is reduced and the Ca:P ratio altered.
4. The carbohydrate content is increased by addition of lactose or maltodextrins (glucose polymers).
5. The fat blend is changed using vegetable oil to reduce saturated fat intake and increase intake of polyunsaturated fat, thus improving fat absorption.
6. Trace minerals are added, particularly iron and copper.
7. Vitamins are added.

'RENAL SOLUTE LOAD'

Both glomerular filtration rate and tubular concentrating power are reduced in the newborn (Ch. 12, Special care – sodium and potassium), limiting the clearance and elimination of solute surplus to growth demands. The *potential renal solute load* (PRSL) of a feed is the amount of solute that would need to be excreted in urine if none were deposited in new tissue or excreted through nonrenal routes.[47] It can be calculated by summing the expected urea production from protein oxidation (approximately 4 mosmol/g protein), sodium, potassium, phosphorus and chloride content. Note that the true renal solute load (RSL) presenting to the kidneys is normally lower than PRSL because a variable proportion of dietary solute, relatively high in the case of human milk, is deposited in new tissue during growth. RSL can be estimated by subtracting from PRSL an amount given by 0.9 × weight gain (in grams per day).

Table 13.6 Composition of cow's milk and infant formula in europe

	Cow's milk	Units	Infant formula Minimum	Maximum	Units
Energy			60	75	kcal/100 ml
Protein	33	g/L	1.8	3	g/100 kcal
Carbohydrate	48	g/L	7	14	g/100 kcal
Fat	38	g/L	4.4	6.5	g/100 kcal
Linoleic acid			300	1200	mg/100 kcal
Linolenic acid			50		
Sodium	59 (35–90)	mg/dl	20	60	mg/100 kcal
Potassium	150 (110–170)	mg/dl	60	145	mg/100 kcal
Chloride	95 (90–110)	mg/dl	50	125	mg/100 kcal
Calcium	120 (110–130)	mg/dl	50	#	mg/100 kcal
Phosphorus	95 (90–100)	mg/dl	25	90	mg/100 kcal
Ca:P ratio	1.2:1		1.2	2	
Magnesium	12 (9–14)	mg/dl	5	15	mg/100 kcal
Iron	50 (30–60)	µg/dl	0.5	1.5	mg/100 kcal
Zinc	350 (200–600)	µg/dl	0.5	1.5	mg/100 kcal
Copper	20 (10–60)	µg/dl	20	80	µg/100 kcal
Vitamin A	31 (27–36)	µg/dl	60	180	µg RE /100 kcal
Vitamin D	0.02	µg/dl	1	2.5	µg/100 kcal
Vitamin E (a tocopherol)	0.09	mg/dl	0.5	#	mg/g of polyunsaturated fatty acid
Vitamin K	1–8.5	µg/dl	4	#	µg/100 kcal
Vitamin C	2	mg/dl	8	8	mg/100 kcal
Thiamine	40 (30–60)	µg/dl	40	#	µg/100 kcal
Riboflavin	190 (150–230)	µg/dl	60	#	µg/100 kcal
Nicotinamide	80 (60–130)	µg/dl	0.8	#	mg/100 kcal
Pyridoxine	40 (21–72)	µg/dl	35	#	µg/100 kcal
Vitamin B_{12}	0.3	µg/dl	0.1	#	µg/100 kcal
Pantothenic acid	0.35 (0.2–0.5)	µg/dl	300	#	µg/100 kcal
Biotin	2 (1.0–1.3)	µg/dl	1.5	#	µg /100 kcal
Folic acid	5	µg/dl	4	#	µg /100 kcal

[†]Data from DHSS 1980;[56] *Infant formula regulations 1995;[57] # no value stated.

Human milk has a PRSL of 93 mosmol/L and unmodified cows' milk 308 mosmol/L. A nongrowing infant with maximal tubular concentrating power of 600 mosmol/L of urine would therefore require at least 513 (or 308/600 × 1000) ml of water to eliminate the solute load generated by 1 L of cows' milk. This explains why infants fed unmodified cow's milk may become hypernatremic. During illness a high nonrenal water loss caused by diarrhea or fever may particularly constrain water available for solute excretion. Energy density also has a bearing on solute load because it affects milk intake, and thus water available for urine formation.

MILK CONSUMPTION

The intake of both breast- and bottle-fed babies is extremely variable and the oft-quoted 'requirement' of 150 ml/kg/d merely a guideline. The intakes of healthy American formula-fed infants 0–2 months old fed ad libitum were 169 ± 25 (1 standard deviation [SD]) ml/kg/d (boys) and 157 ± 22 ml/kg/d (girls).[48] Similarly, although the average breast milk intake of 3-month-old infants is 700–800 ml/d, there is approximately 100% difference between the extremes.

Consequently the 'normal' milk intake for an individual infant cannot be predicted. Acceptable intake is reflected in satisfactory growth. If the baby is not growing, the baby should be fed ad libitum or intake increased to the upper end of the normal range (mean + 2 SD) before seeking other causes.

SOYA FORMULA AND OTHER MILKS

Soya formula is unsuitable for the prophylaxis or treatment of cows' milk protein allergy because cross-sensitivity to soya protein occurs in

15–43% of affected children. A formula based on cows' milk protein hydrolysate is preferable both in proven cows' milk protein intolerance (CMPI) and post gastroenteritis lactose intolerance because CMPI often coexists. Concern about the very high phytoestrogen content of soya formula underpins Department of Health advice that soya formulas should not be used. However they have advantages in the management of galactosemia (Ch. 26) because they are lactose free and more palatable than alternatives.

COMPLEMENTARY FEEDING – 'WEANING'

The term 'weaning' is commonly used to describe the gradual introduction of foods (or 'solids') other than breast milk or formula, though it more correctly describes a reduction in the number of breast-feeds. The phrase 'complementary feeding' is therefore preferred, to indicate the important role played by continued breast-feeding.

Nutritionally, complementary feeding increases the energy, vitamin and mineral (especially iron) density of the diet as demands outstrip milk supply. However it should be considered in the wider context of development because it encourages tongue and jaw movements in preparation for speech, introduces new tastes and textures, and increases social interaction with carers. It is important that complementary feeding is paced to accord with developmental changes in gross, fine motor and oral motor function. Infants must not be 'pushed' if later behavioral eating problems are to be avoided.

By custom most British mothers have commenced complementary feeding by offering relatively bland (unseasoned), single ingredient foods (such as thinly puréed rice, fruit or vegetables) once- or twice-daily from a spoon after breast-feeds. As the spoon is accepted, thicker purées may be offered, with progression to lumps and small finger foods as fine motor skills progress. Such an approach may be less appropriate for infants

Table 13.7 Suggestions for vegetarian weaning diets. After Poskitt[49]

Nutrient	Problem	Solution
Energy	Energy density reduced by water absorption and fiber content. Most fruit low in energy	Use oils in cooking and spreading fats on food. Cereals, pulses, bananas and avocados are energy dense
Protein	Quality variable	Mix complementary food groups to achieve balanced intake, i.e. milk (dairy), legumes, grains, green vegetables
Vitamins	Low B_{12}, D and riboflavin	Use eggs, vitamin D-supplemented margarine or fish oils (if permissible). Consider oral B_{12} supplement
Minerals	Phytates reduce availability (especially of iron). Zinc and calcium intakes may be low	Green leaf vegetables rich in iron. Vitamin C increases uptake. Dairy products important as calcium/zinc source

weaned from 6 months in line with current advice. Oral and manual manipulative skills are more dexterous at this age, suggesting that dietary texture might be more rapidly advanced. However the acceptability of alternative regimens has not been systematically studied. By about 1 year of age the infant should be receiving (chopped) family foods at about three main meals with intervening snacks. Breast milk should remain the principal source of fluid, though formula (in amounts of no more than 500–600 ml/d) may now be replaced by pasteurized whole cows' milk.

WEANING PROBLEMS
Vegetarian and ethnic minority diets
Certain minority ethnic groups (e.g. vegans, Rastafarians) have limited choice of weaning foods threatening protein quality, zinc, iron and vitamin B_{12} intake. Phytates may reduce mineral availability (especially calcium and iron) and increase dietary bulk, compromising energy intake. Suggestions for a suitable vegetarian weaning diet are summarized in Table 13.7.[49]

Asian babies in the UK, particularly those of Bangladeshi and Pakistani background, tend to be weaned later than Caucasian ones.[50] They are more likely to be breast-fed initially, but also more likely to receive cows' milk in the first year of life, often with complementary foods such as rusk added to the feeding bottle. Amongst children of Indian background 38% of 9-month-olds in a national survey had never eaten meat, which may help to explain the higher incidence of iron deficiency anemia. Early supplementation with vitamin D, coupled with supplementation for the mother during pregnancy and breast-feeding is also important (vide supra). Although more Asian mothers (> 50% at 9 months) than Caucasian ones (20%) give vitamins,[50] there is room for improvement. There has been no national study of black, Afro-Caribbean babies in the UK but they are likely to be at increased risk of vitamin D deficiency also, particularly if Rastafarian.

VITAMIN SUPPLEMENTS
Formula is fortified with vitamins, and supplementation is unnecessary until cows' milk is introduced at about 1 year of age. Breast-fed babies should receive vitamin supplements (e.g. *Abidec*™, *Dalavit*™) from 6 months of age or in some cases earlier (vide supra). Vitamin supplements should be continued until at least 2 years of age, and preferably until the age of 5. Under the *Healthy Start* scheme (which has recently replaced the Welfare Food Scheme[51] in the UK), parents on income support can obtain vitamin supplements free of charge until their child is 4 years old.

DENTAL HEALTH
Caries in pre-school children is strongly linked to socioeconomic status; by the age of 5 years children living in the most deprived areas have three times more caries than those in the most affluent areas. Fluoridation of the water supply is an effective public health measure but fluoride supplements (other than toothpaste) should only be used on an individual basis as prescribed by a dentist. Brushing after drinking or eating should commence with emergence of the first teeth, using a smear of fluoridated toothpaste. Excessive dosing may cause enamel mottling. Drinks containing nonmilk extrinsic sugars (including natural juices) should be avoided, especially between meals, and water or milk given instead. Using a cup from about 6 months also helps to prevent caries; infants must never be left unsupervised or left to sleep with a bottle or feeder cup.[52]

DRINKS AND WATER
Boiled tap water is sufficient, if required, for formula-fed babies under 6 months of age. Flavored drinks are unnecessary. Natural mineral water, or water drawn through a domestic softener may be of unsuitable electrolyte content and should not be given to babies. Displacement of milk with flavored drinks during weaning is a common cause of failure to thrive; it is important to ensure that adequate milk intake (breast-feeds or about 500–600 ml formula) is maintained.

PASTEURIZED COWS' MILK
Pasteurized whole cows' milk should not be given to infants under 1 year of age (see Ch. 16) and semi-skimmed milk should be avoided in children under 2 years. Other milk products, such as cheese and yoghurt, may be used from 6 months onwards.

REFERENCES (*Level 1 Evidence)

1. BMRB Social Research. Infant feeding survey 2000. 2001;1–15.
2. World Health Organization DoDaARDC. Indicators for assessing breastfeeding practices. WHO/CDD/SER/91. 1991; 14:1–14.
3. WHO Collaborative Study Team. Effect of breastfeeding on infant and child mortality due to infectious diseases in less developed countries: a pooled analysis. WHO Collaborative Study Team on the Role of Breastfeeding on the Prevention of Infant Mortality. Lancet 2000; 355:451–455.

4. Edmond KM, Zandoh C, Quigley MA, et al. Delayed breastfeeding initiation increases risk of neonatal mortality. Pediatrics 2006; 117:e380–e386.
5. Kramer MS, Chalmers B, Hodnett ED, et al. Promotion of breastfeeding intervention trial (PROBIT). JAMA 2001; 285 (January 24/31):413–420.
6. Owen CG, Whincup PH, Odoki K, et al. Infant feeding and blood cholesterol: a study in adolescents and a systematic review. Pediatrics 2002; 110:597–608.
7. Owen CG, Whincup PH, Gilg JA, et al. Effect of breast feeding in infancy on blood pressure in later life: systematic review and meta-analysis. BMJ 2003; 327:1189–1195.

8. Owen CG, Martin RM, Whincup PH, et al. Effect of infant feeding on the risk of obesity across the life course: a quantitative review of published evidence. Pediatrics 2005; 115:1367–1377.
9. Harder T, Bergmann R, Kallischnigg G, et al. Duration of breastfeeding and risk of overweight: A meta-analysis. Am J Epidemiol 2005; 162:397–403.
10. Anderson JW, Johnstone BM, Remley DT. Breastfeeding and cognitive development: a meta-analysis. Am J Clin Nutr 1999; 70:525–535.
11. Collaborative Group on Hormonal Factors in Breast Cancer. Breast cancer and breastfeeding: collaborative reanalysis of individual data from 47 epidemiological studies in 30 countries, including

50,032 women with breast cancer and 96,973 women without the disease. Lancet 2002; 360:187–195.

12. Eisman J. Relevance of pregnancy and lactation to osteoporosis. Lancet 1998; 352:504–505.

13. Abrams SA. Editorial: Bone turnover during lactation – Can calcium supplementation make a difference? J Clin Endocrinol Metab 1998; 83:1056–1058.

14. Vallenas C, Savage F. Evidence for the Ten Steps to successful breastfeeding. World Health Organization; 1998; 1–111.WHO/CHD/98.9 Geneva.

15. Renfrew M, Dyson L, Wallace L, et al. Breastfeeding for longer: what works? London: National Institute for Health and Clinical Excellence; 2005.

16. Coutinho SB, de Lira PIC, Carvalho Lima M, et al. Comparison of the effect of two systems for the promotion of exclusive breastfeeding. Lancet 2005; 366:1094–1100.

17. Broadfoot M, Britten J, Tappin DM, et al. The Baby Friendly Hospital Initiative and breast feeding rates in Scotland. Arch Dis Child Fetal Neonatal Ed 2005; 90:F114–F116.

18. Woolridge MW. The 'anatomy' of infant feeding. Midwifery 1986; 2:164–171.

19. Woolridge MW. The aetiology of sore nipples. Midwifery 1986; 2:172–176.

20. Nicoll A, Ginsburg R, Tripp JH. Supplementary feeding and jaundice in newborns. Acta Paediatr Scand 1982; 71:759–761.

21. Williams AF. Hypoglycaemia of the newborn: a review. Bull World Health Org 1997; 75:261–290.

22. Gatrad A, Sheikh A. Muslim birth customs. Arch Dis Child Fetal Neonatal Ed 2001; 84:F6–F8.

23. Woolridge MW, Ingram JC, Baum JD. Do changes in pattern of breast usage alter the baby's nutrient intake? Lancet 1990; 336:395–397.

24. Jones E, Dimmock PW, Spencer SA. A randomised trial to compare methods of milk expression after preterm delivery. Arch Dis Child Fetal Neonatal Ed 2001; 85:F91–F95.

25. Collins CT, Ryan P, Crowther CA, et al. Effect of bottles, cups, and dummies on breast feeding in preterm infants: a randomised controlled trial. BMJ 2004; 329:193–198.

26. Pembreya L, Newella ML, Tovob PA. The management of HCV infected pregnant women and their children European paediatric HCV network. J Hepatol 2005; 43:515–525.

27. World Health Assembly. Infant and young child nutrition. Global strategy on infant and young child feeding. Report by the Secretariat 2002; A55:15.

28. Hale TW. Medications and mothers' milk. 11th edn. Amarillo, Texas: Pharmasoft Medical Publishing; 2004.

29. Dewey KG, Peerson JM, Brown KH, et al. Growth of breast-fed infants deviates from current reference data: A pooled analysis of US, Canadian and European data sets. Pediatrics 1995; 96:495–503.

30. Waterlow JC, Thomson AM. Observations on the adequacy of breast-feeding. Lancet 1979; ii:(4 August):238–242.

31. Cole TJ, Paul AA, Whitehead RG. Weight reference charts for British long-term breastfed infants. Acta Paediatr 2002; 91:1296–1300.

32. WHO Multicenter Growth Reference Study Group, De Onis M. WHO Child Growth Standards based on length/height, weight and age. Acta Paediatr–Int J Paediatr 2006; (Supplements):76–86.

33. Kramer MS, Kakuma R. Optimal duration of exclusive breastfeeding (Cochrane Review). The Cochrane Library. Oxford: Update Software; 2002.

34. Cohen RJ, Brown KH, Canahuati J, et al. Effects of age of introduction of complementary foods on infant breast milk intake, total energy intake, and growth: a randomised controlled study in Honduras. Lancet 1994; 344:288–293.

35. Department of Health. Infant feeding recommendations. 1–4 London: Department of Health; 2004.

36. Puckett RM, Offringa M. Prophylactic vitamin K for vitamin K deficiency bleeding in neonates. Cochrane Database Syst Rev 2000; CD002776.

37. Wharton B, Bishop N. Rickets. Lancet 2003; 362:1389–1400.

38. Lawson M, Thomas M, Hardiman A. Dietary and lifestyle factors affecting plasma vitamin D levels in Asian children living in England. Eur J Clin Nutr 1999; 53:268–272.

39. Datta S, Alfaham M, Davies DP, et al. Vitamin D deficiency in pregnant women from a non-European ethnic minority population – an interventional study. BJOG: an International Journal of Obstetrics & Gynaecology 2002; 109:905–908.

40. Gartner LM, Greer FR. Section on Breastfeeding, Committee on Nutrition. Prevention of Rickets and Vitamin D Deficiency: New Guidelines for Vitamin D Intake. Pediatrics 2003; 111:908–910.

41. Idradjinata P, Watkins WE, Pollitt E. Adverse effects of iron supplementation on weight gain of iron-replete young children. Lancet 1994; 343:1252–1254.

42. Sazawal S, Black RE, Ramsan M, et al. Effects of routine prophylactic supplementation with iron and folic acid on admission to hospital and mortality in preschool children in a high malaria transmission setting: community-based, randomised, placebo-controlled trial. Lancet 2006; 367:133–143.

43. Committee on Medical Aspects of Food Policy (COMA) WGotNAoIF. Guidelines on the nutritional assessment of infant formulas. Report on Health and Social Subjects [47]. London: The Stationery Office; 1996.

44. Committee on Medical Aspects of Food Policy (COMA). The composition of mature human milk. Report on Health and Social Subjects [12]. London: Her Majesty's Stationery Office; 1977.

45. Simmer K. Longchain polyunsaturated fatty acid supplementation in infants born at term. (Cochrane Review). Cochrane Library; 2001.

46. Moffatt MEK, Longstaffe S, Besant J, et al. Prevention of iron deficiency and psychomotor decline in high-risk infants through use of iron-fortified infant formula: A randomised clinical trial. J Pediatr 1994; 125:527–534.

47. Fomon SJ, Ziegler EE. Renal solute load and potential renal solute load in infancy. J Pediatr 1999; 134:11–14.

48. Fomon SJ, Thomas LN, Filer LJ, et al. Food consumption and growth of normal infants fed milk based formulas. Acta Paediatr Scand Suppl 1971; 223:1–36.

49. Poskitt EME. Vegetarian weaning. Arch Dis Child 1988; 63:1286–1292.

50. Thomas M, Avery V. Infant feeding in Asian families. London: The Stationery Office; 1997.

51. Committee on Medical Aspects of Food and Nutrition Policy PoCaMN. Scientific review of the Welfare Food Scheme. Report on Health and Social Subjects 2002; 51:1–147.

52. Scottish Intercollegiate Guidelines Network (SIGN). Prevention and management of dental decay in the pre-school child, 83rd edn. Edinburgh: NHS Quality Improvement Scotland; 2005.

53. NHS Centre for Reviews and Dissemination. Promoting the initiating of breast-feeding. Effective Health Care 2000; 6:1–12.

54. WHO/UNICEF. Protecting, promoting and supporting breast-feeding: The specific role of maternity services. Geneva: WHO; 1989.

55. Department of Health and Social Security. The Composition of Mature Human Milk. Report on health and social subjects 12. London: HMSO; 1977.

56. Committee on Medical Aspects of Food Policy (COMA) WPotCoFflaYC. Artificial feeds for the young infant. Report on Health and Social Subjects [18]. London: Her Majesty's Stationery Office; 1980.

57. Her Majesty's Government. The infant formula and follow-on formula regulations. Statutory Instruments 1995; 77.

Section 3
The specialities

14

Genetics

Michael A Patton

INTRODUCTION

There has been an exponential increase in the understanding of human genetics and it would not be possible to discuss all genetic disorders in children, so the purpose of this chapter is to present some of the basic concepts of genetics in relation to pediatric practice.

Traditionally diseases were divided into those due to 'nature' and those due to 'nurture' but it is more fruitful to consider human disease as a spectrum from those conditions like Duchenne muscular dystrophy and Down syndrome, which are purely genetic, through to those which are purely environmental such as scurvy and tuberculosis (Fig. 14.1).[1,2] Between the two extremes are many common diseases like diabetes mellitus, ischemic heart disease and congenital malformations in which both genetic and environmental factors are involved. Such conditions may be referred to as multifactorial. Disorders at the genetic end of the spectrum are due either to changes in a single gene or to visible changes in the chromosomes.

EPIDEMIOLOGY

The frequency of genetic disorders has not increased, but they have become relatively more important with the decline in mortality from infectious diseases and the rapidly increasing knowledge of medical genetics. The number of human chromosomes was only established in 1956 and since then our knowledge of genetics has advanced at an exponential rate with the first draft of the human genome being completed in 2001. Prenatal diagnosis has offered the opportunity of preventing an increasing number of serious handicaps, and the developments in DNA technology have meant that many of the genes that predispose to common adult disorders such as heart disease and cancer have now been identified and play a role in identifying predisposition and developing strategies for the prevention of these disorders.

Genetic disorders are a major component in childhood mortality with up to half of childhood deaths in hospital having a genetic or partly genetic cause. In addition to mortality, genetic disorders produce a substantial morbidity. They often require frequent hospital admissions

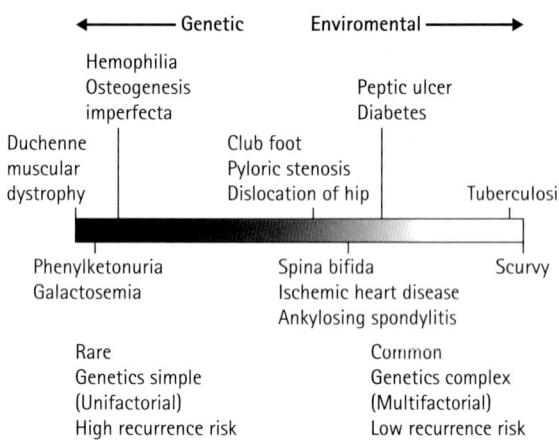

Fig. 14.1 Human disease may be seen as being on a spectrum from those diseases which are exclusively genetic to those which are exclusively environmental. (From Emery & Mueller 1988[1].)

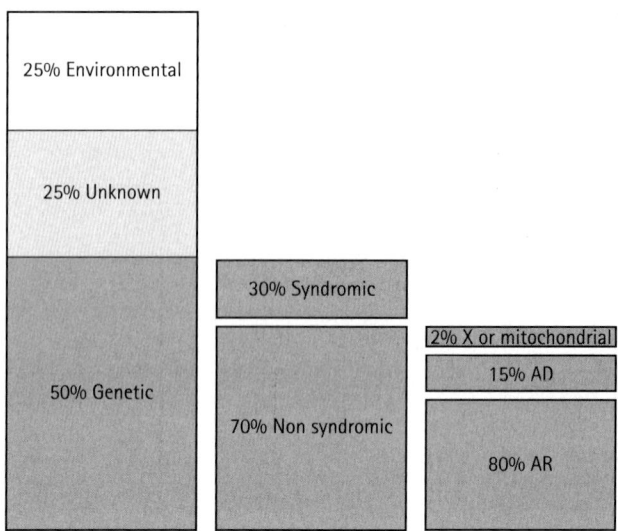

Fig. 14.2 Etiology of deafness. AD, autosomal dominant; AR, autosomal recessive.

or complex surgery and the incidence of genetic or partially genetic disease amongst pediatric inpatients has been found to be between 11 and 27%.[3] It should also be noted that many chronic genetic disorders may place a considerable financial strain on health resources.

In the field of intellectual disability the genetic contribution is even greater. Chromosome abnormalities are the most significant cause and with newer chromosome techniques coming into diagnostic testing the proportion of intellectual disability due to visible chromosome abnormalities or microdeletions will increase. There is also an increasing number of X-linked forms of intellectual disability in which genes are being identified and these may account for the excess of males affected.

The same situation applies in visual handicap and profound childhood deafness. In previous generations retrolental fibroplasia and ophthalmia neonatorum contributed significantly to childhood blindness but the frequency of these disorders is declining with improved medical care. One survey[4] conducted in a national school for children who are registered blind has shown that about 50% of childhood blindness has a genetic basis and that this is largely due to single gene disorders (Table 14.1).[3] In studies on congenital sensorineural deafness around 50% has been attributed to genetic factors and over half of these are due to autosomal recessive genes (Fig. 14.2).

Even before birth, chromosome abnormalities are a major cause of fetal wastage with between 15 and 30% of all human conceptions having an abnormal karyotype and being spontaneously aborted or failing to implant.

The overall incidence of genetic disorders is roughly comparable in different parts of the world, but the frequency of specific disorders may vary for reasons such as inbreeding, selective advantage and genetic isolation.[2] The frequency of sickle cell disease mirrors the frequency of malaria since carriers of sickle cell trait have a greater resistance to *Plasmodium falciparum* malaria. This frequency has taken many generations to develop from a relatively small selective advantage and will remain in those racial groups for a very considerable

Table 14.1 99 Children in blind school, Edinburgh (1988). (Modified from Philips et al 1987[4])

Genetic = 50%	Nongenetic = 50%
Congenital cataract	Birth asphyxia
Anophthalmos	Optic nerve hypoplasia
Leber's amaurosis	Cortical blindness
Laurence – Moon – Biedl	Retrolental fibroplasia
Retinitis pigmentosa	Hydrocephalus
Retinal dystrophy	Non-accidental injury

Table 14.2 Racial and geographic differences in the frequency of genetic disease

Disease	Racial/geographic group	Birth incidence
Sickle cell disease	African	1 in 50
Thalassemia	Mediterranean	1 in 100
Oculocutaneous albinism	Hopi Indians	1 in 250
	N. Europeans	1 in 40 000
Congenital adrenal hyperplasia	Yupik Eskimos	1 in 500
	N. Europeans	1 in 10 000
Cystic fibrosis	N. Europeans	1 in 2000
	Orientals	Very rare
Tay–Sachs disease	Ashkenazi Jews	1 in 3600
Neural tube defects	N. Ireland	1 in 300
Ellis–van Creveld syndrome	Amish	1 in 200
	N. European	1 in 60 000

number of generations even after they have moved to countries without malaria. Cystic fibrosis is one of the most frequent single gene disorders in Western Europe, and although this is probably attributable to a selective advantage in gene carriers, the mechanism has yet to be demonstrated. For other recessive disorders in small isolated communities the frequency of affected children may be increased by inbreeding, e.g. oculocutaneous albinism in the Hopi Indians, congenital adrenal hyperplasia in the Yupik Eskimos and Ellis–van Creveld syndrome in the Amish community (Table 14.2). It should be noted that genetic disease may pose a major health problem even in resource limited countries where infections are still a major cause of childhood deaths, e.g. in Thailand up to 500 000 children suffer from variable degrees of chronic ill health due to the interaction of different thalassemia genes.

MITOSIS AND MEIOSIS

Chromosomes are the means whereby the genes are transmitted from one cell generation to the next. This transmission of genetic information must be precise and accurate and is achieved via one of the two mechanisms of cell division, either mitosis which is the division of somatic cells resulting in the growth of specific organs or the overall body, or meiosis which is the specialized cell division resulting in gamete formation and may be referred to as 'reduction division' since it involves the reduction of the original *diploid* (2n) complement of 46 chromosomes to the *haploid* (n) complement of 23 chromosomes.

MITOSIS: CELL DIVISION

Somatic cell division is a cyclical procedure, the length of the total cycle varying from organism to organism and between cell types. Essentially the cell cycle can be divided into a number of steps. During the resting or *interphase* stage the chromosomes are not visible other than as a mass of chromatin. At *metaphase* the chromosomes are maximally contracted with two sister chromatids held together at the centromere and aligned along the equatorial plate of the cell. At this stage the chromosomes can be visualized and examined under the microscope. The chromatids are then separated by the 'spindle apparatus' to opposite ends of the cell, where they are included in separate daughter nuclei (*telophase*). The products of mitotic division, therefore, are two daughter cells identical in all respects with the parent cell from which they have arisen.

MEIOSIS: PRODUCTION OF GAMETES

Meiosis comprises a reduction of the diploid chromosome number (46) to a haploid chromosome number (23) through two successive nuclear divisions. In the early stages the homologous chromosomes pair closely with one another, and exchange segments of genetic material in a process known as *meiotic recombination* (Fig. 14.3). This recombination ensures the individuality of the offspring in much the same way as shuffling a pack of cards in each game ensures that the players will receive a different combination of cards. After recombination the paired chromosomes separate and eventually two daughter chromosomes of differing genetic constitution from each parent are formed (*metaphase I*). The second stage is a straightforward mitotic division in which the centromeres of the daughter chromosomes divide and their attached chromatids travel to opposite cell poles.

The outcome of this two-stage division process is a quartet of nuclei, each with half (n) the original number (2n) of chromosomes, and with new combinations of parental genes.

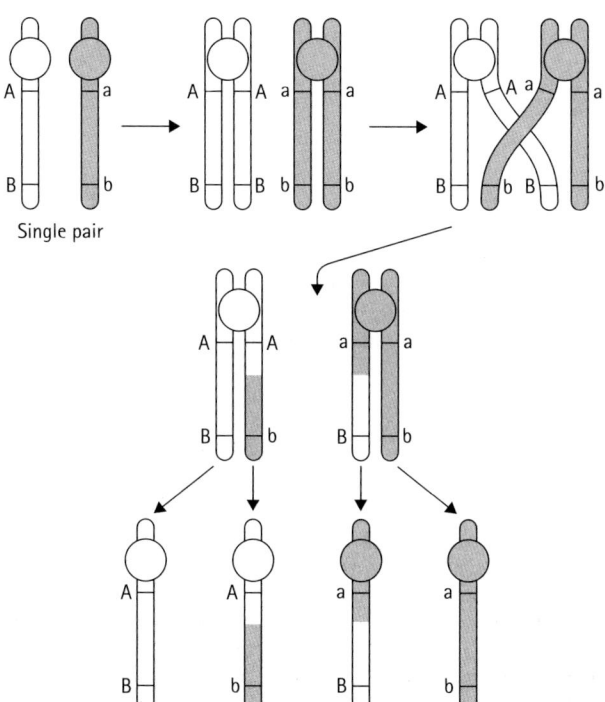

Fig. 14.3 'Crossing over' – the exchange of genetic material between homologous chromosomes.

Spermatogenesis and oogenesis

The basic pattern of chromosome behavior is the same during meiosis in both male and female gametogenesis, but there are differences in timing of the various stages. Spermatogenesis begins around puberty and continues throughout life, with spermatozoa produced by continuing meiotic division of primary spermatocytes. On the other hand, oogenesis commences in intrauterine life but is arrested at a very early stage in meiosis I, with completion of the cycle only when ovulation occurs, anything up to 50 years later.

Spermatogenesis and oogenesis also differ in that, while the former gives rise ultimately to four functional sperm, the latter normally yields only a single functional ovum, with the other three products of the division process forming 'polar bodies', each with its haploid chromosome constitution, but with only a relatively small amount of cytoplasm. The polar bodies are nonfunctional and do not contribute to the future offspring.

CHROMOSOMES

PREPARATION OF BLOOD CHROMOSOMES

The original demonstration that there are 46 chromosomes in the human cell was made using fibroblast cultures from fetal lung.[5] In routine clinical practice, however, it is human lymphocytes that are used for the standard chromosome analysis since a blood sample is convenient to obtain and relatively easy to prepare.

The standard preparation of chromosomes from a blood sample is illustrated in Figure 14.4. The first stage of the process (i) is to separate the white cells from the rest of the blood sample. This is done by centrifugation using a medium such as Ficoll, which leaves the lymphocytes in a buffy coat at the top of the tube. The second stage (ii) is to cultivate the lymphocytes in vitro. The lymphocyte rarely divides in circulation but when a *mitogen* (a chemical which stimulates mitosis or cell division) such as phytohemagglutinin is added the lymphocytes undergo a cell division in about 48–72 h. The third stage (iii) is to arrest the cell division in metaphase when the chromosomes are at their most contracted and are best visualized. This is done by adding colchicine to the culture at 69–70 h. The fourth stage (iv) is to release the chromosomes from the nucleus and spread them on a microscope slide. This is carried out by placing the cultured cells in hypotonic saline and dropping the solution carefully onto a microscope slide from a sufficient height to give a reasonable spread of chromosomes. The fifth stage (v) is to fix and stain the spread for microscopic analysis. The normal staining process is using a Giemsa stain that shows a light and dark banding appearance (Fig. 14.5). Most of the analysis is carried out under the microscope, but a photograph of the spread may be taken and a mounted karyotype prepared as a permanent record or for further analysis. It is usual to analyze several cells in preparing a report.

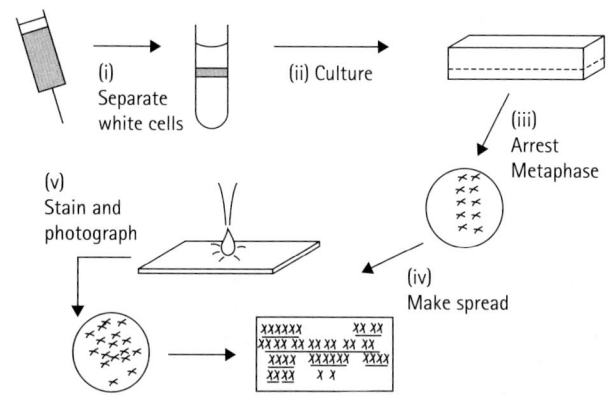

Fig. 14.4 Preparation of a chromosome karyotype from a blood sample.

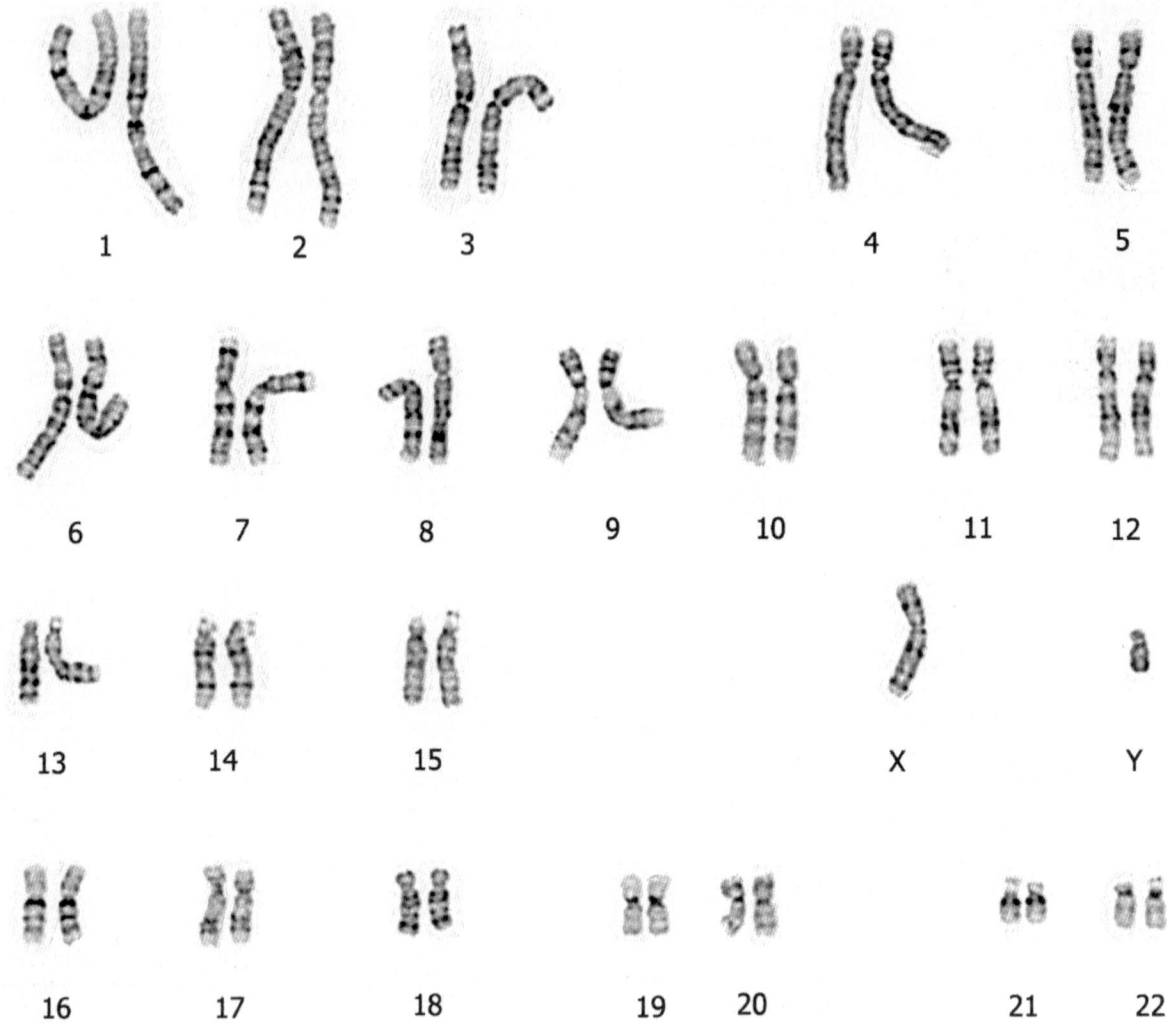

Fig. 14.5 Standard chromosome karyotype.

BONE MARROW

Bone marrow contains many rapidly dividing cells. It is therefore possible to locate cells that are already in metaphase and thus a direct preparation may be obtained. However, short term culture is generally performed and is used in leukemias where chromosome abnormalities may be of value both for diagnosis and prognosis.

FIBROBLASTS

Culture of connective tissue in vitro will result in the growth of fibroblasts, which may be used for chromosome culture. The most common source of fibroblasts is from a skin biopsy. It may be useful to look for mosaicism in a different tissue from blood. At postmortem connective tissue may be obtained from many different sources, but usually it is adequate to take a sample of skin under sterile conditions for culture.

AMNIOCENTESIS

Fluid taken at amniocentesis between 12 and 16 weeks' gestation contains skin cells shed from the fetus and amniotic membranes. These cells are not very numerous in the sample but may be cultured up in a similar way to fibroblasts. It takes 2–3 weeks to culture and analyze the cells.

CHORIONIC VILLUS SAMPLES

Another approach to prenatal diagnosis is to obtain a sample of chorionic villi from the membranes surrounding the fetus at 9–11 weeks' gestation. This material is fetal in origin, but has to be separated from maternal tissue under the dissecting microscope before analysis. Chorionic villi are rapidly dividing and it is possible to obtain direct preparations without culture. However, because of the possibility of maternal contamination and mosaicism, most diagnostic laboratories prefer to wait until culture is also available at 1–2 weeks before giving a definitive result.

FLUORESCENT IN SITU HYBRIDIZATION (FISH)

There has been a considerable gap between cytogenetic analysis at the microscopic level and molecular genetics at the gene level, but it is now possible to combine a gene specific probe with a fluorescent dye and to demonstrate the location of that gene on the chromosome spread.

The FISH technique has wide applications. It has been very valuable in looking for small chromosome deletions such as in Williams syndrome and DiGeorge syndrome (Fig. 14.6) and has greatly extended the ability to make such diagnoses. It has also been used with chromosome specific probes on the uncultured cells to get rapid chromosome diagnosis, e.g. in prenatal diagnosis or for a rapid diagnosis of chromosome abnormalities in the neonatal unit. Another role has been to develop

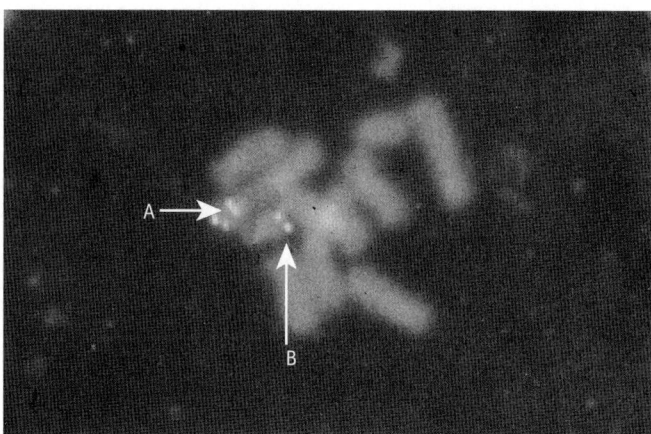

Fig. 14.6   Fluorescent in situ hybridization using probes for chromosome 22q. On chromosome A both the control and the 22q probe show fluorescence, but on chromosome B only the control probe shows up indicating a deletion of 22q seen in DiGeorge syndrome. (Courtesy of Dr J. Taylor.)

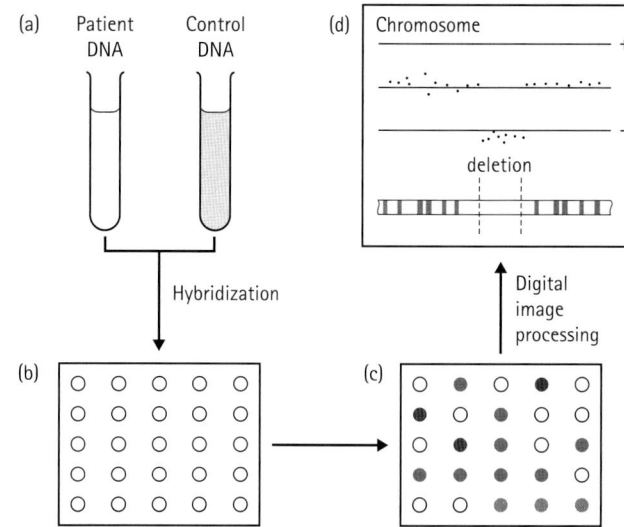

Fig. 14.7   Comparative genomic hybridization (CGH) microarray is a recent technique that will greatly increase our resolution in chromosome analysis. (a) Single stranded fluorescent labeled DNA from the patient (green) is mixed with single stranded control DNA (red) and mixed on a slide (b) with up to 3000 DNA clones covering all the chromosomes at 1 Mb intervals. Where hybridization takes place a yellow color will appear, but where there is a deletion of the patient's DNA only the red color of the control appears (c). The slide is then scanned by an automated microscope and the image processed to show the spread of hybridization reactions across each chromosome and presented against the chromosome karyotype. A small interstitial deletion is seen in (d).

'chromosome paints' with fluorescent gene probes specific to individual chromosomes. Initially this technique was limited by the relatively small number of fluorescent dyes but by using the spectral division of color and computer enhancement it is now possible to assign a separate color to each chromosome and make the analysis of complex chromosomal translocations easier.

One area of the chromosome that is relatively difficult to visualize is the end or telomere, and as a consequence chromosome deletions at the subtelomeric region may be missed on conventional analysis. Knight & Flint[6] developed a range of subtelomeric gene probes that have in clinical practice allowed the identification of chromosome abnormalities in another 7% of children with mental retardation and apparently normal chromosomes on routine analysis.

FISH techniques also have an important role in gene mapping and the identification of chromosome imbalance in malignancy.

COMPARATIVE GENOMIC HYBRIDIZATION MICROARRAY

A new technique that has great promise for future diagnostic work is the comparative genomic hybridization (CGH) microarray. The technique depends on the relative hybridization between the green fluorescent labeled patient's DNA and the red fluorescent labeled reference DNA (Fig. 14.7). Where hybridization takes place a standard yellow fluorescent color will appear; if there is a deletion in the patient's DNA then only the red color will appear; if there is a duplication in the patient's DNA then a green color will appear. This process can be repeated for up to 3000 known markers spread at 1 Mb intervals across the chromosomes. As the microarray is very small it has to be read by a scanning microscope and the image translated into an overview of the chromosome karyotype. Preliminary studies have suggested that it may pick up de novo abnormalities in up to 15% of children with previously undiagnosed mental retardation.[7]

INDICATIONS FOR CHROMOSOME STUDIES

The indications for chromosome studies in pediatric practice include:
1. Intellectual disability, especially when associated with physical abnormalities. It should be borne in mind that there are specific tests now for some forms of mental handicap, e.g. fragile X, Prader–Willi syndrome, Williams syndrome, and these will need to be requested separately with appropriate samples.
2. Multiple congenital abnormalities as many of the malformation syndromes have a chromosomal basis.
3. Intersex conditions manifesting as the presence of ambiguous genitalia in the newborn, inguinal herniae in a girl or the failure of development of secondary sexual characteristics at adolescence. Cryptorchidism or minor degrees of hypospadias alone are unlikely to be manifestations of a chromosome abnormality.
4. Congenital lymphedema may be a manifestation of Turner syndrome and Noonan syndrome, and part of the investigation should include chromosome analysis.
5. Gross failure to thrive which is prenatal in origin may be due to a chromosome abnormality, especially when accompanied by minor physical abnormalities or intellectual disability.
6. Childhood leukemias and malignancies will often reveal major chromosomal rearrangements in the cancerous cells and these may be an indicator of the prognosis.

TYPES OF CHROMOSOME ABNORMALITY

The chromosome abnormalities fall into two categories: (a) abnormalities of number, and (b) abnormalities of structure.

NUMERICAL ABNORMALITIES

Euploidy describes chromosome constitutions which are multiples of the haploid (n) number (23 in man), thus diploid, 2n = 46, triploid, 3n = 69, or tetraploid, 4n = 92. Multiples greater than 2n are designated by the general term *polyploidy*. In clinical practice these are exceptionally rare but *triploidy* is occasionally seen with severe abnormalities at birth. It usually arises from the fertilization of a single ovum by two spermatozoa (*dispermy*).

Aneuploidy refers to those karyotypes in which the chromosome complement is not an exact multiple of the haploid number and includes both the trisomic and monosomic states.

Nondisjunction is the term used to describe the failure of homologous chromosomes or sister chromatids to separate and migrate to opposite poles of the nucleus during cell division and is the major mechanism by which monosomic and trisomic states originate. The consequences of nondisjunction vary depending on whether the event occurs during meiosis or mitosis. Nondisjunction occurring in meiosis will give rise to trisomy or monosomy, but nondisjunction taking place in mitosis in the early embryo will give rise to mosaicism with a mix of abnormal and normal cell lines.

There seems no doubt that in some families there is a predisposition towards nondisjunctional events. The number of families in which aneuploidy recurs and the occurrence of individuals who possess two different aneuploidy states, e.g. both Down and Klinefelter syndromes, are suggestive evidence of this predisposition. The mechanism for this is not understood.

STRUCTURAL ABNORMALITIES IN CHROMOSOMES

Structural chromosome abnormalities include those involving a definite loss or gain of genetic material, and those in which the existing genetic material is rearranged in some way. Structural rearrangements arise from one or more breaks in the chromosomes. Figure 14.8 presents in diagrammatic form the mechanisms of origin of the common structural abnormalities.

Deletions

Deletions (Fig. 14.8a) result when one or more breakages occur along the chromosome with subsequent loss of the resulting fragment, and may be either terminal or interstitial.

Ring chromosomes

Ring chromosomes (Fig. 14.8b) result from simultaneous breakage in both long and short arms of a chromosome with subsequent fusion of the ends of the remaining centric fragment and loss of the acentric terminal segments. Ring chromosomes are notoriously unstable during cell division and break down readily so that the proportion of cells with a clear ring may vary considerably in cultures from the same individual, as also may the actual form and number of the rings observed.

Inversions

Inversions (Fig. 14.8c), as their name suggests, result from a reversal of the sequence of genes in a segment of chromosome lying between two points of breakage. Inversions may be either *paracentric* involving double breakage in only one arm of a chromosome without any alteration in arm ratio, or *pericentric* involving breakage on either side of the centromere.

The clinical significance of inversions is a subject for debate. The vast majority of paracentric inversions are likely to be harmless; however, the risk of having an unbalanced rearrangement in offspring would be increased if there were a family history of recurrent miscarriage or congenital malformations. Small pericentric inversions, including the relatively common pericentric inversions of chromosomes 2 and 9, also seem to be associated with a relatively small risk of unbalanced chromosome arrangements in offspring, and in some cases might be regarded as normal variants. However, the effects of inversions can be unpredictable and the risks in the individual case should be assessed in the light of the family history and cumulative experience from the medical literature.

Isochromosomes

An isochromosome is a chromosome in which the two arms are genetically and structurally identical, e.g. two short arms from the same chromosome. Such chromosomes are thought to arise as a direct result of misdivision of the centromere in the transverse rather than the longitudinal plane, with subsequent reunion of the centric elements of sister chromatids (Fig. 14.8d). In clinical practice this may be seen when an isochromosome X causes Turner syndrome.

Translocations

A translocation is a transfer of genetic material from one chromosome to another. When there is a mutual exchange of segments with no associated loss of genetic material this is termed a *balanced reciprocal translocation*. Such translocations may involve either homologous or nonhomologous chromosomes and can be the result of no more than two breaks, one in each of the chromosomes involved (Fig. 14.8e).

Provided that the translocation does not result in the loss or gain of genetic material there will be no harm to the carrier, although the potential effect for the offspring of carriers may be considerable. Many carriers are first identified following the detection of one or other product of a reciprocal rearrangement in an abnormal infant, in a stillbirth, or in an early abortus. Family studies frequently uncover a history of previously unexplained miscarriages in phenotypically normal individuals, who are found subsequently to be carriers of the rearrangement. Such translocations can often be traced through many generations of a large pedigree. Translocations involving chromosome 9 and those between chromosomes 11 and 22 appear to carry a particularly high risk of an unbalanced defect.

One of the most commonly occurring structural rearrangements in man is the centric fusion or Robertsonian translocation, involving, by definition, only acrocentric chromosomes. The breakpoints occur close to the centromere, either one in the short arm and one in the long arm, in which case the metacentric chromosome formed has a single centromere, or in both short arms with a resultant dicentric chromosome (Fig. 14.8f). The deleted short arm material is generally lost without any apparent effect on phenotype, presumably because it is heterochromatin without structural genes.

A Robertsonian translocation between chromosomes 13 and 14 is thought to be one of the most common structural rearrangements in man, with a frequency of 0.05–0.08% in the newborn population. This rearrangement usually functions more or less normally during meiosis but there is a small risk of trisomy 13 in the offspring of carriers.

Robertsonian translocations involving chromosome 21 such as 14,21 translocations are of considerable clinical significance since they may give rise to Down syndrome and have a high chance of recurrence. There are differences in the risk of recurrence of Down syndrome depending on the sex of the carrier parent. Recurrence is higher if the carrier is female (10–15%) and lower if the carrier is male (< 5%).

MOSAICISM

Mosaicism occurs where there are two or more genetically different cell lines in an individual derived from a single zygote, *chimerism* where an individual has arisen from the fusion of two zygotes or exchange of cells between two zygotes. Chimerism is extremely rare and not usually of clinical significance whereas mosaicism is relatively frequent and may be a cause of diagnostic difficulty.

Significant levels of chromosome mosaicism may be demonstrated by examining a reasonable number of cells. The examination of 30 metaphases will be sufficient to demonstrate mosaicism at the 10–15% level, but many more metaphases would be needed to exclude lower levels of mosaicism. It may be difficult to completely exclude mosaicism as a diagnosis, and failure to demonstrate mosaicism in blood need not necessarily exclude the diagnosis as a possibility in other less available tissues. One of the clinical indicators of chromosome mosaicism is the appearance of linear areas of pigmentary abnormality in the skin. In such cases a skin biopsy including both normal and abnormal skin may be used to look for mosaicism.

NOMENCLATURE[8]

Chromosomes can be arranged in pairs on the basis of certain morphological features. Such morphological features include size, centromere position, and the presence of satellites or secondary constrictions.

The *centromere* is the point of union of the two chromatids. The position of the centromere in relation to the *telomeres* (or chromosome ends) determines the actual shape of the chromosome and divides it into two *arms* which vary in length, being either short (p), or long (q). Where

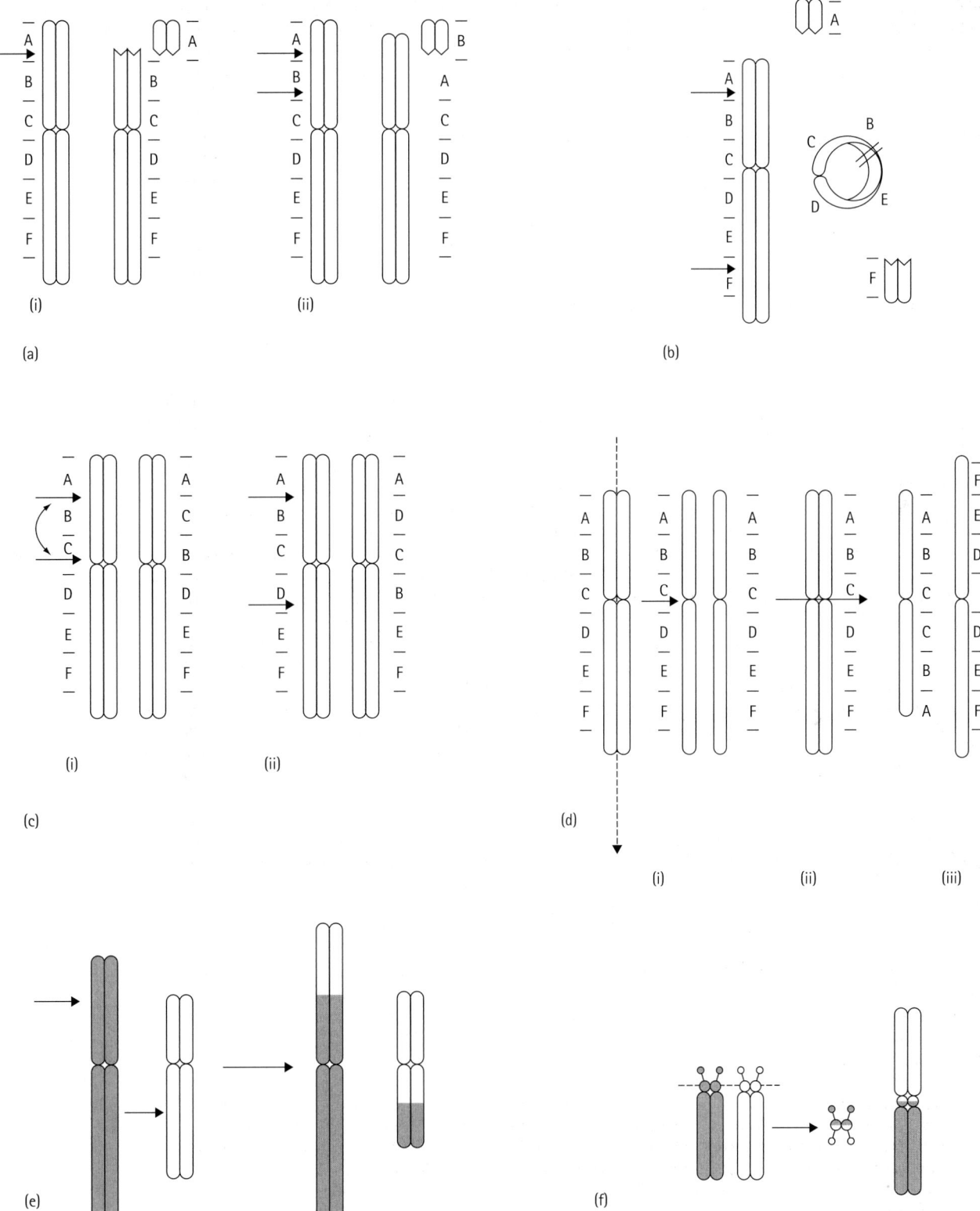

Fig. 14.8 Structural rearrangements in chromosomes. (a) Deletions may be (i) terminal or (ii) interstitial. (b) Ring chromosome. (c) Inversions may be (i) paracentric or (ii) pericentric. (d) Isochromosome formation: (i) normal mitosis with longitudinal division of the centromere; (ii) misdivision of the centromere in the transverse plane leading to the products (iii) of either isochromosome of the short arm. (e) Balanced reciprocal translocation. (f) Robertsonian or centric fusion translocation.

the centromere is median in position and the arms are of approximately equal length, the chromosome is described as *metacentric*. Where the arms are of unequal length, the chromosome is described as *submetacentric*. Where the centromere is more nearly terminal so that the short arms are minute, the chromosome is described as *acrocentric*. Small condensations of heterochromatin or satellites may occur on the short arms of acrocentric chromosomes.

The International Conferences on Standardization in Human Cytogenetics provide a standardized system of chromosome nomenclature and symbols (Table 14.3).[8] The conventions which apply in use of

Table 14.3   Table of nomenclature symbols[9,10]

1–22	The autosome numbers
X, Y	The sex chromosomes
Diagonal (/)	Separates cell lines in describing mosaicism
Plus sign (+) or minus sign (–)	When placed immediately before the autosome number or group letter designation indicates that the particular chromosome is extra or missing; when placed immediately after a symbol it means an increase or decrease in length of the chromosome
cen	Centromere
dic	Dicentric (presence of two centromeres)
h	Secondary constriction or negatively staining region
i	Isochromosome
inv	Inversion
mar	Marker chromosome
mat	Maternal origin
p	Short arm of chromosome
pat	Paternal origin
q	Long arm of chromosome
r	Ring chromosome
s	Satellite
t	Translocation
del	Deletion
der	Derivative chromosome
dup	Duplication
ins	Insertion
inv ins	Inverted insertion
rep	Reciprocal translocation
rec	Recombinant chromosome
rob	Robertsonian translocation ('centric fusion')
ter	Terminal or end (pter = end of short arm; qter = end of long arm)
:	Break (no reunion, as in a terminal deletion)
: :	Break and join
–	From – to

All symbols for rearrangements are placed before the designation of the chromosome or chromosomes involved and the rearranged chromosome or chromosomes should always be placed in parentheses.

this nomenclature are as follows. The number of chromosomes is given first followed by the sex chromosome constitution, e.g. 45X in Turner syndrome and 47XXY in Klinefelter syndrome. Autosomal aneuploidies are indicated by a numerical alteration, the extra or deficient chromosome being designated by a + or − before the chromosome involved, e.g. 47XX,+21, a female with Down syndrome, or 45XX,−21, a female missing a 21 chromosome. When placed after a symbol a + or − means an increase or decrease in the length of a chromosome, e.g. 18p− represents deletion of the short arm of chromosome 18. Diagonals are used in the description of mosaicism, e.g. 45XO/46XX represents a Turner mosaic and 46XX/47XX,+21 a female with mosaic Down syndrome. Translocation is designated by the letter t followed in parentheses by an indication of the nature of the translocated chromosome. An isochromosome is indicated by the letter i before the chromosome arm involved, e.g. 45X,i(Xq) represents an isochromosome for the long arm of one X chromosome. Ring chromosomes are designated by the letter r placed before the chromosome involved, e.g. 46X,r(X). Bands on chromosomes are numbered outwards from the centromere and are represented by a number written after p or q representing the short or long arms, e.g. 8q24 represents a region on the long arm of chromosome 8 and t(8;14)(q24;q32) a translocation between chromosome 8 and 14 involving region 24 on the long arm of chromosome 8 and region 32 on the long arm of chromosome 14.

CHROMOSOMAL SYNDROMES

DOWN SYNDROME

Incidence

Since the original description of the condition by Langdon Down in 1866, this disorder has been recognized to be the commonest single cause of mental handicap, occurring in approximately 1 in 700 of all live births in all populations. However, the incidence varies with the age of the mother: the incidence for mothers aged 25 years is 1 in 1400 and increases to reach an incidence of 1 in 46 for mothers aged 45 years (see Fig. 14.9).

Clinical features

In most instances Down syndrome is recognizable at birth by the craniofacial features (Fig. 14.10). The head circumference is small with a brachycephalic skull. The neck is short and thick. The palpebral fissures slope upwards (i.e. the outer canthus is higher than the inner canthus) and there may be marked epicanthic folds. Brushfield's spots (whitish spots scattered round the periphery of the iris) are found more frequently in Down syndrome than in the general population. There is an increased incidence of lens opacities. The ears are small with an overfolding helix. The nasal bridge is flat. The tongue appears large and may protrude because the mouth is relatively small. Eruption of the teeth is frequently delayed with abnormalities in dental positioning. The hair may be fine and sparse.

The hands are short and broad. The fifth finger is short and incurved (clinodactyly). Radiologically this feature is accompanied by shortening of the shaft of the middle phalanx. A single transverse palmar crease (or simian crease) is seen in both hands in at least 50% of children with Down syndrome. A unilateral transverse palmar crease may be demonstrated in 2–5% of chromosomally normal infants. A deep plantar crease ('sandal gap') between the first and second toe may also be a helpful diagnostic sign.

Congenital heart disease occurs in between 40 and 60% of infants with Down syndrome. Atrioventricular canal and ventricular septal defects are the commonest types of cardiac lesion seen. Intestinal atresia, in particular duodenal atresia, is also considerably more common in Down syndrome. One third of cases of congenital duodenal atresia occur in Down syndrome.

Initially a child with Down syndrome may be hypotonic, but the early developmental milestones are eventually reached. The ultimate

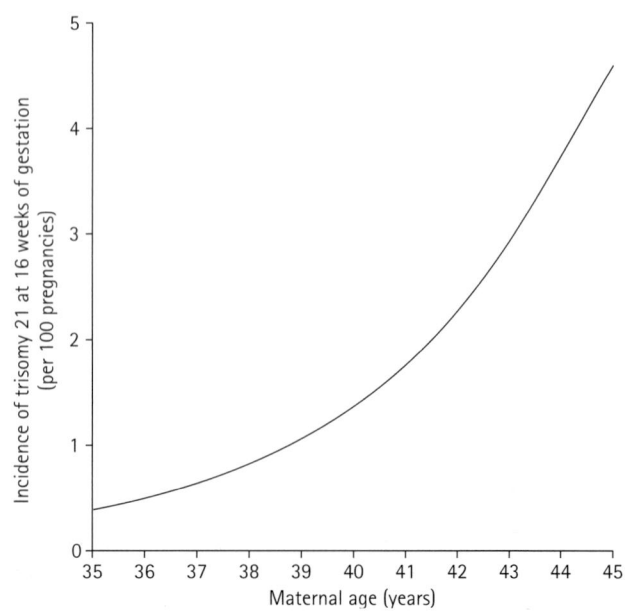

Fig. 14.9   The frequency of Down syndrome increases with maternal age.

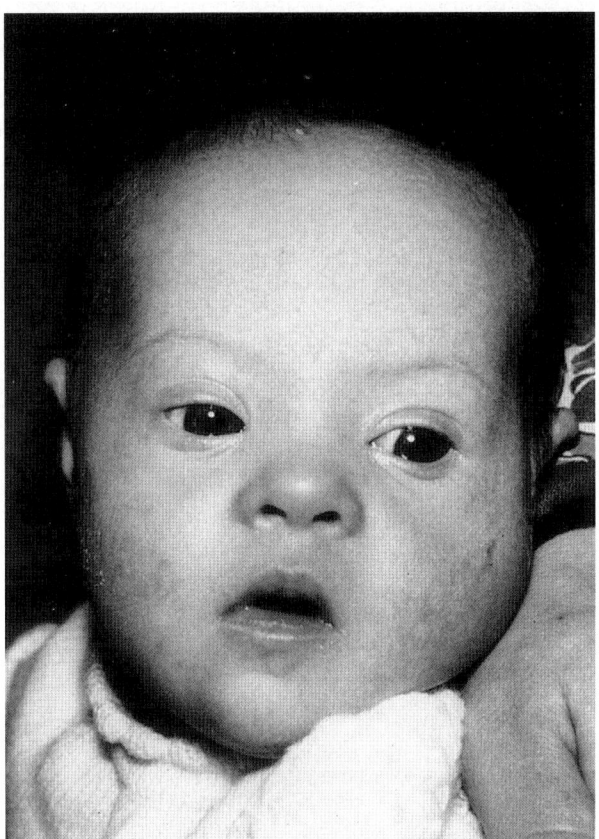

Fig. 14.10 Facial features of Down syndrome.

Cytogenetics
Full trisomy 21
Approximately 95% of children with Down syndrome have a full trisomy 21. Trisomy 21 arises as a result of meiotic nondisjunction, usually from the maternal side.

Translocation as a cause of Down syndrome
Translocations account for 2–3% of Down individuals. The most frequent cause is from a Robertsonian 14,21 translocation (Fig. 14.11). In this form the carrier would have one 14 chromosome, one 21 chromosome and one fused 14,21 chromosome giving a total of 45 chromosomes and would be phenotypically normal. However, when a carrier produces offspring there is a risk of producing an unbalanced karyotype.

In Figure 14.11, when an individual with a 14,21 translocation produces offspring with an individual with a normal karyotype then three viable chromosome arrangements may be produced: (i) a normal karyotype, (ii) a balanced translocation and (iii) an unbalanced translocation giving 46 chromosomes with trisomy 21. Other arrangements can be produced, but these will be nonviable or lead to early miscarriage, e.g. monosomy 21, monosomy 14 or trisomy 14. While in theory it may appear that one third of pregnancies would produce an unbalanced translocation with trisomy 21, this does not take into account the selective disadvantage that acts on gametogenesis, fertilization or the early zygote. From analysis of pooled family data the likelihood of a female carrier producing an unbalanced trisomic child is 15%, and the likelihood of a male carrier producing an unbalanced trisomic child is 2.5%. The different risks may be explained by selective disadvantage in the sperm carrying the extra 21 chromosome.

A 21,22 Robertsonian translocation may also give rise to Down syndrome in a similar way. Very rarely a 21,21 translocation may arise. Carriers of this 21,21 translocation can only produce zygotes that are either monosomic or trisomic for chromosome 21, and since monosomy 21 would almost always be lethal their risk of producing a child with trisomy 21 is 100%.

IQ ranges from 20 to 75 with a mean around 50. The earlier assessment of development tends to be more favorable than the formal measurement of IQ in later childhood. Children with Down syndrome are often affectionate and good humored but like all stereotypes this tends to underestimate the range of personality and behavioral traits seen in a defined group.

Intellectual function shows a decline with age in adults with Down syndrome due to an increased incidence of early onset dementia of the Alzheimer type. Decline may start in the third decade of life but becomes frequent by the fifth decade.[11] The neuropathology in Down syndrome is similar to Alzheimer disease with the presence of amyloid plaques and neurofibrillary tangles. Gene mapping studies have found mutations in the amyloid precursor protein gene on chromosome 21 in some early onset familial cases of Alzheimer disease suggesting a causative link with Down syndrome.

The development of secondary sexual characteristics is delayed in Down syndrome. Adult males with Down syndrome are infertile and in females there may be delayed puberty but they will usually be fertile. The incidence of leukemia, but not other malignancies, is greater in Down children. A transient leukemoid reaction may occur in newborns with Down syndrome. In the first year of life acute nonlymphoblastic leukemia predominates, but in older children it is predominantly acute lymphoblastic leukemia. Overall the incidence is 10–18 times greater than that in the general childhood population.

A generation ago, two thirds of children with Down syndrome died in early childhood, usually from the associated congenital abnormalities. Now only about 20% die in the first year and 45% of individuals with Down syndrome will survive to 60 years of age.[12,13] This improved survival will represent a greater burden of care for those families facing the diagnosis today.

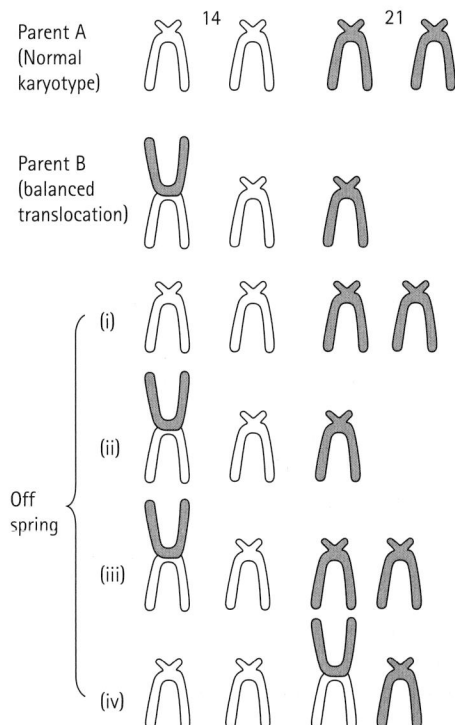

Fig. 14.11 Segregation of a 14,21 translocation. Four combinations may be produced: (i) normal karyotype; (ii) balanced translocation; (iii) unbalanced trisomy 21; (iv) unbalanced trisomy 14 (lethal).

Mosaic trisomy 21

In about 2.5% of individuals with Down syndrome there is a mosaic combination of cells with a normal karyotype and cells with trisomy 21. The phenotypic variation produced may range from apparently normal individuals to those with typical Down syndrome.

Genetic counseling and screening

It is essential to determine the chromosome karyotype in the affected child prior to genetic counseling, since the recurrence risks are different for standard trisomy 21 and translocation trisomy 21.

In the case of a child with a standard trisomy 21 the chance of recurrence in further children is 1% in mothers under 35 years and twice the maternal age risk in mothers over 35 years.

When Down syndrome has arisen as a result of an unbalanced translocation, it is necessary to check both parents' chromosomes and if one is found to be a carrier, then further family studies are necessary to determine if other members of the family are also carriers. The recurrence risks for carriers of a 14,21 translocation carrier are given above. In some instances neither parent is found to be a translocation carrier and the unbalanced translocation has arisen de novo. In such situations the chance of recurrence in further pregnancies is equivalent to the population risk.

Since Down syndrome is a major cause of mental handicap, pregnancy screening and chromosome analysis have been incorporated into various public health programs. Since the incidence of Down syndrome increases with increasing maternal age, amniocentesis was initially offered to mothers aged 35 and above. This approach, if fully taken up by all mothers, would diagnose 30% of all pregnancies with Down syndrome, and the remaining 70% would occur in younger mothers. The next refinement was to use maternal blood markers that indicated a higher risk of Down syndrome and offer amniocentesis to those at higher risk. The blood markers used were alpha-fetoprotein, estriol and human chorionic gonadotrophin. Now most centers use earlier ultrasound scanning as the preliminary screen. If there is an increased amount of thickening over the back of the neck or *nuchal translucency* then there is a greater risk of chromosome abnormalities and chorionic villus sampling may be carried out. This approach will diagnose up to 80% of Down syndrome in the early stages of pregnancy.

TRISOMY 18 (EDWARDS SYNDROME)

This was first described by Edwards.[14] Although much rarer than Down syndrome, it is the second commonest autosomal trisomy with an incidence between 1 in 3500 and 1 in 7000. It is also associated with increased maternal age. Of the affected infants some 80–90% die within the first week, usually from cardiopulmonary failure. A few cases have been reported surviving into the teens, but they have all been profoundly retarded.

There is often polyhydramnios and intrauterine growth retardation. The cranium is long and narrow with a prominent occiput. The ears are low set and frequently underdeveloped. The facies characteristically shows micrognathia and narrow sloping palpebral fissures. The hands are clenched with the second and fifth fingers overlapping the third and fourth fingers (Fig. 14.12a). There may be other flexion deformities. The nails are hypoplastic. The feet show a 'rocker bottom' appearance like the shape of the runners of a rocking chair (Fig. 14.12b).

A variety of congenital malformations are present. Anomalies of the gastrointestinal tract are particularly common, e.g. intestinal atresias, malabsorption and exomphalos. Around one third of cases of exomphalos detected prenatally on ultrasound have trisomy 18. Renal abnormalities are also frequent with renal hypoplasia or cystic dysplasia being one of the commoner and more serious abnormalities. Congenital heart defects, ocular abnormalities and neural tube defects can also occur.

In the past a number of conditions which clinically appeared similar to trisomy 18 but showed normal karyotypes were described as pseudotrisomy 18. Some of these cases were probably Pena–Shokeir

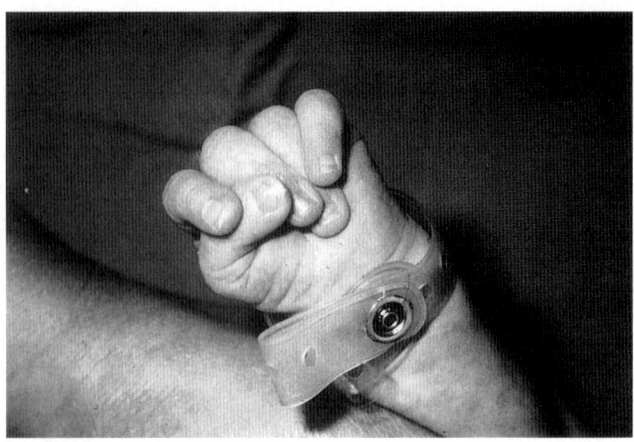

(a)

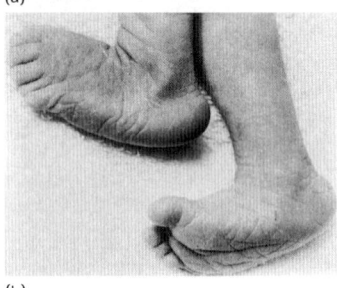

(b)

Fig. 14.12   The typical appearance of the (a) hands and (b) feet in trisomy 18 (Edwards syndrome).

syndrome[15] which is autosomal recessive. It presents with a combination of microcephaly, joint contractures, pulmonary hypoplasia and cataracts, and should be considered in the differential diagnosis when the karyotype is normal.

The vast majority of cases arise as a result of primary nondisjunction and have a regular trisomy 18. Like trisomy 21, it is associated with increased maternal age and thus may be diagnosed on screening prenatally. After the diagnosis of one affected pregnancy the chance of recurrence is 0.5% in younger mothers.

TRISOMY 13 (PATAU SYNDROME)

This syndrome has an incidence of around 1 in 6000. The majority of affected children have multiple malformations and die shortly after birth. The few cases reported with longer survival have all been severely retarded. There is some maternal age effect, but probably not as significant as that seen in trisomy 21 or trisomy 18.

The affected children show intrauterine growth retardation. There may be marked microcephaly. Structural malformations of the brain are common and this may alter facial development. Instead of two cerebral hemispheres with lateral ventricles, a single forebrain with a single ventricle may form. This malformation sequence is known as holoprosencephaly (Fig. 14.13). The process alters the development and separation of optic vesicles from the forebrain and the migration of the median process from the forehead to form the nose. In its most extreme form the optic vesicles may fuse to give cyclopia. More usually (Fig. 14.14) there is marked hypotelorism with a small nose and cleft lip and palate. Ocular abnormalities such as microphthalmos are common, often reflecting the underlying cerebral abnormality.

In the hands, postaxial polydactyly is frequent. Flexion contractures and 'rocker bottom' feet may also be present. Scalp defects may be helpful diagnostically as they rarely appear in other abnormalities. Internally, in addition to cerebral malformations, renal and cardiac abnormalities are also frequent.

The majority of cases of trisomy 13 arise as a result of primary nondisjunction and there is a low chance of recurrence (0.5%).

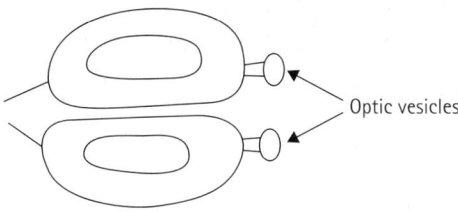

Normal development

Optic vesicles

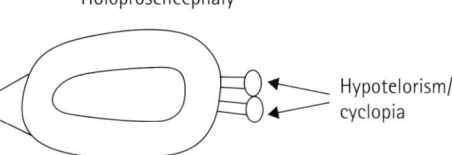

Holoprosencephaly

Hypotelorism/
cyclopia

Fig. 14.13 Holoprosencephaly sequence. The forebrain divides into two hemispheres and the optic vesicles develop from these to form the eyes. In holoprosencephaly the forebrain divides incompletely and the optic vesicles develop in close proximity, leading to hypotelorism or cyclopia.

It may occasionally arise from an unbalanced chromosome translocation t(13q,14q). In the vast majority of cases carriers of a t(13q,14q) do not produce unbalanced progeny, but in practice it is appropriate to counsel such carriers with a small recurrence risk and offer amniocentesis.

1p36 DELETION

This small telomeric deletion is being increasingly recognized with newer laboratory techniques and gives rise to a severe neurological phenotype with severe intellectual disability and seizures. There are deep set eyes and straight eyebrows and there may also be congenital heart disease.[16]

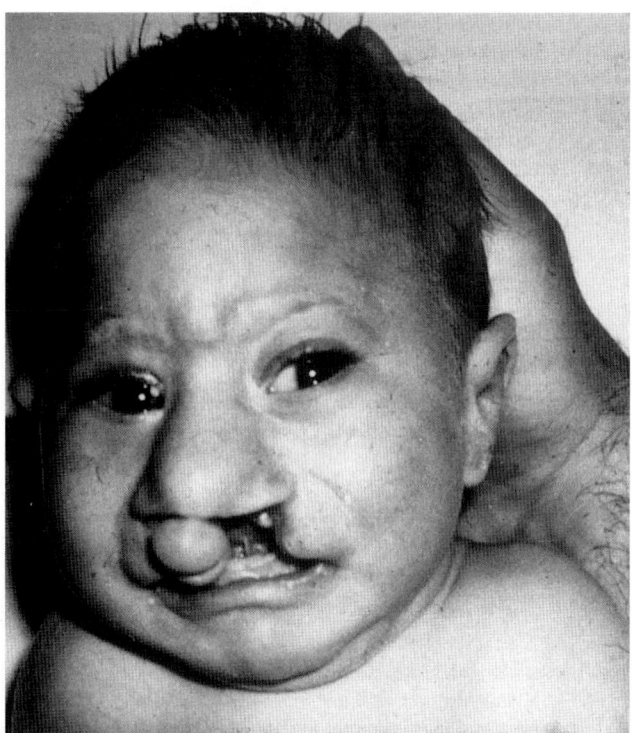

Fig. 14.14 Facial features of trisomy 13 (Patau syndrome).

4p⁻ (WOLF–HIRSCHHORN) SYNDROME

This syndrome gives a clearly recognizable phenotype. The features include microcephaly, hypertelorism, low set simple ears, coloboma (25%), cleft palate (30%), renal abnormalities, heart defects (50%) and intrauterine growth retardation. The facial features (Fig. 14.15) are described as resembling a Greek helmet since the flat nasal bridge appears to run in continuity from the glabella in much the same way that the protective nosepiece is incorporated into a Greek helmet.

The natural history is known.[17] Death usually occurs in early childhood (at least one third die in the first year of life) and survivors invariably show profound mental retardation with seizures. As 10% arise from balanced translocations it is important to examine the parents' chromosomes. The deletion required to produce this syndrome may be very small and may require specific cytogenetic tests to identify it.

5p⁻ (CRI DU CHAT) SYNDROME

This was one of the first autosomal deletions to be recognized. The syndrome derives its name from the striking cat-like cry that is heard in infancy. This cry is related to the hypoplastic larynx and tends to lessen with increasing age and growth of the larynx. In the newborn the face is round with microcephaly, micrognathia and down-slanting palpebral fissures. With further growth the microcephaly remains but the face becomes long and narrow. Survival into adult life with severe mental retardation has frequently been described.

The deletion may involve a variable amount of the short arm of chromosome 5 but band 5p15 is invariably involved.[18] About 15% of cases arise from a balanced reciprocal translocation.

DELETIONS OF 13q

Deletions of 13q14 (Fig. 14.16) are associated with retinoblastoma. The dysmorphic features associated with this deletion are variable. Further genetic analysis of the interstitial 13q14 deletions has led to recognition that this chromosomal region contains an anti-oncogene responsible for inhibiting the proliferation of embryonic retinal cells. In the presence of a homozygous deletion or a deletion in one allele with a mutation in the other allele, retinal cells continue to proliferate in a malignant fashion producing a retinoblastoma. Inherited forms of retinoblastoma are usually bilateral whereas isolated cases of retinoblastoma are usually unilateral and are the result of a somatic mutation in the retinoblastoma gene that has arisen in one eye.

Terminal deletions of 13 may also produce eye abnormalities but not retinoblastoma. These children also characteristically have hypoplastic thumbs and anal atresia. Most die in the neonatal period.

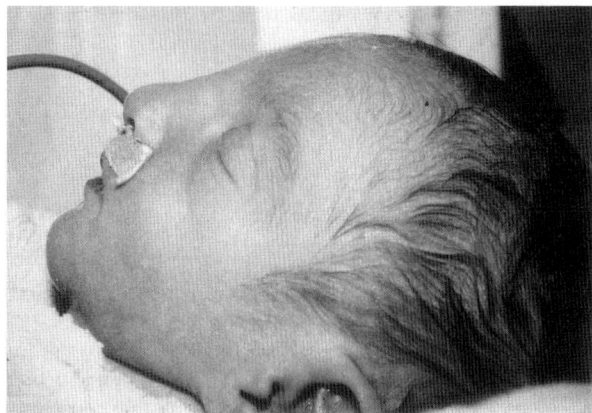

Fig. 14.15 Facial features of 4p⁻ (Wolf–Hirschhorn) syndrome.

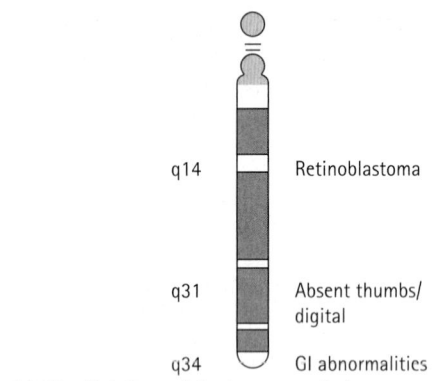

Fig. 14.16 Deletions of the long arm of chromosome 13.

q14   Retinoblastoma

q31   Absent thumbs/digital

q34   GI abnormalities

DIGEORGE SYNDROME (22q11 DELETION)

Prior to the discovery of the underlying chromosome defect this disorder was described with different emphasis and with different names, e.g. velocardiofacial syndrome, Sprintzen syndrome or CATCH 22. With the advent of fluorescent gene probes this has become one of the commonest chromosomal microdeletion syndromes.

About 75% of patients with 22q11 deletion will have significant congenital heart defects.[19] The range of defects is wide but tetralogy of Fallot and abnormalities in the main arteries are most frequently seen. About 50% of patients will have defects of the palate. This is often velopharyngeal insufficiency rather than overt cleft palate. Hypocalcemia may also occur and is a cause for fits. Developmental delay tends to be mild and a significant number of affected children have normal development. In the original description of this syndrome there was severe immunodeficiency with T cell depletion and although this is infrequent, care should be given with live immunization.[20]

The main indication for requesting a 22q deletion test is the presence of congenital heart defect or facial clefting but it is appropriate to consider it with any feature of the syndrome. The facial features include a long bulbous nose and a small mouth but are relatively subtle. When a deletion is identified it is important to carry out testing in the parents as around 30% of cases are inherited.

By dissecting out the critical region of the deletion it has been possible to identify a T box developmental gene as the primary cause of heart defects in the syndrome.[21]

WILLIAMS SYNDROME

Williams syndrome was initially referred to as infantile hypercalcemia as the biochemical change was the usual presentation. It is now recognized to be a more generalized syndrome with 'elfin facies', short stature, supravalvar aortic stenosis, hyperacusis and developmental delay. After autosomal dominant supravalvar aortic stenosis was recognized to be due to a defect in elastin, it was found that there is a deletion of elastin and contiguous genes in Williams syndrome. It is now easily diagnosed by a FISH probe for elastin on chromosome 7, but obviously the features such as learning difficulties and the characteristic behavior are due to the adjacent genes in the deletion rather than elastin alone.[22]

ANIRIDIA–WILMS

The association of bilateral aniridia and Wilms tumor is due to a deletion of chromosome 11p13. It is a good example of a contiguous gene deletion in which a gene involved in eye development (Pax 6) is deleted together with an oncogene WT1. There is often developmental delay and growth retardation as well due to deletion of other genes in the area. This concept of a contiguous gene deletion syndrome will probably be found to be a cause of many other apparently unrelated features in malformation syndromes.

ANGELMAN SYNDROME AND PRADER–WILLI SYNDROME

Although these are very different clinical disorders it is important to consider these two syndromes together as they can both be due to deletions of chromosome 15 and illustrate an important biological principle known as genetic imprinting.

Prader–Willi syndrome usually presents with neonatal hypotonia with feeding difficulties and in males undescended testes.[23] As the affected child becomes older the muscle tone and feeding difficulties improve but the child develops a voracious appetite (hyperphagia) and becomes obese. Affected children will also have developmental delay and in later life may suffer from the complications of obesity. Angelman syndrome presents with severe developmental delay, inappropriate laughter and complex seizures. There may be a characteristic electroencephalogram (EEG) in early life[24] and later absence of speech and ataxia.

The commonest cause of these syndromes is deletion of 15q11–13 but it was found that Prader–Willi syndrome was due to paternal deletions and Angelman syndrome was due to maternal deletions. This phenomenon would not be predicted by Mendelian inheritance, where the parental origin of a mutation does not usually matter, and is an example of *genetic imprinting*. It appears that both paternal and maternal chromosome 15s are required in early embryonic development and that paternal and maternal chromosome 15q12 have different functions. Thus genetic imprinting may be defined as the determination of gene expression depending on the parental origin.

The situation became more complex with analysis of other cases. In some cases there was no deletion but two copies of chromosome 15 from the same parent, which is referred to as uniparental disomy.[25] In the case of Prader–Willi syndrome this would have started with trisomy 15 in which there were two copies of the maternal 15 and one of paternal 15; then, if the paternal chromosome 15 is lost, the child effectively has two maternal chromosome 15s and no paternal 15. The net effect is the same as a deletion on the paternal chromosome 15. The situation is now more complicated as there can also be mutations affecting the imprinting mechanism and in Angelman syndrome point mutations in the UBE3A gene at 15q12.

A number of other genetic disorders involve genetic imprinting, e.g. transient neonatal diabetes, Russell–Silver syndrome and Beckwith–Wiedemann syndrome.

KILLIAN–PALLISTER SYNDROME

Most chromosomal disorders can be diagnosed on blood analysis. However this is not the case in the Killian–Pallister syndrome. It is unusual in that a mosaic cell line containing tetrasomy 12p is found in the skin fibroblasts but not in the blood. Although the mosaicism is relatively tissue specific the effects are generalized.[26] There is severe mental retardation with coarse facial features and a characteristic bitemporal loss of hair growth (Fig. 14.17).

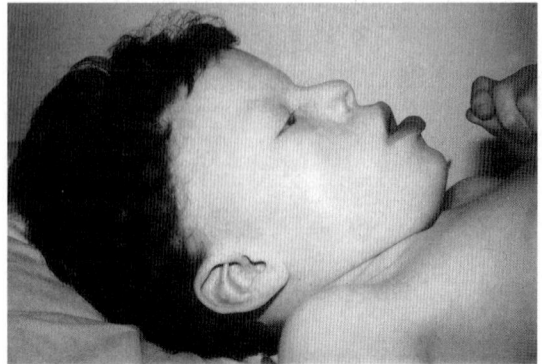

Fig. 14.17 Killian–Pallister syndrome is caused by a mosaic isochromosome 12p, which is present in skin culture but not in blood culture. The syndrome has a characteristic coarse facies.

OTHER AUTOSOMAL ABNORMALITIES

Many other aberrations involving the autosomes have been described. As a general rule they are associated with low birth weight, mental retardation and physical malformations. In many instances a specific phenotype cannot be delineated because gene dosage will depend on the exact breakpoints and, in the case of unbalanced translocations, which other chromosome is involved. It is recommended that the reader refers to a chromosomal atlas such as de Grouchy & Turleau,[27] Gardner & Sutherland[28] or Schnizel[29] for details of other autosomal abnormalities.

SEX CHROMOSOME ABNORMALITIES

TURNER SYNDROME

The syndrome was first described in 1938 and subsequently became the first disorder recognized to have a chromosomal basis. It is a frequent finding in first trimester abortions, but, as many 45X conceptuses are non-viable, the frequency at birth is 1 in 3000 live-born females.

Clinical features

At birth there is lymphedema (Fig. 14.18) especially in the dorsum of the hand and there may be redundant skin over the back of the neck. Hydrops and cystic hygroma are seen in utero and may occasionally be present in the neonate.

In childhood, Turner syndrome may present with short stature. There is a short webbed neck with low posterior hairline. The chest is shield shaped with widely spaced nipples. The carrying angle at the elbow is increased (cubitus valgus). Pigmented nevi and a tendency to keloid scarring are frequently found. Coarctation of the aorta may also be present. Around 60% will have renal tract abnormalities, which include horseshoe kidneys and duplex ureters, but these do not usually compromise renal function. Mental development is normal although detailed psychometric testing may demonstrate a minor defect in spatial perception.

At puberty Turner syndrome may present for the first time with primary amenorrhea and failure of secondary sexual development. Streak gonads are found with ultrasound and at laparotomy. The patients are usually infertile, but menstruation and secondary sexual development may be induced by estrogen replacement (see Ch. 15).

Girls with Turner syndrome have a normal life span. It is now recognized that hypertension may be a complication in adult life, and in the absence of hormone replacement osteoporosis may also develop.

Cytogenetics

Although 60% of patients with Turner syndrome have a 45X karyotype, a variety of chromosome abnormalities are seen with the syndrome (Table 14.4).

Mosaic cell lines arise from mitotic nondisjunction in early embryogenesis. On the whole the phenotype with mosaicism is similar to the classic features of Turner syndrome. When the mosaicism involves an XY cell line there is an increased risk of gonadoblastoma, and the streak ovaries should be removed. In the rare situation of an unbalanced X: autosome translocation and in some cases of ring X, mental retardation may occur.

Turner syndrome is not associated with increased maternal age and as it usually arises from mitotic rather than meiotic error is not associated with an increase of recurrence in further pregnancies.

47XXX

The majority of girls with triple X (47XXX) will not have been brought to medical attention and have had their chromosomes tested. However prospective studies have identified some potential differences. Their height tends to be greater than average and in statistical terms there is a slight lowering of mean IQ, but no specific abnormal behavioral patterns. Fertility is normal. In theory there should be an increased risk of sex chromosome aneuploidy in the offspring of these girls, but in practice the risk appears to be insignificant.

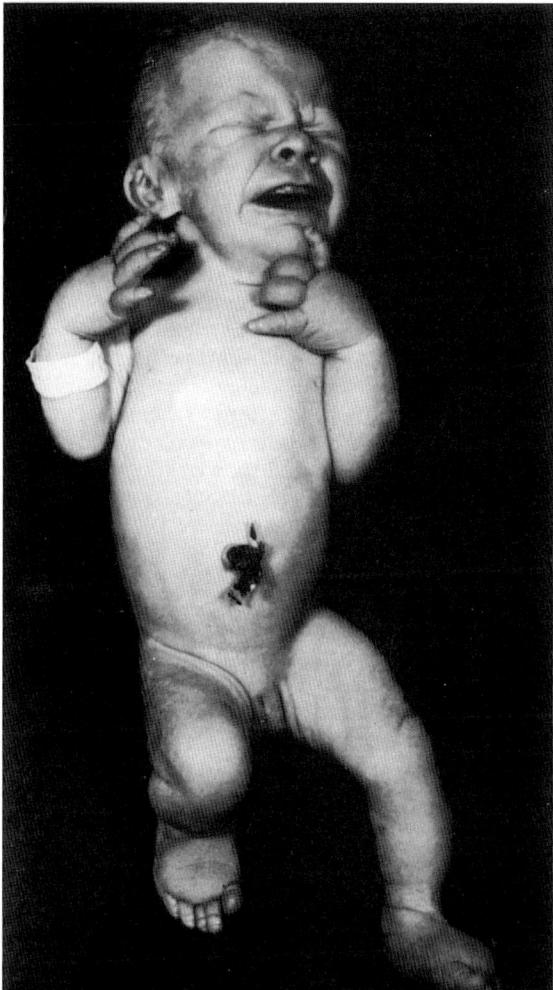

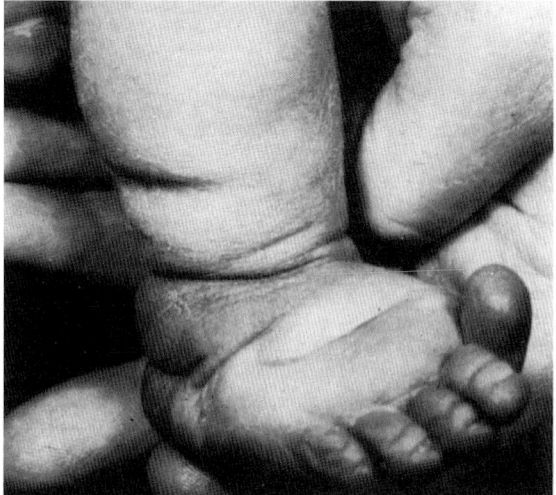

Fig. 14.18 Turner syndrome in the neonate may present with edema of the hands and feet.

Table 14.4 Chromosome abnormalities in Turner syndrome

Chromosome abnormality	Percentage
45XO	60
Mosaic XX/XO	20
Isochromosome Xq or Xp	5
46X del (X)	5
46X ring (X)	5
With Y chromosome	5

KLINEFELTER SYNDROME (47XXY)

Klinefelter syndrome of gynecomastia, small atrophic testes and absent spermatogenesis (azoospermia) in phenotypic males is associated with an abnormal karyotype (47XXY). The incidence is around 1 in 1000 live-born males.

The clinical features are not usually evident in the first few years of life although it may be discovered coincidentally in apparently normal male infants. When the syndrome is diagnosed early there are often considerable parental anxieties and careful counseling will be required. At puberty, however, the secondary sexual characteristics develop poorly and body fat tends to take on a feminine distribution with gynecomastia. Beard growth is minimal and in adult life patients will rarely need to shave more than twice a week. The testes remain small and infertility may be the presenting feature in adult males. Sexual function is normal although the libido is reduced. The testosterone levels are low and the gonadotrophin levels elevated, and testosterone replacement may be helpful. Testicular histology shows an increase in Leydig cells and interstitial fibrosis. Height is usually increased with relatively long limbs. The mean intelligence is on average slightly reduced in Klinefelter syndrome, but this rarely poses a problem.

Cytogenetics

The extra X chromosome usually arises from disjunctional errors during oogenesis. As would be predicted from this, the incidence of Klinefelter syndrome increases with maternal age. In about 15% of patients with Klinefelter's there is a mosaic XY/XXY form but even in mosaic forms infertility would usually occur.

48XXXY AND 49XXXXY

These sex chromosome abnormalities are more severe than Klinefelter syndrome and should not be referred to as Klinefelter syndrome. Mental retardation is frequent and there may be skeletal abnormalities, especially radioulnar synostosis (leading to inability to supinate the forearm). The facies may also be dysmorphic with hypertelorism, epicanthic folds, broad nose and large open mouth.

XX MALES

Very rarely patients have been identified who have an essentially male phenotype with an apparently normal 46XX karyotype. This has led to further basic research into the embryological determination of sex. On molecular analysis these males will almost invariably be found to have the SRY gene. This gene is now known to be the main genetic switch in determining whether a fetus becomes male or female. After the SRY gene has been expressed there may still be other hormonal and genetic factors which will modify the sexual phenotype. Amongst the hormonal factors are congenital adrenal hyperplasia in which an overproduction of androgens will lead to virilization, and testicular feminization in which the absence of testosterone receptors prevents the development of the external genitalia. There are also other modifying genes on the autosomes found through the analysis of malformation syndromes, e.g. the gene responsible for sex reversal in camptomelic dysplasia is the SRY related gene SOX9,[30] and the gene responsible for ovarian dysgenesis in blepharophimosis–ptosis syndrome is the forkhead transcription factor FOXL2.[31] A good review of the role of SRY in sexual differentiation is given by Goodfellow & Lovell-Badge.[32]

XYY SYNDROME

The initial reports of males with 47XYY came from studies of males in institutions for mentally ill criminals and this biased ascertainment initially distorted the understanding of this chromosomal abnormality.

It is relatively common with an incidence of 1 in 1000 males. In order to obtain a truer picture of the syndrome a number of prospective studies have been carried out looking, for example, at the karyotypes of all newborn children in a particular area and following those with sex chromosome abnormalities through childhood.[33] The XYY karyotype is associated with a normal birth weight but increased growth in early to mid-childhood. About a third are in the 90th centile for height. Intelligence is not significantly different from their chromosomally normal siblings. Detailed psychological testing does reveal a tendency to compulsive behavior, which in certain settings may lead to socially deviant behavior, but in the presence of a stable family background this can be more appropriately channeled. It should be remembered that the vast majority of males with 47XYY remain undetected in the community.

FRAGILE X MENTAL RETARDATION

It has long been recognized that there is a considerable excess of males in the mentally handicapped population, and it is now realized that this is due to a considerable number of X-linked forms of mental retardation. Systematic research studies of these families have revealed a large number of new genes but as yet testing for the genes is not available. There are a number of good reviews available.[34,35] At present the most significant of form of X-linked mental retardation is fragile X mental retardation.

In 1969 Lubs demonstrated a fragile site on culture of the X chromosome in a family with mental retardation, but it was initially regarded as an isolated curiosity. Around the same time Dr Gillian Turner studied a number of X-linked mental retardation families in a mental handicap institution and described their relatively 'normal looking' appearance together with large testes. Lubs had described the cytogenetic finding and Turner the phenotypic appearance of fragile X mental retardation. Several years later the connection between the clinical and laboratory findings was firmly established and the condition is now recognized as the second commonest cause of mental handicap in males after Down syndrome. The incidence of fragile X mental retardation is 1 per 1000 males. In a study of autism 5% of the male patients were found to have fragile X mental retardation.

Clinical features

The phenotype of fragile X mental retardation is not as striking as that of Down syndrome, but with experience can be recognized (Fig. 14.19). Fragile X males have a large forehead, large head, long nose, prominent chin and long ears. The facial phenotype, however, becomes more obvious with age and is not easily recognizable in younger children.

Fragile X males tend to be larger at birth and taller than other children, but do not achieve the full growth predicted by the centile chart. In adult life fragile X males tend to be short. The head circumference is increased, with many having a head circumference greater than the 97th centile. Similarly the ear length is increased. This is an extremely useful clinical sign and may be measured and compared with a centile chart prepared from a normal population.[15]

Macro-orchidism is present in 80% of adult fragile X males and 15% of prepubertal fragile X boys. The size of the testes may be considerably enlarged. In one series the range was 15–127 ml (the standard orchidometer can only be used for testicular volumes up to 25 ml!). The large testes are functionally normal and the increased size may be due to an increase in interstitial edema or connective tissue. Large testes are a relatively rare feature in other syndromes with mental handicap.

It has been suggested that there may be a connective tissue abnormality in fragile X. There is a slight increase in the frequency of mitral valve prolapse. More striking clinically is the soft skin and joint hypermobility, which may be helpful diagnostically.

The range of intellectual handicap in fragile X males varies but most are moderately to severely retarded. Females tend to be more mildly affected. There is also a suggestion that intelligence may decline with age. Speech development is particularly affected in fragile X males and behavioral changes and seizures may occur.

Molecular genetics

The fragile site in the X chromosome was initially used to diagnose this disorder but in affected males only 5–20% of cells will

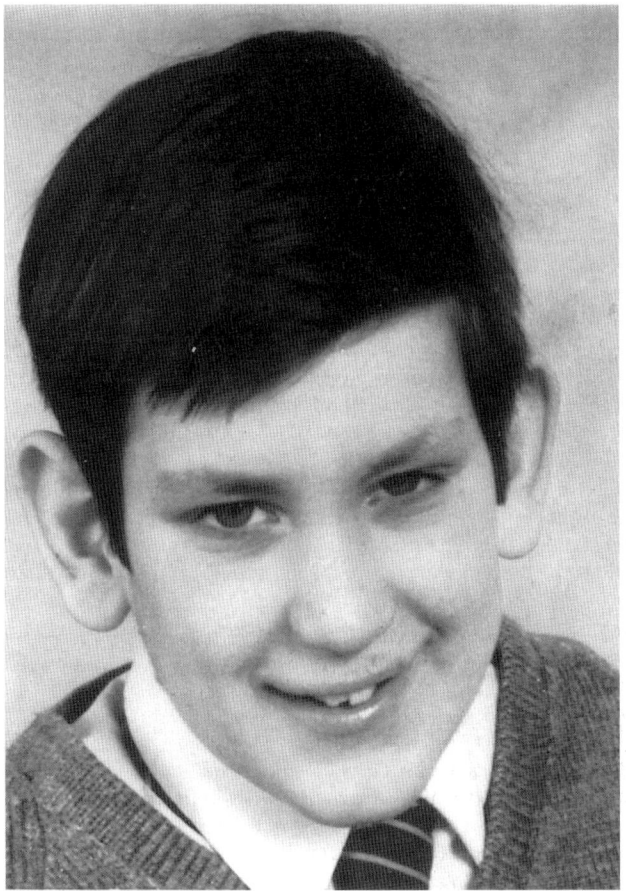

Fig. 14.19 Facial features of fragile X mental retardation (reproduced with permission).

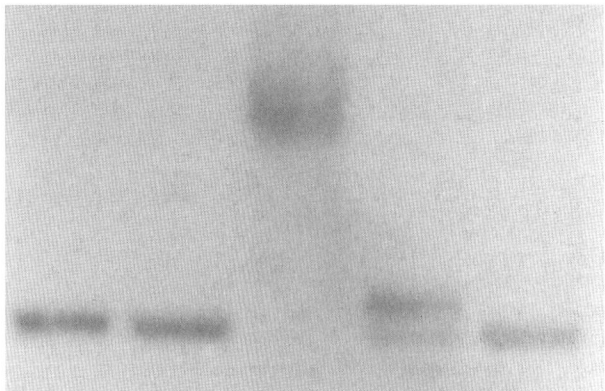

Fig. 14.20 Autoradiograph of Southern blot looking for fragile X. The DNA has been digested by the restriction enzyme Eco R1 and probed with FMR-1 probe OX1.9. The normal fragment size is seen in lanes 1, 2 and 5. In lane 3 there is an expanded fragment (< 500 repeats) indicating an affected boy. In lane 4 there is a female with a normal band and a slightly larger band above, indicating a carrier of a premutation. (Courtesy of R. Taylor.)

SINGLE GENE DISORDERS: INHERITANCE

Distributed amongst the 46 chromosomes, there are approximately 45 000 structural genes, which code for specific proteins. The position at which the gene lies on the chromosome is referred to as the *locus*. At the locus there is a pair of alleles. If an individual possesses two alleles that are the same, the individual is said to be *homozygous* for that particular trait. If the two alleles are different, the individual is said to be *heterozygous*. A gene which is manifest in the heterozygote is *dominant*, whereas a gene which is only manifest in the homozygote is *recessive*. These terms do not refer to the characteristics of the genes, but only to their manifestations. It is, therefore, more correct to refer to a 'dominant disorder' rather than a 'dominant gene'.

A trait or disorder which is determined by a gene on an *autosome* is said to be inherited as an autosomal trait and may be dominant or recessive. A trait or disorder that is determined by a gene on one of the *sex chromosomes* is said to be sex linked and may also be either dominant or recessive.

DRAWING THE PEDIGREE

The first stage in analyzing the pattern of inheritance in a family is to draw up a pedigree. This is a shorthand method of putting all the relevant family information together in a systematic way. The symbols used in drawing up a pedigree are illustrated in Table 14.5. Each individual

demonstrate the fragile site and in female carriers only half of the carriers could be detected by the cytogenetic test. It is now recognized that the fragile site is a marker for the disease rather than its cause.

The diagnostic difficulties were resolved by the identification of the FMR-1 gene at Xq27. The gene has within it a repeating sequence of three nucleotides CGG. Normal individuals have up to 45 copies of the nucleotide repeat. If the number of repeats is greater than 45–55 it becomes unstable in meiosis and can then increase in repeat number. The initial increase to between 55 and 200 repeats is referred to as the *premutation*. It may be found in intellectually normal males and female carriers. However, after passing through meiosis in the female the size of the repeats increases to the *full mutation* of greater than 200 repeats and can then produce learning difficulties in both males and females. Repeat number may increase or decrease in the full mutation during somatic cell division and therefore somatic mosaicism can be detected in some affected individuals. The full mutation affects the methylation of the DNA and this in turn switches off the FMR-1 gene and will affect both intellectual function and the cytogenetic fragility.

In terms of inheritance therefore it appears very similar to X-linked recessive inheritance as the condition is passed through females and will affect males, but up to a third of carrier daughters may also be affected with learning difficulties and the mutation can arise from unaffected males.

The discovery of the FMR-1 gene has meant that accurate follow-up and counseling of families is possible (Fig. 14.20). Prenatal diagnosis using chorionic villus sampling (CVS) and molecular analysis is possible in the first trimester of pregnancy.

Table 14.5 Pedigree symbols

□	Male unaffected
○	Female unaffected
■	Male affected
●	Female affected
▱	Deceased unaffected
◇	Sex unknown
↓	Miscarriage or termination
⚭	Dizygotic twins
⚭	Monozygotic twins
▮	Heterozygote
●	Propositus or index case
⚬⚬	Consanguineous marriage
□	Illegitimate or adopted
○	Female without offspring
②	Two unaffected females

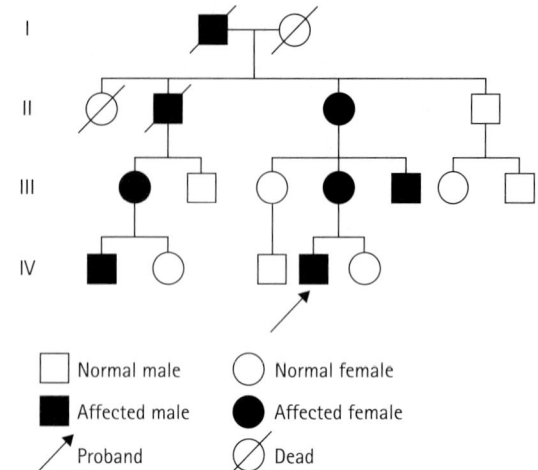

Fig. 14.21   Pedigree pattern of an autosomal dominant trait.

in a pedigree is identified from his generation (Roman numerals) and his location in the generation (Arabic numerals). Thus the index case or proband in Figure 14.21 is IV.4. It is usually necessary to ask specifically about consanguinity and miscarriages as most patients will not realize that these details are relevant.

AUTOSOMAL DOMINANT INHERITANCE

In an autosomal dominant disorder an affected individual possesses the abnormal (mutant) gene and its normal allele. When an affected individual marries a normal person, on average half their children will be affected. This is because an affected person produces gametes that have either the mutant allele for the disorder or the normal allele. If the normal allele is represented as 'a' and the abnormal allele as 'A' then the various combinations are illustrated in Table 14.6.

Classically an autosomal dominant disorder can be traced back through several generations, but if the condition is severe, affected individuals may not survive to have children and transmit the disease to subsequent generations. In such cases the affected individual is 'sporadic', as the condition in the individual has arisen as a new mutation and they will not live to reproduce. The frequency of new mutations arising varies from condition to condition, e.g. about 50% of cases of neurofibromatosis arise from new mutations whereas new mutations are rare in Huntington disease.

Autosomal dominant traits affect both males and females (Fig. 14.21). They may show great variation in severity (= *expressivity*) as in neurofibromatosis, which may range from being a relatively mild pigmentary skin disorder to a cause of severe deformity. Sometimes the gene may not express itself at all, in which case it is said to be nonpenetrant. This phenomenon explains apparent skipped generations in certain pedigrees. The *penetrance* of the trait is the proportion of heterozygotes who express a trait.

Some autosomal genes are expressed more frequently in one sex than in the other. This is referred to as sex-influenced inheritance or, in the extreme case in which only one sex is affected, as *sex-limited inheritance*. Possible examples of sex-influenced autosomal traits include hemochromatosis, gout and male pattern baldness. The underlying difference in expression may be due to the different hormonal background.

In myotonic dystrophy it was suggested that the severity of the condition tended to increase with each generation, e.g. the grandparent could have had cataracts only, while the mother had myotonia and muscle weakness and the affected child had the disorder in its congenital form with developmental delay. This was referred to as *anticipation*. It was initially thought that the cause of this was a bias in ascertainment but it is now clear that the underlying mutation is a triplet repeat in the myotonin kinase gene. Triplet repeats within a gene may become unstable at a critical size and at this point there may be an increase in the repeat size number during meiosis leading to an increasing severity in the next generation.

Occasionally it is known that a particular disorder is autosomal dominant and fully penetrant, and yet an unaffected parent will have two affected offspring. It is very unlikely that this was due to two independent de novo mutations and the most likely explanation is *germinal* or *gonadal mosaicism*. In this situation the unaffected parent carries the mutation only in the testis or ovary and not in the other tissues of the body.

AUTOSOMAL RECESSIVE INHERITANCE

Autosomal recessive traits affect both sexes and only homozygotes are affected. The affected individuals in a family are all in one sibship, i.e. they are brothers and sisters (Fig. 14.22). The parents of an affected child or children are both heterozygotes and are perfectly healthy. It is, therefore, not possible to trace the disease through several generations unless there is complex inbreeding. With rare recessive traits the parents of affected individuals are often related, the reason being that cousins are more likely to carry the same genes because they inherited them from a common ancestor.

When parents have a child affected by an autosomal recessive disorder the likelihood of the next pregnancy being similarly affected is 1 in 4. The risk remains 1 in 4 for each successive pregnancy no matter how many children may be affected in the family. If the normal allele is represented as 'A', and the abnormal allele as 'a', then the possible combinations are illustrated in Table 14.7.

Nowadays, since families tend to be small, it frequently happens that an autosomal recessive condition appears sporadic with only one affected person in the family.

The majority of inborn errors of metabolism are due to deficiencies of specific enzymes and are inherited as autosomal recessive traits. In some instances it may be possible to demonstrate that individuals are heterozygotes in these disorders by finding an intermediate level of enzyme activity.

Table 14.6   Autosomal dominant inheritance

| | | Affected parent (Aa) ↓ gametes | |
		A	a
Normal parent (aa) → gametes	a	Aa affected	aa normal
	a	Aa affected	aa normal

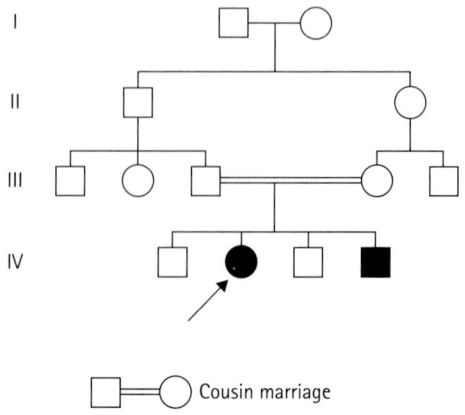

◻—◯ Cousin marriage

Fig. 14.22   Pedigree pattern of an autosomal recessive trait.

Table 14.7 Autosomal recessive inheritance

		Normal heterozygous parent (Aa) gametes ↓ gametes	
		A	a
Normal heterozygous parent → (Aa) gametes	A	AA normal	Aa unaffected heterozygote
	a	Aa unaffected heterozygote	aa affected

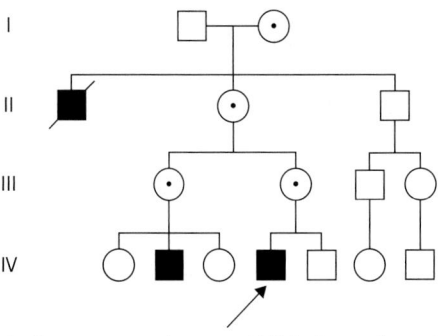

Fig. 14.24 Pedigree pattern of a severe X-linked recessive trait in which affected males do not survive to have children.

Where a number of different mutant alleles exist it is occasionally possible to find an individual who is heterozygous for two different mutant alleles. An example of this is seen in the hemoglobinopathies. An individual may be heterozygous for both HbS and HbC. Such double heterozygotes or 'genetic compounds' have a disease intermediate in severity between sickle cell disease and HbC disease.

CODOMINANCE

Codominance is the term used for two traits, which are both expressed in the heterozygote. An example of codominance is the inheritance for the blood groups A and B. An individual with both alleles will have the blood group AB.

X-LINKED RECESSIVE INHERITANCE

In theory sex-linked inheritance could be either X-linked or Y-linked, but as there are no structural genes other than those determining sexual development on the Y chromosome, sex linkage is effectively the same as X linkage.

An X-linked recessive trait is one which is due to a mutant gene on the X chromosome, and is carried by females to affect males (Figs 14.23 and 14.24). The affected males are *hemizygous* (with the mutant gene on their single X chromosome) while the carrier females are heterozygous and are usually perfectly healthy. X-linked disorders may also be transmitted by affected males through their daughters unless the disorder is so severe that affected males do not survive to have children (e.g. Duchenne muscular dystrophy). Hemophilia is an X-linked recessive disorder in which improvements in medical treatment and surgical techniques have led to affected males often surviving into adult life. If an affected male marries a normal female

and if the hemophilia gene is represented as X^h and the normal gene as X, then the various gametic combinations that can occur are represented in Table 14.8. Thus, all daughters of an affected male are carriers and all his sons are normal. In the case of a woman who is a carrier (XX^h) and who marries a normal male then half her sons will be affected and half her daughters will be heterozygote carriers (Table 14.9).

Quite often in serious X-linked conditions there is only one affected boy in a family. Such a sporadic case may be the result of a new mutation in the affected boy's X chromosome and in such cases recurrence would not occur in the family. It is also possible that the mother might be a carrier, and by chance the mutant gene has not been transmitted to any of her other male offspring. In families with predominantly female offspring an X-linked mutation may be inherited through the female line for a few generations without affected males. In one third of isolated cases of Duchenne muscular dystrophy the mutation occurs in the affected boy, and in two thirds of cases the mother is a carrier. It is obviously of vital

Table 14.8 X-linked inheritance: the offspring of affected males

		Affected male (X^hY) ↓ gametes	
		X^h	Y
Normal female (XX) → gametes	X	XX^h carrier daughter	XY normal son
	X	XX^h carrier daughter	XY normal son

Table 14.9 X-linked inheritance: the offspring of affected females

		Normal male (XY) ↓ gametes	
		X	Y
Carrier female (XX^h) → gametes	X	XX normal daughter	XY normal son
	X^h	XX^h carrier daughter	X^hY hemophiliac son

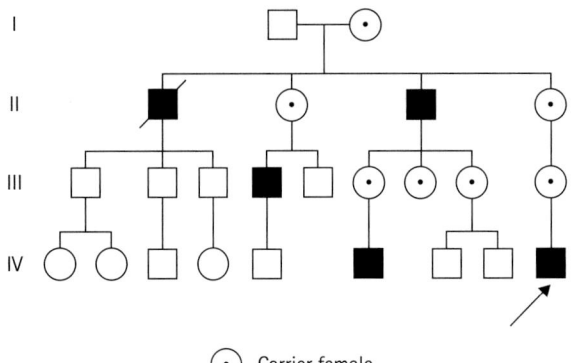

⊙ Carrier female

Fig. 14.23 Pedigree pattern of an X-linked recessive trait in which affected males reproduce.

importance to determine if the mother is a carrier in order to provide accurate information about recurrence risks. The probability of the mother being a carrier can be calculated using knowledge of the numbers of unaffected males in the family (the more unaffected males the less chance the mother is a carrier), the level of creatine kinase (female heterozygotes have slightly higher levels than female controls from the general population) and using information from DNA studies.

In a number of special circumstances a female may exhibit manifestations of an X-linked recessive trait. It may occur as a result of random inactivation or *lyonization* of the X chromosome. In early embryogenesis in the female zygote one of the X chromosomes is inactivated in each cell. This process is random so that on average half the cells in a female will have one X chromosome inactivated and half will have the other X chromosome inactivated. However, occasionally by chance the majority of cells will have the X chromosome with the normal allele inactivated and the mutant allele will be partially expressed. This situation is seen in female carriers of Duchenne muscular dystrophy where about 5% of female carriers may show some muscle weakness. It may also occur in the rare situation when a female is both a carrier of an X-linked mutation and has a 45X karyotype (Turner syndrome). Finally it can also occur in common X-linked disorders such as red–green color blindness where an affected male marries a female heterozygote and produces a daughter in whom both X chromosomes possess the mutant allele.

X-LINKED DOMINANT INHERITANCE

An X-linked dominant disorder is one which is manifest in the heterozygous female as well as in the hemizygous male. The pedigree pattern superficially resembles that of autosomal dominant inheritance, but in an X-linked dominant disorder an affected male transmits the disease to all his daughters and to none of his sons. Affected females transmit the disease equally to sons and daughters, half of whom, on average, will be affected (Fig. 14.25).

There are relatively few X-linked dominant disorders. One example is vitamin D-resistant rickets (hypophosphatemia). In some X-linked dominant disorders the condition is lethal in males and so only females are affected (e.g. incontinentia pigmenti, Rett syndrome).

MITOCHONDRIAL INHERITANCE

While the vast majority of genes are located in the nuclear genome there are a small number of genes located on the mitochondrial DNA (mtDNA). The mitochondrial DNA consists of 16.5kb of circular DNA and accounts for 1% of the total DNA. mtDNA encodes for the proteins essential for aerobic respiration, and defects in mtDNA reflect abnormalities in this function.[36] Each cell contains between 1000 and 100000 copies of mtDNA. In the vast majority of cells the functional mtDNA will be identical. This is referred to as *homoplasmy*. However, where there is a mutation in the mtDNA it will not usually be present in all mitochondria and cells will have a mixture of mitochondria with the 'wild type' gene and mitochondria with the mutation. This is referred to as *heteroplasmy*. The proportion of the mitochondria with the mutation will determine whether there is a phenotypic effect from the mutation. In practice over 85% of the mitochondria would need to have the mutation before there was a phenotypically significant defect in the enzymes of the respiratory chain.

In mitochondrial diseases there may also be variation among tissues in the body. This may have considerable practical implications in diagnosis since a blood sample may not give an accurate reflection of abnormalities in other tissues. For this reason muscle biopsy is the mainstay of diagnosis of mitochondrial diseases rather than blood sampling. In many mitochondrial diseases there will be characteristic 'ragged red fibers' on Gomori staining and a nonspecific elevation of lactate and pyruvate in the blood. It also follows from these tissue differences that prenatal diagnosis may be difficult, as the proportion of a mitochondrial mutation in a chorionic villus sample may not reflect the proportion of the mutation in other parts of the fetus.

The segregation of mitochondrial genes does not follow Mendelian inheritance. Mitochondrial genes are not passed paternally as the mitochondria are in the tail of the sperm and only the nucleus of the sperm penetrates the ovum at fertilization. The ovum on the other hand has a relatively large volume of cytoplasm and thus contains many mitochondria. The exact proportion of offspring affected will depend on the proportion of mitochondria containing the specific mutation in the fertilized ovum. It is thus very difficult to give accurate recurrence risks for mitochondrial disorders and the best guide at present is to rely on the statistical data from family studies.

Another complication in mitochondrial disease is that some of the enzymes in the respiratory chain and hence some of the mitochondrial functions are not coded for in the mtDNA but are coded for in the nuclear DNA. Mutations in these genes affecting mitochondrial function are inherited in a Mendelian pattern. One example of such a disorder is Barth syndrome (endocardial fibroelastosis, neutropenia and muscle weakness) which is due to a mutation in the G-45 gene on the X chromosome and is therefore inherited as an X-linked recessive disorder.[37]

There are a number of characteristic mitochondrial disorders which are important in clinical practice:
- Kearns–Sayre syndrome: this is a progressive external ophthalmoplegia with ptosis and muscle weakness.
- MERRF: myoclonic epilepsy with ragged red fibers.
- MELAS: mitochondrial encephalomyopathy with lactic acidosis and stroke-like episodes.
- Leber's hereditary optic neuropathy (LHON) which presents as acute or subacute visual failure in the second or third decade.[38]

However in many cases the clinical phenotype will not fit into a characteristic presentation and the possibility of mitochondrial disease should be considered in cases of lactic acidosis, muscle weakness, cardiomyopathy, deafness or pigmentary retinopathy.

In clinical practice pathological mutations are most significant, but there is also a wide range of harmless variation in the mtDNA. Such genetic variations are similar to the variation seen in blood groups and are known as *polymorphisms*. The mitochondrial polymorphisms have been used to study human evolution and the spread of different populations.[39]

DNA AND GENE ACTION

STRUCTURE AND FUNCTION OF GENES

The genetic material that is capable of providing a perfect replica in cell division is in the form of a molecule of DNA. While it is possible to study chromosomes at a microscopic level, the genes are well below the resolution of the microscope. Looking at the chromosomes under the microscope is rather like looking at the wrapping around the genes. In rough terms a 5cm length of DNA is compressed into a chromosome 10000 times smaller by tight coiling and packing with proteins called *histones*.

DNA consists of long chains of molecules called *nucleotides*. Each nucleotide consists of a nitrogenous base (*adenine, thymine, guanine* or

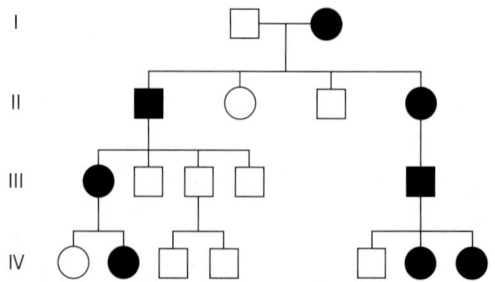

Fig. 14.25 Pedigree pattern of an X-linked dominant trait.

cytosine), a pentose sugar and a phosphate group. The pentose sugar in DNA is deoxyribose. The DNA (unless denatured) is in the form of two polynucleotide chains arranged in a double helix (Fig. 14.26a). The arrangement of the bases in the double helix is not random since adenine in one chain always pairs with thymine, and in the other cytosine always pairs with guanine. Thus the arrangement of nucleotides in the two chains is *complementary*, and in cell division using one chain a complementary chain may be synthesized, thus preserving the sequence of bases in each daughter cell.

The sequence of bases is important, because the arrangement of the bases provides the genetic code from which proteins may be made (Fig. 14.26b). The genetic information in the DNA is first *transcribed* with messenger ribonucleic acid (mRNA) and this in turn is *translated* into the synthesis of a polypeptide chain. RNA is very similar to DNA in structure except (i) the thymidine is replaced by uracil, (ii) the deoxyribose is replaced by ribose and (iii) it is a single-stranded rather than a double-stranded polynucleotide chain.

The DNA, which is responsible for the synthesis of specific proteins, forms the structural genes. The information is in the form of a *triplet code*, a sequence of three bases or a *codon* determines one amino acid. Since there are four bases involved the possible combination that could be provided is $4^3 = 64$. Since there are only 20 amino acids this code is said to be degenerate and most amino acids can be coded for by more than one triplet sequence. The code also provides codons to initiate and terminate synthesis.

In the first stage of protein synthesis the DNA sequence between the initiation codon and the stop codon is transcribed into mRNA. The mRNA then moves from the nucleus to the ribosomes in the cytoplasm. Here the second stage takes place, viz. the translation of mRNA into a polypeptide chain. The ribosome binds to the initiation site on the mRNA and for each codon an amino acid is added on using transfer RNA (tRNA). Transfer RNA is another form of RNA, which because of its molecular configuration is able to carry an amino acid and match it to the appropriate codon.

It has become apparent that the majority of DNA does not code for proteins and is not transcribed at all. The total amount of human DNA is 3 billion bases and if each gene were around 2000 bases in length this would allow for 1.5 million genes. Instead it is estimated that there are around 45 000 structural genes and 90% of the genome is DNA which does not code for proteins. Much of this is highly repetitive in its sequences and may have some as yet undefined function in the control of gene action. There are various classes of noncoding DNA. One form of the highly repetitive DNA known as microsatellite DNA is widely distributed throughout the genome and also because it is variable between individuals it can be used by researchers in mapping genes in family linkage studies. In another form there are also copies of genes which are nonfunctional and are known as pseudogenes. There are also inactivated DNA sequences known as transposable sequences which resemble the sequence found in retroviruses and indeed may have entered the human DNA from viral infection.

The structural gene has an ordered sequence that is illustrated in Figure 14.27. Upstream of the structural gene there is highly repetitive DNA and within this there are two promoter regions which regulate gene transcription. The beginning of the structural gene is marked by an initiation codon, AUG, which indicates where transcription begins. Within the region that is transcribed, the DNA may be divided into *exons* and *introns*. The exons mark the regions of DNA that code for the amino acids in the translated protein, whereas the introns or intervening sequences are spliced out of the processed RNA before it migrates to the cytoplasm as mRNA. The introns probably have a role in gene

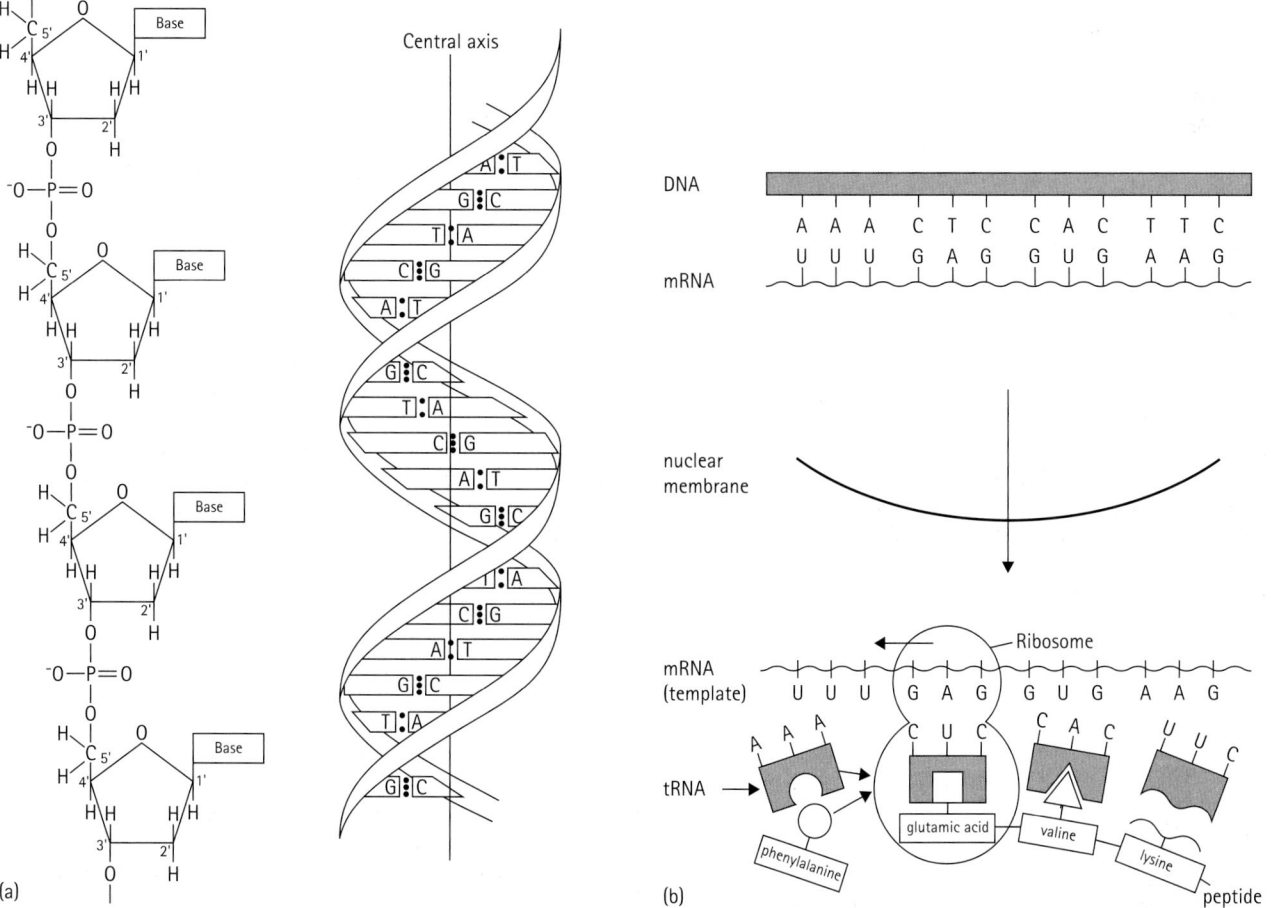

(a)

(b)

Fig. 14.26 (a) The structure of DNA. (From Weatherall 1986[40] with permission.) (b) The production of proteins from DNA. (Modified from Emery 1983[41] with permission.)

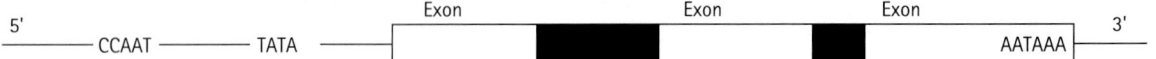

Fig. 14.27   The structural gene consists of promoter and terminator sequences that are located at either end of the gene. The coding sequence of the gene is made up of exons and introns (the mRNA of which will eventually be spliced out before translation into a protein).

regulation. The complexity of genes varies, e.g. insulin has two introns, whereas some collagen genes may have as many as 50 introns. At the end of the transcribed gene there is a stop codon and further downstream an AATAAA sequence that allows the release of the RNA.

This description of one gene producing one protein has been derived from biochemical studies in bacteria and it is often more complex than this in human genetics. In some cases such as the hemoglobin genes or some developmental genes there is a cluster of genes closely positioned together and the genes will work together to produce a complex protein or sequence of changes. In the case of the muscle protein dystrophin involved in Duchenne muscular dystrophy there is a very large gene measuring 2.5 million bases and within this gene there are several tissue specific promoters which produce different forms of dystrophin in different tissues. With immunoglobulins there is enormous diversity that comes from the alternative splicing of the RNA and DNA. With insulin the gene produces a precursor protein, preproinsulin, which is subsequently cleaved enzymatically after protein translation leaving the physiologically active insulin and its protein precursors.

At a disease level there are now many examples of one gene being associated with more than one disease. Most mutations in the androgen receptor gene will cause differing degrees of androgen insensitivity, but a CAG repeat mutation in the same gene produces X-linked spinomuscular atrophy and gynecomastia. Similarly, different mutations in the cystic fibrosis transmembrane receptor (CFTR) gene may produce the classic features of cystic fibrosis at one end of the spectrum and bilateral absence of the vas deferens without respiratory disease at the other end of the spectrum.

MUTATIONS AT A MOLECULAR LEVEL

A *mutation* represents a change in the genomic material. Mutations may occur in somatic cells or germinal cells. Somatic cell mutation may predispose to malignancy but will not be inherited. Mutations in the germinal cells, on the other hand, may be transmitted in the form of genetic disease. Mutations may be in the form of large chromosomal rearrangements as described in the earlier part of the chapter or may occur at molecular level in a single gene.

At a molecular level the main types of structural mutation are:

1. *Single base substitutions ('point mutations').* These involve the substitution of one base for another but may have different effects.
   - Missense mutations: the replacement of one amino acid for another in the gene product. A good example of such a mutation is sickle cell disease in which an A to T substitution in the 6th codon of the globin gene changes GAG to GTG and hence leads to the substitution of valine for glutamic acid and the subsequent physiological effects on the hemoglobin molecule.
   - Nonsense mutations: the replacement of an amino acid codon with a stop codon (UAA or UAG or UGA) which leads to a truncation of the gene product.
   - Splice site mutations: a single base substitution which creates or destroys an intron–exon splice site.
2. *Deletions.* Deletions may vary in size from single bases to megabase lengths of DNA. There are many examples of molecular deletions, e.g. over 60% of mutations in Duchenne muscular dystrophy are due to deletions in the dystrophin gene. One specific type of deletion is that which occurs in the promotor sequence of the gene;

these will affect the rate of synthesis of the gene product rather than its structure, e.g. promoter deletions have been reported in thalassemia.
3. *Insertions and duplications.* These mutations may arise from unequal crossing over at meiosis and can disrupt the gene.
4. *Frameshift mutations.* These can be produced by deletions or single base substitution and as a result all the subsequent codons in the gene are misread as the nucleotides must be read in 'threes'.
5. *Dynamic mutations.* When there are trinucleotide or triplet repeats in a gene the transmission of the exact number of repeats may become genetically unstable and may increase further in subsequent generations, e.g. fragile X mental retardation, myotonic dystrophy and Huntington disease.

In addition to the structural classification for mutations it is possible to classify mutations in functional terms. Some mutations will produce no change in the function of the gene and thus will not be selected against in evolutionary terms. These nonpathological changes become variations or *polymorphisms* in the population. When a new change is found in a gene it is important to determine whether it is pathological or simply a polymorphism.

Mutations may produce loss of function. In many cases this loss of function is not critical unless both alleles have a loss of function and then the level of the gene product becomes critically low. This is the situation in autosomal recessive disorders. Other genes may serve a more critical role and the loss of function in one allele will be sufficient to produce an effect. This is referred to as haploinsufficiency and is the situation that is found in autosomal dominant inheritance. If a chromosome deletion in the same area produces the phenotype then haplosufficiency of critical genes is likely to be the molecular mechanism.

Collagen is made up of three strands of procollagen polypeptides in a triple helix. The procollagen polypeptides are produced by several collagen genes. A heterozygous mutation in one of these collagen genes may produce serious abnormalities in collagen because the abnormal procollagen polypeptide produced binds abnormally with the other procollagen polypeptides and leads to major disruption in the final collagen product. The effect of this mutation has been described as 'protein suicide' or a dominant negative effect. This is the underlying molecular pathology in some forms of osteogenesis imperfecta.

Mutations can produce a gain of function. The gain of function may be due to the overproduction of a protein such as the peripheral myelin protein (PMP22) in Charcot–Marie–Tooth disease or the accumulation of protein aggregates in Huntington disease. It may also be due to a receptor being switched on permanently, such as the GNAS subunit of the G protein in McCune–Albright syndrome.

Genetic heterogeneity underlies much of the complexity of inherited disease. The term may be used to describe how similar conditions may have different patterns of inheritance, e.g. Noonan syndrome and Turner syndrome both have short stature and a webbed neck but Noonan syndrome is autosomal dominant and Turner syndrome is chromosomal. It may also apply at the molecular level. *Locus heterogeneity* describes the situation where the same disease may be caused by mutations in different genes, e.g. osteogenesis imperfecta may be caused by mutations in either the COL1A1 on chromosome 17 or the COL1A2 gene on chromosome 7. *Allelic heterogeneity* describes the situation where the same disease may be caused by different mutations in the same gene, e.g. there are now over 700 recognized mutations in the CFTR gene causing cystic fibrosis.

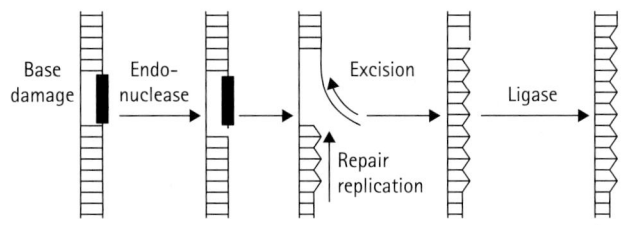

Fig. 14.28 DNA may be damaged but has a capacity to repair itself. (From Bundey 1985[42] with permission.)

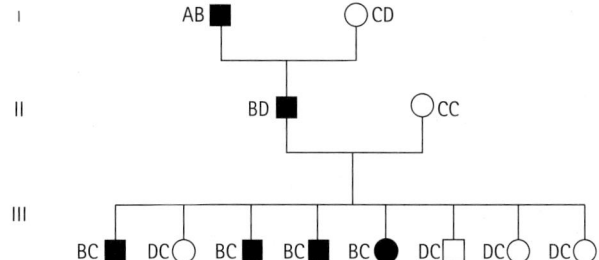

Fig. 14.29 Gene mapping by linkage analysis. In this pedigree the polymorphic marker B is segregating with the disease, with the exception of III.7 where a meiotic recombination between the polymorphic marker and the disease has occurred.

Mutations usually produce a permanent change in the gene, but DNA has some ability to repair itself. This has been studied largely from disorders where DNA damage leads to malignancy. Ultraviolet exposure leads to the formation of pyrimidine dimers binding the nucleotide bases. In the rare skin disorder xeroderma pigmentosum such abnormal dimers cannot be repaired because of an enzyme deficiency and ultimately skin tumors develop. The stages in normal repair are illustrated in Figure 14.28. Firstly, the single strand of DNA with the dimer formation is excised and removed, then using a DNA replicase a new strand is synthesized using the complementary strand as a template; finally the new strand is fixed into strands of the original using a DNA ligase. Some of the other inherited disorders leading to premature aging are also due to defects in DNA repair.

THE HUMAN GENOME MAPPING PROJECT

One of the most important events in human biology has been the mapping of genes to their chromosome location which started in the mid-1980s; by February 2001 the first draft of the human genome was published.[43,44] To understand the process it is necessary to look at the classic approaches to gene mapping and also the more automated approach.

TRADITIONAL GENE MAPPING

Gene mapping has depended on finding gene loci that are linked. When two genetic loci are close together on the same chromosome they are said to be *linked*. If two loci are at different ends of the chromosome then it is very likely that they will be separated during meiosis since there are two or three crossovers for each chromosome (see Fig. 14.3). The closer together they are, the less likely that they will be separated during meiosis. Thus a measure of how close gene loci are to each other is the frequency of recombination. This is measured in *map units* or *centiMorgans* where 1 centiMorgan is equivalent to a 1% chance of recombination.

Gene mapping has been of considerable practical value in medical genetics as it has been possible to progress from gene localization to sequencing the gene and to identifying the gene product. A good example of this was the research that led to the discovery of dystrophin as the altered gene product in Duchenne muscular dystrophy.[42,45] This approach is known as *reverse genetics*, since it reversed the traditional approach of identifying the gene mutation from the enzyme or protein abnormality.

Genes have sometimes been mapped by finding an association between a disorder and a specific chromosome rearrangement, then the gene for that disorder may be located at the chromosome breakpoints. For example, patients were found with retinoblastoma and deletions of 13q14, and further research has identified the gene responsible for retinoblastoma to be located in this region.

The other technique commonly used is *linkage analysis*. If a specific genetic marker segregates in a family with a single gene disorder, then the gene for that disorder will be located on the same chromosome as the marker and the position of two genes can be estimated from the frequency of crossovers. For example, in Figure 14.29, a large family with an autosomal dominant disorder is studied with a DNA polymorphism which gives four alleles, A, B, C and D. In the first generation the disease is inherited with the B allele from the grandfather (I.1) to his son (II.1).

In other words the DNA polymorphism B and the disease allele are on the same particular chromosome and the linkage phase is established. In the third generation it is possible to see if any recombination takes place. In all but one of the eight children the B polymorphism segregates with the disease and the D polymorphism segregates with the normal allele. The exception is III.7 in whom there has been a recombination. Thus there has been one recombination out of eight meioses and the recombination rate is 12.5% or 0.125. Obviously not all families are so obligingly large and informative, but it is still possible to carry out linkage analysis with smaller families because the number of meioses may be added together.

The usual way of expressing linkage is as the log of the odds of linkage or the *lod score*, and this is expressed in terms of genetic distance by the recombination fraction θ. A recombination fraction of 0.05 represents a 5% chance of recombination. A lod score of 3 or over, for a recombination fraction of 0.05 or less, is significantly close linkage for prenatal diagnosis.

AUTOMATED APPROACH

While the traditional approaches have continued to prove useful in mapping diseases it was realized that a more industrialized approach using banks of automated gene sequencers could be used to systematically identify all the genes. The DNA is basically cut into small sections and cloned and then the fragments are sequenced. The order of the fragments can be worked out if they have overlapping sequences and eventually all the DNA in the human genome can be sorted into these overlapping fragments. The structural genes can be identified by relating the DNA to expressed sequences (ESTs) and from this the total number of genes can be identified. One of the first surprises from the Human Genome project was the finding that humans did not have 100 000 genes, as had been previously predicted, but probably only have 45 000 genes or less. This gives us only twice as many genes as the nematode worm and might be taken to indicate we are not as complex or advanced in evolutionary terms as we had thought. It is, however, probably not correct to equate biological complexity with the number of genes. An analogy could perhaps be taken from literature. Everyone writes with the same number of letters in the alphabet but that does not stop Shakespeare from writing great sonnets. In the same way it may be the complexity of gene expression that distinguishes humans from other species. One of the most challenging questions that comes from the genome project is the fact that the difference between some primates and humans comes down to a mere 1% of genes. Perhaps determining what difference this makes will help to define the essential qualities that make the human species different and define the biological basis of humanity.

At present there is only a draft of the genome available and many gaps to fill in with further sequencing. At the time of writing about 17 000 disease genes have been identified. This is just a beginning and there will need to be an enormous amount of research to determine the clinical significance of the genes in relation to disease and normal function.

Already there are a number of new developments in human genetics which will develop the discoveries of the human genome:

- *Bioinformatics.* The amount of information that has to be analyzed is staggering, and making sense of the interrelationship between genes will be even more challenging. This has led to the development of new information technology systems to handle the data.
- *Comparative genomics.* The genome mapping project is not confined to analyzing the human genome and the genomes of other species are being analyzed using the same technology. This has already meant that the location of human diseases can be identified by finding a similar defect in the mouse and working back from the knowledge of the position of the defect on the mouse chromosomes to the homologous position on the human chromosome.
- *Transgenic animals.* It is often necessary to test out treatments in animals but difficult to find the appropriate animal model. Now it is possible to take a gene mutation causing human disease and to insert the mutated human gene into a mouse embryo and construct a transgenic mouse model that matches the human disease very accurately.
- *Gene expression and proteomics.* Having found a disease causing gene it is then necessary to see how that gene is expressed and what the protein it produces is like. The studies will therefore move from the gene (genomics) to the protein (proteomics).
- *Pharmacogenomics.* At present it costs up to £500 million to develop a new drug and along the way there will be many potential drugs which might be effective but cannot be used because a small number of people will develop severe side-effects from the potential drug. It has been discovered that many of these side-effects are determined by genetic variation. Therefore if those who might develop side-effects could be identified genetically before the drug was used then it would be possible to bring many new drugs safely to the market and possibly to reduce the enormous cost of development. Another approach that might be used in pharmacogenomics is to define the heterogeneity within a disease and to target drug treatment more specifically, e.g. rather than treating all individuals with high blood pressure with the same drugs it might be possible by genetic analysis to identify those with abnormal salt metabolism from those with abnormal vascular responses.
- *Gene therapy.* Although gene therapy is the ultimate aim for genetic research it is likely to take some time for this to be more widely successful. There are many technical problems to solve. At present the correct gene is usually introduced into the patient using a viral vector, but this is relatively inefficient and even when it does correctly enter the disease tissue it is lost rapidly. There are also problems about using a virus even when it has been biologically inactivated and the use of a viral vector would probably never be acceptable in the treatment of neurological disease since it might well cause serious complications. There is considerable knowledge of the genetic defect in cystic fibrosis and a number of attempts have been made to use gene therapy to treat cystic fibrosis with rather disappointing results so far.[46] Because of the risks involved it may well be malignant disease rather than chronic genetic disease where the first major successes take place.

THE USE OF MOLECULAR GENETICS IN DIAGNOSIS

The recent rapid advances in medical genetics have come about largely because of the development of DNA technology. Some knowledge of the technology is helpful in understanding its practical application in the diagnosis of genetic disease. A more detailed review of the laboratory techniques may be found in Strachan & Read.[47]

DNA extraction

DNA may be extracted from many different tissues. In most clinical work blood samples will be used as a source of DNA but in population studies buccal scrapes or mouthwashes may be useful for limited DNA testing. It may also be possible to extract DNA from the dried blood spots used for neonatal screening and this may be a source of archival DNA from a child who has subsequently died. Pathology samples are more difficult to analyze as the DNA is often broken down in the fixation process and only short DNA sequences may be analyzed. In prenatal diagnosis chorionic villi provide the best source of DNA.

The DNA is obtained by lysing the cells, digesting the proteins by a proteinase and purifying the DNA by serial extractions with phenol and chloroform. The purity of the DNA obtained is then determined by spectroscopy and running an electrophoretic gel. Extracted DNA may be stored for many years at $-80°C$.

Southern blotting

The first widespread use of DNA hybridization was Southern blotting, but this is now being superseded by new techniques. The DNA is extracted and cut into small fragments with a *restriction enzyme* which will recognize specific DNA sequences and cleave the DNA at these points. The DNA may then be separated by electrophoresis so that the smallest fragments move fastest through the gel. If this is compared to a control sample, the specific size of the DNA fragment may be estimated. Throughout the genome there will be variations or polymorphisms in the cutting sites for the restriction enzymes [*restriction fragment length polymorphisms* (RFLPs)] and therefore it will be possible to study the pattern of inheritance of these RFLPs within a family. If a particular RFLP is located close to a disease gene locus, it will be possible to follow the segregation through the family and make use of this in predicting whether or not a disease has been passed on within the family. The main disadvantages of using Southern blotting are that it takes relatively large amounts of DNA and involves the use of radioisotopes, which require some days to develop on the X-ray plate.

It should be noted that this technique is named after its originator (Southern[48]), but rather confusingly a geographical nomenclature has been applied to other techniques, e.g. a DNA–RNA blot is known as a Northern blot, and a protein–monoclonal antibody analysis is known as a Western blot!

Polymerase chain reaction

The polymerase chain reaction (PCR) is now the most frequently used technique in molecular biology. It is used to study a specific area of DNA using short complementary sequences of DNA (*oligonucleotides*) from both the 3′ and the 5′ ends of the DNA to be studied. These oligonucleotides build copies of the DNA using a *heat stable polymerase* (Taq 1). It is then possible to heat the mixture and the DNA strands will separate. On cooling, the DNA can once more be duplicated and the process repeated again and again leading to an exponential increase in the copies of the two fragments. The main advantages of this technique are that it is very quick, highly sensitive and very robust and it can be used to study mRNA as well as DNA. It can also be used to study very small amounts of almost any tissue, e.g. the blood spots on a Guthrie card or the cells found in a mouthwash sample. The technique is widely used in molecular diagnosis of genetic disease (Figs 14.30 and 14.31). It is also being used in infectious disease to confirm the presence of infectious agents and in immunology to identify the human leukocyte antigen (HLA) haplotype.

Gene sequencing

There are a number of techniques available to decode or sequence a gene into its component nucleotide bases. Originally the process of sequencing a gene might have taken a PhD student 3–4 years but now semi-automated sequencers are available. In theory it may appear that the best way to identify gene mutations is to fully sequence the gene but this is still a major task and full exclusion of mutations causing the disease will still be very difficult, expensive and time consuming. Figure 14.32 illustrates the use of a gene sequencer in identifying a mutation in the ROR2 gene in a patient with Robinow syndrome and shows a point mutation in the gene sequencer printout.[49]

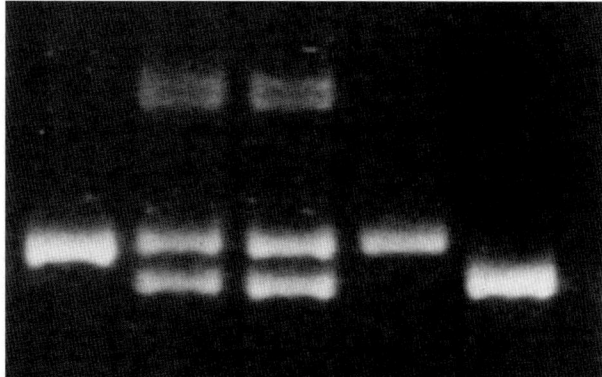

Fig. 14.30 PCR of exon of CFTR gene. Lanes 1 and 4 show homozygous normal individuals. Lanes 2 and 3 show heterozygous carriers of the ΔF508 mutation and lane 5 shows an affected homozygous ΔF508 individual. (Courtesy of R. Taylor.)

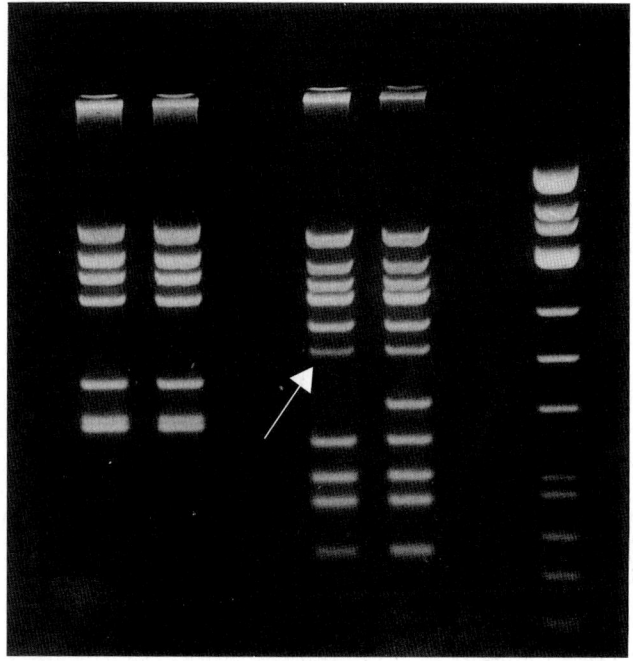

Fig. 14.31 Multiplex PCR testing for deletions in the dystrophin gene. The third lane from the left shows a band missing in amplifying exons from the 3′ end of the gene, indicating a patient affected with Duchenne muscular dystrophy. (Courtesy of R. Taylor.)

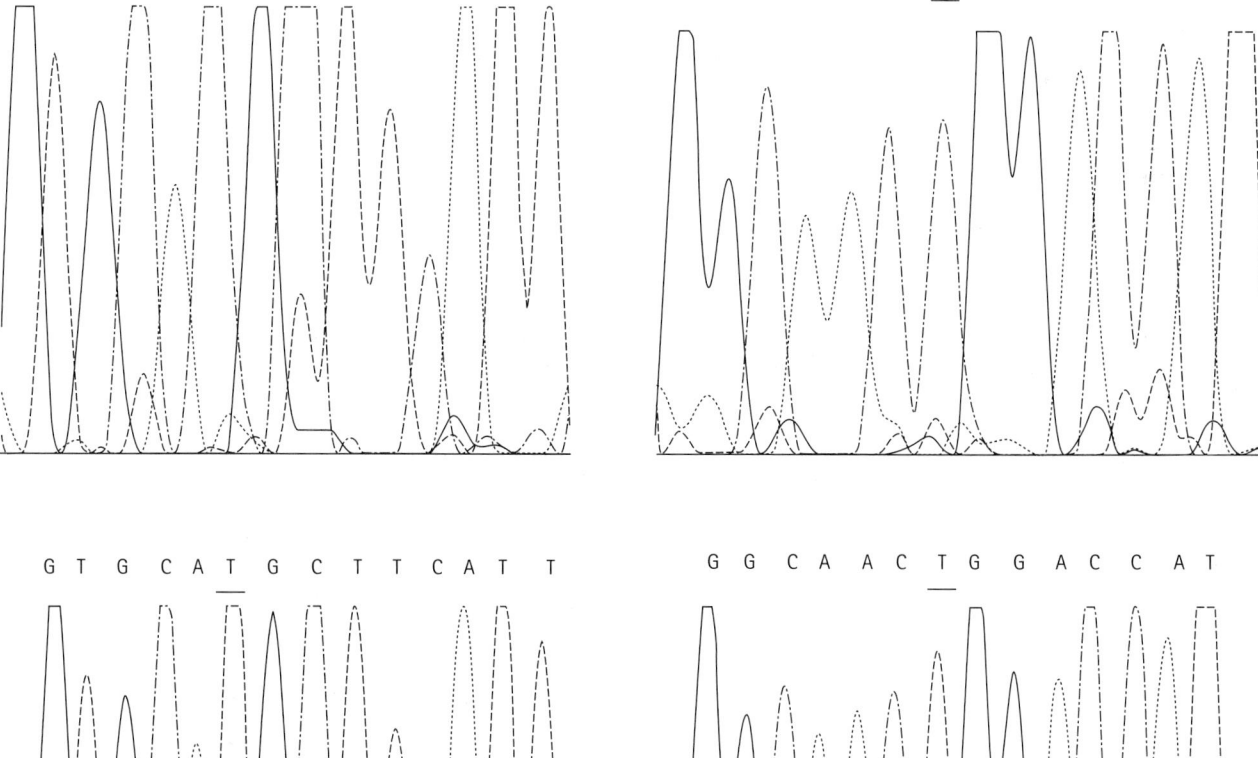

(a)

(b)

Fig. 14.32 Gene sequencing of the ROR2 gene in Robinow syndrome. The bases are labeled fluorescently and scanned. The upper printout shows the normal sequences and the lower printout shows two point mutations: (a) is a 550C → T and (b) is a 565C → T change. (Courtesy of Dr Afzal.)[49]

A different strategy is to take a two step approach and to carry out a screen for mismatch between the known DNA sequence and the patient's DNA first and then to look at any areas of mismatch with full sequencing. A number of techniques have therefore been evolved to screen for mismatching between the known gene sequence and the patient's DNA. Single stranded conformation polymorphism (SSCP) analysis is relatively inexpensive but has limited sensitivity. Another technique known as denaturing high performance liquid chromatography (HPLC) requires relatively expensive equipment but is very sensitive and can be used with a high throughput of samples. A protein truncation test may be used to screen for mutations that lead to terminating mutations which shorten the gene product.

Some researchers have looked to the computer industry for inspiration and have tried to develop a DNA chip consisting of a microarray of literally thousands of individual DNA hybridization reactions on a small silicon wafer (see CGH microarray). Each reaction would cause a color change and the whole chip would be read by an automated scanning microscope. By further analogy with the computer industry, further development may increase the number of reactions per chip and bring the cost per test down.

The techniques of molecular genetics have moved out of the research laboratory into the diagnostics laboratory. There are now many diseases in which gene analysis may help in diagnosis, but it is still necessary to recognize the limitations of the present technology. A summary of these is given in Table 14.10. The tests roughly fall into two groups:

1. *Fully diagnostic.* In these diseases there is only one mutation and analysis of this will give a clear and conclusive result which may be used to confirm or exclude the disorder. Examples of these are sickle cell disease where the only mutation is the point mutation in position 6 of the beta globin chain, and in myotonic dystrophy and fragile X where there is an expansion of a triplet repeat sequence.
2. *Partially diagnostic.* In these disorders there is more than one mutation that may cause the disorder and while it may be possible to make a clear positive diagnosis it is more difficult to exclude the diagnosis without fully sequencing the whole gene. There are many examples of this, but two will illustrate the point.
   - In cystic fibrosis around 70–80% of patients have a deletion of the codon for phenylalanine at position 508 (ΔF508) and if a patient is found to be homozygous for this mutation the diagnosis is confirmed (Fig. 14.30). If, however, the patient without a family history of cystic fibrosis is tested for ΔF508 and is found not to have it, the diagnosis is not completely excluded as it is possible to have any one of several hundred other mutations. Rather than trying to test for such a large number of mutations it is possible to test for the commonest 32 mutations using a multiplex PCR test and this will give a 95% exclusion which is sufficient in most cases. The problem also exists if the patient is found to be heterozygous for ΔF508. The patient might be an unaffected heterozygote carrier or could be an affected homozygote with another rarer mutation on the other chromosome 7.
   - The other example is Duchenne muscular dystrophy. By using a combination of gene probes it is possible to look for several possible deletions in the dystrophin gene. If a deletion is found the diagnosis is confirmed (Fig. 14.31). However, the absence of the deletion only provides a 60% exclusion of the diagnosis.

MULTIFACTORIAL INHERITANCE

Many common disorders, including congenital malformations, show some increase in frequency within families, but follow no simple Mendelian pattern of inheritance. In these disorders the condition becomes manifest when there is a sufficient combination of genetic predisposition and environmental factors. These disorders are thus referred to as multifactorial.

One way of understanding multifactorial inheritance is to consider an individual's *liability* to a particular disorder to be a combination of genetic and environmental factors. Liability in the general population will have a normal distribution and it is only those whose liability goes beyond a certain threshold who will show the disease or malformation (Fig. 14.33). This would be a relatively small proportion of the general population. First degree relatives of those who manifest the disorder will have half the genes in common with their affected relatives and therefore have a greater proportion of the genetic predisposition than the general population. If one then looked at the distribution of liability in first degree relatives it would be shifted away from the distribution in the general population, so that a greater proportion of first degree relatives would be affected than in the general population (Fig. 14.33).

While the mathematical model of liability may be helpful in understanding the principles of multifactorial inheritance, it is not of practical value in providing information on recurrence risks for genetic counseling. These are best provided by the statistical analysis of family studies. For example the recurrence of neural tube defects in those families who have already had an affected child is around 5% or 15 times the risk for the general population. Similar studies looking at the offspring of those affected by spina bifida have shown a 5% risk for their offspring. Table 14.11 gives some of the empiric risks

Table 14.10 Single gene disorders with their chromosome locations and approaches to diagnostic testing

Disease	Location(s)	Molecular tests
Adrenoleukodystrophy	Xq27	Mutation or biochemical
Adult polycystic kidney disease	16p13, 4q13	Clinical or mutation
Alpha thalassemia	16p13	Mutation
Beta thalassemia	11p15	Mutation
Charcot–Marie–Tooth disease	17p11, 1q21, Xq13	Mutation
Color blindness	Xq27	Research
Congenital adrenal hyperplasia	6p21	Mutation
Cystic fibrosis	7q31	Mutation
Duchenne muscular dystrophy	Xp21	Mutation or FISH
Emery–Dreifuss muscular dystrophy	Xq27	Mutation
Facioscapulohumeral muscular dystrophy	4q34	Linkage
Fragile X mental retardation	Xq27	Mutation
Friedreich's ataxia	9q13	Mutation
Galactosemia	9p13	Biochemical
Hemophilia A & B	Xq28	Mutation/hematological
Hypertrophic cardiomyopathy	14q12	Mutation
Marfan syndrome	15q21	Mutation or linkage
Myotonic dystrophy	19q13	Mutation
Neurofibromatosis type 1	17q11	Clinical or mutation
Neurofibromatosis type 2	22q11	Mutation
Noonan syndrome	12q23	Mutation
Oculocutaneous albinism	11q14	Mutation
Osteogenesis imperfecta	7q21, 17q21	Radiological or mutation
Phenylketonuria	12q24	Biochemical/mutation
Polyposis coli	5q21	Mutation
Sickle cell disease	11p15	Mutation
Tuberous sclerosis	9q34, 16p13	Mutation
Von Hippel–Lindau syndrome	3p25	Mutation
Werdnig–Hoffmann disease	5q13	Mutation

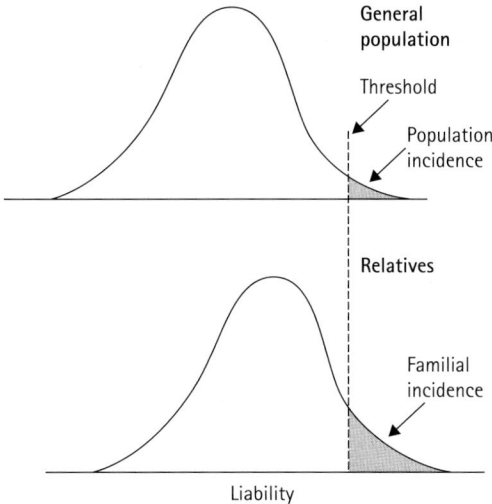

Fig. 14.33 Hypothetical curve of liability in the general population and in relatives for a hereditary disorder in which the genetic predisposition is multifactorial.

for common disorders calculated from family studies. With new techniques in molecular biology it may become possible to identify the genetic factors in multifactorial disorders. This has to some extent already been achieved in Hirschsprung disease where many of the predisposing genes have been identified.[50]

With multifactorial inheritance there are some general rules which are helpful.

1. The risk for sibs is approximately equal to the risk for offspring. On the whole the risks are lower than those for Mendelian inheritance.
2. The risk for second degree relatives (uncles, aunts, nephews and nieces) is considerably smaller than for first degree relatives. The risks for third degree relatives (cousins) are for practical purposes more or less the same as those for the general population.
3. If the frequency of a multifactorial disorder is q, then the risk for first degree relatives is approximately the square root of q, e.g. esophageal atresia occurs in 1 in 10 000 births; the risk for further offspring is the square root of 0.0001 = 1/100.
4. If there is a sex difference in the frequency of the disorder, then the risks are greater for further relatives of the rarer sex. For example, with pyloric stenosis males are affected five times as frequently as females. After an affected male the risk of further affected children is 2%, but after an affected female the risk is 9%.
5. The risks increase with the number of affected individuals in the family. The risk after a second affected child is more than twice the risk after a single affected child. For example after one child with a cleft lip and palate the risk is 4%, but after two affected children it is 10%.
6. In theory the recurrence data collected from family studies are only relevant for the same racial group and geographical area. If there are differences in the incidence of a disorder in different racial groups and countries, then care must be taken in applying the data, e.g. the recurrence risk for anencephaly and spina bifida is less in blacks than whites.

The epidemiological studies in neural tube defects have shown the value of looking at both the environmental and genetic aspects of multifactorial disease. The studies looked at the geographic variation of spina bifida and also looked at environmental factors that might explain this variation. It was suspected that dietary factors and especially vitamin intake were important. Eventually trials with periconceptual supplementation of folic acid to pregnant mothers at higher risk of having a child with a neural tube defect demonstrated that the predicted rate of the malformation could be reduced by 60%. This, together with the use of rubella vaccination, is an excellent example of the primary prevention of congenital abnormalities.

Table 14.11 Recurrence risks (%) for some common disorders. (From Emery 1983[41] with permission)

Disorder	Incidence	Sex ratio M:F	Normal parents having a second affected child	Affected parent having an affected child	Affected parent having a second affected child
Anencephaly	0.20	1:2	5*	–	–
Asthma	3–4	1:1	10	26	–
Cleft palate only	0.04	2:3	2	7	15
Cleft lip ± cleft palate	0.10	3:2	4	4	10
Club foot	0.10	2:1	3	3	10
Congenital heart disease (all types)	0.50	–	1–4	1–4	–
Diabetes mellitus (early onset)	0.20	1:1	8	8	10
Dislocation of hip	0.07	1:6	4	4	10
Epilepsy ('idiopathic')	0.50	1:1	5	5	10
Hirschsprung disease	0.02	4:1		–	–
Male index			2	–	–
Female index			8	–	–
Mental retardation ('idiopathic')	0.30–0.50	1:1	3–5	–	–
Profound childhood deafness	0.10	1:1	10	8	–
Pyloric stenosis	0.30	5:1			
Male index			2	4	13
Female index			10	17	38
Renal agenesis (bilateral)	0.01	3:1			
Male index			3	–	–
Female index			7	–	–
Schizophrenia	1–2	1:1	10	16	–
Scoliosis (idiopathic, adolescent)	0.22	1:6	7	5	–
Spina bifida	0.30	2:3	5*	3*	–

*Anencephaly or spina bifida.

MALFORMATION SYNDROMES

The majority of single congenital malformations has a multifactorial inheritance and a relatively low risk of recurrence. In the case of multiple malformations or the combination of mental handicap and congenital abnormalities, considerable care needs to be exercised since a proportion of such cases are caused by single gene mutations and consequently have a high risk of recurrence.

Another reason why it is important to recognize when a malformation is part of a syndrome is that it may give a better indication of the ultimate prognosis or likelihood of subsequent complications. For example, Stickler syndrome is an autosomal dominant disorder with variable expression. It may present in the newborn with a cleft palate and micrognathia and a characteristic facial appearance with a flat nasal bridge (Fig. 14.34). There is often severe myopia and possibly retinal detachment; by anticipatory follow-up the retinal detachment can be prevented by early treatment.

The clinical approach to the diagnosis and study of malformations and birth defects is known as *dysmorphology*.[15] There are a number of concepts that are useful in delineating patterns of malformation.

1. A *syndrome* is a recognized pattern of clinical abnormalities that have a single cause, e.g. Meckel syndrome is an autosomal recessive disorder in which postaxial polydactyly, encephalocele, cystic dysplastic kidneys and hepatic fibrosis occur together.
2. An *anomalad* is a recognized pattern of congenital abnormalities that may have several different causes, e.g. the Robin anomalad of micrognathia, cleft palate and posteriorly displaced tongue may be a feature of Stickler syndrome, fetal compression, cerebrocostal syndrome and others.
3. An *association* is a combination of congenital abnormalities that occur together at a frequency greater than by chance alone, but do not appear to recur in families, e.g. the VATER association is a combination of Vertebral abnormalities, Anal atresia, TracheoEsophageal fistula, Radial and Renal abnormalities. The combination of abnormalities might represent an insult at a specific point in embryonic development which affects all systems developing at that particular time in embryogenesis.
4. A *sequence* is a series of malformations that arise secondary to one specific developmental incident, e.g. in the prune belly sequence urethral or bladder neck obstruction leads to bladder distension which in turn leads to abdominal distension, hydronephrosis and possibly interference with testicular descent and the iliac blood supply. When the pressure is sufficient to overcome the obstruction the bladder may deflate leaving the characteristic wrinkled prune belly appearance.
5. A *deformation* arises not from an error in embryological development but because normal fetal growth is restricted, e.g. the low set ears, micrognathia and joint contractures seen with oligohydramnios in utero.

THE CLINICAL APPROACH TO THE DIAGNOSIS OF A DYSMORPHIC SYNDROME

With the exception of radiological and cytogenetic investigations the diagnosis of a dysmorphic syndrome rarely depends on laboratory investigations. It is primarily a clinical diagnosis based on the assessment of the clinical signs and knowledge of the pattern of abnormalities seen in the dysmorphic syndromes.

In trying to weigh up the significance of specific dysmorphic features it is helpful to consider whether they are relatively common or rarely seen outside the context of a dysmorphic syndrome. Abnormalities such as a single palmar crease or partial syndactyly between the second and third toes are commonly seen in the general population and therefore are relatively minor clinical signs. Features like retinitis pigmentosa, cleft lip and polydactyly are rare in the general population as single abnormalities, and are frequently a feature of syndromes and therefore are relatively major clinical signs. Occasionally there is a specific feature that is diagnostic such as the 'hitchhiker thumb' seen in the autosomal recessive diastrophic dwarfism (Fig. 14.35).

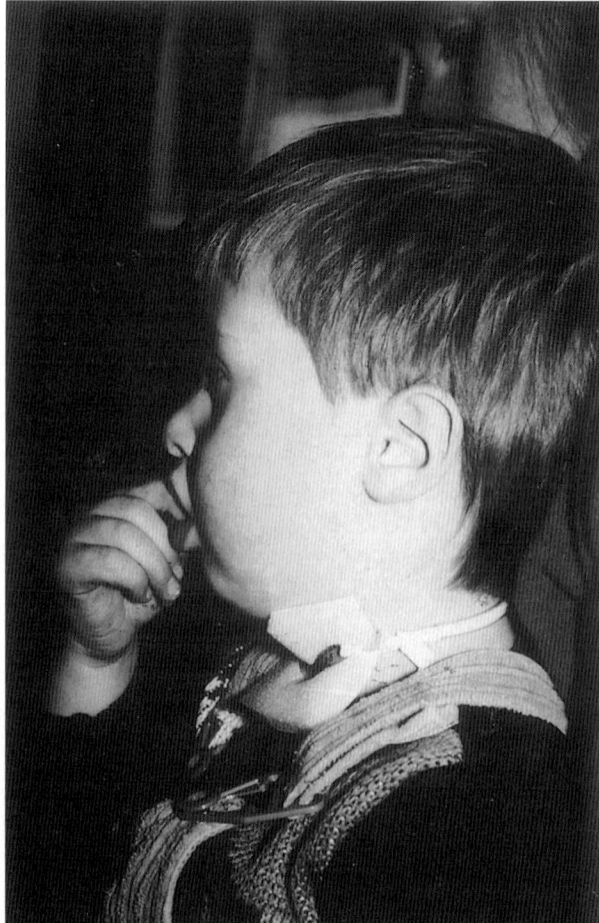

Fig. 14.34   Stickler syndrome.

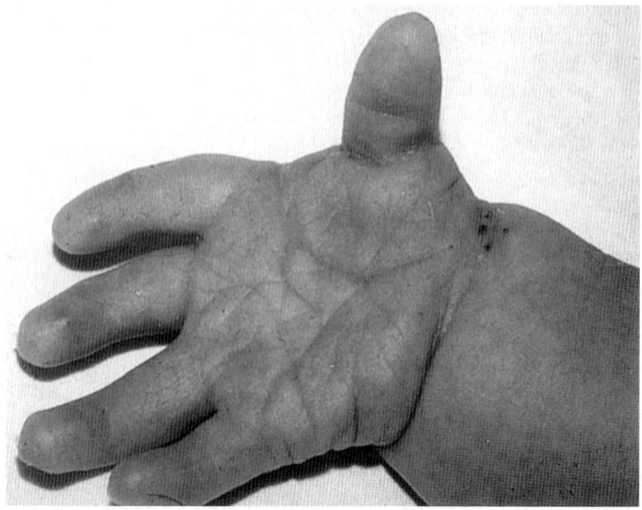

Fig. 14.35   'Hitch-hiker thumb' in diastrophic dwarfism.

Table 14.12 Descriptive terms used in dysmorphology

Hypertelorism	Increased distance between the eyes
Hypotelorism	Decreased distance between the eyes
Blepharophimosis	Narrowed palpebral fissures
Synophrys	Medial fusion of the eyebrows
Nasal bridge	Upper part of nose between eyes
Alae nasi	Lateral border of nostril
Columella	Medial part or septum of nostril
Philtrum	Vertical folds on upper lip
Pterygium	Webbing, e.g. webbing of neck = pterygium colli
Syndactyly	Fusion of digits
Preaxial polydactyly	Extra digit(s) on lateral border of limb
Postaxial polydactyly	Extra digit(s) on medial border of limb
Clinodactyly	Incurving usually of 5th digit
Brachydactyly	Short fingers or toes
Camptodactyly	Bent and contracted digits
Ectrodactyly	Cleft hand or foot
Symphalangism	Fusion of phalanges
Phocomelia	Absence of limb
Rhizomelia	Shortening of proximal segment of limb
Mesomelia	Shortening of middle segment of limb
Acromelia	Shortening of distal segment of limb
Dysplasia	Generalized abnormality of development, e.g. skeletal dysplasia

In trying to describe dysmorphic features, in particular facial characteristics, everyday language may be very imprecise and subjective so it is helpful to use defined terms (Table 14.12) as far as possible and to keep photographic records. The objectivity may also be improved by anthropometric measurements. There is a considerable literature on the use of anthropometric measurements in dysmorphology but some of the more useful measurements are listed in Jones.[15]

The diagnosis of a dysmorphic syndrome depends primarily on pattern recognition and knowledge. The task has been helped by the publication of some excellent photographic atlases.[51] As there are now over 2000 malformation syndromes described, a computerized database is a great asset in the recognition of rare syndromes which may have been described on only a few occasions.[52,53]

The subject of dysmorphology has proven itself in identifying the genes that control normal development. Genetic studies in Waardenburg syndrome (deafness, heterochromia and depigmentation) have led to the identification of a developmental gene responsible for the migration of cells from the neural crest.[54] Studies on craniosynostosis syndromes such as Pfeiffer and Apert syndrome have identified a group of genes such as fibroblast growth factor or fibroblast growth factor receptor which play a very significant part in skeletal development.[55]

COUNSELING AND GENETIC SERVICES

ORGANIZATION OF SERVICES

While all pediatricians and other doctors will be involved in providing some genetic information and counseling to their patients, the increasing complexity of medical genetics has led to the development of a new specialty which links the clinical and laboratory aspects. In England each regional health authority (population 1.5–4.5 million) has a regional genetic service, which combines clinical and laboratory skills. One of the important aspects of such a service is that it is orientated towards the extended family rather than the individual, and as such can provide the follow-up required for chromosome translocations or single gene disorders. Separate family records are kept on a long term basis as opposed to the relatively short periods for which individual records are kept in most general hospitals. In addition to this, DNA may be 'banked' from family blood samples and be available for family studies in the future. Coordinating this may require a computerized follow-up or genetic register. The philosophy of family orientated screening can provide a highly personalized service which is very cost effective in terms of preventing handicap.

APPROACHES TO GENETIC COUNSELING

As in all areas of medicine the first stage of genetic counseling is to establish an accurate diagnosis. Without accurate diagnosis the counseling may be erroneous. There are a number of problems in establishing a diagnosis which are unique to medical genetics. The first is the enormous number of genetic disorders which have now been described. There are over 17 000 single gene traits or disorders.[56] In addition to this, there are many chromosomal abnormalities and malformation syndromes, and the number of disorders described is increasing exponentially. The second problem is that the disorders are often very rare and thus even a specialist covering a relatively large population cannot rely solely on his own personal experience, but must be familiar with the medical literature. A third problem is heterogeneity. *Heterogeneity* may be at the clinical or molecular level. At the clinical level it means that two or more disorders may have the same phenotype, e.g. both Marfan syndrome and homocystinuria have dislocation of the lenses with a similar physical habitus, but Marfan syndrome is autosomal dominant, whereas homocystinuria is autosomal recessive. At a molecular level it means that a number of different allelic mutations can cause the same disease. This point is of considerable practical significance if a specific DNA diagnosis is to be made. Fourthly, the individuals who come to the genetic clinic may not themselves have any clinical features of the genetic disorder in question and so clinical examination will not necessarily provide the appropriate diagnosis. It is essential before seeing the individual in the clinic to obtain as much background medical information about the family as possible. This may mean a careful search of hospital records and considerable ingenuity in tracking the results of autopsies or laboratory investigations.

Having established the correct diagnosis it is then necessary to discuss the prognosis and likelihood of recurrence. It is particularly important to discuss the prognosis in the case of parents whose experience of a disorder may be limited because, for example, the disease has not yet progressed to any significant extent in their affected child. It should also be remembered that some conditions, such as neurofibromatosis, may show a considerable range of expression and this should be taken into account in giving advice. The risk of passing on the gene for neurofibromatosis is 1 in 2, but as only about one third of patients have serious medical complications from the disease the risk of serious complications in offspring is $1/2 \times 1/3$ or 1 in 6.

Having diagnosed the disorder and given guidance about recurrence and prognosis, the next stage is to discuss the options that may be available to the couple (Table 14.13). It must be stressed that these reproductive discussions are personal choices rather than medical decisions and the counselor's approach should remain nondirective. The immediate aim of genetic counseling is to inform and support families faced with genetic disease rather than reduce the frequency of genetic handicap per se.

Table 14.13 Options which may be available for couples receiving genetic counseling

No further action
Restrict family size
Adoption
Artificial insemination by donor
Ovum donation or preimplantation diagnosis

With advances in technology accurate prenatal diagnosis can be offered for most genetic disorders and malformations. This may be by ultrasound or by an invasive test such as amniocentesis or chorionic villus sampling. For severe handicaps the option of termination of pregnancy is welcomed by many couples but in some cases prenatal diagnosis may also be used to guide and improve early neonatal treatment such as corrective surgery. In these instances it is very helpful for the couple to have the opportunity to discuss the surgical management with the pediatric surgeon when a diagnosis is made during pregnancy.

Choosing the right time for genetic counseling is very important. The couple whose child has just died from a major congenital malformation will usually want to come to terms with their loss before considering the recurrence in further pregnancies. On the other hand, leaving genetic counseling until pregnancy is advanced may produce an emotional crisis that could have been avoided by anticipation. It is to the advantage of the family and the geneticist if the initial referral is made before pregnancy.

While the above description outlines one approach to genetic counseling, it is important that the counselor's approach should be flexible. It is important to allocate sufficient time for the counseling session and to be able to elucidate the couple's feelings with open ended questions. It should be noted that a report from a working party of the Clinical Genetics Society in the UK (endorsed by the Royal College of Paediatrics and Child Health) regarded genetic screening of children for late onset disorders when there is no treatment for the disorder screened (e.g. Huntington disease) to be unethical.[57]

It has been shown that a patient's comprehension of the genetic information is limited by anxiety and the counselor must ensure that the patient is given every opportunity to express feelings and be put at ease as far as possible. It is often helpful to follow the session with a letter to the family outlining the important pieces of information and give them the opportunity of a further session or sessions to discuss the matter further. The consequences of genetic counseling can be profound and far reaching and so such advice should not be given lightly. Further information on genetic counseling is given elsewhere.[58]

GENETIC SCREENING IN THE POPULATION

The usual provision of genetic services is on an individual or family basis. The follow-up in families may be extended to the wider family and may be on a long term basis. This approach is difficult using the normal hospital record systems, and a computerized genetic register may be developed. The genetic register can program follow-up for screening tests and make appointments for counseling when children grow up and want to make their own decisions.

It has also been recognized that genetic testing might be very effective for public health screening and the prevention of inherited disease. The development of genetic services for population screening requires a different approach (Ch. 10). The development of a population screening program should meet certain criteria:

1. The screening test should allow a useful outcome either because early diagnosis will improve treatment or because genetic testing allows reproductive choice.
2. The testing should be socially and ethically acceptable which means that issues of consent and discrimination need to have been fully considered.
3. The screening test must be accurate with a high sensitivity and specificity.
4. The screening program should be cost effective with the benefits outweighing the costs.

In many inherited diseases the rarity of the condition will not justify specific screening in the population but there is the possibility of adding many other tests onto the present neonatal blood spots as many different PCR tests can be undertaken with the same sample. Such an approach would widely increase the opportunity for screening but would require a great deal more information to be given with a consent process. There is considerable debate at present about the possibility of neonatal screening for cystic fibrosis. It appears that early diagnosis will improve the prognosis, so there is a benefit, but there is no consensus on the most appropriate approach to testing.[59] It is relatively easy to include a DNA test on the Guthrie card but the genetic tests for cystic fibrosis cannot be used alone as they are relatively expensive and only pick up 90% of the known mutations. The pilot studies are evaluating using IRT (immunoreactive trypsin) measurement on the Guthrie card as the first step of screening. This may be followed by a DNA test for cystic fibrosis mutations. One of the problems with this is that the test cannot easily distinguish between a heterozygote carrier and an affected child with a known mutation and a second rare unidentified mutation. Further help may come from a second IRT measurement as the level of trypsin declines with age in the first few weeks of life and a persistently high level is strongly suggestive of cystic fibrosis. Neonatal screening for cystic fibrosis is being piloted in a number of studies at present and is likely to become universal across the UK when the testing dilemmas are resolved.

Several screening tests are routinely used in pregnancy (see also Ch. 11). Screening for rubella, venereal disease and rhesus incompatibility has long been established. Screening for Down syndrome is also widely used although different approaches may be taken. The use of fetal ultrasound has also allowed many fetal malformations to be recognized at an early stage, but there may be difficulties in considering this as a screening test. The test is usually used to monitor normal fetal growth, and formal consent for screening for malformations is not always requested. This may be a problem for couples who would not consider the option of termination of pregnancy. Similarly some of the ultrasound findings are also difficult to interpret and unnecessary anxieties may be raised.

With carrier screening for genetic disorders there is often difficulty in knowing which stage of life is best for screening. The neonatal period may be relatively easy from the organization point of view but the knowledge of carrier status is not needed at that stage and results will often be lost before the individual starts a family. Premarital counseling and testing may seem to be the best option but not all pregnancies are planned and such programs have had very low levels of recruitment. Testing in pregnancy may also seem relatively easy as all mothers come to the antenatal clinic but it may be a very emotional time to test and puts a great time pressure on the laboratory for rapid test results.

Many genetic screening programs will take a two stage approach. One example of this would be to take a family history asking about bowel cancer and only to offer screening to those with a first degree relative whose cancer came on before the age of 45 years. The family history is easy to take and only identifies those with a 10% or greater risk of bowel cancer, and then the use of resources for colonoscopy or gene testing is concentrated on those with highest risk. A similar approach in screening for Down syndrome in pregnancy is to use maternal age as the first risk stratification and then use biochemical or ultrasound screening as a second risk stratification with chromosome testing only offered to those at highest risk.

In some populations the risk of genetic disease may be confined to specific ethnic groups and knowing ethnic origin may be the first stage in screening. Such programs need to be carefully designed to avoid discrimination issues. Often the best approach is to make screening 'bottom up' rather than 'top down'. Rather than impose a program with government directives it is better to provide the screening resources to the specific ethnic group so that they may organize their own program. This approach has worked very successfully in screening for Tay–Sachs disease in the Ashkenazi Jewish populations.

Another two stage approach is *cascade screening*. This is effectively a systematic follow-up from the procedure already used in the genetic clinic. For example children with cystic fibrosis are identified and genotyped and counseling is offered to their immediate family. From this the screening can be offered to members of the extended family out to cousins. This means that the population that is screened is at high risk of being carriers and there is already knowledge of the disorder within the population screened. It obviously falls short of comprehensive population screening but can still be very economic and effective.[60]

REFERENCES (* Level 1 evidence)

1. Emery AEH, Mueller RF. Elements of medical genetics, 7th edn. Edinburgh: Churchill Livingstone; 1988.

2. Ellard S, Turnpenny P. Emery's Elements of medical genetics, 9th edn. Edinburgh: Churchill Livingstone; 1995.

3. Emery AEH, Rimoin DL, eds. Principles and practice of medical genetics, 2nd edn. Edinburgh: Churchill Livingstone; 1990.

4. Philips CI, Levy AM, Newton M, et al. Blindness in schoolchildren: importance of heredity, congenital cataract and prematurity. Br J Ophthalmol 1987; 71:578–584.

5. Tijo JH, Levan A. Chromosome number in man. Hereditas 1956; 42:1–6.

6. Knight SJ, Flint J. Perfect endings: a review of subtelomeric probes and their use in clinical diagnosis. J Med Genet 2000; 37:401–409.

7. Shaw-Smith C, Redon R, Rickman L, et al. Microarray based comparative genomic hybridization (array CGH) detects submicroscopic chromosomal deletions and duplications in patients with learning disability/mental retardation and dysmorphic features. J Med Genet 2004; 41:241–248.

8. Mitelman F, ed. ISCN. An international system for human cytogenetic nomenclature 1995. Basel: S Karger; 1995.

9. Chicago Conference. Standardization in human genetics. Birth Defects 1966; ii, no. 2.

10. Paris Conference. Standardization in human cytogenetics. Birth Defects: original article series, viii, 1972 & Supplement 1975, xi. New York; 1971.

11. Bush A, Beail N. Risk factors for dementia in people with Down syndrome: Issues in assessment and diagnosis. Am J Ment Retard 2004; 109:83–97.

12. Baird PA, Sadovnick AD. Life expectancy in Down syndrome adults. Lancet 1988; ii:1354–1356.

13. Glasson EJ, Sullivan SG, Hussain R, et al. The changing survival profile of people with Down's syndrome: implications for genetic counseling. Clin Genet 2002; 62:390–393.

14. Edwards JH, Harnden DG, Cameron AH, et al. A new trisomic syndrome. Lancet 1960; i:787–790.

15. Jones KL. Smith's Recognisable patterns of human malformation, 5th edn. Philadelphia: WB Saunders; 1997.

16. Slavotinek A, Shaffer LG, Shapira SK. Monosomy 1p36. J Med Genet 1999; 36:657–663.

17. Battaglia A, Carey JC. Health supervision and anticipatory guidance of individuals with Wolf-Hirschhorn syndrome. Am J Med Genet 1999; 89:111–115.

18. Mainardi PC, Perfumo C, Cali A, et al. Clinical and molecular characterisation of 80 patients with 5p deletion: genotype-phenotype correlation. J Med Genet 2001; 38:151–158.

19. Ryan AK, Goodship JA, Wilson DA, et al. Spectrum of clinical features associated with interstitial chromosome 22q11 deletions: a European collaborative study. J Med Genet 1997; 34:798–804.

20. Greenhalgh KL, Aligianis IA, et al. 22q11 Deletion: a multisystem disorder requiring a multidisciplinary input. Arch Dis Child 2003; 88:523–524.

21. Merscher S, Funke B, Epstein JA, et al. TBX1 is responsible for cardiovascular defects in velo-cardio-facial/DiGeorge syndrome. Cell 2001; 104:619–629.

22. Donnai D, Karmiloff-Smith A. Williams syndrome: from genotype through to the cognitive phenotype. Am J Med Genet 2000; 97:164–171.

23. Butler MG, Meaney FJ, Palmer CG. Clinical and cytogenetic survey of 39 individuals with the Prader-Labhart-Willi syndrome. Am J Med Genet 1986; 23:793–809.

24. Boyd S, Harden A, Patton MA. The EEG in early diagnosis of the Angelman (Happy Puppet) syndrome. Eur J Pediatr 1988; 147:508–513.

25. Malcolm S, Clayton-Smith J, Nichols M, et al. Uniparental paternal disomy in Angelman's syndrome. Lancet 1991; 337:694–697.

26. Reynolds JF, Daniel A, Kelly T, et al. Isochromosome 12p mosaicism (Pallister mosaic aneuploidy of Pallister-Killian syndrome): report of 11 cases. Am J Med Genet 1987; 27:257–274.

27. Grouchy J, Turleau C. Clinical atlas of human chromosomes, 2nd edn. Chichester: John Wiley; 1984.

28. Gardner RJM, Sutherland GR. Chromosome abnormalities and genetic counseling, 3rd edn. Oxford: Oxford University Press; 2004.

29. Schnizel A. Catalogue of unbalanced chromosome aberrations in man, 2nd edn. Berlin: Walter de Gruyter; 2001.

30. Foster JW, Dominguez-Sterglich MA, Guioli S, et al. Campomelic dysplasia and autosomal sex reversal caused by mutations in an SRY related gene. Nature 1994; 372:525–530.

31. Crisponi L, Deiana M, Loi A, et al. The putative forkhead transcription factor FOXL2 is mutated in blepharophimosis/ptosis/epicanthus inversus syndrome. Nat Genet 2001; 27:159–166.

32. Goodfellow PN, Lovell-Badge R. SRY and sex determination in mammals. Ann Rev Genet 1993; 27:71–92.

33. Ratcliffe SG, Paul N. Prospective studies on children with sex chromosome aneuploidy. Birth defects: original articles series. Vol 22, No 3. New York: Alan Liss; 1985.

34. Ropers HH, Hamel BC. X-linked mental retardation. Nat Rev Genet 2005; 6:46–57.

35. Raymond FL. X linked mental retardation: a clinical guide. J Med Genet 2006; 43:193–200.

36. Chinnery PF, Howell N, Andrews RM, et al. Clinical mitochondrial genetics. J Med Genet 1999; 36:425–436.

37. D'Adamo P, Fassone L, Gedeon A, et al. The X-linked gene G4.5 is responsible for different infantile dilated cardiomyopathies. Am J Hum Genet 1997; 61:862–867.

38. Riordan-Eva P, Harding AE. Leber's hereditary optic neuropathy: the clinical relevance of different mitochondrial DNA mutations. J Med Genet 1995; 32:81–87.

39. Cavalli-Sforza LL, Cavalli-Sforza F. The great human diasporas: the history of diversity and evolution. Massachusetts: Addison-Wesley; 1995.

40. Weatherall DJ. The new genetics and clinical practice, 2nd edn. Oxford: Oxford University Press; 1986.

41. Emery AEH. Principles and practice of medical genetics. Edinburgh: Churchill Livingstone; 1983.

42. Bundey S. Genetics and neurology. Edinburgh: Churchill Livingstone; 1985.

43. The human genome. Nature 2001; 409: 813–957.

44. The human genome. Science 2001; 1291: 1145–1434.

45. Witkowski JA. The molecular genetics of Duchenne muscular dystrophy: the beginning of the end. Trends Genet 1988; 4:27–30.

46. Griesenbach U, Alton EW. Recent progress in gene therapy for cystic fibrosis. Curr Opin Mol Ther 2001; 3:385–389.

47. Strachan T, Read AP. Human molecular genetics, 2nd edn. Oxford: BIOS Publications; 1999.

48. Southern EM. Detection of specific sequences among DNA fragments separated by gel electrophoresis. J Mol Biol 1975; 98:503–517.

49. Afzal AR, Rajab A, Fenske CD, et al. Recessive Robinow syndrome – allelic to dominant brachydactyly type B is caused by mutations in ROR2. Nat Genet 2000; 25:419–422.

50. Brooks AS, Ostra BA, Hofstra RM. Studying the genetics of Hirschsprung's disease: unraveling an oligogenic disorder. Clin Genet 2005; 67:6–14.

51. Gorlin RJ, Cohen M, Levin LS. Syndromes of the head and neck, 3rd edn. New York: Oxford University Press; 1990.

52. Winter RM, Baraitser M, Douglas JM. A computerized database for the diagnosis of rare dysmorphic syndromes. J Med Genet 1984; 21:121–124.

53. Patton MA. A computerized approach to dysmorphology. MD Computing 1987; 4:33–39.

54. Tassabehji M, Read AP, Newton VE, et al. Waardenburg's syndrome patients have mutations in the human homologue of the Pax 3 paired box gene. Nature 1992; 355:635–636.

55. Park WJ, Bellus GA, Jabs EW. Mutations in the fibroblast growth factor receptors: phenotypic consequences during eukaryotic development. Am J Hum Genet 1995; 57:748–754.

56. McKusick VA. Mendalian inheritance in man. Catalogs of autosomal dominant, autosomal recessive and X linked phenotypes, 10th edn. Baltimore: Johns Hopkins University Press; 1992. Available online: www.ncbi.nlm.gov/Omim

57. Clarke A. The genetic testing of children – Report of a working group of the Clinical Genetics Society – Chairman, Dr Angus Clarke. March 1994. J Med Genet 1994; 34:785–797.

58. Harper PS. Practical genetic counselling, 5th edn. Oxford: Butterworth Heinemann; 1996.

59. Price JF. Newborn screening for cystic fibrosis: do we need a second IRT? Arch Dis Child 2006; 91:209–210.

60. Super M, Schwarz MJ, Malone G, et al. Active cascade testing for carriers of cystic fibrosis gene. BMJ 1994; 308:1462–1467.

15

Endocrine gland disorders and disorders of growth and puberty

Christopher JH Kelnar, Gary E Butler

MECHANISMS OF HORMONE ACTION

DEFINITION

Hormones are chemical substances secreted directly into the bloodstream that affect the specific functioning of a cell or system in some other part of the body. They are produced from endocrine glands. The integration of hormone activity is of vital importance for the maintenance of a stable and appropriate internal environment and for the response to external environmental changes. Few hormones have unique actions and few bodily processes are determined by one hormone.

TYPES OF HORMONE

Hormones can be divided into four distinct broad categories in terms of glands of origin, basic chemical nature, mode of synthesis, transport in the circulation, half-life, mode of action, metabolism and excretion. The properties of these groups – peptides, steroids, iodothyronines and catecholamines – are summarized in Table 15.1. Actions at cellular level are summarized in Figures 15.1 and 15.2.

ORGANIZATION OF THE ENDOCRINE SYSTEM

The biological effects of hormones are regulated within well-defined physiological limits by a complex system of stimulation, inhibition and feedback control – secretion, delivery to target cells, recognition by receptors, exertion of a specific biological action, appropriate degradation and feedback to secretory cells to inhibit further production. Control mechanisms are complex and may involve other hormones (facilitative, additive or antagonistic), neurotransmitters and metabolic substrates. The principles are summarized schematically in Figure 15.3.

Interrelationships between environment and endocrine and central nervous systems are close. Physiological states, such as sleep, are important in the hypothalamic control of growth, and sex steroids modify behavior at puberty. The hypothalamus, situated between brain and pituitary gland, has an important integrative and regulatory role, exerting effects on the pituitary adenohypophysis via a series of small peptides secreted from the ventromedial nucleus near the median eminence. Their synthesis and release is determined by neurotransmitters such as dopamine, serotonin and noradrenaline, and others such as acetylcholine, melatonin and gamma-aminobutyric acid (GABA) may

Table 15.1 Categories of hormone

	Peptides	Steroids	Iodothyronine	Catecholamines
Synthesis	From large precursors (prohormones) via enzymatic reactions	From common precursor (cholesterol) via enzymatic reactions	In thyroid gland from iodine and tyrosine via enzymatic reactions	In adrenal medulla and in sympathetic and central nervous tissues and chromaffin tissue from phenylalanine and tyrosine via enzymatic reactions
Storage (gland of origin)	High proportion	Very little	High proportion	Very little
Solubility	Aqueous	Lipid	?	?
Circulation	Unbound	Plasma protein bound	Plasma protein bound	Unbound
Half-life	Minutes	Hours	Days	? (short)
Periphery	Little transformation	Transformation ++ increasing biological activity	Little transformation	Little transformation
Action	Via specific plasma membrane receptors and cyclic AMP (cAMP)	Via binding to cytoplasmic receptors and stimulating nuclear messenger ribonucleic acid (mRNA) and protein synthesis	As steroids (no cytoplasmic receptor for T3)	Via alpha-, beta- and dopaminergic cell surface receptors

cAMP, cyclic adenosine monophosphate.

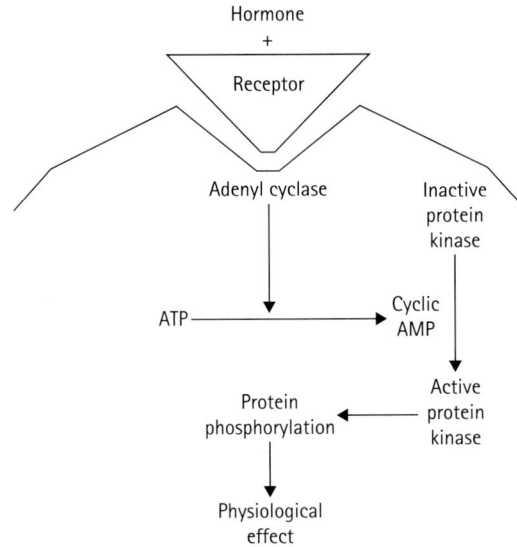

Fig. 15.1   Cellular mechanism of action of peptides.

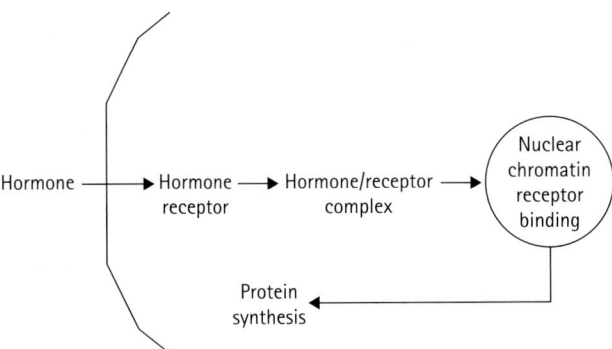

Fig. 15.2   Cellular mechanism of action of steroids.

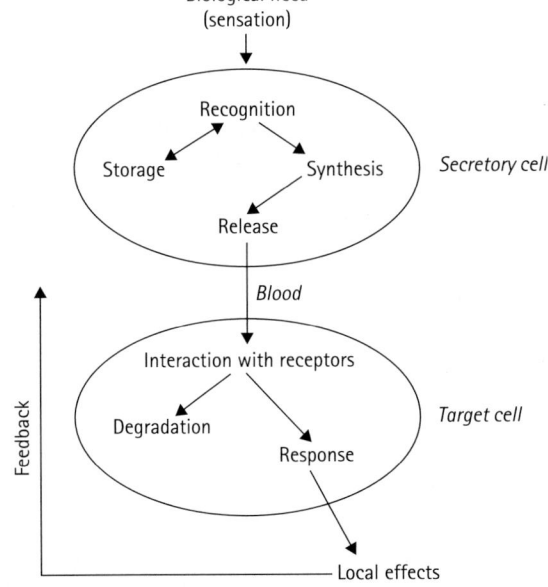

Fig. 15.3   Organization of the endocrine system.

also be important. Some peptides have stimulatory and some inhibitory activity in terms of pituitary hormone secretion.

Neurosecretory cells producing neurotransmitters are in close anatomical relationship with hypothalamic secretory neurones whose axons anastomose with portal blood vessels traversing the pituitary stalk and transporting hypothalamic peptides to the pituitary. Blood-borne anterior pituitary hormones in turn control secretion by a number of glands – thyroid, adrenals and gonads – as well as physiological processes such as growth and lactation. The ontogeny of fetal pituitary hormone secretion and brain – hypothalamo – pituitary connections is discussed on p. 415. Other endocrine systems are independent of hypothalamo-pituitary axis control – serum calcium is the major controlling mechanism for parathyroid hormone (PTH) secretion as is plasma glucose for pancreatic insulin secretion.

Hormone receptors on cell surfaces mediate the activities of water soluble protein hormones (e.g. growth hormone, IGF-1, ACTH) by signal transduction through second messenger systems. Lipid soluble hormones (e.g. thyroid hormones, steroids) act through nuclear receptors where ligand-bound receptors act at target gene promotor sequences to activate gene transcription. There are three classes of cell surface receptors: those with intrinsic tyrosine kinase activity (e.g. insulin receptor), those that recruit tyrosine kinase activity (e.g. GH receptor) and G-protein coupled receptors (e.g. ACTH receptor).

Biorhythms are a common feature of endocrine systems with periodicities of minutes or hours (e.g. LH, testosterone), a day (cortisol), weeks (menstrual cycle), seasons and life span.

Laboratory-based advances are having important impacts on endocrine practice: protein chemistry is increasing understanding of how GH regulates growth, differentiation and metabolism; transmembrane signaling can now 'explain' such pediatric endocrine disorders as McCune–Albright syndrome, pseudohypoparathyroidism (PHP) type 1, acromegaly, and many thyroid, adrenocortical and ovarian granulosa cell tumors as disorders of heterotrimeric 'G' (Gsalpha) proteins which are important for GTP binding and hydrolysis that amplifies hormonal signals. In particular, two G proteins have been identified which are susceptible to naturally occurring mutations: Gsalpha, the activator of adenylyl cyclase, and Gi2alpha, involved in adenylyl cyclase inhibition and ion channel modulation. The gene encoding Gsalpha (GNAS1) may be altered by functional loss or gain mutations. Thus heterozygous inactivating germ line mutations cause PHP type 1a in which physical features of Albright's hereditary osteodystrophy (AHO) are associated with resistance to several hormones, i.e. PTH, TSH and gonadotropins, that activate Gs-coupled receptors, or pseudopseudohypoparathyroidism in which AHO is the only clinical manifestation.[1]

Advances in molecular genetics are enabling recognition of the genetics and biochemistry of sex determination and there appears to be a major susceptibility locus for sex reversal/gonadal dysgenesis on Xp.[2] New disease mechanisms are being described – mosaicism in pseudoachondroplasia and McCune–Albright syndrome, placental mosaicism in some forms of IUGR; imprinting (parental origin effects) in Prader–Willi and Angelman syndromes, PHP, Beckwith–Wiedemann syndrome, and, possibly, Silver–Russell syndrome. Whilst genetic defects have 'explained' many eponymous syndromes, it is clear that genotype/phenotype correlations are often poor: one gene abnormality may only explain a minority of cases and mutations in one gene can cause different syndromes. Indeed even very disparate syndromes can share a common molecular genetic defect.[3]

In addition, it is clear that fetal and childhood growth may have important implications not only for the child but also for adult health and disease (see pp. 416–7).

Endocrine disorders may be due to subnormal hormone production or hormone deficiency, hormone excess, production of abnormal hormones, resistance to hormone action, abnormalities of hormone transport or metabolism or multiple hormone abnormalities. A working classification of pediatric endocrine disorders is available.[4]

HISTORY TAKING AND EXAMINATION

FAMILY HISTORY

Many endocrine disorders are familial with clear mendelian patterns of inheritance and a history of unexplained neonatal deaths may be significant in this context, particularly in parts of the world where neonatal pediatric services are poorly developed.

Genetic contributions may be less clear cut as for example in insulin dependent diabetes where the HLA identical sibling of an already affected child has about a 90-fold increased risk of developing the disease before 15 years. However, less than 1% of genetically susceptible children in the general population will ever develop diabetes. Autoimmune processes are important in pathogenesis and a family history of autoimmune disease (e.g. candidiasis, pernicious anemia, alopecia or vitiligo) should alert the clinician to disorders such as diabetes mellitus, Addison's disease, hypothyroidism or hypoparathyroidism. Growth hormone (GH) deficiency can be familial.

A family history of early or late puberty may be relevant (ask about age of menarche in mother and older girl siblings; ask fathers whether they were growing fast after they left school and when they started shaving) but there is considerable variation in the timing of puberty amongst normal family members.

Sometimes a child of normal stature is short for the parents (e.g. a girl with Turner syndrome and tall parents). An unusually short parent can have an undiagnosed disorder such as GH deficiency, skeletal dysplasia or pseudohypoparathyroidism (Fig. 15.4) which the child has inherited.

PREGNANCY

Maternal illness during pregnancy may have significant effects on endocrine function in the fetus and neonate. Neonatal hyperthyroidism is seen in about 1.5% of infants born to mothers with Graves' disease. This relates to placental transfer of human thyroid-stimulating immunoglobulins. In the first trimester, 19-norprogestogens (e.g. norethisterone) for recurrent abortion are associated with masculinization of a female fetus. In the second or third trimesters, carbimazole and thiouracil are associated with neonatal goiter and hypothyroidism; chlorpropamide may cause neonatal hypoglycemia.

NEONATAL HISTORY

Breech delivery, micropenis, hypothermia and hypoglycemia are all commoner in infants with GH insufficiency or panhypopituitarism. Birth asphyxia may be associated with subsequent precocious puberty.

Ambiguous genitalia suggest congenital adrenal hyperplasia (CAH, most commonly 21-hydroxylase deficiency in a genotypic female) or an androgen biosynthetic defect (in a phenotypic male). Severe vomiting, hyponatremic dehydration and excessive urinary sodium loss suggest a form of CAH, hypoplasia or pseudohypoaldosteronism (or renal disease). Hypertension can develop in the 11beta-hydroxylase form of CAH.

Prolonged jaundice is a clue to congenital hypothyroidism. Other clinical signs may not be present until later. Even where screening programs are in operation false negatives can occasionally occur.

PAST MEDICAL HISTORY

Very poor feeding in infancy may be associated with prolonged intrauterine growth retardation and later short stature. Recurrent hypoglycemia may be due to GH deficiency, panhypopituitarism or adrenal problems (e.g. Addison's disease). Insidious fall off in school performance is often a feature of acquired hypothyroidism.

CLINICAL EXAMINATION

Accurate height measurements (Fig. 15.15; p. 430), repeated to determine growth velocity, are important in the diagnosis of endocrine (and many other) childhood disorders. Many cause slow growth (and, ultimately, short stature) and are associated with mild or moderate obesity (best assessed using skinfold calipers (Fig. 15.5) in addition to weighing to calculate body mass index (BMI). In contrast, obesity due to an excessive food intake causes rapid growth and tall stature in childhood. Endocrine causes of abnormally rapid growth in childhood include precocious puberty, thyrotoxicosis and gigantism.

Disproportionate stature (abnormal body proportions) is seen in long-standing panhypopituitarism, hypothyroidism and GH deficiency, skeletal dysplasias and some inborn metabolic errors. Short fourth and fifth metacarpal bones are characteristic of pseudohypoparathyroidism (Fig. 15.6) and Turner syndrome.

Delayed puberty in girls may be due to Turner syndrome. Primary amenorrhea may be associated with CAH, Turner syndrome or rarer disorders of sexual differentiation.

Hirsutism (reviewed by Rosenfield[5]) may be due to a variety of causes of adrenal and ovarian dysfunction including CAH, obesity-related polycystic ovarian syndrome (PCOS) and Cushing syndrome. The last is often associated with temporarily rapid growth, truncal obesity, striae

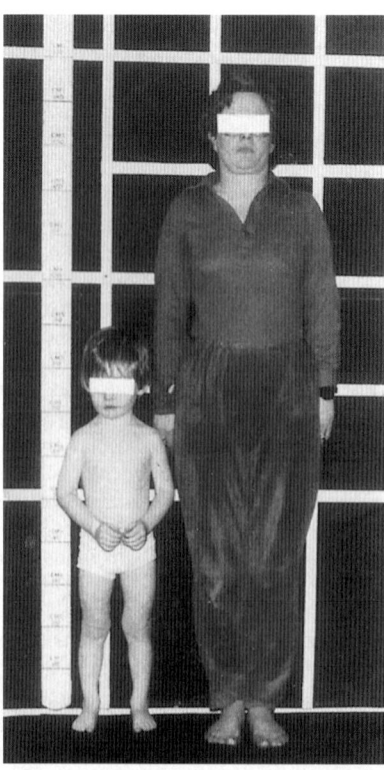

Fig. 15.4   Pseudohypoparathyroidism in mother and child (see also Fig. 15.6).

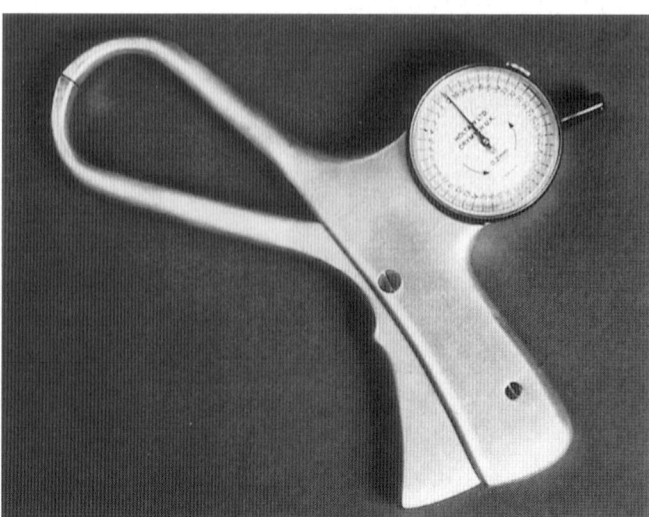

Fig. 15.5   Skinfold calipers.

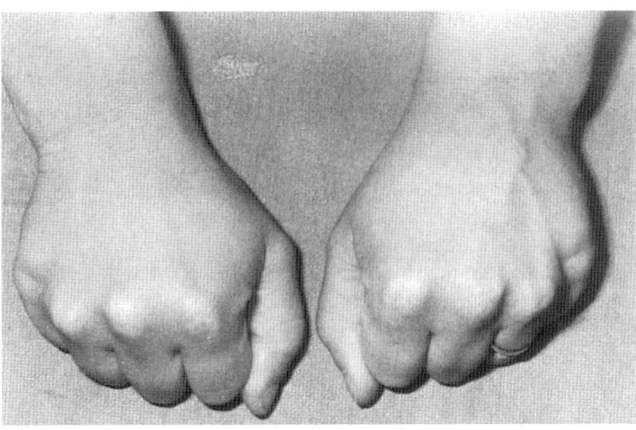

(a)

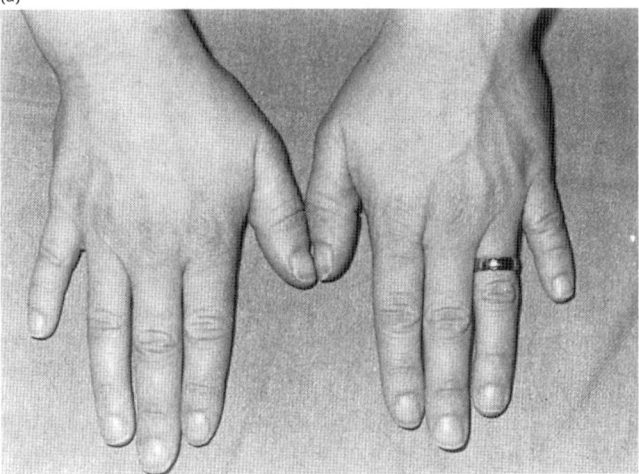

(b)

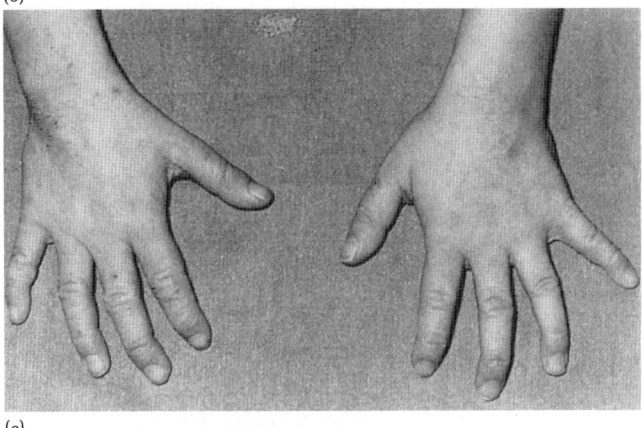

(c)

Fig. 15.6   Short fifth metacarpal in a mother (a, b) and child (c) with pseudohypoparathyroidism (see also Fig. 15.4).

and moon face. Secondary hypertension can be due to endocrine disease (usually adrenal cortical mineralocorticoid excess).

Fundal examination and visual fields assessment is vital in any child with abnormal growth or recurrent headache. Craniopharyngioma (see Ch. 24) commonly presents in this way. Dysmorphic features (especially midline abnormalities) may be associated with hypothalamo-pituitary or other endocrine disorders.

ENDOCRINE TESTS

Diagnosis can often be suspected on the basis of history and clinical findings. In puberty, clinical staging of secondary sexual characteristics is an excellent 'bioassay' of hormone function. A girl of 14 years with stage

2[6] breast development can be reassured that puberty is underway, without measuring estradiol or LH – indeed a 'random' clinic measurement would suggest the opposite (see below).

Nevertheless, biochemical assessment is often necessary, either to confirm or refute a diagnosis or to assess the appropriateness and effectiveness of treatment but the information obtained must be assessed critically if misleading conclusions are not to be drawn (see Appendix).

As many hormones are secreted episodically in pulses or may vary diurnally, a single measurement may be meaningless or misleading. Dynamic tests to assess maximum secretory capacity will give different normal values to physiological secretory profiles.

BLOOD

Stress from cannulation (or the thought of it) will affect levels of hormones such as cortisol, GH and prolactin (PRL). Baseline samples must be obtained before suppression or stimulation tests commence. A sample 30 min before baseline may, for example, help to quantify and reduce stress effects or indicate that a spontaneous pulse of growth hormone has just been secreted which will result in a blunted response to a stimulus because of the lack of a readily releasable GH pool.

It may be necessary to measure simultaneously hormones at both ends of a feedback system: ACTH levels will be inappropriately high for the normal cortisol levels in untreated CAH; raised TSH levels with normal T4 levels indicate developing (compensated) primary hypothyroidism.

Overnight fasting does not preclude day case tests if the family live nearby. Those traveling far are best admitted the previous evening. Fasting from midnight (water only allowed) is generally safe in the older child provided testing starts before 9 a.m. but is dangerous in a child with GH deficiency or panhypopituitarism. If this is suspected blood glucose levels should be checked at regular intervals overnight. Younger children are particularly vulnerable to fasting hypoglycemia.

URINE

Urine sampling is atraumatic in children (less so in infants). 24-h collections can reflect overall production of (e.g.) steroids more accurately than isolated plasma samples but can be difficult to obtain, even in hospital. Expressing results per 24 h per gram excreted creatinine may not control for incomplete timed collection[7] and even distort results.

SALIVA

Many hormones (e.g. peptides) cannot be assayed in saliva but the technique is useful for steroids, e.g. cortisol, progesterone and testosterone – concentrations are independent of flow rate and reflect free plasma levels. Most children over about 6 years can produce saliva. Specimens can be collected easily and non-invasively, serially or during dynamic tests.

ERRORS
Specimen collection, labeling, transport
Liaise with the laboratory beforehand if samples need special handling such as for example ACTH assay samples which must be collected in cooled lithium heparin tubes, centrifuged immediately at 4°C and plasma stored at 20°C until assay.

Interpreting results
For larger polypeptides, including many hormones (whose structure cannot be physicochemically characterized), values are sometimes reported in terms of 'units' calibrated in terms of 'standards' derived from specific assays from material that may have different biological or immunological properties.

Hypersecretion is easier to diagnose than hyposecretion – a concentration half the mean of values in the normal population is more likely to fall within the 'normal range' than a concentration that is twice normal (Fig. 15.7) and it is more difficult analytically to measure low hormone levels.

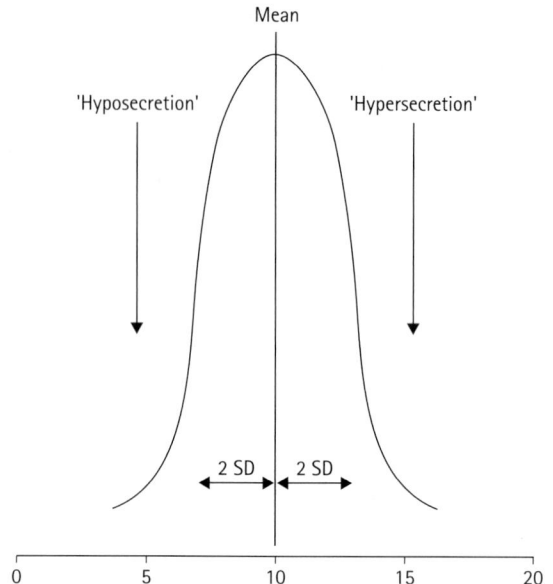

Fig. 15.7 Hypo- and hypersecretion – see text. (After Jeffcoate 1981[8])

This is important for screening tests (e.g. T4 or TSH for congenital hypothyroidism) or choosing particular assay techniques – TSH immunoradiometric assays (IRMA) give added precision at low levels compared to radioimmunoassay (RIA) (helpful in managing thyroxine replacement) and make the TRH test obsolete. LH and FSH IRMA and ultrasensitive immunofluorometric assays (IFA) are providing insights into the evolution of the hypothalamo-pituitary–gonadal axis during childhood and puberty control mechanisms for puberty (see pp. 447–9).

The prevalence of a condition is important in determining the likely significance of an abnormal result in individual patients. Screening for congenital hypothyroidism (1 in 4000) with a TSH assay with 0.1% false positive rate will yield 4 out of 5 positive results in babies without the disease.

HORMONE ACTION AND MEASUREMENT

Many assays measure total hormone plasma levels of which only a small amount may be free, unbound and metabolically active. Direct measurement of the free, active hormone is of more value in diagnosis and treatment and abnormal hormone levels due to abnormalities of the binding protein can be more easily detected. It is invalid to extrapolate from isolated plasma samples to overall secretion or production rates. Circulating hormone levels may not reflect activity at tissue level. Many hormones have paracrine activity locally at tissue level and are not released in measurable quantities into the peripheral circulation.

Many laboratory assays are based on immunoassay techniques. These have, in many areas, replaced pre-existing bioassay (in vivo) techniques. However many commercial immunoassays are less than ideally reliable because of cross-reactivity or matrix effects and, for steroid analysis for example, liquid chromatographic/tandem mass spectrometry techniques will often be preferable.

What is measured in an immunoassay may not always have biological significance. For example, in mild acromegaly GH levels as measured by RIA may be very high, suggesting that GH molecular forms with low biological activity may be present.

CIRCULATING HORMONE LEVELS AND RECEPTORS

Endocrine disorders may not only result from hormone under- or over-production but also from lack of tissue response to normal circulating concentrations. Receptor or postreceptor defects ('end-organ unresponsiveness') may be important, e.g. bone or renal unresponsiveness to PTH in pseudohypoparathyroidism, pseudohypoaldosteronism, partial insensitivity of androgen-dependent structures causing incomplete masculinization in some genotypic males or, as seems increasingly possible, in some children with 'idiopathic' growth failure.

Receptor assays, when available, may provide an indicator of biological activity. However structural and functional properties of receptors may not be the same: in a given disorder they could be abnormal in number, function or both. In clinical practice, many defects must be inferred from finding functional inadequacy in clinical terms with abnormally high circulating levels of the hormone(s) that stimulate that tissue activity.

FETAL ENDOCRINOLOGY

FETAL ENDOCRINE FACTORS

Profound perinatal changes occur in many endocrine glands. Progress in understanding fetal endocrine functioning has come from increased access to wide ranges of abortus material from normal pregnancies, animal studies (which must be interpreted carefully in applying results to man), tissue culture experiments, advances in non-invasive (ultrasound) assessment of fetal growth and techniques such as fetoscopy.

Although fetal growth is ultimately controlled by genetic endowment, it is influenced by a number of fetal factors (including hormones and growth factors), uterine environment and other environmental factors. Control of fetal growth is by complex interaction between an evolving central nervous system, endocrine maturation, local tissue (paracrine) growth factors and placental and maternal hormone secretion – within environmental constraints which may impair fetal growth (Table 15.2).

Organogenesis occurs at a variety of times and tempos: organ embryogenesis and functional cell differentiation during the first trimester; rapid growth largely due to cell hyperplasia during the second; further functional maturation during the third. It is likely that endocrine factors, fetal, maternal and placental, are more involved with nonspecific growth stimulation or maturation and that specific stimuli to growth in individual cells and cell systems result from paracrine peptide growth factors derived locally. Positive and negative feedback loops are important in the dynamic regulation of developmental signaling and feedback failure can cause disease.[9] Measurable hormone levels in fetal circulation do not necessarily indicate a functional role at that time; target organ receptors may only appear later.

Table 15.2 Factors reducing fetal growth

Maternal illness during pregnancy
Chronic maternal disease
Maternal age (less than 20, over 35 years)
Increased parity
Maternal short stature
Ethnic group
Birth weight of other family members
Lower social class
Smoking
Poor nutrition
Alcohol
Poor weight gain
Multiple pregnancy
High altitude
Genetic factors
Fetal disease
Fetal abnormalities

ONTOGENY OF FETAL HORMONE SECRETION

Anterior pituitary

The anterior pituitary is of ectodermal origin arising from Rathke's pouch, an evagination from the roof of the primitive buccal cavity appearing from about 3 weeks post conception. After 2 months, pouch anterior wall cells proliferate and differentiate to form the pituitary anterior lobe. Growth hormone (GH) is found in the fetal pituitary and circulation by 10 weeks' gestation and levels are very high (greater than 200 mU/L) by mid-pregnancy.[10]

Extrinsic and intrinsic signaling gradients determine expression patterns of pituitary-specific factors in the developing anterior pituitary gland.[11]

In man, no anterior pituitary hormone crosses the placenta in physiologically significant amounts. Fetal growth continues relatively normally with absent GH secretion – anencephalics are only slightly small for gestational age (SGA).[12] However there is a small reduction in birth length for weight in babies with congenital GH deficiency[13] – postnatal growth failure is more marked. GH receptors do not appear before the second trimester. In vitro, GH stimulates insulin-like growth factor 1 (IGF-1) release from isolated fetal hepatocytes by 12 weeks' gestation[14] but has no effect on fetal muscle growth. GH promotes beta cell replication and insulin release in pancreatic islet cell cultures from 12 to 25 week fetuses[15] and any effects of GH in utero may be via insulin (see below). Nevertheless, the human growth hormone (hGH)/human placental lactogen (hPL) gene family, which consists of two GH and three PL genes, is important in the regulation of maternal and fetal metabolism and the growth and development of the fetus.[16] However it seems that prenatal IGF-1 production is largely independent of GH and that IGF-1 (and not GH) is the major factor in intrauterine growth regulation.

PRL [198 amino acids structurally related to GH, molecular weight (MW) 22 500] is synthesized by the fetal anterior pituitary from about 7 weeks postmenstrual age[17] and the pituitary content increases subsequently. Fetal plasma levels rise during the third trimester to peak just before term. Cord blood levels are higher than maternal and normal in anencephalics (cf. GH). Its physiological role in man (other than in the initiation and maintenance of lactation in women) is unknown.

ACTH is present in fetal pituitary by 10 weeks and responsible for adrenal cortical steroidogenesis and growth.[18]

LH and FSH may be present from as early as 5 weeks.[19] At each stage, gonadotrophin (GT) levels are higher in female than male fetuses. They are probably more important for later gonadal development than for early sexual differentiation.

The cytokine receptors for growth hormone (GH), prolactin and leptin probably have a critical role in regulating embryo, placental and fetal development.[20]

Posterior pituitary

In the 6-week embryo, a downward extension of neural tissue from the floor of the diencephalon has formed the infundibulum. This gives rise to the stalk and neurohypophysis (posterior pituitary). From 12 weeks, the 9-amino-acid peptides vasopressin and oxytocin are synthesized in and secreted from the supraoptic and paraventricular hypothalamic nuclei and transported via axons in the supraopticohypophyseal tract to capillaries drained by inferior hypophyseal veins. They have no known fetal function. Vasotocin seems to be concerned with water shifts across fetal membranes.

Thyroid

Fetal thyroid is active from mid-gestation and develops autonomously from the mother. Thyroxine (T4) is present at low but increasing levels from about 20 weeks but the more physiologically active metabolite tri-iodothyronine (T3) is present only in persisting low levels from about 30 weeks. Reverse T3 (rT3) levels are high due to active conversion from T4 in fetal liver, and placenta which also deiodinates T4 and T3 to inactive rT3 and T2 respectively.

Maternal thyroid hormones exert important developmental effects on the fetal brain[21] and protect the human fetus from adverse effects of fetal thyroid hormone deficiency.[22] Maternal thyroxine plays a crucial role in the development of the fetal brain in early pregnancy. This has implications for fetal development in iodine deficient areas and underlies limitations to effectiveness of screening programs in preventing adverse neurological sequelae in every case even with early thyroxine substitution.

Adrenal

During the second month adrenal cortical tissue differentiates into peripheral neocortex and active inner fetal zone. Rapid fetal zone hyperplasia and hypertrophy occurs[23] to comprise 85% of total adrenal size and is the major site of dehydroepiandrosterone sulfate (DHAS) and 16-hydroxy DHAS production. As there is little fetal zone 3beta-hydroxysteroid dehydrogenase (3betaOHSD) activity, these compounds are produced in large quantities (equal to cortisol production) and placentally aromatized to estrogen, especially estriol. Fetal cortisol synthesis is maintained from placental progesterone and, possibly under the influence of progesterone, increased fetal zone 11beta-hydroxylase and 21-hydroxylase activity leads to considerable cortisol production. Progesterone and PRL, as well as estrogens, are implicated in fetal 3betaOHSD inhibition and thus fetal zone maintenance.

A high rate of DHAS secretion is an intrinsic property of human adrenocortical cells and ACTH is the only hormone required for its synthesis. In tissue culture, even fetal zone cells increase 3betaOHSD activity in response to ACTH to levels of definitive zone cells and distinction between zonae fasciculata and reticularis is lost. ACTH stimulation increases intra-adrenal blood flow leading to enhanced zonae fasciculata and reticularis activity but has no effect on zona glomerulosa function. Zonal differences in blood flow may therefore have important consequences on zonal function – adrenarche (see p. 480) may be a by-product of the need of the inner cells of the fetal adrenal to respond to the hormonal milieu of pregnancy by developing an androgen (i.e. estrogen precursor) synthesizing zone.

It is speculated that fetal adrenal steroidogenic patterns, which could reflect placental and fetal growth (see below), might provide a link with the development of adult hypertension.[24]

Within a few days of birth the fetal zone rapidly begins to atrophy. By 3 months the adrenal weight has halved and the weight at birth is not regained until puberty.

Gonads

Primitive gonads appear in the fourth week as a longitudinal ridge of proliferating celomic epithelium and underlying mesenchyme between mesonephros and dorsal mesentery. Primordial germ cells appear in the yolk sac wall by 3 weeks and migrate towards and enter the ridges by 6 weeks until when male and female human fetal gonads are morphologically identical. Primitive, undifferentiated gonads will develop in a female manner unless directed towards male differentiation by the presence of the sex-determining region of the Y chromosome – SRY (see below).

In females, proliferating epithelial cords surround primordial germ cells in the mesenchyme. These cords subsequently degenerate and are replaced by others which remain near the surface of the gland whilst the surface epithelium thickens. Germ cells develop into oogonia surrounded by follicular cells derived from surface epithelium.

From the third month, oogonia undergo meiosis to form primary oocytes which, by birth, have completed prophase of the first meiotic division and entered a resting stage. At sexual maturity, they complete the first meiotic division to form secondary oocytes which are extruded into the Fallopian tube at ovulation. Primary oocytes are surrounded by a layer of flat epithelial cells, later to form the granulosa cells – the complex is known as the primordial follicle. This is surrounded by a basal lamina and, externally, a layer of thecal cells. In the maturing follicle there is oocyte enlargement, granulosa cell proliferation and thecal differentiation into inner vascular and outer fibrous layers. Some 6–7 million oogonia are present by 6 months post conception but only 2–4 million primordial follicles at birth and less than half a million by menarche. Most follicles degenerate – only a few are lost by ovulation during reproductive life.

In males, in the presence of a Y chromosome carrying a testis determining gene – sex-determining region of the Y chromosome (SRY) – on its short arm and cell membrane histocompatability (H-Y) antigen, normally the primitive sex cords proliferate and differentiate to form testis cords. These become separated from surface epithelium by a layer of dense fibrous connective tissue (tunica albuginea) which, with the degeneration of the surface epithelium, forms the testis outer surface (capsule).

The testis cords differentiate to form the rete testis and straight and convoluted tubules. They remain solid until puberty when they develop a lumen and form seminiferous tubules. In the fetus they comprise primitive germ cells surrounded by supporting cells which will eventually develop into Sertoli (sustentacular) cells. Leydig (interstitial) cells develop from mesenchyme.

The major hormonal stimulus for fetal Leydig cells is testosterone, and for primitive seminiferous tubule, germ cell and Sertoli cell formation it is placentally derived human chorionic gonadotrophin (HCG). At this stage, there is little pituitary GT secretion – anencephalic male genital tract development is normal.

Before gonadal differentiation, Wolffian ducts have already developed (by 4 weeks). Müllerian ducts appear at about 7 weeks. In males, in the presence of a testis, degeneration of Müllerian structures occurs by 9 weeks under the influence of anti-Müllerian hormone (AMH), a high molecular weight glycoprotein secreted by the Sertoli cells.[25] AMH is a member of the transforming growth factor beta (TGFbeta) family (like the inhibins and activins). The human AMH gene has been cloned and mapped to the short arm of chromosome 19. There is a critical period during which Müllerian tissue is sensitive to inhibition by AMH – although AMH is now known to be produced by Sertoli cells until puberty, no postnatal physiological effects have been identified. In women, AMH is produced by the granulosa cells of preantral and small antral follicles and may be a useful marker of ovarian aging and follicular reserve.[26]

Leydig cell testosterone secretion is responsible for persistence of the Wolffian ducts and their differentiation into epididymis, vas deferens, seminal vesicles and ejaculatory ducts. Male external genitalia are sensitive to dihydrotestosterone (DHT) rather than testosterone and the enzyme which converts the latter to the former, 5alpha-reductase, is present in high concentrations in these tissues. DHT is responsible for fusion of labia, growth of the phallus and formation of the scrotum.

In females, in the absence of Leydig cell testosterone secretion, Wolffian ducts virtually completely disappear. The Müllerian system, in the absence of Sertoli cell AMH secretion, differentiates into upper vagina, uterus and Fallopian tubes.

In humans, it now seems that testis development depends on a regulated genetic hierarchy initiated by the Y-linked SRY gene. Several components of the testis determining pathway have been identified and it seems that early gonadal development is the result of a network of interactions instead of the outcome of a linear cascade.[27]

Development of a fetus into a phenotypic male thus depends, first, on testis formation and second, on hormone production by the fetal testis. Disorders of testicular hormone production or action can lead in severe cases to phenotypic abnormalities or can predispose towards impaired reproductive health. There is evidence, of variable quality, for deteriorating human male reproductive health, including an increase in testicular cancer and falling sperm counts. It seems likely that sperm production in adulthood is susceptible to 'hormonal' disruption in fetus and neonate, perhaps in relation to estrogenic and (especially) anti-androgenic environmental chemicals.[28]

Parathyroid

The fetus accumulates calcium rapidly. Maternal PTH and 1,25-dihydroxy cholecalciferol (1,25-DHCC) levels are high during pregnancy and there is active calcium (and phosphate) transfer to the fetus. 25-HCC crosses the placenta and preterm infants have lower levels than term infants, by when levels are comparable to those in the mother. PTH and 1,25-DHCC levels are low at birth but calcitonin levels are high. Calcitonin reduces fetal bone resorption; low PTH levels aid bone calcification.

Pancreas

Insulin is present in fetal pancreas by 8 weeks and plasma by 12 weeks and is an important anabolic factor in response to maternal glucose concentrations with major, particularly last trimester, influence on somatic size and growth. Fetal hyperinsulinemia causes adiposity and has little effect on lean body mass but there is a permissive effect on protein synthesis and hepatic glycogen deposition. Insulin does not cross the placenta in physiologically significant amounts. In normal pregnancy, fetal plasma glucose levels are modulated by maternal homeostatic mechanisms. The fetus of a poorly controlled diabetic mother has greatly increased adipose tissue stores, organomegaly and increased birth size. Other disorders associated with hyperinsulinism [e.g. persistent hyperinsulinemic hypoglycemia of infancy (HI) and Beckwith–Wiedemann syndrome] are associated with fetal overgrowth. Monogenic diseases that impair glucose sensing, lower insulin secretion or increase insulin resistance are associated with impaired fetal growth.[29] Insulin appears to have no direct action on release of IGF from human fetal connective tissue or hepatocytes in tissue culture and may act through stimulation of nutrient uptake and utilization (see below).

Glucagon is present in human fetal pancreatic tissue from 10 weeks and cannot cross the placenta. Its fetal metabolic role is still largely unknown but there is a high overall circulating insulin:glucagon ratio in the fetus favoring anabolism.[30]

Human pancreatic polypeptide (HPP) secreting cells are present in the pancreatic head by 18 weeks but sparse in the adult organ. HPP may have a role in liver glycogenolysis. The physiological role of pancreatic D (somatostatin secreting) cells, present from 10 weeks, is unknown.

Growth factors

By the second trimester, insulin-like growth factors are present in many fetal tissues including liver, kidneys, gut, lung, cardiac and skeletal muscle, fetal zone adrenal, hemopoietic cells and dermis. They are regulated independently of GH and are important for fetal growth regulation. IGF-1 is particularly important in muscle fibre, ovarian granulosa cells (causing LH receptor and sex steroid accumulation) and brain astrocyte differentiation. IGF-2, like IGF-1, has metabolic, mitogenic and differentiative actions in a wide range of fetal tissues, is highly expressed in growth plate germinal and proliferative zones and increases extracellular connective tissue matrix synthesis, especially in chondrocytes. It synergizes with nerve growth factor in promoting neurite outgrowth from sensory and sympathetic ganglia.

Epidermal growth factor (EGF) and its probable fetal form, transforming growth factor-alpha (TGF-alpha), influences the growth, differentiation and function of epithelial cells, including lung and gut. It modulates trophoblast differentiation and function in tissue culture with release of human placental lactogen (HPL) and human chorionic gonadotrophin (HCG) via placental receptors and may be important in fetal growth retardation.

Overall late gestational fetal growth is primarily determined by the functional status of the pathways by which nutrients are transferred from the mother across the placenta and taken up by fetal tissues. Both maternal and fetal endocrine systems can influence this pathway at several levels, including regulation of placental metabolism.[31]

LONG TERM IMPLICATIONS OF FETAL GROWTH

Most small for gestational age (SGA) babies are appropriately grown for their small parents, and maternal size in particular is an important determinant of birth weight. Some babies seem small because the expected date of delivery is incorrect. However, at any gestational age, babies can also be born small either because of (1) underlying pathology in the fetus (chromosomal or other genetic factors) or (2) intrauterine starvation due to abnormal placental function causing intrauterine growth retardation (IUGR). This uteroplacental insufficiency may relate to reduced maternal and placental perfusion and is associated with low PO_2, low pH and raised lactate levels in the fetus and neonate and redistribution of fetal blood flow from the thoracic aorta to the middle cerebral artery to protect, as far as possible, the growing and maturing fetal brain.

IUGR is now thought to be important not just in the short (e.g. neonatal hypoglycemia) or medium term (e.g. difficult feeding in infancy and poor growth) but because of possible long term (adulthood) consequences. Epidemiological evidence suggests that small fetuses are more likely in adulthood to develop premature adrenarche,[32] hypertension and other cardiovascular diseases and type 2 diabetes mellitus[33] and, in girls, ovarian hyperandrogenism and polycystic ovarian syndrome.[32] Babies most at risk of subsequent hypertension are those born small with large placentae[34] and it is not yet clear how this relates to a pathophysiological classification of small babies nor whether, for example, 'normal' birth weight babies lighter than they should have been for their tall parents (and thus also starved in utero) are at risk.

Early nutrition is undoubtedly important for long term outcomes, i.e. it has biological as well as nutritional effects, and fetal malnutrition is likely to result in life-long metabolic dysregulation.[33] Preterm appropriate for gestational age babies could also be at risk of later insulin resistance.[35]

A suggested explanation for the association between low birth weight and hypertension, coronary artery disease, and insulin resistance and type 2 diabetes is thus intrauterine programming in response to maternal malnutrition. Such infants could have been exposed to excessive cortisol in utero due to relative placental 11beta-OHSD deficiency[36]. However it is possible that the link could be genetically determined insulin resistance resulting in impaired insulin-mediated growth in the fetus associated with insulin resistance in adult life.[29]

PLACENTAL HORMONE SECRETION

The placenta is the source of a hormone structurally similar to pituitary GH (differing by 13 amino acids) coded by a variant GH gene (human growth hormone V) inactive in the pituitary. Placental GH appears to be secreted into the maternal circulation in large amounts towards full term but has disappeared within 1 h of delivery.[37] Thus during pregnancy, pituitary GH (hGH-N) expression in the mother is suppressed and hGH-V, the GH variant expressed by the placenta, becomes the predominant GH in the mother.

The placenta also secretes HCG (structurally similar to thyrotrophin but with significant thyroid stimulating activity) which is more likely than fetal pituitary derived LH to be the important stimulus to fetal Leydig cell testosterone production.

MATERNAL DISEASE AND ENDOCRINE FUNCTION

Maternal thyrotoxicosis occurs in about 1 in 2000 pregnancies but hyperthyroid women seldom become pregnant unless treated, and miscarriage commonly occurs. After the first trimester there is relative independence of fetal and maternal pituitary – thyroid axes. Iodine, antithyroid drugs and human thyroid stimulating immunoglobulins (TSI) cross the placenta from mother to fetus. Neonatal thyrotoxicosis occurs in about 1.5% of infants born to mothers with Graves' disease (see later). The risk relates more to the presence of TSI than to disease activity and the disease may have been inactive for many years.

Hypocalcemia used to occur in full-term infants fed with high phosphate load cows' milk preparations. The same problem occurring in some babies on low phosphate milks suggests that maternal factors such as osteomalacia due to vitamin D deficiency (or rarer conditions such as pseudohypoparathyroidism with maternal hypocalcemia) may be important.

Fetal effects from poor maternal diabetic glycemic control are described above. Fetal hyperinsulinism causing neonatal hypoglycemia is seen there and in hyperinsulinemic hypoglycemia of infancy (HI, formerly labeled nesidioblastosis).

MATERNAL DRUGS AND ENDOCRINE FUNCTION

In second and third trimesters, substances of MW ≤ 600 cross the placenta including most drugs which are often more toxic to fetus than mother. Examples of drugs affecting endocrine function include iodides (cough mixtures, radiographic contrast media) which cause hypothyroidism with neonatal goiter, carbimazole and thiouracil (similar effects), and glucocorticoids.

NEONATAL ENDOCRINOLOGY

By late gestation, the fetus has developed significant endocrinological autonomy. Nevertheless, profound hormonal changes occur during and shortly after birth. This has implications for newborn screening: transient abnormalities may be misinterpreted as permanent, or vice versa.

Important endocrine disorders may present in the newborn. In this section, clinical and biochemical clues and general principles are discussed.

HYPOGLYCEMIA

Hypoglycemia is a common finding in the neonate although the definition of clinically significant hypoglycemia remains controversial. Pragmatic recommendations for blood glucose levels at which clinical interventions should be considered are given by Cornblath et al.[38] Fetal metabolism is essentially anabolic: enzymes concerned with formation of glycogen, fat and protein are increasingly active with advancing gestation in mammalian liver – glycogenolytic and gluconeogenic enzymes appear relatively inactive before birth. At delivery, transplacental glucose ceases. Full-term infants experience falls in blood glucose during the early hours after birth to about 2.5 mmol/L. Normal feeding is important for the subsequent rise in blood glucose levels as are hormonal changes stimulating liver glycogenolysis and gluconeogenesis and lipolysis. Glucagon levels rise, GH levels are high and there is a surge in TSH, T3 and T4 secretion.

Birth asphyxia is an important cause of neonatal hypoglycemia causing rapid depletion of glycogen stores. Glucose is the most important substrate for brain metabolism. The large neonatal brain:body mass ratio largely explains the increased susceptibility to hypoglycemia – prolonged or recurrent hypoglycemia is a preventable cause of long term neurological damage and mental retardation.

Neonatal hypoglycemia may be an important clue to endocrine disorders such as HI or insulinoma, congenital hypopituitarism (panhypopituitarism or isolated ACTH or GH deficiency) and adrenal disease causing glucocorticoid deficiency (e.g. congenital adrenal hypoplasia, hyperplasia or following bilateral adrenal hemorrhage).

Hypoglycemia, at any age, is not a diagnosis in itself (see p. 503).

MICROPENIS

Small penis and under-developed genitalia without hypospadias are characteristic findings in a male infant with pituitary disease – generalized, GT deficiency or GH deficiency – or rudimentary testes. The association with hypoglycemia is characteristic of hypothalamo-pituitary disorders; hypotonia and feeding difficulties suggest Prader–Willi syndrome. Other congenital abnormalities may suggest other syndromes in which hypogonadism is a feature.

AMBIGUOUS GENITALIA

The cause of ambiguity, and sex of the infant, cannot be identified by clinical examination alone (see Fig. 15.52) – an urgent karyotype must be obtained. If both gonads are palpable in the labioscrotal folds the baby is likely to be a male with XY karyotype in whom there is a defect in testosterone biosynthesis or tissue insensitivity to androgen. If no gonads are palpable the most likely diagnosis is congenital adrenal hyperplasia (CAH) – watch for possible salt loss in the commonest type (21-hydroxylase deficiency). Rarely hypertension will develop (11beta-hydroxylase deficiency).

Fetal androgen deficiency in a male may result in appearances anywhere between severe hypospadias and a 'normal female'. Exposure of a female fetus to androgen may result in appearances between clitoromegaly and 'normal male'. It is important, therefore, to try to classify disorders etiologically rather than descriptively.

Gender depends on a number of features which are normally self-consistent in any one individual: genetic sex – XX or XY; gonadal sex – presence of ovaries or testes; phenotypic sex – internal and external genital structures.

PROLONGED JAUNDICE

Primary hypothyroidism was a common cause of prolonged jaundice in the UK. Even now, no screening program is problem free; check TSH levels again if there is clinical suspicion.

SALT WASTING

Vomiting, diarrhea and dehydration in the early days or weeks of life is seldom due to endocrine disease; sodium and water loss in the stool from gastroenteritis or vomiting associated with pyloric stenosis are much more common. Sodium loss in the urine is due to renal or adrenal disease. Aldosterone levels will be high in renal disease but are generally low in adrenal disease (usually CAH). In pseudohypoaldosteronism, aldosterone levels will be very high. If appropriate and prompt treatment is not given, symptoms can rapidly progress to vascular collapse with severe hyperkalemia and hyponatremia, hypoglycemia, metabolic acidosis, coma and death.

HYPOTHERMIA

Preterm babies are at particular risk of hypothermia. The SGA infant is also at increased risk because of high surface area and lack of subcutaneous fat. Suspect hypothalamo-pituitary disease with persisting hypothermia, particularly in association with hypoglycemia or micropenis.

THE SMALL-FOR-GESTATIONAL-AGE (SGA, LOW BIRTH LENGTH) BABY

Some SGA babies have grown slowly for much of pregnancy while others only more recently. These situations can be distinguished by serial ultrasound measurements of biparietal diameter and lower thoracic circumference. The prognosis for growth and development varies with the time of onset of poor growth. Babies who have grown slowly before ~35 weeks are increasingly likely to be not only light- but also short-for-gestational age at birth and to have a low head circumference. They characteristically feed extremely poorly in infancy and later may show characteristic dysmorphic features: body asymmetry, clinodactyly, triangular 'elfin' facies – the Silver–Russell syndrome – and present in childhood with short stature (see p. 439).

Some SGA babies have specific reasons for slow intrauterine growth, e.g. congenital rubella, chromosome disorders or major congenital abnormalities. Suspect Turner syndrome in a SGA female baby with peripheral edema.

UNDESCENDED TESTES

Cryptorchidism, in the context of otherwise normal external male genitalia, is much less common than normally retractile testes. Normal testes have usually descended by 36 weeks' gestation due to GT-induced testosterone. They will not do so if there is GT deficiency, defective testicular testosterone production or anatomical impediment in the line of descent (much more commonly a unilateral problem). Even in cases of unilateral cryptorchidism, the contralateral (descended) testis is now known to be frequently abnormal and cryptorchidism to be usually due to an endocrine abnormality at pituitary or testicular level or both. Karyotype and endocrine investigation should be undertaken, and hormonal treatment and, if necessary, orchidopexy during the early months of life are

now thought to be essential to optimize fertility[39]. Environmental and genetic causes for the increasing frequency of the problem are a current area of scientific interest.

SCREENING

Few infants show diagnostic features of hypothyroidism at birth and screening programs in the USA and Europe have suggested an incidence of about 1 in 4000, double that expected from results of retrospective surveys.

Congenital hypothyroidism is an excellent disease for which to screen – it is common, unreliably diagnosed clinically until too late, detectable with simple and cheap biochemical tests on small amounts of easily stored blood, and prompt and adequate treatment usually prevents significant neurodevelopmental deficit. It is generally thought that adequate treatment within 4 weeks leads to normal overall development; subtle perceptual and hearing/speech deficits may remain.[40]

There are two alternative strategies for the screening program. If T4 alone is used, there is too much overlap between normal and hypothyroid values at the end of the first week. TSH must be measured in addition in those babies where the T4 is 'low'. In many countries (including the UK) TSH is measured as the primary test – there is no overlap between normal and high levels, high levels are easier to interpret as abnormal (a level twice normal is less likely to fall within the 'normal range' – see Fig. 15.7, p. 414) and are easier to measure reliably. Hypothyroidism due to pituitary or hypothalamic disease is missed (TSH levels are low) but these babies usually have clinical features associated with other pituitary hormone deficiencies (e.g. micropenis, hypoglycemia) and thyroid function is usually sufficiently preserved to prevent neurological and intellectual problems even with later diagnosis.

Screening has shown transient abnormalities, previously unrecognized, to be almost as common in many countries. In particular, preterm infants may have temporary functional abnormalities and clear-cut diagnosis may be difficult. Any abnormal screening result must be confirmed by definitive tests before diagnosis and commitment to long term therapy but the results should not be awaited before treatment is started. Generally good results (normal mental and psychomotor development) are achieved in congenital hypothyroidism following prompt detection (by newborn screening) and early postnatal thyroxine treatment in adequate dosage.

It is possible to screen newborn babies for 21-hydroxylase deficiency for raised 17OH progesterone levels using the 'Guthrie' test filter paper. The incidence is between 1 in 5000 and 1 in 23 000 (gene frequency in Europe and USA ~1 in 100). Boys do not have significant abnormalities at birth and there may be significant morbidity or even mortality if they present without warning with salt wasting. The non-salt losing boy (around 50% in the UK) presents late with pseudoprecocious puberty, rapid growth and tall stature but a short final height prognosis. Despite significant morbidity from late diagnosis and many newborn screening programs worldwide, in the UK it is generally considered unnecessary or 'uneconomical' to screen even though this would only add a small additional unit cost in the screening laboratory already measuring TSH and phenylalanine.

DISORDERS OF SEX DIFFERENTIATION (DSD)

Normal fetal sexual differentiation is described earlier. Currently, further insights are being developed into the control of testis maturation in man using a primate (marmoset) rather than a rodent model.[41] It is increasingly possible to determine underlying molecular genetic and pathophysiological processes that have led to inappropriate virilization or its inappropriate lack and a novel human sex-determining gene has been recently linked to Xp11.21–11.23.[2] Nevertheless descriptive terms are sometimes of value (if they are not used simply to hide ignorance).

Abnormal external genitalia may be found in many dysmorphic syndromes and an international consensus statement on the nomenclature and management of disorders of sex differentiation has been published.[42] Specific disorders of fetal sex differentiation have been descriptively categorized on the basis of gonadal (dys)morphology into the following three groups:

46XX DSD (formerly known as female pseudohermaphroditism)

There is virilization of *external* genitalia with XX karyotype and normal ovaries and Müllerian structures. Important causes are summarized in Table 15.3. Virilization may be due to excessive fetal androgen production or exposure to increased transplacental androgen (maternal or iatrogenic). Some remain idiopathic.

Preterm female infants have underdeveloped labia mimicking 'clitoromegaly'. Clitoromegaly is found in some rare dysmorphic syndromes (e.g. Beckwith, Seckel and Zellweger).

Virilization by fetal androgens
Virilizing congenital adrenal hyperplasia
See p. 480.

21-hydroxylase (P450c21) deficiency

This is the commonest cause of virilization in the genotypic female. The degree of intrauterine virilization may depend on the completeness of the block, but the degree of salt loss, when present, correlates poorly with the degree of virilization.

Some females have relatively normal looking genitalia at birth but in the majority there is clitoromegaly and variable labial fusion. There may be a urogenital sinus with common opening for urethra and vagina. In severely affected cases, appearances are 'normal male' with a 'penile' urethra but with no testes in the 'scrotum'. Ovarian and Müllerian development (upper vagina, cervix, uterus and Fallopian tubes) is normal. Most males appear normal at birth – the scrotum may occasionally appear pigmented and the penis large.

11beta-hydroxylase (P450c11) deficiency

Virilization is variable but may be severe enough for females to be brought up as males. It is much less common than 21-hydroxylase deficiency but relatively common in the Middle East. Hypertension, which occurs in some, takes time to develop. Males appear normal at birth.

3beta-hydroxysteroid dehydrogenase deficiency

Ambiguous genitalia occur in either sex. Males are incompletely virilized (see below). Females are virilized by excessive production of the (weak) adrenal androgen dehydroepiandrosterone (DHA). There is usually severe associated salt wasting in early infancy.

Other causes of fetal androgen overproduction, for example adrenal adenoma or congenital nodular adrenal hyperplasia, seem excessively rare.

Transplacental virilization
Maternal androgens
Variable fetal virilization from maternal ovarian and adrenal tumors has been described.[43]

Iatrogenic
During the 1950s recurrent spontaneous abortion was treated with natural (progesterone, 17OH progesterone) and synthetic (medroxy-progesterone, norethynodrel) progestogens with androgenic properties resulting in significant virilization of female fetuses. Such treatment is now almost never used.

46XY DSD (formerly known as male pseudohermaphroditism)

Incomplete virilization of the *external* genitalia, XY karyotype and normally differentiated testes occurs for one of three reasons (see Table 15.4): abnormality of AMH secretion or action, deficient fetal testosterone synthesis due to Leydig cell hypoplasia or an inborn metabolic error, or impaired peripheral androgen metabolism. There is an association with other abnormalities in rare dysmorphic syndromes (e.g. Meckel, Opitz and Smith–Lemli–Opitz). The genetics of undermasculinization is reviewed by Ahmed and Hughes.[44]

Persistent Müllerian structures

This is a rare familial condition in which Müllerian structures (Fallopian tubes and uterus) may be found in males whose genitalia may generally look normal apart from cryptorchidism.

Deficient fetal testosterone biosynthesis
Leydig cell hypoplasia

This is another rare disorder, probably autosomal recessive (but obviously male limited) with defective Leydig cell differentiation and testosterone response to HCG. The phenotype is female but Müllerian structures are absent because of normal Sertoli cell AMH production.

Inborn errors of testosterone biosynthesis (see Fig. 15.8)

These result in defective virilization of the male's internal and external genitalia. Adrenocortical steroid biosynthesis is affected when the defect is at an early stage in the pathway so that hypoglycemias and salt loss may occur. AMH synthesis is unaffected; Müllerian structures are absent.

Cholesterol desmolase deficiency [(P450scc) cholesterol side chain cleavage deficiency, lipoid adrenal hyperplasia]

This is due to deficiency of any of the microsomal enzymes 20alpha-hydroxylase, 20,22-desmolase (the rate limiting step) or 22alpha-hydroxylase converting cholesterol to pregnenolone, causing defective androgen, glucocorticoid (GC) and mineralocorticoid (MC) biosynthesis with cholesterol accumulation in the gland. The P450scc gene is located in the q23 to q24 region of chromosome 15. In surviving cases, genitalia appear female and there is severe salt loss and hypoglycemia, often with fatal outcome; prompt treatment may be life saving.

3beta-hydroxysteroid dehydrogenase deficiency (3beta-HSD)

Two genes encode for 3beta-HSD: type I (placental) and type II (adrenal and gonadal). Patients with classical 3beta-HSD deficiency have type

Table 15.3 Causes of female pseudohermaphroditism

Virilization by:
1. Fetal androgens – congenital adrenal hyperplasia (21-hydroxylase, 11beta-hydroxylase, 3beta-hydroxysteroid dehydrogenase deficiencies)
2. Maternal androgen-secreting tumor
3. Iatrogenic (progestational abortifacients)
4. Miscellaneous (see text)
5. Idiopathic

Table 15.4 Causes of male pseudohermaphroditism

Impaired Leydig cell activity
  Leydig cell hypoplasia
  Inborn errors of testosterone biosynthesis (see Fig. 15.8)
Impaired peripheral tissue androgen metabolism
  5alpha-reductase deficiency
  Receptor defects
    Testicular feminization (complete)
    Testicular feminization (incomplete)
    Reifenstein syndrome
    Infertile male syndrome
Postreceptor defects
Abnormal secretion or action of AMH (persistent Müllerian duct syndrome)
Associated with dysmorphic syndromes (e.g. Opitz, Smith–Lemli–Opitz)

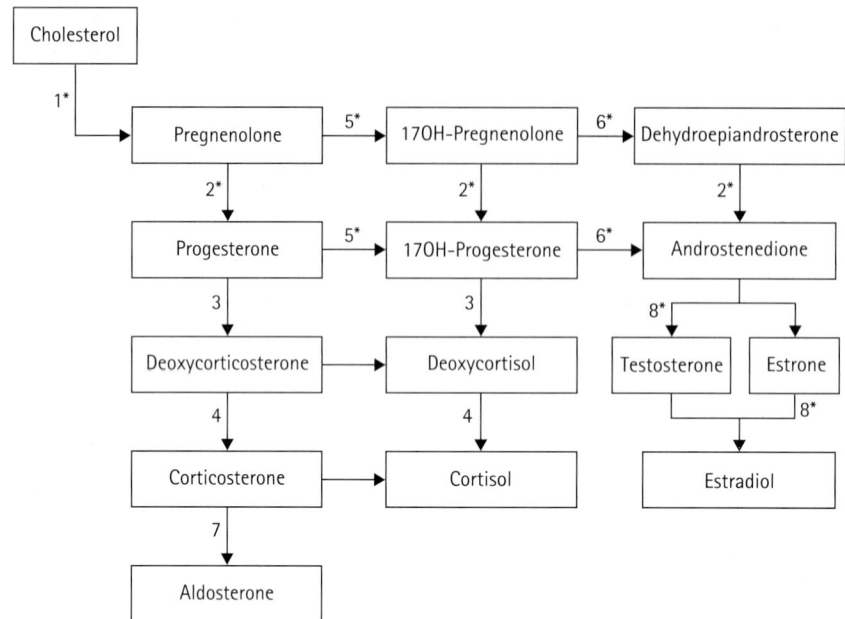

Fig. 15.8 Inborn errors of testosterone biosynthesis – marked with an asterisk (compare with Fig. 15.50). 1* – cholesterol side chain cleaving system (20alpha-hydroxylase, 20,22-desmolase, 22alpha-hydroxylase); 2* – 3beta-hydroxysteroid dehydrogenase; 3 – 21-hydroxylase; 4 – 11beta-hydroxylase; 5* – 17alpha-hydroxylase; 6* – 17,20-lyase (desmolase); 7 – 18-hydroxylase and 18-hydroxysteroid dehydrogenase; 8* – 17beta-hydroxysteroid dehydrogenase.

II gene point mutations. Genotypic males are incompletely (variably) virilized. Wolffian structures are normal. Salt loss and hypoglycemia are generally severe with high mortality.[45]

17alpha-hydroxylase deficiency (P450c17)

This results in GC and androgen deficiency (hypoglycemia and complete lack of virilization) plus mineralocorticoid excess due to ACTH drive (Fig. 15.8) resulting in hypokalemic alkalosis and hypertension. At puberty there may be virilization with gynecomastia.

17,20-desmolase (P450c17 17,20-lyase deficiency)

This is characterized by inadequate virilization and excessive urinary pregnanetriolone excretion. Gluco- and mineralocorticoid pathways are intact. Nevertheless, a single gene encoding cytochrome P450c17 controls both 17alpha-hydroxylase and 17,20-desmolase activities – combined defects have been reported regardless of phenotype.

17beta-hydroxysteroid dehydrogenase deficiency

There is defective conversion of androstenedione to testosterone and estrone to estradiol.[46] Adrenal steroidogenesis is normal. In most cases, male infants are sufficiently poorly virilized to be reared as females but there is significant virilization at puberty.

Impaired peripheral androgen metabolism

There are three types, collectively constituting the commonest group of male pseudohermaphrodite patients:
1. 5alpha-reductase deficiency;
2. X-linked abnormalities of the androgen receptor (including complete or incomplete androgen insensitivity, Reifenstein and the infertile male syndromes);
3. postreceptor (receptor-positive) resistance (a similar clinical spectrum to 2 but normal receptor function).

5alpha-reductase deficiency

Virilization of external genitalia in the male fetus requires testosterone and dihydrotestosterone (DHT). DHT is formed from testosterone by the action of 5alpha-reductase type 2 (5alphaR-2) Two human cDNA clones for 5alpha-reductase have been isolated and the 5alpha-reductase 2 gene mapped to band 23 of the short arm of chromosome 2 (2p23).

Mediation of androgenic effects requires a functional androgen receptor (AR) located in the cytoplasmic compartment of target cells. Any event which impairs DHT formation (mutation within the 5alphaR-2 gene or 5alphaR-2 inhibitors) or normal function of the AR (mutation in the AR gene, anti-androgens) may result in insufficient androgen action in the male fetus and in subsequent undervirilization in the newborn.[47]

5alpha-reductase deficiency is an autosomal recessive defect. The biochemical defect is in the conversion of testosterone to dihydrotestosterone (DHT) in the androgen target cell characterized by a high plasma testosterone:DHT ratio (after HCG stimulation in prepuberty). Definitive diagnosis is by finding diminished 5alpha-reductase activity in genital skin fibroblast cultures. Newborn external genitalia appear female (fetal DHT deficiency produces a very small phallus and perineal hypospadias) but the testosterone-dependent internal (Wolffian) genital structures develop normally with testes capable of spermatogenesis.

At puberty considerable, but incomplete, virilization occurs spontaneously with male body habitus, psychosexual orientation and gender conversion. External genitalia remain small but large testosterone doses may produce cosmetic improvement. DHT therapy has proved disappointing.

Androgen receptor defects

These may result either from major structural abnormalities of the androgen receptor (AR) gene or point mutations altering either AR messenger RNA or single amino acids causing a spectrum of appearance from 'female' (complete and incomplete testicular feminization) to 'male' (Reifenstein syndrome and infertile male syndrome). The AR gene has been cloned and is located on Xq11–12. Mutations in exon 2 and 3 code for the DNA region have been identified in patients with 'receptor positive' androgen insensitivity. However most mutations are in exons 4–8 which code for the steroid binding domain – 'receptor negative' androgen insensitivity.

As well as natural mutations in the 5alphaR-2 gene and AR gene, recent attention is being focused on environmental endocrine disruptors that are able to mimic steroid 5alpha-reductase deficiency or partial androgen insensitivity syndrome. Any event which impairs DHT formation (mutation within the 5alphaR-2 gene or 5alphaR-2 inhibitors) or normal function of the AR (mutation in the AR gene, anti-androgens) may result in insufficient androgen action in the male fetus and in subsequent undervirilization in the newborn. Hypospadias may be due to a defect in androgen action due to mutation of the 5alphaR-2 or of the AR gene and mutation of unidentified genes may underlie displacement of the urethral meatus from the tip to the ventral side of the phallus. An etiological role for environmental industrial and agricultural chemical products has also been postulated, since ethnic as well as geographical differences in the incidence of hypospadias have been noted.[48] Thus cryptorchidism and micropenis may represent a distinct phenotype, even if they are isolated, and etiological factors include 5alpha-reductase 2 gene, AR gene mutation or environmental hormonal disruptors (chemicals or phytoestrogens).[28] The hypothesis of the testicular dysgenesis syndrome (TDS) proposes that several disorders of the male reproductive system such as infertility, hypospadias, cryptorchidism and testicular cancer are all manifestations of TDS, which is most likely initiated during early fetal development and may be provoked by external factors such as endocrine disruptors in addition to genetic predisposition.[49]

Complete testicular feminization: patients generally present after puberty with primary amenorrhea but normal breast development, scanty pubic and axillary hair, and female body habitus and psychosexual orientation. There is a short blind-ending vagina as Müllerian structures have regressed. Gonads show Leydig cell hyperplasia with defective spermatogenesis and may undergo malignant change if they are not removed. In *incomplete testicular feminization* there is more virilization with prepubertal clitoromegaly and variable labial fusion. There may be a mixture of virilization and feminization at puberty.

In *Reifenstein syndrome* appearance is generally male but with severe (perineal) hypospadias. Virilization at puberty may be significant but still inadequate and associated with gynecomastia. There is male psychosexual orientation and infertility. In the *infertile male syndrome* there is a normal prepubertal male appearance although penis and testes may be rather small. Gynecomastia develops at puberty and there is oligospermia and infertility.

ABNORMAL GONADAL DIFFERENTIATION

This is a clinically heterogeneous group, including true hermaphroditism and syndromes of dysgenetic gonadal development. In most there is ambiguity of external genitalia in the newborn.

True gonadal disorder ('true hermaphroditism') usually presents with abnormal external genitalia (e.g. phallus with urogenital sinus at the base). Testicular and ovarian tissue are present, more commonly as ovotestes than as separate gonads. The commonest karyotype is 46XX (58%), 10% are XY and the remainder mosaics, of which the commonest is 46XX/46XY (13%). If the diagnosis is made neonatally, testicular tissue should be removed, and gender assignment should be female – there is good feminization at puberty with menstruation and fertility is possible.

XX males usually present with hypogonadism as adults but genital ambiguity may occur.

Klinefelter syndrome may be suspected in a neonate with hypospadias, small testes and extension of the scrotal skin onto the shaft of a small penis or found by serendipity at antenatal screening but is seldom diagnosed before the time of puberty (see p. 459).

Mixed gonadal dysgenesis: generally there is a testis with Wolffian (and absent Müllerian) structures on one side, with streak gonad and Müllerian (but poorly developed Wolffian) development on the other. Karyotype is generally 46XY or 45XO/46XY mosaic – the latter associated with clinical features and the growth pattern of Turner syndrome. Bilaterally dysgenetic testes are less common. In both groups there is a high risk of malignant change in the gonads.

Turner syndrome. See pp. 455–6.

Pure gonadal dysgenesis seldom presents before puberty. There are normal female external genitalia but the karyotype may be 46XX or 46XY. Gonadal malignant change is common.

Agonadism presents in a variety of clinical guises depending on the timing of testicular involution. There may be normal female appearances with absent Müllerian and Wolffian structures, micropenis with rudimentary testes or anorchia in an otherwise normal male.

CLINICAL MANAGEMENT
Initial assessment

Uncertainty as to the sex of their newborn baby is extremely distressing to parents. Emphasize that their baby's sex will be swiftly determined, the baby is either male or female (and not 'somewhere in between') and that the cause of the problem will be discovered. Birth should not be registered until sex of rearing is decided. Appearance of external genitalia is important in this decision – an adequately functional phallus cannot be created out of very little tissue – but is unhelpful in reaching an etiological diagnosis.

Check the family history and for any hormone treatment during the pregnancy. Look for associated abnormalities or dysmorphic features. The most important aspect of clinical examination is for the presence of gonads – a clinical classification, based on the number of abnormalities or dysmorphic features, is useful for planning immediately relevant investigations[50]:

In *all* patients, an urgent karyotype is indicated for diagnostic purposes

If *no* gonads are palpable: the most likely diagnosis is the 21-hydroxylase deficiency in a genotypic female – salt loss may occur. Measurement of plasma 17OH progesterone will confirm the diagnosis; urinary pregnanetriol levels are high. 11-Deoxycortisol levels are high in 11beta-hydroxylase deficiency. Male pseudohermaphroditism with intra-abdominal testes is much less common and true hermaphroditism very rare.

If *one* gonad is palpable, mixed gonadal dysgenesis (usually with XO/XY karyotype) is least uncommon. Pelvic ultrasound and genitogram, HCG test, gonadal biopsy and exploratory laparotomy may be necessary.

If *two* gonads are palpable, male pseudohermaphroditism is likely. An HCG test measuring testosterone, DHT, DHA and androstenedione will help distinguish 5alpha-reductase deficiency, testosterone biosynthetic disorders and androgen receptor or postreceptor defects. In vitro androgen binding studies and measurement of 5alpha-reductase activity in genital skin fibroblast cultures may be necessary. A genitogram may be helpful in imaging internal genitalia and lower urinary tract.

MANAGEMENT: CHOICE OF GENDER/GENDER IDENTITY

Choice should normally be based on appearance of external genitalia and functional possibilities in the context of information (cytogenetic, biochemical and radiological) about the nature of the underlying defect and implications for pubertal development. The decision should be made jointly by parents (whose ethnic background may be important in determining their views), pediatric endocrinologist and surgeon. The karyotype is not always of fundamental importance in this context. In cases where the phallus seems inadequate but there are pressures for male gender assignment, information about likely growth of the phallus in response to androgen can be predicted with depot testosterone (50 mg once monthly i.m. for 3 months).

It used to be thought that psychosexual orientation was dependent on sex of rearing but some of this work has been discredited[51] (for a journalistic but interesting account see Colapinto[52]) and from observations in the 'natural history' of patients with 5alpha-reductase deficiency[53] and those with 17beta-hydroxysteroid dehydrogenase deficiency,[54] it seems that the role of the fetal testis and androgens in 'imprinting' male gender identity is crucially important.

Nevertheless, ideally, sex of rearing should be decided as early as possible. Conventionally, surgery has been carried out so as to achieve cosmetically acceptable external genitalia by 2 years. However parent/patient organizations (such as the Disorders of sex differentiation Society of North America) have been outspoken in their view that surgery should be carried out only if and when the person with a DSD requests it, and then only after she/he has been fully informed of the risks and likely outcomes.

Sometimes, because of late presentation or late diagnosis in the older child, or if there is spontaneous 'inappropriate' feminization or virilization at puberty, gender reassignment is indicated. With expert psychiatric support and counseling this can be satisfactorily achieved but cultural considerations may again be important.

The status of the empirical evidence for the development of gender and sexuality in 46XX persons with classical CAH and its implications for clinical practice has been reviewed by Meyer-Bahlburg[55] and outcomes reviewed by Warne et al.[56]

Incidence of tumors in DSD

Patients with a Y chromosome but androgen insensitivity or a disorder of gonadal differentiation are at increased risk of neoplasia in an intra-abdominal gonad by adolescence or early adulthood. The risk with scrotal gonads is probably much less, particularly with regular clinical and ultrasound follow-up.

Carcinoma in situ, benign hamartomas and seminomas are reported in complete gonadal dysgenesis patients. In them, therefore, testes should be removed, but some argue that this should be done after spontaneous feminization has taken place at puberty. [In contrast, virilization at puberty will occur in incomplete testicular feminization (incomplete androgen insensitivity) or an androgen biosynthetic defect and the testes should be removed in childhood.]

Tumors are common in dysgenetic gonads. Benign gonadoblastomas may be endocrinologically functional, and malignant seminomas, dysgerminomas, choriocarcinomas or yolk sac tumors are reported. Unless there can be careful observation of scrotal gonads through childhood and puberty (with subsequent removal), they are best removed in childhood.

PHYSICAL GROWTH AND DEVELOPMENT

ASSESSMENT

Historical aspects

Within the last century it has been appreciated that assessment of a child's growth is the best marker of their well-being. The repeated measurement of groups of children from particular populations over the course of time has made it possible to pass comment about the influence of social changes on the health of children as this is reflected directly in growth of stature and the timing of sexual maturation. The average height of populations in resource rich countries is increasing generation upon generation but in resource limited countries inadequate nutrition with its intermittent supply still has a profound adverse effect on physical growth and on the health of children. Growth velocity remains one of the most useful indices of public health and economic well-being in both resource limited and socially heterogeneous resource rich countries[57] and the importance of this has inspired the World Health Organization to a new venture with the production in 2006 of the first set of international standards reflecting how children should grow in optimal conditions (www.who.int/childgrowth/en/ and see below).

The normal pattern of growth

The normal pattern of expected growth is traditionally displayed on a growth chart. Growth charts show the range of growth of a reference population and consequently do not describe exactly the growth curve of any individual child. Nevertheless they are important tools, but it must be remembered that each child has their own individual pattern of growth and timing of the events of puberty. This is called their 'tempo' of growth.

Which growth chart?

Two types of growth chart produced from United Kingdom data, each with a different form of construction, are currently available. The UK 1990 standards[58] are recommended for general use.[59] These are cross-sectional charts based largely on single measurements of many thousands of children at different ages, and the LMS statistical method[60] is employed to produce the mean and multiples of the standard deviation at each age and thus the smooth curves found on the growth charts (Figs 15.9–15.12). The nine centile bands are equally spread, interval 0.67 standard deviations (SD), and range between $-2\,SD$ (2nd centile) and $+2\,SD$ (98th centile). In an attempt to quantify extremes of variation, two further centile lines (0.4th and 99.6th which is $\pm 2.67\,SD$) are provided with shaded areas above and below respectively. The measurements of 1 in 250 normal children lie above and below these lines but the chances of finding a pathological cause for abnormal growth in a child is greater outwith these boundaries. The Buckler–Tanner charts are of the tempo-conditional type; they are constructed with a greater influence from longitudinal data, i.e. serial measurements from the same child, and the shape of the curve reflects the growth pattern of an individual child more closely.[61] These charts are only recommended for height measurements beyond the age of 2 years, weight standards already being outmoded for the UK population. Consequently they are best reserved for the longitudinal follow-up of the growth in height of an individual child. The variations in growth particularly at puberty can be followed more easily, and the additional colored lines assist in determining whether the growth of an adolescent with onset of puberty not at the 50th centile is normal or otherwise (Figs 15.13, 15.14).

Racial, ethnic and national factors

UK growth charts have mainly been constructed from measurements from the indigenous white population, whereas today's population is multiracial. There are differences in body proportions between the main three human races. People of African origin have longer legs, with the opposite being true for those of Mongolian racial origin. The pattern and tempo of growth is similar across mankind, however. Although African origin and Mongolian origin children start puberty and mature earlier than Caucasian children, individual differences do not fall outside of expected norms. Even if standards particular to each racial group were available, with so much social integration they would be little use in practice. Consequently UK 1990 charts are valid both before and during puberty for all children irrespective of ethnic background. It is the calculation of a child's target height which needs to be considered in determining whether the child is of abnormal stature, not their ethnic background per se. The WHO has considered this issue in considerable detail and commissioned the WHO Multicentre Growth Reference Study. Longitudinal growth data were collected prospectively in 8440 children from birth to 5 years, breast-fed and reared in optimal circumstances, from six countries worldwide (India, Norway, USA, Ghana, Oman and Brazil). The resulting standards are intended to represent ideal growth in healthy children irrespective of racial or ethnic origin. The charts are available in either standard deviation or centile format and can be downloaded for use from the WHO website www.who.int/childgrowth/en/.

Decimal ages and decimal charts

The year time scale on a growth chart may be divided according to weeks or months, or can have a decimal scale (i.e. thousandths of a year, usually rounded to 2 decimal places). For routine use the standard weekly or monthly subdivisions are preferable as this helps with accurate plotting. Decimal ages are advantageous when the calculation of height velocity is required and when more precise plotting of the growth chart is necessary, for example in long term follow-up. Decimal ages are calculated according to the following example (see Table 15.5 for decimal age conversion):

a.	Date of examination:	12th May 2007	Decimal date from table: 2007.359
b.	Date of birth:	23rd September 1998	Decimal date 1998.726
	Subtracting b from a:		Decimal age: 8.633 year

Height velocity can be calculated as the height increment (cm) divided by interval between measurements in decimal years:

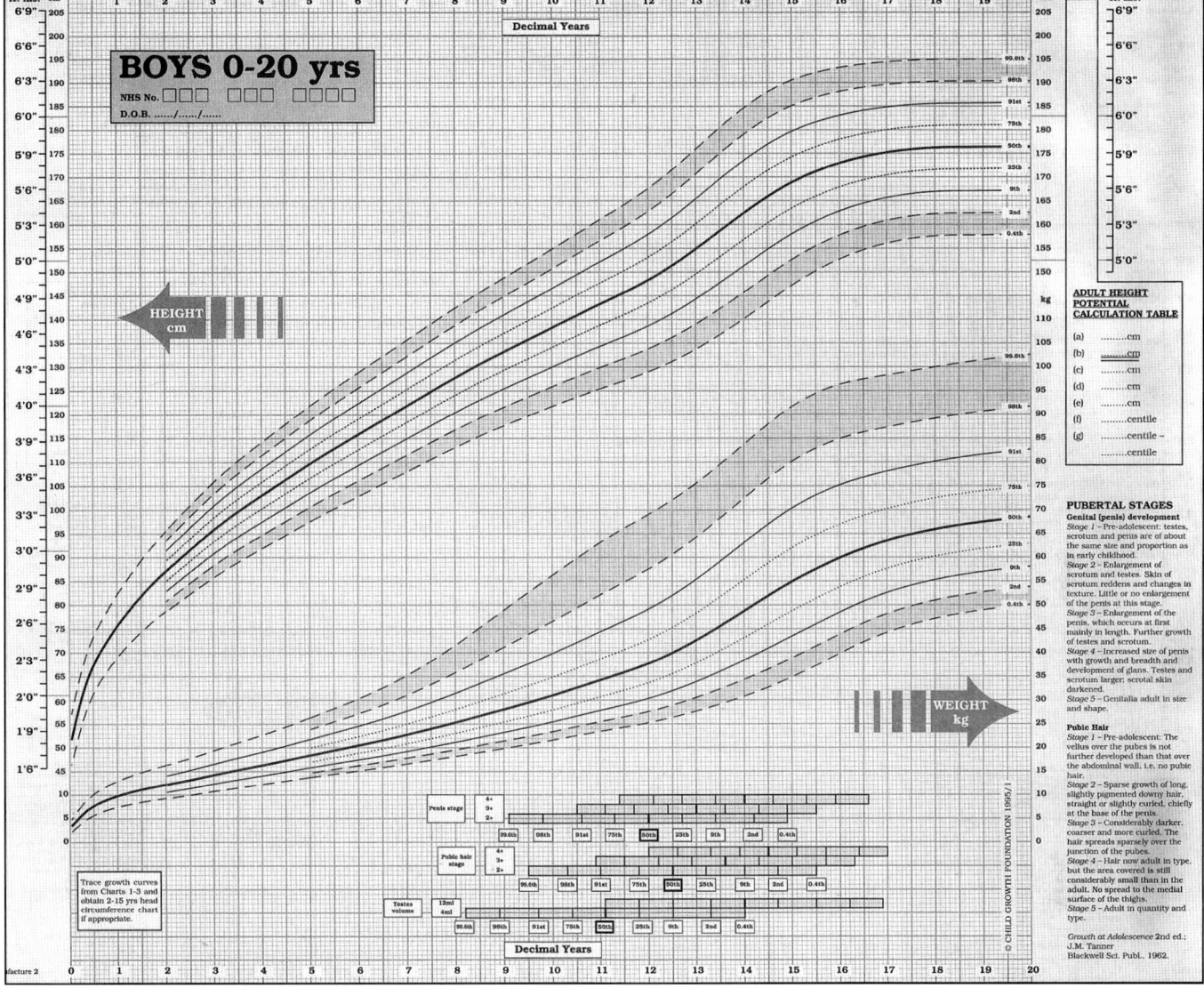

Fig. 15.9 UK1990 standard centile chart for height, weight and pubertal staging in boys (© Child Growth Foundation).

c. Decimal age at examination:	8.633 years
d. Decimal age at previous examination:	7.876 years
Height increment over interval c–d 0.757 years:	4.2 cm
Height velocity (annualized, see below):	5.5 cm/year

Plotting growth charts

Mis-plotting is a common error even by experienced personnel, so care should be taken and the plot reviewed with reference to previous plots when available. A precise dot, uncircled, provides maximum clarity on the chart as this will not overlap with previous or subsequent points. Plots of weight in very obese children sometimes stray onto the height centile spread, so these points should be clearly indicated as being weight not height.

Screening for growth disorders in the community (growth monitoring)

Screening for growth and other disorders by height and weight measurement assists in the diagnosis of problems which would otherwise be missed or come to light at a later stage when the outcome of treatment may be less favorable. Growth monitoring is important in the early detection of disease in children and of particular value in detecting a wide variety of endocrine abnormalities in which poor growth may be the earliest, or only, sign of a problem. After considerable debate as to the prac-

ticality and economics of measuring all children, it has recently been demonstrated to be a very cost-effective intervention.[62] Currently in the UK growth is assessed at primary school entry and close to exit (ages 4 and 10 years) as a minimum, but any changes in policy need to be evidence based. Measurements should be conducted by trained staff using reliable and calibrated equipment. Regular updates on training are required.

Which measurement?

Standard measurements include supine length and weight with head circumference up until 2 years of age. Beyond that, height and weight are the norm. The British Society for Paediatric Endocrinology and Diabetes recommends that recording and plotting of a child's height and weight at every encounter is an example of best clinical practice. Body mass index charts (weight in kg/height in meters squared) are now available and can be used to assess a child's body composition and follow any changes (Figs 15.11, 15.12). However as an approximation, a child's weight centile should not be more than 2 centile bands above or below their height centile. This approximates to the 98th and 2nd centiles for body mass index (BMI) respectively, i.e. the determinants of obesity and underweight. Skinfold thickness may be assessed to determine the degree and pattern of obesity and to calculate body composition (percentage body fat). Skinfold thickness can also be measured

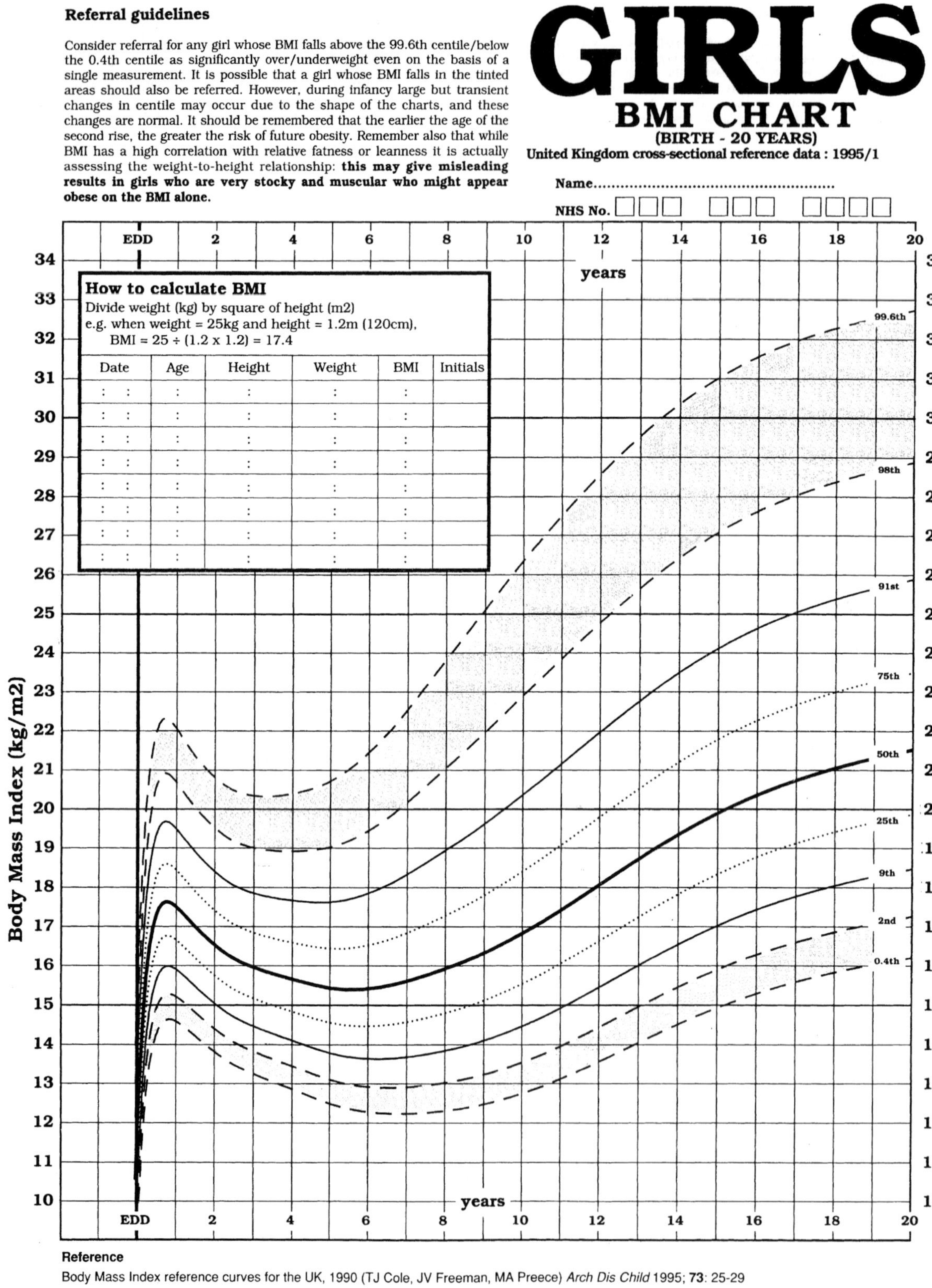
Referral guidelines
Consider referral for any girl whose BMI falls above the 99.6th centile/below the 0.4th centile as significantly over/underweight even on the basis of a single measurement. It is possible that a girl whose BMI falls in the tinted areas should also be referred. However, during infancy large but transient changes in centile may occur due to the shape of the charts, and these changes are normal. It should be remembered that the earlier the age of the second rise, the greater the risk of future obesity. Remember also that while BMI has a high correlation with relative fatness or leanness it is actually assessing the weight-to-height relationship: this may give misleading results in girls who are very stocky and muscular who might appear obese on the BMI alone.
GIRLS
BMI CHART
(BIRTH - 20 YEARS)
United Kingdom cross-sectional reference data : 1995/1
Name
NHS No.
How to calculate BMI
Divide weight (kg) by square of height (m2)
e.g. when weight = 25kg and height = 1.2m (120cm),
BMI = 25 ÷ (1.2 x 1.2) = 17.4
Date
Age
Height
Weight
BMI
Initials
EDD
years
Body Mass Index (kg/m2)
99.6th
98th
91st
75th
50th
25th
9th
2nd
0.4th
Reference
Body Mass Index reference curves for the UK, 1990 (TJ Cole, JV Freeman, MA Preece) Arch Dis Child 1995; 73: 25-29

Fig. 15.12 Body mass index reference centile chart for girls (© Child Growth Foundation).

head against the headboard in the Frankfurt plane as above, while the other straightens the legs and moves the footboard up against both heels firmly. The measurement can then be taken. Children with unequal leg length should be measured on the longest leg, but the frequent practice of measuring one leg only can give inaccurate readings because of pelvic tilt.

Sitting height

The child is positioned on the sitting height table as upright as possible with the legs fully in contact with the table (Fig. 15.15c). Back and foot supports are adjusted to support the child. Head positioning and measurement technique is the same as for height (see above). Sitting height may also be measured by placing a flat-topped stool of known height below the stadiometer and subtracting this amount from a measurement of the child sitting on the stool.

Weight

Infants should be weighed naked. Older children can be weighed in light underclothes and with shoes removed. Uncooperative toddlers

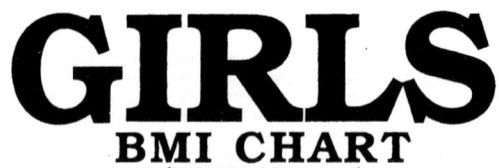

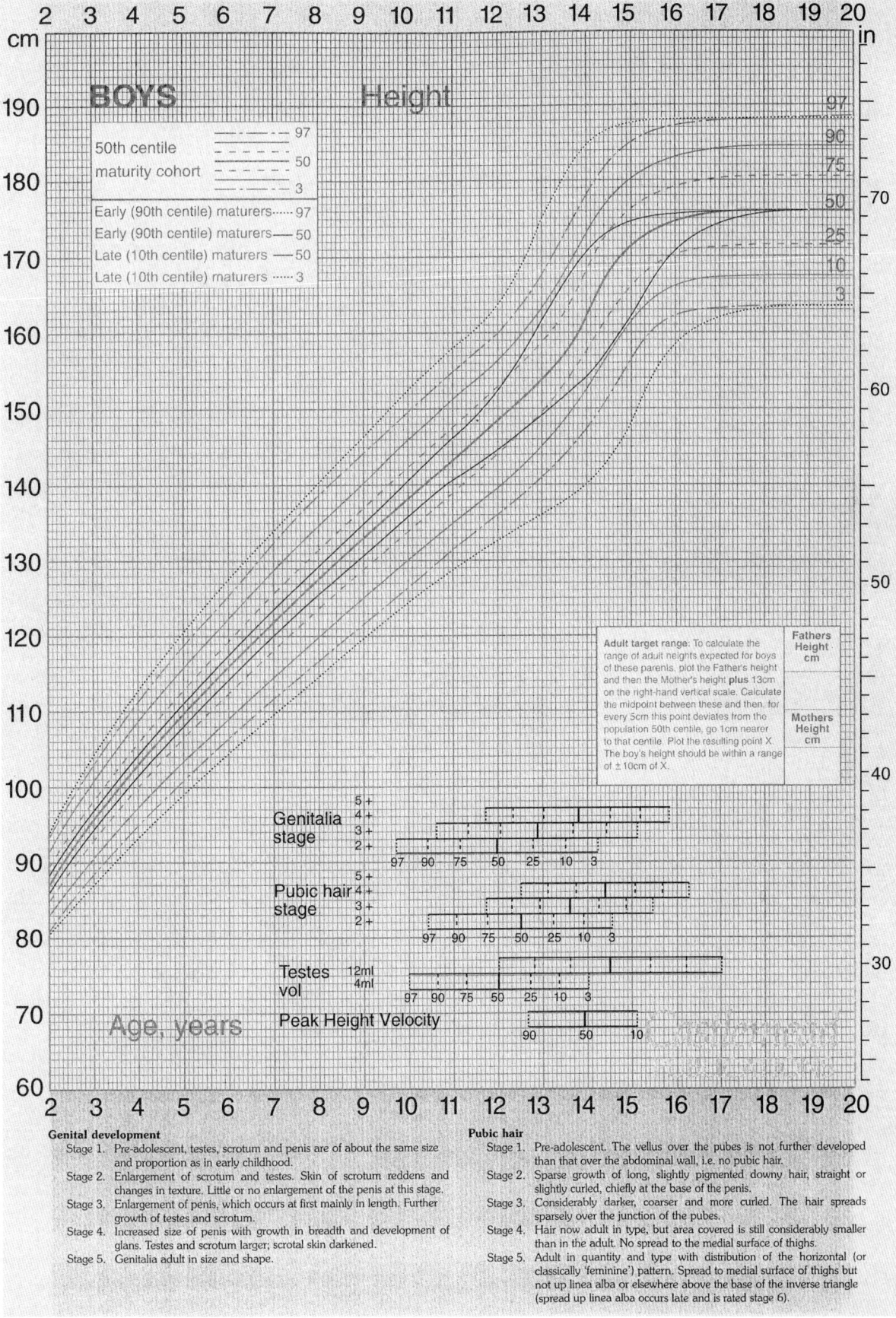

Genital development

Stage 1. Pre-adolescent, testes, scrotum and penis are of about the same size and proportion as in early childhood.

Stage 2. Enlargement of scrotum and testes. Skin of scrotum reddens and changes in texture. Little or no enlargement of the penis at this stage.

Stage 3. Enlargement of penis, which occurs at first mainly in length. Further growth of testes and scrotum.

Stage 4. Increased size of penis with growth in breadth and development of glans. Testes and scrotum larger; scrotal skin darkened.

Stage 5. Genitalia adult in size and shape.

Pubic hair

Stage 1. Pre-adolescent. The vellus over the pubes is not further developed than that over the abdominal wall, i.e. no pubic hair.

Stage 2. Sparse growth of long, slightly pigmented downy hair, straight or slightly curled, chiefly at the base of the penis.

Stage 3. Considerably darker, coarser and more curled. The hair spreads sparsely over the junction of the pubes.

Stage 4. Hair now adult in type, but area covered is still considerably smaller than in the adult. No spread to the medial surface of thighs.

Stage 5. Adult in quantity and type with distribution of the horizontal (or classically 'feminine') pattern. Spread to medial surface of thighs but not up linea alba or elsewhere above the base of the inverse triangle (spread up linea alba occurs late and is rated stage 6).

Fig. 15.13   Buckler Tanner height centile chart for boys (© Castlemead Publications).

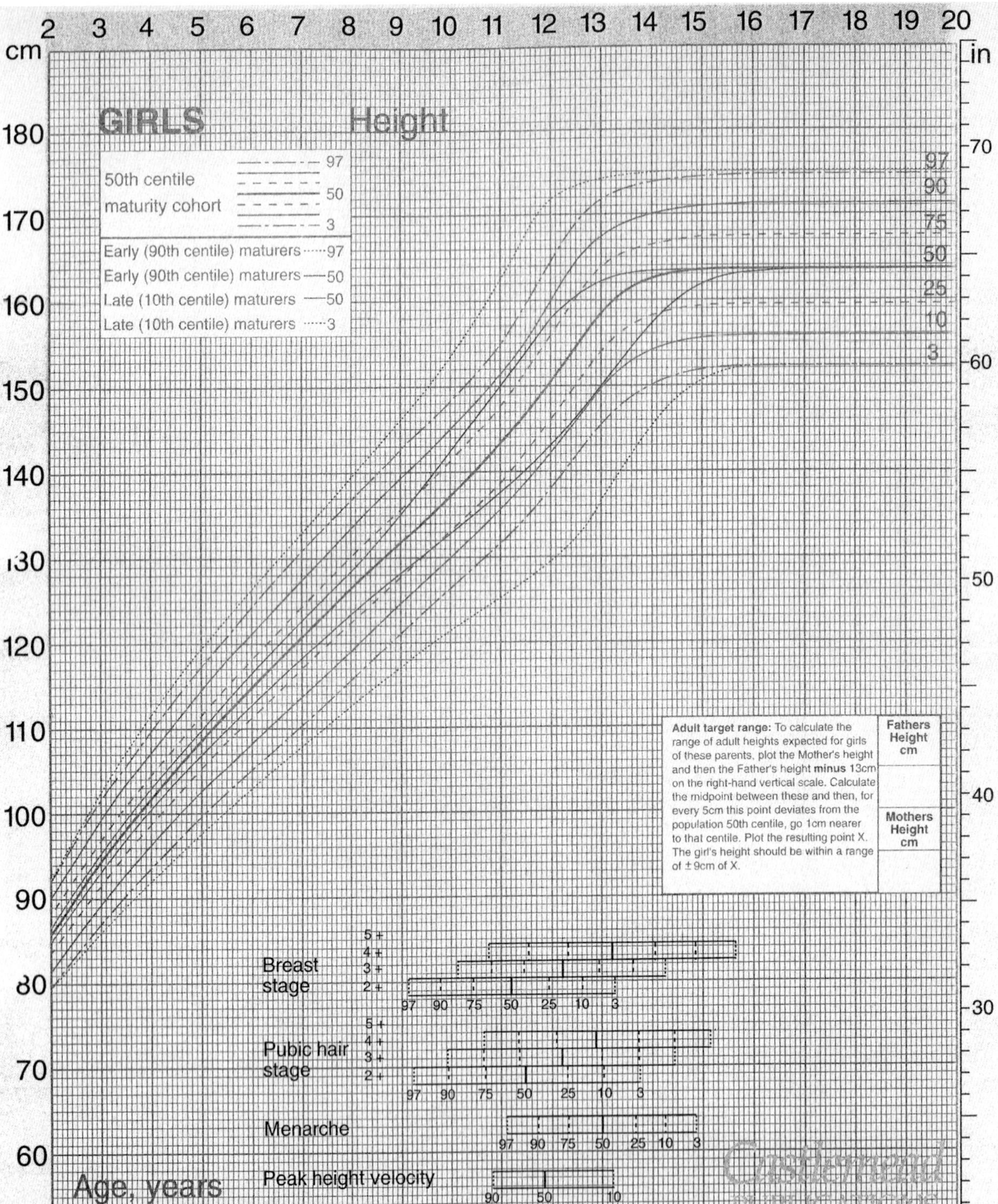

GIRLS   Height

50th centile	----- 97
maturity cohort	----- 50
	----- 3
Early (90th centile) maturers ······97
Early (90th centile) maturers ——97
Early (90th centile) maturers ——50
Late (10th centile) maturers ——50
Late (10th centile) maturers ······3

Adult target range: To calculate the range of adult heights expected for girls of these parents, plot the Mother's height and then the Father's height **minus** 13cm on the right-hand vertical scale. Calculate the midpoint between these and then, for every 5cm this point deviates from the population 50th centile, go 1cm nearer to that centile. Plot the resulting point X. The girl's height should be within a range of ± 9cm of X.

Fathers Height cm

Mothers Height cm

Age, years

Breast stage

Pubic hair stage

Menarche

Peak height velocity

Breast development
Stage 1. Pre-adolescent: elevation of papilla only.
Stage 2. Breast bud stage: elevation of breast and papilla as small mound. Enlargement of areola diameter.
Stage 3. Further enlargement and elevation of breast and areola, with no separation of their contours.
Stage 4. Projection of areola and papilla to form a secondary mound above the level of the breast.
Stage 5. Mature stage: projection of papilla only, due to recession of the areola to the general contour of the breast.

Pubic hair
Stage 1. Pre-adolescent. The vellus over the pubes is not further developed than that over the abdominal wall, i.e. no pubic hair.
Stage 2. Sparse growth of long, slightly pigmented downy hair, straight or slightly curled, chiefly along labia.
Stage 3. Considerably darker, coarser and more curled. The hair spreads sparsely over the junction of the pubes.
Stage 4. Hair now adult in type, but area covered is still considerably smaller than that in the adult. No spread to the medial surface of thighs.
Stage 5. Adult in the quantity and type with distribution of the horizontal (or classically 'feminine') pattern. Spread to medial surface of thighs but not up linea alba or elsewhere above the base of the inverse triangle, (spread up linea alba occurs late and rated stage 6).

Fig. 15.14   Buckler Tanner height centile chart for girls (© Castlemead Publications).

Table 15.5 Decimal year calculation

	1	2	3	4	5	6	7	8	9	10	11	12	13	14	15	16	17	18	19	20	21	22	23	24	25	26	27	28	29	30	31
JAN	000	003	005	008	011	014	016	019	022	025	027	030	033	036	038	041	044	047	049	052	055	058	060	063	066	068	071	074	077	079	082
FEB	085	088	090	093	096	099	101	104	107	110	112	115	118	121	123	126	129	132	134	137	140	142	145	148	151	153	156	159			
MAR	162	164	167	170	173	175	178	181	184	186	189	192	195	197	200	203	205	208	211	214	216	219	222	225	227	230	233	236	238	241	244
APR	247	249	252	255	258	260	263	266	268	271	274	277	279	282	285	288	290	293	296	299	301	304	307	310	312	315	318	321	323	326	
MAY	329	332	334	337	340	342	345	348	351	353	356	359	362	364	367	370	373	375	378	381	384	386	389	392	395	397	400	403	405	408	411
JUN	414	416	419	422	425	427	430	433	436	438	441	444	447	449	452	455	458	460	463	466	468	471	474	477	479	482	485	488	490	493	
JUL	496	499	501	504	507	510	512	515	518	521	523	526	529	532	534	537	540	542	545	548	551	553	556	559	562	564	567	570	573	575	578
AUG	581	584	586	589	592	595	597	600	603	605	608	611	614	616	619	622	625	627	630	633	636	638	641	644	647	649	652	655	658	660	663
SEP	666	668	671	674	677	679	682	685	688	690	693	696	699	701	704	707	710	712	715	718	721	723	726	729	731	734	737	740	742	745	
OCT	748	751	753	756	759	762	764	767	770	773	775	778	781	784	786	789	792	795	797	800	803	805	808	811	814	816	819	822	825	827	830
NOV	833	836	838	841	844	847	849	852	855	858	860	863	866	868	871	874	877	879	882	885	888	890	893	896	899	901	904	907	910	912	
DEC	915	918	921	923	926	929	932	934	937	940	942	945	948	951	953	956	959	962	964	967	970	973	975	978	981	984	986	989	992	995	997

can be weighed with an adult, subtracting the adult's weight measured separately (the buddy-weighing technique).

Head circumference

This measurement is the maximum occipitofrontal circumference with the reading taken on three occasions (Fig. 15.15d). A thin specially constructed tape measure is required (see above).

Height velocity

Much has been written on the use of height velocity as part of the assessment of the growth of a child. Appreciation of the total amount grown at each age for any child is important as part of their assessment. However the individual pattern of growth of any child can show daily, weekly and seasonal variations. Height velocity is usually assessed over periods of not less than one year to avoid seasonal effects and to minimize the effect of measurement error, but increments of less than one year can be 'annualized' for comparative purposes and this is often sufficient to recognize growth problems quickly. (For the method of calculation of height velocity see decimal ages, above.) Even so, annual height velocity tends to oscillate with the periodicity of approximately 2 years[67] and this needs to be taken into consideration during interpretation of growth patterns (Fig. 15.16). Rhythms of growth have been reviewed by Wales and Gibson.[68] Measurement of height velocity is an accurate, cheap and non-invasive contribution to assessing the need for and adjustment of endocrine replacement therapy. This can be assisted by the regular assessment of skeletal maturation (bone age) where appropriate.

Biochemical markers of growth

In certain circumstances, carefully chosen biochemical markers of growth may overcome some of these disadvantages. Biochemical markers are free from observer bias and their precision is independent of frequency of sampling. Bone alkaline phosphatase (BALP) is found in hypertrophic chondrocytes of the epiphyseal growth plate, in matrix vesicles associated with bone mineralization and in mature osteoblasts. There is a close quantitative relationship between serial measurements of BALP and height velocity in short normal children undergoing GH treatment.[69,70]

Mid parental height

In the assessment of a child's growth potential, calculation of mid parental (or target) height is essential. The difference between the male and female 50th centile heights in the UK is 14 cm. For a boy, mid parental height is calculated as the simple average of parents' height + 7 cm, for a girl average of parents' height − 7 cm. The mid parental height (MPH) can be plotted on the growth chart (Fig. 15.9) and 90% of children will achieve an adult height within + or − 10 cm of that value (the target centile range). Caution needs to be exercised when predicting adult height if one parent is of extreme stature. A chart to help assess whether a child's short stature is of familial origin or not is also available.[71]

Standard deviation scores

Standard deviation scores (SDS or Z-scores) have traditionally been used to monitor individual and group variations in height or any other growth parameter over time, as the function of age is excluded, and this makes statistical analysis possible. Height measurements are normally distributed and SDS can be estimated from the UK 1990 charts, each centile band being equally spaced 0.67 SD apart. For more accurate calculation and for measures such as weight and body mass index which are in a positively skewed distribution, the methodology of Cole[60] should be used.

VARIATIONS IN GROWTH
Postnatal adjustment

Weight at birth generally reflects the intrauterine environment and nutrition, and most if not all infants will show a degree of tracking, i.e. a shift across centiles for height weight and head circumference within the first 6 months after birth. The challenge here is to differentiate between a normal growth variant and failure to thrive or another pathological process. However normal variation, i.e. adjustment to the genetic growth pattern, will show a shift upwards

or downwards by as much as 2 centile bands, followed by stabilization of growth and subsequent following of the child's genetically determined centile band. Abnormal growth patterns will continue to show centile shift beyond the first 6 months, and further investigation should take place. Weight gain is more susceptible to the influence of feeding problems and intercurrent illnesses. The regular and accurate assessment of supine length in an infant will help distinguish between normal variation and true failure to thrive and as in the normal situation will demonstrate less fluctuation than weight.

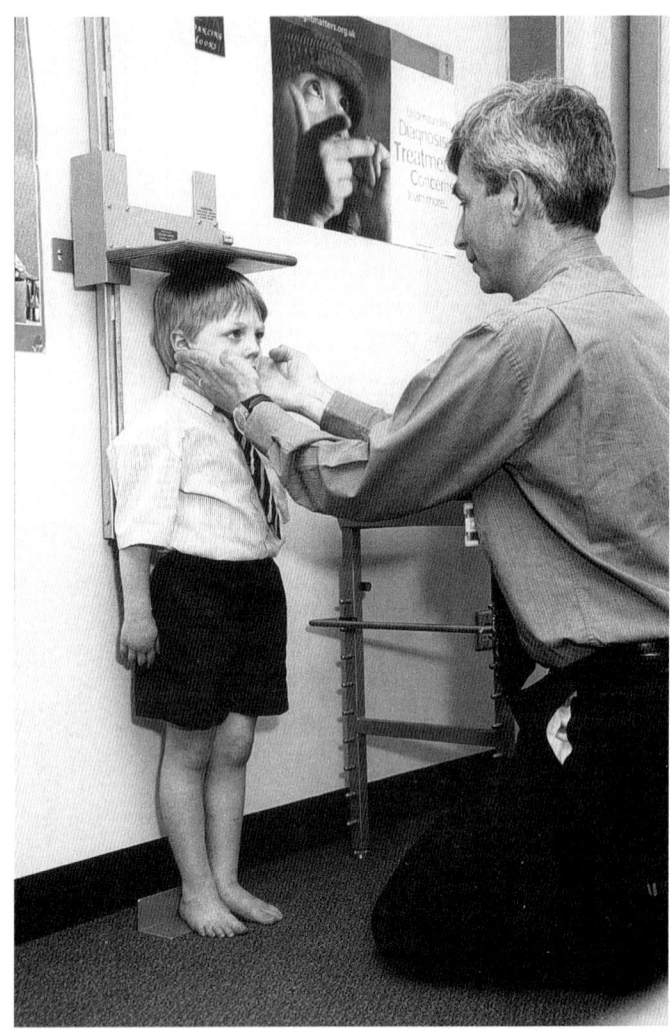

(a)

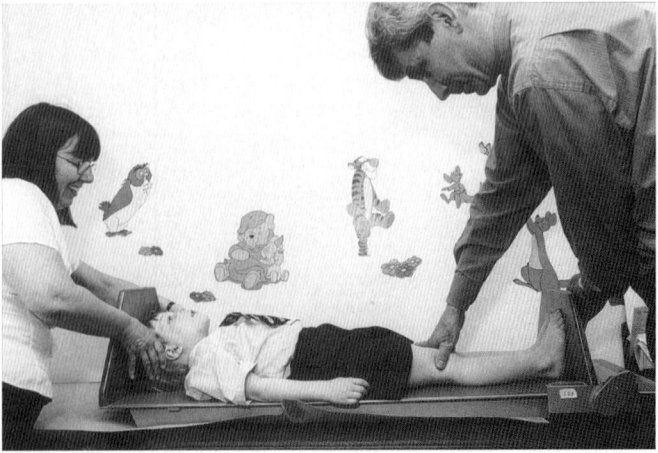

(b)

Fig. 15.15   Correct positioning and technique for accurate measurement of (a) height, (b) supine length.

(Continued)

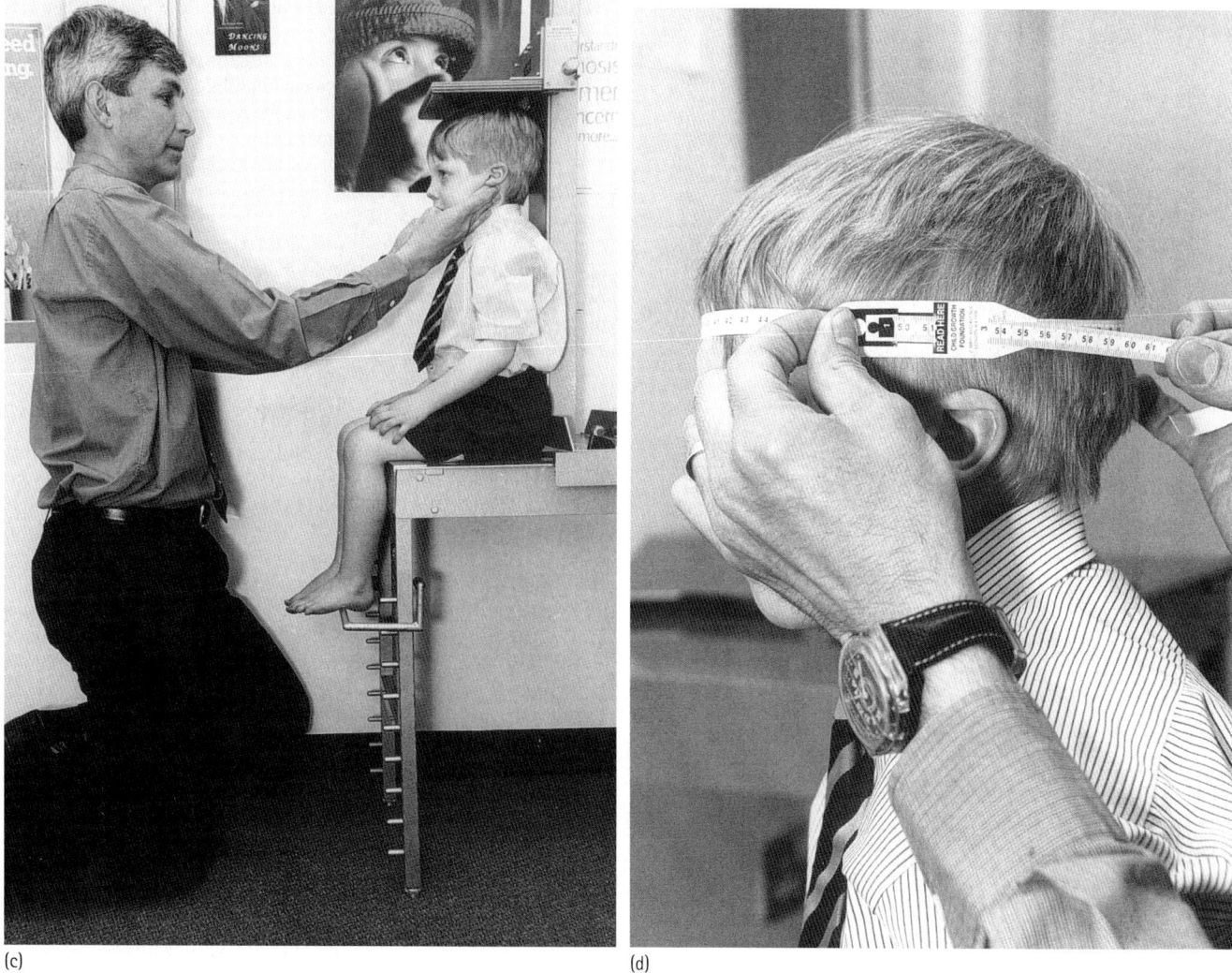

(c)　　　　　　　　　　　　　　　　　　　　(d)

Fig. 15.15 Continued　(c) sitting height, (d) head circumference. For description see text.

Intrauterine growth retardation and catch-up growth

Low birth weight (defined as below 2nd centile or − 2 SD for gestational age) may originate as a result of poor fetal growth throughout pregnancy or just in the last trimester. Both are of different causality and produce a different outcome. The latter arises as a result of maternal factors such as placental failure or pre-eclampsia. An otherwise normal fetus is starved of nutriments and fails to gain weight but grows in length near-normally, so-called asymmetrical growth retardation. After birth, these infants almost always show complete catch-up growth with rapid weight gain within the first 6–12 months. Research based on midwifery record archives suggests that this rapid gain in weight might be associated with a higher predisposition to diseases such as coronary artery disease, hypertension and type 2 diabetes later in life – the metabolic syndrome or syndrome-X.[33]

Symmetrical growth retardation is shown by those fetuses which grow poorly throughout all three trimesters and who are born at low birth weight and with reduced length and head circumference. The etiology is fetal rather than maternal and although this is likely to be multifactorial, endocrine factors such as insulin and glucocorticoid resistance have been implicated, and the phenomenon of genetic imprinting may also be responsible. Imprinting of certain paternal growth genes appears to be required for normal growth. Deletions and uniparental disomy can account for the growth retardation in about 10% of infants with Russell–Silver syndrome (see p. 439 and Fig. 15.24). Most infants with this form of growth retardation either catch up either very slowly (3 years or more) or never catch up fully.

Growth during the prepubertal years and referral criteria

Once set on a particular trajectory, a child's growth in height will deviate little from its centile band until the onset of puberty. So predictable is this pattern that concern should be raised if height drifts up or down by as little as one height centile band, even within the designated normal range (i.e. 2nd to 98th centiles), and an explanation sought. This is the basis of the advice given to those conducting community growth screening programs.

Syndrome specific charts

The pattern of growth is so reproducible in certain conditions that specific growth charts are available, e.g. for Down[72] and Turner[73] syndromes. They serve a very useful purpose in allowing correct judgments to be made about the growth of children with these conditions, and whether other external factors such as poor nutrition or ill health are affecting a child's growth adversely. In addition they assist with the prediction of adult height and in quantifying the effect of any treatments, such as the use of growth hormone in Turner syndrome.

Medical conditions which affect growth

Previously, chronic ill health from conditions such as cystic fibrosis, diabetes mellitus, inflammatory bowel disease, chronic renal failure and asthma could be associated with poor growth and weight gain and a delay in the onset of puberty, although with modern treatment regimens and much more careful attention to nutrition this is rarely seen. However, poor growth can still be associated with severe forms of inflammatory bowel disease, juvenile chronic arthritis, chronic renal failure and congenital adrenal

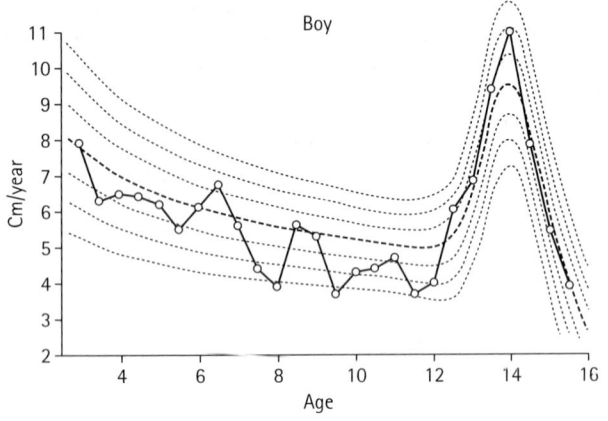

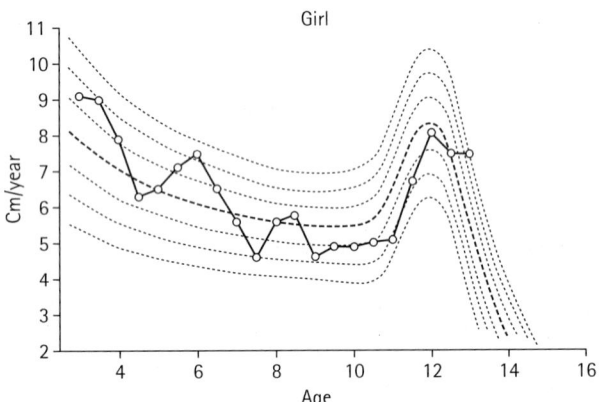

Fig. 15.16 Height velocity standards for boys and girls (redrawn from Tanner 1976) showing a height velocity curve for a typical normal boy and girl, both demonstrating the cyclical nature of growth. (From Butler et al 1990[67])

hyperplasia, even when the associated glucocorticoid therapy is reduced to a minimum. The most frequently seen cause of iatrogenic growth failure is in the survivors of childhood malignancy. Treatment regimens including cranial and total body irradiation and high dose chemotherapy, often with stem cell rescue or bone marrow transplant, usually cause growth and thyroid hormone deficiencies, and steroidogenesis from the adrenals and gonads is frequently impaired. Hormone replacement may restore growth, but the success of treatment depends on how much primary damage is caused to the tissues of the body by the oncological regimens.

BONE AGE

The bone age is a useful guide to an individual child's growth potential but the value of this investigation as a diagnostic tool is frequently overestimated, its main place being in adult height prediction. A bone age radiograph when scored according to current techniques gives a value (the 'bone age') which represents the 50th centile for a child of that age with that degree of skeletal maturation. This result can be interpreted in the same way as any measurement plotted on a reference chart. The 3rd and 97th centiles of skeletal maturity correspond to approximately 2 years either side of the child's chronological age, but whether a bone age is 'advanced' or 'delayed' its main value is estimating completed, and hence residual growth.

Conventionally X-rays of the left wrist are used because there is a large aggregation of long and round bones in this single area which can be imaged at minimal radiation dose. The Greulich and Pyle system[74] provides pictorial standards for direct comparison with the individual child's X-ray and the best fit determines the bone age. The Tanner–Whitehouse system (currently TW3[75]) requires the scoring of epiphyseal maturation of 13 individual bones (radius, ulna, 1st, 3rd and 5th

metacarpals and phalanges) and is more accurate and more suitable for longitudinal follow-up of the individual child. Bone ages can be performed serially, especially when monitoring response to treatment or an intervention, but as the rating system imposes artificial stages on a continuous biological process, it is not recommended to perform the investigation at less than 6 monthly intervals.

Epiphyseal fusion and growth cessation are now known to be related to estrogen secretion in both sexes. Thus estrogen deficiency due to mutations in the aromatase gene (CYP19) and estrogen resistance due to disruptive mutations in the estrogen receptor gene have no effect on normal male sexual maturation in puberty. However, these mutations result in an absent pubertal growth spurt, delayed bone maturation, unfused epiphyses, continued growth into adulthood and very tall adult stature in both sexes.[76]

PREDICTION OF ADULT HEIGHT

It is helpful to plot the child's height for bone age on the height chart, and following the bone age/height centile through to maturity can give a reasonable approximation of the child's projected adult height. Figure 15.17 gives examples of height for chronological age and height for bone age plots in two boys, one early maturing and one late maturing, both however achieving 50th centile adult height. Although adult height prediction can be used for children with parents within the population norms it is far less reliable in extremes of stature and where pathology exists or treatment is given. Predicted adult height can be estimated based on the two principal bone age rating systems (TW3[75] and Greulich and Pyle[74]) with a margin of error in normal sized children of approximately + or − 4 cm. Reference should be made to the accuracy of height prediction from methods of bone age estimation in different disease states as margins of error vary greatly.

Mathematical description of growth and growth curves has frequently been undertaken, but the Infant–Childhood–Puberty model of Karlberg et al[77] provides the best description of growth during the three postnatal phases: infantile – principally under nutritional influence; childhood – growth being predominantly controlled by growth hormone secretion; and puberty – where both sex steroids and growth hormone drive growth. More recently, mathematical models have been derived to predict the response to an intervention, e.g. growth hormone treatment.

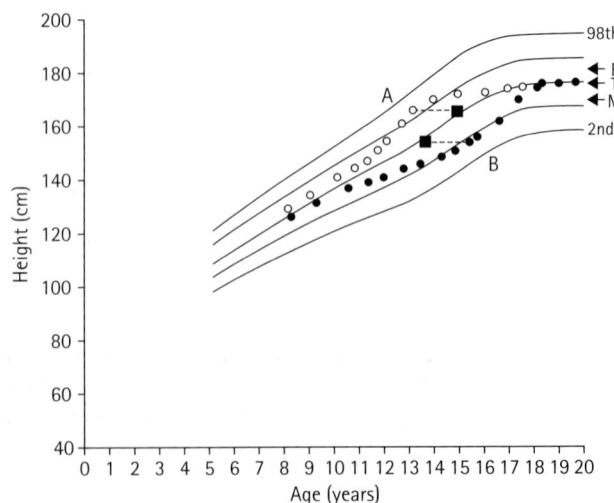

Fig. 15.17 Examples of the use of mid-parental height and bone age in the prediction of adult height in an early maturing (A) and a late maturing (B) boy. For details see text. Circle = height plot for chronological age, square = height plot for bone age, F = father's height, M = mother's adjusted height, T = target height.

ASSESSMENT OF PUBERTY

The adolescent years are manifested by fundamental changes to the physical and psychological functioning of a person. To a pediatrician the process of puberty may influence the pathological process or management of some conditions and conversely a number of chronic conditions influence, usually adversely, the process of puberty, either in consonant way (the normal pattern of development but accelerated or delayed in time) or in a dissonant way (disruption of the normal pubertal process). Consequently an assessment of pubertal staging should be part of the clinical examination of any adolescent patient. The universally accepted method of pubertal staging is according to Tanner.[6]

Clinical staging of puberty

Boys

In the male, ratings are expressed as stages of genital (penis) development, pubic hair development and testicular volume. Knowledge of these standards is extremely important when assessing growth in adolescents. They are shown in Figures 15.19–15.21 and are described below.

Genitalia (penis) development stages (Fig. 15.18)

Stage G1: Preadolescent. Testes, scrotum and penis are about same size and shape as in early childhood.

Stage G2: Scrotum slightly enlarged, with reddening of the skin and changes in the texture. Little or no enlargement of the penis at this stage.

Stage G3: Penis slightly enlarged, at first mainly in length. Scrotum further enlarged than in stage G2.

Stage G4: Penis further enlarged, with growth in breadth and development of glans. Further enlargement of scrotum and darkening of scrotal skin.

Stage G5: Genitalia adult in size and shape.

Testicular volume. Testicular volumes are assessed by palpation in comparison with a string of plastic models of testicular shape known as the Prader orchidometer (Fig. 15.19). Although this principally measures spermatic tubular growth, testicular volume correlates closely with testosterone secretion. The models are marked according to their volumes in milliliters.

1–2 ml are prepubertal;

3–4 ml mark the beginning of puberty;

8–10 ml are associated with the beginning of height acceleration in mid-pubertal boys, usually at stage G3;

12–15 ml coincide with the maximum growth velocity, usually at stage G4;

20 ml (usually at stage G5) signifies that most boys have passed the peak of their growth spurt and are beginning to fuse their epiphyses on account of higher levels of testosterone secretion.

The majority of adult males reach volumes of 15–25 ml. Testicular volumes of less than 12 ml in adulthood may be associated with reduced fertility.

Pubic hair stages for boys and girls (Fig. 15.20)

Stage PH1: Preadolescent. The vellus over the pubes is not further developed than that over the abdominal wall, i.e. no pubic hair.

Stage PH2: Sparse growth of long, slightly pigmented downy hair, straight or slightly curled, chiefly at the base of the penis or along labia.

Stage PH3: Considerably darker, coarser and more curled. The hair spreads sparsely over the junction of the pubes.

Stage PH4: Hair now adult in type, but area covered is still considerably smaller than in adults. No spread to medial surface of thighs.

Stage PH5: Adult in quantity and type with distribution of the horizontal (or classically 'feminine') pattern. Spread to medial surface of thighs, but not up the linea alba.

Stage PH6: Spread upwards along the linea alba (the typical male escutcheon).

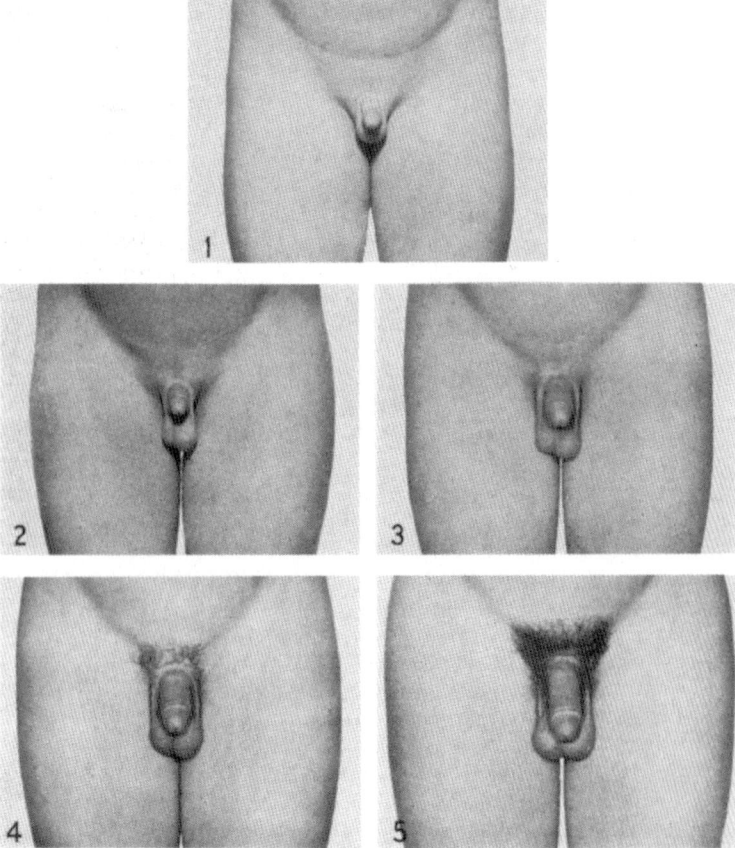

Fig. 15.18 Standards for genital (penis) development. (From Tanner 1962[6] with permission)

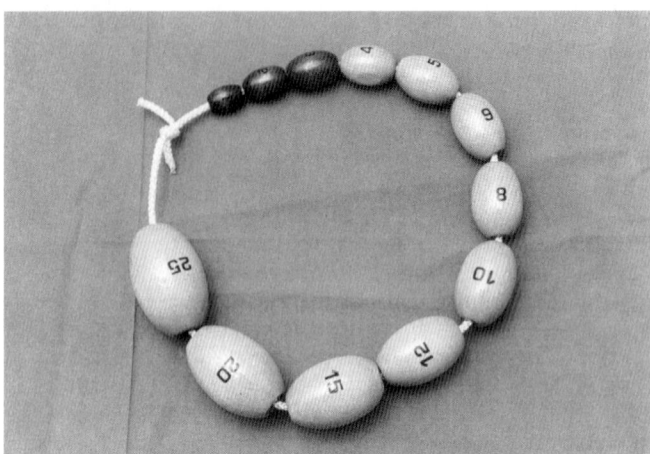

Fig. 15.19   The Prader orchidometer for the assessment of testicular volume.

Girls

In girls it is the development of the breast which provides the best marker as to girls' progress through puberty (Fig. 15.21).

Breast development

Stage B1: Preadolescent: elevation of papilla only.

Stage B2: Breast bud stage: elevation of breast and papilla as small mound. Areolar diameter enlarged over stage B1.

Stage B3: Breast and areola both enlarged and elevated more than in stage B2, but with no separation of their contours.

Stage B4: The areola and papilla form a secondary mound projecting above the contour of the breast.

Stage B5: Mature stage: papilla only projects, with the areola recessed to the general contour of the breast.

The timing of puberty

In almost all children the pattern of progress through puberty is constant but the timing of attainment of each stage can be considerably variable. Centile bands for boys and girls at each stage of puberty are found beneath the weight curves on standard growth charts (see Figs

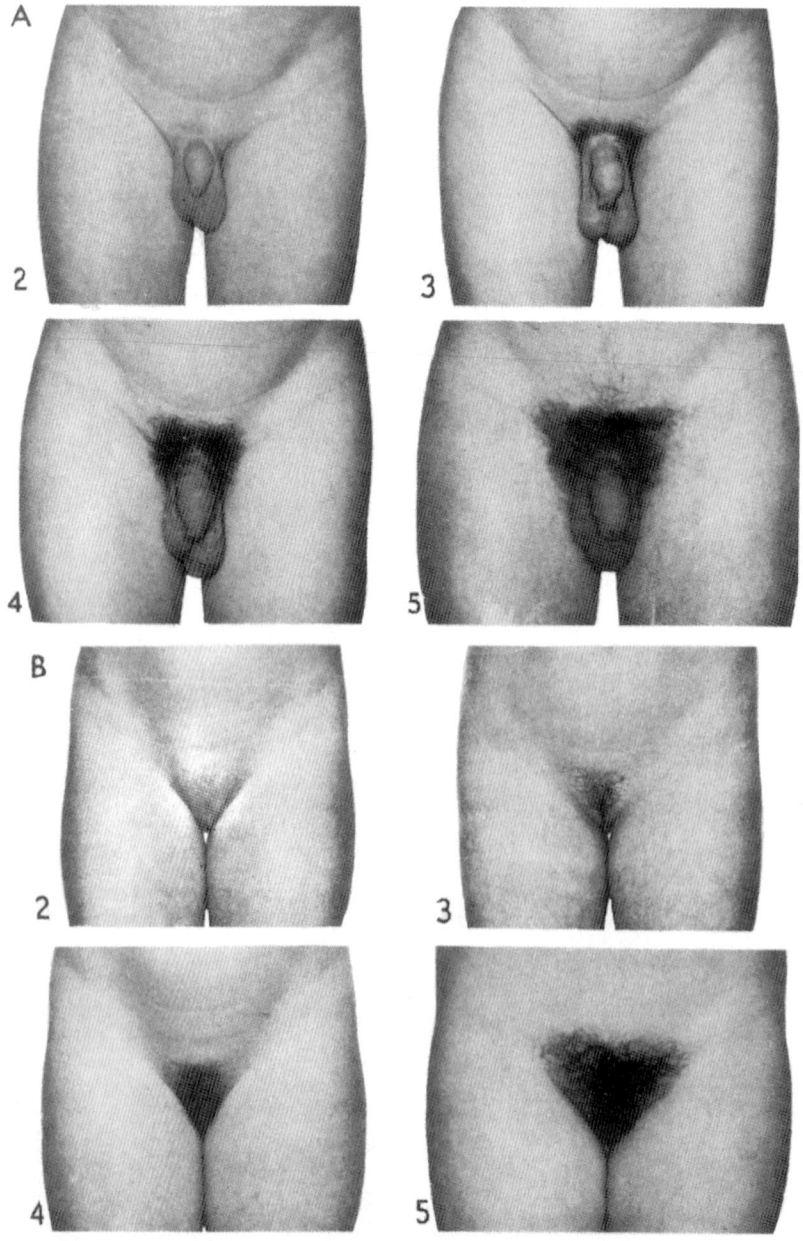

Fig. 15.20   Standards for pubic hair development in boys and girls. (From Tanner 1962⁶ with permission)

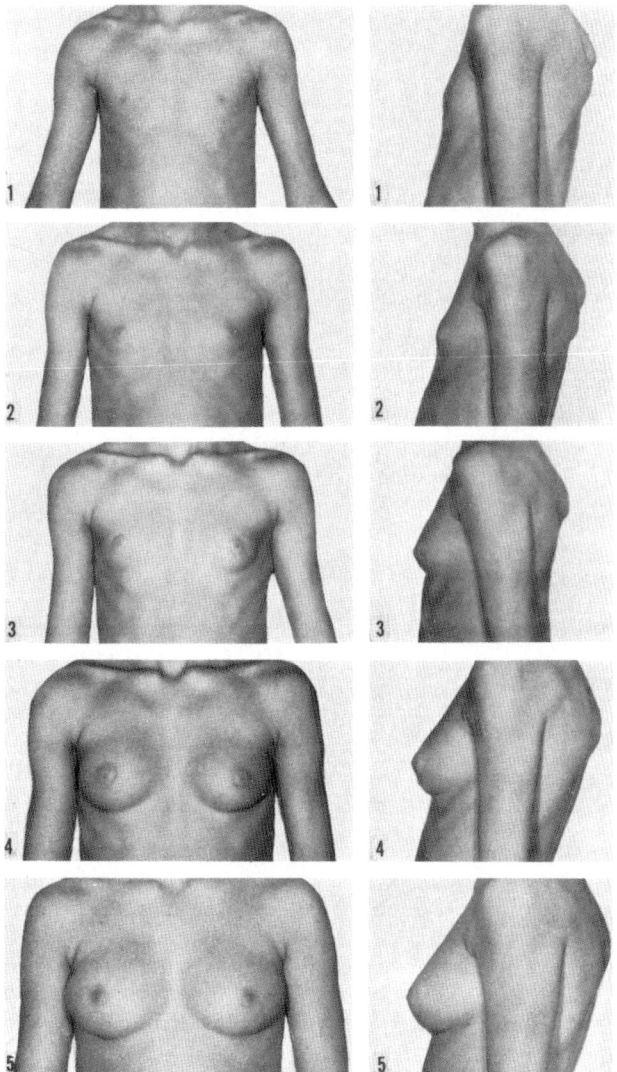

Fig. 15.21   Standards for breast development. (From Tanner 1962[6] with permission)

15.9 and 15.10). The onset of puberty G2 in boys occurs at the mean age of 12.0 years (range 98th centile 9.8 years to 2nd centile 14.2 years), and in girls the mean age at B2 is 11.0 years (range 98th centile 8.2 years to 2nd centile 13.8 years). The mean age at menarche is 13.0 years (range 98th centile 11.0 years to 2nd centile 15.0 years). The duration of puberty (stage G/B2 to stage G/B5) may unusually take less than 2 years and more than 5 years, but on average is 3.0 years (2.3 years B2 – menarche in girls). A very rapid, delayed or halted passage through puberty especially with an attenuated adolescent growth spurt should be of major concern and a search for systemic or intracranial pathology should be conducted.

Other markers of puberty

Often it is not possible to perform a formal Tanner pubertal staging due to inappropriate circumstances or refusal. Adolescents may be prepared to self-rate themselves if provided with line diagrams and simple descriptions or an orchidometer for boys. Axillary hair begins to appear 2 years after pubic hair. Facial hair grows initially above the upper lip (moustache area) at about G4. By the time sideburns begin to appear, a boy will have reached G5. The voice begins to break at G3–4. The timing of the first conscious ejaculation is very variable, but occurs in 90% boys by age 14 years. Sperm can be detected in early morning urine samples as early as 12 years of age and in early puberty (G2) before any other clinical features

are apparent. Menarche occurs by the time 90% of girls have reached B4 and PH4.

GROWTH DURING PUBERTY

Prior to the onset of puberty height velocity gradually declines to between 4 and 6 cm/year (the prepubertal growth lag) and this is much more marked in boys than girls, especially when the onset of puberty is delayed (constitutional or maturation delay). The endocrinology of puberty gives a different tempo in boys compared with girls (Fig. 15.22). As soon as puberty begins with breast development in girls, height acceleration occurs and body shape changes become apparent. Maximal growth (peak height velocity) is achieved one year after the onset of puberty (mean 8 cm/year, range 6–10 cm/year) but the intensity of the spurt, i.e. maximal velocity achieved, is greater in early maturers and lower in later maturers. Menarche occurs 2.3 years (mean) subsequently when growth is on its decline. Girls gain on average 20–25 cm during puberty and average growth post menarche is 6 cm.

In boys peak height velocity is attained usually 2 years after the onset of puberty with maximum strength spurt following this. Peak height velocity is on average 9 cm/year ranging from 6 to 13 cm, the later maturers growing less intensely. Boys grow on average between

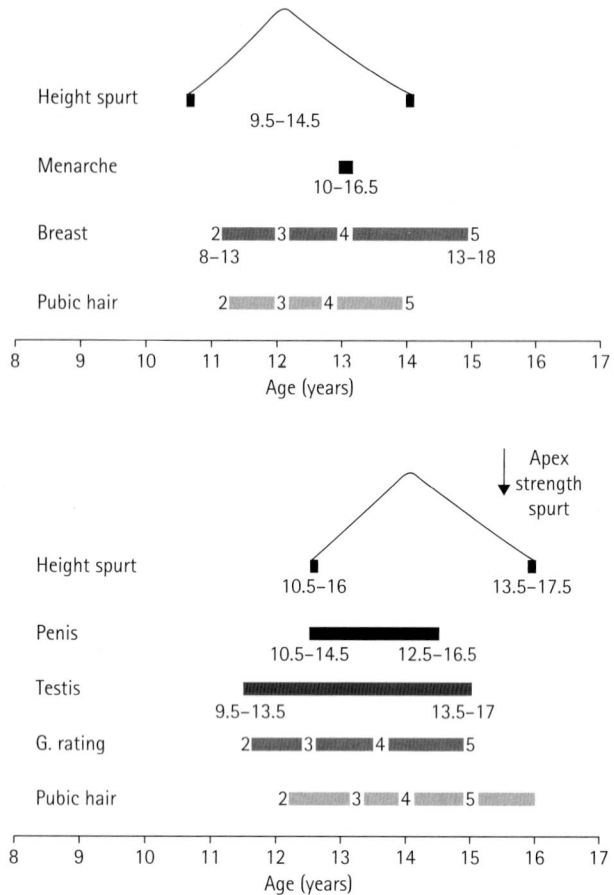

Fig. 15.22 Diagram of sequence of events in normal male and female puberty. Numbers indicate age ranges of each landmark stage. (From Marshall & Tanner 1970[78] with permission of the BMJ Publishing Group)

25 and 30 cm although the total growth during puberty is unpredictable and is the principal source of error of height prediction methods.

COMMON ERRORS IN PUBERTAL ASSESSMENT

The method of construction of the UK 1990 growth charts reflects average population growth in children of average age at puberty (see above) so it is normal to see crossing of centile lines during the teenage years. This should not cause alarm and can be interpreted by knowing the adolescent's pubertal stage. The onset of puberty in boys is frequently missed as early scrotal and testicular changes are subtle and require careful inspection. Accurate documentation of pubertal stages is important, as 'false starts' can be common. Testicular volume is often overestimated, the orchidometer representing testicular size only, and not accessory structures such as the epididymis and scrotal skin.

PUBERTAL VARIATIONS
Precocious adrenarche

Adrenarche, the awakening of the adrenal cortex to produce adrenal androgens, commences from around the age of 6 years and can be more pronounced in some children causing the appearance of pubic and axillary hair, greasiness of the skin and adult body odor. This proceeds only very slowly and in general is felt to be a variant of normal although links have been made in girls with hyperinsulinism and polycystic ovarian syndrome later on in life. For more detail see adrenarche, p. 480.[32]

Isolated menarche

Rarely an apparently prepubertal girl may present with a vaginal bleed of a few days' duration which sometimes can be repeated at monthly intervals. Exclusion of intrapelvic pathology is necessary by pelvic ultrasound and measurement of estradiol and gonadotrophins, after which this feature can be regarded as a variant of normal. A thin endometrial echo may be seen on the pelvic ultrasound scan. A single isolated vaginal withdrawal bleed (dark blood) in an otherwise prepubertal girl may be due to involution of a dominant follicular ovarian cyst. (See pseudopuberty, p. 451.)

Adolescent gynecomastia

Gynecomastia, either unilateral or bilateral, occurs in 40% of normal boys as a result of a testosterone/estrogen imbalance. The commonest time of onset is between Tanner stages G3 and G4, and it usually disappears 1–2 years later when testosterone levels rise (Tanner stage G4 to G5). In most situations no treatment, only reassurance, is required. Persistent discs of breast tissue may require surgical removal for cosmetic reasons. (See gynecomastia, p. 459.)

GROWTH REGULATION AND DISORDERS OF GROWTH

THE GROWTH HORMONE (GH) AXIS AND GROWTH

GH, a 191 amino acid anterior pituitary polypeptide, is secreted episodically throughout 24 h, but predominantly at night during slow wave sleep during which there are usually three to five discrete pulses, and is of cardinal importance in the control of growth. Release is mediated by the two hypothalamic peptides: GH releasing hormone (GHRH) – stimulatory, and somatostatin (SRIH) – inhibitory.

The hypothalamic release of GHRH and SRIH is regulated by a complex network of brain neurotransmitters and neuropeptides. Dopaminergic, serotonergic and noradrenergic pathways impinge on the GH regulatory neurone system, but cholinergic neurotransmitter pathways seem particularly important in controlling GHRH and somatostatin release. Hippocampal impulses, perhaps sleep-related, are stimulatory whilst impulses from the amygdala may be either stimulatory or inhibitory. Somatostatin secretion is mediated via the hypothalamic ventromedial nucleus.

A number of drugs induce changes in GH secretion via specific neurotransmitter pathways: clonidine is stimulatory via alpha-adrenergic and diazepam via GABA pathways; bromocriptine, propranolol and cholinergic agents probably inhibit somatostatin release. This is relevant in understanding pharmacological stimulation tests and, potentially, for therapy to stimulate GH secretion.

GH releasing hormone (GHRH) was first identified from the pancreas of a woman with Turner syndrome who developed acromegaly which failed to resolve after transsphenoidal pituitary surgery. Full bioactivity resides in its first 29 amino acids. Recently, a long-recognized family of potent small synthetic GH-releasing peptides, GH releasing hexapeptide (GHRP) and its analogues, have become important for their potential future therapeutic roles. GHRPs are active given by intravenous, subcutaneous, intranasal and oral routes, releasing GH via a specific, non-opiate, non-GHRH pituitary receptor – GHRPs do not interact with GHRH and somatostatin (SRIH) receptors. An additional, hypothalamic, site of action is possible as they require intact GHRH secretion to be effective. Continuous GHRP administration leads to pulsatile GH release.

Analogues such as GHRP6 (hexarelin) and GHRP2 have been under investigation as are nonpeptide orally active mimetics such as L-692,429. At equivalent (near-maximal) intravenous doses, hexarelin is a more potent GH secretagogue than GHRH. Intranasal hexarelin is also a potent GH secretagogue in prepubertal children with constitutional short stature. GHRPs given intravenously and orally are currently under investigation in a variety of groups of short stature children. Their potent ability to stimulate GH synthesis and release plus their effectiveness when given orally make them potentially useful, both as diagnostic agents in the evaluation of pituitary disorders and as oral GH secretogogues in 'short normal' children and those in whom 'GH deficiency' is largely hypothalamic rather than pituitary in origin (e.g. post radiotherapy). They are ineffective in children with organic pituitary disease. For a review see Gigho and Broglio.[79]

Ghrelin, a 28 amino acid peptide, has been identified as the natural ligand of the GH secretogogue receptor in the hypothalamus and pituitary.[80] In humans, the serum GH response to intravenous ghrelin is greater than that observed with GHRH, and when ghrelin and GHRH are co-administered, the response is augmented. Ghrelin has been isolated from the arcuate nucleus, but the gastrointestinal tract, and particularly the stomach, appears to be a major site of production. Plasma ghrelin-like immunoreactivity is increased by fasting, reduced by feeding and correlates negatively with BMI.[81] Pharmacological studies suggest that ghrelin is involved in integrating hormonal and metabolic responses to fasting, producing an increase in GH secretion, increased drive to eat, inhibition of insulin secretion and activation of mechanisms directed at maintaining blood glucose levels.[82] Abnormalities of the growth hormone secretagogue receptor may be a cause of short stature in man.[83]

The effective therapeutic use of GHRH itself, potentially a physiological way of treating GH deficiency when the pituitary is intact, has been hampered by the lack of a depot preparation. However subcutaneous GHRH (given twice daily) has been shown to be effective at stimulating growth, e.g. in children treated with cranial irradiation-induced GH deficiency.[84]

Yet other peptides are also important in the regulation of GH secretion: endorphins, neurotensin and vasoactive intestinal peptide (VIP) are stimulatory whilst substance P and central TRH pathways are inhibitory. VIP may have an important role in the release of GH and prolactin in health and disease (e.g. obesity, anorexia nervosa).

GH regulates its own secretion by feedback directly or via effects mediated by the insulin-like growth factors (IGFs) and (probably) metabolic factors such as free fatty acids, insulin and glucose. This results in the characteristic pattern of episodic pulsatile secretion with amplification during the early hours of sleep. New techniques are beginning to reveal the complex functional organization of GH-secreting cells in effecting coordinated pulsatile GH secretion.[85] Disruption of such a coordinated network may explain such slowly developing GH deficiency states as 'neurosecretory dysfunction' or GH insufficiency following traumatic brain injury[86,87] or cranial irradiation.

GH is unusual in being species specific. Two forms are present in man and it is secreted as a heterogeneous molecular species. The predominant, and presumably more bioactive, form is of MW 22000 (22K). An approximately 20K form is present in smaller amounts. Structurally abnormal GH variants with varying bioactivity could be important in the etiology of growth failure in certain rare conditions but are unlikely to be common reasons for poor growth in the population as a whole.

GH is not inhibited by feedback from peripheral endocrine glands although thyroxine and glucocorticoids influence its secretion. Regulation is by GH itself (at hypothalamic and pituitary levels), peripheral GH-dependent growth factors (e.g. IGF-1), GHRH and somatostatin and metabolic factors such as free fatty acids and glucose. The physiological role of GHRPs is still unclear. The integration of this control with physiological states – sleep, exercise, appetite and nutrition – is via the monoaminergic and peptide systems described above.

The plasma half-life of exogenously administered GH is 20–25 min; that of endogenous GH is thought to be similar or shorter although this remains controversial. GH affects linear growth directly by stimulating early epiphyseal growth plate precursor cell differentiation but and it is probable that it has anabolic effects independent of IGF-1. Paracrine IGF-1, produced locally in proliferating chondrocytes of the growth plate, is more important than liver-derived circulating IGF-1 in stimulating epiphyseal cartilage growth. Receptors for many hormones, including estrogen, glucocorticoids and GH, are present in the growth plate which suggests that they directly influence local growth plate processes together with IGF-1 and other growth factors such as Indian hedgehog (Ihh), parathyroid hormone-related peptide (PTHrP), fibroblast growth

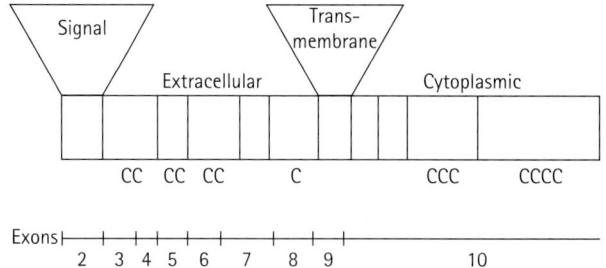

Fig. 15.23   The growth hormone receptor.

factors, bone morphogenic proteins and vascular endothelial growth factor.[88]

In the interaction between GH and tissue growth, the GH receptor is of crucial importance. The GH receptor was cloned from rabbit liver based on amino acid sequence data and from human liver by cross hybridization and consists of a 620 amino acid (AA) peptide situated astride the target cell membrane with a single transmembrane domain. The extracellular hormone-binding domain consists of approximately 245 AAs and there is a cytoplasmic region of 350 residues (Fig. 15.23).

Laron dwarfism[89] is the classical form of GHIS resulting from molecular defects in the GH receptor caused by gene deletions or point mutations. Evidence[90] that heterozygous expression of GH receptor mutations may be associated with growth failure raises questions not only as to whether heterozygotic expression of Laron dwarfism results in a clinically important phenotype but also whether a significant minority of children with 'idiopathic short stature' could be heterozygous for mutations of the GH receptor[91] with abnormal receptor signaling.[92] This also has implications for investigation and diagnosis of short stature and GH 'deficiency'.

Current GH signal transduction models[93] involve activation by GH of a GH receptor-associated tyrosine kinase (GHRTK), an important early (and perhaps initiating) step in signal transduction. GHRTK is stimulated within less than 30 seconds of GH binding to the receptor by very low GH concentrations and is likely to stimulate a variety of cellular responses including kinase activity and gene expression. In particular, GH stimulates tyrosyl phosphorylation and kinase activity of a GH dependent GH receptor-associated kinase JAK 2 (one of a family of Janus kinases). JAK 2 probably serves as a signaling molecule for multiple members of a cytokine/hematopoietin family which includes GH, PRL, erythropoietin, interleukin-3, etc. GHRTK functions both to activate other proteins by phosphorylation and to phosphorylate tyrosine residues in itself and the GH receptor. These phosphorylated tyrosines may serve as docking sites for proteins in other signaling pathways. Such studies should lead to the identification of new cellular actions for GH.

To be biologically active, GH must bind to a transmembrane receptor, which must dimerize and activate an intracellular signal transduction pathway causing IGF-1 synthesis and secretion. However, IGF-1 which, in blood, is itself bound to members of a family of binding proteins (IGFBPs), must bind to the IGF-1 receptor, in turn activating its own signal transduction pathways producing mitogenic and anabolic responses and tissue growth. Thus GH effects its action on target tissues by binding to specific receptors expressed both in the liver and other target tissues throughout the body. This activates genes which include those which code for IGF-1 which stimulates tissue growth by endocrine and (largely) paracrine and autocrine activity. The complexity of these pathways (together with the vagaries of GH assays and the pulsatile nature of GH release) helps to explain the difficulties in measuring 'GH secretory ability' or 'GH sensitivity' in many short stature children.

The clinical phenotypes of GH insensitivity reflect the effects of postnatal IGF deficiency and are broadly identical to the phenotype of complete congenital GH deficiency. This phenotype differs somewhat from that of defects of the IGF-1 gene[94,95] indicating that prenatal IGF-1 production is largely independent of GH and that IGF-1 (and not GH) is a major factor in intrauterine growth regulation.

GROWTH REGULATION

The determination of the somatotroph cell line is dependent on various transcription factors: Prop-1, Pit-1, HesX-1, Lhx-3, Lhx-4. Mutations in all of these have now been identified in patients with hypopituitarism. Defective Prop-1 function causes combined pituitary hormone deficiencies. Hypogonadism represents the major difference between the Pit-1 and Prop-1 hormone phenotype. HesX-1 is necessary for the normal development of the forebrain, eyes, olfactory placodes and anterior pituitary. Mutations result in variable hypopituitarism ranging from isolated GH deficiency to panhypopituitarism.[96] Sox 3 mutations in humans may also account for some sporadic forms of GH deficiency.[97] Pit-1 also plays a role in the activation and regulation of the somatotroph gene product, GH. Additional factors such as CREB and the GHRH receptor may be important for somatotroph determination, while Zn-15 and Pitx2 are thought to be involved in GH gene activation.[11]

A gene thought to be critical for normal growth, the 'short stature homeobox-containing gene' (SHOX), has been identified on the pseudo-autosomal region of the sex chromosomes (a region of the X chromosome which normally escapes X inactivation). SHOX may have a general role in determining chondrocyte function (and perhaps differentiation in particular) in the growth plate, and is expressed there from 12 weeks' gestation until epiphyseal fusion in late adolescence.[98]

SHOX mutations have been occasionally found in children with idiopathic short stature, more commonly in Leri–Weill dyschondrosteosis – an autosomal dominant form of mesomelic dysplasia which has a number of features in common with Turner syndrome (e.g. wide carrying angle, scoliosis and palatal abnormalities) implicated in both the short stature and skeletal dysplastic abnormalities of Turner syndrome. Phenotypes associated with SHOX deficiency are reviewed by Ross et al[99] and the genetic background to cellular expression of the hormonal control of growth regulation by Mullis.[100]

Mechanisms by which physiological states, GH regulation and genetic determination of growth potential are integrated to achieve appropriate stature are largely unknown. Tanner has proposed[101] that the CNS contains a 'sizostat' – the rate of synthesis or release of a specific molecule could decrease as maturity increases and another molecule could be synthesized in proportion to the amount of growth. A 'mismatch' would be sensed by the sizostat and growth adjusted accordingly. This concept, and 'catch-up'[102] and 'catch-down' growth questions whether exogenous hormone therapy in some categories of short children would necessarily increase final height significantly – predictions that do seem to be the case in various pathological conditions and so-called 'idiopathic short stature' (see below).

'Catch-up' growth, rather than CNS-dependent, is more likely intrinsic to the growth plate as suggested in a number of elegant laboratory animal experiments by Baron et al.[103]

The 'infancy–childhood–puberty' model of growth suggests that the infancy component (which is a continuation of fetal growth) is primarily determined by nutritional factors, the childhood component by GH and the puberty component by sex steroids. The infancy component is initially rapid but decelerates as the influence of GH appears by the end of the first year. The effect of GH is sustained but in the absence of adequate sex steroid secretion the pubertal growth spurt is blunted or absent. The combined input of the three components results in the normal pattern of growth to final height. Although simplistic, such a model enables effects of different insults which may affect growth and different treatment modalities to be studied more effectively. Thus epiphyseal fusion is thought to be estrogen mediated (in both sexes) and growth stimulating estrogen effects (in early puberty) to be mediated largely via GH. Estrogen also has direct effects on bone cross-sectional development mainly by suppressing bone resorption at the endocortical surface.[104]

Tall children secrete more GH than their short peers, and GH secretory pulse amplitude correlates with growth velocity although not very strongly.

'Growing pains' appear to be a frequent form of pain in otherwise healthy schoolchildren. However, they probably have little to do with growth. The pain or ache is usually bilateral, commonly situated in the front of the thighs, in the calves and behind the knees, and never situated at or near any joints. There is never any limp, tenderness, redness or swelling. The groin is sometimes affected. Discomfort may come on suddenly or gradually and does not usually occur every day; it usually occurs late in the day and in the evening. When the child wakes in the morning, the pain has usually disappeared. It was once said that emotional growth can be painful but physical growth is not. Perhaps it is simply best to admit ignorance about the cause(s) of 'growing pains' and recognize that they are harmless and self-limiting. They may also be part of the migraine/periodic syndrome spectrum (see migraine in Ch. 22).

THE SHORT OR SLOWLY GROWING CHILD

The 'normality' of a child's height is determined by reference to growth charts showing population norms. Ideally each country and ethnic group should have its own growth standards. In practice, UK charts serve well even in resource limited countries and for ethnic minorities within the UK as differences in final stature reflect minor differences in growth velocity over the whole growing period. Introduction in the UK of nine centile growth charts, based on seven largely cross-sectional local growth surveys between 1978 and 1990,[58] should help to facilitate the appropriate referral of children with growth disorders following community height *screening* (see above). The lowest centile is the 0.4 line – only one normal child in 250 will fall below that line, which is a clear indicator for referral. The interval between each provided pair of centile lines is the same – two thirds of a standard deviation. Two percent of the normal population will have a height below the second centile. It is recommended that any child between the 2nd and 0.4 centiles be monitored to see whether their growth is normal. Versions are available for community and hospital use.

The WHO Multicentre Growth Reference Study (MGRS) is described on page 422. The new growth curves are expected to provide a single international standard that represents the best description of physiological growth for all children from birth to 5 years of age and, importantly, to establish the breast-fed infant as the normative model for growth and development.[105]

Revised charts based on the Tanner–Whitehouse growth standards (determined in a longitudinal study of South of England children in the 1960s) have been produced – the Buckler–Tanner 1995 longitudinal standards.[61] Height revision is adjusted to take account of the recent cross-sectional studies and of Buckler's longitudinal study of adolescent growth.[106] For *monitoring* the growth pattern in an individual child such charts are preferable. Three percent of normal children will, by definition, be below the third centile on a distance (height for age) chart yet a child with a growth disorder of recent onset will be of normal stature. Only serial measurements and calculation of growth velocity will distinguish normality from abnormality.

Parental genetic contributions reduce the population standard deviation of height by about 30%. Ninety-five percent of the children of given parents will have a height prognosis within ± 8.5 cm of the mid parental *centile*. Children also 'inherit' an environment from their parents. A child's shortness, whilst 'appropriate' for his short parents, may reflect poor nutrition or emotional deprivation continuing down the generations with no family member achieving their true genetic height potential.[57]

The possibility of an unrecognized and untreated growth disorder in an unusually short parent must be excluded before attributing a child's shortness to constitutional reasons – pathology, e.g. GH deficiency, a skeletal dysplasia or pseudohypoparathyroidism, may also be genetically transmitted.

Growth retardation affects about one third of children younger than 5 years of age in resource limited countries and is associated with poor cognitive, neurodevelopmental and educational outcomes.

The differential diagnosis of short stature or slow growth is summarized in Table 15.6. Whatever their ultimate height prognosis, many short children may suffer emotionally and underachieve. 'Western' society views tallness as a positive attribute and the social consequences of short stature are not dependent on the presence of underlying pathol-

Table 15.6   Differential diagnosis of short stature and slow growth

Short with currently normal growth velocity
Constitutional short stature, short normal parent(s)

Previous problem affecting growth, now cured or no longer operative
Prolonged intrauterine growth retardation – light for gestational age, low birth length and head circumference, difficult feeders in infancy, including Silver–Russell syndrome – triangular facies, clinodactyly, facial and limb length asymmetry
Congenital heart disease

Physiological growth delay (delayed bone age, normal height prognosis)

Growing slowly (whether already short or still of normal stature)
With increased skinfold thicknesses
Endocrine disease (e.g. panhypopituitarism, severe growth hormone insufficiency – idiopathic or secondary to tumor or irradiation, hypothyroidism, pseudohypoparathyroidism, Cushing syndrome)

Disproportionate
Short limbs for spine (the dyschondroplasias, e.g. achondroplasia, hypochondroplasia, multiple epiphyseal dysplasia)
Short limbs and spine (spine relatively shorter, e.g. mucopolysaccharidoses, metatropic dwarfism)

Often without other obvious signs of disease (see text)
Chromosomal abnormalities (e.g. Turner syndrome – other signs variable)
Unrecognized asthma (may be misdiagnosed)
Malabsorption due to celiac disease, ulcerative colitis, Crohn's disease (bowel habit may be normal)
Psychosocial deprivation
Malnutrition
Cardiovascular or renal disease

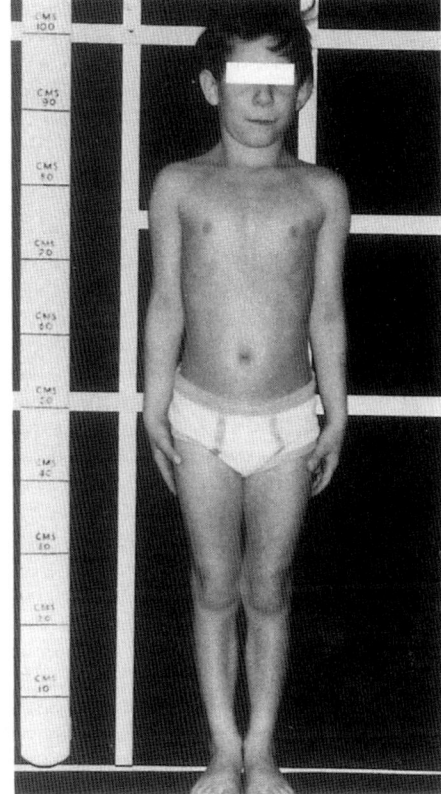

(a)

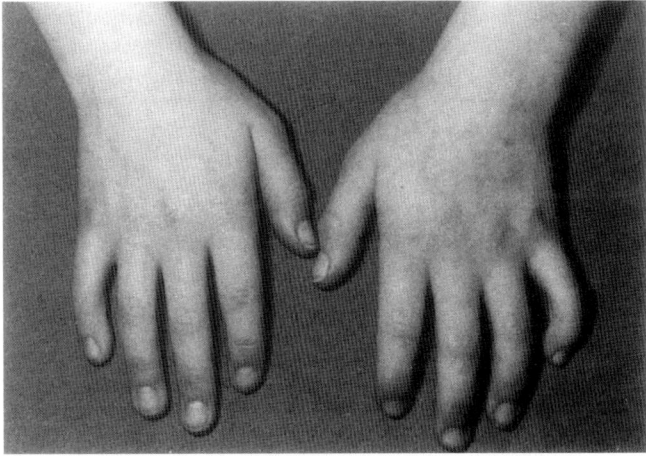

(b)

Fig. 15.24   A child with prolonged intrauterine growth retardation (Silver–Russell) syndrome presenting with short stature. Note the triangular facies, low-set ears, asymmetry (a) and clinodactyly (b).

ogy, which must be sought if growth velocity is inadequate. Without diagnostic clues from history or examination, the screening test for a child presenting with short stature is calculation of growth velocity.

A small child who is growing normally may have small parents (constitutional short stature, but see above), growth (and likely maturational) delay, a previous period of poor growth (for example due to prolonged IUGR, e.g. Silver–Russell syndrome, see Fig. 15.24) or a combination of these factors.

There are currently many children who are short without a recognized cause. These so-called 'idiopathic short stature' (ISS) children can be considered either as part of the continuum between complete growth hormone deficiency (GHD) and normality, or as short stature in the absence of a demonstrable abnormality of the GH–IGF-1 axis. Synonyms of the condition have included normal short stature, primary or constitutional short stature, normal-variant short stature, constitutional delay of growth and adolescence (CDGA) and familial short stature (FSS).

The definition of ISS cannot be refined until we have an adequate definition of GHD. An agreed current working definition is that ISS is a heterogeneous state that encompasses individuals of short stature, including those with FSS, for which there is no currently recognized cause.

Many children referred to as having ISS will undoubtedly have some undiagnosed underlying pathology within the GH–IGF-1 axis, and increasing understanding of the pathophysiology of growth disorders will reduce the number of children categorized as having ISS. Licensing arrangements within the UK and EU refer to 'non-GHD short stature' rather than 'ISS'.

The relatively poor sensitivity and specificity of GH stimulation tests means that many patients currently labeled as having idiopathic GHD would probably be better categorized as having ISS. Many of these 'misdiagnosed' patients are currently responding well to GH therapy. Significant increases in final height have been reported after treatment of ISS with GH although many of the studies have involved small numbers of patients and have suffered from significant methodological faults. A recent randomized double-blind, placebo-controlled study has now been reported[107] in which despite a suboptimal treatment regimen and late age for starting treatment, a mean increase of (only) 3.7 cm was found. Another recent study[108] has also shown small but dose-related increases in final height.

However the clinical significance of the reported increases is doubtful and, in any case, final height is not a validated proxy for quality of life. Whilst some patients with ISS may show psychological stress, they do not appear to have clinically significant behavioral or emotional problems, and it needs to be established whether being taller produces measurable psychological benefit. There is no strong evidence that GH therapy improves psychological adaptation in children with ISS and from a socioeconomic perspective, more evidence of the effectiveness of GH therapy in individual patients with ISS is required before the use of pooled funds can be justified. However, any treatment recommendations based on socioeconomic considerations should be tempered by the fact that it is still not possible to discriminate clearly between partial GHD, subtle abnormalities of the GH–IGF-1 axis and many cases of ISS.

The differential diagnosis of causes of slow growth, whatever the current height, is wide (see Table 15.6).

Endocrine causes
Impaired GH secretion
A few children lack the gene for making GH, demonstrate prenatal GH deficiency, respond to GH therapy with the major antibody response expected to a foreign protein and cannot be treated with any form of GH. Otherwise there is a wide spectrum of GH and IGF-1 secretory ability, which, within the normal population, is likely to be largely genetically determined (see above). At one end of the spectrum are children, perhaps 1 in 4000, with severe GH insufficiency ('GH deficiency'). They grow slowly (Fig. 15.25), demonstrate characteristic clinical features – truncal obesity with characteristic fat 'marbling' (Fig. 15.26), crowding of mid-facial features with immature appearance and small genitalia with micropenis in boys – and show an inadequate (< 7 mU/L) response to a pharmacological stimulus to GH secretion.

There is a continuum from lack of the GH gene at one end of the spectrum through ISS (see above), moderate GH insufficiency (so-called 'partial' GH deficiency), short normal children, those of average height, tall normal individuals, to those with gigantism (Fig. 15.27). Some short, slowly growing children have what is considered to be an abnormal pattern of GH pulsatile release but normal GH responses to stimulation – 'neurosecretory dysfunction'. It is possible that genetic polymorphism for the GH or IGF-1 receptor, IGF-1 or IGFBP3, could also underlie the spectrum of height seen in a normal population, and heterozygosity for classical autosomal recessive disorders could explain growth abnormalities in many children with 'idiopathic' short stature.

Severe GH insufficiency may be congenital, acquired, isolated or associated with other pituitary hormone deficiencies. Many children with 'idiopathic isolated GH deficiency' have a hypothalamic disorder of GHRH release responding to a GHRH bolus by secreting GH normally

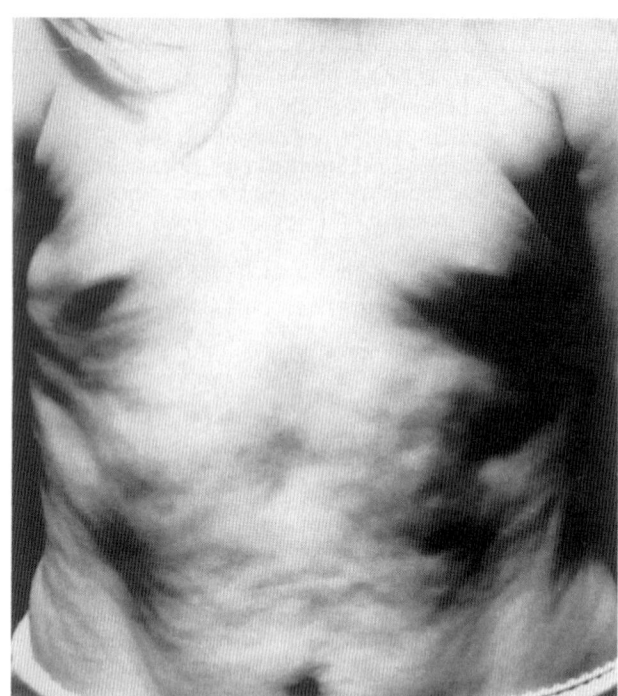
Fig. 15.26 Characteristic 'marbling' of fat in severe GH insufficiency.

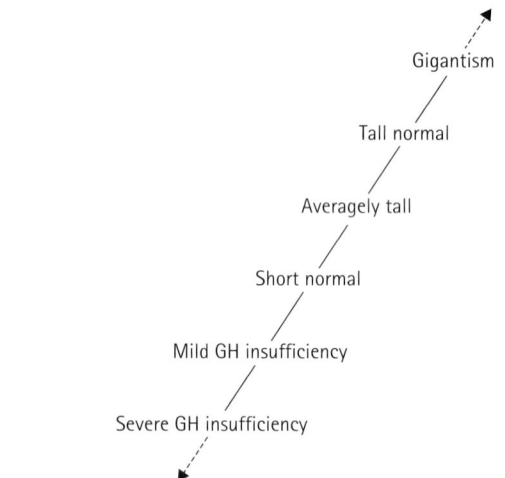
Fig. 15.27 The spectrum of growth hormone secretory ability.

(see below). In others, high resolution CT or MR scanning demonstrates abnormalities ranging from absent septum pellucidum associated with other midline defects (septo-optic dysplasia) to pituitary hypoplasia.

Acquired GH 'deficiency' may result from intracranial tumor (e.g. craniopharyngioma) or from cranial irradiation for medulloblastoma or acute lymphoblastic leukemia. The effects of chemotherapy on growth (and endocrine function) are increasingly recognized. Temporary GH deficiency is seen in children with psychosocial deprivation (see below) and occurs physiologically in late prepuberty and early male puberty. GH biosynthesis and release is also impaired in other conditions (e.g. primary hypothyroidism or coeliac disease) – secretion normalizes with treatment of the underlying disorder.

Hypothyroidism
Acquired primary hypothyroidism is usually autoimmune (Hashimoto thyroiditis) and poor growth velocity and school performance often precede the well-known symptoms and signs by many months.

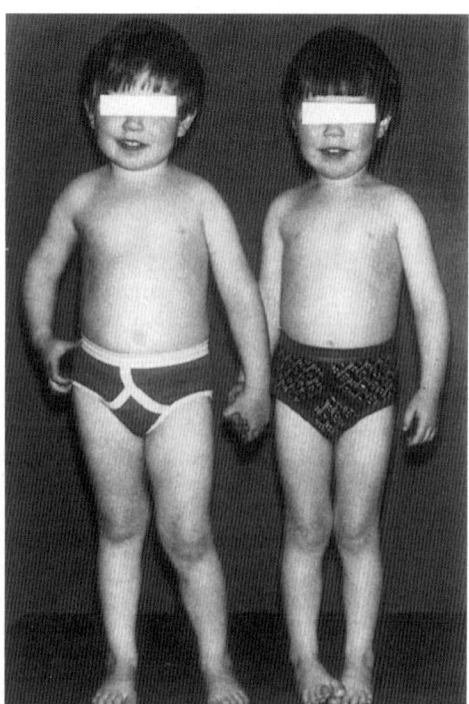
Fig. 15.25 A boy with severe GH insufficiency (right) who is shorter than his 2 years younger brother. Triceps and subscapular skinfold measurements were 97th centile.

Steroids (see also below)

Growth failure from glucocorticoids is usually iatrogenic (excessive medication) rather than due to pituitary dependent Cushing disease (excess ACTH secretion), adrenal tumor (benign or malignant) or ectopic tumor ACTH production which are all rare in children. Alternate day steroid regimens seem less growth suppressing.

Disproportionate short stature

Most constitutional disorders of bone involve long bones and spine to a different extent leading to disproportionate short stature. This may be obvious clinically when there is gross disproportion but may need to be specifically identified from sitting height measurements (subischial leg length equals standing height minus sitting height) and reference to standard charts.

The most important group of skeletal dysplasias affecting cartilage and/or bone growth and development are the osteochondrodysplasias (see Ch. 29).

It is important to recognize disproportionate short stature so that accurate diagnosis can be made without unnecessary investigation. In general, biochemical investigation is unhelpful other than when a mucopolysaccharidosis or disorder of calcium metabolism is suspected and bone biopsy is rarely diagnostic. A full or selective skeletal survey with expert radiological interpretation generally yields most helpful diagnostic information although in the main only in older children.

In general specific therapy is unavailable (although there can be a short term response to GH therapy) and accurate diagnosis is necessary for genetic counseling and accurate prognosis. Limb lengthening orthopedic procedures are reviewed by Saleh et al.[109]

Chromosomal abnormalities

Many chromosomal disorders are associated with poor growth and short stature, particularly absence, partial deletion or translocations of the X chromosome (Turner syndrome and its mosaic forms – Fig. 15.28) (see below). Turner syndrome girls with tall parents may not become conspicuously short until puberty fails to start. Growth charts for Turner syndrome[73] and Down syndrome[110] are available.

Inheritance of two maternal alleles from the same parent (uniparental disomy), in this case on chromosome 7, may be a feature in around 10% patients with severe IUGR (Silver–Russell syndrome or 'primordial dwarfism'). There are several potentially relevant genes which map to the long arm of chromosome 7, e.g. those for IGFBP1, IGFBP3 and

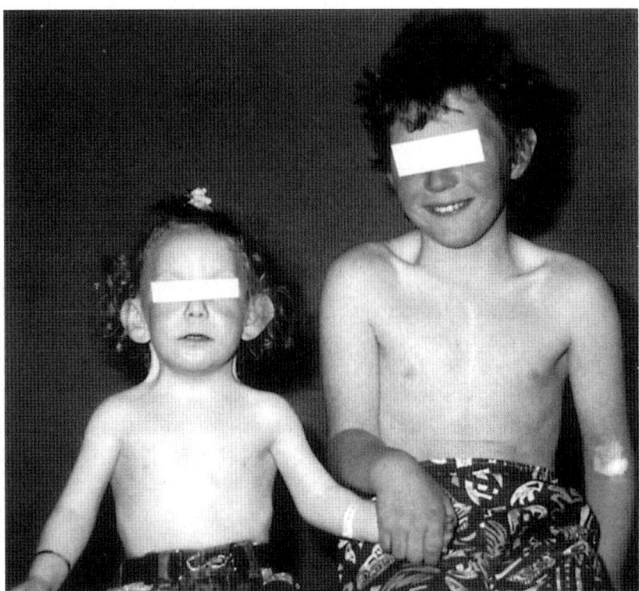

Fig. 15.28 Two unrelated girls with Turner syndrome.

the EGF receptor. Whether any are influenced by the disomy, and thus involved in the pathogenesis of Silver–Russell syndrome, remains to be determined. In addition the chromosome 11p15 region contains a cluster of imprinted genes important for fetal growth, including IGF-2, and partial loss of paternal methylation at various loci has been found to decrease IGF-2 expression and result in clinically typical Silver–Russell syndrome.[111] Some children with postnatal short stature following IUGR appear to have alterations in IGF-1 receptor (IGF-1R) binding[112] and associations have been found between IGF-1 polymorphisms and pre- and postnatal growth in small-for-gestational-age populations.[113]

Chronic disease

Differential diagnosis of the short but not fat child covers virtually the whole field of chronic disorders. Some may be suspected from history or clinical findings but poor growth is often the major diagnostic clue to psychosocial deprivation (see below), unrecognized or undertreated asthma, renal tubular acidosis and malabsorption syndromes such as celiac disease, Crohn disease or ulcerative colitis. Worldwide, protein/calorie deprivation is the commonest cause of growth failure; GH levels are high but peripheral growth factor synthesis and IGF-1 levels are low. Similar effects have also been associated with renal, cardiac and neurological diseases and with hemoglobinopathies.

Whereas it can be difficult to disentangle the relative contributions to impaired growth from the disease process itself and drugs, such as glucocorticoids (GC), data from an in vitro organ culture mouse model suggest that IGF-1 stimulation of chondrocyte hypertrophy (rather than proliferation) may result in reversibility of GC-induced growth retardation.[114] In clinical terms GH therapy may reverse GC-induced growth failure but will have little effect if the chronic disease process remains active.

Psychosocial deprivation

Psychosocial deprivation often causes poor growth, may mimic idiopathic hypopituitarism in terms of GH responses to conventional stimuli and abnormal overnight GH secretory profiles may return to normal rapidly following admission to hospital. Any child growing poorly at home who thrives in hospital or when fostered (Fig. 15.29) should be suspected of being emotionally deprived (see Ch. 5).

Laron syndrome[89]

Laron syndrome is an autosomal recessively inherited syndrome associated with molecular defects in the GH receptor caused by gene deletions or point mutations. These children, whose GH is active in in vitro GH receptor assays, characteristically demonstrate severe postnatal growth failure, secrete abundant GH (with normal or elevated serum levels) but have markedly reduced serum concentrations of IGF-1 and IGFBP3 and do not respond to GH therapy. Some respond well to IGF-1 therapy, and pharmacokinetic studies of recombinant human IGF-1/recombinant IGFBP3 complex are encouraging.[115] Such therapy has potential application in acquired (and much commoner) GH resistance states such as severe catabolism.

Early cases demonstrated low serum GHBP concentrations indicating abnormalities of the extracellular domain of the GH receptor, i.e. circulating GHBP. Many may have deletions or point mutations of the GH receptor gene [nine coding regions (exons) occupying an 87 kilobase segment of chromosome 5] coding for the GH-binding domain. However, it now seems that a minority of the several hundred cases identified worldwide have normal circulating GHBP levels suggesting a degree of heterozygosity and defects in either the portion of the extracellular domain of the GH receptor molecule needed for dimerization or intracellular defects affecting signal transduction. There is now debate as to whether heterozygotic expression of Laron dwarfism results in a clinically important phenotype.

INVESTIGATION OF POOR GROWTH

This is summarized in Table 15.7. Random determination of serum GH levels is unhelpful – pulsatile release and short serum half-life often

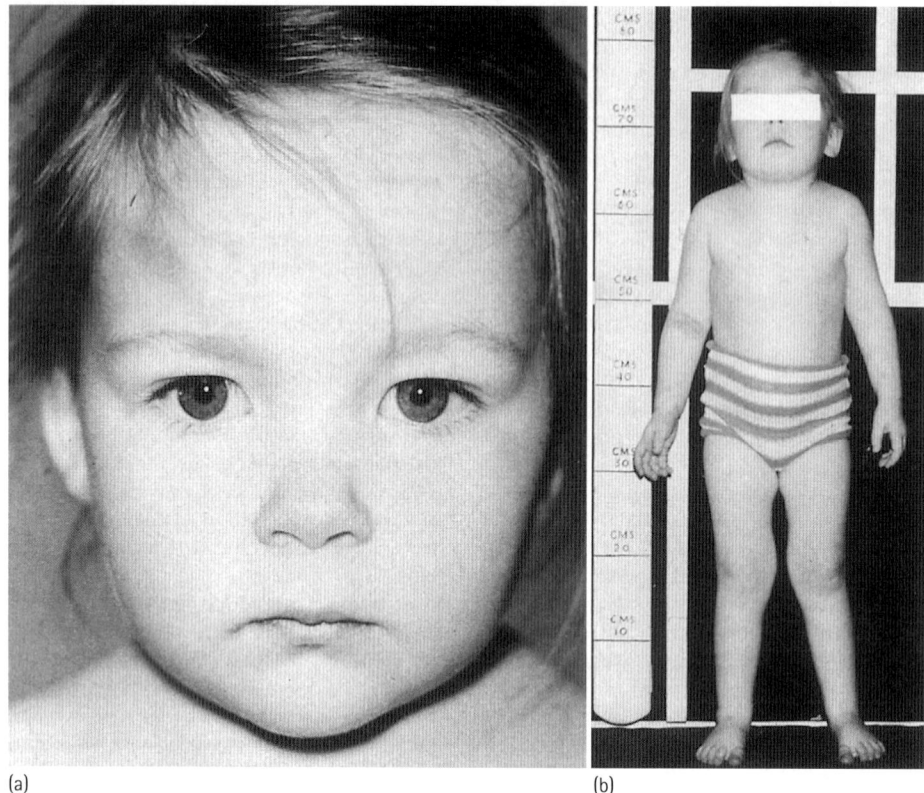

(a)   (b)

Fig. 15.29 An emotionally abused child (note the characteristic expression of 'frozen watchfulness'), photographed on the day of admission to hospital. In the ward environment she showed remarkable 'catch-up' growth and growth hormone secretion normalized. She has since been successfully adopted.

result in low levels in normal children. Establishing a reasonable assessment of GH secretory ability or a firm diagnosis of GH deficiency can be difficult because of the pulsatile, and predominantly nocturnal, nature of GH secretion, variability of GH assays (monoclonal, polyclonal, RIA, IRMA which recognize different circulating forms of GH to varying

Table 15.7 Investigation of poor growth

Full medical and social history
Accurate measurement of the child and his parents
Thorough clinical examination (including measurement of blood pressure, fundi, visual fields)
Bone age
Karyotype (girls)
Specific investigation (when indicated)
    Hematological (e.g. Hb, FBC, ESR)
    Biochemical (e.g. Ca, PO$_4$, alkaline phosphatase, urea and electrolytes)
    Cardiac
    Respiratory
    Renal
    Gastrointestinal including jejunal biopsy
    Endocrine (e.g. T4, prolactin, GnRH, TRH tests, growth hormone provocation test*)
    Skeletal (e.g. radiograph of pituitary fossa, skeletal survey)

*Growth hormone 'provocation' tests (see text):
post-exercise
3–4 h postprandial ⎫ 'screening'
1 h after sleep onset ⎭
clonidine ⎫
ITT ⎬ 'pharmacological'
arginine ⎭
glucagon
physiological sleep studies
urinary GH.

extents) and the complexity of the control of GH secretion and the GH–IGF-1 growth metabolic pathways.

All GH provocation tests may give false negative or positive responses. Screening tests are difficult to standardize and response is variable. The insulin hypoglycemia (tolerance) test (ITT) remains the standard for confirming a diagnosis of severe GH insufficiency. Adequate (symptomatic) hypoglycemia must be obtained if results are to be meaningful (blood glucose < 2.2 mmol/L). Following adequate hypoglycemia, 85% of 'normal' children will produce a serum GH level of over ~ 15 mU/L (usually after 30–60 min, but this cut-off is arbitrary and test stimulus- and assay-dependent). In conjunction with an ITT, the GH response to GHRH is useful for determining whether 'GH insufficiency' is due to a pituitary defect or hypothalamic disorder of GHRH synthesis or release. In the latter case the GH response to GHRH will be normal indicating that pituitary somatotrophs are functional, e.g. in many children with 'isolated GH insufficiency' or 'GH insufficiency' secondary to cranial irradiation.

Tests of GH secretion must be performed only when indicated (and when other possible causes of poor growth have been considered). An ITT is potentially dangerous and requires supervision by competent and experienced junior pediatric staff working from clear and understood protocols and guidelines. These should ensure that glucose and hydrocortisone are drawn up in readiness, there is checking of insulin and glucose dosages, continual presence of a dedicated and experienced member of nursing staff present throughout for monitoring of blood glucose and conscious level, adequate and secure venous access established before insulin is administered and detailed instruction for management of hypoglycemia. It should only be undertaken in specialist endocrine units experienced with its performance.

Spontaneous nocturnal pulsatile GH release measurement provides greater insight into secretory control mechanisms, although their relevance to short stature assessment or as a predictor of response to therapy remains controversial, and this test is impracticable for 'screening' large numbers of children.

Urinary GH levels vary considerably day by day, are approximately 1000-fold lower than in plasma, and accuracy and reproducibility are poor.

Measurement of serum IGF-1 may be a useful screening test for identifying short children who need more complex investigations of GH secretory ability, and theoretical algorithms for the biochemical diagnosis of GH deficiency and insensitivity disorders have been proposed (e.g. Ranke[116]).

TREATMENT OF POOR GROWTH

Treatment aims to correct the underlying problem where possible (e.g. gluten-free diet in celiac disease, thyroxine in hypothyroidism) and can only maximize remaining growth potential. The sooner poor growth is recognized and its cause diagnosed and treated, the better the height prognosis.

Growth hormone
Preparations
From 1958 to 1985, pituitary derived GH was available in limited quantities for children with GH 'deficiency'. These preparations were withdrawn because some batches could have been contaminated with Creutzfeldt–Jacob disease (CJD) 'prion' and current purity could not be guaranteed. Biosynthetic GH, E. coli synthesized and produced by recombinant DNA technology, became available in the UK by late 1985. This was initially with an additional amino-terminal methionine (192 amino acids). Since December 1988, natural sequence 191 amino acid biosynthetic GH has been prescribable in the UK. This is physicochemically identical to natural human hormone. No brain tissue is involved in its production and its administration cannot transmit CJD.

Indications for use
Children with severe GH insufficiency (GH 'deficiency') and moderate GH insufficiency should be treated with GH provided other causes of impaired GH secretion have been excluded. Treatment with a physiological replacement dose of 15–21 units (5–7 mg)/m^2/wk in daily s.c. doses will result in > 90% achieving an adult height within their genetic target height range.[117] Larger (pharmacological – 30 U/m^2/wk, 10 mg/m^2/wk) doses are appropriate in Turner syndrome and chronic renal failure.[118] It is inappropriate to prescribe GH indiscriminately to short children, and GH therapy is of proven benefit in fewer situations than had been predicted when biosynthetic GH first became available.[119] The improved psychological state resulting from knowledge that treatment is being given could itself have a growth-stimulating effect via hypothalamic pathways – children with psychosocial deprivation secrete more GH and grow better when in a normal emotional environment. Postponing puberty in children with GH deficiency is not generally appropriate.[120]

Although a social class-related and socially desirable attribute in 'developed' societies, tall stature does not confer innate biological advantage in all societies. In disadvantaged environments (e.g. the Peruvian Andes), small mothers have more surviving offspring;[121] in an agricultural peasant economy, a small man is more efficient than a tall one, requiring to do less work to feed himself.[122,123] Even if GH therapy increases the height of a normally growing short child, will taller stature in itself contribute to academic or material success or psychological contentment? Leaving aside methodological problems in assessing possible psychological disadvantage from short stature in childhood, it seems probable that there are genuine cultural differences in the psychological effects of short stature even between 'developed' countries (e.g. USA and UK).[124,125]

GH therapy seems to be of particular benefit to children with Turner syndrome and could also benefit those with prolonged IUGR (who often remain short despite normal postnatal growth). The variable outcomes of studies of GH in IUGR probably reflect their heterogeneity of etiology of growth retardation. There is controversy over whether catch-up growth in SGA children has adverse metabolic consequences (e.g. insulin resistance), particularly if high GH doses are used.[126] There is encouraging growth improvement in children with chronic renal failure treated with GH.[118] Infants with chronic renal failure have also been found to benefit in the short and longer term.[127]

GH has been evaluated in the treatment of some skeletal dysplasias but outcomes are generally disappointing and in these groups, surgical limb lengthening may be indicated once the postpubertal patient is able to decide whether they wish to undergo these major and prolonged procedures.[109]

Due to the shortage of available pituitary GH over many years, the dose used in severe GH insufficiency was the most 'cost effective' (in terms of increase in growth velocity achieved per unit GH given) rather than that which would maximally stimulate growth so that, even now, the optimal treatment regimen is not clearly established. A GH dose of 6–8 mg (18–24 units)/m^2/week divided into daily (bedtime) subcutaneous injections may be most effective. Higher (pharmacological) doses [~ 10 mg (30 units)/m^2/week] are more effective in chronic renal disease, Turner syndrome[128] and IUGR. Optimal regimens during puberty have not been established although there is some evidence that mimicking the increase in endogenous GH secretion at the pubertal growth spurt produces a better height outcome.[129] The role of short bursts of GH therapy in a variety of situations remains to be evaluated.

GH antibodies could result in severe growth restriction in a previously normal child but antibodies of sufficient specificity and binding capacity to produce growth attenuation are rare. Potential metabolic side-effects include glucose intolerance, hyperinsulinism, hyperlipidemia and hypertension. Reports of an increased risk of type 2 diabetes[130] are controversial. Benign intracranial hypertension[131] and slipped capital femoral epiphysis are associations but the latter is found in GH deficient children prior to GH treatment. Leukemia may be more common in GH deficient children treated with GH but there is no evidence causally linking GH treatment with leukemia. GH is best avoided in syndromes with chromosomal fragility such as Fanconi syndrome. Psychological harm could result if treatment expectations are not fulfilled.

As with most other drugs, there is wide variation in the treatment efficacy and side-effects profile of GH therapy in individual patients and pharmacogenomic studies are now underway in pediatric endocrinology, particularly in evaluating responsiveness to GH therapy.

GHRH therapy may be appropriate in many 'GH insufficient' children when the problem is at hypothalamic, rather than pituitary, level but optimal treatment regimens are unclear. Although it is possible that future growth promoting treatment modalities could include intranasal GH, intranasal GHRH, depot (intramuscular) GHRH, and IGF-1 in particular circumstances, with several of these preparations bioavailability, practical production difficulties and costs or possible side-effects remain problematic. The most promising developments in the therapeutic application of growth stimulating compounds seem currently to be in the use of depot GH preparations and GH releasing peptides which may impinge significantly on the management of certain types of growth disorder in the future.

Anabolic steroids
Synthetic steroids with enhanced anabolic but little androgenic activity are valuable in growth delay, increasing (normal) slow growth in early male puberty and in Turner syndrome (see pp. 455–6). As with GH therapy, the decision to use these preparations should generally be the province of the specialist in growth disorders.

Emotional support
Emotional support is particularly important for short stature children and their families. Specific treatment may not be available, may be of unproven benefit or may start too late to achieve adequate stature. Any child physically different from his or her peers will attract attention: a short child has to cope with an identity which is determined primarily (and seen by others) in terms of their size. Growth related changes in body shape and size are important determinants of perceived age and adult care-giving responses. Short children must be treated appropriately

for their chronological age, emotionally, intellectually and practically. Teasing, bullying and expectations based on physical size rather than on intrinsic abilities will cause immature behavior, underperformance at school and may impair growth further. They are likely to be aggressive to siblings and peers and more anxious and depressed than controls. Poor exam results cause the small school-leaver to have particular difficulties finding employment.

Children treated with GH should not routinely stay on GH therapy once they reach adulthood. Nevertheless, there is evidence that untreated GH deficiency in adulthood is associated with reduced muscle strength and increased fatigue, a high fat to muscle ratio, reduced bone mineral content with increased risk of osteoporosis and fractures, and adverse cardiovascular risk factors (dyslipidemia and increased fibrinogen levels). All children who have received GH replacement therapy should have their GH status reassessed in young adulthood. A consensus statement is now available with a suggested algorithm for the investigation and treatment of the GH 'insufficient' child at final height at the end of puberty.[132] Patients with clear structural lesions of the hypothalamus/pituitary (organic GHD secondary to a mass lesion, pituitary surgery or radiotherapy) are likely to remain GH deficient and should be considered for GH treatment in adulthood,[133] but others (e.g. with 'idiopathic isolated' GH deficiency) frequently have a normal GH secretory capacity on retesting. Untreated adolescents with reconfirmed 'partial' GH deficiency have altered body composition[134] but it is not known whether this worsens with age or is specifically associated with increased cardiovascular risk.

IGF-1 has important cardioprotective actions through stimulating nitric oxide production in endothelium and vascular smooth muscle and improving cardiac muscle cell survival and function.[135] However it is also mitogenic and antiapoptotic, important actions for tumor genesis, and this has led to concerns (also fueled by overinterpretation in some epidemiological studies) that if GH therapy results in persistently 'high' circulating IGF-1 levels there is an increased risk of developing some cancers in later life. However those at risk epidemiologically have high IGF-1 and low IGFBP3 levels whereas GH therapy results in increases in both. In addition, circulating IGF-1 levels do not reflect tissue IGF-1 (secreted in an autocrine and paracrine manner). A meta-analysis of high quality studies has concluded that, whilst circulating concentrations of IGF-1 and IGFBP3 are associated with modest and variable increased risks for prostate and premenopausal breast cancer, the 3–4-fold increases in cancer risk quoted by narrative reviews are exaggerated.[136]

THE TALL OR RAPIDLY GROWING CHILD (Table 15.8)

Tall stature presents less often than short: syndromes causing tallness are rare whereas poor growth is a common result of childhood disease, and childhood tallness, unless extreme, is socially advantageous. Nevertheless, a tall child is often taken for older and expectations may be greater than can be met. Clumsiness and gangliness may result from neurological immaturity for size.

Advanced skeletal maturation may be associated with tallness in childhood (and a normal growth velocity) but this rarely results in problems or medical help being sought (cf. growth delay).

Constitutional tall stature infrequently presents but tall mothers sometimes worry about their normal daughters' heights. In this situation, drug treatment – attempting to limit GH secretion whilst allowing normal sex steroid mediated skeletal maturation [e.g. with bromocriptine somatostatin analogue (octreotide) or anticholinergic drugs such as pirenzepine or rapidly advancing skeletal maturation (using sex steroids)] – is generally unsatisfactory. Estrogen therapy causes an initial increase in growth velocity, and potential side-effects from the high doses necessary, both short term (headaches and nausea) and long term (diabetes mellitus, hyperlipidemia, hypertension, endometrial carcinoma), limit its usefulness particularly as there has never been a randomized controlled trial to determine its efficacy. It cannot be used much earlier than normal pubertal onset and treatment after the growth spurt

Table 15.8 Differential diagnosis of tall stature or rapid growth

Tall with currently normal growth velocity
Constitutional tall stature (tall normal parent(s))
Previous rapid growth (usually due to overeating)
Physiological growth advance

Currently rapid growth (whether already tall or still of 'normal' stature)
Associated with precocious puberty
Idiopathic (physiological)
Pathological
   Intracranial space-occupying lesions
   Gonadal tumors
   Ectopic gonadotropin-producing tumor (e.g. hepatoblastoma)
   Adrenal
      Congenital adrenal hyperplasia (21-hydroxylase deficiency, 11beta-hydroxylase deficiency)
      Cushing syndrome
      Neoplasia
   Estrogen ingestion (e.g. mother's oral contraceptives)
   Primary hypothyroidism
   Undefined mechanisms
      Birth asphyxia
      Mental retardation, including tuberous sclerosis
      Neurofibromatosis, McCune–Albright syndrome

Not associated with signs of puberty
Hyperthyroidism
Growth hormone excess (gigantism)

With obesity: currently excessive food intake

With dysmorphic features or disproportion
Marfan syndrome
   Long, narrow limbs (dolichostenomelia)
   Arachnodactyly
   Scoliosis
   Aortic incompetence – dissecting aneurysm
   Myopia, retinal detachment, upward lens dislocation
   Autosomal dominant (often new mutation)

Homocystinuria
   Marfanoid body habitus
   Mental retardation
   Stiff joints with knock knee
   Downward lens subluxation
   Urine positive for homocystine
   Autosomal recessive

Congenital contractural arachnodactyly
   Kyphoscoliosis
   Joint contractures
   No ocular or CNS problems
   Autosomal dominant

Sotos syndrome (cerebral gigantism)
   Large size at birth
   Hypertelorism, downslanting palpebral fissures, prominent forehead
   Large hands and feet
   Large male external genitalia
   Mental retardation ± hypotonia, ataxia

Klinefelter syndrome
   Disproportionately long legs
   Small firm testes
   Hypogonadism, infertility, with or without gynecomastia

is underway (early in female puberty) would have only a small effect on reducing final height. Recent data suggest that there are additional deleterious effects on fertility.[137]

When height prognosis remains unacceptably high to child and family, surgical epiphysiodesis, an established procedure for reducing moderate leg length discrepancy[138] may be indicated. Surgical management of tall stature is reviewed by Macnicol.[139]

Tall stature syndromes

These are outlined in Table 15.8. Gigantism due to excessive GH secretion is extremely rare in pediatric practice (cf. acromegaly after epiphyseal closure).

Tallness and obesity

Tallness in childhood is commonly associated with food intake that is, or has been, excessive for growth and energy requirements. In wealthy societies, eating is a social as well as nutritional activity and moderate fatness in a baby may be seen as proof of mother love. Fat babies tend to be placid and little trouble. Once a child is overweight, calorie intake need not be excessive to maintain the situation. Continuing overeating causes rapid growth, skeletal maturational advance, earlier puberty and early epiphyseal closure – adult height is not increased. If overeating stops but calorie reduction is insufficient to lose weight, growth velocity is normal but the child is tall and bone age remains advanced.

Rapid growth and precocious puberty

If nutrition has been normal, rapid growth is most commonly due to precocious puberty (see p. 451). Final height may be significantly short (depending on etiology and duration) due to early epiphyseal closure in pathological precocious puberty but in children with constitutional advance of growth and puberty their genetic adult height potential will be reached.

Endocrine causes of rapid growth

These are either uncommon (thyrotoxicosis) or rare (gigantism, excess androgen secretion from an adrenal tumor).

OBESITY AND THINNESS

Malnutrition leading to obesity or thinness is discussed in Chapter 16. Discussion here is limited to some general comments and consideration of endocrine disorders which may be associated with each nutritional state.

Mechanisms of body mass regulation include genetic, environmental and behavioral factors. Genetic studies in obese mice have revealed the ob gene, its products leptin and the leptin receptor to be important factors in the regulation of both appetite and energy expenditure. In rodents as well as in humans, homozygous mutations in genes encoding leptin or the leptin receptor cause early-onset morbid obesity, hyperphagia and reduced energy expenditure.[140]

Leptin concentrations correlate with adipose tissue mass and are regulated by feeding and fasting, insulin, glucocorticoids and other factors. Leptin acts via the CNS to reduce food intake and increase energy expenditure. Overweight children generally have leptin concentrations raised in proportion to their fat mass, and leptin deficiency or insensitivity is an extremely rare cause of obesity.

Leptin is thought to play a role as an endocrine mediator in sexual development and reproduction (see below). In addition, SGA children have both low cord blood and plasma leptin levels with a predisposition to adverse metabolic outcomes in later life. Some gut hormones have been shown to be important in influencing food intake and body weight. For a review see Druce et al.[141]

Weight in itself is a poor guide to nutrition – the interpretation of a high weight for a child's height as 'obesity' may be seriously misleading at times when growth and fatness are varying in opposite directions: a normal early pubertal boy is growing slowly but increasing body fat rapidly. Poor weight gain in a baby may be normal if the mother is tall and the father short as the maternal environment (in addition to genetic factors) is important in determining birth weight. In infancy weight gain largely reflects fluid flux; in the older child differences between normal and abnormal rates of weight gain are smaller than the reproducibility of weight measurements obtained some months apart even on sophisticated (and well-maintained and balanced) weighing scales.

The use of body mass index (BMI) – weight (kg)/height (m)^2 – provides a practical clinical tool for identification of adults with different degrees of obesity which carry particular adverse risks, for example hypertension, hypercholesterolemia and type 2 diabetes. However use of a stable height as a basis for calculation, inapplicable to growing children, had limited its usefulness in pediatric practice. BMI changes substantially in children, rising steeply in infancy, falling during pre-school years (from around 2 years of age) and rising again (between 5 and 8 years – the 'adiposity rebound') and into adulthood.[60]

Children accumulate fat free mass as they grow and muscle is denser than fat. Thus BMI underestimates the percentage of lean body mass by taking no account of variations in muscularity: particularly fit and muscular individuals will have a relatively high BMI.

In normal and underweight individuals between one quarter and one half of total body fat is subcutaneous – most excess fat in the obese is deposited there. Thus the adequacy, inadequacy or overadequacy of nutrition is effectively assessed from skinfold measurements using calipers comparing results with available standards for age.[142] Measurement of limb circumference assesses muscle and bone as well as fat. Measurements of triceps and subscapular skinfolds are representative of total body fat[143] and show least between observer error.[144]

Care must be taken in interpretation: standards will depend on racial, maturational and genetic factors[145] as well as age, and change as nutritional recommendations and feeding policies vary. British children were fatter in 1975[142] than 1962 and there is evidence that this trend is continuing.[146] Standards reflect what is present in the 'normal' population, not necessarily what is optimally physiological. Despite this, skinfold measurements provide quick, easy and reproducible estimates of nutritional state and are particularly useful in longitudinal assessment of an individual child.

Mesenteric fat thickness (assessed by ultrasound) is an important determinant of metabolic syndrome[147] and, despite concerns about its reproducibility, waist circumference measurement (in addition to BMI) significantly increases information about the obesity-related health risks in children and adolescents.[148]

OBESITY

In 'normal' children

A standard definition of 'overweight' and 'obesity' in children and young people is desirable. In adults, cut-off points for overweight and obesity are based on morbidity and mortality associated with excessive weight. In the absence of such data in children, the International Obesity Task Force defined the cut-offs for young people by back-extrapolating from the BMI centile corresponding to values of > 25 kg/m^2 (overweight) and 30 kg/m^2 (obese) at age 18.[71] Simply defining overweight as > 85th BMI centile and obesity as > 95th centile means that as standards are updated the nature of any secular trend to increasing obesity is obscured (15% and 5% will always be overweight or obese respectively) and international comparisons are obscured.[149]

The prevalence of overweight and obesity amongst children has trebled in 20 years[150] and is now a global epidemic.[151] The increase is not only in industrialized but also in resource limited countries. Overeating and increases in sedentary behavior are the commonest causes of childhood obesity. Energy intake surplus to requirements for growth, thermogenesis, basal metabolism and activity results in fat deposition (Fig. 15.30). It is likely that some, but not all, obese individuals eat, or have been eating, excessively. Nevertheless, observed variation between individuals in energy intake necessary to achieve normal fat deposition is likely to reflect genetic factors as well as differences in energy expenditure. Relative contributions of environmental and genetic factors remain poorly understood and certainly differ between different obese individuals.

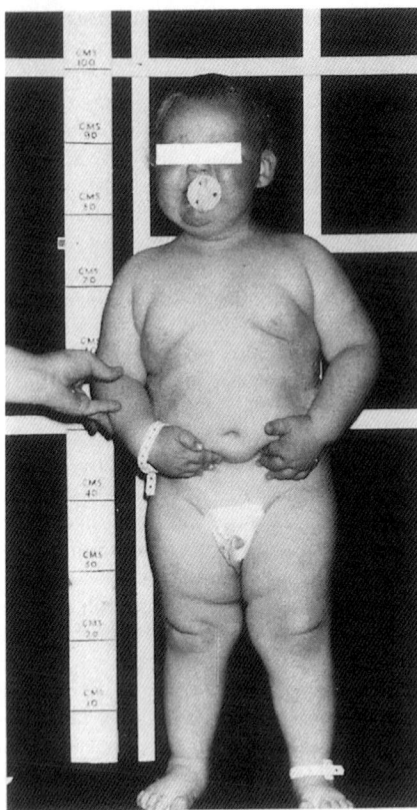

Fig. 15.30 Gross obesity in a toddler due to excessive food intake.

The first year of life is not critical for determining adipocyte numbers, which are related to the degree and duration of obesity rather than age at onset. Nevertheless, fat infants are 2–3 times likelier to become obese children than their normal peers.[152] A childhood BMI > 85th centile, an obese parent and an early recurrence of the adiposity rebound (at about 5 years) may predict adult obesity,[153] and overweight and obesity in adolescents lead to a significant and (in health terms) meaningful increase in obesity and mortality in mid-adulthood.[154]

There are three groups of children who are at particular risk of obesity in later life: (1) low birth weight (mainly SGA but also probably some pre-term) infants with rapid early infancy catch-up growth; (2) normal birth weight infants with an early adiposity rebound; and (3) infants with increased body weight and faster growth during infancy.[155] Metabolic complications seem more common in the first two groups.

Although mild overweight seems unlikely to be associated with short or long term ill health, childhood obesity may affect educational attainment and interpersonal relationships adversely,[156] especially in boys, will probably persist into adulthood and is associated with an increased risk of hypertension, stroke, myocardial infarction or type 2 diabetes mellitus, osteoarthritis, breast and bowel cancers, skin disorders and asthma and other respiratory problems.[157]

The most important treatment goal is sustainable healthy eating (rather than 'dieting') and habitual reasonable levels of physical activity (e.g. walking and cycling). Young obese children should aim to maintain their weight (which they will 'grow into') rather than lose weight. Interventions involving parents and behavior modification may be effective.[158] Advice is only likely to be successful if the child and whole family are involved and motivated. Evidence-based management of childhood obesity is summarized by Edmunds et al.[159]

Sibutramine, which inhibits the reuptake of noradrenaline and serotonin in the CNS, results in reduced energy intake and increased thermogenesis and appears safe and effective in producing short term weight loss in obese adolescents.[160] However, pharmacological treatment of obese adolescents remains experimental as is bariatric surgery (stomach stapling or gastric banding) which has been little studied in children. Despite the risks, surgery for extremely obese children (BMI > 40) may have to be considered .

Secondary endocrine effects

'Simple' obesity (due to large appetite and excessive food intake) is associated with a number of minor (secondary) endocrine abnormalities. Increased adrenal androgen secretion for chronological (but not for bone) age could be a factor influencing the early onset of puberty in such children[161] but increased GC metabolite excretion may reflect increased liver cortisol metabolism. There is frequently hyperinsulinemia, more marked in girls, older children and long-standing obesity, and unrelated to adipocyte size.[162] It is thought to be related to both insulin resistance (with a fall in the concentration of adipocyte insulin receptors) and excessive carbohydrate intake.[163] A low sex hormone binding protein level for age is a useful biochemical marker for insulin resistance. A low calorie diet results in a rapid fall in insulin levels (before there are changes in weight, body fat mass or adipocyte size) with a rapid rise once dieting ceases, again preceding these other changes.[164]

The risk of developing overt type 2 diabetes mellitus increases with age and degree of obesity but is still an uncommon complication in children, although now less so in adolescents in the UK and particularly ethnic minority groups.[165] Impaired glucose tolerance is certainly common amongst obese adolescents but changes in insulin secretion and sensitivity that precede its development are still poorly understood. There is evidence that altered fat partitioning in abdominal adipose tissue and skeletal muscle is an early metabolic change in obese adolescents progressing to impaired glucose tolerance.[166]

As Part of genetic/endocrine disorders

Obesity can be genetic or endocrine in origin. Height measurement is an important screening test. Overeating in normal children causes an increase in growth velocity and these children are generally tall for age with bone age advance. There is early epiphyseal closure and usually no final height increase. Some adolescent boys, in particular, may present with obesity, below average height and delayed puberty. Acceleration of height velocity is seen with rapid weight gain, and strict dieting is associated with slowing of linear growth. Thus if overeating stops but there is insufficient reduction in calorie intake to lose weight, growth velocity may be normal but the child is tall and bone age remains advanced.

In contrast, virtually all endocrine and hypothalamic causes of obesity are associated with poor linear growth, short stature and bone age delay. Endocrine causes include excessive corticosteroid administration, GH insufficiency, hypopituitarism, hyper- or hypogonadotrophic hypogonadism, hypothyroidism, pseudohypoparathyroidism and craniopharyngioma. Cushing syndrome may initially cause rapid growth. Obesity also occurs with hyperinsulinism.

Hypothalamic damage from tumors, meningitis, encephalitis, radiotherapy or trauma may cause obesity. Possible mechanisms underlying the obesity include endocrine factors (hyperinsulinism – but this could be cause or effect, hyperprolactinemia, GH deficiency – but suppressed GH secretion may also be due to obesity) and nutritional and psychological factors.

Hypothalamic syndromes associated with mental retardation and obesity include Laurence–Moon–Biedl, Bardet–Biedl and Prader–Willi. Craniopharyngioma may be associated with obesity after surgery or radiotherapy even if vision and activity are normal, food intake is appropriate and endocrine replacement therapy optimal. It seems likely that 'Fröhlich syndrome' (one case of blindness, short stature, obesity and pubertal failure with a cyst in the region of the sella turcica) was due to craniopharyngioma.

The obesity of Down and other mental handicap syndromes may relate both to underlying genetic or metabolic abnormalities and physical inactivity – the latter is a major cause of obesity in physically handicapped children (e.g. spina bifida, muscular dystrophy).

Diagnosis of Prader–Willi syndrome (PWS) is based on the characteristic history and clinical features (see Ch. 14) Diagnosis may often be made at birth from the association of characteristic facial features with history of poor fetal movements, hypotonia and poor feeding.

Endocrine features include hypogonadism (micropenis, hypoplastic scrotum and bilateral cryptorchidism in males), normal or increased

GT secretion, poor secondary sexual development and delayed menarche, insulin resistance and diabetes mellitus and growth failure. Energy requirements are abnormally low and appetite insatiable. Growth may be particularly poor when appetite is most successfully controlled and during adolescence. Scoliosis may impair spinal growth and, with gross obesity, predisposes to respiratory failure and death. There is a suggestion (largely from uncontrolled cohort studies) that GH therapy is effective in stimulating growth if started in the young child and can result in a height within the parent-based target range within 3 years of treatment. However the main benefit is metabolic (body composition, fat utilization) and in improving muscle tone and power. Current studies are focusing on GH treatment in younger patients, including infancy, tempered by anecdotal reports of sudden death during GH therapy, the pathogenesis of which remains unclear.[167,168]

There have been recent advances in the molecular genetics of obesity risk including the suggestion that GAD2 on chromosome 10p12 is a candidate gene for human obesity and that genetic variation in GABA metabolism may influence obesity risk.[169] Further obesity candidate genes include loci on 6q.[170]

THINNESS

Skinfold measurements and BMI, not weight, are best guides to thinness and undernutrition. A healthy child who is offered appetizing food in adequate amounts and variety in an emotionally supportive environment will eat enough to enable him to grow normally. This may be much less than mother (or granny) feels should be eaten. A thin child who is growing normally and not getting thinner should not be investigated or treated; one who is growing slowly or getting thinner needs investigation, diagnosis and treatment.

The battle to get a healthy child to eat more than necessary is one that parents are likely to lose and can produce emotional problems in both child and parents then or later. Reassurance that a thin child is healthy and growing normally will often, in itself, defuse an emotionally strained family situation. In other circumstances, treatment of the underlying cause of the thinness is necessary but may be easier with organic than emotional disorders.

Recognizable syndromes (e.g. lipodystrophy, Marfan syndrome) and malignancies are rare, but unrecognized organic disease (e.g. asthma, malabsorption due to celiac disease, ulcerative colitis or Crohn's disease) may present with few overt signs and commonly causes poor growth and thinness. Calories may be too few (worldwide the most important cause of poor growth and thinness, particularly in association with recurrent infection) but some children are on inadequate diets for ethnic or cultural reasons and some mothers are so concerned to prevent obesity that calorie intake is deficient. In the UK, emotional problems are common causes of thinness and poor growth. Anorexia nervosa may be life threatening in an adolescent.

Acute malnutrition causes loss of fat and muscle; chronic malnutrition causes stunting but thinness may be masked by fat deposition.[171] Secondary endocrine responses to malnutrition result from the need to conserve the limited energy intake available. Cortisol, TSH, T3, GT and IGF-1 levels are low.

IGF-1 is controlled to a major extent by nutrition. In kwashiorkor and marasmus growth slows because of end-organ unresponsiveness to the action of GH; GH levels are high[172] and IGF-1 levels low.[173]

Acute fasting in the human is associated with a reduction in GH receptor numbers and receptor loss can be prevented with GH infusion, suggesting that resistance is at the post-receptor level. Zinc deficiency is associated with reduced IGF-1 levels and supplementation may stimulate catch-up growth.[174]

Anorexia nervosa patients have normal cortisol production but decreased clearance rates[175] due to low liver 11betaOHSD activity. 5alpha-reductase levels are also reduced[176] – this enzyme is also present in the liver. The secretory pattern of LH is immature and pubertal development either does not begin, halts (and may regress) or there is amenorrhea, depending on age at onset of anorexia and its degree. Estrogen deficiency is likely to reduce GH pulsatile release and this may be an additional

mechanism by which growth slows. Multicystic ovaries (a normal phase in ovarian maturation) are seen during recovery, and vomiting, hypotension and cachexia may suggest Addison disease but are generally much more severe in anorexia nervosa – hirsutism may also occur in both.

ENDOCRINOLOGICAL ASPECTS OF PUBERTY AND ADOLESCENCE

THE GONADS

Ovaries and testes have two main functions: development and maintenance of secondary sexual characteristics, and reproductive capability. Sex steroidogenic pathways in adrenals and gonads are identical – relative differences in types and quantities of individual androgens and estrogens reflect different enzymic activities.

Physiology

The ovary

Endocrine functions reside in ovarian follicles. Luteinizing hormone (LH) binds to theca cells to stimulate androstenedione and testosterone biosynthesis from cholesterol. These diffuse into granulosa cells which convert them to estrone (E1) and estradiol (E2) respectively (aromatization) under the influence of follicle stimulating hormone (FSH). E1 and E2 interconversion also takes place in the granulosa cells. E1 is largely albumin bound; E2 is also bound to a specific globulin which also binds testosterone.

Estrogens stimulate secondary sex character development and, in the sexually mature, estrogens and progestogens ensure fertility by releasing ova and regulating the menstrual cycle. Estrogens are responsible for growth of vagina, uterus and Fallopian tubes, and have a major role in the normal pubertal growth spurt and fusion of epiphyses at the end of puberty. They are metabolized in liver and excreted in urine.

The mechanism by which the dominant follicle suppresses others in both ovaries is unclear. 'Inhibin' is found in follicular fluid, is thought to be secreted by granulosa cells and may have local effects as well as affecting feedback inhibition of FSH.

The testis

Both LH and FSH are required for spermatogenesis. FSH is necessary for initial establishment of mature germinal epithelium and initiation of spermatogenesis. LH effects are mediated through Leydig cell testosterone secretion. Spermatogenesis duration is approximately 74 days. Thus testosterone has both endocrine (secondary sexual characteristics and libido development) and paracrine effects (a permissive effect on spermatogenesis in the presence of FSH).

Two percent of testosterone in the mature male is in free active form, one third is bound to a specific beta-globulin – sex hormone binding globulin (SHBG) – and the remainder to albumin. In the target organs which require dihydrotestosterone (DHT) (scrotum, phallus, prostate), testosterone is converted to DHT by 5alpha-reductase; in other tissues (e.g. bone, muscle, internal genitalia) testosterone acts directly.

Testosterone exerts negative feedback on LH secretion mainly at hypothalamic level but has little effect on FSH. However FSH levels are high in the castrate. There is also a family of gonadal peptides which have inhibitory ('inhibin') and stimulatory ('activin') feedback effects at pituitary level and important gonadal (paracrine) effects. Modulation of FSH secretion at pituitary level is by mechanisms distinct from the GnRH receptor on the pituitary gonadotroph. Inhibins are now known to be secreted in a variety of forms from the testis (Sertoli cells), placenta and ovary (granulosa cells).

The inhibins may be important in normal puberty (see below).

The adrenals produce quantitatively more androgens than testes and these are of importance in childhood in physiological and pathological situations. In puberty and subsequently, the role of the testes is qualitatively paramount because testosterone is much more potent than androstenedione or dehydroepiandrosterone (DHA) – testicular failure causes hypogonadism despite normal adrenal function. Small quantities of estrogen are produced by normal testes by Sertoli cell aromatization of androgen. Testosterone is also metabolized to estrogen in some peripheral tissues (notably adipose cells) and the liver prior to urinary excretion.

ENDOCRINE BACKGROUND TO NORMAL PUBERTY

Individual secondary sexual characteristics result from different hormonal events and must be assessed independently. Over the last century, children have tended to become taller and reach physical and sexual maturity earlier but whether this process is continuing is more contentious.[177]

Reports of, and recommendations based on, data which purport to show that African–American and White American girls are showing secondary sexual development respectively 2 years and 1 year earlier than was the case a generation ago[178,179] may well be the result of methodological (selection and observer) bias. Early breast development may be mimicked superficially by obesity which will bias self-reported data.

Although an increasing prevalence of obesity in the population might be an explanation for a genuine advance in the timing of puberty onset, the age of menarche (a much more robust maturational marker) does not seem to be lowering comparably further in industrialized nations.[180] This implies either significant methodological flaws in the study of Herman-Giddens et al[178] [and in unpublished UK data from the Avon Longitudinal Study of Parents and Children (ALSPAC)] or that the tempo of pubertal progression is slower than was previously the case (for which there is no evidence or obvious physiological explanation at a population, as opposed to individual, level).[177]

Accurate national registry population-based data from Denmark have estimated that 0.2% of Danish girls and 0.05% of Danish boys had some form of precocious pubertal development and, importantly, that the incidence was unchanged over the 9 years of the study (1993–2001).[181] In this context, the claim that similar differences in the timing of male puberty (onset of genital and pubic hair growth) have been occurring[182] must be treated with caution.

Although puberty timing and duration are very variable between normal individuals, pubertal development is a harmonious process: marked discrepancies from the normal sequence of events (loss of consonance) should lead to suspicion of pathology. In contrast, adolescence is sometimes far from harmonious – social pressures may be particularly marked in many who are sexually mature but still growing emotionally and intellectually, and emotional problems seen in those with the timing of puberty at either end of the normal spectrum.

CHANGES IN FETUS, INFANT AND CHILD AND THEIR RELEVANCE TO PUBERTY INITIATION

Fetal GT production occurs from the fifth week, rising until 20 weeks. Levels are higher in females, perhaps because of feedback inhibition by fetal testosterone in males. Placental human chorionic gonadotrophin (HCG) is secreted from implantation onwards and is the major stimulus for fetal Leydig cell testosterone; it seems unlikely that the fetal hypothalamo-pituitary–gonadal axis is fully functional by postpubertal standards. After delivery, a rise in GT levels persists for several months in both sexes. Total testosterone levels are high in males partly due to high SHBG levels. During the first year, the axis becomes quiescent. There is little evidence for the existence of specific inhibitory hormones (see pineal, p. 464) although CNS inhibitory influences could be important – precocious puberty is common following cranial irradiation for acute lymphoblastic leukemia (ALL).

Pulsatile gonadotrophin releasing hormone (GnRH) secretion is of paramount importance in primate sexual maturation although there is increasing biochemical and ultrasound evidence for activity well before the onset of clinical gonadarche. During childhood, there is gradual amplification of GnRH signals with pulses of low frequency and amplitude, and from well before the clinical onset of puberty, around adrenarche, nocturnal pulsatile GnRH secretion is detectable with increasing pulse frequency[183] associated with multicystic prepubertal ovaries on ultra-

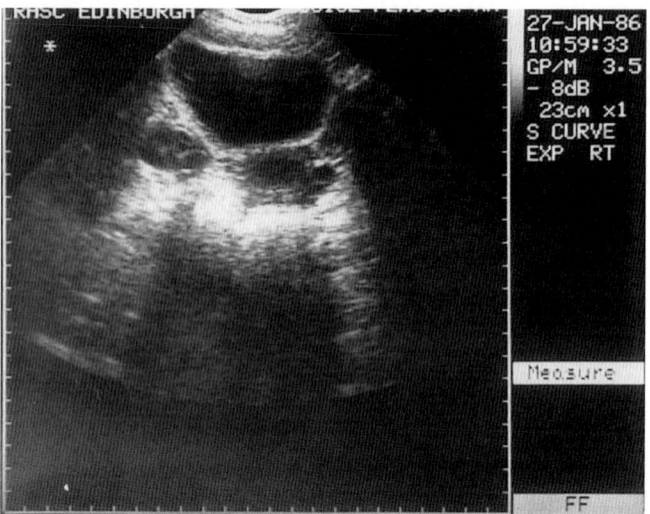

Fig. 15.31   The multicystic appearance of late prepubertal ovaries.

sound (Fig. 15.31). This normal stage of development (characterized by the presence of > 6 follicles of diameter > 4 mm) is associated with activation of the axis resulting in nocturnal pulsatile GnRH secretion without (as yet) estrogen-mediated positive feedback. For normal ranges of ovarian and uterine size during childhood see Neu.[184]

Modulation of pituitary LH secretion resulting from increased GnRH pulse frequency is an important characteristic of transition between juvenile and peripubertal stages in man (Fig. 15.32). A crucial condition for normal pubertal development may involve organization of neuronal circuits which not only maintain synchronized pulsatile GnRH release but enable their incorporation into the daily sleep – wake rhythm.[186] It is likely that continuing pubertal transition to adult pituitary – gonadal function involves gradual further recruitment, organization and synchronization of GnRH neuronal discharge over an increasing proportion of the evening/night and resetting of gonadal negative feedback. Clinically, an early morning testosterone measurement is a useful predictor of the imminence of puberty.[187]

Sensitive and specific assays to distinguish different inhibin forms have shown that in normal boys testicular production of inhibin B increases as puberty progresses and that the initiation of puberty is accompanied by a dramatic switch from a positive to a negative relationship between inhibin B and FSH.[188] Inhibin B may also be a more sensitive predictor than testosterone of clinical pubertal onset. The two peaks of inhibin B (during infancy and early puberty) appear to reflect the two periods of Sertoli cell proliferation in normal human males. During mid-childhood a relatively constant amount of inhibin B is secreted. The early FSH-independent increase in inhibin B that precedes clinical puberty and continues to stage G2[6] may be stimulated by testosterone or other Leydig cell factors. The inverse relationship between inhibin B and FSH that develops from mid-puberty onwards is consistent with the establishment of the negative feedback loop at this stage.[189]

Although median levels of inhibins A and B remain low until after age 10 years in girls, there is evidence, from sporadically increased levels in normal prepubertal girls and their positive correlation with FSH levels, of sporadic FSH-dependent follicular development in infancy and childhood.[189] In puberty, the increase in inhibins A and B and their lack of positive correlation with FSH from stage B3[6] onwards, suggests that follicular growth is dependent more on the duration of FSH elevation above a critical threshold than the levels per se.[189]

As puberty progresses, GnRH (and thus GT) pulse frequency remains at about 2 h but with increasing amplitude and daytime as well as nocturnal pulses (Fig. 15.33).[185] Twenty-four hour pulsatile release is necessary for full pubertal development, menarche and ovulation. In the follicular phase of the menstrual cycle, GnRH pulse frequency increases to approximately hourly and falls to 3 hourly in the luteal

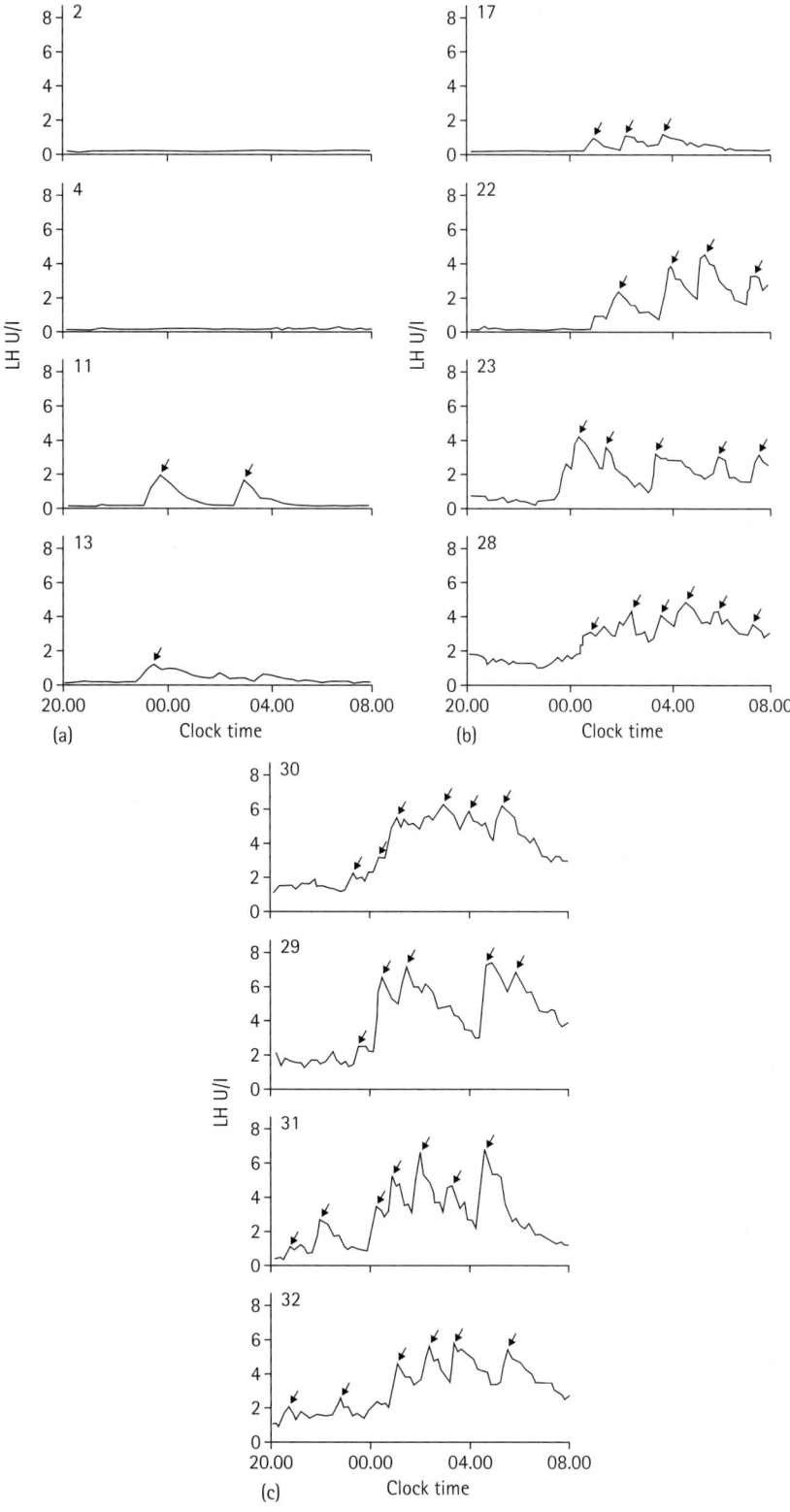

Fig. 15.32 Evolution of GT secretory profiles (1). Profiles of plasma LH between 20.00 and 08.00 h in (a) four young prepubertal subjects (G1 PH1 testicular volume = 2 ml); arrowheads indicate a significant LH pulse; none of these patients progressed into puberty during the following 12 months; (b) four prepubertal subjects: two with G1 PH1 testicular volume = 2 ml at time of study, but progression into puberty with testicular volume = 4 ml within 12 months (subjects 15 and 13); two in earlier puberty at study (G1 PH1–2 testicular volume 3–4 ml); (c) four pubertal subjects (G2–3 PH1–3 testicular volume 6–10 ml). (From Wu et al 1990[185])

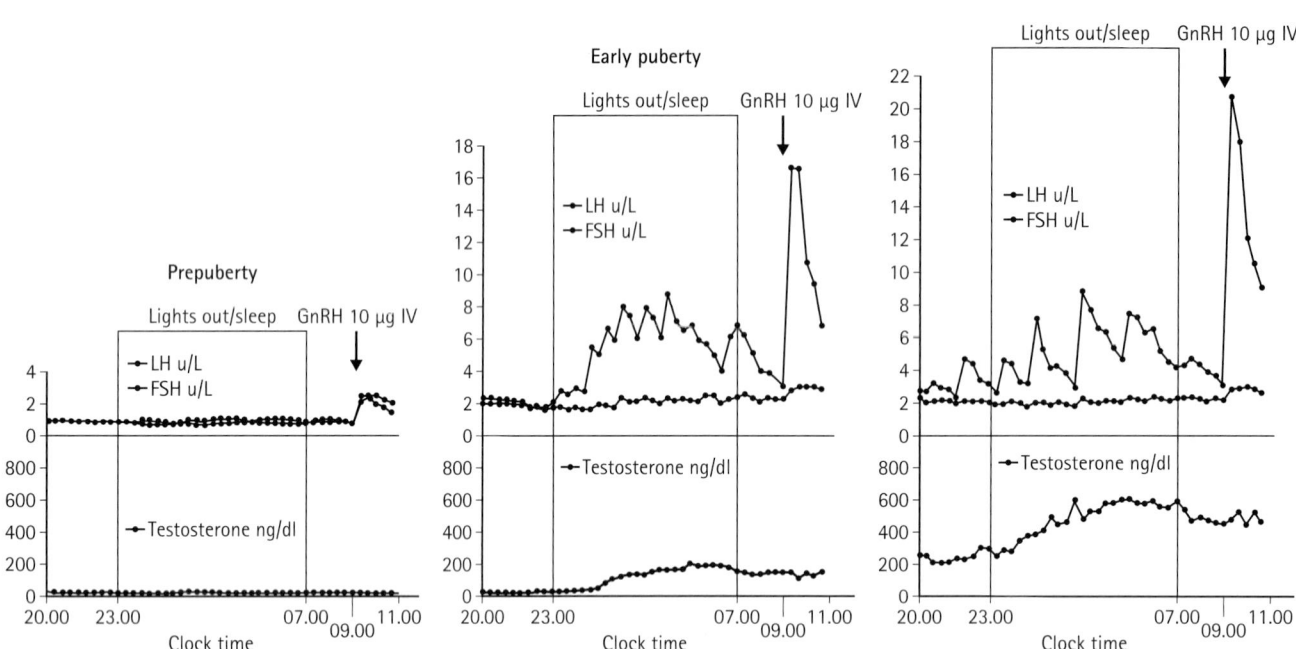

Fig. 15.33 Evolution of GT secretory profiles (2) and response to exogenous GnRH at different stages of pubertal development. (Data by courtesy of Dr FCW Wu[185])

phase. Increasing sex steroid secretion resulting from increasing pulsatile GnRH secretion produces the physical changes of puberty and all pubertal events can be induced by pulsatile administration of exogenous GnRH, even if this is a cumbersome way to do so in clinical practice.

ADRENARCHE AND GONADARCHE

See p. 480.

CHANGES OF BODY COMPOSITION AND METABOLIC SIGNALS FOR PUBERTY ONSET

Although in pathological situations (e.g. anorexia nervosa, excessive exercise) nutritional factors are important for pubertal development and menarche, evidence for the hypothesis that menarche depends on attainment of a critical weight for height is poor. For a given body weight, the proportion of girls reaching menarche increases with age and the relative weight (weight as a percentage of standard weight) at 11 years explains less than 5% of variation in the age of menarche.[190] It is likely that in normally nourished populations genetic factors are of paramount importance for the timing of menarche – this is probably true of pubertal onset and events in general.

This does not mean that metabolic factors and signals are unimportant for pubertal development although circumstantial evidence in man suggests that it is brain (rather than pituitary) maturation which is of primary importance for puberty onset. Are there simply genetically determined biological clocks which, in the absence of pathological modulators, trigger puberty or could there be metabolic or other cues which signal into the CNS? In anorexia nervosa or severe malnutrition there are low GT levels, menstruation ceases and puberty regresses as a way of conserving energy – the likely outcome of maintenance of reproductive capacity in such circumstances would be disastrous for mother and fetus. Although anorexics who regain ~75% of ideal body weight resume menstrual cycling with normal pituitary responsiveness to GnRH,[191] leanness alone cannot account for the reproductive disturbances: sustained exercise (in female distance runners) affects GnRH pulse amplitude and amenorrheic ballet dancers who stop training resume normal menstruation within a few months without

detectable changes in body weight or composition suggesting that metabolic signals are important in controlling reproductive function in these situations and, speculatively, in the control of normal pubertal development.

The discovery of leptin, the ob gene product, has now provided a molecular basis for the lipostatic theory of the regulation of energy balance. By modulating the hypothalamo – pituitary – gonadal axis both directly and indirectly, leptin may serve as an important signal from fat to the brain about the adequacy of fat stores for pubertal development and reproduction. Normal leptin secretion is necessary for normal reproductive function to proceed and leptin may be a signal allowing for the point of initiation of and progression toward puberty.[192]

ABNORMAL PUBERTY

As with other normally distributed characteristics (e.g. height or IQ) there is no absolute age at which pubertal timing becomes abnormal. Pubertal onset at an 'average' time does not necessarily exclude a pubertal disorder. The mean UK age of onset is such that 3% of boys or girls will have started puberty by 9 and 8 years and only 3% will have no pubertal signs by 13.8 and 13.4 years, respectively. A useful clinical rule is that puberty should be investigated if there is an abnormal sequence of pubertal changes (i.e. loss of consonance), any abnormal sign or symptom of underlying pathology and if signs have or have not (respectively) appeared outwith the above age limits. Studies purporting to show that the age of onset of secondary sexual development is lowering further are likely to be methodologically flawed [see above (p. 448) and Viner[177]].

Children with precocious puberty may simply have early onset of normal (central) mechanisms (which may be idiopathic or secondary to underlying pathology) or may have an abnormal mechanism causing development (pseudopuberty). Children with no signs by 14 years may have delay in maturation (on a background of constitutional growth delay – see p. 451) but may permanently lack ability to develop spontaneously. Investigations, potential outcomes and management are different in each situation and depend on not only presence or absence of underlying pathology but also emotional and psychological consequences. A clinical classification of disorders of puberty or its timing is given in Table 15.9.

Table 15.9 A simplified classification of disorders of puberty (see text)

Precocious puberty DMUD
Consonance:
Idiopathic central precocious puberty
Central precocious puberty due to, e.g.
Intracranial tumors
Cranial irradiation
Raised intracranial pressure
Gonadotrophin-independent precocious puberty (GIPP, testotoxicosis)
Loss of consonance (pseudopuberty)
Isolated premature thelarche
Thelarche variant
Adrenal causes
Premature pubarche
Congenital adrenal hyperplasia
Cushing syndrome
Adrenocortical tumors
Gonadal causes
Ovarian cysts
Ovarian or testicular tumors
Ingestion of sex steroid (accident or child abuse)
Primary hypothyroidism
McCune–Albright syndrome
Extrapituitary tumors (e.g. hepatoblastoma)

Delayed puberty
Consonance
Constitutional delay of growth and puberty
Chronic systemic disease
Idiopathic hypogonadotropic hypogonadism
Hypogonadotropic hypogonadism due to, e.g.
Kallmann syndrome
Craniopharyngioma
Cranial irradiation
Panhypopituitarism
Primary hypothyroidism
Loss of consonance
Turner syndrome
Ovarian agenesis with normal karyotype
Polycystic ovaries
Anorchia (primary or secondary to testicular irradiation)

PRECOCIOUS SEXUAL MATURATION

It was conventionally considered that there were only two distinct conditions resulting in premature sexual maturation from a gonadal axis etiology: central precocious puberty and isolated premature thelarche, of which the latter is a benign condition not requiring treatment. However, there is no pathognomonic endocrinological distinction between these two conditions; LH and FSH secretion represent a complete spectrum with girls with isolated premature thelarche (see below) having predominant FSH secretion and those with central precocious puberty predominant LH secretion.[193]

The concept of loss of consonance is particularly useful in the differential diagnosis of precocious puberty[194] but initiation of normal pubertal events can be due to underlying pathology and gonadotrophin-independent precocious puberty (GIPP, an important cause of precocious puberty in boys) may be clinically identical to 'consonant' precocious puberty.

Pseudopuberty (loss of consonance)
Isolated premature thelarche
This consists of breast development in the absence of any other pubertal signs although vaginal bleeding may occur. Onset is usually in the first year and uncommon after 2 years. There is usually cyclical waxing and waning of mild breast development (stage < B3)

which may have persisted from postnatal breast enlargement (potentially in both sexes) due to placental maternal estrogen transfer. In contrast to true precocious puberty, pubic and axillary hair does not develop, growth velocity is normal for age and skeletal maturation is not advanced.

There is evidence for increased estrogen production, high basal and GnRH-stimulated FSH levels, pulsatile nocturnal GT, predominantly FSH, secretion and increased ovarian follicular activity. Ultrasound may show several ovarian cysts whose size changes with breast size and moderate uterine enlargement.

A primary abnormality in GnRH pulse generation resulting predominantly in FSH secretion is unlikely as there is no response to GnRH analogues (see p. 453). The activin/inhibin system may be important for pathogenesis – inhibin B as well as FSH levels are high[195] – potentially exerting effects both at pituitary level, on FSH independently of the gonadotroph GnRH receptor, and at gonadal level by paracrine regulation.

There is waxing and waning of breast enlargement with gradual disappearance over months or years. Puberty generally takes place normally at appropriate age. Treatment consists of explanation and reassurance. Pelvic ultrasound and measurement of GTs basally and following a low dose (0.25 mcg/kg i.v.) GnRH test may be helpful in doubtful cases. Occasionally, particularly in girls presenting after 2 years, there may be confusion with early true precocious puberty and a 'non-classical' variant[196] has a high incidence of progression to central precocious puberty.

The variation in gonadotrophin secretion in this situation represents a spectrum of disorders of gonadal maturation which have received different names depending on the countries in which they were reported: unsustained central sexual precocity, slowly progressive precocious puberty, thelarche variant and exaggerated thelarche. It is probable that all four conditions are identical. There is a normal height prognosis and no response to gonadotrophin releasing hormone analogue treatment.[197]

Adrenal causes
The normal rise in adrenal androgens in mid-childhood (adrenarche, see p. 480) sometimes manifests with appearance of pubic (and less commonly axillary) hair – 'premature' pubarche' – without breast development but with increased height velocity. Such children are particularly sensitive to adrenal androgens or at the upper end of a secretory spectrum. The timing of true pubertal onset is generally unaffected. In occasional children with true precocious puberty, pubic hair development may be the first sign. Other causes of adrenal androgen secretion must be considered in the differential diagnosis and excluded.

Congenital adrenal hyperplasia (CAH), specifically non-salt-losing 21-hydroxylase deficiency in boys, is the commonest cause of precocious pseudopuberty. There is virilization in early childhood but testes classically remain prepubertal – adrenals are the androgen source. Occasionally ACTH-responsive adrenal rests will cause some testicular growth but significant enlargement signifies secondary central precocious puberty (Fig. 15.34) – a common consequence of GC therapy on the pre-existing advanced skeletal maturation. Mild or late-onset forms of 21-hydroxylase or 3beta-hydroxysteroid dehydrogenase deficiencies may present with pubic hair growth in girls mimicking premature pubarche.

Cushing syndrome and adrenocortical tumors
See p. 484.

Gonadal causes (see also Ch. 24)
Testicular tumors are uncommon in children and (usually benign) Leydig cell androgen-secreting lesions are rare. Clinically, presentation may be with normal pubertal development but the affected testis is enlarged and the contralateral small and atrophic from suppression of the hypothalamo-pituitary–gonadal axis. Enlargement may be uniform or with a palpable nodule, causing confusion with enlargement due to ACTH-responsive adrenal rests in CAH. Rapid onset of true pubertal onset may follow surgical removal.

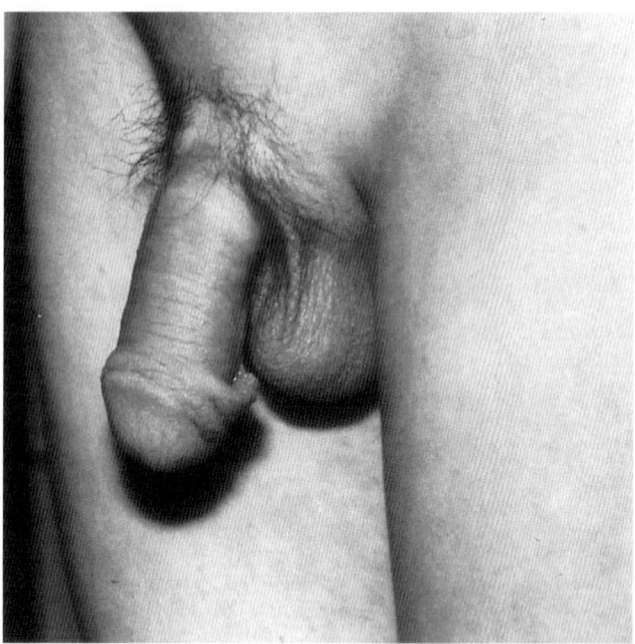

Fig. 15.34 True precocious puberty following glucocorticoid treatment of congenital adrenal hyperplasia. Note the testicular enlargement (same child as Fig. 15.53).

Ovarian tumors, usually benign in childhood, are also rare causes of precocious pseudopuberty, accounting for only around 1%. Least uncommon is the granulosa-theca cell tumor. Presentation is rarely before 4 years. Distinguishing features include early (in context of other pubertal signs) irregular vaginal bleeding or regular anovulatory cycles, marked areolar pigmentation and abdominal pain. A pelvic or abdominal mass is usually palpable.

Ovarian cysts are found in normal and precocious puberty. Multicystic appearances of late prepubertal and early pubertal ovaries are described above. Isolated follicular cysts may cause breast development, can be a feature of isolated premature thelarche and may regress spontaneously with conservative management.[198] Chronic estrogen secretion and large size may necessitate surgical removal. Polycystic ovaries may be common in puberty and late prepuberty and can be associated with pubertal delay.

Ingestion of sex steroid

Most commonly there is accidental ingestion of mother's contraceptive pills. Estrogen will cause slight breast enlargement and, often, an estrogen withdrawal bleed.

Child abuse

Sex steroids may be administered deliberately and chronically as a form of child abuse.[199] Sexual abuse (and pelvic neoplasia) must be excluded when vaginal bleeding is the presenting feature of precocious pseudopuberty. Factitious vaginal bleeding may be caused by presentation of mother's menstrual blood as though it came from the child. The laboratory can determine its origin.

Thyroid disease

Primary hypothyroidism may be associated both with delayed and precocious puberty. Unusually (in the context of precocity) growth velocity will not have been rapid, stature may be short and bone age is characteristically delayed. It is usually seen in girls (in whom autoimmune hypothyroidism is commoner). Breast development is the main feature (sometimes with galactorrhea) but there is usually little (androgen dependent) pubic or axillary hair development. In boys enlarged testes consist of seminiferous tubules without Leydig cells, consistent with the postulated mechanisms (p. 416). Pulsatile FSH release is common in primary hypothyroidism but only results in precocious pseudopuberty

in a few. Follicular cysts are seen on ovarian ultrasound in association with FSH predominance and suppressed GH pulsatility during overnight sampling. The latter may contribute to slower height velocity.

The child may be clinically euthyroid at presentation in puberty with normally maintained TSH and thyroid hormone levels. The pituitary fossa may be enlarged (Fig. 15.35) due to pituitary hyperplasia – the pituitary gland shrinks rapidly on thyroxine therapy. Ultimately, secondary pituitary failure may result, with an empty but still enlarged fossa on CT or MRI scan. Menarche may occur early while growth is still accelerating (cf. normal puberty and central precocious puberty). Treatment is with thyroxine.

McCune–Albright syndrome

The original descriptions were of hyperpigmented macules, precocious sexual development and thinning and sclerosis of bone with fractures in young children without systemic disease. Macular brown skin hyperpigmentation with characteristic ragged edges may not be present, and areas of rarefaction, commonly in long bones and elsewhere (polyostotic fibrous dysplasia; Fig. 15.36), may not develop until later childhood.

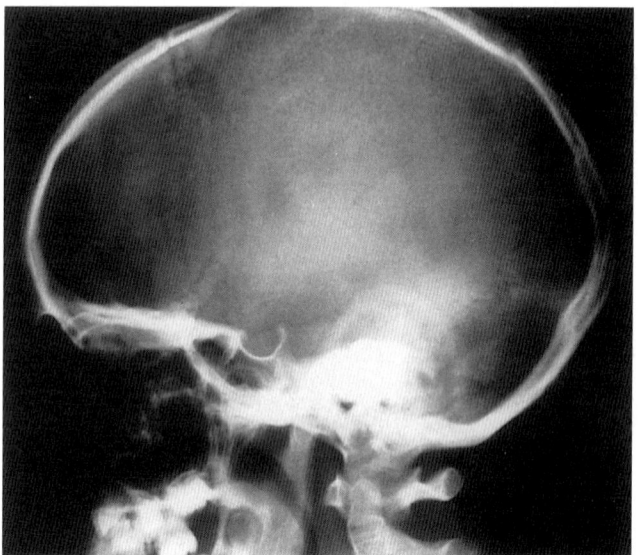

Fig. 15.35 Enlarged pituitary fossa due to pituitary (thyrotroph) hyperplasia in a child with primary hypothyroidism presenting with precocious puberty.

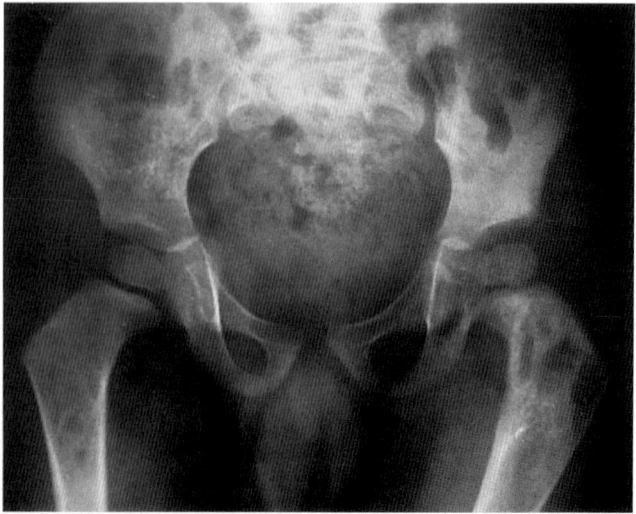

Fig. 15.36 Polyostotic fibrous dysplasia of bone in the McCune–Albright syndrome.

Multiple endocrinopathies with glandular hyperfunction (thyrotoxicosis with goiter, GH hypersecretion, Cushing syndrome, hyperprolactinemia, hyperparathyroidism and hyperphosphaturic rickets) may develop subsequently.

Endocrine hyperfunction is autonomous and not secondary to central trophic hormone stimulation. The syndrome is due to activating missense mutations in GNAS1, the Gs protein involved in G-protein-coupled receptor signaling, that stimulates cyclic AMP formation.[200,201] The mutation is variably expressed in different tissues consistent with a mosaic distribution of aberrant cells from a somatic cell mutation.[201]

Precocious puberty is the usual presentation, sometimes with early vaginal bleeding (cf. central precocious puberty). Bone lesions may not develop for many years and the skin pigmentation is inconstant. In girls, ovaries may be asymmetrically enlarged[202] by isolated follicular cysts. The GT response to exogenous GnRH is 'prepubertal' with absent GT pulsatility. As would be expected, suppression of puberty with GnRH agonists is ineffective. Cyproterone acetate or medroxyprogesterone are drugs of choice.

Extrapituitary tumors

These may cause precocious puberty as a result of the ectopic secretion of GT-like substances. Least uncommon are hepatoblastomas in boys and ovarian chorionepitheliomas and teratomas in girls; extrapituitary intracranial malignant teratoma and pineal choriocarcinoma have been reported. In boys testicular enlargement is rapid, and vaginal bleeding often occurs early in girls.

Central precocious puberty

Normal activation of the hypothalamo-pituitary–gonadal axis may occur abnormally early secondary to an underlying disorder or idiopathically. The pattern of secondary sexual characteristic development and endocrine findings are as in puberty developing at a more average time ('consonance') except that growth acceleration may occur relatively early in boys. This, plus more rapid epiphyseal maturation in boys in early puberty, may compromise final height more than expected in boys even with early presentation. In general, early age at onset and short parents imply a worse height prognosis but accurate individual prediction is difficult – predictive equations are most accurate for children of 'average' height developing normally at an average' time – and will tend to underestimate adult height in this context.[203]

Mechanisms initiating normal pubertal development are still not clearly understood, perturbations in timing even less so. Central precocious puberty presents much more frequently in girls (female:male ratio of about 10:1) and in the majority (> 80%) of girls no sinister underlying cause is found. With high resolution neuroradiological scanning, hypothalamo-pituitary hamartomas have been reported[204] but their incidence in the normal population at equivalent age is unclear. In boys, however, there is a high incidence of intracranial pathology, especially tumors such as teratomas, astrocytomas or gliomas causing pineal destruction – neuroradiological investigation is necessary even without abnormal signs. The sex difference in incidence of idiopathic precocious puberty may relate to lower GT release thresholds to endogenous pulsatile GnRH in girls. GIPP (see below) may account for precocious puberty in a significant number of boys in whom normal central mechanisms had previously been implicated.

In girls, investigation is necessary to confirm the mechanism and to exclude an underlying cause. Ovarian ultrasound, which will show characteristic multicystic appearances, and low dose (0.25 mcg/kg i.v.) GnRH test (more practical than overnight GT profiling)[205] will confirm central precocious puberty and exclude primary ovarian pathology. Neuroradiological investigation may be necessary (mandatory in boys). In addition to tumors, important central pathologies include CNS infection, raised intracranial pressure, trauma (during birth or childhood head injury) and previous cranial irradiation

Silver–Russell syndrome

Abnormalities of sexual development, including precocious puberty, can be associated with this prolonged IUGR syndrome.[206]

Gonadotrophin-independent precocious puberty (GIPP, testotoxicosis)[207]

Incidence, importance and classification are controversial – characteristically there are normal somatic consequences (consonance) from abnormal mechanisms (pseudopuberty). Patients have accelerated growth, early development of secondary sexual characteristics and usually reduced adult height. Diagnostic criteria are absent GT spontaneous pulsatility, poor but variable GT response to GnRH, no clinical response to GnRH analogue therapy and cyclical steroidogenesis. In reported studies there is a strong family history of precocious puberty but the etiology is unknown. Nearly all cases have been boys – girls may have the McCune–Albright syndrome. Maturation of testicular steroidogenesis and spermatogenesis is normal but GnRH/GT-independent. Testotoxicosis is caused by an activating mutation of the luteinizing hormone (LH) receptor, leading to increased levels of sex steroids in the context of low LH. Therapy has traditionally targeted steroidogenesis but drugs used have had significant side-effects. Combinations of oral antiandrogens and aromatase inhibitors seem more promising.[208]

Investigation and diagnosis

In summary it is reasonable to investigate any girl < 8 and boy < 9 years with secondary sexual characteristics. Where a girl's development is harmonious and proceeds at a normal tempo (consonance) and clinical examination is normal, invasive investigation to exclude pathology is unnecessary but basal TSH, estradiol and PRL measurement with skull X-ray, low dose GnRH test and pelvic ultrasound will give valuable information about the mechanism and underlying pathology. Overnight profiling of GT secretion is essentially a research tool. If no underlying cause is found which itself requires treatment, the need to suppress GT secretion and further development is considered below. Adrenal or intracranial pathology must be actively sought in boys by steroid profiling and neuroradiological (CT or MRI) investigation.

Clinical consequences and management

Management of precocious pseudopuberty is of the underlying cause. In central precocious puberty, an underlying cause requires treatment and pubertal suppression may be necessary also. In idiopathic cases, suppression may be indicated on social and psychological (rather than medical) grounds (see below).

Treatment of central precocious puberty was traditionally with progestogen-like drugs such as cyproterone acetate and medroxyprogesterone. Cyproterone was widely used in the UK for many years and is generally effective and free from significant side-effects in a dose of 75–100 mg/m²/day given twice daily. It has progestational, antiandrogenic, antigonadotrophic and adrenal suppressive activities – the precise mechanism by which GT secretion is suppressed is unclear.

Problems with cyproterone relate to adrenal suppression. Treated children must carry a steroid 'card' or talisman and need steroid cover during major stress, illness or surgery. Cortisol deficiency in other situations is uncommon unless high doses are used. Adults treated with cyproterone (for prostatic carcinoma) have altered lipid metabolism[209] which may be of concern if childhood treatment is prolonged. Taking the natural history of central precocious puberty into account, there is no evidence for improvement in height prognosis. Although still widely used, cyproterone has been replaced as treatment of choice by GnRH analogues (see below). It remains important for treatment of GIPP and may be used to cover the initial (stimulatory) phase of GnRH analogue therapy (see below).

GnRH analogues are specific and effective in suppressing central precocious puberty and are the treatment of choice. Some analogues are now available in the UK as depot preparations which are administered about every 10–12 weeks.[210]

Although they act by desensitizing the pituitary to GnRH and inhibiting pulsatile GnRH secretion, analogues have an initial stimulatory effect (lasting several weeks) on sex steroid secretion. This is of most practical relevance in a girl sufficiently advanced for a menstrual bleed to occur. In this situation, particularly, additional treatment with cyproterone for the first 4 weeks of analogue therapy is appropriate. Height velocity may initially increase further due to the effect of sex steroids on spinal growth. Sometimes GnRHa therapy decreases height velocity to below normal rates and this may be due to a prior acceleration of growth plate senescence secondary to the prior exposure to unphysiologically high estrogen levels.[211]

Effectiveness of therapy is best assessed by serial pelvic ultrasound in girls (assessing ovarian morphology and volume, uterine cross-sectional area and endometrial thickness), by clinical assessment of testicular volume in boys, plasma estradiol and testosterone measurements (respectively) and (if necessary) GT responsiveness to GnRH (0.25 mcg/kg i.v.). There is no effect on the adrenal axis (cf. cyproterone) but (as with cyproterone) probably no effect also on improving height prognosis.[203] Slowing of epiphyseal maturation on treatment is mirrored by a slowing of height velocity (perhaps due to reduced GH pulsatile secretion secondary to sex steroid suppression).

In the absence of underlying pathology, there is no *prima facie* reason why those who, for genetic or constitutional reasons, are destined to reach adult height earlier than average should fail to reach their genetically determined adult height. There are also methodological reasons for being cautious about the conclusions from many studies which purport to show that interventions with GnRHa increase adult height. Many studies include patients in the 'precocious puberty' group who probably have thelarche variant.[203] In addition, most studies fail to recognize that in comparing adult height achieved with predicted adult height (PAH) at the start of treatment, skeletal maturational (bone age) estimations on the same individual repeated through puberty do not show increments of 1 'year' bone age (BA) per year chronological age (CA) because BA accelerates and deviates from a cross-sectional-based centile in a way similar to that for height. BA standards are based on those with puberty at an average age, thus in those entering puberty at an age younger than average, a rapid acceleration and progressive advancement of BA occurs – at peak height velocity BA velocity can be up to 2.5 'years' per year.[106] As a result, predicted adult height at the start of treatment is misleadingly low and any treatment effect on adult height (e.g. from GnRHa treatment) will be overestimated.[203]

It is on this theoretical background that specific growth stimulation using GH therapy in addition to pubertal suppression is being assessed but it is best reserved for those in whom final height is particularly reduced due to underlying pathological causes of precocious puberty.[203]

Whatever the therapy, secondary sexual development will seldom diminish significantly and families must be warned not to expect dramatic cosmetic improvement. GnRH analogues may allow further long-term progression of pubic and axillary hair. There is evidence in girls for reversibility of inhibition[212] and for recovery of hypothalamo-pituitary–gonadal function and ovarian activity occurring from the pre-treatment stage of puberty.[213,214] There is little experience of long-term outcomes of GnRH analogue therapy in boys – observed effects on inhibition of seminiferous tubule activity could impair subsequent fertility if irreversible.

Emotional problems are often considerable in these children who are already tall for age. They appear clumsy and, in association with precocious puberty, may be more aggressive with undesirable social consequences. They feel different both because of size and precocious development and are often ill equipped to cope with psychological aspects of adolescence, particularly if parents and teachers are uncomprehending or embarrassed. Ultimate short stature may be particularly emotionally disabling against this background. However the indication for suppressing puberty with gonadotrophin releasing hormone analogues is for psychological or psychosocial reasons and not to achieve an improvement in final stature.[203]

The decision to treat idiopathic central precocious puberty thus depends on age at onset, rate of progression, level of emotional support provided by parents and other social and psychological factors. Menarche in primary school can cause additional psychological problems. In every case emotional support must be given.

DELAYED SEXUAL MATURATION

Late puberty, particularly when accompanied by short stature and delayed skeletal maturation, is the commonest reason for referral to a pediatric endocrinologist. This 'constitutional delay of growth and puberty' (CDGP) is seen more commonly in boys, who are also more stressed by it as growth deceleration continues until puberty is well advanced. Pathological causes of late puberty are much more common in girls (e.g. Turner syndrome); central causes are equally common in both sexes. A karyotype is an important early investigation in any slowly growing girl and mandatory if puberty is delayed even without any syndromic 'stigmata'. Virtually any chronic systemic disease may be associated with both growth retardation and pubertal delay.

Constitutional delay of growth and puberty (CDGP)

This is the likely diagnosis in a healthy adolescent short for the family but not for pubertal stage and skeletal maturation, giving a normal height prognosis. There is often a family history of CDGP in parents or siblings but its presence does not make the diagnosis and absence does not exclude it. CDGP is more common and often more stressful in boys. Emotional, psychological and social consequences may be severe despite absence of underlying pathology. Aspects of treatment which require consideration are puberty induction, growth stimulation and emotional support. Individual treatment modalities interact with each other in terms of their psychological and physical effects.

Chronic systemic disease

Chronic systemic disease may cause slowing of growth which may or may not be reversible (see Ch. 34) and is often associated with subsequent maturational delay or pubertal failure. Anorexia nervosa results in secondary endocrine disturbances (see thinness, p. 455) whilst pubertal delay causes secondary psychological disturbances. A sympathetic clinical psychologist or child psychiatrist is helpful in providing evidence of underlying emotional disturbance and managing primary or secondary emotional problems.

Causes of growth and maturational delay or failure in these conditions may be explicable in nutritional, secondary hormonal, metabolic or therapeutic (e.g. glucocorticoid treatment) terms. However in many conditions the etiology is both multifactorial and poorly understood.

Malnutrition and weight loss

Undernutrition is the commonest worldwide cause of growth failure and pubertal delay and may occur in resource rich countries, for example with inappropriate 'faddish' diets or emotional deprivation. Whatever the specific relevance of metabolic signals for the onset of puberty, it is likely that growth retardation and pubertal delay or failure are a secondary adaptation to the need to conserve energy and to prevent reproduction in suboptimal circumstances.

Exercise

Intensive training (e.g. in female gymnasts) can lead to delayed sexual maturation, and amenorrhea occurs in female distance runners. Amenorrheic ballet dancers who stop training resume normal menstruation within a few months without detectable changes in body weight or composition.

Hypothalamo–pituitary disorders

Puberty is initiated when GnRH begins to be secreted by the hypothalamus but many of the genetic factors involved with the onset of puberty remain to be determined. Hypogonadotrophic hypogonadism may cause pubertal delay, arrest or infertility depending on age at onset and severity. The cause is usually a hypothalamic disturbance in GnRH pulsatile release.

Several genes have been identified as causes of 'idiopathic' hypogonadotrophic hypogonadism (IHH) in the human accounting for 10–20%

of cases described: KAL, the gene for X-linked Kallmann syndrome (IHH and anosmia), DAX1, the gene for X-linked adrenal hypoplasia congenita (IHH and adrenal insufficiency), GnRHR (the GnRH receptor), and PC1 (the gene for prohormone convertase 1, causing a syndrome of IHH and defects in prohormone processing).[215]

Mutations in GPR54, which encodes a novel G-protein receptor activated by the ligand KiSS-1, can cause autosomal recessive IHH and the KiSS-1/GPR54 system is now thought to be an important system for the regulation of puberty and reproduction.[216] Mutations in GPR54 affect receptor signaling and probably regulate the reproductive axis at hypothalamic level by direct stimulation of GnRH release via G-protein-coupled receptor 54.[217] Galanin-like peptide (GALP) may mediate the effects of leptin on the reproductive system.[218] It seems increasingly likely that the KiSS-1/GPR54 system could, in the future, be a target for therapies in children with disorders of sexual development.

Primary GT deficiency is usually associated with pituitary tumors (e.g. craniopharyngioma) and other pituitary hormone deficiencies. Cranial irradiation is associated with (hypothalamic) GT deficiency. Prolactinomas are rarely associated with delayed puberty – moderately elevated PRL levels are due to stress.

In contrast to CDGP, a child with hypogonadotrophic hypogonadism is generally normal or tall for the family and bone age is arrested at around 13 'years' in the older child. A family history of delay with hypogonadism (cryptorchidism or micropenis) and anosmia suggests *Kallmann syndrome* – inherited as an autosomal dominant with relative male limitation. Features may include color blindness, other midline craniofacial abnormalities, nerve deafness, mental retardation and renal anomalies. Differentiation from CDGP is generally possible at presentation and molecular genetic abnormalities (in the KAL gene) have been described.[215]

Mental retardation syndromes associated with GT deficiency and obesity include Laurence–Moon–Biedl (with polydactyly and retinitis pigmentosa) and Prader–Willi.

Hypothyroidism

Acquired hypothyroidism is often associated with pubertal delay but may cause precocious puberty.

Gonadal

Disorders of ovarian function

These may relate to defective estrogen secretion or action (hypogonadism), androgen overproduction (hirsutism, amenorrhea or virilization), ovulatory failure (infertility) or menstrual abnormalities (amenorrhea and infertility).

Turner syndrome (TS). Primary gonadal dysgenesis is much more common in girls because of the high incidence of Turner syndrome. Although diagnosis is usually possible well before the age when puberty should occur, even in those with no dysmorphic features, few children are now measured regularly and accurately by primary carers so that presentation with delayed puberty is common. There is a poor correlation between physical manifestations (Figs 15.37, 15.38) – neonatal lymphedema, broad ('shield') chest with widely spaced nipples, webbed neck, high arched palate, low posterior hair line, wide carrying angle, short fourth metacarpals and hypoplastic or malformed (spoon-shaped) nails (Fig. 15.39), cardiac and renal abnormalities – and the precise genetic abnormality.

One to two percent of all conceptuses have TS but rates of early spontaneous miscarriage are very high so the birth prevalence is about 1 in 2500. About half have a single X chromosome and the remainder have one normal X and one abnormal because of partial deletions, ring formation or

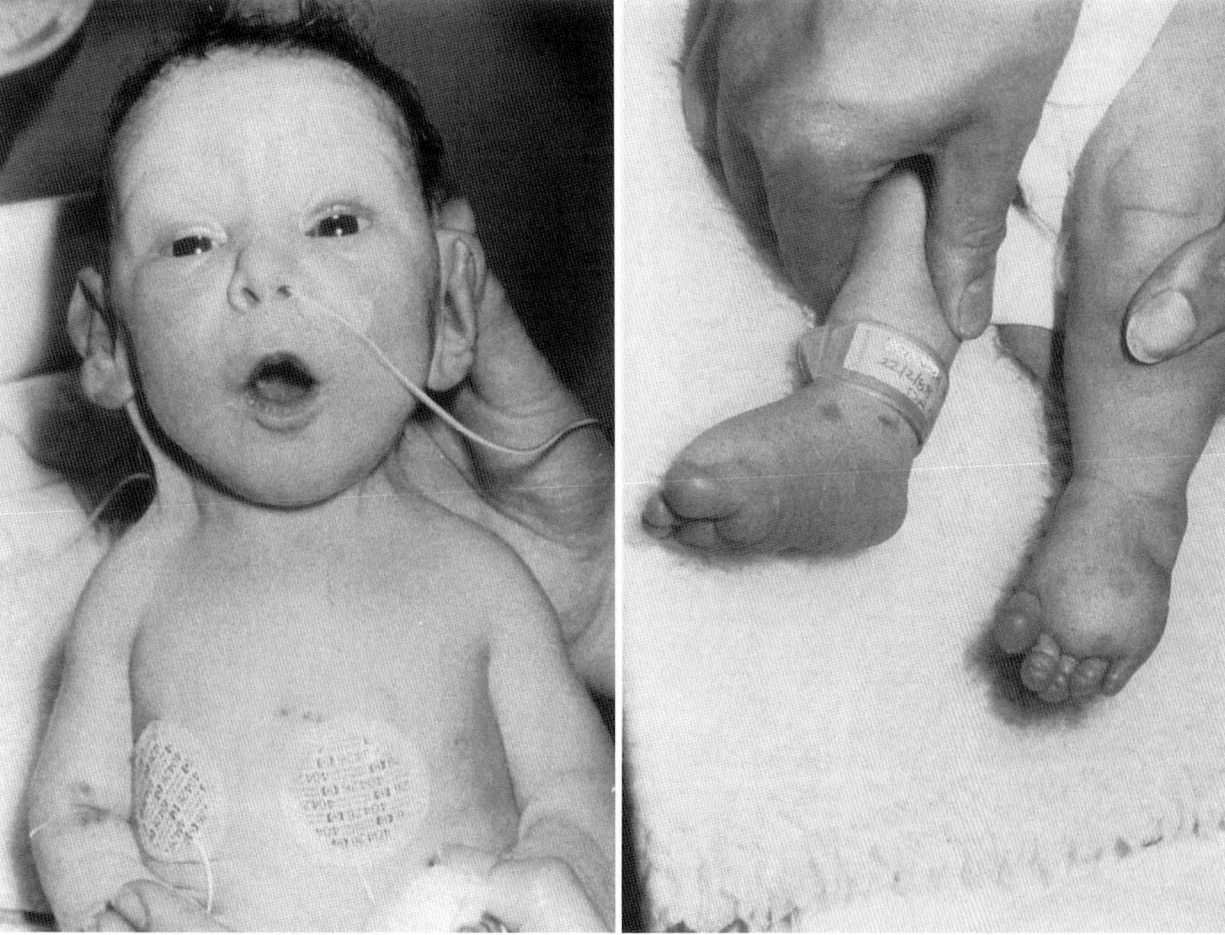

(a)   (b)

Fig. 15.37 Turner syndrome diagnosed at birth – note the peripheral edema in a small-for-gestational-age infant.

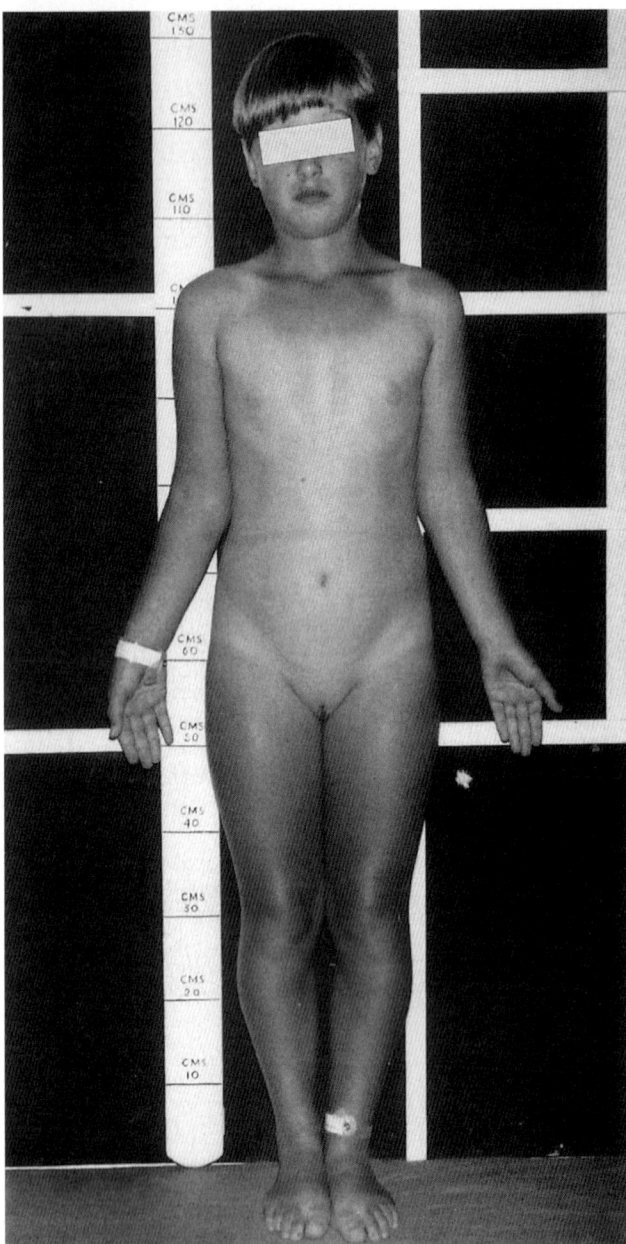

Fig. 15.38 Turner syndrome presenting with pubertal delay in a 14-year-old girl.

occurs before puberty in the majority. Some will enter puberty spontaneously – this is more common with 'mosaicism' (but see above). With partial deletions, long arm preservation may be important for ovarian function and short arm deletions are associated with the growth deficit.

There is defective end-organ responsiveness to growth factors at cartilage and collagen level and a spectrum of GH secretory insufficiency. Intrauterine growth is poor, growth velocity declines progressively after infancy and the pubertal growth spurt is absent. As the height relationship with parents is maintained, TS girls with tall parents (or, more specifically, a tall parent from whom their normal X chromosome has been inherited) may not become conspicuously small until they fail to enter puberty when their normal peers are growing rapidly. Approximately 20 cm in height is lost compared to relevant population means – the mean adult UK height is about 143.0 cm although it may be a little more in 'mosaics' and when short arm material is present. Thus about 20% of TS girls will achieve a spontaneous final height above the 3rd centile for the normal population. Specific growth charts for Turner syndrome are available.[73] Significant deviation from syndrome specific centiles necessitates a search for additional pathology (e.g. hypothyroidism or Crohn's disease).

Mean IQ is 95 and the majority have IQs within the normal range. Many have specific difficulties with visuospatial perception and full psychometric assessment will allow specific remedial help. Autoimmune disease is more common in TS: autoimmune thyroiditis has an increasing risk with age and particularly by adolescence.[219] The frequency of antithyroid antibodies also increases with age as it does in the normal population – elevated antibody titers indicate the need for regular evaluation of thyroid function.

Ideally estrogen replacement must be initiated to keep the TS girl in line with her peers and increased at a physiological rate. An appropriate regimen is described below. This produces good cosmetic breast appearances and allows normal psychological maturation and bone mineralization. Oral estrogen enters the portal circulation and exposes the liver to high levels – transdermal natural estrogen patches will be preferable in the future. Estrogen replacement therapy is necessary at least until menopausal age and probably beyond.

Ultra-low dose estrogen in early childhood cannot be routinely recommended on present evidence although estrogen has an important role in bone mineral accrual prepubertally and there are data supporting its use.[5] GH therapy (see below) can normalize bone mineralization.[220] Delaying estrogen therapy much beyond 13 years may increase social isolation, stigmatization and psychological distress and reduce life-long bone mineralization, and recent data suggest that delay is unnecessary from a height point of view also.[221]

Growth-promoting therapy with GH with or without additional anabolic steroid (oxandrolone) has been widely assessed in TS but many studies have significant methodological flaws. Pharmacological doses of GH produce a dose-related increase in height to socially acceptable levels in many TS girls; most gain is during the first 3 years of therapy; individual responses are variable and unpredictable; combining GH with oxandrolone increases the tempo of growth, thus shortening the duration of GH therapy to final height, and may contribute extra height gain – androgenic side effects of oxandrolone are dose related whereas the growth-promoting effect is not and thus very low doses (0.0625 mg/kg daily) are optimal.

The first high quality (Canadian) trial of GH therapy in Turner syndrome has now been reported[221] and shows an average adult height gain (over predicted/controls) of around 7 cm. However, in view of the high dropout rate, lack of data for starting GH therapy at less than 7 years, variable individual responses and increase in some side-effects, there are still a number of unanswered questions. Height is not a validated proxy for psychological well-being or quality of life and, based on French population TS data, two thirds of the TS patients treated with GH in the Canadian study would not have considered the treatment to have been worthwhile based on these results.[222]

TS women are candidates for in vitro fertilization using donated ova. In future, they, and perhaps women with acquired gonadal dysgenesis who have had abdominal irradiation in childhood, will be candidates for cryopreservation and ovarian autografts, although the latter group, unlike TS women, will have compromised uterine function.

Rarely ovarian agenesis occurs with a normal female karyotype. Stature is normal and there are no dysmorphic features. The presence of an XY cell line necessitates removal of dysgenetic gonads.

short or long arm isochromosomes. At least 10% have mosaicism (different proportions of abnormal cells in different tissues) and molecular analysis suggests that the proportion is much higher. In children with mixed karyotypes, there is an equal abnormal genetic contribution from mother and father whereas in the 45X karyotype the missing chromosome is paternal in origin. The presence of Y chromosomal material can also be detected by karyotype and molecular genetic techniques. If it is found, gonads should be removed to prevent possible malignant change (e.g. gonadoblastoma).

Short stature homeobox-containing (SHOX) gene mutations have been implicated in both the short stature and skeletal dysplastic abnormalities of Turner syndrome. Genomic imprinting (differential expression of genetic material depending on whether it originates from father or mother) is important in several disorders (e.g. Prader–Willi/Angelman syndromes) and is relevant in determining some aspects of the TS phenotype (e.g. cardiac abnormalities, neck webbing) when the normal X chromosome is maternal in origin (see Ch. 14).

The fetal ovary forms normally and germ cell numbers are normal until the end of the second trimester. These then decline to birth and subsequently at a variable but increased rate so that a 'menopause'

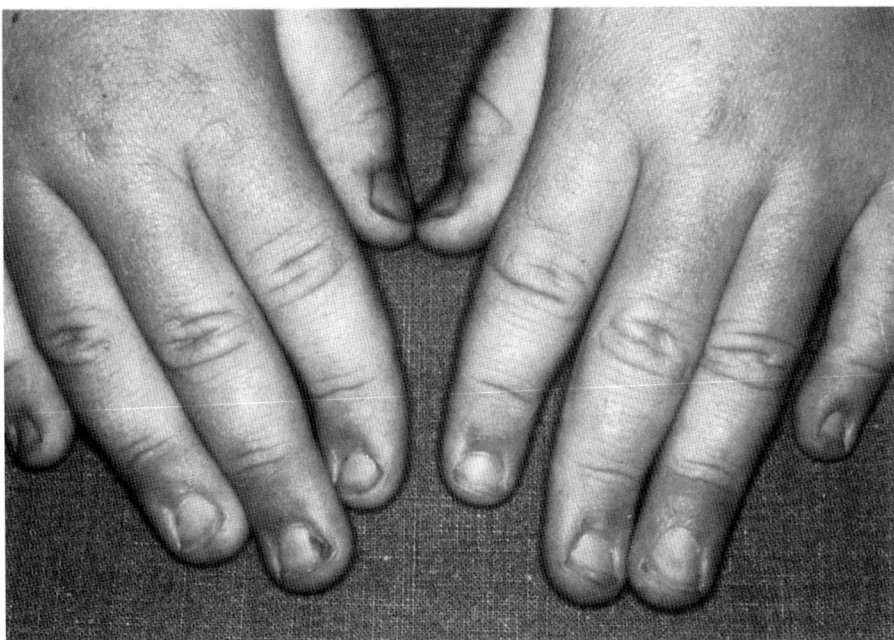

Fig. 15.39 The nails in Turner syndrome (the same girl as in Fig. 15.38).

Disorders of testicular function

These are uncommon. Anorchia is usually detected prepubertally but may be secondary to testicular irradiation in the treatment of ALL or follow suboptimal management of testicular torsion.

Polycystic ovarian syndrome

Menstrual disturbances in many adult women presenting with polycystic ovarian syndrome (hirsutism, obesity and menstrual irregularities) had been thought to date from puberty but ultrasonic appearances (enlarged ovaries with many small circumferential cysts surrounding increased stromal tissue) may be common in prepuberty and an important pathological cause of pubertal delay. There is an association with premature pubarche and prepubertally detectable hyperinsulinemia and dyslipidemia. Birth weight SD scores have been found to be lower in premature pubarche girls than in controls, and particularly so in those with hyperinsulinemia and subsequent ovarian hyperandrogenism. This suggests that these associations may result, at least in part, from a common prenatal origin.[32]

Investigation

Distinguishing physiological from pathological delay may be impossible clinically. Assessment must include physical examination (nutritional state, fundal and visual field assessment) and calculation of height velocity. Loss of 'consonance' – tall stature for the family associated with pubertal delay and delayed bone age – is incompatible with CDGP and may be due to Klinefelter syndrome, hypogonadism or GT deficiency; marked pubic or axillary hair growth in a girl with absent breast development suggests Turner syndrome. The appropriateness or otherwise of height velocity can only be determined in the context of pubertal stage, e.g. growth should be accelerating in a girl with stage 2 breast development but slow growth is normal in a boy until 8–10 ml testicular volumes. Assessment of skeletal maturity may indicate likely delay before puberty starts spontaneously (if it will do so) but seldom distinguishes pathology from physiological delay.

Children with loss of consonance should be investigated at any age, as should those with signs or symptoms attributable to an underlying pathological process. Where height and degree of skeletal maturational delay seem appropriate for the family in terms of final height prediction, delay is probably physiological. Three percent of normal boys and girls will have no signs of puberty by 13.8 and 13.4 years respectively and it is reasonable to investigate those presenting after this. Even if delay is physiological it is unkind (in emotional and psychological terms) and

inappropriate (in growth terms) to allow too much delay in relation to the child's peers, and pubertal induction may be indicated.[223]

Raised GT levels are diagnostic of primary gonadal failure but are not elevated before about 10 years. At any age, normal testes will respond to stimulation by LH (given as HCG) by secreting testosterone. In hypogonadotrophic hypogonadism there is a presumed lack of LH receptors in the testis, basal and stimulated GT levels will be low and the testosterone response to HCG is absent. Pubertal imminence can be assessed by measuring nocturnal GTs – pulsatile nocturnal GnRH release occurs well before clinically detectable signs – or more practically by measuring the GT response to a small (0.25 mcg/kg i.v.) dose of GnRH.[205] If puberty is imminent, LH responsiveness will exceed that of FSH and rise significantly. Where available, skilled ultrasound assessment is helpful in girls and non-invasive. An 8 a.m. plasma testosterone level may be a useful simple guide in boys[187] but inhibin B may be a more sensitive predictor than testosterone of clinical pubertal onset.[224]

Moderately raised basal PRL levels may be due to stress but higher levels are a sensitive indicator of reduction in its dopaminergic inhibitory control secondary to hypothalamic lesions or those causing portal compression (e.g. craniopharyngioma, radiotherapy, histiocytosis X). Hyperprolactinemia is itself a cause of delayed puberty. Prolactinomas are rare in children – PRL levels are generally very high (> 3000 mU/L). A significantly elevated PRL is thus a sensitive indicator of intracranial pathology as a cause of delayed puberty and an indication for neuroradiological investigation which is important if an evolving endocrinopathy is suspected – hypogonadotrophic hypogonadism may be the first sign of panhypopituitarism.

There is physiological blunting of GH secretion in late prepuberty in both sexes and in early male puberty so that, if pharmacological testing of GH secretion is deemed necessary and is to be interpreted correctly, sex steroid priming is necessary. Stilbestrol was originally studied in both sexes but depot testosterone or oral estrogen are used in boys and girls respectively.

If pathology is suspected, investigations should be carried out urgently (treatment of underlying pathology may be necessary) and puberty induced at normal time and tempo. Otherwise, although much can be learnt by several months' observation of growth and for early signs of puberty, the psychological pressures on some can be considerable.[223] The short, undeveloped and poorly qualified 16-year-old school-leaver may find it particularly hard to obtain employment. It is inappropriate to induce puberty late to maximize prepubertal growth because continuing late prepubertal growth deceleration is leading to a lower point from which to accelerate and the magnitude of the pubertal growth spurt in a late developer is generally smaller. It is also unkind to subject a child to unnecessary social and emotional pressures.

With optimal treatment, puberty can be started at an appropriate time and progressed at a physiological tempo. In girls, too large a starting dose and too rapid escalation of estrogen therapy will reduce the magnitude of the growth spurt, produce cosmetically unattractive 'cylindrical' breasts and potential difficulties in important emotional and psychological aspects of adolescent development. A boy may have 2 years or more from early testicular enlargement until he notices height acceleration. Meanwhile his more average peers are both more developed and growing 3–4-fold faster. Stimulation of growth during early male puberty is thus of considerable potential psychological benefit. Possible therapies (anabolic steroid, androgen or GH) are reviewed by Kelnar.[223]

Clinical consequences and management

Emotional and psychological consequences of delay are not dependent on the presence of underlying pathology: the most common group, boys with CDGP, may suffer considerably yet are entirely normal. Where an underlying non-endocrine condition is responsible, diagnosis and optimal management may facilitate spontaneous development. When pubertal induction is necessary, it should mimic closely normal pubertal progression to optimize growth, cosmetic appearances and psychological maturation. Too rapid induction is disadvantageous and is unnecessary if induction is not unduly delayed.

Puberty induction

Induction in girls is with estrogen whatever the precise nature of pubertal failure. An appropriate starting regimen is ethinylestradiol 1–2 mcg orally daily, increasing to 10 mcg over 18–24 months. At that dose, or before if breakthrough bleeding occurs, a progestogen (e.g. norethisterone 350 mcg) should be added for 5 days every 4 weeks. Unopposed estrogenic endometrial stimulation otherwise increases risks of endometrial or breast carcinoma. Full secondary sexual development will generally occur with ethinylestradiol 20–30 mcg – a low estrogen combined contraceptive pill may then be conveniently substituted. If hypogonadism is permanent, estrogen/progestogen therapy must be maintained to enable sexual intercourse to be enjoyed without discomfort and prevent osteoporosis and, perhaps, early atherosclerosis. Transdermal natural estrogen, when available in low enough dosage for pubertal induction, will be preferable.

Many different regimens are used for hormone replacement therapy in young women, and it is likely that optimal HRT in young women (in terms of bone strength, cardiovascular protection, feminization, etc.) is different from that appropriate for older women who are 'conventionally' postmenopausal.

In boys, physiological sex steroid replacement is even more difficult. Conventionally, depot preparations of testosterone esters (e.g. Sustanon 50–100 mg i.m. once every 6 weeks increasing gradually over 2 years to 250 mg i.m. twice weekly) are used. Oral testosterone (undecanoate, TU) was considered too variably and excessively absorbed for pubertal induction but experience suggests that resulting high total testosterone levels reflect changes in SHBG on treatment, and that appropriate free (active) testosterone levels for pubertal induction are achievable with TU 40 mg alternate daily – TU may be the treatment of choice for the short, sexually immature adolescent boy where explanation and reassurance alone are not enough.[223] Long term androgen replacement will probably be best given using testosterone implants or transdermally – patches are now available in the UK and suitably low dose regimens for pubertal induction need evaluation.

In future, recombinant human chorionic gonadotrophin (rHCG) therapy may be a suitable alternative in boys with hypogonadotrophic hypogonadism; in girls HCG may cause abdominal pain, ascites and hemorrhagic rupture of ovarian cysts. Spermatogenesis would be induced by recombinant FSH (rFSH). Optimal fertility in both sexes requires eventual low dose pulsatile GnRH therapy.

The physician will need to assess carefully individual underlying psychological and social pressure before deciding on the optimal management of CDGP, which might comprise anabolic steroid (oxandrolone) or testosterone therapy.[223] The role of aromatase inhibitors in increasing adult height in adolescent boys by inhibition of estrogen action is under evaluation.[225]

Emotional support is always important whatever other treatment modalities are used but the morale boost from an increase in growth velocity in early male puberty is often dramatic with improvement in school attendance and performance.

OTHER DISORDERS RELATED TO FEMALE AND MALE REPRODUCTION

AMENORRHEA

Amenorrhea may be secondary (absent menstruation with previously normal menstrual history) – causes include pregnancy, anorexia nervosa, intense training or chronic underlying disease – or primary (menstrual bleeding has never occurred). Primary amenorrhea may be a consequence of abnormal GnRH pulsatile secretion or release – a middle stage between GnRH deficiency causing delayed or arrested puberty or infertility due to anovulatory cycles. Other important causes include primary ovarian failure (often in TS), gonadal dysgenesis with absent uterus (e.g. the XY girl) or imperforate hymen. Hypertension suggests 17alpha-hydroxylase deficiency.

NOONAN SYNDROME

In this syndrome, which is thought to have an incidence of 1 in 1000 to 1 in 2500 live births, there is frequently variable hypogonadism associated with characteristic features such as pulmonary valvular stenosis, a broad forehead with hypertelorism, epicanthic folds, ptosis and downward slanting palpebral fissures, abnormal or low-set ears, neck webbing, low posterior hair line, shield chest or kyphoscoliosis, deafness, visual problems, clotting disorders and short stature (Fig. 15.40). However, as in TS, all these are inconstant and diagnosis has been clinical, with the typical facial features and at least two other features as key elements. The phenotype changes with age.

Cryptorchidism is found in about two thirds of boys; sexual development generally occurs spontaneously but is delayed. Infertility is

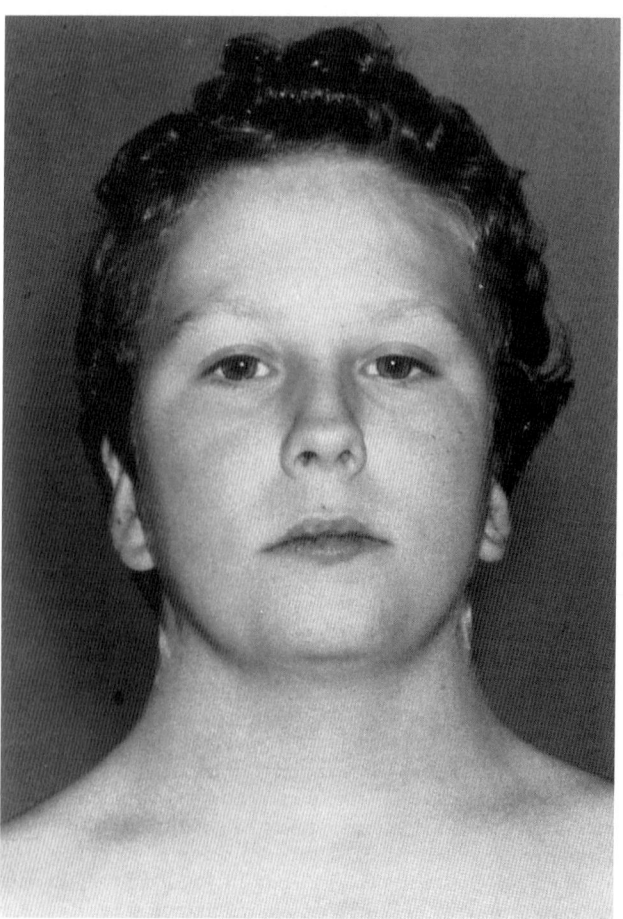

Fig. 15.40 Noonan syndrome.

usual. In girls (whose karyotype is normal) puberty and menarche can be delayed (presentation may be with primary amenorrhea) but fertility seems common. Mean adult height is approximately 162.5 cm (males) and 153 cm (females) although standards are based on relatively small numbers and largely cross-sectional data. GH treatment improves medium term height velocity, and theoretical adverse effects on cardiac ventricular wall thickness (potentially leading to hypertrophic obstructive cardiomyopathy) have not been seen.

Noonan syndrome is associated with germline gain-of-function mutations in the PTPN11 gene which encodes the protein tyrosine phosphatase Shp2 (a protein that controls cardiac semilunar valvulogenesis) on the long arm of chromosome 12 (12q24.1)[226] but only in about 40–50% of those identified clinically. The presence or absence of these mutations influences responses to GH therapy.[227]

The recent finding of germline oncogene (KRAS) mutations in some patients with Noonan syndrome, cardio-facio-cutaneous syndrome and Costello syndrome (which have some phenotypic features in common) suggests a common underlying molecular basis and may explain the reported increased tendency to malignancy in these conditions.[228]

Further knowledge of the true incidence and phenotypic diversity may allow the design of appropriately controlled studies of the efficacy of GH therapy with sufficiently large numbers of subjects defined on a molecular genetic basis and followed to final height.

KLINEFELTER SYNDROME (KS) (47XXY)

There is tall stature for the family with disproportionately long legs from childhood (Fig. 15.41), small testes for apparent virilization (Fig. 15.42) and azoospermia. Presentation is usually with tall stature, hypogonadism (often with marked pubertal gynecomastia) or infertility. The incidence is about 1 in 500 to 1 in 1000 live births. Prepubertal faster than average growth relates to the extra 'dose' of the SHOX gene. Extremely tall ultimate height with increasingly disproportionately long legs relates to testosterone secretion inadequate for conversion to estrogen and epiphyseal closure at the appropriate time or for normal rapid late pubertal spinal growth – GH predominantly stimulates long bone growth. Spontaneous pulsatile GT secretion in pre- and peripubertal 47XXY boys may be normal, cf. the usual GT elevation in adults. Pubertal onset is generally not delayed. Mean IQ is below the population mean, but most are within the normal range. If the diagnosis is made sufficiently early, excessive stature can be prevented, or at least reduced, by high dose testosterone treatment (but see below) or epiphysiodesis.[139] There is now the potential to achieve fertility by testicular sperm extraction and intracytoplasmic sperm injection techniques, particularly in the young adult with KS.[229] Whilst the outcome seems less favorable in those who had high dose testosterone supplementation in puberty it is unclear as to whether this is causative or simply reflects the greater need for such supplementation in those worse affected.

GYNECOMASTIA

Hormonal effects on breast structures are complex. In males androgens are important in inhibiting stimulatory estrogenic effects on breast tissue: breast development occurs in pubertal girls at estrogen levels comparable to those in adult males. It also occurs in androgen insensitivity syndromes, where testosterone is inactive because of androgen receptor deficiency, at normal male estradiol levels.

Thus a degree of gynecomastia occurs in < 50% of normal boys during early to mid-puberty when estrogen levels are high in relation to androgens. It is usually mild, resolving spontaneously within 12–18 months, but sometimes subareolar mastectomy is necessary if the condition is distressing and persistent. Gynecomastia is a particular feature of Klinefelter syndrome (see above). Gross pubertal gynecomastia, prepubertal gynecomastia or persistence in late puberty requires investigation.

Prepubertal gynecomastia may be unilateral, can cause discomfort and is usually benign, self-limiting and idiopathic. Exposure to exogenous estrogen or endogenous production by adrenal, testicular or other tumors

must be excluded. Drugs such as digoxin, methyldopa, ketoconazole and cannabis and amphetamine abuse have been associated.

UNDESCENDED TESTES

This common problem is considered elsewhere (see Ch. 37, p. 1620.). Many 'undescended' testes are simply retractile, can be manipulated into the scrotum and will descend (and stay in the scrotum) at puberty. Hypogonadotrophic hypogonadism is the most common cause of cryptorchidism which is now known to be an important cause of infertility secondary to impaired hormonal priming in infancy; genetic defects have been described in minority of subjects.[215] In bilateral cryptorchidism fertility is likely to be severely compromised. Cryptorchidism and micropenis may represent a DSD phenotype, even if they are isolated, and a karyotype should always be checked. In unilateral cryptorchidism the undescended testis fails to establish an adequate adult stem cell pool by 2–3 months of age and similar (if less severe) changes occur in the contralateral (descended) testis. To enhance the chance of adult fertility, hormonal treatment (GnRH analogue over 4 consecutive weeks) should start by 6 months of age. If there is no response HCG should be given (500 IU

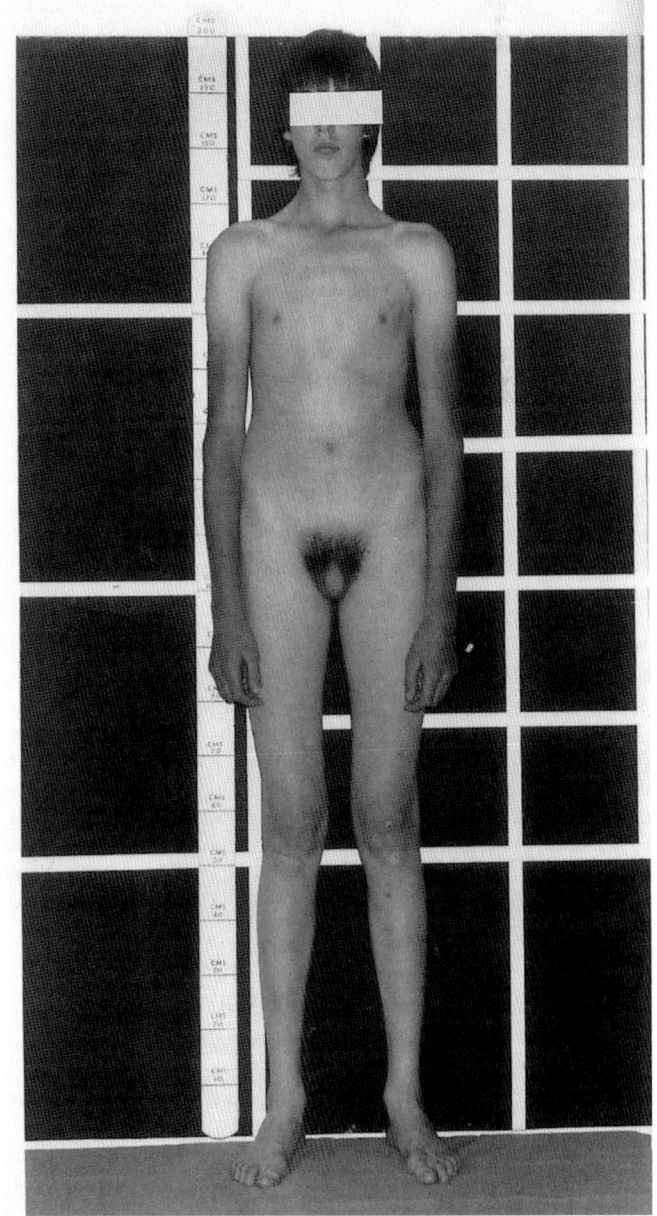

Fig. 15.41 Klinefelter syndrome – note the disproportionately long legs in this 202 cm 18-year-old.

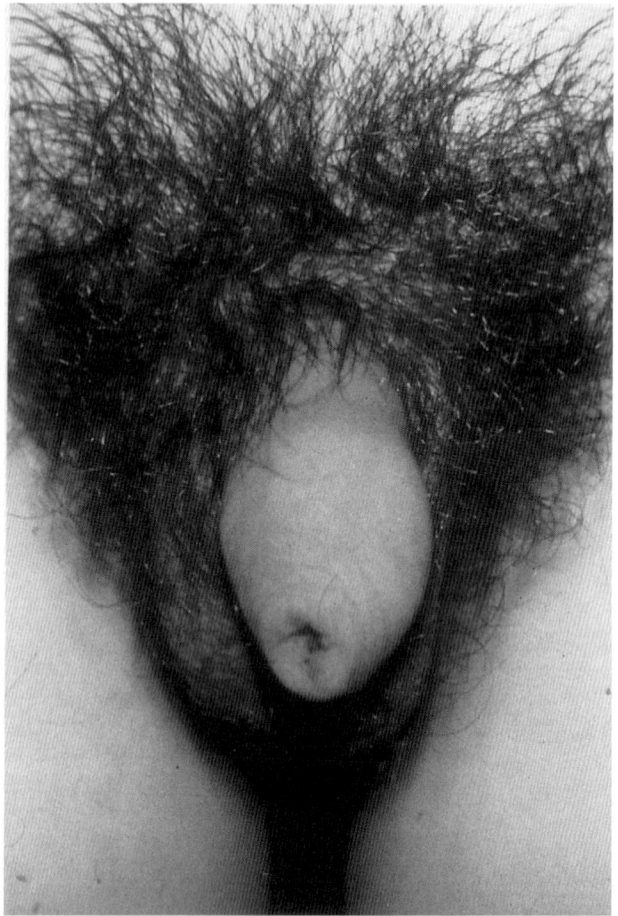

Fig. 15.42 Genitalia in Klinefelter syndrome – note the small testes for the degree of virilization (the same subject as in Fig. 15.41).

i.m. weekly for 3 consecutive weeks). If there is still no response, orchidopexy and testicular biopsy should be carried out. The biopsy will identify those with a germ cell count <0.2/tubule and/or no adult dark (Ad) spermatogonia. They should be treated with a further course of a GnRH analogue (10 mcg every other day for 6 months). GnRHa has been shown to induce increased numbers of germ cells and their differentiation from gonocytes into Ad spermatogonia which improves the chance of fertility.[39]

Scrotal testes are necessary functionally (testosterone biosynthesis, spermatogenesis/fertility), cosmetically and because of the (difficult to quantify) risk of malignant change in functional intra-abdominal testes. A testis not in the scrotum by infancy is now thought unlikely to show adequate spermatogenesis. Functional but ectopic tissue which cannot be brought into the scrotum surgically is probably best removed unless it is easily accessible to clinical examination and follow-up can be assured. Nonfunctioning intra-abdominal testicular tissue is probably best left – it carries extremely low risk of malignant change and may be impossible to locate at laparotomy or laparoscopy.

THE HYPOTHALAMO–PITUITARY UNIT

CONNECTIONS/ANATOMY/PHYSIOLOGY

Ontogeny of fetal hypothalamo-pituitary hormone biosynthesis is described on p. 415. By 15 weeks' gestation the hypothalamus is anatomically mature and functionally active and by 18 weeks pituitary vascularization is complete. The hypothalamo-pituitary axis is functional by 20 weeks with development of the portal system. Functional maturity is important for normal development of thyroid (secondary to TSH secretion), external genitalia in the male (GH and GTs) and adrenal (ACTH and related peptides).

The pituitary gland is situated within the pituitary fossa, directly below and in close relationship with the hypothalamus. Laterally are

Table 15.10 Hypothalamic regulatory peptides and their properties

Regulatory peptide	Amino acids	Molecular weight
Growth hormone releasing hormone	40/44	4545/5040
Somatostatin (growth hormone release inhibiting hormone)	14	1638
Gonadotropin releasing hormone/ luteinizing hormone releasing hormone	10	1182
Thyrotropin releasing hormone	3	362
Corticotropin releasing hormone/factor	41	4758

the cavernous sinuses, the internal carotid arteries, the 3rd, 4th and 6th cranial nerves and temporal lobes. Above lie arachnoid and subarachnoid spaces and above them the optic chiasma and hypothalamus.

The hypothalamus has afferent connections with frontal cortex, thalamus, amygdala, hippocampus and anterior thalamic (autonomic) nuclei and can integrate and respond to a wide range of physiological and behavioral inputs. Efferent pathways also connect with midbrain, pons, medulla, amygdala and hippocampus and there are specific pathways to adenohypophysis via the portal system and to neurohypophysis via the supraopticohypophyseal tract.

Neuroendocrine control of hypothalamic secretion is by CNS neurotransmitters including dopamine, noradrenaline, serotonin, acetylcholine, gamma-aminobutyric acid (GABA), melatonin and histamine. Anterior pituitary hormone secretion is directly controlled by hypothalamic factors (regulatory peptides) that affect hormone synthesis and release (Table 15.10).

ANTERIOR PITUITARY HORMONES
Corticotrophin (ACTH)

ACTH is a single chain 39 amino acid polypeptide. The first 24 N-terminal amino acids are identical in most species and produce the biological (adrenocortical) activity. However ACTH is one of a group of related pituitary peptides which originates from a common large molecular weight (31 000) glycosylated precursor molecule, pro-opiomelanocortin (POMC). Glycosylation accounts for basophil staining of pituitary corticotrophs.

The bovine precursor protein (Fig. 15.43) consists of 265 amino acids encoding three peptides: ACTH, beta-lipotrophin (beta-LPH) and a 105 amino acid N-terminal sequence N-POMC. Human N-POMC is a 76 amino acid peptide of molecular weight 11 200. All three POMC-derived peptides are found in the same secretory granules within the cell, are released concomitantly into the circulation in equal concentrations, become undetectable after hypophysectomy and their plasma concentrations rise after adrenalectomy. Secretion is stimulated by median eminence extracts containing CRF activity and suppressed by dexamethasone. Plasma concentrations of N-POMC and ACTH correlate closely, reflecting coordinated synthesis and secretion.

The principal modulator of ACTH secretion is CRF but vasopressin also has a stimulatory effect on ACTH secretion, directly and by potentiating the actions of CRF. Neurotransmitter pathways important in ACTH secretion are alpha-adrenergic (perhaps most important), cholinergic, serotoninergic and histaminergic (all excitatory) and via GABA (inhibitory).

ACTH release is circadian, resulting in the early morning peak of ACTH and cortisol in association with more frequent ACTH pulses. Factors modulating its secretion are cortisol [by negative feedback at hypothalamic (mainly) and pituitary levels via fast and slow feedback loops] and ACTH itself at pituitary level.

ACTH stimulates adrenal growth and cortisol synthesis and release. Plasma half-life is about 10 minutes. Mechanisms stimulating adrenocortical steroidogenesis are complex: ACTH binds to its adrenal cell membrane receptor, in the presence of calcium ions, to generate cyclic AMP; cyclic AMP activates, by phosphorylation, enzymes which stimulate hydrolysis of cholesterol esters (first steps in adrenal steroidogenesis). Rapid steroid production follows (p. 479 and Fig. 15.50). There is also

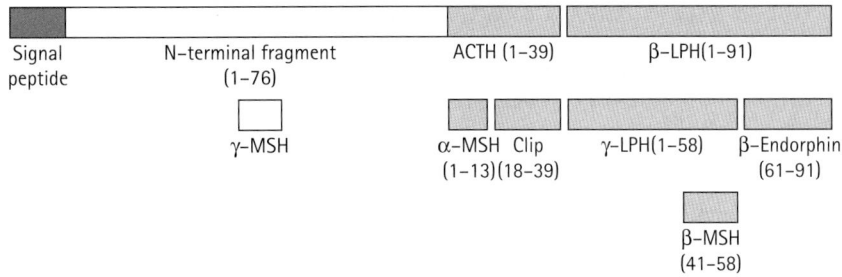

Fig. 15.43 Structure of bovine pro-opiomelanocortin (POMC). (After Nakanishi et al 1979[230]) (The connecting peptide N-POMC 79–109 has been omitted.)

a slower, chronic effect on protein synthesis in the cytochrome P450 dependent enzyme systems (11beta-, 17alpha- and 21-hydroxylases).

ACTH acutely stimulates aldosterone release from zona glomerulosa cells – this has important practical implications for managing of salt-losing CAH – and modulates adrenal androgen secretion. It stimulates amino acid and glucose uptake by muscle and lipolysis in adipose cells and inhibits thymic growth.

The 13 ACTH N-terminal amino acids are identical with alpha-MSH (see Fig. 15.43) and homologous with amino acids 7–13 of beta-MSH. Beta-MSH is not present in the pituitary or circulation in man and may not exist in discrete form. The etiology of skin pigmentation in pathological states is unclear – ACTH itself is probably causative in some situations.

Somatotrophin (growth hormone)
See p. 436.

Gonadotrophins (GTs – LH, FSH)
LH and FSH are glycoproteins (MW 30000 and 32000 respectively), each with identical A but different B chains and possibly stored within the same secretory granules in pituitary gonadotrophs. Release is controlled by a single hypothalamic hormone, GnRH (see Table 15.10). GnRH is released in a pulsatile manner.

In men, LH stimulates testicular Leydig cell testosterone secretion and FSH stimulates spermatogenesis. In women, LH induces ovulation, maintains the corpus luteum and stimulates it to produce progesterone and estrogens. Ovarian follicles secrete estrogens in response to FSH and endometrial gland growth and secretion result from estrogen and progesterone secretion, respectively. In men, LH secretion is under negative feedback control from testosterone and FSH secretion is regulated by inhibin B secreted by testicular Sertoli cells. In the female, estrogens exert either positive feedback at pituitary level (before ovulation) or negative feedback (at other times). For further details on the inhibins, see p. 447.

Prolactin (PRL)
PRL (198 amino acids, MW 22500) is strikingly homologous with GH. Its major role is in initiation and maintenance of lactation. Its role in childhood, when levels are low and constant, is unknown although it rises in response to stress. There is no evidence that slight rises during normal puberty are important in pubertal onset or control. Transiently high levels in neonates secondary to feto-placental estrogen may cause galactorrhea ('witch's milk') from engorged breasts in either sex.

PRL is predominantly under inhibitory dopaminergic control and hyperprolactinemia is an important early nonspecific sign of neuroendocrine disturbance and intracranial pathology. A PRL inhibiting factor (PIF) has been postulated but has not been characterized. GABA may also have some inhibitory effect but TRH and VIP are stimulatory.

Thyrotrophin (TSH)
TSH is a glycoprotein, MW 26600. It shares a common A chain with LH and FSH. TRH stimulates TSH synthesis and release which increases thyroid vascularity and stimulates follicular cell hypertrophy. TSH stim-ulates iodine uptake, organification, coupling of tyrosines and the synthesis and release of thyroxine (T4) and triiodothyronine (T3). Feedback inhibition is by T3, both directly and via deiodination of T4 within the pituitary. In man dopaminergic inhibition may occur at the level of the thyrotroph; the inhibitory role of somatostatin is unclear in normal physiology. Glucocorticoids inhibit TSH release at hypothalamic level.

After birth, there is a large rise in TSH release followed by a more gradual rise in circulating T4 and T3 levels. TSH levels return to normal by the end of the first week but thyroid hormone levels may be elevated for up to several weeks.

Melanocyte-stimulating hormones (alpha- and beta-MSH)
See above under ACTH.

POSTERIOR PITUITARY HORMONES

Arginine vasopressin (antidiuretic hormone, AVP) and oxytocin
Vasopressin and oxytocin are 9 amino acid peptides differing from each other at two sites (amino acids 3 and 8). They are synthesized in the supra-optic (mainly vasopressin) and paraventricular (mainly oxytocin) hypothalamic neurones bound to proteins (neurophysins I and II) whose function is unknown. Both hormones reach the posterior pituitary, where they are stored in secretory granules, via the supraopticohypophyseal tract.

The principal stimulus to vasopressin (AVP) release is rising plasma osmolality, but plasma volume and blood pressure may exert independent effects. Some physiological states (e.g. pain, stress, sleep) also stimulate vasopressin release. The most important physiological action is to cause water reabsorption by renal distal tubules and collecting ducts – water is reabsorbed in excess of sodium resulting in concentrated urine. Plasma osmolality is normally kept within the range 275–290 mosmol/kg throughout life.

The principal stimulus to oxytocin release is suckling. Oxytocin stimulates the 'let-down' reflex during lactation and uterine contractility. It has weak antidiuretic activity. Except in pregnancy and the puerperium, its physiological role in man is unknown. Neither excess nor deficiency is associated with any syndrome in children (or adults).

DISEASES OF THE HYPOTHALAMO-NEUROHYPOPHYSEAL UNIT

Diabetes insipidus (DI)
Hypothalamic AVP deficiency leads to voiding of inappropriately large volumes of dilute urine (polyuria). If thirst sensation is normal, fluid lost is replaced and there is excessive drinking (polydipsia) to maintain normal plasma osmolality. Nocturia is invariable and may present as secondary enuresis in older children. If thirst recognition is defective (usually due to extensive hypothalamic damage to both AVP and thirst osmoreceptors) or there is no access to adequate or appropriate fluid (e.g. in neonate or infant), hypernatremic dehydration may result in fever, irritability, vomiting and failure to thrive, and polyuria may be absent.

Polyuria and polydipsia may result from renal unresponsiveness to AVP (nephrogenic DI, see Ch. 18). Sometimes primary polydipsia ('compulsive water drinking') may develop in children (leading to secondary polyuria). Both these situations must be considered in the differential diagnosis as must other causes of polyuria (e.g. urinary tract infection, diabetes mellitus). Defects in AVP release are usually due to hypothalamic dysfunction – more than 75% of secretory capacity must be lost before symptoms develop. Removal of, or damage to, the neurohypophysis does not cause DI.

DI is rare in childhood: the incidence in Finland is 5 cases per million per year up to 14 years of age.[231] Causes are listed in Table 15.11.

Primary DI may be familial or sporadic, and families with dominant or X-linked inheritance have been described.

Familial AVP deficiency (DI) is of variable severity which increases with age and may not manifest itself clinically until adolescence. It is probably due to a degenerative process in the cells of the hypothalamus that produce antidiuretic hormone (AVP). As there is high redundancy of function (more than 75% of secretory capacity must be lost before symptoms develop) it is not surprising that, despite being inherited, the condition may take many years to develop.

AVP deficiency is found in 25–50% of children with Langerhans' cell histiocytosis and may precede other evidence of the disease by months or years (see Ch. 24, p. 1030). Other rare infiltrative causes include Hodgkin disease, leukemias and sarcoidosis but transient DI is common after head injury and pituitary surgery. It may complicate severe neonatal infections and may be associated with autoimmune states with AVP antibodies.

Differential diagnosis of polyuria depends on history, examination and laboratory tests. Osmotic diuresis (e.g. due to salt or glucose) is readily excluded from the history and by testing the urine for glucose. Habitual polydipsia most often develops in response to fluids being offered to pacify a demanding infant or young child. Such primary polydipsia of 'psychogenic' origin is suggested by fluctuating symptoms, evidence of psychological difficulties in the child or family, and a refusal of water (as opposed to juice) if waking thirsty at night. A morning plasma osmolality in the normal range (cf. in DI) often contrasts with a low value in the evening.

History of head injury, meningitis or encephalitis should be sought. Poor growth suggests either inadequate appetite or food intake relating to the polydipsia or an associated anterior pituitary lesion with TSH, GH, GT or ACTH deficiencies. TSH or ACTH deficiency may temporarily conceal DI until thyroxine or cortisol replacement is given. Headaches, vomiting and visual disturbances indicate raised intracranial pressure secondary to tumor.

Synchronous measurements of plasma and urinary osmolality are valuable provided accurate assays are available. If not, plasma sodium (not specific gravity) should be substituted. Inappropriately low urinary osmolality with raised plasma osmolality confirms DI – charts aiding interpretation have been produced for children.[236] To achieve this mismatch a water deprivation test may be necessary. Plasma AVP assays are increasingly available but their value in diagnosis of central DI in children is not established (high, diagnostic values are found in nephrogenic DI).

Water deprivation tests are potentially both dangerous and misleading if inadequately supervised and a strict protocol should be followed. Several protocols are available: Czernichow[237] is readily accessible. Specific additional endocrine and neuroradiological investigations may be necessary.

Provision of adequate water with free access to solute-free fluid at all times is vitally important. Treatment with AVP has been much simplified by the availability of a synthetic AVP analogue 1-desamino-

8D-arginine vasopressin (DDAVP, desmopressin) which has a longer duration of action than AVP itself. It can be administered intranasally – a reasonable starting dose is 0.25 mcg (in neonates), 0.5–1.0 mcg (infants) and 2.5 mcg (children). Therapeutic effect is seen within 1 h. The 2 or 3 times daily dose is adjusted to provide an antidiuretic effect for 8–12 h and may need increasing during rhinitis. DDAVP, like other small peptides, is orally active and can now be given orally – initially 100 mcg tds; maintenance 200–600 mcg per day in divided doses as above.

Special care must be taken with infants who do not have free access to water and children with an impaired sense of thirst (adipsic DI) who can be extremely difficult to manage. Water intoxication is a risk with overdosage or if water is given inappropriately. A talisman detailing the disease and its therapy should be carried or worn at all times.

Poor control of DI is associated with nocturia, enuresis, irritability and poor behavior and school performance. Appetite and growth velocity may be poor. Polyuria may lead to secondary enuresis. If treatment is optimal, prognosis reflects the underlying condition in secondary DI; in treated primary DI growth and development should be normal.

DI, diabetes mellitus, optic atrophy, deafness syndrome ('DIDMOAD' syndrome, Wolfram syndrome)

See p. 503.

Syndrome of inappropriate secretion of antidiuretic hormone (SIADH)

Causes are listed in Table 15.12. Excessive AVP secretion results in water retention, hypo-osmolality and dilutional hyponatremia. Inhibition of aldosterone with continuing AVP secretion leads to paradoxically high urinary sodium levels and concentrated urine. AVP levels may not be supranormal but are inappropriately high for the expanded extracellular volume and hypo-osmolality.

In pediatric practice, SIADH is usually seen either in neonates following birth asphyxia, hyaline membrane disease or intraventricular hemorrhage, or in older children in association with meningitis, encephalitis or CNS tumors. It occasionally complicates pneumonia or pulmonary

Table 15.11 Causes of diabetes insipidus (data from Crawford & Bode 1975, Czernichow et al 1985, Niaudet et al 1985, Perheentupa 1995)[232–235]

Hypothalamic tumor 38% – craniopharyngioma 23% (usually postoperative); germinoma 6.5%; optic neuroma rarely
Idiopathic 23% – autoimmune factors may be important
Congenital renal 23%
Histiocytosis X 8%
Cerebral malformations 3%
Primary polydipsia 3%
Traumatic 2%

Table 15.12 Causes of inappropriate ADH secretion

CNS disease/disorder
Meningitis/encephalitis
Trauma
Tumor
Hemorrhage
Hypoxia
Ischemia
Malformation
Guillain–Barré syndrome
Obstructed ventriculoatrial shunt
Lung disease
Pneumonia
Tuberculosis
Pneumothorax*
Asthma*
Cystic fibrosis*
Ventilation
Postoperative (including mitral valvotomy*, ductus arteriosus ligation*)
Drugs (e.g. analgesics, sedatives, anesthetics)
Malignancy
Trauma/burns
Endocrine/metabolic
Hypothyroidism
Adrenocortical failure
Hypoglycemia
Idiopathic

*May be secondary to reduced left atrial filling.

tuberculosis, vincristine or cyclophosphamide therapy, and is a common, temporary (up to several days) complication of surgery requiring general anesthesia. It may be a particular problem in burns and trauma patients. SIADH may be iatrogenic, due to inappropriate intravenous fluid therapy.

The first signs and symptoms are often masked by, or taken as manifestations of the underlying problem – anorexia, confusion, headaches, muscle weakness and cramps. Eventually, there is vomiting, convulsions or coma. There is no edema. Diagnosis depends on clinical suspicion and the above biochemical findings.

Treatment is by water restriction to between 30% and 50% maintenance and sodium replacement to compensate for secondary sodium losses. Correction should be gradual (over several days). In situations where this cannot be achieved drug therapy may be indicated. Lithium and demethylchlortetracycline have serious side-effects in children and should not be used. Furosemide (with slow infusion of hypertonic saline) may be indicated. AVP antidiuretic analogues which, it was hoped, would become the treatment of choice, have all had significant vasopressor activity.[238]

DISEASES OF THE ADENOHYPOPHYSIS

ACTH excess

Hypercortisolism in children usually results from excessive GC medication. Endogenous adrenocortical overactivity is rare, whether due to adrenal tumor (benign or malignant), hyperplasia, ectopic tumor ACTH production or pituitary dependent ACTH secretion (Cushing disease). Cushing syndrome includes all pathological states secondary to excessive GC production. Cushing found a basophil pituitary adenoma in only six of his original 12 patients[239] – it is now thought that bilateral adrenal hyperplasia secondary to excessive ACTH secretion of pituitary origin is not a single entity and may be due to a variety of hypothalamic, pituitary or even CNS (neurotransmitter) abnormalities.

Classical clinical features of hypercortisolism (hypertension, striae, truncal obesity, moon face, osteoporosis) are less obvious in children than in adults. Growth failure is usually marked but there can be temporary adrenal androgen-mediated acceleration. Investigation with low and high dose dexamethasone suppression tests and hCRH test will identify the etiology[240] – Cushing disease itself is probably the commonest cause in children and adolescents.

The aim in treating Cushing disease is to control cortisol overproduction (if appropriate by removing the source of ACTH hypersecretion) whilst avoiding permanent endocrine deficiencies and dependence on replacement therapy. In practice, treatment of Cushing syndrome in children is still controversial given its poorly understood and diverse etiological basis. Options include surgery to adrenals or pituitary, pituitary irradiation (conventional or with radioactive implants), or medical management with dopaminergic agents or serotonin antagonists. Collaboration between pediatric and adult endocrinologists, an experienced neurosurgeon and a radiotherapist is essential for a successful therapeutic outcome.

ACTH deficiency

ACTH deficiency is usually associated with other anterior pituitary hormone deficiencies which may be congenital, idiopathic, due to brain malformations or pituitary hypoplasia or to tumors such as craniopharyngioma (especially following surgery and/or radiotherapy). Hypothalamic CRF/pituitary ACTH secretion is more resistant to irradiation than the GH or GnRH axes. Secondary or tertiary adrenal insufficiency can be difficult to diagnose and assess but ACTH deficiency is rarely found in patients with a normal MRI and TSH levels.[241] Isolated ACTH deficiency is rare, may be congenital and can be associated with primary hypothyroidism – thyroxine therapy precipitates adrenal insufficiency by increasing cortisol clearance.

Congenital panhypopituitarism (see Fig. 15.44) is associated with severe neonatal hypoglycemia but isolated ACTH deficiency does not usually produce as severe adrenal hypofunction as in primary adrenal insufficiency. GC and adrenal androgen secretion are impaired; aldosterone secretion is normal. Collapse with salt loss may occur during severe intercurrent illness or general anesthesia. Treatment is with appropriate GC replacement.

TSH deficiency

Congenital hypothyroidism due to decreased TSH stimulation of thyroid hormone secretion may be due to abnormalities of hypothalamic or

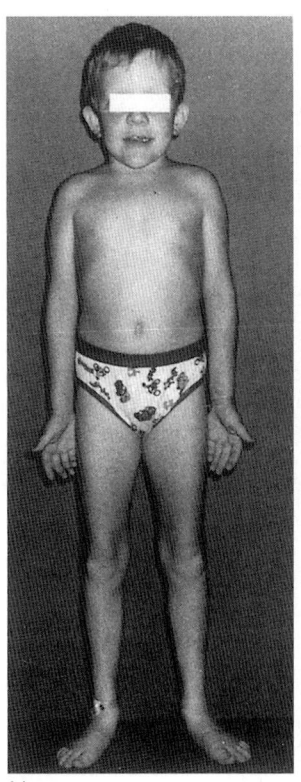
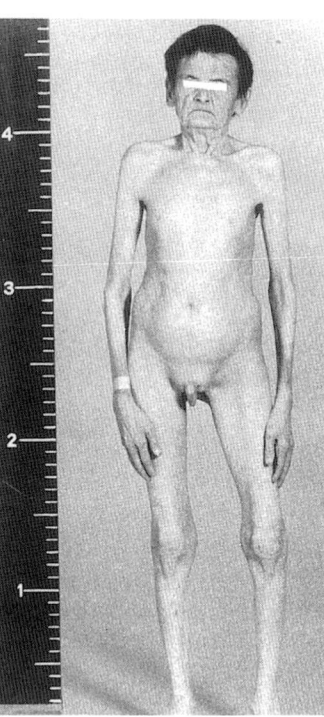
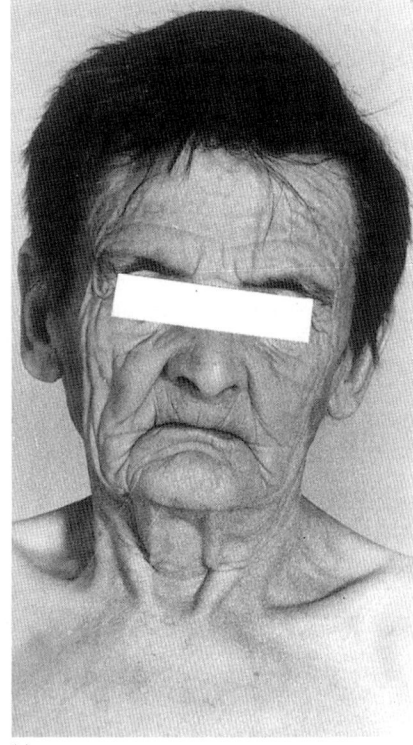

(a)   (b)   (c)

Fig. 15.44   Untreated panhypopituitarism (a) at age 11 years, (b) and (c) at age 71 years.

pituitary development, isolated TRH or TSH deficiency (familial or idiopathic) or panhypopituitarism. Congenital primary hypothyroidism is 15–30-fold more common.

TSH deficiency may present in later childhood, usually in association with other anterior pituitary hormone deficiencies and secondary to tumors (especially craniopharyngioma), cranial irradiation (to which the thyroid axis is relatively resistant) or meningitis. Symptoms and signs due to associated deficiencies usually predominate.

Differential diagnosis of primary, secondary (pituitary) and tertiary (hypothalamic) hypothyroidism and management is discussed below.

Gonadotrophin (GT) deficiency

Isolated GT deficiency may occur without underlying anatomical abnormality. Usually congenital abnormalities of brain development give rise to hypothalamic GnRH deficiency, either isolated (e.g. Kallmann syndrome) or associated with other hypothalamic disturbances. GT deficiency may be associated with other pituitary hormone deficiencies in pituitary aplasia or hypoplasia, craniopharyngioma, etc.

Hyperprolactinemia

Moderately raised PRL levels are an early nonspecific sign of neuroendocrine disturbance and particularly of suprasellar or hypothalamic space-occupying lesions. Stress also causes a moderate rise in PRL levels. Very high levels result from PRL-secreting micro- or macroadenomas but these are rare in children. They may cause delayed puberty. Raised PRL in association with raised GT (and especially FSH) levels causes precocious puberty in primary hypothyroidism.

Intracranial space-occupying lesions

These are the second commonest neoplasms in children (after leukemia) accounting for 20% of the total. Endocrine aspects are of practical importance in a variety of ways:

As 'early warning' signs of intracranial pathology

1. Moderately raised PRL levels in the absence of stress (see above).
2. Slow growth or signs of precocious or delayed puberty resulting from endocrine dysfunction may precede more specific clinical manifestations by many months.

In pre-, peri- and postoperative management

1. Hydrocortisone cover must be adequate for the stress of surgery, irradiation or radioactive implant.
2. Transient DI is common after surgery to the pituitary area but temporary inappropriate ADH secretion may occur (management is reviewed by Albanese et al[242]).

Permanent hormone replacement therapy after surgery and/or radiotherapy

1. The need for therapy should be reassessed in terms of adeno- and neurohypophyseal function after these procedures – variable deficiencies of any or all hormones may be found.
2. Some tumors are particularly associated with endocrine dysfunction. These include craniopharyngiomas (see below), hypothalamic and optic nerve gliomas, third ventricular tumors and pituitary adenomas. Third ventricular tumors and hamartomas and other tumors of the pituitary stalk region may result in hypofunction, but may, like many pituitary adenomas, be functional. They seem to be more common in boys and precocious puberty may be the earliest sign.

Craniopharyngioma (see Ch. 24, p. 1011)

This is the commonest tumor affecting the hypothalamo – pituitary region in childhood and accounts for 8–13% of all intracranial tumors in those under 14 years of age. The endocrine situation is never improved by surgery or radiotherapy (usually it is made worse) and endocrine disturbance alone is not an indication for either form of treatment.

Pre-, peri- and postoperative management and fluid balance must be meticulous. Pre-existing hormone deficiency should be corrected but hydrocortisone to cover the stress of the procedure must always be given even if ACTH reserve seems adequate. The need for long-term replacement therapies should be assessed several weeks postoperatively. DI may only become obvious after cortisol replacement. Occasional damage to the thirst center causes major management problems. In many cases, GH, thyroxine, hydrocortisone (certainly to cover stress and sometimes regularly), DDAVP and pubertal induction will be necessary. Despite appropriate hormone replacement, obesity can be a major long term problem in many patients. The prognosis is improved with early diagnosis and careful initial management.[243]

OTHER DISORDERS

Septo-optic dysplasia

Septo-optic dysplasia (SOD) is a condition characterized by midline neurological abnormalities associated with pituitary and optic nerve hypoplasia. The abnormalities and their manifestations are variable but a presentation may be with disturbed hypothalamic function and resulting hypopituitarism (usually GT, GH and AVP deficiencies) in infancy with hypothermia, hypoglycemia and blindness. CT or MR scanning shows variable hypoplasia of the optic nerves, chiasma and hypothalamic infundibular region, often with an absent septum pellucidum. Similar endocrine consequences are sometimes seen in other midline developmental abnormalities such as corpus callosum agenesis.

The homeobox gene Hesx1/HESX1 was initially implicated in pituitary development through loss-of-function studies in the mouse. Although the etiology of SOD is unknown, a homozygous missense point mutation in the gene resulting in a single amino acid substitution, Arg160Cys (R160C), is associated with a heritable form of human SOD.[244] Numerous other Hesx1/HESX1 gene mutations are now described and are important in providing a genetic basis for more general midline defects associated with an undescended or ectopic posterior pituitary.

Empty sella syndrome

Pituitary hypoplasia is associated with a small fossa. The infundibulum and pituitary stalk are normal but the chiasmatic cistern may extend into the small sella and appear empty with the stalk outlined by CSF. Enlargement of the sella and pituitary has been found in some cases of primary hypothyroidism, see Figure 15.35. Decreasing pituitary size on thyroxine replacement may give the appearance of an empty sella with the small pituitary gland situated posteroinferiorly within the enlarged fossa.

Diencephalic syndrome

This is usually due to an anteriorly growing hypothalamic glioma which presents in infancy or early childhood with excessive alertness and hyperexcitability, pallor, vomiting, gross wasting and failure to thrive. CSF protein levels are raised and tumor cells may be present. CT or MR scanning will confirm the diagnosis.

Sotos syndrome (cerebral gigantism)[245]

Prenatal overgrowth occurs in several syndromes, including the Sotos and Weaver syndromes which are probably closely related. Birth weight and length are high reflecting the rapid intrauterine growth. This continues until by middle childhood growth velocity is normal. As puberty occurs early, final stature is seldom excessive. Mental retardation is common but may be mild or absent. Associated cardiac defects are common and there are increased malignancy risks. There are also similarities with another tall stature syndrome, Beckwith–Wiedemann, and excessive secretion of fetal growth factors could be etiologically important.

THE PINEAL GLAND

The pineal, like the hypothalamus, develops from the diencephalon. Ependymal cells and vascular mesenchyme from the anterior part of the diencephalic roof plate form the choroid plexus. Caudally, the roof plate of the diencephalon thickens, evaginates by about 7 weeks and forms an ultimately cone-shaped solid organ, the pineal, attached by a peduncle to the posterior border of the third ventricle. It lies in the quadrigeminal cistern between the superior colliculi covered by the splenium of the corpus callosum and is innervated by postganglionic sympathetic superior cervical ganglionic nerve fibers. Pinealocytes form a mosaic pattern around capillaries, astrocytes and ganglion cells.

At one time thought to be the seat of the soul, seen as guiding the cerebral hemispheres or, more mundanely, being important in the control of the onset of human puberty, the pineal role remains speculative. Pinealocytes convert tryptophane via serotonin to melatonin which is primarily produced by the pineal gland during the dark period of the light–dark cycle.

It had been conjectured that endocrine pubertal events are inhibited prepubertally by melatonin. However, there appears to be no inhibitory effect of melatonin on GT secretion: 24-hour melatonin profiles are similar in prepuberty, puberty and adulthood (low daytime levels, high nocturnal levels). Blindness, which would upset the pineal circadian clock, is associated with early menarche.

Melatonin may have a role in inhibiting gonadal development – levels decrease significantly with sexual maturation and age. There is evidence for a decline in the day to night increment of serum melatonin concentrations from infancy to childhood, that children with early puberty have lower melatonin day to night increments than age matched controls, and that those with constitutionally delayed puberty show increments comparable to those of preschool children.[246]

This implies a relationship between maturation and the mechanisms controlling pineal gland secretion whether or not melatonin plays any significant role in the onset of puberty. Certainly, in seasonal breeders melatonin regulates reproductive physiology and influences the age of sexual maturation in laboratory rodents. In the human, melatonin rhythms are closely related to those of reproductive hormones during infancy and reciprocally correlated during puberty. There are melatonin receptors in the brain and gonads, and sex hormone receptors in the pineal gland but functional relationships have not been demonstrated.

In pediatric practice the pineal is important in two, sometimes related, contexts: rare pineal tumors and precocious puberty. Pineal tumors comprise < 1% of all intracranial tumors, are associated with precocious, delayed or absent puberty, but classically cause precocious puberty in boys. Lesions can be multifocal. About half are radiosensitive germinomas; astrocytomas, gliomas, germ cell teratomas and carcinomas also occur. Pineal destruction is usually associated with precocious puberty. Germinomas sometimes secrete HCG and alpha-fetoprotein, and secreting pineoblastomas and pineocytomas (pinealomas) occur.

Signs of raised intracranial pressure are common due to aqueduct compression. Visual loss, paresis of upward gaze and hypothalamic dysfunction (obesity, loss of temperature control, DI) may occur. Surgery is hazardous. Most pineal tumors recur after radiotherapy but germinomas are curable.

The pineal normally calcifies to varying extent with age. It is rarely seen radiographically before 6 years, is found in 2% by 8 years and 10% by 15 years (30% on CT scan). CT or MRI is indicated if calcification is seen on skull radiographs up to about 10 years and in any boy with central precocious puberty.

THE THYMUS

The thymus comprises cells of two origins. The epithelial component derives from 3rd and 4th pharyngeal pouches, the same embryological origin as the parathyroids. Thymic migration to the thorax from about 6 weeks is associated with parathyroid migration and branchial (pharyngeal) arch organization to form the aortic arch and other structures. Abnormal thymic stromal differentiation results in DiGeorge syndrome, where disruption of TGF-beta signaling in neural crest stem cells may be responsible for at least some of the phenotypic features.[247]

T-lymphocyte progenitors travel from fetal liver and, postnatally, from bone marrow and undergo maturation within the thymus to form T lymphocytes – the lymphoid component. Thymic stromal cells manufacture humoral substances, thymosin and thymopoietin, thought to be important in this maturational process. The thymus is the major site of production of immunocompetent T lymphocytes from their hematopoietic stem cells. Thymic hormones induce in situ T-cell marker differentiation, expression and functions. These polypeptide hormones localize in the reticulo-epithe-

lial (RE) cells of the thymic cellular microenvironment. Thymosin derivatives have been detected as products of neoplastically transformed cells and employed in the early diagnosis of neoplasms. In clinical trials, thymic hormones strengthen the effects of immunomodulators in immunodeficiencies, autoimmune diseases and neoplastic malignancies.[248]

Thymus and other lymphoid tissues reach their greatest proportion of body weight at birth, and by puberty are nearly twice their size in the young adult. The decline to adult size is probably sex steroid mediated. Adrenalectomy delays involution and severe infection or stress hastens it. In addition to its central role in immune regulation, the thymus may influence non-immunological components of the body, including the neuroendocrine system.

Cellular immune deficiencies of aging correspond to decline in function of the hypothalamo-pituitary–endocrine axis. Recent studies point to important roles for the pituitary, the pineal and the autonomic nervous system as well as the thyroid, gonads and adrenals in thymus integrity and function. Thymic function at the local level requires complex cellular interactions among thymic stromal cells and developing thymocytes, involving paracrine and autocrine mediators including interleukins and interferon-gamma. An important endocrine function of the thymus is to package zinc in zinc-thymulin for delivery to the periphery.[249]

Thymic tumors are rare but may arise from either tissue component. There is an association with myasthenia gravis, and tumors secreting an ACTH-like substance causing Cushing syndrome are described.

THE THYROID GLAND

EMBRYOLOGY

The thyroid gland develops as an epithelial proliferation in the pharyngeal gut floor at 17 days between what will become the body and root of the tongue – the foramen caecum. It descends as a bilobed diverticulum in front of the pharyngeal gut, still connected to it by a canal – the thyroglossal duct. This normally disappears but cystic remnants may persist – a thyroglossal cyst. Migration continues in front of hyoid bone and laryngeal cartilages to the definitive position in front of the trachea by 7 weeks.

PHYSIOLOGY

By 30 min post delivery, TSH levels surge, perhaps reacting to the cooler extrauterine environment. In response, within 28 h, total and free T3 and T4 levels rise – TBG levels do not change. High rT3 levels fall gradually over weeks. The importance of 'physiological neonatal hyperthyroidism' is not known, but animal data suggest a role in catecholamine-mediated brown fat and nonshivering thermogenesis.

Normal thyroid function is crucial in infancy and childhood because of its importance for normal somatic and brain growth and development. Thyroid hormone actions include protein synthesis, cholesterol turnover, water and ion transport and thermogenesis. There are direct and indirect (growth factor synthesis) effects on growth and CNS and skeletal development.

The thyroid concentrates iodide from blood (as do other tissues – salivary and mammary glands, placenta, uterus, stomach and small bowel) and (uniquely) combines it with tyrosine to form metabolically active derivatives. Endemic dietary iodine deficiency is the commonest cause of hypothyroidism and affects some 300 million people worldwide. This has implications for fetal CNS development[250] – see below.

Steps in thyroid hormone biosynthesis are summarized in Figure 15.45. Inborn errors of each step are described and comprise about 10% of neonates with congenital non-endemic hypothyroidism. Transport of iodide into thyroid cells is rate limiting. Iodide oxidation (activation) is followed by peroxidase-catalyzed tyrosine iodination and iodotyrosine coupling to form T3 and T4. Thyroglobulin (TG), a high molecular weight iodinated glycoprotein, provides tyrosyl residues for iodotyrosine synthesis (any other physiological role is speculative) and reaches the circulation via thyroid lymphatics. Mono- and di-iodo tyrosines (MIT and DIT), T3 and T4 are stored as extracellular colloid. Thyroid hormone secretion involves formation of intracellular colloid droplets, fusion with lysosomes, proteolytic digestion and hydrolysis of thyroglobulin to form free

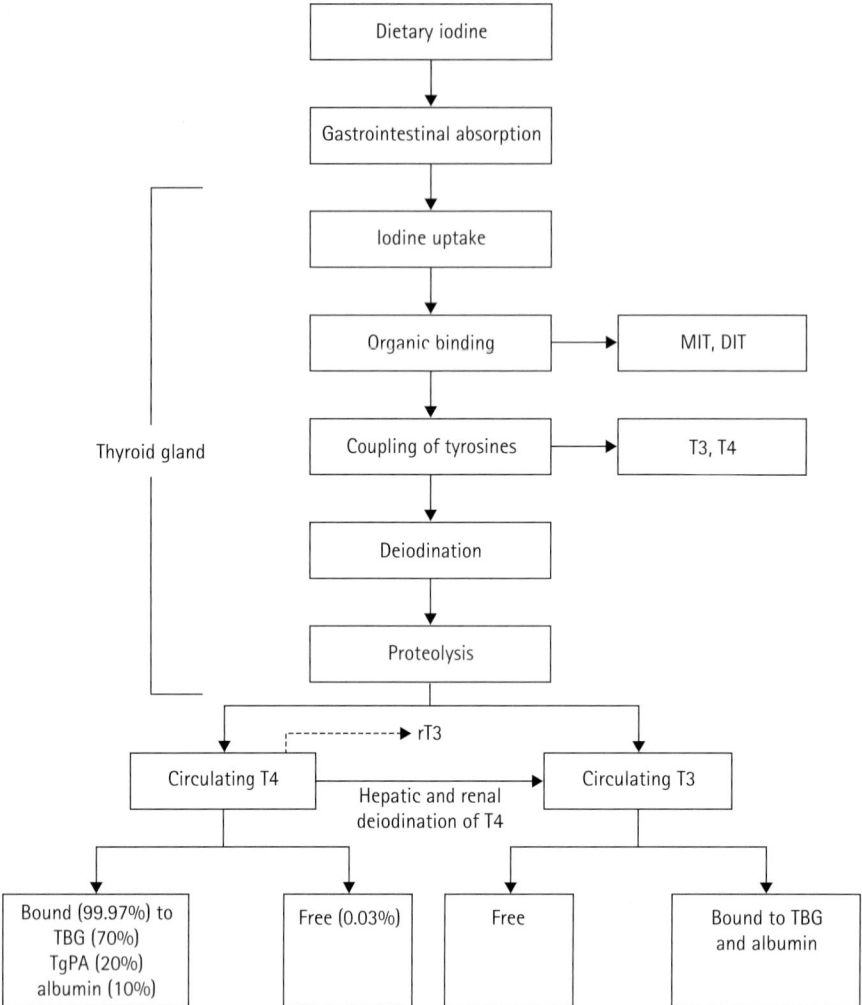

Fig. 15.45 Thyroid hormone biosynthesis. DIT, di-iodo tyrosine; MIT, mono-iodo tyrosine; TBG, thyroxine binding globulin; TgPA, thyroglobulin antibody by passive agglutination.

MIT, DIT, T3 and T4. T3 and T4 are released into the circulation; MIT and DIT are deiodinated and free iodide is reutilized for hormone synthesis.

Physiological thyroid hormone action at cellular level is by binding to a specific nuclear plasma membrane and mitochondrial receptors. T3 binding to nuclear receptors seems most important.

For many years it was believed that maternal thyroid hormones did not reach the developing embryo and fetus throughout gestation. More recent research has shown that this is not the case and that these hormones, derived from the mother, probably do exert important developmental effects on the fetal brain.

There is evidence from animal (largely rat) experiments that if the fetal thyroid gland is underactive (congenital hypothyroidism), the transfer of normal amounts of maternal thyroxine (T4) is crucial and protects the fetal brain until birth.[22] Most of the results from animal experiments seem relevant in man, and some, such as the transfer of maternal hormones from mother to fetus during pregnancy and their protective effects on the fetal brain of infants with congenital hypothyroidism, have also been directly demonstrated in man.[21]

Specifically, current evidence suggests that if fetal thyroid secretion is impaired (congenital hypothyroidism), transfer of maternal thyroid hormone (thyroxine, T4) is normally sufficient to enable the fetal brain to convert this thyroxine to triiodothyronine (T3) upon which fetal brain growth and development is dependent, and thus to avoid major subsequent neurodevelopmental problems until birth. The protective effect of normal maternal circulating T4 concentrations ends at birth and cerebral T3 deficiency in the newborn follows, which is why treatment with thyroxine must be started in the congenitally hypothyroid baby within a few weeks of birth.

In some parts of the world, severe iodine deficiency is endemic amongst the population and can result in low maternal T4 levels during early pregnancy. In that situation even prompt treatment of the congenitally hypothyroid baby with thyroxine following birth does not prevent the child from having neurological problems and cognitive and intellectual impairment. This emphasizes the crucial role of maternal thyroxine in the development of the fetal brain in early pregnancy.[250]

Thus the effects of congenital hypothyroidism alone on fetal brain growth and development do not result in significant or irreversible neurodevelopmental abnormalities. The central nervous system damage in congenital hypothyroidism is preventable by adequate early postnatal thyroxine treatment provided maternal thyroid status has been adequate during the pregnancy. This is also demonstrated by the generally good results (normal mental and psychomotor development) achieved in this condition following prompt detection (by newborn screening) and early postnatal thyroxine treatment in adequate dosage (see below).

REGULATION OF FUNCTION

Plasma iodide and circulating TSH levels regulate thyroid follicular cell function. Circulating FT4 exerts negative feedback on TSH release. Seventy-five to eighty percent of circulating FT3 is produced by deiodination of T4 in peripheral tissues. The control mechanism for production of T3 in nonthyroidal tissue is poorly understood but during many disease states or fasting T4 conversion to T3 is reduced and (inactive) rT3 accumulates. T3 has 3–4 times the potency of T4 and binds to cell membrane receptor proteins with 10-fold greater affinity.

THYROID FUNCTION TESTS (TFTs)

Normal ranges for TFTs are age related and vary between laboratories. The most sensitive single test of primary thyroid disease is plasma TSH immunoradiometric assay (IRMA). In primary hypothyroidism levels are raised; in hyperthyroidism (or overtreatment of hypothyroidism) levels are suppressed, usually to below the assay detection limit (< 0.1 mU/L). RIA TSH measurement will not reliably distinguish appropriate from excessive replacement.

Total T3 (TT3) and T4 (TT4) levels reflect TBG levels; free (active) hormone measurements (FT3, FT4) reflect functional thyroid status more accurately. T3 may be a more sensitive guide to developing thyrotoxicosis than T4 if TSH IRMA assays are unavailable, but diagnosis on clinical examination is seldom problematic.

Biochemical assessment strategies are reviewed by Vanderscheuren-Lodeweyckx.[251] It is good practice to measure TSH and FT4 simultaneously to assess the whole axis. TRH tests are no longer considered useful in assessing hypothalamo-pituitary function, and they are not of practical use either for diagnosing central hypothyroidism or discriminating between hypothalamic and pituitary disorders.[252]

Most specific situations where nonthyroidal illness, pregnancy or drug treatment causes abnormal TFTs (e.g. malnutrition, anorexia nervosa) are uncommon in pediatric practice provided tests are not performed during severe intercurrent illness. During the acute phase of such illnesses (e.g. severe burns or trauma, diabetic ketoacidosis, liver or renal failure), TT3, TT4 and FT3 levels are often low, FT4 may be low or normal (depending on assay methodology); TSH may also be low or normal. During recovery, thyroid hormone levels gradually normalize, but persisting low levels, even with raised TSH levels, do not necessarily indicate hypothyroidism.

Drugs affecting TFTs include estrogens, salicylates, phenytoin, carbamazepine, glucocorticoids and propranolol. Iodide (in expectorants) can cause clinical, as well as biochemical, hypothyroidism.

Apparent thyroid disorders in euthyroid patients due to abnormal carrier proteins will not cause confusion if free hormone and IRMA TSH assays are available. Children with hereditary TBG deficiency (X-linked dominant inheritance, incidence 1 in 10 000, males:females 9:1) will have low TT4 and TT3 levels; high levels of TBG, and thus of TT4 and TT3, are seen during estrogen therapy. In both situations, FT4, FT3 and TSH levels are normal and the patient is clinically euthyroid.

Raised TSH levels with normal FT4 levels in treated hypothyroidism may indicate poor compliance (other than just before a clinic visit). TFTs must always be considered in the context of growth velocity and skeletal maturation and not in isolation (see earlier). Clinical examination alone for signs of hypothyroidism or thyrotoxicosis is a very insensitive guide.

FUNCTION IN PRETERM INFANTS

TT4 and FT4 levels increase with gestation – ~25% of preterm infants have low levels by term standards (50% at less than 30 weeks). FT4 levels are never as low as in congenital hypothyroidism. There is presumed hypothalamic immaturity: TSH levels may be normal or low; TSH and T4 levels rise normally following TRH. T4 levels correct spontaneously with maturation over 4–8 weeks, postnatal growth and development are normal and treatment is unnecessary. This has implications for screening programs and the timing of retesting of preterm babies so that cases of congenital hypothyroidism in the preterm are not missed and whether this should be postnatal age- or birth weight-related.

There are babies (term or preterm), however, with significantly reduced FT4 levels (into the congenital hypothyroidism range). This seems much more common in Europe than the USA (perhaps reflecting relative iodine availability). Prevalence in Belgium is 20% in the preterm and related to gestational length.[253] Cord blood T4 and TSH levels are normal for gestation. In many, thyroid function quickly normalizes; in others, recovery may take 1–2 months and treatment has been thought to be necessary (based on observational studies) in order to prevent abnormal neurodevelopmental outcomes. Although a Cochrane review[254] does not support the use of thyroid hormones in preterm infants to reduce neonatal mortality, improve neurodevelopmental outcome or reduce the severity of respiratory distress syndrome, a further study with 10 year follow-up[255] shows benefit in those less than 28 weeks' gestation but a worse outcome at 29 weeks' gestation. The influences of many postnatal illnesses and drug usage are important in the preterm[256] and further large scale studies are warranted.

Transient hypothyroidism may occur in preterm infants exposed in utero to maternal iodine-containing drugs or following injection of radiographic contrast agents. Low T3 levels are commonly seen in preterm infants and may persist for 1–2 months. They are due to the lower T3 postnatal surge and reduced conversion of T4 to T3 in peripheral tissues resulting from, e.g. birth asphyxia, hypoglycemia, hypocalcemia and relative malnutrition. FT4 and TSH levels are usually normal for gestational age and no treatment is necessary.

HYPOFUNCTION

Congenital

Thyroid dysgenesis

The commonest cause of congenital hypothyroidism is aplastic, hypoplastic or ectopic thyroid tissue – thyroid dysgenesis – occurring with consistent prevalence worldwide: 1 in 3500 to 4500 births. Females are twice as commonly affected but familial cases are rare – nearly all occur sporadically and idiopathically although there is increased incidence in Down syndrome babies and seasonal variation. In 50% there is some functioning thyroid tissue resulting in a spectrum of severity of hypothyroidism. There is generally no relationship with maternal thyroid function, treatment with thyroxine or thyroid autoimmune status. A role for immunoglobulins which block TSH-stimulated thyroid cell growth in vitro in pathogenesis remains speculative.

Dyshormonogenesis (inborn errors of thyroid hormone biosynthesis)

Autosomal recessively inherited defects in thyroid hormone biosynthesis are the second commonest causes of congenital hypothyroidism, accounting for about 10% of those identified on screening (i.e. about 1 in 40000 births). Presence of a goiter at birth is strongly suggestive but may not develop for months or years. There is a spectrum of hypofunction but it is generally less severe than in the dysgenetic group. Sex incidence is equal.

A defect may occur at any biosynthetic step (Fig. 15.45):
1. Decreased TSH responsiveness – very rare.
2. Decreased trapping of iodide: thyroid enlargement and reduced (or virtually absent) radioiodine (RAI) uptake by thyroid and tissues such as salivary glands and gastric mucosa.
3. Defective organification: peroxidase deficiency (defective oxidation of thyroidal iodide to reactive iodine). The association with high tone or complete nerve deafness (Pendred syndrome, 2 per 100000 children of school age) is not due to peroxidase deficiency – the precise etiology of the thyroid biosynthetic defect (and deafness) is unknown. Together, these are the commonest dyshormonogenetic defects. In peroxidase deficiency (and most Pendred patients) there is a rapid fall in thyroid radioactivity with thiocyanate or perchlorate after radioiodine administration.
4. Defective iodotyrosine coupling or deiodination: nondeiodination of MIT and DIT leads to their leakage from the gland, urinary excretion and iodine loss.
5. Abnormal thyroglobulin synthesis, storage or release.

Hypothalamo-pituitary (tertiary/secondary) congenital hypothyroidism

Congenital hypothyroidism due to TRH or TSH deficiency may be familial or sporadic, isolated or associated with other hypothalamo-pituitary deficiencies and can be associated with anatomical defects (e.g. absent pituitary or sella turcica). Prevalence is about 1 in 100000 births. Associated hypothyroidism will be missed by TSH screening. This is not critically important – there are often associated features (dysmorphism, micropenis, hypoglycemia) drawing attention to the differential diagnosis. Hypothyroidism is generally mild and treatment can be unnecessary for some months.

Clinical and laboratory features

During the early weeks of life, babies are usually asymptomatic and early clinical signs are nonspecific (Fig. 15.46): even in resource rich countries only about 5% are diagnosed before the positive screening result and only ~50% can be diagnosed reliably before 3 months, by when subsequent neurodevelopmental problems are much more likely. No screening program is totally reliable – there must still be clinical suspicion in certain circumstances. Important features include: umbilical hernia, wide posterior fontanelle or goiter at birth, a placid, sleepy, 'good' baby, poor feeding, constipation, hypothermia, peripheral cyanosis, edema, prolonged physiological jaundice. More specific features such as the coarse facies, large tongue, hoarse cry, dry skin and low hair line are late signs.

Biochemically, both dysgenetic and dyshormonogenetic groups have low T4 and high TSH levels after neonatal changes have settled. About 1 in 6 will have T4 levels in the lower part of the normal range.

Screening

Although clinical detection of congenital hypothyroidism is unreliable, no screening program is 100% specific and sensitive: there may be laboratory error or communication breakdown between laboratory and clinician, and there is a minority of affected babies in whom the screening result will be normal. Up to 10% of babies with congenital hypothyroidism will not have grossly elevated screening TSH values. Where TSH is used for screening, hypothyroidism due to hypothalamic or pituitary disease will be missed; where T4 (followed by TSH for the lower range of T4 values) is used, a 10th centile or absolute T4 level of 130–140 nmol/L cut-off is used as < 20% of affected babies have low normal (90–140 nmol/L) T4 levels.

All abnormal or suspicious screening results must be confirmed before the infant is committed to long term therapy but it is safer to start thyroxine whilst definitive results are awaited. If they are normal, full reassessment is necessary.

Scanning

Thyroid scans using ^{99m}Tc-pertechnetate or ^{123}I-labeled sodium iodide (the latter has the advantage of shorter half-life and better concentration in the thyroid) may be helpful in the newborn for detection and anatomical localization of functioning thyroid tissue and to exclude the commonest dyshormonogenetic defect (organification). The technique is relatively invasive, time-consuming and expensive, and results can be unreliable, especially when tests are performed by inexperienced investigators. Misleading results can also result from maternal blocking immunoglobulins or perinatal iodine contamination.

Such 'functional' scans may be supplemented by 'structural' ultrasound scanning (inexpensive and rapid) which will provide complementary information in skilled hands. Ultrasound can reveal whether thyroid tissue is present in the normal position but is poor at detecting ectopic thyroid tissue. If no gland is detectable with normal T3 but low T4 levels and measurable levels of thyroglobulin, an ectopic rest of thyroid tissue is likely. From a practical management perspective, the need for scanning (either or both modalities) remains controversial.

Following ^{123}I-labeled sodium iodide scanning, most dyshormonogenetic defects (other than of iodide trapping) will show high or normal isotope uptake and normal thyroid position and anatomy. In the commonest defect (peroxidase deficiency) there is discharge of 60–70% of radioactive iodide within 1 h following perchlorate. If organification is normal, less than 5–10% is discharged within 1 h. Frequencies of different possible biosynthetic defects are unknown although molecular genetic studies have revealed mutations in the thyroid peroxidase (TPO) and thyroglobulin genes in some familial cases.[257]

Treatment

Once the diagnosis is suspected, treatment is urgent and should be started immediately blood has been taken for definitive testing without waiting for those results. Sodium-l-thyroxine (l-T4) is the treatment of choice as it is reliably absorbed and its peripheral endogenous conversion to T3

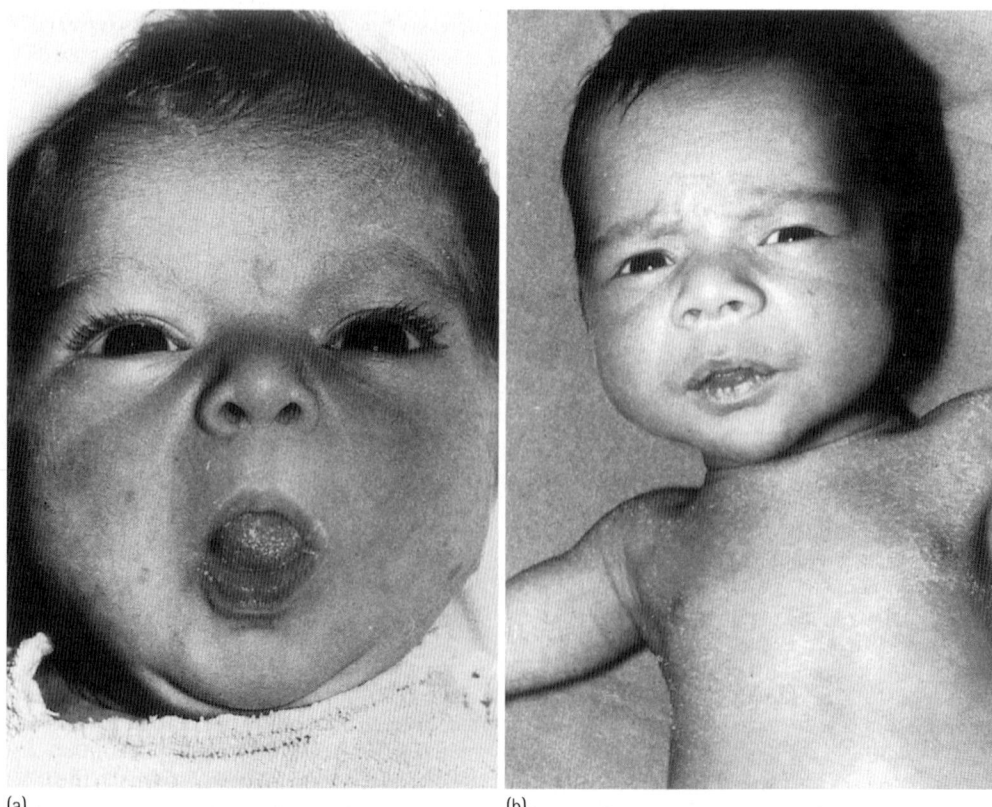

(a)   (b)

Fig. 15.46   Congenital hypothyroidism presenting (a) at 3 months in 1978 (prior to UK screening) and (b) at 10 days following a raised level of TSH screening (1983).

allows automatic 'fine tuning' of function. In infancy, T4 levels should be in the upper normal range and T3 levels normal. TSH levels must not be used as a guide to treatment efficacy in infancy – in > 50% the feedback set point is abnormal and TSH levels remain high in the presence of adequate replacement and normal T4.

A starting dose of l-T4 of 15 mcg/kg orally (or, conveniently, 50 mcg) once daily is appropriate and ~15 mcg/kg is usually appropriate throughout infancy. Recent data confirm that it is better to suppress TSH levels as quickly as possible (using higher doses than previously recommended) rather than simply normalizing free T4 levels.[258,259] Marginal over-replacement can generally be compensated for by endogenous deiodination but under-replacement may result in significant long term neurological impairment.

After infancy, the required daily dose is ~100 mcg/m^2/24 h. Overtreatment will cause symptoms and signs of thyrotoxicosis but clinical-assessment alone only detects significant under- or over-replacement.

Growth, TFTs, bone age maturation and clinical progress (including psychomotor development) should be checked regularly during the first year. Assessment should be at 1 month and then every 3 months. It is essential that parents know the importance of giving the l-T4 regularly and do not forget or stop treatment because their baby seems normal.

By the third year of life, briefly interrupting medication will have no long term effects on brain growth and development and it is necessary to assess the need for permanent treatment. So as to minimize the time off treatment, T3 (with its shorter half-life) can be substituted for l-T4 therapy (100 mcg l-T4 is equivalent to 20 mcg T3) for 2 weeks, all treatment stopped for 7 days, thyroid function checked (and an isotope scan performed if indicated) and the previous l-T4 dose restarted immediately whilst results are awaited and assessed. Alternatively l-T4 can simply be discontinued for 2 weeks.

Outcome

'Not the magic wand of Prospero or the brave kiss of the daughter of Hippocrates ever effected such a change as that which we are now enabled to make in these unfortunate victims, doomed heretofore to live in hopeless imbecility, an unspeakable affliction to their parents and their relatives' William Osler wrote in 1897[260] on the transforming effects of the then recently introduced thyroid replacement therapy. However, although gross physical manifestations of congenital hypothyroidism are abolished by treatment, significant neurodevelopmental and intellectual deficits remain unless treatment is started during the early weeks of life.

Delay beyond 3 months is particularly serious: in one study[261] the mean IQ with treatment before 3 months was 89, 70 if started between 3 and 6 months and 54 after 6 months. With screening programs, sufficiently early diagnosis is almost always possible and neurodevelopmental prognosis good. At 2 years, children adequately treated before 4 weeks show no differences from controls on the Bayley mental development index, and at 3, 4 and 5 years, in Stanford Binet IQ assessment in contrast to those inadequately treated.[262] However, there may be subtle deficiencies in hearing/speech performance scales at 1 year and practical reasoning at 18 months and 3 years and, possibly, in motor and perceptual abilities, speech, behavior and personality.[258]

It seems that a low T4 level (< 30–40 nmol/L) at diagnosis is associated with a deficit in mental development.[263] A recent comprehensive UK survey[264] has demonstrated a discontinuous effect of severity of congenital hypothyroidism with a risk of a 10 point IQ deficit with initial thyroxine level of < 40 nmol/L. Lower social class (perhaps also associated with poorer compliance) accounted for another 10 point IQ decrement. Up to 10% needed special education[40] in contrast to other studies.[265] Surprisingly, timing of onset of treatment did not seem important.

Acquired

Hypothyroidism may develop, usually insidiously, at any age. Important causes are summarized in Table 15.13.

Endemic iodine deficiency

Worldwide, ~300 million people have endemic goiter. Simple iodine deficiency is generally responsible but genetic factors may predispose and environmental goitrogens (e.g. *Brassica* vegetables) potentiate the

Table 15.13 Important causes of acquired hypothyroidism in childhood

Autoimmune thyroiditis
Thyroid dysgenesis
Endemic iodine deficiency
Exposure to goitrogens
Hypothalamo–pituitary disease (TRH/TSH deficiency)

effects. Iodine deficiency leads to deficient thyroid hormone production, TSH hypersecretion and increased iodide trapping with goiter and raised T3:T4 ratio. Such compensatory mechanisms can result in euthyroidism with goiter or varying degrees of goitrous hypothyroidism. In endemic areas < 8% of the population may be affected.

The problem is still common in some areas of Europe, Scandinavia and the Middle East including Switzerland, Finland, Austria, Germany, Italy, Spain, Greece, Lebanon and Iraq. In Switzerland and Finland iodination of salt is effectively reducing the prevalence – endemic cretinism is now uncommon.

In the context of low maternal T4 levels during early pregnancy, even prompt treatment of the baby with thyroxine following birth does not prevent the child from having neurological problems and cognitive and intellectual impairment (see above). The introduction of iodized salt in Denmark (where iodine intake was low) has resulted in a small increase in the incidence of autoimmune hypothyroidism, predominantly in young people against a background of low rates of overt hypothyroidism.[266]

Autoimmune (Hashimoto) thyroiditis

This commonest cause of acquired hypothyroidism in non-endemic areas of iodine deficiency was described by Hashimoto in 1912. Girls are much more commonly affected; a family history of thyroid disorders is found in about one third.

The gland, infiltrated by lymphocytes and plasma cells (delayed hypersensitivity) with fibrosis and degeneration, is generally irregularly enlarged and firm. There is prominence of normal architecture but usually no nodules. Acinar regeneration can occur – growth immunoglobulins and TSH may be important for this. One or more of several possible types of circulating antithyroid antibodies are found in about 95% at presentation but such antibodies also occur in up to 20% of the 'normal' population (some of whom may eventually develop thyroiditis). The commonest antibodies are against thyroglobulin and microsomes but antiperoxidase (now commonly available), TSH-receptor blocking or stimulating, colloid and thyroid growth inhibiting or stimulating antibodies may occur. Antinuclear factor (ANF) is particularly likely to be positive in children.

Presentation may be with euthyroid goiter, goiter with hypothyroidism or in the context of pre-existing autoimmune disease. In < 10%, and particularly at adolescence, presentation may be with signs of thyrotoxicosis. Usually, however, onset is with insidious hypothyroidism (Fig. 15.47) – classical myxedema may not occur for many months. School performance frequently deteriorates but can be attributed to other problems. Height velocity slows but this may not be recognized if children are not measured regularly – slow growth must be prolonged before a single measurement or simple observation detects conspicuous short stature.

In a still euthyroid child, diagnosis can be made on the basis of goiter, increased antiperoxidase, antithyroglobulin or antimicrosomal antibody titers, abnormal thyroid scan with positive perchlorate discharge test and biochemical signs of compensated hypothyroidism.

Associated multiple endocrine deficiency disease includes diabetes mellitus with or without adrenal insufficiency (Schmidt syndrome), hypoparathyroidism, candidiasis, pernicious anemia and thrombocytopenia. Fewer than 30% of children with type 1 diabetes mellitus will have detectable thyroid antibodies and 10% will have raised TSH levels. There is an association between autoimmune thyroid disease and a variety of cytogenetic disorders including Down, Turner, Klinefelter and Noonan syndromes. All children with diabetes mellitus and cytogenetic disorders should be screened regularly for thyroid disease.

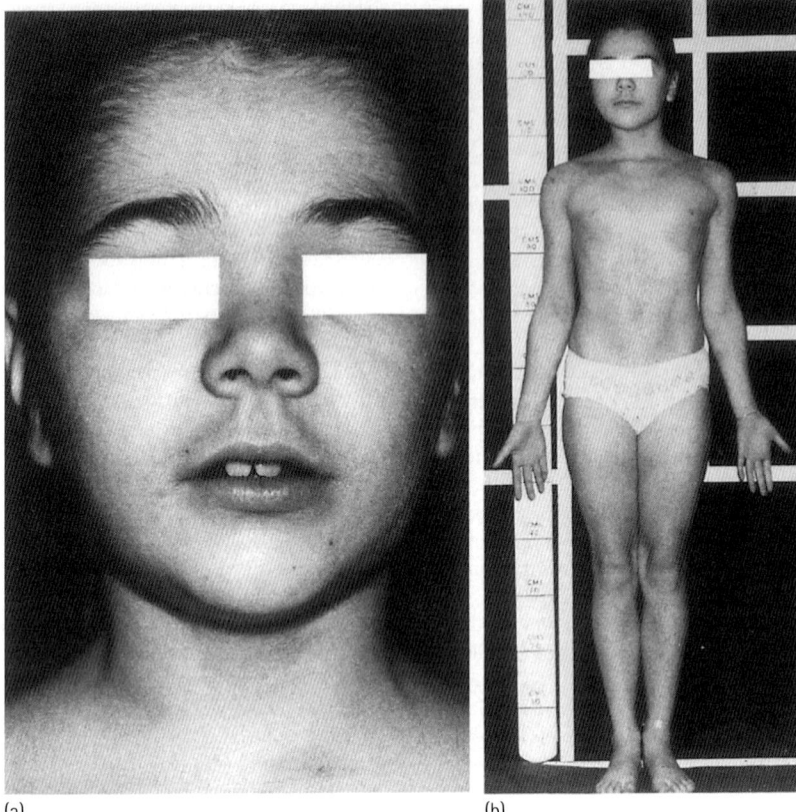

(a)   (b)

Fig. 15.47 The result of insidious development of hypothyroidism over several years.

There is usually progressive thyroid atrophy and treatment, once started, is generally life-long. If there is initial hyperfunction, euthyroidism and eventual hypothyroidism will probably develop. Spontaneous remission is said to occur in < 30% of adolescents. Nodules in Hashimoto thyroiditis are due to lymphoid or thyroid hyperplasia and only rarely indicate malignancy.

Diffuse goiter in a euthyroid adolescent occurs commonly in non-endemic areas. Some have Hashimoto thyroiditis but in others aspiration biopsy shows a colloid goiter with no evidence of the characteristic lymphocytic infiltration and there may be autosomal dominant transmission. Although, in the medium term, the goiter usually regresses untreated, the common finding of thyroid-stimulating immunoglobulins (TSI) and the fact that a significant number of adults presenting with nodular goiters have a history of diffuse adolescent goiter suggest that autoimmune mechanisms are important for pathogenesis.

Ultrasound measurement of thyroid volume is preferable to palpation for grading goiters, and normative data for thyroid volume by ultrasound in iodine-sufficient school children are now available.[267]

Thyroid dysgenesis
Most inborn errors of biosynthesis present in the newborn or by infancy. However, with mild compensated defects, goiter develops slowly and hypothyroidism may not develop until childhood. There is an increased incidence of thyroid dysgenesis in Down syndrome.

Ectopic and inadequately functional thyroid may present as an enlarging mass at the base of the tongue or along the course of the thyroglossal duct ('cryptothyroidism'). Removal of a 'thyroglossal cyst' may result in severe hypothyroidism if that is the only functional thyroid tissue present.

Thyroid destruction due to infiltration with cystine crystals may cause eventual hypothyroidism in children with cystinosis.

Exposure to goitrogens
Foods interfering with thyroid hormone biosynthesis include cabbage, cassava and soybeans. Ingestion of a goitrogen in the context of a genetically predisposed population or iodine deficiency is more likely to result in frank hypothyroidism. Drugs acting similarly include iodide (in proprietary expectorants), perchlorate and thiocyanate, lithium, amiodarone, phenylbutazone, aminoglutethimide, aminosalicylic acid and the specifically antithyroid drugs, carbimazole and propylthiouracil.

Hypothalamo-pituitary dependent hypothyroidism
Slowing of linear growth due to TSH or associated GH deficiency is the usual presentation with a history of head injury, cranial irradiation for leukemia or medulloblastoma, meningitis or granulomatous disease. Craniopharyngioma must be excluded. There may be associated neurological signs, and symptoms or signs relating to underlying disease, or hypothalamo-pituitary dysfunction. Latent hypothalamo-pituitary hypothyroidism may develop in 'isolated' GH deficiency treated with GH and may prevent growth acceleration.

Thyroid hormone unresponsiveness
Families with goiter and variable thyroid hormone unresponsiveness have been described with possible autosomal dominant or recessive inheritance. The defect may be at receptor or postreceptor level.

Presentation and diagnosis
Slowing of height velocity is the earliest sign. Retrospectively, growth data (or holiday photographs) will help pinpoint age at onset. Skinfold measurements are usually increased and bone age delayed but both are common in many childhood endocrinopathies. Very delayed skeletal maturation (> 3 years over chronological age) is a particular feature. Muscle weakness is common on testing but is seldom a presenting complaint. Muscle atrophy, hypertrophy and dysfunction have been described. Classical signs of myxedema develop gradually with infiltration of many tissues (including skin) by mucopolysaccharides, hyaluronic acid and chondroitin sulfate (Fig. 15.47). Skin becomes yellow from high carotene levels and there may be tiredness (with poor school

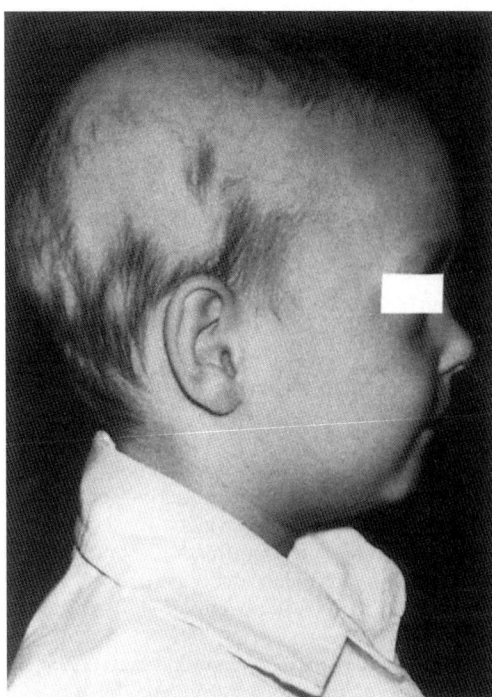

Fig. 15.48 Alopecia associated with autoimmune hypothyroidism.

performance), cold intolerance and characteristically slow relaxation of tendon reflexes. Hypertrichosis with low hair line may occur, as may hair loss with alopecia (Fig. 15.48).

Classically pubertal delay occurs, but a significant minority develop precocious puberty and this may occur whilst the child is still clinically euthyroid. A failing thyroid gland causes hypothalamic release of TRH; consequent high TSH levels initially maintain euthyroidism but TRH also stimulates PRL and GT (LH and FSH) release causing ovarian estradiol secretion and breast development in girls and testicular (and sometimes penile) enlargement in boys. PRL may cause inhibition of gonadal stimulation by LH but not FSH resulting in sustained gonadal stimulation. A direct effect of TSH on the HCG receptor has also been described.[268] Clinically there is loss of consonance with breast development with or without galactorrhea in girls. Testicular (with or without penile) enlargement occurs in boys due to the FSH-dependent seminiferous tubule development. LH-dependent Leydig cell development does not occur and there is little (androgen-dependent) pubic or axillary hair development. There is no increase in height velocity, short stature and (pathognomonic) BA delay. The sella turcica may be enlarged. Why a minority of children with acquired hypothyroidism develop sexual precocity rather than pubertal delay is unexplained. On thyroid replacement therapy pubertal development arrests and there may be some regression until puberty recommences at a time appropriate to bone age maturity.

Clinical diagnosis of acquired hypothyroidism must be confirmed biochemically before treatment is started. Low total or free T4 or T3 levels confirm hypothyroidism, raised TSH levels that the defect is at thyroid level. A goiter necessitates thyroid and other autoantibody measurement. If there is no goiter, or no evidence of autoimmune disease, thyroid scanning to exclude dysgenesis is valuable.

Inappropriately low (i.e. low or normal) TSH levels for low T3 or T4 levels suggest hypothalamic or pituitary disease. With acquired TSH deficiency, pituitary function and neuroradiological tests are necessary to identify other pituitary hormone deficiencies and exclude a pituitary tumor.

Treatment

The drug of choice is sodium-1-thyroxine (l-T4) – usually ~100 mcg/m²/24 h once daily but precisely adjusted individually. Catch-up growth usually follows onset of treatment and height prognosis is favorable in comparison with most growth disorders. However, it is important to interpret height velocity on treatment in the context of accurate assessment of rate of bone age maturation. Inappropriately rapid skeletal maturation for height velocity indicates overtreatment and will result irretrievably in stunting due to early epiphyseal fusion. IRMA TSH levels are sensitive markers of over-replacement, under-replacement or noncompliance (except in hypothalamo-pituitary disease).

There is still controversy about whether to treat euthyroid patients with compensated autoimmune hypothyroidism. Treatment does not alter the natural progression of the disease and chronic oversecretion of TRH/TSH is not generally associated with problems (although there are theoretical risks in children treated with radiotherapy for brain tumors), but enlarged pituitary fossa and secondary pituitary failure have been described. Often free T4 levels are low and treatment should certainly start if so or growth velocity is slow.

Outcome

Mental retardation does not occur in late onset hypothyroidism. School performance and growth improve on appropriate replacement therapy. Final height is normal for the family.

HYPERFUNCTION
Neonatal

Neonatal thyrotoxicosis is rare and usually due to transplacental passage of TSI from a mother with active or inactive Graves' disease or Hashimoto thyroiditis. High maternal antibody titers are strong predictors of neonatal disease in a clinically euthyroid mother whose disease has been inactive for many years. Only 1.5% of mothers with thyrotoxicosis due to Graves' disease will have affected babies. Thyrotoxicosis is nevertheless rare in pregnancy – autoimmune disease tends to remit during pregnancy and anovulatory cycles are common in thyrotoxic women.

Goiter may be present at birth and an irritable infant rapidly develops tachycardia, dysrhythmias, flushing, hypertension and weight loss (until cardiac failure supervenes) despite ravenous hunger. There may be associated jaundice, hepatosplenomegaly and a bleeding tendency due to thrombocytopenia and low prothrombin levels. In some, symptoms and signs are delayed for 7–10 days either because of transplacental passage of maternal antithyroid drugs or postnatal T4 to T3 conversion.

Total and free T4 and T3 levels are high and TSH suppressed within a few days – cord blood levels may be normal. The half-life of TSI is 2–3 weeks and clinical resolution of the disorder mirrors their degradation – the condition is generally self-limiting over 4–12 weeks. In severely affected babies, mortality may be as high as 25% due to cardiac arrhythmias or high output failure. Propranolol (1–2 mg/kg/24 h) with carbimazole (0.5–1 mg/kg/24 h) and Lugol's iodine (5% iodine, 10% potassium iodide, 8 mg tds) to inhibit thyroid hormone synthesis and secretion may be life saving. Satisfactory response is usually seen within 24–36 h. As thyrotoxicosis comes under control, iodine and propranolol can be gradually withdrawn and carbimazole gradually discontinued from about 6 weeks. Rarely, persisting hyperthyroidism suggests early onset Graves' disease.

Graves' disease

In children, thyrotoxicosis is nearly always due to Graves' disease, is much rarer than hypothyroidism and rarer than in adults – only about 5% of patients with Graves' disease present in childhood or adolescence, usually in the second decade. It is 3–5-fold more common in girls. As in Hashimoto thyroiditis, there is evidence of an autoimmune disorder on a background of genetic (HLA A1, B8, DR3) predisposition and positive family history of thyroid disease in about 60%.

The thyrotoxicosis is due to thyroid follicular cell TSH receptor IgG antibodies – thyroid stimulating immunoglobulins (TSI) – which bind to the extracellular receptor domain stimulating thyroid hormone release analogously to TSH via the adenyl cyclase cAMP system. They do not cause the eye signs although these too are immunologically mediated.

The TSH receptor is a 744 amino acid, single chain, polypeptide glycoprotein member of the guanine-nucleotide binding (G) protein-coupled receptor family and represents the primary target antigen for autoantibodies mediating the hyperthyroidism and goiter of Graves' disease. Glycosylation is necessary for receptor expression and hormone – receptor interactions.

Clinical features

The onset may be insidious and is usually well established before presentation to a physician. As in hypothyroidism, poor school performance may be marked, but usually from poor concentration, tiredness and behavior disturbances with temper tantrums and emotional lability. There is marked weight loss despite rapid growth and enormous appetite. The gland is usually diffusely enlarged and often with a bruit. Many systemic (tachycardia, tremor and sweating) and eye (staring due to lid retraction, wide palpebral aperture and lid lag) signs reflect sympathetic overactivity. Periorbital puffiness, exophthalmos, chemosis and squint due to infiltration of the orbit, lacrimal glands and ocular muscles occur less commonly and severely than in adults, but exophthalmos in particular may persist once euthyroidism is established. Pretibial myxedema characteristic of adults is rare in children.

Diagnosis

In children, a clinical diagnosis can usually be made confidently, but there must be biochemical confirmation and hyperthyroidism secondary to TSH hypersecretion must be excluded. Usually free and total T4 levels are high (occasionally they are normal but T3 levels are raised) and TSH is suppressed even using a sensitive (IRMA) assay. TSI are positive. Skeletal maturity is generally advanced disproportionately for the rapid growth.

Treatment

Treatment aims to reduce excessive thyroid hormone secretion and blunt the somatic consequences (largely mediated via beta-adrenergic pathways). The former may be achieved with antithyroid drugs (e.g. carbimazole or propylthiouracil), surgery (subtotal thyroidectomy) or radioactive iodine (^{131}I). In childhood, in most centers, antithyroid drugs are the initial treatment of choice. These inhibit diiodotyrosine and iodothyronine formation and, to some extent, tyrosine iodination. Thyroid function normalizes by 3–4 weeks. The initial dose of carbimazole in childhood is 0.5 mg/kg/24 h and of propylthiouracil 5 mg/kg/24 h, both in three divided doses.

Skin rashes occur in 2–3% on either drug but are usually transient and a change of therapy is not usually necessary, particularly if antihistamine is used symptomatically. More seriously, agranulocytosis may occur idiosyncratically, unpredicted from serial blood counts. Full recovery usually occurs on stopping treatment and the alternative generally substituted as cross-reactivity is rare. Progressive neutropenia can also occur: symptoms such as sore throat must be taken seriously and blood count checked regularly.

Once clinical and biochemical euthyroidism is achieved, it is probably beneficial (in terms of reducing both the goiter and necessity for frequent monitoring of thyroid function for developing hypothyroidism) to add l-thyroxine to an appropriate (usually half to one third of initial dose) antithyroid medication. Combination therapy has also been reported to decrease production of TSI and the frequency of thyrotoxicosis recurrence in adults.

Although antithyroid drugs do not alter the natural disease process, they do, in most children, allow maintenance of euthyroidism until spontaneous remission occurs (usually after about 2 years). Signs that this is not the case include persisting goiter and continuing presence of TSI. In any case there is a high relapse rate (50–70% within 2 years).

Beta-blockers (e.g. propranolol) are valuable during the first 2–3 weeks of treatment in providing symptomatic relief of tachycardia, nervousness and tremor and can then be discontinued as the specific antithyroid drug becomes clinically effective.

Subtotal thyroidectomy may be the treatment of choice in young adults in whom hyperthyroidism has returned after > 2 years of medical treatment or if compliance with treatment is poor – and, because of high relapse rates on medical treatment, is the primary treatment of choice in some centers with a surgeon experienced in thyroid surgery. Patients must be made euthyroid before surgery, in which case morbidity and mortality are comparable to other major procedures. Specific complications include laryngeal nerve palsy (transient or permanent), transient hypocalcemia (~10%) and permanent hypoparathyroidism (~1%). One year post surgery, 80% are euthyroid, 15% have permanent hypothyroidism (easily treated with thyroxine) and 5% are still thyrotoxic. Either thyrotoxicosis or hypothyroidism may develop many years after surgery in a previously euthyroid patient.

Radioactive iodine (^{131}I iodide) is the treatment of choice if judged by ease of administration, efficacy, short term safety and cost.[269] UK use has traditionally been restricted to adults > 40 years because of fears (based on few data) that risks of congenital malformations in subsequent pregnancies are increased or, if used in younger patients, leukemia or thyroid cancer could result – radiation is indeed an important cause of thyroid cancer in children[270] as the short-lived radioactive fallout caused by the 1986 Chernobyl nuclear power plant accident demonstrated.[271] However the evidence suggests that treating young people, including pediatric patients, with radioiodine is effective and safe in the long term (> 30 years follow-up).[272] A lower age cut-off of 17 years is still recommended in the USA.[273]

Generally, use in UK pediatric practice has been restricted to poorly compliant adolescents who cannot be rendered euthyroid for surgery, but with increasing long term experience practice may change. There is a high incidence of hypothyroidism (25% in the first year, a subsequent annual rate of 24% and an incidence of 80% by 15 years post treatment).

Hashimoto thyroiditis

About 5–10% of children with Hashimoto thyroiditis present with hyperthyroidism, particularly in adolescence. Occasionally Graves' disease and Hashimoto thyroiditis coexist: there are clinical and laboratory features of the latter with TSI antibodies present. Treatment is as for Graves' disease.

TSH hypersecretion

This is a rare cause of thyrotoxicosis, described either with a pituitary TSH-secreting tumor or a defect in TSH feedback inhibition by T3 causing goitrous hyperthyroidism associated with high TSH levels – an indication for neuroradiological evaluation.

Autonomous functioning nodules

These are uncommon in children and adolescents, usually occurring after ~35 years. Occasionally, single nodules of follicular adenoma (diameter > 3 mm) are found in association with thyrotoxicosis. Diagnosis is by isotope scanning. Carcinoma occurs in less than 1% of functional nodules (see below).

NEOPLASIA (Table 15.14)

A history of head and neck irradiation was common in children presenting with thyroid neoplasia and the latter is common following

Table 15.14 Types of thyroid neoplasia

Follicular (epithelial) tumors
  Follicular adenoma
  Follicular carcinoma
  Papillary carcinoma
  Anaplastic carcinoma

Nonfollicular tumors
  Medullary carcinoma
  Lymphoma
  Teratoma
  Miscellaneous

Chernobyl[271] – see above. Palpable thyroid nodules must be taken seriously – the prevalence of malignancy in childhood thyroid nodules is probably less than 15–20% but still higher than in adults.

Thyroid neoplasia may arise from follicular epithelium (follicular adenoma and carcinoma, papillary carcinoma, anaplastic carcinoma) or other tissue (medullary carcinoma, lymphoma, teratoma, metastatic tumor). More than 50% of solitary thyroid nodules in childhood are cystic lesions or benign adenomas. Hyperfunctioning adenomas are rare and 90% of malignant nodules consist of well-differentiated follicular carcinomas. In this group, prognosis is better than for rarer types.

Features suggestive of malignancy include history of head and neck irradiation, a hard or rapidly enlarging nodule, lymphadenopathy, hoarseness, dysphagia or metastases. Nodules in Hashimoto thyroiditis rarely represent carcinomatous change. In other situations, radioisotope and ultrasound scanning are valuable for differential diagnosis. Ultrasound identifies cystic lesions (usually benign); if iodide is concentrated by the nodule(s), carcinoma is rare. Small needle aspiration biopsy[274] may aid further diagnosis of cystic lesions and distinguish benign from malignant lesions.

Treatment (where possible following needle biopsy histology) is surgical removal of the affected thyroid lobe and subsequent total thyroidectomy if frozen sections reveal malignancy. Radioiodine treatment postoperatively is reserved for metastatic disease or distant lymph node involvement. Prognosis is excellent even with metastatic well-differentiated follicular carcinoma. TSH must be fully suppressed chronically by adequate thyroxine therapy so as not to stimulate tumor growth or regrowth. Life expectancy is normal with follicular carcinoma but not with rarer carcinomas despite radical surgery, radiotherapy and chemotherapy.

An important rare thyroid carcinoma [medullary thyroid carcinoma (MTC), accounting for < 10% of thyroid carcinomas] arises from parafollicular (C) cells and nearly always secretes calcitonin and sometimes other hormones (e.g. ACTH, serotonin, prostaglandins). Although often sporadic, they are associated with syndromes involving tumors of neuroectodermal origin (multiple endocrine neoplasia – MEN) inherited autosomal dominantly. MEN type 2 (MEN 2) comprises three syndromes: medullary thyroid carcinoma alone (familial MTC); MTC, pheochromocytoma and hyperparathyroidism (MEN 2A); and MTC, pheochromocytoma, ganglioneuromatosis and a Marfanoid habitus (MEN 2B). (MEN 1 comprises hyperparathyroidism, pancreatic islet cell tumors and pituitary adenomas.)

These familial endocrine neoplasia syndromes (MEN 1, MEN 2 and von Hippel–Lindau) can now be diagnosed genetically in childhood. The MEN 1 gene is on chromosome 11, the MEN 2 gene on chromosome 10, and children with a mutation and all offspring of affected subjects where the mutation is unknown should be screened on a regular basis (for protocols, see Johnston et al[275] and Brandi et al[276]).

The aggressive nature of the thyroid lesion, which may develop in childhood or adult life (usually before pheochromocytoma), has led to a search for markers of its presence whilst still microscopic. Calcitonin levels are usually normal at this stage but may rise significantly following pentagastrin infusion. Previously, annual stimulation tests provided the best monitor in affected children – rising levels with time as well as raised absolute values may be suspicious.[275]

In a family with MEN 2 cases, a predisposing RET proto-oncogene abnormality on chromosome 10 indicates whether a child (at 50% risk) has inherited the condition and will guide the timing of prophylactic thyroidectomy to prevent progression to thyroid carcinoma and lymph node metastases. Codon-specific timing of thyroidectomy may be indicated, with some (e.g. with codon 634 mutations) needing surgery well before 5 years of age.[277]

MEN 1 is caused by germline mutations of a tumor suppressor gene MEN1 at 11q13 coding a protein, menin, which is involved in the regulation of gene expression at the level of transcription and important for maintaining TGF-beta signaling.[278]

Prophylactic thyroidectomy may be justified – therapy (as well as diagnostic) consensus guidelines for MEN 2 (and MEN 1) are available.[276]

PARATHYROID GLANDS AND CALCIUM METABOLISM

There are two pairs of parathyroid glands, superior and inferior, although two, five or six glands may be present in normal individuals. Paradoxically, the inferior pair originates (at ~ 5 weeks) from the 3rd pharyngeal pouch (endodermal) tissue, the superior pair from the 4th pouch. The inferior pair are pulled medially and caudally by the migrating thymus to the thyroid; the superior attach higher on its dorsal surface. There are two cell types: chief cells secreting parathyroid hormone (PTH) and oxyphil cells (function unknown).

Although the major function is contributing to calcium and phosphate homeostasis by PTH production, the role of the parathyroid in health and disease must be considered in conjunction with other hormones and metabolic factors.

PHYSIOLOGY OF CALCIUM HOMEOSTASIS

Calcium must be accumulated by a growing child – 99% of total body calcium is present in the skeleton. Nevertheless, as well as for bone mineralization, calcium is important for normal endocrine and neuromuscular function at plasma membrane level, enzymatic reactions and blood coagulation, so that the 1% in extra- and intracellular fluids must be closely regulated within narrow concentration limits. Thus homeostatic control mechanisms are inevitably complex. Serum calcium concentration is maintained within normal limits by the interaction of vitamin D, PTH and calcitonin acting at three target tissues: bone, kidneys and gastrointestinal tract. Unlike calcium, normal serum inorganic phosphate levels are age related during childhood (declining from high levels in infancy).

Calcium is present in serum in three fractions in dynamic equilibrium: 50% ionized (metabolically active), 40% protein bound (inactive), the remainder complexed to phosphate, citrate, etc. The proportion of ionized calcium is controlled by vitamin D, PTH and calcitonin but is affected by acid–base changes (acidosis increases and alkalosis decreases ionized calcium levels as hydrogen ions compete with calcium for albumin binding sites). Vitamin D itself is biologically inactive and must be hydroxylated to active metabolites.

Total serum calcium is measured routinely – ionized levels may be measured directly using ion-selective electrodes. Indirect estimation of biologically active calcium using a formula may be misleading if serum protein concentrations are low. In hypoproteinemic states total calcium may be low but ionized calcium normal. Diet and diurnal variation will influence many indices of mineral and bone metabolism.

Although hypo- or hypercalcemia may be associated with disorders of vitamin D metabolism or parathyroid disease, non-endocrine disorders (e.g. chronic renal failure) may be etiologically important. Specific disorders of mineral and bone metabolism occur in infants, occasionally secondarily to maternal hyperparathyroidism.

Peak bone mass accumulation and mineralization occurs during puberty, continues into early adult life and is influenced by genetic (racial) factors, body mass, adequate calcium intake during growth and physical activity. A current recommendation for dietary calcium intake in children between 9 and 18 years so as to maximize peak bone mass and minimize fracture risk and osteoporosis in later life is 1300 mg per day.[279] Peak calcium accretion is attained at 12.5 years in girls and 14 years in boys. Only around 10% of adolescent girls in the USA achieve the recommended intake but separate supplementation has been reported to lower the age of menarche[280] which may have an adverse effect on bone mineral accretion overall.

Reduced peak bone mass occurs in GH deficiency, GT deficiency, male hypogonadism, Turner syndrome and delayed puberty. Bone mass is also reduced by malnutrition, chronic illness and anorexia nervosa. Appropriate management of these conditions will reduce risks of clinically significant osteoporosis from middle age.

CALCIUM REGULATION IN THE FETUS AND NEONATE

Normal fetal bone mineralization requires considerable net calcium and phosphorus transfer from mother to fetus. There is active placental transport of calcium and some 80% of the total accumulates in the third trimester. Fetal blood total and ionized calcium levels exceed those in the mother by about 0.5 and 0.25 mmol/L respectively and absolute values have doubled from mid-gestation to a mean of 2.75 mmol/L at term.

PTH and calcitonin do not cross the placenta but it is not clear whether active vitamin D metabolites do. Both fetal kidney and placenta can synthesize the active metabolite 1,25-dihydroxy vitamin D. Although their importance compared with that of the maternal kidney is uncertain, it seems likely that that fetal 1,25-dihydroxy D is the major stimulus to placental calcium transfer, perhaps analogously to its effect on intestinal calcium absorption.

To accommodate fetal transfer, there is increased maternal intestinal calcium absorption – calcium loss to the fetus stimulates maternal PTH secretion and maternal 1,25-dihydroxy vitamin D levels are raised. In the fetus, conversely, PTH levels are suppressed and calcitonin levels high encouraging bone mineralization.

At birth, cessation of transplacental calcium and these hormonal changes cause significant lowering of serum calcium. Lowest levels are reached, in the term neonate, between 24 and 48 h after birth; by 5 days rising PTH and falling calcitonin levels have established 'normal' serum calcium levels. Intestinal absorption of calcium and phosphate (very low in the fetus) is, suddenly, the sole mechanism and source – 1,25-dihydroxy vitamin D_3 secretion increases sharply.

As with other physiological changes from fetal to extrauterine life (e.g. circulatory, respiratory, bilirubin metabolism), these complex adaptations lead potentially to a variety of neonatal disorders, especially in the preterm.

Vitamin D

Vitamin D (calciferol) is a collective term for two steroid-related, cholesterol-derived naturally occurring compounds, vitamin D_2 (ergocalciferol) – derived from the plant sterol ergosterol, and vitamin D_3 (cholecalciferol) – produced in skin by the effect of ultraviolet irradiation on a precursor (7-dehydrocholesterol) in the epidermal Malpighian layer (Fig. 15.49). In man D_2 and D_3 are equally active biologically. Serum D_3 levels are higher in summer than winter (reflecting differences in sunlight exposure). Pigmented skin synthesizes it less efficiently.

Plant and animal foods (e.g. fish, eggs, butter and margarine) are important sources of D_2 and D_3 respectively. Absorption is via upper small intestine and lymphatic system in chylomicrons. Normal bile salt secretion is necessary – absorption is impaired by steatorrhea. In blood, ~98% is bound to a high MW liver-derived protein which also transports and binds active vitamin D metabolites and acts as a buffer against vitamin D toxicity.

The first step in vitamin D activation (Fig. 15.49) is 25-hydroxylation in liver microsomes but bowel and kidney may contribute. 25-Hydroxy D is the major circulating metabolite but is metabolically inactive and converted in mitochondria of the proximal renal tubule to two major metabolites, proportions depending on physiological requirements: active 1,25-dihydroxy D and 24,25-dihydroxy D (some, but much less, biological activity). Other metabolites of uncertain pathophysiological significance and with varying biological activities can be formed. Placenta and bone can also hydroxylate at C1.

1,25-dihydroxy D has major effects on intestinal villus and crypt cells, osteoblasts and osteoclasts and distal renal tubular cells. The net effect is to increase serum calcium and phosphate by stimulating intestinal absorption and mobilization from bone, and reducing renal excretion. Calcium mobilization from bone is also PTH dependent.

Average total serum concentrations of 1,25-dihydroxy D are 1000-fold lower than those of 25-hydroxy D but there is only a 10-fold difference in relative concentrations of the free (metabolically active in the case of 1,25-dihydroxy D) components.

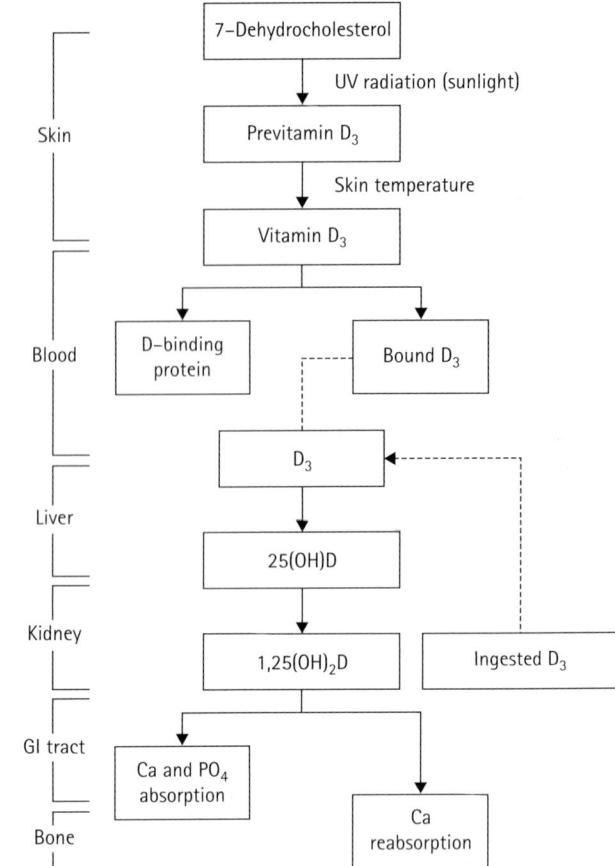

Fig. 15.49 Vitamin D metabolism and its regulation.

Parathyroid hormone (PTH)

PTH is an 84 amino acid peptide, MW 9500; 34 amino acids at the amino- (N-) terminal are essential for receptor binding and activation and thus biological activity. The PTH gene is close to the insulin gene on the short arm of chromosome 11. PTH is synthesized by parathyroid chief cells and cleaved from higher molecular weight biologically inactive precursors which are not released into the circulation. Both intact PTH and carboxy- (C-) terminal fragments are released into the circulation and the proportion of the latter is increased in primary hyperparathyroidism. Intact PTH is metabolized by liver (predominantly) and kidney and fragments returned to the circulation. Intact PTH and N-terminal fragments are cleared rapidly (< 10 min); C-terminal fragments (mainly metabolized by kidney) are cleared more slowly (2 h). Thus circulating PTH is a heterogeneous mixture of intact hormone together with N-, C-terminal and intermediate fragments.

Serum calcium concentration is the major regulator of PTH synthesis and release. There is a greater response to evolving hypocalcemia than to falling levels within the normal range. Hypercalcemia suppresses PTH secretion. Catecholamines, vitamin D metabolites and cortisol increase PTH secretion but their physiological function is doubtful.

The major role of PTH is prevention of hypocalcemia by three main mechanisms: calcium resorption from bone, renal calcium reabsorption and, indirectly, increasing intestinal calcium absorption by stimulating renal 1,25-dihydroxy D synthesis.

In bone, PTH regulates the movement of calcium between lacunar osteocytes and extracellular fluid, and influences remodeling. Osteoblasts (not osteoclasts) have PTH receptors and it is presumably release of an osteoblast factor which promotes osteoclast activation. A factor of MW 500–1000 has been postulated. PTH has several effects on renal tubules, acting distally to promote calcium and inhibit phosphate and bicarbonate reabsorption and proximally to stimulate hydroxylation at C1 to form 1,25-dihydroxy D.

Heterogeneity of circulating PTH forms makes measurement difficult. There is cross reactivity of RIAs against the intact molecule, the N- and C-terminal and the intermediate region. Because serum half-lives of intact PTH and N-terminal fragments are shorter than those of the C-terminal or intermediate fragments, the latter account for 80% of immunoreactive material measured and better reflect PTH secretion rates. Except in chronic renal failure (where C-terminal and intermediate fragments accumulate because of impaired glomerular filtration), assays specific for C-terminal or intermediate fragment PTH provide better discrimination between normal and raised PTH levels. Some PTH RIAs (and bioassays) are too insensitive to distinguish between normality and hyposecretion.

There is diurnal circadian variation in serum PTH secretion with higher values in early morning. For correct interpretation, simultaneous serum calcium and phosphate concentrations should be measured. Renal phosphate reabsorption and urinary cyclic adenosine monophosphate (cAMP) may need assessment. The ratio of tubular maximal rate of phosphate reabsorption to glomerular filtration rate is calculated from simultaneous fasting serum and urinary phosphate and creatinine concentrations and reference to nomograms – ratios are high in hypoparathyroidism and low in hyperparathyroidism. cAMP is important in PTH release into the circulation in response to hypocalcemia; measurement is useful for indirectly assessing circulating active PTH, evaluating the renal response to exogenous PTH and distinguishing pseudohypo- from hypoparathyroidism.

Calcitonin

Calcitonin is synthesized in and secreted by thyroid parafollicular (C) cells of neuroectodermal origin. It is discussed here because of its importance in calcium metabolism.

As for insulin and PTH, the gene encoding calcitonin is on the short arm of chromosome 11. Calcitonin is a 32 amino acid peptide, MW 3500, derived from a polypeptide precursor by loss of N- and C-terminal fragments. Species differences derive from mid-molecule amino acid sequences. The entire sequence is required for biological activity. Calcitonin-like bioactive material has been identified in thymus, lung, adrenal medulla, brain and parathyroid glands but none are major sources of circulating calcitonin.

As with PTH, serum calcium concentration is the major regulator of calcitonin secretion but with opposite effect: hypercalcemia stimulates and hypocalcemia suppresses calcitonin secretion. Gastrointestinal hormones such as gastrin, glucagon and cholecystokinin stimulate calcitonin secretion as do estrogens, beta-adrenergic agonists and 1,25-dihydroxy D, but none seem physiologically important. Pentagastrin (a synthetic gastrin derivative) is used to stimulate calcitonin secretion in the diagnosis of medullary thyroid carcinoma.

More sensitive assays are helping to define calcitonin changes with age and deficiency states. In children, monomeric calcitonin (the major active circulating form) is present in very low concentrations – levels are higher in infancy.

Like PTH, calcitonin influences serum calcium levels by action on bone, kidneys and bowel. It inhibits bone resorption by reducing osteoclast cytoplasmic motility. In kidney it binds to specific receptors to increase calcium, phosphate, magnesium, sodium and potassium excretion and stimulates 1-hydroxylation in the proximal tubule to produce 1,25-dihydroxy D. This promotes intestinal calcium reabsorption indirectly but it may also have a direct, but inhibitory, effect.

The importance of calcitonin for physiological calcium metabolism regulation remains uncertain. Neither thyroidectomy nor calcitonin hypersecretion from medullary thyroid carcinoma affects serum calcium levels. Its major inhibitory effect on bone resorption is directly antagonistic to PTH and 1,25-dihydroxy D and its role in that context may be prevention of excessive resorption. It is secreted in response to eating calcium-rich food secondarily to secretion of various gastrointestinal and pancreatic hormones which itself inhibits. The net effect is delayed calcium absorption which may be important in preventing postprandial hypercalcemia and hypercalciuria.

A major physiological role may be in situations (fetal life, infancy, pregnancy and lactation) with extra needs for calcium and when calcitonin and 1,25-dihydroxy D levels are high – calcitonin may prevent unwanted bone resorption whilst allowing the stimulatory effect of vitamin D on intestinal calcium absorption.

DISORDERS OF CALCIUM AND BONE METABOLISM

Metabolic and hormonal interactions in many of these disorders are complex.

Advances in understanding the molecular pathogeneses of disorders of calcium, vitamin D and bone, including the roles of the extracellular calcium sensor, the vitamin D receptor, and new factors for bone cell embryogenesis and function, are reviewed by Langman.[281]

Significant diagnostic pointers can be obtained from a full history (including family history) and specific abnormalities found on examination. To minimize effects of food and diurnal changes, blood is ideally taken in the fasting state in the morning and, when possible, without compression of the arm (venous stasis also influences calcium levels).

The important basic laboratory measurements are of serum calcium (Ca), phosphate (P) and alkaline phosphatase (ALP) which should be interpreted in the context of simultaneously estimated serum total protein and albumin, electrolytes, creatinine, magnesium and pH. Urine measurements (early morning or 24 h collections) of calcium, phosphate, creatinine and hydroxyproline (a measure of bone turnover) may be valuable. If significant abnormalities are found, more complex investigations can be instigated assessing aspects of parathyroid function, vitamin D metabolism and bone turnover as indicated.

INFANCY

See also Ch. 12.
1. Hypocalcemia: early and late neonatal hypocalcemia
2. Hypercalcemia
   a. Idiopathic infantile hypercalcemia (see below)
   b. Familial hypocalciuric hypercalcemia (see below)
   c. Neonatal primary hyperparathyroidism
   d. Hypervitaminosis D (see below)
   e. Other associations: fat necrosis; phosphate deficiency
3. Metabolic bone disease in the preterm infant.

ABNORMAL 1,25–DIHYDROXY VITAMIN D SECRETION OR ACTION

Increased intake (hypervitaminosis D)

Vitamin D intoxication usually results from excessive treatment of hypoparathyroidism, rickets, renal osteodystrophy, etc. with concentrated preparations – it is available in proprietary multivitamin preparations without prescription in many countries and may also be prescribed inappropriately. 'Stoss therapy' – administration of 600 000 units for the prevention of rickets – is not now used but was formerly a cause. Toxicity may persist for many weeks because of adipose tissue storage. Despite its potency, an advantage of the synthetic analogue of 1,25-dihydroxy D (1alpha-hydroxy D) is its short half-life with more rapid return to normocalcemia after inadvertent overdose.

Clinical signs reflect hypercalcemia from excessive intestinal calcium absorption and bone resorption. Initially, there is nausea and vomiting with anorexia, constipation and polyuria. Infants fail to thrive and become irritable. Ultimately, there may be nephrocalcinosis with renal insufficiency and ectopic calcification. Investigation confirms hypercalcemia with hypercalciuria: serum PTH will be suppressed – normal or elevated PTH with hypercalcemia indicates hyperparathyroidism.

Treatment is by withdrawing the vitamin D preparation and calcium supplements (if any), saline infusion and furosemide (to increase urinary calcium loss) and glucocorticoids (e.g. hydrocortisone 4 mg/kg/24 h 6 hourly) which gradually reduces intestinal calcium absorption.

Idiopathic hypercalcemia of infancy was though to be due to excessive vitamin D administration. This is unlikely to be the case, although it remains a heterogeneous and poorly understood condition. The fall in incidence of the mild form observed in the UK preceded the reduction in vitamin D supplementation of artificial infant feeds. Incidence of the severe form often associated with mental retardation, cardiovascular abnormalities (supravalvar aortic stenosis or peripheral pulmonary stenosis) and facial and other dysmorphic features has not changed. The mild form is now rarely seen. The severe form (Williams syndrome – see Ch.14, p. 390) may be due to a defect in calcitonin synthesis or release resulting from a neural crest developmental anomaly affecting face, heart and thyroid C-cell (calcitonin-producing) precursors which would explain the variable relationship between somatic developmental abnormalities and degree of calcium homeostatic disturbance (calcium levels may be normal). The molecular genetic defect in Williams syndrome is a deletion of the elastin gene and other contiguous genes at 7q11.23.

Increased synthesis

Hypercalcemia from raised 1,25-dihydroxy D levels (with suppressed PTH) is seen in granulomatous disease (sarcoidosis, tuberculosis, etc.) due to conversion of 25-hydroxy D into the active metabolite by 1-hydroxylation in granulomatous cells. Similar findings in some patients with lymphoma are unusual – most patients with hypercalcemia due to malignant disease have low 1,25-dihydroxy D levels and reduced intestinal calcium absorption, and other mechanisms are presumably involved.

Increased secretion and/or responsiveness (absorptive hypercalciuria)

This specific type of 'idiopathic' hypercalciuria is thought to be due to a primary abnormality of secretion of, or responsiveness to, 1,25-dihydroxy D. It may be transmitted autosomal dominantly and cause renal stones or hematuria. A form secondary to a renal tubular defect is also found (see renal hypercalciuria below) and may share a common pathogenesis.

Decreased formation or action (calciopenic rickets)

Rickets (Table 15.15) is caused by defective growth plate mineralization and may be due to decreased calcium and phosphate availability in extracellular fluid at those sites (deficiency or malabsorption of vitamin D, defective formation or action of 1,25-dihydroxy D – calciopenic rickets; increased renal phosphate excretion or decreased intake – phosphopenic rickets). Phosphopenic rickets is usually due to renal phosphate loss (see below) but hypophosphatemia, commonly seen in low birth weight preterm infants, is due to inadequate phosphate intake – see also Chapters 12, 16 and 18.

Table 15.15   Classification of rickets

'Classical': lack of sunshine, diet deficient in vitamin D	Immigrants (pigmented skin); during rapid growth (infancy/puberty)
Malabsorption	Celiac disease; giardiasis; hepatobiliary disease (biliary atresia/fistula; cirrhosis; neonatal hepatitis)
Hereditary renal (mainly tubular)	Hypophosphatemic; vitamin D dependency; fibrous dysplasia/neurofibromatosis (with hypophosphatemia); Fanconi syndrome (including cystinosis, tyrosinemia, Lowe syndrome, Wilson disease); distal renal tubular acidosis
Acquired renal (mainly tubular)	Chronic renal failure (glomerular); hypophosphatemia; hypercalciuria

ABNORMAL PTH SECRETION OR ACTION

Increased secretion (primary hyperparathyroidism)

Increased PTH secretion may be a normal physiological compensatory response to hypocalcemia (secondary hyperparathyroidism). Primary hyperparathyroidism is due to abnormally increased secretion of PTH, is rare in childhood and uncommon even by adolescence with an overall prevalence of 25 per 100 000.

The etiology is unknown but cases may be sporadic (nearly always associated with a solitary adenoma, rarely with carcinoma) or familial (usually due to hyperplasia of all four glands). Familial cases may be isolated (autosomal dominant and recessive forms are reported), but may be associated with autosomal dominant multiple endocrine neoplasia syndromes: MEN 1 (see below) in association with pancreatic tumors or gastrinoma and pituitary adenomas; and MEN 2 with medullary thyroid carcinoma and pheochromocytoma, see p. 473. There is also an association with autosomal dominant hypocalciuric hypercalcemia syndrome where there is defective renal calcium excretion (see below).

Heterozygous germline mutations of the tumor suppressor gene MEN1 (on chromosome 11) are responsible for multiple endocrine neoplasia type 1 (MEN 1), a dominantly inherited familial cancer syndrome characterized by the combined occurrence of pituitary, parathyroid and enteropancreatic tumors.[282] It typically presents with clinical signs or symptoms in the middle decades of adult life but intractable peptic ulceration (Zollinger–Ellison syndrome due to a gastrin secreting pancreatic tumor) is reported by adolescence and raised gastrin and calcium levels may be found in asymptomatic family members by then. Hypercalcemia occurs in about 97% and the serial fasting serum calcium measurement is a valuable screening test. For a screening protocol see Johnston et al.[275]

The clinical spectrum of primary hyperparathyroidism ranges from asymptomatic to lethal. There may be fatigue, anorexia, constipation, polyuria, polydipsia, renal stones, bone pain and pathological fractures. Diagnosis depends on demonstration of inappropriately high PTH levels for hypercalcemia on three separate occasions. This is found otherwise only in familial hypocalciuric hypercalcemia (see below) where urinary calcium excretion is low for the hypercalcemia. Antibody against the C-terminal or intermediate PTH fragments is more sensitive to high PTH levels. Radiographically, there is usually generalized bone demineralization, osteolysis and subperiosteal bone resorption, especially of the phalanges and, occasionally, cysts.

Once diagnosis is secure, surgical parathyroid exploration by an experienced surgeon is necessary. Preoperative localization of the responsible gland is unreliable (although ultrasound may detect enlargement < 1 cm) – hyperplasia of all four is common. In this situation total parathyroidectomy with autotransplantation of tissue into the forearm is the treatment of choice. Other family members should be screened for hypercalcemia.

Decreased secretion (hypoparathyroidism – HP)

HP is much more common than hypersecretion but less common than decreased peripheral hormone action ['end-organ resistance' due to receptor or postreceptor abnormalities – pseudohypoparathyroidism (PHP)].

Cases may be sporadic or familial. Presentation can be in the neonate and may be transient, permanent (autosomal dominant, recessive, sex-linked recessive and sporadic forms have all been described) or part of DiGeorge syndrome – see Chapter 14, p. 390. Postneonatal onset may be idiopathic or occur secondarily to neck surgery, irradiation, hemosiderosis, hypomagnesemia, etc.

A familial (autosomal recessive) form may be associated with autoimmune disease affecting other endocrine glands (especially Addison disease) and mucocutaneous candidiasis [polyglandular autoimmune disease (PGAD) type 1] or autoimmune polyendocrinopathy – candidiasis – ectodermal dystrophy (APECED). Presentation is with severe candidiasis (due to a defect in cellular immunity) followed, successively, by HP and Addison disease (rarely before mid-childhood). Other autoimmune manifestations include alopecia, vitiligo, thyroiditis, chronic hepatitis and pernicious anemia. Parathyroid antibodies cause glandular destruction.

APECED results from loss-of-function mutations in the Aire gene which controls expression of self antigen in thymic epithelial cells and thus prevents autoimmunity.[283] Growth failure may result as the growth plate (particularly in early life) may be an additional target.

Clinical signs and symptoms of HP are from hypocalcemia due to decreased renal calcium reabsorption, bone resorption and, indirectly, decreased intestinal calcium absorption. Manifestations depend on age, severity and speed of onset and relate to the neuromuscular system (latent tetany – positive Chvostek and Trousseau signs; overt tetany – paresthesiae, muscle cramps, carpopedal spasm), brain (focal or grand mal convulsions, papilledema, basal ganglia calcification, eventual mental retardation), heart (prolonged QT interval), eyes (lenticular cataracts) and ectodermal changes (dry skin, coarse hair, brittle nails, tooth enamel hypoplasia).

Treatment aims to correct hypocalcemia and prevent recurrence (treatment of associated problems may also be indicated). A vitamin D preparation is currently the long term treatment of choice – PTH is expensive and must be given parenterally daily.

Acute hypocalcemia is treated with 10% calcium gluconate (9.4% calcium by weight) 1–2 ml/kg by slow i.v. injection repeated, as necessary, 6 hourly, or carefully and slowly infused (in dilute form). Oral calcium supplements (e.g. calcium gluconate) and a vitamin D analogue (e.g. 1alpha-hydroxy D 25–50 ng/kg/24 h) should be started and serum and urinary calcium levels checked 3 monthly. Vitamin D will not correct renal calcium loss – although there is reduced urinary calcium excretion, there is relative hypercalciuria due to deficient (PTH mediated) renal tubular calcium reabsorption and thus serum calcium levels should be maintained in low normal range to avoid nephrocalcinosis and renal stones. Treatment with a thiazide diuretic and sodium restriction may be necessary.

Decreased peripheral action (pseudohypoparathyroidism – PHP)

Uncommon causes of PTH-resistant HP include severe hypomagnesemia (which causes resistance to and decreased secretion of PTH) and calciopenic rickets (due to low 1,25-dihydroxy D levels). Receptor or postreceptor defects of response to PTH at the target organ (especially the renal tubule) are more common, first described by Albright – pseudohypoparathyroidism.[284] This heterogeneous condition has been divided into several types:

Type 1 (originally described by Albright)

There is often symptomatic hypocalcemia in mid-childhood on a background of variable mental retardation and characteristic (but inconstant) somatic features ('Albright's hereditary osteodystrophy', AHO) including short stature, obesity, round face, short neck (Fig. 15.4) and marked metacarpal and metatarsal shortening (especially 4th and 5th – see Fig. 15.6). There is no phosphaturic response to PTH administration and a blunted urinary cyclic AMP increase in comparison with both normals and patients with HP. This type has been further subdivided on the basis of decreased (type 1a) or normal (type 1b) amounts of a protein membrane component that couples the PTH receptor to the catalytic unit of the adenylate.

Type 2

In this rarer form,[285] the defect is thought to be due to an intracellular defect beyond cyclic AMP generation – cyclic AMP responses to PTH are normal but the phosphaturic response is defective.

These differences do not entirely explain the very variable clinical manifestations (see below). Some patients with somatic features show no renal resistance to PTH – pseudopseudohypoparathyroidism (pPHP). In some families, PHP type 1 and pPHP coexist and individuals may fluctuate between normo- and hypocalcemia.

PTH activates the adenylate cyclase system via the Gs alpha member of the 'G' protein family, a heterotrimeric guanine nucleotide binding protein. The gene encoding Gs alpha is GNAS1. The Gs alpha protein membrane component is deficient in PHP type 1a/pPHP.[286] Numerous GNAS1 mutations have been identified in PHP-1a and pPHP.[287] Patients with either disorder show skeletal and developmental defects (AHO). Owing to paternal imprinting with inactivation of the paternal allele, which may be tissue- or cell-specific, resistance toward PTH and, often, other hormones is only observed in patients with PHP-1a, i.e. the variable and tissue-specific hormone resistance observed in PHP 1a may result from tissue-specific imprinting of the GNAS1 gene.[1] Patients with PHP-1b show PTH-resistant hypocalcemia and hyperphosphatemia but no AHO. The abnormal regulation of mineral ion homeostasis, such as in PHP-1a/pPHP kindreds, is paternally imprinted. Recent linkage studies have mapped the genetic defect responsible for PHP-1b to chromosome 20q13.3, making it likely that mutations in distinct regions of the GNAS1 gene are the cause of at least three different forms of PHP.[288]

The G protein family mediates numerous transmembrane hormone and sensory transduction processes in eukaryotic cells including LH, GH and TSH synthesis and release.[1] Unsurprisingly, therefore, abnormalities of other peptide hormones, particularly thyroid and GT, have been described in these patients. It is likely that abnormalities of GH secretion also occur – the GRF/receptor complex on the somatotroph activates a similar coupling ('G') protein to stimulate adenylate cyclase and hence GH synthesis and release. Thus in PHP there could be a defect in GRF binding and/or activation of its regulatory protein similar to that postulated for the defect in PTH regulatory protein.

Although these individuals are a heterogeneous group, some grow better on GH treatment. Indeed GH deficiency as a consequence of GHRH resistance in the context of PHP-1a is consistent with Gs-alpha imprinting in the human pituitary.[289] Treatment of hypocalcemia in PHP is analogous to treatment in HP (see above).

ABNORMAL CALCITONIN SECRETION
Increased

Hypocalcemia is almost never a feature of calcitonin excess. High calcitonin levels are seen in *medullary thyroid carcinoma* (sporadic or in MEN 2, see p. 473) and a variety of nonthyroid tumors in adults but have not been described in children. Levels are high in the rare autosomal recessive condition pyknodysostosis and may be raised in pancreatitis. High levels, presumably due to a normal physiological response, are described in hypercalcemic states and renal insufficiency.

Decreased

A number of congenital and acquired hypocalcitoninemic conditions are described, including primary hypothyroidism or post-thyroidectomy, anticonvulsant treatment (phenytoin or primidone) and Williams syndrome (see Chapter 14, p. 390).

ABNORMALITIES OF PHOSPHATE EXCRETION
Increased

Phosphopenic rickets results from excessive urinary phosphate excretion with resulting hypophosphatemia (Table 15.15) and only rarely from inadequate intake (other than in the preterm infant – see above and Ch. 12). Familial forms of primary hypophosphatemia secondary to renal phosphate loss have been described including X-linked (dominant) hypophosphatemic rickets (Albright's vitamin D resistant rickets) and autosomal dominant and recessive forms. Phosphopenic rickets is a feature of Fanconi syndrome (sporadic or familial, idiopathic or secondary to a number of inborn metabolic errors); it has been described in rare (usually benign mesenchymal) tumors and is a feature of distal renal tubular acidosis (sporadic and familial).

Decreased

Decreased renal phosphate excretion is important in the pathogenesis of *renal osteodystrophy* – other factors such as altered vitamin D metabolism become increasingly important as renal failure worsens (see Ch. 18). *Tumor calcinosis* (deposition of calcium phosphate around large joints due to increased phosphate reabsorption) is rarely seen outside Africa and may be familial or sporadic.

ABNORMALITIES OF CALCIUM EXCRETION
Increased
Hypercalciuria may be associated with hypercalcemia (e.g. vitamin D intoxication, primary hyperparathyroidism), normocalcemia (e.g. distal renal tubular acidosis, following corticosteroid, furosemide or immobilization) or may be 'idiopathic'. Absorptive (see above) and renal forms (renal hypercalciuria) of this last group occur but may share a common pathogenesis.

Decreased (familial hypocalciuric 'benign' hypercalcemia)
There are inappropriately raised (normal or high) PTH levels with hypercalcemia (see above). Inheritance is autosomal dominant. Hypercalcemia results from increased tubular calcium reabsorption, but there are no consequent symptoms of chronic hypercalcemia. There is a presumed abnormal set point for calcium mediated PTH suppression but no abnormalities of vitamin D metabolism, calcitonin secretion or parathyroid histology have been found. Parathyroid surgery is ineffective and contraindicated.

PRACTICAL DIFFERENTIAL DIAGNOSIS
Rickets
Initial clinical assessment, characteristic radiographic changes and raised ALP, decreased P and normal (especially in phosphopenic rickets) or decreased Ca in serum usually make diagnosis straightforward. It is important to determine etiology (Table 15.15) and further tests will usually be necessary.

Normal PTH and cyclic AMP levels are characteristic of phosphopenic rickets (usually familial X-linked hypophosphatemic, but associated hypercalciuria suggests the rarer autosomal recessive type unless there is inadequate phosphate intake in, for example, the preterm infant). Tumor rickets should be considered in sporadic cases presenting in late childhood or adolescence. Renal function must be assessed to exclude primary renal causes such as chronic renal failure and Fanconi syndrome (which may be secondary to other inborn metabolic errors) and is characterized by glycosuria and aminoaciduria.

Secondary hyperparathyroidism (i.e. secondary to calcium malabsorption) with raised PTH levels suggests calciopenic rickets, usually due to lack of vitamin D or impaired synthesis or action of the active metabolite 1,25-dihydroxy D. Further differential diagnosis necessitates measurement of individual vitamin D metabolites: low levels of 25-hydroxy D are found in all acquired forms (nutritional, liver disease, malabsorption, anticonvulsants). If 25-hydroxy D levels are normal, low 1,25-dihydroxy D levels indicate vitamin D deficient rickets type 1 and high levels indicate end-organ resistance to its action (type 2).

Hypocalcemia
In the presence of normal total protein, albumin and magnesium levels and renal function, repeated fasting early morning hypocalcemia is interpreted in the context of serum phosphate levels. If these are high, HP or PHP is likely and can be differentiated on the basis of PTH and cyclic AMP measurements: in PHP, PTH levels are high and, in type 1 – the common form – there is blunted cyclic AMP response to PTH infusion; in HP, PTH levels are low and the cyclic AMP response is normal.

Low or normal serum phosphate levels suggest calciopenic rickets; elevated ALP and PTH levels will confirm the diagnosis, which should be further elucidated as above.

Hypercalcemia
Confirmed raised fasting early morning hypercalcemia on at least three occasions with normal renal function and serum protein and albumin levels is uncommon in childhood. Raised or even detectable PTH levels in the presence of hypercalcemia are inappropriate and indicate primary hyperparathyroidism. MEN syndromes (see p. 478) should be excluded and family members screened for hypercalcemia. Detectable PTH levels with hypercalcemia but hypocalciuria are characteristic of familial hypocalciuric hypercalcemia.

Suppressed PTH levels suggest vitamin D intoxication (most commonly), idiopathic infantile hypercalcemia, malignancy, sarcoidosis or Addison disease.

HP from PHP
Hypomagnesemia, because of its dual effect on PTH secretion and resistance to PTH action, may produce features of both HP and PHP – serum magnesium must be checked in hypocalcemia. Somatic features of Albright hereditary osteodystrophy (see above) and radiographic changes of hyperparathyroidism indicate PHP. In HP, PTH levels are inappropriately low for hypocalcemia; PTH levels are high in PHP. Deficient cyclic AMP generation after PTH infusion is characteristic of PHP. Measurement of plasma cyclic AMP has replaced the older tests which measured urinary cyclic AMP excretion.

OTHER THERAPIES – BISPHOSPHONATES
Bisphosphonates are synthetic analogues of inorganic pyrophosphate and have been used in adults to treat osteoporosis (mainly), but also Paget's disease, metastatic breast carcinoma and hypercalcemia. They are being used more extensively in pediatric practice, particularly for the treatment of osteogenesis imperfecta (reducing fracture risk), juvenile or glucocorticoid-induced osteoporosis and fibrous dysplasia despite a variable (and sometimes minimal) evidence base for their efficacy and concerns regarding their safety.[290,291] More data are needed before their role in these conditions can be established (see also Chapter 29).

THE ADRENAL GLANDS

The adrenal glands are formed from mesodermal and ectodermal components which form cortex and medulla respectively. During the fifth week, mesothelial cells migrate and proliferate to form large acidophilic cells which comprise the fetal cortex. These become surrounded by smaller cells which later make up the definitive cortex. Meanwhile, sympathetic neural crest neuroblasts invade the medial aspect of the fetal cortex forming the adrenal medulla rather than nerve processes and known as chromaffin cells.

For ontogeny of fetal adrenal steroidogenesis see p. 415. The neonatal adrenals are comparable in size to the kidneys. After birth, there is rapid atrophy of the fetal zone of the cortex and adrenal weight at birth is only regained by late puberty. The definitive cortex secretes glucocorticoids (GC) affecting carbohydrate metabolism, mineralocorticoids (MC) affecting electrolyte balance, and androgens (which are also estrogen precursors). The medulla secretes catecholamines (adrenaline and noradrenaline).

THE ADRENAL CORTEX
Morphology and steroidogenesis
The cortex comprises three histologically distinct zones but cells appear to migrate through them changing function as they do so. This has important implications for control of steroidogenesis. The outer (subcapsular) zone, the zona glomerulosa, consists of balls of small cells and overlies the radially arranged cord-like bundles of larger cells of the zona fasciculata. The innermost area, the zona reticularis, consists of a network of short cords with capillaries. It only gradually becomes a distinct zone from ~6 years and largely accounts for the pubertal adrenal size and weight spurt. In contrast, there is relatively little change in postnatal morphological glomerulosa and fasciculata appearances.

In tissue culture, fasciculata and reticularis cells differ functionally as well as histologically, preferentially synthesizing GC (cortisol) and androgens respectively. Dehydroepiandrosterone (DHA) is a marker of zona reticularis function. Increasing production of androgens by reticularis from about 5 or 6 years and peaking around 12 or 13 years – 'adrenarche' – is synchronous with morphological and functional reticularis development. Aldosterone, the main MC, is produced in the zona glomerulosa (but also in other organs including the CNS).[292]

Plasma measurements reflect one moment in time, but many steroids are released episodically in relation to circadian rhythms and to environmental stimuli, often in sudden bursts at intervals.

Cortisol is secreted intermittently in response to pulsatile ACTH release. Most secretory activity occurs during sleep but there are, on average, about nine episodes of cortisol secretion through a 24 h period in adults under basal conditions. The circadian diurnal cortisol rhythm results from maximal duration and number of ACTH secretory episodes between 3 a.m. and 8 a.m. Circadian cortisol rhythm is present by ~6 months and is abolished in Cushing syndrome.

ACTH binds to receptors on the adrenal cell membrane, activating adenylate cyclase (a calcium dependent step); cyclic AMP activates enzymes (mainly intracellular protein kinases) which stimulate hydrolysis of cholesterol esters. Steroidogenesis is initiated in mitochondria by cholesterol binding to a C27 side chain cleavage enzyme which starts its stepwise conversion to pregnenolone, a necessary step in biosynthesis of all three groups of adrenal cortical hormones.

There are acute and chronic responses to ACTH in terms of GC biosynthesis. In contrast, the glomerulosa only seems to produce aldosterone acutely – chronic ACTH stimulation is not generally associated with sustained hyperaldosteronism. ACTH is probably the most, and perhaps only, important adrenal androgen modulator. It is likely that changes in adrenal androgen production with age (cf. unchanging cortisol levels for surface area) result from ACTH-mediated intrinsic local vascular and morphological changes, and children with familial glucocorticoid deficiency demonstrate diminished adrenal androgen secretion implicating a significant role for ACTH, rather than a specific, unidentified, pituitary adrenal androgen stimulating hormone, in the induction of adrenarche.

Physiological ACTH levels regulate acute aldosterone fluctuations – ACTH is important in the pathogenesis of GC-suppressible hyperaldosteronism.[293,294] Although the primary control mechanism is the renin–angiotensin system, this ACTH role is important in managing salt losing CAH (p. 483).

GCs such as cortisol and corticosterone are fast feedback antagonists of ACTH secretion; other steroids [e.g. deoxycorticosterone (DOC), deoxycortisol (S) and synthetic GCs] show delayed feedback inhibition. The relative importance of these responses in normal physiological control of ACTH is unclear.

Simplified steroidogenic pathways are summarized in Figure 15.50. For the clinician, working knowledge of the pathways will aid understanding of physical and biochemical consequences of various types of congenital hyperplasia.

Approximately 70% of circulating cortisol is bound to a 52 000 molecular weight alpha-2 globulin, transcortin (corticosteroid binding globulin – CBG) and ~20% albumin bound. Aldosterone, other GCs and precursors are less strongly bound to CBG and synthetic steroids only weakly. CBG is synthesized in liver; levels are increased by estrogen and decreased in cirrhosis. Binding sites are saturated when total plasma cortisol levels exceed about 600 nmol/L; at normal concentrations very little free cortisol is in plasma or excreted in urine. Urinary free cortisol is thus a sensitive screening test for Cushing syndrome (p. 484). Cortisol plasma half-life is 60–90 min; that of aldosterone is only ~20 min because proportionately much less is protein bound. Important adrenal androgens include DHA and its sulfated form (DHAS) which is also synthesized by the gland. DHAS half-life is 10–20 h; DHA secretion is episodic and concurrent with cortisol. Aldosterone levels show marked circadian changes which follow cortisol but are significantly influenced by posture.

Normal values for individual steroids and urinary metabolites in infancy, childhood and puberty are available[295] based on cross-sectional and mixed longitudinal studies.

Urine sampling is atraumatic and 24 h collections are more likely than isolated plasma samples to reflect accurately overall steroid

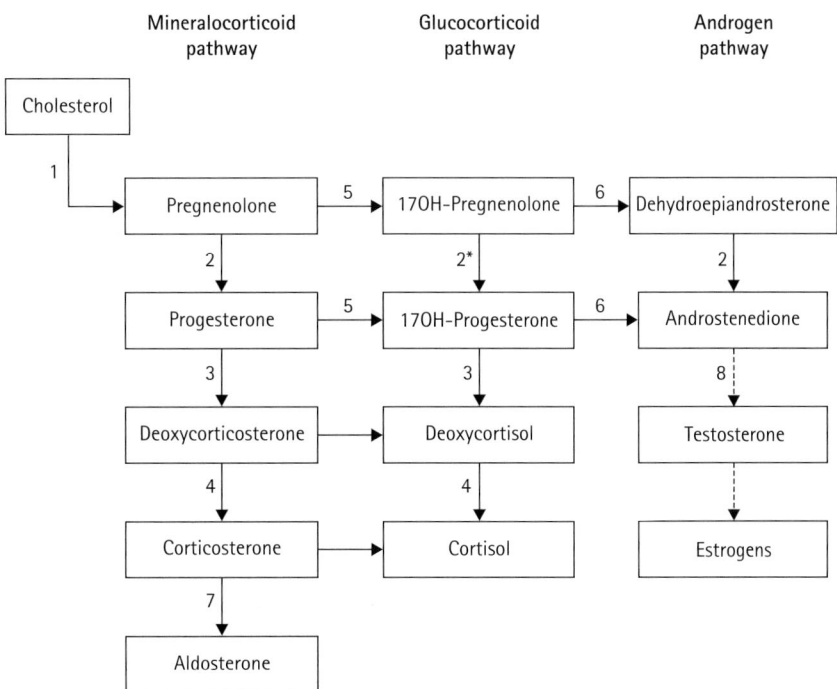

Fig. 15.50 Pathways of adrenal biosynthesis. 1 – cholesterol side chain cleaving system (20alpha-hydroxylase, 20,22-desmolase, 22alpha-hydroxylase); 2 – 3beta-hydroxysteroid dehydrogenase; 3 – 21-hydroxylase; 4 – 11beta-hydroxylase; 5 – 17alpha-hydroxylase; 6 – 17,20-lyase; 7 – 18-hydroxylase and 18-hydroxysteroid dehydrogenase; 8 – 17beta-hydroxysteroid dehydrogenase.

production. However, such collections may be difficult and unreliable in infants and young children. In general steroids are present in urine in about 1000 times their plasma concentrations. However, because of the complexity of metabolic pathways via which adrenal (and gonadal) steroids are excreted (and influences of disease or drugs) there can be uncertainty about clinical significance, relationship to gland of origin or even specific steroid from which they derive. Nevertheless, steroid profiles obtained by gas chromatography are valuable in complementing plasma steroid assays, e.g. studying normal children longitudinally to determine changes with age and the mechanism of adrenarche, detecting abnormal metabolites (e.g. secreted by tumors), metabolite ratios (e.g. in 5alpha-reductase deficiency), differential diagnosis of rarer or less clear-cut forms of CAH and differential diagnosis of salt losing states in infancy due to aldosterone biosynthetic defects.

Adrenarche

Adrenarche, the awakening of the adrenal cortex to produce adrenal androgens, commences from around the age of 6 years. During the early months of life the fetal zone rapidly atrophies so that high fetal and neonatal DHAS levels [reflecting low 3beta-hydroxysteroid dehydrogenase (3beta OHSD) fetal zone activity] fall and remain low for ~6 years. During mid-childhood adrenal androgen secretion rises steeply ('adrenarche') (Fig. 15.51) – coincident with zona reticularis development.

Adrenarche is important because of (1) its role in precocious sexual (pubic and axillary) hair development in mid-childhood; (2) possible relevance to triggering normal puberty, although underlying mechanisms and relationship to subsequent rises in GT and gonadal steroids at clinical puberty onset ('gonadarche') are controversial; (3) the association between premature adrenarche and subsequent functional ovarian hyperandrogenism, polycystic ovarian syndrome, and insulin resistance in later life ('syndrome X') but which may present by childhood or adolescence, and an association with previous intrauterine growth retardation; (4) potential etiological relevance to concomitant steep rise in normal blood pressure (BP) centiles and the mid-childhood growth spurt.

The adrenal androgen rise is not accompanied by significant increases in intermediate metabolites in cortisol or corticosterone biosynthesis for body surface area.

In some children, predominantly girls, the rise manifests as appearance of pubic, and sometimes axillary, hair ('premature pubarche'). These children probably represent one end of a spectrum of adrenal androgen secretion or perhaps of sensitivity to its action as plasma levels are not always high for age. It must be distinguished from nonclassical, late onset or missed CAH and (rare) adrenal tumors (in which, in contrast, androgens are not dexamethasone suppressible) as well as from true precocious puberty. In one clinic, a 30% incidence of nonclassical 21-hydroxylase deficiency was found

in those presenting with premature pubarche.[297] Although premature pubarche per se is probably physiological and has no adverse effect on the onset and progression of gonadarche and final height (puberty timing is normal or slightly early), hirsutism or polycystic ovarian disease may develop at puberty. Thus 'exaggerated' adrenarche can be a forerunner of syndrome X in some children (see above – Ibanez et al[32]). The association of these endocrine – metabolic abnormalities with reduced fetal growth and their genetic basis remain to be elucidated.[32]

The role of adrenarche in man remains controversial – it is difficult to extrapolate from pathological situations to normal gonadarche control. Adrenarche may be delayed in children with CDGP and isolated GH deficiency but not in hypergonadotrophic hypogonadism (e.g. Turner syndrome). Children with Addison disease enter puberty normally and in diabetic adolescents gonadarche may proceed normally despite delayed adrenarche. Children with congenital adrenal hypoplasia all have hypogonadotrophic hypogonadism and do not enter puberty normally.

Adrenarche is coincident with the preadolescent fat spurt and with the (disputed) mid-childhood growth spurt. The latter could reflect a bone and muscle response to adrenal androgens, directly or indirectly by influencing GH secretion.

Adrenarche could simply be a by-product of the need of inner fetal adrenal cells to respond to the hormonal milieu of pregnancy by developing an androgen (i.e. estrogen-precursor) synthesizing zone. Other than man, only the chimpanzee has adrenarche, which therefore occurs in two species which have the most prolonged interval between birth and puberty. Adrenarche may merely be revealed by such an interval. However, the more complex the organism the greater the advantage in prolonging the period between birth and reproductive activity to allow brain growth and childhood learning. If during that period androgens are required for continuing skeletal and muscular growth, this could be achieved by transferring androgen biosynthesis from gonad to adrenal – adrenarche.

Congenital adrenal hyperplasia (CAH)

CAH describes collectively a group of autosomal recessively inherited disorders of adrenal corticosteroid biosynthesis due to deficiency of one of five enzymes in the cholesterol to cortisol biosynthetic pathway – 21-hydroxylase (21OH, P450c21), 11beta-hydroxylase (11betaOH, P450c11), 3beta-hydroxysteroid dehydrogenase (3betaOHSD), 17alpha-hydroxylase (17alphaOH, P450c17) and cholesterol desmolase (P450scc) (see Fig. 15.50). Deficiencies of other enzymes such as 17,20-desmolase (P450c17 17,20-lyase), 17beta-hydroxysteroid dehydrogenase (17betaOHSD) and 5alpha-reductase have effects limited to the adrenal androgen (and gonadal) biosynthetic pathway.

The steroidogenic block due to a specific enzyme deficiency will have potential clinical effects by two types of mechanism: (1) distal hormone deficiency and (2) the effect of ACTH drive, a compensatory response in CRF–ACTH release secondary to the defect in cortisol biosynthesis and reduced feedback inhibition of ACTH, leading to (a) proximal metabolite accumulation and (b) abnormal production of steroids whose biosynthesis is unaffected by the primary enzyme deficiency (Table 15.16).

Thus in the commonest form of CAH (21OH deficiency, P450c21 deficiency) there is, potentially, cortisol deficiency (in practice unstressed cortisol levels are normal as the enzyme deficiency is seldom complete), aldosterone deficiency and salt loss (when the defect is also present in the zona glomerulosa); plasma 17-hydroxyprogesterone (17OHP), and its principal urinary metabolite, pregnanetriol, levels are raised (and conveniently measured to confirm the diagnosis) and ACTH hypersecretion results in excess adrenal androgen and virilization (by birth in females, during early childhood in undiagnosed males).

Inappropriately raised plasma ACTH levels for plasma cortisol are pathognomonic of CAH – measuring cortisol alone is useless for diagnosis. Although the clinical picture may suggest the specific underlying enzyme defect, definitive diagnosis is dependent on detecting raised plasma levels of precursors in plasma by RIA or IRMA and

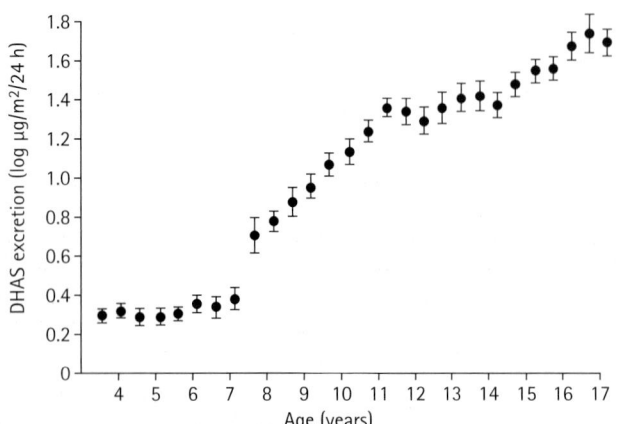

Fig. 15.51 Urinary excretion of dehydroepiandrosterone sulfate (DHAS) in childhood. (From Kelnar 1985[296])

characteristic urinary metabolites. Occasionally, measurement following ACTH stimulation may be necessary if the situation is not clear-cut. Pointers to the possibility of CAH include ambiguous genitalia in the newborn, vomiting with dehydration and urinary salt wasting during early days or weeks of life, collapse during stress (e.g. severe intercurrent illness or general anesthesia) at any age, hypertension, hirsutism or inappropriate virilization, primary amenorrhea, unexplained previous neonatal death (particularly if parents are consanguineous) and a family history of CAH.

21-Hydroxylase (21OH, P-450c21) deficiency

This is by far the commonest form of CAH worldwide although there are considerable ethnic differences. The frequency of the homozygous state varies from 1 in 5000 (Europe) to 1 in 23 000 and is particularly common in Alaskan Eskimos (1 in 700). Nonclassical 21OH deficiency (see below) seems more common and may affect 1 in 30 Jews of Eastern European (Ashkenazi) origin and 1 in 100 other whites.[298]

Genetics

Molecular genetic techniques have localized two genes encoding the 21OH enzyme, CYP21B (active) and CYP21A (inactive), to the short arm of chromosome 6 either side of the genes for the fourth component of complement – there is close linkage with the HLA complex. Deletion of CYP21B is associated with severe, salt-wasting disease and the HLA B47, DR7 haplotype; deletion of CYP21A seems not to cause any hormonal abnormality.[299] Most affected individuals are compound heterozygotes. HLA associations with nonclassical 21OH deficiency vary between ethnic groups.

Obligate heterozygote parents of salt-losing and simple virilizing patients show identical sodium, aldosterone and renin responses to a low sodium diet, and some infants with aldosterone biosynthetic defects subsequently develop normal glomerulosa 21OH activity suggesting that other (non-HLA linked) mechanisms are involved in enzyme expression.

The importance of these molecular genetic developments lies in the practical ability to confirm (pre- or postnatally) whether family members are affected or unaffected and in advancing understanding of pathogenesis.

Prenatal diagnosis of 21OH deficiency was first reported in 1965[300] on the basis of elevated 17-ketosteroids and pregnanetriol levels in amniotic fluid (i.e. dilute fetal urine) of an affected fetus. Raised 17OHP and androstenedione levels have since been found in many studies and HLA genotyping of amniotic cells was used in addition. Chorionic villus sampling, and molecular typing for restriction fragment length polymorphisms of the chromosome 6 loci, 21-hydroxylase gene and HLA, is now possible by 8–11 weeks' gestation and has replaced HLA genotyping of amniotic cells. Rapid early prenatal diagnosis by direct assay of specific mutations using DNA amplification by polymerase chain reaction (PCR) is feasible.

Antenatal diagnosis (AND) and treatment

Where there has been a previously affected female child, the possibility of prenatal treatment to reduce or prevent significant neonatal virilization in a second affected female fetus and obviate the need for surgery in infancy and beyond is potentially attractive. Dexamethasone (which crosses the placenta) is used in a dose not exceeding 20 mcg/kg/day of the prepregnancy weight in 2–3 divided doses to suppress the excessive ACTH/androgen induced virilization. Fetuses in whom therapy would be appropriate are affected females – a one in eight possibility with each pregnancy. However dexamethasone must be started very early in pregnancy because sexual differentiation starts at 6 weeks' gestation, and significantly before antenatal diagnosis is possible. Thus 7 out of 8 infants will have treatment unnecessarily for a number of weeks. In affected female infants treatment is continued to term.

Although data from uncontrolled studies are available concerning prenatal diagnosis and dexamethasone therapy, the degree of benefit (reduced virilization) compared to potentially significant maternal side-effects is unclear – possible long term childhood side-effects have not been studied. Substantial adverse effects on neuromotor and cognitive function at school age have been found after postnatal dexamethasone therapy for lung disease of prematurity[301] and transient variations in glucocorticoid status may have profound and long term programming effects in later life[302] by influencing the number and morphology of corticotrophs as well as the hypothalamo-pituitary–adrenal axis.[303]

At present, therefore, there seems insufficient evidence regarding the safety of mother and fetus to recommend general dexamethasone use outwith controlled scientific studies.

Heterozygote detection and neonatal screening

Stimulated 17OHP levels after ACTH will distinguish classical 21OH deficiency patients from heterozygotes for classical or nonclassical disease and from HLA-typed normal family members but HLA typing cannot be used on a population basis to detect heterozygosity (e.g. in the spouse of a potential carrier).

Newborn screening is probably desirable. Male infants (with normal genitalia) may give no warning of a salt-losing crisis with higher morbidity and mortality.[304] Females may be sufficiently virilized to be thought normal males leading to later gender reassignment or hysterectomy and sterility. Non-salt-losing males may be late diagnosed, by when secondary true precocious puberty and ultimate short stature may be inevitable. In a retrospective study covering the last 30 years in five middle European countries there was a 4-fold higher mortality amongst siblings and salt-wasting males in the first year of life compared with the general population. It was calculated that 2–2.5 salt-wasting and up to 5 simple virilizing infants stay undiagnosed out of 40 expected CAH patients per year in the countries investigated. Both clinical detection and treatment of CAH patients, at least in males, were insufficient.[304]

Classical 21OH deficiency is more common than phenylketonuria and, in Europe, is nearly as common as congenital hypothyroidism. A reliable and cheap (in centers already providing a neonatal screening service) screening test is available[305] using heel-prick capillary blood samples taken onto filter paper to measure 17OHP, easily done as part of the 'Guthrie test' procedure.

Significant mortality and serious physical and emotional morbidity consequent on late diagnosis has led to many screening programs worldwide, e.g. Italy, France, Japan, Ireland, New Zealand and a number of USA States.[306] Experience from screening more than 1 000 000 neonates in over 13 screening programs in 6 countries confirms that screening improves detection of salt-wasting newborns whose diagnosis is otherwise delayed or missed and in whom there is significant mortality and morbidity.[307] Morbidity in non-salt-losing males presenting in mid-childhood is also considerable.

However, current screening programs yield a high proportion of false positive results and the future use of tandem mass-spectometry to evaluate positives found in the initial Delfia screen may significantly improve the effectiveness of a screening program.[308] False negative results seem to be more common in girls.[309]

Genotyping may be a helpful diagnostic tool and a good complement to neonatal screening, especially in confirming or discarding the diagnosis in cases with slightly elevated 17OHP levels. It also provides information on disease severity, which reduces the risk of overtreatment of mildly affected children.[310]

In the UK it is generally considered unnecessary or 'uneconomical' to screen the whole newborn population even though this would add only a small additional unit cost in screening laboratories already measuring TSH and phenylalanine. There may be insufficient acknowledgment of considerable potential morbidity and concentration on mortality statistics. However, there are, to date, few published data on improvements in morbidity resulting from early detection and treatment.

Clinical presentation

Classical simple virilizing 21OH deficiency in a karyotypic female results in masculinization generally leading to ambiguous external genitalia recognized at birth (Fig. 15.52) but occasionally so severe that the

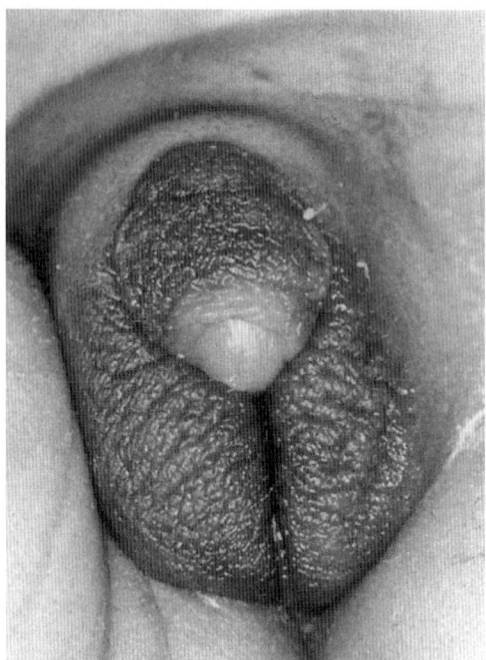

Fig. 15.52 Ambiguous genitalia in a 10-day-old genotypic female due to 21-hydroxylase deficiency.

infant is thought to be a normal male. Internal female structures including ovaries, Fallopian tubes and uterus are normal (there are no testes to elaborate AMH) but there is variable labioscrotal fold fusion with a urogenital sinus, genital pigmentation and clitoromegaly. Males usually appear normal at birth but present with penile enlargement, rapid growth (and tall stature) and advanced skeletal maturation (leading to eventual short stature) within a few years (Fig. 15.53). Finding small testes with clinical signs of precocious puberty suggests the adrenals as the androgen source but skeletal maturational advance can be marked so that true precocious puberty develops when treatment starts (see Fig. 15.34).

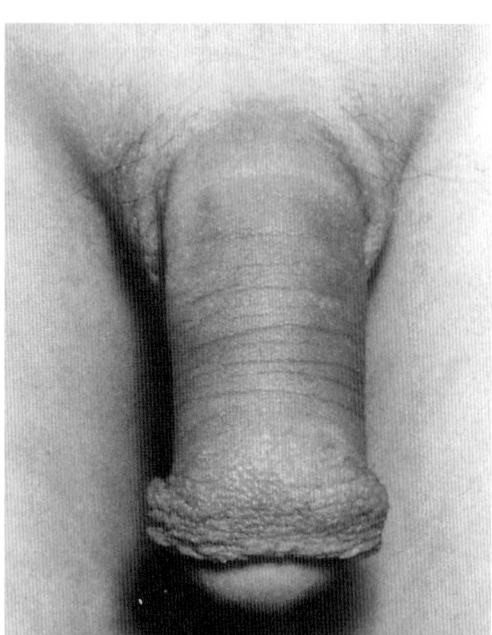

Fig. 15.53 Precocious pseudopuberty – a boy with non-salt-losing 21-hydroxylase deficiency at presentation at 5 years – testicular volume 2 ml (see also Fig. 15.34).

In the classical salt-wasting form (50–75%) there is an additional defect in mineralocorticoid biosynthesis with aldosterone deficiency due to an inability to convert progesterone to deoxycorticosterone in the glomerulosa. Presentation in both sexes is with severe renal wasting of sodium, dehydration and vomiting within a few days or weeks of birth – this should be foreseen as a possibility in a baby with ambiguous genitalia.

Nonclassical ('mild, late-onset') 21OH deficiency was suspected in women presenting with hirsutism and infertility, and family studies in classical 21OH deficiency characterized it as having different (and differing) HLA associations from classical forms but also autosomal recessive. It may present as early as 6 months or later with premature pubarche, rapid growth (and reduced height prognosis), acne, male-type baldness in the female, delayed menarche or secondary amenorrhea. There is an association with polycystic ovarian disease – infertility may result and respond to GC therapy.

Laboratory diagnosis

17OHP measurement in the newborn is reliable for screening and diagnosis but false positives are reported in preterm or sick neonates. Plasma ACTH, androstenedione and urinary pregnanetriol levels will also be raised. In the salt-wasting form, there is urinary sodium loss (cf. the gut in gastroenteritis); aldosterone levels are low for the high renin levels (cf. renal disease). Clinical and laboratory features of this and the other least uncommon forms of CAH are summarized in Table 15.16. Management is discussed below.

11beta-hydroxylase (11betaOH, P450c11) deficiency

This accounts for some 5% of CAH. There is no HLA association (cf. 21OH deficiency). Clinical manifestations are, as predicted from biosynthetic pathways (Fig. 15.50), identical to 21OH deficiency from the virilizing point of view – in some affected individuals there is restriction of the defect to the glucocorticoid pathway. In over 50%, however, the glomerulosa is also affected but the consequences differ from 21OH deficiency (Table 15.16) because there is accumulation of deoxycorticosterone (DOC) which has significant MC (salt-retaining) properties and, in excess, causes hypertension. DOC may not be directly responsible for hypertension in all cases as some patients with 11betaOH deficiency with raised DOC levels are normotensive and others are hypertensive with normal or only slightly raised DOC levels. Other DOC metabolites such as 18-hydroxy DOC have been implicated.

18-hydroxylation (the next step in the aldosterone biosynthetic pathway) is a function of the same mitochondrial enzyme – a defect in 18-hydroxylase is often seen with 11betaOH deficiency. Milder (late onset) forms and even salt-wasting patients have been reported – clinically 11betaOH deficiency is as heterogeneous as 21OH deficiency.

Hypertension, when present, is characteristic and may be extreme; hypokalemic alkalosis is common. Virilizing effects are as described under 21OH deficiency above. DOC and deoxycortisol (S) levels are raised, as are their respective urinary tetrahydro (TH) metabolites (THDOC and THS), and rise further following ACTH, but their proportional elevations vary between subjects. Prenatal diagnosis has been carried out using a combination of amniotic fluid studies and maternal urinary THS measurement. Management is discussed below.

3beta-hydroxysteroid dehydrogenase (3betaOHSD) deficiency

This is also associated with ambiguous genitalia in newborns but the site of the block (Fig. 15.50) results in potential ambiguity both in genotypic males and females (Table 15.16): high levels of DHA and its peripheral conversion to potent androgens result in variable clitoromegaly in females but are insufficient to fully masculinize a male infant, resulting in variable hypospadias (often the severe perineo-scrotal form) with palpable testes. The defect in MC biosynthesis usually causes severe salt wasting. Mild defects are important causes of hirsutism presenting in young adult women so that, as in 21OH deficiency, mild, late onset

Table 15.16 Clinical and laboratory features in the commonest forms of congenital adrenal hyperplasia

Enzyme deficiency	Sexual ambiguity in newborn	Salt-wasting	Hypertension	Blood	Urine
21-hydroxylase (simple virilizing)	Female	−	−	17OHP ++ An ++ DHA n/+ Renin n/+	PT ++ Aldo n
21-hydroxylase (salt-wasting)	Female	+	−	17OHP ++ An ++ DHA n/+ Renin ++	PT ++ Aldo −
11beta-hydroxylase	Female	−	+	17OHP + An ++ DHA + Renin −−	PT + THS ++ Aldo −
3beta-hydroxysteroid dehydrogenase	Male and female	+	−	17OHP n/+ An ++ DHA +++ Renin +	PT n/+ Aldo −

17OHP = 17alpha-hydroxyprogesterone, An = delta-4-androstenedione, DHA = dehydroepiandrosterone, THS = tetrahydrodeoxycortisol, Aldo = aldosterone, PT = pregnanetriol. +++ = very high, ++ = high, + = moderately high, n = normal, − = low, −− = very low.

forms are apparently more common than the classical severe type. There is no HLA association and neither ethnic nor geographical clustering. Prenatal diagnosis is impossible because of low 3betaOHSD fetal zone activity.

17alpha-hydroxylase (17OH, P450c17) deficiency

Mineralocorticoid biosynthesis is intact (Fig. 15.50) and ACTH drive may result in neonatal hypertension and hypokalemic alkalosis. Deficient adrenal (and gonadal) sex steroid secretion means that karyotypic females usually present with failure of puberty and primary amenorrhea; males have ambiguous genitalia or virilize inadequately at puberty with gynecomastia. Recently described CYP17 mutations correlate poorly with phenotypic features (degree of virilization, blood pressure, etc.).[311]

P450 oxido-reductase deficiency (POR)[312]

Formerly known as 'apparent combined P450c17 and P450c21 deficiency' this newly characterized variant of CAH is associated with cranio- and radiofemoral synostosis and mid-facial hypoplasia (and is distinct from other craniosynostosis syndromes caused by FGFR mutations).

Cholesterol desmolase deficiency (P450scc, cholesterol side chain cleavage deficiency, lipoid adrenal hyperplasia)[313]

This was originally described as lipoid adrenal hyperplasia because of adrenal accumulation of cholesterol. Pregnenolone is the precursor of all MCs, GCs and androgens (Fig. 15.50) and complete deficiency is presumably incompatible with life. In contrast to congenital adrenal hypoplasia (see below), gonadal steroids are also deficient. The P450scc gene has been located in the q23 to q24 region of chromosome 15.

Management of CAH

The basic defect (in cortisol biosynthesis) has wide repercussions including survival itself, sexual differentiation, growth, pubertal development and adult sexual functioning. Management potentially involves sex assignment, hormone therapy, surgery and psychological and emotional support with attention to growth and puberty and not merely adrenal steroid levels.

Hormone replacement is aimed at appropriately suppressing excessive ACTH drive rather than simply replacing cortisol; cortisol levels are often normal in the unstressed situation. In a baby with salt loss, titration of the appropriate GC replacement dose (against ACTH, adrenal androgen or 17OHP levels) is misleading until there is sodium balance (evidenced by normal plasma renin and plasma and urinary sodium). In the older child also, raised ACTH levels may be due to inadequate MC replacement.

The normal cortisol production rate is lower than previously thought: approximately 6–7 mg/m²/day. Appropriate GC replacement will allow normal growth, skeletal maturation and puberty – hydrocortisone (HC) 12–15 mg/m²/day in 2–3 divided doses is usually appropriate. However, larger doses (< 20–25 mg/m²/day) may be necessary to suppress androgen levels and a combination regimen of physiological GC replacement with antiandrogens or aromatase inhibitors[225] has been suggested[314] as has carbenoxolone as an 11betaOHSD inhibitor[315] – or bilateral laparoscopic adrenalectomy for difficult to control cases.[316]

To mimic normal diurnal rhythms, approximately two thirds of the total HC dose is usually given first thing in the morning and the last dose at bedtime. In some it is necessary to give a longer acting steroid (e.g. prednisone or dexamethasone) at bedtime if early morning ACTH and 17OHP levels are not to be too high – once-daily dexamethasone may be appropriate for adolescents and adults and may also improve ovarian function in women.

The correct GC dose must be determined for each individual. Too low a dose will allow androgen-mediated excessively rapid growth, disproportionate bone age advance and eventual stunting. Too much will cause slowing of linear growth and delay (but not comparable delay) in bone maturation, also resulting ultimately in short stature. Swinging from one extreme to the other causes cumulative deficits in height prognosis.

Monitoring is by accurate growth and bone age assessment supplemented by home finger-prick blood spot 17OHP profiles four times daily approximately monthly. Abnormally rapid growth and bone age maturation is associated with nonsuppressed 17OHP levels (> 40 nmol/L), whereas GC over-replacement, evidenced by pathologically slow growth, is associated with levels < 10 nmol/L.

GC therapy must be increased 2–3-fold during stress such as significant infection or general anesthesia which could otherwise precipitate hypoglycemia and collapse. The family should be provided with, and instructed in the use of, home blood glucose monitoring strips, and injectable hydrocortisone in case the child is vomiting or becomes rapidly ill at home. A Medicalert bracelet or talisman should be worn, as with other patients on steroid medication.

Mineralocorticoid (MC) replacement is necessary in salt-losing forms of CAH, given as the synthetic analogue 9alpha-fluorocortisol (fludro-cortisone) 0.1–0.15 mg/m²/day in one or two daily doses. However the salt-losing crisis cannot be treated with fludrocortisone (nor with hydro-cortisone which has limited MC activity) – emergency treatment with sodium replacement and i.v. normal or even hypertonic saline will be necessary as the total body sodium deficit is considerable. Once sodium balance is restored, fludrocortisone is introduced (and GC dose titra-tion can begin) but oral sodium supplements (initially 2 mmol/kg/day) may also be required during infancy. Regular BP and urinary electro-lyte measurements are sufficient to check that MC replacement is appro-priate. Renin and aldosterone clinic measurements may not be very meaningful. After infancy, children can adjust their salt intake and the-oretically do not require long term MC replacement. In practice, health and growth seem better if MC therapy is continued. The hypertension found in some forms of 11betaOH and 17OH deficiencies responds to GC suppression of ACTH/MC overproduction.

Sex assignment seldom poses problems but for a review of the devel-opment of gender and sexuality in 46XX persons with classical CAH and its implications for clinical practice see Meyer-Bahlburg.[55] In 21OH and 11betaOH deficiencies karyotypic females with ambiguous genitalia should normally be reared as girls – internal sexual organs are normal female and with appropriate therapy there is a significant chance of fertil-ity. Clitoral reduction is sometimes appropriate for cosmetic reasons (see below). Assignment in rarer forms (3betaOHSD, 17OH and cholesterol desmolase deficiencies) where males may be very poorly virilized depends on functional possibilities after potential reconstructive procedures.

In severely virilized females, clitoral reduction is widely felt to be best undertaken before 6 months. The vascular and neural supply to the glans is maintained to aid later sexual functioning and pleasure. Labial separation, if necessary, may be carried out simultaneously. Vaginal reconstruction has been thought best delayed until after puberty – often simple stretching will allow estrogen-mediated development at puberty obviating the need for major surgery, and early reconstruction has been more commonly associated with discomfort at intercourse. However, there are contrary views in favor of early one stage reconstructive sur-gery.[317] Fertility prospects are generally good in males, but abnormal sonogram findings of testicular adrenal rests are more frequent in the salt-wasting form and are associated with a higher risk for infertility.[318] Fertility is reduced in affected women.[319]

Emotional support is necessary for families of children with ambig-uous genitalia particularly in the neonatal period and adolescence. Reports of high rates of homosexuality in female CAH patients may reflect inadequate vaginoplasty and difficult heterosexual relationships but effects of high androgen levels on the female fetal cerebral cor-tex could be important. Psychosexual outcomes in individuals treated prenatally will help to resolve the question but are not yet available.

Because standard and indeed 'optimal' GC therapy may result in Cushingoid side-effects and suboptimal growth and height prognosis, several supplementary approaches including GnRH analogues, aro-matase inhibitors and antiandrogens have been proposed in order to reduce the GC dose. However, as compliance (concordance) with pre-scribed medication(s) is generally the biggest cause of suboptimal treat-ment outcomes, it is doubtful whether the need to take additional tablets will improve control. Similarly, bilateral adrenalectomy has been tried in patients with CYP21 null mutations or difficulty in achieving good con-trol on conventional therapy[320] and found (in a small cohort) to be safe and effective. The advantages of easier therapeutic management (no hyperandrogenism) must be balanced against an increased risk of adrenal crises and Nelson syndrome. All such treatments remain experimental.

Hyperadrenocorticism

Adrenal hypercorticism is commonly secondary to trophic hormone stimulation causing adrenal hyperplasia and hypersecretion and rarely primary (usually due to adrenal tumor). Clinical features are mimicked

Table 15.17 Important causes of adrenocortical hyperfunction

Glucocorticoids	Iatrogenic (glucocorticoid therapy); Cushing syndrome; carcinoma/adenoma; bilateral hyperplasia (Cushing disease/pituitary tumor/ectopic ACTH-secreting tumor)
Mineralocorticoids	Primary hyperaldosteronism; Conn syndrome (adenoma); Bartter syndrome; congenital adrenal hyperplasia (17alpha-hydroxylase and 11beta-hydroxylase deficiencies); deoxycorticosterone- (DOC) or corticosterone-secreting tumors
Sex steroids	*Androgens* Congenital adrenal hyperplasia (21-hydroxylase and 11beta-hydroxylase deficiencies); 'premature' adrenarche (pubarche); virilizing carcinoma/adenoma *Estrogens* Feminizing carcinoma/adenoma

by (and in practice much more commonly due to) excessive GC admin-istration (iatrogenic Cushing syndrome – see below). Causes are listed in Table 15.17.

Cushing syndrome

Cushing syndrome (disorders due to chronic excessive GC production) is uncommon in childhood – only 5–10% of reported cases – and rare in young children. It may be due to: (1) benign or malignant adrenal tumor; (2) pituitary ACTH hypersecretion (Cushing disease); (3) ACTH or CRF hypersecretion from malignant extrapituitary tumors (ecto-pic ACTH syndrome); (4) supraphysiological parenteral, oral, nasal or topical GC or ACTH therapy for other medical conditions – most frequently.

Clinical features are due to cortisol excess resulting in protein catabolism, increased carbohydrate production, fat accumulation and potassium wasting. In children, classical signs and symptoms (hyper-tension, truncal obesity, moon face, striae, proximal muscle weakness, osteoporosis, psychiatric symptoms) are usually less clear-cut than in adults, and combined growth effects of hypercortisolism and excess adre-nal androgen secretion may cause growth failure or temporarily rapid growth. The former is more common, however, and hirsutism, progres-sive truncal obesity and growth failure (cf. obesity due to overeating), make up the most common presenting triad. Hypertension is usually only moderate and of multifactorial pathogenesis.

Iatrogenic disease must be specifically sought. ACTH is used to treat hypsarrhythmia and oral GC is used for a variety of chronic renal and connective tissue disorders (now less commonly for asthma). Large doses of inhaled steroids can be associated with significant adrenal suppres-sion and growth failure as can nasal drops and topical steroids, depend-ing on the extent of surface treated, frequency of application, potency of drug, use of occlusion and the age of the child. Infants, treated for seborrheic dermatitis/eczema, and adolescents are relatively sensitive to topical steroid side-effects – an infant's (wet and occluded) napkin area has relative absorption 42-fold higher than the forearm; adolescents' increasing fat deposits and muscle mass inducing dermal remodeling makes them particularly susceptible to striae particularly around breasts and buttocks. If the hypothalamo–pituitary–adrenal axis is suppressed, treatment must be withdrawn gradually if acute adrenal insufficiency (see below) is not to be precipitated.

No single screening test is reliable in detecting Cushing syndrome at an early stage or in differentiating it from exogenous obesity. A nor-mal plasma cortisol diurnal rhythm, with normal urinary free cortisol levels and a normal short (overnight) dexamethasone suppression test (0.3 mg/m² orally at midnight measuring 8 a.m. plasma cortisol) will reasonably exclude the diagnosis. A 2-day low dose (6 mg/kg every 6 h) dexamethasone suppression test measuring plasma cortisol at 48 h, or urinary free cortisol corrected for creatinine, is necessary if results are equivocal.

Once the diagnosis is established, further differential diagnosis of the cause may also be difficult. Rapidly evolving symptoms, palpable abdominal mass and virilization at any age make adrenal carcinoma most likely and this is relatively common in infancy, but generally diagnosis depends on imaging techniques (e.g. adrenal ultrasound, pituitary and adrenal CT scanning, adrenal iodocholesterol scintigraphy) and further dynamic hormone tests (e.g. response to metyrapone, high dose dexamethasone, CRF). Petrosal sinus sampling seems not to be a reliable test for lateralization of a pituitary adenoma.[321] Diagnostic algorithms are available[240] – investigation should be carried out in specialist centers.

Treatment depends on the cause and may be medical, surgical (to pituitary or adrenals), radiotherapy or radioactive implants. Medical treatment (e.g. with drugs blocking cortisol biosynthesis or GC antagonists) is of value in many patients prior to surgery, if inoperable lesions are found and in Cushing disease. In virtually all situations, however, treatment is urgent because of the progressive and severe natural course if untreated.

Hyperaldosteronism

Primary MC hypersecretion is very rare in childhood and usually due to a zona glomerulosa adenoma (Conn syndrome) or bilateral hyperplasia. There is sodium retention and hypertension with hypokalemia, renin suppression and hyperaldosteronism which fails to suppress with dexamethasone. In addition to hypertension, there may be muscle weakness, polyuria and impaired growth. Treatment is medical (long term spironolactone) in hyperplasia and surgical in adenoma.

Familial forms of hyperaldosteronism

Dexamethasone-suppressible hyperaldosteronism is clinically and biochemically indistinguishable from primary hyperaldosteronism but aldosterone levels suppress rapidly on dexamethasone. Hypertension can be controlled by GC therapy. Autosomal dominant inheritance (not HLA linked) has been proposed. *Bartter syndrome* is discussed in Chapter 18, p. 551. *Apparent mineralocorticoid excess (AME) syndrome* is often familial – aldosterone levels are low and there is no evidence for overproduction of other MCs. The pathogenesis is now known to be primary *11beta-hydroxysteroid dehydrogenase (11betaOHSD) deficiency* resulting in defective cortisol metabolism to cortisone. The resulting prolongation of cortisol half-life and bioactivity may result in sufficient MC activity to cause hypertension. Diagnosis depends on the finding of a raised (> 1) ratio of the main urinary metabolite of cortisol (tetrahydrocortisol, THF) to that of cortisone (THE) on gas chromatography, in association with low renin hypertension and normal or low aldosterone levels.

11betaOHSD is a widely distributed enzyme which exists in two types – type II is found in the placenta and distal renal nephron, is NAD dependent and converts the (active) glucocorticoid cortisol (F) to (inactive) cortisone (E) (Fig. 15.54). The mineralocorticoid receptor (MR) has little affinity for E whereas aldosterone cannot be inactivated in this way and retains full access to the MR.[322] Increased availability and binding of cortisol at the MR at the renal distal tubule is the currently accepted pathophysiological mechanism underlying AME.

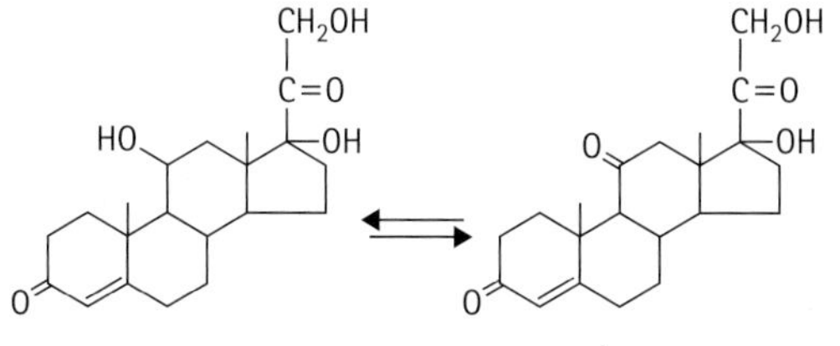

Fig. 15.54 Cortisol–cortisone interconversion (see text).

11betaOHSD may be of wider importance than simply in the etiology of AME. It is plentiful in the placenta and could be important in protecting the fetus from maternal cortisol. It is speculated that the growth-retarded human fetus has been exposed to excessive cortisol in utero due to relative placental 11betaOHSD deficiency which could reflect placental and fetal growth and that this has long-lasting effects (e.g. adult hypertension) by imprinting via brain receptor or neurochemical mechanisms.[36]

Secondary hyperaldosteronism may be due to various causes, most importantly renin-secreting tumors either of the juxtaglomerular apparatus or from ectopic sites such as pancreatic adenocarcinoma. Renin levels are very high.

Pseudohypoaldosteronism due to end-organ resistance to aldosterone is characterized by high levels of urinary aldosterone metabolites which distinguish it from 18-hydroxylase and dehydrogenase deficiencies. Clinical presentation is identical and it is discussed under sodium-losing states (see below).

Insufficiency

Adrenocortical hypofunction may result from primary adrenal disorders or may be secondary to hypothalamo–pituitary disorders. Hypofunction may be complete or affect specific functions – GC, MC or androgen biosynthesis. Chronic conditions may present with dramatic symptoms relating to acute adrenal insufficiency ('Addisonian crisis') but may remain asymptomatic and diagnosis may be long delayed. Causes are listed in Table 15.18.

Congenital adrenal hypoplasia

After CAH, this is the commonest neonatal cause of adrenal hypofunction. Sporadic cases are associated with anencephaly or other congenital (e.g. renal and cardiac) malformations and maternal pre-eclampsia. Familial forms are sex-linked or autosomal recessive. Adrenocortical failure presents with adrenal hypoplasia or atrophy – combined adrenal autopsy weight < 1 g or < 1% of total body weight

Table 15.18 Important causes of adrenocortical hypofunction

Primary complete (glucocorticoids/mineralocorticoids/androgens)
  Congenital adrenal hypoplasia
  Lipoid adrenal hyperplasia (cholesterol desmolase deficiency)
  Addison disease
  Adrenal apoplexy (Waterhouse–Friderichsen syndrome)
  Adrenal hemorrhage/cysts
  Adrenoleukodystrophy
  Autoimmune multiple endocrinopathy syndromes

Primary selective – glucocorticoids
  Congenital adrenal hyperplasia (21-hydroxylase, 17alpha-hydroxylase and 11beta-hydroxylase deficiencies)
  Iatrogenic
  Hereditary unresponsiveness to ACTH

Primary selective – mineralocorticoids
  Pseudohypoaldosteronism
  Aldosterone biosynthetic defect (18-hydroxylase and 18-dehydrogenase deficiency)

Primary selective – androgens
  17,20-desmolase deficiency

Secondary
  Iatrogenic (glucocorticoid therapy)
  Hypothalamo–pituitary dysfunction
    Panhypopituitarism
    Isolated ACTH deficiency
    Craniopharyngioma
    Structural midline defects

is characteristic. It is a rare cause of low maternal estriol levels during pregnancy.

Histological findings are heterogeneous but of three main types: (1) primary (cytomegalic) – a rare form in males, with poorly differentiated cortex, disordered architecture and giant cells; (2) secondary (anencephalic) – the commonest in sporadic and familial cases – the fetal zone is reduced or absent but definitive cortex is well differentiated, mimicking the appearance in anencephalics; (3) miniature, comprising about one third of cases – the glands are small but normally differentiated. All three types occur sporadically.

Two hereditary forms have been characterized: (1) autosomal recessive, usually associated with the miniature histological type; (2) X-linked, usually associated with the cytomegalic form and affecting boys. The latter type is now known to be due to mutations in the DAX-1 gene – DAX-1 is a member of the orphan nuclear hormone receptor family expressed in the adrenal gland, gonads, ventromedial hypothalamus and pituitary gonadotrophs. There is an association with hypogonadotrophic hypogonadism and with X-linked glycerol kinase deficiency.

In all types and forms, clinical presentation is within the first few hours or days of life with vomiting, diarrhea, apnea, hypoglycemia with convulsions, hyponatremic dehydration, hyperkalemia and metabolic acidosis. Plasma cortisol and aldosterone levels are very low with high renin. ACTH levels are very high (cf. adrenal failure secondary to pituitary disorders but not differentiating it from CAH). In karyotypic females it is indistinguishable from cholesterol desmolase deficiency but other forms of CAH can be identified as described above. Treatment is analogous to that of salt-losing CAH. Prognosis was poor but is now much improved, particularly in those surviving the first few days.

Familial GC deficiency (hereditary unresponsiveness to ACTH)

Onset is after the first year, sometimes with recurring hypoglycemia but often merely with a history of prostration during intrinsically mild intercurrent illness. There is hyperpigmentation and tall stature is common. Inheritance is probably autosomal recessive. The pathogenesis is unknown but may be degenerative – the glomerulosa is broad but fasciculata and reticularis are reduced to a fibrous band.

There is a defect in cortisol production with high ACTH levels, and also diminished adrenal androgen secretion implicating a significant role for ACTH in the control of adrenal androgen secretion. MC production is normal under basal conditions but may not remain so, making the distinction from Addison disease particularly difficult. Treatment is with GC, which must be increased during severe intercurrent illness.

Addison disease

This primary chronic form of adrenal insufficiency first described in 1855 is rare in childhood affecting ~ 1 in 10 000. Hypoadrenalism much more commonly results from corticosteroid medication suppressing the pituitary–adrenal axis (see below). Variations in incidence – historically, geographically and in age of onset – probably represent changes in the epidemiology of the primary causes of adrenal damage and failure: until the 1950s, tuberculosis was overwhelmingly the commonest cause but 20 years later it accounted for only about 1 in 5 UK cases.

The commonest cause is now autoimmune (AI) adrenal disease. As with other AI diseases there is a familial incidence and female preponderance. Adrenalitis is characterized by lymphocyte infiltration and adrenal microsomal and mitochondrial autoantibodies are found. The medulla is unaffected. There are associations with other autoimmune conditions including hypoparathyroidism (in about 1 in 3 cases) and mucocutaneous candidiasis [polyglandular autoimmune disease (PGAD) type 1], thyroid disease and/or diabetes mellitus (PGAD type 2) and a range of other autoimmune endocrinopathies (PGAD type 4). Antibody titers are generally low, decrease further with age and do not correlate with the severity of the endocrinopathies. Cell-mediated (T-lymphocyte) processes are more likely to be responsible for the adrenal cortical destruction. Familial (autosomal recessive) occurrence probably relates to the inheritance of the underlying tendency to AI disease – there is an association with HLA A1, A3 or B8.

There is GC and MC deficiency which may not develop simultaneously. In childhood, presenting features are usually hypoglycemia, progressive lassitude and muscle weakness, gastrointestinal disturbances (including constipation or diarrhea, vomiting and abdominal pain), associated with mild hyperpigmentation (classically of buccal and vaginal mucosa, nipples and palmar creases and pressure areas – axillae and groin – due to pituitary beta-lipotropin secretion). In practice, pigmentation may simply appear as excellent suntan or 'dirt' over extensor surfaces exposed to friction (e.g. knees, knuckles, elbows).

Major symptoms result from cortisol deficiency and consequent high plasma ACTH elevation. Glycogen stores are low – severe hypoglycemia may occur during fasting or intercurrent stress or illness. Hyponatremia results from aldosterone deficiency and reduced plasma volume induced vasopressin secretion causing water retention.

Characteristic laboratory findings are hyponatremia, hyperkalemia, raised urea, fasting hypoglycemia and anemia. Basal cortisol, aldosterone and adrenal androgen levels are commonly normal but with raised ACTH levels. Cortisol levels do not rise 60 or 120 minutes after a 'short' ACTH test (i.v. 1,24-ACTH 500 ng/1.73 m^2) – although the sensitivity of this test is still debatable – or after i.m. ACTH 25 mg/m^2 (8 hourly for 3 days). Low T4 with raised TSH levels may be found but often correct rapidly with GC treatment without thyroxine. Adrenal autoantibodies are characteristically present even before clinical onset and should lead to regular testing of adrenal function in patients with other AI disorders or siblings of affected individuals.

Acute 'Addisonian' crisis may occur as the presenting feature in a previously unsuspected case precipitated by intercurrent illness or stress. There is hypotension (otherwise uncommon in children with Addison disease), dehydration, prostration and collapse, with hypoglycemia and the classical electrolyte disturbances described above, superimposed on symptoms and signs of the precipitating cause. Treatment with intravenous hydrocortisone and plasma or normal saline with 5 or 10% dextrose is urgent. Intravenous or intramuscular hydrocortisone must be continued whilst oral GC replacement is started. With adequate sodium replacement, MC treatment is not usually necessary acutely.

GC therapy must be increased 2–3-fold during stress such as significant infection or general anesthesia which could otherwise precipitate hypoglycemia and collapse. Instruction should be given in the use of home blood glucose monitoring strips and injectable hydrocortisone provided for home use in case the child is vomiting or becomes rapidly ill at home. A Medicalert bracelet or talisman should be worn.

Long term treatment is with oral hydrocortisone, usually 10–15 mg/m^2/24 h – the dose individually adjusted based on disappearance of symptoms, normal growth and skeletal maturation and normal diurnal ACTH levels. MC dosage (fludrocortisone 0.1–0.15 mg/m^2/24 h) is less critical provided it is adequate and assessed as in salt-losing CAH. Treatment must be life-long. Adrenal androgen therapy is unnecessary in childhood but a mild androgenic preparation may improve libido and pubic hair growth in adolescent and adult women. It is usually considered that puberty is normal in timing and progression (cf. congenital adrenal hypoplasia). Prognosis is normal in terms of health and life span presupposing optimal prevention and treatment of acute crises.

Sodium-losing states

These may be due to renal disease (e.g. dysplasia, tubular disease, Bartter syndrome – see Ch. 18, p. 551) or adrenal insufficiency. Adrenal urinary sodium wasting is characterized by hyperkalemia and due to defective aldosterone biosynthesis (congenital adrenal hypoplasia, salt-wasting forms of CAH – see above – or isolated aldosterone biosynthetic defects) or impaired action at the renal tubule (pseudohypoaldosteronism – see below and Ch. 18, p. 552).

Isolated defects of aldosterone biosynthesis may result from defective 18-hydroxylation or 18-dehydrogenation in conversion of corticosterone to aldosterone (see Fig. 15.50). Both are due to deficiency of corticosterone methyloxidase (CMO) which converts corticosterone to

18-hydroxycorticosterone – defective hydroxylation is known as CMO I, defective dehydrogenation as CMO II.

Inheritance is autosomal recessive. Presentation is with marked salt wasting, hyperkalemia and failure to thrive usually in early infancy. GC and androgen function are normal. Although, as in 21OH deficiency, there can be self-regulation of salt intake and proximal renal tubular maturation, the salt-wasting tendency is life-long and MC replacement should be for life.

Pseudohypoaldosteronism is due to a primary renal tubular sodium/potassium ATPase defect. The effects of aldosterone are mediated largely through activation of the epithelial sodium channel, and inactivating mutations of this channel lead to pseudohypoaldosteronism with signs of mineralocorticoid deficiency. Clinical presentation is identical to the 18-oxidation (CMO) defects (see above) but aldosterone is markedly elevated and MC therapy ineffective as the proximal renal tubule is unresponsive to its action. Treatment is with sodium supplements. Transient pseudohypoaldosteronism has been reported with the renal tubular resistance to aldosterone secondary to renal disease (see also Ch. 18).

Adrenoleukodystrophy (ALD)
Various uncommon associations between chronic adrenal insufficiency and progressive brain demyelinization are described with differing inheritance but have in common the abnormal accumulation of saturated unbranched or monosaturated very long chain fatty acids due to a defect in their catabolism. The ALD gene maps to the long arm of the X chromosome (Xq28) and adrenal insufficiency is secondary to cortical destruction – treatment is with GC and MC. The neurological disorder is progressive – these and related conditions (e.g. Zellweger syndrome) are further discussed in Chapter 26, p. 1114.

Other causes of acute adrenal insufficiency include adrenal destruction, e.g. hemorrhage due to birth trauma and Waterhouse–Friderichsen syndrome (sepsis and collapse, often associated with meningococcemia).

Steroid withdrawal
Most commonly, adrenal crisis results from abrupt withdrawal of GC medication when the axis is suppressed from chronic GC administration (oral, inhaled, intranasal or topical) or failure to increase GC during severe intercurrent illness or stress (see above). Alternate day GC causes less hypothalamo – pituitary – adrenal axis suppression and appears more growth sparing. ACTH treatment is associated with more rapid current growth than is high dose GC, but this probably results from additional secondary adrenal androgen secretion and, if bone age advances disproportionately rapidly, ultimate stature may be just as impaired.

Tumors
Adrenal cortical tumors are rare in children. Virilizing tumors[323] are relatively more common than feminizing or nonsecreting tumors and are usually carcinomas rather than adenomas although their malignancy can be difficult to determine. They are histologically identical to those causing Cushing syndrome but differ in secretory pattern and thus clinical manifestations. Predominantly androgen hypersecretion produces pseudoprecocious puberty – tall stature with growth acceleration and precocious pubic and axillary hair; in boys growth of the penis with prepubertal size testes, in girls clitoromegaly and labial enlargement. Adrenocortical carcinomas are aggressive and tumor size relates poorly to malignancy. Treatment other than by surgical removal is disappointing and the prognosis often poor. Tumor morphology is a better predictor of metastatic risk than biochemical markers or immunohistochemistry.[324]

THE ADRENAL MEDULLA
The medulla comprises cells of neuroectodermal origin which synthesize and secrete catecholamines, hormones containing a dihydroxylated phenolic ring. The most active compounds, adrenaline and noradrenaline, are both secreted by the medulla and noradrenaline is also produced in sympathetic ganglion cells.

Catecholamine biosynthesis
Catecholamines are synthesized (Fig. 15.55) from dietary tyrosine and tyrosine converted from phenylalanine by liver hydroxylation. Tyrosine is converted to dihydroxyphenylalanine (DOPA) in brain and sympathetic tissue as well as adrenal medulla. There is then conversion to dihydroxyphenylethylamine (dopamine) and to noradrenaline and, only in the adrenal medulla and the organ of Zuckerkandl at the aortic bifurcation, to adrenaline. Catabolism and excretion (Fig. 15.55) is via vanillylmandelic acid (VMA) and homovanillic acid (HVA), urinary markers for catecholamine hypersecretion. Hypoglycemia, hypoxia, hypovolemia and exercise stimulate catecholamine release. Adrenaline has alpha- and beta-adrenergic effects but noradrenaline is mainly alpha-adrenergic. Vasoconstriction is alpha receptor mediated; cardiac stimulation is via the beta receptor. Dopaminergic effects also occur.

Hypofunction
Adrenomedullary hypofunction is seldom important clinically. Adrenomedullary unresponsiveness is a rare cause of hypoglycemia in children but might be found less infrequently if catecholamines were measured more often during hypoglycemia. Sweating and pallor do not occur. The disorder may be of primarily hypothalamic origin as adrenocortical responsiveness may also be impaired and there is an association with perinatal problems.

In familial dysautonomia (Riley – Day syndrome), an autosomal recessive condition most common in Ashkenazi Jews, there is disturbed autonomic function due to dopamine-beta-hydroxylase deficiency resulting in impaired noradrenaline biosynthesis. Urinary VMA is decreased and urinary levels of HVA, a dopamine metabolite, are high. There is impaired swallowing in infancy with aspiration pneumonia, excessive sweating and salivation, defective lacrimation, labile BP, indifference to pain, loss of taste buds and corneal insensitivity and ulceration. Treatment is symptomatic and the majority die in childhood.

Hyperfunction
Catecholamine hypersecretion is usually associated with hypertension due to a neural crest catecholamine-secreting tumor – pheochromocytoma, neuroblastoma, ganglioblastoma or ganglioneuroma, although the mechanism of hypertension in neuroblastoma patients may be renovascular in origin – and discussed below.

ENDOCRINE HYPERTENSION

IMPORTANCE OF HYPERTENSION IN CHILDHOOD
The majority of children with higher than average blood pressure (BP) for age are part of a normal spectrum and those above the 95th centile will, in general, come within the category of essential hypertension although many will simply be obese.[325] BP tracking occurs from an early age in normal children[326] – there are steeper rises in normal levels from ~7 years of age. The pathogenesis of essential hypertension is poorly understood – primary endocrine abnormalities seem unlikely to be of paramount significance. Until pathogenesis is clearer, preventive measures aimed at children in the upper BP centiles will remain controversial. Mass BP screening of children is probably unjustified.[327] Aldosterone levels have been found to predict development of hypertension in normotensive subjects and increased aldosterone action may contribute to hypertension and cardiovascular damage in around 10% of patients with established hypertension.[292]

In contrast, children with sustained and very high BP are likely to have hypertension secondary to specific, and treatable, causes – overwhelmingly (~90%) renal disease (see Chapter 18). Diagnosis and treatment are urgent because, in this group, there is high morbidity and mortality from untreated hypertension. Too few ill children have BP measured. Regular measurements should be made in those

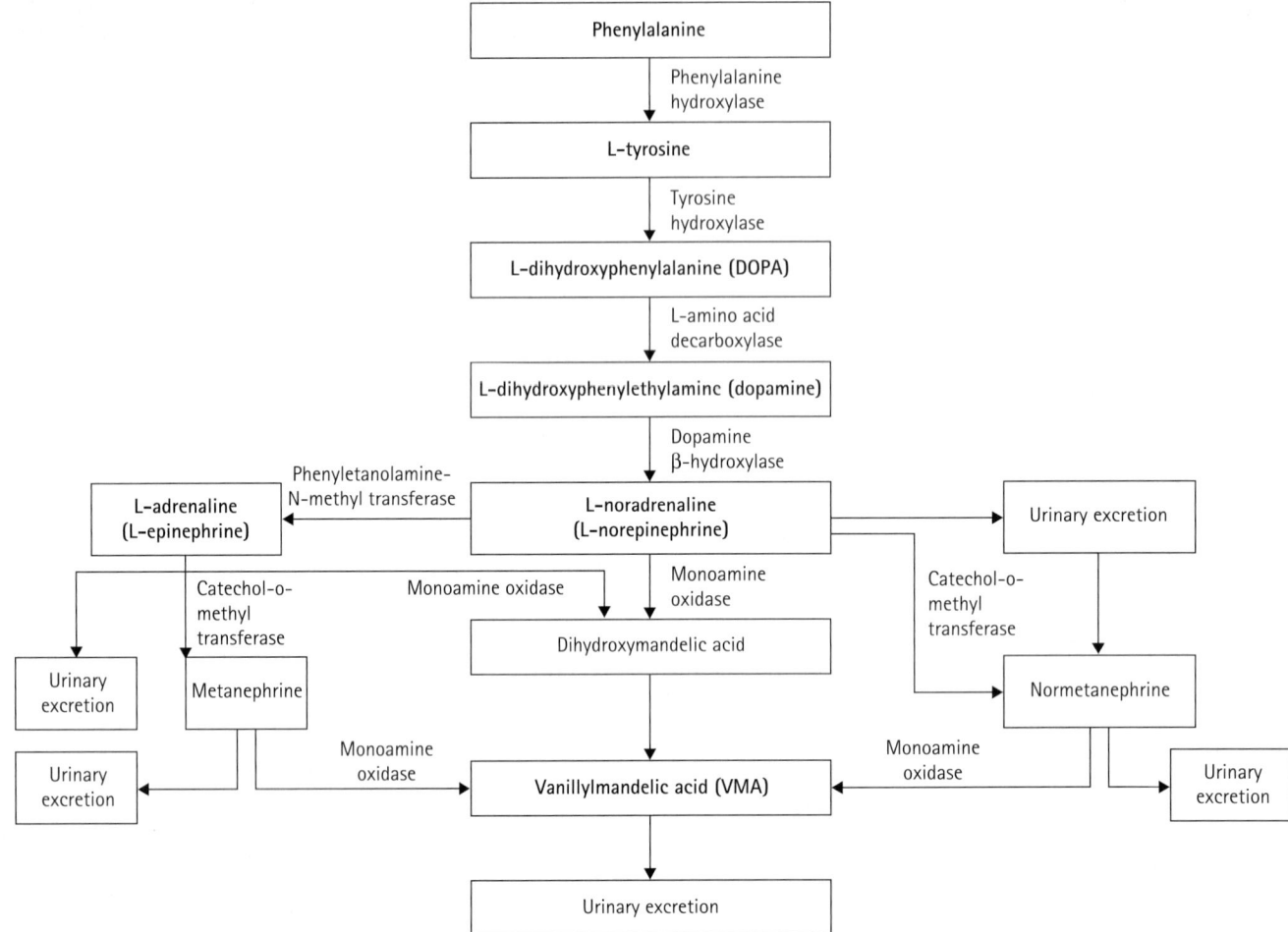

Fig. 15.55   Catecholamine biosynthesis and metabolism.

with renal disease or diabetes and if previously high BP has been found.[327]

Endocrine hypertension usually results from corticosteroid excess (with low renin levels, cf. renal causes) or, less commonly, from catecholamine excess.

ENDOCRINE CAUSES OF HYPERTENSION
Corticosteroid excess
Congenital adrenal hyperplasia (CAH)
Some patients with 11betaOH deficiency and all with 17OH deficiency are hypertensive from ACTH-stimulated mineralocorticoid overproduction secondary to impaired cortisol biosynthesis. In both, excessive DOC levels are generally thought to be responsible for the hypertension (but see above). Appropriate GC treatment returns BP to normal.

Primary and familial forms of hyperaldosteronism
Although rare, their study has increased understanding of mechanisms which may have much wider significance (see above).

Cushing syndrome
Hypertension is common in children with Cushing syndrome but BP may be only moderately elevated. Its etiology is multifactorial including the significant mineralocorticoid effect of excessive cortisol secretion, increased renin substrate and, perhaps, increased vascular reactivity to vasoconstrictors (see above).

Exogenous excessive administration of glucocorticoid is a much commoner cause of hypertension than any of the above.

Catecholamine excess
Pheochromocytomas are rare causes of secondary childhood hypertension. They develop from chromaffin cells. Two thirds are from the adrenal medulla but they can also arise from the sympathetic chain in the abdomen, the mediastinum or the neck. They are usually sporadic but may be familial and associated with MEN 1 and MEN 2 (p. 473) and von Hippel – Lindau syndrome (pheochromocytoma, retinal hemangioblastoma, renal cysts and carcinoma) or neurofibromatosis.[275] The tumors can be bilateral and multiple. In childhood, hypertension is nearly always sustained rather than paroxysmal, and headaches, sweating, nausea and vomiting are common. There may be visual disturbances, abdominal pain, polydipsia and polyuria, convulsions and acrocyanosis.

Diagnosis depends on raised plasma catecholamine levels and increased urinary excretion of catecholamines and their metabolites (metanephrines, VMA and HVA). Repeated collections and estimations may be necessary. Localization of the tumor(s) may be possible by non-invasive techniques [ultrasound, CT scan, [131]I- or [23]I-metaiodobenzylguanidine (MIBG) scintigraphy].

If invasive techniques (e.g. arteriography or vena caval catecholamine sampling) are planned there must be full alpha- and beta-sympathetic blockade, careful BP monitoring and drugs which will acutely lower BP immediately available. Blockade is necessary preoperatively to prevent severe hypertension, hypotension and dysrhythmias during definitive surgical removal. Complete surgical removal results in BP normalization and, usually, 'cure' – only 5–10% are malignant. Analogous pharmacological blockade is necessary in children with hypertension associated with neuroblastoma.

THE ENDOCRINE CONSEQUENCES OF CURING CHILDHOOD CANCER

Long-term effects of radiotherapy (RT) and chemotherapy (CT) on growth and endocrine function have become more obvious and important as survival following childhood cancers has improved. The incidence of childhood cancer is 100–130 per 10^6 per annum and 1 in 600 children under the age of 15 years will develop cancer which is now curable in 65–70%. One in 1000 young adults are now childhood cancer survivors. Leukemia (predominantly lymphoblastic) makes up approximately one third of childhood cancers and brain and spinal tumors about one quarter. Treatment-induced late effects are potentially manifested in a number of areas including growth and puberty, endocrine dysfunction, infertility, cognitive dysfunction and the risk of second tumors.

The risk relates to treatment modality and the challenge remains to further improve survival rates whilst reducing the incidence and severity of treatment-induced late effects. These can be anticipated and monitored to optimize prevention and treatment – ideally through multidisciplinary follow-up involving pediatric oncologist, pediatric endocrinologist, pediatric neurologist, radiation oncologist, pediatric neurosurgeon, clinical psychologist and social worker.

Adverse effects on growth may result from radiation-induced hormone deficiencies, impaired spinal growth from spinal RT (and from CT), primary hypothyroidism from spinal RT, precocious or delayed puberty from abnormal GT secretion, gonadal failure (puberty/fertility) from RT or CT, and problems with nutrition or obesity.

At diagnosis of acute lymphoblastic leukemia (ALL), there is already low bone turnover with reduced levels of collagen formation and resorption markers (PICP, PIIINP and ICTP). In remission, there is further bone synthesis suppression (low levels of PICP and PIIINP) and growth suppression[328] which probably relates to glucocorticoid (prednisolone) and high dose methotrexate therapies. This suggests that there may be an increased risk of long term osteoporosis and fractures. Comparison between countries suggests that the degree of growth impairment is proportional to the intensity of the CT regimen. CT has a disproportionate effect on spinal growth impairment, perhaps because of the large numbers of spinal epiphyses. High dose cranial irradiation is associated with a significant potential height deficit because of the combined effects of precocious puberty and an impaired pubertal growth spurt (see below). Chemotherapy also causes abnormalities of growth and bone turnover in children with solid tumors.[329]

The hormone deficiency effects of RT will depend on the site of irradiation, total dose of irradiation, fractionation schedule and the child's age at treatment. Growth impairment will result from RT to the hypothalamo-pituitary axis (the hypothalamus is more radiosensitive than the pituitary and the GH axis the most radiosensitive followed by the gonadal axis). RT to the spine (in the treatment of medulloblastomas, ependymomas, germinomas) will result in late pubertal growth failure (the spinal growth spurt occurs towards the end of secondary sexual development) and primary hypothyroidism due to a direct effect on the thyroid gland. CT (glucocorticoids, methotrexate) will also impair growth (see above). Tumor recurrence should always be considered as a cause of growth failure in these patients.

RT doses of > 24 Gy will be associated with precocious (especially in young girls) or delayed puberty and GH deficiency within 5 years.[330] Very high RT doses [e.g. ~ 54 Gy (used in craniopharyngioma)] will cause GH deficiency within 2 years. Lower doses (< 24 Gy) may be associated with precocious puberty, an impaired pubertal growth spurt due to relative GH insufficiency and reduced pubertal spinal growth. Total body irradiation (TBI) used as preparation for bone marrow transplantation (~ 7.5–15.75 Gy) may also be associated with pubertal GH insufficiency, thyroid dysfunction and a radiation-induced skeletal dysplasia. In the medium term, impaired beta-cell function seems often to result from TBI resulting in degrees of insulin resistance, impaired glucose tolerance or even frank diabetes.[331]

The same total dose of RT given in several fractions minimizes GHD and growth impairment and fractionated TBI produces less damage to normal tissues. Younger children (especially girls) are more likely to develop precocious puberty and a pubertal growth spurt can be mistaken for 'catch-up' growth. Obesity can normalize growth at the expense of disproportionate bone age advance and reduced height prognosis.

Clinical growth assessment should consist of the regular measurement of sitting and standing height, skinfolds, weight and calculation of BMI, and puberty staging. Laboratory assessment (baseline free thyroxine, cortisol, testosterone/estradiol, IGF-1, etc.), physiological profiles (GH, GTs, cortisol, etc.) and dynamic tests (insulin hypoglycemia, GNRH, HCG, TRH, Synacthen, etc.) will be relevant. Integrating the information as a prelude to appropriate investigation and treatment is an important role for the pediatric endocrinologist in the multidisciplinary team. Much information can be gleaned from careful anthropometry and pubertal assessment in the context of knowledge about the anticancer treatment received so as to minimize investigations in children who have already been through many unpleasant treatments and investigations.

Available treatment modalities include the use of GH for growth failure, pubertal suppression and thyroxine, glucocorticoid and sex steroids as indicated.

If a child has a good prognosis from the underlying condition 2 years from treatment, GH therapy should be given when indicated on biochemical and anthropometric grounds. There is no evidence that GH is associated with reactivation of the primary lesion.

The majority of childhood cancer survivors are fertile. There are low risks of infertility following chemotherapy for Wilms' tumor and ALL and following cranial RT < 24 Gy. Infertility or subfertility is common after CT for Hodgkin disease or RT (TBI, testicular or pelvic). Thus ovarian failure after TBI is common with the risk relating to age at treatment (younger children are at lower risk). Physiological sex steroid replacement therapy improves uterine function (blood flow, endometrial thickness) so that these women could potentially benefit from assisted reproductive technologies. However they have reduced uterine distensibility with increased risk of IUGR and miscarriage or preterm delivery.

In boys, the germinal epithelium is much more sensitive to radiation than Leydig cells – 1.2 Gy to the testis will result in azoospermia, whereas > 20 Gy (in prepuberty) or > 30 Gy (postpuberty) is necessary before Leydig cell function is damaged significantly. Thus spontaneous progression through puberty does not necessarily indicate subsequent fertility. Inhibin B is a potential marker of gonadotoxicity in prepubertal children treated for cancer.[332]

As part of their monitoring, childhood cancer survivors should have routine assessment of gonadal function. The majority will be fertile and the risk of infertility relates to the treatment received. In some situations hormonal manipulation may restore fertility. Counseling is necessary for young people at high risk of infertility and sperm cryopreservation is available for postpubertal boys. Ovarian cortical strip cryopreservation is one current research technique in girls. Strategies to protect the prepubertal testis from damaging effects of CT or RT are under investigation.

An evidence-based guideline for the long term follow-up of child and adult survivors of childhood cancer is available.[333]

THE PANCREAS AND CARBOHYDRATE METABOLISM

PANCREATIC MORPHOLOGY

The pancreas forms by proliferation of endodermal duodenal epithelium at the end of the fourth week of development as separate dorsal and ventral pancreatic buds. The ventral bud migrates posteriorly from a position close to the primitive liver bud and bile duct to lie in close contact with the dorsal bud. The duct systems and parenchyme subsequently fuse and the definitive (common) pancreatic duct is formed by the distal part of the dorsal and entire ventral duct. Failed fusion is a common normal variant. The pancreas is supplied by the splenic and superior mesenteric arteries and drained by the splenic and superior mesenteric veins into the portal vein. The islets of Langerhans, the pancreatic endocrine units, develop from the parenchymatous pancreatic tissue during the third month, are scattered throughout the gland and secrete insulin by about 5 months. There is a rich blood supply to and rich sympathetic and parasympathetic (vagal) innervation in contact with the islet cells.

Exocrine pancreatic function is discussed in Chapter 19. The main endocrine secretions, insulin and glucagon, are intimately concerned in glucose homeostasis. Insulin is secreted from islet beta cells, glucagon from alpha cells. There are also delta cells (thought to secrete somatostatin and perhaps gastrin) and a fourth cell type, F cells, which secrete pancreatic polypeptide (PP). The physiological importance of PP is unclear although it is secreted in response to food. Somatostatin's role in this context is in downregulating the rate of entry of nutrients from the gut by delaying gastric emptying, decreasing duodenal motility, altering splanchnic blood flow, suppressing pancreatic exocrine and endocrine (insulin and glucagon) secretion and gastrin and secretin production from the gut. Thus integration of islet cell hormone and portal vein hormonal secretions is influenced by nutritional state, extrapancreatic hormones (especially gastrointestinal inhibitory polypeptide – GIP) and autonomic input.

INSULIN

Insulin is formed in beta cells from a 9000 molecular weight precursor, proinsulin, itself derived from a larger polypeptide precursor, preproinsulin. Proinsulin is an 86 amino acid linear molecule with three peptide chains – A, B and (intermediate) C (Fig. 15.56). A and B peptides are joined by two disulfide bonds. C peptide is cleaved in Golgi apparatus by proteolytic enzymes leaving the covalently bonded A and B peptides (chains) – the definitive insulin molecule (MW 6000) (Fig. 15.56) – stored in cytoplasmic granules. Insulin and C peptide are thus present in granules in equimolar concentrations and expelled together into the draining capillary (emiocytosis). Circulating C peptide is a marker for endogenous insulin secretion, disappearing at the end of the partial remission ('honeymoon') period of diabetes mellitus.

Insulin is the major metabolic hormone. Factors modulating secretion include glucose, amino acids, glucagon, secretin, gastrin and GIP. During feeding, rising blood glucose and amino acid concentrations stimulate release – there are two phases in the response, a short-lived burst as preformed insulin is released and a slower and more sustained phase of de novo synthesis.

Insulin stimulates glucose uptake by muscle and fat cells, its conversion to glycogen and triglycerides and amino acid incorporation into muscle protein. Lipolysis, glycogenolysis, gluconeogenesis and muscle breakdown are inhibited and hepatic glycogen synthesis stimulated. The net effect is a fall in blood glucose associated with low circulating levels of free fatty acids, ketone bodies and branched chain amino acids. As plasma glucose levels fall below normal (e.g. during starvation), insulin secretion diminishes and secretion of glucagon and other hormones which increase blood glucose levels (catecholamines, GH, glucocorticoids) is stimulated ('counter-regulation') leading to stabilization of blood glucose levels. Insulin is mainly degraded in liver and kidney but also in pancreas and other tissues.

GLUCAGON

Glucagon is a single chain 29 amino acid polypeptide (MW 3485) secreted by islet alpha cells. Plasma levels increase during starvation – falling blood glucose levels are probably the major release stimulus but protein ingestion stimulates secretion through release of gut hormones such as pancreozymin. Anxiety and exercise increase secretion via sympathetic pathways. Somatostatin suppresses secretion.

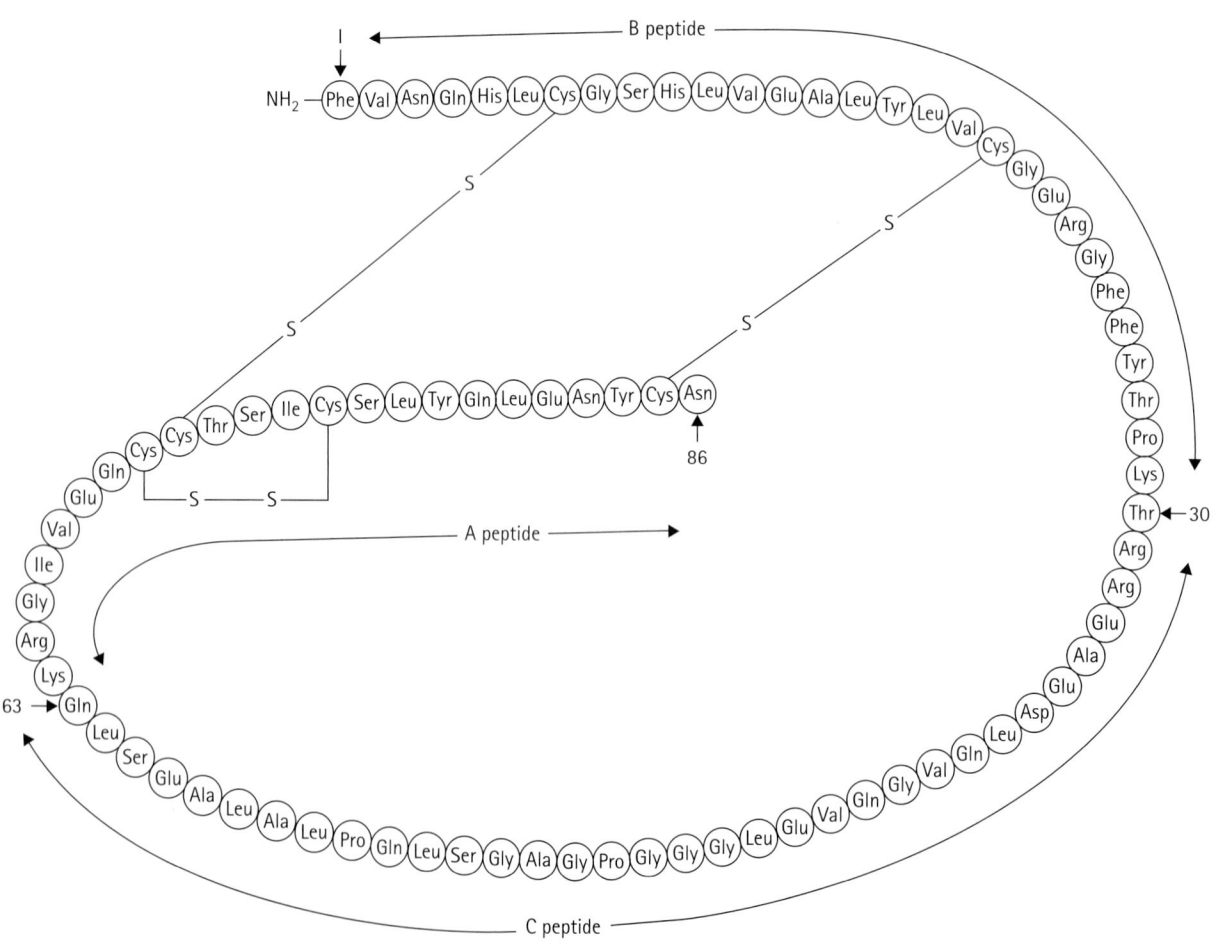

Fig. 15.56   Structure of proinsulin.

Glucagon increases glucose levels by liver glycogenolysis and gluconeogenesis and stimulates fat cell lipolysis (increasing free fatty acids and ketones) and insulin, catecholamine, GH and calcitonin release. Circulatory half-life is only about 10 min – degradation is mainly in liver and kidney.

Integration

Interaction between insulin, glucagon and other counter-regulatory hormones is crucial in glucose and protein homeostasis, to provide sufficient and constant supply of glucose substrate to brain and for growth and energy requirements in infancy and childhood. The liver is particularly important for glucose homeostasis – liver gluconeogenesis, glycogen synthesis and glycogenolysis are summarized in Figure 15.57.

During *starvation*, two thirds of daily glucose production is directly utilized by the brain as an energy source, insulin secretion falls and counter-regulation follows. This produces increased proteolysis, lipolysis, glycogenolysis and gluconeogenesis with reduced tissue glucose uptake resulting in increasing blood glucose levels. There are increased plasma fatty acids (used as an additional energy source), glycerol, ketone bodies and branched chain amino acids associated with high levels of glucagon, cortisol, GH and catecholamines and low or undetectable insulin levels (Fig. 15.58).

In the *fed* state, circulating glucose stimulates insulin secretion and suppresses counter-regulation. Proteolysis, lipolysis, glycogenolysis and gluconeogenesis are suppressed, tissue glucose uptake increases and blood glucose levels fall (Fig. 15.58).

Understanding glucose homeostasis is necessary for rational differential diagnosis, investigation and treatment of hypoglycemia (see p. 490).

Surprisingly little is known about overnight blood glucose levels in normal children. Cyclical variation, periodicity 80–120 min, is described with a gradual fall until wakening with no evidence of a dawn blood glucose rise. In some children levels fall to < 3 mmol/L. Maintenance of normoglycemia seems largely mediated through free fatty acid metabolism (with significant differences between 8 p.m. and 8 a.m. beta-hydroxybutyrate levels) whereas lactate levels suggest that glycogen stores are relatively protected overnight but available for acute hypoglycemic crises.

DIABETES MELLITUS (DM)

DM is defined as a metabolic disorder of multiple etiology characterized by chronic hyperglycemia with disturbances of carbohydrate, protein and fat metabolism resulting from defects in insulin secretion, insulin action or both. Consensus guidelines discussing the epidemiology, classification and management details have been published by the International Society for Paediatric and Adolescent Diabetes (ISPAD)[334] and evidence-based guidelines, with a section on diabetes in children and young people, have been published by the Scottish Intercollegiate Guidelines Network.[335]

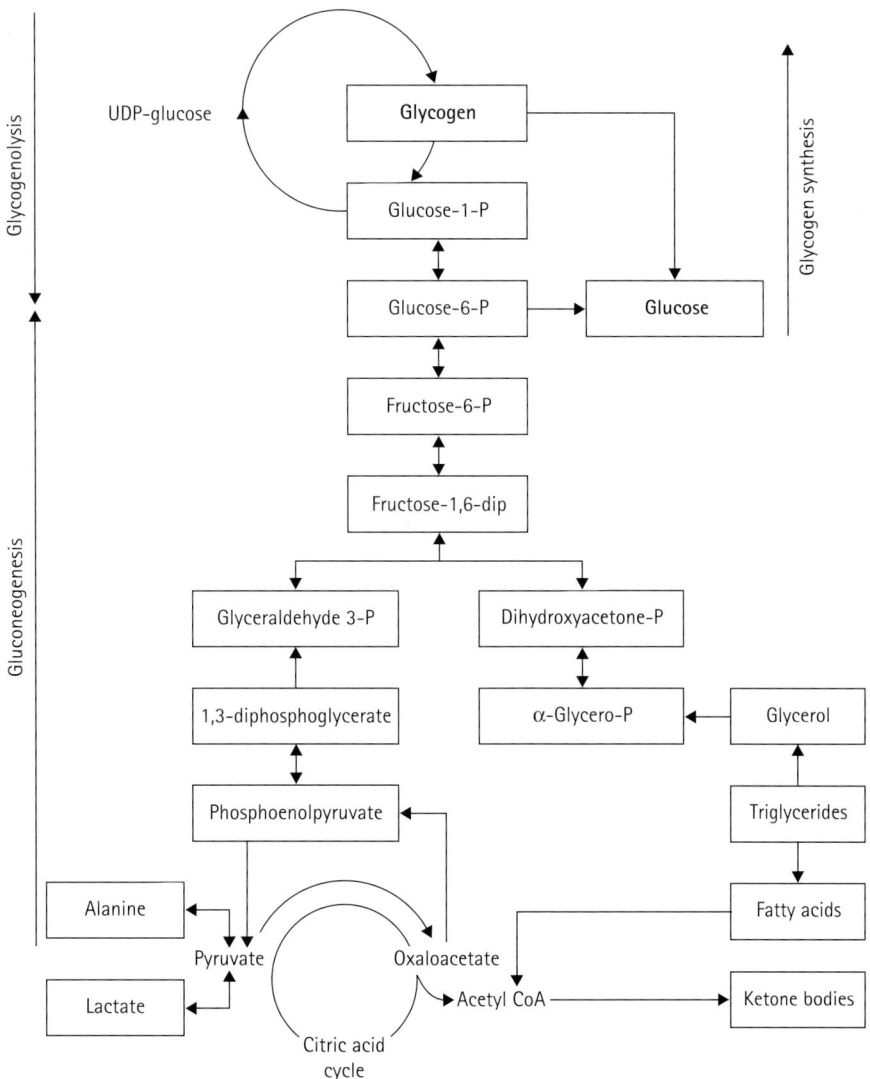

Fig. 15.57 Metabolic pathways of liver gluconeogenesis, glycogenolysis and glycogen synthesis.

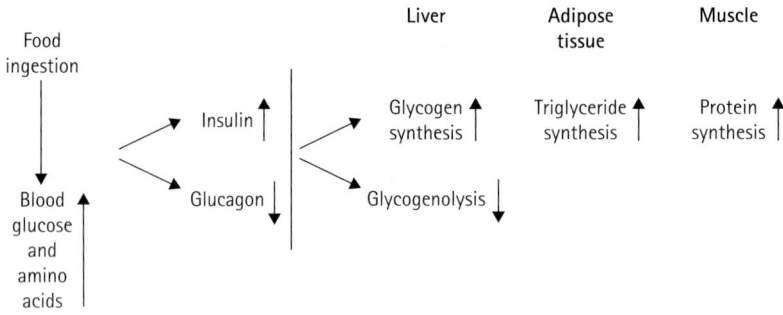

Effects: nitrogen sparing; triglycerides saved for future needs; low circulating levels of ketone bodies, free fatty acids and branched chain amino acids

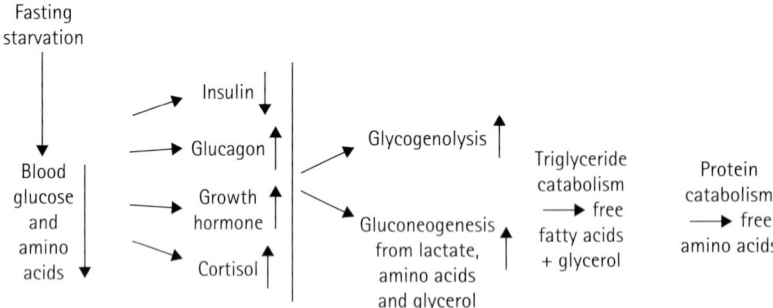

Effects: free fatty acids as energy source; ketone bodies generated from fatty acids; amino acids released by proteolysis for hepatic gluconeogenesis

Fig. 15.58   Metabolic and endocrine characteristics of fed and fasted states.

HISTORICAL INTRODUCTION

Diabetes mellitus (DM) was first mentioned (though not by name) in the 'Ebers' papyrus (about 1550 BC). 'Diabetes' (siphon or diuresis) was first used by the Turkish physician Aretaeos of Capadokia (AD 130–200): 'Diabetes is an awkward affection melting down the flesh and limbs into the urine patients never stop making water life is short and painful they are affected with nausea, restlessness and a burning thirst and at no distant term they expire.' (Aretaeos 1554). The sweetness of diabetic urine ('mellitus' = sweet), first mentioned in sixth century AD Indian Vedic literature was rediscovered by Thomas Willis (1674).[336] Matthew Dobson (1775) showed that the sweet taste was due to sugar and that serum also tasted sweet.[337]

For 1500 years it was thought that the kidney's inability to retain water caused diabetes. Von Mering & Minkowski[338] showed that total pancreatectomy in dogs resulted in diabetes mellitus and, within 10 years, islet function was becoming understood and fasting and dietary treatment introduced. The discovery of insulin by Banting and Best in 1922[339] led to early development of insulin for treatment of human diabetes.

DISEASE SPECTRUM

Recognition of the spectrum of diabetes and its manifestations led to a WHO classification: primary diabetes mellitus is insulin dependent (IDDM) – type 1, or non-insulin-dependent (NIDDM) – type 2, irrespective of age of onset.

DM is the commonest metabolic or endocrine disorder in children and adolescents and was almost invariably type 1. In the past, the diagnosis (as opposed to the management) of DM in children and adolescents has not been complex. However, the current etiological diversity of DM in the young makes their differential diagnosis (suspected clinically and confirmed on a molecular genetic basis) very important for determining prognosis and appropriate treatment.[340]

Non-insulin-dependent DM occurs temporarily in the partial remission ('honeymoon') phase of type 1 DM and permanently in type 2 DM, genetic syndromes accompanied by DM, and 'maturity onset diabetes in the young' (MODY). The overall UK prevalence in young people of non-type 1 DM is currently around 3% of the total, with type 2 making up less than 0.5%. In a largely Caucasian population, MODY is over 10 times more common than type 2 DM. However, type 2 DM predominates in areas with large ethnic minority (e.g. Asian Indian) populations.[340]

Typical phenotypic features in type 1, type 2 DM and MODY are summarized in Table 15.19 – based on referrals to a specialist genetics of diabetes unit in Exeter UK,[340] and ISPAD.[334] There is no single phenotypic marker that is pathognomonic for non-type 1 DM making both individual diagnosis and epidemiological study difficult.[340]

TYPE 2 DM

Type 2 DM has become very much more common in adolescents and children in association with the dramatically rising prevalence of obesity in these age groups but still has a low prevalence in childhood in the UK overall, apart from ethnic minorities who are at increased risk.[165] In Europe as a whole, type 2 DM and impaired glucose tolerance in children and adolescents with obesity is an increasing problem.[342] In contrast to the USA,[343] severe disorders of glucose tolerance are still uncommon even in a UK at risk population.[156]

Intrauterine growth retardation may increase the risk of type 2 DM[33] as may maternal smoking during pregnancy.[344] Many genes are involved in the etiology of type 2 DM, each contributing a small amount to the overall risk. Certain ethnic indigenous populations seem particularly at risk of type 2 DM (e.g. Pima Indians, Australian Aboriginals, Tonga Islanders). Among 15–19-year-old North American Indians, the prevalence of type 2 diabetes per 1000 is 50.9 for Pima Indians, 4.5 for all US American Indians. From 1967–1976 to 1987–1996, the prevalence increased 6-fold for Pima Indian adolescents. Among African Americans and whites aged 10–19 years in Ohio, type 2 diabetes accounted for 33% of all cases of DM.[345]

Table 15.19   Characteristics of pediatric DM patients (After Hattersley 2000[340], 2001[341])

	Type 1	MODY GCK	MODY HNFalpha-1	Type 2	Diabetes + syndromes
Age of diagnosis in pediatric clinic	11 (0–16)	5 (0–16) = age of testing	15 (4–16)	15 (10–16) usually postpubertal females	Variable
Severity of glycemia	Progressive 11–50 mmol/L	Mild 5.5–14 mmol/L	Variable, progressive 5–25 mmol/L	Variable 5–25 mmol/L	Variable 5–25 mmol/L
Ketosis	Ketosis prone, insulin dependent by 5 yr post diagnosis	No ketoacidosis, not insulin dependent	Ketoacidosis rare, not insulin dependent	Ketoacidosis rare, not insulin dependent	Ketosis in DIDMOAD, not in others
Optimal treatment	Insulin	Diet	Sulfonylureas	Metformin	Variable
Parents affected	0–1	1 (often not diagnosed)	1	1–2	Rarely
Obesity	+/–	+/– (5% BMI > 30)	+/– (5% BMI > 30)	++++	Variable + to +++
Acanthosis nigricans	–	–	–	++	Variable
Racial	Low type 2 prevalence	Low type 2 prevalence	Low type 2 prevalence	High type 2 prevalence	All
Islet antibodies	++++	–	–	–	–
Biochemical features		Small increment OGTT	Large increment OGTT, high HDL, low renal threshold	Variable	Low HDL, high TG
Genetic test specificity	+	++++	++++	–	+++

BMI, body mass index; DIDMOAD, DIDMOAD syndrome; GCK, glucokinase; HDL, high density lipoprotein; HNF, hepatic nuclear factor; MODY, maturity onset diabetes in the young; OGTT, oral glucose tolerance test; TG, thyroglobulin.

In Japanese adolescents, type 2 DM is four times more common than type 1. In the USA, young people with type 2 DM are most commonly obese girls from minority populations with insulin resistance, acanthosis nigricans and a family history of type 2 DM. This is becoming a major health problem with up to 45% of children diagnosed with DM in parts of the USA now having type 2. Currently, in the UK, type 2 DM is also becoming much more common, especially in early postpubertal obese girls. There is seldom ketosis at presentation, fasting insulin levels are raised (with low SHBG levels – a marker of insulin resistance), and there is often dyslipidemia and hypertension. Chronic microvascular complications are at least as severe and often occur earlier and more rapidly than in type 1 DM.

There can be diagnostic confusion with type 1 and MODY, but there is, in contrast with type 1, obesity and a stronger family history (an 80% chance of one or both parents having type 2 DM). The obesity and family history do not help the differential diagnosis from MODY where there is a similar family history and age of onset.

Treatment with diet, exercise and, often, metformin is indicated. Metformin is also being used in adolescents with severe insulin resistance and impaired glucose tolerance but its overall effectiveness and safety profile remains unclear.

MATURITY ONSET DIABETES IN THE YOUNG (MODY)

MODY is a heterogeneous group of autosomal dominantly inherited, young-onset beta-cell disorders (Table 15.19). Characteristically, two or more consecutive generations are affected with individuals diagnosed before 25 years of age. MODY comprises two discrete clinical syndromes (Table 15.19): glucokinase MODY [caused by mutations in the glucokinase (GCK) gene on chromosome 7p, MODY 2] and transcription factor MODY [caused by mutations in the genes encoding hepatocyte nuclear factor (HNF)-1alpha (chromosome 12q, MODY 3 – the commonest form), HNF-1beta (MODY 5), HNF-4alpha (chromosome 20q, MODY 1) and insulin promoter factor (IPF)-1 (MODY 4)].[340,341]

In white UK children with non-type 1 diabetes MODY is as common as type 2 DM, and MODY should be particularly suspected if there are three consecutive generations with DM, insulin requirements persistently < 0.5 U/kg/day and no tendency to ketosis. GCK MODY is mild and nonprogressive with hyperglycemia caused by a resetting of the pancreatic glucose sensor. It is treated with diet, and complications are rare.

In contrast, transcription factor MODY results in a progressive beta-cell defect with a high incidence of diabetic complications. Sulfonylureas are the treatment of choice for patients with HNF-1alpha mutations and very good control is achievable. HNF-1beta mutations are associated with DM and renal cysts and HNF-1beta has a critical role in renal development.[346] Mild mutations in IPF-1 predispose to type 2 DM but most transcription factor mutations result in monogenic DM.[341]

TYPE 1 DM

The remainder of this section refers to type 1 DM unless otherwise stated.

Incidence and pathogenesis of type 1 diabetes mellitus

Prevalence (sum of patients related to total age-related population) and incidence (age-related annual manifestations) show wide variations worldwide. Incidence rates for type 1 DM show a 400-fold variation and there are intriguing findings: annual incidence rates broadly increase with distance (north and south) from the equator both within Europe (3.7 per 100 000 in France, 45 per 100 000 in Finland) and within quite small distances within countries (about 2-fold higher in Scotland than England and higher in northern Scotland than southern).[347] Within individual areas, incidence is higher in whites than non-whites and in boys (M:F ratio about 1.1:1) and increases with age, peaking at adolescence. In many studies in geographically disparate countries an increasing incidence of between 2 and 5% per annum is reported (a rise in 50% over 10 years).

Incidence and prevalence differences reflect the complex interaction of genetic and environmental factors (e.g. temperature, nutrition, viruses, chemical toxins) in the development of diabetes. *Genetic factors* are clearly important as there is an increased incidence in parents and siblings of index cases: the risk to a sibling is 15–50-fold that in the normal population and 12–15% of young people under the age of 15 years with diabetes mellitus have an affected first degree relative.[348] Children are three times more likely to develop diabetes if their father has diabetes rather than their mother.[349]

Monozygotic twins are concordant for type 1 DM five times more frequently than dizygotic twins but the rate is much lower than in type 2 diabetes and a discordance rate of nearly 50% over a 30-year follow-up suggests the importance of environmental factors in clinical manifestation of the genetically susceptible individual.

Type 1 DM is a T cell mediated autoimmune disease involving beta cell damage from inflammatory cytokines and autoaggressive T lymphocytes. A large number of chromosomal regions have been identified as containing potential diabetes susceptibility genes although the IDDM1 locus, which encompasses the major histocompatibility (HLA) complex on chromosome 6p, is the major genetic risk factor. The HLA DQ genes are the primary susceptibility genes within this region – loci DR3 and DR4 have particularly strong associations and increase the relative risk for developing diabetes between 3-fold (DR3) and 14-fold (DR3/DR4 heterozygosity). The IDDM2 locus maps to a variable number of tandem repeats in the insulin gene region on chromosome 11.[350]

The HLA identical sibling of a child with type 1 diabetes has about a 90-fold increased risk of developing the disease before 15 years. The risk is hardly increased at all if the sibling is HLA non-identical. Ninety to ninety-eight percent of all type 1 diabetics express DR3, DR4 antigens or both, but fewer than 1% of healthy subjects with such markers will ever develop diabetes.

Environmental factors are crucial for disease expression and clinical diabetes development and may be either causative or protective. Epidemiological data indicate that such factors operate from early in life. The search for preventable environmental triggers for autoimmune destruction and acute decompensation precipitating clinical diabetes onset (by when > 90% of beta cell function is destroyed) continues.

Viruses can cause diabetes in animals, and in humans there is seasonal variation of clinical onset in association with high viral prevalence with a particular association with Coxsackie B4.[351] However, it is known that beta cell destruction, ultimately leading to decompensation and clinical onset of diabetes, occurs over many years prior to presentation. A virus or other 'insult' such as early exposure to cows' milk protein, chemical toxin, certain foods or cooking products, or even stressful life events have been postulated as being responsible for triggering autoimmune (AI) beta cell destruction in genetically susceptible individuals. Childhood vaccinations do not increase the risk of developing type 1 DM in childhood.[352] Acute decompensation, up to many years later and leading to clinical presentation, is often due to an intercurrent infection when insulin requirements rise and cannot, by then, be met.

Histopathological studies indicate that AI mechanisms are paramount in diabetes pathogenesis which has implications for its prevention or modification by immunosuppression. There is a strong association between type 1 diabetes and other AI disease (e.g. thyroid, adrenal, parathyroid).

Although a number of specific genetic, immune and metabolic markers have been identified as significant risk factors there is as yet no evidence for effective prevention.[353] In particular, high dose nicotinamide[354] and low dose oral or parenteral insulin[355,356] have failed to halt beta cell damage in individuals at increased risk for type 1 DM. Screening (whether in the general population or in high risk children and young people) is currently unethical and not recommendable except in the context of future randomized trials of prevention therapy strategies.

Clinical onset and diagnosis

Although, in retrospect, parents may feel their newly diagnosed diabetic child has not been 'right' for several months with poor appetite and malaise, the clinical onset in most children is usually relatively acute: increasing polyuria (due to osmotic glucose load), secondary polydipsia, weight loss, anorexia and fatigue develop over days or weeks.[334] Some children present particularly acutely with rapid onset of ketoacidosis and coma. This may be more common in DR3/DR4 heterozygotes, DR3 patients presenting less. More acute onset is also reported in younger children perhaps because of lack of awareness by parents or health professionals, or pre-existing enuresis, hence the importance of testing the urine for glucose in any child with secondary enuresis.

Once suspected, diagnosis is not usually difficult, but too often there is delay because urine is not tested (for glucose and ketones) when a child presents with nonspecific symptoms or signs – anorexia, vomiting, abdominal pain, tachypnea (assumed to be 'pneumonia'), vaginal candidiasis, fatigue or irritability or recurrent skin infections.[334] Finding glycosuria or hyperglycemia (random level = 11.1 mmol/L) is an emergency – the child should preferably be seen the same day and certainly within 24 h and never simply referred by letter to an outpatient clinic. If diagnosis and treatment are not prompt, further catabolism may rapidly cause increasing ketosis and acidosis (Fig. 15.59) with coma and death. There is still significant morbidity and mortality in children who present with severe ketoacidosis and dehydration, and children unconscious at presentation have a 12-fold increase in mortality compared to those not in coma.[357]

If the diagnosis is in doubt, criteria are the same in children as for adults[358,359]:

- symptoms (polyuria, polydipsia or unexplained weight loss) plus random venous plasma glucose $\geq$ 11.1 mmol/L; *or*
- fasting venous plasma glucose $\geq$ 7 mmol/L [impaired fasting glycemia (IFG) is indicated by a level $\geq$ 6.1 and < 7 mmol/L]; *or*
- plasma glucose $\geq$ 11.1 mmol/L at 2 hours after a 75 g oral glucose load (impaired glucose tolerance is indicated by levels of 7.75 mmol/L up to 11.1 mmol/L).

Normal values 2 hours following the glucose load are < 7.75 mmol/L.

In asymptomatic patients, the diagnosis should only be made on the basis of at least two abnormal measurements of significant hyperglycemia on separate days.

Improvements in health education (of parents and professionals) and prompt access to a specialist pediatric unit will help reduce the incidence of severe ketoacidosis.

Morbidity and mortality will be reduced if specific well-tried, well-understood and adequately supervised management guidelines are followed. An integrated care pathway (ICP) for management of diabetic ketoacidosis[360] (DKA) heightens awareness of optimal diabetes management, increases confidence in management by staff and reduces inappropriate treatment variation leading to improvements in clinical practice (see below). Such ICPs are also of potential benefit in other areas of diabetes management (e.g. the management of the newly diagnosed child without ketoacidosis, hypoglycemia, children undergoing emergency or elective surgery, etc.).

Initial management of the child without ketoacidosis

Most children who have developed diabetes have only mild symptoms and are not ketoacidotic. With a network of primary carers (e.g. diabetes specialist nurses) nearly all such children can be successfully managed at home. Careful continuing assessment – frequent telephone contact and at least daily home visits – is necessary to prevent onset of ketoacidosis at home and to provide basic information.

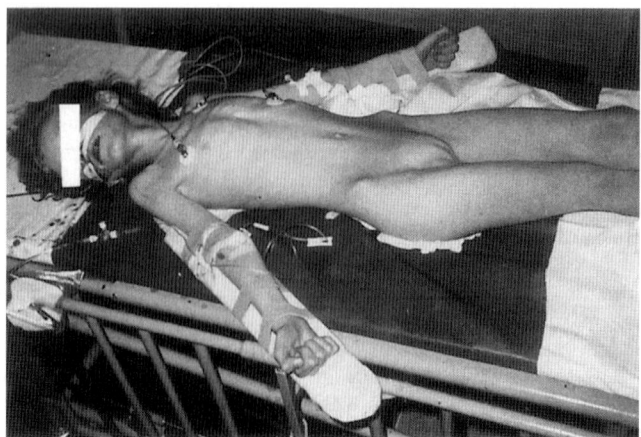

Fig. 15.59 A newly (and 'late') diagnosed diabetic with severe ketoacidosis and dehydration.

This approach is being increasingly adopted in many UK centers and is cost-effective but may be inappropriate for socially deprived families, rural settings a long way from the hospital or, particularly, in areas where adequate community-based personnel with specialist training are unavailable. Some parents are so distressed at diagnosis that admission is desirable. A home-based program of management and education for children and their families is an appropriate alternative to a hospital-based program (Grade C recommendation[335]) but potential benefits of home management – greater acceptance by the family and a quick return to 'normal' family life – can also be achieved if the child's hospital admission is sensitively handled. There is no evidence that either home or hospital initial management and education is superior – the appropriate choice should depend on local circumstances and resources.

Whatever strategy is adopted, several days will be necessary for unhurried education of child and family in basic diabetic care. It is a mistake to try and impart too much early information – upset, anxious, grieving or frightened parents and children are not receptive learners. Simple practical information and instruction about insulin, injection techniques and dietetic principles are important with a positive emphasis that, provided simple guidelines are followed, their child will soon be feeling better than for some weeks and will be able to take part in all the activities enjoyed. Availability of a personal diabetes handbook with written information is helpful.

Recognition and treatment of ketoacidosis

A child with ketoacidosis and severe dehydration (Fig. 15.59) is dangerously ill and requires emergency treatment. Vomiting and abdominal pain with tenderness and guarding may mimic an acute abdomen whilst hyperventilation may be misdiagnosed as pneumonia. There may be circulatory collapse, oliguria and coma. Salicylate poisoning should be considered in the differential diagnosis.

In children known to have type 1 DM on insulin, ketoacidosis is usually precipitated by intercurrent infection (fever is not part of DKA), but may occur if too little insulin is given (perhaps because of fear of hypoglycemia), insulin is omitted altogether (e.g. by an emotionally disturbed adolescent) or with menstruation or severe emotional upset. In this group, there may not be pronounced hyperglycemia, particularly if insulin has been (correctly) continued or increased but vomiting has led to inadequate carbohydrate (CHO) intake. For this reason, urinary ketones should always be tested for by the established diabetic when there is significant hyperglycemia on home blood glucose testing as metabolic decompensation may be more severe than realized. Near patient plasma ketone testing is proving valuable in monitoring the adequacy of treatment and, for example, 'sick day' management at home.

DKA management is facilitated by the use of an integrated care pathway to reduce inappropriate treatment variation leading to improvement in clinical practice.[360] The priority is appropriate *volume repletion* – rehydration is more crucial than insulin in the early stages. Initial fluid should be isotonic (0.9%, 150 mmol/L) saline, or PPS if there is circulatory collapse or unconsciousness – 10–20 ml/kg within the first 30–60 min for initial volume expansion. A rapid history, clinical examination and blood glucose (by indicator stick) will confirm the diagnosis and a sample for true blood glucose, urea and electrolytes, plasma osmolality and arterial blood gas estimation should be obtained as the infusion is set up. Full blood count, hematocrit, platelets and an infection screen (blood culture, urine microscopy and culture, viral cultures, swabs) should be obtained and the ECG monitored.

Dehydration should be assessed clinically:
- mild (3–5%) – dry mucus membranes, reduced skin turgor;
- moderate (6–8%) – the above plus sunken eyes and poor capillary return;
- severe (≥ 9%) – shock with poor perfusion, hypotension, thready pulse, tachycardia;

and, if possible, by weighing and comparing with average weights for age or previous records. PPS should be given if there is severe dehydration and/or marked acidosis.

Whilst hypernatremia is due to severe water loss (exceeding sodium loss), hyponatremia is usually factitious – high glucose levels increase extracellular tonicity and draw water out of cells thereby diluting the extracellular sodium content – and often associated with hyperlipidemia. Empirically derived equations have been developed to calculate the 'true' sodium value which results when all excess glucose is removed from the extracellular fluid: either divide the plasma [glucose] (mmol/L) by 4 and add the result to the measured plasma [Na] (mmol/L), or subtract 5 from the plasma [glucose] mmol/L, divide the result by 3 and add this figure to the plasma [Na] (mmol/L). It can be helpful to apply one or other when managing DKA with initial hyponatremia to identify the [Na] which will be reached with approaching normoglycemia a number of hours later. Plasma sodium levels should rise as ketoacidosis is corrected. If levels are > 150 mmol/L 0.45% saline should be substituted for 0.9% saline. If the plasma sodium is falling rapidly, fluid replacement should be recalculated to be given over 48 hours or longer.

Creatinine levels may be spuriously high due to assay interference by acetoacetate and hematocrit may be falsely elevated by osmotic swelling of erythrocytes in the Coulter counter.

Dehydration should generally be corrected over 24 hours or longer with 0.9% saline. The deficit (ml) is calculated as % dehydration × weight (kg) × 10. Normal fluid requirements are calculated as 100 ml/kg for the first 10 kg body weight, 50 ml/kg for the second 10 kg and 20 ml/kg for the remainder. The hourly infusion rate is then calculated as

$$\frac{\text{maintenance requirements} + \text{deficit}}{24}$$

The volume of any albumin that may have been given during resuscitation should be ignored.

Indications for correcting over 48 hours are pH < 7.1, initial plasma [Na] < 128 or > 150 or any child aged 5 years or less.

A short acting *insulin* must be used and is best given as a continuous intravenous infusion by syringe pump. Conventionally a rate of 0.1 units/kg/h is recommended but a rate of 0.03–0.05 units/kg/h (50 units of a short-acting insulin in 50 ml of 0.9% saline produces a solution containing 1 unit/ml of insulin) has proved safe and effective in our hands over many years. The aim is to decrease the blood glucose gently (by about 2–3 mmol/L/h) and the rate of insulin infusion adjusted in aliquots of 0.1 ml (= 0.1 units) / hour (0.03 units/kg/h should be the minimum infusion rate). This regimen results in a smooth and steady fall whilst being sufficient to switch off ketone production. The infusion should be changed 12 hourly.

Acidosis will almost always correct with correction of fluid balance. Correction should not be too rapid, and as pH is a log scale small changes are significant. If the acidosis is not correcting, resuscitation may have been inadequate and more PPS may need to be given.

Bicarbonate should be considered only with severe acidosis (pH < 7.0), impending circulatory collapse (requiring inotrope support) or respiratory depression and used only on advice of senior medical staff as a slow i.v. infusion. In less severe ketoacidosis it may increase the risk of cerebral edema (due to the large sodium load) and hypokalemia (more rapid shift of potassium into cells) with increased morbidity and mortality. It must be infused slowly intravenously (over 30–60 min) and separately. The amount needed is derived from the formula:

$$\text{mmol bicarbonate (ml of 8.4\% NaHCO}_3\text{) required}$$
$$= \text{wt (kg)} \times \text{base deficit (mmol/l)} \times 0.1$$

Once blood glucose levels are ≤ 13 mmol/L, 0.45% saline/5% dextrose is substituted for 0.9% saline. The insulin infusion rate is then adjusted to maintain blood glucose levels between 7 and 13 mmol/L. If blood glucose levels fall to 7 mmol/l or less, 10% dextrose and 0.45% saline should be substituted without decreasing the rate of insulin infusion further as adequate insulin is necessary to switch off ketosis.

Potassium. There is always substantial depletion of total body potassium whatever the initial plasma level, which will fall once insulin is commenced. KCl (20 mmol/500 ml saline) should be added once the child has passed urine (or in the knowledge that urine has been passed in the previous 4 hours). Potassium replacement can be adjusted to maintain normal plasma levels. A cardiac monitor (observing for T wave changes) is important if levels are abnormal.

If no urine is passed by 4 hours, catheterization may be necessary. Inappropriate ADH secretion may develop (low urine output, high urinary and falling plasma osmolalities) necessitating fluid restriction to prevent cerebral edema. Low plasma sodium levels may be factitious (see above) – plasma osmolality is a better hydration guide. All urine passed should be tested for glucose and ketones.

Neurological observations, including Glasgow Coma Score (GCS – see Table 22.48), should be frequent and changes or development of headache reported to medical staff immediately. A nasogastric tube should be passed if there is vomiting or drowsiness (the stomach will be dilated and aspiration can be fatal), aspirated hourly, and gastric losses included in an accurate fluid balance record. Intravenous ranitidine (1 mg/kg t.i.d) should be given if the aspirate is positive for blood. Antibiotics may be necessary if infection is suspected once bacteriology specimens are obtained. Fluid balance should be calculated hourly and near patient blood glucose should be monitored hourly using a strip test read on a glucose meter. Capillary or venous blood gas measurements, plasma glucose (measured in the laboratory) and urea and electrolytes should be checked 4 hourly until the pH reaches 7.3. The aim should always be to correct metabolic abnormalities slowly – too rapid changes are thought to contribute to the risk of cerebral edema (see below) with significant morbidity and mortality.

Once the fluid deficit is corrected, maintenance requirements should be recalculated and given. The nasogastric tube is removed when bowel sounds are present. Oral fluids can be started gently as tolerated from 12 to 18 hours onwards once pH is > 7.3 and urinary ketones are moderate or less. Intravenous fluids are discontinued when the child is rehydrated, drinking, eating a light diet and ketone free. Intravenous insulin is continued until ketones are absent and just prior to a meal. If the insulin infusion is stopped prematurely, ketonuria and anorexia will take longer to resolve and acidosis may persist.

A suitable initial s.c. insulin regimen is 0.8 units/kg/day given as $\frac{2}{3}$ daily dose pre-breakfast [of which $\frac{1}{3}$ as short acting (soluble) insulin and $\frac{2}{3}$ as intermediate acting (isophane) insulin], and $\frac{1}{3}$ total daily dose split as short acting insulin pre-tea (evening meal) and $\frac{1}{3}$ as intermediate-acting insulin pre-bed. Thirty to sixty minutes after s.c. insulin is given the i.v. insulin infusion is discontinued and the child fed. Potassium should be given orally (as KCl 1 mmol/kg/24 h) for 2 days. Children with DKA are best managed on a high dependency unit and high quality, appropriately experienced nursing care is essential. After recovery, diabetes education begins.

In many countries there are major issues with regard to the provision of skilled medical services to remote and rural communities and this is a particular issue for children with DKA.

Cerebral edema

Cerebral edema is the main cause of morbidity and mortality and single commonest cause of death in children with diabetes. It is a feared complication of DKA, often developing several hours after starting treatment in a context of apparent biochemical and clinical improvement. Over a 3 year period in the mid to late 1990s in the UK, the calculated risk of developing cerebral edema was 6.8 per 1000 episodes of DKA. The risk is higher in new (11.9 per 1000 episodes) as opposed to established (3.8 per 1000) diabetes. Within childhood, there are no sex or age differences but children are more susceptible than adults (in whom hypoglycemia is a much commoner context for cerebral edema to develop).[361] Little is known of the etiology of cerebral edema in DKA – over-rapid fluid replacement and insulin infusion, hypoxemia and injudicious bicarbonate use[362] may increase its likelihood, but it is unlikely to be due solely to management factors – changing management practices have not been associated with a drop in the incidence – and biological patient variables may be important. There may be an association with low arterial partial pressures of carbon dioxide and high urea levels (reflecting the degree of dehydration) at presentation.[362]

Signs and symptoms of cerebral edema consist of headache, irritability, decreasing conscious level (falling GCS) and convulsions. Danger signs are a falling plasma sodium concentration, poor urine output, bradycardia and hypertension. Papilledema is a late sign. Hypoglycemia should be excluded. Diagnosis and treatment are urgent.[361] Mannitol 20% (2 g in 10 ml) 0.5 g/kg should be given i.v. over 30–60 minutes but needs to be started within a few minutes of the diagnosis of cerebral edema if it is to be effective. Mannitol may need to be repeated and there should be urgent discussion with senior medical and ITU/anesthetic staff about the need for intubation and hyperventilation. Any child with a GCS falling below 12 should be observed carefully where there are facilities and expertise for intubation. A GCS of less than 8 will need urgent elective intubation and ventilation which may be life saving. MR scanning is helpful if available. Fluid should be restricted to $\frac{2}{3}$ maintenance and the fluid deficit corrected over 48–72 (rather than 24) hours. Unfortunately, cerebral edema occurs even when management of DKA follows current 'best practice' guidelines and mortality (24%) and morbidity (35% of survivors) rates remain high.[363] Subclinical brain swelling may be common during even optimal treatment[364] and seems generally not to be of long term consequence.

Whilst most increased mortality in diabetes is related to long term complications, there is also a significantly increased mortality in young people, with a 4-fold increase in the age- and sex-specific standardized mortality rate for those diagnosed before the age of 2 years and a 2-fold increase for those diagnosed between 3 and 15 years, in many cases due to ketoacidosis (with or without presumed cerebral edema).[365]

Long-term management

There is irrefutable epidemiological evidence (at least in those aged 13 years or over) from the American 10 year prospective Diabetes Control and Complications Trial[366,367] that if good long term glycemic control is achieved, risks of microangiopathic complications (retinopathy, nephropathy and neuropathy) are greatly reduced. The question is therefore not 'why' or 'whether' to maintain good glycemic control but 'how'.

Other questions remain. Pediatricians seldom see complications silently bequeathed with their patients to adult diabetologists. What level of childhood or adolescent glycemic control constitutes 'sufficiently good' or optimal control? Is prevention of complications by establishment of good control in childhood and adolescence a realistic goal? How is it to be achieved in the context of normal physical and emotional growth and normal daily activities and family lifestyle? Will it be at the expense of more hypoglycemia? If so, how frequent or severe must it be in children of different ages before it affects cognitive function long term? Does more education or new or improved skills in family or clinician necessarily produce better control?

There is now no doubt that better metabolic control is associated with fewer and delayed microvascular complications.[366] This applies to younger children, and suboptimal metabolic control at all ages is likely to be associated with higher risks of acute (DKA, severe hypoglycemia) and long term complications. However, in very young children, the achievement of very tight glycemic control must be balanced against the increased risks of severe, and potentially damaging, hypoglycemia. Basal insulin analogues may be particularly helpful in this regard (see below).

Optimal control must also be achieved in the context of normal family and school life and normal physical and emotional growth. Diabetes is a largely self (child and family) managed condition and successful care models need to focus on strategies that promote and maintain improved self-care behaviors. Children, young people and their families need to be empowered to control diabetes. Specific attempts to increase the effectiveness of education in diabetes care can improve short term control. Focuses need increasingly to be on insulin regimens that are flexible and fit the demands of school and social life. New technologies [continuous subcutaneous insulin infusion (CSII), inhaled insulin, continuous glucose monitoring systems, etc.][368] have the potential to allow young people with type 1 DM to take control of their diabetes.

Motivation derives from encouragement and explanation, not coercion and arbitrary rules. Diabetes must not be ignored but should not need to preoccupy the child or family. Goals need to be framed from the perspective of the person with diabetes and their family. Education (instruction) is a partnership between health care professionals and families which attempts to achieve this through increased understanding of diabetes, empowerment and self-confidence in management.[369] Specific management aims and decisions will reflect the child's age, the family's diverse abilities, motivation and psychosocial backgrounds and personnel and resources available in hospital and community. A consistent approach by all members of the team is vital and will do much to create an environment in which the quality of control can improve.

Normoglycemia is dependent on an appropriate balance between calorie (carbohydrate, fat and protein) intake necessary for normal growth and energy expenditure and insulin. Diverse uncontrollable or unpredictable factors affect glycemia, e.g. intercurrent infection, a birthday party, attending the clinic, exams, GH, puberty, menstruation. Living with diabetes may require support which can be derived from involvement with self-help organizations.

Achieving 'tight' glycemic control in the context of a 'normal' lifestyle remains difficult for many families – in many children control is inadequate – but is helped by the multidisciplinary approach of the pediatric diabetes clinic: doctors have specialist knowledge of pediatrics, growth and diabetes; there is a dietitian present with expertise in pediatric dietetics and diabetes; a psychologist or child psychiatrist may sit in or be readily available. Family emotional problems may be precipitated by diabetes impacting on parents or other siblings; the child's and family's emotional responses to diabetes will themselves have major effects on glycemic control. Omission of insulin, simulating hypoglycemia or making up test results is common and an understandable response in many situations either to gain reward or avoid reprimand. This does not represent severe underlying psychopathology but should prompt a re-evaluation of management and a consistent parental and professional approach with proactive psychological involvement (see below).

Diabetes nurse specialists (DNS) are important assets to a clinic as key members of the multidisciplinary diabetes team linking family, home, school, community and hospital in a way that other health professionals cannot. They provide specific support in hospital and at home at diagnosis and at times of crisis, visit schools to talk to teachers, provide continuing support, advice and education, by telephone and through home and school visits, and discuss specific problems with the hospital-based team.

Insulin regimens

Insulin is vital for glucose transport, storage and disposal. Glucose transport into cells provides energy, conversion to glycogen provides storage in liver and muscle, excess glucose is converted into fat, and protein catabolism is inhibited. The body's insulin requirements are continually fluctuating. In normal individuals, glucose is the main stimulus to insulin release from pancreatic beta cells; insulin is secreted into the portal vein and is immediately physiologically available. Insulin levels thus rise rapidly after meals and snacks with equally rapid falls to basal secretory rates between meals and at night. The main aim in type 1 DM management is to reproduce physiological insulin secretion with the aim of optimizing glycemic control. Most currently practicable regimens do so relatively poorly, but modern molecular engineering techniques – leading to the development of extremely short acting and extended action (true basal/background) insulin analogues – together with developments in continuous subcutaneous insulin infusion (CSII) pump technology are providing opportunities for young people with type 1 DM to take more informed control of their diabetes and achieve improved glycemic control[368] – see below. However, improvement in metabolic control can be related to intensified education and training rather than to pump therapy itself. Patient satisfaction, and perhaps metabolic control,[370,371] may be better with pump therapy than with

multiple injections but it is considerably more expensive financially and in terms of time and resources needed from the diabetes team. Results of research studies may not be directly applicable to a particular clinical setting and patient population, and intensified education with appropriate psychological motivational and dietetic input may still be the most effective and cost-effective way to improve metabolic control in children and adolescents with type 1 DM.

The regimen chosen must be individualized for child and family. Traditional examples are shown in Figure 15.60. Conventional therapy for type 1 diabetes has consisted of twice daily soluble and isophane insulin regimens with support from a multidisciplinary health care team and regular diabetes and health monitoring. Such twice daily regimens are still frequently used by many children and young people and are simple but inflexible (meals need to be eaten on time and have a relatively fixed carbohydrate content). A relatively physiological split is 30% soluble (short acting)/70% isophane (long acting). The insulins can either be premixed and injected using an insulin 'pen' or mixed by the patient (necessitating use of a syringe and needle).

Alternatively, a generally more satisfactory regimen, which reduces the risk of nocturnal hypoglycemia, consists of the pre-breakfast insulin given as above (either free mixing or premixed) but the evening soluble and isophane insulins split with soluble insulin given before the evening meal (supper, Scottish 'tea') and the isophane before bed. Short acting analogue insulin can be substituted for soluble insulin in these regimens and may be valuable in managing some patients, e.g. toddlers whose appetite is unpredictable and who can be injected after the meal.[372] Lente insulin is far from ideal as a 'background' – it has a peak in action between 2 and 6 hours after injection and even ultralente has a significant peak at 8–12 hours. Basal analogue insulins are preferable.

More intensive multiple daily injection (MDI) basal–bolus regimens are also used. In one regimen, soluble insulin is given preprandially and isophane insulin at bedtime. The soluble insulin provides sufficiently

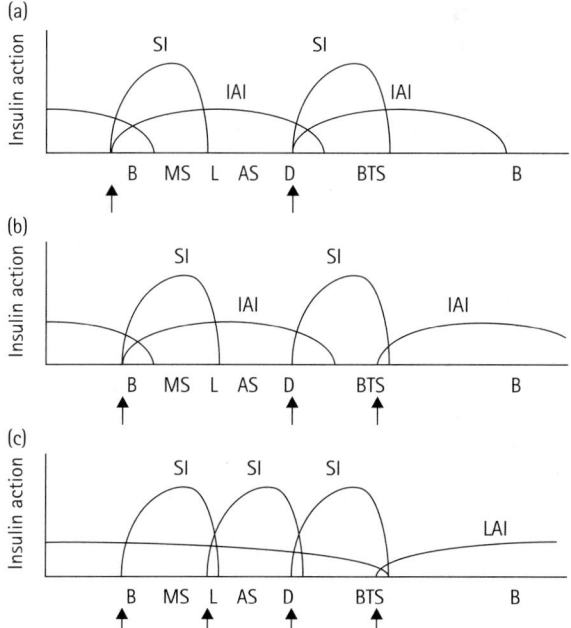

Fig. 15.60 Examples of insulin regimens: (a) two daily doses of short and intermediate acting insulins; (b) as (a) but the evening intermediate acting insulin delayed until bedtime; (c) insulin pen regimen – combination of preprandial short acting insulin with long acting insulin at bedtime. Key: B = breakfast; MS = mid-morning snack; L = lunch; AS = afternoon snack; D = dinner (Scottish tea); BTS = bedtime snack; SI = short acting insulin; IAI = intermediate acting insulin; LAI = long acting insulin; ↑ = insulin injection.

sustained action over the day to provide basal as well as bolus (meal-time) insulin availability. The main disadvantage is the need for four injections daily but this is compensated for by flexibility of lifestyle, meal sizes and times and exercise. Better, and obviating the need for snacks between meals, boluses of rapid acting insulin analogues (see below) can be given up to five times daily preprandially with a basal analogue insulin at bedtime. The bolus analogue can be given immediately before (or even during or immediately after) a meal (obviating the need to wait 20–30 minutes with soluble insulin). There is a reduced risk of nocturnal hypoglycemia and improved postprandial control with analogue[373,374] rather than soluble insulin[367] regimens with the added potential for improved glycemic control.

CSII regimens deliver insulin via an indwelling subcutaneous (usually abdominal) fine cannula, powered by microprocessor controlled pump devices which allow variable and programmable basal infusion rates between meals and overnight together with boluses of insulin when food is taken. This is undoubtedly the regimen which currently approximates most closely to physiological insulin delivery in people who do not have diabetes, with the potential for optimal glycemic control and reduced risk of hypoglycemia. Missing a meal or unexpected exercise can be adjusted for much more readily.

In contrast to the situation when insulin pump therapy was first introduced in the 1970s, current CSII and pumps seem well tolerated by children and young people because of their small size and flexible programmability which puts them in control of their diabetes – sporting activities without hypoglycemia, flexible meals in keeping with their peer group and less nocturnal hypoglycemia. However, there are still few published randomized trial data on the efficacy and safety of CSII versus MDI regimens. Evidence regarding the impact of an intensive insulin regimen (four or more injections or CSII) on long term control is derived principally from the Diabetes Control and Complications Trial (DCCT) which also involved a comprehensive patient support element (diet and exercise plans, monthly visits to the health care team, etc.).[367] Thus although intensive insulin therapy (MDI or CSII) significantly improved glycemic control over a sustained period compared with conventional insulin therapy (two injections per day), DCCT did not include children aged less than 13 years and, due to the study design, it is impossible to separate the benefits of intensive insulin therapy from intensive support.

In any case, intensive insulin therapy should only be delivered as part of a comprehensive support package (Grade B recommendation[335]). Thus CSII has resource implications – not only are insulin pumps and their consumables expensive but intensive support is necessary from diabetes teams (increased patient and family contact and support at least in the early stages, continuous blood glucose monitoring downloading and advice, etc.).

The insulin regimen should be tailored to the individual child to achieve the best possible glycemic control without disabling hypoglycemia (Grade C recommendation[335]). The number of daily insulin injections does not necessarily correlate with excellence of glycemic control. In a study from Sweden,[375] mean HbA$_{1c}$ levels of 7% and a low incidence of severe hypoglycemia have been reported with such an intensive regimen, but in Belgium[376] similar results have been reported using a twice daily insulin regimen. Other important factors for good glycemic control include continuing support from the health care team, psychosocial factors and blood glucose self-monitoring.

Insulin Analogues. There are currently several rapid acting insulin analogues available: insulin lispro (reversed proline and lysine at positions B29 and B30), insulin aspart (aspartate substituted for proline at B28) and insulin glulisine (lysine replacing asparagine at B3, glutamate replacing lysine at B29). Plasma insulin concentrations peak more rapidly and higher and decrease more rapidly than following soluble s.c. insulin. The peak action is approximately one hour after injection and there is no activity by 3–4 hours. A virtually peakless long acting insulin analogue (glargine insulin) has recently become available[377] – there is C terminal elongation of the insulin beta chain by two arginines and replacement of asparagine by glycine in position A21 – and experience

is developing in its use.[378–381] Hypoglycemia risks may be reduced using glargine compared to NPH (lente) insulin in adults[382] and similar data are now available in children and adolescents.[383]

A further long acting insulin analogue (insulin detemir) has now been introduced. Its pharmacokinetic profile suggests that its action may be slightly shorter than that of glargine but it too may decrease hypoglycemia risk in children with type 1 DM.[384] Indeed it may be superior in that regard as it has a significantly more predictable glucose-lowering effect than both NPH insulin and insulin glargine.[385] More studies and wider experience are necessary before the definitive role of these basal insulins in children and adolescents with type 1 DM can be determined but they are likely to increasingly replace NPH insulin and are particularly valuable in very young children.

With a combination of rapid and basal analogue insulins it is potentially possible to achieve improved ('tighter') control without problematic hypoglycemia. This reflects both the reduced variability of absorption of the basal analogue insulins and an awareness that bolus insulin analogues must be adjusted on the basis of postprandial plasma glucose increments.

Insulin requirements

About 30–60% of children and adolescents demonstrate a partial remission ('honeymoon') phase (insulin requirements <0.5 units/kg/day) for up to 6 months (sometimes longer) after diagnosis. Subsequently average insulin requirements are in the order of 0.6–0.8 units/kg/day although considerably higher doses are necessary during the adolescent growth spurt (in early female and late male puberty).

Insulin requirements will vary according to activity levels, intercurrent illness, etc. Insulin resistance will develop when blood glucose levels have been high over a period of days or weeks (perhaps due to injecting into lipohypertrophic sites, eating inappropriately or intercurrent infection or omitting insulin). Increased insulin doses may be necessary for several weeks but it is important then to reduce the dose once more to avoid a vicious cycle of eating more to prevent hypoglycemia, resulting in weight gain and further increased insulin requirements and appetite.

Insulin adjustments are ideally based on home self-monitoring of blood glucose (see below). With consistent abnormalities at a particular time of day the appropriate insulin is adjusted up or down by child or parent, if necessary after consultation by phone with a member of the diabetes team. Development of skills in independent adjustment of insulin varies considerably between individuals and their families but adjustment only every few months in clinic is very unsatisfactory. Written information should be given for 'sick day' management and discussed at annual review appointments.

Subcutaneously injected insulin bioavailability is very variable but basal analogues seem superior in this regard. Absorption varies with injection site – fastest from the abdomen and slower from the thigh than the arm – and with exercise (see below) or if the site is rubbed after injection. If the same injection site is used repeatedly (because the injection becomes painless) lipohypertrophy (Fig. 15.61) is likely and injecting into lipohypertrophic injection sites is an extremely common cause of poor and unpredictable insulin absorption and erratic glycemic control amongst children and young people with type 1 DM.

Of the continuing developments in alternative insulin delivery routes (including oral, transdermal, intranasal), inhaled insulin, absorbed across the alveolar surface of the lungs, is now available for use in adults. Both liquid and dry powder formulations have been developed. There is a rapid onset and early peak action (similar to the time course of s.c. rapid acting analogue insulin) but with a longer period of action (more comparable to s.c. soluble insulin).[386] Insulin could be given by inhalation as often as necessary as preprandial boluses – injections would still be required for basal insulin administration. The relative efficiency of insulin delivery by aerosol, compared to s.c. injection, has been estimated as between 8 and 25%.[387] Initial studies in children and adolescents seem promising[368] but there remain significant anxieties about the use of inhaled insulin in children with still developing lungs and especially in those with common respiratory conditions such as asthma. Observations

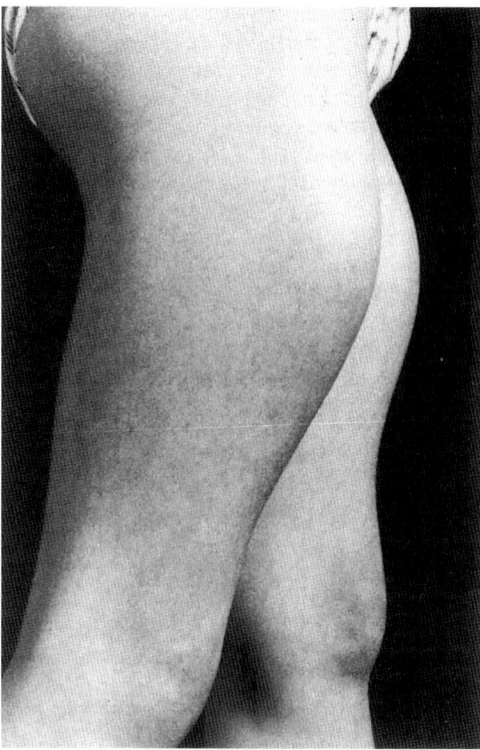

Fig. 15.61 Severe lipohypertrophy in a diabetic child on human insulin who was not adequately rotating the injection sites.

including alterations in pulmonary function tests,[388] a higher frequency of severe hypoglycemia[389] and increased insulin antibody formation[388,389] give particular cause for concern.

If a child with type 1 DM requires emergency or elective surgery, clear protocols or an integrated care pathway should be in place to facilitate safe management. In the perioperative period, additional metabolic demands contributing to unstable glycemic control potentially include preoperative fasting and dehydration, the stress response to surgery and anesthesia and postoperative calorie and fluid deficits. With careful management, mortality and morbidity should be no higher than in children without diabetes.

Emerging options

By clinical presentation more than 90% of beta cell function is already destroyed. Nonspecific immunosuppressive therapy at diagnosis, with toxic drugs such as cyclosporin A, has been shown to prolong the partial remission period, but no case of total remission or with normal glucose tolerance has been reported[390] and renal toxicity was common. Nevertheless, less toxic immunosuppressive agents have been developed and the possibility of a potential 'cure' for diabetes by pancreatic islet cell transplantation to secrete insulin physiologically in response to endogenous metabolic signals is an extremely attractive proposition if it could be realized.

However, despite the successful reversal of diabetes in small animal models, insulin independence after islet allotransplantation has been very difficult to achieve in the human with the use of diabetogenic immunosuppressive agents to suppress both islet alloimmunity and autoimmunity, the critical islet mass to achieve insulin independence and the detrimental effects of transplanting islets in an ectopic site and loss of graft function with time.[391] Promising approaches to these problems, including xenogeneic sources of cells, engineering islet cells with genes that induce expression of immunoprotective molecules, and neogenesis factors that may sustain populations of transplanted beta cells, are demonstrating that islet allotransplantation still has great potential to become an established treatment option.

Human beta cell lines derived from pancreatic tissue obtained from infants with persisting hyperinsulinemic hypoglycemia of infancy (PHII) which respond to physiological glucose levels are of potential use both in gene therapy for PHII and in cell transplantation studies for administering insulin for the treatment of diabetes mellitus.

Diet

If it is to be acceptable to child and family and followed in practice, diet should be closely related to recommendations for nondiabetics, but is inevitably tempered by the family's eating habits which may fall short of that ideal. Rigid and dogmatic rules encourage noncompliance. In the past, diets have involved 'quantitative' advice with a 'stable' carbohydrate intake at regular intervals: breakfast, mid-morning snack, lunch, mid-afternoon snack, evening meal, bedtime snack.

A regimen which includes dietary management has been shown to improve glycemic control and is recommended (Grade B recommendation[335]). Specialist dietetic advice should be given by a dietitian with expertise in childhood diabetes wherever possible. Until the 1980s, counting of carbohydrate exchanges was recommended. The carbohydrate (CHO) exchange system (one exchange = 10 g CHO) has the virtue of dogmatic simplicity allowing a wide variety of foods to be eaten, but all nutrients can, of course, be converted directly or indirectly to glucose. The previously conventional guide to CHO intake (100 g per day for a 1 year old plus an extra 10 g per day for each additional year of age) needed to be varied considerably to meet growth and energy requirements of the individual. The proportion of CHO was high enough (40–50%) to enable fat intake to be reasonably low – less than 35% of calories should be from fat, which should be polyunsaturated to reduce long term risks of hyperlipidemia and cardiovascular disease.

The recognition that not all types of carbohydrate have the same effect on blood glucose levels and of the potentially restrictive nature of counting CHO exchanges had led to a change in focus to 'healthy eating'. However, the emphasis has shifted again towards the view that flexible intensive insulin treatment combining dietary freedom and insulin adjustment can improve both glycemic control and quality of life.[392] Such approaches are being studied in children, and newer insulin regimens (MDI or CSII) require CHO intake assessment once again if short or rapid acting insulin is to be given in appropriate dosage.

CHO type remains important: concentrated, rapidly absorbed, sugary food taken in significant and regular amounts precludes stable glycemic control and should be confined to occasional treats before exercise, or at the end of a meal. Starchy, low fiber foods are acceptable, but starchy high fiber foods (Table 15.20) are best, because of their gradual

Table 15.20 Some high fiber foods

Wholemeal bread
Wholemeal spaghetti
Wholemeal cereals
Weetabix
Jacket potatoes
Ryvita
Oatcakes
Dried beans
Lentils
Fruits
Apples
Bananas
Blackberries
Pineapple
Strawberries
Vegetables
Brussels sprouts
Cabbage
Peas
Sweetcorn

absorption and metabolism. With education of the general population towards 'healthy eating' these foods are now more socially accepted and more easily obtainable cheaply.

Dietary management is therefore the 'art of the possible' and involves educating the whole family's eating habits. A pediatric dietitian with an interest in diabetes is a crucial part of the management team. A sensible approach to 'treats', fast foods and reasonable flexibility over timing is more likely to lead to cooperation; psychological benefit (not being different to family and friends) is likely to benefit lifestyle and control.

Exercise

Exercise has major effects and in children is variable and capricious. Regular exercise allows participation in peer group activities and improves self-confidence and physical fitness. Strenuous exercise usually results in rapid but unpredictable falls in blood glucose (increased insulin mobilization results from increased blood flow and muscular activity). Energy stores (and particularly muscle glycogen) are depleted during medium to long duration exercise and hypoglycemia can occur up to many hours afterwards. Before activity, an extra 10–30 g CHO may be necessary depending on age, blood glucose level and the intensity of exercise planned (best taken as pure fruit juice or an isotonic sport drink). Such drinks are best taken during and after exercise as well, rather than loading with carbohydrate before the exercise starts. It is sensible to have a snack within an hour of completing the activity and post- (as well as pre-) exercise insulin doses may need to be reduced.

On a background of under-insulinization, exercise results in counter-regulation and hyperglycemia with ketosis. It is important not to exercise in the presence of ketones – exercise is not a replacement for insulin. On activity holidays it is often sensible to cut insulin by < 50% if severe hypoglycemia is not to result on the first day even with additional snacks.

Psychological interventions

In the past, there has been a tendency to expect children with diabetes to take on too much responsibility for their diabetes management at too young an age. As they grow older, children with diabetes pass through a stage of 'interdependence' (between total dependence on parents and full independence) where they know what to do and how to do it, in terms of the practicalities of, for example, drawing up and injecting insulin and self blood glucose monitoring (SBGM), but are not ready to take responsibility for injections or monitoring. Maintaining parental involvement improves glycemic control.[393,394]

Managing diabetes is inevitably stressful at times, both for the children with diabetes themselves and for their families. Factors contributing to an increased risk of young people with diabetes developing psychological problems include: too much responsibility being placed on the child; avoidance coping (never coming to terms with diabetes emotionally or developing conscious or unconscious strategies which do not address the problem faced); family conflict or lack of communication both within the family and with the diabetes team; low socioeconomic status or a nontraditional family structure;[395] poor maternal health, especially depression.[396]

Eating disorders are more common in adolescents with diabetes compared with nondiabetic peers, especially in girls, adversely affect glycemic control and can be difficult to treat.[397] Specific psychological problems linked potentially to future poor glycemic control (e.g. maladaptive coping strategies) can be identified at diagnosis and 1–2 years later, using validated tools performed by a trained practitioner.[398] Regular assessment for psychological problems, especially maladaptive coping strategies and eating disorders, is desirable (Grade B recommendation[335]).

Psychological or educational interventions have positive effects on psychological outcomes and knowledge about diabetes and glycemic control.[399] Interventions which promote diabetes-specific coping skills are effective and add to the effectiveness of intensive management.[400] Thus the use of cognitive coping strategies targeted at diabetes-specific problems is recommended (Grade A recommendation[335]) and parental support and family communication should be encouraged, with targeted psychological treatment of family disruption and related stress factors (Grade B recommendation[335]). Education programs, computer-assisted packages and telephone prompting should be considered as part of a multidisciplinary lifestyle intervention program (Grade B recommendation[335]). It is desirable that health care professionals should receive training in patient-centered interventions in diabetes (Grade B recommendation[335]).

Glycemic control and its assessment

Many children with type 1 DM enjoy active and healthy lives but some are poorly controlled requiring frequent hospital admissions for ketoacidosis, hypoglycemia or stabilization. Poor control may reflect unhappiness or instability in the family (see above), particularly if there has never been emotional (as opposed to intellectual) acceptance of diabetes.

'Brittle' diabetes[401] is now accepted to be overwhelmingly due to insulin omission – injection sites should be checked for lipohypertrophy, but fruitless searches for underlying metabolic abnormalities are counterproductive. Long term poor control causes severe stunting of growth and pubertal development and may be associated with 'Cushingoid' obesity and hepatomegaly (Mauriac syndrome). Gross abnormalities are now seldom seen and assessment of physical and emotional growth and well-being while essential are, in themselves, insufficient – normal growth and no reported symptoms of hypo- or hyperglycemia may be found even when glycemic control is far from ideal.

Insulin adjustments are ideally based on home self-monitoring of blood glucose (SBGM). Checking for glycosuria gives limited retrospective information about likely previous blood glucose levels (has the level been high enough to exceed the renal threshold for glucose since the bladder was last emptied?), do not warn of impending hypoglycemia, and are valueless with normoglycemia as the optimal therapeutic goal. Even early morning glycosuria may be misleading, reflecting early morning hyperglycemia (excessive insulin the previous evening with counter-regulation, the Somogyi effect), too little insulin, or the 'dawn phenomenon' – decreased insulin sensitivity due to nocturnal GH peaks.

Immediate knowledge of blood glucose levels is only of practical benefit if child and parents understand their significance and relevance and are motivated to take appropriate action on the basis of consistent abnormalities. That SBGM monitoring does not, in itself, lead to better control[402] is not surprising. Blood tests done in rotation once or twice daily just before main meals and at bedtime, and occasionally 60–90 min after main meals, an acceptable regimen for many, will provide most information from fewest tests. Blood glucose estimation is of particular value during illness or symptoms that could relate to hypoglycemia. Nevertheless blood tests are uncomfortable and a chore. Education and motivation will reduce the number omitted, done inaccurately or of results made up to 'keep the doctor happy'. Intensive treatment of type 1 DM (using MDI or CSII) requires more frequent measurements (post- as well as preprandially – '8 point profiles') for optimal glycemic control.

However, conventional daytime SBGM provides incomplete information on nocturnal (hypo)glycemia for which the development and availability of continuous glucose monitoring systems (CGMS) is a major advance. The glucose sensor is inserted (via a needle which is then withdrawn) into s.c. tissue, usually of the anterior abdominal wall. An electrical signal is generated by the oxidation (catalyzed by glucose oxidase in the sensor) of glucose in the interstitial fluid. Systems providing 'real-time' data are available. Patterns of hypo- and hyperglycemia not detectable by conventional SBGM will become apparent in young people using CGMS[403] and improvement in glycemic control can be expected (it has already been documented in adults[404]). As with conventional SBGM, the relative error of the measurements is likely to increase at levels in the hypoglycemia range[404] and the relative importance of pressure or temperature changes (especially overnight) remains to be determined.

Amongst available technologies, the combination of CSII therapy with glucose sensor data from CGMS currently provides the nearest approach to mimicking physiological insulin secretion and allowing motivated children and young people to achieve and maintain optimal control of their diabetes whilst minimizing hypoglycemia (not least at night).

Glycosylated hemoglobin (HBA$_{1c}$). Hemoglobin forms a non-enzymatic link with glucose – percentage of glycosylated hemoglobin (HbA$_{1c}$) is an objective measure of integrated glycemic control over the previous 6–8 weeks. Assessed in this way, the majority of diabetic children are less than ideally controlled[405] and in some control is abysmal. Identifying this group is easier than improving the situation. There has been doubt as to the appropriateness of some laboratory quoted normal ranges for HbA$_{1c}$ and the 'target range' (6–8% with a DCCT-equivalent method) is lower than previously considered desirable. It is likely that the risk of microvascular complications rises sharply above mean HbA$_{1c}$ levels > 9%.[406] This has implications for children, at greater risk of hypoglycemia and its consequences, when 'tight' glycemic control is the aim (see below). Finding high values is helpful when home monitoring results apparently indicate excellent control – either monitoring technique is faulty or, commonly, there is deliberate manipulation due to emotional disturbance.

The ideal HbA$_{1c}$ value (between 6% and 8%) reflects average blood glucose levels since the last estimation of approximately 6.5 mmol/L and 10.5 mmol/L respectively. A 1% increase in HbA$_{1c}$ reflects an average increase in blood glucose levels of 2 mmol/L in the preceding period – a mean HbA$_{1c}$ value of 10% will reflect prior mean blood glucose levels of around 14.5 mmol/L, i.e. very poor control.

HbA$_{1c}$ estimation is much more valuable if the current result is available in clinic so that appropriate discussion can take place with the child and parent(s) and appropriate advice given. In many clinics, portable or fixed analyzers are available to provide such a service; if that is not the case, capillary blood samples on filter paper or in special containers can be obtained at home shortly before the next clinic visit and posted to the laboratory. Shorter term indices of glycemic control, e.g. plasma proteins such as fructosamine, may be useful when assessing, for example, the efficacy of a specific therapeutic intervention.

Hypoglycemia

Parents, and many children, worry particularly about 'hypos' and, especially, nocturnal hypoglycemia which is likely to be more common with the quest for tighter glycemic control. Recently introduced basal analogue insulins reduce the variability of blood glucose levels, and thus achieve significant relative risk reductions for hypoglycemia, particularly at night.

There are few long term neurophysiological and psychometric studies of effects of frequent mild hypoglycemia. Children's hypoglycemic symptoms differ from those of adults. In very young children, neuroglycopenic symptoms (dizziness, poor concentration, drowsiness, weakness) and nonspecific symptoms (tearfulness, confusion, tiredness, irritability, aggression) are reported more frequently than autonomic symptoms (hunger, trembling, pallor). Sweating is absent during the early stages of hypoglycemia in prepubertal children with type 1 DM and other symptoms may be minimal. This is despite the fact that children (with and without diabetes) have a much more pronounced catecholamine response to hypoglycemia than do adults. However, the prolonged nature of nocturnal hypoglycemic episodes in children may be explained in part by defective counter-regulation. Weakness is the symptom most commonly reported by children, and the sign most frequently reported by their parents is pallor. Severe hypoglycemia can be associated with transient hemiparesis.[407]

Children diagnosed before 3 years potentially have particular problems with hypoglycemia. This relates both to the common occurrence of hypoglycemia in the children with type 1 DM (the normal young child has a relative inability to maintain normoglycemia during even periods of 6–12 h without food) and to the increased sensitivity to hypoglycemia of the still maturing brain. Children with type 1 DM can have episodes of profound and prolonged hypoglycemia with glucose nadirs of < 2 mmol/L and yet no effect on sleep.[408]

Occasional mild hypoglycemia – a feeling of hunger with faintness, headache or belligerency if a meal is delayed (but see above) – indicates tight control and seems harmless. Hypoglycemia is usually caused by delayed or missed food, unexpected (or unexpectedly strenuous) exercise or excess insulin administration (by mistake, or, more rarely, deliberately). There is particular risk after diagnosis when endogenous insulin secretion is temporarily partially re-established if exogenous insulin is not reduced.

Both stress and early stages of an intercurrent viral illness can cause hypo- rather than hyperglycemia. Children and young people with diabetes should always carry extra glucose: 3 glucose tablets should be taken at early signs of hypoglycemia (alternatives are 50 ml of Lucozade or 2 teaspoons of glucose powder added to juice) and followed by food. 'Hypo' management must be available to families in written form and specifically discussed at annual review clinic appointments.

A child having a moderate or severe hypo will require assistance. A semiconscious or uncooperative child who cannot coordinate swallowing a sweet drink should be given a glucose gel product. This is available on prescription in the UK as GlucoGel and is rubbed into the inside of the cheek but should not be given to an unconscious child unless by a health care professional. In the unconscious or fitting child at home, glucagon (available as a GlucaGen kit, 1 mg i.m. or s.c.) should be given. Both will improve neuroglycopenia and the conscious level sufficiently for oral sugary carbohydrate (e.g. sugary juice plus toast and jam) to be given. If it is not, glucose levels will fall again – sometimes a problem with glucagon as it can induce vomiting. Blood glucose levels should be checked at home every 15 minutes for an hour to ensure that they return to normal. The next dose(s) of insulin may need to be reduced depending on the cause.

Prolonged severe hypoglycemia resulting in cerebral edema is seen following deliberate and massive insulin overdose and in adolescents after significant alcohol intake and can cause death or permanent brain damage. Hypoglycemia may be the major contributing factor to 'unexplained' death in otherwise healthy young people with type 1 DM.[365] Young people, including students, who live alone, abuse drugs or have had a previous psychiatric referral are particularly at risk.

ADOLESCENCE (see also Ch. 35)

Adolescence is characterized by major changes in energy intake, growth and hormonal maturation as well as by profound changes in cognitive function, lifestyle, mood and coping. In nondiabetic adolescents, fasting insulin levels increase in both sexes through puberty until Tanner stages 3 or 4, with higher levels in girls reflecting their earlier growth spurt and marginally earlier pubertal maturation. These increases in both basal and stimulated insulin levels reflect and compensate for decreased insulin sensitivity during puberty which is partly due to the significant increase in growth hormone (GH) secretion.

Optimal glycemic control may be particularly difficult to achieve in adolescents: rapid growth necessitates a high calorie intake and must be paralleled by sufficient increases in insulin at that pubertal stage. Many adolescents are underinsulinized on conventional regimens and the daily insulin dose may need to be increased to around 1.5 units/kg during the pubertal growth spurt. Menstruation may precipitate ketoacidosis; important exams cause stress; emotional lability may cause rebelliousness against dietary restrictions, the need for monitoring control or insulin injections. Eating disorders (anorexia nervosa, bulimia) are also common (see above).

Standard insulin regimens through puberty will not correct all the metabolic abnormalities or maintain optimal glycemic control. However, in practical terms these considerations are overshadowed for many young people by lifestyle and behavior which characterize adolescence (see Ch. 35) and militate against good glycemic control in adolescents with type 1 diabetes.

Psychological transition from childhood to adolescence and beyond requires new approaches to motivation and education, flexible diet, insulin regimens and lifestyle. Maintaining parental involvement through the adolescent stage of 'interdependence' (see above) improves glycemic control[393,394] and improved control leads to better quality of life.[409]

Seeking excitement and involvement in risk-taking behaviors is the norm during adolescence. This extends from music and dance to sexual behavior and the use of drugs. The impact of drug use on diabetes is relatively unknown with most of the evidence anecdotal, apart from information on alcohol and tobacco. Cigarette smoking greatly increases the microvascular risks to the diabetic. Alcohol use, in particular binge drinking which is common in adolescents, potentiates hypos. Adolescents must be aware of these risks and how to avoid the dangers and pitfalls. Health professionals should avoid being judgmental and encourage their patients to discuss these issues openly so that appropriate advice can be given. Drug taking should always be taken into consideration when trying to identify reasons for admission with DKA or severe hypos in this age group. Young female patients need to be very aware of the risks of unplanned pregnancy and health professionals should seek opportunities to discuss contraception and preconception care with adolescent girls with diabetes.

Coping strategies adopted by adolescents with diabetes range from obsessional control to denial of diabetes. Those using denial will generally come to the attention of health professionals reasonably quickly but those who are obsessional may never be recognized and may be seen as 'good diabetics'. Chronic insulin omission ('brittle diabetes') will be reflected in weight loss and is associated with episodes of DKA and poor glycemic control.[410]

Glycemic control is better in adolescents who have supportive families.[411] The adolescent with diabetes may feel isolated and not know anyone else with the condition. Many adolescents appear to benefit from sharing experiences with others in a variety of contexts – diabetes holiday camps and Youth Diabetes projects can be helpful in this regard and health professionals should encourage families to join the appropriate national support organization (Diabetes UK in the UK).

Special adolescent needs are often poorly met. Specific adolescent clinics, jointly staffed by pediatricians and adult diabetologists with empathy for the adolescent and his or her 'world-view', may be the ideal – a paternalistic approach is doomed to failure. Annual screening should be carried out to detect early manifestations of complications (see below). Psychological care should be an integral part of the support offered, particularly in view of the fact that psychological problems are more common where chronic illness exists. Integrated home-based, family-centered community-delivered interventions can result in improved metabolic control, treatment adherence and reduced hospitalization rates but are intensive and costly.[412] There is probably no 'right' time for transition or transfer from pediatric to adult clinic and the timing must both be individualized and determined by local arrangements and resources.

Clinics should be run separately from other diabetes clinics. There are some adolescents who do not attend clinic and refuse support in the community. It is important that these patients are identified and some form of contact, no matter how minimal, should be maintained – ideally with a diabetes nurse specialist with specific responsibilities for the adolescent service.

The overall aims of a service for young people with diabetes should be to ensure normal growth and development, minimize episodes of DKA and hypoglycemia, screen for and minimize the risks of complications (see below), promote social and psychological well-being, reduce risk-taking behavior and give support and education to empower the patient to become independent and in control of their diabetes.

Complications

Complications are seldom seen before puberty even in long-standing diabetes. Sex steroid secretion at puberty could be important in their development and progression but pathogenesis is still poorly understood.

Early abnormalities in children and adolescents (e.g. microalbuminuria, background retinopathy) predict later development of long term microvascular complications[367,413] and maintaining glycemic control to as near normal as possible significantly reduces the long term risk of microvascular diseases.[367] An HbA$_{1c}$ >10% over time in young people with diabetes increases the risk of the development of retinopathy by approximately 8-fold.[367] Thus with the aim of management of type 1 DM to reduce the risk of long term microvascular complications, the target

for all young people with diabetes is the optimizing of glycemic control towards a normal level (Grade A recommendation[335]).

Microalbuminuria is a marker for early nephropathy in diabetic children and adults. Using the first morning urine sample and relating concentration to creatinine is probably appropriate but its presence is likely to be related to such factors as acute glycemic control, posture, exercise, hydration and BP. It remains unclear how persistent and at what level it must be to cause concern or how justifiable is long term antihypertensive therapy in a child with a raised diastolic BP and microalbuminuria. BP rises concurrently with the onset of microalbuminuria and is also closely related to BMI.[414]

The evidence is unclear about the timing of commencing screening in young people with diabetes – age and puberty are reported without any strict definition. For clarity and simplicity 12 years of age in both boys and girls has been suggested.[335] However, early microvascular abnormalities may occur before puberty, which then appears to accelerate these abnormalities.[415]

The following can be detected and should be screened for in young people with diabetes: retinopathy (by ophthalmoscopy or fundal photography); microalbuminuria (by albumin excretion rate (AER) or albumin/creatinine ratio (ACR); and hypertension. Young people with diabetes from the age of 12 years should annually receive examination of the retina (Grade C recommendation[335]), have their urine tested for microalbuminuria (overnight AER or first morning ACR) (Grade C recommendation[335]) and have blood pressure measured (Grade D recommendation[335]). There is no evidence that routine screening for autonomic neuropathy or hyperlipidemia is beneficial.[335]

Every effort should be made to optimize glycemic control in young people with diabetes who have abnormal levels of microalbuminuria or elevated blood pressure for age so as to minimize the chance of progression to microangiopathic disease (retinopathy, nephropathy and neuropathy). There are encouraging data demonstrating that efforts to improve glycemic control can, when successful, halve the cumulative incidence of severe retinopathy and nephropathy over a 25 year follow-up period.[416]

In type 1 diabetes, preproliferative retinopathy has been identified within 3.5 years of diagnosis in postpubertal patients[417] and within 2 months of the onset of puberty. Ideally retinal photography or slit lamp biomicroscopy utilized by trained individuals should be employed in a program of systematic screening for diabetic retinopathy, with dilated direct ophthalmoscopy used for opportunistic screening.[335]

The role of statins and/or ACE inhibitors in the management of adolescents with microalbuminuria is under investigation.

ASSOCIATIONS – THYROID DISORDERS AND CELIAC DISEASE

Both thyroid[418] and celiac disease[419] are more common in young people with type 1 DM compared with nondiabetic subjects – both may occur with minimal or no symptoms and thus be missed during routine care. It is recommended that young people with diabetes should be screened for thyroid and celiac disease at diabetes onset and at intervals throughout their lives (Grade C recommendation[335]). Screening for other autoimmune endocrine disorders has also been suggested. Standard blood tests exist to screen for thyroid and celiac disease, but there are limited data to support the specific frequency of screening. There are also few data as to which screening tests should be used – the authors measure TSH levels (by capillary sample at the same time as an HbA$_{1c}$ check) as part of the annual review.

Dietary management of young people with type 1 DM and celiac disease is complex and can be difficult for the family.

OTHER DIABETIC SYNDROMES IN CHILDHOOD
Secondary diabetes mellitus

Diabetes may occur with islet damage secondary to other factors, e.g. pancreatitis and pancreatic disease in cystic fibrosis (see below), thalassemia and certain drug or poison ingestion. It may occur in association with individually rare genetic syndromes (e.g. Prader–Willi, Down, Alstrom, DIDMOAD – see below) or with abnormalities of insulin or its receptors. It may be secondary to other endocrine disorders (e.g. Cushing syndrome, pheochromocytoma).

DIDMOAD (diabetes insipidus, diabetes mellitus, optic atrophy and deafness) syndrome, wolfram syndrome[420]

Optic atrophy (OA) and diabetes insipidus (DI) usually present on a background of established diabetes mellitus. The bilateral progressive OA is present in nearly all by young adulthood causing eventual blindness. DI occurs in about one third and the (high tone) deafness is usually not severe. Inheritance is autosomal recessive and a nuclear gene at chromosome 4p16.1 (WFS1/wolframin), has been identified that segregates with disease status. Mutation analysis of the WFS1 gene in Wolfram syndrome patients has identified mutations in 90% of patients but their biological or clinical significance is not yet established.[421]

Cystic fibrosis (CF) and diabetes (see also Ch. 20, p. 660)

Longer survival is resulting in diabetes being seen increasingly in CF patients. Although no evidence exists that the presence of diabetes or its treatment affects long term survival, it is recommended that patients with CF should be screened annually for diabetes (testing for hyperglycemia, glycosuria and/or a raised HbA_{1c}) from 10 years of age (Grade C recommendation[335]).

Neonatal diabetes mellitus

Transient neonatal diabetes mellitus is a rare condition (the UK national incidence is 1 in 400 000 live births[422]) generally seen in SGA infants. Presentation is with rapid weight loss, severe dehydration, fever and vomiting without diarrhea. Thirst and polyuria are usually unnoticed. Babies appear pale and lively. Blood glucose is very high with glycosuria but only mild (if any) ketonuria and acidosis. There is extreme insulin sensitivity – treatment is with 0.01 unit/kg/h continuous infusion and normal saline initially. The condition is self-limiting, resolving before 1 year of age (median 3 months). Subsequent glucose tolerance is normal but there is a predisposition to later type 2 diabetes, perhaps because of reduced beta cell functional capacity. Seventy-five percent of cases are associated with either paternal uniparental disomy of chromosome 6 or an unbalanced duplication of paternal chromosome 6 – the imprinted gene responsible maps to chromosome 6q24 and may be important for normal pancreatic development.[423,424]

Infants with permanent neonatal diabetes usually present within the first 3 months of life. Cerebellar hypoplasia, developmental delay, muscle weakness, epilepsy and Walcott–Rallison syndrome are associations, suggesting an autosomal recessive inheritance pattern. A mutation in the insulin promoter factor 1 gene has been identified as a cause of the pancreatic agenesis,[424] and a number of heterozygous missense activating mutations in the gene encoding Kir6.2 (important for ATP-sensitive potassium channels which mediate glucose-stimulated insulin secretion from the pancreatic beta cells) have been identified, leading to the hope that treatment of the disease may be possible with oral sulfonylurea therapy.[425]

HYPOGLYCEMIA

Hypoglycemia is a common, but often poorly investigated and managed, metabolic abnormality in infancy and childhood but not a diagnosis in itself. If prolonged or recurrent it can result in severe neuroglycopenia, potentially irreversible brain damage and long term mental handicap, particularly in the very young.

Blood glucose regulation and the metabolic consequences of starvation are discussed above (see also Figs 15.57 and 15.58).

Normal neonates (see Chapter 12) and young children tolerate fasting less well than adults. Blood glucose levels may start to fall after

periods as short as 6–12 h which has implications for the preoperative management of children requiring surgery. Glucose levels appear to fall in a cyclical fashion overnight in normal children, some falling into the 'hypoglycemic' range before compensation.

Neonatal symptoms are nonspecific and include 'jitteriness', hypotonia, feeding difficulties, pallor, apnea, tachypnea, convulsions and coma. In older children, symptoms and signs are attributable to neuroglycopenia (confused or bizarre behavior, bad temper, irritability, headache, visual disturbances, hunger, abdominal pain, convulsions, coma) or to counter-regulation (pallor, sweating, nausea, vomiting).

Blood glucose levels below which there is arbitrarily defined hypoglycemia (e.g. 2.2 mmol/L) are controversial – it is unclear whether 'low' but asymptomatic blood glucose levels cause short or long term problems in different age groups. Prolonged or recurrent symptomatic hypoglycemia is undoubtedly associated with permanent neurological damage.

ETIOLOGY

There are many potential causes of hypoglycemia – the most important are classified by age at presentation in Table 15.21. Endocrine causes are discussed in the section relating to the relevant gland; causes of hyperinsulinism are discussed below.

Persistent neonatal hypoglycemia is usually due to hyperinsulinism, deficiency of a counter-regulatory hormone or of a gluconeogenic or glycogenolytic enzyme. Recent onset recurring hypoglycemia is most commonly due to hyperinsulinism, 'accelerated starvation', defective hepatic gluconeogenesis or GH and/or glucocorticoid deficiency. Accidental or nonaccidental administration of hypoglycemic agents must be considered and hypoglycemia anticipated in any child who has ingested alcohol.

DIFFERENTIAL DIAGNOSIS

History and examination may provide diagnostic clues, for example a family history of neonatal death or acidosis in an inherited metabolic disorder, short stature with micropenis in hypopituitarism, hepatomegaly in galactosemia or gluconeogenic or glycogenolytic disorders, macroglossia and transverse ear lobe creases in Beckwith–Wiedemann syndrome (see Chapter 12, p. 337).

Essential diagnostic information is obtained from blood and urine samples taken *when there is hypoglycemia* and before treatment commences. Blood glucose, ketone bodies, lactate, free fatty acids, branched chain amino acids, insulin, GH, cortisol and catecholamines and urinary ketone bodies, catecholamine metabolites and reducing substances should ideally be measured. If sampling is difficult the most important assays are for blood glucose, plasma insulin and cortisol and urinary ketone bodies, and samples should be deep frozen for future analysis.

The metabolic consequences of starvation with counter-regulation are increased plasma fatty acids, glycerol, ketone bodies, and branched chain amino acids associated with high levels of cortisol, GH and catecholamines. Insulin levels will be low or undetectable. Significant ketosis excludes hyperinsulinism as the cause for hypoglycemia but 'ketotic hypoglycemia' is not a diagnosis in itself and requires further elucidation to find the cause. Important endocrine causes of ketotic hypoglycemia include deficiencies of counter-regulatory hormones (GH and ACTH deficiencies, CAH – especially during intercurrent stress or infection – Addison disease, familial glucocorticoid deficiency and adrenomedullary unresponsiveness).

Hyperinsulinism results in hypoglycemia without ketonuria because insulin inhibits lipolysis. Plasma insulin levels may not be elevated but will be high for plasma glucose; plasma ketone bodies may be detectable but will be low for the glucose level.

Further differential diagnosis may necessitate 24 h metabolic profiles, calculation of the glucose infusion rate necessary to maintain

Table 15.21   Causes of hypoglycemia by age

Transient neonatal
Decreased glucose production
    Birth asphyxia
    Small for gestational age
    Sepsis
    Starvation
    Hypothermia

Hyperinsulinism
    Infant of diabetic mother
    Erythroblastosis
    Beckwith–Wiedemann syndrome (usually)
    Maternal glucose infusions
    Idiopathic

Persistent neonatal and infancy
Hyperinsulinism
    PHHI (nesidioblastosis)
    Islet cell adenoma/hyperplasia/leucine sensitivity
    Beckwith–Wiedemann syndrome (sometimes)

Hormonal
    Growth hormone deficiency
    Hypopituitarism
    Glucocorticoid
    Congenital adrenal hyperplasia
    ACTH deficiency
    Glucagon deficiency
    Hypothyroidism (?)

Inborn errors of metabolism (enzyme deficiency – see Fig. 15.57)
    Glucose-6-phosphatase – glycogen storage disease (GSD) type I*
    Amylo-1,6-glucosidase (GSD III)*
    Debrancher*
    Phosphorylase (GSD VI)*
    Phosphorylase kinase*
    Glycogen synthetase*
    Fructose-1,6-diphosphatase*
    Phosphoenolpyruvate carboxykinase*
    Pyruvate carboxylase*
    Galactose-1-phosphate uridyl transferase (galactosemia)
    Beta-oxidation defects*
    Fructose intolerance
    Maple syrup urine disease

Later childhood
    Accelerated starvation

Hormonal
    As above
    Addison's disease
    Familial glucocorticoid deficiency

Enzyme deficiency
    Those marked* above
    Adrenomedullary hyporesponsiveness

Liver disease
    Fulminant hepatitis
    Reye syndrome
    Jamaican vomiting sickness

Hyperinsulinism
    Insulin administration (including Munchausen by proxy syndrome)
    Oral hypoglycemics (including Munchausen by proxy syndrome)

Ingestion
    Alcohol
    Salicylates

normoglycemia and assessment of glycogen reserve by glucagon provocation tests and of gluconeogenesis.

After exclusion of other causes of ketotic hyperglycemia, there remains a group of children who regularly develop hypoglycemia during periods of fasting – 'accelerated starvation'. Jewish children are absolved from fasting on Yom Kippur (Day of Atonement) until they are 'adult' (13 years). More severe hypoglycemia with convulsions may occur during intercurrent infection (particularly with vomiting), after pronounced physical activity or during preoperative starvation. There is often a history of difficult delivery or intrauterine growth retardation and the child (usually a boy) may be underweight. The hypoglycemic tendency is usually outgrown by later childhood. It is likely that these patients represent one end of a normal distribution of ability to maintain normoglycemia during fasting.

Defects in beta oxidation of fatty acids (see Chapter 26, p. 1067) are increasingly recognized as important causes of hypoglycemia in previously 'idiopathic' groups. Ketone levels are low (cf. ketotic hypoglycemia including 'accelerated starvation'), plasma fatty acid levels are high (cf. hyperinsulinism). Medium chain acyl CoA dehydrogenase (MCAD) deficiency may now be specifically diagnosed by molecular genetic studies and by measuring urinary phenylpropionyl glycine levels which are high following an oral phenylpropionic acid load due to inability to convert phenylpropionic acid to hippuric acid, an essential step in fatty acid oxidation.

ENDOCRINE PANCREATIC ABNORMALITIES CAUSING HYPOGLYCEMIA

These are almost always due to hyperinsulinism – glucagon deficiency seems very rare. Transient neonatal hypoglycemia due to hyperinsulinism is seen in the infant of a poorly controlled diabetic mother (fetal hyperinsulinism secondary to maternal hyperglycemia) and is found in erythroblastosis fetalis (cause unknown) and Beckwith–Wiedemann syndrome (see Chapter 12, p. 337).

In a minority of infants of diabetic mothers hypoglycemia is delayed, but persisting neonatal hypoglycemia is usually associated with an underlying structural pancreatic abnormality. These conditions may not present until later in the first year, making hyperinsulinism the commonest cause of persistent hypoglycemia in infants below 1 year of age or even in childhood.

It is likely that the spectrum of histological findings, from discrete beta cell adenoma(s) through diffuse beta cell hyperplasia, microadenomatosis and nesidioblastosis to functional beta cell disorder alone, and perhaps also 'leucine sensitive hypoglycemia', all result from the same pathological process, probably in the control of pancreatic endocrine secretion.

Persistent hyperinsulinemic hypoglycemia of infancy

Persistent hyperinsulinemic hypoglycemia of infancy (HI) is a rare disorder which may be familial or sporadic, and which is characterized by unregulated secretion of insulin and profound hypoglycemia in the neonate (see Chapter 12). Cases may be sporadic, autosomal recessive, dominant or syndromic.

The majority of infants present neonatally with symptoms (including convulsions) of intractable hypoglycemia. Occasionally presentation is later in the first 6 months. There may be a positive family history. The infants are obese, resembling the infant of the poorly controlled diabetic mother (hyperinsulinism is common to both). There may be a history of maternal glucose intolerance during previous pregnancies.

Diagnosis is dependent on demonstrating hyperinsulinemic hypoglycemia without significant ketosis. Very high glucose infusion rates (> 15 mg/kg/min) may be necessary to maintain normoglycemia – rates above 6–9 mg/kg/min are highly suggestive of hyperinsulinism. The demonstration, when hypoglycemic, of a glycemic response to glucagon, low branched chain amino acid levels, and insulin suppression following somatostatin infusion will confirm the diagnosis.

The management priority is to correct hypoglycemia but this can be difficult because of the high glucose infusion rates necessary and technical problems with siting infusion lines.

If a discrete adenoma is found it should be resected – this will be curative. Otherwise, if medical therapies are unsuccessful, surgery is indicated: subtotal (98%) pancreatectomy (more effective than less radical removal) is performed. This may, commonly, result in 'cure' – normoglycemia without medical therapy, or normoglycemia on diazoxide. If the infant remains glucose infusion-dependent, total pancreatectomy is performed. Postpancreatectomy diabetes is generally easy to manage on small doses of insulin because of associated alpha cell loss causing glucagon deficiency and altered CHO absorption secondary to pancreatic exocrine deficiency.

REFERENCES (* Level 1 evidence)

1. Lania AG, Mantovani G, Spada A. Mechanisms of disease: mutations of G proteins and G-protein-coupled receptors in endocrine diseases. Nat Clin Pract Endocrinol Metab 2006; 2:681–693.

2. Rajender S, Thangaraj K, Gupta NJ, et al. A novel human sex-determining gene linked to Xp11. 21–11.23. J Clin Endocrinol Metab 2006; 91: 4028–4036.

3. Baujat G, Rio M, Rossignol S, et al. Paradoxical NSD1 mutations in Beckwith–Wiedemann syndrome and 11p15 anomalies in Sotos syndrome. Am J Hum Genet 2004; 74:715–720.

4. Ranke MB, Wit J-M, Kelnar CJH, eds. Classification system for paediatric endocrine diseases, 2nd edn. (in press). 2007. Hormone Research Special Edition 68 (suppl 2):1–120.

5. Rosenfield RL. Clinical practice. Hirsutism. N Engl J Med 2005; 353:2578–2588.

6. Tanner JM. Growth at adolescence. 2nd edn. Oxford: Blackwell Scientific Publications; 1962.

7. Petersen KE. The production of cortisol and corticosterone in children. Acta Paediatr Scand 1980; 281:(suppl):2–38.

8. Jeffcoate SL. Efficiency and effectiveness in the endocrine laboratory. London: Academic Press; 1981.

9. Freeman M. Feedback control of intercellular signalling in development. Nature 2000; 408:313–319.

10. Kaplan SL, Grumbach MM, Shepard TH. The ontogenesis of human fetal hormones. 1. Growth hormone and insulin. J Clin Invest 1972; 51:3080–3093.

11. Cohen LE. Genetic regulation of the embryology of the pituitary gland and somatotrophs. Endocrine 2000; 12:99–106.

12. Honnebier WJ, Swaab DF. The influence of anencephaly upon intrauterine growth of the fetus and placenta and upon gestation length. Br J Obstet Gynaecol 1973; 80:577–588.

13. Gluckman PD, Gunn AJ, Wray A, et al. Congenital idiopathic growth hormone deficiency associated with prenatal and early postnatal growth failure. J Pediatr 1992; 121:920–923.

14. Strain AJ, Hill DJ, Swenne I, et al. The regulation of DNA synthesis in human fetal hepatocytes by placental lactogen, growth hormone and insulin-like growth factor 1/somatomedin C. J Cell Physiol 1987; 132:33–40.

15. Sandler S, Andersson A, Korsgren O, et al. Tissue culture of human fetal pancreas: growth hormone stimulates the formation and insulin production of islet-like cell clusters. J Clin Endocrinol Metab 1987; 65:1154–1158.

16. Handwerger S, Freemark M. The roles of placental growth hormone and placental lactogen in the regulation of human fetal growth and development. J Pediatr Endocrinol Metab 2000; 13:343–356.

17. Siler-Khodr TM, Morgenstern LL, Greenwood FC. Hormone synthesis and release from human fetal adenohypophysis in vitro. J Clin Endocrinol Metab 1974; 39:891–905.

18. Kahri AI, Huhtaniemi F, Salmenpetra M. Steroid formation and differentiation of cortical cells in tissue culture of human fetal adrenals in the presence and absence of ACTH. Endocrinology 1976; 98:33–41.

19. Kaplan SL, Grumbach MM, Aubert ML. The ontogenesis of pituitary hormones and hypothalamic factors in the human fetus: maturation of central nervous system regulation of anterior pituitary function. Recent Prog Horm Res 1976; 32:161–234.

20. Symonds ME, Mostyn A, Stephenson T. Cytokines and cytokine receptors in fetal growth and development. Biochem Soc Trans 2001; 29:33–37.

21. Darras VM, Hume R, Visser TJ. Regulation of thyroid hormone metabolism during fetal development. Mol Cell Endocrinol 1999; 25:37–47.

22. Calvo R, Obregon MJ, Ruiz de Oña C, et al. Congenital hypothyroidism as studied in rats. Crucial role of maternal thyroxine but not of 3,5,3'-triiodothyronine in the protection of the fetal brain. J Clin Invest 1990; 86:889–899.

23. Idelman S. The structure of the mammalian adrenal cortex. In: Chester Jones I, Henderson IW, eds. General, comparative and clinical endocrinology of the adrenal cortex. London: Academic Press; 1978: vol 2:1–199.

24. Seckl JR, Cleasby M, Nyirenda MJ. Glucocorticoids, 11beta-hydroxysteroid dehydrogenase, and fetal programming. Kidney Int 2000; 57:1412–1417.

25. Josso N, Picard J-Y. The antimullerian hormone. Physiol Rev 1986; 66:1038–1090.

26. van Rooij IA, Broekmans FJ, te Velde ER, et al. Serum anti-Mullerian hormone levels: a novel measure of ovarian reserve. Hum Reprod 2002; 17: 3065–3071.

27. Migeon CJ, Wisniewski AB. Human sex differentiation: from transcription factors to gender. Horm Res 2000; 53:111–119.

28. Sharpe RM. Pathways of endocrine disruption during male sexual differentiation and masculinisation. Best Pract Res Clin Endocrinol Metab 2006; 20:91–110.

29. Hattersley AT, Tooke JE. The fetal insulin hypothesis: an alternative explanation of the association of low birthweight with diabetes and vascular disease. Lancet 1999; 353:1789–1792.

30. Aynsley-Green A. Metabolic and endocrine interrelations in the human fetus and neonate. Am J Clin Nutr 1985; 41:399–417.

31. Gluckman PD. Endocrine and nutritional regulation of prenatal growth. Acta Paediatr Suppl 1997; 423:153–157.

32. Ibanez L, Dimartino-Nardi J, Potau N, et al. Premature adrenarche – normal variant or forerunner of adult disease? Endocr Rev 2000; 21:671–696.

33. Barker DJ, Hales CN, Fall CH, et al. Type 2 (non-insulin-dependent) diabetes mellitus, hypertension and hyperlipidaemia (syndrome X): relation to reduced fetal growth. Diabetologia 1993; 36:62–67.

34. Barker DJP, Bull AR, Osmond C, et al. Fetal and placental size and risk of hypertension. BMJ 1990; 301:259–262.

35. Hofman PL, Regan F, Jackson WE, et al. Premature birth and later insulin resistance. N Engl J Med 2004; 351:2179–2186.

36. Seckl JR. Glucocorticoid programming of the fetus; adult phenotypes and molecular mechanisms. Mol Cell Endocrinol 2001; 185:61–71.

37. Frankenne F, Closset J, Gomez F, et al. The physiology of growth hormone in pregnant women and partial characterisation of the placental GH variant. J Clin Endocrinol Metab 1988; 66:1171–1180.

38. Cornblath M, Hawdon JM, Williams AF, et al. Controversies regarding definition of neonatal hypoglycemia: suggested operational thresholds. Pediatrics 2000; 105:1141–1145.

39. Hadziselimovic F. Cryptorchidism, its impact on male fertility. Summary of the 4th International Symposium on Pediatric Andrology. Basel, Switzerland, November 10–11, 2000. Hormone Res 2001; 55:55.

40. Simons WF, Fuggle PW, Grant DB, et al. Intellectual development at 10 years in early treated congenital hypothyroidism. Arch Dis Child 1994; 71:232–234.

41. Sharpe RM, Fraser HM, Brougham MFH, et al. Role of the neonatal period of pituitary–testicular activity in germ cell proliferation and differentiation in the primate testis. Hum Reprod 2003; 18:2110–2117.

42. Lee PA, Houk CP, Ahmed SF, et al. Consensus statement on management of Disorders of sex differentiation. Pediatrics 2006; 118:e488–e500.

43. Verhoeven ATM, Mostblum JL, Van Lonsden HAIM, et al. Virilization in pregnancy coexisting with an ovarian mucinous cystadenoma: a case report and review of virilizing ovarian tumours in pregnancy. Obstet Gynecol Surv 1973; 28:597–622.

44. Ahmed SF, Hughes IA. The genetics of male undermasculinization. Clin Endocrinol 2002; 56: 1–18.

45. Parks GA, Bermudez JA, Anast CS, et al. Pubertal boy with the 3-beta-hydroxysteroid dehydrogenase defect. J Clin Endocrinol Metab 1971; 33:269–278.

46. Saez JM, de Peretti E, Morera AM, et al. Familial male pseudohermaphroditism with gynaecomastia due to testicular 17-ketosteroid reductase defect. 1 Studies in vitro. J Clin Endocrinol Metab 1971; 32:604–610.

47. Sultan C, Paris F, Terouanne B, et al. Disorders linked to insufficient androgen action in male children. Hum Reprod Update 2001; 7:314–322.

48. Boisen KA, Chellakooty M, Schmidt IM, et al. Hypospadias in a cohort of 1,072 Danish newborn boys: prevalence and relationship to placental weight, anthropometrical measurements at birth, and reproductive hormones at three months of age. J Clin Endocrinol Metab 2005; 90:4041–4046.

49. Skakkebaek NE, Rajpert-De Meyts E, Main KM. Testicular dysgenesis syndrome: an increasingly common developmental disorder with environmental aspects. Hum Reprod 2001; 16:972–978.

50. Ahmed SF. Gonadal disorders. In: Kelnar CJH, Savage MO, Cowell C, et al. eds. Growth disorders – pathophysiology and treatment, 2nd edn. London: Arnold; 2007.

51. Diamond M, Sigmundson HK. Sex reassignment at birth. Long-term review and clinical implications. Arch Pediatr Adolesc Med 1997; 151:298–304.

52. Colapinto J. As nature made him: the boy who was raised as a girl. New York: HarperCollins; 2000.

53. Savage MO, Preece MA, Jeffcoate SL, et al. Familial male pseudohermaphroditism due to deficiency of 5-alpha-reductase. Clin Endocrinol 1980; 12:397–406.

54. Imperato-McGinley J, Peterson RE, Stoller R, et al. Male pseudohermaphroditism secondary to 17-beta-hydroxysteroid dehydrogenase deficiency – gender role change with puberty. J Clin Endocrinol Metab 1979; 49:291–295.

55. Meyer-Bahlburg HF. Gender and sexuality in classic congenital adrenal hyperplasia. Endocrinol Metab Clin North Am 2001; 30:155–171.

56. Warne G, Grover S, Hutson J, et al. A long-term outcome study of Disorders of sex differentiation conditions. J Pediatr Endocrinol Metab 2005; 18:555–567.

57. Floud R, Gregory A, Wachter K. Height, health and history: nutritional status in the United Kingdom 1750–1980. Cambridge: Cambridge University Press; 1990.

58. Freeman JV, Cole TJ, Chinn S, et al. Cross-sectional stature and weight reference curves for the UK 1990. Arch Dis Child 1995; 73:17–24.

59. Wright CM, Booth IW, Buckler JMH, et al. Growth reference charts for use in the United Kingdom. Arch Dis Child 2002; 86:11–14.

60. Cole TJ, Freeman JV, Preece MA. Body mass index reference curves for the UK 1990. Arch Dis Child 1995; 73:25–29.

61. Tanner JM, Buckler JM. Revision and update of Tanner–Whitehouse clinical longitudinal charts for height and weight. Eur J Pediatr 1997; 156:248–249.

62. Fayter D, Nixon J, Hartley S, et al. A systematic review of the effectiveness and cost-effectiveness of growth monitoring programmes in primary school aged children. Arch Dis Child (in press). 2007.

63. Buckler JMH. A reference manual of growth and development. 2nd edn. Oxford: Blackwell Scientific Publications; 1987.

64. Hall JG, Froster-Iskenius UG, Allanson JE. Handbook of normal physical measurements. Oxford: Oxford Medical Publications; 1989.

65. Wolthers OD, Pedersen S. Short term linear growth in asthmatic children during treatment with prednisolone. BMJ 1990; 301:145–148.

66. Wales JKH, Milner RDG. Knemometry in the assessment of linear growth. Arch Dis Child 1987; 62:166–171.

67. Butler GE, McKie M, Ratcliffe SG. The cyclical nature of prepubertal growth. Ann Hum Biol 1990; 17:177–198.

68. Wales JK, Gibson AT. Short-term growth: rhythms, chaos, or noise? Arch Dis Child 1994; 71:84–89.

69. Crofton PM, Stirling HF, Kelnar CJH. Bone alkaline phosphatase and height velocity in short normal children undergoing growth-promoting treatments: a longitudinal study. Clin Chem 1995; 41:672–678.

70. Crofton PM, Stirling HF, Schönau E, et al. Bone alkaline phosphatase and collagen markers as early predictors of height velocity response to growth-promoting treatments in short normal children. Clin Endocrinol 1996; 44:385–394.

71. Cole TJ, Bellizzi MC, Flegal KM, et al. Establishing a standard definition for child overweight and obesity worldwide: international survey. BMJ 2000; 320:1240–1243.

72. Styles ME, Cole TJ, Dennis J, et al. New cross sectional stature, weight, and head circumference references for Down's syndrome in the UK and Republic of Ireland. Arch Dis Child 2002; 87:104–108.

73. Lyon AJ, Preece MA, Grant DB. Growth curve for girls with Turner syndrome. Arch Dis Child 1985; 60:932–935.

74. Greulich WW, Pyle SI. Radiographic atlas of skeletal development of the hand and wrist, 2nd edn. Stanford: Stanford University Press; 1959.

75. Tanner JM, Healy MJR, Goldstein JM, et al. Assessment of skeletal maturity and prediction of adult height. London: WB Saunders; 2001.

76. MacGillivray MH, Morishima A, Conte F, et al. Pediatric endocrinology update: an overview. The essential roles of estrogens in pubertal growth, epiphyseal fusion and bone turnover: lessons from mutations in the genes for aromatase and the estrogen receptor. Horm Res 1998; 49:(Suppl 1):2–8.

77. Karlberg J, Engstrom I, Karlberg P, et al. Analysis of linear growth using a mathematical model. Acta Paediatr Scand 1987; 76:478–488.

78. Marshall WA, Tanner JM. Variations in the pattern of pubertal changes in boys. Arch Dis Child 1970; 45:13–23.

79. Gigho E, Broglio F. Growth hormone-releasing peptides/secretogogues. In: Kelnar CJH, Savage MO, Cowell C, et al, eds. Growth disorders – pathophysiology and treatment, 2nd edn. London: Arnold; 2007.

80. Kojima M, Hosoda H, Date Y, et al. Ghrelin is a growth-hormone-releasing acylated peptide from stomach. Nature 1999; 402:656–660.

81. Ariyasu H, Takaya K, Tagami T, et al. Stomach is a major source of circulating ghrelin, and feeding state determines plasma ghrelin-like immunoreactivity levels in humans. J Clin Endocrinol Metab 2001; 86:4753–4758.

82. Broglio F, Arvat E, Benso A, et al. Ghrelin, a natural GH secretagogue produced by the stomach, induces hyperglycemia and reduces insulin secretion in humans. J Clin Endocrinol Metab 2001; 86:5083–5086.

83. Pantel J, Legendre M, Cabrol S, et al. Loss of constitutive activity of the growth hormone secretagogue receptor in familial short stature. J Clin Invest 2006; 116:760–768.

84. Ogilvy-Stewart AL, Stirling HF, Kelnar CJH, et al. Treatment of radiation-induced growth hormone deficiency with growth-hormone releasing hormone (GHRH). Clin Endocrinol 1997; 46: 571–578.

85. Bonnefont X, Lacampagne A, Sanchez-Hormigo A, et al. Revealing the large-scale network organization of growth hormone-secreting cells. Proc Natl Acad Sci USA 2005; 102:16880–16885.

86. Agha A, Rogers B, Mylotte D, et al. Neuroendocrine dysfunction in the acute phase of traumatic brain injury. Clin Endocrinol (Oxf) 2004; 60:584–591.

87. Agha A, Rogers B, Sherlock M, et al. Anterior pituitary dysfunction in survivors of traumatic brain injury. J Clin Endocrinol Metab 2004; 89:4929–4936.

88. van der Eerden BC, Karperian M, Wit J-M. Systemic and local regulation of the growth plate. Endocrinol Rev 2003; 24:782–801.

89. Laron Z. Laron syndrome: from description to therapy. Endocrinologist 1993; 3:21–28.

90. Goddard AD, Covello R, Luoh S-M, et al. Mutations of the growth hormone receptor in children with idiopathic short stature. N Engl J Med 1995; 333:1093–1098.

91. Rosenfeld RG. Broadening the growth hormone insensitivity syndrome. N Engl J Med 1995; 333:1145–1146.

92. Salerno M, Balestrieri B, Matrecano E, et al. Abnormal GH receptor signaling in children with idiopathic short stature. J Clin Endocrinol Metab 2001; 86:3882–3888.

93. Baumann G. Growth hormone binding protein. J Pediatr Endocrinol Metab 2001; 14:355–375.

94. Woods KA, Fraser NC, Postel-Vinay M-C, et al. A homozygous splice site mutation affecting the intracellular domain of the growth hormone (GH) receptor resulting in Laron syndrome with elevated GH-binding activity. J Clin Endocrinol Metab 1996; 81:1686–1690.

95. Woods KA, Camacho-Hubner C, Savage MO, et al. Intrauterine growth retardation and postnatal growth failure associated with deletion of the insulin-like growth factor-I gene. N Engl J Med 1996; 335:1363–1367.

96. Cohen RN, Cohen LE, Botero D, et al. Enhanced repression by HESX1 as a cause of hypopituitarism and septo-optic dysplasia. J Clin Endocrinol Metab 2003; 88:4832–4839.

97. Rizzoti K, Brunelli S, Carmignac D, et al. Sox3 is required during the formation of the hypothalamo-pituitary axis. Nat Genet 2004; 36:247–255.

98. Munns CJF, Haase HR, Crowther LM, et al. Ex- pression of SHOX in human fetal and childhood growth plate. J Clin Endocrinol Metab 2004; 89:4130–4135.

99. Ross JL, Scott C, Jr Marttila P, et al. Phenotypes associated with SHOX deficiency. J Clin Endocrinol Metab 2001; 86:5674–5680.

100. Mullis PE. Genetic control of growth. In: Kelnar CJH, Savage MO, Cowell C, et al, eds. Growth disorders – pathophysiology and treatment, 2nd edn. London: Arnold; 2007.

101. Tanner JM. The regulation of human growth. Child Dev 1963; 34:817–847.

102. Prader A, Tanner JM, von Harnack GA. Catch-up growth following illness or starvation. J Pediatr 1963; 62:646–659.

103. Baron J, Klein KO, Colli MJ, et al. Catch-up growth after glucocorticoid excess: a mechanism intrinsic to the growth plate. Endocrinology 1994; 135:1367–1371.

104. Wang Q, Nicholson PHF, Suuriniemi M, et al. Relationship of sex hormones to bone geometric properties and mineral density in early pubertal girls. J Clin Endocrinol Metab 2004; 89:1698–1703.

105. de Onis M, Garza C, Victora CG, et al. The WHO Multicentre Growth Reference Study (MGRS): Rationale, planning, and implementation. Food Nutr Bull 2004; 25:(suppl 1):S3–S84.

106. Buckler JMH. A longitudinal study of adolescent growth. London: Springer Verlag; 1990.

107. Leschek EW, Rose SR, Yanovski JA, et al. Effect of growth hormone treatment on adult height in peripubertal children with idiopathic short stature: a randomized, double blind, placebo-controlled trial. J Clin Endocrinol Metab 2004; 89:3140–3148.

108. Wit JM, Rekers-Mombarg LT, Cutler GB, et al. Growth hormone (GH) treatment to final height in children with idiopathic short stature: evidence for a dose effect. J Pediatr 2005; 146:45–53.

109. Saleh M, Bomd J, Fletcher S. Limb-lengthening techniques. In: Kelnar CJH, Savage MO, Stirling HF, et al, eds. Growth disorders – pathophysiology and treatment. London: Chapman and Hall; 1998.721–744.

110. Cronk CE, Crocker AC, Pueschel SM, et al. Growth charts for children with Down's syndrome: 1 month to 18 years of age. Pediatrics 1988; 81:102–110.

111. Gicquel C, Rossignol S, Cabrol S, et al. Epimutation of the telomeric imprinting center region on chromosome 11p15 in Silver-Russell syndrome. Nat Genet 2005; 37:1003–1007.

112. Abuzzahab MJ, Schneider A, Goddard A, et al. IGF-1 receptor mutations resulting in intrauterine and postnatal growth retardation. N Engl J Med 2003; 349:2211–2222.

113. Johnston LB, Dahlgren J, Leger J, et al. Association between insulin-like growth factor 1 (IGF-1) polymorphisms, circulating IGF-1 and pre- and post-natal growth in two European small for gestational age populations. J Clin Endocrinol Metab 2003; 88:4805–4810.

114. Mushtaq T, Bijman P, Ahmed SF, et al. Insulin-like growth factor-1 augments chondrocyte hypertrophy and reverses glucocorticoid-mediated growth retardation in fetal mice metatarsal culture. Endocrinology 2004; 145:2478–2486.

115. Camacho-Hubner C, Rose SR, Preece MA, et al. Pharmacokinetic studies of recombinant human insulin-like growth factor 1 (rhIGF-1)/rhIGF-binding protein-3 complex administered to patients with growth hormone insensitivity syndrome. J Clin Endocrinol Metab 2006; 91:1246–1253.

116. Ranke MB. Growth hormone insufficiency: clinical features, diagnosis and therapy. In: de Groot L, ed. Endocrinology. Philadelphia: Saunders; 1994.330–340.

117. Thomas M, Massa G, Bourguignon JP, et al. Final height in children with idiopathic growth hormone deficiency treated with recombinant human growth hormone: the Belgian experience. Horm Res 2000; 55:88–94.

118. Vimalachandra D, Craig JC, Cowell CT, et al. Growth hormone treatment in children with chronic renal failure: A meta-analysis of randomized controlled trials. J Pediatr 2001; 139:560–566.

119. Paterson WF, Donaldson MDC, Greene SA, et al. The boom that never was: results of a 10 year audit of paediatric growth hormone prescribing in Scotland. Health Bull 2000; 60:457–466.

120. Kelnar CJH. Postponing puberty in children with growth hormone deficiency. J Pediatr Endocrinol Metab 2005; 18:533–534.

121. Frisancho AR, Sanchez Z, Pollardel D, et al. Adaptive significance of small body size under poor socioeconomoic conditions in southern Peru. Am J Phys Anthropol 1977; 39:255–262.

122. Malcolm LA. Monograph no. 1. Madang: Institute of Human Biology; 1971.

123. Stini WA. Malnutrition, body size and proportion. Ecol Food Nutr 1972; 1:121.

124. Stabler B, Clopper RR, Siegel PT, et al. Academic achievement and psychological adjustment in short children. The National Cooperative Growth Study. J Dev Behav Pediatr 1994; 15:1–6.

125. Skuse DH, Gilmour J, Tian CS, et al. Psychosocial assessment of children with short stature: a preliminary report. Acta Paediatr Scand 1994; 406:11–16.

126. Cianfarani S, Geremia C, Germani D, et al. Insulin resistance and insulin-like growth factors in children with intrauterine growth retardation. Is catch-up growth a risk factor? Horm Res 2001; 55:(suppl 1):7–10.

127. Maxwell H, Rees L. Recombinant human growth hormone treatment in infants with chronic renal failure. Arch Dis Child 1996; 74:40–43.

128. Donaldson MDC. Growth hormone therapy in Turner syndrome – current uncertainties and future strategies. Horm Res 1997; 48:(suppl 5):35–44.

129. Mauras N, Attie KM, Reiter EO, et al. High dose recombinant human growth hormone (GH) treatment of GH-deficient patients in puberty increases near-final height: a randomized, multicenter trial. Genentech, Inc., Cooperative Study Group. J Clin Endocrinol Metab 2000; 85:3653–3660.

130. Cutfield WS, Wilton P, Bennmarker H, et al. Incidence of diabetes mellitus and impaired glucose tolerance in children and adolescents receiving growth-hormone treatment. Lancet 2000; 355:610–613.

131. Malozowski S, Tanner LA, Wysowski DK, et al. Benign intracranial hypertension in children with growth hormone deficiency treated with growth hormone. J Pediatr 1995; 126:996–999.

132. Clayton PE, Cuneo RC, Juul A, et al. Consensus statement on the management of the GH-treated adolescent in the transition to adult care. Eur J Endocrinol 2005; 152:165–170.

133. Leger J, Danner S, Simon D, et al. Do all patients with childhood-onset growth hormone deficiency (GHD) and ectopic neurohypophysis have persistent GHD in adulthood? J Clin Endocrinol Metab 2005; 90:650–656.

134. Murray RD, Adams JE, Shalet SM. Adults with a partial growth hormone deficiency have an adverse body composition. J Clin Endocrinol Metab 2004; 89:1586–1591.

135. Laughlin GA, Barrett-Connor E, Criqui MH, et al. The prospective association of serum insulin-like growth factor 1 (IGF-1) and IGF-binding protein-1 levels with all cause and cardiovascular disease mortality in older adults: the Rancho Bernardo Study. J Clin Endocrinol Metab 2004; 89:114–120.

136. Renehan AG, Zwahlen M, Minder C, et al. Insulin-like growth factor (IGF)-1. IGF binding protein-3 and cancer risk: systematic review and meta-regression analysis. Lancet 2004; 363:1346–1353.

137. Venn A, Bruinsma F, Werther PG, et al. Estrogen treatment to reduce the adult height of tall girls: long term effects on fertility. Lancet 2004; 364:1513–1518.

138. Alexceff M, Macnicol MF. Epiphysiodesis in the management of limb length inequality. Curr Orthopaed 1995; 9:178–184.

139. Macnicol MF. Surgical management of tall stature. In: Kelnar CJH, Savage MO, Cowell C, et al, eds. Growth disorders – pathophysiology and treatment. London: Arnold; 2007.

140. Janeckova R. The role of leptin in human physiology and pathophysiology. Physiol Res 2001; 50:443–459.

141. Druce MR, Small CJ, Bloom SR. Minireview: Gut peptides regulating satiety. Endocrinology 2004; 145:2660–2665.

142. Tanner JM, Whitehouse RH. Revised standards for triceps and subscapular skinfolds for British children. Arch Dis Child 1975; 50:142–145.

143. Parizkova J, Roth Z. The assessment of depot fat in children from skinfold thickness measurements by Holtain (Tanner-Whitehouse) caliper. Hum Biol 1972; 44:613–620.

144. Womersley J, Durnin JV. An experimental study on variability of measurements of skinfold thickness on young adults. Hum Biol 1973; 45:281–292.

145. Owen GM. Measurement, recording and assessment of skinfold thickness in childhood and adolescence: report of a small meeting. Am J Clin Nutr 1982; 35:629–638.

146. Hughes JM, Li L, Chinn S, et al. Trends in growth in England and Scotland, 1972 to 1994. Arch Dis Child 1997; 76:182–189.

147. Liu KH, Chan YL, Chan WB, et al. Mesenteric fat thickness is an independent determinant of metabolic syndrome and identifies subjects with increased carotid intima-media thickness. Diabetes Care 2006; 29:379–384.

148. Jannsen I, Katzmarzyk PT, Srinivasan SR, et al. Combined influence of body mass index and waist circumference on coronary artery disease risk factors among children and adolescents. Pediatrics 2005; 115:1623–1630.

149. Jebb SA, Prentice AM. Single definition of overweight and obesity should be used. BMJ 2001; 323:999.

150. Chinn S, Rona RJ. Prevalence and trends in overweight and obesity in three cross sectional studies of British children, 1974–94. BMJ 2001; 322:24–26.

151. WHO. Obesity: preventing and managing the global epidemic. Geneva: WHO; 1998.

152. Poskitt EME, Cole TJ. Do fat babies stay fat? BMJ 1977; i:7–9.

153. Parsons TJ, Power C, Logan S, et al. Childhood predictors of adult obesity: a systematic review. Int J Obes Relat Metab Disord 1999; 23:(suppl 8):S1–107.

154. Engeland A, Bjorge T, Tverdal A, et al. Obesity in adolescence and adulthood and the risk of adult mortality. Epidemiology 2004; 15:79–85.

155. Baird J, Fisher D, Lucas P, et al. Being big or growing fast: systematic review of size and growth in infancy and later obesity. BMJ 2005; 331:929–931.

156. Viner RM, Cole TJ. Adult socioeconomic, educational, social and psychological outcomes of childhood obesity: a national birth cohort study. BMJ 2005; 330:1354.

157. Reilly JJ, Methven E, McDowell ZC, et al. Health consequences of obesity. Arch Dis Child 2003; 88:748–752.

158. Campbell K, Waters E, O'Meara S, et al. Interventions for preventing obesity in children (Cochrane Review). Cochrane Database Syst Rev 2001; 3:CD001871.

159. Edmunds L, Waters E, Elliott EJ. Evidence based management of childhood obesity. BMJ 2001; 323:916–919.

160. Godoy-Matos A, Carraro L, Vieira A, et al. Treatment of obese adolescents with sibutramine: a randomized, double-blind, controlled study. J Clin Endocrinol Metab 2005; 90:1460–1465.

161. Savage DCL, Forsyth CC, Cameron J. Excretion of individual adreno-cortical steroids in obese children. Arch Dis Child 1974; 49:946–954.

162. Lestradet H, Deschamps I, Giron B, et al. Relationship between the size of the adipocytes, blood glucose, plasma insulin, NEFA and the degree of obesity in children. In: Howard A, ed. Recent advances in obesity research. London: Newman Publishing; 1975.167–169.

163. Grey N, Kipnis DM. Effect of diet composition on hyperinsulinaemia of obesity. N Engl J Med 1971; 285:827–831.

164. Brook CGD, Lloyd JK. Adipose cell size and glucose tolerance in obese children. Arch Dis Child 1973; 48:301–302.

165. Ehtisham S, Hattersley A, Dunger DB, et al. First UK survey of paediatric type 2 diabetes and MODY. Arch Dis Child 2004; 89:526–529.

166. Weiss R, Dufour S, Taksali SE, et al. Prediabetes in obese youth: a syndrome of impaired glucose tolerance, severe insulin resistance, and altered myocellular and abdominal fat partitioning. Lancet 2003; 362:951–957.

167. Eiholzer U. Deaths in children with Prader–Willi syndrome. A contribution to the debate about the safety of growth hormone treatment in children with PWS. Horm Res 2005; 63:33–39.

168. Nagai T, Obata K, Tonoki H, et al. Cause of sudden, unexpected death in Prader–Willi syndrome patients with or without growth hormone treatment. Am J Med Gen A 2005; 136:45–48.

169. Boutin D, Dina C, Vasseur F, et al. GAD2 on chromosome 10p12 is a candidate gene for human obesity. PLoS Biol 2003; 1:E68.

170. Meyre D, Lecoeur C, Delplanque J, et al. A genome-wide scan for childhood obesity-associated traits in French families shows significant linkage on chromosome 6q22.31-q23.2. Diabetes 2003; 53:803–811.

171. Cutting WAM, Elton RA, Campbell JL, et al. Stunting in African children. Arch Dis Child 1987; 62:508–509.

172. Pimstone B, Barberazat G, Hansen J, et al. Studies on growth hormone secretion in protein-calorie malnutrition. Am J Clin Nutr 1968; 21:482–487.

173. Mohan PS, Rao KSJ. Plasma somatomedin activity in protein calorie malnutrition. Arch Dis Child 1979; 54:62–64.

174. Doherty CP, Crofton PM, Sarkar MAK, et al. Malnutrition, zinc supplementation and catch-up growth: changes in insulin-like growth factor I, its binding proteins, bone formation and collagen turnover. Clin Endocrinol 2002; 57:391–399.

175. Boyar RM, Hellman LD, Roffward H, et al. Cortisol secretion and metabolism in anorexia nervosa. N Engl J Med 1977; 296:190–193.

176. Bradlow HL, Boyar RM, O'Connor J, et al. Hypothyroid-like alterations in testosterone metabolism in anorexia nervosa. J Clin Endocrinol Metab 1976; 43:571–574.

177. Viner R. Splitting hairs. Is puberty getting earlier in girls? Arch Dis Child 2002; 86:8–10.

178. Herman-Giddens ME, Slora EJ, Wasserman RC, et al. Secondary sexual characteristics and menses in young girls seen in office practice: a study from the Pediatric Research in Office Settings network. Pediatrics 1997; 99:505–512.

179. Kaplowitz PB, Oberfield SE. Reexamination of the age limit for defining when puberty is precocious in girls in the United States: implications for evaluation and treatment. Drug and Therapeutics and Executive Committees of the Lawson Wilkins Pediatric Endocrine Society. Pediatrics 1999; 104:936–941.

180. Whincup PH, Gilg JA, Odoki K, et al. Age of menarche in contemporary British teenagers: survey

of girls born between 1982 and 1986. BMJ 2001; 322:1095–1096.

181. Teilmann G, Pedersen CB, Jensen TK, et al. Prevalence and incidence of precocious pubertal development in Denmark: an epidemiologic study based on national registries. Pediatrics 2005; 116:1323–1328.

182. Herman-Giddens ME, Wang L, Koch G. Secondary sexual characteristics in boys: estimates from the national health and nutrition examination survey III, 1988–1994. Arch Pediatr Adolesc Med 2001; 155:1022–1028.

183. Wu FCW, Borrow SM, Nicol K, et al. Ontogeny of pulsatile gonadotrophin secretion and pituitary responsiveness in male puberty in man – a mixed longitudinal and cross-sectional study. J Endocrinol 1989; 123:347–359.

184. Neu A. Sonographic size of endocrine tissue. In: Ranke MB, ed. Diagnostics of endocrine function in children and adolescents, 2nd edn. Heidelberg: Barth Verlag; 1996.44–60.

185. Wu FCW, Butler GE, Kelnar CJH, et al. Patterns of pulsatile LH secretion before and during the onset of puberty in boys – a study using an immunoradiometric assay. J Clin Endocrinol Metab 1990; 70:629–637.

186. Wu FCW, Butler GE, Kelnar CJH, et al. Ontogeny of pulsatile gonadotrophin releasing hormone (GnRH) secretion from midchildhood through puberty to adulthood in the human male: a study using deconvolution analyses and an ultrasensitive immunofluorometric assay. J Clin Endocrinol Metab 1996; 81:1798–1805.

187. Wu FCW, Butler GE, Brown DC, et al. Early morning testosterone is a useful predictor of the imminence of puberty. J Clin Endocrinol Metab 1993; 76:26–31.

188. Crofton PM, Evans AE, Wallace AM, et al. Nocturnal secretory dynamics of inhibin B and testosterone in pre-pubertal boys. J Clin Endocrinol Metab 2004; 89:867–874.

189. Crofton PM, Evans AEM, Groome NP, et al. Dimeric inhibins in girls from birth to adulthood: relationship with age, pubertal stage, follicle stimulating hormone and oestradiol. Clin Endocrinol 2002; 56:223–230.

190. Stark O, Peckham CS, Moynihan C. Weight and age at menarche. Arch Dis Child 1989; 64:383–387.

191. Warren MP, Jewelewicz R, Dyrenfurth I, et al. The significance of weight loss in the evaluation of pituitary responsiveness to LH-RH in women with secondary amenorrhea. J Clin Endocrinol Metab 1975; 40:601–611.

192. Kiess W, Muller G, Galler A, et al. Body fat mass, leptin and puberty. J Pediatr Endocrinol Metab 2000; 13:(suppl 1):717–722.

193. Pescovitz OH, Hench KD, Barnes KM, et al. Premature thelarche and central precocious puberty: the relationship between clinical presentation and the gonadotrophin response to luteinizing hormone-releasing hormone. J Clin Endocrinol Metab 1988; 67:474–479.

194. Bridges NA, Christopher JA, Hindmarsh PC, et al. Sexual precocity: sex incidence and aetiology. Arch Dis Child 1994; 70:116–118.

195. Crofton PM, Evans AEM, Groome N, et al. Plasma inhibin in healthy girls and in girls with disorders of puberty. Horm Res 2000; 53:(suppl 2):80.

196. Stanhope R. Premature thelarche: clinical follow-up and indication for treatment. J Pediatr Endocrinol Metab 2000; 13:827–830.

197. Stanhope R, Brook CGD. Thelarche variant: a new syndrome of precocious sexual maturation? Acta Endocrinol 1990; 123:481–486.

198. Lyon AJ, DeBruyn R, Grant DB. Transient sexual precocity and ovarian cysts. Arch Dis Child 1985; 60:819–822.

199. Meadow R. Munchausen syndrome by proxy. Arch Dis Child 1982; 57:92–98.

200. Mauras N, Blizzard RM. The McCune-Albright syndrome. In: Illig R, Visser HKA, eds. Paediatric endocrinology. Copenhagen: Acta Endocrinologica Supplementum 1986; 279: 207–217.

201. Shenker A, Weinstein LS, Moran A, et al. Severe endocrine and non-endocrine manifestations of the McCune–Albright syndrome associated with activating mutations of stimulatory G protein Gs. J Pediatr 1993; 123:509–518.

202. Foster CM, Feuillan P, Padmanabhan V, et al. Ovarian function in girls with McCune–Albright syndrome. Pediatr Res 1986; 20:859–863.

203. Kelnar CJH, Stanhope R. Height prognosis in girls with central precocious puberty treated with GnRH analogues. Clin Endocrinol 2002; 56:295–296.

204. Cacciari E, Frejauille E, Cicognani A, et al. How many cases of true precocious puberty in girls are idiopathic? J Pediatr 1983; 102:357–360.

205. Zevenhuijzen H, Kelnar CJH, Crofton PM. Diagnostic utility of a low-dose gonadotropin releasing hormone test in the context of puberty disorders. Horm Res 2004; 62:168–176.

206. Silver HK. Asymmetry, short stature and variations in sexual development: a syndrome of congenital malformations. Am J Dis Child 1964; 107:495–515.

207. Rosenthal SN, Grumbach MM, Kaplan SL. Gonadotrophin independent sexual precocity with premature Leydig and germinal cell maturation (familial testotoxicosis): effects of a potent luteinising hormone-releasing factor agonist and medroxyprogesterone acetate therapy in four cases. J Clin Endocrinol Metab 1983; 57:571–579.

208. Reiter EO, Norjavaara E. Testotoxicosis: current viewpoint. Pediatr Endocrinol Rev 2005; 3:77–86.

209. Paisey RB, Kadow C, Bolton C, et al. Effects of cyproterone acetate and a long acting LHRH analogue on serum lipoproteins in patients with carcinoma of the prostate. J Roy Soc Med 1986; 79:210–211.

210. Paterson WF, McNeill E, Reid S, et al. Efficacy of Zoladex LA (goserelin) in the treatment of girls with central precocious or early puberty. Arch Dis Child 1998; 79:323–327.

211. Weise M, Flor A, Barnes KM, et al. Determinants of growth during gonadotropin-releasing hormone analog therapy for precocious puberty. J Clin Endocrinol Metab 2004; 89:103–107.

212. Ward PS, Ward I, McNinch AW, et al. Reversible inhibition of central precocious puberty with a long-acting GnRH analogue. Arch Dis Child 1986; 60:872–874.

213. Stirling HF, Butler GE, Glasier A, et al. Hypothalamo-pituitary-ovarian function after D-ser LHRH agonist (Buserelin) treatment for central precocious puberty. J Endocrinol 1989; 121:(suppl):A153.

214. Stirling HF, Kelnar CJH, Wu FCW. What happens after treatment of precocious puberty? Eur J Pediatr 1989; 149:150.

215. Seminara SB, Oliveira LM, Beranova M, et al. Genetics of hypogonadotropic hypogonadism. J Endocrinol Invest 2000; 23:560–565.

216. Seminara SB, Messager S, Chatzidaki EE, et al. The GPR54 gene as a regulator of puberty. N Engl J Med 2003; 349:1614–1627.

217. Messager S, Chatzidaki EE, Ma D, et al. Kisspeptin directly stimulates gonadotropin-releasing hormone release via G-protein-coupled receptor 54. Proc Natl Acad Sci USA 2005; 102:1761–1766.

218. Seth A, Stanley S, Jethwa P, et al. Galanin-like peptide stimulates the release of gonadotropin-releasing hormone in vitro and may mediate the effects of leptin on the hypothalamo-pituitary gonadal axis. Endocrinology 2004; 145:743–750.

219. Pai GS, Leach DC, Weiss L, et al. Thyroid abnormalities in 20 children with Turner syndrome. J Pediatr 1977; 91:267–269.

220. Neely EK, Marcus R, Rosenfeld RG, et al. Turner syndrome adolescents receiving growth hormone are not osteopenic. J Clin Endocrinol Metab 1993; 76:861–866.

221. Stephure DK. Canadian Growth Hormone Advisory Committee. Impact of growth hormone supplementation on adult height in Turner syndrome: results of the Canadian randomized controlled trial. J Clin Endocrinol Metab 2005; 90:3360–3366.

222. Carel JC, Ecosse E, Bastie-Sigeac I, et al. Quality of life determinants in young women with Turner syndrome after growth hormone treatment: results of the StaTur population-based cohort study. J Clin Endocrinol Metab 2005; 90:1992–1997.

223. Kelnar CJH. Does the short, sexually immature adolescent boy need treatment and what form should it take? Arch Dis Child 1994; 71:285–287.

224. Crofton PM, Evans AEM, Groome NP, et al. Inhibin B in boys from birth to adulthood: relationship with age, pubertal stage, follicle stimulating hormone and testosterone. Clin Endocrinol 2002; 56:215–221.

225. Dunkel L. Use of aromatase inhibitors to increase final height. Mol Cell Endocrinol 2006; 254–255:207–216.

226. Tartaglia M, Mehler EL, Goldberg R, et al. Mutations in PTPN11, encoding the protein tyrosine phosphatase SHP-2, cause Noonan syndrome. Nat Genet 2001; 29:465–468.

227. Limal JM, Parfait B, Cabrol S, et al. Noonan syndrome: relationships between genotype, growth and growth factors. JCEM 2006; 91:300–306.

228. Schubbert S, Zenker M, Rowe SL, et al. Germline KRAS mutations cause Noonan syndrome. Nat Genet 2006; 38:331–336.

229. Schiff JD, Palermo GD, Veeck LL, et al. Success of testicular sperm extraction and intracytoplasmic sperm injection in men with Klinefelter syndrome. J Clin Endocrinol Metab 2005; 90:6263–6267.

230. Nakanishi S, Inove A, Kita T, et al. Nucleotide sequence of cloned cDNA for bovine corticotrophin–lipoprotein precursor. Nature 1979; 278:423–427.

231. Bode HH, Crawford JD, Danon M. Disorders of antidiuretic hormone homeostasis: diabetes insipidus and SIADH. In: Lifshitz F, ed. Pediatric endocrinology. New York: Marcel Dekker; 1996.731–752.

232. Crawford JD, Bode HH. Disorders of the posterior pituitary in children. In: Gardner LI, ed. Endocrine and genetic diseases of childhood and adolescence, 2nd edn. Philadelphia: Saunders; 1975:126–158.

233. Czernichow P, Pomerade R, Brauner R, et al. Neurogenic diabetes insipidus in children. In: Czernichow P, Robinson AG, eds. Diabetes insipidus in man. Basel: Karger; 1985: 190–209.

234. Niaudet P, Dechaux M, Lercy D, et al. Nephrogenic diabetes insipidus in children. In: Czernichow P, Robinson AG, eds. Diabetes insipidus in man. Basel: Karger; 1985:224–231.

235. Perheentupa J. The neurohypophysis and water regulation. In: Brook CGD, ed. Clinical paediatric endocrinology, 3rd edn. Oxford: Blackwell; 1995:560–615.

236. Richman RA, Post EM, Notman DD, et al. Simplifying the diagnosis of diabetes insipidus in children. Am J Dis Child 1981; 135:839–841.

237. Czernichow P. Testing water regulation. In: Ranke MB, ed. Diagnostics of endocrine function in children and adolescents, 2nd edn. Heidelberg: Barth Verlag; 1996:230–240.

238. Hofbauer KG, Marr SC. Vasopressin antagonists: present and future. Kidney Int 1987; 31:521.

239. Cushing H. Basophil adenomas of the pituitary body and their clinical manifestations

(pituitary basophilism). Bull Johns Hopkins Hosp 1932; 50:137–195.

240. Weber A, Trainer PJ, Grossman AB, et al. Investigation, management and therapeutic outcome in 12 cases of childhood and adolescent Cushing's syndrome. Clin Endocrinol (Oxf) 1995; 43:19–28.

241. Walvoord EC, Rosenman MB, Eugster EA. Prevalence of adrenocorticotropin deficiency in children with idiopathic growth hormone deficiency. J Clin Endocrinol Metab 2004; 89:5030–5034.

242. Albanese A, Hindmarsh P, Stanhope R. Management of hyponatraemia in patients with acute cerebral insults. Arch Dis Child 2001; 85:246–251.

243. Karavitaki N, Brifani C, Warner JT, et al. Craniopharyngiomas in children and adults: systematic analysis of 121 cases with long-term follow up. Clin Endocrinol (Oxf) 2005; 62:397–409.

244. Dattani ML, Martinez-Barbera J, Thomas PQ, et al. Molecular genetics of septo-optic dysplasia. Horm Res 2000; 53:(suppl 1):26–33.

245. Sotos JF, Dodge PR, Muirhead D, et al. Cerebral gigantism in childhood: a syndrome of excessively rapid growth with acromegalic features and non-progressive neurologic disorder. N Engl J Med 1964; 271:109–116.

246. Attanasio A, Borelli P, Marina R, et al. Serum melatonin in children with early and delayed puberty. Neuroendocrinol Lett 1983; 5:387–392.

247. Wurdak H, Ittner LM, Lang KS, et al. Inactivation of TGFβ signaling in neural crest stem cell leads to multiple defects reminiscent of DiGeorge syndrome. Genes Dev 2005; 19:530–535.

248. Bodey B, Bodey Jr B, Siegel SE, et al. Review of thymic hormones in cancer diagnosis and treatment. Int J Immunopharmacol 2000; 22:261–273.

249. Hadden JW. Thymic endocrinology. Ann N Y Acad Sci 1998; 840:352–358.

250. Kooistra L, Crawford S, van Baar AL, et al. Neonatal effects of maternal hypothyroxinaemia during early pregnancy. Pediatrics 2006; 117:161–167.

251. Vanderscheuren-Lodeweyckx M. Thyroid function tests. In: Ranke MB, ed. Diagnostics of endocrine function in children and adolescents, 2nd edn. Heidelberg: Barth Verlag; 1996:107–127.

252. Mehta A, Hindmarsh PC, Stanhope RG, et al. Is the thyrotropin-releasing hormone test necessary in the diagnosis of central hypothyroidism in children. J Clin Endocrinol Metab 2003; 88:696–703.

253. Delange F, Henderson P, Bourdoux P, et al. Regional variations of iodine nutrition and thyroid function during the neonatal period in Europe. Biol Neonate 1986; 49:322–330.

254. Osborn DA. Thyroid hormones for preventing neurodevelopmental impairment in preterm infants (Cochrane Review) Cochrane Database Syst Rev 2001; 4:CD001070.

255. van Wassenaer AG, Westera J, Houtzager BA, et al. Ten-year follow-up of children born at <30 weeks' gestational age supplemented with thyroxine in the neonatal period in a randomized, controlled trial. Pediatrics 2005; 116:613–618.

256. Williams FL, Ogston SA, van Toor H, et al. Serum thyroid hormones in preterm infants: associations with postnatal illnesses and drug usage. J Clin Endocrinol Metab 2005; 90:5954–5963.

257. Bikker H, Vulsma T, Baas F, et al. Identification of five novel inactivating mutations in the human thyroid peroxidase gene by denaturing gradient gel electrophoresis. Hum Mutat 1995; 6:9–16.

258. Bongers-Schokking JJ, de Muinck Keizer-Schrama SM. Influence of timing and dose of thyroid hormone replacement on mental, psychomotor and behavioural development in children with congenital hypothyroidism. J Pediatr 2005; 147:768–774.

259. Selva KA, Harper A, Downs A, et al. Neurodevelopmental outcomes in congenital hypothyroidism: comparison of initial T4 dose and time to reach target T4 and TSH. J Pediatr 2005; 147:775–780.

260. Osler W. Sporadic cretinism in America. Transactions of the Congress of American Physicians and Surgeons 1897; 4:169–206.

261. Klein AH, Meltzer S, Kenny FM. Improved prognosis in congenital hypothyroidism treated before age 3 months. J Pediatr 1972; 81:912–915.

262. New England Congenital Hypothyroidism Collaborative. Characteristics of infantile hypothyroidism discovered on neonatal screening. J Pediatr 1984; 104:539–544.

263. Fuggle PW, Grant DB, Smith I, et al. Intelligence, motor skills and behaviour at 5 years in early treated congenital hypothyroidism. Eur J Pediatr 1991; 159:570–574.

264. Tillotson SL, Fuggle PW, Smith I, et al. Relation biochemical severity and intelligence in early treated congenital hypothyroidism: a threshold effect. BMJ 1994; 309:440–445.

265. New England Congenital Hypothyroidism Collaborative. Elementary school performance of children with congenital hypothyroidism. J Pediatr 1990; 116:27–32.

266. Carle A, Laurberg P, Pedersen IB, et al. Epidemiology of subtypes of hypothyroidism in Denmark. Eur J Endocrinol 2006; 154:21–28.

267. Zimmermann MB, Hess SY, Molinari L, et al. New reference values for thyroid volume by ultrasound in iodine-sufficient schoolchildren: a World Health Organization/Nutrition for Health and Development Iodine Deficiency Study Group Report. Am J Clin Nutr 2004; 79:231–237.

268. Hidaka A, Minegishi T, Kohn LD. Thyrotropin, like luteinizing hormone (LH) and chorionic gonadotropin (CG) increases cAMP and onositol phosphate levels in cells with recombinant human LH/CG receptor. Biochem Biophys Res Commun 1993; 196:187–195.

269. Hamburger JI. Management of hyperthyroidism in children and adolescents. J Clin Endocrinol Metab 1985; 60:1019–1024.

270. Brill AB, Becker DV. The safety of 131 I treatment of hyperthyroidism. In: Van Middlesworth L, Givens JR, eds. The thyroid gland: a practical clinical treatise . Chicago: Year Book; 1986.347–362.

271. Shibata Y, Yamashita S, Masyakin VB, et al. 15 years after Chernobyl: new evidence of thyroid cancer. Lancet 2001; 358:1965–1966.

272. Read CH, Jr Tansey MU, Menda Y. A 36-year retrospective analysis of the efficacy and safety of radioactive iodine in treating young Graves' patients. J Clin Endocrinol Metab 2004; 89:4229–4233.

273. Wartofsky L. Radioiodine therapy for Graves' disease: case selection and restrictions recommended to patients in North America. Thyroid 1997; 7: 213–216.

274. Corrias A, Einaudi S, Chiorboli E, et al. Accuracy of fine needle aspiration biopsy of thyroid nodules in detecting malignancy in childhood: comparison with conventional clinical, laboratory, and imaging approaches. J Clin Endocrinol Metab 2001; 86:4644–4648.

275. Johnston LB, Chew SL, Lowe D, et al. Investigating familial endocrine neoplasia syndromes in children. Horm Res 2001; 55:(suppl 1):31–35.

276. Brandi ML, Gagel RF, Angeli A, et al. Guidelines for diagnosis and therapy of MEN type 1 and type 2. J Clin Endocrinol Metab 2001; 86:5658–5671.

277. Machens A, Niccoli-Sire P, Hoegel J, et al. Early malignant progression of hereditary medullary thyroid cancer. N Engl J Med 2003; 349:1517–1525.

278. Dreijerink KM, Hoppener JW, Timmers HM, et al. Mechanisms of disease: multiple endocrine neoplasia type 1-relation to chromatin modifications and transcription regulation. Nat Clin Pract Endocrinol Metab 2006; 2:562–570.

279. Institute of Medicine, Food and Nutrition Board. Dietary reference intakes for calcium, phosphorus, magnesium, vitamin D and fluoride. Washington: National Academy Press; 1997.

280. Chevalley T, Rizzoli R, Hans D, et al. Interaction between calcium intake and menarcheal age on bone mass gain: an 8-year follow-up study from pre-puberty to postmenarche. J Clin Endocrinol Metab 2004; 90:44–51.

281. Langman CB. New developments in calcium and vitamin D metabolism. Curr Opin Pediatr 2000; 12:135–139.

282. Tsukada T, Yamaguchi K, Kameya T. The MEN1 gene and associated diseases: an update. Endocr Pathol 2001; 12:259–273.

283. Harris M, Kecha O, Deal C, et al. Reversible metaphyseal dysplasia, a novel bone phenotype in two unrelated children with auto-immunepolyendocrinopathy-candidiasis-ectodermal dystrophy: clinical and molecular studies. J Clin Endocrinol Metab 2003; 88:4576–4585.

284. Albright F, Burnett CH, Smith PH. Pseudohypoparathyroidism: an example of "Seabright-Bantam syndrome". Endocrinology 1942; 30:922–932.

285. Drezner MK, Neelon FA, Lebovitz HE. Pseudohypoparathyroidism type II. A possible defect in the reception of the cyclic AMP signal. N Engl J Med 1973; 289:1056–1060.

286. Levine MA, Jap T-S, Mauseth RS, et al. Activity of the stimulating guanine nucleotide-binding regulatory protein in erythrocytes from patients with pseudohypoparathyroidism and pseudopseudohypoparathyroidism: biochemical, endocrine and genetic analysis of Albright's hereditary osteodystrophy in six kindreds. J Clin Endocrinol Metab 1986; 62:497–502.

287. Ahmed SF, Dixon PH, Bonthron DT, et al. GNAS1 mutational analysis in pseudohypoparathyroidism. Clin Endocrinol 1998; 49:525–532.

288. Bastepe M, Juppner H. Pseudohypoparathyroidism. New insights into an old disease. Endocrinol Metab Clin North Am 2000; 29:569–589.

289. Mantovani G, Maghnie M, Weber G, et al. Growth hormone-releasing hormone resistance in pseudohypoparathyroidism type 1a: new evidence for imprinting of the Gs alpha gene. J Clin Endocrinol Metab 2003; 88:4070–4074.

290. Sakkers R, Kok D, Engelbert R, et al. Skeletal effects and functional outcome with olpadronate in children with osteogenesis imperfecta: a 2 year randomised placebo-controlled study. Lancet 2004; 363:1427–1431.

291. Whyte MP, Wenkert D, Clements KL, et al. Bisphosphonate-induced osteopetrosis. N Engl J Med 2003; 349:457–463.

292. Connell JM, Davies E. The new biology of aldosterone. J Endocrinol 2005; 186:1–20.

293. Giebink GS, Gothin RW, Bighen EG, et al. A kindred with familial glucocorticoid-suppressible aldosteronism. J Clin Endocrinol Metab 1973; 36: 715–723.

294. New MI, Siegal EJ, Peterson RE. Dexamethasone suppressible hyperaldosteronism. J Clin Endocrinol Metab 1973; 37:93–100.

295. Honour JW, Kelnar CJH, Brook CGD. Urine adrenal steroid excretion rates in childhood reflect growth and activity of the adrenal cortex. Acta Endocrinol 1991; 124:219–224.

296. Kelnar CJH. Adrenal steroids in childhood. MD thesis, University of Cambridge; 1985.

297. Temeck JW, Pang S, Nelson C, et al. Genetic defects of steroidogenesis in premature pubarche. J Clin Endocrinol Metab 1987; 64:609–617.

298. Speiser PW, Dupont B, Rubinstein P, et al. High frequency of nonclassical steroid 21-hydroxylase deficiency. Am J Hum Genet 1985; 37:650–667.

299. White PC, Grossberger D, Onufer BJ, et al. Two genes encoding steroid 21-hydroxylase are located near the genes encoding the fourth component of complement in man. Proc Natl Acad Sci USA 1985; 82:1089–1093.

300. Jeffcoate TNA, Fliegner JRH, Russell SH, et al. Diagnosis of the adrenogenital syndrome before birth. Lancet 1965; ii:553–555.

301. Yeh TF, Lin YJ, Lin HC, et al. Outcomes at school age after postnatal dexamethasone therapy for lung diseases of prematurity. N Engl J Med 2004; 350:1304–1313.

302. Bertram CE, Hanson MA. Prenatal programming of postnatal endocrine responses by glucocorticoids. Reproduction 2002; 124:459–467.

303. Theogaraj E, John CD, Christian HC, et al. Perinatal glucocorticoid treatment produces molecular, functional and morphological changes in the anterior pituitary gland of the adult male rat. Endocrinology 2005; 146:4804–4813.

304. Kovacs J, Votava F, Heinze G, et al. Lessons from 30 years of clinical diagnosis and treatment of congenital adrenal hyperplasia in five middle European countries. J Clin Endocrinol Metab 2001; 86: 2958–2964.

305. Pang S, Hotchkiss J, Drash AL, et al. Microfilter paper method for 17alpha-hydroxy progesterone radioimmunoassay: its application for rapid screening for congenital adrenal hyperplasia. J Clin Endocrinol Metab 1977; 45:1003–1008.

306. Pang S, Wallace AM, Hofman L, et al. Worldwide experience in newborn screening for classical congenital adrenal hyperplasia due to 21-hydroxylase deficiency. Pediatrics 1988; 81:866–874.

307. Pang S, Dobbins RH, Kling S, et al. Worldwide newborn screening update for classical congenital adrenal hyperplasia. In: Schmidt BJ, ed. Current trends in infant screening. Amsterdam: Elsevier Science; 1989.307–312.

308. Lacey JM, Minutti CZ, Magera MJ, et al. Improved specificity of newborn screening for congenital adrenal hyperplasia by second tier steroid profiling using tandem mass spectrometry. Clin Chem 2004; 50:621–625.

309. Varness TS, Allen DB, Hoffman GL. Newborn screening for congenital adrenal hyperplasia has reduced sensitivity in girls. J Pediatr 2005; 147: 493–498.

310. Nordenström A, Thilén A, Hagenfeldt L, et al. Genotyping is a valuable diagnostic complement to neonatal screening for congenital adrenal hyperplasia due to steroid 21-hydroxylase deficiency. J Clin Endocrinol Metab 1999; 84:1505–1509.

311. Costa-Santos M, Kater CE, Auchus RJ, et al. Two prevalent CYP17 mutations and genotype-phenotype correlations in 24 Brazilian patients with 17-hydroxylase deficiency. J Clin Endocrinol Metab 2004; 89:49–60.

312. Miller WL, Huang N, Pandey AV, et al. P450 oxidoreductase deficiency: a new disorder of steroidogenesis. Ann NY Acad Sci 2005; 1061:100–108.

313. Richmond EJ, Flickinger CJ, McDonald JA, et al. Lipoid congenital adrenal hyperplasia (CAH): patient report and a mini-review. Clin Pediatr (Phila) 2001; 40:403–407.

314. Cutler GB, Jr Laue L. Congenital adrenal hyperplasia due to 21-hydroxylase deficiency. N Engl J Med 1990; 323:1806–1813.

315. Irony I, Cutler GB. Effect of carbenoxolone on the plasma renin activity and hypothalamic-pituitary-adrenal axis in congenital adrenal hyperplasia due to 21-hydroxylase deficiency. Clin Endocrinol (Oxf) 1999; 51:285–291.

316. Meyers RL, Grua JR. Bilateral laparoscopic adrenalectomy: a new treatment for difficult cases of congenital adrenal hyperplasia. J Pediatr Surg 2000; 35:1586–1590.

317. Schnitzer JJ, Donahoe PK. Surgical treatment of congenital adrenal hyperplasia. Endocrinol Metab Clin North Am 2001; 30:137–154.

318. Cabrera MS, Vogiatzi MG, New MI. Long term outcome in adult males with classic congenital adrenal hyperplasia. J Clin Endocrinol Metab 2001; 86:3070–3078.

319. Mulaikal RM, Migeon CJ, Rock JA. Fertility rates in female patients with congenital adrenal hyperplasia due to 21-hydroxylase deficiency. N Engl J Med 1987; 316:178–182.

320. van Wyk JJ, Ritzen EM. The role of bilateral adrenalectomy in the treatment of congenital adrenal hyperplasia. J Clin Endocrinol Metab 2003; 88:2293–2298.

321. Batista D, Gennari M, Riar J, et al. An assessment of petrosal sinus sampling for localization of pituitary adenomas in children with Cushing's disease. J Clin Endocrinol Metab 2006; 91:221–224.

322. New MI, Crawford C, Virdis R. Low-renin hypertension in childhood. In: Lifshitz F, ed. Pediatric endocrinology. New York: Marcel Dekker, 1996:775–790.

323. Wolthers OD, Cameron FJ, Scheimberg I, et al. Androgen secreting adrenocortical tumours. Arch Dis Child 1999; 80:46–50.

324. Stojadinovic A, Brennan MF, Hoos A, et al. Adrenocortical adenoma and carcinoma: histopathological and molecular comparative analysis. Mod Pathol 2003; 16:742–751.

325. de Swiet M, Dillon MJ. Hypertension in children. BMJ 1989; 299:469–470.

326. de Swiet M, Fayers P, Shinebourne EA. Blood pressure in 4 and 5 year old children: the effects of environment and other factors in its measurement. The Brompton Study. J Hypertens 1984; 2:501–505.

327. de Swiet M, Dillon MJ, Littler W, et al. Measurement of blood pressure in children. BMJ 1989; 299:497.

328. Crofton PM, Ahmed SF, Wade JC, et al. Bone turnover and growth during and after continuing chemotherapy in children with acute lymphoblastic leukaemia. Pediatr Res 2000; 48:490–496.

329. Bath LE, Crofton PM, Evans AE, et al. Bone turnover and growth during and after chemotherapy in children with solid tumors. Pediatr Res 2003; 55:224–230.

330. Ahmed SR, Shalet SM, Beardwell CG. The effects of cranial irradiation on growth hormone secretion. Acta Paediatr Scand 1986; 75:255–260.

331. Mohn A, Di Marzio A, Capanna R, et al. Persistence of impaired pancreatic beta-cell function in children treated for acute lymphoblastic leukaemia. Lancet 2004; 363:127–128.

332. Crofton PM, Thomson AB, Evans AE, et al. Is inhibin B a potential marker of gonadotoxicity in prepubertal children treated for cancer? Clin Endocrinol 2003; 58:296–301.

333. SIGN. Long term follow up care of survivors of childhood cancer sign. SIGN 76: 2004; www.sign.ac.uk

334. Swift PGF, ed. ISPAD Consensus Guidelines for the management of type 1 diabetes in children and adolescents. Zeist, Netherlands: Medical Forum International; 2000.

335. SIGN Guideline 5. Diabetes Mellitus Scottish Intercollegiate Guidelines Network. 2001. www.sign.ac.uk.

336. Willis T. Practice of physick. London: 1684.

337. Dobson M. Experiments and observations on the urine in diabetes. London: Medical observations and enquiries 5; 1776.

338. Von Mering J, Minkowski O. Diabetes mellitus nach panceasextirpation. Archiv fur experimentalische Pathologie und Pharmacologie 1890; 25:371–387.

339. Banting FG, Best CH, Collip JB, et al. Pancreatic extracts in the treatment of diabetes mellitus. Can Med Assoc J 1922; 12:141–146.

340. Hattersley AT. Diagnosis of maturity-onset diabetes of the young in the pediatric diabetes clinic. J Pediatr Endocrinol Metab 2000; 13:(suppl 6):1411–1417.

341. Hattersley AT. Transcribing diabetes. J Pediatr Endocrinol Metab 2001; 14:(suppl 3):1025.

342. Reinehr T, Andler W, Kapellen T, et al. Clinical characteristics of type 2 diabetes mellitus in overweight European Caucasian adolescents. Exp Clin Endocrinol Diabetes 2005; 113:167–170.

343. Weiss R, Dziura J, Burgert TS, et al. Obesity and the metabolic syndrome in children and adolescents. N Engl J Med 2004; 350:2362–2374.

344. Montgomery SM, Ekbom A. Smoking during pregnancy and diabetes mellitus in a British longitudinal birth cohort. BMJ 2002; 324:26–27.

345. Fagot-Campagna A, Pettitt DJ, Engelgau MM, et al. Type 2 diabetes among North American children and adolescents: an epidemiologic review and a public health perspective. J Pediatr 2000; 136:664–672.

346. Kolatsi-Joannou M, Bingham C, Ellard S, et al. Hepatocyte nuclear factor-1beta: a new kindred with renal cysts and diabetes and gene expression in normal human development. J Am Soc Nephrol 2001; 12:2175–2180.

347. Rangasami JJ, Greenwood DC, McSporran B, et al. Rising incidence of type 1 diabetes in Scottish children, 1984–93. The Scottish Study Group for the Care of Young Diabetics. Arch Dis Child 1997; 77:210–213.

348. DIABAUD. Factors influencing glycemic control in young people with type 1 diabetes in Scotland: a population-based study (DIABAUD2). Diabetes Care 2001; 24:239–244.

349. Gale EA, Gillespie KM. Diabetes and gender. Diabetologia 2001; 44:3–15.

350. Kelly MA, Mijovic CH, Barnett AH. Genetics of type 1 diabetes. Best Pract Res Clin Endocrinol Metab 2001; 15:279–291.

351. Banatvala JE, Bryant J, Scherntaner G, et al. Coxsackie B. mumps, rubella and cytomegalovirus-specific IgM responses in patients with juvenile-onset insulin-dependent diabetes in Britain, Austria and Australia. Lancet 1985; i:1409–1412.

352. Hviid A, Stellfeld M, Wohlfahrt J, et al. Childhood vaccination and type 1 diabetes. N Engl J Med 2004; 350:1398–1404.

353. Rosenbloom AL, Schatz DA, Krischer JP, et al. Therapeutic controversy: prevention and treatment of diabetes in children. J Clin Endocrinol Metab 2000; 85:494–522.

354. ENDIT Group. European Nicotinamide Diabetes Intervention Trial (ENDIT): a randomized controlled trial of intervention before the onset of type 1 diabetes. Lancet 2004; 363:925–931.

355. Diabetes Prevention Trial – Type 1 Diabetes Study Group. Effects of insulin in relatives of patients with type 1 diabetes mellitus. N Engl J Med 2002; 346:1685–1691.

356. Schatz D, Gale EAM, Atkinson MA. Why can't we prevent type 1 diabetes? Diabetes Care 2003; 26:3226–3228.

357. Tjima N. Coma at the onset of young insulin-dependent diabetes in Japan: the result of a nationwide survey. Diabetes 1985; 34:1241–1246.

358. American Diabetes Association. Report of the Expert Committee on the Diagnosis and Classification of Diabetes Mellitus. Diabetes Care 1997; 20: 1183–1197.

359. WHO. Definition, diagnosis and classification of diabetes mellitus and its complications. Geneva: WHO; 1999 (Available from URL http://whqlibdoc.who.int/hq/1999/WHO_NCD_NCS_99.2.pdf)

360. Noyes KJ, Henderson A, Hughes H, et al. An integrated care pathway for the management of diabetic ketoacidosis. J Pediatr Endocrinol Metab 2001; 14:(suppl 3):PP-120 1064.

361. Strachan MW, Nimmo GR, Noyes K, et al. Management of cerebral oedema in diabetes. Diabetes Metab Res Rev 2003; 19:241–247.

362. Glaser N, Barnett P, McCaslin I, et al. Risk factors for cerebral edema in children with diabetic ketoacidosis. The Pediatric Emergency Medicine Collaborative Research Committee of the American Academy of Pediatrics. N Engl J Med 2001; 344: 264–269.

363. Edge JA, Hawkins MM, Winter DL, et al. The risk and outcome of cerebral oedema developing during diabetic ketoacidosis. Arch Dis Child 2001; 85:16–22.

364. Krane EJ, Rockoff MA, Wallman JK, et al. Subclinical brain swelling in children during treatment of diabetic ketoacidosis. N Engl J Med 1985; 312:1147–1151.

365. Dahlquist G, Kallen B. Mortality in childhood-onset type 1 diabetes: a population-based study. Diabetes Care 2005; 28:2384–2387.

366. Diabetes Control and Complications Trial Research Group. The effect of intensive treatment of diabetes on the development and progression of long term complications in insulin-dependent diabetes mellitus. N Engl J Med 1993; 329:977–986.

367. Diabetes Control and Complications Trial Research Group. The effect of intensive treatment of diabetes on the development and progression of long term complications in insulin-dependent diabetes mellitus. J Pediatr 1994; 125:177–188.

368. Tamborlane WV, Bonfig W, Boland E. Recent advances in treatment of youth with Type 1 diabetes: better care through technology. Diabet Med 2001; 18:864–870.

369. Ross LA, Frier BM, Kelnar CJH, et al. Child and parental mental ability and glycaemic control in children with type 1 diabetes. Diabet Med 2001; 18:364–369.

370. DiMeglio LA, Pottorff TM, Boyd SR, et al. A randomized, controlled study of insulin pump therapy in diabetic preschoolers. J Pediatr 2004; 145:380–384.

371. FAX LA, Buckloh LM, Smith SD, et al. A randomized controlled trial of insulin pump therapy in young children with type 1 diabetes. Diabetes Care 2005; 28:1277–1281.

372. Tupola S, Komulainen J, Jaaskelainen J, et al. Post-prandial insulin lispro vs. human regular insulin in prepubertal children with Type 1 diabetes mellitus. Diabet Med 2001; 18:654–658.

373. Gale EA. A randomized, controlled trial comparing insulin lispro with human soluble insulin in patients with Type 1 diabetes on intensified insulin therapy. The UK Trial Group. Diabet Med 2000; 3:209–214.

374. Brunelle BL, Llewelyn J, Anderson JH Jr, et al. Meta-analysis of the effect of insulin lispro on severe hypoglycemia in patients with type 1 diabetes. Diabetes Care 1998; 10:1726–1731.

375. Nordfeldt S, Ludvigsson J. Severe hypoglycemia in children with IDDM. A prospective population study. 1992–1994. Diabetes Care 1997; 20:497–503.

376. Dorchy H, Roggemans MP, Willems D. Glycated hemoglobin and related factors in diabetic children and adolescents under 18 years of age: a Belgian experience. Diabetes Care 1997; 20:2–6.

377. McKeage K, Goa KL. Insulin glargine: a review of its therapeutic use as a long-acting agent for the management of type 1 and 2 diabetes mellitus. Drugs 2001; 61:1599–1624.

378. Lepore M, Pampanelli S, Fanelli C, et al. Pharmacokinetics and pharmacodynamics of subcutaneous injection of long-acting human insulin analog glargine, NPH insulin, and ultralente human insulin and continuous subcutaneous infusion of insulin lispro. Diabetes 2000; 49:2142–2148.

379. Heinemann L, Linkeschova R, Rave K, et al. Time-action profile of the long-acting insulin analog insulin glargine (HOE901) in comparison with those of NPH insulin and placebo. Diabetes Care 2000; 23:644–649.

380. Ratner RE, Hirsch IB, Neifing JL, et al. Less hypoglycemia with insulin glargine in intensive insulin therapy for type 1 diabetes. U.S. Study Group of Insulin Glargine in Type 1 Diabetes. Diabetes Care 2000; 23:639–643.

381. Pieber TR, Eugene-Jolchine I, Derobert E. Efficacy and safety of HOE 901 versus NPH insulin in patients with type 1 diabetes. The European Study Group of HOE 901 in type 1 diabetes. Diabetes Care 2000; 23:157–162.

382. Schober E, Schoenle E, Van Dyk J, et al. Comparative trial between insulin glargine and NPH insulin in children and adolescents with type 1 diabetes. Diabetes Care 2001; 24:2005–2006.

383. Chase P, Dixon B, Pearson J, et al. Reduced hypoglycaemic episodes and improved glycemic control in children with type 1 diabetes using insulin glargine and neutral protamine Hagedorn insulin. J Pediatr 2003; 143:737–740.

384. Danne T, Lüpke K, Walte K, et al. Insulin detemir is characterized by a consistent pharmacokinetic profile across age-groups in children, adolescents and adults with type 1 diabetes. Diabetes Care 2003; 26:3087–3092.

385. Heise T, Nosek L, Ronn BB, et al. Lower within-subject variability of insulin detemir in comparison to NPH insulin and insulin glargine in people with type 1 diabetes. Diabetes 2004; 53:1614–1620.

386. Heinemann L, Traut T, Heise T. Time-action profile of inhaled insulin. Diabet Med 1997; 14:63–72.

387. Patton JS, Bukar J, Nagarajan S. Inhaled insulin. Adv Drug Deliv Rev 1999; 35:235–247.

388. Teeter JG, Riese RJ. Dissociation of lung function changes with humoral immunity during inhaled human insulin therapy. Am J Respir Crit Care Med 2006; 173:1194–1200.

389. Skyler JS, Weinstock RS, Raskin P, et al. Use of inhaled insulin in a basal/bolus insulin regimen in type 1 diabetic subjects: a 6-month, randomized, comparative trial. Diabetes Care 2006; 28:1630–1635.

390. Rubenstein AH, Pyke DA. Immunosuppression in the treatment of insulin-dependent (type 1) diabetes. Lancet 1987; i:436–437.

391. White PC. Congenital adrenal hyperplasias. Best Pract Res Clin Endocrinol Metab 2001; 15:17–41.

392. DAFNE Study Group. Training in flexible, intensive insulin management to enable dietary freedom in people with type 1 diabetes: dose adjustment for normal eating (DAFNE) randomised controlled trial. BMJ 2002; 325:746.

393. Satin W, La Greca AM, Zigo MA, et al. Diabetes in adolescence: effects of multifamily group intervention and parent simulation of diabetes. J Pediatr Psychol 1989; 14:259–275.

394. Anderson BJ, Brackett J, Ho J, et al. An office-based intervention to maintain parent–adolescent teamwork in diabetes management. Impact on parent involvement, family conflict, and subsequent glycemic control. Diabetes Care 1999; 22:713–721.

395. Overstreet S, Goins J, Chen RS, et al. Family environment and the interrelation of family structure, child behavior, and metabolic control for children with diabetes. J Pediatr Psychol 1995; 20:435–447.

396. Blankfield DF, Holahan CJ. Family support, coping strategies and depressive symptoms among mothers of children with diabetes. J Fam Psychol 1996; 10:173–179.

397. Jones JM, Lawson ML, Danman D, et al. Eating disorders in adolescent females with and without type I diabetes: cross-sectional study. BMJ 2000; 10:1563–1566.

398. Grey M, Cameron ME, Lipman TH, et al. Psychosocial status of children with diabetes in the first two years after diagnosis. Diabetes Care 1995; 18:1330–1336.

399. Hampson SE, Skinner TC, Hart J, et al. Effects of educational and psychosocial interventions for adolescents with diabetes mellitus: a systematic review. Health Technol Assess 2001; 5:1–79.

400. Grey M, Boland EA, Davidson M, et al. Coping skills training for youth with diabetes mellitus has long-lasting effects on metabolic control and quality of life. J Pediatr 2000; 137:107–113.

401. Tattersall RB. Brittle diabetes. Clin Endocrinol Metab 1977; 6:403–419.

402. Hermansson G, Ludvigsson J, Larsson Y. Home blood glucose monitoring in diabetic children and adolescents. A 3 year feasibility study. Acta Paediatr Scand 1986; 75:98–105.

403. Kaufman FR, Gibson LC, Halvorson M, et al. A pilot study of the continuous glucose monitoring system: clinical decisions and glycemic control after its use in pediatric type 1 diabetic subjects. Diabetes Care 2001; 24:2030–2034.

404. Gross TM, Bode BW, Einhorn D, et al. Performance evaluation of the MiniMed continuous glucose monitoring system during patient home use. Diabetes Technol Ther 2000; 2:49–56.

405. Danne T, Mortensen HB, Hougaard P, et al. Persistent differences among centers over 3 years in glycemic control and hypoglycemia in a study of 3,805 children and adolescents with type 1 diabetes from the Hvidore Study Group. Diabetes Care 2001; 24:1342–1347.

406. Krolewski AS, Laffel LM, Krolewski M, et al. Glycosylated hemoglobin and the risk of microalbuminuria in patients with insulin-dependent diabetes mellitus. N Engl J Med 1995; 332:1251–1255.

407. Spallino L, Stirling HF, O'Regan M, et al. Transient hypoglycaemic hemiparesis in children with IDDM. Diabetes Care 1998; 21:1567–1568.

408. Matyka KA, Crawford C, Wiggs L, et al. Alterations in sleep physiology in young children with insulin-dependent diabetes mellitus: relationship to nocturnal hypoglycemia. J Pediatr 2000; 137: 233–238.

409. Hoey H, Aanstoot HJ, Chiarelli F, et al. Good metabolic control is associated with better quality of life in 2,101 adolescents with type 1 diabetes. Diabetes Care 2001; 24:1923–1928.

410. Morris AD, Douglas IR, Boyle AD, et al. Adherence to insulin treatment, glycaemic control, and ketoacidosis in insulin-dependent diabetes mellitus. Lancet 1997; 350:1505–1510.

411. Hentinen M, Kyngas H. Diabetic adolescents' compliance with health regimens and associated factors. Int J Nurs Stud 1996; 33:325–335.

412. Ellis DA, Frey MA, Naar-King S, et al. Use of multisystemic therapy to improve regimen adherence among adolescents with type 1 diabetes in chronic poor metabolic control: a randomized controlled trial. Diabetes Care 2005; 28:1604–1610.

413. Holl RW, Lang GE, Grabert M, et al. Diabetic retinopathy in pediatric patients with type-1 diabetes: effect of diabetes duration, prepubertal and pubertal onset of diabetes, and metabolic control. J Pediatr 1998; 132:790–794.

414. Schultz CJ, Neil HA, Dalton RN, et al. Blood pressure does not rise before the onset of microalbuminuria in children followed from diagnosis of type 1 diabetes. Oxford Regional Prospective Study Group. Diabetes Care 2001; 24:555–560.

415. Schultz CJ, Konopelska-Bahu T, Dalton RN, et al. Microalbuminuria prevalence varies with age, sex, and puberty in children with type 1 diabetes followed from diagnosis in a longitudinal study. Oxford Regional Prospective Study Group. Diabetes Care 1999; 22:495–502.

416. Nordwall M, Bojestig M, Arnqvist HJ, et al. Declining incidence of severe retinopathy and persisting decrease of nephropathy in an unselected population of type 1 diabetes – the Linkoping Diabetes Complications Study. Diabetalogia 2004; 47:1266–1272.

417. Bonney M, Hing SJ, Fung AT, et al. Development and progression of diabetic retinopathy: adolescents at risk. Diabet Med 1995; 12:967–973.

418. Radetti G, Paganini C, Gentili L, et al. Frequency of Hashimoto's thyroiditis in children with type 1 diabetes mellitus. Acta Diabetol 1995; 32:121–124.

419. Carlsson AK, Axelsson IE, Borulf SK, et al. Prevalence of IgA-antiendomysium and IgA-antigliadin autoantibodies at diagnosis of insulin-dependent diabetes mellitus in Swedish children and adolescents. Pediatrics 1999; 103:1248–1252.

420. Cremers CW, Wijdeveld PG, Pinckers AJ. Juvenile diabetes mellitus, optic atrophy, hearing loss, diabetes insipidus, atonia of the urinary tract and bladder, and other abnormalities (Wolfram syndrome). A review of 88 cases from the literature with personal observations on 3 new patients. Acta Paediatr Scand 1977; 264:(suppl):1–16.

421. Khanim F, Kirk J, Latif F, et al. WFS1/Wolframin mutations, Wolfram syndrome, and associated diseases. Hum Mutat 2001; 17:357–367.

422. Shield JP, Gardner RJ, Wadsworth EJ, et al. Aetiopathology and genetic basis of neonatal diabetes. Arch Dis Child Fetal Neonatal Ed 1997; 76:F39–F42.

423. Gardner RJ, Mungall AJ, Dunham I, et al. Localisation of a gene for transient neonatal diabetes mellitus to an 18.72 cR3000 (approximately 5.4 Mb) interval on chromosome 6q. J Med Genet 1999; 36:192–196.

424. Shield JP. Neonatal diabetes: new insights into aetiology and implications. Horm Res 2000; 53:(suppl 1):7–11.

425. Gloyn AL, Pearson ER, Antcliff JF, et al. Activating mutations in the gene encoding the ATP-sensitive potassium-channel subunit Kir6.2 and permanent neonatal diabetes. N Engl J Med 2004; 350:1838–1849.

16

Nutrition

Barbara Golden, John Reilly

NUTRITION, GROWTH, DEVELOPMENT AND DISEASE

Optimal nutrition is the foundation of good health. Malnutrition implies both under- and overnutrition, and is a consequence of disturbance of energy and nutrient balance, between supply and demand. Undernutrition is often manifest as growth failure, which may be due to insufficient energy or nutrient intake, disordered digestion, absorption or metabolism, or excessive losses.[1] Foods deficient in specific nutrients may cause specific diseases (such as scurvy or anemia). Chronic disease is frequently associated with undernutrition and nutrient deficits. However, nutrient deficiencies lead to depletion of tissue stores, derangement of normal biochemistry and disordered tissue function before they are manifest as anatomical changes, and may easily go unrecognized. Awareness of poor nutrition is critical to the effective management of many childhood diseases, particularly those that are chronic, and there is growing evidence that undernutrition in early life may play a part in the genesis of chronic adult disease.

This chapter aims to summarize the knowledge required to evaluate the nutritional needs of normal and sick children and to provide them with a healthy diet or nutritional support. A summary of nutrient requirements is presented, how they are defined and how they should be properly used. Nutritional assessment is an essential prerequisite to the provision of nutritional support and the principal methods used are outlined. Healthy diets for the infant, toddler, child and adolescent are then described briefly. The next section summarizes how nutritional support can be provided to the sick child and is followed by an account of some of the main causes of over- and undernutrition. A trained nutrition team should work together in the clinic, ward and community to provide nutritional support for sick children. The basic science of nutrition (composition of food, metabolic pathways, gastrointestinal physiology, body composition, etc.) is not covered in detail in this chapter, but references to textbooks on nutritional science are provided.[2,3]

NUTRITIONAL REQUIREMENTS

PRINCIPLES AND DEFINITIONS

Figures for nutrient requirements set by expert committees emphasize the avoidance of nutrient deficiency. They generally do not concern themselves with the safety of excess intake. Underlying the concept of requirement is the assumption that, for most nutrients, need is approximately normally distributed in any population. To recommend requirements of nutrients that are sufficient to meet the needs of almost the entire population, they have been set 'high' in the distribution, at approximately two standard deviations (SDs) above the mean requirement. With the exception of energy (excess energy intake leads to obesity), consumption of a nutrient in excess of requirements of this magnitude is not harmful and setting a high value as a reference nutrient intake (RNI) or recommended daily allowance (RDA) entails minimal risk for most nutrients.

In the UK, the term 'dietary reference values' (DRVs) is used rather than 'recommendations', and DRVs have been in place since 1991.[4] Three reference values are set for each nutrient. These values reflect the range of nutrient requirements (low, medium and high) rather than just one reference value. The three DRVs are:

1. 'estimated average requirement' (EAR), the mean requirement;
2. 'reference nutrient intake' (RNI), the mean requirement +2 SD; and
3. 'lower reference nutrient intake' (LRNI), the mean requirement −2 SD.

For some nutrients the 1991 UK report set a 'safe intake' if there were insufficient data upon which to set DRVs. This was judged to be an intake at which there was no risk of deficiency and below a level where there was a risk of adverse effects.

APPLICATIONS AND LIMITATIONS OF DIETARY REFERENCE VALUES

There are three main applications of DRVs:
1. to assess the adequacy of the dietary intake of individuals or groups. For example, if a hospital population of children consume a diet below the LRNI for a particular nutrient, their diet is probably deficient in that nutrient.
2. as a guide to prescribing or designing the diet of individuals or groups. The DRVs (often the EAR) can be a useful starting point in setting a diet prescription, in the absence of any other information on the requirements of the patient, and DRVs are also used in the design of infant milk formulae.
3. food labeling. A food might be described as containing X% of the EAR for iron, for example.

When applying DRVs, their limitations must be borne in mind. In childhood, estimates of requirement are usually based on limited data. They change over the years and DRVs should be regarded as best estimates at the time that they were set. There are also variations in the values agreed for the RNI or RDA between different national committees, and estimates in the light of new evidence. For example, older estimates of energy requirements during infancy have been shown to be too high.[5]

NUTRITIONAL REQUIREMENTS DURING INFANCY AND CHILDHOOD

ENERGY

Energy is required for physical activity, thermogenesis, tissue maintenance and growth. Dietary energy is consumed in the form of fat, protein and carbohydrate. Dietary protein does not simply build new tissue but is also oxidized to provide energy. In the UK and in most Western countries dietary surveys of children of school age show that they consume about 35–40% of dietary energy in the form of fat, 10–15% as protein and 45–50% as carbohydrate. The main food sources of dietary fat are milk and milk products, fried foods and meat products.[6,7] In developing countries and in vegetarian children the contribution to energy intake of carbohydrate is much higher and the contribution of fat is generally much lower.

In infants and children, the energy requirement is the amount of dietary energy needed to balance energy expended and energy deposited in new tissue (growth). Energy expenditure can be subdivided into basal (BMR) or resting metabolic rate (RMR, around 65% of total energy expenditure [TEE] in most healthy children); energy expended on physical activity (around 25% of TEE in most healthy children) and thermogenesis (approximately 8% of TEE) (Fig. 16.1). BMR or RMR can be considered to be a 'maintenance' cost since it is the energy cost of biosynthesis, turnover, cellular ion pumps, physical work (respiratory and cardiac function). The energy expended on physical activity varies widely between children and is generally reduced when they are sick. The energy expended in thermogenesis is primarily the cost of digesting, absorbing and resynthesizing nutrients ('diet-induced thermogenesis'). Growth demands some energy expended on biosynthesis and the energy content of newly synthesized tissue. This represents up to about 35% of energy intake in rapidly growing infants, but falls for the rest of childhood and adolescence (to < 2% of energy intake) because growth rate is so much slower thereafter.

In clinical or dietetic use the EAR can provide a basis for estimating the energy requirements of individual infants and children. Alternatively a more considered approach involves estimating BMR[4] from equations based on age, weight and gender and multiplying this by a factor to take

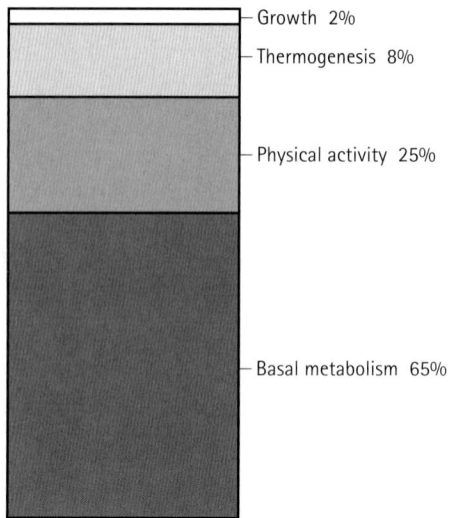

Fig. 16.1   Components of total energy expenditure in childhood.

into account physical activity. In most children 1.5–2 times BMR will meet requirements for growth and TEE. Estimation of minimum energy requirements using this approach, though better than depending on the EAR, can lead to large errors for individual children and so the adequacy of diet prescriptions for children with chronic disease should be 'titrated' against clinical observations of growth and weight change.

PROTEINS AND AMINO ACIDS

Proteins are essential components of every living cell and subserve numerous biological functions. Dietary protein is essential to maintain nitrogen balance in the body and to provide sources of sulfur. All amino acids provide nitrogen for synthesis of human proteins but some dietary amino acids are 'essential' as they cannot be synthesized de novo. Adequate intake of these essential amino acids is achievable only with a diet containing a wide variety of protein sources. Average requirements increase with age in absolute terms (EAR at 4 months is 10.6 g/d and at 18 years is 46.1 g/d) but decrease per kg body weight (EAR is 120 mg N/kg/d at 1 year and 96 mg N/kg/d in adults). In Western societies most diets, including the diets of undernourished children, contain protein well in excess of requirements.

FATS

Fats are a major energy source with an energy density of approximately 37 kJ (9 kcal)/g and they are also essential for the formation of membranes and neural tissue. Different types of fat play particular roles in the structure and function of cell membranes and neural tissue and the quality as well as the quantity, of fat intake is important. Dietary fats (lipids) are mostly triglycerides containing a wide variety of fatty acids. Where a fatty acid is replaced with phosphate a phospholipid is produced and substitutions with other compounds produce other structural and functional lipids such as sphingolipids and glycolipids.

Fats from animal produce tend to contain saturated fatty acids with no double bonds and those from plants and fish tend to contain mono- or polyunsaturated fatty acids (PUFAs). This is not universally true: some plants, such as coconut, produce saturated fat. It is recommended that children over 5 years should adopt a diet with a similar fat content to that recommended for adults. Thus 10% of daily energy needs should be from saturated fat, 12% from monounsaturated fats, 6% from polyunsaturated, with a mixture of n-6 and n-3 fatty acids (with at least linoleic 1%, alpha-linolenic 0.2%) and trans fatty acids 2%, giving a total fatty acid intake of 30% dietary energy or 33% including dietary glycerol.

There are two essential fatty acids – linoleic (C18:2n-6) and alpha-linolenic (C18:3n-3) – which the human body cannot synthesize. These are precursors of phospholipids, prostaglandins, thromboxane, leukotrienes and arachidonic (AA), eicosapentaenoic (EPA) and docosahexaenoic (DHA) acids. Young infants have limited ability to transform linolenic acid to DHA and linoleic to AA, which are both present in human milk. Many infant formulae do not contain DHA and the membrane phospholipids in the brains of infants whose intake of DHA is deficient have substituted saturated fatty acids for DHA. While some infant formulas have been supplemented with PUFAs their impact on neurodevelopment, except in the preterm, is unproven.[8]

CARBOHYDRATES

Carbohydrates in the diet provide energy of approximately 17 kJ (4 kcal)/g and are also an important component of structural and functional glycoproteins and glycolipids. Glucose is an essential fuel for the brain, which cannot metabolize fat for energy. It can be synthesized by the liver from amino acids and propionic acid, but a minimum amount of dietary carbohydrate is necessary to inhibit ketosis and to allow complete oxidation of fat.

Carbohydrates can be divided into sugars (up to three residues), oligosaccharides (up to 10 residues) and complex carbohydrates (polysaccharides) on the basis of chain length. It is recommended that intake of extrinsic sugar is restricted to less than 10% of energy intake to prevent dental caries and, possibly, obesity.

Some oligosaccharides are undigestible in the human small intestine. These include fructo-oligosaccharides such as raftilose from inulin, and galactosyl-oligosaccharides such as raffinose in beans. Similar oligosaccharides are present in human milk. These pass to the colon, where they are rapidly fermented to short chain fatty acids (SCFAs) and gases and may produce flatulence if eaten in excess. These oligosaccharides are believed to have 'probiotic' properties: that is they promote the growth of beneficial bacteria, mainly bifidobacteria and lactobacilli, in the colon.

Complex carbohydrates include starch and dietary fiber. Starch is found in several forms in food, some of which are less digestible than others. Starch cooked under normal conditions can be rapidly or slowly digestible, but is mostly digested and absorbed in the small intestine, whereas raw starches, as found in unripe bananas or raw potato and some processed starches (retrograded amylose) may be resistant to human enzymes ('resistant starch') and pass into the colon undigested. Other modified starches, included in many foods during manufacture and processing, are also resistant to digestion to some degree. More starch may escape small intestinal digestion in young children than in adults, owing to immaturity of digestion in early life, and this will influence colonic function and the energy absorbed from food.

Nondigestible carbohydrates include nonstarch polysaccharides and lignin. Dietary fiber polysaccharides are undigested in the small intestine and are fermented by the colonic microflora to SCFA and gases. These SCFAs are rapidly absorbed, resulting in an average energy value of 8.4 kJ (2 kcal)/g for dietary fiber.

Because diets high in dietary fiber are less energy dense and more satiating than the converse, it is not recommended that infants and young children consume high-fiber diets. Nevertheless dietary fiber plays an important part in normal large bowel function and is an essential constituent of the healthy diet from an early age. Older children, however, who do not need such an energy-dense diet, should be encouraged to eat foods rich in complex carbohydrates.

VITAMINS AND MINERALS: STRUCTURE, FUNCTION, DIETARY SOURCES

Vitamins are a group of naturally occurring organic nutrients that have little in common except that they are essential in the diet. They can be divided into water-soluble and fat-soluble vitamins (Tables 16.1 and 16.2). The major dietary sources of vitamins are summarized in Table 16.3. Water-soluble vitamins are easily absorbed, sometimes by active transport, and are not stored in the body to any great extent. Excessive intake normally results in excretion of the excess in the urine.

Fat-soluble vitamins, on the other hand, are absorbed with fat and thus any factor reducing the amount of fat digested and/or absorbed will reduce their absorption. Fat-soluble vitamins are also stored in the body and thus deficiencies in the diet may take some time to affect nutritional status, but they are more likely to have toxic effects if eaten in excess.

Minerals are the inorganic elements (other than carbon, hydrogen and nitrogen) that are found in the body and which are essential constituents of diet. The major dietary sources of minerals are summarized in Table 16.4. They include the 'trace elements' which are required in very small, but vital amounts. Minerals serve many different biological functions ranging from structural (calcium in bone), transport (iron in hemoglobin), energy metabolism (phosphorus in adenosine triphosphate [ATP]), endocrine (iodine in thyroid), neurotransmission (magnesium) and enzyme action (molybdenum).

The dietary sources, function and requirements of vitamins and minerals are provided elsewhere.[2-4] Deficiency and toxicity diseases associated with these micronutrients are described later.

NUTRITIONAL ASSESSMENT

Nutritional assessment is the evaluation of an individual's nutritional status. It is a means by which the undernourished (or overnourished) child can be identified, the nutritional effects of therapy and the efficacy of nutritional interventions monitored, and the prevalence of under- or overnutrition in a group determined. Undernutrition is common, particularly among sick children in hospital,[9] and evidence that it has important clinical consequences has led to increasing interest in methods for assessing nutritional status in sick children.[10,11]

There are five principal approaches to nutritional assessment: anthropometric; dietary; biochemical; clinical; functional.[11] Each evaluates a different aspect of nutritional status. All have limitations, and there is still much debate over choice of methods, reference values, and interpretation of measurements. Functional assessment, the use of functional deficits (e.g. deficits in immune function or muscle function) to identify or measure undernutrition, is not discussed here since it is so rarely used in children and remains largely restricted to research applications.[11]

ANTHROPOMETRIC NUTRITIONAL ASSESSMENT

Anthropometry is the measurement of physical dimensions of the human body at different ages. Typically, the measurements are compared with population reference data to identify abnormalities that may result from nutrient deficiencies or excess (usually energy deficiency, with protein deficiency in developing countries).[11]

The body mass index (BMI) – weight (kg)/height (m)^2 – is a simple and useful tool for assessing or monitoring the overweight and underweight which is gradually superseding more traditional indices such as weight for height and weight for age. Many countries have population reference data for BMI from birth to adulthood, and these are available as BMI charts for clinical use. BMI can be expressed as a SD score or as a centile, and a cut-off is often used to define over- or undernutrition. To avoid the problem of changes in population distribution of BMI over time it has been agreed in the UK to 'freeze' the charts based on the 1990 growth charts.[12] In the UK it is suggested that children who cross two centile 'spaces' or who are below the 2nd or above the 98th centile for BMI should be considered as likely to be under- or overnourished and at least require further assessment. It is important to note that the meaning of a particular approach depends on using cut-off points in this way carries the risk of misclassifying individual children, but this is reduced if there is other (e.g. biochemical or clinical) evidence of nutritional abnormalities, or if serial measures of BMI are available.

In clinical practice these whole-body anthropometric indices are useful, but can be limited, as for instance, when a child has ascites, fluid retention, or a large solid tumor. Such conditions can confound weight-based anthropometric indices, and the most useful and widely used alternatives are mid upper arm circumference (MUAC – related to

Table 16.1   Structure, function and mode of absorption of water-soluble vitamins

Vitamin	Chemical structure	Functions	Absorption
Thiamin	Pyrimidine ring joined to thiazole ring	Thiamin pyrophosphate coenzyme for many reactions in carbohydrate metabolism	Active transport or passive transport at concentration 1 µmol or 5 mg/d
Vitamin B$_{12}$	Cobalamin, porphyrin like ring containing cobalt; 5-deoxyadenosylcobalamin, methyl cobalamin, hydroxycobalamin	Co-factor for methionine synthetase, methylmalonyl-CoA mutase	Absorbed bound to various carrier proteins; R protein in stomach, IF protein in small intestine. Transcobalamin in basolateral membrane, 70% efficient
Folic acid	Folate, substituted pteridine ring linked to p-aminobenzoic acid. Exists as polyglutamated reduced or substituted forms of folic acid	Coenzyme for several reactions, transfer of single carbon units in reactions essential to metabolism of several amino acids and nucleic acid synthesis	Various dietary forms need to be hydrolyzed before absorption as monoglutamyl folate by active transport
Vitamin B$_6$	Pyridoxine, pyridoxal, pyridoxamine, pyridoxine HCl	Pyridoxal phosphate coenzyme for reactions related to protein metabolism, amino transferase decarboxylase and for amine synthesis, e.g. 5HT, heme synthesis, glycogen metabolism, sphingolipid and niacin synthesis	Hydrolyzed and absorbed passively
Niacin	Nicotinamide	NAD, NADP for oxidoreductases	Absorbed as nicotinic acid, nicotinamide, NMN
Riboflavin	Isoalloxazine ring with ribityl side chain. Flavin mononucleotide, flavin adenosine	Flavoprotein enzymes in oxidative reductive reactions, in metabolic pathways and cellular respiration	By sodium-dependent saturable proteins
Biotin	Imidazole ring fused to tetrahydrothiophene ring with valeric acid side chain	Co-factor for carboxylases in fatty acid synthesis, metabolism, gluconeogenesis branched chain amino acid metabolism	Actively absorbed as free biotin in small intestine
Pantothenic acid	Dimethyl derivative of butyric acid linked to beta-alanine	Constituent of CoA and esters essential for lipid and carbohydrate metabolism	Ingested as part of CoA released by intestinal phosphatase absorbed as pantothenic acid
Vitamin C	Ascorbic acid	Essential for hydroxylation of proline and lysine in collagen synthesis, needed for carnitine and noradrenaline synthesis	Active sodium-linked absorption

IF, intrinsic factor; NAD, nicotinamide adenine dinucleotide; NADP, nicotinamide adenine dinucleotide phosphate; NMN, nicotinamide mononucleotide.

Table 16.2   Structure, function and mode of absorption of fat-soluble vitamins

Vitamin	Chemical structure	Functions	Absorption
Vitamin A	Retinol, beta-carotene, six beta-carotene = one retinol	Cellular differentiation, vision, fetal development, immune system, spermatogenesis, appetite, hearing, growth	With fat 80% absorbed
Vitamin D	Calciferol, ergocalciferol, cholecalciferol. Metabolized in skin, liver and kidneys to active forms	Essential for calcium absorption, regulates calcium metabolism, involved in immune system	With fat 80% absorbed
Vitamin E	Tocopherols, tocotrienols; 8 naturally occurring forms	Antioxidant prevents lipid peroxidation	With fat absorption
Vitamin K	2 metholnaphthoquinone rings, with side chains. Phylloquinone, menaquinone, menadione	Needed for gla-proteins. Catalyzes synthesis of prothrombin in liver for clotting factors VII, IX and X	With fat 50–80% absorbed

muscle mass and fat mass, an index of 'protein/energy' status), skin-fold thickness (notably over the triceps: an index of fatness), and indices derived from these (arm muscle area or arm muscle circumference), which are more specific indices of muscle bulk and are particularly useful in measuring small changes.[11]

When reporting and interpreting raw or derived anthropometric indices (e.g. BMI, weight-for-height, height-for-age) relative to a reference population there are three principal approaches: (1) classification with reference to centiles, (2) use of percentage of reference median,

and (3) use of SD or 'Z' scores. While the first two approaches are most commonly used in clinical nutritional assessment, there is now a consensus that the third approach, the calculation of SD scores, is more clinically informative.[13]

DIETARY NUTRITIONAL ASSESSMENT

Assessment of nutritional status based on dietary intake should take into account current and past food intake. Dietary assessments

Table 16.3   Dietary sources of vitamins

Vitamin	Food sources
Thiamin	Cereals (breakfast cereals, bread), vegetables (potatoes), milk and milk products, meat and meat products, cereal products
Vitamin B$_{12}$	Milk and milk products, meat and meat products, cereals (alternative source: yeast extract for vegetarians)
Folic acid	Cereals, vegetables, milk products, liver *Breakfast cereals, bread, vegetables, milk products*
Vitamin B$_6$	Vegetables, cereal products, milk products, meat products *Milk and milk products, vegetables, breakfast cereals* (Alternative sources: poultry, fish, eggs, nuts)
Niacin	Cereal products (bread, breakfast cereals), meat products, milk and milk products. *Vegetables*
Riboflavin	Milk products, cereal products (bread, breakfast cereals), meat products. *Cereals, milk*
Biotin	(Good sources: liver, egg, cereals, yeast)
Pantothenic acid	(Good sources: widely distributed, meat, cereals, legumes)
Vitamin C	Beverages (fruit juice), vegetables (potatoes), fruit and nuts. *Vegetables, beverages*
Vitamin A	Retinol: vegetables, milk products, fat spreads, cereal products. *Milk products, meat products, vegetables* Beta-carotene: vegetables, meat and meat products. *Vegetables*
Vitamin D	Cereal products, fat spreads, meat products (Alternative source: oily fish) *Fat spreads, breakfast cereals, milk and milk products*
Vitamin E	Vegetables, fat spreads, cereal products *Fat spreads, vegetables, meat and meat products, cereal products*
Vitamin K	(Good sources: vegetables, margarines, but synthesized in colon)

Sources of nutrients for infants are shown in italics.
From UK National Diet and Nutrition Surveys[6,7]

Table 16.4   Dietary sources of minerals

Minerals	Food sources of major minerals	Alternative good sources
Iron	Cereal products (bread, breakfast cereals), vegetables, meat/meat products. *Cereals, meat, vegetables*	
Calcium	Milk and milk products, cereal products *Milk, milk products, cereals*	
Phosphorus	Milk products, cereal products, meat products, vegetables *Milk and milk products, cereal products, meat*	
Potassium	Vegetables, milk products, cereal products, meat products *Milk and milk products, vegetables, cereal products*	
Copper	Cereal products, vegetables, milk products, fruit *Cereal products, meat and meat products, vegetables*	
Iodine	Milk products, cereal products *Milk and milk products, cereal products*	Shellfish, legumes, cereals, liver, seafood, seaweeds, iodized salt
Zinc	Meat and meat products, milk, cereal products, vegetables	
Selenium	(Good sources: cereals, meat, fish)	Amount in foods depends on soil quality Deficiency may occur where soil is poor
Magnesium	Cereals, milk products, vegetables, meat products *Cereals, milk products*	
Chromium	(Good sources: yeast, meat, cereals, legumes, nuts)	

Sources of nutrients for infants are shown in italics.
From UK National Diet and Nutrition Surveys[6,7]

should be done by a pediatric dietitian who has the skills to ensure that all aspects of intake are considered, including assessment of the quantities of food eaten. All methods of dietary assessment have limited accuracy and the data obtained should always be interpreted with caution. Dietary assessment in children is best viewed as a means of explaining or solving a nutritional problem, rather than definitively identifying or confirming it. Detailed descriptions of methodology for obtaining dietary and nutrient intakes are provided elsewhere.[2,3,11]

For nutritional assessment of infants (excluding those who are exclusively breast-fed), dietary assessment methods are more accurate, since much food is provided by milk feeds and most mothers can readily provide a fairly accurate record of the number and volume of feeds and the amount of solids taken.

BIOCHEMICAL NUTRITIONAL ASSESSMENT

Biochemical nutritional assessment requires measurement of nutrient concentrations in the blood, urine, other fluids or tissues. There is an optimal concentration of nutrients within the body, below and above which deficiency and toxicity can occur. However circulating concentrations of nutrients are not an accurate measurement of tissue stores and reflect the immediate availability of particular nutrients. In the blood some nutrients are found 'free' (e.g. vitamin C), some 'bound' (e.g. calcium, iron) to carrier proteins, and some as 'precursors' (e.g. beta-carotene). Each nutrient has its own site of storage and function and so universally applicable statements about biochemical nutritional assessment are not possible.

In pediatric practice, measurements of nutrient concentrations or biochemical markers of nutritional status and/or growth are made most commonly in the blood or urine. In certain nutritional deficiency or toxicity states, and in some metabolic diseases, measurements of concentrations of particular nutrients in specific tissues should be made. Changes in circulating concentrations of many nutrients occur only when tissue stores have been depleted and normal blood concentrations do not necessarily indicate normal nutritional status. The nutrients that are commonly measured in the blood are discussed here.

Blood urea reflects not only renal function but also protein intake. It can be low in rapidly growing neonates and in children with hepatic failure. High blood urea can be a marker of the infant or toddler with a high cows' milk intake. Low urea is not an early or a sensitive sign of undernutrition. Plasma amino acids measured quantitatively may show low glutamine. In the fasting state, hepatic uptake of alanine for gluconeogenesis causes blood levels of this amino acid to fall. In patients on vegan diets or where severely reduced protein intake limits lysine availability for its synthesis, carnitine deficiency may develop. In these circumstances clinical effects are rare.

Alkaline phosphatase is a sensitive indicator of nutritional rickets and osteomalacia. Measurement of vitamin D level is not indicated in the presence of normal calcium and phosphate. Prevalence studies have shown how difficult it is to make absolute definitions of iron deficiency. Hemoglobin and red cell indices may not fully reflect iron stores. Ferritin reflects total body iron stores but is also an acute phase protein and concentrations may be falsely high in acute infection. Serum iron, total iron binding capacity (TIBC) and free erythrocyte protoporphyrin (FEP) may be measured: iron falls, and TIBC and FEP rise in iron deficiency anemia.

Deficiency of water-soluble vitamins is rare in developed countries, although this may develop rapidly in patients who are receiving inadequately supplemented i.v. fluids or total parenteral nutrition (PN). Red cell transketolase activity gives an indirect indication of thiamine deficiency, which can occur because of the demands of a high glucose intake for thiamine pyrophosphate cofactor. Deficiency of vitamin B_{12}, vitamin A or vitamin E develops late because of large tissue stores. Prothrombin time reflects vitamin K status if liver function is normal.

Circulating concentrations of trace elements (copper, zinc, selenium) decrease late in deficiency. Zinc or magnesium deficiency occurs in Crohn's disease and other causes of chronic diarrhea. Low glutathione peroxidase activity in red cells indirectly indicates selenium deficiency but a direct selenium assay may be preferable.

CLINICAL NUTRITIONAL ASSESSMENT

Clinical nutritional assessment is limited by its subjectivity, even when performed by specialists.[14] More structured, and objective, forms of clinical assessment are likely to become valuable in clinical practice, but are based on limited evidence at present.[15] Signs of 'pure' or single nutrient deficiencies rarely occur alone and physical signs such as glossitis or angular stomatitis are nonspecific. Physical examination should ideally be interpreted in association with anthropometric, dietary and biochemical nutritional assessment.

The 'classical' physical signs of protein-energy malnutrition, some vitamin and mineral deficiencies are described later. It should be remembered, however, that physical signs are a late manifestation of nutrient deficiency, occurring after tissue stores have been depleted and adaptive changes have failed to maintain normal nutrient homeostasis and function.

HEALTHY DIET: INFANCY, CHILDHOOD AND ADOLESCENCE

INFANT

Milk is believed to be the sufficient and sole source of energy and nutrients for about the first 6 months of life.[16] Complementary (nonmilk, weaning) foods should be introduced at around this time, to fill the gap between the energy and nutrient needs provided by milk and those that the infant requires to maintain normal growth and development.

Human milk

Human milk is a complex blend of nutrients and immunological and other bioactive substances. The former provide the energy, macronutrients (carbohydrates, fats and proteins) and micronutrients (vitamins and minerals) that the baby needs to grow, develop and function (physical activity, thermogenesis, essential organ function – BMR). The latter confer protection from bacterial and viral infections and assist adaptation to life outside the womb.

Formula milk

Approved infant formulas provide safe but inferior alternatives to breast milk. They broadly resemble human milk in terms of their chemical composition but lack the enzymes, immunological or other bioactive substances found in human milk. The majority of formulas is based on cows' milk and are either whey or casein predominant. The former have a protein content based on demineralized whey with a whey:casein ratio similar to breast milk (60% whey:40% casein). The protein source of casein-predominant formulas is skimmed cows' milk with a ratio of 80% casein:20% whey. Ideally infants should remain on the formula first used until the end of the first year of life but a follow-on formula may be used from the age of 6 months. Whole cow's milk should not be used as the main milk drink for infants until the age of 1 year.[16]

Soya formulas should be used only for infants with proven intolerance to cows' milk formulas or lactose and for infants of vegetarian mothers who have elected not to breast-feed. Although satisfactory growth has been achieved in babies fed formulas based on cows' milk and soya, their nutritional composition differs from that of human milk, for example in their essential fatty acid contents, non-nutritional factors, and bioavailability of some micronutrients such as iron. Short- and long-term studies on risk of infection, growth and neurological outcome of children who have received these formulas show that human milk is preferable to 'artificial' formulas for the infant.[16]

Complementary foods

At about 6 months of age complementary foods (nonmilk, 'solids') should be introduced into the diet. The infant's iron stores are becoming depleted, chewing needs to be developed, and milk alone is insufficient to meet the growing nutritional requirements of the infant.[16] In addition to a nonmilk diet, infants should continue to receive at least 500–600 ml of breast milk or formula daily. Nonwheat cereals, fruit, vegetables and potatoes are all suitable first weaning foods. Between 6 and 9 months of age, meat, fish, all cereals, pulses, fish and eggs can be introduced. No salt should be added to home-prepared foods, and only enough sugar used to make sour fruits palatable. Complementary foods should aim to have an energy density of at least 1 kcal/g (4.2 kJ/g).

TODDLER

By the end of the first year infants are taking a widening range of foods and beginning to share those eaten by the rest of the family. The feeding of the preschool child progresses through many skill-learning processes, from the semi-solid/liquid diet of the weanling, through finger-feeding of bits of food which require chewing at around 1 year of age, to spoon-feeding by the age of 2 years, to mastering child-sized cutlery and adult-type food by the age of 5 years.

Nutritionally, toddler foods bridge the gap between the energy-dense diet of the infant, which provides around 50% of energy from fat, and that of the adult, where around 35% of energy should be derived from fat. Toddlers, however, have smaller gastric capacities than adults, and a balance must be struck between the gradual reduction of energy-dense, fat-containing foods and the introduction of lower fat foods. Toddlers are at risk of iron deficiency and care should be taken that foods containing adequate iron are used. The toddler should continue to consume around 500 ml of milk daily (or equivalent from other foods such as yoghurt and cheese). Full-fat milk should be used from 1–2 years of age. Thereafter, as long as growth and energy intake are satisfactory, semi-skimmed milk can be given from 2–5 years of age. After 2 years of age other lower fat dairy products such as yoghurt, spreads and cheese may be used. Many toddlers become fussy and difficult with meals and it may be more appropriate to follow a feeding regimen based on three small meals and three snacks daily. Some young children begin to prefer easily assimilated liquids, particularly if given from bottles, for solid food, which requires chewing and the use of cutlery. After the first year all drinks taken during the day should be taken from a cup. National surveys have shown that some toddlers and young children are at risk of inadequate energy, vitamin A, iron and zinc intakes.[6,7] There has also been concern about the risk of rickets in Asian children, who should receive vitamin D supplementation up to the age of 5 years.

SCHOOLCHILD

After the age of 5 years the diet can change towards that advised for adults. Fiber intake should increase with generous consumption of fruits, vegetables and high fiber cereals such as wholemeal bread, pasta and breakfast cereals. Saturated fat intake should be moderated by the use of skimmed or semi-skimmed milk, low fat or polyunsaturated spreads, low fat dairy products and eating fish, poultry and lean meats. The intake of non-milk extrinsic sugar should be avoided because of its association with dental caries and possibly obesity.

ADOLESCENT

The timing of the adolescent growth spurt varies between individuals so that nutrient requirements should be related to weight and height rather than age.[4] Weight gain during puberty in girls is mainly due to fat deposition whereas boys accumulate more muscle and skeletal tissue.

Eating habits show a trend to persist with time and a healthy adolescent diet should anticipate and minimize the long-term risks of chronic cardiovascular diseases, obesity, diabetes and other adult conditions associated with a poor diet.

Many adolescents will experiment with different diets. 'Vegetarian' diets which include some animal foods such as milk, cheese or eggs usually achieve adequate nutrient intakes. Teenagers who elect to follow a vegan regimen should take supplements of vitamin B₁₂, calcium, vitamin D, iron and zinc. Avoidance of specific foods on religious or cult grounds may result in severe nutrient deficiencies unless the dietary regimen has been based on long established traditional practices.

PRINCIPLES OF NUTRITIONAL SUPPORT

The skills required to deal with assessment, prescription, administration and monitoring of treatment increasingly fall outside the expertise of a single practitioner. Nutritional support should be provided by a team, led by a pediatrician trained and experienced in clinical nutrition, comprising dietitians, nutrition nurse specialists, a pharmacist in charge of the preparation and prescription of parenteral solutions, a biochemist responsible for monitoring biochemical outcome and a surgeon with experience of gastrostomies and insertion of i.v. long lines for PN (Table 16.5). Introduction of nutrition teams is associated with a reduction of mechanical, metabolic and infection-related complications of PN, shorter duration in hospital and decline in the cost of nutrition

Table 16.5 Composition and functions of members of a hospital nutrition team

Dietitian	Assesses nutritional status Calculates nutritional requirements Designs enteral or parenteral feeding regimens
Nurse specialist	Acts jointly with clinician, dietitian and pharmacist in practical aspects of nutrition support Patient and community care training Care of enterostomy tubes and central venous lines
Clinician	Overall responsibility for nutritional care Monitors outcome and liaises with medical/surgical team Diagnosis and management of underlying conditions and of complications of nutritional support
Pharmacist	Responsible for provision of enteral and parenteral nutrition solutions Advises on compatibility and drug interactions
Surgeon	Fashions enterostomies and inserts i.v. catheters
Biochemist	Monitors biochemical indices of nutritional status
Bacteriologist	Detection and advice on treatment of i.v. line infections

support. Nutrition support may be provided either enterally or parenterally. Before starting nutrition support it is essential to properly assess the patient's nutritional status and nutritional needs (see before and Bresson et al[17]).

ENTERAL NUTRITION

Enteral feeding should be used if the gastrointestinal tract is accessible and functional. PN should be reserved for conditions where enteral nutrition cannot meet energy and nutrient requirements via the gut alone. There are many indications for enteral tube feeding (Table 16.6), and this form of feeding has a number of advantages and disadvantages, summarized in Table 16.7.

Delivery routes and systems

Enteral feeding is a means by which nutrients can be delivered to the gastrointestinal tract by tube or enterostomy. This can be done continuously, as bolus feeds or as intermittent continuous feeds. In continuous feeding the enteral feed is infused over a period of hours (usually from 8–24 h) using a pump, which regulates the volume administered. Bolus feeding simulates the usual pattern of feeding, generating a postprandial metabolic response that is greater than that when continuous feeds are given. Feeds can be given at intervals from hourly to 4 hourly. Intermittent continuous feeding combines the feeding techniques of bolus and continuous feeds.

The choice of mode of delivery can be made using the algorithm shown in Figure 16.2. Nasogastric tubes are easy to introduce and have fewer complications than nasojejunal tubes. Nasogastric tube feeding is also more 'physiological' in that the defense and digestive functions of the stomach are utilized, but gastroesophageal reflux and aspiration are more likely to occur. Nasojejunal tubes are used when these risks are high, such as in children with neuromuscular disease, severe neurological handicap and gastrointestinal motility disorders.

Enterostomies offer a means of delivering enteral feeds directly into the stomach or jejunum, bypassing proximal mechanical, surgical or pathological obstructions. They are also preferred when pharyngeal discomfort is intolerable or the risk of aspiration high. Percutaneous endoscopic gastrostomy (PEG) is an increasingly popular technique of tube placement, and the gastrostomy button is a useful innovation for long-term feeding. Flush with the skin the button can be connected to a

Table 16.6   Conditions in which nutrition support may be indicated

Gastrointestinal disease
- Short bowel syndrome
- Inflammatory bowel disease
- Following gastrointestinal surgery
- Chronic liver disease
- Glycogen storage disease types I and III
- Fatty acid oxidation defects
- Severe enteropathies and disorders of digestion

Neurological disease
- Coma and severe facial and head injury
- Severe mental retardation and cerebral palsy
- Dysphagia secondary to cranial nerve palsy, muscular dystrophy, myasthenia gravis

Malignant disease
- Obstruction of esophagus and upper gut
- Head and neck
- Abnormality of deglutition following surgical intervention
- Gastrointestinal side-effects from chemotherapy and/or radiotherapy
- Terminal support care

Pulmonary disease
- Bronchopulmonary dysplasia
- Cystic fibrosis
- Chronic lung disease

Congenital anomalies
- Tracheoesophageal fistula
- Esophageal atresia
- Cleft palate
- Pierre Robin syndrome

Other
- Primary malnutrition
- Anorexia nervosa
- Cardiac failure
- Chronic renal disease
- Severe burns
- Severe sepsis
- Severe trauma

Enteral formulas

There is a range of enteral feeds available for children. Many are based on cows' milk and are suitable for children with an intact and functional gastrointestinal tract. These whole protein formulas are used to provide full or partial nutritional support and can be supplemented with extra energy (in the form of a glucose polymer or fat emulsion) and protein. Specialized formulas are designed to meet the altered nutrient needs and gastrointestinal and/or metabolic problems of children with different diseases. These include: (1) elemental formulas based on amino acids, vegetable oils (composed of a mixture of medium chain and long chain triglycerides) and glucose, designed for children with protracted diarrhea and severe enteropathies; (2) protein hydrolysates for children with sensitivity to food proteins; (3) formulas that are lactose-free by substitution of lactose with another carbohydrate; and (4) feeds based on soya, which are free of lactose and cows' milk protein. Modular feeds allow each macronutrient to be combined in amounts and source appropriate for the special needs of the child. Almost all clinical needs can be met by ready-prepared, commercially available formulas, and the reader should consult the literature produced by the manufacturers for full details of their composition and indications.

Home-prepared feeds and liquidized foods should not be used for enteral nutrition of children because of uncertain nutrient quality, a risk of bacterial contamination and of the feeding tube becoming blocked with food particles. During the first year of life infants who require enteral feeding and have a normal functioning gastrointestinal tract and require no nutrient modification, should receive one of the standard infant formulas.

Home enteral tube feeding

Home enteral feeding (HEF) should be considered when the sole reason for the child being in hospital is enteral nutritional support.[1] It has been estimated that the expense and effort (of providing equipment, feeds and training) is justified by a minimum of 10 d of HEF. Children with chronic diseases, such as cystic fibrosis, neuromuscular disorders, malignant disease and renal failure, can greatly benefit from HEF; some have received it for more than 10 years, and its use is growing. Many children who are happy and able to pass their own nasogastric tubes, prefer night-time HEF. Children with enterostomies may also receive HEF.

feeding tube at the child's convenience and avoids a long tube protruding from the abdomen. Many children who require long-term enteral nutrition have gastrostomies, including many who receive home enteral feeding. In some children a fundoplication may be required to prevent gastric regurgitation.

PARENTERAL NUTRITION

PN is a means by which nutrients are delivered to the patient via the vein. It may provide complete nutritional support – total parenteral nutrition (TPN) – or be combined with enteral feeding. The administration and monitoring of PN is complex and should be undertaken by

Table 16.7   Advantages and disadvantages of enteral feeding methods

Feeding method	Advantages	Disadvantages
Continuous infusion	Larger volumes of feed can be administered Smaller bore tubes can be used Less gastric distension Less 'dumping' so that feeds with higher nutrient densities can be given	Tube may become dislodged during feed administration with risk of aspiration Electric feeding pumps, reservoirs and giving–sets are expensive Some feeds containing insoluble substances cannot be given
Bolus feeds	Mimics the normal feeding gut hormonal response Position of feeding tube can be checked prior to each feed Simple procedure only: a syringe required for feed to be administered Contact with child at each feed time	Gastric distension and vomiting A wider bore feeding tube may be required, which may cause discomfort in nasopharynx if nasogastric feeding route used 'Dumping' may be experienced especially if high nutrient dense feeds given Adequate fluid requirement may be difficult to achieve
Intermittent continuous feeds	Larger volumes can be tolerated Fine-bore tubes can be used The feeding tube position can be checked Nutrient-dense feeds can be administered	Requires a great deal of supervision Electric feeding pumps, reservoirs and giving–sets are expensive prior to each feed

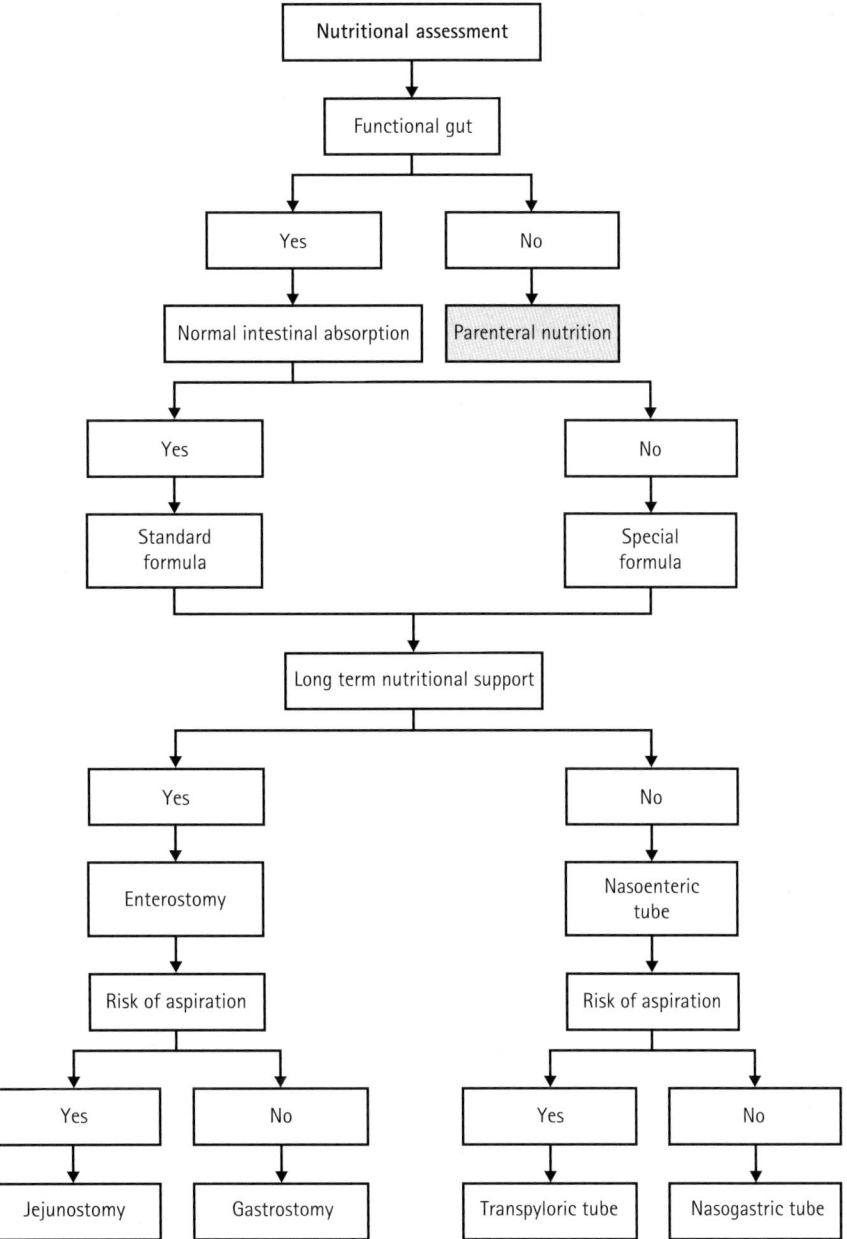

Fig. 16.2 Algorithm for choice of route of delivery of enteral feeds.

the nutrition support team. The process by which energy and nutrient requirements are calculated, techniques of delivery and assessment of PN are described in greater detail elsewhere.[10,11]

Indications and complications of PN

The principal indications for PN are shown in Table 16.8. Although sometimes life-saving, PN has been subjected to few controlled clinical trials and its precise benefits remain unclear. PN is both complex and expensive when compared with enteral nutrition, and because of the risk of serious complications (summarized in Table 16.9) and evidence that enteral nutrition helps to maintain gastrointestinal structure and function, there has been a reappraisal of its use in some groups of patients, for example in those receiving intensive care. Whilst there can be little doubt that gastrointestinal 'failure' (from whatever cause) is an absolute indication for PN, complete exclusion of luminal nutrients is frequently neither essential nor desirable. When planning nutritional intervention it is important to use the gastrointestinal tract if possible. Total enteral nutrition may be feasible if a transpyloric or jejunostomy tube is used. Even if only minimal volumes of enteral feed can be given

in addition to PN, this can help to prevent cholestasis by stimulating bile flow and pancreatic secretions, maintaining splanchnic blood flow and providing mucosal nutrition.

Overall, the most frequent recipients of PN are preterm infants. Infants with surgical problems comprise the next largest group, and are fed parenterally usually because of gut failure following surgery for congenital or acquired gastrointestinal disease, and PN has undoubtedly had a major impact on survival in children with short bowel syndrome. Children undergoing gastrointestinal surgery, those with protracted diarrhea or severe dysmotility, and others receiving intensive care often with multiorgan failure account for much of the remaining PN usage.

Ethical dilemmas arise in relation to the care of children in whom there is little or no prospect of establishing full enteral feeding at any time in the future, such as those with congenital enteropathies. The prognosis in short bowel syndrome has improved considerably. Small bowel transplantation offers hope for some children who are chronically dependent on TPN.

For children receiving PN for more than a few weeks, cyclical nutrition should be considered. This involves a gradual decrease in the time

Table 16.8   Common indications for parenteral nutrition

	Neonates	Older infants and children (relative)	
Absolute indications	Intestinal failure (e.g. functional immaturity, short bowel, pseudo-obstruction) Necrotizing enterocolitis	Gastrointestinal failure	Short bowel syndrome Protracted diarrhea Chronic pseudo-obstruction Postoperative gastrointestinal surgery Radiation/cytotoxic drug therapy (e.g. bone marrow transplantation)
Relative indications	Respiratory failure requiring IPPV Promotion of growth in preterm infants	Intensive care and multiorgan failure	Severe IBD Acute pancreatitis Acute renal failure Acute liver failure Extensive burns Severe trauma

IBD, inflammatory bowel disease; IPPV, intermittent positive pressure ventilation.

over which it is given, so that eventually the PN can be infused overnight and the central venous line left clamped for 12 h during the day. This helps to encourage mobility and psychomotor development and reduce the adverse effects of prolonged hospitalization. Oromotor skills should be promoted with comforters and, when possible, small amounts of enteral feed by mouth. The expert advice of a speech therapist should be sought at an early stage. Cyclical PN may help protect against cholestasis and hepatic dysfunction.

Catheter-related sepsis is a serious complication of PN and its incidence is greatly reduced by scrupulous attention to sterile procedures and minimal handling of i.v. lines. Other complications of long-term PN include electrolyte and micronutrient disturbances, thromboembolism and pulmonary hypertension.

Home parenteral nutrition

For those children committed to long-term PN, home treatment should be considered. The nutritional support industry and hospital outreach services should together provide the organizational and support infrastructure. Home PN offers children who would otherwise become hospitalized the possibility of realizing growth and developmental potential, a good quality of life, and a reduced risk of complications such as i.v. line

Table 16.9   Complications of parenteral nutrition

Phlebitis

Infection

Hypo- and hyperglycemia

Electrolyte disturbance

Fluid overload, dehydration

Hypophosphatemia

Anemia

Platelet and neutrophil dysfunction

Trace element deficiencies

Trace element excess

Vitamin deficiencies

Hyperammonemia

Essential fatty acid deficiency

Cholestasis and hepatic dysfunction

Metabolic acidosis

Hypercholesterolemia

Hypertriglyceridemia

Air and thromboembolism

sepsis. Suitable patients are those with long-term gastrointestinal failure who are medically stable and have adequate home circumstances. The carers must be highly motivated, well supported by the nutrition support team and capable of becoming expert in home care including sterile technique, setting up infusions, managing lines, setting pumps, and recognizing and reacting appropriately to problems. The most frequent diagnoses in children receiving home PN are short bowel, severe dysmotility, congenital enteropathy, and Crohn's disease.

OBESITY

PREVALENCE AND DIAGNOSIS

Obesity is now a major pediatric health problem. In England, for example, in 2004 16% of 2–10-year-olds and 25% of 11–15-year-olds were obese (defined as BMI > 95th percentile[17]).

Systematic reviews have consistently concluded that obesity must be assessed using objective measurements.[18] Measuring body weight alone is inadequate: weight must be adjusted for height. This adjustment is best done by calculating BMI, weight (kg) divided by height squared (m^2). Since BMI changes with age and differs between the sexes, interpretation of a single value requires a comparison to population reference data, i.e. a cut-off point in the BMI distribution must be applied to define overweight and obese. A high BMI for age and sex identifies the fattest children with moderate sensitivity and high specificity (low false-positive rate), and this definition has clinical/biological significance: children with high BMI for age and sex have a high probability of remaining obese, and of experiencing the morbidity associated with obesity.[18] Clinically there are limitations to the interpretation of BMI for individual children: while BMI is highly correlated with body fat (and with visceral fat mass, which is probably the best predictor of adverse effects) on a population basis, a particular BMI may be associated with a wide range of body fat in different individuals; there appear to be significant ethnic differences in the relationship between BMI and body fat; body composition may change as a result of exercise or dieting without change in BMI.[19]

CLINICAL CONSEQUENCES

A systematic review concluded that childhood obesity causes morbidity in childhood, and increases morbidity and mortality in adulthood.[20] Psychosocial morbidity is common, and a range of other problems (respiratory, metabolic, hepatic, orthopedic) less common. In adolescents and young adults, obesity has adverse 'social' effects, particularly in girls. These include reduced educational attainment and income in both the UK and the USA.[20] Cardiovascular risk factors are associated with obesity, even in childhood, and they tend to 'cluster' in the obese child. Childhood obesity has a strong tendency to persist after the age of about

3 years, and it probably increases morbidity and premature mortality in adult life, particularly from cardiovascular disease and diabetes.

CAUSES

Obesity is a disorder of energy balance. Excess dietary (food) energy is stored as fat *and* lean tissue, so that obese children have both a larger fat mass and lean body mass than their non-obese peers. Larger fat-free mass and body mass means that the energy requirements of the obese child are considerably *higher* than those of the non-obese child. Obese patients tend to report low food intakes, implying reduced metabolic rate as a cause of obesity. This is rarely the case and most obese children and adolescents substantially under-report their true dietary intake.[21] One consequence is that dietary intakes reported by obese patients/their families must be viewed with caution, and can only provide a crude estimate of eating habits.

TREATMENT

Detailed descriptions of therapeutic strategies for treating childhood obesity are provided elsewhere.[21,22] Recent systematic reviews of both treatment[23–25] and preventive interventions[23,26] have concluded that we lack good evidence on generalizable intervention strategies from high-quality, long-term, randomized, controlled trials (RCTs). More recent RCTs have been of higher quality and have generally had longer term follow-up, but the effects of pharmacological treatment (adolescents) and lifestyle therapy have usually been modest.[27] The systematic reviews have concluded that the 'best bets' in therapy are: modest dietary restriction and 'healthy eating' (to reduce energy intake), reductions in sedentary behavior (TV viewing and other screen time, to less than 2 h/d, to increase energy expenditure and reduce energy intake), and increases in 'lifestyle physical activity' (such as walking, to increase energy expenditure). As in adults, childhood obesity is often resistant to treatment so therapy should be offered only where the child/family perceive the need to make lifestyle changes, or where there is severe obesity-related co-morbidity (such as sleep apnea). Therapy should involve changing family lifestyle and not simply focus on the child.

SECONDARY OBESITY

Careful history and examination will usually differentiate between 'simple obesity' and any underlying pathology which may be responsible[21–23] (usually very rare). The child with simple obesity often has relatively tall stature. In contrast children with Cushing's syndrome and hypothyroidism have relative or short stature, and growth failure. Hyperphagic dysmorphic syndromes include the Prader–Willi and Laurence–Moon–Biedl syndromes, but many dysmorphic syndromes with learning disability can be associated with voracious appetite. Some chromosomal abnormalities (Down and Klinefelter's syndromes) are associated with obesity. Recurrent headaches with recent increases in severity and frequency may indicate a hypothalamic or pituitary tumor. Severe mood disturbance, unstable temperature, polyuria and polydipsia and visual disturbance support this diagnosis. It is vital to identify causes of secondary obesity early. Management of secondary obesity involves treatment of the underlying disease.

MALNUTRITION

'Malnutrition' describes conditions that result from a diet (supply) that does not satisfy nutritional requirements (demand). 'Secondary malnutrition' refers to malnutrition resulting from disease or trauma, such as inflammatory bowel disease or severe burns.[28] Primary malnutrition, which accounts for the vast majority of cases, is associated with poverty, involving inter alia inadequate food, recurrent infections and lack of health care. It is extremely common, affecting a quarter of the world's children[29] because so many live in poverty in the 'developing' world. It contributes to almost 60% of all child deaths.[30] Lack of effective prevention and treatment accounts for almost all of these unnecessary deaths. In the survivors, malnutrition leads to permanent suboptimal physical and mental development affecting billions of adults mainly in south and south-east Asia, Africa and South America. Fortunately, in most of the world except sub-Saharan Africa, the prevalence of malnutrition is falling slowly.[29]

CLASSIFICATION OF MALNUTRITION

When nutritional supply fails to meet demand, reductive adaptation occurs: in children, weight gain and development are abnormally slow and sometimes negative, and physiological functions become impaired. Malnutrition is characterized initially by thinness (wasting) and later, by shortness (stunting), and there is often evidence of specific nutrient deficiencies. Bilateral (nutritional) edema is a less common complication associated with characteristic abnormalities of metabolism and a poor prognosis. Its cause is unclear.

Malnutrition is most easily diagnosed and classified using anthropometry, measuring the child's dimensions and weight, and relating them to what would be expected normally, based on reference data. Several classifications of malnutrition have been proposed over 50 years. The Wellcome and Waterlow classifications are useful together as they identify which children need which treatment and the degree of urgency (Table 16.10). Recently, the WHO[31] classified moderate malnutrition as wasting (weight −3 to −2 standard deviation score [SDS] or 70–79% of reference weight for height) or stunting (height −3 to −2 SDS or 85–89% height for age); and severe malnutrition as severe wasting (weight lower than −3 SDS or < 70% of reference weight for height) or/and nutritional edema or/and severe stunting (height lower than −3 SDS or < 85% of reference height for age). Supine length, rather than height, is measured in children up to 2 years and those unable to stand. Without appropriate intervention, children with severe wasting or nutritional edema usually deteriorate rapidly until they are at high risk of imminent death. Even more recently,[32] mid-upper arm circumference (MUAC) has emerged as the most useful index of the severity of malnutrition when large numbers are affected, as in complex emergencies. Its particular value is its ease of measurement and classification (Table 16.10).

Wasting and edema can develop rapidly and resolve rapidly: measurable stunting develops slowly and, even with intervention, usually carries on until puberty in a poor environment. Although puberty tends to be delayed, final height is usually less than predicted. This applies to whole populations living in poverty. Stunting is associated with lower than expected IQ. The combination reduces the chances of having normal pregnancies, births and birth weights; good employment and prosperity; and improved life opportunities in the next generation.

CLINICAL FEATURES

Clinical features of malnutrition vary enormously and none distinguishes primary from secondary malnutrition. In an infant, because head size is better preserved than length or weight, the trunk and limbs often appear relatively small. Abdominal girth is variable and sometimes relatively large. The older child, on the other hand, may appear well-proportioned and healthy but diminutive. This implies predominant stunting and thus mild to moderate problems over a long period. However, an acute severe problem in a previously well-nourished child may be visible first as wasting alone. Severely malnourished children are usually wasted and stunted.

In general, edema is less common in very young infants. It often arises over a few days, when a child, already compromised nutritionally and failing to thrive, develops an infection like measles or gastroenteritis. If at the walking stage, edema is first noted on both feet; if younger, it may be seen first in the hands or around the eyes. The child usually appears ill, and is apathetic, irritable and anorexic. Skin lesions tend to be more common and more severe in the edematous child. Typically, they start as a darkening and thickening of the keratin layer which when damaged splits or flakes off, leaving patches of hypopigmented thin skin

Table 16.10   Some classifications of childhood malnutrition

Classification	Variable	Grade	Nutritional edema
Wellcome	Weight for age % 60–80	Undernourished Kwashiorkor	Absent Present
	< 60 (≈ –4 SDS)[a]	Marasmus Marasmic-kwashiorkor	Absent Present
Waterlow	Weight for height[2,3] % 80–90 70–80 < 70 (≈ –3 SDS) Height[b,c] for age % 90–95 85–90 < 85 (≈ –3 SDS)	Mild wasting Moderate wasting Severe wasting Mild stunting Moderate stunting Severe stunting	
CTC[4]	Mid upper arm circumference (6 months to 5 years old only) < 110 mm	Acute malnutrition	

[a]SDS = standard deviation score = number of standard deviations from median of reference data (NCHS/WHO).
[b]'Height', for standing children, 'length' for those unable to stand.
[c]Weight for height = child's weight × 100/weight of 'reference' child of same height; Height for age = child's height × 100/height of 'reference' child of same age.
WHO;[31] Valid International.[32]

and sometimes oozing sores that refuse to heal. Such skin damage tends to occur round the orifices (mouth, perianal and perineal), over joints and on the extremities. It also occurs where edema stretches the skin, as on the foot and lower leg. Firm, smooth hepatomegaly, associated sometimes with vast deposits of lipid, is also frequent in the edematous child. However, abdominal distension, which is common, is usually mainly gaseous. Ascites is rare in children. Stools tend to be frequent, small and often loose, green and mucusy.

Other clinical features include depigmentation, thinning and straightening of the hair associated with increased fragility and pluckability. In contrast, in longstanding malnutrition, eyelashes tend to be long and silky and in some children, lanugo hair grows luxuriantly. Many of these clinical signs can be recognized in Figures 16.3 and 16.4, which show infants with kwashiorkor (edematous malnutrition) and marasmus (severe wasting), respectively. Clinical features of specific

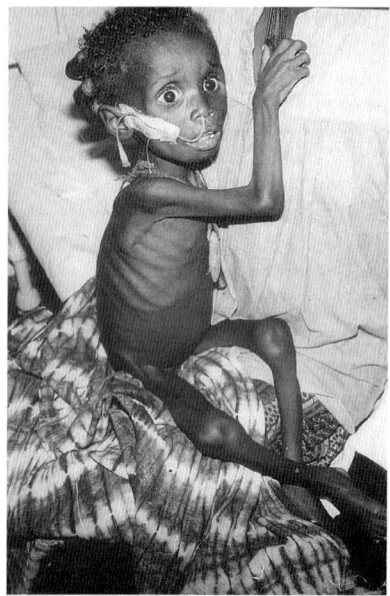

Fig. 16.4   Child with nutritional marasmus. (With permission of R.G. Whitehead)

nutrient deficiencies may also be present, such as rickets, scurvy, keratomalacia, etc. (see later). When a child is severely malnourished, he or she may develop any or all of the following: extreme apathy, hypotonia, pallor, hypothermia, cold extremities with prolonged capillary refill time, a weak pulse, dyspnea, petechiae, purpura and jaundice. They are, in their various ways, evidence of sepsis, cardiac and hepatic failure and eventually, loss of cell homeostasis which, untreated, is fatal.

LABORATORY INVESTIGATIONS

Laboratory investigations are generally unhelpful. Hemoglobin falls but serum ferritin tends to rise and there is anisocytosis. Severely malnourished children, with their damaged skin and mucosae, prolonged intestinal transit time and reduced secretions, are very susceptible to skin,

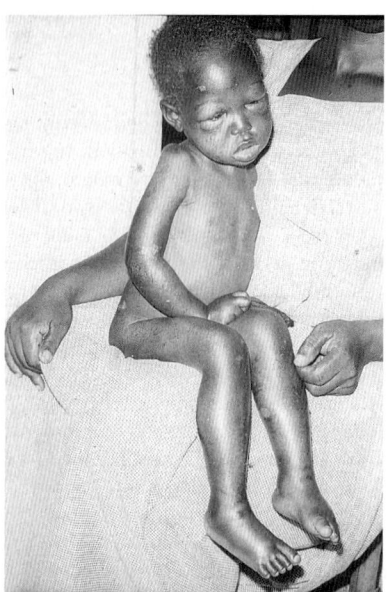

Fig. 16.3   Child with kwashiorkor. (With permission of R.G. Whitehead)

gastrointestinal and respiratory infections. They also have impaired resistance to infection, in particular, their acute phase and cell-mediated immune responses. Fever and the cardinal signs of inflammation tend to be slight or absent. White cell counts and C-reactive protein (CRP) rise little. In very ill children, neutropenia may occur, with hypothermia and hypoglycemia when feeding has been withheld for only a couple of hours. Serum electrolytes do not reflect body content, only circulating concentrations. Thus, high serum potassium masks intracellular potassium deficiency, and in hospital, is most likely due to i.v. delivery and impaired cellular uptake. A low serum sodium masks sodium overload and the only useful interpretation is that the child is very ill. Magnesium deficiency occurs. Serum urea tends to be low, reflecting low protein intake and reduced catabolism. Serum albumin is almost invariably low in edematous children. This finding led the way to the protein deficiency theory of development of nutritional edema in some children. However, edema is not due to low serum albumin alone, protein deficient diets are not limited to those children who develop edema and dietary protein repletion does not cure it.[33] At present, the most likely pathogenesis of edematous malnutrition involves extensive membrane dysfunction associated with lipid peroxidation, a product of antioxidant deficiency in the face of acute oxidative stress.[34] As evidence of this, red blood cell glutathione and plasma zinc, copper, selenium and glutathione peroxidase, vitamin E and carotene are all particularly low in edematous children while *free* iron, a major pro-oxidant, circulates because transferrin concentrations are very low.

MANAGEMENT

Successful management of malnutrition should mean complete catch-up followed by sustained normal growth, health and development. This is rarely achieved. Effective home management should be widely implemented for children with less than severe wasting (weight for height above −3 SDS of WHO reference values) and those with stunting. Continuing poverty means this is also rarely achieved. It requires education and practical help to ensure exclusive breast-feeding to 6 months; continued breast-feeding to 2 years; good hygiene; more energy-dense diets containing all essential nutrients, taking into account their bioavailability; regular monitoring of body weight; early, appropriate treatment of complications like infections; and mental and physical stimulation to allow normal development.

Community-based therapeutic care, when feasible and carried out according to specific guidelines[32] can also be successful for many severely malnourished children including some with nutritional edema. Those who respond well are the uncomplicated ones who still have good appetites. However, for the more severely affected, and all anorexic children, a period of specialized treatment within a well-staffed and equipped specialized unit, or 'stabilization center', is essential to prevent early death, treat infection successfully and repair the child's metabolism in preparation for catch-up growth. Thus, in complex emergencies, when vast numbers of children are acutely malnourished, triage is essential to distinguish those in need of early specialized management. The same principles of management apply to all. Provided they are adhered to, the mortality from severe malnutrition should be less than 5%,[35] a vast improvement over traditional hospital figures of 20–30%.[30]

Phases of treatment

Management of severely wasted or/and edematous children is described in detail in a WHO manual[31] and several other publications.[32,36] It is best divided into phases. Following triage and, if necessary, resuscitation, the *Initial phase* involves treatment of infection and correction of disordered metabolism. The latter requires prevention and often treatment of electrolyte imbalance, specific deficits, hypoglycemia, hypothermia, dehydration, heart failure and shock, all of which will continue until death or their successful treatment. Bacterial infection must be assumed and treated with broad-spectrum antibiotics unless and until specific infections are diagnosed which require different, available therapy.

Intravenous fluids pose a major risk (cardiac failure or arrest) and should be avoided if possible. Oral or nasogastric rehydration is recommended for dehydration. However, compared with the standard WHO Oral Rehydration Solution, the solution should contain less sodium but more potassium and magnesium, zinc and copper, all of which are grossly deficient in the malnourished child with acute diarrhea. Such a solution is available commercially (ReSoMal) but this can also be prepared from WHO ORS.[31] Frequent breast-feeding is encouraged. Instead of or in addition to this, a special cows' milk based formula, 'F-75' (0.31 MJ [75 kcal]/100 ml) with relatively low protein, fat and sodium contents and osmolarity is recommended, to provide minimal stress. In the absence of F-75, recipes, from ingredients likely to be available, are also provided in the WHO manual.[31] In this initial phase, every effort is made to ensure that children receive sufficient intake for maintenance of body weight (0.42 MJ [100 kcal]/kg/d) but not growth. This may require very frequent, small tube-feeds if anorexia and vomiting are major problems. It is very important to feed regularly throughout the night to avoid hypoglycemia. Hypothermia also tends to occur then, and both of these suggest that sepsis may not have been treated successfully. F-75 contains extra minerals and vitamins but further supplements of vitamin A and folic acid are also recommended initially. Iron is contraindicated because of its potential toxicity and aggravation of infection.

Usually within a week, the second or *Rehabilitation phase* is heralded by increased appetite and improvement of mood and major abnormalities including loss of edema. The principles of management change to include feeding for growth, and stimulating mental and physical development. The transition between the first and second phases is a period of risk when 'refeeding syndrome' tends to occur. This may resolve on returning to the Initial phase and proceeding more slowly. Depending on circumstances, in particular, the availability of trained support within the community, the child may now be better managed at home. At this stage, the formula feed is changed to one that provides more energy and protein. Commercially available F-100 contains 0.42 MJ/100 ml, 12% energy from protein and 53% from fat. Like F-75, it also provides extra minerals and vitamins but not iron. However, supplementary iron is necessary during this phase for new hemoglobin synthesis. Like F-75, F-100 can also be prepared from usually available ingredients but both 'home-prepared' feeds benefit from the addition of extra minerals and vitamins. These are best provided as a commercial preparation whose composition is given in the WHO manual.[31] Another product, ready-to-use-therapeutic food (RUTF),[32] which is a vegetable oil (originally peanut)-based feed of similar nutrient and energy content to F-100, is now available within many malnourished populations, mainly in African countries. This is a welcome substitute for F-100 as it is much easier to store safely for long periods, needs no preparation and is popular among older infants and children. Like F-100, it can often be manufactured locally according to the 'free' recipe.

During this *Rehabilitation phase*, the child should be offered increasing amounts of feed until some is left at each meal – 'ad libitum' feeding. The frequency of feeding is reduced. Provided there are no setbacks, dietary intake increases steadily, and weight gain is rapid, up to 20 times normal, on average 10 g/kg/d. The child's mother or closest carer must be taught how to make home as conducive as possible to continuing catch-up growth and development of her child. This includes teaching nutrition, hygiene, play for mental and physical development, and also when and how to get help. Depending on circumstances, 'cure' may be defined as attainment of 80% (−2 SDS), 85% or 90% (−1 SDS) of reference weight for height or a MUAC, in 6-month to 5-year-old children only, of for example 110 mm or 125 mm. Ideally, a final *Follow-up phase* ensues in which the child is reviewed at increasing intervals to ensure that recurrence of malnutrition is prevented and health and normal development are promoted, supported and achieved.

PREVENTION

A few severely malnourished children in a poor community imply a large number of moderately malnourished children. If the moderately malnourished are ignored, as usually happens, some deteriorate, some die and all are blighted for the rest of their lives by not realizing their potential. The ideal solution to primary malnutrition is prevention. However, this requires what we are presently unwilling or unable to provide to a large section of the world's population, improved standards of living: health care, education, sanitation, security, sufficient good quality food and more, to permit the birth of healthy well-nourished infants, tolerable burdens of infection during childhood and hence, normal growth and development. In the 'resource rich' world, however, prevention of secondary malnutrition is achieved to varying extents within good health care systems in, for example, children with inflammatory bowel disease, cystic fibrosis and those with various inborn errors of metabolism.

MICRONUTRIENT DEFICIENCY AND EXCESS

Micronutrients are generally recognized as the vitamins and essential trace elements. Vitamins are preformed organic compounds required in the diet each within a given physiological range to ensure optimal health. The same requirement applies to the 10–17 essential trace elements[37] which, in total, comprise about 0.03% of body weight. The most abundant and best known is iron while one of the least abundant but also well known, is iodine. Cobalt, a less obvious essential trace element, is required at only one hundred-thousandth the intake of iron and, in humans but not ruminants, has to be supplied within vitamin B_{12}.

Nutrients essential for optimal health can be divided into type I and type II nutrients, distinguished by their roles.[37] Type I nutrients include all of the vitamins and essential trace elements except zinc. Each has a limited number of specific functions and most have body stores. After the stores are depleted, specific signs of deficiency appear, which makes specific diagnosis relatively easy. Type II nutrients include major body elements such as potassium, calcium and the essential amino acids – also zinc, which is a micronutrient. These are required for maintenance and growth of all cells and they tend not to have effective stores. Deficiency limits, first and foremost, cell hyperplasia and hypertrophy. In childhood, the consequence is growth failure. This, in turn, reduces the requirement for all nutrients. Thus deficiencies of type II nutrients are difficult to diagnose and often overlooked. However, they are no less important than type I nutrient deficiencies and should be considered as possible contributors to growth failure, particularly when the diet is monotonous or specialized.

Interactions among nutrients and other components within diets influence the final balance of nutrients absorbed. This is particularly important when therapeutic diets, enteral feeds or food supplements are prescribed, or when the diet is monotonous. For example, a diet with a high phytate content (the storage form of phosphate in plants) reduces the availability of nutrients such as zinc, iron and copper; a diet high in ascorbic acid content increases iron but decreases copper absorption, and many trace elements interfere with one another's absorption. Thus, the intake of a particular micronutrient does not necessarily reflect its bioavailability. Important characteristics of a few of the essential micronutrients are summarized below and further information can be found elsewhere.[37]

IRON

For body iron, 70% is contained within heme, where it is intimately involved in O_2 carriage. Iron is a highly reactive element as ferrous ion releases an electron to become ferric ion. The freed electron takes part in many normal metabolic events such as electron transfer in the mitochondrial respiratory chain and free radical production which, on the one hand, is used to kill pathogens but on the other, may result in peroxidation of membrane lipids, a highly dangerous complication. This hazard is reduced by an elaborate system of iron-binding proteins, the main ones being heme, which holds ferrous iron, ferritin (which binds stored ferric iron), and transferrin (which carries ferric iron between cells).[38]

Iron deficiency causes a microcytic, hypochromic anemia after iron stores are depleted. This is a particular hazard of preterm birth because iron stores accumulate first in the fetal liver in late gestation. Iron deficiency anemia in infants also occurs when they are fed largely cows' milk mainly because it is a poor source of iron.[39] Appropriate advice is to introduce heme-containing foods like meat and liver, replace cow's milk with breast milk or formula and, if necessary, provide iron supplements. Iron deficiency is also relatively common in adolescent boys and girls. Vegetarians are at higher risk than omnivores because non-heme iron is less bioavailable than heme iron and their phytate intake tends to be high. As well as anemia, which is probably a late manifestation, iron deficiency is associated with reduced exercise tolerance, impaired resistance to infection and poor psychomotor development.

Iron toxicity can occur. Acute iron poisoning is less common than it used to be. Hemochromatosis and multiple blood transfusions are relatively rare in childhood but malnutrition is commonly complicated by iron excess and toxicity.[38] In edematous malnutrition, although anemia is usual, plasma ferritin and hepatic iron content are high while plasma transferrin, but not plasma iron, is low. This leads to an increased risk of circulating free iron which, together with antioxidant deficiencies, may lead to lipid peroxidation in membranes and contributes to at least some of the features of edematous malnutrition. Iron supplementation may also increase the severity of infection in malnourished children. Thus, although the treatment of anemia with iron is usually appropriate, it may be deleterious in children with malnutrition or if the anemia is not due to iron deficiency.

Iron status can be measured in different ways, some more specific than others. For example, anemia is a nonspecific measure, which may be due to many nutrient deficiencies or indeed, other non-nutritional causes. In contrast, low plasma ferritin and high transferrin receptor concentrations are quite specific, each for a different aspect of iron status: the former implies low iron stores, the latter, low uptake of iron for heme synthesis.

COPPER

Though the dietary requirement for copper is only about one tenth that of iron or zinc, it is also crucial to normal metabolism. Copper shares several features with iron. It is reactive, cuprous copper releasing an electron to become cupric copper and vice versa. It circulates bound largely within caeruloplasmin, otherwise known as ferroxidase I, which catalyzes the oxidation of ferrous to ferric iron. Thus copper deficiency interferes with iron metabolism. Located at the active site of several other oxidases, copper is also involved in the crosslinking of connective tissue proteins such as collagen and elastin and responsible for end-oxidation in the respiratory chain. The main features of copper deficiency are microcytic, hypochromic anemia indistinguishable from that of iron deficiency, neutropenia, tortuous dilatations of blood vessels, herniae, 'osteoporosis' clinically not unlike infantile rickets, skin and hair hypopigmentation and neurological problems.

Like iron, copper stores accumulate in the fetal liver in late gestation. Similarly, cows' milk is a poor source of copper. Thus, copper deficiency tends to occur in preterm infants and infants fed largely cows' milk. It also accompanies malnutrition, particularly edematous malnutrition.

Copper toxicity is usually insidious, most commonly from chronic ingestion associated with copper piping or utensils carrying relatively acidic fluids. The excess copper ends up in the liver and cirrhosis ensues. Two inherited inborn errors of metabolism involve copper transporting ATPases, Wilson disease and Menkes syndrome. Wilson disease, an autosomal recessive defect, usually presents in adolescence with cirrhosis associated with excessive hepatic copper. High concentrations of copper in the brain, eye and kidneys also occur: biliary excretion of copper and plasma caeruloplasmin are low (see Chapter 26). Treatment with copper chelators or zinc, which inhibits copper absorption, is partially effective in controlling copper accumulation. Menkes, or steely hair syndrome, is also autosomal recessive in origin but more like copper deficiency in presentation in that progressive anemia, hypopigmentation, hypothermia, osteoporosis, cardiovascular abnormalities and mental deterioration occur from infancy and plasma copper is low. However, this syndrome is unresponsive to copper (see Chapter 26).

Plasma copper is a poor measure of copper status because it follows closely plasma caeruloplasmin, which is an acute phase protein whose concentration rises during an acute phase response. Erythrocyte superoxide dismutase level reflects copper status more reliably.

IODINE

Iodine plays its major role in the hormone thyroxine, whose function and disorders are covered in Chapter 15. Iodine deficiency disorders are of worldwide importance accounting for stunting and suboptimal mental development in many millions of children and, subsequently, adults in developing regions with low iodine water supplies. Selenium deficiency, which is also widespread, may influence the response to iodine deficiency, particularly in regions within China.[37] Iodine excess also impairs thyroid function in communities with a high intake of food of marine origin.

ZINC

The dietary requirement for zinc is similar to that of iron and its body content is about half as much. However, unlike iron or copper, zinc is relatively unreactive. About 60% of plasma zinc is bound loosely to albumin, about 25% is bound to alpha-2 macroglobulin and the rest to amino acids and other small molecules. Zinc is a classic type II nutrient without an effective store. Its association with several hundred ubiquitous enzymes, including those necessary for DNA, RNA and protein synthesis, means that it is necessary for normal cell metabolism, hyperplasia and hypertrophy. Zinc deficiency decreases growth until the demand for zinc meets the supply. Clinically this means that zinc deficiency in childhood presents with growth failure. Other features are skin lesions in areas subject to trauma, poor wound healing, impaired cell mediated immunity and diarrhea associated with intestinal mucosal atrophy.

Conditions in which zinc deficiency is common include poverty and thus, inadequate, monotonous, relatively low protein, low zinc diets; increased zinc loss from burns or protein losing enteropathies; and increased zinc demand for healing or for rapid growth. The autosomal recessive inherited disease, acrodermatitis enteropathica, appears to involve reduced zinc absorption. Its clinical features are those of simple zinc deficiency as described earlier. It can be treated successfully with zinc supplements thereby overcoming the intestinal block (see Chapters 19 and 30).

Zinc status is particularly difficult to define or measure because intracellular concentrations are controlled within narrow limits and there is no store to sample. In zinc deficiency, hair and plasma zinc fall. However, hair zinc is hard to measure accurately. Low plasma zinc often implies an ongoing acute phase response rather than zinc deficiency. Thus its interpretation requires an independent measure of the acute phase response and preferably knowledge of zinc intake and demand. In practice, a trial of zinc supplementation is often the most helpful test provided that its endpoint is defined at the outset. If zinc deficiency is present the child should respond within a month by, for example, gaining weight more rapidly than before supplementation.

Zinc toxicity is very unusual in childhood because homeostatic mechanisms prevent excess intestinal absorption. A recent syndrome featuring hyperzincemia with clinical features of persistent, gross inflammation has been described. There is no evidence however that zinc excess causes the clinical features.[40]

VITAMIN A

The vitamin A family is headed by all-*trans* retinol and includes all naturally occurring compounds with the biological activity of retinol, as well as the provitamin A carotenoids, such as beta-carotene. Preformed vitamin A is found in liver, dairy products and oily fish and over 80% may be absorbed (Table 16.2). The carotenoids are present in many plant foods and absorption varies from 5 to 50%. They act as anti-oxidants themselves and are also converted to vitamin A by oxidative cleavage. The vitamin A family members are fat soluble and bound in plasma to specific retinoid-binding proteins (RBPs), which protect them from oxidation. They are stored mainly in the liver.

In childhood, vitamin A is best known for its roles in vision, in immunity and in cell differentiation. Vitamin A deficiency is a major public health problem, affecting at least 200 million of the world's children, particularly malnourished children.[39] Only a small proportion has overt clinical signs. These start with night blindness, photophobia and Bitot's spots on the conjunctivae, which result from squamous metaplasia, then xerophthalmia, keratomalacia and eventually blindness. At the same time children suffer increased severity of infections and mortality is high. Prevention is possible using a 'massive dose' approach, which depends on the ability of vitamin A to be stored and used slowly. A large oral dose is also used for xerophthalmia.

Vitamin A toxicity can occur, which can be acute or chronic. Both are usually iatrogenic, resulting from gross overdoses of vitamin preparations. Typically the former resolves completely on stopping supplementation but the chronic form, which is more common, occasionally causes permanent damage to liver, muscle, vision and bones.

Vitamin A status is assessed by different methods in different situations, often by serum retinol in hospital; and by presence or absence of Bitot's spots or conjunctival impression cytology in populations. Serum retinol is depressed in the acute phase response and affected by protein and zinc intake, therefore relative dose response tests are becoming more popular where serum retinol is measured before and after a supplement of vitamin A.

VITAMIN D

This comprises vitamins D_2 and D_3, which are both fat soluble and stored within adipose tissue. D_3 is hydroxylated in the liver to 25-hydroxyvitamin D, which is further hydroxylated in the kidney to 1,25-dihydroxyvitamin D, which acts as a hormone and is the most biologically active form of the vitamin. It stimulates calcium absorption in the small intestine and calcium resorption from bone. It also promotes cell maturation within the intestine and it increases bone formation and growth plate mineralization by providing sufficient circulating calcium. The vitamin has several other roles including improving resistance to infections.

Egg yolk, fortified margarines and spreads and especially cod liver oil are rich in vitamin D (Table 16.3): breast milk is a poor source. By far the major source is photoconversion of 7-dehydrocholesterol, through exposure of the skin to ultraviolet B light. This means that breast-fed infants in the UK who are mostly indoors or covered up, or whose mothers are vitamin D deficient, are at particular risk of deficiency. Daily supplementation is recommended. Very preterm infants are also prone to deficiency signs but other factors contribute as well as vitamin D deficiency. Fat malabsorption for any reason is associated with vitamin D deficiency.

In early life, deficiency results in rickets, which is characterized by failure of skeletal growth, poor bone mineralization and muscle weakness. In infancy, frontal bossing, craniotabes and rachitic rosary are typical: later, short stature, bowed legs and swollen wrists are more distinctive. Bone pain, anemia and respiratory infections are common. Plasma 25-hydroxyvitamin D is low: plasma alkaline phosphatase is high but this is not specific for vitamin D deficiency. Radiological changes include poor mineralization, delayed epiphyseal development and marked metaphyseal changes including cupping, fraying and splaying (Fig. 16.5).

Vitamin D toxicity usually results from injudicious supplementation and is associated first with failure to thrive and gastrointestinal features including constipation, and later, urinary tract features with

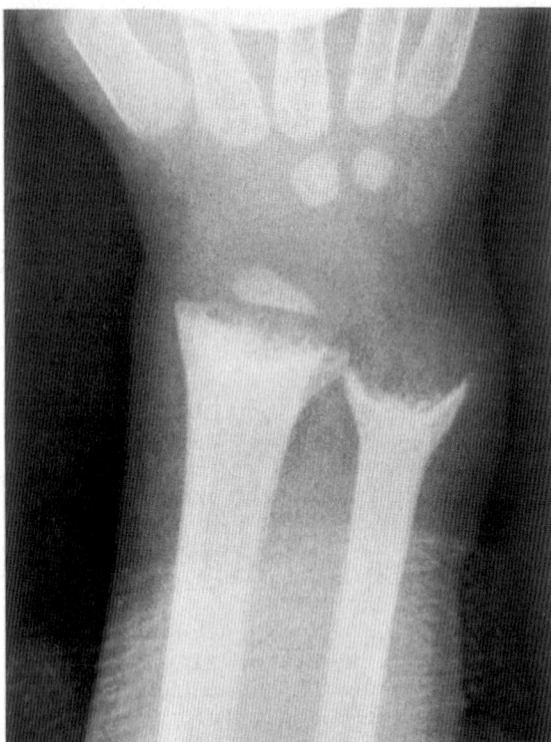

Fig. 16.5 Rickets: X-ray of wrist showing frayed radial and ulnar metaphyses with slight expansion.

nephrocalcinosis and eventually renal failure. Hypercalcemia and increased bone mineralization occur. Therapy includes glucocorticoids and a low-calcium diet.

FOLATE

Folate comprises the double aromatic ring of a pteridine linked to para-aminobenzoate and glutamate. It is water soluble and functions as a coenzyme receiving and donating single carbon fragments. It provides methylene groups for pyrimidine synthesis and formyl groups for purine synthesis for DNA and RNA biosynthetic cycles. It also participates in methylation of a variety of substrates, for example, DNA, myelin and phospholipids.[17] Over half of natural folates are in the 5-tetrahydrofolate form attached to a polyglutamyl chain. The best dietary source is liver (Table 16.3). Synthetic folic acid is twice as bioavailable as natural folates.

Marginal folate deficiency is very common but the extent to which this contributes to suboptimal health is not yet clear. However there is good evidence that high maternal folate status during the first few weeks after conception reduces the risk of neural tube defects in their offspring (see Chapter 11). Folate deficiency accompanies malnutrition and also occurs as a complication of increased requirements for growth or erythropoiesis, malabsorption syndromes, impaired utilization due to vitamin B_{12} deficiency and as a result of prolonged treatment with methotrexate, trimethoprim and some anticonvulsants. Overt folate deficiency is characterized by megaloblastic anemia with thrombocytopenia, leukopenia and increased segmentation of polymorph nuclei.

The risk of folate toxicity has become an important issue since recognition of the need for relatively high doses of folic acid to prevent neural tube defects. High doses may mask vitamin B_{12} deficiency, allowing the neuropathy induced by the latter to progress. They *may* also interfere with anticonvulsive therapy and with anti-folate therapy for malignancies.

Folate status is best estimated as erythrocyte folate concentration but, due to the long life of erythrocytes, this does not change quickly in response to deficiency or excess. In contrast, serum folate falls quickly when folate absorption falls but this is not necessarily associated with folate deficiency.

REFERENCES (* Level 1 evidence)

1. Doherty CP, Reilly JJ, Paterson WF, et al. Growth failure and malnutrition. In: Walker W A, et al, eds. Pediatric gastrointestinal disease, 3rd edn. Hamilton, Ontario: Decker; 2000.12–27.
2. Mann J, Truswell AS. Essentials of human nutrition. 3rd edn. Oxford: Oxford University Press; 2006.
3. Gibney MJ, Kok FJ, Vorster HJ. Introduction to human nutrition. London: Blackwell Publishing; 2002.
4. Department of Health. Dietary reference values for food energy and nutrients for the UK. Report on health and social subjects. No. 41 London: HMSO; 1991.
5. FAO/WHO/UNU. Expert consultation. 2002. Human energy requirements.
6. National diet and nutrition survey: young people aged 4–18 years. London: HMSO; 2000.
7. National Diet and Nutrition Survey. Children aged 11/2 to 41/2 years. In: Report of the Diet and Nutrition Survey. London: HMSO; 1995.
8. Koletzko B, Agostoni C, Carlson SE, et al. Long chain polyunsaturated fatty acids and perinatal development. Acta Paediatr 2001; 90:460–464.
9. Hendrikse WW, Reilly JJ, Weaver LT. Malnutrition in a children's hospital. Clin Nutr 1997; 16:13–18.
10. Goulet O. Assessment of nutritional status in clinical practice. Baillieres Clin Gastroenterol 1998; 12:647–669.
11. Gibson RS. Principles of nutritional assessment. 2nd edn. Oxford: Oxford University Press; 2005.
12. Cole TJ, Freeman JV, Preece MA. Body mass index reference curves for the UK, 1990. Arch Dis Child 1995; 73:25–29.

13. Krick J. Using the Z score as a descriptor of discrete changes in growth. Nutr Supp Serv 1986; 6:14–21.
14. Cross JH, Holden C, Macdonald A, et al. Clinical examination compared with anthropometry in evaluating nutritional status. Arch Dis Child 1995; 72:60–61.
15. Secker DJ, Jeejeebhoy KN. Subjective global nutritional assessment in children. Am J Clin Nutr 2007; 85:1083–1089.
16. Michaelsen KF, Weaver LT, Branca F, et al. Feeding and nutrition of infants and young children. Copenhagen: WHO; 2000.
17. Bresson JL. Protein and energy requirements in healthy and ill paediatric patients. Baillieres Clin Gastroenterol 1998; 12:631–645.
18. Reilly JJ. Diagnostic accuracy of the BMI for use in pediatrics. Int J Obes 2006; 30:595–597.
19. Hall DM, Cole TJ. What us is BMI? Arch Dis Child 2006; 91:283–286.
20. Reilly JJ, Kelnar CJ, Alexander DW, et al. Health consequences of obesity: systematic review. Arch Dis Child 2003; 88:748–752.
21. Reilly JJ, Wilson D. Childhood obesity: ABC of Obesity. Br Med J 2006; 333:1207–1210.
22. Kopelman PG, Caterson ID, Dietz WH, eds. Clinical obesity in adults and children. 2nd edn. London: Blackwell Publishing; 2005.
23. Scottish Intercollegiate Guidelines Network (SIGN). 2003 Management of obesity in children and young people: a national clinical guideline. SIGN 69.www.sign.ac.uk.

24. Summerbell CD, Kelly S, Waters E. Interventions for treating obesity in children. The Cochrane Library. 2003.
25. National Institute for Health and Clinical Excellence, 2006. Obesity: the prevention, identification, assessment and management of overweight and obesity in adults and children, NICE December 2006. www.nice.org.uk.
26. Summerbell CD, Waters E, Edmunds L. Interventions for preventing obesity in children. The Cochrane Library. 2005.
27. Reilly JJ. Tackling the obesity epidemic: new approaches. Arch Dis Child 2006; 91:724–726.
28. Elia M. Nutrition. In: Kumar P, Clark M, eds. Clinical medicine. 5th edn. Bath: WB Saunders; 2002.221–231.
29. de Onis M, Monteiro C, Akré J, et al. The worldwide magnitude of protein-energy malnutrition: an overview from the WHO Global Database on Child Growth. Bull World Health Organ 1995; 71:703–712.
30. Jackson AA, Ashworth A, Khanum S. Improving child survival: Malnutrition Task Force and the paediatrician's responsibility. Arch Dis Child 2006; 91:706–710.
31. World Health Organization. Management of severe malnutrition: a manual for physicians and other senior health workers. Geneva: WHO; 1999.
32. Valid International Community-based Therapeutic Care (CTC). A field manual. Oxford: Valid International; 2006.
33. Golden MH. Protein deficiency, energy deficiency and the oedema of malnutrition. Lancet 1982; i:1261–1265.

34.   Golden MH. Oedematous malnutrition. Br Med Bull 1998; 54:433–444.

35.   SPHERE Project Team. The SPHERE Humanitarian Charter and Minimum Standards in Disaster Response. Geneva: The SPHERE Project; 2004.

36.   Ashworth A, Burgess A. Caring for severely malnourished children. London: Macmillan; 2003.

37.   Hallberg L, Sandstrom B, Ralph A, et al. Iron, zinc and other trace elements. In: Garrow JS, James WPT, Ralph A, eds. Human nutrition and dietetics, 10th edn. London: Harcourt; 2000.177–205.

38.   Ramdath DD, Golden MHN. Non-haematological aspects of iron nutrition. Nutr Res Rev 1989; 2:29–49.

39.   Lawson M. Infancy and childhood. Task Force Report of the British Nutrition Foundation eds. In: Iron: Nutrition and physiological significance. London; Chapman & Hall 1995:93–105. World Health Organization. Indicators for assessing vitamin A deficiency and their application in monitoring and evaluating intervention programmes. Micronutrient Series. Geneva: WHO; 1996.

40.   Sampson B, Richmond P, Golden BE, et al. Identification of the zinc binding protein in a child with hyperzincaemia as calprotectin (MRP8/ MRP14). In: Roussel AM, Anderson RA, Favrier AE, eds. Trace element metabolism in man and animals – 10. London: Plenum; 2000.1031–1034.

17

Fluid, electrolyte and acid–base disturbances

Gale A Pearson

INTRODUCTION

Disturbances of the 'internal milieu' are common in pediatric illness. This chapter will focus mainly upon the background (i.e. the reasons why they are so common) and the associated clinical issues that arise as a consequence. Two appendices are also provided as references for the less clinical material. The 'Physical and physiological influences on the internal distribution of water and electrolytes' and 'Acid–base chemistry and blood gas measurement' are nonetheless essential knowledge for the clinician. Otherwise the layout of the chapter is intended to provide the reader with the information required to deal with clinical situations of increasing complexity as the chapter proceeds. Wherever possible, generic descriptions have been favored over specific diseases since the intended focus is not upon the differential diagnosis of deranged laboratory results. This is because in the first instance and to a large extent, abnormalities of fluid balance, electrolytes and acid–base can be characterized, assessed and treated on their own merits. Clinical situations often arise where this approach is necessary whilst the diagnosis is still being determined. Nevertheless the best clinical solution will always involve treatment of the cause.

Careful assessment is an essential prerequisite to proper management of fluid, electrolytes and acid–base in children. In this respect clinical judgment and laboratory assessment are complementary to each other. Therapeutic decisions should not be made on laboratory findings alone though in hospital, patients cannot be managed to modern clinical standards without appropriate measurement and monitoring.

The first priority when a patient presents, is a rapid assessment of the need for resuscitation following an 'ABC' approach (see Ch. 35). Then a comprehensive history of the disorder should be taken and skilled clinical examination performed to determine the speed and extent of investigation and the intensity of treatment. The patient should be weighed at this point. Biochemical investigation also forms part of the assessment and should be performed whenever fluid therapy is contemplated, particularly if by the intravenous (i.v.) route. Baseline investigations should include the determination of serum urea, creatinine, electrolytes, osmolality and some indication of acid–base status such as serum bicarbonate along with the hematological profile. Patients with abnormalities of acid–base detected by this screening and those with significant respiratory problems should be further investigated with arterial blood gases. Urine electrolyte content, urea, pH and osmolality should be measured if there is a clinical suspicion of an abnormality of fluid balance or renal function. During the subsequent care of acutely unwell babies and children, the volume of urine production should be monitored, with repitition of laboratory urinary analysis where relevant. While it is helpful if accurate urine collections can be obtained to calculate electrolyte excretion, measurements performed on casual spot urine specimens can be interpreted by relating sodium and potassium concentrations to the urinary creatinine content (see 'Fractional sodium excretion' below). Further assessment both clinically and biochemically should be made as soon as the response to treatment can be assessed.

The body content and internal distribution of fluid and electrolytes are subject to tight physiological controls and are conveniently interpreted using 'compartment' models. The most important distinction for fluid, electrolyte and acid–base is between the intra- and extracellular environment, which is preserved by the cell membrane. Likewise the composition of the various extracellular fluids depends heavily on the integrity and function of epithelia and the vascular endothelium. The extracellular fluid (ECF) consists of intravascular fluid (plasma) and extravascular fluid. The latter includes 'tissue' or 'interstitial' fluid as well as specialized collections of transcellular fluids formed by secretory activity which include gastrointestinal (GI) secretions, synovial fluid, ocular and cerebrospinal fluids. Body compartments can also be 531 conceptualized if not defined anatomically, by the behavior/distribution of solutes within them. This latter approach is more commonly applied in pharmacology than physiology but it usefully defines some aspects of the behavior of the body as a compartmentalized vessel. In a 'one-compartment' model the drug, once administered, is assumed to instantly distribute homogeneously throughout the volume of distribution. In a two-compartment model the drug distributes rapidly through a small-volume, central compartment that usually corresponds to blood and the ECF of highly vascular organs and more slowly through a larger compartment, which usually includes adipose tissue and intracellular fluid (ICF).

Both total ECF volume and the distribution of fluid between extracellular compartments can vary widely in disease. Furthermore, one of the main consequences of ECF changes is corresponding or consequential change within the ICF. These changes are dictated by the interplay of hydrostatic, oncotic and osmotic forces, endothelial and cell membrane permeability and the integrity of active homeostatic systems such as membranous Na^+/K^+ ATPase.

DIFFERENCES AMONG BABIES, CHILDREN AND ADULTS

The physiological differences between premature and term neonates and among babies, older children and adults are extreme. From a constitutional perspective, neonates have proportionally the greatest water content and obese adults the least. The 'total body water' accounts for 80% of mass at birth and this percentage falls to 60% by 1 year of age. The change is the result of a disproportionate increase in cell mass (due to growth) compared to the volume of ECF. The percentage of water in postpubertal females is lower than males due largely to their higher percentage of body fat. In both sexes, throughout adulthood, the body water content falls with advancing age.

Children need higher water and electrolyte intakes than adults, making them more susceptible to dehydration. Their increased water losses are due to the:
- caloric expenses of a high metabolic rate;
- high insensible loss (high minute ventilation, high surface area: volume ratio, immature epidermis in premature babies);
- decreased ability to concentrate urine.

The distribution of water between the 'compartments' also differs between infants and adults (Table 17.1). During the first few days of life there is a transfer of water from ICF to ECF. This mechanism, which may protect the infant against the effects of dehydration, increases the already large ECF volume and could be a factor in the occurrence of edema sometimes observed at this time. After this the ICF accounts for an increasing percentage of total body water up to 1 year of age but this is mostly a reflection of the reduction in ECF volume. The ratio of ICF:ECF volume increases from unity, nearing the adult value of 2:1 some time after the age of 1 year.

The sodium content per kilogram body weight is 35–50% higher in the infant than in the adult due to the greater amount of extracellular fluid. With the relative reduction of ECF with growth, adult values are reached at about 2 years of age. Neonatal calcium and phosphate levels are higher than maternal levels, the former as a result of active placental

transfer and the latter as a consequence of the resulting fetal parathyroid hormone levels. Intracellular calcium stores are lower however, making muscle function (particularly myocardium) more dependent upon the serum ionized calcium.[1] The average plasma concentration of chloride is also higher in babies, like the phosphate levels. Anion/cation balance must exist for there to be electroneutrality and both are balanced by a lower bicarbonate level. Age- and gender-related reference ranges should be available from the laboratory for each electrolyte being measured.

As already stated, babies have a higher obligatory urinary water loss than older children and adults, a consequence of a higher urinary solute load and a decreased concentrating ability (to about 600 mosm/L).[2] These features are a consequence of tubular immaturity, one aspect of which is that fewer nephrons have loops which extend into the renal medulla. The result is a much higher flux of water and electrolytes. A term infant exchanges about one half of his ECF in the day whilst an adult exchanges only one seventh. Renal immaturity is accentuated in the premature infant.[2] It manifests in a number of ways including a tubular leak of bicarbonate creating a tendency towards metabolic acidosis and an almost unique ability to develop genuine sodium depletion through urinary losses even in the absence of diuretics.

Babies also have a reduced ability to deal with a water load,[2] a consequence of a low glomerular filtration rate (GFR). The GFR subsequently increases over the first 6 months of life.

MAINTENANCE FLUID AND ELECTROLYTE REQUIREMENTS

The prescription of fluids for children has three components:
1. meeting maintenance requirements;
2. coping with ongoing losses;
3. correcting fluid and electrolyte deficits.

The first two components will be dealt with here. The correction of fluid and electrolyte deficits is covered under 'Fluid and electrolyte disturbances' below.

Normal water requirement is closely linked to energy requirements, both on account of the associated heat production and the urinary solute load resulting from the diet. A normal infant requires 110 cal/kg body weight/day and, it is claimed, approximately 150 ml fluid (i.e. solution) per 100 cal expended. For babies an enteral food source is available which balances calories and volume perfectly. A breast-fed term newborn drinks approximately 150 ml/kg/day. This gives the baby 100 kcal/kg/day of energy (the creamatocrit of breast milk increases during a feed but on average it contains 67 kcal/100 ml or 20 kcal/ounce). This ratio of water to energy promotes optimum growth. As milk has a significant fat content, 150 ml of milk is not the same as 150 ml of water and the volume requirement of enteral milk (150 ml/kg/day) does not transpose to the prescription of parenteral fluids. In contrast to fats, carbohydrates and salts dissolve in solution.

When parenteral fluids and nutrition are limited to a few days in a previously healthy child, a calorie intake of 20–35% of the average normal requirement will suffice. After a few days a more comprehensive approach is required. Catabolism due to illness is unresponsive to hyperalimentation and feeding in excess of metabolic requirements during illness increases morbidity.[3,4] Fluid provision needs to be adapted to the

Table 17.1 Partition of body fluids (average figures)

	Adult (70 kg; 1.85 m²)			Infant (3 kg; 0.2 m²)		
	% Body weight	Liters	Liters/m²	% Body weight	Liters	Liters/m²
Intracellular	40	28	15.2	38	1.14	5.70
Extracellular						
Interstitial*	16	11.2	6.0	33	0.99	4.95
Plasma	4	2.8	1.5	5	0.15	0.75
Total	60	42	22.7	76	2.28	11.4

*Includes transcellular fluids.

circumstances. Even when water intake is zero during illness, appreciable quantities of water are being produced by the oxidation of the hydrogen content of tissues undergoing catabolism. Water is also preserved by increased antidiuretic hormone (ADH) levels. Baseline 'maintenance' fluids are a considerable overestimation of water requirement for most hospitalized patients. Indeed unrestricted fluid regimens should only be allowed in enterally fed patients when relying on satiety. Mandatory reductions to baseline fluids apply for patients receiving i.v. fluids, nursed in bed, paralyzed, breathing humidified gases or being nursed in a humidified environment. All fluids administered must be taken into account in the fluid balance, including drugs, flushes for i.v. and intra-arterial (i.a.) lines, etc. A regimen for making interactive decisions about fluid management is summarized in Table 17.2.

For example, using this regimen, a 10-kg child being ventilated for bacterial pneumonia might be prescribed an i.v. fluid regimen of 100 ml/kg × 0.75 (for breathing humidified gases) × 0.7 (if paralyzed) × 0.7 (for the risk of high ADH levels) = 37 ml/kg/day. Subsequent provision would be judged in the light of fluid balance (weight), plasma urea and electrolytes and urinalysis. A normal dietary sodium intake ranges between 1 and 4 mmol (23–92 mg)/kg body weight/day. The normal daily dietary potassium intake ranges between 1 and 3 mmol (39–117 mg)/kg body weight. To administer these quantities of electrolytes within the fluid restrictions that are commonly required may necessitate the use of tailor made solutions. However 40 ml/kg/day of 0.45% saline and 5% dextrose with 20 mmol of potassium added to each 500 ml bag provides 3 mmol/kg/day of sodium and 1.6 mmol/kg/day of potassium (but only 8 calories/kg/day).

ONGOING LOSSES

Stipulated 'normal' maintenance requirements include an allowance for natural sensible and insensible losses. To prospectively compensate for abnormal fluid and electrolyte losses, the volumes involved must be measured and recorded and the composition of the fluid determined (Table 17.3). At first the primary fluid loss is always from the extracellular compartment and its composition can often be anticipated according to its origin. Acute losses from the intravascular compartment can be replaced directly. With time and continuing losses, there is equilibration of fluid and electrolytes occurs between compartments (particularly between the ICFs and ECFs). As the ICF is not directly accessible, replacement regimens devised to compensate for previous (as opposed to current) losses are different to simple plasma/ECF and are considered in more detail below under 'Fluid and electrolyte disturbance'.

Table 17.2 Volume of Intravenous fluid administered. (From Shann 1999[5] with permission)

		Fluid regimen/adjustment
Baseline	1 day of age	50 ml/kg/day
	2 days of age	75 ml/kg/day
	3+ days of age	100 ml/kg/day
	<10 kg	100 ml/kg/day
	10–20 kg	1000 ml/day + 50 ml/kg/day for every kg >10 kg
	>20 kg	1500 ml/day + 20 ml/kg/day for every kg >20 kg
Decreases	Humidified gases	× 0.75
	Paralyzed	× 0.7
	High ADH (e.g. IPPV or coma)	× 0.7
	Hypothermia	− 12% per °C core temp. is <37
	High ambient humidity	× 0.7
	Renal failure	× 0.3 (+ urine output)
Increases	Full activity and oral feeds	× 1.5/free fluids
	Fever	+ 12% per °C core temp. is >37
	Room temp. >31°C	+ 30% per °C
	Hyperventilation	× 1.2
	Preterm neonate (< 1.5 kg)	× 1.2
	Radiant heater	× 1.5
	Phototherapy	× 1.5
	Burns day 1	+ 4% per 1% of body surface area affected
	Burns day 2+	+ 2% per 1% of body surface area affected

ADH, antidiuretic hormone; IPPV, intermittent positive pressure ventilation.

MONITORING

The intensity with which patients are monitored in respect of fluid electrolytes and acid–base is, like other aspects of their care, based primarily on the clinical impression of illness severity. At the highest levels of intensity, intake and sensible losses may be monitored to allow fluid balance to be determined several times per hour. Electrolyte levels and acid–base status may also be measured as frequently. At the other end of

Table 17.3 Composition of solutes in body fluids

	Na+ (mmol/L)	K+ (mmol/L)	Cl- (mmol/L)	HCO-3 (mmol/L-1)
Plasma	135–145	3.5–5	98–110	18–25
Interstitial fluid	145	4.1	117	27
Intracellular fluid	10	159	3	7
Saliva	10–25	20–35	10–30	2–10
Gastric	20–80	5–20	100–150	0
Jejunal	130–150	5–10	100–130	10–20
Ileal	50–150	3–15	20–120	30–50
Diarrheal	10–90	10–80	10–110	20–70
Sweat (normal)	10–30	3–10	10–35	0
Sweat (cystic fibrosis)	50–130	5–25	50–110	0
Burn exudate (includes 30–50 g/L of protein)	140	5	110	20

the spectrum an experienced clinician, given a good history of a child with reasonable renal function, can treat the majority of cases effectively with limited resources and little or no laboratory help. On a normal pediatric ward, the sickest patients and those exclusively dependent upon i.v. fluids should have their weight, fluid balance and serum urea electrolytes and bicarbonate determined daily.

Monitoring fluid balance by means of daily weight measurements is considered the practical standard when issues of fluid balance are of importance. It has the advantage that it includes the impact of abnormal insensible losses, which are otherwise difficult to quantify. Clearly strict attention to technique should be maintained to provide interpretable results. Patients should not be clothed during measurement and the weight of any medical kit that is attached to them should be the same at each measurement. The results should be graphed with particular attention to the accuracy of the plot. The relationship between total body water and body weight is linear over short time scales within an individual, but there is considerable variation between individuals. This is largely accounted for by variation in the amount of adipose tissue (which contains < 10% water). Hence at the point of clinical presentation with significant illness, the patient's weight must be measured and recorded so that subsequent changes can be correctly interpreted.

TOTAL BODY WATER AND SODIUM BALANCE

The proportion of body weight that is attributable to its water content varies with age, sex and the amount of adipose tissue present. Total body water can be measured by indicator dilution methods (e.g. deuterium) or bioimpedance. For dilution methods the results differ between the chosen solutes according to their true distribution and the relative truth of the assumption that the material will diffuse rapidly throughout the water of the body before significant metabolism or excretion occurs. The results obtained from bioimpedance measurements are also dependent upon scrupulous technique. Water loss from the body occurs by various routes such as insensible perspiration, transpiration from lungs, and loss in urine, feces and sweat. Normally losses in feces and sweat are minimal. Insensible perspiration is essential to dissipate heat generated by metabolism and is augmented as required by sweating.

Of the sensible water losses, the principal physiological control is over the volume and content of urine production. This is reduced by ADH, which works on the collecting duct and increased by atrial natiuretic peptide (ANP), which is released from the heart when the ECF is expanded. ANP inhibits sodium reabsorption in the distal nephron and increases GFR by increasing blood pressure and the filtration fraction. There are however obligatory water losses in the urine – the volume required to excrete the solute load – which are higher in babies. ADH release occurs in response to osmoreceptors in the hypothalamus and baroreceptors (really stretch receptors) in the circulation. The osmoreceptors are by far the more sensitive, enabling fine control over plasma osmolality, but the ADH response that they initiate is muted compared to that caused by a fall in plasma volume. Strong releases of ADH occur in response to reduced plasma volume irrespective of the tonicity of the plasma. Water balance naturally fluctuates with the dictates of sodium balance (renin–angiotensin system). The urine sodium content can be used to differentiate oliguric states since it is a reasonably reliable predictor of ECF. If renal perfusion pressure falls to levels short of those that produce acute renal failure, the kidneys produce good 'quality' concentrated urine (osmolality > 300 mosm/L, urine:plasma urea ratio > 5) with a urine sodium <20 mmol/L. The fractional sodium excretion = (urinary sodium × plasma creatinine)/(plasma sodium × urinary creatinine) is also low ≈0.4. These findings are negated by diuretic therapy. In acute tubular necrosis the urine 'quality' is poor, urine sodium is > 40 mmol/L and fractional sodium excretion is ≥ 7.

Most of the sodium excretion from the body occurs via the kidney which can compensate within wide limits for variation in the dietary intake. Normal glomerular filtrate has an osmolality of 300 mosmol/kg but the osmolality of the urine excreted by adolescents and adults may range from 30 to 1200 mosmol/kg (specific gravity 1.001–1.035).

The infant kidney is unable to form such concentrated or dilute urine, a more realistic range being 100–600 mosmol/kg (specific gravity 1.003–1.023). Sodium depletion (unlike water depletion) does not occur under conditions of reduced intake but requires some abnormal loss – in sweat, alimentary secretions or urine.

The regulation of body sodium is closely linked to water.[6] Control of the osmolality of the ECF through changes in thirst and renal water excretion would otherwise lead to large changes in body volume in the face of sodium imbalance. Control over absorption and excretion of sodium is mediated primarily by the renin–angiotensin system. Adequacy of circulating blood volume and blood pressure affect perfusion of the juxtaglomerular apparatus, which if inadequate leads to the production of renin and thus aldosterone. The principal site of sodium control by alsosterone is the distal nephron (after the essential resorption of the majority of the sodium in the glomerular filtrate which occurs in the proximal tubule). In hypervolemia, renin production is decreased and atrial natriuretic peptide is released. The GFR increases, supplying more sodium (and water) to the distal convoluted tubule where it passes on into the urine.

COMPARTMENTAL DISTRIBUTION OF WATER AND ELECTROLYTES

The physical and physiological influences on the internal distribution of water and electrolytes are described in Appendix 1. Figure 17.1 highlights the difference in composition between various ECFs and ICF. In essence, ECF is rich in sodium and chloride with relatively small amounts of potassium. The reverse applies to ICF where potassium, protein and phosphate predominate. Indeed the internal distribution of potassium is related to cell mass, about 70% of the total body content being found in muscle. The concentration of magnesium is also greater in ICF, with 50% of the body's content being in the cells of soft tissue and

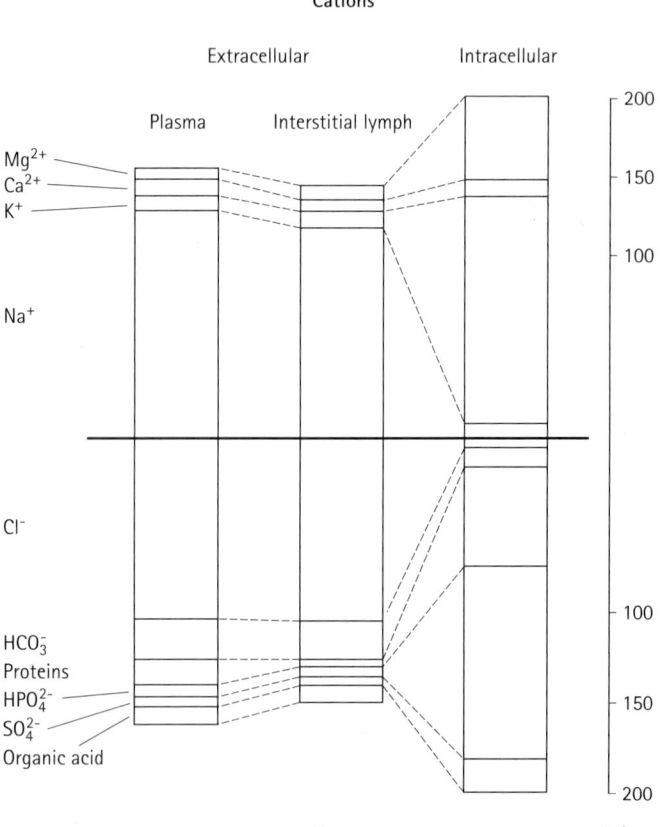

Fig. 17.1 Ionic composition of body fluids. The ionic composition of intra- and extracellular fluids. Cations are displayed above the dark horizontal line and anions below it. (From Ichikawa 1990[7] with permission)

most of the remainder in bone. The sum of anions and cations in ICF is greater than that in ECF. Normal osmotic equilibrium *is* present however, because there is an excess of divalent and polyvalent anions in ICF each contributing several electrical charges but only one osmotic particle. Secondly, some intracellular univalent ions (especially potassium) are not in free ionic form, but in combination with anions.

The two divisions of ECF most frequently involved in the understanding of disease states are plasma and interstitial fluid. Normally, plasma water accounts for approximately 93% of the plasma volume. The remaining 7%, although predominantly proteins, includes lipids, electrolytes, glucose and urea. The plasma volume occupied by electrolytes is always insignificant.

ACID–BASE

Most disturbances of fluid and electrolyte metabolism are associated with changes in the acid–base state of the blood. For example reduction in ECF volume leads to circulatory failure or 'shock'. The associated cellular hypoxia causes acidosis predominantly by the production of lactate. Some relevant details of acid–base chemistry and blood gas measurement are contained in Appendix 2.

Hydrogen ion concentration ([H$^+$]) within the body is closely controlled under normal conditions but the extreme concentrations that can arise during illness can range from 40 to 400% of the normal mean. Thus the body can be considered tolerant of changes in hydrogen ion concentration even if these conditions are not favored. The normal [H$^+$] is 37–48 nmol/L in babies corresponding to pH 7.43–7.32. The normal [H$^+$] range in infants and children is 37–46 nmol/L corresponding to a pH of 7.43–7.34. Values higher than the upper limit of normal [H$^+$] (lower pH) are acidotic and values lower than the lower limit (higher pH) are alkalotic.

For there to be long term stability of [H$^+$], metabolic production of acid must be balanced by respiratory and renal excretion. Respiration controls [H$^+$] by clearing carbon dioxide. The kidney controls urinary excretion of [H$^+$], the resorption of bicarbonate and the excretion of the nonvolatile acids that are produced during metabolism. The latter are derived principally from the sulfur contained in the methionine and cysteine of protein and form the titratable acid and ammonium in the urine.

Fluctuations in acid–base are tempered by:
- dilution of any acid produced;
- buffering;
- regulation of respiratory rate to control plasma CO_2 tension;
- renal resorption of filtered bicarbonate, and excretion of excess hydrogen ion (Fig. 17.2).[8]

Derangements of acid–base that are due primarily to fluctuations in PaCO$_2$ (and hence carbonic acid) are termed 'respiratory', all others are 'metabolic'. These acid–base fluctuations have a variety of consequences:
- Serum potassium levels change: Acute rises in [H$^+$] (acidosis) equilibrate across the cell membrane. An efflux of intracellular potassium ions preserves the transmembrane electrical potential but results in hyperkalemia. Similarly alkalosis from any cause results in an influx of potassium into the cells and hypokalemia. These changes occur without perturbing the whole body potassium. The relationship between acid–base and potassium flux is complicated if insulin is being administered since it promotes potassium movement into cells along with glucose.
- Albumin binding is affected: For example, alkalosis increases the ratio of bound to unbound (ionized) Ca^{2+} and can lead to tetany.
- Hemoglobin dissociation is affected: Acidosis increases the P50 of the hemoglobin dissociation curve creating potential problems with oxygen delivery, and alkalosis decreases it creating potential problems with oxygen uptake.
- Regional blood flow may change: [H$^+$] fluctuations (especially those caused by CO_2) affect vascular tone. Hypercapnic acidosis causes cerebral vasodilatation and pulmonary vasoconstriction.[9]
- Pharmacodynamic and pharmacokinetic effects occur: For a variety of drugs, e.g. weak acids and alkalis, tissue penetration is affected by ionization.

Most importantly a level of compensation is achieved via the alternate mechanism (changing levels of CO_2 or bicarbonate respectively). The rapid respiratory compensation for metabolic derangements is mediated by changes in respiratory drive and is effected as altered minute ventilation controls the PaCO$_2$. Metabolic compensation for respiratory acidosis is much slower and is effected by renal conservation of bicarbonate. In either case, full compensation is unusual but would bring the [H$^+$] right back into the normal range if it worked.

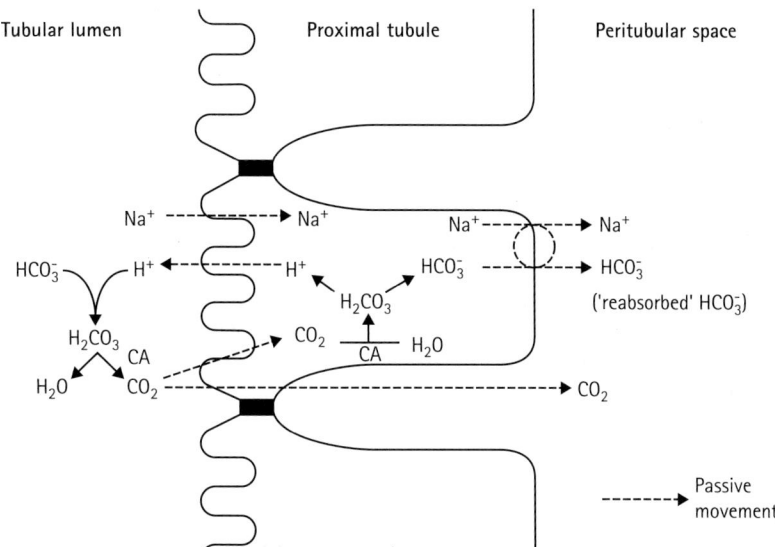

Fig. 17.2 Reabsorption of filtered bicarbonate. Reabsorption of filtered bicarbonate is achieved via H$^+$ secretion. The secreted H$^+$ (derived from carbonic acid) reacts with bicarbonate in the tubular fluid to reform carbonic acid which dissociates into carbon dioxide and water. Hence a bicarbonate anion is lost from the tubular fluid. But since the hydrogen ion came from a reaction which also generated a bicarbonate anion in the peritubular fluid, the net result is bicarbonate reabsorption. This figure illustrates the situation in the proximal convoluted tubule where 90% of filtered bicarbonate is reabsorbed. CA, carbonic anhydrase. (From West 1989[8] with permission)

DISTURBANCE OF ACID–BASE

RESPIRATORY ALKALOSIS

Hyperventilation causes a reduction in $PaCO_2$ and acute changes in $PaCO_2$ have a linear effect on $[H^+]$ (1 kPa to 5.5 nmol/L). Thus $[H^+]$ is low and $PaCO_2$ is low. Common causes include excessive mechanical ventilation, central hyperventilation associated with encephalopathy, central nervous system (CNS) infection, trauma, etc. Acutely hypoxic and acidotic patients can hyperventilate. In the latter case some degree of compensation for the high $[H^+]$ is achieved. One would expect the calculated bicarbonate and base excess from the blood gas machine to be normal. Treatment is directed at the specific cause.

RESPIRATORY ACIDOSIS

Hypoventilation causes a rise in $PaCO_2$. Acute changes in $PaCO_2$ have a linear effect on $[H^+]$ (1 kPa to 5.5 nmol/L). Thus $[H^+]$ is high and $PaCO_2$ is high. Common causes include respiratory depression, obstructive and restrictive respiratory diseases, terminal exhaustion, inadequate mechanical ventilation, etc. Similar derangements may be caused by muscle weakness and increased CO_2 production (malignant hyperthermia, seizures, ...). One would expect the calculated bicarbonate and base excess to be normal. Treatment is directed at improving respiratory function/support and to a lesser extent minimizing CO_2 load, e.g. by lowering the metabolic rate and providing fat as a metabolic substrate. If it is unsuccessful then compensation occurs over several days through renal conservation of bicarbonate. A compensated respiratory acidosis therefore has a near normal (but high) $[H^+]$ and a high $PaCO_2$ and one would expect the bicarbonate level calculated by the blood gas machine to be high.

METABOLIC ALKALOSIS

An acute fall in hydrogen ion concentration without a fall in CO_2 may be due to a rise in bicarbonate concentration or, less commonly, a loss of $[H^+]$ ions. Some compensatory CO_2 retention may occur and reduced respiratory drive should be anticipated, for example if one is attempting to wean mechanical ventilation. The calculated base excess would be expected to be high (see below) but under most circumstances confusion should not occur with a compensated respiratory acidosis because the $[H^+]$ will be near normal (but low). If the patient is being mechanically ventilated to a low $PaCO_2$ then the true interpretation of the blood gas may only be possible when placed in the wider clinical context.

During potassium deficiency renal conservation of K^+ occurs at the expense of H^+ which creates a metabolic alkalosis with a paradoxically acid urine. The problem is aggravated by hyponatremia. Intracellular acidosis occurs by a similar mechanism (lost K^+ replaced by H^+ and Na^+).

Chloride depletion is a common consequence of loop diuretic therapy but can also occur from gastrointestinal losses or as a secondary consequence of chronic respiratory acidosis. It is associated with increased sodium reabsorption in the proximal convoluted tubule and excess H^+ and K^+ loss, the former resulting in increased bicarbonate absorption from the filtrate. Chloride-sensitive causes of metabolic alkalosis are associated with low urinary chloride (< 20 mmol/L) and chloride-insensitive forms with higher urinary chloride. The former include diuretic therapy, vomiting and chloridorrhea and the latter, citrate poisoning. Diminished ECF volume will perpetuate a metabolic alkalosis because it is associated with an obligatory increase in proximal tubular Na^+ reabsorption.

By analogy, a metabolic alkalosis can be produced by the loss of hydrogen ion by vomiting, or by the introduction of bicarbonate-containing material into the body. In either event the blood pH tends to increase. In the former case an increase in total buffer base occurs and a reduction in H_2CO_3. In the latter an increase in total buffer base occurs but with an increase in H_2CO_3. Renal compensation corrects both imbalances.

In the rare circumstances where a metabolic alkalosis requires treatment it is important to treat the cause rather than the effect. Treat hypokalemia with potassium supplements and hypochloremia with saline infusion. Acid loads can be delivered where necessary however in the form of ammonium chloride (avoid in liver failure in favor of dilute hydrochloric acid 200 mmol/L in 5% dextrose).

METABOLIC ACIDOSIS

An acute rise in $[H^+]$ with a normal or even reduced $PaCO_2$ (attempted compensation) results from an abnormal bicarbonate loss or excess H^+. The calculated base deficit (negative base excess) would be expected to be high and the calculated bicarbonate would be expected to be low. Treatment must be directed at the cause. Routine investigation of a metabolic acidosis in order to determine the cause includes measurement of urine pH, anion and osmolar gaps and measurement of the serum lactate and/or arteriovenous oxygen difference as markers of the adequacy of tissue perfusion/oxygen delivery.

The anion gap is calculated according to the formula:

$$[Na^+] - ([Cl^-] + [HCO_3^-])$$

An anion gap greater than 12 implies the presence of a 'non-Henderson–Hasselbalch' source of acid. The osmolar gap is the difference between measured and calculated osmolality. If measured osmolality is > 15 mosm/L higher than calculated then this implies the presence of additional osmotically active solutes:

$$\text{Calculated osmolality} = (2 \times [Na]) + [glucose] + [urea] \text{ mmol/L}$$

Under certain circumstances it is justifiable to attempt to compensate a metabolic acidosis therapeutically by administering exogenous base such as sodium bicarbonate, for example to supplement recognized bicarbonate losses (e.g. urine, ileostomy fluid) or to treat drug overdoses involving agents that are weak acids. Bicarbonate can also be used as emergency therapy if there is associated symptomatic hyperkalemia or an inadequate response to inotropic support in the context of severe acidosis ($[H^+] > 63$ nmol/L, pH < 7.2). This bicarbonate rapidly forms CO_2 because of the prevailing pH. It thus creates a respiratory load. Furthermore although CO_2 diffuses fairly freely across the various membranes in the body, the bicarbonate ion may take several hours to attain access to all phases. It is possible therefore for exogenous bicarbonate to aggravate intracellular acidosis and similarly to lower the pH of cerebrospinal fluid. This latter effect explains the persistent respiratory alkalosis which occurs when metabolic acidosis is artificially corrected rapidly by administration of exogenous bicarbonate.

MIXED DISTURBANCES

A number of mixed acid–base disturbances are worthy of mention. For example mixed metabolic and respiratory acidosis is common in critical illness. Disease processes that cause combined effects such as these inevitably limit or curtail physiological compensation, causing more severe and persistent increases in $[H^+]$. Similarly the combination of heart failure (hence diuretic therapy) and chronic respiratory disease can cause hypokalemic/hypochloremic metabolic alkalosis and compensated respiratory acidosis, in which case $[H^+]$ levels fall, bicarbonate levels rise and CO_2 retention may be exacerbated.

Severe vomiting (e.g. in pyloric stenosis) causes loss of hydrogen and chloride ions causing hypochloremic alkalosis. Concurrent hypokalemia can lead to production of a paradoxically acid urine. In diabetic ketoacidosis complicated by severe vomiting the concurrent loss of hydrogen ions may lead to an apparent discordance with the severity of hyperglycemia and dehydration.

In salicylate poisoning the initial upset is usually respiratory alkalosis, partly compensation for the acid load but mostly from direct stimulation of respiratory drive. The supervening metabolic acidosis is due to uncoupled oxidative phosphorylation and increased metabolism of lipid, carbohydrate and amino acids. Blood gases show a high anion gap metabolic acidosis due to the salicylic acid, ketones, free amino acids and lactate. Respiratory alkalosis which is commonly associated with low ionized calcium levels gives way to respiratory acidosis as the conscious level is reduced. Hyperglycemia is common and may mimic diabetic ketoacidosis. Hypoglycemia may occur in small children.

CAUTIONARY NOTES ON LABORATORY TESTS OF FLUID AND ELECTROLYTES

The diagnosis of dehydration is essentially a clinical one. The total body water is not a particularly useful measurement under most circumstances since it is hard to standardize between individuals. The common assumption in clinical practice is that uremia indicates dehydration (and usually a contraction of the ECF volume) or renal failure. There are other causes of uremia however, such as excessive protein catabolism and the metabolism of ingested blood. In water depletion, the packed cell volume (PCV) tends to remain normal, whilst the concentrations of hemoglobin and plasma proteins show only slight increases. Unfortunately these observations are usually obscured because the predehydration figures are not known.

In hyperlipidemia, uremia or diabetes mellitus, the amount of lipids, urea or glucose may be large enough to produce a reduction in sodium concentration per unit volume. In hyperlipidemia the amount of water in plasma may be reduced to 75% of the norm and consequently the concentration of sodium apparently reduced. Nevertheless when expressed per liter of water (rather than solution) it is normal.

Serum potassium measurements must be interpreted in context since levels may not reflect total body levels. Beta-adrenergic stimuli, alkalosis or insulin therapy all lower serum potassium. However confidence that total body levels have not changed should not translate to a reticence to treat the serum level whether it is high or low because of the physiological consequences.

Serum phosphate levels like those of potassium are poor predictors of body levels since it is principally an intracellular anion. Plasma levels fluctuate as the result of shifts between ECF and ICF, they are also closely linked to ionized calcium levels. False low values/assay interference occur after mannitol administration or in the presence of lipemia, free hemoglobin (hemolysis) or bilirubinemia.

Calcium and magnesium homeostasis are closely linked to phosphate levels. Interpretation of total calcium levels must also be put into context with the serum albumin although it is more physiological to look directly at the ionized (free) component. Albumin binding of all species (drugs, bilirubin, calcium, ...) changes radically with acid–base. Respiratory alkalosis is capable of inducing tetany.

FLUID AND ELECTROLYTE DISTURBANCE

EDEMA

Edema is common in a variety of clinical situations particularly in the severely ill and malnourished. It is a common manifestation of a systemic inflammatory response and is therefore not necessarily a manifestation of fluid overload. Indeed in many clinical situations the edematous patient has a reduced intravascular volume. Indicators of hypervolemia such as hepatomegaly, high pulmonary blood flow and pulmonary edema make the clinical diagnosis of fluid overload more likely. However water intoxication causes hyponatremia long before significant edema occurs. Diuretic-resistant edema may occur in renal or cardiac failure: the implication is that renal excretion is impaired in spite of the possible presence of an increased ECF volume. The total body sodium under these circumstances may be increased but water retention is even more marked, resulting in hyponatremia.

Where capillary endothelial damage has occurred, for example as a consequence of a systemic inflammatory response, then the resultant edema may again be resistant to treatment with diuretics and fluid restriction. Hypernatremia may occur due to the associated leak of protein into the interstitial fluid. Treatment with supplemental i.v. infusion of albumin under such circumstances contributes to the interstitial albumin load unless endothelial repair has occurred. The sequence of events leading to this syndrome is complicated and involves excessive secretion and/or diminished inactivation of aldosterone and ADH together with the changes in capillary permeability. The outcome is an increase in the volume of interstitial fluid but a decrease in plasma volume. This results in prerenal uremia which is further aggravated by sodium restriction. Hypoalbuminemia such as occurs in nephrosis causes edema by altering the balance between hydrostatic and colloid osmotic pressures.

CLINICAL SIGNS OF DEHYDRATION

A history of increased thirst and oliguria implies dehydration, the clinical signs of which include reduced skin turgor, dry mucous membranes, sunken eyes and a sunken fontanelle. In the extreme case, signs of shock are present such as poor peripheral perfusion (prolonged capillary refill), cold peripheries, poor peripheral pulses, Kussmaul respiration (from metabolic acidosis) and ultimately hypotension and prostration. The clinical severity of dehydration can be matched to a pragmatic scale (mild, moderate, severe) (Table 17.4). This can then be used as a guide to the proportion of the premorbid weight that has been lost as fluid (e.g. 3%, 6%, 9%) and subsequently the fluid deficit that needs to be replaced (30 ml/kg, 60 ml/kg or 90 ml/kg). Dehydration severe enough to cause weight loss of 15% of the premorbid weight (as water) can reputedly occur and does not preclude successful salvage. However there is good evidence that even relatively experienced pediatricians overestimate the degree of dehydration during clinical examination. The danger is that this overestimate will then lead to excessive fluid administration. Furthermore individual clinical signs such as dry mucous membranes and a sunken fontanelle prove to be remarkably poor objective predictors of dehydration as determined retrospectively.[10]

Table 17.4 Fluid deficit in dehydration

	% Body weight	Adult (70 kg)	Infant (6 kg)	Signs and symptoms
Mild	3	2.0	0.18	Thirst; oliguria; dry mucous membranes
Moderate	6	4.0	0.36	Thirst; oliguria; restlessness; weakness and tachycardia
Very severe	7–14	5–10	0.42–0.84	Collapse, convulsions, blood pressure low; sunken eyeballs and fontanelle; loss of skin turgor with 'doughy' feeling; plasma sodium, urea and osmolality all raised

DEHYDRATION

Water and electrolyte losses occur in tandem but not always in strict proportion depending upon the source of the fluid loss and the nature of intake or replacement at the time. Thus the result may leave the plasma isotonic with respect to normal values, hypertonic or hypotonic. The loss of water and sodium in proportion leads to isotonic dehydration. An excess loss of water or the use of hypertonic fluids as intake leads to hypertonic dehydration. An excess loss of electrolyte or the use of hypotonic fluids as intake leads to hypotonic dehydration.

Hyperosmolar dehydration can result from the provision of incorrectly reconstituted feed or hyperosmolar (e.g. sugary) drinks. The infant's inability to handle the solute load causes an osmotic diuresis and the hyperosmolar intake compounds the situation. Water is lost initially from the ECF but the hyperosmolal plasma equilibrates with the intracellular environment. ECF volume is hence relatively preserved and the ICF experiences a greater fluid loss than in other forms of dehydration. Thus more of the total body water is lost for the same degree of hemodynamic compromise. Thrombosis, most notably of intracranial venous sinuses and renal veins, may occur. More importantly, rehydration involves re-expansion of the ICF volume and carries a high risk of cerebral swelling. It should therefore be performed slowly (over at least 48 h). Hyperosmolality is usually but not exclusively recognized by hypernatremia. It is also present in hyperglycemic dehydration due to diabetic ketoacidosis.

By contrast in hypo-osmolar dehydration the predominant water loss is from the extracellular (hence including the vascular) space and so hypotension and shock occur earlier and are more severe for a given amount of water loss. Relative preservation of intracellular turgor may increase the risk of cerebral ischemia during hypotension.

In all forms of dehydration, shock, acidosis and hypoglycemia are treated aggressively but rehydration should be more controlled, using normal saline initially irrespective of the serum sodium.

Thus salt is replaced in hypo-osmolal dehydration and in hyperosmolal dehydration the serum osmolality is sustained during the early stages of rehydration – reducing the risk of cerebral edema. A policy of aiming to replace water deficit over at least 48 h in all forms of dehydration protects against the common tendency to overestimate the water deficit. Replacement of potassium stores may take days as the rate of administration has to be limited to allow time for redistribution into the ICF. The associated protein calorie deficit may take weeks to correct.

ENTERAL REHYDRATION

When dehydration complicates illness in children, hospital admission is reserved for the younger patients and the more severe cases. There is therefore a tendency towards i.v. rehydration regimens for these patients. This may not always be appropriate. For example, from a wider perspective oral rehydration regimens for diarrhea are appropriate in over 90% of cases and most do not require hospitalization. The therapeutic effects of oral rehydration solutions (ORS) include facilitation of sodium transport across the bowel wall driven by glucose. A variety of proprietary preparations are available. Those intended for pre-emptive use contain less sodium than those designed specifically for rehydration of the dehydrated patient. Preference should be given to those in which the carbohydrate content is provided as monosaccharides (glucose), since disaccharidases are brush border enzymes which may be depleted by the illness. Loss of brush border lactase is the cause of postenteritic lactose intolerance which, when present, causes osmotic diarrhea if dairy products are introduced too early during recovery.

The principles of enteral fluid management in treating diarrhea are:

1. It is usually wrong to interrupt breast-feeding.
2. Supplemental water is allowed during treatment with ORS provided sufficient ORS has been administered.
3. A guide to the required volume of ORS is that it should normally equal the volume of stool produced.

When dehydration is evident at presentation as much as 50–100 ml/kg of ORS can be given enterally over 4–6 h depending upon its severity.

Subsequent treatment with as much as 200–300 ml/kg/day is usually well tolerated, if faced with equivalent losses.

HYPONATREMIA

Hyponatremia causes ileus, listlessness and ultimately cerebral edema and convulsions, the extent of the symptoms being more closely related to the rapidity of change in serum sodium than the absolute value. There are some patients whose plasma sodium concentrations remain below the lower limit of the normal range (e.g. 132 mmol/L) without symptoms and who excrete supplemental sodium to maintain this 'new' steady state.

Hyponatremia can occur in the face of normal total body sodium [syndrome of inappropriate secretion of antidiuretic hormone (SIADH), glucocorticoid deficiency, water overload ...], raised total body sodium with greater retention of water (heart failure, cirrhosis, nephrotic syndrome and sequestration) or decreased total body sodium (increased losses – particularly enteral, diuretic therapy or inadequate intake). Sodium loss is usually associated with a concomitant water loss and, as described above, the resultant serum sodium depends upon the balance between the two. Hyponatremia is common in preterm infants because of their high urinary losses. Breast milk on its own contains inadequate amounts of sodium for their needs.

Hyponatremia occurs as the result of water intoxication in a variety circumstances including:

- the prescription of hypotonic i.v. fluids particularly if too much fluid is prescribed (see Table 17.2);
- SIADH;
- missed cases of acute renal failure, e.g. in hemolytic uremic syndrome.

Babies are susceptible to water intoxication because of their relatively low GFR. Clinical manifestations may appear when water amounting to as little as 5% of body weight is retained. The excess water is widely distributed between both ECF and ICF.

SIADH is well recognized but it is frequently a misnomer. ADH secretion can be considered an appropriate evolutionary physiological response to injuries/illnesses which are of sufficient severity to preclude drinking for several days. The most common causes are CNS injury and bacterial pneumonia. The retained water however often does not come from a physiological source but from a prescription to administer fluid in quantities that did not anticipate the ADH secretion.[11] In any case the clinical picture of water intoxication (hyponatremia) develops. The diagnosis is made by proving that urine osmolality exceeds that of a hypo-osmolar plasma (i.e. inappropriate retention of water by the kidney) and the treatment is usually fluid restriction (see below and Table 17.2).

Two 'salt wasting' syndromes are worthy of individual mention because of the extraordinary scale of the sodium loss involved. In the salt-losing forms of congenital adrenal hyperplasia, deficiency of cortisol and aldosterone leads to natriuresis in the neonatal period. The clinical presentation however is with vomiting and weight loss. 'Cerebral salt wasting' is a condition which can appear in the first week after brain injury and spontaneously resolves in 2–4 weeks. It is characterized by natriuresis and subsequent hyponatraemic dehydration. It can be confused with SIADH in its early stages. Both conditions display coincident urine hyperosmolarity and hypo-osmolar plasma. The distinction is made by 24 h urinary sodium content which is high in salt wasting and normal in SIADH. The pathogenesis is unclear but it may prove to be a dopaminergic phenomenon or related to other circulating natriuretics such as atrial natriuretic peptide.[12] The treatment is to supply adequate salt *and water* (as opposed to fluid restriction in SIADH) but fludrocortisone may also be required.

Euvolemic hyponatremia with or without hyperkalemia can occur in a variety of critical illness states in the absence of renal dysfunction. Known precipitants include anoxia, septicemia and malnourishment. Pragmatically these should be assumed to be Addisonian crises (i.e. they should prompt the administration of steroids) but some may be due to failure of the Na^+/K^+ ATPase, the so called 'sick cell syndrome'.[13]

Rapid correction of hyponatremia is justified in circumstances where severe symptoms have resulted from a rapid fall in serum sodium. If a good history is not available, symptoms are severe and serum Na[+] is < 120 mmol/L, a rapid initial correction is justifiable to values of 125 mmol/L. To increase the serum sodium by 2 mmol/L/h (maximum safe rate):[14]

$$\text{Infusion rate (ml/h)} = 8 \times \text{wt (kg)}/(\% \text{ saline being used)}.$$

Further increase in serum sodium is best achieved more gradually with fluid restriction. In all other circumstances slow correction is advisable by fluid restriction alone and the provision of normal rather than increased sodium supplements.[15] Acute hyponatremia causes cerebral edema which may improve with the hypertonic saline as the brain shrinks.[16] The rapid correction of chronic hyponatraemia can lead to 'central pontine myelinosis' which can lead to quadriplegia.

HYPERNATREMIA

Hypernatremia can occur in association with low total body sodium, in which case the salt loss has occurred in the context of a greater water loss (e.g. osmotic diuresis, vomiting/diarrhea). When losses are predominantly water, total body sodium balance may be close to normal (e.g. fever, radiant heater, phototherapy, diabetes insipidus) as is the case when the interstitial fluid space expands at the expense of the plasma volume (e.g. capillary leak). True excess of sodium can also occur (e.g. when i.v. sodium bicarbonate is used to repeatedly correct metabolic acidosis without treating the cause or when malreconstituted formula is fed to a baby).

In all hyperosmolar states, water moves from ICF to ECF and so the ICF is dehydrated. Neurological symptoms predominate (irritability, seizures and coma). The loss of volume of brain cells can even cause cerebrovascular disruptions and bleeding. Treatment of hypernatremia should be aimed at the primary cause and any necessary rehydration should be slow because of the risks of cerebral edema. These risks are compounded by the formation of idiogenic osmoles within the cell. This term is used to describe additional osmotically active substances formed apparently in response to the hyperosmolal ECFs that serve to counter the shrinkage of the cell volume. The term 'idiogenic' has persisted since it was originally coined, despite the fact that at least some of the molecular species concerned have been established.[17]

True sodium overload without dehydration can be recognized by acute changes in weight (up in response to the overload and down as normality is restored) combined with calculation of the fractional sodium excretion. It requires removal with loop diuretics or renal replacement therapy as required. [Renal replacement therapy now includes hemofiltration (both low and high flow), hemodiafiltration, plasma filtration, plasmapheresis, peritoneal dialysis and hemodialysis.]

There is no such thing as pure water depletion; however excessive fluid losses from very high in the GI tract (saliva) and diabetes insipidus can lead to severe water depletion in the face of trivial sodium losses. Diabetes insipidus describes a situation where there is inadequate ADH resulting from injuries to the neurohypophysis, or alternatively there is resistance to the effects of ADH on the kidney (nephrogenic). The diagnosis is usually made when polyuria is recognized in association with hypernatremia. If necessary a dehydration test exaggerates the discrepancy between urine and plasma tonicity. Central causes can be treated with vasopressin (1 unit/kg in 50 ml at 1 ml/h). Nephrogenic causes necessitate treatment with dietary sodium restriction and if necessary deliberate sodium depletion induced by thiazide diuretics (presumed to enhance sodium and therefore water absorption in the proximal convoluted tubule).

HYPOKALEMIA

Hypokalemia without a true deficit in potassium can result from redistribution into the cells in response to a beta-adrenergic stimulus, alkalosis, excess insulin or rarer causes like familial hypokalemic periodic paralysis. Since the body potassium level is closely linked to muscle mass, reduction in muscle mass is associated with reduction in total body potassium but the relative amount of potassium and nitrogen remains constant. Hypokalemia with a deficit in potassium can result from inadequate intake, or increased renal (diuretic) or GI losses introducing a host of potential diagnoses including endocrine disturbances such as Cushing's syndrome and primary hyperaldosteronism. One situation that requires clinical caution is where i.v. therapy is employed to correct severe dehydration and associated acidosis (e.g. diabetic ketoacidosis). The patient's initial plasma potassium concentration is artificially elevated due to compartment shifts that have occurred as a consequence of the acidosis. A whole body potassium deficit means that, in the absence of renal failure, hypokalemia is inevitable during rehydration unless potassium supplements are included in the regimen.

Irrespective of the cause, hypokalemia has cardiovascular, neuromuscular and metabolic consequences including a propensity for dysrhythmias, ileus, muscle weakness and effects on carbohydrate and protein metabolism. Electrocardiograph (ECG) changes include ST depression, flattening or inversion of the T wave, prolonged Q–T interval and prominent or even bifid U waves. Potassium replacement has to be given into the ECF even though the principal destination is the ICF. Infusion rates should never exceed 0.5 mmol/kg/h for fear of deranging the myocardial membrane potential and hence causing lethal arrhythmia. The ECG changes associated with serum potassium levels reflect the cell membrane potential and so hyperkalemic changes may be seen with a normal serum potassium if correction of hypokalemia is performed too rapidly. Adequate replacement may take days where there is whole body depletion. Potassium supplements/replacement should not be given in the presence of oligo/anuria without regular monitoring of serum levels.

HYPERKALEMIA

Hyperkalemia without true overload (or even deficit) may result from measurement error (e.g. hemolysis in the sample), acidosis, insulin deficiency, or drugs such as digoxin, beta blockers and depolarizing muscle relaxants. There is also a hyperkalemic form of familial periodic paralysis. High serum potassium occurs in instances of increased load (e.g. iatrogenic infusion, tissue destruction, GI bleed and tumor lysis syndrome) usually in combination with decreased excretion (e.g. renal failure or mineralocorticoid deficiency). Significant elevation of the whole body potassium:nitrogen ratio is rare since fatal hyperkalemia occurs early. Hyperkalemia is dangerous because of its effects upon cell membrane potential and therefore upon cardiac rhythm (sinus arrest and ventricular fibrillation). The point at which such rhythm supervenes is unpredictable but depends upon the rate of rise of the serum level and the age/maturity of the patient. Neonates are far more tolerant of hyperkalemia than older children and adults, particularly in relation to the propensity for ventricular dysrhythmias. The normal range of serum level extends higher in preterm babies.

The principal recognizable ECG changes, where rhythm is preserved, are tall peaked T waves and prolonged p waves.

In acute renal failure hyperkalemia may be dramatic and easily aggravated by simultaneous injury to other organs and tissues increasing the load. In chronic renal failure GFR has to get down to 5–10% before hyperkalemia results although the 'renal reserve' for potassium excretion is reduced before this. The most severe consequence of hyperkalemia is cardiac arrest, which can occur at any point in the progression of the ECG abnormalities and arrhythmias. If the problem is detected before cardiac arrest then possible emergency therapeutic measures cause compartment shifts from ECF to ICF:

- correction of acidosis (mild acidosis 1 mmol/kg, severe acidosis 2–3 mmol/kg of $NaHCO_3$);
- salbutamol administration (2.5–5 mg nebulized or i.v. 1–5 μg/kg/min);
- glucose and insulin (2 ml/kg of 50% dextrose and 0.1 U/kg of soluble insulin).

A slower response can be obtained using ion exchange resins such as calcium polystyrene sulfonate (Resonium) 0.5 g/kg dose per rectum. An i.v. bolus of calcium (0.1 mmol/kg to a maximum of 5 mmol) can temporarily stabilize the heart rhythm whilst other treatments are initiated. Renal replacement therapy (dialysis) is indicated if the hyperkalemia is recalcitrant (as it will be if it is due to renal failure).

CALCIUM AND MAGNESIUM

Parathormone (PTH) increases calcium by promoting bone resorption, increasing calcium reabsorption from the renal tubule and increasing activation of vitamin D, which increases enteral absorption of calcium and phosphate. Calcitonin is secreted by the thyroid and thymus in response to hypercalcemia and lowers both calcium and phosphate levels.

Hypocalcemia is common in sick infants due to high levels of PTH antagonists like glucocorticoids and calcitonin. It may also be due to i.v. bicarbonate therapy or the use of citrated blood products. If persistent in the newborn it may be due to DiGeorge syndrome, maternal vitamin D deficiency, cows' milk feeding or magnesium deficiency. It causes jittery symptoms in babies, multifocal clonic convulsions and rarely ECG abnormalities, dysrhythmias or heart failure. Normal requirements are 0.3 mmol/kg/day increased to 1 mmol/kg/day when treating deficiency. Calcium infusion has vasoconstrictive and inotropic effects of greater significance in children than in adults. Vasoconstriction predominates in hypomagnesemic states. Calcium opposes the negative inotropic effects of hyperkalemia.

Hypomagnesemia usually occurs in the context of parenteral nutrition because of solubility problems caused by the concurrent administration of phosphate. Clinical problems are rare until levels fall below 0.5 mmol/L but do include lethal arrhythmias such as ventricular fibrillation/ventricular tachycardia (VF/VT) and torsade de pointes. Deficiency also reduces cardiac contractility but during infusion, magnesium salts are reasonably potent vasodilators and will drop the blood pressure. Magnesium has also been used to treat pulmonary hypertension and asthma. Hypocalcemia and hypokalemia may not respond to supplementation if concurrent hypomagnesemia is uncorrected.

Hypercalcemia is rare but occurs in the recovery phase of acute renal failure, a variety of endocrine diseases, hypervitaminosis D and granulomatous disorders. Idiopathic hypercalcemia is a feature of Williams syndrome. Most cases of hypercalcemia are iatrogenic. Symptoms include neurological problems (hypotonia, seizures and coma), cardiovascular problems (tachyarrhythmias) and in chronic cases hypertension. Severe cases are treated with renal replacement therapy (dialysis).

Hypermagnesemia occurs when excessive administration (cathartics or enemas) coincides with renal failure. Symptoms are similar to hypercalcemia but include bradyarrhythmias with first degree block and broad QRS complexes. Treatment is again focused upon enhanced excretion. Serious arrhythmias may respond to calcium.

PHOSPHATE

Phosphate excretion involves free filtration at the glomerulus with passive reabsorption of 80% in the proximal convoluted tubute (PCT) as a symport with sodium. [A symport is a membrane carrier that combines the movement of more than one type of molecule (species) in a given direction. Both species bind on one side of the membrane and are then translocated to the other side.] Although PTH results in phosphate release from bone and increased phosphate absorption from the gut, its net effect at high levels is to decrease plasma phosphate because it inhibits its renal tubular reabsorption. The fetus is relatively hypoparathyroid in response to active calcium influx across the placenta.

Hypophosphatemia occurs from:
- inadequate intake: e.g. breast-fed preterm infants;
- impaired GI absorption: e.g. as a consequence of antacids containing calcium, magnesium or aluminum (such as sucralfate);
- cellular redistribution: e.g. alkalosis, therapy for diabetic ketoacidosis, beta 2-adrenergic stimulation;
- carbohydrate infusions and other forms of hyperalimentation which can lead to hypophosphatemia by stimulating insulin release (phosphate moves into cells with glucose in response to insulin) (successful stimulation of an anabolic state after critical illness can be associated with a profound and symptomatic hypophosphatemia);
- excessive losses: e.g. as a consequence of diuretics, steroids, cytotoxic regimens or paracetamol poisoning;
- trauma (including burns);
- hereditary hypophosphatemic rickets.

The most important feature of phosphate physiology is the formation of adenosine triphosphate (ATP). Symptomatic hypophosphatemia occurs in severe depletion and causes muscle weakness that can aggravate respiratory failure and reduce myocardial contractility. When necessary, phosphate supplementation should aim to provide a dose of up to 1 mmol/kg/day (max 20 mmol) (beware some proprietary phosphate supplements have a high potassium content).

Hyperphosphatemia occurs in neonates fed cows' milk or inadequately adjusted formula feed, tumor lysis syndrome and renal failure, severe hemolysis, hyperthyroidism, acromegaly, hypoparathyroidism and phosphate poisoning. Symptoms are those of the consequent hypocalcemia and deposition of hydroxyapatite crystals in cornea, lungs, heart, etc. Treatment includes resuscitation to restore ECF volume. In the absence of renal failure, phosphate binders and alkaline diuresis may be used.

CONCLUSION

The intention of this chapter has been to cover fluid, electrolyte and acid–base from a clinical perspective. This has necessarily led to the omission of some essential basic science, some of which is contained in the following two appendices. However the key point is that while fluid, electrolyte and acid–base disturbances can and should be evaluated and treated on their own merits, they should be considered as effects of illness. To 'cure' them the cause must be treated.

APPENDIX 1: PHYSICAL AND PHYSIOLOGICAL INFLUENCES ON THE INTERNAL DISTRIBUTION OF WATER AND ELECTROLYTES

MEMBRANE PROPERTIES AND FUNCTION

The homeostasis of body fluids is intricately related to the integrity and function of their adjacent membranes. An 'ideal' membrane permits only water to pass through, and is impermeable to dissolved substances. Membranes resemble molecular sieves with the added influence of the solubility of substances in the membrane lipids. Isolated cellular membranes are partially permeable. They are fully permeable to water and small crystalloid molecules but will not permit the passage of larger molecules such as proteins and mucopolysaccharides. The metabolic activity of the cell also maintains differences between the intracellular and extracellular concentrations of various ions. This ability decreases if the cell is cooled or poisoned. Cell membranes carry negative internal and positive external charges and the membrane potential is governed by the ratio of internal to external concentration of ions.

Substances cross membranes in several ways. Water or solutes may simply flow through pores. Solutes may also dissolve in the membrane and diffuse through it in solution or they may be actively transported from one side to the other. Potassium penetrates cells more rapidly than sodium, probably in part due to the smaller diameter of the potassium ion. At equilibrium the rate of movement of any material across a membrane is equal in both directions.

Under normal circumstances exchange between physical compartments in the body is tightly regulated by both steroid hormones (cortisol, aldosterone) and peptide hormones (ADH and thyroxine). Water and small solutes pass freely through intercellular pores in endothelium and in and out of cells through a facilitative transport mechanism in the cell membrane mediated by specialized transmural proteins – 'aquaporins'. The expression of aquaporins within a membrane may provide a mechanism for physiological control of the movement of small solutes as well as water.[18] The nature of such transcellular transport mechanisms, which also include epithelial sodium channels (ENaC), and their role in health and disease is only now becoming apparent.

The structure of the capillary endothelium varies according to site but there are common features in the basic structure that persist throughout. A layer of thin endothelial cells, one cell thick, lines the luminal surface of a basement membrane. The luminal surfaces of these cells bear a negative charge, imparted by a layer of glycosaminoglycans. These species restrict the permeability of the membrane with regard to negatively charged molecules such as albumin. The cellular lining may be fenestrated (depending upon the site) and there are numerous clefts between cells and tubular channels that traverse the epithelial cells themselves. Endothelial cells may change shape with changes in pressure and they have physiological responses to blood flow and shear stress, which include the release of vasoactive mediators and anticoagulants.

For the diffusion of small water-soluble molecules (e.g. sodium, chloride and glucose) across capillary endothelium, the size and number of the pores (which vary depending upon the site) is not rate limiting and movement is dictated by blood supply, i.e. is 'flow limited'. These movements are dictated by the Fick equation (diffusion rate = blood flow/arteriovenous concentration difference) and Fick's law of diffusion which relates the diffusion rate:

- directly to the diffusion coefficient of the solute (related to molecular size and therefore weight);
- directly to the area of the capillary membrane;
- directly to the concentration gradient;
- inversely to the thickness (and hence permeability) of the membrane.

Capillary diffusion gradients depend on capillary size. As intercapillary distances increase, there will be islands of tissue where supply or removal of solutes becomes inadequate.

In addition to solute diffusion, bulk movement of fluid across membranes (filtration) also carries solutes across the membrane or through its pores. This occurs irrespective of whether it is initiated by hydrostatic or osmotic influences. The anatomical variation in the size and number of clefts between endothelial cells is related to their filtration properties. By far the most important homeostatic mechanism controlling this process is the vasomotor control of precapillary vessels. Glomeruli are specialized exceptions where control is exerted over pre- and postcapillary vessels. The filtration of fluid is a passive process proceeding at a rate dictated by:

- the filtration coefficient of the membrane (influenced by its surface area and permeability);
- the hydrostatic pressure gradient (greater within the arterial end of the capillary but consistent across a glomerulus);
- the colloid osmotic pressure gradient;

in a relationship described by Starling's law of ultrafiltration. The net filtration is out of the capillary at the arterial end and into the capillary at the venous end.

Epithelial and endothelial function are profoundly affected by the processes of acute inflammation in which both cell destruction and damage to basement membranes occur. Endothelial damage can be initiated and/or aggravated by activated neutrophils, which degranulate releasing proteolytic enzymes such as elastase, and reactive oxygen species in addition to cationic proteins. Activated platelets also contribute. Further endothelial cell destruction involves the stripping of glycosaminoglycans from the luminal surface of capillaries. The loss of their negative luminal charge increases the permeability of the endothelium to albumin. An interstitial edema of relatively protein rich fluid results.

The physical factors that govern transport across all membranes (cell membrane, capillary endothelium, etc.), include total osmotic pressure, hydrostatic pressure, colloidal (oncotic) pressure of proteins, Donnan

equilibrium and the law of electroneutrality. (Properties that are determined by the number rather than the nature of the particles present are termed 'colligative'. One of the most important points about colligative properties is that they are interrelated. They include such characteristics as the lowering of vapor pressure, the elevation of boiling point, the reduction of freezing point and osmotic pressure.)

The equivalent weight (gram equivalent) of an electrolyte

$$= \frac{\text{molecular weight in grams}}{\text{valency}}$$

e.g. sodium $\frac{23}{1} = 23$, calcium $\frac{40}{2} = 20$.

In the SI system (Système International d'Unités), the preferred unit for chemical measurement, is the mole (the amount of a substance with a mass equal to its molecular weight expressed in grams). According to this system concentrations are expressed in millimoles/liter (mmol/L) rather than as milliequivalents/litre. The relationship between the numerical values is:

$$\frac{\text{mEq /L}}{\text{valency}} = \text{mmol/L}$$

therefore for monovalent species $\text{mEq L}^{-1} = \text{mmol L}^{-1}$

MOLARITY

Molarity is defined as the gram molecules (moles) of solute *per liter of solution*.

MOLALITY

Molality is defined as the gram molecules (moles) of solute *per kilogram of solvent*.

At all body temperatures 1 kg of water is regarded as occupying 1 liter.

The terms molarity and molality should not be confused. For dilute aqueous solutions they are approximately equal, but in the body the distinction is marked.

OSMOLARITY

One liter of solution containing 1 mole of undissociated solute represents an osmolarity of 1 osmol/L or 1000 mosmol/L. An aqueous solution of such concentration will exert an osmotic pressure of 22.4 atmospheres under ideal conditions and with an ideal membrane.

OSMOLALITY

Osmolality is applicable when the concentration of solute is molal. This term, unlike osmolarity, takes account of the solute volume.

For undissociated non-electrolyte solutions the molarity (molality) and osmolar (osmolal) concentrations are identical. For a substance dissociating fully into ions, however, each ion has the same osmotic effect as an undissociated molecule (i.e. dissociation increases the osmotic effect beyond that expected in terms of the molar content of the undissociated solute). A molar solution of sodium chloride (Na^+Cl^-) has, therefore, an ideal osmotic pressure of 2×22.4 atmospheres (2 osmoles). Calcium chloride ($Ca^{2+}2Cl^-$) yields three osmotically active ions if fully dissociated. In practice it is only with very dilute solutions that full dissociation occurs and the appropriate correction factor (osmotic coefficient) must be applied to calculate the osmolality when only the molality is known. Conversely association of macromolecules will result in a lowering of the theoretical osmotic pressure.

Solutions with the same osmotic pressure are termed isosmotic, and if separated by an 'ideal' membrane are termed isotonic when no net transfer of water occurs between them. Naturally most compartments in the body are in osmotic equilibrium although this does not apply to fluids such as urine and saliva. It is most convenient to determine osmolality by using an osmometer which actually measures the freezing point of plasma. Normal plasma osmolality is approximately 285 mosmol/kg body water.

Plasma and extracellular osmolality are closely related to the concentration of the major cation, sodium. A similar relationship exists between the osmolality of ICF and intracellular potassium concentration. The polyvalent protein anions contribute about 16 electrical milliequivalents per liter of plasma water but they only represent approximately two osmotically active particles per liter.

PHYSIOLOGICAL MOVEMENTS OF WATER AND ELECTROLYTES

When a solute is added to a solution on one side of a membrane there is a potential difference in concentration between the phases. Equilibrium can be established by:

- free distribution of the solute on both sides of the membrane (this is possible only with a diffusible solute and permeable membranes);
- passage of water through the membranes, thereby eliminating the potential difference by equalizing the number of water molecules per unit area on each side of the membrane;
- applying pressure to the solution to increase the potential again to that of pure water.

The addition of a diffusible solute to one compartment thus results in an increase of total osmolality in both compartments without net water transfer. A nondiffusible solute increases the effective as well as total osmolality and results in a transfer of water from one compartment to the other (Fig. 17.3).

Physiologically, urea may be regarded as being a freely diffusible (penetrating) solute, and increasing the concentration of urea in the body causes no transfer of water between the phases. An exception is when urea is rapidly removed from the plasma by hemodialysis, when water moves into the ICF before outward diffusion of intracellular urea can occur. In diabetes mellitus the elevated plasma glucose concentration causes intracellular water loss, because glucose is not a diffusible solute in the absence of insulin.

Although sodium, potassium and chloride are freely diffusible, the fact that most of the sodium and chloride are found in the ECF and that the potassium is mainly intracellular demonstrates the presence of an active transport mechanism. The distribution of potassium between the ICF and ECF is heavily dependent upon the action of the Na$^+$/K$^+$ ATPase. This latter enzyme imports 2 × K$^+$ from the ECF and exports 3 × Na$^+$

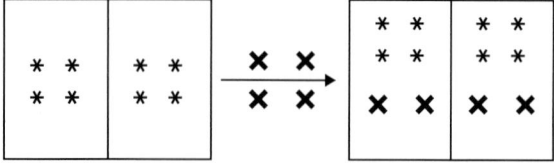

Diffusible solute and permeable membrane

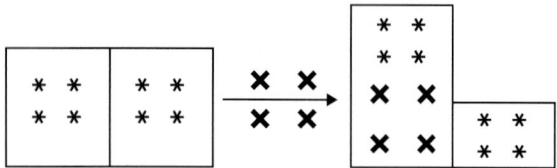

Non-diffusible solute

Fig. 17.3 Water distribution in response to changes in tonicity. In each example two fluid spaces are separated by a membrane which is permeable to water. The effect of adding solute to the left hand compartment is displayed on the right. Relative changes in volume accompany the movement of water.

from the ICF. Electrical neutrality may be preserved by the efflux of a Cl$^-$, which adds to the osmotic effect leading to a reduction of the ICF volume. The balance of potassium across the cell membrane otherwise contributes to the resting membrane electrical potential. Acid–base status, insulin and catecholamines all exert effects upon the distribution of potassium across the cell membrane. Acidosis causes an efflux of potassium from the cell and alkalosis the reverse. The greatest effect occurs with mineral acids rather than lactic or keto acids where the cell is more permeable to the accompanying anions and the effects on potassium levels lag behind those of pH.

The fixed intracellular anions (protein and phosphate) are unable to traverse the membrane and their concentrations will largely determine the concentration of potassium in the ICF. Inhibiting cellular metabolism by cooling or by enzyme inhibitors results in the disappearance of the sodium and potassium gradients normally present. The maintenance of a high intracellular potassium content by cells in a saline medium requires the presence of oxygen, glucose and L-glutamate. The absence of any one of these materials results in entry of sodium into the cell and diffusion of potassium into the ECF. Thereafter, application of Donnan equilibrium (see below) allows entry of water and further sodium ions, causing swelling, and finally rupture of the cell.

The diffusion of chloride ions into or out of the cell is intimately related to the membrane potential.

Membrane potential

The cell membrane may be regarded as being permeable to water, potassium and chloride, but impermeable to protein, phosphate and sodium. An electrochemical potential difference exists between the two sides of the membrane, referred to as the membrane potential. This has been measured in various cells and within experimental error the relationship for calculating its value depends upon the relative concentrations of diffusible ions in the ECF and in the ICF.

A potential difference also exists across the membrane separating the intravascular phase of ECF (plasma) from the extravascular phase (interstitial fluid). This E$_m$ is small since the gradients exhibited by sodium, potassium and chloride are not great. This is because sodium ions can penetrate capillary membranes freely, there being no active transport, and the electrolyte gradients result only from the presence of nondiffusible protein anions in plasma.

Donnan membrane equilibrium

When a diffusible solute is added to water on one side of a partially permeable membrane, rapid diffusion of the solute and water occurs between the phases. Small electrolyte differences occur when a nondiffusible ion (e.g. a plasma protein with anionic charge) is present on one side of the membrane. The drive to maintain electrical neutrality then causes movement of diffusible ions (Na$^+$ in our example) against their own concentration gradient. The number of diffusible ions that move increases disproportionately as the concentration gradient of protein rises and the result is a greater concentration of osmotically active particles in the phase containing the nonpenetrating protein ion. The movement of protein itself across capillary membranes is resisted by a negative charge on the luminal surface of the vascular endothelium largely generated by glycosaminoglycan molecules. The osmotic effect exerted by colloids (colloid osmotic pressure or oncotic pressure) is quantitatively small but nevertheless it may be crucial in the fine balance of fluid movement across capillary beds.

These conditions exist even in the absence of active transport such as between plasma and interstitial fluid but can be magnified or opposed by active transport, which can maintain an intracellular ion at a constant concentration as though it were a nonpenetrating ion. Unless opposed, there is a tendency for water to move into the compartment containing the constrained anion. The metabolic process preventing the entry of water into cells is directly related to the extrusion of sodium (Na$^+$/K$^+$ ATPase).

Hydrostatic and colloid osmotic pressure

Equilibrium in plasma is established between the formation and the reabsorption of interstitial fluid by the interplay of hydrostatic and colloid osmotic pressures.

The total osmotic pressure of plasma (285 mosmol/kg body water) is equivalent to about 6.5 atmospheres (5000 mmHg), but the proportion due to the colloid osmotic pressure of the proteins is small, being less than 30 mmHg. Since the interstitial fluid contains only small amounts of protein, the difference in colloid osmotic pressure (oncotic pressure) is equivalent to about 25 mmHg.

Although it is small, this figure is of fundamental physiological importance in controlling the flow of water between plasma and tissue fluids.

Since albumins have smaller molecular weights than globulins, approximately 80% of the plasma protein osmotic effect is due to albumin. Thus hypoalbuminemia predisposes to the formation of increased amounts of interstitial fluid, causing clinically detectable edema.

APPENDIX 2: ACID–BASE CHEMISTRY AND BLOOD GAS MEASUREMENT

An 'acid' is any molecule or ion which tends to donate a proton (H^+) and a 'base' is any molecule or ion which tends to accept a proton. Hence (as implied) the acidity of a solution is its hydrogen ion concentration:

acid   proton   base

In general: HB H^+ B^-

B^- is referred to as the conjugate base of the acid HB (conjugate acid).

The more readily an acid donates a proton the stronger it is. The more readily a base accepts a proton the stronger it is. The dissociation of a conjugate acid to produce a proton occurs as part of an equilibrium described by an equilibrium constant 'K'

$$\text{where } K = \frac{[H^+][B^+]}{[HB]}$$

K is large for strong acids and small for weak acids. Hence pK [the negative logarithm (to base 10) of K] is low for strong acids and high for weak acids. Biological acids may be neutral molecules, cations or anions. Biological bases may be anions or neutral molecules. Water is amphoteric (i.e. acts either as an acid or a base).

Sorensen introduced the term pH, which is the negative logarithm (to base 10) of the molal hydrogen ion activity. The term simplifies the appreciation of hydrogen ion concentration in relation to the behavior of buffers. Its use however can be misleading in clinical situations and the hydrogen ion concentration is the preferred nomenclature (see below).

Hydrogen ion activity$(H^+) = [H^+] \times f$, where f = activity coefficient.

In dilute aqueous solution f tends to 1.0 and (H^+) tends to $[H^+]$. It is, therefore, justifiable to derive the equation:

$$pH = pK + \log \frac{[\text{conjugate base}]}{[\text{conjugate acid}]}$$

In clinical practice acid–base discussions are conducted using a shorthand based upon the carbonic acid/bicarbonate system which is quantitatively the most important buffer in plasma and whole blood. All the buffer systems are however in equilibrium so the approach may have some shortcomings. With these provisos the Henderson–Hasselbalch equation applies:

$$pH = pK + \log \frac{[HCO_3]}{[H_2CO_3]}$$

When considering the roles of respiratory and renal physiology on acid–base the equation may be considered as:

$$pH = pK + \log \frac{\text{renal component}}{\text{respiratory component.}}$$

'Buffers' are substances which tend to prevent a change in pH occurring within a system when either an acid or a base is added. Biological buffer systems are composed of a solution of weak acids together with their conjugate bases. Increases in the $[H^+]$ of the system cause conjugation of the buffer and vice versa. For any given addition of acid or base the change in ratio will be least (most efficient buffering) when:

[conjugate base] = [conjugate acid],

$$\text{i.e. when } \log \frac{[\text{conjugate base}]}{[\text{conjugate acid}]} = 0 \text{ and pH = pK}$$

Chemically, the carbonic acid bicarbonate buffer system is not ideal for maintaining pH = 7.40, since the pK $\approx$ 6.1 and the ratio of buffer base:buffer acid is 20:1.

Fortunately the respiratory center is extremely sensitive to changes both in the CO_2 tension and the pH of plasma. This is the main reason why the system is effective physiologically in conserving blood pH within narrow limits.

BIOLOGICAL BUFFER SYSTEMS (Table 17.5)

The relative importance of the various buffers depends both upon their concentrations in the body compartments concerned and on the prevailing pH values. The bicarbonate system is the most important in plasma, with proteins and phosphate making smaller contributions. Hemoglobin is the most important buffer within erythrocytes, whilst within other cells the major buffers are phosphates and proteins.

Blood gas machines measure pH, PCO_2 and PO_2 and it is best to limit one's interpretation to these parameters. The machines however can perform calculations using assumptions (that may be erroneous) to derive other parameters such as the base excess. The sort of assumptions made in these calculations are: the relevant hemoglobin concentration (if it has not been measured), the solubility coefficient of carbon dioxide in plasma (which is assigned a designated value whereas it may vary) and constancy of the pK of the Henderson–Hasselbalch equation (which again may vary significantly). Given these assumptions, the following parameters may be presented:

- Base excess. The difference between the observed buffer base and the normal buffer base. The base excess is a measure of the metabolic contribution to the hydrogen ion concentration. It is an empirical expression which approximates (by calculation) the amount of acid (or base for a 'base deficit') which would be needed to titrate 1 liter of blood to a $[H^+]$ of 40 nmol/L (pH 7.4). The base excess of blood with a $[H^+]$ of 40 nmol/L, $PaCO_2$ 40 mmHg (5.33 kPa), total [Hb] 15 g/dl at 37°C is zero. In a metabolic acidosis where nonvolatile acids such as lactic acid have accumulated, a negative base excess or base deficit results. Conversely, in a metabolic alkalosis the buffer base may increase, giving a positive base excess. In respiratory acidosis, for each moiety of H^+ produced, a corresponding increase in HCO_3^- occurs and total buffer base remains unaltered. A comparable situation occurs in respiratory

Table 17.5 Biological buffer systems

Approximate % contribution to buffering of whole blood	Buffer acid (HB)	H^+	+	Buffer base⁻ (B⁻)
64	H_2CO_3	H^+	+	HCO_3^-
1	$H_2PO_4^-$	H^+	+	HPO_4^{2-}
6	HPr	H^+	+	Pr⁻
29	HHB	H^+	+	Hb⁻

Hb, hemoglobin; Pr, protein.

alkalosis. Respiratory acidosis and alkalosis thus produce no change in the base excess unless renal compensation occurs.

- Standard bicarbonate. This is another index of the metabolic component. It is the calculated concentration of plasma bicarbonate in fully oxygenated blood at a PCO_2 of 40 mmHg and at 37°C. Normal range = 22–26 mmol/L plasma.
- Actual bicarbonate (mmol/L plasma) is the calculated bicarbonate content of the plasma.
- Total CO_2 content = actual bicarbonate + (PCO_2 mmHg × 0.03). This parameter is by definition a measure of both the metabolic and respiratory components of blood acid–base status. It is of interest to consider the possible effect of PCO_2 on the actual bicarbonate and total CO_2 content values, and to compare these with the unaltered standard bicarbonate.

The strong ion theory has been proposed as a more comprehensive approach towards interpretation of acid–base.[19–21] The term 'strong ion' is used to describe species which are almost entirely dissociated at physiological pH (Na^+, K^+, Ca^{2+}, Mg^{2+}, Cl^-, lactate). The 'strong ion difference' is essentially a more comprehensive 'anion gap' calculated as the charge difference between the sum of measured strong cations and that of strong anions. It is regarded as an independent variable determining [H^+] and as such is comparable to the 'buffer base' (the sum of the buffer anions in the blood). Hence falls in strong ion difference have an acidifying effect. The two other independent variables regarded as affecting [H^+] are the PCO_2 and the charge from weak acids, increases of which also increase [H^+]. All three effect their influence on [H^+] by altering the degree of dissociation of water (which is amphoteric) into hydrogen ions and hydroxyl groups. Other variables such as the concentration of bicarbonate ions are regarded as dependent variables to be, in essence, ignored. Changes in dependent variables are impossible without changes in independent ones. Thus if PCO_2 and the charge from weak acids remain constant, hydrogen ion and bicarbonate can only be changed by altering the concentration of strong ions. The latter maneuver requires their movement between compartments or out of the body.[20,21]

To use the strong ion difference as an analytical approach in clinical practice requires more extensive laboratory activity. It has been asserted to be useful in some acid–base derangements such as hyperchloremic acidosis.[22]

PH VERSUS [H⁺]

Hydrogen ion concentration ([H^+]) has been used in place of pH in this chapter because in clinical practice physiological measurements and therapeutic influences create changes that are linear in [H^+] (as opposed to inverse logarithmic in pH) and therefore more easily interpreted.[23] For example, acute changes in $PaCO_2$ affect [H^+] in the ratio 1 kPa to 5.5 nmol/L. Tracking the [H^+] is intuitively easier and makes it easier to monitor the effect of therapeutic interventions, which have their effects primarily on the molar [H^+].

A change of 0.3 pH units is equivalent to a twofold change in the concentration of hydrogen ion because $\log_{10}2$ is 0.3. A pH of 7.4 corresponds to a [H^+] of 40 nmol/L. An increase of 40 nmol/L reduces the pH to 7.1. A similar numerical change in pH towards alkalosis (pH 7.7) involves a reduction in [H^+] of only 20 nmol/L (to halve the concentration). A drop in pH from 7.4 to 6.8 involves a sixfold increase in [H^+].

There is a counter to this argument which is becoming less relevant as the technology of blood gas machines improves. It is again linked to the linear versus logarithmic nature of the variables. When using ion specific electrodes (like a pH electrode) a precise value for the potential difference being measured is necessary to minimize error in the calculation of ionic concentration. The logarithmic transformation hides the errors in measurement of the potential difference in the decimal places of the pH. For example each millivolt error in measurement creates a 4% error in the calculated [H^+], whereas an error of more than 5 millivolts creates a change of only 0.1 pH units. Thus, when using [H^+] for clinical decisions, greater technical precision may be required and therefore better performance of the electrode in terms of drift and other errors.

FURTHER READING

Ganong WF. Review of medical physiology. Los Altos: McGraw Hill; 1999.
Halperin MLG. Fluid, electrolyte, and acid–base physiology: a problem-based approach. Philadelphia: WB Saunders; 1999.

REFERENCES (*Level 1 evidence)

1. Anderson PA. Maturation and cardiac contractility. Cardiol Clin 1989; 7:209–225.
2. Aperia A, Broberger O, Herin P, et al. Postnatal control of water and electrolyte homeostasis in pre-term and full-term infants. Acta Paediatr Scand Suppl 1983; 305:61–65.
3. Jaksic T, Shew SB, Keshen TH, et al. Do critically ill surgical neonates have increased energy expenditure? J Pediatr Surg 2001; 36:63–67.
4. Shew SB, Jaksic T. The metabolic needs of critically ill children and neonates. Semin Pediatr Surg 1999; 8:131–139.
5. Shann F. Paediatric fluid and electrolyte therapy. In: Oh TE, ed. Intensive care manual. Hong Kong: Butterworth-Heinemann; 1999.
6. Carlotti AP, Bohn D, Mallie JP, et al. Tonicity balance, and not electrolyte-free water calculations, more accurately guides therapy for acute changes in natremia. Intensive Care Med 2001; 27:921–924.
7. Ichikawa I. Pediatric textbook of fluids and electrolytes. Philadelphia: Williams & Wilkins; 1990.
8. West JB. Best and Taylor's physiological basis of medical practice. Philadelphia: Williams & Wilkins; 1989.
9. Domino KB, Swenson ER, Hlastala MP. Hypocapnia-induced ventilation/perfusion mismatch: a direct CO_2 or pH-mediated effect? Am J Respir Crit Care Med 1995; 152 (5pt 1):1534–1539.
10. Mackenzie A, Barnes G, Shann F. Clinical signs of dehydration in children. Lancet 1989; 2 (8663):605–607.
11. Halberthal M, Halperin ML, Bohn D. Lesson of the week: acute hyponatraemia in children admitted to hospital: retrospective analysis of factors contributing to its development and resolution. BMJ 2001; 322 (7289):780–782.
12. Maesaka JK, Gupta S, Fishbane S. Cerebral salt-wasting syndrome: does it exist? Nephron 1999; 82:100–109.
13. Gill G, Leese G. Hyponatraemia: biochemical and clinical perspectives. Postgrad Med J 1998; 74 (875):516–523.
14. Shann F. Drug doses, 10th edn. Melbourne: Collective Pty; 1998.
15. Gross P, Reimann D, Neidel J, et al. The treatment of severe hyponatremia. Kidney Int Suppl 1998; 64:S6–S11.
16. Porzio P, Halberthal M, Bohn D, et al. Treatment of acute hyponatremia: ensuring the excretion of a predictable amount of electrolyte-free water. Crit Care Med 2000; 28:1905–1910.
17. Arieff AI, Kleeman CR. Studies on mechanisms of cerebral edema in diabetic comas: effects of hyperglycemia and rapid lowering of plasma glucose in normal rabbits. (J Clin Invest 1973; 52:571–583). J Am Soc Nephrol 2000; 11:1776–1788.
18. Cooper GJ, Boron WF. Effect of PCMBS on CO_2 permeability of Xenopus oocytes expressing aquaporin 1 or its C189S mutant. Am J Physiol 1998; 275 (6pt 1) C1481–C1486.
19. Kellum JA. Metabolic acidosis in the critically ill: lessons from physical chemistry. Kidney Int Suppl 1998; 66:S81–S86.
20. Wooten EW. Strong ion difference theory: more lessons from physical chemistry. Kidney Int 1998; 54:1769–1770.
21. Wooten EW. Analytic calculation of physiological acid–base parameters in plasma. J Appl Physiol 1999; 86:326–334.
22. Kellum JA, Bellomo R, Kramer DJ, et al. Etiology of metabolic acidosis during saline resuscitation in endotoxemia. Shock 1998; 9:364–368.
23. Hooper J, Marshall WJ, Miller AL. Log-jam in acid–base education and investigation: why make it so difficult? Ann Clin Biochem 1998; 35 (pt 1): 85–93.

18

Disorders of the urinary system

Moin A. Saleem, Jane Tizard, Jan Dudley, Carol Inward, Richard Coward, Mary McGraw

Online Mendelian Inheritance in Man (OMIM) is a freely accessible source of information which communicates the recent advances in the discovery of important genes and proteins responsible for inherited diseases. The reference numbers for inherited renal diseases described in this chapter are shown in brackets after the disease is mentioned. This should allow the reader to access up-to-date information regarding the molecular biology of the disease of interest. Web page: http://www. ncbi.nlm.nih. gov/entrez/query.fcgi?db=OMIM

RENAL PHYSIOLOGY

The kidneys comprise of two organs located posteriorly in the extraperitoneal space of the abdomen. Each kidney normally contains approximately 1 million nephrons, which are the functional units of this organ. There are seven major physiological functions of the kidney, which are shown in Table 18.1. The nephron for simplicity can be considered functionally in five parts (Fig. 18.1), each of which will be discussed in turn:

1. *Glomerulus.* This is the filtering unit of the kidney and allows a massive amount of water and small molecules to freely pass across the filtration barrier from the circulation into Bowman's capsule (equivalent to approximately 25–35 times the entire circulating

Table 18.1 Functions of the kidney

1. Water removal
2. Potassium excretion
3. Blood pressure control
4. Stimulation of the production of red blood cells
5. Acid–base control
6. Toxin excretion
7. Bone modeling

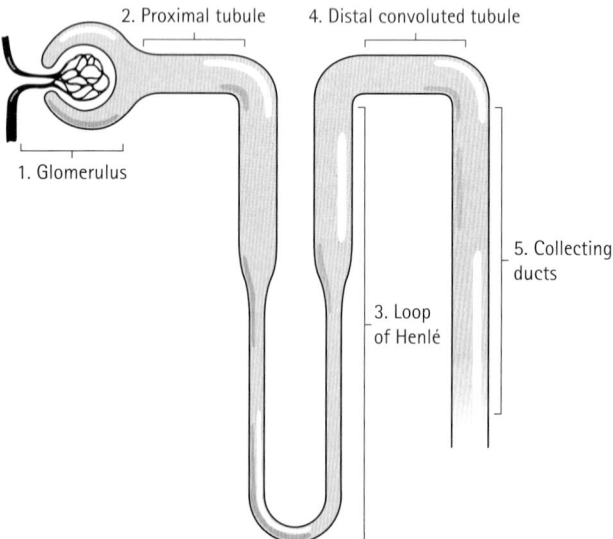

Fig. 18.1 Simplified drawing of a nephron. Isonatremic reabsorption of tubular fluid takes place in the proximal tubule in the cortex. The thick ascending limb of the loop of Henlé is a diluting segment in which sodium chloride is avidly recovered but water does not follow. All the distal nephron can be regarded as a functional whole. It is derived from the original ureteric bud. It is responsive to hormones that regulate volume osmolality and potassium concentrate. Note that the junction between the diluting and concentrating segments meets at the juxtaglomerular apparatus of the self-same nephron providing a point at which tubular performance regulates the rate of glomerular filtration.

volume a day in a child, or in an adult 180 L/d). However very little protein traverses the filtration barrier. The glomerular filtration barrier (GFB) consists of three layers: the capillary endothelial cell, the glomerular basement membrane and adjacent to the urinary space the podocyte (Fig. 18.2). The negatively charged 50 kDa protein *albumin* is one of the first proteins to leak into the urine when the glomerular filtration barrier breaks down and is used as a marker in glomerular disease. In recent years the importance of the podocyte in the prevention of proteinuria has become obvious, as at least six different inherited human forms of nephrotic syndromes have been described, all of which have genetic mutations of genes coding for proteins expressed almost exclusively in the podocyte in the kidney (see Nephrotic syndrome section and Table 18.14).

Filtration across the GFB is passive and is driven by the glomerular intracapillary pressure, the work for which is generated by the left ventricle. The glomerular filtration rate (GFR) is closely regulated by adjusting intracapillary pressure through afferent and efferent arteriolar tone. Autoregulation keeps the GFR constant over a wide range of blood pressure. Superimposed on this there is also a circadian rhythm, which has an amplitude of about 25%. GFR also responds to physiological events, such as a high protein meal and pregnancy. In early infancy, the GFR, whether standardized for body surface area or for weight, is a fraction of that in older children and adults. Outside of the neonatal period it is conventional to express GFR per body surface area as this relationship holds constant from about 3 years of age until late adulthood, the normal being between 85 and 140 ml/min/1.73 m².

2. *Proximal tubule.* At least 80% of filtered salt and water is recovered in the proximal tubule in the cortex of the kidney. This requires

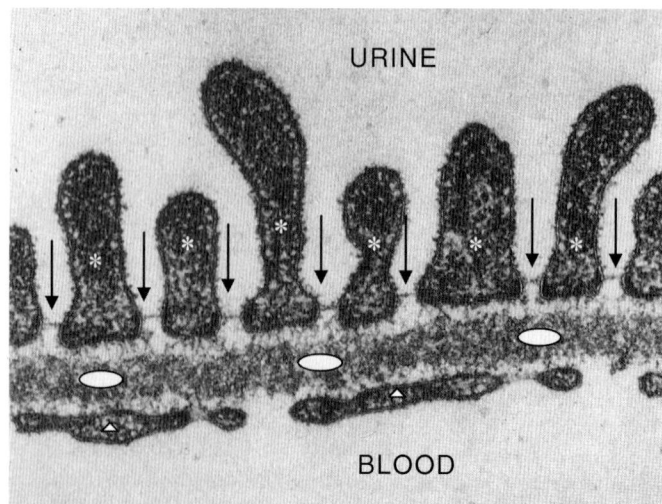

Fig. 18.2 Transmission electron microscopy through the GFB of the glomerulus. From blood to urine the three layers are fenestrated endothelial cells (△), glomerular basement membrane (◯), and the foot processes of podocytes (*). Between the foot processes are the slit diaphragms, which restrict albumin passage into the urine (arrowed).

energy expenditure through Na⁺–K⁺–ATPase, however the process is facilitated by the fact that plasma in the peritubular capillaries has a high oncotic pressure. The plasma leaving the glomerulus, which goes on to supply the peritubular capillaries, is hyperoncotic and contributes an additional driving force for water reabsorption. The active export of sodium from the basolateral surface of the proximal tubular cells by Na⁺–K⁺–ATPase creates an ionic and sodium gradient across the epithelium. This gradient is responsible for the co-transport systems, which recover glucose, phosphate and amino acids. Hydrogen ion secretion by the proximal epithelium is essential for the recovery of filtered bicarbonate. In the presence of apical carbonic anhydrase, H^+ and HCO_3^- combine to form carbonic acid. This dissociates to carbon dioxide, which can readily enter the cell and is converted back to bicarbonate. The essential luminal hydrogen ion secretion, which permits this process, also depends on the sodium gradient. Failure of the sodium gradient for any reason gives rise to the Fanconi syndrome of impaired proximal tubular reabsorption of bicarbonate, glucose, phosphate and amino acids (see Fanconi syndrome).

3. **Loop of Henlé.** In the thick ascending limb of the loop of Henlé sodium is actively pumped into the renal interstitium. However, owing to the waterproofing effect of Tamm–Horsfall protein, uniquely secreted into the lumen of this part of the nephron, water cannot follow. Nascent urine flowing along this section of the nephron therefore becomes increasingly dilute, achieving an osmolality of < 80 mOsm/kg. Meanwhile the renal interstitium becomes hyperosmolar, reaching 1400 mOsm/kg in the renal papillae, the deepest part of the medulla. This is important for water resorption from the collecting ducts.

An important anatomical feature is that at the end of the diluting section, the nephron is reflected back to pass by the hilum of its own glomerulus. Here the specialized tubular cells of the macula densa relate intimately with the juxtaglomerular apparatus and both the afferent and efferent arterioles. At this site tubular performance is policed, and filtration regulated by a process referred to as tubuloglomerular feedback. If there is a major failure of tubular reabsorption upstream of the macula densa there will be increased sodium chloride delivery to this site which in turn signals for downregulation of filtration. The kidney fails safely. It can be appreciated that the low GFR observed in infancy is an appropriate response to the smaller capacity for salt and water recovery by the relatively short proximal tubules. Newborns are much more dependent on the distal nephron for electrolyte reabsorption. This is one of the reasons why mineralocorticoid deficiency has such profound effects in the newborn compared to older subjects.

4. **Distal convoluted tubule.** This region of the nephron is responsible for fine tuning the acid–base regulation of the body and also for further reabsorption and secretion of salts. The distal convoluted tubule (DCT) is found beyond the macula densa the distal nephron, and is derived originally from the ureteric bud. Three cell types are particularly worthy of review in this region as their transport systems have important homeostatic roles in salt and acid–base regulation. The first transport system is located in the principal cell of the DCT. This cell regulates potassium secretion into, and sodium resorption from the urine. For potassium this is the principal route of excretion into the urine, as the potassium freely filtered through the glomerulus is re-absorbed (predominantly in the proximal tubule) prior to reaching the DCT. This transport system is dependent on the hormone aldosterone and on the delivery of sodium to the lumen of the distal convoluted tubule to be exchanged with potassium. A number of channels on the apical (urine) and basal (blood) side of the principal cell regulate the movement of potassium out of, and sodium into, the cell. The epithelial sodium channels (EnaC) are located on the apical aspect of the cell. EnaC are the rate-limiting step for sodium recovery and are synthesized in response to aldosterone. The second important cell is the intercalated cell. This regulates the secretion of hydrogen ions into the urine in exchange for potassium.

In conditions of decreased aldosterone production (e.g. congenital adrenal hyperplasia due to 21 hydroxylase deficiency) or end organ resistance (pseudohypoaldosteronism) there is reduced secretion of potassium into the tubular lumen of the DCT at the principal cells, which then results in less potassium to exchange with hydogen ions in the intercalated cells. The net end result is decreased excretion of potassium and hydrogen ions from the body (hyperkalemic metabolic acidosis). The combined effect of both cells is shown pictorially in Figure 18.3. The final cell type worthy of note is the sodium chloride co-transporter (NCCL) cell which contains the Na–Cl cotransporter channel. At this channel sodium and chloride are resorbed from the tubular fluid (Fig. 18.4). It is here that the thiazide diuretics exert their action by inhibiting this channel. Furthermore this channel is mutated in the hypokalemic metabolic alkalotic condition known as Gitelman syndrome. This cell also has an important role in the resorption of calcium from the urine.

Healthy children exposed to salt restriction can almost fully recover sodium in the nephron, with less than 1% of the sodium filtered at the glomerulus being excreted in the urine (fractional sodium excretion). However, newborns commonly have a fractional excretion of 1%, and in preterm infants as much as 5% of the filtered sodium load. Aldosterone is stimulated not only by the renin–angiotensin system but also directly by the plasma potassium concentration, a feature which assists in excretion of a potassium load.

5. **Collecting ducts.** Collecting ducts are embryologically derived from the ureteric bud. They are responsible for the resorption of water

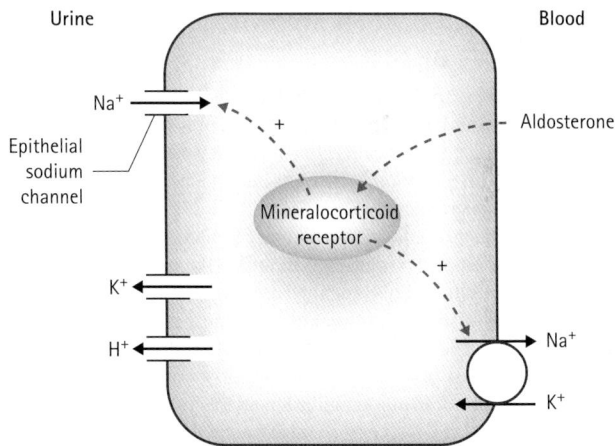

Fig. 18.3 Simplified diagram illustrating the important physiological effects of the principal and intercalated cells of the kidney.

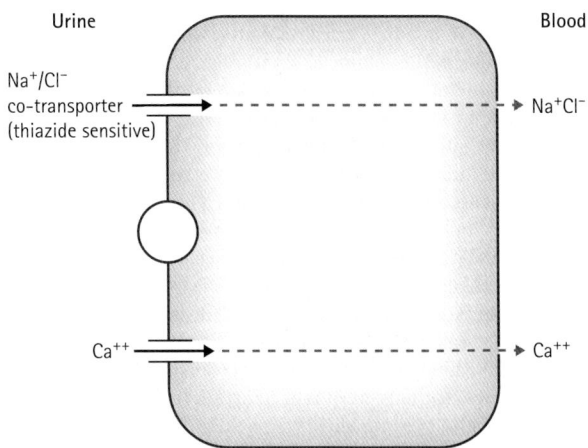

Fig. 18.4 Simplified diagram illustrating the physiologically important ion channels in the NCCT cells of the kidney.

through the action of vasopressin (also known as anti-diuretic hormone [ADH]) on water-permeable channels called aquaporins. Aquaporins (particularly aquoporin 2) are able to rapidly move from intracytoplasmic vesicles into the plasma membrane of the collecting ducts in response to vasopressin. After this occurs, water moves down an osmotic gradient from the dilute urine arriving in the distal nephron to the hyperosmolar medullary interstitium surrounding the collecting ducts, which has been generated by the loop of Henlé. The maximum urine concentration capacity thus depends on the presence of vasopressin, the integrity of vasopressin-2 receptor and aquaporin assembly, as well as a high medullary interstitial solute (sodium and urea). In breast-fed infants, whose dietary protein is efficiently used for anabolism, there is proportionately less for urea generation. Thus the maximal medullary concentration and urine concentration capacity is reduced. In health, and with adequate protein intake, children over 6 months of age can generate urine concentration > 870 mOsm/kg and figures approaching this can be achieved from the early weeks of life.

At least 80% of the filtered salt and water is recovered in the proximal tubule.

Over 6 months of age urine concentrations of > 800 mosmol/kg can be generated and this concentration would be the end point in a water deprivation test for diabetes insipidus.

Predicted GFR ml/min/1.73m² = 40 × ht(cm)/plasma creatinine µmol/L (Schwartz formula).

ASSESSMENT OF RENAL FUNCTION

MEASUREMENT OF GFR

It is helpful to measure the GFR in children as it is predictive of renal damage and informative of when renal support may be necessary. A GFR of < 60 ml/L.73 m²/min indicates chronic kidney disease (CKD) and the need for medical intervention to prevent metabolic bone disease, acidosis, anemia and hypertension. When the GFR is less than 15 ml/1.73 m²/min pharmacological medical management is often inadequate and the child needs renal support by dialysis (hemodialysis or peritoneal dialysis) or renal transplantation. This is defined as end stage renal failure.

Unfortunately there are no easy and accurate methods of measuring the GFR in a child. The ideal filtration marker is a substance that is freely filtered by the glomerulus and then not reabsorbed or secreted along the nephron. A time-honored marker is inulin, an inert sugar with a molecular weight of 5500 Da which can be measured with accuracy in plasma and urine. After an i.v. loading dose, an infusion is maintained to provide a constant plasma concentration of inulin (P). Then either the mass of inulin excreted over a fixed time (urine volume × urine concentration, UV), or, assuming a steady state the dose of inulin infused must be known, which should be the same. The theoretical volume of plasma that contains the mass of inulin excreted per minute using the formula: (UV)/P can then be deduced. The volume of plasma cleared of its inulin can then be regarded as the net volume of water that has been filtered; the glomerular filtration rate. It is convention to express this rate per 1.73 m², the average body surface area of an adult man. This allows comparison of rate between individuals of different stature and holds true down to 3 years of age. Other methods that can be used include the use of exogenous markers including Chromium-51 Ethylenediamine tetra-acetic acid (EDTA), diethylene triamine penta-acetic acid (DTPA) and iohexol.

In clinical practice, the precision of inulin clearance methods are seldom required and such tests are best reserved for specialist departments. The same can be said for slope clearance methods, although they have the important advantage that timed urine collections are not required. In slope clearance methods, a bolus of a marker (inulin, ⁵¹Cr edetic acid, or ⁹⁹ᵐTc DTPA) is injected rapidly into a vein. Following this there is a complex distribution into the extracellular fluid space, as well as clearance from the circulation by glomerular filtration. After approximately 1h, the plasma concentration falls exponentially. Two or more plasma samples are then taken over the next few hours and from the slope of the declining concentration the following can be estimated: the theoretical volume of distribution at the moment of injection and the half-time when 50% of the marker has been cleared. From this information, GFR can be estimated. Precision of this method is excellent except at very high filtration rates.

Endogenous creatinine is a useful, although imperfect, marker with which to measure clearance. Formal creatinine clearance studies relying on timed urine samples have poor precision, probably because children are unable to void to completion on demand. There is *no* place for such tests in routine pediatric practice. More accurate, reproducible and user friendly is the interpretation of plasma creatinine in relation to a child's height. In the steady state creatinine excretion (UV creatinine) is matched by creatinine synthesis in muscle and is thus related in turn to muscle mass and body weight. Body weight and height also feature in the calculation of surface area in the denominator of the GFR expression. Although the logic is tortuous this conveniently resolves to the formula which is known as the Schwartz equation:

$$\text{GFR/body surface area} = (\text{body height/plasma creatinine}) \times \text{constant (40)}$$

Much hinges on the accuracy of plasma creatinine measurement, especially at the low concentrations of normal range. New automated methods overcome errors from drugs or non-creatinine chromogens. Using these methods, and with the child's height in cm and plasma creatinine expressed in µmol/L, the constant in the above equation is approximately 40. The formula performs well when used sequentially to follow GFR in an individual. Recently there has been interest in the use of serum cystatin A as a marker of GFR. This is a small molecule (molecular weight 13 KD) which is synthesized in a less variable manner in the body, and is less dependent on the height or sex of the child, compared with creatinine. It is freely filtered by the glomerulus and then metabolized by the tubules, with very little escaping in the urine. A number of groups have demonstrated that estimation of a child's GFR can be improved by measuring cystatin A on its own or in combination with the serum creatinine.[1]

Given that tubular performance upstream of the macula densa governs filtration rate by tubular glomerular feedback mechanisms, clinicians are able to use estimates of GFR as a guide to whole kidney performance. It is not surprising that some of the most abrupt and severe reductions of GFR are caused by interstitial or tubular injury rather than isolated glomerulonephritis. The corollary of this is that extensive glomerular destruction may occur with little, if any, change in plasma creatinine. In a disorder, which gives a progressive loss of nephrons over time, surviving nephrons will exhibit hyperfiltration. Thus considerable nephron loss has to occur before there is any downward trend in GFR; renal impairment is a late indicator. It is helpful to correlate impaired GFR with kidney size as determined, for example, by ultrasound. If kidney size is normal, or perhaps increased, while GFR is impaired, it is likely that the nephron population is intact but parenchymal injury has induced a shutdown of filtration. The causes may be inflammatory, drug induced, metabolic as in hypoxia or recent ischemia, or secondary to malignant infiltration. By contrast, if both kidneys are small it is likely that the nephron population is reduced because of some previous destructive process. Small echobright kidneys with normal contours might suggest a previous glomerulonephritis. Small kidneys with an irregular outline are seen following the coarse scarring of pyelonephritis or secondary to renal dysplasia.

PROXIMAL TUBULAR FUNCTION

Glucose is not normally detected by conventional glucose oxidase strip reagent until the plasma glucose concentration exceeds 10 mmol/L, the renal threshold for glucose. Glycosuria occurring at a lower threshold may indicate an isolated transport defect, idiopathic renal glycosuria. If this occurs in conjunction with other markers of proximal tubular dysfunction it implies either renoparenchymal injury, chronic renal failure or the Fanconi syndrome.

Amino acids are readily filtered in the glomerulus and extensively reabsorbed in the proximal tubule by five separate cotransport systems:

1. basic amino acids and cystine;
2. glutamic and aspartic acids;
3. neutral amino acids;
4. imino acids;
5. glycine.

At very high plasma concentrations an amino acid may overspill into the urine. With normal plasma concentrations, newborns frequently have mild generalized aminoaciduria as a transient event. Otherwise, generalized aminoaciduria with normal plasma concentrations indicates tubulopathy in exactly the same way as glycosuria (above). Specific patterns of aminoaciduria imply isolated transport defects, e.g. cystinuria.

Phosphate is extensively recovered in the proximal tubule. However, the amount of phosphate filtered is close to the maximum rate of recovery, so that small changes in recovery rate govern plasma phosphate concentrations. Under normal conditions phosphate reabsorption will exceed 80% and the fractional excretion will therefore be less than 20% of filtered load. The fractional excretion can be calculated easily for any compound freely filtered at the glomerulus by comparing its clearance with that of creatinine:

$$\text{Fractional excretion of x (\%)} = (\text{urine x/plasma x}) \div (\text{urine creatinine/plasma creatinine}) \times 100$$

Calcium is partly bound to protein and only the ionized fraction, about 50% of the total, is available for filtration. In the proximal tubule calcium reabsorption is proportionate to salt and water reabsorption. Thereafter there is both passive and active reabsorption in the loop of Henlé. Ten percent of the filtered calcium then reaches the distal nephron and of this two thirds will be reabsorbed. Hypercalciuria can be readily diagnosed by urine calcium/creatinine ratio. The 95th centile for children is given below:

Age range	Urine calcium/creatinine (molar)
0–6 months	< 2.0 mmol/mmol
7–18 months	< 1.4 mmol/mmol
1½ > –6 years	<0.78 mmol/mmol
7 years–adult	0.56 mmol/mmol

TESTS OF URINE CONCENTRATION CAPACITY

Although the ability to excrete a water load can be tested, it has little clinical relevance. Impairment of water excretion occurs in the syndrome of inappropriate antidiuretic hormone (ADH) secretion and an extremely rare familial condition that mimics it in which ADH is not the cause. These conditions are suggested by a low plasma sodium concentration in the absence of dehydration.

Tests of urine concentration capacity, by contrast, are important. A simple screening test is to measure the urine osmolality on the first urine sample voided in the morning after fluids are restricted at bedtime. A urine osmolality value of 600 mosmol/kg is generally taken as excluding significant impairment of urinary concentration. However, in a study in 318 apparently healthy children with a median age of 9.8 years the median osmolality was 845 mOsm/kg (range 275–1344). Only 82% of males and 75% of females had an osmolality of 600 mosmol or more.[2]

If the diagnosis of diabetes insipidus is entertained, a water deprivation test should only be undertaken in hospital with close observation of hydrational status. The end point is either a urine concentration capacity > 800 mosmol/kg or a 3% body weight loss, by which time the plasma osmolality should be rising and in excess of 295 mOsm/kg. If the latter, the final urine osmolality would be accepted as the concentration capacity. In fully expressed diabetes insipidus a urine osmolality will remain lower than that of plasma. As well as the obvious risks, young children find water deprivation disagreeable. A screening test for the ability to concentrate urine is to administer DDAVP 20 μg nasally (10 μg for infants) in the normally hydrated state. At 1 h children are asked to void and that urine sample is discarded. Between 1 and 5 h after DDAVP normal children will produce a urine osmolality in excess of 800 mOsm/kg (infants <600 mosml/kg). Patients with pituitary diabetes insipidus will respond to this test either normally or they will achieve osmolalities close to normal. Failure to respond implies either nephrogenic diabetes insipidus, in which case the urine osmolality will be below that of plasma, or chronic renoparenchymal disease, where the urine osmolality will be similar to plasma concentrations. Normality and fully expressed diabetes insipidus are easy to distinguish. Problems arise when the urine osmolality falls between 300 and 870 mOsm/kg. Often this is because the water deprivation study has not been conducted rigorously. Also habitual water drinkers, especially those with poor dietary protein intake, have a reduced medullary solute concentration and underachieve for this reason. Reductions in maximal urine concentration capacity may be seen in any renoparenchymal disorder, including recent upper urinary tract infection. As chronic renal failure progresses, concentrating and diluting capacity is lost and urine osmolality approaches that of plasma.

TESTS OF RENAL TUBULAR ACIDOSIS

The kidney is responsible for the excretion of a small proportion of the total acid production of the body, this being those acids which cannot be metabolized to carbon dioxide and water and eliminated by respiration. Thus in severe renal failure patients develop a moderate acidosis with an *increased* anion gap. The anion gap is a measurement of the interval between the sum of the 'routinely' measured cations minus the 'routinely' measured anions in the blood, i.e. $(Na+K) - (Cl + HCO_3)$. The acidosis of chronic renal failure is readily corrected by 1–2 mmol/kg/d of administered bicarbonate. Renal tubular acidosis describes the hyperchloremic acidemia with a *normal* anion gap, $(Na + K) - (Cl + HCO_3) = < 20$ mmol/L, which occurs with normal glomerular function. There is either a failure to recover filtered bicarbonate, an inability to secrete hydrogen ion, or both.

In the proximal tubule H^+ is buffered by bicarbonate and leads to net bicarbonate recovery via the formation of carbon dioxide. Less than 10% of the filtered bicarbonate is presented to the distal nephron. In the distal nephron, where luminal bicarbonate is at a low concentration, two other buffering systems are proportionately more important. One is the tubular secretion of ammonia (NH_3) generated by the deamination of glutamine. In the presence of H^+ an ammonium (NH_4^+) ion forms which is unable to diffuse back across the tubular epithelium. The second is the conversion of filtered alkaline phosphate HPO_4^{2-} to acid phosphate $H_2PO_4^-$. These buffers allow the urine to 'carry' more hydrogen ions. In health, the actual H^+ gradient becomes apparent in that the urine can be made acid with a pH as low as 4.5.

To test the maximum H^+ gradient delivered by the distal nephron it may be necessary to induce a metabolic acidemia by administration of ammonium chloride enterically, although this is rarely clinically required. In distal renal tubular acidosis (*type 1 RTA*) urine pH remains above 6.5 even if the plasma bicarbonate is reduced to < 22 mmol/L. This test is seldom required as type 1 RTA patients typically present with sufficient systemic acidosis to observe the inappropriately alkaline urine. As a general rule if the urine pH < 5.5 when the serum bicarbonate is < 16 mmol this excludes a distal renal tubular acidosis as the kidney is able to appropriately acidify the urine in response to systemic acidosis. Moreover, correction of acidosis occurs at modest doses of sodium bicarbonate such as 3–5 mmol/kg body weight per day.

90% of bicarbonate is recovered in the proximal tubule and the remainder distally, so that the threshold at which bicarbonate normally starts to appear in the urine is a plasma concentration of 25–26 mmol/L. In infants this threshold is rather lower at approximately 22 mmol/L. In patients presenting with hyperchloremic acidosis in whom proximal renal tubular acidosis is suspected, sodium bicarbonate is infused intravenously to lift the plasma concentration of bicarbonate. The bicarbonate concentrations in paired plasma and urine samples are plotted, thus determining the renal threshold. Note that while the plasma bicarbonate concentration is below the threshold for bicarbonate recovery it is possible for normal distal mechanisms of urinary acidification to produce an acid urine. A simple clue to proximal renal tubular acidosis is the very large requirement for replacement bicarbonate to improve the acidemia. Often this amounts to more than 10 mmol/kg/d which is quite unlike that required to control the acidemia of chronic renal failure or distal (type 1) renal tubular acidosis.

RENAL TUBULAR DISORDERS

Defects in renal tubular transport may result in marked derangements in electrolyte and mineral homeostasis with significant morbidity. Within the past decade advances in understanding of the molecular genetics and biology of a number of inherited renal tubular disorders have provided exciting new insights into the function of specific transport proteins and the physiology of renal tubular handling of solutes.[3]

FANCONI SYNDROME

The Fanconi syndrome consists of a generalized failure of proximal tubular reabsorption. This leads to glycosuria, phosphaturia, calciuria, bicarbonaturia and generalized hyperaminoaciduria. Proximal sodium and potassium reabsorption also fails and the distal nephron, driven by aldosterone, attempts to recover sodium, but only at the expense of potassium and hydrogen ion secretion, potentiating severe hypokalemia. The salt and water wasting gives rise to polyuria, polydipsia and failure to thrive. Usually children exhibit a metabolic acidosis secondary to the urinary loss of bicarbonate (type 2 renal tubular acidosis). However, distal hydrogen ion secretion in most forms of Fanconi syndrome is normal, and during periods of hypovolemia and reduced glomerular filtration, the pH of urine may actually fall below 5.5. In states of extreme dehydration hypokalemic alkalosis may be seen. At other times hypokalemia with *acidosis* is a strong pointer to a proximal tubular lesion. The hypokalemia itself may aggravate the proximal tubular nephropathy as well as giving rise to muscle weakness, growth retardation and constipation. The glycosuria and aminoaciduria, in themselves have little in the way of clinical sequelae. The hypercalciuria is not associated with urinary stone formation, probably because of the very high urine flow rate. Plasma calcium concentrations tend to be normal. By contrast hypophosphatemia is the principal cause of the osteopenia and rickets of the Fanconi syndrome.

In clinical practice Fanconi syndrome is rare. The causes are legion and include primary disorders, sometimes familial with a variety of inherited patterns. Some of these are likely to prove to be secondary to respiratory chain defects and one type has been described in which the brush border of the proximal tubular cell is absent. The condition can arise secondarily due to intoxication by heavy metals or drugs and in relation to other inborn errors of metabolism (see Table 18.2). However, by far the commonest single cause of the Fanconi syndrome is *nephropathic cystinosis* and this condition is therefore dealt with in more detail.

Table 18.2   Associations with Fanconi syndrome

Inborn errors of metabolism
Nephropathic cystinosis
Lowe syndrome (oculocerebrorenal dystrophy)
Glycogen storage
Galactosemia
Fructose intolerance
Tyrosinemia type 1
Wilson disease (hepatolenticular dystrophy)

Tubulotoxic events
Drugs, e.g. tetracycline, ifosfamide
Heavy metals, e.g. lead, cadmium, uranium, mercury, thallium
Maleic acid (experimental)

Cystinosis (OMIM #219800)

Cystinosis[4] is a rare metabolic disorder inherited as an autosomal recessive trait. The gene responsible for the condition lies on chromosome 17p, and codes for cystinosin, a lysosomal transmembrane protein essential for the transport of cystine. In the disorder cystine is stored intracellularly in lysosomes and there is a defect in the ability to transport cystine back into the cytoplasm. How this disrupts tubular function is unknown at present. Various patterns of cystinosis have been described. In the benign adult form cystine crystals are deposited only in the cornea, bone marrow and leukocytes; there appears to be no renal involvement. A juvenile form of the disorder includes a slowly progressive nephropathy, which becomes manifest in the second decade of life. By contrast, infantile nephropathic cystinosis is the most severe form. These infants appear normal at birth and the disorder becomes apparent at around 6 months of age with failure to thrive, polyuria, polydipsia, episodes of dehydration and unexplained fever. Rickets occurs early.

Over the first few years the glomerular filtration rate remains normal, and it is during this early stage that abrupt episodes of dehydration and electrolyte disturbance precipitated by intercurrent infective illnesses can prove fatal. The GFR declines with time so that end-stage renal failure is reached in untreated patients within 10 years of diagnosis. There is profound growth retardation and photophobia is a universal complaint due to cystine deposition in the eye. In later childhood, children have biochemical evidence of hypothyroidism and hypercholesterolemia.

The diagnosis is confirmed by the positive identification of cystine deposition within cells. In the first months of life the kidneys look histologically normal, but later the birefringent crystals of cystine can be seen in the interstitial tissue between tubules. Interstitial fibrosis then occurs so that the kidneys in time become small and contracted. Crystals can be seen in the cornea by slit lamp examination of the eye. The cystine concentration of leukocytes can be measured, and this test can be applied shortly after birth. Antenatal diagnosis is also possible, cystine measurements being made on fibroblasts obtained from amniotic fluid or chorionic villus sampling. It may also be diagnosed by genetic testing in informative families.

Cystinosis patients are difficult to manage and require careful electrolyte supplementation. Many need tube feeding to ensure an adequate salt, water and calorific intake.[5] Attempts to reduce the glomerular filtration rate, and thus the electrolyte loss, using indomethacin are advocated. Cysteamine treatment can mobilize intralysosomal cystine and deplete cystine in cells. Cysteamine has a foul taste and compliance with this therapy is often poor. However, where cysteamine therapy or phosphocysteamine therapy has been given early with rigid compliance, children have retained kidney function longer than expected.

Once end-stage renal failure is reached, renal transplantation is an effective treatment. The transplant may become colonized by host cells, which will store cystine, but the tubular cells of the donor do not have the underlying biochemical defect and long-term kidney function is satisfactory. Concern is raised, however, that long-term survivors risk previously unrecognized complications such as corneal degeneration, diabetes mellitus, and cerebral atrophy.

Renal tubular disorders are rare but important causes of failure to thrive and electrolyte disturbances.

Cystinosis is the commonest cause of a Fanconi syndrome.

Nephrocalcinosis is an early complication of type 1 renal tubular acidosis but does not occur in type 2 proximal RTA.

RENAL TUBULAR ACIDOSIS

Renal tubular acidosis refers to conditions in which there are defects in the tubular reabsorption of bicarbonate, the excretion of hydrogen ion or both. They can be primary disorders, or secondary to a wide range of pathogenic insults to the tubular cells. Four types are described (Table 18.3).

Table 18.3 Classification of renal tubular acidosis (RTA)

Type 1 – Distal RTA
Primary
— sporadic, familial (autosomal dominant)
— transient infantile

Secondary
— interstitial nephritis, hypergammaglobulinemia, transplant rejection
— hypercalciuria, nephrocalcinosis
— drugs, lithium, amphotericin

Type 2 – Proximal RTA
Primary
Secondary – Fanconi syndrome

Type 3 – Mixed proximal and distal RTA

Type 4 – Hyperkalemic RTA
Hypoaldosteronism, Addison disease, congenital adrenal hyperplasia
Pseudohypoaldosteronism
Distal tubular dysfunction, e.g. obstructive uropathy
Hyperreninemia, hypoaldosteronism in chronic renal failure
Angiotensin-converting enzyme inhibitors
Early childhood hyperkalemia RTA (transient)

Type 1 renal tubular acidosis

Permanent distal renal tubular acidosis (*type 1 RTA*) is more often a sporadic disease, although families with autosomal dominant and recessive inheritance are described. The nature of the cellular defect is known in some cases. For example, an autosomal recessive form with accompanying sensorineural deafness is caused by a mutation in the beta subunit of H^+-ATPase located in the apical membrane of intercalated cells of the distal nephron.[5] A mutation of a 116 kDa subunit of H^+-ATPase is found in autosomal recessive type 1 RTA without hearing loss.[6] The resulting functional defect prevents active hydrogen ion secretion. Defects in anion exchange mechanisms have been found in autosomal dominant forms of type 1 RTA.[7] Infants present with growth retardation, vomiting, polydipsia, constipation and dehydration, although these symptoms may be mild and in sporadic or autosomal dominant cases the diagnosis is often not made until the child is more than 2 years of age. Osteomalacia and rickets do not occur, with the exception of the autosomal recessive form with normal hearing, but nephrocalcinosis is an early complication secondary to the accompanying hypercalciuria and hypocitraturia. Treatment demands life-long therapy with bicarbonate or citrate. While the acidosis is readily correctable with modest doses of bicarbonate, 3–5 mmol/kg body weight per day, higher doses of 5–7 mmol/kg and good compliance with therapy is essential if progressive nephrocalcinosis is to be avoided. The long-term stability of renal function depends on control of nephrocalcinosis.

Type 2 renal tubular acidosis

Proximal renal tubular acidosis (*type 2 RTA*) occurs because of failed bicarbonate reabsorption in the nephron. As a primary disorder both autosomal recessive and autosomal dominant inheritance patterns have been described. The molecular mechanisms are less well understood than in type 1 RTA, but abnormalities in the Na/HCO_3 cotransporter have been found in a case with ocular lesions. A transient form of type 2 RTA occurs in infants. In any child suspected of having type 2 RTA it is important to look for other evidence of proximal tubular dysfunction as bicarbonate wasting occurs as part of the Fanconi syndrome. Patients with type 2 RTA present with growth retardation and vomiting. Because they have normal urine acidification mechanisms in the distal nephron nephrocalcinosis does not occur. The low bicarbonate threshold means that the more the plasma concentration is increased therapeutically, the greater the urine loss. Thus massive bicarbonate replacement is needed to control the acidemia, often more than 10–15 mmol of bicarbonate/kg body weight/d.

Type 3 renal tubular acidosis

The term *type 3 RTA* is used to describe a mixed picture of both proximal and tubular defects and can occur with almost any renoparenchymal injury.

Type 4 renal tubular acidosis

Type 4 RTA is probably the most common subtype in children. In this there is hyperchloremic acidosis with hyperkalemia and usually an acid urine during acidosis. The pathogenesis is linked to $H^+/K^+/Na^+$ exchange in the collecting duct. It is therefore seen in states of mineralocorticoid deficiency such as congenital adrenal hyperplasia and Addison disease. Similarly it is seen in pseudohypoaldosteronism in which there is end organ unresponsiveness to aldosterone, for example with mutations causing loss of function of the epithelial sodium channel, or occasionally in conditions where there is direct damage to the renal medulla as in obstructive uropathy. In all these cases there is accompanying salt wasting which is most evident in the very young child who relies heavily on the distal nephron for physiological sodium reabsorption. Type 4 RTA can also occur with hyporeninism and hypoaldosteronism in chronic renal failure patients who are not volume depleted. An isolated early childhood form of type 4 RTA has been described. This occurs without salt wasting and the condition resolves by 5 years of age. Both sexes are affected and the disorder appears in siblings. High-dose alkaline therapy may be required (up to 20 mmol/kg/d), but this dose independently corrects the hyperkalemia. Nephrocalcinosis does not occur and the underlying nature of the defect is not known.

HYPOKALEMIC ALKALOSIS

Severe potassium chloride wasting can occur from either the gastrointestinal tract or from the kidney. Examples of the first include pyloric stenosis, laxative abuse or familial chloride diarrhea. In these situations the kidney will initially respond appropriately by avid electrolyte conservation and a reduction in urine output. However, if potassium deficiency is severe enough, proximal tubular cells become vacuolated and lose their ability to reabsorb salt and water. In this situation, there can be an additional proximal tubular defect causing inappropriate salt and water loss – hypokalemic nephropathy.

Renal potassium wasting occurs in covert diuretic abuse, notably with furosemide (frusemide), or as a group of primary disorders generally referred to as *Bartter syndrome*. The hypokalemic alkalosis of all of the above disorders is accompanied by various degrees of *extracellular fluid volume depletion*. It is this feature that distinguishes them from the hypokalemia and alkalosis of actual or apparent mineralocorticoid excess, in which there is enhanced sodium and water reabsorption in the distal nephron giving rise to *extracellular sodium expansion* and hypertension (see later).

Bartter syndrome

Bartter syndrome is a rare disorder, either familial or sporadic, which can affect both children and adults. The pathogenesis is best explained by a failure of chloride reabsorption in the thick ascending limb of the loop of Henlé, thus resembling the pharmacological effect of furosemide (frusemide). Three subtypes have been described with loss of function mutations in the furosemide (frusemide)-sensitive Na–K–2Cl cotransporter (type 1) (OMIM #601678), the potassium channel regulator ROMK (type 2) (OMIM #241200) or the basolateral chloride channel CLCNKB (type 3) (OMIM #607364). However there are cases where the molecular abnormality has not been found. As a secondary response to salt wasting, there is activation of the renin–angiotensin–aldosterone pathway in an attempt to recover sodium chloride in the distal nephron. This is achieved at the expense of increased potassium and hydrogen ion secretion, which largely explains the hypokalemic alkalosis.

Children present with failure to thrive, hypotonia, lethargy, poor feeding, polydipsia and polyuria. There is a wide spectrum of disease expression with a severe form presenting in the neonatal period. Such infants are usually born prematurely after a pregnancy complicated by polyhydramnios. In early life they may become so volume depleted as to experience secondary oliguric renal failure, during which time the hypokalemic alkalosis is masked. Dehydration also gives rise to episodes of fever and developmental delay. In this group, there is hypercalciuria and bone demineralization, which may be secondary to the increased production of prostaglandins PGE$_2$ and PGI$_2$, which are found in this and other forms of Bartter syndrome. Nephrocalcinosis is a serious and early complication except in type 3. The neonatal form of Bartter syndrome, first described by Fanconi in 1971, has at times been inappropriately titled 'calcium losing tubulopathy', or 'primary hyperprostaglandin E syndrome'.

Management consists of potassium, sodium and chloride replacement. Prostaglandin inhibitors such as indometacin 3 mg/kg daily in divided dose are indicated, and angiotensin-converting enzyme inhibitors such as captopril may give additional control.

Bartter syndrome presenting in older children may run a relatively mild course without hypercalciuria or nephrocalcinosis. Simple potassium supplementation may be all that is required.

Gitelman syndrome
Gitelman syndrome (OMIM #263800) is a distinct autosomal recessive disorder in which there is renal loss of both potassium and magnesium so that hypokalemia and hypomagnesemia are combined with metabolic alkalosis and hypocalciuria. If Bartter syndrome is analogous to the effects of furosemide (frusemide), Gitelman syndrome mimics the effects of thiazide diuretics, and mutations have been confirmed in the thiazide sensitive cotransporter gene (NCCT). These patients present with muscle weakness, particularly after exercise. Many patients come to medical attention incidentally when they are investigated for intercurrent illnesses. The salt wasting is mild in comparison to Bartter syndrome and growth and renal function are unaffected. Potassium and/or magnesium supplements help to ameliorate symptoms.

Hypokalemic alkalosis with extracellular sodium expansion
Hypokalemic alkalosis, with volume expansion and hypertension, can occur because of increased sodium recovery by the epithelial sodium channel with consequent secretion of potassium and hydrogen ions. An obvious cause of this is mineralocorticoid excess, as in *Conn syndrome*; vanishingly rare in childhood. However, there are other conditions with similar dynamics of increased distal sodium recovery in which plasma aldosterone concentrations are suppressed or normal. These are referred to as disorders of *apparent mineralocorticoid excess*. One of these is 11beta-hydroxysteroid dehydrogenase deficiency, a rare inherited disorder in which the conversion of cortisol to cortisone at the site of the mineralocorticoid receptor is defective. As a result, physiologically normal amounts of cortisol can directly activate the mineralocorticoid receptor in the collecting duct, thus driving distal sodium reabsorption. Children present with severe labile hypertension and failure to thrive. Hypercalciuria and nephrocalcinosis occur. It is inherited as an autosomal recessive condition. Another is *Liddle syndrome* (OMIM #177200). In this, mutations in the beta or gamma subunit of the amiloride-sensitive epithelial sodium channel give rise to a constitutive gain of function; the opposite of pseudohypoaldosteronism type 1. The syndrome is autosomal dominant and can present clinically either in childhood or adult life. Treatment of both these disorders consists of amiloride to reverse the salt and water retention. This controls blood pressure and normalizes plasma potassium.

Renal tubular hyperkalemia
This refers to the failure of the tubules to secrete potassium in conditions other than chronic renal failure. This can occur if there is a failure in the renin–angiotensin–aldosterone pathway. Examples would include treatment with angiotensin-converting enzyme inhibitors such as captopril and the failure to synthesize mineralocorticoid in the salt-losing forms of congenital adrenal hypoplasia. In these situations, there will also be reduced ability to secrete hydrogen ion resulting in type 4 renal tubular acidosis (see earlier).

Primary pseudohypoaldosteronism type I
An abnormality in the end organ receptor responsiveness to aldosterone results in primary pseudohypoaldosteronism (PHA) type 1. *Renal type 1 PHA* is inherited in an autosomal dominant fashion with variable penetrance (OMIM #177735). It is caused by abnormality of the mineralocorticoid receptor and predominantly affects the distal tubular cells of the kidney. Infants classically present with salt losing states, dehydration and failure to thrive early in life, but clinical features are variable. It is treated with sodium chloride and sodium bicarbonate supplementation normally with good effect. In severe cases dietary potassium restriction and potassium exchange resins may be necessary. Improvement in this condition commonly occurs as the child grows enabling cessation of medication as the proximal tubule matures and is able to increase its reabsorption of sodium. A much rarer form of type 1 PHA affects multiple organs (*multiple type 1 PHA*) (OMIM #264350). This is normally inherited in an autosomal recessive manner and is due to a mutation in the gene coding for the epithelial sodium channel (EnaC) resulting in the lack of its function. As this channel is widely expressed in other tissues in the body it results in a more severe phenotype of children affected. Children again present with salt losing crisis in the neonatal period but also suffer from lower respiratory tract infection which may result in confusion with cystic fibrosis. Multiple type 1 PHA is much less responsive to the supplements used in the dominant form and often requires the addition of indomethacin and thiazide diuretics. It rarely improves with age and is associated with considerable mortality.

Gordon syndrome
Pseudohypoaldosteronism type II, or 'chloride shunt' syndrome; OMIM #145260) is a rare autosomal dominant disorder of hyperkalemia, hyperchloremic metabolic acidosis, volume expansion and hypertension. Plasma renin activity and aldosterone levels are suppressed. Patients may also have hypercalciuria and a tendency to stone formation. The molecular basis of this condition has recently been unraveled. Mutations of either WNK4 kinase (17q21) or WNK1 kinase (12p)[8] result in the increased action of the Na–Cl thiazide channel which causes increased tubular resorption of sodium and chloride (with resulting volume overload). This results in less sodium delivery to the principal and intercalated cells of the distal tubule with less sodium to be exchanged with potassium and hydrogen ions. Treatment is with a thiazide diuretic.

Action of diuretics on the kidney
There are three broad mechanisms by which diuretics affect the kidney (Table 18.4). Oncotic diuretics decrease the resorption of water from the nephron and effectively 'pull' water with them. Osmotic diuretics include Mannitol and glucose. The majority of diuretics used in clinical practice prevent the resorption of sodium from the nephron, which results in increased water clearance. These diuretics effect different sodium channels in the kidney and inherited loss of function mutations in all of these channels result in tubulopathies. The final group of drugs that result in increased water clearance from the kidney effect the collecting tubules and mimic the effects of nephrogenic diabetes insipidus. Drugs that cause this include lithium and amphotericin B.

Cystinuria causes renal calculi and is associated with excess excretion of cystine, ornithine, lysine and arginine ('cola') amino acids.

Severe primary hyperoxaluria may require liver and kidney transplantation.

Nephrogenic diabetes insipidus can cause hypernatremia and mental retardation if not recognized.

HEREDITARY TUBULAR DISORDERS
Cystinuria
Cystinuria (OMIM #220100) is a complex genetic disorder involving at least three alleles governing dibasic amino acid (lysine, orthnithine, arginine) and cystine transport.[9] It is more common in Japanese and

Table 18.4 Mechanisms of action of diuretics on the kidney, and genetic diseases which physiologically affect the same region of tubule

Location in nephron	Class of diuretic or drug side-effect	Known inherited condition mimicking effect
A. Proximal tubule	Carbonic anhydrase inhibitors	Osteopetrosis
B. Loop of Henlé	Loop	Bartter syndromes
C. Distal tubule – NaCl channel	Thiazide	Gitelman syndrome
D. Distal tubule – ENaC channel	Amiloride	Liddle syndrome, Autosomal recessive pseudohypoaldosteronism type 1
E. Distal tubule – mineralocorticoid receptor	Spironolactone	Autosomal dominant pseudohypoaldosteronism type 1
F. Collecting duct	Lithium	Nephrogenic diabetes insipidus
G. Throughout the nephron (Osmotic effects)	Mannitol Glucose	Fanconi syndrome

Caucasians, with an incidence of 1:18 000 in Japan and 1:20 000 in the UK. Defects are seen in both renal tubular and intestinal epithelial transport. Nutritional disturbances probably do not arise because amino acids are absorbed from the gut as oligopeptides rather than free amino acids. Renal tubular cells demonstrate an inability to take up cystine from their brush border, but can do so from the basolateral surface. Because the excretion of cystine can exceed the amount filtered, there is evidence of net cystine secretion by the tubule.

The clinical manifestations are confined to individuals in whom the cystine concentration in urine exceeds its solubility product and leads to calculus formation. This occurs in homozygotes and in those heterozygous for the type II allele.[10] Family studies show that heterozygotes excrete different amounts of cystine depending on the allele type (see later). Two genes have been found to be mutated in this condition SLC3A1 (rBAT), which codes for the heavy subunit of the renal aminoacid transporter and is found on chromosome 2p, together with SLC7A9, which codes for the light subunit of the transporter and is found on chromosome 19. Almost all untreated homozygotes will experience calculi at some time in their lives, a quarter of them before 20 years of age. Obstruction and infection cause lasting damage to the urinary tract. Patients present with renal colic or episodes of hematuria. The stones are radiopaque because of their high sulfur content. Ultrasound is a good way of identifying calculi in both the renal collecting system and the bladder but often misses calculi in ureters. Microscopy of the urine reveals flat hexagonal birefringent crystals under polarized light, and the nitroprusside test for urinary disulfides is positive. Confirmation is by quantification of urinary cystine secretion:

Cystine excretion as urinary cystine/creatinine ratio

Normal		<100 μmol/g creatinine
Heterozygote	type I	<100 μmol/g creatinine (recessive)
	type II	>1000 μmol/g creatinine (dominant)
	type III	100–1000 μmol/g creatinine (partially dominant)
Homozygous cystinuria		>2000–5000 μmol/g creatinine

This classification is not perfect but it does give some clues to the underlying genetic defect the child has inherited. Heterozygous rBAT mutations always excrete cystine in the normal range (phenotype 1) and homozygotes excrete cystine in the range of 200–500 mmol/mmol. Heterozygous SLCA9 mutations cause the majority of partially dominant cystinuria (80%). However the genotype–phenotype association with SLCA9 mutations is not consistant with mutations in this gene also resulting in type I and type III cystine excretion in probands. A number of series have been unable to identify both of the above described gene mutations in their cystinuric patients suggesting that other cystinuria causing genes exist.

The mainstay of treatment is to keep the urine volume sufficiently high that cystine is kept below its solubility maximum of 1.25 mmol/L (300 mg/L). This necessitates fluid loading, especially at night to overcome the normal night-time antidiuresis. The solubility maximum of cystine increases to 2.0 mmol/L (500 mg/L) where the urine pH exceeds 7.5. A second line of treatment, additional to and not a substitute for the first is to prescribe bicarbonate or citrate to ensure that the early morning urine pH is alkaline.

Family members should be screened so that presymptomatic, affected members can be treated early. It is easier to prevent stone formation than to dissolve existing stones. In difficult cases with existing calculi a further increase in cystine solubility can be achieved by forming a thiol-cysteine disulfide with agents such as D-penicillamine.

Hyperoxaluria

Hyperoxaluria is a rare but important metabolic disorder to consider in a child with renal calculi or nephrocalcinosis. The majority of urine oxalate is derived from the hepatic metabolism of glyoxalate and ascorbate with a small proportion being ingested with diet. Oxalate is a metabolic end product, which is excreted via the kidneys, and its relative insolubility may lead to nephrocalcinosis or stone formation.

Enteric hyperoxaluria can occur in patients with chronic diarrhea due to short gut syndromes or other enteropathy.

Primary hyperoxaluria is a rare autosomal recessive disorder of oxalate metabolism due to a deficiency of hepatic alanine glyoxylate transferase (AGT) (type 1) (OMIM #259900) or glycerate reductase/D-glycerate dehydrogenase (type 2) (OMIM #260000). Both types lead to excessive urine oxalate excretion. In type 1 there is excess urinary glycolic acid, whereas type 2 is characterized by increased urinary L-glycerate.

Random urine samples for urine oxalate:creatinine ratio is part of the standard workup for children with renal stones but the normal ranges vary considerably with age and it is important to consult the laboratory for age-specific reference data. Normal results require measurement of 24-hour urinary oxalate and glycolate excretion and organic analysis of urine (for L-glycerate).

Treatment of hyperoxaluria includes high fluid intake, crystal inhibitors such as citrate, orthophosphate, magnesium and pyridoxine to act as a co-factor for AGT deficient type 1 patients. Dietary advice should aim to avoid high oxalate foods and beverages such as black tea or cocoa as part of a high fluid intake. Patients with obstructing stones require urgent urological assessment to avoid renal damage due to obstruction and infection.

Anyone with significant renal impairment, i.e. GFR < 75 ml/min/1.73 m^2 should undergo specialist review. Oxalosis is a term used to describe the final stage of primary hyperoxaluria when reduction of glomerular filtration rate produces systemic oxalate excretion, with crystals being deposited in bone, muscles, artery walls, eyes, skin and nerves. Isolated renal transplantation has now been replaced by combined liver and kidney transplantation with good results.[11]

Oculocerebrorenal (Lowe) syndrome

Oculocerebrorenal (Lowe) syndrome (OMIM #309000) describes a rare syndrome of mental retardation, excess aminoaciduria, cataract and glaucoma. It is transmitted as an X-linked recessive trait mapped to Xp24–24. Most carriers are normal, or at worst have early onset of cataract, but several female cases have been reported. The gene appears to code for a phosphatidyl inositol biphosphate phosphatase localized in the Golgi complex.

Clinical features

Boys present from 2 months of age with the facial features of large ears, prominent forehead, flattened nasal bridge and prominent scalp veins in a pale skin. Cataract is typical and in the early stages may only be detected by slit lamp examination. The severity of the cataract varies, as does its distribution. Buphthalmos and congenital glaucoma may be present.

Intermittent pyrexia and failure to thrive are usual, and growth retardation, osteoporosis and rickets often occur. The mental deficiency is usually severe, with loss of muscle tone, hypermobility of joints and absent or greatly diminished tendon jerks. The eyes often roll in pseudonystagmus and it is commonly noted that children press on their eyeballs with their fingers to produce visual 'hallucinations'. The EEG may show the fast 24 cycles per second general activity. The blood pressure is normal and ultrasound of the kidneys is often normal. Proteinuria occurs with complex tubular dysfunction, which may not manifest itself until the second year of life. Tubular acidosis, usually of classical 'distal type' is present and there is hyperphosphaturia with hypophosphatemia, normocalcemia and elevated levels of alkaline phosphatase.

Treatment

Treatment is supportive with adequate replacement of bicarbonate, potassium, phosphate and vitamin D metabolites. As with all rare conditions, parents may obtain benefit from contact with other families.

Hereditary hypophosphatemic rickets (vitamin D–resistant rickets)

Hypophosphatemic rickets is a rare dominantly transmitted X-linked disease, for which the affected gene (PHEX, phosphate regulating gene; OMIM #307800), has recently been identified. Hypophosphatemia is due to a urinary leak of phosphate, which is itself secondary to a defect of proximal tubular sodium/phosphate co-transport.

Clinical signs are rickets in a child, and sometimes osteomalacia or bone deformities in the adult. Hypophosphatemia is associated with hyperphosphaturia, elevated serum alkaline phosphatase but with normal plasma calcium, calcitriol and PTH levels. No other tubular defects can be found and there is never the aminoaciduria associated with nutritional rickets or Fanconi syndrome.

Treatment is with phosphate supplements which, if given on a regular basis, should improve bone mineralization and prevent bony deformities. Oral neutral phosphate (Phosphate Sandoz) should be pushed to the limit of tolerability in a dose of 50–100 mg/kg/d given as at least four, preferably five, doses. High doses produce diarrhea and compliance with the medication must be constantly encouraged. Alfacalcidol is also introduced in an initial dose of 20–40 ng/kg/d but a careful watch must be kept for hypercalcemia and hypercalciuria.[12] Hypophasphatemic rickets can also be inherited in an autosomal dominant (OMIM #193100) and recessive (OMIM 241520) manner. Interestingly these conditions can often be treated with either phosphate supplemenation (autosomal recessive) or vitamin D supplementation (autosomal dominant) alone.

Nephrogenic diabetes insipidus

Nephrogenic diabetes insipidus (NDI) is the isolated inability of the kidney to concentrate urine in response to circulating arginine vasopressin. Although acquired forms exist, the disorder mostly occurs in infants and is congenital. At a molecular level, two disease mechanisms have been found. In 90% of congenital cases NDI is an X-linked disorder so that the full expression of the disease is confined to males (OMIM #304800). Mutations can occur in the arginine vasopressin-2 receptor (AVP2R) encoded at Xq28. AVP2R is normally located in the basolateral membrane of the collecting duct epithelial cell. On recognizing AVP the receptor signals to the cell nucleus through cyclic AMP leading to

synthesis of the water channel aquaporin-2 and its insertion into the apical membrane. In this way, vasopressin regulates the ability of water to flow down the osmolar gradient from the dilute tubular fluid to the hyperoncotic medullary interstitium. Among the remaining families with congenital nephrogenic diabetes insipidus, mutations have been found in the gene coding for aquaporin-2 on 12q13 (OMIM #125800). These can be inherited in an autosomal dominant or recessive manner. It appears that the aquaporin molecule is synthesized, but not routed to its apical destination, resulting in a loss of water transport. It is possible to distinguish between these forms, in that those with an aquaporin-2 defect show a rise in urinary cyclic AMP with vasopressin stimulation, while those with the receptor defect do not.

Clinical features

The condition usually presents in infancy but a late recognition can occur. Polyuria and polydipsia are prominent features but difficult to recognize in infancy, although a preference for water rather than milk feeds may be evident. Water loss leads to recurring episodes of hypernatremic dehydration, fever, constipation and vomiting. Episodes of dehydration can seriously compromise intellectual development, and many cases exhibit growth retardation. The renal defect is permanent, but with increasing age water intake spontaneously increases to compensate for the persistent polyuria so that patients learn to avoid episodes of dehydration.

Diagnosis and differential diagnosis

Plasma sodium and chloride concentrations are increased and, when dehydration is severe, renal plasma flow falls leading to raised blood urea and serum creatinine levels. The osmolality of the urine is commonly less than 100 mOsm/kg. If a paired plasma and urine osmolality is obtained as soon as an infant presents with a dehydrational state, this is often sufficient to lead to the diagnosis. Always ensure that the kidneys are structurally normal by ultrasound. Renal dysplasia and reflux nephropathy may present with a water losing crisis in infancy. In apparently normally hydrated children fluid restriction to test renal concentrating ability must be carried out with very careful inpatient supervision, as severe dehydration may rapidly ensue. DDAVP has no effect on urine concentration and this forms the basis for the diagnosis.

Treatment

Replacement of urinary water losses, by increasing the fluid intake, is the basis of treatment. This may need to be by nasogastric tube feeding in the very young, although most infants will readily drink extra water given between milk feeds, even when appetite is poor. Paradoxically, thiazide diuretics have been shown to decrease free water clearance and urine flow rate in this condition. This action depends on the induction of a state of salt depletion, which causes an increase in proximal tubular reabsorption, and therefore diminished excretion of sodium and water to the distal nephron. The effect can be maintained by a low-salt diet, when thiazide diuretics are stopped. Unfortunately, the urine volume may decrease only by about one third. The addition of prostaglandin synthetase inhibitors such as indometacin to this treatment causes a further fall in urine volume. It does not enhance urine concentration but, by reducing GFR and enhancing tubular sodium reabsorption, restricts salt (and thus water) delivery to the collecting duct, reducing total water losses. Provided adequate supplies of water are maintained from early infancy, mental development is preserved but physical growth often remains a problem. The prognosis depends on making the diagnosis early and fastidious parental supervision of hydration.

In later childhood it is often preferable to discontinue the thiazide/indometacin therapy because it carries significant hazards, particularly peptic ulceration and haemorrhage, and interstitial renal fibrosis. Most older children adapt well to the inconvenience of polydipsia and polyuria. Therapy can be reintroduced for longer or shorter periods as needed – for example during a holiday to a hot climate where excessive thirst could be a serious problem.

CONGENITAL ABNORMALITIES OF THE URINARY TRACT

Development of the renal tract has been described in Chapter 12. The increasing use and accuracy of obstetric ultrasound has added considerably to our recognition of urinary tract abnormalities (see neonatal renal). This is a family of disorders with a diverse anatomical spectrum including kidney anomalies, pelvi-ureteric anomalies, ureterovesical junction abnormalities, duplex systems and anomalies of the bladder and urethra. These abnormalities often occur concurrently in a variable pattern. Abnormalities in the genetic mechanisms underlying renal tract development may explain how many of these arise.[13]

Some of these are obviously important to recognize, because of their potential for causing considerable renal damage, e.g. posterior urethral valves in a male infant, but others produce no symptoms in infancy or childhood and their natural history is still being defined, e.g. unilateral multicystic dysplastic kidney.

RENAL AGENESIS, ECTOPIA AND FUSION

These anomalies may occur in isolation but may also be associated with a large number of chromosomal and nonchromsomal syndromes. A careful clinical assessment should be made in all individuals with these anomalies. If there are other associated malformations an evaluation for a specific diagnosis should be made. In all cases evaluation for any other renal or urological problem should be made. This may include a renal tract ultrasound, a micturating cystogram and a MAG3 or a DMSA scan. A check of renal function is often made at the time of the isotope scan unless there is an indication to do so sooner.

RENAL AGENESIS

Bilateral renal agenesis is incompatible with prolonged life, due to the associated pulmonary hypoplasia and oligohydramnios sequence.

Unilateral renal agenesis occurs in about 0.1% of the infant population, is more common in males and has been described in association with abnormalities of the external ear on the ipsilateral side. Atresia of the corresponding ureter is frequent and supports the view that unilateral renal agenesis is commonly the result of failure of formation of the ureteric bud or its inability to stimulate differentiation of the nephrogenic mesoderm. There is now a strong suspicion that many cases of unilateral renal agenesis are due to multicystic dysplastic kidneys, which have become involuted in utero.

Ultrasound and dimercaptosuccinic acid (DMSA) scan, including views of the whole abdomen to exclude ectopic location, should be undertaken. The presence of a normal hypertrophied kidney on the contralateral side should lead to reassurance and there is no need for long-term follow-up unless there are associated abnormalities.

RENAL FUSION AND ECTOPIA

The metanephric blastema is originally sited in the pelvis and ascends to its subdiaphragmatic position during early fetal life. During the ascent, some rotation occurs, so that the renal pelvis, which originally lies anterior to the disc-shaped pelvic metanephros, comes to lie medial to the lumbar kidney. Moreover, the kidney assumes its reniform shape by virtue of its lumbar position and the rotation it undergoes. An ectopic non-ascended kidney is therefore likely to be non-reniform in shape, being usually discoid, and to have a pelvis and ureter arising anteriorly. The ureter may have a normal vesical opening but may also open in an ectopic position in the bladder, bladder neck, urethra or vaginal vault. The blood supply is derived from nearby arteries such as the common iliac. A frequent site for the ectopic kidney is in the pelvis but it may be higher up the posterior abdominal wall or crossed to the opposite side. Such 'crossed' ectopia is more often than not fused with the normal kidney – 'crossed fused ectopia'. Fusion of normally placed kidneys may also occur – commonly

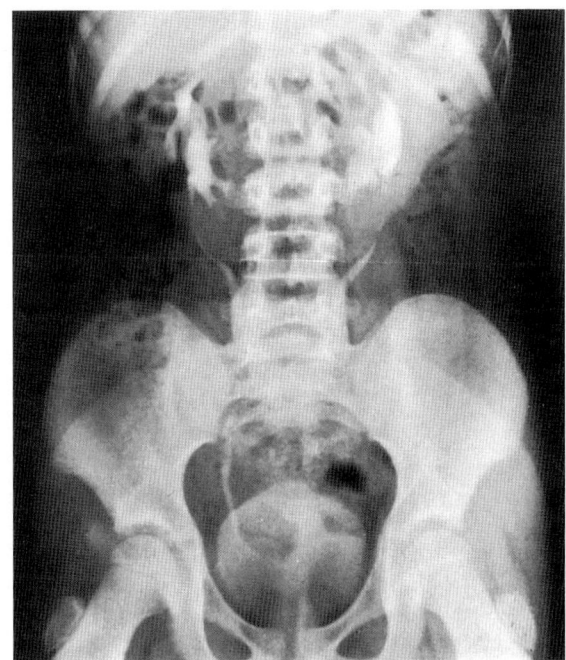

Fig. 18.5   Horseshoe kidney. I.v. urogram showing rotated kidneys with calyces overlying pelves and ureters running inferiorly and then medially to produce 'flower vase' configuration.

at the lower poles – and gives rise to the 'horseshoe kidney' (Fig. 18.5). The fusion of such kidneys prevents normal medial rotation, and the ureters arise from an anterior or lateral, rather than medial, position relative to the renal parenchyma.

The site of an ectopic kidney may render it more vulnerable to trauma or liable to obstruct the delivery of an infant (although most pelvic kidneys do not). The usual route of the ureter may impede urinary drainage and lead to stasis and dilatation with subsequent infection. Dysplastic tissue is not infrequently also found, increasing the risk of infection. An ectopic ureteric orifice in the bladder may lead to vesicoureteric reflux. If the ureter opens into the urethra or vagina there may be incessant urinary incontinence. Despite these problems many malpositioned or fused kidneys function well and are quite unproductive of symptoms.

Diagnosis is made by appropriate radiological investigations, particularly ultrasound and radionuclide imaging.

DUPLEX SYSTEMS

Varying degrees of duplication occur. Double and completely separate pelves may occur (on one or both sides), draining via separate ureters to separate ureteric orifices in the bladder. There may be two pelves and one ureter or the two ureters may unite in Y fashion during the descent to the bladder. Such duplication is sometimes associated with vesicoureteric reflux or other abnormalities and this gives rise to problems such as recurrent infection.

However, a duplex kidney is probably one of the commonest abnormalities detected on imaging of the urinary tract and in the absence of other urinary tract disease requires no treatment. Occasionally one of the ureters is associated with a ureterocele (cystic dilatation of the intravesical portion of the ureter), which can lead to obstruction and hydronephrosis (Fig. 18.6).

The ureter leading from the lower pelvis to the upper ureteric orifice is most often the abnormal one. Either ureteric orifice may open ectopically elsewhere in the bladder, urethra or vagina. It can give rise to the problem of continued wetting and is one of the conditions to consider when a child is referred with a wetting problem and has never apparently had a dry day.

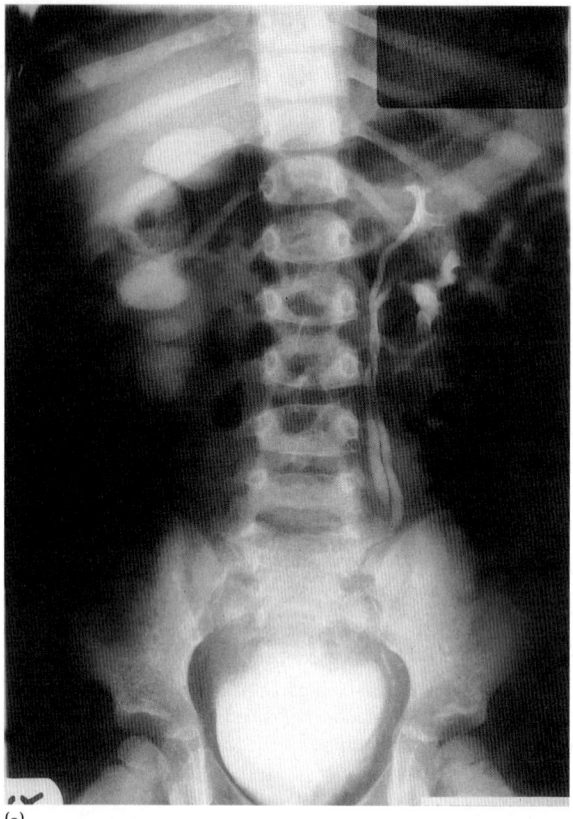

(a)

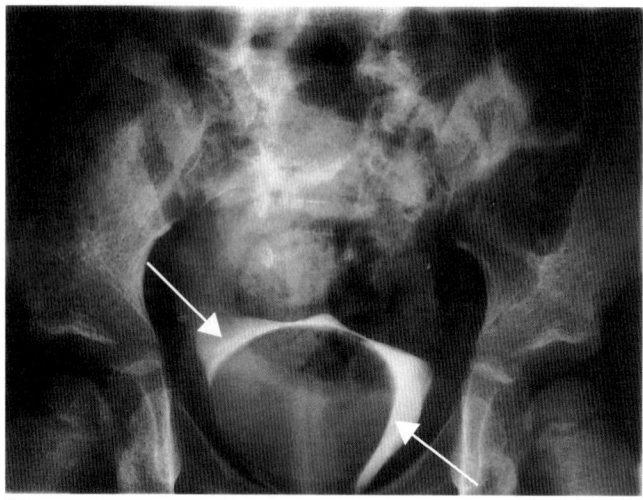

(b)

Fig. 18.6 (a) IVU in a 3-year-old girl with UTI, duplex system of left side and gross hydronephrosis on right side. (b) Hydronephrosis associated with large ureterocele seen as filling defect in bladder.

RENAL DYSPLASIA AND HYPOPLASIA

It is unlikely that these two conditions should be separated. True hypoplasia (i.e. a normally developed but unduly small kidney) is rare. It is best identified by its small size and diminution of the number of papillae and calyces present. Most cases are associated with some degree of dysplasia as well. Renal dysplasia may produce diminution or increase in total renal size, but its characteristic is the presence of pluripotent undifferentiated mesenchyme which may give rise to aberrant tissue such as cartilage and smooth muscle within the kidney. Cyst formation is common and has been attributed to premature cessation of branching by the ureteric bud which, being unable to induce nephron formation, degenerates and becomes cystic. Obstruction to the ureter in fetal life is also a factor in pathogenesis, and causes well marked dilatation of Bowman's capsule in some cases. The dysplasia may be unilateral when the opposite kidney functions normally, or may be bilateral. Gene mutations that have dominant inheritance and cause renal hypodysplasia, urinary tract anomalies, and defined extrarenal symptoms have been identified in *TCF2* (renal cysts and diabetes syndrome, OMIM #137920), *PAX2* (renal-coloboma syndrome, OMIM #120330), *EYA1* and *SIX1* (branchio-oto-renal syndrome, OMIM #113650, #608389), and *SALL1* (Townes-Brocks syndrome, OMIM #107480). It has been estimated that 17% of patients with renal hypodysplasia have one of these mutations.

Renal hypodysplasia contributes significantly to the causes of chronic renal failure in childhood, especially now that dialysis and transplantation are possible, even for small infants. Many children may go undetected but progress into chronic renal failure at the end of the first decade when their body size begins to outgrow their kidney reserve.

Oligomeganephronia is one form of dysplastic kidney when there is a reduced number of very large nephrons, which undergo progressive focal sclerosis.

MULTICYSTIC DYSPLASTIC KIDNEY

The most common cystic lesion recognized antenatally is a multicystic dysplastic kidney (MCDK) disease (Fig. 18.7). In this disorder renal dysplasia is associated with a variable number of cysts and is believed to result from failed coordination development of the metanephros and the branching ureteric bud. Al-Khaldi et al[14] reported 44 fetuses with MCDK disease. In 14 fetuses the disease was bilateral and there were associated lethal abnormalities or syndromes. All 30 surviving infants had unilateral disease, six (20%) having significant reflux into the normal contralateral kidney. Although there have been occasional reports of sepsis, hypertension and even malignancy in association with cystic dysplastic kidneys, in many centers current management is conservative as many MCDK kidneys involute with time.[15]

POSTERIOR URETHRAL VALVES

This affects male infants with an incidence of approximately 1 in 12 000 pregnancies.[16] The back pressure produced by the valves results in vesico-ureteric reflux, hydronephrosis, renal dysplasia and impaired renal function. This most commonly presents antenatally although the scan appearances may vary from an apparently normal 18–20-week scan to severe bilateral hydronephrosis and hydroureter with renal parenchymal loss. Even with antenatal detection and, occasionally, intervention with vesicoamniotic shunts in utero, many fetuses do not survive to term, or die in the neonatal period, because of the associated oligohydramnios and the severe lung abnormalities.

However, posterior urethral valves represent a spectrum of disorders, with some neonates presenting with bladder outflow obstruction, infection and acute renal failure (ARF) in the newborn period in association with urosepsis (Fig. 18.8). Other children present later with apparently minor symptoms. When the diagnosis of posterior urethral valves is suspected a urethral catheter should be passed and an ultrasound and a micturating cysto-urethrogram (MCUG) arranged urgently. After relief of obstruction there will often be a diuretic phase resulting in electrolyte and water loss which require careful monitoring and replacement. Most cases are managed in conjunction with a pediatric urologist and the prognosis will depend upon the degree of associated renal dysplasia and bladder abnormality. The reported experience of one tertiary referral center suggests that the long-term outcome is good for approimately two thirds of patients but a poor outcome, i.e. death in childhood or end-stage renal failure occurs in one third.[17]

PELVIURETERIC JUNCTION (PUJ) AND VESICOURETERIC JUNCTION OBSTRUCTION (VUJ)

These two conditions cause hydronephrosis antenatally and have provided some of the biggest dilemmas in respect of postnatal management.

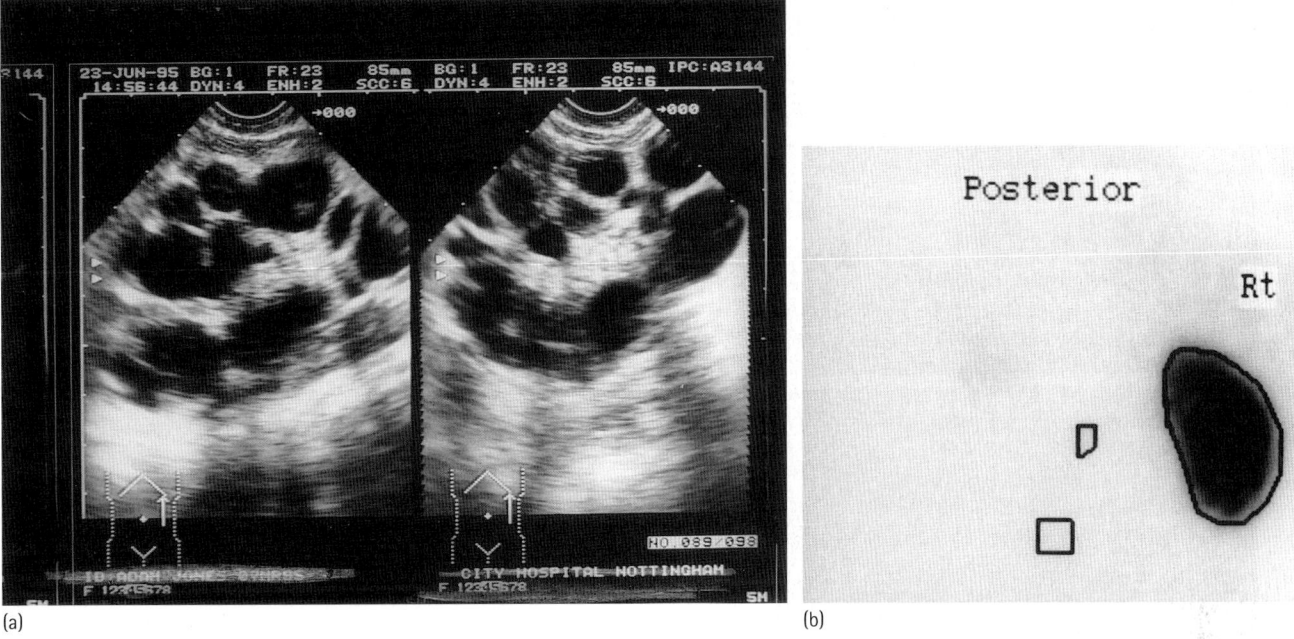

(a)   (b)

Fig. 18.7 (a) Postnatal ultrasound of infant with left MCDK showing numerous cysts in enlarged kidney. (b) Nonfunction confirmed on DMSA scan.

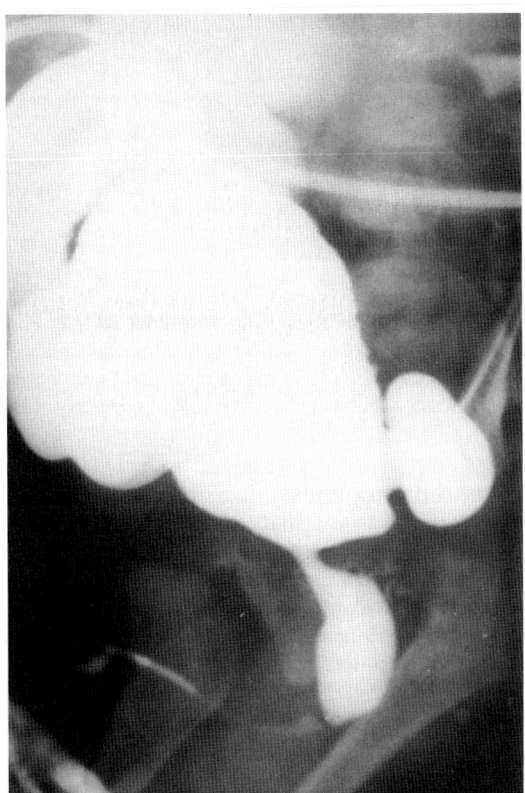

Fig. 18.8 Micturating cystourethrogram in a male infant presenting with septicemia and acute renal failure. Gross dilatation of posterior urethra, bladder diverticulum and reflux into dilated ureter.

PUJ and VUJ can occur at any time of life in association with intermittent abdominal pain, hematuria, urinary tract infection and asymptomatic flank mass. Such symptoms or signs are justification for a pyeloplasty or reimplant operation.

However, most infants with antenatally detected hydronephrosis have little in the way of signs or symptoms postnatally. In the rare instances where there is a large tense kidney, with much diminished function, then an initial nephrostomy is undertaken. Most infants are assessed by a combination of ultrasound, micturating cystourethrogram (MCUG) (to exclude associated reflux) and a radionuclide scan, which is preferably MAG 3 (⁹⁹ᵐTc-labeled mercaptoacetyltriglycine), rather than DTPA (⁹⁹ᵐTc-labeled diethylenetriamine-pentaacetic acid). The general consensus is that a combination of significant calyceal, as well as pelvic, dilatation, accompanied by a reduction of differential function below 40% on the radionuclide scan, are indicators for an operative approach (Fig. 18.9).[18] There are no controlled trials to guide us and information concerning patients with significant dilatation is best reviewed by pediatric nephrologists, pediatric urologists and pediatric radiologists in combined nephrouroradiology meetings.

MCDK is usually a unilateral condition and most involute with time.

Posterior urethral valves must always be considered in a male infant with urosepsis.

Severe vesicoureteric reflux can be associated with small dysplastic kidneys and apparent global 'scarring' in the absence of infection.

VESICOURETERIC REFLUX (see later)

Even minimal hydronephrosis on the antenatal or postnatal scan may be associated with gross degrees of reflux on the MCUG (Fig. 18.10). Care should be taken in neonates, where gross reflux is detected on the MCUG, to ensure that a 5-day course of full-dose antibiotics is prescribed before recommencing prophylactic antibiotics, as fatal urosepsis has occurred after this investigation.

RENAL CYSTIC DISEASE

There are a number of disorders that share renal cysts as a common feature (Table 18.5).

These disorders may be inherited or acquired in the clinical context and associated systemic manifestations may help distinguish cystic disorders one from another. A solitary cyst in a young child may indicate a calyceal diverticulum rather than a simple cyst, which is more common in adult life. Bilateral enlarged kidneys in a neonatal infant would raise the suspicion of autosomal recessive polycystic kidney disease, which is more likely in this context than of autosomal

558 THE SPECIALITIES

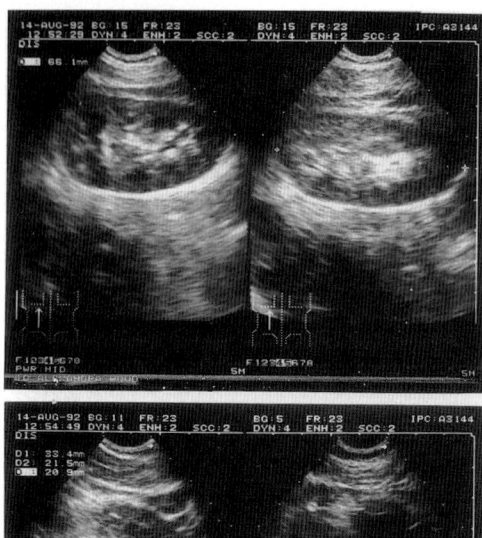

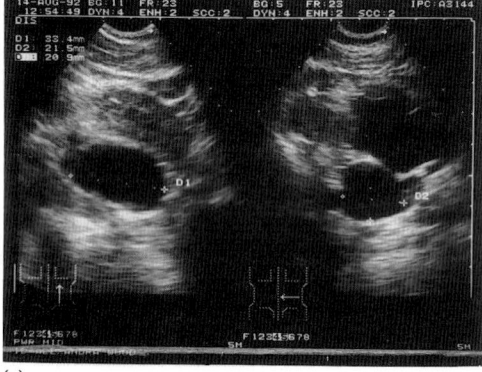

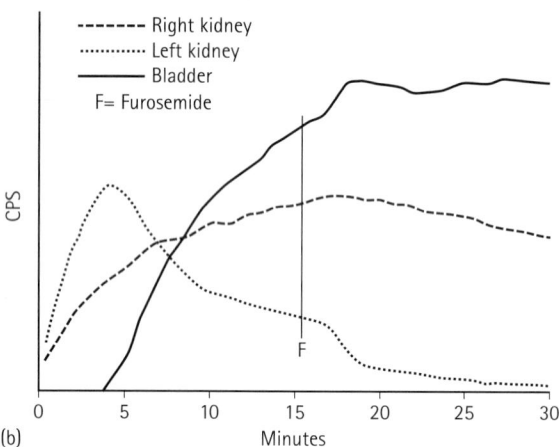

Fig. 18.9 (a) Ultrasound of 1-month-old infant with antenatally detected right hydronephrosis showing normal left kidney and dilatation of pelvis and calyces on right side. (b) Excretion curves of MAG 3 scan in the same infant showing normal excretion left kidney and delayed excretion right side with poor response to furosemide (frusemide). Differential function: right 36%, left 64%.

dominant polycystic kidney disease or tuberous sclerosis complex. Renal insufficiency in an adolescent might suggest juvenile nephronophthisis or autosomal recessive polycystic kidney disease as possible etiologies.

AUTOSOMAL RECESSIVE POLYCYSTIC KIDNEY DISEASE (OMIM #263200)

Autosomal recessive polycystic kidney disease (ARPKD) is an inherited malformation complex with varying degrees of renal collecting duct dilatation and biliary ectasia.[19] There is an estimated incidence of 1 in 20 000 live births and it appears to occur more frequently in Caucasians than in other ethnic populations.

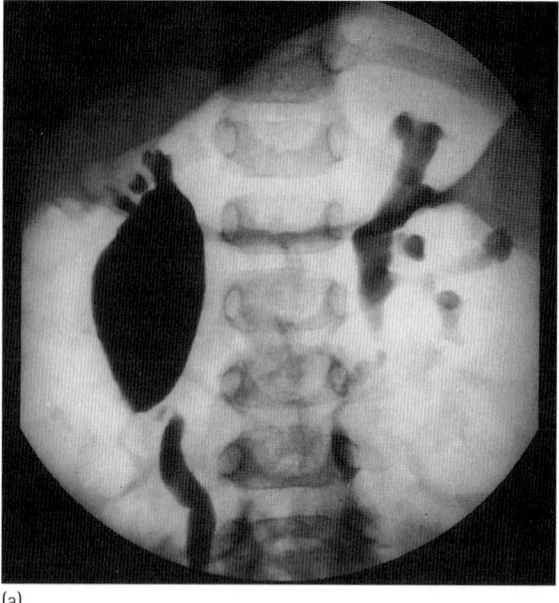

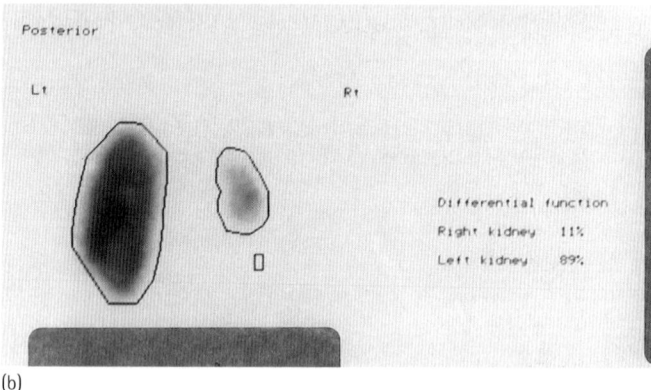

Fig. 18.10 (a) Postnatal MCUG on infant with antenatally detected hydronephrosis showing gross reflux bilaterally with pseudo PUJ appearance on right side. (b) DMSA scan in same infant showing very poor function on right side suggesting dysplastic kidney (no history of infection).

Etiology and pathogenesis

Genetic linkage studies indicate that mutations at a single locus, PKHD1 (polycystic kidney and hepatic disease 1), located on human chromosome region 6p21.1-p12, are responsible for all phenotypes of ARPKD. The gene product, polyductin/fibrocystin, is located in the primary cilium, an epithelial cell organ sensing fluid movement.

Late in the 1970s ARPKD was subdivided into four distinct phenotypes according to the age of presentation and the proportion of dilated renal collecting ducts (perinatal, neonatal, infantile, and juvenile). However, the process typically begins in utero and the renal cystic lesions appear to be superimposed on a normal developmental sequence. The tubular abnormality primarily involves fusiform dilatation of the collecting ducts. The early liver lesion appears to involve defective remodelling of the ductal plate in utero such that primitive bile duct configurations persist and progressive portal fibrosis evolves.

Clinical features

The clinical spectrum of ARPKD is variable and depends on the age at presentation. Most patients are identified either in utero or at birth. The most severely affected fetuses present in pregnancies with oligohydramnios and have enlarged echogenic kidneys. They may die at birth because of pulmonary hypoplasia. Those infants who survive the perinatal period have hypertension, renal failure and portal hypertension. Renal

Table 18.5   Renal cystic disorders

Genetic disorders
Autosomal dominant
Autosomal dominant polycystic kidney disease (ADPKD)
Von Hippel–Lindau disease (VHL)
Tuberous sclerosis complex (TSC)
Adult-onset medullary cystic disease

Autosomal recessive
Autosomal recessive polycystic kidney disease (ARPKD)
Nephronophthisis (NPHP)
Other rare syndromes associated with multiple malformations

X-linked
Orofaciodigital syndrome type 1

Nongenetic disorders
Developmental
Medullary sponge kidney
Renal cystic dysplasia; multicystic dysplasia; cystic dysplasia associated
with lower urinary tract obstruction, diffuse cystic dysplasia (syndromal
and nonsyndromal)

Acquired
Simple cysts
Hypokalemic cystic disease
Acquired cystic disease (in advanced renal failure)

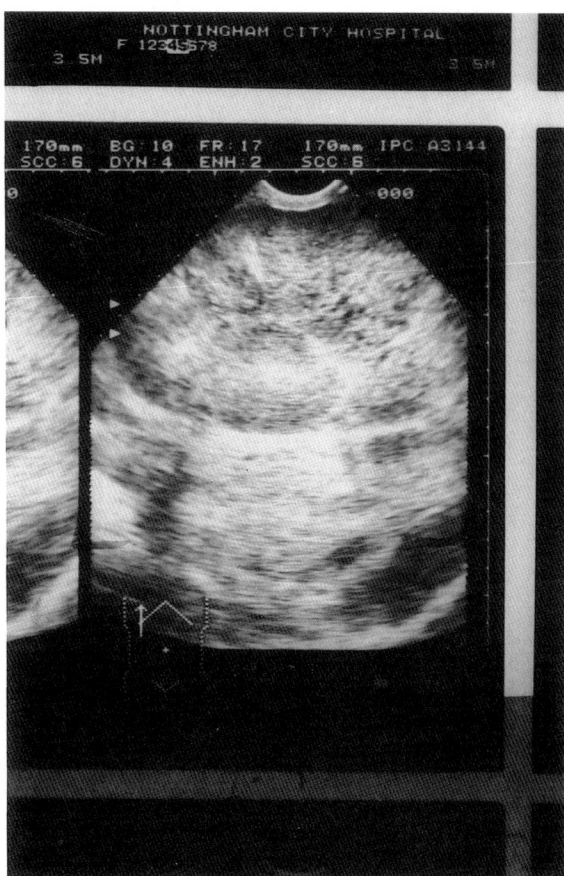

Fig. 18.11   Ultrasound showing diffuse increase in echogenicity. Bilateral enlargement in newborn with ARPKD.

hypertension usually develops in the first few months and ultimately affects 70–80% of patients. There is also an increase in the incidence of urinary tract infections.

Portal hypertension can be the predominant clinical abnormality in older children and adolescents with ARPKD. These children typically present with hepatosplenomegaly and bleeding esophageal or gastric varices as well as hypersplenism. Hepatocellular function is usually preserved but ascending suppurative cholangitis is a serious complication and can cause hepatic failure.

Diagnosis

In the antenatal period, oligohydramnios or enlarged echogenic kidneys suggest ARPKD. Postnatally, ultrasound can reveal symmetrically enlarged diffusely echogenic kidneys, with poor demarcation from surrounding tissues, as well as cortex, medulla and renal sinus (Fig. 18.11). With high resolution ultrasound the regular ray of dilated collecting ducts may be imaged and i.v. urography and computed tomography scanning will show similar features. In older children the development of scattered small cysts and progressive fibrosis can alter the reniform character and ARPKD in older children can be mistaken for ADPKD.

The liver may be normal in size or enlarged and is usually less echogenic than the kidneys. Prominent intrahepatic bile duct dilatation suggests associated Caroli disease. With age, the portal fibrosis tends to progress and there may be hepatosplenomegaly and a patchy increase in hepatic echogenicity.

Genetic testing

Although haplotype-based analysis is feasible in most cases, it is associated with a risk of misdiagnosis in families without patho-anatomically proven diagnosis. Linkage analysis is impossible in families where DNA of the index patient is not available. Direct mutation analysis of the PKHD 1 gene opens new options in families for prenatal diagnosis, though this is not yet widely available, partly because this is an exceptionally large gene to screen, with hundreds of described mutations.

Outcome

The estimated perinatal mortality is 30–50%. For those who survive the first month of life the reported mean 5-year patient survival rate is 80–95%.[20] The prognosis outside the perinatal period is improved, because of the availability of aggressive interventions such as unilateral or bilateral nephrectomy, and the availability of dialysis and transplantation for this group of children. For those with end-stage renal failure and severe portal hypertension, combined liver and kidney transplantation may be indicated.

AUTOSOMAL DOMINANT POLYCYSTIC KIDNEY DISEASE (OMIM #173900)

ADPKD is a multisystem disorder characterized by multiple bilateral renal cysts and associated with cysts in other organs such as liver, pancreas and arachnoid membranes. It is one of the most common hereditary diseases affecting approximately 1 in 400 to 1 in 1000 individuals.

Etiology and pathogenesis

The genes responsible for ADPKD have provided a major breakthrough in the study of the disease. PKD1 is the gene on chromosome 16 and is responsible for 85% of clinically detected cases and PKD2 has been identified in the long arm of chromosome 4 and there is likely to be a third gene. Proteins encoded by PKD1 and PKD2 are named polycystin 1 and polycystin 2, respectively. Recently, biologic evidence documented the crucial role of the renal primary cilia on the formation of polycystins to induce cystogenesis. Molecular genetic work has stimulated a great deal of research into variation in disease progression between patients and this appears to depend upon underlying mutations, modifying genes, somatic mutations and environmental factors.[21]

Clinical features

It is very rare for ADPKD to manifest clinically in childhood, but an occasional child may have significant renal enlargement with hypertension. Urinary tract infections are also known to exacerbate kidney disease in adults. Although ADPKD may be recognized incidentally on renal ultrasound scans done for urinary tract infection (UTI) investigation etc., there is a general consensus that asymptomatic children from affected families should not be routinely screened for this condition either by ultrasound or genetic studies. They should be free to make their own autonomous decision as to whether they want to be investigated when they reach adulthood.

FAMILIAL JUVENILE NEPHRONOPHTHISIS AND MEDULLARY CYSTIC DISEASE COMPLEX

Juvenile nephronophthisis (NPHP) and medullary cystic disease complex are histologically similar diseases differing in their mode of transmission and age of onset. They are now shown genetically to be distinct diseases. Medullary cystic kidney disease (MCKD; OMIM #174000) is an autosomal dominant form of tubulointerstitial nephropathy characterized by formation of renal cysts at the corticomedullary junction. Progression to end-stage renal failure occurs in the third to fourth decade of life.

Three loci have been mapped for nephronophthisis, the leading genetic cause of chronic renal failure in young adults: juvenile NPHP1 (OMIM #256100) on 2q13; infantile nephronophthisis (NPHP2; OMIM #602088) on 9q22-q31; and adolescent nephronophthisis (NPHP3; OMIM #604387) on 3q21-q22. By renal histology the three forms of the disease are indistinguishable, all three exhibiting a triad of interstitial-cell infiltrates, renal tubular-cell atrophy with cysts arising from the corticomedullary junction of the kidneys, and renal interstitial fibrosis. Clinically, there is a statistically different age at onset at end-stage renal disease: terminal renal failure develops at median ages of 1 year, 13 years, and 19 years, in NPHP2, NPHP1, and NPHP3, respectively. The chromosomal localization of a fourth gene locus, NPHP4 has been reported, in which end-stage renal disease commences within a wide age range, 11–34 years.

Clinical features

Reduced urinary concentrating capacity is common in patients with NPHP and this usually precedes a decline in renal function. The mean age of onset is 4 years. Polyuria and polydipsia are common symptoms and the patients may be anemic, even before the onset of renal insufficiency. Growth retardation, out of proportion with the degree of renal insufficiency, is a common finding.[22] A gradual decline in renal function is typical and end-stage renal failure usually develops by adolescence. The disease is not known to recur in renal allografts.

In 10–15% of NPHP, now shown to link to NPHP4, there is an association with retinitis pigmentosa caused by retinal degeneration (Senior–Loken syndrome) and presents with coarse nystagmus and early blindness. NPHP associated with ocular motor apraxia and coexisting retinal degeneration (Cogan syndrome) has been reported in several kindreds and a subset of these patients has also had mental retardation. Congenital hepatic fibrosis occurs occasionally in patients with NPHP

MEDULLARY SPONGE KIDNEY

This developmental disorder is characterized by cystic anomalies of precalyceal ducts, which is frequently associated with nephrocalcinosis and renal stones. Again this condition more commonly comes to light in adult life, when calcification in the renal pyramids may give rise to calculi, abdominal pain and hematuria. It is occasionally identified in childhood for the same reasons, but more often because of the urographic appearance of streaky opacification in the renal pyramids.

TUBEROUS SCLEROSIS COMPLEX (OMIM #191100)

Tuberous sclerosis complex (TSC) is an autosomal dominant disorder in which tumor-like malformations, called hamartomas, develop in multiple organ systems. This affects 1 in 10 000 individuals but spontaneous mutations appear to occur at high frequency and are estimated to account for 60% of new cases.

Renal cystic disease is the earliest finding in TSC and may be the presenting manifestation in infants and children before even the seizures and mental retardation have become manifest alongside the facial angiofibromas, hypomelanotic macules and periungual fibromas.

The principal hamartomas in TSC are angiomyolipomas. They rarely occur before 5 years of age but increase in frequency and size and give rise to hemorrhage or mass effects leading to severe hypertension and progressive decrease in renal function. Malignant tumors, found in TSC patients, were originally thought to be a renal cell carcinoma but are now regarded as malignant epithelioid angiomyolipomas.[23]

URINARY TRACT INFECTIONS

EPIDEMIOLOGY

Urinary tract infections are common in childhood and adolescence. Up to 7% of girls and 2% of boys will have a symptomatic, culture confirmed UTI by 6 years of age.[24]

RISK FACTORS ASSOCIATED WITH THE DEVELOPMENT OF UTI

1. *Age and sex.* The highest rates of childhood UTI are reported in males younger than 1 year of age and females younger than 6 years of age.[24] The prevalence of UTI in febrile infants is higher than that in older children and increases with younger age. In a recent prospective, multicentre, cross-sectional study the highest rate of UTI in febrile infants was seen in uncircumcised male infants (21.3%) compared with female (5.0%) and circumcised male (2.3%) infants.[25] In males, circumcision is reported to significantly reduce the risk of UTI.[26]
2. *Race.* Higher rates of UTI have been reported in Caucasian children as compared to African-American children.[27]
3. *Family history.* There is an increased incidence of UTI in children whose first-degree relatives have had UTIs.[28]
4. *Constipation* in children increases the likelihood of urinary incontinence, dysfunctional voiding, a large capacity, poorly emptying bladder, and UTI.
5. *Sexual activity.* Adolescents with UTIs have a significant frequency of sexual activity and information pertaining to this should be sought in this group of patients.[29]
6. *Bladder catheterization* may predispose to UTI, although this is generally asymptomatic bacteriuria.[30]
7. *Abnormalities of the urinary tract.*
   a. *Vesico-ureteric reflux* (VUR) is present in 30–40% of children investigated for UTI.[31] The importance of VUR as a causative factor in the initiation of UTIs with consequential renal scarring is controversial. Historically it was widely held that the combination of VUR and UTI resulted in renal damage in the form of scarring. More recently these assumptions have been challenged. This is explored in more detail in the section on vesicoureteric reflux.
   b. *Obstruction.* Anatomical defects of the urinary tract that predispose to obstruction are infrequent causes of UTI. These include pelvi-ureteric junction (PUJ) obstruction, vesico-ureteric junction (VUJ) obstruction, ureterocoele, posterior urethral valves and myelomeningocele with neurogenic bladder. Renal stones may also (rarely) present as UTIs.

PATHOPHYSIOLOGY OF UTIs

Infection of the urinary tract is related to both the characteristics of the invading bacteria and those of the host urinary tract. The most common bacterial species to invade the urinary tract is *Escherichia coli* (*E. coli*), which accounts for up to 92% of UTI in children.[32] Other organisms include *Klebsiella, Proteus, Enterobacter, Enterococcus, Pseudomonas* and *Citrobacter.* Virulence factors have been well studied in *E. coli* and most strains isolated from patients with suspected upper UTIs have pili or fimbriae, which are polypeptides with tubular receptors specific for glycolipid components of human cell membranes. Such fimbriae allow attachment to receptors expressed on uroepithelial cells, enabling bacteria to ascend into the bladder and kidney. *P. fimbriae* expression is associated with increased severity of infection. Over 90% of *E. coli* isolated from children with a first episode of pyelonephritis expressed *P. fimbriae* compared with 19.2% of isolates of children with cystitis.[32]

CLINICAL PRESENTATION OF UTI

The younger the child the more nonspecific the symptoms:
1. **Neonates**. Prolonged jaundice is a classical association of bacteriuria in the newborn. A high index of suspicion should be maintained in any baby 'going off', or who has abdominal distension, disturbance of temperature regulation, changing ventilation requirements or metabolic disturbance.
2. **Infants and toddlers** may present with vomiting, diarrhea, poor feeding and failure to thrive or fever. UTI should be excluded in any infant with an unexplained temperature.
   a. Young infants with an abnormal urinary tract can present with acute renal failure and gross electrolyte abnormalities.
3. **Preschool and older children** may have cystitis-like symptoms such as frequency and dysuria, often accompanied by 'new' bed-wetting and daytime accidents. There may be mild lower abdominal discomfort and hematuria. Such symptoms do not exclude involvement of the upper urinary tract.

The classical symptoms of high fever, vomiting, abdominal or loin pain and rigors in the child is suggestive of acute pyelonephritis. The presence of such symptoms, or septicemia, in a young infant will influence subsequent management and intensity of the investigations.

PHYSICAL EXAMINATION OF INFANTS AND CHILDREN WITH SUSPECTED UTI

This should include:
1. *Abdominal palpation* for renal masses and fecal loading:
   a. A palpable bladder combined with a poor urinary stream may indicate neuropathic bladder.
2. *Examination of the spine and lower limb reflexes* should be undertaken to examine for the presence of spina bifida occulta with associated neuropathic bladder.
3. *Examination of the anal and genital areas* may be appropriate and might suggest signs of sexual abuse in a female infant.
4. *Height, weight and blood pressure* should be recorded.

INVESTIGATION OF INFANTS AND CHILDREN WITH SUSPECTED UTI

1. urine dipsticks incorporate strips for the detection of white blood cells (leukocyte esterase) and nitrite production (by reduction of nitrate). These are increasingly used as a first-line investigation of UTI. Dipstick analysis for nitrite and leukocyte esterase has similar sensitivity to gram stain in the detection of UTI in children.[33] Hence a urine specimen obtained in an asymptomatic child in the outpatient department which is clear and negative on dipstick does not need laboratory assessment and culture. Conversely, a positive nitrite and leukocyte result is an indication for urine culture and empirical treatment with antibiotics, while awaiting culture, if the child is symptomatic;
   Dipstick analysis may not be reliable in the following situations:
   a. in infants, due to frequent micturition and dilute urine, there may be insufficient leukocytes and nitrates to cause a positive reaction;
   b. in patients with inadequate dietary nitrate there may be a low sensitivity rate;
   c. infection with enzyme deficient bacteria.
2. urinalysis;
3. C-reactive protein, full blood count, blood cultures and urea and electrolytes if the child is systemically unwell.

METHODS OF URINE COLLECTION:

1. *Suprapubic aspirate* (SPA). This is the 'gold standard' against which all other sampling methods are compared.[34–36] Although SPC can be undertaken in people of all ages, it is usually only attempted in infants under 6 months in whom the bladder is an abdominal organ. If performed correctly, aspirating the needle while advancing, the sample should be uncontaminated and any organisms seen should be regarded as significant.[34] The procedure may be unsuccessful if the bladder is empty and It may be worthwhile confirming that the bladder is full by ultrasound examination prior to commencing the procedure. We would recommend that SPA should be performed in unwell neonates and infants under 6 months with a suspicion of UTI unless the child's clinical condition allows for collection of urine by the 'clean-catch' method.
2. *Catheter specimen of urine* (CSU) is generally undertaken when an urgent sample is required and a suprapubic sample is not practical because of age/parental wishes. CSU is often more acceptable to parents than SPA and has a low false-positive rate.[35] However there is a risk of introducing an infection if one isn't already present.
3. *Clean catch urine* (or mid-stream urine in continent children). These are reliable methods of collecting urine with lower contamination rates than bag urines. They are recommended by the Royal College of Paediatrics and Child Health as the preferred non-invasive methods of urine collection.[36] If possible, two samples should be sent prior to commencing treatment. In the infant, micturition can be encouraged by tapping in the suprapubic region, stroking alongside the spine or even exposure to cold while undressing. Sterile trays should always be to hand and parents should be encouraged to participate in this method of urine collection. The older continent boy can easily introduce a sterile container into the urinary stream and there is no need for specific cleansing of the glans or withdrawal of the prepuce. Similarly the vulva does not require cleansing (antiseptics are to be avoided) in older girls, but cleaning with sterile water may be required in younger girls where a sterile container placed inside a potty is usually employed. Using the child's own potty is not satisfactory and is a common reason for erroneous results in general practice.
4. *Bag urine samples* are a commonly used method of collecting urine in non-toilet trained children. However, the current authors would not recommend their use routinely due to high contamination rates of up to 40%.[37] If bag urine samples are to be used, sending a second sample (prior to the commencement of treatment) has been reported to reduce the contamination rate to 12%.[38]
5. *Pad urine collection*. This is an easy but unreliable method of collecting urine. The pad is easily applied to the nappy and urine is removed from the pad by syringe. The current authors would not recommend their use routinely due to high contamination rates.[39]
6. *Dip slides* for transmitting urine specimens or bottles containing boric acid have been promoted as a means of collecting specimens at home where there are transport difficulties to the laboratory. However, technical failures with dip slides may be disappointingly high and if the container with boric acid is not filled with urine to the appropriate level then growth may be inhibited.[40]

HANDLING OF URINE CULTURE SPECIMENS

Since practitioners are so reliant upon urine culture to confirm the UTI, it is important that all urine cultures should be submitted to the laboratory with the minimum delay. If there is any delay, storage at 4 °C will still permit accurate diagnosis for 24 h and possibly longer.

MICROSCOPY

Although the finding of pyuria is good supportive evidence of UTI, up to 50% of patients with significant bacteriuria will not demonstrate a significant number of white cells (> 5 white cells per high powered field) in the centrifuged urine specimen. Furthermore, pyuria may be present in sepsis and does not always imply a UTI.[41] Gram stain at the time of urgent microscopy may help direct antibiotics, however negative gram stain is unhelpful in refuting a UTI.

CULTURE

The classical definition of significant bacteriuria [10^5 organisms per ml (10^8/L) of urine] is still applied in childhood with the proviso that any bacteriology reports should always be interpreted in the clinical context. It is possible that a lower colony count, especially with a pure growth on repeated samples, is clinically important. Any growth obtained on a suprapubic urine sample or 'in-out' catheter specimen urine is regarded as significant. Growth of more than one strain of bacteria is an indication of contamination and if not already done a repeat sample should be obtained.

TREATMENT OF UTIs

Empiric antibiotic therapy is recommended while awaiting culture results if there is a high clinical suspicion of UTI (Table 18.6). If there is no clinical improvement within 2 d of commencing antibiotic therapy, repeat urine culture should be undertaken and consideration given to renal/bladder ultrasound.[42]

In two randomized controlled trials[43,44] comparing oral and parenteral regimens in children with fever and positive urine cultures, there were no differences in cure rates or speed of improvement between the two regimens. Parenteral antibiotics may be indicated in cases of suspected septicemia, or where there is intolerance to oral administration (e.g vomiting). Neonates should be treated as per local unit protocols.

Trimethoprim is commonly used as first-line oral therapy for urinary tract infections, however choice of therapy will depend upon information from the local microbiology laboratory about changing patterns of antibiotic resistance locally. Patients on trimethoprim prophylaxis with 'breakthrough' infection suggestive of resistant organisms are often treated with third or fourth generation cephalosporins, nitrofurantoin or augmentin. Amoxicillin has also been used, however, resistance rates of over 70% have been reported.[45,46] Ciprofloxacin is the antibiotic of choice for *Pseudomonas* infections.

Parenteral agents include second- and third-line cephalosporins and aminoglycosides, as directed by local policy.

One-day courses of antibiotics should not be used to manage UTI in children.[47] Shorter courses (3–5 d) are reported to be as effective longer courses for uncomplicated UTIs without systemic features and in the absence of structural anomalies of the urinary tract.[47,48] We would recommend a 3–5-day course in these children and a 7–14 day course in children with features suggestive of acute pyelonephritis.

There is no evidence to support a recommendation for routine post-treatment urine cultures in children with UTIs.[49]

Children with obstructive uropathy such as posterior urethral valves should be managed in centers where there is both nephrology and urology expertise.

IMAGING IN CHILDREN WITH UTI

At present the consensus is that all children, boys and girls, should undergo imaging of the urinary tract after the first proven urinary tract infection. This is in line with the published guidelines of the Royal College of Physicians (UK).[50] However, these recommendations are followed in a minority of cases, as the assumptions upon which they were based have been challenged in recent years.[51] There is increasing evidence that imaging for children with a first uncomplicated UTI may not improve patient care.[52,53]

The following imaging techniques are employed for the investigation of children with proven UTI:

1. Ultrasound will provide basic information on the structure of the urinary tract (Fig. 18.12). Kidney sizes should be recorded with reference to centile charts based on the child's height. Ultrasound is useful in the detection of obstruction of the urinary tract and bladder abnormalities as well as stones and gives an estimation of postmicturition residual volumes. It is relatively cheap and requires no radiation. However, ultrasound is operator-dependent and is difficult in uncooperative children. It is not useful for the detection of subtle renal scars and does not detect vesicoureteric reflux, which may be present with a normal ultrasound especially in the newborn period.[54]

2. Dimercaptosuccinic acid (DMSA) demonstrates acute renal involvement in UTIs and is the best technique for detection of scars and determining differential renal function (Fig. 18.13). A DMSA scan performed during or soon after the acute illness may show acute defects of the renal parenchyma, which do not necessarily result in permanent scars[55] and DMSA should therefore be delayed for 6 months after the infection if using this technique to determine permanent renal damage.

3. Micturating cystourethrogram (MCUG) is the 'gold standard' for detecting and grading vesicoureteric reflux. MCUG permits identification of posterior urethral valves and bladder anomalies (e.g. ureterocoeles, diverticulae). The MCUG is the most traumatic of the imaging investigations for UTI[56] and carries a significant radiation burden.[57] There is also a risk of introducing infection and antibiotic prophylaxis should be prescribed for 24 h prior to the MCUG and for 48 h following the MCUG (usually trimethoprim).

4. Abdominal X-ray (AXR) is generally only indicated where stones are suspected from the history, or there is the suggestion of a spinal abnormality on abdominal examination.

5. Isotope renography (MAG 3 or DTPA) is useful for detecting VUR in cooperative children, usually age 3+ (Fig. 18.14). This is the basis of indirect micturating cystography, which has a lower radiation dose than the direct MCUG. Although catheterization is avoided, the technique still requires i.v. injection of isotope. MAG 3 and DTPA will give information on drainage and therefore urinary tract obstruction. Excretion curves permit calculation of differential kidney function. MAG 3 is favored over DTPA as the resolution of the former is better. MAG 3 is useful for the detection of large scars but is less sensitive than DMSA in the detection of smaller scars.

Table 18.6 Antibiotics used in the treatment and prophylaxis of UTIs

	Treatment (dose in mg/kg/d)	Dose interval (h)	Prophylaxis (dose in mg/kg/d)
Co-amoxiclav	75 mg i.v.	8	NR
	20–40 oral amox content	8	NR
	25–45 oral amox content	12 (duo suspension)	NR
Amoxicillin	25 oral	8	NR
Trimethoprim	8 oral	12	2
Nalidixic acid	50 oral	6	12.5
Nitrofurantoin	3–5 oral	6	1
Cefotaxime	100 i.v.	12	NR
Cefradine	25–50 oral	8–12	NR
Cefuroxime	60 mg i.v.	8	NR
	6.25–25 oral	12	NR
Gentamicin	2 mg/kg/dose i.v.	Depends upon renal function and levels	NR

NR, not recommended for prophylaxis

PREVENTION OF FURTHER INFECTION

Recurrence of UTI is common in children, with about 30% of girls having another UTI within 1 year[58] Look for and treat constipation.

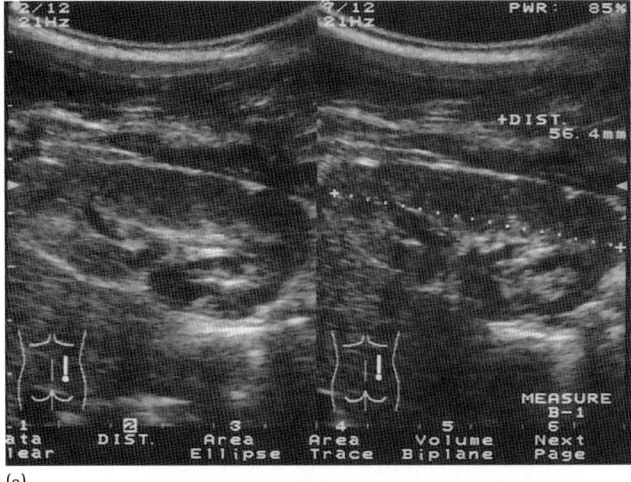

(a)

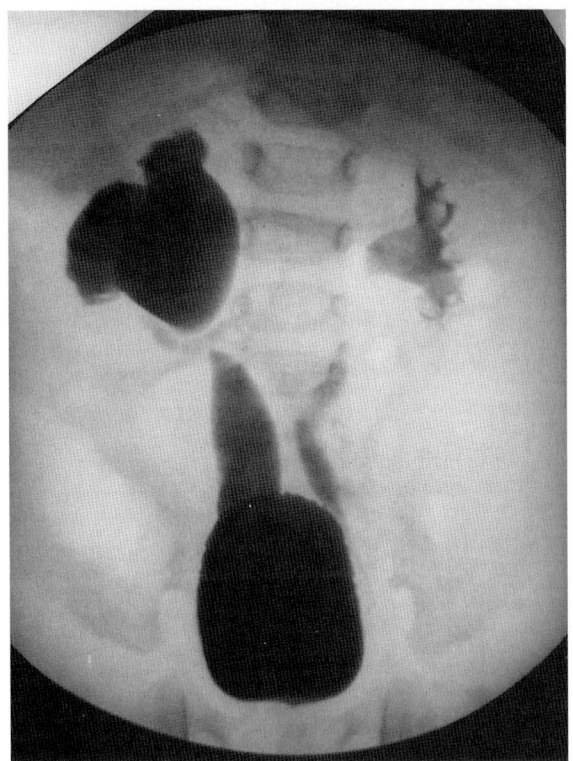

(b)

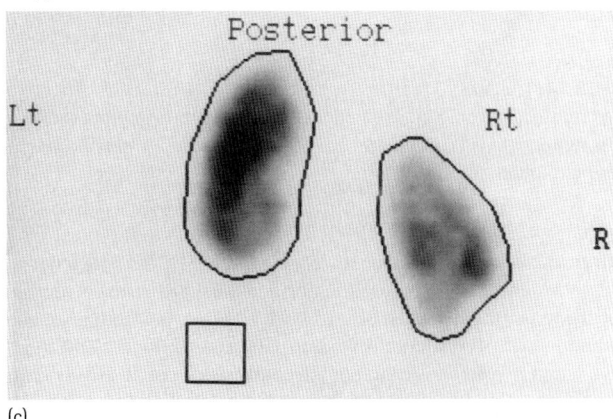

(c)

Fig. 18.12 Investigation in a 2-year-old boy with proven UTI: (a) ultrasound revealed normal left kidney (6.6 cm) with right kidney (shown) 5.6 cm and extensively scarred, especially at lower pole; (b) MCUG showed bilateral vesicoureteric reflux, gross right side; (c) DMSA shows scarring at both poles laterally of right kidney (40% of differential function).

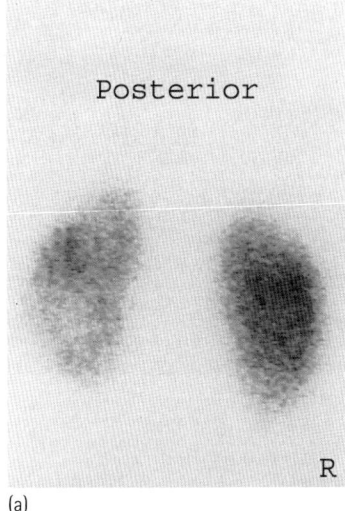

(a)

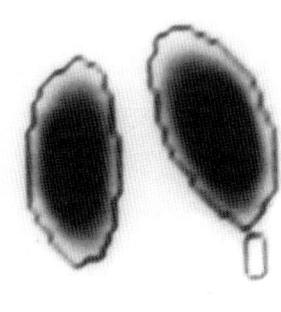

(b)

Fig. 18.13 (a) DMSA scan showing parenchymal defects in left kidney of 3-year-old with pyelonephritis. (b) DMSA scan in the same child 4 months later showing resolution of acute changes.

The following simple measures should be discussed at consultations to reduce the risk of further infections:
1. avoid local irritants (bubble bath, soaps);
2. avoid excessive clothing and nylon underwear;
3. maintain a good fluid input;
4. avoid excessive 'holding on' and not emptying the bladder adequately;
5. cranberry juice has been reported to prevent (not treat) UTIs in women with recurrent UTI.[59,60] There are no data in children;
6. live yoghurt/lactobacillus has also been shown in adults to prevent UTI.[61] Again, there are no conclusive data in children, however it would seem reasonable to consider for older children;
7. prompt treatment of UTI is likely to be as beneficial as prophylaxis.[34,62] Therefore the importance of early recognition and treatment of UTI should be stressed to the child's parents.

Uncircumcised febrile male infants have a higher prevalence of UTIs than circumcised male infants. In a recent meta-analysis, circumcision was associated with a significantly reduced risk of UTI.[26] These data do not, however, support the routine circumcision of boys to prevent UTI, rather, support the principle that circumcision should be considered in those with recurrent UTI or significantly increased risk of UTI.

Prophylaxis

Antibiotic prophylaxis, given as a single dose at night has been shown to be beneficial in reducing risk of recurrent infections to 36% of the control group.[63] However, a recent systematic review suggests that most published studies to date have been poorly designed with biases known to overestimate the true treatment effect. Large, properly randomized, double-blinded trails are still needed to determine the efficacy of long-term antibiotics for the prevention of UTI in susceptible children.[64]

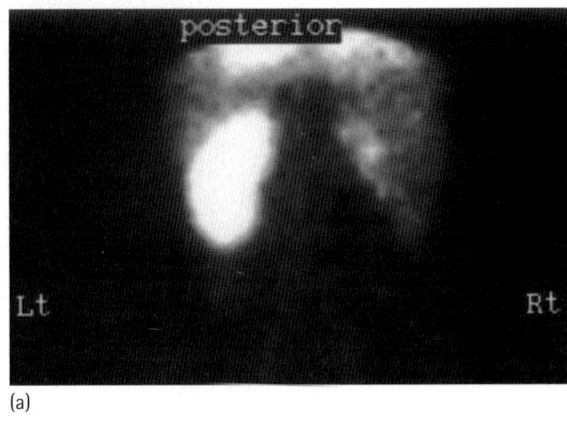

(a)

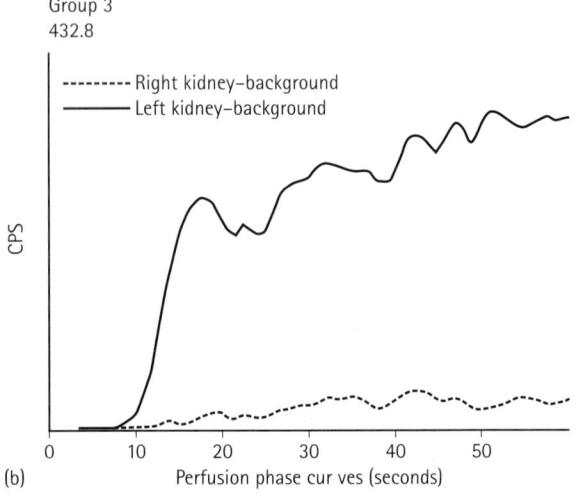

(b)

(c)

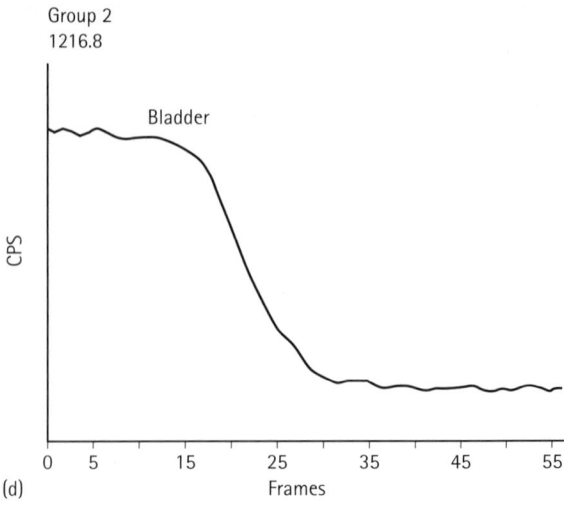

(d)

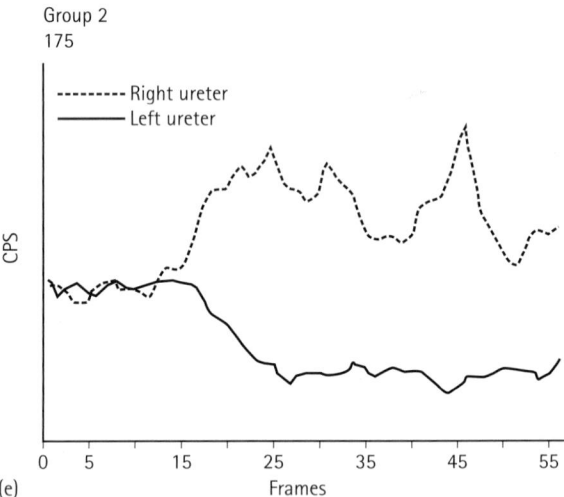

(e)

Fig. 18.14 (a) MAG 3 scan in 6-year-old boy with history of UTI and small right kidney on scan. (b–e) Indirect micturating cystogram showing gross reflux right side, as bladder empties, reflected in increased counts over right ureter and kidney.

Trimethoprim and nitrofurantoin are common choices for prophylaxis, trimethoprim seems to be better tolerated.[63,65]

Screening for bacteriuria

There is no evidence that screening for bacteriuria in healthy children is of value in preventing renal disease and general screening programs are not advocated.[66]

FURTHER MANAGEMENT OF CHILDREN WITH UTI

This will depend in part on the results of investigations. In the unusual situation where a child presents with an obstructive uropathy or stones,

a surgical consultation will be required. Children with suspected neurogenic bladder require further imaging, such as MRI scans of the spine and urodynamic evaluation of the bladder.[58] There is a significant group of children with dysfunctional voiding patterns (see under Wetting problems) who are prone to recurrent infections. Such children may require assessment of bladder emptying by ultrasound and stressing the importance of double or triple voiding. Children with recurrent UTIs may benefit from prophylactic antibiotics given for 6–12 months to break the vicious cycle of re-infection. The risk of 'breakthrough' infections due to antibiotic resistance can be reduced by 'rotating' trimethoprim (single dose at night) for 3 months, followed by nitrofurantoin (single dose at night) for 3 months.

SUMMARY: MANAGEMENT OF UTI IN CHILDHOOD

Guidance for the management of Urinary Tract Infection in Childhood has been produced in 2007 by the National Institute for Clinical Excellence (UK) (NICE). This guidance, currently in draft form, can be found at www.nice.org.uk. In developing this guidance it has been acknowledged that further research is required to better understand the epidemiology of UTI in children and provide a robust evidence base for the management of UTI in children. In particular, well-designed randomized, double blinded, placeb controlled trials are now urgently required to determine the effectiveness of prophylactic antibiotics in the prevention of renal parenchymal defects in children with UTIs. The following algorithms in Figures 18.15 and 18.16 detail the proposed NICE guidance for diagnosis and management of UTI in children.

VESICOURETERIC REFLUX

Vesicoureteric reflux (VUR) is the retrograde passage of urine from the bladder into the kidneys and/or ureters. Primary VUR is likely to be due to a maturational abnormality of the vesicoureteric junction. VUR may also occur as a secondary effect of anatomical or neurological bladder outflow obstruction.

VUR is most commonly detected during the course of investigation of urinary tract infection in children, where it is reported to be present in 30–40% of cases.[67,68] VUR is also detected in 15–40% of infants investigated for antenatal hydronephrosis.[69-71] Primary VUR is associated with other anomalies of the urinary tract (duplex systems, renal aplasia and multicystic dysplastic kidney)[72,73] implying a common pathogenic link between these conditions.

INHERITANCE OF VUR

Hereditary factors are strongly implicated in the development of VUR, which has been reported to occur in up to 65% of first-degree relatives of affected individuals.[74,75] On the basis of these data, it has been proposed that VUR is inherited in an autosomal dominant manner. However, the search for the responsible gene(s) has, to date, proved elusive. Candidate loci have been identified on chromosomes 1p13, 6p21, 10q26, and 19q13[76-82] and a further search for candidate genes in sibling pairs is currently underway. The variable severity of VUR even in affected individuals within the same family, together with the association of VUR with diverse and complex anomalies of the urinary tract implies that VUR may be genetically heterogeneous.

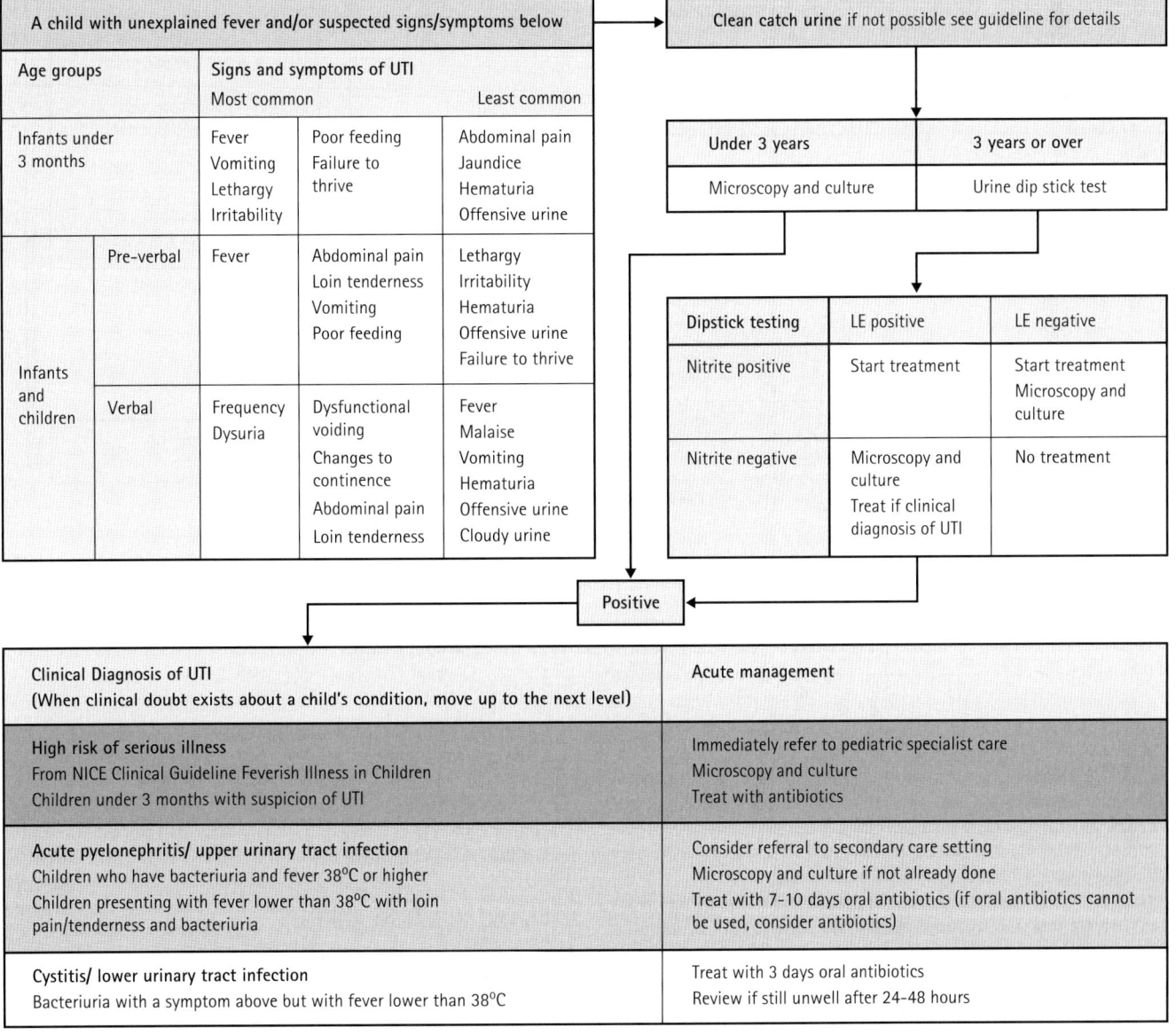

Fig. 18.15   NICE Clinical Guideline 'UTI in children'. Diagnosis and acute management for first time UTI (with permission). See www.nice.org.uk/nicemedia/pdf/cg54algorithm for latest update.

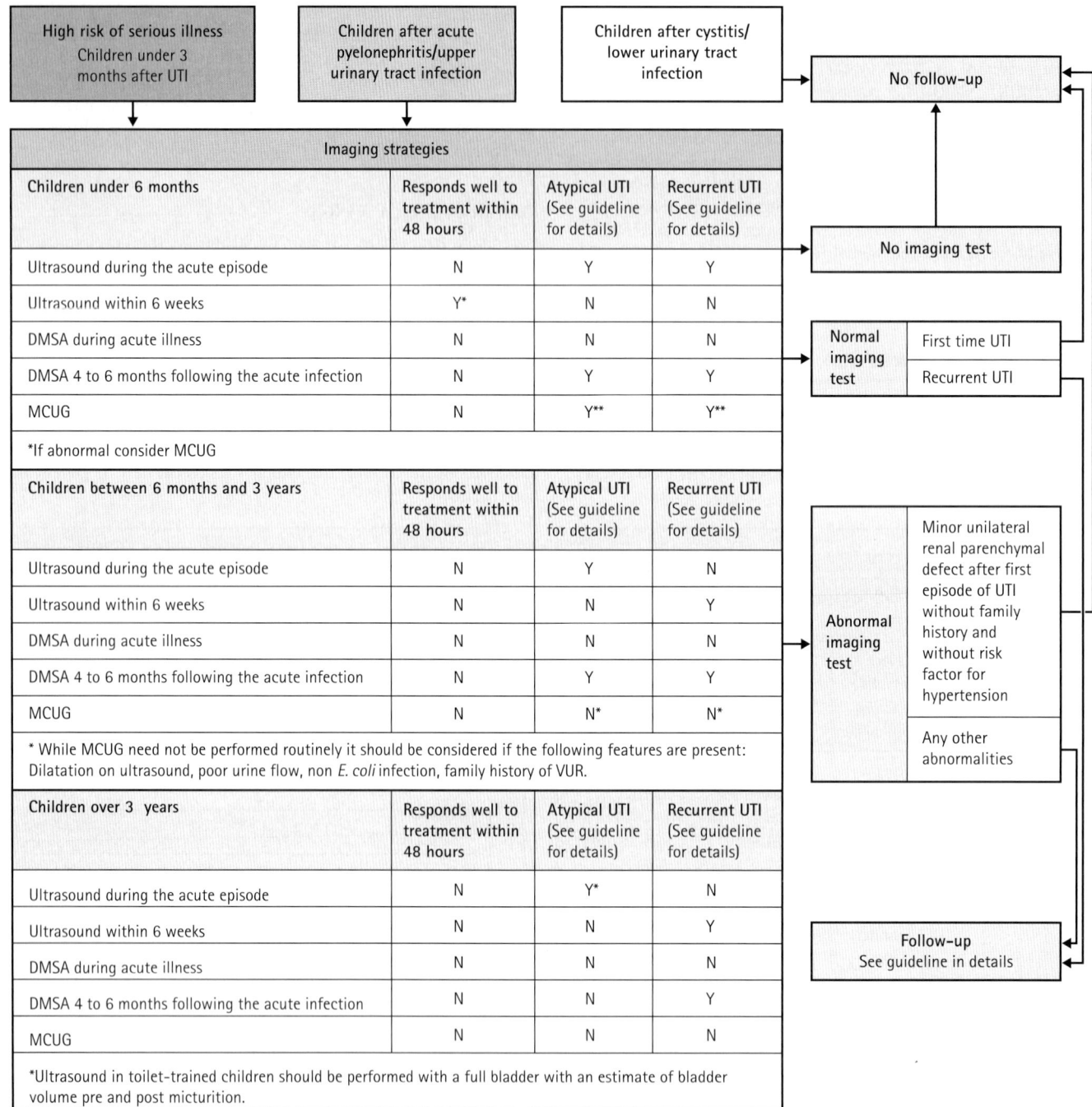

Children under 6 months	Responds well to treatment within 48 hours	Atypical UTI (See guideline for details)	Recurrent UTI (See guideline for details)
Ultrasound during the acute episode	N	Y	Y
Ultrasound within 6 weeks	Y*	N	N
DMSA during acute illness	N	N	N
DMSA 4 to 6 months following the acute infection	N	Y	Y
MCUG	N	Y**	Y**

*If abnormal consider MCUG

Children between 6 months and 3 years	Responds well to treatment within 48 hours	Atypical UTI (See guideline for details)	Recurrent UTI (See guideline for details)
Ultrasound during the acute episode	N	Y	N
Ultrasound within 6 weeks	N	N	Y
DMSA during acute illness	N	N	N
DMSA 4 to 6 months following the acute infection	N	Y	Y
MCUG	N	N*	N*

* While MCUG need not be performed routinely it should be considered if the following features are present: Dilatation on ultrasound, poor urine flow, non *E. coli* infection, family history of VUR.

Children over 3 years	Responds well to treatment within 48 hours	Atypical UTI (See guideline for details)	Recurrent UTI (See guideline for details)
Ultrasound during the acute episode	N	Y*	N
Ultrasound within 6 weeks	N	N	Y
DMSA during acute illness	N	N	N
DMSA 4 to 6 months following the acute infection	N	N	Y
MCUG	N	N	N

*Ultrasound in toilet-trained children should be performed with a full bladder with an estimate of bladder volume pre and post micturition.

Fig. 18.16 NICE Clinical Guideline 'UTI in children' Imaging tests (with permission). See www.nice.org.uk/nicemedia/pdf/cg54algorithm for latest update.

DIAGNOSIS OF VUR

VUR is currently best detected by a MCUG, which is regarded as the 'gold standard' for assessing the presence of VUR. Radiopaque contrast medium is instilled into the bladder producing images of the bladder and renal fossae during filling and voiding.

Nuclear cystography is at least as sensitive for the detection of reflux as a standard VCUG and exposes the child to less radiation.[83] However, grading of reflux is less precise, and associated bladder abnormalities cannot be excluded with nuclear cystography. Therefore, a VCUG is preferred as the initial study for the initial detection of VUR. Nuclear cystography is used in follow-up of patients with known VUR.

CLASSIFICATION SYSTEM FOR GRADING
VUR (FIG. 18.17)

The classification of grading of VUR is based upon the extent of filling and dilatation by VUR of the ureter, the renal pelvis and the calyces.[67]

VUR AND RENAL SCARRING

Renal parenchymal defects or scars are reported in approximately one third of children with VUR detected during the course of investigation of urinary tract infection.[84] The association of VUR and bilateral renal scarring is called 'reflux nephropathy'. This association was initially described by Hodson and colleagues in 1960 in children during

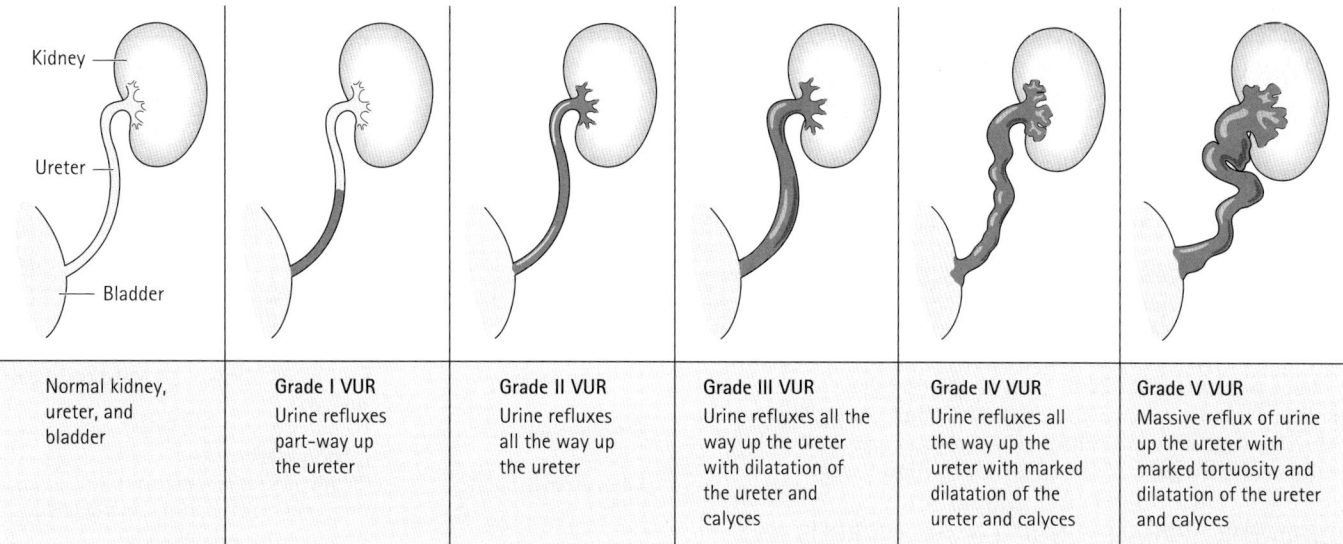

| Normal kidney, ureter, and bladder | Grade I VUR Urine refluxes part-way up the ureter | Grade II VUR Urine refluxes all the way up the ureter | Grade III VUR Urine refluxes all the way up the ureter with dilatation of the ureter and calyces | Grade IV VUR Urine refluxes all the way up the ureter with marked dilatation of the ureter and calyces | Grade V VUR Massive reflux of urine up the ureter with marked tortuosity and dilatation of the ureter and calyces |

Fig. 18.17   VUR grading, reproduced with kind permission from Pamela Lally.

the course of investigation of children with UTI.[85] As a result of this and other observations, there was a call for the investigation of all children with their first UTI to look for the presence of VUR. During this period and subsequently, reflux nephropathy has been identified as the cause of up to 25% of cases of end stage renal failure in children and young adults.[86] Between 10 and 23% of children with VUR and scarring (either unilateral or bilateral) are reported at risk of developing hypertension.[87] There are, however important issues to consider pertaining to these outcomes:

Firstly, the risk of such adverse outcomes may have been overestimated in these reports for the following reasons:

1. Many children had secondary VUR as a cause of their end-stage renal failure (ESRF) in association with obstructive uropathy and other abnormalities of the urinary tract.[88] In a recent analysis of causes of ESRF in 686 UK children reflux nephropathy accounted for 7.2% of cases.[89]

2. The incidence of hypertension in association with renal scars may be overestimated as the reports are from specialist centers. Wolfish and colleagues reported a lack of association between hypertension, renal scarring and primary vesicoureteric reflux.[90]

Secondly, there is an historic assumption that renal scarring is both acquired and preventable. The evidence to support this assumption is sparse. In the last two decades antenatal ultrasound has led to the identification of infants with vesicoureteric reflux, with associated 'scars' in up to 30% of cases in the absence of infection, suggesting underlying dysplasia.[71,91] Similar rates of renal scarring have been reported in asymptomatic siblings of children with VUR.[92] Thus, rates of renal scarring are similar in children with confirmed VUR whether or not there has been an associated UTI. These observations, together with the finding that the development of new scars is very unusual after the first UTI raise the possibility that many children with assumed 'acquired' renal scars, in fact have 'congenital' reflux nephropathy that is not amenable to modification by treatment.

MANAGEMENT OF CHILDREN WITH VUR
Conservative management of VUR
The majority of children will have resolution of their VUR over time.[93,94] Infants with confirmed VUR receive antibiotic prophylaxis, generally until potty trained. At this stage prophylaxis is discontinued if the child has been free of infections. Many clinicians will undertake nuclear cystography to ensure that the VUR has resolved prior to discontinuing the antibiotics.

Even after resolution of VUR, children with confirmed scars will need regular review to monitor for hypertension and in the case of bilateral renal scarring, progressive renal damage leading to chronic renal failure.

MCUG is an invasive procedure that generates distress in the child and parents and carries a significant radiation burden. Therefore the only indication to repeat this should be where surgery is contemplated.

Surgical management of VUR
In children with VUR identified following UTI, no significant differences in the risk for UTI or renal parenchymal injury were found in a meta-analysis of seven trials comprising 833 patients comparing antibiotic prophylaxis with combined surgery and antibiotics.[95] Surgical intervention should therefore be restricted to difficult cases with complex anomalies of the urinary tract. Such children are best referred to a unit where there is joint discussion between a pediatric urologist, nephrologist and radiologist. The standard reimplantation procedure is the Cohen or Leadbetter Politano technique, which involves changing the intramural segment of ureter through the bladder wall.[96] Newer, less invasive techniques, which involve endoscopic periureteral injection of polytetrafluoroethylene, glutaraldehyde cross-linked bovine collagen, dextranomer/hyaluronic acid copolymer, or polydimethylsiloxane have been trialled with promising results.[97–99]

SCREENING OF ASYMPTOMATIC SIBLINGS FOR VUR
In any family where VUR is detected parents are advised to keep a close eye out for UTI in other children. Ultrasound and MCUG are currently offered to newborn siblings of children with known VUR.

SUMMARY
At the present time, the diagnosis of VUR is most commonly made after urinary tract infection in childhood. The exact prevalence of VUR in childhood is unknown but is estimated to be in the region of 1–3%.[100] Although there is a strong association between VUR, UTI and renal scarring, evidence that vesicoureteric reflux is a modifiable risk factor in the development of kidney damage is weak. The effectiveness of antibiotic prophylaxis in the prevention of renal scarring has never been proven and urgently needs to be evaluated in a prospective, placebo-controlled trial.

ENURESIS (WETTING)

BLADDER MATURATION

Normal bladder function is established through a complex arrangement of autonomic and somatic nerves, integrated at various sites in the spinal cord, brainstem, midbrain and cerebral cortex.

In the neonatal period, micturition occurs in the region of 20 times per day due to uncontrolled detrusor contractions in a small capacity bladder. Bladder capacity increases during early childhood from 60–70 ml in the neonatal period to 120–140 ml at 4 years.[101] Bladder 'awareness' or sensation of bladder fullness develops in the first few years of life. Approximately 30% of 2-year-olds, 80% of 3-year-olds and 100% of 4-year-olds are able to indicate bladder awareness.[101] Concomitantly, children acquire the ability to suppress detrusor contractions voluntarily and coordinate sphincter and detrusor function. Daytime bladder control is achieved in most children by 4 years of age, while night-time bladder control is generally achieved by 5–7 years of age.[102,103]

IDIOPATHIC (PRIMARY) NOCTURNAL ENURESIS (bed wetting)

Nocturnal enuresis is the involuntary loss of urine at night, in the absence of structural abnormality of the urinary tract, at an age when a child could reasonably be expected to be dry (by consensus, at a developmental age of 5 years).[104] Nocturnal enuresis is often termed primary in children who have never achieved a satisfactory period of night-time dryness (approximately 80%). The remaining 20% have secondary enuresis, in that they have had a period of dryness, usually for at least 6 months, before the onset of wetting. Secondary enuresis is often ascribed to an unusually stressful event (e.g. parental separation, birth of a sibling).

Diurnal enuresis (daytime wetting) is often associated with bedwetting, however, the two conditions are generally considered separately. Daytime symptoms should prompt investigations to identify underlying causes such as congenital malformations and neurogenic disorders (see later).[105]

In the UK nocturnal enuresis is reported to be prevalent in approximately 15–20% of 5-year-olds, 7% of 7-year-olds, 5% of 10-year-olds, 2–3% of 12–14-year-olds and 1–2% of those aged 15 and over.[106,107]

PATHOPHYSIOLOGY OF NOCTURNAL ENURESIS

The pathophysiology of nocturnal enuresis is not clear, however the following factors alone, or in combination have been proposed to play a role (Table 18.7):

1. *Genetics.* There is often a family history of nocturnal enuresis in close relatives. Epidemiological studies show that if one parent has a history of nocturnal enuresis, his/her children are five to seven times more likely to have the disorder than those without an affected parent. Recent genetic studies in families with nocturnal enuresis have located two markers known as ENUR1 which flank the enuresis gene on chromosome 13.[108] Additional genetic loci for enuresis have been identified on chromosomes 12q and 22q11.[109]
2. *Delayed bladder maturation.* The high spontaneous resolution rate (approximately 15%/year[110]) of nocturnal enuresis implies a role for delayed maturation of a normal developmental process.[111] Nocturnal enuresis has been described as a genetically determined maturational disorder of the central nervous system due to an inhibition defect of the micturition reflex combined with a failure of conscious arousal in response to the sensation of bladder fullness.[111]
3. *Small bladder capacity.* Children with nocturnal enuresis have been noted to have a smaller bladder capacity than age-matched children who do not have nocturnal enuresis.[112]
4. *Decreased nocturnal antidiuretic hormone (ADH) secretion and polyuria.* Some children with nocturnal enuresis have decreased nocturnal secretion of ADH and increased urine production at night.[113] Since ADH secretion is thought to increase with bladder distension, small bladder capacity may contribute to this.[114]

Table 18.7 Differential diagnosis of enuresis

Diagnosis	Clinical indicators
Urinary tract infection	Other urinary tract symptoms, secondary onset wetting
Detrusor instability	Daytime symptoms of urinary frequency, urgency and urge incontinence usually with a minor degree of wetness and worse in the afternoons
Neuropathic bladder	Constant severe daytime wetting, soiling, lumbosacral dimple or nevus, abnormal gait, abnormal perianal or lower limb neurology, palpable bladder
Ectopic ureter	Constant dribble of urine between voidings
Posterior urethral valves	Poor urinary stream, daytime wetting, palpable bladder
Chronic renal disease	Chronic ill health, hypertension, palpable kidneys or bladder, anemia, polydipsia
Diabetes mellitus	Recent illness with weight loss, thirst and polydipsia

5. *Sleep disorders.* Elevated arousal thresholds have been reported in boys with nocturnal enuresis compared with non-enuretic boys,[115,116] however, sleep studies show that sleep patterns among children with and without enuresis are similar.[117]

MANAGEMENT OF NOCTURNAL ENURESIS

This should include a careful history and physical examination. The history should attempt to:
1. establish toileting history and distinguish primary from secondary enuresis;
2. identify predisposing environmental factors such as stress and emotional disturbances (particularly important in secondary enuresis);
3. establish the frequency of wet nights, fluid intake (day and night), the presence of daytime wetting or symptoms (frequency, dribbling) and the presence of constipation;
4. ascertain whether there is a family history of nocturnal enuresis.

The physical examination of the child with nocturnal enuresis should include:
1. documentation of growth and blood pressure (poor growth and/or hypertension may indicate renal disease);
2. abdominal palpation (assessment of constipation, enlarged bladder, renal masses);
3. examination of the spine and lower limb reflexes (spina bifida occulta).

Urinalysis may be useful to evaluate the presence of diabetes mellitus, diabetes insipidus, water intoxication, and urinary tract infection.

If no underlying pathology is suggested from the history and examination ('isolated' nocturnal enuresis), imaging of the urinary tract is not generally required. Children with concomitant kidney disease, urinary tract infection, neurogenic bladder or daytime bladder problems and children with refractory nocturnal enuresis that has failed to respond to treatment[118] should be referred to a pediatrician/pediatric nephrologist/urologist for further evaluation.

TREATMENT OF NOCTURNAL ENURESIS

In children aged between 5 and 7 years, the strategy of explanation, reassurance, star charts and praise or small rewards for dry nights is usually all that is necessary. For older children conditioning therapy with an enuresis alarm is the most effective treatment.[119] However, it is hard work and the child and family need to be closely supervised and supported.[120]

The role of medication remains controversial but may give some short-term relief. Desmopressin, a synthetic analogue of antidiuretic hormone, can be given as a nasal spray or tablet but relapse is usual when treatment finishes.[121] Imipramine is also effective but has a higher incidence of side-effects and is potentially lethal to children in accidental overdose.[122] There may be benefit from combining desmopressin with an alarm but again there are significant relapse rates.[123]

DIURNAL ENURESIS DUE TO BLADDER INSTABILITY

Wetting occurs during the day (and night), due to a functional disturbance of the detrusor muscle, which intermittently contracts during the filling/storage phase of the bladder at a time when the muscle is normally relaxed. The child has difficulty suppressing these contractions (normally an involuntary reflex), which therefore results in leakage of urine and urgency/urge incontinence before the child contracts the pelvic floor to stop micturition. The condition has a strong association with urinary tract infection and constipation, and emotional stresses may precipitate the problem in some children. Ectopic ureter is a rare cause of day- and night-time wetting and is suggested by a history of never having been dry in the day and dribbling of urine.

Treatment is again aimed at providing information and support along with establishing a routine of complete and regular emptying of the bladder to restore the child's confidence. Star charts and rewards may be helpful. Constipation must be vigorously treated and urine infection eradicated. If infections are proven, then the child will justify an ultrasound of the urinary tract with a check on bladder emptying. Day case assessment by experienced urology nurses may help to promote biofeedback training and promote compliance. An anticholinergic drug such as oxybutynin is usually effective but more conservative measures should be tried first. Some families require the support of a psychologist.

NEUROPATHIC BLADDER

Myelomeningocele is the main cause of neuropathic bladder in the pediatric population. Although children with myelomeningocele are usually born with normal kidneys, the function of the obstructed neuropathic bladder can result in chronic kidney damage if unrecognized.[124] Neuropathic bladder/sphincter dysfunction is complex and these children require careful assessment in specialist centers with expertise in urodynamics. The detrusor and/or striated pelvic floor muscles may lack spinal motor innovation (inactivity); with lesions above the level of the spinal motor neuron pelvic floor muscles are overactive during filling and voiding. This dyssynergic pelvic floor activity constitutes a functional infravesical obstruction during voiding, implying a high risk of kidney damage because of high emptying pressures.

Clean intermittent catheterization has been the major advance in the management of children with neuropathic bladders. It provides a means of both promoting continence as well as safeguarding kidney function. Oxybutynin to inhibit detrusor overactivity is often combined with intermittent catheterization.

Small capacity bladders may require augmentation procedures using the patient's own ureter or bowel. At the same time, the appendix can be used to fashion a Mitrofanoff channel to the umbilicus or laterally for intermittent catheterization. Patients and families derive great benefit from close support by a specialist nurse.

HEMATURIA

Children may present with gross (or macroscopic) hematuria, in which case they are usually quickly brought to medical attention, or they may be found to have microscopic hematuria on routine urinalysis using one of the many types of urinary testing strips (dipsticks). The degree of hematuria is a poor guide to the severity of any underlying disease, but careful examination of the urine is an important non-invasive diagnostic tool (Fig. 18.18).

Urinary dipsticks are very sensitive for blood and it is important that the manufacturer's instructions are followed closely and the test repeated on further samples. Microscopic hematuria may be transient and can occur in the context of exercise or stress. Urine could also be contaminated with blood from the external genital area, urethral meatus or menstrual blood.

Gross hematuria may be described as coke- or tea-colored due to the oxidized heme pigment, but it may also be bright red, suggesting an extrarenal or lower urinary tract source. Inquiry should be made of other possible causes of red urine, such as foods (beetroot, berries and food dyes) and drugs (e.g. rifampicin). Hemoglobinuria and myoglobinuria should also be considered (Table 18.8). Urate crystals may give the urine a pinkish tinge when present in high concentration, particularly in young infants.

URINE MICROSCOPY

Microscopy of fresh urine should be performed in all cases of hematuria to confirm the presence of red blood cells. Red cells hemolyze in standing urine, and fresh urine is also better for the identification of red cell or heme granular casts, which are strong pointers to a renal source for the hematuria (Fig. 18.19). Microscopy may also reveal pyuria and/or motile bacteria (suggesting infection) or crystals (using contrast microscopy). It may be possible to differentiate glomerular bleeding, when the red cells appear dysmorphic, from bleeding originating from the lower urinary tract, when the red cells tend to be of uniform shape and size.[125]

CAUSES OF HEMATURIA

The causes of hematuria are listed in Table 18.9. Many of the causes can be differentiated on the basis of the history, examination and urinalysis. If gross hematuria is reported, then the child or observer should be asked if it is more prominent in the initial or terminal parts of the urinary stream. Initial hematuria suggests a urethral cause, but this line of questioning is unlikely to be as relevant as it is in the adult patient, where bladder tumors and stones are much more prominent causes of hematuria.

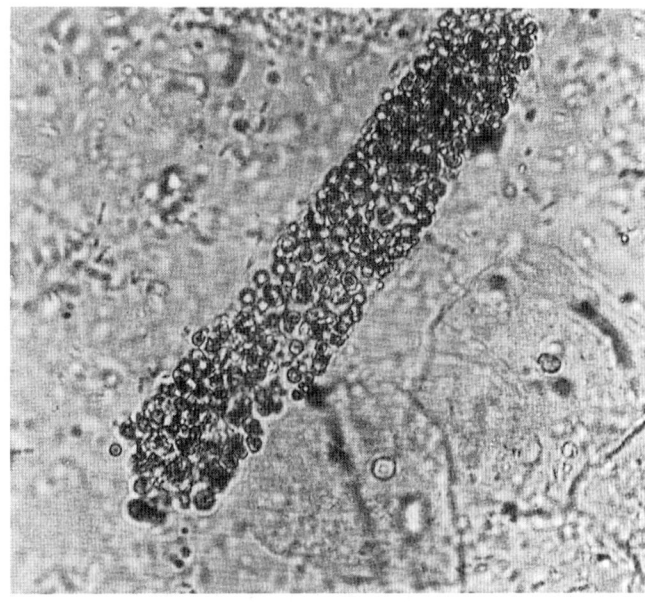

Fig. 18.18 Red cell granular cast. The outlines of many erythrocytes can still be made out clearly (× 400).

Table 18.8 Interpretation of urine dipsticks in renal disease

Feature	Method	Comment
pH	Methyl red Bromothymol blue	Normal range 4.5–8; typically in early morning urine pH 8: renal tubular acidosis, infection with urea-splitting organisms
Hemoglobin	Ortholidine + peroxidase	Detects hemoglobin and myoglobin; does not distinguish hemoglobinuria from hematuria False negative: ascorbic acid, rifampin (rifampicin) False positive: iodine, hypochlorite
Protein	Protein binding to tetrabromophenol blue	Only detects albumin, does not detect light chains False positive: alkaline urine
Glucose	Glucose oxidase peroxidase	Also detects fructose, lactose, galactose False negative: ascorbic acid
Leukocyte esterase	3-Hydroxy-5-phenolpyrrole + leukocyte esterase Griess's test	Detects intact or lysed leukocytes; sensitivity/specificity contentious False positive: vaginal contamination
Nitrite		Some organisms do not reduce nitrate Urine in bladder > 4 h for accurate result

Infection

Hematuria associated with dysuria, frequency, enuresis and suprapubic discomfort suggests a hemorrhagic cystitis, while systemic upset, fever, abdominal pain or loin tenderness suggest pyelonephritis. Urinary tract infection, either proven or suspected, remains a common cause of hematuria. Since other symptoms and signs may be minimal, it is essential that appropriate urine cultures are taken before treatment is initiated.

Viral infections can result in acute hemorrhagic cystitis, particularly adenovirus types 11 and 21. This is usually a self-limiting illness with resolution towards the end of the first week.

Persistent dysuria, hematuria and sterile pyuria would suggest tuberculosis, in the right clinical context, but this would be a very rare cause of hematuria in children in Western countries. Infection with *Schistosoma haematobium* is an important cause of hematuria in endemic areas such as the Middle East and Africa. The ova can cause a granulomatous reaction in the bladder wall and lower ureter, and prompt treatment is essential (see Ch. 28).

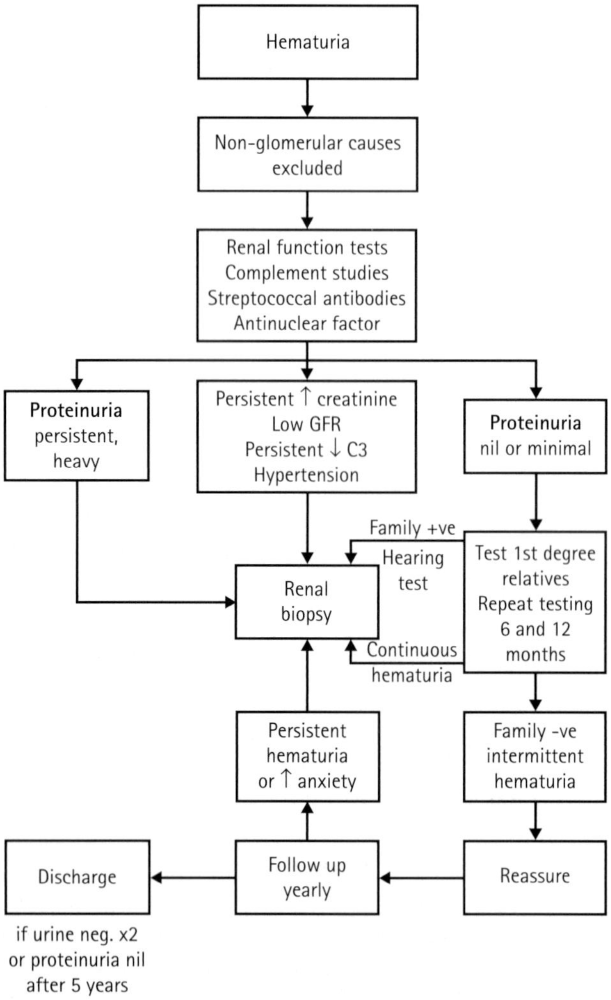

Fig. 18.19 A scheme for the management of children with hematuria.

Table 18.9 Causes of hematuria

1. Infection	a. Bacterial b. Viral c. Schistosomiasis d. Tuberculosis
2. Glomerular diseases	
3. Stones	a. Urolithiasis b. Idiopathic hypercalciuria
4. Trauma	
5. Anatomic abnormalities	a. Congenital abnormalities, e.g. pelviureteric junction obstruction b. Polycystic kidneys c. Tumor
6. Vascular	a. Arteritis b. Infarction and thrombosis c. Loin pain–hematuria syndrome
7. Hematological	a. Coagulopathies b. Sickle-cell disease
8. Drugs	e.g. Cyclophosphamide
9. Exercise-induced	
10. Factitious	

Table 18.10 Investigations for children with renal calculi

1. Urinalysis including pH and urine for amino acids
2. Urine culture
3. Plasma biochemistry including creatinine, chloride, bicarbonate, calcium, phosphate, urate, magnesium levels
4. Second morning urine sample for calcium:creatinine and oxalate: creatinine ratios (24 h urine collections to confirm hypercalciuria or hyperoxaluria in older children)
5. Analysis of calculus if available

Glomerulonephritis

The history of an upper respiratory tract or other infection, particularly if associated with gross hematuria, is suggestive of some form of acute postinfectious glomerulonephritis. Recurrent macroscopic hematuria in the older child raises the suspicion of IgA nephropathy.

A positive family history of renal disease with or without deafness suggests the possibility of hereditary nephritis (see section on Glomerulornephritis).

Renal calculi

Incidence

The incidence of urinary tract calculi in children is approximately 1–5/100 000 in resource rich countries. It is much higher in areas of the world where stone disease is endemic, e.g. the Middle East. In these areas, there are more likely to be urate calculi, whereas in Europe most children with stones will have them as a result of infective causes. These are more likely to occur in the presence of obstruction to the urinary flow combined with infection, reduced fluid intake and episodes of dehydration. Stone formation may also occur due to underlying genetic factors such as hyperoxaluria or tubular transport problems such as cystinuria and hypercalciuria syndromes.

Clinical features

The classical presentation of renal colic, common in adult patients, is rare in childhood. More often calculi are recognized as a result of investigations in children for urinary tract infection or hematuria. Many children are diagnosed incidentally when imaging techniques such as ultrasound are carried out for investigation of abdominal pain. Certain children are at high risk of renal calculi and these include ex-premature babies (risk factors include transient hypercalciuria and/or furosemide use), those who are immobilized or who have a neuropathic bladder. A family history of renal calculi should always be sought.

Investigation

Most stones are associated with infection and magnesium/ammonium phosphate complex. However, screening investigations, as listed in Table 18.10, are necessary, as hypercalciuria and hyperoxaluria may both need treatment, and the amino acid profile should define cystinuria.[126] Rare inborn errors of purine metabolism, xanthinuria and 2,8-dihydroxyadenine due to adenine phosphoribosyl transferase deficiency need to be remembered.

Management

This will depend upon the severity of the presentation, but percutaneous nephrostomy to treat an obstructed kidney, due to stones, is rarely required. Renal ultrasound is the most sensitive method for identifying stones within the kidney or renal pelvis, as these will show as echo-bright densities casting acoustic shadows. Occasionally, ultrasound will miss ureteric calculi in a child with acute renal colic with or without hematuria. A plain abdominal X-ray and Intravenous Urogram (IVU) will possibly be required.

Extracorporeal shockwave lithotripsy (ESWL) can be successfully performed under general anesthesia in children, but may be less successful if the stone is very hard (e.g. cystine), if it is located at the lower pole calyx or if it is very large and fragments are likely to obstruct the ureter. There is some evidence that ESWL causes a short term of reduction in renal function and may have long-term effects on developing kidneys.

Direct nephrolithotomy may be required for a large staghorn calculus in the renal pelvis. Other urological techniques such as percutaneous nephrolithotomy and ureteroscopy may be attempted in some children.

Trauma

Hematuria is associated with an obvious history of a damaging event. There is often bruising and other signs of external injury. With increasing recognition of the spectrum of sexual abuse, it is important that a careful history be taken if the injury involves the anogenital region.

Anatomic abnormalities

Although it is sometimes hard to equate abnormalities on X-ray with hematuria, there is no doubt that problems such as hydronephrosis, due for example to pelviureteric junction obstruction, can be a cause of hematuria. Although autosomal dominant polycystic kidney disease is increasingly recognized in childhood by the use of ultrasound scanning, it very rarely results in hematuria in the pediatric population.

The major kidney tumor of childhood is nephroblastoma (Wilms' tumor), and this usually presents as an abdominal mass, with one third of patients having associated hematuria, mainly microscopic. Bladder tumors are very rare in childhood[127] and so cystoscopy is rarely indicated, unlike the case in the adult population.

Vascular and hematological causes

Hematuria may occur in the context of any child with a problem such as hemophilia, leukemia or sickle-cell disease. The hematuria in the latter condition is presumably due to sickling of erythrocytes in the hypertonic, hypoxemic medulla, with resulting local papillary infarcts. It is unlikely to be the initial presentation.

Gross hematuria, associated with a palpable mass, in a newborn infant, would suggest renal vein thrombosis. Hematuria may be part of the symptom complex in a multisystem disorder such as polyarteritis.

The loin pain–hematuria syndrome, which predominantly affects young women, is rare in childhood and requires renal angiography in suspected cases.

Drugs

There is an extensive list of drugs, poisons and ingested substances which can give rise to hematuria.[128] Cyclophosphamide is a well-recognized cause of a sterile hemorrhagic cystitis, and a high fluid intake should be maintained during the use of this drug. Other drugs such as sulfonamides can cause crystalluria.

Exercise-induced

Hematuria may occur after severe exercise and has usually disappeared within 48 h. It would appear to have a glomerular origin and is an accentuation of the small amount of blood excreted by a number of people after heavy exercise.

Factitious hematuria

This may be part of the spectrum of Munchausen syndrome by proxy, where the child's carer (usually the mother) adds blood to the urine sample after it has been passed. There may be other pointers in the history or behavioral observations, which suggest this diagnosis.[129] A forensic laboratory may be able to determine whether the origin of the blood is from the parent or child.

INVESTIGATIONS IN A CHILD WITH HEMATURIA

The tests performed will depend upon the information provided from the history, examination and urinalysis (Fig. 18.19). Again, it should be stressed that *microscopy* on a fresh urine sample can be invaluable, as identification of dysmorphic red cells and heme granular or red cell casts (the urine should be centrifuged for 3 min at 3000 rev/min) strongly suggests a nephritic process and the child will be investigated accordingly. A *familial* condition may be detected by testing the urine of all immediate family members, particularly in cases of persistent microscopic hematuria.

Urine culture

A proven bacterial infection will lead to the appropriate investigations. Urine is rarely cultured for viruses, but should be considered in epidemics.

Hematology

Full blood count and film. Coagulation tests if appropriate.

Biochemistry

1. plasma urea, electrolytes, creatinine, calcium, phosphate, alkaline phosphatase, albumin, total protein;
2. urine calcium/creatinine ratio on second morning sample (if > 0.7 mmol/mmol confirm with a 24-hour collection).

Radiology

1. An ultrasound of the urinary tract in experienced hands should define any hydronephrosis, masses, renal calculi, etc. A plain abdominal X-ray is not required routinely.
2. An i.v. urogram may be ordered to confirm any suspicion raised on the initial screening ultrasound or to define the level of obstruction if ureteric stones are suspected.
3. An MCUG or cystoscopy is *rarely* necessary in childhood, but may be indicated based on the history. If there is recurrent or persistent gross unexplained hematuria then cystoscopy during an episode may localize the bleeding to one kidney (in which an anatomic abnormality is probably present) or to both kidneys (making glomerulonephritis more likely).
4. Further radiological investigations may include CT scanning or MRI for renal masses, radionuclide scans to define parenchymal masses or rarely renal arteriography.

Further tests for glomerulonephritis

Glomerulonephritis should be suspected if there are characteristic urinary changes or if the hematuria is persistent and no other cause can be found. The appropriate investigations will be discussed in detail later but should include:

1. throat swab for bacteria and viruses;
2. antistreptolysin O titer and other streptococcal antigens;
3. complement studies;
4. autoantibody screen including antinuclear factor antibody;
5. viral titers including screening for hepatitis B surface antigen.

Hearing test

In cases of suspected familial nephritis (Alport syndrome), in which a high tone sensorineural deafness is present.

Renal biopsy

This is never routine and is only performed when there are indications of a more serious and potentially progressive disease, such as: progressive or persistent renal impairment; hypertension; persistent hypocomplementemia; heavy proteinuria; a familial disease that has not been characterized; or a systemic disorder where therapy may be influenced by the histopathological findings, e.g. systemic lupus erythematosus (SLE). Renal biopsies are also carried out in children with persistent microscopic hematuria (usually of greater than 1 year's duration), often because of the family's request to know a specific diagnosis and prognosis (Fig. 18.19).

Only nephrologists or radiologists experienced in the technique should carry out a renal biopsy. They should have access to expert pathology advice, based on light and electron microscopy as well as immunofluorescence (or immunohistochemistry). In most instances, the biopsy is performed under ultrasound guidance in the sedated child. The biopsy can be carried out as a day case procedure with appropriate preparation of the child and family.[130] An open renal biopsy under general anesthetic is only necessary in the very young child. In expert hands the morbidity associated with renal biopsy is low.

The commonest cause of hematuria in childhood is infection

Children with macroscopic hematuria and persistent microscopic hematuria should undergo a renal tract ultrasound but rarely need cystoscopy

Hypercalciuria can cause hematuria and can be screened for by a second morning urine calcium/creatinine ratio

GLOMERULONEPHRITIS

Glomerulonephritis, or more simply nephritis, is both a generic term for several diseases, and a histopathological term signifying inflammation and proliferation of cells within the glomerulus. In many instances the inflammatory changes are initiated by immunological mechanisms, but in others the pathogenesis is unknown.

Injury may be limited to the kidney alone, or the immune or non-immune mechanisms may be part of a systemic disorder (Table 18.11).

There is still very little understanding of the specific events involved with glomerulonephritis, and so when therapy has been employed it has tended to be 'blunderbuss' in nature, with broad-spectrum immunosuppressive drugs such as corticosteroids, azathioprine and cyclophosphamide, or other therapies such as plasma exchange.

PATHOLOGY

Many of the categories of so-called primary glomerulonephritis (Table 18.11) are based on histopathological descriptions obtained from renal biopsy specimens. The terminology is derived from changes that are found on light, electron and immunofluorescent microscopy (Figs 18.20, 18.21).

CLINICAL PATTERNS OF GLOMERULONEPHRITIS

Patients with glomerulonephritis may present with:

1. asymptomatic *hematuria* and/or proteinuria;
2. *acute nephritic syndrome* characterized by hematuria, oliguria, edema and hypertension. The hematuria is heavy with red cell casts on microscopy. Proteinuria is variable;

Table 18.11 Classification of glomerular disorders

Primary glomerulonephritis
1. Immune complex glomerulonephritis
   a. Postinfectious acute glomerulonephritis
   b. IgA nephropathy (Berger disease)
   c. Membranoproliferative glomerulonephritis (types I to III)
   d. Membranous glomerulonephritis (idiopathic)

2. Anti-GBM-antibody-mediated glomerulonephritis

3. Uncertain etiology, e.g. minimal lesion glomerulonephritis, focal segmental glomerulosclerosis

Glomerulonephritis associated with systemic disorders
1. Immunologically mediated
   a. Henoch–Schönlein purpura
   b. Systemic lupus erythematosus and other collagen disorders, e.g. scleroderma
   c. Polyarteritis nodosa, Wegener's granulomatosis and other vasculitides
   d. Mixed cryoglobulinemia
   e. Systemic infections (subacute bacterial endocarditis, shunt nephritis, syphilis, malaria, hepatitis B, HIV)

2. Hereditary disorders
   a. Familial nephritis, e.g. Alport syndrome
   b. Sickle cell anemia

3. Other conditions
   a. Diabetes mellitus
   b. Amyloidosis

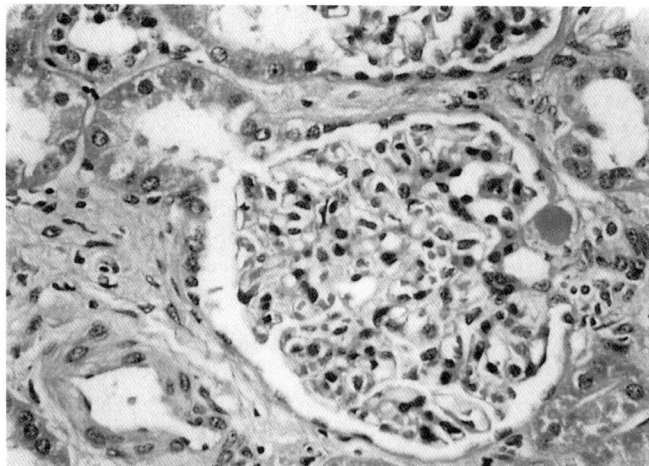

Fig. 18.20 Light microscopy of a normal glomerulus. Part of the proximal tubule at upper left-hand corner and hilum on the right.

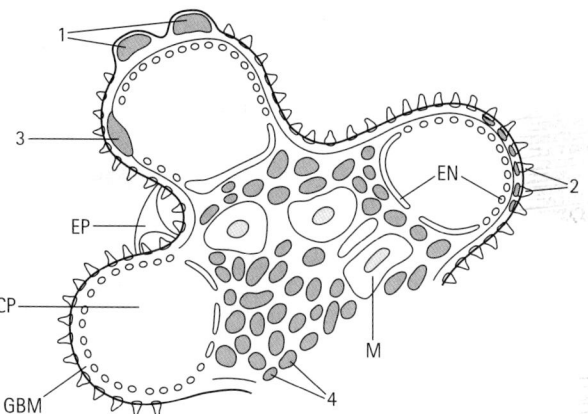

Fig. 18.21 Schematic depiction of the anatomy of the glomerulus and possible sites of immune complex deposition (CP, capillary space; EN, endothelial; EP, epithelial; GBM, glomerular basement membrane; M, mesangial cell). Deposits are in the following locations: 1, subepithelial lumps; 2, intramembranous; 3, subendothelial; 4, mesangial.

3. *nephrotic syndrome* characterized by heavy proteinuria leading to hypoalbuminemia and edema with hyperlipidemia. The urinalysis shows heavy proteinuria (+++ or > 5 g/L) with variable hematuria. Microscopy may show fatty casts and free fat droplets.

It is important to appreciate that there is a spectrum of clinical presentation and patients may have a mixed picture of nephritis/nephrosis. For example, the majority of children with Henoch–Schönlein purpura (HSP) have nephritis with asymptomatic hematuria and/or proteinuria, which usually resolves, but may progress into a nephritic syndrome. If the proteinuria is so heavy that hypoalbuminemia results, then the patient may have the clinical picture of nephrotic syndrome.

ACUTE GLOMERULONEPHRITIS

Acute glomerulonephritis usually presents as acute nephritic syndrome. This is a constellation of clinical signs including acute fluid overload, hematuria (often 'coca cola'-colored urine) and hypertension. Proteinuria is often present as is some degree of renal insufficiency. The etiology of acute nephritic syndrome is varied but is most commonly due to post-infectious glomerulonephritis of which group A beta hemolytic *Streptococcus* is the most frequent organism involved. Other

causes include SLE, antineutrophil cytoplasmic antibody (ANCA)-associated vasculitis, and Goodpasture syndrome (Anti-GBM disease) but any of the more chronic forms of glomerulonephritis may present with acute nephritis.

Initial investigations should therefore include the following:
- urine;
- urine microscopy: red cells and casts;
- protein/creatinine ratio;
- hematology;
- full blood count and film (for example to exclude haemolytic uremic syndrome);
- CRP/ESR;
- biochemisty;
- renal function: urea, creatinine, electrolytes (including calcium status) and acid–base status;
- immunology;
- C3, C4;
- antinuclear antibody (ANA), dsDNA (double-stranded DNA) Ab;
- ANCA;
- anti-glomerular basement membrane (GBM) Ab;
- microbiology;
- throat swab;
- ASOT (anti-streptolysin-O-titre);
- anti-DNAse B;
- urine culture.

ACUTE POST-STREPTOCOCCAL GLOMERULONEPHRITIS (APSGN)

Group A beta hemolytic *Streptococcus* is the most common organism implicated in post infectious glomerulonephritis. In resource rich countries it usually follows a nasopharyngeal infection whilst in developing countries antecedent skin infections are more common.[131] Although the disease is uncommon in Western countries, it is still prevalent in many parts of the world where overcrowding, poor nutrition and widespread skin sepsis still prevail.

Other organisms that have been implicated in post infectious glomerulonephritis include *Staphylococcus aureus*, *Streptococcus pneumoniae*, *Haemophilus influenzae*, *Escherichia coli*, *Salmonella* and *Mycoplasma* species. Viruses such as Coxackie, ECHO, Epstein–Barr, varicella, hanta and influenza as well as rickettsial, fungal and parasitic organisms have also been etiological agents.

Clinical features

Acute post streptococcal glomerulonephritis (APSGN) usually affects children aged 5–15 years but can occur at any age. The nephritic complication of streptococcal infection is commoner in males. The onset on symptoms usually occurs about 7–14 d after the pharyngeal infection but several weeks after skin infection (Fig. 18.22). Children present with features of an acute nephritic syndrome. There is often a history of general malaise, anorexia, abdominal pain and headache but the development of frank hematuria and generalized edema are often the features that bring the child to medical attention. Oliguria may only be revealed on direct questioning.

Examination may reveal signs of fluid overload including generalized edema, pulmonary edema, pleural effusions and occasionally congestive cardiac failure. Hypertension is found in 60–80% and rarely patients develop hypertensive encephalopathy with headaches, alteration in mental state, convulsions and coma.

Investigations

The investigations are as for acute glomerulonephritis (p. 573)

Urinary abnormalities include hematuria, microscopic and macroscopic and variable proteinuria. Urine microscopy reveals numerous dysmorphic red cells and heme granular casts. Other findings include pyuria, white cell, granular and hyaline casts.

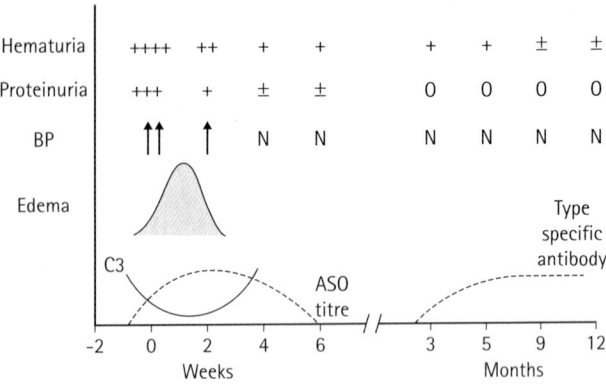

Fig. 18.22   Course of acute poststreptococcal glomerulonephritis.

A full blood count may demonstrate a mild normochromic, normocytic anemia due to dilution. Renal function tests including plasma electrolytes, bicarbonate, urea and creatinine may show a variable degree of renal impairment, hyperkalemia and acidosis. Serum albumin levels and total protein may be low but generally not to levels seen in nephrotic syndrome.

The diagnosis is confirmed by the association of evidence of a previous streptococcal infection together with the presence of hypocomplementemia. Throat swabs should be cultured but in addition blood should be sent to identify antibody titers to streptococcal antigens. The antistreptolysin O (ASO) titer is present in 16–18% of healthy children and may not rise after skin infections and therefore anti-DNAse B and hyaluronidase antibodies may be useful in making the diagnosis. Measurement of total hemolytic complement and C3 and C4 are essential in making the diagnosis. C3 is nearly always significantly low in APSGN, often to levels < 50% of normal. C4 is usually normal or very mildly depressed. Other immunological tests including antinuclear antibodies, anti-neutrophil cytoplasmic antibody, anti-glomerular basement membrane antibody (anti-GBM), immunoglobulin and cryoglobulin titers are done to exclude other diagnoses.

Radiological investigations include a chest X-ray to assess for cardiomegaly, pleural effusions and pulmonary edema and a renal ultrasound, which may show large bright kidneys in support of the diagnosis.

Renal biopsy is indicated only if there is significant deterioration of the renal function, nephrotic syndrome or other atypical features, particularly if any of the other immunological tests are abnormal, suggesting an alternative diagnosis. In rapidly progressive glomerulonephritis (a rapid progression of renal failure) renal biopsy may demonstrate extensive crescent formation. In APSGN the C3 levels normalize within 6–8 weeks and failure to do so would be another indication for renal biopsy at this stage to assess for an alternative diagnosis (usually membranoproliferative glomerulonephritis).

Treatment

A 10-day course of penicillin is prescribed for the patient and any culture-positive family members. Although there is no evidence that it affects the natural history of the glomerulonephritis, it is known to limit the spread of the nephritogenic strains. The management of the acute nephritis is otherwise supportive and depends on the degree of renal impairment and hypertension. It may include careful fluid balance, diuretics, antihypertensives and management of electrolyte imbalance. In a small number who develop a rapidly progressive nephritis dialysis is required, although most can be managed conservatively.

Prognosis

Children with APSGN can usually be discharged once renal function is improving and hypertension is controlled. Complement levels need to be rechecked at 6–8 weeks to confirm that these have normalized. Complete recovery occurs in over 95% of children with APSGN.[132] The incidence

of chronic renal insufficiency post APSGN is <1% although a small number may have persistent hypertension or proteinuria. Microscopic hematuria may last up to 1–2 years. Some patients with a pre-existing chronic glomerulonephritis may present with an exacerbation secondary to a streptococcal illness and persistence of urinary abnormalities may be an indication for renal biopsy, which can identify an underlying diagnosis.

Second attacks of APSGN are rare and there is no evidence that penicillin prevents future recurrences. Once the urinalysis, blood pressure and renal function have normalized the patient can be discharged from long-term follow up.

IgA NEPHROPATHY

IgA nephropathy was first described in 1968 and is thought to be the most common primary glomerulonephritis worldwide. There is marked geographical variation in the incidence, IgA nephropathy accounting for 18–40% of glomerulonephritides in Japan, France, Italy and Australia compared with 2–10% in the UK, US and Canada.[133] Part of this variation may be due to the regional difference in practice. For example in Japan all children aged 6–18 have routine urinalysis screening thus identifying patients who might otherwise have failed to present to medical services for investigation. There is a 2:1 to 6:1 male-to-female ratio for IgA nephropathy, with the peak incidence in the second and third decades of life.

Clinical features

The commonest feature is macroscopic hematuria, which has been reported in more than 80% of children from Europe and the USA. Asymptomatic microscopic hematuria with or without proteinuria is the second most common method of presentation with acute nephritic syndrome, nephrotic syndrome or a mixed picture being relatively unusual. The classical picture is of recurrent episodes of macroscopic hematuria occurring 1–3 d after an upper respiratory tract infection. This is in contrast with APSGN, where the latent period is about 7 d. Following acute episodes the macroscopic hematuria resolves but microscopic hematuria may persist with or without proteinuria. Acute renal failure, if present, usually resolves.

Diagnosis

The condition is often recognized from the typical clinical pattern of recurrent episodes of macroscopic hematuria. Laboratory investigations are necessary to exclude other causes of hematuria: In particular, normal complements and ANA/dsDNA to exclude postinfectious glomerulonephritis and SLE, respectively. Serum IgA levels are only elevated in 6–16% of children and therefore not helpful in making the diagnosis. There is therefore no specific diagnostic test apart from the histological findings on renal biopsy.

Renal biopsy

The diagnostic finding on renal biopsy is the presence of mesangial IgA, immunofluorescent deposits together with lesser amounts of IgG, IgM and C3. Light microscopy usually reveals mesangial proliferation and increased mesangial matrix. These findings also occur in HSP, which is histopathologically indistinguishable although clinical features differentiate the two. However, IgA nephropathy and HSP have been known to occur in the same patient separated by several years or in members of the same family, suggesting that the two conditions do have a common immunopathological basis.

Treatment

There is a lack of multicentre randomized, controlled trials to assess the efficacy of treatment modalities in children with IgA nephropathy. Some small studies on the use of tonsillectomy have found a reduction in episodes of macroscopic hematuria but none have shown an effect on the progression of renal disease. There is some evidence in adults that fish oil supplements (FOS) may delay the loss of renal function but this has not been demonstrated in children to date.[134]

In children with significant proteinuria and/or progressive renal disease, angiotensin-converting enzyme (ACE) inhibitors +/− angiotensin II receptor antagonists[135] and rigorous control of hypertension are advocated.

The use of immunosuppression in the management of chronic IgA nephropathy remains controversial due to the lack of randomized, controlled studies but for those with a rapidly progressive glomerulonephritis small studies have shown a benefit from high-dose methylprednisolone, cyclophosphamide and plasma exchange.

The results of further trials involving ACE inhibitors, fish oils and mycophenolate are awaited.

Prognosis

In the past it was thought that IgA nephropathy in childhood was a benign disease. It is known that about 25% of adults develop renal failure over 20 years. A long-term follow-up study of 241 Japanese children showed that 5% of children developed chronic renal failure by 5 years, 6% by 10 years and 11% by 15 years from the onset of the disease. Another study of 103 children found predicted kidney survival to be 94% at 5 years, 87% at 10 years and 70% at 20 years. The difference in outcome may relate to different populations. Poor prognostic features include older age at onset, proteinuria, hypertension, renal impairment and glomeruolsclerosis on renal biopsy.

In children with intermittent macroscopic hematuria with or without persistent microscopic hematuria there is little to be gained from renal biopsy as no specific treatment is available. If proteinuria is present then biopsy is advised to make the diagnosis and exclude other diagnoses which may benefit from treatment. Some advocate renal biopsy if microscopic hematuria persists for more than 1–2 years in order to give a clearer prognosis and to allay parental anxiety. The results may also be relevant for future employment counseling, particularly with respect to the Armed Forces.

HENOCH-SCHÖNLEIN PURPURA NEPHRITIS

HSP is the commonest vasculitis of childhood with an incidence of 10–20/100 000 per year. It is a small vessel vasculitis with characteristic skin involvement of a vasculitic rash on the extensor surfaces, particularly on the lower limbs, gastrointestinal symptoms and joint manifestations. Renal involvement is usually reported in between 28 and 60% of cases. This develops within 3 months in 97% of cases but may occur years later in a small number. Features include microscopic hematuria, proteinuria, a nephrotic/nephritic picture, renal impairment and hypertension.[136]

The natural history is that most patients make a good recovery with the incidence of severe long-term renal morbidity/mortality being about 1–2%.[137] The presence of a nephrotic or nephritic picture or renal impairment is a poor prognostic indicator and these patients should be considered for renal biopsy. The severity of the histological changes is a guide to appropriate therapy.

The histological changes vary from mild mesangial proliferation to diffuse proliferative changes with crescent formation or membranoproliferative changes. Immunofluorescence shows mesangial IgA deposits and is indistinguishable from IgA nephropathy.

The treatment of HSP remains controversial. There is some evidence to suggest that steroids may prevent development of renal involvement when given early in the disease course although this has not been confirmed by recent prospective randomized, controlled[138] studies. There is a lack of clear data on the treatment of established nephritis. However, as with IgA nephropathy, in those with severe disease there are reports of good outcomes using intensive immunosupression.

Children with a history of HSP nephritis should be followed up long term. Although most will not have severe long-term sequelae there is a risk of hypertension and renal impairment even in those with mild disease at onset and girls are at increased risk of hypertension in pregnancy.[139] Therefore at minimum an annual check of BP and urinalysis is recommended.

MEMBRANOPROLIFERATIVE (MESANGIOCAPILLARY) GLOMERULONEPHRITIS

This condition is uncommon in children and usually presents in the second decade of life. The clinical presentation includes asymptomatic microscopic hematuria +/− proteinuria, frank hematuria, nephrotic syndrome, renal impairment and hypertension. In about one third of children hypertension and elevated creatinine are evident at presentation.

Investigations may reveal similar features to that of post-streptococcal glomerulonephritis including a low C3 in over 50% of cases and raised ASO titer levels in some. However in APSGN C3 levels return to normal in 6–8 weeks. Therefore both the persistence of a low C3 and/or persistent heavy proteinuria/impaired renal function are indicators that a renal biopsy should be performed to distinguish these conditions.

There is also an association between partial lipodystrophy, low C3 and the presence of a C3 nephritic factor (autoantibodies that bind to and stabilize the C3 convertase of the alternative or classical pathway, thus resulting in continued complement activation).

Renal biopsy identifies three distinct types of membranoproliferative glomerulonephritis:

Type 1 MPGN

This is the most common form with glomeruli revealing an accentuation of the lobular pattern due to a generalized increase in mesangial cells and matrix. The glomerular capillary walls appear thickened and in some areas duplicated or split due to interposition of mesangial cytoplasm and matrix between the endothelial cells and glomerular basement membrane. Crescents may be present and may be associated with a rapidly progressive glomerulonephritis. Deposition of C3 and a lesser amount of immunoglobulin may be shown on immunofluorescence. Electron microscopy confirms the presence of deposits in the subendothelial and mesangial regions.

Type 2 MPGN

In this type the capillary walls demonstrate irregular, ribbon-like thickening due to the dense deposits. Electron microscopy reveals extensive homogenous electron dense material in the glomerular basement membrane in the region of but distinct from the lamina densa.

Type 3 MPGN

This is sometimes considered a variant of type 1. There are contiguous subepithelial and subendothelial deposits associated with disruption of the basement membrane.

Treatment and prognosis

Overall this is a chronic progressive disease with 50% of patients progressing to end-stage renal disease within 10 years of diagnosis. The outcome for type 2 appears to be worse than for types 1 or 3. In view of the rarity of the condition large randomized trials are difficult to perform. However studies have shown a probable benefit in those treated with long-term alternate-day steroids in those with MPGN types 1 and 3.[139,140] Treatment with steroids should probably be reserved for those with nephrotic syndrome or renal impairment. There may be a benefit in using an ACE inhibitor in those with lesser degrees of proteinuria.

Membranoproliferative glomerulonephritis associated with systemic disease

MPGN is usually a primary kidney disease without systemic manifestations. However the features of MPGN may be seen on the renal biopsies of patients with other conditions such as HSP, SLE or polyarteritis.

MPGN features may also accompany chronic infections such as subacute bacterial endocarditis, infected ventricular-atrial shunts, syphilis, hepatitis C, hepatitis B, candidiasis and malaria. The infecting organisms usually have low virulence and the host is chronically seeded with foreign antigen. The combination with host antibodies results in complexes being deposited in the glomerular mesangium, producing mesangial proliferation and interposition. Immune deposits are subendothelial and in the mesangium. Hence, the disease is like type I MPGN with hypocomplementemia. If elimination of the infecting agent is achieved then the lesion may heal, but with scarring and there is a possibility of progression to renal failure.

Chronic infections may also produce the pathological changes of membranous glomerulopathy, focal glomerulosclerosis and focal and segmental proliferative glomerulonephritis.

MEMBRANOUS GLOMERULONEPHRITIS

Membranous glomerulonephritis (MGN) is the commonest cause of nephrotic syndrome in adults, but is uncommon in childhood, accounting for less than 5% of pediatric patients undergoing biopsy for nephrotic syndrome. It very rarely causes hematuria alone. Membranous glomerulonephritis is defined by the histological appearances on light microscopy of diffuse thickening of the glomerular basement membranes without significant proliferative changes. On silver staining, the continuous subepithelial deposits give a spike appearance to the glomerular basement membrane, and immunofluorescent microscopy demonstrates granular deposits of IgG and C3, which can be also identified by electron microscopy.

Clinical features

The disease can occur at any age, but is most common in the second decade of life. The presentation may be covert, with disease discovered at routine urinalysis, or it may present with nephrotic syndrome and, less often, macroscopic hematuria. The blood pressure and C3 levels are normal.

There is a lower threshold for biopsying children who present with nephrotic syndrome over 10 years of age, because of the likelihood of finding a condition other than minimal lesion glomerulonephritis, such as MGN. In practice, unless there are other unusual features such as hypertension children may be treated with a month of daily steroids and steroid resistance is the indication for renal biopsy. Membranous glomerulonephritis may occasionally be seen in association with SLE, drug therapy, such as gold or penicillamine, syphilis, hepatitis B virus infection and some cancers.

Treatment and prognosis

Spontaneous remission is quite common with this pathology, and the present consensus is that children who are not clinically nephrotic are at only slight risk of developing renal failure in the long term and do not require treatment. However, children with a prolonged nephrotic syndrome may have a poor prognosis and alternate-day steroid therapy has been suggested. The small numbers of patients make randomized, controlled trials very difficult to perform in children. The persistent nephrotic state is best controlled with salt restriction, diuretics, lipid-lowering drugs and ACE inhibitors and sometimes anticoagulation.

SYSTEMIC LUPUS ERYTHEMATOSUS

SLE is a disease of immune dysregulation that affects about 1 in 2000 individuals (see also Ch. 29 on bones and joints etc.) Children represent about 15–20% of all SLE patients. It is a multisystem disease that has a wide spectrum of manifestations. Diagnosis is based on the presence of four or more of the 11 identified criteria. These include clinical features together with immunological findings of a positive ANA and as DNA and hematological abnormalities such as hemolytic anemia, leucopenia and thrombocytopenia. Lupus is rare before puberty although onset in the first year of life has been recorded. The female-to-male ratio rises from 2:1 in prepubertal children to 4.5:1 in adolescents and 8–12:1 in adults. Black and Hispanic children have a higher incidence. Black children have a greater prevalence and more severe renal and neuropsychiatric disease.

Renal involvement varies from microscopic hematuria and mild proteinuria to nephrotic syndrome, renal impairment and hypertension. Since the overall prognosis of childhood and adult SLE is closely correlated with the nature of the pathological renal lesions, it is recommended that a kidney biopsy be performed on all patients presenting with renal involvement to establish the severity of the histological changes. These range from normal, through mesangial hypercellularity to proliferative changes (focal or diffuse) and membranous changes.

Treatment and prognosis

Mild nonrenal lupus such as skin and joint manifestations may be managed with nonsteroidal anti-inflammatories or hydroxychloroquine. For those with moderate disease but with mild renal disease corticosteroids are used. More aggressive therapy is required for major organ involvement with renal, cardiac or central nervous system involvement. This may include high-dose methyprednisolone, mycophenolate, cyclophosphamide, immunoglobulin and more recently rituximab, a monoclonal anti-CD 20 antibody. Plasma exchange has also been used in some patients with life-threatening disease. Azathiaprine has been used as a steroid sparing agent in the long term to prevent steroid toxicity.

The prognosis has improved dramatically over the past 2 decades. In 1968 the 10-year survival was reported as 20%. In the last 10 years, 5-year survival of 78–92% and 5-year kidney survival of 44–93% are reported.[141] Survival rates of 94% after a mean follow up of 11 years in patients with biopsy proven lupus nephritis have also been reported. Following renal transplantation allograft survival is no different but children are 1.8 times more likely to die compared with patients without SLE.

RAPIDLY PROGRESSIVE GLOMERULONEPHRITIS

Rapidly progressive glomerular nephritis (RPGN) is a description of the clinical course of several forms of nephritis where there is acute renal insufficiency associated with the presence of extensive crescents on the renal biopsy. Such crescents may be found in poststreptococcal, membranoproliferative, lupus and HSP nephritis, ANCA-associated vasculitis such as Wegener's granulomatosis and microscopic polyangiitis as well as the glomerulonephritis of Goodpasture disease.

After the earlier mentioned forms of glomerulonephritis have been excluded, there remains a small group of patients with so-called idiopathic rapidly progressive disease. Since the identification of ANCA the truly idiopathic groups are less common. Often there is no evidence for immunological mechanisms and the C3 level is normal. All forms of RPGN have crescents, which are found on the inside of Bowman's capsule and are composed of fibrin, proliferating epithelial cells of the capsule, basement-membrane-like material and macrophages. The stimulus for crescent formation is believed to be the deposition of fibrin in Bowman's space as a result of necrosis or disruption of the glomerular capillary wall.

Severe crescentic nephritis is associated with ARF in association with a nephritic or nephrotic syndrome. Although there have been well-documented spontaneous recoveries of renal function with poststreptococcal and HSP nephritis, about 50% of patients will progress to end-stage renal failure within weeks or months after onset.[142] With such a rare condition it is hard to mount a controlled trial, but some patients improve with aggressive therapy combining immunosuppressive agents with anticoagulation and plasma exchange.

ANCA-ASSOCIATED GLOMERULONEPHRITIS
Wegener's granulomatosis

Wegener's granulomatosis (WG) is a systemic vasculitis associated with granuloma formation. It is a distinct clinicopathological entity characterized by the classical triad of necrotizing granulomas of the upper and lower respiratory tract, a disseminated small vessel vasculitis involving arteries and veins together with a necrotizing glomerulonephritis. It has been found to be associated with the presence of c-ANCA, a typical cytoplasmic immunofluorecence pattern of antineutrophil cytoplasmic antibodies. Renal involvement is variable but may include a RPGN picture which requires intensive immunosupression.[143]

Microscopic polyangiitis

Microscopic polyangiitis is a small vessel vasculitis associated with a focal segmental necrotizing glomerulonephritis. Histologically, it is similar to WG without the evidence of granulomas. It has also been associated with the finding of ANCA but with a different perinuclear immunofluoresence staining pattern (p-ANCA). The renal manifestations predominate and this diagnosis may include what was previously considered to be idiopathic crescentic glomerulonephritis. Immunosuppression is again the treatment.[144]

GOODPASTURE SYNDROME

Goodpasture syndrome is the association of pulmonary hemorrhage, glomerulonephritis and the presence of anti-glomerular basement membrane antibodies (anti-GBM antibodies) which are typically in a continuous linear pattern along the GBM. It is one form of a rapidly progressive glomerulonephritis which is extremely rare in childhood.

Hemoptysis is the usual presenting feature and pulmonary hemorrhage may be fatal. The finding of anti-GBM antibodies in the serum support the diagnosis but this is confirmed on renal biopsy. Treatment includes intensive immunosuppression with methylprednisolone and cyclophosphamide together with plasma exchange. The prognosis is worse for those with advanced renal disease at presentation but treatment is still required to treat pulmonary hemorrhage.[145]

A Goodpasture-like syndrome also occurs in patients with WG and microscopic polyangiitis but the diagnosis is supported by the identification of the associated antibodies (i.e. c-ANCA or p-ANCA).

HEREDITARY NEPHRITIS (ALPORT SYNDROME)

Hereditary nephritis is not a homogeneous entity, as the clinical expression of the disease and the mode of inheritance can vary widely between families. The classic description of Alport syndrome was of a progressive hematuric nephritis associated with sensorineural deafness and ocular abnormalities such as anterior lenticonus and cataracts. In familial cases about 80–90% are X-linked dominant, 10–20% of cases are autosomal recessive and a few are transmitted in an autosomal dominant pattern. New mutations account for up to one fifth of individuals. The most common abnormality is the inheritance of mutations in the COL4A5 gene encoding the alpha-5 (IV) collagen chain which is found on chromosome Xq26–48. Patients with an autosomal recessive form are either compound hetrozygotes or have homozygous mutations in the COL4A3 or the COL4A4 gene encoding the alpha-3 (IV) or alpha-4 (IV) chain, respectively on chromosome 2q35–37.[146]

The condition is generally more severe in male members of the family, with most (but not all) females remaining in good health throughout life. The prognosis is best based upon the progress of other affected family members, as there appears to be a correlation between deafness, ocular abnormalities, proteinuria and chronic renal failure.

Renal biopsy in the early stages of Alport syndrome shows only focal mesangial hypercellularity. There is progressive glomerular sclerosis, tubular atrophy, interstitial inflammation and foam cells (non-specific lipid-laden tubular or interstitial cells). Immunofluorescence is unrewarding, but electron microscopy may reveal irregular thickening, thinning, splitting and layering of the basement membrane of the glomeruli, with a lattice work appearance described as 'basket weave' (Fig. 18.23). These findings are very suggestive of Alport syndrome of the classical type but may occur in patients without an abnormal family history, suggesting a new mutation.

Clinical features

The disease is characteristically silent during childhood, but may present as an episode of macroscopic hematuria, an incidental finding of microscopic hematuria with or without proteinuria or following family screening after an affected individual has been identified. There is progression in the second decade of life, as sclerosis proceeds, and the proteinuria becomes heavier, with hypertension and renal failure. Nephrotic syndrome can occasionally occur at presentation, or late in the disease process. There is no effective treatment but careful control of blood pressure and the use of ACE inhibitors may delay the progression

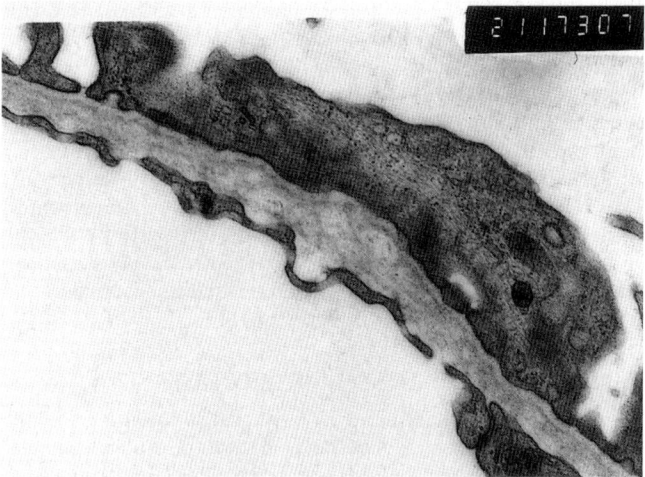

Fig. 18.23 Electron microscopy of basement membrane in a child with Alport syndrome. Lattice work appearance.

of renal failure. Dialysis and transplantation will be required as early as the second or third decade of life. Anti-glomerular basement membrane nephritis is a rare but dramatic manifestation occurring in 3–4% of Alport syndrome transplanted patients.

The deafness is initially high frequency, but is progressive and may ultimately be quite profound, especially in males. It is wise to carefully assess the hearing of children with any type of inherited nephritis. This may be of more initial importance than the renal disease.

Female carriers of mutations in the COL4A5 gene may occasionally progress to renal failure and should also be followed up particularly to monitor blood pressure and proteinuria.

Genetic counseling is an important part of the overall management.

A pattern of painless recurrent macroscopic hematuria after infections and persistent microscopic hematuria suggests IgA nephropathy.

Partial lipodystrophy is associated with membranoproliferative glomerulonephritis.

A family history of chronic renal failure and deafness strongly suggests Alport syndrome.

BENIGN HEMATURIA: SPORADIC AND FAMILIAL

In any child with persistent microscopic hematuria it is important to test the urine of all first-degree family members even though there is no clear history of familial nephritis. A familial recurrent hematuria syndrome is generally inherited as an autosomal dominant trait, but recessive examples may occur. The microscopic hematuria may sometimes be accompanied by short-lived episodes of frank hematuria with mild proteinuria. However, there is usually no impairment of renal function.

The condition is generally regarded as benign (synonym: benign familial hematuria) and hence not all children have been subjected to renal biopsy. Part of the reluctance to do so is because of the absence of therapeutic measures and the lack of a history of progressive nephritis.

However, even if the biopsy is normal on light microscopy and immunofluorescence, it may be possible to demonstrate changes in the GBM on electron microscopy.[147] Basement membrane nephropathy has been grouped into:

1. **Group 1:** Lamellation type, with features indistinguishable from Alport syndrome.
2. **Group 2:** Extensive thinning, commonly found in children with mild microscopic hematuria (thin glomerular basement membrane disease).[148]
3. **Group 3:** Idiopathic hematuria, with minimal basement membrane alteration.

The long-term outcome for types 2 and 3 is still uncertain but in the absence of a positive family history is usually regarded as benign.

However, cases of renal insufficiency have been described, even with minor GBM changes and so follow-up every 1–2 years with urinalysis, blood pressure and creatinine measurements is justified. In some patients with thin basement membrane disease COL4A3 and COL4A4 mutations have also been identified suggesting that these patients may have a variant of Alport syndrome.[148]

Children with hematuria *and* proteinuria have renal parenchymal disease until proven otherwise. However, the child with asymptomatic, low-degree, isolated hematuria and a negative family history is likely to have a favorable prognosis, and a renal biopsy is not initially warranted. However, prolonged clinic supervision can generate its own anxiety and a suggested approach is shown in Figure 18.19.

FABRY DISEASE (ANDERSON–FABRY DISEASE)

Fabry disease is an X-linked disorder associated with deficiency of the enzyme alpha-galactosidase A, resulting in the intracellular accumulation of neutral glycosphingolipids with terminal alpha-linked galactosyl moieties. Fabry coined the term 'angiokeratoma corporis diffusum'. The angiokeratomas usually appear during the second decade of life presenting as dark red macules or papules of various size.

The nephropathy of Fabry disease typically manifests as mild to moderate proteinuria, sometimes with microhematuria, and end-stage renal failure usually develops by the fourth or fifth decade of life. Fabry disease is a multisystem disorder with involvement of the heart, kidneys, skin, peripheral and central nervous systems. Enzyme replacement therapy with i.v. agalsidase beta appears to control symptoms but also potentially reverses the disease process.

NAIL–PATELLA SYNDROME

Nail–patella syndrome (NPS) is an autosomal dominant disorder consisting of hypoplasia or absence of the patellae, dystrophic nails, dysplasia of the elbows and iliac horns, and renal disease.

The nephropathy is usually benign and includes microhematuria and mild proteinuria, which usually appear in adolescence or young adulthood. Some patients develop nephrotic syndrome and mild hypertension and are at risk of progression to end-stage renal failure. The risk of renal disease is about 10%. Mutations in the LMXIB gene on 9q34 cause nail–patella syndrome but to date there are no correlations between phenotype and genotype.[149]

OTHER SYSTEMIC DISORDERS ASSOCIATED WITH GLOMERULAR DISEASE

Scleroderma

Scleroderma, or progressive systemic sclerosis, is a rare multi-system disorder in children. Renal involvement is unusual at the outset, but can occur with progression of the disease, and is characterized by proteinuria, hypertension and renal insufficiency. Scleroderma renal crisis occurs, with the abrupt onset of malignant hypertension and oliguric renal failure. The angiotensin-converting enzyme inhibitor, captopril, has been used successfully in its treatment.

Vasculitis

Vasculitis is characterized by inflammation of small, medium or large blood vessels. Classification is difficult because of the heterogeneous nature of many of these conditions and the overlapping clinical features.[150] A new consensus classification of childhood vasculitides has recently been developed.[151] Vasculitis of small vessels occurs with HSP, microscopic polyangiitis and WG.

Kawasaki disease is the second commonest vasculitis of childhood affecting the medium and large arteries. Renal disease is unusual and is generally related to vascular disease. However hematuria and proteinuria may be present and acute renal failure associated with interstitial nephritis has also been reported. Takayasu's arteritis is not associated with glomerular disease but hypertension can be a feature and renal insufficiency may occur secondary to poor blood flow.

Polyarteritis nodosa

This is a necrotizing vasculitis of medium-sized muscular arteries with associated aneurysm formation. There is multiple organ involvement with angiographic features of aneurysms in hepatic, renal and abdominal vessels. In contrast to microscopic polyangiitis elevated antineutrophil cytoplasmic antibodies (p-ANCA) are usually absent. The prognosis will depend upon the organ systems involved, and can be improved with the use of corticosteroid and immunosuppressive therapy such as cyclophosphamide.

Diabetic nephropathy

Diabetic nephropathy is a leading cause of ESRF in adult patients in Western societies and accounts for 16% of end-stage renal disease in the UK. Diabetic nephropathy develops slowly over 10–15 years. Diabetes mellitus in childhood is rarely associated with overt manifestations of renal disease but microlbuminuria (an excretion of 30–300 mg/d in an adult) is reported in up to 20% of children and this may progress into overt nephropathy.

The highest long-term incidence of nephropathy is found in those who develop type 1 diabetes between the ages of 11 and 20 years. The median time between the onset of proteinuria and ESRF is 14 years, for those diagnosed under the age of 12, and 8 years for those diagnosed between the ages of 12 and 20. Mogensen[152] described five distinct stages of renal dysfunction: renal hypertrophy and hyperfiltration; microalbuminuria; incipient nephropathy; overt nephropathy and ESRF.

Children should commence annual screening for microalbuminuria from 3 to 5 years after the onset of diabetes or from puberty. If microalbuminuria is identified management strategies should include tighter glycemic control, ACE inhibition and management of hypertension.

Amyloidosis

Juvenile idiopathic arthritis (JIA) has become a common cause of secondary amyloidosis in children following the eradication of tuberculosis and chronic osteomyelitis in Western countries. However, it is very rare in childhood and only occurs after many years of severe disease. Renal vein thrombosis is a well-documented complication of renal amyloidosis. Confirmation of the diagnosis requires biopsy material. Immunosuppressive agents such as busulfan may be of benefit.

PROTEINURIA

Although proteinuria is one of the cardinal features of renal disease, and a risk factor for deterioration in most renal conditions, its isolated occurrence may be a transient finding in healthy children. Proteinuria combined with hematuria is much more significant.

In the normal individual, minimal protein is filtered, because of the charge and size selectivity of the glomerular filtration barrier (which consists of capillary endothelial cells, the GBM, and glomerular podocytes on the outside). Proteins are negatively charged and are repelled by the filtration barrier, which contains sialoproteins and proteoglycans, such as heparan sulfate, which are negatively charged. In addition, the tight collagen meshwork within the GBM, and the overlying podocytes (also known as visceral glomerular epithelial cells) with their interdigitating foot processes, act as an effective size barrier, with little protein passing through the filtration slit diaphragms. Proteinuria may result from increased glomerular permeability due to:

1. loss of the negative charges in the filtration barrier;
2. An increase in the effective pore size or number due to direct damage to components of the filtration barrier;
3. The hemodynamic effects of angiotensin II and other vasoactive amines, which may explain the mild proteinuria seen with heart failure.

Albumin (MW = 69 000) is the predominant protein lost in the urine, but globulin excretion may also be increased.

Another type of proteinuria, *tubular* proteinuria, occurs when there is increased excretion of the normally filtered low-molecular weight proteins, such as immunoglobulin light chains and beta$_2$-microglobulin (MW < 50 000). Tubular proteinuria occurs when proximal tubular reabsorption is impaired, as in Fanconi syndrome, or when the production is increased to a level exceeding tubular reabsorption capacity, e.g. in multiple myeloma.

NORMAL VALUES

Most of the filtered protein is reabsorbed, and the normal daily protein excretion in a child is < 4 mg/h/m^2, or < 150 mg/24 h in an adult. Albumin accounts for about 25% of the normal protein excretion, and after severe exercise, proteinuria may increase several fold, with the albumin excretion representing up to 80% of total urinary protein. 40% of normal urinary protein is of tissue origin, and the major protein in this group is the uromucoid or Tamm–Horsfall protein, which is produced in the distal tubule.

DETECTION

Testing for proteinuria has been simplified by the use of dipsticks, which are impregnated with a dye, tetrabromophenol blue, and change color according to the quantity of protein present. The strips detect predominantly albuminuria, but a negative dipstick does not exclude the presence in the urine of low concentrations of globulins, hemoglobin, Bence Jones protein or mucoproteins. These would be detected by 3% sulfosalicylic acid, which detects all proteins. However, dipsticks predominate in clinical practice. It is important to appreciate that false-negative results can also occur with very acid or dilute urine, whereas false-positive results may occur in the presence of highly concentrated or alkaline urine (pH > 8) along with gross hematuria, pyuria and contamination with antiseptics, such as chlorhexidine.

Dipsticks are highly sensitive and cannot accurately measure protein excretion, which is best quantified using timed (preferably 24-hour) urine collections. However, obtaining accurate 12- or 24-hour urine collections in children can be difficult to accomplish. Single voided urine samples, which relate the concentration of both the protein and creatinine in the same sample, have a high correlation with 24-hour urine excretion rates. The urine protein:creatinine ratio can be used to estimate the severity, and follow the progress, of proteinuric patients. The normal urine protein:creatinine ratio is < 20 mg/mmol in the early morning urine sample.[153]

Protein selectivity index

This has usually been measured by comparing the clearances of small and large molecular weight proteins, on the basis that diseases such as glomerulonephritis, which cause severe histological change to the glomeruli, are more likely to result in the urinary loss of large plasma proteins than are diseases such as minimal change nephrotic syndrome, in which there is no obvious glomerular injury. However, there is considerable overlap in the results and the test is no longer performed routinely. It is preferable to rely on clinical features and/or the response to corticosteroids in children with nephrotic syndrome.

The causes of proteinuria are listed in Table 18.12.

INTERMITTENT PROTEINURIA

Transient proteinuria may be found in patients with high fevers in excess of 38.5 °C. The mechanism is unknown and the proteinuria usually resolves as the fever abates.

Proteinuria, like hematuria, may also follow vigorous exercise and usually resolves within 48 h of rest.

Postural or *orthostatic* proteinuria is important because it is a relatively frequent cause of referral to pediatric clinics. It is suggested by finding normal protein excretion (< 20 mg/mmol) in the first morning

Table 18.12   Causes of proteinuria

Intermittent proteinuria
1. Postural (orthostatic)

2. Nonpostural
   a. Exercise
   b. Fever
   c. Anatomic abnormalities, e.g. urinary tract
   d. Glomerular lesions, e.g. IgA nephropathy
   e. Random finding; no known cause

Persistent proteinuria
1. Glomerular
   a. Isolated asymptomatic proteinuria
   b. Damage to glomerular basement membrane, e.g. acute or chronic glomerulonephritis
   c. Loss or reduction of basement membrane anionic charge, e.g. minimal change and congenital nephrosis
   d. Increased permeability in residual nephrons, e.g. chronic renal failure

2. Tubular
   a. Hereditary, e.g. cystinosis, Wilson disease, Lowe syndrome, proximal tubular acidosis, galactosemia
   b. Acquired, e.g. interstitial nephritis, acute tubular necrosis, post renal transplantation, pyelonephritis, vitamin D intoxication, penicillamine, heavy metal poisoning (gold, lead, mercury, etc.), analgesic abuse, drugs

urine after being supine overnight and increased protein excretion in the upright collection. Long-term follow-up has suggested that orthostatic proteinuria, as an isolated finding, is benign. These patients do not need prolonged follow-up in the clinic, if the history and examination and other urinary findings are normal. However, it is important to note that patients with glomerular disease will often have an orthostatic component to their proteinuria, so that true orthostatic proteinuria should not be diagnosed unless the urine collected in the supine position has no protein detectable by routine methods.

PERSISTENT PROTEINURIA

In these patients, the amount of protein present in the individual samples may vary considerably, but is persistent, unless it resolves as in acute glomerulonephritis. If the proteinuria is associated with additional evidence for renal disease, e.g. microscopic hematuria, then these patients are most likely to have significant pathology in the kidney or urinary tract.

GLOMERULAR PROTEINURIA

In the majority of cases, persistent proteinuria is of glomerular origin. The degree of proteinuria may range from > 4 mg/h/m^2, to < 400 mg/h/m^2, when it is usually associated with altered levels of protein in the plasma and nephrotic syndrome. Acute and chronic glomerulonephritis are believed to produce proteinuria as a result of damage to the glomerular basement membrane, which increases the permeability to plasma proteins to a degree which overwhelms the tubular absorptive mechanisms. In conditions such as minimal change or congenital nephrotic syndrome, it is usually a highly selective loss of albumin as a result of loss of the glomerular anionic charge for reasons still to be elucidated.

There has been a great deal of interest in recent years in patients who develop proteinuria with a reduced renal mass. Evidence has accumulated that the remaining nephrons, in such patients, are subject to hyperfiltration damage, which produces progressive glomerulosclerosis.[154] Hence several long-term studies are evaluating the use of ACE inhibitors or angiotensin II, receptor antagonists to ameliorate the progression of renal disease.

TUBULAR PROTEINURIA

The amount of protein in the urine resulting from tubular damage is usually not as great as with glomerular disease but it has occasionally been sufficient to result in a nephrotic syndrome. Transient overflow proteinuria may occur after repeated blood or albumin infusions, and increased secretion of tubular proteins may occur with urinary tract infection or transiently in the neonatal period. Many hereditary causes of tubular proteinuria are part of a Fanconi-type syndrome.

PERSISTENT ASYMPTOMATIC PROTEINURIA

This is defined as proteinuria, in apparently healthy children, occurring without hematuria, but persisting on repeated testing over 3 months. Significant proteinuria (Uprot/Ucr > 20 mg/mmol) is usually an indication for proceeding with further investigations. These would include urine culture, full blood count, and blood chemistry including electrolytes, urea, creatinine, albumin and an accurate measurement of glomerular filtration rate. The serological tests are performed at the same time and will include antistreptolysin O, antinuclear antibodies, immunoglobulins and complement studies. A renal tract ultrasound and plain abdominal X-ray will usually exclude any significant urinary tract pathology. A renal biopsy will only be considered in those with confirmed proteinuria or when there are other abnormal tests, such as a decreased GFR, abnormal urinary sediment, hypocomplementemia or evidence of generalized vascular disease.

NEPHROTIC SYNDROME

The nephrotic syndrome is characterized by:
1. heavy proteinuria (> 40 mg/h/m^2 or protein/creatinine ratio > 200 mg/mmol);
2. hypoalbuminemia (< 25 g/L);
3. edema (Fig. 18.24).

It should be noted that this definition is distinct from a nephritic 'syndrome' (i.e. glomerulonephritis), which is defined by glomerular hematuria +/− hypertension. It is possible for a patient to be nephrotic, nephritic or nephrotic/nephritic depending on the underlying cause, and the following section describes diseases that cause primarily (or solely) a nephrotic state.

The incidence of all forms of nephrotic syndrome in childhood is 2–4 per 100 000 population, but this figure will vary according to the ethnic mix of the population. For instance, the incidence amongst Asian children in two cities in the UK was reported to range from 9 to 16 per 100 000, respectively.[155]

The predominant pathology is minimal change disease (MCD), with contributions from other pathologies such as focal segmental glomerulosclerosis (FSGS) and MPGN. This applies only in Caucasian populations, as around the world the pathology varies. For instance, in Africa it has long been thought that 'tropical nephropathy' (malaria, HIV, hepatitis B etc.) predominates, though this has been challenged,[156] with schistosomiasis being responsible for the majority of the cases in South America.

Nephrotic syndrome could be subdivided into congenital, idiopathic (primary) or secondary. Many of the secondary causes have already been mentioned, and include HSP nephritis, acute post-streptococcal nephritis, connective tissue disorders (e.g. SLE), toxic causes (e.g. drugs and heavy metal poisoning), sickle-cell disease, and amyloidosis.

IDIOPATHIC NEPHROTIC SYNDROME

Minimal change disease accounts for approximately 85% of cases presenting in childhood but only 10% of cases in adults. The other histological types of mesangial proliferative and FSGS may well represent the spectrum of a single disorder with varying histological features. There are familial cases of MCD, but these appear to be very rare in the UK. The gene locus for steroid sensitive idiopathic nephrotic syndrome appears to be distinct from the NPHS2 gene, located on chromosome 1q25 that

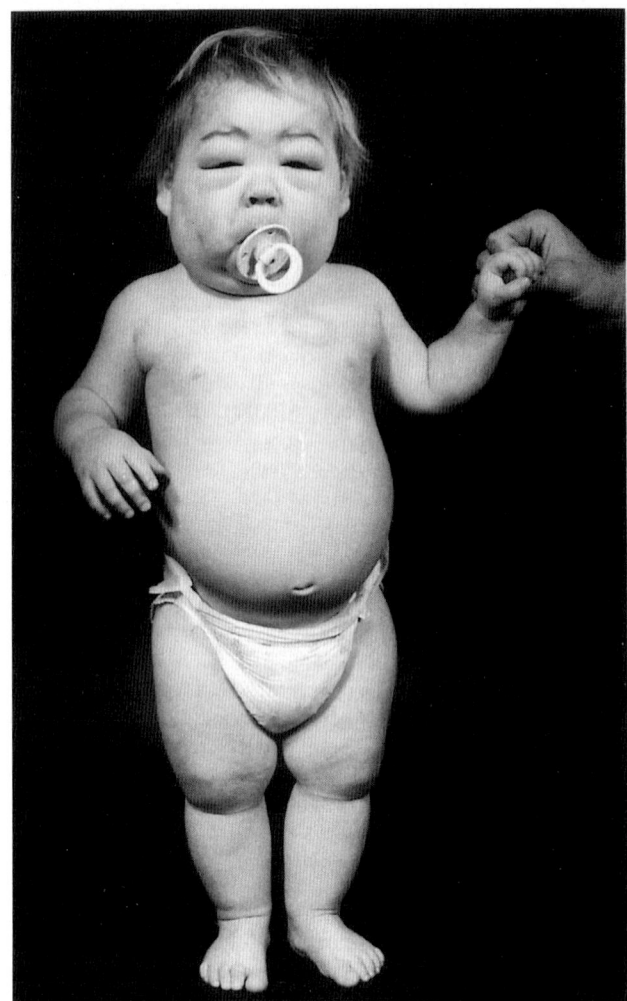

Fig. 18.24 17-month-old male infant with nephrotic syndrome and gross generalized edema (anasarca).

has been found to be mutated in a subset of patients with early onset autosomal recessive FSGS (see p. 584).

The cause of minimal change nephrotic syndrome (MCNS) remains unknown. It is more prevalent in families with an atopic history, and some studies have suggested an abnormality of T cell function. Although broad-spectrum immunosuppressive drugs have been used to control the disease, there is lack of evidence for classical mechanisms of immunological injury.

In minimal change disease, the glomeruli appear normal or show a minimal increase in mesangial cells and matrix. The immunofluorescence studies are negative, and electron microscopy reveals gross podocyte foot process fusion, which is a nonspecific finding in any patient with heavy proteinuria.

Clinical features

Minimal change nephrotic syndrome is more common in boys than girls (2:1) and usually occurs between the ages of 2 and 6 years. There may be an antecedent history of an upper respiratory tract infection and, certainly, these are well known to precipitate relapses in this condition. The presenting feature is usually edema, which is first noticed around the eyes (Fig. 18.24). Since the condition is so uncommon in general practice, many children are treated for allergic conditions before the true nature of the condition is appreciated. The edema may become generalized, with swollen limbs, ascites and pleural effusions with diminishing urine output. There may be lethargy, poor appetite, mild diarrhea and, sometimes, abdominal pain.

Investigations

The diagnosis is suggested by simple urinalysis, which will show heavy proteinuria (+++ or > 5 g/L). About 30% of patients will have transient microscopic hematuria, but gross hematuria is rare. Heavy proteinuria can be confirmed by timed urine collections or by early morning urine protein/creatinine ratio (> 200 mg/mmol). Renal function is usually normal, but there will be a low serum albumin (< 25 g/L), with raised serum cholesterol and triglyceride levels. Swabs should be taken from the throat and any skin lesions, as well as a urine culture. Overt or covert infection can be the cause of steroid resistance. Serological tests such as complement studies, an ASO titer, hepatitis B surface antigen and antinuclear factor antibodies need only be measured in patients when there is a mixed nephritic/nephrotic picture. The traditional urine protein selectivity index can be omitted, because in terms of prognosis, the response to corticosteroids is more important.

Children between the ages of 1 and 10 years are very likely to have *steroid-responsive minimal change disease* and so prednisolone therapy is usually initiated without a renal biopsy. This latter procedure is recommended *before* treatment with corticosteroids when the nephrotic syndrome occurs:

1. onset at less that 6 months of age (congenital nephrotic syndrome types);
2. evidence of a mixed nephritic/nephrotic picture with hypertension and/or low plasma C3 (pathology other than MCD more likely);

A biopsy may be *considered* in children with nephrotic syndrome and:

1. onset between 6 and 12 months of age;
2. onset over 12 years of age (other pathology may be more likely);
3. persistent hypertension, microscopic hematuria, or low plasma C3;
4. renal failure – persistent and not attributable to hypovolemia.

Complications

Children with nephrotic syndrome still have a 1–2% mortality rate. The two major complications are infection and thrombosis.

Peritonitis is the most frequent type of infection and *Streptococcus pneumoniae* is the most common organism. Gram-negative bacteria are also encountered. The reasons for the susceptibility may be multifactorial and include decreased immunoglobulin levels, ascitic fluid acting as culture medium and immunosuppressive therapy. While on corticosteroids the clinical findings may be masked, and so any child with nephrotic syndrome and abdominal pain should be carefully evaluated in conjunction with a surgeon. Although there are instances where an unnecessary laparotomy has been carried out on a child with primary peritonitis, before the edema and nephrotic state has been recognized, there are also instances of children with nephrotic syndrome and appendicitis. In the very edematous state, penicillin prophylaxis may be considered, but antibiotics to cover Gram-negative organisms should be used for any suspected peritonitis, until the cultures and sensitivities are known. Many authors now advocate polyvalent pneumococcal vaccine when the child is in remission, but this does not appear to be fully effective, as not all the serotypes are covered.

Chickenpox and measles are major threats to the immunocompromised child. It is likely that the child has received MMR, but if not, measles and varicella immunity status should be checked as part of the routine evaluation. Zoster immune globulin should be given if there is chickenpox exposure while taking high-dose prednisolone or alkylating agents and aciclovir given promptly if the condition develops.

Nephrotic children also have a tendency to arterial and venous thrombosis. The nephrotic syndrome is a hypercoagulable state with high levels of fibrinogen, factor VIII:R:AG and alpha-2-macroglobulin with a decrease of both functional and immunological antithrombin III.[158] The greatest risk of thrombosis appears to be when the albumin level is very low. Children with nephrotic syndrome should be seen for prompt assessment if they have a potentially dehydrating state such as vomiting and diarrhea.

Thyroid function should be checked in all children with persistent hypoalbuminemia, as loss of thyroid binding globulin can lead to low levels of available T3 and T4.

Treatment

Hospitalization should only be required for the initial attack, when the diagnosis can be established, treatment initiated and the response evaluated. It will also give an opportunity to educate the patient and the family in what may be a frustrating chronic illness. Good education and efficient communication should enable further problems to be assessed and treated on an outpatient basis.

Bed rest does not need to be enforced, as the child will determine their appropriate activity level.

Dietary advice

The traditional high-protein, no-salt-intake diet should be abandoned in favor of trying to maintain the recommended daily allowances of calories and protein in a child whose appetite is likely to be markedly diminished until on steroids.[159] When edema is present, a no-added-salt diet is advised, with avoidance of foods known to be high in sodium, particularly snack or processed foods.

Diuretics

A moderate fluid restriction of 750–1000 ml is advocated in the edematous state. Diuretics should be used with caution in plasma-volume-depleted nephrotic patients, as they may be predisposed to fluid and electrolyte disturbances. Thiazide diuretics have little effect. Cautious use of loop diuretics such as furosemide (frusemide) (1–2 mg/kg/24 h), in combination with an aldosterone antagonist such as spironolactone 0.5–5 mg/kg/24 h (which may take several days to act), can be used to control the edema, until there is a diuretic response to the corticosteroids. Occasionally, metolazone (0.2–0.4 mg/kg/24 h), in combination with furosemide (frusemide), may be needed to induce a diuresis, but careful biochemical monitoring is required.

If there are signs of hypovolemia, such as abdominal pain (due to a contracted plasma volume), hypertension, oliguria, low urinary sodium excretion (<10 mmol/L) or evidence of renal insufficiency, then an i.v. 4.5% albumin infusion (1 g/kg) given over 3–4 h with careful monitoring and followed by furosemide (frusemide) (1–2 mg/kg) may replenish intravascular volume. For diuretic-resistant symptomatic edema, 20% albumin infusion (1 g/kg) can be added if intravascular volume is adequate, to promote loss of peripheral fluid. Albumin infusions are both expensive and potentially hazardous, as pulmonary edema could be precipitated if the volume status has been misjudged. Since most of the infused albumin is rapidly lost in the urine, there is little place for their routine use. Mannitol (5 ml/kg of 20% solution) and furosemide (frusemide) (2 mg/kg/dose) have also been used to treat diuretic-resistant edema.[160]

Corticosteroid therapy

Corticosteroid therapy has been used in childhood nephrotic syndrome since the 1950s. Of those children who present with a typical illness, 95% will respond to steroid therapy within the first 4 weeks. Nephrotic syndrome is potentially a chronic disease with about 70% of patients suffering a relapsing course and therefore being at risk of adverse effects of repeated steroid treatment.

A number of steroid regimens have been suggested. The consensus regimen proposed by the British Association for Paediatric Nephrology[161] was prednisolone 60 mg/m²/d until the urine was protein-free for 3 d, followed by 40 mg/m² for 4 weeks. In a national audit conducted in the UK in 1998, this was found to be associated with a high relapse rate.

The current consensus on management is shown in Figure 18.25, the major change being that daily prednisolone is now given in a dose of 60 mg/m² (maximum 80 mg) for a full 28 d followed by a further month of alternate day therapy at 40 mg/m² (maximum 60 mg). The increase in the initial steroid dose acknowledges the evidence that the relapse rate is reduced with increased duration of initial therapy.[162] However, it falls short of the 3-month duration of initial prednisolone therapy recommended by Hodson et al[163] in a meta-analysis of randomized, controlled trials. Nephrologists remain concerned about the possibility of

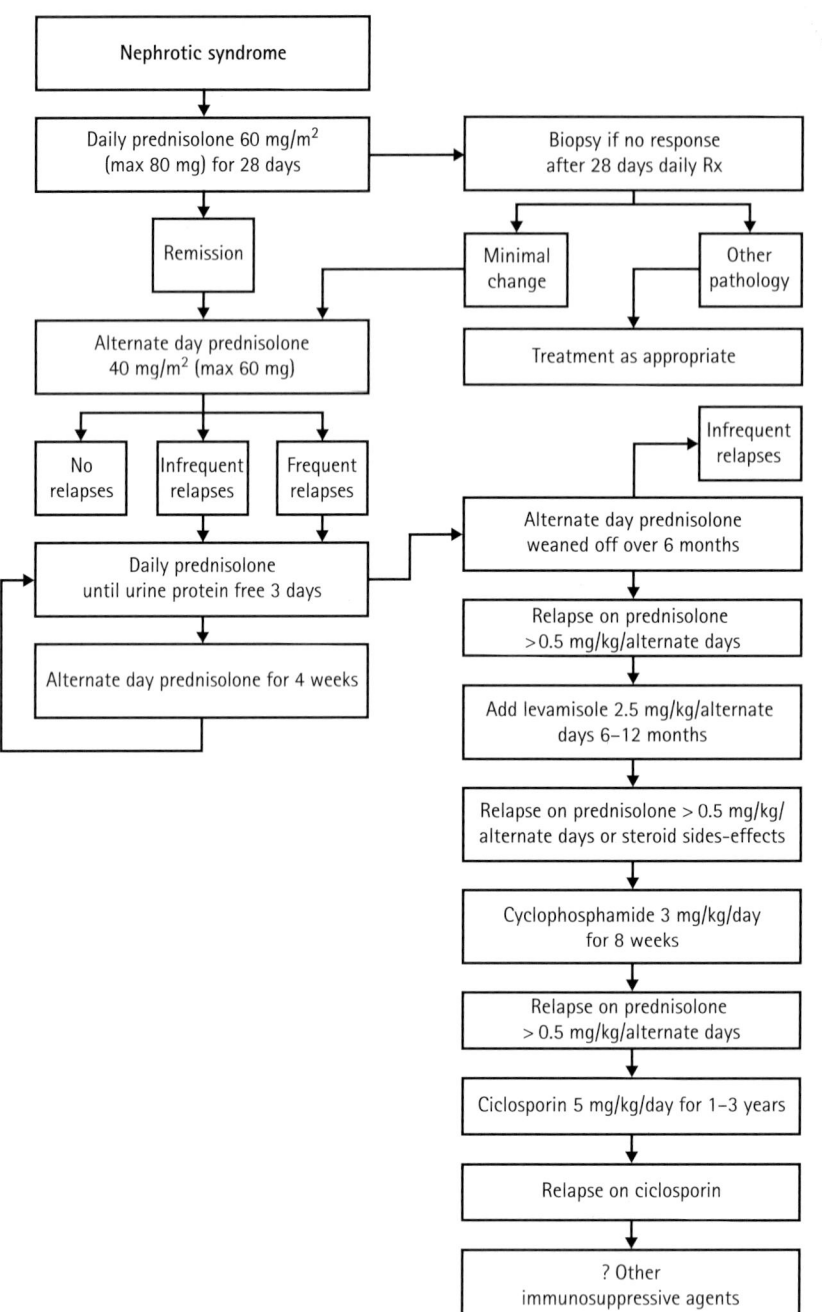

Fig. 18.25   Scheme for the management of children with nephrotic syndrome.

steroid side-effects, with this large initial dosage, and their effect on the hypothalamic pituitary axis.

Surprisingly, there is usually little gastric upset from the use of soluble prednisolone in children, and the more expensive enteric coated forms or drugs to control gastric acidity are not routinely prescribed. Children who have problems with vomiting or diarrhea should receive i.v. methylprednisolone in an equivalent dose to the oral prednisolone dosage and additional care should be taken to monitor blood pressure. It is important to exclude occult infection such as UTI as a cause of steroid resistance.

The parents should be told daily steroids may well alter the child's behavior as well as increasing the appetite. General dietary advice about avoiding excess consumption of snacks, etc. should be given. A steroid warning card should be issued, and the parents should report if the child is exposed to infections such as measles or chicken-pox, while on daily steroids. Immunization using live vaccines should

be avoided until the child has been off daily steroids for at least 3 months, but are permissible if the child is on alternate-day steroids (< 0.5 mg/kg body weight/d). It should be noted that there is a reported increased risk of NS recurrence after meningococcal conjugate C vaccination. Overall, vaccines are best given when the child has been in remission for some months and inactivated, rather than live, polio should be utilized.

Steroid-responsive patients

The family is instructed in the use of dipsticks for recording the first morning urine protein results, which should be carefully logged in a diary. This can serve as an individual record of the child's condition over a number of years.

When there is a relapse of proteinuria (3 consecutive days of heavy proteinuria [+++ or greater]), treatment may be withheld for up to 5 d (or possibly 10 if variable proteinuria) unless the child becomes edematous. This is because some children will spontaneously remit during this period. If proteinuria persists, then remission is induced with daily steroids as before until the urine is protein free for 3 d, and then alternate-day corticosteroids are continued for 28 d. More than 75% of children with minimal change nephrotic syndrome will have at least one relapse.

Frequent relapses or steroid dependency

If the child has two or more relapses within 6 months of initial treatment, or four or more relapses within any 12-month period (frequent relapser), then a slow weaning dose of alternate-day prednisolone may be considered, after inducing remission with daily steroids as mentioned earlier. The prednisolone may be weaned off over 6 months, and by this means steroid toxicity may be minimized.

Steroid dependency may be defined as those who relapse on two consecutive occasions as prednisolone is being decreased, or within 2 weeks of it being discontinued. If a child requires more than 0.5 mg/kg of prednisolone on alternate days to remain protein free, and particularly if there are signs of steroid toxicity, then alternative therapy should be considered. Such steroid side-effects would include stunting of growth, cataracts, obesity and behavioral changes, but alternative therapy to corticosteroids and/or the advice of a pediatric nephrologist will, preferably, have been sought before many of these side-effects are manifest. Alternative therapy consists of levamisole, cyclophosphamide, chlorambucil and ciclosporin (Fig. 18.25) which all reduce the risk of relapse in children with relapsing steroid-sensitive nephritis compared with prednisolone alone.[164]

Cyclophosphamide

When cyclophosphamide was originally used in MCNS it was prescribed for 6–12 months and achieved 90% long-term remission. However, this was before gonadal toxicity was appreciated, and many young men were subsequently rendered oligo- or azoospermic. Consequently, the course of cyclophosphamide has been restricted to 8 weeks and is given after remission has been induced with daily steroids, which are then usually tapered off over 4–6 weeks. The restriction to shorter courses of 8 weeks means the remission rate has been reduced to approximately 50% at 2 years.

The potential toxic effects of bone marrow depression, hemorrhagic cystitis and mild alopecia can be minimized by close monitoring of weekly blood counts and clinic visits. Although there is no firm guarantee of future fertility, restriction of therapy to less than 16 weeks or 300 mg/kg body weight appears to be safe.[165,166] Nevertheless, this point needs to be discussed at length with the parents, as a prolonged remission cannot be guaranteed and there may still be long-term effects from the use of this drug. Chlorambucil does not appear to be superior to cyclophosphamide and its use has been more limited.

It was once customary to perform a renal biopsy on all nephrotic children *prior* to cyclophosphamide therapy. However, this is probably no longer justifiable if the patient is still *steroid responsive*. Even if FSGS changes are found on biopsy, the best prognostic indicator remains *steroid responsiveness*.

Psychosocial

The current authors have found it helpful to provide the family of a child with nephrotic syndrome with an information booklet about the condition, as a great deal of anxiety can result with the clinical course of relapse and remission. In addition, the parents have benefited from attending a local parents' group, where they can discuss and share many of their anxieties.[167]

If a nephrotic child has been free of relapses for 5 years, then there is a strong chance of a long-term remission. However, some children may continue to relapse into adult life, and those who develop nephrosis earlier in life are likely to relapse more often.[168] With a decreasing relapse rate the urine tests can be performed less frequently, but the family should be cautioned to test urine at times of stress such as incidental infection.

FOCAL SEGMENTAL GLOMERULOSCLEROSIS

Focal segmental glomerulosclerosis (FSGS) is characterized on light microscopy by sclerosis or hyalinosis of glomeruli in a focal and segmental distribution. The involved area obliterates Bowman's space and is adherent to the capsule without epithelial cell proliferation. Epithelial foot process fusion is similar to that seen in MCD and electron microscopy should confirm the sclerosing nature of the lesion. There may be nonspecific deposition of IgM and C3 in the affected segments. Tubular atrophy and interstitial fibrosis are proportional to the extent of glomerular damage.

The typical features of FSGS may be missed if the renal biopsy is too superficial, as the changes are more likely to be seen in the juxtamedullary region. FSGS usually carries with it an entirely different prognosis from minimal lesion, especially if the patient is steroid resistant. Again, the important practice point is that, if the patient responds to steroids, then whether the histology shows MCD and FSGS is generally irrelevant as long as steroid resistance does not develop. If the patient is steroid resistant, the best evidence is to use calcineurin inhibitors (ciclosporin A, or FK506) in conjunction with alternate-day steroids. Alternative immunosuppressives such as cyclophosphamide have a less consistent benefit. These agents may reduce the proteinuria sufficiently for the patient to remain edema free, with the attendant benefits.

Another mandatory investigation now becoming increasingly available is to screen for *NPHS2* mutations in any child with steroid resistance (see later), as these children will not respond to immunosuppression, and have a far smaller risk of post-transplant recurrence of disease.[169–171]

Orthostatic (postural) proteinuria should be proven by finding no significant protein in the first morning compared to the afternoon sample.

Steroid responsiveness, not the underlying pathology, suggests a better outcome in idiopathic nephrotic syndrome.

Children with nephrotic syndrome are susceptible to life-threatening events such as thrombosis and infection.

FAMILIAL NEPHROTIC SYNDROME

An exciting development in recent years has been the elucidation of the genetic bases for many inherited cases of nephrotic syndrome. According to the molecular defect, these can present during the first year of life (congenital nephrotic syndrome), in early childhood, or in adolescence and adulthood. Congenital nephrotic syndrome was predominantly described in children of Finnish extraction (hence 'Finnish type') and is an autosomal recessive disorder. The major pathological feature is dilatation of the proximal convoluted tubules (microcystic disease), but this is very variable. The glomeruli may initially appear quite normal by light microscopy, but later show mesangial hypercellularity with an increase in matrix. Most glomeruli are immature. Both sexes are equally affected, and prematurity, with a placenta which weighs more than 25% of the infant's birth weight, is typical. Proteinuria is usually present at birth, and a frank nephrotic syndrome is usually apparent within 3 months of life. The clinical course is one of persistent edema and recurrent infections.

This condition was previously almost invariably fatal before 2 years of age. However, more aggressive feeding regimens with unilateral or bilateral nephrectomy and the appropriate management for end-stage renal disease has resulted in increasing numbers of children being successfully transplanted with normal growth and development.[172] Genetic counseling is very important, as antenatal diagnosis is possible by measuring the alpha-fetoprotein level in the amniotic fluid, as early as 15 weeks of gestation, or by screening for the gene mutation. The gene for the Finnish type is termed *NPHS1* and the protein product of this gene is called nephrin (see later).

Other histological types have been described in association with nephrotic syndrome in the first year of life (Table 18.13). Diffuse mesangial sclerosis is a steroid-resistant lesion with progressive loss of renal function, and renal replacement therapy may be required in the second

Table 18.13   Causes of infantile nephrotic syndrome

Primary		
	a.	Congenital nephrotic syndrome – NPHS1; NPHS2 mutations
	b.	Diffuse mesangial sclerosis
	c.	Minimal change nephrotic syndrome
	d.	Focal segmental glomerulosclerosis
	e.	Denys–Drash syndrome
	f.	Nail–patella syndrome; Pierson syndrome; Galloway–Mowatt syndrome
Secondary		
	a.	Syphilis
	b.	Toxoplasmosis
	c.	Cytomegalovirus
	d.	Mercury
	e.	Hodgkin's lymphoma or T cell malignancies

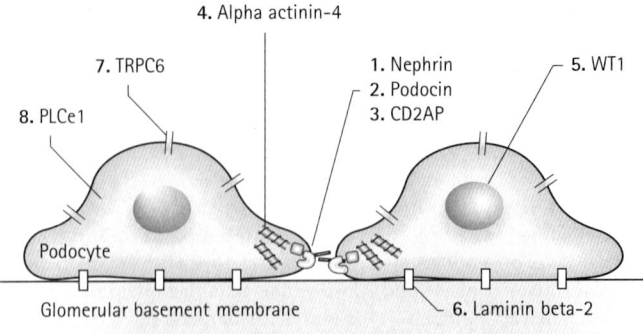

Fig. 18.26   Schematic representation of podocyte anatomy, showing adjacent podocyte foot processes on the glomerular basement membrane – indicating location of proteins mutated in familial nephrotic syndromes (see text for details).

year of life. The gene defect responsible for this variant has not yet been identified. Patients with the histological appearances of minimal change NS have also been described in very young patients, and biopsy is essential, in order to predict which patients are likely or not likely to respond to a course of steroids.

In any female infant with early-onset nephrotic syndrome, chromosome analysis should be considered, as there is an association between nephrotic syndrome, pseudohermaphroditism and Wilms' tumor (Drash syndrome). Older female children with FSGS should be similarly screened, because of an association with pseudohermaphroditism and gonadal dysgenesis (Frasier syndrome).

Molecular basis of familial nephrotic syndromes

One of the first genes identified as a cause for familial nephrotic syndrome was *NPHS1*, encoding nephrin (OMIM #602716), in the 'Finnish' type of nephrotic syndrome.[173] Subsequently patients have been described from many diverse populations around the world with a variety of mutations in this gene. A molecule which interacts with nephrin, called podocin (the gene is termed *NPHS2*), has been found to be mutated in congenital and early onset FSGS (OMIM #604766). In fact it is estimated that around 10–18% of children with 'acquired' FSGS in childhood have a podocin gene defect,[172] hence the importance of genetic screening to avoid heavy immunosuppression of children with mutations, who will be unresponsive.[171]

Autosomal dominant gene mutations in two familial nephrotic syndromes that present typically later in life (beyond childhood) have been identified. *ACTN4* coding for α-actinin-4 was identified in patients with slowly progressive adult-onset FSGS (OMIM #604638), and the cation channel protein TRPC6 is mutated in late teenage and adult patients presenting with FSGS (OMIM #603965). Intriguingly, a signaling protein potentially in the TRPC6 pathway called phospholipase epsilon 1 (PLCε1, OMIM #608414) has been discovered to be mutated in a pedigree of early onset NS patients, some of whom responded to immunosuppression. The common link between all these proteins is that they are expressed almost exclusively in the podocyte, within the glomerulus (Table 18.14), thus emphasizing the importance of this cell in maintenance of an intact filtration barrier (Fig. 18.26).

SYNDROMIC NEPHROTIC SYNDROMES

A number of syndromes present with nephrotic syndrome as a significant component. Different mutations in the WT1 transcription factor gene (expressed in the podocyte), are responsible for Denys Drash syndrome and Frasier syndrome, respectively (see earlier, and Table 18.13). Pierson syndrome (OMIM #609049) is severe oculorenal syndrome, with early lethality, although milder nonlethal phenotypes have been reported. The mutation is in the laminin-β2 (LAMB2) gene, an essential component of the glomerular basement membrane. Microcephaly associated with congenital nephrotic syndrome, occasionally with hiatus hernia, has been described as the Galloway–Mowatt syndrome. Nail-Patella Syndrome (NPS) is characterized by developmental defects of dorsal limb structures (dysplasia of the nails, patellar aplasia or hypoplasia), nephropathy (about 22% have proteinuria), and glaucoma and is caused by heterozygous mutations in the transcription factor LMX1B (OMIM #161200).

SECONDARY CAUSES OF NEPHROTIC SYNDROME

Secondary causes of infantile nephrotic syndrome are shown in Table 18.13. Syphilis can cause a membranous type of glomerular nephropathy, while cytomegalovirus and toxoplasmosis may be coincidental rather than causative agents. Mercury intoxication can cause a nephrotic syndrome, which usually responds to withdrawal of the toxic agent. Patients have been reported with lymphoma or other T-cell malignancies, and have developed MCNS.

RENAL HYPERTENSION

MEASUREMENT OF BLOOD PRESSURE

The gold standard method of blood pressure measurement is with the mercury sphygmomanometer. The blood pressure should be measured with the weight of the arm supported after the child has been sitting quietly for at least 3 min using an appropriately sized cuff.[174] Oscillometric machines are also widely used in clinical practice. They may be preferred

Table 18.14   Proteins expressed in the podocyte, mutated in congenital nephrotic syndromes

Mutated protein	Inheritance	Region of podocyte affected	Typical age of presentation
Nephrin	Recessive	Slit diaphragm	Infancy
Podocin	Recessive	Slit diaphragm	Infancy/early childhood
WT1	X-linked	Nuclear transcription factor	Infancy
α-actinin-4	Dominant	Actin cytoskeleton cross-linker	Adulthood
TRPC6	Dominant	Calcium channels	Late adolescence/adulthood
β-laminin-2	Recessive	Anchorage to glomerular basement membrane	Childhood
PLCε1	Recessive	Cell signaling	Infancy/early childhood

for measurement of blood pressure in BP in newborns and young infants in whom auscultation is difficult.[175]

Since blood pressure increases with height and age the value of the blood pressure must be interpreted by comparison with normal data.[175,176] The trend of rising levels of blood pressure in populations as a consequence of the increasing prevalence of obesity leads to questions to about which 'normal' data is the most appropriate to use.

Ambulatory blood pressure monitoring (ABPM) can also be used to assess blood pressure in children and adolescents and provides information about the presence or absence of a normal diurnal variation. The values obtained should be compared with published normal data.[177] Absence of a night-time dip in blood pressure is associated with a greater risk of cardiac events in adults and is more common in children with secondary hypertension than primary hypertension. However based on the data presently available ABPM is too insensitive to allow primary hypertension to be distinguished from secondary hypertension.[178]

Hypertension is defined as an average systolic or diastolic BP greater than the 95th centile for age, gender and height on at least three separate occasions. Tables of normal values for blood pressure in children are presented in Chapter 21 (Cardiology). Decisions about the child's management should not be made on the basis of single measurements. The timespan over which the three measurements are taken depends on clinical circumstances. Reactive causes of hypertension for example emotion, activity or pain should be excluded.

White coat hypertension, a phenomenon well documented in adults also occurs in children. This is a phenomenon in which blood pressure that is elevated when measured in a clinical environment is normal when measured in the child's home. The significance of white coat hypertension is uncertain – there is evidence to suggest that some individuals with white coat hypertension will go on to develop essential hypertension.[179]

ASSESSMENT OF THE HYPERTENSIVE CHILD

An accurate medical history and full clinical examination are essential to the evaluation of the child with elevated blood pressure. The purpose is to identify underlying causes, to detect any end-organ damage and to search for other cardiovascular risk factors.

History

Important features in the history include the following:
- *Presenting symptoms:* headache, epistaxis, vertigo, impaired vision, abdominal pain, polyuria, muscle weakness, weight loss, palpitations, flushing, chest pain and breathlessness should be sought;
- *Previous history:* urinary tract infection, renal, cardiac or endocrine disorders and any history of neonatal intensive care should be documented;
- *Drug history:* prescribed and recreational drugs may be of relevance;
- *Family history:* hypertension, premature cardiovascular disease, diabetes and renal disease.

Examination

Physical examination is normal in the majority of children with hypertension. However a careful examination should be undertaken. Centiles for height, weight and BMI should be documented. Particular attention should be paid to the cardiovascular system, seeking evidence of cardiomegaly and coarctation of the aorta. The blood pressure should be measured in two arms and a thigh. The child's volume status should be assessed. On abdominal examination abdominal masses and renal bruits should be sought. The examination of the CNS should include the cranial nerves and fundoscopy. Turner syndrome, Williams syndrome, neurofibromatosis, tuberose sclerosis and Cushing syndrome may all be associated with hypertension so their clinical features should be sought.[180,181]

If the child is symptomatic immediate referral to a specialised center and prompt treatment is indicated.[176]

Investigation

The extent of the investigation is determined by the severity of the hypertension and the presenting clinical features. Initial investigation consists of urinalysis, urine culture, FBC, urea and electrolytes, creatinine, calcium, albumin and phosphate, supine renin, CXR, cardiac echo, renal USS. Plasma lipid profile and fasting glucose measurement may be indicated to evaluate co-morbidity that may contribute to overall cardiovascular risk.

Further investigation is indicated in those cases in which the blood pressure is greater than the 99th centile or clinical presentation or initial investigations suggest an underlying cause.

Urinary catecholamines, plasma aldosterone, plasma cortisol, thyroid function, DMSA or Mag 3 scan, magnetic resonance angiography, renal angiography (Fig. 18.27) with renal vein renin sampling, cerebral imaging and angiograph.[176]

PREVALENCE AND CAUSES OF HYPERTENSION

The estimated prevalence of hypertension in children is 1–2%. Most studies indicate that of these approximately 70% have a detectable cause and 30% primary hypertension (Table 18.15). The most likely cause of hypertension depends on the age of the child. In all age groups secondary hypertension is most commonly due to renal disease (Table 18.16).

TREATMENT OF CONFIRMED HYPERTENSION

The aims of treatment are to reduce blood pressure below the 95th centile and to prevent the long-term adverse effects of sustained hypertension. For children with renal disease, diabetes or evidence of target organ damage the aim should be to reduce blood pressure below the 90th centile.

The families of all hypertensive children should receive advice about lifestyle modifications that may offer benefits of reducing blood pressure. These include healthy eating to reduce excessive weight gain, reducing dietary sodium intake and taking part in regular physical activity. These measures may be sufficient to treat children with primary hypertension.

Indications for antihypertensive drug therapy include severe hypertension at presentation, secondary hypertension, evidence of target organ damage and inadequate response to lifestyle modifications. Controlling the blood pressure is important even if the etiology is not established.

There are six classes of oral antihypertensive agents for long-term treatment: diuretics, beta-blockers, ACE inhibitors and angiotensin–receptor antagonists, calcium channel blockers and alpha-blockers (Table 18.17).

In choosing an antihypertensive agent it is important to consider the child's volume status, cardiac and renal function. Diuretics and calcium channel blockers are useful agents in children with salt and water overload. It is good practise to avoid the use of ACE inhibitors in children with renal impairment until the presence or absence of renovascular disease has been evaluated. In specialized centers these drugs may occasionally be used successfully to control blood pressure in children with small vessel-renovascular disease. Hypertension caused by renovascular disease or phaeochromocytoma may cause increased peripheral vascular resistance and a pressure natriuresis leading to hypovolemia. Vasodilators are useful in treating these children but concomitant fluid replacement may be needed to maintain tissue perfusion and avoid precipitous falls in blood pressure. In severe heart failure beta-blockers and vasodilators may further compromise cardiac function. Diuretics or ACE inhibitors may be preferable in this situation.

The selected agent should be started at a low dose and increased gradually until blood pressure is controlled. If blood pressure control

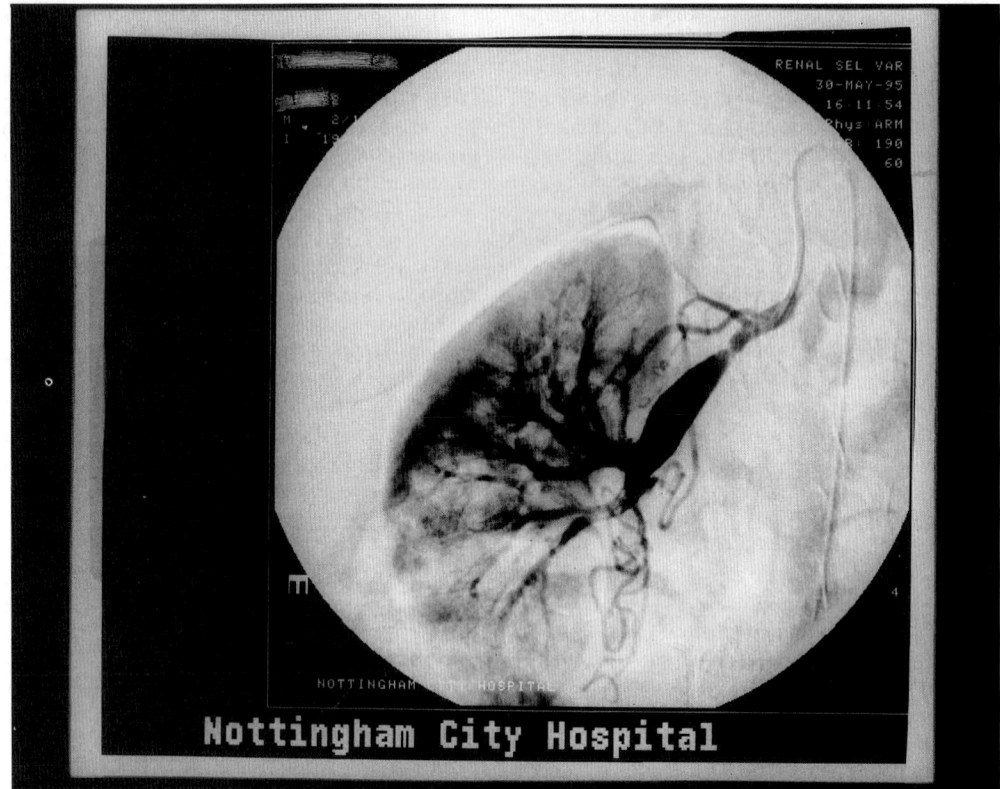

Fig. 18.27   Renal angiogram in 13-year-old female with sustained hypertension and abnormal spectral Doppler flow on ultrasound. 33% stenosis of the mid portion of the main renal artery.

Table 18.15   Causes of hypertension (from Varda & Gregoric[180])

Age	Newborn	First year	1–6 years	6–12 years	12–18 years
Causes of hypertension	Renal artery thrombosis, renal artery stenosis, renal venous thrombosis, congenital renal abnormalities, coarctation of the aorta, bronchopulmonary dysplasia, patent ductus arteriosus, intraventricular hemorrhage	Coarctation of the aorta, renovascular disease, renal parenchymal diseases	Renal parenchymal diseases, renovascular disease, coarctation of the aorta, endocrine causes, essential hypertension	Renal parenchymal diseases, renovascular disease, essential hypertension, coarctation of the aorta, endocrine causes, iatrogenic (e.g. medications, postoperative hypertension)	Essential hypertension, iatrogenic, renal parenchymal diseases, renovascular disease, endocrine causes, coarctation of the aorta

Table 18.16   Causes of renal hypertension

1. Chronic renal failure and post renal transplant
2. Renal parenchymal disease
   a. Scarring due to reflux nephropathy or obstructive uropathy
   b. Acute or chronic glomerulonephritis
   c. Hemolytic uremic syndrome
   d. Renal dysplasia
   e. Polycystic kidneys
3. Renovascular disease
   a. Renal artery stenosis
   b. Renal artery thrombosis
   c. Renal artery aneurysm
   d. Arteriovenous fistula
   e. Vasculitis, e.g. polyarteritis nodosa
4. Renal tumors
   a. Nephroblastoma
   b. Hamartoma
   c. Hemangiopericytoma

Table 18.17   Maintenance oral therapy for treatment of hypertension

Vasodilators		
Nifedipine	0.25–2 mg/kg/24 h	2 divided doses
Hydralazine	1–8 mg/kg/24 h	2–3 divided doses
Prazosin	0.05–0.4 mg/kg/24 h	2–3 divided doses
Minoxidil	200 µg–1.0 mg/kg	Single dose
Beta-blockers		
Propanolol	1–10 mg/kg/24 h	2–3 divided doses
Atenolol	1–4 mg/kg/24 h	Once/day if adequate renal function
Diuretics		
Frusemide	1–5 mg/kg/24 h	1–2 divided doses
Spironolactone	1–3 mg/kg/24 h	1–2 divided doses
ACE inhibitors		
Captopril	0.5–5 mg/kg/24 h	2–3 divided doses
Enalapril	0.1 mg–1 mg/kg/24 h	Single dose

is inadequate and the upper dose limit is reached or side-effects are encountered another agent from a different class is added.

The agents are often combined as follows: beta-blocker + diuretic, ACE inhibitor + diuretic, calcium channel blocker + beta-blocker, calcium channel blocker + ACE inhibitor.[176]

Beta-blockers have been considered the preferred first-line agent in children but data from adults indicating that ACE inhibitors are more effective in controlling blood pressure and beta-blockers are associated with a greater risk of non-insulin-dependent diabetes may lead to a change in prescribing for children.[181]

Emergency treatment

Severe hypertension may cause hypertensive encephalopathy, cerebral infarction and hemorrhage, facial palsy, visual disturbance, cardiac and renal failure. These clinical situations constitute a medical emergency. Antihypertensive therapy must be introduced promptly but with intensive monitoring to produce a gradual reduction in blood pressure, allowing preservation of target organ function (Table 18.18). Every effort should be made to avoid abrupt falls in blood pressure, as these are hazardous, particularly for neurological function. The aim is to reduce the blood pressure by one third of the total desired reduction over the first 12–24 h. This is usually best achieved using i.v. infusion of short-acting antihypertensive agents in a pediatric intensive care unit. Severe hypertension should be treated with labetalol as an i.v. infusion, which will lower blood pressure in a controlled manner. I.v. alternatives include nicardipine, or nitroprusside, although with the latter cyanide levels need to be monitored after 24 h. If i.v. access is difficult, sublingual nifedipine 0.25 mg/kg has been used, but carries the risk of too rapid a fall in BP. Once the blood pressure is under control oral agents can be introduced.

Follow-up

Regular follow-up is important in the care of children with hypertension. This is to monitor blood pressure control and adjust treatment accordingly. It also provides an opportunity to undertake surveillance for the side-effects of treatment and to look for the emergence of previously undetected causes of high blood pressure. Rarely the need for antihypertensive medication diminishes and treatment can be withdrawn.

ACUTE RENAL FAILURE

ARF is a sudden decrease in renal function resulting in an accumulation of nitrogenous wastes and associated with fluid and electrolyte imbalance. A urine output of 300 ml/m^2/24 h (or 1.0 ml/kg/h) is required to excrete the daily solute output. ARF is therefore usually associated with oliguria, although it may be associated with polyuria, particularly in the neonate.

EPIDEMIOLOGY

The incidence of ARF in children varies according to the population studied. In the UK, data from children referred to regional nephrology units for further management, suggested an incidence of 7.5 children per million population per year.[182] Most of the data is from single-center

studies and as a result the etiology largely reflects the population seen at that center with considerable inter-center variations; for example in one study[183] those with hemolytic uremic syndrome (HUS) accounted for 45% whereas in another study those with primary renal disease including HUS was only 7%.[184] The more recent studies suggest an epidemiologic shift towards an increase in renal failure resulting from complications of other systemic diseases resulting from advancements in congenital heart surgery, neonatal care, bone marrow and solid organ transplantation. Aggregate data from two large single-center studies[184,185] showed the commonest causes to be congenital heart disease (20%), acute tubular necrosis (18%), bone marrow transplantation/malignancy (16%), nephrotoxins (13%), and sepsis (13%).[186]

In neonates again the incidence varies mainly because of differences in the criteria used to define renal failure and ranges from 8 to 24% of all admissions to neonatal intensive care units.[187] Acute renal failure is often transient and related to hypovolemia, hypotension or hypoxemia or drug nephrotoxicity and is reversible with the resolution of the underlying problems causing hypoperfusion or the suspension of certain treatments. In one study[188] up to 60% of severely asphyxiated infants were shown to have renal failure, but none required dialysis. Very low birthweight infants are at particular risk of developing renal failure and in one study 79% of those developing neonates in the neonatal period were under 1500 g.[187]

PATHOGENESIS
Prerenal

If renal perfusion pressure falls, renal blood flow and GFR decline but there is excretion of good-quality urine (see Table 18.19). Causes include:

1. Excess losses:
   - gastroenteritis;
   - diabetes;
   - burns;
   - ileus;
   - hemorrhage.

These children appear dehydrated with signs including sunken fontanelle, poor peripheral perfusion with wide peripheral core temperature gap, tachycardia, and hypotension.

2. Impaired cardiac output:
   - congestive heart failure;
   - pericardial tamponade;
   - sepsis/shock.

Table 18.19 Biochemical urine indices in renal failure

	Prerenal	Renal
Urine osmolality (mOsm/kg)	> 500	< 350
Urine Na (mmol/L)	< 20	> 40
U/P creatinine	> 40	< 20
U/P urea	> 15	< 5
$FeNa^+ = \dfrac{UNa \times PCr}{PNa \times UCr}$	< 1%	> 3%

Table 18.18 Drug therapy of hypertensive crisis

Drug	Administration	Onset of effect	Side-effects
Nifedipine	Sublingual hourly p.r.n. 0.2–0.5 mg/kg	Minutes	Headaches, tachycardia
Sodium nitroprusside	0.5–10 mcg/kg/min as infusion	Seconds/minutes	*Very* rapid effect, titrate dose, cyanide accumulates after 48 h of use
Labetalol	1–3 mg/kg/h	10–30 min	Postural hypotension
Hydralazine	Slow i.v. 0.1–0.5 mg/kg	10–30 min	Tachycardia, flushing, headaches
Phentolamine	0.02–0.1 mg/kg	Minutes	Use in catecholamine excess states

3. Hypoalbuminemic states:
   - nephrotic syndrome;
   - liver failure.

These children are often edematous but have intravascular volume depletion with signs including poor peripheral perfusion with wide peripheral core temperature gap and tachycardia. Blood pressure, particularly in nephrotic syndrome, is variable.

Renal

Intrarenal causes of renal failure may be vascular, glomerular or tubular. These children are more likely to present with oliguria and signs of fluid overload, although those with tubular damage may present with polyuric renal failure. Causes include:

1. Vascular:
   - renal vein thrombosis;
   - arterial occlusion;
   - arteritis;
   - hemolytic uremic syndrome.
2. Glomerular:
   - acute glomerulonephritis.
3. Tubular:
   - nephrotoxins (especially drugs);
   - acute interstitial nephritis;
   - myoglobinuria;
   - crystal nephropathy;
   - secondary to prerenal failure.

Postrenal

Many children with obstructive causes present acutely with infection associated with obstruction and have signs of septicemia. A poor urinary stream or a palpable bladder is highly suggestive of bladder outflow obstruction. Causes include:

- posterior urethral valves;
- pelviureteric junction obstruction;
- vesicoureteric junction obstruction;
- neuropathic bladder;
- nephrolithiasis.

HISTORY AND EXAMINATION

Often the diagnosis may be clear, e.g. after cardiac bypass surgery, burns, or in association with multiorgan failure as in septicemia. In less obvious cases important clues in the history may include a history of diarrhea and vomiting, a poor urinary stream or exposure to drugs. Important features to note on examination include the state of hydration, blood pressure and other features including the presence of enlarged kidneys or a palpable bladder.

INVESTIGATIONS

Initial investigations should include full biochemical indices, including renal function and acid–base status together with hematological indices, including a blood film, and in many cases a blood culture. Dipstick urinalysis for blood and protein, microscopy and culture of the urine should also be performed and in some cases urine electrolytes may be helpful in differentiating prerenal and renal failure (see Table 18.19). A renal tract ultrasound will give information on renal size and will exclude obstruction.

All other investigations ordered will depend on these initial screening results. If the ultrasound suggests bladder outflow obstruction a micturating cystogram will be necessary to demonstrate the presence of urethral valves. If the ultrasound suggests pelviureteric obstruction a percutaneous nephrostomy together with a nephrostogram (or antegrade pyelogram) will be both therapeutic and diagnostic.

If the clinical picture is that of acute glomerulonephritis then further serological investigations and a renal biopsy will help to elucidate the cause and also guide further management with respect to immunosuppressive therapy (see Glomerulonephritis section).

MANAGEMENT

Fluids and circulation

Volume overload with hypertension, raised central venous pressure and edema may be treated with a diuretic *volume depletion* with a low blood pressure, low central venous pressure and a wide peripheral core temperature gap requires resuscitation with either volume expanders, e.g. isotonic saline, or 4.5% albumin 20 ml/kg. However the observation that fluid overload is associated with increased mortality in acute renal failure in children with multi-organ dysfunction supports the recommendation of goal-directed fluid resuscitation support with less post resuscitation fluid and increased use of inotropic support together with early renal replacement therapy.[189]

Low-dose dopamine was commonly administered to critically ill patients because it increased renal blood flow and induced diuresis in healthy volunteers. Clinical trials[190] and a systematic review of the literature[191] have shown no significant effect on overall patient survival/outcome or delay in dialysis. Similarly diuretics have been used in patients with oliguric renal failure to improve output, but have not been shown to prevent or facilitate recovery from acute tubular necrosis, and may cause renal function to deteriorate further.[192]

If poor peripheral perfusion remains, i.e. a wide peripheral core temperature gap, despite an adequate circulating volume and perfusion pressure, a vasodilator, hydralazine 0.2 mg/kg, may reverse the peripheral vasoconstriction such as furosemide 1–5 mg/kg/intravenously. If there is no response dialysis is indicated.

Maintenance fluids should be calculated as insensible losses together with continuing losses. Daily fluid requirements are directly related to energy expended. In practice, insensible losses are calculated as approximately 400 ml/m^2 body surface area. Modifications are required in the presence of fever (an increase of 12% of calculated insensible losses per degree above 37.5 °C), tachypnea (an increase of 20–25%), or in neonates nursed under radiant heaters (an increase of 25%).

Electrolyte disturbances

Hyperkalemia

- Salbutamol (alpha-2 adrenoceptor stimulant) as the first-choice treatment.[193] Salbutamol can be given intravenously (4 μg/kg in 10 ml of water over 10 min) or more commonly by nebulizer (2.5 mg < 25 kg body weight or 5 mg > 25 kg body weight).
- 10% calcium gluconate 0.5 ml/kg over 5–10 min antagonizes the effect of hyperkalemia on cells and is useful for prevention, or treatment of cardiac dysrhythmias.
- 8.4% sodium bicarbonate 1–2 mmol/kg may lower serum potassium in the presence of acidosis.
- Glucose 0.5 g/kg/h with insulin 0.1 u/kg/h intravenously acts rapidly (within 1 h) to lower potassium but has been superseded by salbutamol.
- Calcium resonium 1 g/kg orally or rectally acts more slowly.
- Salbutamol, the correction of acidosis and insulin shift potassium intracellularly, and should only be regarded as temporary measures until dialysis can be established.

Hyponatremia

Hyponatremia may be associated with neurological disturbances and convulsions particularly with values less than 120 mmol/L. This is often due to fluid overload and therefore treatment should be aimed at fluid removal. However, excess losses, particularly gastrointestinal, are associated with true sodium deficits, which should be replaced. Sodium deficit may be calculated as follows:

$$\text{mmol sodium deficit} = (140 - \text{actual serum sodium}) \times 0.6 \times \text{body weight in kg}$$

Half the deficit should be replaced in the first 24 h and the situation reviewed.

Hypocalcemia

Symptomatic patients may be given a bolus of 10% calcium gluconate 0.5 ml/kg intravenously over 5–10 min. Slower correction may be achieved by an infusion of 10% calcium gluconate, 0.1 mmol/calcium/kg body weight/h. The dose should be adjusted by frequent blood monitoring at least 6-hourly. Reduction of high phosphate levels may also improve plasma calcium levels.

Hypomagnesemia

50% magnesium sulfate 0.1 ml/kg intramuscularly.

Acidosis

Sodium bicarbonate 2 mmol/kg should be given intravenously as immediate treatment. The total deficit may be calculated as follows:

$$(24 - \text{the actual bicarbonate}) \times 0.6 \times \text{body weight in kg}$$

Half this amount may be given as an infusion over 4–6 h, and the acid–base status rechecked. Sodium bicarbonate needs to be given with caution, particularly in neonates and infants, as it may cause sodium, and thus fluid, overload as well as precipitating hypocalcemic symptoms.

Hyperuricemia

Uric acid levels are elevated in ARF and no specific treatment is usually given. Tumor lysis syndrome with grossly elevated uric acid levels can occur in the treatment of lymphomas and leukemia and a high fluid intake, allopurinol and an alkali therapy are usually employed.[194] However, the production of uric acid may be switched to that of xanthine and hypoxanthine, which can also cause a crystalline nephropathy. Recently rasburicase has been introduced, an agent that will oxidize uric acid to allantoin, a metabolite with 5–10-fold greater solubility than uric acid, and reduces serum uric acid levels within 4 hours of i.v. administration.

Convulsions

Convulsions may be due to electrolyte disturbances, uremia, hypertension, or the underlying disease such as hemolytic uremic syndrome. Many anticonvulsants tend to accumulate in renal failure. The safest emergency treatment is diazepam 0.25 mg/kg intravenously.

Hypertension

Hypertension may be due to fluid overload, which should be treated appropriately. Severe hypertension should be treated as an emergency as outlined in the section Renal hypertension. For sustained moderate hypertension a suitable regimen is a beta-blocker (e.g. propranolol) with or without a vasodilator (e.g. hydralazine) and/or calcium channel blocker (e.g. nifedipine).

Nutrition

Adequate nutrition is essential to prevent catabolism and the child should receive at least the estimated average requirement (EAR) for energy for chronological age. Energy is best provided as a combination of carbohydrate and fat, often using glucose polymers exclusively or in combination with fat emulsions. Protein intake will depend upon whether the child is being managed conservatively or is on dialysis.[195] Enteral feeding should be used whenever possible, although i.v. feeding may on occasions be necessary. Fluid restriction may limit the amount of nutrition that can be administered and this may be an indication to institute dialysis or increase ultrafiltration on dialysis. Specialized renal feeds often contain a high energy density and may need to be introduced gradually to prevent gastrointestinal intolerance. The protein, phosphate, sodium and potassium content of feeds need to be analyzed carefully as many are unsuitable for use in renal failure.

Anemia

This is inevitable in ARF but transfusion is only indicated if there are symptoms or the hemoglobin concentration is less than 6 g/dl or falling rapidly. Caution is required in transfusing a child who is not on dialysis as hyperkalemia and fluid overload may be precipitated.

Renal replacement therapy

The need for renal replacement therapy will in part be guided by the anticipated prognosis for recovery. If a quick return of renal function seems likely then the child may be managed conservatively. However, if a prolonged period of oliguria seems likely it is better to dialyze earlier and be able to ensure adequate nutrition as well as maintain metabolic balance. Guidelines on the indications for dialysis may be:

1. uncontrollable fluid overload/hypertension;
2. uncontrollable acidosis;
3. symptomatic electrolyte disturbances not controlled by above measures;
4. symptomatic uremia;
5. presence of a dialyzable toxin;
6. established anuria, even if 1–5 not present, provided obstruction excluded.

Because of the complexity of the fluid and electrolyte imbalance in acute renal failure dialysis remains the definitive treatment with the mode of dialysis chosen being dependent on the patients' needs and limitations and the local resources. Good practice requires early discussion of patients with ARF with pediatric nephrology staff and transfer for investigation and management in those with rapidly deteriorating renal function.[196,197]

Peritoneal dialysis

Peritoneal dialysis is the preferred option for neonates and is particularly useful in the hemodynamically unstable patient, who may tolerate hemodialysis, or even hemofiltration, poorly.

A soft Silastic catheter may be placed surgically or a more rigid polyethylene catheter inserted percutaneously into the abdomen using a Seldinger technique, though this technique is now seldom used. Commercially available dialysis solutions containing electrolytes, and glucose as an osmotic agent, are then introduced into the abdominal cavity. The volume and duration of the cycles of fluid are adjusted according to the ultrafiltration and clearance requirements of the patient.

Hemodialysis

Hemodialysis may be used in patients in whom there are technical difficulties encountered in running peritoneal dialysis, for example catheter blockage or leakage. It may also be used in those children in whom peritoneal dialysis is contraindicated, for example children with intra-abdominal sepsis, major intra-abdominal pathology or following recent abdominal surgery. It is the treatment of choice for acute poisoning with nonprotein-bound drugs or metabolic derangements such as hyperammonemia where high flux filters provide the most effective rapid removal of toxins. Vascular access is usually obtained via a venous catheter inserted percutaneously into a large vessel (either subclavian or femoral vein), to permit the necessary rapid blood flow rates required. Commercially available filters and lines are available to enable hemodialysis to be undertaken even in neonates, but such children need to be managed in specialist nephrology centers where nephrology nursing expertise is available.

Hemofiltration

The shift towards an increasing number of children requiring renal replacement therapy for acute renal failure in association with multi-organ dysfunction, together with the production of hemofiltration machines with volumetric control has led to an increase in the use of continuous renal replacement therapy in the form of continuous arteriovenous hemofiltration (CAVH), continuous veno-venous hemofiltration (CVVH) continuous veno-venous hemodialfiltration (CVVHD). These modalities have been used even in very small infants.[198] All provide controlled ultrafiltration and safe removal of fluid, which is particularly useful in unstable critically ill patients. Small molecular weight clearance (i.e. urea) has similar removal with CVVH and CVVHD but larger molecular weight clearance is enhanced by diffusive clearance (CVVHD) compared to convective clearance (CVVH).[199] One of the major disadvantages of continuous renal replacement therapies is the need for anti-coagulation.

Drugs

The kidney is the major route of elimination of many drugs and their metabolites. Decreased renal function leads to both predictable and unpredictable changes in the pharmacokinetic profiles of various drugs. Many drugs will also be removed by dialysis although as peritoneal and hemodialysis remove different sized molecules, the elimination of drugs may be different with the two forms of dialysis. It is therefore essential to refer to either drug data sheets or a reference text[200,201] to ensure the correct dosages of drugs are administered.

Outcome

Patient survival rates from ARF although 10–20% higher than in adults are around 30–58% with no change in recent years.[184,185,189] Mortality is the highest with multi-organ dysfunction syndrome and survival best in those with primary renal disease. The incidence of chronic renal failure or markers suggesting an uncertain prognosis (proteinuria, hypertension) in those surviving acute renal failure is not known[202] as follow-up studies are often limited and incomplete.[203]

Family support

ARF is an uncommon problem in resource rich countries. When dialysis is anticipated or a biopsy is necessary the child is transferred to a designated pediatric nephrology center, which can be some distance away from the patient's home, and this adds to the family's stress. Appropriate information and psychosocial support from the center's multidisciplinary team are very necessary.

Hyperkalemia is a medical emergency if ECG changes are present

I.v. labetalol or sodium nitroprusside is required for hypertensive encephalopathy but blood pressure reduction should be gradual

Patients with rapidly deteriorating renal function should be discussed early with the pediatric nephrology team

HEMOLYTIC UREMIC SYNDROME

The hemolytic uremic syndromes (HUSs) comprise a heterogeneous group of disorders in which a triad of features, microangiopathic hemolytic anemia, thrombocytopenia and ARF occur together. The average annual incidence in the UK is 0.7 per 100 000 children,[204,205] which is similar that seen in North America.[206] HUS has many different causes.

Epidemiology and pathogenesis
Shiga toxin producing E. coli
90% of childhood HUS follows a colitis prodrome with a Shiga toxin (Stx) producing E. coli. The reported risk of developing HUS with toxin associated diarrhea is very variable although is probably around 5–8%.[207]

In Canada and the USA > 80% of cases[208] are associated with E. coli O157 and in a UK survey in children with diarrhea associated HUS 83% had E. coli O157, in 15% no organism was isolated and in the remaining a variety of organisms were cultured including Campylobacter, Shigella, Salmonella, Rotavirus, staphylococci, streptococci and cryptosporidia.[205] In Australia O157 is rare and O111 strains are more common. The reason O157 may be the most prevalent is because it possesses certain virulence factors including virulence genes.[209] It is also an extremely hardy organism.[210] There are two main toxins, Stx1 and Stx2. Strains that produce only Stx1 have the lowest risk of producing HUS and strains that produce only Stx2 have the highest risk.[211]

The pathogenic cascade begins with the ingestion of the E. coli, which causes a colitis; the inflamed colon facilitates transmural absorption of Shiga toxins and lipopolysaccharide into the circulation. These Stxs then bind to genetically determined surface expressed glycolipid (Gb3) receptors on target cells. Renal tubular and glomerular Gb3 expression may be higher in infants than in adults and is one hypothesis to explain the age-related susceptibility.[212] This toxin-mediated injury model hypotheses that these toxins induce pro-inflammatory cytokines that upregulate Gb3 receptors on vascular endothelial cells allowing Stx to bind and subsequently injure endothelial cells. It is injury of the vascular endothelial cell which appears to be central in the pathogenesis of HUS,[213] although the contributions of host immunity, toxin receptor expression and development of intravascular coagulation in the development of that injury are uncertain.

The pathogenesis of the thrombotic disturbances in HUS is complex and remains incompletely understood. Current theory favors the concept that HUS is a pro-thrombotic disturbance in which a limited form of disseminated intravascular coagulation takes place. However unlike the consumptive coagulopathies the concentration of fibrinogen is normal or elevated, and the pro-thrombin time and the partial thromboplastin time are normal or only slightly prolonged. Elevation of plasma-plasminogen activator inhibitor activity and increased levels of tissue plasminogen activator antigen and D-dimer are also characteristic.[214] Thrombin generation and impaired fibrinolysis have been found, even in children with Stx colitis, without signs of HUS and it has been suggested these findings even may precede the development of HUS.[214,215]

There is good evidence that a pro-inflammatory cytokines play an important role. TNF alpha and certain other cytokines are known to activate the p38MAP kinase cascade and in animal studies administration of an inhibitor to p38MAP prevents the thrombotic microangiopathy.[216] Recent evidence suggests that the action of Stx and cytokines on the vascular endothelium is followed by secondary activation of platelets and coagulation cascade. The activated platelets further bind to the Shiga toxin amplifying the pro-thrombotic state.[217]

Stxs also cause release of von Willebrand factor (vWf), which mediates platelet adhesion to the endothelium and promotes the formation of platelet thrombi. Raised factor VIII-related antigens, together with an abnormal multimer pattern have been shown in some patients with HUS, although it is clear that the role of vWf is not the same in HUS as in thrombotic thrombocytopenic purpura (TTP). The deficiency of vWf cleaving metalloprotease (ADAMTS 13) resulting in elevated factor VIII levels seen in TTP is not typical of HUS. Renal tissue findings, however, suggest there may be a role for Stx-mediated intrarenal vWf release in the acute nephropathy of shiga toxin associated HUS.[218]

Prostacyclin is produced by normal endothelial cells and is a powerful inhibitor of platelet aggregation. Its precise role in the pathogenesis of HUS remains controversial, although prostacyclin activity has been shown to be low in some patients, either due to accelerated prostacyclin degradation or to a reduction in production. Animal studies have demonstrated normal biosynthesis[219] and other work in animal models suggest that prostacyclin is unlikely to be central to the pathophysiology. More recently the observation in animal models that the surface expression of thrombomodulin, which is a protein that normally inhibits coagulation,[220] is reduced offers another speculative explanation of the pathogenesis of the coagulation abnormalities seen.

Stx-induced HUS occurs most commonly in the summer months, affects younger children and is associated with a prodromal illness, usually of bloody diarrhea. The prognosis for a full recovery in this group is excellent. Survival is > 95%, and up to 75% of children will have no long-term sequelae.

Neuraminidase-producing organisms
Neuraminidase is an enzyme produced by a number of microorganisms, although in many it is cell bound and not released. It removes sialic acid from erythrocytes, platelets and glomeruli exposing the hidden Thomsen–Friedenreich antigen (T-cryptantigen). Anti-T, an IgM antibody present in most adult plasma, can then react with this exposed antigen leading to all the clinical manifestations of HUS. This phenomenon has been described in association with HUS in association with, most

commonly, *Streptococcus pneumoniae* but also other infections including influenza, parainfluenza, *Clostridium perfringens*, and *Bacteroides fragilis*. HUS complicating invasive pneumococcal disease is uncommon but often severe.[221,222] It is less common after meningitis than pulmonary disease, although that complicating meningitis has a poorer prognosis. In the largest series reported to date[223] 84% of children required dialysis, 12% died and 14% of the survivors developed chronic renal failure. It is anticipated that changes in immunization policies to include routine pneumococcal vaccination will alter the incidence of this condition.

Factor H and the complement pathway

There are many reports of decreased C3 levels in children with HUS, and in some cases, this is permanent, suggesting primary complement activation. Some cases are linked to abnormalities of complement Factor H, an important regulator of the alternative complement pathway. Following the observation of Warwicker,[223] several studies have linked mutations in the Factor H gene with familial or sporadic HUS. Complement levels should be checked in all children with atypical HUS but interpreted with caution. Abnormal levels which return to normal can be seen in Stx-associated HUS and those with abnormalities of factor H may have normal complement levels. Factor H can be measured quantitatively although determining functional abnormalities are more difficult and at present available only in a few research laboratories. The defect in factor H can be inherited as a heterozygous or homozygous disorder and is the result of a variety of nucleotide substitutions, insertions or deletions, which makes molecular genetic diagnosis challenging[224] and may explain the variability in clinical expression. Reduced expression of membrane co-factor, a widely expressed trans-membrane complement regulator has also been recognized as a cause of familial HUS.[225] Children with factor H associated HUS tend to have hypertension early in the course of the disease, tend to relapse and have a poor prognosis.[226]

Other causes

There is increasing awareness that there is a wide variety of other causes of HUS. Bone marrow transplantation is a well recognized cause and this may be aggravated by both *H. pylori* infection[227] and cyclosporine. A variety of other drugs,[228] malignant hypertension, malignancy and a wide range of infections have also been associated with the syndrome.

Clinical features

The commonest presentation is with gastrointestinal symptoms, usually bloody diarrhea. This prodrome may last for up to 2 weeks before the onset of the triad of features comprising the syndrome. Increasing pallor and mild jaundice due to hemolysis are noted, together with decreasing urine output. Typical hematological features are then present, the blood film revealing a microangiopathic hemolytic anemia, with thrombocytopenia and the presence of fragmented red cells. Biochemical changes are indicative of renal dysfunction together with macroscopic or microscopic hematuria and variable proteinuria. There is often no correlation between the severity of the hemolysis and the renal failure. Other nonrenal features include:

Gastrointestinal

Colitis is a feature of the disease and it may be difficult to distinguish between the prodrome and the onset of the disease itself. Although fever is not typical of acute colitis when it is seen there is an increased likelihood of developing HUS.[229] The presence of abdominal pain, and the passage of blood and mucus per rectum may lead to misdiagnosis as intussusception, ulcerative colitis or even Henoch–Schönlein syndrome. The acute colitic phase is usually self-limited although rectal prolapse and intussusception can occur and in more severe cases bowel ischemia can lead to bowel perforation or colonic stenosis. Cholethiasis has also been described as a complication.[230]

Pancreatic

Mild pancreatic involvement is common but in severe cases can lead to necrosis of the panceas or pseudocysts. Diabetes can be a long-term complication and is seen in the course of the disease in 1–2% of patients. Exocrine involvement is rare.

Cardiovascular

Most of the cardiovascular manifestations are due to volume overload. However, there are reports of cardiac involvement with thrombotic microangiopathy resulting in myocarditis, cardiomyopathy and cardiac failure. This life-threatening complication has been treated with ECMO.[231] Hypertension is also common and seen in between 23 and 32% of cases, more commonly in the nondiarrhea-associated HUS.

Neurological

Minor neurological disturbances of irritability, drowsiness, myoclonic jerks and tremor or ataxia are common. These may be due to metabolic derangements, or accelerated hypertension as well as a result of neurological involvement in the disease. More major neurological involvement such as coma, focal neurological deficit or decerebrate rigidity occurs less frequently although seizures may occur in up to 30% of patients.[232] Early regional EEG abnormalities, especially those in the occipital and temporal areas, are potentially useful in identifying those who might subsequently develop visual problems and epilepsy.[233] Neuroimaging typically shows basal ganglia involvement but in itself does not have a predictive value as the prognosis has been shown to be favorable even in those with severe changes.[234]

Investigations

Close monitoring of renal function and full blood count are necessary and blood glucose should be checked regularly. The neutrophil count can be a useful indicator as neutrophilia indicates both the likelihood of developing HUS and the severity of HUS once it has occurred.[235] A high neutrophil count, $> 20 \times 10^9$, is associated with an adverse prognosis.[236] Of patients with a neutrophil count $< 20 \times 10^9$, 93% have a good outcome compared to 33% of those with a neutrophil count $> 20 \times 10^9$. Neutrophils from patients with HUS have been shown to have increased adhesion to endothelium and are able to induce endothelial injury in vitro. It is postulated that these activated neutrophils degranulate onto endothelium causing damage by local release of proteases such as elastase, which has been found to be elevated in patients with HUS.

Stool should be sent for culture, even in the absence of diarrhea and serum should also be sent to look for antibodies to *E. coli* O157 as this increases the diagnostic identification above that of stool culture alone. Latex agglutination and immunoassays are also available to detect toxin in the stool.[237] Complement studies should be followed by further studies on factor H if abnormal or the history atypical. Factor VIII levels and measurement of ADMTS13 should also be sent if the history is atypical. Troponin subtype cTnI,[238] useful in detecting myocardial injury, should be sent in children with cardiological features.

Management

Many children with hemolytic uremic syndrome can be successfully managed with supportive therapy and careful attention to fluid balance, without the need for dialysis. However, it is essential to arrive at the diagnosis as soon as possible, as much morbidity can be induced by inappropriate fluid therapy, in patients whose renal function is compromised. Children with deteriorating renal function, oliguria/anuria or poor prognostic features should be referred early to a pediatric nephrology center. Poor prognostic features would include older children without a diarrheal prodrome, evidence of nonrenal involvement including encephalopathy or cardiomyopathy, or those children with a high neutrophil count $> 20 \times 10^9$/L. A prospective study of children with HUS showed that 57% of children received dialysis.[204]

A wide variety of treatments have been used in HUS. Anticoagulants such as heparin, prostacyclin, fibrinolytics such as streptokinase, i.v. immunoglobulin, steroids, antiplatelet agents and high doses of i.v. infusions of frusemide have all be tried but the evidence is insufficient to recommend their use.[239–243] None has been shown by controlled studies to affect prognosis, with the exception of the use of plasma infusion in a multicenter study.[244] Unfortunately this study is disadvantaged by the inclusion of children with epidemic HUS, who would be expected to have a good prognosis, together with those with sporadic HUS, who would be expected to have a poorer prognosis. The benefits of plasma, therefore, need to be weighed against the disadvantages. Such disadvantages would include the risk of volume overload, the transmission of blood-borne viral diseases and the potential for worsening hemolysis in those patients with neuraminidase-associated HUS. Plasma exchange has also been advocated and although it has been shown to be of benefit in thrombotic thrombocytopenic purpura in both the acute illness and in patients with recurrent episodes, there are insufficient data on children with HUS. There are theoretical reasons why it may be beneficial and its use may therefore be justified in the child with a severe deteriorating course, particularly with neurological involvement. In children with factor H deficiency, plasma exchange and replacement with plasma product containing factor H seems a reasonable option in the absence of better evidence.[226]

The role of antibiotics in influencing the clinical course is unclear, with studies showing both an increase and a decrease in the incidence of HUS in Stx-associated infections.[245,246] A recent meta-analyis[247] suggests that the issue remains unresolved.

A number of methods of prevention are being explored and include infusion of monoclonal antibodies to Stx,[248] administration of Gb3 receptor analogues[249] inhibiting the p38MAP pathway,[215] immunization[250] and development of medications to sequester Stx in the gastrointestinal lumen and prevent absorption.[251]

However currently best supportive therapy with dialysis and plasma exchange where indicted remains the mainstay of treatment.

Influencing long-term outcome

The acute mortality of HUS is around 5% in most series, although a recent survey in the UK comparing the mortality between 1985 and 1987 with that from 1999 to 2001 showed a fall in overall mortality from 5% to 2.5% between the two cohorts.[205] Mortality is higher in the nondiarrhea-associated HUS, and renal recovery is 88% in those with diarrhea-associated HUS compared to 56% in those with nondiarrhea-associated disease.[205]

Evidence of hypertension or impaired glomerular filtration rate is seen in between 11 and 25% of patients, with hypertension being more common in the nondiarrhea-associated disease and severe hypertension being particularly associated with Factor H associated HUS. Although children who remain on dialysis longer have a higher risk of long-term renal problems, the long-term sequelae cannot be reliably predicted by the acute clinical course. Persistent proteinuria is associated with a less good prognosis. A positive correlation between microalbuminuria and systolic blood pressure and a negative correlation between microalbuminuria and glomerular filtration rate[252] suggests that those children with albuminuria should receive longer and closer follow-up to identify occult nephropathy earlier. It has been suggested that long-term follow-up should be carried out on all children with proteinuria, hypertension, abnormal ultrasound or an impaired GFR at 1 year.[253] The full implications of the long-term sequelae of HUS may not yet have been realized, as a study on renal functional reserve demonstrated that all patients who had apparently made a complete recovery presented abnormalities in their renal functional reserve similar to that seen in children with a single kidney. However, the patients with HUS showed in addition an increase in microalbuminuria after a protein load, which may imply a poorer long-term prognosis.[254]

There is evidence that for those who develop chronic renal failure with proteinuria ACE inhibitors are useful for slowing progression due to hyperfiltration injury.[255] For those who develop chronic renal failure, renal transplantation is available. The prognosis for those with diarrhea-associated HUS is excellent and recurrence rate low.[256] For those with factor H associated HUS there is a high risk of recurrence and a potential definitive therapy that has been suggested in combined kidney–liver transplant although to date the outcomes have been poor.[257]

Hemolytic uremic syndrome associated with shiga toxin producing _E. coli_ is a major cause of acute renal failure in childhood.

Atypical or familial HUS has a poorer prognosis and may be associated with mutations in Factor H associated with the alternative complement pathway.

Persistent proteinuria, hypertension and/or reduced GFR are poor prognostic features after any acute or chronic renal insult.

CHRONIC RENAL FAILURE

Data on the prevalence of chronic renal failure are uncertain, at least in part as a result of the differing definitions of the level of renal dysfunction. European data[258] suggest a prevalence of between 25 and 50 children per million child population with a GFR less than $25-50 \, ml/min/1.73 \, m^2$.

End-stage renal failure is defined as the stage at which dialysis and renal transplantation are required (Table 18.20). There is no absolute level of renal function at which this is required although in practice it is usually a GFR $< 10 \, ml/min/1.73 \, m^2$. There are national and international renal registries for end-stage renal failure, which are important for identifying changes in incidence, treatment modalities and outcome. The European Dialysis Transplant Association (EDTA) register of children under 15 years of age accepted for renal replacement therapy each year suggested an incidence increasing from 4.6 per million child population in 1971 to 7–8 per million child population per annum in 1991.[259] In the UK, the national renal registry[260] reveals a take-on rate of under 15-year-olds is similar at 9 per million childhood population. The prevalence of renal failure rises steadily with age throughout childhood, the overall prevalence in under 15-year-olds being 51.4 per age-related population. There is however a wide ethnic variation with prevalence being twice as high in the Asian population compared to the white population. The etiology of renal failure varies also according to the child's country of origin, and age at presentation. In the UK renal dysplasia and glomerular diseases rank evenly in the UK, followed by obstructive uropathy and reflux nephropathy (Table 18.21).

Table 18.20 Stages of chronic renal failure

	GFR (ml/min/1.73 m²)	
Mild	50–75	Asymptomatic
Moderate	25–50	Metabolic abnormalities
Severe	< 25	Progressive growth failure
End-stage renal failure	< 10	Require renal replacement therapy

Table 18.21 Primary renal disease causing end-stage renal failure in 845 patients in UK[89]

	%
Primary renal dysplasia	23.4
Renal dysplasia	23.0
Obstructive uropathy	15.5
Reflux nephropathy	7.9
Tubulo-interstitial diseases	7.4
Congenital nephrotic syndrome	5.3
Metabolic diseases	4.8
Renovascular problems	3.7
Polycystic kidney disease	2.8
Chronic renal failure etiology unknown	2.7
Drug nephrotoxicity	2.0
Malignancy and associated disease	1.2

CLINICAL PRESENTATION

In many children, chronic renal failure will be the end result of known progressive renal disease. More recently, antenatal diagnosis has led to detection of renal tract malformations before symptoms develop. Other children may present with signs and symptoms associated with renal failure. These may be nonspecific symptoms, including lethargy, poor appetite and nausea, together with urinary symptoms, including polyuria or enuresis.

Growth

Growth failure is a major problem for children with chronic renal failure. The severity of the growth failure is related to the age at presentation: 50% of children with renal failure since infancy have growth failure, with a height of > 2 SD below the mean height for age, in contrast to 10% of those with acquired disease. Important factors contributing to the growth failure include: acidosis, salt depletion, other biochemical abnormalities, renal osteodystrophy, and energy malnutrition. Estimation of renal function would be a routine investigation in a child presenting with unexplained growth failure.

Renal osteodystrophy

Phosphate retention, secondary hyperparathyroidism and skeletal resistance to parathyroid hormone, intestinal malabsorption of calcium leading to hypocalcemia and altered vitamin D metabolism all contribute to the disturbances in bone and mineral metabolism associated with renal osteodystrophy. The severity of the bone disease is related to age at onset and underlying renal disease, together with the level of renal function and duration of renal failure. It is more common with the congenital and obstructive uropathies and rarely manifests clinically with a GFR of above $25\,ml/min/1.73\,m^2$ although biochemical abnormalities are seen with a GFR between 50 and $80\,ml/min/1.73\,m^2$.[261] Symptoms may include poor growth, bone pain, skeletal deformities, and slipped epiphyses.

Anemia

Anemia secondary to a lack of erythropoietin is also a well-recognized complication of renal failure and may be the presenting feature of the condition.

Hypertension

Renin-dependent hypertension is the commonest cause of hypertension in childhood and may be associated with renal failure. The presentation of renal failure may therefore be with the symptoms of hypertension including headache, visual disturbances or hypertensive encephalopathy.

MANAGEMENT
Fluid and electrolyte therapy

Many children with congenital renal diseases, in particular dysplasia, obstructive uropathy and nephronophthisis, have poor renal concentrating capacity with polyuria and salt loss. Salt supplementation is often necessary and salt deficiency is an important cause of poor growth in these infants. Children with acquired diseases, in particular focal glomerulosclerosis and other forms of glomerulonephritis, may have salt and water retention and therefore require salt restriction. Acidosis is common and should be corrected with sodium bicarbonate.

Infection

Urine cultures should be checked, especially in those with abnormalities of the urinary tract, as repeated infection may hasten progression of CRF.

Renal osteodystrophy

The impairment of excretion of phosphate and the decreased renal production of 1,25-dihydroxycholecalciferol together play important roles in the development of renal osteodystrophy and secondary hyperparathyroidism. Initially, dietary phosphate restriction may be sufficient to control hyperphosphatemia, although this can be difficult in young infants on a predominantly milk diet and the use of phosphate binders may become necessary. Calcium carbonate and calcium acetate are the most commonly used phosphate binders but the use of these may result in hypercalcemia. Noncalcium-containing phosphate binders are available although the aluminum containing compounds are best avoided in children because of the potentially neurotoxic effects.

Pharmacologic replacement, with 1-alpha-hydroxycholecalciferol, should be commenced when there are biochemical features of altered mineral metabolism or if the GFR falls below $25\,ml/min/1.73\,m^2$. The phosphate should be controlled before it is introduced as vitamin D causes an increase in phosphate absorption. If secondary hyperparathyroidism remains uncontrolled then success has been achieved with the use of the newly introduced calcimimetic agents.[262] There are no data on the use of these in children at present.

Data from adults has demonstrated that control of phosphate and parathyroid hormone is important not only for control of renal osteodystrophy but has important implications for long-term cardiovascular health.[263,264]

Erythropoietin

The production of human erythropoietin (rhEPO), by recombinant DNA techniques, has made possible the treatment of the anemia of chronic renal failure and significantly improved the quality of life for many patients. The use of rhEPO, usually given subcutaneously, has been shown to be effective in raising the hematocrit of children with end-stage renal failure. It is also effective in predialysis patients. RhEPO may result in hypertension and changes in renal function so both of these should be monitored closely. Standards for management of anemia, mineral metabolism and various other aspects of renal failure are published in national guidelines.[265,266]

Growth hormone

Short stature is a serious problem for children with chronic renal failure. Endogenous growth hormone secretion is normal, as are serum levels of insulin-like growth factors I and II. However, exogenous growth hormone has been shown to increase the height velocity in a number of conditions in which growth hormone secretion is not impaired including renal failure. Growth hormone does increase the short-term growth velocity of prepubertal children with chronic renal failure. Long-term use of growth hormone for up to 9 years is associated with persistent catch-up growth and an improvement in final height was demonstrated compared with untreated children.[267] However, one study[268] suggested that the improvement in height, obtained after a limited course of growth hormone, was maintained after discontinuation of treatment. The optimal treatment regimen of growth hormone therefore remains unknown. Of concern is that growth hormone may accelerate renal functional decline by increasing renal plasma flow and glomerular hyperfiltration and thus concerns have been expressed on the use of growth hormone post renal transplantation. However it has been shown to be effective and not associated with any increased adverse effects.[269] In view of the possible side-effects growth hormone use should be restricted to children who are below the third centile for height and in whom all other abnormalities such as electrolyte and acid–base balance, renal osteodystrophy and nutritional deficiencies have been corrected.

Nutrition

General recommendations for children with chronic renal failure suggest that children should have at least the EAR for chronological age for energy, although many will need additional energy to promote growth. Protein intake should be based on the reference nutrient intake (RNI) for height age. However, individual dietary and biochemical assessment will determine requirements, as well as the stage of management.[270] Large reliance is placed upon nutritional supplements to achieve nutritional goals in infants and children with chronic renal failure and the assistance of an experienced pediatric dietitian is essential. In many infants and young children the supplements are delivered either nasogastrically or via the gastrostomy route. Each child will need assessing individually, with respect to fluid and electrolyte needs, along with adequacy of micronutrient intake. These children require frequent and repeated assessments of their dietary prescriptions, if growth is to be maintained or promoted.

In adults attention has focused on dietary modifications to retard the progression of chronic renal failure. Of particular interest has been the role of restriction of dietary phosphate and protein in retarding the progression of chronic renal failure. Both the efficacy and safety of severe protein restriction in growing children requires evaluation, because of the concern regarding the effect of protein restriction on growth. The results from trials in children using protein restriction of 1 g/kg/d have shown conflicting results in the effect on GFR, although no adverse effect on growth has been demonstrated.[271] Compliance with dietary manipulations in childhood is often poor and in the European study on protein restriction only 76% of children adhered to their dietary prescription. Further studies are needed before such treatments are recommended for widespread clinical use in children.

Dialysis

Dialysis does achieve satisfactory control of fluid and biochemistry, but is an incomplete form of renal replacement therapy, and is therefore considered a stepping-stone to renal transplantation in most children. The two main forms of dialysis are chronic peritoneal dialysis and hemodialysis. The choice between peritoneal dialysis and hemodialysis will depend on patient preference, geographical and practical considerations.

Chronic peritoneal dialysis

Access to the peritoneal cavity is by way of a surgically implanted permanent Silastic catheter.[272] When chronic peritoneal dialysis (CPD) was first introduced, children underwent continuous ambulatory peritoneal dialysis (CAPD), where the dialysis fluid was exchanged three or four times via 'bag changes'. The advent of automated peritoneal dialysis (APD), in the 1980s, meant that children could receive most of their dialysis overnight (nocturnal intermittent peritoneal dialysis, NIPD) or mostly overnight with daytime dwell as well (continuous cycling peritoneal dialysis [CCPD]). APD is now the preferred modality in many Western countries, with the obvious benefit of freedom from daytime exchanges at school.

The disadvantages of CPD are the risk of peritonitis and other abdominal complications such as hernias.

Hemodialysis

Hemodialysis requires adequate vascular access either via an arteriovenous fistula, or more commonly, via an indwelling vascular catheter, usually in the subclavian or jugular vein. Although the technical principles of hemodialysis are similar in adults and children, because of the challenges presented by the smaller intravascular volumes of children and the potential hemodynamic instability, together with the psychological issues it is recommended that children be treated in units with pediatric expertise. Difficulties with vascular access, including infection, are a disadvantage of the technique.

Transplantation

Renal transplantation is the best mode of renal replacement therapy for children and adolescents.[273] In the UK[260] 76% of children with end-stage renal failure has a functioning graft. At all ages pediatric renal transplant recipients have better survival than do dialysis patients of the same age. Moreover, successful transplantation confers a degree of physiological and psychological rehabilitation not seen with any form of dialysis. Whilst most children undergo transplantation following the commencement of dialysis, in the UK about 20% of children receive transplantation prior to this (pre-emptive transplantation). Not only do results demonstrate improved growth and psychosocial development, the long-term outcome may be superior and peritoneal and hemodialysis access is preserved for future use in childhood or adult life.[274,275] A child is generally considered for pre-emptive transplantation once the glomerular filtration rate (GFR) has fallen below 10–15 ml/min/1.73 m², and dialysis is anticipated within 18–24 months and/or a significant complication of renal failure is present, for example, growth failure.

Graft survival

Registries held by UK Transplant in the UK and the North American Pediatric Renal Transplant Cooperative Study (NAPRTCS) in North America provide good quality data on the outcomes of renal transplantation. Graft survival rates in the UK suggest 1-year graft survival of 90% for cadaveric renal transplantation, with over 93% survival for live donor grafts. Longer term follow-up results need to be interpreted with caution as treatment modalities and immunosuppressive regimens have changed considerably over the last decade but UK 5-year survival is 72% in cadaveric donors and 85% in live donors.[276] The use of live donor grafts between countries is very variable. In the UK currently 25% of those with grafts are from living donors whereas in North America rates of 50%[277] have been reported and in the Nordic countries even higher.

Graft success rates are dependent on a wide variety of factors including tissue matching, donor age, storage time of the kidney, immunosuppression regimens, previous transplantation and original and associated diseases. There was concern about outcomes in the younger renal transplant recipient, as early European and North American data tended to suggest that graft survival was lower in children less than 2 years old compared to older children. Recent reports are more encouraging.[278,279] A study on children developing end-stage renal failure under 2 years of age and receiving grafts at a median age of 2.6 years demonstrated a 10-year graft survival of 78%.[280] Results from live donation are consistently superior and comparable with other age groups.[281,282] There is a highly significant increased risk of graft failure associated with donors under 5 years of age.[283] In cadaveric transplantation there was a tendency to use young donors in young recipients and when stratified for donor age, recipient age does not seem to influence outcome and it is anticipated that policies involving not using organs from young donors in young recipients will improve the outcome of this group. More recent concern has focused on the outcome of renal transplantation in adolescents,[284,285] in whom long-term outcome lags significantly behind that of younger children. Poor compliance is a major contributory factor in these young people.

Immunosuppression

All transplanted children will remain on immunosuppressive therapy with a calcineurin inhibitor, either ciclosporin or tacrolimus, usually with steroids and, in some, also azathioprine. Induction therapy with monoclonal antibodies may be used in some children and mycophenolate mofetil may be used particularly in those children with calcineurin inhibitor toxicity. In the UK national guidelines on immunosuppression therapy in children have recently been produced.[286] It is important to consider the side-effects of these medications, including risk of infection, hypertension, hirsutism and other cosmetic side-effects, which may influence compliance, particularly in adolescents. The long-term risks of steroids are particularly well known and there are some early encouraging reports of steroid-free immunosuppression.[287] With further medications being developed in future it may be possible to provide immunosuppression with greater specificity and fewer toxic effects.

Rehabilitation

Growth is improved after renal transplantation, with a significant increase in growth velocity in prepubertal children. However, perhaps one of the most important issues when considering the quality of life following renal transplantation is the neurodevelopmental and psychological outcome.

Early reports of children with chronic renal failure, particularly those who had had renal failure since infancy, showed a worrying proportion of those children having significant developmental delay.[288] The etiology was felt to be multifactorial, including: poor biochemical control, inadequate nutrition, the use of aluminum-containing phosphate binders and psychosocial factors. However, recent studies have been more encouraging, with the authors suggesting that the marked improvement in neurodevelopmental outcome was due to a shift in emphasis in renal failure management, with a more aggressive approach to nutrition and biochemical parameters.[289,290]

Studies on older children with renal failure have demonstrated effects on cognitive development, but despite these deficits there is no difference in grades achieved at school. Studies on the psychosocial adjustment of adult survivors of pediatric dialysis and transplant programs have shown that although the educational and employment achievements of those with renal disease are less than those of controls, two thirds of the patients leave school with qualifications and two thirds are in employment.[291] In conclusion, therefore, dialysis and transplantation enable the majority of children with end-stage renal failure to enter adulthood in good physical health and well adjusted socially. However, the burden for families caring for children with renal failure, as with many other chronic illnesses is considerable. It is essential that such families have the benefits of support from an experienced multidisciplinary team which includes nursing and medical staff, dietitians, social workers, teachers, play leaders, psychologists and psychiatrists who are able to work not only in hospital but also support the families in their own communities.

Renal dysplasia/hypoplasia and glomerulopathies are the commonest categories of conditions causing chronic renal failure (CRF) in childhood.

Recombinant erythropoietin by subcutaneous or i.v. injections can correct the anemia of CRF.

Renal transplantation is the treatment of choice for children with end-stage renal failure and is increasingly performed before dialysis is necessary.

REFERENCES

1 Stevens LA, Coresh J, Greene T, et al. Assessing kidney function – measured and estimated glomerular filtration rate. N Engl J Med 2006; 354:2473–2483.

2 Skinner R, Cole M, Pearson ADJ, et al. Specificity of pH and osmolality of early morning urine sample in assessing distal renal tubular function in children: results in healthy children. BMJ 1996; 312:1337–1338.

3 Scheinman SJ, Guay-Woodford LM, Thakker RV, et al. Genetic disorders of renal electrolyte transport. N Engl J Med 1999; 340:1177–1187.

4 Gahl WA, Thoene JG, Schneider JA. Cystinosis. N Engl J Med 2002; 347:111–121.

5 Karet FE, Finberg KE, Nelson RD, et al. Mutations in the gene encoding B1 subunit of H+-ATPase cause renal tubular acidosis with sensorineural deafness. Nat Genet 1999; 21:84–90.

6 Smith AN, Skaug J, Choate KA, et al. Mutations in ATP6N1B, encoding a new kidney vacuolar proton pump 116-kD subunit, cause recessive distal renal tubular acidosis with preserved hearing. Nat Genet 2000; 26:71–75.

7 Bruce LJ, Cope DL, Jones GK, et al. Familial distal renal tubular acidosis is associated with mutations in the red cell anion exchanger (Band 3, AE1) gene. J Clin Invest 1997; 100:1693–1707.

8 Wilson FH, Disse-Nicodème S, Choate KA, et al. Human hypertension caused by mutations in WNK kinases. Science 2001; 293:1107–1112.

9 Goodyer P. The molecular basis of cystinuria. Nephron Exp Nephrol 2004; 98:e45–e49.

10 Goodyer P, Saadi Y, Ong P, et al. Cystinuria subtype and the risk of nephrolithiasis. Kidney Int 1998; 54:56–61.

11 Cochat P. Primary hyperoxaluria type 1. Kidney Int 1999; 55:2533–2547.

12 Reusz GS, Hoyer PF, Lucas M, et al. X-linked hypophosphataemia: treatment height gain and nephrocalcinosis. Arch Dis Child 1990; 65:1125–1128.

13 Ichikawa I, Kuwayama F, Pope JC, et al. Paradigm shift from classic anatomic theories to contemporary cell biological views of CAKUT. Kidney Int 2002; 61:889–898.

14 Al-Khaldi N, Watson AR, Zuccollo J, et al. Outcome of an antenatally detected cystic dysplastic kidney disease. Arch Dis Child 1994; 70:520–522.

15 Sukthankar S, Watson AR on behalf of the Trent and Anglia Paediatric Nephrourology Group. Unilateral multicystic dysplastic kidney disease: defining the natural history. Acta Paediatr 2000; 89:811–813.

16 James CA, Watson AR, Twining P, et al. Antenatally detected urinary tract abnormalities: changing incidence and management. Eur J Pediatr 1998; 157:508–511.

17 Parkhouse HF, Barratt TM, Dillon MJ, et al. Long-term outcome of boys with posterior urethral valves. Br. Journal of Urology 1988; 62:59–62.

18 Ulman I, Jayanthi VR, Koff SA. The long-term follow up of newborns with severe unilateral hydronephrosis initially treated nonoperatively. J Urol 2000; 164(Pt 2):1101–1105.

19 Guay-Woodford LM. Autosomal recessive disease: clinical and genetic profiles. In: Torres V, Watson M, eds. Polycystic kidney disease. Oxford: Oxford University Press; 1996.237–267.

20 Roy S, Dillon M, Trompeter R, et al. Autosomal recessive polycystic kidney disease: long-term outcome of neonatal survivors. Pediatr Nephrol 1997; 11:302–306.

21 Peters DJM, Breuning MH. Autosomal dominant polycystic kidney disease: modification of disease progression. Lancet 2001; 358:1439–1444.

22 Ala-Mello S, Kivivuori S, Ronnholm K, et al. Mechanism underlying early anemia in children with familial juvenile nephronophthisis. Pediatr Nephrol 1996; 10:578–581.

23 Torres V. Tuberous sclerosis complex. In: Torres V, Watson M, eds. Polycystic kidney disease. Oxford: Oxford University Press; 1996.283–308.

24 Marild S, Jodal U. Incidence rate of first-time symptomatic urinary tract infection in children under 6 years of age. Acta Paediatr 1998; 87:549–552.

25 Zorc JJ, Levine DA, Platt SL, et al. Multicenter RSV-SBI Study Group of the Pediatric Emergency Medicine Collaborative Research Committee of the American Academy of Pediatrics. Clinical and demographic factors associated with urinary tract infection in young febrile infants. Pediatrics 2005; 116:644–648.

26 Singh-Grewal D, Macdessi J, Craig J. Circumcision for the prevention of urinary tract infection in boys: a systematic review of randomised trials and observational studies. Arch Dis Child 2005; 90:853–858.

27 Chand DH, Rhoades T, Poe SA, et al. Incidence and severity of vesicoureteral reflux in children related to age, gender, race and diagnosis. J Urol 2003; 170 (Pt 2):1548–1550.

28 Stauffer CM, van der Weg B, Donadini R, et al. Family history and behavioral abnormalities in girls with recurrent urinary tract infections: a controlled study. J Urol 2004; 171:1663–1665.

29 Nguyen H, Weir M. Urinary tract infection as a possible marker for teenage sex. South Med J 2002; 95:867–869.

30 Tambyah PA, Maki DG. Catheter-associated urinary tract infection is rarely symptomatic: a prospective study of 1,497 catheterized patients. Arch Intern Med 2000; 160:678–682.

31 Gauthier M, Chevalier I, Sterescu A, et al. Treatment of urinary tract infections among febrile young children with daily intravenous antibiotic therapy at a day treatment center. Pediatrics 2004; 114:e469–e476.

32 Stull TL, LiPuma JJ. Epidemiology and natural history of urinary tract infections in children. Med Clin North Am 1991; 75:287–297.

33 Gorelick MH, Shaw KV. Screening tests for urinary tract infection in children: a meta-analysis. Pediatrics 1999; 104:54.

34 American Academy of Pediatrics: Committee on Quality Improvement and Subcommittee on Urinary Tract Infection Practice Parameter. The Diagnosis, Treatment, and Evaluation of the Initial Urinary Tract Infection in Febrile Infants and Young Children. Pediatrics 1999; 103:843–852.

35 Report of a Working Group of the Research Unit Royal College of Physicians Guidelines for the management of acute urinary tract infection in childhood. J Roy Coll Phys Lond 1991; 25:36–42.

36 Verrier-Jones K, Hockley B, Scrivener R, et al. Diagnosis and management of urinary tract infections in children under two years: Assessment of practice against published guidelines. R Coll Paediatr Child Health 2001; 1–136.

37 McGillivray D, Mok E, Mulrooney E, et al. A head-to-head comparison: 'clean-void' bag versus catheter urinalysis in the diagnosis of urinary tract infection in young children. J Pediatr 2005; 147:451–456.

38 Li PS, Ma LC, Wong SN. Is bag urine culture useful in monitoring urinary tract infection in infants? J Paediatr Child Health 2002; 38:377–381.

39 Macfarlane PI, Ellis R, Hughes C, et al. Urine collection pads: are samples reliable for urine biochemistry and microscopy? Pediatr Nephrol 2005; 20:170–179.

40 Jewkes FEM, McMaster DJ, Napier WA, et al. Home collection of urine specimens – boric acid bottles or dipslides? Arch Dis Child 1990; 65:286–289.

41 Turner GM, Coulthard MG. Fever can cause pyuria in children. BMJ 1995; 311:924.

42 Committee on Quality Improvement, Subcommittee on Urinary Tract Infection. Practice parameter: the diagnosis, treatment, and evaluation of the initial urinary tract infection in febrile infants and young children. [published corrections appear in Pediatrics 2000;105:141; 1999;103:1052, and 1999; 104:118]. Pediatrics 1999; 103: 843–852.

43 Hoberman A, Wald ER, Hickey RW, et al. Oral versus initial intravenous therapy for urinary tract infections in young febrile children. Pediatrics 1999; 104:79–86.

44 Baker PC, Nelson DS, Schunk JE. The addition of ceftriaxone to oral therapy does not improve outcome in febrile children with urinary tract infections. Arch Pediatr Adolesc Med 2001; 155:135–139.

45 Ladhani S, Gransden W. Increasing antibiotic resistance among urinary tract isolates. Arch Dis Child 2003; 88:444–445.

46 Prais D, Straussberg R, Avitzur Y, et al. Bacterial susceptibility to oral antibiotics in community-acquired urinary tract infection. Arch Dis Child 2003; 88:215–218.

47 Keren R, Chan E. A meta-analysis of randomized, controlled trials comparing short- and long-course

antibiotic therapy for urinary tract infections in children. Pediatrics 2002; 109:E70.

48 Bloomfield P, Hodson EM, Craig JC. Antibiotics for acute pyelonephritis in children. The Cochrane Database of Systematic Reviews 2005; (Issue 1): Art. No.: CD003772. DOI: 10.1002/14651858. CD003772.pub2.

49 Currie ML, Mitz L, Raasch CS, et al. Follow-up urine cultures and fever in children with urinary tract infection. Arch Pediatr Adolesc Med 2003; 157:1237–1240.

50 Royal College of Physicians. Guidelines for the management of acute urinary tract infection in childhood. Report of a working group of the Research Unit. JR Coll Physicians Lond 1991; 25:36–42.

51 Dudley J, Chambers T. Why the resistance to diagnostic imaging in childhood urinary tract infections. Lancet 1996; 348:71–72.

52 Dick PT. Annual Meeting of Canadian Pediatric Society, June 12–16. Pediatric Notes 2002; 26:105.

53 Hoberman A, Charron M, Hickey RW, et al. Imaging studies after a first febrile urinary tract infection in young children. N Engl J Med 2003; 348:195–202.

54 Tibballs JM, De Bruyn R. Primary vesicoureteric reflux – how useful is postnatal ultrasound?. Arch Dis Child 1996; 75:444–447.

55 Jakobsson B, Svensson L. Transient pyelonephritic changes on 99m Technetium-dimercaptosuccinic acid scan for at least five months after infection. Acta Paediatr 1997; 86:803–807.

56 Phillips D, Watson AR, Collier J. Distress and radiological investigations of the urinary tract in children. Eur J Pediatr 1996; 155:684–687.

57 Rothwell DL, Constable AR, Albrecht M. Radionuclide cystography in the investigation of vesicoureteric reflux in children. Lancet 1977; 1:1072–1275.

58 Hansson S, Jodal U. Urinary tract infection. In: Barratt M T, Avner E D, Harmon W E, eds. Pediatric nephrology. Boston: Little, Brown; 1999.1943–1991.

59 Jepson RG, Mihaljevic L, Craig J. Cranberries for preventing urinary tract infections. The Cochrane Database of Systematic Reviews 2004; 2: CD001321

60 Jepson RG, Mihaljevic L, Craig JC. Cranberries for treating urinary tract infections. The Cochrane Database of Systematic Reviews 1998; CD001322

61 Reid G. The potential role of probiotics in pediatric urology. J Urol 2002; 168:1512–1517.

62 Wheeler DM, Vimalachandra D, Hodson EM, et al. Interventions for primary vesicoureteric reflux. The Cochrane Database of Systematic Reviews 2004; 2: CD001532

63 Williams GJ, Lee A, Craig JC. Long-term antibiotics for preventing recurrent urinary tract infection in children. The Cochrane Database of Systematic Reviews 2001; 4: CD001534

64 Williams GL, Lee A, Craig JC, et al. Cochrane Review. The Cochrane Library, 4. Oxford: Update Software; 2002.

65 Ladhani S, Gransden W. Increasing antibiotic resistance among urinary tract isolates. Arch Dis Child 2003; 88:444–445.

66 Kemper KJ, Avner ED. The case against screening urinalyses for asymptomatic bacteriuria in children. Am J Dis Child 1992; 146:343–346.

67 Lebowitz RL, Olbing H, Parkkulainen KV, et al. International system of radiographic grading of vesicoureteric reflux. International Reflux Study in Children. Tamminen-Mobius TE. Pediatr Radiol 1985; 15:105–109.

68 Downs S. Technical report: urinary tract infections in febrile infants and young children. Pediatrics 1999; 103:

69 Phan V, Traubici J, Hershenfield B, et al. Vesicoureteral reflux in infants with isolated antenatal hydronephrosis. Pediatr Nephrol 2003; 18: 1224–1228. Epub 2003 Oct 30

70 Marra G, Barbieri G, Moioli C, et al. Mild fetal hydronephrosis indicating vesicoureteric reflux. Arch Dis Child Fetal Neonatal Ed 1994; 70:F147–F149. discussion 149–150

71 Dudley JA, Haworth JM, McGraw ME, et al. Clinical relevance and implications of antenatal hydronephrosis. Arch Dis Child Fetal Neonatal Ed 1997; 76:F31–F34.

72 Ichikawa I, Kuwayama F, Pope JC, et al. Paradigm shift from classic anatomic theories to contemporary cell biological views of CAKUT. Kidney Int 2002; 61:889–898.

73 Eccles MR, Bailey RR, Abbott GD, et al. Unravelling the genetics of vesicoureteric reflux: a common familial disorder. Hum Mol Genet 1996; 5:1425–1429.

74 Noe HN, Wyatt RJ, Peeden Jr JN, et al. The transmission of vesicoureteral reflux from parent to child. J Urol 1992; 148:1869–1871.

75 Aggarwal VH, Verrier-Jones K. Vesicoureteric reflux – screening of the first degree relatives. Arch Dis Child 1989; 64:1538–1541.

76 Feather SA, Malcolm S, Woolf AS, et al. Primary, nonsyndromic vesicoureteric reflux and its nephropathy is genetically heterogeneous, with a locus on chromosome 1. Am J Hum Genet 2000; 66:1420–1425.

77 Mackintosh P, Almarhoos G, Heath DA. HLA linkage with familial vesicoureteric reflux and familial pelvi-ureteric junction obstruction. Tissue Antigens 1989; 34:185–189.

78 Groenen PM, Vanderlinden G, Devriendt K, et al. Rearrangement of the human CDC5L gene by a t(6;19)(p21;q13.1) in a patient with multicystic renal dysplasia. Genomics 1998; 49:218–229.

79 Eccles MR, Schimmenti LA. Renal-coloboma syndrome: A multi-system developmental disorder caused by PAX2 mutations. Clin Genet 1999; 56:1–9.

80 Ogata T, Muroya K, Sasagawa I, et al. Genetic evidence for a novel gene(s) involved in urogenital development on 10q26. Kidney Int 2000; 58:2281–2290.

81 Groenen PM, Garcia E, Debeer P, et al. Structure, sequence, and chromosome 19 localization of human USF2 and its rearrangement in a patient with multicystic renal dysplasia. Genomics 1996; 38:141–148.

82 Izquierdo L, Porteous M, Paramo PG, et al. Evidence for genetic heterogeneity in hereditary hydronephrosis caused by pelvi-ureteric junction obstruction, with one locus assigned to chromosome 6p. Hum Genet 1992; 89:557–560.

83 Lebowitz RL. The detection and characterization of vesicoureteral reflux in the child. J Urol 1992; 148(Pt 2):1640–1642.

84 Gleeson FV, Gordon I. Imaging in urinary tract infection. Arch Dis Child 1991; 66:1282–1283.

85 Hodson CJ, Edwards D. Chronic pyelonephritis and vesico-ureteric reflux. Clin Radiol 1960; 11:219–231.

86 Ardissino G, Dacco V, Testa S, et al. Epidemiology of chronic renal failure in children: Data from the ItalKid project. Pediatrics 2003; 111:e382–e387.

87 Goonasekera CDA, Shah V, Wade AM, et al. 15-year follow-up of renin and blood pressure in reflux nephropathy. Lancet 1996; 347:640–643.

88 Alexander SR, Arbus GS, Butt KMH, et al. The 1989 Report of the North American Pediatric Renal Transplant Cooperative Study. Pediatr Nephrol 1990; 4:542–553.

89 Lewis M, Watson AR, Clark G, et al. Report of the paediatric renal registry 1999. In: The UK Renal Registry: Second Annual Report. London: Renal Association; 1999.175–187.

90 Wolfish NM, Delbrouck NF, Shanon A, et al. Prevalence of hypertension in children with primary vesicoureteral reflux. J Pediatr 1993; 123:559–563.

91 Yeung CK, Godley ML, Dhillon HK, et al. The characteristics of primary vesico-ureteric reflux in male and female infants with pre-natal hydronephrosis. Br J Urol 1997; 80:319–327.

92 Kenda RB, Fettich JJ. Vesicoureteric reflux and renal scars in asymptomatic siblings of children with reflux. Arch Dis Child 1992; 67:506–508.

93 Ismaili K, Hall M, Piepsz A, et al. Primary vesicoureteral reflux detected in neonates with a history of fetal renal pelvis dilatation: a prospective clinical and imaging study. J Pediatr 2006; 148:222–227.

94 Sjostrom S, Sillen U, Bachelard M, et al. Spontaneous resolution of high grade infantile vesicoureteral reflux. J Urol 2004; 172:694–698.

95 Wheeler D, Vimalachandra D, Hodson EM, et al. Antibiotics and surgery for vesicoureteric reflux: a meta-analysis of randomised controlled trials. Arch Dis Child 2003; 88:688–694.

96 Seseke F, Strauss A, Seseke S, et al. Long-term experience with Cohen ureteral reimplantation in bilateral VUR in childhood. Urologe A 2006; [Epub ahead of print]

97 Frankenschmidt A, Katzenwadel A, Zimmerhackl LB, et al. Endoscopic treatment of reflux by subureteric collagen injection: critical review of five years' experience. J Endourol 1997; 11:343–348.

98 Capozza N, Caione P. Dextranomer/hyaluronic acid copolymer implantation for vesico-ureteric reflux: a randomized comparison with antibiotic prophylaxis. J Pediatr 2002; 140:230–234.

99 Oswald J, Riccabona M, Lusuardi L, et al. Prospective comparison and 1-year follow-up of a single endoscopic subureteral polydimethylsiloxane versus dextranomer/hyaluronic acid copolymer injection for treatment of vesicoureteral reflux in children. Urology 2002; 60:894–897.

100 Hellstrom A, Hanson E, Hansonn S, et al. Association between urinary symptoms at 7 years old and previous urinary tract infection. Arch Dis Child 1991; 66:232–234.

101 Jansson UB, Hanson M, Hanson E, et al. Voiding pattern in healthy children 0 to 3 years old: a longitudinal study. J Urol 2000; 164:2050–2054.

102 Michel RS. Toilet training. Pediatr Rev 1999; 20:240.

103 Stadtler AC, Gorski PA, Brazelton BT. Toilet training methods, clinical interventions, and recommendations. Pediatrics 1999; 103:1359.

104 WHO. Nonorganic enuresis. In: WHO editor(s). The ICD-10 classification of mental and behavioural disorders: Clinical descriptions and diagnostic guidelines, WHO; Geneva: 1992.

105 Djurhuus JC, Norgaard JP, Rittig S. Monosymptomatic bedwetting. Scandinavian Journal of Urology and Nephrology 1992; 141(Suppl):7–19. [MedLine: 92302804]

106 Blackwell C. A guide to enuresis: A guide to treatment of enuresis for professionals. Bristol: ERIC; 1989.

107 Rutter M, Yule W, Graham P. Enuresis and behavioural deviance. Some epidemiological considerations. In: Kolvin I, MacKeith R C, Meadow S R, eds. Bladder control and enuresis. London: William Heinemann Medical Books; 1973.

108 Eiberg H, Berendt I, Mohr J. Assignment of dominant inherited nocturnal enuresis to chromosome 13q. Nat Genet 1995; 10:354–356.

109 Loeys B, Hoebeke P, Raes A, et al. Does monosymptomatic enuresis exist? A molecular genetic exploration of 32 families with enuresis/incontinence. BJU Int 2002; 90:76–83.

110 Forsythe WI, Redmond A. Enuresis and spontaneous cure rate. Study of 1129 enuretis. Arch Dis Child 1974; 49:259.

111 Light L. Children with enuresis. Most cases of primary nocturnal enuresis are caused by isolated developmental immaturity. BMJ 1998; 316:777.

112 Yeung CK, Sit FK, To LK, et al. Reduction in nocturnal functional bladder capacity is a common factor in the pathogenesis of refractory nocturnal enuresis. BJU Int 2002; 90:302–307.

113 Pomeranz A, Abu-Kheat G, Korzets Z, et al. Night-time polyuria and urine hypo-osmolality in enuretics identified by nocturnal sequential urine sampling – do they represent a subset of relative ADH-deficient subjects? Scand J Urol Nephrol 2000; 34:199.

114 Kawauchi A, Watanabe H, Nakagawa S, et al. Development of bladder capacity, nocturnal urinary volume and urinary behavior in nonenuretic and enuretic children. Nippon Hinyokika Gakkai Zasshi 1993; 84:1811.

115 Wolfish NM, Pivik RT, Busby KA. Elevated sleep arousal thresholds in enuretic boys: clinical implications. Acta Paediatr 1997; 86:381.

116 Ritvo ER, Ornitz EM, Gottlieb F, et al. Arousal and nonarousal enuretic events. Am J Psychiatry 1969; 126:77.

117 Bader G, Neveus T, Kruse S, et al. Sleep of primary enuretic children and controls. Sleep 2002; 25:579.

118 Yeung CK, Chiu HN, Sit FK. Bladder dysfunction in children with refractory monosymptomatic primary nocturnal enuresis. J Urol 1999; 162:1049.

119 Lister-Sharpe D, O'Meara, Bradley M, et al. A systematic review of the effectiveness of interventions for managing childhood nocturnal enuresis (CRD report 11). NHS Centre for Reviews. York: University of York; 1997.

120 Evans JHC. Evidence based management of nocturnal enuresis. BMJ 2001; 323:1167–1169.

121 Glazener CMA, Evans JHC. Desmopressin for nocturnal enuresis in children (Cochrane review). The Cochrane Library, 2. Oxford: Update Software; 2000.

122 Glazener CMA, Evans JHC. Tricyclic and related drugs for nocturnal enuresis in children (Cochrane review). The Cochrane Library, 2. Oxford: Update Software; 2000.

123 Bradbury MG, Meadow SR. Combined treatment with enuresis alarm and desmopressin for nocturnal enuresis. Acta Paediatr 1997; 84:1014–1018.

124 Borzykowski M, Mundy AR. The management of neuropathic bladder in childhood. Pediatr Nephrol 1988; 2:56–66.

125 Shichiri M, Oowada A, Nishio Y, et al. Use of autoanalyser to examine urinary-red-cell morphology in the diagnosis of glomerular haematuria. Lancet 1986; I:781–782.

126 Hulton S. Evaluation of urinary tract calculi in children. Arch Dis Child 2001; 84:320–323.

127 Rayner RJ, Watson AR, Bishop MC. Haematuria in an adolescent due to bladder carcinoma. Eur J Pediatr 1988; 147:328–329.

128 Milford D. Haematuria. In: Webb NJA, ed. Clinical paediatric nephrology. Oxford: Butterworth Heineman; 2003.

129 Rinaldi S, Strologo LD, Montecchi F, et al. Relapsing gross haematuria in Munchausen syndrome. Pediatr Nephrol 1993; 7:202–203.

130 Tomsett A, Watson AR. Renal biopsy as a day case procedure. Paediatr Nurs 1996; 8:14–15.

131 Berrios X, Lagomarsino E, et al. Post-streptococcal acute glomerulonephritis in Chile – 20 years experience. Pediatr Nephrol 2004; 19:306–312.

132 Clark G, White RHR, Glasgow EF, et al. Poststreptococcal glomerulonephritis in children: clinicopathological correlations and long-term prognosis. Pediatr Nephrol 1988; 2:381–388.

133 Mitsioni A. IgA nephropathy in children. Nephrol Dial Trans 2001; 16:123–125.

134 Wyatt RJ, Hogg RJ. Evidence-based assessment of treatment options for children with IgA nephropathies. Pediatr Nephrol 2001; 16:156–167.

135 Yang Y, Ohta K, Shimizu M, et al. Treatment with low dose angiotensin-converting enzyme inhibitor (ACEI) plus angiotensin II receptor blocker (ARB) in pediatric patients. Clin Nephrol 2005; 64:35–40.

136 Tizard EJ. Henoch–Schönlein purpura. Arch Dis Child 1999; 80:380–383.

137 Stewart M, Savage JM, Bell B, et al. Long term renal prognosis of Henoch–Schönlein purpura in an unselected childhood population. Eur J Pediatr 1988; 147:113–115.

138 Goldstein AR, White RH, Akuse R, et al. Long-term follow-up of childhood Henoch–Schönlein nephritis. Lancet 1992; 339:282.

139 Tarshish P, Bernstein J, Tobin JN, et al. Treatment of mesangiocapillary glomerulonpehritis in alternate-day prednisolone – a report of the International Study of Kidney Diseases in Children. Pediatr Nephrol 1992; 6:123–130.

140 Yanagihara T, Hayakawa M, Yoshida J, et al. Long term follow up of diffuse membranoproliferative glomerulonephritis type 1. Pediatr Nephrol 2005; 20:585–590.

141 Stichweh D, Arce E, Pascual V. Update on pediatric systemic lupus erythematosus. Curr Opin Rheumatol 2004; 16:577–587.

142 Jardim H, Leake J, Risdon A, et al. Crescentic glomerulonephritis in children. Pediatr Nephrol 1992; 6:231–235.

143 Belostotsky VM, Shah V, Dillon MJ. Clinical features of 17 paediatric patients with Wegener's granulomatosis. Pediatr Nephrol 2002; 17:754–761.

144 Hattori M, Kurayama H, Koitabashi Y, et al. Antineutrophil cytoplasmic antibody-associated glomerulonephritis in children. J Am Soc Nephrol 2001; 12:1493–1500.

145 Phelps RG, Turner AN. Antiglomerular basement membrane disease and Goodpasture's syndrome. In: Johnson R J, Feehally J, eds. Comprehensive Clinical Nephrology. 2nd edn. 2003.331–340.

146 Hudson BG, Tryggvason K, Sundaramoorthy M, et al. Alport's syndrome, Goodpasture's syndrome and type IV Collagen. N Engl J Med 2003; 348:2543–2556.

147 Lang S, Stevenson B, Risdon RA. Thin basement membrane nephropathy as a cause of recurrent haematuria in childhood. Histopathology 1990; 16:331–337.

148 Monnens LAH. Thin glomerular basement membrane disease. Kid Int 2001; 60:799–800.

149 Bongers EM, Gubler MC, Knoers NV. Nail–patella syndrome. Overview on clinical and molecular findings. Pediatr Nephrol 2002; 17:703–712.

150 Ozen S. Problems in classifying vasculitis in children. Pediatr Nephrol 2005; 20:1214–1218.

151 Ozen S, Ruperto N, Dillon MJ, et al. EULAR/PReS endorsed consensus criteria for the classification of childhood vasculitides. Ann Rheum Dis 2006; 65:936–941.

152 Mogensen CE. How to protect the kidney in diabetic patients with special reference to IDDM. Diabetes 1997; (Suppl 2):104–111.

153 Elises JS, Griffiths PD, Hocking MD, et al. Simplified quantification of urinary protein excretion in children. Clin Nephrol 1988; 30:225–229.

154 Kriz W, Lehir M. Pathways to nephron loss starting from glomerular diseases – Insights from animal models. Kidney Int 2005; 67:404–419.

155 Sharples PM, Poulton J, White RHR. Steroid responsive nephrotic syndrome is more common in Asians. Arch Dis Child 1985; 60:1014–1017.

156 Doe JY, Funk M, Mengel M, et al. Nephrotic syndrome in African children: lack of evidence for 'tropical nephrotic syndrome? Nephrol Dial Transplant 2006; 21:672–676.

157 Boute N, Gribouval O, Roselli S, et al. NPHS2, encoding the glomerular protein podocin, is mutated in autosomal recessive steroid-resistant nephrotic syndrome. Nat Genet 2000; 24:349–354.

158 Hoyer PF, Gonda S, Barthels M, et al. Thromboembolic complications in children with nephrotic syndrome. Acta Pediatr Scand 1986; 75:804–810.

159 Watson AR, Coleman JE. Dietary management in nephrotic syndrome. Arch Dis Child 1993; 69:179–180.

160 Lewis MA, Awan A. Mannitol and frusemide in the treatment of diuretic resistant oedema in nephrotic syndrome. Arch Dis Child 1999; 80:184–185.

161 Consensus statement on management and audit potential for steroid responsive nephrotic syndrome. Report of a workshop by the British Association for Paediatric Nephrology and Research Unit, Royal College of Physicians. Arch Dis Child 1994; 70:151–157.

162 Bargman JM. Management of minimal lesion glomerulonephritis: evidence-based recommendations. Kidney Int 1999; (Suppl 70):S3–S16.

163 Hodson EM, Knight JF, Willis NS, et al. Corticosteroid therapy for nephrotic syndrome in children. Cochrane Database Syst Rev. 2005; CD001533.1

164 Durkan AM, Hodson EM, Willis NS, et al. Non-corticosteroid treatment for nephrotic syndrome in children. Cochrane Database Syst Rev 2005; CD002290

165 Watson AR, Rance CP, Bain J. Long term effects of cyclophosphamide on testicular function. BMJ 1985; 291:1457–1460.

166 Watson AR, Taylor J, Rance CP, et al. Gonadal function in women treated with cyclophosphamide for childhood nephrotic syndrome: a long-term follow-up study. Fertil Steril 1986; 46:331–333.

167 Moore EA, Collier J, Evans JHC, et al. Information needs of parents of children with nephrotic syndrome. Child Health 1994; 2:147–149.

168 Lewis MA, Baildom EM, Davis N, et al. Nephrotic syndrome: from toddlers to twenties. Lancet 1989; I:255–259.

169 Weber S, Gribouval O, Esquivel EL, et al. NPHS2 mutation analysis shows genetic heterogeneity of steroid-resistant nephrotic syndrome and low post-transplant recurrence. Kidney Int 2004; 66:571–579.

170 Ruf RG, Lichtenberger A, Karle SM, et al. Patients with mutations in NPHS2 (podocin) do not respond to standard steroid treatment of nephrotic syndrome. J Am Soc Nephrol 2004; 15:722–732.

171 Caridi G, Perfumo F, Ghiggeri GM. NPHS2 (Podocin) mutations in nephrotic syndrome. Clinical spectrum and fine mechanisms. Pediatr Res 2005; 57:54R–61R.

172 Holmberg C, Laine J, Ronnholm K, et al. Congenital nephrotic syndrome. Kidney Int 1996; 49:S51–S56.

173 Kestila M, Lenkkeri U, Mannikko M, et al. Positionally cloned gene for a novel glomerular protein – nephrin – is mutated in congenital nephrotic syndrome. Mol Cell 1998; 1:575–582.

174 de Swief M, Dillan MJ, Littlev W, et al. Measurement of blood pressure in children. Recommendations of a working party of the British Hypertension Society. BMJ 1989; 299:497.

175 De Man SA, Andre JL, Bachmann H, et al. Blood pressure in childhood: pooled findings of 6 European studies. J Hypertension 1991; 9:109–114.

176 National High Blood Pressure Education Program Working Group on High Blood Pressure in Children and Adolescents. Pediatrics 2004; 144(Suppl):555–576.

177 Soergel, et al. Oscillometric twenty-four-hour ambulatory blood pressure values in healthy children and adolescents a multicenter trial including 1141 subjects. J Pediatr 1997; 130:167–169.

178 Seeman T, Palyzova D, Dusek J, et al: Reduced nocturnal blood pressure dip and night-time hypertension are specific markers of secondary hypertension. J Pediatr 147: 366–371.

179 Verdecchia P. White-coat hypertension in adults and children. Blood Pressure Monitoring 1999; 4:175–179.

180 Varda NM, Gregoric A. A diagnostic approach for the child with hypertension. Pediatr Nephrol 2005; 20:499–506.

181 National Institute for Health and Clinical Excellence (NICE) 2006. Clinical Guideline. Hypertension: management of hypertension in adults in primary care.

182 British Association for Paediatric Nephrology. Report of a Working Party: the provision of services in the United Kingdom for children and adolescents with renal disease. BAPN 1991.

183 Moghal NE, Brocklebank JT, Meadow SR. A review of acute renal failure incidence etiology and outcome. Clin Nephrol 1998; 49:91–95.

184 Hui-Sickle S, Brewer ED, Goldstein SL. Paediatric ARF epidemiology at a tertiary centre from 1999 to 2001. Am J Kidney Dis 2005; 45:96–101.

185 Bunchman TE, McBryde KD, Mottes TE, et al. Paediatric acute renal failure: outcome by modality and disease. Paediatr Nephrol 2001; 16:1067–1071.

186 Goldstein SL. Overview of paediatric renal replacement therapy in acute renal failure. Artificial Organs 2003; 27:781–785.

187 Cataldi1 L, Leone R, Moretti U, et al. Potential risk factors for the development of acute renal failure in preterm newborn infants: a case–control study. Arch Dis Childh – Fetal and Neonatal Edition 2005; 90:F514–F519.

188 Karlowicz MG, Adelman RD. Nonoliguric and oliguric renal failure in asphyxiated term neonates. Pediatr Nephrol 1995; 9:718–722.

189 Goldstein SL, Somers MJ, Baum MA, et al. Paedaitric patients with multi-organ dysfunction syndrome receiving continuous renal replacement therapy. Kidney International 2005; 67:653–658.

190 Australia and New Zealand Intensive Care Society (ANZICS). Clinical Trials Group. Low dose dopamine in patients with early renal dysfunction: a placebo-controlled trial. Lancet 2000; 356:2139–2143.

191 Kelleum JA. The use of diuretics and dopamine in acute renal failure: a systematic review of the evidence. Critical Care 1997; 1:53–59.

192 Lassnig A, Donner E, Grubhofer G, et al. Lack of renoprotective effects of dopamine and furosemide during cardiac surgery. J Am Soc Nephrol 2000; 11:97–104.

193 McClure RJ, Prasad VK, Brocklebank JT. Treatment of hyperkalaemia using intravenous and nebulised salbutamol. Arch Dis Child 1994; 70:126–128.

194 Jones DP, Mahmoud H, Chesney RW. Tumour lysis syndrome: pathogenesis and management. Pediatr Nephrol 1995; 9:206–212.

195 Watson AR. Nutrition in renal disease. In: Davies D, ed. Nutrition in child health. London: Royal College of Physicians; 1995.133–142.

196 Strazdins V, Watson AR, Harvey B. European Pediatric Peritoneal Dialysis Working Group. Renal replacement therapy for acute renal failure in children: European guidelines. Paediatr Nephrol 2004; 19:199–207.

197 Maxvold NJ, Bunchman TE. Renal failure and renal replacement therapy. Crit Care Clin 2003; 19:563–575.

198 Symons JM, Brophy PD, Gregory MJ, et al. Continuous renal replacement therapy in children up to 10 kg. Am J Kidney Disease 2003; 41:984–989.

199 Parakininkas D, Greenbaum LA. Comparison of solute clearance in three modes of continuous renal replacement therapy. Paediatr Crit Care Med 2004; 5:269–274.

200 Daschner M. Drug dosage in children with reduced renal function. Paediatr Nephrol 2005; 20:1675–1686.

201 Ashley C, Curry A. The Renal Drug Handbook. UK renal pharmacy group. Oxford: Radcliffe Medical Press; 2004.

202 Radhakrishnan J, Kiryluk K. Acute renal failure outcomes in children and adults. Kidney Int 2006; 69:184–189.

203 Askenazi DJ, Feig DI, Graham NM, et al. 3–5 year follow up of paediatric patients after acute renal failure. Kidney Int 2006; 69:184–189.

204 Milford DV, Taylor CM, Guttridge B, et al. Haemolytic uraemic syndromes in the British Isles 1985–8: association with verocytotoxin producing E. coli. Part 1: Clinical and epidemiological features. Arch Dis Child 1990; 65:716–721.

205 Lynn RM, O'Brien SJ, Taylor CM, et al. Childhood hemolytic uremic syndrome. United Kingdom and Ireland. Emerg Infect Dis 2005; 11:590–596.

206 Cummings KC, Mohle-Boetani JC, Werner SB, et al. Population-based trends in pediatric hemolytic uremic syndrome in California, 1994–1999: substantial underreporting and public health implications. Am J Epidemiol 2002; 5(155):941–948.

207 Ochoa TJ, Cleary TG. Epidemiology and spectrum of disease of Escherichia coli O157. Curr Opin Infect Dis 2003; 16:259–263.

208 Banatvala N, Griffin PM, Greene KD, et al. Hemolytic Uremic Syndrome Study Collaborators. The United States National Prospective Hemolytic Uremic Syndrome Study: microbiologic, serologic, clinical, and epidemiologic findings. J Infect Dis 2001; 183:1063–1070.

209 Werber D, Fruth A, Buchholz U, et al. Strong association between shiga toxin producing E. coli O157 and virulencegenes Stx2 and eae as possible explanation for predominance of serogroup O157 in patients with haemolytic uraemic syndrome. Eur J Clin Mictrbiol Infect Dis 2003; 22:7129–7139.

210 Seigler R, Oakes R. Hemolytic uremic syndrome; pathogenesis, treatment and outcome. Curr Opin Pediatr 2005; 17:200–204.

211 Friedrich AW, Bielaszewska M, Zhang WL, et al. Escherichia coli harboring Shiga toxin 2 gene variants: frequency and association with clinical symptoms. J Infect Dis 2002; 185:74–84.

212 Chaisri U, Nagata M, Kurazono H, et al. Localization of Shiga toxins of enterohaemorrhagic Escherichia coli in kidneys of paediatric and geriatric patients with fatal haemolytic uraemic syndrome. Microbiol Pathol 2001; 31:59–67.

213 Kaplan BS, Cleary TG, Obrig TG. Recent advances in understanding the pathogenesis of the hemolytic uremic syndromes. Pediatr Nephrol 1990; 4:276–283.

214 Grabowski EF. The hemolytic-uremic syndrome – toxin, thrombin, and thrombosis. N Engl J Med 2002; 346:23–32.

215 Chandler WL, Jelacic S, Boster DR, et al. Prothrombotic coagulation abnormalities preceding the hemolytic-uremic syndrome. NEJM 2002; 346:23–32.

216 Fu XJ, Iijima K, Nozu K, et al. Role of p38 MAP kinase pathway in a toxin-induced model of hemolytic uremic syndrome. Pediatr Nephrol 2004; 19:844–852.

217 Ghosh SA, Polanowska-Grabowska RK, Fujii J, et al. Shiga toxin binds to activated platelets. J Thromb Haemost 2004; 2:499–506.

218 Pysher TJ, Siegler RL, Tesh VL, et al. von Willebrand factor expression in a Shiga toxin-mediated primate model of hemolytic uremic syndrome. Pediatr Dev Pathol 2002; 5:472–479.

219 Seigler RL, Pyscher TJ, Tesh VL, et al. Renal prostacyclin biosynthesis in a baboon model of shiga toxin mediated hemolytic uremic syndrome. Nephron 2002; 92:363–368.

220 Fernandez GC, Te Loo, van de Veiden TJ, et al. Decrease of thrombomodulin contributes to the procoagulant state of the endothelium in hemolytic uremic syndrome. Pediatric Nephrology 2003; 18:1066–1068.

221 Feld LG, Springate JE, Darragh R, et al. Pneumococcal pneumonia and hemolytic uremic syndrome. Pediatr Infect Dis J 1987; 6:693–695.

222 Kerecuk L, Waters A, Taylor CM, et al: Pneumococcal haemolytic uraemic syndrome: an emerging problem. Arch Dis Child 91(Suppl)1:A33.

223 Warwicker P, Goodship THJ, Donne RL, et al. Genetic studies into inherited and sporadic haemolytic uraemic syndrome. Kidney Int 1998; 53:836–844.

224 Taylor CM. Complement factor H and the haemolytic uraemic syndrome. Lancet 2001; 358:1200–1202.

225 Noris M, Brioschi S, Caprioli J, et al. Familial haemolytic uraemic syndrome and MCP mutation. Lancet 2003; 362:1542–1547.

226 Taylor CM. Hemolytic-uremic syndrome and complement factor H deficiency: clinical aspects. Semin Thromb Hemost 2001; 27:185–190.

227 Takatsuka H, Wakae T, Toda A, et al. Association of Helicobacter pylori with thrombotic purpura/hemolytic uremic syndrome: a concise view. Clin Transplant 2004; 18:547–551.

228 Diott JS, Danielson CF, Blue-Hindy DE, et al. Drug induced thrombotic thrombocytopenic purpura/hemolytic uremic syndrome. Ther Apher Dial 2004; 8:102–111.

229 Ikeda K, Ida O, Kimoto K, et al. Predictions of the development of haemolytic uraemic syndrome with Escherichia coli O157:H7 infections with focus on the day of the illness. Epidemiol Infect 2000; 124:343–349.

230 Brandt JR, Joseph MW, Fouser LS, et al. Cholelithiasis following Escherichia coli O157:H7 associated hemolytic uremic syndrome. Pediatr Nephrol 1998; 12:222–225.

231 Thomas NJ, Messina JJ, DeBruin WJ, et al. Cardiac failure in hemolytic uremic syndrome and rescue with extracorporeal life support. Pediatr Cardiol 2005; 26:104–106.

232 Gallo GE, Gianantonio CA. Extrarenal involvement in diarrhoea associated haemolytic uraemic syndrome. Pediatr Nephrol 1995; 9:117–119.

233 Eriksson KJ, Boyd SG, Tasker RC. Acute neurology and neurophysiology of haemolytic-uraemic syndrome. Arch Dis Child 2001; 84:434–435.

234 Steinborn M, Leiz S, Rudisser K, et al. CT and MRI in haemolytic uraemic syndrome with central nervous system involvement: distribution of lesions and prognostic value of imaging findings. Pediatr Radiol 2004; 34:805–810.

235 Buteau C, Proulx F, Chaibou M, et al. Leukocytosis in children with E. coli O157:H7 enteritis developing the haemolytic-uremic syndrome. Pediatr Infect Dis 2000; 19:642–647.

236 Coad NAG, Marshall T, Rowe B, et al. Changes in the postenteropathic form of hemolytic uremic syndrome in children. Clin Nephrol 1991; 35:10–16.

237 Kehl SC. Role of the laboratory in the diagnosis of enterohemorrhagic Escherichia coli infections. J Clin Microbiol 2002; 40:2711–2715.

238 Askiti V, Hendrickson K, Fish AJ, et al. Troponin I levels in a hemolytic uremic syndrome patient with severe cardiac failure. Pediatr Nephrol 2004; 19:345–348.

239 Van damme-Lombaerts R, Proesmans W, Van Damme B, et al. Heparin plus dipyridamole in childhood hemolytic uremic syndrome: a prospective randomized study. J Pediatr 1988; 113:913–918.

240 Robson WLM, Fick GH, Jadavji T, et al. The use of intravenous gamaglobulin in the treatment of typical hemolytic uremic syndrome. Pediatr Nephrol 1991; 5:289–292.

241 Perez N, Spizziri F, Rahman R, et al. Steroids in hemolytic uremic syndrome. Pediatr Nephrol 1998; 12:101–104.

242 O'Regan S, Chesney RW, Mongeau JG, et al. Aspirin and dipyridamole in the hemolytic uremic syndrome. J Pediatr 1980; 97:473–476.

243 Rousseau E, Blais N, O'Regan S. Decreased necessity for dialysis with loop diuretic therapy in

hemolytic uremic syndrome. Clin Nephrol 1990; 34:22–25.

244   Loirat C, Sonsino E, Hinglais N, et al. Treatment of the childhood haemolytic uraemic syndrome with plasma. Pediatr Nephrol 1988; 2:279–285.

245   Shiomi M, Togawa M, Fujita K, et al. Effect of early oral fluoroquinolones in hemorrhagic colitis *Escherichia coli* O157:H7. Pediatr Nephrol 1999; 41:228–232.

246   Wong CS, Jelacic S, Habeeb RL, et al. The risk of hemolytic-uremic syndrome after antibiotic treatment of O157:H7 infections. New Engl J Med 2000; 342:1930–1931.

247   Safdar N, Said A, Gangnon RE, et al. Risk of hemolytic uremic syndrome after antibiotic treatment of *Escherichia coli* O157:H7 enteritis: a meta-analysis. JAMA 2002; 288:996–1001.

248   Donohue-Rolfe A, Kondova I, Mukherjee J, et al. Antibody-based protection of gnotobiotic piglets infected with *Escherichia coli* O157:H7 against systemic complications associated with Shiga toxin 2. Infect Immunol 1999; 67:3645–3648.

249   Karmli MA. Prospects for preventing serious systemic toxemic complications of Shiga toxin-producing *Escherichia coli* infections using Shiga toxin receptor analogues. J Infect Dis 2004; 189:355–359.

250   Konadu EY, Parke Jr JC, Tran HT, et al. Investigational vaccine for *Escherichia coli* O157: phase 1 study of O157 O-specific polysaccharide-Pseudomonas aeruginosa recombinant exoprotein A conjugates in adults. J Infect Dis. 1998; 177:383–387.

251   Trachtman H, Christen E. Pathogenesis, treatment, and therapeutic trials in hemolytic uremic syndrome. J Am Soc Nephrol 1999; 11:162–168.

252   Fitzpatrick MM, Shah V, Trompeter RS, et al. Long term renal outcome of childhood haemolytic uraemic syndrome. BMJ 1991; 303:489–492.

253   Small G, Watson AR, Evans JHC, et al. Hemolytic uremic syndrome: defining the need for long-term follow-up. Clin Nephrol 1999; 52:352–356.

254   Perelstein EM, Grunfield BG, Simsolo RB, et al. Renal functional reserve in haemolytic uraemic syndrome and single kidney. Arch Dis Child 1990; 65:728–731.

255   Van Dyck M, Proesmans W. Renoprotection by ACE inhibitors after severe hemolytic uremic syndrome. Pediatr Nephrol 2004; 19:688–690.

256   Loirat C, Niaudet P. The risk of recurrence of hemolytic uremic syndrome after renal transplantation in children. Pediatr Nephrol 2003; 18:1095–1101.

257   Cheong HI, Lee BS, Kang HG, et al. Attempted treatment of factor H deficiency by liver transplantation. Pediatr Nephrol 2004; 19:454–458.

258   British Association for Paediatric Nephrology. Report of a Working Party: the provision of services in the United Kingdom for children and adolescents with renal disease. BAPN. 1991.

259   Broyer M, Chantler C, Donckerwolke R, et al. The paediatric registry of the European Dialysis and Transplant Association: 20 years' experience. Pediatr Nephrol 1993; 7:758–768.

260   Renal Association UK Renal Registry The Eighth annual report December 05. Chapter 18 Report of the Paediatric Renal Registry.

261   Norman LJ, Coleman JE, Macdonald IA, et al. Nutrition and growth in relation to severity of renal disease in children. Pediatr Nephrol 2000; 15:259–265.

262   Block GA, Martin KJ, de Francisco AL, et al. Cinacalcet for secondary hyperparathyroidism in patients receiving hemodialysis. N Engl J Med. 2004; 8:1516–1525.

263   Block GA, Hulbert-Shearon TE, Levin NW, et al. Association of serum phosphorus and calcium x phosphate product with mortality risk in chronic hemodialysis patients: a national study. Am J Kidney Dis 1998; 31:607–617.

264   De Boer IH, Gorodetskaya I, Young B, et al. The severity of secondary hyperparathyroidism in chronic renal insufficiency is GFR-dependent, race-dependent, and associated with cardiovascular disease. J Am Soc Nephrol 2002; 13:2762–2769.

265   The Renal Association: treatment of adults and Children with renal failure: standards and audit measures. Third Edition August 2002.

266   The Kidney Disease Outcomes Quality Initiative (K/DOQI) Clinical Practice guidelines accessed May 2005 from www.kidney.org/professionals/kdoqi/

267   Haffner D, Schaeffer F, Nissel R, et al. Effect of growth hormone treatment on adult height of children with chronic renal failure. N Engl J Med 2000; 343:923–930.

268   Rees L, Ward G, Rigden S. Growth over 10 years following a one year trial of growth hormone therapy. Pediatr Nephrol 2000; 14:309–314.

269   Fine RN, Stablein D. Long-term use of recombinant human growth hormone in pediatric allograft recipients a report of the NAPRTCS Transplant Registry. Pediatr Nephrol. 2005; 20:404–408.

270   Coleman JE. The kidney. In: Shaw V, Lawson M, eds. Clinical paediatric dietetics. Oxford: Blackwell Science; 2001.158–182.

271   Wingen AM, Fabian-Bach C, Mehls O. Low protein diets in children with chronic renal failure. Pediatr Nephrol 1991; 5:496–500.

272   Watson AR, Gartland C on behalf of the European Paediatric Peritoneal Dialysis Working Group. Guidelines by an ad hoc European committee for elective chronic peritoneal dialysis in pediatric patients. Peritoneal Dial Int 2001; 21:240–244.

273   Warady BA, Alexander SR, Watkins S, et al. Optimal care of the pediatric end stage renal disease patient on dialysis. Am J Kidney Dis 1999; 33:567–583.

274   Mahmoud A, Said MH, Dawahra M, et al. Outcome of pre-emptive renal transplantation and pretransplantation dialysis in children. Pediatr Nephrol 1997; 11:537–541.

275   Vats AN, Donaldson L, Fine RN, et al. Pretransplant dialysis status and outcome of renal transplantation in North American children: a NAPRTCS Study. Transplantation 2000; 69:1414–1419.

276   http://www.uktransplant.org.uk/ukt/statistics/centre-specific_reports/comparison_of_survival_rates.jsp accessed 26/04/06

277   McDonald R, Donaldson L, Emmett L, et al. A decade of living donor transplantation in North American children: the 1998 annual report of the North American Pediatric Renal Transplant Cooperative Study. Pediatr Transplant 2000; 4:221–234.

278   Vester U, Offner G, Hoyer PF, et al. End stage renal failure in children younger than 6 years: renal transplantation is the therapy of choice. Eur J Paediatr 1998; 157:239–242.

279   Dall'Amico R, Ginevri F, Ghio L, et al. Successful renal transplantation in children under 6 years. Pediatr Nephrol 2001; 16:1–7.

280   Coulthard MG, Crosier J. Outcome of reaching end stage renal failure in children under 2 years of age. Arch Dis Child 2002; 87:511–517.

281   Tyden G, Berg U, Bohlin AB, et al. Renal transplantation in children less than 2 years old. Transplantation 1997; 63:554–558.

282   Kari JA, Romagnoli J, Duffy P, et al. Renal transplantation in children under 5 years of age. Pediatr Nephrol 1999; 13:730–736.

283   Postlethwaite RJ, Johnson RJ, Armstrong S, et al. Paediatric Task Force of United Kingdom Transplant, Bristol. The outcome of pediatric cadaveric renal transplantation in the UK and Eire. Pediatr Transplant 2002; 6:367–377.

284   Smith JM, Ho PL, McDonald RA. North American Pediatric Renal Transplant Cooperative Study Renal transplant outcomes in adolescents: a report of the North American Pediatric Renal Transplant Cooperative Study. Pediatr Transplant. 2002; 6:493–499.

285   Gjertson DW, Cecka JM. Determinants of long-term survival of pediatric kidney grafts reported to the United Network for organ sharing kidney transplant registry. Pediatr Transplantation 2001; 5:5–15.

286   NICE Iimmunosuppressive therapy fore renal transplantation in children and adolescents. http://www.nice.org.uk accessed 24/04/06

287   Sarwal MM, Yorgin PD, Alexander S, et al. Promising early outcomes with a novel, complete steroid avoidance immunosuppression protocol in pediatric renal transplantation. Transplantation 2001; 72:13–21.

288   Geary DF, Haka-Ikse K. Neurodevelopmental progress of young children with chronic renal disease. Pediatrics 1989; 84:68–72.

289   Becker N, Brandt JR, Sutherland TA, et al. Improved neurological outcome of young children on nightly automated peritoneal dialysis. Pediatr Nephrol 1997; 11:676–679.

290   Warady BA, Belden B, Kohaut E. Neurodevelopmental outcome of children initiating peritoneal dialysis in early infancy. Pediatr Nephrol 1999; 13:759–765.

291   Reynolds JM, Garralda ME, Postlethwaite RJ, et al. Changes in psychosocial adjustment after renal transplantation. Arch Dis Child 1991; 66:508–513.

19

Disorders of the alimentary tract and liver

W Michael Bisset, Susan V Beath,
Huw R Jenkins, Alastair J Baker

INTRODUCTION

Optimum growth and development is dependent on the normal functioning of the gastrointestinal tract and of the liver. When this activity is deranged the child will develop symptoms of gastrointestinal disease and as a consequence will frequently fail to grow adequately.

The gastrointestinal tract extends from the mouth to the anus and is structurally and functionally divided into the mouth, oropharynx, esophagus, stomach, small intestine and colon (Table 19.1). Following the ingestion of food by the mouth the bolus is moved by the oropharynx into the esophagus, which acts as a conduit for the transfer of food to the stomach, where it is stored and mixed prior to its controlled passage into the small intestine. In the small intestine the food is digested and absorbed before moving on into the large intestine, where salt and water are conserved prior to excretion. This simplified view of gastrointestinal function disguises the very complex nature of the many systems which interact to give normal intestinal function.

GASTROINTESTINAL FUNCTION

DIGESTION

Ingested food consists almost exclusively of large macromolecules which the intestinal tract is unable to absorb without prior digestion.

Table 19.1 The function of the gastrointestinal tract

Section of gut	Function
Mouth	Grinding of food by teeth Lubrication by salivary secretions
Oropharynx	Move food into esophagus Protect airway
Esophagus	Propulsive conduit for food Clearance of regurgitated food Prevention of reflux
Stomach	Store for food Gastric acid production Pepsin production
Small intestine	Digestion of food Absorption of food Immune tolerance
Terminal ileum	Absorption of vitamin B_{12} Absorption of bile salts
Pancreas	Digestive enzyme production Bicarbonate production
Colon	Reabsorption of luminal fluid Storage and excretion of feces

Complex carbohydrates are broken down into their component monosaccharides; fats, with the help of the emulsifying activity of bile salts, are digested to free fatty acids and monoacylglycerol and proteins are dismantled into dipeptides and amino acids. The digestive enzymes act mainly within the lumen of the stomach and small intestine although the process is completed for carbohydrate by small intestinal brush border disaccharidases.

TRANSPORT

Discrete transport processes are present within the epithelial cells of the intestinal tract to promote the absorption of nutrients, salts and water by some cells and the excretion of salt and water by others. Many of these processes are dependent on the electrochemical gradient across the cell wall created by the Na^+/K^+ ATPase ion pump. This generates a low Na^+ concentration and a negative charge within epithelial cells, which facilitate the movement of specific ions and solutes through transmembrane proteins which traverse the lipophilic cell membrane.

MOTILITY

The movement of food along the gut is integrated with, and related to, the function of each section of the intestine. The rate of emptying of nutrients from the stomach is closely controlled to prevent overloading of the small intestine. Specific patterns of fasting motor activity have developed in the small intestine to clear the lumen of food debris after meals and highly developed control mechanisms are present to facilitate the controlled emptying of the distal colon and rectum at the time of defecation.

IMMUNITY

The gastrointestinal tract serves as the interface between ingested elements from the external environment and the internal milieu of the individual. By a combination of immunological and non-immunological mechanisms the entry of noxious substances such as bacteria, viruses and undigested food protein is prevented. The development of tolerance to the foreign proteins of commonly ingested food is vital to the normal functioning of the gut.

ENDOCRINE

The gastrointestinal tract is a major endocrine organ and many regulatory peptides with endocrine, paracrine and neurocrine functions are released along the length of the intestine. The function of many of these peptides is poorly understood, although it is clear that they have an important role in modulating intestinal secretion, growth and motor function.

A more detailed description of the anatomy and physiology of the intestinal tract[1] is given in subsequent sections of this chapter.

NATURE OF GASTROINTESTINAL DISEASE

Normal intestinal function requires the combined action of each of the functional systems described earlier and if any one should break down intestinal function will be compromised. An understanding of the basic physiology of these systems is important when interpreting symptoms of gastrointestinal disease and planning the rational investigation of these problems.

Diarrheal disease will develop if, as a consequence of maldigestion or active secretion, there is an increased effluent of fluid passing into the colon from the small intestine or if the absorptive capacity of the colon is compromised by disease.[2] Loss of normal intestinal motility will result in the development of symptoms of obstruction and where a defect of mucosal immunity is present recurrent enteric infection is likely to occur. Damage to the digestive or absorptive capacity of the small intestine will result in failure of the patient to grow adequately.

THE MOUTH

The mouth is responsible for the grinding of food into small fragments, through the voluntary action of the tongue and jaw, prior to its passage into the esophagus. In addition, the fragments are mixed with salivary secretions, which help lubricate the food and initiate digestion, through the action of salivary amylase and lingual lipase. Any disease of the mouth which makes feeding painful or compromises the normal process of deglutition is likely to lead to difficulties with feeding.

While most oral lesions are the result of local disease, both gastrointestinal and systemic disease may result in abnormalities within the mouth.[3] It is therefore important to look closely at the mouth in all children undergoing physical examination.

THE LIPS

Unilateral or bilateral clefts of the upper lip are among the most common of congenital malformations and are frequently found in combination with a cleft of the palate (see Ch. 37). Dryness of the lips with cracking may be due to mouth breathing, and fissure formation at the angle of the mouth may result from chronic drooling in children with swallowing disorders. Nutritional deficiencies of iron, zinc and riboflavin may all produce an angular stomatitis.

Edema of the lips may occur as part of an immediate hypersensitivity reaction following the direct contact of the lips with a sensitized protein or as part of the systemic response in anaphylaxis. Intermittent swelling of the lips due to chronic granulomatous infiltration is seen in orofacial granulomatous disease, a condition associated with Crohn's disease in some patients. Exacerbation may be brought on by dietary triggers.[4] Cobblestone ulceration of the buccal mucosa may be seen in Crohn's disease.

THE ORAL MUCOSA

Ulceration to the buccal mucosa occurs most commonly in healthy individuals as a result of recurrent aphthae. These may be precipitated by local trauma and heal spontaneously within 2 weeks. More persistent ulcers may occur in chronically debilitated patients, children with poor dental hygiene and as mentioned earlier in inflammatory bowel disease (IBD). Extensive ulceration of the oral mucosa in association with lesions on the perineum are seen in Stevens–Johnson syndrome and less commonly in Behçet syndrome.

Abnormal pigmentation may be seen in Addison disease and Albright syndrome; in Peutz–Jeghers syndrome there is freckling of the lips and buccal mucosa and in lead, mercury and bismuth poisoning pigmented lines are sometimes seen near the dental margin of the gums. Koplik's spots are characteristically present in measles, palatal petechiae may be seen in rubella and oral vesicles in chickenpox can make feeding very uncomfortable.

The most common infections involving the mucosa are herpes stomatitis and thrush. Primary herpes infection occurs most commonly in children between the ages of 1 and 3 years and presents with pyrexia, lymphadenopathy and the eruption of vesicular lesions on the buccal mucosa, lips and on the skin below the mouth. The vesicles burst, forming painful ulcers, making the ingestion of solids and liquids very uncomfortable. Although the condition is self-limiting, with a course of 7–10 d, this may be shortened by treatment with oral aciclovir.

Oral candidiasis or thrush commonly occurs in young babies who become infected in the neonatal period but may also develop in patients on broad-spectrum antibiotics, inhaled steroids or in patients who are immunosuppressed. Gut carriage may also lead to infection of the napkin area. Treatment is with a topical antifungal such as nystatin. Oral nystatin should also be given where gut carriage is likely to be a source of reinfection.

THE GUMS

Infection of the gums in children most commonly results from poor oral hygiene and leads to inflammation of the free margin of the gingiva. Hypertrophy of the gums is a common side-effect of phenytoin or cyclosporine treatment and may also be rarely seen in Langerhans' cell histiocytosis (see Ch. 24). Bleeding of the gums may be secondary to local infection but will also occur in children with bleeding diatheses and in nutritionally compromised patients who are vitamin C deficient.

THE TONGUE

Macroglossia occurs in hypothyroidism, as part of generalized visceral enlargement in Beckwith syndrome and in glycogen storage disease type II. A normal-sized tongue may appear to be enlarged if the oral cavity is small as in children with Down syndrome. The tongue can also be enlarged by a lymphangioma or a hemangioma and a mass in the region of the foramen cecum may be due to a lingual thyroid.

The surface of the tongue becomes coated in children with poor oral hygiene and in patients with dehydration. In scarlet fever the tongue is first white and coated and then becomes red, hence the name 'strawberry tongue'. In familial dysautonomia the tongue is smooth due to the absence of papillae and in congenital familial telangiectasia the vascular abnormality may be clearly seen. The focal loss of papillae leads to the so-called 'geographical tongue', a benign self-limiting condition.

THE TEETH

The primary dentition usually erupts at about 6 months but in hypothyroidism, hypopituitarism, rickets, congenital syphilis and cleidocranial dysostosis this can be delayed. Premature shedding of these teeth is likely to occur in hypophosphatasia and in mercury poisoning. The enamel of the teeth will become hypoplastic as a result of such insults as prematurity, kernicterus, vitamin D deficiency and from congenital infections such as rubella and syphilis. Similarly the shape of the teeth may be abnormal as a consequence of congenital infection (notched incisors in congenital syphilis) or in ectodermal dysplasias, where the teeth may be peg shaped.

A black staining of the teeth can occur with oral iron, a brown discoloration occurs with congenital defects of enamel and dentine, in congenital porphyria the teeth are a purplish brown and in neonatal unconjugated hyperbilirubinemia a green staining may be left. The administration of tetracycline to a mother after the fourth month of pregnancy or to the infant in the first year of life will result in yellow discoloration of the primary dentition and administration up to the age of 7 years will affect the permanent dentition.

THE SALIVARY GLANDS

With the exception of mumps, inflammation or enlargement of the salivary gland is uncommon in childhood. Acute bacterial parotitis may occur in the neonate or debilitated child and is characterized by a unilateral swollen tender parotid gland. Infection with *Staphylococcus aureus* is generally responsible and treatment with flucloxacillin is required.

Recurrent parotitis either uni- or bilateral may occur where the symptoms are generally mild and not associated with systemic upset.[5] Treatment with parotid massage and stimulants of salivary flow such as chewing gum along with oral penicillin are generally helpful. The condition is self-limiting and generally resolves by puberty. Less commonly, recurrent pain and infection may be precipitated by salivary stones.

THE ESOPHAGUS

STRUCTURE AND FUNCTION

The esophagus is a long, narrow muscular tube which connects the oropharynx and stomach providing a conduit for the passage of food. The lumen of the esophagus is lined by a stratified squamous epithelium and is encircled by an inner circular and an outer longitudinal layer of muscle. The muscle of the upper third of the esophagus is striated and is dependent on extrinsic innervation from the vagus nerve while the muscle in the lower third is smooth muscle and is under the influence of both intrinsic and extrinsic controls. The muscle of the middle third forms a transitional zone. Two high pressure zones are found along the length of the esophagus, one at the proximal end forms the upper esophageal sphincter and the other at the distal end forms the lower esophageal sphincter.

Deglutition

After food has been chewed and mixed with saliva a bolus of food is isolated and pushed back, between the tongue and the hard palate, towards the pharynx at the same time as the soft palate is raised to close off the nasopharynx. As the food enters the oropharynx an involuntary reflex is initiated whose afferent limb is transmitted along the glossopharyngeal nerve and the superior laryngeal branch of the vagal nerve to the medulla. Efferent impulses from the facial, glossopharyngeal, vagus, accessory and hypoglossal nerves result in contraction of the pharyngeal muscles and relaxation of the upper esophageal sphincter with movement of the bolus of food onward into the upper esophagus. Entry of food into the larynx is prevented by cessation of respiration, elevation of the larynx and closure of the glottis.

Given the very complicated nature of this reflex and its reliance on many cranial nerve nuclei within the brainstem it is perhaps not surprising that central nervous system disorders which result in the development of bulbar or pseudobulbar palsies will disturb the swallowing reflex; similarly any anatomical disorder of the pharyngeal apparatus (i.e. Pierre Robin or cleft palate) will disrupt normal feeding (Table 19.2). Disordered deglutition is also likely to result in the nasopharyngeal regurgitation of food and the aspiration of ingested food into the lungs. This reflex develops in the neonate at approximately 34 weeks' gestation.

Oromotor coordination develops throughout the first year of life to accommodate the many food consistencies and textures experienced by the child after weaning. If inappropriate foods are given, which fail to match the child's oromotor development, feeding may become difficult and lead to the development of behavioral problems at meal times.

Esophageal peristalsis

During primary peristaltic activity pressure waves of 50–80 mmHg (7–11 kPa) propagate down the esophagus, pushing the bolus of food at a velocity of 2–5 cm/s. A marked reduction in magnitude and propagation velocity of this activity is seen in cerebral palsied children with severe gastroesophageal reflux. Secondary peristaltic activity which develops in response to distension of the esophagus and plays an important role in clearing regurgitated gastric contents back into the stomach is also compromised in children with neurological disease. Tertiary peristaltic activity occurs spontaneously and may be responsible for the pain induced by esophageal spasm.

Table 19.2 A list of the causes of dysphagia

1. Anatomical abnormalities
   a. Cleft palate
   b. Micrognathia (Pierre Robin)
   c. Macroglossia
   d. Cysts, tumors and diverticula of the pharynx
   e. Esophageal atresia
   f. Esophageal stricture
      (i)   Anastomotic
      (ii) Corrosive
      (iii) Reflux esophagitis
   g. Esophageal compression
      (i)   Aortic arch anomaly
      (ii) Mediastinal tumor
      (iii) Esophageal duplication

2. Neuromuscular
   a. Prematurity
   b. Cerebral palsy of any type
   c. Bulbar or pseudobulbar palsies
   d. Isolated cranial nerve paralysis or agenesis
   e. Familial dysautonomia (Riley–Day syndrome)
   f. Achalasia
   g. Esophageal dysmotility (i.e. spasm)
   h. Myasthenia gravis or dystrophica myotonica

3. Inflammatory/trauma
   a. Stomatitis
   b. Acute tonsillopharyngitis
   c. Esophagitis
      (i)   Reflux
      (ii) Eosinophilic esophagitis
      (iii) Corrosive
      (iv) Infective (i.e. *Candida*)
   d. Foreign body

4. Behavioral
   a. Rumination
   b. Globus hystericus

Lower esophageal sphincter

The lower esophageal sphincter is a zone of raised pressure (20 mmHg; 3 kPa), just proximal to the gastroesophageal junction which has a central role in the control of the reflux of gastric contents into the esophagus.[6]

The effectiveness of the lower esophageal sphincter as an antireflux barrier depends also on a number of anatomical factors which assist the sphincteric smooth muscle. A length of intra-abdominal esophagus potentiates the high pressure zone of the sphincter; the acute angle between the esophagus and fundus of the stomach forms a flap valve which closes as the intragastric pressure rises and the crura of the diaphragm press on the lower esophagus. These mechanisms are illustrated in Figure 19.1. Loss of the normal anatomy of the gastroesophageal

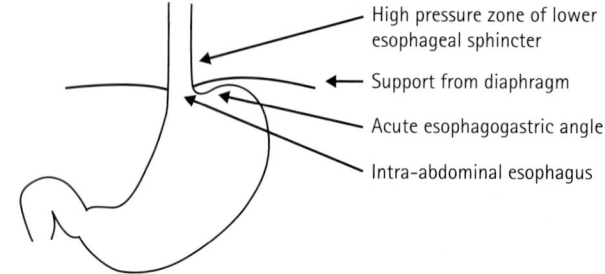

Fig. 19.1 The factors contributing to the normal function of the lower esophageal sphincter.

junction as occurs in patients with sliding hiatus hernias severely disrupts these mechanisms and increases the likelihood of gastroesophageal reflux.

DYSPHAGIA

Diagnosis

The diagnosis of dysphagia can be made by taking a detailed clinical history and by careful observation of the child feeding. Nasal regurgitation of liquids in the absence of vomiting is suggestive of nasopharyngeal reflux and coughing and choking during feeding is very suggestive of aspiration into the larynx. As a consequence the child may develop recurrent chest infections due to aspiration or, because of the difficulty in ingesting an adequate calorie intake, the child may fail to thrive.

Many of the anatomical abnormalities will be obvious on inspection (Table 19.2) and most neuromuscular disorders will be associated with other neurological sequelae such as cerebral palsy. Assessment of feeding and swallowing by a speech therapist will give insight into the level of oromotor coordination; video fluoroscopy (except esophageal atresia) will define the degree of pharyngeal coordination during swallowing and the motility of the esophagus and will determine whether aspiration or nasopharyngeal regurgitation has occurred. A chest X-ray will show signs of aspiration pneumonia or mediastinal space occupation and laryngoscopy and esophagoscopy will allow direct visualization of any motor incoordination, foreign bodies or strictures that may be present.

Treatment

The management of dysphagia depends very much on the underlying cause. Thickening of liquids or giving solids as a puree are often found to be easier and also safer to swallow than liquids alone. Great care and attention is needed with feeding technique but in some patients the airway has to be protected by instituting nasogastric or gastrostomy feeding. Neuromuscular disorders of swallowing are also frequently associated with severe gastroesophageal reflux and in conditions such as cerebral palsy and familial dysautonomia an antireflux procedure such as a Nissen fundoplication is frequently required in addition to a gastrostomy.

GASTROESOPHAGEAL REFLUX

Gastroesophageal reflux is the passive regurgitation of gastric contents into the esophagus and should not be confused with vomiting, which is an active process and requires the contraction of the diaphragm and abdominal muscles to initiate the event.[7] Gastroesophageal reflux will result if there is incompetence of the sphincteric mechanisms at the gastroesophageal junction or if raised intragastric or intra-abdominal pressures are able to overcome this mechanism. It is clear that the lower esophageal sphincter is poorly developed in the very young infant and that the formation of a sliding hiatus hernia severely limits the competence of the sphincter. Similarly in conditions where gastric emptying is delayed or in chronic respiratory diseases such as cystic fibrosis, where coughing increases intra-abdominal pressure, gastroesophageal reflux is exacerbated. In atopic children, dietary protein intolerance may be a significant factor in the development of reflux symptoms.[8]

With prolonged ambulatory recordings of intraesophageal pH (Fig. 19.2) it has become clear that gastroesophageal reflux is a physiological phenomenon which occurs in most children for between 1% and 5% of any 24 h period, with the majority occurring in the postprandial periods. Whether gastroesophageal reflux is deemed to be trivial or pathological is dependent on many factors of which the parents' perception of the problem, the absolute level of reflux and the development of any complicating sequelae are important. It has been shown that in normal individuals reflux most commonly occurs as the child is swallowing and the lower esophageal sphincter is relaxing to allow the passage of food into the stomach. During these brief 'unguarded moments' ingested food and acid pass into the lower esophagus, where a secondary peristaltic

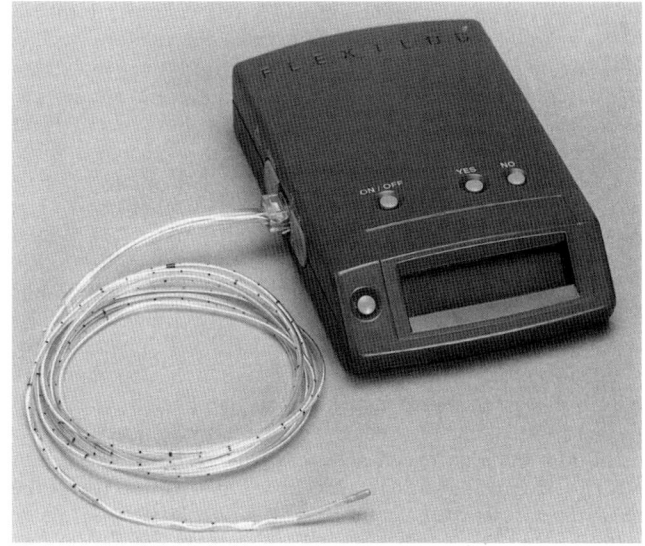

(a)

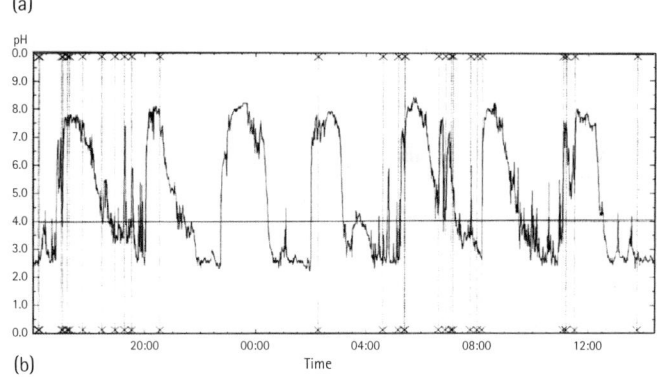

(b)

Fig. 19.2 (a) A solid state 24 h pH recorder with recording electrode. (b) A trace from a 24 h pH recording showing prolonged reflux episodes (pH < 4) after feeds. The time is shown on the horizontal axis.

wave promptly clears the food back into the stomach. If, however, esophageal peristalsis is deranged the contact time of gastric acid on the esophageal mucosa will be prolonged. In a patient with very severe reflux, spontaneous relaxations of the lower esophageal sphincter occur throughout the day, leading to many more 'unguarded moments'. The most troublesome reflux occurs in patients with cerebral palsy or previous esophageal surgery where disordered innervation of the esophagus leads to increased spontaneous relaxation of the sphincter and poor peristaltic clearing mechanisms.[9]

Clinical features

The passive regurgitation of milk occurs in up to half of newborn babies and is accepted by most mothers as being a normal feature of infancy. With time the problem steadily improves and with the introduction of solids and the development of a more upright posture the problem clears in almost all cases. Problems, however, develop where the mother is inexperienced or stressed and has difficulty coping with the problem or where complications such as esophagitis, aspiration or failure to thrive occur.[10]

In most children with reflux the volume of milk which is lost with each regurgitation is insignificant but in some children the intake is severely compromised and as a consequence weight gain is poor. With the prolonged contact of gastric acid on the esophageal mucosa an esophagitis may develop. This may present clinically as blood in the vomit or more insidiously with the development of anemia or stricture. Older children may complain of heartburn with reflux while smaller infants may develop feeding difficulties due to esophageal discomfort.

Aspiration in cerebral palsied children is very common, due to an inability to protect the upper airway from food during both swallowing and regurgitation. When considering the differential diagnosis for children with recurrent cough or respiratory tract infections, gastroesophageal reflux must be included. Aspiration is thought to be a cause of 'near-miss episodes' and in some circumstances may present with the sudden death of the infant. A bizarre presentation of gastroesophageal reflux has been described (Sandifer syndrome) where reflux episodes are associated with dystonic movements of the neck.[11] The clinical clue is that these episodes occur after meals and it has been postulated that stimulation of vagal afferents by the falling esophageal pH results in reflex stimulation of the spinal accessory nerve with the resulting contraction of the sternomastoid.

Although most children with reflux present in the first year of life there are some who present later with symptoms of heartburn or vomiting and a small group who though apparently symptom free through most of their lives present with a peptic stricture of the esophagus (Fig. 19.3). Chronic irritation by acid reflux may lead to replacement of the esophageal mucosa with a columnar epithelium (Barret's esophagus). This metaplastic change can lead to increased risk of adenocarcinoma in later life. There is also the occasional child who will present outwith the first 2 years of life with the precipitous development of severe gastroesophageal reflux in whom detailed investigation may reveal the presence of a posterior fossa tumor.

In children with reflux there may also be longer term behavioral sequelae which can frequently lead to major management problems. Some children are reluctant to eat, particularly solids, and as a consequence feeding problems develop which may last long after the reflux has apparently cleared. Other children who find it easy to reflux are able to regurgitate at will and use this as a powerful attention-seeking tool. A small number of children develop the ability to ruminate, a condition which is generally associated with prolonged periods of reflux.

Diagnosis

In the majority of cases the diagnosis is made clinically from the history of effortless vomiting occurring after meals and no further investigations are required. The family history is often positive in children with severe reflux who do not have neurological disease. Where the clinical picture is unclear or where symptoms suggest a more severe problem,

further investigation is required. Unfortunately no single investigation provides all the information which is required. A 24 h pH study will quantify the degree of acid reflux (Fig. 19.2); a barium meal will tell if there is a hiatus hernia or more distal obstruction (i.e. malrotation) but it has poor sensitivity and frequently misses short reflux episodes. If esophagitis is suspected an endoscopy is required and a full blood count may show evidence of anemia secondary to blood loss. The presence of fat-laden macrophages in the sputum may help in the detection of aspiration. A fuller discussion of esophageal investigations is given later in this section.[12,13]

Treatment (Table 19.3)

Although it is possible to differentiate between physiological and pathological reflux by using 24-hour pH studies, it is likely that in most children treatment decisions will be determined largely on clinical grounds. In an otherwise well baby who is growing adequately and who is free of any complicating features it is likely that the condition will follow a benign course and will resolve spontaneously. The mother should be reassured and advised of simple measures to help with the problem. If the infant is being overfed this should be stopped and if over 3 months of age the introduction of solids should be encouraged. There is generally no need to alter the child's feed but where there is a strong family history of atopy or signs of eczema the introduction of a hypoallergenic feed may be indicated. In addition a small but significant number of children who fail to respond to medical treatment improve dramatically with dietary exclusion. Some of these children will have eosinophilic oesophagitis (see p 607). As the consistency of the feed seems to influence the degree of reflux, thickening agents are found to be helpful in many babies. Alginate compounds are sometimes also found to relieve symptoms.

Traditionally it was advised that children with reflux should be kept sitting upright in a chair but it is likely that this may increase intra-abdominal pressure and exacerbate the problem. Babies should sleep in the supine position to reduce the risk of sudden infant death syndrome.

Where these simple measures fail to reduce reflux, the use of prokinetic agents should be considered. Domperidone and metoclopramide can be used but the former is not licensed to treat reflux in children and the latter can be associated with extrapyramidal side-effects. Additionally domperidone may cause prolongation of the QTc, as has previously been reported with cisapride, and as such a pretreatment electrocardiogram should be considered. They both act by increasing the rate of gastric emptying and it has been postulated that they also increase the lower esophageal sphincter pressure. They do, however, have to be taken continuously to be effective.

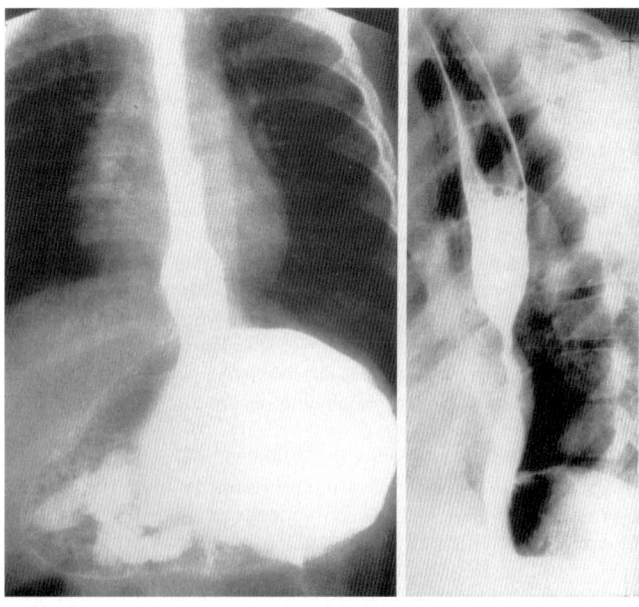

Fig. 19.3 (a) (left) A barium meal showing gross gastroesophageal reflux. (b) (right) A lateral view of the esophagus showing a peptic stricture with proximal dilatation.

Table 19.3 Treatment for children with gastroesophageal reflux (see text for details)

Clinical condition	Treatment
Very mild reflux	Mother reassured Simple feeding advice
Mild reflux	Thickened feeds
Moderate reflux	Prokinetic drugs (consider risk versus benefit)
Reflux with esophagitis	Add histamine 2 blockers Proton pump inhibitor
Severe reflux	Consider continuous nasogastric tube feeding in children less than 1 year as an alternative to fundoplication
Failure of medical treatment	Fundoplication
Esophagitis with stricture	Fundoplication with dilation (Consider a trial of exclusion diet if there is an atopic history)

In patients with crying, irritability or persistent discomfort due to esophagitis, measures to control gastric acid output are required. Histamine 2 (H2) blocking drugs such as ranitidine, or proton pump inhibitors such as omeprazole, will raise the pH of the regurgitated food and seem to help in the healing of esophagitis. In the screaming baby the empirical trial of a H2 blocking drug can if successful, and be a helpful diagnostic test to confirm reflux as the cause of the child's discomfort. It is, however, unclear how long and in what dose this treatment should be continued as suitable controlled trials have yet to be carried out. Antacids have no place in the long-term treatment of esophagitis as the amount required to adequately alkalinize the gastric juices would be likely to lead to salt overload. Their occasional use may be helpful in the older symptomatic child with heartburn.

In young children with reflux there is an expectation that spontaneous clinical improvement is likely up to about 18 months of age. Continuous nasogastric feeding significantly reduces the amount of reflux and in some children with severe symptoms, may be preferable to fundoplication. Although this treatment needs a high degree of motivation from the parents it may adequately control symptoms until the child spontaneously improves.

Where medical management, including a trial of exclusion diet, fails to control complications and gastroesophageal reflux persists, a surgical antireflux procedure is indicated. Where stricture formation has already occurred this should be combined with dilatation of the stricture. It is important that an experienced pediatric surgeon carries out these procedures as the operation may be complicated by retching or gas bloat syndromes. Careful preoperative assessment of patients is required to try and minimize subsequent complications.[14]

A suggested plan of treatment for patients with gastroesophageal reflux is shown in Table 19.3.

EOSINOPHILIC ESOPHAGITIS

Eosinophilic esophagitis is a condition that has only been recognized in children over the last 10–20 years and in adults for an even shorter time.[15] These children present with many of the symptoms of gastroesophageal reflux such as vomiting, nausea and abdominal pain but fail to respond to conventional medical treatment for reflux. Diagnosis is made by esophageal biopsy which frequently shows small macroscopic white 'candida-like' patches. Microscopically the biopsies show more than 20 eosinophils per high power field. If left untreated, this can lead to symptoms of dysphagia with the eventual development of esophageal stricture.

The cause is thought to be due to food allergens such as milk, soya, egg and wheat although in some patients respiratory allergies such as pollen have been implicated. IgE, radioallergosorbent testing (RAST) and skin prick measurement is generally unhelpful as the allergic reactions which may involve all layers of the esophagus are not IgE mediated.

Exclusion diets based on liquid amino acid feeds have been shown to be successful in treating this condition but in all but the youngest patients the feed needs to be given by nasogastric tube. Other treatments such as steroid administration, sodium chromoglycate or leucotriene receptor antagonists have all been tried with varying degrees of success.

The natural history of this condition remains unclear and until this is clarified and high-quality treatment trials are carried out, the best management for this condition will be open to debate.

ACHALASIA

Achalasia of the cardia results from a failure of the lower end of the esophagus to relax with swallowing, resulting in the development of dysphagia, aspiration, retrosternal discomfort and weight loss. This functional obstruction is caused by neurodegenerative changes in the enteric nerves of the lower end of the esophagus.

The condition is very uncommon in childhood and may be confused with gastroesophageal reflux or peptic stricture in young children and

anorexia nervosa in older children. An autosomal recessive form called the triple A syndrome occurs when achalasia is associated with addisonism (hypoadrenalism), alacrima and in some patients neurological deterioration.

The diagnosis is confirmed by the barium swallow appearance of esophageal dilatation with a funnel-shaped narrowing at the lower end and by esophageal manometry which demonstrates disturbed peristaltic activity in the body with increased basal tone and failure of relaxation of the lower esophageal sphincter.

The condition is generally progressive and is treated either by pneumatic dilatation of the lower esophageal sphincter or by Heller's cardiomyotomy.[16] Dilatation procedures frequently have to be repeated more than once and effective treatment of achalasia may lead to the development of gastroesophageal reflux. For this reason in the long term a myotomy and fundoplication procedure is frequently also necessary.

ESOPHAGEAL INVESTIGATIONS

A number of esophageal investigations are available but unfortunately no single test is likely to give all the information that is required to resolve a clinical problem. Each test gives information on a specific aspect of esophageal structure or function and it is necessary for tests to be combined for an overall picture to be obtained (Table 19.4).

Barium studies

Traditionally the barium swallow has been the investigation of choice in children with gastroesophageal reflux. While it is true that contrast studies give good information on the anatomy of the esophagus and the gastroesophageal junction it is a very insensitive test for reflux and the mucosal changes of esophagitis will only show if they are well advanced (see Fig. 19.3). Video studies are useful in detecting abnormalities of swallowing and motility disturbances of the body of the esophagus. It is important that screening is continued until contrast has passed into the jejunum as abnormalities of gastric emptying or malrotation will otherwise be missed.

Gastroesophageal scintigraphy

Scintiscanning using technetium-99m (^{99}Tc)-labeled milk has been shown to be more sensitive in detecting reflux than barium studies and with prolonged scans gastric emptying can be measured and bronchial aspiration of the milk can be detected. The method, however, requires the patient to remain still for up to 30 min on a gamma camera and gives very little anatomical information.

Esophageal manometry

This technique is presently available in only a few pediatric centers and its clinical uses are limited to the diagnosis of the less common conditions such as achalasia and esophageal spasm. The measurement of

Table 19.4   Investigations of esophageal structure and function

Test	Uses
Barium studies	Define anatomy of upper GI tract
Scintiscanning	For the detection of reflux and aspiration (not as sensitive as pH studies)
Manometry	Detect achalasia or esophageal spasm
pH monitoring	Most sensitive test for acid reflux
Esophagoscopy	Detect esophagitis and allows mucosal biopsy
Trial of NG feeding	Unmasked reflux in patients with poor oral intake

GI, gastrointestinal; NG, nasogastric

lower esophageal sphincter pressure is a very insensitive indicator of gastroesophageal reflux.

Esophageal pH monitoring

The prolonged ambulatory recording of esophageal pH using catheter-mounted electrodes is a very sensitive means of quantifying acid gastroesophageal reflux (Fig. 19.2). Modern computerized systems allow the length of time and the number of episodes of acid reflux to be measured and their division between awake, asleep, postprandial and fasting periods can be derived. Unfortunately it fails to detect non-acid reflux and with the realization that up to 50% of reflux in some patients may be non-acid, the potential limitations of this investigation are becoming clear. Newer impedence techniques when combined with pH measurement should hopefully help overcome this problem as all liquids refluxed are detected.

Esophagoscopy

If significant reflux is found or peptic or eosinophilic esophagitis is suspected it is important that an esophagoscopy is carried out. This is the only method which allows accurate assessment of esophagitis both visually and histologically and mucosal inflammation can be detected at a very early stage long before any radiological changes are found. With modern pediatric endoscopes the procedure can be carried out as a day case under sedation or a short general anesthetic.

Trial of nasogastric tube feeding

The assessment of children with cerebral palsy is often compromised by the fact that their oral intake is significantly reduced and reflux may not be seen during barium studies. The passage of a nasogastric tube and the administration of appropriate feed volumes often unmasks symptoms of reflux and facilitates the administration of contast during barium studies.

THE STOMACH AND DUODENUM

STRUCTURE AND FUNCTION

The stomach is a J-shaped organ which lies obliquely across the midline in the upper abdomen. It is covered by an inner oblique, middle circular and outer longitudinal layer of smooth muscle and is lined by a columnar epithelium which is indented with gastric pits. The muscular layer is thickened at the pylorus, which acts as a valve to control the rate of emptying from the stomach. The columnar epithelium produces mucus, which forms a protective layer over the mucosa. The pits in the antrum, body and distal fundus are short and contain the parietal cells which produce hydrochloric acid and intrinsic factor, the chief cells which synthesize and secrete pepsinogen, endocrine cells and mucus-producing cells which are located at the neck of the glands. The pyloric glands which also contain endocrine cells are more tortuous and secrete large amounts of mucus.

Gastric motility

Following the ingestion of food, the body and fundus distend greatly and act as a reservoir for the storage of food. In contrast the antrum is a more muscular organ which, working in concert with the pylorus, produces propagative, segmenting and retrograde activity to break the food down into small, easily digested pieces.

Liquids generally empty very rapidly from the stomach with the rate being determined by the pressure gradient across the pylorus. A typical half emptying time for a drink of orange squash is 15 min. Solids in contrast empty much more slowly with a half emptying time being more typically between 90 and 120 min. The rate of emptying is very closely controlled by mechanoreceptors in the antrum and chemorecepters in the duodenum which feed back to the gastric smooth muscle to limit the rate of emptying. As a consequence of this a homogenized meal will empty more rapidly than a solid meal and a low energy meal will empty faster than a more energy-dense meal. The rate of emptying is also inhibited by the presence of undigested fat in the ileum and by distension of the rectum due to fecal loading. The nongastrointestinal factors which influence gastric emptying are discussed further in the section on vomiting.

Digestion

Pepsinogen is released from zymogen granules in the chief cells of the gastric glands in response to the ingestion of food. Under the influence of hydrochloric acid and then by the autocatalytic action of free pepsin the active pepsin is formed. This enzyme has a pH optimum of 1.0–1.5 and initiates proteolysis in the stomach by hydrolyzing peptide bonds at the amino groups of aromatic or acidic amino acids.

It is also likely that triglyceride hydrolysis starts in the stomach with the activation of the acid-stable lingual lipase and possibly also by the action of gastric lipase. In the preterm infant, because of the very low activity of pancreatic lipase it is likely that this mechanism is of some importance.

Gastric acid production

Hydrochloric acid is actively secreted by the parietal cells of the gastric glands maintaining the pH of the stomach at approximately 1. The rate of acid production is modulated by circulating levels of the gut hormone gastrin, which is produced by G cells within the antrum of the stomach. The acid environment of the stomach has an important defensive role against ingested pathogens and as mentioned earlier provides the optimal environment for activity of the gastric digestive enzymes. The low pH facilitates the absorption of inorganic iron by preventing its precipitation. Excessive acid production, however, is likely to lead to an increasing incidence of duodenal ulceration.

The parietal cells are also responsible for the secretion of the glycoprotein intrinsic factor which stabilizes vitamin B_{12} during intestinal transit and binds to specific receptors in the terminal ileum prior to absorption. In autoimmune gastritis where the parietal cells are destroyed, hydrochloric acid and intrinsic factor production cease, resulting in achlorhydria and vitamin B_{12} deficiency.

GASTRITIS

Acute gastritis

Acute inflammation of the stomach may arise from conditions as diverse as irritation from nonsteroidal anti-inflammatory drugs (NSAIDs), chemical ingestion or the duodeno gastric reflux of bile. Many of these conditions are self-limiting and may resolve spontaneously if the insult is removed. If the cause of the mucosal irritation persists the gastritis may become chronic and in the case of continued NSAID ingestion, may proceed to peptic ulceration.

Chronic gastritis

There are two main forms of chronic gastritis: atrophic and non-atrophic. The former is usually associated with autoimmune disease and leads to loss of glandular tissue with resulting achlorhydria and loss of intrinsic factor production. This condition is very rare in childhood.

Non-atrophic gastritis is most commonly caused by *Helicobacter pylori* although less common causes include Crohn's disease and eosinophilic gastroenteritis.[17] Diagnosis is made by histological examination of mucosal biopsies from the antrum, incisura and body of the stomach. The Syndey classification of gastritis has been devised primarily for adults but it is likely that the general principles also apply to children. In *H. pylori* infection, the gastric antrum frequently has a nodular appearance and histologically acute infection is associated with an increase in intraepithelial neutrophils which progresses to chronic inflammatory changes with an associated increase in lymphoid follicles.

PEPTIC ULCERATION

Acute ulcers

Peptic ulceration can occur acutely in response to stress or the administration of ulcerogenic drugs. Stress ulcers can occur in either the stomach or duodenum and are most common in the neonatal period in response to birth asphyxia or respiratory distress but they can also occur in later childhood following severe burns, meningitis or other major stresses. In patients receiving NSAIDs for conditions such as juvenile arthritis or corticosteroids for severe asthma or IBD, acute ulcers can also occur. It is unlikely that *H. pylori* plays a significant role in acute ulceration.

A stress ulcer is likely to present with intestinal bleeding or acute pain and should be treated with an H2 blocker or proton pump inhibitor but where perforation occurs, surgery is required. In situations where stress ulceration is likely, prophylaxis with gastroprotective drugs should be considered.

Chronic ulcers

Chronic peptic ulceration occurs most commonly in children over the age of 5 years but unlike acute ulcers, which affect the stomach and duodenum equally, chronic ulcers occur 10 times more frequently in the duodenum. As in adulthood there is very frequently a family history of peptic ulcer disease with a slight (3:2) male to female preponderance.

In many older children the classical ulcer symptoms of localized epigastric discomfort, nocturnal wakening and relief of symptoms with food or antacids are present. However, in younger children more non-specific symptoms such as vague abdominal pain, vomiting and nausea may make the diagnosis less clear. Some children may present with an occult anemia or more acutely with a hematemesis or melena. Because of the vague nature of many of these symptoms it is very important to differentiate between peptic ulcer disease and the far more common 'non-organic' recurrent abdominal pain of childhood. The presence of epigastric pain, nocturnal wakening, a progressive worsening of symptoms, an iron deficiency blood picture or a family history should alert the practitioner to the possibility of duodenal ulceration.

While the diagnosis can be made on a barium meal, carried out by an experienced radiologist, the relatively poor sensitivity of this test (50%) means that where a peptic ulcer is suspected upper gastrointestinal endoscopy should be the investigation of first choice. In addition to visualizing the ulcer, endoscopy allows the practitioner to look for *H. pylori* infection in mucosal biopsies.[18] Although the measurement of gastric acid output is a very insensitive way of diagnosing peptic ulcer disease, in the rare situation where multiple ulcers refractory to treatment are present it is important to measure fasting serum gastrin and basal and stimulated gastric acid output levels to exclude the possibility of a gastrin-secreting pancreatic tumor (Zollinger–Ellison syndrome).

Treatment

Much of the advice for treatment of peptic ulceration has been extrapolated from the adult experience as clinical trials in children have been limited by the small number of patients and by ethical constraints. It is likely, however, that a similar condition exists in both groups of patients as the clinical experience of therapeutic regimens is similar in each.

The treatment of chronic peptic ulcer disease is primarily aimed at reducing excess gastric acid production and eradicating *H. pylori* infection, which is invariably present. A 6-week course of treatment with acid suppressive therapy will provide symptomatic relief of dyspeptic symptoms within 1–2 weeks in most patients and by the end of the 6-week course the ulcers will have healed in over 80% of patients. Recurrence of ulcer symptoms is likely to develop unless attempts are made to eradicate *H. pylori* and a course of triple therapy using one of the regimens outlined in the section on anti-*Helicobacter* therapy, is indicated at the time of initial treatment. If symptoms recur after treatment it is likely that the *H. pylori* has not been completely eradicated.

HELICOBACTER PYLORI

Since the identification of *H. pylori* in the mucosa of the gastric antrum there has been an explosion of interest in the role of this small spiral organism and its causal relationship to gastritis, duodenal ulcer, recurrent abdominal pain, lymphoproliferative disorders and gastric cancer.

While *H. pylori* is undoubtedly a causal factor in the pathogenesis of peptic ulcer disease in both children and adults, the presence of infection only leads to active disease in 10% of the population. Up to half of the world's population is infected with *H. pylori*, the majority of whom will have no recognizable disease. Similarly in children the presence of an active gastritis may not lead to the development of any symptoms and the priority when investigating a child is to determine the cause of their symptoms and not whether they are or are not infected with *H. pylori*. Our present understanding remains incomplete and many questions remain unanswered. There have however been consensus statements in recent years from both Europe and North America which begin to answer questions such as, who should be screened for infection, how they should be tested, and who should be treated and what is the optimal method of eradicating *H. pylori*?[18,19] (see Table 19.5).

Pathogenesis

This organism is recognized as the most important cause of non-autoimmune gastritis in both children and adults. It may colonize either the antrum of the stomach, leading to increased acid production, or the body of the stomach, where inflammation may lead to the development of an atrophic gastritis. Normal duodenal mucosa is not colonized unless gastric metaplasia has developed. *H. pylori* lies deep within the mucus layer which covers the gastric mucosa and through the action of the enzyme urease, which produces ammonia and the release of cytotoxins, the underlying mucosa becomes damaged and inflamed. During endoscopy a nodular inflammation of the antrum may be seen and hypertrophy of the gastric mucosal folds has been reported.

Epidemiology

H. pylori is acquired in early childhood and, once infected, children are likely to remain colonized, despite the mounting of a host response, for the rest of their life unless they are inadvertently treated with antibiotics. The incidence of *H. pylori* infection in industrialized countries is approximately 0.5% of the susceptible population per year compared to a rate of 3–10% in developing countries. Spread occurs though close physical contact either by oral–oral or fecal–oral routes with the prevalence increasing where there is social deprivation or institutionalization.

Diagnosis of *Helicobacter pylori*
Biopsy and histopathology

Endoscopy and biopsy is the most reliable method for diagnosing infection. Multiple biopsies from the antrum, incisura and body of the stomach allow the location and severity of inflammation to be defined and the presence of small spiral organisms on specially stained tissue

Table 19.5 Agreed points from consensus statements on *Helicobacter pylori*

1. The aim of diagnosis is to find the cause of the symptoms rather than the presence of *H. pylori*
2. Testing all children and treating those positive for *H. pylori* is not recommended
3. Antibody tests of blood, serum or saliva are not recommended
4. Upper GI endoscopy and biopsy is the best test for a child with chronic upper abdominal pain or suspected peptic ulcer disease
5. A child diagnosed with peptic ulcer disease by barium study should undergo endoscopy if symptoms recur
6. The urea breath test is not a satisfactory alternative to endoscopy for *H. pylori* diagnosis because of the wide differential diagnosis. It can be used for confirming success of treatment
7. Screening for *H. pylori* in asymptomatic individuals is not indicated
8. Treatment should be given when *H. pylori* is causing active disease (i.e. duodenal ulcer). When it is present without associated disease (i.e. asymptomatic child) the need for treatment should be discussed with the parents

sections confirms the presence of infection. In patients with infection that is resistant to treatment, biopsy allows culture and antimicrobial sensitivity to be determined.

The advantages of high sensitivity and specificity and the ability to examine the esophagus and duodenum at the same time have to be balanced against the invasiveness, availability and cost of the procedure.

Rapid urease (CLO) test

A single gastric biopsy is placed in the well of a CLO test slide. If *H. pylori* is present, its urease activity will cleave urea to produce ammonia, which will turn the pH indicator red if left at room temperature for 24 h. This test gives indirect evidence of infection but cannot be relied upon in isolation to make a diagnosis.

Serology

This test is based on the detection of specific IgG to *H. pylori* in serum samples. The tests are cheap and relatively easy to set up. In children however the humoral immune response to infection may be slow to develop and this test is most unreliable in children under 5 years. The accuracy of serum-based kits in symptomatic patients is between 60% and 70%. These tests cannot be used to confirm eradication after treatment as antibodies may remain positive for many months despite successful therapy. The recent consensus reports do not recommend the use of serological testing as the primary means of diagnosing *H. pylori* infection.

Tests using salivary antibodies are not presently recommended but stool tests for *H. pylori* antigens appear a little more promising.

C^{13} urea breath test

This non-invasive test involves the patient taking a small oral dose of C^{13}-enriched urea following a test meal which delays gastric emptying.[20] If *H. pylori* is present within the stomach the urea is cleaved, releasing C^{13}-enriched CO_2, which is then exhaled in the breath. By collecting two breath samples, one before and the other 30 min after taking the oral urea, a rise in C^{13} levels in the breath signifies infection. This test has a sensitivity of 95% and a specificity of almost 100%. The sensitivity is reduced if antibiotics or acid suppressing drugs are not discontinued for 1 month prior to the test. The breath collection may also be technically difficult in young children.

The primary role of breath testing is confirming successful eradication after a course of treatment.

Symptoms

It is likely that the majority of children infected with this organism have no symptoms but, conversely, in children with evidence of chronic peptic ulceration, *H. pylori* is likely to have an important role in its pathogenesis. Why the majority of children has no symptoms and only a small minority develops peptic disease remains unclear. It is not possible to differentiate infected from non-infected patients on the basis of history alone and in infected patients only those with proven ulceration responded well to eradication therapy. This would suggest that *H. pylori* gastritis does not in isolation cause symptoms.

It was initially thought that *H. pylori* infection might be a significant cause of recurrent abdominal pain in childhood. While 5–17% of such children may be infected, it has been found that 5–29% of children without pain also had evidence of infection. It is therefore quite clear that this infection is not a significant factor in children with recurrent

abdominal pain and current recommendations are that such children should not be screened for infection.

Treatment
Who to treat?

Eradication therapy is recommended where *H. pylori* infection and symptoms due to that infection are both present.[21–23] However because infection with *H. pylori* is so common many children in whom infection is found will either be asymptomatic or will have symptoms not directly attributable to the infection. In this latter group the decision to treat is less clear-cut as it may not be of any benefit to the child and may carry the risk of side-effects from treatment.

Treatment is indicated for children with *H. pylori* infection and gastric or duodenal ulcer. In the rare patient with mucosa-associated lymphoid tissue (MALT) lymphoma or atrophic gastritis with intestinal metaplasia eradication therapy is also indicated.

Many children with *H. pylori* infection have evidence of gastritis without either gastric or duodenal ulceration. Under such circumstances treatment is unlikely to benefit the child. There is at present no convincing evidence that eradication therapy will reduce the risk of later peptic ulceration, adenocarcimoma or lymphoma. The clinician should discuss the pros and cons of treatment with the child and his/her parents before making a decision on whether to treat or not.

At present there is no evidence that children with recurrent abdominal pain or asymptomatic children benefit from eradication therapy.

Drug therapy

No properly controlled trials of *H. pylori* eradication therapy in children have been carried out and most of the available information is extrapolated from adult studies. A number of factors however are clear. Firstly the most important determinant of the success of therapy is compliance with treatment and secondly it is recommended that three medications are given twice daily for 1–2 weeks. The use of one or two medicines is likely to be ineffective and will increase the risk of drug resistance developing. The recommended first-line treatment for *H. pylori* eradication is given in Table 19.6.[19] It is suggested that successful eradication is confirmed by C^{13} breath testing and where reinfection occurs the use of alternative antibiotics such as tetracycline (over 12 years) or bismuth salts should be considered.

UPPER GASTROINTESTINAL BLEEDING

Bleeding from the upper gastrointestinal tract may present either as a hematemesis or melena depending on the site and severity of the bleeding. In the majority of cases the bleeding has little hemodynamic effect but major bleeds warrant urgent treatment. It is important, however, when taking a history to be sure that the child has in fact passed blood. The swallowing of bloodstained liquor, sucking on a cracked nipple, a recent nose bleed and the recent ingestion of beetroot can all mimic an intestinal hemorrhage.[24,25]

Diagnosis

The most likely cause for a bleed can be determined from the age of the child and by searching for clues from the history and examination. A history of previous gastrointestinal symptoms, recent drug ingestion, umbilical catheterization as a neonate, stigmata of chronic liver disease or a bleeding diathesis, or evidence of subcutaneous or cutaneous hemangioma should be sought (Table 19.7). In children with forceful

Table 19.6 Recommended first-line eradication therapy for *Helicobacter pylori* in children. Gold et al 2000[19]

Medication	Dose
Omeprazole (or equivalent proton pump inhibitor)	1 mg/kg/day up to 20 mg twice a day
Give two } amoxicillin	50 mg/kg/d up to 1 g twice a day
of three } metronidazole	20 mg/kg/d up to 500 mg twice a day
antibiotics } clarithromycin	15 mg/kg/day up to 500 mg twice a day
Treatment should be as a twice-daily regimen (to aid compliance) for 7–14 d.	

Table 19.7 Causes of upper gastrointestinal bleeding

1. Hemorrhagic disease of the newborn
2. Stress peptic ulcer
3. Blood dyscrasia
4. Esophagitis
   a. Peptic
   b. Caustic
5. Esophageal varices
6. Mallory–Weiss tear
7. Chronic ulcers
   a. Gastric
   b. Duodenal
8. Gastric erosions
   a. Salicylates
   b. Nonsteroidal anti-inflammatory drugs
   c. Corticosteroids
9. Infantile hypertrophic pyloric stenosis
10. Foreign body
11. Vascular malformations
12. Intestinal polyps

vomiting due to gastroenteritis, Mallory–Weiss tears are the likely cause if specks of blood are present in the vomitus.

A full blood count will give an indication of the duration and severity of the bleed but may be misleading in the acute situation. A clotting screen will define the nature of any bleeding disorder that may be present. Direct visualization of the upper gastrointestinal tract by endoscopy should be carried out within 24 h of the bleed or whenever the patient is hemodynamically stable. This investigation will allow the detection of esophagitis, esophageal varices, gastric and duodenal ulcers and vascular malformations of the intestine proximal to the third part of the duodenum. If bleeding persists and these initial investigations are negative, a small bowel meal should be carried out and if negative a capsule endoscopy should be considered.[26] The direct visualization afforded by this technique is ideal for the detection of polyps, ulcers and vascular malformations. If bleeding persists and no cause can be found a laparotomy may be indicated.

At times it can be very difficult to distinguish between upper and lower tract bleeding and it is suggested that this section is read in conjunction with the section on rectal bleeding (see p. 638).

Treatment

The initial treatment of the shocked patient is resuscitation, ensuring the patient has a secure airway and is breathing adequately with maintenance of the circulation by the rapid infusion of 10–30 ml/kg initially of saline and then whole blood when available. Any bleeding diathesis should be corrected and attempts should be made to define the underlying cause. If varices are found the patient should be treated by a team experienced with this type of problem. A description of the management of a variceal bleed is given in the section on liver disease (see p. 651). Most patients stop bleeding with simple medical management, and treatment should be aimed at the underlying cause of the bleeding.

VOMITING

Vomiting is a very common symptom of disease in childhood and should not be confused with the regurgitation of food, which occurs in conditions such as gastroesophageal reflux. The vomiting reflex is the body's response to noxious stimuli, which may reside within the gastrointestinal tract or result from some systemic disturbance and act directly or indirectly on the 'vomiting center' in the area postrema of the brainstem. The act of vomiting can be divided into three phases. In the pre-ejection phase the patient feels nauseous, looks pale, salivates and through the action of visceral efferent nerves develops a tachycardia with relaxation of the proximal stomach. This is followed by a period of retching and

then, with synchronous contractions of the intra-abdominal muscles and diaphragm with an open glottis, upper esophageal sphincter and mouth, the contents of the stomach are ejected.

In the neonate, vomiting may be the first symptom of an intestinal obstruction, although any infection, metabolic disturbance or cerebral insult may present in an identical manner. The presence of bile in the vomit would suggest an obstruction distal to the duodenum. As the child becomes older the range of conditions causing obstructive and metabolic problems will change and in addition dietary indiscretions or intolerances may develop. The possibility of idiopathic hypertrophic pyloric stenosis should be considered in any baby of 1–4 months of age who develops projectile vomiting. In the older child drugs taken either accidentally or therapeutically may result in vomiting. A history of recurrent episodes of severe vomiting punctuated by asymptomatic periods should alert the practitioner to the possibility of cyclical vomiting. The symptoms of vomiting and diarrhea are frequently combined during enteric infections and it is likely that on a worldwide scale this is the most common cause of vomiting.

Diagnosis

A good history and examination will often give strong pointers to the most likely cause for the vomiting. A pyloric tumor or the mass of an intussusception may be palpable on abdominal examination. In some patients, particularly the very young, clues may be few and far between and it must also be remembered that the differential diagnosis varies greatly depending on the age of the patient and on whether any associated features such as diarrhea are present (Table 19.8).

An erect and supine abdominal X-ray will show multiple air–fluid levels in intestinal obstruction but it must also be remembered that a

Table 19.8 Causes of vomiting in infancy

Cause	First week of life	After first week
Alimentary tract	Duodenal atresia	Malrotation/volvulus
	Jejunal atresia	Hirschsprung disease
	Malrotation/volvulus	Intussusception
	Duplication of bowel	Strangulated hernia
	Diaphragmatic hernia	Pyloric stenosis
	Meconium ileus	Functional obstruction
	Hirschsprung disease	Peptic ulceration
	Anal atresia	Appendicitis
	Functional obstruction	Bezoar
		Crohn's disease
Metabolic	Galactosemia	Organic acidemia
	Organic acidemia	Hyperammonemia
	Hyperammonemia	Hypoadrenalism
	Hypercalcemia	Diabetic ketoacidosis
	Hypoadrenalism	Drug intoxication
		Reye syndrome
		Uremia
Dietetic	Cow's milk intolerance	Cow's milk intolerance
		Celiac disease
		Overeating
Infection	Any infection	Gastroenteritis
		Tonsillitis
		Otitis media
		Urinary infection
		Meningitis
		Septicemia
Cerebral	Birth trauma	Head injury
	Hydrocephalus	Cerebral tumor
		Encephalitis
		Increased intracranial pressure
Others		Motion sickness
		Cyclical vomiting

functional obstruction due either to some intrinsic abnormality of the gut or to the toxic effect of sepsis or metabolic derangement may also give a similar picture. Barium contrast studies will define the nature of surgical causes of vomiting which are not clear from plain films. Where appropriate, detailed infection and metabolic screens should be carried out and signs of raised intracranial pressure should be sought. The serum electrolytes will give information on the extent of the vomiting and may even, as in the case of hypochloremic hypokalemic alkalosis of pyloric stenosis, give clues to the underlying cause.

If a non-organic cause for the vomiting is suspected or if a behavioral element is thought to be present, referral to a psychiatrist or psychologist for a diagnostic assessment should be considered.

Treatment

The treatment should be aimed at the resuscitation of the patient in the first instance and then more specifically at the underlying cause of the vomiting. Electrolyte losses should be corrected with i.v. fluids and oral fluids should be stopped. If vomiting persists a nasogastric tube should be passed and where an obstructive lesion seems likely a pediatric surgeon should be consulted. As an adjunct to the treatment of the underlying problem, antiemetic drugs may be useful in modifying the emetic response. Given the wide variety of stimuli which can produce vomiting and the varying mode of actions of these drugs it is perhaps not surprising that these agents are not universally effective.

INFANTILE HYPERTROPHIC PYLORIC STENOSIS

Pyloric stenosis develops in approximately 3 per 1000 live births with a male-to-female preponderance of 4:1. The cause of the condition is unclear although a reduced number of cases occur in babies with blood group A and there is also a strong familial pattern of inheritance. A thickening of the pyloric muscle results in gastric outlet obstruction with resulting vomiting.[27]

Symptoms of projectile vomiting occurring 10–20 min after a feed, develop between the second and fourth week of life, although they can occasionally occur either sooner or at up to 4 months of age. With progressive vomiting the infants lose weight and may eventually become dehydrated and alkalotic. On clinical examination gastric peristaltic activity may be seen, and palpation of the right upper quadrant of the abdomen during a test feed will reveal the pyloric tumor in most cases. If the mass cannot be felt diagnosis can be aided by a barium meal, which will show a narrow elongated pyloric canal or by ultrasound, which should also define the mass.

The initial management of the patient after the diagnosis has been confirmed is i.v. rehydration and correction of any acid–base disturbance. The patient should then undergo a Ramstedt's pyloromyotomy where the pyloric muscle is split down to the mucosa. Oral feeds can be restarted 24 h after surgery (see Ch. 37).

Other surgical causes of vomiting are discussed more fully in Chapter 38.

CYCLICAL VOMITING

Cyclical vomiting is defined as three or more periods of intense nausea and unremitting vomiting with intervening periods free of symptoms in a child without metabolic, gastrointestinal or central nervous system disease.[28,29] The attacks, which can occur as frequently as once a week in some children and as infrequently as every 6 months in others, are generally preceded by a prodromal phase when the child is pale and withdrawn with the attack lasting anything from 12–72 h. The vomiting may also be associated with features of the periodic syndrome such as abdominal pain or headache.

The vomiting may be exacerbated by the child's desire to drink large amounts of fluid; persistent vomiting can lead to Mallory–Weiss tears, dehydration, electrolyte imbalance and eventually coma. It is frequently difficult to define the factors which precipitate each attack but a careful history may reveal stress factors, the most common being marital conflicts and school-based problems. The children require a full blood count, the measurement of serum electrolytes and a urine culture. Where symptoms persist or bilious vomiting occurs, a contrast study should be done to exclude malrotation. It is important also to exclude raised intracranial pressure as a cause of the vomiting. Rare metabolic problems such as medium chain acyl CoA dehydrogenase deficiency (MCAD) or ornithine transcarbamylase deficiency in girls need to be considered and excluded. In a small number of children an intercurrent viral infection may appear to initiate the episode.

If left untreated the majority of children will grow out of the problem but this may take many years. In others, headache may become a prominent feature and a picture of migraine may develop later. If stress factors have been revealed from the history, psychological therapy may be of benefit in preventing further attacks while in those with migraineous features, dietary exclusion of cheese, chocolate, caffeine or citrus fruits should be considered. During acute attacks the child may require hospital admission for i.v. fluids. The 5 hydroxy tryptophan three ($5HT_3$) antagonist ondansetron given with a benzodiazepine such as lorazepam may be helpful in shortening the length of attacks. I.v. dexamethasone may potentiate this effect. Good control of the raised blood pressure associated with this condition is also required.

FOREIGN BODIES

Children between the ages of 1 and 4 are particularly liable to swallow foreign bodies. The majority of these cause very few problems and simply pass straight through the intestine but long pointed objects such as fish bones or needles can become lodged in the pharynx, esophagus or occasionally in the duodenal loop. If the foreign body becomes lodged in a high position, coughing and choking may occur but frequently there may be no initial symptoms. Perforation of the mucosa will result in the development of a mediastinitis or peritonitis and where a battery becomes lodged a caustic stricture or mucosal erosion may develop.

Bezoar

The repeated ingestion of hair or paper or fibers from clothing or blankets can result in the formation of a large non-opaque foreign body in the stomach. These masses can grow to quite a large size but frequently there are very few symptoms other than vague abdominal pain or halitosis. The bezoar may be felt by abdominal palpation or outlined on a contrast study where the barium adheres to the fibrous mass.

Treatment

Small foreign bodies without sharp edges should be left to pass through the intestine. If they do not appear within 72 h a plain X-ray should be taken to check on their position. Sharp foreign bodies should be removed endoscopically under direct vision. If endoscopic removal from the stomach is not possible a laparotomy will be required.

GASTRIC INVESTIGATIONS
Barium studies

In patients with chronic nausea and vomiting a barium meal will define the anatomy of the stomach and detect the presence of a hiatus hernia, reflux, if it occurs during the examination, malrotation or any space occupation due to a bezoar. Although duodenal ulcers may be detected, endoscopy is the investigation of choice where a mucosal lesion is suspected.

Gastroscopy

Fiberoptic endoscopy is the preferred investigation for detecting duodenal or gastric ulcers or the antral gastritis associated with *H. pylori* infection. The method can be used in infants of all ages allowing histological and microbiological confirmation of the suspected diagnoses.

THE SMALL INTESTINE

STRUCTURE OF THE SMALL INTESTINE

In man the small intestine occupies the major length of the gastrointestinal tract and is the major organ of digestion and absorption. In the adult the small intestine varies in length from 3 to 5 m depending on the state of contraction, while in the term infant the length is probably nearer 1.5 m. The small intestine is divided into the duodenum, which extends from the pylorus to the duodenal–jejunal flexure at the ligament of Treitz, and the remaining small intestine is arbitrarily divided into the jejunum and ileum, which represent the proximal two fifths and distal three fifths, respectively.

In cross-section the structure of the small intestine is grossly similar throughout. The inner circular lumen is lined by a highly convoluted mucosa which exposes a large surface area for the absorption of nutrients. Underneath the surface epithelium lies the submucosa, which in turn is encircled by the muscularis, which comprises an inner circular and an outer longitudinal layer. The outermost layer is the serosa, which is in continuity with the peritoneum. The mesentery of the small intestine is inserted diagonally across the posterior abdominal wall from the ligament of Treitz to the cecum. When this mesentery is shortened by malrotation of the small intestine it becomes unstable and is liable to twist.

Mucosa

The mucosa consists of the surface epithelium and the lamina propria. The mucosal surface is covered by villi which project into the lumen and greatly increase the surface area and by the crypts of Lieberkühn, which lie between the villi and form a depression in the mucosa (Fig. 19.4). In the jejunum the villous:crypt ratio is 3:1 but this decreases more distally to 1–2:1 in the ileum. Underneath the surface epithelium lies the lamina propria, which contains a connective tissue core for the villi along with the vascular, lymphatic and neural networks which serve the nutrient and transport needs of the surface epithelium.[30]

The surface epithelium

The crypts and villi should be thought of as the functional unit of the surface epithelium. The crypts contain paneth, goblet, endocrine and undifferentiated cell types. Goblet cells which lie on the lateral wall of the crypts produce large amounts of protective mucus and the endocrine cells, which are neuroectodermal in origin, synthesize and secrete gastrointestinal hormones. Rapidly dividing undifferentiated cells migrate up the length of the crypts and on to the villi, where they transform into

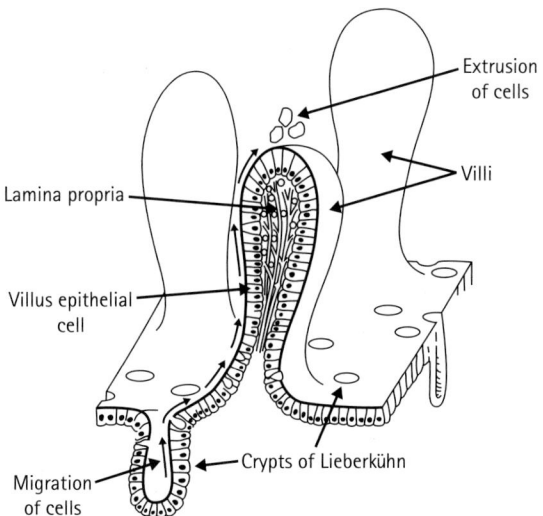

Fig. 19.4 A diagrammatic view of the surface of the small intestine. (Reproduced from *Harries' Paediatric Gastroenterology*[30] by kind permission of the publisher.)

mature villus cells (Fig. 19.4). The rate of division of these cells and their speed of migration is under the control of the trophic effect of enteral nutrients and a number of gut hormones. When enteral nutrients are removed as a result of starvation or the prolonged use of parenteral nutrition (PN), mucosal hypoplasia results while during the adaptation process that follows small intestinal resection, the rate of cell turnover increases resulting in mucosal hypertrophy and increased villous length.

As the epithelial cells reach the villous tip they degenerate and fall off into the lumen. This rapid turnover of the villous epithelium takes between 4 and 6 days and explains both why the intestinal mucosa is on the one hand very susceptible to the toxic effects of ionizing radiation and chemotherapeutic drugs and why on the other its rate of repair and recovery from serious insult can be very rapid. The enterocytes have a well-developed brush border which further increases the surface area of the mucosa to luminal nutrients and supports the enzymes responsible for the final digestion of nutrients prior to absorption.

The cells in the crypts play an important role in the secretion of water and electrolytes into the lumen in contrast to the villous cells, which largely absorb water, electrolytes and nutrients. In health the small intestine is a net absorber of water but in situations where the villous structure is damaged (i.e. celiac disease) or where mucosal inflammation stimulates the activity of the secretory crypt cells (i.e. Crohn's disease) this situation is reversed, leading to active mucosal secretion. A similar situation occurs in rotavirus gastroenteritis, where the rapid turnover of regenerative cells results in villi populated with immature cells which have yet to develop significant absorptive capacity.

The muscularis

The motor activity of the small intestine is provided by the inner circular and outer longitudinal muscle layers which are present along the whole length of the small intestine. Nerve fibers freely travel between these layers with extension distally onto the mucosa and proximally through afferent and efferent fibers which project both to and from the brainstem and cerebral cortex.

DIGESTION

Digestion of carbohydrates

Starch, the main form of ingested carbohydrate, is a mixture of long chains of glucose units linked at the alpha-1,4 position (amylose), and shorter chains of alpha-1,4-linked glucose units connected by alpha-1,6 links to give a branched structure (amylopectin). As the intestine is only able to absorb monosaccharide units these large molecules require digestion by hydrolytic enzymes.

This digestion takes place in two steps: the first, occurring within the lumen of the gut, breaks the starch into oligosaccharides and the second, which occurs on the brush border of the small intestine, further digests these carbohydrates to their component monosaccharides. The luminal digestion is carried out by amylase from the salivary glands and the pancreas, which hydrolyzes alpha-1,4 bonds, breaking the amylose into maltose (two glucose units) and maltotriose, and amylopectin into limit dextrins with on average eight glucose units and one or more alpha-1,6 branching points. In the adult approximately 15% of duodenal amylase activity is salivary in origin but in the newborn infant, where pancreatic exocrine function is very poorly developed, this may increase to 50%.

Dietary disaccharides and the products of amylase digestion are further hydrolyzed by the enzymes of the enterocyte brush border membrane. These include the alpha-glucosidases sucrase, isomaltase, maltase and trehalase, the latter having no functional significance in the human. The beta-galactosidase lactase is also present. The substrate and product of each of these enzymes is outlined in Table 19.9. These enzymes are all high molecular weight glycoproteins which are synthesized in the endoplasmic reticulum, processed in the Golgi and inserted into the plasma membrane. The sucrase and isomaltase activities originate from a large molecule which is synthesized in continuity

Table 19.9   Carbohydrate digestion by the brush border

Enzyme	Substrate	Product
Lactase	Lactose	Glucose Galactose
Sucrase	Sucrose	Glucose Fructose
Maltase	Maltose	Glucose
Isomaltase	Isomaltose Limit dextrins	Glucose Glucose
Glucoamylase	Maltose Glucose oligomers	Glucose Glucose

and subsequently split, after insertion in the brush border, into two separate functional units. Damage to the villi results in loss of disaccharidase activity with lactase being the most susceptible enzyme.

Undigested carbohydrate is fermented by colonic bacteria and salvaged as short chain fatty acids. If however the carbohydrate load is large, the osmotic pull will draw fluid into the lumen, causing diarrhea.

Digestion of proteins

Ingested proteins are all very large molecules which must be broken down to their constituent amino acids or di- and tripeptides before absorption can occur. The process of protein digestion involves the initial extraction of protein from food due to mastication and the mechanical activity of the stomach and denaturation of the protein, which is promoted by the low pH of the stomach. The subsequent hydrolysis of the denatured protein is brought about by four major groups of enzymes: the pepsins secreted by the chief cells of the gastric glands and trypsins, elastase and chymotrypsins, which are all secreted by the acinar cells of the pancreas. All four enzymes are secreted as proenzymes with hydrogen ions promoting the activation of pepsin and the enzyme enterokinase and trypsin activating the other three. The presence of enterokinase, which is found on the brush border membrane of the proximal small intestine, is vital for the activation of these pancreatic proteinases. Luminal digestion is completed by the action of amino- and carboxypeptidases which cleave the terminal amino acids of the peptides. This results in a mixture of small peptides and free amino acids being presented to the brush border membrane. The larger peptides are further hydrolyzed by brush border-bound peptidases leaving free amino acids, dipeptides and tripeptides for absorption.

Digestion of lipids

Dietary lipids are mainly in the form of triglycerides but phospholipids and cholesterol esters are also present in smaller amounts. Lipid digestion occurs mainly in the small intestine under the influence of bile salts, which form an emulsion of the ingested fat and of pancreatic lipase, which hydrolyzes the ester links at the 1 and 3 position of the triacylglycerol to yield monoacylglycerol and free fatty acid.

The presence of an adequate concentration of bile salts in the lumen of the small intestine (> 2 mmol/L) is of vital importance, as a failure to form a fat emulsion with small micelles (approximately 1 μm in diameter) severely reduces the surface area of contact between the lipase and the fat with resulting maldigestion. Inadequate bile salt concentrations can occur where there is an obstruction to biliary flow, deconjugation by luminal bacteria or where the total bile salt pool is depleted by bile salt malabsorption due to ileal resection.

Pancreatic lipase is quantitatively the most important enzyme in the digestion of triacylglycerols but lingual and gastric lipase are also present. Gastric lipase may be important in the hydrolysis of lipids with short and medium chain fatty acids, and in the preterm and newborn infant; where pancreatic exocrine function is very poorly developed it is likely that lingual and gastric lipase are the major enzymes of lipid digestion, helped in breast-fed babies by breast milk lipase. Ingested phospholipids

are hydrolyzed by pancreatic phospholipase and cholesterol esters are hydrolyzed by pancreatic cholesterol esterases.

The resulting monoacylglycerols, free fatty acids and cholesterol are absorbed by the epithelial cells of the small intestine. The fat-soluble vitamins A, D, E and K are absorbed from micelles and where the production of micelles is compromised by low bile salt concentrations, fat-soluble vitamin malabsorption is likely to occur. Following the digestion and absorption of the lipid from the micelles the bile salts are reabsorbed by the terminal ileum and recycled through an enterohepatic circulation.

INTESTINAL ABSORPTION

The absorptive surface area of the small intestinal mucosa is greatly enhanced by the mucosal folds and by the presence of villi. The differentiated villous cells are responsible for the absorption of electrolytes and the products of the luminal and brush border digestion of food. Water is transported passively and moves down its osmotic gradient through a paracellular path. The epithelial cells are polarized with a brush border membrane facing the lumen of the intestine, a tight junction joining the lateral border of adjacent enterocytes and a basolateral membrane which is in close contact with the vasculature of the villi (Fig. 19.5).

The membranes of cells are very rich in lipid and thus while free fatty acids and monoacylglycerols can readily pass into epithelial cells, water-soluble compounds such as monosaccharides, amino acids, dipeptides and electrolytes all require specific transport processes to facilitate absorption.

Electrolyte absorption

The direction of movement of an electrolyte across a cell membrane is determined by the electrical and chemical gradient which exists across that membrane. In the villous cells of the small intestine there is a strong electrochemical gradient for Na^+ across the brush border membrane with the inside of the cell -40 mV relative to the luminal surface and the intracellular Na^+ concentration being much lower than that found externally (Fig. 19.5). This gradient is maintained by the activity of the basolateral membrane Na^+/K^+ ATPase which pumps Na^+ out of the cell at the expense of the hydrolysis of ATP.

Sodium absorption may be either electroneutral when the absorption of Na^+ and Cl^- is coupled, or electrogenic when it is linked to the absorption of a solute such as glucose or an amino acid. Once absorbed the Na^+ is actively pumped out of the cell by Na^+/K^+ ATPase and the Cl^- is able to leave down its electrochemical gradient. K^+ is transported across the small intestine by a passive process while HCO_3^- is absorbed across the jejunum by a Na^+-dependent process.

Solute absorption

The absorption of glucose and galactose across the brush border membrane occurs by a carrier-mediated process which is driven by the Na^+ gradient across the cell, while fructose is absorbed by a Na^+-independent

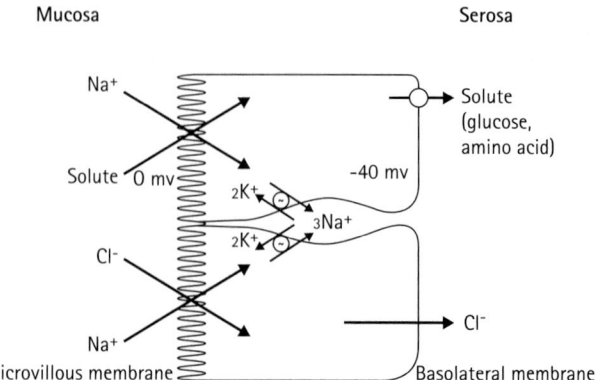

Fig. 19.5   A diagrammatic view of the Na^+, Cl^- and solute absorption across the enterocyte of the small intestinal villi. Water moves passively between the cells down an osmotic gradient.

mechanism. Similarly group-specific active Na$^+$-coupled cotransport is responsible for the absorption of free amino acids and unhydrolyzed short peptides.

The presence of a luminal solute enhances the absorption of Na$^+$ and water by the small intestine. This explains the success of glucose electrolyte solution in the oral rehydration of children with diarrheal disease.

SMALL INTESTINAL MOTILITY

In the fasting state small intestinal motor activity is characterized by a highly organized band of propagative activity which moves down the intestine from the stomach to the ileum, called the migrating motor complex.[31] This activity develops between 2 and 4 h after a meal and recurs, every 25 min in the term infant and every 90 min in the older child, until disrupted by the next meal. The exact role of the migrating motor complex is uncertain but it has been postulated that it helps clear the small intestine of undigested food debris between meals and this may in part explain the very high incidence of bacterial overgrowth in patients where this activity is absent.

Following the ingestion of food the rate of transit through the small intestine is slowed to allow the complete digestion and absorption of the luminal contents. The rate of slowing is dependent on the energy density of the meal with lipids exerting a greater inhibitory effect than carbohydrates or protein. If undigested lipid reaches the ileum a powerful entero-entero reflex called the 'ileal brake' reflexly decreases the rate of gastric emptying and the degree of propagated intestinal motor activity, a situation which might pertain in patients with cystic fibrosis. Mouth to cecal transit time as measured by the breath hydrogen method is increased from 60 to 90 min in the fasting state to 3–4 h postprandially.

IMMUNE DEFENCES

The gastrointestinal tract, as with other mucosal surfaces, acts as an important interface between the external environment and the internal milieu of the individual. On the one hand it has to allow the uninterrupted passage of nutrients while on the other it acts as a major barrier to the entry of toxic macromolecules derived from the microbiological flora of the gut or from ingested food (Table 19.10).

Non-immunological mechanisms

Gastric acid has an important role in initiating the digestion of ingested protein and in activating the intraluminal proteases. The colonization of the small intestine by bacteria may be enhanced by reduced gastric acidity and the failure to fully digest large macromolecules may facilitate the absorption of large unaltered proteins. Normal peristaltic small intestinal motor activity is required to clear the small intestine of food debris between meals and to prevent colonization by bacteria. The mucosal

surface, which comprises the microvillous membrane and overlying mucus, acts as a physical barrier to the attachment and uptake of luminal antigen and bacteria.

Immunological mechanisms

The specific immunological response to absorbed antigen is expressed by the production of secretory antibodies, systemic antibodies and by activation of the cellular immune system.

The secretory response is initiated by the absorption of antigen across specialized epithelial cells (M cells) which over lie lymphoid aggregates in the small intestine. This antigen is then passed to the underlying lymphoid tissue where, with the help of T lymphocytes, B lymphocytes are activated to become IgA-producing cells. These cells initially proliferate and then migrate through the thoracic duct into the systemic circulation. The plasma cells then move back into the lamina propria where dimeric IgA, and to a lesser extent IgG, is produced prior to processing by the epithelial cells and secretion into the lumen in their secretory form. Secretory IgA is also produced by the salivary and mammary glands. A systemic immune response will occur in response to some antigens with the production of IgG, IgE and IgD.

T cells are also activated by the absorption of foreign antigen and these follow a path similar to that described earlier, back into the lamina propria. Along with these activated lymphocytes, mast cells and macrophages are also available to initiate a cell-mediated response within the intestinal mucosa.

A failure of activation or conversely an overactivation of these immune defences will result in the development of gastrointestinal disease.

MALABSORPTION

Malabsorption may result either from a failure of the intraluminal digestion of food or from a defect of mucosal function which prevents the absorption of nutrients. The range of conditions which can cause malabsorption is extensive and is listed in Table 19.11. The presenting signs and symptoms are also very variable and may include diarrhea, vomiting, abdominal distension and weight loss. Some children, however, do not have symptoms directly referable to the gastrointestinal tract and may present with evidence of nutritional or other deficiency states.

A good history, with particular reference to the dietary and family history, is vital in assessing any child with suspected malabsorption. The age of the child is also important as food allergy is most likely to present in the first 6 months of life while celiac disease can only develop after gluten products have been introduced into the diet. One might expect diarrhea to be a universal feature in a child with malabsorption but such is the reserve capacity of the small intestine and the ability of the colon to absorb fluids and electrolytes, that this is not always the case. Failure to thrive, anemia and nongastrointestinal symptoms such as chest problems in cystic fibrosis should be sought. The sections below outline the major causes of malabsorption along with a guide to diagnosis and treatment.

CELIAC DISEASE

Although first described in children over 100 years ago it was only in 1950 that Dicke noticed the association between celiac disease and the dietary protein gluten, and it was still later in 1957 that the enteropathy associated with this condition was first described following peroral jejunal biopsy. The enteropathy associated with celiac disease involves predominantly the proximal small intestine and following the removal of gluten from the diet it resolves completely.

In the last decade there has been a dramatic change in our understanding of celiac disease brought about largely by the introduction of screening tests which have unmasked a large population with lesser symptoms or sometimes none at all.[32]

Table 19.10 Gastrointestinal defense mechanisms

1. Nonimmunological mechanisms
   a. Intraluminal
      (i) Gastric acid
      (ii) Pancreatic proteases
      (iii) Intestinal motility
   b. Mucosal
      (i) Mucin
      (ii) Microvillous membrane
      (iii) Lysozyme
2. Immunological mechanisms
   a. Mucosal immune system
      (i) Secretory antibody production
      (ii) Cellular immunity
   b. Systemic antibody production

Table 19.11   Causes of malabsorption

Disorders of intraluminal digestion
1. Congenital
   a. Pancreatic
      (i)   Cystic fibrosis
      (ii) Shwachman disease
   b. Hepatic
      (i)   Neonatal hepatitis
      (ii) Hepatocellular failure
      (iii) Cholestasis
   c. Intestinal
      (i)   Enterokinase deficiency
2. Acquired
   a. Pancreatic
      (i)   Chronic pancreatitis
   b. Hepatic
      (i)   Neonatal hepatitis
      (ii) Hepatocellular failure
      (iii) Cholestasis
   c. Intestinal
      (i)   Bacterial overgrowth

Disorders of intestinal mucosal function
1. Congenital
   a. Carbohydrate absorption
      (i)   Glucose/galactose malabsorption
      (ii) Sucrose isomaltase deficiency
      (iii) Alactasia
   b. Amino acid absorption
      (i)   Cystinuria
      (ii) Hartnup disease
   c. Fat absorption
      (i)   Abetalipoproteinemia
      (ii) Lymphangiectasia
   d. Electrolyte absorption
      (i)   Chloride-losing diarrhea
      (ii) Primary hypomagnesemia
      (iii) Acrodermatitis enteropathica
   e. Enteropathies
      (i)   Microvillous atrophy
      (ii) Idiopathic
2. Acquired
   a. Enteropathies
      (i)   Celiac disease
      (ii) Food allergic
      (iii) Autoimmune
      (iv) Postgastroenteritis
   b. Infections
      (i)   Tuberculosis
      (ii) Giardiases
      (iii) Hookworm
   c. Infiltrations
      (i)   Crohn's disease
      (ii) Reticuloses
   d. Anatomical
      (i)   Intestinal fistulae
      (ii) Short gut syndrome
   e. Drugs
      (i)   Chemotherapeutic agents

Pathophysiology

Celiac disease is a multifactorial condition where environmental, genetic and immunological factors interact to produce damage to the mucosa of the proximal small intestine.

Genetic

The human leukocyte antigen (HLA) DQ2 is found in 80% of patients with type I diabetes who develop celiac disease and in almost 100% of Down syndrome children who have celiac disease. HLA DQ8 is found in almost all the remaining patients. HLAs DQ2 or DQ8 occur in about 30% of the general population. The prevalence of celiac disease is approximately 10% in first-degree family members with 40% concordance in HLA matched siblings and 70% in monozygotic twins.

Environmental

The exposure of the small intestine to gluten from wheat, barley or rye is a prerequisite for the development of celiac disease. The small amount of gluten found in oats may also cause problems for some patients. The amount of gluten in the diet is also a factor in the time of presentation and the type of symptoms the patient may experience. In Sweden where the weaning diet contains large amounts of gluten, children with celiac disease present most commonly with classical symptoms of diarrhea and failure to thrive between the age of 1 and 2 years. In contrast in Denmark, where the weaning diet has much less gluten, children present between 7 and 9 years with milder symptoms such as anemia or abdominal pain.

Immunological

The contact of gluten with the small intestinal mucosa activates a cellular immune response in which T cells are activated and cytokines are released. The net result of this is that the mucosa is damaged and heavily infiltrated with inflammatory cells. The villus structure is completely lost and the crypts hypertrophy in an attempt to repair the damage. This transformation is outlined in Figure 19.6. There is also a humoral immune response which leads to the production of antibodies against

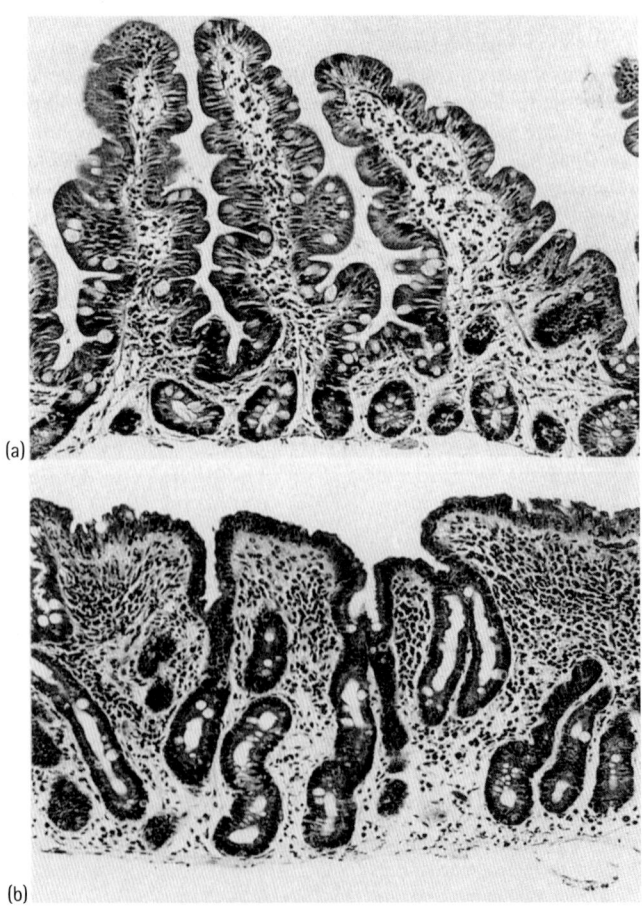

(a)

(b)

Fig. 19.6   A light micrograph (magnified × 240, stain hematoxylin and eosin) of a jejunal biopsy in (a) a normal child and (b) a child with untreated celiac disease. (Reproduced by kind permission of G. Anderson)

grain peptides (antigliadin) and connective tissue autoantigens (antiendomysial, antireticulin). It is unlikely that these play a part in the tissue damage.

Presenting symptoms

The classical form of celiac disease presents with severe diarrhea, abdominal distension, weight loss, anemia and a general debilitation. This is most commonly found in younger patients while in older children there is a tendency for symptoms to be milder. Such symptoms might include abdominal pain, mild anemia, linear growth failure, delayed menarche or pubertal delay. The older child is often free of diarrhea.

Celiac disease can be present in association with enamel defects of the teeth or with dermatitis herpetiformis, an itchy vesicular rash of the skin. There is now an irrefutable association between celiac disease and other autoimmune conditions such as type 1 diabetes mellitus[33,34] and hyperthyroidism and with genetic abnormalities such as Down syndrome and Turner syndrome. Frequently it is the associated condition that is diagnosed first and it has been suggested that patients with the above conditions should all be screened for celiac disease at diagnosis. Before screening these at-risk groups, it is important to fully counsel the children/families as to the relative risk of untreated celiac disease and the need for a confirmatory biopsy and gluten-free diet if testing is positive.

Epidemiology

Generally celiac disease is uncommon in black African, Japanese and Chinese populations. Previously it was thought that the prevalence of celiac disease in Europe was about 1 in 2000. With the possibility of screening populations for celiac antibodies it is now being realized that the true prevalence is probably 10–20 times higher at approximately 1 in 100–200. This situation has been described as the 'celiac iceberg' in which only a small percentage of patients are diagnosed and 'visible above the waterline' while the majority are undiagnosed and 'hidden' from view. This is illustrated schematically in Figure 19.7. Silent celiac patients will have positive celiac antibodies and histological evidence of celiac disease but will not have overt symptoms. These children are often labeled asymptomatic but when diagnosed and started on treatment, many feel better and only report symptoms in retrospect. Other children, so-called latent celiacs, have positive celiac antibodies but have a normal or near-normal duodenal mucosa. If followed, many of these children go on to develop classical histological changes in their small intestine in subsequent years.

Screening tests

The starting point is either with a patient in whom there is a clinical suspicion of celiac disease or a patient diagnosed as having a condition which is associated with a greatly increased risk of developing celiac

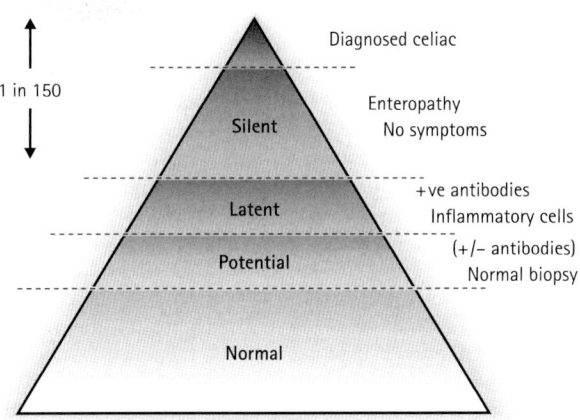

Fig. 19.7 The 'celiac iceberg'. Approximately 90% of people with celiac disease are presently undiagnosed.

Table 19.12 Conditions associated with an increased prevalence of celiac disease

Condition	Percentage
Type 1 diabetes	1–10%
Autoimmune thyroid disease	
Children	8%
Adults	3%
Turner syndrome	8%
Down syndrome	4–12%
First-degree relative of known celiac	6%
General population	0.2–1%

disease (see Table 19.12). The former group all need further investigation while screening of the latter at-risk groups requires full counseling of the child and families as to the relative risk of untreated celiac disease (see page 618) and the need for a confirmatory biopsy and gluten-free diet if testing is positive. Up to 50% of so-called 'asymptomatic' patients, identified from screening programs as having celiac disease, receive benefit in terms of improved symptoms and quality of life from treatment of their celiac disease.

The preferred screening test for celiac disease is the measurement of the IgA anti tissue transglutaminase (anti-tTG) combined with total IgA estimation. If the anti-tTG assay is not available the measurement of the IgA antiendomysial antibody (AEA) can be substituted. 0.3% of the general population is IgA deficient although this rises 10-fold in patients with celiac disease to 3%. This association between celiac disease and IgA deficiency means that screening with a single IgA antibody will lead to false-negative results in deficient patients. In IgA-deficient patients there is the option of testing for IgG anti t-TH or IgG AEA but these tests are less readily available and less sensitive and specific than the IgA antibodies. Where a strong clinical suspicion exists the practitioner should proceed to biopsy even in the presence of negative antibodies. The sensitivity and specificity results with these tests are over 90% but this will vary depending on the reagent kits used and on the laboratory. At present none of the screening regimens have 100% sensitivity and specificity and as such **all positive results require confirmation with a small bowel biopsy**.

In type I diabetes screening is generally recommended, with full consent, at the time of diagnosis and at 2-yearly intervals thereafter. It is known that celiac disease may still develop may years after the initial presentation. In the asymptomatic, antibody-negative child HLA typing may help to clarify which patients may subsequently develop celiac disease. Patients who are HLA DQ2/DQ8 positive should continue to undergo surveillance or if symptomatic undergo biopsy. Alternatively those who are negative are most unlikely to develop celiac disease and do not require further screening. This also applies to all at-risk groups.

Diagnosis

The only diagnostic test for celiac disease is small intestinal biopsy. From the time of their introduction in the 1950s biopsies of the jejunum were carried out using Crosby or Watson capsules. This technique, which required the capsules to be swallowed and the child sedated, was very unpleasant for the child and due to problems with the capsule firing, was not always successful. Now all pediatric centers have adopted upper intestinal endoscopy as the primary method for intestinal biopsy. This is a relatively rapid and reliable method of collecting mucosal samples from the distal duodenum and if four or more biopsies are taken from the second part of the duodenum or beyond, the diagnostic yield is comparable to the traditional capsule biopsy.

Because of our changing understanding of celiac disease guidelines for diagnosis and management are constantly evolving. The North American Society of Pediatric Gastroenterology Hepatology and Nutrition (NASPGHAN) published updated guidelines in 2005 which represents the first major guideline revision since the widespread use of antibody screening.[35]

The primary criterion for making a diagnosis of celiac disease is the presence of the characteristic crypt hyperplastic subtotal villus atrophy on small intestinal mucosal biopsy (see Fig. 19.6b). It is vitally important that the child has an adequate amount of gluten in the diet and under no circumstances should a gluten-free diet be started prior to biopsy. In symptomatic patients a clear-cut clinical remission on starting a gluten-free diet should be seen. In all patients the anti-tTG or AEA should become negative 6–12 months after starting treatment and if this is not the case it implies that dietary exclusion of gluten has been incomplete.

In patients where there is diagnostic doubt or no initial biopsy has been taken, a gluten challenge is required. This is often the case in children under 2 years of age where other causes of enteropathy such as food allergy can confuse the diagnostic picture. After 3 months on gluten the antibodies should be rechecked. If positive or if symptomatic earlier, the biopsy should be done. If negative the challenge should be continued. The gluten challenge should be carried out between the ages of 6–10 years or after the pubertal growth spurt.

Treatment

The treatment of celiac disease is with life-long exclusion of gluten from the diet. This essentially means avoiding all wheat, barley and rye products. Tolerance of oats is generally good if products free from contamination with other cereals can be provided. The education of the child and their parents in this diet needs the expert help of a pediatric dietitian. Many gluten-free products are commercially available and this goes some way to making what is essentially a very restrictive diet, a little easier to tolerate.

Some newly diagnosed children, particularly those with a classical presentation, may be severely malnourished at the time of diagnosis. Addition nutritional supplementation will be required and in the very lethargic child, short-term nasogastric feeding may be required until the child is able to feed. Because of the risk of osteoporosis, all patients with celiac disease require a good calcium intake and often require calcium supplements.

Consequences of untreated celiac disease

Because most patients with celiac disease are presently undiagnosed (nine out of 10) and many may have little in the way of symptoms, it has been argued by some that there is little point in screening at-risk groups. Untreated celiac disease however can lead to anemia, osteoporosis, reproductive problems and worryingly an increased risk of intestinal malignancy. In children who do not comply with their gluten-free diet school performance is poorer.

Untreated celiac disease does appear to be linked to an increased incidence of gastrointestinal neoplasm (1.8-fold risk) although the rate from recent studies is not as high as previously reported.[36,37] Most of this risk appears to be in the first year after diagnosis of celiac disease with lymphoproliferative (4.8-fold risk) disorders being the most common. Interestingly the risk of breast cancer (0.35-fold risk) is reduced in patients with celiac disease.

FOOD ALLERGY

Food allergy most commonly develops in the first few months of life with the most common allergens being cows' milk protein, although soya protein and a wide range of other dietary proteins may also be responsible. This sensitization develops most commonly in atopic individuals with a family history of food allergy or clear evidence of another atopic symptom such as eczema, asthma and urticaria. In many of these children, although their intolerance generally resolves between the age of 18 months and 5 years, symptoms of asthma and hay fever frequently follow. In older patients sensitization may follow an enteric infection leading to persistent intestinal symptoms long after the pathogen has been cleared.

In healthy individuals oral tolerance to dietary protein develops through the suppression of lymphocytes within the intestinal mucosa.[38]

This occurs when a large antigen load is presented to the immune system by the epithelium without co-stimulation and in the case of low-dose antigen, processing by the M cell from the Peyer's patches leads to the production of suppressor lymphocytes which home in on the lamina propria. Where mucosal integrity is compromised these mechanisms break down and sensitization to food allergens may develop. Mucosal integrity will be disrupted by enteric infection but it is clear that a close interaction between the epithelial cell and the gut flora is also important in maintaining integrity. It has recently been shown that the administration of the probiotic *Lactobacillus* GG, which promotes the colonization of the gut by 'healthy bacteria', to the mother before and the infant after birth, reduced the subsequent development of atopic disease.[39,40]

Cows' milk protein intolerance

This condition develops most commonly within the first 6 months of life and occurs predominantly in formula-fed babies or babies receiving cows' milk in weaning foods. Breast-fed babies are also at risk as cows' milk protein is secreted at lactation if the mother's diet contains cows' milk. The most common symptoms at presentation are of vomiting, diarrhea and poor weight gain with eczema frequently present in babies and asthma or hay fever in older children.[41] Rectal bleeding due to an allergic colitis may be a presenting symptom in some infants.

Diagnosis

The diagnosis is made from the history and from the characteristic improvement in symptoms with exclusion of cows' milk protein from the diet. Jejunal biopsy is likely to reveal a patchy partial villous atrophy with eosinophilic infiltrate, although in some patients the enteropathy may be more severe and be difficult to distinguish histologically from celiac disease. Jejunal biopsy however is not required in most patients as the condition usually responds well to an exclusion diet and is self-limiting, but if there is severe failure to thrive or a failure to respond to a cows' milk-free diet a jejunal biopsy is essential to exclude any other more serious pathology. A full blood count may reveal evidence of a peripheral eosinophilia, serum immunoglobulins may show a raised IgE and a low IgA and skin test or RAST may reveal positive reactions to food and environmental allergens. RAST has a poor sensitivity in childhood food allergy as up to 50% of allergic reactions are non-IgE mediated. There is also a high false-negative rate and in many patients who are quite clearly food allergic they may still be negative. This can be improved significantly by skin patch testing, which will detect non-IgE-mediated allergy. The clinical response to challenge and withdrawal remains the gold standard for diagnosing allergic disease in children.

Management

It is usual to exclude cows' milk protein from the diet and as many atopic children also react to egg protein a combined milk and egg exclusion is frequently required. In breast-fed babies the mother should be put on a milk-free diet and started on a calcium supplement. It is essential that the diet is supervised by a dietitian to ensure that adequate calories and calcium remain in the diet. A complete milk substitute based on a whey or casein hydrolysate should be prescribed, and where the infant has been weaned the mother should be instructed on a diet containing milk- and egg-free solids. The use of soya formula can lead to sensitization as 30% of children allergic to cows' milk protein also react to soya and such formulae are generally not recommended in young children under 6 months of age, because of their phytosterols content. A small number of patients will even fail to tolerate a hydrolyzed formula and an elemental feed may be substituted. Some older children refuse to take these milk substitutes because of the taste and under such circumstances, if the diet is otherwise adequate, an oral calcium substitute should be prescribed. Alternatively if the intake is poor, the feed can be given by nasogastric tube.

Most children will improve quickly after starting their diet but it may take many months for full catch-up growth to occur in children who have been failing to thrive. The natural history of this condition is one of spontaneous remission but in some children further intolerances may develop.

Multiple food intolerances

Although cows' milk protein, soya and egg are most commonly responsible for food intolerances in children, wheat, colorings, preservatives and sugar have all been implicated. In the very atopic child almost any dietary intolerance is possible. In addition to the gastrointestinal and atopic symptoms described earlier for cows' milk protein intolerance, behavior disturbance and hyperactivity may occur in some children.

It should be possible to discover which foods are responsible for the symptoms by taking a good dietary history, and an appropriate exclusion diet should be devised. In some children, however, it is difficult to isolate which foods are causing the problem and under these circumstances two further dietary options are available. The diet can be restricted to five or six foods which are felt least likely to cause allergic reactions. If symptoms resolve, new foods can then be introduced one at a time at weekly intervals. Alternatively the patient can proceed straight to an elemental, amino acid based feed which in older children will almost certainly have to be administered by nasogastric tube. Both of these diets are a very major undertaking for the family and where symptoms are less severe the use of oral sodium chromoglycate may be helpful in suppressing allergic symptoms.

Eosinophilic gastroenteritis

It is likely that a fair degree of overlap exists between the allergic conditions described earlier and eosinophilic gastroenteritis. The condition is characterized by an eosinophilic infiltrate which can involve the stomach and/or small intestine and which appears to be triggered by the presence of dietary antigens. Three forms of the condition, each involving a different layer of the intestine, have been described.

The mucosal form is characterized by protein loss with hypoalbuminemia and edema. Damage to the antral and duodenal mucosa will result in blood loss and anemia while jejunal damage leads to an enteropathy with malabsorption. Where the muscle layer is involved symptoms of intestinal obstruction occur and in the serosal form of the condition an eosinophilic ascites may develop. Most patients are likely to have the markers of atopy, which are outlined earlier.

Diagnosis will be suggested by the history of atopy with abdominal pain, diarrhea, vomiting, weight loss and edema. Some patients, however, may have no abdominal symptoms. Upper gastrointestinal endoscopy is invaluable for detecting antral and duodenal lesions and for confirming the diagnosis by mucosal biopsy. Barium contrast studies may show evidence of inflammation in the mucosal form or luminal obstruction in cases involving the enteric smooth muscle. Protein loss from the intestine may be detected by measuring the level of alpha-1 antitrypsin in the stool.

Treatment with dietary exclusion is frequently all that is required in the mucosal form but where there is transmural or serosal inflammation, oral corticosteroids may also be required. The level of therapy required will vary from patient to patient but those with mucosal disease are likely to be the most responsive to therapy. Where intestinal obstruction occurs, surgery with local resection is likely to be required.

POSTENTERITIS ENTEROPATHY

While most enteric infections are self-limiting and are free of long-term sequelae, some organisms damage the mucosal surface of the gut, resulting in a persistence of symptoms long after the original infective organism has been cleared. This postenteritis syndrome can be caused by viruses such as adenovirus or by bacterial pathogens such as the enteropathogenic *Escherichia coli* which totally denude the mucosa of villi. The consequences of acute enteric infections and their management are discussed more fully later in this chapter (see p. 627).

CONGENITAL ENTEROPATHIES

Intractable diarrhea presenting from the time of birth may be caused by inborn errors which result either in a disruption of enterocyte absorptive or secretory function, or where structural genes are damaged, leading to an enteropathy of the small intestinal mucosa. Microvillus inclusion disease (microvillus atrophy) is the best characterized of these congenital enteropathies but other forms include intestinal epithelial dysplasia (tufting enteropathy) and syndromic forms which are associated with dysmorphic features.[42]

Microvillus atrophy is characterized by a hypoplastic villous atrophy associated with depletion and shortening of the microvilli over the villous epithelium. This condition can be differentiated from other congenital enteropathies by the presence of smudging of stains which outline the microvillous membrane and by electron micrographs which show the presence of characteristic microvillous inclusions in the villous enterocytes. Patients who survive with this condition are likely to remain dependent on PN for a prolonged period as no specific treatment other than intestinal transplantation is available.

For children with the other forms of congenital enteropathy the lack of understanding of the underlying cause makes treatment and prognostication difficult. Nutritional support with predigested hypoallergenic feeds and i.v. alimentation can greatly prolong life but will frequently not alter the underlying disorder.

AUTOIMMUNE ENTEROPATHY

In a small number of patients with intractable diarrhea and an enteropathy the presence of enterocyte autoantibodies has been described. Autoimmune enteropathy presents with intractable watery and sometimes bloody diarrhea between 3 months and 2 years of age.[43] In some of these patients other organ-specific autoantibodies or autoimmune diseases have also been found, making it likely that the intestinal disease is caused by an autoimmune process. Treatment of these children with hypoallergenic diets, steroids and immunosuppressive drugs, such as azathioprine, cyclosporin or tacrolimus, is successful in some cases.

PROTEIN-LOSING ENTEROPATHY

Small amounts of albumin pass into the gut each day and under the influence of pancreatic enzymes are digested and reabsorbed. In response to an increased loss into the gut the liver is able to compensate by increasing the rate of albumin synthesis by up to a factor of two. Above this level, however, the patient becomes increasingly hypoproteinemic. Albumin and IgG are the first to fall and in severe protein-losing enteropathies between 10% and 50% of the plasma albumin pool may be lost into the gut each day.

Etiology

Protein-losing enteropathy may arise either as a consequence of the increased permeability of the intestine to plasma proteins or as a result of disordered intestinal or mesenteric lymph flow which leads to the loss of lymphocytes and fat, in addition to protein, into the intestine. Protein loss due to increased permeability is most marked in hypertrophic gastritis, eosinophilic gastroenteritis and in some forms of intestinal polyposis but any condition which results in severe damage or inflammation to the lining of the gut is likely to result in increased luminal protein loss. Lymphangiectasia is the most common cause of disordered lymph flow. The conditions associated with protein-losing enteropathy are listed in Table 19.13.

Clinical features and diagnosis

The clinical features are of peripheral edema and ascites, when the serum albumin falls below 20 g/L, in addition to those of the underlying condition. The diagnosis of a protein-losing enteropathy is confirmed by the detection of increased amounts of protein in the stool in the face of a low serum albumin. The increased losses can be shown by increased levels of fecal alpha-1 antitrypsin. The cause of the protein loss, which may be from the stomach, small intestine or large intestine, can best be defined by endoscopy and biopsy.

Table 19.13   Causes of protein-losing enteropathy

1. Increased mucosal permeability to protein
   a. Hypertrophic gastritis
   b. Eosinophilic gastroenteritis
   c. Polyposis
   d. Inflammatory disease
      (i) Crohn's disease
      (ii) Ulcerative colitis
      (iii) Enterocolitis
      (iv) Pseudomembranous colitis
      (v) Radiation enteritis
      (vi) Graft-versus-host disease
      (vii) Autoimmune enteropathy
   e. Celiac disease
   f. Nephrotic syndrome
   g. Esophagitis

2. Altered lymph flow
   a. Primary intestinal lymphangiectasia
   b. Secondary intestinal lymphangiectasia
      (i) Congestive cardiac failure
      (ii) Constrictive pericarditis
      (iii) Lymphoma
      (iv) Tuberculous adenitis
      (v) Volvulus

The treatment is that of the underlying condition but 20% albumin infusion may be required in the short term to correct the hypoalbuminemia and edema.

INTESTINAL LYMPHANGIECTASIA

The lymphatics of the small intestine play a vital role in the absorption of fat, being responsible for the transport of chylomicrons from the mucosal cells, via the thoracic duct to the venous system. This lymphatic fluid is also rich in protein and in lymphocytes. In intestinal lymphangiectasia these lymphatic channels become blocked, and as a consequence protein and lymphocytes are lost into the gut while fat and fat-soluble vitamins are malabsorbed.

The condition may be either congenital when it is frequently associated with other abnormalities of lymphatic development, such as peripheral lymphedema, or it may arise secondary to acquired lymphatic obstruction from congestive cardiac failure, constrictive pericarditis, malrotation or infiltration of the lymphatics by neoplastic processes. Examination of the jejunal mucosa under a dissecting microscope reveals pale villi of normal length. On higher magnification the lymphatics of the lamina propria and submucosa are distended and filled with lipid staining material.

Patients are likely to present with diarrhea, abdominal distension with hypoproteinemia leading to edema and ascites. The loss of lymphatic cells will result in lymphopenia and an increased susceptibility to infections. Fat-soluble vitamin deficiencies are likely to lead to rickets and clotting abnormalities. The diagnosis is confirmed by the characteristic jejunal biopsy findings in a patient with lymphopenia and a protein-losing enteropathy.

If the primary cause of the lymphangiectasia cannot be remedied treatment involves the use of a high-protein diet to compensate for the large stool losses. The substitution in the diet of long-chain by medium-chain fats which are absorbed directly into the portal venous circulation reduces the protein loss. In some patients regular albumin infusions may be required to control hypoproteinemia.

IMMUNE DEFICIENCY AND GUT DISEASE

The normal immune function of the small intestine plays a major part in preventing both the absorption of foreign proteins and the penetration of enteric pathogens across the lining of the gut. While the immunodeficiencies

Table 19.14   Immune deficiency leading to gastrointestinal disease

1. Antibody defect
   a. X-linked agammaglobulinemia
   b. IgA deficiency
2. Combined immunodeficiency
   a. Common variable immunodeficiency
   b. Severe combined immunodeficiency
3. Defect of phagocytosis
   a. X-linked chronic granulomatous disease
4. Immunodeficiency as part of a syndrome
   a. Wiskott–Aldrich syndrome
   b. DiGeorge syndrome
   c. IPEX syndrome
5. Acquired immune deficiency syndrome

themselves very rarely cause any primary damage to the gut, the consequences of the sensitization of the gut to foreign proteins or of recurrent enteric infections can lead to structural damage to the small intestinal mucosa with the development of malabsorption and diarrhea and as a consequence, failure to thrive. The immunodeficiencies which can lead to compromised intestinal function are listed in Table 19.14.

While the majority of children with IgA deficiency may have no symptoms, the incidence of food allergy and of celiac disease is increased as is infection with *Giardia lamblia*. In agammaglobulinemia and common variable immundeficiency (CVI), as well as giardiasis, bacterial overgrowth and nonspecific colitis can occur. Where T cell function is compromised in CVI, chronic fungal infection and a nonspecific enterocolitis may develop. Chronic granulomatous disease can cause liver and perianal abscesses, and an enterocolitis which can mimic Crohn's disease; a granulomatous narrowing of the gastric antrum has also been reported.

In both Wiskott–Aldrich and DiGeorge syndrome there is T cell dysfunction, the former associated with severe eczema and thrombocytopenia and the latter associated with esophageal, parathyroid and cardiac defects. A less common immunodeficiency associated with gastrointestinal disease is the IPEX syndrome, an X-linked condition with severe autoimmune enteropathy, autoimmune polyendocrinopathies and hemolytic anemia. Acquired immune deficiency syndrome (AIDS) frequently presents with opportunistic intestinal infection with *Cryptosporidium*, *Candida*, *Salmonella* or cytomegalovirus.

The diagnosis and treatment of these immune deficiencies is more fully described in Chapter 27. When gut disease occurs, therapy should be aimed at the primary disorder, at treating the enteric infection and at supporting nutrition with elemental feeds or even PN.

Immunodeficiencies may themselves occur as a consequence of primary gastrointestinal disease and this in turn can feed back to potentiate the initial disorder. This can occur in any severely malnourished child, in patients where gut protein loss results in hypoproteinemia and hypogammaglobulinemia, and in acrodermatitis enteropathica where zinc deficiency suppresses immune function.

SHORT GUT SYNDROME

Resection of part of the small intestine is not uncommonly required in neonates who develop an acute surgical problem (Table 19.15). Similarly

Table 19.15   Causes of the short bowel syndrome in the neonate

1. Small intestinal malrotation with volvulus
2. Jejunal and ileal atresias
3. Meconium ileus
4. Omphalocele or gastroschisis with volvulus
5. Internal hernias
6. Necrotizing enterocolitis
7. Congenital short small bowel

in the older child intestinal resection may be required following trauma or volvulus formation. The consequences of such a resection depend very much on the length of gut resected, the part of the small intestine resected, whether the ileocecal valve and colon are still present and on the nutritional state of the patient.[44] Loss of more than 30 cm of intestine is likely to have nutritional consequences to the infant. The remaining bowel, however, has great powers of adaptation and it is possible for as little as 20 cm of small intestine with an intact ileocecal valve to adapt adequately over many months or years to support life by enteral nutrition.

Clinical features

As a consequence of the loss of intestinal surface area the child develops diarrhea and the absorption of all nutrients, minerals and vitamins is reduced. This is likely to lead to weight loss and the development of specific nutritional deficiencies.

Loss of the terminal ileum will lead to malabsorption and depletion of the bile salt pool and failed vitamin B_{12} absorption will over a period of years lead to the development of a deficiency state. If duodenal bile salt concentration falls below 2 mmol/L, micelle formation may be inhibited, leading to malabsorption of long chain fats, and the passage of bile salts into the colon will result in intestinal secretion, which will compound the diarrhea. The ileum is also rich in enteroglucagon, a potent trophic factor in intestinal adaptation, and where the ileum has been resected the adaptive response may be further delayed or blunted.

The ileocecal valve has a vital role in preventing the reflux of colonic flora into the small intestine and when the valve is resected bacterial overgrowth of the small intestine is an almost inevitable sequela. This leads to mucosal damage and the deconjugation of bile salts with resulting disruption of lipid solubilization and intestinal secretion. Without an ileocecal valve the length of gut that is needed to support life is probably more than doubled and this is further increased if the colon has also been extensively resected.

The small intestine also has an important role in the metabolism of gastrin and where a large length of jejunum is resected hypergastrinemia with increased gastric secretion can occur. This not only increases the fluid load on the intestine but also lowers the duodenal pH and as a result reduces bile salt solubility and the activity of the digestive enzymes.

Management

During the period of adaptation which follows an intestinal resection the turnover of regenerative cells in the crypts of the small intestine increases and as a consequence the length of villi increases. With time this leads to an increase in the absorptive capacity of the residual small intestine. This process, however, may take many months and the mainstay in management is the promotion of the adaptive response and the nutritional support of these patients during this period.

One of the most potent trophic factors in promoting adaptation is the presence of food within the gastrointestinal tract. Starvation is known to produce a partial villous atrophy which is reversed by re-feeding. In short gut syndrome it is therefore most important that enteral feeding is maintained at a level which is able to stimulate the adaptive response while at the same time not causing torrential diarrhea. Because of the reduced digestive and absorptive capacity of the small intestine it is usual to feed these infants with a predigested feed, synthetic elemental feed or a modular feed to which carbohydrate and fat can be added individually as tolerated.

There is also a need to control the many complications of short gut syndrome in order to further increase the absorptive and digestive capacity of the gut. These treatments are listed in Table 19.16. In some infants where very little small intestine remains, or where the adaptive response has been blunted by loss of the ileum and ileocecal valve, the child may remain dependent on PN and under such circumstances efforts should be made to institute this therapy at home. These most severe patients may also be candidates for intestinal transplantation (see pp. 632–33).

Table 19.16   Complications in short gut syndrome and their treatment

Complications	Treatment
Bacterial overgrowth	Antibiotics Resect stricture or stagnant loop
Gastric hypersecretion	Histamine 2 blockers
Rapid transit	Loperamide
Malabsorption of fats	Medium chain triglycerides in feeds
Bile salt diarrhea	Bile salt chelator: cholestyramine
Poor growth	Increase parenteral/enteral nutrition

INBORN ERRORS OF DIGESTION AND ABSORPTION

Although most causes of gastrointestinal disease are acquired, there are a number of specific inborn errors of intestinal function which interfere with the normal digestion and absorption of nutrients. Although these disorders are generally uncommon it is important to be aware of their existence as failure to recognize their signs and symptoms may have severe consequences for the child. A knowledge of normal intestinal physiology is important if the clinical consequences of these defects are to be understood.

CARBOHYDRATE MALABSORPTION

Carbohydrates will be malabsorbed if there is a failure of luminal or brush border digestion or a defect in the transport proteins which facilitate the absorption of monosaccharides. The most common inborn error involving carbohydrate digestion is cystic fibrosis, in which luminal levels of pancreatic amylase are markedly reduced. Of the disaccharidases outlined in Table 19.9, specific defects of lactase, sucrase–isomaltase and trehalase have all been reported although the latter defect is of no clinical significance.

The presence of increased concentrations of disaccharides in the lumen of the small intestine leads to an osmotic diarrhea that results in abdominal distension with large water and electrolyte losses which can be life threatening in young infants.

Lactase deficiency

Primary lactase deficiency is very uncommon and presents with profuse watery diarrhea soon after the introduction of milk feeds. The diagnosis can be suspected from the clinical history and the response to a lactose-free diet, although it can only be confirmed by the measurement of brush border lactase activity. The condition is thought to be inherited in an autosomal recessive fashion.

In many African and Asian races, adult levels of lactase activity fall far below those found in European races. This has previously been labeled 'late-onset lactase deficiency', but given that most of these individuals do not have any symptoms, it is probably incorrect to say that they are deficient. Transient lactase deficiency commonly occurs as a result of damage to the intestinal mucosa from a primary infective agent.

Sucrase–isomaltase deficiency

The incidence of this deficiency is probably very low although it is said to affect up to 10% of Greenland Eskimos. The condition probably occurs in a number of distinct genetic forms and this may in part explain the variability in its clinical presentation.[45] Symptoms of diarrhea and failure to thrive usually develop following the introduction of sucrose or complex carbohydrate into the diet, but in some children the symptoms may be very mild and the condition goes undiagnosed. As sucrase also contributes to a large part of the brush border maltase activity the use of refined formula feeds which all contain glucose polymer invariably results in an increase in the diarrhea.

In response to an oral sucrose load, exhaled breath hydrogen rises and sucrose can be detected by sugar chromatography of the loose stools. Jejunal biopsy will show normal mucosal morphology but histochemical studies reveal low or absent enzyme activity. Dietary removal of sucrose and complex carbohydrate results in an immediate symptomatic recovery.

Glucose–galactose malabsorption

The condition results from a defect in the transport protein which is responsible for sodium–glucose and sodium–galactose linked co-transport.[46] Diarrhea develops shortly after the first feed and persists until glucose and galactose are removed from the diet. In contrast fructose absorption is normal and sodium–amino acid co-transport is preserved. In some children the degree of glucose intolerance decreases with increasing age. The inheritance is autosomal recessive and is treated with the fructose-containing feed, Galactamin 19.

LIPID MALABSORPTION

Lipid malabsorption with steatorrhea will result from failed luminal solubilization and digestion of triglycerides, as occurs in pancreatic insufficiency, biliary disease and short gut syndrome, and from failure of mucosal fat transport as occurs in abetalipoproteinemia and hypobetalipoproteinemia.

Abetalipoproteinemia

This autosomal recessive condition which was first described in 1950 is characterized by the presence from birth of steatorrhea, acanthocytosis on the peripheral blood film and failure to thrive. If diagnosis is delayed signs of ataxia and retinopathy may develop in the second decade.

Failure to synthesize apoprotein B means that chylomicrons cannot be manufactured and exported into the lymphatics. Lipid electrophoresis reveals absent serum low density lipoprotein (LDL), very low density lipoprotein (VLDL) and chylomicrons and as a consequence serum triglyceride and cholesterol levels are low. Jejunal biopsy reveals fat-laden enterocytes.

There is now strong evidence that the neurological signs result from chronic vitamin E deficiency and if treatment is started promptly with a low-fat diet, large oral supplements of vitamin E (100 mg/kg/24 h) along with supplements of the other fat-soluble vitamins, the development of ataxic symptoms and mental deterioration can be prevented.

PROTEIN MALABSORPTION

The digestion of proteins is dependent on the action of proteases which are secreted by the stomach, pancreas and the intestinal mucosa. Inborn errors of these enzymes are very uncommon although specific deficiencies of trypsinogen and enterokinase have been reported. Both these conditions result in failure to thrive, hypoproteinemia, edema, anemia and neutropenia, and following the introduction of a protein hydrolysate feed with oral pancreatic supplements there is a marked improvement in symptoms.

Defects of brush border amino acid absorption tend to have few clinical consequences as the particular amino acid can still be absorbed as part of a dipeptide. This explains why cystinuria and iminoglycinuria do not result in the development of any nutritional deficiencies and why in Hartnup disease symptoms tend to develop only when the diet is otherwise compromised. Defects of basolateral transport appear, however, to have more severe clinical consequences.

Hartnup disease

A defect in the transport of free neutral amino acids across the brush border of the small intestine and the proximal renal tubules of the kidney leads to a pellagra-like skin rash in areas exposed to sunlight with associated diarrhea and a dementing psychiatric illness. These features are the result of low levels of tryptophan leading to the decreased production of nicotinamide. Treatment with nicotinamide supplementation controls the symptoms of pellagra, which spontaneously become less severe with increasing age.

Lysinuric protein intolerance

In this disorder there is impaired absorption of the dibasic amino acids lysine, ornithine and arginine across the basolateral membrane of intestinal, hepatic and renal tubular cells. The patients present with severe failure to thrive, diarrhea, hepatosplenomegaly and aversion to high protein foods by 1 year of age. Developmental delay and mental retardation occur if there have been prolonged episodes of hyperammonemia. This can occur following a protein load due to the low level of urea cycle intermediates, and as a consequence treatment with oral citrulline can in part prevent this problem arising.

DISORDERS OF ELECTROLYTE AND MINERAL ABSORPTION

Congenital chloride diarrhea

This condition is characterized by severe watery diarrhea with hypochloremia, hypokalemia and metabolic alkalosis.[47] This autosomal recessive condition is characterized by a defect in Cl^-/HCO_3^+ transport in the ileum and colon with the resulting loss of large amounts of Cl^- in the stool. Na^+ is also lost in the stool and as a consequence the patients develop secondary hyperaldosteronism with urinary sparing of Na^+ and loss of K^+. This secretion starts in utero and is associated with maternal polyhydramnios, which frequently results in premature delivery. In the neonatal period the presence of diarrhea may be missed, leading to confusion with Bartter syndrome, in which the Cl^- loss is primarily renal and not intestinal. If the salt losses are not corrected the infant will become increasingly dehydrated and may die. Alkalosis is not present at birth and only develops over the subsequent weeks. Those infants who survive without adequate electrolyte replacement are invariably growth retarded with hypotonia and developmentally delayed as a consequence of chronic salt depletion.

The diagnosis is made from the high Cl^- content of the stool with levels > 90 mmol/L exceeding the sum of the Na^+ and K^+ concentrations. Blood gases will show a metabolic alkalosis, serum Cl^- and K^+ are low while the Na^+ level is likely to be normal. Urinary electrolytes will show very low or absent Na^+ and Cl^- excretion with markedly raised K^+ losses in the face of hypokalemia.

Treatment is with oral electrolyte supplements in the form of both NaCl and KCl given in amounts large enough to suppress the hyperaldosteronism, maintain urinary Cl^- excretion and correct the electrolyte deficiency. This treatment does not influence the diarrhea but results in the normal growth and development of the child.

Congenital sodium diarrhea

Diarrhea secondary to a defect of Na^+/H^+ exchange can present in newborn babies in a manner very similar to congenital chloride diarrhea. The watery stools however contain more sodium than chloride and the child will develop a metabolic acidosis. Treatment with sodium citrate and oral rehydration solutions maintains fluid and electrolyte balance.

Acrodermatitis enteropathica

This is an autosomal recessive condition characterized by a specific defect in the absorption of zinc by the histologically normal small intestinal mucosa. The resulting zinc deficiency leads to a florid rash over the perineum (Fig. 19.8), buttocks and oral region with associated diarrhea, infection, alopecia and behavioral disturbance. The clinical features are reversed promptly by treatment with oral zinc supplements, which need to be taken life-long.

Primary hypomagnesemia

This autosomal recessive condition results from the defective absorption of magnesium by the small intestine and leads in the first few weeks of life to tetany and generalized convulsions associated with hypomagnesemia and hypocalcemia. On a normal diet the patient is in negative magnesium balance but this can be reversed by giving oral magnesium supplements. These supplements increase serum levels of both magnesium and calcium but unfortunately frequently induce diarrhea.

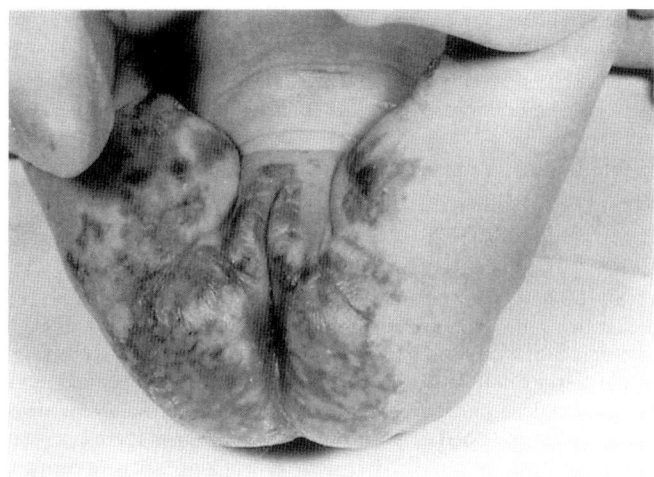

Fig. 19.8 The napkin area of a child with acrodermatitis enteropathica. (Reproduced by kind permission of P J Milla)

INVESTIGATIONS OF THE SMALL INTESTINE

A wide range of tests are available to look at the structure and function of the small intestine. Each test has its own specific indications and limitations and with the correct choice of investigations the maximum relevant information can be obtained with the minimum of invasive investigations.

RADIOLOGY

Plain abdominal X-ray is of value in detecting intestinal obstruction and the presence of free gas will also be seen if perforation has occurred. The barium follow-through or small bowel enema is the investigation of choice to define the anatomy of the small intestine and to demonstrate the gross mucosal pattern. This examination will define the rotation of the small intestine and allow the detection of blind loops, strictures and duplication cysts. Contrast studies are also invaluable in detecting small bowel involvement in Crohn's disease, intestinal polyps and infiltrative lesions of the small bowel such as non-Hodgkin's lymphoma.

The ectopic gastric mucosa in Meckel's diverticulum can be outlined with a ^{99}Tc pertechnetate scan and mucosal inflammation can be detected with the autologous labeling of leukocytes with ^{99}Tc hexametazime (HMPAO).

Celiac axis angiography is only very rarely required to define the site of intestinal hemorrhage from a vascular malformation.

SMALL INTESTINAL BIOPSY

The development of peroral small intestinal biopsy using the Watson or Crosby capsule in the late 1950s led to major advances in the diagnosis and management of small intestinal disease. This method has now been largely superseded by the use of upper gastrointestinal endoscopy for small bowel biopsy. Biopsies need to be taken from the distal second or third part of the duodenum in order to avoid the presence of Brunner's glands, which are found more proximally. This technique has the advantage that the area for biopsy can be directly visualized, other pathologies may be detected at endoscopy and with the development of small instruments, biopsies in preterm infants are now possible. A limitation is that biopsies tend to be small and more difficult to orientate but this problem can be largely overcome by taking multiple biopsies.

If the biopsy material is correctly stored it is possible to carry out the quantitative measurement of brush border disaccharides by histochemical methods, to characterize the infiltrate in the lamina propria with immunostaining, and with electron microscopy the characteristic lesion of microvillous atrophy can be seen.

Serial mucosal biopsy is also valuable in monitoring the therapeutic response to therapy.

CAPSULE ENDOSCOPY

Traditional endoscopic techniques allow direct examination of the duodenum at upper endoscopy and of the terminal ileum during colonoscopy. Push endoscopy, a technique used more widely in adult practice, should allow direct examination beyond the duodeno-jejunal flexure. Direct visualization of the entire length of the small intestine is now available using the technique of capsule ensocopy, where a video camera 'pill' is swallowed and continuous images are transmitted to a data recording device as it passes along the length of the small intestine.[26] This technique is particularly valuable in the detection of intestinal polyps, small bowel Crohn's disease and occult intestinal bleeding. In younger children down to the age of about 6 years the capsule can be passed during an endoscopic procedure if it cannot be swallowed.

NUTRIENT LOSS IN STOOL

Alpha-1 antitrypsin is a protein which is resistant to digestion by the gut and excretion in the feces is a reliable marker of stool protein loss. Fat loss can be quantified by the homogenization and separation of fat within fecal material by centrifugation of spot stool samples. The steatocrit refers to the fat content as a percentage of the total solid matter in the stool. Carbohydrate loss in the stool is discussed more fully in the section on stool chromatography.

BREATH HYDROGEN

When bacteria in the colon come in contact with undigested carbohydrate it is fermented with the production of hydrogen, which is exhaled in the breath. By the use of a suitable carbohydrate load this phenomenon can be used to measure mouth to cecal transit time, the absorption of a range of mono- and disaccharides and to detect colonization of the small intestine by bacteria.

Lactulose is a naturally occurring carbohydrate which is not absorbed or digested by the human small intestine but is readily fermented by colonic bacteria to produce hydrogen. Therefore the time between an oral dose (250 mg/kg) and a rise in the basal level of breath hydrogen is an indication of mouth to cecal transit time. If an oral load of glucose (2 g/kg) is given to a healthy fasting subject the monosaccharide should be completely absorbed by the small intestine and no breath hydrogen peak will occur. In a patient with glucose–galactose malabsorption the glucose will pass straight into the colon causing a large peak in breath hydrogen along with abdominal pain and diarrhea. Finally, in a patient with bacterial overgrowth the glucose will be fermented almost immediately it leaves the stomach producing a very brisk and early rise in breath hydrogen.

STOOL CROMATOGRAPHY

Whenever a patient has osmotic diarrhea it is likely that the stool will contain sugars. While reducing sugars can be crudely detected using clinitest tablets, the quantification and characterization of these sugars by stool chromatography can be very useful, when taken along with the carbohydrate content of the child's feed or a specific oral load, in defining the cause of the underlying disorder. Two classic examples are the child with sucrase–isomaltase deficiency who, following the ingestion of complex carbohydrate, has loose stool containing limit dextrins, maltotriose and maltose and the baby with glucose–galactose malabsorption who, following a milk feed, has diarrhea containing glucose and galactose.

Specimens require immediate transport to the laboratory so that further digestion of sugars by colonic bacteria is prevented.

DUODENAL INTUBATION

When bacterial overgrowth is suspected, intubation with aspiration of duodenal juices is essential to confirm the diagnosis and define the sensitivities of the organisms present. Aspiration will similarly allow the concentration and pattern of luminal bile salts to be measured. The technique used to measure pancreatic function is described in the section on the pancreas.

GASTROINTESTINAL TUMORS

JUVENILE POLYPS

The most common polyp found in childhood is the juvenile polyp. These inflammatory lesions are found most frequently in the rectosigmoid but may develop more proximally and in 50% of cases more than one may be found. They present most frequently with painless rectal bleeding, in children between the ages of 2 and 5, although rarely they may present with recurrent abdominal pain and intussusception. These polyps do not undergo malignant change although if more than 10 lesions are seen, juvenile polyposis coli should be suspected. This condition can be differentiated from familial polyposis coli by the earlier age of onset and the presence of inflammatory, rather than adenomatous, polyps.[48]

The diagnosis can be confirmed by flexible colonoscopy and at the same examination the polyps can be diathermied and removed for histological examination.

FAMILIAL ADENOMATOUS POLYPOSIS (FAP)

This autosomal dominant condition is characterized by multiple adenomatous polyps throughout the large intestine and is likely to present insidiously with diarrhea, blood and mucus in the stools. The polyps, which generally appear after puberty, slowly enlarge with time until they invariably undergo malignant change. The children of affected adults should be offered genetic screening and with the recognition of mutations in the FAP gene on chromosome 5q21 and the association with congenital hypertrophy of the retinal pigment epithelium (CHRPE), patients at high risk of developing the condition can be detected. Those at high risk require regular colonoscopic screening from the age of 12 years. Although the rate of polyp growth may be slowed by nonsteroidal anti-inflammatory drugs (NSAIDs), for the majority of individuals total colectomy in early adulthood is still the treatment of choice.

In Gardner syndrome adenomatous polyps are seen throughout the gut in association with bone osteomas and epidermoid cysts.

PEUTZ–JEGHERS SYNDROME

In this autosomal dominant condition multiple hamartomatous polyps are distributed throughout the jejunum, ileum and large intestine of children in association with pigmentation of the oral mucosa and the skin of the perioral region, the digits and the anus. The condition presents with anemia due to blood loss or with obstruction secondary to intussusception. The risk of gastrointestinal cancer is increased 15-fold in this condition and up to 50% of untreated patients will die of cancer by the age of 57 years.

PSEUDOPOLYPS

In response to any inflammatory reaction the intestinal mucosa may become swollen and a polyp-like structure will be formed. As a result of enteric infections or allergy, lymphoid hyperplasia of the ileum may occur and in conditions such as ulcerative colitis and Crohn's disease exuberant mucosal inflammation leads to pseudopolyp formation. The true nature of the lesions can be defined by mucosal biopsy.

HEMANGIOMAS

Intestinal hemangiomas, which are frequently multiple, are a well-recognized cause of rectal bleeding. Small colonic lesions can be sclerosed during endoscopic examination but laparotomy may be required for large angiomas and small intestinal lesions. In the blue rubber bleb nevus syndrome skin lesions may be associated with luminal lesions within the intestine.

MALIGNANT TUMORS

Fortunately, malignant tumors of the intestine are very rare in childhood and in particular colonic and gastric neoplasms, which are so common in adult life, are hardly ever seen.

Small intestinal lymphoma of the nonHodgkin's type is, however, occasionally seen. These tumors may be unifocal and present with obstruction or intussusception of the ileocecal region, or more commonly they are multifocal and present with ascites. Lymphoma is more likely to occur in children with immunodeficiency or following infection with the Epstein–Barr virus (EBV) while in adults there is a clear association with untreated celiac disease. If a laparotomy is required for intestinal obstruction the diagnosis can be made from the histology of the resected specimen but under other circumstances bone marrow aspiration and cytological examination of ascitic fluid is required.

THE PANCREAS

CYSTIC FIBROSIS

Cystic fibrosis is an autosomal recessive condition which affects approximately 1 in every 2000 live Caucasian births.[49,50] The underlying defect results from one of a number of possible mutations, in a chloride transporter protein which lines ductular epithelium. This results in inspissation of mucus in the ducts of the pancreas and in the bronchial and biliary trees with the resulting development of pancreatic insufficiency, chronic respiratory disease and biliary cirrhosis. In this section discussion will be confined to the effects of cystic fibrosis on the pancreas and intestine (Table 19.17) as the pulmonary (see Ch. 20) and hepatic (see p. 652) consequences are discussed elsewhere.

Pancreatic insufficiency

The inspissated concretions result in distension of the ducts and acini of the pancreas, which with time progress to the formation of small cysts with destruction and fibrosis of the exocrine tissue. As a consequence of this the output of pancreatic enzymes and bicarbonate falls, leading to pancreatic insufficiency. In some patients endocrine pancreatic tissue is also damaged with the development of diabetes mellitus. Approximately 85% of patients with cystic fibrosis have pancreatic insufficiency with resulting malabsorption and steatorrhea, while in the remaining 15%, although not normal, the pancreas has adequate reserve capacity. Signs of pancreatic insuffi-

Table 19.17   Gastrointestinal manifestations of cystic fibrosis

1. Pancreas
   a. Pancreatic insufficiency
   b. Pancreatitis
   c. Diabetes mellitus
2. Hepatobiliary
   a. Biliary cirrhosis
   b. Lobular cirrhosis
   c. Cholelithiasis
   d. Biliary obstruction
3. Intestinal
   a. Meconium ileus
   b. Rectal prolapse
   c. Intussusception
   d. Esophageal reflux
   e. Esophageal varices
   f. Distal intestinal obstruction syndrome

ciency are usually present within the first 2 years of life with the passage of foul, bulky pale stools. In the majority of untreated children, growth is abnormal and fat-soluble vitamin deficiencies are likely to develop.

As a consequence of chronic steatorrhea, bile salts are lost in the stool, leading to depletion of the bile salt pool, which may be further compounded if liver disease reduces the rate of synthesis. The resulting reduction in bile salt concentration will not only reduce the solubilization of lipids in the duodenum but may also reduce the solubilization of cholesterol and predispose to the formation of gall stones.

Meconium ileus

Cystic fibrosis may present in the first day or two of life with vomiting and abdominal distension due to meconium ileus. This obstruction to the small intestine with thick tenacious meconium may be complicated by volvulus, atresia or peritonitis. Plain abdominal X-ray will show dilated loops of intestine with meconium, outlined by trapped air, present in the obstructed segment of bowel and gastrografin enema will reveal a microcolon distal to the obstruction. The enema may be of benefit in the nonsurgical clearance of the meconium (see Ch. 37).

Difficulty in passing stool may also lead to rectal prolapse.

Distal intestinal obstruction syndrome

This condition, which is sometimes also referred to as meconium ileus equivalent, is a common problem known to occur in up to 15% of patients with cystic fibrosis. It is most common in adolescence and is characterized by recurrent episodes of subacute or occasionally acute obstruction with abdominal pain, vomiting and anorexia. Marked fecal loading may be detected by abdominal palpation or plain abdominal X-ray. If treatment with laxatives fails, the use of mucolytic drugs or balanced intestinal lavage should be considered.

Diagnosis of cystic fibrosis

The main diagnostic test for cystic fibrosis is the sweat test, which measures the increased sodium content found in the sweat of children with cystic fibrosis. The vast majority of healthy children have a sweat sodium less than 45 mmol/L while in cystic fibrosis it is greater than 74 mmol/L in 99% of cases. A modification of this test measures the sweat osmolality, which is greater than 125 mOsmol/L in cystic fibrosis.

Many mutations have been described for the cystic fibrosis gene. If the patient's DNA is tested against the most common 20 mutations for the study population, it is possible to get a diagnostic accuracy of about 99%. Screening for cystic fibrosis in newborn babies can be carried out by heterozygote screening of mothers using genetic techniques or by immunoreactive trypsin measurement of a blood spot from a Guthrie card after birth.

Treatment

As far as the intestinal complications of cystic fibrosis are concerned the main treatment for pancreatic insufficiency is with oral pancreatic supplements. Although only 10% of normal lipase activity is required to prevent steatorrhea, the majority of ingested supplements are inactivated by the low pH of the stomach and as a consequence symptoms may persist. This may be overcome by incorporating the pancreatic supplements within a pH-sensitive microsphere. The dose required by each patient is likely to vary greatly, although an inadequate dose will result in a failure to relieve symptoms while an excessive dose may lead to perianal excoriation or some children may develop thickening of the colonic mucosa with the development of obstruction.

The nutritional intake of patients with cystic fibrosis is frequently less than recommended for their age and given that their requirements may be increased due to chronic infestion or the increased work of breathing, it is perhaps not surprising that many children grow poorly. With improved dietary advice and the use of nutritional supplements children with cystic fibrosis are now growing better and as a consequence they are surviving longer. Where supplements cannot be given enterally, nasogastric or gastrostomy feeding may be helpful. Oral fat-soluble vitamin supplements, in particular vitamin E, are also required.

SHWACHMAN SYNDROME

After cystic fibrosis, Shwachman syndrome is probably the next most common cause of pancreatic insufficiency in childhood.[51] This autosomal recessive condition is due to a mutation on chromosome 7q11. Although the gene product is not known, the gene is expressed widely in the pancreas and bone marrow. The condition is characterized by the presence of neutropenia, short stature and bony changes in addition to pancreatic insufficiency. The neutropenia may occur cyclically as may the thrombocytopenia, which is seen in two thirds of patients. Arrest in proliferation of the myeloid series may be seen on bone marrow aspiration and leukemic transformation has been reported in a number of patients. Bony abnormalities with metaphyseal chondrodysplasia are frequently seen with involvement of the femoral neck.

The diagnosis should be considered in any child with pancreatic insufficiency, a normal sweat test and neutropenia. Treatment is with pancreatic supplements and fat-soluble vitamins and where symptomatic neutropenia persists, the use of human granulocyte colony stimulating factor should be considered. The patients are particularly prone to recurrent infections and antibiotic prophylaxis may be of some benefit.

ACUTE AND CHRONIC PANCREATITIS

Pancreatitis is uncommon in childhood with idiopathic (23%) and trauma being the most common causes. Obstruction to the pancreatic duct, loss of vascular integrity and a direct insult to the parenchymal cells are all factors which can lead to the development of pancreatitis. Hereditary causes are the most common reason for chronic pancreatitis; mutations in the cationic trypsinogen gene, the cystic fibrosis transmembrane conductance regulator (CFTR) and the serine protein inhibitor (SPINK1) have all been implicated. Some hereditary cases may be due to a defect which prevents the inactivation of pancreatic enzymes with resulting autodigestion.[52] The causes of pancreatitis are listed in Table 19.18.

Table 19.18 Causes of pancreatitis

1. Acute
   a. Trauma
   b. Infections
      (i) Mumps
      (ii) Coxsackie
      (iii) *Leptospira*
      (iv) *Ascaris*
   c. Gallstones
   d. Drugs
      (i) Valproic acid
      (ii) Cytosine arabinoside
      (iii) L-asparaginase
   e. Inflammatory bowel disease
   f. Metabolic
      (i) Reye syndrome
      (ii) Re-feeding malnutrition
      (iii) Parenteral nutrition
   g. Vasculitis
   h. Duodenal ulcer
   i. Idiopathic

2. Chronic
   a. Hereditary
   b. Metabolic
      (i) Hyperlipidemia
      (ii) Hyperparathyroidism
      (iii) Cystic fibrosis
   c. Duct malformations
   d. Idiopathic

Presentation

Attacks of pancreatitis are characterized by severe epigastric or umbilical pain which tends to be constant rather than colicky and which can radiate to the back or shoulders.[53] The pain is exacerbated by food and is not relieved by antacids. The patient will find abdominal movement uncomfortable and if the pancreatitis is severe, hemorrhagic bruising of the flanks with a paralytic ileus may develop. When the course is prolonged the condition may be complicated by circulatory collapse, hyperglycemia, hypocalcemia or by the formation of pleural effusions and pancreatic pseudocysts. The diagnosis is confirmed by markedly raised levels of serum amylase.

Treatment

The management of acute pancreatitis is conservative. All oral feeds should be stopped and i.v. fluids should be given to correct any fluid losses and to provide normal requirements. Acute pancreatitis can be very painful, requiring adequate analgesia and where the patient is vomiting a nasogastric tube should be passed. An acute attack will normally last for between 3 d and 5 d but if the attack is more prolonged total PN should be started and treatment with a somatostatin analogue should be considered. The patient should be monitored for the development of complications and serial abdominal ultrasounds will allow fluid collections to be detected at an early stage. Pseudocysts which fail to resolve spontaneously will need to be drained.

In both acute and chronic pancreatitis if an underlying cause has been defined, this should be appropriately treated. Where a duct abnormality has been isolated reconstructive surgery may be of benefit and if a localized area of the pancreas is responsible for recurrent attacks, a partial pancreatectomy should be considered.

INVESTIGATION OF THE PANCREAS

The most commonly used indirect measure of pancreatic function in childhood is the sweat test, which was discussed in the section on cystic fibrosis (see p. 625). The remaining investigations can be divided into blood tests which measure the level of pancreatic enzymes (i.e. amylase), tests which measure fecal fat or enzyme activity, more direct measures of pancreatic function and radiological imaging methods.

Pancreatic function tests

These tests can be divided into the traditional tests which require duodenal intubation and the newer tubeless function tests. The traditional tests remain the most accurate although they are also the most invasive. They involve the collection of duodenal juice during a basal fasting period followed by the stimulation of the pancreas with cholecystokinin (1–2 iu/kg) and then secretin (1–2 iu/kg) with the further collection of duodenal juice. In pancreatic insufficiency the stimulated levels of lipase and trypsin are reduced and the juice fails to alkalinize following stimulation with secretin. The tubeless tests rely on the pancreatic enzymes cleaving an ingested compound (bentiromide or fluorescein dilaurate) and the amount subsequently collected in the urine is a measure of pancreatic function.

Stool elastase activity is a non-invasive measure of pancreatic function which although not as accurate as the intubation technique described earlier, is easy to carry out. Pancreatic lipase activity can also be indirectly measured by the labeling of a fatty substrate with C^{13} and measuring the appearance of the stable isotope in the breath.

Radiology

Ultrasound is a very useful non-invasive imaging method in pancreatitis as it will show pancreatic edema during the acute attack, outline any fluid collections and allow gallbladder disease to be excluded. Where more detailed imaging is required of the structure of the pancreas, computerized tomographic (CT) techniques using X-ray and magnetic resonance imaging (MRI) may be used. In chronic pancreatitis where imaging of the pancreatic ducts is required to exclude a malformation or stricture, endoscopic retrograde cholangiopancreatography (ERCP) or magnetic resonance cholangiopancreatography (MRCP) can be used.

Any abnormality of the structure of the duodenum will be seen on a barium study.

DISORDERS OF GASTROINTESTINAL MOTILITY

Disorders of gastrointestinal motility are very common in childhood and are responsible for such diverse conditions as gastroesophageal reflux, irritable bowel syndrome and chronic constipation. Normal contractile activity relies on the coordinated action of the intestinal smooth muscle, its enteric and central neural connections and the humoral environment of the gut. Diseases exist in which damage to the enteric nervous system (Hirschsprung disease) or smooth muscle severely compromises the luminal transit of food and present with the symptoms of intestinal obstruction. The central nervous system has an important role in the modulation of intestinal motility with central insults commonly resulting in vomiting or even paralytic ileus. Lesser disturbances such as stress may lead to vomiting, abdominal pain and diarrhea.[54]

ESOPHAGUS AND STOMACH

Motility disorders of the esophagus and stomach have already been discussed in their respective sections (pp. 604 and 605).

INTESTINAL PSEUDO-OBSTRUCTION

Intestinal pseudo-obstruction is a clinical syndrome characterized by the signs and symptoms of intestinal obstruction in a patient with no evidence of an obstructing lesion. Pseudo-obstruction occurs most commonly as a primary disorder in childhood; it may be familial but may occasionally present in adolescence as a secondary manifestation of some other disease such as diabetes mellitus. The disorder tends to be generalized, involving either the smooth muscle or the enteric nerves of the entire length of the intestine.

A quarter of children present at birth and by 1 year two thirds have developed symptoms of abdominal distension, vomiting, constipation and failure to thrive. Frequently it is only after laparotomy that the condition is diagnosed. Associated abnormalities of the urinary tract such as megacystis and megaureter are found in some patients and an association with malrotation of the small intestine has been reported. Diagnosis can be made from the history and from intestinal manometry, which shows either a disruption or loss of cyclical fasting motor activity. A full-thickness biopsy is required for a definitive diagnosis.

The condition is complicated by bacterial overgrowth of the small intestine and is punctuated by repeated episodes of obstruction. In some patients this can be significantly improved by the formation of a defunctioning ileostomy. Nutrition is frequently compromised and in the most severe cases survival without total PN may not be possible.

LARGE INTESTINE

Colonic motility disorders will present in the neonatal period with the delayed passage of meconium and symptoms of intestinal obstruction if severe, or may be delayed for many months or years when they are more likely to present with chronic constipation. Hirschsprung disease (see Ch. 37), hypo- and hyperganglionosis are now all well-recognized entities but unfortunately the nature of the structural or functional disorder in children with chronic constipation due to other causes is less well defined.

Treatment is symptomatic with oral laxatives in milder cases. In more severe cases, regular enemas may be required and in some patients the use of regular intestinal lavage through a continent cecostomy is effective. Where these techniques fail a defunctioning stoma or resection of the affected bowel may be required.

ACUTE INFECTIVE DIARRHEA

Acute infective diarrhea is one of the major causes of morbidity and mortality in childhood in the world today, killing up to 3 million children each year. In resource rich countries each child under 5 years has one to two episodes each year and over 10% of all hospital admissions in this age group are with acute diarrhea. In developing countries the much higher incidence of diarrheal illness is a consequence of the combined effect of contaminated water supplies, the preparation of bottle feeds under unhygienic conditions and from malnutrition, which frequently occurs in these children at the time of weaning.

Most acute diarrheal illnesses in well-nourished children are self-limiting and resolve within a few days. However, when frequent reinfection occurs, the child may develop a state of chronic diarrhea which will inevitably result in further malnutrition and an increased susceptibility to recurrent infection. It is this vicious cycle of events which along with the acute effects of dehydration leads to the significant mortality from this condition in developing countries.

ETIOLOGY AND PATHOGENESIS

The infective agent in acute diarrhea cannot always be isolated but with improvements in diagnostic techniques a pathogen can be isolated in up to 80% of cases. Viral agents are the most common cause of acute infective diarrhea in childhood, followed by bacteria and then protozoal infection. The causes of acute infective diarrhea are shown in Table 19.19.

In the young infant who is most at risk from the complications of acute diarrhea a number of protective mechanisms exist to limit the effect of infective pathogens. The acid content of the stomach and IgA secreted by the small intestine and in breast milk will limit the growth of bacteria in the upper small intestine and the resulting predominance of bifidobacteria in feces may inhibit colonization by enteric pathogens. These factors all lead to a reduced incidence of acute enteric infection in breast-fed infants. Modification of the intestinal flora with probiotics may be of benefit both in preventing and reducing the severity of acute infective diarrhea.[55]

Viral infection

The agent most commonly responsible for acute infantile gastroenteritis is the rotavirus. The rotavirus selectively attacks the mature enterocytes at the tips of the small intestinal villi, which are killed and shed into the lumen. This leads to the increased production of immature crypt-like cells with shortening of the villi. These cells have greatly reduced absorptive and disaccharidase activity and this loss of normal small intestinal function combined with the active secretion of fluids and electrolytes, leads to the production of diarrhea. Following the clearance of the viral pathogen the functional mucosal abnormalities resolve.

Table 19.19 Causes of acute infective diarrhea

Viruses
  Rotavirus
  Astrovirus
  Adenovirus
  Parvovirus-like (i.e. Norwalk agent)
  Coronavirus

Bacteria
  Campylobacter sp.
  Salmonella sp.
  Escherichia coli
  Shigella sp.
  Yersinia enterocolitica
  Vibrio cholerae
  Clostridium difficile

Protozoa
  Giardia lamblia
  Cryptosporidium
  Entamoeba histolytica

Bacterial infection

Four major mechanisms are responsible for the effects of bacterial pathogens. Organisms such as *Vibrio cholerae* and some strains of *Escherichia coli* synthesize proteins called enterotoxins, which are able to promote intestinal secretion. The preservation of electrogenic sodium-linked solute co-transport in these patients is exploited by the use of sodium- and glucose-containing oral rehydration solutions (ORSs), which are able to promote net intestinal absorption in the face of active secretion.

Enteropathogenic organisms such as some strains of *E. coli* adhere to the brush border membrane of the small intestine causing severe mucosal damage which may take many weeks to recover and such children may require parenteral nutritional support during the intervening period. *Shigella* species and *E. coli* serotypes O124 and O164 possess enteroinvasive properties leading to the development of watery diarrhea and dysentery with bacterial invasion of the colonic mucosa, while some bacteria, such as *Clostridium difficile* also produce cytotoxins, which have a direct toxic effect on enterocytes.

CLINICAL FEATURES

Acute infective diarrhea characteristically results in a combination of nausea, vomiting, abdominal pain and diarrhea. In some children the symptoms may be relatively trivial while in others dehydration and metabolic disturbances may be life threatening. Symptoms appear generally to be most severe in younger and in malnourished infants who also run the risk of becoming septicemic with some bacterial pathogens. Bloody diarrhea frequently occurs in *Shigella, Salmonella, Campylobacter* and *E. coli* O157 infection. In children infected with *E. coli* O157 monitoring for signs of hemolytic uremic syndrome (HUS) and renal failure are required, particularly those under the age of 5 years, who are most vulnerable to this complication. Diarrhea and vomiting may also occur in a number of other medical conditions and it is important to consider systemic infection, metabolic disorders, surgical problems and other gastrointestinal disorders in the differential diagnosis of such patients.

The most serious consequence of acute diarrhea and vomiting is dehydration. The severity of the dehydration (see Table 19.20), which can be assessed clinically, determines the best treatment for the child. Children on high-solute diets, who develop diarrhea, may develop hypernatremic dehydration in which case the signs of dehydration are less obvious although lethargy and irritability may develop earlier.

Loss of bicarbonate and potassium in the stool, poor tissue perfusion, hypoglycemia, ketosis and renal failure may all lead to severe metabolic derangement. Symptoms of lethargy and irritability are particularly marked in hypernatremic dehydration and its rapid correction with i.v. fluids may lead to cerebral edema as a result of fluid shifts across the blood–brain barrier. This can result in convulsions or even death.

MANAGEMENT

The management of children with acute infective diarrhea hinges upon the treatment of their dehydration.[56–59] The treatment required depends very much on the severity of their dehydration and on the facilities

Table 19.20 Assessment of the severity of dehydration

	No dehydration	5% dehydration	10%+ dehydration
Condition	Well, alert	Restless, irritable	Lethargic, unconscious
Eyes	Normal	Sunken	Very sunken and dry
Tears	Present	Absent	Absent
Mouth and tongue	Moist	Dry	Very dry
Thirst	Not thirsty	Thirsty, drinks eagerly	Drinks poorly
Skin pinch	Goes back quickly	Goes back slowly	Goes back very slowly

which are available. Most mild cases can be treated at home by their family practitioner with ORS but where dehydration is more severe, social circumstances are poor or where other complicating medical factors are present, hospital admission is required. Even in moderate dehydration, ORS remains the treatment of choice although this therapy is underused in developed countries, where i.v. therapy is often used inappropriately. Additionally the practitioner has to consider how best to feed these infants during both the acute and recovery phase of their illness. Generally drug therapy has no role in the management of acute diarrhea.

Oral rehydration therapy

The management of acute diarrhea was revolutionized by the introduction of ORS over 30 years ago. This treatment continues to be the mainstay of therapy and by preventing the patient becoming dehydrated; it has greatly reduced the morbidity and mortality. While most children with acute diarrhea will have active intestinal secretion, their ability to absorb fluid and electrolytes is largely preserved. As outlined in Figure 19.5, the absorption of sodium and glucose across the luminal surface of the enterocyte is facilitated by a transmembrane cotransport system. Solutions containing sodium and glucose in an optimum concentration are absorbed at an accelerated rate and where this is greater than the fluid losses incurred by the diarrheal process, dehydration can be prevented. It must be remembered that ORS does not stop the diarrhea and this is probably one of the reasons why its acceptance in developed countries is sometimes poor, as parents want any treatment to be a 'quick fix' to their child's problems.

The main recommendations for the treatment of acute diarrhea have come from the World Health Organization (WHO). Their oral rehydration solution contained 111 mmol/L of glucose and 90 mmol/L of sodium (Table 19.21). There has however been concern that in developed countries where cholera is an uncommon cause of diarrhea, this sodium concentration is too high and a concentration of 60 mmol/L has been suggested by the European Society for Pediatric Gastroenterology and Nutrition. It has also recently been shown that the traditional ORS, which has a slightly hyperosmolar osmolality of 311 mOsmol/L, may not be as effective as solutions with a lower osmolality of 210–260 mOsmol/L. This has resulted in revised recommendations by the WHO suggesting that rehdration solutions should contain 75 mmol/L of sodium and 75 mmol/L of glucose with a resulting osmolality of 245 mOsmol/L.[57] It must be remembered that fruit juices and colas are entirely unsuitable as ORS as they contain large amounts of sugar and very small amounts of electrolytes.

Fluid replacement therapy

When assessing how best to treat a child with infective diarrhea, first severity of the patient's dehydration should be assessed (Table 19.20). The majority of children presenting for medical attention in resource rich countries are not yet dehydrated and the aim of treatment should be to prevent this occurring. Such children are often reluctant to take ORS and a normal age-appropriate diet should be continued. Unweaned infants should continue either with breast-feeding or undiluted formula feed. The diet of older children should contain complex carbohydrate and meat but large amounts of fat or simple sugars should be avoided. There is increasing evidence that not only is the continued use of diet safe in children with infective diarrhea but through the trophic effect on the intestinal mucosa, a more rapid recovery of symptoms is promoted.

Children who are dehydrated and not shocked should be rapidly rehydrated with ORS. They should receive 50 ml/kg in the first 4 h with an additional 10 ml/kg for each stool and supplements for vomiting. In the more severely dehydrated child up to 100 ml/kg can be given in the first 4 h. By giving frequent small sips, vomiting can be reduced. If the child will not take adequate volumes of ORS, administration by nasogastric tube is preferable to i.v. administration in the nonshocked child who is not vomiting. Once the child is rehydated, normal diet should be resumed as for the nondehydrated child.

I.v. rehydration is required if the patient is shocked or where repeated vomiting prevents adequate oral rehydration. The shocked patient should receive 20 ml/kg boluses of normal saline until the signs of shock resolve. ORS should be introduced at the earliest opportunity to continue the rehydration of the patient and food intake should be started as soon as it is likely to be tolerated. If continued i.v. rehydration is required, a 5% deficit should be corrected over 24 h and a 10% deficit (Table 19.20) over 48 h with a 0.45% saline/dextrose solution.

Other therapies

Generally antibiotics have no place in the management of acute infective diarrhea, the exception being *Shigella, V. cholerae, Clostridium difficile* and *Giardia*. Similarly antimotility drugs, many of which are opiate derivatued, should not be given. There is now increasing evidence that probiotic therapy is beneficial in the treatment of acute infective diarrhea. A large European multicenter study has shown that *Lactobacillus rhamnosus* strain GG given with ORS reduces the length of diarrhea and the time of hospital stay.[55]

Complications

Acute infective diarrhea may be complicated by the extraintestinal spread of the infection with the development of intestinal perforation, abscess formation, septicemia and meningitis. If dehydration is pronounced acute renal failure may develop and if hypernatremia is corrected too rapidly cerebral edema with convulsions is likely to occur. This complication is less common when ORS is used as fluid shifts occur more slowly. In some children severe damage to the intestinal mucosa will lead to the development of diarrhea which persists long after the original pathogen has been cleared.

CONCLUSIONS

There have been many changes and advancements in the management of acute infective diarrhea in the last 10 years. There is clear agreement that ORS is the preferred method of rehydration, that diet should be introduced at an early stage and that drugs have very little role in the treatment of this problem. These points are summarized in Table 19.22.

Table 19.21   Major constituents of appropriate oral rehydration solutions (mmol/L) compared to inappropriate preparations. World Health Organization (WHO), European Society of Paediatric Gastroenterology Hepatology and Nutrition (ESPGHAN)

	Glucose (or other sugar)	Sodium	Potassium	Base	Osmolality
WHO (original)	110	90	20	30	311
ESPGHAN	74–111	60	20	10	225–260
WHO (revised 2001)	75	75	20	10	245
Solution not suitable for ORS					
Cola	700	2	0	13	750
Apple juice	690	3	32	0	730

Table 19.22 Principles of treatment of acute gastroenteritis (Adapted from Szajewska, 2000[56])

1. Use of ORS for dehydration
2. Use hypotonic ORS, Na 60–75 mmol/L (see Table 19.21)
3. Fast oral rehydration, over 3–4 h
4. Rapid realimentation with normal feeding thereafter
5. Use of special formula is unjustified
6. Use of diluted formula is unjustified
7. Continuation of breast-feeding at all times
8. Supplementation of ORS for ongoing losses
9. No unnecessary medications

PROTRACTED DIARRHOEA IN EARLY INFANCY

Protracted diarrhea may be defined as the passage of four or more watery stools per day persisting for at least 2 weeks. This definition encompasses a wide variety of disorders (Table 19.23) and a definitive diagnosis may only be made in approximately 70% of cases. In most instances, the protracted diarrhea appears to follow an episode of acute gastroenteritis in early infancy, although by the time of presentation to hospital it may be impossible to isolate an infective agent from the stool. Furthermore, unless the situation is managed effectively at an early stage, a cycle of malabsorption and malnutrition may result which will further compromise intestinal function and perpetuate the diarrhea.[42]

One proposed sequence of events is that an acute infective insult may sensitize the intestine to foreign proteins (usually cows' milk protein), and subsequent ingestion of the offending food antigen causes further damage to the intestinal mucosa thus continuing the diarrhea (see also Ch. 33). Although the resulting enteropathy may be caused primarily by the protein content of the milk feed, disaccharide intolerance (particularly lactose) may also develop and the institution of an appropriate exclusion diet will often result in resolution of the diarrhea. In this situation, an exclusion diet may be necessary only for 2 or 3 months, after which a normal weaning diet can be reintroduced. In some cases, particularly in the developing world, bacterial overgrowth of the small intestine may be an added complication and bacterial toxins themselves may impair mucosal function.

Celiac disease, cystic fibrosis, selective inborn errors of absorption and immunodeficiency states may all present with intractable diarrhea of infancy. These conditions are discussed elsewhere in this chapter.

Less common causes include autoimmune enteropathy, while in some children there may be a family history suggesting an inborn error

Table 19.23 Causes of protracted diarrhea in early infancy

1. Food sensitivity/postenteritis syndrome
2. Cystic fibrosis
3. Celiac disease
4. Microvillous inclusion disease
5. Congenital chloride losing diarrhea
6. Congenital short bowel
7. Inborn error of carbohydrate absorption
   a. Sucrase–isomaltase deficiency
   b. Glucose–galactose malabsorption
8. Immunodeficiency
9. Hormone-secreting tumor (i.e. VIPoma)
10. Autoimmune enteropathy
11. Bacterial overgrowth
12. Nonaccidental injury (laxative administration)
13. Idiopathic

as a causative factor. A proportion of these infants may suffer from congenital chloride-losing diarrhea or intestinal microvillus inclusion disease.[60] Where intestinal secretion is present in utero there may be a history of polyhydramnios or premature labor.

INVESTIGATIONS

Collection and examination of the stool is vital and a careful search for intestinal pathogens (bacteria, viruses, parasites) should be undertaken at an early stage. The stools should be analyzed for the presence of reducing substances (> 1%) and stool electrolytes and osmolality should be measured to determine whether the diarrhea is osmotic or secretory in nature (Table 19.24). Chromatography of a fresh stool specimen may help in the diagnosis of inborn errors of carbohydrate absorption and in determining the osmotically active substances within the stool. Valuable information may also be obtained by fasting the child as this is likely to result in a marked diminution of osmotic diarrhea with little change in secretory diarrhea. It is essential to collect and measure the volume of all stools as this will influence the amount and the nature of fluid replacement therapy.

Jejunal biopsy is invaluable in detailing the morphology of the small intestinal epithelium and a sweat test can rule out cystic fibrosis. Blood tests are of limited value although peripheral blood eosinophilia may be present in children with food protein sensitivity and investigation of immune function may reveal specific abnormalities in the child with diarrhea due to immunodeficiency. Measurement of electrolytes and acid–base balance is important in the day-to-day management of fluid balance and may be abnormal in children with congenital chloride-losing diarrhea. If the cause of the diarrhea is not immediately evident serum should be sent for gut-autoantibody estimation to exclude gut autoimmune disease, and circulating gut hormones should be measured to exclude a hormone-secreting tumor. Serum and urine toxicology should be checked if laxative abuse by the mother is suspected.

Radiological studies are rarely informative but barium meal and follow-through will exclude malrotation and may occasionally demonstrate a blind loop. Endoscopic evaluation of the upper and lower gastrointestinal tract is often helpful and multiple biopsies may be taken for examination by light and electron microscopy in addition to obtaining fluid from the lumen of the gut, which should be screened for the presence of pathogens.

TREATMENT

The management of the infant with protracted diarrhea depends on the cause and the severity of the condition. In many cases dietary manipulation is the mainstay of management as appropriate exclusion diets often reduce the volume of diarrhea. A hypoallergenic feed should be used, either as a complete amino acid based feed (Neocate, Scientific Hospital Supplies), peptide based (Nutramingen, Mead Johnston) or as a modular feed where the protein, carbohydrate and fat content can be varied independently. The assistance of an experienced pediatric dietitian is essential in the management of any infant with protracted diarrhea. Those infants who are severely malnourished or who do not respond to enteral feeding and dietetic management may, in addition, need a period of i.v. feeding. If this fails to resolve the problem, long-term PN or even gut transplantation need to be considered.

In certain situations drug therapy may be beneficial. If there is evidence of bacterial overgrowth and bile salt degradation, colestyramine and antibiotics may help the situation. Antisecretory agents such as

Table 19.24 Stool analysis in osmotic and secretory diarrhea

	Osmotic	Secretory
Osmolality (mOsmol/L)	400	290
Na$^+$ (mmol/L)	30	105
K$^+$ (mmol/L)	30	40
(Na$^+$ + K$^+$) × 2	120	290
Solute gap (mmol/L)	280	0

chlorpromazine, octreotide and loperamide may be beneficial in some cases where the primary pathology is not reversible.

In general terms, for those children who present several weeks or months after birth the prognosis is good, while for those who present at birth with an intractable secretory diarrhea the prognosis is poor and the mortality rate high.

INTESTINAL FAILURE

DEFINITION AND PREVALENCE

Intestinal failure is defined as the inability of the alimentary tract to digest and absorb sufficient nutrients to maintain normal fluid balance, growth and health. Acute intestinal failure is relatively common and self-limiting, for example, surgical treatment for an ileal atresia, or an episode of rotavirus gastroenteritis. Chronic intestinal failure resulting in dependence on i.v. feeding/PN is less common and is variously defined as intestinal failure persisting for 4, 6 or 8 weeks. In the United Kingdom period prevalence varies from 4.5 per million population in Wales to 14.3 per million in Scotland, 12.5 per million in Northern Ireland and 9.5 per million in England. This does not take account of the number of patients, especially children, who remain hospitalized long term, because of social factors or complications related to intestinal failure. Whatever the precise number of children affected, the prevalence of treated intestinal failure is increasing. The administration of PN either at home or in hospital is complex with many potential, even life-threatening complications, which means that patients with intestinal failure benefit from early referral to a multidisciplinary team experienced in the management of this highly technical therapy.[61-63]

ETIOLOGY

The vast range in functions and huge physical dimensions of the gastrointestinal system, mean that the possible causes of intestinal failure are numerous and often overlap with disorders in other systems. Broadly, there are three categories of intestinal failure: disorders related to reduced surface area or intestinal mass (e.g. short gut syndrome), disorders of motility (e.g. Hirschsprung disease) and disorders of the mucosa (e.g. microvillus inclusion disease) (Table 19.25). Intestinal failure may be caused by a primary disease of the gastrointestinal tract or it may be secondary to disease in other systems (e.g. immunodeficiency).

Clinical presentation at different ages
Congenital

Intestinal failure may present antenatally or in the neonatal period, where it tends to have a congenital cause. Polyhydramnios is an important sign common in conditions in which the gastrointestinal tract produces excess secretions as in microvillus inclusion disease. The antenatal ultrasound may show distended loops of bowel in the second trimester in babies who develop features of pseudo-obstruction, and gastroschisis can be diagnosed from 12 to 14 weeks' gestation. Antenatal diagnosis is important as it allows the parents to be prepared and for delivery to take place in a unit with rapid access to a neonatal surgical facility.

The cardinal symptoms of intestinal failure are vomiting (with or without bile), abdominal distension, protracted diarrhea, and constipation. These symptoms will be rapidly followed by dehydration, weight loss, shock and renal failure (Table 19.26). Perhaps the most sinister symptom in babies is that of a secretory diarrhea such as occurs in microvillus inclusion disease. In this condition large volume watery diarrhea is uninfluenced by restricted intake. Such diarrhea can be mistaken for urine, with the result that the severity of illness is not recognized until renal failure develops. Another diagnostic pitfall is when the symptoms are intermittent, as can occur in midgut malrotation and which may present at any age with pain and vomiting with spontaneous remissions when the associated volvulus untwists and frees the mesenteric blood supply. Once a midgut volvulus is recognized it is usual to proceed to an operation to fix the bowel (Ladds procedure) and prevent ischemia of the midgut.

Malabsorption may be the predominant problem in children with short gut or mucosal disorders; this is manifested by diarrhea which is exacerbated by feeding. Clinical signs of malabsorption include: excoriated perineum secondary to carbohydrate malabsorption, edema secondary to protein-losing enteropathy and bulky offensive stools secondary to fat malabsorption.

The presence of opportunistic infections such *Candida* species and *Cryptosporidium parvum* indicates the possibility of immune deficiency either primary or acquired as a result of infection by human immunodeficiency virus (HIV). Granulomas may be present on mucosal biopsy, which may suggest an autoimmune enteropathy if Crohn's disease and mycobacterial infection have been excluded.

Acquired

During infancy and childhood the causes of intestinal failure are usually of an acquired nature such as ischemia, trauma and food antigen intolerance (celiac disease usually presents in patients from 9 months of age and older). Fabricated or induced illness is an important diagnosis to consider in a child whose symptoms were not apparent until months or years after birth and in whom the disease appears to be relentlessly progressive despite visits to more than one expert center. Usually such cases do not have a clear diagnosis, but have been labeled 'atypical pseudo-obstruction' or 'protracted diarrhea'.[64]

INVESTIGATIONS

A detailed history and examination including height, weight, midarm circumference, triceps skin fold and head circumference should be carried

Table 19.25 Causes of intestinal failure. Examples in brackets (also see Table 19.23)

	Primary gastrointestinal disorders	Secondary gastrointestinal disorders
Reduced surface area or mass	Gastroschisis Small bowel atresia Mid-gut volvulus Necrotizing enterocolitis Crohn's disease	Gardener syndrome Meconium ileus equivalent (cystic fibrosis) Vascular accident (mesenteric artery thrombosis)
Motility disorder	Aganglionosis (Hirschsprung disease) Megacystis microcolon syndrome	Tumors secreting vasoactive substances (VIPoma) Inappropriate use of purgatives (Munchausen by proxy)
Mucosal lesion	Microvillous inclusion disease Abnormal electrolyte or solute transporters Congenital disaccharidase deficiency Lymphangiectasia Enteropathies (celiac disease, autoimmune) Crohn's disease	Postgastroenteritis viral disease (rotavirus) Ischemia re-perfusion injury after cardiac bypass Mucositis secondary to chemotherapy Graft versus host disease Immune deficiency (see also Table 19.14)

Table 19.26 Symptoms and signs of intestinal failure

Early	Late
Polyhydramnios	Weight loss
Vomiting	Malabsorption (see also Table 19.11)
Diarrhea	Food aversion
Perineal ulceration	Micronutrient deficiency including zinc
Abdominal distension (and pain)	Water and fat-soluble vitamin deficiency
Weight loss	Abdominal pain (colicky)
Electrolyte imbalance	Edema
Convulsions	Opportunistic infection

out. Blood and urine tests should be done with the aim of identifying the extent of illness, devising a management plan and making a diagnosis (Table 19.27). In addition radiology, histopathology and evaluation of intestinal motility are key investigations in arriving at a diagnosis.[63]

MANAGEMENT
Multidisciplinary team

Children with intestinal failure will require urgent resuscitation, initially rehydration with saline and glucose and usually followed by PN if it is clear that intestinal failure is either life threatening or likely to persist for some weeks. Most hospitals have guidelines for prescribing PN which should avoid over- and underprovision of calories since both can cause liver dysfunction. After initial resuscitation a team consisting of dietitian, specialist nurse, pharmacist, pediatric gastroenterologist, radiologist and surgeon should establish the diagnosis, prognosis and plan treatment. For patients with a purely medical cause for intestinal failure, the role of the surgeon will be limited to careful placement of central venous feeding catheters to minimize trauma to major veins

and the superior vena cava in particular. However, patients with short gut will require frequent review by the multidisciplinary team as the maturing and adapting intestine becomes capable of absorbing greater volumes of feed, which should be supervised by a pediatric dietician. If intestinal adaptation does not occur, the presence of strictures, blind ending loops and dilated nonpropulsive bowel should be considered, since well-timed surgery will facilitate reduced dependency on parenteral nutrition.[62]

Dietetic management

In brief four main themes can be identified:

1. Establish oral feeding including sucking and chewing as soon as practical. Even if the quantity of nutrition consumed is negligible, the positive effects on development in speech, social skills and physiology of the upper intestinal tract are great. When it is available, breast milk is ideal, otherwise a hydrolysate is frequently used initially (e.g. Peptijunior, Pregestimil, Neocate) for neonates who have immature pancreatic function and an intestinal mucosal barrier which is still highly permeable to foreign proteins.

2. Initiate continuous nasogastric tube feeding in short gut patients in order to promote intestinal adaptation. Oral feeding is also important and the usual compromise is to offer bottle or bolus feeds during the day and feed by infusion pump for 12–18 h overnight.

3. If feed tolerance is poor consider the use of a modular feed in which the carbohydrate, fat and protein components can be varied independently of each other to achieve a more digestible feed (e.g. less carbohydrate for infants with short gut, medium chain fat for children with lymphangiectasia). Pharmaceutical agents to improve gastric emptying (e.g. domperidone), or to slow transit time (e.g. loperamide 50–200 μg per kg per dose, two to four times per day) can be used in conjunction with manipulations to the feed.

4. Keep micronutrient balance (e.g. fat-soluble vitamins and trace elements) and sodium balance under regular review in case supplements to the feed are necessary.

Table 19.27 Investigations in intestinal failure: acute (less than 4 weeks old); chronic (more than 4 weeks old)

		Acute (less than 4 weeks old)	Chronic (more than 4 weeks old)
Key clinical facts to be elicited		Vomiting related to feeding or not Bile present in vomitus? Presence of pain Nature of diarrhea: watery, offensive, blood present?	Symptoms are static, improving worsening? Which is the dominant symptom? Does the diarrhea reduce when nil by mouth (osmotic), or is it similar in fasting and fed state (secretory)
Biochemistry	Blood Urine Stool	Electrolytes, chloride, acid–base, amylase Acidification, laxative screen Microscopy including electron microscopy Culture, ELISA test for rotavirus and adenovirus Reducing substances, electrophoresis Chymotrypsin, steatocrits	Liver function tests, parathyroid hormone Urinary sodium:potassium ratio Stool electrolytes (? sodium losing diarrhea; see also Table 19.24) Intestinal transit time by the appearance of orally administered pigment in stool (e.g. Carmine red) Fecal alpha-1 antitrypsin concentration
Hematology		Full blood count (polycythemia ?dehydrated) blood film (?fragmented cells as in hemolytic uremic syndrome)	Full blood count, anemia, also note neutropenia (Shwachman syndrome), lymphopenia (lymphangiectasia) Coagulation profile (? vitamin K malabsorption)
Radiology		Plain abdominal X-ray (gas pattern, intramural gas?, calcification) Abdominal ultrasound to identify cystic lesions, e.g. pancreatic pseudocyst	Small bowel contrast study (provides information about malrotation, reflux, motility disorders) Scintiscanning (gastric emptying) Abdominal ultrasound to identify portal hypertension Venogram if difficulty with central venous access
Manometry			Esophageal, upper small bowel and rectal manometry, depending on likely site of lesion
Histopathology		Mucosal biopsy Full thickness biopsy of large bowel and proximal bowel if indicated	Duodenal or jejunal tissue for disaccharidase measurement Liver biopsy, repeat intestinal mucosal biopsy

Avoidance of complications

Infection

The child with intestinal failure is susceptible to serious infections mainly via the i.v. feeding catheter. Skin organisms which have colonized the catheter via the hub and access ports can cause major systemic upset in the presence of the PN solutions. Less frequently bacteria from the bowel appear to translocate to the circulation. Infection from any source however is a risk factor for hepatic impairment, especially in the preterm infant who will become chronically cholestatic after two or three infections when such infections occur within months of birth.[65] Sepsis at any age diminishes transport of bile from hepatocytes into bile canaliculi, leading to retention of bile salts, which itself leads to disruption of hepatocyte function.[66] Other risk factors include overprovision of nutrients, which is associated with depletion of glutathione, induction of steatosis, and lipids especially if the daily infusion rate exceeds 3.5 g/kg. Avoiding sepsis depends on good hygiene and restricting the number of individuals who have access to the feeding catheter. In France it has been shown that patients discharged home on PN had one tenth the incidence of central line infections compared to hospitalized patients.

Hepatic

In patients fed by the i.v. route, purified nutrients consisting of simple glucose, essential amino acids, and triglyceride (derived from soya oil) are delivered to the hepatic sinusoids via the hepatic artery without the benefit of intestinally derived growth factors. This may explain the frequently observed phenomenon of fatty liver in parenterally fed patients (see also Table 19.28). Patients who are fed exclusively by the parenteral route are more likely to experience cholestasis. Total enteral starvation deprives the liver of intestinally derived growth factors and hormones including cholecystokinin and is associated with reduced portal blood flow, reduced bile secretion at canalicular level and impaired motility of the large bile ducts. Other risk factors for cholestasis include:

1. Prematurity since the immature liver is unsuited structurally (paucity of bile ductules) and physiologically (detoxification and conjugation and transulfuration pathways are inadequate[66]) to handle nutrients which have not been processed by the placenta or only partly digested in the immature intestine. The majority of babies less than 28 weeks' gestation who receive PN after surgery become cholestatic;[65]
2. Emergency abdominal surgery, especially if it leads to short gut syndrome;
3. Lack of a multidisciplinary care team.[61,67]

Avoiding liver damage therefore depends on establishment of oral feeding as soon as possible, rigorous hand washing routine and a low threshold for suspecting and treating infection.

Thromboembolism and thrombosis

This is more commonly a complication of long-term PN, although there are case reports of extensive thrombosis of the inferior vena cava occurring a few days after insertion of a femoral line. A review of patients at Great Ormond Street Hospital, England showed that 30% of patients on long-term PN had evidence of pulmonary embolus, and around 10% of children referred for small bowel transplantation had superior vena cava thrombosis; most such children have a history of 10 or more insertions of the feeding catheter.[68] Strategies for avoiding this complication have been reviewed by European Society of Paediatric Gastroenterology Hepatology and Nutrition (ESPGHAN) and the following treatments

Table 19.28 Complications of parenteral nutrition upon the liver

Biliary sludge, gall stones and occasionally cholecystitis
Steatosis which may be intense and lead to hepatomegaly and fibrosis
Fibrosis which may be portal and within the parenchyma ('pericellular fibrosis')
Cirrhosis and portal hypertension

are used: oral warfarin, oral aspirin, heparin added to the vamin compent of the PN solution. The use of ultrasound to locate veins, and the designation of a senior surgeon to be responsible for line insertion are recommended good practice.

Social isolation

The nursing skills which parents are obliged to learn and the need to protect their child from accidental damage to his feeding catheter mean that some families are disinclined to travel outside their home except for hospital visits. The involvement of a social worker, specialist nurse and play specialist are vital in encouraging the child and family to integrate in society, to benefit from education and to make adequate developmental progress despite the restrictions of PN. Contact with self-help groups such as Patients on Intravenous and Nasogastric Nutrition Therapy (PINNT), who have a children's section, Half-PINNT and the Children's Liver Disease Foundation (CLDF) can be encouraged (see Charities and Organizations, p. 654).

Surgical

Nontransplant surgery

This consists of a range of surgical operations ranging from those which are consequent on the primary procedure such as closure of a stoma previously created to treat a bowel perforation, to identification and repair of strictures, to reconstruction of residual intestine. The indications and timing for reconnection surgery are usually clear, but intestinal lengthening and tapering operations remain somewhat controversial. Since some poor early experiences in which prolonged surgery was carried out in infants already experiencing hepatic complications, it is now recognized that longitudinal intestinal lengthening and tapering operations (the Bianchi procedure) are more successful in children with dilated nonpropulsive bowel who are at least 12 months old and in whom intestinal adaptation appears to be static. Nontransplant surgery for short gut is likely to proliferate as innovative surgeons describe techniques such as the creation of artificial strictures and reverse segments for expanding the residual bowel prior to lengthening and tapering.[69] Patients who have been referred for possible small bowel transplantation may be suitable for this kind of nontransplant surgery, so it is important for specialist teams to network even when operating in different institutions.[62]

Isolated liver transplantation in short bowel syndrome

For a small group of patients who could be expected to be weaned off PN by the the age of 5 years because they have at least 40 cm residual small bowel and have tolerated significant amounts of enteral nutrition, the option of isolated liver transplant rather than combined liver and bowel transplant, could be considered if they develop liver failure whilst still dependant on PN. This is a challenging group with a prolonged postoperative recovery time who require careful selection and the involvement of a multi-disciplinary team.[62,63,66,67,69]

Small bowel transplantation

The small bowel, being a hollow viscous contaminated with bacteria, liable to autolysis and prone to intense rejection, has proved to be difficult to transplant, but experience is increasing rapidly with 180 patients per year receiving grafts, and results are improving to the point where they are starting to parallel the outcome of i.v. nutrition.[70] Since 2000, breakthroughs in the form of monoclonal antibodies targeting the receptors for triggering rejection (anti-CD 25 receptors on T lymphocytes) and the other therapies for depleting lymphocytes such as: (1) administering humanized monoclonal anti-thymocyte globulin, (2) pre-treatment of the recipient with Campath, and (3) pre-treatment of the small bowel allograft with anti-lymphocyte globulin have been described. The main gain in these new approaches is the reduction in tacrolimus and steroid exposure and is associated with 1-year survival rates in the order of 80–100%.

The 3- and 5-year survival reported from the Intestinal Transplant Registry remains at 50%; however, results are somewhat better in individual busier centers (Pittsburgh, Omaha, Miami) where 25–50 transplants per center are performed annually and in which 3-year survival has exceeded 65% since 2001.[70,71] Nevertheless, this still means that the transplant option is generally reserved for patients with life-threatening complications such as PN-related liver disease or recurrent line sepsis.

Indications for referral. Most transplant centers are prepared to review patients with intestinal failure at any stage, but recommend early referral if the child is becoming progressively jaundiced (i.e. if plasma bilirubin is in excess of 100 μm/L), where there are problems with maintaining fluid balance despite the provision of PN, or if there are complications associated with placing a feeding catheter.[72] Results from the international transplant registry and the UK[67] clearly show that delayed referrals have an adverse impact on survival: the difference in survival between adult patients who are hospitalized (40–60%) versus those who are still at home (80–100% survival) when called to transplant makes it almost unethical to delay evaluating patients for small bowel transplantation once they start experiencing complications on home PN. Patients who have developed a thrombosis of the superior vena cava may become impossible to cannulate safely and require stenting of the superior vena cava[68] to maintain them prior to isolated bowel transplant provided their liver function is satisfactory. Failure to progress with intestinal adaptation and tolerance of enteral feeds in patients with short gut may also prompt a referral.

Types of intestinal transplants (see Fig. 19.9). Of the 989 intestinal transplants carried out in 923 individuals and reported to the Intestinal Transplant Registry 2003 (http://www.intestinaltransplantregistry.org/), 606 were children. Half (n = 306) were combined procedures with liver and bowel, 37% were isolated small bowel transplants and about 13% multivisceral involving variously stomach, colon, pancreas, kidney combined with small bowel and liver grafts. In infants for whom small donors are very scarce, a technique to cut down the size of organs from donors up to five times the size of the patient has been developed[73] (see Fig. 19.9c). The survival after isolated bowel transplant is better in the first 12 months (90% compared with 70% for combined liver and bowel transplants), but the long-term complications of rejection and opportunistic infections are similar, resulting in a 3–5-year graft survival, which is no different when compared to combined liver and bowel grafts.

Complications. The complications related to small bowel transplantation are numerous.[74] Early complications are generally related to the surgery and the consequences of organ preservation and reperfusion. These include perforation of native bowel and transplanted bowel (30% in pediatric series), bile leaks, pancreatitis, stomal prolapse, ileus and translocation of enteric bacteria to the liver and systemically via the portal vein. Unlike isolated liver transplantation, thrombosis of the splanchnic vasculature (i.e. portal vein, hepatic artery) is almost unheard of because the anastomoses are large, usually being made between the aorta on the arterial side and inferior vena cava on the venous side.

Early medical complications include generalized edema secondary to fluid retention, ileus secondary to morphine, acute cellular rejection of the small bowel allograft and infection by enteric bacteria. Rejection of the small bowel is common and causes fever, deterioration in absorption of feed and changes in the morphology of the mucosa (apoptosis combined with a mixed inflammatory infiltrate). Severe rejection is less common since the advent of monoclonal antibodies active against T cell receptors which mediate rejection, but it is important to treat promptly as untreated rejection may progress rapidly to severe rejection in 12–48 h. This can be life threatening with full-thickness lesions associated with bloody diarrhea, peritonitis and systemic sepsis from escaping enteric bacteria.

The long-term complications are mainly related to opportunistic infections including cytomegalovirus, cryptosporidiosis, mucosal fungal infections and EBV. The EBV is a particularly important complication for children after intestinal transplantation in whom it is often a primary infection. In the context of selective T lymphocyte inhibition induced by tacrolimus treatment, the B lymphocytes infected with the EBV proliferate greatly and may become malignant, resulting in post-transplant lymphoproliferative disease (PTLD). Up to 30% of small bowel transplant recipients in the transplant program in Pittsburgh developed PTLD within 2 years of transplantation with half (15% overall) eventually died from this complication. Optimal management requires routine testing for EBV genome copies in blood using PCR techniques and the use of antiviral agents such as ganciclovir and rituxamab (an anti-CD20 antibody which destroys B lymphocytes) which has brought about an improvement in the outcome of PTLD since 2000. Chronic rejection appears to be a vascular phenomenom in which the mesentery of the distal bowel in particular becomes infiltrated with inflammatory cells, leading to occlusion and ischemia. The early symptoms are subtle, resembling an intermittent distal ileal obstruction syndrome. Small bowel transplant recipients also experience the usual childhood infections such as otitis media and viral gastroenteritis, notably rotavirus and adenovirus; the latter can be severe and necessitate a temporary resumption of PN to hasten recovery.

Outcome. Historically, one in five small bowel transplant recipients did not survive the early postoperative period, reflecting their poor condition at the time of surgery. However, those children who are discharged from hospital do well, with 90% completely independent of PN and maintaining normal growth rates. The number of appliances such as Broviac lines, nasogastric tubes, gastrostomy tubes, and stoma bags reduces steadily in the 3 years after transplant. Most families report a sense of greater freedom and improved quality of life compared with that which they experienced with i.v. feeding before the transplant.

INTESTINAL FAILURE AND QUALITY OF LIFE

Measurement tools for quality of life are numerous,[75] but the most commonly used ones appear to be questionnaires in which the subject chooses one of five possible choices in response to questions about emotions (hopes and fears), physical function, pain, relationships (e.g. The General Health Questionnaire [GHQ], The Nottingham Short Form-36, The Euro-Qol Questionnaire), and semi-structured questionnaires which allow a more individualized response by the subject. In children on PN, it is clear that families cope with the demands of home PN by developing obsessive/neurotic traits and that there is a high incidence of depression among them compared with the general population. In the case of children after small bowel transplant, a study from the Nebraska medical center showed an improved quality of life as rated by the children themselves after the transplant, although their parents expressed different perceptions and did not score so highly for quality of life.[76]

PROGNOSIS

Although chronic intestinal failure is a disabling condition with long-term implications for the child's development and carers, medical

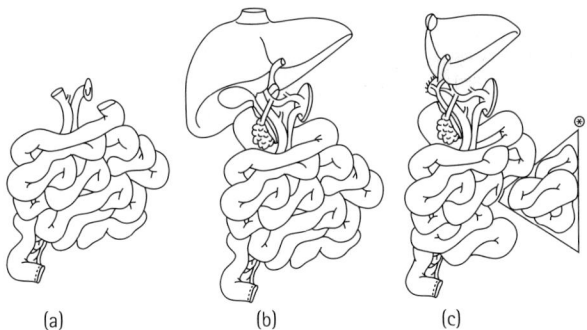

Fig. 19.9 Anatomical sketch of (a) isolated small bowel allograft, (b) combined liver and small bowel allograft, and (c) reduced en-bloc liver and small bowel allograft. (Line drawing by J de Ville de Goyet)

(a)   (b)   (c)

advances have improved survival and allowed such children to be kept alive and even discharged home with good quality of life.[63] In children without major complications the 5-year survival rate is around 95%.[67] In contrast, children who develop serious complications, especially cholestasis, are at risk of early death from overwhelming sepsis. Of 55 children assessed at the Birmingham Children's Hospital (England) and considered to fulfill criteria for intestinal transplantation between 1993 and 2003, 20 died of infection and or liver failure before they could be transplanted. Children with intestinal failure who are experiencing a delay in being discharged on home PN, or deteriorating despite home PN, should be referred for assessment by a multidisciplinary team, which includes gastroenterologists working with a transplant team, to allow them to have the opportunity to have their intestinal failure treated by the full range of medical and surgical options in an integrated manner up to and including intestinal transplantation.[62,70]

THE COLON

STRUCTURE

The colon is a long hollow tube which, with the exception of the sigmoid, which has a short mesentery, lies retroperitoneally. Along its length from the ileocecal valve to the anus the mucosa is lined by a cuboidal epithelium which is indented with crypts. The mature colon has no villi and no brush border disaccharidase activity. Submucosal and myenteric nerve plexuses are present, similar to those in the small intestine, but the smooth muscle layers differ in that the longitudinal layer is incomplete, forming three tenia coli.

FUNCTION

The large intestine fulfills both storage and salvage functions. The colon stores the intestinal contents prior to excretion, but it is also an organ of conservation which reduces liquid ileal effluent to solid feces excreted via the anus. It plays an important role in the salvage of electrolytes and water, and in addition, the salvage of nutrients in the form of short chain fatty acids.

Absorption

Although it is clear that the majority of water and electrolyte absorption occurs in the small intestine, it is often the adequacy of colonic function which determines whether the child experiences diarrhea, and whether or not there is net loss of water and electrolytes from the body. In small intestinal disease there is an increase in the volume of fluid arriving at the ileocecal valve but the colon has a reserve reabsorptive capacity which can adequately absorb the excess ileal effluent. When there is massive small intestinal secretion, the reserve reabsorptive capacity of the colon may be overwhelmed, resulting in diarrhea. In addition, in disorders which compromise colonic function such as inflammatory bowel disease (IBD), diarrhea may occur as a result of either reduced colonic absorptive capacity or frank colonic secretion.[77]

The importance of the colonic sodium absorptive mechanism is demonstrated clinically by the high rate of sodium supplementation necessary for normal growth in infants with ileostomies. The majority of sodium absorption occurs via an active, electrogenic mechanism, while chloride is absorbed down its electrochemical gradient. Potassium is secreted into the lumen, largely in response to electrochemical gradients and, in older children bicarbonate is secreted into the colonic lumen via an exchange mechanism with chloride. It has previously been shown that colonic sodium absorptive processes are already highly efficient in preterm infants and there is evidence that circulating aldosterone levels may be important in the regulation of these mechanisms.[78] In addition to its role in the absorption of water and electrolytes, the colon may also salvage extra nutrient energy from the contents of the gastrointestinal tract via the absorption of short chain fatty acids such as acetate, butyrate and propionate. These are produced by colonic bacterial fermentation of unabsorbed dietary carbohydrate and studies have shown that they are rapidly absorbed from the large intestine, providing a significant additional source of energy, and also that they promote further colonic salt and water absorption.

The salvage of electrolytes, water and nutrients requires sophisticated integration of the functions of bacterial digestion, epithelial transport and motor activity of the colonic muscle layers. Details of colonic motility patterns are scanty in childhood, although a major proportion of the total mouth to anus transit time occurs in the large intestine.

INFLAMMATORY BOWEL DISEASE

Although infective agents are the commonest cause of IBD in a worldwide context, the term will be used in this section to describe chronic inflammation of the gastrointestinal tract in the absence of a detectable pathogenic agent. Included in this definition in descending order of importance are Crohn's disease, ulcerative colitis and allergic colitis. In addition, the term 'indeterminate colitis' has been employed to describe children with colitis which is impossible to precisely categorize at presentation: the final diagnosis may often only become evident in these patients with the lapse of time and further, or repeated, investigation.

EPIDEMIOLOGY

The prevalence of Crohn's disease in both Wales and Scotland[79,80] appears to have increased in the 1980s and 1990s, with the incidence of Crohn's being at least twice as common as ulcerative colitis. In Sweden, the incidence of pediatric IBD has also increased over a 10-year period,[81] although in contrast to the UK this was primarily an increase in ulcerative colitis. A prospective study of pediatric IBD in the British Isles, from the British Paediatric Surveillance Unit (BPSU), has suggested an estimated incidence of IBD of 5.3 per 100 000 children under the age of 16, equivalent to about 700 new cases per annum in the UK, with Crohn's disease again being twice as common as ulcerative colitis.[82] This study suggests that 10% of patients may be of Asian origin (an over-representation compared with the overall population) with some 5% of patients from the Afro-Caribbean population. There is a slight male preponderance (58%). In childhood the peak in incidence is between 11 and 13 years, although 13% of cases in the recent BPSU study developed in children aged less than 10 years. Although Crohn's disease and ulcerative colitis may present in early childhood, it seems likely that many cases of colitis presenting in the first 2 years of life may be related to food allergy that responds to an appropriate exclusion diet, and with a favorable long-term prognosis.[83]

ETIOLOGY/PATHOPHYSIOLOGY

The etiology and pathogenesis of Crohn's disease and ulcerative colitis are unknown despite many theories and much painstaking research work.[84,85] There is no doubt that there is a genetic preponderance for both diseases and twin studies suggest a much higher concordance in monozygotic than in dizygotic twins. It is likely that Crohn's disease and ulcerative colitis are related polygenic diseases,[86] and genome-wide linkage studies have identified a number of possible susceptibility genes, involving several chromosomes with some loci being more specific for UC and some for CD including the CARD15 gene (previously known as NOD2) on chromosome 16q.[87] Some genes influence disease susceptibility while others only affect the course of the disease and more research is needed on the significance of the genotype and phenotype interactions.

Multiple immunological abnormalities have been described in patients with IBD but none has convincingly been shown to be a primary pathogenetic event. Environmental factors such as bacterial pathogens or their products, dietary components and intercurrent infections appear necessary to trigger and maintain the diseases and may well interact with specific genes. The basic problem appears to be an over-stimulation or over-reaction of the mucosal immune system to a particular antigenic stimulus in genetically susceptible individuals although the antigenic stimulus, such as a microorganism or food antigen, may vary from case to case. Though there has been controversy over the role of the measles virus, and indeed the measles mumps rubella (MMR) vaccine, there is no convincing evidence that this is related to the development of IBD. Infectious agents have been postulated as playing a major role but so far the evidence is inconclusive. There is no conclusive evidence for causal associations for any environmental exposure in the etiology of Crohn's disease or ulcerative colitis, although there is strong evidence incriminating dietary allergens, particularly dairy produce and soya milk, in the pathogenesis of allergic colitis in younger children.

Studies have, however, shown that intestinal permeability may be increased in Crohn's disease and it is conceivable that this could result in an increase in absorption of antigens from the gut, which may be important in the pathogenesis of the disease. Finally, it has been suggested that psychosomatic factors may be important and a 'colitis personality' was previously defined. However, several studies have not supported this concept and it is hardly surprising that there may be a higher incidence of emotional problems and depression found in sufferers and their families as a consequence of their chronic, debilitating disease. Thus adequate psychological and emotional support from health care staff is of paramount importance in the management of children with IBD. Adequate communication is vital, and several self-help groups publish helpful booklets and can provide additional support and information for the child and family (see Charities and Organizations, p. 654).

CROHN'S DISEASE

Pathology

The disease may involve any part of the gastrointestinal tract from the lips to the perianal area, and normal bowel may be found in between affected areas. The inflammation is transmural, often extending from the mucosa to the serosal surface, resulting in sinus tracts or fistulae formation. In childhood disease, terminal ileitis is common with variable involvement of the colon in 50–70% and the recent UK British Paediatric Surveillance Unit study[82] suggested that one third of patients have small intestinal disease, one third ileocolitis and one third colitis, with total colitis being more common (50%) than segmental colitis or isolated proctitis. Macroscopically, the bowel mucosa may look inflamed, and small shallow, aphthoid or linear ulcers may be present. Later on in the disease, deeper fissures may occur, leading to the classic 'cobblestone' appearance of the mucosa, as well as stricturing of the bowel. Histologically, there is transmural inflammation and the diagnostic hallmark is the finding of noncaseating epithelioid granulomata with giant cells which may not be present in all affected tissues.

Clinical features

The insidious onset and subtle nature of the symptoms and signs of Crohn's disease often result in a considerable delay in diagnosis with left-sided colonic disease being usually diagnosed more rapidly than diffuse small intestinal disease. The manifestations of the disease depend upon the site of involvement but periumbilical, colicky abdominal pain, diarrhea with or without blood and growth failure are the commonest forms of presentation. Occasionally more subtle manifestations, such as oropharyngeal disease, perianal skin tags and fissuring or growth failure, may be the first signs of the disorder in the absence of overt gastrointestinal symptoms. The diarrhea in Crohn's disease is likely to be due to a combination of several factors which may include mucosal dysfunction, bile acid malabsorption, bacterial overgrowth and protein exudation from inflamed bowel.

On examination, it is important to ascertain whether extraintestinal manifestations of Crohn's disease are present. Thus there may be intermittent pyrexia, clinical anemia, arthralgia and arthritis, uveitis, finger clubbing, perianal disease (skin tags, bluish discoloration, fissures, fistulae), oral ulceration, skin manifestations (erythema nodosum and pyoderma gangrenosum), signs of liver dysfunction and evidence of growth failure and delayed sexual maturation. Examination of the abdomen may reveal generalized or localized tenderness and occasionally an ill-defined palpable mass. The importance of growth retardation and pubertal delay must be emphasized as it may occur in up to 30% of children with Crohn's disease and may be present well before the diagnosis is made.[88] There is little evidence that this is due to a primary endocrine disturbance

and the most likely reason for growth failure is nutritional deprivation or a direct effect of inflammatory molecules such as cytokines on the growing skeleton. Growth failure must be detected earlier as there is evidence that this can be successfully reversed by prompt treatment.[89]

Osteopenia has been recognized as an important complication of IBD, particularly in children with Crohn's disease and, although the mechanisms are not yet fully elucidated, the cause appears to be a combination of both the disease itself and drug treatment with steroids.[90]

Diagnosis

Laboratory assessment involves the search for infective agents in the stools of patients with Crohn's disease presenting with diarrhea. Hematological investigation often reveals iron-deficiency anemia and acute phase reactants such as erythrocyte sedimentation rate (ESR) and C reactive protein (CRP) may be elevated, although not universally. Thrombocytosis and hypoalbuminemia may also be present and these appear to be more reliable markers of disease activity. Plasma zinc levels are frequently low and liver function tests may be abnormal. It should, however, be remembered that alkaline phosphatase is a zinc-dependent enzyme which may be spuriously depressed in the presence of zinc deficiency. Recent studies also suggest that measurement of stool calprotectin, a protein secreted into the gut by lymphocytes, is a reliable indicator of intestinal inflammation.[91]

Radiological assessment is important and plain abdominal X-rays may reveal evidence of intestinal obstruction or bowel dilatation. A barium meal and follow-through is vital in order to assess the small bowel and, although a small bowel meal (via a transpyloric tube) is the most sensitive technique, this is not always acceptable as it may be particularly uncomfortable for the child. The presence of skip lesions, with narrowing of the lumen, thickening and fissuring ('rose-thorn ulcers') of the bowel wall and fistulae formation are all highly suggestive of Crohn's disease (Fig. 19.10).

Technetium white cell scanning has been suggested as a useful investigation for initial screening/follow-up but there is continued debate about the sensitivity and specificity of this investigation.[92] With proper bowel preparation, magnetic resonance imaging of the small intestine is possible and virtual colonoscopy using computerized tomographic scan-

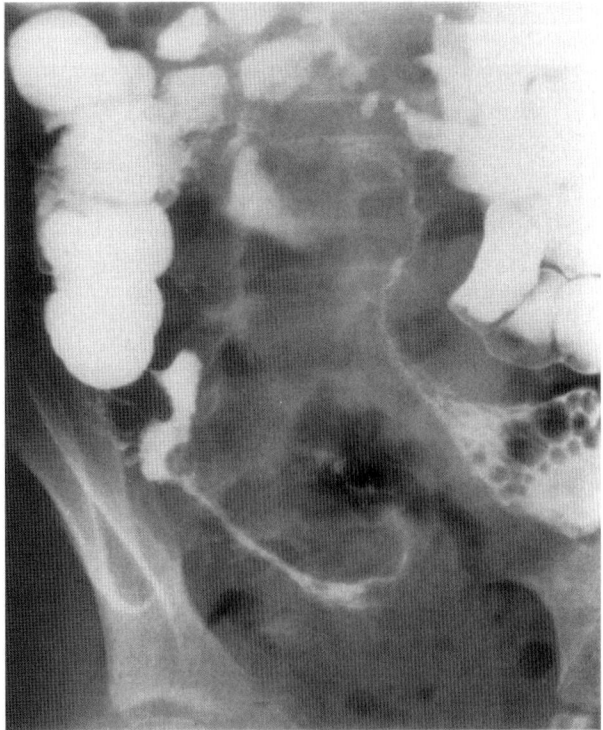

Fig. 19.10 Extensive narrowing of the ileum in a child with small intestinal Crohn's disease. (Reproduced by kind permission of P J Milla)

ning is available in some centers. Small bowel disease may be detected by capsule endoscopy although this investigation is contraindicated if a stricture is present. The main weakness of all these techniques is that they do not allow mucosal biopsy.

Endoscopy remains the most important tool for assessing both the upper gastrointestinal tract and colon (Fig. 19.11), and colonoscopy has superceded the barium enema as the primary investigation of the lower bowel. Several authors have suggested that upper intestinal endoscopy should be performed at the same time as colonoscopy, as a majority of patients with IBD may show histological abnormalities in the upper gastrointestinal tract, which may be useful in diagnosis.

Treatment

The goal of therapy is both to induce and maintain a remission of active disease and also to correct malnutrition and promote growth. Two main treatment modalities are available, one being drug therapy and the other nutritional therapy. They can if necessary be combined. They are

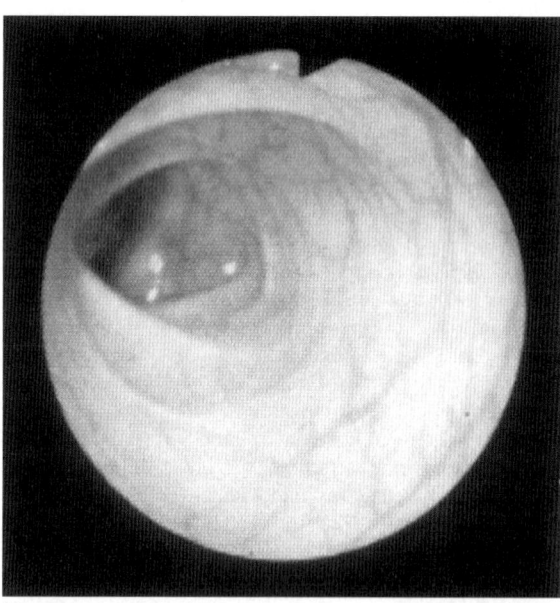

(a)

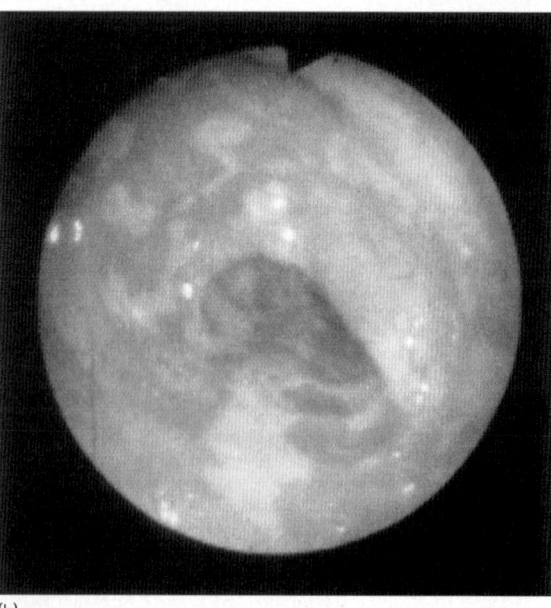

(b)

Fig. 19.11 The colonoscopic appearance in (a) a normal child with the mucosal blood vessels clearly seen and (b) in a child with Crohn's disease showing 'snail tract' ulceration and loss of the vascular pattern of the mucosa. (Reproduced by kind permission of P J Milla)

probably both equally effective with drug therapy being preferred where disease is localized to the colon, weight has been maintained and compliance with nutrional therapy is likely to be problematic. Where there has been significant weight loss prior to diagnosis and small bowel disease is present, nutritional therapy is to be encouraged. Where these treatments fail surgical intervention may be required.

Drug therapy

There is no convincing evidence that any drug alters the long-term natural history of Crohn's disease, but several agents have a place in the treatment of the disorder. Steroids may induce remission in over 70% of patients and prednisolone should be given in an initial dose of 2 mg/kg/d (max. 40–60 mg) with a gradual reduction after 2–4 weeks, preferably to an alternate-day regimen in order to minimize the growth-suppressive side-effects. There is no good evidence that low-dose steroid therapy can maintain remission and, if possible, steroid therapy should be gradually reduced over a further 6–8 weeks and stopped if the disease is quiescent.[93]

5 amino salicylic acid (5ASA) drugs such as mesalazine slow release (15–20 mg/kg [max. 1 g] three times a day) and sulfasalazine (50–80 mg/kg/d) are useful in the treatment of active Crohn's colitis in inducing remission, although there is little evidence that continuous therapy will maintain remission. The pure 5ASA preparations such as mesalazine have fewer site-effects than sulphasalazine and are therefore now used as the preparation of first choice. There is an increasing use of immunomodulatory drugs, such as azathioprine and 6-mercaptopurine, which allow reduction or cessation of steroids and also help to maintain remission. However, although very useful, such drugs are potentially hazardous and their use should be monitored carefully. Metronidazole may be effective in colonic and particularly perianal disease although peripheral neuropathy may develop with its long-term use. In children who are acutely toxic and systemically unwell on presentation, it is reasonable to start i.v. broad-spectrum antibiotics, including metronidazole, in addition to i.v. steroids until the disease begins to remit. Where perianal diasease is troublesome topical treatment with tacrolimus 0.1% may be helpful.

There are potential advances in the use of new biological drugs such as anti-TNF alpha monoclonal antibodies. Inflammatory cytokines (such as TNF alpha) tend to be consistently elevated in the mucosa and the anti-TNF alpha monoclonal antibody shows promise as an agent which, through blockage of TNF, will reduce disease activity in patients resistant to conventional treatment. However, its place in the treatment of children with Crohn's disease is presently being established and concerns still remain about its long-term safety.

Nutritional therapy

Nutritional therapy is recognized as a very important therapeutic modality in Crohn's disease, not only in the correction of specific nutrient deficiencies, but also in the reduction of disease activity and the reversal of growth failure. Patients may need specific therapy with iron, folate, vitamin B_{12} and zinc in addition to ensuring an adequate energy intake via the oral or nasogastric route or indeed via i.v. feeding. Furthermore, nutritional therapy has been shown to be effective in inducing remission of active disease[94] and both enteral and parenteral routes may be used. Over the last decade, there has been increasing use by pediatric gastroenterologists (though less use by adult gastroenterologists) of enteral nutrition as a primary therapy to induce remission. An analysis of five randomized clinical trials comprising 147 children showed that enteral nutrition was as effective as corticosteroids in inducing remission;[95] however there is still debate as to the appropriate place of enteral therapy in the treatment of Crohn's disease and randomized trials involving large numbers of patients are necessary. Several questions remain unanswered, i.e. how the enteral therapy works, whether a polymeric diet is as effective as an elemental diet, whether or not large intestinal disease is treated as effectively as small intestinal disease and the role of on-going maintenance – there is some evidence that intermittent periods of enteral feeding may maintain remission, but these results need to be confirmed.

Surgical treatment

The indications for surgical intervention in Crohn's disease include intestinal obstruction, fistula formation, hemorrhage and perforation, and a failure of medical therapy, particularly where there is growth failure. The surgical results in Crohn's disease are most encouraging in children with localized ileal disease,[96] although children with both large and small bowel disease may require reoperation at a later date. Elective surgery is perhaps most important in children nearing puberty with specific growth problems and it is very important to use as an option when the disease is not too extensive and it is feasible to resect the diseased bowel. The early use of surgery can be vital during the narrow window of therapeutic opportunity before the pubertal growth spurt is complete. Colectomy in ulcerative colitis is curative while in Crohn's disease, although surgery may modify the immediate outcome, it does not prevent recurrence.

Prognosis

The prognosis for childhood Crohn's disease is reasonably optimistic and, although the morbidity is relatively high, the mortality is low. Psychosocial aspects particularly those influencing quality of life are being investigated in the childhood IBD population.

The risk of colorectal carcinoma in children with Crohn's colitis is not well defined although there is a suggestion that the incidence is slightly increased when compared with a control population. Long-term follow-up studies are needed to clarify this point and in the meantime the large intestine in patients with persistent colitis should be inspected regularly by colonoscopy through adult life.

ULCERATIVE COLITIS

Pathology

Ulcerative colitis is an inflammatory disease of the large intestinal mucosa and the abnormal changes are seen most commonly in the rectum and distal colon, although the whole colon may be affected. Indeed, pancolitis is the most common form (62%) while disease of the left colon (22%) or rectum (16%) occurs less frequently. Unlike Crohn's disease, the inflammation is continuous and it is usually limited to the colonic mucosa. Macroscopically the mucosa is friable and granular, and ulceration may be present in association with a bloody or mucopurulent exudate. The ulceration, which is often patchy, may be interspersed with areas of regenerating epithelium, resulting in pseudopolyp formation. In addition, there may be an inflammatory reaction in the distal ileum, so-called 'backwash ileitis'. The characteristic histological features are an acute and chronic inflammatory cell infiltrate in the lamina propria, distortion of crypt architecture, the presence of crypt abscesses and goblet cell depletion.

Clinical features

The commonest presenting features are diarrhea, often associated with blood and mucus, and tenesmus with lower abdominal pain, which is relieved by defecation. Attacks may be graded as mild, moderate or severe depending upon stool frequency, abdominal tenderness, fever and the degree of anemia and hypoalbuminemia. It is important to recognize that 5–10% of patients with ulcerative colitis may present with fulminating colitis associated with toxic megacolon, and a plain abdominal X-ray should be performed to look for the presence of a dilated colon (usually exceeding 6 cm in diameter).

On examination the only positive findings may be minimal lower abdominal tenderness, although in severe disease the child may be pyrexial, dehydrated, anemic and profoundly toxic. It is important to look carefully for evidence of extraintestinal manifestations which are similar to those of Crohn's disease, although growth retardation occurs less frequently in ulcerative colitis and affects less than 20% of patients at presentation.

Diagnosis

Infective agents such as *Shigella*, *Salmonella*, *Campylobacter*, *Yersinia* and *Entamoeba* may cause an acute or chronic colitis, and it is vital to look carefully for pathogens in the stool and perform appropriate serological tests. Further laboratory assessment may reveal anemia, raised levels of ESR and CRP, leukocytosis and hypoalbuminemia which may reflect the disease activity. Radiological investigations should include plain abdominal X-ray, in patients with severe disease, and a good colonoscopy examination makes barium enema examination unnecessary. Endoscopic evaluation of the whole colon is very useful in assessing both the severity and extent of inflammation. However, the procedure should be deferred, or at least limited, in patients with acute severe colitis because of the risk of toxic megacolon and perforation.

Treatment

Therapy is directed towards inducing and maintaining remission in mild or moderate disease and may be life saving in fulminating colitis. Patients with mild disease are best treated with mesalazine slow release (15–20 mg/kg [max. 1 g] three times a day) or sulfasalazine (50–80 mg/kg/d) and, in those children with disease confined to the distal colon, a topical steroid or 5ASA preparation may be useful. Moderately severe disease (bloody diarrhea five times/d, abdominal pain, fever) may require the addition of oral steroids (prednisolone 1–2 mg/kg/d, max. 40–60 mg) in order to induce remission, and this dose should be gradually reduced after 2 weeks if the child's condition is improving. Antispasmodic medication and agents which decrease gut motility should not be given as they may precipitate the development of toxic megacolon.

Severe, fulminating colitis is a medical emergency which is easily underestimated. The child should receive nothing by mouth and i.v. therapy is always indicated. The patient will usually need rehydration and blood transfusion, and regular albumin infusions are often required. All children should receive i.v. hydrocortisone (10 mg/kg/d) and broad-spectrum antibiotics (ceftriaxone and metronidazole) and, if malnourished, PN should be instituted at an early stage. Many children with severe colitis will respond to this aggressive medical therapy within 7–10 d, but if by this time there is no improvement rescue therapy with i.v. cyclosporin should be considered. If the child develops a complication such as toxic megacolon, colonic hemorrhage or perforation, then surgery is necessary. In addition to emergency surgery for complications of acute disease, elective surgery may be required if there is a failure of medical therapy, severe growth retardation unresponsive to improved nutrition or severe colonic dysplasia with the risk of adenocarcinoma formation in long-standing colitis. The surgical procedures available for the child include a proctocolectomy with ileostomy or ileal reservoir, or a colectomy with rectal mucosectomy and endorectal pull-through.

As regards the maintenance of remission, there is good evidence that continued therapy with a 5ASA is superior to placebo in preventing relapse although, in some patients, alternate-day steroids may also be required. Immunosuppressive drugs are proving to be useful in patients with intractable disease.

In contrast to Crohn's disease, there is less compelling evidence that aggressive nutritional therapy alone, either enteral or parenteral, is effective in inducing remission in ulcerative colitis, although the correction of malnutrition and specific nutritional deficiencies is mandatory in all patients.

Prognosis

Approximately 90% of patients with ulcerative colitis presenting in childhood or adolescence will experience one or more relapses of their disease after initial treatment. The majority will be able to lead a relatively normal life despite chronic disease but some 20% will be chronically incapacitated. The prognosis is best for isolated, distal colitis, with only 10% progressing to pancolitis; overall, approximately 30% of patients will eventually require colectomy. There is an increased risk of developing large intestinal adenocarcinoma in patients with long-standing ulcerative colitis, although the risk is probably considerably less than previously thought.[97] The advent of flexible endoscopy has made possible careful, regular surveillance of the colonic mucosa and colonoscopy and biopsy should be performed at regular intervals in older patients with long-standing colitis.

RECTAL BLEEDING

The passage of small amounts of blood per rectum is not uncommon in childhood and is rarely of sinister significance, being often due to a simple anal fissure or self-limiting infective colitis. It is important to determine whether it is bright red blood that has been passed, around, after or mingled with the stool as in the case of bleeding from the colon, or whether the blood is altered, or indeed melena, which may signify a more proximal source of bleeding. It is also helpful to determine whether there is mucus or slime in the stool or if there is associated diarrhea or constipation, abdominal pain or perianal pain on defecation.

Clinical examination should attempt to assess the degree of blood loss and whether anemia is present. Adequate visualization of the perianal region is mandatory and the use of a pediatric proctoscope may yield important diagnostic clues. General examination includes a detailed examination of the skin for evidence of purpura and telangiectases, circumoral pigmentation, and evidence of arthritis and renal abnormalities should be sought. Although direct visualization of the stool may reveal fresh blood or melena, chemical testing may be required when occult bleeding from a more proximal source is present. A number of kits are available for the testing of occult fecal blood, although most are highly sensitive and are likely to give false-positive results, particularly if the child is receiving vitamin C supplements or food high in peroxidase activity such as uncooked vegetables.

Etiology

Table 19.29 outlines some of the commoner causes of rectal bleeding in childhood. It is important at any age (particularly in the neonatal period) to exclude swallowed blood as a cause of rectal bleeding. The etiology of bleeding per rectum is influenced by the age of the patient and also by the mode of clinical presentation. Thus, a child with chronic constipation who passes bright red blood on the surface of the stool may have an associated anal fissure, while the infant with intussusception may present with colicky abdominal pain, shock and the passage of 'red currant jelly stools'. Acute vomiting and bloody diarrhea may herald the onset of intestinal infection and the presence of hematuria and proteinuria may suggest Henoch–Schönlein purpura or the hemolytic uremic syndrome. Chronic blood loss with the painless passage of bright red blood is suggestive of a colonic polyp or hamartoma and a detailed family history may be helpful.

Table 19.29 Causes of rectal bleeding in childhood

1. Anal fissure
2. Infective colitis
   a. *Shigella*
   b. *Salmonella*
   c. *Campylobacter*
   d. *Escherichia coli* O157
3. Allergic colitis
4. Intestinal polyps
   a. Juvenile polyps
   b. Familial polyposis coli
   c. Peutz–Jeghers syndrome
   d. Gardner syndrome
5. Generalized bleeding diathesis
6. Inflammatory bowel disease
7. Rectal prolapse
8. Intussusception
9. Meckel's diverticulum/gut duplication
10. Henoch–Schönlein purpura
11. Hemangioma/angiodysplasia/telangiectasia
12. Upper gastrointestinal bleeding

Investigation and treatment

The pattern of investigation will depend upon the urgency of the clinical presentation. Thus an infant who is shocked and passing bright red blood per rectum will need resuscitation and an urgent plain abdominal X-ray or ultrasound and possibly an air contrast enema to exclude intussusception. Usually the presentation is less acute and initial laboratory assessment should include a full blood count, ESR, serum iron and ferritin estimation, serum electrolytes and clotting studies. In cases of bloody diarrhea, stool culture is mandatory and plain abdominal X-ray may be helpful. The most useful investigation is colonoscopy, which after scrupulous bowel preparation will provide direct visualization of the colonic mucosa and allow multiple biopsies to be obtained for histology. Furthermore, the procedure may be therapeutic as smaller polyps may be removed at colonoscopy by diathermy.

Isotope scanning using technetium may identify ectopic gastric mucosa in either a Meckel's diverticulum or in a duplication of the intestine, and labeling of red blood cells with the isotope may also be useful in detecting the site of active, but occult, gastrointestinal blood loss. In the last resort, in selected cases of severe chronic unexplained iron-deficiency anemia associated with positive fecal occult blood, it may be necessary to perform angiography to localize the source of bleeding and rarely laparotomy and intraoperative endoscopy is indicated. Capsule endoscopy may be helpful in visualizing more proximal sources of bleeding.

CHRONIC GASTROINTESTINAL SYMPTOMS

RECURRENT ABDOMINAL PAIN

Recurrent abdominal pain is a relatively common pediatric problem, occurring primarily in older children and adolescents. The term generally describes recurrent and moderately severe episodes of abdominal pain over a period of at least 3 months which may lead to absence from school and may affect the child's lifestyle. Typically the pain is nonspecific although most children describe colicky, periumbilical discomfort. Most importantly the child is healthy in between these episodes and physical examination is normal; 10–20% of schoolchildren are affected.[98]

Etiology and pathogenesis

Although early studies showed that in only 7% of cases is an organic cause found to explain the pain, it is increasingly recognized that many conditions may cause such pain, such as constipation, abdominal migraine,[99] gastritis and peptic ulcer associated with *H. pylori* and the irritable bowel syndrome[100] (Table 19.30). As clinical examination is usually normal, it is vital to take a detailed and comprehensive history which may provide clues as to the etiology of the pain.

Table 19.30 Organic causes of recurrent abdominal pain in childhood

1. Gastrointestinal
   a. Constipation
   b. Peptic ulceration/gastritis
   c. Gastroesophageal reflux
   d. Anatomical abnormalities
      (i) Meckel's diverticulum
      (ii) Malrotation
   e. Inflammatory bowel disease
   f. Food intolerance
   g. Infection (e.g. *Yersinia ileitis*)
   h. Pancreatitis
   i. Hepatobiliary disease
2. Others
   a. Migraine
   b. Urinary tract disorder
      (i) Chronic infection
      (ii) Hydronephrosis
      (iii) Calculi

Where the pain has lasted for more than 6 months with no associated weight loss, bleeding or diarrhoea, a non-organic cause is most likely. Psychological disturbances including over-reaction to normal life events and family dysfunction have often been considered important in the pathogenesis of the symptoms. However, studies have failed to show any psychological differences among children with recurrent abdominal pain compared with control subjects, although a proportion of these children and their families may benefit from psychological or family therapy.

Management

Blanket investigation is no substitute for a careful history and examination although selective laboratory and radiological testing may be necessary, based on the pediatrician's clinical assessment. Routine urine testing and culture is mandatory and a full blood count and ESR may be helpful in excluding anemia and inflammatory conditions. If the child's symptoms are suggestive of pancreatitis, then a serum amylase may be useful when the child is experiencing pain, and liver function tests may be abnormal in children with pain due to hepatobiliary disease. Radiological investigations are usually unhelpful although a plain abdominal film will reveal calcification and gross constipation which may not be evident clinically. An abdominal ultrasound can be of use, particularly if urinary symptoms are suspected, but only rarely is it necessary to perform barium studies in order to exclude malrotation and IBD. Screening for *H. pylori* infection (see pp. 609–10) may not be helpful in children with generalized abdominal pain but where symptoms suggest peptic ulcer disease, upper gastrointestinal endoscopy and biopsy will be required.

Treatment will depend on the clinical assessment and on the results of investigations undertaken. It is important to exclude constipation as therapeutic intervention may alleviate the child's pain. In children where there is a typical history of abdominal migraine,[101] a trial of anti-migraine prophylaxis such as pizotifen and/or the exclusion of cheese, chocolate, citrus fruit and caffeine (the 4Cs) is sometimes justified, particularly if the child is missing a substantial amount of schooling. In the majority of cases, however, none of these measures is indicated and the most important therapeutic maneuver is to reassure the child and his parents that there is no serious organic disease present. It is often helpful to emphasize that the disorder is common in childhood and that the symptoms are likely to improve with age. It is important also to explain that although there is no obvious organic cause for the pain, it is not suggested that the pain is imaginary; rather it can be useful to admit that we as physicians do not understand why the pain is occurring, but do know that stress and emotional upheaval will tend to exacerbate the symptoms. In some children who present with intractable symptoms it is helpful to enlist the services of either a child psychologist or psychiatrist at an early stage so that a joint approach can be made in the exclusion of organic and non-organic causes for the recurrent abdominal pain.

Prognosis

Prospective follow-up studies have been undertaken in children with recurrent abdominal pain and these suggest that a substantial proportion of children may continue to suffer in adult life from the symptoms of IBS. Furthermore it has been suggested that in children who develop symptoms at an early age and in whom treatment is delayed, the prognosis may be worse. It is tempting to speculate that recurrent abdominal pain in childhood and the IBS found in later life are manifestations of the same condition, although further large prospective studies are needed to clarify this point.

INFANTILE COLIC

Infantile colic is a condition which is difficult to classify and define. It is used to describe the baby who, in the first few weeks of life, has frequent spells of inconsolable crying, usually occurring in the evening, and often associated with excessive flatus. The infant appears to be suffering abdominal pain although the 'colic' is intermittent and usually self-limiting, often subsiding after 3 months of age. The disorder occurs equally in boys and girls and may occur in up to 20% of all babies in the first few months of life. The pathogenesis of the disorder is still unclear and several etiologic theories have been proposed including psychosocial factors, a failure of parent–infant interaction and milk allergy.[102]

Although the pathogenesis of the disorder is unclear, all the evidence points to an intestinal origin for the discomfort, and fundamental physiological and clinical research needs to be undertaken in order to understand the phenomenon more clearly.

As regards management, the most important therapeutic maneuver is to carefully examine the baby and reassure the parents that colic is common, self-limiting and without harmful long-term effects. Many remedies have been tried but the sheer number of treatment options testifies to the fact that none works particularly well. However, for the parents who are at the end of their tether, it may be worth a trial of simple measures such as gripe or peppermint water, and where a child is clearly atopic a cows' milk exclusion may be of benefit; a whey-based hydrolysate formula is the feed of choice. Counseling and support of the parents, however, remains the mainstay of management.[103]

Although the condition is usually self-limiting by 3 months of age, some children continue to experience colic throughout the first year of life and go on to develop recurrent abdominal pain and the irritable bowel syndrome in later life.

CHRONIC CONSTIPATION

Although often regarded as a less than glamorous and rather insignificant problem by many physicians, chronic constipation is of great importance to the child and his family. It should be stressed that early accurate assessment and prompt treatment of constipation is vital to the child's well-being and lifestyle, as delays in management will only exacerbate the problem and perpetuate the child's lack of self-esteem and feelings of hopelessness. Furthermore it has been shown that constipation may cause reversible urinary tract abnormalities that may predispose the child to urinary tract infection and enuresis.[104]

The term 'constipation' is used to describe difficulty or delay in the passage of stools, which may progress to a chronic state where defecation is infrequent and the bowel motions passed are hard pellets or firm and very bulky; in addition there may be leakage of fecal liquid around the hard compacted stools in the dilated rectum causing soiling, which is distressing for the child and may result in inappropriate referral to a child psychiatrist. It is important to distinguish chronic constipation and associated overflow incontinence from true encopresis, which is the voluntary passage of normal stools in an inappropriate fashion or place. Normal bowel frequency varies widely although the average baby passes three to six stools per day in the neonatal period, one to two stools per day at 1 year of life and approximately one stool per day, or every other day, in the preschool years.[105]

Pathophysiology and clinical features

Although the vast majority of children presenting with constipation have no serious underlying organic pathology, it is generally true that the younger the child, the more likely it is that the problem is due to a congenital abnormality of the lower bowel. It is particularly important to diagnose Hirschsprung disease (see Ch. 37) at an early stage, as the infant is at risk from developing an associated and severe life-threatening enterocolitis. Such children almost always have symptoms of constipation dating from before 3 months of age with the majority presenting in the first few days of life. Most children with chronic constipation, however, present in the preschool years with symptoms that may have been present for several months and sometimes several years. In these children it is unlikely that organic disease is present although the organic pathologies shown in Table 19.31 should be considered. A careful history and examination, particularly of the perianal region, is crucial in the evaluation of the problem, and the need for further investigation is dictated by the clinical assessment.

Table 19.31 Organic causes of constipation

1. Dietary
2. Dehydration
3. Intestinal obstruction
4. Anal fissure/stenosis
5. Hirschsprung disease
6. Hypo/hyperganglionosis
7. Cerebral palsy
8. Spinal cord lesion
9. Cystic fibrosis
10. Food allergy
11. Hypothyroidism
12. Hypercalcemia
13. Hypokalemia
14. Lead poisoning
15. Renal failure

By the time most children present to the pediatrician, an enlarged megacolon full of hard feces is present. The child is usually otherwise well although abdominal pain and occasionally nausea and vomiting may be associated with chronic constipation. The original genesis of the constipation is often difficult to pinpoint and several initiating factors may have been involved such as a loss of appetite during an acute illness, the prescription of constipating medications following a bout of diarrhea, pain from an anal fissure, a stressful life event, difficult toilet training made worse by inadequate facilities at school or aggressive management by parents determined to see their child toilet trained at a very early age. It has also become clear that chronic constipation may be a manifestation of food intolerance and this should be considered in a child or family with a strong history of atopy.

Chronic constipation is most often the end result of a sequence of events which starts with an episode of acute constipation which is inadequately treated. Adequate bowel evacuation relies on the child experiencing the urge to defecate consequent on the distension of the rectum with feces. If this urge is suppressed, for whatever reason, retained feces become hard and painful to expel, the rectum becomes distended, reducing rectal sensation, and the urge to defecate is diminished. A consequence of this chain of events is persistent fecal loading, a capacious rectum and frequent overflow soiling caused by fluid stool passing around the hard feces and staining the child's pants. As a result of these symptoms the parents may adopt a punitive approach towards the child which may compound an already unfortunate situation.

The problem of chronic constipation in children with neurological disability such as cerebral palsy, or spinal cord abnormalities such as myelomeningocele, is especially intractable due to a combination of reduced sensation, weakness of the muscles of the pelvic floor and abdominal wall, and also particular abnormalities of gastrointestinal motility in these patients. These difficulties should be anticipated and appropriate measures taken at an early stage.

Management
Prompt management of children with acute constipation may prevent the development of chronic constipation and the vicious cycle outlined earlier.[106] In the baby with delayed passage of meconium and continuing constipation, Hirschsprung disease should be excluded by rectal suction biopsy at an early stage. Investigation of older children and exclusion of the rare organic causes of chronic constipation will depend on the clinical features following a careful history and examination. Laboratory assessment is usually not warranted, but a plain abdominal film may occasionally be helpful in assessing the degree of constipation and the size of the rectum, and also to demonstrate the fact to the child and his parents. General measures such as ensuring an adequate fluid and fiber intake are important and the advice of a pediatric dietitian is helpful in this regard. If anal stenosis is present, then repeated gentle anal

dilatation, or an anal stretch under anesthesia, may be of benefit. It is important to carefully examine the perianal region for the presence of an anal fissure as the application of local anesthetic preparations may encourage the child to open his bowels.

It is important to explain to the child and his parents the sequence of events leading to chronic constipation and to outline the aims of therapy, which are designed to clear the enlarged rectum and distal colon of feces, and subsequently keep it empty. It should be stressed that the situation is not the child's or family's fault and that treatment may involve many months of therapy. It is vital to provide a reassuring approach that the situation will improve, although setbacks and further bouts of constipation may be encountered during this period. It is not adequate to prescribe a 2-week course of laxatives and tell the family that the situation will improve with time. In practical terms, the initial therapeutic goal is to empty the rectum and distal colon and this can usually be achieved by oral disimpaction regimens although occasionally there is a need for enemas. This can often be undertaken on an outpatient basis if the general practitioner or health visitor is enthusiastic, but sometimes it is necessary to admit the child to hospital for 2 or 3 days for the disimpaction regimen and also to establish that the bowel is empty with an abdominal radiograph prior to starting maintenance laxative therapy. Once the large intestine is empty, oral laxatives should be prescribed in adequate doses to ensure that the child's bowels are open at least once a day. This can be achieved by a combination of a stool softener such as lactulose with a stimulant aperient such as senna, although a macrogol preparation such as Movicol (Norgine) is becoming the treatment of choice. If the initial dose of laxatives is inadequate, it should be increased; if the laxatives result in diarrhea the dose should be reduced. With time, however, sensation will return to the rectum as its size decreases, and the amount of laxative medication can eventually be decreased and finally stopped.

In addition to medical therapy, it is usually beneficial to institute a behavioral program based on simple rewards such as a modified star chart, where the child is rewarded for a normal, daily bowel action. This is coupled with advice that the child should be able to visit the toilet in a relaxed atmosphere at regular times and it is helpful to see the child regularly in the outpatient clinic, initially at fortnightly intervals, to provide continuing support and encouragement. The child should be encouraged to drink plenty of fluids and to eat a good balanced diet containing fruit and vegetables.

Treatment of children with chronic neurological disease and spinal cord lesions poses particular difficulties and early institution of regular suppositories and oral laxative therapy may be helpful. Furthermore, the development of an enema continence catheter or the use of an anterior continence enema (ACE procedure) whereby the colon is emptied on a regular basis is providing a useful adjunct in patients with constipation and fecal incontinence who experience little or no rectal sensation.

Overall the long-term prognosis for functional chronic constipation is excellent and this should be emphasized to the child, the parent and the physician.

Short segment Hirschsprung disease
In a small proportion of children who present in childhood with a history of chronic constipation dating from birth and associated with the delayed passage of meconium, a diagnosis of short segment Hirschsprung disease is made. In these children anorectal manometry is abnormal but rectal biopsy may be unremarkable. The term 'internal sphincter spasm' may be a more appropriate term for this condition with treatment involving a full anal sphincter stretch and internal sphincterotomy performed under general anesthesia.

In some children with chronic constipation rectal biopsy may show either an increase or decrease in the number of ganglion cells. Such hypo- or hyperganglionosis undoubtedly can result in altered colonic motility which leads to chronic constipation and the development of a megacolon.

CHRONIC NONSPECIFIC DIARRHEA

The syndrome of chronic nonspecific diarrhea (CNSD, previously known as toddler diarrhea or irritable colon of childhood) is now recognized to be the commonest cause of diarrhea without failure to thrive in early childhood; the mechanisms underlying the disorder are largely unknown and speculative, thus making it difficult to advise with confidence about management. It has been suggested that CNSD is self-limiting in 90% of cases, although others have reported a high incidence of constipation on follow-up and a significant history of functional bowel disorders in close family members.[107] Indeed it seems likely that CNSD may be merely part of a spectrum of gastrointestinal motility disorders that includes colic in infancy, recurrent abdominal pain in older children and IBS in adults.

Clinical features

Children with CNSD present with loose stools usually between the ages of 6 months and 5 years. The condition is commoner in boys and a careful history will usually elicit the characteristic features of a variable pattern of stool consistency and frequency, often following an initial episode of acute gastroenteritis, with firmer stools passed in the morning and decreasing in consistency later in the day. Occasionally there may be a history of alternating diarrhea and constipation and the presence of undigested foods (especially peas and carrots), with or without mucus, is typical of the disorder. The diarrhea is often exacerbated by a high roughage diet, fruit and sugary drinks. The absolute characteristic of the condition is the absence of faltering growth, and it is of paramount importance to carefully document the child's height and weight on presentation and at subsequent follow-up. If the child is failing to gain weight and height, the diagnosis must be suspect and further investigation is then warranted.

Etiology and pathogenesis

Although the precise pathophysiological mechanisms operating in CNSD are unknown, several possible etiological factors have been suggested. It is important to exclude excessive intake of fruit juices as a cause of diarrhea. Food allergy can cause similar symptoms in childhood and, although circumstantial evidence for this may be present in the form of a strong personal or family history of atopy, the most important diagnostic test is the response to an elimination diet and challenge. It has been suggested that a low dietary fat intake is a possible cause of CNSD as gastric emptying and gut transit time may be slowed by increasing dietary fat intake. It is thus conceivable that a diet low in fat causes rapid gastric emptying with increased propagative motor activity resulting in the formation of loose stools.

Abnormal intestinal secretion has been implicated in the causation of CNSD as has a primary motility disturbance. It has been suggested that some children with CNSD may demonstrate a significantly higher incidence of environmental indicators of personal or family stress compared with matched controls,[108] which is in keeping with the anecdotal experience of many clinicians.

Diagnosis

CNSD is primarily a diagnosis of exclusion although there are certain positive clinical features, already described, which may provide a pointer to the diagnosis. The prime feature is that the child is healthy and growing normally. In some children there may be a family history of functional bowel disorders, or indeed a personal or family history of food intolerance. It is important to exclude both urinary and enteric infection although food intolerance and the postenteritis syndrome are the main differential diagnoses. Any evidence of malabsorption, atypical clinical features or failure to thrive should prompt further investigation.

Treatment

In the majority of cases, simple reassurance is all that is required. It is important to explain to the parent that, apart from the loose stools, the child is otherwise well and thriving, and the problem is likely to improve.

It is also useful to explore the probable etiology of the disorder, which may be explained in terms of deranged motility which will improve with time. It is very important to emphasize that growth and general health will be normal in the future, and there will be no delay in achieving continence. Most parents will accept with relief the fact that their child has no serious disease, but for parents who feel that the problem is too difficult to manage, further measures may be necessary.

It is important to advise the parents to avoid giving an excessive intake of fruit juices or squash. Dietary treatment may be beneficial and, in those children with a strong personal or family history of atopy or in whom chronic diarrhea was manifested following an episode of acute gastroenteritis, a trial of an exclusion diet (usually cows' milk and egg free) may be helpful. The services of an experienced pediatric dietitian are invaluable, and the diet must be adhered to for at least 1 month before any decisions are taken about its efficacy. If there is an improvement in symptoms, the diet is continued for at least 3 months before trying to gradually reintroduce the excluded foods. Some pediatricians have achieved success by increasing the child's fat intake so that 50% of the calories are derived from fat.

There is evidence that loperamide may provide symptomatic improvement and it can be used intermittently. All drugs, however, have significant side-effects and they should be prescribed only in carefully selected cases.

Prognosis

Overall parents can be reassured that the prognosis for their child with CNSD is very good. In the past, the condition has been described as benign and self-limiting and although it is known that diarrhea may persist after toilet training, it usually becomes less obvious to the parents who no longer have to change dirty nappies. It is possible that a proportion of children who manifest CNSD may represent one end of a spectrum of familial functional bowel disorders which will re-emerge as continuing gastrointestinal complaints as they become older.

INVESTIGATION OF THE COLON

Investigation of colonic anatomy and physiology has in the past been difficult, largely owing to the relative inaccessibility of the large intestine and the fact that investigation has involved the use of invasive techniques and exposure to radiation. Those investigative techniques in most common usage are described later.

Radiology

The plain abdominal film (supine and/or erect) can be very useful in the investigation of acute and chronic gastrointestinal disease. Thus the presence of fluid levels may indicate intestinal obstruction, and free gas in the peritoneal cavity may represent intestinal perforation. Repeated plain abdominal films are an essential part of the management of toxic megacolon associated with colonic inflammatory disease such as fulminant ulcerative colitis.

Barium enema examination is now used much less frequently to study colonic anatomy since the advent of colonoscopy, although it may yield useful diagnostic information as well as being potentially therapeutic in cases of intussusception. The indications for barium enema examination include neonatal intestinal obstruction and intussusception. The use of double contrast barium enema technique is preferable for demonstrating colonic polyps or subtle mucosal disease, although it can be an uncomfortable examination for the child and almost all the indications for such investigation have been superceded by colonoscopy. The need for barium enema examination in Hirschsprung disease has largely been replaced by the use of rectal suction biopsy.

Radioisotopic scanning after injection of technetium-labeled leukocytes may have a part to play in the diagnosis of the site and extent of inflammatory disease[109] and occasionally patients with unexplained lower gastrointestinal blood loss may require investigation by a ^{99m}Tc-labeled red blood cell scan or selective angiography of the inferior mesenteric artery.

Rectal suction biopsy

Biopsy of the rectal mucosa and submucosa is the most useful technique for diagnosing Hirschsprung disease but it also may be helpful in the diagnosis of neural lipidoses and amyloidosis. The technique is usually carried out under sedation, and multiple biopsies at varying intervals from the anal margin can be taken. The biopsies are studied for the presence or absence of ganglion cells and for the activity of cholinesterase.[110]

Colonoscopy

The use of flexible endoscopy in pediatric practice has revolutionized the investigation of large intestinal disease in childhood.[111] Using the technique it is possible to traverse and visualize the whole colon and also to obtain multiple biopsies for histological assessment.

Proctoscopy can be performed easily at the bedside in older children and the use of an auroscope may be useful in neonates. Rigid sigmoidoscopy is uncomfortable for the child and this technique has been superseded by the use of small diameter flexible pediatric colonoscopes. Colonoscopy may be performed under sedation using a combination of pethidine and midazolam given intravenously immediately prior to the procedure. Alternatively a short general anesthetic may be more comfortable for the patient, easier for the operator and reduce recovery time. For an adequate inspection of the colon to be undertaken, it is vital that bowel preparation is effective and this may require the administration of 'clear fluids' for 24 h before the examination in addition to generous doses of laxatives and occasional recourse to rectal washouts. The procedure is generally well tolerated and the experience of centers using the technique in childhood has been that the complication rate is minimal.

Virtual colonoscopy using magnetic resonance imaging is not yet widely used in children with colonic disease. The inability to directly visualize the mucosa and to take mucosal biopsy means that endoscopic colonoscopy is likely to remain the gold standard for the investigation of intestinal inflammation.

Motility studies

Anorectal manometry is a useful technique for distinguishing the different causes of constipation and is particularly helpful in the diagnosis of short segment Hirschsprung disease where the characteristic abnormality of failed internal sphincter relaxation is seen. Large bowel transit can be measured by the ingestion of multiple radio-opaque markers followed by a plain abdominal film at 48 h and 72 h. More detailed investigation of colonic motility is at present only available in research centers.

HEPATIC AND BILIARY DISEASE

ANATOMICAL STRUCTURE AND FUNCTION OF THE LIVER

The anatomical site and structural organization of the liver are designed to maintain close homeostatic control of the constituents of portal blood when returned to the hepatic venous system. Substrates from the portal system are rapidly taken into the liver cells, metabolized, and their products stored or transferred as required into the blood and bile. Blood-, bile- and lymph-containing channels transport nutrients, metabolites, antigens, antibodies, hormones and drugs to and from hepatocytes, and also to the other specialized liver cells, the Kupffer cell, the sinusoidal endothelial cell, the stellate cells and to the cells of the biliary tree.

The basic functional unit of the liver is the acinus, being the parenchyma receiving its blood supply from a hepatic artery and portal vein in a single portal tract. Traversing the sinusoids, specialized capillaries lined by Kupffer and endothelial cells which contain fenestra allow ready access of plasma and its contents to the surface of the hepatocyte (Fig. 19.12).[112] The sinusoids drain to the central vein of the hepatic lobule, and into the inferior vena cava. The hepatocytes near the portal tracts receive more oxygen, nutrients and hormones, have a higher metabolic rate, synthesize more proteins and regenerate more rapidly than those nearer the central vein, which are particularly susceptible to hypoxic and toxic injury. This structure can regain its pristine condition when

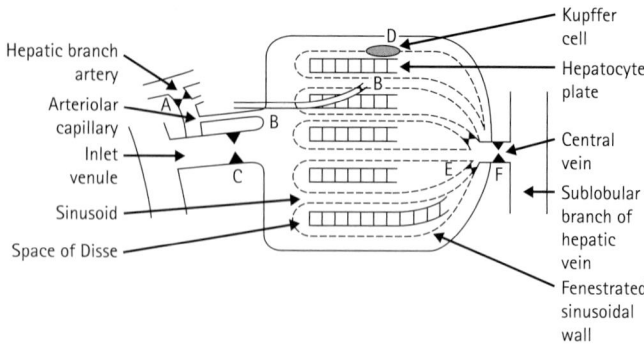

Fig. 19.12 A diagrammatic representation of the liver sinusoids and their blood supply. A–F represent sites of possible sphincters involved in controlling blood flow through the hepatic sinusoids. (Reproduced from *Liver Disorders in Childhood*[112] by kind permission of Elsevier Science Ltd.)

destroyed by acute toxins such as paracetamol or type A viral hepatitis but persisting injury with infiltration by cells of the reticuloendothelial system sets in train deposition of extracellular matrix components leading ultimately to irretrievable disruption of the acinar relationships by cirrhosis, with consequences for homeostatic function.

CLINICAL ASSESSMENT OF LIVER DYSFUNCTION

Unfortunately, the sensitivity and specificity of many clinical symptoms and signs in liver disease are low so disease may be present without detectable signs or symptoms and those present may not be specific to liver disease. Thus, for example, it is possible to have chronic viral hepatitis B for decades proceeding to cirrhosis without any external or even biochemical evidence. Features with some degree of sensitivity in established liver disease are:

- Jaundice with dark urine implies cholestasis. The urine of infants should not contain significant color or stain the nappy. Yellow sclerae also suggest cholestatic jaundice but are often difficult to detect in small infants and those with scleral pigment.
- Liver palms are not often seen in the first year of life.
- Splenomegaly indicating portal hypertension, although as children get older a larger spleen can be accommodated beneath the ribs, further reducing the sensitivity of this sign.
- Coagulopathy in the context of cholestasis may represent failure of absorption of sufficient vitamin K particularly leading to vitamin K deficiency bleeding of the newborn when intracranial bleeding is associated with severe long-term morbidity. Infants should not normally suffer spontaneous bleeding and fresh blood from sites such as the umbilicus or nares should always prompt a search for evidence of liver disease. Jaundice may be so mild as to be disregarded in such cases. When coagulopathy is not responsive to vitamin K, coagulation factors are being consumed intravascularly or not being formed. Thus in the patient with liver disease and coagulopathy unresponsive to vitamin K but without consumptive coagulopathy liver synthetic failure must be present. This criterion is the most sensitive for liver failure in children. Hypoglycemia and encephalopathy are less so.
- White stools, or stools the color of cream cheese or uncooked pastry are clearly abnormal. Those with mild degrees of green pigment or pale yellow or a pale buff brown color may also evidence reduced bile flow. Particular emphasis should be placed on examining stool and urine personally, as the history particularly from first-time parents can be misleading.
- Hepatomegaly is likely to be associated with liver disease, hepatic mass, infiltration or cardiac failure. Normal infants may have up to 2 cm of liver edge palpable parallel to and below the costal margin with soft texture. Riedel's lobe is seldom encountered

in practice. Firm/hard texture and an irregular inferior margin strongly suggest established liver disease with fibrosis/cirrhosis. Changed liver conformation with prominence in the midline but an impalpable right lobe suggests collapse, regeneration and the development of cirrhosis. A liver of this shape is also found in the Budd–Chiari syndrome as a consequence of caudate hypertrophy. Tenderness of a smooth liver suggests rapid recent increase in liver size, e.g. acute hepatitis or cardiac failure.

Severity of liver dysfunction can be considered in three broad categories. These are:

1. cholestasis, implying impairment of bile flow with reduction of intraluminal bile salt concentration, conjugated hyperbilirubinemia and raised serum bile acids causing pruritus;
2. portal hypertension (PHT) with associated hypersplenism and the effects of porto systemic shunting (if present);
3. hepatocellular impairment with evidence of failure of synthetic and homeostatic function.

Clinical and basic laboratory findings can be interpreted according to this classification although some such as ascites are represented in more than one category (Tables 19.32 and 19.33). Transudative ascites can result from a combination of increased portal pressure and low plasma oncotic pressure (implying low serum albumin). Serum albumin reflects liver synthetic function but also depends on nutritional status and losses, e.g. via the gastrointestinal tract or kidneys. Thus it is necessary to consider all clinical features supported by laboratory parameters in order to evaluate the severity of liver disease.

Table 19.32 The clinical features of liver disease and their significance

Clinical features	Cholestasis	PHT	Cell function
Jaundice	Conjugated	–	Mixed if severe
Pruritus	+	–	–
Leuconychia	+	–	–
Clubbing	+	–	–
Fat-soluble vitamin deficiency	+	–	–
Xanthomas	+ but not in PFIC	–	–
Splenomegaly	–	–	+
Clubbing	+	–	–
Cutaneous shunts	–	+	–
Other cutaneous stigmata	–	+	+
Hypersplenism	–	+	–
Cyanosis – hepatopulmonary syndrome	–	+	–
Esophageal varices	–	+	–
Ascites	–	+	+
Encephalopathy	–	+	+
Dependent edema	–	–	+
Malnutrition	+	+	+

PFIC, progressive familial intrahepatic cholestasis; PHT, portal hypertension

Ultrasound

Ultrasonography has become a mainstay in examining liver parenchyma texture, anatomical structures, portal and arterial blood flow and intrahepatic lesions. Particular examples are cysts, abscesses, solid tumors, hemangioendotheliomas, dilatation of the biliary tree from choledochal cysts and tumors. Calculi, sludge and polyps in the gallbladder can be visualized. Parenchymal echotexture may be altered with cirrhosis, edema in acute hepatitis, in storage disorders and with fatty or malignant infiltration. Splenomegaly and portal and hepatic arterial flow patterns can be evidence of portal hypertension. It is unhelpful in diagnosing biliary atresia other than it may show an absent or irregular small gallbladder.

Other imaging

CT scanning, MRI, cholangiography and angiography, percutaneous transhepatic cholangiography (PTC) and endoscopic retrograde cholangiopancreatography are informative although their safe and/or effective use requires specialist diagnostic imaging expertise.

Percutaneous liver biopsy

Skilled histological interpretation, histochemical and biochemical analysis and bacterial, fungal or viral culture of liver biopsy tissue may be of crucial diagnostic importance, giving information on the severity of liver damage and also in assessing the requirements for therapy in chronic hepatitis. An ultrasound scan, to exclude a focal liver lesion or bile duct dilatation, is required before a biopsy. If the following contraindications are observed the risk of significant bleeding is of the order of 1 in 5–10 000:INR (international normalized ratio for prothrombin time) greater than 1.3, platelet count of less than 70×10^9/L, the presence of clinical ascites, hydatid cyst or abscess in the right lobe of liver, angiomatous malformation of liver and hepatocellular carcinoma but not hepatoblastoma. It should only be undertaken with adequate vascular access by trained personnel having immediate surgical support.

NEONATAL CHOLESTASIS SYNDROME

Hepatitis in infancy is characterized by clinical and laboratory features of hepatic inflammation with conjugated hyperbilirubinemia.[113] It must be suspected in any jaundiced infant, particularly if the urine is yellow, or if jaundice persists beyond 14 days of age. Specimens of stool must be saved in a container excluding light and examined for pigment by the clinician personally according to the description earlier (Clinical assessment, p. 642). If the stools contain no yellow or green pigment, cholestasis is complete and biliary atresia must be suspected.

Occasionally, infants will present with bleeding diathesis, hypoglycemia, fluid retention or malabsorption. The most important investigation is INR following administration of parenteral vitamin K, which if it remains abnormal indicates acute liver failure (ALF).

The prognosis is that of the associated disorder (see remainder of chapter), with positive family history, consanguinity and normal serum gamma-glutamyltranspeptidase (gamma-GT) predictors of the development of progressive intrahepatic cholestasis. Chronic liver disease rarely occurs in cholestasis associated with acute infections, or when disease remains cryptogenic after full investigation.

Table 19.33 Laboratory features of liver disease and their significance

Laboratory features	Cholestasis	PHT	Cell function
Serum bilirubin	Conjugated	–	Mixed
Serum albumin	N	N (low in severe enteropathy)	Low
Serum cholesterol	High except in FIC	N	Low
Prothrombin time/ratio	N if vitamin K replete	N*	Prolonged if severe

N, normal; PHT, portal hypertension
*Implies minor prolongation seen in portal vein thrombosis

Differential diagnosis

Three management priorities can be identified:

1. to prevent complications such as vitamin K deficiency bleeding and hypoglycemia;
2. to identify treatable bacterial, metabolic, endocrine or hematological disorders and initiate treatment (Tables 19.34 and 19.35);
3. to diagnose biliary atresia as early as possible so as to optimize the surgical outcome.

Biliary atresia must be considered in any infant remaining jaundiced beyond 14 days of age. Evidence of consanguinity or liver disease in siblings suggests the possibility of familial, genetic, metabolic or hemolytic disease. Physical abnormalities are occasionally very helpful (Table 19.36).

Vitamin K deficiency bleeding, hypoglycemia, septicemia, urinary tract infection, syphilis and herpes simplex infections, listeriosis and toxoplasmosis all have effective treatments. Galactosemia (low RBC galactose-1-phosphate uridyl transferase activity), fructosemia (often a history of dietary exposure to honey can be obtained) and tyrosinemia (urinary succinylacetone excretion) should also be excluded immediately since dietary treatment is available. Inborn errors of bile acid

Table 19.34   Disorders associated with neonatal cholestasis

1. Intrahepatic disorders
   a. Inherited disorders
   b. Endocrine abnormalities
   c. Vascular abnormalities
   d. Severe hemolytic disease
   e. Chronic hypoxia and circulatory abnormalities
   f. Chromosomal anomalies
   g. I.v. nutrition
   h. Drugs
   i. Alagille syndrome
   j. Sclerosing cholangitis
   k. Maternal systemic lupus erythematosus
   l. Variants of progressive intrahepatic cholestasis
   m. Idiopathic
2. Extrahepatic disorders
   a. Biliary atresia
   b. Choledochal cyst
   c. Spontaneous perforation of the bile duct
   d. Inspissation in the biliary system
      (i)   Hemolytic disorders
      (ii) Cystic fibrosis
      (iii) Total parenteral nutrition
      (iv) Congenital infections
   e. Gallstones
   f. Malignant nodes
   g. Tumor of the duodenum or pancreas
   h. Hemangioendotheliomata

Table 19.35   Inherited disorders associated with neonatal cholestasis

1. Galactosemia
2. alpha-1-antitrypsin deficiency
3. Cystic fibrosis
4. Tyrosinemia
5. Niemann–Pick types A&C
6. Gaucher disease
7. Wolman disease
8. Zellweger syndrome
9. Polycystic disease (ARPKD)
10. Erythrophagocytic reticulosis
11. Neonatal hemochromatosis
12. Defects in synthesis of primary bile acids
13. Variants of progressive intrahepatic cholestasis (PFIC)

Table 19.36   Helpful physical findings in neonatal cholestasis

Physical signs	Disorder suggested
IUGR, skin lesions, purpura, choroidoretinitis, myocarditis	Congenital infections
Cataracts	Galactosemia, hypoparathyroidism
Multiple and characteristic abnormalities	Trisomy 21, 18, 13, Lawrence–Moon–Biedl, Beckwith–Wiedemann syndromes
Mass beneath liver	Choledochal cyst
Ascites, bile stained hernia and umbilicus	Spontaneous perforation of the bile ducts
Murmur, characteristic facies, embryotoxon	Alagille syndrome
Cutaneous hemangioma	Hemangioendothelioma of liver
Situs inversus, cardiac defect 'cor triatum'	Biliary atresia
Optic nerve hypoplasia, wandering eye movements, micropenis	Hypopituitarism

synthesis can respond to primary bile acid treatment. Early diagnosis of alpha-1 antitrypsin deficiency (see Ch. 20 p 648) cystic fibrosis and Niemann–Pick C clarifies the prognosis and allows genetic counseling. Associated endocrine disorders (Table 19.37) must also be excluded on the basis of the clinical findings and appropriate laboratory investigations. Current subgroups of progressive familial intrahepatic cholestasis (PFIC)[114] appear in Table 19.38.

A percutaneous liver biopsy is usually required for diagnosis. Some of the material obtained must be frozen at −70 °C for subsequent biochemical analysis for inherited disorders (Table 19.35) if indicated by the liver histology or other investigations. Outstanding results of investigations for conditions including congenital infections (Table 19.39) should not delay diagnosis of surgically correctable disorders, particularly biliary atresia.

If percutaneous liver biopsy shows increased edema, fibrosis and bile duct reduplication with bile plugs, biliary atresia is highly likely although this appearance can also be found in some genetic and endocrine disorders and after PN, in some infants who will ultimately develop bile duct hypoplasia and in some of the conditions within the spectrum of intrahepatic cholestasis shown in Table 19.38.

Paucity of interlobular bile ducts (intrahepatic biliary hypoplasia)

The above diagnosis is based on a decrease in the number of interlobular bile ducts seen in portal tracts (ratio < 0.06) on liver biopsy. It is found in prematurity, with neonatal hepatitis of CMV inter alia. and with right-sided cardiovascular anomalies, classically peripheral pulmonary stenosis, skeletal and ocular anomalies defining Alagille syndrome (AS). Diagnosis of AS is supported by the typical facies: triangular face shape, deep-set eyes, overhanging forehead, a straight nose which in profile is in the same plane as the forehead and a small pointed chin, posterior embryotoxon and vertebral arch defects on spinal radiographs. Long-

Table 19.37   Endocrine disorders associated with hepatitis syndrome in infancy

1. Hypopituitarism
2. Diabetes insipidus
3. Hypoadrenalism
4. Hypothyroidism
5. Hypoparathyroidism
6. Growth hormone deficiency may become evident toward the end of infancy

Table 19.38 Currently recognized variants of progressive familial intrahepatic cholestasis (PFIC) (Shneider, 2004 187/id)

Clinical variant	Genetic marker or locus	Features
Byler disease or PFIC1	Ch 20 autosomal recessive	Low gGT, Diarrhea, FTT, Byler bile on EM
BSEP deficiency or PFIC 2	Ch 2 autosomal recessive	Low gGT
Other low gGT variants	Unknown	29% of low gGT PFIC have no Ch 2 or 18 marker
Aagenaes syndrome	Ch 17 autosomal recessive	High gGT, lymphoedema, seen in South Norway
American Indian cholestasis	Ch 16 autosomal recessive	High gGT, otitis media, paper money skin
Neonatal sclerosing cholangitis	Unknown	High gGT, clinically similar to biliary atresia
MDR3 deficiency	Ch 7 autosomal recessive	High gGT, bile phospholipid transport defect
With renal polycystic disease ARPKD, Caroli disease	Ch 4 autosomal recessive	High gGT, renal failure

Table 19.39 Infections causing hepatitis in infancy

1. Viral infections
   a. Cytomegalovirus
   b. Epstein–Barr virus
   c. Rubella virus
   d. Varicella zoster virus
   e. Hepatitis A
   f. Hepatitis B virus (+ delta virus)
   g. NonA, nonB hepatitis
   h. Herpes simplex virus
   i. Coxsackie A9, B
   j. Echo virus 9, 11, 14, 19
   k. Adenovirus
   l. Reovirus Type III
2. Nonviral infections
   a. Bacterial infection
   b. Psittacosis
   c. *Listeria*
   d. *Treponema pallidum*
   e. *Toxoplasma gondii*
   f. Tuberculosis
   g. Malaria

standing cholestasis causes jaundice, pruritus, hypercholesterolemia and xanthelasma. AS is inherited in an autosomal dominant fashion, with one of a wide variety of Jagged 1 mutations on chromosome 20q shown in most affected families studied. Phenotypic expression is variable. Jaundice is usually evident from the neonatal period. The long-term prognosis is uncertain but 30% may progress to cirrhosis and 5–10% die from liver disease.[115,116] In one series 25% died from cardiac involvement or infection. The treatment is that of chronic cholestasis with particular emphasis on adequacy of vitamin E replacement and the control of pruritus. Intolerably low quality of life may be an indication for liver transplantation.

Liver disease associated with parenteral nutrition

Prolonged i.v. PN, particularly in early infancy causes cholestasis and hepatocellular damage which may progress if PN cannot be stopped.[117] The mechanism remains unclear. Prevalence increases with the degree of prematurity, growth retardation before birth sepsis, hypoxia, shock, cardiac failure, intra-abdominal surgery and potentially hepatotoxic drugs, the duration of PN and the absence of enteral intake. Inspissated bile syndrome is an important complication, when ursodeoxycholic acid and cholecystokinin may be beneficial in promoting bile flow.

Clinical features and laboratory findings

Infants show early conjugated hyperbilirubinemia with elevated biochemical tests of liver function. It is important to consider other causes of cholestasis before incriminating PN. If it can be withdrawn the jaundice settles, although liver function tests may remain abnormal for over 6 months.

Disorders requiring urgent surgical treatment

Biliary atresia (BA) is a destructive sclerosing inflammatory process with onset about the time of birth. Obstruction of the extrahepatic bile ducts extending into the major intrahepatic bile ducts leads to severe progressive cholestasis and cirrhosis. If surgery is to be successful it must be performed before complete intrahepatic occlusion occurs. By 6–10 weeks of age the portal blood pressure is increased by incipient or established cirrhosis. The mean age at death in untreated cases is 11 months, with less than 5% surviving beyond 2 years.

Clinical features

Prolonged jaundice while always present may be very mild, and urine is always yellow. The stools contain no yellow or green pigment, but in up to 30% of infants with BA, stools are pigmented in the first weeks after birth before bile flow is completely obstructed. There is hepatomegaly often with splenomegaly. All too frequently the infant's apparent well-being causes health workers to overlook biliary atresia in the early weeks, when surgery is most likely to be successful. The incidence in the prematurely born or light-for-gestational age infant is the same as full term.

Laboratory investigations

There is no single test to guarantee a pre-laparotomy diagnosis of BA. Percutaneous liver biopsy showing the features described earlier in all portal tracts is over 90% sensitive and specific if alpha-1 antitrypsin deficiency, cystic fibrosis and AS have been excluded. Radionuclide studies such as ^{99m}Tc-tagged iminodiacetic acid derivative (IDA) are only of value in excluding biliary atresia by showing continuity between the biliary system and gastrointestinal tract. ERCP is helpful in diagnosing ambiguous cases.

Diagnosis of BA is confirmed at laparotomy, which should only be undertaken by a surgeon performing at least five Kasai portoenterostomies per year who can assess changes in the porta hepatis and proceed to portoenterostomy. Currently there are only surgeons in three such centers in the UK. An anastomosis is fashioned between the area of the porta hepatis from which the inflamed bile duct remnants have been resected and a Roux-en-Y loop is fashioned, allowing bile to drain from the main hepatic bile ducts directly into the bowel. Good bile flow can be achieved in 70% operated on by 60 days of age but in only 20–30% following later surgery.[118]

Complications

Cholangitis occurs in a significant minority of cases in the first 2 years after surgery, characterized by fever, recurrence or aggravation of jaundice and occasionally features of septicemia. Blood culture, ascitic aspirate and possibly liver biopsy to identify the organism responsible, should precede i.v. antibiotic therapy, which is continued for 7–14 d. Recurrent cholangitis has an adverse effect on liver function and prognosis indicating early and aggressive treatment. Prophylactic antibiotics are of no proven value.

Portal hypertension is present in almost all cases of BA at the time of initial surgery. At 5 years of age approximately 50% will have esophageal varices but only 10–15% will have alimentary bleeding when band ligation is the treatment of choice. All patients have a degree of malabsorption in the first year indicating dietary supplements with medium chain triglycerides and glucose polymers. Supplements of fat-soluble vitamins E, D, K and A are essential.

Prognosis

The prognosis of BA has been transformed by the Kasai operation followed by liver transplantation if necessary. Following the Kasai procedure a normal serum bilirubin is found in 65% of patients with approaching 90% 10-year survival and a good quality of life. Overall there is no evidence of portal hypertension in 25%, 10% with normal transaminases and 15% with abnormal transaminases, 40% will have varying degrees of portal hypertension, almost all with good quality of life. Subsequent liver transplantation will be required by 35% and with this combined approach mortality can be reduced to less than 5% compared with universal mortality 30 years ago.[119]

Choledochal cyst

In this disorder there is enlargement or dilatation of part or all the extrahepatic +/− intrahepatic biliary system. Bile flow may be obstructed causing histological changes similar to those of BA. Cholangitis, cyst rupture, pancreatitis, gall stones and carcinoma of the cyst wall are important complications. Incidental antenatal diagnosis by ultrasound occurs infrequently. In infancy it presents with features of neonatal cholestasis. In older children there may be recurrent upper abdominal pain, recurrent jaundice and/or a palpable cystic mass but the classical triad is rare. Diagnosis is by ultrasonography and other imaging, usually MRCP. The treatment is surgical removal with biliary drainage via a Roux-en-Y loop. Intrahepatic elements of the cyst are associated with a poorer prognosis with increased risk of developing biliary cirrhosis.

Spontaneous perforation of the bile duct

Perforation occurs at the junction of the cystic duct and common hepatic duct in infants. The etiology is unclear but may represent the consequence of a choledochal malformation. Mild jaundice, acholic stools, failure to thrive and biliary ascites with bile-stained hernia and umbilicus are the clinical features. Treatment entails surgical drainage of the biliary system into a Roux-en-Y loop.

HEPATITIS AND LIVER INFECTIONS

Acute and chronic inflammation of the liver with varying degrees of hepatocellular necrosis may be due to a wide range of causes including viral infections, drugs and toxins, metabolic and infiltrative conditions, and autoimmunity. Chronic low-grade hepatitides may progress to cirrhosis despite repeatedly measured normal serum transaminases.

Viral hepatitis (see also Ch. 28)

The term 'viral hepatitis' is usually applied to infections caused by viruses with a high degree of hepatotrophism. Five distinct agents can be identified at present.

Acute viral hepatitis type A (HAV)

Following ingestion of enterovirus type 72 (picorna), the virus becomes established in the liver, spills into the biliary system and is excreted in the stools. Stool virus concentration is highest 7 d before the onset of biochemical hepatitis, falls rapidly but may still be detected months later in patients with a relapsing course. The diagnosis is confirmed by finding specific HAV IgM antibodies appearing as early as 7 d after exposure, reaching peak concentrations at 20–40 d and usually clearing by 60 d. Infection occurs predominantly in early childhood and is related to overcrowding and poor hygiene. In northern Europe only 10–15% becomes infected in childhood. Children under 2 years are very unlikely to become icteric; the likelihood of severe hepatitis increases with age.

Clinical features

The incubation period varies from 15 to 40 d, followed by a preicteric stage which may be accompanied by anorexia, nausea, vomiting, fever, headache, lassitude, dull intermittent upper abdominal pain and loose stools. The liver may be enlarged and tender, and the spleen enlarged. Jaundice and pruritus may develop with dark urine and pale stools. Jaundice usually lasts for 2 weeks, but may persist for months or follow a relapsing course. Chronic liver disease does not occur although transient liver nodularity with portal hypertension can occasionally persist for up to 1 year. Rare complications include ALF, bone marrow aplasia, pancreatitis, myocarditis and polyneuropathy.

Prevention

Provision of drinking water uncontaminated by feces and safe disposal of sewage are essential in the prevention of this disorder. Person-to-person spread may be minimized by scrupulous hand washing after defecation and before handling food. Two doses of hepatitis A vaccine 14 d apart are extremely safe, providing over 95% protection.

Viral hepatitis type B (HBV)

Hepatitis B (HBV) is a DNA-containing virus of the hepadna group that can integrate into the hepatocyte genome.[120] In up to 10% of adults, less than 20% of 2–3-year-olds, 80% of infants aged 6 months or less and up to 90% of newborns, infection leads to a chronic infective carrier state, associated with normal liver structure and function or a range of pathological abnormalities including chronic hepatitis, cirrhosis and hepatocellular carcinoma. Patients with HBV may be superinfected by the delta virus (HDV).

Serological responses in HBV infection

Viral antigens and antibodies to them may be present so transiently that they are never detected or they may persist in high concentrations indefinitely. The antigens and antibodies used in clinical practice are given in Table 19.40. There may be an interval following the disappearance of an antigen before its antibody becomes detectable or both may be present together. Immunosuppressed children with hepatitis B infection usually have massive viral replication within the liver but may lack serological responses. HBV DNA may be detectable by very sensitive techniques even after successful anti-e seroconversion occurring spontaneously or induced by interferon treatment.

Clinical features

The acute and chronic responses to HBV infection in childhood are given in Table 19.41. The risk of serious sequelae is higher in males than in females. Those with anicteric hepatitis and minimal elevation of serum transaminases appear to be at greater risk of becoming chronically infected. The population chronic carrier rate varies from 0.1% in northern Europe and North America to 10% in southern European

Table 19.40   Serological markers in viral hepatitis type B

Marker	Clinical significance
HBsAg	Acute or chronic hepatitis B infection
HBsAb	Immunity to hepatitis B, postinfective or with active or passive immunization
HBcAb IgM	High titer: acute hepatitis, recent infection Low titer: chronic infection
HBcAb IgG	Past exposure to hepatitis B
HBeAg	Highly infectious state, high risk of progressive liver disease
HBeAb	Less infective state in the HBsAb-positive patient with low risk of progressive liver disease
HBV DNA by direct DNA hybridization	Quantification of viral replication

Table 19.41 Clinical expression of hepatitis B virus in childhood

1. Asymptomatic development of HBsAb
2. Acute hepatitis, anicteric or icteric
3. Papular acrodermatitis
4. Acute liver failure
5. Acute hepatitis proceeding to chronic hepatitis or cirrhosis
6. Disorders associated with circulating immune complexes
   a. Glomerulonephritis
   b. Periarteritis
   c. Pericarditis
   d. Arthritis
7. Chronic hepatitis
8. Cirrhosis
9. Hepatocellular carcinoma
10. 'Healthy' carrier state
11. Carrier state with immune disorders
    a. Down syndrome
    b. Malignant disease and its treatment
    c. Renal failure
    d. Immunosuppression with transplantation

and Mediterranean countries and as high as 20% in parts of Africa and South-East Asia.

Only 5% of infections in early infancy are symptomatic, as opposed to 40% in later life. The clinical features of acute HBV are similar to those of HAV but the incubation period ranges from 30 to 180 d and the onset more insidious. Often infection is asymptomatic and the carrier state is only detected by serological testing.

Natural history of HBV infection
It has been estimated that 20–25% of those infected in infancy are still positive in the fourth decade. HBe clearance rate varies between 2% per year for those infected in earlier infancy to 20% of children infected later in life. The conversion to anti-HBs in carriers is much rarer at between 0% and 2% per year.

Neither the clinical features nor biochemical tests of liver function predict the histological findings. Cross-sectional studies of children with HBV in Europe show 'interface' hepatitis in about 50%, with portal hepatitis in 33%, the remainder having chronic lobular hepatitis or minimal changes. Histological diagnosis of cirrhosis is made in approximately 5% but as many as one third may become cirrhotic. Those with active CAH are more prone to develop cirrhosis with complications, particularly if super-infected by delta virus. Hepatocellular carcinoma, associated with HBV infection, accounted for 13% of childhood cancers in Taiwan seen in children as young as 8 months but has almost disappeared since the introduction of neonatal vaccination against HBV. Children with chronic persistent hepatitis or chronic lobular hepatitis have a good prognosis over a period of 15 years in terms of developing cirrhosis.[121]

Prevention of HBV
Blood, saliva, urine and other secretions are infectious. All blood and blood-derived products should be screened for hepatitis B. Wearing disposable gloves and hand washing after handling blood or excretions minimize the risk of infection. Highly immunogenic synthetic vaccines should be used to protect family members of index cases and medical and paramedical personnel. Hyperimmune gamma-globulin to HBV (HBIG) must be given immediately after accidental inoculation of hepatitis B-positive blood.

The combined use of HBIG in a dose of 200 iu, with active immunization starting within 48 h of delivery with further doses at 1, 2 and 12 months, is very effective in producing high anti-HBs titers. Further doses are recommended later if the anti-HBs titer falls below 100 iu/L. This schedule is applied in the UK to all infants of mothers who are found to be HBsAg positive by screening during pregnancy, including those who

are HBe antibody positive. In areas of high prevalence it is cost effective to protect all newborns with vaccination alone rather than set up a system to identify those at risk and this regimen has been recommended universally by the WHO. Where infection is acquired after the neonatal period, vaccination at 3 months would seem to be cost effective. Instead of the UK recommended dose of 20 mg, doses as low as 2 mg given intradermally or intramuscularly are almost as effective.

Therapy of chronic hepatitis
In European children, treatment with interferon alpha 2b, 3 MU/m² for 3 months increased anti-HBe seroconversion rates over 12 months from 13% in controls to 40%. Pretreatment with steroids is not beneficial. The long-term clinical and histological benefit is assumed but unproven. No benefit has been shown of combined lamivudine interferon treatment. Lamivudine may have a role in reducing viral load in patients with abnormal immunity or those who cannot tolerate interferon. The role of other antivirals in children is under evaluation.

Viral hepatitis delta (HDV)
HDV is a defective RNA virus that requires HBV core Ag to replicate. It may be transmitted by parenteral inoculation or close body contact but is rare in the UK and in children. Subjects may be simultaneously infected with HBV or HBV carriers may be superinfected. When acquired simultaneously with HBV it may cause acute hepatitis from asymptomatic infection to ALF. Usually a chronic HBV carrier state does not follow. Superinfection of HBV carriers causes a serious exacerbation with progression to ALF, chronic active hepatitis or cirrhosis. It is confirmed by detecting antibodies to the delta virus. There is no effective treatment. HBV vaccination should limit its spread.

Viral hepatitis type C (HCV)
It has been shown that this 9500-RNA-base Flavivirus was responsible for up to 90% of post-transfusion hepatitis in North America prior to the screening of blood products. Infection in childhood was almost entirely acquired from unscreened blood products before 1989. It has now become rare with new infections by vertical transmission occurring in 5% of pregnancies of infected mothers. No vaccine is currently available.[122]

Natural history of HCV infection
The consequences of infection for adults are becoming clearer and it is assumed that they are similar for children. A mild hepatitis typically follows infection and an incubation period of about 60 d. Only 30% are icteric and ALF occurs exceedingly rarely. Perhaps 30–40% of immunocompetent patients will clear the virus while developing anti-HCV antibodies. The remainder will have chronic infection with anti-HCV antibodies and RNA polymerase chain reaction (PCR) positivity. Of these the majority will have mild liver disease such as minimal change or chronic persistent hepatitis with normal or occasionally abnormal transaminases. Liver disease is slowly progressive with cirrhosis developing over 20 years in 5–25% with one third taking 50 years or longer to develop cirrhosis. Concomitant liver diseases such as drug-induced, iron overload, HBV or alcohol will increase the rate of progression. Genotype 1 tends to progress more quickly and hepatocellular carcinoma occurs in 1–10%. Non-immunocompetent patients are more likely to develop chronic infection with antibodies to HCV being negative. The presence of HCV RNA can be used to demonstrate infection and the response to treatment.[123]

Treatment
Interferon with ribavirin treatment has been used with benefit in adults, but should only be undertaken by specialist centers under a research protocol in children. Sustained virological response (SVR), implying lack of viremia with associated improvement of inflammatory liver damage at least 12 months after completion of treatment, is the current outcome measure. Virus genotype 1 or 4 should be treated for 48 weeks and 2 or 3 for 24 weeks. SVR for genotype 1 is 30–40% and for 2 and 3

60%+. Side-effects with both drugs are frequent. Pegylated interferon promises even better results.[124]

Prevention of cross-infection

HCV is blood borne and despite being less infectious than HBV requires scrupulous antisepsis for spilled blood. Patients' razors and toothbrushes should be separated from others'. Counseling of sexual infectious risk, as 5% per partner, is required. HCV can also be detected in breast milk but breast-feeding is not contraindicated.

Viral hepatitis E (HEV)

This enterically transmitted 30 nm RNA virus is responsible for epidemics of hepatitis in the Middle East and Asia. Icteric disease occurs in 1–3% of infections. The prognosis is usually good but mortality is recognized in pregnant women and in association with other liver diseases including Wilson disease. Chronicity has not been documented but a relapsing course may occur.

NONVIRAL INFECTIONS

Hepatic abscesses

Hepatic abscesses may be caused by almost any bacteria or fungi, in association with any septicemic state, particularly with portal pyemia from appendix abscess and Crohn's disease that may be associated with portal vein thrombosis. Patients at risk include those with primary or secondary immune deficiencies, particularly chronic granulomatous disease. Secondary infection of another hepatic lesion such as bile duct obstruction, or sickle cell infarct may occur.

Clinical features

There are frequently no clinical or biochemical features of liver disease, but high spiking fever is universal and abdominal pain frequent. Diagnosis rests on ultrasonic detection of the lesion but CT scan is necessary to demonstrate possible appendix abscess and exclude associated malignancy. Successful management requires prolonged appropriate antibiotics as determined by culture of material aspirated from the lesion with ultrasonically guided drainage. Surgical drainage is required if there is associated peritonitis, bile duct obstruction or if chronic abscesses with established walls are present.

Hepatic amebiasis

This disorder has a high prevalence in children in endemic areas. Malaise, fever, rigors and tender hepatomegaly are usual. It is unusual to obtain a history of diarrhea. Secondary bacterial infection may be present. Diagnosis is based on finding living ameba in the stools or gut biopsy and positive serological tests.

Treatment

Metronidazole (50 mg/kg/24 h in three doses for 10 d) is the treatment of choice. Therapeutic needle aspiration or surgical drainage may be necessary when rupture of the abscess seems imminent or the liver lesion enlarges in spite of drug treatment.

Hydatid disease

Hydatid disease is usually caused by the larval stage of the dog tapeworm *Echinococcus granulosus*. Rarely the fox tapeworm, *Echinococcus multilocularis*, may be responsible.

Clinical features

Infection is usually acquired asymptomatically in early childhood. Earlier signs are discomfort in the right hypochondrium or hepatomegaly. Rarely rupture into the biliary system may cause cholangitis; sudden collapse may be caused by rupture into the peritoneum. Diagnosis is based on serological tests. Secondary bacterial infection may produce a liver abscess. Treatment is surgical resection. Patients with *E. multilocularis* or those too ill for surgery may respond to mebendazole or albendazole.

Schistosomiasis

Hepatic features are firm hepatomegaly, portal hypertension with splenomegaly, ascites and/or Hematemesis. Liver disease may occur as early as 2 years after initial infection. The recovery of ova in stools or rectal mucosa proves infection as positive serology does not distinguish past from present infection. The treatment is praziquantel. Alimentary bleeding due to portal hypertension should be treated by injection sclerotherapy or banding, not by portosystemic shunting.

Liver infestations

The liver and biliary system may be damaged by infestation with *Fasciola hepatica* (sheep), *Clonorchis sinensis* (freshwater fish), *Opisthorchis felineus* and *Opisthorchis viverrin* (cat) and by larvae of the roundworm *Ascaris*. All cause cholangitis which may become suppurative and be complicated by bile duct obstruction, calculus formation, bile duct carcinoma, biliary cirrhosis and portal hypertension.

CHRONIC LIVER DISEASE

Chronic liver disease implies evidence of liver damage persisting longer than 6 months likely to lead to cirrhotic change and its complications. It may develop asymptomatically, insidiously and without physical signs. Paradoxically, the presentation may appear acute when features of decompensation appear suddenly or when a relapsing course presents with severe exacerbation. Liver biopsy to aid in etiological diagnosis and assess progress of disease should be performed unless there is a specific contraindication. If there is evidence of hepatitis B infection biopsy should be delayed for 6 months to allow spontaneous remission.

Features suggesting chronicity

Chronic hepatitis should be suspected in the following situations:
1. relapse of an apparent acute hepatitis;
2. clinical or biochemical features of hepatitis persisting beyond 8 weeks;
3. hepatitis occurring after a history of neonatal cholestasis;
4. signs such as a small or hard liver, enlarged left or collapsed right lobe of liver, or others shown in Table 19.32.

Autoimmune liver diseases

Autoimmune chronic active hepatitis (AIH) and sclerosing cholangitis (AISC) are recognized to be part of an overlap syndrome.[125] At presentation, when patients may have aggressive hepatitis, occasionally ALF, or cirrhosis, it may be difficult to distinguish from Wilson disease. High serum immunoglobulins with IgG greater than 16 g/L, low concentrations of C4, and the presence of one or more non-organ-specific antibodies, particularly anti-nuclear, anti-smooth muscle are found in SMA/ANA antibody-positive AIH (type 1) and AISC. Anti-liver/kidney microsomal (LKM) antibodies define type 2 AIH, very rarely associated with AISC and occasionally with normal serum IgG level. IBD may be present in up to 30% of all patients. Presence of anti-gastric parietal cell antibodies is a marker of possible autoimmune polyendocrinopathy.

Drug treatment

Prednisolone in a dose of 2 mg/kg/d up to a maximum 50 mg/kg/d is given initially and continued until serum transaminase values fall by 80% or to less than 100 IU/L. Over the course of 2–3 months the dose is gradually reduced to that which will have no side-effects whilst maintaining normal transaminases, typically 0.1 mg/kg/d. Ursodeoxycholic acid 15–20 mg/kg/d is given for AISC. If the reduction of the steroid dose is associated with a rise in transaminase level, azathioprine 0.5 mg/kg/d is added and the dose increased gradually to 1.5 mg/kg/d. Weekly full blood counts and platelet counts are essential early in azathioprine therapy. Mycophenolate mofetil is a powerful second-line steroid sparing alternative to azathioprine. LKM antibody-positive patients will require indefinite treatment, while a minority of SMA/ANA-positive patients can slowly reduce and stop steroids after 2–4 years of normal transaminase levels.

The majority of patients have cirrhosis at the time of diagnosis but over 90% can be maintained in biochemical remission by immunosuppressive therapy with stable liver function and without side-effects of medication over a 20-year period. Patients with AISC have a marginally increased risk of need for liver transplantation during that period.

Sclerosing cholangitis

Sclerosing cholangitis is a chronic obliterative inflammation in the intrahepatic and/or extrahepatic biliary system shown as irregularities in the outline of the ducts with areas of stricturing and dilatation (beading) on cholangiography. The various types are listed in Table 19.42.

Treatment

Symptomatic treatment includes adequate replacement of fat-soluble vitamins and cholestyramine for pruritus. Ursodeoxycholic acid may be beneficial. Dietary, drug and/or surgical treatment of bowel disease associated with AISC and AIH is necessary but does not influence the biliary pathology.

Wilson disease

This inborn error of metabolism is characterized by defective biliary copper excretion. The spectrum of mutations causing a defective transport protein, ATP7B has been described.[126] Wilson disease may simulate virtually any form of liver disease from the age of 2 years onwards but typically presents in adolescence with ALF or severe hepatitis. Coombs negative hemolytic anemia or evidence of renal tubular damage often with hypophosphatemia suggests the diagnosis. In 80% the serum ceruloplasmin value is less than 20 g/dl (1.25 μmol/L). Biopsy liver copper concentration is > 250 mg/g of dry weight. Kayser–Fleischer rings may be identified by slit lamp examination in children over the age of 7. The gold standard for diagnosis is urinary copper excretion requiring both 1.2 mmol/24 h and more than 25 mmol/24 h with 1 g of penicillamine.

Treatment

The prognosis of Wilson disease at treatment is predicted by the total score according to Table 19.43. A score > 9 is associated with an early death (< 2 months) without liver transplantation. Patients with score < 6 should respond satisfactorily to penicillamine (5 mg/kg/d increased by 5 mg/kg/d at 2-weekly intervals to 20 mg/kg/d) and zinc sulfate 100–300 mg three times a day after meals given at different times from the penicillamine. Patients with scores of 6–9 require close monitoring. Recovery on treatment may take 12 months or longer.

It is *essential* to screen families of patients with Wilson disease to enable early treatment. Serum transaminases, copper, ceruloplasmin and urinary penicillamine challenge are required for all first-degree relatives. Genetic markers are available, but with more than 100 alleles described genetic tests are frequently uninformative.

Table 19.42 Classification of sclerosing cholangitis

1. Autoimmune (with or without chronic inflammatory bowel disease) with high serum immunoglobulins and non-organ-specific autoantibodies, C4 concentration normal and circulating T lymphocytes displaying IL-2R < 5%
2. Following cholestasis in infancy or with family history or consanguinity (neonatal sclerosing cholangitis)

Associated with:

3. Langerhans' cell histiocytosis
4. Immune deficiency states, particularly HIV and CD40 ligand deficiency
5. Cystic fibrosis
6. Biliary surgery, or trauma
7. Ischemia after liver transplantation or in sickle cell disease
8. Primary (with or without chronic inflammatory bowel disease with normal serum immunoglobulins and no autoantibodies)

Table 19.43 Prognostic score in Wilson disease

Bilirubin (μmol/L)	Aspartate amino-transferase	Prothrombin time INR (u/L)	Prognostic score
N < 20	N < 40	N < 1.3	
< 100	< 100	<1.3	0
101–150	101–150	1.3–1.6	1
151–200	151–200	1.7–2.0	2
201–300	201–300	2.1–2.5	3
> 300	> 300	> 2.5	4

N, normal

Other copper-associated liver diseases

Indian childhood cirrhosis was largely confined to the Indian subcontinent and was characterized by necrosis of hepatocytes containing Mallory's hyaline and orcein-staining copper-associated protein due to accumulation of copper in the liver. Over 80% died within 6 months. Elimination of exposure to dietary copper has resulted in near elimination of the disease. Rare non-Indian cases have been described both with and without excessive environmental exposure to copper but with similar poor prognosis.

Non-alcoholic steatohepatitis (NASH)

This condition, long recognized in adult practice, is becoming increasingly prevalent in children.[127] Presentation is with incidentally discovered raised serum transaminases or fat as brightness on liver ultrasound. Children are usually obese with a high fat and refined carbohydrate diet and sedentary lifestyle. The diagnosis is by exclusion of other liver disease associated with fat in the liver and by the characteristic liver biopsy features of inflammation, macrovesicular fat and occasional fibrosis. Other causes of fatty infiltration include Wilson disease, alpha-1 antitrypsin deficiency, HCV, and milder forms of glycogen storage disease. A glucose tolerance test is mandatory. Treatments suggested have included antibiotics against bacterial translocation, antioxidants and metformin, but dietary and lifestyle changes to reduce weight are the mainstay of management. Progressive liver fibrosis will be found in 5–10%.

ACUTE LIVER FAILURE

The adult terminology 'fulminant liver failure' based on the onset of encephalopathy is not helpful in pediatrics as in infants and small children severe liver failure may occur without apparent encephalopathy.[128] ALF is preferred for children with a 'de novo' liver injury causing coagulopathy without disseminated intravascular coagulation or vitamin K deficiency. Two minority subgroups may be defined, one with hyperacute presentation of duration less than 1 week and typically low levels of jaundice, and one with subacute presentation of more than 8 weeks. ALF is a rare, complex, multisystem disorder with a mortality of 30–100%. Life-threatening complications include septicemia, especially from fungi, and raised intracranial pressure secondary to encephalopathy proceeding to impaired cerebral blood flow. In ALF, but possibly not the subacute subgroup, if the patient survives, the liver usually regains normal histology and function.

Diagnosis

The differential diagnosis of ALF is shown in Table 19.44. Although no diagnosis is possible in up to 40% of cases the search for a diagnosis should not delay transfer of the patient to a center with facilities and experience of managing ALF.

Clinical features

The grades of hepatic encephalopathy are shown in Table 19.45. Prognostic features for ALF other than paracetamol toxicity and Wilson disease appear in Table 19.46. The prognosis for ALF from Wilson disease appears in Table 19.43. Adverse prognostic markers for paracetamol toxicity include metabolic acidosis, renal dysfunction and encephalopathy

Table 19.44   The causes of acute liver failure

1. Infective
   a. Viral hepatitis
      (i)   A, B, B+ Delta, C, enteric or blood borne NANB
      (ii)   Epstein–Barr virus
      (iii) Cytomegalovirus
      (iv)   Herpes virus
      (v)   Adenovirus
      (vi)   Echovirus
      (vii) Yellow fever
      (viii) Lassa fever
      (ix)   Ebola
      (x)   Marburg
   b Leptospirosis
   c Septicemia

2. Toxic
   a. *Amanita phalloides*
   b. Carbon tetrachloride
   c. Paracetamol
   d. Halothane
   e. Valproate
   f. Carbamazepine
   g. Phenytoin
   h. Isoniazid
   i. Amiodarone
   j. Cytotoxics
   k. Monoamine oxidase inhibitors
   l. Chemotherapy particularly actinomycin D causing veno-occlusive disease

3. Metabolic
   a. Galactosemia
   b. Fructosemia
   c. Tyrosinemia
   d. Familial erythrophagocytic reticulosis (hemophagocytic lympho-histiocytosis)
   f. Neonatal hemochromatosis
   e. Wilson disease
   f. Niemann–Pick type C
   g. Mitochondrial respiratory chain defects

4. Ischemia
   a. Budd–Chiari syndrome
   b. Acute circulatory failure
   c. Septicemia with shock
   d. Heat stroke
   e. Leukemia

5. Cryptogenic in 40%

NANB, non-A non-B

Table 19.45   The grade of hepatic encephalopathy

Grade of encephalopathy	Features
1	Lethargy, minor reductions in consciousness or motor function, vomiting
2	Stupor, irrational hyperactivity, combative behavior
3	Unresponsive to command but responds to pain
4	Unresponsive to command, extensor posturing and rigidity, brainstem depression with respiratory and vasomotor failure

Table 19.46   Prognostic markers in acute liver failure

Prognostic factor	Risk of mortality
INR ≥ 4.0	93%
Serum bilirubin > 235 µmol/L	92%
Age < 2 years	96%
WBC $\geq 9 \times 10^9$/L	93%
Encephalopathy grade 3 or 4	90%+
Drug etiology	90%+
Etiology unknown	90%+
HBV	70–90%
HAV	50–70%
3 or more adverse factors	100%

but not transaminase level. Unlike ALF of other causes, INR of > 4.0 does not necessarily herald a poor prognosis in paracetamol toxicity.

Indications for liver transplantation

Since the 5-year survival following liver transplantation for children with ALF is approximately 70%, transplantation is indicated when the prognosis of the liver failure is worse than that of transplantation,[129] assuming no other influences on the overall prognosis of the underlying condition, e.g. respiratory chain disorders with central nervous system complications.

Treatment

Intensive care aimed at preventing and treating complications is essential until the liver function recovers or transplantation can be performed. Early arrangements should be made to transfer the child to a pediatric intensive care unit (PICU) with the experience to manage the multisystem complications and to proceed to liver transplantation if indicated. *Sedatives must not be given unless patients are to be ventilated.* Vitamin K is given to optimize coagulation. Hypoglycemia must be prevented by i.v. glucose. Protein intake is restricted to 0.5 g/kg/d. Lactulose may precipitate diarrhea without altering the outcome. Ranitidine given intravenously may prevent bleeding from gastric erosions. Prophylactic antibiotics and antifungals are indicated as 40% of cases have early covert sepsis.

Reye syndrome and Reye-like ALF

Reye syndrome is an increasingly rare, acute, frequently fatal encephalopathy of unknown cause occurring in children of any age characterized by a self-limiting abnormality of mitochondrial structure and function. It occurs following an unremarkable viral infection of the respiratory or gastrointestinal tract. Aspirin may play a role although Reye syndrome has been disappearing in countries where aspirin is still given to children at a similar rate as in countries where it has been prohibited. Reye syndrome must be distinguished from an increasing range of inborn errors of metabolism that present in a similar fashion, particularly urea cycle disorders, fatty acid oxidation disorders, e.g. medium chain acyl CoA dehydrogenase deficiency, organic acidemias and mitochondrial respiratory chain disorders (see Ch. 26). Respiratory chain disorders are increasingly recognized as causing encephalopathy often with fits followed by ALF perhaps precipitated by sodium valproate. They are often distinguished by high serum transaminases and mild or initially absent jaundice.[130] Classical Reye syndrome does not have very high serum transaminases. In all these conditions liver transplantation is not usually required despite the severity of the initial coagulopathy and may be contraindicated in view of the neurological sequelae. Prevention of further episodes and genetic counseling are required after diagnosis.

In Reye syndrome encephalopathy with prominent vomiting may proceed over 4–60 h to brain death. Diagnosis of Reye syndrome or Reye-like conditions must be suspected in any encephalopathy if there is laboratory evidence of liver involvement such as raised serum transaminases, hyperammonemia, hypoglycemia or prolonged INR.

Treatment

Mortality is as high as 40% with a considerable proportion of survivors being left with brain damage or with progressive encephalopathy in those with respiratory chain disorders. The patient should be nursed in a fashion that minimizes increases in intracranial pressure while being transferred to a specialist PICU. At presentation it is essential to collect and store serum (at $-70\,^{\circ}$C) and urine in order to diagnose Reye-like disorders.

Hemophagocytic lymphohistiocytosis

This rare condition is due to uncontrolled activation of the immune system, particularly by viral infection, and results in aggressive tissue damage by histiocytes and possible liver failure. Lymphadenopathy and hepatosplenomegaly are frequently present. Inflammatory markers particularly triglycerides and ferritin are elevated, fibrinogen is low, and cytopenia is indicative of disseminated intravascular coagulation and bone marrow involvement.[131] Recent work has shown abnormalities of apoptosis in infected cells being the primary defect with perforin gene abnormalities in 30%. Treatment includes anti-T cell globulin and etoposide. Prognosis is poor and particularly grave in infants.

CIRRHOSIS

The main pathophysiological effects are impaired hepatic function and portal hypertension. Hepatocellular carcinoma may develop. Although the diagnosis of cirrhosis implies an irreversible and usually progressive pathological change, it may be compatible with normal growth and activity for many years. There are two broad pathological categories: biliary cirrhosis and so-called postnecrotic cirrhosis. Genetic factors contribute to both pathological varieties (Table 19.47).

Table 19.47   Causes of cirrhosis in childhood

1. Biliary
   - a. Biliary atresia
   - b. Intrahepatic biliary hypoplasia
   - c. Choledochal cyst
   - d. Cystic fibrosis
   - e. PFIC
   - f. Bile duct stenosis or obstruction
   - g. Choledocholithiasis
   - h. Sclerosing cholangitis
   - i. Cholangitis due to:
     - (i) *Fasciola*
     - (ii) *Clonorchis sinensis*
     - (iii) *Ascaris*
   - j. Pancreatic tumors
   - k. Langerhans' cell histiocytosis

2. Postnecrotic
   - a. Hepatitis in infancy
   - b. Auto-immune chronic active hepatitis
   - c. Acute viral hepatitis (viral hepatitis, B, C, delta, non-A non-B)
   - d. Hepatitis due to drugs, e.g. actinomycin D, methotrexate
   - e. Toxins, e.g. aflatoxin, copper, copper associated liver diseases

3. Genetic disorders
   - a. Wilson disease
   - b. Galactosemia
   - c. Fructosemia
   - d. Glycogen storage disease type IV
   - e. Hurler syndrome
   - f. alpha-1-antitrypsin deficiency
   - g. Tyrosinemia
   - h. Cystinosis
   - i. Gaucher disease
   - j. Wolman disease
   - k. Niemann–Pick disease type C
   - l. Defects in fatty acid oxidation
   - m. Sickle cell disease
   - n. Thalassemia
   - o. Hepatic porphyria
   - p. Hemochromatosis, idiopathic
   - q. Hemochromatosis secondary to chronic hemolytic disease
   - r. Defects in primary bile salt synthesis

4. Venous congestion
   - a. Constrictive pericarditis
   - b. Ebstein's anomaly
   - c. Congestive cardiac failure
   - d. Budd–Chiari syndrome
   - e. Venacaval webs
   - f. Veno-occlusive disease
   - g. Radiation

PFIC, progressive familial intrahepatic cholestasis

Clinical and laboratory features

Clinical and nonspecific laboratory features are described earlier. Five disorders may cause particular diagnostic difficulty: extrahepatic portal hypertension, congenital hepatic fibrosis, constrictive pericarditis, sclerosing cholangitis and infiltrative disorders such as reticuloses.

Management

Based on the history, examination findings and standard investigations listed in Table 19.48, a differential diagnosis may be possible prior to performing a liver biopsy. In considering the genetic disorders, consideration must be given to those with effective treatment, e.g. Wilson disease and AIH, and to identify surgically correctable abnormalities of the biliary tree, e.g. choledochal cyst. The further aim of management is to minimize further liver damage by treating the cause of liver disease and preventing or controlling complications (Table 19.49).

Portal hypertension (see later) causes splenomegaly, ascites and alimentary bleeding. Splenomegaly and hypersplenism rarely require intervention. Ascites may respond to spironolactone 4–7 mg/kg/d. If there is hyponatremia, water restriction is essential. It is rarely possible to reduce the sodium intake to less than 0.5 mmol/kg/d. If these measures are unsuccessful albumin infusions with furosemide (frusemide) 0.5–1 mg/kg/d may control ascites for 7–21 d. Paracentesis may be necessary if there is severe abdominal distension or respiratory embarrassment, followed by 20% i.v. albumin 5 ml/kg. It is essential to monitor the patient's weight, abdominal girth, urinary output of water and sodium and to measure the serum urea and creatinine when managing ascites.

Treatment of alimentary bleeding

Following small initial bleeds, shock requiring rapid blood transfusion may occur. The child should be immediately admitted to the nearest hospital with resuscitation facilities. Bleeding decreases hepatic perfusion

Table 19.48   First-line investigations in children with evidence of chronic liver disease

FBC reticulocytes, film, INR, APTT, fibrinogen, cross match, Coombs test
Renal, bone, liver, lipid profiles, amylase, CK, blood glucose, lactate urate
Blood gases
Ferritin, copper, caeruloplasmin, zinc
Alpha-fetoprotein
Alpha-1-antitrypsin phenotype
CF alleles, sweat test
Immunoglobulins, complement C3 & C4, autoantibody screen
Serology for hepatitis B HBSAg, eAg, HCV Ab, HCVRNA PCR, CMV, EBV
24-hour urine copper collection and penicillamine challenge
CXR (cardiac echo if constrictive pericarditis is possible)
Liver and spleen ultrasound

Table 19.49   Complications of cirrhosis

1. Portal hypertension and hypersplenism
2. Bleeding diathesis
3. Hypoxemia
4. Increased susceptibility to infection
5. Hyperdynamic circulation (cardiac failure)
6. Ascites
7. Spontaneous bacterial peritonitis
8. Pulmonary hypertension
9. Hepatoma
10. Malnutrition
11. Gallstone formation
12. Renal failure
13. Hepatic encephalopathy
14. Endocrine changes
15. Impaired hepatic metabolism of drugs and hormones
16. Impaired neurodevelopment, particularly gross motor

with the possibility of ischemic hepatitis and hepatic encephalopathy. On admission, a baseline assessment of the clinical state should be made, blood cross-matched, and a secure i.v. line established. I.v. octreotide 25 µg/h is indicated. A Sengstaken–Blakemore tube of suitable size should be available and chilled to facilitate insertion by an experienced operator. Oral ranitidine and sucralfate reduce the risk of bleeding from gastric erosions. I.v. vitamin K should be given. As soon as the patient is stable, transfer to a unit equipped to manage the causes and complications of portal hypertension is required. Endoscopy is essential to determine the cause and source of bleeding, which may be gastric erosions or peptic ulceration rather than varices with band ligation or injection sclerotherapy if necessary.[132] Propranolol 1 mg/kg/d in two doses may reduce the frequency of subsequent bleeds. Emergency portosystemic shunting is rarely required.

Spontaneous bacterial peritonitis

This potentially lethal complication of ascites may present with signs of peritonitis and fever. Blood culture and diagnostic ascitic tap are required for early diagnosis and antibiotics against *Streptococcus pneumoniae* and Gram-negative organisms are given. With high risk of recurrence prophylactic antibiotics and consideration of liver transplantation are required.

Chronic hepatic encephalopathy

Chronic hepatic encephalopathy is a complex neuropsychiatric syndrome with major portosystemic shunting usually complicating cirrhosis with portal hypertension.[133] It is characterized by intellectual impairment, personality change and clouding of consciousness. Sleep patterns may be disturbed. Causes of hepatic encephalopathy and compounding factors are given in Table 19.50.

Treatment

The objectives of treatment are to prevent accumulation of ammonia and other vasoactive or false neurotransmitter substances in the gut, to remove or correct identifiable precipitating factors and to try to improve liver function. Protein intake should be reduced to 0.5–1 g/kg of body weight initially but then increased if tolerated. Sodium benzoate may be beneficial.

Nutritional complications of severe liver disease

Cirrhosis and portal hypertension may be associated with a characteristic habitus having a full abdomen with thin limbs. Body weight underestimates the severity of derangement of body composition. Anorexia and fluid retention complicate management.[134]

Dietary management of cholestasis and cirrhosis

The calorie requirements may be up to 40% above recommended daily intake for weight. The diet must contain sufficient protein (up to 4 g/kg/d), essential fatty acids, minerals, trace elements and vitamins. Anorexia is frequently a problem, which may be aggravated by restricted fluid and/or salt intake. Fat malabsorption of varying severity is frequent. Water- and fat-soluble vitamin supplements are required. If hepatic

encephalopathy develops, dietary protein should be stopped and gradually reintroduced up to the maximum tolerated, while sodium benzoate is given. There is no proven advantage in using branched chain amino acids. Nutritional requirements are shown in Table 19.51.

Pulmonary complications

Hepatopulmonary syndrome (HPS) presents insidiously as exertional dyspnea followed by cyanosis.[135] Type 1 HPS implies pulmonary capillary vasodilatation and type 2 new vessel intrapulmonary shunts both with ventilation/perfusion mismatch. The degree of shunting does not correlate with the severity of the liver damage or portal hypertension but may relate to the degree of portosystemic shunting. Hypoxia is only partially relieved by increasing inspired oxygen concentration but is cured by liver transplantation. Portopulmonary hypertension may develop due to pulmonary vasoconstriction, the converse of the dilatation of HPS.[136]

Hepatorenal failure

Oliguric renal failure without structural abnormalities in the kidney (functional renal failure) is frequently a terminal event in advanced cirrhosis. There is a slow development of uremia, oliguria, and hyponatremia with a low urinary sodium concentration. Glomerular filtration may show transient improvement with inotropes or vasopressin analogues. Liver transplantation is the definitive treatment.

PORTAL HYPERTENSION
Portal vein obstruction

The portal vein may be obstructed by infective or thrombotic disorders or by a congenital abnormality. The presenting features are asymptomatic splenomegaly, alimentary bleeding with portal hypertension at any age throughout childhood or adult life, and rarely ascites and failure to thrive. The diagnosis is suspected by the finding of portal hypertension or esophageal varices in a patient with splenomegaly without clinical or biochemical evidence of liver disease. The diagnosis is confirmed by ultrasonography or angiography. The treatment is that of bleeding esophageal or rectal varices.[132] There is an increased frequency of bleeding during adolescence.[137]

Congenital hepatic fibrosis

The clinical features are those of portal hypertension, hepatomegaly and occasionally cholangitis. Liver function tests are usually normal. Diagnosis requires an adequate liver biopsy showing wide bands of fibrous tissue linking portal tracts but clearly demarcated from the hepatic parenchyma. The bands contain irregularly shaped clefts lined by bile duct epithelial cells. Portal veins are sparse. There is little inflammatory cell infiltrate unless there is associated cholangitis. There is frequently significant associated renal disease, particularly infantile polycystic disease and renal excretion scans are essential. A wide range of dysmorphic syndromes is associated including Senior–Loken syndrome, Lawrence-Moon–Biedl syndrome and neurofibromatosis. Alimentary bleeding from varices is treated by band ligation, and cholangitis with appropriate antibiotics. Rarely liver transplantation is indicated for biliary cirrhosis secondary to chronic cholangitis.

Cystic fibrosis (see Ch. 20)

Clinical syndromes include:
1. prolonged conjugated hyperbilirubinemia in infancy presenting as a hepatitis syndrome sometimes difficult to distinguish from biliary atresia;
2. massive hepatic steatosis which reverses as nutrition improves;
3. cirrhosis with portal hypertension and variceal hemorrhage, hypersplenism or splenic pain;
4. biliary abnormalities take the form of micro gallbladder present in up to a third, with gallstones in as many as 12%. Up to 40% of patients with CF have evidence of liver disease.

Table 19.50   Causes of hepatic encephalopathy

1. End-stage chronic parenchymal disease
2. Acute or subacute liver failure
3. Liver disease with severe portosystemic shunting
4. Precipitating factors
    a. Sedative medications
    b. Hypoglycemia
    c. Hypokalemia
    d. Hypovolemia
    e. Sepsis
    f. GI bleeding
    g. Hypoxia
    h. High-protein diet

Table 19.51 Nutritional requirements – vitamins and minerals

Nutritional element	Daily requirement	Products/source	Means of administration	Comments/monitoring
Vitamin A	<10 kg 5000 IU >10 kg 10 000 IU IM – 50 000 IU	Ketovite liquid & tabs, Abidec	Oral	IM supplement only in severe refractory deficiency Serum retinol/ RBP ≥ 0.8
Vitamin D	25-OHD: 2–5 µg/kg IM – 30 000 IU 1–3 monthly	Ketovite liquid & tabs, Abidec have calciferol 400 iu/d IM calciferol	Oral/IM	Supplementation with oral products containing calciferol may suffice. Refractory cases may require 25–OHD or IM preps 25-OHD serum levels > 20 ng/ml
Vitamin E	TPGS* 25 iu/kg IM 10 mg/kg (max. 200 mg) every 3 weeks	TPGS from Eastman–Kodak or Orphan Europe. Others include Ketovite liquid & tabs, Abidec, Ephynal	Oral	Vit. E/total lipids ≥ 0.6 mg/g Vit. E < 30 µg/ml Look for reflexes!
Vitamin K	2 mg/d Weekly 5 mg: 5–10 kg 10 mg > 10 kg IM – 5–10 mg every 2 weeks	Konakion MM Micellar formulation or menadiol Phytomenadione	Oral IM	Prothrombin time PIVKA II < 3 ng/ml
Water-soluble vitamins	Twice RDA	Children's multivitamins, Ketovite liquid & tabs	Oral	Supplement as needed
Minerals Calcium Selenium Zinc Phosphate	 25 –100 mg/kg 1–2 µg /kg 1 mg/kg 25–50 mg/kg		Oral	Supplement as needed
Total lipid/MCT	30–50% of energy of which 30–70% MCT	Depending on product and level of malabsorption	As formula	
PUFA/LCP	Probably > 10% total energy	Rapeseed oil Egg yolk Walnut oil Fish oil Sunflower oil Soybean oil	Walnut oil added to feed/given separately	Products unpalatable Levels difficult to measure and interpret. Most centers lack access to clinical measurement
Protein	2–4 g/kg (min. 2 g/kg)	Whey protein	As formula	Avoid semi-elemental diet/ hydrolysates if not necessary. Treat hyper-ammonemia instead of reducing protein intake
BCAA	10% total AAs			
Energy	RDA for age or up to 150% of requirement for weight	2/3 as CHO and 1/3 as lipids approx.	As formula	
Carbohydrate		CHO polymer	As formula	Usually lactose free
Na/K	Minimum/2–3 mmol/kg		As formula	

Treatment is aimed at improving nutrition, particularly deficiency of fat-soluble vitamins, and the management of portal hypertension. Ursodeoxycholic acid (15–20 mg/kg/d) improves transaminases, serum bile acids and ultrasound findings but is of uncertain effect on prognosis.[138] Surgery may be required for symptomatic gall stones. Liver transplantation has also been performed with good results but no large series has clarified indications and outcomes.

LIVER TUMORS

Primary liver tumors are rare and occur at approximately one tenth of the frequency of neuroblastoma. Malignant tumors include hepatoblastoma and hepatocellular carcinoma, both of which are usually accompanied by a high alpha-fetoprotein level, fibrolamellar hepatoma (accompanied by transcobalamin markers), rhabdomyosarcoma and cholangiocarcinoma. Other tumors appear in Table 19.52.[139] Infantile hemangioendothelioma may present in two forms: 'sump' effect with consumptive features of Kasabach–Merritt syndrome and 'shunt' like with high output cardiac failure. The others present with abdominal distension, hepatomegaly, abdominal pain or rarely complications of the tumor, such as virilization. Diagnosis is supported by the demonstration of a space-occupying lesion within the liver by imaging.

Malignant tumors are treated with appropriate chemotherapeutic agents followed by resection. Hemangioendothelioma is treated by surgical hepatic artery ligation in congestive cardiac failure. Such surgery should be confined to specialist centers.

Table 19.52 Tumors of the liver in childhood

	Benign/malignant
Hepatoblastoma[141]	M
Hepatoma/HCC including fibrolamellar HCC	M
Small cell tumor of infancy	M
Biliary rhabdomyosarcoma	M
Lymphoma	M
Neuroblastoma (including 4S)	M (spontaneous remission)
Secondary carcinomas/sarcomas	M
Hemangioendothelioma/angiosarcoma	B/M
Mesenchymal hamartoma	B
Adenoma	B
Focal nodular hyperplasia/nodular regenerative hyperplasia	B
Inflammatory pseudotumor	B

Table 19.53 Indications for liver transplantation

Indications for liver transplantation	Examples
Decompensation of cirrhosis	Uncontrollable ascites Encephalopathy Failure to thrive Coagulopathy unresponsive to vitamin K
Untreatable complications of portal hypertension	Hepatorenal syndrome Hepatopulmonary syndrome
Poor quality of life	Pruritus Lethargy
Life-threatening complications	Varices refractory to all other treatments
Selected liver tumors	Unresectable chemosensitive hepatoblastoma Benign but unresectable tumors
Extra-hepatic manifestations of hepatic inborn errors of metabolism	Crigler–Najjar type 1 Primary oxaluria Propionic acidemia
Acute liver failure	INR > 4 Grade 3 or 4 encephalopathy Children under 2 years

LIVER TRANSPLANTATION

With 5-year survival rates as high as 90% for chronic liver diseases, orthotopic liver transplantation should be considered in any child with acute or chronic liver disease if death within 1 year is likely, or as a consequence of liver disease when the quality of life has deteriorated to unacceptable levels, or if irreversible damage to the central nervous system or other organs is likely as a consequence of liver disease. Transplantation must be considered in ALF or subALF and in selected children with an increasing range of metabolic disorders (Table 19.53). Auxiliary transplants may be most suitable for some of these latter indications. Full consideration must be given to other forms of treatment and the presence of relative contraindications. The results are better in children transplanted in a good nutritional state and if the procedure is elective.[140]

Complications

Complications are those of major surgery involving multiple vascular and biliary anastomoses, of rejection and the effects of long-term anti-rejection drugs. Rejection occurs in up to 70% but is resistant to treatment with steroids in about 15%. In patients with poor graft function, opportunistic infections remain a high risk while those on modest doses of anti-rejection drugs are at risk of infections with community-acquired and gastrointestinal organisms. Between 1 and 6 months, cytomegalovirus, and opportunistic infection with organisms such as *Nocardia* and *Pneumocystis* may occur. EBV infection may lead to post-transplant lymphoproliferative disease, particularly but not exclusively in patients who have received exceptional total immunosuppression for rejection. Tacrolimus and cyclosporine have reduced the risk of infective complications but with major side-effects including chronic renal dysfunction, neurotoxicity, glucose intolerance and cosmetic considerations.

The longest survivor to date remains well 25 years after transplant, and the majority of survivors have a good quality of life. Life-long immunosuppressive therapy with expert medical supervision is required. The supply of suitable donor organs remains a major limiting factor in liver transplantation in childhood despite improvements from reducing organs, splitting organs between two recipients and using part of the liver of live related donors. Selecting the appropriate time for surgery can be difficult, being a compromise between early enough to receive a liver while in good condition and not undertaking transplant with its risks of complications before it is clearly necessary. Thus, it is essential that patients who may become candidates for transplantation should be referred at the earliest possible stage to units with the expertise to advise on the optimum timing.

CHARITIES AND ORGANIZATIONS

British Society of Pediatric Gastroenterology, Hepatology and Nutrition E-mail. secretary@bspghan.org.uk Website: http://bspghan.org.uk
Children's Liver Disease Foundation, 36 Great Charles Street, Birmingham B3 3JY, UK. Tel: 0121 212 3839; Fax: 0121 212 4300. E-mail: info@childliverdisease.org; Website: http://www.childliverdisease.org
Coeliac UK, Suites A–D Octagon Court, High Wycombe, Bucks HP11 2HS, UK. Tel: 01494 437278; Fax: 01494 474349; E-mail: adminsec@coeliac.co.uk; Website: http://www.coeliac.co.uk
Crohn's in Childhood Research Association, Parkgate House, 356 West Barnes Lane, Motspur Park, Surrey KT3 6NB, UK. Tel: 020 8949 6209; Fax: 020 8942 2044; E-mail: support@cicra.org; Website: http://www.cicra.org
Cystic Fibrosis Trust, 11 London Road, Bromley, Kent BR1 1BY, UK. Tel: 020 8464 7211; Fax: 020 8313 0472; Website: http://www.cftrust.org.uk

European Society for Paediatric Gastroenterology, Hepatology and Nutrition. Website: http://www.espghan.med.up.pt/
Gut Motility Disorders Support Network, Westcott Farm, Oakford, Tiverton, EX16 9EX, UK. Tel: 01398 351173 (mornings only); E-mail: help@gmdnet.org.uk; Website: http://www.cafamily.org.uk/Direct/g42.html
Ileostomy and Internal Pouch Support Group, Peverill House, 1–5 Mill Road, Ballyclare, County Antrim, BT39 9DR, UK. Tel: 028 9334 4043; Fax: 028 9332 4606; E-mail: info@the-ia.org.uk Website: http://www.the-ia.org.uk/
National Association for Crohn's and Colitis, 4 Beaumont House, Sutton Road, St Albans, Herts AL1 5HH, UK. Tel: 0845 130 2233; Fax: 01727 862550; E-mail: nacc@nacc.org.uk; Website: http://www.nacc.org.uk
The North American Society for Pediatric Gastroenterology, Hepatology and Nutrition NASPGHAN, PO Box 6, Flourtown, PA 19031, USA. Tel: (215) 233 0808; Fax: (215) 233 3918; E-mail: naspghan@naspghan.org; Website: http://www.naspghan.org/

Patients on Intravenous & Nasogastric Nutrition Therapy, PO Box 3126, Christchurch, Dorset BH23 2XS, UK. E-mail: pinnt@dial.pipex.com; Website: http://www.pinnt.com

REFERENCES

1. Johnston L, Barrett K, Ghishan F, et al. Physiology of the Gastrointestinal Tract, 1–2. 4th edn. Academic Press; 2006.
2. Bisset WM. Understanding diarrhoea. Current Paediatrics 2001; 11:291–295.
3. Porter S, Speight PM. Disorders of the oral cavity. In: Walker WA, Hamilton JR, Watkins JB, et al, eds. Pediatric gastrointestinal disease. 3rd edn. Hamilton: BC Decker; 2000:257–265.
4. Leao JC, Hodgson T, Scully C, et al. Review article: orofacial granulomatosis. Aliment Pharmacol Ther 2004; 20:1019–1027.
5. Stong BC, Sipp JA, Sobol SE. Pediatric parotitis: a 5-year review at a tertiary care pediatric institution. Int J Pediatr Otorhinolaryngol 2006; 70:541–544.

6. Omari TI, Miki K, Davidson G, et al. Characterisation of relaxation of the lower oesophageal sphincter in healthy premature infants. Gut 1997; 40:370–375.

7. Omari TI, Barnett C, Snel A, et al. Mechanisms of gastroesophageal reflux in healthy premature infants. J Pediatr 1998; 133:650–654.

8. Kelly KJ, Lazenby AJ, Rowe PC, et al. Eosinophilic esophagitis attributed to gastroesophageal reflux: improvement with an amino acid-based formula. Gastroenterology 1995; 109:1503–1512.

9. Suwandhi E, Ton MN, Schwarz SM, et al. Gastroesophageal reflux in infancy and childhood. Pediatr Ann 2006; 35:259–266.

10. Rudolph CD, Mazur LJ, Liptak GS, et al. Guidelines for evaluation and treatment of gastroesophageal reflux in infants and children: recommendations of the North American Society for Pediatric Gastroenterology and Nutrition. J Pediatr Gastroenterol Nutr 2001; 32(Suppl 2):S1–S31.

11. Frankel EA, Shalaby TM, Orenstein SR, et al. Sandifer syndrome posturing: relation to abdominal wall contractions, gastroesophageal reflux, and fundoplication. Dig Dis Sci 2006; 51:635–640.

12. Vandenplas Y, Salvatore S, Hauser B, et al. The diagnosis and management of gastro-oesophageal reflux in infants. Early Hum Dev 2005; 81:1011–1024.

13. Hassall E, Hassall E. Decisions in diagnosing and managing chronic gastroesophageal reflux disease in children. J Pediatr 2005; 146(3 Suppl):S3–S12.

14. Hassall E, Hassall E. Outcomes of fundoplication: causes for concern, newer options. Arch Dis Child 2005; 90:1047–1052.

15. Liacouras CA, Ruchelli E. Eosinophilic esophagitis. Curr Opin Pediatr 2004; 16:560–566.

16. Karnak ISM. Achalasia in childhood: surgical treatment and outcome. Eur J Pediatr Surg 2001; 11:223–229.

17. Horvitz G, Gold BD, Horvitz G, et al. Gastroduodenal diseases of childhood. Curr Opin Gastroenterol 2006; 22:632–640.

18. Drumm B, Day AS, Gold B, et al. Helicobacter pylori and peptic ulcer: Working Group Report of the second World Congress of Pediatric Gastroenterology, Hepatology, and Nutrition. J Pediatr Gastroenterol Nutr 2004; 39(Suppl 2):S626–S631.

19. Gold BD, Colletti RB, Abbott M, et al. Helicobacter pylori infection in children: recommendations for diagnosis and treatment. J Pediatr Gastroenterol Nutr 2000; 31:490–497.

20. Koletzko S, Koletzko S. Noninvasive diagnostic tests for Helicobacter pylori infection in children. Can J Gastroenterol 2005; 19:433–439.

21. Malfertheiner P, Megraud F, O'Morain C, et al. Current concepts in the management of Helicobacter pylori infection – the Maastricht 2–2000 Consensus Report. Alimentary Pharmacology & Therapeutics 2002; 16:167–180.

22. Mourad-Baars P, Chong S, Mourad-Baars P, et al. Helicobacter pylori infection in pediatrics. Helicobacter 2006; 11(Suppl 1):40–45.

23. Czinn SJ, Czinn SJ. Helicobacter pylori infection: detection, investigation, and management. J Pediatr 2005; 146(3 Suppl):S21–S26.

24. Fox VL. Gastrointestinal bleeding in infancy and childhood. Gastroenterol Clin N Am 2000; 29:37–66.

25. Chawla S, Seth D, Mahajan P, et al. Upper gastrointestinal bleeding in children. Clin Pediatr (Phila) 2007; 46:16–21.

26. Seidman EG, Sant'Anna AM, Dirks MH, et al. Potential applications of wireless capsule endoscopy in the pediatric age group. Gastrointestinal Endoscopy Clinics of North America 2004; 14:207–217.

27. Hernanz-Schulman M, Hernanz-Schulman M. Infantile hypertrophic pyloric stenosis. Radiology 2003; 227:319–331.

28. Andrews PL. Cyclic vomiting syndrome: timing, targets, and treatment – a basic science perspective. Dig Dis Sci 1999; 44(8 Suppl):31S–38S.

29. Lindley KJ, Andrews PL, Lindley KJ, et al. Pathogenesis and treatment of cyclical vomiting. J Pediatr Gastroenterol Nutr 2005; 41(Suppl 1):S38–S40.

30. Milla PJ, Muller DPR. Harries paediatric gastroenterology. 2nd edn. Edinburgh: Churchill Livingstone; 1988.

31. Milla PJ. The physiology of gastrointestinal motility. J Pediatr Gastroenterol Nutr 2001; 32(Suppl 1):S3–S4.

32. Ravikumara M, Tuthill DP, Jenkins HR. The changing clinical presentation of coeliac disease. Arch Dis Child 2006; 91:969–971.

33. Freemark M, Levitsky LL, Freemark M, et al. Screening for celiac disease in children with type 1 diabetes: two views of the controversy. Diabetes Care 2003; 26:1932–1939.

34. Holmes GK, Holmes GKT. Screening for coeliac disease in type 1 diabetes. Arch Dis Child 2002; 87:495–498.

35. Hill ID, Dirks MH, Liptak GS, et al. Guideline for the diagnosis and treatment of celiac disease in children: recommendations of the North American Society for Pediatric Gastroenterology, Hepatology and Nutrition. J Pediatr Gastroenterol Nutr 2005; 40:1–19.

36. West J, Logan RF, Smith CJ, et al. Malignancy and mortality in people with coeliac disease: population based cohort study. BMJ 2004; 329:716–719.

37. Card TR, West J, Holmes GK, et al. Risk of malignancy in diagnosed coeliac disease: a 24-year prospective, population-based, cohort study. Alimentary Pharmacol Therapeutics 2004; 20:769–775.

38. Murch SH, Murch SH. Clinical manifestations of food allergy: the old and the new. Eur J Gastroenterol Hepatol 2005; 17:1287–1291.

39. Host A, Halken S, Host A, et al. Primary prevention of food allergy in infants who are at risk. Curr Opin Allergy Clin Immunol 2005; 5:255–259.

40. Vanderhoof JA, Young RJ, Vanderhoof JA, et al. Role of probiotics in the management of patients with food allergy. Annals Allergy Asthma Immunology 2003; 90(Suppl 3):99–103.

41. Vanderhoof JA, Young RJ, Vanderhoof JA, et al. Allergic disorders of the gastrointestinal tract. Curr Opin Clin Nutr Metabol Care 2001; 4:553–556.

42. Sherman PM, Mitchell DJ, Cutz E, et al. Neonatal enteropathies: defining the causes of protracted diarrhea of infancy. J Pediatr Gastroenterol Nutr 2004; 38:16–26.

43. Murch SH, Murch SH. Toward a molecular understanding of complex childhood enteropathies. J Pediatr Gastroenterol Nutr 2002; 34(Suppl 1):S4–S10.

44. Vanderhoof JA, Vanderhoof JA. New and emerging therapies for short bowel syndrome in children. J Pediatr Gastroenterol Nutrit 2004; 39(Suppl 3):S769–S771.

45. Baudon JJ, Veinberg F, Thioulouse E, et al. Sucrase-isomaltase deficiency: changing pattern over two decades. J Pediatr Gastroenterol Nutr 1996; 22:284–288.

46. Wright EM, Hirayama BA, Loo DF, et al. Active sugar transport in health and disease. J Intern Med 2007; 261:32–43.

47. Hihnala S, Hoglund P, Lammi L, et al. Long-term clinical outcome in patients with congenital chloride diarrhea. J Pediatr Gastroenterol Nutr 2006; 42:369–375.

48. Erdman SH, Barnard JA, Erdman SH, et al. Gastrointestinal polyps and polyposis syndromes in children. Curr Opin Pediatr 2002; 14:576–582.

49. Durie PR. Inherited and congenital disorders of the exocrine pancreas. Gastroenterologist 1996; 4:169–187.

50. Eggermont E. Gastrointestinal manifestations in cystic fibrosis. Eur J Gastroenterol Hepatol 1996; 8:731–738.

51. Rothbaum R, Perrault J, Vlachos A, et al. Shwachman–Diamond syndrome: report from an international conference. J Pediatrics 2002; 141:266–270.

52. Cavestro GM, Comparato G, Nouvenne A, et al. Genetics of chronic pancreatitis. Jop: J Pancreas [Electronic Resource] 2005; 6(1 Suppl):53–59.

53. Benifla M, Weizman Z, Benifla M, et al. Acute pancreatitis in childhood: analysis of literature data. J Clin Gastroenterol 2003; 37:169–172.

54. Hyman PE, Milla PJ, Benninga MA, et al. Childhood functional gastrointestinal disorders: neonate/toddler. Gastroenterology 2006; 130:1519–1526.

55. Guandalini S, Pensabene L, Zikri MA, et al. Lactobacillus GG administered in oral rehydration solution to children with acute diarrhea: a multicenter European trial. J Pediatr Gastroenterol Nutr 2000; 30:54–60.

56. Szajewska H, Hoekstra JH, Sandhu B. Management of acute gastroenteritis in Europe and the impact of the new recommendations: a multicenter study. The Working Group on acute Diarrhoea of the European Society for Paediatric Gastroenterology, Hepatology, and Nutrition. J Pediatr Gastroenterol Nutr 2000; 30:522–527.

57. World Health Organisation. Expert consultation on oral rehydration salts (ORS) formulation. 2001. Geneva

58. Hoekstra JH, European Socirty of Paediatric Gastroenterology HaNWGoAD, Hoekstra JH, et al. Acute gastroenteritis in industrialized countries: compliance with guidelines for treatment. J Pediatric Gastroenterol Nutr 2001; 33(Suppl 2):S31–S35.

59. Armon K, Stephenson T, MacFaul R, et al. An evidence and consensus based guideline for acute diarrhoea management. Arch Dis Child 2001; 85:132–142.

60. Goulet OJ, Brousse N, Canioni D, et al. Syndrome of intractable diarrhoea with persistent villous atrophy in early childhood: a clinicopathological survey of 47 cases. J Pediatr Gastroenterol Nutr 1998; 26:151–161.

61. Beath SV, Booth IW, Murphy MS, et al. Nutritional care and candidates for small bowel transplantation. Arch Dis Child 1995; 73:348–350.

62. Sudan D, DiBaise J, Torres C, et al. A multidisciplinary approach to the treatment of intestinal failure. J Gastrointest Surg 2005; 9:165–176.

63. Gupte GL, Beath SV, Kelly DA, et al. Current issues in the management of intestinal failure. Arch Dis Child 2006; 91:259–264.

64. Ginies JL, Goulet O, Champion G, et al. Munchausen's syndrome by proxy and chronic intestinal pseudo-obstruction. Arch Fr Pediatr 1989; 46:267–269.

65. Beath SV, Davies P, Papadopoulou A, et al. Parenteral nutrition-related cholestasis in postsurgical neonates: multivariate analysis of risk factors. J Pediatr Surg 1996; 31:604–606.

66. Buchman AL, Iyer K, Fryer J. Parenteral nutrition-associated liver disease and the role for isolated intestine and intestine/liver transplantation. Hepatology 2006; 43:9–19.

67. Gupte GL, Beath SV, Protheroe S, et al. Improved outcome of referrals for intestinal transplantation in the UK. Arch Dis Child 2007; 92:147–152.

68. Rodrigues AF, van M, I, Sharif K, et al. Management of end-stage central venous access in children referred for possible small bowel transplantation. J Pediatr Gastroenterol Nutr 2006; 42:427–433.

69. Hassan KO, Beath SV, McKiernan PJ, et al. Difficult management choices for infants with short bowel syndrome and liver failure. J Pediatr Gastroenterol Nutr 2002; 35:216–219.

70. Grant D, bu-Elmagd K, Reyes J, et al. 2003 report of the intestine transplant registry: a new era has dawned. Ann Surg 2005; 241:607–613.

71. Tzakis AG, Kato T, Levi DM, et al. 100 multivisceral transplants at a single center. Ann Surg 2005; 242:480–490.

72. Kaufman SS, Atkinson JB, Bianchi A, et al. Indications for pediatric intestinal transplantation: a position paper of the American Society of Transplantation. Pediatr Transplant 2001; 5:80–87.

73. de Ville de GJ, Mitchell A, Mayer AD, et al. En block combined reduced-liver and small bowel transplants: from large donors to small children. Transplantation 2000; 69:555–559.

74. Beath SV, deVilledeGoyet J, Kelly DA. Risk factors for death and graft loss after small bowel transplantation. Curr Opin Organ Transplant 2003; 8:195–201.

75. Sudan D. Cost and quality of life after intestinal transplantation.Gastroenterology 2006;130(Suppl 1): S158–S162.

76. Sudan D, Horslen S, Botha J, et al. Quality of life after pediatric intestinal transplantation: the perception of pediatric recipients and their parents. Am J Transplant 2004; 4:407–413.

77. Jenkins HR, Milla PJ. The effect of colitis on large-intestinal electrolyte transport in early childhood. J Pediatr Gastroenterol Nutr 1993; 16:402–405.

78. Jenkins HR, Fenton TR, McIntosh N, et al. Development of colonic sodium transport in early childhood and its regulation by aldosterone. Gut 1990; 31:194–197.

79. Armitage E, Drummond HE, Wilson DC, et al. Increasing incidence of both juvenile-onset Crohn's disease and ulcerative colitis in Scotland. Eur J Gastroenterol Hepatol 2001; 13:1439–1447.

80. Cosgrove M, Al-Atia RF, Jenkins HR. The epidemiology of paediatric inflammatory bowel disease. Arch Dis Child 1996; 74:460–461.

81. Lindberg E, Lindquist B, Holmquist L, et al. Inflammatory bowel disease in children and adolescents in Sweden, 1984–1995. J Pediatr Gastroenterol Nutr 2000; 30:259–264.

82. Sawczenko A, Sandhu BK, Logan RF, et al. Prospective survey of childhood inflammatory bowel disease in the British Isles. Lancet 2001; 357:1093–1094.

83. Hill SM, Milla PJ. Infantile colitis. BMJ 1991; 302:545–546.

84. Beattie RM, Croft NM, Fell JM, et al. Inflammatory bowel disease. Arch Dis Child 2006; 91:426–432.

85. Fiocchi C. Inflammatory bowel disease: etiology and pathogenesis. Gastroenterology 1998; 115:182–205.

86. Russell RK, Wilson DC, Satsangi J. Unravelling the complex genetics of inflammatory bowel disease. Arch Dis Child 2004; 89:598–603.

87. Gaya DR, Russell RK, Nimmo ER, et al. New genes in inflammatory bowel disease: lessons for complex diseases? Lancet 2006; 367:1271–1284.

88. Motil KJ, Grand RJ, vis-Kraft L, et al. Growth failure in children with inflammatory bowel disease: a prospective study. Gastroenterology 1993; 105:681–691.

89. Walker-Smith JA. Management of growth failure in Crohn's disease. Arch Dis Child 1996; 75:351–354.

90. Sylvester FA, Sylvester FA. IBD and skeletal health: children are not small adults! Inflamm Bowel Dis 2005; 11:1020–1023.

91. Bunn SK, Bisset WM, Main MJ, et al. Fecal calprotectin as a measure of disease activity in childhood inflammatory bowel disease. J Pediatr Gastroenterol Nutr 2001; 32:171–177.

92. Shah DB, Cosgrove M, Rees JI, et al. The technetium white cell scan as an initial imaging investigation for evaluating suspected childhood inflammatory bowel disease. J Pediatr Gastroenterol Nutr 1997; 25:524–528.

93. Rufo PA, Bousvaros A, Rufo PA, et al. Current therapy of inflammatory bowel disease in children. Paediatric Drugs 2006; 8:279–302.

94. Kleinman RE, Baldassano RN, Caplan A, et al. Nutrition support for pediatric patients with inflammatory bowel disease: a clinical report of the North American Society for Pediatric Gastroenterology, Hepatology and Nutrition. J Pediatr Gastroenterol Nutr 2004; 39:15–27.

95. Heuschkel RB, Menache CC, Megerian JT, et al. Enteral nutrition and corticosteroids in the treatment of acute Crohn's disease in children. J Pediatr Gastroenterol Nutr 2000; 31:8–15.

96. Davies G, Evans CM, Shand WS, et al. Surgery for Crohn's disease in childhood: influence of site of disease and operative procedure on outcome. Br J Surg 1990; 77:891–894.

97. Hudson B, Green J, Hudson B, et al. British Society of Gastroenterology guidelines for ulcerative colitis surveillance: creating consensus or confusion?. Gut 2006; 55:1052–1053.

98. Apley J. The child with abdominal pains. 2nd edn. Oxford: Blackwell Scientific; 1975.

99. Chitkara DK, Rawat DJ, Talley NJ, et al. The epidemiology of childhood recurrent abdominal pain in Western countries: a systematic review. Am J Gastroenterol 2005; 100:1868–1875.

100. Walker LS, Lipani TA, Greene JW, et al. Recurrent abdominal pain: symptom subtypes based on the Rome II Criteria for pediatric functional gastrointestinal disorders. J Pediatr Gastroenterol Nutr 2004; 38:187–191.

101. Russell G, bu-Arafeh I, Symon DN. Abdominal migraine: evidence for existence and treatment options. Paediatr Drugs 2002; 4:1–8.

102. Hill DJ, Hosking CS. Infantile colic and food hypersensitivity. J Pediatr Gastroenterol Nutr 2000; 30(Suppl):S67–S76.

103. Wade S, Kilgour T. Extracts from 'clinical evidence': Infantile colic. BMJ 2001; 323:437–440.

104. Dohil R, Roberts E, Jones KV, et al. Constipation and reversible urinary tract abnormalities. Arch Dis Child 1994; 70:56–57.

105. Weaver LT, Steiner H. The bowel habit of young children. Arch Dis Child 1984; 59:649–652.

106. North American Society for Pediatric Gastroenterology HaN, North American Society for Pediatric Gastroenterology HaN. Evaluation and treatment of constipation in children: summary of updated recommendations of the North American Society for Pediatric Gastroenterology, Hepatology and Nutrition. J Pediatr Gastroenterol Nutr 2006; 43:405–407.

107. Davidson M, Waserman R. The iritable colon of childhood (chronic nonspecific diarrhea syndrome). J Pediatr 1966; 69:1027–1038.

108. Dutton PV, Furnell JR, Speirs AL. Environmental stress factors associated with toddler's diarrhoea. J Psychosom Res 1985; 29:85–88.

109. Jobling JC, Lindley KJ, Yousef Y, et al. Investigating inflammatory bowel disease – white cell scanning, radiology, and colonoscopy. Arch Dis Child 1996; 74:22–26.

110. Qualman SJ, Murray R. Aganglionosis and related disorders. Hum Pathol 1994; 25:1141–1149.

111. Thomson M. Colonoscopy and enteroscopy. Gastrointest Endosc Clin N Am 2001; 11:603–639.

112. Mowat AP. Liver disorders in childhood. 3rd edn. Oxford: Butterworth & Heinemann; 1994.

113. Roberts EA, Roberts EA. Neonatal hepatitis syndrome. Semin Neonatol 2003; 8:357–374.

114. Shneider BL, Shneider BL. Progressive intrahepatic cholestasis: mechanisms, diagnosis and therapy. Pediatric Transplantation 2004; 8:609–612.

115. Emerick KM, Rand EB, Goldmuntz E, et al. Features of Alagille syndrome in 92 patients: frequency and relation to prognosis. Hepatology 1999; 29:822–829.

116. Lykavieris P, Hadchouel M, Chardot C, et al. Outcome of liver disease in children with Alagille syndrome: a study of 163 patients. Gut 2001; 49:431–435.

117. Btaiche IF, Khalidi N, Btaiche IF, et al. Parenteral nutrition-associated liver complications in children. Pharmacotherapy 2002; 22:188–211.

118. Baker A, Dhawan A, Hadzic N, et al. Biliary atresia. In: David T J, (ed). Recent Advances in Paediatrics. vol. 16 London: Churchill Livingstone; 1988.25–40.

119. Davenport M, Davenport M. Biliary atresia. Semin Pediatr Surg 2005; 14:42–48.

120. Dumas L, Vergani D, Mieli-Vergani G, et al. Hepatitis B virus: something old, something new. J Pediatr Gastroenterol Nutr 2007; 44:14–17.

121. Fujisawa T, Komatsu H, Inui A, et al. Long-term outcome of chronic hepatitis B in adolescents or young adults in follow-up from childhood. J Pediatr Gastroenterol Nutr 2000; 30:201–206.

122. Hochman JA, Balistreri WF, Hochman JA, et al. Chronic viral hepatitis: always be current!. Pediatr Rev 2003; 24:399–410.

123. Rerksuppaphol S, Hardikar W, Dore GJ, et al. Long-term outcome of vertically acquired and post-transfusion hepatitis C infection in children. J Gastroenterol Hepatol 2004; 19:1357–1362.

124. Manns MP, McHutchison JG, Gordon SCM, et al. Peginterferon alfa-2b plus ribavirin compared with interferon alfa-2b plus ribavirin for initial treatment of chronic hepatitis C: a randomised trial. Lancet 2001; 358:958–965.

125. Gregorio GV, Portmann B, Karani J, et al. Autoimmune hepatitis/sclerosing cholangitis overlap syndrome in childhood: a 16-year prospective study. Hepatology 2001; 33:544–553.

126. Ala A, Walker AP, Ashkan K, et al. Wilson's disease. Lancet 2007; 369:397–408.

127. Patton HM, Sirlin C, Behling C, et al. Pediatric nonalcoholic fatty liver disease: a critical appraisal of current data and implications for future research. J Pediatr Gastroenterol Nutr 2006; 43:413–427.

128. Rivera-Penera T, Moreno J, Skaff C, et al. Delayed encephalopathy in fulminant hepatic failure in the pediatric population and the role of liver transplantation. J Pediatr Gastroenterol Nutr 1997; 24:128–134.

129. Durand P, Debray D, Mandel R, et al. Acute liver failure in infancy: a 14-year experience of a pediatric liver transplantation center. J Pediatr 2001; 139:871–876.

130. Kayihan N, Nennesmo I, Ericzon BG, et al. Fatal deterioration of neurological disease after orthotopic liver transplantation for valproic acid-induced liver damage. Pediatr Transplant 2000; 4:211–214.

131. Janka GE, Schneider EM, Janka GE, et al. Modern management of children with haemophagocytic lymphohistiocytosis. Br J Haematol 2004; 124:4–14.

132. McKiernan PJ, McKiernan PJ. Treatment of variceal bleeding. Gastrointestinal Endoscopy Clinics of North America 2001; 11:789–812.

133. Blei AT, Cordoba J. Hepatic encephalopathy. Am J Gastroenterol 2001; 96:1968–1976.

134. Novy MA, Schwarz KB. Nutritional considerations and management of the child with liver disease. Nutrition 1997; 13:177–184.

135. Gupta D, Vijaya DR, Gupta R, et al. Prevalence of hepatopulmonary syndrome in cirrhosis and extrahepatic portal venous obstruction. Am J Gastroenterol 2001; 96:3395–3399.

136. Salvi SS. Liver disease and pulmonary hypertension. Gut 2000; 47:595.

137. Lykavieris P, Gauthier F, Hadchouel P, et al. Risk of gastrointestinal bleeding during adolescence and early adulthood in children with portal vein obstruction. J Pediatr 2000; 136:805–808.

138. Colombo C, Battezzati PM, Crosignani A, et al. Liver disease in cystic fibrosis: A prospective study on incidence, risk factors, and outcome. Hepatology 2002; 36:1374–1382.

139. Emre S, McKenna GJ, Emre S, et al. Liver tumors in children. Pediatric Transplantation 2004; 8:632–638.

140. Muiesan P, Vergani D, Mieli-Vergani G, et al. Liver transplantation in children. J Hepatol 2007; 46:340–348.

141. Stringer MD, Hennayake S, Howard ER, et al. Improved outcome for children with hepatoblastoma. Br J Surg 1995; 82:386–391.

20

Respiratory disorders

Edited by Peter Helms, John Henderson

INTRODUCTION

Acute respiratory illness is among the most common reasons for admission to medical pediatric beds in industrialized countries and, together with acute gastroenteritis, acute respiratory infections (ARIs) remain among the most common causes of death and serious morbidity in young children in resource limited and emerging economies (Fig. 20.1). Despite a high worldwide prevalence of ARIs, the infective agents differ in that bacterial infections, including tuberculosis, are common in resource limited countries while viral infections are more commonly associated with ARIs in resource rich economies. In temperate countries there is also a marked seasonality of ARIs with a significant rise in prevalence in the winter months, falling to relatively low levels in

the summer – so much so that many acute medical pediatric units have low occupancy rates in the summer months. This seasonal pattern of illness is most dramatically seen for respiratory syncytial virus (RSV) bronchiolitis (Fig. 20.2). Whereas serious morbidity and mortality from respiratory disease has fallen to very low levels in resource rich economies, the total burden of respiratory disease remains high with a shift from life threatening ARIs to an increased incidence of asthma and related atopic disease. Worldwide comparisons of asthma prevalence using carefully standardized methodology have shown a high prevalence in resource rich, industrialized countries and generally low prevalence in resource limited countries.[1] The increasing prevalence of asthma and allergic disorders that was consistently reported over several decades in a number of resource rich countries, including the UK,[2,3] with some, although not all, recent studies suggesting that the rate of increase is slowing in the UK,[4] Europe[5] and elsewhere.[6] The reasons for what has been termed the 'asthma epidemic' have still not been fully elucidated but, since the proposition that a rise in allergic diseases could be linked to reductions in the burden of infections – the so-called hygiene hypothesis,[7,8] there has been accumulating evidence to support a role for bacterial-derived endotoxin exposure in programming the developing immune system to reduce the risk of allergic disease,[9] possibly by interactions with specific genetic polymorphisms in the innate immune system.[10] This raises the possibility of development of targeted interventions for the primary or secondary prevention of asthma in genetically predisposed individuals.

IN RESOURCE RICH ECONOMIES

The marked reduction in the prevalence of life threatening ARIs in resource rich countries in the last 50 years reflects an improved standard of living, immunization against tuberculosis, pertussis, diphtheria, measles and *Haemophilus influenzae*, and the introduction of effective

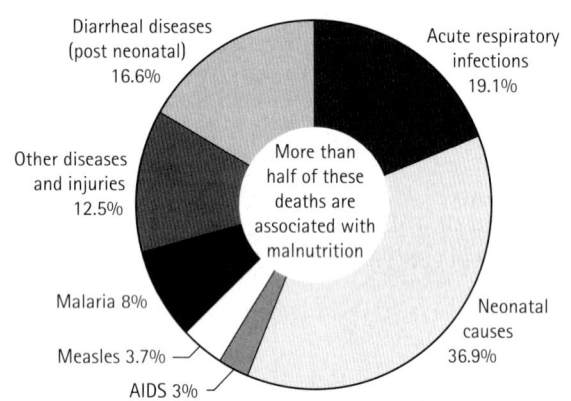

Fig. 20.1   Causes of death in children under 5 years. UNICEF under 5 mortality statistics, 2000–2003. (www.childinfo.org/areas/childmortality/)

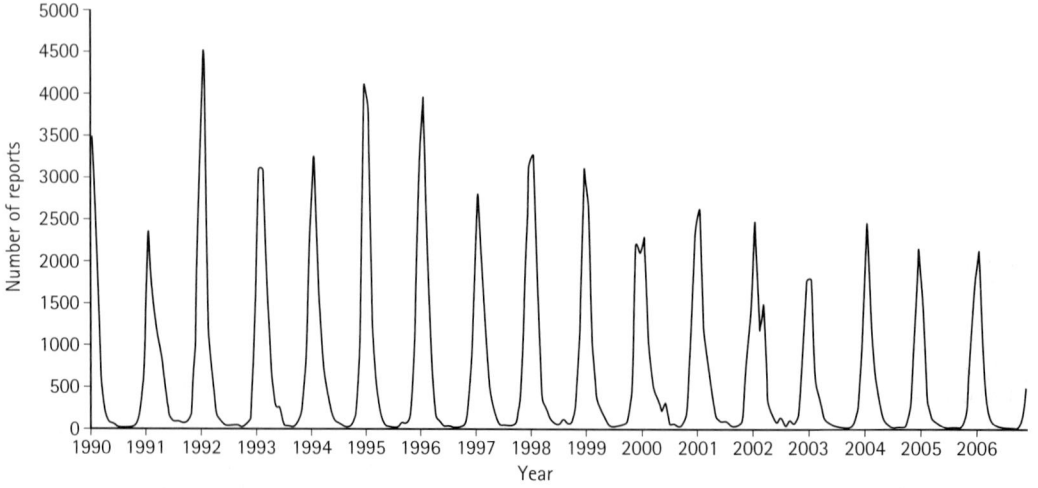

Fig. 20.2   Laboratory reports to CDSC of infections due to respiratory syncytial virus, England and Wales. RSV laboratory reports, 4-weekly by date of report 1990–2006. Source: UK Health Protection Agency (www.hpa.org.uk/infections/topics_az/rsv/graphmenu.htm).

antimicrobial drugs. For those children with life threatening disease, technological advances in managing respiratory failure have also had their impact. Targets for further reductions in the burden of illness, particularly in the youngest age groups, would be the elimination of RSV infection by an effective vaccine and a reduction in exposure to cigarette smoke in utero and in early childhood. Whereas the work load for acute asthma in hospitals has been diminishing, the burden in primary care remains at high levels with the highest annual incidence, in proportion to the at risk population, in the youngest age groups (Fig. 20.3). Ecological analyses have suggested that the early and sustained use of prophylactic therapy, particularly inhaled corticosteroids (ICSs), has contributed to this reduction in hospital admissions, although this beneficial outcome needs to be balanced by concerns about the possible systemic effects of long term use of ICSs.[11] Recent controlled trials of inhaled corticosteroids for infant wheeze have not demonstrated that this is an efficacious strategy to alter the natural history of asthma after treatment is stopped.[12–14]

In resource rich economies improvements in therapeutic options, including age appropriate inhalation delivery devices, antibiotics and organization of care, have resulted in increasing actuarial survival for conditions that in previous generations and epochs were invariably fatal in childhood. This increased survival applies to a number of conditions, including cystic fibrosis, unusual congenital anomalies such as congenital diaphragmatic hernia and respiratory complications of other conditions such as extreme prematurity and neuromuscular disorders (see p. 727 – Chronic lung disease of prematurity, and p. 687 – Sleep and respiratory disorders). In cystic fibrosis, for example, a strong cohort effect on actuarial survival, although modulated by socioeconomic factors, has become apparent since the disease was first characterized in the 1940s (Fig. 20.4).[15,16] The recent introduction in the UK of universal newborn screening for cystic fibrosis may also contribute to improved survival during childhood.[17] The increased survival of children with significant lung disease, or with neuromuscular disorders and associated respiratory impairment, has effectively exported much morbidity and mortality into adult life. These medical 'successes' have placed increased burdens on affected individuals and their families and, in order to maintain a satisfactory quality of life, more attention is now being given to psychosocial aspects of disease and to palliative care (see Ch. 35). Quality of life instruments are being increasingly used to assess the impact of disease and in assessing therapeutic interventions.[18,19]

IN RESOURCE LIMITED AND EMERGING ECONOMIES

Respiratory disease is a prevalent cause of mortality in resource limited countries and a major contributor to child deaths in Africa and South East Asia (see Fig. 20.1). In a global health context these potentially avoidable causes of death have moved up the political agenda and the UN Millennium Summit in 2000 agreed a number of goals to reduce the burden of infectious diseases, including ARIs, setting defined targets for

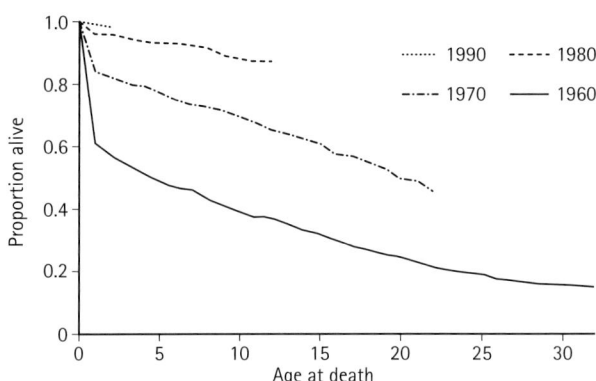
Fig. 20.4 Actuarial survival of patients with cystic fibrosis by birth cohort. Source: Elborn et al.[16]

their reduction. One such target is to combat HIV/AIDS, malaria and other infectious diseases, including tuberculosis (TB). The World Health Organization (WHO) declared TB a global emergency in 1993 and set targets to detect 70% of new infectious (smear positive) cases of TB worldwide, to successfully treat 85% of all cases detected and to halve TB prevalence and death rates. Although progress has been made on mortality using strategies such as directly observed treatment strategy (DOTS), factors such as the AIDS epidemic and the emergence of drug resistant strains of Mycobacterium tuberculosis have contributed to the still growing burden of new cases worldwide (Fig. 20.5).

Deaths from pneumonia can also be significantly reduced if the WHO guidelines are fully implemented. The WHO program requires identification of children with clinical evidence of pneumonia followed by early introduction of antibiotics and advice on use of fluids and adequate nutrition. This program can be delivered relatively inexpensively by village health workers who are trained to identify signs of pneumonia, including rapid breathing and chest indrawing, and who use appropriate antibiotics and discourage the use of commercial cough remedies, some of which contain harmful ingredients. The benefits of such programs can be dramatic (Fig. 20.6).

FETAL PROGRAMMING OF LUNG DISEASE IN CHILDREN AND ADULTS

There is growing evidence that fetal life and early childhood are critical periods of development for many diseases that present during childhood and adult life. In humans and other long-gestation species, the development of lung architecture occurs during fetal and early postnatal life. A number of epidemiological studies have demonstrated associations between prenatal factors that restrict intrauterine growth and respiratory symptoms in infancy. This observation led to speculation that factors which impair fetal growth may also constrain fetal lung development, resulting in permanent changes to lung architecture. Longitudinal follow-up of birth and childhood cohorts to adolescent and adult life has suggested that pulmonary function decrements that are established in early childhood track with somatic growth to adulthood,[20,21] suggesting that some late-onset diseases, such as chronic obstructive pulmonary disease (COPD), may have their origins in childhood.[22] Work in fetal lambs with imposed growth restriction during late gestation has demonstrated structural and mechanical abnormalities of the lungs but no effects on surfactant protein expression in these animals.[23] Barker et al[24] described an association between low birth weight and lung function decrements in over 5000 adult males. Furthermore, respiratory infection during early childhood was associated with further decrements in adult lung function in this population, suggesting that either impaired lung function at birth was associated with predisposition to pulmonary infections during infancy or that respiratory infections, such as pneumonia and whooping cough, cause airway and lung remodeling which further impairs lung function. A follow-up study of lung function in

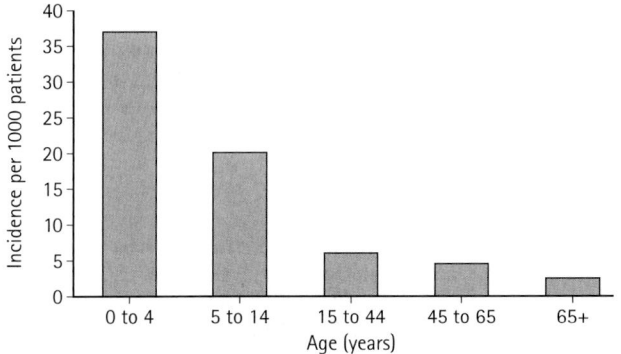
Fig. 20.3 Annual incidence of physician-diagnosed asthma in Scottish General Practices 1998. Data from the General Practice Data Evaluation Project (GDEP) Scotland.

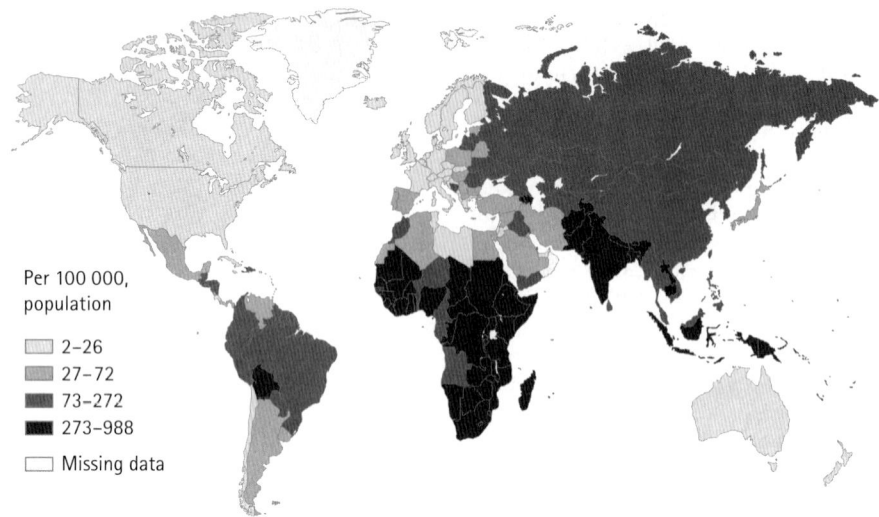

Fig. 20.5   Tuberculosis prevalence worldwide (2003). Source: UN Statistics Division 'Millenium Indicators Database' (July 2005).

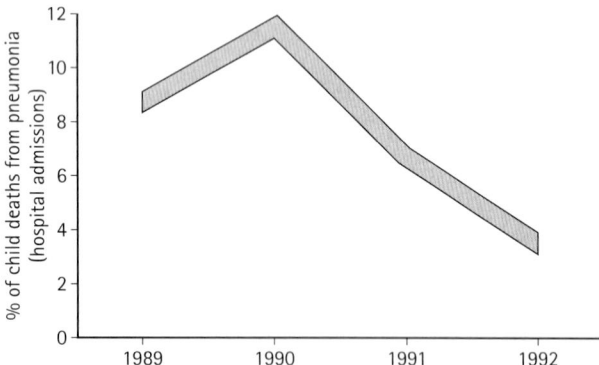

Fig. 20.6   Reduction in hospital deaths attributable to pneumonia after the introduction of the WHO guidelines for identifying and managing acute respiratory infection in childhood (www.who.int/inf-new/child3.htm).

infancy has demonstrated reduced forced expiratory flows at the age of 2 months in infants who subsequently developed pneumonia,[25] supporting a role for predisposition to infections in infants who already have pre-existing lung function impairment. Other epidemiological studies have confirmed an association between respiratory infections during infancy and early childhood and later functional abnormalities consistent with airway obstruction in adults.[26]

GENETIC DETERMINANTS

Cystic fibrosis

Pulmonary disease may accompany a number of genetic disorders in children and some pulmonary diseases have a genetic basis, although this is seldom based on simple Mendelian inheritance but may have polygenic or multifactorial etiology. A clear exception to this is cystic fibrosis, which results from a variety of mutations in a single gene located on chromosome 7q (see p. 706 – Cystic fibrosis).

Asthma

Asthma is a complex, polygenic disease that results from the exposure of genetically susceptible individuals to environmental triggers, possibly at critical stages of development. Linkage studies and genome-wide searches have identified a number of potential candidate genes for asthma and atopy.[27,28] Although variants in over 60 genes have been associated with asthma and related traits, candidate gene studies have demonstrated considerable heterogeneity of associations with asthma and many have failed to replicate in independent samples.[29] Also, the rate of increase in asthma prevalence in the UK and other Western countries is inconsistent with major shifts in population genetics. Therefore, attention has focused on identification of environmental exposures that may be causally implicated in the etiology of asthma and atopy.

Non-cystic fibrosis bronchiectasis

The approach to bronchiectasis in children without cystic fibrosis (non-CF bronchiectasis) has changed in emphasis from the role of childhood infections, such as pertussis, tuberculosis and complicated measles, to the role of intrinsic defects with an inherited basis. Although deficiency of protease inhibitors, primarily alpha1-antitrypsin, is often included in the work-up of these children, it is not a condition that presents in this way. Primary ciliary dyskinesia (PCD), however, is increasingly recognized in children with chronic suppurative lung disease and bronchiectasis. PCD is generally observed to follow an autosomal recessive mode of inheritance, although dominant and X-linked inheritances have been described. Linkage studies of separate populations with PCD have mapped loci to a number of chromosomes and a genome-wide screen has demonstrated extensive locus heterogeneity in PCD.[30] Candidate genes for the disease include those encoding the intermediate and heavy dynein chains, e.g. DNAI2 and DNAH5.[31] There is also increasing recognition of the importance of nodal cilia in determining laterality,[32] underpinning the observed association of PCD with congenital heart disease, including atrial isomerism and disorders of laterality, such as situs inversus.

Immune deficiency is another important risk factor for bronchiectasis. A survey of 150 patients, mainly adults, with bronchiectasis, during which systematic investigations for possible heritable causes were performed, identified 12 subjects with abnormalities of immune function, including common variable immune deficiency (CVID), IgM deficiency and isolated IgG subclass deficiencies.[33]

Other lung disorders

Other pulmonary diseases that have a genetic basis but rarely present during childhood include interstitial lung disease in association with collagen disorders, such as lupus erythematosus, and sarcoidosis. There is increasing interest in the origins of COPD, which has been demonstrated in several studies to cluster within families, independent of smoking status. It is possible that mechanisms such as oxidative lung injury due to deficiencies of components of the antioxidant defenses, such as superoxide dismutase and glutathione-S-transferases, are responsible for respiratory morbidity in childhood that is the antecedent of COPD in adults. Increasing knowledge of the genetic and cellular regulation of pulmonary inflammation and defense is likely to lead to new insights into the origins of pulmonary diseases. The challenge will be to recognize individuals at risk and to develop effective interventions to prevent the onset or alter the natural history of some of these conditions.

ENVIRONMENTAL RISK FACTORS

Tobacco smoke exposure

A series of systematic reviews demonstrated consistent relationships between parents' smoking and respiratory illnesses and symptoms and middle ear disease in children with odds ratios between 1.2 and 1.6.[34] The odds were greater for preschool children and higher for maternal compared with paternal smoking. The latter observation might be explained by increased exposure to maternal rather than paternal smoking among preschool children. Alternatively, a prenatal effect of maternal smoking on the developing fetal lungs might be responsible. One of the difficulties of disentangling the interrelationships of prenatal and postnatal tobacco smoke exposure on children's respiratory symptoms in epidemiological studies is the observation that prenatal maternal smoking is almost always associated with postnatal tobacco smoke exposure.

Several studies have demonstrated an association between prenatal tobacco smoke exposure and decrements in pulmonary function in infants soon after delivery and before the onset of symptoms. Such decrements appear to be associated with respiratory symptoms during the first year after birth[35-37] and it seems likely that in utero smoke exposure causes growth restraint of fetal airways. The longer term effects of such fetal growth restraint have yet to be determined. Recent studies have attempted to examine the differential effects of intrauterine and postnatal tobacco smoke exposure on the outcomes of asthma and wheezing in later childhood. Gilliland et al[38] have demonstrated associations between in utero exposure and physician diagnosed asthma in later childhood but, although current or past environmental (postnatal) exposure was related to wheezing symptoms, there was no significant relationship with asthma. The authors speculated that environmental exposure may act as a cofactor for attacks of wheezing but did not appear to be a factor that induced asthma in this population.

Parental smoking has also been demonstrated in several case control and cohort studies[39] to be significantly associated with sudden infant death syndrome. Maternal smoking was associated with increased risk and a dose response effect has been demonstrated in several studies, suggesting a casual relationship, and, although smoking rates vary with socioeconomic status, the risk appears to be consistent across socioeconomic groups. Fleming et al in a study of sudden infant death after the 'Back to Sleep' campaign in the UK calculated an odds ratio of sudden infant death syndrome (SIDS) for maternal smoking during pregnancy of 2.1 with an additional independent effect of paternal smoking.[40] The mechanisms for this effect have not been elucidated but fetal lung growth restraint or effects of smoking on neurological responses to thermal, hypoxic or hypercapnic stress have been postulated. Recent pathological studies of infants dying of SIDS have demonstrated increased thickness of the airway wall in infants of mothers who smoked compared with infants of nonsmoking mothers, suggesting that airway obstruction may be an important mechanism.

Many studies have concentrated on the respiratory health effects of passive exposure to tobacco smoke in children. However, active smoking by children remains a significant health problem. In the UK, smoking becomes detectable in the 10–12 year age range and approximately one quarter of 15 year olds are reported to smoke.[41] A survey of 14–16-year-old children revealed that 30% had been active smokers in the previous 12 months, with 14.1% reporting regular smoking.[42] Similar figures are reported from the USA, although with encouraging signs of a downward trend in recent years.[43] Trials of smoking cessation targeted specifically at adolescents have recently been reviewed, suggesting that complex approaches may be required for these to be effective.[44]

Social deprivation (see also Chs 2 and 3)
Resource limited countries

Using the World Bank definition of $1/person/day, it is estimated that 2.1 billion of the world's population live in conditions of absolute poverty below this threshold. Diseases associated with poverty are primarily infectious diseases, which are linked to inadequate income, lack of access to clean water and sanitation, malnutrition and poor access to medical services. In resource limited countries the commonest causes of death in children under 5 years of age are lower respiratory infections, diarrheal illnesses and measles. In 2000, acute lower respiratory tract infections accounted for 1.89 million deaths in children under 5 in the resource limited world,[45] with approximately 40% estimated to be related to malnutrition. Some resource limited countries have achieved lower rates of poverty-related ill health by government interventions in health, education and social security, and also by active programs to increase the level of female literacy in their populations.

Resource rich countries

In the UK, adults and children of lower socioeconomic status have also been demonstrated to be at higher risk of communicable diseases, particularly respiratory infections.[46] A longitudinal study of a UK cohort born in 1946 demonstrated that a poor home environment, parental bronchitis and atmospheric pollution were the best predictors of lower respiratory tract infections in the first 2 years after birth and these factors, together with later smoking and childhood respiratory infections, were the best predictors of lower respiratory tract diseases in adults.[47] It is possible that increased infections in socially disadvantaged populations are related to crowding and increased exposure to infectious agents or to alterations in host immunity, possibly related to nutritional status. One of the characteristic diseases of social deprivation, tuberculosis (see Ch. 28) has shown a reversal of the decline in notified cases in the UK (Public Health Laboratory Service; www.phls.co.uk) with the largest number of cases reported from urban regions, particularly London. The annual incidence of tuberculosis in children in the UK is currently around 3.5 per 100 000 with a doubling of cases in London reported between 1993 and 1998.[48] In contrast to the adult population in which the majority of cases occur in males, the sex distribution in children appears to be even. Studies of variations in tuberculosis rates between electoral wards in inner cities have suggested that the country of birth was the single most explanatory variable, with measures of poverty being of only secondary importance.[49,50]

Early respiratory infections

In addition to potential protective effects on later development of asthma and related allergic disease (see p. 690 – Asthma), viral respiratory infections have also been proposed as contributors to the development of obstructive airways disease. A number of studies have reported persistent or recurrent wheezing after RSV bronchiolitis in infants. Sigurs et al[51] demonstrated a significant risk of asthma and allergic sensitization at the age of 7½ years in children who had been hospitalized with RSV bronchiolitis during infancy compared with matched controls. However, there is still debate about whether RSV causes asthma or whether severe RSV infection is a manifestation of pre-existing risk factors for both bronchiolitis and asthma.[52] It is hoped that randomized controlled trials (RCTs) of RSV prophylaxis will be able to address some of these questions but these are currently restricted to high risk infants.

Diet

The prenatal effects of maternal famine were studied in a Dutch population exposed to the famine of 1944–45. The prevalence of obstructive airways diseases in the offspring of famine-exposed mothers was higher, particularly when the exposure occurred in early gestation. This effect did not appear to be mediated through increased prevalence of atopic disease in this population, suggesting that impairment of fetal lung development was an important factor.

A number of dietary constituents have been examined in relation to their potential role in the etiology of lung diseases, including fatty acids, antioxidants and sodium intake. The observation that Eskimos had a low prevalence of lung disease and a diet high in oily fish prompted speculation that *n*-3 fatty acids, which competitively inhibit the metabolism of arachidonic acid, may be protective against asthma.[53] However, there is only weak evidence for this and no intervention studies have yet been done.

Oxidative damage to the lungs, mediated through oxygen free radicals, is believed to be important in the pathogenesis of asthma and COPD. Fruit is a major source of antioxidant vitamins and epidemiological associations between fruit intake and lung function in adults have been established. A positive association between fresh fruit consumption and lung function has also been demonstrated in children.[54] Selenium is essential to the activity of glutathione peroxidase enzymes that are involved in the lung's antioxidant defenses. Low serum concentrations of selenium have been demonstrated in subjects with asthma but it is unclear whether selenium deficiency contributes to the development of asthma or if selenium consumption occurs as a consequence of oxidant injury. An ecological study of asthma and allergy (ISAAC) did not demonstrate an increased prevalence in countries in which selenium deficiency is endemic[55] compared with areas with abundant dietary selenium sources. A systematic review of selenium supplementation in asthma identified only one RCT. This suggested improvements in clinical control when asthma treatment was supplemented by selenium but there were no objective correlates of this improvement.[56] Low dose vitamin A supplementation has been examined for its possible protective role in the development of lower respiratory infections in children. Intervention studies in resource limited countries had suggested that this effect was strongly related to nutritional status with decreased acute lower respiratory infections observed in underweight children only.[57,58] However, a recent review of vitamin A supplementation in nonmeasles-related pneumonia concluded that there was no evidence of reduction in mortality or measures of morbidity.[59]

Regional differences in asthma mortality have been correlated with table salt purchase, leading to the possibility that dietary sodium may be an important factor in asthma pathogenesis. However, dietary salt intake in children has been associated with increased bronchial responsiveness to methacholine but not with a diagnosis of asthma or with exercise induced bronchospasm.[60] A recent systematic review of a number of small trials of dietary salt reduction or exclusion in asthma concluded that there was insufficient evidence on which to base current recommendations.[61]

Atmospheric pollution (including indoor pollution)

There is clear evidence that atmospheric pollution may exacerbate respiratory symptoms in human subjects but what is less clear is whether specific pollutants have a causal role in the pathogenesis of respiratory diseases. The principal pollutants of the external (outdoor) environment include nitrogen oxides (NO, NO_2), ozone, sulphur dioxide (SO_2) and particulates from the burning of fossil fuels. Hospital admission rates for respiratory diseases, especially pneumonia, have been demonstrated to be correlated with high atmospheric concentrations of particulates (PM_{10}), NO_2 and ozone[62] and effects of NO_2, carbon monoxide (CO) and SO_2 on general practice consultations for asthma have been found to be stronger in children than adults.[63] The well documented rise in the prevalence of asthma in industrialized countries has coincided with a general increase in the density of road traffic in the majority of these countries. Therefore, a number of studies have investigated the possibility that traffic pollution is an exposure that initiates asthma in previously unaffected individuals but with conflicting results. A landmark study of this aspect of lung disease in children was undertaken following the German reunification in 1989. This allowed a study of two genetically similar populations exposed to different levels of atmospheric pollution with higher concentrations of industrial pollutants (SO_2 and particulates) in Leipzig, East Germany compared with Munich, West Germany where traffic density was higher. The results of this study demonstrated a higher lifetime prevalence of asthma and a greater prevalence of sensitization to common aeroallergens in the West

German population compared with the East German population, suggesting that prolonged exposure to industrial pollutants was not associated with the development of asthma or allergy.[64] The same group studied the relationships between traffic density and respiratory health of children in several school districts in Munich and, although demonstrating associations between traffic density and small decrements in lung function, found no association between high traffic density and either lifetime prevalence of asthma or bronchial responsiveness to cold air.[65] It should be borne in mind that geographical comparisons such as this are prone to confounding by other differences in exposures between the populations, such as indoor environment and lifestyle variations. The importance of the indoor environment for respiratory diseases has been highlighted in observational studies of populations in resource limited countries that rely on burning fossil fuels for domestic energy: this practice appears to be associated with increased respiratory infections and obstructive airways diseases in children,[66] although no controlled studies have been done and few have measured exposures directly. An association between gas cooking and asthma in children has been described[67] and Burr et al[68] have described an increased 12-month prevalence of wheeze in 12–14 year olds in association with the use of bottled gas, paraffin and other unusual domestic fuels for heating. However, of all the potential indoor pollutants to which children may be exposed, it is likely that parental tobacco smoke exposure has the single greatest effect on their respiratory health.

DEVELOPMENT OF THE RESPIRATORY SYSTEM

FETAL AND PERINATAL DEVELOPMENT
Structural development
Lung growth and development commences in early intrauterine life with the development of the trachea from the primitive esophagus at approximately 5 weeks of gestational age. The right and left lung buds develop at about 7 weeks and the formation of the main lobar structures is already evident by 9 weeks. This process of branching airway development continues through the first trimester of pregnancy and is largely complete by 16 weeks of gestational age. By this time the lungs have a glandular appearance with alveoli emerging over the next 8–10 weeks, increasing in complexity and surface area up to and beyond term.[69,70] Arguments concerning the duration of alveolar development have depended on the distinction of saccules and alveoli and on techniques for counting alveolar number in postmortem lungs. Approximately 50% of alveoli are present at term with 85% complete by 2–3 years of age, a process accompanied by a reduction in interstitial tissue and the remodeling of capillaries into a single network, and with an enormous thinning of the blood–gas barrier. A network of elastin strands form the 'skeleton' (likened to a fishnet) between which the new alveoli are formed. Normal fetal breathing movements are important in promoting this growth. Adverse influences on this ordered sequence of development will have important and different consequences for future respiratory health of the individual depending on their timing and duration. Generally the earlier the insult the more profound the long term consequences.

Implications for disease
Many adverse intrauterine influences, e.g. congenital diaphragmatic hernia[71] and renal agenesis and oligohydramnios[72] can have devastating effects on subsequent lung growth and development. Insults during the early phase of airway development will reduce branching and will inevitably lead to reductions in the number of alveoli that can bud from a reduced number of terminal bronchioles (Fig. 20.7). This can also be inferred from physiological measurements in infants with impairment of intrauterine growth due to diaphragmatic hernia or reduced fetal breathing movements associated with spinal muscular atrophy of intrauterine origin.[73] The importance of fetal breathing movements has been demonstrated in a series of elegant experiments in laboratory animals in which the relative contributions of fetal breathing and the volume of amniotic fluid have been demonstrated.[74] As pulmonary vascular

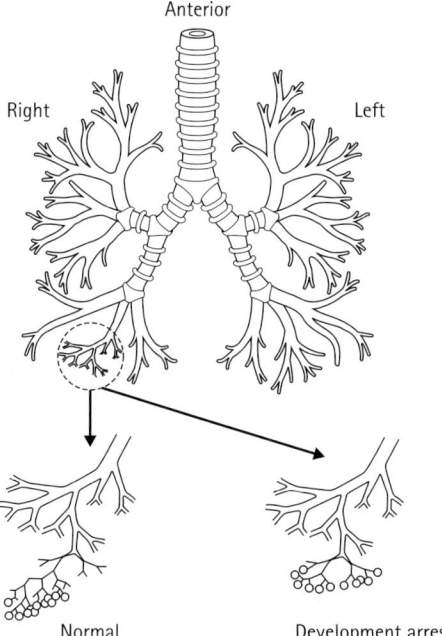

Fig. 20.7 Representation of the bronchial tree in a normal newborn infant and in an infant with intrauterine pulmonary hypoplasia in whom peripheral airways development has been impaired. Note the implication for reduced alveoli.

development follows the development of the airways it is hardly surprising that pulmonary perfusion anomalies have also been observed in the survivors of diaphragmatic hernia repair despite what appears to be a satisfactory radiological outcome.[75] Although the intrauterine insults described above are dramatic, they are thankfully relatively rare in population terms. What may be more relevant for population respiratory health are the more subtle influences on lung growth and development in utero and in early life. Such associations between early respiratory symptoms and adverse environmental exposures have been inferred by the association between low birth weight and subsequent respiratory health and in particular chronic respiratory lung disease of adulthood.[24] The most clearly identified adverse exposure at a whole population level is fetal tobacco smoke exposure associated with maternal smoking in pregnancy. Whereas postnatal or environmental tobacco smoke (ETS) exposure has a significant influence on respiratory morbidity in the young,[76] the effects of prenatal exposure are likely to be more long lasting. Studies which have assessed lung function soon after birth, when the effects of ETS would be expected to be small, have shown evidence of reduced airway function.[77,78] Whereas it is clearly not possible to identify the exact mechanisms of these effects in humans, animal studies have shown that fetal ETS significantly reduces cell division in the lung (as evidenced by reduced DNA), alveolar number and the amount of connective tissue within the lung.[79,80]

The structures of the airways themselves also have important functional consequences. Cartilaginous structures appear in segmental bronchi at 10–12 weeks of gestational age but continue to develop in small bronchi until after birth. Generalized bronchomalacia or local disorders affecting the trachea and bronchi are associated with several important disorders, including tracheomalacia, stovepipe trachea and lobar emphysema. Airway smooth muscle, contrary to popular belief, is found at term down to the smallest terminal and respiratory bronchioles and consequently failure of wheezing illnesses to respond to bronchodilators cannot be ascribed to the absence of smooth muscle at this level. Vascular modeling after birth may be disturbed as a result of widespread perinatal lung damage such as chronic lung disease of prematurity (see p. 727), or in association with congenital heart disease (see Ch. 21, p. 765), leading to persistence of high pulmonary vascular resistance

and pulmonary hypertension. A number of major developmental defects in the nasopharynx may lead to respiratory obstruction, infection or recurrent aspiration. These include choanal atresia or stenosis, palatal anomalies and, at a cellular level, ciliary dyskinesia. These, as well as mid-facial syndromes, Down syndrome and neuromuscular disorders, can lead to obstructive apnea or sleep-disordered breathing problems (see p. 687 – Sleep and respiratory disorders).

The chest wall

The chest wall is defined as the structures which surround the lung and which have significant influences on lung growth and function. It includes the rib cage, the diaphragm and the abdominal contents together with the paraspinal and accessory muscles of respiration. The diaphragm becomes a complete membrane by 8 weeks of gestation and the abdominal wall is complete at 9 weeks, allowing the establishment of effective fetal breathing. At birth, however, the proportion of fatigue resistant (Type 1) striated muscle fibers is approximately 10%, much less than the 50% found in adults. The proportion is even less in preterm infants and along with the instability of the chest wall explains in part the tendency of preterm infants to develop respiratory failure and to suffer from apnea. The diaphragm is also inserted more directly into the chest wall with a reduced area of apposition (or alignment with the lower rib cage) than that found in mature subjects and this again results in a relative functional impairment in the infant and very young child. The chest wall has important influences on the function of the underlying lungs both in maintaining lung volume at rest (the lung tends to seek a lower volume whereas the chest wall recoils outwards) and in its role as the 'respiratory pump'. During growth and development important changes occur in the function of the chest wall, not only at rest but also during respiratory efforts that affect underlying lung function (see below).

POSTNATAL DEVELOPMENT

Alveolization is virtually complete by 3 years of age, after which the lungs grow as a result of stretch, mainly due to the associated growth of the rib cage. This can be seen in the different patterns of alveolar growth assessed from postmortem pathological studies and physiological lung volumes measured during respiratory maneuvers (Fig. 20.8). This disparity emphasizes the significant influence of the chest wall on the function of the underlying lung. The stretch and subsequent growth of volume of the lung results in what has been termed 'dysnaptic' growth. In infancy the airways are relatively large in relation to the total lung volume, a ratio which falls progressively during subsequent

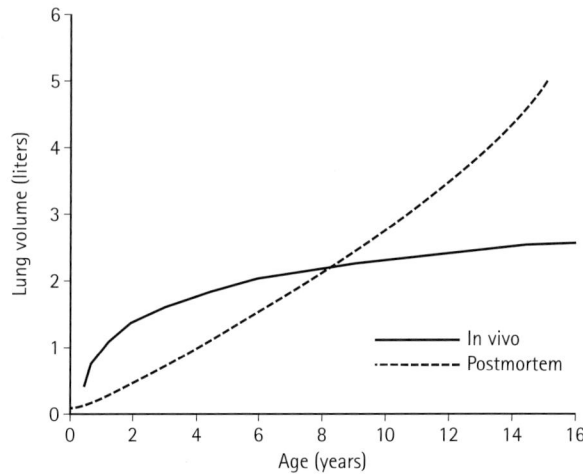

Fig. 20.8 Increase in lung volume in boys contrasting in vivo to post mortem measurements. Measurements in vivo are of total lung capacity and are influenced by increasing inspiratory effort with age. Measurements post mortem made at the same distending pressure of 3.3 kPa.

growth. This feature of physiological lung growth results in a gradual fall in the contribution of peripheral airway resistance to overall airway resistance, a feature which also contributes to the severe nature of lower respiratory illnesses and an increased tendency to develop symptomatic airway obstruction in infancy and early childhood. Another feature during growth and development is that females appear to have more patent airways (lower resistance) than males, as seen in physiological measurements,[81,82] and in the increased risk of significant respiratory morbidity in boys. This relative female advantage reverses during puberty and is in part explained by the increased stretch of the underlying lung that is associated with increased muscular development and thoracic expansion in males at that time.

Large airways are supported by cartilage in order to resist collapse during expiration whereas smaller peripheral airways within the lung have no such support but rely on the distending pressure within the lung parenchyma to remain patent. In infancy and early childhood this distending pressure is low and in the region of 0.15 kPa at the end of quiet expiration. In the young healthy adult these pressures increase to between 0.5 and 1.0 kPa, differences which can be largely attributed to increasing chest wall recoil associated with maturation. A highly compliant (or floppy) chest wall is an advantage in utero in that the low lung distending pressure reduces the amount of lung liquid that needs to be cleared by lymphatic drainage soon after birth. However, in the transition to air breathing the highly compliant and unstable ribcage has significant functional consequences. Whereas it is the chest wall that determines the distribution of ventilation and airway function in infancy and early childhood, it is the gradual loss of the elastic recoil of structures within the lungs themselves that is associated with increasing peripheral airway closure and reduced airway function in the elderly (Fig. 20.9).

The thoracic configuration is also different in infants and young children in that the ribs are more horizontally placed with less potential for thoracic expansion than in older children and adults.[83] As a consequence infants and very young children rely more on diaphragmatic activity and this, in combination with a more direct insertion into the ribcage and a reduced number of Type 1 muscle fibers (slow twitch high oxidative fibers), places the infant and young child at significant risk of developing respiratory failure when presented with an added respiratory load. Any additional impairment of the chest wall itself, e.g. in association with scoliosis or neuromuscular disorders, will only augment this relative inefficiency of the respiratory system in early life.

The upper airway of the infant and young child is also structurally different from that of the mature child or adult in that the posterior

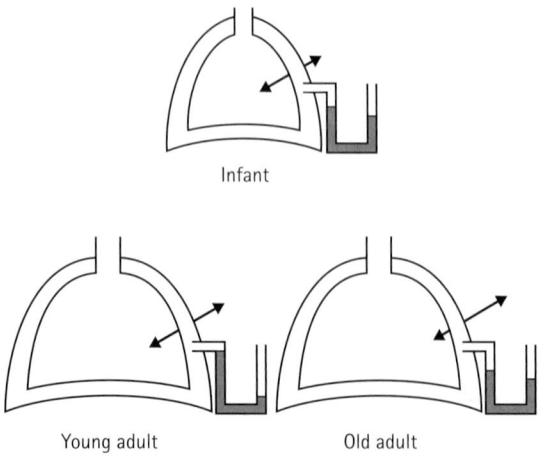

Fig. 20.9   Interaction between outward recoil of chest wall and inward recoil of the underlying lung. The reduced chest wall recoil in the infant results in low transpulmonary pressures whereas in the elderly reduced lung recoil has the same effect. Low transpulmonary pressures result in increasing risks of peripheral (small) airways closure.

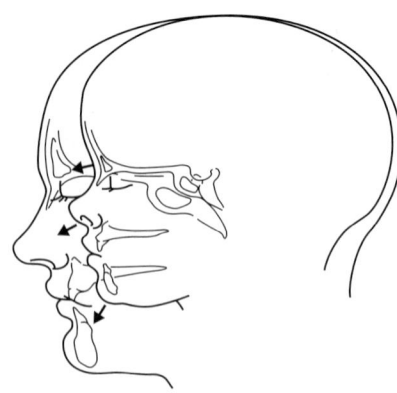

Fig. 20.10   Growth of facial skeleton from childhood to adult life. The relative hypoplasia of the facial skeleton and sinuses renders the infant and very young child prone to upper airway obstruction as a consequence of a crowded hypopharynx.[84]

nasopharynx is relatively crowded and therefore vulnerable to obstruction. The immaturity of the facial skeleton, particularly the mid-facial skeleton in the infant and young child, results in the relative backward displacement of the tongue. Together with the hypertrophy of the tonsilar tissue that occurs in early childhood, it is hardly surprising that upper respiratory airway obstruction is a common clinical feature in early life (Fig. 20.10).

Gas exchange

The immediate process of adaptation at birth takes about 5 h but in premature infants a significant alveolar to arterial oxygen difference [(A–a) DO_2] persists up to term largely due to intrapulmonary anatomical shunt through non-alveolized vessels. Persistence of a significant (A–a) DO_2 through the first year is largely due to the ventilation/perfusion imbalance described below. Thus the mean arterial oxygen tension PO_2 for a term infant for the first week of life is 10 kPa, giving an approximate (A–a) DO_2 of 4 kPa compared with 1 kPa for an adult. Oxygen consumption per kg and hence alveolar ventilation in the newborn is two to three times adult values. The suboptimal gas exchange in subsequent infancy and early childhood is largely due to the poor support offered by the compliant chest wall to the underlying lungs (see Fig. 20.9) with subsequent closure of small airways in dependent parts of the lungs (the lung bases when posture is upright) and shunting of blood through nonventilated areas.[85]

Developmental disorders of gas exchange are not common. Severe lung hypoplasia may impose limits in the newborn period which diminish with growth. Incomplete collateral ventilation (the canals of Lambert are not apparent in lungs from preschool children) may lead to atelectasis and hence impaired gas exchange in disease.

RESPIRATORY PHYSIOLOGY, PATHOPHYSIOLOGY AND THE MEASUREMENT OF RESPIRATORY FUNCTION

The principal function of the respiratory system is gas exchange: oxygenation of the blood and the removal of carbon dioxide. A knowledge of the means whereby this is achieved forms the basis for understanding many of the clinical features of respiratory disease and of lung function tests. Although the principles of disturbed pathophysiology are no different in children and adults, growth and development add further dimensions both to the interpretation of data and to the challenge of making the measurements.

RESPIRATORY FUNCTION TESTS

A decision to carry out respiratory function tests will generally have followed clinical assessment and can often usefully be combined with other investigations. The tests should be performed by an operator experienced in dealing with children, who can allay their anxiety and turn natural inquisitiveness and playfulness to advantage. A positive approach, with lots of encouragement and the insight to abandon a session before failure to cooperate turns into panic, are essential virtues.

For most simple procedures the equipment found in any adult lung function laboratory will be adequate. In infancy most measurements can only be made in specialized laboratories and will not be dealt with here. Preschool children form another challenging group, where specially adapted equipment may be needed and where the repeatability of measurements is not as good as in older children and adults. However, spirometric measurements, for example, can be performed in children as young as 4 years of age with suitable equipment and experience and peak flow can occasionally be measured in 3 year olds. In view of these challenges there is a burgeoning interest in tidal breathing techniques in this young age group.[86,87]

Interpretation

Lung function is most closely related to body length or height but with small additional effects of age and sex, particularly around puberty, and of ethnic group. In the presence of scoliosis, arm span can be substituted directly for length. Body weight is a poor reference standard, since its variation in disease can be extreme. The significance of individual measurements in relation to the population is found by reference to a graph, table or appropriate prediction equations.[81,82] For sequential measurements in an individual, the confidence limits or coefficient of variation for repeated measurements must be sought.

AIRWAY FUNCTION

As most lung problems in infancy and childhood are associated with airway obstruction, measurements that reflect airway caliber and function are of particular relevance.

The conducting airways extend from the tip of the nose to the terminal bronchioles and are physiologically very active, constantly varying their caliber and the nature of their secretions in response to changing environmental exposures.

The volume of the conducting airways constitutes a dead space (i.e. the volume of the lungs which although ventilated does not contribute to alveolar gas exchange; it measures about 2.2 ml/kg throughout life[80]). Disorders of airway structure such as bronchiectasis lead to an increase in anatomical dead space. In addition, the ventilation of underperfused regions of the lung, such as the apices in the erect posture, leads to another form of dead space referred to as physiological dead space.

Airway resistance (R_{aw}) is a function of gas flow and pressure: airway resistance = pressure/flow. The reciprocal of R_{aw}, airway conductance

(G_{aw}), is often used, since its relationship with lung volume is linear, rather than curvilinear as with R_{aw}. In peripheral airways, because the total cross-sectional area of the enormous number of airways is large, gas velocity and resistance is low. In the most distal respiratory bronchioles, alveolar ducts and alveolar spaces, gas molecules move by diffusive processes. In the larger central airways, where flow rates are high, the pattern of gaseous movement is transitional (somewhere between ordered laminar and turbulent flow) with a consequent steep increase of resistance with increasing flow. In nose-breathing infants, about 50% of the total resistance is nasal, 25% is in the glottis and large central airways, and the remainder in the peripheral airways. This distribution of resistance together with the relatively crowded upper airway (see p. 663 – Postnatal development) renders infants particularly prone to develop upper airway obstruction. The highly compliant chest wall and consequent tendency to peripheral airway closure, particularly at lung bases (see p. 663 – Postnatal development) also renders the infant prone to small airway obstruction (e.g. bronchiolitis) in contrast to older children and adults in whom the small airways represent a clinically 'silent zone'.

During forced expiration intrapulmonary airways progressively close as lung volume falls. Towards the lung periphery small airway patency relies on the tension within the surrounding connective tissue elements, a tension which in turn is dependent on the degree of lung stretch or inflation. During forced expiration a point is reached where the pressures within and surrounding the airway reach equality, the equal pressure point (EPP), and when flow becomes effort independent. EPP is usually reached somewhere near the mid-point of a forced expiratory effort whereas in diseases associated with increased lung compliance (reduced lung recoil), or in airway obstruction, the EPP occurs closer to the lung periphery and expired flow rates become limited earlier during expiration. This produces the concave flow volume curve so characteristic of moderate to severe asthma or cystic fibrosis (Fig. 20.11) whereas obstruction in larger airways reduces peak expiratory flow rates (Fig. 20.11). During forced inspiration the airways remain widely patent throughout and as a consequence inspiratory flow is more symmetrical. The exceptions to this rule are in fixed large airway obstruction, in profound neuromuscular weakness, or where the site of the obstruction is extrathoracic. Variable large airway obstruction such as in obstructive sleep apnea may be associated with characteristic oscillations (Fig. 20.11).

Inflammation, excessive mucus secretion and active contraction of airway smooth muscle all lead to increased airflow obstruction. Although these processes may be part of normal defense mechanisms in the lungs, one of the characteristic features of asthma is an exaggerated airway responsiveness (i.e. reversible airway narrowing in response to either allergic or non-immunological irritant factors). The degree of airway responsiveness can be measured by standardized challenge procedures

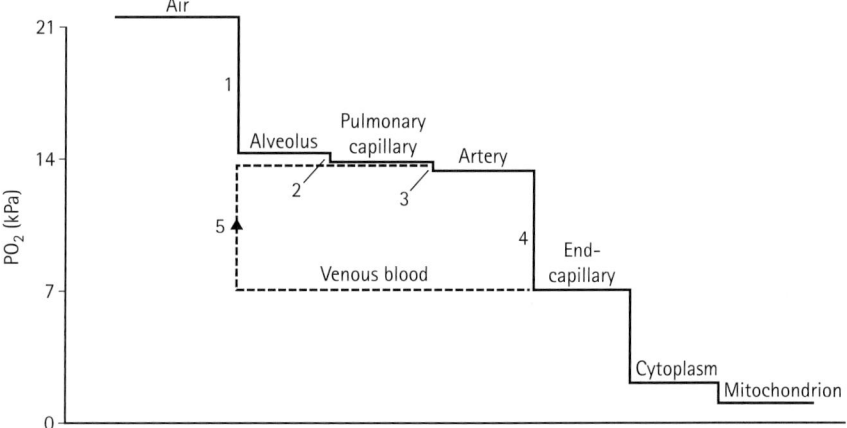

Fig. 20.11 Flow–volume curves. Maximum forced expiratory and inspiratory flow volume curves, showing patterns characteristic of airflow obstruction at various sites.

based, for instance, on exercise or inhalation challenge with cold dry air, hypertonic or hypotonic saline or with pharmacological agents such as histamine or methacholine (see p. 689 – Asthma).

Measurement of airflow obstruction

Forced expiratory maneuvers, which require a maximum expiratory effort from total lung capacity, form the basis of the most useful tests of airway obstruction. The peak expiratory flow (PEF), the forced expiratory volume in the first second of expiration (FEV_1) and the indices derived from the maximum expiratory flow volume (MEFV) curve are the most commonly performed. The best of three efforts (after two practice blows for novices) should be recorded, the two most important features being the completeness of the maximum expiratory effort at the start of each procedure and whether the effort is sustained to residual volume (RV), as evidenced by a smooth progress of flow until it meets the volume axis (Fig. 20.11). Most children from 4 years old can perform a PEF maneuver, although they may not be able to meet the recommended adult standards of less than 5% viability for other forced measurements (FEV_1, MEFV curve). In young children, the whole vital capacity may be exhaled in under 1 s and in this group, $FEV_{0.75}$ or $FEV_{0.5}$ have been suggested as more sensitive indices of obstruction.

Airway obstruction is indicated by a reduction in the ratio FEV_1/ forced vital capacity (FVC) (or $FEV_{0.75}$/FVC) since airway obstruction will prolong the expiratory time constant of the lungs and reduce the rate of emptying. The FEV_1/FVC ratio normally decreases with age, from over 90% in the youngest children in whom it can be measured to over 75% in young adults.

The shape of the expiratory flow–volume curve provides additional information, which is not available from the traditional volume–time plot (Fig. 20.11). Compensatory changes in lung volume with airways disease or its treatment may explain apparent changes in forced flow expiratory rate as airway caliber is modified by lung stretch. The maximal expiratory procedure itself may induce airway obstruction in children with reactive airways although this effect is transient and is responsive to inhaled bronchodilators.

Methods for measuring airflow obstruction which do not depend on respiratory effort, and which have therefore been adapted for use in infants and young children, include the plethysmographic determination of airway resistance and the measurement of total respiratory system resistance (impedance) by a forced oscillation and interrupter techniques.[84] Like PEF these methods mainly reflect large airway function and are especially sensitive to glottic narrowing and (in nose-breathing infants) to nasal obstruction.

Peak flow measurements

Objective evidence of the severity and nature of airway obstruction in wheezy children of school age can be obtained from twice-daily peak flow measurements that can easily be made at home using a peak flow meter. Although this kind of monitoring can be useful in assessing responses in clinical trials and in large scale epidemiological studies, its contribution to asthma management at the individual patient level is disappointing (see p. 689 – Asthma). However, peak flow measurements made at home can be of value in providing objective evidence of the severity or absence of reported asthma. A single isolated value of peak flow (or of any other measure of lung function) is of little use in the assessment of severity since variability, even within a 24-h period, can be considerable.

Measurement of bronchial responsiveness (bronchial provocation tests)

Bronchial provocation tests rarely help in the diagnosis of asthma as they are neither specific nor sensitive for asthma. They may be used in order to assess the importance of airway responsiveness in a patient with atypical symptoms (e.g. chronic cough) or in patients with other forms of airway obstruction (e.g. cystic fibrosis, bronchiectasis). Their main use is as a research tool in whole population studies or in assessing

the response to prophylactic anti-asthma therapy. Children under the age of 6 can be tested only under the conditions of a research laboratory. Simple, repeatable measurement techniques (FEV_1, PEF) are the reference norms for bronchial provocation tests but increasingly techniques that reflect airways resistance, including specific resistance, and interrupter techniques are being employed.[84]

There are three broad categories of challenge test: pharmacological challenge by aerosol, bronchial provocation with aerosolized antigen and exercise (or isocapnic hyperventilation) challenge. In order to determine the degree of responsiveness, pharmacological or exercise challenge are usually used. Exercise is said to be specific for asthma, whereas a response to pharmacological challenge also occurs in other lung disorders. Antigen provocation is a risky procedure confined to research laboratories.

Pharmacological challenge with solutions of histamine, methacholine or adenosine is performed by administering increasing concentrations of aerosol by jet nebulizer at regular intervals, until at least a 20% fall in PEF or FEV_1 has been produced (or the maximum concentration has been reached). By interpolation on a graph the concentration which provokes a 20% fall in PEF or FEV_1 (PC_{20}) can be calculated. The PC_{20} or the cumulative dose (PD_{20}) is an index of bronchial responsiveness. There is a continuum of values of PC_{20} from the lowest in severe, labile asthma to the highest in normal individuals. Many factors influence asthmatics, such as environmental antigen exposure (pollen, dust mite), time of day and recent medication. In children with other forms of chronic bronchial obstruction (e.g. cystic fibrosis), bronchial responsiveness appears to become greater as their airway obstruction worsens.

Exercise-induced asthma (EIA) can be reproducibly induced by having a child run for 5–6 min at a rate sufficient to produce a heart rate of > 170 beats/min, ideally on a treadmill in an air-conditioned laboratory. The fall in PEF or FEV_1 can be expressed as a percentage of the baseline value, to provide an index of EIA (upper limit of normal about 15%). Again, a number of clinical variables (a recent cold) and laboratory conditions (air temperature and humidity) may affect the result; outdoor tests of a similar type are very poorly repeatable. Used as a diagnostic aid, EIA has poor sensitivity and specificity. Exercise tests can be used to study the protective effects of drugs given before challenge and to demonstrate their value to the child and family. They can also be used to show that some children get 'short of breath' when they exercise, not because of EIA but simply because they are unfit!

Normal (reference) values

The choice of reference norms remains controversial. Whereas many equipment manufacturers use composite reference values,[81] there may be important racial and regional differences that need to be accounted for. For example, reference values for Caucasian European children may not be appropriate for children of African origin[88] and even within Europe differences in flow rates have been reported between studies from Northern and South-Eastern Europe.[89] Another particular problem is in predicting expected values in children and adolescents who fall between the published reference norms for children, usually up to 18 years of age, and those of adults, usually starting at about 18 years. A possible solution to these problems has been suggested by the European Respiratory Society Standardisation Report of 1989 which provided all the summary equations up to that point in time. This report suggested that individual centers should perform lung function measurement in a sample of 50–100 normal, healthy children from their own population and then identify and use the published norms that most closely fit these local values.

THE AIRSPACES: LUNG VOLUME AND COMPLIANCE
Physiology

As described above (p. 663 – Postnatal development) the elasticity of the lung and chest wall (i.e. compliance: change in volume for a given change in pressure) is such that at high volumes, the respiratory system tends to deflate and at low volumes to expand, reaching equilibrium at

Table 20.1 Lung function patterns (for spirometry)

Setting	Vital capacity	Peak flow	FEV_1/FVC	MEF_{50}	MIF_{50}
Poor effort/weakness	Reduced	Reduced	Normal	Normal	Reduced
Mild asthma/cystic fibrosis	Normal	Normal	Normal	Reduced	Normal
Severe asthma/cystic fibrosis	Reduced	Reduced	Reduced	Reduced	Normal

the functional residual capacity (FRC) where the outward recoil of the chest wall and inward recoil of the lungs are at equilibrium.

In pulmonary fibrosis where the lungs are less compliant (stiffer), the inward recoil forces of the lungs are greater and FRC is reduced. Conversely in emphysema (where the lungs are 'stretched') the inward recoil forces are lower and hence FRC is increased. Peripheral airway obstruction with 'gas trapping', as seen in chronic asthma and cystic fibrosis, results in overstretch of the lung and an increase in FRC. Static lung volumes, total lung capacity (TLC) and residual volume (RV) depend on several factors including lung compliance, chest wall compliance, respiratory muscle strength and the caliber of the small intrapulmonary airways. These may all be important in relation to changes in the vital capacity (VC) in disease and need to be interpreted together with expiratory flow rates (Table 20.1).

Measurement of lung volume and compliance

Lung volume is most commonly estimated by clinical examination aided by chest radiography. On formal laboratory testing, the distinction is often made between dynamic lung volumes produced by respiratory effort (e.g. FVC) and static lung volumes measuring absolute lung volumes (e.g. FRC, RV and TLC). Static lung volumes and lung compliance are less often measured and require a specialized lung function laboratory.[82]

The VC is a most useful, repeatable measurement, although almost any disturbance of lung function will lead to its reduction (Fig. 20.12). FVC can be reduced by poor or inefficient inspiratory or expiratory efforts due to chest wall disorders, such as scoliosis, to neuromuscular disorders or as a consequence of premature airway closure resulting in gas trapping and an elevated RV (Table 20.1; Fig. 20.12). Lung volumes may also be valuable in following the course of patients with these disorders. There are two methods of measuring static lung volumes: by the plethysmographic technique and by dilution of an inert non-absorbable gas such as helium. The former technique measures all the gas in the thoracic cage, whether or not it is in communication with airways, using

simple physical principles (Boyle's law). The latter technique, relying on equilibration of gas concentrations between the gas in the lungs and in a mixture of air and a known initial concentration of helium, tends to underestimate the volume of those parts of the lung which are very poorly ventilated (i.e. in the presence of obstructed airways). Both techniques require cooperative subjects and are rarely reliable under the age of 6 apart from in sleeping or sedated infants.

VENTILATION AND PERFUSION
Physiology

During tidal breathing, air is distributed within the lungs according to local variations in airway resistance and lung compliance. In the upright subject, because of the weight of the lungs (density about 0.2 g/ml), the pleural pressure is more negative near the apex so that the airspaces are relatively overdistended compared with those near the base. In infants the low chest wall recoil results in a reversal of the normal apex to base gradient in ventilation (see p. 663 – Postnatal development). Disease may also affect the regional distribution of ventilation by affecting the chest wall (e.g. spinal muscular atrophy, severe rickets in infancy), the diaphragm (e.g. congenital diaphragmatic hernia, eventration or paralysis), the airways (e.g. bronchiectasis, asthma) or the airspaces (e.g. lobar pneumonia, pulmonary edema).

The matching of ventilation to pulmonary perfusion mainly takes place at alveolar level with the airways playing a smaller part in this homeostatic mechanism. Alveolar hypoxia induces local pulmonary arteriolar constriction by a nitric oxide-dependent mechanism, cutting down the local blood supply. The effect is amplified by acidosis. The particular problems of the perinatal period are described in Chapter 12.

In older children, a sustained increase in pulmonary resistance, usually associated with severe chronic and generalized disease (e.g. chronic lung disease of prematurity, terminal cystic fibrosis), may lead to cor pulmonale.

Mismatching of ventilation ($\dot{V}$) and perfusion ($\dot{Q}$) occurs in acute lung disease before adaptation has occurred and in severe chronic disease, beyond the limits of adaptation. Its effects are wasted ventilation (excessive dead space ventilation) on the one hand, and hypoxemia (due to right-to-left intrapulmonary shunting) on the other. Hypoxemia due to mild $\dot{V}/\dot{Q}$ imbalance, as well as that due to alveolar hypoventilation, is largely corrected by increased inspired oxygen concentrations.

Tests of the distribution of ventilation and perfusion

Regional distribution of ventilation and perfusion can be studied fairly simply in standard nuclear medicine facilities, using radionuclide-labeled gas and microspheres and a gamma camera (see p. 671 – Special investigations – imaging). Other tests remain research procedures.

GAS TRANSFER AND GAS TRANSPORT
Physiology

Within the alveoli, gas movement takes place by diffusion. Transfer of oxygen from alveolus (PaO_2 14 kPa) into the pulmonary capillary and of carbon dioxide in the reverse direction ($PaCO_2$ 5 kPa) take place by passive diffusion down partial pressure gradients.

The gradient of PO_2 can be thought of as running from alveolus to mitochondrion. Oxygen is transported as oxyhemoglobin. The quantity of oxygen carried depends on the PaO_2 (and its characteristic sigmoid relationship with oxygen saturation), the hemoglobin concentration

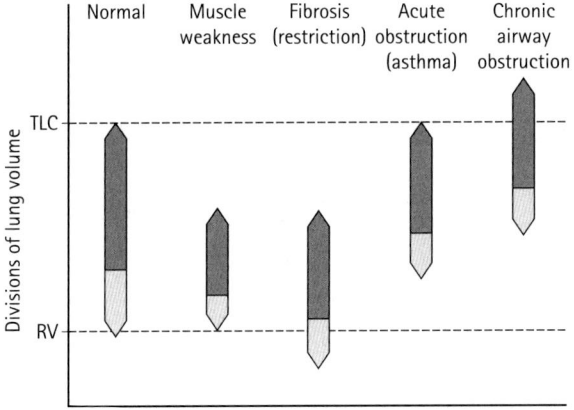

Fig. 20.12 Causes of reduced vital capacity. The length of the arrows indicates the vital capacity and the position indicates the changes in total lung capacity (TLC) and residual volume (RV) for each condition in relation to normal. The horizontal line across each arrow indicates the usual end-expiratory curve (functional residual capacity, FRC).

and the cardiac output: oxygen delivered = oxygen content of blood × cardiac output. Thus oxygen delivery will be reduced by anemia, hypoxemia or diminished cardiac output. Metabolic acidosis (anaerobic metabolism leading to lactic acid production) is one consequence of impaired oxygen delivery.

The oxygen dissociation curve is also affected by a number of other factors: the dominant class of hemoglobin (e.g. HbF in the newborn), adaptive variations in intracellular 2,3-diphosphoglycerate (2,3-DPG) concentration with chronic anemia and arterial pH and $PaCO_2$ (the Bohr effect).

The transport of CO_2 is much more robust, since the CO_2 content of blood is almost linearly related to PCO_2 over the clinical range. Respiratory acidosis results from hypercapnia.

Respiratory failure is a general term used to imply a breakdown of the supply of oxygen and removal of CO_2. A single definition which covers the whole pediatric range would be inappropriate, since degrees of acute disturbance of blood gases which may have dire clinical consequences in a preterm neonate may have little effect in a chronically sick older child. In newborns when the labile fetal circulation shunts through fetal channels, a low PaO_2 may indicate a complex failure of ventilation and circulation which it would be inappropriate to label as 'respiratory' (see Ch. 12).

Terminology

Hypoxemia

Hypoxemia (PaO_2 at sea level in postneonates of < 12 kPa) may have several causes (Fig. 20.13; Table 20.2). At altitude the oxygen content of inspired air is reduced and the PO_2 will fall. However, acclimatization principally by hyperventilation and the development of polycythemia preserves the oxygen content of arterial blood.

Alveolar hypoventilation, with resultant hypoxemia and hypercapnia, may be due to mechanical factors (stiff or obstructed lungs), weakness of respiratory muscles or a defect of the control of breathing.

Shunt refers to systemic venous blood which effectively bypasses ventilated portions of lung. There are two main varieties of right-to-left shunt: intracardiac shunt and intrapulmonary shunt. In childhood, the main extrapulmonary cause of shunt is cyanotic congenital heart disease. Breathing 100% oxygen for at least 5 min (the nitrogen washout test) is useful for diagnosing this 'central' shunting. In order to understand this test, the shape of the hemoglobin–oxygen dissociation curve should be borne in mind. Even if the PO_2 of pulmonary venous blood is > 55 kPa (400 mmHg), the content of oxygen in that blood will be hardly greater than if the PO_2 is 13 kPa (100 mmHg). When mixed with shunted blood of low oxygen content the PO_2 will fall dramatically. Even when the lungs are completely normal, the presence of a very small central shunt will prevent a significant rise in PO_2 when breathing 100% oxygen. A rise in PaO_2 to 20 kPa (150 mmHg) makes cyanotic heart disease an unlikely cause of hypoxemia. On the other hand, if breathing 100% oxygen (for a minimum of 5 min) does successfully elevate the PaO_2 the hypoxemia in air is likely to have been due to intrapulmonary shunting (regions of low $\dot{V}/\dot{Q}$ ratio) or hypoventilation. A specific exception to this rule is the situation of pulmonary hypertension in the newborn, when oxygen therapy, by reducing pulmonary vascular resistance, can abolish the extrapulmonary right-to-left shunt through fetal channels, causing the hypoxemia to resolve for 'vascular' rather than 'pulmonary' reasons.

Ventilation perfusion $\dot{V}/\dot{Q}$ mismatching is by far the commonest cause of hypoxemia in pulmonary disease. Blood leaving alveolar units which are underventilated but well perfused will have a low O_2 content and a raised CO_2 content. For the reasons mentioned above, the total PaO_2 will fall and hyperventilation results. CO_2 is washed out of the well-ventilated lung units. As the CO_2 content of blood bears an almost linear relationship to $PaCO_2$, the reduction in CO_2 content of blood leaving well-ventilated units offsets the rise in that leaving poorly ventilated alveoli. However, no matter how good the ventilation of healthy alveolar units, the O_2 content of blood leaving them remains the same and does not offset the reduced content of those leaving poorly ventilated alveoli. Hypoxemia due to $\dot{V}/\dot{Q}$ imbalance will therefore be unaltered by hyperventilation, an increased ventilatory drive will persist and the $PaCO_2$ may fall. (This is sometimes referred to as type I respiratory failure.)

This is the situation in the early stages of acute asthma and bronchiolitis. Increasing the inspired oxygen concentration will improve the oxygen content of poorly ventilated areas and the PaO_2 will rise as a result. Patients are able to compensate for the increase in dead space initially by increasing overall minute ventilation but eventually they may become exhausted or, because of worsening disease, the dead space may rise. In either case alveolar hypoventilation results and the $PaCO_2$ will eventually rise (type II respiratory failure).

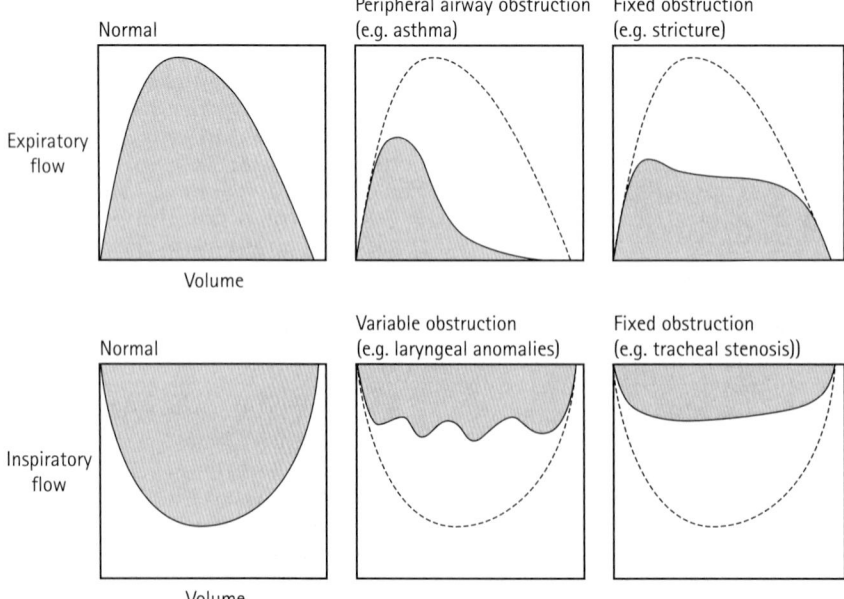

Fig. 20.13 Oxygen 'waterfall' in health and disease. Under normal circumstances oxygen is transported down a gradient between atmospheric air and the mitochondria where it is consumed.

Table 20.2 Oxygen 'waterfall' in disease: hypoxia. Various causes of hypoxemia have their effect at different steps in the waterfall. Increase in inspired oxygen concentration (FiO_2; the hyperoxia test) will usually correct the first two causes of hypoxemia. The level of $PaCO_2$ depends on the degree of compensatory hyperventilation which is possible; in severe lung disease, hypercapnia may develop

Cause of hypoxia	Effect of increase in FiO_2	Value of $PaCO_2$
1. Decreased alveolar ventilation	Correction of hypoxemia	Increase
2. Impaired diffusion	Correction of hypoxemia	Decrease (unless severe imbalance)
3. Right–left shunt and ventilation/perfusion imbalance	No change if pure right–left shunt	Decrease (unless severe shunting)
4. Decreased oxygen delivery*	No change	Decrease (due to metabolic acidosis)
5. Demand for oxygen exceeding supply**	Depends on cause	Increased mixed venous PCO_2

* PaO_2 may be normal under these circumstances; not true for hypoxemia
** Refers to the fall in mixed venous (pulmonary artery) PO_2; PaO_2 may be normal

Alveolar hypoventilation

Alveolar hypoventilation in the presence of normal lungs or severe ventilation perfusion mismatching, as described under hypoxemia, results in *hypercapnia*, a rise in $PaCO_2$. Hypercapnia should always be taken very seriously. In acute respiratory disease the $PaCO_2$ may remain normal or low for some time but may eventually rise very quickly. Children in whom this happens are very often exhausted and may well require ventilatory support. With chronic hypercapnia, central insensitivity results as cerebrospinal fluid (CSF) pH is buffered by a rise in bicarbonate. Administration of an oxygen-enriched gas to a patient not receiving assisted ventilation may result in a further dangerous increase in $PaCO_2$ because of removal of the hypoxemic drive to respiration. In practice this is extremely uncommon in children as chronic type II respiratory failure is rare. Oxygen should therefore never be withheld from children with acute respiratory disease.

Alveolar–arterial PO_2 difference

(A–a) DO_2 is a measure of the degree of right-to-left shunt (of all types).

In respiratory failure of whatever cause the PaO_2 falls while the patient is breathing air. When accompanied by alveolar hypoventilation the $PaCO_2$ rises. An assessment of respiratory failure may be made by use of the alveolar air equation:

$$P_AO_2 = P_IO_2 - (P_ACO_2/R) + F$$

where P_AO_2 is the partial pressure of oxygen in the alveoli, P_IO_2 is the partial pressure of inspired oxygen (minus water vapor) (partial pressure: 6 kPa at body temperature), P_ACO_2 is the mean alveolar PCO_2, R is the respiratory quotient (approximately 0.8 in healthy individuals) and F is a small correction factor which for clinical purposes can be omitted. P_ACO_2 in most clinical situations is equal to $PaCO_2$. Normally with a $PaCO_2$ of 5 kPa and a barometric pressure of 100 kPa breathing air (O_2 content = 0.21) and a water vapor pressure of 6 kPa, P_AO_2 = 0.21 (100 – 6) – (5/0.8) = 13.5 kPa.

In a healthy child breathing air the difference between the P_AO_2 and the PaO_2 is 1–2 kPa. In pure alveolar hypoventilation this difference does not change or become smaller. In the presence of shunt or $\dot{V}/\dot{Q}$ imbalance the difference rises. Hence the (A–a) DO_2 is an index of severity of mismatching of gas and blood.

Example 1. A baby with severe bronchiolitis may have a PaO_2 of 10 kPa in 70% oxygen and a $PaCO_2$ of 8 kPa. The (A–a) DO_2 = 0.7 (100 – 6) – (8/0.8) – 10 = 46 kPa. He has both $\dot{V}/\dot{Q}$ mismatching, resulting in a rise in (A–a) DO_2, and alveolar hypoventilation, resulting in a rise in $PaCO_2$.

Example 2. A child with infective polyneuritis breathing 30% oxygen has a $PaCO_2$ of 7 kPa and a PaO_2 of 18 kPa. The (A–a) DO_2 = 0.3 (100 – 6) – (7/0.8) – 18 = 1.5 kPa. This child has pure alveolar hypoventilation as the (A–a) DO_2 is normal and the $PaCO_2$ is raised.

In rare disorders which affect the alveolar membrane, where clinical disability is mainly reduced exercise tolerance and airway function is normal, oxygen transport across the membrane may be adequate at rest but not during exercise. The (A–a) DO_2 may become abnormally wide only during exercise.

Acid–base abnormalities

These relate to disturbed hydrogen ion homeostasis in body fluids. The maintenance of a normal blood pH is a function of lung and kidney which together control the buffering capacity of the blood. The most important physiological buffer is bicarbonate, because of its relationship with CO_2 which is excreted through the lungs. The Henderson–Hasselbalch equation describes the relationship:

$$H^+ + HCO_3^- \rightleftharpoons H_2CO_3 \rightleftharpoons CO_2 + H_2O$$

From this:

$$H^+ \propto CO_2/HCO_3^-$$

and:

$$pH = -\log H^+ = \log (HCO_3^-/CO_2)$$

Provided the ratio of HCO_3/CO_2 remains constant, the pH will remain constant.

When the acid–base balance is disturbed and the normal values of pH and PCO_2 are altered it is helpful to know something of the status of the buffering system in the blood in order to unravel the sequence of events. The *base excess* is a useful parameter which reflects the metabolic component of the abnormality under steady state conditions (*not* during rapid changes in acid–base status). When the blood gases are analyzed the pH of the sample is determined. The CO_2 electrode is calibrated with gases of high and low CO_2 concentrations and the $PaCO_2$ of the sample determined. Blood pH and log $PaCO_2$ have a linear relationship whose slope varies according to whether there is an excess or deficit of base. The line which describes the relationship when there is neither excess nor deficit is known as the 'normal buffer baseline'. The amount of base which has to be added to or removed from this 'ideal' sample to reach the line which describes the actual sample is referred to as the base excess or deficit (see also Ch. 17).

In *respiratory acidosis* the $PaCO_2$ rises and the pH falls, and in order to maintain the ratio HCO_3/CO_2 the kidney conserves bicarbonate.

Metabolic acidosis in pulmonary or cardiac disease reflects tissue hypoxia due to poor oxygen delivery, resulting in local lactic acid production. Other important causes include renal failure, severe infection and acute diabetic ketoacidosis. In these settings bicarbonate falls as it buffers the rise in hydrogen ions while a simultaneous increased drive to breathe results in increased CO_2 removal and a return towards a more normal HCO_3/CO_2 ratio.

Respiratory alkalosis occurs when the $PaCO2$ falls due to voluntary or artifactual hyperventilation or hyperventilation due to CNS pathology (e.g. meningoencephalitis). The hydrogen ion concentration falls and to conserve the HCO_3/CO_2 ratio and hence the pH, the kidney sheds bicarbonate.

Metabolic alkalosis occurs in children when acid is lost through vomiting, as in pyloric stenosis. Hydrogen ions are lost and the bicarbonate rises. Hypoventilation produces a compensatory rise in CO_2.

Mixed respiratory and metabolic acidosis is a common situation in pediatric practice. Tissue hypoxia results in metabolic acidosis and inadequate ventilation results in respiratory acidosis. The $PaCO_2$ is elevated and the bicarbonate and pH are low. There will be a base deficit.

The administration of bicarbonate in this situation is tempting, particularly when the pH is below 7.2. However, in order for bicarbonate to correct the metabolic component, CO_2 must be formed and excreted from the lungs and in the presence of respiratory failure with an already elevated $PaCO_2$ this may not be possible. Administration of bicarbonate may therefore elevate the $PaCO_2$ even further. The blood–brain barrier is much more permeable to CO_2 than it is to bicarbonate and the effect on the CSF will be to paradoxically reduce pH with serious consequences for the child who is not receiving ventilatory support. Even in pure metabolic acidosis such as occurs in diabetic ketoacidosis, rapid administration of bicarbonate can have this effect (see Ch.15).

The treatment for mixed acidosis is the correction of the respiratory component first of all by increasing ventilation. The metabolic component may respond to better oxygenation, improved circulation or correction of anemia. When the $PaCO_2$ has returned to normal, bicarbonate may be given if the metabolic component persists.

Measurement of gas transfer

Gas transfer at alveolar level can be studied by measuring the diffusing capacity for carbon monoxide (D_{co}). By measuring the FRC by helium dilution simultaneously, the diffusing capacity can be normalized for variation in lung volume (K_{co}). The test has its main use in detecting the response to treatment of interstitial lung diseases (e.g. those associated with connective tissue disorders) in older children.

Measurement of arterial blood gases and acid–base balance

Oximetry has largely replaced arterial blood gas measurement for most children. Blood gas measurements are indicated for worsening acute lung disease where exhaustion (muscle fatigue) suggests the need for mechanical ventilation and in chronic lung disease as a guide to progress. Sampling of arterialized capillary blood (i.e. after warming or application of histamine cream) may be adequate for pH monitoring, but in general arterial sampling is preferable for postneonatal patients.

Blood should be collected from a radial artery cannula or, if impossible to site, by arterial puncture from the radial artery. This vessel is preferred for three reasons. First, the chance of sampling venous blood in error is small as no major veins lie nearby. Second, there is a good collateral circulation to the hand should circulation be compromised in any way as a result of the procedure. Third, the vessel is accessible. If pulsation is difficult to feel, as in shock, it may be approached blindly. The femoral artery, on the other hand, has a direct medial relation to the femoral vein. Infection may be introduced into the femoral sheath or into the hip joint from the groin. Collaterals will not compensate for femoral artery thrombosis, a particular hazard if the vessel is damaged in the presence of hypovolemia. It is also worth remembering that the femoral vessels may be used for cannulation at cardiac catheterization and it is particularly annoying for the cardiologist if the site has been traumatized.

As the walls of arteries are particularly sensitive and more than one attempt may be necessary to obtain blood, local anesthetic cream should be applied to the site 30 min before starting and local anesthetic should be injected around the site. As well as being a kindness, this should allow the blood to be collected under conditions which are as stable as possible although admittedly anxiety is not always avoided. Hyperventilation will reduce the $PaCO_2$ and consequently the pH will rise; crying in a child who has a right-to-left intracardiac shunt may increase the shunt and reduce the PaO_2.

Non-invasive methods of measuring oxygenation include the transcutaneous PO_2 electrode, which is at best a trend indicator in

Table 20.3 Typical arterial blood gas values for adolescents and young adults in room air at sea level. All values tend towards the lower ranges in younger children and are lower still in infants

pH	7.35–7.45
PaO$_2$ (kPa)	11.5–13.5
PaCO$_2$ (kPa)	4.7–6.0
HCO$_2$ (mEq/L)	22–28

Data adapted from Cassels & Morse[90] and Gaultier et al[91]

postneonatal patients, and the pulse oximeter for monitoring oxygen saturation (e.g. in acute severe asthma and during sleep studies). For PCO_2, transcutaneous measurements again provide trends while end-tidal sampling using an infrared CO_2 meter gives a useful assessment of alveolar breath (and hence arterial) CO_2 only when lung disease is mild and during mechanical ventilation. 'Normal' values for adolescents and young adults are given in Table 20.3.

BREATHING
Physiology
The principal muscle of inspiration is the diaphragm, innervated by the phrenic nerve (C2–5). As with other skeletal muscles, within its usual working range the tension it can generate is proportional to its length. Because the diaphragm adopts a curved shape, when it contracts the pressure difference across it is proportional to the tension developed and inversely proportional to the radius of the curvature. Thus as a pressure generator, the diaphragm works best near its end expiratory position, where its radius of curvature is smallest (more domed). Hyperinflation by flattening the diaphragm, and increasing the radius of curvature, reduces the effective pressure generated for any particular muscle tension, reduces efficiency and may lead to muscle fatigue. The resulting alveolar hypoventilation, whose onset can be quite sudden, is the major contributory factor to respiratory failure in severe bronchiolitis.

Because of its tangential insertion, normal diaphragmatic contraction causes the chest wall to expand laterally ('bucket handle' effect) and anteriorly ('pump handle' effect). Scoliosis, for example, disturbs normal integrated movements of the diaphragm and chest wall and may lead to respiratory failure, presenting initially during sleep, when the diaphragm may be the sole muscle of breathing.

The phasic action of the intercostal muscles plays a part in stabilizing the chest wall, as illustrated by the indrawing (recession) which occurs during inspiration in patients with intercostal weakness (e.g. acute polyneuritis, spinal muscular atrophy) or in normal infants during rapid eye movement sleep (when the intercostal muscles remain passive). The intercostal muscles are particularly important in infancy, as the chest wall is inherently unstable and the expanding action of the diaphragm is less effective because of its less acute, more direct insertion into the rib cage and because of the more horizontal arrangement of the ribs.[83]

Expiration is normally a passive function, dependent on the elastic recoil of the lungs and chest wall. The elastic work normally carried out by the diaphragm during inspiration is almost totally 'recovered' during expiration and the work expended in overcoming frictional forces (the resistance to air flow) is dissipated as heat. However, active expiratory effort, applied mainly by the muscles of the anterior abdominal wall, may be needed if ventilatory demands are great (e.g. during exercise), if there is increased resistance to expiratory airflow (e.g. laryngeal edema) or if the natural recoil of the lungs is reduced (as in emphysema). The diaphragm may be used as a brake during expiration, although when a more effective brake is required (e.g. in neonatal respiratory distress or infantile bronchiolitis), the variable resistance of the glottis may be used, resulting in characteristic expiratory grunting.

From the point of view of the respiratory physician, the brain is part of the respiratory system! Apart from recognized CNS disorders which can affect the respiratory centers (e.g. Leigh disease) and congenital central hypoventilation (see p. 684 – Congenital hypoventilation syndrome), altered central respiratory drive is especially dependent on sleep state (see p. 683 – Sleep and respiratory disorders). Rapid eye movement (REM) sleep is normally associated with a small drop in PaO_2. However, when upper airway obstruction is present (e.g. due to weakness or to tonsillar or adenoidal hypertrophy) or in the presence of severe lung disease (e.g. cystic fibrosis, severe scoliosis), the degree of hypoventilation may be profound, leading to periods of extreme hypoxemia. The consequences may be severe (pulmonary hypertension, hypoxic fits or brain damage) or limited to sleep disturbance as a consequence of repeated waking, leading to excessive somnolence (or paradoxically in children, hyperactivity) the following day.

Control of breathing may become clinically important in chronic respiratory failure with hypercapnia (e.g. terminal lung disease, chronic neuromuscular disorders) when renal compensation for respiratory acidosis leads to an increase in plasma and CSF bicarbonate concentration. This acts as a buffer, blunting the sensitivity of the respiratory center to further rises in PCO_2, again leading to severe hypoventilation during REM sleep, when the metabolic control of breathing is paramount.

Measurement of respiratory muscle strength

The function of the respiratory muscles is best assessed by clinical observations assisted (in the absence of gross lung disease) by comparison of supine and standing vital capacity. Diaphragmatic paralysis will be accompanied by a fall in vital capacity of more than 10% and by paradoxical respiratory movements of the rib cage and abdomen in the supine posture. Direct measurements by mouthpiece and transducer of the maximum pressure which can be generated at the mouth during inspiratory effort from residual volume, and expiratory effort from total lung capacity, allow precise quantitations of respiratory muscle strength. Unfortunately, if weakness affects the facial muscles, children find it impossible to maintain an airtight seal around a mouthpiece.

SPECIAL INVESTIGATIONS – IMAGING

Despite recent advances in imaging (see also Ch. 8), the plain chest radiograph (CXR) continues to play a fundamental role in the evaluation of the pediatric respiratory system. Many diagnoses are confirmed or excluded by a simple CXR without recourse to other complex imaging modalities. When pleural fluid or a pneumothorax is suspected an additional decubitus film (with the patient positioned on his/her side) or a horizontal shoot through lateral film are also occasionally useful.

Apart from ultrasound (US) examination and magnetic resonance imaging (MRI), all thoracic imaging techniques involve irradiation. Certain images involve exceedingly low radiation doses, e.g. krypton 81m ventilation lung scan (^{81m}Kr V); others may be more invasive and have significantly high inherent radiation, e.g. cardiac catheterization, computed tomography (CT) or bronchography. It is therefore important to consider the invasiveness, the radiation dose and the potential discomfort to the patient when planning detailed pulmonary investigations.

The importance of the esophagus in particular should not be forgotten when chest disease in young patients is being investigated. Diseases of the upper gastrointestinal tract, e.g. hiatus hernia, gastroesophageal reflux or recurrent aspiration, may all manifest with chest signs or symptoms.

RADIOGRAPHY OF UPPER AIRWAYS

The lateral neck/postnasal space and sinuses are frequently included on the same lateral radiograph. The palatine tonsils as well as the adenoidal area can be studied on this film. The adenoids may be quite large in normal children, making the diagnosis of adenoidal hypertrophy difficult. The relationship of the trachea to the cervical spine as well as the general tracheal caliber should be well visualized. The lateral view has certain technical limitations and it is important to be sure that the projection is adequate, i.e. the floors of the anterior, middle and posterior fossae of the skull are overlapping, and that the cervical spine is truly lateral. The normal space between the trachea and the cervical spine is

approximately the diameter of one vertebral body. An apparent increase in this space may be pathological but may also be due to the radiograph being taken in expiration – in this latter situation the trachea may show some buckling or the hyoid bone may be elevated.[92]

The frontal projection visualizes the facial sinuses but in children under 5–6 years of age the relatively small size of the facial bones makes it exceedingly difficult to interpret plain sinus views. Although the antra are usually aerated sufficiently by the age of 18–24 months to be seen on a radiograph, diagnosing sinusitis from plain radiographs is notoriously unreliable. In older children the ethmoid and frontal sinuses, the nasal septum and turbinate bones should be seen. There is a wide age range in the normal development of these sinuses such that when sinusitis needs to be diagnosed or excluded with certainty most radiologists recommend CT or MRI.

CHEST RADIOGRAPHY

For a frontal posteroanterior (PA) chest radiograph [anteroposterior (AP) in younger children], the patient must be straight. This is best evaluated on the film by either the relationship of the medial ends of the clavicles to the pedicle of the vertebral body or by the symmetry of the anterior ribs on each side. Even slight rotation can cause unusual appearances in a normal patient. The medial ends of the clavicles should lie at the level of the fourth vertebral body. Radiographs in inspiration are generally preferred, the degree of inspiration judged by counting either the anterior rib ends in the mid-clavicular line down to the level of the diaphragm (there should be 5–6 ribs present) or counting the posterior aspect of the ribs where down to the tenth rib should be seen on inspiration above the hemidiaphragm. A film in expiration is often regarded as being of little value although it infers that no overinflation or air trapping is present and this film may permit exclusion of lobar consolidation. A film in expiration should not be disregarded but rather carefully reviewed to consider whether it needs to be repeated. Pathological conditions which result in a loss of lung compliance, e.g. opportunistic infection in the immunosuppressed child, cause repeated 'expiration films' to be obtained. It is worth noting that the normal pediatric cardiothoracic ratio of 60% may be exceeded on an expiratory radiograph in a normal child, leading to the erroneous impression of cardiomegaly.

In the infant or sick child, supine AP chest radiographs are commonly carried out. Here the classic signs of well-known pathological conditions alter, e.g. a pleural effusion may only be seen as an 'apical cap'; a pneumothorax may not appear as a peripheral lung edge; and a pneumomediastinum may appear only as a vague transradiancy in the mediastinum. A lateral chest radiograph with a horizontal beam or a decubitus film may be useful when doubt persists following the AP view.

The normal visualization of the cardiac outline as well as the diaphragm is due to an aerated lung being adjacent to a more solid non-aerated organ. Loss of the normal outlines means that the adjacent lung tissue is no longer aerated; this can occur with consolidation (i.e. fluid in the alveolar spaces due to infection, inflammation, hemorrhage or pulmonary edema). If the airway remains patent throughout, then consolidation without major collapse may occur. If there is collapse in a lobe of lung, i.e. loss of volume, then bronchial pathology, e.g. foreign body, mucus or extrinsic compression, must be borne in mind. When consolidation occurs first it is not possible for this solid pulmonary parenchyma to lose volume to any major extent. The diagnosis of a collapsed lobe is made by either identifying a displaced fissure or displaced hilum.

The lateral chest radiograph requires a greater exposure than the frontal film and because the two lungs are superimposed, interpretation is difficult. This film is no longer part of the 'routine' chest radiograph in pediatrics but is rather reserved for specific clinical situations such as persistent post-pneumonic change (Fig. 20.14). In children with known solid tumors, in whom initial screening with CT and CXR is normal, follow-up may be with repeat CXR, usually including a lateral film also, at intervals determined by protocol. When a suspicious new lesion is seen, CT is required. In a child with recurrent chest pathology undergoing

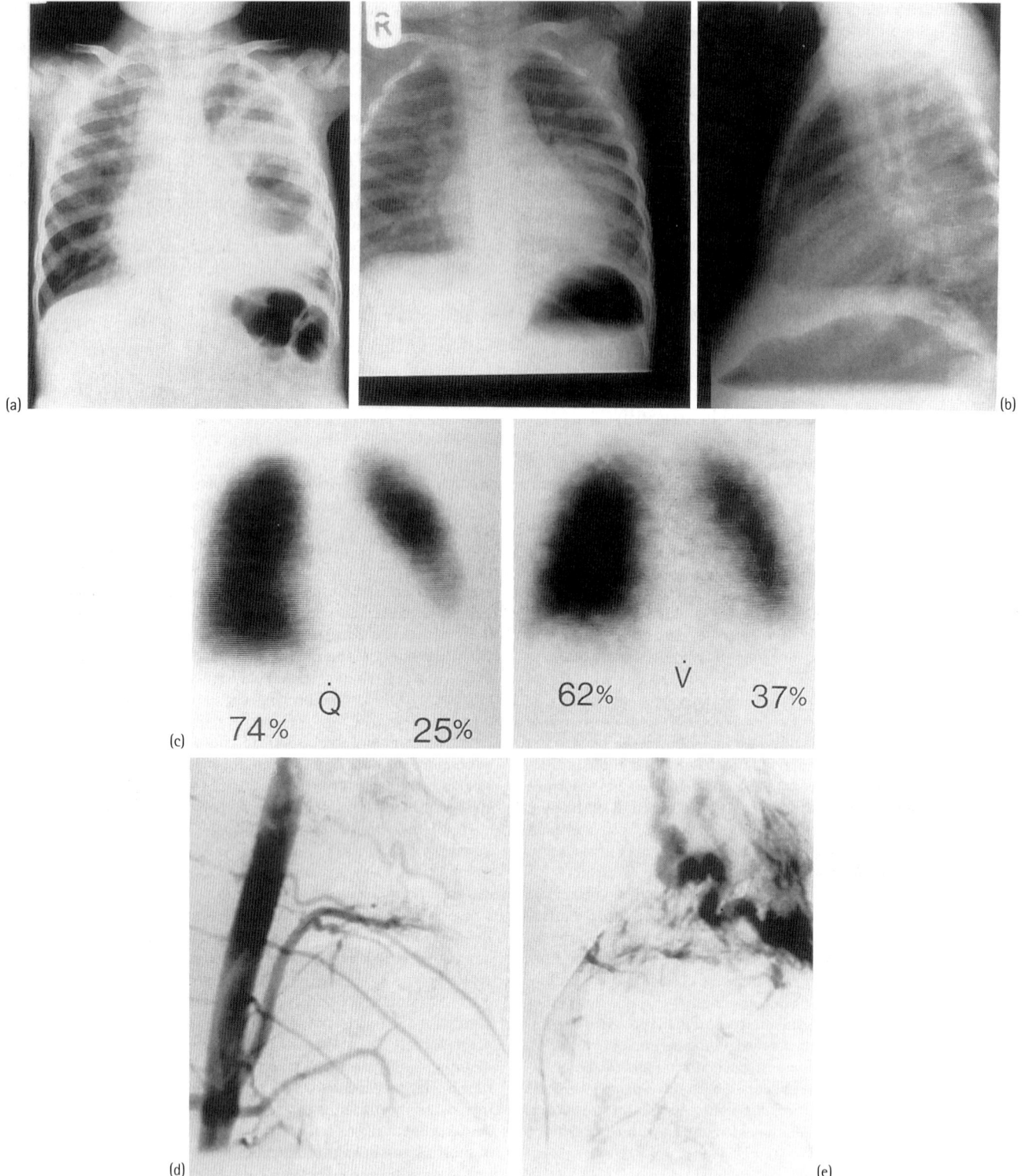

Fig. 20.14   A 3-year-old girl with unresolved pneumonia in the left lower lobe. (a) PA chest radiograph at 3 months of age. (b) Following recovery from the acute episode the routine follow-up chest radiograph 6 months later showed persistent shadowing in the left lower lobe. Persisting post-pneumonic lower lobe changes like these raise the possibility of an underlying sequestration, as proven subsequently in this case. An abdominal ultrasound should be performed to search for an anomalous feeding artery from the abdominal aorta to the lesion, in addition to lung CT in this context. (c) A ^{99m}Tc macroaggregate perfusion scan (Q) and a krypton 81m ventilation scan (V) were obtained 1 year following the acute episode. The left lung shows decreased perfusion compared to the right with the left lung only contributing 25% of overall perfusion. On ventilation the left lung contributes 37% and there is a segment in the left lower zone which is relatively well ventilated but not perfused. The diagnosis of a sequestrated segment was suggested. (d) A digital subtraction angiogram was carried out. The arterial phase shows a vessel arising from the abdominal aorta going cranially into the thorax to supply the abnormal area on chest radiograph. (e) The venous phase shows the drainage from the sequestrated segment all going cranially. At surgery a sequestrated segment in the left lower lobe was resected.

investigation, a lateral film at the time of the first chest radiograph is recommended. In the long term follow-up of chronic chest disease, e.g. cystic fibrosis, many would recommend that a lateral view is carried out whenever the PA film is obtained. The normal lateral chest radiograph should show progressive transradiancy over the dorsal spine, i.e. the lower vertebral bodies are blacker than the upper ones. The trachea is well seen; displacement and narrowing are easily detected on this projection whereas tracheal compression is seldom visible on the frontal view.[92]

When the patient is too unwell to sit upright, a horizontal beam radiograph can be useful. For this the patient is placed supine or in a decubitus position and the horizontal X-ray beam allows the effect of gravity to be maximized in order to demonstrate air–fluid interfaces or positional shifts of fluid. Thus either a frontal or a lateral film can be obtained. This technique is useful to demonstrate a small pleural effusion, the presence of pneumomediastinum or pneumothorax and, with intrapulmonary pathology, to demonstrate air–fluid interfaces such as in an abscess. Oblique radiographs, done to search for rib fractures, are recommended as part of a skeletal survey in the context of suspected non-accidental injury.

FLUOROSCOPY

Examination of the esophagus is the major role for fluoroscopy of the chest. Additional information to be gained during an esophagogram includes evaluation for tracheomalacia (when the trachea, viewed from a lateral position, collapses in expiration by > 50%). If present, a pleural effusion or consolidation may also be noted.

Evaluation of the motion of both hemidiaphragms to assess for suspected immobility or paradoxical motion secondary to phrenic nerve injury is easily performed, although particularly in smaller children, the same information can be achieved with US, thereby avoiding irradiation.

A fully distended esophagus is essential for an adequate examination by contrast or barium. An esophagogram can show extrinsic lesions such as a vascular ring – a double aortic arch causes a posterior impression on the esophagus whilst an aberrant left pulmonary artery (so-called pulmonary sling) typically indents the anterior esophagus posterior to the trachea (Fig. 20.15). Intrinsic diseases such as hiatus hernia, gastroesophageal reflux or incoordinate swallowing with aspiration can also be diagnosed.

A dedicated esophagogram is necessary in those patients with a normal barium swallow in whom an H-type tracheoesophageal fistula is suspected. This usually requires an injection of contrast via an esophageal tube which is gradually withdrawn with the child in the prone position. Prone positioning allows the dependent anterior esophagus to be well coated which, with the aid of gravity, helps improve the likelihood of finding a small fistula to the trachea.

BRONCHOGRAPHY

High-resolution CT (HRCT) is very accurate in defining bronchiectasis, such that the indications for bronchography have reduced considerably. Furthermore, surgical treatment for bronchiectasis is now uncommon. The current major indication for bronchography is for suspected localized bronchomalacia, particularly in ventilator dependent children. However, it is an invasive procedure and should only be undertaken by an experienced pediatric radiologist. Bronchoscopy is also useful in the investigation of localized tracheobronchomalacia (see p. 683 – Bronchoscopy).

ANGIOGRAPHY

This is the most invasive radiological investigation in the cardiorespiratory system and is therefore reserved for those patients in whom the diagnosis is unconfirmed by any other technique. Digital subtraction angiography allows a small volume of contrast to be used and provides high quality imaging with a lower radiation burden to the child (Fig. 20.16). With the advent of multidetector CT (MDCT) and more recently fast gadolinium-enhanced dynamic MRI sequences, the need for

pulmonary angiography continues to reduce. Increasingly angiography is performed not for diagnostic purposes but for intervention and embolization, e.g. arteriovenous malformation or a sequestrated lung segment.

ULTRASOUND

Aerated lung prevents the propagation of an ultrasound beam. Pathology, e.g. pleural fluid or other collection, must lie adjacent to the pleura to be visualized. In the opaque hemithorax on CXR, i.e. so-called lung white-out, US can easily distinguish between the presence of fluid, a mass or lung collapse and can give a useful guide as to how much fluid is present. When a peripheral lung mass is present, then US can determine if this is predominantly cystic or solid. Occasionally in a child with pneumonia it is difficult both clinically and radiologically to assess how much fluid is present in addition to the consolidation; US is particularly useful if the consolidation is basal in location. Effusion and empyema may require tapping or draining and in this context US is very useful in defining the appropriate site for chest tube insertion. The diaphragm is well visualized by US, especially on the right, and therefore may be useful when defects are suspected. In cases of suspected diaphragmatic palsy subsequent to surgery US can be as accurate as fluoroscopy in assessing diaphragmatic motion and has the advantage that it can be performed in the intensive care setting. Antenatal diagnosis by US of diaphragmatic hernia or an adenomatoid malformation in the chest may alert the pediatrician to the birth of an infant who may require the facilities of a neonatal intensive care unit.

Children with stridor in whom the diagnosis of extrinsic compression is being considered should undergo US (echocardiographic) examination. Ultrasound in experienced hands can detect the site of the aortic arch and may thus pick up a right-sided arch or double aortic arch. The detection of an aberrant left pulmonary artery arising from the right pulmonary artery and swinging back to the left between the esophagus and trachea may be missed, however, on echocardiography.[92]

The normal thymus can have a variety of appearances on CXR, being particularly prominent in children under 3 years of age. A large thymus can be mistaken for a mediastinal mass or upper zone pneumonia. A large normal thymus can be easily identified with US corresponding to the apparent CXR abnormality, ruling out more sinister pathology. In cases of suspected sequestrated segment, US may show the feeding vessel arising from the abdominal aorta coursing upwards into the chest.

RADIOISOTOPE INVESTIGATIONS

Ventilation/perfusion lung scans

Sequential images of both ventilation and perfusion can be obtained in children of any age. $\dot{V}/\dot{Q}$ scans even have been carried out in the newborn. Multiple views are obtained so that a three-dimensional image of the lungs is built up. ^{81m}Kr is an inert radioisotope gas with a half-life of 13 s. The inspired air/^{81m}Kr mixture never reaches equilibrium in the alveolar airspaces. The image is therefore of alveolar ventilation and not lung volume. This holds true for all children over 1–2 years but in an infant the high respiratory rate may invalidate this situation so that the ^{81m}Kr V scan may reflect a complex lung volume/specific ventilation situation. Xenon-133 (^{133}Xe) is used in many institutions where Kr is unavailable. The advantages of this gas are its ready availability and relatively long half-life of 5.3 days; the disadvantages are the relatively high radiation dose. As it requires very good patient cooperation it is used with difficulty in the child under 6 years old. Only a single posterior view can be obtained and therefore it is difficult to compare the ^{99m}Tc perfusion image with the ^{133}Xe image.

^{99m}Tc MAA Technetium Labeled macroaggregated albumin are injected intravenously and are stopped by the first capillary bed, normally the lungs. This gives images of pulmonary perfusion. In pulmonary hypertension caution should be exercised but a perfusion scan may be undertaken if clinically indicated. In the presence of right-to-left shunts perfusion lung scans should ideally be avoided but have been used without ill effect; the ^{99m}Tc MAA are then seen in the systemic circulation (mainly kidneys and brain).

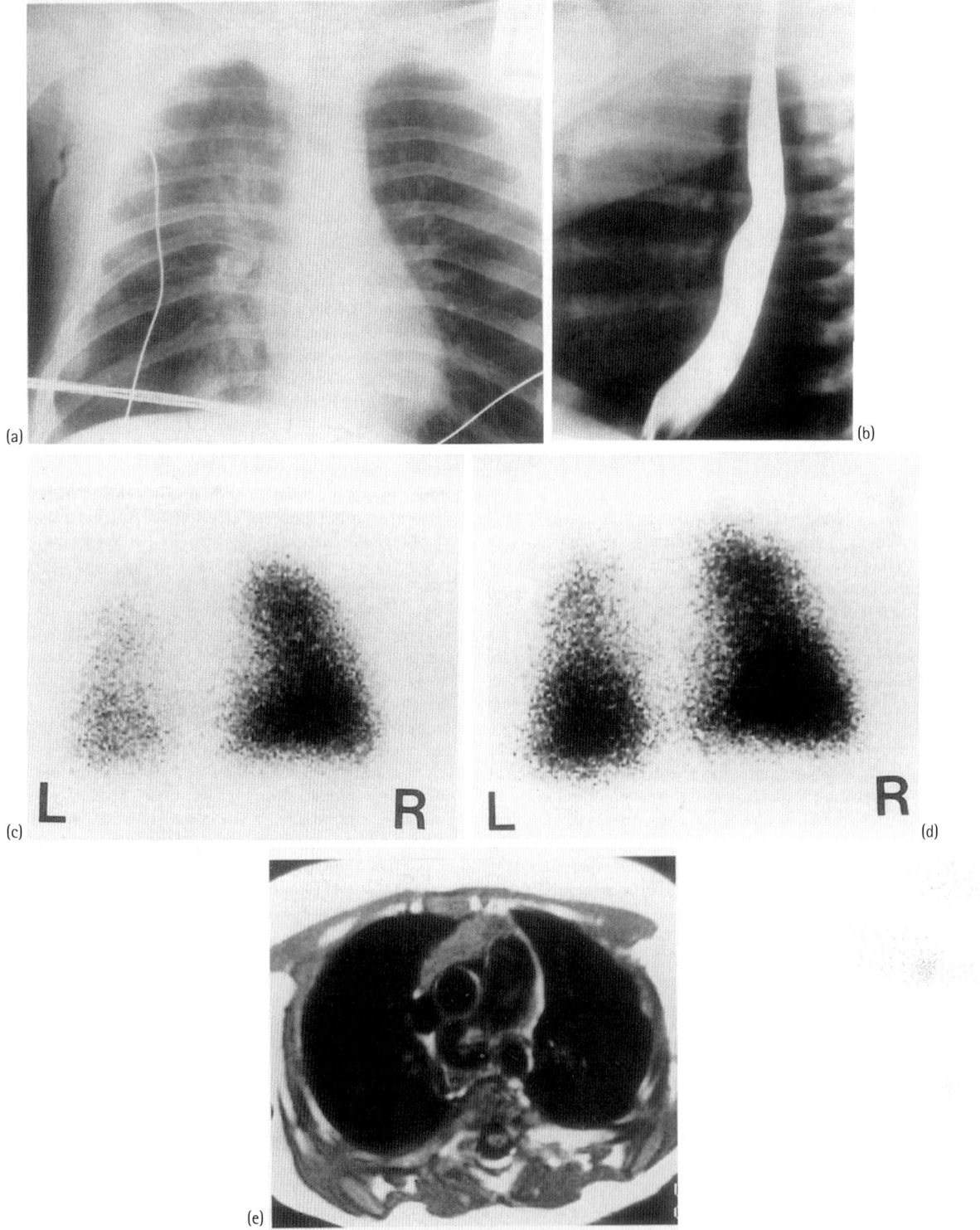

Fig. 20.15   A 6-month-old boy with stridor. (a) The PA chest radiograph shows evidence of overinflation in both lung fields. The left upper zone shows fewer vessels than on the right. There is a deformity of the posterior aspect of the 7th rib but no previous surgery had been undertaken. (b) The lateral project of the barium swallow shows clear indentation on the anterior wall of the esophagus at the level of the carina. This is a typical appearance of an aberrant left pulmonary artery which is only seen in the true lateral projection on barium. (c) Krypton 81 m ventilation lung scan shows normal ventilation of the right lung with decreased ventilation of the left upper lobe. (d) ^{99m}Tc macroaggregate perfusion scan reveals a normal right lung with decreased perfusion of most of the left lung. The left lung contributed 32% to overall perfusion and 39% to overall ventilation. (e) MRI scan of the mediastinum shows the aberrant left pulmonary artery arising from the right pulmonary artery and curling around behind the trachea but in front of the esophagus. This child underwent resection and anastomosis of the left pulmonary artery to the main pulmonary artery. The postoperative $\dot{V}/\dot{Q}$ lung scan revealed a normally perfused and ventilated left lung (not illustrated).

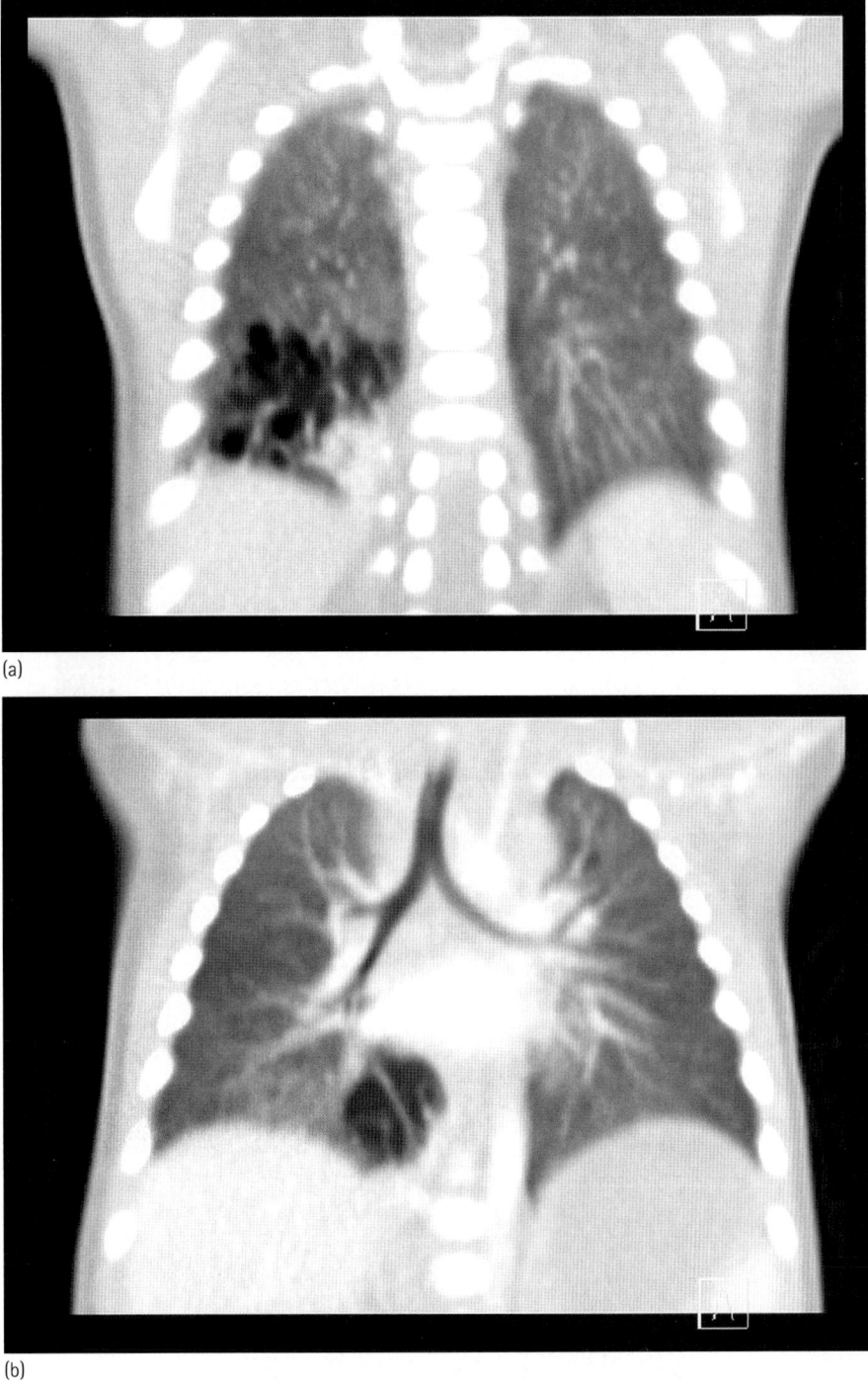

(a)

(b)

Fig. 20.16   Hybrid congenital pulmonary malformation. (a) Coronal CT image at lung window settings showing a cystic lesion in the right lower lobe typical of a congenital cystic adenomatoid malformation (CCAM). (b) Adjacent slices showed more normal lung parenchyma with apparent air trapping. Blacker (lower attenuating) lung with fewer vessels visible in the parenchyma is more characteristic of air trapping as seen with congenital lobar emphysema (CLE) (although this lesion is in a lower lobe which is unusual for CLE).

(*Continued*)

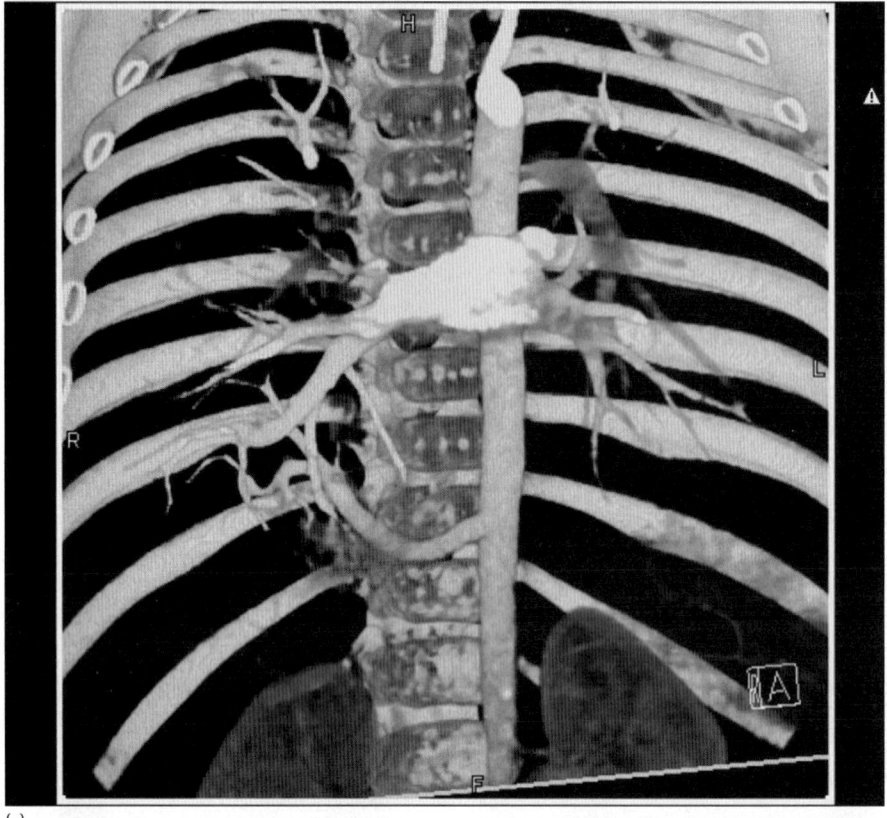

(c)

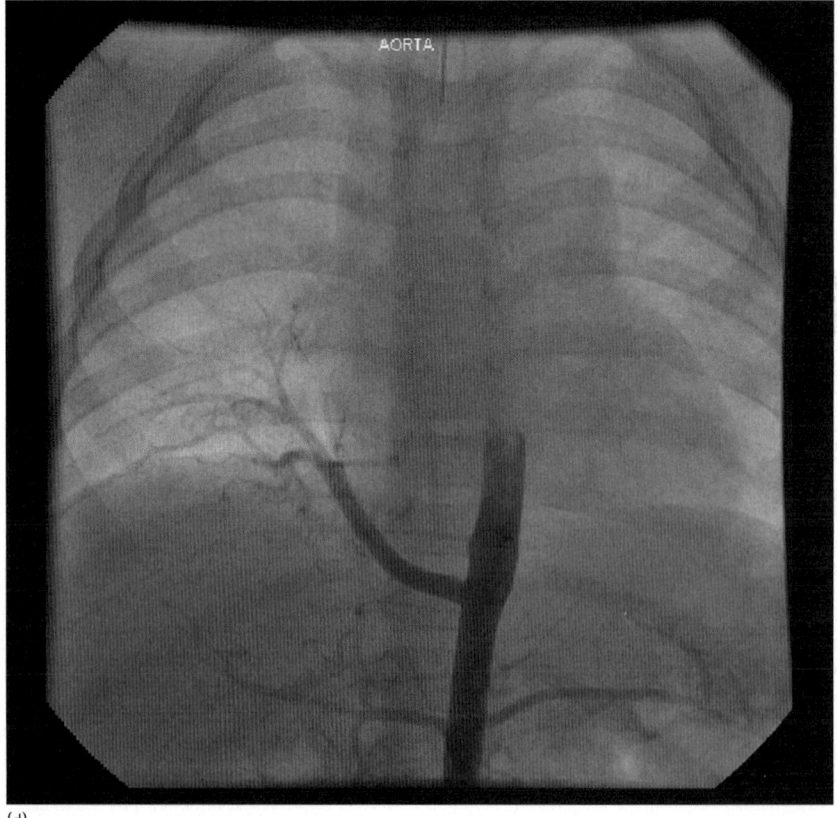

(d)

Fig. 20.16 (cont'd)   (c) Volume-rendered reformatted CT image, after contrast administration, showing a large vessel arising from the lower thoracic aorta on the right which supplied the lesion in the right lower lobe. Systemic arterial supply to a lung abnormality is characteristic of a pulmonary sequestration. (d) Conventional angiography confirms the large feeding vessel prior to embolization. This congenital pulmonary malformation can thus be regarded as a hybrid lesion containing elements of a CCAM, CLE and sequestration within it.

The $\dot{V}/\dot{Q}$ images reflect regional lung function. The main indication for $\dot{V}/\dot{Q}$ scanning now is in suspected pulmonary embolism with $\dot{V}/\dot{Q}$ studies being occasionally useful in children with established disorders such as obliterative bronchiolitis in whom regional lung function warrants assessment.

Radioisotope milk scan

This is used for evaluation of gastroesophageal reflux (see Ch 19, p. 605) and pulmonary aspiration. ^{99m}Tc-sulfur colloid is added to a normal feed (10 MBq/100 ml). Following the feed a small volume of nonradioisotope fluid is given to clear any activity from the esophagus. Infants are cuddled for 5 min; all children are placed supine over the gamma camera. Continuous imaging for 1 h then takes place with delayed images of the lungs 3–5 h after completion of the feed. The Tc-sulfur colloid has a small particle size and is not absorbed by gut mucosa. When aspiration occurs the activity may be seen in the lung. This test is more sensitive than a barium swallow in detecting gastroesophageal reflux since the esophagus is studied for up to 60 min continuously rather than intermittently as with barium studies.

COMPUTED TOMOGRAPHY

As CT scanning times reduce, particularly with the introduction of fast MDCT scanners, the indications for thoracic CT in children have increased.[93] CT affords excellent anatomical detail, particularly in older children who can suspend respiration. MDCT has the added advantage, when contiguous (adjacent) images are taken, that sagittal and coronal reconstructions are possible with similar resolution to standard axial imaging (see Fig. 20.16). There are essentially two types of chest CT studies generally performed. Standard, contiguous 1–2 mm sections are used when the whole chest or mediastinum is examined in detail. Indications here would include assessment of the pulmonary vasculature,[94] empyema (Fig. 20.17) or suspected adenopathy, typically performed after intravenous contrast enhancement. Standard contiguous slices would also be used in staging for suspected lung metastases in children with known solid tumors. HRCT involves using fine sections, usually 1 mm slices at 10–20 mm intervals through the lungs to assess for diffuse lung disorders such as an interstitial disease or bronchiectasis. The very fine detail of selected areas of the lung that is achievable with HRCT can help characterize unusual processes, define their extent and in certain cases plan an appropriate area for biopsy. The major disad-

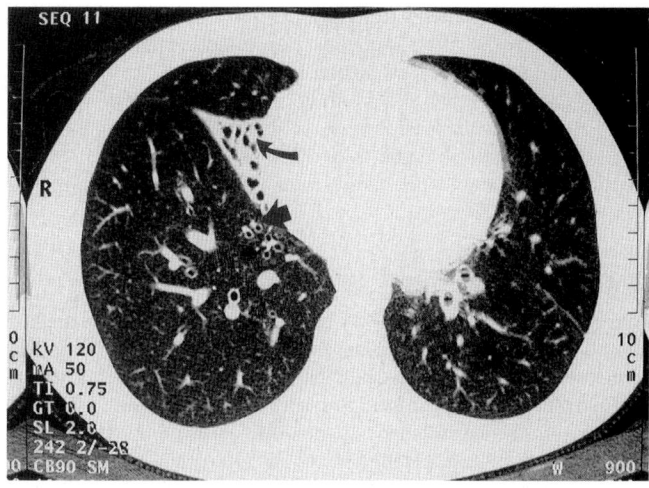

Fig. 20.18 High resolution chest CT image showing chronic right middle lobe collapse with airways dilatation, i.e. bronchiectasis (curved arrow). In addition, bronchial wall thickening is seen in the right lower lobe with the classic *signet ring* sign of bronchiectasis, which is due to a dilated airway adjacent to a more normal sized pulmonary artery, also evident (thick arrow). Normal cardiac pulsation has resulted in blurring of the cardiac outline.

vantage of CT is that it carries a large radiation burden and so should be used sparingly in young patients. Most pediatric centers now routinely utilize low dose (low mA) techniques to keep radiation to a minimum. As only selected areas through the lungs are examined, HRCT involves a relatively low radiation dose in comparison to standard CT. HRCT is very accurate in the assessment of bronchiectasis (Fig. 20.18). A normal HRCT essentially excludes this diagnosis assuming the study is of a reasonable quality. Expiratory images in cooperative older children can be very useful in showing air trapping with small airways disease, e.g. obliterative bronchiolitis (Fig. 20.19). Decubitus positioning mimics expiration (in the dependent lung) in sedated younger children. The role of HRCT is controversial in cystic fibrosis, but routine CT assessments are certainly justifiable in the context of clinical trials.

Virtually all solid tumors with the exception of neuroblastoma (which characteristically metastasizes to bone) require a chest CT at presentation. If the initial CT is negative for metastases, most cancers

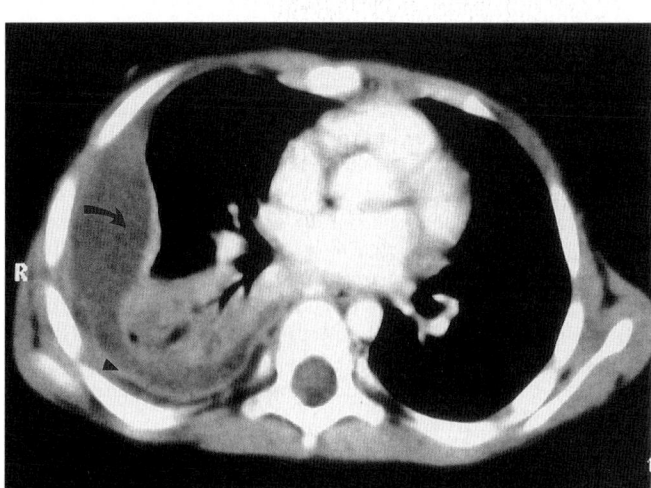

Fig. 20.17 Axial CT after intravenous contrast enhancement showing a moderate sized, low attenuating right-sided pleural effusion (curved arrow), proven to be an empyema at drainage. Note the adjacent area of consolidation, some thickening of the parietal pleura (arrowhead) and edema of the extrapleural space. Intravenous contrast administration has resulted in dense opacification of the cardiac chambers and descending aorta.

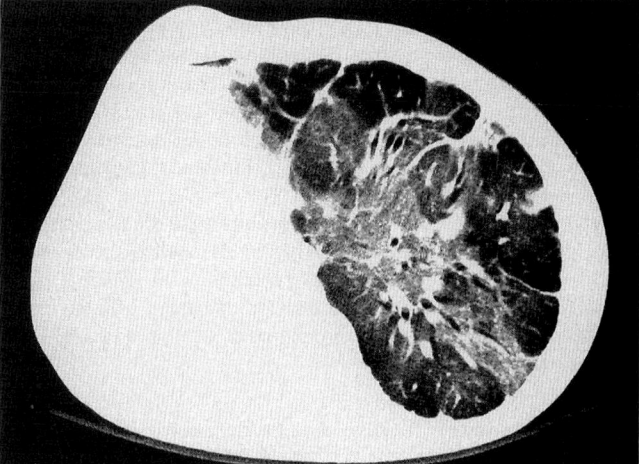

Fig. 20.19 Axial high resolution CT post single lung transplant in a child who had had a previous right pneumonectomy for cystic fibrosis. Obliterative bronchiolitis is evident in the left lung transplant, manifesting as areas of varying attenuation and curvilinear interstitial septal thickening. The peripheral blacker or low density foci represent areas of air trapping which become more conspicuous in older, cooperative patients who can breath hold for expiratory images.

are followed up thereafter with serial CXRs – except osteosarcoma which has a high propensity for pulmonary relapse and so merits repeated CT studies in the first few years from diagnosis.

In cases of suspected sequestration, CT after contrast enhancement often reveals the feeding vessel arising from the abdominal aorta although the venous drainage is less often seen. Mediastinal pathology is well visualized and tissue characterization allows some differentiation of solid from cystic lesions.

MAGNETIC RESONANCE IMAGING

The role of MRI in chest pathology is still being established. The mediastinum and airways are well visualized but negative (black) signal from aerated lung precludes good pulmonary imaging for the foreseeable future. MRI is highly accurate in assessing vascular anatomy and so can easily demonstrate a vascular ring or double aortic arch.[92] The increasing availibility of fast gadolinium-enhanced angiographic sequences has reduced the indications for arteriography of the lungs and great vessels.[95] A cooperative, still patient is an absolute prerequisite; hence there is a continuing need for sedation or anesthesia in smaller children.

ENDOSCOPY OF THE AIRWAY

BACKGROUND

The passage of instruments through the larynx to visualize, sample and manipulate the lower airways is a procedure with many applications in pediatric respiratory medicine.

Bronchoscopy has a long history. It was first developed nearly 100 years ago for the diagnosis and removal of foreign bodies from the trachea or bronchus. Early instruments were rigid and had a low level of illumination and a limited visual field. With better illumination and improved optics wider applications became possible.

The first flexible fiberoptic bronchoscope was developed in Japan in 1966. This instrument made it possible to see easily parts of the airway that were difficult to visualize using the rigid bronchoscope. It also became possible to perform bronchoscopic examinations without the need for general anesthesia, and with a significant reduction in operative morbidity. This led to a dramatic increase in the usefulness of bronchoscopy as a diagnostic and therapeutic tool. The application of fiberoptic bronchoscopy to pediatrics had to await the development of smaller instruments. Wood and Fink first described the use of the flexible bronchoscope in children in 1978.[96] Fiberoptic bronchoscopes small enough for use in children only became widely available in 1981. Technical progress has allowed a greater number of fiberoptic bundles per unit area, increasing the flexibility of the bronchoscope while retaining and even enhancing light transmission. Smaller bronchoscopes with a wider field of vision, providing a sharper, less grainy picture, are now being manufactured. Developments in instrumentation have made bronchoscopy an increasingly useful diagnostic and therapeutic tool in the newborn, infants and children.

While adult physicians are frequently looking for evidence of malignancy, pediatricians are usually looking for anatomical airway abnormalities or inflammatory or infective conditions. In children, upper airway problems are a common reason for endoscopic evaluation and 'bronchoscopy' often involves examination of the upper as well as the lower airway.

TECHNIQUES USED IN PEDIATRICS

Endoscopes

In order to perform bronchoscopy in children, the bronchoscope must meet some specific technical requirements. First, the instrument must be sufficiently small that it can safely enter the trachea (in a full-term newborn infant the trachea is approximately 5 mm in diameter). Second, it must have suitable optical characteristics and provide for illumination of the airway.

Rigid bronchoscopes

Small rigid bronchoscopes meet these criteria and are available in sizes from 2.5 mm (the nominal size of a rigid bronchoscope refers to the smallest internal diameter through which instruments may be passed, not to the outer diameter which may be several millimeters greater because of the thickness of the material). Endoscopes suitable for use in infants are 2.8 or 3.5 mm in external diameter.

Rigid bronchoscopy in children requires a general anesthetic, the bronchoscope functioning as an artificial airway allowing effective ventilation either with positive pressure inflation or with a Venturi jet injection device. With appropriate anesthetic technique, spontaneous respiration through the bronchoscope allows for assessment of laryngo-, tracheo- or broncho-malacia.

The optical properties of the rigid bronchoscope alone are poor but when a Hopkins glass rod telescope is passed through the bronchoscope, the optical resolution is excellent. Rigid bronchoscopy is particularly good at visualizing the posterior wall of the larynx such as when looking for a laryngeal cleft or H-type tracheoesophageal fistula. In children, although angulated telescopes can be used to look into the upper airways, direct access to more distal bronchi and to the upper lobes using a rigid bronchoscope is limited.

The main advantage of the rigid bronchoscope is that it provides complete airway control during the procedure. The excellent view and the extensive range of instruments available mean that a wide variety of therapeutic maneuvers can be carried out. Rigid bronchoscopy remains the procedure of choice for foreign body removal, tissue resection and biopsy where there is a risk of copious hemorrhage.

Flexible bronchoscopes

In the flexible fiberoptic bronchoscope light to visualize the airway is transmitted via a solid bundle of glass fibers. The child has to breathe around rather than through the endoscope.

There is now a range of endoscopes suitable for use in smaller children and neonates from a number of manufacturers (Table 20.4). The distal tip can be flexed by the operator in a single plane with side to side movement brought about by rotation of the shaft of the instrument made possible when the proximal shaft forms a looped shape. All but the smallest flexible endoscopes incorporate a small suction channel.

The standard pediatric endoscope has an external diameter of 2.8 mm with a 1.2 mm suction channel. The suction channel can be used to perform bronchoalveolar lavage, or to pass small instruments for bronchial brushings or bronchial biopsy. In older children, a small adult endoscope with an external diameter of 4.9 mm can be used. This has a larger working channel, enabling more effective suctioning and the use of larger biopsy forceps for epithelial or transbronchial biopsy (TBB).[97]

In infants less than 3000 g, an endoscope will nearly totally obstruct the airway. Bronchoscopy can be performed by pre-oxygenating the

Table 20.4 Examples of flexible endoscopes commonly used in the examination of the pediatric airways

Model*	Outer diameter (mm)	Angulation	Suction channel (mm)	Comments
BF-XP40	2.8	Up 180°, down 130°	1.2	Can pass through a 3.5 mm ET tube
BF3C40	3.3	Up 180°, down 130°	1.2	Previous versions were the standard flexible instrument used in children
BFP30	4.9	Up 180°, down 140°	2.2	

* All these instruments are manufactured by the Olympus Optical Company, but other manufacturers make instruments of similar specifications

infant with 100% oxygen and limiting the time below the glottis to 30–40 s. Alternatively, the airways of small neonates can be visualized with the 2.2 mm 'ultra thin' bronchoscope which lacks a suction channel. Endoscopes can be passed through a connector placed between the endotracheal tube and the ventilator, allowing uninterrupted ventilation and oxygen delivery during the procedure.

Video recording

Video recording is an important part of any endoscopic procedure in children. With a video monitor, the operator's assistants can view the findings and anticipate the operator's needs. The use of video also facilitates training by allowing trainees either to watch the procedure or to be carefully supervised performing the procedure. Recording improves documentation of endoscopic findings and facilitates communication with other members of the clinical team. Reviewing the video with a child's parents can be particularly helpful in explaining the study findings to them.

Setting and techniques

There are two general approaches to performing bronchoscopy in children: using either conscious sedation in an older child or adolescent, or under general anesthesia. Rigid bronchoscopy invariably requires a general anesthetic.

General anesthesia is not essential for flexible bronchoscopy in children. In many cases, airway endoscopy can be safely performed under conscious sedation and topical anesthesia. Adequate conscious sedation has most frequently been achieved using a combination of a short acting benzodiazepine and an opiate. A topical vasoconstrictor, applied to the nasal passages before the procedure, enlarges the nasal passages and decreases the risk of epistaxis. Lignocaine is applied to the same nostril and then delivered directly via the endoscope's suction channel above the vocal cords and below in the trachea and main bronchi. There is evidence that topical anesthesia in infants and children exaggerates the findings commonly associated with laryngomalacia. Because overestimation of these findings might lead to unnecessary treatment, it is important to examine the larynx and contiguous structures before applying topical anesthesia.[98]

While flexible bronchoscopy under sedation and topical anesthesia can provide excellent airway access, it is often difficult to be precise about the level of sedation achieved and the child is often sedated to a deeper level than is consistent with conscious sedation. The benefits of general anesthesia in terms of child safety and comfort, as well as the ease of examination, have been increasingly recognized and, in most circumstances, are now preferred.

When general anesthetic is employed for flexible endoscopy, or bronchoscopy performed on a ventilated patient, the flexible bronchoscope is passed down an endotracheal tube or through a laryngeal mask airway (LMA). An LMA has the important advantage of allowing the use of a larger diameter bronchoscope with a larger suction channel than could be passed through an endotracheal tube on the same child. This can make direct removal of foreign bodies possible or allow larger biopsies to be obtained through the use of larger instruments or biopsy forceps. Increasingly, the use of general anesthesia via an LMA is becoming the standard approach for children.[99]

Patient monitoring

It is essential that one person other than the endoscopist is solely responsible for observing and monitoring the child during the procedure. Many centers will have an anesthetist responsible for the sedation and monitoring of the child even in the absence of the need for a general anesthetic. Before the procedure, children undergoing endoscopy should have an i.v. line placed. Monitoring during the procedure should always include continuous pulse oximetry as well heart rate, respiration and color. Access to appropriate resuscitation equipment including suction and supplemental oxygen, and antagonists for any sedative agents used, must be immediately available and staff involved in airway endoscopy must be fully trained in resuscitation.

Contraindications and complications of airway endoscopy

Contraindications to bronchoscopy are largely relative. When performed by properly trained personnel in carefully controlled conditions, bronchoscopy is a low-risk procedure. Nevertheless, bronchoscopy should only be performed if the relative benefits of the procedure outweigh the risks. Complications are more likely in children with:

1. bleeding diatheses that cannot be corrected;
2. massive hemoptysis;
3. severe airway obstruction;
4. severe hypoxia;
5. pulmonary hypertension;
6. lung abscess where there is a risk of pus spreading throughout the lung if the cavity is ruptured.

Anklyosis of the jaw or neck may preclude rigid bronchoscopy.

The complications of airway endoscopy can generally be divided into those associated with the medications used before and during the endoscopic procedure, and those related to the instrumentation.[100]

Inadequate topical analgesia may lead to laryngospasm or other vagally mediated phenomena. Inadequate sedation may lead to patient discomfort; alternatively, too much sedation may lead to respiratory depression and apnea. Episodes of hypoxemia, bradycardia or apnea are common but usually transient and self-limiting.

Transient high fever is common within 24 h after a bronchoalveolar lavage. Small hemoptyses commonly follow biopsy procedures. The risk of trauma to the oropharynx or airway is greater with the rigid bronchoscope. More serious problems, including laryngospasm and pneumothorax, can occur, but are rare. Airway instrumentation may exacerbate airway narrowing in children with already compromised airways such as those with subglottic stenosis. Nebulized adrenaline (epinephrine) or intravenous corticosteroids may tide the child over but, rarely, intubation may be necessary. The reported incidence of pneumothorax following TBB is up to 8%.[101]

With careful attention to detail, the safety record of airway endoscopy in children is excellent and bronchoscopy can now be performed easily and safely even in small premature neonates, and ventilated children in the pediatric intensive care unit (PICU).

Infection control

Spread of infection during bronchoscopy has been suggested to be both under-recognized and under-reported.[102] Unless proper infection control procedures are followed, the greater number of procedures now being undertaken is likely to be associated with more frequent episodes of infection attributable to bronchoscopy. Accordingly, clinical staff involved in endoscopic procedures should be educated in infection control procedures. Those who may be exposed to body secretions during bronchoscopy should use universal precautions.

To prevent cross-infection between children or contamination of specimens collected, endoscopes must be scrupulously cleaned and disinfected after each use. Rigid bronchoscopes can be autoclaved. Flexible bronchoscopes must first be cleaned with detergent (including the suction channel) to remove any residue before being placed in a suitable sterilizing solution. Detailed guidelines have been published on the appropriate duration of sterilization, particularly for high-risk infections such as TB or HIV.[103] The instrument used for each procedure should be identified in the case sheet to enable tracking if there is future suspicion of cross-infection.

USES AND INDICATIONS FOR AIRWAY ENDOSCOPY IN CHILDREN

Clinical use of airway endoscopy in children falls into two broad categories: diagnostic and therapeutic.

Diagnostic uses

Nowadays, the flexible bronchoscope is the instrument of choice for most diagnostic purposes.[104]

Direct observation of intranasal, laryngeal, intratracheal and intrabronchial abnormalities

Endoscopy allows direct visualization of the nasal passages, pharynx, larynx and vocal cords, glottis, trachea, carina, lobar bronchus and more peripheral bronchi. Abnormalities of airway structure, size or patency, including congenital anomalies, stenosis or extrinsic airway compression, and endobronchial masses, particularly foreign bodies or mucus plugging, can all be seen. If an obstructing lesion pulsates it may point to the presence of a vascular abnormality such as a vascular ring. In children with TB, evidence of airway compression or granulation tissue may guide the need for steroid therapy or for the resection of granulation tissue.[105] In children with stridor or persistent wheezing, abnormal airway dynamics can be visualized. Areas of inflammation or bleeding may be directly identified.

Direct suction and bronchoalveolar lavage

Samples may be collected by suction either directly or after lung washings with saline. Bronchoalveolar lavage (BAL) is a method of collecting fluid through the suction channel of a wedged fiberscope after saline has been injected. This method is commonly used for collection of material for the analysis of cellular or biochemical components.[106]

Usually, BAL is carried out in the most affected area identified radiologically or by endoscopy. In diffuse lung disease, the right middle lobe is preferred because fluid recovery is better. BAL is carried out using sterile normal saline solution warmed to body temperature. Various protocols for determining the amount of fluid to be lavaged are available but there is limited information on which is optimal. Fluid is instilled in between two and four aliquots. The first aliquot collected is of more bronchial origin; subsequent aliquots, which are usually pooled, sample more distal airspaces. Generally, the initial fraction is used for culture while later fractions are submitted for cytological and biochemical analysis. A BAL can be considered technically satisfactory if fluid recovery is greater than 40% of the volume instilled and the lavage fluid (except for the first sample) contains few epithelial cells.

Bronchial biopsy

Areas in the airway that look abnormal can potentially be biopsied using endoscopic biopsy forceps. This may be useful if there is suspicion of a granulomatous disease (e.g. caseating tuberculosis). In children with poorly controlled asthma, mucosal biopsies have been used to investigate the extent of bronchial inflammation.[107] With infiltrative lung disorders, TBB may provide an alternative to open or percutaneous lung biopsy, although the small samples obtained are not always sufficient to make a diagnosis.

With an endobronchial brush inserted through the suction channel, it is easy to collect ciliated epithelium from the lower airways for assessment of cilial function and structure.

Bronchography

Although bronchography has largely been superseded by the development of HRCT, it is easy and safe to obtain a precise bronchogram by injection of contrast medium through the suction channel into the desired lobe or segment. This technique can produce very high quality bronchograms while minimizing the volume of contrast material used.

Therapeutic uses
Endoscopic removal of material

Operative procedures such as the extraction of foreign bodies are difficult with flexible instruments and rigid instruments are almost always used for this purpose. Material obstructing the airway, such as a foreign body, mucus plug or tissue mass, can be removed endoscopically. Mucus plugs can usually be aspirated through the suction channel of flexible instruments.

Placing of endobronchial stents

Stents have been widely used in adults for palliation of inoperable tracheobronchial malignancies. In children, tracheobronchial stenoses are usually congenital. Surgical treatment has been unsatisfactory, largely because of the occurrence of recurrent stenoses.

There is growing experience with the use of balloon-expandable, metal stents and silicone stents placed under combined bronchoscopic and fluoroscopic guidance. Such procedures have been used for the treatment of airway compression in pediatric patients, especially severe tracheal stenosis, either congenital or after tracheoplasty for congenital tracheal stenosis repair, and for severe tracheobronchomalacia in children as young as 2 months.

Complications, especially with metal stents, are not uncommon. A stent may migrate (often distally) or produce reactive granulation tissue formation (leading to subsequent airway stenosis). It may erode the mucosa or cause problems during attempted removal. If left in situ permanently, the stent may well lead to a fixed narrowing in the context of a growing child.[108-110]

SPECIFIC CLINICAL INDICATIONS FOR AIRWAY ENDOSCOPY (TABLE 20.5)[111-113]

STRIDOR[114]

Chronic stridor is the commonest indication for examination of the airway in infants and children. If stridor is mild and/or intermittent then a conservative approach may be appropriate. Even with mild stridor, an endoscopy may be useful if the parents are very anxious. Showing the parents the abnormality may be particularly valuable in helping them to understand their child's problem.

When the stridor is severe, persistent, associated with apnea, failure to thrive or an abnormal cry, or is present in a child who has previously been ventilated, then chances of a structural abnormality are high and endoscopy is indicated.[113]

The flexible bronchoscope is well suited for the evaluation of stridor. Because the instrument is passed through the nose, the entire airway can be examined. More importantly, a transnasal approach in a spontaneously ventilating sedated child leaves the laryngeal structures in their natural state, without any distorting forces being applied. This allows an evaluation of the 'normal' airway dynamics. If the child has stridor at the time of the examination, then the vibrating structures giving rise to the noise can be identified.

Table 20.5 Indications for bronchoscopy

Stridor
Unexplained or persistent wheeze
Unexplained or persistent cough
Unexplained hemoptysis
Possible tracheobronchial foreign body aspiration
Investigation of chest radiograph abnormalities
Persistent/recurrent lobar consolidation or atelectasis
Recurrent or persistent infiltrates
Lung lesions of unknown etiology
Pulmonary infection – to identify pathogens
In infection unresponsive to antibiotics
In a child with cystic fibrosis to identify pathogens
In an immunosuppressed child
Recurrent infection
Intensive care/anesthetic room
Examine for the position, patency or airway damage due to ET or tracheostomy tube
Facilitate difficult intubations
Airway injury
Assessment of injury from toxic inhalation or aspiration
Other therapeutic and diagnostic indications
Endobronchial stent placement
Sampling and/or removal of airway secretions and mucus plugs
Endobronchial and transbranchial biopsy

Laryngomalacia

Laryngomalacia is the commonest cause of persistent non-infective stridor, accounting for over 75% of cases, and is easily diagnosed endoscopically.

Stridor is usually evident in the first few days of life but may not be evident until later in the first month. The noise is a fairly characteristic jerky, inspiratory crowing noise which varies in intensity from breath to breath, commonly being loudest when the infant is crying or in the supine position. The noise may disappear when the infant is quiet, asleep or prone. Usually there is no respiratory distress or cyanosis. Stridor may worsen during an upper respiratory tract infection (URTI). Feeding difficulties and failure to thrive are very uncommon except in severe cases. The noise usually lessens gradually as the child becomes older and in the majority of children has disappeared by about 2 years.

The endoscopic findings of laryngomalacia are characteristic. The epiglottis is long and omega-shaped (Ω). The tissues of the larynx are floppy so that the epiglottis, arytenoids and aryepiglottic can be seen collapsing inwards on inspiration, prolapsing into and narrowing the glottic opening. The floppy tissues vibrate during inspiration causing the stridor, while on expiration the positive pressure of air blows them apart. Concomitant lesions below the cord are not uncommon. Accordingly, it is important that bronchoscopy is performed in addition to laryngoscopy.

Subglottic stenosis

Subglottic stenosis may be congenital or acquired. It is characterized by a narrowing in the subglottic region such that a bronchoscope appropriately sized for the child's age cannot pass through the subglottic area or passes snugly. Clinically, children may present with stridor, cough or recurrent croup.

Congenital subglottic stenosis is secondary to a small cricoid or thick submucosa. The prognosis is good, with fewer than 50% of cases coming to tracheostomy. Acquired subglottic stenosis is most commonly secondary to prolonged endotracheal intubation in the neonatal period. It may coexist with damage to other parts of the larynx and trachea.

Vocal cord paralysis

Vocal cord paralysis, unilateral or bilateral, is the second most common laryngeal anomaly in neonates and may be either congenital, secondary to central nervous system disorders, or iatrogenic, usually after surgical repair of cardiovascular disorders. In iatrogenic cases, unilateral paralysis is more frequent and the paralysis is temporary, usually recovering within 2–4 weeks. Children with vocal cord paralysis have a weak or absent cry, respiratory obstruction and difficulty in feeding. The diagnosis is made at endoscopy when passive, paradoxical movements of the vocal cord are observed.

Subglottic hemangiomata

Although rare, subglottic hemangiomata may be life threatening. Typically, an afebrile infant presents with increasing biphasic inspiratory and expiratory stridor. The voice is typically normal and there is commonly no swallowing difficulty. In most cases, symptoms are present before 16 weeks of age. The initial presentation may mimic croup but rather than resolving, stridor is progressive. Diagnosis may be difficult because of the rarity of the lesion and the overlap in presentation with other commoner illnesses such as croup. The presence of skin hemangioma should alert the clinician. An association between extensive hemangioma present in a cervicofacial 'beard' distribution and subglottic hemangioma has been noted. If present, the early evaluation of the airway may be appropriate.[115] Diagnosis is confirmed by the presence of a characteristic red or blue lesion seen at endoscopy. Regression usually begins by 2 years of age and thus a conservative approach is preferred. Other than this, treatment options include systemic steroids (prednisolone 2–4 mg/kg for 4–6 weeks, tapering the dose with response), direct steroid injection into the lesion or CO_2 laser excision. For steroid resistant lesions and in the presence of life threatening symptoms, interferon alpha-2a may be effective but has substantial side-effects. Another option in steroid-resistant lesions is vincristine. If the airway is compromised, tracheostomy may be necessary until regression occurs.

Tracheomalacia and bronchomalacia

Congenital malacia of the large airways is one of the few causes of irreversible airway obstruction in children.[116] In children, malacia has been defined as a collapse of at least 50% in the airway lumen during expiration, cough or spontaneous breathing.

As bronchoscopy has been used more often in children, it is clear that malacia of the large airways is not a rare problem with an estimated incidence of primary malacia of at least 1 in 2100.[117]

Expiratory stridor and a cough, often described as barking, are common symptoms in children with malacia.[117] However, symptoms may vary depending on severity and the presence or otherwise of associated conditions. Severe cases will usually present in the neonatal period with ventilator dependency or severe obstructive episodes with cyanosis ('near death episodes'). Those associated with specific syndromes or congenital heart disease (secondary malacia) may be detected early because of selective screening. Children with milder airway malacia without other clinical features ('primary malacia') often present later with more nonspecific respiratory symptoms such as cough, recurrent lower respiratory infections, shortness of breath, wheeze, rattling or stridor. One series noted stridor in only 18% with cough the most common problem, present in 83%. Not infrequently, children with airway malacia are wrongly diagnosed as severe persistent or therapy resistant asthma because of the lack of response to standard asthma therapy or evidence of irreversible airway obstruction. In children with primary airway malacia, the diagnosis was not suspected before bronchoscopy in half of cases.

At bronchoscopy, abnormalities of the tracheal cartilage may be seen, most typically with anterior flattening of the usual horse-shoe shape. Dynamic movement of the airway during the respiratory cycle produces anteroposterior narrowing in expiration, often more pronounced to one side. Extreme cases will demonstrate a touching, or kissing, of the anterior and posterior parts. With associated anomalies such as tracheoesophageal atresia, the tracheomalacia may be localized, while in other primary cases it can affect most of the trachea and bronchi.

PERSISTENT OR UNILATERAL WHEEZING

Persistent wheezing unresponsive to bronchodilators or unilateral wheezing is an important indication for bronchoscopic examination. Lower airway problems were found in 79% of one large series. Tracheomalacia, compression of the left main bronchus usually in association with cardiac anomalies and tracheal compression due to vascular structures were the commonest structural findings. However, previously unsuspected foreign bodies were also surprisingly common.[118]

PERSISTENT COUGH

If persistent cough is unresponsive to treatment, bronchoscopy may be indicated although the diagnostic yield may be low in the absence of other symptoms and signs. It can, however, be reassuring if the airways are normal.

UNEXPLAINED HEMOPTYSIS

Hemoptysis is an unusual symptom in children. If the bleeding is of significant size or is persistent and a careful history and examination, including a careful examination of the mouth and nose, fails to identify a cause, then bronchoscopy is indicated. The chances of finding a cause are greater if the bleeding is active at the time of the examination. Rigid bronchoscopy with its better suction is safer if hemoptysis is brisk. Heavily blood-stained BAL fluid raises the possibility of pulmonary hemosiderosis. The demonstration of hemosiderin-laden macrophages in the lavage fluid confirms the diagnosis. If hemoptysis persists after a normal bronchoscopy, a pulmonary origin for the blood is unlikely.[113]

PERSISTENT ATELECTASIS

If atelectasis persists despite adequate treatment, bronchoscopy should be considered to exclude a foreign body, remove mucus plugs and obtain pathological specimens. In one large series, around 60% of children with persistent atelectasis had a diagnostic abnormality.[118] While the causes were diverse, the commonest finding was the presence of a central mucus plug. Removal of large plugs by lavage and suction frequently can lead to complete and immediate resolution, particularly in young children with massive atelectasis.

RECURRENT/PERSISTENT PULMONARY INFILTRATES

Bronchoscopy combined with BAL can provide valuable information in the assessment and treatment of a child with pulmonary infiltrates and should be considered in every child suspected of interstitial lung disease.

In an immunocompetent child

When a child with pulmonary infiltrates fails to respond to a broad spectrum antibiotic or where an atypical pneumonia is suspected and other techniques of collecting airways secretions are not practical, bronchoscopy with BAL can be used to collect specimens for microbiological and cytological analysis. However, samples collected by BAL can be contaminated by bacteria normally present in the respiratory tract. Interpretation of cultures, therefore, may need to be based on quantitative cultures with appropriate thresholds and/or identification of intracellular bacteria on direct examination of the sample in conjunction with the clinical picture. Newer molecular techniques are extending the range of organisms that can be detected.

In children with alveolar proteinosis, alveolar hemorrhage and pulmonary histiocytosis, BAL may be diagnostic. In other situations, even if not diagnostic, BAL cell profiles may help orientate further investigations.[106] Once a diagnosis of an alveolar inflammatory process has been reached, inflammatory markers in BAL fluid may help monitor disease activity and progression, although there is as yet no general consensus on the measurement or interpretation of such markers.

Finally, bronchoscopy and BAL may have a therapeutic role in the removal of material present in the airways resulting from lipoid material in alveolar structures. Several reports have shown that whole lung lavage may be an effective treatment in some children with alveolar proteinosis.[119]

In an immunocompromised child

In the immunocompromised child with pulmonary infiltrates, bronchoscopy and BAL have an important role. In children with primary or secondary immunodeficiency who develop pneumonitis, BAL should ideally be performed soon after clinical and radiological signs develop, before any antibiotic therapy is started. Where antibiotics are started empirically, bronchoscopy and BAL may be informative in those who do not improve despite adequate antibiotic therapy.

The identification of primary pathogens, such as *Mycobacterium tuberculosis*, *Pneumocystis jiroveci* (formerly *P. carinii*), or respiratory syncytial virus (RSV) not usually isolated from BAL fluid, may be diagnostic. Where the organisms may also be present as airway commensals or contaminants (e.g. Aspergillus, atypical mycobacteria, cytomegalovirus), interpretation is more difficult.

Children with HIV can develop a range of respiratory presentations ranging from acute pneumonia to interstitial pneumonitis (see Ch. 27, p. 1155). Bronchoscopy and BAL may help differentiate infectious causes such as *P. jiroveci* from non-infectious pulmonary complications such as lymphoid interstitial pneumonitis.

BAL and TBB are frequently used in the monitoring of children after lung transplantation, either routinely or as a result of clinical and/or radiological deterioration.[101,120] TBB is necessary to establish a histological diagnosis of rejection while BAL fluid can be used for microbiological studies to exclude infection.

INHALATION OF FOREIGN MATERIAL

Foreign body aspiration

Aspiration of a foreign body in a child is among the most important indications for bronchoscopy. Indeed, the presence of a foreign body cannot be reliably excluded without a bronchoscopy.

The typical history is of the sudden onset of choking, coughing or wheezing. A careful history will identify a choking episode in most cases. After the initial period, a symptom free interval may follow. Some patients with foreign bodies have chronic or subtle clinical features (atelectasis, recurrent or persisting pneumonia, persistent wheezing unresponsive to bronchodilators, diminished local breath sounds) and radiological changes (hyperinflation or atelectasis of an affected segment), but no history of foreign body aspiration. Others may have no physical or radiological signs.

Peanuts (ground nut) and other nuts are the most common objects inhaled in the UK. These materials are highly irritating to bronchial epithelium and can lead to florid local inflammation and necrosis if not rapidly removed. Grass seeds and seed husks are commoner in other parts of the world and may be especially troublesome because their barbed nature prevents expectoration or removal by bronchoscopy. The most common site of impaction of a foreign body is in a segmental bronchus on the right side.

In the many cases where history, physical examination and radiographic studies suggest a diagnosis of foreign body aspiration, the child should have rigid bronchoscopy without delay.

When there is doubt about foreign body aspiration, a flexible bronchoscopy may be diagnostically valuable. In some children, foreign body aspiration may be totally unsuspected. Wood found a previously unsuspected foreign body in nearly 1% of children undergoing flexible bronchoscopy.[118] If a foreign body is identified, then the child should have a rigid bronchoscopy to remove it. Occasionally when removal of a foreign body has been unusually delayed, it may be necessary to resect an irretrievably damaged lung segment.

Recurrent aspiration

Bronchoscopy and BAL can be useful in the investigation of a child suspected of recurrent aspiration. Chronic pulmonary aspiration of oral and/or gastric contents occurs when normal airway protective mechanisms are impaired, bypassed or overwhelmed. The resulting airway contamination causes lung injury which may lead to bronchospasm, atelectasis, pulmonary edema, pneumonia or bronchiectasis, depending on the frequency and quantity of aspiration, the composition and pH of aspirated material and the efficacy of the lung clearance response. Thus, there may be a range of clinical presentations ranging from wheezing, through recurrent episodes of pneumonia to chronic inflammation with eventual interstitial fibrosis and bronchiectasis. Children with neurodevelopmental problems are particularly susceptible. The predominant site of pathology depends on the patient's habitual posture: upper lobes in infants nursed supine; basal disease for older children propped in a semi-recumbent position.

There are three main groups of pathophysiological processes that interfere with normal airway protective mechanisms and lead to recurrent aspiration (Table 20.6). Anatomical abnormalities such as cleft palate or laryngeal cleft can lead to pooling of food or saliva in the pharynx. Abnormal swallowing coordination occurring in children with neuromuscular disorders such as cerebral palsy or dysautonomia results in aspiration of material with symptoms likely to occur during feeding. Esophageal disorders cause aspiration by a number of mechanisms. Fistulous connections will lead to lower airway soiling, particularly during feeding. There may be soiling of the lower airway from overspill of contents refluxed from the stomach or more rarely from overspill from a dilated esophagus in conditions such as achalasia or with esophageal strictures.

The diagnosis of recurrent aspiration can be surprisingly problematic. Associated disorders, varying clinical presentations and lack of specific diagnostic criteria all contribute to frequent diagnostic difficulties. Diagnosis starts with a careful history and examination (including a careful dental inspection) combined with observation

Table 20.6   Causes of recurrent aspiration

Swallowing disorders
Anatomical disorders
    Cleft palate
    Macroglossia
    Laryngeal cleft
Neuromuscular disorders
    Cerebral palsy
    CNS degenerative disorders
    Congenital neuromuscular disorders
    Dysautonomia

Esophageal lesions
    Obstruction
    Stricture or compression
    Systemic sclerosis
    Achalasia
    Tracheoesophageal fistula
    Gastroesophageal reflux
    Hyperinflation (severe asthma, cystic fibrosis)

of the child feeding, followed by imaging studies including a CXR, barium swallow and video recording of the child swallowing. If a fistula is suspected, specific lateral X-ray views are taken while injecting contrast rapidly to distend the esophagus through a slowly withdrawn, gastric tube with side holes. The gold standard for demonstrating gastroesophageal reflux has been a 24-h pH probe study. Gastroesophageal scintiscans using radiolabeled milk may provide direct evidence of aspiration (see p. 673 Radioisotope investigations). While positive studies are highly suggestive of chronic aspiration false positives may occur and none of these tests may rule out aspiration.

Bronchoscopy may provide direct evidence of anatomical abnormalities such as the presence of a tracheoesophageal fistula. Dye can be introduced via the endoscope into the airway with simultaneous esophageal observation endoscopically to observe leakage through a fistulous connection. The semi-quantitative estimation of lipid-laden alveolar macrophages (LLMIs) in bronchoalveolar fluid has been used as a marker of chronic aspiration. While more recent studies suggest that LLMIs alone cannot be used to diagnose chronic aspiration, they may be a useful adjunct when taken in combination with other investigations.[121]

BRONCHOSCOPY IN INTENSIVE CARE AREAS AND ANESTHETIC ROOMS

There are a number of important uses for airway endoscopy in neonatal and pediatric intensive care units and in pediatric anesthesia.[122,123] Documentation of abnormal anatomy and airway injury secondary to intubation and suction is part of the full assessment of each child. Specific indications for endoscopy in neonatal and pediatric intensive care are discussed below.

Intubation

Endoscopic intubation is a useful method in difficult to intubate children whose larynx is otherwise impossible to visualize. Following a nasal approach and passage of the endoscope into the trachea, an endotracheal tube (ETT) is passed over the endoscope and directly positioned in the airway under direct visualization. Custom-made intubation endoscopes have a small battery light source and are stiffer and more robust than diagnostic endoscopes, but with care the ultra-thin 2.2 mm bronchoscope can aid intubation with ETTs as small as 3.0 mm.

Problems with ventilation

Abnormal gas exchange may be due to an ETT problem. Bronchoscopy can quickly confirm ETT patency and position. Children in the PICU with congenital abnormalities (e.g. Di George syndrome, myelomeningocele, congenital heart disease) may have a low placed ETT at bronchoscopy despite an apparent satisfactory position on CXR, due to an associated short trachea.[124,125] Occasionally endoscopy can assist in selective placement of the ETT into a main stem bronchus in the treatment of persistent contralateral air leak.

Unsuspected congenital airway abnormality (malacia, stenosis, compression, tracheal bronchus) or acquired pathology (granulation tissue, mucus or blood plugs) can also cause difficulty with assisted ventilation, and in an unstable newborn infant or child in intensive care the diagnostic procedure of choice will be an endoscopy. Ventilation can be continued during the examination using a bronchoscope swivel adaptor, with the procedure being well tolerated by the majority of patients.

Bronchomalacia, while often causing a ventilation problem, is unlikely to need any specific treatment. Tracheomalacia may require aortopexy, while tracheal stenosis causing significant ventilation problems may require a slide tracheoplasty. Major airway compression most commonly occurs in conjunction with congenital cardiac disease, which may not be treatable or may even be made worse by corrective surgery. Positioning an expandable metallic stent for a short period can be considered in an attempt to enable extubation in a child who remains dependent on positive pressure ventilation due to a discrete narrowing of a main airway.[126]

Persistent or recurrent atelectasis

In intensive care, persistent atelectasis can be caused by a congenital lung abnormality or an acquired problem such as airway compression or plugging. In the latter case, bronchoscopy with BAL can remove the obstruction allowing re-inflation of the affected lung. On occasions, a foreign body may be the cause of the consolidation secondary to airway inflammation and obstruction, though the more usual clinical scenario would be one of increased airway obstruction on expiration causing a 'ball valve' effect with resulting lung hyperinflation and airleak.

Sampling of airway secretions

Flexible bronchoscopy can enable collection of lower airway secretions for analysis in different clinical situations. Current technology limits specimen collection to an ETT large enough to enable the passage of a 2.8 mm diameter scope, which is the smallest instrument available with a suction channel.

Even the sickest child will tolerate quickly passing the bronchoscope into the lower airway to lavage either a lobe identified as abnormal on a CXR, one with thick infected secretions seen at the time of the examination, or alternatively the Right middle lobe (RML) or lingula. While ETT secretions have traditionally been used for antibiotic targeting in nosocomial pneumonia, bronchoscopic BAL is more likely to differentiate bacterial colonization from infection.[127]

Staining for lipid- or hemosiderin-laden macrophages can be an important diagnostic investigation in a ventilated child with unexplained respiratory disease. At times a newborn child will become ventilator dependent due to a surfactant protein B deficiency or alveolar proteinosis. BAL will demonstrate large volumes of cloudy lung fluid, which can be analysed for surfactant.

CONCLUSIONS

Airway endoscopy is firmly established as an important tool in the investigation and management of respiratory disorders in children. New developments and wider use of the technique mean that the full potential of the technique is still being realized.

SLEEP DISORDERED BREATHING

Humans spend approximately one third of their lives asleep, yet many of the functions of sleep remain poorly understood,[128] but probably include neocortical maintenance, energy conservation, memory consolidation, neurodevelopmental roles and effects on immunoregulation. Despite its essential role in mammalian function (total sleep deprivation can result in the rapid death of small mammals) and ancestral origins, the structure of sleep has been elucidated only in relatively modern times. Prior to the use of EEG to decipher different stages of sleep in 1937,[129] sleep was believed to represent a homogeneous state of inertia. Rapid eye movement (REM) sleep was first described in 1953[130] and conventional sleep staging as currently applied is based on the work of Rechtschaffen and Kales,[131] which categorizes sleep into REM and four stages of non-REM (nREM) sleep based on electrophysiological criteria. Sleep is organized into a number of 'sleep cycles' with slow wave sleep predominating during the early part of sleep and REM periods becoming more prolonged in the latter half of a night's sleep. Typically, once adult-type sleep patterns are established, there will be four to five nREM/REM cycles during a night and REM will occupy approximately 20% of the total sleep time. In contrast, sleep in the newborn does not have such clearly defined electrophysiological features that distinguish REM from nREM sleep. Instead, a behavioral state that shares many features of adult REM sleep, active sleep (bAS), is distinct from the nREM equivalent, quiet sleep (bQS). These stages are organized as a number of much shorter sleep cycles than in the adult, each of approximately 1 h duration and comprising equivalent periods of bAS and bQS, such that the neonatal equivalent of REM sleep occupies almost 50% of total sleep time. A diurnal pattern of sleep behavior emerges in the infant at around 16 weeks of age and habitual daytime sleep gradually diminishes over the first 2 years of life.

Sleep is a metabolically active process and is associated with the pulsatile release of a number of important hormones, including growth hormone (see Ch. 15, p. 436). Physiological changes in respiration also occur during sleep and in general these are state dependent, varying between REM and nREM sleep. Minute ventilation falls by about 8–15% during sleep compared with wakefulness. In adults, this is largely due to decreased tidal volume. However, in infants and children, the respiratory rate decreases during sleep, possibly in association with a decrease in tidal volume. During REM sleep, breathing becomes irregular with frequent central apneas, intercostal muscle activity decreases and there is an increase in upper airway resistance. These changes are important in early childhood as infants spend a proportionately greater period in REM or REM-equivalent (bAS) sleep compared with adults. Also, as infants have markedly greater chest wall compliance than adults, the loss of postural muscle tone during REM sleep leads to paradoxical inward rib cage motion during inspiration that is typically associated with airway obstruction in older children.[132] In contrast, during quiet sleep, intercostal muscle activity is maintained and thoracic and abdominal movements are coupled and in phase.

Infants and children have greater ventilatory drive relative to body size than adults.[133] Infants also have an exaggerated biphasic response to hypoxia with an initial increase in ventilation followed by a decrease, often in association with apnea. This is coupled with a higher arousal threshold to hypoxia in children compared with adults, resulting in moderate hypoxemia being a poor stimulus to arousal. In contrast, hypercapnea and increased upper airway resistance are potent stimuli for arousal during sleep in all age groups.

Respiration during quiet sleep is largely determined by autonomic control through chemoreceptor inputs. Thus failure of chemoreceptor control mechanisms, e.g. congenital central hypoventilation, results in hypoventilation that is most marked in, but not confined to, quiet sleep. During REM sleep, infants and children have frequent central apneas. In asymptomatic infants, these have been demonstrated to exceed 20 s duration and to be associated with desaturations to below 81%.[134] Therefore, their clinical significance remains uncertain. The physiological changes occurring during REM sleep also contribute to increased upper airway resistance associated with obstructive sleep apnea syndrome, in which loss of genioglossus tone is an important factor, and to hypoventilation in cases of diaphragmatic paresis or palsy, when ventilation during wakefulness and quiet sleep is maintained by intercostal and accessory muscle activity. Thus, investigation of children with damage to or disorders of any component of the respiratory musculature must include measurements of respiration during sleep, particularly during intercurrent illnesses associated with increased work of breathing. Abnormal respiratory muscles that provide adequate alveolar ventilation when a child is well may not be able to cope under conditions of increased load.

CONGENITAL CENTRAL HYPOVENTILATION SYNDROME
Prevalence
Congenital central hypoventilation syndrome (CCHS), previously commonly known as 'Ondine's curse' is a rare (between 1 in 50 000 and 1 in 200 000) congenital condition in which there is an abnormality of control of respiration in the absence of any identifiable primary CNS, neuromuscular, lung or cardiac disease. Approximately 800 cases of CCHS have been identified worldwide.

A Strategic Health Authority, with a population of 1–1.5 million and 10 000–15 000 births per year, will have 3–4 children with CCHS. In the past many children with CCHS may have died in early infancy, but increased awareness of the condition in recent years has led to an increased number of children being diagnosed within a few days of birth.[135–138]

Because of the extreme rarity of this condition, virtually all published studies are based upon case reports, case series and expert opinion (i.e. evidence levels 3 or 4).

Consequences and benefits of identification
Affected children show hypoventilation during sleep, especially non-REM sleep, but some severely affected patients may also hypoventilate while awake. Untreated children with the more severe forms of CCHS are likely to die within the first few weeks after birth. If not recognized in early infancy, children with the milder forms of CCHS may present with cyanosis, edema and right heart failure with pulmonary hypertension as a consequence of recurrent or chronic hypoxemia. Some children may present with apparently life threatening episodes or apneas necessitating resuscitation. Untreated mild to moderate CCHS is compatible with survival for several months, and it is possible for subtle disease to go unnoticed. In the late-onset variant that presents around 2–4 years of age there are commonly associated hypothalamic disorders, particularly endocrine dysfunction. Several cases have now been reported of presentation of CCHS in adult life, commonly with symptoms dating to early childhood, though in others these are only recognized on the diagnosis of CCHS in a child of the affected adult.[135–140]

Prevention
Although the great majority of children with CCHS will be the first affected person in the family, recent studies have identified heterozygous de novo mutations of the PHOX2B gene in > 90% of children with CCHS,[141–143] raising the possibility of prenatal diagnosis. Genetic investigation and counseling should be offered to all newly diagnosed families.

Identification and diagnosis
Diagnostic criteria
The clinical and physiological diagnosis of CCHS has been considered to require the following criteria:[144,145]

1. persistent evidence of hypoventilation during sleep [$PaCO_2$ > 60 mmHg (8 kPa)];
2. onset of symptoms usually in the first year after birth;
3. absence of primary pulmonary or neuromuscular disease;
4. no evidence of primary heart disease.

However, the clinical presentation of CCHS is variable and may reflect the severity of the underlying disorder. Children typically present in the newborn period with duskiness or cyanosis when falling asleep, but no associated increase in respiratory effort. These infants may not awaken during these episodes. Hypoventilation may be present during waking but is generally worse during sleep. Presentation may be with apparent life threatening events (ALTEs), or it may be delayed until adult life, as noted above.[140]

CCHS is associated with a number of other conditions affecting or derived from the autonomic nervous system. These include neurocristopathies such as Hirschsprung disease, abnormalities of a range of autonomic functions (e.g. temperature control, pupil size, heart rate variability) and tumors, including ganglioneuroma, neuroblastoma and ganglioneuroblastoma.[135–137,141–143]

In the evaluation of children with sleep hypoventilation, it is important to exclude primary neuromuscular, cardiac or pulmonary disease or any identifiable brainstem lesions. Other conditions that may cause sleep hypoventilation include congenital myopathy, myasthenia gravis, abnormalities of the airway or intrathoracic anatomy, diaphragm dysfunction, congenital cardiac disease, structural hindbrain or brainstem abnormalities and metabolic disorders.

Assessment

The identification of characteristic abnormalities of the PHOX2B gene – either polyalanine insertions, frameshift or mis-sense mutations,[140–143] in >90% of children with clinically diagnosed CCHS allows the rapid identification of the diagnosis in the great majority of affected individuals. In the UK, investigation of the PHOX2B gene is available through the UK clinical genetics testing network (www.geneticstestingnetwork. org.uk).

Definitive physiological evaluation of CCHS includes a detailed assessment of spontaneous breathing during sleep and wakefulness in a reference sleep physiology laboratory. Good quality polysomnography, including an adequate period during both REM and non-REM phases of sleep, is essential. The measurements should include at a minimum, tidal volume and flow (pneumotachograph), movement of the chest and abdomen (respiratory inductance plethysmography), pulse oxymetry, end-tidal CO_2 and ECG, together with EEG and electro-oculogram (EOG) for sleep state determination. This may be supplemented by invasive blood gas measurements, preferably obtained from an indwelling arterial line, to objectively quantify hypoxemia and hypercarbia. Careful observation of tidal volume and respiratory rate of infants during endogenous hypercarbia during sleep and wakefulness may be sufficient to assess central chemoreceptor function. Peripheral chemoreceptor sensitivity to hypoxia may be assessed by measurement of the ventilatory depression caused by hyperoxia from the administration of increased inhaled oxygen concentration. More detailed assessment of chemoreceptor ventilatory responses to hypercarbia may be performed using a rebreathing or steady state challenge with 5% CO_2 administered via a head box. Functional MRI has shown abnormalities of CNS responses to both hypoxia and hypercapnia in multiple CNS sites, including the frontal cortex, cerebellar cortex and basal ganglia, as well as the midbrain, pons and ventral and dorsal medulla.[137,144–154]

Management

Ventilatory support is necessary in almost all children with CCHS. This may be continuous or during sleep only. In contrast to the generally poor prognosis of untreated infants, >60% of patients receiving ventilatory support will survive to later childhood.[135–138] Most such children with CCHS have an overall high quality of life, though many have persisting hypotonia with varying degree of neurocognitive deficits, and many have multiple autonomic deficits, particularly affecting heart rate variation, blood pressure control and thermal responses.[146–154] Many children with CCHS suffer from seizure disorders and some show evidence of poor growth and delayed puberty. It is difficult to separate the effects of intrinsic CNS abnormalities from the effects of intermittent hypoxemia in determining the neurodevelopmental outcome. Pulmonary hypertension and cor pulmonale occur in some children with CCHS and may be fatal; it is not yet clear whether these can be completely prevented by rigorous ventilatory management, but in order to minimize the risk of cor pulmonale, current recommendations are to aim to maintain normal levels of both CO_2 and O_2 during all periods on ventilatory support.[137,138,145]

Conventional management of infants with CCHS has been to maintain ventilation via a tracheostomy, but recent reports have shown the feasibility of non-invasive ventilatory support from early infancy for selected infants.[135,136,155,156] With adequate education, support and resources provided to the family and the primary health care team almost all children with CCHS can be safely and effectively cared for at home in the longer term.[135–138,155,156] The practicalities of discharging a child home on ventilation in the UK have been dealt with elsewhere.[157,158]

Several ventilatory options are available for these children. With increasing age and as the infant becomes ambulatory, diaphragmatic pacing using phrenic nerve stimulation is an option for children with CCHS who are ventilator dependent for 24 h a day and who have no evidence of ventilator-related lung disease.[159–161] Phrenic nerve electrodes may be bipolar (relatively easier insertion through the neck but somewhat less reliable because of possible displacement) or more recently quadripolar (more difficult transthoracic insertion but more stable position and hence more reliable). The aim is to ensure adequate alveolar ventilation and oxygenation. Because of the more natural breathing pattern, with negative inspiratory intrathoracic pressure, pulmonary ventilation perfusion matching is improved in some patients by the use of phrenic stimulators. Adverse effects of phrenic nerve stimulators include permanent phrenic nerve damage, diaphragmatic fatigue, discomfort associated with surgical implantation, accidental displacements in ambulatory children and the potential need for repeated surgical revisions. The quadripolar electrodes offer greater duration of pacer support, diminished risk of phrenic nerve damage and diaphragmatic fatigue, and allow optimization of the pacing activity during exercise. Despite limitations, parents and children have emphasized the improvements in mobility and quality of life after phrenic nerve stimulator insertion in CCHS.[159] Despite the very high cost of phrenic nerve stimulators and their insertion and maintenance, this option should be explored for all children who require awake as well as asleep ventilatory support. Phrenic nerve stimulators are usually used only during the daytime, with positive pressure ventilation by a ventilator at night, to minimize the risk of phrenic nerve damage from continuous electrical stimulation, although some patients have chosen to use nerve stimulators round the clock for prolonged periods.[159]

Children who require ventilatory support only during sleep and who are able to cooperate may be considered for non-invasive facemask ventilation with bilevel positive pressure ventilation. Non-invasive ventilation is generally not recommended for children younger than 6–7 years of age, partly because of the likely need for continuous ventilatory support with intercurrent illness, and partly because of the risk of midfacial growth abnormalities as a consequence of a tightly placed face mask. Some authors have reported successful use of such techniques in early infancy, however.[135,136,155] If non-invasive ventilation is successfully instituted, tracheal decannulation may be performed.

Negative pressure ventilation has been used successfully in one center in the UK.[156] However, this is cumbersome and may need significant equipment adjustment over time. In addition negative pressure ventilation may aggravate any coexisting upper airway obstruction in these children.

Other general supportive measures are also important as many children with CCHS suffer from feeding difficulties and severe gastroesophageal reflux necessitating nutritional support, antireflux medications and in extreme cases antireflux surgery.

Well coordinated multidisciplinary care involving members of the primary, secondary and tertiary health care teams, and regular review in a pediatric sleep physiology laboratory, are central to the successful care of children with CCHS. The monitoring required is well described in the American Thoracic Society guidelines.[145]

Unlike other children on home ventilation, children with CCHS do not show ventilatory responses to hypoxemia or hypercarbia, and may hypoventilate more severely when unwell, with increased right-to-left intrapulmonary shunting. They may show minimal or absent increase in ventilation with exercise, and with infection may develop relative hypothermia rather than fever.

Continuous monitoring of blood oxygen saturation is recommended whenever children with CCHS are on the ventilator, and when they are unwell periodic checks of oxygen saturation are required when awake, as well as assessments of CO_2 levels.

Due to their reduced perception of hypoxia and hypercarbia, and the absence of any appreciation of dyspnea, together with depressed ventilatory responses to exercise, children with CCHS may exert themselves beyond physiological limits and come to harm. Children with CCHS should be allowed to participate in noncontact sports with a moderate level of activity and frequent rest periods. Swimming may be hazardous for these children – the lack of hypoxic response may put them at risk. Underwater swimming is particularly hazardous, but with very careful supervision gentle swimming may be acceptable. Rhythmic activity with the opportunity to develop a learned increase in ventilation may be of value. Dance is particularly helpful in developing appropriate rhythmic increased ventilation with exercise.[135-138,145]

Children and adolescents with CCHS are at particular risk of severe and potentially fatal hypoventilation on ingestion of alcohol or use of cannabis. Affected children and their families must be informed and warned of these potential dangers.[137,162]

OBSTRUCTIVE SLEEP APNEA SYNDROME AND RELATED PROBLEMS

Upper airway resistance increases during sleep due to a reduction in the tonic activation of pharyngeal dilator muscles, especially during REM sleep when postural muscle activity is inhibited. When this is associated with situations that increase the upstream resistance in the airway, there is a tendency for airway collapse to occur, which results in a spectrum of clinical manifestations from simple snoring through upper airway resistance syndrome (UARS) to obstructive sleep apnea syndrome (OSAS). These in turn are associated with a range of adverse outcomes that are related, at least in part, to the disturbances of gas exchange and sleep structure that occur in response to upper airway obstruction with or without frank apnea.

Snoring is a cardinal symptom of upper airway obstruction during sleep and occurs in approximately 10% of children on a regular and frequent basis,[163] although only a small proportion of children who habitually snore will have obstructive sleep apnea.[164] In contrast to experience in adults, the single commonest association with OSAS in children is adenotonsillar hypertrophy with peak incidence in the preschool years when adenotonsillar size is maximal in relation to airway cross-sectional area. Other groups of children at increased risk from OSAS include those with craniofacial anomalies, e.g. Robin sequence, Treacher–Collins syndrome, Down syndrome, achondroplasia and mucopolysaccharoidosis. Increased awareness of the adverse consequences of occult OSAS in such children has led to calls for screening of high-risk groups, such as those with Down syndrome,[165] but this is still not universally practised. Another population of children at risk of OSAS and one that is likely to represent an increasing proportion of children with sleep disordered breathing is those who are obese.[166] Additionally there are interesting associations of sleep disturbance with control of appetite and weight gain,[167] such that OSAS may also be a risk factor for obesity. There have been case reports of an association between the initiation of growth hormone treatment in children with Prader Willi syndrome (see Ch. 15, p. 503) and a risk of apnea and sudden death,[168,169] but systematic polygraphic evaluation of children with Prader Willi syndrome has indicated that sleep-related problems are common and are probably unrelated to growth hormone treatment.[170] However, consideration should be given to regular assessment of this group of patients.

Although OSAS in children is clearly associated with conditions that increase upper airway resistance, this is an oversimplification of the problem and by no means all children with adenotonsillar hypertrophy will develop clinically significant OSAS. This reflects the balance between forces tending to exacerbate airway collapse during inspiration and the distending forces of pharyngeal dilators. Although there appears to be a positive association between pharyngeal size and severity of sleep disordered breathing,[171] variations in airway neuromotor control during wakefulness have been correlated with the presence of sleep disordered breathing in children,[172] familial aggregation of OSAS has been described[173] and a proportion of children with OSAS in association with adenotonsillar hypertrophy fail to improve after adenotonsillectomy.[174]

Presentation of OSAS in children may be with habitual snoring, with or without a parental description of apneic events, restless sleep or sleeping in an unusual posture, nocturnal enuresis, daytime somnolence, although this is less commonly described in children than in adults with

OSAS, and problems with daytime learning and behavior. A link between sleep disordered breathing and attention deficit hyperactivity disorder (ADHD)[175] and autism[176] has been proposed but the causal relationship remains to be established and there are clearly complex reasons for sleep disturbance in these spectra of disorders. Clinical examination during wakefulness in an otherwise healthy child with OSAS due to adenotonsillar hypertrophy may be unremarkable. However, attention should be paid to ENT examination, careful evaluation of growth and assessment of cardiovascular status, including systemic blood pressure and signs of pulmonary hypertension.

The earliest descriptions of OSAS in children reported strong associations with growth failure and cor pulmonale,[177,178] but these are now uncommon outcomes in the majority of otherwise healthy children who present with OSAS in association with adenotonsillar hypertrophy. Recent attention has focused on the neurocognitive, developmental and behavioral consequences of OSAS and the gathering speculation that adverse consequences in these modalities may not be limited to children with frank OSAS but may occur in association with milder states, including UARS and primary snoring.[167] Several studies have reported decrements in IQ and other measures of cognitive performance, including memory and attentiveness in children with OSAS compared with otherwise healthy children.[179] School performance has been shown to be poorer in children with OSAS and the converse, children with low school performance are more likely to have OSAS, has also been reported. Additionally, treatment of OSAS in this group of children has been demonstrated to improve academic performance.[180] However, although the effects of gas exchange abnormalities and sleep fragmentation that occur in association with OSAS may be largely reversible, there is evidence that longer lasting deficits in neurocognitive performance may also occur.[181] The potential for long term neurological sequelae of sleep disordered breathing has been exemplified by the description of neuronal injury on MRI brain scans in association with OSAS in children.[182]

As well as effects on cognition, OSAS in children has also been implicated in behavioral disturbance, but although sleep disordered breathing has been reported to be associated with daytime hyperactivity disorders[183] and parent-reported sleep disturbance is very common in children with ADHD, a relatively small proportion of children with stringent diagnostic criteria of ADHD have polysomnographic evidence of sleep disordered breathing.[184]

BREATHING DURING SLEEP IN NEUROMUSCULAR AND RESTRICTIVE DISEASES

Conditions associated with restrictive impairment of ventilatory function are relatively uncommon in childhood but contribute substantially to the burden of sleep-related breathing disorders and the provision of long term domiciliary respiratory support (see p. 687 – Long term ventilation) to such children is increasing rapidly in many countries. Examples of disorders in which nocturnal hypoventilation may be a consequence are neuromuscular diseases, including Duchenne muscular dystrophy, spinomuscular atrophy types I and II, and some congenital myopathies, e.g. nemaline myopathy (see Ch. 22, p. 909), traumatic cervical spinal cord injury, severe kyphoscoliosis, which often coexists with severe neuromuscular weakness, and some restrictive lung diseases, including chronic lung disease of prematurity (see p. 727). In some of these conditions, respiratory failure is a progressive and relatively predictable sequel, such as in Duchenne muscular dystrophy, while in others it is a less consistent or predictable feature. The importance of breathing during sleep in these conditions is that, due to the physiological changes in respiration that occur in sleep, dysfunctional breathing usually predates the occurrence of symptomatic hypoventilation during wakefulness.[185] Symptoms might include apneas, restless or disturbed sleep, feeling unrefreshed after sleep, and problems with concentration, fatigue and sleepiness during the day. Morning headaches may be reported as a consequence of CO_2 retention and a loss of appetite for breakfast is a relatively frequent symptom in children who develop nocturnal hypoventilation. Frequent respiratory infections in these patients are also common, due to a combination of depressed cough and pulmonary atelectasis associated with chest wall weakness or deformity leading to an inability to preserve functional residual capacity.[186] Bulbar dysfunction and gastroesophageal reflux leading to aspiration may exacerbate these problems. It should be borne in mind that many children who are at risk of nocturnal hypoventilation are likely to have comorbidities and the symptoms associated with these may be difficult to distinguish from those associated with sleep-related breathing disturbance.

INVESTIGATION AND TREATMENT OF SLEEP DISORDERED BREATHING

The frequency and importance of sleep-related breathing disturbances in children for health, neurocognitive development and behavior should prompt a sleep history in all children, but particularly those in the high-risk groups identified above. This should include questions about sleep onset, quantity and quality (restlessness, arousals, awakenings), how the child appears on waking, and daytime symptoms, including excessive daytime sleepiness or somnolence and problems with concentration, learning and behavior. As mentioned above, although excessive daytime somnolence is a characteristic feature of OSAS in adults, it is less commonly described in children.[187] Symptoms of snoring and other respiratory sounds, descriptions by parents of unusual sleeping postures and careful description of any apneic events should be documented. A history of nocturnal enuresis can be associated with sleep fragmentation due to sleep disordered breathing, and morning headaches and loss of appetite may be symptomatic of nocturnal hypoventilation. Sleep questionnaires have been devised as screening tools for sleep disordered breathing in children,[188] particularly in association with OSAS,[189] but the utility of these is limited by the inconsistent relationship between reported symptoms and objective measurements.[190–193]

The recommended investigation for the detection of obstructive sleep apnea is the sleep polysomnogram (PSG). Criteria for diagnosis of sleep disordered breathing based on polysomnography have been published,[194,195] and it is important to note that these vary considerably from their adult equivalents due to the different spectrum of disorders associated with the condition in childhood. As the name implies, a PSG comprises a variable (but large) number of channels of physiological recordings made continuously during sleep. Typically these will include a measure of breathing movement of the chest and abdomen, often using inductance plethysmography, electrocardiogram, body position and limb motion sensors, pulse oximetry with or without capnography measured either transcutaneously or by end-tidal sampling,[196] an indication of nasal and oral gas flow, and neurophysiological measurements, which include a minimum of two channels of EEG, electro-oculogram (EOG) and electromyogram (EMG), usually measured submentally. These last variables are primarily used for sleep staging and, as obstructive events are more abundant in REM sleep, some authorities argue that a diagnosis of OSAS cannot be excluded without demonstration that the child has spent time in REM. This is one argument against so-called nap studies,[197] as REM is more abundant towards the end of a usual night's sleep. Although PSG can be performed unattended and in the patient's home, the majority are carried out in hospitals or designated sleep laboratories to ensure adequate quality of data recording. However, this has the detriment of putting the child in an unfamiliar sleeping environment, which is likely to alter sleep quality and therefore may in some cases lead to problems with interpretation of data.[198,199] Polysomnography is a resource-intensive investigation that requires specialized equipment and substantial staff time. Therefore, there have been numerous investigations of more limited diagnostic techniques that are suitable for home or unattended use and which may at least serve as screening investigations. These include pulse oximetry,[200] abbreviated polysomnography[201] and video/audio[202,203] recordings. In general, these options are relatively specific and, in the context of a suggestive clinical history of OSAS, an abnormal oximetry or abbreviated PSG study can form the basis for management decisions. In practice, many clinicians will base a decision to proceed to adenotonsillectomy on clinical history alone in otherwise uncomplicated cases.[204] When there is doubt and a screening study is negative, or in the context of more complicated situations, e.g. when parasomnias or seizures are suspected or when there is excessive daytime sleepiness and sleep fragmentation needs to be assessed, consideration should be given to referral for PSG. In control of breathing disorders, such as CCHS, it is important to measure ventilation during different behavioral states, in which case PSG is again the appropriate investigation. The limited availability of facilities for PSG in some countries has led to the use of more limited studies, such as oximetry and capnography, for the assessment of nocturnal hypoventilation in children with neuromuscular and chest wall disorders, but these have not been subjected to formal validation against the gold standard PSG and will inevitably lead to loss of information.

A variety of surgical approaches to the management of OSAS has been devised, mainly in adult practice, although many have not been subjected to formal RCTs and there is a paucity of evidence for surgical management of OSAS in adults.[205] The majority of otherwise healthy children with OSAS have adenotonsillar hypertrophy and adenotonsillectomy is an effective treatment with a reported success rate in normalizing PSG abnormalities of 83%[206] and substantial improvements in quality of life scores post surgery in both mild and severe disease.[207] Intranasal corticosteroids have been reported to improve symptoms of OSAS in children and are likely to be of benefit when the syndrome is exacerbated by seasonal rhinitis.[208] Other surgical procedures include mandibular distraction, which has a place in the management of even very young children with craniofacial abnormalities in association with OSAS.[209,210] For children who have persistent OSAS after adenotonsillectomy and other patient groups in which OSAS is not accompanied by adenotonsillar hypertrophy, such as morbidly obese children, continuous or bilevel positive airway pressure has been shown to be highly efficacious in reducing the number of apneas or hypopneas but adherence may be suboptimal even in children.[211,212] The management of sleep disordered breathing in children with neuromuscular disease and nocturnal hypoventilation includes long term positive pressure ventilation, which is considered below.

LONG TERM VENTILATION OF CHILDREN

Home mechanical ventilation (HMV) is a treatment option that is becoming increasingly available and one that is being chosen by families with increasing frequency as an alternative to prolonged hospitalization and institutional care. The goals of HMV in children include extending duration of life and enhancing its quality. Additionally, the use of HMV should reduce morbidity, improve the child's physiological function, help to achieve normal growth and development whenever possible, and also reduce overall health care costs.[213] The ethical and moral issues surrounding long term mechanical ventilation are complex. A useful starting point is to have a methodological framework to help analyze specific situations in order to arrive at a morally justifiable endpoint. Such a framework, based upon principles of respect for autonomy (the obligation to respect the decision making capacities of autonomous persons), nonmaleficence (the obligation to avoid causing harm), beneficence (obligations to provide benefits and to balance benefits against risks) and justice (obligations of fairness in the distribution of benefits and risks), has been reviewed.[214] In this context, for many clinicians, the most challenging patients are those with severe neuromuscular weakness such as spinal muscular atrophy and Duchenne muscular dystrophy. In the end, the decision to ventilate or provide positive pressure support for a child at home will depend upon locally available resources, access to appropriate technology and the attitudes of physicians, caregivers, patients and other health staff.

Children requiring home ventilation or positive pressure support are managed best by a multidisciplinary team and an appropriate care plan must be developed with the patient and caregivers before discharge from hospital. The plan should consider availability of working utilities, i.e. power and telephone services, and ease of access to emergency and respite care and technological support.

The prevalence of HMV in Europe in 2001 has been estimated at 6.6 users per 100 000 population,[215] although there are no recent prevalence data for children. However, a number of reports from centers that care

for children ventilated at home indicate the type of patients who are now being managed in this way.[216–221] There are four main diagnostic groups:
- disorders of the respiratory pump (including neuromuscular diseases, diseases of the chest wall and spinal cord injury);
- obstructive diseases of the airways (including those associated with craniofacial anomalies);
- parenchymal lung diseases (particularly cystic fibrosis and bronchopulmonary dysplasia);
- disorders of the control of respiration (notably CCHS).

Neuromuscular diseases are the largest single group, accounting for between 28% and 51% of cases.

Generally, children are commenced on home ventilation by one of two pathways. First, mechanical ventilation may be started as a result of an acute illness and the child is unable to be successfully weaned from ventilation. Alternatively a decision may be made, in a child with chronic respiratory failure, to electively commence ventilation. Patients ventilated via tracheostomy are usually stabilized in the intensive care unit either during an acute episode of respiratory failure or following an elective tracheostomy. In either case, the ventilatory requirements can be relatively easily assessed because of the stable patient interface and the use of versatile ventilators with a range of modes that further facilitate stabilization. However, for patients requiring non-invasive ventilation (NIV) by nasal or oro-nasal mask the situation is more complex. For example, the patient interface is less stable and prone to leaks and the flow generators commonly used for inspiratory and expiratory support ventilation are relatively unsophisticated. A wide variety of machines that support ventilation are available. The type of machine and settings should be tailored to the patient's characteristics, goals of ventilation and the experience of the center managing the child. Flow generators used for non-invasive positive pressure (NIPP) support might not be suitable for home ventilation in some children because of the low maximum back-up ventilation rates, rudimentary trigger algorithms, high flows and inability to accurately set or determine FiO_2.

For patients requiring long-term NIV the establishment of ventilation is best done in hospital with careful attention paid to mask fitting and titration of ventilatory variables. Initially a crude titration can be performed at the bedside but a formal titration PSG should be performed at discharge or, alternatively, soon after discharge for stable patients with straightforward ventilation requirements. Recent evidence supports regular 6–12 monthly titration PSGs for most patients requiring long term NIV, and more frequent assessment in patients with evolving conditions, complex respiratory diseases or difficult interface issues. Prior to titration care should have been taken to fit an appropriate and comfortable mask and then a time is chosen for titration when the child is likely to be asleep. The aims of titration are to establish optimal ventilation and sleep (Fig. 20.20).

Other important considerations before discharge are the need for humidification, airway clearance and alarms that indicate power failure and circuit disconnection. The provision of further home monitoring, such as pulse oximetry and capnography, should be considered on a case-by-case basis. While pulse oximetry, particularly in a child with a supplemental oxygen requirement, may be useful for assessment purposes, it is seldom indicated continuously.

Children ventilated at home via tracheostomy have prolonged survival.[117,222–224] Despite some deaths directly related to the intervention,[225] mortality is generally determined by the underlying disease.[226] Although data for children ventilated non-invasively are few, the same effect on survival is likely since NIV improves respiratory function and delays the onset of daytime respiratory failure.[227,228] Furthermore, after commencing home ventilation, children with neuromuscular diseases have reduced hospitalizations, reduced days spent in intensive care units[229] and improved quality of life.[230] However, global quality of life is difficult to assess, particularly in adolescent patients and families of patients ventilated at home. This is due to complex, dynamically changing interactions between developmental, social and disease factors.[231–234] Improvements in technology, in particular that required for successful

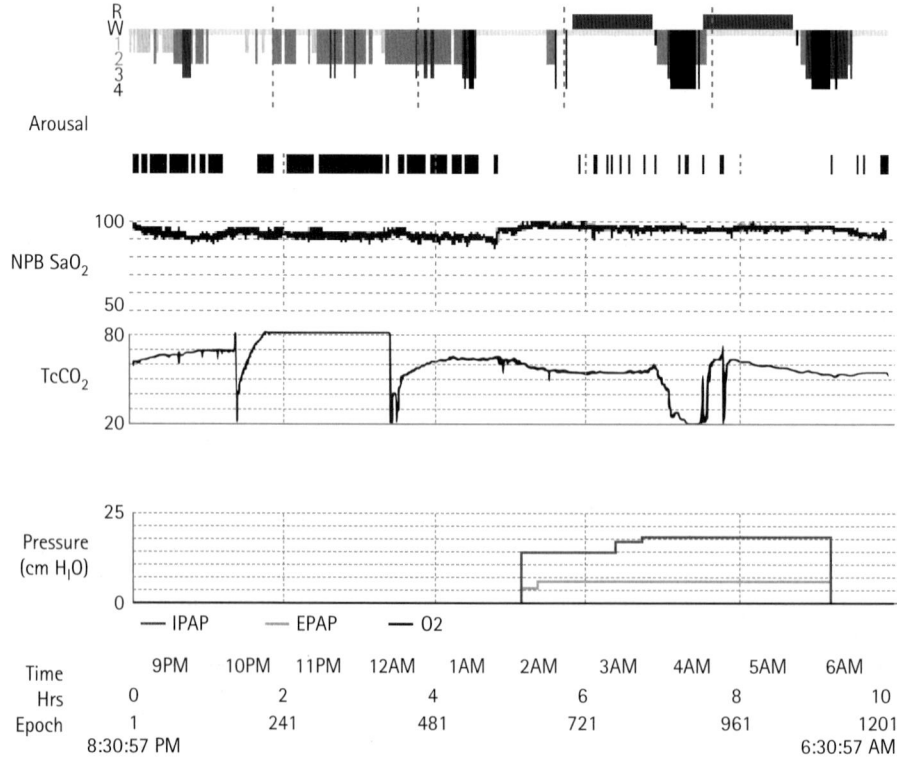

Fig. 20.20 A split night sleep study performed in a 16-year-old boy with Duchenne muscular dystrophy. In the first part of the night he is breathing spontaneously in room air; non-invasive ventilation (NIV) via nasal mask is commenced just before 2 a.m. In the first part of the night there is severe sleep fragmentation, oxygen desaturation and hypercarbia. Once NIV is commenced, oxygenation, ventilation and sleep quality improve. There is an increased percentage of time spent in REM sleep once adequate ventilation is restored – 'REM rebound'.

non-invasive ventilation, will inevitably result in more families and children seeking home ventilation as a management option. The extent to which this is viable will depend upon the availability of resources locally and within individual families.

ASTHMA

Asthma is the most common chronic disease of childhood, with up to 20% of children being affected. The variability in disease prevalence between countries most likely reflects the major role played by the gene–environment interaction in disease expression. Although asthma can be well controlled by highly effective anti-inflammatory therapy [mainly inhaled corticosteroids (ICSs)] in the large majority of children, optimal asthma control is not achieved in about 50% of all asthmatic children in daily practice. Asthma is still a leading cause of emergency department visits, hospital admission, absence from school, limitations in activity and sleep, and hence imposes a huge burden on the individual, the caregiver and the society.

Definition

There is no universally accepted clinical definition of asthma.[235] The definition can be physiological, pathophysiological or symptom based and can therefore be purely subjective or include some objective measurement. Several descriptive definitions have been devised and used in a variety of studies. Epidemiological studies tend to focus on recurrent *wheeze* as the most prominent symptom or on *variation of airway caliber* as the major physiological expression of the disorder. On the other hand, guidelines such as the Global Initiative for Asthma (GINA) define asthma in pathophysiological terms as a *chronic inflammatory disorder* of the airways which causes the airways to be *hyperresponsive* to stimuli which, in turn, causes variable airway obstruction (www.ginasthma.com). These differences in definitions and hence in outcome measures may explain the controversy around studies on asthma in general and on asthma epidemiology in particular.

It is agreed that asthma is not a homogeneous disease, but a heterogeneous group of wheezing syndromes.[236] This agreement is mainly based on observations from clinical and epidemiological studies,[237] and is increasingly supported by physiological and pathophysiological data. The group of wheezing or asthma syndromes can be distinguished by risk factors, pathophysiology, treatment response and natural history. Therefore, for educational purposes, it is pertinent to distinguish different phenotypes within the asthma syndromes. It should be emphasized, however, that mixed or overlap syndromes are more common than pure phenotypes,[238] and that patients may change from one phenotype to another over time.

Wheezing syndromes in childhood are usually divided into those observed in children under 6 years of age and those in children aged 6 years and older (Table 20.7). Multi-triggered wheezing syndromes (asthma) have been subdivided into separate descriptive phenotypes according to their most prominent trigger, such as exercise-induced asthma. However, because most children with exercise-induced asthma

Table 20.7 Descriptive definitions of clinical wheezing syndromes

Preschool children (< 6 years)
- *Episodic viral wheeze:* episodes of wheezing associated with upper respiratory tract infections (URTIs), interspersed with completely symptom-free intervals
- *Persistent or multi-trigger wheeze:* as above, but with occasional or frequent wheezing between acute episodes associated with URTIs
- *Allergic asthma:* multi-trigger wheeze *plus* evidence of sensitization to one or more inhalant or food allergens (see p. 691)

School-aged children and adolescents (6–18 years)
- *Allergic asthma:* multi-trigger wheeze *plus* evidence of sensitization to one or more inhalant or food allergens (see p. 690)
- *Non-allergic asthma:* multi-trigger wheeze without evidence of sensitization to one or more inhalant or food allergens
- *Episodic viral wheeze:* episodes of (mostly mild) wheezing associated with URTIs, with symptom-free intervals

(and other such descriptive labels) also have wheeze or airway obstruction brought about by other stimuli, a judgement has to be made as to the major disease feature in such cases.

Table 20.7 contains the descriptive definitions of wheezing syndromes used in this section.

CAUSATIVE FACTORS

All phenotypes of asthma are multifactorial disorders which are the result of a complex interplay between genetic and environmental factors. These factors are thought to lead to inflammatory and structural changes which cause asthma symptoms. The variability in etiology and pathophysiology explains why overlap syndromes are more common than the pure phenotypes.

Genetic factors

Asthma runs in families. The risk of asthma in children increases if either parent has asthma or atopy. Most studies suggest that maternal asthma confers greater risk than paternal asthma.[239] However, paternal asthma appears to be the most important risk factor in some populations.[240] In addition, the parental type of obstructive airways disease is an important determinant of disease expression in children. Offspring from parents with a history of preschool wheeze have fewer symptoms than those from parents with asthma.[241] No single gene accounts for the familial segregation of asthma. The model that best explains data from family studies is one of oligogenic loci, i.e. a handful of genes are responsible for the large majority of genetic control, all of which are under strong environmental influences.

Genome screens and linkage studies have identified numerous genes involved in different aspects of asthma syndromes in children, including atopic sensitization, serum IgE levels, airway hyperresponsiveness (AHR), level of lung function, and different cytokines and their receptors. There is strong evidence that genes identified as being important in one population may not be as important in other populations. For example, a disintegrin and metalloproteinase 33 gene (ADAM33) was strongly related to the diagnosis of asthma and to bronchial hyperresponsiveness in a British/US population of families.[242] Studies on the functional properties of this gene brought about the speculation that ADAM33 not only determined the responsiveness of airway smooth muscle cells but also the tissue response to injury, thus linking the gene to inflammation.[243] However, in a more recent and larger American study, no association between asthma and ADAM33 was found.[244]

Although the field of asthma genetics is expanding rapidly, the clinical applicability of this research is limited. So far, only the increased risk of asthma in children of asthmatic parents is used for counseling, mainly to recommend preventive measures to be taken in early life (see p. 694 – Nonpharmacological management).

Recent studies have shown that the response to certain medications is genetically determined and this may have therapeutic implications in the future. For example, the response to bronchodilators is influenced by polymorphisms in the beta-2 adrenergic receptor.[245]

Environmental factors
The 'asthma epidemic'

Environmental factors are of major importance in the development of asthma. This concept was already apparent from the complex inheritance patterns of asthma in families. The investigation of environmental risk factors became more important when it was recognized that the steep increase in the prevalence of asthma in children in the last 20 years of the 20th century could not be explained by genetic factors.[246] As with all studies on asthma in general and genetic studies in particular, this research endeavor was hampered by the lack of uniformly accepted definitions of wheezing syndromes, and hence the likelihood of different phenotypes, each with different interactions with differing environmental factors in different populations. In addition, enormous pressure has been put on the scientific community by government agencies and public opinion to identify and eliminate causative factors to turn around the 'asthma epidemic'. This has likely induced publication bias (with positive associations more likely to be published than negative ones), over-interpretation of study findings (risk factors viewed as causes of asthma instead of epidemiological associations with multiple possible explanations) and exaggerated expectations of asthma prevention programs. Despite these shortcomings, research on asthma risk factors has considerably increased the knowledge on the origins of asthma. It is quite clear, however, that no single most important factor which is responsible for the rise in asthma prevalence has so far been identified. As a result, primary prevention of asthma is not an easy task. The only really evidence-based advice that can be given to parents of children at high risk of asthma (because of parental asthma) is to avoid exposure to cigarette smoke as much as possible. Exclusive breast-feeding also confers a certain degree of protection,[247] but it will never be possible to examine breast-feeding in an RCT in order to achieve level 1 evidence. There also seems to be consistent evidence that hypoallergenic formula for the first 4 months of life (when breast-feeding is not possible or when weaning from breast-feeding) reduces the risk of asthma in children,[248] but methodological problems in these studies limit their applicability in routine practice.[249]

Since the turn of the century, the increase in asthma prevalence has been leveling off or declining in many countries,[250] without any clues as to what environmental changes could explain these trends.

International comparisons

The International Study of Asthma and Allergies in Children (ISAAC) was designed to study prevalence of asthma and other allergic diseases throughout the world with identical epidemiological methods. Large differences in asthma prevalence rates were found between countries, with the highest prevalence rates in resource rich countries, in particular the UK, Australia and New Zealand.[251] Thus, aspects of Western lifestyle were investigated as possible risk factors. Whilst air pollution was more severe in East Germany before the fall of the iron curtain, prevalence of asthma was much higher in West Germany, suggesting that air pollution was not an important risk factor for the development of asthma.[252] After the two countries were united and the East adopted a more Western lifestyle, the prevalence of asthma and allergic rhinitis rose rapidly to 'Western' levels in the East.[253]

The hygiene hypothesis

By far the most influential theory on the cause of the 'asthma epidemic' has been the hygiene hypothesis. Coined in the late 1980s after finding that asthma and allergy prevalence were inversely related to family size, it states that a lack of immunological stimuli (infections) in early life deviates the immune system into the allergic state. This hypothesis is supported by numerous observations, including lower asthma prevalence rates in children raised on farms, differences in fecal microflora between atopic and non-atopic children, and lower risk of asthma in children attending kindergarten.[254] The hypothesis has, however, been criticized for a number of reasons:

- The most dramatic improvement in hygiene in the 20th century (clean drinking water) occurred at least half a century before the increase in asthma began.[255]
- There is no association between the rise in asthma prevalence and two major infection reduction measures: childhood immunizations and the use of antibiotics.[255,256]
- It has been shown that the 'asthma epidemic' has at least partly been a self-perpetuating process, with increased awareness of asthma leading to increased willingness to make the diagnosis in wheezy children.[250]

The current version of the hygiene hypothesis is that early-life immunological stimuli (including infections and exposure to gut flora) are important in priming and activating antigen-presenting cells and regulatory T lymphocytes. Proper stimulation of these cells is thought to result in a normal balance of immune responses; disturbances of this process by insufficient or improper immunological stimuli could then cause immune deviation to allergy (and allergic asthma),[257] but also to episodic viral wheeze[258] and to autoimmune diseases such as diabetes and rheumatoid arthritis. The factors that determine which unfavorable turn the immune system is going to take as a result of insufficient stimulation are as yet unknown.

Risk factors

With the limitations of observational studies and the variability of study results in mind, Table 20.8 summarizes the most extensively studied risk factors for asthma in children.

The most consistent and best modifiable risk factor for all asthmatic phenotypes in children is exposure to cigarette smoke, both in utero and after birth. It is disturbing to observe that so many parents continue to smoke despite the overwhelming evidence of its deleterious effects on their children's health. Although allergic sensitization is a strong risk factor for childhood asthma and allergen exposure is thought to be a prerequisite for sensitization, studies have found no direct relationship between allergen exposure and the development of asthma.[259] Accordingly, although able to delay symptoms of eczema, allergen avoidance studies have been disappointing in preventing asthma.[260]

PATHOPHYSIOLOGY

As stated above, the GINA guidelines define asthma in pathophysiological terms as a chronic, eosinophilic inflammatory disorder of the airways which causes the airways to be hyperresponsive to stimuli, which, in turn, causes variable reversible airway obstruction and symptoms of wheeze, dyspnea and cough.

Airway inflammation
Asthma in school-aged children and adolescents

Most of the knowledge of inflammation as the key pathophysiological mechanism in asthma comes from studies in young, otherwise healthy, adults with allergic asthma. The limited evidence on inflammation in general and on eosinophilic inflammation in particular in childhood asthma can be summarized as follows:

- Eosinophilic infiltration is not a consistent finding in mucosal biopsies of children with asthma;[261] neutrophilic infiltration and activation are commonly found.[262]
- The only consistent finding in the few children undergoing biopsy studies has been thickening of the reticular basement membrane (RBM) (Fig. 20.21).[263]
- Studies are hampered by the small sample sizes and highly selected nature of cohorts (patients with troublesome disease or other abnormalities where bronchoscopy is clinically indicated).
- Although there are differences in inflammatory cell profiles in bronchoalveolar lavage fluid between children with allergic asthma, Non-atopic asthma (NAA) and episodic viral wheeze, a great deal of overlap exists between these groups.[264]

Table 20.8 Risk factors for childhood asthma

Risk factor	Preschool wheeze	Asthma in children 6 years of age or older
Parental smoking (both prenatally and after birth)	+++	++
Sensitization to allergens	+	++
Exposure to allergens	–	–
Breastfeeding	+ (protective)	+ (protective)
RSV infection	+	–
Family history	+	++
Obesity	+	+
Prematurity	+	–

+ indicates a positive association; ++ and +++ strong positive associations;
– indicates absence of association

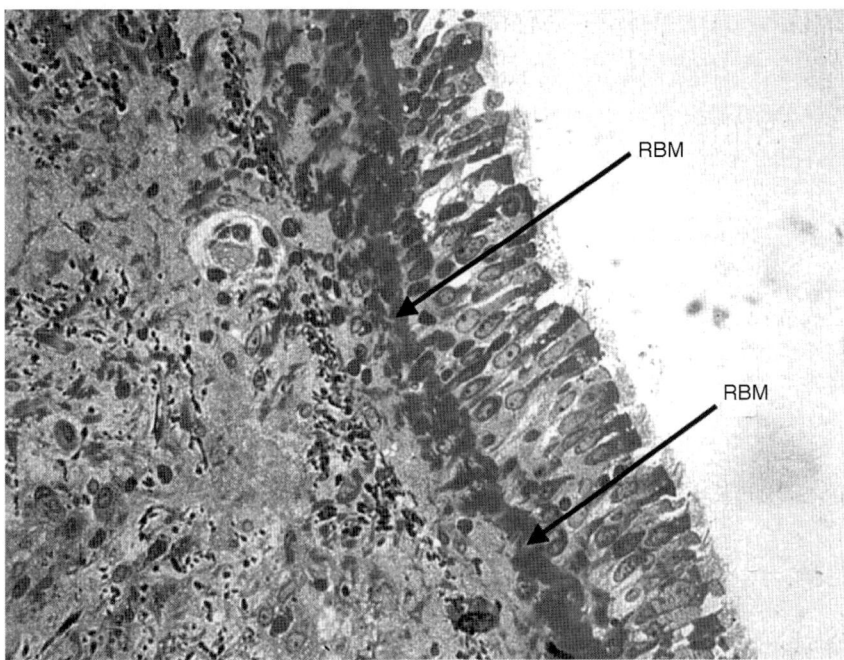

Fig. 20.21   Bronchial biopsy specimen of a child with asthma showing reticular basement membrane (RBM) thickening. (From Payne et al[263] with permission)

Thus, asthma in school-aged children and adolescents, as in adults, is characterized by airway inflammation and structural changes, in particular RBM thickening. However, the nature of the inflammation differs from that in adults and appears to be of a mixed eosinophilic–neutrophilic origin.

Wheeze in preschool children

Very few studies have examined airway inflammation in preschool wheezy children. Markers of eosinophil activation correlate with wheeze, irrespective of atopy.[265,266] In preschool children with recurrent wheeze, increased levels of eosinophilic cationic protein (ECP) in plasma indicate a higher risk of persistent wheeze.[267] These indirect observations suggest that eosinophils are involved in the pathophysiology of persistent preschool wheeze. The very few bronchial biopsy studies of early childhood wheeze, however, show different findings, with neutrophil dominated inflammation in toddlers,[268] and lack of inflammation and RBM thickening in infants with recurrent wheeze and documented reversible airway obstruction.[269]

Increasingly, the immune response to viral infection is being considered as an important determinant of recurrent wheeze, AHR and asthma.[270] It has been proposed that early childhood recurrent wheeze is an immunodeficiency disorder, with delayed maturation of Th1 function putting the infant at risk for both sensitization to aeroallergens and severe viral airway infections causing inflammation and lung injury.[271,272] This is supported by observations showing that increased levels of tumor necrosis factor (TNF)-alpha and interleukin (IL)-10 are associated with recurrent wheeze after RSV infection,[273,274] and that severe rhinovirus infections in early life predict recurrent wheezing at the age of 3 years.[275]

Airway hyperresponsiveness

AHR, exaggerated airway response to exogenous stimuli, is considered to be one of the hallmarks of asthma. It is thought that this is caused by chronic airway inflammation (see above). The exaggerated response of the airways to stimuli consists of swelling of airway mucosa, mucus hypersecretion and contraction of bronchial smooth muscle, thus causing airway obstruction and symptoms of wheeze, cough and dyspnea.

It has been suggested that the combination of wheeze and AHR best identifies asthma in population studies;[276] however, AHR can be detected in completely asymptomatic individuals, and no test of AHR will perfectly discriminate children with and without asthma.

AHR can be measured directly (with agents that interact with airway smooth muscle, such as histamine or methacholine) or indirectly (with agents that induce airway inflammation, such as hypertonic saline or adenosine). Perhaps the most convenient way to assess AHR in children is the exercise test. Exercise tests can be performed either by free running for 6 min,[277] or by running on a treadmill at submaximal heart rate for 5 min.[278] A 15% fall in PEF or a 10% fall in FEV_1 indicates a positive test.

Reversible airway obstruction

The key physiological phenomenon of childhood asthma is airway obstruction, which is reversible, both spontaneously and as a result of treatment. This can be reproducibly measured by spirometry in school-aged children (see p. 692; Fig. 20.22) but is much more difficult to assess in preschool children. The degree of airway obstruction is highly variable: a child with asthma may display perfectly normal lung function at one time and have severe airway obstruction only hours later. Thus, an isolated measurement of airway obstruction is of limited diagnostic value in asthma. On the other hand, normal lung function and absence of response to bronchodilator when a child is symptomatic reasonably excludes asthma. A recent study showed that an improvement of 9% in FEV_1 (as a percentage of the predicted value) after bronchodilator was 50% sensitive and 86% specific for previous wheeze, and increased the odds of subsequent wheeze by a factor of 3.6.[279]

Reduced baseline expiratory flows are assumed to reflect relatively small airway size which is thought to be a key pathophysiological feature of early childhood wheeze.[280] Children with episodic viral wheeze are thought to have smaller airways to nonwheezy children, which are further narrowed when viral infections cause airway mucosal swelling.

DIAGNOSTIC APPROACH TO ASTHMA IN CHILDREN

According to the definition of asthma, the diagnosis can be based on physiological or pathophysiological measures or it can be based on the clinical judgement of the physician (doctor diagnosed asthma). The

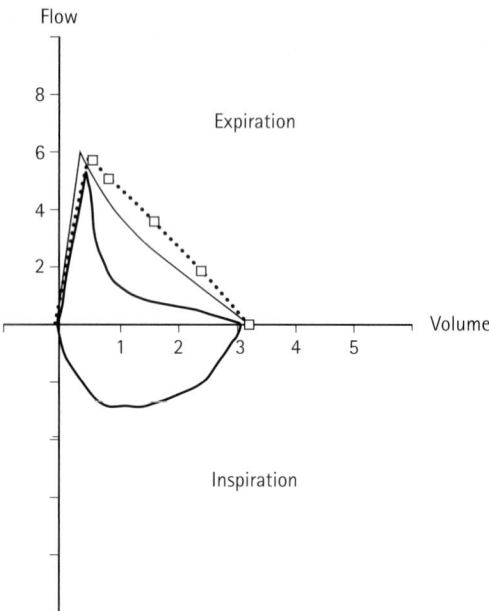

Fig. 20.22 Flow–volume curve of a child with asthma, showing the characteristic concave expiratory pattern with markedly reduced mid-expiratory flow rates (thick line) and the almost complete reversibility to normal values after bronchodilator (thin line). The reference values for peak expiratory flow (PEF), mid-expiratory flows at 25%, 50%, and 75% (MEF$_{25–75}$) of forced vital capacity (FVC), and the FVC itself are represented by squares, and are connected by a dotted line representing a hypothetical 'normal' expiratory flow–volume curve. The FEV$_1$ can not be read directly from a flow–volume curve because there is no time axis, but the spirometer software will provide it. Note that despite considerable airways obstruction, PEF is normal.

latter is primarily based on asthma history (reported symptoms) and to a lesser extent on physical examination, although according to the GINA guideline (www.ginasthma.com) documented wheeze, preferably on chest auscultation, is a requirement for secure diagnosis. Physiological measurements include the assessment of baseline airway function (lung function: spirometry), the reversibility of reduced airflow and the degree of AHR to nonspecific challenges such as histamine, methacholine, cold air or exercise. Pathophysiological measurements include invasive and non-invasive assessments of airway inflammation.

Asthma history

Children with asthma almost invariably present with recurrent wheeze, dyspnea and cough. A detailed history is the most important diagnostic tool for asthma in children. It helps in differential diagnosis, in classification of the type of asthma (see Table 20.7) and in the assessment of asthma severity. Although taking a good asthma history is time consuming, it is justified because in most cases the diagnosis of asthma can be reliably made or rejected by history alone.

The asthma history focuses on the nature of symptoms, their pattern, triggering factors, influence on daily activitites, and response to treatment, environment and family history (Table 20.9).

Nature of symptoms

Wheeze. Wheeze is the key symptom in asthma. However, patients and parents differ in their description and understanding of wheeze.[281] There is no universally accepted way to circumvent this problem in history taking. Expiratory wheeze should be differentiated from inspiratory noises (see p. 698 – Stridor). Wheeze is caused by turbulent airflow in obstructed intrathoracic airways. Lower airway obstruction can have several causes; hence all that wheezes is not asthma. However, asthma is by far the most common cause of recurrent wheeze in childhood.

Table 20.9   Items to evaluate in asthma history

Nature of symptoms
    Wheeze
    Cough
    Shortness of breath (dyspnea)
Pattern of symptoms
    Episodes (how often, how long)
    Only with upper respiratory tract infections (URTIs)?
    Symptoms between episodes?
    If interval symptoms, evaluate triggering factors
Triggering factors
    Specific (allergic): dust, pets, animals, pollen, plants and flowers
    Nonspecific: fog, damp weather, cigarette smoke, changes in
        temperature, 'smells' (perfumes, vapors), stress (emotion)
    Exercise
    URTIs
Influence on daily activities
    Absence from school, parental absence from work
    Limitations in sports and play
    Nocturnal awakening
Response to treatment
    Improvement of symptoms when taking reliever?
    Improvement of (pattern of) symptoms when using controller for several
        weeks?
Environment
    Home: pets, cigarette smoke, house dust mite control measures
    Local environment: traffic, factories, pollution
Family history
    Asthma, allergic rhinitis or eczema in parents and siblings

Cough. Although most asthmatic children cough, most children with recurrent cough do not have asthma. The most common cause of recurrent cough is frequently recurring upper respiratory tract infections (URTIs), particularly in toddlers.[282] Parents of children with asthma do not report cough alone as a symptom.[281] Irrespective of its cause, cough tends to be more troublesome at night, consequently, in contrast to popular belief, isolated nocturnal cough is not an indicator for asthma. Children with isolated cough do not benefit from ICSs or from bronchodilators.[283,284]

Chronic wet (productive) cough is unusual in asthma, and should prompt further evaluation for other causes, including bronchiectasis, ciliary dyskinesia and cystic fibrosis.[285] Other history warning signs ('red flags') that should prompt further investigations for other causes are listed below (adapted from British guideline on the management of asthma[235]):

- diagnosis unclear or in doubt;
- symptoms present from birth;
- excessive vomiting or posseting;
- severe URTI;
- persistent wet cough;
- family history of unusual chest disease;
- failure to thrive;
- unexpected clinical findings such as stridor, dysphagia, unusual voice or cry.

Shortness of breath (dyspnea). Most children with asthma complain of dyspnea (shortness of breath) when they are wheezy. It is not uncommon, however, that children with obvious wheeze and considerable airway obstruction do not complain of dyspnea. Such poor perception of dyspnea is thought to be caused by adaptation to chronic airway obstruction. This can only be assessed by reviewing the sensation of dyspnea in the presence of wheeze or airway obstruction. Hence, a provocation test to assess AHR may be required to address this issue (see p. 691).

Exercise is a common trigger of symptoms in asthmatic children. However, most complaints of exercise-induced dyspnea are not caused by asthma,[277] but by physiological limitation, dysfunctional breathing (hyperventilation), vocal cord dysfunction or poor exercise condition.[278] These can sometimes already be distinguished from asthma by the absence of wheeze or the presence of other symptoms such as stridor.

Because shortness of breath is so unspecific for asthma, this symptom should always be assessed in more detail by asking further questions.

Pattern of symptoms

Evaluating the pattern of symptoms is not only important in distinguishing different wheezing phenotypes (see Table 20.7) but also as an assessment of the effects of treatment. Children with purely episodic wheeze will likely first present during an episode, and will be perfectly normal once the episode has ceased, irrespective of treatment given. Children with infrequent symptoms will be less easily motivated to take daily controller medication than children with daily complaints. It is important to distinguish purely episodic viral wheeze in a child with a negative family history of asthma and atopy, because this particular phenotype is unlikely to benefit from ICS therapy.[286]

Triggering factors

These are divided into specific (allergic) and non-specific stimuli. Although occasional high dose exposure to allergens such as pets and house dust mite can cause immediate symptoms, the most common pattern of exposure is a chronic one which is usually not recognized as a trigger factor by patients or parents. For example, a child living in a house with a cat will not easily recognize the cat as a trigger factor because he/she is exposed on a daily basis.

Influence on daily activities

This important feature of asthma can be best evaluated by using validated quality of life questionnaires.[287] If these are not available, the key questions in taking this part of the history are school absence, limitations in play and exercise, and nocturnal awakening with wheeze, dyspnea and cough.

Response to treatment

Although rapid resolution of symptoms after taking reliever medication is suggestive of asthma, the physician should consider what would have happened if no medication had been taken. For example, the physiological sense of shortness of breath after exercise is commonly perceived as 'dyspnea'. If a bronchodilator is taken, this sensation will subside, as it would have done with rest alone.

Environment

Home exposure to dust can be assessed by asking about carpeting, upholstered furniture and house dust mite control measures taken. Exposure to pets (including birds) and animals should be recorded. Smoking habits of parents, other caretakers and home visitors must also be assessed.

Family history

As stated above, asthma is caused by complex gene–environment interactions. Parental asthma and allergy, particularly maternal asthma, determines the risk of asthma in a child and its phenotypic expression. Therefore, in order to take appropriate prevention measures, it is important to know the family history in parents and siblings.

Physical examination

Physical examination in children with asthma is usually unremarkable. Uncommon findings such as chest hyperinflation and Harrison sulci (Fig. 20.23) indicate chronic airway narrowing.

If the history is insufficient reliably to make or exclude the diagnosis of asthma, a useful approach is to perform a physical examination when the patient is symptomatic. The absence of wheeze in the presence of symptoms reasonably excludes asthma. Conversely, the presence of wheeze on auscultation, preferably supported by a lung function measure of airway obstruction, strongly supports the diagnosis of asthma.

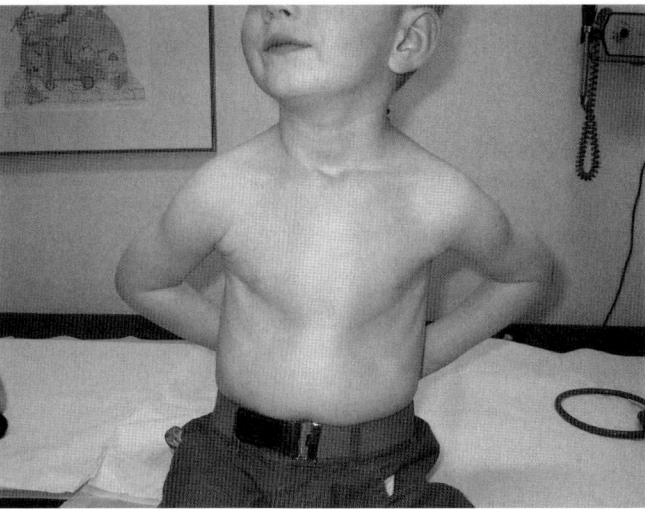

Fig. 20.23   Harrison's sulci in a child with chronic airway narrowing due to severe untreated asthma.

Investigations

Investigations are usually not needed to make the diagnosis of asthma. Chest films and routine laboratory studies are unhelpful in the diagnostic work-up of asthma. They may be helpful, however, in the differential diagnosis of asthma, either in initial work-up, or when patients respond poorly to treatment (see p. 693). The most common differential diagnoses of asthma are:[288]

- tracheo- or broncho-malacia (particularly in preschool wheeze);
- vocal cord dysfunction or dysfunctional breathing ('hyperventilation');
- recurrent lower respiratory infections (immunodeficiency, cystic fibrosis);
- vascular ring.

Lung function measurements

Lung function measurements can be useful to demonstrate airway obstruction, response to bronchodilator and AHR (see p. 691), but an isolated measure is of limited usefulness due to the variability of the disease.[289] Although an improvement in FEV_1 of 12% or more after bronchodilator is considered to be highly sensitive for asthma, the scientific basis for this assumption is weak. Most children with persistent symptoms referred for evaluation will nowadays already be using ICSs, and are likely to show normal lung function and absence of bronchodilator response.[290] Although most of these patients have reduced mid-expiratory flow rates, and although increased residual volume levels and air trapping have been demonstrated in children with stable asthma, the usefulness of these measurements in the diagnosis of asthma has never been properly tested.

Measurement of airway inflammation

Measurement of exhaled nitric oxide (eNO) is a non-invasive way to quantify airway inflammation. The test is easy to perform in children from the age of 4–5 years, is reproducible, and provides a reasonable separation of children with asthma from those without in population studies.[291] During treatment with ICS, however, eNO values tend to return to normal levels (< 10 ppb) rapidly, reducing the usefulness of the test in children using this treatment.

Tests for allergic sensitization

Although most preschool children with episodic viral wheeze and a considerable proportion of school-aged children with asthma are non-atopic, an assessment of sensitization to aeroallergens is useful, both for diagnostic and therapeutic purposes. Although many clinicians tend to avoid sensitization tests in preschool children because of the low pretest probability of atopy, this is probably not correct. UK studies have shown general population sensitization rates of 5% in 2 year olds and 20% at 4 years of age.[292]

Total serum IgE levels are of no use in the diagnosis of asthma. Specific IgE tests and skin prick tests are of comparable diagnostic usefulness in determining sensitization. The usual approach is to perform a screening test for the most common aeroallergens in the area. Because food allergy is an unusual trigger factor in asthma, testing for food allergy is not routinely recommended in the diagnostic work-up of asthma.

Based on the results of skin prick or specific IgE tests, asthmatic children are divided into allergic asthma (one or more test positive) or nonallergic asthma. Recent studies show that, in general populations, not only the presence but also the degree of sensitization determines the risk and severity of asthma in children.[293]

TREATMENT

Comprehensive guidelines for the management of childhood asthma are available in the UK and are updated regularly.[235] Although these guidelines are derived by principles of evidence-based medicine, much less high-quality evidence in many areas is available in children than in adults. Despite this shortcoming, the asthma management guidelines provide an excellent overview of the current treatment options in childhood asthma. The principles of asthma management are given in Table 20.10.

Nonpharmacological management

Once the diagnosis of asthma has been established, a number of nonpharmacological interventions should be considered. The most important of these is education. In addition, environmental control is important, in particular avoidance of active and passive tobacco smoke exposure. Although increasing evidence suggests that air pollution (in particular from motor vehicle exhaust fumes) may aggravate asthma, no studies aimed at reducing such exposure have been carried out to date.

Education of patients and parents

As with any chronic disease, careful and extensive patient and parent education is of key importance in determining the success of asthma management. There is strong and consistent evidence that education is effective in reducing asthma morbidity in children.[294] Education should be aimed at both patients and parents, and should comprise a discussion of disease mechanisms, causative and triggering factors, and explanation of the difference between controller and reliever medication. The treatment plan should be reviewed and a personalized written action plan be provided.[235] The exact content of this written action plan (what to do in what circumstances) seems to be less important than the fact

Table 20.10   Principles of asthma management

Education and self-management
• Explanation of disease mechanisms, triggering factors and pattern of symptoms
• Explanation of difference between preventer and controller medication
• Inhalation instruction
• Regular check-up and correction of inhalation technique
Nonpharmacological interventions
• Smoking cessation counseling
• Allergic asthma: reduction of allergen exposure (if possible and feasible)
• Consider immunotherapy
Determine asthma severity
Choose an age appropriate inhaler device
• Inhalation instruction
• Regular check-up and correction of inhalation technique
Prescribe reliever to each patient
Prescribe controller to each patient with persistent asthma

that the patient has such a plan, and much of the advice given in such written action plans is not evidence based, e.g. the largely ineffective advice to double the dose of ICS during a symptomatic episode.[295]

Correct inhalation technique is critically important in assuring that prescribed medication actually reaches the lower airways.

Smoking cessation

The association between passive smoking and respiratory health in children has been extensively reviewed. There is a direct and strong causal relationship between parental smoking and wheeze, asthma, lower lung function, exacerbations of asthma and school absence due to asthma.[296] Parents who smoke should not only be advised to stop smoking because of the dangers to themselves and their children, but also be offered appropriate support to stop smoking. In addition, children should be strongly encouraged and supported not to commence smoking, because this doubles the risk of developing asthma.

If smoking cessation is not feasible, the best advice to parents is to only smoke outdoors.[297]

Allergen avoidance

In patients with allergic asthma, reducing exposure to relevant allergens may improve considerably symptoms, lung function and AHR. This has been shown convincingly by transferring patients to low allergen exposure areas, such as hospital rooms or high altitude, for prolonged periods of time. There is no doubt, therefore, that aeroallergen avoidance is useful; the problem is that it is difficult to achieve in practice.

The most common aeroallergen in asthmatic children in Western Europe is the house dust mite. An extensive package of measures is needed to reduce exposure to levels below which symptoms no longer occur, including a mite impermeable mattress, pillow and duvet cover, removing carpets and upholstered furniture, and assuring proper cleaning and ventilation methods.[298] A large US study showed that such an approach in urban children improved asthma outcomes considerably.[299] It has also been shown, however, that applying house dust mite impermeable bed covers alone is not useful.[300] The clinically relevant consideration, therefore, is not whether or not reduction of allergen exposure is effective, but whether or not achieving effective allergen exposure reduction is feasible.

In children allergic to pets, removal of the pet is the only effective way to reduce allergen exposure. Washing the animal or application of high-efficacy vacuum cleaners or air cleaners are not effective.[301]

Immunotherapy

Immunotherapy is effective in reducing allergic sensitization and the symptoms associated with it.[302] Although there is strong evidence that immunotherapy is effective in improving symptoms and lung function in asthma,[303] this treatment option is not very popular in Western Europe because of the high efficacy of pharmacological management (see p. 694) in asthma, and the burden of repeated subcutaneous injections in children that may have to be sustained for many years. At present there is insufficient evidence to support sublingual immunotherapy for childhood asthma.

Influenza vaccination

A large RCT showed no benefit of influenza vaccination on symptoms and exacerbations of asthma in children.[304] Although influenza vaccination is highly effective in preventing influenza-associated morbidity in children, asthma should no longer be considered an indication for influenza vaccination.

Pharmacological management

Based on the pathophysiology of asthma with chronic airway inflammation and intermittent bronchial smooth muscle constriction as key features, the pharmacological treatment is based on anti-inflammatory (controller medication) and bronchodilator (reliever medication) therapy. This treatment is preferably administered directly to the airways by inhalation.

Most children with persistent asthma can be well controlled by treatment with inhaled controller medication alone. The goal of pharmacological management is total control of symptoms (including nocturnal and exercise-induced symptoms), prevention of exacerbations, allowance of normal daily activities including sports and play, and achievement of best possible lung function with minimal side-effects. This goal should be reached and maintained with the lowest effective dose of controller medication.

Grading asthma severity

In all recent evidence-based management guidelines, the pharmacological management of asthma is presented in a stepwise fashion, from the mildest cases of intermittent asthma (step 1) through the most therapy-resistant cases of severe asthma (step 5). The first step in pharmacological management, therefore, is to assess asthma severity (Table 20.11). However, because asthma is a variable disease, asthma severity should be re-evaluated on a regular basis and treatment should be adjusted accordingly.

This grading of asthma severity was originally devised for children and adults who did not receive controller medication. Later, when the use of daily ICS therapy became generally accepted, the definitions used for steps 2–4 were generally as follows:

- Step 2: mild persistent asthma: well controlled on ICS therapy alone.
- Step 3: moderate persistent asthma: not well controlled on ICS therapy alone, requires additional treatment for good control.
- Step 4: severe persistent asthma: not well controlled despite 'step 3' therapy.
- Step 5: refractory severe asthma: severe symptoms and limitations despite high-dose intensive therapy.

In the American guidelines, levels of lung function abnormality and peak flow variation are given for each severity level; these are based on expert opinion and there is no independent evidence to support them. Most children with persistent asthma and established on ICSs have normal levels of lung function;[290] hence grading of severity based on lung function measurements is not appropriate for children.

Choosing an appropriate inhaler device

The majority of medications used to treat childhood asthma are given by inhalation. Children should be prescribed an inhaler device that is suitable for their age (Table 20.12).[305]

After choosing the appropriate inhaler device, children and their parents should be instructed extensively in the correct inhalation technique. This is difficult and time consuming, but extremely important. If inhalation instruction is performed perfunctorily, half of patients will use their inhaler incorrectly.[306] This can be improved by repeated instructions and by having the child demonstrate his/her ability to use the inhaler correctly.[307]

Table 20.11 Grading asthma severity

Severity	Symptoms/day	Symptoms/night
Mild intermittent (step 1)	< 1 time/week Asymptomatic and normal lung function between attacks	<2 times per month
Mild persistent (step 2)	>1 time/week but <1/day Attacks may affect activity	>2 times per month
Moderate persistent (step 3)	Daily Attacks affect activity	>1 time per week
Severe persistent (step 4)	Continuous Limited physical activity	Frequent
Refractory (step 5)	As in step 4 despite high-dose therapy	

Table 20.12 Inhaler devices for children of different ages[305]

0–2 years	Metered dose inhaler with valved spacer with facemask Second choice: nebulizer
3–6 years	Metered dose inhaler with valved spacer with mouthpiece Second choice: nebulizer
>7 years	Dry powder inhaler Second choice: metered dose inhaler with valved spacer with mouthpiece; metered dose inhaler with breath actuation

Choosing appropriate medication

Reliever therapy (short acting beta-2 agonists) (Fig. 20.24). Every child with asthma should be given an inhaled short-acting beta-2 agonist (salbutamol, terbutaline) for relief of acute symptoms of wheeze and dyspnea. These should only be used on demand. As their effects subside after approximately 4 h, they may be given up to six times per day. There is good evidence that adding anticholinergic agents such as ipratropium is not needed for relief of symptoms in outpatients,[308] or in preschool children with recurrent wheeze.[309]

Controller therapy: inhaled corticosteroids. In patients who experience symptoms or use their reliever agents two or more times per week, daily use of a controller agent is indicated. Inhaled corticosteroids are the drugs of first choice for the treatment of mild persistent asthma in children 5 years of age or older. There is strong evidence that these agents improve symptoms and quality of life, lung function and AHR, and reduce exacerbations and school absence. In most patients with asthma, ICSs alone at dosages of 200 mcg/day (given in two doses) are able to control the disease and normalize lung function, provided that the patient is adherent to medication and inhalation technique is correct.[290,310] Starting with a high dose is not superior to starting with a regular dose.[311]

Different ICSs are available, the oldest ones being beclometasone dipropionate (BDP) and budesonide. Fluticasone and ciclesonide are approximately twice as potent as BDP, hence lower doses of the latter two ICSs should be used.

Side-effects of ICSs are very rare at regular doses, but may occur at doses exceeding 800 mcg/day of BDP equivalent.[312,313] Adrenal suppression is the most threatening side-effect to be have been described repeatedly in high-dose treatment, in particular with fluticasone. Although growth of asthmatic children is slightly reduced during the first year of ICS therapy, final adult height is normal, even after treatment with ICSs for many years.[314]

ICSs are more effective than the leukotriene receptor antagonist montelukast in controlling asthma in school children.[315] In preschool children with recurrent wheeze, however, the situation is slightly more complex. Although ICSs are effective in preschool children with multi-trigger wheeze and in allergic asthma,[286,316,317] they are not effective in preschool children with episodic viral wheeze.[286,318,319] As montelukast reduces exacerbation rates and improves lung function and eNO levels in preschool children with episodic viral wheeze,[320,321] this agent may be particularly useful in this clinical setting.

Step 3 therapy: when ICSs alone are not enough. In contrast to the situation in adults, limited evidence is available to guide 'step 3' therapy in children with asthma who remain symptomatic despite low dose ICS treatment. Although guidelines recommend addition of long-acting beta-2 agonists (LABAs; salmeterol or formoterol) as the treatment option of choice,[235] this has not been substantiated in children.[322] A systematic review and a RCT have shown that addition of LABA to ICS in children has no effect on exacerbation rates.[323,324] Clinical experience suggests that children may, however, respond favorably to the combination of ICS and LABA. A recent study using a combination of budesonide and formoterol, both as maintenance and reliever

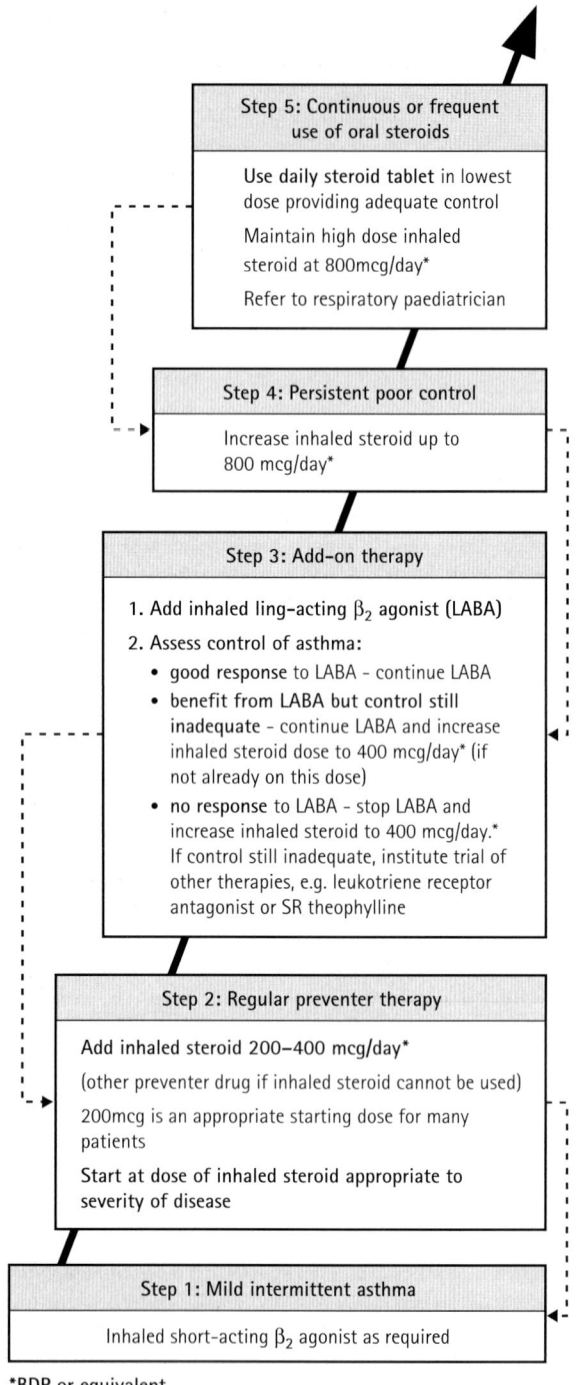

Step 5: Continuous or frequent use of oral steroids

Use **daily steroid tablet** in lowest dose providing adequate control

Maintain high dose inhaled steroid at 800mcg/day*

Refer to respiratory paediatrician

Step 4: Persistent poor control

Increase inhaled steroid up to 800 mcg/day*

Step 3: Add-on therapy

1. Add inhaled ling-acting β₂ agonist (LABA)

2. Assess control of asthma:

• **good response** to LABA - continue LABA

• **benefit from LABA but control still inadequate** - continue LABA and increase inhaled steroid dose to 400 mcg/day* (if not already on this dose)

• **no response** to LABA - stop LABA and increase inhaled steroid to 400 mcg/day.* If control still inadequate, institute trial of other therapies, e.g. leukotriene receptor antagonist or SR theophylline

Step 2: Regular preventer therapy

Add inhaled steroid 200–400 mcg/day*

(other preventer drug if inhaled steroid cannot be used)

200mcg is an appropriate starting dose for many patients

Start at dose of inhaled steroid appropriate to severity of disease

Step 1: Mild intermittent asthma

Inhaled short-acting β₂ agonist as required

*BDP or equivalent

Fig. 20.24 Stepwise management of asthma in school-aged children and adolescents.[235] BDP = beclometasone dipropionate. Doses are given for BDP; same doses apply for budesonide. Use half dosages for fluticasone, ultrafine BDP solution or ciclesonide.

therapy, did show reduction of asthma exacerbations in children.[325] A recent meta-analysis of LABAs in children and adults concluded that LABAs increase severe and life threatening exacerbations, and in adults increase the risk of death.[326] However, these conclusions have been challenged and do not appear to be congruent with falling asthma admission rates and stabilization of asthma deaths in countries with high use of ICSs and LABAs in combination. A LABA should never be used without a concomitant ICS.

Given the observation that the majority of children with asthma can be well controlled on ICSs alone, it is useful to consider possible explanations for poor treatment response to ICSs before stepping up to add-on 'step 3' therapy:

• ongoing exposure to triggering factors:
  • cigarette smoke;
  • allergens;
  • allergic rhinitis.
• poor adherence to therapy;
• poor inhalation technique;
• other diagnosis than asthma (see p. 693 – Investigations).

If 'step 3' therapy is truly indicated, the British guidelines propose addition of a LABA on a trial basis (see Fig. 20.24). Other treatment options include doubling the dose of ICS or addition of montelukast.[327] Comparative trials between these options in children have not been performed.

There is no good evidence to support decisions regarding the treatment of asthma in cases who remain symptomatic despite 'step 3' therapy; all recommendations in the guidelines are based on Level 3 evidence. Truly severe asthma is a rare but disabling disorder in children, for which referral to tertiary pediatric respiratory care is indicated. Data on the pathophysiology of severe asthma in childhood are slowly emerging.[261] Inflammation is not a consistent feature of severe asthma, neither in bronchial biopsies nor in eNO levels, but thickening of RBM is.[261,328]

Treatment options in severe asthma include combination of high-dose ICS, LABA and montelukast, addition of sustained-release theophylline or subcutaneous terbutaline, and maintenance therapy with systemic anti-inflammatory agents such as prednisolone or ciclosporin. A relatively new and promising treatment option is anti-IgE (omalizumab) which reduces asthma exacerbation rates and improves lung function.[329] Unfortunately, apart from being very expensive, omalizumab requires 2-weekly subcutaneous injections and the effects subside rapidly after discontinuation of therapy.

Monitoring and follow-up

Although not supported by Level 1 evidence, there is ample circumstantial evidence that close monitoring and follow-up improves asthma outcomes in children. First, it has been shown that poor adherence and poor monitoring is associated with troublesome symptoms, restricted activities and school absence.[330] Perhaps the most convincing data are that once close monitoring and follow-up is instituted, the ICS dose can be reduced by 25% whilst maintaining asthma control.[310] Such follow-up should include re-inforcement of education and inhalation instruction, review of symptoms, exacerbations, school absence and quality of life, and adaptation of maintenance (controller) therapy when needed. Follow-up can be performed safely and (cost)effectively by specialized nurses once the diagnosis and a treatment plan have been established.[310]

Although guidelines recommend close monitoring of lung function in children with asthma, there is no evidence to support this practice.[331] In particular, the recommendation to record peak expiratory flow at home on a regular basis in children with asthma is based on belief and dogma and not on evidence. Written peak flow diaries are very unreliable.[332] In addition, clinical trials show that monitoring peak expiratory flow at home does not improve asthma control, even when the data are recorded electronically.[333] Thus, although it is probably useful to monitor lung function during scheduled follow-up visits to avoid overestimation of asthma control,[334] home monitoring of peak flow can not be recommended.[331]

Monitoring of eNO levels may be useful to predict asthma relapse after discontinuation of ICS, and perhaps in titrating ICS dose.[335]

Although still quite popular, the advice to double the dose of ICS during an (impending) exacerbation of asthma is not proven and should no longer be recommended.[295] Instead, patients should be encouraged to use reliever medication as needed, and to seek medical help when this is insufficient to control symptoms.

PROGNOSIS

Approximately two thirds of cases of episodic viral wheeze recover completely before the age of 6 years.[280] Because such 'transient wheeze' can only be recognized in retrospect, and because overlap syndromes between wheezing phenotypes in early childhood are common, the need for maintenance therapy with daily controller agents should be reconsidered from time to time in preschool children. The most common approach to this is to step down and discontinue controller therapy in children in whom asthma control is achieved and maintained for prolonged periods of time. However, as symptoms are frequently worse during the winter, it may not be best practice to withdraw controller therapy after an apparent resolution of symptoms during the summer months.

Although a similar approach to the step down of the maintenance dose of ICS to the lowest effective dose is recommended for school-aged children and adolescents, truly withdrawing such treatment in children aged 5 years or older is not a treatment goal per se. Complete remission of asthma in this age range is possible, although rare. Approximately 50% of children with asthma become symptom-free during their teenage years, but half of these will have a recurrence of asthma symptoms during the third or fourth decade.[336] As it appears that 'growing out of asthma' once established in school-aged children is a relatively rare event, the current perspective is to consider childhood asthma as a life-long chronic disease. It is important to review these data with asthmatic children and their parents when discussing withdrawing ICS therapy, and to strongly discourage them from smoking. As the likelihood of young people taking up smoking is increased if their parents smoke, encouraging parental cessation is a worthwhile target for prevention.

ACUTE SEVERE ASTHMA

Although rare in children, fatalities from asthma do occur, and every effort should be made to avoid these. The most important factors associated with fatal asthma are poor asthma education, insufficient or absent use of controller medication, food allergy and the lack of monitoring and follow-up. The most important 'red flags' indicating increased risk of dying from asthma are heavy use of reliever medication, repeated A&E attendance for asthma or a history of a severe attack requiring intensive care or mechanical ventilation.

Causes and pathophysiology

Although acute exacerbations of asthma can be provoked by multiple triggers (see Table 20.9), viral URTI remains the single most common trigger.[337] More than half of cases of acute severe asthma presenting to hospital are preschool children.

During an asthma attack, smooth muscle constriction causing bronchial narrowing, inflammation leading to airway mucosal edema, and excess mucus secretion contribute to airway obstruction. There is reduced ventilation in some areas and absent ventilation in others, because of airway closure. This results in ventilation/perfusion mismatching and hypoxemia, which in turn stimulates ventilation. Carbon dioxide is extremely diffusible and is rapidly washed out of normally ventilated alveoli. As alveolar minute ventilation rises as a result of hypoxemic drive, $PaCO_2$ will fall. However, with continued increased work of breathing, exhaustion sets in and minute ventilation falls, leading to a rise in $PaCO_2$. The treatment of acute asthma is directed at stopping this happening.

Assessment

At presentation with an exacerbation, a brief history should include details of usual medication, extra medication and outcomes of previous episodes. Physical examination is often of limited value as it is difficult to categorize severity of wheeze according to physical signs. There is poor correlation between the severity of airway obstruction and physical signs. Nasal flaring, use of accessory muscles and sternal recession all reflect an increased work of breathing. A silent chest, reflecting exhaustion, altered level of consciousness and cyanosis are late signs. Pulsus paradoxus is difficult to measure in children and is not very informative.

Measuring oxygen saturation is useful as an $SaO_2 < 92\%$ in air confers increased risk of severe exacerbations requiring hospital admission.[338]

Table 20.13 Treatment for acute severe asthma in the emergency department

Oxygen: high-flow, humidified, by nasal canula or nonbreathing mask
Bronchodilators: either high-dose β_2 agonist by metered dose inhaler/spacer
- Salbutamol 100 µg per puff: 1–5 years 6 puffs × 3; > 5 years 12 puffs × 3
- Or combination of β_2 agonist and ipratropium by nebulization

Prednisolone: initial dose of 1 mg/kg (max 30 mg)

If possible, an FEV_1 or peak expiratory flow should be assessed. Other investigations are not useful in assessing the severity of the attack or predicting outcome.

Treatment in hospital

Initial treatment in hospital should include supplemental oxygen, inhaled bronchodilators and systemic corticosteroids (Table 20.13).

Supplemental oxygen reduces hypoxemia and improves outcome.[339] Bronchodilators should be given frequently until dyspnea improves. In preschool children, beta-2 agonists by metered dose inhaler/spacer are more effective than by nebulization.[340] It has also been shown, however, that adding anticholinergics to beta-2 agonists improves symptoms and lung function in acute severe asthma.[308] Nebulization can then be a practical way to give oxygen, anticholinergics and beta-2 agonists in a single intervention. Observation for a few hours is recommended to recognize rapid deterioration after initial improvement.

Systemic corticosteroids improve outcome of asthma exacerbations in children.[341,342] Oral prednisolone is the drug of choice; an oral solution or syrup is better tolerated than crushed tablets.[343] There is no evidence to support the use of systemic steroids in acute severe wheeze in children younger than 6 months of age,[344] or to support the home use of prednisolone in episodic viral wheeze in young children.[345]

Most cases of acute severe asthma can be discharged home after this initial treatment, but children who do not improve considerably should be admitted to hospital and followed up closely. This can be done clinically; only if work of breathing and oxygen saturation deteriorate is arterial blood gas analysis indicated.

Refractory cases of acute severe asthma can be treated with intravenous salbutamol,[346] magnesium sulfate,[347] or aminophylline.[348] There is no good evidence to guide the choice between these different treatment strategies.

CONGENITAL ABNORMALITIES

Congenital lung malformations have assumed increased importance as a result of routine detailed antenatal ultrasound scanning. Pediatricians may be involved in counseling pregnant women about the prognosis for the fetus, as well as in the postnatal management of an apparently normal baby with a small malformation which in past years would have escaped discovery. It is a field in which there is little evidence base, and in which the nomenclature is confusing and used differently ante- and postnatally. There is also increasing interest in the longer term consequences of all congenital lung malformations as greater numbers survive into adult life; follow-up studies have been reviewed.[349]

GENERAL PRINCIPLES

It is better to describe the abnormality as seen, in simple English, without speculating as to the embryology, since such speculation will almost inevitably be proved wrong in the future.[350] Table 20.14 illustrates this approach. A detailed justification of this nomenclature can be found elsewhere.[350] Two new terms deserve further elaboration. Congenital large hyperlucent lobe (CLHL) is a factual description of an appearance on a CXR or CT scan, whereas congenital lobar emphysema is a frightening and wrong allusion to a condition of elderly smokers, when the

Table 20.14 Comparison of new nomenclature with old terms, based on the principles of describing what is seen, in clear language, without embryological speculation

New nomenclature	Old terms superseded
Congenital large hyperlucent lobe (CLHL)	Congenital lobar emphysema Polyalveolar lobe
Congenital thoracic malformation (CTM) – described as solid or cystic; if cystic; the cysts are described as single or multiple, thin or thick walled, and the contents described (either from CXR and other imaging, or from pathological examination of excised specimens)	Cystic adenomatoid malformation Congenital pulmonary airway malformation Malinosculation Sequestration (intra- and extra-pulmonary) Bronchogenic cyst Reduplication cyst Foregut cyst
Congenital small lung (CSL)	Pulmonary hypoplasia
Absent lung, absent trachea	Agenesis of lung, tracheal aplasia
Absent bronchus	Bronchial atresia
Narrow bronchus, narrow trachea	Bronchial stenosis, tracheal stenosis
Bilateral right lung, bilateral left lung	Right isomerism, left isomerism

pathology may be too many, not too few alveoli. Congenital thoracic malformation (CTM) is used to describe both sequestration and cystic adenomatoid malformation because they are ends of a spectrum and not discrete entities. Either may have a systemic arterial supply, and pathological features of both may be found in the same lesion.

A further important principle is to describe the lung systematically. For these purposes, the lung is broken into six trees (bronchial, systemic and pulmonary arterial, systemic and pulmonary venous, and lymphatic). Other relevant systems should be described (chest wall, heart and mediastinum, abdomen) and all other systems reviewed, because, as with other congenital abnormalities, there may be coexistent problems elsewhere.

NASOPHARYNGEAL ABNORMALITIES

Babies are preferential nose breathers, so bilateral choanal stenosis or atresia presents with respiratory distress at birth. Milder forms may present with difficulty feeding. Unilateral disease may present later in childhood, sometimes with a unilateral nasal discharge. Diagnosis is suspected if a nasogastric tube cannot be passed into the pharynx. Management is surgical. Pierre Robin syndrome results in the tongue obstructing breathing secondary to micrognathia. The baby should be nursed prone but if this is unsuccessful a carefully positioned nasopharyngeal tube or tracheostomy may be necessary until the mandible grows sufficiently to accommodate the tongue, usually before the age of 1 year. Babies with congenital syndromes associated with midfacial hypoplasia (e.g. Apert) should also be considered at risk for obstruction to breathing, at least during sleep. Congenital tumors and cysts, such as teratoma, hemangioma, ectopic thyroid and cystic hygroma, are unusual causes of pharyngeal obstruction, all of which require surgical treatment. Crowding of the pharynx occurs in Down syndrome and in disorders associated with a large or abnormally positioned tongue. Sleep-disordered breathing may result from airways obstruction as muscle tone falls during sleep, and polysomnography is indicated for diagnosis. If obstructive sleep apnea is present, adenotonsillectomy may relieve symptoms (for cleft lip and palate, see Ch. 32, p. 1516).

CONGENITAL STRIDOR
Laryngomalacia

This accounts for over 75% of stridor in infancy. On endoscopy, the arytenoids, epiglottis and aryepiglottic folds are sucked inwards on inspiration; there may be associated pharyngomalacia and tracheomalacia. Presentation is with isolated stridor in an otherwise well baby in the first days of life, but usually not at birth, but may be delayed until over 1 month of age. The inspiratory stridor is worse during periods of agitation and upper respiratory tract infection.

If the clinical presentation is characteristic, and the infant is improving, no investigation is needed. If there are any atypical features, including growth failure, bronchoscopy should be performed to exclude other or multiple causes of stridor. This investigation requires skilled anesthesia and the occasional child may require short term ventilation after the procedure. The stridor usually disappears by the age of 2 years, but sometimes continues into early childhood and rarely beyond 5 years of age.

Laryngeal stenosis

This is the second commonest cause of congenital stridor and may be caused by supraglottic, glottic or subglottic webs or subglottic stenosis. The most severe form of congenital laryngeal disease is absent larynx. This results in normal appearances from above, but intubation is impossible. The lungs are normal or large. Most laryngeal webs are glottic and present with stridor and a poor cry at or shortly after birth. The severity of the symptoms depends on the size of the web, which may cause complete airways obstruction, a condition incompatible with life unless diagnosed and treated within minutes of delivery. Many of these babies have other severe abnormalities. Treatment is surgical.

Subglottic stenosis is usually the result of soft tissue thickening of the subglottic area, usually acquired following prolonged intubation during the neonatal period. Occasionally laser resection of the granulation tissue or tracheostomy is required but most improve as the larynx grows. Localized tracheo- or broncho-malacia resulting from damage in the neonatal period due to ventilatory assistance may also cause stridor with or without wheeze in the first few years of life. These babies are more likely to require hospital admission if they acquire a respiratory infection as they will almost certainly have associated lower respiratory tract damage.

Subglottic hemangiomata

These become obvious before 6 months and 50% of babies have hemangiomata elsewhere, usually on the skin. Presentation may be with recurrent croup, improving as the usual prescription for corticosteroids leads to temporary shrinkage of the hemangioma. The diagnosis is confirmed at endoscopy. Most regress during the first 2 years and thus a conservative approach is preferred. If medical treatment is indicated for severe obstruction or complications, prednisolone or interferon may shrink the hemangioma. Severe cases may need laser surgery or even tracheostomy.

Vocal cord paralysis

This can be unilateral or bilateral. Unilateral is more frequent. Paralysis may be associated with other abnormalities, especially in the cardiovascular and respiratory systems. In most cases the paralysis is temporary with recovery within 4 weeks. Birth trauma with stretching of the neck and the recurrent laryngeal nerve may be a factor. Bilateral paralysis is usually associated with central nervous system disorders, such as hydrocephalus, which may themselves have a poor prognosis. Diagnosis is made at laryngoscopy.

Laryngeal clefts

Laryngeal clefts are associated with tracheoesophageal fistulae in about 20% and hydramnios in 30%. The infant presents with a toneless cry, choking and cyanosis on feeding, and aspiration pneumonia. Later in childhood a chronic cough or recurrent lower respiratory tract infection may be the only clue. Diagnosis is at laryngoscopy; inexperienced operators may miss a small cleft, particularly if a flexible, rather than a rigid endoscope is used. Surgical repair can be extremely difficult.

Laryngeal cysts

Laryngeal cysts are very rare and cause stridor and a poor cry in the neonatal period. Endoscopy should be performed cautiously, and no attempt should be made to approach or go past the cyst if the airway is critically narrowed. Laser de-roofing of the cyst is curative.

Vascular abnormalities

Vascular abnormalities include abnormalities of the vessels of the aortic arch which cause tracheal compression ('vascular ring'), usually presenting during the first year of life, but not uncommonly later as a prior diagnosis of steroid resistant asthma. Stridor, wheezing and a barking cough are the commonest presenting symptoms. Since the larynx is not involved, the tone of the cry is normal. Excessive secretions, difficulty with feeding and apneic episodes are sometimes associated.

TRACHEOESOPHAGEAL FISTULA (see also Ch. 37)

The preoperative pulmonary problems associated with tracheoesophageal fistula (TEF) are related either to aspiration of secretions or food through the larynx if, as is usual, the upper end of the esophagus is blind, or to reflux of stomach and duodenal secretions through the distal end of the esophagus into the tracheobronchial tree.

In the rare H-type fistula (4%) aspiration of food may cause recurrent chest infection. The underlying abnormality may even not be diagnosed until adult life. The diagnosis of the H-type TEF is not easy and rests on the demonstration of contrast medium flowing through the fistula. Seventy percent of lesions lie high in the esophagus and since the fistula passes obliquely upwards from the esophagus a tube esophagram (not a barium swallow) should be carried out with the child lying prone. Late presentation may occur with coughing after drinking, hemoptysis, retrosternal pain and recurrent infection.

Prognosis of TEF is related to the gestational maturity of the baby, the presence of pulmonary disease before surgery, the incidence of postoperative pulmonary disease and the presence of associated abnormalities. TEF has a reported association with other congenital abnormalities of 50–70% and 2% of these are associated abnormalities of the respiratory tract.

Long term follow-up of survivors of surgery suggests that airway disease is common. This may be related to disorders of esophageal motility and repeated small aspirations or to the severity of the initial respiratory disease. In addition, at the site of the fistula, tracheal cartilage is inadequately formed or missing and there is an absence of normally ciliated respiratory epithelium. Tracheomalacia accounts for the brassy cough, worse during upper respiratory tract infections. Apneic episodes following feeding are a problem in a small number of babies and the incidence of sudden unexpected death is increased. Whether this is due to aspiration or associated with the tracheomalacia is debated. A mild restrictive pattern of pulmonary physiology is not uncommon in survivors. Some children develop scoliosis, which is a well described complication of thoracotomy,[351] although probably much less frequent with modern surgical techniques.

LOWER AIRWAY ABNORMALITIES

Trachea

With total or partial absence of the trachea ('tracheal aplasia'), the main bronchi either communicate only with each other or with the esophagus. The trachea may be smaller than normal in both the sagittal and coronal planes in Down syndrome. Congenital intrinsic tracheal narrowing (stenosis) may take the form of a gradual tapering, an isolated segmental narrowing or a membranous web, or be due to a nodule of ectopic esophageal tissue. Congenital extrinsic compression may be due to a vascular ring or pulmonary artery sling (see p. 701 – Pulmonary arterial abnormalities).

Bronchial tree
Bronchial arrangement and connections

Airway morphology is defined by the number of lobes (three for right sided, two for left) and the length of the main bronchus before the first bifurcation (short for right sided, long for left). The commonest abnor-

mal bronchial arrangement is a mirror image, which may be associated with primary ciliary dyskinesia. This must be distinguished from a right-sided congenital small lung (CSL), which may have a systemic arterial supply. In 80% of cases, bilateral right lung is associated with asplenia and hence the risk of overwhelming pneumococcal disease, bilateral left lung (BLL) with polysplenia. Both are associated with abdominal visceral malrotation and complex congenital heart disease.[352,353] A syndrome of BLL, normal atrial arrangement and severe tracheobronchomalacia presenting as steroid resistant wheeze has been described.[354] Other variants are indeterminate morphology; bronchi crossing the mediastinum to supply the contralateral lung (cross-over) and even a tongue of lung crossing the mediastinum (horseshoe lung).[356]

Congenital absence of a lobe or lung

Absent lung ('aplasia') is not uncommon but absence of a lobe or of both lungs is rare. There may be a rudimentary bronchial stump. In bilateral absent lungs the trachea ends blindly and the pulmonary artery arises from the aorta. Unilateral absent lung is often associated with other ipsilateral malformations.

Congenital small lungs

Small ('hypoplastic') lungs may be normal or abnormal in form. Alveoli are reduced in number or size. Normal right and left lung weights at term are 21 and 18 g, respectively; the lungs are small if the lung-to-body weight ratio is < 0.012.[357] The reduction in alveoli may be associated with fewer airway generations. Small lungs may be isolated with no underlying cause, but are more usually associated with a variety of other malformations. These include diaphragmatic defects, renal anomalies, extralobar pulmonary parenchymal malformations, and severe neuromuscular and musculoskeletal disorders. Most of these associations have a causal relationship but some, such as that with Down syndrome, are puzzling. Lung growth before birth is dependent upon blood supply, availability of space, respiratory movements taking place in utero and fluid filling the airways. The causes of bilateral small lungs (BSL) are summarized in Table 20.15.

Disorders of the bronchial walls

Airway caliber abnormalities may result in all or part of the bronchial tree being too large or too small. Congenital tracheobronchomegaly (Mounier–Kuhn syndrome) is associated with tracheomalacia and bronchiectasis. There are saccular bulges between the cartilages. An autosomal recessive connective tissue defect has been postulated.[358] This is supported by the occasional association of Mounier–Kuhn syndrome with Ehlers–Danlos syndrome, cutis laxa or Kenny–Caffey syndrome.

Localized narrowing and in particular obstruction due to an absent bronchus often results in cystic degeneration of the lobe distal to the obstruction before birth, as fetal lung liquid continues to be secreted and

Table 20.15 Causes of bilateral congenital small lungs. Occasionally no underlying cause is found

Underlying problem	Example
Abnormal thoracic contents	Diaphragmatic hernia, pleural effusion, large congenital thoracic malformation
Thoracic compression from below	Abdominal tumors, ascites
Thoracic compression from the sides	Amniotic bands, oligohydramnios, asphyxiating thoracic dystrophy, scoliosis
Abnormal vascular supply	Pulmonary valve or artery stenosis, tetralogy of Fallot
Neuromuscular disease	CNS, anterior horn cell, peripheral nerve muscle disease reducing fetal breathing movements

cannot drain into the amniotic cavity. Absent bronchus may be detected radiographically in an asymptomatic individual and presentation may be late. The radiological appearances are virtually diagnostic, consisting of an ovoid hilar opacity, most commonly in the left upper lobe, with branches radiating out into a distal area of hyperlucency. The opacity represents a distended, mucus-filled bronchus that is continuous with the distal airways but has no connection with the more proximal, blind ending airway. The interruption to the airway may take the form of a membrane, a fibrous cord or a gap. The focal opacity seen in absent bronchus is not present in a congenital large hyperlucent lobe (CLHL). The continuity of the cyst with the distal airways and the hyperinflation of the distal lung distinguish absent bronchus from 'bronchogenic cyst'.[359] True congenital bronchiectasis is much rarer than previously thought, but may be found within a CTM.

Congenital bronchomalacia may be isolated, generally with a good prognosis, at least in the short term, and has been described in association with other congenital abnormalities, including connective tissue disorders, and Larsen and Fryn syndrome. Williams and Campbell described a syndrome of generalized bronchomalacia affecting the second to the seventh generations of the bronchial tree. The occurrence in two siblings and the very early onset of symptoms suggests a congenital etiology. Finally, bronchomalacia may be secondary to other congenital abnormalities, such as vascular ring. Fixed bronchial narrowing may be due to defects in the wall (e.g. complete cartilage rings) or extrinsic compression by an abnormal vessel or cyst.

Abnormal bronchial connections

The separation of those parts of the primitive foregut to become esophagus and trachea may be incomplete resulting in TEF (see p. 700). Communication between the trachea and a CTM is also recorded.

Alveolar disorders

Counting alveolar numbers requires an open lung biopsy, and is usually of theoretical importance only. CLHL is an example of a disorder of alveoli. CLHL may be diagnosed antenatally, or presents with tachypnea and respiratory distress in the newborn period, or is a chance finding on a CXR later in life. In some cases it is due to partial obstruction of the lobar bronchus leading to air trapping. The obstruction may be caused by external compression, e.g. by a cyst or abnormal blood vessel; alternatively, intrinsic abnormalities such as mucosal flaps, mucus plugs or twisting of the lobe on its pedicle may be responsible.[360] A deficiency of bronchial cartilage is a diagnosis of exclusion; in practice the cause is frequently not identified. Some patients also have congenital cardiac anomalies. CLHL affects the left upper lobe in about half the cases, the right middle and right upper lobes in most of the remainder and the lower lobes in < 10%. Curiously, it almost never becomes infected; if CLHL is the seat of recurrent infection, suspect that the appearances are secondary to bronchial stenosis. Diagnosis should be confirmed on a CT scan, which distinguishes CLHL from a thin walled cystic CTM. If the infant is symptomatic and fails to thrive, then surgical removal is advised. If the child is well, no treatment is needed; even a quite dramatic looking CLHL becomes less prominent over time. Another cause of CLHL is a polyalveolar lobe, which is a pathological, not a clinical, diagnosis. A polyalveolar lobe has a normal number of conductive airways but an increased number of normal sized alveoli in each acinus.

Solid and cystic thoracic lesions: clinical approach

When assessing patients with a suspected congenital lung malformation, it is more logical to describe abnormalities by their appearance, whether on images (CXR, CT or MRI) or pathologically. The use of terms like 'reduplication cyst' and 'bronchogenic cyst' in clinical practice, *prior to the resection of the abnormality,* imply embryology and/or pathology, and should be discarded. A better term to use in clinical practice, which makes no assumptions, is CTM, some forms of which were previously described as a congenital cystic adenomatoid malformation (CCAM) or congenital pulmonary airway malformation (CPAM). CTM encompasses a spectrum of conditions, clinically described as cystic, intermediate or solid. It will be seen that the clinical definition of CTM includes what the pathologist may previously have described as a CCAM, or a bronchogenic or reduplication cyst, or other more specific term.

Solid and cystic lesions: pathological approach

The same constraints of clarity outlined above should apply to the pathologist. CTM should be used in pathological descriptions, attaching the term cystic, intermediate or solid as above, and describing the tissue in terms of what is seen on microscopy.

Bronchogenic and other foregut cysts are one type of CTM recognizable by cartilage and glands in their wall and a lining of respiratory epithelium. They are usually situated in the mediastinum close to the carina (51%) but may be found in the right paratracheal region (19%), alongside the esophagus (14%), the hilum of the lung (9%) or a variety of other locations (7%) including the substance of the lungs, and even beneath the diaphragm.[361] Cysts may be lined by respiratory-type epithelium but lack cartilage in their walls. Cysts may also have a gastric, intestinal or squamous epithelial lining and a muscle coat. These types of cyst are usually situated in the posterior mediastinum or, as they may be associated with vertebral malformations, even within the spine. They may also be associated with abdominal cysts.

Pathologically, five patterns of 'CPAM' have been recognized, which *clinically* may also be mimicked by other conditions such as pulmonary hamartoma or ectopic tissue (below), which are readily distinguished pathologically. The blood supply may be from either or both of the pulmonary artery and the aorta. Some workers incorporate 'sequestration' into the 'CPAM' spectrum. The fact that 'extralobar sequestrations' may contain tissue identical to CCAM underscores the logic of combining not separating these two conditions and dropping the terms 'sequestration', 'CPAM' and 'CCAM' in favor of the single, catch-all term CTM.[362-364] The five pathological types formerly described as CPAM are overlapping entities. Type 0 ('acinar dysplasia') is incompatible with life. Microscopically, bronchial-type airways that have cartilage, smooth muscle and glands are separated by abundant mesenchymal tissue. Type 1 ('cystic CCAM') is the commonest. The boundary between the lesion and the adjacent normal lobe is sharply delineated but there is no capsule. Radiographically, air-filled cysts that are usually limited to one lobe compress the rest of the lung, depress the diaphragm and cause mediastinal shift. The cysts range in size from 1 to 10 cm. They are lined by pseudostratified ciliated columnar epithelium interspersed with rows of mucus cells of pyloric type. The relevant bronchus is often absent, yet the cysts are usually radiolucent, presumably due to collateral ventilation. Type 2 (intermediate type 'CCAM') is sponge-like, consisting of multiple small cysts as well as solid pale tumor-like tissue. Microscopically the cysts are seen to be dilated bronchioles separated by normal alveoli. Occasional examples contain striated muscle. This type of lesion also may be identified within 'extralobar sequestrations'. Type 3 (solid type 'CCAM') is a large, bulky lesion that typically involves and expands a whole lobe, the others being compressed and the mediastinum displaced. Microscopically, an excess of bronchiolar-like structures are separated by small airspaces which have a cuboidal lining, with no cystic change. Type 4 is characterized by large air-filled cysts which are peripheral and thin walled. They have a simple squamous epithelium composed of alveolar type I cells resting upon loose mesenchymal tissue.

A further type of CTM is 'mesenchymal cystic hamartoma' (MCH). The lesions may be supplied by bronchial, intercostal or phrenic arteries. Pathological examination shows them to consist of multilocular, thin-walled cysts lined by primitive mesenchymal cells that support a ciliated cuboidal epithelium. Muscular hamartomas, which are small focal proliferations of smooth muscle, are occasionally observed incidentally in the lung, sometimes associated with similar lesions in the bowel and liver.

The sequestration spectrum has been used to indicate that a portion of lung exists without appropriate bronchial and vascular connections. Classically, no airway connects the lesion to the tracheobronchial tree and the blood supply is systemic; however, in some there may be a normal airway. Alternatively, an 'airway' may connect the sequestration to the esophagus or stomach in a complex 'bronchopulmonary–foregut malformation'. Occasionally, 'sequestration' is associated with duplication of the esophagus, stomach or pancreas. There is therefore a spectrum of abnormalities associated with 'pulmonary sequestration'.[365,366] Conventionally, two forms have been recognized: extralobar, which has its own covering of visceral pleura, and intralobar, which is embedded in otherwise normal lung. Both should be considered part of the CTM spectrum. There is often a defect in the diaphragm and about 15% of 'extralobar sequestrations' are abdominal. The veins leaving an 'extralobar sequestration' generally join the azygos or other systemic veins, whereas an 'intralobar sequestration' usually has normal pulmonary venous connections, but as with all CTMs, any combination of arterial supply and venous drainage is possible. The lung tissue in a 'sequestration' is often poorly developed and cystically dilated. The cysts are lined by columnar or cuboidal epithelium, or the 'sequestered' lung may be entirely composed of structures resembling alveolar ducts. Mucus distends the multiple intercommunicating spaces and the lesion appears solid radiographically, unless air enters through a bronchial connection or, in the case of 'intralobar sequestration', by collateral ventilation, when fluid levels are often seen.

Management of congenital thoracic malformations

A CTM most commonly presents as an antenatal ultrasound finding. Antenatal management is beyond the scope of this chapter. It should be noted that the majority of antenatally diagnosed malformations do well, and surgery (if performed) is usually elective.[367,368] The postnatal management of antenatally diagnosed CTM is fraught with difficulty, because of a lack of good information about natural history. If a baby has had a CTM diagnosed antenatally, then a CXR and a thoracic CT scan should be performed. Even quite large malformations may not be apparent on a CXR alone.[368] If the presence of a CTM is confirmed, there is no evidence base on which to offer advice. Reasons for operative removal would be the (currently unquantifiable) risk of infection; risk of malignancy; and (if there is a large systemic arterial supply) risk of high output heart failure. It should be noted that malignancy has been reported even after complete removal of congenital cysts.[369] If operation is contemplated, then it is important to delineate the vascular supply (below) to minimize the risk of severe bleeding. An option for selected malformations with a systemic arterial supply may be coil embolization of the feeding vessels. The author's practice is to offer surgical treatment for all but the smallest CTMs, usually carried out in the second year of life. Others would operate on even the smallest malformation. CTM may also present later in life as a chance finding, with recurrent infection, hemoptysis or steroid unresponsive wheeze due to compression of a large airway. Treatment considerations for the asymptomatic CTM diagnosed later in childhood are largely the same as for antenatally diagnosed ones; symptomatic CTM should be excised. In particular, once a CTM becomes infected, recurrence is inevitable and operation should be advised. Excision may also be needed to confirm the diagnosis and exclude more sinister causes such as a malignancy. Increasingly, excision is performed using video-assisted thoracoscopic surgery (VATS).

Abnormally placed pulmonary tissue and abnormal intrapleural tissue

Abnormal intrapleural tissue of adrenocortical tissue, thyroid (lacking C cells) and liver has been described in the lung and pancreatic tissue has been noted within so-called 'intralobar sequestrations' with gastrointestinal connections. Rarely, a whole kidney may be found above the diaphragm but outside the lung. There may be ectopic lung tissue in the neck, the abdomen or the chest wall, often associated with skeletal or diaphragmatic abnormalities.

The arterial trees

There are two arterial trees (pulmonary and systemic), which are considered separately. Systemic arterial abnormalities of the great vessels of the mediastinum can be subdivided from those of the bronchial circulation. Finally, the pulmonary capillary bed may be bypassed leading to direct arteriovenous communication; or absent, resulting in minimal pulmonary arteriovenous connections.

Pulmonary arterial abnormalities

In general, the pulmonary arteries and veins follow the bronchial anatomy, and thus pulmonary arterial and venous arrangement mirrors bronchial arrangement. There are important exceptions. The first of these is congenital origin of the left pulmonary artery from the right ('pulmonary artery sling'), sometimes with a cross-over arterial segment, with the right upper lobe supplied by a branch from the left pulmonary artery. Surgical repair of a sling with a cross-over may result in infarction of the right upper lobe if the abnormal vessel has not been discovered. Isolated cross-over pulmonary artery branches in the absence of bronchial cross-over are occasionally seen. They cross the mediastinum to supply lung segments which often are abnormal in other ways.

Lobar and segmental vessels as well as the main pulmonary arteries may be narrowed, and there may be multiple constrictions. Unilateral absence of a pulmonary artery leads to the lung on that side receiving only systemic blood, either through anomalous systemic arteries or enlarged bronchial arteries. The defect may be isolated or associated with other cardiovascular anomalies.

Anomalous systemic arteries supplying the lung may be associated with any CTM, or even be an isolated finding.[370] When operation is contemplated for any CTM, it is important that abnormal vasculature is detected. Inadvertent severance of anomalous systemic arteries has led to fatal hemorrhage, whilst ligation of anomalous veins from adjacent nonsequestered lung has led to infarction of normal tissue. Anomalous systemic arteries are also found if the pulmonary artery is absent and they may also be part of complex arteriovenous malformations. One or both pulmonary arteries may take origin from the aorta. Bilateral origin from the aorta is part of the spectrum of common arterial trunk. Unilateral origin of pulmonary artery from the aorta may be an isolated abnormality.

Congenitally small unilateral pulmonary artery is usually seen in association with an ipsilateral CSL. Normal pulmonary blood flow is needed for normal lung development. Bilateral small or absent pulmonary arteries are usually part of the spectrum of pulmonary valve atresia/tetralogy of Fallot. Very large pulmonary arteries which compress the central airways are seen in absent pulmonary valve syndrome.

Abnormalities of the systemic arteries

Two groups of abnormalities are relevant to the lung. The first group is those producing a vascular ring. There are a number of different variants, which present with stridor, cough, wheeze, and sometimes with recurrent infection or feeding difficulty. Diagnosis is by barium swallow, echocardiogram, bronchoscopy or CT or MRI angiography. Treatment is surgical, but prolonged postoperative symptoms due to the chronic effects of airway compression are common. The second group is the collateral vessels which may arise from the aorta and supply all or part of one or both lungs, or a CTM. These may be hypertrophied bronchial arteries or abnormal nonbronchial vessels; there may be multiple collaterals. This last group may be seen in association with direct pulmonary arteriovenous connections ('pulmonary arteriovenous malformations'). Aneurysm of aortopulmonary collateral vessels has been described.

The venous trees

Anomalous pulmonary veins result in blood from the lungs returning to the right side of the heart. The anomalous veins may join the inferior caval vein or hepatic, portal or splenic veins below the diaphragm, or above the diaphragm they may drain into the superior caval vein or its tributaries, the coronary sinus or the right atrium. The anomaly may be total or partial, unilateral or bilateral, and isolated or associated with other cardiopulmonary developmental defects. Anomalous pulmonary venous connections are often narrow and this may cause relatively mild pulmonary hypertension.

A particular clinical problem is the 'scimitar' syndrome; this is characterized by a small right lung, resulting in the heart being in the right chest (cardiac dextroposition), and an abnormal band shadow representing the abnormal venous drainage to the systemic veins, fancifully compared to a scimitar (which in fact is often absent). Initial treatment which may need consideration is coil occlusion of aortopulmonary collaterals and occasionally of an abnormal vein if venous drainage is double-arched (to both caval vein and left atrium). This intervention may be followed by surgical correction. The results are unlikely to be perfect; some blood supply may be restored, but the ultimate functional result will depend on the normality of the underlying lung. In view of evidence in other contexts that normal intrauterine blood supply is essential for normal lung development, it would be naïve to suppose that a perfect functional result could be achieved whatever treatment is given. Pulmonary venous obstruction is a not infrequent late complication of surgery, particularly if surgery is carried out in infancy. Occasionally lobectomy or pneumonectomy is performed, usually in the context of severe pulmonary hypertension; this operation should only be a last resort.[372,372]

Absence of the pulmonary veins or narrowing of their ostia into the left atrium similarly results in pulmonary venous obstruction. Partial anomalous pulmonary venous drainage may be obstructed or unobstructed. Unilateral anomalous venous drainage may be part of complex lung malformations; it may also be seen in association with what appears to be a simple lung cyst. This underscores the need for accurate delineation of all abnormalities in even straightforward appearing cases. Minor abnormalities of venous connection, such as of a segment direct to the azygos system, are not uncommon and are usually not of practical significance.

No congenital disorders of the systemic (bronchial) venous tree have been described.

Disorders of connection between the pulmonary and venous trees

An important group of abnormalities which potentially involves systemic and pulmonary arterial and venous trees are the various forms of 'pulmonary arteriovenous fistulae'. They range from the diffuse, microscopic to the single or multiple large abnormality. The large connections may have both a systemic and a pulmonary arterial supply. There may be arteriovenous malformations elsewhere in the body, and they may be part of Osler–Weber–Rendu disease. Presentation is with cyanosis, the chance discovery of an asymptomatic mass on CXR, or with a complication such as systemic embolization or abscess. Confirmation of the diagnosis is with contrast echocardiography. Treatment of discrete lesions is with transcatheter embolization.[373] Medium term follow-up has confirmed that the results are good. Multiple diffuse lesions in both lungs cannot be embolized, and may lead to progressive cyanosis and polycythemia. If symptoms are severe, lung transplantation may need to be considered, but this is a last resort, and is inferior in results to those of multiple embolization, when this is feasible.

Congenital alveolar capillary dysplasia (misalignment of lung vessels) represents a failure of capillaries to extend into the alveolar tissue of the lung, and presents initially as persistent fetal circulation, but which relentlessly progresses to death whatever treatment is given. Histology shows increased septal connective tissue and pulmonary veins accompanying small pulmonary arteries in the centers of the acini rather than occupying their normal position in the interlobular septa (misalignment of lung vessels). The pulmonary arteries are decreased in number and show increased muscularization. Pulmonary lobules are small and radial alveolar counts may be decreased. Alveoli are decreased in complexity, their walls contain few capillaries and there is poor contact of capillaries with alveolar epithelium. The primary fault is poorly understood. The relationship of congenital alveolar capillary dysplasia to a condition previously described as congenital alveolar dysplasia is unclear.

Lymphatic tree

Congenital lymphangiectasia may be isolated, associated with abdominal lymphangiectasia, or found with congenital heart disease. It usually presents with relentlessly worsening respiratory distress which does not respond to any treatment; however, it is becoming clear that the prognosis is not uniformly gloomy.[374] Rarely, milder localized cases may present in adolescence.[375] Diagnosis is by HRCT scan appearances, which may be confirmed by open lung biopsy.

Congenital chylothorax may be an isolated abnormality, or associated with congenital abnormality of the main lymphatic duct or pulmonary lymphatics. Associations with Noonan, Ullrich, Turner and Down syndrome, fetal thyrotoxicosis, H-type TEF and mediastinal neuroblastoma have been described; familial cases have been reported.

RELEVANT CARDIAC ABNORMALITIES

Cardiac malformations may be coincidental, or a fundamental part of the malformation. They are sufficiently common that echocardiography should be a routine part of the work-up of congenital lung disease. Coincidental malformations are seen with, for example, a congenital large hyperlucent lobe ('congenital lobar emphysema'). Lung abnormalities in which heart disease is fundamental include those with the pulmonary atresia spectrum. By definition, lung blood supply is abnormal. These however usually present to the pediatric cardiologists.

DIAPHRAGM AND CHEST WALL ABNORMALITIES
Diaphragmatic anomalies

Diaphragmatic hernia occurs in about 1 in 3600 live births. Classification is according to position – 70–90% occur through the left diaphragm, most commonly posterolaterally between the lumbar and costal muscle fibers (the foramen of Bochdalek).

Usually the diagnosis is made antenatally. Postnatally the infant presents with respiratory distress and physical examination suggests displacement of the heart, and ipsilaterally reduced breath sounds and bowel sounds in the chest. Bowel is seen in the chest on a chest radiograph. Treatment is surgical (see Ch. 37) and it is the degree of pulmonary hypoplasia and iatrogenic ventilator induced lung damage that largely determines outcome. Both lungs exhibit abnormal airway branching and alveolization, although this is more severe in the ipsilateral side.

When the hernia is small presentation may be delayed. These are often anterior and may mimic a cystic CTM on the CXR. The possibility of this diagnosis should be considered in any child presenting with an air–fluid level on a chest radiograph, cystic lesion or where the diaphragm is ill defined. A coexisting pneumonia may further confuse the issue. A barium meal will confirm the diagnosis and operation should proceed immediately diagnosis is made as there is a very real risk of strangulation.

Long term follow-up of successful neonatal surgical repair shows that although lung volumes may be normal, morphologically the lungs probably remain small (with reduced alveolization). Pulmonary perfusion to the ipsilateral lung remains reduced even in adolescence. Long term, most survivors do well, although a few have recurrent respiratory infections and a small minority have severe respiratory disability.[349]

Although most diaphragmatic hernias present antenatally or immediately after birth, a few present in mid-childhood. Whether this is truly a congenital defect, or is in fact an acquired diaphragm rupture, is disputed. In most cases, pulmonary hypoplasia is minimal if present at all, and this suggests that these children in practice have a very different disease.

If the substance of the diaphragm is deficient, usually on one side, the abdominal viscera are elevated (eventration of the diaphragm). Eventration is believed to result from failure of all or a portion of the normal muscularization of the developing diaphragm which remains thin and translucent. It is usually unilateral and isolated, but occasionally other abnormalities are associated. Isolated unilateral eventration rarely needs treatment; occasionally plication of the diaphragm may be indicated if there are recurrent infections in the associated lung. Fluoroscopy will help to distinguish phrenic nerve palsy where there is paradoxical movement of the diaphragm. In eventration there is little or no movement. Duplication of the diaphragm results in a fibromuscular septum dividing one pleural cavity in two, usually between the right upper and middle lobes.

Asphyxiating thoracic dystrophy (Jeune syndrome)

This is a rare autosomal recessive disorder of generalized chondrodystrophy in which the costal cartilages in which the ribs are shortened and the rib cage narrowed so that lung development is retarded and the lungs are small. Other manifestions include pelvic and phalangeal anomalies and rarely hepatic, renal and neurological disorders. Those who survive the neonatal period usually succumb to respiratory failure in infancy and early childhood.

ABDOMINAL DISEASE

Any large abdominal mass or fluid may compress the lungs, thus impairing development. Congenital absence of the kidneys causes oligohydramnios and small lungs (above). Rare CTMs may connect with the stomach and be associated with abdominal visceral malrotation.

MULTISYSTEM DISEASE

Most congenital lung abnormalities are isolated, but a few are part of a more generalized disorder, e.g. tuberose sclerosis may affect the lung as well as kidneys, heart and brain. Complex abnormalities of lung development may be associated with chromosomal abnormalities.

RARE LUNG DISEASES

The majority of these conditions are so rare that they will be encountered but once in a lifetime by the general pediatrician. Thus, early referral for specialist review is recommended in suspected cases.

THE TRUE INTERSTITIAL PNEUMONITIDES

About 50% of children with these conditions present at under 1 year of age. The spectrum includes chronic pneumonitis of infancy (CPI), desquamative interstitial pneumonitis (DIP, the 'usual' pattern of adults, which rarely if ever occurs in children), pulmonary interstitial glycogenosis (PIG), neuroendocrine cell hyperplasia of infancy (NEHI)[376] and nonspecific interstitial pneumonitis (NSIP), the last of which may be subclassified by the presence or absence of a fibrotic component.[377] The cause of many of these conditions is unknown, but mutations of the surfactant proteins (see p. 705) account for some cases; genetic studies should always be considered. Presentation is similar and nonspecific, with cough, tachypnea, respiratory distress, failure to thrive and sometimes cyanosis. The physical signs may include digital clubbing and fine crackles. The CXR appearances are nonspecific, and include generalized ground glass shadowing, reticular nodular infiltrates and honeycombing. HRCT is performed to confirm that an interstitial disease is present; but unlike in adults, it is relatively rare for a specific diagnosis to be made on the scan alone.[378] Diagnosis requires a lung biopsy; transbronchial biopsy gives only small samples, which may be sufficient for the rare diseases with highly specific histological features such as pulmonary alveolar microlithiasis, and is the investigation of choice in the transplant recipient with possible rejection.[379] Some advocate CT guided, percutaneous needle biopsy, but the complication rate is thought by many to be unacceptable.[379] Open lung biopsy (OLB) through a mini-thoracotomy is safe in experienced hands and has a high diagnostic yield.[380] In older children, a VATS procedure may be preferred. However, it has to be said that there seems to be little relationship between biopsy appearances and response to treatment or prognosis. These conditions are so rare that treatment recommendations are scanty. Most pediatricians would treat with hydroxychloroquine alone, or in combination with prednisolone.[381] If there is no response, recommendations are even more anecdotal; pulse methylprednisolone, azathioprine and ciclosporin have all

been tried. Prognosis is variable and unpredictable from either radiology or histological features; in general, the younger the age of onset the poorer the prognosis, but spontaneous and complete resolution of even severe disease is well described. There is a rare autosomal dominant, familial form of DIP for which the gene is currently not identified.

RARE SINGLE SYSTEM DISORDERS

Interested readers are referred to a comprehensive narrative review.[382]

Extrinsic allergic alveolitis

The allergen is usually pigeon or budgerigar excreta or moldy hay. Exposure to bird allergen may be indirect via the clothes of a parent. Presentation is with chronic respiratory distress (birds) or acute symptoms within hours of exposure (moldy hay), confirmed by positive serology. Treatment is allergen avoidance; oral steroids are given for severe acute or chronic progressive disease.

Pulmonary alveolar microlithiasis

This condition, which may be inherited, has a nonspecific presentation but a classical sandstorm appearance on CXR. Calcium carbonate stones are formed within the alveoli; the differential diagnosis is other forms of pulmonary calcification. Pulmonary fibrosis may develop many years later when the patient becomes symptomatic. A narrative review discusses these unusual problems in greater depth.[383]

THE LUNG AS PART OF A MULTISYSTEM DISORDER

Causes include conditions thought to be autoimmune (scleroderma, systemic lupus erythematosus, rheumatoid disease); inherited conditions (sickle cell disease, Riley–Day syndrome, mucopolysaccharidoses); and those of unknown cause (sarcoidosis, Langerhans' cell histiocytosis, and the disorders of the pulmonary lymphatics).[383] More details on these rare conditions are reviewed elsewhere.[384]

The lung in connective tissue diseases

The lung may be affected as part of a systemic vasculitis, such as Wegener granulomatosis or Churg–Strauss syndrome. Systemic lupus erythematosus may cause a variety of manifestations, including interstitial pneumonitis, obliterative bronchiolitis, respiratory muscle weakness, pulmonary hemorrhage and pleural effusion. Scleroderma is associated with pulmonary fibrosis, and pulmonary hypertension. All these conditions are so rare that referral to a pediatric respiratory center is advisable if they are suspected.

Histiocytosis

Lung involvement is usually part of a multisystem disease in children, but in young adults who smoke it may be confined to the lungs. Presentation is with respiratory distress, or sometimes with acute and non-resolving pneumothorax. CXR shows interstitial changes, and HRCT shows characteristic nodules which cavitate, allowing the diagnosis to be made without recourse to further tests. If in doubt, BAL shows increased numbers of Langerhans' cells, and biopsy is definitive. Treatment is smoking cessation, and sometimes prednisolone or a cytotoxic agent. Multisystem disease requires combination chemotherapy usually with inclusion of vinblastine or etoposide (see Ch. 24). The disease may progress to respiratory failure, and recurs in the transplanted lung.

Sarcoidosis

Pulmonary disease is very rare in children; presentation is more usually with bilateral anterior uveitis, skin rashes and tendon sheath effusions. Diagnosis is on biopsy and is suggested by a high serum level of angiotensin-converting enzyme. Treatment is with steroids, to which may be added hydroxychloroquine and other steroid sparing agents. For refractory cases, a combination of methotrexate and the TNF-alpha blocker etanercept may be considered.

Pulmonary lymphangiomatosis

Pulmonary lymphangiomatosis is a manifestation of a systemic lymphatic malformation which may also affect the spleen, heart and bone. It is usually fatal over 5–7 years, whatever treatment is tried.[385]

Alpha1-antitrypsin deficiency

The fully expressed disease requires two copies of the protease inhibitor (Pi) Z allele, hence PiZZ, and such individuals usually have serum levels of <2mg/ml (<20% of normal). The incidence in Caucasian populations is between 1 in 2000 and 1 in 4000 and the pulmonary manifestations usually present in adult life with emphysema or sometimes bronchiectasis. In childhood, however, it presents as a neonatal hepatitis as the site of production is in the liver (see Ch. 19). Pulmonary disease is usually not evident until late in adolescence. Antitrypsin and other proteases help defend the lung from damage associated with the release of proteases such as elastase released from neutrophils which would otherwise cause digestion of lung interstitial tissue and the subsequent development of emphysema. Children who are known to have this disorder should be advised never to smoke, as smoking is a potent stimulus to protease activity in the lung. Many nonsmokers with this condition remain asymptomatic for many years, but prognosis for pulmonary function is poor in smokers. Replacement therapy with alpha1-antitrypsin is now available.

RARE DISORDERS OF THE BRONCHIOLES

The most distal airways are the physiologically silent areas of the lungs, and are notoriously difficult to investigate. Currently, patchy air trapping in the absence of overt large airways bronchiectasis, best demonstrated with inspiratory and expiratory HRCT, is the best diagnostic pointer.

Obliterative bronchiolitis

Obliterative bronchiolitis (OB) has been described in association with infections caused by adenovirus types 3, 7 and 21; measles, pertussis, influenza A, mycoplasma; after lung transplantation; and secondary to chronic aspiration.[386] Often the cause remains conjectural. The clinical course is one of cough, wheeze and tachypnea in an infant or young child which may be static if the cause is an infection, or progress at a variable rate to respiratory failure and failure to thrive if there is ongoing aspiration. Chest radiography initially shows generalized hyperinflation. HRCT demonstrates patchy air trapping, particularly if the scan is expiratory. Focal hyperlucency involving a lobe or a whole lung represents the radiological appearance of Macleod syndrome, in which the affected lung appears small and hyperlucent. This represents long term damage to lung development, both parenchymal and vascular. HRCT will usually show ipsilateral bronchiectasis, and contralateral, albeit less severe, areas of air trapping. This radiographic appearance should not be confused with other causes of hyperlucency such as hypoplastic pulmonary artery, congenital large hyperlucent lobe (congenital lobar emphysema) or ball valve obstruction to a large airway (see p. 697 – Congenital abnormalities). Radioisotope split lung function studies examining both ventilation and perfusion may help to clarify equivocal radiographic features. In Macleod syndrome the affected lung is small and both poorly perfused and ventilated.

Lung function studies show severe airways obstruction, and, in pure OB, large static lung volumes. Underlying diseases such as cystic fibrosis, immunodeficiency, ciliary dyskinesia and chronic aspiration may need to be ruled out. The main differential diagnosis is fibrosing alveolitis, which should easily be distinguished by HRCT. Management is supportive. Steroids have no proven value. Individuals may find bronchodilators helpful.

The prognosis for OB is most serious after adenoviral disease. Long term oxygen dependency is common.[387] Improvement after 2–3 years may be seen. The condition is usually stable once the initial effects of the devastating infection have burnt out, but some may go on to require lung transplantation. OB developing after lung transplant is eventually fatal, and the results of a second transplantation are very poor.

Follicular bronchiolitis

Follicular bronchiolitis (FB) is part of the spectrum of lymphoid disorders of the lung, which includes lymphoid interstitial pneumonia (LIP). There is a polyclonal expansion of lymphoid tissue, probably part of the bronchus associated lymphoid tissue (BALT), which causes small airways obstruction. Presentation is with chronic respiratory distress, and HRCT demonstrates air trapping, sometimes with associated infiltrates. Such a finding should prompt a full immune work-up, including HIV testing (see Ch. 27). If no immune defect is found, anecdotal evidence suggests that treatment with inhaled steroids and long term macrolide antibiotics (clarithromycin, azithromycin) for their anti-inflammatory effects may be worthwhile.

SPONTANEOUS AIR LEAKS

Air leaks such as pneumothoraces, subcutaneous emphysema and pericardial and mediastinal air are very unusual outside the neonatal period, and are usually seen as a complication of positive pressure ventilation. Children with airways obstruction such as asthma or cystic fibrosis are at relatively higher risk. A spontaneous pneumothorax in a previously healthy child is extremely rare, and more often is a sign of an underlying lung disease than in adults.[388] Apical bullae or an isolated lung cyst are sometimes identified on a chest radiograph or CT scan. Rare causes include pulmonary Langerhans' cell histiocytosis and lung metastases from a primary sarcoma. Presenting features include sudden chest pain and breathlessness. There are reduced breath sounds over the affected side. In the management of a first episode the options are observation alone, simple aspiration or tube drainage with pleurodesis, depending on the size of the pneumothorax and on risk factors such as distance from hospital or future air travel, as well as any underlying disease. In spontaneously breathing children with acute asthma, an air leak may be identified quite unexpectedly on a chest radiograph; the majority resolves without intervention. Pneumothorax in a patient with cystic fibrosis is usually a sign of severe underlying disease and carries a poor prognosis. Treatment should be discussed with the local transplant center, to avoid prejudicing lung transplantion by too aggressive a pleurodesis.

PULMONARY HEMORRHAGIC DISORDERS

The spectrum of these disorders has been reviewed.[389] Idiopathic pulmonary hemosiderosis is characterized pathologically by recurrent alveolar bleeding. Presentation is either as an iron deficiency anemia or with respiratory distress. The anemia may respond to oral iron, and the child has frequently been subjected to numerous invasive gastrointestinal investigations before a CXR is inspected. The respiratory presentation is with tachypnea, cough and sometimes but not invariably, hemoptysis. There may be digital clubbing and crackles, and hepatosplenomegaly in up to 20% of children. Gastric aspirates may be positive for hemosiderin-laden macrophages, and the stools positive for occult blood. CXR may show ground glass opacification, or blotchy shadowing. HRCT may strongly suggest the diagnosis, which may also be confirmed by finding hemosiderin-laden macrophages in BAL fluid; open lung biopsy is rarely necessary. An association with IgD milk antibodies (Heiner syndrome) is in fact rarely if ever seen today. Secondary causes of pulmonary hemorrhage, e.g. pulmonary venous hypertension, must be excluded. Treatment is with hydroxychloroquine,[390] to which prednisolone may need to be added. Relapse is common, and death may be from acute massive bleeding or chronic respiratory failure. Treatment should probably be continued for at least 2 years after the last relapse. Cases apparently resistant to therapy should be referred for open lung biopsy, which may not show the expected normal lung architecture with intra-alveolar blood and hemosiderin-laden macrophages, but a neutrophilic vasculitis. This very rare picture is important to identify as it responds to cyclophosphamide.

PULMONARY VASCULAR DISEASES CHARACTERIZED BY PULMONARY HYPERTENSION

Primary pulmonary hypertension

Primary pulmonary hypertension (PPH) is a diagnosis of exclusion. Presentation is with nonspecific symptoms such as breathlessness and syncope, and the physical signs of pulmonary hypertension (loud pulmonary component of the second heart sound, parasternal heave) may be elicited. Secondary causes such as congenital heart disease are excluded by echocardiography and are discussed in Chapter 21 (p. 765). PPH may be isolated, or inherited as an autosomal dominant disorder, or associated with liver or autoimmune disease, or HIV infection. The gene accounting for some cases of familial PPH has been localized to chromosome 2.[391] Treatment advice is largely based on adult guidelines,[392] which assumes that the adult and pediatric diseases are the same. Possible lines of treatment include oxygen, at least overnight, to maintain normal arterial saturation; anticoagulation; oral pulmonary vasodilators such as the calcium channel antagonists; and, for those rare children who can tolerate it, a continuous intravenous infusion of epoprostenol (prostacyclin, PGI_2). Alternative modes of delivery are preparations that are active orally, by nebulizer, or by subcutaneous infusion. Recently, these patients have been treated with combinations of the selective phosphodiesterase 5 inhibitor, sildenafil; and the endothelin receptor antagonist, Bosentan. Patients with pulmonary hypertension should be referred to specialist centers for consideration of such therapy. If these fail, lung transplantation is the only other option.

Embolic pulmonary hypertension

This presents in a similar manner to PPH. Spiral CT with contrast or angiography may lead to suspicion of the diagnosis by the demonstration of large pulmonary artery filling defects. OLB may be needed to confirm the presence of microemboli. Thromboembolic disease is the commonest cause. It may be a manifestation of an underlying congenital or acquired coagulopathy. Other predisposing factors include immobility, and a sluggish circulation, as for example after a Fontan procedure or secondary to right atrial stasis in dilated cardiomyopathy. Tumor emboli are another cause, with Wilms tumor or hepatoblastoma the commonest primary sources. Talc microemboli should be considered in adolescents who abuse substances intravenously; crushed up injected tablets result in talc microemboli. Worldwide, schistosomal disease must be the commonest cause of nonthrombotic embolic disease.

Pulmonary veno-occlusive disease

This condition presents as chronic pulmonary venous hypertension, with pulmonary edema resistant to diuretics. Cases are usually isolated, but may rarely be familial, or a complication of cytotoxic chemotherapy. Diagnosis may be confirmed at cardiac catheterization or OLB. There is no known effective treatment, and most cases die of severe pulmonary hypertension unless transplanted.

Invasive pulmonary capillary hemangiomatosis

This is due to proliferating sheets of thin walled capillary channels infiltrating blood vessels and causing secondary vascular occlusion. Familial cases have been described. Diagnosis is by OLB, and the condition is usually fatal.

PULMONARY VASCULAR DISEASES CHARACTERIZED BY CYANOSIS WITHOUT PULMONARY HYPERTENSION

Macroscopic pulmonary arteriovenous malformations

Pulmonary arteriovenous malformations (PAVMs) are large malformations which typically present with cyanosis, and sometimes a bruit may be heard over the lung field. There may be an associated cerebral AVM with a bruit heard over the cranium. There is an obvious mass on CXR, and contrast echocardiography or peripheral injection of technetium-labeled albumin microspheres confirms a large intrapulmonary right-to-left shunt. Most such PAVMs consist of a direct connection between the pulmonary arterial and venous circulations, but some also have a systemic arterial supply. Treatment is with transcatheter embolization using a balloon or coil. Untreated, complications include polycythemia, systemic embolization and abscess formation, these last complications being the result of the systemic venous return bypassing the filtration function of the pulmonary capillary bed. Cerebral abscess or embolic stroke are the most feared complications of PAVM.

Microscopic pulmonary arteriovenous malformations

These may be an isolated finding or a manifestation of Osler–Weber–Rendu disease [hereditary hemorrhagic telangiectasia (HHT)], liver disease, or as a complication of some congenital heart diseases. Mutations in two genes leading to Osler–Weber–Rendu disease, ENG (HHT type 1) and ACVRL1 (HHT type 2) have recently been described.[393] Presentation is with cyanosis without respiratory distress, and a clear CXR. There is no treatment other than lung transplantation.

INHERITED DISORDERS OF SURFACTANT PROTEINS

There are four surfactant proteins, lettered A to D. Surfactant proteins A and D are more properly considered as members of the collectin family, with important functions in host defense but with little surface active function. Inherited disorders of proteins B and C, with a respiratory presentation, have been described. Additionally, abnormalities in the ATP-binding cassette transporter (ABCA3) gene cause a similar picture. The lung histology is very variable, and surfactant genetic studies should be considered part of the work-up of the child with an interstitial lung disease.

Congenital surfactant protein B (SpB) deficiency

This condition presents as relentlessly progressive respiratory distress, usually in a term baby.[394] It is inherited as an autosomal recessive disorder. CXR shows a ground glass appearance. Open lung biopsy shows alveoli filled with lipoproteinaceous material, and special stains confirm the absence of SpB. A few mild cases with prolonged survival have been reported. Successful treatment with granulocyte-colony stimulating factor has been reported. If this fails, lung transplantation is the only other option.

Congenital surfactant protein C (SpC) deficiency

SpC deficiency was first described in a woman with an interstitial lung disease, who gave birth to an infant with respiratory distress.[395] The mother subsequently died. Molecular studies established the diagnosis. Some children previously given the diagnosis of CPI and nonspecific interstitial pneumonitis (NSIP) have subsequently been shown to have inherited defects of surfactant proteins.

Congenital ABCA3 deficiency

The intracellular processing of surfactant proteins is very complex, so it is unsurprising that an alveolar proteinosis-like disease can be produced by mutations in genes encoding processing proteins. This is exemplified by ABCA3 deficiency.[396] This protein is confined to lamellar bodies, implying a role in surfactant protein handling.

Pulmonary alveolar proteinosis

Pulmonary alveolar proteinosis (PAP) is characterized histologically by alveoli which are filled with granular, eosinophilic material staining with periodic-acid Schiff, with preservation of lung architecture. Initially, two forms were recognized; 'idiopathic', responding very well to whole lung, large volume lavage, and secondary to conditions associated with functional impairment of the macrophage (such as hematological cancers and some infections). The possible role of granulocyte–macrophage-colony stimulating factor (GM-CSF) in PAP was highlighted when the GM-CSF knockout mouse was found to have a PAP-like illness with normal surfactant synthesis, and with recovery after GM-CSF replacement. Subsequently, late-onset 'idiopathic' PAP was found to be an autoimmune disease, with autoantibodies targeting GM-CSF, or rarely, with a defect in GM-CSF/IL-3/IL-5 receptor common beta chain. Treatment with aerosolized or subcutaneous GM-CSF has been successful in some late-onset cases.[397,398]

In some children PAP may be related to a form of immune deficiency such as thymic atrophy, lymphopenia and immunoglobulin deficiency. CXR shows a ground glass appearance and HRCT a typical cobblestone appearance. Unlike adult PAP, whole lung, large volume lavage is usually only of transient benefit, and the prognosis is very poor.

THORACIC TUMORS

Primary and secondary tumors within the thorax are very rare;[399] even within tertiary specialist pediatric pulmonology practice, thoracic malignancy is usually diagnosed only once or twice a year. Possible presentations include airways compression and stridor; chest wall invasion with either or both of pleuritic chest pain and pleural effusion; systemic symptoms such as fever, malaise and weight loss; or, in the case of a primary tumor, with the effects of secondary systemic disease. The rarity of tumors leads to the very great danger that the possibility is not even considered. Although measurement of catecholamine metabolites, alpha-fetoprotein or beta human gonadotrophin in serum may reveal the diagnosis, surgical biopsy is usually needed. Treatment of all such lesions is the province of the pediatric oncologist (see Ch. 24, p. 1015 for neuroblastoma and p. 1027 for mediastinal tumors).

Benign tumors

These include true benign lesions such as pulmonary hamartomas and pseudotumors, e.g. plasma cell granuloma. Carcinoid tumors present as an endobronchial mass which may bleed profusely if biopsied. Some behave as true malignancies.

Primary malignant lung tumors

Less than 2% of childhood cancers are lung primaries. Endobronchial cancer should at least be considered as a possibility in an otherwise unexplained bronchial obstruction. The intrathoracic sarcomas enter the differential diagnosis of large mass lesions within the chest. Whether intrathoracic lymphoma is a true primary pulmonary malignancy is a matter of semantics; suffice it to say that T-cell lymphoma may present as a rapidly progressive upper airway obstruction. Emergency control of the airway may be necessary to prevent asphyxia.

Metastatic tumors

These usually present in the context of a known primary tumor, most commonly osteo- or other sarcoma, Wilms tumor, germ cell tumors, neuroblastoma or hepatoblastoma. Presentation as pulmonary vascular disease is discussed above. Occasionally metastatic disease is found de novo as multiple round lesions on CXR; the differential diagnosis includes multiple lung abscesses and hydatid disease. Occasionally, pulmonary metastases may be cured surgically; specialist advice should always be sought before recommending such a course.

Mediastinal tumors

These may be benign or malignant, and there is an extensive differential diagnosis. Presentation is with compression of the central airways leading to stridor; compression of the superior caval vein; and as the chance finding of mediastinal widening on the CXR. Although clues as to the likely histology may be obtained from CT and MRI, most lesions will need a surgical biopsy to establish the exact diagnosis (see Ch. 24, p. 1027).

CYSTIC FIBROSIS

EPIDEMIOLOGY

Cystic fibrosis (CF) is the commonest, life-limiting, autosomal recessive disorder of Caucasians. The condition was first described by Dorothy Anderson in 1938. The incidence in the UK is 1 in 2500 live births and approximately 1 in 25 individuals in the general population are carriers for the condition. There are almost 7000 individuals with CF in the UK[400] and an estimated 30 000 in the USA.[401] Survival has improved steadily over the last four decades. Survival curves run nearly parallel after the first year of life, suggesting that much of the increase in life expectancy is due to improvements in care in the first year.[402] Data from the Danish CF clinics (which have some of the best survival figures in the world) show that there is now an 80% chance of a newborn baby with CF reaching his/her 45th birthday.[403] Survival after infancy is consistently worse in girls with CF than it is in boys.[404] The reasons for this are not clear. The incidence of CF is lower in the black population in the USA (1 in 15 000 live births).[405] CF is seen in the Asian community in the UK and there is a more severe clinical phenotype in this group.[406]

PATHOGENESIS

CF is caused by an abnormality in a protein, known as the cystic fibrosis transmembrane conductance regulator (CFTR). This protein is a cyclic AMP (cAMP)-dependent chloride channel. In the lung, the protein is located on the apical membrane of respiratory epithelial cells. When CFTR function is impaired, chloride ions cannot pass from the cell cytoplasm into the airway surface liquid layer. This defect in the chloride channel is accompanied by overactivity of the epithelial sodium channel (EnaC) with the passage of sodium ions into the cell cytoplasm. These ion transport abnormalities together lead to a reduction in salt levels in the airway surface liquid and the loss of water from this layer by osmosis. This reduces the thickness of the airway surface liquid layer. The cilia can no longer beat freely because they have become entangled in the raft of mucus and particulate matter which forms the mucociliary escalator (Fig. 20.25). Consequently the mucociliary escalator does not function. Mucus plugging of small airways occurs, bacterial organisms in the lower respiratory tract are no longer cleared and secondary bacterial infection occurs. This leads to the release of inflammatory cytokines such as IL-8 and neutrophil driven inflammation. The cycle

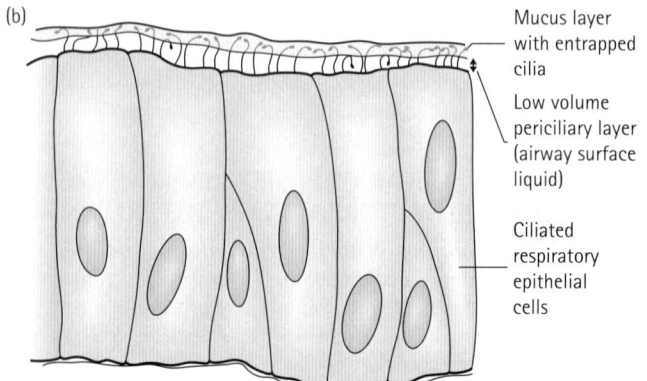

Fig. 20.25   (a) The normal mucociliary escalator with normal airway surface liquid volume. (b) In CF the airway surface liquid layer is diminished and the cilia become entrapped in the mucus layer, preventing the cilia from beating in a coordinated fashion.

of infection, inflammation and lung damage eventually leads to permanent dilatation of the subsegmental airways or bronchiectasis. Severe bronchiectasis can ultimately lead to death from respiratory failure. In the upper airway, abnormalities of CFTR, leading to impaired mucociliary clearance, can lead to chronic sinusitis and the formation of nasal polyps.

The effects of abnormal CFTR are not only seen in the respiratory tract. In the normal sweat gland, salt is removed from sweat in the sweat duct, resulting in sweat which is low in salt. In CF this does not occur because of a failure of CFTR function and excessively salty sweat is produced. This is the basis of the sweat test (see below). Abnormalities of CFTR in intestinal epithelial cells result in thick sticky meconium and meconium ileus in the newborn infant with CF. In the pancreas, the pancreatic duct cells are responsible for the production of bicarbonate rich fluid, which dilutes the pancreatic enzymes, produced by the acinar cells. The defect in CFTR impairs water secretion into the pancreatic duct by interfering with chloride–bicarbonate exchange.[407] These thick secretions block the pancreatic ducts, leading to back pressure and destruction of the acinar cells, pancreatic enzyme deficiency and malabsorption. With increasing age, destruction of the pancreatic islet cells also occurs, leading to CF-related diabetes (CFRD). In the liver, CFTR dysfunction in the intra- and extra-hepatic bile ducts leads to bile which has increased viscosity and is depleted in bicarbonate. This leads to obstruction of the ducts and to focal biliary cirrhosis. What is not clear is why the process should be focal, if it affects bile ducts throughout the liver, and why not all patients with CF develop liver disease.[408] In males, CFTR dysfunction leads to absence of the vas deferens and male infertility.

There has been some debate over whether pulmonary inflammation in CF is the result of infection or whether CF itself is a pro-inflammatory condition. Where bronchoscopy and BAL have been performed in infants as young as 3 months with CF, a high proportion (31%) have been found to have lower respiratory tract infection with *Staphylococcus aureus*. In contrast, samples from non-CF control infants did not show significant levels of bacterial pathogens. Levels of IL-8 were high in infants with infection but not in controls or in non-infected CF infants, suggesting that infection is the most important driver of inflammation.[409] The CF airway shows inflammatory dysregulation, with the same amount of bacterial endotoxin leading to significantly more IL-8 release and neutrophil infiltration.[410]

GENETICS

The gene for CFTR is located on the long arm of chromosome 7. The commonest gene mutation is termed delta F508 and results in the loss of a phenylalanine residue at position 508 in the first nucleotide binding fold of CFTR (Fig. 20.26).[411] Over 50% of individuals with CF are homozygous for the delta F508 and, in the UK, over 90% will have at least one copy of delta F508. However, more than 1000 different mutations of the CF gene have been identified. Some (termed 'dominant mild mutations') seem to confer a milder phenotype when they occur as compound heterozygotes with delta F508. Mutations of the CF gene can cause a number of distinct defects of CFTR, which are categorized as follows:[412]

- *Class I:* a defect in protein synthesis and no production of CFTR. In the mutation W1282X, the mutant allele has a stop codon which prevents full transcription of mRNA. Some drugs such as gentamicin show promise in preventing this premature termination of translation.
- *Class II:* trafficking defects (includes delta F508). Misfolded CFTR is produced which does not leave the endoplasmic reticulum.
- *Class III:* CFTR is present in the apical membrane but there is a defect of regulation, e.g. G551D where CFTR in the apical membrane does not respond to elevated cAMP.
- *Class IV* (e.g. R117H): CFTR is present in the membrane but does not conduct chloride ions normally.
- *Class V:* Low levels of CFTR are produced or there is a defect of mRNA splicing, e.g. 5T or 7T thymidine tract variant (see below).

The class IV mutation R117H may occur on the same chromosome as either the 5T or 7T thymidine tract variant of intron 8. (The intron represents 'redundant DNA'.) The number of thymidine residues in intron 8 will affect the splicing (removal of bases) of exon 9 (functional DNA) when transcription takes place to form mRNA. Individuals with R117H and 5T on the same chromosome will have a mild CF phenotype whereas 7T is associated with congenital bilateral absence of the vas deferens alone.

The dominant mild mutations are mainly class IV or V. Patients with class IV and V defects have a lower mortality and a milder phenotype than patients who are homozygous for delta F508.[413] Patients with R117H are more likely to be pancreatic sufficient.[414] It is clear that 100% CFTR function is not essential for health as heterozygote carriers do not have clinical manifestations of CF and these individuals express only 50% of normal CFTR. It is thought that CFTR expression of > 10% of normal may result in a normal clinical phenotype.[413]

There are great differences in the severity of lung disease, even in individuals who are homozygous for delta F508. This may be due to environmental differences such as viral infection in early life, passive smoking exposure or social deprivation. However, it has been suggested that a number of other genes can act to modify the severity of mutations of the CF gene. A recent study has looked at the effects of polymorphisms in 10 candidate modifier genes in a large sample of CF patients, with a second validation study in a separate large population.[415] This has implicated polymorphisms in the transforming growth factor beta1 (TGF-beta1) gene in more severe lung disease in both delta F508 homozygotes and patients with other genotypes. TGF-beta1 is a signal molecule which influences cell growth and differentiation, inflammation and the immune response. In contrast to its association with more severe disease in CF, it is linked to milder disease in chronic obstructive pulmonary disease.

MICROBIOLOGY

As mentioned above, pulmonary infection with *S. aureus* occurs in early life in individuals with CF. In older children, other organisms, such as *Haemophilus influenzae*, are found more frequently. By the late teens the majority of CF patients in the UK will have pulmonary infection with *Pseudomonas aeruginosa*.[400] Patients with CF who are homozygous for the delta F508 mutation appear to be hypersusceptible to pulmonary infection with *P. aeruginosa*, due to increased adherence of the organisms to respiratory epithelial cells.[416] Initially the organism is present in the respiratory tract in its free living or planktonic form. However, *P. aeruginosa* has the ability to form bacterial communities or biofilms in the lungs. In the biofilm the organisms are surrounded by an exopolymeric substance, rich in alginate, and can communicate by means of signal molecules, which control the expression of virulence factors. In this form *P. aeruginosa* is protected from neutrophil phagocytosis and from the actions of

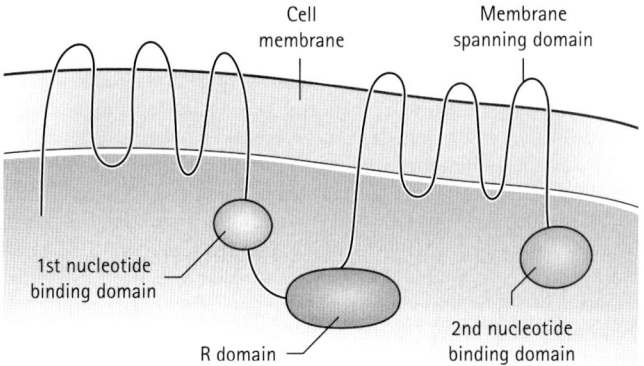

Fig. 20.26 Schematic diagram of the CFTR showing the two nucleotide binding domains. The delta F508 mutation is due to deletion of a phenylalanine residue in the first nucleotide binding domain.

antibiotics. The biofilm mode of growth ensures that some organisms will always persist after antibiotic treatment and hence there is selective pressure, favoring the emergence of antibiotic resistance. Furthermore, resistant organisms can be transmitted between patients.[417] A much less common, but clinically important, group of pathogens in CF patients is the *Burkholderia cepacia* complex – a group of environmental organisms which have found a niche in the CF lung. They are highly antibiotic resistant and are transmissible between patients. Acquisition of *B. cepacia* complex is associated with a more rapid deterioration in lung function and increased mortality.[418]

DIAGNOSIS

The diagnosis of CF is based on the presence of phenotypic features of CF, a history of CF in a sibling or a positive screening test plus evidence of CFTR abnormality, as shown by an abnormal sweat chloride, two mutations in the CFTR gene known to cause CF or abnormal nasal potential difference.[419] The sweat test is the most commonly used test of CFTR function and detailed guidelines are available, describing the correct procedure for the test.[420] The sweat test should not be performed on infants who are < 7 days old; who weigh < 3 kg; in children who are systemically unwell or who have eczema or edema. Sweat production is stimulated by means of pilocarpine iontophoresis and sweat is collected on a piece of sodium-free filter paper, under an occlusive dressing. The amount of sweat collected should equate to $1 g/m^2/min$ and the usual collection period is 30 min. This is then analyzed for seat chloride and sodium concentration. A sweat chloride of > 60 mmol/L supports the diagnosis of CF and a chloride of < 40 mmol/L is normal. Values of 40–60 mmol/L are suggestive of CF but are not diagnostic. There are variations on this technique, such as capillary duct systems, which also produce reliable results.

Newborn screening

There has been controversy over whether CF meets the criteria for a screening program, particularly over whether early intervention affects the natural history of the disease. In a pivotal study, Farrell et al described a controlled trial, conducted over 9 years and involving over 650 000 newborn infants.[421] Infants with an abnormal screening test (initially trypsinogen and subsequently trypsinogen and DNA) were recalled for sweat testing only if their specimen number ended in an odd digit. When children in the control group reached the age of 4 years, a sweat test was performed on those who had not been diagnosed clinically beforehand. The outcomes in children in the early screening group and the control group were compared. A significantly greater proportion of children in the screened group were homozygous for delta F508 and were pancreatic insufficient. However, the children in the early screening group had better nutrition at diagnosis and this was maintained over a 10 year follow-up period, as measured by weight and height centiles. Screening is also associated with an improvement in cognitive function, thought to be related to earlier treatment of vitamin E deficiency.[422] However, screened children acquired chronic pulmonary infection with *P. aeruginosa* significantly earlier than the control group.[423] The investigators attributed this to inadequate precautions against cross-infection. From 10 years onward, the CXR scores were significantly worse in the early screening group and this was partly explained by *P. aeruginosa* status.

Newborn screening has been practiced in parts of the UK for many years. However since 2007, the screening program has been extended to all of the UK.[424] The protocol, which will be used throughout the UK, initially uses an immune reactive trypsin (IRT) measurement on a dried blood spot collected on day 5. Trypsin is raised in blood of newborn infants with CF as a result of pancreatic exocrine failure. Where the IRT test is positive (> 99.5 centile) the sample is tested against a panel of CF gene mutations. This may identify two genes, in which case the child is referred with a presumptive diagnosis of CF. If one gene is identified or none but the initial IRT is very high (i.e. > 99.9 centile), then a repeat IRT is performed at between 21 and 28 days. The cut-off for this sample is set lower than those used earlier in the process and infants are referred with a 'high likelihood of CF' if their IRT value is above the cut-off.

Genetic counseling

When an infant is diagnosed as having CF, the parents should be offered genetic counseling. The timing of this may be difficult. When their baby is first diagnosed, parents will have to cope with the demands of a new baby and the therapeutic burden of CF care, and they may not want to see the genetics team right away. However, some couples will wish to have another child after a short interval and it is important to offer the opportunity of genetic counseling before the next pregnancy. In contrast to carriers identified by antenatal screening (see below), parents who already have a child with CF are less likely to have antenatal testing in a subsequent pregnancy.[425] Of those who do, fewer opt for a termination. There may be other family members who may be CF carriers and are also contemplating pregnancy, and antenatal screening can be offered to these couples ('cascade screening').

Antenatal screening

Although newborn screening is now offered throughout the UK, there has been no population-based implementation of antenatal screening. There are two possible approaches to screening in pregnancy, where there is no family history of CF: 'stepwise' and 'couple' screening. With stepwise screening a genetic test for CF is offered to women attending the antenatal booking clinic (usually before 17 weeks' gestation). If she is shown to be a carrier, then her partner is offered testing. With couple screening, samples are taken from both partners at the same time. The stepwise approach has the disadvantage that a woman will experience unnecessary anxiety, while awaiting the result of her partner's test, if she has been found to be a carrier and her partner subsequently is shown not to be a carrier.[426] However, if couple screening is offered, either the man must attend with his partner or a DNA sample must be provided by post. The uptake for antenatal screening is between 70 and 90%. If both partners are identified as carriers the risk of CF in the fetus is 1 in 4. In the first trimester the diagnosis can be made in the fetus by chorion villus biopsy or, after 12 weeks, by amniocentesis or placental biopsy. Each of these procedures carries a risk of miscarriage. Where an antenatal screening program is in place, the uptake of a diagnostic test on the fetus by high risk couples is high (> 90%). Where CF is diagnosed in the fetus, most couples opt for termination.[427] Where antenatal screening has been practiced, there has been a 65% reduction in the birth incidence of CF.[428] Antenatal diagnosis may also be made following abnormal appearances on fetal ultrasound (see below).

CLINICAL FEATURES
Meconium ileus

Meconium ileus is acute small bowel obstruction in a newborn infant due to sticky meconium. It occurs in about 15% of infants with CF. Increasingly the diagnosis is suspected antenatally, because of the finding of echogenic bowel on detailed ultrasound, which confers a risk of CF in the fetus of around 3%.[429] Where bowel dilation is also present, the risk increases to 17%. Genotyping of the parents and the fetus (following amniocentesis) may allow the diagnosis of CF to be made antenatally (where two CF genes are identified in the fetus) or a more precise estimate of the risk of CF in the fetus (where only one gene is found). In some cases meconium ileus will progress to perforation in utero, with abdominal calcification on the plain abdominal radiograph at birth. Where the diagnosis is not made antenatally, the infant may fail to pass meconium in the first 24 h and develops progressive signs of small bowel obstruction. Appropriate supportive care is essential. A nasogastric tube should be passed, hypovolemia should be managed with appropriate fluid replacement and any electrolyte imbalance corrected. In some cases, a hydrostatic reduction of meconium ileus can be achieved by means of a contrast enema. This may reveal an associated microcolon (Fig. 20.27). However, in most cases surgical reduction is unavoidable, with either an ileostomy or a primary anastomosis. Prolonged periods of total parenteral nutrition should be avoided because of the associated cholestasis.

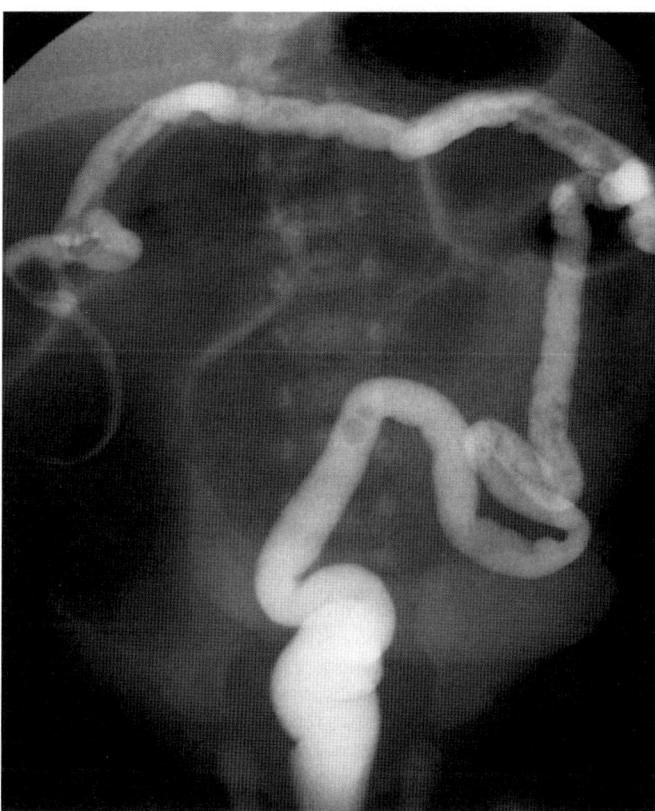

Fig. 20.27 A contrast enema in an infant with meconium ileus showing microcolon. Contrast would not pass beyond the ascending colon and the terminal ileum is not visible. The diagnosis was suspected antenatally due to bowel dilatation. Placental biopsy at 22 weeks showed that the fetus was homozygous for delta F508.

Infants who present with meconium ileus are at greater risk of subsequent CF-related liver disease, poor nutrition (at 13 years)[430] and worse lung function (at 8–10 years).[431]

Gastrointestinal features outside the neonatal period

In many parts of the world, the diagnosis of CF is made through newborn screening programs and so it is now uncommon to see infants with CF presenting with severe failure to thrive as a result of pancreatic malabsorption. Similarly, complications such as rectal prolapse are uncommon in a screened population. Infants with CF have a lower birth weight and, in early infancy, the mean weight is more than one standard deviation below normal.[432] Catch-up growth is seen in the first year, although the mean weight remains below the population mean. Infants diagnosed by newborn screening are in a better nutritional state at diagnosis and remain so over a 10 year follow-up period.[421] Much of this benefit is attributed to instituting pancreatic enzyme supplementation, a high calorie diet and supplements of fat soluble vitamins early in life. Vitamin E deficiency causes hemolytic anemia in around 4% of infants with CF.[433] There are reports of both vitamin A deficiency (with xerophthalmia or poor dark adaptation) and hypervitaminosis (as a result of vitamin A supplementation) in CF.

Nutrition in children with CF depends on the balance between energy expenditure and energy intake. Resting energy expenditure in CF can be up to 150% of that seen in unaffected individuals.[434] Much of this increased energy requirement is due to the chronic inflammatory response and energy requirements are increased further during pulmonary exacerbations. Energy intake may be compromised by vomiting, related to coughing or swallowed sputum; gastroesophageal reflux, anorexia or abnormal eating behavior. Malabsorption due to failure of pancreatic exocrine function can be exacerbated by loss of bile salts in the gut, previous small bowel resection (related to meconium ileus), lack

of pancreatic bicarbonate secretion and decreased small bowel pH, liver disease and CFRD.

Distal intestinal obstruction syndrome occurs when the terminal ileum and ascending colon become blocked with fecal material, high in fat. The condition may be brought on by inadequate dosing or poor adherence to pancreatic enzyme supplements and reduced fluid intake or hot weather. Clinically there is intermittent abdominal pain which may progress to intestinal obstruction with abdominal distention and constipation. Vomiting is a late feature and it is important to intervene before this occurs. A mass may be palpable in the right iliac fossa. Mild symptoms may be treated with a simple laxative such as lactulose. For more severe obstruction, treatment with the oral radiological contrast medium gastrograffin may result in the passage of stool and the relief of symptoms. Where this fails, surgical management may be necessary, but this should be avoided where possible.

In the early 1990s, a group of CF patients, presenting with intestinal obstruction, was found to have a histologically distinct form of bowel disease, characterized by mucosal and submucosal fibrosis. This new entity was termed fibrosing colonopathy. A subsequent case control study demonstrated a relationship between the dosage of high strength pancreatic enzyme supplements and the risk of colonopathy.[435] This led to a recommendation by the UK Committee on Safety of Medicines that the dose of any enzyme preparation should be restricted to no more than 10 000 lipase units/kg/d.[436]

Respiratory features

Cough is an unusual symptom in infants under 4 weeks old and its presence should alert the clinician to the possibility of underlying disease such as CF, primary ciliary dyskinesia or immune deficiency. Wheezing (which is usually persistent rather than intermittent) may be a presenting symptom of CF in the young infant or toddler. In areas where there is newborn screening, it is unusual for children to present with features of advanced chest disease such as chronic productive cough, chest deformity or finger clubbing.

In children with an established diagnosis of CF, the objective is to minimize respiratory symptoms and allow full attendance at school and participation in physical activity. Many children will be symptom free when well. Pulmonary exacerbations (see below) are periods when respiratory symptoms appear in a previously well patient or worsen in children who already have chronic symptoms. These exacerbations are associated with a deterioration in quality of life[437] and reduced life expectancy.[438]

Children who have a productive cough frequently have blood stained sputum or small hemoptyses. These are thought to be due to a localized area of infection eroding a small bronchial vessel. They are managed by treating the underlying infection. Rarely, there may be severe, uncontrolled bleeding into the airway, with life threatening airways obstruction and hypovolemia. A major hemoptysis is defined as bleeding of more than 240 ml in 24 h or 100 ml/d over several days.[439] This complication affects around 1% of patients per year with the vast majority occurring in patients over 16 years. Children who have a major hemoptysis will need high flow face mask oxygen and may require intubation and ventilation. Where there are signs of hypovolemic shock, vigorous fluid resuscitation and blood transfusion are essential. Blood should be sent urgently for hemoglobin, platelets, clotting and group and save. Where the child is shocked, type specific uncross-matched blood can be given to avoid delay. Clotting abnormalities should be corrected. Rigid bronchoscopy may allow the bleeding point to be identified. Definitive treatment through bronchial artery embolization is usually successful, though resection of the segment of lung containing the bleeding vessel may be necessary in some cases.

Similarly, spontaneous pneumothorax occurs in around 1% of CF patients per year, with the incidence increasing with age and severity of lung disease.[440] Pneumothorax may be asymptomatic, being detected on a routine CXR, or may cause chest pain and respiratory distress. If the pneumothorax is < 20% of the volume of the affected hemithorax, or if the patient is asymptomatic, then conservative treatment with

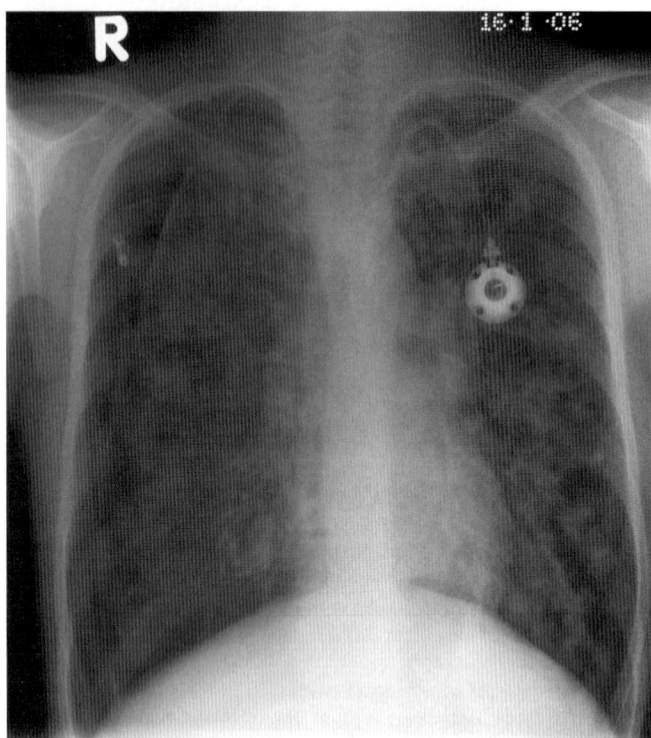

Fig. 20.28 Chest radiograph of an 18 year old with CF showing a right-sided pneumothorax and a chest drain in situ. There is underlying severe bronchiectasis and an indwelling intravenous access device.

face mask oxygen is appropriate. If not, a chest drain should be inserted (Fig. 20.28). A small diameter drain will be more comfortable for the child, may cause fewer adhesions and can be inserted using the less invasive Seldinger technique. Adhesions are commonly seen in patients who have had chest drainage for pneumothorax but do no preclude the possibility of lung transplantation.[441] Underwater drainage is maintained until the drain has stopped bubbling and a CXR has shown the lung to be re-inflated, whereupon the drain is removed. Pneumothorax which persists in spite of adequate chest drainage or recurs may require pleurodesis.

Liver disease (see also Ch. 19)
The hallmark of CF-related liver disease is focal biliary fibrosis. This may progress to multilobular biliary cirrhosis and portal hypertension. Cirrhosis or advanced fibrosis is seen in about 10% of patients who undergo liver biopsy.[441] The peak incidence is before or at puberty, and it is uncommon for previously unaffected adults with CF to develop liver disease. Meconium ileus and pancreatic insufficiency are risk factors for the later development of liver disease. There is no genotype–phenotype correlation with CF liver disease.

In the neonatal period, cholestatic jaundice may be seen in CF, though this is rare. Gall stones or biliary sludge are usually an incidental finding on routine ultrasound. The diagnosis of CF liver disease is frequently made late. Liver function as measured by transaminase levels are an insensitive test for CF liver disease. Children with liver disease usually develop hepatomegaly but this may be confused with a liver which is palpable as a result of air trapping in the chest and downward displacement of the diaphragm. Parenchymal changes on liver ultrasound are often noted when the diagnosis of CF is first made. Liver disease may progress to portal hypertension and splenomegaly, with thrombocytopenia. Esophageal varices can occur, leading to life threatening upper gastrointestinal bleeding. The enlarged liver and spleen can lead to pressure on the diaphragm, in turn leading to retention of secretions and mucus plugging in the lower lobes.

Some clinicians would start treatment in the presence of mild liver abnormalities on ultrasound or persistently raised transaminase levels. Ursodeoxycholic acid is a soluble bile acid which improves the flow of bile. One study has demonstrated that it improves biliary excretion in CF[441a]. However, although lifelong therapy is recommended, once significant liver disease has been shown, there is no evidence that ursodeoxycholic acid improves long term outcomes such as nutrition, death or the need for liver transplantation.[442] Patients with liver disease are usually given vitamin K supplements in an effort to reverse clotting abnormalities. Banding of eosphageal varices and transjugular intrahepatic portasystemic shunting (TIPS procedure) are temporizing measures in patients with portal hypertension, which may prevent upper gastrointestinal bleeding. Patients who do bleed should be managed with high flow oxygen, correction of hypovolemia, transfusion and correction of clotting abnormalities. In addition to these general resuscitative measures, an intravenous infusion of octreotide is indicated. Octreotide is a somatostatin analog which reduces variceal bleeding by reducing the pressure in the portal vein. Liver transplantation is the only definitive treatment for cirrhosis and portal hypertension associated with CF liver disease.

Diabetes
In the USA, 16% of patients with CF have CFRD.[401] The prevalence increases with age, rising to almost 30% of adults with CF. In the UK, the figure is 1% for the under 5s rising to 12% by the late teens.[400] Girls are affected more frequently as are patients with pancreatic insufficiency.[443] Patients with CFRD also have more severe lung disease, more frequent pulmonary exacerbations and poorer nutritional status.

As there is often residual islet cell function, the onset may be insidious and frank polyuria and polydipsia may be absent. CFRD should be suspected in any patient with an unexplained decline in pulmonary function or weight loss not responding to nutritional support. An annual oral glucose tolerance test is recommended as part of the annual assessment in patients over the age of 12 years.[444] CFRD is characterized by post-prandial hyperglycemia more frequently than by fasting hyperglycemia.

Most patients benefit from treatment with insulin, though often a once daily, long acting insulin analog such as glargine can be used alone, to aid adherence. In patients who cannot or will not take insulin, then the oral hypoglycemic agent repaglinide (which stimulates the release of insulin from the remaining islet cells) can be used but is less effective than insulin.[445]

Low bone mineral density
Over half of young patients with CF have reduced bone mineral density.[446] This is associated with poor lung function, treatment with oral corticosteroids and CF liver disease. In CF the increase which normally takes place in bone mass in adolescence is inadequate and puberty may be delayed, leading to reduced bone mineral density in adulthood.[447] This can in turn lead to an increased incidence of fractures, particularly vertebral compression fractures and rib fractures.

Good nutritional care is essential to allow the physiological increase in bone mass to take place in adolescence. (A quarter of adult bone mass is acquired during the pubertal growth spurt.) Thorough dietary assessment should be undertaken to ensure good intake of energy and calcium. Vitamin D levels should be measured annually (preferably in the autumn) and vitamin D supplemented if levels are low. Adolescents should have regular pubertal assessment as part of their annual assessment. Dual energy X-ray absorptiometry (DEXA) scanning should be considered for adolescents at risk of bone disease. DEXA scanning measures bone mineral content/unit bone area and so must be corrected for height and age. Although a recent trial has demonstrated the effectiveness of the antiresorptive agent alendronate in adults with reduced bone mineral density,[448] this indication is not licensed in children and adolsescents.

Salt depletion
Salt depletion in young children with CF was first reported by Di Sant'Agnese in 1953 following a New York heat wave.[449] Di Sant'Agnese

attributed this to loss of salt in sweat and described abnormal sweat electrolyte concentrations. Salt depletion may be associated with other biochemical abnormalities which constitute pseudo-Bartter syndrome (a combination of hypochloremic, hyponatremic dehydration, with metabolic alkalosis and hypokalaemia) (see Ch. 18, p. 554). Salt supplements should be prescribed for children with CF during periods of prolonged hot weather. In young children oral rehydration solution is a suitable salt supplement.

Other complications

Children with CF may have transient flitting joint pain. This is caused by a nondestructive arthritis, thought to be related to immune complex formation. It usually responds to simple analgesic or anti-inflammatory treatment. It should be distinguished from hypertrophic pulmonary osteoarthropathy in patients with severe supportive lung disease and marked finger clubbing.

TREATMENT

Parents of a baby diagnosed as having CF will have to cope with the anxiety for their child's future wellbeing, the practical demands of caring for an infant with CF (such as achieving good nutrition and giving chest physiotherapy), and the 'ordinary' stresses of coping with a young infant (sleep deprivation and social isolation). Where the diagnosis has been made by newborn screening, the parents may have had no prior inkling that their baby had a medical problem. It is therefore important to introduce CF therapy in a stepwise fashion to avoid imposing an excessive initial burden of care.

Nutritional management

Nutrition must be the first priority. Approximately 83% of infants identified by newborn screening will be pancreatic insufficient.[421] At the first visit, a test for pancreatic insufficiency should be performed, such as stool pancreatic elastase. Even where the genotype is almost invariably associated with pancreatic insufficiency (such as infants homozygous for delta F508) there are exceptions. In spite of early diagnosis through screening, infants may have signs of nutritional deficiency. A mean weight Z score of −0.5 was found at the time of diagnosis in the screened group in one study, with around two thirds of screened infants having vitamin E deficiency and one third vitamin A deficiency.[421]

The use of pancreatic enzyme replacement therapy (PERT) in an enteric coated microsphere formulation has revolutionized the nutritional management of children with CF. These formulations are resistant to gastric acid and therefore much more effective in reducing pancreatic malabsorption. Capsules may be opened and the granules administered to infants, mixed with a small amount of apple pureé or fromage frais. Approximately 2500 U of lipase/100 ml of milk is a suitable starting dose. Mothers should be encouraged to breast-feed if they wish to do so and breast-feeding infants with CF has nutritional, immunological and psychological advantages. The dosage of PERT in breast-fed infants is as above, given with each breast-feed. Initially, infants should be reviewed very 1–2 weeks to ensure good weight gain and to troubleshoot any problems with enzyme replacement. Once steady weight gain has been achieved the interval between appointments is gradually extended, to

approximately every 8 weeks. The dose of PERT is gradually increased as the infants grows, with the weight gain and stool appearance used as a guide as to whether an effective dose is being given.

Supplements of the fat soluble vitamins A and E should be introduced early on. Vitamin A can be administered as a liquid multivitamin formulation such as Abidec®. A suitable dose for a preschool child is 0.6 ml once daily. For vitamin E supplementation, alpha tocopheryl in a 100 mg/ml suspension is suitable and 50 mg (0.5 ml) should be administered once daily.

Specific dietary advice will be needed at the time of weaning and parents may need support when the child reaches the toddler age group, when difficult eating behavior is common. Parents of young children with CF may feel very guilty when their child refuses to eat. Giving in to 'toddler blackmail' may lead to more difficult behavioral problems later on and sometimes a period of indifferent weight gain must be accepted at this age. Most school-aged children will be able to swallow pancreatic enzymes as capsules and this will increase their effectiveness in overcoming pancreatic malabsorption. Maximal doses of lipase should not exceed 10 000 U/kg (see p. 709 – Gastrointestinal features outside the neonatal period).

There is controversy regarding the best way of monitoring growth in children, with some units using body mass index (BMI) and others percentage weight for height. Although the absolute value for BMI is useful in adults, normal values in children change with age and the results should be recorded on a centile chart. Percentage weight for height has the disadvantage that children whose height is restricted by poor nutrition (nutritional stunting) may appear to have a near normal percentage weight for height. Current recommendations for nutritional intervention in CF are based on percentage weight for height[451] and are summarized in Table 20.16.

Where children with CF are failing to grow there should be a thorough re-evaluation of the child's condition, looking specifically for the following factors:

- *Non-adherence to diet or enzyme supplements.* In the parents of young children (who adhere to treatment plans on behalf of their child) this may be due to a lack of a full understanding of CF or due to difficult social circumstances. Make sure that explanations have been given with the help of an interpreter where the parents' first language is not English, and that illiteracy is not the reason for poor understanding. Social support and welfare advice should be followed and, where there is clearly neglect, local child protection procedures should be followed (see Ch 5). School-aged children may not take their enzymes with their school lunch because of teasing or because they do not wish other pupils to know about their CF. Teenagers may be non-adherent because they are asserting their independence – support the young person (and their parents) through the process of transition. Consider the possibility of an eating disorder in this age group.
- *Comorbidity.* Poor weight gain may be the first sign of evolving CFRD. Children may lose weight acutely during a pulmonary exacerbation. Gastroesophageal reflux is more frequent in children with CF.
- *Inadequate enzyme dosage or action.* The dose of enzyme supplements prescribed should be carefully reviewed. An upper dosage limit of

Table 20.16 Levels of nutritional deficiency with appropriate nutritional support

Percentage weight for height (0–18 years)	Body mass index (> 18 years)	Action
90–110%	19–25	Routine support and advice
85–89% or weight loss for 4 months (< 5 years) or 6 months (5–18 years) or weight static for 6 months	< 19 or 5% weight loss over > 2 months	Refer to dietitian and consider supplements
< 85% or falling two centiles and no response to supplements	< 19 or 5% weight loss over > 2 months and no response to supplements	Vigorous nutritional support

10 000 U/kg has been recommended by the Committee on Safety of Medicines to reduce the risk of fibrosing colonopathy.[436] Fat-based dosing may give better control of malabsorption.[450] Enzymes work most effectively when taken before and during meals. Enzyme supplements may be inactivated in children with CF because the duodenum is relatively acid, due to the lack of bicarbonate in pancreatic secretions. This can be overcome by prescribing a proton pump inhibitor such as omeprazole.

Where each of these factors has been considered and addressed, nutritional supplements should be considered if appropriate. A recent study of oral calorie supplements has shown that the use of supplements over a 1 year period does not improve nutrition (as measured by BMI centile).[451] However, supplements may have a role in short term supplementation.

Where there is severe nutritional failure, then nasogastric tube or gastrostomy feeding is indicated. Nasogastric tubes are unsightly for older children. They may be passed in the evening for an overnight feed and removed in the morning but this approach suits relatively few children. 'Button type' gastrostomies are more popular than the traditional gastrostomy tube as they cannot be seen under clothing. A gastrostomy can be inserted endoscopically, in which case a tube is inserted initially and a second procedure under anesthetic is usually needed to change to a button. A gastrostomy button can be inserted as a single procedure using a laparoscopic technique. In most cases a polymeric rather than an elemental feed is appropriate. Overnight feeds are often most convenient, though smaller boluses can be given during the day. For overnight feeds, enzyme doses should be divided with half given before the feed starts and the remainder given in the morning. Care must be taken to ensure the gastrostomy is a good fit to avoid leakage of gastric juice and irritation of the surrounding skin. Conversely, children who put on weight rapidly may find that the gastrostomy becomes 'buried' in subcutaneous fat. With any form of overnight feeding, vomiting due to sputum swallowed overnight can be a problem during pulmonary exacerbations. In these circumstances the feed volume should be reduced or the feed temporarily stopped. The volume is then gradually increased once antibiotics and physiotherapy have begun to take effect.

Chest physiotherapy

Chest physiotherapy, aimed at the clearance of airway secretions, is recommended for all children with CF from diagnosis. For young infants twice daily chest physiotherapy, using percussion and postural drainage, has previously been recommended. Recently, practice has changed, as newborn screening has become more widespread, and babies rarely have chest symptoms at diagnosis. Currently once daily physiotherapy is recommended for young children who are asymptomatic, with therapy given more frequently if the child develops a cough or appears chesty. Parents are taught to perform chest physiotherapy on their children shortly after diagnosis. There is an urgent need for a large, well designed RCT of chest physiotherapy for infants with CF diagnosed by newborn screening. A systematic review which looked at cross-over studies of physiotherapy techniques, has shown that physiotherapy increases clearance of secretions from the airway in CF.[452] There is evidence that percussion and postural drainage is associated with gastroesophageal reflux in infants and some authorities recommend modified chest physiotherapy for infants with CF where the child is not 'tipped'.[453]

As children mature and become more independent, they should be encouraged to use physiotherapy techniques which do not need to be administered by an adult. There are a number of approaches and the technique selected should be tailored to the individual. Techniques include: active cycle of breathing, autogenic drainage, positive end expiratory pressure and oscillatory techniques. There appears to be no difference in outcome when conventional physiotherapy is compared to these contemporary techniques and patients often prefer the more independent approach. Both conventional chest physiotherapy and airway clearance techniques are associated with improved lung function

during exacerbations.[454] It is sensible to combine physiotherapy with physical exercise as this introduces a fun element for younger children (trampolines and dance mats) and improves wellbeing in young people.

Treatment of pulmonary infection

As noted above (see p. 707 – Microbiology), pulmonary infection occurs in young infants with CF, initially with S. aureus. In order to interrupt the cycle of infection, inflammation and lung damage which leads to bronchiectasis, some CF centers recommend prophylactic antistaphylococcal antibiotics from first diagnosis. There are marked international variations in the use of prophylactic antibiotics. In the UK prophylaxis is recommended in national guidelines[455] whereas, in contrast, in the USA prophylaxis has been discouraged because a RCT found an association with acquisition of P. aeruginosa.[456] A subsequent Cochrane review has found that prophylaxis is associated with fewer isolates of S. aureus from respiratory secretions when given continuously for the first 3 years of life[457] and with no significant association with P. aeruginosa. However, there are few data on the use of prophylaxis beyond 3 years of age and longer term data are required in order to resolve this issue. In children over the age of 3 years, intermittent infection with S. aureus or with other organisms such as H. influenzae should be treated with an appropriate course of oral antibiotics. Similarly, children with a persistent cough and negative cough swab or sputum samples should receive empiric antibiotic treatment based on the last positive respiratory culture.

Where P. aeruginosa is found either for the first time or in patients not chronically infected with P. aeruginosa, then vigorous attempts should be made to eradicate the organism. Treatment with nebulized tobramycin has been shown to be effective, though the duration of treatment has varied from 1 to 12 months.[458] Treatment with a 3-week course of oral ciprofloxacin and nebulized colistin is also effective, with benefit seen up to 2 years after treatment.[458] The Danish center, where this combination eradication treatment was developed, recommends 3 months of treatment for isolates of P. aeruginosa in patients not chronically infected.[459]

Chronic pulmonary infection with P. aeruginosa will eventually occur in most CF patients and when it does, patients should receive vigorous early treatment for respiratory exacerbations. It has been difficult to find a consensus over what should be considered the most important features of such an exacerbation. However, in a prospective study the following clinical features were found to be important predictors, when compared with a 'gold standard' of physician diagnosis:[460]

- decreased exercise tolerance;
- increased cough;
- increased sputum;
- decreased appetite;
- absence from school or work;
- increased adventitial sounds.

Strenuous efforts should be made to prevent pulmonary exacerbations in children with CF and a number of preventative strategies are supported by good evidence. Much of the viscosity of sputum is attributable to DNA, mostly derived from neutrophils. The recombinant enzyme dornase alfa ('DNase'), given in nebulized form, will break down DNA and produce less viscous sputum, which is easier for children to expectorate. When given once daily to young children over a 2 year period, this reduced the number of exacerbations significantly (by approximately one third).[461] Nebulized tobramycin, given as a maintenance therapy on a '4 weeks on'/'4 weeks off' basis has been shown to reduce hospitalizations by a quarter.[462] Although there is better evidence for the use of nebulized tobramycin in CF, many children with chronic P. aeruginosa infection receive maintenance treatment with nebulized colistin. An advantage of this approach is that resistance of P. aeruginosa to colistin is very uncommon. Azithromycin, although not active against P. aeruginosa in a conventional sense, also significantly reduces the number of exacerbations over a 6 month period.[463] Azithromycin is thought to have an anti-inflammatory action and to inhibit P. aeruginosa within the biofilm. It can be taken in a single dose three times per week and so does not add greatly to the therapeutic burden. Nebulized hypertonic saline helps restore the airway surface liquid layer and encourages patients to cough. Over a 1 year period, it has been shown to reduce the number of pulmonary exacerbations,[464] although there is more experience with its use in adults than in children.

As well as these maintenance therapies, annual immunization against influenza is recommended in CF, though properly designed studies are lacking. There is no consensus on passive immunization against RSV in infants with CF and this is expensive. A vaccine against infection with *P. aeruginosa* is currently in phase III clinical trials.

There has been much debate as to when patients with chronic *P. aeruginosa* infection should receive intravenous antibiotics, with some centers favoring regular treatment every 3 months. This policy is not supported by evidence from RCTs,[465] although when regular treatment and symptomatic treatment have been compared the number of courses which patients receive is very similar, suggesting a convergence of these clinical approaches.[466] When intravenous antibiotics are administered, it is recommended that two antipseudomonal antibiotics are used to prevent the emergence of antibiotic resistance.[455] In patients with strains of *P. aeruginosa*, which show some antibiotic resistance, the choice of which antipseudomonal antibiotic to use is not easy. Laboratory sensitivities do not predict clinical response.[467] Commonly, two antibiotics with different and synergistic mechanisms of action are recommended, e.g. a beta-lactam (such as ceftazidime) and an aminoglycoside (such as tobramycin).[455] It is known that pulmonary exacerbations in patients with chronic pseudomonas infection are usually caused by the 'resident' strains of *P. aeruginosa* rather than a new strain and so initial treatment can be based on previous microbiology results, while current microbiology is awaited.[468] Conventionally, antibiotics are administered for between 10 d and 2 weeks. For patients who are well enough, intravenous antibiotics can be administered at home, with less disruption to schooling and reduced costs.[469] In recent years efforts have been made to simplify antibiotic regimens. Once daily aminoglycoside dosing is more convenient to administer than conventional three times daily dosing (particularly for patients receiving intravenous antibiotics at home) and has been shown to be equally effective with less renal toxicity in children.[470] Whichever antibiotic regimen is chosen, good supportive therapy must be ensured, with chest physiotherapy targeted at areas of consolidation and mucus plugging, and good nutritional support. Children who are admitted for treatment of pulmonary exacerbations of CF spend a long time in hospital compared to children admitted for other reasons. A pleasant and appropriate ward environment, with the opportunity to continue schooling (or for preschool children to take part in play activities), are crucial to a good recovery. Young people with CF benefit from peer support in these circumstances. Where this cannot be from other young people with CF (because of the risk of cross-infection), then support from young people with other chronic illness can be just as helpful.

When the response to conventional antibiotic therapy for a pulmonary exacerbation is poor, a thorough review of clinical status and treatment is required. Mucus plugging can lead to lobar collapse and a CXR is indicated. Initial treatment of mucus plugging is with continuing antibiotics and physiotherapy with the addition of oral steroids and dornase alfa. Bronchoscopy and suction of mucus plugs under direct vision may be needed.

Clinical review should include the search for other organisms. Children with pulmonary infiltrates on the CXR and a poor response to antibiotics should be investigated for allergic bronchopulmonary aspergillosis. This is likely where there has been a four-fold rise in total IgE (particularly to above 500 IU/ml) and there are positive aspergillus precipitins.[471] Treatment is with prednisolone 0.5–1 mg/kg once daily for 2–3 weeks, combined with itraconazole (3–5 mg/kg once daily or 200–400 mg for children over 12 years), changing to the same dose of prednisolone alternate daily for 2–3 months. A good response to treatment is indicated by improved symptoms, resolution of CXR changes and a fall in the total IgE level.

Nontuberculous mycobacterial lung infection can occur in children with CF (primarily with *Mycobacterium avium* and *M. abscessus*). These infections become more common as patients get older, with an estimated prevalence of 13% in CF patients who are over the age of 10.[472] Prolonged treatment is required with a combination of agents determined by the organism identified.

Effective antibiotic therapy of *B. cepacia* complex is difficult. Meropenem has some activity and should be combined with a second antibiotic.[473]

MONITORING PROGRESS
Annual assessment
The annual assessment is an opportunity to step back and take an overview of the progress that a child or young person has made in the last year. This is a multidisciplinary process, with assessments (where appropriate) made by the clinician, CF dietician, physiotherapist, specialist nurse, pharmacist, social worker and clinical psychologist. It is also a two-way process with the child and his/her family given the chance to discuss the results of investigations and any concerns.

The following investigations are recommended at annual assessment:
- weight, height and BMI. These should be plotted on the appropriate centile chart and progress over the last year reviewed;
- CXR, scored using a recognized scoring system;
- Shwachman Kulczycki score;[474]
- spirometry with more detailed pulmonary function (e.g. bronchodilator test) if indicated;
- blood tests including: full blood count; prothrombin time; liver and renal function; vitamin A, D and E levels; total IgE and aspergillus-specific IgE;
- glucose tolerance test in patients over 12 years;
- sputum for routine pathogens and atypical mycobacteria.

Conventional liver function tests are relatively insensitive for detecting CF liver disease and clinicians should have a low threshold for requesting a liver ultrasound.

It has been suggested that an annual HRCT scan may allow early diagnosis of mucus plugging and bronchial thickening in CF, which may be missed on a conventional CXR. Scans may be limited to six slices to reduce radiation exposure. However, limited CT scans still involve a higher radiation burden than a conventional CXR and an annual CT scan would only be justified if there were evidence that this approach will change management and improve outcome.[475]

Monitoring response to treatment during a pulmonary exacerbation
As well as the overview provided by the annual assessment, it is helpful to monitor the short term response to treatment, particularly for pulmonary exacerbations. All CF centers will measure pulmonary function and weight before and during intravenous antibiotic treatment. New inflammatory markers such as serum calprotectin and human neutrophil lipocalin (both of which measure neutrophil driven inflammation) are being evaluated in CF. Sputum markers such as arginase may also be useful.

MANAGEMENT OF ADVANCED DISEASE
Artificial ventilation
While ventilation cannot be recommended for end-stage lung disease it may be considered during severe pulmonary exacerbations, when recovery is considered likely or as a bridge to transplantion. Non-invasive ventilation is preferable to endotracheal intubation, as children receiving non-invasive ventilation can talk, can perform chest physiotherapy and the ventilatory support can be given intermittently, with rest periods. If non-invasive ventilation is likely to be necessary, it is essential to prepare for this possibility in advance, in order to identify a correctly fitting mask and allow the child to become familiar with the technique. The outcome of any form of ventilation in children is better than in adults.[476]

Lung transplantation

Lung transplantation is the only definitive treatment for end-stage CF lung disease. Many clinical and psychosocial factors should be considered when referring for transplant assessment. However, patients with a FEV_1 of less than 30% predicted have a 50% risk of dying within 2 years[477] and when lung function deteriorates to this level, transplantation should be discussed with the family. Sequential double lung transplantation is currently the procedure performed most frequently. Figure 20.29 shows the CXR appearance in a child before and after transplantation. Figures from the International Society for Heart and Lung Transplantation (www.ishlt.org) give a 5 year survival after lung transplantation of around 40%, but 5 year survival of up to 57% is reported by some centers.[478]

Although CF causes generalized bronchiectasis, in some patients one lobe or one lung is more severely affected. This area of the lung can act as a reservoir of infection, which can spread to other, less severely affected lobes. The disproportionate inflammatory response, due to uncontrolled infection in this area, may lead to anorexia, malaise and cachexia, attributable to inflammatory cytokine production. In selected cases, lobectomy or pneumonectomy may be an acceptable alternative to transplantation (Fig. 20.30).[479]

Palliative care

After a full discussion of treatment options for advanced disease, some children or young people and their families may not wish to be evaluated for lung transplantation or other interventions such as non-invasive ventilation or major lung surgery. In these cases comprehensive and well planned palliative care is essential. This will usually be delivered by the CF team alone or in collaboration with a generic palliative care team. The aim of treatment is no longer to arrest the decline in pulmonary function but to provide good symptom relief. Many of the treatment options will be the same as those used during the active phase of treatment – antibiotics and physiotherapy are an excellent way of relieving symptoms of cough and dyspnea. However, the setting for treatment (hospital vs home) and its duration will be determined by the wishes of the patient and family. Opiates may be helpful for the management of chest pain and dyspnea and, if the child or young person is in hospital, clear advanced directives describing the resuscitation plan to be followed in the event of a sudden deterioration or respiratory arrest need to be agreed with the patient, his/her family and the caring team. Local practice guidelines should be followed.

THE FUTURE

There are undoubtedly many reasons for the improvements in survival in CF seen over the last four decades. These include: the establishment of CF centers[480] (including shared care with local hospitals); improved formulations of pancreatic enzyme supplements; vigorous antibiotic therapy to eradicate or treat *P. aeruginosa*; and the establishment of dedicated adult CF centers. However, these improvements in survival have been achieved at a price. Center care is associated with improved nutrition but patients may acquire chronic infection with *P. aeruginosa* earlier in life.[480] Some units which practice regular intravenous antibiotic treatment have better survival[403] but antibiotic treatment exerts selective pressure and produces resistant organisms which may be transmissible between patients. Adverse effects of intravenous antibiotic treatment include allergy, renal failure and deafness. Diabetes and reduced bone mineral density cause substantial morbidity in adults with CF.

Although the CF gene was identified in 1989, there is still no practical therapy based on this discovery which can be used in the clinic. However, a phase II clinical trial of liposome based gene therapy is now ongoing, and the Therapeutic Development Network, of the US CF Foundation is undertaking high throughput screening for novel compounds which may modify CFTR function. Whether or not these developments deliver practical therapies for people with CF, the quality of life and life expectancy for CF patients will still depend on ensuring that current best practice is followed. Accreditation or peer review of CF units will help ensure a uniform high standard of care for patients, irrespective of where they live, and will help the CF team make the case

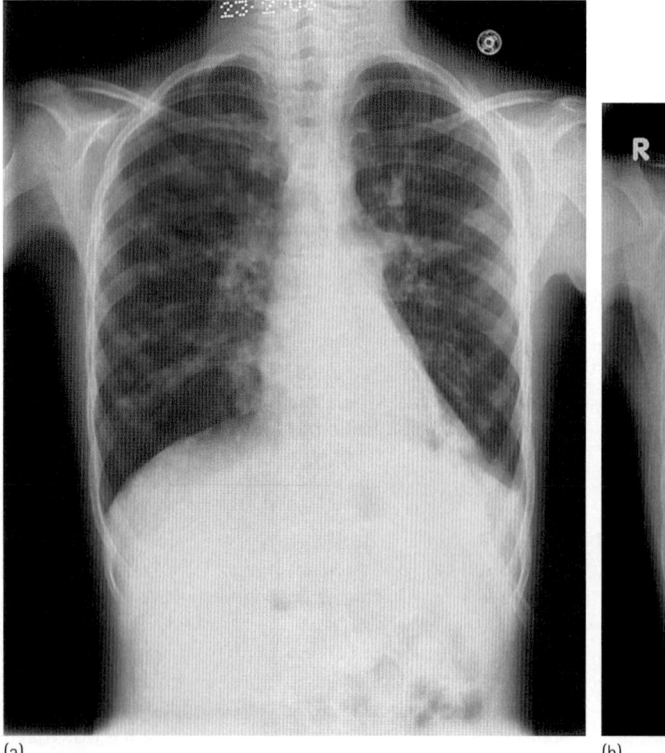
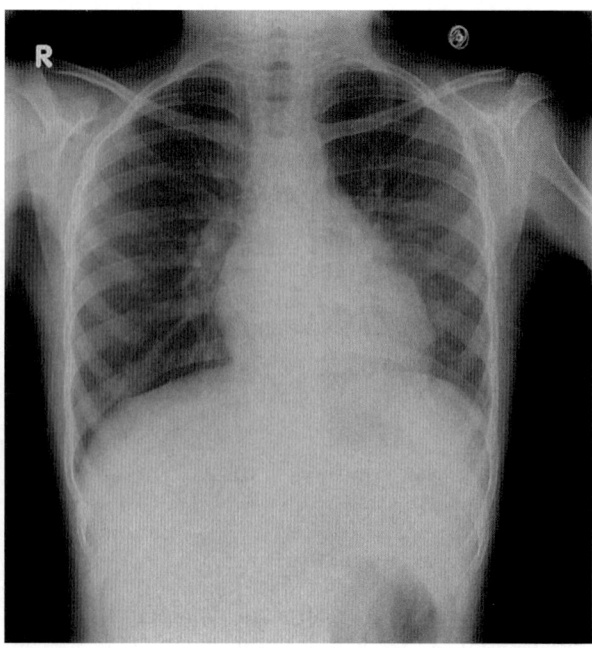

(a)   (b)

Fig. 20.29 Chest radiographs of a 13-year-old patient with CF. (a) Before transplantation, showing widespread nodular–cystic shadowing and complete collapse of the left lower lobe due to mucus plugging. (b) After transplantation.

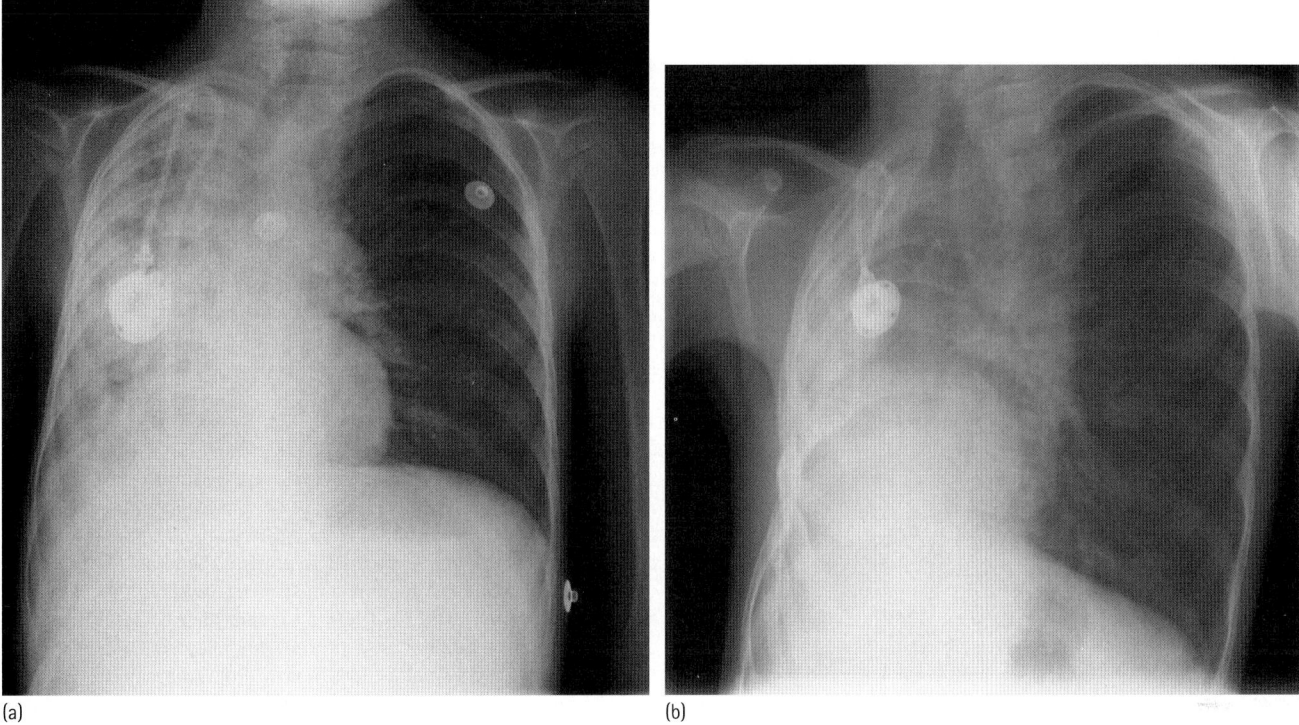

(a)   (b)

Fig. 20.30 Chest radiographs of a CF patient who had a right pneumonectomy at the age of 7 years. (a) Before pneumonectomy (aged 6 years) showing complete collapse of the right lung due to mucus plugging. (b) After pneumonectomy (aged 12 years) showing mediastinal shift to the right and scoliosis.

for adequate funding of their services. Newborn screening allows therapy to be started early and it would be hoped that this can be linked to a program of RCTs and cohort studies so that therapies where evidence is inadequate can be fully assessed. This should reduce the burden of care by discarding ineffective or harmful interventions whilst concentrating on effective therapies.

RESPIRATORY INFECTIONS

Although mortality from respiratory infections in previously healthy children is now rare in the UK, respiratory infections continue to account for a large number of hospital admissions, one half of all illnesses in preschool children and one third of GP attendances. A preschool child has, on average, six to eight respiratory infections per year, ranging in severity from mild colds to severe lower respiratory infections, such as bronchiolitis. Lower respiratory tract infections (LRTIs) are commonest in the first year of life and then decline in incidence during subsequent years.

UPPER RESPIRATORY TRACT INFECTIONS

Upper respiratory tract infections (URTIs) are common and, although rarely fatal, are a source of considerable morbidity, especially in young children. URTIs account for 95% of all respiratory infections and include colds, pharyngitis, tonsillitis, otitis media, sinusitis, croup and epiglottitis.

The common cold

The common cold is a short, mild and usually self-limiting illness. However, it has a substantial impact in terms of school absence and complications, including secondary bacterial infection and exacerbation of underlying respiratory conditions such as asthma and CF. Children may have up to 12 colds per year, usually acquired from day care or from siblings. The causative organisms of the common cold are viruses of which there are more than 200 types, the most common being rhinovirus, responsible for up to 40% of cases.

Clinical features

The common cold is characterized by rhinorrhea, sore throat, cough, fever and malaise lasting up to 7 d and often a lingering mucopurulent nasal discharge. Otitis media may be a complicating feature, often with secondary bacterial infection. In infants colds may manifest as irritability, snuffles and difficulty with feeding. Infants under 3 months of age are particularly susceptible to rapidly evolving secondary bacterial LRTI, and other infections such as septicemia, meningitis and pneumonia should be considered in infants with poor feeding. Allergic rhinitis is sometimes difficult to distinguish from the apparent permanent colds of toddlers, but is characterized by a clear watery nasal discharge with a pale nasal mucosa. The discharge associated with a foreign body is unilateral, purulent, foul-smelling and blood-stained. Other diseases may present with a nasal discharge, including primary ciliary dyskinesia and immune deficiencies.

Treatment

Many interventions for the treatment and prevention of colds have been studied since the 1940s. There is no evidence to support treatment with antibiotics to hasten clinical improvement or to reduce the number of days missed from school or work.[481] Some antiviral agents have been shown to be useful in prevention of colds and further assessment of these agents, focusing on non-virus-specific compounds, is necessary. Evaluations of nonspecific measures such as Echinacea, humidified air, nasal decongestants, vitamin C and zinc have reported some positive results but there is insufficient evidence to recommend any of these for the treatment or prevention of colds.

Acute otitis media (see also Ch. 32)

Acute otitis media is one of the most frequent diseases in early infancy and childhood. The peak incidence is between 6 and 15 months. Although for most children acute otitis media is a disease which resolves spontaneously, it represents a large health burden and a substantial amount of money is spent on antibiotics to treat this disease. Secondary bacterial infection is common following a viral URTI. *H. influenzae, Streptococcus pneumoniae*, *Moraxella catarrhalis*, *M. pneumoniae* and occasionally Gram negative bacteria, particularly in the neonatal period, are the most likely bacterial pathogens.

Symptoms and signs

Non-specific symptoms such as fever, poor feeding, irritability, diarrhea and vomiting are presenting features of an infant with otitis media. An older child will complain of earache. On examination, a red, dull, bulging tympanic membrane suggests acute suppurative otitis media. Hemorrhagic bullae on the surface of the eardrum suggest *M. pneumoniae* infection. Rupture of the membrane may follow, often with dramatic relief of pain.

Complications

Meningitis and mastoiditis are rare but important complications. Chronic suppurative otitis media has in the past been attributed to inadequate treatment of the acute infection but this relationship remains unclear. Temporary hearing loss at all sound frequencies is common.

Treatment

Analgesia and antipyretics should be used for symptomatic relief. Topical analgesia may be useful.[482] Although there is limited evidence to support this intervention, one RCT reported a 25% reduction in pain 30 min after instillation of anesthetic ear drops compared with placebo.[483]

Despite a large number of published clinical trials, there is no consensus on the use of antibiotic therapy for acute otitis media. The primary considerations are whether treatment with antibiotics is justified and, if so, what is the optimal duration of treatment. As most cases will resolve spontaneously, any benefit must be weighed against possible adverse reactions and the emergence of bacterial resistance.

The decline in suppurative complications of otitis media in North America and Europe during the 1940s and 1950s was attributed to antibiotic therapy. However, evidence since then suggests that long term outcomes are similar in antibiotic treated and untreated children with acute otitis media living in resource rich countries.[484]

A recent meta-analysis that pooled the results of 10 studies suggested that, in comparison with placebo, antibiotic treatment of acute otitis media in children is associated with a small benefit in reduction of pain at 2–7 d into the illness.[485] A semi-randomized trial in Sweden in 1954[486] reported a rate of mastoiditis of 17% in an untreated group compared with none in the penicillin treated group. However, this was excluded from the above meta-analysis because of significant methodological flaws. Another systematic review concluded that 60% of children will improve spontaneously after 24 h without any treatment and 80% of cases will resolve within 3 d.[487] A further review has reported that a short course of antibiotics (< 7 d) is as effective as a longer course (7 d or longer) for the treatment of uncomplicated acute otitis media in children.[489]

In cases where the child is not toxic and the parents are in agreement, it may be reasonable to delay antibiotic prescribing unless pain and/or fever persist for 2 d. This practice has resulted in a decreased use of antibiotics in children without significant adverse effects.[489,490] The American Academy of Pediatrics and the American Academy of Family Physicians have recently published a clinical practice guideline recommending this approach in selected children over 6 months old.[491]

Current evidence does not support the use of decongestants or antihistamines for otitis media. No additional benefit has been demonstrated in terms of symptom relief or prevention of complications and an increased risk of adverse effects has been reported.[492]

Pharyngitis and tonsillitis

Sore throat is a common complaint and is usually associated with URTIs. Although it is usually a self-limiting problem, it causes significant morbidity, school absence and high consultation rate in general practice, resulting in a large number of antibiotic prescriptions.

Etiology and diagnosis

Most sore throats have a viral etiology, especially in children under the age of 3 years. Viral pathogens include adenovirus, influenza and parainfluenza, Coxsackie A and Epstein–Barr virus (EBV), which are the causes of herpangina and glandular fever respectively. The primary bacterial etiology is Group A beta-hemolytic streptococcus. It is difficult to distinguish clinically between viral and bacterial sore throat and results of throat swab culture correlate poorly with symptoms. A purulent exudate over the tonsils does not signify a bacterial etiology, but a membrane may be suggestive of EBV or diphtheria. Petechial hemorrhages on the palate and cervical lymphadenopathy are nonspecific signs which often accompany pharyngitis. Interpretation of throat swabs is complicated by the 40% asymptomatic carriage rate in the general population. Rapid antigen tests may be used but these tests have low sensitivity and have not changed practice in primary care.[493]

Treatment

The majority of children with sore throats require only symptomatic treatment with simple analgesia. A recent meta-analysis concluded that antibiotic treatment of sore throats reduced the number of complications, including glomerulonephritis, rheumatic fever, acute otitis media, acute sinusitis and quinsy.[494] However, the incidence of these complications in the UK is low and the evidence does not support the routine use of antibiotics to prevent complications. Penicillin has been shown to have a small benefit in providing symptomatic improvement in children with severe symptoms of sore throat, but is not recommended for routine use.[495] If Group A beta-hemolytic streptococcus has been isolated, a 10 d course of penicillin or a shorter course of a cephalosporin or macrolide may be effective. The convenience of once or twice daily dose regimens of cephalosporins should be balanced against the potential for the emergence of resistant strains of streptococcus.

The effectiveness of tonsillectomy for the treatment of recurrent tonsillitis has not been formally evaluated.[496] Tonsillectomy has a significant perioperative complication rate of around 1–2%, but there are suggested benefits for children, not only in reducing the number of sore throats, but for general health including growth. Tonsillectomy is generally considered if a child has had more than six to seven significant recurrences over 1–2 years despite antibiotic treatment, has significant obstructive sleep apnea, or has had two or more peritonsillar abscesses.

Diphtheria (see also Ch 28, p. 1213)

Diphtheria is an acute, communicable disease caused by *Corynebacterium diphtheriae*. Despite the success of mass immunization in many countries, diphtheria remains an important cause of mortality. Early, accurate microbiological diagnosis and identification of contacts and carriers are imperative since delay in specific treatment may result in death. Recent developments have focused on methods of detection of the potent exotoxin produced by *C. diphtheriae*, the definitive test for the diagnosis of diphtheria.

Symptoms and signs

The possibility of diphtheria should be considered in the differential diagnosis of sore throat, especially in patients traveling from Eastern Europe, the Indian subcontinent and South East Asia. The incubation period is 1–6 d and it is possible that travelers may arrive in the early stages of the disease. Diphtheria is characterized by local growth of the bacterium in the pharynx with pseudomembrane formation. The membrane becomes greenish–black and firmly adherent and can involve the tonsillar zones, larynx, soft palate, uvula and nasal cavities. Less commonly, bacterial growth can occur in the stomach or lungs; systemic dissemination of toxin then invokes lesions in distant organs. When the membrane involves only the nasal septum the disease is relatively minor. However, extension to the larynx causes stridor and upper airway obstruction. Prior to immunization, laryngeal diphtheria was the commonest indication for tracheostomy in Britain. The patient presents with a sore throat, stridor, fever and general malaise. The clinical features may be indistinguishable from epiglottitis.

Treatment

Infected children should be isolated and urgent attention should be given to protecting the airway, with a team on standby for tracheostomy if necessary. Treatment is with antitoxin 5000–30 000 U intravenously and systemic penicillin 4 hourly. Erythromycin can be used to treat carriers. More details are given in Chapter 28.

Whooping cough (see also Ch. 28)

Whooping cough, or pertussis, is a respiratory infection caused predominantly by the bacterium *Bordetella pertussis*. A wide range of other respiratory pathogens can cause a similar illness, including *Bordetella parapertussis*, RSV, adenovirus, *M. pneumoniae* and *Chlamydia trachomatis*. *B. pertussis* is transmitted by respiratory droplets and causes disease only in humans. The incubation period is around 7–10 d.

Whooping cough is underdiagnosed by pediatricians and family doctors. Early diagnosis and prompt public health notification allows review of vaccination programs and can lead to more effective treatment and control measures, such as prophylaxis for contacts at risk, thus preventing further cases and avoiding inappropriate investigations.

Symptoms and signs

The onset of cough is preceded by a catarrhal stage of fever and coryza, which can be easily missed. The catarrhal prodrome is the most infectious stage of the illness. The onset of a hacking cough is often nocturnal before becoming constant and occurring in paroxysms, classically rising in pitch and terminating with a whoop and/or vomiting. Between coughing spasms, the child may look well, but the cough can be forceful enough to precipitate petechiae, subconjunctival hemorrhages, pneumothorax and subcutaneous emphysema, rib fractures or rectal prolapse. After the acute phase of the disease, many patients continue to cough for prolonged periods, sometimes for several months. Adolescents and adults may present with typical disease but more frequently with isolated prolonged cough. Complications include pneumonia, failure to thrive from post-tussive vomiting, seizures, encephalopathy, secondary bacterial infection and pulmonary hypertension.

Infants are a particularly vulnerable group. There is little placental transfer of passive immunity to pertussis and, until primary vaccination is completed at 4 months, this age group is at risk if exposed. There is often a household contact with pertussis, often the mother, which may be proven by culture, or detailed enquiry may reveal a history of concurrent paroxysmal cough. Presenting features in infants include nonspecific cough, poor feeding, vomiting, cyanosis, apneas and bradycardia, usually without the characteristic paroxysmal cough or whoop. This can make the diagnosis difficult and it is often confused with bronchiolitis. Despite intensive care treatment, there is still significant mortality, particularly in infants requiring mechanical ventilation. There is a high rate of major complications such as bacterial pneumonia, pulmonary hypertension, air leaks, seizures and encephalopathy. Pertussis can occasionally be the cause of sudden infant death.

Diagnosis

The gold standard for the diagnosis of *B. pertussis* is culture of the organism from pernasal swab or nasopharyngeal aspirate. The sensitivity of this technique decreases the later the sample is taken after the onset of the illness, but can be increased by using the PCR technique. If more than 2 weeks after disease onset, serology for pertussis toxin IgG may be more useful. There is a characteristic peripheral blood lymphocytosis and extreme leukocytosis may be an independent predictor of mortality in the neonatal age group.[497] Chest X-rays may demonstrate pulmonary infiltrates, particularly in the perihilar region. These may represent excess secretions, which can lead to areas of atelectasis and compensatory hyperinflation of other lung regions.

Treatment

Pertussis is highly infectious and barrier nursing of hospitalized patients must be enforced. Assisted ventilation may be needed for respiratory failure or prolonged apnea.

A macrolide is the antibiotic of choice for clearance of *B. pertussis* infection on culture; however, it is most effective during the catarrhal stage of the disease. There is probably no effect on outcome if started more than a week after onset of the illness. A 14 d course of erythromycin has been the treatment of choice but shorter-course macrolide antibiotics (e.g. azithromycin, clarithromycin) may be as effective with fewer adverse effects and improved adherence to therapy.

Early phase I clinical trials of an intravenous pertussis immunoglobulin have indicated that this preparation is safe and achieves high levels of pertussis toxin antibody titers in infants.[498] There is no RCT evidence to support the use of salbutamol (albuterol) for the treatment of pertussis.[499]

In view of the high rate of secondary transmission of the organism to household members, macrolide antibiotics have been used as chemoprophylaxis for close contacts of the primary case to protect non-immunized or partially immunized infant contacts, who are at risk of severe disease. A review of the evidence for the use of erythromycin in preventing secondary transmission showed very little benefit, compared with the protection conferred by the vaccine.[500] Therefore, it should probably be reserved for vulnerable contacts only. Further blinded RCTs of erythromycin prophylaxis should consider shorter courses of erythromycin as well as the newer macrolide antibiotics, which have fewer adverse effects. For prevention see Chapter 28, p. 1197.

INFECTIONS CAUSING UPPER AIRWAY OBSTRUCTION

The major infective causes of upper airway obstruction are croup, epiglottitis and bacterial tracheitis (Table 20.17). Rarer causes include retropharyngeal abscess, cellulitis or severe tonsillitis. Other causes of stridor include foreign body aspiration, angioneurotic edema, vallecular cyst or abscess, inhalational burns, diphtheria, epiglottic hemangiomas or other congenital abnormalities.

Croup

Croup (laryngotracheobronchitis) is a common cause of airways obstruction in children. The term croup refers to a clinical syndrome characterized by a barking cough, inspiratory stridor and hoarseness of the voice. These symptoms are thought to be due to edema of the larynx, trachea and bronchi as a result of a viral infection, hence the term laryngotracheobronchitis. Parainfluenza types 1 and 2 are the most common infecting organisms, but rhinovirus and RSV can also cause croup. Although croup is a self-limiting illness, it causes frequent visits to GPs and hospital emergency departments and often results in hospitalization. Although severe croup occurs infrequently, early recognition of the signs of severe airways obstruction is important.

Symptoms and signs

Coryzal symptoms are followed over 12–24 h by a harsh, barking cough. Stridor is most evident when the child is upset and the parents often report that the onset of symptoms is at night, when the child is woken in the early hours of the morning by cough and stridor. The symptoms may reach a peak on the second or third night. Usually, croup resolves spontaneously over a 3–4 d period. Certain groups of children such as those with pre-existing subglottic stenosis following prolonged neonatal ventilation or those with Down syndrome may be at greater risk of severe croup. In patients with atypical features, e.g. those aged over 6 years or with a high fever, alternative diagnoses such as epiglottitis, bacterial tracheitis, retropharyngeal abscess or inhaled foreign body should be considered.

Assessment of severity

Laboratory and radiological investigations are unhelpful. The decision to treat or admit to hospital is based on clinical features and an assessment of the severity of the croup. Signs of a severe episode of croup include evidence of hypoxemia such as restlessness and cyanosis, and signs of airways obstruction such as subcostal and intercostal recession. The intensity of the stridor itself is a poor indicator of severity. A child with a low oxygen saturation in air is likely to have severe upper airway

Table 20.17   Clinical presentations of upper airway obstruction due to infections

	Croup	Epiglottitis	Bacterial tracheitis
Age	1–2 years	2–6 years	Throughout childhood
Causative organism	Parainfluenza	*Haemophilus influenzae*	*Staphylococcus aureus* *Steptococcus pneumoniae* *Haemophilus influenzae*
History	Onset 1–2 d Coryza Barking cough	Onset <24 h Sore throat Dysphagia	Onset <24 h Rattling cough Sore throat
Signs	Fever <38.5°C Nontoxic Harsh stridor Hoarse voice	Fever 38–40°C Toxic Upright position Open mouth, drooling Muffled stridor	Fever 38–40°C Toxic Mucopurulent secretions Absent or soft stridor
Course	Resolves 4–10 d Intubation <3%	All need intubation	Intubation in >80%, often >1 week
Treatment	Steroids Adrenaline (epinephrine)	Cephalosporin	Cephalosporin

obstruction. Some units use croup scores to grade the severity and to guide treatment and the decision to admit to hospital.[501]

Management

The most important aspect in the management of children with croup is airway maintenance.

Children with mild croup, i.e. barking cough with no clinical signs of obstruction, require reassurance. There is no evidence that steroids have a place in the management of this group. Recent trials have shown that mist/humidified air provides no additional symptom improvement, nor does it alter the overall cause of the disease process.[502,503]

Steroids. The results of meta-analysis have shown that treatment with steroids is effective in improving the symptoms of croup in children, with improvement in croup severity scores, shorter hospital stay, fewer admissions to intensive care units (ICUs) and decreased use of adrenaline (epinephrine).[504] The evidence supports all children with croup and increased effort of breathing, i.e. accessory muscle use and/or stridor at rest, being treated with corticosteroids.[505]

The most frequently studied classes of steroids in croup have been dexamethasone and budesonide. Dexamethasone is a potent steroid with an anti-inflammatory ratio of 5:1 compared with prednisolone. It can be administered either by mouth or intramuscular injection. Budesonide is a synthetic glucocorticoid with a lower bioavailability than beclomethasone because of its hepatic first-pass clearance. Most of the nebulized dose is deposited in the upper airway, the point of maximal inflammation in croup. No significant difference in efficacy has been demonstrated comparing oral or intramuscular dexamethasone with nebulized budesonide[506] and both treatments are effective as early as 6 h and for up to at least 12 h after administration. Oral dexamethasone (0.6 mg/kg) may be the best treatment option because of its ease of administration, widespread availability and lower cost. In a child who is vomiting, nebulized budesonide (2 mg) or i.m. dexamethasone may be preferable.

Adrenaline (epinephrine). Adrenaline is a potent stimulator of alpha- and beta-adrenergic receptors. In patients with croup, it is believed to provide short term benefit due to its ability to reduce bronchial and tracheal secretions and mucosal edema. It is not a definitive treatment but may allow time for the underlying pathology to resolve. Nebulized adrenaline (5 ml of 1:1000 solution) should be considered for children with croup who have moderate to severe respiratory distress, i.e. accessory muscle use, stridor at rest and/or signs of hypoxemia. The onset of action has been observed as early as 30 min after treatment and its duration is around 2 h.[507] Because of the relatively short duration of action, patients may have rebound symptoms as the effects of the drug wane, although this may also indicate progressive worsening of the croup.

Glucocorticosteroids should therefore be given contemporaneously with adrenaline to attenuate rebound and patients given adrenaline should be observed carefully for at least 2 h. There is some evidence that it is safe to discharge improved patients after a period of observation.[508]

Epiglottitis

Epiglottitis is an airway emergency with a high risk of acute complete obstruction of the upper airway. Its primary cause is *H. influenzae* type b (Hib). The epiglottis is characteristically swollen, edematous and cherry red. The introduction of the conjugate Hib vaccine to the UK primary immunization schedule in October 1992 has substantially reduced the incidence of epiglottitis. However, there continue to be sporadic cases due to vaccine failure[509] and clinicians should continue to have a high index of suspicion, even in a fully vaccinated child. Other pathogens include *Streptococcus*, *Staphylococcus* and *Klebsiella*.

Hib has been shown to be an important cause of life threatening childhood infections worldwide. Epiglottitis is the second most common of these in industrialized countries and accounts for 10% of Hib infections worldwide with meningitis being the most common (52%). Epidemiological data from 19 countries before implementation of routine immunization showed average incidences of epiglottitis of 13 per 100 000 in children aged 0–4 years and 5 per 100 000 in those aged 0–14 years, with higher rates in Sweden and parts of Australia and lower rates in resource rich countries. Worldwide there were 12 000 cases per year and 400 deaths, i.e. a 2.5% mortality.

Prevention

Conjugate vaccines against Hib were introduced in the late 1980s and have been shown to have an efficacy exceeding 90% from the first months of life.[510]

Introduction of the vaccine has been associated with a dramatic decline in the incidence of Hib over a short period. This is partly due to the ability of the vaccine to prevent nasopharyngeal Hib colonization and thus confer herd immunity. From September 2006, children in the UK receive a dose at 2, 3 and 4 months of age and a booster at 12 months as part of the standard vaccination program. Ninety percent coverage has been achieved and the incidence of all Hib infections is now 2 per 100 000 or less in children aged 0–4 years, which represents a decline of over 97%.

Clinical features

Differences between the presentation of croup and epiglottitis are presented in Table 20.18. Epiglottitis generally affects slightly older children, usually aged 2–6 years, although it has been reported in infants and is being increasingly recognized in adults. It may occur at any time

Table 20.18 Features of bacterial and viral pneumonias

	Bacterial	Viral
Fever	>38.5°C	<38.5°C
Respiratory rate	>50/min	Normal or raised
Recession	Present	Marked
Wheeze	Not usually an early sign	Often present
CXR	Consolidation	Hyperinflation Segmental collapse in 25%
Coexisting disease	Consider influenza, measles, other viruses; cystic fibrosis, immune problem if recurrent	Consider bacterial infection; aspiration if recurrent

of year, but more often in spring and winter. Children usually lack a viral prodrome and complain of a sore throat which progresses within hours to a toxic illness in which the child appears irritable, pyrexial and dyspneic. The child has dysphagia and prefers to sit forward with the neck extended and the arms forward for support to optimize the patency of the airway. There is marked intercostal and subcostal recession and use of the accessory muscles of respiration. A soft inspiratory stridor results from edema of the supraglottic mucosa and physical obstruction of the airway results in drooling and muffled voice. Fatigue develops if the obstruction is not relieved. Cyanosis and deteriorating conscious level are precursors of impending complete obstruction and respiratory arrest.

Diagnosis
The diagnosis is made on clinical grounds and ensuring an adequate airway takes precedence over all investigations. Airway radiology should never delay definitive diagnosis and management of the airway. The full blood count shows a characteristic immature polymorphonuclear leukocytosis and blood cultures are positive for *H. influenzae* in around 50% of cases.[511] The yield of positive culture results from pharyngeal swab is lower than that of blood.

Treatment
As soon as epiglottitis is suspected, preparations should be made to protect the airway and the child should be given 100% humidified oxygen. Any procedure that may cause distress to the child, such as examination of the throat, should be avoided as this may precipitate sudden occlusion of the airway due to intense vagal discharge and laryngeal spasm. Attempts should be made to provide a comfortable environment for the child with the parent present. Observation of the child or radiological confirmation of the diagnosis are not appropriate and can be dangerous, due to rapid progression of the airway occlusion. Intravenous access should be obtained only after stabilization of the airway and fluid resuscitation may be required for the toxic child.

Airway management. Direct examination of the larynx is indicated to exclude other causes of laryngeal obstruction such as abscesses or foreign bodies. This should be carried out under inhalational anesthesia, with a team on standby prepared for immediate airway intervention with either an endotracheal tube or tracheostomy. This team should include a pediatrician, anesthetist and ENT surgeon and preferably the examination is carried out in the anesthetic room with the child breathing spontaneously. Nebulized adrenaline (epinephrine) may provide temporary relief, but should not be used unless measures for protecting the airway are already available and should be abandoned if it causes distress to the child. Inhalation of sevoflurane has been reported to be a safe and effective anesthetic induction agent and is better tolerated than the traditional agent halothane.[512]

Antimicrobial therapy. In addition to airway management, antibiotics are the definitive treatment for epiglottitis. Third generation cephalosporins such as cefotaxime and ceftriaxone are usually recommended to cover the increasing emergence of beta-lactamase producing strains of *H. influenzae* that are resistant to treatment with ampicillin or chlor-

amphenicol. Rifampicin prophylaxis (20 mg/kg daily for 4 d in children aged 3 months–12 years) may be recommended for non-immunized contacts and to the index case to eradicate carriage of the organism.

Complications
Pulmonary edema following relief of the upper airway obstruction is a recognized complication and is probably due to alterations in capillary wall permeability. This can be managed by using a moderate level of continuous positive airway pressure (CPAP) or positive pressure ventilation with positive end expiratory pressure (PEEP). Other manifestations of Hib infection such as exudative tonsillitis, otitis media, pneumonia, meningitis, pericarditis and septic arthritis have been observed to coexist with epiglottitis.

Bacterial tracheitis
Bacterial tracheitis is a severe condition characterized by acute upper airway obstruction and purulent secretions within the trachea. Affected children can present at any age with a fever, sore throat, hoarse voice and soft stridor. The onset of symptoms is often acute. Prolonged endotracheal intubation is often required and severe septicemia may follow with associated high mortality and morbidity. *S. aureus* is the commonest organism involved, with Group A *Streptococcus* and *H. influenzae* also identified. There is a suggestion of an epidemiological change in recent years towards a less morbid condition in which children are less toxic and require intubation less frequently, with *M. catarrhalis* and viral causes becoming more common.[513] Diagnosis is usually made at laryngoscopy by visualization of the inflamed trachea and the presence of purulent secretions and a pseudomembrane. Secretions can be collected for culture. Treatment is with supportive airway management with intensive care if necessary and a broad spectrum, intravenous antibiotic.

LOWER RESPIRATORY TRACT INFECTIONS
Lower respiratory tract infections (LRTIs) are a common cause of mortality in developing countries and represent a major cause of morbidity among children worldwide. LRTIs account for 5% of all respiratory infections and include bronchiolitis, pneumonias and exacerbations of respiratory exacerbations in bronchiectasis. One in four children has a LRTI in the first year of life. Differential diagnoses include CF, aspiration associated with gastroesophageal reflux or H-type tracheoesophageal fistula.

Bronchiolitis
Bronchiolitis is the commonest cause of lower respiratory tract illness in infants and is an important cause of acute and long term morbidity. The infecting organism in around 75% of cases is RSV; others include adenovirus and rhinovirus. RSV causes annual winter epidemics of respiratory disease and can also manifest as pneumonia, otitis media, croup or mild URTIs. During a single epidemic, over 70% of infants become infected with the virus and almost all infants are infected by the end of their second winter. Thirty percent of these develop lower respiratory tract symptoms and between 0.5 and 1.5% are admitted to hospital with RSV bronchiolitis.

Infants at high risk of severe RSV bronchiolitis include those born prematurely, and those with cardiovascular disease, chronic respiratory disease including bronchopulmonary dysplasia (BPD) and CF or immunosuppression.

Clinical features
Acute. The peak age of infants hospitalized with RSV bronchiolitis is around 3 months. The clinical features of the illness reflect the plugging of small airways with inflammatory exudates leading to a large increase in airway resistance and a corresponding increase in work of breathing, leading to fatigue of the respiratory muscles. Characteristically there is a short prodromal upper respiratory tract illness with coryzal symptoms and low-grade pyrexia, followed by rapid onset of tachypnea, hypoxia, moist cough and difficulty feeding. Increased work of breathing is reflected by

suprasternal, subcostal and intercostal recession with head bobbing and nasal flaring. The predominant feature on auscultation is crackles with or without the presence of wheeze. As the chest becomes hyperinflated, the liver is displaced and is often easily palpable in the abdomen.

Signs of more severe illness include apnea, especially in young and preterm infants, irritability, listlessness, cyanosis and reduced conscious level. Approximately 2% of infants who are hospitalized with RSV bronchiolitis require assisted ventilation because of either an obstructive bronchiolitis or, more unusually, a restrictive pneumonia or acute respiratory distress syndrome (ARDS).

Chronic. Lower respiratory tract RSV infections are associated with increased respiratory morbidity in the early years of life. At 9–10 years of age, those who had RSV infection as babies have an increase in respiratory symptoms[514] but the mechanisms contributing to this chronic respiratory morbidity are unclear. RSV does not itself appear to lead to atopic asthma. The long term outcome can in part be predicted by the presence of wheeze during the acute illness, with those in whom wheeze is the dominant symptom having a much greater likelihood of having asthma later in life than those with classical bronchiolitis. Factors such as a family and personal history of atopy and esoinophilia appear to be the best guide to predicating who will exhibit asthmatic symptoms. In the group with acute bronchiolitis (i.e. predominantly crackles) there is an excess of symptoms generally associated with intercurrent viral infections compared with controls, but these appear to have a much better prognosis with prevalence falling rapidly through early childhood.[515]

Diagnosis

Rapid identification of RSV infection can be confirmed by immunofluorescence on nasopharyngeal aspirate samples, which gives a result within hours, or by viral culture.

Radiology

Chest radiology is unhelpful in typical cases of bronchiolitis and should be avoided unless there is an underlying illness or deterioration in clinical status suggesting the need for intensive care. Chest X-rays show hyperinflation with multiple areas of interstitial infiltration. Signs of segmental or subsegmental collapse occur in 25% and this often leads to the inappropriate use of antibiotics.

Treatment

Current therapy for RSV bronchiolitis is primarily supportive, involving maintenance of hydration and oxygen status. Nasogastric or intravenous feeding is required if the baby is unable to suck. Oxygen saturation monitoring is necessary and oxygen should be administered via nasal prongs or headbox if the oxygen saturation falls below 92%. An increasing oxygen requirement indicates worsening disease with increasing ventilation/perfusion imbalance. Hypercapnia is a sign of exhaustion and alveolar hypoventilation and if this develops the baby should be moved to a high-dependency area or intensive care for ventilatory support.

Overall, evidence from RCTs does not support the use of additional therapies. Bronchodilators, including adrenaline (epinephrine), have not been shown to be helpful, except perhaps in reducing a clinical severity score,[516,517] and desaturations have been reported after salbutamol (albuterol) nebulization.[518] The majority of studies have demonstrated no benefit from inhaled or oral corticosteroid therapy either in the acute phase or in the prevention of post-bronchiolitic wheezing.[519,521] Antibiotics are not indicated except in the case of secondary bacterial infection which is rare in babies who do not need ventilatory support.

Ribavirin inhibits viral replication and is the only available antiviral agent active against RSV. Although early studies of the effect of ribavirin found some benefit, a systematic review of 10 trials showed no reliable evidence of efficacy.[521,522] For infants who require respiratory assistance, there is a paucity of evidence to support modes of non-invasive ventilation such as CPAP or continuous negative extrathoracic pressure (CNEP).[523] In severe cases, particularly infants with chronic lung disease, conventional ventilation alone may be insufficient. Extracorporeal membrane oxygenation (ECMO) has been shown to be associated with a survival of over 50%.[524] Nitric oxide may improve the respiratory status of those infants with restrictive lung disease or pre-existing pulmonary hypertension by improving gas exchange, although its long term influences remain unproven. DNAse may be efficacious and exogenous surfactant can improve oxygenation and may lead to a shorter duration of ventilatory support and ICU care,[525] although further RCTs to confirm these findings are awaited.

Prevention

RSV is spread by direct contact with infected secretions and contaminated objects and this may be reduced by effective and appropriate hand-washing and cohort nursing. The importance of these measures in the prevention of RSV transmission should not be underestimated. There is as yet no safe and effective vaccine for use in infants. A formalin-inactivated vaccine was introduced in the 1960s but this led to more severe respiratory disease in vaccinated infants during the following season. Until an effective vaccine is developed, alternative prophylactic measures must be optimized.

Palivizumab is a humanized monoclonal antibody that provides immunoprophylaxis against serious LRTIs caused by RSV. In a double-blind, placebo-controlled trial,[526,527] intramuscular palivizumab 15 mg/kg every 30 d for 5 months significantly reduced RSV-related hospitalizations by 55% in infants with prematurity and/or BPD/chronic lung disease (CLD) and by 45% in infants with hemodynamically significant congenital heart disease, and was most effective in infants under 6 months born at or before 35 weeks' gestation. The number needed to treat was 17, i.e. 17 patients would need to be given monthly injections to prevent one RSV-related hospital admission. There were also fewer admissions to ICU, fewer total hospital days and fewer days with supplementary oxygen. The administration of the product appears to be safe and is easy to administer but it is costly and should therefore be reserved for infants at highest risk of severe RSV infection. Other high-risk infants in whom palivizumab has not been formally assessed, such as those with immunodeficiency and CF, might potentially benefit from palivizumab.

Pneumonia

LRTIs are a common cause of morbidity among children in resource rich countries and a major cause of mortality in resource poor countries. Of these infections, pneumonia is the most serious and can still be difficult to diagnose because of lack of reliable diagnostic methods. The epidemiological pattern of pneumonia is constantly altering because of changes in patient characteristics, altered immune status and changes in medical practice. There is an increasing level of resistance to antibiotics by the more common pathogens such as S. pneumoniae. For these reasons, accurate identification and treatment of the individual etiological organisms causing pneumonia is important.

Community acquired pneumonia

Community acquired pneumonia is defined clinically as the presence of symptoms and signs of pneumonia in a previously healthy child due to an infection that has been acquired outside of hospital.[528] The diagnosis can be verified radiologically by demonstrating consolidation on CXR if available.

Etiology

Identification of the responsible organism is a challenge because of difficulty in obtaining adequate samples, lack of reliable diagnostic methods and difficulty in differentiating infection from colonization. In 20–60% of cases a pathogen is not identified and in those that are, around 14–35% appear to be caused by viruses alone and a substantial proportion (8–40%) represent a mixed infection. Age is a good predictor of likely pathogens with viruses being the most frequently identified cause in younger children. In older children, when a bacterial cause is found, it is most commonly S. pneumoniae (pneumococcus), followed by Mycoplasma and chlamydial pneumonia.

Overall, *S. pneumoniae* is the most common bacterial cause of pneumonia in childhood. The commonest viral cause is RSV with others including influenza A, influenza B, parainfluenza and adenovirus. Respiratory syncytial virus and influenza viral infections typically peak in late autumn and winter, whereas bacterial pneumonias exhibit less marked seasonal fluctuations. *Chlamydia pneumoniae* and *M. pneumoniae* occur commonly in children older than 4–5 years and increase in incidence over the age of 10 years. Nonserotypable *Haemophilus* and *M. catarrhalis* were previously considered nonpathogenic for the respiratory tract but do occasionally cause pneumonia. Enterobacteriaceae, Group A *Streptococcus* and *S. aureus* are uncommon in the immunocompetent host, but when they occur can cause severe disease including lung abscesses, empyema and pneumatoceles. Atypical organisms such as *Chlamydia* and *Legionella* species can cause disease of the lower respiratory tract in children, although these organisms are seen more commonly in adults.

Clinical features

Pneumonia is classically characterized by rapid onset of fever, tachypnea, cough and difficulty with feeding or difficulty in breathing in the older child. These symptoms are frequently preceded by a relatively minor upper respiratory tract illness with coryza and low-grade fever. It is often difficult to distinguish those children with viral pneumonia from those with bacterial disease (see Table 20.18) and there is considerable overlap in the clinical findings in young children and infants with pneumonia and other LRT illnesses such as bronchiolitis. Bacterial pneumonia should be considered in children under 3 years of age when there is a fever of > 38.5 °C with chest recession and a respiratory rate of > 50/min. On examination, crackles on auscultation are classical, and bronchial breathing is a late sign indicating consolidation. Wheeze may also be present in viral or mycoplasma pneumonia but the presence of wheeze in the preschool child makes bacterial pneumonia unlikely. Symptoms of lower lobe pneumonia in older children may include abdominal pain, reflecting referred pain from the diaphragmatic pleura, and can occasionally lead to a paralytic ileus with abdominal distention. Upper lobe consolidation may be associated with neck pain and apparent neck stiffness. Chest pain is common and is due to accompanying pleuritis. Pulse oximetry should be performed on every child admitted to hospital with pneumonia.

Laboratory investigations

Blood cultures should be collected on all children suspected of having bacterial pneumonia but yield an organism in only around 10–15% of cases. Only a small number of bacterial pneumonias are accompanied by bacteremia and many children receive antibiotics before reaching hospital.

Culture of respiratory specimens is the best method for identifying organisms causing pneumonia on culture. However, small children are unable to expectorate sputum and procedures such as BAL are generally regarded as too invasive to be used routinely, other than on an ICU.

Nasopharyngeal specimens for viral antigen detection (such as immunofluorescence) and/or viral culture should be collected from all children under the age 18 months as soon as possible, as viral shedding is maximal at the time of onset of symptoms. The presence of a virus in the upper respiratory tract does not necessarily imply that this is the cause of the pneumonia.

Serology can be useful in cases where no microbiological diagnosis was reached during the acute illness. Acute serum samples should be saved and a specimen for convalescent titers at 2–4 weeks is necessary, leading to a delay, and can be complex due to multiple serotypes. This method is useful for the detection of atypical species such as mycoplasma and chlamydia.

PCR is a technique used to amplify deoxyribonucleic acid (DNA) from microorganisms in either blood or respiratory secretions. This technique offers the possibility of a rapid bacteriological diagnosis and may be more sensitive than bacterial culture, especially if antibiotics have already been given.

Other laboratory investigations include full blood count and C-reactive protein (CRP). A high white cell count and CRP may be more suggestive of bacterial pneumonia, although there is considerable overlap so that confident prediction of the microbiological diagnosis is not possible on these variables alone and they should not be measured routinely.

Radiology

Because the clinical features of pneumonia may be nonspecific, CXRs are often used to confirm the presence and determine the location of a pulmonary infiltrate. CXRs do not reliably distinguish between bacterial and viral pneumonias, although interstitial shadowing or peribronchial infiltrates are said to be more characteristic of a viral infection and lobar consolidation of pneumococcal disease. The radiological features of segmental consolidation are difficult to distinguish from those of segmental collapse seen in around 25% of viral LRTIs. Complete resolution of radiographic changes may take several weeks. CXRs are also used to identify associated air leaks, effusions and abscesses. Follow-up CXRs should only be performed after lobar collapse, an apparent round pneumonia, or for continuing symptoms.

Treatment

For the management of pneumonia in children, it is important first to assess the severity of the illness and second to direct treatment against the identified or likely pathogen. These factors are important in deciding whether to withhold or to prescribe antibiotic therapy, whether the child requires admission to hospital and whether therapy should be given via the oral or intravenous route. As outlined above, definitive information about the causative organism is rarely available, and therefore empirical treatment is often necessary.

The majority of children with community acquired pneumonia can be managed in primary care. In the mildly unwell, ambulatory child, infection is most likely to be viral and therefore antibiotics can be withheld. Children with difficulty breathing, poor feeding or vomiting, intermittent apnea or grunting or who are in need of supplementary oxygen require hospital admission. Supportive measures include adequate hydration and nutrition. Antipyretics and analgesia may also be required.

Because of concerns about antimicrobial resistance, it is preferable that effective narrow spectrum agents are used wherever possible. Penicillin remains the treatment of choice for *S. pneumoniae*, and amoxicillin is the first choice oral antibiotic for children under the age of 5 years or if *S. pneumoniae* is suspected because it is effective, well tolerated and cheap. Both mycoplasma and chlamydia are susceptible to macrolide antibiotics such as erythromycin, azithromycin and clarithromycin[529] and these are the drugs of choice if either of these infections is suspected and in cases of penicillin-resistant strains of *S. pneumoniae*. Because mycoplasma pneumonia is more prevalent in older children, macrolide antibiotics may be used as first line empirical treatment in children aged 5 years and older. RCT evidence has also shown that an early switch to oral therapy after a short (2 d) course of intravenous therapy has comparable efficacy to a full week's course of intravenous therapy, and can reduce hospital stay and costs, with no increased adverse patient outcome.[530] If the child remains pyrexial or unwell 48 h after admission with pneumonia, re-evaluation is necessary with consideration given to possible complications such as a parapneumonic effusion or lung abscess.

Prevention

The improvement in uptake of routine vaccines against Hib, *Bordatella pertussis* and influenza has had an impact on both prevention of cases of these infections in children and helping to reduce spread of cases in the community. Pneumococcus is known to be the most common bacterium isolated from children with pneumonia. The existing capsular polysaccharide vaccine (Pneumovax) is ineffective in younger children but the new conjugate vaccine (Prevenar) is immunogenic in children from 2 months of age (see Ch. 4, p. 35). This vaccine was licensed for use in infants and young children in the USA in 2000. The subsequent introduction of the vaccine into the childhood immunization schedule led to a significant decrease in pneumococcal disease.[531] The vaccine is effective against invasive and non-invasive pneumococcal infection and, like all conjugate vaccines, provides long-lasting immunity. On 8 February 2006, the Departments of Health in England, Scotland and Wales announced the inclusion of Prevenar in the childhood immunization schedule. This has important implications for the future prevention of pneumococcal infection in the UK.

Staphylococcus aureus pneumonia

S. aureus is an organism that is causing increasing concern as a cause of both hospital- and community-acquired pneumonia. Carriage rates in adults are around 10–40%, although this figure is lower in children. The organism produces coagulase and is also capable of producing toxins which cause different clinical presentations with varying degrees of severity.

A new pattern of severe disease due to the Panton–Valentine leukocidin (PVL) toxin is emerging in the UK, Europe and the USA.[532,533] PVL is a toxin which destroys white blood cells and is rare but can be found in both methicillin sensitive and resistant strains of *S. aureus*. PVL-positive *S. aureus* can be associated with necrotizing skin lesions, cellulitis or septic arthritis but can also cause a highly lethal form of community-acquired necrotizing pneumonia carrying a mortality rate of around 40%.

PVL-associated *S. aureus* infection should be considered in cases of community acquired pneumonia in young immunocompetent, previously well adults or children presenting with fever, hemoptysis, severe sepsis and often a preceding flu-like illness. There is typically a marked leukopenia, high CRP, multilobar infiltrates on CXR and rapid clinical progression to ARDS.

Clinical management is supportive, usually requiring intensive care, in addition to early aggressive antibiotic therapy with combinations including vancomycin, clindamycin, linezolid, rifampicin and co-trimoxazole in high doses. The combination used will reflect susceptibility of individual isolates. Linezolid and clindamycin have the added advantage of suppressing toxin production. Other therapies such as intravenous immunoglobulin and activated protein C may be appropriate because of the high mortality rate. The care of the patient should include strict infection control measures.

Atypical pneumonia

Mycoplasma

Mycoplasma is a common cause of pneumonia in schoolchildren and young adults. Epidemics tend to occur in 4–7 year cycles with a peak incidence in autumn, thought to correspond with children returning to school. In early school years it is responsible for about 12% of pneumonia, rising to 20% in older schoolchildren and over 30% in young adults. The incubation period is 2–3 weeks. The symptoms associated with pneumonia are often much worse than the physical signs would suggest. Classically, a dry cough develops over 1–2 d with a low-grade fever. The cough can be debilitating and may be confused with pertussis. Often severe, systemic complaints such as weakness, headache, sore throat, arthralgia and chest or abdominal pain predominate. Signs in the chest are often subtle but auscultation may reveal fine crackles, either localized or multifocal, and wheeze may be present in up to 30%. Rashes are common in association with *M. pneumoniae* and Stevens–Johnson syndrome, hemolytic anemia, polyarthritis, pericarditis, hepatitis, pancreatitis, myocarditis and encephalitis have all been described as rare complicating features. CXR changes are nonspecific and variable. Interstitial infiltrates, multifocal or lobar shadowing, hilar adenopathy and effusions have all been described. A rise in paired specific antibody titer is regarded as the gold standard for the diagnosis of *M. pneumoniae*. Cold agglutinins are often used as an acute test but their value is limited as they are neither fully sensitive nor specific for mycoplasma infection and may also occur in cytomegalovirus (CMV) and EBV infection. Culture of the organism takes about 3 weeks and is therefore not of clinical use. PCR can be applied to blood or nasal secretions and may increase diagnostic yield in combination

with serology. Macrolide antibiotics such as erythromycin, azithromycin or clarithromycin are effective treatments for mycoplasma.[529]

Chlamydia

Chlamydia is an obligate intracellular parasite. Three species of chlamydia are pathogenic in man.

Chlamydia trachomatis is a cause of pneumonia in the newborn and can be recovered from 25% of infants of mothers who have been identified positive for chlamydial antigen. It can be acquired across intact amniotic membranes and so babies delivered by Cesarean section can be infected as well as those delivered vaginally. About 15% of infected infants develop signs of pneumonia, from 4–6 weeks of age, a dry, 'staccato' cough being a classical feature. Crackles are described more frequently than wheeze. There is a history of sticky eye in 50%. Chlamydia is isolated by cell culture from respiratory secretions or conjunctival scrapings. Chlamydia may also be isolated from high vaginal swab from the mother in whom carriage may be asymptomatic. The respiratory disease is generally mild and responds poorly to erythromycin. Respiratory symptoms can persist for at least 7 years afterwards but it is difficult to know whether this is because chlamydial infection identifies a host susceptibility or because it leads to permanent damage.

Chlamydia pneumoniae, identified in 1986, is a common cause of community acquired pneumonia in school-aged children. Symptoms are initially upper respiratory followed by a prolonged hoarse cough which may persist for months after treatment. Treatment is with erythromycin or another macrolide antibiotic.

Chlamydia psittaci is the cause of psittacosis, a rare and potentially fatal zoonosis acquired from birds. Most wild urban birds are infected but the infectivity of birds to man is variable: pigeons are poorly infective but parakeets and budgerigars are highly infective. The symptoms and signs range from a mild 'flu-like' illness to pulmonary involvement with a mild to moderately severe pneumonia. The diagnosis rests on a history of contact with infected birds in the presence of respiratory infection and with rising titers to chlamydial antigen. Treatment is with a macrolide antibiotic, or a tetracycline in children over 12 years. Extrapulmonary manifestations include myocarditis, nephritis, thrombophlebitis and meningoencephalitis.

Legionnaires' disease

Legionnaires' disease is an unusual disorder in childhood. It occurs either sporadically or in epidemics in communities. *Legionnella pneumophila* is a Gram negative, aerobic organism. It survives in warm water and is harbored in water supplies and water-cooled air-conditioning systems and transmission is either by inhalation or by ingestion of contaminated water. Infected infants and children suffer from widespread and sometimes life threatening pneumonia. Serological studies demonstrate raised titers to *L. pneumophila* and the organism can be identified at lung biopsy. Treatment is with macrolides, quinolones or co-trimoxazole.

Q fever

This is caused by infection with the rickettsial organism *Coxiella burnetii* acquired from livestock such as cattle and sheep. Animal to animal transmission is via ticks; however, infection to humans is airborne from contaminated feces, urine and birth products such as placenta. It is a frequent cause of 'flu-like' symptoms and when the organism causes pneumonia, fever is universal and is accompanied by a dry cough. Diagnosis is serological and if erythromycin is ineffective it usually responds to treatment with quinolones or rifampicin.

Fungal infections

Despite the prevalence of fungi in the environment fungal disease is rare. Fungi cause both pathogenic and opportunistic infections and in the UK the latter, affecting children with altered host defense mechanisms, are by far the most prevalent.

Histoplasmosis, blastomycosis and *coccidioidomycosis* are exceptionally rare in children outside the US and South America. All cause illnesses which range from asymptomatic infection to disseminated disease and all have clinical features which are very similar to tuberculosis. In the lung, granulomas associated with hilar lymphadenopathy can progress to pneumonia, cavitating pulmonary lesions and pleural disease. Diagnosis rests on appropriate skin testing and sputum culture. Amphotericin B is used to treat severe blastomycosis and coccidioidomycosis but the treatment of histoplasmosis is extremely difficult.

Aspergillus causes two forms of respiratory disease in childhood: allergic bronchopulmonary aspergillosis (see p. 712 – Treatment of pulmonary infection) caused by hypersensitivity in children with underlying lung conditions such as asthma, CF and invasive pneumonitis, usually in immunocompromised hosts.

Actinomycosis is due to species of *Actinomyces* which live in the mouth, in dental plaque and calculus. As mouth hygiene has become better actinomycosis, in which organisms reach the chest by inhalation, has become rare.

Parasites

Pulmonary eosinophilia or Loeffler syndrome is believed to be caused by *Ascaris*, *Toxocara*, hookworms or *Strongyloides*, although drugs such as aspirin, penicillin and the sulfonamides have been implicated. Pulmonary involvement includes cough, wheezing, shortness of breath, hemoptysis, fever and weight loss. Diagnosis is suggested by migratory pulmonary infiltrations and a high eosinophil count in the peripheral blood. Identification of the offending parasite can be made by stool examination and by serological methods.

Persistent bacterial bronchitis

Persistent bacterial bronchitis (PBB), sometimes termed persistent endobronchial infection or chronic suppurative lung disease, is a condition characterized by a persistent, wet cough present for longer than 1 month that resolves with appropriate antibiotic therapy. The majority have onset of symptoms in the first year of life and the commonest precipitating event is probably a viral LRTI which leads to disruption of the normal mucociliary clearance mechanism, making the airways more susceptible to bacterial infection. The commonest organisms to be isolated are *H. influenzae* and *S. pneumoniae*.

Recent reports have emphasized the importance of making a specific diagnosis in children with a chronic cough and in particular have highlighted the important prognostic implications of an ongoing wet cough and the importance of PBB as the commonest cause of a chronic cough.[534,535] If untreated, the condition is likely to lead to damaged airways, and may be a precursor to bronchiectasis. The condition is often misdiagnosed as 'difficult asthma', although the two can coexist causing significant challenges in diagnosis and management.

Currently there is no consensus regarding treatment. Appropriate and aggressive medical treatment has been reported to lead to a dramatic reduction in morbidity and complete resolution of symptoms in the vast majority of patients. However, a small number have a more protracted course and underlying causes such as CF, primary ciliary dyskinesia or significant immunodeficiency should be excluded. A suggested approach is the use of an appropriate high-dose antibiotic and review of the response at 2 weeks. Typically the cough takes 10–14 d to resolve. If there has been a clear response to this intervention the treatment is continued for a further 4–6 weeks or up to 6 months in some centers in order to keep the airways free from colonization and permit repair of the affected airways. For those with persistent symptoms, physiotherapy is an important part of the treatment regimen. Intravenous or nebulized antibiotics may be needed for those with more troublesome symptoms. The accurate identification and development of RCTs of management of children with PBB and 'pre-bronchiectasis' remain challenges for the future.

Parapneumonic effusion and empyema

Parapneumonic effusion and empyema are parts of a continuum of pleural complications of bacterial pneumonia. In the initial stages of development of parapneumonic effusion there is pleural inflammation with leakage of fluid and protein into the pleural space. Bacterial invasion ensues, followed by leukocytes and then activation of fibroblasts with the formation of loculations. If the inflammatory process continues, a thick peel is formed on both pleural surfaces with pleural fluid becoming a gelatinous mass. The visceral peel can contract and entrap the underlying lung. There may be fever, cough, chest or abdominal pain and dyspnea. The usual clinical signs are reduced breath sounds and dullness to percussion on the affected side, and children with empyema usually look unwell. There is often anemia, leukocytosis, thrombocytosis and raised inflammatory markers such as CRP.

The bacteria most frequently responsible are *S. pneumoniae*, *S. aureus*, and Group A *Streptococcus*. Recently, PCR on pleural fluid has identified the responsible organism in culture negative cases.[536] After CXR, ultrasound is very useful and can identify fibrinous septation, rind formation and also lung mobility. Computed tomography (CT) can be used as an additional mode of imaging.

Blood cultures should be taken and appropriate intravenous antibiotics started. Guidelines for the management of pleural infection in children have been published.[537] Small uncomplicated effusions may be managed with antibiotic therapy alone, but larger effusions are best managed with closed chest tube drainage. The place of intrapleural fibrinolytic therapy in childhood empyema has become clearer in recent years. A randomized placebo controlled trial showed that 3 d of urokinase therapy was associated with a significantly shorter hospital stay, which was further reduced if a small percutaneous drain was used.[538] The use of video-assisted thoracoscopic surgery (VATS) as an alternative method of debridement of the pleural space has been increasingly used in some centers. However, a randomized trial of urokinase versus VATS as a primary procedure showed no difference in outcomes between the two therapies.[539]

Imaging can be used to assess response to treatment but should not dictate therapy alone. Multiloculated effusions and organizng empyemas may not resolve with chest tube placement and fibrinolysis and may need operative intervention. Thoracotomy with removal of fibrinopurulent debris and if necessary decortication of thickened parietal pleura to release entrapped lung can however produce rapid recovery with a short hospital stay.[540]

Intravenous antibiotics should be continued until there is clinical improvement with defervescence, guided by change in inflammatory markers. Oral antibiotics should be given for at least another 2 weeks. Chest radiography may show pleural thickening for several months. With appropriate management most children make a good recovery.

RESPIRATORY DEFENSES AND INFECTION IN THE COMPROMISED HOST

The lungs are continuously exposed through respiration to a multitude of airborne particles and microorganisms. A complex system of host defense exists for protection against this repeated challenge, but when this breaks down significant and recurrent infection can occur.

PULMONARY HOST DEFENSE

There are both physical and immune defenses. Immune defense mechanisms are either innate or specific, although there is considerable interaction between the two.[541]

Physical and innate immune defense

The upper airway and branching airways in the lung are the first line of defense with airborne particle deposition dependent on particle size, flow rates during inspiration, and age. Large particles (> 10 microns) are usually trapped in the upper airway whereas smaller particles may be able to penetrate beyond the terminal bronchioles. Particulate or chemical stimulation may trigger the neurally mediated protective reflexes of sneeze, cough and bronchoconstriction. Cough is also an adjunct to the normal mechanism of mucociliary clearance and is particularly important when the latter is defective. Laryngeal integrity and competence of airway protective reflexes are important further defense mechanisms.

The bronchial tree down to the 16th bronchial division at the terminal bronchioles is lined by ciliated columnar epithelium. This is covered by a layer of mucus which is propelled by ciliary movement to the oropharynx where it is swallowed or expectorated. Small particles and organisms are thereby cleared from the airways. Each epithelial cell has around 200 cilia composed of nine interconnected doublet microtubules surrounding and joined to two centrally positioned microtubules. Cilia start beating with a slow recovery stroke by bending sideways and backwards, followed by an effective stroke which propels mucus in a cephalad direction.[543] Ciliary beating results from ATP driven sliding of microtubules via dynein arms, and is coordinated locally in metachronal waves. Normal ciliary beat frequency is 11–16 Hz.

Tracheobronchial mucus is produced by the submucosal glands, goblet cells and Clara cells, and through transudation from the vascular space and alveolar fluid. It consists of glycoproteins (mucins), proteoglycans, lipid and water. The airway surface liquid consists of two layers: an inner periciliary liquid layer in which the cilia beat, and an outer mucus layer, which is viscous and into which the tips of the cilia just penetrate.[542]

The lungs however provide an additional chemical defense. Airway surface fluid contains a variety of antimicrobial molecules, including lysozyme, complement, fibronectin, transferrin, lactoferrin, lipopolysaccharide binding protein, defensins, cathelicidins and collectins. There has been much recent interest in the role of these substances in health and disease states.[543] The collectins include surfactant proteins A and D and mannose-binding lectin, synthesized by the distal airways and alveolar type II cells. The epithelium appears to be able to respond to the presence of pathogens by induction of these antimicrobial factors, as well as by secretion of cytokines for recruitment of inflammatory cells.[544]

Macrophages are present in large numbers throughout the lung, in alveoli, airways and in the interstitium. They play an important role in defense against agents that have escaped clearance by the above mechanisms, through phagocytsis but also by activating other inflammatory cells. Mast cells and polymorphonuclear leukocytes can also be activated through non-immunological mechanisms. Neutrophils can be recruited and activated in the lung, and kill pathogens by phagocytosis and mechanisms including the respiratory burst. This is more effective if they are opsonized with specific antibody.[545] Some encapsulated organisms are not susceptible unless opsonization occurs.

Specific immune defense

The predominant antibody in respiratory secretions in the upper airway is secretory IgA, which is synthesized locally in the submucosa and is dimeric in structure. IgA can activate the alternative complement pathway and can inhibit viral binding to epithelial cells and neutralize toxins. Conversely IgG relies on transudation from the bloodstream with an increased concentration in the lower airway where it exceeds IgA concentration in bronchoalveolar fluid. IgG activates complement via the formation of immune complexes and acts as an opsonin facilitating phagocytosis. IgM and IgE are also present in respiratory secretions.

Lymphocytes are the main effector cells in the specific immune response, comprising approximately 10% of the cells in bronchoalveolar fluid.[542] Pulmonary macrophages, dendritic cells and B cells act as antigen presenting cells, interacting with CD4+ T cells, leading to secretion of IL-1. This activates CD4+ cells further to produce IL-2 which induces proliferation of both CD4+ and CD8+ cells. CD4+ cells can stimulate B cells to produce immunoglobulin and also produce lymphokines such as interferon-gamma which activates macrophages and natural killer cells in delayed-type hypersensitivity.[545] CD8+ cells effect cell-mediated cytotoxicity which destroys virus-infected cells.

IMPAIRED HOST DEFENSE

Impairment of any of the above mechanisms can lead to infection. This applies to innate physical defenses as well as to the specific immune pathways. Compromise of the upper airway defenses, such as bypassing the upper airway by tracheostomy or in children with neurological disability associated with impaired cough or laryngeal reflexes, leads to recurrent respiratory infections. Mucociliary clearance is affected by a variety of environmental pollutants as well as by disease states. It is also impaired in CF, mainly due to abnormal amounts of viscous mucus, asthma and respiratory infection.[542] Recent viral and bacterial infections can induce temporary ciliary dysfunction.

Primary ciliary dyskinesia

Cilia line the nasal cavity, paranasal sinuses, middle ear, eustachian tube and parts of the male and female genital tracts. The term primary ciliary dyskinesia (PCD) refers to all congenital abnormalities of ciliary function. If ciliary beating is slow or uncoordinated then mucociliary clearance will be impaired. The incidence of PCD is at least 1 in 20 000, but there is probably considerable underdiagnosis.[546] The clinical features are variable but the main feature is chronic sinopulmonary infections. It can present in the neonatal period with unexplained tachypnea or pneumonia, particularly when there are no other risk factors, or rhinitis. In the older child there may be apparent asthma that responds poorly to treatment, or chronic wet cough with sputum production. There may be a history of chronic secretory otitis media with continuous discharge after grommet insertion. Purulent rhinitis and sinusitis are common. Adult males are usually infertile due to defective sperm motility or dyskinetic cilia in the vas deferens and there is associated female subfertility. Repeated respiratory infection can lead to bronchiectasis.

Fifty percent of patients with PCD have malrotation of the internal viscera with dextrocardia or complete mirror image arrangement. The absence of normal ciliary activity is thought to allow random rotation of the thoracic and abdominal viscera early in development. Kartagener syndrome refers to a triad of situs inversus, sinusitis and bronchiectasis, but this term is no longer used. Inheritance of PCD is generally autosomal recessive through a number of gene mutations that are reflected in the range of structural defects observed. There has been significant recent progress in the elucidation of the molecular basis of PCD, with mutations identified in DNAI1 and DNAH5.[547]

Guidelines for diagnosis and standards of care have been published.[548] The clinician should have a high index of suspicion and a child should be investigated if there is any combination of the above clinical problems. However, it may be appropriate to investigate for other disorders first. Nasal nitric oxide is abnormally low in PCD and, where available, this can be used as a screening test.[549] Ciliated cells can be obtained from the nasal mucosa using a cytology brush. These should be examined in a center with appropriate equipment and expertise by direct inspection and quantification of ciliary beat frequency (CBF). If CBF is low or the beat pattern is abnormal, ciliary ultrastructure should be assessed using electron microscopy.

Ciliary abnormalities in PCD include defects in the dynein arms, radial spokes, microtubules, nexin links between microtubules and ciliary disorientation.[550] Secondary ciliary abnormalities can occur, mostly with microtubular defects. Unless the ultrastructure is completely diagnostic of PCD, a repeat sample should be taken.

Daily physiotherapy is recommended with increased frequency during exacerbations of respiratory infection. Exercise should be encouraged and bronchodilator therapy may be useful. There should be regular monitoring of pulmonary function and sputum surveillance. Prolonged oral and, if necessary, intravenous antibiotics should be given early in any respiratory infection. Children should be referred to an otolaryngologist and for hearing assessment. Nasal steroids, or novel therapies such as DNase, hypertonic saline, beta-adrenergic agonists, uridine-5'-triphosphate or arginine, may prove to be useful.[551] Generally the prognosis is good with appropriate management.

Bronchiectasis

Bronchiectasis has been defined as permanent dilatation of the subsegmental airways. Its incidence in developed countries has decreased over recent decades with the decline in incidence of infections associated with the development of bronchiectasis, including measles, pertussis and pulmonary tuberculosis. It is now mostly associated with an underlying condition. Recognized causes of bronchiectasis are listed in Table 20.19. There has been recent recognition of an increase in the identification of non-CF bronchiectasis using CT imaging.[552]

The underlying pathophysiology appears to be accumulation of purulent secretions and obstruction of the airway leading to dilatation. There is loss of the ciliated epithelium and the airway elastic tissue together with edema and chronic inflammation. Classification into cylindric, varicose and saccular types has been described but this does not generally correlate with the underlying etiology. There is a rare congenital form (Williams–Campbell syndrome) in which the airway cartilage is abnormal. Bronchiectasis may follow the right middle lobe syndrome, in which there is chronic atelectasis. Young syndrome comprises bronchiectasis, sinusitis and obstructive azoospermia, but with normal ciliary function.

Symptoms are chronic cough, purulent sputum and recurrent respiratory infections. There may be crackles over affected lobes, wheeze and digital clubbing. Chest radiography may show nonspecific changes such as peribronchial thickening, atelectasis and persistent infiltrates. High resolution CT is the investigation of choice to identify bronchiectasis. This can show thick walled and dilated bronchi that are larger than their accompanying pulmonary artery (the 'signet ring' sign), and associated lobar or segmental collapse. Pulmonary function tests usually show an obstructive defect with combined obstructive and restrictive patterns in advanced disease.

Underlying conditions should be identified and have been found in up to 70% of series.[552] Appropriate investigations are directed towards the conditions listed in Table 20.19, and include sweat test, immune function studies, ciliary brushing and esophageal pH monitoring. Flexible bronchoscopy can be used to look for bronchial stenosis, compression or foreign body, as well as directing antibiotic therapy on the basis of culture of BAL fluid.

Sputum cultures commonly yield *S. aureus*, *S. pneumoniae*, *H. influenzae* and possibly *P. aeruginosa* or *E. coli*. Oral and occasionally intravenous antibiotics should be given during exacerbations guided by sputum surveillance. Regular physiotherapy is an important aid to mucus clearance. Treatment should be given for the underlying cause if identified.

Table 20.19   Causes of bronchiectasis

Cystic fibrosis
Immunodeficiency
Primary ciliary dyskinesia
Bacterial pneumonia
Foreign body aspiration
Allergic bronchopulmonary aspergillosis
HIV infection
Gastroesophageal reflux
Mycobacterium tuberculosis endobronchitis
Bordetella pertussis
Adenovirus pneumonia
Measles pneumonitis
α1-Antitypsin deficiency
Marfan syndrome
Ehlers–Danlos syndrome
Autoimmune disorders
Asthma
Young syndrome
Bronchogenic carcinoma
Williams–Campbell syndrome
Mounier–Kuhn syndrome

Bronchodilators may be of benefit, as directed by spirometry. Surgical resection may be helpful, particularly if the bronchiectasis is limited to one lobe. Repeated CT imaging has recently shown that some changes of bronchiectasis can resolve over time.[552,553]

Immunodeficiency (see also Ch. 27)

Respiratory tract infections are common in childhood and most children do not have an immunodeficiency. However, if there is a defect in immune defense then respiratory infection can be one of the first and most serious clinical manifestations. This may either be a primary immunodeficiency, an acquired disorder or from immunosuppressant therapy for another condition. Any of the following presentations may be an indicator that there is a problem in the immune system and that investigation may be warranted:

- recurrent bacterial respiratory infections;
- persistent respiratory infection not responding to appropriate therapy;
- severe infection with an organism of low pathogenicity;
- presence of an opportunistic pathogen;
- unexplained bronchiectasis;
- family history of primary immunodeficiency or unexplained infant deaths;
- features of a syndrome associated with immunodeficiency.

It is important to be aware of and to look for other features that are associated with immunodeficiency disorders, e.g. growth failure, chronic diarrhea, skin infections and rashes, and hepatosplenomegaly. The possibility of more common conditions should be entertained first. Immune function investigations should be conducted in a stepwise fashion, starting with a full blood count and differential, and serum concentrations of IgG, IgM, IgE and IgA. Depending on these results, the persistence of symptoms and the degree of suspicion, further investigations may include the following: serum concentrations of IgG subclasses, HIV status, quantification of specific antibody responses, e.g. to tetanus toxoid or pneumococcal vaccination, complement studies, lymphocyte phenotype and function, and neutrophil function. The clinical presentation and the organisms involved can be a guide to the most appropriate investigations.

Primary immunodeficiencies

These have been recently classified into broad categories including:[554]

- predominantly antibody defects;
- combined B- and T-cell immunodeficiencies;
- congenital defects of phagocyte number and/or function;
- complement deficiencies;
- other well-defined immunodeficiency syndromes (e.g. Wiskott-Aldrich syndrome, Di George syndrome, ataxia-telangiectasia).

There has been significant recent progress in the identification of the molecular basis of many of the primary immunodeficiency diseases.[555,556]

Predominantly antibody defects

X-linked agammaglobulinemia usually presents in early childhood with recurrent respiratory infections, with a particular susceptibly to encapsulated bacteria such as *S. pneumoniae* and *H. influenzae*. Serum concentrations of IgG, IgA and IgM are absent or very low and there is a decrease in circulating B lymphocytes.

Common variable immunodeficiency (CVID) usually presents later in childhood or adulthood, usually with recurrent pyogenic respiratory infection. There is a progressive decline in levels of IgG, IgA and often IgM. Both conditions should be treated with immunoglobulin replacement. Bronchiectasis can result from recurrent infection.

Selective IgA deficiency is present in 1 in 700 Caucasians but in many individuals it is asymptomatic. However, in some it may be related to recurrent sinopulmonary infections and autoimmune disease. Replacement therapy is not usually required.

It is also sometimes difficult to establish the clinical significance of selective IgG subclass deficiency. IgG2 antibodies are primarily directed against polysaccharide-encapsulated bacteria and this response is poor under the age of 2 years, predisposing this group to infection with these organisms. Some children with IgG subclass deficiency may have recurrent infections, particularly if there is associated IgA deficiency, but others are asymptomatic. Specific antibody response may be of greater clinical importance.

Combined B- and T-cell immunodeficiencies

Severe combined immunodeficiencies (SCIDs) often present in the first 6 months of life with persistent respiratory infections, particularly with viruses, fungi or intracellular bacteria.[555] *Pneumocystis jiroveci* (formerly *carinii*) is the most common respiratory pathogen. Other important features are failure to thrive, recurrent oral candidiasis and persistent diarrhea. The absolute lymphocyte count is usually low. Early diagnosis is extremely important with bone marrow transplantation a potentially curative procedure. Successful gene therapy has been reported in some patients.

In X-linked hyper-IgM syndrome B lymphocytes are unable to switch immunoglobulin production from IgM to IgG, IgA or IgE, due to a deficiency of the CD40 ligand normally found on activated T cells. There is also neutropenia and infants are prone to opportunistic infection.

Congenital defects of phagocyte number and/or function

These give particular susceptibility to *S. aureus*, *P. aeruginosa*, enteric Gram negative bacteria and fungi. Neutropenia may be isolated or part of a wider disorder. Respiratory infection often occurs in association with involvement of the skin and gastrointestinal tract. Chronic granulomatous disease (CGD) results from a deficiency in intracellular killing of ingested microorganisms through a failure of production of superoxide. Chronic infected granulomas may form in the lungs, lymph nodes, liver, urogenital and gastrointestinal tracts. There are X-linked and autosomal recessive forms, with onset of symptoms usually before 1 year of age.[555] Diagnosis is by demonstration of failure of phagocytes to produce a normal respiratory burst, e.g. with the nitroblue tetrazolium (NBT) test, or by assessment of superoxide production with flow cytometry. Treatment includes prophylaxis with cotrimoxazole and itraconazole, prompt empirical therapy for acute infections, interferon-gamma and potentially bone marrow transplantation.

Secondary immunodeficiency (see also Ch. 27)

Acute respiratory infections are a leading cause of death worldwide, with many due to immunodeficiency from malnutrition. All aspects of immune defense may be compromised by malnutrition leading to infection from both common and opportunistic organisms. Infections themselves may cause immunosuppression, e.g. pneumonia following measles. Many chronic conditions can also lead to a secondary immunodeficiency. Immunoglobulins can be lost in nephrotic syndrome or protein losing enteropathy. Children who have had a splenectomy or who have functional hyposplenism from sickle cell disease are at increased risk of infection with encapsulated organisms.

Respiratory tract infection is one of the main manifestations of HIV infection. Upper and lower respiratory tract infections are common, not only with usual bacteria and viruses such as *S. pneumoniae*, *H. influenzae* and RSV, but also opportunistic organisms. *Pneumocystis jirovecii* pneumonia (PCP) is a common first AIDS indicator illness. The pattern of PCP in HIV infection has changed with prophylactic therapy and highly active antiretroviral therapy, but considerable associated mortality remains.[557] *Mycobacterium tuberculosis* is an extremely important pathogen worldwide. Lymphocytic interstitial pneumonitis (LIP) is a non-infectious complication of HIV, with characteristic diffuse reticulonodular infiltrates on CXR. It can present with a gradual onset of cough, tachypnea and hypoxemia, and may respond to systemic corticosteroids.

Cytotoxic therapy in the treatment of malignancy or immunosuppressant therapy for bone marrow or solid organ transplantation is the commonest cause of secondary immunodeficiency. Although its incidence has decreased, infection is a major reason for treatment-related death in childhood leukemia, particularly with bacterial sepsis.[558] The main risk factor is chemotherapy-induced neutropenia, underlying the need for prompt antibiotic treatment in febrile neutropenia, with the use of empirical antifungal therapy if it is prolonged. The causative organisms in respiratory infection following bone marrow transplantation vary with time after transplantation. An initial period of neutropenia induced by the conditioning regimen predisposes towards bacterial and fungal pneumonias. With engraftment there is the risk of acute graft versus host disease, with the need for immunosuppressive therapy with corticosteroids and ciclosporin A, associated with viral (particularly CMV), fungal and *P. jirovecii* infection. Late pneumonias (> 4 months post transplant) are related to humoral defects to encapsulated organisms. Bronchiolitis obliterans can occur during this period. CMV is the major organism causing pulmonary infection in recipients of solid organ transplants.

GENERAL APPROACH TO PNEUMONIA IN THE IMMUNOCOMPROMISED

It is important to have a low threshold for investigation and treatment in immunocompromised children. Similarly a respiratory tract infection that is unusually prolonged or has atypical features should raise the suspicion of an immunodeficiency. Children with significant immunocompromise will often present for the first time with respiratory disease, and common respiratory pathogens can be devastating. Likely organisms can be predicted in a known defect but any infection is potentially possible and microbiological investigation should be conducted carefully in order to obtain a diagnosis. In addition mixed infection is not uncommon. There are also non-infectious processes that may either simulate or complicate infection, including pulmonary edema, atelectasis, hemorrhage, drug- or radiation-induced pneumonitis, and tumor infiltration.

Fever is a sensitive sign of infection, but clinical and other features may vary due to the abnormal host response. An interstitial pneumonitis may present with a dry cough, tachypnea and dyspnea, but there may be few findings on auscultation. Chest radiography can show variable abnormalities and is not specific but there are some recognizable patterns. Diffuse interstitial changes are associated with infection with *P. jirovecii*, and viral infections such as CMV and adenovirus. Lobar consolidation can be caused by common bacteria, but can also be seen in some fungal infections. A nodular appearance, cavitation or abscess formation occurs in bacterial infection with *S. aureus* and anaerobes, and fungal infections. Computed tomography, particularly high resolution, can provide extra information, and is a more sensitive investigation for other complications, e.g. bronchiectasis or bronchiolitis obliterans.

Blood cultures should be obtained before empirical treatment is started. Treatment protocols will vary between centers and with the clinical setting, but usually include broad-spectrum antibiotic cover of Gram negative and Gram positive organisms. A macrolide may be added to cover *M. pneumoniae*, high-dose cotrimoxazole for *P. jirovecii*, and potentially antifungal therapy. Urine or blood can be sent for bacterial antigen detection but serology is rarely helpful due to limited antibody response. Nasopharyngeal aspirates are useful in the younger child with urgent immunofluorescence for respiratory viruses, CMV and *P. jirovecii*. Sputum collection is often difficult, but in the older child sputum can be induced by the nebulization of hypertonic saline. Gastric aspirates are helpful in the diagnosis of *M. tuberculosis*.

Further investigation is necessary when there is failure to respond to empirical therapy and when the causative organism is not identified. Flexible bronchoscopy with BAL is a safe procedure that is often used in immunocompromised children.[559] However, even this technique has limitations in identifying pathogens, particularly after empirical treatment or with the use of prophylactic therapy. If children are intubated, an alternative is nonbronchoscopic BAL. Transbronchial biopsy is useful following lung transplantation. Open lung biopsy is generally reserved for both treatment and diagnostic failure despite BAL, and can identify both infection and non-infectious conditions.[560]

PNEUMOCYSTIS PNEUMONIA

P. jirovecii is now regarded as an atypical fungus and is the leading opportunistic pathogen, particularly in those with impaired cell mediated immunity. It can cause a severe interstitial pneumonitis presenting with nonspecific features including cough, tachypnea, fever, hypoxia and often no added sounds on auscultation. It is common in HIV infection when its presentation may be more insidious and it is often the first AIDS indicator disease.[561] Chest radiography typically shows diffuse bilateral infiltrates that spread outwards from the perihilar areas (Fig. 20.31). Several morphological forms of *P. jirovecii* are recognized.[562] Cysts contain sporozoites and are identified with most of the traditional staining techniques, whereas the smaller trophozoite forms are more abundant and attach themselves to type I pneumocytes. The host inflammatory response plays a significant part in the lung damage in infection. The organism cannot be cultured but can be identified in sputum, nasopharyngeal aspirate, BAL fluid or lung biopsy using immunofluorescent techniques or PCR.

Treatment is high dose co-trimoxazole. Intravenous pentamidine is an alternative if there is treatment failure or if co-trimoxazole is not tolerated. Respiratory support may be necessary. Corticosteroids have reduced the need for mechanical ventilation and mortality in randomized studies.[563] Children at risk of *Pneumocystis* infection should have prophylaxis with co-trimoxazole; other options are dapsone or inhaled pentamidine.

VIRAL PNEUMONIAS

Cytomegalovirus

Like other herpes viruses, CMV can become latent following primary infection. Pneumonitis can occur following reactivation in CMV positive patients with secondary immunodeficiency or with primary infection. It is a particular problem in HIV infection and in bone marrow, renal and lung transplantation. The clinical features of CMV pneumonitis are similar to PCP with a diffuse reticulonodular pattern on CXR. There may be extrapulmonary involvement, such as hepatitis, colitis or retinitis. CMV can be identified in urine, blood, nasopharyngeal aspirates and BAL fluid by using immunofluorescence and PCR techniques. However, these results may need to be interpreted with caution. A definitive diagnosis of

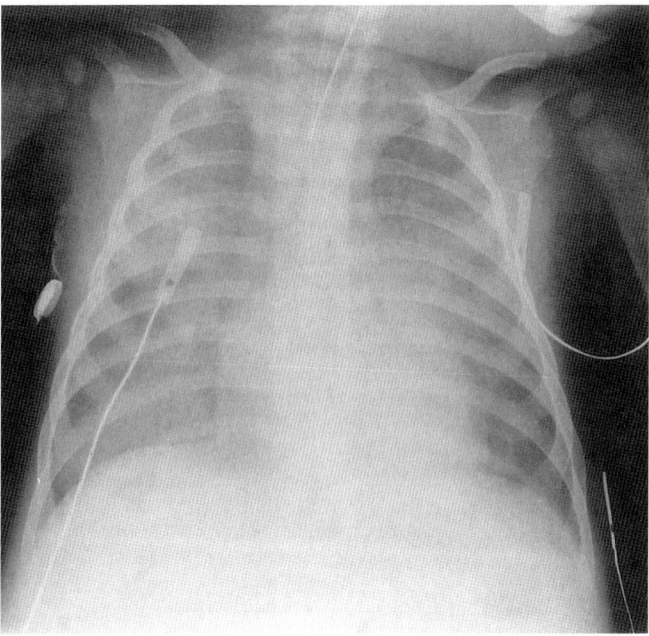

Fig. 20.31 Bilateral interstitial pneumonitis due to *Pneumocystis jejuni* in an infant with vertically acquired HIV infection.

CMV pneumonitis is made with lung biopsy, with characteristic intranuclear and intracytoplasmic inclusions and positive immunohistochemistry. Significant recent progress has been made with quantitative PCR for CMV plasma viral load, as well as RNA and antigen detection, in guiding treatment and prophylaxis.[564] Treatment includes intravenous ganciclovir and foscarnet, but mortality is significant. Those at high risk can receive prophylaxis with ganciclovir or aciclovir.

Varicella zoster

Primary varicella infection in the immunocompromised, particularly lymphopenic, patient can produce overwhelming disease with visceral dissemination and pneumonitis. There may be cough, dyspnea and chest pain, with bilateral nodular infiltrates on chest radiography that may coalesce. Varicella in the immunocompromised child should be treated promptly with intravenous aciclovir. Varicella-zoster immunoglobulin (VZIG) should be given within 72 h to at risk patients who have had exposure to varicella.

Herpes simplex

Mucocutaneous herpes simplex infection is common in severe immunodeficiency. More severe infection can progress to involve the upper airway, including the trachea, and can cause a pneumonitis. Prophylaxis and treatment is with aciclovir.

Adenovirus

Adenoviruses commonly cause respiratory infections in immunocompetent children, but can result in a severe pneumonia in the immunocompromised. There may be associated renal or hepatic involvement. There is no specific antiviral therapy but ribavirin may be used.

Measles

Bacterial pneumonia can complicate measles infection and this is a major cause of death of children in resource poor countries. There is insufficient evidence to support the use of antibiotics in all children with measles to prevent pneumonia.[565] With immunocompromise, measles can cause a progressive giant cell pneumonia that may be fatal. There may be an atypical rash, and coarse nodular infiltrates on CXR. Prior exposure to measles or vaccination is usually protective and with good uptake of immunization it is fortunately rare.

FUNGAL INFECTIONS

Aspergillus

Invasive pulmonary aspergillosis, usually due to *Aspergillus fumigatus*, can occur in prolonged neutropenia, bone marrow transplantation and HIV infection. Clinical features include fever, cough, chest pain, tachypnea and rapid deterioration. A chronic necrotizing form also exists. Chest radiography can show nodular changes and cavitation, but CT imaging is more sensitive at detecting suggestive abnormalities. BAL may be useful but definitive diagnosis is with lung biopsy. Treatment includes amphotericin, voriconazole or caspofungin. Further therapy may include the use of granulocyte colony stimulating factor and surgery on focal lung lesions.[566]

Candida spp

Prolonged neutropenia, HIV infection, combined immunodeficiencies and prolonged presence of a central venous catheter are the major risk factors for deeply invasive *Candida* infection. Pulmonary infection can result from hematogenous spread or aspiration from the oropharynx. Treatment is with amphotericin B or fluconazole.

CHRONIC LUNG DISEASE OF PREMATURITY

Although chronic lung disease (CLD) is usually ascribed to preterm infants, hence CLD of prematurity, it may also affect older more mature infants (Table 20.20). The early course of CLD whilst the infant is in the neonatal intensive care unit is described in Chapter 12. This section

Table 20.20 Diseases which may lead to a prolonged requirement for oxygen. By far the commonest is oxygen dependency due to prematurity

Preterm	Chronic lung disease of prematurity
	Wilson–Mikity syndrome
	Chronic pulmonary insufficiency of prematurity
Term	Meconium aspiration
	Respiratory infections
	Pulmonary hyperplasia
	Muscular disorders
Surgical	Tracheoesophageal fistula
	Congenital diaphragmatic hernia
Congenital abnormalities	Cystic adenomatoid malformations
	Congenital lobar emphysema
	Sequestration of the lung
	Chylothorax

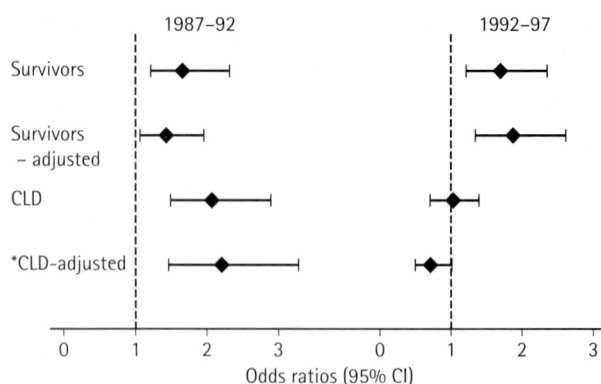

Fig. 20.32 Odds ratios for survival and CLD at 28 d of age between 1987–1992 and 1992–1997. Note improvement in survival between both time periods but with increased incidence of CLD during the first period. *Odds ratios corrected for gestation and birth weight. **(Adapted from Manktelow 2001).**

considers the features associated with CLD after discharge from hospital. Since CLD predominantly affects the preterm child, most definitions have focused on this group of infants. The earliest definitions described the different stages through which the infant progressed during development of his/her disease and the extreme stage (IV on Northway's original classification[567]) with large cystic changes interspersed with areas of collapse was termed bronchopulmonary dysplasia (BPD). Although the term BPD or new-BPD is widely used, the preferred term remains chronic lung disease of prematurity or CLD, since it embraces a wide range of diseases which may lead to the development of oxygen dependency. Many definitions have been proposed (see Ch. 12) but the most commonly used are oxygen dependency beyond 28 d of age with chest radiological changes or oxygen dependency at 36 weeks' post-conceptional age.[568] A more recent report from a meeting sponsored by the NICHD has proposed yet another definition in the face of extremely preterm infants surviving the early neonatal period, to facilitate comparisons between units.[569] This definition is based on whether the infant is greater or less than 32 weeks' gestation at birth and also attempts to classify the severity based on respiratory support including oxygen and ventilation requirements. Regardless of the definitions of CLD, it is clearly important to determine why the definition is required in the first instance.[570] For mechanistic studies, the definition is likely to be oxygen dependency at 28 d but for epidemiological studies oxygen dependency at 36 weeks' corrected gestation is more likely to be more relevant.

INCIDENCE

Estimating the incidence of CLD is problematical because of inconsistencies in case definition between different studies. Furthermore, incidence is often quoted for individual units which is subject to referral bias and to local practices. Varying approaches between individual units, for example the approach to extremely preterm infants, will markedly influence the local incidence. There are few comprehensive population-based studies which are essential to precisely estimate the incidence of CLD. In the Trent region of the UK, systematic data have been collected since 1987 for infants born at less than 32 weeks' gestation. Analysis of these data suggested that, despite falling birth rates, the number of babies of < 32 weeks' gestation admitted to neonatal units increased significantly.[571] For the two consecutive 5-year periods 1987–1992 and 1992–1997, during which a number of therapeutic modalities, including regular use of antenatal corticosteroids, exogenous surfactant therapy, high frequency ventilation and postnatal corticosteroids, were introduced, the survival improved for both time periods (Fig. 20.32). [Odds ratios adjusted for gestation and birth weight for survival at 28 d of age: 1.69 (1.23–2.33) between 1987 and 1992 and 1.90 (1.36–2.64) between 1992 and 1997.] During the first of these periods, the odds ratio for

CLD, defined as oxygen dependency at 28 d of age, increased [2.20 (1.47–3.30) adjusted for gestation and birth weight]. However, during the second period the odds ratio was 0.72 (0.5–1.03), suggesting no further increase despite a further improvement in survival. Taken together these data suggest that the survival of increasingly preterm infants in recent years has not resulted in an increased incidence of CLD.

The reported incidence of CLD (whether defined as oxygen dependency at 28 d or 36 weeks' postconceptional age) varies from 18% to 36% between centers.[572–574] In Trent, the unadjusted incidence has remained remarkably stable at 40–45% for infants born at < 32 weeks' gestation and who required mechanical ventilation.[575] This is despite interunit differences in practices and approaches to care of extremely preterm infants. Factors which may affect the reporting of the prevalence and incidence of CLD from different units are given in Table 20.21.

PATHOPHYSIOLOGY

The risk factors which lead to the development of CLD are described below. However, it is worth re-iterating that although the risk factors associated with the development of CLD have been accurately described, the mechanisms which lead to the development of CLD remain largely unknown. Antenatal and postnatal factors contribute to the development

Table 20.21 Factors that may affect the reported incidence and prevalence of chronic lung disease

Population base of community
- Social factors
- Environmental factors
- Age and health structure of community
- Ethnic mix of population

Referral patterns of neonatal unit
- Obstetric population (high/low risk)
- Obstetric practices
- Postnatal referral from less expert units

Morbidity of patients
- Early morbidity
- Maturity of population
- Complication rate
- Early mortality

Quality of care
- Quality and quantity of medical and nursing staff
- Quality of equipment
- Use of protocols based on scientific data

From Kotecha & Silverman[571]

of lung injury in infants destined to develop CLD.[576] Mechanical ventilation and oxygen therapy have received much attention in the past. More recently, antenatal factors, especially infection, have assumed more prominence, particularly as antenatal infection is also associated with preterm labour.[577] It is now thought that antenatal infection may trigger pulmonary inflammation in the fetus and that the resulting lung injury can be exacerbated by oxygen therapy and mechanical ventilation.

With the survival of extremely preterm infants, the pathological changes observed in infants who do not survive the neonatal course have altered over the years. When CLD affected more mature infants, both lung fibrosis and atelectatic areas were regularly seen.[578] With CLD now largely confined to the smallest immature infants, the picture has changed to one of decreased alveolization rather than lung fibrosis. The final number of alveoli is decreased markedly and associated with rudimentary air sacs of increased diameter and decreased gas exchanging surface area.[579,580] Whether dysregulated lung growth is due to arrest of normal lung growth[581] or due to accelerated lung growth resulting in reduced final numbers of alveoli[576] is unknown. The decrease in alveolar number is associated with abnormal deposition of extracellular matrix components, including elastin.[582] Abnormalities are also seen in the larger airways with smooth muscle extending more distally in infants with CLD compared with normal lung development.[583] It is likely that this last observation is responsible for the airways obstruction that is described in infants with CLD. Initially the airways may respond to bronchodilators but with subsequent remodeling and fixed airways obstruction, the response to such treatment becomes less predictable. Whether similar changes of smooth muscle hypertrophy occur in the airways of infants with 'new' CLD is currently unknown.

CLINICAL FEATURES

The clinical features of infants developing CLD in the neonatal intensive care unit are discussed in detail elsewhere (see Ch. 12). A typical infant with CLD will have been born prematurely and may have received mechanical ventilation and oxygen therapy either from birth or at some stage during the neonatal course.[571] Prolonged oxygen requirement is the most consistent feature and clinical signs of respiratory distress,

including an increased respiratory rate, inter- and sub-costal recession, may be evident even at rest. At the more severe end of the spectrum, the infant may develop chest deformities, including a barrel chest reflecting air trapping and Harrison's sulci indicating increased diaphragmatic workload. Some of these infants may be discharged home on oxygen. Associated problems include poor appetite and reduced weight gain despite increased energy intake. Vomiting and feeding difficulties may be present due to gastroesophageal reflux. Other features of being born too early include poor sucking, retinopathy of prematurity and early evidence of neurodevelopmental delay.

On examination, besides an increased respiratory rate and the features mentioned above, widespread wheezing and/or crackles may be present throughout the lung fields on auscultation especially in those at the extreme end of severity. In most infants, however, tachypnea without added breath sounds is the norm. Pulmonary hypertension when present may manifest with signs of right ventricular hypertrophy and tricuspid regurgitation. If prolonged endotracheal intubation has been necessary, signs of upper airway obstruction due to subglottic stenosis may also be present.

Chest radiographs are likely to show abnormalities ranging from mild haziness of type I disease (Fig. 20.33a)[584] to large cystic areas interspersed with areas of atelectasis of type 2 or Northway Stage IV BPD (Fig. 20.33b). Lung function testing in infancy (which remains largely a research tool) may demonstrate evidence of gas trapping. In addition, decreased dynamic and static lung compliance and increased airway resistance are commonly reported. Response to bronchodilators is variable but may provide a guide to future treatment of the child. Electrocardiography and echocardiography (discussed below) are indicated, particularly when pulmonary hypertension is suspected.

Causes of oxygen dependency other than prematurity are likely to have been excluded by the time the child is discharged from the neonatal unit. Nevertheless, there are a number of associated differential diagnoses that should be sought and treated as appropriate (Table 20.22). Obstructive disorders are discussed in pp. 689–697 (Asthma) but other disorders including laryngo-, tracheo- and broncho-malacia, subglottic stenosis, laryngeal webs and granulomas, vascular rings and enlarged

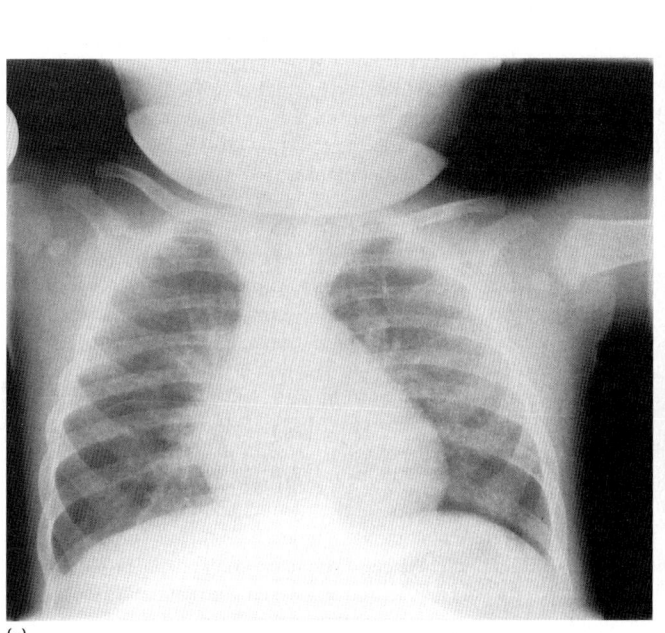

(a)

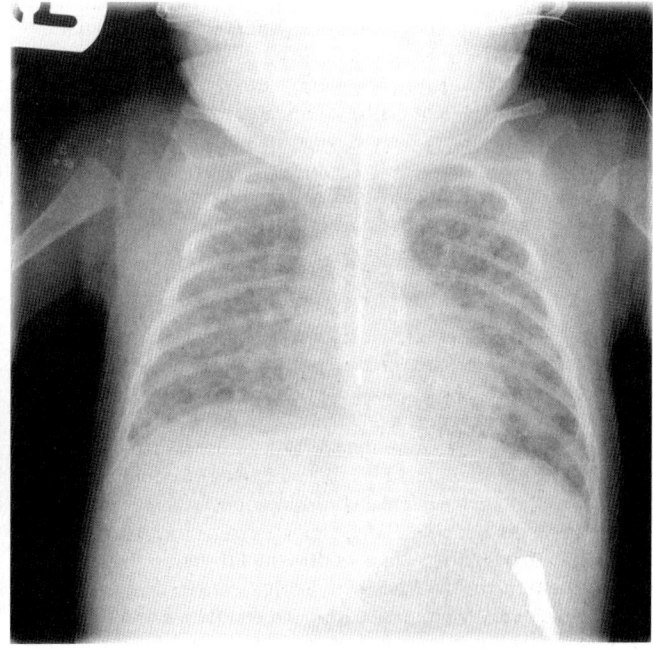

(b)

Fig. 20.33 Chest radiograph showing (a) haziness of both lung field with oxygen dependency typical of type I CLD (Hyde 1989), and (b) more cystic changes associated with CLD typical of Type II (Hyde 1989) or Stage 4 CLD (Northway 1967). Note also presence of pH probe for assessing presence of gastroesophageal reflux.

Table 20.22 Conditions which may be associated with chronic lung disease

System	Clinical manifestation
Respiratory	Oxygen dependency for hypoxia
	Airways obstructive disease
	Laryngo-, tracheo- or broncho-malacia
	Subglottic stenosis
	Acquired bronchial stenosis
	Respiratory viral infections
	Aspiration pneumonitis
Cardiovascular	Pulmonary hypertension
	Cor pulmonale
	Arterial hypertension
Gastrointestinal system and growth	Gastroesophageal reflux
	Malabsorption
	Poor growth
Renal	Renal calculi
Central nervous system	Developmental abnormalities
	Behavioral abnormalities
Ophthalmology	Retinopathy of prematurity
Metabolism	Rickets
	Electrolyte imbalance

tonsils should be sought and treated. In one study, 30% of low birth weight infants underwent surgery for upper airway abnormalities.[585]

Exacerbations of respiratory disease may occur as a result of respiratory infections, gastroesophageal reflux with or without pulmonary aspiration, airways obstruction and heart failure. Of particular importance are viral respiratory infections which remain a common cause of morbidity in children with CLD. Because of decreased respiratory reserve, many infants with CLD present with severe exacerbations of their respiratory status during viral respiratory infection. Of particular note is RSV. In one retrospective study of hospitalizations for RSV in Tennessee, USA, there were 40.8 hospitalizations for RSV per 1000 infants under 1 year of age.[586] For infants with medical factors the estimated number of hospitalizations per 1000 infants under 12 months of age were: 388.4 for infants with CLD and 92.2 for infants with congenital heart disease. The rates also increased with decreasing gestation: 57.2 per 1000 children if born between 33 and 36 weeks' gestation, 65.9 if born between 29 and 32 weeks' and increasing to 70.0 if born at < 28 weeks' gestation. Clearly, respiratory viruses, particularly RSV, place a great burden on both human and economic resources. Therefore considerable effort has been directed to both prevention and treatment of this infection. Ribavirin has not been as efficacious as initial expectations predicted and intravenous pooled immunoglobulins have had variable success reported. The IMPACT study, an RCT of the monoclonal antibody palivizumab in infants < 35 weeks' gestation, showed a 55% reduction of the proportion of preterm infants admitted to hospital from 10.6% in the placebo group to 4.8% in the treated group. In infants with CLD the reduction was 39%, from 12.8% in the placebo group to 7.9% in the treated group.[587] On this evidence, the American Academy of Pediatrics recommends this drug for infants at risk of acquiring RSV. In Europe, cost and case-mix considerations restrict the use of palivizumab to infants at risk of severe exacerbations of respiratory status. A recent statement from the Joint Committee of Vaccination and Immunisation (JCVI) in the UK recommended palivizumab prophylaxis for: (a) children under 2 years of age with CLD, on home oxygen or who have had prolonged use of oxygen; (b) infants under 6 months of age who have left-to-right shunt, hemodynamically significant congenital heart disease and/or pulmonary hypertension; (c) children under 2 years of age with severe congenital immunodeficiency.[588] However, it was interesting that the definition of CLD suggested by the JCVI was oxygen dependency at 28 d, which substantially increases the number of infants recommended for palivizumab treatment. Reassuringly, data from the PICNIC study in Canada demonstrated that infants with CLD who acquired RSV

and required mechanical ventilation did not fare worse than children with other respiratory disorders (CF, congenital lung malformations, respiratory disease associated with CNS disorders).[589]

EXTRAPULMONARY COMPLICATIONS
Growth and nutrition
Many other systems may be affected in children with CLD either directly as a result of developing CLD or indirectly due to being born prematurely (see Table 20.22). Gastroesophageal reflux is common. It may exacerbate respiratory disease if recurrent aspiration occurs or can provoke airways obstruction via reflex neural pathways. Gastroesophageal reflux may present with vomiting, failure to thrive, cough, poor feeding and in the worst cases recurrent lower respiratory tract infections or aspiration pneumonitis. Twenty-four hour esophageal pH monitoring and an upper gastrointestinal tract contrast study are the investigations of choice to confirm gastroesophageal reflux (see Ch. 19, p. 605). Medical treatment with a prokinetic agent together with a feed thickener or alginate are the drugs most often used and in the worst cases reduction of gastric acid by H_2 blockers or proton pump inhibitors is useful. Erythromycin has been used in low doses for its prokinetic action. Fundoplication is required in some children in whom medical treatment fails, as evidenced by failure to thrive, continuing respiratory exacerbations or rare complications of gastroesophageal reflux including hematemesis, anemia or strictures. The diagnosis and management of gastroesophageal reflux in infants has been extensively reviewed by Vandenplas et al.[590]

Growth failure is common in infants with CLD due to a number of reasons that may include increased work of breathing, hypoxemia, gastroesophageal reflux, neurodevelopmental abnormalities resulting in poor feeding, heart failure and other complications of prematurity including necrotizing enterocolitis. Groothuis et al reported that oxygen therapy appeared to improve growth as its discontinuation was associated with poor growth which did not improve to previous levels with the re-introduction of oxygen treatment.[591] However, more recent data from the BOOST trial suggest that oxygen saturations of between 91% and 94% did not affect growth when compared with oxygen saturations of between 95 and 98%.[592] Nevertheless, increased energy intake is indicated in these children to promote growth and high calorie supplements are often necessary. In some cases enteral feeds may have to be given or supplemented via a nasogastric or gastrostomy tube.

Cardiovascular system
Cardiac abnormalities are often seen in children with CLD. These include increased pulmonary vascular resistance due to respiratory disease, right-to-left shunting, left ventricular hypertrophy most likely due to corticosteroid treatment during the neonatal period, patent ductus arteriosus (which will have been treated in the neonatal period) and fluid overload. One or a combination of these features may result in heart failure manifested as poor feeding and failure to thrive, tachypnea, hypoxemia and worsening respiratory disease, and inappropriate weight gain.

Pulmonary hypertension remains the commonest association with CLD and markedly improves with oxygen treatment.[593,594] Cor pulmonale is now uncommon especially since the introduction of home oxygen programs. Electrocardiographs may demonstrate right heart strain or hypertrophy and echocardiography may be used to estimate the degree of pulmonary hypertension in the presence of tricuspid regurgitant flow. Indirect methods of assessing pulmonary arterial pressures by echocardiography and Doppler have also been used (e.g. the ratio of pulmonary arterial acceleration-to-right ventricular ejection time).[594] Such measurements may be used to determine the fixed and reversible components of pulmonary hypertension with the child on and off oxygen. The data may be useful in determining when to wean an infant from supplemental oxygen.

Neurodevelopmental complications
It is almost impossible to attribute the risk of developing neurodevelopmental abnormalities exclusively to CLD as sick extremely preterm

infants are at risk of developing both conditions. Of particular note is that systemic corticosteroid administration in the early neonatal period has been associated with neurodevelopmental delay.[595] Majnemer et al reported the results of a case control study of 27 children with CLD and a similar number of preterm controls matched for gestational age, birth weight and year of birth.[596] Neurological abnormalities were more prevalent in the CLD group (71%) compared with the controls (19%). A variety of disorders were described including cerebral palsy, subtle neurological disorders, microcephaly and behavioral difficulties. Feeding disorders including dysphagia and sleep disorders are also more prevalent in these children. Retinopathy of prematurity leading to visual impairment, in some cases blindness, and hearing abnormalities are more common in infants with CLD. Respiratory responses to hypoxia may be blunted in infants with CLD when compared with non-oxygen-dependent preterm infants, at least in the early stages after weaning from oxygen.

MANAGEMENT

General aspects

The management of the oxygen-dependent child with CLD can be divided into pulmonary and nonpulmonary aspects. The latter should focus on maximizing the growth of the child and on treating conditions such as gastroesophageal reflux which may exacerbate existing respiratory disease. Cardiovascular abnormalities should be sought and treated as necessary. Pulmonary hypertension is likely to respond to oxygen therapy and is discussed below. Full immunization of these infants is essential and live vaccines should be avoided if there has been prolonged corticosteroid treatment. Multivalent pneumococcal vaccination is now included in UK routine immunization for all infants.[597] Influenza vaccination is recommended but not licensed for infants below 6 months of age.[598] Input from relevant agencies, including community pediatricians, health visitors, dieticians, physiotherapists, speech and occupational therapists, and educational psychologists, is often necessary, especially if neurodevelopmental abnormalities are evident.

For established CLD, the mainstays of therapeutic treatment remain:

- domiciliary oxygen;
- corticosteroids;
- bronchodilators;
- diuretics.

Due to the small numbers of infants with established CLD in any one center, there have been very few adequately powered, controlled evaluations of the above treatments in this group of children. Most studies have been uncontrolled observational studies or have included only small numbers of patients. Almost all studies of these treatments have been confined to the neonatal period and are discussed in Chapter 12. Many of these studies have evaluated only short term outcomes and their relevance to longer term outcomes is unknown. The variations of treatment, particularly the use of corticosteroids, diuretics and bronchodilators between the continents was recently described in a series of articles describing the treatment of CLD.[599–602] As a result most treatment which is described below is empirical and founded on 'best practice' rather than evidence.

Domiciliary oxygen

By definition children with CLD are hypoxemic in room air and their wellbeing, particularly with regard to growth, development, work of breathing and pulmonary hypertension, may depend on achieving normoxemia using oxygen therapy. The criteria for prescribing domiciliary oxygen vary between units but, generally speaking, an infant with an oxygen requirement, i.e. supplemental oxygen is required to achieve arterial PaO_2 of $>8\,kPa$ or arterial oxygen saturation (SaO_2) of 94%, should be considered for domiciliary oxygen if attempts to wean the child from oxygen have failed. Particular attention should be paid to hypoxemia during periods of feeding orally by bottle or breast.

More recent data have challenged the optimal target oxygen saturations: the BOOST and STOP-ROP trials suggest that oxygen saturations of lower than 94% may not result in poor growth, neurodevelopmental outcomes or increased pulmonary hypertension.[602,603] Nasogastric feeding may not preclude the child from going home on oxygen but may place a greater burden and stress on the family. Clearly the family should be willing and capable of looking after the child on oxygen. A stable oxygen requirement and a thriving child are ideal but changes to respiratory treatment, particularly the recent cessation of corticosteroids, may result in a rebound increase in oxygen requirements.

Oxygen is most often given by nasal cannulae[604] and is most commonly delivered by an oxygen concentrator.[605] Portable cylinders, especially the lighter versions, allow greater mobility and are helpful for emergency use. Liquid oxygen is sometimes necessary if flow rates higher than 1 L/min are required. Oxygen is now prescribed by the attending pediatrician and provided regionally by a limited number of commercial companies which provide a 24 h service.[606] The oxygen provider will install and provide initial training for the parents. It is usual to provide two outlets – one in the living room and one for the child's sleeping area.

Monitoring of oxygenation is essential. Pulse oximeters have transformed the monitoring of these children. A small number of units have used *continuous* monitoring with transcutaneous monitors but few have used pulse oximeters in this way, partly due to movement artefacts and partly due to the poor quality probes of portable machines for small infants. Therefore, most units have relied on intermittent oxygen saturation measurements on a regular basis. Monitoring should be frequent early after discharge, during intercurrent infections and during weaning of oxygen. Specialist respiratory nurses provide a vital link between the hospital environment (to which the family should have 'open' access) and the community. Infants should also be evaluated regularly within the hospital environment in the presence of all relevant agencies. Weaning from oxygen can commence once the child is stable and thriving.[606] Usually by this stage the oxygen saturations are ≥94% and only insignificant drops occur during feeding and sleep (≤4%). Where available, echocardiography can be used to determine the reversible component of pulmonary hypertension by assessing the pulmonary arterial pressures on and off oxygen. Rates of weaning vary greatly, from increasing time off oxygen gradually, e.g. 15–60 min every week, to completely stopping the oxygen abruptly. Regardless of rates of weaning, it is essential to monitor the child's oxygen saturations once off oxygen and at times of intercurrent infections. The duration of oxygen dependency varies widely but in one study of infants with CLD discharged at a mean age of 3.7 months, mean duration of oxygen therapy was 97 d (range 15–320 d), and the mean age of discontinuation of oxygen was 6.9 months (range 3–14.7 months).[607] It is necessary to continue to monitor after weaning, especially at times of viral URTIs.

The challenge over the next few years is to assess and identify the optimal oxygen saturations for preterm infants at which adverse events such as poor growth, increased pulmonary arterial hypertension and neurodevelopmental delay are avoided.

Corticosteroids

The only clear evidence for the use of corticosteroids for CLD remains the ability of these drugs to facilitate extubation of ventilator dependent infants. Most clinicians are much more cautious than previously due to the association of these drugs with adverse neurodevelopment.[595,608,609] In contrast to ventilated preterm infants, adequate studies of the use of both systemic and inhaled corticosteroids in established CLD are lacking. Caution with the use of dexamethasone, the most frequently used corticosteroid for CLD, was reported by Noble-Jamieson et al in 1989.[610] They treated 18 non-ventilated infants with CLD with either dexamethasone or placebo, and reported that, although there was an initial decrease in oxygenation requirements with steroid treatment, the overall duration of oxygen dependency was similar in both groups. Of particular note was the observation that the treated group had an apparent increase in periventricular abnormalities. In the most recent Cochrane review of the use of inhaled corticosteroids in established CLD by Lister et al,[611] only one study published as an abstract was included in their analysis. In that study,[612] nonventilated infants of at least 36 weeks' corrected gestation and who were oxygen dependent were included. Budesonide (1 mg) was administered by an Airlife Misty-Neb jet nebulizer three times a day for 7 d. A significant reduction in oxygen requirements was observed by the authors. In another study of 18 preterm infants at a mean postnatal age of 10.5 months, the use of inhaled beclomethasone for 6 weeks was associated with an improvement in respiratory tract symptoms and functional residual capacity.[613] Since this study did not specify the number of infants with oxygen dependency, it is difficult to extrapolate the results to infants with established CLD.

In practice, the approach adopted by most is to consider the clinical need (e.g. wheezing) and clinical response to the use of inhaled corticosteroids in infants with CLD and to continue treatment in those who respond, but to actively cease treatment when an adequate response is not observed. Pulmonary function tests may be useful but remain largely a research tool for this group of infants. As this set of children form a large group in the community, there is a clear need for adequately powered RCTs to examine the role of both systemic and inhaled corticosteroids in infants with established CLD.

Bronchodilators

Several studies have shown that preterm infants who are mechanically ventilated have an improvement in lung compliance and resistance following the administration of bronchodilators.[614] Whether these agents have a beneficial effect on longer term outcomes, including symptoms or oxygen dependency, is unknown. In established CLD, marked airway smooth muscle hypertrophy is seen.[583,615] It is likely that this increased smooth muscle stabilizes the compliant infant airway but whether relaxation of airway smooth muscle by bronchodilators leads to increased airway resistance by increasing dynamic airway compression is speculative. Few studies have investigated bronchodilators in infants with CLD beyond the neonatal period. A Cochrane review could identify only one study of prevention by salbutamol (albuterol).[616] Most studies have examined a small number of children in short term, observational studies. In one study of 1-year-old infants with CLD treated with inhaled salbutamol, decreased airway resistance was reported in half the group with no improvement in the remainder.[617] Similarly in older children, functional small airways abnormalities remain and a favorable response to salbutamol is seen in some but not all children.[618] Taken together, these data suggest that there is a subgroup of children who had CLD in infancy who have reversible airways obstruction. However, routine use of salbutamol in all children with CLD is not recommended but should be assessed clinically. If no response is observed, the treatment should be stopped.[618]

Similarly, few studies have evaluated the benefits of inhaled ipratropium bromide in infants with CLD, especially beyond the neonatal period. Benefit from ipratropium has been noted in small studies of ventilated neonates and during early infancy with improvement observed in some children.[619] As with salbutamol, not all children with CLD respond to ipratropium. Another poorly studied area is the optimal method of administering bronchodilators. A metered-dosed inhaler is most frequently used with a spacer device such as the Aerochamber. Questions remain regarding the optimal dose, timing and assessment of clinical response when bronchodilators are used in children with established CLD.

Diuretics

There have been few studies investigating the role of diuretics in CLD beyond the neonatal period. Even those in the neonatal unit have investigated only short term pulmonary outcomes such as decreased pulmonary resistance, improved compliance and reduced oxygen requirements. Cochrane reviews of the use of diuretics have concluded that studies of longer term outcomes are necessary.[620–622] Clearly diuretics are indicated for cardiac failure diagnosed by excessive weight gain, tachypnea, tachycardia, hepatomegaly and peripheral edema. The short-term benefits on respiratory mechanics from diuretics are likely to result from a direct action on pulmonary vascular resistance and on extracellular pulmonary water. Whether there are longer term benefits, e.g. decreased numbers of days of oxygen dependency, is currently unknown. In addition, adverse effects of long term diuretic treatment may be clinically important. The use of diuretics, especially loop diuretics such as furosemide, can result in renal calcification and calculi which often but not always resolve on cessation of therapy. It is usual practice to use loop diuretics in the short term and to change over to a combination of a thiazide and spironolactone to decrease the risks of adverse effects, although electrolyte imbalance with hyponatremia and hypokalemia may still be troublesome.

PROGNOSIS

There has been great improvement in survival of preterm infants and, with home oxygen programs, the outlook for children with CLD has also improved vastly. However, although there is improvement in the respiratory status of preschool children following CLD as infants, as they reach adolescence there remains a degree of respiratory morbidity as evidenced by increased cough, wheezing and decreased exercise tolerance. Lung function improves with time but, compared with healthy controls or preterm controls without CLD, persisting abnormalities, particularly of FEV_1, more peripheral airway function (FEF_{25-75}) and gas trapping have been reported.[623–625] The decreased alveolar numbers described in infants with CLD is of concern.[580] Whether these children are candidates for chronic pulmonary dysfunction in later life remains to be seen.

THE FUTURE

Despite improvements in prognosis for infants with CLD, there are a number of areas which need to be refined over the next few years. The optimal oxygen saturation range clearly needs to be identified. The role of therapeutic agents such as systemic and inhaled corticosteroids, bronchodilators and diuretics in children with established CLD clearly needs clarification. Further information regarding efficacy, doses and their timing and routes of administration is required urgently. The role of supportive therapies, such as the effects of nutrition on lung growth, need to be clarified further. Since candidates for developing CLD are preterm and at an early stage of lung development, we need a better understanding of both normal lung development in the fetus and also after the infant is delivered. Only by understanding the underlying mechanisms, including the role of antenatal factors such as infection in the development of CLD, are we likely to develop specific targeted therapies for developing or established CLD which do not have adverse effects, including poor neurodevelopment.

REFERENCES (*Level 1 evidence)

1. Beasley R, ISAAC Steering Committee. Worldwide variation in prevalence of symptoms of asthma, allergic rhinoconjunctivitis, and atopic eczema: ISAAC. Lancet 1998; 351:1225–1232.
2. Omran M, Russell G. Continuing increase in respiratory symptoms and atopy in Aberdeen schoolchildren. BMJ 1996; 312:34.
3. Burr ML, Watt D, Evans C, et al. British Thoracic Society Research Committee. Asthma prevalence in 1973, 1988 and 2003. Thorax 2006; 61:296–299.
4. Devenny A, Wassall H, Ninan T, et al. Respiratory symptoms and atopy in children in Aberdeen: questionnaire studies of a defined school population repeated over 35 years. BMJ 2004; 329:489–490.
5. Galassi C, De Sario M, Biggeri A, et al. Changes in prevalence of asthma and allergies among children and adolescents in Italy: 1994–2002. Pediatrics 2006; 117:34–42.
6. Asher MI, Montefort S, Bjorksten B, et al; ISAAC Phase Three Study Group. Worldwide time trends in the prevalence of symptoms of asthma, allergic rhinoconjunctivitis, and eczema in childhood: ISAAC Phases One and Three repeat multicountry cross-sectional surveys. Lancet 2006; 368:733–743.
7. Strachan DP. Hay fever, hygiene and household size. BMJ 1989; 299:1259–1260.

8. Strachan DP. Family size, infection and atopy: the first decade of the "hygiene hypothesis". Thorax 2000; 55(Suppl 1):S2–S10.

9. Stern DA, Riedler J, Nowak D, et al. Exposure to a farming environment has allergen-specific protective effects on T(H)2-dependent isotype switching in response to common inhalants. J Allergy Clin Immunol 2007; 119:351–358.

10. Simpson A, John SL, Jury F, et al. Endotoxin exposure, CD14, and allergic disease: an interaction between genes and the environment. Am J Respir Crit Care Med 2006; 174:386–392.

11. Helms PJ. Corticosteroid-sparing options in the treatment of childhood asthma. Drugs 2000; 59(Suppl 1):15–22.

12. Guilbert TW, Morgan WJ, Zeiger RS, et al. Long-term inhaled corticosteroids in preschool children at high risk for asthma. N Engl J Med 2006; 354:1985–1997.

13. Bisgaard H, Hermansen MN, Loland L, et al. Intermittent inhaled corticosteroids in infants with episodic wheezing. N Engl J Med 2006; 354:1998–2005.

14. Murray CS, Woodcock A, Langley SJ, et al. IFWIN study team. Secondary prevention of asthma by the use of inhaled fluticasone propionate in Wheezy Infants (IFWIN): double-blind, randomised, controlled study. Lancet 2006; 368:754–762.

15. Britton JR. Effect of social class, sex and region of residence on age at death from cystic fibrosis. BMJ 1989; 298:483–487.

16. Elborn JS, Shale DJ, Britton JR. Cystic fibrosis: current survival and population estimates to the year 2000. Thorax 1991; 46:881–885.

17. Grosse SD, Rosenfeld M, Devine OJ, et al. Potential impact of newborn screening for cystic fibrosis on child survival: a systematic review and analysis. J Pediatr 2006; 149:362–366.

18. Eiser C, Morse R. A review of measures of quality of life for children with chronic illness. Arch Dis Child 2001; 84:205–211.

19. Reichenber K, Broberg AG. The Paediatric Asthma Caregiver's Quality of Life Questionnaire in Swedish parents. Acta Paediatr 2001; 90:45–50.

20. Morgan WJ, Stern DA, Sherrill DL, et al. Outcome of asthma and wheezing in the first 6 years of life: follow-up through adolescence. Am J Respir Crit Care Med 2005; 172:1253–1258.

21. Sears MR, Greene JM, Willan AR, et al. A longitudinal, population-based, cohort study of childhood asthma followed to adulthood. N Engl J Med 2003; 349:1414–1422.

22. Smith OO, Helms PJ. Genetic/environmental determinants of adult chronic obstructive pulmonary disease and possible links with childhood wheezing. Paediatr Respir Rev 2001; 2:178–183.

23. Harding R, Cock ML, Louey S, et al. The compromised intrauterine environment: implications for future lung health. Clin Exp Pharmacol Physiol 2000; 27:965–974.

24. Barker DJ, Godfrey KM, Fall C, et al. Relation of birth weight and childhood respiratory infections to adult lung function and death from chronic obstructive airways disease. BMJ 1991; 303:671–675.

25. Castro-Rodriguez J, Holberg C, Wright A, et al. Association of radiologically ascertained pneumonia before age 3 years with asthma like symptoms and pulmonary function during childhood: a prospective study. Am J Respir Crit Care Med 1999; 159:1891–1897.

26. Shaheen SO, Barker DJ, Holgate ST. Do lower respiratory tract infections in early childhood cause chronic obstructive pulmonary disease? Am J Respir Crit Care Med 1995; 151:1649–1651.

27. Hoffjan S, Ober C. Present status on the genetic studies of asthma. Curr Opin Immunol 2002; 14:709–717.

28. Anderson GG, Morrison JFJ. Molecular biology and genetics of allergy and asthma. Arch Dis Child 1998; 78:488–496.

29. Hoffjan S, Nicolae D, Ober C. Association studies for asthma and atopic diseases: a comprehensive review of the literature. Respir Res 2003; 4:14.

30. Blouin JL, Meeks M, Radhakrishna U, et al. Primary ciliary dyskinesia: a genome-wide linkage analysis reveals extensive locus heterogeneity. Eur J Hum Genet 2000; 8:109–118.

31. Hornef N, Olbrich H, Horvath J, et al. *DNAH5* mutations are a common cause of primary ciliary dyskinesia with outer dynein arm defects. Am J Respir Crit Care Med 2006; 174:120–126.

32. Okada Y, Takeda S, Tanaka Y, et al. Mechanism of nodal flow: a conserved symmetry breaking event in left-right axis determination. Cell 2005; 121:633–644.

33. Pasteur MC, Helliwell SM, Houghton SJ, et al. An investigation into causative factors in patients with bronchiectasis. Am J Resp Crit Care Med 2000; 162:1277–1284.

34. Cook DG, Strachan DP. Summary of effects of parental smoking on the respiratory health of children and implications for research. Thorax 1999; 54:357–366.

35. Martinez FD, Morgan WJ, Wright AL, et al. Diminished lung function as a predisposing factor for wheezing respiratory illness in infants. N Engl J Med 1988; 319:1112–1117.

36. Stick SM, Burton PR, Gurrin L, et al. Effects of maternal smoking during pregnancy and a family history of asthma on respiratory function in newborn infants. Lancet 1996; 348:1060–1064.

37. Dezateux C, Stocks J, Dundas I, et al. Impaired airway function and wheezing in infancy: the influence of maternal smoking and a genetic predisposition to asthma. Am J Respir Crit Care Med 1999; 159:403–410.

38. Gilliland FD, Li Y-F, Peters JM. Effects of maternal smoking during pregnancy and environmental tobacco smoke on asthma and wheezing in children. Am J Resp Crit Care Med 2001; 163:429–436.

39. Mitchell EA. Smoking: the next major and modifiable risk factor. In: Rognum TO, ed. Sudden infant death syndrome. New trends in the nineties. Oslo: Scandinavian University Press, 1995:114–118.

40. Fleming PJ, Blair P, Bacon C, et al. Environment of infants during sleep and risk of the sudden infant death syndrome: results of the 1993–5 case-control study for confidential enquiry into stillbirths and deaths in infancy. BMJ 1996; 313:191–198.

41. Office for National Statistics. Drug use, smoking and drinking among young teenagers in 1999. www.statistics.gov.uk/pdfdir/drugs0500.pdf2000 (accessed 4th March 2005); Vol. 189.

42. Withers NJ, Low JL, Holgate ST, et al. Smoking habits of a cohort of UK adolescents. Respir Med 2000; 94:391–396.

43. National Institute on Drug Abuse. Teen smoking dropped dramatically in 2003. www.drugabuse.gov/NIDA_notes/NNVol17N6/tearoff.html (accessed 4th March 2005).

44. Grimshaw GM, Stanton A. Tobacco cessation interventions for young people. Cochrane Database Syst Rev 2006 Oct 18; (4): CD003289.

45. Williams BG, Gouws E, Boschi-Pinto C, et al. Estimates of world-wide distribution of child deaths from acute respiratory infections. Lancet Infect Dis 2002; 2:25–32.

46. Cohen S. Social status and susceptibility to respiratory infections. Ann N Y Acad Sci 1999; 896:246–253.

47. Mann SL, Wadsworth ME, Colley JR. Accumulation of factors influencing respiratory illness in members of a national birth cohort and their offspring. J Epidemiol Comm Health 1992; 46:286–292.

48. Rose AMC, Watson JM, Graham C, et al. Tuberculosis at the end of the 20th century in England and Wales: results of a national survey in 1998. Thorax 2001; 56:173–179.

49. Beckhurst C, Evans S, MacFarlane AF, et al. Factors influencing the distribution of tuberculosis cases in an inner London borough. Commun Dis Public Health 2000; 3:28–31.

50. Bennett J, Pitman R, Jarman B, et al. A study of the variation in tuberculosis incidence and possible influential variables in Manchester, Liverpool, Birmingham and Cardiff in 1991–1995. Int J Tuberculosis Lung Dis 2001; 5:158–163.

51. Sigurs N, Bjarnason R, Sigurbergsson F, et al. Respiratory syncytial virus bronchiolitis in infancy is an important risk factor for asthma and allergy at age 7. Am J Respir Crit Care Med 2000; 161:1501–1507.

52. Sigurs N. Clinical perspectives on the association between respiratory syncytial virus and reactive airway disease. Respir Res 2002; 3(Suppl 1):S8–S14.

53. Schwartz J. Role of polyunsaturated fats in lung disease. Am J Clin Nutrition 2000; 71(Suppl 1):393S–396S.

54. Cook D, Carey I, Whincup P, et al. Effect of fresh fruit consumption on lung function and wheeze in children. Thorax 1997; 52:628–633.

55. Moreno-Reyes R, Suetens C, Mathieu F, et al. Kashin-Beck osteoarthropathy in rural Tibet in relation to selenium and iodine status. N Engl J Med 1998; 339:1112–1120.

56. Allam MF, Lucane RA. Selenium supplementation for asthma. Cochrane Database Syst Rev 2004; (2): CD003538.

57. Sempertegui F, Estrella B, Camaniero V, et al. The beneficial effects of weekly low-dose vitamin A supplementation on acute lower respiratory infections and diarrhea in Ecuadorian children. Pediatrics 1999; 104:e1.

58. Fawzi WW, Mbise R, Spiegelman D, et al. Vitamin A supplements and diarrheal and respiratory tract infections among children in Dar es Salaam, Tanzania. J Pediatr 2000; 137:660–667.

59. Ni J, Wei J, Wu T. Vitamin A for non-measles pneumonia in children. Cochrane Database Syst Rev 2005 Jul 20; (3): CD003700.

60. Demissie K, Ernst P, Donald K, et al. Usual dietary salt intake and asthma in children: a case-control study. Thorax 1996; 51:59–63.

61. Ram FS, Ardern KD. Dietary salt reduction or exclusion for allergic asthma. Cochrane Database Syst Rev 2004; (3): CD000436.

62. Gouveia N, Fletcher T. Respiratory diseases in children and outdoor air pollution in Sao Paulo, Brazil: a time series analysis. Occup Environ Med 2000; 57:477–483.

63. Hajat S, Haines A, Goubet SA, et al. Association of air pollution with daily GP consultations for asthma and other lower respiratory conditions in London. Thorax 1999; 54:597–605.

64. von Mutius E, Fritzsch C, Weiland SK, et al. Prevalence of asthma and allergic disorders among children in united Germany: a descriptive comparison. BMJ 1992; 305:1395–1399.

65. Wjst M, Reitmeir P, Dold S, et al. Road traffic and adverse effects on respiratory health in children. BMJ 1993; 307:596–600.

66. Bruce N, Perez-Padilla R, Albalak R. Indoor air pollution in developing countries: a major environmental and public health challenge. Bull WHO 2000; 78:1078–1092.

67. Dekker C, Dales R, Bartlett S, et al. Childhood asthma and the indoor environment. Chest 1991; 100:922–926.

68. Burr ML, Anderson HR, Austin JB, et al. Respiratory symptoms and home environment in children: a national survey. Thorax 1999; 54:27–32.

69.   Cooney TP, Thurlbeck WM. The radial alveolar count method of Emery and Mithal: a reappraisal 1–Postnatal lung growth. Thorax 1982; 37:572–579.

70.   Hislop A, Muir DC, Jacobsen M et al. Postnatal growth and function of the pre-acinar airways. Thorax 1972; 27:265–274.

71.   Thurlbeck WM, Kida K, Langston C, et al. Postnatal lung growth after repair of diaphragmatic hernia. Thorax 1979; 34:338–343.

72.   Wigglesworth JS, Desai R, Guerrini P. Fetal lung hypoplasia: biochemical and structural variations and their possible significance. Arch Dis Child 1981; 56:606–615.

73.   Helms P, Stocks J. Lung function in infants with congenital pulmonary hypoplasia. J Pediatr 1982; 101:918–922.

74.   Wigglesworth JS, Winston RML, Bartlett K. Influence of the central nervous system on fetal lung development. Arch Dis Child 1977; 52:965–967.

75.   Falconer AR, Brown RA, Helms P, et al. Pulmonary sequelae in survivors of congenital diaphragmatic hernia. Thorax 1990; 45:126–129.

76.   Taylor B, Wadsworth J. Maternal smoking during pregnancy and lower respiratory tract illness in early life. Arch Dis Child 1987; 62:786–791.

77.   Hanrahan JP, Tager IB, Segal MR, et al. The effect of maternal smoking during pregnancy on early infant lung function. Am Rev Respir Dis 1992; 145:1129–1135.

78.   Young S, Le Souef PN, Geelhoed GC, et al. The influence of a family history of asthma and parental smoking on airway responsiveness in early infancy. N Engl Med 1991; 324:1168–1173.

79.   Collins MH, Moessinger AC, Kleinerman J, et al. Fetal lung hypoplasia associated with maternal smoking: a morphometric analysis. Pediatr Res 1995; 19:408–412.

80.   Vidic B, Ujevic N, Shabahang MM, et al. Differentiation of interstitial cells and stromal proteins in the secondary septum of early postnatal rat: effect of maternal chronic exposure to whole cigarette smoke. Anat Rec 1989; 223:165–173.

81.   Polgar G, Weng TR. The functional development of the respiratory system. Am Rev Respir Dis 1979; 120:625–695.

82.   Quanjer PH, Helms P, Bjure J, et al. Standardization of lung function tests in paediatrics. Eur Respir J 1989; 54:54.

83.   Openshaw P, Edwards S, Helms P. Changes in rib cage geometry during childhood. Thorax 1984; 39:624–627.

84.   Proctor DF. Physiology of the upper airway. In: Fenn W O, Rahn H, eds. Respiration. American Physiological Society. Baltimore: Williams & Wilkins Baltimore; 1964.

85.   Davies H, Kitchman R, Gordon I, et al. Regional ventilation in infancy. N Engl J Med 1985; 313:1626–1628.

86.   Nielsen KG, Bisgaard H. Discriminative capacity of bronchodilator response measured with three different lung function techniques in asthmatic and healthy children aged 2 to 5 years. Am J Respir Crit Care Med 2001; 164:554–559.

87.   Vilozni D, Barak A, Efrati O, et al. The role of computer games in measuring spirometry in healthy and "asthmatic" preschool children. Chest 2005; 128:1146–1155.

88.   Wang XB, Dockery DW, Wypij D, et al. Pulmonary-function between 6 and 18 years of age. Pediatr Pulmonol 1993; 15:75–88.

89.   Tsanakas JN, Primhak RA, Milner RD, et al. Unexpectedly high peak expiratory flow rates in normal Greek children. Eur J Pediatr 1983; 141:46–49.

90.   Cassels DE, Morse M. Arterial blood gases and acid-base balance in normal children. J Clin Invest 1953; 32:824–836.

91.   Gaultier C, Boule M, Allaire Y, et al. Determination of capillary oxygen tension in infants and children. Bull Eur Physiopathol Respir 1978; 14:287–297.

92.   McLaren CA, Elliott MJ, Roebuck DJ. Tracheobronchial intervention in children. Eur J Radiol 2005; 53:22–34.

93.   Daltro P, Fricke BL, Kuroki I, et al. CT of congenital lung lesions in pediatric patients. AJR Am J Roentgenol 2004; 183:1497–1506.

94.   Siegel MJ. Pediatric CT angiography. Eur Radiol 2005; 15(Suppl 4):32–36.

95.   Boechat MI, Ratib O, Williams PL, et al. Cardiac MR imaging and MR angiography for assessment of complex tetralogy of Fallot and pulmonary atresia. Radiographics 2005; 25:1535–1546.

96.   Wood RE, Fink RJ. Applications of flexible fiberoptic bronchoscopes in infants and children. Chest 1978; 73:737–740.

97.   Midulla F, de Blic J, Barbato A, et al. Flexible endoscopy of paediatric airways. Eur Respir J 2003; 22:698–708.

98.   Nielson DW, Ku PL, Egger M. Topical lidocaine exaggerates laryngomalacia during flexible bronchoscopy. Am J Respir Crit Care Med 2000; 161:147–151.

99.   Nussbaum E, Zagnoev M. Pediatric fiberoptic bronchoscopy with a laryngeal mask airway. Chest 2001; 120:614–616.

100.   Flexible endoscopy of the paediatric airway. Am Rev Respir Dis 1992; 145:233–235.

101.   Whitehead B, Scott JP, Helms P, et al. Technique and use of transbronchial biopsy in children and adolescents. Pediatr Pulmonol 1992; 12:240–246.

102.   Mehta AC, Prakash UBS, Garland R, et al. American College of Chest Physicians and American Association for Bronchology Consensus Statement: Prevention of flexible bronchoscopy-associated infection. Chest 2005; 128:1742–1755.

103.   British Thoracic Society guidelines on diagnostic flexible bronchoscopy. Thorax 2001; 56(Suppl 1):i1–i21.

104.   Barbato A, Magarotto M, Crivellaro M, et al. Use of the paediatric bronchoscope, flexible and rigid, in 51 European centres. Eur Respir J 1997; 10:1761–1766.

105.   de Blic J, Azevedo I, Burren CP, et al. The value of flexible bronchoscopy in childhood pulmonary tuberculosis. Chest 1991; 100:688–692.

106.   ERS Task Force on bronchoalveolar lavage in children. Bronchoalveolar lavage in children. Eur Respir J 2000; 15:217–231.

107.   Payne D, McKenzie SA, Stacey S, et al. Safety and ethics of bronchoscopy and endobronchial biopsy in difficult asthma. Arch Dis Child 2001; 84:423–426.

108.   Nicolai T, Huber RM, Reiter K, et al. Mal airway stent implantation in children: follow-up of seven children. Pediatr Pulmonol 2001; 31:289–296.

109.   Fayon M, Donato L, de Blic J, et al. French experience of silicone tracheobronchial stenting in children. Pediatr Pulmonol 2005; 39:21–27.

110.   Vinograd I, Keidar S, Weinberg M, et al. Treatment of airway obstruction by metallic stents in infants and children. J Thorac Cardiovasc Surg 2005; 130:146–150.

111.   Wood RE, Postma D. Endoscopy of the airway in infants and children. J Pediatr 1988; 112:1–6.

112.   Barbato A, Novello Jr A, Tormena F, et al. Use of fiberoptic bronchoscopy in asthmatic children with lung collapse. Pediatr Med Chir 1995; 17:253–255.

113.   Brownlee KG, Crabbe DC. Paediatric bronchoscopy. Arch Dis Child 1997; 77:272–275.

114.   Zalzal GH. Stridor and airway compromise. Pediatr Clin North Am 1989; 36:1389–1402.

115.   Orlow SJ, Isakoff MS, Blei F. Increased risk of symptomatic hemangiomas of the airway in association with cutaneous hemangiomas in a "beard" distribution. J Pediatr 1997; 131:643–646.

116.   Carden KA, Boiselle PM, Waltz DA, et al. Tracheomalacia and tracheobronchomalacia in children and adults: an in-depth review. Chest 2005; 127:984–1005.

117.   Boogaard R, Huijsmans SH, Pijnenburg MW, et al. Tracheomalacia and bronchomalacia in children: incidence and patient characteristics. Chest 2005; 128:3391–3397.

118.   Wood RE. Spelunking in the pediatric airway: explorations with the flexible fibreoptic bronchoscope. Pediatr Clin North Am 1984; 31:785–799.

119.   Mahut B, Delacourt C, Scheinmann P, et al. Pulmonary alveolar proteinosis: experience with eight pediatric cases and a review. Pediatrics 1996; 97:117–122.

120.   Kurland G, Noyes BE, Jaffe R, et al. Bronchoalveolar lavage and transbronchial biopsy in children following heart–lung and lung transplantation. Chest 1993; 104:1043–1048.

121.   Colombo JL, Hallberg TK. Pulmonary aspiration and lipid-laden macrophages: in search of gold (standards). Pediatr Pulmonol 1999; 28:79–82.

122.   Bar-Zohar D, Sivan Y. The yield of flexible fiberoptic bronchoscopy in pediatric intensive care patients. Chest 2004; 126:1353–1359.

123.   Manna SS, Durward A, Mo1ganasundram S, et al. Retrospecptive evaluation of a paediatric intensivist-led flexible bronnchoscopy service. Intensive Care Med 2006; 32:1432–1438.

124.   Wells AL, Wells TR, Landing BH, et al. Short trachea, a hazard in tracheal intubation of neonates and infants: syndromal associations. Anesthesiology 1989; 71:367–373.

125.   Wells TR, Jacobs RA, Senac MO, et al. Incidence of short trachea in patients with myelomeningocele. Pediatr Neurol 1990; 6:109–111.

126.   Mizikov VM, Variushina TV, Kirimov I. [Fiberoptic bronchoscopy via laryngeal mask in children]. Anesteziol Reanimatol 1997; 78–80.

127.   Mayhall CG. Ventilator-associated pneumonia or not? Contemporary diagnosis. Emerg Infect Dis 2001; 7:200–204.

128.   Siegel JM. Clues to the functions of mammalian sleep. Nature 2005; 437:1264–1271.

129.   Loomis AL, Harvey EN, Hobart GA. Cerebral states during sleep as studied by human brain potentials. J Exp Psychol 1937; 21:127–144.

130.   Aserinsky E, Kleitman N. Regularly occurring periods of eye motility, and concomitant phenomena, during sleep. Science 1953; 118:273–274.

131.   Rechtschaffen A, Kales A. A manual of standardized terminology, techniques, and scoring system for sleep stages of human subjects. US Department of Health, Education, and Welfare Public Health Service – NIH/NIND; 1968.

132.   Gaultier C, Praud JP, Canet E, et al. Paradoxical inward rib cage motion during rapid eye movement sleep in infants and young children. J Dev Physiol 1987; 9:391–397.

133.   Marcus CL, Glomb WB, Basinski DJ, et al. Developmental pattern of hypercapnic and hypoxic ventilatory responses from childhood to adulthood. J Appl Physiol 1994; 76:314–320.

134.   Hunt CE, Hufford DR, Bourguignon C, et al. Home documented monitoring of cardiorespiratory pattern and oxygen saturation in healthy infants. Pediatr Res 1996; 39:216–222.

135.   Trang H, Dehan M, Beaufils F, et al. The French Congenital Central Hypoventilation Syndrome Registry. General data, phenotype and genotype. Chest 2005; 127:72–79.

136.   Vanderlaan M, Holbrook CR, Wang M, et al. Epidemiologic survey of 196 patients with congenital central hypoventilation syndrome. Pediatr Pulmonol 2004; 37:217–229.

137.   Maitra A, Shine J, Henderson J, et al. The investigation and care of children with congenital

central hypoventilation syndrome. Curr Paediatr 2004; 14:354–360.

138. Chen ML, Keens TG. Congenital central hypoventilation syndrome: not just another rare disorder. Pediatr Respir Rev 2004; 5:182–189.

139. Katz E, McGrath S, Marcus C. Late-onset central hypoventilation with hypothalamic dysfunction: a distinct clinical syndrome. Pediatr Pulmonol 2000; 29:62–68.

140. Antic NA, Malow BA, Lange N, et al. PHOX2B Mutation-confirmed congenital central hypoventilation syndrome. Presentation in adulthood. Am J Respir Crit Care Med 2006; 174:923–927.

141. Weese-Mayer DE, Berry-Kravis EM, Marazita ML. In pursuit (and discovery) of a genetic basis for congenital central hypoventilation syndrome. Respir Physiol Neurobiol 2005; 149:73–82.

142. Amiel J, Laudier B, Attie-Bitach T, et al. Polyalanine expansion and frameshift mutations of the paired-like homeobox gene PHOX2B in congenital central hypoventilation syndrome (see comment). Nat Genet 2003; 33:459–461.

143. Berry-Kravis EM, Zhou L, Ransd CM, et al. Congenital central hypoventilation syndrome. PHOX2B Mutations and phenotype. Am J Respir Crit Care Med 2006; 174:1139–1144.

144. Keens T. Congenital central hypoventilation syndrome. In: Association DcscotASD (ed): The international classification of sleep disorders: Diagnostic and coding manual. Lawrence, Kansas: Allen Press, Inc; 1990.205–209.

145. American Thoracic Society. Idiopathic congenital central hypoventilation syndrome. Diagnosis and management. Am J Respir Crit Care Med 1999; 160:368–373.

146. Gozal D, Marcus CL, Shoseyov D, et al. Peripheral chemoreceptor function in children with the congenital central hypoventilation syndrome. J Appl Physiol 1993; 74:379–387.

147. Fleming PJ, Cade D, Bryan MH, et al. Congenital central hypoventilation and sleep state. Pediatrics 1980; 66:425–428.

148. Paton JY, Swaminathan S, Sargent CW, et al. Hypoxic and hypercapnic ventilatory responses in awake children with congenital central hypoventilation syndrome. Am Rev Respir Dis 1989; 140:368–372.

149. Harper R, Macey PM, Woo MA, et al. Hypercapnic exposure in congenital central hypoventilation syndrome reveals CNS respiratory control mechanisms. J Neurophysiol 2005; 93:1647–1658.

150. Woo MA, Macey PM, Macey KE, et al. FMRI responses to hyperoxia in congenital central hypoventilation syndrome. Pediatr Res 2005; 57:510–518.

151. Macey PM, Macey KE, Woo MA, et al. Aberrant neural responses to cold pressor challenges in congenital central hypoventilation syndrome. Pediatr Res 2005; 57:500–509.

152. Kumar R, Macey PM, Woo MA, et al. Neuroanatomic deficits in congenital central hypoventilation syndrome. J Comp Neurol 2005; 487:361–371.

153. Kumar R, Macey PM, Woo MA, et al. Elevated mean diffusivity in widespread brain regions in congenital central hypoventilation syndrome. J Magn Reson Imaging 2006; 24:1252–1258.

154. Gaultier C, Gallego J. Development of respiratory control: evolving concepts and perspectives. Respir Physiol Neurobiol 2005; 149:2–15.

155. Tibballs J, Henning RD. Noninvasive ventilatory strategies in the management of a newborn infant and three children with congenital central hypoventilation syndrome. Pediatr Pulmonol 2003; 36:544–548.

156. Hartmann H, Jawad MH, Noyes J, et al. Negative extrathoracic pressure ventilation in central hypoventilation syndrome. Arch Dis Child 1994; 70:418–423.

157. Jardine E, Wallis C. Core guidelines for the discharge home of the child on long term assisted ventilation in the United Kingdom. Thorax 1998; 53:762–767.

158. Edwards E, O'Toole M, Wallis C. Sending children home on tracheostomy dependent ventilation: pitfalls and outcomes. Arch Dis Child 2004; 89:251–255.

159. Weese-Mayer DE, Silvestri JM, Kenny AS, et al. Diaphragm pacing with a quadripolar phrenic nerve electrode: an international study. Pacing Clin Electrophysiol 1996; 19:1311–1319.

160. Flageole H, Adolph VR, Davis GM, et al. Diaphragmatic pacing in children with congenital central alveolar hypoventilation syndrome. Surgery 1995; 118:25–28.

161. Weese-Mayer DE, Morrow AS, Brouillette RT, et al. Diaphragm pacing in infants and children. A life-table analysis of implanted components. Am Rev Respir Dis 1989; 139:974–979.

162. Chen ML, Turkel SB, Jacobson JR, et al. Alcohol use in congenital central hypoventilation syndrome. Pediatr Pulmonol 2006; 41:283–285.

163. Ali NJ, Pitson DJ, Stradling JR. Snoring, sleep disturbance, and behaviour in 4–5 year olds. Arch Dis Child 1993; 68:360–366.

164. Gislason T, Benediktsdottir B. Snoring, apneic episodes, and nocturnal hypoxemia among children 6 months to 6 years old. An epidemiologic study of lower limit of prevalence. Chest 1995; 107:963–966.

165. Shott SR, Amin R, Chini B, et al. Obstructive sleep apnea: Should all children with Down syndrome be tested? Arch Otolaryngol Head Neck Surg 2006; 132:432–436.

166. Tauman R, Gozal D. Obesity and obstructive sleep apnea in children. Paediatr Respir Rev 2006; 7:247–259.

167. Taheri S, Lin L, Austin D, et al. Short sleep duration is associated with reduced leptin, elevated ghrelin, and increased body mass index. PLoS Med 2004; 1:e62.

168. Eiholzer U, Nordmann Y, L'Allemand D. Fatal outcome of sleep apnoea in PWS during the initial phase of growth hormone treatment. A case report. Hormone Res 58 Suppl 2002; 3:24–26.

169. Grugni G, Livieri C, Corrias A, et al. Death during GH therapy in children with Prader-Willi syndrome: description of two new cases. J Endocrinol Invest 2005; 28:554–557.

170. Festen DA, de Weerd AW, van den Bossche RA, et al. Sleep-related breathing disorders in prepubertal children with Prader-Willi syndrome and effects of growth hormone treatment. J Clin Endocrinol Metab 2006; 91:4911–4915.

171. Fregosi RF, Quan SF, Kaemingk KL, et al. Sleep-disordered breathing, pharyngeal size and soft tissue anatomy in children. J Appl Physiol 2003; 95:2030–2038.

172. Gozal D, Burnside MM. Increased upper airway collapsibility in children with obstructive sleep apnea during wakefulness. Am J Respir Crit Care Med 2004; 169:163–167.

173. Redline S, Tishler PV, Tosteson TD, et al. The familial aggregation of obstructive sleep apnea. Am J Respir Crit Care Med 1995; 151:682–687.

174. Tauman R, Gulliver TE, Krishna J, et al. Persistence of obstructive sleep apnea syndrome in children after adenotonsillectomy. J Pediatr 2006; 149:803–808.

175. Owens JA. The ADHD and sleep conundrum: a review. J Dev Behav Pediatr 2005; 26:312–322.

176. Liu X, Hubbard JA, Fabes RA, et al. Sleep disturbances and correlates of children with autism spectrum disorders. Child Psychiatry Hum Dev 2006; 37:179–191.

177. Guilleminault C, Eldridge FL, Simmons FB, et al. Sleep apnea in eight children. Pediatrics 1976; 58:23–30.

178. Brouillette RT, Fernbach SK, Hunt CE. Obstructive sleep apnea in infants and children. J Pediatr 1982; 100:31–40.

179. Kheirandish L, Gozal D. Neurocognitive dysfunction in children with sleep disorders. Dev Sci 2006; 9:388–399.

180. Gozal D. Sleep-disordered breathing and school performance in children. Pediatrics 1998; 102:616–620.

181. Gozal D, Pope Jr DW. Snoring during early childhood and academic performance at ages thirteen to fourteen years. Pediatrics 2001; 107:1394–1399.

182. Halbower AC, Degaonkar M, Barker PB, et al. Childhood obstructive sleep apnea associates with neuropsychological deficits and neuronal brain injury. PLoS Med 2006; 3:e301.

183. Blunden S, Lushington K, Kennedy D. Cognitive and behavioural performance in children with sleep-related obstructive breathing disorders. Sleep Med Rev 2001; 5:447–461.

184. O'Brien LM, Holbrook CR, Mervis CB, et al. Sleep and neurobehavioral characteristics of 5- to 7-year-old children with parentally reported symptoms of attention-deficit/hyperactivity disorder. Pediatrics 2003; 111:554–563.

185. Bourke SC, Gibson GJ. Sleep and breathing in neuromuscular disease. Eur Respir J 2002; 19:1194–1201.

186. Dohna-Schwake C, Ragette R, Teschler H, et al. Predictors of severe chest infections in pediatric neuromuscular disorders. Neuromuscul Disord 2006; 16:325–328.

187. Arens R. Obstructive sleep apnea in childhood: clinical features. In: Loughlin G M, Carroll J, Marcus C L, eds. Sleep and breathing in children: A developmental approach. New York, NY: Marcel Dekker; 2000.575–600.

188. Owens JA, Spirito A, McGuinn M. The Children's Sleep Habits Questionnaire (CSHQ): psychometric properties of a survey instrument for school-aged children. Sleep 2000; 23:1043–1051.

189. Chervin RD, Hedger K, Dillon JE, et al. Pediatric sleep questionnaire (PSQ): validity and reliability of scales for sleep-disordered breathing, snoring, sleepiness, and behavioral problems. Sleep Med 2000; 1:21–32.

190. Carroll JL, McColley SA, Marcus CL, et al. Inability of clinical history to distinguish primary snoring from obstructive sleep apnea syndrome in children. Chest 1995; 108:610–618.

191. Montgomery-Downs HE, O'Brien LM, Holbrook CR, et al. Snoring and sleep-disordered breathing in young children: subjective and objective correlates. Sleep 2004; 27:87–94.

192. Chervin RD, Weatherly RA, Garetz SL, et al. Pediatric sleep questionnaire: prediction of sleep apnea and outcomes. Arch Otolaryngol Head Neck Surg 2007; 133:216–222.

193. Brietzke SE, Katz ES, Roberson DW. Can history and physical examination reliably diagnose pediatric obstructive sleep apnea/hypopnea syndrome? A systematic review of the literature. Otolaryngol Head Neck Surg 2004; 131:827–832.

194. Cardiorespiratory sleep studies in children. Establishment of normative data and polysomnographic predictors of morbidity. American Thoracic Society. Am J Respir Crit Care Med 1999; 160:1381–1387.

195. Standards and indications for cardiopulmonary sleep studies in children. American Thoracic Society. Am J Respir Crit Care Med 1996; 153:866–878.

196. Kirk VG, Batuyong ED, Bohn SG. Transcutaneous carbon dioxide monitoring and capnography during pediatric polysomnography. Sleep 2006; 29:1601–1608.

197. Saeed MM, Keens TG, Stabile MW, et al. Should children with suspected obstructive sleep

apnea syndrome and normal nap sleep studies have overnight sleep studies? Chest 2000; 118:360–365.

198. Verhulst SL, Schrauwen N, De Backer WA, et al. First night effect for polysomnographic data in children and adolescents with suspected sleep disordered breathing. Arch Dis Child 2006; 91:233–237.

199. Scholle S, Scholle HC, Kemper A, et al. First night effect in children and adolescents undergoing polysomnography for sleep-disordered breathing. Clin Neurophysiol 2003; 114:2138–2145.

200. Brouillette RT, Morielli A, Leimanis A, et al. Nocturnal pulse oximetry as an abbreviated testing modality for pediatric obstructive sleep apnea. Pediatrics 2000; 105:405–412.

201. Jacob SV, Morielli A, Mograss MA, et al. Home testing for pediatric obstructive sleep apnea syndrome secondary to adenotonsillar hypertrophy. Pediatr Pulmonol 1995; 20:241–252.

202. White JE, Smithson AJ, Close PR, et al. The use of sound recording and oxygen saturation in screening snorers for obstructive sleep apnoea. Clin Otolaryngol Allied Sci 1994; 19:218–221.

203. Sivan Y, Kornecki A, Schonfeld T. Screening obstructive sleep apnoea syndrome by home videotape recording in children. Eur Respir J 1996; 9:2127–2131.

204. Mitchell RB, Pereira KD, Friedman NR. Sleep-disordered breathing in children: survey of current practice. Laryngoscope 2006; 116:956–958.

205. Sundaram S, Bridgman SA, Lim J, et al. Surgery for obstructive sleep apnoea. Cochrane Database Syst Rev 2005; (4): CD001004.

206. Brietzke SE, Gallagher D. The effectiveness of tonsillectomy and adenoidectomy in the treatment of pediatric obstructive sleep apnea/hypopnea syndrome: a meta-analysis. Otolaryngol Head Neck Surg 2006; 134:979–984.

207. Mitchell RB, Kelly J. Quality of life after adenotonsillectomy for SDB in children. Otolaryngol Head Neck Surg 2005; 133:569–572.

208. Nixon GM, Brouillette RT. Obstructive sleep apnea in children: do intranasal corticosteroids help? Am J Respir Med 2002; 1:159–166.

209. Mandell DL, Yellon RF, Bradley JP, et al. Mandibular distraction for micrognathia and severe upper airway obstruction. Arch Otolaryngol Head Neck Surg 2004; 130:344–348.

210. Lin SY, Halbower AC, Tunkel DE, et al. Relief of upper airway obstruction with mandibular distraction surgery: Long-term quantitative results in young children. Arch Otolaryngol Head Neck Surg 2006; 132:437–441.

211. Marcus CL, Rosen G, Ward SL, et al. Adherence to and effectiveness of positive airway pressure therapy in children with obstructive sleep apnea. Pediatrics 2006; 117:e442–e451.

212. O'Donnell AR, Bjornson CL, Bohn SG, et al. Compliance rates in children using noninvasive continuous positive airway pressure. Sleep 2006; 29:651–658.

213. O'Donohue WJ, Jr, Giovannoni RM, Goldberg AI, et al. Long-term mechanical ventilation. Guidelines for management in the home and at alternate community sites. Report of the Ad Hoc Committee, Respiratory Care Section, American College of Chest Physicians. Chest 1986; 90(Suppl 1):1S–37S.

214. Beauchamp TL. Methods and principles in biomedical ethics. J Med Ethics 2003; 29:269–274.

215. Lloyd-Owen SJ, Donaldson GC, Ambrosino N, et al. Patterns of home mechanical ventilation use in Europe: results from the Eurovent survey. Eur Respir J 2005; 25:1025–1031.

216. Nelson VS, Carroll JC, Hurvitz EA, et al. Home mechanical ventilation of children. Dev Med Child Neurol 1996; 38:704–715.

217. Appierto L, Cori M, Bianchi R, et al. Home care for chronic respiratory failure in children: 15 years experience. Paediatr Anaesth 2002; 12:345–350.

218. Sakai H, Kobayashi K, Miyasaka K. [Current status of pediatric home mechanical ventilation in Japan]. Nihon Kyobu Shikkan Gakkai Zasshi 1992; 30:1274–1279.

219. Fauroux B, Sardet A, Foret D. Home treatment for chronic respiratory failure in children: a prospective study. Eur Respir J 1995; 8:2062–2066.

220. Jardine E, O'Toole M, Paton JY, et al. Current status of long term ventilation of children in the United Kingdom: questionnaire survey. Br Med J 1999; 318:295–299.

221. Fauroux B, Boffa C, Desguerre I, et al. Long-term noninvasive mechanical ventilation for children at home: a national survey. Pediatr Pulmonol 2003; 35:119–125.

222. Frates RC, Jr. Splaingard ML, Smith EO, et al. Outcome of home mechanical ventilation in children. J Pediatr 1985; 106:850–856.

223. Gilgoff RL, Gilgoff IS. Long-term follow-up of home mechanical ventilation in young children with spinal cord injury and neuromuscular conditions. J Pediatr 2003; 142:476–480.

224. Nelson VS, Dixon PJ, Warschausky SA. Long-term outcome of children with high tetraplegia and ventilator dependence. J Spinal Cord Med 2004; 27(Suppl 1):S93–S97.

225. Schreiner MS, Donar ME, Kettrick RG. Pediatric home mechanical ventilation. Pediatr Clin North Am 1987; 34:47–60.

226. Teague WG. Long-term mechanical ventilation in infants and children. In: Hill N S, ed. Long-term mechanical ventilation. New York: Marcel Dekker; 2001.177–213.

227. Sritippayawan S, Kun SS, Keens TG, et al. Initiation of home mechanical ventilation in children with neuromuscular diseases. J Pediatr 2003; 142:481–485.

228. Hukins CA, Hillman DR. Daytime predictors of sleep hypoventilation in Duchenne muscular dystrophy. Am J Respir Crit Care Med 2000; 161:166–170.

229. Katz S, Selvadurai H, Keilty K, et al. Outcome of non-invasive positive pressure ventilation in paediatric neuromuscular disease. Arch Dis Child 2004; 89:121–124.

230. Simonds AK, Elliott MW. Outcome of domiciliary nasal intermittent positive pressure ventilation in restrictive and obstructive disorders. Thorax 1995; 50:604–609.

231. Carnevale FA, Alexander E, Davis M, et al. Daily living with distress and enrichment: the moral experience of families with ventilator-assisted children at home. Pediatrics 2006; 117:e48–e60.

232. Wegener DH, Aday LA. Home care for ventilator-assisted children: predicting family stress. Pediatr Nurs 1989; 15:371–376.

233. Lumeng JC, Warschausky SA, Nelson VS, et al. The quality of life of ventilator-assisted children. Pediatr Rehabil 2001; 4:21–27.

234. Abresch RT, Seyden NK, Wineinger MA. Quality of life. Issues for persons with neuromuscular diseases. Phys Med Rehabil Clin N Am 1998; 9:233–248.

235. *British Thoracic Society, Scottish Intercollegiate Guidelines Network. British guideline on the management of asthma. Thorax 2003; 58(Suppl 1):i1–i94.

236. Silverman M. Out of the mouths of babes and sucklings: lessons from early childhood asthma. Thorax 1993; 48:1200–1205.

237. Silverman M, Wilson N. Wheezing phenotypes in childhood. Thorax 1997; 52:936–937.

238. Bush A. Coughs and wheezes spread diseases: but what about the environment? Thorax 2006; 61:367–368.

239. Kurukulaaratchy RJ, Matthews S, Arshad SH. Does environment mediate earlier onset of the persistent childhood asthma phenotype? Pediatrics 2004; 113:345–350.

240. Alford SH, Zoratti E, Peterson EL, et al. Parental history of atopic disease: disease pattern and risk of pediatric atopy in offspring. J Allergy Clin Immunol 2004; 114:1046–1050.

241. Christie GL, Helms PJ, Godden DJ, et al. Asthma, wheezy bronchitis, and atopy across two generations. Am J Respir Crit Care Med 1999; 159:125–129.

242. Van Eerdewegh P, Little RD, Dupuis J, et al. Association of the ADAM33 gene with asthma and bronchial hyperresponsiveness. Nature 2002; 418:426–430.

243. Shapiro SD, Owen CA. ADAM-33 surfaces as an asthma gene. N Engl J Med 2002; 347:936–938.

244. Raby BA, Silverman EK, Kwiatkowski DJ, et al. ADAM33 polymorphisms and phenotype associations in childhood asthma. J Allergy Clin Immunol 2004; 113:1071–1078.

245. Israel E, Chinchilli VM, Ford JG, et al. Use of regularly scheduled albuterol treatment in asthma: genotype-stratified, randomised, placebo-controlled cross-over trial. Lancet 2004; 364:1505–1512.

246. Peat JK, van den Berg RH, Green WF, et al. Changing prevalence of asthma in Australian children. Br Med J 1994; 308:1591–1596.

247. Gdalevich M, Mimouni D, Mimouni M. Breastfeeding and the risk of bronchial asthma in childhood: a systematic review with meta-analysis of prospective studies. J Pediatr 2001; 139:261–266.

248. Hays T, Wood RA. A systematic review of the role of hydrolyzed infant formulas in allergy prevention. Arch Pediatr Adolesc Med 2005; 159:810–816.

249. Custovic A, Simpson A. Environmental allergen exposure, sensitisation and asthma: from whole populations to individuals at risk. Thorax 2004; 59:825–827.

250. Russell G. The childhood asthma epidemic. Thorax 2006; 61:276–278.

251. The International Study of Asthma and Allergies in Childhood (ISAAC) Steering Committee. Worldwide variation in prevalence of symptoms of asthma, allergic rhinoconjunctivitis, and atopic eczema: ISAAC. Lancet 1998; 351:1225–1232.

252. von Mutius E, Martinez FD, Fritzsch C, et al. Prevalence of asthma and atopy in two areas of West and East Germany. Am J Respir Crit Care Med 1994; 149:358–364.

253. von Mutius E, Weiland SK, Fritzsch C, et al. Increasing prevalence of hay fever and atopy among children in Leipzig, East Germany. Lancet 1998; 351:862–866.

254. von Mutius E. The increase in asthma can be ascribed to cleanliness (pro/con editorial). Am J Respir Crit Care Med 2001; 164:1106–1107.

255. Bloomfield SF, Stanwell-Smith R, Crevel RWR, et al. Too clean, or not too clean: the Hygiene Hypothesis and home hygiene. Clin Exp Allergy 2006; 36:402–425.

256. Marra F, Lynd L, Coombes M, et al. Does antibiotic exposure during infancy lead to development of asthma?: a systematic review and metaanalysis. Chest 2006; 129:610–618.

257. Romagnani S. Regulatory T cells: which role in the pathogenesis and treatment of allergic disorders? Allergy 2006; 61:3–14.

258. Kuehni CE, Davis A, Brooke AM, et al. Are all wheezing disorders in very young (preschool) children increasing in prevalence? Lancet 2001; 357:1821–1825.

259. Lau S, Illi S, Sommerfeld C, et al. Early exposure to house-dust mite and cat allergens and development of childhood asthma: a cohort study. Lancet 2001; 356:1392–1397.

260. Arshad SH. Primary prevention of asthma and allergy. J Allergy Clin Immunol 2005; 116:3–14.

261. Payne DN, Qiu Y, Zhu J, et al. Airway inflammation in children with difficult asthma: relationships with airflow limitation and persistent symptoms. Thorax 2004; 59:862–869.

262. Najafi N, Demanet C, Dab I, et al. Differential cytology of bronchoalveolar lavage fluid in asthmatic children. Pediatr Pulmonol 2003; 35:302–308.

263. Payne DN, Rogers AV, Ädelroth E, et al. Early thickening of the reticular basement membrane in children with difficult asthma. Am J Respir Crit Care Med 2003; 167:78–82.

264. Stevenson EC, Turner G, Heaney LG, et al. Bronchoalveolar lavage findings suggest two different forms of childhood asthma. Clin Exp Allergy 1997; 27:1027–1035.

265. Gore C, Peterson CG, Kissen P, et al. Urinary eosinophilic protein X, atopy, and symptoms suggestive of allergic disease at 3 years of age. J Allergy Clin Immunol 2003; 112:702–708.

266. Azevedo I, de Blic J, Vargaftig BB, et al. Increased eosinophilic cationic protein levels in bronchoalveolar lavage from wheezy infants. Pediatr Allergy Immunol 2001; 12:65–72.

267. Koller DY, Wojnarowski C, Herkner KR, et al. High levels of eosinophil cationic protein in wheezing infants predict the development of asthma. J Allergy Clin Immunol 1997; 99:752–756.

268. Krawiec ME, Westcott JY, Chu HW, et al. Persistent wheezing in very young children is associated with lower respiratory inflammation. Am J Respir Crit Care Med 2001; 163:1338–1343.

269. Saglani S, Malmstrom K, Pelkonen AS, et al. Airway remodeling and inflammation in symptomatic infants with reversible airflow obstruction. Am J Respir Crit Care Med 2005; 171:722–727.

270. Holtzman MJ, Tyner JW, Kim EY, et al. Acute and chronic airway responses to viral infection: implications for asthma and chronic obstructive pulmonary disease. Proc Am Thorac Soc 2005; 2:132–140.

271. Holt PG, Upham JW, Sly PD. Contemporaneous maturation of immunologic and respiratory functions during early childhood: implications for development of asthma prevention strategies. J Allergy Clin Immunol 2005; 116:16–24.

272. Wark PA, Johnston SL, Bucchieri F, et al. Asthmatic bronchial epithelial cells have a deficient innate immune response to infection with rhinovirus. J Exp Med 2005; 201:937–947.

273. Balfour-Lynn IM, Valman HB, Wellings R, et al. Tumour necrosis factor-α and leukotriene E₄ production in wheezy infants. Clin Exp Allergy 1994; 24:121–126.

274. Bont L, Heijnen CJ, Kavelaars A, et al. Monocyte IL-10 production during respiratory syncytial virus bronchiolitis is associated with recurrent wheezing in a one-year follow-up study. Am J Respir Crit Care Med 2000; 161:1518–1523.

275. Lemanske RF, Jr, Jackson DJ, Gangnon RE, et al. Rhinovirus illnesses during infancy predict subsequent childhood wheezing. J Allergy Clin Immunol 2005; 116:571–577.

276. Peat JK, Toelle BG, Salome C, et al. Predictive nature of bronchial responsiveness and respiratory symptoms in a one year cohort study of Sydney schoolchildren. Eur Respir J 1993; 6:662–669.

277. De Baets F, Bodart E, Dramaix-Wilmet M, et al. Exercise-induced respiratory symptoms are poor predictors of bronchoconstriction. Pediatr Pulmonol 2005; 39:301–305.

278. Seear M, Wensley D, West N. How accurate is the diagnosis of exercise induced asthma among Vancouver schoolchildren?. Arch Dis Child 2005; 90:898–902.

279. Dundas I, Chan EY, Bridge PD, et al. Diagnostic accuracy of bronchodilator responsiveness in wheezy children. Thorax 2005; 60:13–16.

280. Martinez FD, Wright AL, Taussig LM, et al. Asthma and wheezing in the first six years of life. N Engl J Med 1995; 332:133–138.

281. Cane RS, Ranganathan SC, McKenzie SA. What do parents of wheezy children understand by "wheeze"? Arch Dis Child 2000; 82:327–332.

282. de Jongste JC, Shields MD. Cough. 2: Chronic cough in children. Thorax 2003; 58:998–1003.

*283. Tomerak AA, McGlashan JJ, Vyas HH, et al. Inhaled corticosteroids for non-specific cough in children. Cochrane Database Syst Rev 2005; Oct 19(4): CD004231.

*284. Chang AB, Phelan PD, Carlin JB, et al. A randomised, placebo controlled trial of inhaled salbutamol and beclomethasone for recurrent cough. Arch Dis Child 1998; 79:6–11.

285. Marchant JM, Masters IB, Taylor SM, et al. Evaluation and outcome of young children with chronic cough. Chest 2006; 129:1132–1141.

286. Kaditis AG, Gourgoulianis K, Winnie G. Anti-inflammatory treatment for recurrent wheezing in the first five years of life. Pediatr Pulmonol 2003; 35:241–252.

287. Juniper EF, Guyatt GH, Feeny DH, et al. Measuring quality of life in children with asthma. Quality Life Res 1996; 5:35–46.

288. Rosenthal M. Differential diagnosis of asthma. Pediatr Respir Rev 2002; 3:148–153.

289. Brand PLP. The practical interpretation of lung function tests in asthma. Recent Adv Pediatr 1999; 18.

290. Baatenburg de Jong A, Brouwer AFJ, Roorda RJ, et al. Normal lung function in children with mild to moderate persistent asthma well controlled by inhaled corticosteroids. J Allergy Clin Immunol 2006; 118:280–282.

291. Nordvall SL, Janson C, Kalm-Stephens P, et al. Exhaled nitric oxide in a population-based study of asthma and allergy in schoolchildren. Allergy 2005; 60:469–475.

292. Arshad SH, Tariq SM, Matthews S, et al. Sensitization to common allergens and its association with allergic disorders at age 4 years: a whole population birth cohort study. Pediatrics 2001; 108:E33.

293. Simpson A, Soderstrom L, Ahlstedt S, et al. IgE antibody quantification and the probability of wheeze in preschool children. J Allergy Clin Immunol 2005; 116:744–749.

*294. Guevara JP, Wolf FM, Grum CM, et al. Effects of educational interventions for self management of asthma in children and adolescents: systematic review and meta-analysis. BMJ 2003; 326:1308–1313.

295. Keeley D. Higher dose inhaled corticosteroids in childhood asthma: what we do doesn't work and what we don't do does. BMJ 2001; 322:504–505.

296. Cook DG, Strachan DP. Summary of effects of parental smoking on the respiratory health of children and implications for research. Thorax 1999; 54:357–366.

297. Johansson A, Hermansson G, Ludvigsson J. How should parents protect their children from environmental tobacco-smoke exposure in the home? Pediatrics 2004; 113:e291–e295.

298. O'Connor GT. Allergen avoidance in asthma: what do we do now? J Allergy Clin Immunol 2005; 116:26–30.

*299. Morgan WJ, Crain EF, Gruchalla RS, et al. Results of a home-based environmental intervention among urban children with asthma. Inner-City Asthma Study Group. N Engl J Med 2004; 351:1068–1080.

*300. Custovic A, Wijk RG. The effectiveness of measures to change the indoor environment in the treatment of allergic rhinitis and asthma: ARIA update (in collaboration with GA(2)LEN). Allergy 2005; 60:1112–1115.

*301. Gore RB, Durrell B, Bishop S, et al. High-efficiency particulate arrest-filter vacuum cleaners increase personal cat allergen exposure in homes with cats. J Allergy Clin Immunol 2003; 111:784–787.

302. Norman PS. Immunotherapy: 1999–2004. J Allergy Clin Immunol 2004; 113:1013–1023.

*303. Abramson M, Puy R, Weiner J. Immunotherapy in asthma: an updated systematic review. Allergy 1999; 54:1022–1041.

*304. Bueving HJ, Bernsen RM, de Jongste JC, et al. Influenza vaccination in children with asthma: randomized double-blind placebo-controlled trial. Am J Respir Crit Care Med 2004; 169:488–493.

305. O'Callaghan C, Barry PW. How to choose delivery devices for asthma. Arch Dis Child 2000; 82:185–187.

306. Kamps AWA, van Ewijk B, Roorda RJ, et al. Poor inhalation technique, even after inhalation instruction, in children with asthma. Pediatr Pulmonol 2000; 29:39–42.

307. Kamps AW, Brand PL, Roorda RJ. Determinants of correct inhalation technique in children attending a hospital-based asthma clinic. Acta Paediatr 2002; 91:159–163.

*308. Plotnick LH, Ducharme FM. Should inhaled anticholinergics be added to β₂ agonists for treating acute childhood and adolescent asthma? A systematic review. Br Med J 1998; 317:971–977.

309. Everard ML, Bara A, Kurian M, et al. Anticholinergic drugs for wheeze in children under the age of two years. Cochrane Database Syst Rev 2005; Jul 20(3): CD001279.

*310. Kamps AW, Brand PL, Kimpen JL, et al. Outpatient management of childhood asthma by paediatrician or asthma nurse: randomised controlled study with one year follow up. Thorax 2003; 58:968–973.

*311. Visser MJ, Postma DS, Arends LR, et al. One-year treatment with different dosing schedules of fluticasone propionate in childhood asthma. Effects on hyperresponsiveness, lung function, and height. Am J Respir Crit Care Med 2001; 134:2073–2077.

312. Leone FT, Fish JE, Szefler SJ, et al. Systematic review of the evidence regarding potential complications of inhaled corticosteroid use in asthma: collaboration of American College of Chest Physicians, American Academy of Allergy, Asthma, and Immunology, and American College of Allergy, Asthma, and Immunology. Chest 2003; 124:2329–2340.

313. Visser MJ, Van DV, Postma DS, et al. Side-effects of fluticasone in asthmatic children: no effects after dose reduction. Eur Respir J 2004; 24:420–425.

314. Pedersen S. Do inhaled corticosteroids inhibit growth in children? Am J Respir Crit Care Med 2001; 164:521–535.

*315. Ostrom NK, Decotiis BA, Lincourt WR, et al. Comparative efficacy and safety of low-dose fluticasone propionate and montelukast in children with persistent asthma. J Pediatr 2005; 147:213–220.

*316. Teper AM, Kofman CD, Szulman GA, et al. Fluticasone improves pulmonary function in children under 2 years old with risk factors for asthma. Am J Respir Crit Care Med 2005; 171:587–590.

*317. Guilbert TW, Morgan WJ, Zeiger RS, et al. Long-term inhaled corticosteroids in preschool children at high risk for asthma. N Engl J Med 2006; 354:1985–1997.

318. Wilson N, Sloper K, Silverman M. Effect of continuous treatment with topical corticosteroid on episodic viral wheeze in preschool children. Arch Dis Child 1995; 72:317–320.

319. Barrueto L, Mallol J, Figueroa L. Beclomethasone dipropionate and salbutamol by metered dose inhaler in infants and small children with recurrent wheezing. Pediatr Pulmonol 2002; 34:52–57.

*320. Bisgaard H, Zielen S, Garcia-Garcia ML, et al. Montelukast reduces asthma exacerbations in 2- to 5-year-old children with intermittent asthma. Am J Respir Crit Care Med 2005; 171:315–322.

*321. Straub DA, Moeller A, Minocchieri S, et al. The effect of montelukast on lung function and exhaled nitric oxide in infants with early childhood asthma. Eur Respir J 2005; 25:289–294.

322. Bisgaard H, Szefler S. Long-acting beta2 agonists and paediatric asthma. Lancet 2006; 367:286–288.

*323. Bisgaard H. Effect of long-acting beta2 agonists on exacerbation rates of asthma in children. Pediatr Pulmonol 2003; 36:391–398.

*324. Verberne AAPH, Frost C, Duiverman EJ, Dutch Paediatric Asthma Study Group et al. Addition of salmeterol versus doubling the dose of beclomethasone in children with asthma. Am J Respir Crit Care Med 1998; 158:213–219.

*325. O'Byrne PM, Bisgaard H, Godard PP, et al. Budesonide/formoterol combination therapy as both maintenance and reliever medication in asthma. Am J Respir Crit Care Med 2005; 171:129–136.

326. Salpeter SR, Buckley NS, Ormiston TM, et al. Meta-analysis of long-acting beta-agonists on severe asthma exacerbations and asthma-related deaths. Ann Internal Med 2006; 144:904–912.

327. Simons FER, Villa JR, Lee BW, et al. Montelukast added to budesonide in children with persistent asthma: a randomized, double-blind crossover study. J Pediatr 2001; 138:694–698.

328. de Blic J, Tillie-Leblond I, Emond S, et al. High-resolution computed tomography scan and airway remodeling in children with severe asthma. J Allergy Clin Immunol 2005; 116:750–754.

329. Milgrom H. Is there a role for treatment of asthma with omalizumab? Arch Dis Child 2003; 88:71–74.

330. Kuehni CE, Frey U. Age-related differences in perceived asthma control in childhood: guidelines and reality. Eur Respir J 2002; 20:880–889.

331. Brand PLP, Roorda RJ. Usefulness of monitoring lung function in asthma. Arch Dis Child 2003; 88:1021–1025.

332. Kamps AWA, Roorda RJ, Brand PLP. Peak flow diaries in childhood asthma are unreliable. Thorax 2001; 56:180–182.

333. Wensley D, Silverman M. Peak flow monitoring for guided self-management in childhood asthma: a randomized controlled trial. Am J Respir Crit Care Med 2004; 170:606–612.

334. Nair SJ, Daigle KL, DeCuir P, et al. The influence of pulmonary function testing on the management of asthma in children. J Pediatr 2005; 147:797–801.

335. Pijnenburg MW, Bakker EM, Hop WC, et al. Titrating steroids on exhaled nitric oxide in children with asthma: a randomized controlled trial. Am J Respir Crit Care Med 2005; 172:831–836.

336. Oswald H, Phelan PD, Lanigan A, et al. Outcome of childhood asthma in mid-adult life. Br Med J 1994; 309:95–96.

337. Murray CS, Poletti G, Kebadze T, et al. Study of modifiable risk factors for asthma exacerbations: virus infection and allergen exposure increase the risk of asthma hospital admissions in children. Thorax 2006; 61:376–382.

338. Geelhoed GC, Landau LI, LeSouëf PN. Predictive value of oxygen saturation in emergency evaluation of asthmatic children. Br Med J 1988; 297:395–396.

339. Inwald D, Roland M, Kuitert L, et al. Oxygen treatment for acute severe asthma. Br Med J 2001; 323:98–100.

*340. Castro-Rodriguez JA, Rodrigo GJ. β-agonists through metered-dose inhaler with valved holding chamber versus nebulizer for acute exacerbation of wheezing or asthma in children under 5 years of age: a systematic review with meta-analysis. J Pediatr 2004; 145:172–177.

341. FitzGerald M. Extracts from clinical evidence. Acute asthma. Br Med J 2000; 323:841–845.

*342. Smith M, Iqbal S, Elliott TM, et al. Corticosteroids for hospitalised children with acute asthma. Cochrane Database Syst Rev 2003; (2): CD002886.

343. Lucas-Bouwman ME, Roorda RJ, Jansman FGA. et al. Crushed prednisolone tablets or oral solution for acute asthma?. Arch Dis Child 2001; 84:347–348.

344. Csonka P, Kaila M, Laippala P, et al. Oral prednisolone in the acute management of children age 6 to 35 months with viral respiratory infection-induced lower airway disease: a randomized, placebo-controlled trial. J Pediatr 2003; 143:725–730.

345. Oommen A, Lambert PC, Grigg J. Efficacy of a short course of parent-initiated oral prednisolone for viral wheeze in children aged 1–5 years: randomised controlled trial. Lancet 2003; 362:1433–1438.

346. Roberts G, Newsom D, Gomez K, et al. Intravenous salbutamol bolus compared with an aminophylline infusion in children with severe asthma: a randomised controlled trial. Thorax 2003; 58:306–310.

347. Chipps BE, Murphy KR. Assessment and treatment of acute asthma in children. J Pediatr 2005; 147:288–294.

*348. Mitra A, Bassler D, Goodman K, et al. Intravenous aminophylline for acute severe asthma in children over two years receiving inhaled bronchodilators. Cochrane Database Syst Rev 2005; Apr 18(2): CD001276.

349. Zach MS, Eber E. Adult outcome of congenital lower respiratory tract malformations. Thorax 2001; 56:65–72.

350. Bush A. Congenital lung disease: a plea for clear thinking and clear nomenclature. Pediatr Pulmonol 2001; 32:328–337.

351. Durning RP, Scoles PV, Fox OD. Scoliosis after thoracotomy in tracheoesophageal fistula patients. J Bone Joint Surg 1980; 62:1156–1159.

352. Landing BH, Lawrence TK, Payne CV, et al. Bronchial anatomy in syndromes with abnormal visceral situs, abnormal spleen and congenital heart disease. Am J Cardiol 1971; 28:456–462.

353. McCartney FJ, Zuberbuhler JR, Anderson RH. Morphological considerations pertaining to recognition of atrial isomerism. Consequences for chamber localisation. Br Heart J 1980; 44:657–667.

354. Bush A. Left bronchial isomerism, normal atrial arrangement and bronchomalacia mimicking asthma: a new syndrome? Eur Respir J 1999; 14:475–477.

355. Kramer MS. 'Horseshoe' lung: report of five new cases. AJR Am J Roentgenol 1986; 146:211–215.

356. Reale FR, Esterly JR. Pulmonary hypoplasia: a morphometric study of the lungs of infants with diaphragmatic hernia, anencephaly, and renal malformations. Pediatrics 1972; 51:91–96.

357. Johnston RF, Green RA. Tracheobronchio-megaly: report of five cases and demonstration of familial occurrence. Am Rev Respir Dis 1965; 91:35–50.

358. Williams AJ, Schuster SR. Bronchial atresia associated with a bronchogenic cyst. Evidence of early appearance of atretic segments. Chest 1985; 87:396–398.

359. Hislop A, Reid L. New pathological findings in emphysema in childhood: 2. Overinflation of a normal lobe. Thorax 1971; 26:190–194.

360. Aktogu S, Yuncu G, Halilcolar H, et al. Bronchogenic cysts: clinicopathological presentation and treatment. Eur Respir J 1996; 9:2017–2021.

361. Samuel M, Burge DM. Management of antenatally diagnosed pulmonary sequestration associated with congenital cystic adenomatoid malformation. Thorax 1999; 54:701–706.

362. Aulicino MR, Reis ED, Dolgin SE, et al. Intra-abdominal pulmonary sequestration exhibiting congenital cystic adenomatoid malformation – report of a case and review of the literature. Arch Pathol Lab Med 1994; 118:1034–1037.

363. Fraggetta F, Cacciaguerra S, Nash R, et al. Intra-abdominal pulmonary sequestration associated with congenital cystic adenomatoid malformation of the lung: just an unusual combination of rare pathologies? Pathol Res Pract 1998; 194:209–211.

364. Heithoff KB, Sane SM, Williams HJ, et al. Bronchopulmonary foregut malformations: a unifying etiological concept. AJR Am J Roentgenol 1976; 126:46–55.

365. Sade RM, Clouse M, Ellis FH, Jr. The spectrum of pulmonary sequestration. Ann Thorac Surg 1974; 18:644–655.

366. Dommergues M, Louis-Sylvestre C, Mandelbrot L, et al. Congenital diaphragmatic hernia: can prenatal ultrasonography predict outcome? Am J Obstet Gynecol 1996; 174:1377–1381.

367. Abel RM, Bush A, Chitty LS, et al. Congenital lung disease. In: Chernick V, Boat T F, Wilmott R W, Bush A, eds. Kendig's Disorders of the respiratory tract in children. Philadelphia: Elsevier, 2006:280–316.

368. dell'Agnola C, Tadini B, Mosca F, et al. Advantages of prenatal diagnosis and early surgery for congenital cystic disease of the lung. J Perinat Med 1996; 24:621–631.

369. Papagiannopoulos KA, Sheppard M, Bush A, et al. Pleuropulmonary blastoma: is prophylactic resection of congenital lung cysts effective? Ann Thorac Surg 2001; 72:604–605.

370. Yamanaka A, Hirai T, Fujimoto T, et al. Anomalous systemic supply to normal basal segments of the left lower lobe. Ann Thorac Surg 1999; 68:332–338.

371. Schramel FM, Westermann CJ, Knepen PJ, et al. The scimitar syndrome: clinical spectrum and surgical treatment. Eur Respir J 1995; 8:196–201.

372. Najm HK, Williams WG, Coles JG, et al. Scimitar syndrome: twenty years' experience and results of repair. J Thorac Cardiovasc Surg 1996; 112:1161–1168.

373. Saluja S, Sitko I, Lee DW, et al. Embolotherapy of pulmonary arteriovenous malformations with detachable balloons: long-term durability and efficacy. J Vasc Interv Radiol 1999; 10:883–889.

374. Barker PM, Esther CR, Jr, Fordham LA, et al. Primary pulmonary lymphangiectasia in infancy and childhood. Eur Respir J 2004; 24:413–419.

375. White JES, Veale D, Fishwick D, et al. Generalised lymphangiectasia: pulmonary presentation in an adult. Thorax 1996; 51:767–768.

376. Bush A. Paediatric interstitial lung disease. Breathe 2005; 2:17–29.

377. Nicholson AG, Kim H, Corrin B, et al. The value of classifying interstitial pneumonitis in childhood according to defined histological patterns. Histopathology 1998; 33:203–211.

378. Copley SJ, Coren M, Nicholson AG, et al. Diagnostic accuracy of thin-section CT and chest radiography of pediatric interstitial lung disease. AJR Am J Roentgenol 2000; 174:549–554.

379. Bush A. Diagnosis of interstitial lung disease. Pediatr Pulmonol 1996; 22:81–82.

380. Coren ME, Nicholson AG, Goldstraw P, et al. Open lung biopsy for diffuse interstitial lung disease in children. Eur Respir Dis 1999; 14:817–821.

381. Sharief N, Crawford OF, Dinwiddie R. Fibrosing alveolitis and desquamative interstitial pneumonia. Pediatr Pulmonol 1994; 17:359–365.

382. Spencer D. Rare single system diseases. Pediatr Respir Rev 2001; 2:63–69.

383. Dinwiddie R. The lung in multisystem disease. Pediatr Respir Rev 2000; 1:58–63.

384. Chernick V, Boat TF, Wilmott RW, et al. Kendig's Disorders of the respiratory tract in children. 7th ed. Philadelphia: Elsevier; 2006.

385. Shah AF, Dinwiddie R, Woolf D, et al. Generalised lymphangiomatosis and chylothorax in the pediatric age group. Pediatr Pulmonol 1992; 14:126–130.

386. Chan PW, Muridan R, Debruyne JA. Bronchiolitis obliterans in children: clinical profile and diagnosis. Respirology 2000; 5:369–375.

387. Becroft DM. Bronchiolitis obliterans, bron-chiectasis, and other sequelae of adenovirus type 21 infection in young children. J Clin Pathol 1971; 24:72–82.

388. Davis AM, Wensley DF, Phelan PD. Spontaneous pneumothorax in pediatric patients. Respir Med 1993; 87:531–534.

389. Avital A, Springer C, Godfrey S. Pulmonary hemorrhagic syndromes in children. Pediatr Resp Rev 2000; 3:266–273.

390. Bush A. Pulmonary hypertensive disorders. Pediat Respir Rev 2000; 1:361–367.

391. Deng Z, Haghighi F, Helleby L, et al. Fine mapping of PPH1, a gene for familial primary pulmonary hypertension, to a 3-cM region on chromosome 2q33. Am J Respir Crit Care Med 2000; 161:1055–1059.

*392. Paramothayan S, Wells A, Lasserson T, et al. Prostacyclin for pulmonary hypertension. [Protocol] Cochrane Airways Group. Cochrane Database of Systematic Reviews, Issue 1; 2002.

393. Bossler AD, Richards J, George C, et al. Novel mutations in ENG and ACVRL1 in a series of 200 individuals undergoing clinical genetic testing for hereditary hemorrhageic telangiectasia (HHT): correlation of genotype with phenotype. Hum Mutat 2006; 27:667–675.

394. Nogee LM, deMello DE, Dehner LP, et al. Deficiency of surfactant protein B in congenital alveolar proteinosis. N Engl J Med 1993; 328:406–410.

395. Nogee LM, Dunbar E, 3rd , et a et all. A mutation in the surfactant protein C gene associated with familial interstitial lung disease. N Engl J Med 2001; 344:573–579.

396. Shulenin S, Nogee LM, Annilo T, et al. ABCA3 gene mutations in newborns with fatal surfactant deficiency. N Engl J Med 2004; 350:1296–1303.

397. Yenkateshiah SB, Yan TD, Bonfield TL, et al. An open-label trial of granulocyte-macrophage colony stimulating factor for moderate symptomatic pulmonary alveolar proteinosis. Chest 2006; 130:227–237.

398. Price A, Manson D, Cutz E, et al. Pulmonary alveolar proteinosis associated with anti-GM-CSF antibodies in a child: successful treatment with inhaled GM-CSF. Pediatr Pulmonol 2006; 41:367–370.

399. Hartman GF, Shochat SJ. Primary pulmonary neoplasms of childhood: a review. Ann Thorac Surg 1983; 36:108–119.

400. UK CF Trust. UK Cystic Fibrosis Database Annual Report 2003. Dundee: University of Dundee; 2005.www.cystic-fibrosis.org.uk/pdfs/Annual Report/AnnualReport2003.pdf.

401. US CF Foundation. Patient registry. Annual Data Report 2004. Bethesda: Cystic Fibrosis Foundation, 2005.www.cff.org/UploadedFiles/publications/files/2004%20Patient%20Registry%20Report.pdf.

402. Dodge JA, Morison S, Lewis PA, et al. Incidence, population, and survival of cystic fibrosis in the UK, 1968–95. UK Cystic Fibrosis Survey Management Committee. Arch Dis Child 1997; 77:493–496.

403. Frederiksen B, Lanng S, Koch C, et al. Improved survival in the Danish center-treated cystic fibrosis patients: results of aggressive treatment. Pediatr Pulmonol 1996; 21:153–158.

404. Kulich M, Rosenfeld M, Goss CH, et al. Improved survival among young patients with cystic fibrosis. J Pediatr 2003; 142:631–636.

405. Hamosh A, FitzSimmons SC, Macek M, et al. Comparison of the clinical manifestations of cystic fibrosis in black and white patients. [see comment]. J Pediatr 1998; 132:255–259.

406. Bowler IM, Estlin EJ, Littlewood JM, et al. Cystic fibrosis in Asians. Arch Dis Child 1993; 68:120–122.

407. Taylor CJ, Aswani N. The pancreas in cystic fibrosis. Paediat Respir Rev 2002; 3:77–81.

408. Colombo C, Crosignani A, Battezzati PM. Liver involvement in cystic fibrosis. J Hepatol 1999; 31:946–954.

409. Armstrong DS, Grimwood K, Carzino R, et al. Lower respiratory infection and inflammation in infants with newly diagnosed cystic fibrosis. Br Med J 1995; 310:1571–1572.

410. Muhlebach MS, Noah TL. Endotoxin activity and inflammatory markers in the airways of young patients with cystic fibrosis. Am J Respir Crit Care Med 2002; 165:911–915.

411. Southern KW. Delta F508 in cystic fibrosis: willing but not able. Arch Dis Child 1997; 76:278–282.

412. Zeitlin PL. Novel pharmacalogic therapies for cystic fibrosis. J Clin Invest 1999; 103:447–42.

413. McKone EF, Emerson SS, Edwards KL, et al. Effect of genotype on phenotype and mortality in cystic fibrosis: a retrospective cohort study. Lancet 2003; 361:1671–1676.

414. The Cystic Fibrosis Genotype–Phenotype Consortium. Correlation between genotype and phenotype in patients with cystic fibrosis. N Engl J Med 1993; 329:1308–1313.

415. Drumm ML, Konstan MW, Schluchter MD, et al. Genetic modifiers of lung disease in cystic fibrosis. N Engl J Med 2005; 353:1443–1453.

416. Zar H, Saiman L, Quittell L, et al. Binding of Pseudomonas aeruginosa to respiratory epithelial cells from patients with various mutations in the cystic fibrosis transmembrane regulator. J Pediatr 1995; 126:230–233.

417. Cheng K, Smyth RL, Govan JRW, et al. Spread of beta-lactam-resistant Pseudomonas aeruginosa in a cystic fibrosis clinic. Lancet 1996; 348:639–642.

418. Gallagher MJ, Jackson M, Hart CA, et al. Outcome of Burkholderia cepacia colonisation in an adult cystic fibrosis centre. Thorax 2002; 57:142–145.

419. Rosenstein BJ, Cutting GR for the Cystic Fibrosis Foundation consensus panel. The diagnosis of cystic fibrosis: A consensus statement. J Pediatr 1998; 132:589–595.

420. Multi-Disciplinary Working Group. Guidelines for the performance of the sweat test for the investigation of cystic fibrosis in the UK. 2003. www.ukneqas.org.uk/nov2003guideline.pdf.

421. Farrell PM, Kosorok MR, Laxova A, et al. Nutritional benefits of neonatal screening for cystic fibrosis. Wisconsin Cystic Fibrosis Neonatal Screening Study Group. N Engl J Med 1997; 337:963–969.

422. Koscik RL, Farrell PM, Kosorok MR, et al. Cognitive function of children with cystic fibrosis: deleterious effect of early malnutrition. Pediatrics 2004; 113:1549–1558.

423. Farrell PM, Li Z, Kosorok MR, et al. Bronchopulmonary disease in children with cystic fibrosis after early or delayed diagnosis. Am J Respir Crit Care Med 2003; 168:1100–1108.

424. UK Newborn Screening Programme Centre. 2006. www.newbornscreening-bloodspot.org.uk.

425. Polnay JC, Davidge A, Lyn UC, et al. Parental attitudes: antenatal diagnosis of cystic fibrosis. Arch Dis Child 2002; 87:284–286.

*426. Miedzybrodzka ZH, Hall MH, Mollison J, et al. Antenatal screening for carriers of cystic fibrosis: randomised trial of stepwise v couple screening. BMJ 1995; 310:353–357.

427. Brock DJ. Prenatal screening for cystic fibrosis: 5 years' experience reviewed. [see comment]. Lancet 1996; 347:148–150.

428. Cunningham S, Marshall T. Influence of five years of antenatal screening on the paediatric cystic fibrosis population in one region. Arch Dis Child 1998; 78:345–348.

429. Muller F, Simon-Bouy B, Girodon E, et al. Predicting the risk of cystic fibrosis with abnormal ultrasound signs of fetal bowel: Results of a French molecular collaborative study based on 641 prospective cases. Am J Med Genet 2002; 110:109–115.

430. Lai HC, Kosorok MR, Laxova A, et al. Nutritional status of patients with cystic fibrosis with meconium ileus: a comparison with patients without meconium ileus and diagnosed early through neonatal screening. Pediatrics 2000; 105:53–61.

431. Li Z, Lai HJ, Kosorok MR, et al. Longitudinal pulmonary status of cystic fibrosis children with meconium ileus. Pediatr Pulmonol 2004; 38:277–284.

432. Morison S, Dodge JA, Cole TJ, et al. Height and weight in cystic fibrosis: a cross sectional survey. Arch Dis Child 1997; 77:497–500.

433. Wilfond BS, Farrell PM, Laxova A, et al. Severe hemolytic anemia associated with vitamin E deficiency in infants with cystic fibrosis. Implications for neonatal screening. Clin Pediatr 1994; 33:2–7.

434. Vaisman N, Pencharz PB, Corey M, et al. Energy expenditure of patients with cystic fibrosis. J Pediatr 1987; 111:496–500.

435. Smyth RL, Ashby D, O'Hea U, et al. Fibrosing colonopathy in cystic fibrosis: results of a case-control study. Lancet 1995; 346:1247–1251.

436. Committee on Safety of Medicines MCA. Fibrosing colonopathy associated with pancreatic enzymes: dose related strictures in children with cystic fibrosis. Curr Prob Pharmacovigil 1995; 21:11.

437. Britto MT, Kotagal UR, Hornung RW, et al. Impact of recent pulmonary exacerbations on quality of life in patients with cystic fibrosis. Chest 2002; 121:64–72.

438. Liou TG, Adler FR, FitzSimmons SC, et al. Predictive 5-year survivorship model of cystic fibrosis. Am J Epidemiol 2001; 153:345–352.

439. Schidlow DV, Taussig LM, Knowles MR, et al. Cystic Fibrosis Foundation consensus conference report on pulmonary complications of cystic fibrosis. Pediatr Pulmonol 1993; 15:187–198.

440. Curtis HJ, Bourke SJ, Dark JH, et al. Lung transplantation outcome in cystic fibrosis patients with previous pneumothorax. J Heart Lung Transpl 2005; 24:865–869.

441. Lindblad A, Glaumann H, Strandvik B, et al. Natural history of liver disease in cystic fibrosis. Hepatology 1999; 30:1151–1158.

441a. O'Brien S, Fitzgerald MX, Hegarty JE. A controlled trial of ursodeoxycholic acid treatment in cystic fibrosis-related liver disease. Eur J Gastroenterol Hepatol 1992; 4: 857–63.

*442. Cheng K, Ashby D, Smyth R. Ursodeoxycholic acid for cystic fibrosis-related liver disease. Cochrane Database of Systematic Reviews 1999.

443. Marshall BC, Butler SM, Stoddard M, et al. Epidemiology of cystic fibrosis-related diabetes. J Pediatr 2005; 146:681–687.

444. CF Trust Clinical Standards & Accreditation Group. Standards for the Clinical Care of Children and Adults with Cystic Fibrosis in the UK 2001. London: UK Cystic Fibrosis Trust, 2001.

445. Moran A, Phillips J, Milla C. Insulin and glucose excursion following premeal insulin lispro or repaglinide in cystic fibrosis-related diabetes. Diabetes Care 2001; 24:1706–1710.

446. Bianchi ML, Romano G, Saraifoger S, et al. BMD and body composition in children and young patients affected by cystic fibrosis. J Bone Mineral Res 2006; 21:388–396.

447. Buntain HM, Schluter PJ, Bell SC, et al. Controlled longitudinal study of bone mass accrual in children and adolescents with cystic fibrosis. Thorax 2006; 61:146–154.

*448. Aris RM, Lester GE, Caminiti M, et al. Efficacy of alendronate in adults with cystic fibrosis with low bone density. Am J Respir Crit Care Med 2004; 169:77–82.

449. di Sant'Agnese PA, Darling RC, Perera GA, et al. Abnormal electrolyte composition of sweat in cystic fibrosis of the pancreas; clinical significance and relationship to the disease. Pediatrics 1953; 12:549–563.

450. UK Cystic Fibrosis Trust Nutrition Working Group. Nutritional management of cystic fibrosis. Bromley: Cystic Fibrosis Trust, 2002.

*451. Poustie VJ, Russell JE, Watling RM, CALICO Trial Collaborative Group et al. Oral protein energy supplements for children with cystic fibrosis: CALICO multicentre randomised controlled trial. BMJ 2006; 332:632–636.

*452. van der Schans C, Prasad A, Main E. Chest physiotherapy compared to no chest physiotherapy for cystic fibrosis. Cochrane Database Syst Rev 2000; Issue 2. Art. No.: CD001401. DOI: 10.1002/14651858. CD001401.

453. Button BM, Heine RG, Catto-Smith AG, et al. Chest physiotherapy, gastro-oesophageal reflux, and arousal in infants with cystic fibrosis. Arch Dis Child 2004; 89:435–439.

*454. Main E, Prasad A, van der Schans C. Conventional chest physiotherapy compared to other airway clearance techniques for cystic fibrosis. Cochrane Database Syst Rev 2005; Issue 1. Art. No.: CD002011.pub2. DOI: 10.1002/14651858. CD002011.pub2.

455. UK Cystic Fibrosis Trust Antibiotic Group. Antibiotic treatment for cystic fibrosis (amended 2004). Bromley: UK CF Trust, 2002.www.cftrust.org.uk/scope/documentlibrary/Publications/Antibiotic.pdf

*456. Stutman HR, Lieberman JM, Nussbaum E, and The Antibiotic Prophylaxis in Cystic Fibrosis Study Group et al. Antibiotic prophylaxis in infants and young children with cystic fibrosis: A randomised controlled trial. J Pediatr 2002; 140:229–305.

*457. Smyth A, Walters S. Prophylactic antibiotics for cystic fibrosis. The Cochrane Database of Systematic Reviews 2003; Issue 3. Art. No.: CD001912. DOI: 10.1002/14651858.CD001912.

*458. Wood DM, Smyth AR. Antibiotic strategies for eradicating Pseudomonas aeruginosa in people with cystic fibrosis. Cochrane Database of Syst Rev 2006; Issue 1. Art. No.: CD004197.pub2. DOI: 10.1002/14651858.CD004197.pub2.

459. Frederiksen B, Koch C, Hoiby N. Antibiotic treatment of initial colonization with Pseudomonas aeruginosa postpones chronic infection and prevents deterioration of pulmonary function in cystic fibrosis. Pediatr Pulmonol 1997; 23:330–335.

460. Rosenfeld M, Emerson J, Williams-Warren J, et al. Defining a pulmonary exacerbation in cystic fibrosis. J Pediatr 2001; 139:359–365.

461. Quan JM, Tiddens HA, Sy JP, et al. A two-year randomized, placebo-controlled trial of dornase alfa in young patients with cystic fibrosis with mild lung function abnormalities. J Pediatr 2001; 139:813–820.

*462. Ramsey BW, Pepe MS, Quan JM, et al. Intermittent administration of inhaled tobramycin in patients with cystic fibrosis. N Engl J Med 1999; 340:23–30.

*463. Saiman L, Marshall BC, Mayer-Hamblett N, et al. Azithromycin in patients with cystic fibrosis chronically infected with Pseudomonas aeruginosa: a randomized controlled trial. JAMA 2003; 290:1749–1756.

*464. Elkins MR, Robinson M, Rose BR, et al. A controlled trial of long-term inhaled hypertonic saline in patients with cystic fibrosis. N Engl J Med 2006; 354:229–240.

*465. Breen L, Aswani N. Elective versus symptomatic intravenous antibiotic therapy for cystic fibrosis. The Cochrane Database of Systematic Reviews 2001; Issue 4. Art. No.: CD002767. DOI: 10.1002/14651858.CD002767.

*466. Elborn JS, Prescott RJ, Stack BHR, et al. Elective versus symptomatic antibiotic treatment in cystic fibrosis patients with chronic Pseudomonas infection of the lungs. Thorax 2000; 55:355–358.

*467. Smith AL, Fiel SB, Mayer-Hamblett N, et al. Susceptibility testing of Pseudomonas aeruginosa isolates and clinical response to parenteral antibiotic administration: lack of association in cystic fibrosis. Chest 2003; 123:1495–1502.

468. Aaron SD, Ramotar K, Ferris W, et al. Adult cystic fibrosis exacerbations and new strains of Pseudomonas aeruginosa. Am J Respir Crit Care Med 2004; 169:811–815.

469. Elliott RA, Thornton J, Webb AK, et al. Comparing costs of home- versus hospital-based treatment of infections in adults in a specialist cystic fibrosis center. Int J Technol Assess Health Care 2005; 21:506–510.

*470. Smyth A, Tan KH, Hyman-Taylor P, et al. Once versus three-times daily regimens of tobramycin treatment for pulmonary exacerbations of cystic fibrosis – the TOPIC study: a randomised controlled trial. Lancet 2005; 365:573–578.

471. Marchant JL, Warner JO, Bush A. Rise in total IgE as an indicator of allergic bronchopulmonary aspergillosis in cystic fibrosis. Thorax 1994; 49:1002–1005.

472. Olivier KN, Weber DJ, Wallace Jr RJ, et al. Nontuberculous mycobacteria. I: multicenter prevalence study in cystic fibrosis. [see comment]. Am J Respir Crit Care Med 2003; 167:828–834.

473. Pitt TL, Kaufmann ME, Patel PS, et al. Type characterisation and antibiotic susceptibility of Burkholderia (Pseudomonas) cepacia isolates from patients with cystic fibrosis in the United Kingdom and the Republic of Ireland. J Med Microbiol 1996; 44:203–210.

474. Shwachman H, Kulczycki LL. Long term study of one hundred five patients with cystic fibrosis. Am J Dis Child 1958; 96:6–15.

475. Langton Hewer SC. Is limited computed tomography the future for imaging the lungs of children with cystic fibrosis? Arch Dis Child 2006; 91:377–378.

476. Slieker MG, van Gestel JPJ, Heijerman HGM, et al. Outcome of assisted ventilation for acute respiratory failure in cystic fibrosis. Intensive Care Med 2006; 38:754–758.

477. Kerem E, Reisman J, Corey M, et al. Prediction of mortality in patients with cystic fibrosis. N Engl J Med 1992; 326:1187–1191.

478. Burch M, Aurora P. Current status of paediatric heart, lung, and heart-lung transplantation. Arch Dis Child 2004; 89:386–389.

479. Lucas J, Connett GJ, Lea R, et al. Lung resection in cystic fibrosis patients with localised pulmonary disease. Arch Dis Child 1996; 74:449–451.

480. Mahadeva R, Webb K, Westerbeek RC, et al. Clinical outcome in relation to care in centres specialising in cystic fibrosis: cross sectional study. Commentary: Management in paediatric and adult cystic fibrosis centres improves clinical outcome. BMJ 1998; 316:1771–1775.

481. Arroll B, Kenealy T. Are antibiotics effective for acute purulent rhinitis? Systematic review and meta-analysis of placebo controlled randomised trials. BMJ 2006; 333:279.

482. Foxlee R, Johansson A, Wejfalk J, et al. Topical analgesia for acute otitis media. Cochrane Database of Systematic Reviews 2006, Issue 3. Art. No.: CD005657. DOI: 10.1002/14651858.CD005657.pub2.

483. Hoberman A, Paradise JL, Reynolds EA, et al. Efficacy of Auralgan for treating ear pain in children with acute otitis media. Arch Pediatr Adolesc Med 1997; 151:675–678.

484. Burke P, Bain J, Robinson D. Acute red ear in children: controlled trial of non-antibiotic treatment in general practice. Br Med J 1991; 303:558–562.

485. Glasziou PP, Del Mar CB, Sanders SL, et al. Antibiotics for acute otitis media in children. Cochrane Database of Systematic Reviews 2004, Issue 1. Art. No.: CD000219. DOI: 10.1002/14651858. CD000219.pub2

486. Rudberg R. Acute otitis media: comparative therapeutic results of sulphonamide and penicillin administered in various forms. Acta Otolaryngol 1954; 113:71–79.

487. Rosenfeld RM. Natural history of untreated otitis media. Laryngoscope 2003; 113:1645–1657.

488. Kozyrskyj A, Hildes-Ripstein G, Longstaffe S, et al. Short course antibiotics for acute otitis media. Cochrane Database Syst Rev 2000; (2): CD001095.

489. Spurling GKP, Del Mar CB, Dooley L, et al. Delayed antibiotics for symptoms and complications of respiratory infections. Cochrane Database of Systematic Reviews 2004, Issue 4. Art. No.: CD004417. DOI: 10.1002/14651858.CD004417.pub2

490. Little P, Gould C, Williamson I, et al. Pragmatic randomised controlled trial of two prescribing strategies for childhood acute otitis media. BMJ 2001; 322:336–342.

491. American Academy of Pediatrics Subcommittee on Management of Acute Otitis Media. Diagnosis and management of acute otitis media. Pediatrics 2004; 113:1451–1465.

492. Flynn CA, Griffin GH, Schultz JK. Decongestants and antihistamines for acute otitis media in children. Cochrane Database of Systematic Reviews 2004, Issue 3. Art. No.: CD001727. DOI: 10.1002/14651858. CD001727.pub2.

493. Burke P, Bain J, Lowes A, et al. Rational decisions in managing sore throat: evaluation of a rapid test. Br Med J 1998; 296:1646–1649.

494. Del Mar CB, Glasziou PP, Spinks AB. Antibiotics for sore throat. Cochrane Database of Systematic Reviews 2004, Issue 2. Art. No.:CD000023. DOI: 10.1002/14651858.CD000023.pub2.

495. Royal College of Paediatrics and Child Health. Guidelines for good practice: management of acute and recurring sore throat and indications for tonsillectomy. London: RCPCH; 2000.

496. Burton MJ, Towler B, Glasziou P. Tonsillectomy versus non-surgical treatment for chronic/recurrent acute tonsillitis. Cochrane Database of Systematic Reviews 1999, Issue 3. Art. No.: CD001802. DOI: 10.1002/14651858.CD001802

497. Ranganathan S, Tasker R, Booy R, et al. Pertussis is increasing in unimmunized infants: is a change in policy needed? Arch Dis Child 1999; 80:297–299.

498. Bruss J, Malley R, Halperin S, et al. Treatment of severe pertussis: a study of the safety and pharmacology of intravenous pertussis immunoglobulin. Pediatr Infect Dis 1999; 18:505–511.

499. Mertsola J, Viljanen M, Ruuskanen O. Salbutamol in the treatment of whooping cough. Scand J Infect Dis 1986; 18:593–594.

500. Dodhia H, Miller E. Review of the evidence for the use of erythromycin in the management of persons exposed to pertussis. Epidemiol Infect 1998; 120:143–149.

501. Canciani M, Morittu A, Del Pin B. Croup: Diagnosis and treatment. Breathe 2006; 2:333–338.

502. Scolnik D, Coates AL, Stephens D, et al. Controlled delivery of high vs low humidity vs mist therapy for croup in emergency departments: a randomized controlled trial. JAMA 2006; 296:393–394.

503. Moore M, Little P. Humidified air inhalation for treating croup. Cochrane Database of Systematic Reviews 2006, Issue 3. Art. No.: CD002870. DOI: 10.1002/14651858.CD002870.pub2.

504. Ausejo M, Saenz A, Pham B, et al. The effectiveness of glucocorticoids in treating croup: meta-analysis. Br Med J 1999; 319:595–600.

505. Russell K, Wiebe N, Saenz A, et al. Glucocorticoids for croup. Cochrane Database of Systematic Reviews 2004, Issue 1. Art. No.: CD001955. DOI: 10.1002/14651858.CD001955.pub2.

506. Cetinkaya F, Tufekci BS, Kutluk G. A comparison of nebulised budesonide and intramuscular and oral dexamethasone for treatment of croup. Int J Pediatr Otorhinolaryngol 2004; 68:453–456.

507. Waisman Y, Klein B, Boenning D, et al. Prospective randomized double-blind study comparing L-epinephrine and racemic epinephrine aerosols in the treatment of laryngotracheitis (croup). Pediatrics 1992; 89:302–306.

508. Prendergast M, Jones J, Hartman D. Racemic epinephrine in the treatment of laryngotracheitis. Can we identify children for outpatient therapy? Am J Emerg Med 1994; 12:613–616.

509. Kessler A, Wetmore R, Marsh R. Childhood epiglottitis in recent years. Int J Pediatr Otorhinolaryngol 1993; 25:155–162.

510. Booy R, Hodgson L, Carpenter L, et al. Efficacy of *Haemophilus influenzae* type b conjugate vaccine PRP-T. Lancet 1994; 344:362–366.

511. Murrage K, Janzen V, Ruby R. Epiglottitis: adult and pediatric complications. Otolaryngology 1988; 17:194–198.

512. Sobolev I, Plunkett N, Barker I. Acute epiglottitis, sevofluorane and Hib vaccination. Anesthesia 2001; 56:799–820.

513. Bernstein T, Brilli R, Jacobs B. Is bacterial tracheitis changing? A 14 month experience in a pediatric intensive care unit. Clin Infect Dis 1998; 27:458–462.

514. Noble V, Murray W, Webb MS, et al. Respiratory status and allergy nine to 10 years after acute bronchiolitis. Arch Dis Child 1997; 76:315–319.

515. Everard ML. The relationship between respiratory syncytial virus infections and the development of wheezing and asthma in children. Curr Opin Allergy Clin Immunol 2006; 6:56–61.

516. Gadomski AM, Bhasale AL. Bronchodilators for bronchiolitis. Cochrane Database of Systematic Reviews 2006; Issue 3. Art. No.: CD001266. DOI: 10.1002/14651858.CD001266.pub2.

517. Hartling L, Wiebe N, Russell K, et al. Epinephrine for bronchiolitis. Cochrane Database of Systematic Reviews 2004; Issue 1. Art. No.: CD003123. DOI: 10.1002/14651858.CD003123.pub2.

518. Ho L, Collins G, Landau L, et al. Effect of salbutamol on oxygen saturation in bronchiolitis. Arch Dis Child 1991; 66:1061–1064.

519. Cade A, Brownlee K, Conway S, et al. Randomized placebo controlled trial of nebulized corticosteroids in acute respiratory syncytial viral bronchiolitis. Arch Dis Child 2000; 82:126–130.

520. Richter H, Seddon P. Early nebulized budesonide in the treatment of bronchiolitis and the prevention of postbronchiolitis wheezing. J Pediatr 1998; 132:849–853.

521. Randolph A, Wang E. Ribavirin for respiratory syncytial virus infection of the lower respiratory tract. Cochrane Database Systematic Reviews 2000; Issue 2: CD000181

522. Ventre K, Randolph AG. Ribavirin for respiratory syncytial virus infection of the lower respiratory tract in infants and young children. Cochrane Database of Systematic Reviews 2004; Issue 4. Art. No.: CD000181. DOI: 10.1002/14651858. CD000181.pub2.

523. Shah PS, Ohlsson A, Shah JP. Continuous negative extrathoracic pressure or continuous positive airway pressure for acute hypoxemic respiratory failure in children. Cochrane Database Systematic Reviews 2005; Issue 3:CD003699

524. Steinhorn R, Green T. Use of extracorporeal membrane oxygenation in the treatment of respiratory syncytial virus bronchiolitis: the national experience, 1983 to 1998. J Pediatr 1990; 116:338–342.

525. Luchetti M, Casiraghi G, Valsecchi R, et al. Porcine-derived surfactant treatment of severe bronchiolitis. Acta Anaesthesiol Scand 1998; 42:805–810.

526. IMpact-RSV Study Group. Palivizumab, a humanised respiratory syncytial virus monoclonal antibody, reduces hospitalisation from respiratory syncytial virus infection in high risk infants. Pediatrics 1998; 102:531–537.

527. Fenton C, Scott LJ, Plosker GL. Palivizumab: a review of its use as prophylaxis for serious respiratory syncytial virus infection. Paediatr Drugs 2004; 6:177–197.

528. British Thoracic Society Standards of Care Committee. BTS guidelines for the management of community acquired pneumonia in childhood. Thorax 2002; 57:1–24.

529. Block S, Hedrick J, Hammerschlag M, et al. *Mycoplasma pneumoniae* and *Chlamydia pneumoniae* in pediatric community-acquired pneumonia: comparative efficacy and safety of clarithromycin vs. erythromycin ethylsuccinate. Pediatr Infect Dis J 1995; 14:471–477.

530. Omidvari K, de Boisblanc B, Karam G, et al. Early transition to oral antibiotic therapy for community-acquired pneumonia: duration of therapy, clinical outcomes and cost analysis. Respir Med 1998; 92:1032–1039.

531. Black S, Shinefield H, Baxter R, et al. Impact of the use of heptavalent pneumococcal conjugate vaccine on disease epidemiology in children and adults. Vaccine 2006; 24(Suppl 2):79–80.

532. Gillet Y, Issartel B, Vanhems P, et al. Association between *Staphylococcus aureus* strains carrying Panton–Valentine leukocidin and highly lethal necrotising pneumonia in young immunocompetent patients. Lancet 2002; 359:753–759.

533. Klein JL, Petrovic Z, Treacher D, et al. Severe community acquired pneumonia caused by Panton–Valentine leukocidin-positive *Staphylococcus aureus*: first reported case in the United Kingdom. Intensive Care Med 2003; 29:1399.

534. Marchant JM, Masters IB, Taylor SM, et al. Evaluation and outcome of young children with chronic cough. Chest 2006; 129:1132–1141.

535. Donnelly D, Critchlow A, Everard ML. Outcomes in children treated for persistent bacterial bronchitis. Thorax 2007; 62:80–84.

536. Eastham KM, Freeman R, Kearns AM, et al. Clinical features, aetiology and outcome of empyema in children in the north east of England. Thorax 2004; 59:522–525.

537. Balfour-Lynn IM, Abrahamson E, Cohen G, et al. BTS guidelines for the management of pleural infection in children. Thorax 2005; 60(Suppl 1): i1–21.

538. Thomson AH, Hull J, Kumar MR, et al. Randomised trial of intrapleural urokinase in the treatment of childhood empyema. Thorax 2002; 57:343–347.

539. Sonnappa S, Cohen G, Owens CM, et al. Comparison of urokinase and video-assisted thoracoscopic surgery for treatment of childhood empyema. Am J Respir Crit Care Med 2006; 174:221–227.

540. Hilliard TN, Henderson AJ, Langton Hewer SC. Management of parapneumonic effusion and empyema. Arch Dis Child 2003; 8:915–917.

541. Wilmott RW, Khurana-Hershey G, Stark JM. Current concepts on pulmonary host defense mechanisms in children. Curr Opin Pediatr 2000; 12:187–193.

542. Knowles MR, Boucher RC. Mucus clearance as a primary innate defense mechanism for mammalian airways. J Clin Invest 2002; 109:571–577.

543. McCormack FX, Whitsett JA. The pulmonary collectins, SP-A and SP-D, orchestrate innate immunity in the lung. J Clin Invest 2002; 109:707–712.

544. Diamond G, Legarda D, Ryan LK. The innate immune response of the respiratory epithelium. Immunol Rev 2000; 173:27–38.

545. Parkin J, Cohen B. An overview of the immune system. Lancet 2001; 357:1777–1789.

546. Meeks M, Bush A. Primary ciliary dyskinesia (PCD). Pediatr Pulmonol 2000; 29:307–316.

547. Noone PG, Leigh MW, Sannuti A, et al. Primary ciliary dyskinesia: diagnostic and phenotypic features. Am J Respir Crit Care Med 2004; 169:459–467.

548. Bush A, Cole P, Hariri M, et al. Primary ciliary dyskinesia: diagnosis and standards of care. Eur Respir J 1998; 12:982–988.

549. Wodehouse T, Kharitonov SA, Mackay IS, et al. Nasal nitric oxide measurements for the screening of primary ciliary dyskinesia. Eur Respir J 2003; 21:43–47.

550. Chodhari R, Mitchison HM, Meeks M. Cilia, primary ciliary dyskinesia and molecular genetics. Paediatr Respir Rev 2004; 5:69–76.

551. Yoo Y, Koh YY. Current treatment for primary ciliary dyskinesia conditions. Expert Opin Pharmacother 2004; 5:369–377.

552. Eastham KM, Fall AJ, Mitchell L, et al. The need to redefine non-cystic fibrosis bronchiectasis in childhood. Thorax 2004; 59:324–327.

553. Spencer DA. From hemp seed and porcupine quill to HRCT: advances in the diagnosis and epidemiology of bronchiectasis. Arch Dis Child 2005; 90:712–714.

554. Anonymous. Primary immunodeficiency diseases. Report of an IUIS Scientific Committee. International Union of Immunological Societies. Clin Exp Immunol 1999; 118(Suppl 1):1–28.

555. Buckley RH. Pulmonary complications of primary immunodeficiencies. Paediatr Respir Rev 2004; 50(Suppl A):S225–S233.

556. Bonilla FA, Geha RS. 2. Update on primary immunodeficiency diseases. J Allergy Clin Immunol 2006; 117:S435–S441.

557. Morris A, Lundgren JD, Masur H, et al. Current epidemiology of Pneumocystis pneumonia. Emerg Infect Dis 2004; 10:1713–1720.

558. Hargrave DR, Hann II, Richards SM, et al. Progressive reduction in treatment-related deaths in Medical Research Council childhood lymphoblastic leukaemia trials from 1980 to 1997 (UKALL VIII, X and XI). Br J Haematol 2001; 112:293–299.

559. De Blic J, Marchac V, Scheinmann P. Complications of flexible bronchoscopy in children: prospective study of 1,328 procedures. Eur Respir J 2002; 20:1271–1276.

560. Stefanutti D, Morais L, Fournet JC, et al. Value of open lung biopsy in immunocompromised children. J Pediatr 2000; 137:165–171.

561. Williams AJ, Duong T, McNally LM, et al. *Pneumocystis carinii* pneumonia and cytomegalovirus infection in children with vertically acquired HIV infection. AIDS 2001; 15:335–339.

562. Wazir JF, Ansari NA. *Pneumocystis carinii* infection. Update and review. Arch Pathol Lab Med 2004; 128:1023–1027.

*563. Briel M, Boscacci R, Furrer H, et al. Adjunctive corticosteroids for *Pneumocystis jiroveci* pneumonia in patients with HIV infection: a meta-analysis of randomised controlled trials. BMC Infect Dis 2005; 5:101.

564. Ison MG, Fishman JA. Cytomegalovirus pneumonia in transplant recipients. Clin Chest Med 2005; 26:691–705, viii.

565. Duke T, Mgone CS. Measles: not just another viral exanthem. Lancet 2003; 361:763–773.

566. Yao Z, Liao W. Fungal respiratory disease. Curr Opin Pulm Med 2006; 12:222–227.

567. Northway Jr W, Rosan R, Porter D. Pulmonary disease following respirator therapy of hyaline-membrane disease: Bronchopulmonary dysplasia. N Engl J Med 1967; 276:357–368.

568. Shennan AT, Dunn MS, Ohlsson A, et al. Abnormal pulmonary outcomes in premature infants: prediction from oxygen requirement in the neonatal period. Pediatrics 1988; 82:527–532.

569. Jobe AH, Bancalari E. NICHD, NHLBI, ORD Workshop Summary: Bronchopulmonary dysplasia. Am J Respir Crit Care Med 2001; 163:1723–1729.

570. Kotecha S, Silverman M. Chronic respiratory complications of neonatal disorders. In: Landau L I, Taussig L M, eds. Textbook of pediatric respiratory medicine. St Louis: Mosby; 1999.488–521.

571. Manktelow BN, Draper ES, Annamalai S, et al. Factors affecting the incidence of chronic lung disease of prematurity between 1987, 1992 and 1997. Arch Dis Child 2001; 85:F33–F35.

572. Fenton AC, Mason E, Clarke M, et al. Chronic lung disease following neonatal ventilation. II.

Changing incidence in a geographically defined population. Pediatr Pulmonol 1996; 21:24–27.

573. Farstad T, Bratlid D. Incidence and prediction of bronchopulmonary dyplasia in a cohort of premature infants. Acta Paediatr 1994; 83:19–24.

574. Fanaroff AA, Wright LL, Stevenson DK, et al. Very-low-birth-weight outcomes of the National Institute of Child Health and Human Development Neonatal Research Network, May 1991 through December 1992. Am J Obstet Gynecol 1995; 173: 1423–1431.

575. Field D. Trent neonatal survey. Department of Epidemiology and Public Health, University of Leicester; 2000.

576. Kotecha S. Lung growth: implications for the newborn infants. Arch Dis Child Fetal Neonatal Ed 2000; 82:F69–F74.

577. Maxwell N, Davies PL, Kotecha S. Review of the role of antenatal infection in the pathogenesis of chronic lung disease of prematurity. Curr Infect Dis. Curr Opin Infect Dis 2006; 19:253–258.

578. Stocker JT. The respiratory tract. In: Stocker J T, Dehner L P, eds. Pediatric pathology. Philadelphia: JB Lippincott; 1992.533–541.

579. Margraf LR, Tomashefski JF, Bruce MC, et al. Morphometric analysis of the lung in bronchopulmonary dysplasia. Am Rev Respir Dis 1991; 143:391–400.

580. Husain AN, Siddiqui NH, Stocker JT. Pathology of arrested acinar development in postsurfactant bronchopulmonary dysplasia. Hum Pathol 1998; 29:710–717.

581. Jobe AJ. The new BPD: an arrest of lung development. Pediatr Res 1999; 46:641–643.

582. Thibeault DW, Mabry SM, Ekekezie II, et al. Lung elastic tissue maturation and perturbations during the evolution of chronic lung disease. Pediatrics 2000; 106:1452–1459.

583. Pandya HC, Kotecha S. Chronic lung disease of prematurity: clinical and pathophysiological correlates. Monladi Arch Chest Dis 2001; 56:270–275.

584. Hyde I, English RE, Williams JD. The changing pattern of chronic lung disease of prematurity. Arch Dis Child 1989; 64:448–451.

585. Fan LL, Flynn JW, Pathak DR. Risk factors predicting laryngeal injury in intubated neonates. Crit Care Med 1983; 11:431–433.

586. Boyce TG, Mellen BG, Mitchel EF, et al. Rates of hospitalisation for respiratory syncyticial virus infection among children in Medicaid. J Pediatr 2000; 137:865–870.

587. Anonymous. Palivizumab, a humanized respiratory syncytial virus antibody, reduces hospitalisation from respiratory syncytial virus infection in high-risk infants. The Impact-RSV Study Group. Pediatrics 1998; 102:531–537.

588. Joint Committee on Vaccination and Immunisation (JCVI) 2004. http://www.advisorybodies.doh.gov.uk/jcvi/mins111104rvi.htm Accessed July 3rd 2006.

589. Arnold SR, Wang EE, Law BJ, et al. Variable morbidity of respiratory syncytial virus infection in patients with underlying lung disease: a review of the PICNIC RSV database. Pediatric Investigators Collaborative Network on Infections in Canada. Pediatr Infect Dis J 1999; 18:866–869.

590. Vandenplas Y, Salvatore S, Hauser B. The diagnosis and management of gastro-oesophageal reflux in infants. Early Hum Dev 2005; 81:1011–1024.

591. Groothuis JR, Rosenberg AA. Home oxygen promotes weight gain in infants with bronchopulmonary dysplasia. Am J Dis Child 1987; 141:992–995.

592. Askie LM, Henderson-Smart DJ, Irwig L, et al. Oxygen-saturation targets and outcomes in extremely preterm infants. N Engl J Med 2003; 349:959–967.

593. Abman SH, Wolfe RR, Accurso FJ, et al. Pulmonary vascular response to oxygen in infants with severe bronchopulmonary dysplasia. Pediatrics 1985; 75:80–84.

594. Benatar A, Clarke J, Silverman M. Echocardiographic studies in chronic lung disease of prematurity. Arch Dis Child 1995; 72:F14–F19.

595. Grier DG, Halliday HL. Corticosteroids in the prevention and management of bronchopulmonary dysplasia. Semin Neonatol 2003; 8:83–91.

596. Majnemer A, Riley P, Shevell M, et al. Severe bronchopulmonary dysplasia increases risk of later neurological and motor sequelae in preterm survivors. Dev Med Child Neurol 2000; 42:53–60.

597. Joint Committee on Vaccination and Immunisation (JCVI). http://www.advisorybodies.doh.gov.uk/jcvi/childhoodimmunisationoc05.pdf Accessed July 3rd 2006.

598. Balfour-Lynn IM, Primhak RA, Shaw BN. Home oxygen for children. Thorax 2005; 60:76–81.

599. Kotecha S. Management of infants with chronic lung disease of prematurity in various parts of the world. Early Hum Dev 2005; 81:133–134.

600. Banacalari E, Wilson-Costello D, Iben SC. Management of infants with bronchopulmonary dysplasia in North America. Early Hum Dev 2005; 81:171–179.

601. Thomas W, Speer CP. Management of infants with bronchopulmonary dysplasia in Germany. Early Hum Dev 2005; 81:155–163.

602. Askie LM, Henderson-Smart DJ, Jones RA. Management of infants with chronic lung disease of prematurity in Australasia. Early Hum Dev 2005; 81:135–142.

603. STOP ROP Multicenter Study Group. Supplemental therapeutic oxygen for prethreshold retinopathy of prematurity (STOP-ROP), a randomized, controlled trial. I. primary outcomes. Pediatrics 2000; 105:295–310.

604. Frey B, Shann F. Oxygen administration in infants. Arch Dis Child 2006; 88:F84–F88.

605. Dunbar H, Kotecha S. Domiciliary oxygen for infants with chronic lung disease of prematurity. Care Crit Ill 2000; 16:90–93.

606. Wedzicha JA, Calverley PMA. All change for home oxygen services in England and Wales. Thorax 2006; 61:7–9.

607. Baraldi E, Carra S, Vencato F, et al. Home oxygen therapy in infants with bronchopulmonary dysplasia: a prospective study. Eur J Pediatr 1997; 156:878–882.

608. Yeh TF, Lin YJ, Huang CC, et al. Early dexamethasone therapy in preterm infants: a follow-up study. Pediatrics 1998; 101:E7.

609. Shinwell ES, Karplus M, Reich D, et al. Early postnatal dexamethasone treatment and increased incidence of cerebral palsy. Arch Dis Child 2000; 83:F177–F181.

610. Noble-Jamieson CM, Regev R, Silverman M. Dexamethasone in neonatal lung disease: pulmonary effects and intracranial complications. Eur J Pediatr 1989; 148:365–367.

611. Lister P, Iles R, Shaw B, et al. Inhaled steroids for neonatal chronic lung disease (Cochrane Review). In: The Cochrane Library. Oxford: Update Software; Issue 1, 2006.

612. Dunn M, Pandit P, Magnani L, et al. Inhaled corticosteroids for neonatal chronic lung disease: a randomised, double-blind cross-over study. Pediatr Res 1992; 31:201A.

613. Yuksel B, Greenough A. Ipratropium bromide for symptomatic preterm infants. Eur J Pediatr 1991; 150:854–857.

614. Wilkie RA, Bryan MH. Effect of bronchodilators on airway resistance in ventilator-dependent neonates with chronic lung disease. J Pediatr 1987; 111:278–282.

615. Hislop AA, Haworth SG. Airway size and structure in the normal fetal and infant lung and the effect of premature delivery and artificial ventilation. Am Rev Respir Dis 1989; 140:1717–1726.

616. Ng GYT, da Silva O, Ohlsson A. Bronchodilators for the prevention and treatment of chronic lung disease in preterm infants. Cochrane Database of Systematic Reviews 2001; (3): CD003214.

617. De Boeck K, Smith J, Van Lierde S, et al. Response to bronchodilators in clinically stable 1-year old patients with bronchopulmonary dysplasia. Eur J Pediatr 1998; 157:75–79.

618. Koumbourlis AC, Motoyama EK, Mutich RL, et al. Longitudinal follow-up of lung function from childhood to adolescence in prematurely born patients with neonatal chronic lung disease. Pediatr Pulmonol 1996; 21:28–34.

619. Yuksel B, Greenough A. Randomised trial of inhaled steroids in preterm infants with respiratory symptoms at follow up. Thorax 1992; 47:910–913.

620. Brion LP, Primhak RA. Intravenous or enteral loop diuretics for preterm infants with (or developing) chronic lung disease. Cochrane Database of Systematic Reviews (2): CD001453, 2000.

621. Brion LP, Primhak RA, Ambrosio-Perez I. Diuretics acting on the distal renal tubule for preterm infants with (or developing) chronic lung disease. Cochrane Database of Systematic Reviews ; (2): CD001817, 2000.

622. Brion LP, Primhak RA, Yong W. Aerosolized diuretics for preterm infants with (or developing) chronic lung disease. Cochrane Database of Systematic Reviews (2): CD001694, 2000.

623. Doyle LW, Cheung MMH, Ford GW, et al. Birth weight < 1501 g and respiratory health at 14. Arch Dis Child 2001; 84:40–44.

624. Doyle LW, the Victorian Infant Collaborative Study Group. Respiratory function at 8–9 years in extremely low birth weight/very preterm children born in Victoria in 1991–92. Pediatr Pulmonol 2006; 41:570–576.

625. Gross SJ, Iannuzzi DM, Kveselis DA, et al. Effect of preterm birth on pulmonary function at school age: a prospective controlled study. J Pediatr 1998; 133:188–192.

21

Cardiovascular disease

Edited by Denise J Kitchiner

CLINICAL ASSESSMENT OF HEART DISEASE

Detailed clinical evaluation is essential in the assessment of a child suspected of having a cardiac lesion. A comprehensive history provides information on the nature and severity of the condition. It also helps to establish a rapport with the child and family. A thorough physical examination is also necessary. If suspicion of a cardiac lesion exists, an electrocardiogram may give additional information. Chest radiography is seldom helpful in the diagnosis of a specific cardiac lesion. It remains useful in differentiating heart disease from other conditions and in assessing the severity of some lesions. Echocardiography has revolutionized the diagnosis and management of children with heart disease. It must be carried out and interpreted in conjunction with the clinical findings, if errors in diagnosis are to be avoided.[1] Cardiac catheterization is less frequently used in diagnosis, but transcatheter intervention is performed for a range of conditions. Other investigations are helpful in evaluating some children.

HISTORY

Symptoms can give important clues to the diagnosis and severity of heart disease. The history can also help to differentiate cardiac lesions from other conditions.

Infants with heart failure present with feeding difficulties and symptoms of respiratory distress. The infant takes frequent small feeds, rapidly becoming exhausted. This results in poor weight gain, which in some children is also due to increased energy expenditure.[2] It is important to assess the volume of feed, or the time taken if breast-feeding. Infants may perspire profusely, particularly with feeds. Parents may notice that their baby breathes rapidly and suffers from recurrent chest infections. Cyanosis may not be recognized until it is quite severe.

Children often present with an asymptomatic murmur. Heart failure manifests as breathlessness and reduced exercise tolerance. Orthopnea and nocturnal dyspnea indicate severe heart failure. Cyanosis rarely presents in children over a year of age. A history of 'blueness around the lips' is most likely to be due to cold, crying or breath-holding episodes.

A detailed history is also essential when assessing a child with palpitations, dizziness or syncope. In childhood, chest pain is rarely cardiac in origin and is more likely to be musculoskeletal, pulmonary or due to anxiety. Angina occurs during intense physical activity and is relieved by rest. It is a crushing central chest pain, not related to breathing.[3] It lasts some minutes, unlike muscular pain, which is often fleeting and sharp. Symptoms associated with acquired heart disease such as rheumatic fever, Kawasaki disease and myocarditis are discussed later.

Children may also have symptoms that are unrelated to a cardiac lesion. Nonspecific symptoms, such as tiredness, can cause concern in a child with a cardiac lesion. Reassurance may be necessary if this is not due to the heart condition. A history of prematurity, fetal distress or other congenital anomalies may have a bearing on diagnosis. A maternal history of diabetes, systemic lupus erythematosus, phenylketonuria or drug ingestion (p. 765) results in a higher incidence of congenital heart disease. A family history of heart disease, arrhythmias or sudden death, particularly in first-degree relatives[4] or parental consanguinity, results in an increased risk.[5]

CLINICAL EXAMINATION

A detailed examination provides essential information for diagnosis, assessment of severity and monitoring of children with heart disease. Systematic examination is preferable but may be adjusted to obtain the maximum information in young children. It is sensible to listen to the heart with a toddler seated on the parent's lap before attempting to feel the femoral pulses or measuring the blood pressure.

GENERAL FEATURES

Children with some congenital abnormalities have a 20–40% incidence of heart disease and 20% of children with a cardiac lesion will have

Table 21.1   Normal values of respiratory and heart rates in infants and children[1,7]

	Birth–6 weeks	6 weeks–2 years	2–6 years	6–10 years	Over 10 years
Respiratory rate/min	45–60	30–40	20–30	15–25	12–20
Heart rate/min	125 ± 30	115 ± 25	100 ± 20	85 ± 20	75 ± 20

an extracardiac anomaly.[6] Chromosomal abnormalities are the most common, occurring in 10% of children with congenital heart disease and this will increase as more are identified. Down, 22q11 deletion, Williams, Noonan and Turner syndromes are most commonly associated with congenital heart disease, but many other associations have been reported.[1]

Weight and height should be plotted on a growth chart together with birth weight, to assess growth. Poor growth is associated with heart failure and cyanosis. It may also be unrelated to the cardiac lesion, particularly in children with dysmorphic features. The respiratory rate should be recorded. Normal values are shown in Table 21.1.[1,7] Tachypnea may be cardiac or respiratory. Upper airway obstruction with stridor can occur in association with a vascular ring. Chronic upper airway obstruction can cause pulmonary hypertension. Estimation of the jugular venous pressure is difficult in young children, and hepatomegaly is a more reliable indicator of systemic venous congestion.

CARDIOVASCULAR EXAMINATION
Heart failure
Signs of heart failure should be sought in any child suspected of having a cardiac lesion (p. 762). Particular attention should be paid to peripheral perfusion, edema and respiratory distress.

Cyanosis and clubbing
Mild central cyanosis may be difficult to detect. It must be distinguished from peripheral cyanosis (acrocyanosis) that does not involve well-perfused areas such as the tongue and mucous membranes. Central cyanosis requires the presence of more than 5 g/dl of reduced hemoglobin in the arterial circulation, so anemia will affect the recognition of cyanosis. With the advent of pulse oximetry it has become clear that cyanosis with an oxygen saturation in the region of 85% can be detected clinically in children in good light. Clubbing of the digits takes months to develop, and is not seen in young infants.

Pulses
Pulses should be evaluated for rate, rhythm, volume and character. Rate varies with age, and ranges are shown in Table 21.1. Faster rates are normal during crying or activity, but persistent tachycardia (> 200 beats/min in neonates, 150/min in infants or 120/min in older children), bradycardia (< 70 in under young children, < 50 in older children) and irregular rhythms should be evaluated with an electrocardiogram. Sinus tachycardia is usually present with heart failure. The volume of both arms and femoral pulses should be assessed to exclude coarctation and other arterial anomalies. Radiofemoral delay is difficult to appreciate in children with a rapid pulse, but a difference between the volume of the right axillary and femoral pulse is significant. Femoral pulses should be checked at the postnatal examination, but if the arterial duct is still patent, the pulse may be palpable in the presence of coarctation. The femoral pulses should be checked again at routine assessments, and if there is a suspicion of heart disease. Poor volume of all pulses reflects a reduced cardiac output indicating hypoplastic left heart syndrome, critical aortic stenosis, severe heart failure, shock or cardiac tamponade. A wide pulse pressure (the difference between systolic and diastolic pressure) produces a collapsing (bounding) pulse in children with a large arterial duct, arteriovenous malformation, severe anemia and severe aortic regurgitation. A slow rising (plateau) pulse is found in severe aortic stenosis.

Blood pressure
Blood pressure should always be recorded in *the right arm*, as the measurement in the left may be lower if coarctation is present.[8] Blood pressure should be measured with the child lying or sitting comfortably with the sphygmomanometer at heart level. The inflatable cuff should cover two thirds of the upper arm from shoulder tip to elbow and completely encircle the arm. A smaller cuff will give a falsely high reading. If there is any suspicion of aortic coarctation, both arm and leg pressures should be measured. The blood pressure in the leg is normally higher than the arm. A measurement in the leg that is 10 mmHg or more lower than in the arms is abnormal.

Blood pressure in children is labile, and measurements above the 95th percentile on at least three different occasions are necessary to diagnose hypertension.[8] Taller children have higher blood pressures than smaller ones. Charts of the 50th, 90th, 95th and 99th percentile for blood pressure, related to sex, age and height, are shown in Tables 21.2 and 21.3.[8] Twenty-four hour ambulatory blood pressure monitoring can be performed on older children. It is useful in those whose readings are affected by anxiety.

Automated oscillometric methods with digital readout of systolic, diastolic and mean pressure are increasingly used. These are reasonably reliable, but inaccuracies occur with movement. Measurement done in this way is approximately 10 mmHg higher than that obtained by auscultation.[9] Comparisons are not available for infants and young children. Measurements obtained by oscillometric devices that exceed the 90th percentile should be repeated by auscultation.[8]

Precordial examination
This may reveal a bulge indicating chronic cardiac enlargement. Scars from previous surgery should also be noted. The apex beat is felt at the fourth left intercostal space within the midclavicular line. It is produced by the left ventricle and is displaced laterally and inferiorly with cardiomegaly. It is palpable on the right in dextrocardia. Left ventricular hypertrophy produces a forceful impulse that is usually not displaced. Right ventricular enlargement produces a diffuse impulse at the lower half of the sternum and in the epigastrium. A poorly felt apex beat suggests a pericardial effusion or severe heart failure. Dextrocardia should be excluded by palpating the right precordium. Thrills are palpable over the site of maximum intensity of loud murmurs, but the thrill of aortic stenosis is felt in the suprasternal notch. Thrills are usually systolic. Rarely diastolic thrills occur in severe mitral or tricuspid stenosis. The loud second heart sound of severe pulmonary hypertension is sometimes palpable.

Auscultation
Auscultation of all phases of the cardiac cycle should be systematic and include the whole precordium, axilla and the back. Note changes during inspiration and expiration, and with the child sitting and lying. The heart sounds and high-pitched murmurs are best heard with the diaphragm of the stethoscope, and low-pitched ones with the bell.

The *first heart sound* is caused by mitral and tricuspid valve closure and is best heard at the apex. It is louder with tachycardia, as the valve leaflets are further apart in early systole. It is usually single, reflecting mitral closure but split if tricuspid closure is delayed. The *second heart sound* is caused by aortic and pulmonary valve closure and is best heard at the upper left and right sternal borders. During inspiration, pulmonary valve closure is delayed because of the increased volume

Table 21.2 Blood pressure levels for boys by age and height percentiles (adapted from Falkner et al[8])

Age, (y)	BP percentile	SBP, mmHg Percentile of height							DBP mmHg Percentile of height						
		5th	10th	25th	50th	75th	90th	95th	5th	10th	25th	50th	75th	90th	95th
1	50th	80	81	83	85	87	88	89	34	35	36	37	38	39	39
	90th	94	95	97	99	100	102	103	49	50	51	52	53	53	54
	95th	98	99	101	103	104	106	106	54	54	55	56	57	58	58
	99th	105	106	108	110	112	113	114	61	62	63	64	65	66	66
2	50th	84	85	87	88	90	92	92	39	40	41	42	43	44	44
	90th	97	99	100	102	104	105	106	54	55	56	57	58	58	59
	95th	101	102	104	106	108	109	110	59	59	60	61	62	63	63
	99th	109	110	111	113	115	117	117	66	67	68	69	70	71	71
3	50th	86	87	89	91	93	94	95	44	44	45	46	47	48	48
	90th	100	101	103	105	107	108	109	59	59	60	61	62	63	63
	95th	104	105	107	109	110	112	113	63	63	64	65	66	67	67
	99th	111	112	114	116	118	119	120	71	71	72	73	74	75	75
4	50th	88	89	91	93	95	96	97	47	48	49	50	51	51	52
	90th	102	103	105	107	109	110	111	62	63	64	65	66	66	67
	95th	106	107	109	111	112	114	115	66	67	68	69	70	71	71
	99th	113	114	116	118	120	121	122	74	75	76	77	78	78	79
5	50th	90	91	93	95	96	98	98	50	51	52	53	54	55	55
	90th	104	105	106	108	110	111	112	65	66	67	68	69	69	70
	95th	108	1.09	110	112	114	115	116	69	70	71	72	73	74	74
	99th	115	116	118	120	121	123	123	77	78	79	80	81	81	82
6	50th	91	92	94	96	98	99	100	53	53	54	55	56	57	57
	90th	105	106	108	110	111	113	113	68	68	69	70	71	72	72
	95th	109	110	112	114	115	117	117	72	72	73	74	75	76	76
	99th	116	117	119	121	123	124	125	80	80	81	82	83	84	84
7	50th	92	94	95	97	99	100	101	55	55	56	57	58	59	59
	90th	106	107	109	111	113	114	115	70	70	71	72	73	74	74
	95th	110	111	113	115	117	118	119	74	74	75	76	77	78	78
	99th	117	118	120	122	124	125	126	82	82	83	84	85	86	86
8	50th	94	95	97	99	100	102	102	56	57	58	59	60	60	61
	90th	107	109	110	112	114	115	116	71	72	72	73	74	75	76
	95th	111	112	114	116	118	119	120	75	76	77	78	79	79	80
	99th	119	120	122	123	125	127	127	83	84	85	86	87	87	88
9	50th	95	96	98	100	102	103	104	57	58	59	60	61	61	62
	90th	109	110	112	114	115	117	118	72	73	74	75	76	76	77
	95th	113	114	116	118	119	121	121	76	77	78	79	80	81	81
	99th	120	121	123	125	127	128	129	84	85	86	87	88	88	89
10	50th	97	98	100	102	103	105	106	58	59	60	61	61	62	63
	90th	111	112	114	115	117	119	119	73	73	74	75	76	77	78
	95th	115	116	117	119	121	122	123	77	78	79	80	81	81	82
	99th	122	123	125	127	128	130	130	85	86	86	88	88	89	90
11	50th	99	100	102	104	105	107	107	59	59	60	61	62	63	63
	90th	113	114	115	117	119	120	121	74	74	75	76	77	78	78
	95th	117	118	119	121	123	124	125	78	78	79	80	81	82	82
	99th	124	125	127	129	130	132	132	86	86	87	88	89	90	90
12	50th	101	102	104	106	108	109	110	59	60	61	62	63	63	64
	90th	115	116	118	120	121	123	123	74	75	75	76	77	78	79
	95th	119	120	122	123	125	127	127	78	79	80	81	82	82	83
	99th	126	127	129	131	133	134	135	86	87	88	89	90	90	91
13	50th	104	105	106	108	110	111	112	60	60	61	62	63	64	64
	90th	117	118	120	122	124	125	126	75	75	76	77	78	79	79
	95th	121	122	124	126	128	129	130	79	79	80	81	82	83	83
	99th	128	130	131	133	135	136	137	87	87	88	89	90	91	91
14	50th	106	107	109	111	113	114	115	60	61	62	63	64	65	65
	90th	120	121	123	125	126	128	128	75	76	77	78	79	79	80
	95th	124	125	127	128	130	132	132	80	80	81	82	83	84	84
	99th	131	132	134	136	138	139	140	87	88	89	90	91	92	92
15	50th	109	110	112	113	115	117	117	61	62	63	64	65	66	66
	90th	122	124	125	127	129	130	131	76	77	78	79	80	80	81
	95th	126	127	129	131	133	134	135	81	81	82	83	84	85	85
	99th	134	135	136	138	140	142	142	88	89	90	91	92	93	93

(Continued)

Table 21.2   Blood pressure levels for boys by age and height percentiles (adapted from Falkner et al[8])—cont'd

Age, (y)	BP percentile	SBP, mmHg Percentile of height							DBP mmHg Percentile of height						
		5th	10th	25th	50th	75th	90th	95th	5th	10th	25th	50th	75th	90th	95th
16	50th	111	112	114	116	118	119	120	63	63	64	65	66	67	67
	90th	125	126	128	130	131	133	134	78	78	79	80	81	82	82
	95th	129	130	132	134	135	137	137	82	83	83	84	85	86	87
	99th	136	137	139	141	143	144	145	90	90	91	92	93	94	94
17	50th	114	115	116	118	120	121	122	65	66	66	67	68	69	70
	90th	127	128	130	132	134	135	136	80	80	81	82	83	84	84
	95th	131	132	134	136	138	139	140	84	85	86	87	87	88	89
	99th	139	140	141	143	145	146	147	92	93	93	94	95	96	97

The 90th percentile is 1.28 SD, the 95th percentile is 1.645 SD, and the 99th percentile is 2.326 SD over the mean.

Table 21.3   Blood pressure levels for girls by age and height percentiles (adapted from Falkner et al[8])

Age, (y)	BP percentile	SBP, mmHg Percentile of height							DBP, mmHg Percentile of height						
		5th	10th	25th	50th	75th	90th	95th	5th	10th	25th	50th	75th	90th	95th
1	50th	83	84	85	86	88	89	90	38	39	39	40	41	41	42
	90th	97	97	98	100	101	102	103	52	53	53	54	55	55	56
	95th	100	101	102	104	105	106	107	56	57	57	58	59	59	60
	99th	108	108	109	111	112	113	114	64	64	65	65	66	67	67
2	50th	85	85	87	88	89	91	91	43	44	44	45	46	46	47
	90th	98	99	100	101	103	104	105	57	58	58	59	60	61	61
	95th	102	103	104	105	107	108	109	61	62	62	63	64	65	65
	99th	109	110	111	112	114	115	116	69	69	70	70	71	72	72
3	50th	86	87	88	89	91	92	93	47	48	48	49	50	50	51
	90th	100	100	102	103	104	106	106	61	62	62	63	64	64	65
	95th	104	104	105	107	108	109	110	65	66	66	67	68	68	69
	99th	111	111	113	114	115	116	117	73	73	74	74	75	76	76
4	50th	88	88	90	91	92	94	94	50	50	51	52	52	53	54
	90th	101	102	103	104	106	107	108	64	64	65	66	67	67	68
	95th	105	106	107	108	110	111	112	68	68	69	70	71	71	72
	99th	112	113	114	115	117	118	119	76	76	76	77	78	79	79
5	50th	89	90	91	93	94	95	96	52	53	53	54	55	55	56
	90th	103	103	105	106	107	109	109	66	67	67	68	69	69	70
	95th	107	107	108	110	111	112	113	70	71	71	72	73	73	74
	99th	114	114	116	117	118	120	120	78	78	79	79	80	81	81
6	50th	91	92	93	94	96	97	98	54	54	55	56	56	57	58
	90th	104	105	106	108	109	110	111	68	68	69	70	70	71	72
	95th	108	109	110	111	113	114	115	72	72	73	74	74	75	76
	99th	115	116	117	119	120	121	122	80	80	80	81	82	83	83
7	50th	93	93	95	96	97	99	99	55	56	56	57	58	58	59
	90th	106	107	108	109	111	112	113	69	70	70	71	72	72	73
	95th	110	111	112	113	115	116	116	73	74	74	75	76	76	77
	99th	117	118	119	120	122	123	124	81	81	82	82	83	84	84
8	50th	95	95	96	98	99	100	101	57	57	57	58	59	60	60
	90th	108	109	110	111	113	114	114	71	71	71	72	73	74	74
	95th	112	112	114	115	116	118	118	75	75	75	76	77	78	78
	99th	119	120	121	122	123	125	125	82	82	83	83	84	85	86
9	50th	96	97	98	100	101	102	103	58	58	58	59	60	61	61
	90th	110	110	112	113	114	116	116	72	72	72	73	74	75	75
	95th	114	114	115	117	118	119	120	76	76	76	77	78	79	79
	99th	121	121	123	124	125	127	127	83	83	84	84	85	86	87
10	50th	98	99	100	102	103	104	105	59	59	59	60	61	62	62
	90th	112	112	114	115	116	118	118	73	73	73	74	75	76	76
	95th	116	116	117	119	120	121	122	77	77	77	78	79	80	80
	99th	123	123	125	126	127	129	129	84	84	85	86	86	87	88

Since it is now such a crucial aspect of pediatric cardiology, it is important to know of its indications, strengths and limitations. A knowledge of cardiac anatomy is also necessary.

CROSS-SECTIONAL (2D) ECHOCARDIOGRAPHY

Echocardiographers usually use a sector scan; the image that results is shaped like a section of a pie. This sector is built up of many individual lines of ultrasound, sweeping across the sector. Since the heart rate is high in pediatrics, the frame rate (the number of completed sectors per minute) must be high to avoid a jerky appearance to the heart movement. The best definition is achieved by using ultrasound with higher frequencies, but the higher the frequency, the poorer the tissue penetration. The best compromise between these two factors means a frequency of 8–12 MHz can be used for preterm infants with often extremely good image quality, but a frequency of 2–3 MHz is needed for larger children and adults.

Echocardiographic windows

Since ultrasound cannot pass through the air within the lungs, the ultrasonic approach to the heart is through echocardiographic 'windows' where there is little or no air between the transducer and heart. These are subcostal, apical, parasternal and suprasternal (see Figs 21.5–21.9). In the newborn there are large echo windows making imaging easier than in older children and adults, and it is often possible to do most of the scan subcostally.

Imaging axes

Since the heart lies at an angle within the chest, the apex pointing caudal and leftward, the 'standard' anatomical cuts (coronal, sagittal, etc.)

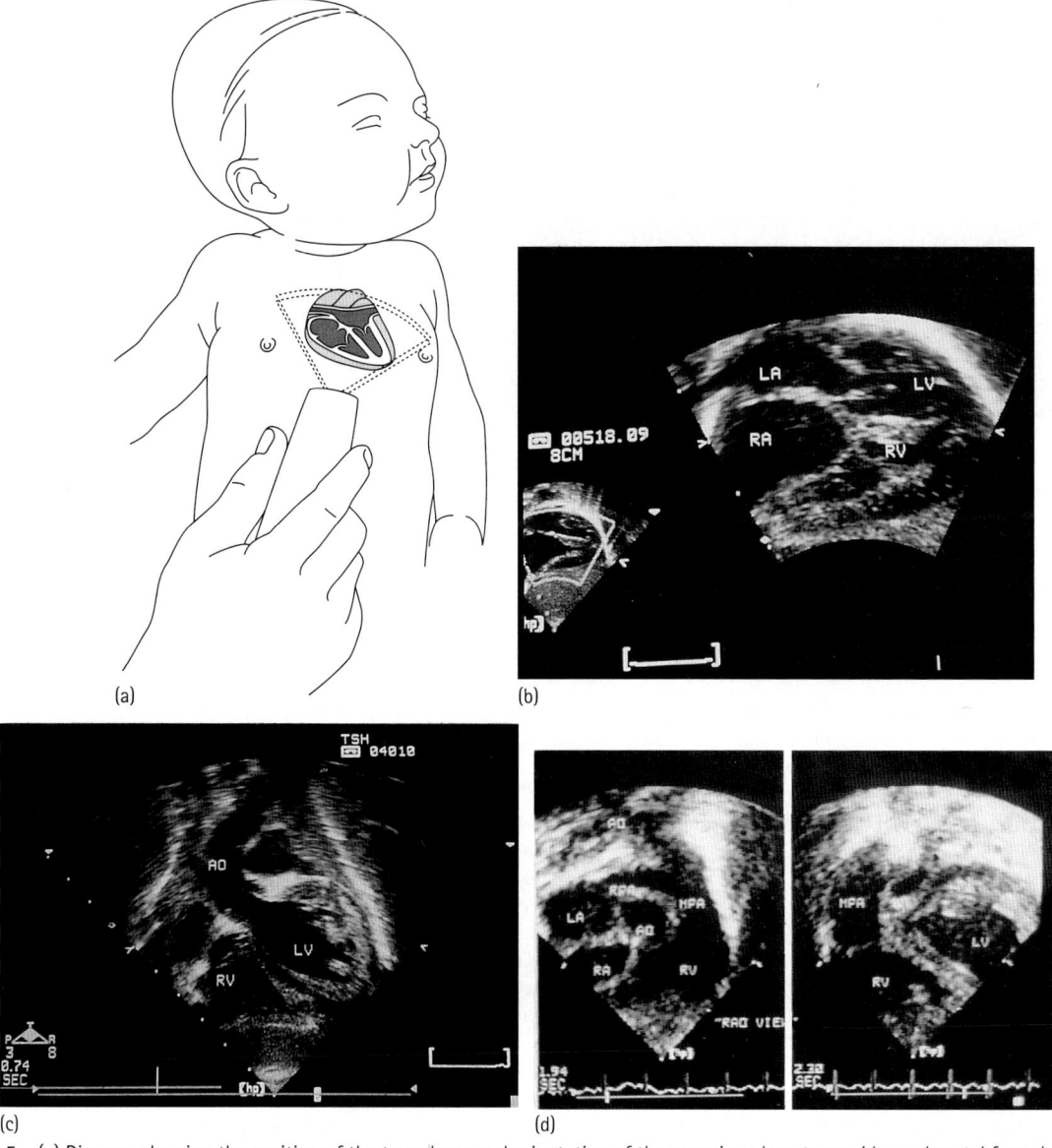

Fig. 21.5 (a) Diagram showing the position of the transducer and orientation of the scanning plane to provide a subcostal four chamber image of the heart. (b) Subcostal four chamber image demonstrating the four chambers. This is an ideal view to see atrial septal defects. (c) Tilting the probe anteriorly brings the ascending aorta into view. (d) Left: rotating anticlockwise brings the right ventricular outflow tract and pulmonary arteries into view [subcostal short-axis or 'RAO' (right anterior oblique) view]. MPA, main pulmonary artery; RPA, right pulmonary artery. Right: rotating clockwise shows the interventricular septum and another view of the right ventricular outflow tract. These views are especially useful in tetralogy of Fallot to assess obstruction of the right ventricular outflow tract. (From Skinner et al 2000[23].)

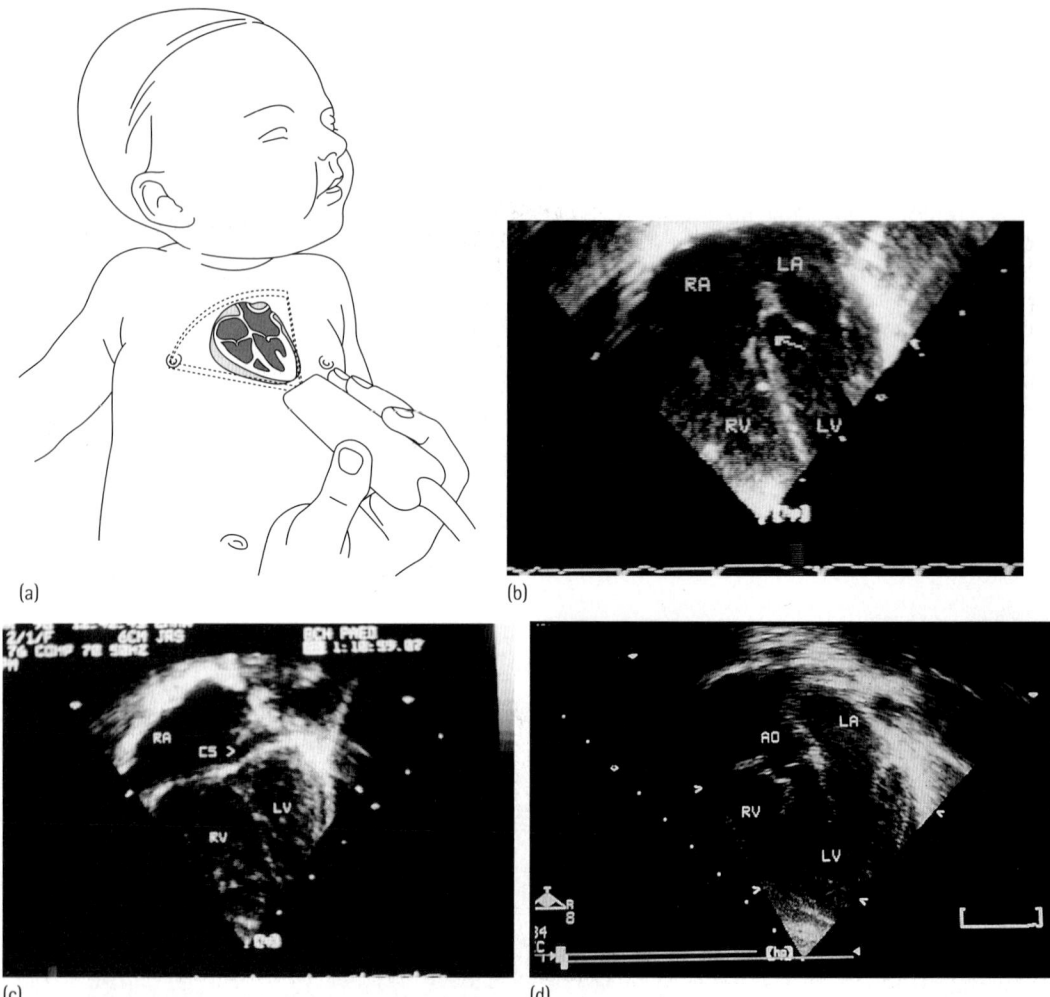

Fig. 21.6 (a) Diagram showing the position of the transducer and orientation of scanning plane to provide an apical four chamber view of the heart. (b) Apical four chamber echocardiogram. Note that the screen has been inverted. The arrow indicates the lower position of the tricuspid valve as it arises from the septum. This region between the two atrioventricular valves is known as the atrioventricular septum, dividing the left ventricle from the right atrium. (c) Apical view of the heart with the probe angled posteriorly to bring the coronary sinus (CS) into view (not to be confused with a low atrial septal defect!). (d) Apical view of the heart with the probe angled anteriorly and rotated to the right bringing the left ventricular outflow tract and aortic valve into view – this is an apical long-axis image. (From Skinner et al 2000[23].)

are not used. Instead the scanning planes are related to the axis of the heart. There are three axes that form the majority of standard views. They correspond to the mathematical x, y and z axes and are at right angles to each other. They create the long axis, short axis and four chamber views. Examples from the normal infant's heart are shown in Figures 21.5–21.8.

Relating normal cardiac anatomy to the standard echocardiographic views

The four chamber views

The plane of this cut through the heart is parallel to the bed upon which the patient is lying. These views, from the apex or subcostal regions (Fig. 21.5b and 21.6b), show that the ventricles are caudal and leftward of their corresponding atria. The most caudal valve in the heart is the tricuspid, which is attached to the septum closer to the cardiac apex than the mitral valve. This offsetting of the tricuspid valve (Fig. 21.6b) means that there is an atrioventricular septum dividing the left ventricle from the right atrium; this part of the septum is absent in atrioventricular septal defects. Since a tricuspid valve is always associated with a right ventricle and a mitral valve with the left, this offsetting is used to identify left and right ventricles.

The atrial septum lies obliquely at 45° to the sagittal plane of the body and is best examined from the subcostal approach (Fig. 21.5). However, the ventricular septum curves in a complex way from a plane which is nearly sagittal to one which is nearly coronal, separating respectively the inlet and outlet portions of the two ventricles. Because of this complex shape, the search for ventricular septal defects needs to include all available views. There is also a tiny component of the septal wall which is not muscular and is known as the membranous septum, closely related to the tricuspid and aortic valves. It has atrioventricular and interventricular portions separated by the attachment of the septal leaflet of the tricuspid valve.

With posterior tilt of the probe in the four chamber plane, the entry of the pulmonary veins into the back of the left atrium can be seen, as can the coronary sinus running in the atrioventricular groove behind the left atrium and opening into the right atrium.

Short axis views

These cut through the heart like transverse slices through a green pepper, and can be obtained from the left parasternum (Fig. 21.7) or subcostally (Fig. 21.5d – left). They show that the right heart 'wraps' around the left heart. The right heart chambers are anterior to the left

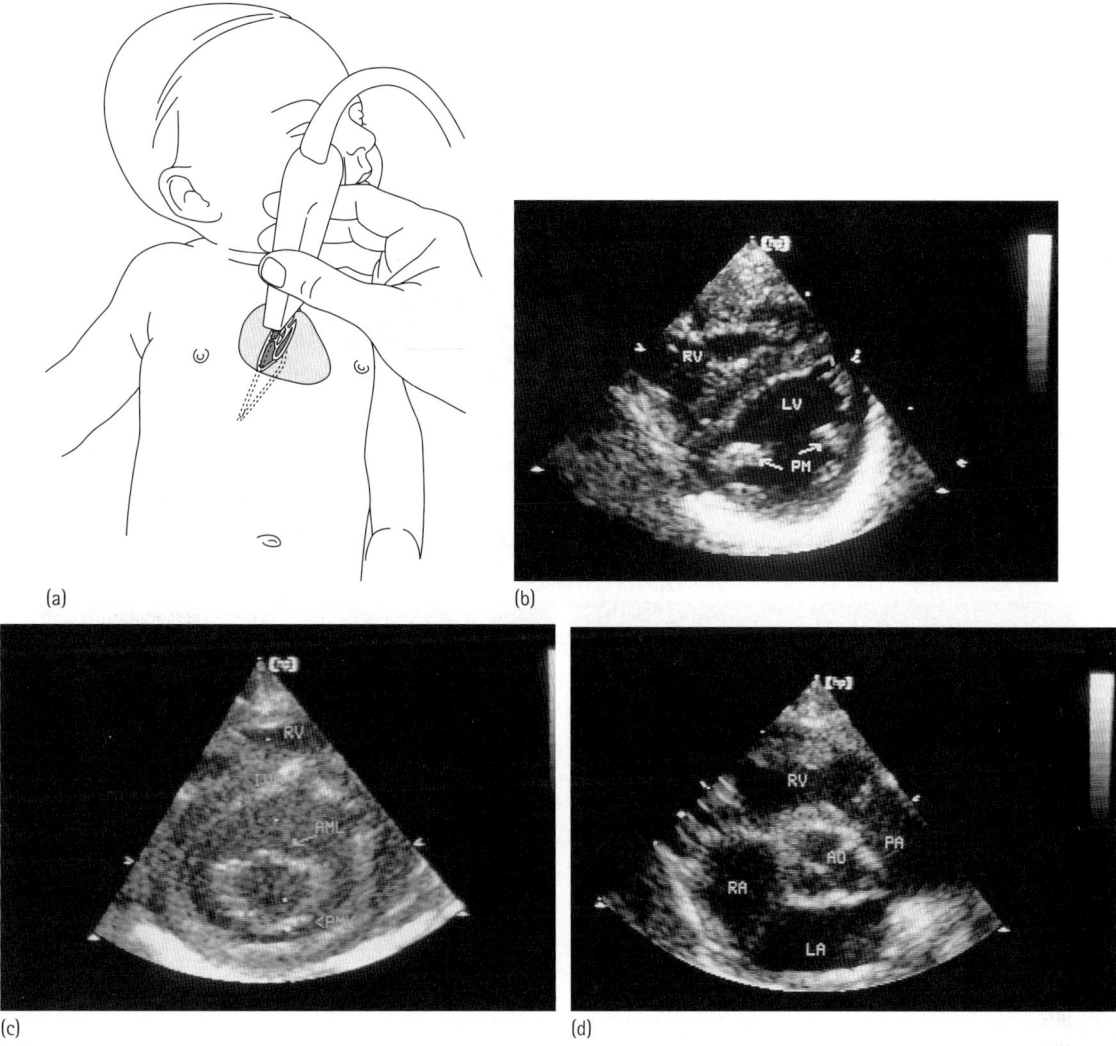

Fig. 21.7 (a) Diagram showing the position of the transducer and orientation of the scanning plane to provide a parasternal short-axis image of the heart at the aortic valve level. (b) Parasternal short-axis echocardiograph at the level of the papillary muscles (towards the apex of the left ventricle). This image is used to obtain an M-mode cut through the left ventricle to assess left ventricular function (see text). (c) Tilting away from the apex (towards the right shoulder) brings this view of the mitral valve. AML, anterior mitral valve leaflet; PML, posterior mitral valve leaflet. (d) Further tilt shows this cut at the aortic valve [as in (a)]. Note here how three aortic valve leaflets are seen, and how the right heart wraps around the aorta. Tilting the probe further still away from the apex demonstrates the pulmonary artery bifurcation. (From Skinner et al 2000[23].)

heart chambers. The left atrium is the most posterior cardiac chamber directly anterior to the esophagus at the bifurcation of the trachea, and has the pulmonary veins draining into the back of it. The right atrium is rightward and anterior, and the tricuspid valve is in a nearly vertical plane.

The aortic valve is seen to lie in a central position (Fig. 21.7d). The pulmonary valve lies anterior and cranially and the atrioventricular valves flank the posterior and caudal margins of the aortic valve. The pulmonary trunk comes from the anterior aspect of the heart, swings to the left side of the ascending aorta, heading posteriorly, bifurcating into the left and right pulmonary arteries. This posterior course of the main pulmonary artery explains why pulmonary valve stenotic murmurs are transmitted to the back.

Angling the short axis cut down towards the apex of the left ventricle brings first the mitral valve structures into view, gaping like a 'fish mouth' as the leaflets open and close (Fig. 21.7c). The cut nearer the apex shows that the mitral valve is tethered and supported by two groups of papillary muscles: the anterolateral and posteromedial groups (Fig. 21.7b).

Long axis views

These views (imagine a cut through the stalk and extending into a green pepper) can be obtained from the left parasternum (Fig. 21.8) or the apex (Fig. 21.6c). They show the relatively straight outflow from the left ventricle to the aorta (compare this to the angled outflow of the right ventricle seen in the short axis view). The anterior leaflet of the mitral valve is in fibrous continuity with the aortic valve, whereas there is a muscular infundibulum between the tricuspid valve and the pulmonary valve. The ascending aorta passes superiorly, obliquely to the right and slightly forwards towards the sternum.

Suprasternal views

These views (Fig. 21.9) demonstrate the arch of the aorta which supplies origins to the brachiocephalic (innominate) artery and the left common carotid artery as it runs superiorly for a short distance before passing backwards and to the left. The arch finishes on the lateral aspect of the vertebral column after the origin of the left subclavian artery. Aortic coarctation most commonly appears just after this point.

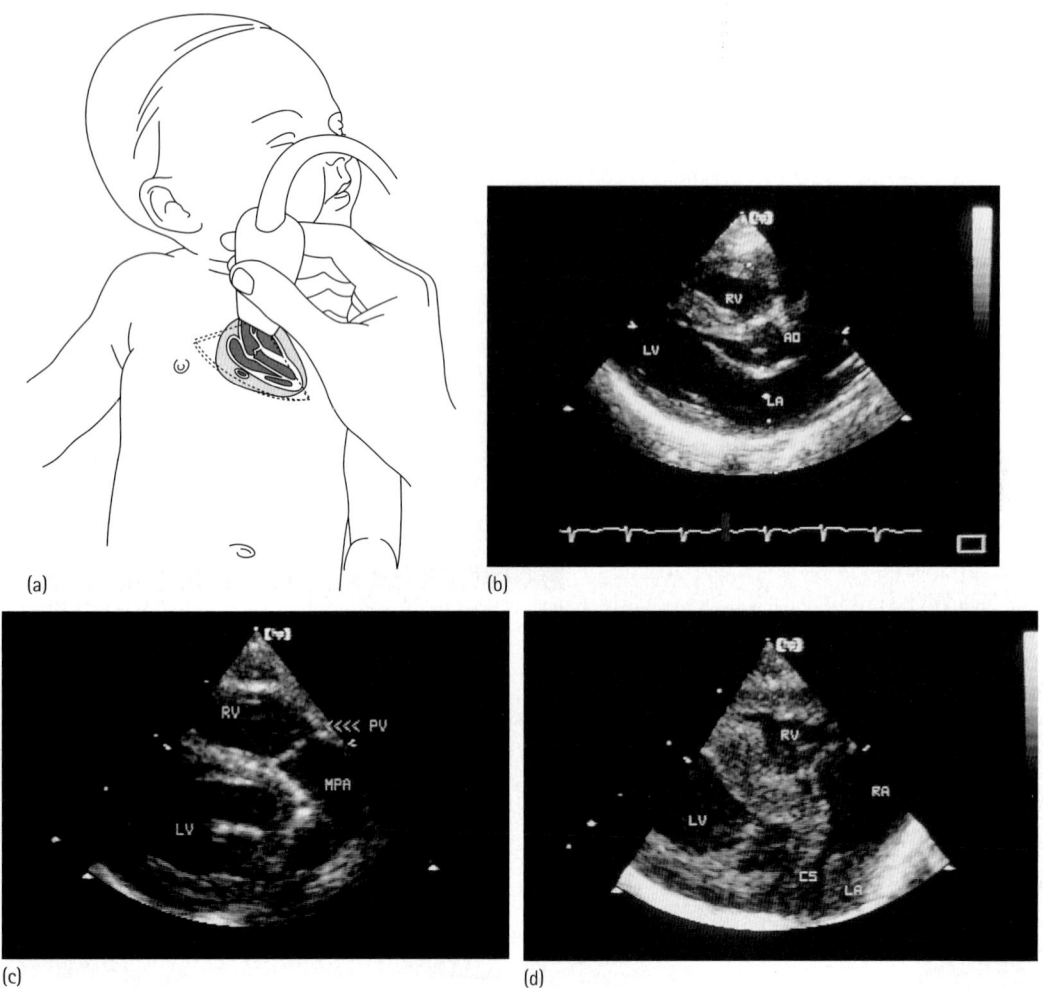

Fig. 21.8 (a) Diagram showing the position of the transducer and orientation of scanning plane to provide a parasternal long-axis image of the heart. (b) Echocardiogram showing a standard parasternal long-axis image of the heart, ideal for demonstrating the left heart. The mitral valve is widely open in this diastolic frame. Ao, aorta; LV, left ventricle; RV, right ventricle. (c) Tilting towards the left shoulder reveals a long-axis view of the main pulmonary artery (MPA) and pulmonary valve (PV). (d) Tilting to the right, away from the left shoulder, reveals the tricuspid valve between the right atrium (RA) and right ventricle (RV). The coronary sinus (CS) is seen draining into the right atrium. LA, left atrium. (From Skinner et al 2000[23].)

THREE-DIMENSIONAL ECHOCARDIOGRAPHY

Increased computer power means that freehand real-time three-dimensional echocardiography will begin to move from the research laboratory into clinical practice. Early signs are that this will improve diagnostic accuracy in congenital heart disease.[24]

NOMENCLATURE IN CONGENITAL HEART DISEASE

There is a trend to avoid eponyms and Latin terms in congenital heart disease because they may mislead and are confusing to nonspecialists; 'solitus' doesn't mean solitary for instance, but 'usual'. 'Inversus' doesn't mean mirror imaged, it actually means 'upside down'. Another essential and helpful part of new cardiac anatomical nomenclature is 'sequential chamber localization' or 'sequential segmental analysis'[25] where congenital heart disease is characterized descriptively using anatomical and physiological terms in a sequential fashion.

SEQUENTIAL CHAMBER LOCALIZATION

If you wish to build a safe house, you first consolidate the foundation before proceeding to the subsequent floors. Taking the same approach to help understand and describe complex heart diseases,

the floors, or segments, of the heart are the atria, the ventricular mass and the great arteries. The type of connection between each segment is also described. The possibilities for each segment are shown in Table 21.5.

Thus a normal heart has the usual atrial arrangement, atrioventricular concordance and ventriculo-arterial concordance. A cyanosed newborn with transposed great arteries has isolated ventriculo-arterial discordance. The condition formally known as 'congenital corrected transposition' is now described as atrioventricular discordance with ventriculo-arterial discordance. The infant is not cyanosed, but the morphological right ventricle is the systemic ventricle. Most pediatric cardiologists start scanning from venous inflow and end with arterial outflow, noting abnormalities along the way. This means starting with subcostal views and ending with the suprasternal views.

Venous inflow and the atria

In the transverse abdominal cut, the inferior caval vein is normally to the right and the aorta to the left. This is reversed when there is abdominal situs inversus (mirror image position). If the thoracic contents are also mirror-imaged, the apex of the heart is seen pointing to the right. The incidence of congenital heart disease is not increased in such cases. It is, though, if the heart and the stomach are not on the same side.

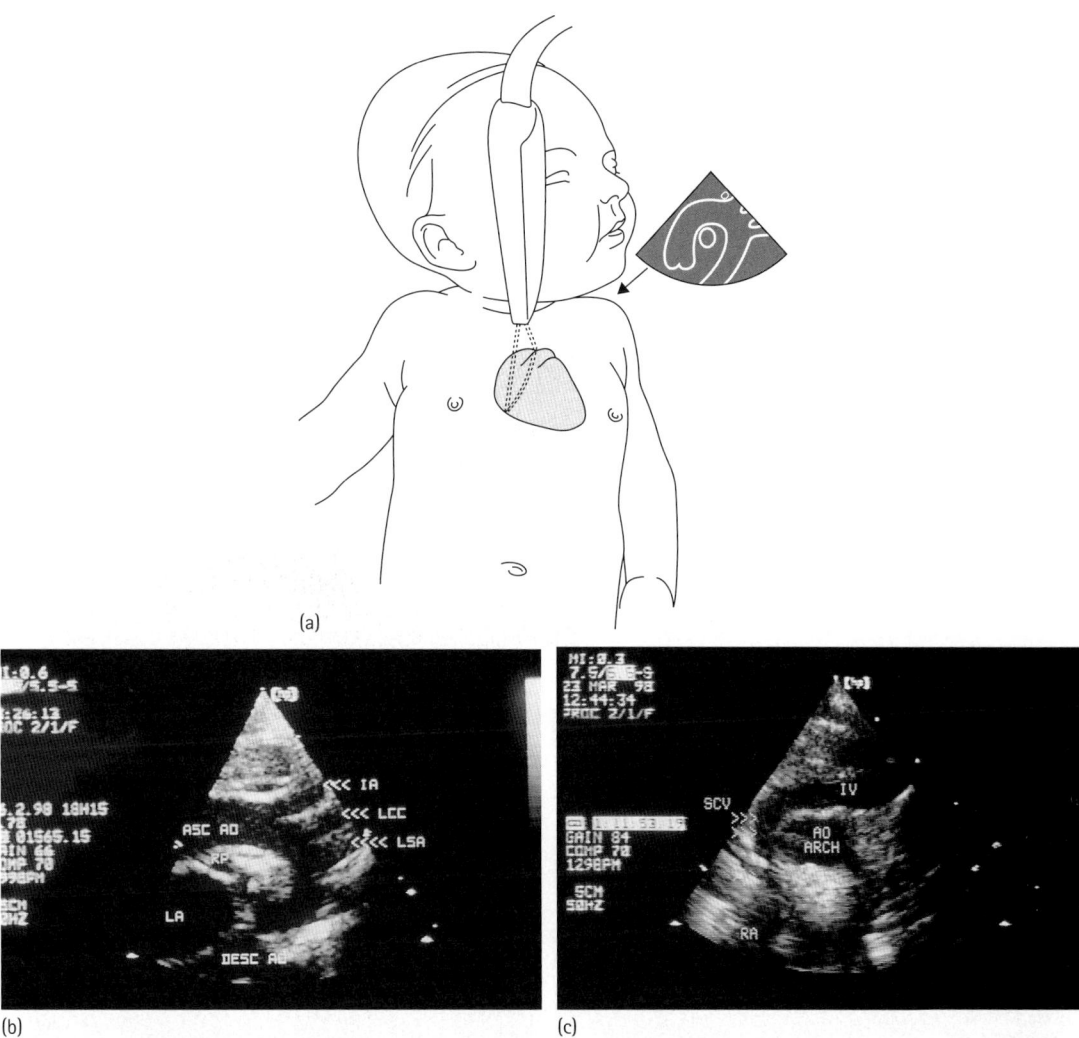

Fig. 21.9 (a) Diagram showing the position of the transducer and orientation of the scanning plane required to obtain views of the aortic arch with a conventional left-sided aorta. Note that a roll has been placed behind the shoulders to extend the neck. (b) Image of the aortic arch and branches obtained from the suprasternal window. IA, innominate artery (or right brachiocephalic artery); LCC, left common carotid artery; LSA, left subclavian artery. Arch interruptions and coarctations are best viewed like this. (c) With a transverse scanning plane, the innominate vein (IV) drains to the superior caval vein (SCV). (From Skinner et al 2000[23].)

Table 21.5 Possible sequential segmental arrangements in congenital heart disease

Segment	Possibilities	Examples/comments
Great veins	Describe abnormalities of position and connection	e.g. Anomalous pulmonary venous drainage, left superior caval vein connecting to coronary sinus
Atria	Usual arrangement	
	Mirror image (left atrium on the right side)	'Situs inversus'
	Two right atria (right atrial isomerism)	Asplenia is common, pulmonary veins connect abnormally
	Two left atria (left atrial isomerism)	Often no inferior caval vein present
Atrioventricular connection	Concordant (RA–RV, LA–LV)	
	Discordant (RA–LV, LA–RV)	
	Ambiguous (if the two atria are the same morphology)	
	Absent right connection	e.g. Tricuspid atresia
	Absent left connection	e.g. Mitral atresia
	Double inlet	
Ventricular mass	Two ventricles (biventricular connection)	
	'Single' ventricle (univentricular connection)	
	LV with a rudimentary RV	This is the most common form
	RV with rudimentary LV	
	Solitary indeterminate ventricle	
Ventriculo-arterial connection	Concordant (RV–PA, LV–Aorta)	
	Discordant (RV–Aorta, LV–PA)	
	Double outlet	Most common is double outlet RV
	Single outlet	e.g. Common arterial trunk, pulmonary atresia
Great arteries	Describe abnormalities	e.g. Patent arterial duct, aortic coarctation, branch pulmonary artery stenosis

Totally anomalous pulmonary venous drainage is seen as failure of the pulmonary veins to connect to the back of the left atrium (Fig. 21.10a).

The echocardiogram is not reliable in deciding on the atrial arrangement. The appearances of the atrial appendages are the only reliable way of differentiating the atria, and they are often not well seen. Fortunately the plain chest X-ray can help. The atria and lung always go together. On chest radiography, a short bronchus on the right suggests a three-lobed right lung on that side with early branching, and a right atrium on the right. On the left, the bronchus is normally longer and bifurcates to supply a two lobed lung indicating that the morphological left atrium lies on the left. Mirror imaging of the lungs will give a long bronchus on the right and a short one on the left. Two long bronchi means two left lungs and two short bronchi means two right lungs – left atrial isomerism and right atrial isomerism respectively. Atrial septal defects are best defined from the subcostal position.

Atrioventricular connection

The connection may be 'concordant' when right atrium leads to right ventricle and left atrium to left ventricle (Fig. 21.6b), or 'discordant' when right atrium leads to left ventricle and left atrium to right ventricle. A 'univentricular connection' occurs when both atria drain to one ventricle, either a double inlet left or right ventricle (Fig. 21.10c). There is another form of univentricular connection where either the right or left connection is absent, either mitral or tricuspid atresia (Fig. 21.10b) ('absent left' or 'absent right AV connection' respectively). In the presence of atrial isomerism, the atrioventricular connection is of necessity 'ambiguous', as it cannot be either truly concordant or discordant.

Ventricles

To define atrioventricular concordance the ventricles need to be positively identified, not by position (since a morphological right ventricle can be on the left for example), but by morphology. If there are two ventricles in the heart, the tricuspid valve is always in the right ventricle and the mitral always in the left ventricle. The atrioventricular valve anatomy is, therefore, the most reliable way of identifying the ventricle.

The right ventricle is identified by its heavy trabeculation, a muscular 'moderator band' across its apex, an infundibulum (muscular section

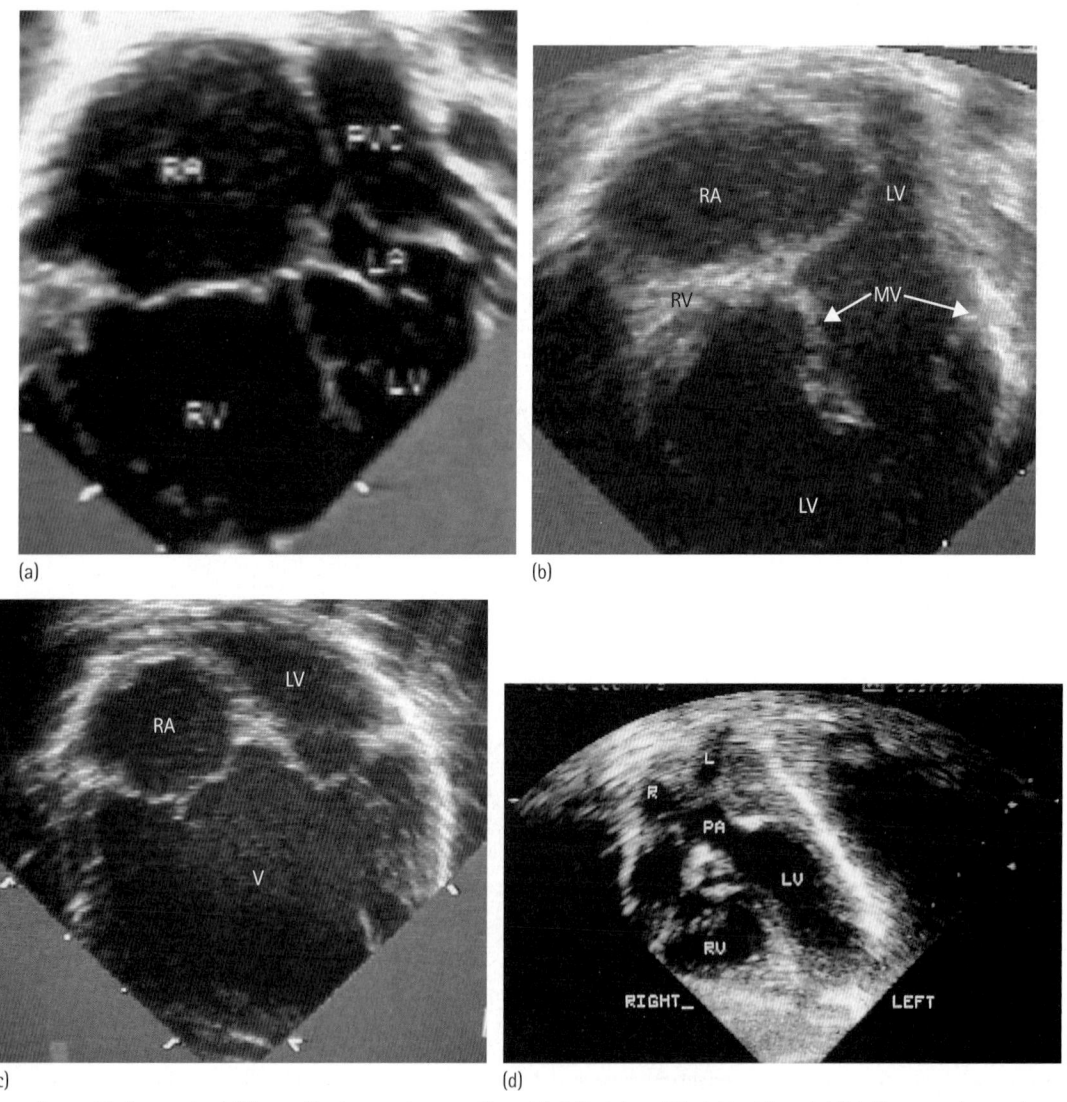

(a)   (b)   (c)   (d)

Fig. 21.10   Echocardiographic images in children with abnormal connections. LA, left atrium; RA right atrium. (a) Totally anomalous pulmonary venous drainage. The pulmonary veins drain into a pulmonary venous chamber (PVC) which does not communicate with the left atrium. (b) Absent right atrioventricular connection (tricuspid atresia). The diminutive right ventricle is hardly visible. The interatrial septum bows across to the left, since in this case the atrial septal defect was restrictive. MV, mitral valve. (c) Double inlet ventricle. Both atrioventricular valves enter into a single large ventricle (V). (d) Ventriculo-arterial discordance. The left ventricle connects with an artery that bifurcates early and is hence the pulmonary artery (PA). This infant was cyanosed due to transposition of the great arteries. (From Skinner et al 2000[23].)

dividing inlet from outlet) and a tricuspid valve which attaches directly to the septum and inserts more apically than the mitral valve. The left ventricle has finer trabeculations, no infundibulum and the mitral valve attached to (usually) two papillary muscles but never attached to the septum.

One or other of the ventricles may be small or even absent. Patients with double inlet left ventricle usually have a small anterior right ventricle connected to the main chamber by a ventricular septal defect and leading to a great artery, frequently the aorta. Double inlet right ventricles with smaller posterior left ventricles are excessively rare. Very occasionally there are truly single ventricle hearts.

Practical point
Features that help to differentiate the right from the left ventricle in complex congenital heart disease:

The tricuspid valve
- Is always associated with the morphological right ventricle.
- Is supported in part from the septum.
- Is not in fibrous continuity with the outlet valve.
- Arises from further down the septum than the mitral valve.

The mitral valve
- Is always associated with the morphological left ventricle.
- Is in fibrous continuity with the outlet valve.
- Has no support from the septum.

Ventriculo-arterial connections
The aorta is identified by not branching early, and having coronary arteries arising from it. The pulmonary artery bifurcates early into two branches. The connection can be 'concordant' when the right ventricle leads to the pulmonary artery and left ventricle to the aorta, or 'discordant' when the right ventricle leads to aorta and left ventricle to pulmonary artery (complete transposition) (Fig. 21.10d). 'Double outlet' can be present from either right or left ventricle and 'single outlets' of the heart describe pulmonary atresia, aortic atresia and common arterial trunk.

Associated lesions such as ventricular and atrial septal defects, valve stenosis or regurgitation, and great arteries abnormalities such as patent arterial duct or aortic coarctation must be identified.

DOPPLER ECHOCARDIOGRAPHY
The speed of blood flow is determined by the Doppler shift created by moving red cells reflecting back ultrasound waves at a different frequency from that which was transmitted by the transducer/receiver. If our brains were programmed like an echocardiography machine, we would be able to determine the speed of an ambulance, with siren blazing, by the increase in pitch as it raced towards us.

The speed of blood flow calculated is relative to the transducer/receiver. Blood flowing at ninety degrees will cause no frequency shift. It is therefore essential to align with flow in order to determine the true speed. From blood flow velocity it is possible to derive volume of blood flow (cardiac output) and pressure gradients (see below). There are three modes of Doppler ultrasound: pulsed wave, continuous wave and color Doppler.

Pulsed wave Doppler ultrasound
Low velocities can be sampled in discrete positions around the heart using pulsed-wave Doppler ultrasound. A small sampling gate is superimposed on the imaging screen. The receiver only listens for its transmitted pulse when it expects the sound waves to have returned (according to the speed of sound and the distance away).

High velocities cannot be measured reliably with pulsed wave Doppler due to a problem relating to the sampling frequency needing to be at least half the wavelength of the frequency shift (the Nyquist limit). Instead, high velocities are measured with continuous wave Doppler ultrasound.

Continuous wave Doppler ultrasound
This form of Doppler ultrasound continuously sends and receives its signals. It is not subject to the Nyquist limit and can measure very high velocities accurately. However, since it receives signals back from all along its course, and not at one particular depth, care has to be taken not to be confused by high velocities coming from a valve or vessel further away or closer than that being imaged. An example of a high velocity is shown in Figure 21.11.

Colour Doppler ultrasound
This is created by the computerized ultrasound machine placing hundreds of pulsed wave Doppler sample gates all over the cardiac chamber, and color coding the speed and direction at that point. For example, red and yellow are slow and fast towards the probe respectively, and blue and green are slow and fast away from the probe. Areas of turbulence and high velocity are shown by a mosaic of mixed colors. This technique is especially useful in detecting ventricular septal defects, valvar or arterial stenosis, and regurgitation (Fig. 21.11).

Determination of pressure gradient
The simplified Bernoulli equation can be used to estimate pressure drop across a stenosis, across a shunt lesion such as a ventricular septal defect, or across a regurgitant valve. The peak velocity is measured with continuous wave Doppler:

$$P_1 - P_2 = 4V^2$$

$P_1 - P_2$ is the pressure drop across the obstruction (mm Hg) and V is the peak velocity (m/s). It is imperative that the Doppler beam is aligned with flow, to avoid underestimation of the peak velocity.

Valvar stenosis
This technique means that cardiac catheterization is no longer needed to determine pressure gradients across valves. However, the Doppler gradient is consistently higher than that measured at catheterization. This is because the Doppler gradient is the maximal instantaneous pressure gradient (the largest difference before and after the stenosis at any time in the cardiac cycle), whereas catheter gradients are expressed as the peak to peak gradient (the difference between the highest pressure before and the highest pressure after the stenosis).

Pulmonary arterial (PA) pressure
Pulmonary arterial pressure can be estimated by determining the pressure drop between the right ventricle (RV) and the right atrium (RA) by measuring peak velocity of tricuspid regurgitation (TR). Thus:

$$\text{RV systolic pressure} = 4 \times \text{TR jet velocity}^2 + \text{RA pressure}$$

Right ventricular systolic pressure approximates to pulmonary arterial systolic pressure (if the pulmonary valve is not stenotic), and right atrial pressure varies little and can in most circumstances be assumed to be 5 or 10 mmHg. The technique is remarkably accurate at all ages and is valuable because of the high incidence of trivial or mild tricuspid regurgitation in the normal population and in many congenital heart diseases. Pulmonary artery pressure can also be estimated by measuring the peak velocity across a ventricular septal defect or arterial duct.

Determination of cardiac output
It is possible to determine left and right ventricular output reasonably reliably in the absence of turbulence in either outflow tract. Cardiac output is equal to stroke volume × heart rate. Left ventricular stroke volume (LVO) is determined by multiplying the flow velocity integral at the aortic valve (measured with Doppler) and the cross-sectional area of the aortic valve (AoCSA) (determined from the valve diameter measured with cross-sectional echocardiography). The flow velocity integral is the area under the velocity curve, and is often known as the 'stroke distance'

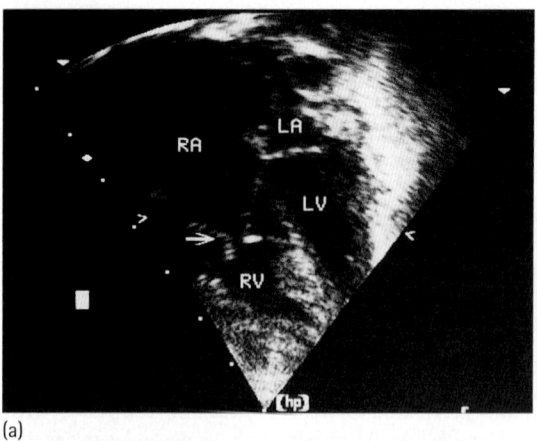

(a)

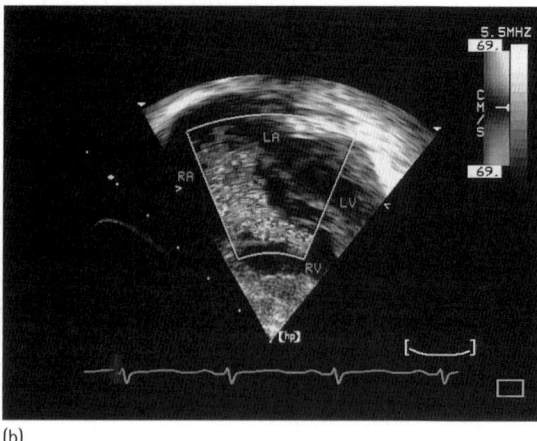

(b)

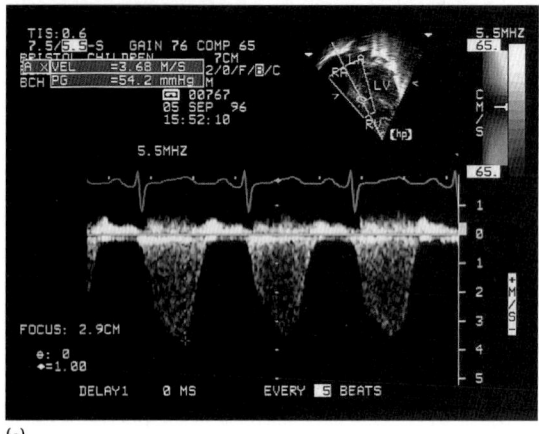

(c)

Fig. 21.11 This example of severe tricuspid regurgitation in a newborn infant demonstrates how several features of echocardiography can be put together in assessing a lesion. (a) The cross-sectional image shows that the tips of the tricuspid valve leaflets do not touch ('coapt') in systole, leaving a large hole for regurgitation. The right atrium (RA) is very dilated. (b) The color Doppler jet (reproduced here in black and white) shows that the regurgitant jet is wide – the width of the jet helps differentiate grades of severity. (c) The velocity of the jet (3.68 m/s) is high. When the simplified Bernoulli equation $(P = 4V^2)$ is applied to this velocity, the systolic RV–RA pressure drop is 54.2 mmHg. To obtain systolic pulmonary arterial pressure a RA estimate of 10 mmHg is added to the RV–RA pressure drop, so that PA systolic pressure is approximately 64 mmHg. There was significant pulmonary arterial hypertension – near to the aortic pressure in this infant of 80 mmHg at the time. As the pulmonary hypertension resolved the regurgitant jet velocity decreased; it was 2.4 m/s the next day, though the degree of regurgitation remained severe. (From Skinner et al 2000[23].)

(AoSD), since it represents the distance the column of blood ascends the aorta in systole.

$$\text{LV stroke volume(cc)} = \text{AoSD(cm)} \times \text{AoCSA(cm}^2)$$

$$\text{LV cardiac output(cc/min)} = \text{Ao SD(cm)} \times \text{AoCSA(cm}^2) \times \text{heart rate}$$

It is usual to represent ventricular output indexed to body surface area (litres/min/m²). The technique is of research interest, especially in intensive care, but is not widely used due to concerns of repeatability error in measurements.

Assessment of valvar regurgitation

Color Doppler is of immense value in identifying valve regurgitation, but the assessment is not precisely quantifiable. Other semiquantitative measurements are added to a visual assessment of the color jet. The more severe the regurgitation, the wider the color jet at the valve. The method is more sensitive than auscultation. Trivial valvar regurgitation is a normal finding in all except the aortic valve. Severe atrioventricular valve regurgitation is associated with dilatation of the respective atrium, and reverse flow in the caval or pulmonary veins. Severe aortic or pulmonary valve regurgitation leads to dilatation of the corresponding ventricle, and reverse flow in the distal pulmonary arteries or descending aorta, respectively.

Assessment of ventricular function

Right ventricle. Visual assessment of ventricular function from cross-sectional images (normal, hyperdynamic, mild, moderate or severe depression) is still the best method of evaluating right ventricular function. This is because the complex shape of the right ventricle makes it difficult to obtain repeatable measurements and accurate mathematical algorithms.

Left ventricle. The left ventricle is more amenable to mathematical algorithms to determine ejection fraction. However, the single most useful

and repeatable technique avoids such complex formulae and employs M-mode echocardiography to measure the *fractional shortening* (FS) or percentage reduction of the left ventricular diameter in systole. Thus:

$$\text{FS}(\%) = \frac{\text{LV diastolic dimension} - \text{LV systolic dimension}}{\text{LV diastolic dimension}} \times 100$$

The normal value lies between 28% and 44% and is reduced with poor myocardial function and increased with volume overload, such as with a left to right shunt through a ventricular septal defect or arterial duct. The measurements are made just beyond the tips of the mitral valve, from the parasternal position, and accurate measurements of septal and posterior wall thickness can be made in assessing ventricular hypertrophy (Fig. 21.12).

CARDIAC CATHETERIZATION

Diagnostic cardiac catheterization and angiocardiography are undertaken to obtain detailed information on the anatomical abnormality and its hemodynamic effects. The indications for diagnostic catheterization have changed with the widespread availability of high resolution echocardiography. With hemodynamic information from spectral Doppler studies and color Doppler mapping to assist in shunt detection, most congenital heart disease can be diagnosed and managed using echocardiography alone.[26] Cardiac catheterization is necessary to obtain accurate assessment of pulmonary vascular disease and for accurate shunt calculations.[27] Angiography is useful for coronary and distal pulmonary artery imaging and clarification of more complex arterial or venous abnormalities. However, computerized tomography and magnetic resonance imaging provide excellent images of vascular structures.

Cardiac catheterization is usually performed under general anesthesia, although occasionally procedures in infants and adolescents may be

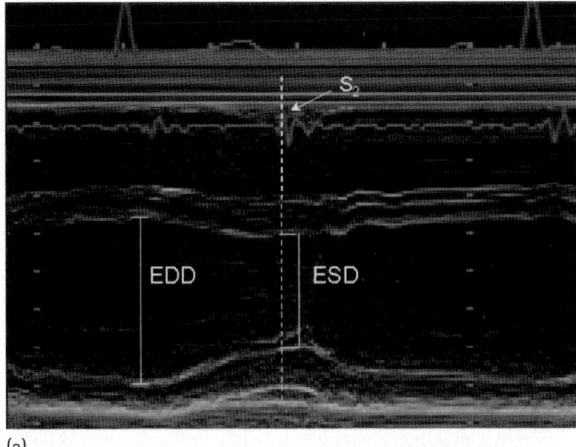

(a)

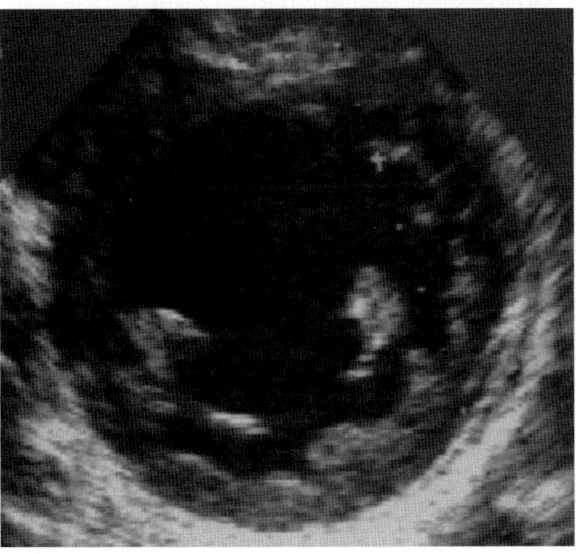

(b)

Fig. 21.12 The M-mode images across the short axis of the left ventricle (a) with the cross-sectional image (b) showing the position from which the M-mode image is derived. Fractional shortening is calculated as end diastolic diameter (EDD) − end systolic diameter (ESD) divided by end diastolic diameter × 100.

undertaken with local anesthesia and sedation. The approach is generally percutaneous through the femoral vessels, although the brachial, axillary or internal jugular routes are occasionally used. Arterial catheterization may be avoided if the venous catheter can be passed into the left side of the heart through an atrial or ventricular septal defect. An atrial septostomy can be performed through the umbilical vein in the first few days of life.

Calculating the left to right shunt

The oxygen saturation is measured in the large veins, atria, ventricles and great arteries. A significant left to right shunt is suggested by a rise in oxygen saturation of 5% or more in the right atrium (atrial septal defect), right ventricle (ventricular septal defect) or pulmonary artery (persistent arterial duct). Systemic and pulmonary output can be calculated from the Fick principle[27] and the pulmonary to systemic flow ratio (Qp:Qs) is calculated from the oxygen saturation values in the aorta (Ao), pulmonary artery (PA), pulmonary vein (PV) and the mixed venous saturation (MV) from the formula:

$$Qp:Qs = \frac{Ao-MV}{PV-PA}$$

While these figures give results sufficiently accurate for clinical management, they are not absolute values and will vary with time and hemodynamic status. A shunt ratio of more than 1.8:1 is likely to require intervention, whereas one of less than 1.5:1 is insignificant.

Pressure gradients

Pressures are measured in the atria, ventricles, great arteries and occasionally veins. Peak pressures in the ventricles and arteries measure transvalvar or arterial gradients. In children, the gradient rather than valve area is generally used in deciding on the need for intervention. Pressure gradients show considerable variation with time or sedation. Consideration must be given to whether the need for intervention should be based on a Doppler measurement with the patient awake, rather than a lower one obtained at catheterization with the child sedated or anesthetized.

Pulmonary vascular resistance

The mean pressure in the atria and great arteries is required for estimation of pulmonary and systemic vascular resistance, which is indexed for body surface area.[27] The pulmonary vascular resistance, rather than the pulmonary artery pressure, is the main determinant of the prognosis and the operability of a child with a left to right shunt. When it is elevated, it is appropriate to assess whether it is fixed or can be reduced by the administration of a pulmonary vasodilator such as 100% oxygen or nitric oxide[27] at the time of the catheter procedure.

Angiography

This is performed by the injection of radiological contrast into the chamber or vessel immediately proximal to the abnormality, e.g. left ventricle for ventricular septal defect, right ventricle for pulmonary stenosis, and ascending aorta for coarctation. Angiography is now less important for the definition of cardiac and vascular abnormalities as echocardiography, computerized axial tomography and magnetic resonance imaging provide similar information less invasively.

Complications

Although cardiac catheterization is a relatively safe procedure, death can occur, most commonly in patients with severe pulmonary hypertension. Complications include femoral artery occlusion, hemorrhage (from cardiac structures or traversed vessels), arrhythmias, cardiac or vessel damage, and cerebral embolism.

INTERVENTIONAL CARDIAC CATHETERIZATION

More than half of all pediatric cardiac catheterization is now related to interventional procedures and is a crucial part of the management of heart disease in children. Balloon atrial septostomy (Fig. 21.13) was the first pediatric interventional catheter procedure and it remains life saving for infants with inadequate intracardiac mixing, as in transposition of the great arteries. It can be performed using ultrasound or radiographic imaging.[28]

Opening procedures

Balloon Valvuloplasty (Fig. 21.14) is now the accepted treatment for pulmonary valve stenosis.[29] It is safe and effective (unless there is severe valve dysplasia) and seldom requires reintervention.[30,31] It can be performed in the neonatal period.[32] Aortic balloon valvuloplasty is an alternative to surgery for aortic stenosis[33] unless there is additional significant regurgitation. The results are comparable[34-36] but both are palliative, and progression of aortic stenosis always occurs.

Balloon dilatation, with or without stenting, is used for a wide variety of arterial and venous narrowing.[28] Balloon dilatation is the treatment of choice for residual or recurrent coarctation following surgery.[37,38] However, there is a higher risk of aneurysm and residual hypertension in young children who have not had previous surgery.[39] Balloon dilatation does not appear to be effective in the treatment of

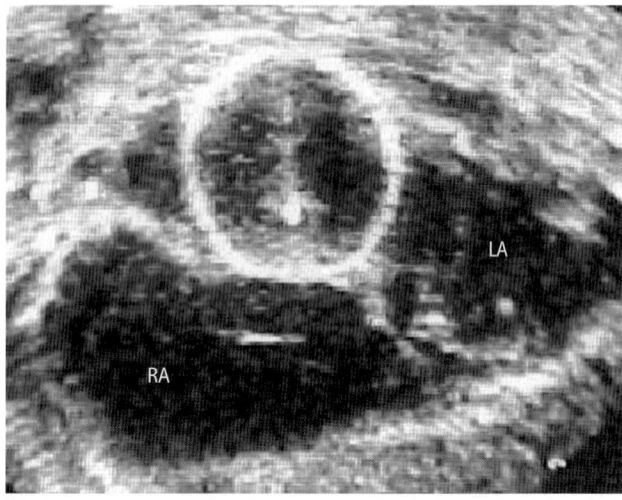

(a)

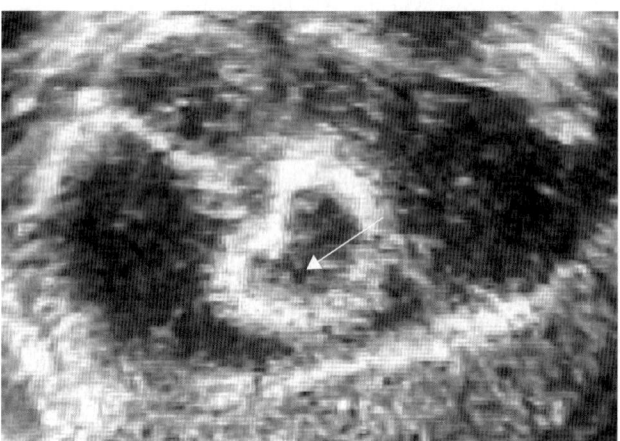

(b)

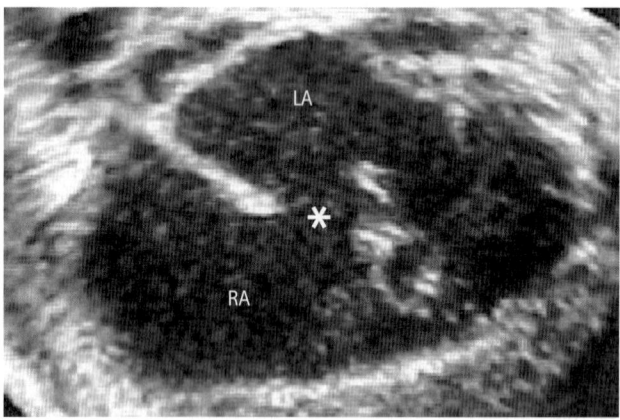

(c)

Fig. 21.13   Balloon atrial septostomy using echocardiographic imaging. (a) A balloon septostomy catheter is advanced from the umbilical or femoral vein into the right atrium and across into the left atrium. (b) The balloon is inflated in the left atrium and pulled across the atrial septum. (c) The atrial septal defect created is identified with the asterisk. LA, left atrium; RA, right atrium.

neonatal coarctation.[40] Balloon dilatation is also used to improve narrowing of pulmonary arteries.[41] In smaller children, balloon dilatation alone is usually performed, but in older children and adolescents, stent placement, although technically challenging, may provide more effective and longer lasting relief of stenoses. Balloon expandable metallic stents are used for treatment of both recurrent and native

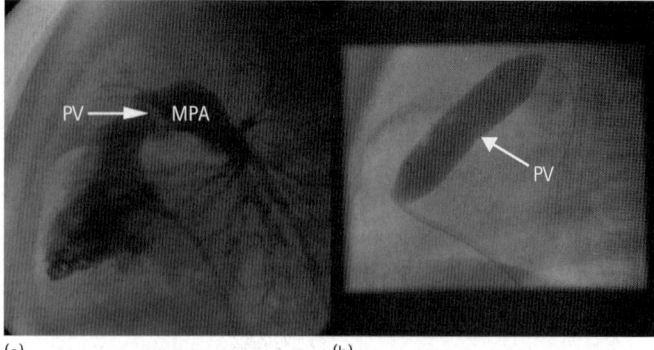

(a)   (b)

Fig. 21.14   (a) Right ventricular (RV) angiogram of a child with pulmonary valve stenosis showing a thickened pulmonary valve (PV) and post-stenotic dilatation of the main pulmonary artery (MPA). (b) The balloon catheter is inflated across the valve resulting in relief of the stenosis.

coarctation in an attempt to produce more 'permanent' results and reduce the risk of aortic rupture or aneurysm formation. Similar stents have also been used to improve narrowing in pulmonary arteries. There are concerns regarding the use of stents in young children, because growth will not occur.[40]

Radiofrequency energy can be applied to intravascular tissues, using specially designed catheters, to perforate occluded valves or vessels to allow subsequent balloon dilatation. This is most commonly performed for relief of valvar pulmonary atresia.[42]

Closing procedures

Closure of the persistent arterial duct with a coil or device is now the procedure of choice for children over a year of age.[28,43,44] Closure of more than 50% of atrial septal defects[45] is possible with one of a variety of devices, and results are comparable with surgery.[46–48] The surgical approach is still required for some anatomical variants and large defects. Although the vast majority of hemodynamically significant ventricular septal defects still require surgical closure, transcatheter devices are available for defects that are difficult to close surgically.[28,43,49] A wide variety of devices are used to occlude venous collaterals, residual surgical shunts, coronary artery and arteriovenous fistulae. Transcatheter replacement of pulmonic and aortic valves has been achieved in selected patients.[50]

OTHER CARDIAC INVESTIGATIONS

MAGNETIC RESONANCE IMAGING (MRI)

Improvements in imaging quality and acquisition times have resulted in its increased use for the imaging and assessment of congenital heart disease, particularly in complex cases.[51] It provides three-dimensional, dynamic images of cardiac structures and is particular suitable for visualizing the aortic arch (Fig. 21.15), peripheral pulmonary vasculature, and in the assessment of ventricular volumes. All images must be gated to the cardiac cycle and performed during 'breath holding' to minimize respiratory artifact. To obtain optimal image quality, the child must either be old enough to cooperate fully with the examination or ventilated under general anesthesia.[51] Children with pacemakers and some intravascular devices cannot undergo magnetic resonance imaging.

COMPUTERIZED AXIAL TOMOGRAPHY (CT)

CT scan with injection of contrast provides excellent imaging of cardiac and vascular structures. The anesthetic time is shorter than for MRI, but this must be balanced against the radiation dose for CT.

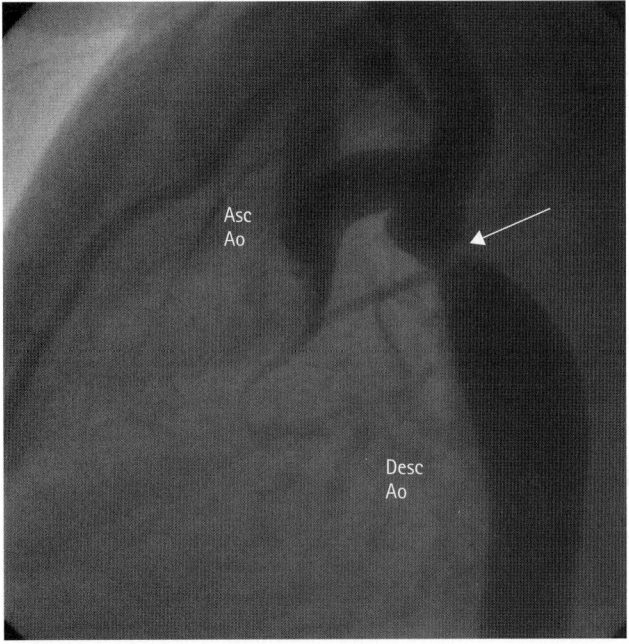

(a)

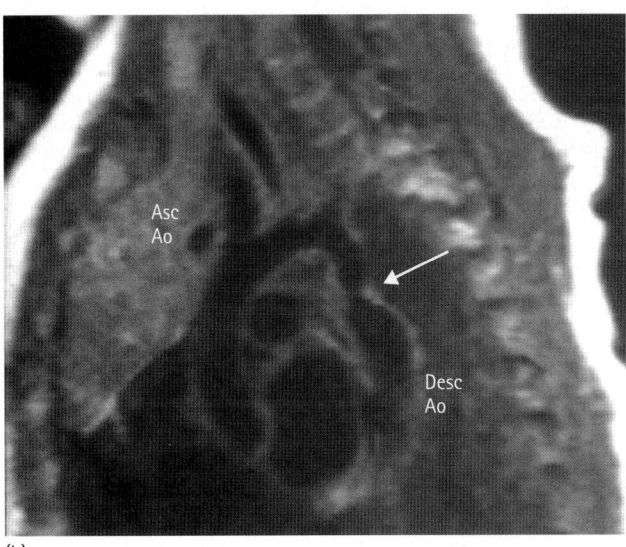

(b)

Fig. 21.15 Lateral projection of an aortogram (a) and magnetic resonance image (b) of coarctation of the aorta. The arrow indicates the coarctation. Asc Ao, ascending aorta; Desc Ao, descending aorta.

RADIONUCLIDE ANGIOGRAPHY

Radionuclide scanning is less frequently performed in children than in adults. However, there are occasions when it may be required (e.g. following Kawasaki coronary arteritis) and it is performed in the same way as in adults. Lung perfusion scanning can assess pulmonary blood flow in children with complex pulmonary vascular abnormalities.

AMBULATORY ELECTROCARDIOGRAPHIC MONITORING

Continuous ambulatory 24 hour electrocardiographic (Holter) monitoring assists in the evaluation of transient events, bradycardia, certain incessant or paroxysmal tachycardias and those associated with symptoms such as syncope. The electrocardiogram is usually recorded continuously for 24–72 hours and provides a printout of any irregularity. Two channel recordings are better than one, and an event marker can be used to correlate symptoms with electrocardiographic events. This technique has clarified the variations in heart rate and rhythm that occur in normal children. The heart rate varies from 45 to 180/min, and may be as low as 30 beats/min during sleep.

Many rhythm disturbances occur infrequently, and the chance of detection from a single 24 hour electrocardiographic recording will be small. An event recorder is activated by the child or parent when the symptom occurs. There are many different types, but most record a short strip in solid state memory. The record is printed and analyzed by transmitting it by telephone or returning it to the cardiac center. Another method of detecting infrequent but potentially serious arrhythmias is with an event or loop recorder implanted under the skin in the left upper chest.[52] This can be programmed to record significant pauses, bradycardia and tachycardia.

ELECTROPHYSIOLOGICAL STUDIES

Arrhythmias may be further evaluated by intracardiac electrophysiological studies in which several electrode catheters are passed transvenously to the right side of the heart and intracardiac potentials are recorded from multiple sites, including the bundle of His. Simultaneous recordings of surface and intracardiac electrocardiograms help to determine more precisely the exact site of origin, delay, and direction of impulse conduction in complex arrhythmias. These techniques have their greatest value in defining the exact mechanism of tachycardia and may result in more appropriate therapy, particularly in children who have drug resistant tachyarrhythmias and who may be candidates for radiofrequency catheter ablation therapy of their arrhythmias.

EXERCISE TESTING

Exercise testing is increasingly used in pediatric cardiac practice. The techniques are similar to those used in adults, although end points and levels of exercise achieved must be adjusted for age. Documentation of peak heart rate, level of exercise achieved and electrocardiographic changes can influence the timing of intervention or evaluate the efficacy of a procedure on effort tolerance. In cyanosed children, saturation monitoring during exercise provides additional information in these situations. Exercise testing can identify and evaluate exercise-related arrhythmias, clarify symptoms in more complex situations and is helpful in long QT syndrome. Measurement of blood pressure response to exercise is important in children following repair of coarctation. Even quite small children can exercise on either the treadmill or a bicycle ergometer, but exercise telemetry or Holter monitoring can also provide useful information.

HEAD-UP TILT TESTING

Syncope is a common problem in childhood, occurring in one in five adolescents.[52,53] Most have 'neurally mediated' syncope related to a disturbance of autonomic control of blood pressure and heart rate. This can sometimes usefully be differentiated from other causes of syncope by head-up tilt testing. Various protocols all involve head-up tilting on a table with foot support to an angle of 60°, for up to 45 minutes after an initial horizontal stabilization period. Continuous electrocardiogram and blood pressure monitoring (usually non-invasive) is performed. A positive response usually consists of hypotension and bradycardia before syncope. This provides an explanation for a child's symptoms and paves the way for more successful management.[52]

THE ASYMPTOMATIC CHILD WITH A MURMUR

The incidental finding of a murmur in an asymptomatic child is common. The clinician must decide whether the murmur is innocent, or if further investigation is required. If the murmur is pathological, the child will need regular follow-up, antibiotic prophylaxis for dental and other surgical procedures, and possibly specialized treatment. A careful history is essential, but children with an innocent murmur may have unrelated symptoms. Innocent murmurs can be diagnosed accurately by their distinctive features. A thorough examination identifies clinical features that are likely to be associated with heart disease. It is much more common to diagnose an innocent murmur as pathological than to call a cardiac lesion innocent.[20]

INNOCENT MURMURS

Innocent murmurs are the most common murmurs in pediatric practice. They occur in the majority of children, usually between 6 weeks and 7 years of age, but they can occur throughout childhood and adolescence.[54] There is a variety of innocent murmurs. A small number of children have more than one, for example a vibratory systolic murmur and venous hum.

Vibratory (Still's) murmur

This accounts for the majority of innocent murmurs.[54] It is characterized by a short vibratory ejection systolic murmur, maximal at the lower left sternal edge and radiating towards the base. It changes in intensity on sitting, and on extending the neck. The exact cause is unknown, but is likely to be due to vibration of structures within the ventricles. The differential diagnosis includes small muscular ventricular septal defect and mitral valve prolapse. If the site of maximal intensity is not accurately defined, it may be confused with mild pulmonary or aortic stenosis or an atrial septal defect.

Pulmonary and aortic flow murmurs

These are soft ejection systolic murmurs maximal in the pulmonary or aortic areas, produced by increased flow across the outlet valves. The common causes are pyrexia, anemia and pregnancy. Review after the fever has subsided prevents referral of a child who no longer has a murmur. The differential diagnosis includes mild aortic or pulmonary stenosis or an atrial septal defect.

Venous hum

This is a continuous murmur maximal in the lower part of the neck and subclavicular area, usually on the right. It is due to turbulence in large veins. It is loudest on sitting up and disappears on lying down, turning or lightly compressing the jugular vein in the neck. The differential diagnosis is a persistent arterial duct or arteriovenous fistula.

Features associated with heart disease in the asymptomatic child

A number of specific clinical features are associated with heart disease.[55] These include a murmur that is:
- pansystolic;
- grade 3 or more in intensity;
- harsh in quality;
- maximal at the left upper sternal border.

The presence of an abnormal second heart sound or a click is also an indication that the murmur is not innocent. Outside the neonatal period, a murmur heard in the back is usually pathological, and diastolic murmurs are always abnormal. Palpation of the femoral pulses is essential. Other clinical features that are more likely to indicate a cardiac lesion are feeding difficulties or failure to thrive in infants, dysmorphic features and noncardiac lesions.

Investigation and management

A complete examination with careful auscultation by a trained clinician is the most useful method of diagnosing an innocent murmur. Chest radiography is likely to be misleading, invasive and unhelpful.[20] An electrocardiogram may be useful in alerting the clinician to the possibility of an atrial septal defect, but may also be misleading. If the murmur is innocent, firm reassurance should be given and the child discharged. Parents should be told that the murmur might be heard intermittently for many years. They should also be reassured that the heart is normal.

If the murmur is not typical of an innocent murmur, or if other features suggest a cardiac lesion, the child should be referred to a pediatric cardiologist. Echocardiographic examination without assessment by a cardiologist or pediatrician competent in echocardiography is not appropriate, as it can be misleading.[1] When a child is referred to a pediatric cardiologist, there is often an expectation that an echocardiogram will be carried out. Although it has been shown that this is usually unnecessary,[54] it may be done to allay fears and prevent further reviews.

HEART FAILURE

Heart failure occurs when the heart:
- Fails to supply sufficient blood for the body's needs.
- Does not allow adequate pulmonary or systemic venous return.

This results in physiological compensatory mechanisms. These include salt and water retention by the kidneys to increase preload, vasoconstriction through the renin–angiotensin axis to increase afterload, and increased catecholamines to improve cardiac output. If the underlying insult continues, these mechanisms overcompensate and heart failure develops. It is most frequently associated with congenital heart disease, usually occurring in the first few months of life. Closure of the arterial duct or fall in pulmonary vascular resistance causes increased pulmonary blood flow, which explains the timing of presentation. Other causes include valvar or myocardial disease, or persistent tachy- or bradyarrhythmia. Noncardiac causes include shock, profound anemia and a large arteriovenous malformation.

CLINICAL FEATURES

The commonest signs are tachycardia, tachypnea and hepatomegaly, the liver size providing an indication of severity. The child appears restless, fretful and pale. Peripheral perfusion may be poor with a capillary refill time of greater than 3 seconds. Measurement of four-limb blood pressure is essential.

In infants combined ventricular failure occurs, with pulmonary and systemic venous congestion. Respiratory symptoms are more marked on feeding. The association of stiff lung parenchyma with soft, flexible ribs causes chest deformity with a deep anteroposterior diameter and flaring of the lower part of the rib cage. This combination produces the 'Harrison's sulcus', the trough created just above the lower ribs anteriorly. There may also be intercostal or subcostal recession during inspiration. With marked respiratory distress there is an audible grunt and flaring of the ala nasi. Pulmonary edema must be differentiated from respiratory infection. Crepitations are not often heard in the chest and marked edema is rare, although some facial puffiness or pitting of the dorsal surfaces of the hands or feet may develop. Pedal edema in newborns is usually lymphedema associated with Turner or Noonan syndrome. Sweating occurs at rest, during feeding or on exertion, and hepatomegaly is common. Chronic heart failure causes feeding difficulties. Initially, weight gain may result from fluid retention, but failure to thrive is seen later. Specific auscultatory signs of the cardiac abnormality causing failure may be detected. Sometimes a gallop rhythm is audible.

In older children, heart failure is relatively uncommon. It usually results from acquired heart disease or arrhythmia and exhibits the clinical features of left or right heart failure as in the adult. These include effort intolerance, dyspnea, cough, ankle edema and abdominal pain.

INVESTIGATIONS

Investigations should be directed at accurately determining the cause, as this is essential for treatment. Electrocardiographic changes may reflect the underlying diagnosis. Sinus tachycardia must be differentiated from an arrhythmia. Chest radiography shows cardiomegaly and prominent vascular markings, due to increased flow or venous obstruction. Echocardiography provides information regarding the cardiac lesion and allows assessment of left ventricular function (Fig. 21.12). If there is a primary myocardial problem, this should be investigated (p. 802).

MANAGEMENT

The primary aim is correction or improvement of the underlying cardiac or noncardiac condition. Supportive therapy is directed at improving myocardial function, reducing preload and afterload, and controlling heart rate. There are no evidence-based guidelines for the management of heart failure in children.[56] Treatment is extrapolated from adult data, despite the difference in causes.

Diuretics remain the initial treatment, most commonly the loop diuretics furosemide or a thiazide. Concomitant use of spironolactone has been shown to be beneficial both for its potassium sparing effect, and the aldosterone receptor blocking action.

Angiotensin converting enzyme (ACE) inhibitors (captopril or enalapril) are widely used[56] and are usually introduced if diuretics are insufficient to control heart failure. They decrease the formation of angiotensin II, resulting in vasodilatation. This reduces left ventricular afterload and facilitates left ventricular function. They have been shown to improve survival in adults. In ventricular septal defect, they reduce the left to right shunt by reducing the systemic, and thus left ventricular pressure. The initial dose should be small and gradually increased to the maintenance dose over a period of time. Observation is required for possible hypotension immediately after the initial dose and each increment. Renal function must be monitored and caution exercised in the presence of renal impairment. Serum potassium must be closely monitored if ACE inhibitors are used with spironolactone because of hyperkalemia. Left sided obstructive lesions such as mitral or aortic stenosis, and coarctation are contraindications to ACE inhibitors. Angiotensin II receptor blockers may be used if side-effects from ACE inhibitors are troublesome.

Beta-blockers are standard therapy for adults with heart failure, where they are used in the management of left ventricular dysfunction and appear to slow left ventricular dilatation and reduce mortality. This suggests that they may be of value in children. They should only be used after stabilization of acute heart failure. The dose must be increased gradually.

Digoxin is occasionally used for its positive inotropic effect, but it also reduces vascular tone. It can be of benefit where there is poor ventricular function but there is no evidence that it improves mortality. It is of doubtful value in situations with volume overload, such as a ventricular septal defect.[57] Serum levels are used to check compliance, or when toxicity is suspected.

Anticoagulants are necessary when severe heart failure could cause thrombus formation in the left ventricle.

Other supportive treatment may include the use of oxygen. Nutrition must be optimized. Anemia should be treated, but caution blood transfusion should only be considered for severe anemia.

Response to treatment

The child should be monitored carefully for response to therapy and side-effects of the drugs used. Daily examination, including weight, respiratory rate and liver size, will assess improvement or deterioration in heart failure. Regular electrolyte, urea and creatinine measurements will detect imbalance, or deteriorating renal function. Echocardiography is used to monitor changes in left ventricular function.

In an intensive care setting

Inotropic agents such as dopamine and dobutamine improve cardiac function and urine output. Afterload can be reduced with vasodilators such as nitroprusside. Phosphodiesterase inhibitors (e.g. milrinone) have potent vasodilator and inotropic effects but have not been shown to improve outcomes. Noradrenaline increases systemic vascular resistance, which is beneficial in the management of septic shock. Mechanical ventricular assist devices may be used to temporarily support ventricular function or as a bridge to transplant.[58]

If intervention is not an option, the child should be assessed for cardiac transplantation when heart failure no longer responds to medication. The 5 year survival following heart transplant is approximately 67%.[59]

INFECTIVE ENDOCARDITIS

Infective endocarditis is rare with an incidence of approximately 0.3 per 100 000 person-years.[60] It is usually superimposed on congenital or rheumatic heart disease, particularly lesions with a high velocity turbulent jet of blood, or cardiovascular prosthetic material. A child with a normal heart can be affected. Mortality remains high, with a late risk of death or significant complications because of valve damage. Primary prevention is therefore important. The Task Force on Infective Endocarditis of the European Society of Cardiology[60] has produced comprehensive guidelines for the prevention, diagnosis and treatment of infective endocarditis.

PROPHYLAXIS AGAINST INFECTIVE ENDOCARDITIS

Antibiotic prophylaxis is advised in children at risk. This is because of the severe cardiac damage and associated mortality that can result from infection within the heart and great vessels. The precise risk of endocarditis is impossible to measure, but cardiac conditions have been grouped into high, moderate and low risk. Children at low risk do not require prophylaxis. This includes those with closed ventricular septal defects and arterial ducts, mitral valve prolapse without regurgitation or valve thickening and 12 months after transcatheter closure of an atrial septal defect or patent foramen ovale. More controversially, prophylaxis is also not recommended for children with a secundum atrial septal defect, isolated pulmonary stenosis, Ebstein's abnormality of the tricuspid valve and following the Fontan or Mustard operations.[60] Most children with congenital and those with rheumatic heart disease or hypertrophic cardiomyopathy fall into the moderate category risk.[60] Antibiotic prophylaxis regimens are shown in Table 21.6.[60,61] Children at high risk include those who have previously had endocarditis and those with prosthetic heart valves, surgically created conduits, intravascular prosthetic material and complex cyanotic congenital cardiac anomalies. These children usually require intravenous antibiotics (Table 21.6).

Indications for prophylaxis are extensive,[60] but endocarditis is such a serious condition that little risk should be taken. Surgical and dental procedures cause transient bacteremia. Poor dental hygiene and inflamed gums predispose to endocarditis. Antibiotics should be given before bacteremia is expected, to reduce the ability of the organism to adhere and multiply (Table 21.6). If given later, antibiotics should be administered intravenously. The probability of bacteremia is highest for dental and other oral procedures, intermediate for procedures of the genitourinary system and lowest for gastrointestinal procedures. It is also likely to be greater for therapeutic than diagnostic interventions. There are a number of procedures that are not regarded as high risk, but bacteremia and/or endocarditis have been reported. These include body piercing and tattooing.[62]

CLINICAL FEATURES OF INFECTIVE ENDOCARDITIS

Early diagnosis depends on a *high index of suspicion* in any child with heart disease and unexplained fever, even when there are no other features of endocarditis. The clinical features and course of the illness vary depending upon the infecting organism and the stage of the illness. Most children present with nonspecific manifestations such as malaise, anorexia, weight loss, arthralgia and backache. A regurgitant murmur may appear or change in character. Splenomegaly may be found and petechiae occur, particularly on the oral mucosa, eyelids or optic fundi (Roth spot). Clubbing or splinter hemorrhages of the nail bed can occur. Osler's nodes are red, indurated, tender lesions on the pulps of fingers and toes and occasionally the palm. These skin lesions, arthralgia and hematuria are immune complex phenomena and not due to emboli. Embolic phenomena have become less common since the introduction of antimicrobial therapy, but occur particularly with staphylococcal or fungal endocarditis. Janeway lesions are thought to be due to septic embolization

Table 21.6   Antibiotic prophylaxis against infective endocarditis (British National Formulary for Children 2006)

Dental, oral or upper respiratory tract procedures

Under local anesthesia (child not allergic to penicillin)

Child under 5 years	oral amoxicillin 750 mg taken under supervision 1 h before procedure
Child 5–10 years	oral amoxicillin 1.5 g taken under supervision 1 h before procedure
Child 10–18 years	oral amoxicillin 3 g taken under supervision 1 h before procedure

Under local anesthesia (child allergic to penicillin)

Child under 5 years	oral clindamycin 150 mg or azithromycin 200 mg taken under supervision 1 h before procedure
Child 5–10 years	oral clindamycin 300 mg or azithromycin 300 mg taken under supervision 1 h before procedure
Child 10–18 years	oral clindamycin 600 mg or azithromycin 500 mg taken under supervision 1 h before procedure

Under general anesthesia (child not allergic to penicillin)

Child under 5 years	i.v. amoxicillin 250 mg intravenously at induction of anesthesia or just before procedure
Child 5–10 years	i.v. amoxicillin 500 mg intravenously at induction of anesthesia or just before procedure
Child 10–18 years	i.v. amoxicillin 1 g intravenously at induction of anesthesia or just before procedure

Under general anesthesia (child allergic to penicillin)

Child under 5 years	i.v. clindamycin 75 mg over at least 10 min at induction of anesthesia or just before procedure
Child 5–10 years	i.v. clindamycin 150 mg over at least 10 min at induction of anesthesia or just before procedure
Child 10–18 years	i.v. clindamycin 300 mg over at least 10 min at induction of anesthesia or just before procedure

Gastrointestinal or genitourinary procedures

Child not allergic to penicillin

Child under 5 years	i.v. amoxicillin 250 mg ± i.v. gentamicin* 1.5 mg/kg at induction of anesthesia or just before procedure
Child 5–10 years	i.v. amoxicillin 500 mg ± i.v. gentamicin* 1.5 mg/kg at induction of anesthesia or just before procedure
Child 10–18 years	i.v. amoxicillin 1 g ± i.v. gentamicin* 1.5 mg/kg at induction of anesthesia or just before procedure

Child allergic to penicillin

Child under 14 years	i.v. teicoplanin 6 mg/kg (max 400 mg) + i.v. gentamicin 1.5 mg/kg at induction of anesthesia or just before procedure
Child 14–18 years	i.v. teicoplanin 400 mg + i.v. gentamicin 1.5 mg/kg at induction of anesthesia or just before procedure
or	
Child under 14 years	i.v. vancomycin 20 mg/kg (max 1 g) over 1–2 h at induction of anesthesia or just before procedure
Child 14–18 years	i.v. vancomycin 1 g over 1–2 h at induction of anesthesia or just before procedure

Child at high risk (previous endocarditis, prosthetic valve, intravascular prosthetic material, complex cyanotic heart disease)

Child not allergic to penicillin

Child under 5 years	i.v. amoxicillin 250 mg + i.v. gentamicin 1.5 mg/kg at induction of anesthesia or just before procedure then 125 mg orally 6 h later
Child 5–10 years	i.v. amoxicillin 500 mg + i.v. gentamicin 1.5 mg/kg at induction of anesthesia or just before procedure then 250 mg orally 6 h later
Child 10–18 years	i.v. amoxicillin 1 g + i.v. gentamicin 1.5 mg/kg at induction of anesthesia or just before procedure then 500 mg orally 6 h later

Child allergic to penicillin

Child under 14 years	i.v. vancomycin 20 mg/kg (max 1 g) over 1–2 h + i.v. gentamicin 1.5 mg/kg at induction of anesthesia or just before procedure
Child 14–18 years	i.v. vancomycin 1 g over 1–2 h + i.v. gentamicin 1.5 mg/kg at induction of anesthesia or just before procedure

*Recommended by British National Formulary for Children[61] but not by The Task Force on Infective Endocarditis of the European Society of Cardiology.[60]

and are transient, non-tender, macular lesions of the palms or soles of the feet. Chest symptoms are common in right heart endocarditis. Heart failure may develop as a result of valve damage. Acute fulminant infection is seen with *Staphylococcus aureus* infections and in young children with overwhelming septicemia.

DIAGNOSIS OF INFECTIVE ENDOCARDITIS

Anemia and leukocytosis are usually present and the erythrocyte sedimentation rate and C-reactive protein are invariably elevated. Microscopic hematuria is common. It is important to identify the organism, so blood cultures must be taken *before* starting antibiotics. Three cultures should be performed over a 24 hour period and a further three after 24 hours, if the initial ones are still negative.[60] Bacteremia is a constant feature in infective endocarditis. This makes timing in relation to fever unimportant. Culture media should include those for aerobes, anaerobes and fungi. Repeated sterile blood cultures are strong evidence against infective endocarditis but do not preclude it since about 10% of cases are negative on culture. Recent antimicrobial treatment is the most common reason for this, and cultures

should be repeated once antibiotics have been discontinued for at least 3 days. Other causes of negative cultures include right-sided cardiac lesions, slow-growing microorganisms or infection with nonbacterial agents such as fungi, Coxiella, Chlamydia or Rickettsia. Arterial blood cultures are unreliable. Demonstration of bacterial DNA by broadspectrum polymerase chain reaction (PCR) aids diagnosis in culture negative endocarditis.

Echocardiography is essential for suspected endocarditis. Identification of a vegetation, peri-valve abscess or fistula, or prosthetic valve dehiscence is diagnostic. Transesophageal echocardiography is necessary if transthoracic views do not show evidence of endocarditis. The absence of echocardiographic findings does not rule out endocarditis.

BACTERIOLOGY OF INFECTIVE ENDOCARDITIS

Streptococcus viridans, Staphylococcus aureus and *coagulase-negative staphylococci* are the common bacteria isolated in children.[63] A wide variety of other organisms cause infection on rare occasions. In neonates, staphylococcal or fungal infections occur in association with central lines and the prognosis is poor.[64]

TREATMENT OF INFECTIVE ENDOCARDITIS

It is important to identify the causative organism before starting treatment. Unless there are signs of fulminant infection, antibiotics should be withheld until the organism is identified. Current guidelines for the treatment of endocarditis have been produced by the Task Force on Infective Endocarditis of the European Society of Cardiology[60] and will be updated as new drugs and further evidence become available. Bactericidal drugs are given intravenously by bolus injection in a dose sufficient to reach therapeutic blood levels and provide a satisfactory minimum inhibitory concentration. The choice of antimicrobials, dosage schedule and duration of therapy will depend on the organism and its sensitivity.[60] It is essential to involve the microbiologist from the beginning regarding choice and duration of treatment. Penicillin is fundamental to the antibiotic treatment of endocarditis, and hypersensitivity seriously compromises the range of antibiotics that can be used. Parents should be closely questioned about the nature of any suspected penicillin hypersensitivity reaction.

Active infective endocarditis is not necessarily a contraindication to cardiac surgery.[65] Valve replacement is indicated when valve damage causes moderate or severe heart failure or when recurrent emboli occur. Fungal or Coxiella infections respond poorly to medical therapy and surgery may be the only way to eradicate infection. When endocarditis occurs following cardiac surgery in a child with a cardiovascular prosthetic material, surgical removal of the foreign material is often necessary.

CONGENITAL HEART DISEASE

INCIDENCE

The incidence of congenital heart disease is approximately 8 per 1000 live births, with a higher rate in stillbirths.[66] Differences in frequencies between studies are due to the method of ascertainment and detection rates of less severe abnormalities. The use of high resolution echocardiography increases detection[67] but increased antenatal diagnosis and termination rates could reduce the incidence of severe lesions. There is no evidence of racial differences in the incidence of congenital cardiac defects, although there are some differences in the type of lesions. The incidence of recessively inherited lesions such as isomerism (heterotaxy) sequences is increased in consanguineous communities.[5] The relative frequency of the most common lesions varies with different reports, but nine common lesions form 80% of congenital heart disease. They can be divided into three hemodynamic groups (Table 21.7) and more than one lesion may coexist. The other 20% of congenital heart disease consists of many rare or complex lesions.[66,68]

The risk of death from congenital heart disease has decreased from 30% in the 1970s to less than 5%. The outlook remains dependent on the severity of the cardiac lesion and other abnormalities. Between 30 and 40% of early deaths are associated with extracardiac malformations. Prematurity and perinatal complications also contribute to outcome. Early deaths are uncommon in acyanotic lesions with the exception of

Table 21.7 Incidence of common congenital cardiac lesions (Jackson et al 1996[68])

	Condition	Incidence
Left to right shunt	Ventricular septal defect	36%
	Atrial septal defect	5%
	Patent arterial duct	9%
	Atrioventricular septal defect	4%
Obstructive lesions	Pulmonary stenosis	9%
	Aortic stenosis	5%
	Coarctation	5%
Cyanotic lesions	Transposition of the great arteries	4%
	Tetralogy of Fallot	4%

coarctation of the aorta and atrioventricular septal defect, and more common in cyanotic lesions, although the outlook is much improved. The majority of survivors enjoy good health but many require life-long expert follow-up and treatment. The incidence of congenital heart disease in adults is now 5 per 1000. As the number of survivors with more complex lesions grows,[69] the requirement for further catheter and surgical interventions, including transplantation, will increase.

ETIOLOGY

In most children, no specific cause is found. However, maternal, environmental and genetic defects can contribute.

Maternal and environmental factors
- Maternal diabetes and phenylketonuria increase the incidence of congenital heart disease. There is some evidence that control of the condition before, and in early pregnancy, decreases the risk.[70,71] Maternal obesity is also a risk factor, but this may be related to diabetes.[72] Maternal connective tissue disease such as systemic lupus erythematosus can result in congenital complete heart block.
- Maternal infection, notably rubella in early pregnancy, results in congenital heart disease.[73]
- Maternal drug ingestion. Fetal alcohol syndrome is a well-recognized association.[74] Lithium,[75] antiepileptics[76] and isotretinoin used for acne[77] are all associated with an increased risk.
- Maternal age is associated with an increased risk of trisomy.

Chromosomal and genetic abnormalities

Cardiac defects are associated with a wide range of chromosomal or genetic abnormalities, other syndromes and associations[78,79] (Table 21.8). Chromosomal abnormalities occur in 10–20% of infants with congenital heart disease. It is thus appropriate to perform chromosomal analysis on infants and children with congenital heart disease who have dysmorphic features, low birth weight, other malformations, developmental delay, failure to thrive or short stature, and those with a cardiac lesion likely to be associated with a chromosomal abnormality. It is also important to involve the clinical geneticist to confirm any syndrome or association. This provides useful information for management and recurrence risk within a family. Autosomal dominant inheritance occurs in a number of conditions that have associated cardiac abnormalities. However, many children with 22q11 deletion, Noonan syndrome and Williams syndrome have a new mutation, resulting in a low recurrence risk. Hypertrophic cardiomyopathy has an estimated prevalence of 1:500 persons.[80] Most patients have a positive family history but sporadic cases occasionally occur. Single gene defects are increasingly being identified and some are associated with heart disease.[80]

RECURRENCE RISK

The recurrence risk for a cardiac defect depends on the nature of the lesion and relationship of the affected person. The risk for another pregnancy rises to about 2% if one previous child is affected; this tends to be highest (3%) for ventricular septal defect, arterial duct and atrioventricular septal defect. There is a tendency for a related anomaly to recur but this is not necessarily the case. The severity of the cardiac lesion may also vary considerably between individuals in a family. If two previous children are affected the risk rises to 6–8% and there is a similar risk if the father has congenital heart disease. If the mother is affected the risk is 5–15%, depending on the lesion.[4]

When counseling parents, consideration must be given to known recurrence risks, maternal age and health, and exposure to possible teratogens, particularly medication. Fetal echocardiography provides an accurate means of diagnosing serious cardiac abnormalities from about 18 weeks' gestation[81] or earlier. In the majority there will be no defect and the family can be reassured. However, the implications for finding an abnormality are serious and should be discussed before the examination.

Table 21.8 Chromosome and genetic associations with congenital heart disease (Harris et al 2003[78], Manning et al 2005[79])

	Chromosome or genetic abnormality	Percentage with heart disease (%)	Common cardiovascular lesions
Chromosome disorders			
Down	Trisomy 21	40–50	AVSD, VSD, ASD, ToF
Edwards	Trisomy 18	90–100	VSD, ASD, PDA, polyvalve disease
Patau	Trisomy 13	80	ASD, VSD, Art Trunk, TGA, ToF
Turner	XO	20–35	Coarct, AS, Bicuspid aortic valve
Autosomal dominant			
22Q11	22Q11 deletion	80–85	Art Trunk, Int Ao Arch, ToF
Alagille	20p12 deletion	90	PPS, PS, ToF, Coarct
Beckwith–Wiedemann	11	15	HCM, ASD, VSD, ToF, PDA
Holt–Oram	12q24.1 mutation	85–95	ASD, VSD, conduction defects
Leopard		50	PS, HCM, conduction defects
Marfan	15q21	80–100	Aortic root dilation, mitral valve prolapse
Noonan	12p24 mutation	80	PS, PPS, ASD, HCM
Tuberose sclerosis		60	Rhabdomyomas
Williams	7q11.23 microdeletion	>80	Supra AS, PPS, renal artery stenosis
Autosomal recessive			
Ellis–van Creveld	4q16	50	ASD, PDA, Coarct, HLHS, TAPVC, TGA
Thrombocytopenia and absent radius	Multiple	30	ASD, ToF
Meckel–Gruber		25	Variable
Smith–Lemli–Opitz	11q12	15	ASD, VSD, PDA
Other associations			
Asymmetric crying facies		44	VSD
CHARGE		85	ToF, DORV, PS, VSD, AVSD
Cornelia de Lange	?3q26	30	VSD, ToF
Cri du chat	5p13.3	30–50	ASD, VSD, PDA, ToF
Diaphragmatic hernia		25	VSD, PDA, TGA, ToF
Intestinal atresia, tracheo-esophageal fistula		10	VSD, ToF
Goldenhar		20–30	ToF
Klippel–Feil	?8q22	25–40	ASD, VSD
Lung agenesis		20	VSD, ToF, PDA, TAPVC
Renal agenesis (unilateral)		17	VSD
VACTRL		73	ASD, VSD, DORV, ToF
Wolf–Hirschhorn	4p16	30	ASD, PS

Note this list is not inclusive, nor are the cardiac lesions always as most commonly seen!
Art Trunk, common arterial trunk; AS, aortic stenosis; ASD, atrial septal defect; AVSD atrioventricular septal defects; Coarct, aortic coarctation; DORV, double outlet right ventricle; HCM, hypertrophic cardiomyopathy; Int Ao Arch, interrupted aortic arch; PDA, patent arterial duct; PPS, peripheral pulmonary artery stenosis, PS, pulmonary stenosis; TAPVC, totally anomalous pulmonary venous connection; TGA, transposition of the great arteries; ToF, tetralogy of Fallot; VSD, ventricular septal defect.

FETAL DIAGNOSIS OF HEART DISEASE

DIAGNOSIS

The most common method of detection of a cardiac lesion is the routine 20 week fetal anomaly scan. The heart is examined in a four chamber view. Normally, the cardiac apex is to the left of the fetus, the cardiothoracic ratio is less than 50%, the two atria and two ventricles are of similar size, and there is normal tricuspid to mitral valve offsetting. This examination should identify most variations of 'single ventricle' such as hypoplastic left or right ventricle, major atrioventricular septal defects (Fig. 21.16) and inlet ventricular septal defects. Disproportion between the atrial sizes can also be identified. However, abnormalities of the cardiac outlets such as tetralogy of Fallot, common arterial trunk, transposition of the great arteries and some ventricular septal defects will not be visible in this view. They can only be detected on more detailed 'outlet screening' where the integrity of the outlet part of the ventricular septum and the ventriculo-arterial connections are also examined. Routine screening of the four chamber view detects 30–50% of fetuses with congenital heart disease.[82,83] Additional examination of the great vessels increases the incidence to more than 70%.[84] This forms part of the routine 20 week scan in some centers. In some conditions, such as aortic or pulmonary stenosis and coarctation, discrepancy in chamber size increases with advancing gestation. Others may only become apparent postnatally when the normal perinatal adaptations fail to occur or develop abnormally as in coarctation of the aorta, atrial septal defect and patent arterial duct. Small septal defects and minor valve abnormalities are outside the resolution and limits of detection of the ultrasound equipment.

If a fetus is thought to be at increased risk of a cardiac abnormality, specialist fetal echocardiography is indicated. Risk includes:
- Maternal diabetes, phenylketonuria, exposure to drugs such as anticonvulsants, lithium, alcohol or retinoic acid.
- Family history of congenital heart disease in a previous child, sibling or parent. History of an inherited condition such as tuberose sclerosis, or 22q11 deletion in a parent. Parental consanguinity increases the risk of complex heart disease.
- Fetal extracardiac or chromosome abnormality, arrhythmia or increased nuchal translucency detected at the 10–12 week scan.

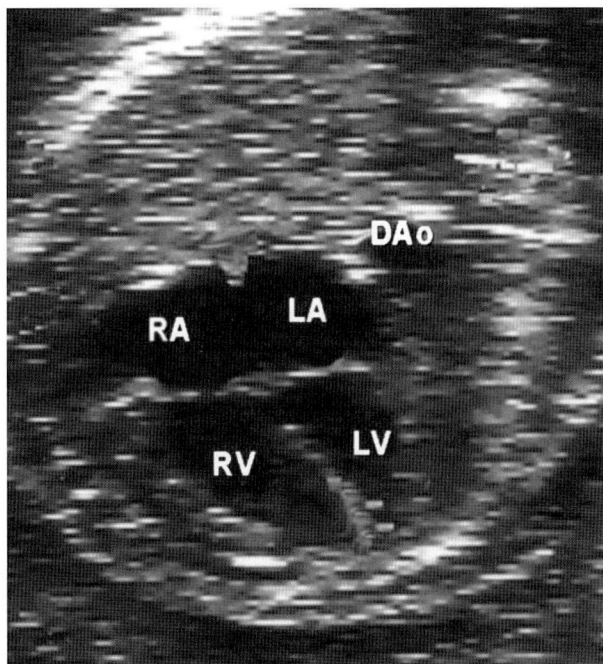

Fig. 21.16 Four chamber view of a fetal heart showing complete atrioventricular septal defect. The left and right components of the atrioventricular valves are at the same level. There is a ventricular septal defect and a primum atrial septal defect. DAo, descending aorta; LA, left atrium; LV, left ventricle; RA, right atrium; RV, right ventricle.

Specialist fetal echocardiography is usually performed at 18–20 weeks' gestation. However, with improved training and equipment, preliminary specialist scans as early as 12–14 weeks may provide some information,[85] although a further scan at 20 weeks is indicated. Further scans beyond 20 weeks are required for conditions that may progress during the pregnancy.

Most fetal cardiac abnormalities occur in 'low risk' pregnancies. The incidence of detection will increase as more ultrasonographers are trained to look at the great vessels as well as the four chamber view at the routine 20 week scan. Increased nuchal translucency at the 10–12 week scan also identifies a large proportion of fetuses at high risk of cardiac lesions.[86]

Once a diagnosis of a fetal cardiac abnormality is made, a detailed examination of the rest of the fetus is essential. Cardiac lesions are commonly associated with extracardiac lesions[87] such as exomphalos or diaphragmatic hernia, or chromosomal abnormalities. This has prognostic implications. Fetal karyotype can be obtained from placental tissue, amniocytes or fetal blood. Chromosomal abnormalities such as trisomy 13, 18 or 21, Turner syndrome and 22q11 deletion can be identified. When fetal heart block is detected, measurement of maternal autoantibodies (anti-Ro antibodies) will inform diagnosis and indicate recurrence risks.

MANAGEMENT

The rationale for prenatal detection of congenital heart disease remains controversial. Detecting a serious cardiac lesion increases parental choice, allowing the option of termination or continuation of the pregnancy. The termination rate is in the region of 30–50%[87,88] and this is often dependent on the severity of the cardiac lesion and the presence of other abnormalities.

Prenatal diagnosis also has implications for perinatal management. Most fetuses with congenital heart disease can be delivered according to normal obstetric parameters, the exceptions being some fetal arrhythmias where intrapartum monitoring may be compromised. Fetuses with known transposition of the great arteries should be delivered in close proximity to a pediatric cardiac center to allow urgent atrial septostomy if the atrial septum is very restrictive. All fetuses must be delivered in a center where adequate neonatal and transport facilities are available for duct-dependent neonates. Such infants should be discussed in advance with both obstetricians and neonatologists.

OUTCOME

Operative mortality for most congenital heart disease, other than hypoplastic left heart syndrome is less than 5%, but this is not reflected in the outcome of prenatally diagnosed lesions.[87–89] Analysis is complicated by the fact that the more severe end of the spectrum of congenital heart disease is diagnosed prenatally, and these infants have a much higher incidence of chromosomal and extracardiac abnormalities[87,89] than children diagnosed with congenital heart disease after birth. Prematurity[89] and fetal growth restriction[90] also increase the risk for infants with complex congenital heart disease, particularly those with a single functioning ventricle. Other risk factors include arrhythmia associated with congenital heart disease. Complete heart block with an atrial rate of less than 100 per minute or a ventricular rate of less than 45 per minute carries a poor prognosis.[91] Most deaths in infants with prenatally diagnosed congenital heart disease occur in the neonatal period.

There is evidence that antenatal diagnosis reduces morbidity.[92] Antenatal diagnosis permits timely and appropriate postnatal management and helps prevent hemodynamic deterioration and acidosis in duct-dependent lesions. There is also some evidence that it reduces mortality in neonates with two functioning ventricles.[93] Mortality in transposition of the great arteries was found to be significantly lower when diagnosed antenatally.[94] With regard to the prognosis of hypoplastic left heart syndrome, the findings are mixed. Brackley et al[95] found that infants with antenatally diagnosed hypoplastic left heart syndrome had lower survival than those diagnosed postnatally. Tworetzky et al[96] found an improved survival and reduced morbidity in an antenatally diagnosed group. Andrews et al[97] found similar survival rates in both groups.

THE NEONATE WITH A CONGENITAL HEART DISEASE

This section describes the timing and mode of presentation of heart disease in the newborn, focusing on the commonest conditions and those that are frequently missed or misdiagnosed. The emphasis is on structural heart disease and the anatomy and physiology of each is described. It discusses the clues and common pitfalls in making the diagnoses and outlines the management.

DIAGNOSIS
Making the diagnosis

Studies of infants with congenital heart disease who died found that in 10–30% of cases the diagnosis of a cardiac lesion was not made during life.[98,99] Some had complex cardiac lesions or severe noncardiac abnormalities, but if the cardiac diagnosis had been made during life, many were likely to have had a good outcome with treatment.[100] Early detection is therefore critical. A neonatal detection rate up to 90% can be achieved with a systematic clinical examination and pulse oximetry check, with a formal very early follow-up protocol for persistent heart murmurs or other physical signs.[101,102] Clinicians must be alert for early signs and refer to the specialist centers quickly, as deterioration can be extremely rapid.

Why is diagnosis delayed?

- *Most infants appear outwardly normal.* Delays in diagnosis occur partly due to false preconceptions that the majority of infants with serious heart disease will have a condition such as Down syndrome, or appear unwell immediately after birth. Most infants with serious heart disease have no associated syndromes or dysmorphic features. They are often well initially and do not have obvious physical signs until the arterial duct begins to close.
- *Cyanosis is not detected.* Transposition of the great arteries and pulmonary atresia have no associated respiratory distress or other clues to the diagnosis. Central cyanosis must be looked for deliberately on every neonatal check. Diagnosis is more difficult with dark skinned races, but the tongue and buccal mucosa are reliable in a well-lit room or with a torch. If there is a suspicion of cyanosis, pulse oximetry should be obtained. Normal values for the neonatal period have been established. Different oximetry machines produce different values[103] but new-generation machines are more accurate. A foot saturation of below 95% is suspicious, and below 90% definitively abnormal. Saturations from both the right hand (pre-ductal) and a foot (post-ductal) are even more accurate and a difference of $\geq 3\%$ is likely to be abnormal.[103]
- *Too much reliance is placed on auscultation.* Shortly after birth, murmurs are common in minor lesions such as small ventricular septal defects, and less common in the most severe conditions such as underdevelopment of the left heart or transposition of the great arteries. Although auscultation is important, serious heart disease is more likely to be revealed by careful observation of the infant's color and respiratory pattern, assessment of peripheral perfusion and palpation of brachial and femoral pulses and of the precordium for a prominent pulsation. A normal neonatal examination does not rule out serious heart disease that may present later, usually when the arterial duct closes.[100] Equally important is to listen to the parents when they express concern. They often know instinctively that something is wrong!

Practical points

- Most infants with life-threatening heart disease have no associated syndrome, a normal outward appearance, are perfectly well and have a normal physical examination for the first day or two after birth.
- Look carefully inside the mouth for central cyanosis.
- Routine use of pulse oximetry in the foot should be encouraged as part of newborn screening for heart disease.
- Rely more on observation and palpation than the stethoscope.
- Always consider heart disease in a sick infant.

Hyperoxia test

The normal newborn should have a PaO_2 greater than 70 mmHg (9 kPa). Cyanosis detected clinically is usually less than 40 mmHg (5 kPa). In a cyanosed infant, if the arterial PaO_2 rises above 150 mmHg (20 kPa) in 90–100% oxygen, a major right to left shunt is unlikely. The test is not completely reliable, but a failure of the PaO_2 to rise strongly suggests a cardiac defect. The PaO_2 can fail to rise for two other reasons:

1. Intrapulmonary shunting in lung disease. Areas of collapsed lung tend to be perfused with blood as well as the well-aerated sections, so some blood returning to the heart is not oxygenated.
2. Failure of the transitional circulation (persistent fetal circulation or persistent pulmonary hypertension of the newborn – see Ch. 12). In this condition, the pulmonary vascular resistance fails to fall normally, and right to left shunting occurs across the fetal channels, the patent oval foramen and arterial duct. It often coexists with severe neonatal lung disease, causing diagnostic and management dilemmas. Once congenital heart disease is excluded, management is aimed at reducing pulmonary vascular resistance by the treatment of acidosis and the use of pulmonary vasodilators, in particular inhaled nitric oxide.

THE IMPORTANCE OF THE OVAL FORAMEN IN NEONATAL HEART DISEASE

Patency of the oval foramen is critical for survival where the mitral or tricuspid flow is absent or inadequate, or when mixing at atrial level is essential as in transposition of the great vessels. In mitral atresia (or hypoplastic left heart), postnatal survival depends on a patent foramen to allow the pulmonary venous blood to enter the right atrium and thence the right ventricle. Blood then reaches the main pulmonary artery and divides between the lungs and the aorta (via the arterial duct). Closure of the oval foramen or arterial duct will result in death. Similarly, in tricuspid atresia, a widely patent foramen is essential for venous return to reach the ventricles via the left atrium. In transposition, the most effective mixing between the systemic and pulmonary circulations is at atrial level and an inadequate or severely restrictive foramen can be life threatening even when the arterial duct is patent.[100] If the oval foramen is inadequate it must be enlarged by cardiac catheter intervention (Fig. 21.13) or surgery.

THE IMPORTANCE OF THE ARTERIAL DUCT IN NEONATAL HEART DISEASE

Prostaglandin E_2 (dinoprostone) is a physiological compound, critical in maintaining duct patency during fetal life. It is used intravenously in duct-dependent cyanotic and left heart obstructive lesions. The starting dose is 5–10 ng/kg/min and this can be increased to achieve duct patency. Although the arterial duct is functionally closed in most healthy term infants by the second day of life and usually completely closed by day 5,[104] persistent or episodic hypoxemia can delay duct closure. Prostaglandin E_2 can be an effective therapy even into the second or third week of life, provided the duct has not completely closed.

Side-effects of prostaglandin therapy

Apnea is a serious side-effect and resuscitation equipment should be available. Doses higher than 10 ng/kg/min may result in apnea. Lower doses can cause apnea in premature infants. If transport to the tertiary center is required, many centers will electively intubate and ventilate such infants.[100] Other common side-effects are jitteriness, pyrexia, hypotension due to systemic vasodilatation, and occasionally hypoglycemia.

PRESENTATION OF HEART DISEASE IN THE NEWBORN
Mode of presentation
Antenatal

As fetal ultrasonographers become increasingly skilled in the detection of heart disease, more than 40% of infants with severe congenital heart disease are born with their diagnosis already made.[83,84] However, the majority still present after birth and rely on the vigilance of the clinicians, parents and midwives to be detected.

Symptoms and signs after birth

Neonates almost always present with one of the following:

- Cyanosis, with or without respiratory distress.
- Heart failure, with or without cyanosis.
- Collapse.
- An associated lesion or syndrome.
- An abnormal clinical sign detected on routine examination such as absent femoral pulses or a heart murmur.

Timing of presentation

The age of presentation depends on the effect that the transition from fetal to postnatal circulation has upon the specific lesion. This relates to how the abnormal heart responds to the high pulmonary vascular resistance at birth, the gradual fall of this resistance, and the closure of the arterial duct. Here are three examples:

1. An infant born with a poorly functioning right ventricle and severe tricuspid regurgitation (as with Ebstein's anomaly of the tricuspid valve) will present at birth. This is because the high pulmonary

vascular resistance prevents the impaired right ventricle from delivering blood effectively into the pulmonary arteries.

2. An infant with pulmonary atresia, despite having no forward flow from the right ventricle into the pulmonary artery, does not present at birth because the arterial duct is open. Blood fills the pulmonary arteries from the aorta. Clinical presentation with severe cyanosis occurs when the duct starts to close a few hours to days after birth.

3. An infant with a large ventricular septal defect has no difficulties at birth because the high pulmonary vascular resistance results in a high systolic pressure in the right ventricle. This prevents excessive flow across the defect from the left to right ventricle. Pulmonary vascular resistance gradually falls after a few weeks and presentation with cardiac failure, due to the large left to right shunt through the defect, typically occurs at 4–6 weeks of age.

When making a diagnosis in a newborn, it is therefore helpful to consider not only the *type* of presentation (cyanosis with or without respiratory distress, cardiac failure, collapse) but also the usual *timing* of presentation (Table 21.9) and the clinical, electrocardiographic and X-ray findings (Table 21.10).

PRESENTATION WITH CYANOSIS WITHOUT RESPIRATORY DISTRESS

The commonest causes of isolated cyanosis are transposition of the great arteries and pulmonary atresia or severe (critical) pulmonary stenosis. Pulmonary atresia can occur with a ventricular septal defect (a variant of tetralogy of Fallot) or without when the right ventricle may be hypoplastic. Other causes include tricuspid atresia and other complex lesions with restricted pulmonary blood flow.

Transposition of the great arteries

This is the most common cyanotic lesion to present in the neonate, accounting for 4–5% of congenital heart disease[66,68] and occurring more commonly in males.

Anatomy and physiology

In this condition, the aorta and pulmonary arteries are transposed. The right ventricle, receiving deoxygenated blood as usual from the right

Table 21.9 Typical timing and mode of presentation of congenital heart disease in the neonate

	EARLY 0–24 hours High pulmonary vascular resistance, arterial duct open	INTERMEDIATE 4 hours–2 weeks Duct closing – 'duct dependent' lesions present	LATE After 2 weeks Duct closed. Pulmonary vascular resistance continues to fall and lesions with left to right shunts present
Cyanosis (without congestive failure or respiratory distress)	TGA	*Duct dependent for pulmonary blood flow*, e.g. Pulmonary atresia with or without VSD Critical pulmonary stenosis (with right to left interatrial flow) Tricuspid atresia with small VSD Complex lesions with severe pulmonary stenosis[b] *Duct dependent for mixing*, TGA (simple and complex)	Tetralogy of Fallot with severe pulmonary stenosis[a] Complex lesions with pulmonary stenosis[b]
Cyanosis with congestive failure or respiratory distress	Obstructed TAPVD (usually infradiaphragmatic) Severe Ebstein's anomaly	Pulmonary arteriovenous fistulae (rare) Partially obstructed TAPVD	*Mixed circulations with unobstructed pulmonary blood flow*, e.g. Unobstructed TAPVD (cardiac or supracardiac) Common arterial trunk Tricuspid atresia with a large VSD Some complex lesions with high pulmonary blood flow[c]
Collapse/shock		*Left heart obstruction*, e.g. Aortic coarctation or interruption HLHS Aortic stenosis	
Congestive cardiac failure (without cyanosis)		Left heart obstruction with a left-to-right shunt e.g. Aortic coarctation ± VSD *Systemic arteriovenous fistulae*, e.g. cerebral	*Left to right shunts*, e.g. Large VSD, complete AV septal defect, PDA, aortopulmonary window Complex lesions[d]

N.B. It is important to use this table as a guideline only – each condition can present unusually late or early! Tachyarrhythmias, usually SVT, can present with heart failure or collapse in any of these age groups, as can myocardial failure due to heart muscle disease such as hypertrophic cardiomyopathy or myocardial ischemia secondary to perinatal distress. Cardiovascular collapse in the first few hours is usually related to such myocardial dysfunction; sepsis and metabolic disease should be considered.

TAPVD, totally anomalous pulmonary venous drainage; HLHS, hypoplastic left heart syndrome; TGA, transposition of the great arteries – those without a VSD and a small oval foramen present earlier; VSD, ventricular septal defect; PDA, persistent ductus arteriosus.

[a] In tetralogy of Fallot, only the most severe present as a cyanotic neonate. The less severe forms present typically with cyanotic spells, or with a loud murmur on routine check.

[b] Examples of complex lesions with low pulmonary blood flow include:
    1. Any single ventricle with severe pulmonary or subpulmonary stenosis.
    2. Double outlet right ventricle with severe pulmonary stenosis.

[c] Examples of complex lesions with high pulmonary blood flow and cyanosis include:
    1. Double outlet right ventricle with transposed great arteries.
    2. Pulmonary atresia with large aortopulmonary collateral arteries or large arterial duct.

[d] Examples of complex lesions with high pulmonary blood flow without cyanosis include:
    1. Single ventricle without pulmonary stenosis.
    2. Double outlet right ventricle with normally related great arteries and *without* pulmonary stenosis.

Table 21.10 Flow chart for the differential diagnosis of central cyanosis. Assessment of whether pulmonary blood flow is increased or diminished combined with the electrocardiographic findings helps to narrow the diagnostic possibilities

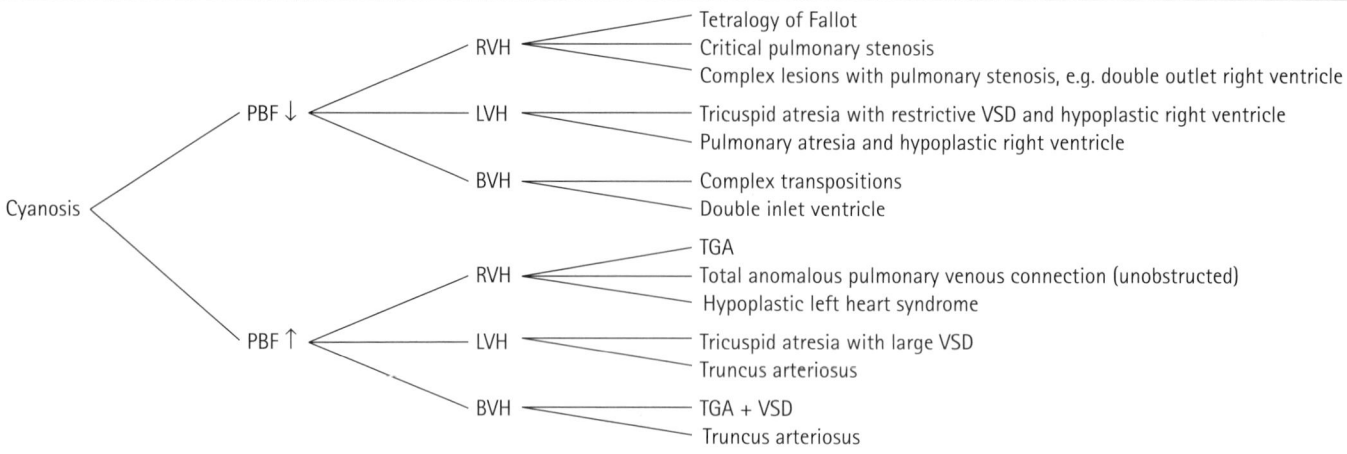

PBF, pulmonary blood flow; RVH, right ventricular hypertrophy; LVH, left ventricular hypertrophy; BVH, biventricular hypertrophy; TGA, transposition of great arteries; VSD, ventricular septal defect.

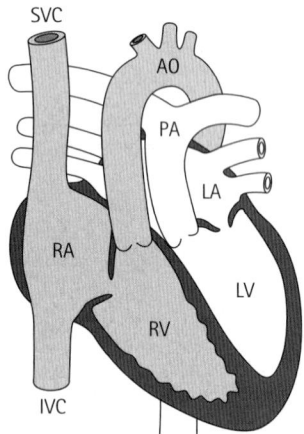

Fig. 21.17 Transposition of the great arteries (atrioventricular concordance, arterioventricular discordance). Shading indicates desaturated/unoxygenated blood. AO, aorta; IVC, inferior vena cava; LA, left atrium; LV, left ventricle; PA, pulmonary artery; RA, right atrium; RV, right ventricle; SVC, superior vena cava.

atrium, delivers this blood into the aorta (Fig. 21.17). The oxygenated blood returning from the pulmonary veins drains into the left atrium and left ventricle but is pumped directly back into the pulmonary arteries (Fig. 21.10d). These two circulations do not mix and this is not compatible with life. Survival in the first few hours is due to mixing at atrial level via a patent oval foramen and at arterial level via the patent arterial duct. Some infants have a ventricular septal defect, pulmonary stenosis or aortic coarctation.

Clinical features
Cyanosis is sometimes detected at birth. More commonly presentation is over the next 1–3 days, the cyanosis becoming more obvious as the arterial duct closes (Table 21.9). If the atrial communication is small, the infant deteriorates rapidly and will die if the duct is not reopened with intravenous prostaglandin therapy or the foramen enlarged by atrial septostomy. No murmurs or other physical signs are present unless there are additional lesions. When there is an associated large ventricular septal defect with pulmonary stenosis, the severity of stenosis determines the degree of cyanosis and timing of presentation.

Investigations
The neonate will fail the hyperoxia test and a metabolic acidosis may be present. Right ventricular hypertrophy on the electrocardiogram becomes more obvious with time. Chest radiography shows increased pulmonary vascularity (Table 21.10). Transposition of the great arteries is unlike most other cyanotic conditions that present early, which have reduced pulmonary blood flow. This is because there is both left to right and right to left shunting at atrial and ductal levels, combined

with hypoxia that causes myocardial dysfunction. The upper mediastinum is narrow because the aorta lies in front, and slightly to the right, of the pulmonary artery. The 'egg on side' appearance of the heart is not usually seen in the neonatal period, as the thymic shadow is often present. Echocardiography shows the pulmonary artery arising from the left ventricle (Fig. 21.10d) and the aorta from the right ventricle. A characteristic finding is the parallel relationship of the great vessels (Fig. 21.18). Additional lesions such as a ventricular septal defect, pulmonary stenosis or aortic coarctation can be identified.

Management and prognosis
Prostaglandin infusion should be commenced immediately without waiting for the diagnosis to be confirmed. Any metabolic acidosis should be corrected.

Balloon atrial septostomy. This is usually performed to enlarge the oval foramen and promote mixing at this level. This can be done with echocardiographic guidance on the intensive care unit, or in the cardiac catheterization theater. A catheter with a balloon mounted on the end is advanced from the umbilical or femoral vein into the right atrium and, via the patent oval foramen, across into the left atrium. The balloon is inflated and pulled back to tear the septum (Fig. 21.13).

Surgical management. The arterial switch operation (Fig. 21.19) is performed within the next few days, using cardiopulmonary bypass. The arterial trunks are transected, the main pulmonary artery pulled forward, and the ascending aorta moved posteriorly such that the branch pulmonary arteries straddle the ascending aorta. The coronary arter-

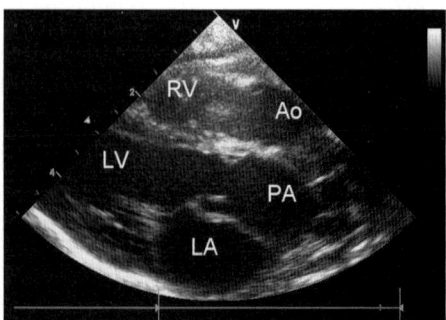

Fig. 21.18 Echocardiogram in long-axis view showing parallel great vessels with the aorta arising anteriorly from the right ventricle and the pulmonary artery arising posteriorly from the left ventricle. Ao, Aorta; LV, left ventricle; PA, pulmonary artery; RV, right ventricle.

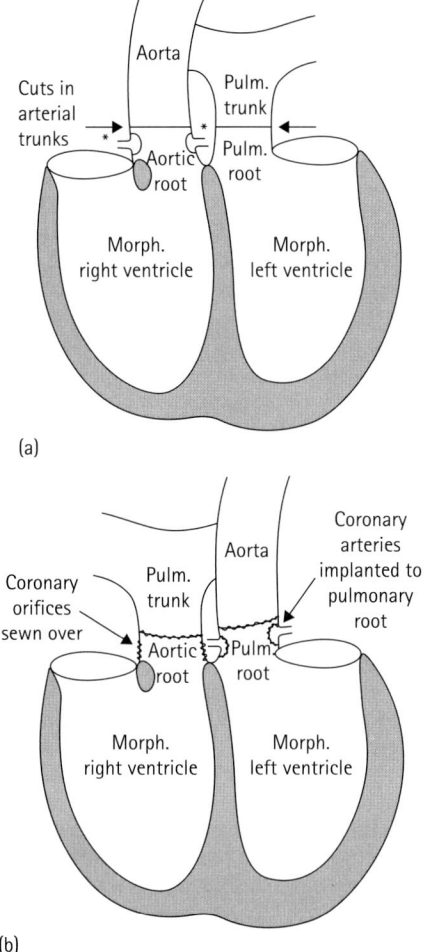

Fig. 21.19 Diagrammatic representations of the arterial switch (a) before and (b) after the procedure. Morph., morphological; Pulm., pulmonary. (From Anderson et al 2002[105].)

ies are removed with a small button of surrounding arterial wall, and re-sutured into the new ascending aorta. This operation is usually performed in the neonatal period, before the left ventricle becomes adapted to pumping against a low pulmonary vascular resistance. This results in thinning of the left ventricular wall, which is then unable to cope with pumping at systemic pressure after the switch operation. In older infants, a band placed around the pulmonary artery will increase left ventricular pressure and 're-train' it to cope with the pressure of the

systemic circulation. Early mortality from the arterial switch operation is now less than 2%, and 10 year survival is 94%.[106] The commonest complication is narrowing of the branch pulmonary arteries as they stretch over the aorta. Myocardial infarction is rare.

Previous surgical procedures. Before the mid-1980s surgery consisted of an atrial re-routing operation, the Senning or Mustard procedure. Systemic venous blood is directed from the right atrium by means of a baffle across the atrial septum to the mitral valve, into the left ventricle and out to the pulmonary arteries. Pulmonary venous blood passes via left atrium to the right atrium, right ventricle and aorta. The morphological right ventricle, designed for pumping through a low pressure circuit to the lungs, pumps blood around the body under high pressure. Although patients do well for the first two decades of life, the right ventricle gradually fails, typically in the third and fourth decade of life, and there is a risk of sudden death from atrial and ventricular arrhythmias. Actuarial survival at 30 years is 80%.[107]

Surgical options for transposition with pulmonary stenosis. It is inappropriate to perform the switch operation when there is significant pulmonary stenosis, as this problem is transferred to the new aorta. Aortic valve stenosis carries a significant lifetime morbidity. If there is an associated large outlet ventricular septal defect, it is sometimes possible to patch the ventricular septal defect so that the left ventricle leads into the aorta anteriorly, and then place a tube graft (conduit) from the right ventricle to the pulmonary artery (Fig. 21.20). This is known as the Rastelli procedure. The conduit must be replaced as the child grows, increasing the cumulative mortality risk.

Tetralogy of Fallot with pulmonary atresia

This condition represents the severe end of the spectrum of this condition. Most children with tetralogy of Fallot have stenosis rather than atresia of the right ventricular outflow tract and, as they present outside the neonatal period, are described later (p. 788).

Anatomy and physiology

Pulmonary atresia is a complete obstruction between the right ventricle and pulmonary arteries. The intracardiac anatomy resembles that of tetralogy of Fallot with a large ventricular septal defect, but the pulmonary arteries are frequently abnormal. The central pulmonary arteries may be confluent and supplied by the arterial duct. Alternatively, or in addition, collateral arteries from the aorta, major aortopulmonary collateral arteries (MAPCAs), supply the lungs and connect with the pulmonary arteries.

Clinical features

When the infant is dependent on the arterial duct, cyanosis develops when it closes in the first days of life (Table 21.9). Major aortopulmonary collateral arteries provide a more stable source of pulmonary blood flow, and cyanosis may be mild. A few infants have exces-

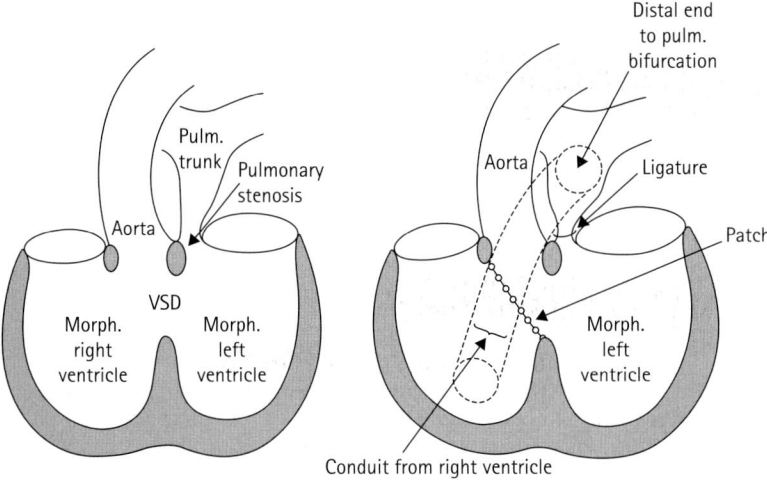

Fig. 21.20 A diagrammatic representation of the steps involved in the Rastelli procedure. Morph., morphological; Pulm., pulmonary; VSD, ventricular septal defect. (From Anderson et al 2002[105].)

sive pulmonary blood flow from these collateral vessels and present in heart failure with minimal cyanosis. The right ventricle is prominent on palpation. The first sound is frequently followed by an aortic ejection click related to the dilated ascending aorta, and the second heart sound is single. Continuous murmurs from the collateral vessels are heard widely over the precordium. Almost 50% of children have 22q11deletion.[108]

Investigations
The electrocardiogram shows right ventricular hypertrophy with persistence of the upright T wave in lead V1. Chest radiography shows pulmonary oligemia (Table 21.10). Right ventricular hypertrophy may produce a 'boot-shaped' cardiac shadow and 25–30% of infants have a right aortic arch. Echocardiography shows the subaortic ventricular septal defect and identifies the central pulmonary arteries. Additional muscular ventricular septal defects and other abnormalities can be identified. Cardiac catheterization or MRI may be needed, prior to definitive surgery, to accurately define the pulmonary arterial anatomy and aortopulmonary collateral arteries.

Management and prognosis
Prostaglandin infusion maintains duct patency until the anatomy of the pulmonary arteries is delineated. The metabolic acidosis should be corrected.

Infants with duct-dependent pulmonary circulation. Stability is usually achieved by creating a shunt, usually a Gore-Tex™ tube, from the innominate or subclavian artery to the pulmonary artery (modified Blalock–Taussig shunt). This encourages pulmonary arterial growth in preparation for definitive surgery. This consists of closing the ventricular septal defect and placing a tissue conduit from right ventricle to pulmonary artery. It is preferable to defer definitive surgery until the child is older to reduce the number of conduit replacements needed during growth.

Infants with major aortopulmonary collateral arteries (MAPCAs). Surgery varies depending on the anatomy of the pulmonary arteries and MAPCAs. The aim is to connect important MAPCAs to the central pulmonary arteries, and to place a conduit between the right ventricle and pulmonary artery. The ventricular septal defect is closed. Several staged operations may be needed.

Prognosis in children without 22q11 deletion is good, with a 90% 5 year survival. However, children with 22q11 deletion have only a 36% 5 year survival, mainly related to less favorable pulmonary artery anatomy.[109]

Pulmonary atresia with intact ventricular septum/ critical pulmonary valve stenosis
This accounts for about 2.5% of all congenital heart defects.

Anatomy and physiology
The pulmonary valve is imperforate (atresia) or has a tiny orifice (critical stenosis). The ventricular septum is intact and the right ventricle is always abnormal, varying in size from slightly small to severely hypoplastic. The tricuspid valve is usually small. Pulmonary blood flow depends on the arterial duct. Cyanosis is caused by right to left shunting at atrial level, through a stretched oval foramen. In some infants with an atretic valve, the muscle-bound, hypertensive right ventricle has fistulous connections to the coronary arteries. The coronary arteries may be stenosed, so that the distal part of the coronary circulation depends entirely on retrograde flow from the right ventricle. Relief of the pulmonary valve obstruction is dangerous, because the right ventricular pressure falls, reducing coronary arterial flow and causing myocardial infarction.

Clinical features
Neonates present with cyanosis when the arterial duct closes (Table 21.9). There is a single second sound and there may be a soft ductal murmur and a systolic murmur of tricuspid regurgitation. Infants with

critical pulmonary stenosis have an ejection systolic murmur audible in the pulmonary area.

Investigations
The electrocardiogram shows right atrial enlargement with tall P waves, and occasionally ST segment changes if there is coronary ischemia. When the right ventricle is hypoplastic, the R wave in V1 is small. Chest radiography shows pulmonary oligemia, with cardiomegaly if tricuspid regurgitation is severe (Table 21.10). Echocardiography shows right ventricular hypertrophy with a varying degree of hypoplasia. The tricuspid valve is abnormal, and pulmonary arteries fill through the arterial duct. Infants with critical stenosis have flow through the pulmonary valve. If coronary fistulae are demonstrated with continuous color Doppler signals within the right ventricular wall, or suspected because of enlarged coronary origins, cardiac catheterization will delineate them more clearly.

Management and prognosis
Prostaglandin infusion should be commenced without waiting for the diagnosis to be confirmed. Any metabolic acidosis should be corrected. Initial intervention consists of transcatheter perforation and balloon dilatation of the stenosed or atretic valve (Fig. 21.21), surgical valvotomy or a systemic to pulmonary shunt. The ultimate clinical course depends on the size of the right ventricle.[110]

Infant with an adequate right ventricle. Infants with critical pulmonary valve stenosis and some with atresia will have a right ventricle of adequate size. With relief of the obstruction, it will eventually function well.[32]

Infant with a severely hypoplastic right ventricle. If the right ventricle is hypoplastic, the heart has functionally only a left ventricle. Palliation for all children with a single ventricle circulation is outlined later (p. 789).

The 5 year survival for pulmonary atresia and intact ventricular septum is approximately 70%.[110] Death is rare following balloon dilatation for critical pulmonary stenosis.[32]

Tricuspid atresia
This spectrum of conditions, accounting for 1% of congenital heart defects, has in common an absent right atrioventricular connection. Survival requires a large oval foramen, allowing systemic and pulmonary venous return to mix in the left atrium. There are many anatomic and hemodynamic variations, producing widely different clinical features. These depend on the atrial and ventricular and septal defects, the size of the right ventricle and the ventriculoarterial connections (Fig. 21.22). If the ventricular septal defect is small, there will be reduced pulmonary blood flow (discussed below). If the ventricular septal defect is large, excessive pulmonary blood flow will result in cyanosis and heart failure (p. 775). When the pulmonary artery arises from the left ventricle and the aorta from the hypoplastic right ventricle, this constitutes a form of hypoplastic 'left' heart syndrome (p. 778).

Tricuspid atresia with reduced pulmonary blood flow
Anatomy and physiology
Flow to the pulmonary arteries is via the left ventricle, either through a restrictive ventricular septal defect to the right ventricle and pulmonary artery or through an arterial duct if the pulmonary valve is atretic (Fig. 21.22).

Clinical features
Infants present, in the first few days, with cyanosis (Table 21.9). There is usually a systolic murmur and the second heart sound is single.

Investigations
The electrocardiogram shows a superior (left) axis, left ventricular dominant forces, and prominent P waves if the right atrium is enlarged. The lung fields are oligemic on chest radiography (Table 21.10).

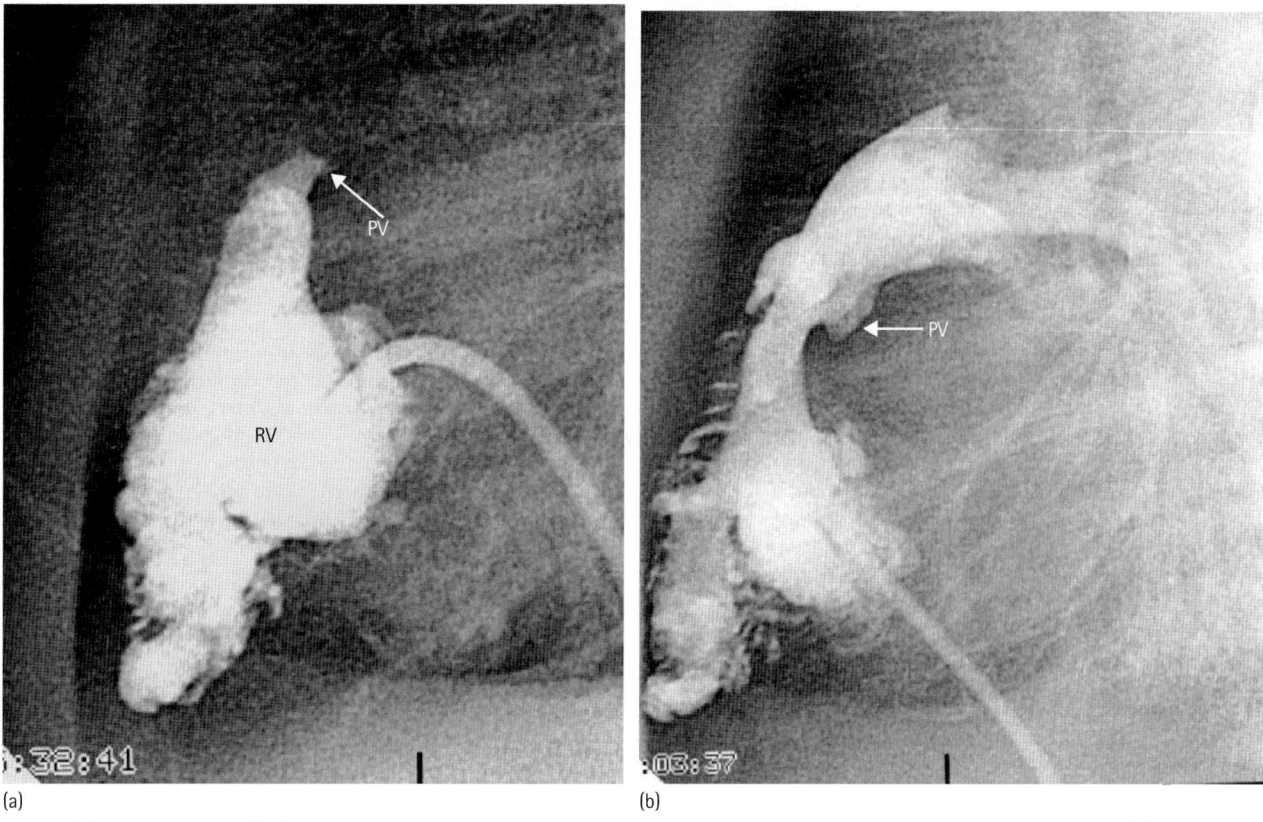

(a)   (b)

Fig. 21.21 (a) Right ventricular (RV) angiogram showing pulmonary atresia with an obstruction of the right ventricular outflow tract. (b) Following radiofrequency perforation and balloon dilatation, there is flow through the pulmonary valve and into the pulmonary arteries. PV, pulmonary valve.

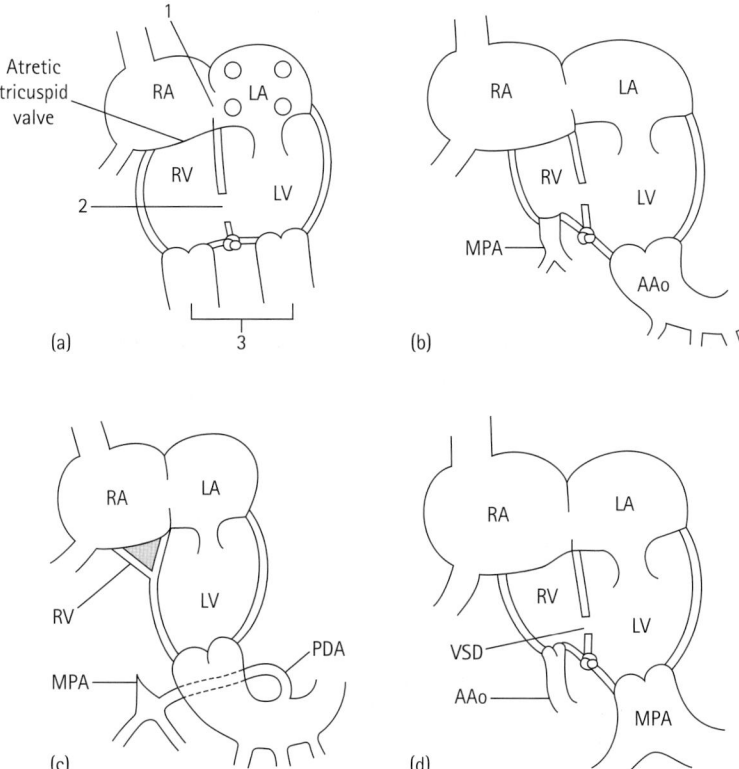

Fig. 21.22 Tricuspid atresia: anatomical variations and physiological implications. (a) The basic structural elements are identified with an atretic tricuspid valve and the three key anatomical–pathophysiological factors: (1) status of the atrial septal defect (ASD), (2) size of the ventricular septal defect (VSD), and (3) great artery connections (normal or transposed).
(b) A common form of tricuspid atresia with a large ASD, small-to-moderate VSD resulting in a small right ventricle (RV) and, with normally related great arteries, a small (stenotic) main pulmonary artery (MPA). This patient is likely to have inadequate pulmonary blood flow and need a neonatal shunt. (c) When there is no VSD and normally related great arteries, the RV is absent and MPA is atretic; pulmonary blood flow is dependent on ductal patency. Such patients always need a systemic-to-pulmonary shunt.
(d) A small VSD and transposition results in hypoplasia of the RV and aorta; effectively, this is hypoplastic left heart syndrome. (From Skinner et al 2000[23].)

Echocardiography demonstrates the absent tricuspid valve (Fig. 21.10b) and other relevant anatomy.[111]

Management and prognosis
The neonate usually requires prostaglandin to maintain duct patency and a systemic to pulmonary shunt to provide a reliable source of pulmonary blood flow. The absent tricuspid valve means that the heart has functionally only a left ventricle. Palliation and prognosis for all children with a single ventricle circulation is outlined under this condition (p. 789).

PRESENTATION WITH CYANOSIS AND RESPIRATORY DISTRESS

The combination of cyanosis with respiratory distress at birth usually indicates a lung rather than a heart problem. These include meconium aspiration syndrome, neonatal pneumonia or surfactant deficiency in the preterm infant. There is often a history suggesting a respiratory problem. Chest radiography may indicate pneumonia or aspiration with areas of focal lung collapse (atelectasis), hyperexpanded or underdeveloped lungs, a pneumothorax or diaphragmatic hernia. However, it is vital not to miss cyanotic heart disease since the management is so different. Persistent cyanosis in a newborn with respiratory distress is a clear indication for echocardiography. A *hyperoxia test* (p. 768) is useful when this is not immediately available.

Two uncommon congenital heart lesions that present in this way are Ebstein's anomaly of the tricuspid valve and obstructed total anomalous pulmonary venous connection. In Ebstein's anomaly there is typically a huge ('wall-to-wall') heart on chest radiography. Total anomalous pulmonary venous connection is, however, often missed or diagnosed late. Differentiation from persistent fetal circulation or primary lung pathology can be difficult.[100] Since the only effective therapy is urgent surgery, late diagnosis may result in death. Delayed diagnosis also occurs when an infant with a lung problem has a coincident cyanotic heart disease.

Ebstein's anomaly of the tricuspid valve
This is uncommon, comprising less than 1% of congenital heart disease.

Anatomy and physiology
The tricuspid valve is displaced down the interventricular septum (Fig. 21.23) towards the apex of the right ventricle, resulting in 'atrialization' of this chamber. The degree of displacement, together with dysplasia and regurgitation of the tricuspid valve, dictates the clinical spectrum. Antenatally, a hugely dilated right heart occupies much of the thorax and the lungs cannot develop normally. Right to left shunting at atrial level and little forward flow across the pulmonary valve may result in pulmonary valve stenosis or atresia.

Clinical features
The most severe form results in marked tricuspid valve regurgitation and a poorly functioning thin-walled right ventricle, causing fetal or neonatal death. At birth, the infant is deeply cyanosed with severe respiratory distress due to the hypoplastic lungs and reduced pulmonary blood flow (Table 21.10). The pansystolic murmur of tricuspid regurgitation, together with tricuspid valve clicks, may be audible. The liver is markedly enlarged.

Mild forms are asymptomatic, presenting with cyanosis, a murmur or supraventricular tachycardia due to the commonly associated Wolff–Parkinson–White syndrome.[112]

Investigations
The electrocardiogram shows right atrial enlargement with large P waves and an incomplete right bundle branch block pattern. Chest radiography shows a markedly enlarged heart and vascularity may be reduced. Echocardiography (Fig. 21.23) defines the severity of the lesion.[111]

Management and prognosis
Fetal and neonatal presentation is associated with a poor outcome as it represents the severe end of the clinical spectrum. Early therapy includes intensive ventilatory support and treatment with nitric oxide to encourage a fall in pulmonary vascular resistance. Early mortality is high although outcome has improved more recently.[112,113] Children with a milder form have a better outlook, but some require surgery to the tricuspid valve in later life.[112,114]

Total anomalous pulmonary venous connection
This is uncommon, accounting for less than 1% of congenital heart disease.[115] The pulmonary veins join to form a confluence or channel behind the left atrium and eventually drain into the right atrium to mix with the deoxygenated blood returning from the body. The route from the pulmonary venous confluence can be of three types (Fig. 21.24), the commonest being the supracardiac.[115,116] The mode and timing of the clinical presentation depend on whether an obstruction prevents free drainage of the pulmonary venous blood into the right heart (Table 21.9). Infants with obstruction present shortly after birth with respiratory distress, cyanosis and cardiac failure. Those without obstruction present at 2–8 weeks of age with mild cyanosis and progressive cardiac failure.

Obstructed total anomalous pulmonary venous connection
Anatomy
The infracardiac type is almost always severely obstructed (Fig. 21.24c). The cardiac and supracardiac types are rarely obstructed but this can occur when narrowing is present in other parts of the channel or when a small foramen prevents right to left flow at atrial level.

Clinical features
The infant becomes unwell shortly after birth as the pulmonary venous obstruction results in severe pulmonary venous hypertension, cyanosis, cardiac failure and respiratory distress, similar to the picture of persistent fetal circulation.

Investigations
Chest radiography shows pulmonary venous hypertension but the heart is often not greatly enlarged. The streaky appearance due to the prominent pulmonary veins can be mistaken for lung disease, particularly meconium aspiration. Once the diagnosis is suspected, echocardiography is extremely urgent. Differentiation from persistent pulmonary hypertension of the newborn is difficult. In both conditions the left atrium and ventricle are under-filled and compressed by the enlarged right ventricle. There is right to left flow across the atrial septum. Diagnosis depends on recognizing the pulmonary venous chamber behind the left atrium but not connecting with it (Fig. 21.10a).[111]

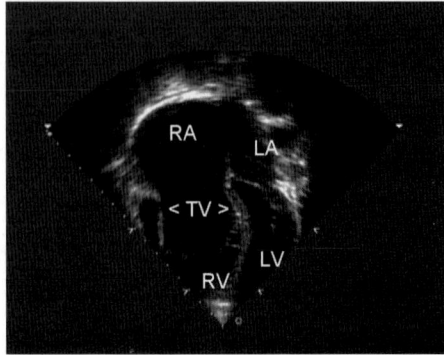

Fig. 21.23   Echocardiogram in four chamber view showing displacement of the abnormal tricuspid valve into the body of the right ventricle. LA, left atrium; LV, left ventricle; RA, right atrium; RV right ventricle; TV, tricuspid valve.

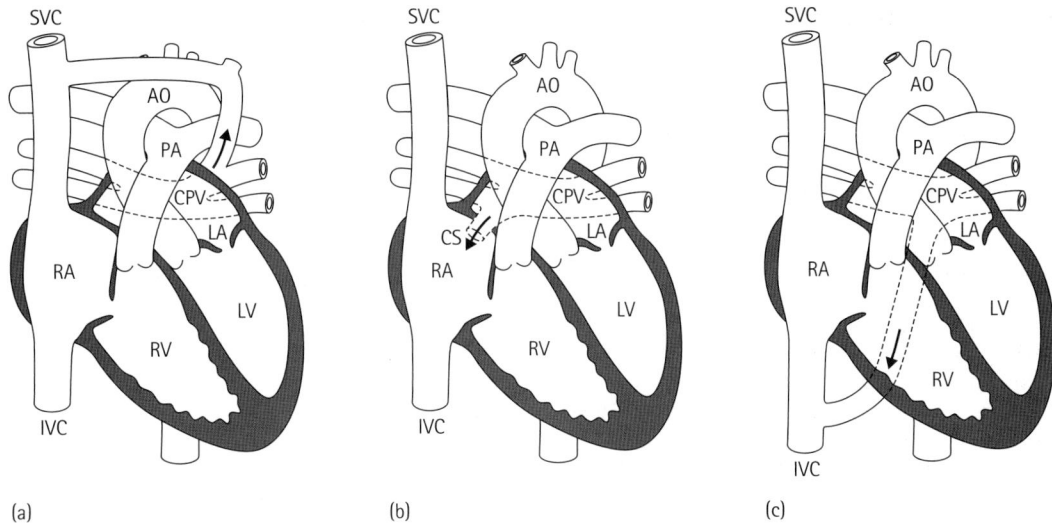

Fig. 21.24 Total anomalous pulmonary venous connection. The three common varieties are shown: (a) supracardiac with the four pulmonary veins draining into a common pulmonary venous channel (CPV) and then via a vertical (ascending) vein to the innominate vein and the right heart; (b) cardiac with the pulmonary veins draining directly to the coronary sinus (CS) as shown or directly to the right atrium (not shown); (c) infracardiac draining into the inferior vena caval or portal vein.

Management and prognosis

Maintaining arterial duct patency with prostaglandin will not help. Ventilatory and circulatory support is necessary and the child must be transferred urgently for surgery, which is performed without delay. The pulmonary venous chamber is opened into the back of the left atrium, and the abnormal connecting vein ligated. Surgical mortality is high if the infant is extremely acidotic prior to surgery, but overall mortality as low as 7% has been reported.[116] There is a risk of later pulmonary vein stenosis (11%) which can be extremely difficult to manage successfully.

PRESENTATION WITH CYANOSIS AND CARDIAC FAILURE

This presentation is rare, and usually caused by unobstructed total anomalous pulmonary venous connection, tricuspid atresia with a large ventricular septal defect or common arterial trunk.

Unobstructed total anomalous pulmonary venous connection

Anatomy and physiology

The majority of supracardiac and intracardiac types (Fig. 21.24 a, b) are unobstructed. Deoxygenated blood from the caval veins mixes with the oxygenated blood from the pulmonary veins in the right atrium. The moderate cyanosis is often not detected clinically. As pulmonary vascular resistance falls, the path of least resistance for the blood is through the tricuspid valve rather than through the oval foramen and the mitral valve. Congestive cardiac failure develops due to excessive pulmonary blood flow.

Clinical features

The infant presents between 2 weeks and several months of age with congestive cardiac failure and moderate cyanosis (Table 21.9). A right ventricular heave is palpable, and the second sound is loud and split. There may be a soft ejection systolic murmur caused by increased pulmonary blood flow.

Investigations

The electrocardiogram shows prominent P waves due to right atrial enlargement, and right ventricular hypertrophy develops. Chest radiography shows cardiomegaly with right atrial dilatation and pulmonary plethora. The supracardiac type frequently has a broad mediastinum due

to the ascending vein, the 'snowman' appearance. Echocardiography shows a dilated right atrium and right ventricle. There is a chamber behind the left atrium (Fig. 21.10a) and a vein draining to superior caval vein or right atrium

Management and prognosis

Initial management includes treatment of heart failure with diuretics (p. 762). Early, but not urgent, surgical correction is performed. The pulmonary venous chamber is opened into the back of the left atrium, and the connecting vein is ligated. The results of surgery are good with few long term complications although early postoperative pulmonary venous obstruction rarely occurs.[116]

Tricuspid atresia with excessive pulmonary blood flow

Anatomy and physiology

There is absence of the right atrioventricular connection and the great vessels are normally related. Systemic venous return passes across the atrial septum to mix with pulmonary venous blood in the left atrium. Flow to the lungs is via the left ventricle, across a large ventricular septal defect to the right ventricle and pulmonary arteries (Fig. 21.22). As the ventricular septal defect is large, pulmonary blood flow is excessive when pulmonary vascular resistance falls.

Clinical features

These infants present with mild cyanosis and congestive cardiac failure after 2 weeks of age (Table 21.9). There may be a soft pulmonary ejection murmur caused by increased blood flow across the pulmonary valve.

Investigations

The electrocardiogram shows a superior axis, and P waves are prominent if the right atrium is enlarged. Chest radiography shows plethoric lung fields (Table 21.10). Echocardiography shows the anatomical features necessary to make the diagnosis (Fig. 21.10b).[111]

Management and prognosis

As the tricuspid valve is atretic, the right ventricle can never function as a normal ventricle. Management and prognosis are those of a child with a single ventricle circulation (p. 789). Initially a pulmonary artery band will be required to limit pulmonary blood flow.

Common arterial trunk (truncus arteriosus)

This comprises about 1% of congenital heart defects.

Anatomy and physiology

The common arterial trunk fails to divide into aortic and pulmonary arteries. There is a large ventricular septal defect below the common outlet (truncal) valve, which overrides the ventricular septum. This valve is usually abnormal, and may have more than three leaflets. It may be stenotic or regurgitant. The condition is subdivided according to the origin of the pulmonary arteries from the arterial trunk (Fig. 21.25).

- Type 1 – common origin of pulmonary arteries.
- Type 2 – pulmonary arteries arise separately but adjacent, from posterior of the trunk.
- Type 3 – pulmonary arteries arise separately, from lateral walls of the trunk.

Aortic coarctation or interruption is occasionally present.

Clinical features

Cyanosis is mild, and congestive cardiac failure occurs after 2 weeks of age due to the high pulmonary blood flow (Table 21.9). Clinical signs include brisk pulses, an ejection click from the abnormal valve and cardiac failure. Systolic or early diastolic murmurs occur with truncal valve stenosis or regurgitation. Approximately 40% of children have 22q11 deletion[117] or other syndromes.

Investigations

The electrocardiogram may show biventricular hypertrophy. Chest radiography shows cardiomegaly and plethora, and > 30% have a right aortic arch. Echocardiography shows the ventricular septal defect with overriding truncal valve similar to that in tetralogy of Fallot, but the pulmonary arteries arise from the arterial trunk.[111] Cardiac catheterization is unnecessary unless there is a suspicion of irreversible pulmonary hypertension.

Management and prognosis

Cardiac failure is managed medically. Prostaglandin is necessary if there is aortic arch obstruction. The large left to right shunt and rapid development of pulmonary vascular disease make early surgery necessary. The ventricular septal defect is closed and a valved conduit is placed from the right ventricle to the pulmonary artery branches after they are detached from the trunk.

Mortality is in the region of 5%[118] and prognosis is worse if there is a stenotic or regurgitant valve, aortic arch obstruction, low weight or older age at intervention. The right ventricle to pulmonary artery conduit will need to be replaced as the child grows. Late mortality is approximately 10%.[118,119]

PRESENTATION WITH CARDIOVASCULAR COLLAPSE

Heart disease, especially left heart obstruction, should always be considered in a shocked infant. It is important to feel all the pulses and examine the heart size on chest radiography. Cardiomegaly is usually present with cardiac causes and rare in other conditions.[120] If there is any suspicion of a cardiac lesion, echocardiography is indicated. Other causes of collapse in the neonate include sepsis,[120] respiratory and metabolic disease.

Common cardiac causes are the left heart obstructive lesions. Supraventricular tachycardia should be considered if the heart rate is over 250 beats per minute.[100] Myocardial disease such as cardiomyopathy (p. 802), either dilated or hypertrophic, myocardial ischaemia following perinatal distress and anomalous origin of the left coronary artery (p. 792) are rare causes. Pericardial effusion with tamponade occasionally presents in this way.

Left heart obstructive lesions

These are due to severe aortic coarctation or arch interruption, hypoplastic left heart or critical aortic stenosis. Mitral stenosis and pulmonary vein stenosis are rare in isolation. Obstructed total anomalous pulmonary venous connection can present with precipitous cardiovascular collapse, but severe cyanosis and respiratory distress due to pulmonary venous hypertension is usually the dominant feature. Pulmonary venous hypertension does not occur to the same degree in left heart obstructive lesions, since the left atrium usually decompresses via the oval foramen into the right atrium.

The importance of the arterial duct with critical left heart obstructive lesions

At birth the arterial duct is widely patent. When there is obstruction within the left heart or aorta, the right ventricle is able to supply blood (albeit deoxygenated) to the descending aorta, and the femoral pulses will be palpable.

- Infants with coarctation or arch interruption usually have a lower saturation in the legs than the right arm.
- In severe aortic stenosis or left heart hypoplasia, the deoxygenated blood from the duct also travels retrogradely around the arch, into the head, arms and down the ascending aorta to the coronary arteries. Oximetry in all limbs will reveal deoxygenation.

When the arterial duct closes

Since neonates are used to lower blood oxygen levels before birth, they remain well until the duct closes. Flow in the aorta falls, with decreased perfusion of vital organs, and the deterioration is often dramatic. This effect is made worse in infants with coarctation, as ductal tissue around the coarctation site in the aorta produces further narrowing.

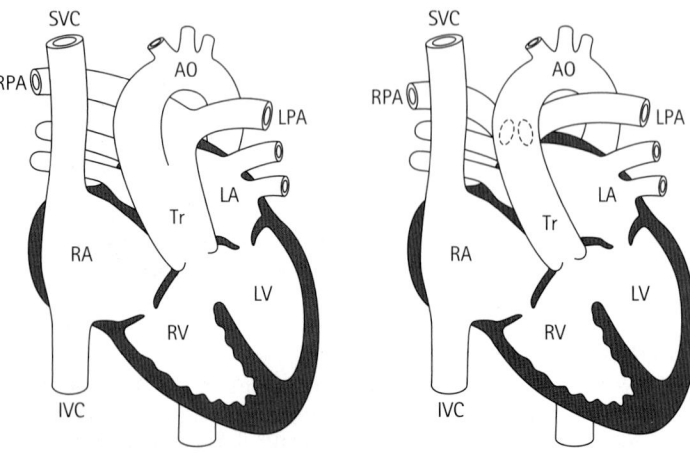

(a)   (b)

Fig. 21.25 Common arterial trunk: (a) in type 1 the pulmonary arteries arise from the truncus (Tr) with a common origin; (b) in type 2 the pulmonary arteries arise separately from the back. In type 3 (not shown) the pulmonary arteries are more widely separate at their origins and arise posteriorly/laterally from the trunk.

Clinical features

All the left heart obstructions share common clinical features related to duct closure (Table 21.9). Presentation is usually within 48 hours of birth and symptoms include poor feeding, lethargy and pallor. Deterioration is extremely rapid with poor peripheral perfusion resulting in delayed capillary refill time and mottled skin. The pulses are poor and the blood pressure is low. The right ventricle is forceful and murmurs are unremarkable. The infant is usually tachypneic with grunting respiration, the liver is markedly enlarged and urine output is poor.

Investigations

There is a marked metabolic acidosis with abnormal renal and hepatic function, which may result in an abnormal coagulation profile. The electrocardiogram shows right ventricular hypertrophy, and there may be ST depression in the left precordial leads from myocardial ischemia. Chest radiography shows cardiomegaly with a combination of pulmonary plethora and edema. The echocardiographic findings are described under the individual lesions.

Management

Intravenous prostaglandin causes the arterial duct to dilate but the precipitous collapse means that these infants often require endotracheal intubation, inotropic and intensive support. Death can occur if acidosis and renal dysfunction are not corrected. The specific management of individual conditions is discussed below.

Aortic coarctation and interruption of the aortic arch

Aortic coarctation accounts for 5% of congenital heart disease. Interrupted aortic arch is extremely rare.

Anatomy and physiology

Narrowing of the aortic arch commonly occurs at its isthmus between the left subclavian artery and the origin of the arterial duct. This is usually due to a shelf-like obstruction but it can be tubular (Fig. 21.26) and is sometimes associated with hypoplasia of the transverse aorta. About 70% of infants with a coarctation have at least one other associated lesion. The most common are ventricular septal defect, left ventricular outflow obstruction and mitral valve anomalies.[121]

Interruption of the aortic arch is a complete occlusion, which can be classified according to the position. Type A is beyond the left subclavian, type B between the left common carotid and the left subclavian arteries and type C between the carotid arteries.

Clinical features

Most infants present in the first 2 weeks with rapid onset of cardiac failure progressing to cardiovascular collapse as described above. In milder forms the presentation is more insidious, with failure to thrive and cardiac failure. The right arm pulse is strong unless the cardiac function is poor, there is coincident aortic stenosis, or the right subclavian artery has an abnormal origin below the coarctation (aberrant right subclavian artery). The left arm pulse is weak if the left subclavian artery

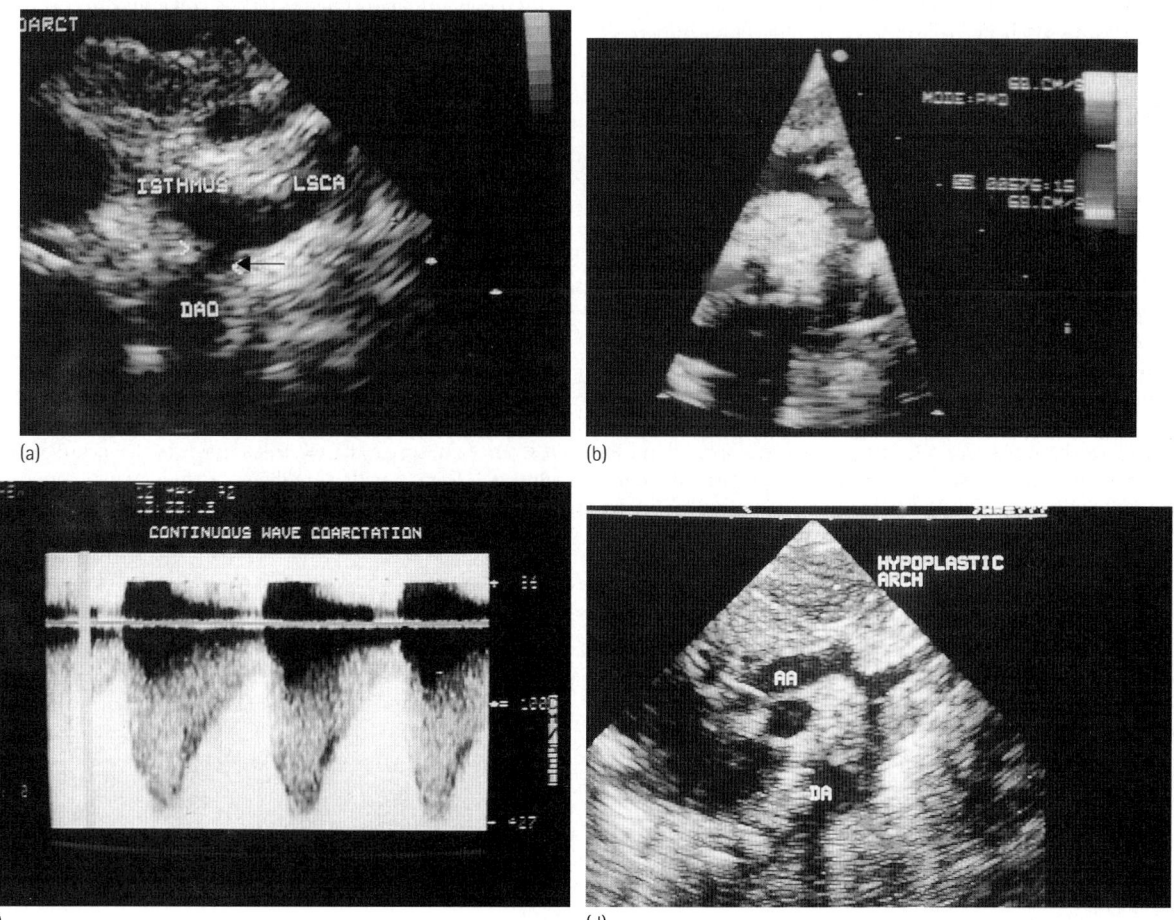

(a)   (b)

(c)   (d)

Fig. 21.26 (a) High parasternal greatly magnified view of the isthmus of the aorta, the origin of the left subclavian artery (LSCA) and the descending aorta (DAO). Narrowed area of coarctation is arrowed. (b) Suprasternal view of a baby with coarctation of the aorta. The arch is of reasonable size and the area of coarctation is only clearly identified by the presence of turbulence on the color flow map. (c) Continuous wave Doppler from descending aorta via the suprasternal approach. The classic continuous flow which is seen in coarctation is present. The peak velocity is high and the diastolic velocity never returns to the baseline. (d) Hypoplastic aorta arch in a child who also had coarctation of the aorta. Coarctectomy has been carried out, but there is still isthmal narrowing. AA, ascending aorta; DA, descending aorta. (From Skinner et al 2000[23].)

arises after the coarctation. The femoral pulses are absent. The right arm blood pressure is high and the blood pressure in the leg is more than 10 mmHg lower. Oscillometric techniques (Dynamap) are not reliable in this setting to record blood pressure in the legs and Doppler sphygmomanometry is more accurate. The right ventricular impulse is prominent and there may be a murmur of mitral regurgitation if the left ventricle is dilated. Murmurs can also be due to associated lesions. Turner syndrome should be considered in girls with coarctation.[79] Over 50% of infants with interruption of the aortic arch have 22q11 deletion.[108,122]

Investigations

In addition to the investigations described, echocardiography defines the lesion. The right ventricle and pulmonary artery are enlarged. In infants with coarctation, an area of narrowing with turbulent flow is seen on color Doppler. The Doppler flow pattern through the coarctation has a characteristic 'saw-tooth' appearance with flow continuing into diastole (diastolic tail) (Fig. 21.26). Left ventricular dysfunction may be present. Associated lesions must be assessed, together with the size of the arterial duct. Interruption of the aortic arch will be visible on echocardiography.

Management and prognosis

Surgery is performed when the infant has been stabilized and the acidosis corrected.

Infants with coarctation usually have repair through a lateral thoracotomy, with excision of the coarctation, ligation of the patent arterial duct and end-to-end anastomosis of the aorta. Cardiopulmonary bypass is required for severe hypoplasia or interruption of the transverse aortic arch. Closure of the associated ventricular septal defect is usually performed.

Prognosis depends on the extent of the aortic obstruction and the associated cardiac[121] and noncardiac lesions. Re-coarctation can occur so long term follow-up is essential. Antibiotic prophylaxis is necessary.

Hypoplastic left heart
Anatomy

This is a group of conditions characterized by underdevelopment of the left ventricle, with mitral and aortic atresia or stenosis to a degree that the left ventricle cannot sustain a systemic cardiac output. It accounts for 4% of congenital heart disease. The ascending aorta is small, and most infants also have coarctation. The milder forms overlap with the severest forms of critical aortic stenosis. Pulmonary venous return is diverted across the oval foramen to the right atrium and ventricle and flow in the aorta is dependent on the arterial duct. As the duct supplies both the systemic and pulmo-

nary circulations, the balance between flow to the body and lungs is critical.[123]

Clinical features

The infant presents acutely with profound collapse (Table 21.9) when the arterial duct closes as described above.

Investigations

The electrocardiogram shows right axis deviation and low left ventricular forces with small R waves in V6. Echocardiography reveals a small left ventricle with stenotic or atretic mitral and aortic valves. The aortic arch is hypoplastic. The right atrium and ventricle are enlarged, as is the pulmonary artery.

Management and prognosis

An increasing number of infants, often with an antenatal diagnosis of this condition, are started on prostaglandin infusion soon after birth. Many are stable enough to undergo the high risk, palliative Norwood operation (Fig. 21.27) in the first days. The aorta is enlarged using part of the pulmonary artery and the distal pulmonary artery is detached and supplied by a modified Blalock–Taussig shunt. Recent modification, using a right ventricle to pulmonary artery conduit instead of a shunt, has improved prognosis.[124] Further surgery is similar to that for other children with a single ventricle circulation (p. 789). One year survival is up to 60% and 10 year as high as 50%.[125,126]

Critical aortic stenosis

This represents approximately 10% of children with aortic stenosis.[127]

Anatomy and physiology

The aortic valve is thickened, dysplastic and often unicuspid. The right heart is enlarged as it supplies both the pulmonary and systemic circulations through the arterial duct.

Clinical features

These are similar to infants presenting with a hypoplastic left heart. A soft ejection murmur may be audible in the aortic area. An aortic ejection click is seldom audible, as the valve is usually thickened and immobile.

Investigations

These are the same as those described for other infants with left heart obstructive lesions, but there may be left ventricular hypertrophy with a strain pattern on the electrocardiogram. Echocardiography distinguishes it from the other conditions, demonstrating an adequate sized left ventricle, which is either hypertrophied or dilated. The function is usually reduced. The aortic valve is thickened with restricted opening,

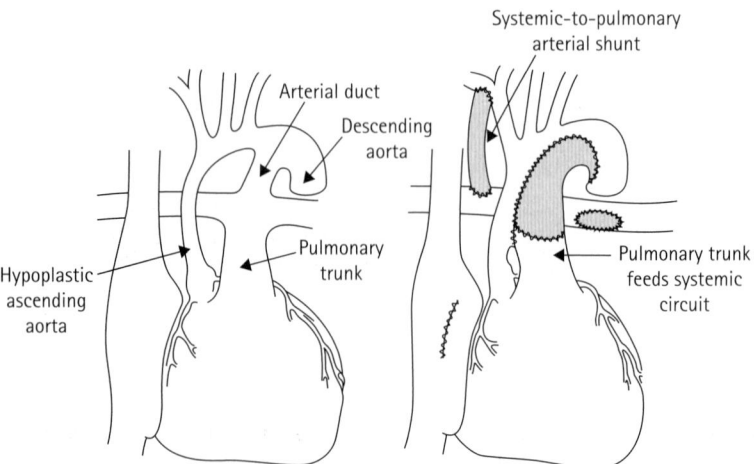

Fig. 21.27 These diagrams show the arrangement of the circulations before and after the classic Norwood procedure, which is the first stage of palliative surgery.

Systemic-to-pulmonary arterial shunt

Arterial duct

Descending aorta

Pulmonary trunk

Hypoplastic ascending aorta

Pulmonary trunk feeds systemic circuit

and turbulence is seen on color Doppler. The Doppler velocity across the valve may be increased, or reduced because of poor ventricular function.

Management and prognosis

Once the infant has been resuscitated and stabilized, transcatheter balloon aortic valvuloplasty or open surgical valvotomy is performed. The results from the two procedures are similar[34,36] but recurrence of the stenosis occurs, requiring further intervention later in life.[127]

PRESENTATION WITH CARDIAC FAILURE WITHOUT CYANOSIS

A number of conditions present in early infancy with cardiac failure. These children usually present outside the neonatal period and are discussed later. These conditions include ventricular septal defect (p. 781), atrioventricular septal defect (p. 783), aortopulmonary window (p. 785), anomalous origin of the left coronary artery (p. 792) and persistent arterial duct (p. 783), which is also covered in the neonatal section. Occasionally infants with cardiomyopathy (p. 802) present in the neonatal period and failure can also be caused by supraventricular tachycardia (p. 793).

PRESENTATION WITH AN ASSOCIATED LESION OR SYNDROME

The more common syndromes associated with congenital heart disease are shown in Table 21.5. Congenital heart disease should always be considered in infants with a syndrome or dysmorphology. These are discussed in the section on the etiology of congenital heart disease (p. 765).

PRESENTATION WITH AN ASYMPTOMATIC MURMUR

Innocent murmurs are common in the first few days, usually related to pulmonary or ductal flow. They are of lower pitch than pathological murmurs, varying with time and heart rate. Physiological branch pulmonary artery stenosis, occurring after duct closure, produces a pulmonary systolic murmur audible in the back. Though more common in the preterm, it can occur in term infants and is usually benign, resolving in a few months.[128]

Less than 5% of neonates with a significant murmur will have life-threatening heart disease.[129] Congenital heart lesions that cause a systolic murmur audible from birth are aortic and pulmonary stenosis and tetralogy of Fallot. Small ventricular septal defects are the most common single lesion causing an asymptomatic murmur. This becomes audible as the right ventricular pressure falls, with postnatal reduction in pulmonary arterial pressure. A patent arterial duct generates a murmur if there is some constriction, allowing the aortic pressure to be higher than pulmonary arterial pressure, but still enough flow through it to generate a noise. In the preterm infant a large left to right ductal shunt typically has a systolic rather than a continuous murmur because the aortic and pulmonary arterial pressures are similar in diastole. Tricuspid or mitral regurgitation causes a pansystolic murmur, most commonly in myocardial ischaemia following perinatal distress but can represent an isolated valve lesion or be part of a more complex condition such as an atrioventricular septal defect. A diastolic murmur is always pathological, most commonly due to a large left to right shunt later in the first month of life.

MISCELLANEOUS COMPLEX LESIONS

Congenitally corrected transposition of the great arteries

This rare lesion accounts for less than 1% of congenital heart disease.

Anatomy and physiology

This condition is characterized by discordance of both the atrioventricular and the ventriculo-arterial connection (Fig. 21.28a). The deoxygenated right atrial blood passes through the mitral valve into a

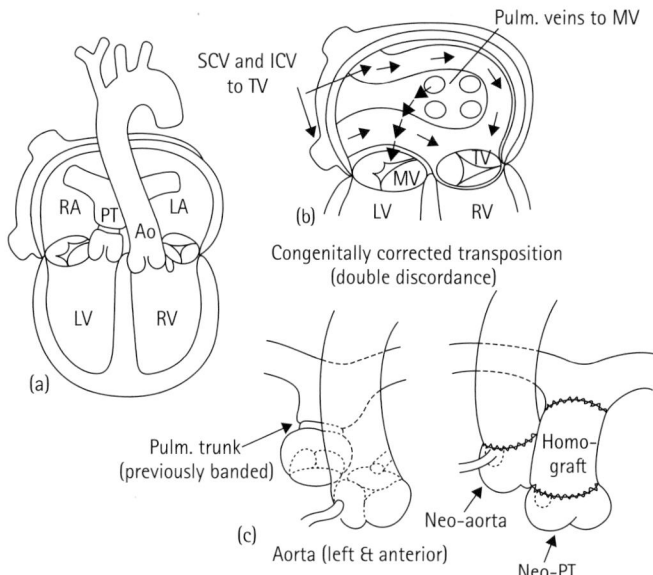

Fig. 21.28 The steps involved in the so-called 'double switch procedure' involve, first, (a) banding of the pulmonary trunk (PT) unless associated lesions have already 'prepared' the left ventricle. (b) An atrial redirection procedure is then combined with (c) an arterial switch. This then produces both physiological and anatomical correction. Ao, aorta; LA, left atrium; LV, left ventricle; MV, mitral valve; Pulm., pulmonary; RA, right atrium; RV, right ventricle; SCV and ICV, superior and inferior caval veins; TV, tricuspid valve.

morphological left ventricle, from which the pulmonary artery arises. The oxygenated pulmonary venous blood passes from the left atrium, through the tricuspid valve, into the morphological right ventricle and thence into the aorta. Thus, although there is transposition, the anatomical fault is functionally corrected by the presence of atrioventricular discordance. The aorta is usually located anterior and to the left of the pulmonary artery. Ventricular septal defect is the most frequently associated lesion and commonly occurs with pulmonary stenosis. This may result in cyanosis from shunting of deoxygenated blood into the aorta. A few patients have no other lesions, and remain pink. The condition is commonly associated with dextrocardia.

Clinical presentation and course

Associated cardiac lesions usually dictate the clinical presentation and course. If a large ventricular septal defect is present, heart failure develops early. Those infants with a ventricular septal defect and pulmonary stenosis present with cyanosis, and clinically resemble tetralogy of Fallot. In the absence of associated defects the condition may not be recognized for many years, but left-sided atrioventricular valve (tricuspid) regurgitation may progress. Tachyarrhythmias and complete heart block are common.

Investigations

Inversion of the ventricles alters the direction of ventricular septal depolarization and produces the characteristic electrocardiographic finding of the absence of Q waves in V5 and V6, and the presence of Q waves in V4R or V1. The electrocardiogram may show heart block, arrhythmias or Wolff–Parkinson–White syndrome. Radiologically, the condition is suspected by the presence of a straight upper left heart border produced by the left-sided anterior aorta. Echocardiography will determine the abnormal atrioventricular and ventriculo-arterial connections and define any associated abnormality.

Management and prognosis

The management is usually that of the associated lesion. Severely cyanosed infants require a systemic to pulmonary shunt. Infants with heart failure secondary to a large ventricular septal defect require pulmonary artery banding. Closure of the ventricular septal defect is associated with a high incidence of complete heart block (30%) and significant mortality. Because of gradual deterioration of the systemic right ventricle and progressive tricuspid regurgitation, surgery can be performed to restore the left ventricle to pump to the systemic circulation. This can be achieved by means of the double switch operation (Figs 21.28b, c).

Prognosis depends on associated lesions and presence of heart block. Anatomic repair (double switch) significantly improves prognosis.[130]

Double inlet (single) ventricle

This condition is more common than previously recognized and may account for up to 2–3% of congenital heart disease. Both atria are connected to a dominant ventricle (Fig. 21.10c), usually the left ventricle, the other ventricle being rudimentary (Fig. 21.29).

The main ventricle usually has the morphology of a left ventricle with two inlet valves, and the right ventricle is a small outflow chamber. The ventriculo-arterial connection can vary, but most commonly the aorta arises from the small right ventricle, and the pulmonary artery from the left ventricle. The small right ventricle communicates with the left ventricle via a ventricular septal defect. The severity of any associated coarctation or pulmonary stenosis determines the initial presentation and treatment. Further management is the same as for other children with a single ventricle circulation (p. 789).

Double outlet right ventricle

Anatomy and physiology. The aorta and pulmonary artery both arise from the right ventricle. There are two common types. In one variation there is a large ventricular septal defect, with no pulmonary stenosis. This is commonly associated with a posterior pulmonary artery and an anterior aorta. The ventricular septal defect is related to the large pulmonary valve and has obvious similarities to transposition with a large ventricular septal defect (known as the Taussig–Bing malformation). In the other variation there is a large ventricular septal defect with pulmonary stenosis and the features mimic the tetralogy of Fallot.

Clinical features

Depending upon the position of the great vessels and associated lesions, the clinical features mimic other lesions such as transposition, ventricular septal defect or tetralogy of Fallot. Echocardiography defines the anatomy and excludes other conditions.

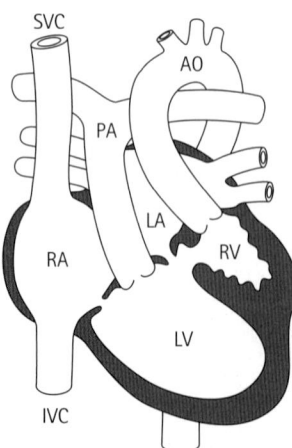

Fig. 21.29   Double inlet ventricle or single ventricle. In the most common variety as here, both atrioventricular valves connect to a morphologically normal left ventricle (LV) and the right ventricle is represented by a small rudimentary outflow chamber from which the aorta arises. There is usually arterioventricular discordance.

Management

Infants with high pulmonary blood flow require pulmonary artery banding whereas those with severe cyanosis, because of restrictive pulmonary blood flow, may require a Blalock–Taussig shunt. Definitive repair depends upon the site of the ventricular septal defect. Occasionally, only an intracardiac patch may be required, but in other children arterial switch and closure of a ventricular septal defect or major reconstruction with the use of a conduit may be necessary.

ABNORMAL CARDIAC POSITIONS

Dextrocardia refers only to the situation in which more than half the heart is situated in the right chest. It does not necessarily have implications for the anatomy of the heart itself. Dextrocardia may thus be a primary abnormality of the heart or secondary to other thoracic pathology. Primary dextrocardia is often associated with abnormal positions of the abdominal organs. Complete situs inversus refers to the mirror image arrangement of the organs. It occurs in approximately 1 per 10 000 of the population and over 90% of these individuals have a normal heart. When dextrocardia is associated with normal abdominal visceral arrangements (i.e. the stomach on the left), or ambiguous visceral arrangement, the heart is usually abnormal. Malformations include atrioventricular discordance, univentricular heart, anomalous pulmonary venous drainage and pulmonary atresia. About one third of patients with asplenia or polysplenia have dextrocardia. The combination of situs inversus, bronchiectasis and paranasal sinusitis (Kartagener syndrome) occurs in 10–15% of patients with mirror-image dextrocardia.

Mesocardia indicates the position of the heart in the center of the thorax, prominent neither to the right nor to the left. It is usually not recognized clinically and is apparent only from chest radiography. The term *levocardia* need be used only when the left-sided heart is associated with abnormal visceral situs.

The possibility of abnormal cardiac position should always be remembered. The cardiac apex and impulse should be palpated over the right chest if it is not apparent on the left side, and heart sounds should be auscultated on both sides. Abnormal location of the liver edge in the midline or the left side, or the stomach resonance on the right side of the abdomen suggests abnormal abdominal situs, often associated with cardiac malposition. Chest radiography confirms the position of the heart. The morphology of the bronchi will suggest the thoracic situs, and the position of the stomach and liver the abdominal situs. Abnormal cardiac or visceral situs is an indication for cardiac review. The electrocardiogram should be performed with the addition of right-sided chest leads (V3R to V7R). In dextrocardia, the QRS complexes are characteristically taller in the right chest leads and become progressively smaller from V3 to V7 in the left-sided chest leads. A negative P wave in lead I indicates reversed atrial arrangement (atrial situs inversus), but does not specify the position of the heart in the chest. Echocardiography provides the best non-invasive means of identifying the arrangements and anatomy of the atria, ventricles and great vessels and any associated malformations.

Mesocardia and levocardia, with abnormal visceral situs, are commonly associated with asplenia or polysplenia.[131] When asplenia or polysplenia is suspected, splenic ultrasound and examination of the peripheral blood for Howell–Jolly bodies are appropriate. Patients with asplenia should receive pneumococcal vaccine and prophylactic antibiotic therapy.

THE INFANT AND CHILD WITH CONGENITAL HEART DISEASE

The range of cardiac lesions, together with their presentation and management, is somewhat different from that of neonates. However, there is overlap with a number of cyanotic and acyanotic lesions presenting in infancy. Acyanotic lesions fall broadly into two groups: those with heart disease that causes an increased volume load, and those with a lesion that results in pressure loading of the heart.

ACYANOTIC HEART DISEASE WITH INCREASED VOLUME LOAD

Increased volume load is usually caused by a left to right shunt, such as an atrial or ventricular septal defect, persistent arterial duct or atrioventricular septal defect. Rare causes include aorticopulmonary window and large arteriovenous fistula. Valvar regurgitation also produces an increased volume load to the heart.

Ventricular septal defect
Anatomy
Ventricular septal defects are usually small and occur in any part of the membranous or muscular interventricular septum (Fig. 21.30). Those in the membranous septum are called perimembranous, as they extend into the adjacent muscle. They are the most common variant and are usually single. They can extend:

- Posteriorly into the muscular inlet between the atrioventricular valves.
- Inferiorly into the trabecular portion of the interventricular septum.
- Anteriorly into the muscular outlet between the right and left ventricular outflow tracts (as in tetralogy of Fallot). Rarely outlet defects are associated with prolapse of the aortic valve into the defect, causing regurgitation.

Muscular defects are completely surrounded by muscle. They occur in the inlet, outlet or trabecular portions of the muscular septum, where they are frequently multiple.

Ventricular septal defects occur in association with other cardiac lesions in 22% of patients.[132] These are most commonly pulmonary stenosis, aortic valve prolapse, atrial septal defect, patent arterial duct or coarctation.

Physiology
The clinical features and prognosis depend on the size and number of defects, and the volume of blood passing into the right ventricle. Small defects limit the shunt, so pulmonary artery pressure and blood flow are close to normal (restrictive defect). If the defect is large, left and right ventricular pressures are equal (nonrestrictive defect) and the volume of shunt depends on the systemic and pulmonary vascular resistances. The fall in pulmonary vascular resistance after birth is delayed and if the pulmonary blood flow remains excessive, irreversible pulmonary hypertension develops (p. 805).

Small ventricular septal defect
Clinical features
Infants present with an asymptomatic murmur, audible in the first few weeks of life, as the pulmonary vascular resistance falls. A perimembra-

nous defect produces a loud, harsh pansystolic murmur at the fourth left intercostal space, usually associated with a thrill. It radiates to the apex and back. A muscular defect gives a short early systolic murmur localized to the fourth left intercostal space that disappears late in systole as the defect closes with ventricular contraction. The rest of the cardiovascular examination is normal unless there are other cardiac lesions.

Differential diagnosis of small perimembranous ventricular septal defect includes mitral regurgitation, where the murmur radiates to the axilla, and tricuspid regurgitation, where the murmur varies in intensity with respiration. The long ejection systolic murmur of tetralogy of Fallot, or severe subaortic aortic stenosis, can mimic a pansystolic murmur and the site of maximum intensity is similar. In severe aortic or pulmonary valve stenosis, the site of maximum intensity is in the second intercostal space.

Differential diagnosis of small muscular ventricular septal defect includes innocent vibratory murmur, mitral valve prolapse, bicuspid aortic valve, mild aortic or pulmonary stenosis and atrial septal defect.

Investigations
The electrocardiogram is normal and chest radiography is not indicated. Echocardiogram confirms the diagnosis. Perimembranous defects often have a small aneurysm of the membranous septum. Color Doppler flow also identifies small muscular defects. The velocity across the defect will be over 4 m/s, indicating that the right ventricular pressure is normal. Echocardiography will also identify additional lesions.[132]

Management and prognosis
Over two thirds of muscular defects and almost one third of perimembranous defects close spontaneously within 6 years.[133] Initially it is necessary to confirm that the pulmonary artery pressure is normal. Thereafter the child is reviewed at infrequent intervals until it has closed. This is most likely in early childhood, but closure into adult life has been reported.[134] Children should be encouraged to lead a normal life. Surgical closure is indicated for patients with aortic regurgitation caused by prolapse of a leaflet into the defect[135] and following endocarditis. A small number of patients (5%) develop subaortic stenosis or right ventricular outflow obstruction (8%). Surgery may be indicated for these or other lesions. Late arrhythmias have been reported[134,136] and sudden death has been described. Antibiotic prophylaxis is necessary for procedures until the defect has closed. Long term survival is excellent with a 96% 25 year survival.[136]

Large ventricular septal defects
Clinical features
Infants present at 2–8 weeks of age as pulmonary vascular resistance falls and blood flow increases. They develop symptoms of heart failure and recurrent respiratory infections. The infant is tachypneic with intercostal and subcostal recession. The left precordium is prominent with a right ventricular lift and displaced apex indicating biventricular enlargement. A thrill may be associated with the pansystolic murmur that is maximal at the fourth left intercostal space and radiates to the apex and the back. A mid-diastolic murmur is caused by excessive pulmonary blood flow returning to the left atrium, resulting in turbulent flow across the mitral valve. It is present at the apex but may be inaudible because of tachypnea and tachycardia. A gallop rhythm may be heard and the liver is enlarged. Some infants, particularly those with Down syndrome, have minimal symptoms because persistently high pulmonary vascular resistance prevents excessive blood flow. Over time, the pulmonary vascular resistance increases, symptoms disappear, the murmur becomes softer and the pulmonary component of the second heart sound louder. Older infants and children have signs of established pulmonary hypertension (p. 805), with reversal of the shunt causing cyanosis (Eisenmenger syndrome).

Differential diagnosis includes a large persistent arterial duct or complete atrioventricular septal defect. Rare conditions include aorticopulmonary window, cardiomyopathy, severe mitral regurgitation, anomalous origin of the left coronary artery from the pulmonary artery,

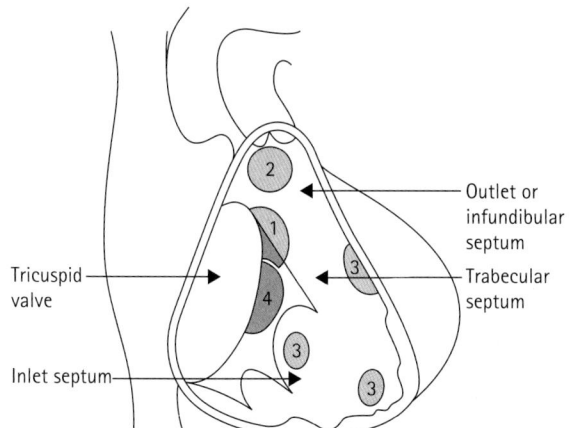

Fig. 21.30 Types of ventricular septal defect: (1) perimembranous; (2) outlet or subarterial; (3) trabecular; (4) inlet.

total anomalous pulmonary venous drainage and complex lesions with unrestricted pulmonary blood flow.

Investigations

The electrocardiogram shows biventricular hypertrophy.[13] The QRS axis is usually normal, but children with inlet or multiple muscular defects may have left axis deviation. The presence of other cardiac lesions may modify the electrocardiogram. When pulmonary hypertension develops, right ventricular hypertrophy is dominant. Chest radiography shows cardiomegaly with biventricular and left atrial enlargement with plethora. As pulmonary hypertension develops, the cardiac shadow becomes smaller, the proximal pulmonary arteries larger and the peripheral vessels less prominent ('peripheral pruning').

Echocardiography identifies the site, size and number of defects[137] and other cardiac lesions. Enlargement of the left atrium, left ventricle and pulmonary artery indicates a large shunt. The Doppler velocity across the defect may be low, reflecting an elevated right ventricular pressure. Cardiac catheterization is rarely performed, as the information necessary for monitoring and surgical closure can be obtained from echocardiography.[138] It is indicated if there is concern about irreversible pulmonary hypertension, especially in a child who presents late, or to obtain information about other lesions. The increase in oxygen saturation between the systemic veins and pulmonary artery allows calculation of pulmonary blood flow, which is more than twice systemic. Measurement of the pulmonary artery pressure allows assessment of pulmonary hypertension. A high concentration of inspired oxygen or nitric oxide will indicate whether pulmonary hypertension is reversible. Angiography in the left ventricle demonstrates the site, size and number of defects. Further angiography may be performed to evaluate other lesions.

Management and prognosis

Treatment is initially for heart failure (p. 762). Nasogastric feeding may help to achieve adequate intake. Added calories are beneficial, but poor weight gain is also due to increased energy expenditure.[2] Limiting the volume of feeds is only necessary for intractable heart failure. Children with large defects can develop pulmonary hypertension in infancy. Surgery is indicated between 2 and 5 months of age to prevent this, and to promote growth. The operative mortality is less than 5%, with a similar risk of re-operation. Children with more complex lesions such as multiple muscular defects or chronic lung disease may be unsuitable for primary repair. This may also not be possible if facilities for infant surgery are unavailable. Pulmonary artery banding is palliative, limiting pulmonary blood flow and preventing irreversible pulmonary hypertension until the defects become smaller or the other problems improve. Transcatheter device closure is available for muscular defects that are difficult to close surgically.[43]

Some children have moderate sized defects without pulmonary hypertension. Intervention can be delayed if weight gain is satisfactory and there are signs of closure on the echocardiogram. If the pulmonary blood flow remains more than twice systemic, the defect should be closed because of the late development of pulmonary hypertension or chronic volume loading of the heart. Transcatheter devices are being developed for use in these children.[28,49]

Rarely a large defect will close spontaneously by apposition of part of the tricuspid valve or prolapse of an aortic leaflet into the defect. Muscular defects are more likely, and outlet defects less likely, to close spontaneously. Antibiotic prophylaxis is essential for procedures until the defect is closed. The long term survival after repair of a ventricular septal defect is excellent, with few late complications.[136]

Atrial septal defect

Anatomy

Atrial septal defects are classified according to their position in the atrial septum (Fig. 21.31). The most common type is the secundum defect, situated in the region of the oval fossa. It is usually single, but may consist of multiple small defects (fenestrated). Sinus venosus

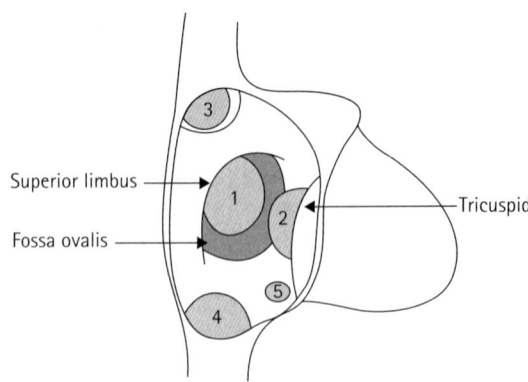

Fig. 21.31   Types of atrial septal defect: (1) ostium secundum; (2) ostium primum; (3) superior sinus venosus; (4) inferior sinus venosus; (5) coronary sinus.

defects occur in the superior part of the atrial septum and are associated with partial anomalous venous drainage of the right upper pulmonary vein to the superior vena cava or right atrium. Ostium primum defects, at the lower margin of the interatrial septum, are partial atrioventricular septal defects (p. 783). Rarely defects are related to the inferior vena cava or coronary sinus. Occasionally there can be an almost complete absence of the atrial septum (common atrium). A patent oval foramen is normal in infancy and occasionally persists into adult life.

Physiology

The volume of the left to right shunt depends on the size of the defect and the relative compliance of the ventricles. This determines the size of the right atrium, right ventricle, pulmonary artery and left atrium that receive the excessive blood flow. Pulmonary hypertension does not develop until adult life. A patent oval foramen is not usually hemodynamically significant, but if the right atrial pressure is increased due to another cardiac abnormality, right to left shunting can occur with systemic desaturation. It may also be a cause of paradoxical systemic emboli.

Clinical features

Most children present between 1 and 5 years of age with an asymptomatic murmur. Rarely this condition is familial. Few have failure to thrive or symptoms of heart failure. The right ventricular enlargement results in a slight precordial bulge and diffuse impulse on palpation. Because of excessive pulmonary blood flow, the pulmonary component of the second heart sound is delayed and does not become single during expiration (fixed splitting). This excessive blood flow also accounts for the murmurs, as flow across the actual defect is silent. The ejection systolic murmur in the pulmonary area is due to flow across the pulmonary valve and is usually audible in the back. The mid-diastolic murmur at the fourth left intercostal space is caused by increased flow across the tricuspid valve.

Differential diagnosis includes innocent murmur, mild pulmonary or aortic stenosis, aortic coarctation and persistent arterial duct with pulmonary hypertension.

Investigations

The electrocardiogram shows incomplete right bundle branch block in over 90% of patients, but this is present in 10% of normal children. Chest radiography shows right atrial, right ventricular and pulmonary artery enlargement with plethora. Echocardiography confirms the size and type of defect, together with a large right atrium, right ventricle and pulmonary artery. The velocity across the pulmonary valve is usually normal, but may be increased due to flow. Cardiac catheterization is unnecessary for diagnosis, except for sinus venosus defects when the pulmonary venous drainage is unclear. Pulmonary artery pressures are normal or slightly elevated. The increase in oxygen saturation between systemic veins and pulmonary artery allows calculation of the left to right shunt. Angiography can identify the site of pulmonary venous drainage. Transesophageal echocardiography also defines the defect and is particularly useful in identifying the pulmonary veins in sinus venosus defects.

Management and prognosis

The majority of secundum defects seen in the neonatal period will close,[139] as will those smaller than 6mm in diameter.[140] Defects more than 8 mm are unlikely to close. It is now possible to close central defects by transcatheter route with various devices.[43,141] This technique carries a low risk in selected patients and results in a high closure rate that is comparable with surgery.[45,46,48] Surgical closure is either by direct suture or patch. Mortality is less than 1%, with a 10% chance of post-cardiotomy syndrome with pericardial effusion, which usually resolves with anti-inflammatory treatment. Closure during early childhood results in long term survival similar to the general population.[142] Closure after 7 years of age results in a progressive increase in the risk of late supraventricular tachycardia, because of chronic right atrial dilatation. Pulmonary hypertension may develop in adult life. Infective endocarditis is rare, and antibiotic prophylaxis for procedures is controversial.[60,62]

Patent arterial duct

Anatomy

The arterial duct connects the pulmonary artery and descending aorta. It closes in the first few days of life by smooth muscle contraction. This is delayed in premature infants (Ch. 12), those with respiratory or cardiac disease, and infants born at high altitudes. It also remains open if there is an abnormality of the duct wall. It may coexist with other cardiac defects. In the presence of inadequate systemic or pulmonary blood flow, it provides a temporary conduit to compensate for the lesion.

Physiology

Flow across an arterial duct depends on its size and the difference between the systemic and pulmonary vascular resistances. The duct is usually constricted and the pulmonary arterial pressure is lower than systemic, producing continuous systolic and diastolic flow. If it remains large, pulmonary arterial and aortic pressures equalize, and flow depends on the relative resistances. The increased pulmonary blood flow results in enlargement of the left atrium and ventricle. A large shunt causes pulmonary hypertension and flow becomes limited to systole or even reversed (Eisenmenger syndrome).

Small patent arterial duct

Clinical features

The child usually presents with an asymptomatic murmur. A history of prematurity or maternal rubella should arouse suspicion of an arterial duct. Rarely it is familial. Pulses and precordial palpation are normal. A continuous murmur is best heard at the left infraclavicular area.

Differential diagnosis includes venous hum (varies with posture and is best heard on the right), arteriovenous connection (e.g. coronary, cerebral, chest wall or pulmonary), ventricular septal defect with aortic regurgitation, and ruptured sinus of Valsalva aneurysm.

Investigations

Electrocardiogram and chest radiography are normal. Echocardiography confirms the presence and size of the duct. There is no chamber enlargement and a high velocity flow across the duct confirms that the pulmonary artery pressure is normal. Cardiac catheterization is not necessary for diagnosis, but transcatheter closure with a device is possible.

Management and prognosis

Arterial ducts are unlikely to close spontaneously in an infant more than a few months after term. Although the risk of endocarditis is small,

closure is usually recommended as this, together with mild left ventricular volume overload, may cause long term problems.[143] Transcatheter closure, by a variety of coils or devices, is the method of choice if this is available, with a successful occlusion rate of over 98%.[43,44,144] Significant complications are rare and embolized coils or devices are usually retrieved by catheter. Alternatively, surgical ligation is performed through a lateral thoracotomy. Echocardiography has allowed visualization of ducts so tiny that they do not produce an audible murmur. The consensus is that they should not be occluded, as this is technically difficult and the risk of endocarditis is remote.[143]

Large patent arterial duct

Clinical features

Large arterial ducts are rare and symptoms are similar to those found in infants with a large ventricular septal defect. The pulse is rapid and bounding with a wide pulse pressure, and there are signs of heart failure. The heart sounds are loud and there may be a third sound at the apex. The murmur is best heard in the pulmonary area but radiates down the left sternal border. It peaks late in systole with a soft, short diastolic component. A mid-diastolic murmur at the apex is caused by increased blood flow returning from the lungs to the left atrium and causing turbulence across the mitral valve. If pulmonary hypertension is present, there will be a right ventricular lift, a short systolic murmur and a loud second heart sound. No mid-diastolic murmur will be heard because pulmonary blood flow is reduced.

Differential diagnosis includes:

- Other conditions presenting with heart failure and a continuous murmur: aorticopulmonary window, pulmonary atresia with major aorticopulmonary collateral arteries, absent pulmonary valve syndrome, arteriovenous connection.
- Other conditions presenting with heart failure and a systolic murmur: as for a large ventricular septal defect.

Investigations

The electrocardiogram shows biventricular hypertrophy.[13] Chest radiography shows left atrial, left ventricular and pulmonary artery enlargement with plethora. As pulmonary hypertension develops, the cardiac shadow becomes smaller, the proximal pulmonary arteries larger and peripheral vessels less prominent ('peripheral pruning'). Echocardiography shows left atrial, left ventricular and pulmonary artery enlargement. The right ventricle is hypertrophied if there is pulmonary hypertension. The duct can be imaged, and Doppler evaluation allows an estimation of pulmonary artery pressure.

Management and prognosis

Initial management includes the treatment of heart failure (p. 762). Surgical ligation is necessary if the duct is too large for transcatheter closure. Risks include recurrent laryngeal nerve damage, recanalization and inadvertent ligation of the left pulmonary artery. The operative mortality is less than 0.5%.[143] Transcatheter device closure is possible in infants over a year of age.[44] If the duct is closed before the development of irreversible pulmonary hypertension, the outcome is excellent.[144]

Atrioventricular septal defect

Anatomy

Atrioventricular septal defects represent a spectrum of conditions that have in common a deficiency of the atrioventricular septum and adjacent valves (Fig. 21.32). A partial atrioventricular septal defect is an ostium primum atrial septal defect. A complete atrioventricular septal defect has both atrial and ventricular components (Fig. 21.16). The atrioventricular valves are always abnormal. Partial defects usually have two separate atrioventricular valves at the same level. In the complete atrioventricular septal defect there is a single (common) atrioventricular valve. Occasionally left ventricular outflow tract obstruction[145] or a hypoplastic ventricle can complicate the clinical picture. Tetralogy of Fallot, coarctation or atrial isomerism

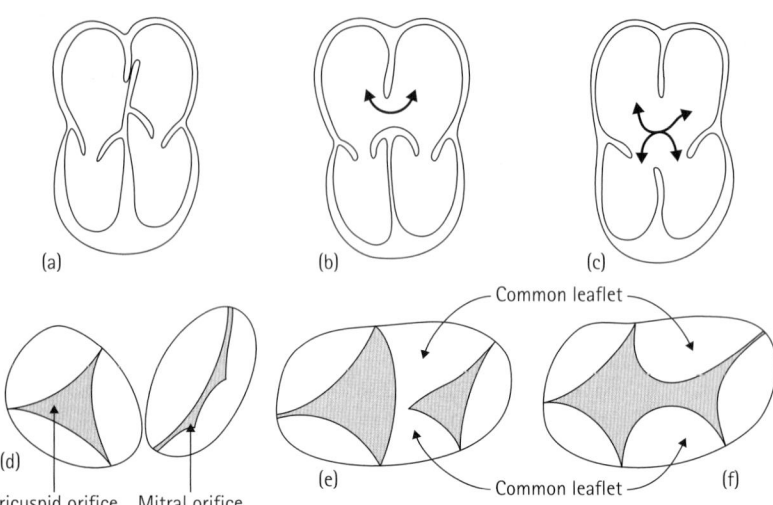

Fig. 21.32 Anatomy of the atrioventricular junction: (a and d) normal septation with no septal communication and separate valve orifices at different levels; (b and e) partial atrioventricular septal defect with atrial shunting, two valve orifices at the same level and a 'cleft' anterior mitral leaflet; (c and f) complete atrioventricular septal defect with interatrial and interventricular communications and a common atrioventricular valve.

with asplenia may coexist. Down syndrome occurs in over 65% of children with a complete atrioventricular septal defect[146,147] and 25% of those with a partial defect. This lesion was previously called an endocardial cushion defect or atrioventricular canal.

Physiology

Children with partial atrioventricular septal defects have hemodynamics similar to an atrial septal defect. Those with a complete atrioventricular septal defect have features of a ventricular septal defect. The atrioventricular valves are always regurgitant. If this is severe, the hemodynamic effect adds to that of the septal defect. Infants with a complete atrioventricular septal defect may have mild desaturation because of common mixing and pulmonary hypertension. Those with Down syndrome develop pulmonary vascular obstructive disease at a younger age.[148]

Clinical features

Infants may present because of the diagnosis of Down syndrome. The other clinical features are those of an atrial or ventricular septal defect. There is also a pansystolic murmur of left atrioventricular valve regurgitation. If this is severe, it will contribute to the clinical features of pulmonary congestion and heart failure.

Investigations

Chest radiography and electrocardiogram correspond to the type of septal defect. There is also left axis deviation on the electrocardiogram. Echocardiography identifies the anatomical type of atrioventricular septal defect and the size of the atrial and ventricular components. It allows evaluation of ventricular size, atrioventricular valve regurgitation and other cardiac lesions. It also provides information on the degree of pulmonary hypertension. Cardiac catheterization may be required to assess pulmonary vascular resistance in older infants and children. Angiography defines the atrial and ventricular septal defects and atrioventricular valve regurgitation.

Management and prognosis

Complete atrioventricular septal defects require surgery at 3–6 months of age[148] to prevent the development of irreversible pulmonary hypertension. Pulmonary artery banding may be performed to defer definitive surgery in infants with other conditions, or when surgery carries a high risk. At the time of repair the left atrioventricular valve is sutured to reduce regurgitation and improve outcome.[145] Early mortality following repair of complete atrioventricular septal defect is less than 5%, with a 10 year survival of over 80%.[146] The prognosis is better for children with Down syndrome, as those who do not have Down syndrome more frequently have complex anatomy with unbalanced ventricles,[149] severely regurgitant atrioventricular valves or atrial isomerism. Partial

atrioventricular septal defects are closed surgically between 2 and 5 years of age. Survival after repair of partial atrioventricular septal defect is excellent with less than 3% early mortality and a 20 year survival of 87%.[145]

Re-operation is occasionally necessary for left atrioventricular valve regurgitation or stenosis, or left ventricular outflow tract obstruction.[149] A few patients require a pacemaker for complete heart block after surgery, or develop late supraventricular tachyarrhythmias.

Mitral regurgitation

Anatomy

Mitral valve prolapse, cleft mitral valve leaflet and atrioventricular septal defect produce mitral regurgitation. A parachute mitral valve, with abnormal papillary muscles that restrict opening, may also cause regurgitation. Left ventricular dilatation, due to cardiomyopathy or certain congenital lesions, may result in stretching of the mitral valve and produce regurgitation. Infants with anomalous origin of the left coronary artery have myocardial ischaemia that results in left ventricular dilatation. Infarction of the papillary muscles of the mitral valve also causes regurgitation.

Physiology

Mild regurgitation has little hemodynamic effect. Increasing severity results in volume loading of the left atrium. Excessive flow returning through the mitral valve into the left ventricle causes dilatation.

Clinical features

Mild regurgitation is asymptomatic. A blowing pansystolic murmur is maximal at the apex, radiating to the axilla. When regurgitation is severe, the child may experience effort dyspnea or palpitation. Severe regurgitation is also associated with a forceful, displaced apex beat, a third heart sound and a mid-diastolic murmur caused by increased blood flow across the mitral valve. Pulmonary hypertension may develop with right ventricular hypertrophy and a loud pulmonary component of the second heart sound.

Investigations

If the regurgitation is severe, the electrocardiogram shows left atrial enlargement and left ventricular hypertrophy. Chest radiography shows cardiomegaly with left atrial enlargement. Echocardiography demonstrates the severity of the regurgitation and the anatomy of the valve. Cardiac catheterization is seldom necessary for diagnosis or management.

Management and prognosis

Mild regurgitation requires only observation for increasing severity and antibiotic prophylaxis for surgical procedures. Moderate regurgitation is treated medically with afterload-reducing drugs such as angiotensin converting enzyme inhibitors and diuretics. Severe regurgitation with symptoms is an indication for surgery. This consists of mitral valve repair or replacement.

Aortic regurgitation

Aortic regurgitation rarely occurs in isolation in children. It is most commonly associated with a bicuspid aortic valve or ventricular septal defect. Aortic regurgitation does not cause symptoms unless there is severe regurgitation with left ventricular dysfunction, when palpitations, sweating and effort dyspnea occur. The pulse is collapsing, the pulse pressure wide, and the apical impulse of left ventricular type. The murmur is a high pitched blowing early diastole murmur, best heard at the upper and middle left sternal edge with the child leaning forward and breath-holding in expiration. Severe regurgitation is associated with an ejection systolic murmur, representing increased flow across the aortic valve. An apical mid-diastolic murmur (Austin Flint) can also be heard with severe aortic regurgitation. This is caused by the mitral valve, which is prevented from opening fully in diastole by the aortic regurgitant jet. It may be indistinguishable from organic mitral stenosis but occurs without mitral valve disease. Signs of pulmonary edema due to left ventricular failure are late features of severe regurgitation.

With moderate or severe regurgitation there will be left ventricular hypertrophy on the electrocardiogram and enlargement on the chest radiograph. Echocardiography will demonstrate a dilated and hypercontractile left ventricle. Color Doppler shows regurgitant flow from the aorta to left ventricle. This may restrict opening of the anterior leaflet of the mitral valve in diastole. Cardiac catheterization adds little further information.

Tricuspid regurgitation

Tricuspid regurgitation is usually associated with Ebstein's anomaly of the tricuspid valve (Fig. 21.23) (p. 776). Occasionally a dysplastic but not displaced tricuspid valve will cause similar hemodynamic and clinical features.

Pulmonary regurgitation

Isolated pulmonary regurgitation is rare. Trivial regurgitation detected on color Doppler echocardiography is a normal finding. Pulmonary regurgitation is usually well tolerated. Severe regurgitation results in right ventricular volume overload with dilatation.

Aorticopulmonary window

This rare condition consists of a direct communication between the ascending aorta and the pulmonary trunk, usually between the left side of the ascending aorta and the right side of the pulmonary artery. Additional cardiac lesions are common.

Most defects are large and increased pulmonary blood flow and pulmonary hypertension occur early. Dyspnea, failure to thrive and congestive heart failure are common in infancy. The pulse is collapsing and there is cardiomegaly on palpation. The pulmonary second heart sound is loud and a systolic rather than continuous murmur is heard over the left sternal border. A mid-diastolic flow murmur may be present at the apex. The findings mimic a large ventricular septal defect or patent arterial duct with pulmonary hypertension.

Chest radiography shows cardiomegaly with prominent pulmonary trunk and plethoric lung fields. The electrocardiogram shows biventricular hypertrophy. The defect is visible on cross-sectional echocardiography and color Doppler imaging. Further definition sometimes requires angiography or MRI. Surgical closure of the defect should be performed early because pulmonary hypertension is likely to develop.

Arteriovenous fistulaa

Fistulaa between a systemic artery and vein can be present anywhere in the body. The common sites are between a cerebral artery and the vein of Galen,[150] the subclavian artery and vein, the hepatic artery and portal vein, the internal mammary artery and the internal mammary vein or the ductus venosus. Cavernous hemangiomas can involve the skin, pelvis or liver. Acquired fistulaa are usually the result of trauma.

The arteriovenous fistula allows run-off of blood from the aorta and increases systemic venous return. Small communications are asymptomatic, but large ones result in high output heart failure. A continuous murmur is audible over the involved area, sometimes accompanied by a palpable thrill. Other signs include bounding pulses, systemic venous congestion, cardiomegaly and hepatomegaly. Hepatic artery fistulaa may produce liver enlargement. In any infant with heart failure and no obvious precordial or echocardiographic findings, a bruit suggestive of an arteriovenous fistula should be sought over the skull, chest wall and abdomen.

Large fistulaa produce cardiomegaly on chest radiography and biventricular hypertrophy on the electrocardiogram. Echocardiography is useful in excluding cardiac pathology, while ultrasound of the affected area may reveal dilated arteriovenous channels. Definitive diagnosis is obtained by MRI or angiography. Aggressive anti-failure treatment and transcatheter occlusion have improved prognosis, but mortality and significant morbidity remain high.[150]

Coronary artery fistula

A coronary artery fistula usually occurs as an isolated malformation. The right coronary artery is more often involved and most commonly drains into the right heart. The left to right shunt is seldom large. However, a large fistula produces exercise intolerance, dyspnea or angina because of the 'stealing' of blood from the normal coronary circulation. Heart failure is rare. The characteristic finding is a continuous murmur heard over the site of drainage into the heart. It is therefore maximal over the lower right or left sternal border when the fistula drains into the right atrium or right ventricle, and over the upper left sternal border when the fistula drains into the pulmonary artery or left atrium. Diagnosis is confirmed by echocardiography. Treatment is by surgery or transcatheter occlusion.[151]

Sinus of Valsalva aneurysm

Congenital aneurysm of the aortic sinus (of Valsalva) may rupture into the right ventricle or atrium producing a left to right shunt. Symptoms of heart failure develop acutely and a continuous murmur is audible over the mid-left sternal area. Diagnosis is made by echocardiography and treatment is surgical.

ACYANOTIC HEART DISEASE WITH INCREASED PRESSURE LOAD

Pulmonary stenosis

Anatomy

Valve stenosis is the most common level of obstruction, but subvalvar or supravalvar stenosis can occur. Thickened and fused valve leaflets open incompletely during systole, producing a jet that causes post-stenotic dilatation of the pulmonary artery. Muscular obstruction develops below a severely narrowed valve. Peripheral pulmonary stenosis consists of single or multiple stenoses of the pulmonary arteries distal to the valve. Rarely rhabdomyomas cause right ventricular outflow obstruction. Associated lesions include atrial and ventricular septal defects.

Physiology

Obstruction to outflow increases right ventricular systolic pressure, causing hypertrophy. Severe obstruction can cause supra-systemic right ventricular pressure. The noncompliant right ventricle causes elevated right atrial pressures, stretching of the oval foramen, and right to left shunting with cyanosis.

Clinical features

Most children present with an asymptomatic murmur before 4 years of age.[152] Supravalvar and peripheral pulmonary stenosis occur with

Williams, Alagille[153] and congenital rubella syndromes.[73] Noonan syndrome is associated with a dysplastic valve.

Mild stenosis. The pulses, precordial pulsation and second heart sound are normal. A short, soft ejection systolic murmur maximal at the second left intercostal space usually radiates to the back. If the valve is mobile, a pulmonary ejection click is heard in the same area. It varies with respiration and is not related to the severity of stenosis.

Differential diagnosis: innocent murmur, atrial septal defect, aortic coarctation, mild aortic stenosis, small muscular ventricular septal defect.[154]

Severe stenosis. Infants may be cyanosed because of right to left shunting at atrial level. Older children are usually asymptomatic, but rarely there is a history of dyspnea, exercise intolerance or syncope. A prominent 'a' wave is seen in the jugular venous pulse. There is a right ventricular lift, and a systolic thrill may be palpable at the second left intercostal space. The long, harsh ejection systolic murmur increases in intensity late in systole, radiating to the back and neck. The pulmonary component of the second heart sound is soft and late, as right ventricular ejection is prolonged. A pulmonary ejection click may be heard.

Differential diagnosis: tetralogy of Fallot, severe aortic stenosis, aortic coarctation, perimembranous ventricular septal defect.

Investigations

Severe obstruction causes right ventricular hypertrophy on the electrocardiogram. Chest radiography may show post-stenotic dilatation of the pulmonary artery. The vascular markings are normal if there is no right to left shunt, as blood returning to the right heart must pass through the lungs. However, substantial right to left shunting at atrial level results in pulmonary oligemia. Echocardiography usually shows a thickened pulmonary valve and pulmonary artery dilatation. Color Doppler shows turbulence distal to the site of obstruction and the measured velocity indicates severity. Severe stenosis is associated with right ventricular hypertrophy, muscular subvalve obstruction, tricuspid regurgitation and right atrial enlargement. Cardiac catheterization is not necessary for diagnosis, but transcatheter balloon dilatation is the treatment of choice (Fig. 21.14). Right ventricular angiography identifies the levels of obstruction and usually shows a thickened, doming pulmonary valve.

Management and prognosis

Pulmonary valve and peripheral pulmonary stenosis often decreases spontaneously over time, but 27% of children have increasing obstruction.[152] This is frequently gradual, but rapid progression occurs in neonates.[155] The electrocardiogram and Doppler echocardiography allow accurate assessment of increasing stenosis. Approximately 17% of children require intervention.[152] This is performed when the pressure gradient exceeds 50 mmHg. Balloon dilatation is the treatment of choice,[29,32] and the gradient is usually markedly reduced or abolished.[30] Pulmonary regurgitation occurs but is well tolerated. The long term results are excellent[31] but repeat balloon dilatation is occasionally necessary. Occasionally a surgical valvotomy is performed, particularly if the valve is dysplastic or other lesions require surgery. Results are similar to balloon dilatation.[156] Infective endocarditis is rare and antibiotic prophylaxis for procedures is controversial.[60,62]

Aortic stenosis

Anatomy

Aortic valve stenosis is the most common level of obstruction. Subaortic or supravalve stenosis occurs less frequently, and occasionally children have more than one level of obstruction.[157]

- *Aortic valve stenosis* is due to a thickened valve that is often bicuspid. Post-stenotic dilatation of the ascending aorta may occur. A bicuspid aortic valve without stenosis occurs in 2% of the population.
- *Subaortic stenosis* is usually due to fibromuscular tissue below the aortic valve which may be damaged by the high velocity jet through the narrowed subaortic area. Muscular subaortic obstruction

occasionally occurs. Rarely cardiac rhabdomyoma or accessory atrioventricular valve tissue causes subaortic obstruction.

- *Supravalve stenosis* is due to localized or diffuse thickening of the ascending aorta. It is associated with Williams syndrome or a positive family history (autosomal dominant inheritance), but 25% of cases are sporadic.[158] Coronary artery abnormalities occur.

Clinical features

Children usually present at about 2 years of age with an asymptomatic murmur and features of mild stenosis.[157] The pulses and apex beat are normal. A systolic thrill may be palpable in the suprasternal notch. An ejection systolic murmur is maximal in the aortic area, with radiation to the neck and left sternal border. If the stenosed valve remains mobile, an ejection click may be audible at the lower left sternal border. The murmur of subaortic stenosis is loudest at the lower left sternal edge. A soft, early diastolic murmur of aortic regurgitation is more common with subaortic stenosis, but may occur with valve stenosis.

Severe aortic stenosis. Symptoms include dyspnea, syncope or angina on exertion but severe stenosis may be asymptomatic. The pulse is weak and slow rising with reduced pulse pressure. The aortic component of the second heart is soft and delayed, resulting in a single second heart sound or paradoxical (expiratory) splitting. The more severe the stenosis, the longer and later the accentuation of the systolic murmur. A long ejection systolic murmur can be difficult to distinguish from the pansystolic murmur of a ventricular septal defect. Most infants with severe (critical) stenosis present with collapse in the neonatal period (p. 780), but some develop heart failure in infancy. The pulses are weak and cardiomegaly is present. A gallop rhythm may be heard, and the ejection systolic murmur is soft if left ventricle function is poor. An ejection click is rare, as the valve is thick and immobile.

Investigations

The electrocardiogram is usually normal but left ventricular strain pattern, with inverted T waves in the left precordial leads, indicates severe stenosis. Chest radiography does not show cardiomegaly in the absence of heart failure. Post-stenotic dilatation of the ascending aorta produces a prominent ascending aorta. Echocardiography shows the site of obstruction and whether left ventricular hypertrophy is present. The Doppler velocity across the outflow tract provides an indication of severity. Turbulence occurs on color Doppler at the level of obstruction. Cardiac catheterization is unnecessary for diagnosis, but is undertaken for therapeutic balloon dilatation of the stenotic valve.

Management and prognosis

- *Aortic valve stenosis* progresses with time. Less than 20% of patients will have mild stenosis after 30 years.[127] Rapid progression may occur in early childhood and adolescence. Surgical valvotomy is undertaken when the pressure gradient across the valve exceeds 50 mmHg, or if there are features of severe stenosis. Transcatheter balloon dilatation is an alternative to surgery.[33,36] Reduction of valve gradient and the incidence of valve regurgitation are comparable to surgery.[34,159] Treatment is palliative as re-stenosis and progressive aortic regurgitation occur. Once severe aortic regurgitation develops, or if obstruction cannot be relieved, valve replacement is necessary. Both aortic homograft and prosthetic valve replacements have potential problems. The Ross procedure appears to carry a lower risk.[160] The aortic valve is replaced by the patient's own pulmonary valve, and a tissue conduit replaces the pulmonary valve.
- *Subaortic stenosis* is rarely significant during infancy but subsequent progression may be rapid, and most children require surgery. Subaortic obstruction is not usually relieved by balloon dilatation and surgery is indicated for increasing gradient or aortic regurgitation.
- *Supravalve aortic stenosis* usually responds well to surgery, and re-operation is rarely necessary.[158,161] Surgery for diffuse narrowing of the ascending aorta produces less favorable results. Balloon

dilatation is not recommended, because of the nature of the narrowing and the proximity of the coronary arteries.

- *Multilevel obstruction* is more severe at presentation and has a worse prognosis than a single level of stenosis. Children are more likely to undergo operation, and have a higher incidence of re-operation.[157] Mortality is higher, emphasizing the difficult surgical problems that these children present.

Sudden death of patients with aortic stenosis is rare, accounting for only 2% of sudden cardiac deaths under 35 years of age.[162] It occurs in less than 2% of patients with aortic stenosis and only in those with severe aortic stenosis.[157] It is unnecessary to restrict activities of children with mild aortic stenosis[163] but regular review and antibiotic prophylaxis for procedures remain essential throughout life.

Coarctation of the aorta

Coarctation most commonly presents acutely in the neonatal period when the arterial duct closes (p. 779). In older infants and children, the signs are more subtle.

Anatomy

The aorta is narrowed at the isthmus between the left subclavian artery and the insertion of the arterial duct. Ductal tissue extending into the aortic wall constricts after birth, producing or increasing an obstruction that is usually discrete. Diffuse hypoplasia of the transverse aortic arch may occur. Rarely constriction occurs in the lower thoracic or abdominal aorta. Collateral vessels from intercostal, mammary and subclavian arteries develop, bypassing the obstruction and augmenting perfusion to the lower body. Associated cardiac lesions are common,[164] including a bicuspid or stenotic aortic valve, ventricular septal defect and mitral stenosis. Shone syndrome consists of left-sided obstructive lesions including supramitral membrane, mitral valve abnormalities, subaortic stenosis and coarctation. More than 15% of girls with Turner syndrome have coarctation.[79]

Physiology

Obstruction of the aorta results in pressure overload of the left ventricle. Systemic hypertension is due to mechanical obstruction and neurohumoral mechanisms related to reduced renal perfusion.

Clinical features

Infants may present with heart failure. More commonly, children have an asymptomatic murmur, weak femoral pulses or systemic hypertension detected on routine examination. The femoral pulses are less easily felt than the right brachial. The blood pressure in the right arm exceeds the 95th percentile for height[8] and is > 10 mmHg higher than in the legs. The left arm blood pressure depends on the site of coarctation. The left ventricular impulse is prominent, with a short ejection systolic murmur maximal at the second left intercostal space and below the left scapula posteriorly. A continuous murmur from the coarctation or collateral arteries may be heard in older children. Murmurs from other cardiac lesions are frequently audible.

Investigations

The electrocardiogram is usually normal, but left ventricular hypertrophy may be present. Chest radiography may show an abnormal aortic contour (3 sign) caused by localized constriction of the aorta at the coarctation site. Dilated intercostal arteries cause rib notching in older children. Echocardiography demonstrates the coarctation site (Fig. 21.26a, b). Hypoplasia of the aortic arch (Fig. 21.26d) and other lesions can also be identified. Turbulence on color Doppler occurs at the obstruction, with increased velocity and continuous flow into diastole (Fig. 21.26c). MRI, CT or angiography demonstrates the anatomy of coarctation (Fig. 21.16).

Management and prognosis

Early treatment improves life expectancy.[165] It is undertaken soon after diagnosis, as the incidence of residual systemic hypertension is related to the age at intervention. Severe hypertension results in premature cardiovascular disease, aortic dissection or cerebrovascular accident. There are no clinical trials which determine the optimum form of treatment.[40,166] Surgical repair consists of excision of the narrowed segment and end-to-end anastomosis of the aorta, or left subclavian flap repair. Rarely a patch or tube graft is used to relieve the obstruction. The risks of surgery include transient severe hypertension, paraplegia from spinal cord ischaemia (1%),[40,164] recurrent laryngeal or phrenic nerve injury, chylothorax and re-coarctation (< 4%). Transcatheter balloon angioplasty has been used as the initial treatment for coarctation[39] and is the treatment of choice for re-coarctation following surgery.[37] Complications include femoral artery damage and aortic aneurysm formation. The risks of surgery and angioplasty are similar and mortality is rare in the absence of other lesions. Balloon-expandable stents have been used to prevent re-coarctation[164] and reduce the risk of aneurysm formation but there are concerns about their use in children.[40]

Hypertension may remain, and other lesions such as left ventricular outflow tract obstruction may require treatment. Follow-up is essential and the risk of infective endocarditis remains.

Left ventricular inflow obstructions

Anatomy

Obstruction between pulmonary venous return and the left ventricle is rare. It is caused by:

- stenosis of pulmonary veins entering the left atrium;
- cor triatriatum, which comprises a fibrous diaphragm dividing the left atrium into two chambers, with a restrictive communication between them;
- supramitral stenotic ring, which is a circumferential ridge of tissue in the left atrium immediately above the mitral valve;
- congenital mitral valve stenosis.

Physiology

Obstructive lesions produce elevated pressure proximal to the site of obstruction and pulmonary venous congestion. Pulmonary hypertension develops, causing right heart failure.

Clinical features

The clinical signs are of pulmonary venous congestion and pulmonary hypertension. When the obstruction at any level is severe, symptoms begin in early infancy with dyspnea, respiratory infections and poor weight gain. Tachypnea, tachycardia, recession and hepatomegaly are present. An apical mid-diastolic murmur is more often audible in mitral valve stenosis or supramitral ring than in cor triatriatum. Children with a mitral valve abnormality frequently present with associated malformations such as aortic coarctation or ventricular septal defect, and the mitral lesion may not be recognized initially.

Investigations

The electrocardiogram shows right atrial and right ventricular hypertrophy. Left atrial enlargement is seen in mitral valve stenosis or supramitral ring but not in cor triatriatum. Chest radiography shows cardiomegaly with left atrial enlargement, producing a double shadow at the right heart border. There is a prominent pulmonary artery and pulmonary venous congestion with 'butterfly wing' distribution of vascular markings or ground glass appearance if pulmonary edema is present. Echocardiography provides definitive diagnosis and Doppler velocity across the obstruction indicates the severity. The tricuspid regurgitant velocity indicates the severity of pulmonary hypertension. Cardiac catheterization is not usually required, but an end-diastolic pressure difference of more than 5 mmHg across the obstruction is significant. Angiography confirms the site of obstruction, but this is better seen on transthoracic or transesophageal echocardiography.

Management and prognosis

Surgical excision of the obstructive membrane is the definitive treatment for cor triatriatum and supramitral ring. For congenital mitral stenosis, the deformity of the valve dictates the surgical approach. Valvotomy, with attempts to conserve the native valve, is preferred to mitral valve replacement.

Double chambered right ventricle

This is a rare condition resulting from a hypertrophied muscular band in the mid-portion of the right ventricle. It may be associated with a ventricular septal defect and is usually not severe at birth, the obstruction developing with time. The clinical features are similar to pulmonary valve stenosis, but there is no ejection click and the murmur is maximal lower down the left sternal border. Diagnosis is confirmed by echocardiography or cardiac catheterization with right ventricular angiography. Surgery is indicated for significant obstruction, and the long term outlook is excellent.

CYANOTIC CONGENITAL HEART DISEASE

The majority of children with cyanotic heart disease present in the neonatal period (p. 769). Tetralogy of Fallot is the commonest cyanotic cardiac defect presenting in infancy.

Tetralogy of Fallot
Anatomy

This condition consists of right ventricular outflow obstruction, right ventricular hypertrophy, a large perimembranous ventricular septal defect and an aorta that overrides the ventricular septal defect (Fig. 21.33). The hilar pulmonary arteries are usually small. When more than 50% of the aorta arises from the right ventricle, it is termed 'double outlet right ventricle'. Other lesions include a right-sided aortic arch (20%), atrial septal defect or persistent arterial duct. Tetralogy of Fallot with an atrioventricular septal defect occurs with Down syndrome. 22q11 deletion is found in 16% of infants.[122]

Physiology

Because the ventricular septal defect is large and nonrestrictive, pressures in both ventricles are similar. The obstruction varies in severity but is always sufficient to result in normal or low pulmonary artery pressure. If it is mild, flow across the ventricular septal defect will be from left to right. Increasing obstruction causes right to left shunting and cyanosis. The hemodynamic effect is labile, depending on the degree of right ventricular outflow obstruction and systemic vascular resistance.

Clinical features

Neonates with severe outflow obstruction present with cyanosis and duct-dependent pulmonary circulation (p. 771). More commonly, infants present with an asymptomatic murmur, minimal cyanosis or heart failure caused by a left to right shunt. As right ventricular outflow obstruction increases, cyanosis becomes more noticeable and clubbing develops. Right ventricular hypertrophy is palpable. The second heart sound is single as the pulmonary component is inaudible. An aortic ejection click is occasionally heard. The long, loud ejection systolic murmur caused by subpulmonary obstruction is maximal at the third left intercostal space, radiating to the back. With increasing obstruction the murmur becomes shorter and the child develops effort intolerance. The characteristic 'squatting' is not seen if children undergo palliative or definitive surgery in infancy. This maneuver increases systemic vascular resistance, promoting pulmonary blood flow.

Differential diagnosis: ventricular septal defect, severe left or right ventricular outflow obstruction, other complex cyanotic lesions with pulmonary stenosis.

Investigations

The electrocardiogram shows right ventricular hypertrophy. Chest radiography shows a normal sized heart with an uptilted apex. Concavity of the left heart border (pulmonary bay) indicates a small pulmonary artery. Oligemic lung fields reflect reduced pulmonary blood flow. A right-sided aortic arch (present in 20%) will cause deviation of the

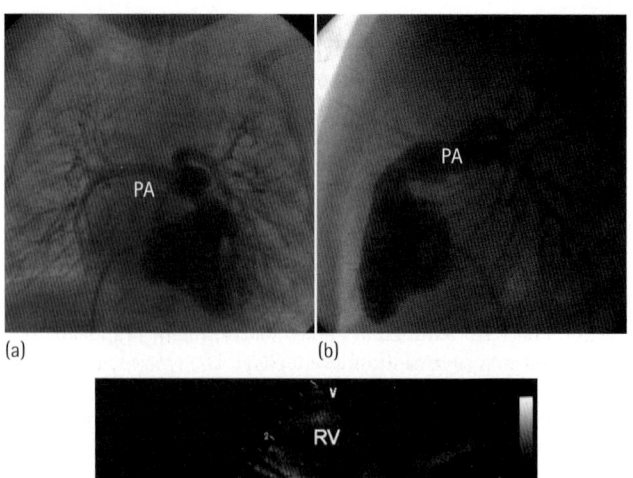
(a)　　　　　　　　　　　(b)

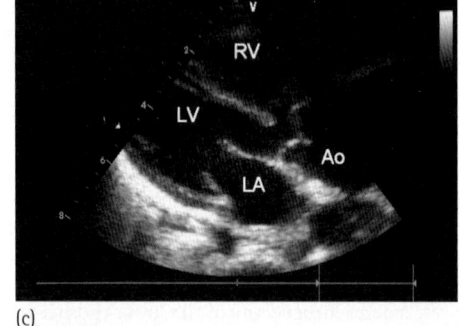
(c)

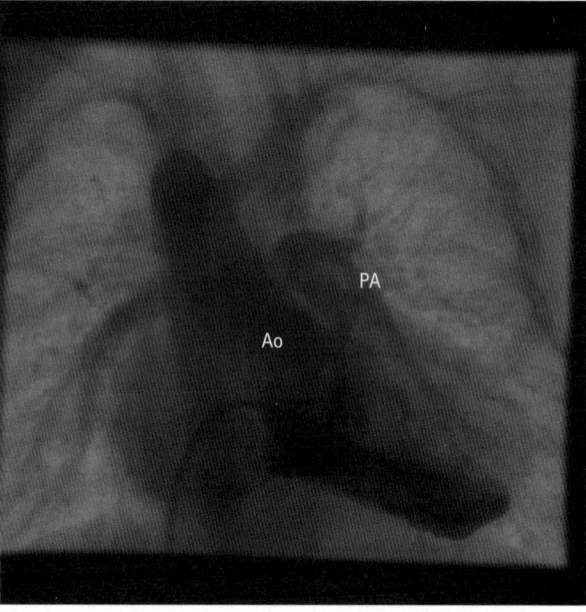
(d)

Fig. 21.33 Tetralogy of Fallot: This demonstrates (a) the anteroposterior and (b) lateral view of the right ventricular angiogram. There is infundibular narrowing below the pulmonary valve and small pulmonary arteries. (c) The echocardiogram in the long-axis view demonstrates the ventricular septal defect with aortic override. (d) Right ventricular angiogram shows opacification of the right-sided aortic arch to the right of the trachea and indicates the reason for the characteristic picture on chest radiography. Ao, aorta; LA, left atrium; LV, left ventricle; PA, pulmonary artery; RV right ventricle.

trachea to the left and a bulge in the right upper mediastinum (Fig. 21.33d). Echocardiography establishes the diagnosis showing the ventricular septal defect, overriding aorta and right ventricular hypertrophy with outflow obstruction. The pulmonary arteries can be measured and a right aortic arch identified. The Doppler velocity will indicate the pressure difference between the right ventricle and pulmonary artery. Color Doppler shows turbulence below the pulmonary valve, extending into the pulmonary arteries. Chromosome analysis for 22q11 deletion should be considered. Cardiac catheterization and angiography provide further information on the anatomy of the coronary and pulmonary arteries if they are not seen on echocardiography.

Complications

With a move to earlier definitive surgery, complications are less common.

- Hypercyanotic attacks (*hypoxic spells*) occur in young children, particularly those with minimal cyanosis. A sudden decrease in pulmonary blood flow causes severe cyanosis and distress. Spells occur in the early morning or after a warm bath and may be initiated by crying, exertion and feeding. The precise cause is unknown but decreased systemic vascular resistance with increased right to left shunting may contribute. The murmur becomes short and soft. The child may lose consciousness and spells are life threatening. Treatment consists of flexing the legs onto the abdomen (knee–chest position) which increases systemic vascular resistance. Administration of oxygen maximizes inspired oxygen. Morphine appears to have a specific effect in addition to sedation. If there is no immediate venous access, intramuscular morphine injection (0.1 mg/kg) helps to relieve the spell, allowing valuable time to site a cannula. Severe metabolic acidosis is common and should be corrected with sodium bicarbonate to prevent further episodes. Intravenous propranolol 0.1 mg/kg is effective but should be used with caution in children on beta-blockers. Intravenous phenylephrine is effective in increasing systemic vascular resistance and promoting pulmonary blood flow, but should only be used with direct arterial pressure monitoring. A hypoxic spell is an indication for urgent surgical intervention to increase pulmonary blood flow. Prevention of spells with regular beta-adrenergic blockade is beneficial prior to surgery.
- Cerebral events. Thrombosis can result from polycythemia, particularly in association with dehydration. The incidence of brain abscess is also increased in children with cyanotic heart disease. Iron deficiency anemia with microcytosis increases the risk of cerebrovascular complications[167] and should be prevented with iron supplements.
- Infective endocarditis is most likely in children with a systemic to pulmonary artery shunt.

Management and prognosis

Palliative surgery may be necessary in symptomatic infants with hypoplastic right ventricular outflow tracts and small pulmonary arteries. This may also be preferred in neonates with a duct-dependent pulmonary circulation. It involves insertion of a Gore-Tex tube between the pulmonary and subclavian arteries (modified Blalock–Taussig shunt) (Fig. 21.34). Complications include chylothorax, diaphragmatic paralysis and Horner syndrome. Definitive repair can then be delayed until the second year of life. Low dose aspirin is necessary to prevent platelet aggregation in the shunt. Clinical findings include cyanosis and a continuous murmur loudest over the site of the shunt.

Definitive surgery is now commonly performed in the first year of life.[168] The ventricular septal defect is closed with a patch and the right ventricular outflow tract is enlarged by muscle resection, pulmonary valvotomy and sometimes patch augmentation. Early mortality is less than 5% and complications include right ventricular dysfunction, pleural effusion and complete heart block. The residual systolic murmur reflects turbulence in the right ventricular outflow tract and the diastolic murmur is due to pulmonary regurgitation. Right bundle branch block may present on the electrocardiogram. Most patients lead normal lives with good effort tolerance. There is a small risk of re-operation for residual ventricular septal defect, pulmonary stenosis or regurgitation.[168] The 20 year survival is over 90%.[169] Patients require follow-up because of a late incidence of ventricular arrhythmias, complete heart block[170] and sudden death. Endocarditis prophylaxis must continue.

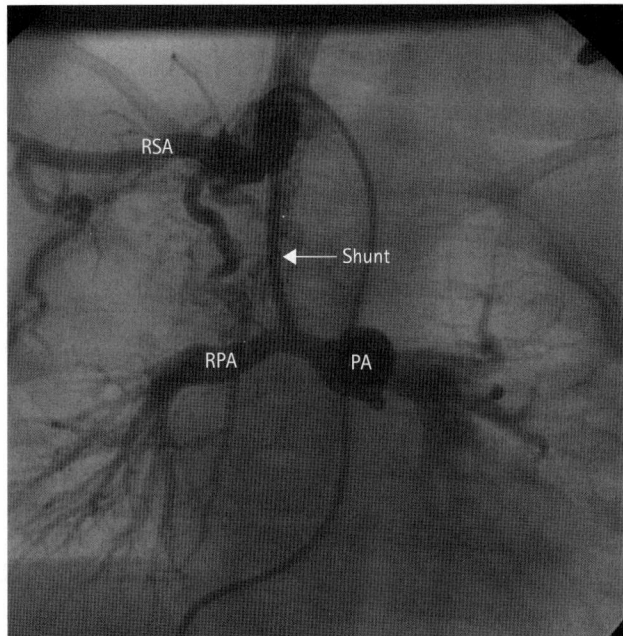

Fig. 21.34 Blalock–Taussig shunt: An angiogram into the right subclavian artery (RSA) at the site of the shunt showing contrast filling the shunt and the pulmonary arteries. The pulmonary valve is atretic. PA, pulmonary artery; RPA, right pulmonary artery.

Pulmonary atresia and ventricular septal defect

Pulmonary atresia with ventricular septal defect is the extreme form of tetralogy of Fallot. Most present in the neonatal period (p. 771), but diagnosis may be delayed when major aortopulmonary collateral arteries (MAPCAs) provide adequate pulmonary blood flow. Clinical features may include heart failure, mild cyanosis and a continuous murmur in the lung fields.

Tetralogy of Fallot with absent pulmonary valve

This occurs in 3–6% of patients with tetralogy of Fallot. A rudimentary pulmonary valve leaflet causes severe regurgitation and the valve ring is narrowed causing stenosis. The pulmonary arteries are usually markedly dilated and compress the bronchi, causing obstruction. The bronchi are also intrinsically abnormal. This may produce severe airways obstruction in infancy with wheeze and recurrent pneumonia. There is mild cyanosis and an ejection systolic murmur is followed by a long diastolic murmur in the pulmonary area. Definitive surgery is similar to that for tetralogy of Fallot.

THE SINGLE VENTRICLE CIRCULATION

This is a complex and diverse group of conditions that have in common only one ventricle, which provides the majority of both the systemic and pulmonary blood flow. Surgical correction is not possible, and effective palliation is directed towards optimizing the circulation. This consists of a series of operations that allow the functional ventricle to supply the systemic circulation. Blood returning from the superior and inferior caval veins is directed into the pulmonary arteries driven by the central venous pressure and the negative forces generated by inspiration and ventricular diastole. This separates the pulmonary and systemic venous returns.

Anatomy

The range of conditions is diverse and the specific abnormality is less important than early identification that the anatomy is unsuitable for two-ventricle repair. It includes conditions with hypoplasia or atresia of the mitral or tricuspid valves, or significant hypoplasia of either ventricle.

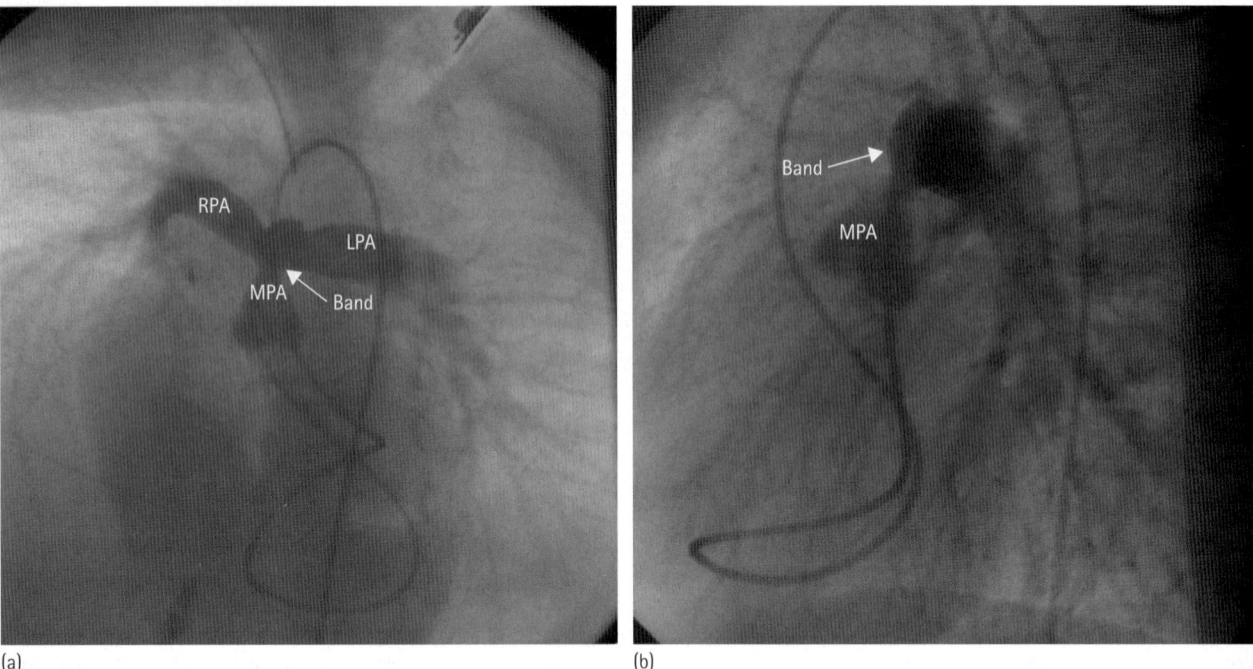

(a)   (b)

Fig. 21.35 Pulmonary artery band: (a) An angiogram into the main pulmonary artery shows the constriction from the pulmonary artery band distal to the pulmonary valve, before the bifurcation into right and left pulmonary arteries. (b) A lateral projection of the same angiogram. LPA, left pulmonary artery; MPA, main pulmonary artery; RPA, right pulmonary artery.

Physiology
Infants may have:

- inadequate pulmonary blood flow (tricuspid atresia with a small ventricular septal defect and pulmonary stenosis, double inlet left ventricle with pulmonary stenosis, pulmonary atresia with intact ventricular septum and hypoplastic right ventricle, severe Ebstein's anomaly of the tricuspid valve);
- inadequate systemic blood flow (hypoplastic left heart, tricuspid atresia with transposition and a small ventricular septal defect);
- unrestricted pulmonary blood flow (double outlet right ventricle with hypoplastic left ventricle).

Clinical features
At birth the arterial duct compensates for inadequate pulmonary or systemic circulation and symptoms only develop when the duct closes. Infants with unrestricted pulmonary blood flow develop symptoms when the pulmonary vascular resistance falls and pulmonary blood flow becomes excessive. The clinical features depend on the physiology. Infants with inadequate pulmonary blood flow present with cyanosis. Those with inadequate systemic blood flow present with cardiovascular collapse. Those with unrestricted pulmonary blood flow present with signs of heart failure. Some infants will be diagnosed antenatally, and others will present with cyanosis, collapse, heart failure, a murmur or poor femoral pulses.

Investigations
Findings on electrocardiogram and chest radiography will depend on the underlying condition. Echocardiography will identify the details of the specific cardiac lesion. The segmental chamber localization (p. 754) will ensure that all details of the cardiac diagnosis are identified.

Management and prognosis
Effective early palliation is critical to achieve a satisfactory long term outcome. It involves at least three staged procedures.
Stage 1: optimizing systemic and pulmonary blood flow. From infancy the blood flow into the lungs must be adequate but at low pressure. Neonates with inadequate pulmonary blood flow require a systemic to pulmonary (modified Blalock–Taussig) (Fig. 21.34) shunt. Those with inadequate systemic blood flow require a Norwood (Fig. 21.27) or similar operation. Those with excessive pulmonary blood flow require a pulmonary artery band to reduce pulmonary blood flow (Fig. 21.35). A few infants have a cardiac lesion that results in optimal systemic and pulmonary blood flow with effective pulmonary stenosis and unobstructed systemic blood flow, and therefore do not require surgery in the neonatal period.

The definitive palliative procedure is the Fontan operation. It is usually carried out in two further stages. This consists of surgery to direct the systemic venous return initially from the superior vena cava, and later from the inferior vena cava, directly into the pulmonary artery to allow oxygenation and separate the pulmonary and systemic blood flow. Successful surgery depends on a low pulmonary vascular resistance as blood returning from the body flows directly into the pulmonary arteries, driven by the systemic venous pressure. Any anatomical or physiological abnormality that impedes this must be corrected and other transcatheter and surgical interventions may be necessary to achieve the optimal hemodynamics. The pulmonary artery pressure must be low and the pulmonary arteries of adequate size without localized narrowing. There must also be unobstructed pulmonary venous return, a normal left atrial pressure, good systemic ventricular function and unobstructed systemic outflow.
Stage 2: superior (bidirectional) cavopulmonary anastomosis. This relieves the systemic ventricle of chronic volume and pressure loads that occur regardless of the type of neonatal palliation. It usually decreases the cyanosis and reduces the risks at subsequent surgery. It is performed at 6–12 months of age. The superior caval vein is anastomosed to the proximal right pulmonary artery (Fig. 21.36). If a left superior vena cava is present, this is anastomosed to the left pulmonary artery at the same procedure. If a Blalock–Taussig shunt is present it is ligated. Forward flow through the main pulmonary artery may also be occluded. Residual lesions that may increase the risk of subsequent surgery, such as pulmonary artery narrowing or re-coarctation, are corrected. The superior cavopulmonary anastomosis is well tolerated, even when combined with other procedures. A superior vena caval syndrome with upper body swelling may occur postoperatively if the pulmonary artery

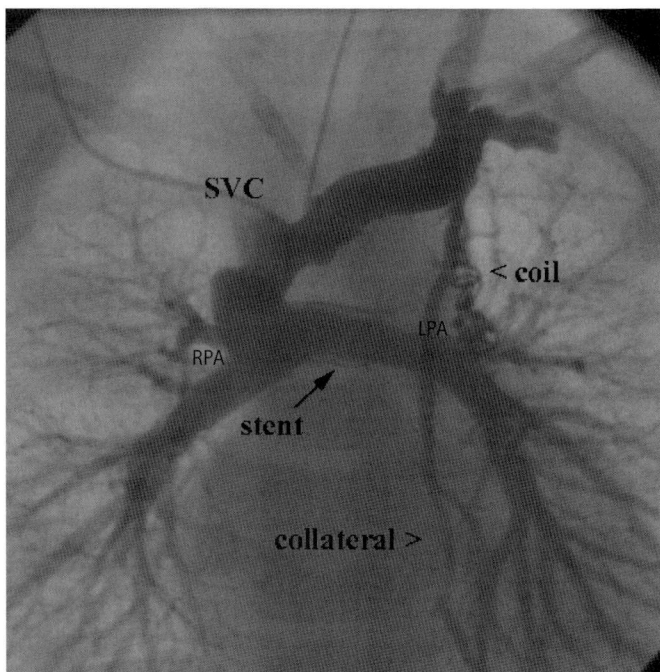

Fig. 21.36 The superior cavopulmonary anastomosis: The angiogram in the superior caval vein shows the connection to the proximal right pulmonary artery. Contrast also fills the innominate vein on the left. Coils have been used to occlude some of the collateral veins from the innominate vein. An intravascular stent was expanded in the proximal left pulmonary artery at the time of surgery. LPA, left pulmonary artery; RPA, right pulmonary artery; SVC, superior caval vein.

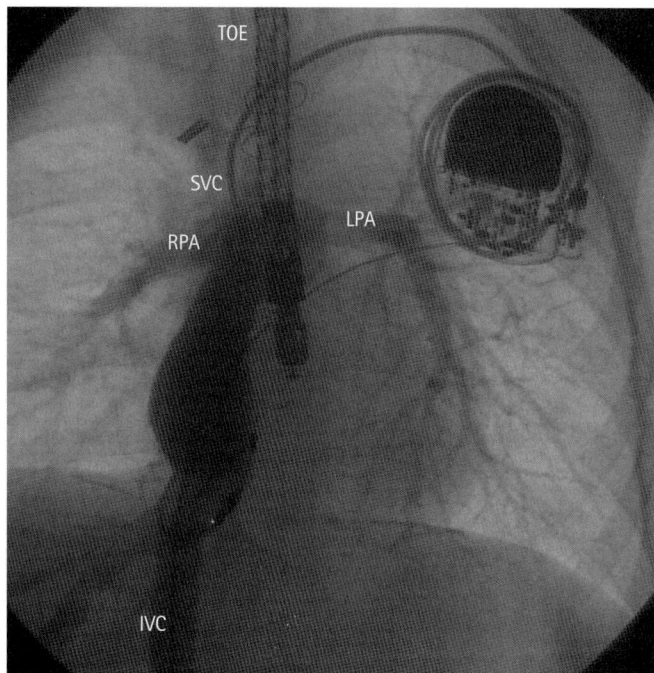

Fig. 21.37 The Fontan operation: The angiogram shows the lateral tunnel connecting the inferior caval vein to the pulmonary arteries. The position of the connection between the superior caval vein and the pulmonary arteries is shown by the pacemaker lead, which passes from the subclavian vein, via the superior caval vein to the atrial wall. The transesophageal probe is visible in the esophagus. IVC, inferior caval vein; LPA, left pulmonary artery; RPA, right pulmonary artery; SVC, superior caval vein; TOE, transesophageal echocardiographic probe.

pressure is elevated. During early childhood the relative size of the lower body increases, and the ratio of blood returning from the inferior and superior caval veins alters. This results in increasing cyanosis, which may also occur due to venous collaterals that develop between the upper and lower body.

Stage 3: completion of modified Fontan operation. This is usually performed at 2–5 years of age. The inferior vena cava is anastomosed to the pulmonary arteries, either by a baffle that is created inside the lateral wall of the right atrium, or an extracardiac conduit (Fig. 21.37). Creation of a small hole or fenestration between this tunnel or conduit and the left-sided (systemic) circulation produces a small right to left shunt. This lowers the central venous pressure, preventing severe venous congestion in the postoperative period but producing systemic desaturation. The fenestration can be closed at a later time if the hemodynamics are suitable.

Prognosis depends on the underlying condition, the success of the various interventions and the long term function of the systemic ventricle. The 30 day mortality is less than 5%, but the postoperative period may be protracted with high central venous pressure, ascites, pleural effusions and poor cardiac output. Atrial arrhythmias can further destabilize the hemodynamics. The highest death rate is in the first year after operation.[171] Recent figures suggest a 5 year survival of more than 70%, but deaths are likely to continue to occur with longer follow-up and the 20 year survival is just under 60%.[171] The quality of life in survivors is satisfactory[172] but a number of late complications account for a continuing mortality. They include cardiac failure, systemic venous obstruction, persistent fluid accumulation and protein-losing enteropathy. Reports of thromboembolism, both pulmonary and systemic (if a fenestration is present), have resulted in the common practice of long term anticoagulation. Arrhythmias can produce significant hemodynamic deterioration and need urgent treatment. Some children will not be suitable for the procedure because of adverse risk factors such as poor sys-

temic ventricular function or elevated pulmonary artery pressure. The only option for a child with a failing 'Fontan' circulation is heart transplantation.

MISCELLANEOUS CARDIOVASCULAR LESIONS
Vascular ring
Anatomy
A vascular ring is a malformation of the aortic arch or its brachiocephalic branches encircling and compressing the trachea and esophagus. Double aortic arch is the most common type. The ascending aorta divides into two vessels that reunite to form the descending aorta. A pulmonary artery sling is the anomalous origin of the left pulmonary artery from the right pulmonary artery crossing the midline between the trachea and esophagus and producing tracheal compression.

Clinical features
Airway obstruction resulting from tracheal compression is progressive and causes inspiratory stridor, which is usually present soon after birth. Wheezing, cough and recurrent respiratory tract infections are common. Dysphagia due to esophageal compression is rare. The diagnosis is often delayed because of the failure to consider it in the child with respiratory difficulties.

Investigations
A barium swallow demonstrates an indentation of the posterior aspect of the esophagus by a vascular ring. A pulmonary artery sling characteristically produces an anterior indentation, sometimes accompanied by a posterior impression on the air column in the trachea at the same level. Echocardiography may show a double arch or pulmonary sling, but a more complete diagnosis requires further investigation such as MRI, CT or angiography.

Treatment

Surgery is always indicated. Outcome is generally good although persistent respiratory symptoms may result from tracheomalacia.

Anomalous origin of the left coronary artery from the pulmonary artery

Anomalous origin of a coronary artery (usually the left) from the pulmonary artery is rare. Perfusion of the left ventricle depends on pulmonary artery pressure and collateral circulation from the right coronary artery. Ischemia occurs with the postnatal fall in the pulmonary pressure, its severity depending on the amount of collateral circulation. The infant usually presents in the second month of life with 'anginal attacks', manifested as acute distress with crying, sweating and pallor, often during feeding or defecation. Heart failure develops, the heart is enlarged and a gallop rhythm is common. There is often a murmur of mitral regurgitation secondary to left ventricular dilatation. There is marked cardiomegaly and pulmonary venous congestion on chest X-ray. The electrocardiogram characteristically shows an anterior infarction pattern with T wave inversion and deep Q waves in the left chest leads, lead I and aVL. Echocardiography reveals a dilated and poorly contractile left ventricle, with an enlarged right coronary artery. The abnormal origin of the left coronary artery may be visualized causing turbulence on color Doppler as it drains into the pulmonary artery. Angiography is necessary if ultrasound studies are inconclusive. An aortogram shows a large right coronary artery and its distal anastomosis with the left coronary artery, which then drains into the pulmonary artery.

Marfan syndrome

This is an autosomal dominant inherited disorder of connective tissue (see also Ch. 29, p. 1398). It is characterized by musculoskeletal, cardiovascular and ocular abnormalities, two of which should be present to make the diagnosis. It is caused by various mutations in the FBN1 gene on chromosome 15q and is inherited in about 75% of children, the rest arising because of a new mutation.[173]

Clinical features

Cardiovascular manifestations include dilatation of the ascending aorta (and occasionally the descending) due to medial necrosis, aortic regurgitation and mitral valve prolapse and regurgitation. Disturbances in cardiac rhythm can occur. A family history should always be sought.

Investigations

Children should be reviewed regularly with echocardiography to measure the aortic root dimensions and these should be plotted against normal values. Transesophageal echocardiography or MRI gives additional information, particularly when dissection is suspected.

Management

Beta-blockers have been shown to slow the aortic root dilatation.[174] Children should be advised against competitive and contact sports. Surgical aortic root replacement should be considered when the aortic diameter reaches 5 cm, with earlier surgery if there is a rapid increase in diameter, and in families with a history of aortic dissection.

CARDIAC ARRHYTHMIAS

The past few years have seen significant advances in our understanding and treatment of cardiac arrhythmias in children. There is now widespread awareness amongst pediatricians that most arrhythmias result from primary electrical abnormalities of the heart. We also have a greater understanding of the anatomical substrates and electrophysiological mechanisms of arrhythmia. There are now available better non-invasive diagnostic techniques, safer and more effective drugs for acute and long term treatment and the possibility of cure by catheter ablation.

IDENTIFICATION OF THE ARRHYTHMIA

Cardiac arrhythmias usually affect children with otherwise normal hearts but they may also develop in those with cardiovascular malformations. They make up a significant proportion of the work of pediatric cardiologists and are one of the more common ways in which babies and children with cardiac problems present to the general pediatrician. For this reason it is important for pediatricians to have some understanding of the types of arrhythmia, and familiarity with non-invasive diagnostic techniques and treatment strategies.

Knowing the age at onset of an arrhythmia, with recordings of the electrocardiogram (ECG) in sinus rhythm, during arrhythmia and during adenosine administration we can often predict accurately the mechanism of the arrhythmia. This will help to define the prognosis and will guide the choice of treatment. Available diagnostic techniques include standard surface electrocardiography, ambulatory 24 h electrocardiography (Holter monitoring), patient-activated event recorders, invasive electrophysiology studies and implantable loop recorders. The first three are widely available whilst the last two are reserved for specialist assessment.

CLINICAL PRESENTATION OF ARRHYTHMIAS

Cardiac arrhythmias may occur at any age and their differential diagnosis depends upon the age of onset. The commonest presentation in infancy is with heart failure, usually caused by sustained tachycardia, but arrhythmias may also be noticed incidentally because of bradycardia, tachycardia or an irregular rhythm. The most common presentation in childhood is with palpitations, usually as a result of paroxysmal tachycardia. Some less common, incessant tachycardias may present in childhood with heart failure due to secondary myocardial dysfunction. Arrhythmias presenting with syncope are rare but are important to recognize. A few rare but dangerous arrhythmias may result in (and may even present with) sudden death.[175,176] Some arrhythmic causes of sudden death are familial, so a precise diagnosis is very important. Children who develop arrhythmias after heart surgery should already be under the care of a pediatric cardiologist but may present acutely to a pediatrician.

CLASSIFICATION OF ARRHYTHMIAS

Tachycardias have conventionally been considered as either supraventricular or ventricular but, as there are many mechanisms of each, this broad classification is relatively unhelpful. The ECG in tachycardia will show QRS complexes that are either normal or wide so these are two clinically useful groups. Arrhythmias in infancy differ in important aspects from those seen in children and so it is helpful to consider them separately.

MECHANISMS OF TACHYCARDIAS

Most tachycardias encountered in clinical practice are due to re-entry, by which we mean that there is recirculating electrical activation traveling around an anatomical circuit. Such arrhythmias are often (but not always) paroxysmal. Re-entry tachycardias usually have fairly constant rates and can be started by pacing and stopped by drugs, pacing and electrical cardioversion. The circuit usually involves an anatomically abnormal structure – the best example is the accessory atrioventricular connection in Wolff–Parkinson–White syndrome – which is really a form of structural congenital heart disease.[177] In other cases, the circuit probably develops during growth – as in atrioventricular (AV) nodal re-entry tachycardia. Other examples of re-entry include atrial flutter, permanent junctional re-entry tachycardia and late postoperative ventricular tachycardia.

A less common arrhythmia mechanism is automaticity. Automatic arrhythmias arise from an ectopic focus and overdrive pacing or cardioversion is ineffective. They are usually incessant and may show significant variation in rate. Those most commonly encountered in children are atrial ectopic tachycardia and early postoperative junctional ectopic tachycardia (His bundle tachycardia).

TACHYCARDIA IN INFANCY
Atrioventricular Re-Entry Tachycardia in Infancy

The commonest type of supraventricular tachycardia (SVT) presenting in infancy is orthodromic AV re-entry via an accessory pathway (Fig. 21.38). The term orthodromic implies that there is normal conduction over the AV node and retrograde conduction over an accessory muscular atrioventricular connection (accessory pathway). About a third of accessory connections encountered in infants show anterograde conduction in sinus rhythm, producing ventricular pre-excitation that is recognized as Wolff–Parkinson–White syndrome. More commonly the pathway can only conduct retrogradely so the ECG is normal in sinus rhythm. In tachycardia the QRS is usually normal in infancy although transient rate-related bundle branch block at the onset of tachycardia is not unusual (Fig. 21.39). Tachycardia usually presents with heart failure, more often causing pallor, breathlessness and poor feeding but sometimes severe enough to cause collapse. The differential diagnosis includes infection and metabolic problems. Sinus tachycardia in an ill baby may exceed 200 beats/min but AV re-entry tachycardia in infancy is rarely slower than 270 beats/min. It is difficult or impossible to distinguish between these heart rates clinically and some ECG monitors are unreliable at high heart rates. Recording a 12 lead ECG on paper will allow accurate measurement of the rate and confirmation of the diagnosis.

The treatment of choice for acute termination of AV re-entry tachycardia is intravenous administration of adenosine. The dose is 150–300 mcg/kg/dose (occasionally higher) given by rapid bolus injection followed by a saline flush (Fig. 21.39).[178] Adenosine is metabolized very quickly and the dose can be repeated or increased if necessary. An ECG should always be recorded during administration of adenosine to evaluate the rhythm. Facial immersion in iced water or facial application of an ice pack is also usually effective but is only appropriate in early infancy. Other drugs are not often required for termination of tachycardia in infancy. Verapamil is contraindicated in early infancy because it may cause acute cardiac decompensation and death.[179] Synchronized electrical cardioversion is effective but, because it requires general anesthetic, is not easily repeated.

The baby's condition will improve once sinus rhythm has been restored. Recurrence of tachycardia in the short term is common so prophylactic drug treatment is usually advised. There are no controlled trials of drug treatment in this situation but digoxin seems to have relatively little effect. Treatment with a beta-blocker, flecainide, propafenone, or amiodarone[180] (or a combination of these in difficult cases) will usually prevent recurrence of the arrhythmia. The liability to attacks of tachycardia will resolve in about two thirds to three quarters of babies before the end of infancy so that prophylactic drug treatment is usually withdrawn after 6 or 12 months if there has been good control. Sometimes, when the problem seems to have resolved, there will be a recurrence later in childhood.

Other 'supraventricular' tachycardias in infancy

Other, less common tachycardias may be encountered in infancy. *Atrial flutter* is usually easy to recognize on the ECG at this age as there are often prominent flutter waves with 2:1 AV conduction (Fig. 21.40). Atrial flutter can be terminated by direct current cardioversion or transesophageal overdrive pacing. Recurrence is rare and prophylactic treatment is not usually required. *Chaotic* or *multifocal atrial tachycardia* causes an irregular rhythm with multiple nonconducted P waves of varying morphology (Fig. 21.41). There is usually sufficient AV block to give a more or less normal ventricular rate so treatment may not be necessary. Resolution during early infancy is likely. *Atrial ectopic tachycardia* may present as

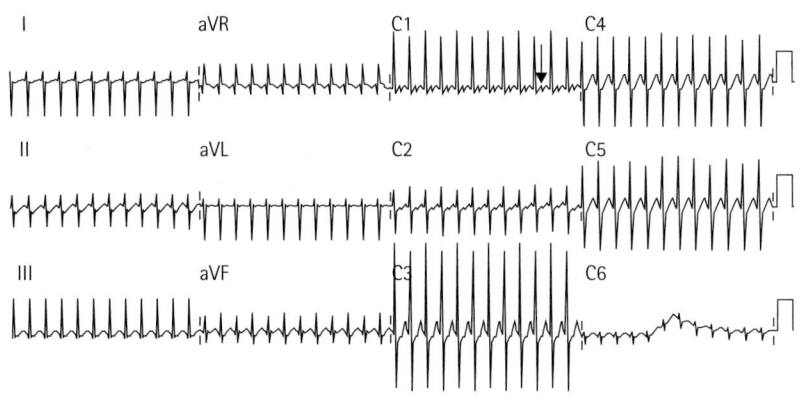

Fig. 21.38 Typical atrioventricular (AV) re-entry tachycardia in a neonate. The ventricular rate is 290 per minute and the QRS is normal. A retrograde P wave is clearly seen in lead C1 (arrow). The timing of the P wave and the age of patient make orthodromic AV re-entry tachycardia via an accessory pathway an almost certain diagnosis.

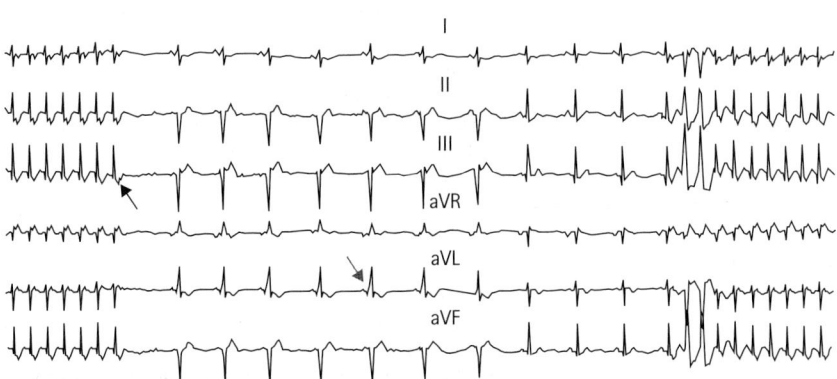

Fig. 21.39 Administration of intravenous adenosine during atrioventricular (AV) re-entry tachycardia in a neonate. Adenosine produces transient AV block and the tachycardia terminates with a non-conducted P wave (black arrow). This is followed by sinus rhythm which for seven beats shows clear evidence of ventricular pre-excitation (gray arrow). As the sinus rhythm speeds up slightly the pre-excitation disappears and there is no delta wave for the next four sinus beats. AV re-entry tachycardia then reinitiates with rate-related bundle branch block during the first two beats of tachycardia.

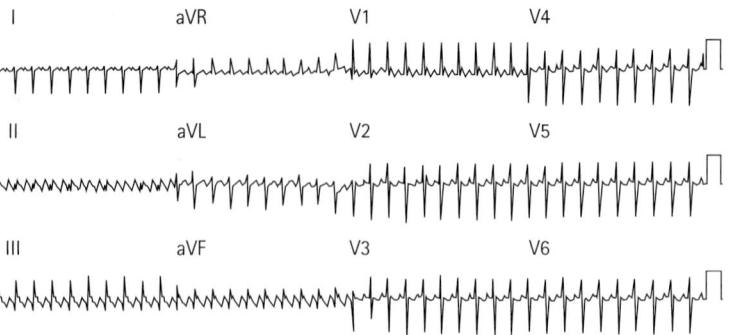

Fig. 21.40 Neonatal atrial flutter. The atrial rate is 460 per minute which, with 2:1 AV conduction, gives a ventricular rate of 230 per minute. Saw-tooth flutter waves are clearly seen in leads II, III, aVF, and V1.

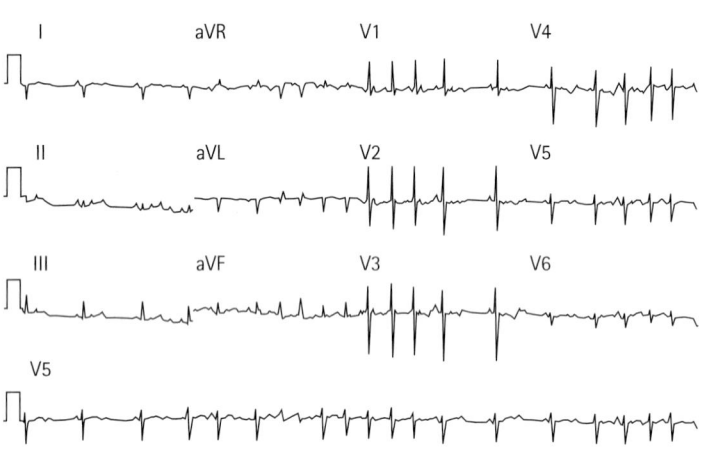

Fig. 21.41 Chaotic atrial tachycardia in infancy. This is also known as multifocal atrial tachycardia. There are several different P wave morphologies and many more P waves than QRS complexes. Many of the P waves are not conducted so the ventricular rate is in fact slightly slow. The extra or early P waves differ in morphology from the sinus beats.

a sustained arrhythmia in early infancy (Fig. 21.42). Drug treatment (beta-blocker, flecainide or amiodarone) may be required in the short term, but the problem usually resolves within a few months.[181]

One unusual but important variety of AV re-entry tachycardia presenting with an incessant tachycardia is *permanent junctional reciprocating tachycardia* (PJRT).[182] It is recognized on the ECG from the long RP interval and the inverted P waves in inferior leads (Fig. 21.43). Treatment with a beta-blocker, flecainide, or amiodarone will suppress the arrhythmia or control the rate. Spontaneous resolution of PJRT is less common and radiofrequency ablation may be required later in childhood (see below). *Congenital junctional ectopic tachycardia* (*His bundle tachycardia*) is rare and is recognized by the presence of slower dissociated P waves. Long term drug treatment is required. This arrhythmia is more common early after infant cardiac surgery.

Ventricular tachycardia in infancy

Pediatricians are often reluctant to consider the diagnosis of ventricular tachycardia (VT) in infants, and most cases are initially mistaken for some form of supraventricular tachycardia. Widening of the QRS can be subtle in infancy but if the QRS is abnormal the diagnosis of VT should be considered. VT may be relatively slow and well tolerated, in which case treatment may not be required and resolution is likely.[183] The most significant type of VT encountered is incessant infant ventricular tachycardia. It usually presents between 3 months and 2 years of age. The QRS most often shows a right bundle branch block pattern with a superior axis indicating a posterior left ventricular origin for the tachycardia (Fig. 21.44). The cause is probably a tiny myocardial hamartoma that is beyond the resolution of imaging techniques. The most effective drug for suppression of incessant VT is amiodarone or flecainide, often used in combination with a beta-blocker. This arrhythmia usually resolves before school age and treatment can be withdrawn without recurrence. Other ventricular tachycardias in infancy are rare and require specialist evaluation.[19]

TACHYCARDIA IN CHILDHOOD WITH NORMAL QRS COMPLEXES

Atrioventricular re-entry tachycardia

As in infancy, the commonest significant arrhythmia in childhood is orthodromic atrioventricular re-entry tachycardia (Fig. 21.38). Few new cases present between 1 and 4 years of age and at this age they are often triggered by fevers. New presentation after early childhood (usually with palpitation) implies only a small chance of long term natural resolution. As in infancy, the ECG may show ventricular pre-excitation in sinus rhythm (Fig. 21.45) but it is more common for the pathway to be 'concealed', that is, to be capable of only retrograde conduction. Most episodes of tachycardia during childhood revert to sinus rhythm spontaneously. In some children vagal stimulation slows AV nodal conduction sufficiently to break tachycardia.[184] The most effective techniques include a Valsalva maneuver (such as trying to blow up a balloon) and other methods of breath-holding, facial application of an ice pack or inversion into a headstand. Carotid sinus massage and eyeball pressure are usually ineffective and the latter may cause injury. If tachycardia is sustained, sinus rhythm can be restored with a rapid intravenous bolus of adenosine 150–500 mcg/kg/dose, or with intravenous verapamil. As AV re-entry tachycardia in childhood is not intrinsically dangerous, the choice of long term treatment depends on the frequency, severity and duration of episodes. If attacks are mild and infrequent, treatment may not be required. Long term treatment involves a choice between prophylactic medication and catheter ablation. Many children and their parents prefer the prospect of a cure with catheter ablation to the alternative of prolonged drug treatment.

Many drugs can be used to suppress AV re-entry tachycardia. The literature relating to their use is mainly a series of retrospective reports. There are no blinded or placebo-controlled trials and very few comparisons between drugs. Most anti-arrhythmic drugs have been tried for control of this common arrhythmia. Those most likely to be effective

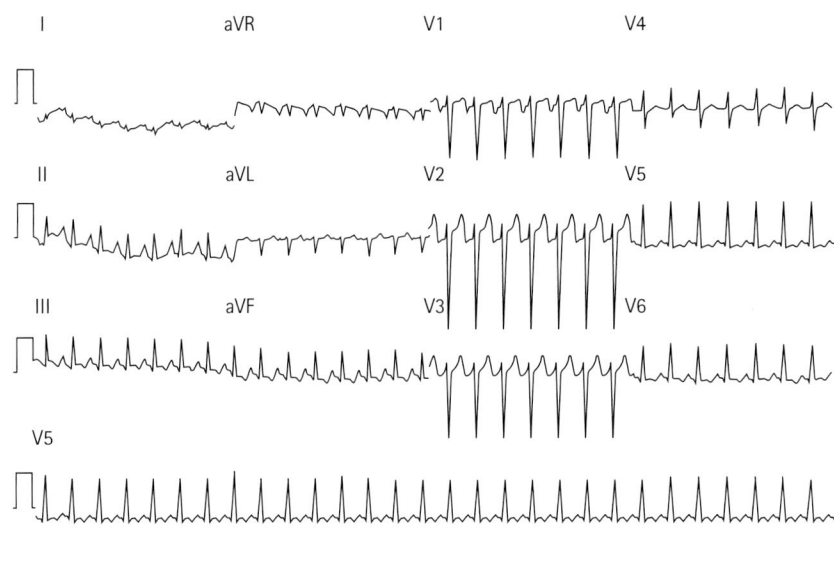

Fig. 21.42 Atrial ectopic tachycardia in a 5-year-old boy. At first glance this looks like a sinus tachycardia but the rate is inappropriately high for the age and clinical situation. The P waves are abnormal and their morphology suggests an ectopic focus in the right atrium. In this example there is 1:1 conduction throughout but transient AV block is not unusual.

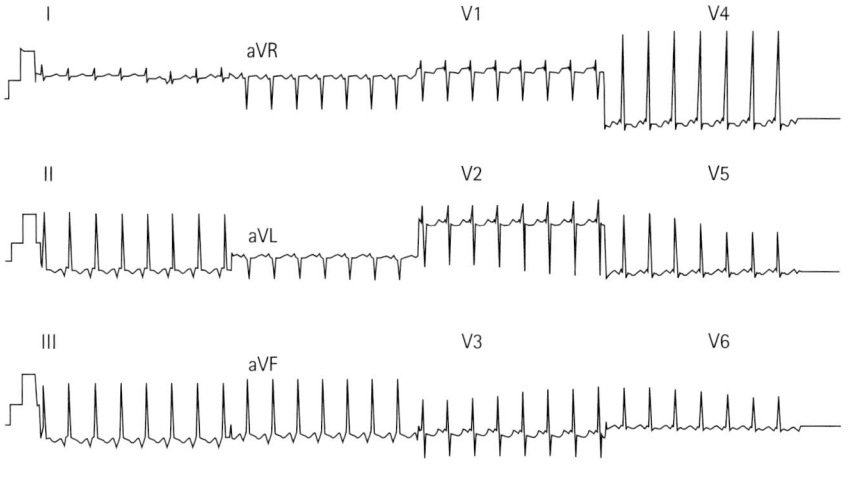

Fig. 21.43 Permanent junctional reciprocating tachycardia. This arrhythmia is characterized by a long RP interval and an abnormal P wave axis with inverted P waves in leads II, III, and aVF. It is usually incessant but will stop transiently with adenosine.

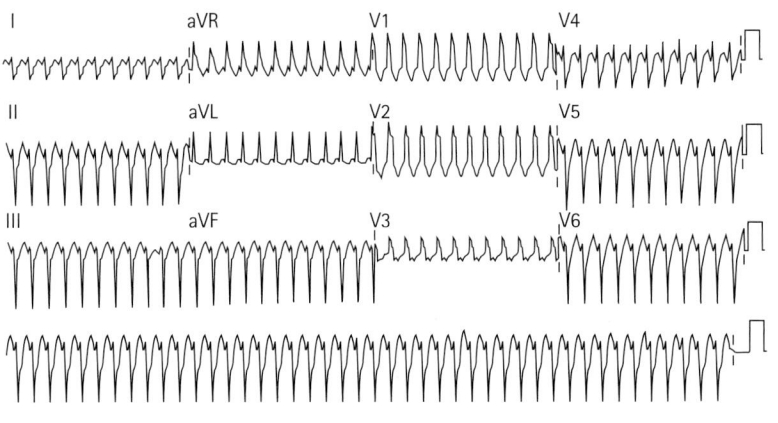

Fig. 21.44 Ventricular tachycardia in an 11-month-old boy. The QRS complexes have an appearance similar to right bundle branch block but the initial R wave in V1 is taller than the secondary R. There is very subtle evidence of ventriculo-atrial dissociation, perhaps best shown by the variable height of the T waves in the rhythm strip at the bottom caused by intermittent superimposition of P waves.

include beta-blockers, flecainide, amiodarone and sotalol. Drug treatment may occasionally produce new arrhythmias, a so-called 'pro-arrhythmic' effect.

Catheter ablation was introduced to clinical practice in the early 1990s and is regarded as the standard treatment for many arrhythmias. In experienced hands, success rates are high and serious complications are rare.[185] The procedure involves the use of a high frequency electric current to induce a small burn at the point of contact between the catheter and the heart. If the catheter is accurately positioned the arrhythmia substrate will be destroyed.

Atrioventricular nodal re-entry tachycardia

This arrhythmia is rare before school age but becomes an increasingly important mechanism of SVT during later childhood (Fig. 21.46). It may be difficult to differentiate from atrioventricular re-entry but the difference is only important if catheter ablation is being considered and diagnosis is easy at electrophysiology study. Both arrhythmias can be stopped with vagal maneuvers or intravenous adenosine. The AV nodal re-entry circuit includes the AV node and adjacent low right atrium[186] (it would perhaps be more accurately termed atrio-nodal re-entry tachycardia). Drug treatment is often relatively ineffective or poorly tolerated.

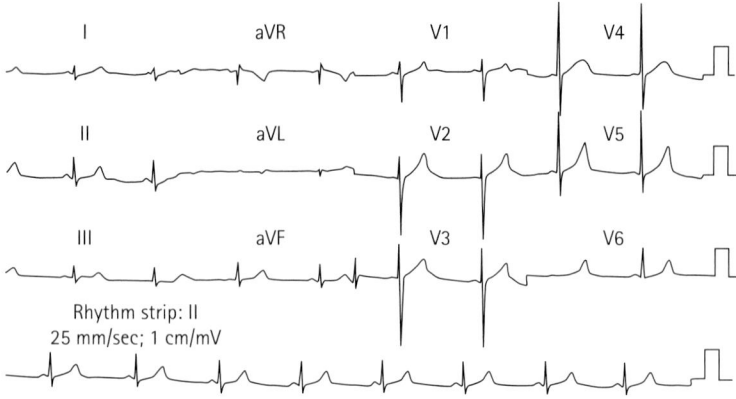

Fig. 21.49   Congenital long QT syndrome. A recording from a 14-year-old boy who presented with syncope. The QT interval is markedly prolonged.

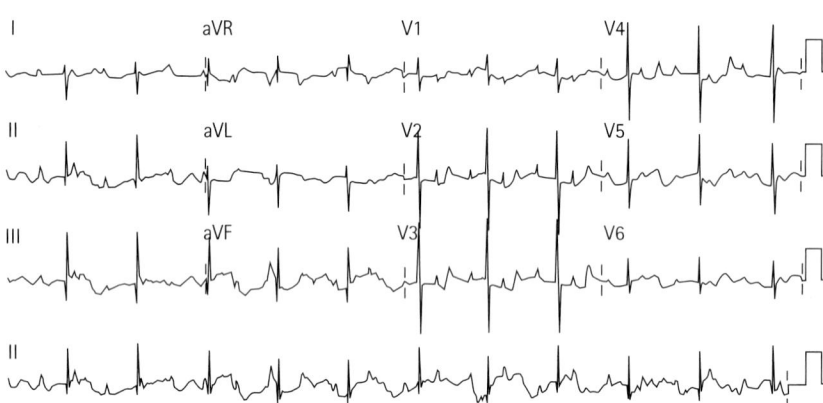

Fig. 21.50   Complete atrioventricular block in a neonate. The atrial rate is 140 per minute. The QRS complexes are regular with a normal morphology at a rate of 67 per minute. The baby's mother has Sjögren syndrome. Pacing was not required during infancy.

implantation.[192] A few infants with complete AV block have underlying structural heart disease, most commonly left atrial isomerism or congenitally corrected transposition (atrioventricular and ventricular arterial discordance). Complete AV block also occurs after surgical repair of heart disease, in which case pacemaker implantation is almost always required.

While AV block in infancy is rare (with a prevalence at live birth of 1:20 000), a much more common arrhythmia, which may be mistaken for AV block, is produced by atrial premature beats or atrial ectopic beats. These are benign, asymptomatic and usually disappear during infancy. Depending on their timing they may be conducted normally, or with a bundle branch block pattern, or may be blocked (Fig. 21.51).

Complete AV block may be detected for the first time in childhood but it is probably most often congenital in origin. An average daytime ventricular rate below 50 per minute may be an indication for pacemaker implantation, even in the absence of symptoms. The presence of symptoms such as syncope, breathlessness or tiredness implies a significant risk and is an absolute indication for a pacemaker.

Other primary bradycardias

Bradycardia may also result from primary failure of impulse formation, known as sinoatrial disease. This is rare in childhood and pacemaker implantation is required only if there are symptoms. It is most often encountered late after cardiac surgery.

CARDIAC ARRHYTHMIAS IN OTHER SITUATIONS

Arrhythmias occurring late after surgery for congenital heart disease

Several cardiac operations are associated with late postoperative arrhythmias that have a significant impact on late morbidity and mortality.[193] Atrial flutter most often complicates atrial repair of transposition of the great arteries (Mustard or Senning operations) or right heart bypass operations for complex malformations (Fontan operation). It may also be a late complication of simpler operations such as repair of atrial septal defect or repair of tetralogy of Fallot. Atrial flutter may be associated with syncope or sudden death and demands expert evaluation and treatment. Postoperative ventricular tachycardia usually complicates

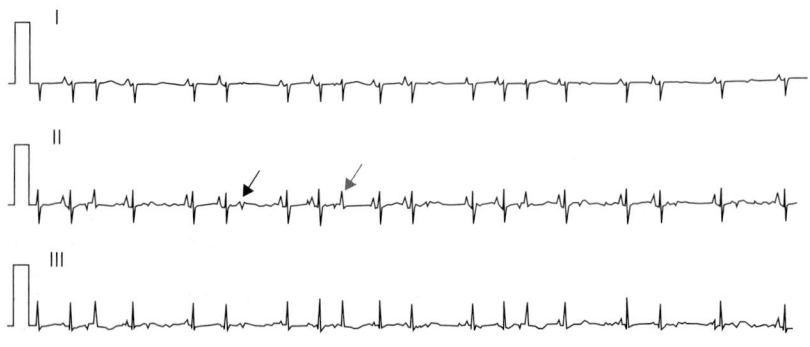

Fig. 21.51   Atrial premature beats in a neonate. The majority of the beats are sinus in origin but several are followed by premature P waves. Some of these are not conducted to the ventricles (black arrow) while others are conducted with a slightly different QRS morphology (gray arrow).

operations that involve surgery on the ventricles such as repair of tetralogy of Fallot or Rastelli operation. Again the arrhythmia is potentially dangerous and requires expert assessment.

Asymptomatic Wolff–Parkinson–White syndrome

Ventricular pre-excitation may be found unexpectedly on an ECG. Population studies have shown that two thirds of children with ventricular pre-excitation have no symptoms. It is likely that the majority will never develop an arrhythmia and the risk associated with asymptomatic ventricular pre-excitation is very small. The consensus at present is that treatment is not required although expert assessment and discussion is appropriate.[194]

SYNCOPE

Syncope is a common symptom in childhood and in most cases is benign.[52] The commonest mechanism is vasovagal syncope (so-called 'simple faint') in which there is a transient vagally mediated bradycardia. Other causes of syncope may be associated with transient bradycardia – such as in reflex asystolic syncope in preschool children and in neurocardiogenic syncope in older children. Documentation of bradycardia during syncope in this situation does not necessarily mean that there is a primary cardiac arrhythmia. In most cases the significance of the syncope and the likely underlying cause will be evident from the history.

A few rare but potentially dangerous arrhythmias may present with syncope. They include polymorphic VT, other types of VT, and atrial fibrillation in the Wolff–Parkinson–White syndrome (all discussed above). An ECG should be part of routine assessment of children with syncope but clinical evaluation is necessary before embarking on further investigation. Children with syncope on exertion, or physical signs of possible cardiovascular abnormality, or a family history of syncope or sudden death, or an abnormal ECG should be referred for expert evaluation.[52]

FAMILY HISTORY OF SUDDEN DEATH

The sudden death of a parent or sibling is a devastating event with many consequences. Some causes of sudden cardiac death are familial. Structural abnormalities include hypertrophic cardiomyopathy, Marfan syndrome, dilated cardiomyopathy and other cardiomyopathies. Primary electrical abnormalities may cause sudden death with an anatomically normal heart. They include long QT syndrome, catecholaminergic polymorphic VT and Brugada syndrome. Although they all have a genetic basis, genetic testing is not widely clinically available, other than for long QT syndrome. All first-degree relatives of victims of sudden cardiac death at a young age should be referred for specialist assessment which will include a detailed history, clinical examination, ECG and echocardiogram. Further assessment may be appropriate if the diagnosis is known in the proband or if initial investigations show abnormalities.[195]

CONCLUSION

Recent years have seen an increased awareness of cardiac arrhythmias amongst pediatricians and pediatric cardiologists and a rapid advance in our understanding of the mechanisms. Non-invasive evaluation will usually identify precisely the type of arrhythmia and will help to define the prognosis and guide treatment. The outlook for most children with arrhythmias is good, especially in the present era of improved acute and long term treatment.

ACQUIRED CARDIOVASCULAR DISORDERS

MYOCARDITIS

Myocarditis is an acute infective, toxic or autoimmune inflammation of the myocardium.[196] Viral infections (coxsackie B and adenovirus) are the most common, but protozoal and bacterial myocarditis occurs. A genetic predisposition with subsequent autoimmune response may be responsible.

Clinical features

The clinical spectrum varies from asymptomatic to severe heart failure. There is frequently a recent history of a flu-like illness or gastroenteritis. There is a persistent, unexplained tachycardia and signs of heart failure (p. 762). Arrhythmias are common. Chest pain may also occur, due to associated pericarditis.

Investigations

The erythrocyte sedimentation rate, C-reactive protein and cardiac muscle enzyme levels are usually elevated. Evidence of viral infection should be sought. Serology with rising or falling titers indicates a viral infection. Electrocardiogram shows a sinus tachycardia, ST segment and T wave changes, and conduction disturbances. Ectopic beats and arrhythmias are common. Decreased QRS voltage with T wave flattening and inversion occur. Chest radiography shows cardiomegaly. Echocardiography demonstrates a dilated, poorly contracting left ventricle. Mitral regurgitation and a pericardial effusion may be present. Myocardial biopsy is rarely performed in children as inflammatory changes are patchy, and the procedure carries a risk of cardiac perforation.

Management and prognosis

Treatment depends on severity of the myocarditis. Cardiac monitoring and rest are advisable. Heart failure is managed as described previously (p. 763). Inotropic support is often necessary. Arrhythmias should be treated aggressively. The use of steroids, other immunosuppressive therapy and immunoglobulin is controversial.[196,197] Mechanical cardiac support can be used as a bridge to recovery or transplant.

If adequate support can be given for the severe heart failure that usually occurs at presentation, the outcome is often favorable.[198] Survivors may recover completely, or develop cardiomyopathy.[197]

PERICARDITIS AND PERICARDIAL EFFUSION
Etiology

Infection, other inflammatory diseases or trauma produce an effusion which may be fibrinous, purulent or hemorrhagic. Viral pericarditis is often associated with a myocarditis caused by similar viruses. Small pericardial effusions occur as part of the pancarditis of rheumatic fever and Kawasaki disease. Large pericardial effusions are most common in children with neoplasia, chronic renal failure, connective tissue diseases, and after cardiac surgery. Purulent or tuberculous pericarditis is rare in resource rich countries. Sometimes no cause is found.

Clinical features

Signs vary with the primary illness, and with the volume and rate of accumulation of pericardial fluid. Rapid accumulation is more likely to produce cardiac tamponade. Chest pain is uncommon in children. Fever is prominent with bacterial infection. A pericardial friction rub may be audible. Signs of tamponade include neck vein distension, hepatomegaly, faint heart sounds and pulsus paradoxus (a fall in systolic blood pressure of >10 mmHg on inspiration).[199] Other signs of cardiac failure are also present. Any underlying cause must be identified. Bacterial pericarditis is usually secondary to other infection such as bronchopneumonia, empyema, lung abscess, osteomyelitis or pyelonephritis.

Investigations

Electrocardiogram shows diminished QRS voltage and diffuse ST segment elevation. There may be cardiomegaly on chest radiography. Echocardiography indicates the size of the effusion (Fig. 21.52). Collapse of the atria and right ventricle indicates tamponade. If infective pericarditis is suspected, a primary focus must be sought and blood cultures and pericardiocentesis performed. The pericardial fluid is examined for cells and organisms and cultured for bacteria, viruses and fungi. When

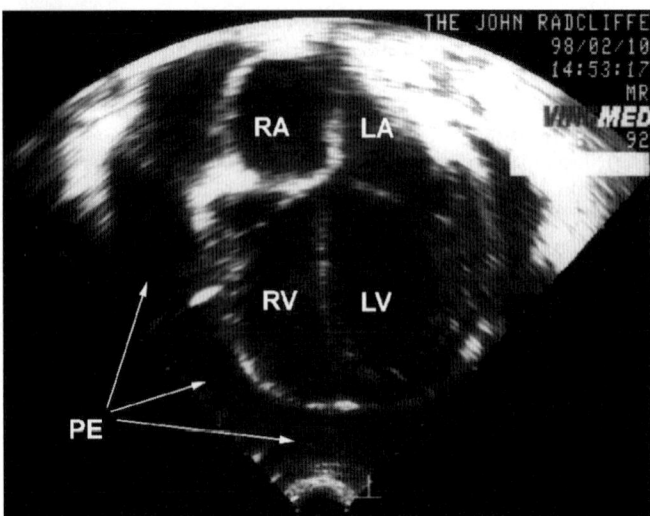

Fig. 21.52 Four chamber echocardiogram view of a pericardial effusion. PE, pericardial effusion; RV, right ventricle; LV, left ventricle; RA, right atrium; LA, left atrium.

appropriate, serological evidence of a viral infection or autoimmune disease should be sought.

Treatment

Symptomatic treatment includes anti-inflammatory drugs. Treatment is also directed at the cause. Purulent or tuberculous pericarditis requires appropriate intravenous antibiotics and surgical drainage may be necessary. Pericardial effusions due to leukemia will usually resolve with appropriate chemotherapy.

Pericardiocentesis is essential for cardiac tamponade. Except in an emergency, this is carried out under ultrasound or fluoroscopic guidance, using a subxiphoid approach. A drain is usually left in situ until the effusion has resolved. Constriction is rare in children and usually due to tuberculous pericarditis.

RHEUMATIC FEVER AND RHEUMATIC HEART DISEASE

Rheumatic fever is an endemic disease in resource limited countries, where it remains a major cause of morbidity and mortality.[200] Acute carditis, with the subsequent development of rheumatic heart disease, is the most serious consequence. The pathogenesis and noncardiac manifestations are discussed in Chapter 29. The most common age of onset is between 5 and 15 years.

Acute carditis

This is a pancarditis, affecting the endocardium with valve involvement, myocardium and pericardium. It occurs in over 50% of children with rheumatic fever, usually within the first 3 weeks of the illness. It is most frequent in younger children, in those who had carditis in the initial attack, and with recurrences. The prime clinical indicator of carditis is a murmur that has developed recently or changed in character. The most common is an apical pansystolic murmur of mitral regurgitation. This may be due to endocarditis with edema of the mitral valve, or myocarditis with dilatation of the left ventricle and stretching of the mitral valve. This murmur must be differentiated from an innocent murmur in association with a febrile illness, and an organic murmur due to pre-existing congenital or rheumatic heart disease. A short apical mid-diastolic flow murmur may be heard. This frequently resolves when the child recovers. Less commonly, the early diastolic murmur of aortic regurgitation is heard in the aortic area and left sternal edge.

Cardiac failure is an uncommon presenting feature but may result from valve regurgitation or ventricular dysfunction caused by myocar-

ditis. Pericarditis, recognized by a friction rub, never occurs in isolation and indicates underlying myocarditis. Sinus tachycardia is also suggestive of carditis, particularly when it occurs during sleep in the afebrile child. Sinus bradycardia occasionally occurs.

Investigations

Electrocardiographic changes include prolongation of the PR interval (first degree heart block), second degree or complete heart block. Flattened or inverted T waves over the left precordial leads are a characteristic finding of myopericarditis. Other investigations are discussed in Chapter 29. Echocardiography may demonstrate a small pericardial effusion. A dilated left ventricle occurs with significant myocardial disease or severe valve regurgitation. Contractility is decreased with myocarditis, but normal or increased with mitral or aortic regurgitation. Approximately 50% of children with rheumatic fever have clinical evidence of carditis, but Doppler and color flow mapping demonstrates valve regurgitation in up to 70%. Echocardiography may be accepted in the future to diagnose carditis[201] but strict criteria must be applied, as minimal mitral regurgitation is physiological.

Treatment

Eradication of streptococcal infection is essential, even in the absence of evidence of active infection. Oral penicillin is given for 10 days. Alternatively a dose of (long-acting) benzathine penicillin 0.6–1.2 million units is given intramuscularly. Erythromycin is used in children allergic to penicillin. Aspirin relieves symptoms, but does not prevent the development of rheumatic heart disease. Steroids shorten the duration of the illness but symptoms often return when they are discontinued. Some clinicians use aspirin as the steroids are reduced. Studies have failed to demonstrate a lower risk of heart disease in children receiving steroids or immunoglobulin.[202] Heart failure is treated as described previously (p. 762).

Rheumatic fever recurs most commonly in young children and in the first 5 years following an episode. Each attack carries an increasing risk of carditis with permanent cardiac damage and death. It is therefore essential that *continuous* antimicrobial prophylaxis against further streptococcal infection be started after the therapeutic course of penicillin. The most effective form of prophylaxis is an intramuscular injection of 0.6–1.2 million units of benzathine penicillin every 3–4 weeks.[203] Alternatively oral phenoxymethylpenicillin (penicillin V) 250 mg is given twice daily. Sulfadiazine is recommended for children allergic to penicillin. Prophylactic therapy must be continued throughout childhood and into early adult life. The decision whether to discontinue prophylaxis thereafter depends on the severity of cardiac involvement, time since the last attack, social circumstances and risk of exposure to further streptococcal infections.

Prognosis

There has been a marked decrease in mortality and morbidity as a result of improved socioeconomic standards and treatment with penicillin, particularly as prophylaxis to prevent recurrences. The prognosis is still much worse in countries where severe rheumatic heart disease develops during childhood. The prognosis is also worse in children who have severe cardiac involvement in the initial attack, and those who have recurrences with carditis. Mitral regurgitation can improve with time but aortic regurgitation is likely to be permanent. The prognosis is excellent for patients who escape carditis during an initial attack of rheumatic fever, but this does not preclude carditis in a subsequent episode, so prophylaxis is indicated.

Rheumatic heart disease

Rheumatic heart disease occurs in childhood in countries where the incidence of rheumatic fever remains high. The prevalence is approximately 6 per 1000 school-aged children.[200] The mitral valve is affected in 85% of children, the aortic valve in 55%, and the tricuspid and pulmonary valves in less than 5%. Isolated aortic valve disease is rare.

Mitral regurgitation is the commonest lesion. The clinical findings are the same as congenital mitral regurgitation (p. 784). In older children it is often associated with mitral stenosis. Echocardiography shows enlargement of the left atrium and left ventricle, and color Doppler confirms the presence of regurgitation and its severity. The mitral valve leaflets are thickened and tethered, with cordal rupture and prolapse. Cardiac catheterization adds little further information, apart from measurement of pulmonary arterial resistance.

Mitral stenosis may be asymptomatic initially but effort intolerance and dyspnea progress to orthopnea, paroxysmal nocturnal dyspnea and hemoptysis. The apex beat is not displaced unless there is significant additional mitral regurgitation. The pulse volume may be reduced and the first heart sound is loud. An opening snap early in diastole is followed by a low-pitched rumbling mitral mid-diastolic murmur. Increasing mitral stenosis causes progressive lengthening of the murmur resulting in presystolic accentuation. Atrial fibrillation is rare in children but, if it occurs, the presystolic component (related to atrial contraction) disappears. A right ventricular parasternal impulse is palpable and the pulmonary second sound is accentuated when pulmonary hypertension occurs.

On chest radiography the cardiothoracic ratio is usually normal, with left atrial enlargement. Increased left atrial pressure causes dilatation of the upper lobe pulmonary veins and edema of the interlobular septa (Kerley B lines). The electrocardiogram demonstrates the broad, notched P waves of left atrial hypertrophy if there is moderate or severe mitral obstruction and right ventricular hypertrophy when pulmonary hypertension develops. Echocardiography shows a large left atrium with thickened and tethered mitral valve leaflets. Fibrosis and calcification of the valve and subvalvar apparatus reduce mobility of the leaflets. The Doppler signal shows an increased velocity and reduced rate of pressure fall across the valve throughout diastole, a quantitative assessment being given by the pressure half-time. This provides some assessment of the severity of the obstruction. Cardiac catheterization is performed to assess pulmonary vascular resistance or as part of therapeutic balloon dilatation of the mitral valve.

Aortic regurgitation has the same clinical features as for congenital causes of aortic regurgitation (p. 785).

Management

Children with mild valve disease require follow-up and antimicrobial prophylaxis. In addition, life-long prophylaxis against bacterial endocarditis is necessary for dental and other surgical procedures (Table 21.6).[60] Indications and timing of mitral and aortic valve surgery remain controversial. Children who are asymptomatic with significant regurgitation and normal left ventricular function on echocardiography should be observed closely. Symptoms, deterioration of left ventricular dysfunction or pulmonary hypertension are indications for surgery. A good result may sometimes be achieved with anuloplasty for mitral regurgitation, or valvotomy for mitral stenosis. Valve replacement is required for severe aortic regurgitation.

KAWASAKI DISEASE

Kawasaki disease is the most common acquired heart disease in children in resource rich countries.[204] The incidence peaks in toddlers, most cases occurring in children under 5 years and rarely in infants under 3 months of age. The cause is multifactorial, probably requiring an infectious agent in association with specific genetic and immunological factors.[204]

Clinical features

Diagnosis is based on the presence of clinical criteria in Table 29.15 *and* the exclusion of other diagnosis.[204,205] The general clinical features are described in Chapter 29, p. 1424.

Cardiac involvement occurs in the second week after the onset of symptoms. In the acute phase, there may be medium and large vessel arteritis with arterial aneurysms, particularly in the coronary arteries.

Coronary aneurysms occur in up to 30% of untreated children. This is significantly reduced by the early administration of immunoglobulin. A friction rub of pericarditis, or gallop rhythm of cardiac failure from myocarditis may be present.

Investigations

Electrocardiographic abnormalities include sinus tachycardia, reduction in QRS amplitude, flattening of T waves, prolongation of rate-adjusted PR and QT intervals and occasional dysrhythmias. Serial echocardiograms are required to evaluate and follow up myocardial and coronary artery abnormalities. The initial echocardiogram should be performed at the time of diagnosis, although aneurysms are rarely seen before the tenth day of illness. Treatment with immunoglobulin should *not be delayed* until after the echocardiogram has been performed. Echocardiograms should be repeated at approximately 14 days into the illness, and at 6–8 weeks.

Acute management

Initial management is described in Chapter 29. The risk of death is greatest in the first 60 days, from coronary artery thrombosis and myocardial infarction.[204] Children with large (giant) aneurysms (> 8 mm) should be started on warfarin in addition to low dose aspirin to prevent clot developing in the aneurysm. If a child has clinical features of coronary thrombosis, thrombolysis with tissue plasminogen activator (tPA) is indicated.[205]

Long term management and prognosis

Approximately 50% of coronary artery aneurysms regress in 5 years following an episode of Kawasaki disease. Small aneurysms (< 5 mm) commonly disappear, but large aneurysms (> 8 mm) seldom resolve completely. Long term morbidity results from initial thickening of the coronary artery wall and accelerated atheroma in later life. These changes may also occur in children who have not had aneurysms during the acute episode.

Risk stratification is carried out after the clinical evaluation and echocardiogram done at 6–8 weeks.[205] If there is:

- *No coronary artery change at any stage of illness.* Discontinue antiplatelet therapy. No further physical restriction. Cardiovascular assessment at 5 year intervals.
- *Transient coronary artery dilatation, disappearing within 6–8 weeks.* Discontinue antiplatelet therapy. No further physical restriction. Cardiovascular assessment at 3–5 year intervals.
- *One small or medium sized coronary artery aneurysm.* Aspirin 3–5 mg/kg/day. Avoid contact and high impact sports. No further physical restriction for patients less than 11 years old. Patients 11–20 years – biennial stress test/myocardial perfusion scan. Annual cardiovascular assessment. Angiography if non-invasive test suggests ischemia.
- *Multiple or giant coronary artery aneurysm* (Fig. 21.53). Aspirin 3–5 mg/kg/day. Additional warfarin if giant coronary artery aneurysm present. Avoid contact and high impact sports. Other physical activity recommendations guided by annual stress test/ myocardial perfusion scan. Biannual cardiovascular assessment. Angiography at 6–12 months. Further angiography if non-invasive test suggests ischemia.
- *Coronary artery obstruction.* Aspirin 3–5 mg/kg/day. Additional warfarin if giant coronary artery aneurysm persists. Avoid contact and high impact sports. Other physical activity recommendations guided by annual stress test/myocardial perfusion scan. Angiography to address therapeutic options.

CONNECTIVE TISSUE DISEASE

Cardiac involvement can occur in all connective tissue diseases, most frequently in systemic lupus erythematosus.

- *Systemic lupus erythematosus.* Small pericardial effusions and valvar lesions (Libman–Sacks) are the most common features. Congenital

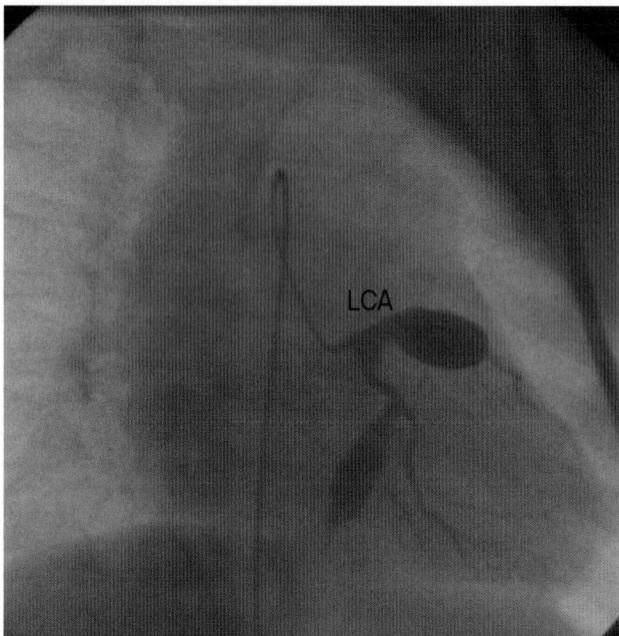

Fig. 21.53 Left coronary arteriogram showing an aneurysm of the main left and anterior descending coronary arteries in a child with Kawasaki disease. LCA, left coronary artery.

complete heart block can occur in infants of mothers suffering from connective tissue disease who are seropositive for anti-Ro.

- *Juvenile rheumatoid arthritis.* Cardiac abnormalities usually occur in the acute systemic form of the disease with pericarditis, myocarditis and occasionally mitral regurgitation. Cardiac failure is an uncommon complication.
- *HLA B27 associated juvenile arthritis.* Aortic regurgitation can occur.
- *Scleroderma.* Diffuse fibrosis within the myocardium can produce ventricular dysfunction.
- *Polyarteritis nodosa.* Coronary artery lesions can result in myocardial ischemia.

CARDIOMYOPATHY

Dilated cardiomyopathy occurs twice as frequently as hypertrophic cardiomyopathy in children. Restrictive cardiomyopathy is rare. Recently, left ventricular noncompaction has been recognized as an important cause of cardiomyopathy, accounting for nearly 10% of cases.[206]

Dilated cardiomyopathy

This is characterized by ventricular dilatation with impaired function. Possible causes are outlined in Table 21.11. Familial cardiomyopathy accounts for up to 30% of patients. Inheritance is usually autosomal dominant, but various other modes have been identified.[207]

Clinical features

Symptoms vary with the age of the child, and severity of dysfunction. Some present with symptoms of easy fatigue and decreased exercise tolerance, while others have severe cardiac failure. Less commonly the child presents with an arrhythmia. Clinical examination shows signs of heart failure (p. 762). Mitral regurgitation can be present, caused by dilatation of the mitral valve ring. Pulmonary or systemic emboli can result from intracardiac thrombosis.

Investigations

A cause should always be sought, and Table 21.12 contains a list of initial investigations. Chest radiography shows cardiomegaly, and there is usually hypertrophy and strain on the electrocardiogram. If there are ischemic changes, an anomalous left coronary artery from the pulmo-

Table 21.11 Conditions producing dilated cardiomyopathy

Cardiovascular
  Anomalous origin of left coronary artery
  Coarctation of the aorta/critical aortic stenosis
  Arrhythmias (SVT/VT)
  Systemic arteriovenous fistula
  Birth asphyxia

Familial – dominant, recessive, X linked or mitochondrial
Drugs and toxins
  Anthracyclines
  Alcohol
  Irradiation

Myocarditis
  Viral/fungal/protozoal
  Rheumatic fever
  Kawasaki disease
  Connective tissue disease

Metabolic: storage
  Mucopolysaccharidoses
  Lipidoses (GM1 gangliosidosis)
  Sialic acid storage disorder
  Fucosidosis
  Hemosiderosis

Metabolic: energy production
  Carnitine, selenium or taurine deficiency
  Fatty acid oxidation defects (usually hypertrophic)
  'Mitochondrial' abnormalities (usually hypertrophic)
  Aminoacidemias
  Malnutrition – vitamin B deficiency (beri-beri), kwashiokor

Neuromuscular disorders
  Muscular dystrophies
  Rare congenital myopathies
  Friedreich's ataxia: (usually hypertrophic)
Chromosomal abnormalities (dysmorphic features)

Table 21.12 Screening investigations for cardiomyopathy

Blood
  Full blood count and film (eosinophilia or neutropenia)
  Erythrocyte sedimentation rate/C-reactive protein
  Carnitine (free and acyl carnitine)
  Fasting sugar and lactate
  Thyroid function
  Calcium/phosphate
  Creatine kinase
  Liver function tests
  Autoimmune/connective tissue screen
  Amino acids
  Vacuolated lymphocytes
  Selenium (if geographical risk)
  Iron and iron binding
  Viral serology (Coxsackie, ECHO, influenza, parainfluenza, mumps, rubella, rubeola and possibly HIV) – acute and convalescent
Urine
  Amino acids
  Organic acids

nary artery should be excluded (p. 785). A 24 hour electrocardiogram should be performed to rule out incessant tachycardia as the cause, and to document arrhythmias secondary to cardiomyopathy. Echocardiography will demonstrate a dilated, poorly contracting left ventricle (Fig. 21.54) and mitral regurgitation.

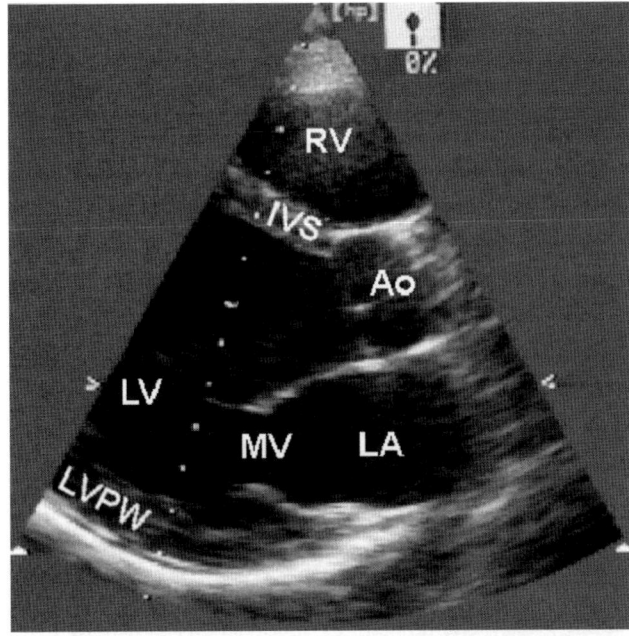

(a)

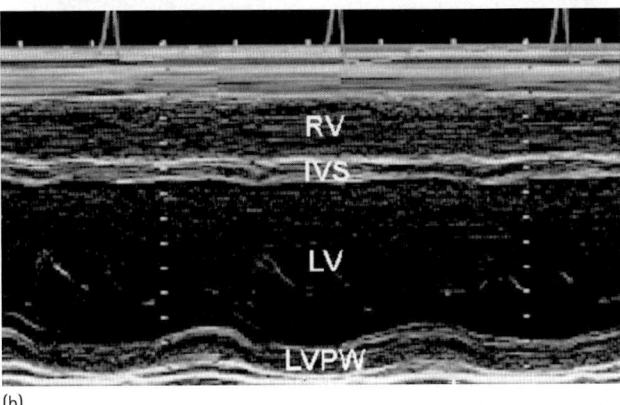

(b)

Fig. 21.54 (a) Parasternal long-axis view of a child with dilated cardiomyopathy demonstrating a dilated left ventricle. The dashed line marks the line through which the (b) M-mode recording was made and demonstrates poor contractility. Ao, aortic root; IVS, interventricular septum; LA, left atrium; LV, left ventricle; LVPW, posterior wall of the left ventricle; MV, mitral valve; RV, right ventricle.

Treatment and prognosis

Initial management is for heart failure (p. 762). Arrhythmias should be treated, avoiding drugs that are negatively inotropic. The outcome is related to severity and whether a cause can be found which is amenable to treatment. Incessant supraventricular tachycardia is treated with radiofrequency ablation, which improves ventricular function. Carnitine deficiency responds to carnitine, with resolution of the cardiomyopathy.[208] Transfusion for anemia must be carried out very cautiously as it can result in acute cardiac decompensation.

Approximately one third of children improve with time, a third stay the same and a third get worse. Older age at presentation and lack of improvement in systolic function are associated with adverse outcome. If ventricular function remains poor, referral for cardiac transplantation should be considered. Left ventricular assist devices may be used as a bridge to transplant.

Hypertrophic cardiomyopathy

Hypertrophic cardiomyopathy is characterized by unexplained ventricular hypertrophy with dysfunction. It is usually inherited as an auto-somal dominant. A number of other conditions are associated with hypertrophic cardiomyopathy (Table 21.13).[209] It is seen in up to 20% of children with Noonan syndrome. Neonatal hypertrophic cardiomyopathy is commonly due to maternal diabetes and is caused by the increased insulin acting as a fetal growth factor. It usually resolves spontaneously. This is also seen in infants with Beckwith–Wiedemann syndrome.

Clinical features

The diagnosis may be made because of the referral of an asymptomatic child for family screening. Infants may present with cardiac failure. In older children, dyspnea or excessive fatigue on exertion is most common but angina, dizziness, syncope and palpitations also occur. An ejection systolic murmur may be audible at the lower left sternal edge or apex and it may be possible to feel a 'jerky' arterial pulse or a double apical impulse.

Investigations

Electrocardiographic changes include left ventricular hypertrophy, ST and T wave abnormalities, deep Q waves, and prolongation of the QT interval. Echocardiography characteristically shows thickening of the septum and posterior left ventricular wall (Fig. 21.55), often with asymmetric septal hypertrophy and systolic anterior motion of the mitral valve. There is also left ventricular diastolic dysfunction with reduced distensibility and impaired relaxation. Doppler ultrasound may demonstrate increased velocity in the left ventricular outflow tract. Typical changes may only become apparent in the teenage years. Genetic testing is becoming possible, to identify children at risk in affected families.

Treatment and prognosis

The course of the disease is variable. Sudden death occurs in 1–6% of patients per year,[210] probably from ventricular tachycardia, and may be the presenting feature. No single feature can reliably predict risk of sudden death. A number have been identified:

- A family history of hypertrophic cardiomyopathy related cardiac arrest or sudden death.
- Nonsustained ventricular tachycardia.
- Severe ventricular hypertrophy.
- Syncope or cardiac arrest.
- Exercise-induced hypotension.

Table 21.13 Conditions associated with ventricular hypertrophy

Cardiovascular
   Coarctation of the aorta/aortic stenosis
   Systemic hypertension
   Tumors

Metabolic: storage
   Glycogenoses (Pompe, GSDIII)
   Mucopolysaccharidoses (ASH in older children)

Metabolic: energy production
   Fatty acid oxidation defects
   'Mitochondrial' cardiomyopathies
   Organic acidurias

Endocrine
   Infant of diabetic mother
   Beckwith–Wiedemann syndrome
   Pancreatic tumors (severe neonatal hypoglycemia)
   Hypothyroidism (ASH)

Neuromuscular disorders
   Friedreich's ataxia
   Rare congenital myopathies (mitochondrial)

Syndromes
   Noonan
   Leopard/neurofibromatosis/Williams
   Chromosomal abnormalities

ASH, asymmetric septal hypertrophy.

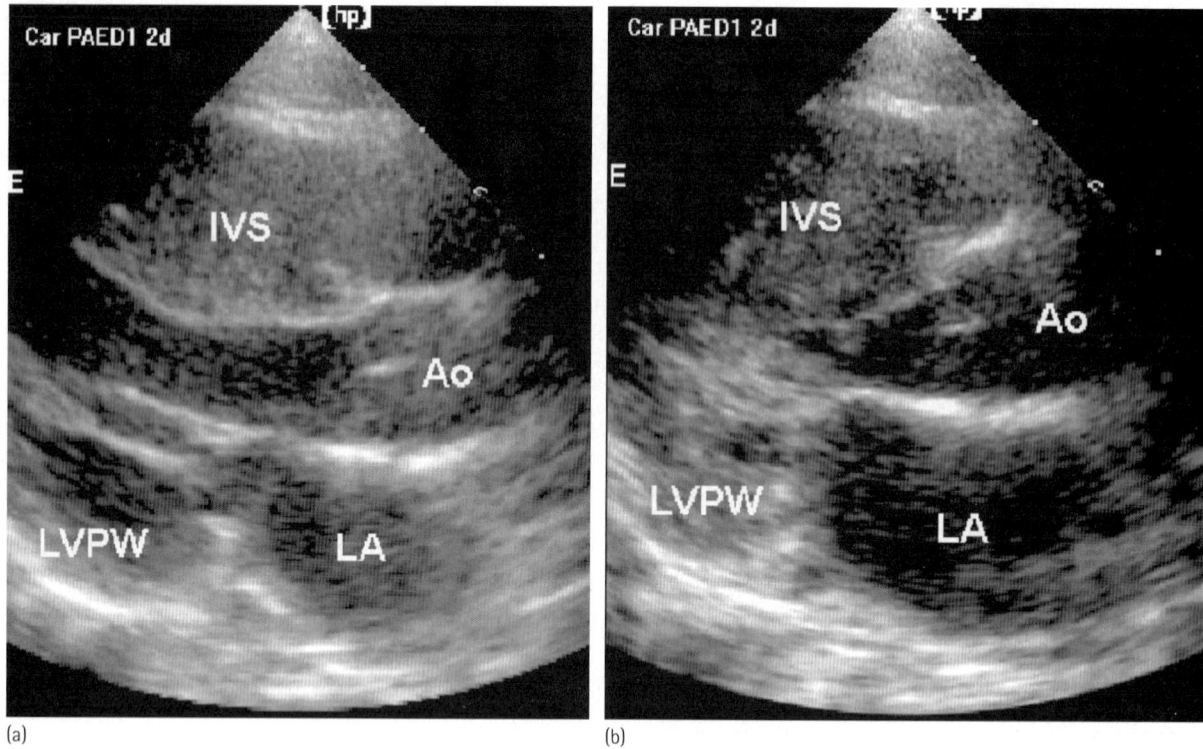

Fig. 21.55 Parasternal long-axis views of a child with hypertrophic cardiomyopathy at (a) end diastole and (b) end systole. Note the marked hypertrophy of the posterior wall of the left ventricle (LVPW) and the interventricular septum (IVS), which results in significant subaortic obstruction at end systole. Ao, aortic root; LA, left atrium.

In adults, two or more risk factors indicate a high risk of sudden death, but in children their predictive value is unknown.[176]

Beta-blockers and verapamil may help with symptoms but they do not prevent sudden death. Amiodarone may be protective but side-effects prevent its long term use.[210] Implantable defibrillators are now small enough to implant in children at high risk of sudden death. Children with severe left ventricular outflow gradients may benefit from a septal myomyectomy. Physical activities should be restricted, as severe exertion is considered a risk factor. However, in most cases, sudden death is unrelated to exertion. Advances in the genetics of hypertrophic cardiomyopathy may identify those most at risk. Screening of first-degree relatives is necessary.

Other cardiomyopathies

Noncompaction of the ventricular myocardium is recognized as an important cause of cardiomyopathy in children.[206] Presentation is in infancy and may be associated with structural heart disease. Some children have dysmorphic features. Echocardiographic features include ventricular dilatation with reduced function. There are alternating finger-like myocardial trabeculations and deep myocardial recesses constituting a large proportion of the myocardium. Either ventricle may be involved. Arrhythmias occur and thrombus may form in the ventricle, with the potential for embolization. Some children improve with time.[211] It may be familial and first-degree relatives should be screened.

Restrictive cardiomyopathies are rare in children. Radiation therapy for malignancies, pseudoxanthoma elasticum and hypereosinophilic syndromes are unusual causes in children. Amyloid, sarcoid and Fabry disease are extremely rare in children.

Endomyocardial fibrosis is a progressive and usually fatal disease of unknown etiology occurring mainly in children and young adults living in specific regions of tropical Africa. The main pathological finding is an endocardial layer of dense fibrous tissue spreading from the apex of the ventricle. Endocardial fibroelastosis has similar clinical features and evolution to dilated cardiomyopathy and may be present as part of that disease. It is also seen secondary to left ventricular outflow tract obstruction or coarctation of the aorta.

Arrhythmogenic right ventricular dysplasia is characterized by fatty infiltration and fibrosis of the free wall of the right ventricle. The disease is familial, and symptoms and risk of sudden death due to ventricular tachycardias increase with age.[212]

CARDIAC TUMORS

Primary cardiac tumors are rare in children.[213] The majority are histologically benign but may cause hemodynamic compromise from obstruction or arrhythmia. Rhabdomyomas are the most common tumor in the pediatric age group.[213] If they are multiple, they usually indicate tuberous sclerosis. Fibromas and teratomas can occur in infants and young children. Hemangiomas and myxomas occur only rarely in older children.

Clinical features depend on the site and size of the tumor. It can cause ventricular outflow obstruction, or obstruction or regurgitation of the atrioventricular valves. Arrhythmias and embolic phenomena can also occur. Echocardiography and MRI are both useful techniques to demonstrate tumors.[213] Surgery is indicated if there is an intractable arrhythmia, or obstruction to the outflow or inflow tracts. Rhabdomyomas usually regress spontaneously during infancy.

SYSTEMIC HYPERTENSION

This is defined as a systolic or diastolic blood pressure that is ≥ 95th percentile for sex, age and height on ≥ 3 occasions (Tables 21.2 and 21.3). Hypertension in children is underdiagnosed and, in adolescents, is frequently primary.[8] Measurement of blood pressure should be part of the clinical examination in all children over 3 years old who are seen in a medical setting. Younger children with specific risk factors should also have their blood pressure measured. Risk factors include:

- prematurity, neonatal intensive care;
- congenital heart disease or family history of heart disease;

- renal disease;
- systemic disease associated with hypertension;
- evidence of raised intracranial pressure;
- malignancy;
- drug treatment which can cause hypertension.

Etiology

Primary hypertension is most common in adolescents, particularly in those who have a hypertensive first-degree relative or who are overweight. Renal disease accounts for about 95% of cases of secondary hypertension (Table 18.12). Other causes include aortic coarctation, Takayashu disease and endocrine conditions (p. 487). Rare causes include neurofibromatosis, familial dysautonomia, porphyria, Turner syndrome and lead poisoning.

Clinical features

Hypertension is frequently discovered on routine examination of a child who has no symptoms directly attributable to it. Techniques of blood pressure measurement are discussed on page 744. In general, the younger the child and the higher the blood pressure, the more likely it is that hypertension is secondary. Children whose blood pressure is consistently above the 95th percentile for sex, age and height (Tables 21.2 and 21.3) should be investigated and treatment should aim to achieve a reduction to below the 95th percentile.[8] Ideally, an obese child with moderate hypertension should be encouraged to lose weight and the blood pressure subsequently repeated before undergoing extensive investigation and treatment.

When symptoms occur, they result from the cause or the complications of hypertension.

Symptoms of the cause. The history may suggest a renal cause (past or present kidney disease), pheochromocytoma (episodes of palpitations, excessive sweating, headache), aldosteronism (weakness, polyuria, muscle cramps) or drug ingestion (corticosteroid, oral contraceptive). Inquiry should be made for a family history of eclampsia, essential hypertension, premature coronary artery or cerebrovascular disease, diabetes mellitus, inherited renal conditions and neurofibromatosis.

Symptoms of the complications. Hypertension may cause raised intracranial pressure resulting in headache or vomiting. Eventually seizures or other neurological disturbances occur. All children should have their blood pressure measured after a first seizure. Visual problems, tiredness, irritability and epistaxis are described. Cardiac failure, respiratory distress, vomiting, irritability or convulsions may be the presenting feature in infants.

Signs of hypertension. Physical examination may be normal initially but with established hypertension changes occur in the optic fundi and evidence of left ventricular hypertrophy becomes apparent. Signs of heart failure may be present.

Signs of the cause of hypertension. Physical examination must include palpation of the femoral pulses and kidneys, and auscultation of the abdomen and flanks for a bruit suggesting renal artery stenosis. The clinical features of Williams and Turner syndromes must be considered. Because primary hypertension has a strong association with obesity, body mass index should be calculated from the height and weight.

Investigation

This will depend on the child's age, blood pressure level, and the clinical findings. Those with severe hypertension, symptoms, or advanced retinopathy require urgent investigation and treatment. A full blood count, urinalysis and culture, serum electrolytes, urea, creatinine and uric acid concentrations should be performed. The presence of associated hyperlipidemia, a further risk factor in coronary artery disease, should be excluded.

Other studies may be warranted on the basis of the history or physical or laboratory findings with the aim of excluding renal and endocrine disease, as detailed in Chapters 18 and 15 respectively. Echocardiography can identify aortic coarctation. Children with established hypertension should have regular cardiac monitoring with echocardiography to assess left ventricular hypertrophy.

Management and prognosis

Borderline hypertension (between the 90th and 95th percentile) does not require drug therapy (Tables 21.2 and 21.3). Obese children should be encouraged to lose weight. All should be advised not to smoke and to avoid excessive salt intake. Girls must be warned of the hypertensive effects of oral contraceptives. Blood pressure should be measured annually. Children with undoubtedly high levels (persistently above the 95th percentile) or symptoms and signs caused by the hypertension must be treated (p. 585).[8] Overweight and hypertension are components of the metabolic syndrome, a condition of multiple risk factors for cardiovascular disease as well as for type 2 diabetes.

PULMONARY HYPERTENSION

Pulmonary hypertension is defined as a mean pulmonary artery pressure > 25 mmHg at rest or 30 mmHg with exercise.[214] The main causes of pulmonary hypertension are listed in Table 21.14. Pulmonary hypertension secondary to congenital heart disease has become less prevalent, as surgery is now usually performed before irreversible pulmonary vascular disease develops. Primary pulmonary hypertension is rare. It can be familial.

Clinical features

Symptoms are nonspecific but breathlessness is a common feature. Cyanosis occurs once the right heart pressure rises above systemic, provided there is communication between the two circulations (Eisenmenger syndrome). The cardiac impulse is hyperdynamic, with a prominent right ventricular impulse, and the pulmonary component of the second heart is loud. A soft pulmonary ejection systolic murmur may be followed by an early diastolic murmur of pulmonary regurgitation. If there is no communication between the systemic and pulmonary circulations, elevated right heart pressures will result in failure

Table 21.14 Causes of pulmonary hypertension

1. Congenital heart diseases
   With increased pulmonary blood flow
   - left to right shunts, e.g. VSD, PDA, truncus arteriosus
   - disconnected pulmonary artery
   - total anomalous pulmonary venous drainage
   - transposition of great arteries

   With pulmonary venous obstruction
   - left ventricular inflow or outflow obstruction
   - obstructed total anomalous pulmonary venous drainage
   - pulmonary vein stenosis or veno-occlusive disease

2. Chronic lung diseases producing hypoxemia
   - airway obstructions, e.g. upper airways obstruction, chronic asthma
   - parenchymal disorders, e.g. cystic fibrosis, neonatal lung disease
   - restrictive disorders, e.g. kyphoscoliosis

3. Pulmonary vascular diseases
   - primary (idiopathic) pulmonary hypertension
   - persistent pulmonary hypertension of the newborn
   - collagen vascular diseases, e.g. systemic lupus erythematosus
   - thromboembolism, e.g. ventriculoatrial shunts for hydrocephalus
   - sickle cell disease

4. Others
   - high altitude
   - drugs and toxins
   - neuromuscular disorders producing hypoventilation
   - familial
   - HIV infection
   - sarcoidosis

PDA, persistent arterial duct; VSD, ventricular septal defect.

with hepatic congestion, elevated jugular venous pressure and peripheral edema.

Investigation

The electrocardiogram demonstrates right ventricular hypertrophy. Chest radiography shows large proximal pulmonary vessels with small distal branches (peripheral pruning of the pulmonary arterial tree). Echocardiography demonstrates the congenital cardiac lesion if present. The Doppler velocity of tricuspid regurgitation reflects right ventricular pressure. Pulse oximetry performed at rest and during submaximal exercise testing demonstrates the degree of desaturation and exercise capacity. Further investigations depend on the most likely cause. Pulmonary function tests, ventilation perfusion scan, CT scan of the lungs and thrombophilia screen may be indicated.[214] Lung biopsy may be indicated.

Cardiac catheterization confirms the diagnosis and measures the response of the pulmonary vascular bed (pulmonary vascular resistance) to vasodilators such as oxygen, prostacyclin and nitric oxide. This identifies patients who may respond to long term oral vasodilator treatment.[214]

Management and prognosis

Children with a large left to right shunt who have a fall in pulmonary vascular resistance in response to an acute vasodilatation are suitable for definitive correction of the underlying lesion.

In all other children, therapy is directed at ameliorating symptoms and improving survival.[215]

- Oxygen therapy may slow the progression of polycythemia and provide symptomatic improvement, especially during intercurrent respiratory infections.
- Digoxin may improve cardiac output in children with right heart failure.
- Diuretics may be useful for severe right heart failure, to relieve hepatic congestion.
- Anticoagulation with warfarin and antiplatelet agents are recommended as patients are at risk of thrombotic events.
- Phlebotomy with replacement fluids is indicated when the hematocrit reaches 65% or if a patient is severely symptomatic. Hypovolemia and iron deficiency must be avoided, as they can increase viscosity.[167]
- Patients should receive immunization against pneumococcal infection and influenza.
- Pulmonary vasodilator therapy. Response is evaluated at cardiac catheterization. The youngest and those without a cardiac lesion are most likely to have a positive response. These children should be treated with chronic oral calcium blockade. Most recently, sildenafil and bosentan have been used with apparent success, but long term studies are awaited.
- Children with right heart failure or syncope should be palliated with an atrial septostomy.[216]
- The results of heart and lung transplantation are poor in children.

REFERENCES (* Level 1 evidence)

1. Pelech AN. Evaluation of the pediatric patient with a cardiac murmur. Pediatr Clin North Am 1999; 46:167–188.
2. Van der Kulp M, Hoos MB, Forget PP, et al. Energy expenditure in infants with congenital heart disease, including a meta-analysis. Acta Paediatr 2003; 92:921–927.
3. Cava JR, Sayger PL. Chest pain in children and adolescents. Pediatr Clin North Am 2004; 51:1553–1568.
4. Burn J, Brennan P, Little J, et al. Recurrence risks in offspring of adults with major heart defects: results from first cohort of British collaborative study. Lancet 1998; 351:311–316.
5. Becker SM, Al Halees Z, Molina C, et al. Consanguinity and congenital heart disease in Saudi Arabia. Am J Med Genet 2001; 99:8–13.
6. Eskedal L, Hagemo O, Eskild A, et al. A population-based study of extra-cardiac anomalies in children with congenital cardiac malformations. Cardiol Young 2004; 14:600–607.
7. Wallis LA, Healy M, Undy MB, et al. Age related reference ranges for respiration rate and heart rate from 4 to 16 years. Arch Dis Child 2005; 90:1117–1121.
8. Falkner B, Daniels SR, Flynn JT, et al. The fourth report on the diagnosis, evaluation and treatment of high blood pressure in children and adolescents. Pediatrics 2004; 114:555–576.
9. Park MK, Menard SW, Schoolfield J. Oscillometric blood pressure standards for children. Pediatr Cardiol 2005; 26:601–607.
10. Pelech AN. The physiology of cardiac auscultation. Pediatr Clin North Am 2004; 51:1515–1535.
11. Garson A Jr. The electrocardiogram in infants and children: a systematic approach. Philadelphia: Lea & Feibiger; 1983.
12. Davignon A, Rautaharju P, Boisselle E, et al. Normal ECG standards for infants and children. Pediatr Cardiol 1979/80; 1:123–152.
13. Rijnbeek PR, Witsenburg M, Schrama E, et al. New normal limits for the paediatric electro-cardiogram. Eur Heart J 2001; 22:702–711.

14. Dickinson DF. The normal ECG in childhood and adolescence. Heart 2005; 91:1626–1630.
15. Tipple M. Interpretation of electrocardiograms in infants and children. Images in Paediatric Cardiology 1999; 1:3–13 available from http://www.health.gov.mt/impaedcard/issue1/ipc00103.htm#top
16. Wren C. The presentation of arrhythmias. In: Wren C, Campbell RWF, eds. Paediatric cardiac arrhythmias. Oxford: Oxford University Press; 1996.
17. Fallah-Najmabadi H, Dahdah NS, Palcko M, et al. Normal values and methodologic recommendations for signal-averaged electrocardiography in children and adolescents. Am J Cardiol 1996; 77:408–412.
18. Rosenstock EG, Cassuto Y, Zmora E. Heart rate variability in the neonate and infant: analytical methods, physiological and clinical observations. Acta Paediatr 1999; 88:477–482.
19. Fogel MA, Lieb DR, Seliem MA. Validity of electrocardiographic criteria for left ventricular hypertrophy in children with pressure or volume loaded ventricles: comparison with echocardiographic left ventricular muscle mass. Pediatr Cardiol 1995; 16:261–269.
20. Gardiner S. Are routine chest X-ray and ECG examinations helpful in the evaluation of asymptomatic heart murmurs?. Arch Dis Child 2003; 88:638–640.
21. Snider AR, Sewer GA. Echocardiography in pediatric heart disease. Chicago: Year Book Medical; 1990.
22. Silverman NH, Hunter S, Anderson RH, et al. Anatomical basis of cross sectional echocardiography. Br Heart J 1983; 50:421–431.
23. Skinner J, Alverson D, Hunter S, eds. Echocardiography for the neonatologist. London: Churchill Livingstone; 2000.
24. Seliem MA, Fedec A, Cohen MS, et al. Real-time 3-dimensional echocardiographic imaging of congenital heart disease using matrix-array technology: freehand real-time scanning adds instant morphologic details not well delineated by conventional 2-dimensional imaging. J Am Soc Echocardiogr 2006; 19:121–129.
25. Anderson RH, Ho SY. Sequential segmental analysis – description and categorisation for the millennium. Cardiol Young 1997; 7:98–116.

26. Khalid O, Koenig P. The use of echocardiography in congenital heart surgery and intervention. Expert Rev Cardiovasc Ther 2006; 4:263–271.
27. Wilkinson JL. Haemodynamic calculations in the catheter laboratory. Heart 2001; 85:113–120.
28. Andrews RE, Tulloh RMR. Interventional cardiac catheterisation in congenital heart disease. Arch Dis Child 2004; 89:1168–1173.
29. Peterson C, Schilthuis JJ, Dodge-Khatami A, et al. Comparative long-term results of surgery versus balloon valvuloplasty for pulmonary valve stenosis in infants and children. Ann Thorac Surg 2003; 76:1078–1082.
30. Garty Y, Veldtman G, Lee K, et al Interventional pediatric cardiology: Late outcomes after pulmonary valve balloon dilatation in neonates, infants and children. J Invasive Cardiol 2005; 17:318–322.
31. Rao PS. Balloon pulmonary valvuloplasty in children. J Invasive Cardiol 2005; 17:323–325.
32. Cheung YF, Leung MP, Lee JW, et al. Evolving management for critical pulmonary stenosis in neonates and young infants. Cardiol Young 2000; 10:186–192.
33. Pedra CA, Sidhu R, McCrindle BW, et al. Outcomes after balloon dilation of congenital aortic stenosis in children and adolescents. Cardiol Young 2004; 14:315–321.
34. McCrindle BW, Blackstone EH, Williams WG, et al. Are outcomes of surgical versus transcatheter balloon valvotomy equivalent in neonatal critical aortic stenosis? Circulation 2001; 104:(Suppl 1): I152–158.
35. National Institute for Clinical Excellence. Balloon valvuloplasty for aortic valve stenosis in adults and children. Interventional Procedure Guidance 2004; 78:www.nice.org.uk
36. Zain Z, Zadinello M, Menahem S, et al. Neonatal isolated critical aortic valve stenosis: Balloon valvuloplasty or surgical valvotomy. Heart Lung Circ 2006; 15:18–23.
37. Agnoletti G, Bonhoeffer P, Borghi A, et al. Age-related aspects of balloon angioplasty for postsurgical aortic recoarctation. Cardiol Young 2002; 12:470–473.

38. National Institute for Clinical Excellence. Balloon angioplasty with or without stenting for coarctation or recoarctation of the aorta in adults and children. Interventional Procedure Guidance 2004; 74:www.nice.org.uk

39. Cowley CG, Orsmond GS, Feola P, et al. Long-term, randomized comparison of balloon angioplasty and surgery for native coarctation of the aorta in childhood. Circulation 2005; 111:3453–3456.

40. Gibbs J. Treatment options for coarctation of the aorta. Heart 2000; 84:1–13.

41. National Institute for Clinical Excellence. Balloon dilatation with or without stenting for pulmonary artery or non-valvar right ventricular outflow tract obstruction in children. Interventional Procedure Guidance 2004; 76:www.nice.org.uk

42. Qureshi SA. Catheterization in neonates with pulmonary atresia with intact ventricular septum. Catheter Cardiovasc Interv 2006; 67:924–931.

43. Piéchaud JF. Closing down: transcatheter closure of intracardiac defects and vessel embolisations. Heart 2004; 90:1505–1510.

44. Pass RH, Hsu DT, Lewis V, et al. Multicenter USA Amplatzer patent ductus arteriosus occlusion device trial: initial and one-year results. J Am Coll Cardiol 2004; 44:513–519.

45. Spence MS, Qureshi SA. Complication of transcatheter closure of atrial septal defects. Arch Dis Child 2005; 91:1512–1514.

46. Du ZD, Hijazi ZM, Kleinman CS, et al. Comparison between transcatheter and surgical closure of secundum atrial septal defect in children and adults: results of a multicenter nonrandomized trial. J Am Coll Cardiol 2002; 39:1836–1844.

47. National Institute for Clinical Excellence. Endovascular closure of atrial septal defect. Interventional Procedure Guidance 2004; 96:www.nice.org.uk

48. Bove T, Francois K, De Groote K, et al. Closure of atrial septal defects: is there still a place for surgery? Acta Chir Belg 2005; 105:497–503.

49. Fu YC, Bass J, Amin Z, et al. Transcatheter closure of perimembranous ventricular septal defects using the new Amplatzer membranous VSD occluder: results of the U.S. phase I trial. J Am Coll Cardiol 2006; 47:319–325.

50. Khambadkone S, Bonhoeffer P. Percutaneous pulmonary valve implantation. Semin Thorac Cardiovasc Pediatr Card Surg Annu 2006; 1:23–28.

51. Baker E. What's new in magnetic resonance imaging? Cardiol Young 2001; 11:445–452.

52. McLeod KA. Dizziness and syncope in adolescence. Heart 2001; 86:350–354.

53. Wieling W, Ganzeboom KS, Saul JP. Reflex syncope in children and adolescents. Heart 2004; 90:1094–1100.

54. Advani N, Menahem S, Wilkinson JL. The diagnosis of innocent murmurs in childhood. Cardiol Young 2000; 10:340–342.

55. McCrindle BW, Shaffer KM, Kan JS. Cardinal clinical signs in the differentiation of heart murmurs in children. Arch Pediatr Adolesc Med 1996; 150:169–174.

56. James N, Smith M. Treatment of heart failure in children. Curr Paediatr 2005; 15:539–548.

57. Salmon AP, Holder R, DeGiovanni JV, et al. Effects of digoxin in infants with ventricular septal defects and cardiac failure. Br Heart J 1989; 61:115.

58. Burch M. Heart failure in the young. Heart 2002; 88:198–202.

59. Boucek MM, Waltz DA, Edwards LB, et al. The registry of the international society for heart and lung transplantation: ninth official paediatric report. J Heart Lung Transplant 2006; 25:893–903.

60. Horskotte D, Follath F, Gutschik E, et al. The Task Force on Infective Endocarditis of the European Society of Cardiology. Guidelines on prevention, diagnosis and treatment of infective endocarditis (Executive Summary). Eur Heart J 2004; 25:267–276.

61. British National Formulary for Children. Endocarditis prophylaxis. In: London: BMJ Publishing; 2006:290.

62. Ramsdale DR, Turner-Stokes L. Prophylaxis and treatment of infective endocarditis in adults: concise guidelines. Clin Med 2004; 4:545–550.

63. Simmons NA, Ball AP, Eykyn SJ, et al. Antibiotic treatment of streptococcal, enterococcal, and staphylococcal endocarditis. Working Party of the British Society for Antimicrobial Chemotherapy. Heart 1998; 79:207–210.

64. Millar BC, Jugo J, Moore JE. Fungal endocarditis in neonates and children. Pediatr Cardiol 2005; 26:517–536.

65. Delahaye F, Célard M, Roth O, et al. Indications and optimal timing for surgery in infective endocarditis. Heart 2004; 90:618–620.

66. Hoffman JIE, Kaplan S. The incidence of congenital heart disease. J Am Coll Cardiol 2002; 39:1890–1900.

67. Samanek M, Voriskova M. Congenital heart disease among 818,5569 children born between 1980 and 19900 and their 15 year survival: a prospective Bohemia survival study. Pediatr Cardiol 1999; 20:411–417.

68. Jackson M, Walsh KP, Peart I, et al. Epidemiology of congenital heart disease in Merseyside – 1979 to 1988. Cardiol Young 1996; 6:272–280.

69. Wren C, O'Sullivan JJ. Survival with congenital heart disease and need for follow-up in adult life. Heart 2001; 85:438–443.

70. Lofreddo CA, Wilson PD, Ferencz C. Maternal diabetes: an independent risk factor for major cardiovascular malformations with increased mortality of affected infants. Teratology 2001; 64:98–106.

71. Lee PJ, Ridout D, Walter JH, et al. Maternal phenylketonuria: report from the United Kingdom Registry 1978–97. Arch Dis Child 2005; 90:143–146.

72. Watkins ML, Rasmussen SA, Honein MA, et al. Maternal obesity and risk for birth defects. Pediatrics 2003; 111:1152–1158.

73. Cooper LZ. The history and medical consequences of rubella. Rev Infect Dis 1985; 7:(Suppl1): S2–10.

74. Beattie JO, Day RE, Cockburn F, et al. Alcohol and the fetus in the west of Scotland. BMJ 1983; 287:17–20.

75. Cohen LS, Friedman JM, Jefferson JW, et al. A reevaluation of risk of in utero exposure to lithium. JAMA 1994; 271:146–150.

76. Meischenguiser R, D'Giano CH, Ferraro SM. Oxcarbazepine in pregnancy: clinical experience in Argentina. Epilepsy Behav 2004; 5:163–167.

77. Lammer EJ, Chen DT, Hoar RM, et al. Retinoic acid embryopathy. N Engl J Med 1985; 313:837–841.

78. Harris JA, Francannet C, Pradat P, et al. The epidemiology of cardiovascular defects, Part 2: A study based on data from three large registries of congenital malformations. Pediatr Cardiol 2003; 24:222–235.

79. Manning N, Kaufman L, Roberts P. Genetics of cardiological disorders. Semin Fetal Neonatal Med 2005; 10:259–269.

80. Vincent GM. Role of DNA testing for diagnosis, management, and genetic screening in long QT syndrome, hypertrophic cardiomyopathy and Marfan syndrome. Heart 2001; 86:12–14.

81. Sharland G. Changing impact of fetal diagnosis of congenital heart disease. Arch Dis Child 1997; 77:F1–F3.

82. Bull C. Current and potential future impact of fetal diagnosis on prevalence and spectrum of serious congenital heart disease at term in the UK. Lancet 1999; 354:1242–1247.

83. Wong SF, Chan FY, Cincotta RB, et al. Factors influencing the prenatal detection of structural congenital heart diseases. Ultrasound Obstet Gynecol 2003; 21:19–25.

84. Carvalho JS, Mavrides E, Shinebourne EA, et al. Improving the effectiveness of routine prenatal screening for major congenital heart defects. Heart 2002; 88:387–391.

85. McAuliffe FM, Trines J, Nield LE, et al. Early fetal echocardiography – a reliable prenatal diagnostic tool. Am J Obstet Gynecol 2005; 193:1253–1259.

86. Devine PC, Simpson LL. Nuchal translucency and its relationship to congenital heart disease. Semin Perinatol 2000; 24:343–351.

87. Fesslova V, Villa L, Kustermann A. Long-term experience with the prenatal diagnosis of cardiac anomalies in high-risk pregnancies in a tertiary center. Ital Heart J 2003; 4:855–864.

88. Brick DH, Allan LD. Outcome of prenatally diagnosed congenital heart disease: An update. Pediatr Cardiol 2002; 23:449–453.

89. Andrews RE, Simpson JM, Sharland GK, et al. Outcome after preterm delivery of infants antenatally diagnosed with congenital heart disease. J Pediatr 2006; 148:213–216.

90. Paladini D, Volpe P, Russo MG, et al. Aortic coarctation: prognostic indicators of survival in the fetus. Heart 2004; 90:1348–1349.

91. Gardner H. Fetal echocardiography: 20 years of progress. Heart 2001; 86:(Suppl2):II12–22.

92. Verheijen PM, Lisowski LA, Stoutenbeek P, et al. Prenatal diagnosis of congenital heart disease affects preoperative acidosis in the newborn patient. J Thorac Cardiovasc Surg 2001; 121:798–803.

93. Copel JA, Tan AS, Kleinman CS. Does a prenatal diagnosis of congenital heart disease alter short-term outcome? Ultrasound Obstet Gynecol 1997; 10:237–241.

94. Bonnet D, Coltri A, Butera G, et al. Detection of transposition of the great arteries in fetuses reduces neonatal morbidity and mortality. Circulation 1999; 99:916–918.

95. Brackley KJ, Kilby MD, Wright JG, et al. Outcome after prenatal diagnosis of hypoplastic left-heart syndrome: a case series. Lancet 2000; 356:1143–1147.

96. Tworetzky W, McElhinney DB, Reddy VM, et al. Improved outcome after fetal diagnosis of hypoplastic left heart syndrome. Circulation 2001; 103:1269–1273.

97. Andrews R, Tulloh R, Sharland G, et al. Outcome of staged reconstructive surgery for hypoplastic left heart syndrome following antenatal diagnosis. Heart 2001; 85:474–477.

98. Abu-Harb M, Hey E, Wren C. Death in infancy from unrecognised congenital heart disease. Arch Dis Child 1994; 71:3–7.

99. Kuehl KS, Loffredo CA, Ferencz C. Failure to diagnose congenital heart disease in infancy. Pediatrics 1999; 103:743–747.

100. Penny DJ, Shekerdemian LS. Management of the neonate with symptomatic congenital heart disease. Arch Dis Child 2001; 84:F141–145.

101. Richmond S, Reay G, Abu Harb M. Routine pulse oximetry in the asymptomatic newborn. Arch Dis Child Fetal Neonatal Ed 2002; 78:F83–F88.

102. Patton C, Hey E. How effectively can clinical examination pick up congenital heart disease at birth? Arch Dis Child 2006; 91:F263–F267.

103. de Wahl Granelli A, Mellander M, Sunnegardh J, et al. Screening for duct-dependent congenital heart disease with pulse oximetry: a critical evaluation of strategies to maximize sensitivity. Acta Paediatr 2005; 94:1590–1596.

104. Skinner JR, Boys RJ, Hunter S, et al. Non-invasive determination of pulmonary arterial pressure in healthy neonates. Arch Dis Child 1991; 66:386–390.

105. Anderson RH, Baker EJ, Macartney FJ, et al, eds. Pediatric cardiology. 2nd edn. Edinburgh: Churchill Livingstone; 2002.

106. Prêtre R, Tamisier D, Bonhoeffer P, et al. Results of the arterial switch operation in neonates with transposed great arteries. Lancet 2001; 357:1826–1830.

107. Moons P, Gewillig M, Sluysmans T, et al. Long term outcome up to 30 years after the Mustard or Senning operation: a nationwide multicentre study in Belgium. Heart 2004; 90:307–313.

108. Iserin L, de Lonlay P, Viot G, et al. Prevalence of the microdeletion 22q11 in newborn infants with congenital conotruncal cardiac abnormalities. Eur J Pediatr 1998; 157:881–884.

109. Mahle WT, Crisalli J, Coleman K, et al. Deletion of chromosome 22q11.2 and outcome in patients with pulmonary atresia and ventricular septal defect. Ann Thorac Surg 2003; 76:567–571.

110. Ashburn DA, Blackstone EH, Wells WJ, et al. Determinants of mortality and type of repair in neonates with pulmonary atresia and intact ventricular septum. J Thoracic Cardiovasc Surg 2004; 127:1000–1007.

111. Waldman JD, Holmes G. The cyanosed newborn: excluding structural heart disease. In: Skinner J, Alverson D, Hunter S, (eds). Echocardiography for the neonatologist. Edinburgh: Churchill Livingstone; 2000:181–195.

112. Celermajer DS, Bull C, Till J, et al. Ebstein's anomaly: presentation and outcome from fetal to adult. J Am Coll Cardiol 1994; 23:170–176.

113. McElhinney DB, Salvin JW, Colan SD, et al. Improving outcomes in fetuses and neonates with congenital displacement (Ebstein's malformation) or dysplasia of the tricuspid valve. Am J Cardiol 2005; 96:582–586.

114. Chauvaud S. Ebstein's malformation. Surgical treatment and results. Thorac Cardiovasc Surg 2000; 48:220–223.

115. Kanter KR. Surgical repair of total anomalous pulmonary venous connection. Semin Thorac Cardiovasc Surg Pediatr Card Surg Annu 2006; 1:40–44.

116. Hyde JA, Stumper O, Barth MJ, et al. Total anomalous pulmonary venous connection and management of recurrent venous obstruction. Eur J Cardiothorac Surg 1999; 15:735–740.

117. McElhinney DB, Driscoll DA, Emanuel BS, et al. Chromosome 22q11 deletion in patients with truncus arteriosus. Pediatr Cardiol 2003; 24:569–573.

118. Thompson LD, McElhinney DB, Reddy M, et al. Neonatal repair of truncus arteriosus: continuing improvement in outcomes. Ann Thorac Surg 2001; 72:391–395.

119. McElhinney DB, Rajasinghe HA, Mora BN, et al. Reinterventions after repair of common arterial trunk in neonates and young children. J Am Coll Cardiol 2000; 35:1317–1322.

120. Pickert CB, Moss MM, Fiser DH. Differentiation of systemic infection and congenital obstructive left heart disease in the very young infant. Pediatr Emerg Care 1998; 14:263–267.

121. Levine JC, Sanders SP, Colan SD, et al. The risk of having additional obstructive lesions in neonatal coarctation of the aorta. Cardiol Young 2001; 11:44–53.

122. Goldmuntz E, Clark BJ, Mitchell LE, et al. Frequency of 22q11 deletions in patients with conotruncal defects. J Am Coll Cardiol 1998; 32:492–498.

123. Salmon AP. Hypoplastic left heart syndrome – outcome and management. Arch Dis Child 2001; 85:450–451.

124. Cua CL, Thiagarajan RR, Taeed R, et al. Improved interstage mortality with the modified Norwood procedure: A meta-analysis. Ann Thorac Surg 2005; 80:44–49.

125. Mahle WT, Spray TL, Wernovsky G, et al. Survival after reconstructive surgery for hypoplastic left heart syndrome: a 15-year experience from a single institution. Circulation 2000; 102:(suppl 3):136–141.

126. McGuirk SP, Griselli M, Stumper OF, et al. Staged surgical management of hypoplastic left heart syndrome: a single institution 12 year experience. Heart 2006; 92:364–370.

127. Kitchiner D, Jackson M, Walsh K, et al. The incidence and prognosis of congenital aortic valve stenosis in Liverpool (1960–1990). Br Heart J 1993; 69:71–79.

128. Arlettaz R, Archer N, Wilkinson AR. Natural history of innocent heart murmurs in newborn babies: controlled echocardiographic study. Arch Dis Child Fetal Neonatal Ed 1998; 78:F166–170.

129. Rein AJT, Omokhodion SI, Nir A. Significance of a cardiac murmur as the sole clinical sign in the newborn. Clin Pediatr 2000; 39:511–520.

130. Alghamdi AA, McCrindle BW, Van Arsdell GS. Physiologic versus anatomic repair of congenitally corrected transposition of the great arteries: meta-analysis of individual patient data. Ann Thorac Surg 2006; 81:1529–1535.

131. Phoon CKL. Where's the spleen. Looking for the spleen and assessing its function in the syndromes of isomerism. Cardiol Young 1997; 7:347–357.

132. Glen S, Burns J, Bloomfield P. Prevalence and development of additional cardiac abnormalities in 1448 patients with congenital ventricular septal defects. Heart 2004; 90:1321–1325.

133. Turner SW, Hunter S, Wyllie JP. The natural history of ventricular septal defects. Arch Dis Child 1999; 81:413–416.

134. Neumayer U, Stone S, Somerville J. Small ventricular septal defects in adults. Eur Heart J 1998; 19:1573–1582.

135. Leung MP, Beerman LB, Siewers RD, et al. Longterm follow up after aortic valvuloplasty and defect closure in ventricular septal defects with aortic regurgitation. Am J Cardiol 1987; 60:890–894.

136. Kidd L, Driscoll D, Gersony W, et al. Second natural history study of congenital heart defects: results of treatment in patients with ventricular septal defects. Circulation 1993; 87:(suppl I):I38–I51.

137. Sutherland GS, Godman MJ, Smallhorn JF. Ventricular septal defects. Two dimensional echocardiographic and morphological correlations. Br Heart J 1982; 47:316–328.

138. Carotti A, Marino B, Bevilacqua M, et al. Primary repair of isolated ventricular septal defect in infancy guided by echocardiography. Am J Cardiol 1997; 79:1498–1501.

139. Riggs T, Sharp SE, Batton D, et al. Spontaneous closure of atrial septal defects in premature vs full-term neonates. Pediatr Cardiol 2000; 21:129–134.

140. Azhari N, Shihata MS, Al-Fatani A. Spontaneous closure of atrial septal defects within the oval fossa. Cardiol Young 2004; 14:148–155.

141. Masura J, Gavora P, Podnar T. Long-term outcome of transcatheter secundum-type atrial septal defect closure using Amplatzer septal occluders. J Am Coll Cardiol 2005; 45:505–507.

142. Murphy JG, Gersh BJ, McGoon MD, et al. Long-term outcome after surgical repair of isolated atrial septal defect: follow-up at 27–32 years. N Engl J Med 1990; 323:1643–1650.

143. Sullivan I. Patent arterial duct: when should it be closed?. Arch Dis Child 1998; 78:285–287.

144. Masura J, Tittel P, Gavora P, et al. Long-term outcome of transcatheter patent ductus arteriosus closure using Amplatzer duct occluders. Am Heart J 2006; 151:755–757.

145. El-Najdawi EK, Driscoll DJ, Puga FJ, et al. Operation for partial atrioventricular septal defect: a forty-year review. J Thorac Cardiovasc Surg 2000; 119:880–889.

146. Najm HK, Coles JG, Endo M, et al. Complete atrioventricular septal defects: results of repair, risk factors, and freedom from reoperation. Circulation 1997; 96:(Suppl):II311–315.

147. Frid C, Bjorkhem G, Jonzon A, et al. Long-term survival in children with atrioventricular septal defect and common atrioventricular valvar orifice in Sweden. Cardiol Young 2004; 14:24–31.

148. Clapp S, Perry BL, Farooki ZQ, et al. Down's syndrome, complete atrioventricular canal, and pulmonary vascular obstructive disease. J Thorac Cardiovasc Surg 1990; 100:115–121.

149. Formigari R, Di Donato RM, Gargiulo G, et al. Better surgical prognosis for patients with complete atrioventricular septal defect and Down's syndrome. Ann Thorac Surg 2004; 78:666–672.

150. Frawley GP, Dargaville PA, Mitchell PJ, et al. Clinical course and medical management of neonates with severe cardiac failure related to vein of Galen malformation. Arch Dis Child Fetal Neonatal Ed 2002; 87:F144–149.

151. Holzer R, Johnson R, Ciotti G, et al. Review of an institutional experience of coronary arterial fistulas in childhood set in context of review of the literature. Cardiol Young 2004; 14:380–385.

152. Gielen H, Daniëls O, van Lier H. Natural history of congenital pulmonary valvar stenosis: an echo and Doppler cardiographic study. Cardiol Young 1999; 9:129–135.

153. Kamath BM, Spinner NB, Emerick KM, et al. Vascular anomalies in Alagille syndrome: a significant cause of morbidity and mortality. Circulation 2004; 109:1354–1358.

154. Danford DA, Salaymeh KJ, Martin AB, et al. Pulmonary stenosis: defect-specific diagnostic accuracy of heart murmurs in children. J Pediatr 1999; 134:76–81.

155. Rowland DG, Hammill WW, Allen HD, et al. Natural course of isolated pulmonary valve stenosis in infants and children utilizing Doppler echocardiography. Am J Cardiol 1997; 79:344–349.

156. Roos-Hesselink JW, Meijboom FJ, Spitaels SE, et al. Long-term outcome after surgery for pulmonary stenosis (a longitudinal study of 22–33 years). Eur Heart J 2006; 27:482–488.

157. Kitchiner DJ, Jackson M, Malaiya N, et al. The incidence and prognosis of left ventricular outflow obstruction in Liverpool (1960–1991). Br Heart J 1994; 71:588–595.

158. Kitchiner D, Jackson M, Walsh K, et al. The long-term prognosis of 81 patients with supravalve aortic stenosis (1960–1992). Heart 1996; 76:395–402.

159. Justo RN, McCrindle BW, Benson LN, et al. Aortic valve regurgitation after surgical versus percutaneous balloon valvotomy for congenital aortic valve stenosis. Am J Cardiol 1996; 77:1332–1338.

160. Karamlou T, Jang K, Williams WG, et al. Outcomes and associated risk factors for aortic valve replacement in 160 children: a competing-risks analysis. Circulation 2005; 112:3462–3469.

161. McElhinney DB, Petrossian E, Tworetzky W, et al. Issues and outcomes in the management of supravalve aortic stenosis. Ann Thorac Surg 2000; 69:562–567.

162. Basso C, Corrado D, Thiene G. Cardiovascular causes of sudden death in young individuals including athletes. Cardiovasc Rev 1999; 7:127–135.

163. Kitchiner D. Physical exertion in patients with congenital heart disease. Heart 1996; 76:6–7.

164. Rosenthal E. Coarctation of the aorta from fetus to adult: curable condition or life long disease process. Heart 2005; 91:1495–1502.

165. Cohen M, Fuster V, Steele PM, et al. Coarctation of the aorta. Long-term follow-up and prediction of outcome after surgical correction. Circulation 1989; 80:840–845.

166. Walhout RJ, Lekkerkerker JC, Oron GH, et al. Comparison of surgical repair with balloon angioplasty for native coarctation in patients from 3 months to 16 years of age. Eur J Cardiothorac Surg 2004; 25:722–727.

167. Linderkamp O, Klose HJ, Betke K, et al. Increased blood viscosity in patients with cyanotic congenital heart disease and iron deficiency. J Pediatr 1979; 95:567–568.

168. Van Arsdell GS, Maharaj GS, Tom J, et al. What is the optimal age for repair of tetralogy of Fallot? Circulation 2000; 102:(Suppl 3):III123–129.

169. Nollert G, Fischlein T, Bouterwek S, et al. Long-term survival in patients with repair of tetralogy of Fallot: 36-year follow-up of 490 survivors of the first year after surgical repair. J Am Coll Cardiol 1997; 30:1374–1383.

170. Gatzoulis MA, Balaji S, Webber SA, et al. Risk factors for arrhythmia and sudden cardiac death late after repair of tetralogy of Fallot: a multicentre study. Lancet 2000; 356:975–981.

171. Freedom RM, Hamilton R, Yoo SJ, et al. The Fontan procedure: analysis of cohorts and late complications. Cardiol Young 2000; 10:307–325.

172. Gewillig M. The Fontan circulation. Heart 2005; 91:839–846.

173. Dean JCS. Management of Marfan syndrome. Heart 2002; 88:97–103.

174. Shores J, Berger KR, Murphy EA, et al. Progression of aortic dilatation and the benefit of long-term adrenergic blockade in Marfan's syndrome. N Engl J Med 1994; 330:1384–1385.

175. Liberthson RR. Sudden death from cardiac causes in children and young adults. N Engl J Med 1996; 334:1039–1044.

176. Wren C. Sudden death in children and adolescents. Heart 2002; 88:426–431.

177. Mazgalev TN, Ho SY, Anderson RH. Anatomic-electrophysiological correlations concerning the pathways for atrioventricular conduction. Circulation 2001; 103:2660–2667.

178. Dixon J, Foster K, Wyllie J, et al. Guidelines and adenosine dosing for supraventricular tachycardia. Arch Dis Child 2005; 90:1190–1191.

179. Garson A. Medicolegal problems in the management of cardiac arrhythmias in children. Pediatrics 1987; 79:84–88.

180. Etheridge SP, Craig JE, Compton SJ. Amiodarone is safe and highly effective therapy for supraventricular tachycardia in infants. Am Heart J 2001; 141:3–5.

181. Baursfeld U, Gow RM, Hamilton RM, et al. Treatment of atrial ectopic tachycardia in infants < 6 months old. Am Heart J 1995; 129:1145–1148.

182. Vaksmann G, D'Hoinne C, Lucet V, et al. Permanent junctional reciprocating tachycardia in children: a multicentre study on clinical profile and outcome. Heart 2006; 92:101–104.

183. Perry JC. Ventricular tachycardia in neonates. PACE 1997; 20:2061–2064.

184. Muller G, Deal BJ, Benson DW. 'Vagal maneuvers' and adenosine for termination of atrioventricular reentrant tachycardia. Am J Cardiol 1994; 74:500–503.

185. Friedman RA, Walsh EP, Silka MJ, et al. NASPE Expert Consensus Conference: Radiofrequency catheter ablation in children with and without congenital heart disease. Report of the writing committee. North American Society of Pacing and Electrophysiology. Pacing Clin Electrophysiol 2002; 25:1000–1017. available from http://www.hrsonline.org/positionDocs/PACE_June02.pdf

186. Delacrétaz E. Supraventricular tachycardia. N Engl J Med 2006; 354:1039–1051.

187. Moss AJ. Long QT syndrome. JAMA 2003; 289:2041–2044.

188. Wilde AAM, Bezzina CR. Genetics of cardiac arrhythmias. Heart 2005; 91:1352–1358.

189. Villain E, Denjoy I, Lupoglazoff JM, et al. Low incidence of cardiac events with β-blocking therapy in children with long QT syndrome. Eur Heart J 2004; 25:1405–1411.

190. Priori SG, Napolitano C, Memmi M, et al. Clinical and molecular characterisation of patients with catecholaminergic polymorphic ventricular tachycardia. Circulation 2002; 106:69–74.

191. Antzelevitch C, Brugada P, Borggrefe M, et al. Brugada syndrome. Report of the second consensus conference. Circulation 2005; 111:659–670.

192. Kertesz NJ, Fenrich AL, Friedman RA. Congenital complete atrioventricular block. Tex Heart Inst J 1997; 24:301–307. Available from http://www.pubmedcentral.nih.gov/articlerender.fcgi?artid=325472

193. Silka MJ, Hardy BG, Menashe VD, et al. A population-based prospective evaluation of risk of sudden cardiac death after operation for common congenital heart defects. J Am Coll Cardiol 1998; 32:245–251.

194. Wellens HJ. Should catheter ablation be performed in asymptomatic patients with Wolff–Parkinson–White syndrome? When to perform catheter ablation in asymptomatic patients with a Wolff–Parkinson–White electrocardiogram. Circulation 2005; 112:2201–2207.

195. Wren C. Screening children with a family history of sudden cardiac death. Heart 2006; 92:1001–1006.

196. Oakley CM. Myocarditis, pericarditis and other pericardial diseases. Heart 2000; 84:449–454.

197. English RF, Janosky JE, Ettedgui JA, et al. Outcomes for children with acute myocarditis. Cardiol Young 2004; 14:488–493.

198. Amabile N, Fraisse A, Bouvenot J, et al. Outcome of acute fulminant myocarditis in children. Heart 2006; 92:1269–1273.

199. Maisch B, Risti AD. Practical aspects of the management of pericardial disease. Heart 2003; 89:1096–1103.

200. Stollermn GH. Rheumatic fever. Lancet 1997; 349:935–942.

201. Vijayalakshmi JB, Mithravinda J, Deva AN. The role of echocardiography in diagnosing carditis in the setting of acute rheumatic fever. Cardiol Young 2005; 15:580–582.

202. Cilliers AM, Manyemba J, Saloojee H. Anti-inflammatory treatment for carditis in acute rheumatic fever (Cochrane Review). The Cochrane Library 2004; (Issue 2):

203. Dajani A, Taubert K, Ferrieri P, et al. Treatment of acute streptococcal pharyngitis and prevention of rheumatic fever: a statement for health professionals. Pediatrics 1995; 96:758–764.

204. Maconochie IK. Kawasaki disease. Arch Dis Child Educ Pract Ed 2004; 89:ep3–ep8.

205. Newburger JW, Takahashi M, Gerber MA, et al. Diagnosis, treatment, and long-term management of Kawasaki disease: A statement for health professionals from the committee on rheumatic fever, endocarditis, and Kawasaki disease, Council on cardiovascular disease in the young, American Heart Association. Pediatrics 2004; 114:1708–1733.

206. Nugent AW, Daubeney PE, Chondros P, et al. The epidemiology of childhood cardiomyopathy in Australia. N Engl J Med 2003; 348:1703–1705.

207. Burkett EL, Hershberger RE. Clinical and genetic issues in familial dilated cardiomyopathy. J Am Coll Cardiol 2005; 45:969–981.

208. Longo N, Amat di San Filippo C, Pasquali M. Disorders of carnitine transport and the carnitine cycle. Am J Med Genet C Semin Med Genet 2006; 142:77–85.

209. Burch M. Hypertrophic cardiomyopathy. Arch Dis Child 1994; 71:488–489.

210. Frenneaux MP. Assessing the risk of sudden cardiac death in a patient with hypertrophic cardiomyopathy. Heart 2004; 90:570–575.

211. Pignatelli RH, McMahon CJ, Dreyer WJ, et al. Clinical characterization of left ventricular noncompaction in children. Circulation 2003; 108:2672–2678.

212. Corrado D, Basso C, Thiene G. Arrhythmogenic right ventricular cardiomyopathy: diagnosis, prognosis, and treatment. Heart 2000; 83:588–595.

213. Shapiro LM. Cardiac tumours: diagnosis and management. Heart 2001; 85:218–222.

214. Rashid A, Ivy D. Severe paediatric pulmonary hypertension: new management strategies. Arch Dis Child 2005; 90:92–98.

215. Berman-Rosenzweig E, Barst BJ. Eisenmenger's syndrome: Current management. Prog Cardiovasc Dis 2002; 45:129–138.

216. Micheletti A, Hislop AA, Lammers A, et al. The role of atrial septostomy in the treatment of children with pulmonary hypertension. Heart 2006; 92:969–972.

22

Neurology

Edited by Colin Ferrie, Richard Newton, Tim Martland

THE NEUROLOGICAL CONSULTATION

THE SETTING

Neurological consultations require time. Our role is to help understand causation, inform on future outlook, deal with the attendant medical problems, give specific treatment where possible, and arrange genetic counseling and supportive services. Special investigation is only part of this process: clinical skills are equally important. A child's appearance, pattern of movement, or mode of presentation all give important diagnostic clues and help shape the approach to investigation.

Histories are often complex; physical examination requires care; and there are often attendant psychological and educational issues which need definition and planned intervention. Consultations need space as gait assessment is an essential feature as is observation of patterns of play. Correct choice of room and a correct scheduling for families therefore demands adequate attention.

First impressions are very important and it is helpful to families to be greeted in a friendly way and for those in the room to be introduced to them. Cunningham and Newton[1] showed that parents and children attending hospital consultations still had difficulty in asking about things that worried them most despite a welcoming environment. These questions are often centered on fears and misunderstandings that would not necessarily be on the doctor's standard consultation agenda. An attractive, clear question sheet proved to be a simple but effective intervention. Parents felt empowered to take control. Its use often led to the adoption of a new consultation format that ensured that all parents' questions were addressed and limited time was used to its best advantage.

THE HISTORY

Good history taking takes time. Concentrate on detail; ask yourself if you would be able to describe all relevant events with all relevant details to a third party at the end. If not, go back and finish off! For paroxysmal events consider the value that video recordings might offer.

In history taking it is important to listen to what the child has to say. In their 1998 study Viswanathan et al[2] showed that children's descriptions of their headaches cannot be tidily 'pigeonholed' into traditionally held views on headache classification. It is important to use language appropriate for the particular age of the child and to acknowledge that some things are difficult to describe. It is therefore perhaps better to note an 'indescribable feeling in the head' than trying to persuade them to accede to a proffered descriptive checklist.

Common clinical scenarios demand individual consideration:

Paroxysmal disorders: including seizure disorders, headaches and paroxysmal movement disorders

In the histories related to paroxysmal disorders an accurate description of the episodes, prodromal features, auras, and situations or activities that trigger the bouts should be taken. The child's views and experiences ought to be sought as well as those of witnesses.

Gait disturbance

For gait disturbance a description of the pattern of early ambulation is necessary along with the evolution of the disorder. For subtle difficulties it is good to ask about when the motor system is put to its greatest test; how is the child able to ascend stairs? How does the child fare in school races? Are they picked for the cricket or rounders teams? Is the disorder intermittent? Is there a hint of fatigability or diurnal variation?

Developmental or speech delay

If there is difficulty with expressive language it is useful to determine whether the child has a good understanding of imitative gesture. This will signify that some fundamental language concept is present. Method of sentence construction will indicate if there is a syntax problem and insight into their sense of humor at a later stage will indicate whether there is a semantic/pragmatic language problem. Speech and language disorders are common in childhood, boys being affected twice as often as girls.[3,4] The history highlights whether the language problem is isolated or associated with global developmental delay. An assessment should be made of language opportunity for the child and whether there is any social disadvantage. Children brought up in a bilingual environment tend to develop speech later, but then catch up. Left handedness or ambidexterity is associated with speech disorder in half the children involved. Elective mutism, commoner in boys, can usually be recognized in the context of unresolved predicament. Children with elective mutism often talk freely in certain situations and continue to communicate with gesture.

For children with suspected global learning difficulties, the consultation enables one to determine whether the problems are indeed global or confined to verbal skills, nonverbal skills and/or social issues. Children with learning difficulties present in relatively few, well circumscribed ways: hypotonia in the newborn period, recognized developmental delay later in infancy or in the early toddler age group, language delay, arrest of development, or difficulties at school (see below). In each of these groups the history should detail the pregnancy, including any drug ingestion or early threatened abortion. A history of fetal distress should lead to careful scrutiny of the obstetric notes, though it is now generally accepted that in order to attribute causation to birth asphyxia the presence of neonatal hypoxic–ischemic encephalopathy must be established and there is nearly always an associated motor difficulty compatible with the type of injury sustained (see section on cerebral palsy below). A record of cord, or early, pH measurements, as well as neonatal behavior are important in this respect as not all early neonatal encephalopathy is due to hypoxic–ischemic insult.[5] Parents, in their own minds, often attribute their child's difficulties to the events of labor and it can be helpful for them to be taken through details of the birth.

A detailed family history is clearly of value especially if supplemented by perusal of the family photograph album. These, together with home video recordings, can give a surprisingly clear idea of the evolution of a disorder. Many motor disorders such as the spasticity in cerebral palsy or the extrapyramidal involvement in Rett syndrome may evolve over a period of time, raising the possibility of a neurodegenerative disorder. Careful scrutiny of the history often reveals that whereas things have changed, skills may not actually have been lost.

All these issues will be dealt with in more detail under separate headings in this chapter, but it is important to say at this early stage that the consultation should give the doctor a clear idea of the pattern of developmental delay, conveniently considered under the headings which follow.

Abnormal behavior in the neonatal period

Dysmorphic features, disordered tone, feeding difficulties, irritability and seizures may all signify continuing neurological abnormality. Hypotonia in the limbs and axis raise the possibility of a neuromuscular disorder, the Prader–Willi syndrome and other causes of learning disability. Where hypotonia is confined to the axis, there is usually a central nervous system abnormality such as a neuronal migration disorder, or hypoxic–ischemic encephalopathy. In the latter cases there may be associated full fontanel (due to cerebral edema), irritability, feeding difficulties and seizures.

The commonest cause of persisting hypotonia or feeding difficulty is the presence of one of the recognizable forms of learning difficulty, of which Down syndrome is the commonest. Of the metabolic disorders, it should be remembered that the cerebrohepatorenal syndrome of Zellweger (one of the peroxisomal disorders) can mimic Down syndrome. It is associated with profound hypotonia as well as a craniofacial dysmorphism, similar to trisomy 21. The use of one of the computer-based databases of dysmorphology can be helpful when attempting to establish a dysmorphic diagnosis.

Arthrogryposis should make one think of a neuromuscular problem or a neuronal migration defect particularly if the hands and arms are held in a 'decorticate' posture. Half of the children with arthrogryposis who are ventilator dependent will have a developmental brain abnormality. The presence of scoliosis and pooling of secretions with aspiration makes a congenital myopathy, and particularly nemaline rod myopathy, likely.

Abnormal head size

This common cause of referrals to pediatricians is dealt with below under 'investigation' – but always start with parental head size![6]

Syndromes of developmental arrest

A number of conditions lead to similar developmental profiles; for example that of a 'ceiling effect'. Here a child will show normal development for a while, learning then slows, arrests, some skills may then actually be lost, and then learning continues at a slower rate. The child with hydranencephaly (e.g. due to pyruvate dehydrogenase deficiency) may well return the mother's smile before this smile is lost. Deaf children may babble but then, lacking input, their language development will subsequently become deviant if the problem is not identified and treated.

Children with autism often make reasonable developmental progress in the first year or so, their problems only becoming evident when there is a greater demand on social contact and language function. Words originally attained may be lost before the depth of communication difficulty is revealed. A very similar profile is seen in the age-related epileptic encephalopathies. West syndrome often begins too early in infancy for much difference with other children to be noticed, but in the Lennox–Gastaut syndrome, which usually presents in the third or fourth year, there is very often an arrest of developmental progress at the time of onset of the seizure disorder. In Rett syndrome, although in retrospect movements may have had a 'jerky' quality throughout infancy, there is often reasonable early developmental attainment before the process slows and the extrapyramidal features and loss of useful hand function become evident.

GENERAL POINTS ON EXAMINATION

Although this is dealt with in detail in Chapter 8 some aspects of clinical examination will be emphasized here: starting with an approach to a shortened neurological examination that can be used in everyday clinical practice. Hopefully this will avoid the practice seen in some clinical records of simply noting, CNS ✓.

Look for dysmorphism, signs of a neurocutaneous syndrome or the visceromegaly, heart murmur or the skeletal abnormality one might associate with a storage disorder. Examination of the eyes should include not only a search for papilledema (which is rare even in the presence of raised intracranial pressure in pediatric practice) but also a careful look at the retina to look for degenerative features or pigmentation that one might associate with a mitochondrial cytopathy, or peroxisomal disorder.

From the age of 5 onwards children will usually cooperate with a formal examination of cranial nerves, coordination and power where required. For the younger child eye movements can be tested through distraction through the various fields of movement. Close inspection of facial expression will reveal any facial weakness. If there is any doubt about hearing, it should be tested formally. Observation of speech and questions about the child's pattern of chewing and swallowing and the ability to handle liquids and solids avoid the need for tongue depressors and more intrusive aspects of physical examination. They will give a good indication of the function of muscles of mastication and the lower brainstem.

Observation of the pattern of movement is more useful than the traditional 'hands-on' approach. Cerebellar function can be tested by holding the arms outstretched and looking for 'drift'. Up to 6% of boys will show choreiform movement of the outstretched hands until the age of about 10. Carrying out the finger/nose test, assessing alternating movements and touching each finger in turn can then further test cerebellar function. The ability to play a musical instrument is a good reflection of coordination.

The gait should be observed with particular features in mind. The first question always is whether this is a heel–toe gait, or a toe–heel gait. If there is any doubt the shoes can be inspected for uneven wear. A toe–heel gait may be due to pyramidal or extrapyramidal motor dysfunction, a foot drop due to a lateral popliteal nerve palsy or tight tendo-Achilles due to a neuromuscular problem. Corticospinal posturing in the upper limb leads to adduction, elbow and wrist flexion and pronation; in the lower limb, adduction, internal rotation and flexion at the hip, knee and plantar flexion at the ankle.

Fog's test may reveal these patterns when subtle. Fog's test involves walking on the heels, then walking on the outside of the feet and then walking on the inside of the feet. At each stage, children are observed for the degree of associated movement in the upper limb. An undue degree of associated movement is often related to poor sequencing and balance and coordination seen in children with a developmental dyspraxia/developmental coordination disorder (see below). Asymmetry over and above what one would see in the dominant hand, as opposed to the non-dominant hand, often reflects contralateral hemisphere dysfunction, which can reflect the presence of a dysgenesis, a space occupying lesion or the site of an epileptogenic focus.

Children with a cerebellar problem have a wide-based gait for additional stability and this is often accompanied by a moderate amplitude truncal tremor, deviations off the path, overcorrection and then restitution. Extrapyramidal disorders will give a paucity of movement with a stiff-legged gait or too much movement, as in a dyskinesia.

A wide base, seen continuing for some months after children first begin to walk, may suggest a cerebellar problem, the general hypotonia of the recognizable forms of learning difficulty or a carbohydrate deficient glycoprotein syndrome.

If learning difficulties are present then think of Duchenne muscular dystrophy. The average age at which boys with this disorder are taken to doctors with developmental concerns is 2.5 years, whereas the average age of diagnosis is 5.5 years. A large contribution to this delay is a misunderstanding of Gower sign.[7] Most clinicians remember the sign as the need to climb up the legs using the hands when rising from a supine to standing position. The most important component, however, is the need to turn prone and in so doing adopting a 'Moslem prayer position' before rising. This overcomes difficulties sustained in attaining a sitting position if the rectus abdominus is weak and furthermore allows the hips to be extended more than is possible in the almost full hip flexion position seen in the normal squatting position. Most children show a Gower or modified Gower maneuver before the age of 3 years. If it is seen after the age of 3 then it is highly likely that there is a neuromuscular problem, or a central nervous system disorder with hypotonia.

Neuromuscular problems leading to proximal weakness often lead to a waddling pattern. The weak gluteal muscles lead the body weight to be transferred outside the weight bearing leg; the resulting mechanical advantage avoids dropping of the pelvis away from the weight bearing side.

The presence of choreoathetosis naturally would lead to investigations for basal ganglia dysfunction, but the erratic movements of Angelman syndrome may certainly imitate this, particularly in infancy and it may also be an early feature of Friedreich ataxia.

If one side of the body 'mirrors' movement seen on the other then agenesis of the corpus callosum should be considered.

Whenever the motor system is examined the examiner should have on their mind, is this normal or abnormal? If it is abnormal is it central nervous or peripheral nervous system, and if it is central nervous system is it corticospinal (voluntary movement), extrapyramidal (where patterns of movement are stored) or cerebellar (the 'air traffic controller')? This in turn will help guide investigation.

Sensory testing is only indicated when the history indicates it should be done (that is sensory symptoms or perhaps features of a peripheral neuropathy or spinal cord lesion). In this eventuality all modalities should be tested working from the point of perceived maximum sensory loss toward more normal areas.

INVESTIGATION OF SUSPECTED NEUROLOGICAL DISORDERS

INVESTIGATION OF NEUROLOGICAL DISEASE

The investigation of a child with suspected neurological disease can be challenging. The differential diagnosis may be very broad . Advances in neuroimaging (primarily MRI), molecular genetics and neurometabolic investigations mean that the label 'undiagnosed neurological disorder' is becoming increasingly rare.

The bewildering number of possible investigations, together with a litigation conscious society, may lead some clinicians to adopt a blanket or fishing net approach to investigation. This is wasteful of resources, subjects the child to unnecessary distress and is intellectually lazy. Many of these 'screening' tests can produce false negatives which will not be recognized as such if the clinician does not recognize the clinical features of a given disorder.

Some investigations are simple and inexpensive whereas others may be invasive, complicated and expensive. For the best results, the clinician should communicate with the laboratory personnel to discuss optimal sample requirements, or local factors that may influence the quality of the sample or procedure. This is as relevant for neuroimaging and neurophysiology as for biochemical or genetic investigations. Where many such investigations are performed, regular meetings between clinicians and nonclinical staff are of great benefit.

Certain principles should underlie the investigation of any child:

- Unfortunately many children have large numbers of investigations performed on the basis of a cursory history or examination (particularly in the investigation of paroxysmal disorders). If the clinical history or signs are unclear, then rather than requesting investigations blindly it may be more appropriate to ask for advice from a more specialized clinician.
- Complete clinical assessment may require evaluation by other professionals such as neuropsychologist, physiotherapist or speech therapist.
- Planning investigations in a logical sequence is important. For example, if the differential diagnosis includes hydrocephalus or a space-occupying lesion in a child with progressive neurological signs or symptoms, neuroimaging should be performed prior to expensive metabolic or genetic investigations.
- Perform simple investigations first. Urea and electrolytes, full blood count and urinalysis are cheap and easy and may suggest the diagnosis, e.g. hyponatremia in coma, leukocytosis in leukemia, or proteinuria due to lupus.
- Investigation often involves building up a picture from multiple clues rather than one single test. While there are exceptions to this, the clinician should not reject a putative diagnosis on the basis of one negative test. For example, a normal blood or CSF lactate does not exclude mitochondrial disease. Evidence of muscle disease might include: clinical signs, blood creatine kinase (CK) level, EMG, muscle imaging or muscle biopsy.
- Repeating tests is important when clinical suspicion is strong.
- Good record keeping with clear summaries of results of investigations facilitates clinical review.
- The purpose of any given investigation should be clear before it is performed. An investigation may be done to help clarify the clinical features, e.g. is there a retinal dystrophy? Is there a peripheral neuropathy? Results from these may then indicate other investigations. Investigation may be seeking a specific etiology, or to monitor the course of a disease or the effects of treatment. It is particularly important that the aim of the investigation is made

clear to the personnel who will be doing the procedure (e.g. biochemist, pathologist, radiologist).

- When the diagnosis is not clear or the results of tests confusing, consultation with colleagues is often helpful. Electronic communication has greatly facilitated this and parents themselves may initiate it. The development of clinical networks and referral pathways should facilitate this. Clinical and scientific meetings also provide an important forum for the discussion of diagnostic problems.
- Psychological disorders commonly present with symptoms or signs that could have a neurological basis. Investigation to exclude increasingly unlikely diagnoses is often inappropriate and will reinforce the notion that there is an obscure or serious underlying disorder in the mind of the child, family or other professionals often delaying appropriate management.

In spite of optimal investigations, the diagnosis in some children with severe neurological disorders remains elusive. Figure 22.1 illustrates how the likely diagnostic yield of investigations becomes less the more investigations that are required and the more invasive or specialized they become.

NEUROIMAGING

In most situations MR is the imaging modality of choice; but the value of imaging has to be balanced against the need in infants and young children for sedation or general anaesthetic.

Consideration needs to be given to 'quality control' and imaging protocols should be agreed with specialist colleagues in the regional neuroscience center (e.g. ILAE protocols for epilepsy). MR imaging is particularly useful in the diagnosis of brain malformations and neurometabolic disease (Figs 22.2, 22.3).

MR angiography allows noninvasive assessment of cerebral arterial and venous anatomy to a high degree of resolution. It does not have the resolution of formal angiography which may still be indicated if there is a high level of suspicion of cerebrovascular disease. Perfusion and diffusion MR imaging are being increasingly used to demonstrate the topography and nature of acute brain insults, particularly ischemic

insults such as stroke. Very early detection may allow appropriate therapeutic interventions.

MR spectroscopy allows in vivo chemical analysis of areas of interest in the brain. It is of particular value in the investigation of neurometabolic disease, some of which can be diagnosed by the MRS pattern. (e.g. Canavan disease and disorders of creatine biosynthesis).

Functional MR (fMR) allows the anatomical location of areas of increased blood flow that have been activated by the initiation of specific functions such as motor, linguistic or visual. This has been of particular value in presurgical evaluation of children with epilepsy and in cognitive research.

The role of MR continues to evolve both as a research and a clinical tool and there are many other potential applications of MR technology which are beyond the scope of this text.

CT scanning remains the imaging modality of choice for immediate assessment of traumatic brain injury, intracranial calcification and for bone imaging (eg craniosynostosis).

NEUROPHYSIOLOGICAL INVESTIGATIONS

The electroencephalogram (EEG) is the most widely used neurophysiological investigation in pediatrics.

Three types of information can be obtained from an EEG: (i) the presence or absence of paroxysmal activity; (ii) the nature of the background activity; and (iii) the topography or asymmetries of any abnormality. The most common reason for requesting an EEG is in the investigation of paroxysmal disorders, especially the epilepsies. It is important to recognize that an EEG is usually unhelpful in the investigation of a paroxysmal disorder when it is unclear from the history whether it is epileptic or non-epileptic.

Both background changes and asymmetries in the EEG are of value in the investigation of acute and chronic neurological disorders, indicating previously unsuspected CNS disturbance (e.g. in organic cognitive or behavioral disorders). In acute disorders they may indicate widespread or focal pathology. The EEG should always be performed in unexplained encephalopathy, particularly to exclude various types of status epilepticus. In coma the EEG is also a good guide to prognosis and very occasionally has a role in the evaluation of brainstem death.

Evoked potentials (EPs) are recordings of EEG waveforms that are seen in response to specific stimuli. The potential recorded is averaged from many single stimuli and considerably amplified. Visual, brainstem (including auditory) and somatosensory EPs provide information on the integrity of pathways within the CNS and on neuronal function in the brainstem or cortex. EPs provide valuable additional information in the investigation of a wide range of acute and chronic neurological disorders. Visual EPs are of most value in assessing potential optic nerve disease (e.g. neuritis or glioma). Serial recordings allow monitoring of response to treatment or disease progression.

Evoked response audiometry is of great value in assessing hearing impairment in small children.

The electroretinogram (ERG) records electrical activity generated from the rods and cones in the retina. Its main role is in the evaluation of possible retinal dystrophies in children with visual impairment or who have a suspected neurodegenerative disease where retinal dystrophy is a prominent feature (e.g. mitochondrial disease, neuronal ceroid lipofuscinoses). While detailed assessment of rod and cone function by ERG studies is possible in older children and adults, this is generally not feasible in infants. In these children it is often only possible to assess whether the ERG is normal or absent; results in between should be interpreted with caution.

Peripheral neurophysiological investigations, electromyogram (EMG) and nerve conduction studies (NCS), are of value in the investigation of suspected neuromuscular disease. In the acute context NCS are of most value in the diagnosis of Guillain–Barré syndrome or other much rarer causes of acute neuropathy. In chronic disorders NCS will identify neuropathy and can indicate whether it is demyelinating or axonal. The EMG is of most value in identifying anterior horn cell disease, disorders

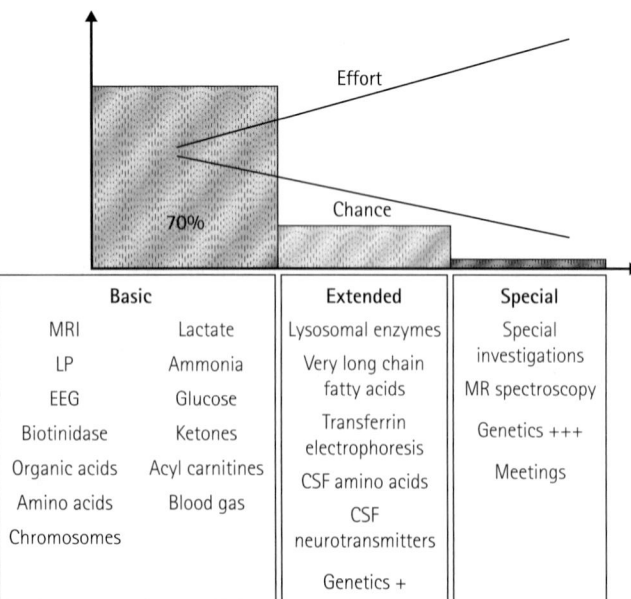

Fig. 22.1 Schematic representation of investigation of neurological disorders. As investigations become more complex and specialized (effort), the likelihood of a final diagnosis becomes smaller (chance). The majority of diagnoses can be made with a comprehensive history, detailed clinical examination and a limited number of relevant tests. (Modified from Dr Joerg Klepper 2006, with permission.)

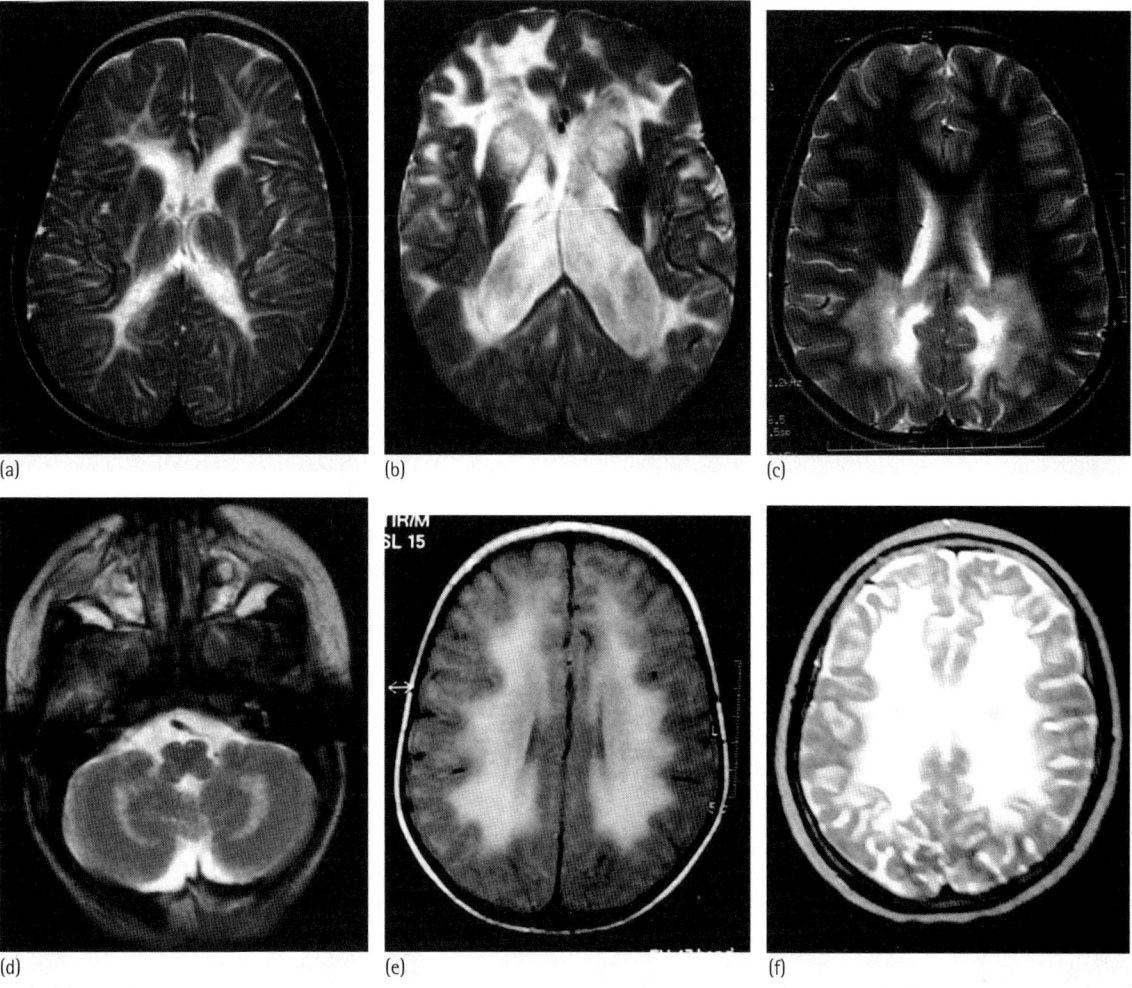

Fig. 22.2 Examples of specific MR patterns in leukodystrophies. (a) Diffuse hypomyelination in recessive Pelizaeous–Merzbacher like disorder. (b) Frontal predominance in Alexander disease. (c) Posterior predominance in X-linked adrenoleukodystrophy. (d) Cerebellar white matter involvement in infantile Krabbe disease. (e) Diffuse white matter involvement in late infantile metachromatic leukodystrophy. (f) Leukodystrophy with vanishing white matter.

of the neuromuscular junction and polymyosistis. It is of less value in primary myopathies.

Quality control is important. The best results come from those laboratories that carry out these procedures on children on a regular basis and that are interpreted by a neurophysiologist familiar with both the technical limitations of these procedures in children and age-related norms. The clinician should always be prepared to question an aparently aberrant result and to consider repeating it if doubt persists.

BIOCHEMICAL INVESTIGATIONS

Specific disorders will be considered in the relevant sections below; however some principles will be considered here. Clinicians often request a 'metabolic screen' without specifying what they are looking for. While most centers now perform a very similar batch of investigations, it is essential to know specifically which tests are included by your local laboratory. Most metabolic screens on urine will include amino acids, organic acids, mucopolysaccharides, oligosaccharides, sugar chromatography and ketones. In general if metabolic disease is suspected several samples should be sent. It is helpful to the biochemist to know if a specific disorder is being considered as they may look at a particular area of the spectrograph in detail (e.g. sulphite oxidase deficiency). It is also important to be aware of diseases where false negatives may occur (e.g. glutaric aciduria type 1).

Acyl carnitine assays on blood (or blood spot) are very useful and may detect fatty acid oxidation disorders, organic acidemias or mitochondrial disease (see Ch. 26, pp. 1067).

Routine analysis of blood amino acids is not usually necessary, although in specific situations it may be helpful.

For most conditions and investigations one negative result does not completely exclude the diagnosis. Screening investigations often look for evidence of abnormalities in the function of an organelle which performs many biochemical activities. Therefore it is often useful to look for several different biochemical clues that point to a given type of metabolic disorder, e.g. peroxisomal or mitochondrial (see Ch. 26, pp. 1081 & 1113). In this context discussing the patient with a specialist colleague before further investigation is advisable.

Lysosomal (or white cell) enzymes are often requested by nonspecialists early in the investigation of neurological disease (see Ch. 26, pp. 1101). Many of these children have none of the clinical features of the conditions that are being tested for or have a static disorder. In general these expensive investigations should not be requested without a specific diagnosis in mind. False positives and negatives may occur which may not be recognized as such if these investigations are used indiscriminately.

An increasing number of conditions can be detected by investigation of the CSF, some of these are simple (CSF sugar), some highly specialized (e.g. neurotransmitters) (Table 22.1).

To diagnose some disorders functional assays of specific biochemical pathways are necessary. For example respiratory chain enzyme activity in muscle or cholesterol handling in fibroblasts in Niemann–Pick type C. Close liaison between the clinicians and laboratory staff is essential for such investigations to be successful.

2. A reactive approach which was more individually tailored but assumes that the doctors involved can intuitively judge parental reactions.

3. A drip feed approach being rather more protective in preselecting topics to meet any given particular situation.

There was little consensus in relation to the use of analogy in explanation and there is often no good knowledge on the usefulness and awareness of available unevaluated literature. All acknowledged the value of a specialist epilepsy nurse, in this context, who is able to visit the family and answer any continuing questions. The doctors involved largely determined consultation content intuitively, rather than on a shared knowledge of the process involved. It is clear that, in this, and in other situations, more study as to the most effective approach is required.

Houston et al[12] studied the information needs and understanding of 5–10-year-old children with epilepsy, asthma or diabetes. They were asked about their knowledge of their condition, psychological effects, medication, restrictions on lifestyle and where they obtained their information if they had unanswered questions. The children with epilepsy had far more unanswered questions and felt excluded from discussions with doctors. They felt reluctant to tell their friends about their diagnosis and often felt stigmatized. The study highlighted a contrast in the understanding of children with epilepsy compared to those with asthma and diabetes. The authors proposed that a simple biological model used to explain epilepsy could aid a child's understanding and reduce their reluctance to disclose the diagnosis.

The subject of written information is important. It is often written using analogy or paradigms that do not specifically relate to biology. It is almost always written without due attention to the reading age of the material involved, and the fact that children at different ages respond to different approaches in this respect. This is an area of research that needs pursuing and with the advent of information technology it should be possible for core information documents to be identified and developed to suit this information need on a national, if not international, basis. Shared web-based sources of information, written to a national standard, are within our grasp.

DEVELOPMENT OF THE HUMAN BRAIN

Knowledge of normal embryogenesis is the key to understanding the myriad of conditions that may present with motor and/or intellectual impairment. It helps us explain to families the biological processes leading to their child's disability. No longer is it acceptable for pediatricians to say, 'We just do not know'; we may not know the particular gene involved but the sort of process that is likely to have occurred and its timing can usually be deduced and a good explanation of that process delivered. This level of understanding should take distress away from many families and help them adjust.

So how do 100 000 million neurones get to the right place? There are a number of well-defined phases:

1. isolation of the neural groove;
2. germinal zone cellular proliferation;
3. neuronal migration;
4. ventral and horizontal organization;
5. synaptogenesis;
6. myelination.

ISOLATION OF THE NEURAL GROOVE

The neural plate begins to form between 18 and 19 days postfertilization. Two neural folds emerge which then fuse at the level of the first pair of somites at 20/21 days, giving the embryonic disc a tubular shape. The neural tube then closes in a zip-like fashion. On day 27 the caudal neuropore closes at what will ultimately become the second sacral segment (Figs 22.4, 22.5).

Rapid differential growth then leads to the emergence of flexures with segmentation. At 35 days a midbrain and pontine flexure are seen. At 29 days three brain vesicles, the prosencephalon, the mesencephalon and the rhombencephalon (Fig. 22.6) appear.

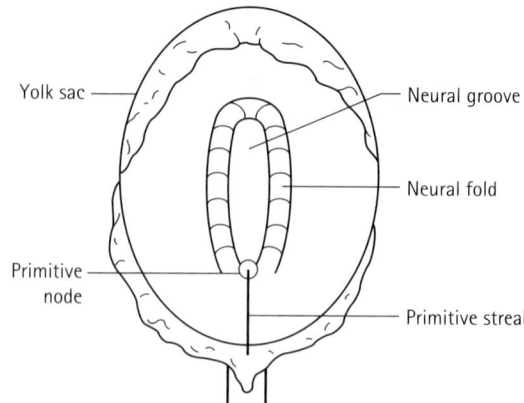

Fig. 22.4 The amnioembryonic vesicle.

At about 29 days postfertilization two telencephalic vesicles appear on the prosencephalon or forebrain, which by the end of the embryonic period (8 weeks' gestation) can be recognized as the developing cerebral hemispheres. After 12 weeks' gestation gyri emerge on the medial aspect.

The mesencephalon changes least but will later contribute the cerebral aqueduct, the cerebral peduncles, and the tegmentum and substantia nigra, which are derived from the basal plate.

The pontine flexure is a prominent feature in the rhombencephalon at 34 days made up by the rhombic lips (destined to form a large part of the cerebellum) at the cephalic end and by the developing floor of the fourth ventricle at its caudal end. Cerebellar foliation follows from 14 weeks' gestation.

GERMINAL ZONE CELLULAR PROLIFERATION OF NEURONES

New neurones then proliferate in cycles involving asymmetrical division from the pseudostratified ventricular epithelium (PVE). One cell migrates, and then ceases to proliferate while another returns to the PVE to undergo a new cell cycle. Most neurones are formed between the 8th and 18th week of gestation and there is probably no significant neurogenesis after birth, in the human. Neuronal and glial lineaging then occurs and specific neurones and glial cells target a particular destination.

The primitive neuroepithelial cells of the embryonic neural tube are the precursors of neurones, astrocytes and oligodendroglia. These cells undergo many proliferation cycles in the ventricular zone and then exit from the cell cycle, leave the ventricular zone and migrate centrifugally in a series of waves. They pass through the intermediate zone to form the layered structure of the cerebral cortex between the 8th and 14th week of postfertilization development (Fig. 22.7).

The earliest migrating neuroblasts form a transient structure, the preplate, and most are lost by programmed cell death (apoptosis). The deep component of the preplate, called the subplate, plays a role in axonal guidance by serving as an intermediate target for the axons of thalamic neurones during their ascent to synapse with cortical plate neurones. The superficial layer of the preplate forms the cells' sparse marginal zone where the Cajal–Retzius neurones lie (see below).

NEURONAL MIGRATION

Later cells migrate into the preplate and split it into an outer marginal zone (or future layer I) and an inner subplate. Later formed cells migrate past these cells. The cells in layer II are therefore formed after those in layer VI (between 12 and 24 weeks).

Migrating neurones advance along columns of radial glial cells between the PVE and the pia. Radial glial cells contain rich amounts of particulate glycogen, an energy source for migrating neurones which depend on anaerobic glycolysis. The migrating neurones then transform

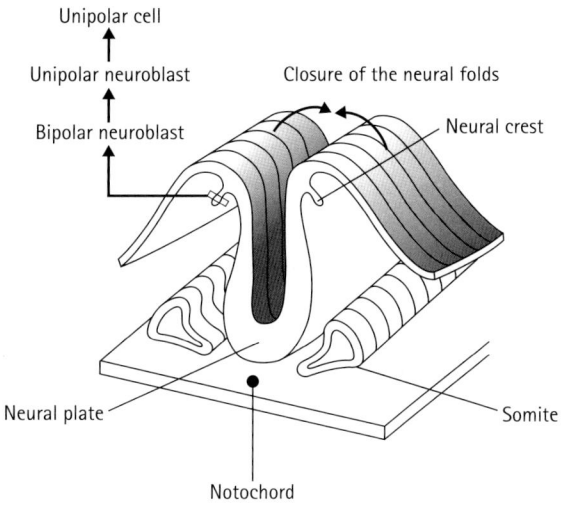

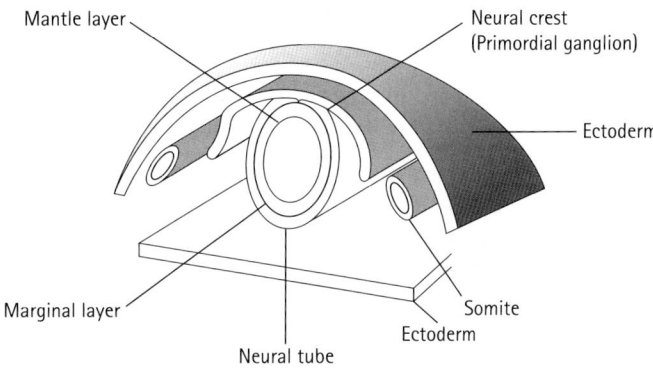

Fig. 22.5 Development of the neural tube from the neural plate 22 days onwards.

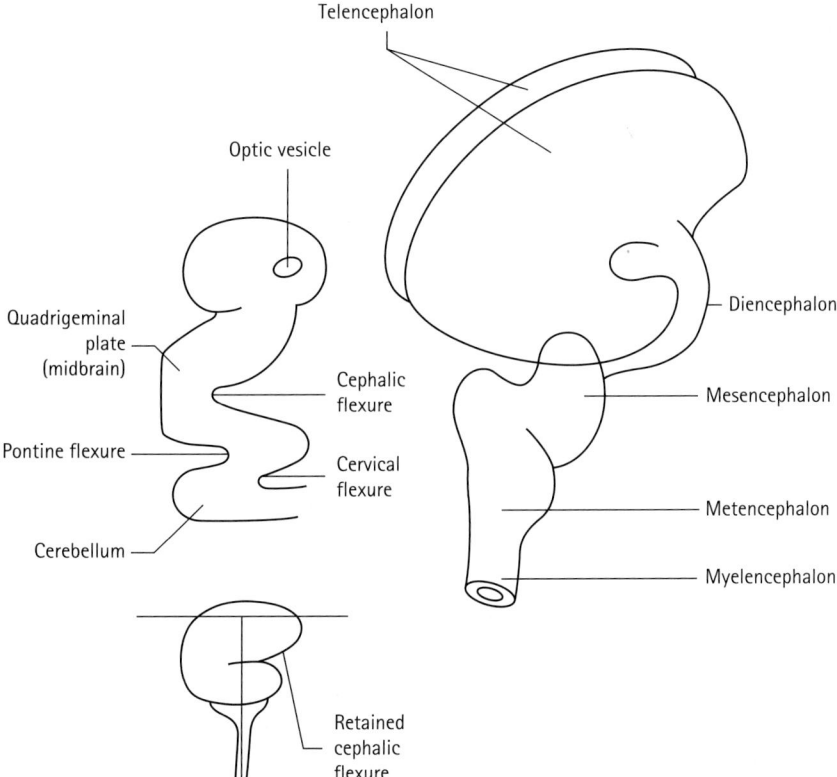

Fig. 22.6 Embryonic flexures of the brain 6 weeks onwards.

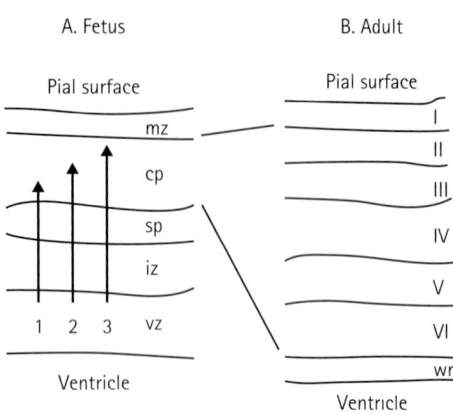

Fig. 22.7 Neuroblasts exit cell cycles and migrate centrifugally along radial glia. Those migrating later pass those migrated earlier to take up more superficial positions. mz, marginal zone; cp, cortical plate; sp, superficial plate; iz, intermediate zone; vz, ventricular zone; wm, white matter.

from anaerobic to aerobic metabolism in the postmigratory settlement areas where they can rely on a vascularized cortical plate.

Some of the neurones formed early in the marginal zone secrete a substance known as reelin. These are the Cajal–Retzius cells. Correct cortical lamination depends on reelin, which appears to instruct neurones on when to cease their migratory activity.

Neurones have differentiated growth cones at their leading end, which respond to signals, categorized as: chemo-attractive, chemo-repellent, contact-attractive or contact-repellent. The chemical signals are diffusable molecules, which create gradients over a distance, whereas contact modulating molecules are cell membrane bound, or in the extracellular matrix.

Many ligand receptor families are known including the semaphorins, with over 30 members. The growth cones probably carry receptors for several classes of these axon guidance molecules.

Nerve growth factors are diffusable peptides acting on specific receptors and define targets for migrating neurones.

Programmed cell death (apoptosis). Most of the subplate neurones are transient and are eliminated by apoptosis. Anomalies of apoptosis have been implicated in the pathogenesis of certain types of neuronal migration disorder, particularly the heterotopias. It seems that 'pro-death' genes (e.g. Bax, Bad) and 'anti-death' genes (e.g. Dcl) are expressed in cells in varying combinations and amounts under exogenous influences such as survival factors. It is the balance between pro- and anti-death genes that determines whether a cell will survive or die. A disruption in this process or an alteration in the local environment leads to the persistence of cells normally destined to die yielding a neuronal heterotopia.

SYNAPTOGENESIS

In monkey experiments, distinct phases have been identified for this process.

In phase 1 (from 6 to 8 weeks' gestation) synaptogenesis is limited to lower structures like the subplate. Phase 2 begins from 12 to 17 weeks, and occurs in the cortical plate. These early synapses are sparse and form contacts in the dendritic shafts of the neurones. Phase 3 is much more rapid and occurs from 20 to 24 weeks and persists up to 8 months after birth. It occurs in conjunction with arborization of axons and dendrites. Phase 4 then proceeds at a very high rate and lasts until puberty. Phase 5 continues up to the age of 70 years, during which time there is also considerable loss. Stage 3 is partially dependent on sensory input, phase 4 much more so.

Excitatory amino acids are the primary neurotransmitter in approximately 50% of mammalian synapses and have an important function in the development of the CNS. They participate in neuronal signal transduction and exert trophic influences on neuronal development. They affect differentiation, growth and survival as well as neuronal circuitry.

Huttenlocher and Dabholkar[13] indicate that maximum synaptic density is not seen until after 15 months of age. It occurs concurrently with dendritic and axonal growth and with myelination of the subcortical white matter. Net synapse elimination occurs late in childhood, often extending to mid-adolescence. Synaptogenesis and synapse elimination in humans occur at different times in different cortical regions. Synapse formation is triggered by the contact of two neurites. Initially this appears to be random but then becomes refined selectively through retrograde and anterograde signaling through neurotransmitter release. Stabilization is activity dependent, so synaptic contacts not included in neuronal circuits are gradually eliminated. Early synaptogenesis is intrinsically regulated and not under environmental control.

MYELINATION

Myelin is formed by oligodendrocytes. Prior to myelin deposition these cells proliferate and there is a marked increase in vascularization. The myelin is laid down first on the fiber close to the nerve cell body, then proceeds along the axon, the oligodendrocyte wrapping its lipoprotein plasma membranes repeatedly around the axon to produce the myelin sheath.

Cycles of myelination progress at different rates and may not be complete for some structures until several years after birth. Table 22.2 summarizes the timetable.[14]

Myelination is a critical process for the development of the brain because it enhances the speed of neural communication. It occurs most rapidly during the first 2 years of life, but probably continues until early adulthood. Klingberg et al[15] studied the degree of myelination of young people's brains with MRI and showed that the maturation of frontal white matter probably continues into the second decade of life.

THE DEVELOPMENT OF SPECIFIC BRAIN STRUCTURES

Forebrain (telencephalon). Initially the cerebral hemispheres are smooth but with growth the sulci and gyri develop. Many gyri are well defined between 26 and 28 weeks' gestation with secondary

Table 22.2 Age (in months) at which myelination becomes apparent. (From Hittmair et al 1994[14])

MR imaging sequence	T1	T2	STIR
Peripheral parts of midcerebellar peduncles	2–3	4	2–3
Folia cerebelli	7[b]	6–7	6–7
Capsula interior			
Posterior limb	0	0	0
Anterior limb	4–5	9–10	5
Corona radiata	0	0–1	0–1
Corpus callosum			
Splenium	4–5	6	5–6
Genu	5–7	7–9	5–9
Optic radiation	0–1	0–1	0–1
Lobar cerebral white matter (central portion)			
Paracentral	2	5–7	5–6
Occipital	4–6	10–12	7–9
Frontal	5–6	11–14	8–12
Completed cerebral white matter Arborization			
Paracentral	3–6	10–12	7–9
Occipital	7–9	18–20	14–16
Frontal	8–10	18–22	14–16

From Hittmair et al 1994[14] T1/T2, T1 or T2 weighted images; STIR, short-inversion-time-inversion recovery images.

and tertiary gyri appearing between 40 and 44 weeks' gestation, initially in the frontotemporal areas and later in the orbital and occipital gyri.

The lateral (sylvian) and central (rolandic) fissures appear in month 4. The callosal sulcus appears around week 14 together with the corpus callosum. At birth the sulci and gyri are similar in arrangement to that of the adult.

The pyramidal tract is the only tract to span the entire length of the central nervous system without synaptic relay. Association fibers connect adjacent areas of the brain while commissures connect equivalent areas on opposite sides (Fig. 22.8).

Diencephalon. This is the posterior part of the forebrain. Three swellings emerge to form:

- The thalami – in the superior diencephalon are the main relay nuclei receiving sensory input and projecting on to the cerebral cortex.
- The epithalamus – incorporates the pineal body, the posterior commissure and the nucleus habenulae (an important relay to the thalamus).
- The hypothalamus – arises in the floor of the diencephalon and from here the mamillary bodies, the tuber cinereum and part of the hypophysial stalk of the pituitary arise.

The medial and lateral geniculate bodies appear later to act as important nuclei for auditory, visual and motor activity caudally to the thalami. The optic vesicles and second cranial nerve grow forward from the diencephalon.

Midbrain (mesencephalon). The lumen of the midbrain is eventually reduced to the narrow cerebral aqueduct of Sylvius connecting the third and fourth ventricles. The dorsal midbrain roof (the tectum) enlarges as two pairs of protuberances, the rostral superior colliculi and the inferior colliculi. The superior colliculi act as relays for visual reflexes and the inferior for auditory reflexes. Several nuclear groups develop from the basal plate in the midbrain floor (the tegmentum): the reticular formation, the red nucleus, the substantia nigra and the nuclei for the third and fourth cranial nerves. The cerebral peduncles develop as small thickenings from the ventral laminae. In the fourth month they increase rapidly in size as the corticopontine, corticobulbar and corticospinal tracts expand and pass through the midbrain area.

Hindbrain (metencephalon). This comprises the cerebellum, the pons and the fourth ventricle lying between the two.

Hindbrain (myelencephalon). This forms the medulla oblongata and is continuous caudally with the spinal cord.

PROTEINS AND GENES ASSOCIATED WITH BRAIN DEVELOPMENT

A number of genes involved in the formation of the brain have been retained phylogenetically and are to be found in insects and lower vertebrates. They are known as homeotic genes and control the orientation of the embryo, segmentation of the body and segment identity. Clustered homeobox-containing genes (the HOX genes) are important. They differentiate the segments of the early embryonic brain. Those expressing many HOX proteins develop as posterior structures, those with lower levels form the anterior part of the axis. EMX and OTX are expressed in the fore- and midbrain region. Mutation of the EMX gene leads to one form of schizencephaly (see below).

Krox-20 is necessary for the development of the cranial nerves in the hindbrain. The Sonic Hedgehog genes determine timing and spacing, for example, which neurones should develop into motor neurones in the spinal cord. If this gene is knocked out all neurones become sensory neurones by default.

Early specification of the forebrain depends on appropriate expression of a number of homeobox and winged helix-containing genes including members of the Otx, Emx, Dlx, BF, Mf, Lhx and Gsh family.

Reelin and Mdab0001 are needed by neuroblasts to pass one another as they migrate centrifugally. With Cdk5 and p35 mutant genes later migrating neuroblasts do not appear to be able to pass early migrating neurones with resulting disruption of the cortical plate. The LIS1 and doublecortin gene are both implicated in the etiology of lissencephaly. Subcortical band heterotopia arises from cortical plate cells that express the mutant doublecortin gene. The protein kinase C substrate MARCKS is needed to define the pial basement membrane that serves as the external anchoring point for radial glial end feet. Without correct functioning of extracellular matrix models including laminin and collagens at pial limiting membranes, determined by MARCKS, layer II neurones are found heterotopically in the marginal zone or in the subarachnoid space.

The interaction between neuroblasts and radial glia is mediated by a number of molecules including astrotactin and neuroregulin (glial growth factor). Patterning of the cerebral cortex depends on interneural signaling and the dynamic response of migrating neurones to the local chemical environment. For example Pax6 and em2 are transcription factors expressed in opposing gradients. This graded concentration of antagonizing diffusible molecules restricts the expression of specific transcription factors, which in turn regulate the expression of downstream target genes specific for regional identity.

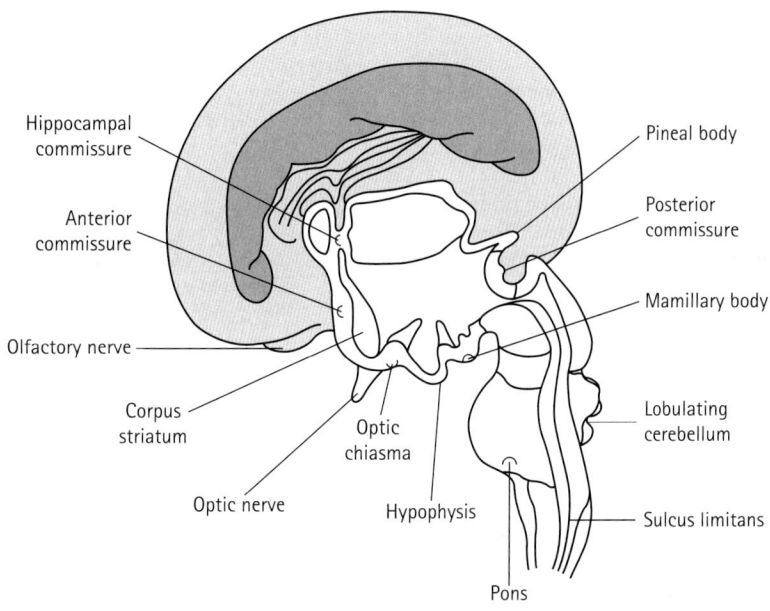

Fig. 22.8 Commissure development at 4 months.

A family of proteins known as the cell adhesion molecules (CAMS) are also important in cell migration. In the cerebellum these have been attributed imaginative names presumably reflecting the likely phenotype when things go wrong!: viz 'reeler', 'weaver', 'staggerer'. Probably the most studied of the cell adhesion molecules is the Down syndrome cell adhesion molecule coded for on chromosome 21. Multiple forms of Dscam are generated through alternative splicing from its four main exons (4, 6, 9 and 17). This gives the amazing possibility of 38 000 possible isoforms indicating what great scope there is for very focused migration targeting. Thus neurones arrive in the target area encouraged by signaling from a variety of growth factors. Having entered the layer they arborize. They are encouraged to enter a specific site and discouraged from leaving, by ephrin and cam gradients which code for different target cells along various axes and layers. The incoming afferents are distinguished by receptors on their surface. These ligand and receptor gradients are the result of very early patterning events in the embryo. Molecular cues from homophilic/heterophilic adhesion molecules aid the process leading to very precise connectivity. Fine tuning then becomes heavily dependent on synaptic activity as previously discussed. Dysplasia may arise when cortical cells mutate and re-express genes normally only seen at an earlier stage of differentiation, or genes that characterize a different cell lineage.

UNDERSTANDING ABNORMALITIES OF CEREBRAL CORTEX DEVELOPMENT

Barkovich and colleagues[16] proposed a rational classification system for malformations of the cerebral cortex in 1996. It is based on three embryological stages of cortical formation:

1. Cellular proliferation within the germinal zone, which occurs between 7 and 16 weeks' gestational age.
2. Migration of neuroblast cells from the germinal matrix to the developing cortex occurring between 12 and 24 weeks' gestational age.
3. Vertical and horizontal organization of cells within the cortex with the establishment of axonal and dendritic ramifications which begins at approximately 22 weeks' gestational age and continues until after birth.

Problems of cellular proliferation

Entities in this category include the following.

Radial micro-brain (also known as lissencephaly type IV) results in a brain of dramatically reduced size but with a normal gyral configuration and cortical thickness. Children with this condition have severe microcephaly and often multiple non-CNS abnormalities.

Microcephalia vera (also called lissencephaly type III) results in severe depletion of neurones in cortical layers 2 and 3. A number of genetic and sporadic abnormalities may lead to this condition, which involves a reduced number of neurones in the germinal zones but no evidence of a migratory disorder. Children with this condition often have moderate developmental delay.

Tuberous sclerosis is a disorder of cellular proliferation that results in hamartomatous growths and, at times, neoplasms. The cortical tuber is composed of bizarre giant cells, heterotopic neurones and glial tissue. Defective stem cells in all germ cell layers may underlie the central nervous system manifestations of tuberous sclerosis. The stem cells differentiate into astrocytes and neurones, which lack the ability to integrate themselves further into the brain structure. Some remain in the germinal zone, resulting in the subependymal hamartomas, whereas others migrate along glial fibers in the white matter to the cortex, where they form the disorganized cellular clusters known as tubers.

van der Knaap and Valk[17] in their categorization included the other phakomatoses, such as neurofibromatosis, Sturge–Weber disease, von Hippel–Lindau disease and ataxia telangiectasia, in the category of abnormalities of neuronal proliferation, differentiation and histogenesis.

Hemimegalencephaly consists of unilateral cerebral enlargement with associated hamartomatous parenchymal overgrowth. Children present with developmental delay and intractable seizures. There may be an association with linear sebaceous nevus syndrome and unilateral hypomelanosis of Ito.

Focal transmantle dysplasia is characterized by abnormal cortical lamination, white matter astrogliosis and balloon cells. It arises from the maldifferentiation of germinal zone stem cells. Children present with a focal epilepsy and the focal dysplasia is demonstrable with MRI.

Disorders resulting from a disorder of migration include classic (type I) lissencephaly, which is also called agyria-pachygyria. There is absent or marked underdevelopment of the gyri and sulci. The cortex comprises only four layers and migration appears to have been arrested sometime between 12 and 16 weeks' gestation. Children are generally hypotonic at birth with the subsequent development of corticospinal tract signs and seizures. The most striking clinical presentations are seen in children with the Miller–Dieker syndrome (17p13.3 microdeletion) and there are relatively milder manifestations in those with isolated lissencephaly.

In type II lissencephaly there is a severely disorganized thickened cortex lacking a normal layered pattern. MRI scanning sometimes gives a 'cobblestone' appearance though the cortex is thinner than seen in type I lissencephaly. There is considerable clinical overlap between type II lissencephaly, the Walker–Warberg syndrome and Fukuyama congenital muscular dystrophy which all have autosomal recessive inheritance. MR imaging reveals a thickened disorganized cortex with shallow sulci and hypomyelinated white matter (Fig. 22.9).

Gray matter heterotopia are foci of normal neurones situated in abnormal locations due to an arrest in the migration process. The heterotopia may be localized or diffuse. Subependymal and band heterotopia are examples of neuronal migration anomalies, which are often diffuse.

Subependymal heterotopia has small ovoid masses of gray matter located along the lateral ventricular walls. Young people with this disorder often have normal development and a seizure onset after the first decade of life. MRI demonstrates the nodules which do not enhance with gadolinium, in contrast to the subependymal nodules seen in tuberous sclerosis.

Band heterotopia, also known as 'double cortex' heterotopia, consists of large circumferential layers of heterotopic neurones that have failed to reach the cortex. The resulting gray matter band is uniform, diffuse and bilateral. Those affected often have moderate to severe learning difficulties and intractable seizures.

It should be noted that all of the above neuronal migration anomalies may be very localized as well as diffuse. They have all arisen between 12 and 16 weeks' gestational age. Subcortical heterotopia may exist as an irregular lobulated mass of gray matter situated in the subcortical white matter. These heterotopia tend to be large, extending between lobes. The overlying cortex is thin, with shallow sulci, and there are

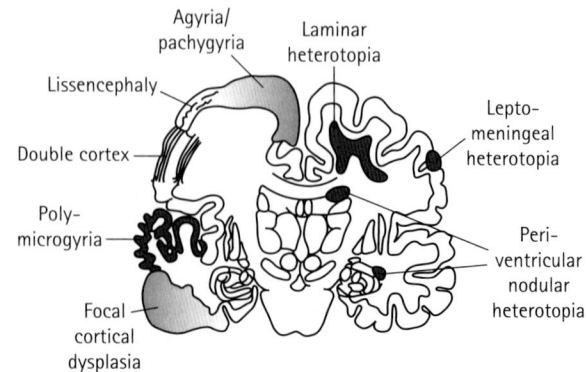

Fig. 22.9 Diagrammatic representation of the more frequent neuronal migration disorders.

often associated dysplastic basal ganglia. Those affected often present with learning difficulties, a hemiplegia, or hemi-hypo-esthesia and localization related epilepsy.

Cortical organization follows 24 weeks of fetal development. Abnormalities occurring in this process include focal or diffuse polymicrogyria and schizencephaly. Polymicrogyria results when neurones reach the cortex but distribute in an abnormal fashion creating multiple small gyri with a deranged sixth layer cortex. It probably represents disruption of cortical maturation and folding in the postmigrational period but does not arise after 28 weeks' gestation. It may be diffuse, symmetrical and bilateral, as in the bilateral opercular syndrome, or focal and unilateral. The clinical presentation depends on the location and extent of involvement but seizures are seen in up to 80% of those affected.

Schizencephaly consists of gray matter lined clefts that extend through the full thickness of the hemisphere from the cortex to the ependymal lining of the ventricles. The gray matter lining the clefts is often polymicrogyric. If the walls of the cleft are fused it is termed 'closed lip' schizencephaly. If not, it is known as 'open lip'. The clinical course often includes seizures, hemiparesis, with the closed lip varieties tending to be associated with the milder clinical course.

Van der Knaap and Valk[17] placed schizencephaly earlier in the migration sequence than polymicrogyria, proposing a time of onset of 2 months' gestational age for schizencephaly and 5 months for polymicrogyria. Whereas mutations of the EMX2 gene have been found in humans with schizencephaly, the lesion may also be due to tissue loss and infarction.

Agenesis of the corpus callosum involves failure of growth of the main forebrain commissure. It is associated with a number of chromosomal abnormalities, drug ingestion, including valproate, and a number of syndromes. Aicardi syndrome is an X-linked dominant condition in which agenesis of the corpus callosum is associated with infantile spasms, intellectual impairment, vertebral anomalies and retinal lacunae.

EARLY DEVELOPMENTAL BRAIN ABNORMALITIES
Abnormalities of dorsal induction
Failure of neural tube fusion results in a range of abnormalities which may also involve adjacent bone and skin coverings. They all arise on or before 28 days of development.

Encephaloceles consist of a bony skull defect through which dura and brain parenchyma protrude. They are identified according to the location of the bony defect, e.g. occipital. The brain parenchyma abnormality reflects many disorders of embryogenesis.

The Chiari II malformation is almost always associated with a spinal myelomeningocele and is a complex hindbrain deformity with caudal displacement of the medulla, pons and portions of the cerebellum through an enlarged foramen magnum. There is often associated callosal dysgenesis and cervicomedullary kinking, which may predispose to hydrocephalus.

Disorders of ventral induction
Ventral induction involves the further growth and development of the three cerebral vesicles between weeks 5 and 10. Congenital abnormalities arising from disorders of ventral induction include holoprosencephaly, the Dandy–Walker syndrome and callosal dysgenesis/agenesis.

Holoprosencephaly results when the prosencephalon fails to cleave laterally and transversely (12 sites on 11 chromosomes have been implicated). The result is varying degrees of hemisphere and ventricular fusion. In alobar holoprosencephaly there is a complete lack of cleavage leading to a horseshoe-shaped monoventricle and absence of the corpus callosum. In semilobar holoprosencephaly there are rudimentary temporal occipital lobes with some differentiation of the ventricular system. In lobar holoprosencephaly there may be very mild appearances on MRI including hypoplasia of the frontal horns or underdevelopment of the anterior aspect of the falx.

The Dandy–Walker complex is a spectrum of hindbrain abnormalities incorporating varying degrees of hypoplasia of the cerebellar vermis and/or enlargement of cisterna magna. There is often associated hydrocephalus.

Callosal development occurs between 8 and 20 weeks of fetal life and proceeds in an anterior to posterior direction. Abnormalities result in complete absence of the corpus callosum or simply underdevelopment. Septo-optic dysplasia associates hypoplasia of the corpus callosum with midline structure abnormalities including optic nerve hypoplasia, hypothalamic and pituitary dysfunction.

FUTURE CLASSIFICATION SYSTEM
Traditionally, morphological classification schemes have focused on anatomical or histological abnormalities identified at postmortem, complemented with the findings of more refined imaging systems, especially MRI. The timing of the interruption of the normal developmental process has then been estimated and the disorder classified (as delineated above) according to whether this was a problem with neurulation, cell migration, axonal projection, synaptogenesis or myelination. As our knowledge of gene receptors and chemotactic agents grows, this system requires refining. A new system for classification of the malformations of the nervous system has been proposed by Sarnat and Flores-Sarnat.[18] They make the point that, whereas traditionally a disorder such as holoprosencephaly was subdivided into alobar, semilobar and lobar forms (see above), this classification does not accommodate the four distinct human genes responsible for various cases of holoprosencephaly. Some of these genes have a ventralizing effect in the vertical gradient (e.g. the Sonic Hedgehog gene, SHH at 7q36) whereas others have a dorsalizing influence (e.g. Z1C2 at 13q32). At least seven other defective chromosomal loci have been associated with holoprosencephaly. Thus, holoprosencephaly is a common end stage of several different disturbances in cerebral development. Severity does not always correlate well with the associated midfacial hypoplasia, which may range from mild hypotelorism to extreme forms of cyclopia, or the correlation with diabetes insipidus, in about one third of affected infants. These correlations most likely relate to the rostrocaudal gradient of the genetic expression, bearing in mind that most rostral neural crest tissue arises in the midbrain and forms not only neural structures but also the membranous bones of the face, orbits and much of the eyeball except the retina, lens and cornea. It must be acknowledged that a scheme purely based on genetic analysis would be very difficult to use for radiologists, pathologists and clinicians. Furthermore, disruption in one gene, particularly one involved in a cascade, may lead to disruption of further genes later in the sequence. For example, defective DAB1 causes underexpression of the downstream genes LIS1, Reelin and EMX2, all of which are important for various stages of neuroblast migration. However nongenetic malformations secondary to acquired lesions in fetal life (e.g. infarction to interrupt radial glial fibers and their guidance of migrating neurones) would not be accommodated within such a genetic scheme.

Sarnat and Flores-Sarnat apply these principles to known patterns of malformation (Table 22.3). A single condition may appear in more than one position in the table, implying that a particular abnormality is a common end point for a number of different mechanisms. Although this proposed classification is likely to change in time, nonetheless it offers clinicians, radiologists and pathologists alike an understanding of some of the complex biological processes involved. It also provides the opportunity to give affected families important understanding and appropriate genetic counseling.

PRENATAL PRESENTATION OF DEVELOPMENTAL BRAIN ABNORMALITIES
Many of the described abnormalities result in motor and/or intellectual impairment and/or epilepsy and the general pediatrician, or pediatric neurologist, may be called upon to advise and counsel families and advise colleagues in radiology on the relevance of brain abnormalities detected by antenatal ultrasound.

Table 22.3 Twelve principles cited by Sarnat and Flores-Sarnat[18] involved in genetic programming of the neural tube

Principle 1:	Development genes are re-used repeatedly. For example, an organizer gene establishing axis of growth may appear later in development as a regulator gene for differentiation and maintenance of specific cellular types
Principle 2:	Domains of organizer genes change in successive stages
Principle 3:	Relative gene domains may differ in various neuromeres
Principle 4:	Some genes activate, regulate, activate, regulate or suppress the expression of others
Principle 5:	Defective homeoboxes usually have reduced domains or result in deletions of entire neuromeres
Principle 6:	Some genes may compensate for the loss of others if their domains overlap: redundancy and synergy
Principle 7:	An organizer gene may be upregulated to be expressed in ectopic domains. For example, epithelial growth regulator-2 may be ectopically expressed with the loss of unique identity of those rhabdomeres in which specific cranial nerve nuclei and other structures are generated
Principle 8:	Developmental genes regulate cell proliferation to conserve constant ratios of synaptically related neurones. For example the regulation of the ratio of Purkinje cells to granule cells is regulated through Sonic Hedgehog (SHH) and the granule cell receptor product of the gene Patched (PTC) and a related additional receptor gene Smoothened. Hemizygous mutations of the PTC gene in mice result in medulloblastoma. Cellular proliferation may be regulated by mitogenic stimulation or by the rate of apoptosis
Principle 9:	Overexpression of genes programming the ventrodorsal or dorsoventral gradients, manifest as hypoplasia or duplication of paramedian structures of the neuroaxis
Principle 10:	Underexpression of genes programming the ventrodorsal or dorsoventral gradients manifests as aplasia, hypoplasia, or midline fusion of paramedian structures of the neuroaxis
Principle 11:	Minor genetic mutations may change cell lineage within or between traditional embryonic germ layers
Principle 12:	Organizer and regulator genes are conserved in a phylogenetic evolution but may form several distinct varieties with related but distinctive functions in more advanced species

Agenesis of the corpus callosum

Up to 0.7% of the general population have complete or partial agenesis of the corpus callosum and 85% of these individuals are asymptomatic. Agenesis may, however, be associated with seizures or learning difficulties and be associated with other CNS abnormalities. Many cases are sporadic, but autosomal recessive or X-linked varieties are also described and there is a 1 in 10 risk of an associated chromosomal abnormality, trisomy being the most common.

Three per cent of all fetuses with ventriculomegaly and 10% of all fetuses with mild ventriculomegaly have agenesis of the corpus callosum. Those features most commonly associated with a poor prognosis include upward displacement of the third ventricle, widened interhemispheric and atrial diameters, absence of the cavum septum pellucidum, the radial array of the medial gyri and dilated occipital horns.

Approximately 80% of children with partial or complete agenesis of the corpus callosum have associated CNS anomalies including ventriculomegaly, porencephaly, microcephaly, encephalocele, holoprosencephaly, lissencephaly, Dandy–Walker malformation and spina bifida. Non-CNS abnormality is also common. Eighty sporadic genetic and chromosomal syndromes have been described with agenesis of the corpus callosum.

Fetal ventriculomegaly

Isolated ventriculomegaly has a prevalence of 1 in 1000 births in the United States. Thirty per cent of fetuses with ventriculomegaly have associated neural tube defects so careful evaluation of the spine should be performed.

Hudgins et al[19] reported that approximately 86% of ventriculomegaly is stable throughout the gestation, 9% progressive and approximately 4–5% resolve. Ventriculomegaly is defined as atrial diameters greater than 10 mm, or above four standard deviations. Measurements are taken at the level of the choroid plexus from the inner border of the medial wall to the inner border of the lateral wall.

Mild idiopathic lateral ventricular dilation defined as atrial dimensions of 10–15 mm encompass approximately 20% of the fetuses with ventriculomegaly and resolution may be seen with ventricular diameters as large as 12 mm. Mild isolated ventriculomegaly during the second trimester has been estimated to occur in 1 in 675 pregnancies. Follow-up shows 80–90% of the fetuses with isolated mild ventriculomegaly develop normally,[20] while up to 50% of fetuses with mild ventriculomegaly and associated congenital defects are developmentally impaired; (seen for example in 23% of children at 2 years of age in a review of 234 reported cases[21] and 12 of 101 fetuses not terminated in a more recent French study of 167 affected pregnancies – assessed after 19 months of age).[22] Fetal hydrocephalus with marked ventriculomegaly is associated with a 55–75% mortality (including elective abortions, intrapartum and postnatal deaths). The prognosis is better where there is no associated abnormality but still 40% survive with severe disability.[23,24] Intrauterine shunting has been shown not to improve outcome.[25] If the ventriculomegaly is due to hydrocephalus infants do best when the shunt is placed postnatally.

Dandy–Walker malformation

This incorporates cystic dilation of the fourth ventricle, an enlarged posterior fossa with upward displacement of the tentorium and cerebellar vermian hypoplasia. A definitive diagnosis cannot be made until after 18 weeks' gestation as normal cerebellar hemisphere fusion is not complete until 17 weeks' gestation. There is an association of Dandy–Walker malformations with chromosomal abnormality in up to 45%. It should be noted that an enlarged cisterna magna in association with a vermian defect or other cerebellar anomaly may be a benign condition. The outcome for Dandy–Walker malformations and its variants ranges from normal to severe disability. All the clinician can offer is detailed screening for associated abnormality and the assessment of any chromosomal abnormality.

Cerebellar hypoplasia

Spinal dysraphism may be associated with cerebellar hypoplasia. Other forms are genetically determined, the most prominent of which is probably Joubert syndrome, whose postnatal clinical features include episodes of overbreathing, ataxia, abnormal eye movements and severe learning difficulties. Cerebellar hypoplasia may be associated with abnormality of gait, eye movement, epilepsy and learning difficulties, but is compatible with normal neurodevelopmental outcome.

Cranial cystic lesions: developmental or destructive in origin

Midline lesions include holoprosencephaly, a Dandy–Walker malformation or cerebral hypoplasia. An arachnoid cyst may also be considered. An arachnoid cyst is often associated with underdevelopment of adjacent brain parenchyma. If a cyst is within the third ventricular region an aneurysm of the great vein of Galen should be considered.

If the cyst is asymmetrical or lateralized this is most often associated with destructive causes, which in turn may result from systemic disease of the fetus, mother or placenta. Prognosis will depend on the site and extent of the lesion.

DEVELOPMENT OF THE SPINAL CORD

The spinal cord extends into the tail of the embryo until days 44–51. Once the filum terminale and conus medullaris have formed the conus assumes a higher and higher position within the vertebral canal. This is thought to be due to differential growth of the vertebrae, which are growing more rapidly than the spinal cord. By week 31 the spinal cord has reached its adult level of L1.

As the neural folds first fuse to form a tube the walls are composed of a single layer of columnar epithelium. These cells proliferate and the neural tube walls become thickened. The central canal is initially relatively large but as the volume of gray and white matter increases they become smaller. A cycle of growth follows so that cells eventually give rise to all the neural and macroglial cells in the CNS.

Once the neural tube has closed the ventricular layer gives rise to neuroblasts and glioblasts. Radial glial cells form the glia limitans, along with guiding neurones. Neuroepithelial cells produce ependymal cells, which will line the ventricular system of the brain, choroid plexuses and the central canal of the spinal cord.

At 33–43 days a second layer, the marginal zone (subpial or molecular layer), appears outside the ventricular zone. This eventually forms the white matter.

The alar plate forms the dorsal gray columns, the basal plates the ventral and lateral gray columns. Axons from unipolar neurones in the spinal ganglia enter the spinal cord and form the dorsal root ganglia, as axons from the ventral horns grow out of the spinal cord and form the ventral roots of the spinal cord.

From the beginning of week 12 ascending, descending and propriospinal fibers invade the marginal zone.

The third layer of the neural tube, the intermediate layer (middle or mantle layer) formed from neurobalasts by 38–40 days is located between the ventricular and marginal zones. This forms the gray matter.

Three periods of synaptogenesis have been described. These include the spinal reflex activities at 8 weeks when the fibrous connections to the spinal reflex arch are complete, the onset of local activities with a rapid increase in axodendritic synapses (9.5 weeks) and multiple responses at 13–15 weeks with a rapid increase in axosomatic synapses. The first observable movements are seen at 7.5 weeks.

NEURAL TUBE DEFECTS

The term includes anencephaly, encephaloceles, cranial meningoceles and the various forms of spinal bifida.

Primary nonclosure of the neural tube is the most likely mechanism in the formation of neural tube defects. The process should be complete by 23–26 days. van Allen et al[26] suggested five separate sites of closure along the length of the neural tube. At the lower sacral end a process of neurulation is followed. There is a condensation of mesenchymal cells arriving from the primitive streak followed by canalization.

Mesodermal defects

There may be bony defects ranging from failure of fusion of the complete spine (total rachischisis) to simple deficiencies of the lower lumbar spinous processes as part of a spina bifida occulta. Hemivertebrae may give a scoliosis and the associated ribs may be absent or fused. Bony spurs occur in diastematomyelia. There may be absence of the sacrum or sacralization of the lower spine. Klippel–Feil anomaly involves fusion of cervical vertebrae, with severe disruption of the cervical spine. This causes marked retroflexion of the head in iniencephalus where there is also complete lack of fusion of the neural tube.

Other mesodermal defects such as angiomas, lipomas, dermoids, renal abnormalities with pelvic kidney or horseshoe kidney may be added to the bony spectrum.

Ectodermal defects

A defect in the neuroectoderm is known as myelodysplasia. This may manifest as disruption of the histological architecture of the spinal cord (multiple anterior horns, several central canals, abnormal neurones), syringomyelia, failure of fusion of the cord so that there is a flat neural plaque rather than a fused tube (myelocele), double neural tube (diplomyelia), tethering of the cord or herniation through the bony defect as a meningocele or myelomeningocoele.

Other ectodermal defects include dimples, sinuses, skin defects, hairy patches, tails and cutaneous capillary hemangiomas that can occur in any combination.

INCIDENCE

Cuckle and Wald[27] showed that the birth prevalence of anencephaly and spinal bifida declined by 80% from 3.15 to 0.6 per 1000 births between 1964 to 1972 and 1985. Prenatal diagnosis followed by termination (achieved by measurement of the serum alpha-fetoprotein and by ultrasound) accounted for 31% of the decline. The increased risk in monozygotic twin pairs and in the siblings and half-siblings of affected children indicate a genetic component to the risk. The 1983 UK Medical Research Council trial of folic acid, mineral and vitamin supplementation indicated that folic acid had a protective effect of 72% at a daily dose of 5 mg. The first genetic risk factor for neural tube defects identified at a molecular level is C677T (alanine to valine), polymorphism in the gene encoding for the folate dependent enzyme 5,10-methylene tetrahydrofolate reductase (MTHFR). Following the work of the MRC Vitamin Study Group[28] it is now recommended that folic acid, 0.4 mg, should be given to all women planning a pregnancy.

SPINA BIFIDA OCCULTA

Spina bifida occulta may present in several ways.

An incidental radiological finding of a narrow split in the fifth lumbar or first sacral spinous process is of no clinical significance. It is very common in young children and the incidence lessens with age.

A cutaneous lesion in the form of a small nevus, hemangioma, tuft of hair, sacral pit or soft lipomatous swelling should be taken as a warning signal that there may be an underlying abnormality. This may consist of a bony abnormality with bifid spinous processes but can also signify an underlying abnormality of the spinal cord with an associated myelodysplasia, lipoma, diastematomyelia or neuroenteric cyst. These cutaneous lesions should be taken as an indication for imaging of the whole neuraxis, using ultrasonography in babies or MRI of the spine in older children, even when there is no neurological deficit.

Myelodysplasia

This term is used to indicate that there is an abnormality in the development of the spinal cord. There may be several central canals, several anterior horns or disorganization of the 'muscle nuclei' so that specific muscles do not form properly. The characteristic clinical findings are often referred to as myelodysplasia. There is usually a cavovarus deformity of the foot, which may be small so that shoe sizes are different. The leg on the affected side is shorter and appears to be the leg of a younger child. It is cold and often shows erythrocyanosis. It may be difficult to demonstrate definite weakness.

Tethering

Tethering of the cord refers to persistent caudal attachment through the filum terminale. It may lead to damage from traction and repeated movement of the spine. The child may present with weakness in one leg or with bladder problems and progressive neurological deterioration is a definite indication for surgery. Whether tethering without neurological deterioration in the legs should be operated upon remains an unanswered question. If operation is not undertaken then careful neurological follow-up is mandatory, especially at peak growth periods. With MRI scanning, it is now possible to diagnose the condition more easily and criteria for operation should become clearer. Serial somatosensory potentials may also assist in diagnosis of progression.

Diastematomyelia

A different cause of tethering is a bony or fibrocartilagenous spur, which arises from a vertebral body and passes between the halves of a bifid cord – diastematomyelia. In some cases this fixes the cord and results in increasing traction with growth. In other cases the cord divides well above the spur and passes around the diastematomyelia in two separate dural canals, i.e. a diplomyelia.

Damage from tethering or compression may cause spastic paraplegia. More frequently, however, the child presents with distal weakness of the foot, with clawing of the toes and equinovarus posture and weakness of the peronei. Dribbling incontinence of urine may be an early feature and there may be sensory loss in the sacral territory, loss of ankle jerk and anal reflexes and trophic changes in the feet. Neurological deterioration in the presence of bony spur is an indication for removal, but removal of any bony spur demonstrated to put the cord at risk during growth should be considered before the development of neurological signs.

Intraspinal lipoma

A cutaneous lipoma or lipomeningocele may penetrate in dumb-bell fashion into the spinal canal. It may cause increase in pressure within the canal. Treatment of a lipoma can be difficult as the cord itself as well as nerve roots may be enmeshed in fatty tissue.

Infection

Infection may be the presenting feature of dermal sinuses. Blind pits over the coccygeal region are rarely associated with communication to the theca but focal infection with abscess formation may be a nuisance. Pits over the sacrum itself, especially at the site of the caudal neuropore, are of much more concern, as there may be a direct communication with the theca and therefore a risk of recurrent meningitis. These should be electively excised in the neonatal period.

SPINA BIFIDA CYSTICA

Meningocele

In this condition there is a defect in the spinous processes (spina bifida), together with herniation of the meninges through the defect to form a cystic mass on the back (Fig. 22.10).

There may be cover by thick skin with little risk of rupture or infection or by a thin transparent membrane; there may be skin at the sides and a thin blue membrane over the top. There is no myelodysplasia or cord within the sac in the pure cases and the child is neurologically completely normal. Hydrocephalus is usually absent and simple repair of the defect can be carried out as an elective procedure. The result should be a normal child. Ultrasound of the head should be performed to be sure that there is no associated hydrocephalus and ultrasound of the abdomen to be sure there is no associated renal abnormality.

Myelomeningocele
Spinal lesion

The spinal cord is an open flat plate on the surface of the bulging meninges. It is not known whether the developmental abnormality itself, intrauterine damage, secondary ischemia, trauma to neural tissue during delivery or postnatal infection is the principal cause of the neurological deficit. Exposure of neural tissue, in normal fetal lambs, to amniotic fluid results in neurological dysfunction of legs and bladder.[29] Stimulation of the exposed neural plate shows that all the muscles of the legs have intact innervation to the exposed plaque. The lower motor neurones are intact but these are not connected to

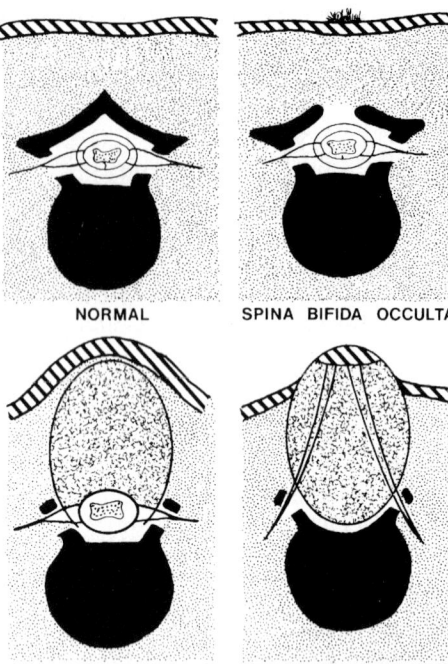

NORMAL   SPINA BIFIDA OCCULTA

MENINGOCELE   MYELOMENINGOCELE

Fig. 22.10   Classification of spina bifida.

higher centers at the upper end of the plaque. These connections are lost as the plaque dries out or is infected. The fetus at 12 weeks of gestation can be shown to have talipes and evidence of neuromuscular imbalance in utero. There is no doubt that secondary postnatal injury may occur, but operation at birth does not reverse all the neurological deficit. An open myelomeningocele is liable to infection (Fig. 22.11). Surface infection leads to meningitis or ventriculitis, which is the usual cause of death in untreated patients. If the open lesion is not closed there is gradual epithelialization of the lesion over a period of weeks or months. The end result is inferior to elective surgical closure; low-grade infection results in further loss of spinal cord function, there is ugly tender scarring on the infant's back and there may be tethering of nerve roots, which can be very difficult to treat at a later date.

Patterns of spinal cord involvement

Type 1 cord lesion. Complete absence of function below a certain segmental level, which results in a flaccid paralysis, loss of sensation and loss of all reflex movement and tendon reflexes below that level. Knowledge of the segmental innervation of the lower limb muscles allows the segmental level to be determined from examination of the lower limbs.

Type 2 cord lesion. Here there is voluntary control of muscles, which have normal innervation and are in direct communication with the long tracts of the brain above the level of the lesion. At the level of the lesion there may be a complete loss of all function, voluntary and reflex, and of sensation. This may extend over a very short area, i.e. one segment, or over several segments of the spinal cord. The cord then resumes reflex function, as an isolated cord segment. There will be no sensation and no voluntary movement of the muscles in this isolated cord segment. Muscles will, however, respond to dermatome stimulation tapping of the muscle, tapping of the tendon and pinprick.

Examination of the lower limbs will determine the neurological level of paraplegia and the prognosis for walking, type of deformity and degree of future handicap. The level of the lesion, level of vertebral abnormality and neurological level are not identical and one should not look at the back lesion and guess the neurology.

Direct stimulation of the muscles which do not move is possible by dermatome-to-myotome stimulation, i.e. as the corresponding

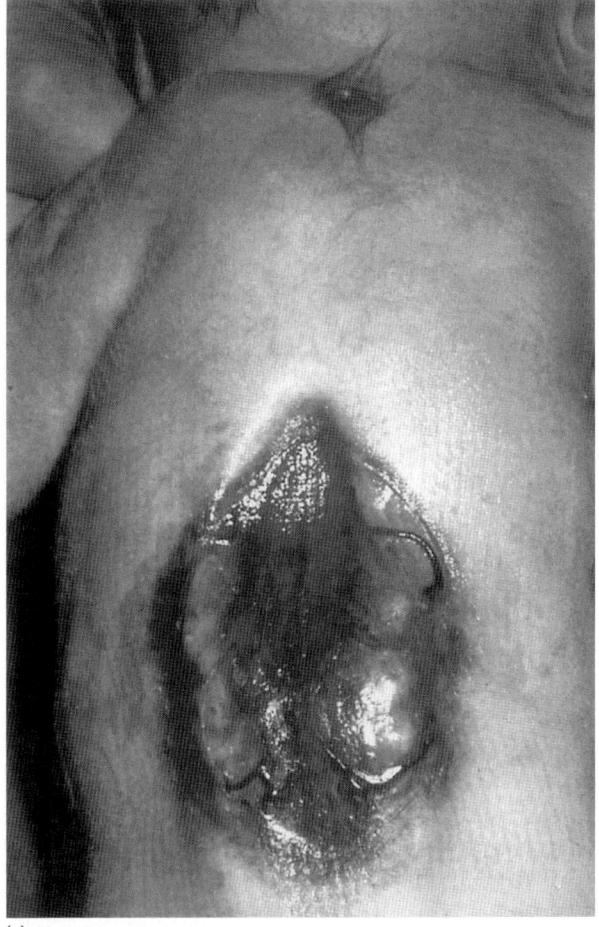

(a)

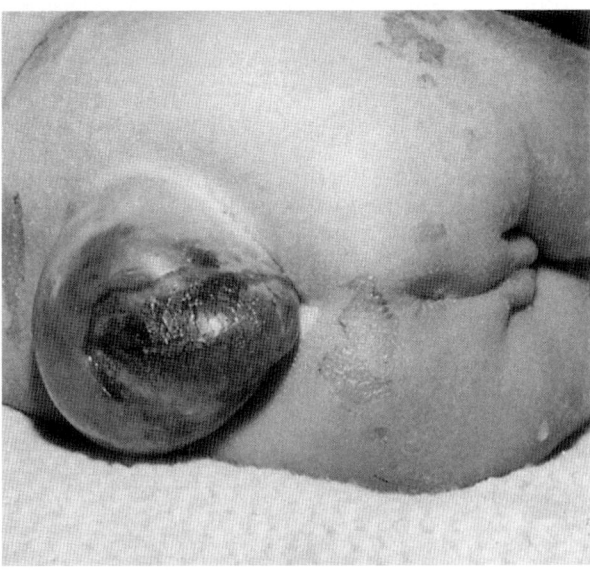

(b)

Fig. 22.11 (a) Meningomyelocele at birth. (b) Bulging meningomyelocele at a few hours of life.

dermatome is stroked, if there is reflex activity the muscle supplied by that segment will contract. In addition to testing the cremasteric reflex (L1), knee jerk (L3–4), ankle (S1–2), anal and bulbocavernosus reflexes (S4–5), for exaggerated flexor withdrawal reflexes, contraction of the muscles of the perineum on stimulating the perianal region and contraction of the short toe flexors by flicking the toes should be assessed.

Reflexes not normally easily elicited, such as tendon jerks of the hamstring muscles, adductors and tibialis anterior, may be elicited, and in very high lesions, adductor and patella clonus may be seen.

If the isolated cord segment is long, then complex reflexes such as flexor withdrawal responses may occur, giving the impression of voluntary leg movement. This has led to confusion in the past as to the degree of paralysis and the tendency to give a misleadingly good prognosis in the neonatal period.

If the area of isolated cord is limited to the sacral segments, then ankle clonus with a brisk ankle jerk and exaggerated anal reflex will be seen together with a spread of the response when stimulating the perianal region to cause toe flexion and flexion of the lateral hamstrings. Equally, tapping the toes in order to elicit the toe jerk will produce flexion of the knee and a contraction of the anus. The segment of cord showing a lower motor neurone loss of activity is more often in the region of the abdominal muscles, which may be completely paralysed, causing a lumbar hernia and a pot belly.

Mechanism of deformity

The level of deformity often determines the neurological level, e.g. involvement below T8 is associated with paralysis of the abdominal walls and all the lower limb muscles. The lower limb deformities arise from two mechanisms:

1. Muscle imbalance, e.g. dislocation of the hip when the flexors and adductors (L1–3) overcome the weak gluteal extensors and abductors (S1–2). Hip adduction is a potent cause of posterior hip dislocation. Involvement below L4 causes the lower limb muscles innervated from above this level (hip flexors, hip adductors, quadriceps and tibialis anterior) to be strong and under voluntary control while their antagonists are paralysed. This causes the characteristic flexed hip, extended knee (genu recurvatum) and equinovarus foot. If the tibialis anterior is active as a dorsiflexor (L4) while the calf muscles as plantarflexors (S1–2) are paralysed, then dorsiflexion and inversion of the foot will occur.
2. Immobility in utero. The fetus may present as a breech and the immobility results in secondary positional deformities adding to the neurogenic deformity (Fig. 22.12).

In 5% of cases the spinal cord is split with only one half of the cord exposed to the surface; the other half remains in the spinal canal and functions normally. In this case only one leg will have a neurological deficit.

Counseling families

Parents are concerned as to whether their child will walk. In a 25-year follow-up of 71 children treated at birth in an aggressive, nonselective manner, Bowman et al[30] observed that 46% of young adults (33/71) walked the majority of the time (75–100%). An additional 13% (9/71)

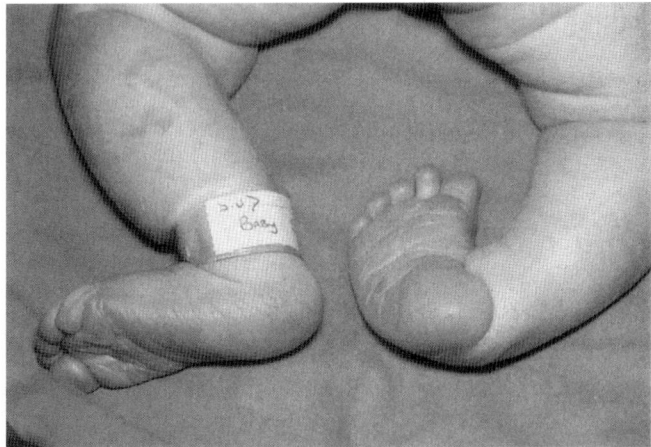

Fig. 22.12 Talipes due to muscle imbalance.

walked 25–50% of the time. Forty-one percent (29/71) got around only with the aid of a wheelchair. As one might expect children with lower defects were more likely to walk the majority of the time [93% of children with a sacral lesion (14/15) walked 100% of the time]. No one with a lesion level of L3 or above walked the majority of the time. These figures closely match those reported from Northern Ireland.[31] Experience shows many, of course, do more than walk, participating in dancing, swimming, basketball, horseback riding, wheelchair sports and so on.

Intelligence
Bowman et al[30] reported that 85% of the 71 young adults followed by their group were attending or had graduated from high school and/or college, and 63% attended regular classes. Forty-five percent were actively employed, and almost 10% worked as volunteers. Most of the 71 lived with their parents, although 11 lived independently and two were married.

Hydrocephalus
Historically, almost all newborns with spina bifida received shunts. Recent data indicate that these rates may be too high. The Children's Hospital of Philadelphia published shunt rates among 189 children treated for spina bifida between 1983 and 2000.[32] One hundred percent (35/35) of children with thoracic level lesions received shunts, compared with 88% (100/114) of children with lumbar lesions and only 68% (27/40) of children with lesions confined to the sacrum. The upper level of the spina bifida lesion appears to be a major determinant of the need for shunt placement. Fewer neurosurgeons are automatically placing shunts at the same time as the spinal lesion is closed.

Continence
Bowman et al[30] noted that 85% of their young adults (60/71) used clean intermittent catheterization (CIC), and 90% of those (54/60) performed their own catheterization. For those on CIC, 15% always had urinary continence, 68% were dry the majority of the time (75–100%) and 7% were dry 50% of the time. Fifty-two percent of the young adults reported bowel control the majority of the time, and 52% reported 100% social bowel continence. McDonnell and McCann[31] reported renal impairment in 48% and 15% were on antihypertensive therapy.

Other problems
McDonnell and McCann[31] reported 50–70% had scoliosis and 9% epilepsy. Pit-ten Cate et al[33] showed how additional medical problems are associated with poorer quality of life, as one might expect. However, the availability of resources to the family was found to help significantly; a clear message for community-based pediatric services.

NEONATAL MANAGEMENT OF THE CHILD WITH A NEURAL TUBE DEFECT
Check for associated abnormalities, such as chromosome disorder or other malformations of the heart and kidney. The face of a child with a meningomyelocele may suggest Down syndrome. The head circumference, sutures and fontanel should be measured and cerebral and renal ultrasound should be routinely performed. X-ray of the spine may show hemivertebrae or gross disruption of the spinal architecture, which would make even sitting eventually impossible.

The lesion is carefully examined for tears in the membranes or leakage of CSF suggesting that operation should be early because of the risk of meningitis. The hips are examined for dislocation.

Detailed neurological examination is carried out with the child warm and recovered from the birth. Sensory testing is carried out first with the child quiet; the skin is stimulated with the end of a straightened paper clip, starting in the saddle area and progressing through the sacral and lumbar territory. Look for facial grimace or a cry.

Following sensory testing, and with the baby active and crying so that there is spontaneous movement of the upper limbs, determine the amount of spontaneous movement in the lower limbs as part of the baby's doggy paddling and cycling movements. It should be possible to give each muscle group an MRC grading of 1–5 and a voluntary motor level down to which the child can move in response to cerebral motor drive can be defined.

Gross hydrocephalus at birth is predictive of severe disability, [an occipitofrontal circumference (OFC) more than 20 cm above the 90th centile or a cortical mantle less than 150 mm]. Serious spinal deformity, absence of voluntary movement below L2 and the presence of other major defects are the factors which help in deciding whether early immediate operation should be performed or whether one should delay surgery to see how the child progresses over the first week or so. Delay does not worsen outcome. Later plastic repair of the back that has granulated is still feasible.

If immediate closure is not undertaken and the spinal lesion granulates without meningitis developing, hydrocephalus may progress. This may lead to impairment of intelligence, and should be prevented by insertion of a ventriculoperitoneal shunt. The parents should be encouraged to feed and handle their baby. During this period many questions can be answered, anxieties are allayed and genetic counseling undertaken. The support of a medical social worker, experienced health visitor or community pediatric nurse is invaluable and the parents can be put in touch with one of the local parent support groups.

Bruner et al[34] reported a 35% reduction in hydrocephalus following intrauterine repair of myelomeningoceles probably linked to a 60% reduction in hindbrain herniation. However the risk of oligohydramnios and preterm labor were significantly increased. Their study compared 29 fetuses operated on between 24 and 30 weeks' gestation with 23 historical controls. Further careful assessment of prenatal intervention is required.

More recently the same group's study[35] of 116 fetuses operated on since 1997 has determined which factors present at the time of intrauterine spina bifida repair predict the need for a shunt in the first year of life. Sixty-one of 116 of the fetuses (54%) required the placement of a ventriculoperitoneal shunt before the age of 1 year. The upper level of the lesion was the strongest predictor of shunt requirement [adjusted odds ratio per 1 level increase with the use of continuous variables (S1 through T10), 1.73 (95% CI, 1.22–2.44)]; followed by gestational age at the time of surgery [adjusted odds ratio per 1 week increase with the use of continuous variables, 1.37 (95% CI, 1.06–1.77)]; and preoperative ventricular size [adjusted odds ratio per 1 unit increase with the use of continuous variables, 1.17 (95% CI, 1.01–1.36)]. This study suggests that, among fetuses who underwent operation in utero for spina bifida, fetuses with a ventricular size of less than 14 mm at the time of surgery, fetuses who had surgery at 25 weeks of gestation or sooner, and fetuses with defects that were located at L4 or lower were less likely to require ventriculoperitoneal shunting for hydrocephalus during the first year of life. Only two intrauterine/neonatal deaths occured. However, clearly this is a specialized intervention and further careful assessment is required.

THE LATER MANAGEMENT OF THE CHILD WITH A NEURAL TUBE DEFECT
Motor problems
It should be possible to make a reasonably accurate prediction of the child's future mobility even in the neonatal period if an accurate clinical neurological assessment is made (Table 22.4).

Orthosis refers to lightweight plastic splints which are malleable when hot, but firm when cool and can be molded to any required position. Reciprocal gait orthoses are hinged splints, which invoke forward momentum when the weight of the wearer is swung from side to side at the hip. They follow the same principle as the toy

Table 22.4 Prediction of walking ability in myelomeningocele

Voluntary motor level	Probable walking ability
T6–L2	Chair Crutches – swing through Parapodium Swivel walker RGO, HGO
L3	HKAFO RGO, HGO with sticks or tripods
L4	KAFO, HKAFO AFO
L5	AFO KAFO
Sacral	nil or AFO

AFO, ankle/foot orthosis; RGO, reciprocating gait orthosis; HGO, hip guidance orthosis; HKAFO, hip/knee/ankle/foot orthosis; KAFO, knee/ankle/foot orthosis.

animals that will 'walk' down a slope, each limb rocking from side to side.

The child with a purely sacral lesion, as for example with sacral agenesis, or a very low meningomyelocele, will have problems with the feet due to paralysis of the intrinsic muscles of the feet, weak calf muscles and weak hip extensors. He will walk with a waddle and will need boots to support the ankles. He will also have a neurogenic bladder and will require a bladder regimen.

Paralysis below L3–4 is compatible with walking aided with sticks and below-knee calipers The effects of the spinal lesion may be compounded by the effects of ataxia from hydrocephalus or hemiplegia as a result of shunt malfunction, ventriculitis or puncture porencephaly. The child with a high lumbar lesion was in the past sentenced to immobility in a wheelchair but the use of reciprocating gait orthoses or hip guidance orthoses means that these children can now be mobile in the erect posture.

It may be necessary for an orthopedic surgeon to perform tenotomies in the neonatal period or later to correct muscle imbalance, for example the very tight tibialis anterior that may occur in an L4 lesion. Talipes will need correcting and hips will need to be released and put back into joint. Scoliosis may require surgery in adolescence.

Nonmotor neurological problems
Sensation
The sensory level in myelomeningocele, i.e. the lowest level of normal sensation, is usually within one or two segments of the motor level. As a result of cutaneous anesthesia there is a constant danger of painless ulceration. Pressure sores may develop over the sacral tuberosity, especially if incontinence has led to maceration of the skin. Sensory loss may become more of a problem in the future with the use of reciprocating gait orthoses when the risk of Charcot joints (i.e. neurogenic arthropathy and painless fractures) is added to the list of problems. The feet are often cold, blue and erythrocyanotic due to poor peripheral perfusion.

Burns may occur from hot-water bottles or sitting on radiators. Shoes which are too tight or failure to recognize the effects of intense cold in the winter can both result in gangrene of the toes.

The neurogenic bladder
The bladder receives its nerve supply from three sources. First, the parasympathetic via the nervi eriginates from the sacral roots S2–4 which control detrusor contraction. Second, a sympathetic component supplies the trigone and internal sphincter and allows opening of the bladder neck during micturition. It is also important in sexual function when the internal sphincter is closed without any contraction of the detrusor. The third supply is via the pudendal nerve, which carries the voluntary control of the striated external sphincter.

The bladder and bowel will be involved in most cases, but the type of bladder involvement depends upon the type of lesion.[36]

If the lower limbs show signs of lower motor neurone denervation in the muscles innervated from S2 to S4 (type 1 lesion), i.e. calf, intrinsic muscles of the foot, anal sphincter and pelvic floor, then a weak or totally paralysed bladder (acontractile) is to be expected. Lack of tone in the anal sphincter shows as a patulous anus and loss of the normal gluteal fold so that the anus appears wide open on top of a mountain rather than in a valley. Depending on the degree of resistance of the bladder outlet, such infants may have constant dribbling of urine with an empty bladder or overflow incontinence from a distended bladder. Ureteric reflux may occur at low pressures from such inert bladders in which the valvular effect of the intramural ureter is lacking.

In infants with an isolated cord lesion (type 2 lesion), where examination of the limb shows purely reflex activity in S2–4 (i.e. spastic calves, toe flexors with exaggerated reflexes, a very brisk anal reflex), a reflex type of bladder (contractile) is to be expected. The ideal automatic bladder, i.e. one with periodic complete reflex emptying, is rare in myelomeningocele. At best an intermittent detrusor contraction results in voiding of up to 100 ml of urine; at worst persistent dribbling may result from constant poorly coordinated detrusor contractions. Despite an active detrusor, which may generate pressures of over 100 mmHg in a small infant, the bladder emptying may be poor because of a high urethral resistance. This outlet obstruction is probably due to failure of relaxation of the striated external sphincter, which is normally under voluntary control via the pudendal nerve. This type of spastic bladder neck responds to stretching by further contraction and very high pressures result in back pressure with acute and severe hydroureter and hydronephrosis. Bladder rupture and urinary ascites can occur in utero. True bladder neck obstruction is relatively uncommon. Dilation of the upper urinary tract may occur in both the flaccid and the high pressure bladder. Stagnation with incomplete bladder emptying and dilation of the upper urinary tract inevitably leads to the risk of infection. Chronic pyelonephritis may lead to renal failure and hypertension before adult life is reached.

Assessment of the upper renal tract
The presence of hydronephrosis is detected using ultrasound. The presence of ureteric reflux and the adequacy of the bladder neck and urethra can all be assessed using cystourethrography. Renal function is assessed using biochemical estimations such as urea, electrolytes and creatinine together with a chromium or DMSA scan.

Assessment of the neurogenic bladder
Clinically the most important part of the assessment is to watch the child actually pass urine. If the urine can be passed in a stream one knows that there must be a coordinated detrusor contraction. If the stream is good, i.e. the child can 'pee in a parabola', there can be no serious bladder neck obstruction. In the older child, the rate of passing urine can be measured as ml/unit time by getting the child to pass urine into a container with an electronic measuring device which draws out a graph of the rate of urination. This is a measure of detrusor contraction and bladder neck obstruction. The infant should be held up to see if there is any dribbling dependent on position and light suprapubic pressure applied to assess effective bladder neck contraction to allow continence and bladder filling.

Investigation of the bladder in the neonatal period is undertaken to decide whether early intervention is necessary or not. If the upper renal tract is normal on ultrasound and the baby passes urine or it can be easily expressed, one can wait until 4 months of age for detailed urinary investigations. If there appears to be bladder outlet obstruction, high pressure bladder and dilation of the upper renal tract then catheterization from birth may be necessary in order to preserve renal function.

Cystometrogram

This is performed either by a urethral catheter into the bladder when the effects of adding small aliquots of saline upon the pressure is monitored or, more physiological but more invasive, a suprapubic cystometrogram is performed using two catheters inserted into the bladder by suprapubic puncture. One of these is used to fill the bladder at the physiological rate of 2 ml/min and the second to measure pressure. The bladder volume, sensation and pressures at which urethral sphincters open can then be measured and it is possible to look at micturition and urethral resistance in a way that is not possible with a catheter per urethra.

Management of the neurogenic bladder

All children with known or suspected spina bifida should have video-urodynamic assessment.[37]

The safe bladder has a normal upper renal tract with normal renal function and no secondary pressure transmitted to the ureter or renal pelvis. There is a residual urine of less than 20 ml with normal pressures and no outlet obstruction, either because the bladder is completely normal (toilet-training program is all that is required), or the child can safely empty the bladder by suprapubic manual pressure. This requires careful monitoring for urinary tract infection as well as regular monitoring of the upper renal tract to be sure that secondary damage is not occurring.

The unsafe bladder has associated hydronephrosis and hydroureter, a high residual urine, a high intravesical pressure and/or the presence of outlet obstruction. Adequate bladder drainage is needed to avoid progressive damage to the kidneys, with resultant renal failure. The unsafe bladder may require catheterization in the immediate neonatal period. A silicone catheter may be changed every 4–6 weeks in the first few years of life after which intermittent self-catheterization can be taught once the child is old enough. Urinary diversions such as ureterostomy or a colonic loop are now only rarely indicated. Bladder neck obstruction can be treated by per urethral resection or pudendal neurectomy or bladder neck Y-V plasty may be required later to try and achieve relief of bladder neck obstruction without producing incontinence.

Toilet training will occasionally achieve continence for the neurogenic bladder not thought to be under voluntary control. There is a need to regulate fluid intake, e.g. at night, and to go to the toilet regularly, utilizing suprapubic pressure to induce voiding, at first hourly. Constipation should be avoided, urinary tract infections should be carefully monitored, and when there is voluntary control, double micturition should be practiced as a routine. Pelvic floor stimulators are not of proven benefit and can have complications.

Most children are managed either by a simple toilet-training regimen or with indwelling and then intermittent catheterization. Drugs may be used to increase or decrease bladder tone and capacity to keep the child dry between catheterizations. Cholinergic drugs such as carbachol, bethanechol chloride or distigmine bromide will increase detrusor contraction while anticholinergic drugs such as propantheline, imipramine and oxybutynin will decrease detrusor contractions. Beta-adrenergic agonists such as ephedrine will increase the tone in the bladder neck while alpha-adrenergic blockers such as phenoxybenzamine will decrease the tone in the bladder neck. These have a useful but limited place in a small percentage of children.

Urinary tract infection is a constant hazard with the risk of pyelonephritis and this, together with the effects of back pressure on the kidney, may result in renal failure by the teenage years.

Sexual function

Motor problems are likely to lead to physical difficulty and result in problems with sexual intercourse. Only small numbers of young adults with spina bifida have any sexual experience and very few females have children even though there is no reason why they should not become pregnant and have a normal delivery. In the male, impotence will depend upon the pattern of sympathetic and parasympathetic involvement. Failure of closure of the bladder neck during ejaculation will cause semen to enter the bladder and not the posterior urethra.

Bowel

Chronic constipation, with gross dilation of the descending colon and overflow incontinence, is common. Prolapse of the rectum may occur in infancy, but rarely remains into school age. Chronic fecal retention may further impede bladder drainage. The anal sphincter, like the bladder neck, may be either patulous and incompetent or tight and spastic. Sensation may be absent so that severe constipation, with retention of feces or fecal incontinence, may occur. In spite of the neurogenic problems, the bowel appears to be more amenable to training than the bladder. The child should take a high-fiber diet and it may be necessary to use stimulative laxatives such as Senokot or fecal softeners such as Dioctyl. The time of day when the bowel would naturally empty should be sought. This need not necessarily be the morning and toilet training with abdominal pressure will be successful in at least half of the cases. Fecal impaction should be avoided as this presses on the bladder neck and may result in both urinary incontinence and secondary spurious diarrhea, which can be cured by emptying the bowel. In occasional patients regular manual evacuation is necessary to maintain continence.

Teenage problems

As the pubertal growth spurt occurs, several problems result other than sexual (see above), and the realization of the degree of disability may lead to a reactive depression. Renal tract problems cause most anxiety, especially if renal damage has progressed to the point of considering the ethics of chronic dialysis or transplantation. Scoliosis may be greatly aggravated by growth and pain at the site of the healed lesion may cause a lot of discomfort. Traction on the nerve roots due to tethering may cause downward pull at the foramen magnum. It is the medullary cervical junction which causes most problems and is the most difficult to deal with. Stretching of the medulla with obstruction at the aqueduct and the fourth ventricular foramina from the Arnold–Chiari formation may cause an isolated fourth ventricular hydrocephalus. This may require separate shunting. The pressure may be projected down the central canal of the spinal cord so that a hydromyelia results with gross distension of the cord, producing a string-of-sausages appearance. A localized dilation may occur as a syringomyelia. These brainstem and cervical spinal abnormalities present as drooling, swallowing difficulties, bilateral sixth and seventh paresis, Erb palsy posture, weakness of shoulder elevation or wasting, weakness and loss of use of the hands. Removal of tethering, shunting fourth ventricles, cerebellar tonsillectomy and removal of the arch of the atlas and part of the foramen magnum-impacted tissue may be attempted to try and prevent progressive loss of function.

HYDROCEPHALUS

DEFINITION

Hydrocephalus denotes an increase in size of the CSF spaces associated with an increase in intracranial pressure (ICP).

INCIDENCE

The incidence of hydrocephalus per 10 000 births around the world is particularly high in Alexandria in Egypt (20.8), and Belfast (12.5) and Dublin (35) in Ireland. A collaborative perinatal survey[38] found an incidence of 15 per 10 000 births, only half of whom were evident at birth. These figures are, however, now too high for the UK, as hydrocephalus associated with spina bifida, secondary to intraventricular hemorrhage in the premature infant and secondary to haemophilus meningitis and tuberculous meningitis, have all declined. The current prevalence[39,40] of congenital and infantile hydrocephalus is between 0.48 and 0.81 per 1000 births (live and still). The ability to diagnose severe hydrocephalus antenatally by ultrasound means that some cases are prevented by termination.

PATHOPHYSIOLOGY
Factors that cause ventricular dilation
The normal intracranial pressure in the human represents a balance between the intracranial contents, i.e. blood, brain and CSF. For the CSF compartment, any increase in production or obstruction of flow or absorption will result in ventricular dilation.

Production of CSF
In normal subjects, CSF is formed at a rate of 0.3–0.5 ml/min. In children with hydrocephalus on external drainage the CSF production rate is similar. CSF production occurs by two mechanisms:

1. That dependent on choroidal capillary blood flow. This is a two-step process with, first, an ultrafiltrate of plasma produced hydrostatically through the lax choroidal capillary endothelium (blood–CSF barrier) and, second, an active process involving secretion of sodium into and out of the apical choroidal villi. The raised osmotic pressure causes water to follow passively.
2. That due to a direct neurogenic stimulation of choroidal villi (which have beta$_2$-adrenergic receptors, cholinergic receptors and GABA receptors), which is independent of choroidal blood flow. Stimulation of adrenergic fibers may reduce CSF flow by approximately one third.

The production rate is similar in newborn and older children, despite the obvious difference in size of the choroid plexus. It is postulated that early maturation of enzyme systems may be responsible for the similar production rates.

A number of factors influence the CSF formation rate. Increased secretion may occur with a choroid plexus papilloma. Furosemide and acetazolamide reduce CSF production. Hypothermia will also reduce the rate of production and although the CSF formation rate is usually independent of the intracranial pressure, when high intraventricular pressures exist the production rate falls, due to decreased choroidal perfusion. Ventricular outflow rates appear to be pulsatile so that peaks and troughs of CSF evacuation occur from the ventricles when measured objectively in children undergoing closed ventricular drainage.[41]

Obstruction
A choroid plexus tumor may not only induce excessive CSF production, but may also block the outlet of the ventricle. Intracranial hemorrhage or meningitis may cause leptomeningeal adhesions and obstruction to the CSF flow as well as impairing absorption by blocking arachnoid granulations. A common site for obstruction is the aqueduct of Sylvius. Congenital atresia may result in an inadequate lumen or a total blind-ending channel with forking of the upper and lower components of the aqueduct. Occasionally there is a filamentous or membranous obstruction, which may be broken down either by an increase in the intraventricular pressure or by surgical bouginage from the fourth ventricle (which rarely succeeds because of inadequate development of the peripheral subarachnoid pathways). The aqueduct of Sylvius may also be occluded by organized blood clot after intracranial hemorrhage, inflammatory exudate following ventriculitis or from an aqueductitis resulting from mumps.

Obstruction to CSF flow at the outlet foramina of the fourth ventricle may be secondary to intracranial hemorrhage or infection or may be due to congenital failure of the foramina of Magendie and Luschka to open during development. Occlusion of the fourth ventricle foramina results in a fourth ventricular cystic dilation with atrophy of the cerebellum (the Dandy–Walker cyst). Tumors or clots, cysts or abscesses within or adjacent to the ventricular system may result in hydrocephalus. Thalamic tumors, and giant cell astrogliomas in tuberous sclerosis may obstruct the foramen of Monro and third ventricle and pontine or brainstem gliomas may distort the aqueduct of Sylvius, although frequently such pontine gliomas are invasive throughout the brainstem and do not usually cause a gross hydrocephalus. Cerebellar tumors will affect the CSF flow from the fourth ventricle. A choroid cyst of the third ventricle may give rise to intermittent high pressure and hydrocephalus, by obstructing the foramen of Monro in a 'ballcock' fashion. During distention of the cyst or venous distention about it there is obstruction of CSF flow through the foramen of Monro. With a possible change of posture, the obstruction may be rapidly released and the pressure decline. Children with cysts of the third ventricle frequently present with a 'bobble-headed doll' syndrome and progressive loss of intellect with frontal horn dilation.

Decreased absorption
Decreased absorption may result from obstruction of the arachnoid villi or other peripheral subarachnoid pathways. Absorption (unlike formation) of CSF is a pressure-dependent phenomenon and increases linearly with CSF pressure. Normally CSF absorption begins at a mean pressure of 5 mmHg.

Factors causing progression of hydrocephalus
Observations in experimental hydrocephalus suggest that after CSF obstruction the ICP rises acutely. This is followed by a stage of periventricular edema with expanded ventricles and subsequently by an increase in CSF absorption. Ventricular dilation and its eventual size depend on the external support of the brain. In infants up to 16 months of age the support of the brain is weak from the poorly myelinated soft parenchyma and there are unfused sutures. Clearly the level of pressure is important at first in the pathogenesis of ventricular dilation, together with the known increase in the outflow resistance and a higher 'pressure volume index' (PVI) than could be predicted from the volume of the cranial and spinal axis.

In term and preterm infants we frequently see levels of intraventricular pressure of 5 mmHg (above normal for age) which are sufficient to interfere with the cerebral blood flow velocity and have the potential to cause ischemia.

A number of physiological buffers come into play in response to the hydrocephalus. There is collapse of cerebral veins, a shunting of CSF from the ventricular to the spinal CSF compartment, expansion of the skull and an increase in the CSF absorption from the raised pressure. There may also be increased CSF absorption about the spinal nerve roots and paranasal sinuses. Once these compensatory mechanisms have been exhausted, then further progression of the hydrocephalus will occur.

The sequence of events is that at first the pressure will increase. The dilation of the ventricles in response to this high pressure is termed 'active or progressive hydrocephalus'. Finally the pressure returns to the normal levels with dilated ventricles, a state of arrest (*compensated or arrested hydrocephalus*). Sometimes the active process may be followed by an intermittent pressure pattern with ventricular dilation until the arrested state is reached. This intermittent pattern may be reversible. However, significant elevation of the pressure with increasing ventricular dimensions to the point where brain perfusion is compromised necessitates CSF diversion procedures before shunt-dependent or compensated arrest occurs.

The effects of raised ventricular pressure
Raised intracranial pressure results in ischemia and/or brain shift. The ischemia results from a reduced cerebral perfusion pressure (CPP – mean arterial blood pressure minus intracranial pressure). At levels of CPP below 60 mmHg, in the older child, there is a progressive reduction in brain perfusion. At 40–50 mmHg, profound ischemia results. In the newborn, cerebral perfusion pressures of 30 mmHg may be associated with a normal neurodevelopmental outcome.

The subarachnoid space and the aqueduct are obliterated after shunting, presumably because they are used less, and the patient becomes totally shunt dependent.

Fourth ventricular entrapment, with ataxia, vomiting, cranial nerve disturbances and headache, is a result of outlet obstruction. Treatment is shunting of the ventricle itself. Fistulous communications and diverticula of the ventricles are usually an accompaniment of severe ventricular dilation. This produces a complex CT scan appearance and intraventricular contrast studies are needed to distinguish these from primary subarachnoid cysts.

CLASSIFICATION AND ETIOLOGY

Terminology

Internal or noncommunicating hydrocephalus: excess of CSF within the ventricular system up to the level of the outlet foramina of the fourth ventricle. The common sites of obstruction are at the outlet foramina of the fourth ventricle, the aqueduct of Sylvius or at the foramen of Monro.

External or communicating hydrocephalus: an increase in the ventricular volume and the subarachnoid spaces of the cranium and spine. The sites of obstruction are at the arachnoid villi or in the basal cisterns.

Panventricular hydrocephalus: dilation of the lateral, third and fourth ventricles (in aqueduct stenosis the fourth ventricle is small or of normal size – 'triventricular hydrocephalus'). An *isolated fourth ventricle* ('double compartment hydrocephalus' or 'trapped fourth ventricle') occurs when there is outlet obstruction from that ventricle and stricture of the aqueduct.

Unilateral hydrocephalus: abnormal dilation of the body, frontal and/or posterior horn of the lateral ventricle on one side. This may be due to compression of the ventricular system on the opposite side, obstruction to one foramen of Monro, slit ventricle syndrome or a hemiparenchymal atrophy.

Slit ventricles: a reduction in the size of the ventricular system seen on CT scan, usually in response to excessive CSF drainage. The slit ventricle *syndrome* is distinguished from radiological slit ventricles by the presence of symptoms and clinical signs attributable to this overdrainage. The etiology of hydrocephalus is given in Table 22.5.

DIAGNOSIS AND ASSESSMENT

Clinical features of progressive hydrocephalus

The symptoms and signs of progressive hydrocephalus in infants are shown in Table 22.6.[42] The symptoms of infantile progressive hydrocephalus are vague and consist of irritability and vomiting but about half are without symptoms. The most common clinical sign is an inappropriately increasing head circumference, followed by a tense nonpulsatile fontanel, then clinical and radiological separation of the sutures, scalp vein distension with taut skin over the scalp. It is important to realize that the classic adult presentation of raised intracranial pressure is rare in children (headache, vomiting, papilledema). Vomiting is a nonspecific symptom in childhood, as are behavioral changes (irritability).

The most common sign of hydrocephalus, 'sunsetting' – the inability to look upwards, with depression of both eyes – may initially be intermittent and later continuous (Fig. 22.13). It is due to pressure on the superior quadrigeminal plate against the free edge of the tentorium causing a supranuclear paresis, which may be accompanied by paralysis of the fourth nerve.

Neurogenic stridor is a result of deranged lower brainstem function caused by bilateral corticobulbar disruption and is a feature of pseudobulbar paresis. Abnormalities of sucking and feeding may also occur with seriously raised intracranial pressure. Papilledema is rare, but distended retinal veins are common.

The symptoms of *chronic hydrocephalus* are an insidious deterioration in school performance, intermittent headaches over many months, behavioral and personality changes, failure to thrive and dizziness. These are distinct from the signs and symptoms of *arrested hydrocephalus* of long standing which include features of ataxic and spastic cerebral palsy, precocious puberty, mental retardation and specific learning problems. The clinical features of hydrocephalus with raised intracranial pressure may be extremely variable and any infant with a rapidly increasing head circumference should have cranial imaging.

Hydrocephalus should be considered in the older infant who presents with a large head and developmental delay (other syndromes of macrocephaly including fragile X and neurofibromatosis should also be considered).

Table 22.5   Etiology of hydrocephalus

Causes of prenatally determined hydrocephalus
Congenital (chromosomal) malformations
Maternal diabetes resulting in holoprosencephaly
Neural tube defects
Occipital meningocele and encephalocele
Cleland–Chiari II malformation
Dandy–Walker syndrome
Hydranencephaly
Multicystic encephalomalacia
Schizencephaly
Achondroplasia
Arachnoid cysts
Quadrigeminal plate cysts, retrocerebellar cysts, cysts of the cerebellopontine angle and supracellar cysts
Congenital craniosynostosis (e.g. Apert syndrome)
Agenesis of the corpus callosum and cysts of the cavum septum pellucidum and cavum vergae
Encephalocraniocutaneous lipomatosis
Isolated stenosis of the aqueduct of Sylvius
Sex-linked stenosis of the aqueduct of Sylvius
Hydrocephalus associated with giant hairy nevus (melanosis of the leptomeninges)
Aneurysm of the great vein of Galen
Hurler disease
Basilar impression
Osteogenesis imperfecta (rarely)
Paget disease
Colpocephaly
Lissencephaly
Say–Gerald syndrome

Causes of acquired hydrocephalus
Posthemorrhagic causes
   Neonatal intraventricular hemorrhage
   Subarachnoid hemorrhage
   Subdural hemorrhage
Postmeningitic
   Toxoplasmosis
   Mumps (aqueductitis, ependymitis)
   Pyogenic organisms (pneumococcus, haemophilus, etc.)
   Cytomegalovirus
   Other viral meningitides
   Rubella
   Tuberculous meningitis and tuberculoma
Space-occupying lesions
   Tumor
   Clot
   Cyst
   Abscess
Postasphyxial
   Injury

Other causes
Stenosis of the aqueduct of Sylvius
1. Due to raised intracranial pressure with secondary kinking of the aqueduct
2. Due to aqueductitis and ependymitis associated with mumps, toxoplasma, tuberculomas, pyogenic meningitis, rarely cytomegalovirus, rubella and tumors
Dystrophia myotonia
Otitic hydrocephalus
Choroid plexus papilloma
Intrathecal contrast agents
Fungal infection (cryptococcus and blastomyces)
Cysticercosis
Sarcoidosis
Spinal tumor
Dural venous thrombosis
Isolated Chiari type I deformity

Table 22.6   Most common clinical features of progressive infantile hydrocephalus (50% of cases are asymptomatic)

Symptoms
Headache or irritability
Vomiting
Anorexia
Drowsiness or lethargy

Signs
Inappropriately increasing occipitofrontal circumference (approx. 75%)
Tense anterior fontanelle
Splayed sutures
Scalp vein distention
Sunsetting (loss of upward gaze)
Neck retraction or rigidity
Pupillary changes
Neurogenic stridor
Decerebration

Table 22.7   Clinical features of decompensated hydrocephalus (children with shunts)

Symptoms
Vomiting
Drowsiness or lethargy
Headache
Behavioral change
Anorexia
Valve malfunction
Sleep disturbance
Seizures

Signs
No clinical signs (approx 25%)
Decreased conscious level
Acute squint
Neck retraction
Distended retinal veins
Sluggish palpable valve mechanism

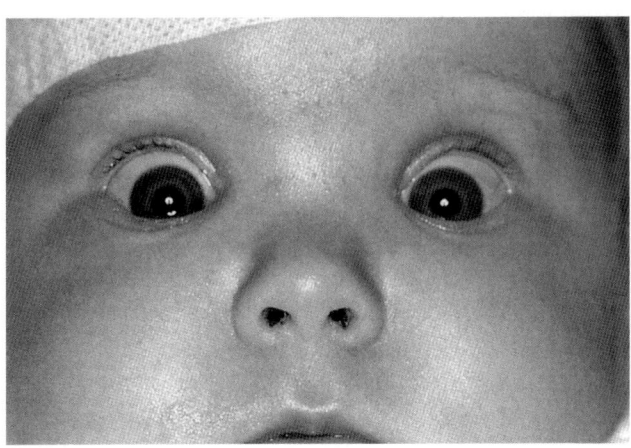

Fig. 22.13   'Sunsetting' due to loss of upward conjugate gaze.

Clinical features of decompensated hydrocephalus

Additional signs of raised pressure (Table 22.7) suggest the possibility of shunt blockage. The median survival time for a ventriculoperitoneal shunt was 4.31 years in the Edinburgh study.[43]

Unusual features of raised ventricular pressure include neurogenic pulmonary edema, profuse sweating, ptosis, neurogenic stridor, pseudobulbar paresis and skin rashes.[42]

Imaging

X-ray examinations of the skull, although not routinely indicated, may show a 'copper-beaten' appearance, shallow orbits and splayed sutures. CT, ultrasound or MRI scans will all define ventricular size. Although repeated ultrasound examinations may show progressive hydrocephalus, it is advisable to have a CT or MRI investigation prior to any surgical intervention. The CT scan provides information about the size and symmetry of the ventricles and whether there is any underlying pathology. A single CT scan, like a single ultrasound or MRI scan, may not reveal whether there is a progressive or an arrested hydrocephalus. When there is significantly elevated intraventricular pressure from progressive hydrocephalus, periventricular lucencies, rounding of ventricles, absence of a cortical subarachnoid space and a spherical appearance of the third ventricle (instead of the usual barrel appearance) is seen on CT scan. It is not sufficient to rely on the skull circumference measurements alone and repeated ultrasound scans are the most useful arbiter. Similarly placed signal changes may be seen with MRI which has the additional advantage that phase-contrast MR may quantify CSF flow rates and give more precise information on etiology.

The most commonly used index of ventricular dilation is the V/P ratio, that is, the ventricular diameter at the mid-portion of the lateral ventricles divided by the biparietal diameter from inner table to inner table. Hydrocephalus is defined as a ratio higher than 0.26.

Antenatal ultrasound for assessment of fetal hydrocephalus is indexed slightly differently. The commonly used parameters are biparietal diameter and the ratio of the lateral ventricular width divided by the width of the head. The latter is approximately 0.61 at 14 weeks, 0.29 at 27 weeks and 0.29 at term. Absolute measurements of ventricular width are done using the atrium as reference point. Ultrasound estimates of ventriculomegaly in utero may be exaggerated by a factor of about 10%, due to the distortion of sound signals passing through two fluids (amniotic and CSF). If hydrocephalus is suspected, ultrasound is done weekly until elective cesarean section at 36 weeks (intraventricular hemorrhage is maximal before 34 weeks). Intracranial Doppler blood flow velocities should be measured in addition to the biparietal diameter.

Intracranial pressure

Ventricular CSF pressure monitoring is the only accurate way of assessing the activity of the hydrocephalus. This can be achieved by direct puncture of the ventricle via the anterior fontanel until it is closed at 18 months. Repeated ventricular punctures should be avoided by placement of a ventricular access device (Rickham or Ommaya reservoir) into the frontal horn of the right lateral ventricle to allow sequential pressure measurements. Repeated brain puncture may cause a puncture porencephaly. A single measurement of intracranial pressure is of limited value. The cerebral perfusion pressure (CPP) should be calculated by subtracting the intracranial pressure (mean ICP) from the mean systemic arterial pressure. For neonates the mean upper normal limit of intracranial pressure is 3.5 mmHg compared to 5.8 mmHg for infants up to 12 months, 6.4 mmHg from 1 to 3 years and 15 mmHg in adults.[44] ($10\,cmH_2O = 7.36\,mmHg$).

For children who present with symptoms of shunt malfunction, due to blockage or infection, and who already have CSF shunting devices in situ, pressure measurements via a 'CSF access device' may be done continuously or overnight. This can indicate when raised pressure should be treated at the bedside and overnight measurements are a way of assessing whether the hydrocephalus is arrested or whether there is an intermittently active component. The rapid eye movement phase of sleep is associated with an increase of cerebral blood flow of about 40% in certain areas of the brain. This increase in intracranial volume has to be buffered if raised pressure is not to occur. In children with abnormal intracranial dynamics, raised pressure is seen particularly during rapid eye movement (REM) sleep and, to a lesser extent, during stage 2 non-REM sleep.

Cerebral blood flow

The cerebral perfusion pressure gives an indication of the potential for ischemic damage to the brain. There are a number of methods available for measuring the blood flow velocity or perfusion to the brain, including flow meters, electrical impedance, autoradiography, washout and wash-in techniques, microspheres, ultrasound, MRI, single photon emission tomography (SPECT), positron emission tomography (PET) and first pass (mean transit time). Our own studies of the first pass method measuring the net mean cerebral transit time use an isotope (sodium pertechnetate or technetium albumin) and were performed on 11 hydrocephalic children. The transit time values correlated with cerebral perfusion pressure values.[45] Children with arrested hydrocephalus had transit times within the normal range, while those with progressive hydrocephalus had up to 15% of their sleep time with a cerebral perfusion pressure of less than 50 mmHg.

It is possible also to use a resistance index (systolic minus diastolic over systolic pressure (S − D)/S) or the area under the curve obtained by pulsed Doppler measurements of the major cerebral arteries as a measure of the cerebral blood flow velocity. The most useful vessel is the middle cerebral artery and an estimate of the velocity is best obtained through the squamous window of the temporal bone, rather than via the open anterior fontanel (Fig. 22.14).

The resistance index correlates significantly with the intracranial pressure[41] and the mean cerebral blood flow velocities fall with elevated ICP measurements. Doppler measurements can be performed intermittently or even continuously in hydrocephalic infants. Since the main effects of raised intracranial pressure are to produce ischemia and brain shifts, an increase in the ventricular pressure sufficient to impair blood flow is an indication for insertion of a CSF shunt or third ventricular ventriculostomy. Despite the low values of ICP in normal newborn infants and the relatively low values in infantile and neonatal hydrocephalus, small rises may be sufficient to impair cerebral blood flow. It is our practice to measure both the pressure and the cerebral blood flow velocity sequentially on these infants and the volume of CSF which needs to be removed in order to produce and maintain a normal resistance index (normal equals 0.68); this will indicate whether the hydrocephalic process is arresting spontaneously or whether it is progressing.[46]

TREATMENTS
Shunts

The usual treatment of progressive hydrocephalus is to divert CSF from the ventricular system to another site. There are numerous valves and shunt systems available, which take CSF out of the head for it to be absorbed elsewhere (Spitz–Holter valve, Pudenz–Hakim, Raimondi, the Indian valve, the Denver, etc.). The author favors the unitised Pudenz with a proximal valve. There are now more sophisticated types (the

Sophy programmable and multiprogrammable and the Cosman ICP telesensor) with various types of opening pressure device incorporated into the shunt system.

The basic shunt system includes a ventricular catheter with a flanged end to cause the choroid plexus to waft away from the drainage holes and so lessen proximal blockage. Some shunt systems have a twin valve, one arranged proximally and another distally, and some include a pump or flushing device. The valve usually has a distinct opening pressure, either 2–4, 4–6 or 6–8 cmH$_2$O, the CSF draining when this pressure is exceeded. In the newborn, a device that opens at low pressure is advisable, but as the child grows, it may be necessary to replace this with one opening at a higher pressure to avoid the development of overdrainage and craniocerebral disproportion. A valve may be incorporated in the pump (Spitz–Holter system) or it may be a distal 'slit valve' at the peritoneal end. It may be a single continuous stiff tube with radiopaque gradations to avoid kinking, such as the Raimondi system. Many different valves and shunt system combinations therefore exist. Our reason for choosing the unitized system with a proximal valve is to avoid the overdrainage, which frequently results by a siphon effect from a long distal catheter.

The potential complications from ventriculoatrial shunts are serious, with infection occurring in between 10% and 30% (Table 22.8). Infection with these shunts is often accompanied by septicemia and

Table 22.8   Complications of CSF shunting

Blockage by choroid plexus, fibrin, neuroglia, blood clot and brain fragments causing raised intracranial pressure

Fractured tubing: fracture of the distal tubing may occur in the neck as a result of direct trauma or kinking of the tubing with repeated movements (fracture can also occur over the surface of the chest and exaggerated flexion/extension movements may result in a crack in the distal tube)

Infection (colonization and ventriculitis) with raised intracranial pressure

Shunt dependence

Slit ventricle syndrome

Other decompressive effects (e.g. subdural hematoma)

Migration of the tubing proximally or distally: cases have been reported of migration of the distal tubing through the gut wall or penetration of other organs. (Cases are known where the tubing has dramatically retracted from the abdominal cavity to the intracranial space. Migration of the distal tubing may cause a volvulus. Commonly if insufficient length is implanted initially, the tubing may retract subcutaneously over the chest wall with growth. Migration of the proximal tubing may result in the proximal catheter extending into a different ventricle or into subcortical structures)

Intestinal obstruction (volvulus)

Peritonitis and peritoneal fibrosis

Endocarditis (VA shunts)

Chronic pulmonary hypertension (VA shunts)

Superior vena caval syndrome (VA shunts)

Arrhythmias (VA shunts)

Shunt nephritis (VA shunts): a case has been reported of shunt nephritis following a VP shunt

Hyperlordosis (TP shunts)

Acute noncommunication (with TP shunts)

Product failure due to mechanical deficiency and a faulty valve

Surgical technique (malplacement or displacement)

Ventricular collapse from excessive drainage causing the tip of the catheter to impinge through the ependyma or brain substance

Pseudocyst formation with defective drainage

VA, ventriculoatrial; VP, ventriculoperitoneal; TP, thecoperitoneal.

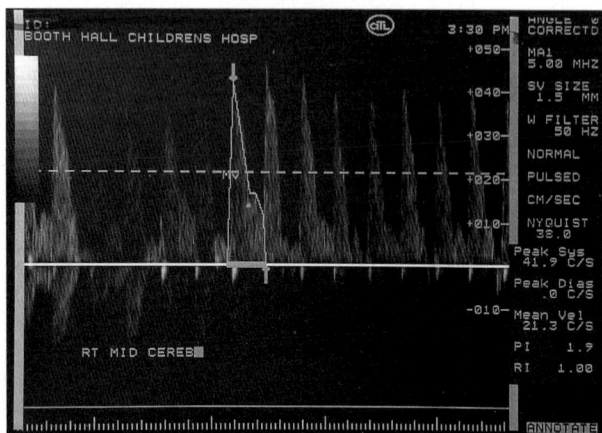

Fig. 22.14   Ultrasound demonstrating flow pattern in left middle cerebral artery with resistance index of 1.22.

chronic infection with shunt nephritis or unexplained rashes of a vasculitic nature due to complement activation from chronic septic emboli. Other chronic effects include right heart failure from pulmonary hypertension and bacterial endocarditis, thrombosis of the superior vena cava with superior vena caval syndrome arrhythmias and possible perforation of the myocardium. Most centers have now turned to the peritoneal route for drainage.

Ventriculoperitoneal shunts also have complications, and on at least one occasion shunt nephritis has been recorded (Table 22.8). More common is distal blockage due to pocketing of CSF from adhesions, preventing CSF spreading through the peritoneum. This may result eventually in pseudocyst formation. Other complications include penetration of the distal end into a viscus or through the gut wall and it has been known for ventriculoperitoneal (VP) shunts to appear per rectum. When infection of the shunt spreads distally, peritonitis may result.

Thecoperitoneal shunts or lumboperitoneal shunts remain useful in the context of benign intracranial hypertension and occasionally posthemorrhagic hydrocephalus. Lumboperitoneal shunt operations can be performed without laminectomy with associated complications.

Shunt and separate reservoir

Separate reservoirs have been used for acute surgical decompression since the early 1960s. They have been used to instil chemotherapeutic agents into the CNS in malignant disease and in the management of preterm intraventricular hemorrhage.

A number of centers use both a shunt and a separate CSF access device (reservoir), which is inserted into the frontal horn of the right lateral ventricle at the same time as the primary shunt surgery. A study to assess the risks attendant on this policy showed no extra mortality or morbidity.[43] The separate reservoir greatly eased the detection and management of raised intracranial pressure, shunt infection and ventriculitis. Children with shunts may have optic discs that become scarred and unreliable as indicators of raised intracranial pressure and frequently the presentation may be subtle with, for example, a decline in school performance. Since there are no absolutely reliable signs or symptoms of raised pressure, the only means of detection is by direct measurement of the intraventricular pressure, which is easy when the reservoir is present.

Many children with shunted hydrocephalus will still present with the usual childhood illnesses and infections and symptoms of these are often impossible to differentiate from those due to shunt malfunction. With the facility for intracranial monitoring via a reservoir, the presence of raised pressure or infection can be detected in a matter of minutes rather than with prolonged inpatient observation and repeated CT scanning, etc. In the Edinburgh study,[43] in 58% of admissions where a tap was thought necessary to exclude raised pressure or infection, normal values for both pressure and cell counts were obtained, thus avoiding the need for unnecessary emergency shunt surgery. If raised pressure is found, it can be lowered by CSF removal via the reservoir. If repeated taps do not effectively normalize the pressure, closed external ventricular drainage can be easily instituted via the reservoir, allowing replacement of the shunt by elective rather than emergency surgery.

The presence of a reservoir also has the advantage of an immediate diagnosis or exclusion of ventriculitis and therapy can be immediately instituted by direct instillation of the appropriate antibiotic into the ventricles, with monitoring of the CSF cell counts and antibiotic levels. With this method of management there is virtually no mortality from ventriculitis and one also expects a near zero infection rate from shunt and reservoir replacement (Table 22.8).

Shunt blockage

The Edinburgh series is shown in Table 22.9.[43] Survival analyses showed no significant relationship between the onset of mechanical blockage and the type of shunt, the age at reservoir insertion, the sex of the child, the etiology of hydrocephalus or the time relationship of the shunt insertion to reservoir insertion. The reduction in complications with the introduction of the reservoir may be due to the ability to measure directly the intracranial pressure and so reduce the number of unnecessary shunt revisions (Table 22.9).

Ventriculitis

Ventriculitis is diagnosed on the basis of a positive ventricular CSF culture with or without pleocytosis. Eighty percent of shunt infections will occur within 9 months of placement. Many factors influence the incidence of shunt infection, such as the length of operation, the skin preparation and the type of shunt, but infection remains a problem in a significant number of children with shunts. It can be difficult to diagnose and there is still controversy about the optimum management. Several different treatment regimens have been suggested, including vancomycin into the shunt and systemic therapy with oral trimethoprim and rifampicin. Others have advocated that infection can only be eradicated successfully by removal of the shunt.

It is our practice to subject the CSF to cytological techniques of cytocentrifugation and millipore filter collection. This improves the identification of cell types in the CSF. It is especially useful in cases of mild CSF pleocytosis. Routine biochemistry is also performed on the separated CSF specimen. The vast majority of episodes of ventriculitis are due to *Staphylococcus albus* with occasional cases of *Escherichia coli*, though any organism commonly found on the skin may be responsible including *Staphylococcus aureus* and streptococci. Neurosurgical intervention increases the number of cells in the CSF transiently but infection may occur in the early postoperative period so the need for accurate cell type identification is clear. Macrophages can persist in the CSF for a long time and these need to be distinguished from the mild persisting pleocytosis of active infection when there are equal numbers of neutrophils, lymphocytes and macrophages. Macrophages indicate that there is an active repair process going on. Intrathecal penicillin and cephalosporins can also produce a CSF pleocytosis, i.e. a chemical ventriculitis.

It is imperative that treatment is begun immediately. Intrathecal and intravenous vancomycin is now preferred to gentamicin, complemented by intravenous rifampicin. Where hypersensitivity or resistance is a problem teicoplanin or meropenem offer useful alternatives. Raised ventricular pressure is controlled. Occasionally there may be organisms present in the CSF which have not yet excited a cellular response, and very few cells are found. In only three episodes of ventriculitis, in our series, were there less than 100 cells/ml. Shunt infections may also be

Table 22.9 Incidence of shunt problems before and after reservoir insertion

Period	Number of episodes (episodes per child shunt year)			
	Serious shunt failure	Blockage	Infection	Ventriculitis
Pre-reservoir period 219 child shunt years	99 (0.45)	75 (0.29)	24 (0.11)	37 (0.17)
Post-reservoir period 269 child shunt years	77 (0.29)*	55 (0.20)*	22 (0.08) ns	28 (0.10) ns

Figures in brackets = per child shunt year.
* = P 0.01 cf. pre- and postreservoir periods.

associated with a negative organism culture. Because many of these children are highly shunt dependent, once the shunt is removed (which is necessary in ventriculitis because the organisms hide within mucoprotein colonies within the shunt tubing) it is imperative that their pressure is managed by tapping or draining CSF from the reservoir. It is also critical that shunt reinsertion is not done before the CSF is sterilized. When CSF infection occurs and a reservoir is not placed the shunt can be externalized. This allows intrathecal antibiotics to be administered and excess CSF to be drained. Subsequently the drain can be removed and the shunt re-inserted.

Slit ventricle syndrome

Effects of acute CSF decompression. This results in a low-pressure headache, delayed valve pump refilling, a depressed fontanel and possibly an upward brainstem cone (apnea, bradycardia, syncope, hypotension, stridor and hemiparesis).

Effects of chronic CSF decompression. These include acquired craniosynostosis, skull deformity, a thickened skull vault, microcephaly, hyperpneumatization of the sinuses, pneumocranium (tension), subdural hematoma, hygroma, cephalocranial disproportion, slit ventricle syndrome (total or partial ventricular collapse), enlarged cortical vascular bed, partial stripped ependymal lining, gliotic scar tissue (subependymal and white matter), wide open Virchow–Robin spaces and decreased intracranial compliance.

In children with normotensive hydrocephalus the normal ICP in the sitting position is negative and approximately −5 mmHg. Following a shunt insertion in the erect position, the pressures are approximately − 18 mmHg. Therefore, in most situations, with the child upright and mobile during the day, the pressures will be negative, but when supine and during REM sleep, there may be significant elevation of pressure. This has given rise to the concept of slit ventricles and the 'slit ventricle syndrome'. Our own studies suggest 10% have radiological slit ventricles, but only 1% were symptomatic.

The slit ventricle syndrome incorporates three components: intermittent or chronic headache secondary to episodic ventricular catheter obstruction; slit-like (Y shaped) ventricles on CT scan; and a slowed refill of the palpable valve mechanism.

The pathogenesis of the slit ventricle syndrome involves a siphon effect of continuing CSF flow down a shunt tubing (particularly with the ventriculoperitoneal route), excessive drainage from thecoperitoneal shunts in patients who are predominantly in the upright posture and the possibility that, with ventriculoatrial shunts, the diastolic phase of blood flow may encourage CSF withdrawal from the distal end of the shunt.

Several procedures have been devised to try and treat the slit ventricle syndrome. These include the use of high-pressure valves, an antisiphon device, a valve upgrade together with an antisiphon device, a subtemporal decompression, a volume-regulated shunt system, an antisiphon ventricular catheter (that is incorporated into the shunt) and lastly the use of steroids and the head-down position.

OTHER TREATMENTS
Choroid plexectomy
This operation reduces CSF production rate by about one third but often offered only temporary relief of symptoms and is no longer used.

Drug effects on CSF production
A number of drugs have been shown to have an effect on the rate of production of CSF, but it is unlikely that even with a substantial reduction in CSF this could be a definitive management for progressive hydrocephalus. However, there may be additional measures to help control CSF pressure in different situations, e.g. with the patient on external ventricular drainage due to ventriculitis. Furosemide and acetazolamide reduce CSF production by virtue of their carbonic anhydrase inhibitory effect. Acetazolamide, while it reduces CSF production, has only a transitory effect and isosorbide (a sorbitol derivative), which acts as an osmotic diuretic, is unpalatable and may produce hypernatremia and metabolic acidosis. For any acute rise in intracranial pressure associated with hydrocephalus, mannitol may reduce the pressure sufficiently to prevent coning. Other drugs with receptor sites on the choroid plexus may also reduce CSF production without diminishing overall choroidal perfusion.

Other procedures
Additional procedures include endoscopic third ventriculostomy – ETV – (the opening of the ventricular CSF system into the subarachnoid space via the lamina terminalis) and ventriculocisternostomy (Torkildsen shunt) between the ventricle and the basal cisterns. These are reliant on a block being present in the CSF outflow from the ventricles with an intact subarachnoid space and surface CSF pathways, with a normal reabsorptive capacity. In purely obstructive hydrocephalus, such as aqueduct stenosis, 70% require no further surgical intervention. Its use in other circumstances, and in particular those under 6 months of age, requires further study and definition.[47] Relative contraindications for an ETV are infants younger than 6-months-old, slit-like ventricles, very thin cortical mantle and communicating hydrocephalus. Nevertheless, some neurosurgeons advocate that it should be considered in all children presenting with hydrocephalus, including those who have previously been treated with a shunt.[48] Complication rates may be as high as 20% and include infection and neurological signs which may reflect pressure shifts, such as third nerve palsy or confusion. The rate seems to reflect the experience of the operator.[49] It is important to remember that previously effective ETV can block, giving rise to the same problems as a blocked shunt.

When there is ventriculitis, meningitis, blood in CSF or other factors making the insertion of a CSF shunt impracticable, then a temporary measure may be necessary, such as ventricular tap through the anterior fontanel. As previously mentioned, a puncture may result in porencephaly and it is preferable to have neurosurgical assistance and have a temporary reservoir implanted.

SPECIFIC TREATMENT REGIMENS
Posthemorrhagic hydrocephalus
This is common in premature infants following periventricular hemorrhage (PVH) but may occur in other age groups as well. Posthemorrhagic ventricular dilation in prematures may be assessed by serial ultrasound to compare the ventricular index (above) to the centiles for age. Approximately one third of infants with a PVH will develop posthemorrhagic ventricular dilation and one fifth of these will require a CSF shunt. Only about one in five cases of dilation are due to outlet obstruction at the fourth ventricle.

Distinguishing progressive hydrocephalus with high pressure, i.e. pressure-driven ventricular dilation, from brain atrophy in such circumstances requires ultrasound or imaging scans and pressure measurements. In atrophy the ventricles retain their usual configuration and do not have loss of the normal angles of the lateral ventricles.

There is no ideal or single method for managing posthemorrhagic hydrocephalus. Repeated lumbar punctures may prevent the need for shunting and will certainly ameliorate progressive ventricular dilation but the pressure should be measured at the same time with CSF removal to reduce the pressure level to normal. It is associated with an increased risk of infection[50] and it has been suggested that it be replaced with alternatives[51] such as early ventriculosubgaleal shunting.[52]

Acetazolamide in a dose 100 mg/kg per 24 h, and furosemide in a dose of 1 mg/kg per day have been shown to be ineffective in decreasing the rate of shunt placement.[53] Ventriculoperitoneal shunting is not done until the CSF hemorrhage has cleared sufficiently to avoid blocking the shunt. Brydon et al[54,55] indicate that it is cells that adversely affect shunt performance rather than CSF protein concentration.

The elective insertion of a ventricular reservoir will allow measurement and treatment of raised pressure by sequential taps. The hydrocephalus may arrest or the patient may subsequently need a ventriculoperitoneal shunt.

Tuberculous meningitis

Details of its presentation and management are given in the central nervous system infection section (see pp. 928–929). Ventricular dilation is uncommon in adults but is seen in nearly 80% of affected children. The immediate management includes CT or MRI scans and to attend to the raised ventricular pressure; the child may sustain serious sequelae, or die, as a result of untreated or unrecognized pressure. The emergency insertion of a ventriculostomy reservoir allows measurement of the ventricular pressure and decompression by CSF removal. A diagnostic lumbar puncture may then be carried out. Pressure is measured at the time of lumbar puncture and comparison can be made with the ventricular measurement to see whether there is any spinal block (Froin syndrome). CSF is then removed for cytocentrifuge cell count, protein, Ziehl–Nielsen, etc. in order to confirm the diagnosis of tuberculous meningitis.

The raised pressure, which may continue for many days, can be treated by intermittent taps of the reservoir, or by closed external ventricular drainage against a pressure head of 10 mmHg. Routine anti-tuberculous chemotherapy is commenced and both the infection and the pressure are monitored and treated carefully over the next 2 weeks. The use of intrathecal steroid preparations may be necessary if there is a spinal block or a basal adhesive arachnoiditis.

Early CSF shunting is an alternative way to control the pressure while treating the infection, but the shunt will need to be replaced if it becomes colonized and shunt dependence continues. Alternatively a temporary shunt may be sufficient to control the pressure while attempting to sterilize the CSF. Although earlier practice was routinely to carry out a lumbar puncture in suspected tuberculous meningitis (in most cases safely), there remains the possibility of coning at the time of diagnosis. These patients, and others who present in coma, must not have a lumbar puncture until a CT scan has been performed and the basal cisterns are seen to be patent.

Fetal hydrocephalus

See above under the 'Prenatal presentation of developmental brain abnormalities' (see p. 823).

Prognosis

Natural history of untreated hydrocephalus

Several studies detail the course of untreated hydrocephalus. An average result from these studies indicates that approximately 50% survive and of the survivors, 25–30% have normal intelligence and 25–30% have severe motor and other handicaps.

Epilepsy

Localized injury to the frontal cortex raises a theoretical risk of precipitating seizures from frontal reservoirs. Also with a reservoir there are two cortical insults. Seizure disorders follow in about one in six children compared with a one in two risk with the siting of a single VP shunt frontally.

Hemiplegia

Hemiplegia is the commonest type of cerebral palsy complicating hydrocephalus associated with spina bifida. This accounts for about 20% of children with congenital hemiplegic cerebral palsy. The hemiplegia in hydrocephalus may be due to the etiology (e.g. prematurity or meningitis) or may be a complication of the hydrocephalus as a result of parenchymal hemorrhage from brain puncture, traumatic puncture of the internal capsule, siting of the shunt to involve the motor strip, subdural hematomata as a result of overdrainage, cortical thrombophlebitis or basilar arachnoiditis or precipitation of status epilepticus with postconvulsive hemiplegia or puncture porencephaly. Occasionally also a mixture of corticospinal and cerebellar signs are seen giving a pattern of movement similar to that seen in the genetically determined ataxic diplegic cerebral palsies.

Vision

Blindness is not a problem of untreated hydrocephalus but sudden total blindness may result from raised pressure due to shunt malfunction. Gaston,[56] in studying a group of spina bifida children, found only 27% of 322 had normal visual function. In the Edinburgh study only one child ($n = 56$ over 12 years) had visual handicap which was of a severity for the child to be registered as blind and 88% had normal visual function. Visual impairment in children with hydrocephalus may result from optic atrophy secondary to chronic papilledema, distension of the third ventricle with chiasmal compression, posterior cerebral artery compression with ischemia of the optic radiation or calcarine cortex or selective posterior horn dilation leading to gross thinning of the calcarine cortex. These are all due to raised pressure with hydrocephalus.

Intelligence

Some 50–60% of shunted hydrocephalic children have normal IQs. In our study group 65% of children were in normal education, 29% were educated in special schools and 6% were in residential care for the severely handicapped. The pathophysiological mechanisms whereby learning is impaired include an associated cortical dysplasia, marked thinning of the cortical mantle (less than 15 mm), ventriculitis, chronically reduced cerebral perfusion pressure and coincidental parenchymatous brain damage (meningitis, asphyxia, etc.).

THE NEUROCUTANEOUS DISEASES

The last decade has seen important advances in the identification of the causes of the neurocutaneous syndromes. Neurofibromatosis 1 (NF1) and NF2 are two diseases caused by separate genes, while tuberous sclerosis (TSC) 1 and 2 is one disease caused by separate genes. Increasing involvement by parents and families, advances in neuroimaging and molecular genetics have all led to important advances in our understanding of these disorders.

NEUROFIBROMATOSIS 1

NF1 is the most common single gene disorder to affect the human nervous system with an estimated incidence of 1 in 3000.

Diagnostic criteria for NF1: Two or more of the following are required:

1. six or more café-au-lait spots (at least 1.5 cm post-puberty, at least 0.5 cm pre-puberty);
2. two or more neurofibromas or one or more plexiform neurofibromata;
3. axillary or inguinal freckling;
4. optic glioma;
5. two or more Lisch nodules (benign iris hamartomas);
6. osseous dysplasia on the sphenoid bone or cortex of a long bone;
7. a first degree relative with NF1.[57]

About a third of young people with NF1 have short stature and almost 50% have a head circumference at or above the 97th centile. NF1 is a multisystem disorder associated with a wide variety of complications. The most common are plexiform neurofibromas, learning disability, optic gliomas and scoliosis occurring in 15–50% of affected individuals. More than 50% of people with NF1 will be mildly affected and may not even know they carry the gene.

Plexiform neurofibromas occur in about 25% of individuals with NF1. They carry the potential for cosmetic disfigurement and malignant transformation often extending deeply into underlying tissues. Here they may cause compression or distortion of adjacent structures.

Specific learning difficulties are most common in NF1 with a frequency of between 30% and 60%. The frequency of global learning difficulties is only slightly higher than in the general population. There is no specific learning disability profile.

Optic nerve gliomas are the most common central nervous system tumors in NF1 occurring in up to 20% but only 30–50% will become symptomatic. They can involve any part of the visual pathway and take the form of low-grade pilocytic astrocytomas. All symptomatic tumors present before 6 years of age but rarely progress. Thus whereas formal ophthalmological assessment is indicated up to the age of 10 years, after this age annual routine clinical assessment of acuity and visual fields is sufficient.

Scoliosis occurs in up to 20% of those with NF1 and usually appears before the age of 10 years of age.

Neuroimaging features

Areas of increased signal intensity on T2-weighted images with magnetic resonance imaging occur in 60–70% of children. They have been referred to as UBOs (unidentified bright objects). They generally disappear during late teenage years or the early 20s.

The genetics of NF1

This is an autosomal dominant disorder although 50% of cases are sporadic. The NF1 gene has been mapped to chromosome 17 and codes the protein neurofibromin. This has a high sequence homology with GAP (GTPase) activator protein. These proteins have an important role in cell growth and differentiation. The genetics of the disorder are dealt with in more detail in Chapter 14.

NEUROFIBROMATOSIS 2 (NF2)

The diagnosis is based on the following criteria:[57]
1. Bilateral VIII nerve masses detected on neuroimaging.
2. A first degree relative with NF2 and either unilateral VIII nerve mass or two of the following:
   neurofibroma;
   meningioma;
   glioma;
   schwannoma;
   juvenile posterior subcapsular lenticular opacity.

NF2 usually presents in adult life, though many childhood cases have been described. Presentation is usually a result of tumors causing progressive loss of hearing, difficulty with walking, loss of sight or chronic pain.

NF2 should be suspected in children presenting with any of the tumors listed above and fewer than six café-au-lait patches.[58] It is unusual for children with NF2 to present with features other than those due to a tumor.

The genetics of NF2

NF2 is very rare with a birth incidence of 1 in 40 000. It shows autosomal dominant transmission with nearly full penetrance. The NF2 gene maps to the long arm of chromosome 22 and codes a member of the protein 4.1 family of cytoskeletal associated elements. For further details see Chapter 14.

Subtle skin tumors often characterized by small well conscribed lesions found on the trunk or face, which after adolescence become roughened with overlying coarse hair, are a clue to the disorder, along with the lenticular opacities.

TUBEROUS SCLEROSIS COMPLEX

Diagnostic criteria for tuberous sclerosis complex (TSC) have been proposed.[59]

Major features:
1. facial or forehead plaque;
2. nontraumatic ungual or periungual fibroma;
3. hypomelanotic macules (more than three);
4. shagreen patch (connective tissue nevus);
5. multiple retinal nodular hamartoma;
6. cortical tuber;
7. subependymal nodule;
8. subependymal giant cell astrocytoma;
9. cardiac rhabdomyoma, single or multiple;

10. lymphangiomyomatosis;
11. renal angiomyolipoma.

Minor features:
1. multiple randomly distributed pits in dental enamel;
2. hamartomatous rectal polyps;
3. bone cyst;
4. cerebral white matter radial migration lines;
5. gingival fibromas;
6. nonrenal hamartoma;
7. retinal achromic patch;
8. 'confetti' skin lesions;
9. multiple renal cysts.

Definite TCS Either two major features or one major feature plus two minor features.

Probable TCS One major plus one minor feature.

Possible TCS Either one major feature or two minor features.

Clinical presentation

Seizures are by far the most common neurological condition in TSC, occurring at some point in up to 90% of young people with the disorder. Infantile spasms occur in about one third. The earlier the onset of seizures, the greater the risk of them being intractable and being associated with cognitive and behavioral impairments. If seizures present after the age of 2 years then attendant learning difficulties may be mild or absent.

The antiepileptic drug vigabatrin is noted to be particularly efficacious in tuberous sclerosis. The risk of associated retinopathy always needs to be considered carefully when this drug is used. As in all children where the epilepsy is intractable the question of the use of surgery for epilepsy needs to be considered. Multifocal lesions are not an absolute contraindication.

Learning difficulties are commonly (probably up to 40%) found in TSC. There is also a strong association between TSC and autism, particularly as an outcome of infantile spasms. Early reported associations between autism and temporal lobe lesions or a high number of tubers seem not to have been borne out.

It is the skin lesions, hypomelanotic (ash leaves) macules, periungual or gingival fibromas and thickened firm areas of subcutaneous tissue often on the lower back (shagreen patch) or forehead and face (fibrous plaques), which offer the most ready diagnostic clue. Adenoma sebaceum does not occur until late childhood or early adolescence. It is an angiofibroma (cutaneous hamartoma) (Figs 22.15, 22.16) which initially appears as flat reddish macular lesions, which become increasingly erythematous. Papular nodules over the bridge of the nose and higher cheek (in a butterfly distribution), often noted in the presence of examination of a child with epilepsy, bring the disorder to the attention of clinicians. MRI usually then confirms the diagnosis by revealing tubers, subependymal nodules or subependymal giant cell astrocytomas. CT scanning is less sensitive and often fails to identify tubers. Subependymal calcification is often not present until the second year of life. In the first year of life ultrasound of the heart will reveal cardiac rhabdomyomas in up to 60% with TCS. Put the other way round any child with a rhabdomyoma in infancy is likely to have TSC. They later regress but occasionally may be the presenting feature due to obstructive cardiomyopathy.

Angiomyolipomas and renal cysts occur in 45–50% of people with TCS. Renal disease is uncommon in childhood except in cases of polycystic disease. Pulmonary involvement is seen exclusively in adult women where cysts or lymphangioliomyomatosis may be associated with respiratory symptoms and hypertension.

Managing people with TS

The management of attendant epilepsy and learning difficulties is discussed in the relevant sections. In relation to problems, which are specific for TSC, it has been recommended that neuroimaging be carried out, perhaps 2-yearly, to check for the growth of subependymal giant cell astrocytomas. The cost effectiveness of the screening examinations

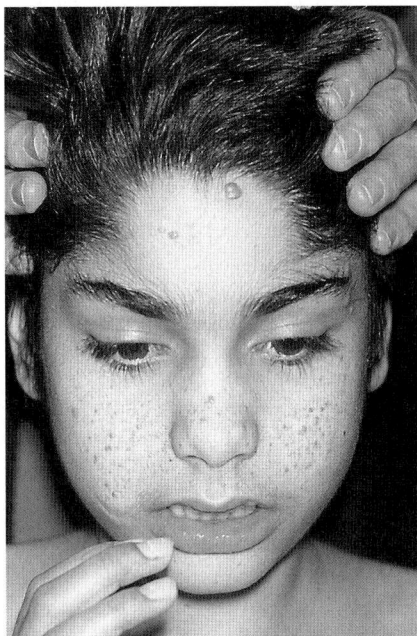

Fig. 22.15 Tuberous sclerosis: adenoma sebaceum.

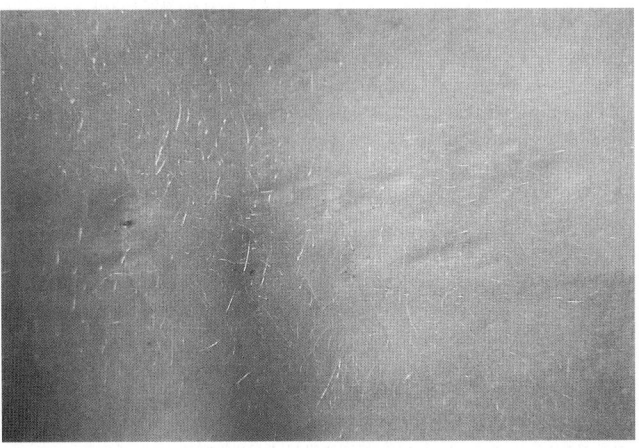

(a)

(b)

Fig. 22.16 Tuberous sclerosis: (a) shagreen patch; (b) depigmented patches.

is not clearly known. Our own policy is to respond to the assessment of new symptoms if they present.

Renal ultrasound needs to be carried out on presentation and then every 2–3 years to assess changes in angiomyolipomas or cysts, hopefully to allow operative intervention before the development of renal failure. An ECG is useful at presentation to screen for the presence of potentially life threatening cardiac arrhythmias.

The genetics of TCS

This is an autosomal dominant condition with a high spontaneous mutation rate. Gene loci for TSC have been identified on chromosome 9q34 (TSC1) and on chromosome 16p13 (TSC2). The TSC1 product is hamartin which may act as a tumor suppressor. TSC2 encodes for tuberin, which has GTPase activating properties and also seems to function as a tumor suppressor. Hamartin and tuberin cooperate to regulate cellular growth and differentiation. The genetics of TSC will be dealt with in more detail in Chapter 14.

ATAXIA TELANGIECTASIA

This is a rare autosomal recessive disorder with an incidence between 1 in 40 and 300 000.

Presentation

The main neurological feature is the ataxia. Children often learn to walk at a normal age, but throughout the toddler years appear to be clumsy. Then, often after entering school, the clumsiness becomes more evident and leads to referral. They have a wide based gait but often demonstrate excessive adduction of the leg during the passing phase on foot strike causing a stagger to the outside of the base. They may choose a toe-walking gait and prefer to run everywhere rather than walk. More typical features of cerebellar ataxia then ensue often superimposed by choreiform movements, the latter being a variable feature.

Very often children lose the ability to walk independently between the ages of 8 years and about 12 years. Similarly after the age of 5 there is a deterioration of speech, the pattern of which carries the features of cerebellar dysfunction. Bulbar function then becomes increasingly involved raising the risk of aspiration. This often, in due course, leads to the requirement for gastrostomy feeding.

Children with the condition also demonstrate an oculomotor dyspraxia. This involves no problem with vertical eye movement, but when trying to follow an object through the horizontal plane the head is moved quickly to follow the object leaving the eyes behind, the latter then restituting on the object once it has stopped moving. This leads to a characteristic flick of the head that is readily perceived.

Around the age of 10 years an axonal polyneuropathy appears with loss of the deep tendon reflexes.

The associated telangiectasia are often evident across the top of the shoulders, on the ears and on the conjunctiva. They tend to become more obvious as children get older.

Premature aging features often appear in people as they move through the teenage years and early adult life with the appearance of gray hairs and aging of the skin with diminution of subcutaneous tissue. Vitiligo may also appear along with hyperpigmented areas.

Up to 80% of children with the condition will have diminished levels of IgA and IgG 2 (less frequently IgE and IgM). They have a diminished cell-mediated response to intradermal antigens and atrophy of the thymus. Infections of the sinuses and lungs are common with bacterial pneumonia being the major cause of death.

The problem with immunity is also associated with malignancy, tending to lymphoreticular disorders in childhood and solid tumors in adult life.

Genetics of ataxia telangiectasia (AT)

The gene known as ataxia telangiectasia mutated (ATM) gene is found at chromosome location 11q22–23. ATM-deficient cells lack sensors (check-point proteins) of double stranded DNA breaks, which would normally suppress the mitotic cycle pending repair. Cell division therefore proceeds and is likely to be directly responsible for the frequent chromosomal rearrangements seen in AT cells.

Diagnostic criteria

The clinical diagnosis is usually straightforward due to the constellation and characteristic features including the oculomotor dyspraxia and deteriorating cerebellar signs. With the identification of the ATM gene a new molecular standard of diagnosis is available. The finding of an elevated alpha-fetoprotein (at least twice the upper limit) along with reduced immunoglobulin levels in the presence of the typical neurological picture, substantiates the case for requesting the genetic study. The gene test has now replaced chromosome fragility studies.

Some children with AT present, before neurological signs have appeared, with acute lymphoblastic leukemia. If these children have an oculomotor dyspraxia then a careful search of the skin ought to be made for the telangiectasis and the ATM gene analyzed.

OTHER DNA REPAIR DISORDERS

Xeroderma pigmentosum

This is also a DNA repair disorder with autosomal recessive inheritance. Its cardinal feature is acute sun sensitivity, often leading in infancy to erythematous and bullous skin lesions. Freckles and hypopigmentation are common, along with dryness, telangiectasis and, at times, skin atrophy. Ectoderm around the eye also shows light sensitivity and may lead to blepharitis, iritis or conjunctivitis with keratitis and edema of the cornea, occasionally leading to ulceration and opacification. Susceptibility to skin neoplasia is very high, and all affected young people should have their eyes and skin inspected weekly for new lesions.

About 20% have associated neurological problems (a much higher percentage in Japan) and, in its severest form, microcephaly, progressive dementia, choreoathetosis, ataxia and spasticity are seen, along with a progressive peripheral neuropathy. Sensorineural deafness may also be progressive. Genetic testing is available with eight mutations in different genes identified to date.

Management is by way of reducing exposure to ultraviolet light as much as possible and the aggressive early treatment of skin cancer.

Cockayne syndrome

This autosomal recessive condition leads to small stature, severe sun sensitivity, ocular, skeletal and neurological abnormalities. The most common findings are optic atrophy, pigmentary retinal degeneration, cataracts, sensorineural deafness and an extrapyramidal movement disorder, in addition to spasticity of the lower extremities with flexion contractures.

At birth, babies are of normal size but significant feeding difficulties and subsequent growth failure leads them to become progressively cachetic. At this time they acquire a distinctive facial appearance with a thin prominent nose and zygomatic processes, prognathism, enophthalmos and absent fat. This appearance is usually well developed by the teens, and neurological abnormalities largely resemble those of xeroderma pigmentosum, which may well exist in some young people. Many young people die in their teens in status epilepticus or with malignant hypertension, or renal and pulmonary dysfunction. Cultured skin fibroblasts lack the ability to form colonies when subjected to UV irradiation and assays are available in specialist laboratories. Mutational analysis of the gene associated with Cockayne syndrome is available on a research basis only.

Incontinentia pigmenti

As this condition predominantly affects girls, it is thought to be an X-linked dominant condition, probably lethal in males in utero. The central nervous system is involved in 30–50%. A cerebral dysgenesis leads to delayed development with seizures, spastic paralysis and cerebellar signs in some. The degree of learning difficulty varies greatly. Associated with this there may be a retinal dysplasia leading to a retrolental mass and skeletal and teeth abnormalities.

The skin abnormality is seen in three distinct stages. In the first 2 weeks of life erythematous, macular, papular, vesicular, bullous or pustular lesions occur proximally in a linear distribution. This is in association with an eosinophilia. In the following 2–3 weeks pustular, lichenoid, verrucous, keratotic and dyskeratotic lesions occur more distally and as they resolve, often leave areas of atrophied skin. In the third stage, areas of pigmentation appear over a period of some weeks.

OTHER NEUROCUTANEOUS SYNDROMES

Sturge–Weber syndrome

This is a sporadic condition involving a malformation of cephalic-venous microvasculature. There is an abnormality in the growth of the primordial vascular plexus in cephalic mesenchyme as it lies between the epidermis and the telencephalic vesicles in close proximity to the optic cup. This leads in its fullest form to a cavernous angioma of the leptomeninges, a facial angiomatous nevus and a choroidal angioma of the eye. The lesion may be unilateral or bilateral and in individual children may affect one or all of brain, eye or skin tissue. The lack of cerebral or ocular symptoms does not preclude them developing at a later date where the facial nevus is present. Sturge–Weber syndrome is not usually applied when neither cerebral nor ocular symptoms have appeared.

The port wine-colored stain on the face is evident at birth and always involves the first division of the trigeminal nerve. Involvement of the skin on that side may be more widespread and there is an association in some with the Klippel–Trenauney syndrome. This syndrome involves angiomatous skin nevi in association with bony hypertrophy, lymphangiomas or varicosities; the genetics are not defined.

In Sturge–Weber syndrome a bilateral facial nevus does not necessarily imply bilateral cerebral involvement. Seizures are seen in up to 90% of those with Sturge–Weber. Abnormal venous return with blood stagnation and hypoxemia coupled with a high metabolic demand of neurones exhibiting seizure activity often lead to a progressive atrophy. Neurological signs emerge, often starting as a postictal paresis contralateral to the cerebral involvement but at times consolidating into a permanent paresis as time goes on. Hemianopias, dysphasias or quadriparesis may also occur. Where the seizures are intractable and infrequent there are very often associated learning difficulties.

Buphthalmos or glaucoma may accompany a choroidal angiomatous lesion and may be present at birth. Rarely, hydrocephalus has been reported but intracranial hemorrhage is exceptionally rare.

In the presence of a facial nevus full radiological assessment of the brain should be carried out to define the extent of any brain lesion. This can be with CT with contrast. MRI is, however, more sensitive. Intracerebral angioma may become more obvious with the passing of time. Calcification of the lesion becomes prominent. Management involves regular assessment of ocular pressure. Seizure control is difficult to attain at times. Where the vascular anomalies and seizure discharge are confined to one hemisphere, an early surgical resection of the lesion may offer benefit. The evidence shows that residual handicap is minimized when lobectomy or hemispherectomy is performed in the early weeks with many children surviving with little sign of a hemiparesis or hemianopia. However, exact criteria for this early intervention have yet to be established, as there are some children in whom a seizure disorder presenting at an early stage stabilizes.

Hypomelanosis of Ito

In some families, this is an autosomal dominant disorder, but in most there is no clear family history. Chromosomal abnormalities including balanced translocation have been described in at least two children. The skin lesion is of linear vorticose or irregular areas of hypopigmentation. These may affect one or both sides of the body and be associated with lesions of the iris or hemihypertrophy.

The central nervous system is affected in at least 50%. Those with seizures in the first year of life are most likely to have a static encephalopathy associated with significant learning difficulties.

The pathology of both skin and brain is very reminiscent of that seen in tuberous sclerosis, neurofibromatosis and in incontinentia pigmenti. They are considered the nonspecific result of a dysplasia or embryopathy affecting the central nervous system and the skin. At about 15 weeks' gestation the melanoblasts migrate from the neural crest and mature to melanocytes in the skin. In the sixth month, the hair anlage is present, accounting for an association between abnormalities of cerebral cortex and hair. The number, size and pigment content of melanocytes in the basal area of the epidermis is generally reduced and in the brain the signs are of a neuronal migration defect, with microcephaly and a rostral displacement.

Linear sebaceous nevus syndrome

In its complete form, this syndrome includes a cutaneous nevus, with neurological and ocular abnormalities. The skin lesion may be of several types. The typical Jadassohn nevus may be visible at birth or in infancy, or become evident only after a few years. It is a slightly raised, yellow-orange, smooth, linear plaque that abuts the midline of the forehead, nose or lips and often involves the scalp. Over years, the lesion tends to become darker and verrucous. Early in life there is little pigment, and sebaceous glands are often not prominent. Later, sebaceous glands proliferate throughout the thickness of the skin.

Neurological manifestations consist mainly of learning disability, seizures and asymmetrical macrocephaly. Seizures are often partial, but infantile spasms have been reported. Hamartomatous tumors may be present and various other abnormalities have been seen including porencephaly arterial aneurysms, abnormal venous return and arachnoid cysts along with hemihypertrophy.

The most common eye abnormalities are dermoids or epidermoids of the conjunctiva and colobomas of the iris, choroid, retina or optic nerve.

The diagnosis may be difficult in early cases without visible nevus. Imaging reveals hypertrophy of one hemisphere, usually on the same side as the nevus, with enlargement of the ipsilateral ventricle and pachygyria with hypodense white matter.

SEIZURES, EPILEPSY AND OTHER PAROXYSMAL DISORDERS

INTRODUCTION

A seizure is any sudden clinical event which is nonspecific in etiology and is a result of a neurological or non-neurological disturbance. However, the term is often used synonymously with epileptic seizure, defined as any clinical event arising as a result of epileptic activity of neurones in the brain. Epileptic activity involves the excessive and/or hypersynchronous electrical discharge of neurones, which, for practical purposes, are located within the cerebral cortex. Epilepsy is the tendency to have recurrent epileptic seizures. The term 'fit' is a lay term whose meaning is almost synonymous with epileptic seizure. A convulsion is any seizure (not necessarily epileptic) characterized by excessive, abnormal muscle contractions, which are usually bilateral. Epileptology abounds with terms many of which, though still used, are now obsolete; included are 'grand mal' (big attack) and 'petit mal' (little attack).

The basic mechanisms which underlie seizure generation are incompletely understood, but involve abnormalities at the cell membrane level (ion channels and receptors) and in neuronal circuits. The electrical behavior of neurones is determined by ion channels in the neuronal membrane, which are either voltage-gated or receptor (ligand)-gated. Voltage-gated ion channels determine the excitability of neurones as well as participating in the release of neurotransmitters. They are membrane-spanning proteins with a pore through which the ion can pass. A voltage sensor controls the opening of the pore and a selectivity sensor determines which type of ion can pass through the pore. Three main classes of voltage-gated ion channels have been described: Na^+, Ca^{2+} and K^+. Sodium currents are involved in the generation of action potentials. Potassium currents cause hyperpolarization and hence

stabilize the neuronal membrane. Both calcium and sodium currents are involved in the generation of burst discharges, generated by certain classes of neurones when excited. They consist of a burst of action potentials produced as an all-or-nothing phenomenon. It is likely that burst discharges and other similar phenomena are important in the generation of some types of seizures. Ligand-gated ion channels are activated by the binding of a neurotransmitter to the ion channel's receptor. Gamma-aminobutyric acid (GABA) and glycine are inhibitory neurotransmitters while glutamate and aspartate are excitatory neurotransmitters. A useful, though simplistic model of epilepsy is that it involves an imbalance of excitatory and inhibitory neurotransmitter systems within the CNS.

Ion channel abnormalities (channelopathies) cause many epilepsies, particularly idiopathic epilepsies. For example, mutations in a neuronal nicotinic acetylcholine receptor have been shown to be associated with familial nocturnal frontal lobe epilepsy, in a potassium channel with benign familial neonatal seizures, and in a sodium channel with generalized epilepsy with febrile seizures and severe myoclonic epilepsy of infancy.[60-63] Many antiepileptic drugs block voltage-gated ion channels. These include carbamazepine and phenytoin, both of which block sodium channels. Other antiepileptic drugs act either at ligand-gated ion channels or else interfere with the production, release, function or catabolism of neurotransmitters. For example, benzodiazepines and barbiturates bind to specific domains on subtypes of the GABA receptor and vigabatrin increases GABA inhibition by preventing the breakdown of GABA at synaptic clefts.[64]

Epileptic seizures involve groups of neurones interacting together abnormally. Neurones within the brain work within physiologically and anatomically defined circuits. Some of these are important in particular types of epilepsy. They include neocortical circuits involved in, for example, frontal and occipital lobe seizures, the limbic system, involved in mesial temporal lobe seizures and thalamocortical circuits involved in generalized epilepsies, particularly absence seizures.

The neocortex comprises six distinct layers. Function occurs within vertically arranged columns. However, there are abundant excitatory horizontal connections. It is thought that it is these connections which allow the rapid seizure propagation, which is a feature of many neocortical epilepsies. Moreover, the neocortex contains intrinsically bursting pyramidal cells, which may be involved in seizure initiation.

At least in adults, mesial temporal lobe epilepsy is the commonest cause of drug-resistant seizures. The mesial temporal lobe structures, including the hippocampus and amygdala, are part of the limbic system. Groups of neurones within parts of the limbic system have relatively low thresholds for seizure generation. Again, this may relate in part to neurones with intrinsic bursting activity and may be augmented by loss of particular classes of neurones caused, for example, by prolonged febrile convulsions. Intimate connections within the limbic system allow seizures to propagate and determine the semiology of mesial temporal lobe seizures.

The thalami have rich connections to the cerebral cortex. Intrinsic membrane properties of thalamic neurones arising as a result of so-called low threshold calcium channels, cause it to generate low frequency oscillatory rhythms which appear to underlie both certain physiological phenomena and also pathological ones such as the 3 Hz spike–wave discharge seen in idiopathic generalized epilepsies. These consist of a spike caused by action potentials in both thalami and cortex followed by an after coming slow wave due to prolonged inhibition within the cortex.

EPIDEMIOLOGY AND NATURAL HISTORY

Epilepsy is the commonest serious neurological condition of childhood. However, it is not a single condition, but comprises many different conditions. Epidemiological studies are bedevilled with problems of subject inclusion. Rates vary according to whether neonatal, febrile and single seizures are included and according to how 'active epilepsy' is defined.[65]

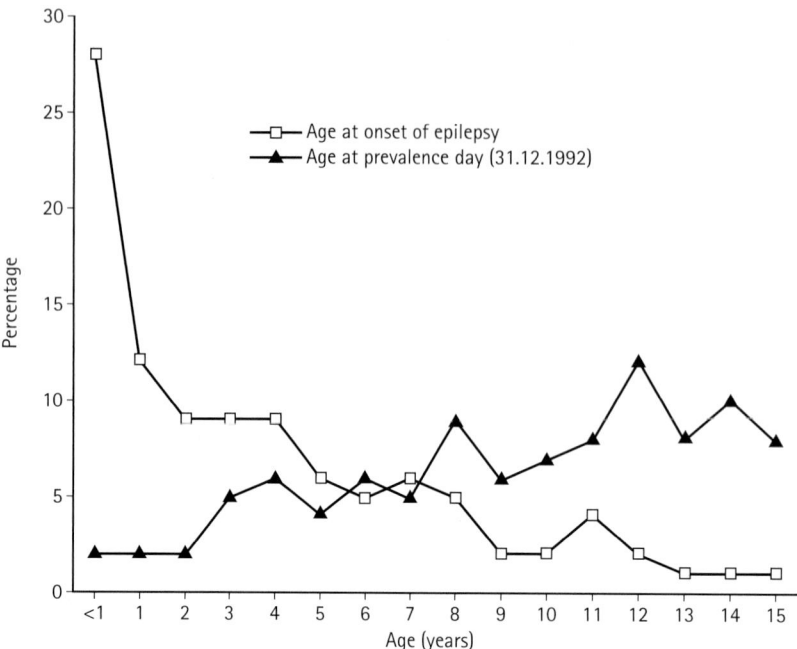

Fig. 22.17   Age specific incidence and prevalence of epilepsy in children. (From Eriksson & Koivikko 1997,[73] reprinted by permission of the journal *Epilepsia*.)

A metanalysis of incidence studies found a median incidence of epilepsy in children (excluding neonates) of 82.2/100000.[66] Rates are lower in resource rich countries compared to resource limited countries. The incidence varies markedly with age (Fig. 22.17).[67] In Europe and North America rates fall from about 150/100000 in the first year of life to around 60/100000 at ages 5–9 years and 45–50/1000000 in older children. Most studies report slightly higher rates in boys. The point prevalence of epilepsy in children is 3–6/1000.[68] Cumulative incidence rates are much higher than annual incidence rates. During childhood, prevalence rates for active epilepsy increase but not as fast as cumulative incidence rates, reflecting the effect of remission (Fig. 22.18). The British National Child Development Study reported cumulative incidence rates for epilepsy of 4, 5, 7 and 8 per 1000 at ages 7, 11, 16 and 23 years respectively and prevalence rates of 4, 4, 5 and 6 per 1000 at the same ages.[69] The lifetime prevalence of nonfebrile seizures is between 1.5% and 5% of the population.[65] In other words, up to 5% of people will have at least one nonfebrile seizure at some point in their life.

Recent data suggest that the incidence of epilepsy is falling in children but rising in the elderly. This may relate to improved standards of pre- and postnatal medical care, to better standards of maternal and child health and to the rise in life expectancy in the elderly coupled with more cerebrovascular disease. Although age-specific incidence and prevalence rates for epilepsy are higher in children than in adults (excluding extreme old age), the rates for treated epilepsy may be higher in adults than in children.[67] The incidence of epilepsy may be increased in those who are socially deprived[70] but the data is conflicting.[71,72] Epidemiological studies in both adults and children, which have taken particular care to classify seizure type, have suggested that focal epilepsies are more common than generalized epilepsies. In the British National Child Development Study after 23 years follow-up about 70% of those whose seizures were classifiable had focal epilepsies and 30% had generalized epilepsy; around 45% of both were symptomatic or probably symptomatic. The type of epilepsy could not be determined in around a fifth of subjects.[69] A number of recent studies have given information on the epidemiology of specific epilepsy syndromes in children.[73–76]

The previous view that epilepsy is a chronic disorder with little prospect of remission was mistaken. The majority of children who have a seizure have a good prognosis both in terms of the likelihood of seizure recurrence and of obtaining remission should recurrent seizures (i.e.

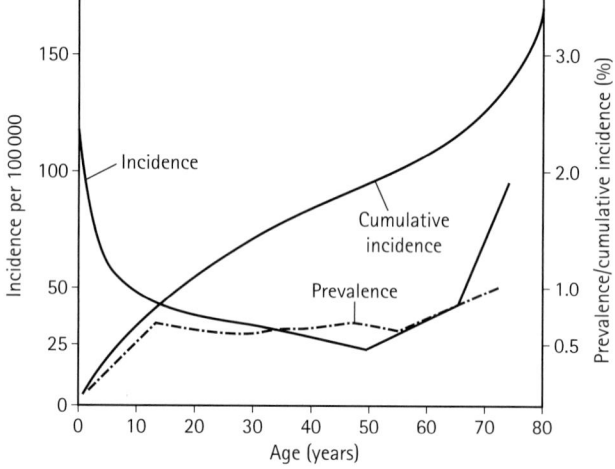

Fig. 22.18   Incidence, prevalence and cumulative incidence rates for epilepsy in an American population. (From Shorvon 1996,[255] reprinted by permission of the journal *Epilepsia*.)

epilepsy) develop. The risk of a further seizure is greatest immediately after the first and declines thereafter. Forty-five percent of children who have a single seizure have a recurrence within 5 years, and once there has been one recurrent seizure further seizures become likely. The risk of having a third after a second, and a fourth after a third seizure at 5 years is 71% and 81% respectively.[77] Etiology is the main determinant of the risk of recurrence.[77–81]

Once epileptic seizures are recurrent, an important issue is the probability of early remission. In a large prospective study 57% of children, 2 years after a diagnosis of epilepsy, had a 'good outcome' (a remission which had lasted more than 12 months), 12% had a 'fair outcome' (a remission which had lasted 6–12 months) and 31% had a 'poor outcome' (a remission which had lasted less than 6 months).[82] Another study reported that at 2 years after diagnosis of epilepsy 53% of children had a 'good outcome' (a remission of more than a year), 8% had a 'bad outcome' (two or more antiepileptic drug failures and at least one seizure per month over an 18-month period) and 38% had an 'intermediate outcome'.[83] In about 80% of children who were followed for 4 or more years the outcome was similar to that at 2 years. However, around half of those with an intermediate outcome at 2 years achieved remission and 8% became intractable. Factors which are associated with the likelihood of a poor outcome include young age at seizure onset, symptomatic etiology, an initial presentation with status epilepticus or infantile spasms and high initial seizure number.[77,78,80]

Information on the long term prognosis of children with epilepsy is provided by the British National General Practice Study of Epilepsy.[84] In this study 86% of children of all ages, with a diagnosis of definite epilepsy, achieved a 3-year remission and 68% a 5-year remission, after 9 years. 'Remission' referred to a remission at any stage in the 3- or 5-year period. The proportions achieving a terminal remission (i.e. seizure free at the end of the follow-up period) of 3 and 5 years were 68% and 54% respectively, indicating that some children with prolonged remission subsequently relapsed. A very long prospective follow-up study of childhood-onset epilepsy found that after a mean of 37 years follow-up 67% were in terminal remission, on or off medication. Overall about a half of children with epilepsy entered terminal remission without relapse and a further fifth did so after a relapse. One third had persistent seizures either without ever having had a remission or after a remission.[85,86] Long-term outcome studies have shown that epilepsy has adverse social outcomes whether or not the epilepsy is symptomatic and whether or not remission is achieved.[85,87] However, the outlook is considerably better in those with idiopathic seizures who achieve remission. Children with idiopathic epilepsies are reported, as adults, to have similar socioeconomic and/or employment status compared to matched controls without epilepsy, but they are less likely to marry.

The standardized mortality ratio of people with epilepsy (children and adults) is two to three times that of the general population.[88] Causes of death in children with epilepsy include accidents, status epilepticus and occasionally idiosyncratic reactions to drugs. As they enter teenage and adult years, suicide becomes increasingly important. Finally seizure-related death (death during or shortly after a seizure when there is no evidence of status epilepticus or when no other explanation for death is found at autopsy) and sudden unexpected death in epilepsy (SUDEP) (a nontraumatic, unwitnessed death occurring in a child with epilepsy who had previously been relatively healthy and for whom no cause of death is found even after postmortem examination) have been the subject of recent interest. By definition, the cause of such deaths is unknown. However, at least some may be caused by seizure-related cardiac arrhythmias. A population-based study of SUDEP found an incidence of 0.27 per 1000 person-years in those under 14 years of age.[89]

The question as to whether antiepileptic drug treatment affects the prognosis for epilepsy (in terms of eventual remission of seizures) has perplexed clinicians and scientists. Although there are theoretical arguments why it might do, there is no evidence that it does.[78,90,91] Antiepileptic drugs may be used to suppress distressing symptoms, but not in the expectation that they are likely to change the natural history of the condition, at least in the large majority of children. Possible exceptions to this are some of the epileptic encephalopathies.

INVESTIGATIONS
EEG and magnetencephalography
Introduction
The EEG is the single most useful investigation in children with seizure disorders. However, it is frequently misused, overinterpreted and, because many clinicians are unaware of its full potential, underutilized.

The EEG gives a visual representation of differences in electrical potential between different areas of the brain. These reflect underlying neuronal activity. Most EEGs are recorded from the scalp using an array of 20 electrodes, although smaller numbers are sometimes used, particularly in young children. The EEG does not record the absolute potential at a particular electrode. Rather differences in potential between

consecutive pairs of electrodes may be recorded (bipolar recordings) or else differences in potential between each electrode may be compared to a common reference electrode (referential recording). The EEG was traditionally recorded on paper, with the potential at each electrode used to cause a deflection of a marker pen. The sequence of electrodes displayed on the EEG trace is called the montage. In any one paper recording, a number of different montages using both bipolar and referential recordings are used in order to best detect normal and abnormal EEG features originating from different parts of the brain. Today most EEGs are recorded digitally and displayed on VDU screens. Other than storage considerations, the advantage of digital recording is that once the data are recorded, computerized reformating and manipulations enable far more information to be obtained than was possible on paper systems. It is, for example, possible to display the same data in numerous different bipolar and referential montages, filters can be added or taken away to remove artefacts which obscure the underlying EEG and EEG features can be precisely timed.

Interictal EEG
Most EEGs are recorded between seizures (interictal recording). A standard interictal EEG is usually recorded for 10–60 min. The EEG trace can be analyzed in terms of ongoing or background activity and episodic or paroxysmal activity. For both, normal and abnormal patterns occur. The background activity includes various physiological rhythms, including the well-known alpha rhythm. It is dramatically different in the premature neonate compared with the mature adult. In general, the EEG becomes increasingly synchronized and physiological rhythms become faster with maturity. The background EEG also changes with the level of arousal. For example, as an older child passes from alert to drowsy to light and then to deep sleep, a drop out in the alpha rhythm occurs, followed by progressive slowing.

Paroxysmal EEG activity is any activity which stands out from the background. There are numerous physiological paroxysmal EEG features which, like background features, are age and state dependent.

Most EEGs also contain artefact, which is not caused by electrical activity of the brain. Some artefacts relate to physiological functions such as eye, head and breathing movements and the electrical activity of the heart. Muscle artefact, which is in effect an EMG recording, is also common. Extraneous artefacts may be caused by poor electrode contact, by the mains electrical source and by nearby electrical equipment. Some artefacts can be very difficult to distinguish from cerebral activity.

Abnormalities of the EEG background are usually rather nonspecific and of limited value when investigating children with seizure disorders. Focal background abnormalities, generally with slowing, reduction in amplitude and loss of physiological rhythms may reflect focal brain abnormalities giving rise to seizures, such as brain tumors, infarcts and abscesses. However, all are better diagnosed by neuroimaging. In children whose epilepsy is part of a static or progressive encephalopathy diffuse slowing and attenuation of the background EEG is expected.

Of most use in the investigation of children with seizure disorders is the detection of abnormal paroxysmal activity. Abnormal paroxysmal activity on interictal EEG can be divided into two broad categories: epileptiform and non-epileptiform abnormalities. Epileptiform abnormalities are those which have an association with the occurrence of epileptic seizures. In addition to being paroxysmal they are also usually abrupt and short-lived giving rise to spikes and sharp waves. Interictal spikes and waves are often followed by slow waves (paroxysmal EEG abnormalities which are of longer duration and blunter), constituting spike–wave complexes.

The nonspecialist is often confused by reports of EEG abnormalities. These are often all incorrectly considered to support or even confirm a diagnosis of epilepsy. Common mistakes are:

- The assumption that focal, paroxysmal, slow wave activity supports the diagnosis of epilepsy. This is a nonspecific finding, occurring frequently in normal children, especially younger children and if the child is drowsy. It can be a postictal phenomenon but this is a relatively rare cause.

- The assumption that all spikes and sharp waves are epileptiform. Although the spike and, to a lesser extent, sharp wave, are considered the paradigm epileptiform abnormality, there are some 'physiological' spike and sharp wave paroxysmal EEG features.
- The assumption that the detection of epileptiform paroxysmal abnormalities necessarily implies that the child has seizures. Some such abnormalities, though more frequent in people with epilepsy than in the general population, are more frequently seen in people with cerebral disease but without seizures. Others have a strong association with epilepsy. They also occur in small numbers of people with other disorders and without seizures. For example, occipital spikes are common in blind people and centrotemporal spikes occur in some children with cerebral palsy and in boys with fragile X syndrome. Finally, a small number of normal children who have never had and never will have a seizure have epileptiform EEG abnormalities.

Certain EEG abnormalities can be activated by physiological maneuvers. These include sleep, hyperventilation and photic stimulation. Sleep (especially light sleep) is a powerful activator of many EEG abnormalities and if an awake recording is unhelpful it is usually worth obtaining a sleep recording. This can be achieved using natural sleep, following partial sleep deprivation or by drug-induced sedation. When sleep is induced by drugs it should be remembered that these may influence the EEG beyond causing sleep. Benzodiazepines and barbiturates often cause excessive fast activity and suppress many EEG abnormalities; they are therefore best avoided. Major tranquilizers such as chlorpromazine can decrease seizure threshold and may activate EEG abnormalities through mechanisms other than by sleep induction. Chloral hydrate and melatonin appear not to have significant effects on the EEG. The recording should be continued while the person is awakening as this may also provoke epileptiform abnormalities.

Hyperventilation, which should be included in the protocol for standard EEG recordings, is of particular use in investigating subjects with idiopathic generalized epilepsies in whom it frequently activates generalized spike–wave discharges. Apparently 'subclinical' discharges can often be shown to be associated with transient cognitive impairment if combined with breath counting during hyperventilation. Other epileptiform abnormalities are less reliably activated by hyperventilation. Hyperventilation often causes bilaterally synchronous slow wave activity in normal children. This physiological response must not be misinterpreted as indicating the likelihood of a seizure disorder.

Photic stimulation should also routinely be applied during standard EEG recordings. 'Photic-driving' or 'following' is a normal response and the 'photomyoclonic response' is a non-epileptiform abnormality often seen in anxious subjects. Photoparoxysmal responses are epileptiform abnormalities in which spikes and/or spike–wave discharges are produced by intermittent photic stimulation (Fig. 22.19). They are usually generalized but can be confined to the occipital regions. Generalized photoconvulsive responses are most often seen in subjects with idiopathic generalized epilepsies but occur in a variety of other epilepsies and rarely in normal children. Occipital photoconvulsive responses are occasionally seen in subjects with occipital lobe seizures.

Ictal EEG

During routine EEG recordings it is rare to record a seizure. An exception to this is in children with typical absences, which often occur during recordings, especially during hyperventilation. Ictal records usually require prolonged recording (24 hours or more) and even then are only likely to be obtained if seizures are frequent. Two types of prolonged EEG are commonly employed. Ambulatory cassette EEG usually records eight channels of EEG using a cassette recorder. The EEG is later analyzed at high speed on a VDU screen with events electronically marked by the child or witness analyzed in detail. Video-EEG telemetry involves the subject staying in hospital while a 20-lead EEG is recorded, usually digitally, with simultaneous time-locked video recording. Again the whole record

can be viewed at high speed with events analyzed in detail. Prolonged recordings are useful to:

- Help decide if paroxysmal clinical events are epileptic.
- Localize the onset of focal seizures. This is usually done as part of a presurgical workup in refractory epilepsy and requires video telemetry rather than a cassette recording.
- Establish the frequency of seizures and interictal epileptiform discharges. This may be useful if a child with epilepsy is performing less well at school than expected and it is considered that this might reflect under-recognized seizure activity.

Special techniques

The sensitivity of EEG recordings can be increased by using additional electrodes. Foramen ovale and sphenoidal electrodes are semi-invasive electrodes used to increase the detection of temporal lobe discharges. They are rarely used in children, in whom cheek electrodes have been suggested as an alternative. Invasive EEG recordings, with recording directly from the surface of the brain (subdural recordings) or from within the substance of the brain (intracerebral recordings), are used in a minority of children undergoing presurgical evaluation. They are employed to precisely localize the onset of seizures and are available only in specialized centers.

Polygraphic recordings, in which a number of physiological variables such as ECG, chest and abdominal wall movements, airflow at the nose and esophageal pH are recorded simultaneously with the EEG, and often video, are particularly useful in investigating children with recurrent apnea and life-threatening events, including Munchausen syndrome by proxy. It should be noted that all EEG recordings should routinely include an ECG lead and if subtle myoclonus is suspected an EMG lead may be useful.

Using the EEG in clinical practice

The EEG is used for six principal purposes:

- to help establish the likely diagnosis of epilepsy;
- to help establish the type of epilepsy;
- to help identify possible precipitants to epileptic seizures;
- to investigate the cause of cognitive decline;
- to help localize the onset of focal seizures;
- to monitor treatment, including the timing of drug withdrawal.

The usefulness of any investigation in helping to establish a diagnosis depends on its sensitivity and specificity. Between 2.2% and 3.5% of normal children have interictal epileptiform abnormalities while, in children with infrequent seizures, the yield of interictal epileptiform EEG abnormalities on initial EEG is probably under 30%.[92] Over-reliance on interictal EEG for diagnosing epilepsy leads to frequent misdiagnoses. The clinical utility of recording interictal epileptiform discharges is exponentially related to the strength of the clinical suspicion of epilepsy.[93]

Some children with epilepsy have persistently normal interictal EEGs. This is often because the epileptiform discharges are infrequent and likely to be missed during a 30–60 min recording. Increasing the length and/or number of recordings or activating discharges, for example, by obtaining a sleep recording will increase the yield in these children. However, in some children, interictal abnormalities may be highly localized and/or attenuated by the dura, skull and scalp and therefore not detected by the standard array of electrodes used with a surface EEG. Many areas of the cortex, including the basal frontal and medial temporal regions, are not directly accessible to scalp recordings and therefore only discharges which propagate will be detected. Obtaining an ictal recording may be the best strategy here. Antiepileptic drug treatment can affect the yield of EEG recordings.[94] Barbiturates and benzodiazepines are reported to reduce the abundance of epileptiform abnormalities and drugs effective in controlling typical absence seizures are likely to reduce epileptiform abnormalities in absence epilepsies. Drugs effective against photosensitive seizures reduce the likelihood of detecting photosensitivity on intermittent photic stimulation. Most antiepileptic drugs have little effect on the EEG of children with focal epilepsies.

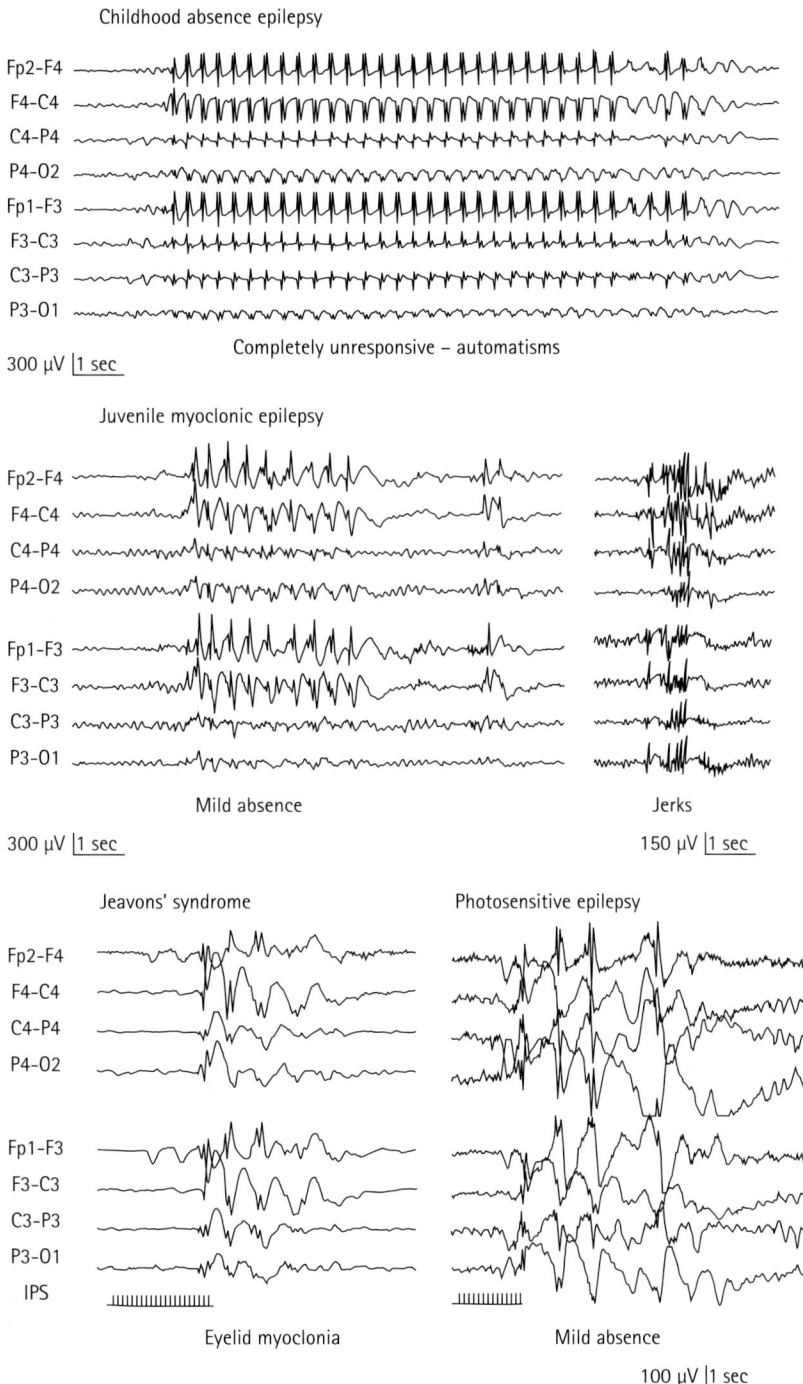

Childhood absence epilepsy

Completely unresponsive – automatisms

300 μV | 1 sec

Juvenile myoclonic epilepsy

Mild absence

Jerks

300 μV | 1 sec

150 μV | 1 sec

Jeavons' syndrome

Photosensitive epilepsy

Eyelid myoclonia

Mild absence

100 μV | 1 sec

Fig. 22.19 Samples of video-EEG in some idiopathic generalized epilepsies of childhood. **Top:** Childhood absence epilepsy, a regular spike–wave discharge at 3 Hz is associated with complete unresponsiveness and automatisms. **Middle:** Juvenile myoclonic epilepsy. Left: An irregular and brief spike and polyspike discharge is associated with mild impairment of cognition. Right: A brief multiple spike discharge associates with myoclonic jerks without absence. **Bottom:** Response to intermittent photic stimulation. Left: A generalized discharge of irregular spike and wave is associated with marked eyelid myoclonia in eyelid myoclonia with absences (Jeavon syndrome). Right: A similar generalized discharge is associated with a mild absence in another child with idiopathic generalized epilepsy and photosensitivity. (With thanks to CP Panayiotopoulos.)

It is unusual for an ictal EEG recording not to show epileptiform activity. However, it may fail to clarify whether a paroxysmal attack is epileptic or not because of obscuration by artefact. Moreover, focal seizures in which there is no disturbance of consciousness (simple focal seizures) often show no EEG changes because of the highly localized nature of the discharges. This is less common in focal seizures in which there is impairment of consciousness (complex focal seizures) but may occur, particularly when the origin is frontal.[95]

In routine clinical practice the EEG is at its most useful in helping to classify the type of epilepsy. Generalized epilepsies and focal epilepsies are commonly associated with generalized and focal interictal epileptiform discharges respectively. However this is not absolute, and in young children in particular, focal epilepsies are not infrequently associated with apparently generalized discharges. In idiopathic epilepsies the background is expected to be normal. Focal background abnormalities are frequent in symptomatic focal epilepsies. Generalized background abnormalities are suggestive of symptomatic generalized epilepsies and epileptic encephalopathies. Finally many more-or-less specific EEG abnormalities have been described for specific epilepsy syndromes (Figs 22.19–22.21). These will be described when the relevant syndrome is discussed.

A small minority of people with epilepsy have specific seizure precipitants. This is exemplified by photosensitive epilepsies, the evaluation of which is greatly aided by photic stimulation. In children in whom other precipitants appear important the recording conditions of the EEG can often be modified to investigate a particular precipitant's role.

Occasionally children with epilepsy show a stagnation or decline in their cognitive performance. The EEG can be useful in investigating the possible role of epileptiform activity in causing this. In some children, especially those with idiopathic generalized epilepsies, frequent interictal and subtle ictal discharges are responsible and can be detected on prolonged EEG recordings, preferably with simultaneous video record-

ing. In others, electrical status during slow wave sleep may be responsible for cognitive problems and this possibility should be investigated by a sleep recording. Finally, some children with apparent cognitive decline are in nonconvulsive status epilepticus. This is usually obvious on a standard EEG.

The EEG has an important role in the localization of the site of onset of focal seizures. However, it is important to remember its limitations. If ictal or interictal discharges originate from areas of the cortex 'hidden' to the scalp EEG, any associated EEG abnormalities will reflect discharge propagation rather than site of origin. Additionally, some discharges rapidly spread giving rise to bilateral EEG abnormalities. Finally, interictal epileptiform abnormalities may originate from sites remote from those giving rise to habitual seizures. For example, in mesial temporal lobe epilepsy it is common to find independent bilateral interictal discharges in people whose seizures all originate from one side.

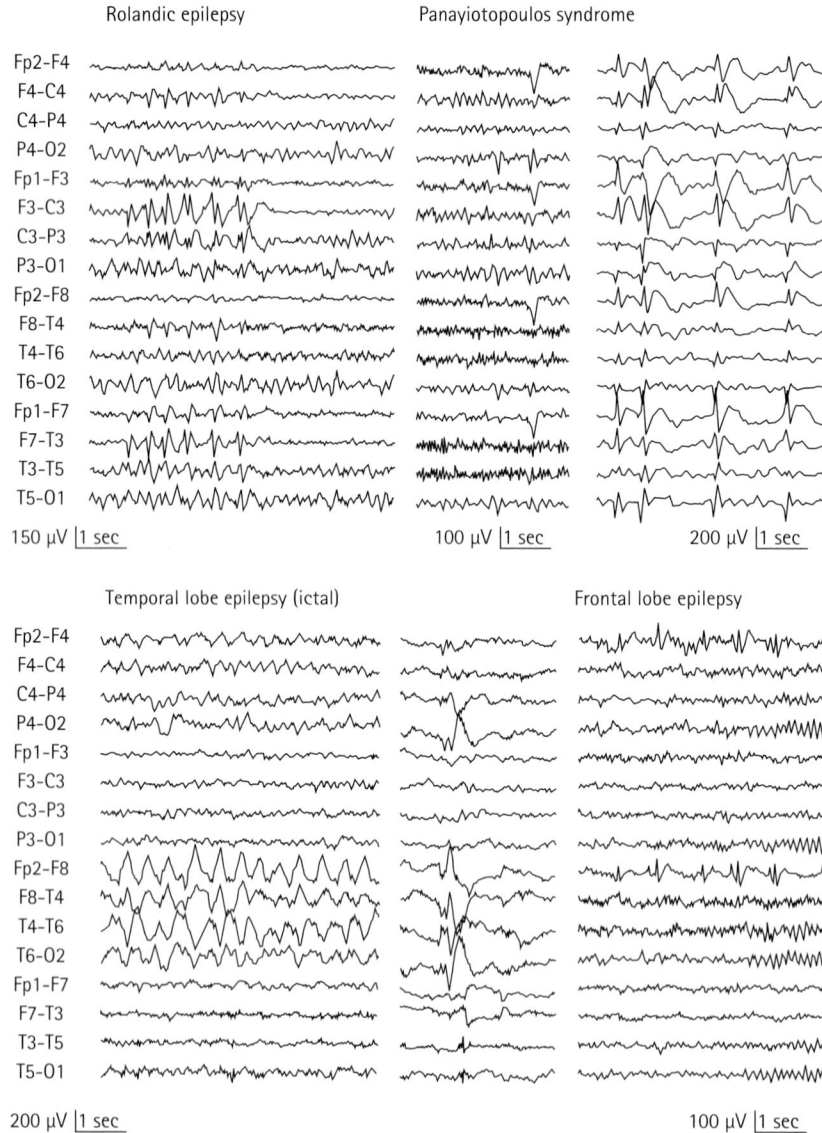

Fig. 22.20 EEGs in some focal epilepsies of childhood. **Top:** Benign childhood epilepsies. Left: Benign childhood epilepsy with centrotemporal spikes (Rolandic epilepsy) – focal high amplitude spike–wave discharges occur mainly in the left centrotemporal regions. These are typical of the EEG abnormalities expected in this syndrome. Some independent sharp waves are also seen in the posterior regions. These are less typical of the syndrome but nevertheless common. Middle and Right: EEG of two different children with Panayiotopoulos syndrome. Despite similar lengthy seizure typical of the syndrome, EEG shows occipital spikes in the first (middle) and cloned-like repetitive multifocal spike–wave complexes, which are mainly frontal in the other (left).
Bottom: Focal symptomatic epilepsies. Left and middle: Temporal lobe seizure of a child with right hippocampal sclerosis. High amplitude rhythmic slow wave activity over the right hemisphere occurred during the seizure; the child complained of 'tummy ache and panic' (left). High amplitude sharp and slow waves in the same regions persisted postictally (middle). Right: Frontal lobe epilepsy. Frequent spike and slow wave complexes are strictly localized in the right frontal regions. (With thanks to CP Panayiotopoulos.)

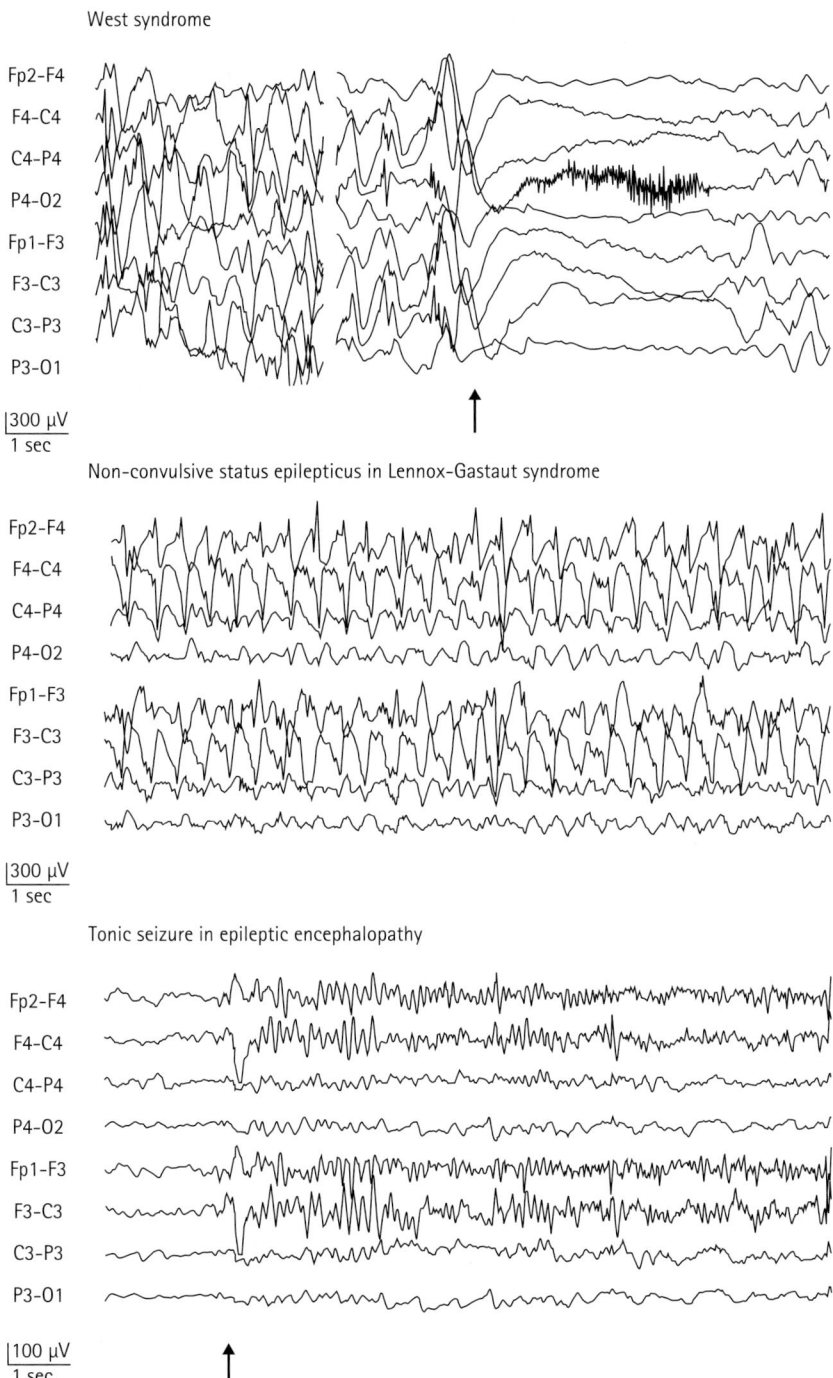

Fig. 22.21 The EEGs in some epileptic encephalopathies of childhood. **Top:** West syndrome showing typical hypsarrhythmia – the arrow indicates the onset of an epileptic spasm. This is accompanied by a high amplitude slow wave followed by flattening of the EEG (an electrodecremental response). **Middle:** Nonconvulsive status epilepticus in Lennox–Gastaut syndrome showing continuous slow spike and wave. **Bottom:** A tonic seizure in Lennox–Gastaut syndrome – the onset of the seizure (arrow) is accompanied by a generalized discharge of spikes (fast spike discharge). (With thanks to CP Panayiotopoulos.)

Intuitively, it would seem likely that the EEG could help predict the likelihood of recurrence after an initial seizure and the prognosis for seizure recurrence after drug withdrawal. Studies have confirmed that this is the case.[92] However, a lack of sensitivity means that, clinically, its role in this regard is limited. The type of epilepsy, including the syndromic diagnosis, is probably a more useful guide. Illustrative examples may be helpful. In benign childhood epilepsy, with centrotemporal spikes, the abundance of interictal discharges varies markedly between EEGs done in the same child. Moreover, they often persist long after clinical remission of seizures has occurred. It would be inappropriate to use the EEG to predict how frequent seizures were likely to be or to help decide when to withdraw antiepileptic drug medication. On the other hand a child with an idiopathic generalized epilepsy whose EEG continues to show frequent spike–wave discharges and a positive response to photic stimulation, despite clinical remission of seizures, would have a high chance of relapse and the EEG result might reasonably help in the decision to continue antiepileptic drug medication.

Magnetencephalography (MEG)

MEG is the newest technique used in the investigation of children with seizure disorders.[96] It is completely non-invasive but requires a degree of cooperation from the child. It is based on the principle that all electric currents, including those produced by neurones, generate a magnetic field, which if large enough can be detected externally using an array of up to 300 sensors distributed over the head. It can be used to localize epileptic activity and when superimposed on MRI (magnetic source imaging) has better spatial resolution than surface EEG. It can also be used to map eloquent cortex during pre-surgical evaluation.

Neuroimaging

For the majority of children with seizure disorders, MRI is the only brain imaging method of importance. Skull X-rays are only now indicated if a child presents with a seizure following a head injury in order to detect skull fractures. The main role of CT is also in the acute situation, in which its ability, unlike MRI, to detect skull fractures, its superior ability to detect fresh blood, and its ready availability, makes it the imaging method of choice when an unwell child presents with seizures of obscure origin. CT may also be useful in young children with seizures in whom neuroimaging is indicated to exclude, for example, space-occupying lesions, but in whom MRI would require a general anesthetic. The reassurance of a normal CT may reasonably enable the clinician to delay obtaining an MRI until this can be obtained without anesthetic. Cranial ultrasound is a useful imaging method in the neonatal period. However, its limitations must be appreciated. In particular it will miss many important lesions encountered in children with seizures.

MRI (Fig. 22.22) enables the following conditions associated with epilepsy to be detected:

- Brain malformations and maldevelopments such as agenesis of the corpus callosum, septo-optic dysplasia, holoprosencephaly, hemimegalencephaly, abnormalities of cortical development and lesions associated with neurocutaneous disorders including tuberous sclerosis and Sturge–Weber syndrome.
- Vascular disorders such as arteriovenous malformations.
- Areas of sclerosis and gliosis associated with old infarcts, hypoxic–ischemic insults and infection.
- Tumors, including low grade gliomas and dysembryoplastic neuroepithelial tumors.

There is an almost limitless number of potential MRI sequences. Close liaison between the clinician and radiologist is essential in order to ensure the most appropriate ones are obtained in an individual child. There are many excellent reviews on the role of MRI in the investigation of children with epilepsy.[97,98] Most brain malformations and maldevelopments comprise 'normal' brain tissue arranged abnormally and are best detected with sequences which give good anatomical definition, such as T1-weighted images. On the other hand 'foreign' tissue including tumors and gliotic tissue is usually best detected with T2-weighted images. The contrast agent gadolinium is rarely helpful and is not indicated as a routine. However, it can be helpful in conditions associated with breakdown in the blood–brain barrier, such as some tumors and vascular malformations. Proton density and fluid attenuated inversion recovery (FLAIR) sequences give improved contrast between brain lesions and CSF.

Detection of mesial temporal sclerosis, the pathological substrate underlying mesial temporal lobe epilepsy, deserves special mention (Fig. 22.22). It is usually not detected with 'standard' T1- and T2-weighted axial images. The important features are decreased volume (atrophy) and increased signal on T2-weighted and FLAIR sequences in the hippocampus and/or amygdala often with dilation of the temporal horn. Its detection requires thin heavily T1-weighted and T2-weighted coronal images taken orthogonal to the long axis of the temporal lobe. More specialist techniques, which may improve detection further but which are not widely available, include T2 relaxometry and volumetric analysis.

An important question for the clinician is which children with epilepsy require neuroimaging. One reasonable approach is to image all children with focal epilepsies except those with a pattern of epilepsy which corresponds clinically and on EEG with the syndrome of benign epilepsy of childhood with centrotemporal spikes. Children with features of one of the idiopathic generalized epilepsies do not require imaging provided they respond as expected to appropriate medication. Another approach is to image children only if there are interictal neurological signs, or if seizures do not come under complete control after the first line antiepileptic drug.

Currently, functional brain imaging's role in the investigation of childhood epilepsy is confined to those in whom epilepsy surgery is being considered. During seizures, seizure foci are metabolically more active and require an increased blood flow. Between seizures, they are often less metabolically active and require less blood. In positron emission tomography (PET) a positron emitting ligand is injected into the subject and is then distributed around the body. In epilepsy studies, the ligand is usually [18]fluorodeoxyglucose (FDG), which is an analog of glucose. FDG enters the glycolytic pathway but cannot proceed beyond the initial steps. It therefore accumulates within tissues, the accumulation being proportional to the metabolic activity of the tissue. The rate of positron emission is detected by the PET scanner. FDG PET is, for a variety of reasons, unsuitable for ictal studies; the vast majority of FDG PET studies are interictal with the aim of detecting focal areas of hypometabolism. Single photon emission tomography (SPECT) is based upon the emission of photons from radioligands. These can be detected using conventional gamma cameras. In epilepsy studies, ^{99m}Tc-hexamethyl-propyleneamine (HMPAO) is the most widely used radioligand. Its distribution around the body reflects blood flow. The main advantage of SPECT over PET is its wider availability, as it utilizes commercially prepared radioligands and conventional gamma cameras which are available in all nuclear medicine departments. In addition, the pharmacokinetics of the distribution of HMPAO make it suitable for injection ictally. Unfortunately interictal SPECT has proved relatively insensitive in the detection of surgical foci and has largely been abandoned. Interictal PET and ictal SPECT appear to have similar sensitivities for the detection of temporal and extratemporal epileptic foci. The reader is referred to recent reviews for more details on these methods.[99-103]

In older children who can undergo MRI without anesthetic or sedation, functional MRI is increasingly used to map eloquent cortex, lateralize language dominance and localize epileptic foci before epilepsy surgery.

Other investigations

Most children with seizure disorders require no investigations other than EEG and structural brain imaging. However, there are children in whom seizures dominate the clinical picture but who have other features which suggest the possibility of an underlying genetic, metabolic or degenerative condition. These include:

- Early onset of refractory seizures in the neonatal or early postnatal period.
- Stormy onset of seizures in the previously well child.
- Occurrence of seizures in children with mental retardation of unknown cause (suggesting the possibility of a genetic or chromosomal disorder).
- Occurrence of seizures in children with dysmorphic features (suggesting genetic and chromosomal disorders; peroxisomal disorders and the carbohydrate-deficient glycoprotein syndrome are also associated with dysmorphism).
- Occurrence of seizures in children with episodes of unexplained drowsiness or confusion (suggesting the possibility of an amino or organic acid disorder, a urea cycle defect or a mitochondrial disorder).
- Occurrence of seizures in children with neurological abnormalities on examination; ataxia should particularly raise suspicion (many degenerative disorders can produce this picture).

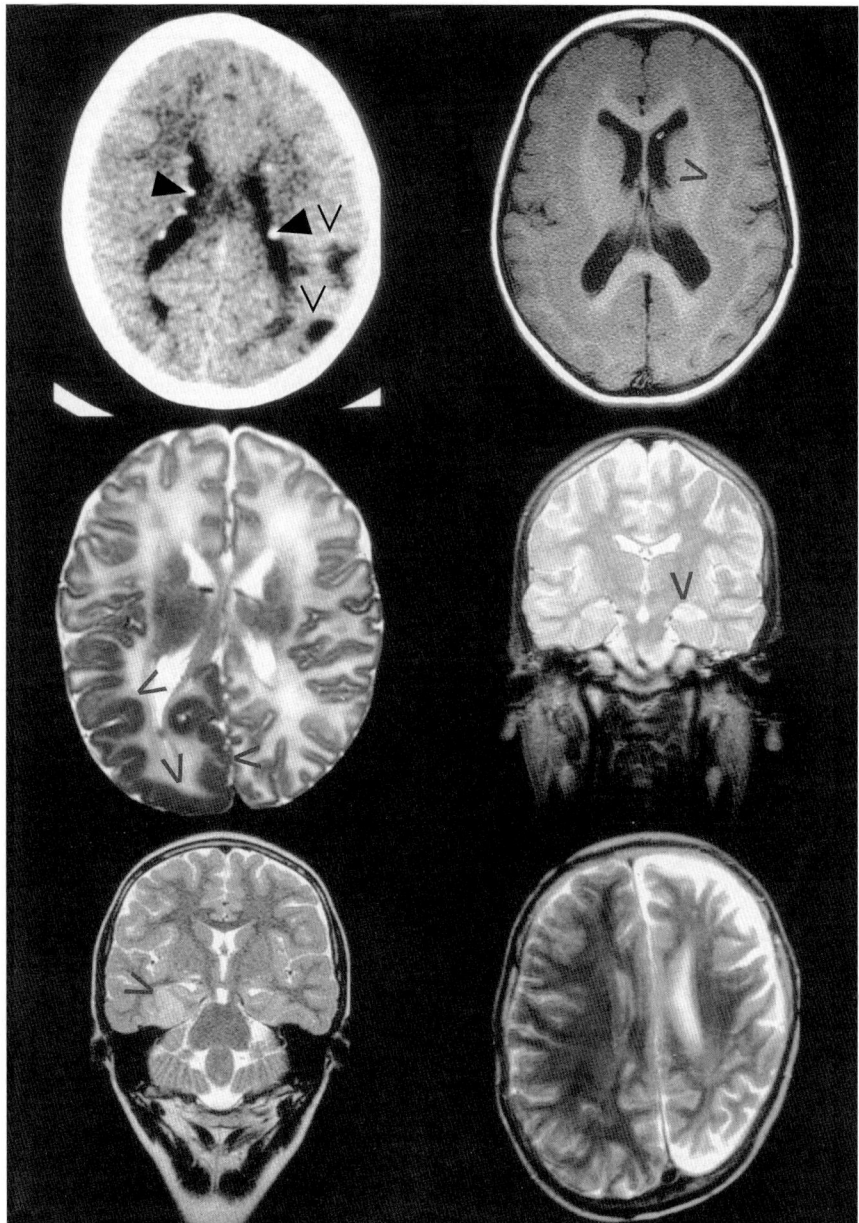

Fig. 22.22   Neuroimaging in some symptomatic childhood epilepsies. **Top left:** Nonenhanced CT showing calcified subependymal nodules (arrowheads) and multiple cortical tubers manifested as low attenuation areas (open arrows). **Top right:** T1-weighted axial MRI image showing subcortical band heterotopia ('double cortex') (arrow). **Middle left:** T2-weighted axial MRI image showing extensive right-sided temporoparieto-occipital polymicrogyria (arrows). The child presented with very frequent occipital seizures and episodes of focal status epilepticus. All seizures ceased following a right temporoparieto-occipital resection. **Middle right:** T2-weighted coronal MRI image showing left mesial temporal sclerosis (arrow). The hippocampus is shrunken and of high signal and there is associated dilation of the temporal horn. **Bottom left:** T2-weighted coronal image showing a right-sided dysembryoplastic neuroepithelial tumor in the right mesial temporal lobe (arrow). The tumor is cortical and of moderately high signal. **Bottom right:** T2-weighted image of a child with hemiconvulsion-hemiplegia-epilepsy syndrome (HHE syndrome) following haemophilus meningitis. There is left hemiatrophy. (With thanks to JH Livingston and S Yeung.)

- Occurrence of seizures in children in whom there is a documented loss of skills, including visual skills (suggesting the possibility of degenerative disorders; the ceroid lipofuscinoses are particularly important to consider in children).
- Occurrence of seizures in children in whom there is evidence of dysfunction in systems outwith the CNS (suggesting mitochondrial disorders in particular).

The investigation of many of these disorders is best undertaken by a pediatric neurologist in conjunction with a metabolic pediatrician and clinical geneticist. However, the general pediatrician will not wish to miss potentially treatable conditions and should understand the rationale for the various investigations performed (Table 22.10).

A genetic etiology is present in about 40% of subjects with epilepsy.[104] The 'genetic epilepsies' include: chromosomal disorders; Mendelian epilepsies;[105] and 'complex epilepsies' in which the interaction of several genetic loci together with environmental factors are thought to lead to the epilepsy phenotype. The first two of these probably account for only about 1% of all epilepsies – hence genetic tests do not currently play a significant role, although this may change.

Seizures are a prominent feature of many chromosomal disorders[106] and therefore chromosomal analysis should be a routine part of the investigation of children in whom seizures are accompanied by learning difficulties and/or dysmorphic features. In addition, there are many

Table 22.10   Investigations useful in children with seizure disorders in whom neurometabolic conditions are suspected

Disorder	Available tests	Comment
Biotinidase deficiency	Plasma biotinidase	Treatable; worth excluding in all refractory childhood epilepsies
Amino acid disorders	Plasma and urine amino acids	Wide range of phenotypes. Worth performing in all children with early onset seizures and in all children in whom seizures are associated with mental retardation or loss of skills
Organic acidurias	Plasma organic acids	Worth performing in all children in whom seizures occur in association with intermittent vomiting and/or lethargy
Peroxisomal disorders	Very long chain fatty acids and phytanic acid	Consider especially in children with 'Zellweger' facies, mental retardation and profound hypotonia
Carbohydrate-deficient glycoprotein syndromes	Transferrin electrophoresis	Wide, incompletely described phenotype. Characteristic dysmorphic features
Menke disease	Serum copper and ceruloplasmin levels	Consider in boys with neonatal and early postnatal seizures
Folate and B_{12} disorders	Plasma and urine amino acids, urine organic acids, blood and CSF folate	Extremely rare; present in infancy
Molybdenum cofactor deficiency	Plasma urate level (low) and urinary sulfite excretion on dipstick test	Extremely rare
Purine and pyrimidine disorders	Urine purine and pyrimidine studies	Extremely rare
Creatine deficiency syndrome	Consistently low plasma creatinine levels	Extremely rare
Mitochondrial disorders	Plasma and CSF lactate levels	Huge variation in clinical phenotype. Suspect when there is evidence of multisystem disease
Storage disorders	White cell enzymes. Specific enzyme assays for the ceroid lipofuscinoses	The main disorders which can present primarily as an epilepsy are the sialidoses, type 3 Gaucher disease and the ceroid lipofuscinoses
Glucose transporter protein deficiency	Paired CSF and blood glucose levels	Extremely rare
Pyridoxine dependency and deficiency	Trial of oral or intravenous vitamin B_6 (pyridoxine)	Consider in neonates and younger children with intractable seizures

other genetic syndromes in whom seizures are prominent and which can now be diagnosed with molecular DNA techniques. These include fragile X syndrome, Wolf–Hirschhorn syndrome, Angelman syndrome, Miller–Dieker syndrome, Smith–Magenis syndrome, Pallister–Killian syndrome and Rett syndrome. There are now a number of disorders of cortical malformation associated with epilepsy caused by specific gene mutations.[107–109] These include X-linked periventricular nodular heterotopia (FLN1 gene), lissencephaly-pachygyria and subcortical band heterotopia (LIS1 or DCX genes), lissencephaly with cerebellar hypoplasia (RELN gene), X-linked lissencephaly (ARX gene) and various patterns of polymicrogyria. Finally, mutations have been described in a number of ion channel genes, mostly giving rise to rare autosomal dominant epilepsies. Diagnostic testing is currently only available for most of these on an ad hoc basis. However, mutations on the sodium channel SCN1A have been described in families and sporadic cases with a number of epilepsy phenotypes, including generalized epilepsy with febrile seizures plus (GEFS+) and Dravet syndrome. Commercial diagnostic testing is becoming available.

CLASSIFICATION

Classification profoundly affects our approach to medical disorders. In the past it was common to confuse classification of epileptic seizure types (i.e. symptoms) with types of epilepsy (i.e. syndromes and diseases). A major advance in the last few decades has been the widespread acceptance of classification schemes for both epileptic seizures and epilepsy syndromes proposed by the International League Against Epilepsy (ILAE). Until recently the classifications of seizures and of syndromes used worldwide were those proposed by the ILAE in 1981 and 1989 respectively.[110,111]

The 1981 classification divided seizures according to whether on clinical and EEG grounds they appeared to begin in a localized group of cortical neurones in one cerebral hemisphere (partial, focal or localization-related seizures) or whether both cerebral hemispheres appeared

to be involved from the start (generalized seizures). The list of generalized epileptic seizures was similar, though not identical, to that in the new system discussed later. Partial epileptic seizures were divided into simple partial (implying no impairment of consciousness), complex partial (implying impairment of consciousness as assessed by the children's reduced reactivity to external stimuli and amnesia for the event) and partial evolving into generalized tonic-clonic seizures. The occurrence of various symptoms (motor, somatosensory, special-sensory symptoms, autonomic and psychic) was the basis for further subdivision.

The 1989 classification of 'epilepsies and epileptic syndromes' introduced a new concept, which has gained widespread acceptance, namely that of epileptic syndromes. This was in recognition of the fact that the etiology, pathogenesis and clinical features were established for very few epileptic conditions and that it was therefore inappropriate to consider them as diseases. An epileptic syndrome is defined by the non-fortuitous clustering of various features of which the most useful are the type(s) of epileptic seizure, EEG features and age of onset. The two main components of the classification were: (i) the division of epilepsies and epileptic syndromes into those with generalized seizures (generalized epilepsies and syndromes) and those with partial seizures (partial epilepsies and syndromes) and (ii) the division of both generalized and partial epilepsies and syndromes according to whether the cause was unknown and there was no suggestion of an underlying cause other than a possible hereditary predisposition (idiopathic epilepsies), whether the cause was unknown but an underlying cause was suspected (cryptogenic epilepsies) or whether the epilepsy occurred as a consequence of a known disorder of the CNS (symptomatic epilepsy).

In 2001 the ILAE published proposals for a 'diagnostic scheme' composed of five axes:[112,113]

1. a glossary of terms used in epileptology;
2. a list of epileptic seizure types;
3. a list of epilepsy syndromes;
4. an etiological classification;

5. a classification of impairments arising as a consequence of the condition.
- The terms 'partial' and 'localization-related' are abandoned in favor of 'focal'.
- The division of focal seizures into simple and complex is abandoned, partly because of conceptual difficulties with the notion of consciousness and the relative lack of importance of this feature anyhow. A new term 'dyscognitive seizure' has been introduced. This is a seizure in which disturbances of cognition are prominent.
- The term 'cryptogenic', which was considered confusing, is abandoned and is replaced by 'probably symptomatic'. A number of new terms are introduced. These include:
i. Epileptic disease. This is a pathological condition with a single specific, well-defined etiology, e.g. tuberous sclerosis.
ii. Epileptic encephalopathy. This is a condition in which the epileptiform abnormalities themselves are considered to cause a progressive disturbance in cerebral function.
iii. Benign epilepsy syndrome. This is a syndrome in which seizures are easily treated, or require no treatment, and remit without sequelae.

Epileptic seizures

Axis 2 of the ILAE proposals classifies seizures into self-limited and continuous seizure types (status epilepticus). Each of these is then subdivided into generalized and focal seizures, whose meaning is unchanged from before.

Generalized, self-limited seizures[112,113]

Generalized tonic-clonic seizures (GTCS) involve an initial, bilaterally symmetrical, sustained contraction of the muscles (tonic phase) followed by bilateral repetitive, rhythmical contractions of the limbs (clonic phase). There is usually a phase of postictal drowsiness, of variable duration. During GTCS, manifestations such as tongue biting, cyanosis of the lips and incontinence are frequent. However, their usefulness in distinguishing between epileptic and non-epileptic seizures has been overemphasized.

Tonic seizures are characterized by sustained muscle contractions lasting a few seconds to minutes. They may involve the whole, or greater part, of the body or be confined to particular parts of the body. For example, tonic seizures may be manifested by opisthotonus or by a subtle elevation of the eyebrows.

Clonic seizures are manifested by rhythmical contractions of the limbs. An alternative term is rhythmic myoclonus.

Myoclonic seizures are characterized by sudden, brief (<100 ms), involuntary, single or multiple contraction(s) of muscle(s) or muscle groups. They may be massive, involving axial and proximal limb muscles, or subtle and fragmentary involving distal muscles. Facial muscles, such as the eyelids, may be involved. A number of special types of myoclonic seizure are described. These include myoclonic absence seizures (characterized by a typical absence seizure with rhythmical myoclonus usually involving the head and proximal muscle of the upper limbs); eyelid myoclonia (characterized by rhythmical myoclonia of the eyelids sometimes accompanied by a brief typical absence seizure) and myoclonic atonic seizures (consisting of a brief jerk followed by a diffuse loss of tone). Negative myoclonic seizures involve an interruption of tonic muscular activity for < 500 ms without any preceding myoclonus.

Atonic seizures are characterized by a sudden diminution of muscle tone lasting a second or longer, and involving the head, trunk, jaw or limb musculature.

An astatic seizure, also called a drop attack, is one in which there is a loss of erect posture resulting from an atonic, myoclonic or tonic mechanism.

Epileptic spasms (previously called infantile spasms) consist of a sudden flexion, extension or mixed extension–flexion of, predominantly proximal and truncal, muscles which is more sustained than myoclonus but briefer than a tonic seizure (approx. 1 s). They frequently occur in clusters and it is now recognized that their occurrence is not limited to infancy or to West syndrome.

Absence seizures are characterized clinically by a brief impairment of consciousness. In typical absence seizures this is of abrupt onset and cessation with no postictal symptoms. In atypical absence seizures the onset and cessation may be less clearly defined, with the person appearing to drift into and out of the seizure. Typical absence seizures are accompanied, on the EEG, by generalized 3-Hz spike–wave discharges. Atypical absence seizures are usually accompanied by generalized spike–wave discharges at frequencies under 2.5 Hz. The depth of impairment of consciousness during absences varies. Unless mild, automatisms (defined as more or less coordinated, repetitive, motor activity usually occurring when cognition is impaired and for which the subject is usually amnesic afterwards) are frequent. They are usually relatively simple, for example lip smacking and fumbling with hands. Mild clonic, myoclonic and atonic phenomena may also occur during absences.

Focal, self-limited seizure[112,113]

Focal motor seizures involve muscle activity in any form, with either an increase or decrease in muscle contraction. Subtypes include:
- Focal motor seizures with elementary clonic motor signs. The term 'elementary' implies that a single type of contraction of a muscle or group of muscles is involved; 'clonic' implies regular repetitive contractions. Such seizures often imply involvement of the primary motor area of the frontal lobe and may include a Jacksonian march with spread of clonic movements through contiguous body parts.
- Focal motor seizures with asymmetrical tonic motor signs. These seizures are characterized by an asymmetrical, sustained increase in muscle contractions, causing, for example, the child to adopt a 'fencing' posture. Such seizures are characteristic of those involving the supplementary motor areas of the frontal lobes although they can arise from other frontal lobe regions and from extrafrontal lobe sites.
- With typical (temporal lobe) automatisms as occurs in mesial temporal lobe seizures (described later).
- With hyperkinetic automatisms (such as pedalling, thrashing and rocking movements). Such seizures usually imply a frontal lobe origin.
- Rarer seizure types include focal negative myoclonus and seizures with inhibitory motor signs (implying a loss of muscle contraction as in motor arrest).

Focal sensory seizures are characterized by a perceptual experience not caused by appropriate stimuli in the external world. Subtypes include:
- Focal sensory seizures with elementary sensory symptoms. Here the term 'elementary' is used to imply a single, unformed phenomenon involving one primary sensory modality, e.g. somatosensory (parietal lobe seizures), visual (occipital lobe seizures), auditory, olfactory, gustatory, epigastric or cephalic.
- With experiential sensory symptoms. By this it is meant affective symptoms (fear, depression, anger, etc.), distortions of reality (déjà vu, jamais vu), feelings of depersonalization and formed illusionary or hallucinatory events. These are characteristic of seizures involving the junction of the temporal, parietal and occipital lobes.

Gelastic seizures are characterized by ictal laughter or giggling, usually without an appropriate affective tone. Such seizures often involve the hypothalamus.

Hemiclonic seizures are characterized by rhythmical clonic jerking involving one side of the body.

Secondary, generalized seizures are seizures whose onset is focal (e.g. motor or sensory) and then becomes generalized, usually as a tonic-clonic seizure.

The term aura, which had recently fallen from use, has now been defined as a subjective ictal phenomenon that, in a given child, may precede an observable seizure; if it occurs alone, it constitutes a sensory seizure.

Autonomic seizures are characterized by altered autonomic function (objective or subjective) of any type (cardiovascular, pupillary, gastrointestinal, sudomotor, vasomotor and thermoregularity) at seizure onset or in which all manifestations are consistent with altered autonomic function.

Continuous seizure types (status epilepticus)

Status epilepticus is defined by the ILAE as 'a seizure which shows no clinical signs of arresting after a duration encompassing the great majority of seizures of that type in most children or recurrent seizures without resumption of baseline central nervous system function, interictally'.[112] However, operationally it is usually defined as 'recurrent epileptic seizures continuing for more than 30 minutes without full recovery of consciousness before the next seizure begins, or continuous clinical and/or electrical seizure activity lasting for more than 30 minutes whether or not consciousness is impaired'.[114] For each type of epileptic seizure it is possible to define a corresponding type of status epilepticus:

- Generalized status epilepticus:
  generalized tonic-clonic status epilepticus;
  clonic status epilepticus;
  absence status epilepticus;
  tonic status epilepticus;
  myoclonic status epilepticus.
- Focal status epilepticus:
  epilepsia partialis continua (of Kozhevnikov);
  aura continua;
  limbic status epilepticus (psychomotor status);
  hemiconvulsive status with hemiparesis.

Some authorities recognize continuous spike and wave during slow sleep and hypsarrhythmia as special forms of 'electrical status'.[115]

A pragmatic clinical classification defines two main groups, convulsive and nonconvulsive status epilepticus. The former includes generalized tonic-clonic, clonic, tonic and myoclonic status epilepticus, epilepsia partialis continua and hemiconvulsive status with hemiparesis as convulsive status epilepticus and the others as nonconvulsive status epilepticus. Status epilepticus can also be defined according to etiology:

- Febrile status epilepticus – essentially a febrile convulsion lasting over 30 minutes. This is the commonest cause in children aged 1–3 years.
- Idiopathic status epilepticus – status epilepticus occurring without evidence of any previous CNS dysfunction (except possible previous seizures), and in the absence of an acute CNS or systemic disorder.
- Remote symptomatic – status epilepticus occurring in the context of a child with pre-existing static or progressive brain damage or dysfunction.
- Acute symptomatic – status epilepticus occurring during the course of an acute brain disorder caused by, for example, infection, trauma, hypoxic–ischemic insults, stroke, intoxication, metabolic and electrolyte disturbances, tumor and drugs, including antiepileptic drug withdrawal.

The clinical features of the different types of status epilepticus can generally be deduced from their names. However, it is worth noting that the clinical manifestations of both convulsive and nonconvulsive forms often become subtle as the seizure progresses. Hence, late in generalized tonic-clonic status, clonic movements may consist of barely perceptible stiffening of the limbs, while long lasting tonic status may mainly be manifested with hypoventilation, salivation and cyanosis. Nonconvulsive status may present with a child who is confused or is performing less well than is usual.

The effects and treatment of status epilepticus are considered elsewhere in this book.

Epilepsies and epilepsy syndromes

The following summarizes the principal features of epilepsies and epilepsy syndromes currently recognized by the ILAE. More detailed accounts are given elsewhere.[116–118]

Syndromes with onset in the neonatal period

The incidence of seizures in the neonatal period is higher than at any time. Neonatal seizures can be classified as:

- Focal clonic – repetitive, rhythmic, unifocal or multifocal contractions of muscle groups of the limbs, face or trunk.
- Focal tonic – sustained posturing of a single limb or asymmetrical posturing of the trunk or sustained eye deviation.
- Myoclonic – generalized, focal or fragmentary arrhythmic shock-like contractions of muscle groups often provoked by stimulation.
- Generalized tonic – sustained symmetrical posturing of limbs, trunk and neck.
- Subtle seizures (often called motor automatisms) – these include random, roving eye movements, sucking, chewing and tongue protrusions and rowing, swimming and peddling movements of the limbs.

There is considerable debate as to whether all of these seizure types are epileptic in origin.[119] Clonic, focal tonic, generalized myoclonic and some subtle seizures are usually accompanied by ictal EEG discharges, are not usually provoked by stimuli and cannot be terminated by restraint or repositioning. They are probably epileptic in origin. Generalized tonic, focal and fragmentary myoclonic, and some subtle seizures, are usually not accompanied by ictal EEG discharges, can often be provoked by stimulation and terminated by restraint and repositioning. Many are probably not epileptic in origin, but may arise due to loss of cortical inhibition on lower centers.

The interictal EEG is of limited value in the investigation of neonatal seizures. Sharp waves, and even spikes, may be normal features and are not regarded as 'epileptiform abnormalities' as in older children. They are unlikely to be of significance, unless markedly asymmetrical in distribution. Asymmetries and absence of normal elements appropriate for the gestational age are of more help, but are indicators of brain dysfunction rather than specifically of seizure activity. Because neonatal seizures are often very frequent, ictal recordings are often obtained. Ictal discharges take many different forms but generally comprise combinations of repetitive sharp waves or spikes and abnormal paroxysmal rhythms. Discharges are often highly localized or may be confined to one hemisphere. They frequently move during the same recording. Generalized discharges are rare. Neonatal seizures are often unaccompanied by EEG discharges; conversely 'ictal' EEG discharges are frequently unaccompanied by clinical seizures. The clinical significance of such events is unclear.

A majority of neonatal seizures are symptomatic arising as a consequence of pre-, peri- or postnatal insults to the brain, including:

- Hypoxic-ischemic insults (including intrapartum hypoxia).
- Infection – including congenital infections, meningitis and encephalitis.
- Hemorrhage – including intraventricular, intracerebral, subdural and subarachnoid.
- Infarction.
- Malformations and maldevelopments of the brain.
- Metabolic problems including hypoglycemia, hypocalcemia, hypomagnesemia and inborn errors of metabolism.

The prognosis for neonatal seizures is heavily dependent on their etiology. It remains controversial as to whether the seizures themselves are damaging. This has led to uncertainty as to how aggressively they should be treated. Many clinicians only treat clinical seizures accompanied by ictal EEG changes (or if no ictal EEG is available, clinical seizures likely to be accompanied by ictal EEG changes).

Two specific symptomatic or probably symptomatic epilepsy syndromes of the neonatal period are described. These are *early myoclonic encephalopathy* and *Ohtahara syndrome*. Both usually have their onset within the neonatal period or first few months of life and are associated with an identical abnormal EEG pattern known as suppression-burst. Early myoclonic encephalopathy is characterized by the occurrence of frequent, refractory generalized, focal or fragmentary myoclonia, focal clonic seizures and epileptic spasms. There is a high frequency of familial cases and the syndrome is often a manifestation of an inborn error of metabolism, especially nonketotic hyperglycinemia. It is highly resistant to treatment, carries a high mortality and survivors are nearly all severely retarded. Ohtahara syndrome is characterized by frequent tonic spasms. The etiology is heterogeneous but structural brain abnormalities are common. It often evolves to West syndrome. Seizures are highly resistant to treatment and again, there is an appreciable mortality with survivors nearly always being severely retarded.

Not all seizures in the neonatal period are a manifestation of a severe underlying problem. Two benign syndromes of neonatal seizure have been described. *Benign familial neonatal seizures* is an autosomal dominant epilepsy syndrome caused by mutations on voltage-gated potassium channels (KCNQ2 and KCNQ3).[61,62,120] The seizures occur in babies, who are otherwise well, and who remain well. They usually begin on the second or third day of life, but can be delayed up to the third month. A variety of seizure types have been described, but most involve an initial tonic component followed by autonomic changes (especially apnea and heart rate changes) and clonic components. Seizures are often initially frequent, but usually abate within a few days or weeks. The interictal EEG is usually normal. The ictal EEG usually shows generalized flattening, often followed by localized or generalized spikes or slow waves. There is no consensus regarding treatment, which is probably not necessary. Although the outlook is good, there is a significantly higher incidence of febrile and nonfebrile seizures in later childhood. *Benign idiopathic neonatal seizures* ('fifth day fits') is a nonfamilial condition occurring in otherwise normal babies.[120] Epidemiological data suggest clustering of cases, with at times epidemics, leading to the hypothesis of an infective etiology. Seizures, often frequent and prolonged, begin between days 1 and 7 of life and are mainly focal clonic in type, often with apnea. Drowsiness and hypotonia are common during the evolution of the disorder. A variety of interictal EEG patterns have been described. Ictal EEGs show rhythmic spikes or slow waves localized to various locations, particularly the rolandic regions. Generalized discharges also occur. As with benign familial neonatal seizures, antiepileptic drug treatment may not be required. The duration of active seizures is short, usually under a day. The long-term outlook is generally considered good, although detailed prospective studies are lacking.

Syndromes with onset in infancy and early childhood

This period is marked by a high incidence of symptomatic and probably symptomatic epilepsies. Nevertheless, benign syndromes do occur, and the most common is that of febrile seizures. A notable feature of this period is the occurrence of the epileptic encephalopathies. These are conditions in which intense epileptiform activity appears to cause or contribute to neurodevelopmental problems.

Benign epilepsies of infancy are rare. The best known is *benign myoclonic epilepsy of infancy*.[121] This is an idiopathic, generalized epilepsy with onset between 4 months and 3 years. The characteristic seizures (indeed the only seizure type considered compatible with the diagnosis) are myoclonic jerks, mainly of the upper part of the body. They can be single or repeated, subtle, for example causing only head nods, or massive, causing falls. Also, in a minority of subjects, they may be precipitated by acoustic and tactile stimuli. Seizures can occur at any time while awake or asleep but often cluster when the infant is tired or on awakening. The seizures are accompanied on the EEG by a generalized discharge of spike or polyspike and waves. The interictal EEG, while awake, is usually normal, but sleep leads to a dramatic activation of spike or polyspike and wave discharges. As expected in an idiopathic epilepsy, neurodevelopmental progress prior to seizure onset is normal and there is often a family history of seizure disorders. Benign myoclonic epilepsy of infancy usually responds well to sodium valproate; treatment is generally recommended and is said in uncontrolled studies to improve prognosis. The period of active seizures probably lasts for up to 3 years. Some children later develop other generalized epilepsies. Although considered a benign condition, around 15% have later learning difficulties.

Benign focal epilepsies in infancy are rare. *Benign infantile seizures (familial and nonfamilial)* occur in otherwise normal infants, with no identifiable predisposing factor, other than, in familial cases, a positive family history. Onset is from 3 to 20 months (usually 4–7 months if familial). Seizures are focal, with rare secondary generalization and often occur in clusters. Interictal EEG is usually normal. The familial form is autosomal dominant and links to chromosomes 2, 16 and 19 are described. *Benign familial neonatal-infantile seizures* is a similar autosomal dominant disorder presenting from day 2 up to 7 months of age. It is caused by mutations in genes for the sodium channel SCN2A.[122] The prognosis for these epilepsies is good. However, a subgroup of benign familial infantile seizures later develop paroxysmal choreoathetosis.[123]

West syndrome (with an incidence of 1.6–4.3 per 10 000 live births) is the best known epilepsy syndrome of infancy. It consists of a triad of epileptic spasms (this term is now preferred to infantile spasms and all other synonyms), hypsarrhythmia and psychomotor regression. Its onset is nearly always within the first year of life, and typically between 3 and 7 months of age.

Epileptic spasms involve a contraction of the axial muscles causing flexion, extension or both. They may be symmetrical or asymmetrical. The latter is a feature of focal brain lesions. Spasms may be single, but more typically occur in clusters and may occur at any time. However, they are particularly likely to occur when drowsy and on arousal and are rare in sleep. Spasms, particularly at onset, may be subtle, causing only brief head nods. Others are massive and cause distress. Other seizure types may precede, accompany or follow spasms. Of particular importance are spasms preceded by focal seizures, as this may indicate an operable lesion.

Typical hypsarrhythmia is defined as a more or less continuously abnormal EEG with high amplitude, irregular and asymmetrical slow wave activity across all leads with random sharp waves and spikes producing a chaotic pattern (Fig. 22.21). Spasms are often accompanied by electrodecremental responses in which the EEG briefly assumes a more normal appearance. Typical hypsarrhythmia occurs in under half of all cases of West syndrome. Modified forms include cases with some preservation of normal background activity, cases with synchronized bursts of generalized spike and wave activity and cases with significant asymmetries. Other EEG patterns which may occur include constant spike foci and burst-suppression. Hypsarrhythmia may be absent during awake recordings, but present in slow wave sleep.

Psychomotor stagnation and regression is extremely frequent, but not constant, in West syndrome. It often precedes the onset of spasms. Particularly prominent is loss, mostly visual, of interest in the environment.

An underlying cause for West syndrome can be identified in 85–90% of cases. Causes include:

- Neurocutaneous syndromes (tuberous sclerosis is the commonest single cause).
- Brain malformations (such as Aicardi syndrome, agyria-pachygyria, laminar heterotropia, hemimegalencephaly and other migrational disorders).
- Chromosomal abnormalities, including Down syndrome.
- Neurometabolic and degenerative diseases, including aminoacidurias, nonketotic hyperglycinemia, organicacidurias, urea cycle defects, mitochondrial disorders, CDG (carbohydrate-deficient glycoprotein) syndrome, pyridoxine dependency, biotinidase deficiency and PEHO (progressive encephalopathy with edema, hypsarrhythmia and optic atrophy) syndrome.
- Pre-, peri- and postnatal destructive lesions of the brain whether due to infection, hypoxic–ischemic insults, hypoglycemia, trauma or hemorrhage.
- Brain tumors.

A number of X-linked conditions causing West syndrome have been described.

The use of the terms 'cryptogenic' and 'idiopathic' are somewhat confusing when applied to West syndrome. Traditionally the former was used if no cause could be found, particularly if development prior to onset of spasms was normal. No idiopathic category was recognized. However, some children with West syndrome of unknown cause are normal prior to onset of spasms, but have spasms (accompanied by typical hypsarrhythmia) for a short period during which development is relatively unaffected. Most authorities now recognize these as true idiopathic cases.[124]

The treatment of infantile spasms is controversial with the debate centered on whether vigabatrin or hormonal treatment should be used first line and the type, dosage and duration of hormonal treatment.[125,126] The efficacy of vigabatrin in treating infantile spasms was first reported in the early 1990s.[127] It has been shown to be more efficacious than placebo[128] and spasms complicating tuberous sclerosis respond much better to vigabatrin than to hormonal treatment. A recent multicenter, randomized controlled trial (UKISS) compared vigabatrin (maximum dose 150 mg/kg/day) with either prednisolone (maximum dose 60 mg/day) or tetracosactide depot (maximum dose 60 IU on alternate days) in children with infantile spasms, except if due to tuberous sclerosis.[129,130] Freedom from spasms on days 13 and 14 was more likely with hormonal treatment (73%) than with vigabatrin (54%). However, at 14 months of age absence of spasms was similar (75% in the hormone group versus 76% in the vigabatrin group). Moreover, development (as assessed by the Vineland Adaptive Behavior Scales (VABS) was similar, although in the subgroup of those with no identified etiology for the spasms there was a significant increase in mean VABS score in those treated hormonally (mean 88.2) compared to those treated with vigabatrin (mean 78.9).

The clinician must make a choice between drugs of similar efficacy but completely different unwanted effects. Whether the evidence suggesting improved adaptive behavior in a subgroup of children is sufficient justification to recommend hormonal treatment over vigabatrin is unclear. The unwanted effects of hormonal treatment are more or less predictable, detectable and reversible but occasionally fatal, while the visual field defects caused by vigabatrin are unpredictable (but probably develop in up to one third) and, in infancy and early childhood, undetectable, but certainly not fatal.

When a response occurs to vigabatrin it is apparent within days. It is usually started at relatively modest doses of around 50 mg/kg/day with the dose increased in nonresponders every few days to around 180 mg/kg/day before concluding that it has been ineffective. It is usually possible to establish efficacy within a period of 2–3 weeks. Significant drowsiness is likely. Subjects who fail to respond to vigabatrin or who relapse often respond to subsequent hormonal treatment.

There are a multiplicity of studies comparing different hormonal regimens for the treatment of infantile spasms. A review concluded that:[131]

- Cessation or improvement in spasms occurs in 50–75% of subjects.
- The effect is apparent within a couple of weeks.
- Studies suggest either that prednisolone and ACTH are equally effective or that ACTH is more effective.
- Subjects who fail to respond to ACTH or prednisolone may subsequently respond to the other agent.
- There is no clear evidence that larger doses (150 U/m²/day) of ACTH are more effective than lower doses (20–30 U/day).
- Longer treatment periods do not usually improve remission rates.

UKISS used oral prednisolone for 2 weeks, starting at 10 mg four times a day and increasing, if necessary, to 20 mg three times a day after a week, subsequently, weaning it off over 15 days. Tetracosactrin was given intramuscularly for 2 weeks starting at 40 IU on alternative days, and increasing, if necessary, to 60 IU on alternative days after a week. A weaning dose of prednisolone was then substituted. Before starting hormonal treatment, infection should be excluded. Frequent monitoring of blood pressure, urine (for glycosuria) and serum electrolytes is important. Hypertensive children should be evaluated for cardiomyopathy. Hypertension and glycosuria may respond to a reduction in dose. Some authorities recommend tapering ACTH and prednisolone over a 1-week period, even when used for only short periods. If high dose and/or prolonged treatment regimens are used longer tapering courses are necessary; evaluation of the hypothalamic–pituitary axis at the end of therapy is advocated by some.

Infantile spasms complicating tuberous sclerosis respond much better to vigabatrin than to hormonal treatment.[132] Otherwise, the response rate is better in those in whom no underlying cause can be found. It is not clear whether it is appropriate to use different first line agents in the treatment of cryptogenic and symptomatic spasms.

Many other agents have been suggested for the treatment of spasms, whether as initial treatment or as add-on therapy. These include: benzodiazepines, especially nitrazepam; sodium valproate (used in doses considerably higher than usual); pyridoxine; topiramate; lamotrigine; zonisamide; and immunoglobulins.

A small, but important, group of children with focal brain lesions develop West syndrome. These may respond best to drugs like carbamazepine. Nonresponders may be candidates for early resective surgery. Suggestive features are: focal neurological signs; focal epileptic seizures, prior to the onset of or concurrent with epileptic spasms; focal onset of spasms or asymmetrical spasms; asymmetrical hypsarrhythmia or fixed EEG foci. All children with West syndrome require early evaluation with structural brain imaging, preferably MRI. Video-EEG may be necessary to detect focal onset of spasms or asymmetrical spasms.

The overall prognosis for West syndrome is poor and it has not been established whether drug treatment has any impact on the ultimate outcome. Spasms usually remit in infancy or early childhood, but may continue. However, 50–75% of children develop other forms of epilepsy, particularly the Lennox–Gastaut syndrome. From 70% to 90% of infants with West syndrome are mentally retarded and a significant minority have cerebral palsy and/or neuropsychiatric disorders, including autism.[131] West syndrome carries an increased mortality of perhaps around 5%. The main determinant of prognosis is etiology. Those with cryptogenic, and especially idiopathic, spasms, have the best prognosis, both in terms of becoming seizure free and in developing normally. However, symptomatic spasms complicating Down syndrome and neurofibromatosis are said to carry a better prognosis. Other good prognostic factors include normal neurodevelopment prior to onset of spasms, older age at onset and short duration of spasms. Early effective treatment is generally felt likely to improve outcome and has been shown to do so in Down syndrome.[133] However, this effect was not apparent in UKISS.

Severe myoclonic epilepsy in infancy (Dravet syndrome) has only been recognized for the last two decades but is among the most distinctive of the severe epilepsies occurring in infants and young children.[134] The key features for its recognition are the occurrence of febrile, or afebrile, clonic, or tonic-clonic, seizures, often unilateral and sometimes prolonged occurring in the first year of life in an otherwise normal infant. Initial development continues to be normal. However, somewhere between the second and fourth years of life, other seizure types occur, notably myoclonic seizures, atypical absences, absence status and focal seizures. This is accompanied by psychomotor delay, with nearly all children eventually being severely retarded. This justifies its inclusion within the epileptic encephalopathies. Ataxia, mild pyramidal signs and behavioral problems are also common. The interictal EEG is initially normal, except for early photosensitivity in a significant minority of children. With the onset of the polymorphous seizures in the second year of life, spike, polyspike and spike and wave discharges occur. The background may remain normal or show progressive slowing. Dravet syndrome is commonly associated with mutations on a sodium channel gene (SCN1A). However, similar mutations are also associated with other epilepsy phenotypes[135] and also with post-pertussis vaccine encephalopathy.[136] It is postulated that the Dravet phenotype results from the cumulative effects or interactions of a few or several genes of which SCN1A is but one. The syndrome is highly resistant to treatment. Given the combination of focal and generalized seizures types, it is probably most appropriate to use antiepileptic drugs with a broad spectrum of activity, such as sodium valproate, topiramate and levetiracetam and to avoid drugs such as carbamazepine which may exacerbate generalized seizures. Lamotrigine may also exacerbate seizures.[137] Efficacy of stiripentol when used with sodium valproate and clobazam was shown in a double blind trial.[138]

Rarer and less well-characterized severe epilepsies occurring in infancy and early childhood include *migrating partial seizures of infancy*, *myoclonic status in nonprogressive encephalopathies* and *hemiconvulsion–hemiplegia syndrome*.[139] The first of these is characterized by an onset at around 3 months of age of intractable and escalating focal seizures (usually focal motor), which characteristically involve one area of the body before shifting to another. Myoclonic status in nonprogressive encephalopathies is characterized by repeated episodes of myoclonic status epilepticus occurring in children with nonprogressive 'static' encephalopathies, including cerebral palsy, Angelman syndrome and Prader–Willi syndrome. Hemiconvulsion–hemiplegia syndrome (HH syndrome) has been long recognized, but appears to be declining in frequency. Its cardinal features are the occurrence, in an otherwise normal child, of a prolonged unilateral, usually clonic, febrile seizure, either in the course of a trivial infection or else symptomatic of a severe acute brain disorder such as meningitis, followed by atrophy of one cerebral hemisphere and hemiplegia. Epilepsy supervenes after a variable period. Both focal and generalized seizures may occur. Prevention with rapid termination of prolonged febrile seizures is important and may help explain its decline in frequency.

Syndromes with onset in mid- and late childhood and adolescence

This age group is associated with a decline in the incidence of epilepsy and by a number of relatively common and well-characterized epilepsy syndromes, which are almost certainly genetic in origin and many of which carry an excellent prognosis. These can be conveniently considered under the categories of the idiopathic focal and generalized epilepsies of childhood and adolescence. Symptomatic and probably symptomatic epilepsies are also important in this age group. They include focal epilepsies, most notably mesial temporal lobe epilepsy, and a number of epileptic encephalopathies such as the Lennox–Gastaut syndrome and the Landau–Kleffner syndrome.

The idiopathic generalized epilepsies.[140] These are characterized by:

- Occurrence in otherwise normal children and adolescents.
- Strong family history of epilepsy, including, but not restricted to, idiopathic epilepsies.
- A preceding history of febrile convulsions in many subjects.
- The occurrence in various combinations of three seizure types: generalized tonic-clonic seizures; typical absence seizures; and myoclonic seizures.
- EEGs in which the background is generally normal with paroxysmal regular or irregular spike or polyspike and wave abnormalities at 3 Hz or greater.

The three best-characterized, idiopathic generalized epilepsies are childhood absence epilepsy, juvenile absence epilepsy and juvenile myoclonic epilepsy.

Childhood and juvenile absence epilepsies are both characterized by the occurrence of typical absence seizures. In both these are relatively prolonged, typically 10–20 seconds, with severe impairment of consciousness such that automatisms are common. Other features during the absences such as eyelid blinking, mild clonic movements around the mouth and head nods may occur but are not prominent. In childhood absence epilepsy, absences are very frequent, occurring many times a day – hundreds may be recorded on video-EEG. In juvenile absence epilepsy they are less frequent, occurring at most a few times a day. Except for febrile convulsions, other seizure types occur only very rarely in childhood absence epilepsy. Occasional myoclonic jerks may occur in juvenile absence epilepsy and up to 80% of subjects with juvenile absence epilepsy have, or develop, generalized tonic-clonic seizures, which are usually infrequent. Many authorities consider that photosensitivity is not compatible with the diagnosis of childhood absence epilepsy, and possibly also juvenile absence epilepsy. Childhood absence epilepsy usually has its onset between 4 and 8 years and generally remits by about the age of 12. Occasional children (no more than 10%) will develop generalized tonic-clonic seizures in their teenage years or adult life. Juvenile absence epilepsy usually has its onset between 7 and 16 years and is usually long lasting with susceptibility to seizures continuing into adult life.

The EEG in childhood and juvenile absence epilepsies is similar and is characterized by regular generalized spike and wave discharges at around 3 Hz (Fig. 22.19). The discharges are increased during sleep and on awakening and are provoked by hyperventilation.

Juvenile myoclonic epilepsy is characterized by a triad of seizure types. Typical absences occur in about one third of children, usually in late childhood or early adolescence. They are usually brief (a few seconds), mild and unaccompanied by automatisms. However, if they start in younger children they may resemble those of childhood absence epilepsy. Myoclonic seizures occur in all individuals, usually starting in early to mid adolescence. They may be massive (causing falls), or confined to the limbs, or extremities. They may be single or multiple and rhythmic. They usually cluster in the period shortly after awakening with a second cluster toward the end of the day. They are often not reported spontaneously, as the child considers them as a normal feature of everyday life. Enquiries should be made as to whether the child is considered 'clumsy' in the morning or has the 'shakes' with a tendency to spill drinks. Generalized tonic-clonic seizures occur in nearly all untreated children, usually a few years after the onset of myoclonic jerks. They usually cluster in the morning and may be heralded by a shower of myoclonic jerks or absences, sometimes leading to an erroneous diagnosis of secondary generalized tonic-clonic seizures. Photosensitivity, both clinical and on EEG, is common. The EEG in juvenile myoclonic epilepsy is characterized by irregular discharges of fast spike, or more often polyspike and wave (Fig. 22.19). Myoclonic seizures are usually accompanied by brief polyspike or polyspike and wave discharges. Although the background EEG is usually normal, focal abnormalities occur in a minority. These have the appearance of abortive generalized discharges and vary in location.

Epilepsy with generalized tonic-clonic seizures only usually begins in adolescence or young adult life. It is characterized by generalized tonic-clonic seizures only. These often occur exclusively, or predominantly, on awakening (hence the old name 'epilepsy with grand mal on awakening'). It should be noted that generalized tonic-clonic seizures, occurring predominantly on wakening, occur in a number of epilepsy syndromes, including juvenile myoclonic epilepsy. It is the lack of other seizure types which distinguishes the syndrome.

The ILAE diagnostic scheme suggests inclusion of two syndromes, *epilepsy with myoclonic astatic seizures and epilepsy with myoclonic absences*, which were previously usually considered amongst the cryptogenic or symptomatic generalized epilepsies, within the idiopathic generalized epilepsies. The former (also known as Doose syndrome) usually has its onset within the first 5 years of life.[141] The defining seizure types are atonic and myoclonic, which are often combined (myoatonic seizure) and are often manifested as drop attacks. Episodes of nonconvulsive status epilepticus are common. The characteristic EEG feature is spike or polyspike and wave discharges, often with photosensitivity. The prognosis is variable. Many children continue to develop normally and seizures eventually remit. However, others, especially those with repeated episodes of nonconvulsive status epilepticus, show cognitive decline. In epilepsy with myoclonic absences, the characteristic seizures are typical absences, accompanied by marked rhythmical myoclonia, mainly affecting the upper limbs and head.[142] These seizures can occur in otherwise normal children, but many have pre-existing neurodevelopmental problems. In children who do not, such problems often supervene. The EEG is very similar to that seen in childhood absence epilepsy. However, video-EEG or an EMG lead applied over the deltoids will reveals myoclonus accompanying each spike–wave discharge.

There are many children with epilepsy with features suggestive of an idiopathic generalized epilepsy who do not fit within the above syndromes. In recent years a number of other syndromes have been suggested and are more or less well characterized. In *eyelid myoclonia with absences* (*Jeavons syndrome*) the characteristic seizure consists of brief episodes of marked jerking of the eyelids usually accompanied by upward deviation of the eyes. These usually start in childhood, are often very frequent, and may be misdiagnosed as tics. On EEG, the seizures occur on eye closure and are associated with generalized polyspike and wave discharges (Fig. 22.19). All children are photosensitive and there is continued debate about the role of self-induction of the seizures. Despite the name, absences are usually inconspicuous. The condition usually continues into adult life and generalized tonic-clonic seizures commonly develop. *Perioral myoclonia with absences* is a syndrome in which typical absences are accompanied by marked rhythmical myoclonia of the perioral and/or jaw muscles. Episodes of absence status appear to be common as are generalized tonic-clonic seizures. The most recently described epilepsy to be placed by the ILAE with the idiopathic generalized epilepsies is *generalized epilepsy with febrile seizures plus (GEFS+)*.[143] This is an autosomal dominant condition in which different family members have variable phenotypes including febrile seizures only, febrile seizures with other, mainly generalized, seizure types, and myoclonic-astatic seizures. It is associated with a number of sodium ion channel mutations (SCN1A, SCN1B and SCN2A) and mutations on a GABA$_A$ receptor gene.

The idiopathic generalized epilepsies usually show an excellent response to sodium valproate, lamotrigine, topiramate and levetiracetam. However, lamotrigine may aggravate myoclonic jerks. Ethosuximide is a useful drug for childhood absence epilepsy, but is considered to be ineffective against generalized tonic-clonic seizures. Combined therapy, with two, or even all three, of these agents, is occasionally useful in refractory cases. Benzodiazepines, including clobazam and clonazepam, are also useful, particularly against myoclonic seizures. Sodium valproate, levetiracetam and lamotrigine are active against photosensitive seizures. Carbamazepine, vigabatrin, tiagabine and probably also phenytoin are generally ineffective and may exacerbate existing seizures and precipitate new seizure types: their use is contraindicated except in exceptional circumstances.[144]

The idiopathic focal epilepsies.[145] These are characterized by:

- Normal preceding neurodevelopment.
- A strong family history of epilepsy including, but not restricted to, idiopathic epilepsies.
- A strong history of preceding febrile seizures.
- Stereotyped seizures reflecting the site of ictal onset and spread.
- EEGs in which the background is normal but in which highly characteristic interictal focal spike and wave abnormalities are frequent.

Benign childhood epilepsy with centrotemporal spikes (commonly called *rolandic epilepsy* or *BECTS*) is the commonest of these epilepsies, and indeed may account for around 20% of all new onset epilepsies in young school-age children who are otherwise normal. The seizures have their onset in the lower rolandic cortex representing the face and oropharynx. Seizure onset peaks between 7 and 10 years. Seizures occur in sleep in only around 70% of children, in both sleep and awake in 15%, and while awake only in 15%. Seizures during sleep often occur shortly after falling asleep or shortly prior to awakening. The seizures are most characteristically unaccompanied by any impairment of consciousness (simple focal in the old terminology), but those during sleep may evolve (often rapidly) with disturbance of awareness and reactivity (complex focal) and/or secondary generalized tonic-clonic or hemiconvulsions. BECTS should always be considered in a child, of appropriate age, who presents with nocturnal generalized seizures. The seizures usually begin with somatosensory symptoms in and around the mouth. The child often complains of paresthesiae, numbness, 'heaviness' or 'thickness' of the lips, gums, inner cheek and tongue. This is often followed by clonic jerking of the perioral muscles, lips and tongue. Salivation is often prominent. Speech arrest may be due to either laryngeal involvement, or to involvement of nearby speech areas. Seizures usually last only a few seconds to a few minutes but status epilepticus has been described. Total seizure count is usually low; many children have a single seizure only. However, some children have numerous seizures, sometimes with more than one in a single night. The EEG is highly characteristic with

interictal sharp and slow wave complexes in the left and/or right central and/or mid temporal region (Fig. 22.20). They may be unilateral or bilaterally synchronous or asynchronous. They are strongly activated by sleep. Similar abnormalities occur in a minority of children in other brain regions. BECTS has an excellent prognosis. It usually remits within 1–2 years of onset and certainly before mid adolescence. It is exceptional for seizures to occur in adult life.

The second most common benign partial epilepsy of childhood is *Panayiotopoulos syndrome (early-onset benign childhood occipital epilepsy)*.[146,147] It is encountered two to three times less frequently than BECTS. It predominantly affects younger children aged 3–6 years old. Seizures manifest with autonomic symptoms, particularly nausea, retching and vomiting. Often the seizure onset is inconspicuous with the child simply appearing unwell, pale, quiet or irritable. They may complain of feeling sick. Other autonomic manifestations include pallor, pupillary, cardiorespiratory and probably thermoregulatory changes. As the seizure progresses, there is frequently deviation of the eyes and head and impairment of consciousness. Unresponsiveness may be accompanied by marked loss of postural tone. The terms 'ictal syncope' or 'syncopal-like episodes' has been suggested for this. Around half of the seizures end in secondary generalization. Two-thirds of seizures start in sleep. An important and unusual feature in Panayiotopoulos syndrome is that around half of all seizures last for more than half an hour (sometimes for many hours) constituting autonomic status epilepticus. During such episodes the child's conscious level fluctuates and there is often intermittent retching and vomiting and eye and head deviation. The status may terminate with a hemiconvulsion or a generalized tonic-clonic seizure. Status in Panayiotopoulos syndrome is frequently not recognized as being epileptic in nature, but may lead to admission to an intensive care unit, with a suspected grave cerebral insult.

The interictal EEG usually reveals abnormalities similar to those seen in BECTS – sharp and slow waves or spikes – but predominating in the occipital regions (Fig. 22.20). As a consequence, Panayiotopoulos syndrome has been classified as an occipital epilepsy. However, this may not be appropriate given the frequency of extraoccipital EEG abnormalities and the predominantly autonomic seizure manifestations. Panayiotopoulos syndrome is among the most benign of all epilepsies. Total seizure count is usually low; many children have only a single seizure and seizures generally remit within 1–2 years of onset.

Late-onset childhood occipital epilepsy (Gastaut type or CEOP) begins predominantly in mid–late childhood with a peak age of onset around the age of 7–9 years. It is characterized by relatively frequent, usually brief, visual seizures occurring while awake. These occur in full consciousness and are mainly manifested by elementary visual hallucinations of, for example, colored balls (Fig. 22.23). By contrast, in migraine, visual hallucinations are usually black and white and jagged or sharp in outline.[148] Less commonly, visual hallucinations in CEOP are complex, e.g. of figures. Visual illusions, such as micropsia, visual field defects and episodes of ictal blindness also occur. Headache, often hemicranial, is common either ictally or postictally and misdiagnosis as migraine is common. The EEG is characterized by occipital paroxysms, which are runs of high-amplitude spike–waves or sharp waves, occurring in the posterior regions. Prognosis is less clear than with either BECTS or Panayiotopoulos syndrome – many individuals continue to have seizures in adolescence and adult life and some develop occasional generalized tonic-clonic seizures.

A third idiopathic occipital epilepsy syndrome in children – *idiopathic photosensitive occipital lobe epilepsy* – is discussed with reflex epilepsies.

A number of other epilepsy syndromes with certain similarities to BECTS and Panayiotopoulos syndrome have been proposed but are less well characterized. These include *benign childhood seizures with affective symptomatology, benign partial seizures in adolescence, benign childhood epilepsy with parietal spikes and frequent giant somatosensory evoked potentials, benign childhood focal seizures associated with frontal or midline spikes, benign focal epilepsy with central and vertex spikes and waves during sleep* and *benign focal seizures of adolescence*. These demonstrate that there are

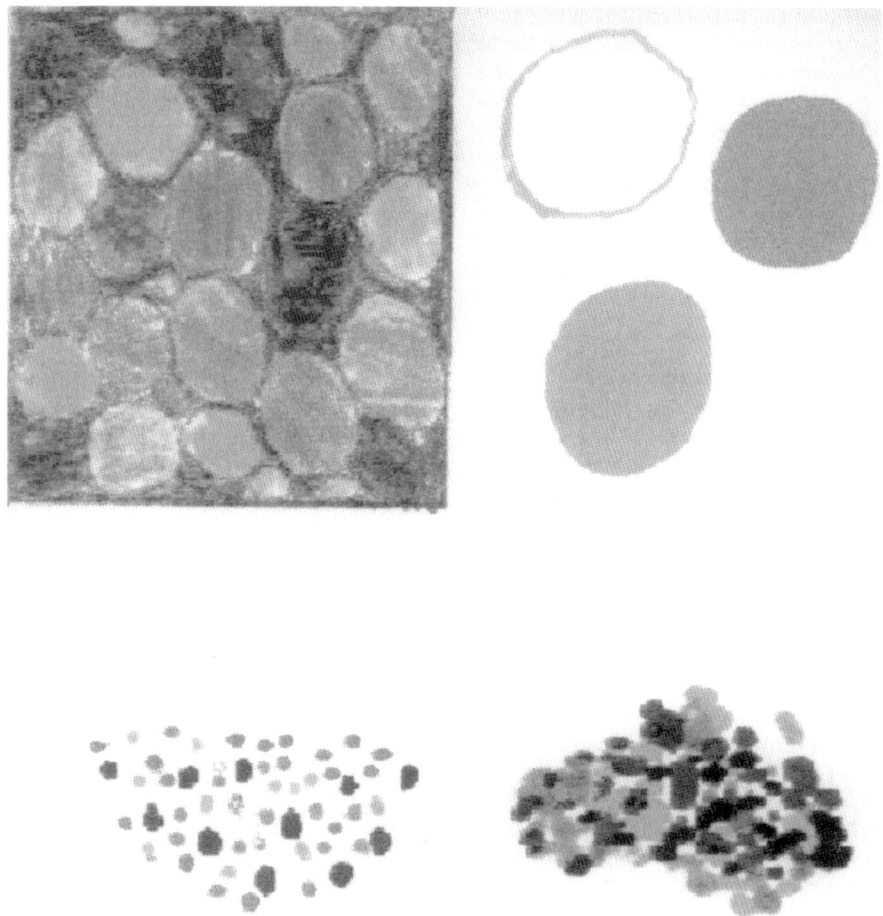

Fig. 22.23 Patient's illustrations of visual hallucinations in childhood occipital epilepsy (Gastaut type).

many children who have features suggestive of benign focal epilepsy, but whose electroclinical features do not fit within existing syndromes.

In recent years, a number of idiopathic focal epilepsies, inherited in an autosomal dominant manner, have been described. The best characterized is *autosomal dominant nocturnal frontal lobe epilepsy*. This usually begins in childhood, but has an exceptionally wide age range of onset. The seizures are characteristically brief and occur during light sleep. They may be repeated many times per night. Motor symptoms predominate. A grunt, groan, or more complex vocalization, often heralds the seizure, followed by hyperkinetic motor behaviors (e.g. thrashing, thrusting and rocking movements) or tonic or dystonic posturing, sometimes with clonic components. The occurrence of dystonic features gave rise to the designation 'nocturnal paroxysmal dystonia', which was previously considered non-epileptic. The EEG is frequently normal, even during attacks. A minority show focal frontal interictal and ictal abnormalities. Neuroimaging is normal. The condition appears to be life-long. A good response to carbamazepine is seen in some, but not all, children. Other autosomal dominant focal epilepsies include *familial temporal lobe epilepsy* and *familial focal epilepsy with variable foci*.[149,150]

In children with benign focal seizures who have few seizures, particularly if seizures cause little distress, and in whom remission is expected (i.e. BECTS and Panayiotopoulos syndrome), it is reasonable not to treat with antiepileptic drugs and to await spontaneous remission. When treatment is given, it is important to ensure that the unwanted effects are not more troublesome than the seizures. Occasionally the idiopathic focal epilepsies can be made more severe with antiepileptic drug treatment. This is particularly described with carbamazepine.[151]

Symptomatic and probably symptomatic focal epilepsies. These epilepsies are mainly defined by their site of origin and, to a lesser extent, by their etiology. A broad distinction is made according to whether the site of origin is in the limbic system or in the neocortex (including the lateral temporal lobes). Of the limbic epilepsies mesial temporal lobe epilepsy is the most important. Neocortical epilepsy syndromes include Rasmussen syndrome.

Mesial temporal lobe epilepsy with hippocampal sclerosis (often referred to simply as *mesial temporal lobe epilepsy*) is of considerable importance because it is the single largest cause of refractory epilepsy in adults and the commonest reason for undertaking epilepsy surgery. Mesial temporal sclerosis consists of severe loss of specific neurones in the hippocampus along with synaptic reorganizations. This probably results from a previous cerebral injury rather than as a consequence of repeated seizures and, at least in adults undergoing epilepsy surgery, is strongly associated with prolonged febrile convulsions in early childhood. It is not established whether these are the cause of mesial temporal sclerosis, or another manifestation of it. Genetic factors are also important and there is an increased incidence of various seizure disorders in the families of subjects with mesial temporal lobe epilepsy.

The following represents the sequence typical in mesial temporal lobe epilepsy, although there is considerable variation:

- Complicated febrile convulsion(s) in infancy/early childhood.
- Later onset of habitual seizures, usually in childhood, which characteristically respond well to initial treatment.
- Return of habitual seizures in adolescence/early adult life, which often become refractory to treatment.

The habitual seizures of mesial temporal lobe epilepsy often begin with an aura, manifestations of which may include autonomic features such as a rising sensation in the epigastrium, psychic features such as fear, déjà vu and feelings of depersonalization, visual illusions such as micropsia and macropsia and olfactory hallucinations such as unpleasant smells. Formed visual and auditory hallucinations are said not to occur. Many seizures do not progress beyond the aura. In the old terminology they were classed as simple focal seizures. However, they often progress such that there is impaired cognition, perception, attention and memory (dyscognitive seizure or 'complex partial' in the old terminology). Motor manifestations are often prominent and include motor arrest, oro-alimentary and manual automatisms and lateralized motor manifestations such as forced head and eye deviation and tonic or dystonic posturing. Language disturbances also occur. Secondary generalization is often not a prominent feature. The postictal period is typically characterized by a variable period of confusion, disorientation, language disturbances and either relaxation or automated semipurposeful movements. Contralateral Todd paresis may occur. More details on the lateralizing features of mesial temporal lobe seizures are to be found elsewhere.[152,153]

The characteristic interictal EEG abnormality is anterior temporal sharp waves, spikes and slow waves (Fig. 22.20). These are quite frequently bilateral, even in children in whom habitual seizures are unilateral. In younger children, bilateral synchronous spike–wave discharges may occur. A repeatedly normal, interictal EEG is common. MRI has revolutionized the detection of hippocampal sclerosis. Thin coronal slices orthogonal to the long axis of the temporal lobes usually reveal hippocampal atrophy, temporal horn dilation (both best appreciated on T1-weighted sections) and, on T2-weighted images, high signal in the hippocampus (Fig. 22.22).

The drug of choice for mesial temporal lobe epilepsy is carbamazepine. Initial response is usually good, but may not be maintained. There is currently no information about what percentage of children gain permanent seizure remission and how many develop refractory epilepsy. When carbamazepine fails, other drugs active against partial seizures should be tried. However, surgery offers the prospect of 'cure' in around 80% of children and should not be unduly delayed through a desire to exhaust all medical options.

Mesial temporal lobe epilepsy can also be caused by cortical dysplasias, tumors (particularly dysembryoplastic neuroepithelial tumors), hamartomas and chronic encephalitis and other destructive lesions.

The neocortical epilepsies are a heterogeneous group of epilepsies arising from the frontal lobes, lateral temporal lobes, parietal and occipital lobes. *Lateral (neocortical) temporal lobe epilepsy* is uncommon. Compared to mesial temporal lobe epilepsy, seizures are more likely to give rise to auditory, vertiginous and complex visual hallucinations and less likely to give rise to motor manifestations.

Frontal lobe epilepsies are relatively common and probably underrecognized. They pose particular diagnostic problems. Three main seizure types have been described:

- Focal clonic seizures. These characteristically occur in clear consciousness and involve localized rhythmical jerking of a limb. A Jacksonian march, consisting of sequential involvement of contiguous areas of the body in a focal motor seizure, may be seen. Such activity implies seizure activity in the primary motor area.
- Focal motor seizures with asymmetrical tonic motor seizures (asymmetrical tonic seizures, supplementary motor seizures). These are characterized by the assumption, usually suddenly, of fixed and abnormal postures, the most classical being the so-called 'fencing posture'. Motor manifestations are often preceded by somatosensory sensations of numbness and tingling. Other ictal features are speech arrest or forced vocalizations and secondary generalization. Asymmetrical tonic seizures are characteristic of seizures arising in the supplementary motor area of the frontal lobes.
- Focal motor seizures with hyperkinetic automatisms (frontal lobe complex partial seizures, hypermotor seizures). These seizures occur in association with impaired cognition and are characterized by complex motor automatisms. Frenetic, agitated, and sometimes sexual, behavior is often seen, along with vocalizations, ranging from humming to the shouting of obscenities. Such seizures can originate from many areas of the frontal lobes.

The reader requiring fuller descriptions is referred elsewhere.[154] Frontal lobe epilepsies are often characterized by frequent, mainly nocturnal, seizures, with little if any postictal drowsiness. The interictal and even ictal EEG is often normal, reflecting the fact that large areas of the mesial and inferior frontal lobes are not directly accessible by scalp EEG. They are often confused with psychogenic seizures, which, however, rarely occur while the child is asleep and usually last longer.

Occipital lobe epilepsies are relatively uncommon. Characteristic ictal features include elementary and sometimes complex visual hallucinations. The most common are hallucinations of colored spots or geometric forms similar to those described for late-onset childhood occipital epilepsy (Gastaut type). Ictal blindness may also occur. Other features are a variety of abnormal eye movements such as tonic deviation, nystagmoid movements, forced blinking and eyelid flutter. Many different patterns of spread can occur, giving rise to features more typical of temporal or frontal lobe seizures. The interictal and ictal EEG is generally useful in the diagnosis of occipital epilepsies. However, occasionally discharges confined to mesial or inferior aspects of the occipital lobes may be undetected by scalp EEG and the propensity of seizures to spread may impede localization. The range of pathologies causing occipital lobe epilepsy is similar to that of other neocortical epilepsies. However, in addition, a syndrome of *occipital lobe epilepsy with bilateral occipital calcifications and celiac disease* has been described.[155] The relationship between occipital lobe epilepsies and migraine has also aroused much debate. Occipital epilepsy and migraine are often confused because both are characterized by visual hallucinations and by headache, often hemicranial. In addition, it is possible that occipital (and other) epilepsies may occasionally trigger migraine attacks. Whether epileptic seizures are ever caused by migraine remains to be established.

Parietal lobe epilepsy is rare. Ictal manifestations include somatosensory symptoms, particularly unilateral paresthesiae and pain (including abdominal pain), speech problems, dyspraxias and agnosias. Many parietal lobe seizures are 'silent' unless they spread. Interictal and even ictal EEG is often unhelpful.

Rasmussen syndrome (often called *Rasmussen encephalitis*)[156] is a symptomatic, neocortical epilepsy syndrome of unknown cause, characterized pathologically by so-called 'chronic encephalitis'. Its onset is usually between 1 and 15 years and may present either with focal seizures, which quickly become more and more frequent, or as status epilepticus, which is usually focal in nature. The most characteristic seizure type is focal motor seizures, often highly localized, for example to an extremity of one limb or around the mouth. However, impaired cognition during seizures is not uncommon, particularly as the condition progresses. Epilepsia partialis continua is seen at some time in the disease in the majority of children. The disease is nearly always strictly unilateral at onset, but 'spread' to the other hemisphere can occur with time. A hallmark of the disease is progressive cerebral atrophy, usually confined to one hemisphere, at least initially. This is accompanied by a progressive hemiparesis whose onset can occur within weeks of the onset of clinical seizures or be delayed for years. It is accompanied by cognitive decline. Interictal EEG may show progressive background slowing of the involved hemisphere. Ictal EEG is often lateralizing but rarely localizing. Structural imaging early in the disease may show focal high signal on T2-weighted images, particularly in the cerebral cortex. Later atrophic changes are seen.

The management of Rasmussen syndrome should involve early referral to an epilepsy surgery center, since early hemispherectomy is considered by many to be the treatment of choice. Localized resections are generally ineffective. Medical therapy with conventional antiepileptic drugs is nearly always unsuccessful in the long term, although short term control of seizure may be achieved. Immunotherapy with either steroid medication or intravenous immunoglobulin may be of benefit in some children and may avoid the need for hemispherectomy.

Epileptic encephalopathies. The best known epileptic encephalopathy of childhood is *Lennox–Gastaut syndrome*. However, there is considerable variation in how this syndrome is defined. At one extreme it has been used to designate virtually any seizure disorder in childhood characterized by drug-resistant seizures and impaired mental abilities. Alternatively, as here, it is used to designate a narrowly defined symptomatic, or probably symptomatic, generalized epilepsy. Its onset is usually between 3 and 5 years of age; onset after 10 years of age is exceptional. The defining features are:

- The occurrence of mixed generalized seizure types of which tonic, atonic and atypical absences are the most prominent.
- Interictal EEG patterns with generalized slow spike and wave discharges and, in sleep, bursts of fast rhythms at 10–12 Hz (Fig. 22.21).
- Psychomotor delay.

Lennox–Gastaut syndrome has multiple causes, similar to those of West syndrome, from which it sometimes evolves. Indeed virtually any cortical brain pathology, whether focal or generalized, can cause it. True idiopathic cases are not generally recognized, children in whom no cause can be found being classified as probably symptomatic.

The characteristic seizures of Lennox–Gastaut syndrome can be present from the start. Alternatively, they may be preceded by other seizure types, including focal seizures. Seizures tend to be frequent, occurring many times a day, and tonic and atonic seizures often cause falls ('drop attacks'). During sleep, tonic seizures are particularly characteristic and are associated with 10–12 Hz fast rhythms. Episodes of nonconvulsive status epilepticus are common. Virtually any other seizure type can occur, including (according to many, but not all authorities), focal seizures. However, myoclonic seizures are not usually prominent. Their occurrence, especially if associated with EEG patterns other than slow spike and wave, should make one consider other severe epilepsies, such as severe myoclonic epilepsy in infancy. However, a myoclonic variant of the Lennox–Gastaut syndrome is recognized. Occasionally, children and adolescents with apparently idiopathic epilepsies develop features of the Lennox–Gastaut syndrome.[157,158] In some cases this may be drug induced.

Mental retardation is often pre-existing. However, the onset of the syndrome is nearly always accompanied by a slowing in development or even apparent regression. This is not of the relentless nature seen in neurodegenerative conditions. It often appears to mirror seizure control, with improvement occurring during quiescent periods. However, a majority of children eventually become mentally retarded, and this is often severe. Behavioral problems, including autistic behaviors, may coexist. A small number of children with otherwise typical Lennox–Gastaut syndrome develop normally.

Lennox–Gastaut syndrome is highly resistant to therapy. There are many different recommendations but in general it is best to use broadspectrum agents such as sodium valproate, lamotrigine, topiramate, levetiracetam and zonisamide rather than narrower spectrum agents such as carbamazepine and vigabatrin. However, there is no doubt that the latter have benefited individual children. Other drugs, usually used as concomitant therapy, which may be useful, include the benzodiazepines, ethosuximide and acetazolamide. Controlled trials have demonstrated efficacy of lamotrigine, topiramate and felbamate in the Lennox–Gastaut syndrome.[159–162] Monotherapy should always be attempted, but many children do best on two, or occasionally three, drugs. Polytherapy carries significant risks of making seizures worse, particularly if they induce drowsiness. In children with Lennox–Gastaut syndrome it is important to define a realistic aim for drug therapy. This will involve accepting that complete seizure control is unlikely and that maximizing function and quality of life is of more importance. The natural history of the disorder is marked by fluctuations in the activity of seizures. This must be recognized when making decisions regarding drug treatment.

Other treatments, which may be helpful in Lennox–Gastaut syndrome, include the ketogenic diet, steroids, intravenous immunoglobulins and surgery. Except on very rare occasions when a focal or strictly hemispheric lesion gives rise to Lennox–Gastaut syndrome, resective surgery is not an option. However, corpus callostomy may be helpful if atonic drop attacks are a major problem. Vagal nerve stimulation may also be useful.[163]

The overall prognosis for Lennox–Gastaut syndrome is poor. A small number of previously normal subjects, particularly those whose condition is of later onset and who have the condition for only a short period

of time, have a favorable outlook. The remainder continue to have seizures for many years. These may continue to show the characteristics of the Lennox–Gastaut syndrome or there may be an evolution into other types of epilepsy.

The Landau–Kleffner syndrome and epilepsy with continuous spike–waves during slow-wave sleep are closely related epilepsy syndromes. The EEG pattern of continuous spikes and waves during slow sleep (CSWS) consists of bilateral generalized spike and wave discharges present for at least 85% of slow-wave sleep. This pattern is occasionally encountered in the course of a number of epilepsies. For example, it is described in children with benign childhood epilepsy with centrotemporal spikes in whom it may be associated with a decline in cognitive performance. It has also been described as a separate, and rather poorly defined, syndrome (epilepsy with continuous spike–waves during slow-wave sleep). Finally it is very common in the Landau–Kleffner syndrome. The latter is an epilepsy syndrome occurring in previously normal children, usually between 3 and 8 years of age, but occasionally younger, who develop an aphasia, which initially is mainly receptive, but often becomes global. Deafness is frequently suspected. Many children become totally mute and may fail to understand environmental noises. A notable feature of the syndrome is severe behavioral problems. Epileptic seizures are usually relatively infrequent and may be totally absent. They can be of various types. The awake EEG may be normal or else show focal, hemispheric or generalized spike–wave abnormalities. The sleep EEG often, but not invariably, shows CSWS. Sophisticated EEG techniques often indicate that the EEG abnormality is maximal in one or other posterior temporal electrodes. MRI is nearly always normal but PET and SPECT often show localized or hemispheric metabolic and perfusion abnormalities. All children with suspected Landau–Kleffner syndrome and/or CSWS require detailed neuropsychological evaluation.

Seizure control in these syndromes may not be difficult and may lead to improved language function. However, the syndrome frequently fails to respond to conventional antiepileptic drug medication. Most authorities appear to treat initially with sodium valproate. However, if an inadequate response is obtained, hormonal treatment (steroids or ACTH) is indicated and the response may be dramatic. Unfortunately relapses are common. The technique of multiple subpial transection has been pioneered for the treatment of Landau–Kleffner and appears to improve the outlook.[164] It is based on the functional organization of the cerebral cortex vertically but with the connections involved in the spread of seizures being arranged horizontally. The horizontal connections are disrupted by making multiple cuts perpendicular to the cortical surface while preserving the vertically orientated fibers. Eventually Landau–Kleffner syndrome remits. This can occur after only a few weeks or after many years. The long-term outlook in Landau–Kleffner syndrome reflects the duration of the condition;[165] most subjects have permanent language problems unless the stage of active disease was very short.

The widespread recognition of the Landau–Kleffner syndrome has lead to renewed interest in the cognitive effect of seizures in other epilepsies.[166] It is now increasingly accepted that specific cognitive and/or behavioral disturbances may have an epileptic basis even when overt seizures are infrequent or absent. Recognition can be a major problem. Clues include fluctuations, sometimes abrupt, in aspects such as mood, attention, memory and performance. Sophisticated EEG techniques coupled with neuropsychological evaluation are necessary to investigate such 'cognitive seizures'. The role of antiepileptic drug treatment is uncertain, but a trial of therapy is probably justified if there is reasonable evidence that cognitive problems are the result of epileptic activity. However, the possibility of inducing cognitive problems with antiepileptic drugs must constantly be borne in mind.

Reflex epilepsies. Reflex seizures are seizures precipitated by sensory stimuli. The stimulus may be simple such as flashes of light, touch or unexpected loud noises, or complex such as colored pictures, eating, etc. Most stimuli inducing reflex seizures are extrinsic. However, intrinsic stimuli such as proprioception can occasionally induce seizures. The 2001 ILAE definition precludes seizures provoked by higher brain functions, such as cognition and specific emotions. However, these have conventionally been considered with reflex seizures. The range of stimuli which have been linked to seizure provocation is wide and the clinician should be alert to the possibility of reflex seizures even if the stimulus seems bizarre and novel. Seizures precipitated by fever, alcohol, drugs and trauma are not considered to be reflex seizures. Reflex seizures occur in many epilepsy syndromes.

Light-induced seizures (photosensitive seizures) are by far the most common reflex seizures. Photosensitivity is a genetically determined trait. It can be assessed in the EEG laboratory by the response to intermittent photic stimulation (IPS). Normally IPS induces so-called 'photic following responses' which must not be interpreted as indicating photosensitivity. A number of abnormalities, both focal (nearly always occipital) and generalized, can be evoked by IPS in susceptible subjects and these may be associated with clinical photosensitivity. Of most significance is generalized spike and wave activity or multiple spikes, which continue for at least 100 ms after the train of flashes ends (Fig. 22.19). Light-induced seizures are most commonly generalized, particularly generalized tonic-clonic seizures, absences and myoclonic jerks. However, partial seizures, often but not exclusively with features suggesting occipital lobe onset, are increasingly recognized. Among the important clinical precipitants of light-induced seizures are television, video-games, VDU screens (which nevertheless are much less provocative than TV screens), discotheques (particularly stroboscopic lights), and natural flickering light, for example caused by light shining through trees or fences or reflected off water. Some people with light-induced seizures are also sensitive to specific patterns such as striped wallpaper and certain patterns on clothing. Very rarely pattern sensitivity can occur without photosensitivity. Some subjects who are photosensitive can, and habitually do, self-induce seizures. This may be achieved by waving the outstretched hand in front of the eyes, viewing provocative patterns, or watching TV sets extremely close up.

Light-induced seizures are particularly common in idiopathic generalized epilepsies. They occur in more than a third of children with juvenile myoclonic epilepsy and are universal in eyelid myoclonia with absences. Photosensitivity is also common in epilepsy with myoclonic-astatic seizures. In addition, many children with idiopathic generalized epilepsies, who have typical absence seizures, and do not fit within the patterns of currently recognized syndromes, have light-induced seizures. Their prognosis, in terms of remission of seizures, is much poorer than children with childhood absence epilepsy. Significant numbers of children and adults have focal seizures provoked by photic factors. *Idiopathic photosensitive occipital lobe epilepsy* is an epilepsy syndrome beginning in late childhood and adolescence. It is characterized by focal seizures with symptomatology suggesting occipital lobe onset (elementary visual symptoms, head and eye deviation, headache), often with secondary generalization. Seizures are provoked by visual stimuli and the interictal EEG shows occipital spike and waves and generalized or occipital photoparoxysmal responses on IPS.

Light-induced seizures are also characteristic of a number of symptomatic epilepsies and epileptic encephalopathies, including severe myoclonic epilepsy of infancy, Unverricht–Lundborg disease and Lafora disease.

Some subjects with photosensitive seizures may be able to avoid the provoking factor. Most, however, will require antiepileptic drug treatment. Sodium valproate is the 'standard' antiepileptic drug for photosensitivity. There is good evidence that levetiracetam, and to a lesser extent lamotrigine, are also effective. Other measures depend on the fact that photically induced seizures are more likely, the larger the area of retina stimulated. Hence TV should be watched from the maximum comfortable viewing distance and a remote control should be used to change channels. Fully covering one eye, or a light-polarizing screen or spectacles may be advised if the child cannot watch a TV or computer screen safely otherwise. Covering one eye may also be useful if the subject is caught unawares, for example at a disco if a strobe is suddenly used. TV should also be watched in a well-lit room. Factors such as fatigue and sleep deprivation are likely to also play a role and therefore photosensitive subjects should be advised to avoid watching TV or playing video-games for prolonged periods and if tired.

Primary reading epilepsy is a rare, probably genetically determined, epilepsy, which usually starts in late childhood and adolescence and is characterized mainly by jaw jerks, sometimes with spread, occurring while reading. Seizures may also be provoked by speaking. Interictal EEG is usually normal; an ictal recording is often easy to obtain.

Seizures evoked by unexpected auditory or somatosensory stimuli are most often encountered in children with symptomatic generalized epilepsies, who usually also have spontaneous seizures. They are sometimes seen in children with Down syndrome. Occasionally all seizures may be provoked by startle (*startle epilepsy*). The seizures are usually tonic but may be atonic or myoclonic. Obtaining an ictal EEG can be very helpful. Clonazepam is probably the most effective drug.

Seizures not necessarily requiring a diagnosis of epilepsy. This inelegant term is used to designate conditions in which recurrent epileptic seizures may occur (the usual pragmatic definition of an epilepsy), but in whom the term 'epilepsy' is, for a variety of reasons, inappropriate. The most important example is febrile seizures (the term 'febrile convulsions' is discouraged), which is distinguished from epilepsy principally to remove the stigma associated with epilepsy when describing a generally benign condition. A similar argument could be made for benign childhood epilepsy with centrotemporal spikes and Panayiotopoulos syndrome, which are equally self-limiting.

Febrile seizures are usually defined as epileptic seizures precipitated by fever (usually defined as above 38°C), not due to an intracranial infection or other definable CNS cause and not preceded by afebrile seizures. They are the most common form of epileptic disorder and affect about 3% of children. They generally occur between 6 months and 4 years of age, although younger and older children may be affected.[167] Prevalence in boys is slightly higher than in girls. Most febrile seizures are generalized tonic-clonic (or purely clonic) seizures. Focal and atonic febrile seizures also occur. A simple febrile seizure is generalized, lasts under 15 min and is not repeated during the same illness. Complex febrile seizures are focal and/or last over 15 minutes and/or recur during the same febrile illness. The focal nature of a febrile seizure may be revealed by a Todd paresis. Febrile status epilepticus is defined as lasting over 30 minutes. Approximately 6% of febrile seizures are prolonged, with 80% of these being the initial seizure.

Genetic factors are important in the etiology of febrile seizures.[168] Children of parents who had febrile seizures have a risk 4 times that of the general population and siblings of probands have a risk 3.5 times that of the general population. There is a high concordance in monozygotic twins. Polygenic inheritance, or autosomal dominant inheritance with reduced penetrance, are considered the most likely modes of inheritance. Although the usual definition of febrile seizures precludes children with known brain disorders, epidemiological studies have shown an increased risk of febrile seizures in children whose developmental milestones are slow (but not necessarily outwith the normal range). All infections which cause fever may be associated with febrile seizures, but some infections are more prominent. Roseola infantum (human herpes virus 6) and shigella dysentery are said to be associated with a particularly high risk of febrile seizures. Vaccinations, especially diphtheria, tetanus and pertussis (DTP) and against measles, may also be associated.[169] A rapid rise in the temperature is said to be important although data to prove this are lacking. However, it is certainly the case that febrile seizures often arise early in the course of the illness; it is often the first indication that the child is unwell.

The clinical skill in managing a child presenting with a suspected febrile seizure involves confirming that the event was probably epileptic, since a number of non-epileptic disorders (syncopes occurring during febrile illnesses, delirium and rigors) are commonly misdiagnosed as febrile seizures. It is important to exclude serious infections (particularly meningitis and encephalitis) in which both fever and seizures may occur. The evaluation must include a detailed history and examination. It is particularly important to obtain a detailed description of the attack and the circumstances in which it took place. Many children, when first seen, will have recovered and will be fully conscious. Febrile seizures are rare under 6 months of age and in this age group examination of the CSF is almost mandatory. Between 6 and 18 months febrile seizures are common but meningitis can present in this age group without meningism. Many authorities advocate lumbar puncture in all children in this age group presenting with a first febrile seizure;[168] meningitis often occurs in children with coexisting respiratory tract infections, including otitis media. However, the value of this approach has been questioned.[170] Beyond 18 months of age lumbar puncture can be avoided if there is no meningism and a clear focus of infection is found. Investigations, other than those looking for sources of infection, are generally not required. Children whose conscious level is impaired when first seen should be assessed along standard lines. The risk of inducing brain herniation is such that lumbar puncture should be delayed unless the subject is localizing pain, has no focal neurological signs and no papilledema. Recovery time following febrile seizures is generally shorter than for other seizures. The median time to full recovery following febrile seizures in a recent study was 18 minutes, compared with 1.35, 1.25 and 4.57 hours following idiopathic, remote symptomatic and acute symptomatic seizures respectively.[171] Apart from etiology, the only other factor which significantly affected (delayed) recovery was administration of 'rescue' medication. It is recommended that a child who has not fully recovered within an hour of a suspected epileptic seizure should be investigated and managed on the assumption that the seizure was acute symptomatic. Children are often admitted to hospital following their first febrile seizure. However, admission is not always necessary.[170] A reasonable alternative is for the child to be observed for several hours. If the child has fully recovered and a source of infection has been identified, s/he can be discharged, with advice given to the parents. Children with complex febrile seizures probably all warrant admission.

The overall prognosis for febrile seizures is excellent.[172] However, around one third will have at least one recurrence and 9% of children will have over three febrile seizures. The majority of recurrences occur within the year following the first seizure. Recurrences are more likely if the seizure has been complex, if there is a family history of febrile or nonfebrile seizures and if the initiating temperature for the seizure was relatively low. Meta-analyses have failed to show any benefit of continuous antiepileptic drug medication in preventing febrile convulsions and there is now almost universal agreement that it is not indicated.[172,173] The parents of children who have had febrile convulsions are generally given antipyretic advice, although this on its own offers poor protection from recurrences. Removal of excessive clothes and blankets is recommended. Occasionally tepid sponging may be useful, but cold baths and fans played directly onto the child should be avoided as they may increase core temperature. Antipyretic agents such as paracetamol and ibuprofen should be given. Intermittent prophylactic therapy with oral or rectal benzodiazepines has been advocated but is rarely used. Most authorities consider the most appropriate management is for the parents to have clear first aid instructions and advice as to when to call for emergency help. Depending on circumstances, it may be appropriate for the family to have a supply of either rectal diazepam or midazolam to be used nasally or buccally for prolonged seizures.[174–176] An important aspect of management is reassurance of the parents, who almost certainly will have been greatly traumatized by the event.

The risk of developing epilepsy in children who have had febrile seizures is increased compared to that of the general population. The risk is 2% at 5 years, 4.5% at 10 years, 5.5% at 15 years and 7% at 25 years.[177] The risk is greater if the febrile seizures started under the age of 1 year, in the presence of any preceding neurodevelopmental problem, if there is a family history of epilepsy and if the febrile seizures have been complex. Generalized epilepsies tend to follow when there is a family history of nonfebrile seizures and a large number of simple febrile seizures. Focal epilepsies are more common if there have been prolonged lateralized seizures. Although it is clear that the overall prognosis for children who have had febrile seizures, even if complex, is excellent, clinicians should avoid overoptimism. They should be particularly wary in cases where prolonged, often asymmetrical, febrile seizures have occurred in association with relatively mild febrile illnesses since this may be the herald of Dravet syndrome. In addition, the majority of children who

subsequently develop refractory mesial temporal lobe epilepsy have had prolonged, often lateralized febrile seizures. The intellectual and behavioral outcome of febrile seizures is excellent.[178]

The EEG has very little role to play in the management of febrile seizures. Within a week of the attack a variety of nonspecific abnormalities may be seen. In addition, various generalized or focal epileptiform abnormalities occur in the EEG of children who have had febrile seizures but are of poor prognostic significance.

Post-traumatic seizures are classified as early (occurring within a week of the trauma) and late. The former include immediate seizures, which occur within 24 hours of the injury. Only recurrent, late, post-traumatic seizures are considered a manifestation of epilepsy. Immediate and early post-traumatic seizures are much more common in children than in adults. They occur in up to 5% of all children and are usually focal, but can be generalized. In up to one fifth of cases they take the form of status epilepticus. Following severe head injuries the risk may be as high as 35%.[179,180] Late, post-traumatic seizures can occur at any time following the trauma but usually within 2 years. They are less common in children than in adults. In a large population-based study they occurred in 7.4% of children following head injury.[179] The risk is determined by the severity and type of head injury. There is no increased risk following mild closed head injuries. The risk is increased by early post-traumatic seizures, intracranial bleeding and depressed skull fracture. Both focal and generalized seizures can occur. Prophylactic antiepileptic drugs probably do not decrease the risk of developing late post-traumatic seizures and are not indicated.[181] Phenytoin is generally used in the acute situation for treatment and prevention of early post-traumatic seizures.

Seizures can occur as a complication of a large number of disturbances in body homeostasis. Generally these only occur while the disturbance persists and hence a diagnosis of epilepsy is inappropriate. They include seizures occurring during hyponatremia, hypocalcemia and hypomagnesemia. Seizures may also be a feature of uremia, the treatment of renal failure with dialysis and during renal transplant rejection. Epileptic seizures are a well-known feature of hypoglycemia; they may also occur during hyperglycemic comas in diabetic children. Epileptic seizures are also an occasional occurrence in individuals with a variety of endocrine disorders.

There are many children and adults who have only a single seizure during their lifetime, or else a cluster of seizures over a short period of time with no further seizures, or else very occasional seizures with long periods between seizures. These individuals do not warrant a diagnosis of epilepsy. They probably represent a heterogeneous group, with the milder forms of different types of epilepsy. Seizures are liable to occur during periods of emotional or physical stress such as at exam times, when sleep deprived, or when drinking unaccustomed alcohol.

DISEASES FREQUENTLY ASSOCIATED WITH EPILEPSY

Epileptic seizures occur in children with a huge range of different diseases and the manifestations of the seizures often show disease-specific characteristics. The following is a survey of some of the clinically relevant features of epileptic seizures as they manifest in diseases encountered in childhood. Comprehensive descriptions of many of these disorders are given elsewhere in this text.

The progressive myoclonic epilepsies[182]

Most pediatricians find the concept of the progressive myoclonic epilepsies a difficult one. Nevertheless they often undertake extensive neurometabolic investigations. These are to a large extent designed to detect the progressive myoclonic epilepsies. The conditions included are so rare that most pediatricians might see only one or two cases throughout their career. Their key characteristics are:

- An epilepsy characterized by myoclonic and other seizure types, including generalized tonic-clonic seizures. The seizures are often precipitated by factors such as touch, action or intention.

- Neurological problems, usually including cerebellar signs, and often progressive.
- Mental deterioration, of varying degrees, but often eventually leading to dementia.

These features typify the 'core group' of progressive myoclonic epilepsies. In other progressive myoclonic epilepsies atypical features are present while in some other progressive epilepsies, myoclonic seizures occur but are overshadowed by other manifestations. In the latter group the epilepsy is almost an incidental problem and its characterization is of limited value in recognizing the disorder. Included are: nonketotic hyperglycinemia; D-glyceric aciduria; Menke disease; Krabbe disease; Tay–Sachs disease; Sandhoff disease; and Niemann–Pick C disease.

The core conditions included in the progressive myoclonus epilepsies are:

- Lafora disease;
- Unverricht–Lundborg disease;
- sialidosis (types I and II);
- Gaucher disease (type III);
- neuroaxonal dystrophy;
- myoclonic epilepsy with ragged red fibers (MERRF);
- dentatorubropallidoluysian atrophy.

Lafora disease is an autosomal recessive disorder, common in the Mediterranean. Mutations on two genes (EPM2A and NHLRC1) have been shown to be responsible for most cases and there is evidence of the involvement of a third gene.[183] It usually presents between 6 and 19 years of age. Two features of the epilepsy are distinctive: (i) the precipitation of myoclonia by action and intention; and (ii) the occurrence of partial seizures with elementary visual phenomena. Mental and neurological decline with pyramidal, extrapyramidal and cerebellar signs appear, leading to early death. Diagnosis by molecular genetics may be possible but identification of so-called Lafora bodies on biopsy, particularly of apocrine sweat glands, may still be required. No specific treatment is available.

Unverricht–Lundborg disease (Baltic myoclonus/Mediterranean myoclonus) is an autosomal recessive disorder caused by a disease causing mutation in the CSTB gene on chromosome 21.[184] The age of onset is similar to that of Lafora disease. The distinctive features of the epilepsy are the precipitation of myoclonic seizures by maintenance of posture or intended movements and photosensitivity. Neurological and mental decline is usually very slow and prolonged survival is expected. Valproate is the treatment of choice; phenytoin is contraindicated as it appears to increase the rate of deterioration.

The *sialidoses* and *Gaucher disease type III* are lysosomal storage disorders caused by deficiencies of alpha neuraminidase and beta-glucocerebrosidase respectively. They present in childhood or adolescence with features of a myoclonic epilepsy and variable evidence of visceral storage and dysmorphism. Cherry red spots may be seen. Gaucher disease type III is characterized by horizontal ophthalmoplegia.

The extremely rare juvenile form of *neuroaxonal dystrophy* causes a progressive myoclonic epilepsy in late childhood or adolescence often with retinal degeneration. The pathological hallmark is the demonstration of axonal spheroids on rectal or skin biopsy.

Epileptic seizures occur in a number of mitochondrial disorders. However, the most characteristic is *MERRF* in which **m**yoclonic **e**pilepsy is associated with cerebellar signs, myopathy and often with other features seen in mitochondrial disorders. **R**agged **r**ed **f**ibers may be seen on muscle biopsy, but it can also be diagnosed on the basis of mitochondrial DNA mutations.

Dentatorubropallidoluysian atrophy (DRPLA) is an autosomal dominant disorder with anticipation due to a trinucleotide repeat on chromosome 12. It is mainly seen in adults from Japan but does occur in children and in non-Japanese. Features of progressive myoclonus epilepsy are combined with an extrapyramidal movement disorder and dementia. If the possibility of Huntington disease is being considered, think also of DRPLA.

Diseases in which features of progressive myoclonus epilepsy occur which are atypical or which are associated with other prominent manifestations include:

- the neuronal ceroid lipofuscinoses;
- poliodystrophies (Alper disease);
- childhood onset Huntington chorea (myoclonic variant);
- Hallervorden–Spatz disease;
- biopterin deficiency;
- other mitochondrial disorders including mitochondrial encephalomyopathy, lactic acidosis and stroke-like episodes (MELAS).

Special mention should be made of the *neuronal ceroid lipofuscinoses*.[185] These disorders were previously diagnosed pathologically and are characterized by the accumulation of ceroid lipofuscin in neurones. All the common forms can now be diagnosed enzymatically or by molecular DNA analysis. Epilepsy occurs in all forms of the disorder, but is a particularly prominent and early feature of the late infantile form which may be mistaken for the Lennox–Gastaut syndrome.

The neurocutaneous disorders

Many neurocutaneous disorders are associated with seizures (e.g. tuberous sclerosis, type 1 neurofibromatosis, Sturge–Weber syndrome, epidermal nevus syndrome, hypomelanosis of Ito and incontinentia pigmenti).

Brain malformations and maldevelopments

One of the major impacts of MRI has been the realization that many epilepsies arise as a consequence of malformations and maldevelopments of the brain (Fig. 22.22). Together these causes probably outweigh perinatal problems in the causation of neurodevelopmental problems. Milder disorders may be silent. When overt they present with combinations of mental retardation, cerebral palsy and epilepsy.

A large number of conditions may be associated with abnormalities of cortical development (previously usually called neuronal migration disorders). These include: metabolic diseases such as peroxisomal disorders and Menke disease; chromosomal disorders including Edwards (trisomy 18), Patau (trisomy 13), Down (trisomy 21), Smith–Magenis (deletion 17p) and Wolf–Hirschhorn (deletion 4p) syndromes; neuromuscular diseases including some forms of congenital muscular dystrophy and myotonic dystrophy; neurocutaneous syndromes; multiple congenital anomaly syndromes and infective and toxic causes. Among the latter prenatal cytomegalovirus infection and fetal alcohol syndrome merit special mention.

Heterotopias, including periventricular, subcortical and laminar (or band) heterotopias; agyria-pachygyria, including lissencephaly types I and II and focal pachygyria; polymicrogyria; schizencephaly and hemimegalencephaly are migrational disorders and are often highly epileptogenic, giving rise to focal or generalized seizure disorders, including epileptic spasms. Agenesis of the corpus callosum is also commonly associated with seizures. Aicardi syndrome is an X-linked dominant disorder almost confined to females. The brain abnormality is complex with agenesis of the corpus callosum (in most but not all cases), periventricular heterotopias, variable dysplasias of the cortex and ependymal cysts. Choroidal lacunae, often with coloboma of the optic discs, are a characteristic feature. Severe mental retardation and epileptic spasms are characteristic.

Cortical microdysgenesis implies a postmigrational defect in cortical organization. It comprises minor malarrangements and malorientations of cells within the cortex and is postulated to be a substrate for seizures in some children. It is not diagnosable in life.

The epilepsy complicating cerebral maldevelopments and malformations is for the most part treated along standard lines. Children with focal cortical malformations may be candidates for resective surgery. Hemimegalencephaly, a cause of catastrophic epilepsy in infancy, may be treated by hemispherectomy.

Brain tumors

Brain tumors are an uncommon, but important and potentially curable, causes of epilepsy in children. Slow growing tumors of the cerebral hemispheres, such as low-grade astrocytomas, oligodendrogliomas, gangliogliomas and gangliocytomas are more likely to present with seizures than are malignant tumors. Diagnosis may be delayed for many years. Seizures are mainly focal, but generalized seizures, with generalized EEG abnormalities, are well recognized. Intellectual ability and neurological examination is often normal. Treatment may be expectant if seizures are controlled by antiepileptic drugs and no tumor growth is observed on serial brain scans. However, surgery often offers a good hope of cure. Gelastic seizures, which often begin in infancy or early childhood, are characterized by laughter, usually without an appropriate affect. They are strongly suggestive of tumors of the floor of the third ventricle, especially hypothalamic hamartomas. Unfortunately these tumors are not easily resected, although there have been encouraging recent reports. Intractable epilepsy, mental retardation, behavioral problems and endocrine problems are frequent. Dysembryoplastic neuroepithelial tumors (DNET) are benign supratentorial tumors which are often located deep in the temporal or frontal lobes and are often associated with intractable focal seizures (Fig. 22.22). Treatment is usually by resection. Recently, angiocentric neuroepithelial tumors (ANET) have been described as a new tumout type associated with childhood seizures.[186] Treatment for brain tumors with surgery and radiotherapy may also give rise to epilepsy.

Although most brain tumors will be apparent on CT, especially if contrast is used, some may be missed. MRI is superior and is the imaging method of choice.

Cavernous angiomas

These are thin-walled clusters of dilated blood vessels whose commonest manifestation is focal epilepsy, often intractable. They may be revealed on CT by areas of calcification. MRI is superior. They are often not apparent on angiograms. Minor bleeding is common; major bleeds are uncommon but occur. Some progressively enlarge and act as space-occupying lesions. Treatment is surgical if the lesion is accessible. Radiotherapy is an alternative.

Genetic or presumed genetic disorders

Numerous chromosomal and other genetic disorders feature seizures as a prominent or occasional manifestation. Some have already been mentioned.

Angelman syndrome is complicated by epilepsy in up to 90% of children. The characteristic jerky movements of the upper limbs and trunk which gave rise to the eponymous name 'happy puppet syndrome' (a term which may cause parents distress) are caused by a unique form of cortical myoclonus which is reported to respond to piracetam. Epileptic seizures can start at any time from childhood to young adult life, but usually begin in infancy and early childhood. Epileptic spasms are rare. Seizure types include generalized tonic-clonic seizures, clonic seizures, myoclonic seizures, atypical absences and focal seizures, possibly with occipital lobe onset.[187] It may present as West or Lennox–Gastaut syndrome. Episodes of nonconvulsive status epilepticus or myoclonic status epilepticus are relatively common and may be recurrent. They are particularly troublesome in early to mid childhood. The severity of the epilepsy often appears to subside in later childhood. A more or less characteristic interictal EEG with high amplitude posterior slow waves with or without spikes has been described but is not always present. Most authorities favor treatment with broad-spectrum antiepileptic drugs or drugs useful against generalized seizures such as sodium valproate, lamotrigine and ethosuximide. Benzodiazepines are useful against episodes of status. Carbamazepine may cause myoclonic and absence seizures.

Rett syndrome is an X-linked dominant mental retardation disorder due to mutations on the MECP2 gene. Epileptic seizures are particularly associated with the third or 'pseudostationary' period of the disease, from about 2 to 10 years of age. Atypical absences are particularly prominent but partial and generalized tonic-clonic seizures also occur. Hyperventilation is a particularly striking feature of the condition. It may provoke atypical absences but many of the phenomena associated with the hyperventilation are probably non-epileptic; certainly the response to antiepileptic drugs is poor. Seizures often show spontaneous improvement or even resolution in later childhood or adolescence. Atypical forms of Rett syndrome may present with epileptic seizures including epileptic spasms.[188]

Fragile X syndrome is associated with epilepsy in about a fifth of affected boys. The epilepsy is usually mild with relatively infrequent seizures and a tendency for remission in the teenage years. Both focal and generalized seizures are described. The EEG often shows paroxysmal abnormalities similar to those seen in benign childhood epilepsy with centrotemporal spikes.

PEHO (progressive encephalopathy with edema, hypsarrhythmia and optic atrophy) syndrome is a rare, probably autosomal recessive, disorder presenting in early life with drug-resistant epileptic spasms, retardation, hypotonia, blindness and optic atrophy. The children are generally almost immobile and have characteristic peripheral edema. Progressive microcephaly and marked cerebellar atrophy are other features. A PEHO-like syndrome, lacking the neuroradiological features and optic atrophy, is also described.

Ring chromosome 20 is now recognized as causing a characteristic epilepsy, often with normal development prior to onset of seizures followed by learning difficulties. These include focal and secondary generalized seizures, seizures with frontal lobe semiology and episodes of nonconvulsive status epilepticus.[106]

Metabolic disorders[189]

Virtually all the metabolic disorders which occur in childhood are associated with seizures. However, these are rarely the major feature and certainly the characteristics of the epilepsy are rarely of significance in establishing the correct diagnosis. Important exceptions to this are:

- *Nonketotic hyperglycinemia* in which early myoclonic seizures and Ohtahara lsyndrome are characteristic. Diagnosis is made by demonstrating a raised absolute or relative (to blood and urine) CSF glycine level.
- *Vitamin responsive seizures* – pyridoxine (vitamin B_6) dependent seizures have been recognized for many years.[190] They typically begin in the neonatal period or infancy, but may begin prenatally (revealed by hiccups) or up to early childhood. Any seizure type, including epileptic spasms, may occur and frequently become intractable. They respond poorly to conventional antiepileptic drugs. Usually a dramatic cessation of seizures occurs on the intravenous administration of pyridoxine (doses of 40–300 mg). However, this may cause profound apnea and some authorities suggest giving a trial of oral pyridoxine. The condition is autosomal recessive but its cause remains elusive. Recently, children have been described with early onset seizures, often with encephalopathic features, who fail to respond to pyridoxine but respond to either pyridoxal phosphate or folinic acid. It is now recommended that trials of these vitamins are given early to neonates and infants with intractable seizures. Diagnosis may be aided by CSF neurotransmitter studies.
- *Biotinidase deficiency*. This autosomal recessive disorder can present in the neonatal period, or beyond, with isolated seizures or seizures in association with skin rashes, alopecia, ataxia and various other neurological abnormalities. It can be detected by the production of a characteristic organic aciduria but more reliable and widely available is testing for deficiency of biotinidase in the blood. Seizures respond to biotin replacement.
- *Glucose transporter deficiency* presents with seizures in infancy and is associated with a deficiency in the transport of glucose across the blood–brain barrier. It is detected by an abnormally low CSF : blood glucose ratio (< 0.45) (preferably tested for after a 4-hour fast) and responds to the ketogenic diet.

Cerebral palsy[191]

Cerebral palsy is not a disease, but a collection of conditions characterized by abnormalities of movement and posture, caused by nonprogressive disorders of the developing brain. Epilepsy has been estimated to occur in 10–40% of cases, but its likelihood depends on the type of cerebral palsy. Cerebral palsy involving damage to the cerebral cortex has a high risk for the development of epilepsy. Hence spastic hemiplegic and quadriplegic cerebral palsy are often accompanied by seizures, while these are rarer in spastic diplegic, dyskinetic and ataxic forms of cerebral palsy. Some studies suggest that nearly all children with spastic quadriplegic cerebral palsy develop epilepsy. Various types of seizure may occur. However, in hemiplegic cerebral palsy, focal motor seizures, often with a Jacksonian march, and secondary generalized tonic-clonic seizures are characteristic. In quadriplegic cerebral palsy generalized seizures (both primarily and secondarily generalized) predominate. Some such children develop epileptic encephalopathies, such as the Lennox–Gastaut syndrome. Startle seizures are relatively common in children with severe forms of cerebral palsy.

MANAGEMENT OF CHILDHOOD EPILEPSY

General principles

In the UK the National Institute for Health and Clinical Excellence (NICE) (www.nice.org.uk) and the Scottish Intercollegiate Guidelines Network (SIGN) (www.sign.ac.uk) provide detailed advice on the diagnosis and management of epilepsy in children.

Education is the cornerstone to the management of children with any form of seizure disorder. Children, and more especially the families of children, who have had a first epileptic seizure, particularly if convulsive, will almost certainly have been extremely frightened. Initial reassurance should allay the fear that seizures are likely to be life threatening and/or cause brain damage. However, it is wrong to trivialize what has occurred. It is also a mistake to suggest that the attack is unlikely to ever happen again. This is a reasonable hope but is an unreasonable expectation. Education should cover the following points:

- An explanation of the terms 'epileptic seizure' and 'epilepsy'. This should stress the multiplicity of conditions covered by the latter and the huge range in their 'seriousness'.
- A specific explanation as to what type of seizure disorder the child has or may have.
- The impact this is likely to have on the child's future. A frank acknowledgment of uncertainties, which are often considerable, is appropriate.
- Treatment options available.
- 'First aid' measures to be taken in the event of further seizures, including detailed advice as to when medical help should be summoned.
- An exploration of the role of possible precipitants and measures which might be taken to reduce the risk of recurrence.
- Sensible restrictions which should be considered to ensure the child's safety and restrictions which are not required.
- What to tell other people, including the child's school.

The clinician should also explore the family's own beliefs about seizures and epilepsy. Highly prejudicial attitudes are surprisingly common and may require to be challenged directly.

Written and video information is usually greatly appreciated and all clinicians involved in treating a child with epilepsy should have access to a range of suitable material. Charities and self-help societies produce high-quality material, which is usually free or obtainable at nominal expense. Guiding families to useful websites is increasingly important as is the need for clinicians to counteract misleading Internet information.

A number of factors are likely to lower the seizure threshold in anyone with a seizure disorder. Knowledge of these is relevant to all children with epilepsies, although they operate most powerfully in the idiopathic generalized epilepsies. They include fatigue, sleep deprivation, emotional stress and anxiety, excitement, hunger and alcohol.

Undue restrictions are often imposed on children with epilepsy.[192] These have the potential to lead to overdependence in later life. The principal dangers are from drowning and falls. A child with continuing seizures (this might reasonably be defined as a daytime seizure within the last year) should be closely supervised during swimming by a responsible adult capable of rescuing the child if a seizure occurs in the water. A 'buddy system' helps supervision. Similarly baths for younger children should be supervised and showers encouraged for older children. Climbing, unless protected, is ill-advised. Cycling on busy roads should be avoided if seizures are active. Otherwise cycling with a helmet poses few additional dangers. Most other sports and leisure activities should be encouraged unless there is clear evidence of an increased risk. Detailed advice about individual sports can be obtained from the websites of Epilepsy Action (www.epilepsy.org.uk) and the National Society for Epilepsy (www.epilepsynse.org.uk).

Teenagers with epilepsy should be given the opportunity to discuss issues regarding sex, genetic implications, fertility, contraception and teratogenicity. The same websites provide up to date information regarding driving and employment issues in the UK.

Finally the clinician should be aware that most parents who have lost a child with epilepsy report that they would have wished to know about the increased mortality of children with epilepsy.

Nondrug treatment and intermittent drug treatment

Although antiepileptic drugs play an important part in the management of children with seizure disorders, there are many children in whom regular antiepileptic drug treatment is not or may not be required. This includes:

- Children who have had a single seizure or who only have infrequent seizures.
- Children whose seizures have occurred in the context of a temporary state, for example during a period of hyper- or hyponatremia, or immediately after a head injury; acute treatment with antiepileptic drugs may be required but these should be withdrawn quickly.
- Children with febrile seizures.
- Children whose seizures are all provoked by a stimulus which can reasonably be avoided.
- Children with certain benign focal epilepsies characterized by infrequent seizures, often at night, causing minimal disturbance and with a high probability of remission. This includes many children with benign childhood epilepsy with centrotemporal spikes and Panayiotopoulos syndrome.

Consideration should be given as to whether, as part of an overall regimen to be followed if seizures occur, an antiepileptic agent should be provided for intermittent use in the event of prolonged convulsive seizures. Diazepam administered rectally has until recently been most often used. Midazolam administered bucally, sublingually or nasally is an alternative and a clinical trial found bucal midazolam to be superior to rectal diazepam.[176] Convulsive seizures generally last less than 2 minutes and it is therefore appropriate to recommend administering the drug either if the seizure lasts longer than usual or after 2 minutes.

Antiepileptic drug treatment

There are a large number of antiepileptic drugs available to treat seizures in children. Before prescribing an antiepileptic drug the prescriber needs to consider:

- its efficacy in the particular type of epilepsy;
- potential adverse effects;
- possible interactions with other drugs, including other antiepileptic drugs and the contraceptive pill;
- route of elimination (essential knowledge if prescribing to children with renal or hepatic impairment);
- its ease of use (related to formulations available, dosing frequency and need for monitoring of levels and other parameters).

Much of our knowledge concerning the efficacy of antiepileptic drugs in humans is derived from clinical observation. The older agents were introduced at a time when classification mainly consisted of a division into grand mal and petit mal seizures. All the new drugs were introduced into clinical practice following trials mainly in adults with focal seizures. These were designed to obtain licensing approval for the drugs rather than to help guide clinical practice. Some antiepileptic drugs have a wide spectrum of action across both generalized and focal epilepsies. These include sodium valproate, lamotrigine, topiramate, levetiracetam and zonisamide. Phenobarbital is also broad spectrum but may exacerbate absences. Other drugs, notably carbamazepine, vigabatrin, gabapentin, tiagabine and probably also pregabalin and, to a lesser extent, phenytoin are narrow spectrum agents with efficacy principally against focal epilepsies; they may exacerbate generalized epilepsies. However, vigabatrin has unique activity against epileptic spasms and all seizure types in tuberous sclerosis. Ethosuximide is active against absences and to a lesser extent atonic and myoclonic seizures. Piracetam is mainly used for cortical myoclonus, for example in Angelman syndrome. The benzodiazepines and acetazolamide are usually used as adjunctive agents in children with refractory focal and generalized epilepsies. Clonazepam may be particularly useful against myoclonic seizures. Historically, nitrazepam has tended to be used for treating epileptic spasms.

All antiepileptic drugs have potentially serious adverse effects. These are reviewed in detail elsewhere.[193] Here, only those adverse effects seen commonly or which are likely to influence prescribing habits are discussed.

All antiepileptic drugs are psychoactive and all have the potential to cause unwanted CNS effects such as drowsiness, sedation, dizziness and ataxia. However, such effects are more likely, even with standard dose regimens, with carbamazepine, phenytoin, phenobarbital, topiramate and the benzodiazepines than with sodium valproate and lamotrigine. Both phenobarbital and phenytoin are considered to impair cognitive function (impaired concentration, decreased motor speed and memory problems) even at normal dosages. Behavioral adverse effects, including hyperactivity and aggression, have been particularly reported with phenobarbital and vigabatrin, one reason for the sharp decline in phenobarbital usage in developed countries. Overall studies on the effects of other agents have been reassuring[194] but the clinician must always be alert to the potential deleterious effect on cognitive function of antiepileptic drugs in individual children. Many antiepileptic drugs, but notably sodium valproate, lamotrigine and ethosuximide, cause gastrointestinal upsets, particularly pain, nausea and vomiting. Hypersensitivity reactions, particularly rash, generally occur within a few weeks of starting the drug, but may occasionally be delayed. There is in particular a problem with lamotrigine, which has been associated with a widespread erythematous rash and Stevens–Johnson syndrome. If this occurs, the drug must be immediately discontinued. The risk of it occurring can be substantially reduced by slow titration, particularly in children also on sodium valproate. Rash is also regularly encountered with carbamazepine, oxcarbazepine, phenytoin, phenobarbital and zonisamide.

A few drugs have more or less unique adverse effects. These include: hair thinning and loss, weight gain and tremor with sodium valproate; appetite suppression and weight loss with topiramate and zonisamide; renal calculi with topiramate, zonisamide and acetazolamide; anhidrosis and hyperthermia with zonisamide and topiramate; and constriction of the visual fields with vigabatrin. The latter appears to be common and irreversible. Because of it, vigabatrin should only be used to treat epileptic spasms, seizures in tuberous sclerosis and those children in whom other options have been exhausted. In those treated and who have a mental age of over 7 years detailed assessment of visual fields every 6–12 months is recommended.[195] Carbamazepine and oxcarbazepine can both cause hyponatremia, although this is rarely severe.

Of the rare, potentially fatal adverse effects of antiepileptic drugs, particular attention has been paid to blood dyscrasias with phenobarbital, phenytoin, carbamazepine and ethosuximide, and to severe hepatic toxicity with sodium valproate. The origin of the latter is poorly understood. It is especially common in infants with developmental delay treated with multiple antiepileptic drugs. An underlying metabolic disorder may be implicated and the drug should be avoided where such conditions seem likely. It is unrelated to the mild hyperammonemia seen in many subjects treated with the drug and cannot be predicted by blood tests taken prior to or after starting the drug.

Long-term cumulative adverse effects do not occur with the commonly prescribed agents but phenobarbital and phenytoin can cause connective tissue disorders and metabolic bone disease with the latter also being associated with a cerebellar syndrome, intellectual blunting, coarsening of the facies, gum hypertrophy (partially avoidable with good oral hygiene) and hirsutism.

Many of the commonly prescribed antiepileptic drugs interact with other antiepileptic drugs and with non-antiepileptic drugs. Many interactions are rarely of clinical importance. In general, interactions between antiepileptic drugs either lower the effective concentration of one or both of the drugs increasing the risk of seizures or raise the plasma level of one of the drugs (or a metabolite) increasing the risk of toxicity. These effects can occur at the time of drug withdrawal as well as when a new drug is introduced. At such times, the clinician must carefully evaluate whether adjustments to the dosages of concomitantly prescribed antiepileptic drugs are needed. Carbamazepine (and oxcarbazepine), phenytoin and phenobarbital are enzyme inducers and increase the metabolism of other drugs eliminated by the liver. The effect is of significance when one or other of these drugs are administered together and also when they are administered with sodium valproate, lamotrigine and topiramate. Carbamazepine also causes significant autoinduction and hence carbamazepine levels often fall after a few weeks treatment. Enzyme inducers may also cause significant interactions with other prescribed drugs; most notably they decrease the effectiveness of the oral contraceptive pill.

Sodium valproate inhibits the hepatic metabolism of many antiepileptic drugs. In most cases this is of little significance. However, it causes an effective doubling of the half-life of lamotrigine. Clinically significant increases in the plasma levels of phenobarbital may also occur.

Phenytoin is a difficult drug to use for a number of reasons. Besides being an enzyme inducer, it has zero order pharmacokinetics, which means that small changes to the dose can lead to marked changes in plasma levels. It is also extensively protein bound. This means that other protein-bound drugs may cause rises in the unbound fraction of the drug by displacing phenytoin.

Unexpected carbamazepine toxicity may arise as a consequence of inhibition of its metabolism by macrolide antibiotics such as erythromycin. It also occasionally occurs due to inhibition of the metabolism of its pharmacologically active epoxide residue by sodium valproate and lamotrigine.

Vigabatrin, gabapentin, tiagabine, piracetam and levetiracetam are relatively free of significant interactions.

Knowledge about the elimination of antiepileptic drugs is useful to the clinician both because it helps predict possible interactions and is essential when treating children with hepatic or renal impairment. Carbamazepine, phenytoin, sodium valproate, lamotrigine, ethosuximide, oxcarbazepine, the benzodiazepines and tiagabine are all exclusively or predominantly eliminated by hepatic metabolism. Vigabatrin, gabapentin, levetiracetam, pregabalin and acetazolamide are excreted unchanged by the kidneys. Phenobarbital, topiramate and zonisamide are eliminated both by hepatic metabolism and by the kidneys.[196]

Although there have been numerous trials, particularly of the newer antiepileptic drugs, many of these were conducted primarily for licensing purposes and have limited relevance to the clinician in helping to choose between available options. To a considerable extent the way in which clinicians use antiepileptic drugs is based upon the results of uncontrolled clinical studies, their own experience and the advice of trusted colleagues. Table 22.11 details the author's practice aided by the published experience of respected experts.[118,197,198]

Using antiepileptic drugs

The decision to initiate treatment with an antiepileptic drug should not be taken lightly. Treatment is likely to be prolonged and the risk of adverse effects is significant. Treatment should only be started after a diagnosis has been made. A therapeutic trial of an antiepileptic drug in children in order to confirm the diagnosis of epilepsy should be avoided. The risk of treating a child who does not have epilepsy with multiple antiepileptic

Table 22.11 Suggested dosage regimens for antiepileptic drugs available in the UK. These are likely to vary from the manufacturers' published information. Many of these drugs are unlicensed or have restricted licences for use in children in the UK

Antiepileptic drug	Initial dose (mg/kg/day)	Usual maintenance dose (mg/kg/day)	Dosage interval	Comments
Carbamazepine	5	10–20; may be up to 30	bd	Liquid and chewtab preparations as well as tablets; slow release preparation has significant advantages
Sodium valproate	10	20–30; occasionally up to 40	bd	'Chrono' preparation has limited advantages
Phenytoin	<3 yr – 8 >3 yr – 5	As determined by response and levels	od or bd	Liquid, tablets and capsules available. Prescribe by brand to avoid bioavailability problems
Phenobarbital	5	5; occasionally up to 10	od	
Ethosuximide	10	30–40	bd	
Acetazolamide	5	0–1 yr – 10 >1 yr – 20–30	bd	
Clobazam	0.25	0.25–1.0; occasionally up to 2.0	bd	
Clonazepam	0.01	0.05; occasionally up to 0.3	bd or tds	
Nitrazepam	0.05	0.25–1.0	bd	
Vigabatrin	40	60–80; up to 180 in epileptic spasms	od or bd	Sachets of dissolvable powder available
Lamotrigine	Monotherapy – 0.5	Monotherapy – 2–10; occasionally up to 15	od or bd	Dispersible tablets available
	With enzyme inducers – 1.0	5–15	bd	
	With sodium valproate – 0.2	1–5	od or bd	
Gabapentin	15	30–90	tds	Only capsules available
Topiramate	1.0	4–10	bd	Sprinkle granules available
Tiagabine	0.1	0.3–1.5	tds	Only tablets available
Oxcarbazepine	20	50–90	bd	Only tablets available
Levetiracetam	10	20–40	bd	
Zonisamide	1	4–8; occassionaly up to 12	bd	

drugs is high. Because of their high prevalence, children with seizure disorders are often treated by clinicians whose knowledge and experience of epilepsy is limited. In developed countries, it should be considered unacceptable to treat a child for epilepsy unless the clinician can recognize the common types of seizure disorders, has access to suitable investigational facilities, including EEG and MRI, and has a reasonable knowledge of the available treatments. All children with rare, atypical or unclassifiable seizure disorders, seizure disorders which require special investigational facilities (such as video-EEG) or treatments (such as steroids) or whose seizures continue despite initial treatment should be assessed by a clinician with a special expertise in the epilepsies.

All children should initially be started on monotherapy. Use of more than one drug increases the risk of adverse effects. Large studies of children with new-onset seizures have failed to show a convincing difference in efficacy between the standard antiepileptic drugs.[199,200] A systematic review concluded that there is no evidence to support the choice of sodium valproate compared to carbamazepine in generalized epilepsies.[201] However, this emphasizes the limitations of overreliance on such studies since there is compelling evidence that carbamazepine may aggravate some generalized epilepsies in which it should be considered contraindicated.[144] Most authorities consider that sodium valproate is the drug of first choice for generalized epilepsies (whether idiopathic or symptomatic). This was supported by a recent randomized controlled trial ('SANAD') comparing sodium valproate with lamotrigine and topiramate in both children and adults.[202] Some authorities recommend lamotrigine in teenage girls because of concerns about weight gain, decreased fertility and the teratogenicity of sodium valproate. However, lamotrigine also has significant adverse effects including teratogenicity.

The wide spectrum of activity shown by levetiracetam, its relative lack of significant adverse effects and its ease of use make it a very attractive choice. However, licencing considerations and the lack of safety data in pregnancy still need to be considered. Ethosuximide is an alternative for childhood absence epilepsy but is less well tolerated. Carbamazepine is generally considered the drug of first choice for most focal seizure disorders, including secondary generalized epilepsies. Some support for this practice was found in a systematic review comparing carbamazepine and sodium valproate monotherapy.[201] However, sodium valproate is a suitable alternative for the benign focal epilepsies of childhood. Recently a randomized controlled study of children and adults (SANAD) concluded that lamotrigine was superior to carbamazpine, lamotrigine, gabapentin, topirmate and possibly oxcarbazepine for focal seizures.[203] However, the numbers of children included appears to have been relatively small since the median age was 38 ± 18 years and only 1.4% had idiopathic focal seizures. Moreover carmamazepine was superior to lamotrigine in terms of efficacy but caused more adverse effects leading to discontinuation. This may have reflected the rapid dose titration recommended for carbamazepine. Sodium valproate is usually the drug of choice for photosensitive seizures; levetiracetam and lamotrigine are alternatives. If it has not proved possible to distinguish focal from generalized seizures reliably it is sensible to treat with a broad spectrum agent such as sodium valproate to avoid the possibility of exacerbating generalized seizures.

When initiating treatment, it is generally advisable to start with modest doses and to build up the dose as required. This reduces the risk of adverse CNS and gastrointestinal unwanted effects. Although many clinicians aim to achieve a 'target dose', seizure control may be achieved at remarkably low doses in some children. The manufacturers of some drugs recommend measurement of various blood parameters prior to initiating, and during, therapy in order to avoid/detect early adverse effects. However, there is no evidence that this is effective and is rarely necessary.[204] Similarly blood monitoring of antiepileptic drug levels, although widely available, is usually unhelpful. The so-called target ranges for individual drugs are defined according to the levels at which a majority of responders to the drug achieved seizure control. Significant numbers of children will respond at lower or higher levels and unwanted effects may occur at levels within the therapeutic range, or may not occur despite levels being considerably above the range. Most epileptologists rarely perform antiepileptic drug levels, relying instead on careful clinical monitoring of wanted and unwanted effects. Exceptions to this are:

- with phenytoin, whose complex pharmacokinetics means that level monitoring can often be helpful;
- in children in whom detection of unwanted effects may be difficult. This is particularly the case in those with severe learning difficulties;
- as a check on compliance.

The limitations of blood levels should be appreciated. For drugs such as phenytoin, in which there is significant binding to plasma proteins, it is the free drug which is of importance both in terms of efficacy and safety. Measurement of the total plasma concentration may be misleading in circumstances in which there is altered protein binding. Saliva levels, though not widely available, may be more relevant.

A majority of children treated with antiepileptic drugs will become seizure free and most should be subsequently withdrawn from antiepileptic medication. However, the maxim of withdrawing treatment after two seizure-free years is an oversimplification.[205] The best predictor of relapse is the epilepsy syndrome. Relapse is rare in benign childhood epilepsy with centrotemporal spikes and benign childhood occipital epilepsy (Panayiotopoulos type) and almost certain in juvenile myoclonic epilepsy. Relapse rates are intermediate for other commonly encountered syndromes. Other predictors, all imperfect, of the likelihood of relapse are age (greater risk with onset of seizures in infancy or very early childhood), symptomatic etiology, EEG abnormalities (photosensitivity appears to be strongly correlated with relapse) and severity of epilepsy prior to control being achieved.[206] The decision as to whether antiepileptic drugs should be withdrawn needs to be an individual one based on a detailed analysis with the child and family which takes into account the likely consequences should a relapse occur. For all children with epilepsies in whom there is a good prospect for successful withdrawal (benign focal epilepsies, childhood and to a lesser extent juvenile absence epilepsy) withdrawal should be attempted after two seizure-free years, or even earlier.[207] Persisting EEG abnormalities, except in the idiopathic generalized epilepsies and if there is photosensitivity, should not unduly influence this decision. For children with epilepsies which have proved difficult to control a longer period free of seizures (perhaps 2–5 years) is advisable. It is probably not justified in recommending drug withdrawal in juvenile myoclonic epilepsy or photosensitive epilepsies in children who remain highly photosensitive on EEG testing.

Children who have been on benzodiazepines and barbiturates for anything other than brief periods are usually withdrawn very slowly over many months or even years as the risk of withdrawal seizure is considered high, although this has recently been questioned.[208] Other drugs are usually withdrawn over short periods such as 1–2 months. The evidence base for these recommendations is poor.[209] Detailed instructions as to what measures to take should a seizure occur during withdrawal should always be given. Some families appreciate being provided with an agent such as diazepam or midazolam for emergency use. However, they should be reassured that status epilepticus is extremely rare during antiepileptic drug withdrawal.[206] Overall the risk of relapse in children withdrawn from antiepileptic drugs is around 20% at 6 months, rising to 35% at 4 years.[206] Relapses usually occur within a year of withdrawal. If seizures recur during or after withdrawal the drug should generally be restarted and the prospect of regaining control is very good but not assured.[209–211]

If the child fails to respond to an antiepileptic drug it is important to reconsider the diagnosis: misdiagnosis of epilepsy remains a major problem. Sometimes a child will have responded to a drug but intolerable unwanted effects cause it to be stopped. It is usually easy in this situation to choose a suitable alternative. If, however, seizures have not been controlled despite pushing the first drug to the limit of tolerability or to the maximum reasonable dose then a second drug should be tried as monotherapy. A study found that 42% of children who failed on initial monotherapy subsequently had a complete remission on other agents.[212] Different clinicians vary in how this is achieved. Some prefer to wean off the first drug as the new drug is being introduced. However, if some response has occurred this may lead to an increase in seizures. The alternative approach is to introduce the second drug while maintaining the child on the first drug. The dose of the first drug may need to be adjusted. When seizures have been controlled the first drug can be withdrawn. The difficulty with this approach is that there is often an understandable reluctance to alter things once seizures have been controlled. For generalized epilepsies, assuming that sodium valproate has been tried initially, appropriate second line choices are lamotrigine, topiramate and levetiracetam.[213] However, for childhood absence epilepsy ethosuximide would be an alternative. Moreover, in juvenile myoclonic epilepsy if absences and generalized tonic-clonic seizures are completely controlled but myoclonic jerks remain problematic a small dose of a benzodiazepine, such as clonazepam, is a suitable alternative. For focal epilepsies, assuming carbamazepine has been the first line drug, a large number of suitable second line agents, including sodium valproate, are now available and it is not possible to give a blanket recommendation. All the recently introduced drugs have been shown in double-blind, placebo-controlled trials to be efficacious against partial seizures. Moreover systematic reviews have concluded that gabapentin, lamotrigine, topiramate, levetiracetam and oxcarbazepine are effective at least in the short term as add-on treatment in children with drug-resistant focal epilepsies.[214–219] However, there are very few studies reported comparing them 'head-to head'. When a child has failed to respond to two suitable major antiepileptic drugs pushed to their maximum dose, the chances of achieving complete seizure control rapidly diminishes. Many different strategies exist but a number of principles should be emphasized:[220]

- There is evidence that control is sometimes better with two and occasionally three antiepileptic agents. However, there is no evidence that four antiepileptic drugs are ever appropriate.
- If more than one drug is to be used the approach taken should be rational. Some combinations of drugs are more appropriate than others. For example when treating drug-resistant focal seizures it may be wise to use combinations of drugs with different modes of action. Moreover, drugs with similar adverse effects such as benzodiazepines and phenobarbital should be avoided.
- Polypharmacy has many potential problems: increased risk of adverse effects; risk of exacerbating seizures, particularly if drowsiness is a problem; risk of drug interactions causing all the drugs to be at subtherapeutic levels – drug levels may be helpful.
- The aim of therapy is to improve quality of life not necessarily to render the child totally seizure free.
- The diagnosis should be re-evaluated periodically. Pseudoseizures should be among the considerations.
- Compliance may need to be checked.
- If seizures are only being reported by one party the possibility of 'misreporting' by the carer to gain attention or benefits should be considered. Seizures are commonly reported in factitious and induced illness.
- A systematic approach should be adopted whereby each agent tried is given an adequate trial before deciding that it is ineffective.

In children with drug-resistant epilepsies thought should be given to trying less conventional medication such as short courses of steroids or ACTH and immunoglobulins. Anecdotal evidence suggests that these may be effective in individual children.

The ketogenic diet[221]

Ketogenic diets have been used in the treatment of drug-resistant epilepsies for decades. It has not been established if they are particularly indicated for any particular seizure or epilepsy syndrome type and have been advocated for children with drug-resistant seizures of any type and from any cause. However, they should be avoided in children with mitochondrial diseases, particularly pyruvate carboxylase deficiency. A recent review concluded that approximately half of children will half their seizures, and about one third will have one tenth their baseline seizures.[221] The mechanism of action remains obscure. All ketogenic diets aim to induce ketosis by providing the child's caloric needs predominantly as ketogenic foods (fats). The classic (4:1) diet uses 4 g of fat to every 1 g of nonketogenic foods (protein and carbohydrate). The medium-chain triglyceride and the modified medium-chain triglyceride diets utilize medium-chain triglycerides, which are more ketogenic and hence allow a lower ratio of fats to other foods to be given. The diet is usually initiated by fasting in hospital with the aim of achieving and maintaining 3–4+ ketonuria. Acetazolamide and topiramate should be withdrawn first because severe acidosis may occur. Other antiepileptic drugs are usually continued, at least initially. A skilled dietitian is essential. Unwanted effects include hypoglycemia (usually only a problem when the diet is first initiated), hunger and thirst, weight problems, antiepileptic drug toxicity and renal stones. The diet must be kept strictly; even sugar-containing medicines can reduce its efficacy. Regular monitoring of growth and of blood electrolytes, liver function tests, lipids, proteins and full blood count is generally advocated. If successful, the diet is usually continued for at least 2 years. It should be stopped gradually.

The Atkin diet is reported to be effective in some children with refractory epilepsy.[222]

The vagal nerve stimulator

This is a relatively new technique involving intermittent stimulation of the left vagus nerve in the neck. A pulse generator is implanted subcutaneously in the upper chest. Leads convey electrical impulses from it to the vagus nerve and are then transmitted up the nerve to the nucleus solitarius. The antiepileptic action of vagal nerve stimulation is poorly understood, but presumably relies on projections from the nucleus solitarius to cortical and subcortical structures. The generator is programmed using a PC and 'wand' to give chronic intermittent stimulation. A systematic review concluded that vagal nerve stimulation appears to be an effective and well-tolerated treatment for focal seizures.[223] There is currently no clear indication as to which children with refractory epilepsy should be offered this treatment. There is as yet no large randomized study reported from children but a median reduction in seizures of up to 43% has been reported in a small group with epileptic encephalopathies.[224] Very few children become seizure free. Efficacy appears to improve with time.

Epilepsy surgery

A significant minority of children with medically refractory epilepsy can benefit from surgery both in terms of improved seizure control and overall quality of life. All children with seizures continuing, despite medical treatment, should be evaluated in a center with the facilities and expertise to assess their suitability for surgical treatment. Epilepsy surgery can be resective or functional. The former involves removing epileptogenic tissue, aiming to 'cure' the epilepsy. The latter modifies brain function in order to interrupt the transmission of epileptic discharges. Its aim is to improve seizure control, to modify seizure type or to minimize the deleterious effects seizures can have on cerebral function.

The evaluation and selection of children for any type of epilepsy surgery is multidisciplinary, involving pediatric neurologists, neurophysiologists, neuropsychologists, neuroradiologists, nuclear medicine physicians and child psychiatrists as well as the neurosurgeon. Severe learning difficulties and behavioral problems are relative, but not absolute, contraindications to surgery.

A prerequisite of resective surgery is that seizures are focal in origin or arise from one cerebral hemisphere. Identification of the seizure focus involves integration of multiple sources of data. In all cases this involves:

- A detailed clinical assessment. Seizure sociology along with the findings on neurological examination may give useful information regarding seizure localization.
- Detailed scalp EEG studies. These will include interictal and ictal recordings with recordings during awake and sleep. Video-EEG is essential and it is usual to try to capture a number of the child's habitual seizures.
- High quality structural imaging with MRI; the prospects for surgery are considerably enhanced if a structural lesion can be identified.
- Neuropsychological evaluation. This may provide further useful information on the likely lateralization and even localization of the epileptic focus. In addition it seeks to identify cerebral dominance for speech and to give a baseline of the child's cognitive abilities.

If the data from these studies are congruent it is often possible to proceed to surgery without further investigations. However, if the site of the epileptic focus is still unclear further investigations are carried out. These may include:

- semi-invasive EEG studies (foramen ovale or sphenoidal electrodes);
- functional neuroimaging usually with ictal SPECT or interictal PET;
- invasive EEG studies using subdural grids of electrodes or depth electrodes.

In older children and teenagers undergoing resective surgery it is usual to establish the dominant hemisphere for language and memory. Traditionally this has been by the invasive carotid amytal test. Increasingly functional MRI and magnetencephalography are being used. Resecting a temporal lobe in which memory resides would result in a dense amnesia.

The majority of resections in both adults and children are of the temporal lobe. However, whereas in adults mesial temporal sclerosis is the predominant pathology, in children, tumors, cortical dysplasias and other focal pathologies are also relatively common.[225] In the Maudsley series of 41 children 15 years or younger 80% became seizure free. There was no mortality and series morbidity occurred in only 1–2%.[225] Extratemporal resections are less commonly performed and the outcome poorer with seizure free rates of well under 50%.[226]

Hemispherectomies and multilobar resections are performed considerably more often in children than in adults. They are indicated for some of the catastrophic epilepsies of infancy such as Sturge–Weber syndrome and hemimegalencephaly. Hemispherectomy is the treatment of choice in Rasmussen disease and has been used to treat severe epilepsies due to extensive unilateral infarctions. It is generally reserved for people with already established hemiplegias. Depending on the underlying pathology, up to 70–80% of children become seizure free.[227]

Functional procedures include callostomy, stereotactic lesioning (e.g. with the gamma knife) and multiple subpial resection. The indications for callostomy are still disputed. However, it is generally reserved for children with seizures presumed to be of focal onset but in whom rapid bilateral synchrony occurs. It seems to be most effective against atonic drop attacks. Few children become seizure free, but in many the seizures postoperatively are less disabling. Significant neuropsychological deficits may occur, particularly if the posterior part of the corpus callosum is divided. Multiple subpial transection involves sectioning horizontal cortical fibers thought to be responsible for seizure propagation, leaving vertically orientated fibers, responsible for normal function, intact. It has mainly been used in the Landau–Kleffner syndrome.

STATUS EPILEPTICUS

This is conventionally defined as an epileptic seizure lasting for more than 30 minutes or frequent seizures for the same period without recovery of consciousness between seizures. Convulsive status epilepticus (CSE) in childhood is a life-threatening condition with serious risk of neurological sequelae[228-230] and constitutes a medical emergency. Although the outcome from an episode of CSE is mainly determined by its cause, the duration of CSE is also important. In addition, the longer the duration of the status, the more difficult it is to terminate.[230,231] Treatment of convulsive seizures lasting more than 5 minutes is recommended in order to prevent the development of CSE.

Data from epidemiological studies suggest that 4–8 children per 1000 have an episode of CSE before the age of 15 years[232] and 17% of children with seizures present with CSE as their first unprovoked seizure.[233] CSE in children has a mortality of approximately 4%.[234] Neurological sequelae of CSE (epilepsy, motor deficits, learning difficulties and behavior problems) are age dependent, occurring in 6% of those over 3 years but in 29% of those under 1 year.[233] Important causes of CSE are febrile seizures and those with epilepsy in whom antiepileptic drug treatment is being modified. Idiopathic CSE is also relatively common.

An evidence-based approach to the prevention/treatment of CSE is shown in Figure 22.24.[235] Initial management should follow the ABC principle of resuscitation. Midazolam, used buccally, is more effective and as well tolerated as rectal diazepam[176] and is preferred by the carers. High flow oxygen should be given and the blood glucose measured by stick testing. It is important to emphasize that not all episodes of apparent status epilepticus are in fact epileptic. A brief history and clinical examination

should therefore be undertaken to confirm that the seizure activity is likely to be epileptic and not, for example, a drug-induced dystonic reaction, a tonic spasm due to raised ICP or a psychogenic (pseudo-epileptic) attack.

If the seizure does not rapidly respond to initial treatments, or if there is significant respiratory, cardiovascular or neurological compromise, the child should be intubated, artificially ventilated and treated in an intensive care setting. Monitoring of vital signs, including pulse, blood pressure and blood gases, is essential to ensure that a hypoxic-ischemic insult is not added to the direct effects of the status epilepticus. A small number of children will continue to convulse despite treatment with thiopental (refractory CSE). The most appropriate subsequent anticonvulsant management is unclear. Regimens using continuous intravenous agents such as midazolam[236] and inhalational anesthetic agents such as isoflurane[237] have been reported but are not fully evaluated.[238] During CSE, depletion of intracellular energy stores in muscle may lead to reduction in muscle activity. This may be misinterpreted as 'the seizure settling down', whereas the cerebral activity and damaging metabolic derangements are continuing. Careful examination, and EEG, if available, will help determine if there is ongoing seizure activity.

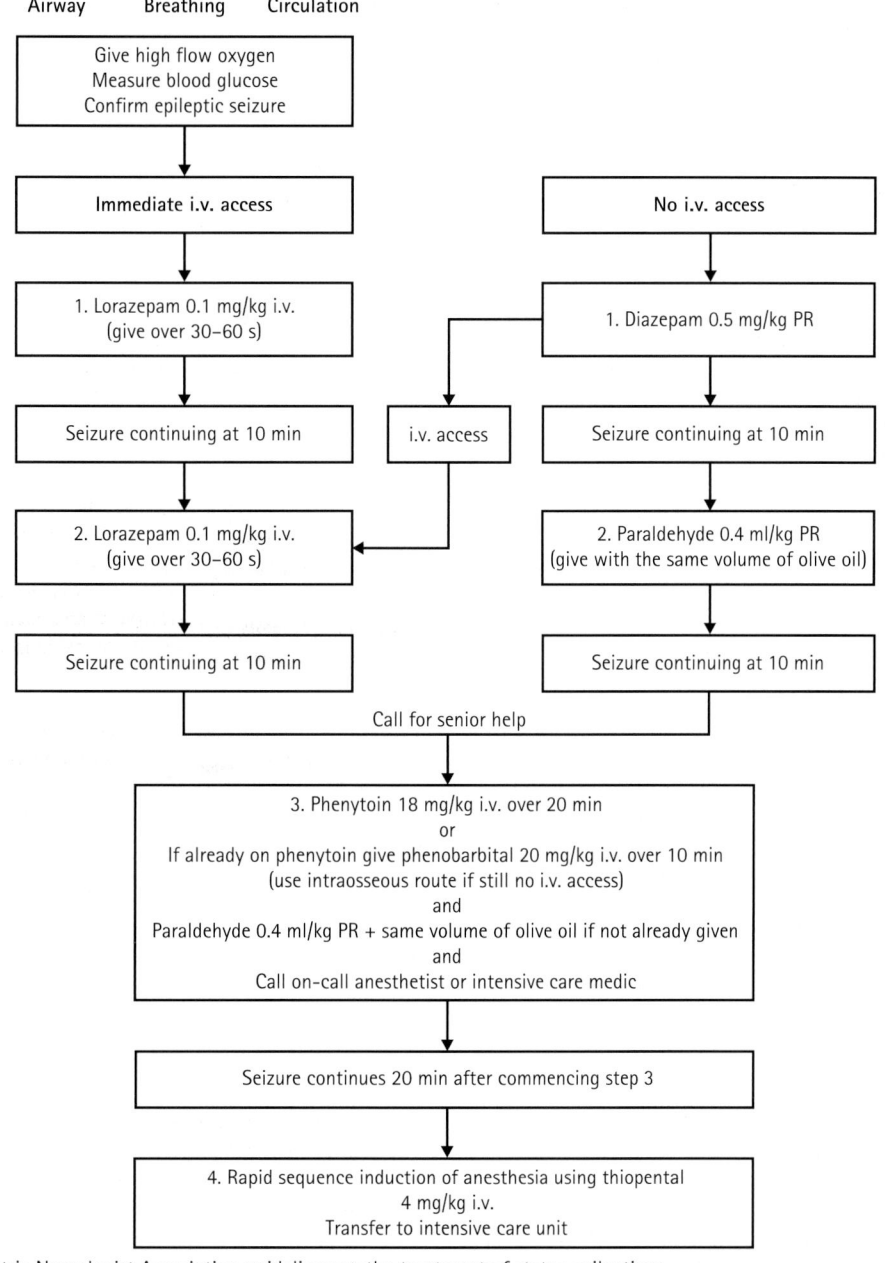

Fig. 22.24 British Paediatric Neurologist Association guidelines on the treatment of status epilepticus.

Impairment of consciousness following a seizure is common. This postictal impairment is easy to diagnose if the seizure has been witnessed, but may present difficulties if it has not. Although the coma score may be very low, supportive care is usually all that is required, provided steady improvement is documented. A cause for the seizure such as hypoglycemia or infection should be sought. Drug treatment with agents such as lorazepam and diazepam will greatly prolong the recovery period.

Nonconvulsive status epilepticus (NCSE) may present as a child with reduced conscious level. The child has continuous, or very frequent absence, atypical absence or complex partial seizures so that an enduring epileptic state is present. The child is unaware, or has severely impaired awareness, is ataxic, drooling and uncommunicative and may manifest minor jerks and myoclonus. This seizure state rarely happens as the first manifestation of epilepsy. It is usually seen as part of an epileptic encephalopathy such as the Lennox–Gastaut syndrome, but can occur in idiopathic epilepsies and may be provoked by inappropriate antiepileptic drug treatment, such as giving carbamazepine to children with absences. The parents or carers will often be aware of the cause of the impaired consciousness. An EEG will usually show continuous spike and wave activity. There is not the same degree of urgency in treating nonconvulsive as compared to convulsive status epilepticus. However, prolonged episodes of nonconvulsive status epilepticus have been linked to intellectual decline. Oral, rectal and intravenous benzodiazepines or steroids are often used. Occasionally benzodiazepines may provoke tonic status epilepticus.

In a child who has had seizures as part of their encephalopathy the possibility that subclinical or subtle seizures are continuing to impair consciousness should be considered. Such seizures may be difficult to detect and an EEG or continuous EEG monitoring may be required. The decision as to whether to treat an abnormal EEG without clear clinical seizure activity is a difficult one. In practice it is often possible to correlate EEG abnormalities with subtle seizure signs or physiological changes. Overtreatment of EEG abnormalities may prolong recovery of consciousness unnecessarily.

NONEPILEPTIC PAROXYSMAL DISORDERS

The conditions described here are frequently misdiagnosed as epilepsy. Their recognition is important, not only to avoid this, but because they are important conditions in their own right, requiring investigation and explanation. Moreover, for many, specific and effective treatments exist. The reader who requires more information is referred to Stephenson unique text.[239]

Syncopes and anoxic seizures

A syncope or faint is a sudden loss of consciousness and postural tone caused by a cessation in the supply of energy substrates to the cerebral cortex. The latter is usually a result of hypoxia or reduced cerebral perfusion or a combination of both. An anoxic seizure is a non-epileptic seizure caused by syncope. In effect, it is a severe form of syncope. The clinical features consist of an initial loss of consciousness and postural tone (this phase may be brief) followed by tonic stiffening and/or clonic movements. If an EEG is recorded during an anoxic seizure it shows slowing, followed by flattening during the tonic phase, followed by the reappearance of slow waves, often coinciding with clonic jerks. No epileptiform abnormalities are seen. It should be noted that there are no unique features of syncopes and anoxic seizures that reliably distinguish them from epileptic seizures: eye rolling, tongue biting and urinary incontinence occur in both. Moreover, although many syncopes are short, both these and reflex anoxic seizures can be prolonged. Postictal drowsiness can follow epileptic seizures, syncopes and anoxic seizures. It is the circumstances in which syncopes and anoxic seizures occur which often allows them to be distinguished from epileptic seizures. However, in some cases definite distinction requires prolonged polygraphic recording.

The commonest forms of syncope are *simple faints* or *vasovagal syncopes*. The most important distinguishing feature is the circumstance of occurrence, which is often stereotyped for the individual. Common provoking factors are stress, emotion and upright posture, especially in confined spaces. Older children may recount initial symptoms of light-headedness, heat and graying of vision. Abdominal pain is also said to be common. During the attack the child is usually pale, limp and the pulse may be slow. Attacks may occur when supine. Clonic limb movements, sometimes asymmetrical, are common and postictal confusion may occur. There is often a family history of similarly affected relatives. Head-up tilt testing may help if the diagnosis remains in doubt. Vasovagal syncopes are considered to arise as a consequence of a vasodepressor mechanism, sometimes combined with vagally mediated cardio-inhibition. *Vagovagal syncopes* in which a reflex bradycardia or asystole follows vagal stimulation by swallowing or vomiting are more rare. Syncopes can also arise due to *orthostatic hypotension*, rare in children but more common in adolescence.

Reflex anoxic seizures (also known as reflex asystolic syncope) are a relatively common form of syncope in young children. The precipitant is usually a minor bump to the head provoking a vagally mediated cardiac asystole, which may last many seconds. Clinically the child simultaneously loses consciousness and becomes floppy and extremely pale (pallid syncope). Subsequent tonic stiffening and clonic movements are common. Although the heart quickly restarts the loss of consciousness may be prolonged. Reflex anoxic seizures should be distinguished from *breath-holding attacks (blue syncopes, prolonged expiratory apnea)*. The pathophysiology of these relatively common attacks is still incompletely understood, but they are not behavioral in origin. They are provoked by fright, pain, anger or frustration. Crying is followed by the breath being held in expiration. Cyanosis and loss of consciousness follows. Although there may be a short period of limpness, characteristically tonic stiffening follows. Iron therapy, especially if there is iron deficiency, may be helpful.

Anoxic seizures, probably of all types, can exceptionally be followed by true epileptic seizures, usually with sustained generalized clonic jerking.[240]

All the syncopes discussed so far are benign, although attacks similar to breath-holding attacks occurring in some neurologically impaired children may not be so. Reassurance and explanation is all that is generally required. Simple faints wax and wane in their frequency, often being particularly troublesome in the teenage years. Most, but not all, infants with reflex anoxic seizures and breath-holding attacks eventually become free of the attacks in mid to late childhood. Specific treatment is not required although some advocate the use of atropine in reflex anoxic seizures. When very severe, these may also be helped by cardiac pacing.[241]

Some forms of syncope are less benign. Retarded children sometimes provoke 'drop-like attacks' by a *Valsalva maneuver*. Occasionally these have been fatal. *Gastroesophageal reflux* occasionally provokes apnea, sometimes followed by an anoxic seizure. The mechanism may be vagally mediated cardiac inhibition or laryngospasm and appears to be a feature of the awake state. Whether this is one cause of apparent life-threatening events and sudden infant death syndrome is controversial. Treatment is of the gastroesophageal reflux.

Cardiac syncopes are important and potentially life threatening.[242] Syncopes and anoxic seizures can be a manifestation of various cardiac arrhythmias and of structural heart disease. Particularly important to recognize are the *prolonged QT syndromes*. These ion channel disorders are characterized by anoxic seizures occurring during exercise and sleep. They are potentially fatal. In most but not all cases the corrected QT interval (QTc) is greater than 440 ms. If the clinical history is suggestive but the QT interval on a standard EEG is normal, prolonged ECG monitoring and exercise ECG is indicated.

Craniocervical junction disorders such as Chiari malformations may be associated with apneas and syncopes occurring during activities which increase intracranial pressure.

Imposed suffocation is a relatively common manifestation of *Munchausen syndrome by proxy*.[243] Attacks all begin in the presence of the perpetrator, usually the mother. Others may witness the conclusion of the attacks.

Movement disorders and related conditions[244]

A large number of paroxysmal movement disorders occur in children and can be mistaken for epilepsy. The *episodic ataxias* are familial ion channel disorders.[80,132,245,246] Episodic ataxia provoked by factors such as startle or exercise often provides the clue to diagnosis and may be isolated or coexist with a variety of other problems, including epilepsy. They may respond to acetazolamide. Two types are distinguished. In type 1 (EA1) attacks last seconds or minutes and myokymia is present between attacks. It is associated with mutations on the potassium channel gene KCNA1. In type 2 (EA2) attacks are longer lasting and there may be associated cerebellar signs. It is associated with mutations on the calcium channel gene CANA1A and is allelic with familial hemiplegic migraine and spinocerebellar atrophy type 6. A variety of conditions are described in which paroxysmal dystonia or dyskinesia or choreoathetosis occurs. The two best characterized conditions are *paroxysmal kinesigenic choreoathetosis* and *paroxysmal nonkinesigenic choreoathetosis*, both of which are autosomal dominant. The former is characterized by very frequent short episodes, unilateral or bilateral, of dystonia or choreoathetosis provoked by sudden movement. Although not an epilepsy, it frequently responds to antiepileptic drugs such as carbamazepine and phenytoin. The nonkinesigenic form is characterized by less frequent, longer attacks precipitated by stress, coffee or alcohol. It may respond to clonazepam. A third type – *paroxysmal exercise-induced dystonia* – is associated with dystonia coming on 10–15 minutes after exercise and lasting 5–30 minutes. It may respond to acetazolamide.

Benign myoclonus of infancy may be mistaken for epileptic spasms. The movements are more sustained than in true myoclonus and benign; non-epileptic infantile spasms and shuddering attacks are alternative names. It is unrelated to *benign neonatal sleep myoclonus* which is relatively common and frequently mistaken as epileptic. It is characterized by repetitive, usually rhythmic jerks of one or more limbs in sleep.

Various abnormal head movements are described. These include repetitive *head bobbing* and *banging*. The latter sometimes occurs in understimulated children. *Tics* are occasionally confused with seizures.

Paroxysmal vertigo, occurring in children between 1 and 5 years of age, and manifest as the child suddenly appearing distressed, pale and unsteady, sometimes with nystagmus, may be related to *benign paroxysmal torticollis of infancy*. In the latter repeated attacks of distress, vomiting and head tilt occur. In turn both conditions may be related to migraine.

Benign paroxysmal tonic up-gaze of childhood is usually seen in infancy and presents with prolonged episodes of sustained or episodic up-gaze. It may respond to L-DOPA. Learning difficulties are very common.

Sandifer syndrome refers to dyskinetic neck movements occurring in children with gastroesophageal reflux often in association with hiatus hernia.

Drug-induced dystonic reactions, including oculogyric crises, are seen with psychotropic drugs, particularly the phenothiazines and metoclopramide. Intravenous benzotropine or a benzodiazepine will abort attacks.

Tetany with carpopedal spasm and laryngospasm is a manifestation of hypocalcemia or hypomagnesemia, both of which can also cause epileptic seizures.

Hyperekplexia

This is usually an autosomal dominant condition; less commonly it is recessive. It is caused by mutations in subunits of the glycine receptor. It is conventionally divided into major and minor forms. The latter is manifested by generalized hypertonia (which may lead to an erroneous diagnosis of cerebral palsy) and excessive startles to auditory, visual and somatosensory stimuli. In the major form there are, in addition, attacks of severe tonic stiffening with apnea. These can be life-threatening. Excess startle can also be symptomatic of a number of other conditions.[247]

A useful diagnostic test is nose-tapping which causes an excessive and reproducible startle. Clonazepam and valproate are useful. In addition, the forced flexion maneuver consisting of sudden flexion of the head and limbs can be life saving during severe apneic attacks.

Paroxysmal extreme pain disorder (previously called familial rectal pain syndrome)

This is a rare, usually autosomal dominant condition, which is probably manifest throughout life and is caused by mutations on genes coding for the sodium channel SCN9A.[248] It is characterized by discrete attacks with marked autonomic features. The most prominent of these is the sudden onset of excruciating pain that can be generalized or localized to sites such as the rectum, genitalia and face. Harlequin color changes may be conspicuous. Some attacks may be associated with severe apnea and asystole. The risk which these pose is unknown. Many attacks are unprovoked but triggers include startles, defecation, wiping of the nappy area, urination, eating and drinking. Carbamazepine is of some benefit.

Sleep disorders

A number of different movement disorders related to sleep are described. These include benign neonatal sleep myoclonus, periodic movements of sleep, restless leg syndrome, jactatio capitis nocturna (repetitive head banging), hypnagogic jactitations (myoclonic jerks, usually of the legs, on falling asleep) and nocturnal myoclonus. These are all benign phenomena and except for restless leg syndrome, require reassurance only.

Night terrors are occasionally confused with frontal lobe seizures. They occur in infancy and early childhood and are associated with partial arousal from deep slow sleep. They usually occur early in the night and are manifested with the child screaming as if terrified. Although appearing awake, the child cannot be consoled and appears not to recognize his parents. There is no recollection next morning. *Nightmares* are a phenomenon of rapid eye movement sleep. *Sleepwalking* and *sleep talking* often occur together, usually in older children and adolescents who previously had night terrors. Again reassurance is all that is required along with advice about sensible safety precautions. *Hypnagogic hallucinations and illusions*, usually visual or auditory, occur in the transitions between wakefulness and sleep and are considered normal phenomena. *Restless leg syndrome* occasionally occurs in children. It usually responds to L-DOPA.

Narcolepsy is usually an autosomal dominant disorder which in its full form features:[249]

- excessive daytime sleepiness with frequent daytime naps;
- cataplexy, i.e. attacks of sudden loss of tone causing falls in full consciousness, often precipitated by laughter or excitement and misdiagnosed as epilepsy;[250]
- hypnagogic hallucinations;
- sleep paralysis manifested by attacks of inability to move or to move a limb occurring as the subject is wakening.

The disorder is probably underdiagnosed in childhood as it is usually manifested only as excessive daytime sleepiness with frequent daytime naps, the other features appearing in adolescence and adult life. However, its recognition is important as it can lead to school failure.

The diagnosis is essentially clinical. However, multiple sleep latency studies can offer confirmatory information. Subjects with narcolepsy have a short latency for entering rapid eye movement sleep and may pass straight into it from the awake state. In addition there is a very strong association with HLA-DQB1 0602, present in up to 98% of subjects. Recently narcolepsy has been shown to be associated with greatly reduced CSF levels of the neuropeptide hypocretin which is produced in the hypothalamus. This is likely to become the preferred diagnostic test. It is important to exclude nocturnal hypoventilation, a much commoner cause of daytime sleepiness than narcolepsy. The most important aspect of management of narcolepsy is ensuring that the family and school understand the nature of the condition and that the child has an appropriate period of night-time sleep (paradoxically night-time insomnia can be a problem), along with daytime naps. It is sensible to present the most important educational material early in the day when the child is likely to be at its brightest. Amphetamines have traditionally been the main pharmacological agent used to treat excessive sleepiness in narcolepsy but modafinil is being increasingly preferred. Imipramine and clomipramine can be useful in cataplexy. More recently sodium oxybate has been shown to be particularly efficacious.[251] There is evidence that eary treatment of narcolepsy/cataplexy with immunoglubulins may be disease modifying.[252]

Psychological and psychiatric disorders

Many different psychological and psychiatric disturbances can present as paroxysmal episodes and are important in the differential diagnosis of epilepsy. *Masturbation* occurs at all ages and may be more or less obvious. In young girls it often involves adduction of the thighs and rhythmic hip flexion. The child is characteristically vacant, rigid and flushed. Other gratification phenomena are described and are manifested with stereotyped behaviors during which the child appears withdrawn. *Daydreams* are particularly prone to misinterpretation by school teachers. They occur when bored or fatigued and generally involve the child's attention gradually drifting away.

Hyperventilation is relatively common, especially in teenage girls. It provokes sensations of light-headedness, chest pain and paresthesiae. It may also be manifested with carpopedal spasm as in tetany. Hyperventilation is often a symptom of anxiety and may be helped by psychological intervention. Milder cases may be helped by rebreathing into a paper bag.

Non-epileptic attack disorder (*pseudoseizures*) occur in mid and late childhood and adolescence. Some are easily distinguished from epileptic seizures while in others the distinction may be extremely difficult. Pseudoseizures may mimic any type of epileptic seizure, including status epilepticus. There are no hard and fast rules whereby epileptic and pseudoseizures can be reliably separated. However, movements in the latter are usually thrashing and semipurposeful rather than rhythmic clonic jerks. In addition, in epileptic seizures the eyes nearly always open within seconds of the attack. Induction by suggestion can be very helpful. A major difficulty is in distinguishing frontal lobe seizures from pseudoseizures. Pseudoseizures are probably most common in children who also have epileptic seizures. However, they also occur in children who had epileptic seizures but whose seizures have stopped and in children who have never had an epileptic seizure, although a friend or relative may.

An ictal EEG recording which shows no epileptiform abnormalities is suggestive, but not conclusive, evidence of pseudoseizures; the ictal EEG is often normal during, for example, frontal lobe seizures and elementary focal seizures. Measurement of serum prolactin levels is occasionally useful, levels increasing after generalized tonic-clonic seizures and some focal seizures, but not usually after frontal lobe seizures or elementary focal seizures. It is crucial to have an accurate baseline measurement and to take the sample at the appropriate time after the start of the seizure.[253]

Confidently distinguishing between epileptic seizures and non-epileptic attack disorder may be impossible, even after extensive history taking and detailed investigations. However, if the latter seems more likely it is inappropriate to treat with antiepileptics in the hope that it might be. It must be accepted that even the best clinician will be mistaken from time to time. What is required is the honesty to review the diagnosis if the management offered fails. All children who have or are suspected of having non-epileptic attack disorder require the input of a child psychologist or psychiatrist. Often there is no serious underlying psychological or psychiatric problem and the prognosis is excellent. However, children who are, or have been, abused physically or sexually may present in this way.

Other conditions to consider in the differential diagnosis of paroxysmal disorders include the effects of *substance abuse, early-onset schizophrenia* with hallucinations and attacks of *rage* seen in older children and adolescents.

Other neurological conditions

Migraine may be confused for epilepsy and vice versa. Some epileptic seizures, particularly of occipital lobe origin, superficially resemble migraine attacks. In addition, given that both conditions are relatively common, it is not surprising that some children will be encountered with both conditions. Both migraine and some forms of epilepsy are regularly provoked by endogenous and exogenous factors. Therefore, it is likely that occasionally a migraine will provoke an epileptic seizure and vice versa. Exceptionally a severe migraine may result in an ischemic lesion, which acts as an epileptic focus.

Alternating hemiplegia of childhood is a rare disorder which begins within the first year of life, usually with brief tonic attacks, often unilateral with eye movement abnormalities, accompanied by general misery.[254] Shortly after attacks of alternating hemiplegia begin and are usually frequent. They may be provoked by various triggers. A striking feature is disappearance of the hemiplegia with sleep, often with its reappearance shortly after awakening. Although some response to flunarizine is reported, the condition is progressive with mental retardation and a variety of motor problems. Structural neuroimaging is normal.

HEADACHE AND MIGRAINE

HEADACHE

Headache is one of the most common health complaints in childhood. It is reported by children from infancy to adolescence and from all ethnic and socioeconomic backgrounds. The predisposition to headache, commonly, continues through adulthood.[256] Population-based studies of schoolchildren, between 5 and 15 years, showed that 66% suffered at least one episode of headache during a 1-year period and in 22% the headache was severe enough to interfere with normal activities.[257] The prevalence of headache increases steadily with age reaching around 90% at age 12–13 years.[258] The prevalence rate in preschool children is difficult to ascertain, but it is not unusual for parents of older children with migraine to describe attacks dating back to the first year of life. The prevalence rate of headache doubled from 13% to 26% between age 3 and 4 years in a population of an urban general practice in the UK[259] reaching a peak of 40–50% during the first year at school followed by a slight drop in the following 1–2 years.[260]

Headache is benign and infrequent in many children. At least 40% of schoolchildren, over the age of 11 years, use over-the-counter painkillers to treat their own headache,[261,262] and parents often treat their children's headaches inappropriately. A study of 100 caregivers showed that only 30% were able to determine the correct dose of paracetamol and to accurately measure the intended dose.[263] Advice may be sought from a wide variety of medical professionals (general practitioners, general pediatricians, pediatric neurologists, neurosurgeons, child psychiatrists, ENT surgeons and ophthalmologists) and from complementary therapists.

Headaches can be classified according to clinical presentation, duration of illness and frequency of attacks as acute, recurrent or chronic (Table 22.12).

Acute headaches

Children often present with single or isolated attacks of headache which are commonly associated with other symptoms indicating an underlying focal or systemic illness. In one survey in 150 unselected children attending an accident and emergency department causes were classified as upper respiratory tract infections (57%), migraine without aura (18%), viral meningitis (9%), brain tumor (2.6%), ventriculo-peritoneal shunt dysfunction (2%), intracranial hemorrhage (1.3%), postictal headache (1.3%), post-concussion (1.3%) and undetermined causes (7%).[264] In a primary care setting febrile illnesses were also the main causes of acute headache in 634 children (56.8%).[265]

Chronic headaches

Children usually present with at least 3 months history of constant headache or a headache with a fluctuating intensity, but with no periods of complete recovery. Chronic headaches are rare in children, but brain tumors are the main concern to the parents and their pediatricians. Headache is rarely the only complaint and other symptoms may be more prominent.

Table 22.12 Main causes of headache in children and adolescents

Acute headaches
Viral illnesses: respiratory, gastrointestinal and flu-like illnesses
Bacterial infections: tonsillitis, pharyngitis, sinusitis, pneumonia
Intracranial infections: viral or bacterial meningitis, encephalitis
Intracranial bleeding
Head trauma
Others

Recurrent headache
Migraine: migraine without aura, migraine with aura, complicated migraine
Tension-type headache: episodic tension headache, chronic tension headache
Short-lasting unilateral headaches: cluster headache, neuralgias
Others

Chronic headache
Raised intracranial pressure: brain tumor, hydrocephalus, idiopathic intracranial hypertension
Hypertension
Substance induced: intoxication, medications

Others

Recurrent headaches

Recurrent headaches are defined as those occurring over a period of at least 3 months. Idiopathic or primary headache is the most common and is separated by periods of complete normality. In a population-based study,[257] migraine (with or without aura) was the most common cause accounting for 77.2% of cases. Other causes were episodic and chronic tension headache in 11.7%, nonspecific headache in 9.7% and headache associated with illnesses such as asthma, hay fever, allergy and constipation in 1.5%. Similar causes, but with different proportions, are reported in children attending specialist clinics; 35% migraine (28% without aura, 5% with aura and 2% hemiplegic migraine), 38% tension headache (22% chronic and 16% episodic), 10% mixed migraine and tension headaches, 12% unclassified and 5% due to other causes or combination of causes.[266]

Clinical classifications of recurrent headache

The 1988 International Headache Society's (IHS) classification of headache and facial pain and the revised second edition in 2004 are the most widely used and tested criteria particularly for migraine and tension headache.[267,268]

The classification and diagnostic clinical criteria suggest a disease continuum[269] with features such as the pain quality, site of maximal intensity, severity and the number and nature of the associated symptoms during attacks determining the clinical diagnosis. Tension type headache is commonly mild to moderate in intensity, dull aching in nature, poorly localized or described as affecting the whole head. It is rarely associated with other sensory, vasomotor or gastrointestinal symptoms. Episodic tension-type headache with its infrequent attacks may represent the mild end of the headache spectrum while at the extreme end of the spectrum the pain during migraine attacks is more intense (moderate or severe), more localized (unilateral or frontal), throbbing or stabbing in character and is associated with a variable number of sensory, vasomotor or gastrointestinal symptoms. Migraine without aura can bear similarities to episodic tension type headache with some blurred borders separating the two conditions midway in the headache spectrum. Migraine with aura at the extreme end of the spectrum has a well-defined symptom constellation that may also include complicated attacks of migraine with dysphasia, hemiplegia or prolonged aura. The concept of the headache continuum encompassing all types of headache into one clinical spectrum has provoked wide interest, but is not universally accepted.[270]

Evaluation of the child with recurrent headaches

A specific diagnosis can be made in the majority of patients on the basis of detailed clinical history and physical examination. Prospective headache diaries provide a reliable source of symptom reporting and also the distinction between several types of headache that may coexist in the same patient. Investigations are only needed occasionally.

Clinical history of headache

Full clinical history is paramount although young children may find difficulties in describing pain and its characteristics (see Ch. 38, p. 1630). The child should be encouraged to use his/her own words and be assisted with visual images to describe certain ideas such as the severity of pain. Assessment of the headache should include the duration of symptoms, of individual attacks, their frequency and severity, the site of maximal intensity and the quality of pain. Possible trigger factors, warning signs and aura symptoms should be recorded. Associated clinical features such as anorexia, nausea, vomiting, light, noise or smell intolerance, pallor, visual disturbances, dizziness, confusion, abdominal pain and motor or sensory deficits should also be carefully assessed and recorded. Assessment should also be made of aggravating and relieving factors and the patients' own treatment strategies. It should also be determined if there are continuing sensory, motor or gastrointestinal symptoms between attacks of headache or a complete resolution of symptoms and a full return to normality. The complete clinical description of these features is best collected prospectively, by using a diary to record the events as they happen.[271]

Physical examination

All patients should have a complete physical examination including the measurement of blood pressure. Neurological examination should be thorough and complete including measurement of the head circumference. Of particular importance is the detection of signs and symptoms of raised intracranial pressure (papilloedema, squints and pupillary abnormalities), cerebellar dysfunction (nystagmus, ataxia, intention tremor or torticollis), focal neurological deficits, brainstem disease and cranial nerve palsies.

Investigations

Investigations are only needed in a minority of children with chronic or recurrent headache. Indications for neuroimaging, with CT or MRI are given in Table 22.13.[266]

Lumbar puncture and measurement of opening CSF pressure is indicated if infection or idiopathic intracranial hypertension is suspected.

CHILDHOOD MIGRAINE

It is estimated that around 1 in 10 schoolchildren suffer from migraine. The prevalence rate is estimated at 1.3% in children between 3 and 5 years of age[259] and 3.4% at age 5 with a steady increase to 19.1% at 12 years of age. After the age of 12 the prevalence rate drops slightly to reach adult prevalence rates.[257] Boys and girls under the age of 12 years are almost equally affected with migraine, but in children older than 12 years migraine is commoner in girls than boys with a transition to adult rates of around 6% in males and 17% in females.

The etiology of migraine is not known, but it has a familial tendency. The risk for first degree relatives of patients is increased above

Table 22.13 Indications for neuroimaging in children with headache

1. Features of cerebellar dysfuction: ataxia; nystagmus; intention tremor
2. Features of increased intracranial pressure: papilloedma; night or early morning vomiting; large head
3. New focal or new neurological deficits including recent squint
4. Seizures, especially focal
5. Personality change
6. Deterioration of school work

general population levels: 1.9-fold for migraine without aura and 4-fold for migraine with aura, indicating that both genetic and environmental factors are probably involved.[272] The concordance rate for migraine without aura is higher in monozygotic (MZ) at 28% than in dizygotic (DZ) twins at 18%.[273] The concordance rates of migraine with aura are also higher in MZ (34%) than in DZ twin (12%).[274] Molecular genetic studies have, to date, identified at least one candidate region (19p13) and in patients with familial hemiplegic migraine the calcium channel gene CACNLA4 has been implicated.[275] Mutations in this same gene have also been associated with familial episodic ataxia.

Pathophysiology of migraine

Migraine attacks are triggered by specific physical or environmental factors in genetically predisposed individuals. The initiating steps may have neural, vascular, autonomic or biochemical origin. Regardless of the exact initiating factors, it seems that the principal pathway in migraine attacks involves the activation of the trigeminovascular system. The interactions between the cranial vascular system and the trigeminal nucleus are complex and interrelated. Stimulation of the trigeminal sensory nerves either naturally by specific trigger factors or experimentally by electrical impulses in laboratory animals may induce the release of vasoactive neuropeptides. The release of vasoactive neuropeptides (substance P, neurokinin A and calcitonin gene-related peptide) initiates a process of microneurogenic inflammation followed by vasodilation, mast cell degradation and plasma extravasation. Dihydroergotamine and sumatriptan as $5HT_{1B/D}$ receptor agonists inhibit this process. As a result of the neurogenic inflammation, nociceptive impulses travel inferiorly to the trigeminal nucleus caudalis and superiorly to the thalamus and the cerebral cortex.[276] Diffuse projections from the locus ceruleus to the cerebral cortex may initiate a process of cortical oligemia that is better known as 'spreading depression of Leo' and may account for the aura symptoms that can occur independently of headache. Interaction of brainstem and afferent impulses from cranial blood vessels may lead to vasomotor changes and the characteristic throbbing headache.

Clinical features and diagnostic criteria

The International Headache Society classifies migraine into two major forms; migraine without aura and migraine with aura. Other less common forms are also recognized. The majority of affected children (75–85%) suffer from migraine without aura although both major forms coexist.

Diagnostic criteria for childhood migraine and related disorders are given in Table 22.14.[268] Migraine headache is typically recurrent in nature with complete recovery between attacks. Stress and anxiety are the most commonly identified trigger factors. Only 10–15% of patients identify a food type (such as cheese, chocolates and caffeine-containing soft drinks) as a trigger factor. Aura symptoms, if present, precede the onset of headache and are commonly visual in nature (blurred vision, tunnel vision, blind spots (scotomata) or zigzag black and white lines in front of the eyes). Rarely the aura symptoms are sensory (tingling or numbness), motor (hemiplegia or speech disturbances), autonomic or nonspecific.

The headache starts as a mild pain that does not interfere with normal activities. It increases in intensity over 30–60 minutes to a moderate intensity that may stop some activities or proceed to a severe intensity that stops all activities. The pain is commonly described as throbbing, but some children may not be able to describe the type of pain, referring to it as 'just sore'. In the majority the site of maximal intensity is more likely to be frontal than unilateral.

During an attack the child is described by parents as pale, quiet and wanting to be left alone. Refusal of food and drink with nausea is common and vomiting may occur. Light, noise, strong smells and physical exercise may aggravate pain. Dizziness (unreal sensation of movement), abdominal pain, visual disturbances and sensory or motor deficits may also be associated, but to a lesser degree. Some patients describe unusual visual hallucination or distortion of images including micropsia (objects appearing small), macropsia (objects appearing very large)

Table 22.14 Diagnostic criteria

IHS criteria for the diagnosis of migraine without aura

A. At least five attacks fulfilling B–D

B. Headache lasting 1–72 hours (untreated or unsuccessfully treated)

C. Headache has at least two of the following characteristics:
1. Unilateral location (frontal and bitemporal locations are common in children)
2. Pulsating quality
3. Moderate or severe intensity (inhibits or prohibits daily activities)
4. Aggravation by walking stairs or similar routine physical activity

D. During headache, at least one of the following:
1. Nausea and/or vomiting
2. Photophobia or phonophobia (symptoms can be inferred from behavior)

E. No evidence of organic disease

IHS criteria for the diagnosis of migraine with aura

A. At least two attacks fulfilling B

B. At least three of the following four characteristics:
1. One or more fully reversible aura symptoms indicating focal cerebral cortical and/or brain stem dysfunction
2. At least one aura symptom develops gradually over more than 4 minutes, or two or more symptoms occur in succession
3. No aura symptom lasts more than 60 minutes. If more than one aura is present, accepted duration is proportionally increased
4. Headache follows aura with a free interval of less than 60 minutes (it may also begin before or simultaneously with the aura)

C. No evidence of organic disease

Criteria for the diagnosis of abdominal migraine

A. At least five attacks fulfilling criteria B–D

B. Attacks of abdominal pain lasting 1–72 hours (untreated or unsuccessfully treated)

C. Abdominal pain has all of the following characteristics:
1. Midline location, periumbilical or poorly localized
2. Dull or 'just sore' quality
3. Moderate or severe intensity

D. During abdominal pain at least two of the following
1. Anorexia
2. Nausea
3. Vomiting
4. Pallor

E. Not attributed to another disorder

Criteria for the diagnosis of cyclical vomiting syndrome

A. At least five attacks fulfilling criteria B and C

B. Episodic attacks stereotyped in the individual patient of intense nausea and vomiting lasting from 1 hour to 5 days

C. Vomiting during attacks occurs at least 4 times/hour for at least 1 hour

D. Symptom-free between attacks

Not attributed to another disorder

or a combination of both: 'The Alice in Wonderland Syndrome'.[277] Sleep, rest and simple analgesics may relieve symptoms. Typical attacks lasts for at least 1 hour followed by gradual resolution.

The clinical features can be dominated by transient symptoms of cerebellar and brainstem dysfunction such as vertigo, ataxia, blurred vision, visual field defects, motor deficits, dysphasia and confusion. These features were attributed to vascular constriction in the territory of the basilar artery and hence described as *basilar migraine*.[278]

Some attacks of migraine are triggered by minor head injury and can be complicated by a disturbed level of consciousness commonly called *confusional migraine.* They occur mainly in children and are commoner in boys than in girls. Features include an aura, followed by headache of variable severity and duration with drowsiness, irritability, agitation, disturbed speech, aggressive behavior and amnesia. Blurred vision, nausea and vomiting are common features and duration can vary from a few hours to several days.

Migraine attacks can be complicated by paralysis or paresis of the extraocular muscles, ptosis and pupillary dilation, but with no associated confusion or loss of consciousness. Such attacks are called *ophthalmoplegic migraine* and the eye features may not resolve for days or occasionally weeks after the resolution of headache. Some cases are indistinguishable from Tolosa–Hunt syndrome with MRI evidence of cavernous sinus dilation and changes consistent with local inflammation .

Attacks of migraine can be complicated by unilateral weakness, impaired speech or sensory loss. The neurological deficits are transient, fully reversible and may start before, with or after the onset of the headache. The neurological deficit may persist after cessation of headache. The disease can be sporadic or familial. In the latter case and when associated with episodic hemiplegia it is called *familial hemiplegic migraine* which has an autosomal dominant inheritance and may be associated with a deletion of the calcium channel gene CACNA 1A on 19p13.

Treatment

The treatment of migraine includes reassurances to the child and the parents about the benign nature of the disorder and education on its natural course of remission and relapse. Satisfactory management may require more than one consultation in order to establish a good understanding of the condition and to address individual concerns. Children should be encouraged to identify their own trigger and relieving factors and explore their own treatment strategies. The judicial use of analgesics and other medications should be discussed early as many children and their parents use over-the-counter medications or have already received advice from their primary care physician.

Management of acute attacks of migraine

In the majority an effective treatment of the acute attacks is the cornerstone of management and prophylaxis is not necessary. The treatment of acute attacks should start as early as possible after the onset of headache. Children should be allowed to rest and lie down in a quiet environment. Early administration of analgesics is commonly associated with good results.

Reviews of evidence-based treatment of migraine in children emphasize that only a few randomized trials are available. Paracetamol and ibuprofen continue to be the first line treatments.[279,280] The analgesic effects of paracetamol are probably mediated centrally with possible indirect action on spinal serotonin receptors. Ibuprofen is a nonsteroidal anti-inflammatory drug (NSAID) that inhibits the cyclo-oxygenase enzyme and hence prostaglandin synthesis. The analgesic effects of ibuprofen may also be mediated through independent spinal mechanisms (see Ch. 38, see p. 1632).

In children under 15 years of age, paracetamol in single doses of 15 mg/kg body weight and ibuprofen (10 mg/kg) were effective and well-tolerated in the treatment of migraine in a double-blind placebo-controlled trial.[281] Paracetamol had a more rapid onset than ibuprofen, but ibuprofen was twice as effective in aborting migraine within 2 hours. Aspirin is an effective analgesic, but its association with Reye syndrome has limited its use in children under the age of 15 years, especially in the presence of symptoms or signs of viral infection. Over-the-counter analgesics may contain combinations of drugs that have not been investigated in children. Occasionally a stronger analgesic such as codeine sulfate may be necessary.

Sumatriptan is a specific antimigraine medication with a good efficacy and safety record in adult patients. It is a selective agonist of 5 hydroxy-tryptamine (5-HT)$_{1B-D}$ receptors. It causes constriction of cerebral blood vessels and blocks nociceptive impulses. Sumatriptan is available by subcutaneous auto injection, oral tablets and as a nasal spray.

Nasal sumatriptan is shown to be effective in the treatment of acute migraine attacks. A large multicenter double-blind placebo-controlled trial of 663 adolescents aged 12–17 years, using 5-, 10- and 20-mg doses, demonstrated that 10- and 20-mg doses were significantly better than placebo in alleviating symptoms after 1 hour and in complete resolution of symptoms after 2 hours.[282] A recent randomized trial of 83 children using nasal sumatriptan 10 mg for children under 40 kg of weight and 20 mg for those above 40 kg, showed similar results.[283] Bad taste was the most commonly reported side-effect.

Oral sumatriptan (doses between 50 and 100 mg) were not effective in children in a placebo-controlled crossover study of 23 children, aged 8–16 years.[284] An open study of subcutaneous injections of sumatriptan (0.06 mg/kg) in 50 children between 6 and 18 years of age showed only limited benefit.[285] Other triptans are available, but their efficacy in childhood is not known.

Metoclopramide or prochlorperazine may alleviate nausea and vomiting during migraine attacks, but there are no controlled trials of their use in children and concerns about extrapyramidal symptoms and dystonic reactions limit their use.

Prevention of migraine

Nonpharmacological strategies for the prevention of migraine attacks should include avoidance of identified specific triggers. Dietary exclusion is only recommended in children with confirmed food triggers. Affected children should be encouraged to assume a healthy lifestyle with a regular pattern of sleep and meals and appropriate balance between rest and exercise. They should avoid spending excessive amounts of time on computer and video-games and be discouraged from smoking.

Pharmacological prophylactic treatment is not reliable and success is not always predictable. There is no consistent evidence for the efficacy and tolerability of any prophylactic agent. Therefore, treatment is only indicated if acute treatment is unsuccessful and migraine attacks are frequent (more than two attacks per month), prolonged and severe enough to interfere with school attendance and education. Prophylactic treatment should be continued for at least 6 weeks before considered ineffective and polytherapy should be avoided. Prophylactic treatment may be discontinued after 6 months, but can be restarted if necessary. Propranolol has been shown to reduce the frequency of migraine attacks in a double-blind placebo-controlled trial,[286] but the results were not confirmed in a similar trial.[287] In children over 7 years of age, propranolol may be given in a dose of 1–2 mg/kg/day in two divided doses. The mechanism of action is not clear, but may involve inhibition of the catecholamine-induced platelet aggregation and release of platelet seratonin. Side-effects may include hypoglycemia, hypotension, tiredness and mood changes.

Topiramate was shown in a large randomized, double-blind and placebo-controlled multicenter trial to provide significant reduction in the number of migraine days per month in children.[288] Doses between 2 and 3 mg/kg/day were reached after a period of 8 weeks' titration.

The evidence for efficacy of other medications (pizotifen, clonidine and valproate) is either inconsistent or based on studies in adults. Pizotifen was found to be effective in the treatment of abdominal migraine only,[289] but not in headache migraine.[290] Flunarizine, a cerebral calcium channel antagonist, may be effective at a dose of 5–10 mg per day,[291] but its use is associated with excessive side-effects such as drowsiness, depression and weight gain. Valproic acid is effective in adults, but has not been studied in children.[292] Amitriptyline was shown to be very effective in prevention of chronic headache, including migraine, in a large open observational study.[293] It may block the re-uptake of both serotonin and norepinephrine (noradrenaline) and its effect in migraine is independent of its antidepressant actions. A study of the efficacy of amitriptyline, (1.5 mg/kg/day) in the prevention of migraine in 19 children (6–12 years of age) has shown only a modest benefit.[294] Unlike in adults, it did not influence the duration of migraine attacks and drowsiness was the most common adverse effect.

Prognosis

The natural course of migraine is that of remission and relapse, but with a tendency for permanent remission with increasing age. Remissions of at least 1 year have been recorded in up to 58% of patients during periods of follow-up of at least 5 years.[295] Long term follow-up studies of 73 children with migraine showed that 34% became headache free after 6 years, 62% after 16 years and 40–47% after 22–40 years.[256,296,297]

Alternating hemiplegia of childhood

Alternating hemiplegia of childhood (AHC) is a progressive disabling disorder of unknown etiology, but has long been considered as a form of 'complicated migraine'.[298] It presents in early infancy and has three distinct clinical phases.[299] During the first year of life (phase I) children show signs of delayed development, abnormal eye movement and episodes of dystonia. During the second year of life (phase II) alternate hemiplegic spells last between a few days to a few weeks. By the age of 5 years (phase III) fixed neurological deficits and variable degrees of disability, with developmental delay, spasticity and epilepsy are evident.

The diagnosis is usually based on the typical clinical course. CT and MRI are usually normal. Long term treatment with flunarizine results in reduced number and severity of hemiplegic spells, but it is unlikely to change the natural course of the disease. The relationship of AHC to migraine is based on its paroxysmal nature, the occurrence of headache during some attacks and the apparent high prevalence of migraine with aura among the relatives. However, the progressive nature of the disease and the permanent neurological and learning disabilities suggest that it is unrelated to migraine.

Benign paroxysmal torticollis of infancy (BPTI)

BPTI is a benign disorder of early childhood characterized by self-limiting episodes of head tilt lasting a few hours to a few days. Attacks start during the first year of life, are sudden in onset and resolution and may alternate between sides.[300] BPTI has been linked to migraine and benign paroxysmal vertigo on clinical and epidemiological basis. The pathophysiology is unclear, but surface electromyography (sEMG) of the sternomastoid muscle during attacks shows dystonic changes.[301] The attacks start suddenly with the head held to one side and neck muscles on the side of the tilt, particularly the sternomastoid, are stiff and tense. During attacks the child may also have pallor, nausea, vomiting, ataxia and irritability. The diagnosis is based on the typical episodic clinical features.

Neuroimaging is indicated in order to exclude intracranial pathology. EEG may be indicated if epilepsy is suspected. A definite diagnosis should be followed by reassurance to parents about the benign nature of the condition. The majority of cases resolve by the age of 3 and almost all by the age of 5 years. No treatment is necessary.

Benign paroxysmal vertigo

Benign paroxysmal vertigo (BPV) is characterized by recurrent episodes of an unreal sensation of movement of the child or his/her surrounding environment (vertigo). Each episode lasts for a few minutes, but occasionally may continue for hours or up to 2 days.

Early onset BPV is uncommon, but affects children between the age of 2 and 4 years. It is characterized by sudden episodes of pallor, screaming, unsteadiness, nystagmus, nausea and occasionally vomiting.[302] The child either sits or clings to his or her parent in fear. The attacks terminate spontaneously and the child returns to normal. There is no loss of consciousness and the child is aware and responsive during the event. Episodes of BPV decrease in frequency by age 5 years and may be replaced by episodes of headache typical of migraine.

Late onset BPV is common among schoolchildren[303] with a prevalence rate of 2.6%. Older children are able to describe the unreal sensation of movement. The attacks last for seconds to minutes with an average frequency of one attack per month and the only abnormal finding during attacks is horizontal nystagmus. Migraine is more common among children with BPV and among their first-degree relatives than in controls.[303]

The diagnosis is based on excluding underlying neurological causes, vestibular disorders, epilepsy, and the effects of medications and toxins by appropriate investigations. Treatment is often not needed, apart from reassurance about the benign nature of the condition. Some children benefit from the antihistamine betahistine.[304]

Abdominal migraine

Recurrent abdominal pain (RAP) is a common problem affecting around 8% of schoolchildren. Half the children with RAP (4%) have abdominal migraine[305] as defined by the clinical criteria in Table 22.14. Abdominal migraine is characterized by recurrent episodes of a dull abdominal pain lasting between 1 and 72 hours. Between attacks the child is completely well. The clinical pattern of trigger factors, associated symptoms and relieving factors is similar to that of migraine headache in children. Attacks have been reported to start at any age from early infancy although the mean age of onset is around 7 years. At least one third of children continue to suffer attacks late into their teenage years and 70% have a current (52%) or past (18%) history of migraine.[306]

Management starts with confirmation of the diagnosis, reassurance to parents and identification and avoidance of trigger factors. Acute attacks should be treated with simple analgesics, rest, and fluid replacement and occasionally with anti-emetics. There is no published data on the use of specific anti-migraine agents such as sumatriptan. Drug prophylaxis has been evaluated in a randomized double-blind placebo-controlled trial of pizotifen and which has been shown to be effective.[289] Evidence for the value of other drugs such as propranolol and cyproheptadine is based on open trials.[307]

Cyclical vomiting syndrome (CVS)

CVS is a disease mainly of early childhood and closely related to migraine. It presents with sudden episodes of anorexia, nausea, vomiting, lethargy and intolerance to light, noise and exercise. During attacks the child looks unwell, pale and miserable which can be severe enough to stop activities and may lead to dehydration if prolonged. The attacks last from a few hours to a few days and the child is completely well between attacks. It is estimated that around 2% of schoolchildren may have unexplained attacks of vomiting that fulfil the criteria for the diagnosis of CVS (Table 22.14).[308] The disease may begin during very early childhood and occasionally during the first year of life. With increasing age typical episodes are associated with headache that fulfils the criteria for the diagnosis of migraine. A follow-up study found a later diagnosis of migraine in 46% of cases compared to 12% in controls and 50% of children continued to suffer from attacks in adolescence and early adult life.[309] The treatment of acute attacks aims to stop vomiting and prevent dehydration. Early administration of oral or intravenous anti-emetic drugs such as ondansetron may abort attacks. Prophylactic treatment with erythromycin as a prokinetic agent may reduce the number and severity of attacks.

TENSION-TYPE HEADACHE

Tension type headache (TTH) is common among children and adolescents who seek medical advice for headache. TTH is also known as psychogenic headache, muscle contraction headache or nonvascular headache. It can be classified as frequent, infrequent or chronic. The prevalence in the general childhood population is not known but in children with headache may be 1%.[257] However, it is common in children and adolescents attending accident and emergency departments, general practice and hospital clinics for headache as their chief complaint. Both male and females are equally affected and it is commoner in older children and adolescents. TTH is rare in children under the age of 6 years.

Etiology and pathogenesis

The etiology is unknown, but there is evidence of a familial tendency, especially in chronic tension type headache (CTTH), and significant environmental influences. CTTH may evolve from episodic tension type headache (ETTH) or may start as chronic from the onset. It may be induced by chronic use of analgesics or high daily caffeine intake. Children with

CTTH have a higher than expected incidence of major life events such as chronic disease, family illnesses and bereavements.[310] Several initiating mechanisms have been suggested including muscle contraction, physical strain, anxiety and stress. No consistent biochemical or EMG changes have been found.

Clinical features of TTH

The attack's duration is usually short, but is continuous in CTTH. The headache is typically described as pressure or tightening and mild to moderate in severity. It is bilateral in location and does not worsen with routine activities. It may be associated with photophobia or phonophobia, but not nausea or vomiting (Table 22.15).[268] The diagnosis is made on the basis of the typical clinical history and normal neurological examination and investigations are not needed in the majority of patients. The clinical features of ETTH can sometimes be indistinguishable from those of migraine without aura. In some patients both migraine without aura and ETTH coexist. The distinction between the two conditions is important in order to plan treatment and predict outcome.

Management of TTH

Management of the child can be complex and multidisciplinary. The child and parents should be reassured of the absence of any sinister cause and offered general advice on healthy lifestyle. Children should be encouraged to adopt predictable patterns of sleep, regular meals, balanced diets, adequate exercise and rest. Successful management will require the co-operation of the children and their parents often with involvement, of schoolteachers, school nurses, and occasionally clinical psychologists. Attention should be paid to possible underlying chronic physical, psychological or emotional problems. The expertise of a clinical psychologist may also help in the management of acute headache attacks and in helping the child and the family to develop their own strategies in dealing with pain in general.

Simple analgesics are often effective and sufficient in ETTH, but are largely unsuccessful and should be discouraged in children with CTTH, as some may develop analgesia-induced headache.

Prophylactic therapy is occasionally needed to reduce distress caused by daily or almost daily attacks. Pain modulating agents such as amitriptyline in dosages between 10 and 50 mg per day (up to 1 mg/kg/day) was shown to be of value in an open trial.[293] The prognosis is variable and patients may run a course of remission and relapse.

CLUSTER HEADACHE

Cluster headache is uncommon in children, but cases have been reported in children as young as 1 year of age.[311] In many adult patients the onset of headache is before the age of 18 years and in some before the age of 10 years.[312] Episodic cluster headache is more common (affecting around 80% of patients) than the chronic form and more males are affected than females.

The cause of cluster headache is not known, but there is a strong familial tendency. The changes during attacks are consistent with neuronal, endocrine and vascular mechanisms involving trigeminovascular activation.[313]

The clinical features of cluster headaches during childhood are similar to those in adults with a tendency for the frequency and duration of cluster periods and the frequency of the individual headache episodes to increase with age. Headache attacks are short (up to 90 minutes) and have a well-defined periodicity. The pain is severe, sharp and reaches its peak intensity within 5–15 minutes and may provoke intense emotions and violent behavior. The pain is almost always unilateral with maximal intensity around the eye and can be associated with nausea and vomiting. Autonomic symptoms (nasal congestion, forehead sweating, conjunctival injection, meiosis, lacrimation and ptosis) are common and are almost always on the same side of the pain and resolve with the resolution of pain.

Atypical attacks (cluster headache-like disorders) have been reported in a small number of children. The headache is bilateral, the pain is not peri-orbital and children exhibit unusual motor behavior consisting of thrashing of limbs and irritability.[314] Early administration of high flow oxygen and subcutaneous injection or nasal administration of sumatriptan may relieve acute attacks. Short course of steroids (prednisolone or dexamethasone) can induce remission and verapamil, valproate, melatonin or topiramate may be given as prophylactic maintenance therapy.

CHRONIC POST-TRAUMATIC HEADACHE (CPTH)

Episodes typically start within 2 weeks after head injury including minor trauma and continue for at least 8 weeks. The prevalence rate of CPTH in children is not known, but a follow-up study, 12–18 months after head injury, has shown that 29% of 138 children (mean age 9.2 years) suffered from recurrent headaches.[315]

The causes of CPTH are not fully understood, but the pathogenesis is likely to be complex and premorbid predisposition to headache and psychosocial factors may contribute.

The clinical features are those of idiopathic recurrent headaches (migraine and tension headache of childhood). Other symptoms of postconcussion syndrome may be present, but physical and neurological examinations are normal.[316] In children with typical presentation neuroimaging is not indicated.

Treatment includes reassurance and appropriate use of simple analgesics as required.

HEADACHE DUE TO INTRACRANIAL DISORDERS
Brain tumors

Headache is a common symptom of brain tumors and hence a common reason for referral to secondary care and neuroimaging. It has been reported in 62% of 3291 children with brain tumors,[317] and almost always associated with at least one other clinical feature such as ataxia, nystagmus, intention tremor, effortless vomiting, headache during sleep, focal neurological deficits, acquired squint, papilloedema, personality change or deteriorating schoolwork. However, headache may be the only initial presenting symptom in a minority (8–10%).[318] In a study of 600 children with migraine and 67 children with brain tumor, the most helpful distinguishing features in children with brain tumors were nocturnal headache and headache present on waking.[319] In a retrospective study of 74 children with brain tumors,[320] the mean duration of symptoms before diagnosis was 20 weeks. When headache is the only presenting symptom of brain tumor or raised intracranial pressure, it may have no specific features or may have features similar to those of migraine or tension-type headache leading to a delay in the diagnosis of

Table 22.15 Diagnostic criteria and clinical spectrum of tension type headache

	Infrequent ETTH	Frequent ETTH	CTTH
A: Frequency	< 12 days/year	12–180 days/year	> 180 days/year
B: Duration	30 minutes	7 days	Hours to continuous
C		At least three of the following: 1. Pressing/tightening quality 2. Mild to moderate severity 3. Bilateral location 4. Not aggravated by walking	
D		All of the following: 1. No nausea (anorexia may occur) 2. No photophobia or phonophobia	
E		Not attributed to any other disorder	

ETTH, episodic tension type headache; CTTH, chronic tension type headache.

Table 22.16 Frequency of associated symptoms in children with brain tumors

Symptom	Headache < 4 months	Headache ≥ 4 months
Vomiting	87%	76%
Visual disturbances	53%	63%
Unsteadiness	49%	45%
Educational or behavioral problems	37%	45%
Disturbed sleep	26%	31%
Growth or endocrine problems	7%	21%
Seizures	7%	8%
None	0	0

the underlying cause. The frequency of associated symptom in 200 children with brain tumors were similar in children with short (<4 months) or long (at least 4 months) history of headache and in no child was the headache the only feature (Table 22.16).[321]

Brain tumors are rare in children with chronic headache and with normal physical and neurological examination. In a large study of 815 children with chronic headache (lasting over 3 months) the prevalence rate of brain tumor was 0.1% suggesting routine neuroimaging in this group of children is not needed.[266] However, neuroimaging is indicated in some children with significant signs and symptoms as shown in Table 22.13.

Idiopathic intracranial hypertension (IIH)

IIH is a rare clinical syndrome of raised intracranial pressure and headache. It occurs in all ages, including infancy. No specific causes have been identified and the pathogenesis is unclear. Clinical features are those of raised intracranial pressure and headache is the most common symptom which is often located at the forehead and is worse on lying down or on awakening in the morning.[322] Other symptoms may include nausea, vomiting, visual disturbances (diplopia, visual loss, blurred vision and visual field defects), lethargy, dizziness and behavioral problems. There is no deterioration in the level of consciousness. On examination, papilledema is the most common sign occurring in the majority of patients followed by VIth cranial nerve palsy and defects of visual acuity.[323]

Ophthalmological examination is an essential part in the assessment and children often present during assessment of visual disturbance by opticians or ophthalmologists.

Neuroimaging with CT or MRI to exclude other causes of increased intracranial pressure is indicated and lumbar puncture shows CSF pressure above 200 mmH$_2$O and a normal CSF analysis.

The criteria of the International Headache Society for the diagnosis of IIH are:[268]

1. cerebrospinal fluid (CSF) pressure above 200 mmH$_2$O water in the recumbent position;
2. normal neurological examination except for papilledema, visual field defect, enlarging blind spot or VIth cranial nerve palsy;
3. normal CSF chemistry and white cell count;
4. no clinical or neuroimaging evidence of venous sinus thrombosis or mass lesion;
5. no metabolic, hormonal or toxic cause for the intracranial hypertension.

IIH is largely self-limiting, although permanent visual field loss and reduced visual acuity occurs in 13–27% of children,[322] hence the need for and early recognition and treatment followed by regular ophthalmological review. A number of treatment measures have been shown to be effective in reducing the intracranial pressure. Single or repeated lumbar puncture with CSF removal may be all that is required. Acetazolamide is useful but large doses may be required in combination with a loop diuretic. Steroids have not been properly evaluated but case reports suggest that the pressure drops within 24 hours. Surgical options include lumboperitoneal or ventricular peritoneal shunt and optic nerve decompression.

HEADACHE DUE TO SINUSITIS

Sinus diseases are unusual during early childhood, as paranasal sinuses are not fully developed before the age of 8 years. In affected children the headache is usually mild and its site of maximal intensity is related to the affected sinuses. The International Headache Society describes the headache of acute frontal sinusitis as 'located directly over the sinus and may radiate to the vertex or behind the eyes'. In maxillary sinusitis 'the headache is located over the antral area and may radiate to upper teeth or to the forehead'. In acute ethmoiditis 'the headache is located between and behind the eyes and may radiate to the temporal area'.[268] The headache of acute sinusitis is almost always associated with other features of upper airway disease: nasal congestion, discharge, sneeze and cough, making the diagnosis of acute sinusitis relatively easy.

Headache due to chronic sinusitis may be present with or without upper respiratory tract symptoms and should therefore be suspected as the cause of chronic headache in the presence of clinical features such as sleep disturbance, nasal discharge, nasal blockage and decreased sense of smell. Headache can be the only symptom of 'silent' sinus disease.

The diagnosis of chronic sinusitis should be confirmed with appropriate imaging. Medical treatment may include antihistamine decongestants, antibiotics and simple analgesia. Surgical treatment is rarely needed except in the presence of underlying predisposing factors or nasal polyps causing obstruction (see Ch. 32, see p. 1514).

DISORDERS OF MOVEMENT

EXTRAPYRAMIDAL DISORDERS, BASAL GANGLIA DISORDERS

Movement disorders (involuntary movements) accompany many diseases thought to originate from the basal ganglia. Some are among the most benign of neurological disorders but others are progressive. There are no clear figures concerning the incidence and prevalence of movement disorders. However, movement disorders are not uncommon.

The underlying causes include infections, metabolic disorders and neurotransmitter imbalance. However, the cause of many is unknown. The basal ganglia are particularly susceptible to hypoxia. This is seen in carbon monoxide poisoning, neonatal asphyxia and post cardiopulmonary bypass. Heavy metals also appear to have a special affinity for this part of the brain (e.g. copper deposition with Wilson disease, iron deposition in Hallervorden–Spatz disease and the dyskinesias of manganese, molybdenum and thallium poisoning). Metabolic diseases such as phenylketonuria, Leigh encephalopathy and glutaric aciduria may present with a predominant dyskinetic clinical picture.

Anatomy of the basal ganglia

The extrapyramidal system in classic neurology consists of part of the cerebral cortex anterior to the motor strip and several masses of gray matter deep in the hemisphere white matter and the upper brainstem. The nomenclature has been rather confusing as words such as basal ganglia, striatum, corpus striatum, and lenticular nucleus are either synonyms or groupings of nuclei. The corpus striatum is the name given to the lentiform nucleus (i.e. the combined putamen and globus pallidus) and the caudate nucleus. It is more appropriate to think in terms of the caudate, putamen and globus pallidus in the cerebral hemisphere together with the substantia nigra in the upper brainstem and the subthalamic nucleus of Luys as constituting together the basal ganglia.

The basal ganglia can be regarded as a major motor computation center receiving information from the cortex about movements being planned together with information from the parietal cortex about body image and from vision. They receive input regarding the force, speed and direction of movement planned by the cerebellum together with information on the position of the head and eyes from the labyrinth and information about body contact and visual information on the position of the body in space. The basal ganglia and extrapyramidal motor cortex inhibit certain primitive brainstem reflexes such as the asymmetrical tonic neck reflex, primitive walking and swimming reflexes and probably store more sophisticated patterns of movement.

Biochemistry of the basal ganglia

The main interest in biochemistry of the basal ganglia stems from the discovery of the dopaminergic pathways from the substantia nigra, the effects of L-DOPA in parkinsonism and the study of the extrapyramidal side-effects of drugs like the phenothiazines.

Classic parkinsonism has three components – tremor, bradykinesia and rigidity – and although the symptoms and signs of basal ganglia disease will be discussed in more detail later (see below), it is necessary to consider some aspects to understand the role of dopamine and L-DOPA in normal basal ganglia function and in disease. The three components appear independently determined because the tremor may be made worse by L-DOPA but helped by surgery; the bradykinesia is helped by L-DOPA but surgery has no effect; the rigidity is helped by L-DOPA and surgery and is especially helped by anticholinergics. Current evidence suggests that cholinergic, serotonergic and gabanergic pathways are normally balanced (inhibited) by dopamine and that while dopamine is important in inhibiting rigidity, it is involved in the causation of the hyperkinetic dyskinesias. Rather confusingly, however, there are some children with dyskinesias involving too much movement who are helped by L-DOPA. In tardive dyskinesia and chorea there should be inherent dopamine excess or drugs that directly stimulate dopamine receptors could be responsible. Drugs which cause tardive dyskinesias, such as the phenothiazines, are known to have anticholinergic, antiserotoninergic and antihistaminergic effects and to leave dopamine unopposed. Drugs which reduce dopamine action, such as tetrabenazine, haloperidol and reserpine, will reduce the involuntary movements in chorea, but are more likely to induce a parkinsonian picture as a side-effect. Parkinsonism can be induced either by depleting the brain's production of dopamine, as occurs with reserpine and tetrabenazine when the dopamine receptors remain free, or alternatively it can be caused by blocking the dopamine receptors by such drugs as haloperidol when L-DOPA cannot reverse the parkinsonism so produced.

Some other drug effects are also important. Thus multiple tics may appear as a complication of chronic amfetamine use or chronic overdose by methylphenidate (Ritalin). Both of these drugs increase brain dopamine as well as having a noradrenergic effect. 5-Hydroxytryptophan has been given to patients with Lesch–Nyhan syndrome, and in this disorder, it appears to lessen self-mutilation. In the past, it has also been used in children with Down syndrome in the hope that it would improve muscle tone and motor performance, but it was found to produce marked rigidity and myoclonic jerks. Cholinergic drugs such as physostigmine will make parkinsonism worse, but will lessen choreiform movements. Together clinical anatomy, physiology, biochemistry and pharmacology help to explain the diverse clinical signs and symptoms which occur in disorders of the basal ganglia.

Movement disorders: general considerations

Many neurological diseases have movement disorders as the main presentation or part of it. These movements are often misdiagnosed as epilepsy, behavioral disorder or tics.

A good eyewitness description is important. However, where possible, it is essential to observe the movements. Videotapes are an excellent way of achieving this especially when they are infrequent or episodic.

Movement disorders may present as more or less continuous abnormal movements or posture or these may fluctuate with time and in relation to emotional state and anxiety. In addition, they may present as paroxysmal episodes mimicking epileptic attacks. Movement disorders may be benign and transient such as benign myoclonus of infancy and dyskinesia after the withdrawal of benzodiazepines (especially intravenous midazolam), or phenytoin in the pediatric intensive care unit (Table 22.17).

Table 22.17 Transient movement disorders in childhood

Benign paroxysmal torticollis of infancy
Benign myoclonus of the newborn
Benign myoclonus of infancy
Jitteriness
Transient paroxysmal dystonia of infancy
Spasmus nutans

It is necessary to observe the child at rest, while sustaining postures, such as outstretching the limbs, during active movement, such as tying shoelaces, and, if possible, under stress. Although involuntary movements often present at rest, they are usually more pronounced with volitional execution of a motor task and may significantly disrupt the motor activities. Children often try to mask abnormal movements by combining them with a normal movement pattern. For example, children with chorea usually mask their abnormal movements by scratching the nose or forehead or by clenching the fingers together. The clinician should not be misled and should notice that these normal movements are not purposeful. Movement disorders are almost always absent during sleep. They are not associated with loss of consciousness and children have full recall of the episodes.

Sometimes, the involuntary movements are a mixture of several types such as choreoathetosis and myoclonic dystonia. The correct classification is often difficult and requires experience and skill. More clinical details will come later regarding specific types of movement disorder and associated conditions.

Investigation of movement disorders

Identification of the movement disorder type should be attempted but is not always possible. Investigations are directed toward the suspected most likely diagnosis. Many diseases may cause more than one type of movement disorder. This includes tumors of the basal ganglia, which makes it reasonable to perform neuroimaging in all children with acquired movement disorder. On the other hand, a single type of movement disorder can be caused by many different diseases. Treatable conditions, such as Wilson disease, should be looked for early as more benefit is obtained with early treatment. Specific investigations for each movement disorder and related conditions will be dealt with in the relevant sections.

Classification of movement disorders

Movement disorders (dyskinesias) can be classified in many ways (Table 22.18). An anatomical classification may conclude that lesions of the globus pallidus cause parkinsonism or a lack of movement,

Table 22.18 Classification of movement disorders

Dyskinesias
Hyperkinetic
Hypokinetic
Akinetic

Anatomical
Lesion of the putamen
Lesion of the caudate
Lesion of the globus pallidus

Clinical presentation
Acute
Progressive
Chronic

Type of predominant movement
Chorea/athetosis
Dystonia
Tremor
Tics

lesions of the putamen cause athetosis and lesions of the caudate cause chorea. However this is a gross oversimplification. Alternatively, they can be classified on the basis of clinical presentation, i.e. whether there is an acute dyskinesia, progressive dyskinesia or chronic nonprogressive dyskinesia. A third method is according to the predominant type of movement, i.e. chorea and choreoathetosis, dystonia and tremor. Also, movement disorders can be classified as hyperkinetic or hypokinetic.

Hyperkinetic dyskinesias

These are typified by the choreas, hemiballismus, tics and orofacial dyskinesias. This group is most often associated with a reduction in muscle tone and the movements disappear in sleep, or if the child is totally relaxed and lying down. Symptomatically there is a close link between this group of disorders and cerebellar dysfunction, e.g. myoclonus can occur in both. In the hyperkinetic dyskinesias the child is restless, fidgety, cannot sit still, stamps his feet, grimaces, shakes his head, may get a constant urge to run, may grunt, make clucking noises and show respiratory irregularity. Difficulty keeping still is referred to as akathisia. The hyperkinetic dyskinesias tend to be associated with high levels of dopamine or noradrenergic substances.

Hypokinetic dyskinesia

In the most severe cases there is akinesia and the child cannot initiate any movement even though not paralyzed. Less severe cases with bradykinesia are associated with difficulty in initiating movements, e.g. difficulty in running is characteristic. The most characteristic hypokinetic state is parkinsonism, which is classically associated with dopamine depletion.

CHOREA AND ATHETOSIS

Definition and general considerations

Chorea is rapid, repetitive, jerky movements affecting any part of the body. It may be unilateral or bilateral and affect the face and trunk as well as the limbs. The movements are neither rhythmic nor stereotyped and they migrate from side to side and limb to limb. True choreiform movements tend to be jerky, unpredictable and random and differ from tics in that they have no pattern of repetition, but the so-called convulsive tic with repeated wild flinging movements of the arms and lateral jerking of the head may resemble hemiballismus. Chorea may be incorporated into a voluntary movement. The sudden wild flinging of the arm or the head in chorea is made semipurposeful by pretending to scratch the head or straighten the hair. The child may sit on the affected hand, or the tongue is held between the teeth to try to lessen the movements. Walking and feeding may become impossible due to the repeated jerks of the head and limbs together with involvement of the lips, tongue and palate.

True choreiform movements can be appreciated most easily by getting the child to stand still, arms outstretched when the jerks appear as a gross caricature of the milder constant readjusting movements seen in pure cerebellar disease, as if there was a total absence of damping, with wild overswings of correction. The head and upper limbs are affected more than the trunk and lower limbs, and total relaxation in the supine position lessens the movements as maintenance of posture and initiation of voluntary movement seems to be important in triggering them off. The face and bulbar muscles are involved when there are bilateral choreiform movements of the arms (a tic may be unilateral and have bulbar involvement). It must be remembered that low amplitude choreiform movement of the outstretched hands as a normal physiological variant is a frequent finding in boys of early primary school age.[324]

Athetosis literally means without posture, i.e. it is a posture that is constantly changing. It is a slow, writhing movement of the limbs that is frequently associated with chorea (choreoathetosis). Isolated athetosis is almost always due to perinatal asphyxia. Previously, kernicterus was the major cause. The movements in the athetoid child are slower than those in a child with pure chorea and they involve gradual changes in posture secondary to changes in muscle tone. The upper limbs appear to be constantly moving between the primitive extensor posture and the hemiplegic flexor posture. The fingers start in the hemiplegic position

with the hand closed across the adducted thumb and flexed at wrist and elbows. The fingers then extend and the arm extends, abducts and internally rotates into the extended (also called avoiding) position. Since the leg is extended in both postures, it remains in equinus and does not show the same movements as occur in the arms. Feeding, especially chewing, is difficult and speech is always affected. Walking may be possible, with a reeling gait and contortions of the trunk, yet surprisingly few falls result.

Athetosis of the hands, dilation of the alae nasae and fanning of the toes is often seen in normal infants at birth and may become very obvious after relatively mild asphyxia. Pathological athetosis rarely appears in the first year of life in brain damage syndromes. Dystonic extension appears at about 4 months of age and athetosis may not occur for a further 2 or 3 years. Grimacing, laughing, crying and inappropriate emotional responses can accompany the fluctuating muscle tone.

Differential diagnosis

The conditions which present with chorea/choreoathetosis may be acute (Table 22.19), chronic and progressive (Table 22.20) or chronic and nonprogressive (Table 22.21). Some conditions are genetic (Table 22.22), systemic, metabolic, or secondary to infections and vascular diseases. Chorea might be the initial or most prominent symptom or may be present as an associated symptom.

Table 22.19   Acute-onset choreiform disease

Sydenham chorea
Toxic dystonic/chorea
Phenothiazines – chlorpromazine (Largactil), trifluoperazine (Stelazine), fluphenazine (Moditen), thioridazine (Melleril)
Phenytoin
Carbamazepine (tics and dystonia)
Maxolon
Prochlorperazine (Stemetil)
Lithium
Tricyclics – amitriptyline
Manganese poisoning
Thallium poisoning
Hydrogen sulfide
Fentanyl
Propofol
Serotonin reuptake inhibitors – paroxetine
Bethanechol
High estrogen contraceptive pill
Lamotrigine
Chorea gravidarum
Chorea and the contraceptive pill
Chorea and lupus erythematosus
Chorea and Henoch–Schönlein purpura
Hemolytic uremic syndrome
Hypoparathyroidism
Paroxysmal kinesiogenic dystonia
DOPA-sensitive dystonia (Segawa)
Carbon monoxide poisoning
Following cardiac bypass surgery
Postdialysis dyskinesia
After burns – burns shakes
Metabolic diseases – Leigh disease
Familial paroxysmal choreoathetosis
Infections
Encephalitis lethargica
Toxoplasmic encephalitis
Coxsackie, echo and varicella encephalitis
Haemophilus influenzae B meningitis
AIDS encephalopathy
Neurosyphilis
Epidemic rubeola

Table 22.20   Progressive diseases associated with chorea

Huntington chorea
Idiopathic torsion dystonia
DOPA-sensitive dystonia of Segawa
Metabolic
Wilson disease
Glutaric aciduria
Phenylketonuria
Leigh encephalopathy
Mitochondrial diseases (MELAS, MERRF)
Homocystinuria
Triosephosphate isomerase deficiency
Sulfite oxidase deficiency
Methylmalonic acidemia
Dihydropteridine reductase deficiency
Hexosaminidase A and B deficiency (onset 10 years with dystonia)
Lesch–Nyhan syndrome
Lysosomal enzyme disorders – G_{M1}, G_{M2}, Krabbe and metachromatic leukodystrophy
Fahr syndrome (basal ganglia calcification)
Hypoparathyroidism
Infectious origin
Subacute sclerosing panencephalitis
AIDS encephalopathy
Infantile bilateral striatal necrosis
Hallervorden–Spatz disease
Ataxia telangiectasia
Ataxia with ocular dyspraxia (Aicardi)
Pelizaeus–Merzbacher disease
Familial dystonic paraplegia
Paroxysmal dystonia with myoclonus
Paroxysmal sleep dystonia
Neuraxonal dystrophy
Parkinson disease
Hunt juvenile parkinsonism (striatonigral degeneration)
Hunt pallidocerebellar degeneration
Pilocytic astrocytomas

MELAS, mitochondrial encephalomyopathy, lactic acidosis and stroke-like episodes; MERRF, myoclonic epilepsy with ragged red fibers.

Table 22.21   Chronic nonprogressive disease (cerebral palsies)

Bilirubin encephalopathy
Hypoxic–ischemic encephalopathy
Autosomal recessive striatonigral dysplasia
Dystonia of prematurity

Table 22.22   Inherited choreas

Benign familial chorea	AD or AR
Dentatorubropallidoluysian atrophy (DRPL)	AD
Familial paroxysmal choreoathetosis	AD
Huntington chorea	AD
Neuroacanthocytosis	AD or AR
Pontocerebellar hypoplasia type 2	AR

AD, autosomal dominant; AR, autosomal recessive.

Specific syndromes
Genetic diseases
Huntington chorea. This dominantly inherited condition characteristically appears in adults around 30 years with dementia, rigidity and chorea as well as psychological and behavior changes. Ten percent of cases start in childhood and inheritance is usually from the father. It is therefore an imprinted disorder with spontaneous mutations being

very rare. It is a triple codon repeat disease; 35–90 repeats of trinucleotide CAG are diagnostic on chromosome 4p16.3. Diagnosis of suspected childhood cases is now possible. Presentation can be with seizures in 50% of cases, thus differing from the adult who presents with dementia or dystonia. However, up to 50% will present with dementia, manifested by a fall off in schoolwork before the rigidity, which is often asymmetrical. MRI scan shows selective atrophy of the head of the caudate nucleus.

Benign familial (hereditary) chorea. This is a rare dominantly inherited disorder. The onset is usually in early childhood. It starts with the child's first steps. Intelligence is usually normal. Chorea may associate with athetosis, hypotonia and tremor. The condition becomes less pronounced by adolescence and may disappear in some affected adults.

It is difficult to distinguish between this condition and other causes of chorea, especially familial paroxysmal chorea. The family history and the continuous, non-episodic chorea are important pointers. Treatment with anticonvulsants, chlorpromazine or haloperidol is beneficial in some.

Hallervorden–Spatz syndrome. The basal ganglia are very rich in iron. The reason for this is not known nor is it understood why the basal ganglia are so selectively vulnerable to heavy metal toxicity. Hallervorden–Spatz syndrome, a recessive condition, is associated with an increase in the amount of stainable iron. The globus pallidus and substantia nigra are affected with accumulation of iron pigments, a decrease in myelin and axonal swellings (spheroids). The clinical picture is not of parkinsonism but of spasticity with brisk reflexes, extensor plantar responses and increasing extrapyramidal rigidity of a hemiplegic dystonic type affecting all four limbs. When progression is very slow, the child may be thought to have cerebral palsy. Usually by the age of 10 years there is fixation of posture with varying degrees of choreoathetosis. Death usually occurs in the early twenties. There is no definitive diagnostic test, but as the condition progresses many children on MRI show an appearance of the basal ganglia which is typical and has been likened to a 'tiger's eye'. Genetically the syndrome appears to be heterogeneous.[325] Brain biopsy does not help unless one is fortunate enough to see circular inclusions known as spheroids. Iron metabolism, as judged by the measurement of serum iron, transferrins or iron absorption, is normal. No treatment is of any avail. The disease is rare and differentiation from metachromatic leukodystrophy, Alexander disease and Pelizaeus–Merzbacher disease can be clinically difficult. All may be misdiagnosed initially as cases of cerebral palsy.

Paroxysmal choreoathetosis. This is an odd condition with grimacing, choreiform movements and abnormal posturing, which occur in episodes. It may be difficult without a continuous 24-hour EEG recording to differentiate sporadic cases from epilepsies manifested with similar abnormal movements. The condition does not progress and is not associated with dementia. Onset may be as early as 6 months of age. Examination between episodes is normal, as is the EEG. It is dominantly inherited and no biochemical abnormality has been found. Sudden movement, or a particular movement, may precipitate bouts of choreoathetosis. The episode may be brief or may last several hours. Consciousness is usually maintained, even in paroxysmal choreoathetosis lasting hours or days. Paroxysmal choreoathetosis can also occur as a consequence of lesions to the basal ganglia, such as low grade astrocytomas. Dystonia or athetoid posturing precipitated by movement, i.e. paroxysmal kinesiogenic dystonia, may be very sensitive to carbamazepine.

Initial treatment is with anticonvulsants, particularly carbamazepine and phenytoin. If unsuccessful, prolonged episodes can be treated with anticholinergics such as benzatropine.

Systemic diseases
Sydenham chorea. This is the most common acquired chorea in children. It is a cardinal feature of rheumatic fever and alone is enough for the diagnosis. The onset is usually 4 months after the initiating streptococcal infection.

The onset is usually insidious and diagnosis is often delayed. Chorea, hypotonia, dysarthria, restlessness and emotional lability are essential features. An early feature is an unexplained deterioration in school work with the affected child being accused of 'messing about'. Obsessive-compulsive behavior may be present.

On examination the child looks fidgety with migratory chorea of limbs and face. This may be unilateral initially but eventually becomes generalized in most. The child tries to mask the chorea with voluntary movements, which gives the appearance of restlessness.

Gradual improvement occurs over several months, and most young people recover completely. Rheumatic valvular heart disease develops in one third of untreated cases.

The diagnosis is essentially clinical. The differential diagnosis includes drug-induced chorea and systemic lupus erythematosus, making measurement of lupus antinuclear antibody titers worthwhile. Antistreptolysin O titer is usually back to normal or only slightly raised by the time of presentation.

All children with Sydenham chorea should be treated with high doses of penicillin for 10 days to eradicate active streptococcal infection and should continue with prophylactic penicillin until the age of 21. Pimozide usually controls the neurological symptoms without sedation. Alternatives are tetrabenazine, benzodiazepines, phenothiazines or haloperidol.

Chorea gravidarum. Chorea can complicate pregnancy. The likely explanation is that it may be the initial attack or recurrence of Sydenham chorea or lupus erythematosus triggered by the pregnancy.[326]

Choreas associated with systemic lupus erythmatosus and hyperthyroidism tumors. Although chorea is a rare presentation of tumors compared with seizures or a slowly evolving paresis, cerebral hemisphere tumors may be associated with any types of movement disorder.

DYSTONIA

Definition

Dystonia is an abnormal posture caused by the simultaneous contraction of agonist and antagonist muscles.

Differential diagnosis

Dystonia may be focal, affecting a single body part, segmental affecting contiguous parts, hemidystonia, affecting one side, or generalized, affecting both sides of the body. The differential diagnosis of dystonia is listed in Table 22.23; other conditions associated with abnormal postures are listed in Table 22.24.

Specific syndromes
Focal dystonias

Benign paroxysmal torticollis. This is a self-limiting, benign condition that starts in the first year of life with repeated attacks of sickness, apparent discomfort and tilting of the head to one side and often associated with eye deviation to the same side. This may be repetitive. The affected side may change from one to another. Occasionally the trunk might incline to the same side and this may be associated with a degree of ipsilateral stiffness. Ataxia is not uncommon, especially later in the course of the disease. Shifting torticollis that occurs in attacks suggests the diagnosis. The combination of head tilt and nystagmus is termed spasmus nutans.

Although the initial presentation may suggest a posterior fossa tumor, the attacks rapidly subside leaving a normal child with no neurological abnormalities.

There is a well-recognized relation between this condition and migraine as with paroxysmal vertigo, and a family history of migraine may be relevant to the diagnosis.

Dystonia associated with hiatus hernia: Sandifer syndrome. Hiatus hernia may be associated with sudden spastic opisthotonic extension of the head, neck and sometimes of the upper part of the trunk. The head may move from side to side with the upper trunk bent to one side. All manner of bizarre posturing predominantly of the upper torso and arms may be seen. These bouts usually cease during sleep and may increase during, or shortly after, feeding. Vomiting and other symptoms of the hernia may be obvious or occult.

Table 22.23 Differential diagnosis of dystonia in children

Focal dystonias
Torticollis
Writer's cramp
Blepharospasm
Drug-induced dystonia
Generalized dystonia present initially with focal dystonia
Drug reaction

Hemidystonia
Basal ganglia tumors
Cerebral tumors
Antiphospholipid syndrome
DOPA responsive dystonia
Glutaric aciduria type 1
Hallervorden–Spatz disease
Idiopathic generalized dystonia
Infantile bilateral striatal necrosis
Wilson disease
Ceroid lipofuscinosis

Generalized symptomatic dystonias
Drug reaction
Post encephalitis/meningitis
Post traumatic
Cerebral palsy
Post stroke
Sandifer syndrome

Table 22.24 Conditions associated with abnormal posture

Dystonia
Myotonia
Spasticity
Neuromuscular conditions
Stiffman syndrome
Hysteria

The condition may be underdiagnosed or misdiagnosed as one of the idiopathic movement disorders leading to unnecessary treatment and intervention. The key is to consider the possibility and then treat the hernia and associated reflux as appropriate.

Generalized dystonias

Flexor dystonia is a feature of carbon monoxide poisoning, head injury and encephalitis. The affected child may lie curled up with marked flexor dystonia and complete akinesia. In less severe cases the child may be stooped, flexed at the elbows, knees and hips with the head bent forward. Classically, the arms are flexed and resist passive extension and the legs are flexed on the abdomen with the toes tending to claw. The asymmetrical tonic neck reflexes and progression reflexes are absent. It is not influenced by anxiety and does not disappear in sleep. Chorea and athetosis are not seen. L-DOPA will release the patient from the flexor rigidity.

Extensor dystonia occurs most commonly in children as the dystonic phase of cerebral palsy. It is not caused by a known neurotransmitter imbalance but may be seen as part of some of the very acute dystonic reactions described later as unwanted effects of certain neuroleptic drugs, in which case they are rapidly abolished by anticholinergics. Extensor dystonia corresponds to the physiological second stage of extension seen in normal child development between 6 weeks and 4 months after birth. In the abnormal or diseased state it is an obligatory exaggeration or caricature of this normal physiological developmental state. It is the hallmark of the cerebral palsies which follow kernicterus before choreoathetosis makes its appearance, of dystonia associated with prematurity or due to basal ganglia damage following perinatal asphyxia.

Juvenile parkinsonism. The clinical picture of tremor, bradykinesia and flexor rigidity has already been outlined. Parkinsonism is a form of dyskinesia rarely seen in children (Table 22.25).

Treatment of parkinsonism consists of L-DOPA combined with inhibition of the peripheral tissue breakdown by a specific carboxylase which increases the concentration of L-DOPA in the brain. This is often combined with an anticholinergic such as benzatropine. Surgery does not have a place in most of the cases of childhood parkinsonism.

Dopa-responsive dystonia. Dopa-responsive dystonia (DRD) is also known as hereditary progressive dystonia with diurnal variation (HPD) and Segawar disease. The onset usually is between 2 and 9 years.

The striking feature of the disease is the fluctuation of dystonia in relation to the sleep–waking cycle. The child may be normal on waking, but after 30–60 minutes the dystonic movements start and increase with time. The response to low dose L-DOPA is dramatic, with restoration of normal mobility.

The initial presentation is with gait disturbance, difficulties walking and frequent falls. Dystonia usually affects one of the lower limbs and then spreads to others. Rarely it involves the truncal muscles.

Sometimes, the diurnal fluctuation might not be prominent, the family history may be absent and the response to L-DOPA may not be dramatic. It is essential to give the medication a full 3 months' trial. It is also very important to consider the diagnosis of a dopa-responsive dystonia in children with a symmetrical cerebral palsy where the investigations, including neuroimaging, are normal and there have been no antenatal/perinatal risk factors (such as prematurity in a child with a diplegia). It is particularly important to think of this possibility where the signs continue to evolve after the first 2 years or so, into later childhood.

In many children in this undoubtedly heterogeneous group, DRD is inherited as a dominant trait with low penetrance. The gene is mapped to chromosome 14 and codes for the enzyme GTP cyclohydrolase 1 which is involved in the synthesis of biopterin. Several different mutations are reported.

Treatment is with L-DOPA along with an inhibitor of peripheral catabolism. The required dose is usually small (50–250 mg/day). Considering the existence of atypical responses, higher doses up to (750 mg/day) may need to be tried. Table 22.26 shows other conditions which respond to L-DOPA. Some people have been treated now for 30 years or so with no reports of long term unwanted effects or signs of tolerance.

Dystonia musculorum deformans. Idiopathic torsion dystonia (ITD) is a severe dystonia that occurs in many of the diseases already described. The term is usually restricted, however, to unilateral torticollis exten-

sion of the leg, torsion of the trunk, extension and internal rotation of the arm (Fig. 22.25).

Although the condition can be seen in some cases of dyskinetic cerebral palsy and in some children with a relatively pure dyskinetic hemiplegia, there are two genetic forms, autosomal recessive and autosomal dominant. The former is more common in Ashkenazi Jews. A large proportion of the early onset dominant form have a coding sequence deletion in the GAG trinucleotide repeat in the DYT1 gene on chromosome 9q34. This offers a useful diagnostic test.[327] Treatment is with L-DOPA, anticholinergics and benzodiazepines (Table 22.27).

A group of children with onset of a paroxysmal dystonia, which is better in the mornings and worsens as the day wears on, has been described. Rest does not reduce the dystonia but rapid eye movement (REM) sleep results in alleviation for a short time. The condition may be associated with a severe generalized dystonia with brisk reflexes and extensor plantar responses and may progress to the point where the child cannot walk. The importance of this subgroup of dystonia musculorum

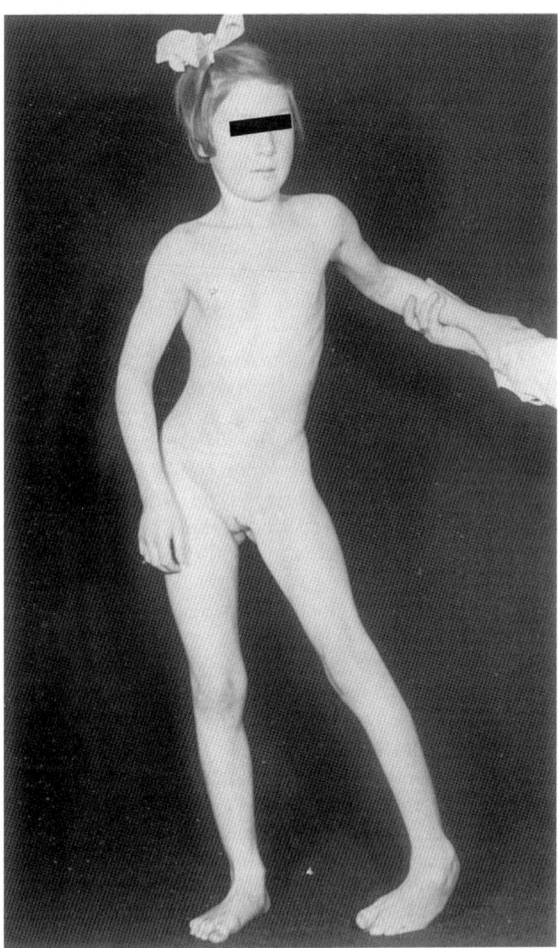

Fig. 22.25 Characteristic posture of the left lower limb in dystonia musculorum deformans. Mother and an uncle also suffered from the condition.

Table 22.25 Causes of parkinsonism in children

Familial striatonigral degeneration of Hunt
Postencephalitic
Drug induced – haloperidol, reserpine, phenothiazine
Subacute sclerosing panencephalitis – measles
Batten disease
Phenylketonuria – lack of tyrosine
Head injury, e.g. boxers
Lewy body idiopathic
Methyl-4–1,2,3,6-tetrahydropyridine (MPTP) toxicity
Manganese toxicity

Table 22.26 Movement disorders which may respond to L-DOPA

DOPA-responsive dystonia
Striatonegral degeneration*
Pallidopyramidal syndrome*
Juvenile idiopathic parkinsonism
Parkinsonism secondary to hydrocephalus*

* Not all the cases, but worth trying.

Table 22.27 Treatment of idiopathic torsion dystonia

Levodopa/carbidopa
Anticholinergics
Benzodiazepines (clonazepam, tetrabenazine)
Others (baclofen, carbamazepine)
Mixed treatments (e.g. anticholinergics + baclofen +/– pimozide and/or tetrabenazine and/or haloperidol)

deformans is that these children are extremely sensitive to L-DOPA and 25 or 50 mg of the drug together with a peripheral carboxylase inhibitor results in very dramatic improvement.

Wilson disease. This is an important cause of dystonia and is discussed in Chapter 26 (see p. 1125).

Glutaric aciduria type 1. In this condition, episodes of crying, cyanosis, pallor, lethargy and hypotonia may commence early in the first year of life. From about 5 months onwards an acute onset with tachypnea, acidosis and stiffness following a minor infection is common. There may be associated seizures, suggesting a diagnosis of febrile convulsions, or encephalitis, in the first instance. The episodes tend to be repeated and dystonia and choreoathetosis, if not present initially, gradually appear. The caudate and putamen show a loss of nerve cells and gliosis. Organic acid analysis shows raised glutaric and betahydroxyglutaric acid excretion in most, but not all cases. Serum L-carnitine is usually reduced. Glutaryl CoA dehydrogenase assay in fibroblasts gives the definitive diagnosis. Treatment with a low lysine and tryptophan diet has been tried without dramatic clinical improvement.

Choreoathetosis can also be a symptom of other metabolic disorders such as D-glyceric acidemia and sulfite oxidase deficiency, underlining the importance of a full metabolic screen with appropriate specialist advice in this group of disorders (see Ch. 26, p. 1062).

Dystonia with basal ganglia calcification. With the advent of modern imaging, basal ganglia calcification is a relatively common finding. There are many causes (Table 22.28) and the movement disorder may not be the initial or sole presentation.

Symptomatic generalized dystonia. Many diseases and disorders such as brain tumors, the effect of hypoxia, stroke, head injury and encephalitis may cause dystonia. The onset of dystonia may be during the acute illness or several years later.

Drug-induced movement disorders

Drug-induced dyskinesias are usually idiosyncratic reactions or the result of toxicity and not related to the principal pharmacological action of the specific causative drug. Drug-induced dyskinesias are particularly likely with major tranquilizers (phenothiazines and butyrophenones) and the newer antipsychotic agents, which may cause parkinsonism, tardive dyskinesia and acute dystonic reactions, the latter presenting as opisthotonos and oculogyric crises. Treatment is with diphenylhydramine (2 mg/kg), tetrabenazine or anticholinergic agents. Metaclopramide can cause an identical clinical picture.

Opisthotonos, muscular rigidity and other extrapyramidal signs association with hypothermia, decreased consciousness and autonomic disturbance occur in the neuroleptic malignant syndrome precipitated by certain inhalational anesthetic agents.

Stimulants (e.g. methylphenidate) cause motor tics and chorea and are a cause of Tourette-like disorder (see below).

The selective serotonin reuptake inhibitors (SSRIs), used in pediatric practice for depression and obsessive-compulsive disorder, may produce a hyperkinetic movement disorder with myoclonus and tremor as part of the serotoninenergic toxic syndrome.

MYOCLONUS

Myoclonus is a brief, sudden, involuntary, shock-like muscle contraction arising from the central nervous system. It is usually associated with co-contraction of agonist muscles. A distinction of practical clinical importance is epileptic versus non-epileptic myoclonus. Both types may be focal or generalized and repetitive or nonrepetitive. Further division into rhythmic myoclonus (of brainstem or spinal origin) and arrhythmic myoclonus (cortical or subcortical in origin and due to lack of inhibition) is useful clinically.[328]

Epileptic myoclonus occurs in many different epilepsies. It is a prominent feature of some idiopathic generalized epilepsies, e.g. juvenile myoclonic epilepsy, of the symptomatic and probably symptomatic encephalopathies of the infant and preschool child and is a prominent feature of the epilepsies associated with inherited metabolic disorders, e.g. mitochondrial disorders.

Benign myoclonus of early infancy very closely resembles infantile spasms but is non-epileptic. The infant is not encephalopathic and the EEG is normal.[329]

In benign neonatal sleep myoclonus focal or generalized myoclonic jerks occur in slow wave sleep. It is a common condition and myoclonus may be very frequent. Anticonvulsants are often prescribed inappropriately. Myoclonus does not occur in wakefulness and may be present for some months beyond the neonatal period into infancy. There may be a family history of the condition.[330]

Essential myoclonus is an extrapyramidal disorder of dominant inheritance and is nonprogressive. Myoclonus is worse on movement. EEG is normal, intellectual impairment absent and the condition is not progressive.

Myoclonus is a feature of a wide range of serious neurological disorders. Metabolic disorders in which myoclonus is a feature include aminoacidopathies (hyperglycinemia, phenylketonuria and maple syrup urine disease), sialidosis – cherry red spot myoclonus, Unverricht–Lundborg disease, mitochondrial cytopathies, the late infantile neuronal ceroid lipofuscinoses, Menke disease, sphingolipidoses and Wilson disease.

A curious form of upper limb myoclonus is seen in slow virus infections, including subacute sclerosing panencephalitis in which the myoclonus is 'hung up', i.e. sudden contraction of muscles followed by delayed relaxation.

Symptomatic myoclonus may occur in conditions characterized by brain malformations, such as Aicardi syndrome, tuberous sclerosis and Sturge–Weber syndrome.

When myoclonus is symptomatic it is never the only neurological symptom, but it may be the only symptom at presentation and for a time thereafter. Symptomatic myoclonus may arise from pathology at any level of the neuroaxis and is the result of hyperexcitability (or lack of suppression) of gray matter in the cortex, basal ganglia, brainstem

Table 22.28   Causes of basal ganglia calcification

Endocrine	Congenital and metabolic disease	Infection	Neoplasms
Hypoparathyroidism	Mitochondrial encephalopathies	Toxoplasmosis	Craniopharyngioma
Pseudohypoparathyroidism	Leigh's encephalopathy	Subacute sclerosing panencephalitis	Optic nerve glioma
Pseudopseudohypoparathyroidism	Hallervorden–Spatz disease	Cytomegalovirus infection	Radiotherapy
Hyperparathyroidism	Chronic methemoglobinemia	Congenital rubella	Methotrexate therapy
Hypothyroidism	Carbon monoxide poisoning	AIDS	for leukemia
	Lead poisoning		
	Systemic lupus		
	Cockayne syndrome		
	Down syndrome		
	Tuberous sclerosis		
	Neurofibromatosis		

and spinal cord. Cortical myoclonus, in which there is increased cortical excitability with giant sensory and action potentials, results from localized brain lesions, e.g. space-occupying lesions of the sensorimotor cortex, or, more frequently, is of multifocal origin following cerebral hypoxia.[331] In the latter situation, the myoclonus may be generalized or focal.

In celiac disease the syndrome of progressive myoclonic ataxia is seen. This is not responsive to a gluten-free diet and an auto-immune etiology has been suggested.

An autoimmune etiology has also been proposed in the opsoclonus-myoclonus (dancing eye) syndrome. This serious disorder presents in the infant or toddler with irritability, loss of skills, generalized myoclonus, ataxia and chaotic eye movements (opsoclonus). The condition has a postinfectious etiology in around 50% of cases but an association with neural crest tumors, particularly neuroblastomas is recognized. The pathophysiology involves binding of specific autoantibodies to the Purkinje cells of the cerebellum. Steroids and intravenous immunoglobulins are effective treatments but the course is often relapsing and half of those affected have persisting neurodevelopmental impairments.[332]

Spinal myoclonus is segmental or involves multiple spinal segments. Segmental myoclonus is usually symptomatic of a structural cord lesion.

Treatment of symptomatic, non-epileptic myoclonus is of the underlying cause. Piracetam, clonazepam and valproate may be helpful but pharmacological treatment of symptomatic myoclonus is often disappointing.

TICS AND TOURETTE SYNDROME

Tics are involuntary, purposeless contractions of functionally related groups of skeletal muscles. They are brief, repetitive, stereotyped, non-rhythmic movements or vocalizations. Motor tics persist in sleep (which is unusual in movement disorders).

Transient tic disorder is common. Estimates vary from 5% to 25% of all children at some time in childhood.[333] Most people have some stereotyped movement that they pursue when tired, bored or stressed. A ride on a bus, a glance around a lecture or committee meeting will reveal an array of hair twiddlers, nail biters or pickers, finger drummers or foot tappers. Most people keep these idiosyncrasies throughout their lives, with periods in which the habit is more or less obvious. The adoption in some diagnostic classifications such as DSM-IV of a fixed time course in some of its definitions (Table 22.29) is therefore problematic.[334]

Those who have movements above the shoulders often get taken to doctors as they are less likely to be accepted in social settings. It is rare to be presented with a finger tapper, much more commonly a blinker. Many children with tics persisting for more than 1 year have Tourette syndrome, which is increasingly recognized as having great variation in severity. Tourette syndrome is a chronic disorder characterized by multiple motor and at least one vocal tic waxing and waning but present for at least 1 year with onset most commonly between 4 and 11 years of age. It is no longer regarded as rare – the prevalence is 1:2000 and the male to female ratio 4:1.[335]

Simple tics presenting to doctors usually involve the face or shoulders – blinking, stretching facial muscles, head flicking, shoulder shrugging, etc. More complex tics include forced touching, sniffing or licking and there is a close association with obsessive-compulsive disorder (OCD). Premonitory sensory sensations preceding the tics are common. Tics can be voluntarily suppressed for a short time but this is distressing if continued. 'Sensory tics' can occur alone.

Simple vocal tics include grunting, throat clearing, coughing, barking and complex vocal tics include echolalia phrases. Coprolalia (obscene words), though well known, is rare, occurring in less than 10% of cases.

Although tics are the most common clinical manifestation of Tourette syndrome, it is often the associated psychopathology that produces most impairment. These include obsessive-compulsive disorder, attention-deficit-hyperactivity disorder (ADHD), depression, anxiety and specific learning difficulties, particularly dyscalculia. There is often a strong family history of tic disorder or psychopathology with OCD being particularly common.

As with most tic disorders people with Tourette syndrome have a lifelong tendency to the disorder with good spells and bad spells and often an exacerbation during adolescence.

Treatment is multidisciplinary. It is important to support the family and the child in education. Occasionally behavioral treatments for tics and obsessive-compulsive symptoms may be helpful. Neuroleptics, sulpiride and haloperidol are highly effective. Tranidine is useful for treatment of ADHD. Drug holidays are indicated and families must be warned about the rare but serious occurrence of tardive dyskinesia with chronic neuroleptic use.

A Tourette-like disorder with tics, but without the psychopathology of Tourette syndrome, may occur secondary to acquired brain injury, such as following head injuries. Pediatric autoimmune neuropsychiatric disorder associated with streptococcal infection (PANDAS) is of interest in that in a significant number of children with Tourette syndrome group A streptococcal infection is associated with antibodies that cross-react with putaminal neurones. Some children in whom traditional pharmacotherapy treatment has failed have responded to steroids or immunomodifying therapy.[336]

TREMOR

Tremor is a continuous rhythmic and involuntary movement disorder of a body part and results in alternating contractions of agonist and antagonistic muscles.

Table 22.29 DSM-IV criteria for tic disorders. (Adapted from APA[334])

Common criteria
The tics occur many times a day (usually in bouts) nearly every day
The disturbance causes marked distress or significant impairment in social, occupational or other important areas of functioning
Onset is before age 18 years
The disturbance is not due to the direct physiological effects of a substance or a general medical condition

Tourette syndrome
Both multiple motor and one or more vocal tics have been present at some time during the illness, although not necessarily concurrently, throughout a period of more than 1 year, and during this period there was never a tic-free period of more than 3 consecutive months

Chronic tic disorder
Single or multiple motor or vocal tics, but not both, have been present at some time during the illness throughout a period of more than 1 year, and during this period there was never a tic-free period of more than 3 consecutive months

Transient tic disorder
Single or multiple motor and/or vocal tics for at least 4 weeks but not longer than 12 consecutive months

Tic disorder not otherwise specified
Cases that do not meet the criteria for a specific tic disorder

A clinically useful classification is tremor at rest, tremor on maintenance of a posture (postural tremor) and action tremor, i.e. tremor occurring on performance of a voluntary activity. It must be noted that action tremor is not synonymous with the intention tremor of cerebellar disease. Intention tremor is one type of action tremor and is characterized by accentuation of tremor just before the target is reached on finger/nose testing. At its most extreme the oscillations in terminal intention tremor, as seen in Wilson disease, may be so violent that there is a risk of self-injury. A similar gross intention tremor can be seen after traumatic brain injury.

Resting tremor is not common in pediatric practice. Causes include Wilson disease, juvenile Parkinson disease and neuroleptic drugs.

Postural tremor is tested by asking the child to stand with arms outstretched or to hold arms abducted and flexed at the elbows, with the hands brought to the midline and the fingers of one hand almost, but not quite touching the fingers of the other hand. The commonest cause of postural tremor is physiological tremor.

Familial essential tremor is often of dominant inheritance and both postural and action tremor are present. While there is a danger of overdiagnosis of essential tremor (particular care is necessary if family history is negative), most high frequency low amplitude tremors are physiological. If an essential tremor is widespread, the legs may be involved, and titubation, producing head nodding, may be present. Shuddering attacks in infants are an early manifestation.[337] Essential tremor may worsen during childhood. Treatment should be considered if writing is seriously impaired. Propranolol and primidone may help but unwanted effects limit usefulness.

Symptomatic causes of tremor include traumatic brain injury (tremor may become evident in the first year post injury and subsides spontaneously in 50% of cases), juvenile Parkinson disease, severe malnutrition with cobalamin deficiency, Wilson disease, hepatic encepalopathy, as a drug side-effect (e.g. sodium valproate), in juvenile multiple sclerosis, galactosemia, hereditary and acquired ataxias, Hartnup disease, hereditary fructose intolerance, thalamic tumor, vascular accidents involving the thalamus and internal capsule, spinal muscular atrophies and occasionally in hereditary motor and sensory neuropathies. Treatment is of the underlying cause.

NYSTAGMUS

Nystagmus is a tremor of the eyes, which may involve rhythmical conjugate oscillatory movement in any plane. It usually involves an initiating component and a fast correcting component. Clinically, different patterns of movement may be recognized. In pendular nystagmus the oscillations are slow in each direction with the eyes in a neutral position but on lateral gaze they may show a jerky quality. Jerk nystagmus indicates a slow phase in one direction followed by a fast corrective jerk in the other. It is the direction of the fast component that conventionally defines the direction of the nystagmus. When gaze is in the direction of the fast phase the intensity of the nystagmus increases.

Nystagmus should be differentiated from the roving eye movements of a blind child or one with significantly reduced acuity, particularly in the first 2 years of life. Opsoclonus involves very fast saccadic eye movement in all directions occurring in sudden bursts. It is associated with the dancing eye syndrome and its underlying causes, notably neuroblastoma. Ocular bobbing and dipping involve downward movement of the eyes with corrective movement to the mid-position. They indicate brainstem dysfunction often seen in comatose children. Oculomotor dyspraxia, commonly associated with ataxia telangiectasia, involves difficulty with horizontal saccadic eye movement. The eyes are often left behind the position of the head, later to be restituted with a characteristic flick of the head.

The most common cause of jerk nystagmus is gaze-evoked nystagmus reflecting dysfunction of the posterior fossa centers responsible for holding the eyes in an eccentric position. Vestibular nystagmus is also a jerk nystagmus resulting from involvement of the vestibular end-organ or its central pathways and nuclei.

Congenital nystagmus may be sensory, due to low acuity, or motor, due to a defect in the slow eye movement system. It is usually evident from birth and dominant, recessive and X-linked inheritance is described. It is usually horizontal (even on upgaze) but may be vertical or rotary. Pendular nystagmus is almost never acquired. Congenital nystagmus is abolished by sleep and increased by attempts at fixation. Up to 8.0% of children may have associated head bobbing.

ATAXIA
Definition and types
Ataxia is incoordination of movement not due to weakness, involuntary movements or abnormal muscle tone and is the major clinical sign of cerebellar disease. Sensory ataxia results when there is impaired afferent input into the cerebellum via the spinocerebellar pathways.

The three types of ataxia resulting from cerebellar disease are gait, truncal and limb and each has anatomical localizing value. Gait and truncal ataxia are due to lesions of the vermis or brainstem cerebellar connections; limb ataxia results from ipsilateral cerebellar hemisphere lesions. The causes are summarized in Table 22.30.

Examination
An infant is best examined on the parent's knee and encouraged to reach out with each hand. Intention tremor is distinctive, of maximum

Table 22.30   Selected causes of ataxia in childhood

Progressive/inherited
Friedreich ataxia
Ataxia telangiectasia
Spinocerebellar degeneration (SCA)/olivopontocerebellar ataxias
Cockayne syndrome
Pelizaeus–Merzbacher disease
Ramsay Hunt syndrome

Metabolic
Any cause of fat malabsorption
Abetalipoproteinemia
Vitamin E deficiency
Mitochondrial cytopathies
Refsum disease
Sialidosis
Neuronal ceroid lipofuscinosis (late infantile)
Biotinidase deficiency
Metachromatic leukodystrophy
Organic acidemias
Urea cycle disorders

Acute/subacute
Acute cerebellar ataxia
Posterior fossa tumor/space occupying lesion
Acute disseminated encephalomyelitis
Miller–Fisher syndrome
Postinfectious polyneuropathy
Acute labyrinthitis
Hydrocephalus
Traumatic brain injury
Toxic/poisoning
Nonconvulsive status

Nonprogressive
Ataxic cerebral palsy
Congenital cerebellar abnormalities

As part of a complex syndrome
Dandy–Walker
Joubert
Angelman
Chiari malformation
Basilar impression

amplitude at the beginning and end of the range of movement and is irregular. Dysmetria is error in the estimation of the amplitude of movement.

In the older infant a delay in gaining independent walking, having cruised at a normal age, may be the first manifestation of gait ataxia. A child with truncal ataxia will not sit without supporting herself or is easily knocked off balance when sitting.

It is important when using the finger/nose test to ensure maximum range of movement, by ensuring that the child's arm is not held adducted against her trunk and that the child's arm is fully extended during finger/nose testing.

A child with gait ataxia stands and walks with feet widely apart and cannot place one foot directly in front of the other (tandem walking). This is best demonstrated to the child. Most 5-year-old children can tandem walk easily, when shown what to do by the examiner.

Rapid alternating movements (dysdiadochokinesis) are tested by rapid pronation and supination of the forearm.

Every ataxic child should have careful fundal examination for papilledema, plotting of head circumference and, in the infant, assessment of fontanel pressure, as posterior fossa space-occupying lesions often present with ataxia.

Other signs of cerebellar dysfunction commonly seen in ataxia are jerk nystagmus, hypotonia and diminished reflexes.

Causes of ataxia
Ataxia is always of significance and requires full investigation. It is rare for a definitive diagnosis not to be made.

Tumors
Infratentorial tumors. Infratentorial tumors often involve the cerebellar vermis producing gait ataxia. Any unsteady child with headache or sleepiness must be assumed to have a posterior fossa tumor. There may be no long tract signs. The commonest tumors are medulloblastoma/primitive neuroectodermal tumors, which produce obstructive hydrocephalus with headache, vomiting and ataxia. Cerebellar hemisphere astrocytomas do not usually produce obstructive hydrocephalus, are indolent, of good prognosis and produce ipsilateral ataxia. Diffuse astrocytomas also occur. Ependymomas produce fourth ventricle obstruction.
Intrinsic brainstem tumors. These present with gait and truncal ataxia, with cranial nerve dysfunction and long tract signs. Cranial nerve dysfunction is often evidenced by dysphagia, lower motor neurone facial palsy and gaze palsy or nystagmus. The duration of ataxia before diagnosis may be as short as a few weeks and a mistaken diagnosis of acute cerebellar ataxia may be made if specific signs, particularly lower motor neurone cranial nerve dysfunction, are not sought.

Cranial MRI is almost invariably abnormal though CT may be normal. Cranial MRI shows an intrinsic brainstem lesion, a cystic mass or an exophytic lesion. Histological diagnosis is difficult because of the site of tumor and danger of brainstem swelling with biopsy. Biopsy is now no longer usually performed in typical cases. Prognosis is generally poor, with death within 2 years, but a small number are long term survivors with only very slow progression.

Acute ataxias
The commonest neurological causes of acute ataxia are infectious or postinfectious.

Acute cerebellar ataxia often follows a viral infection, commonly varicella. It is most common in children under the age of 4 years. It often presents with the child suddenly stopping walking. He may revert to crawling and ataxia may be difficult to demonstrate. The infant is not weak and reflexes are present, although they may be depressed. There is no cranial nerve involvement other than nystagmus (in 50% of cases). However, the child may be dysarthric. Differential diagnosis includes posterior fossa or brainstem tumor and if cranial MRI is available it should be done. CSF is usually normal. It is particularly important to note that CSF protein is normal early in the course of the condition. The importance of this finding is that CSF protein is usually elevated in

postinfectious polyneuropathy, which may present as gait ataxia. The child with acute postinfectious cerebellar ataxia is not encephalopathic and not distressed (pain is an important early feature of postinfectious polyneuropathy). Recovery is rapid (weeks) but occasionally takes months and in a very small number of children ataxia persists.

A rare type of postinfectious polyneuropathy is the Miller–Fisher syndrome, which presents with an acute cerebellar ataxia, ophthalmoplegia and areflexia but with no weakness. CSF protein is elevated and serum antibodies against ganglioside CQ1B may be found. Antibodies against this ganglioside recognize epitopes from *Campylobacter jejuni* indicating crossreactivity. Urgent MRI is indicated by the combination of ophthalmoplegia and ataxia. The cause of ataxia in the Miller–Fisher syndrome is unknown. Recovery is over weeks and is usually complete. Intravenous immunoglobulins may help as in postinfectious polyneuropathy.

Many metabolic disorders include ataxia in their clinical phenotype. In females with X-linked ornithine transcarbamylase deficiency, ataxia (which is often of acute onset) and vomiting occur during metabolic decompensation. Ammonia is elevated. Other metabolic disorders presenting with acute ataxia include mitochondrial cytopathies, maple syrup urine disease and Hartnup disease. Ataxia is a feature of Batten disease and metachromatic leukodystrophy. In these conditions ataxia is of subacute onset.

Distinguishing acute ataxia from acute labyrinthitis is difficult in a young child. The child with labyrinthitis is distressed, vomiting and does not have limb ataxia when encouraged to reach.

Acute ataxia as a result of poisoning or intoxication is caused by anticonvulsants (particularly carbamazepine and benzodiazepines), alcohol and thallium containing insecticides.

In nonconvulsive status epilepticus, and the symptomatic and probably symptomatic age-dependent epileptic encephalopathies ataxia, initially intermittent, may be the presenting feature with regression of speech and cognition.

Inherited ataxias
The inherited ataxias are of recessive, dominant or X-linked inheritance and many are triplet repeat diseases. The commonest is Friedreich ataxia; the others are summarized in Table 22.31.

Friedreich ataxia and other spinocerebellar degenerations
This has a prevalence of 1:48 000 and is a progressive disorder with most children having very severe physical disability by adulthood although survival to the fifth or sixth decade is possible.

Friedreich ataxia is recessively inherited. The gene is mapped to 9q13 and codes for the protein frataxin, an 18-kb soluble mitochondrial protein with 210 amino acids. The GAA triplet repeat expansion produces frataxin deficiency with clinical severity related to the GAA expansion size. The protein function is unknown. Truncal ataxia is the first symptom, with onset as young as 2 years, followed by dysarthria, limb ataxia and evolving kyphoscoliosis. Findings include nystagmus, pes cavus, distal weakness, posterior column dysfunction, areflexia and extensor plantars.

All children require cardiological assessment and review. Hypertrophic cardiomyopathy and ECG abnormalities (T wave abnormalities and heart block) are found. Diabetes and impaired color vision also occur. Friedreich ataxia is relentlessly progressive and there is no specific medical treatment of proven benefit. However, much can be done to help the child and family by rehabilitative management ensuring access to education, independent mobility (often with a powered chair) and help with activities of daily living.

Diagnosis is by determining the number of GAA repeats in a child with progressive ataxia.

All of the inherited spinocerebellar ataxias have varying degrees of pyramidal and extrapyramidal involvement. There are 10 autosomal dominant hereditary ataxias (spinocerebellar ataxias, SCAs) separated by genotype. Most are triplet repeat diseases.[338]

Table 22.31   The spinocerebellar ataxias: genotypes and main clinical features. (After Morrison[338])

Name	Gene locus	Autosomal inheritance	Triplet repeat	Anticipation	Chorea	Dementia	Sensory loss	Retinal degeneration
SCA-1	6p23	AD	CAG	P			+	
SCA-2	12q23	AD	CAG	P	+	+		
SCA-3/MJD	14q32.1	AD	CAG	P			+	
SCA-4	16q24	AD	?	?			+	
SCA-5	11cent	AD	?	M				
SCA-6	19p13	AD	CAG	P			+	
SCA-7	3p12–13	AD	CAG	P			+	+
DRPLA	12p12	AD	CAG	P	+	+		
SCA-?9	13q21	AD	CTG	M			+	
SCA-10	22q13	AD	?	?		+		
SCA-11	15q14–21	AD	?	?		+		
SCA-12	–	AD	CAG	?				
Friedreich	20 9q13	AR	GAA	–			+	
A VED	8q13	AR		–			+	
ABLP	4q22–24	AR		–			+	+
SCA-8/ IOSCA	10q24	AR	?	–	+			+

All show cerebellar ataxia.
P, with paternal transmission; M, with maternal transmission.
?, Not yet identified.
IOSCA, infant onset spinocerebellar ataxia; MJD, Machado–Joseph disease.
AD, autosomal dominant; AR, autosomal recessive.

Ataxia telangiectasia

The second commonest cause of progressive ataxia in childhood is ataxia telangiectasia which is discussed elsewhere in this chapter (see p. 839).

Inherited vitamin E deficiency

Any chronic disorder causing intestinal fat malabsorption may result in vitamin E deficiency and hence features of spinocerebellar degeneration. Vitamin E deficiencies, due to abetalipoproteinemia and familial vitamin E deficiency, are recessive ataxias. The importance of the latter is that the phenotype is of Friedreich ataxia though cardiomyopathy is rare. In hereditary vitamin E deficiency the gene is located on 8q13 and codes for alpha tocopherol transfer protein. Large doses of vitamin E can halt progression and occasionally improve neurological function.

NONPROGRESSIVE ATAXIAS AND ATAXIC CEREBRAL PALSY

Congenital nonprogressive ataxia is synonymous with ataxic cerebral palsy and many nonprogressive ataxias of early onset, particularly if associated with learning difficulties, are inherited. Even if there is a history of intrapartum asphyxia, attributing ataxic cerebral palsy to this cause is likely to be wrong and there may be recurrence in future children. Inheritance is usually recessive, occasionally dominant. All such children should undergo MRI scanning, which often shows congenital cerebellar abnormalities, such as vermian or generalized cerebellar hypoplasia.

In ataxic diplegia there are components of both ataxia and spastic cerebral palsy. The causes are similar to spastic diplegia and both are associated with prematurity. In addition it is a characteristic feature of 'neglected' hydrocephalus. Inherited forms of ataxic diplegia occur.

SYNDROMES FEATURING ATAXIA

Children with Angelman syndrome have severe learning difficulties, a jerky ataxia (hence the former derogatory term 'happy puppet') and (usually) a submicroscopic deletion of maternally derived 15q11-q13.

Ataxia is found in Joubert syndrome, Dandy–Walker cyst and Chiari malformation but in these cases ataxia is but one feature of a complex syndrome. Other causes of ataxia are summarized in Table 22.30.

THE CARBOHYDRATE-DEFICIENT GLYCOPROTEIN SYNDROMES

This group of disorders is dealt with in detail in Chapter 26. The diagnosis should be considered whenever ataxia is accompanied by a learning disability, epilepsy or dysmorphism. Transferrin isoelectric focusing is a useful diagnostic test but will not detect all cases.

CEREBRAL PALSY

DEFINITION

Cerebral palsy is a disorder of posture movement and tone due to a static encephalopathy acquired during brain growth in fetal life, infancy or early childhood. Though the brain disorder is unchanging, the effects are dynamic, as the brain matures, and the child's developmental capabilities extend.

CLASSIFICATION AND EPIDEMIOLOGY

Cerebral palsy syndromes are classified according to the type of motor disorder and the topographical distribution of the condition.[339,340] Spasticity was the commonest motor impairment, reported to be present in 85% of a West Swedish series of 328 children,[341] or about 1:500 children. Dyskinetic cerebral palsy was found in 8.5% and simple ataxia in 6.5%. This means that dyskinetic cerebral palsy occurs in about 1:5000 children and simple ataxia in 1:6500 children. An average general practitioner (GP) in the UK has 25 babies born into the practice per year and the average health visitor (HV) has a caseload of up to 100 new babies per year. So those providing generic services see newly born children with spastic cerebral palsy quite infrequently – a GP once in 20 years and a HV once in 5 years. Only one GP in six and one HV in two will ever have a child patient with dyskinetic cerebral palsy throughout a whole working life. One GP in eight and one HV in three will ever look after a child with simple ataxic cerebral palsy. The diagnosis of cerebral palsy is made by increasing suspicion over time; it is not easy for clinicians who have never seen the condition before.

Cerebral palsy can be classified by its taxonomic distribution. Thus hemiplegia describes cerebral palsy affecting one half of the body predominantly, the upper limb more than the lower limb, normally sparing the bulbar muscles. Quadriplegia, or tetraplegia affects all four limbs, upper limbs more than lower limbs. It is sometimes described as a double hemiplegia and is usually associated with a bulbar palsy. When all four limbs are affected, but the upper limbs are affected less than the legs, this is described as a diplegia. If the part of the body affected predominantly is the bulbar muscles, this is described as congenital suprabulbar paresis or Worster–Drought syndrome.[342] It is helpful to write about functional ability when communicating with colleagues. No two children with cerebral palsy are the same. In recent years improved motor function tools have become available which aid this approach.[343–347]

ETIOLOGY OF CEREBRAL PALSY

Cerebral palsies may arise from genetic causes,[348] developmental brain anomalies, e.g. bilateral perisylvian polymicrogyria in some children with congenital suprabulbar paresis,[349] aqueduct stenosis and Arnold–Chiari malformation of the cerebellum in children with ataxic diplegia, or from a host of acquired causes including intrauterine infection. In a study of 276 term infants with moderate or severe newborn encephalopathy and 564 controls, birth defects were found in 27.5% of the former but only 4.3% of the latter.[350]

Spastic diplegia is the commonest form of cerebral palsy. The children have four-limb cerebral palsy, but the legs are more affected than the arms and bulbar involvement is relatively slight. A minority have ataxia also, mainly truncal (ataxic diplegia). Two thirds of children affected are preterm, but almost always appropriate for gestational age. The characteristic pathology is periventricular leukomalacia (PVL), which occurs when the periventricular structures are particularly vulnerable to hypoperfusion (26–36 weeks' gestation), usually in utero.[351] Birth hypoxia-ischemia is only recorded for a tenth of these children and is never the single risk factor.[352] The response of glial cells to cytokine release triggered by infection in fetus or mother is at least as important.[353] Periventricular venous infarction may coexist with intraventricular hemorrhage in these children, sometimes leading to striking asymmetries of neurological findings in later childhood. In term diplegic infants, with no history of hypoxia-ischemia, it is common to find periventricular myelin defects indicating early prenatal origin from the early third trimester.[354]

Hemiplegia is the commonest form of cerebral palsy in term infants and is second only to diplegia among preterms. The proportion of infants with hemiplegia born at term is about 80%.[355] Hemiplegia derives, usually, from prenatal circulatory disturbances during pregnancy, the commonest, affecting over a third, being periventricular leukomalacia (PVL) due to hypoperfusion of the brain early in the third trimester.[356] Cerebral maldevelopments and major cortical/subcortical lesions each account for about a sixth of cases. Though two thirds of children with hemiplegia have unilateral lesions (rare in other types of cerebral palsy), one third have bilateral lesions.[357] Conversely, children with unilateral lesions, even agenesis of a cerebral hemisphere, do not necessarily show a hemiplegia. The relationship between structural lesions demonstrated by imaging, and neurological function is complex, reflecting the brain's capacity for plasticity in response to dysgenesis or damage.[358]

Spastic quadriplegia (tetraplegia) is a severe form of four-limb cerebral palsy, arms more affected than legs, with bulbar palsy. All have severe or profound learning difficulties; up to 90% have epilepsy; bulbar palsy is often severe and about half have cortical blindness. Currently about a third to 40% are born preterm, including children who would not have survived in the past. Children with acquired spastic diplegia of prematurity almost always show evidence of PVL, whereas those with acquired spastic quadriplegia may show PVL, but more commonly

show full-term-type border zone infarcts, bilateral basal ganglia/thalamic lesions, subcortical leukomalacia and multicystic encephalomalacia.[357] Severe PVL is characteristic of children whose gestational age at birth is between 25 and 32 weeks, whereas term babies tend to have mild PVL. Diplegia (legs are more affected than the arms) should not be loosely confused with quadriplegia (arms more affected) in clinical notes or studies.

Dyskinetic cerebral palsy describes four-limb involvement and bulbar palsy, with fluctuating tone and involuntary movements. Magnetic resonance imaging has helped our understanding of acquired dyskinetic cerebral palsy. Acute near-total intrapartum hypoxia-ischemia for 10–20 minutes causes damage predominantly in the subcortical gray matter.

Affected children should be tested for evidence of congenital rubella, toxoplasmosis or cytomegalovirus (the Guthrie test blood spot taken at birth may be helpful) together with urine culture for rubella and cytomegalovirus, which may be excreted for 3–5 years. Serological tests for syphilis will have been part of the mother's antenatal care but this should be confirmed from the maternity records. Human immunodeficiency virus (HIV) has emerged as an important cause of cerebral palsy (particularly spastic CP) in recent years. This causes a low-grade chronic brain infection, which may not be evident on CT scan. The processes of brain development interact with, and partly overcome, the destructive effects of the encephalopathy so that the child appears to be developmentally delayed, but improving over the first 2 years. Signs of apparent cerebral palsy emerge, but the child may appear to progress up to a point, e.g. sitting and crawling, before regression sets in. Such children do not show signs of full AIDS with a sequence of major infections and bowel upsets. The first serious infection may be *Pneumocystis carinii* pneumonia. This is difficult to diagnose clinically though the chest X-ray is characteristic with a 'ground glass' appearance in the lung fields and a hypoplastic thymus. Opportunistic superinfection, with other organisms such as toxoplasma or cytomegalovirus, may occur and may cause an encephalopathy in their own right. The diagnosis is by detection of HIV antibody titers and characteristic CD4:CD8 lymphocyte counts (see Ch. 28).

Herpes simplex infection can be acquired from the genital tract during birth, leading to a destructive encephalopathy, one consequence of which is a spastic quadriplegia, usually with cortical blindness and epilepsy. The acronym 'TORCH screen' is an aide-mémoire although toxoplasma, rubella and cytomegalovirus cause intrauterine infection whereas herpes simplex virus causes brain damage in an acute, usually obvious, illness after birth. Perhaps the 'H' should now be for HIV.

One mechanism proposed for causing cerebral palsy is the effect of the vanishing twin.[359,360] The proposal is that twin-to-twin transfusion occurs in the first trimester in monochorionic twins through a vascular anastomosis. Following the death of one twin, thromboplastin-like material passes through the vascular connection into the survivor's circulation resulting in end organ damage (the embolic theory). Alternatively the survivor's blood may be shunted into the low-resistance vascular system of the dead fetus causing acute hypovolemia, ischemia and end-organ damage (the ischemic theory). A 'prevanishing twin' syndrome before sonographic detection of two gestational structures may be supported by chorionic villus sampling (CVS). Cytogenetic evidence for this syndrome has been found in 1:2000 singleton pregnancies undergoing CVS.[361] The combination of placental chimerism (rather than mosaicism) and unlike-sexed cell lines, including cells with a chromosome abnormality not found in the surviving fetus, is suggestive of twin-to-twin transfusion early in the first trimester in dichorionic twinning.

PREVENTION OF CEREBRAL PALSY

Stanley et al[362] reviewed causal pathways to the cerebral palsies, a new etiological model and also possibilities for the prevention of the cerebral palsies, i.e. social and medical factors. They quote Hill and Hill's[363] criteria suggesting a causal link should be:

- Strong: high relative risks or odds ratios.
- Consistent: cohorts from different geographic populations/time periods show the same patterns of causal associations.
- Specific: the disease occurs only following exposure to the putative cause and not to other exposures. The exposure is followed by one specific disease, rather than by many diseases.
- Time sequence: the putative cause precedes the outcome.
- Dose dependent, or with a biological gradient: the degree of association increases with increasing intensity of exposure.
- Biological plausibility: a biologically plausible mechanism for the causal association exists.
- Coherence of evidence: the proposed mechanism is consistent with current biological wisdom.

These, often called the Bradford Hill criteria, and the analytical methods to measure the associations, such as multivariate analyses, are largely based on *single and sufficient* or, less often, *multiple independent* causal models. Links between factors on a causal pathway operate in two ways:

1. Independent but their coincidence is necessary for the consequence, e.g. a Rh−ve mother has a Rh+ve partner hence the possibility of a Rh incompatible fetus.
2. Cascade: A causes, or predisposes, to B, which causes or predisposes to C, e.g. a multiple pregnancy predisposes to premature delivery and higher risk for intracerebral hemorrhage.

There are many interventions which could prevent cerebral palsy. These may be considered as follows:

- Proven: MMR vaccination, iodine supplementation in iodine-deficient areas, anti-D for RH−ve women, reducing risk of methylmercury exposure, transfer of the very preterm infant in utero to a tertiary center, reducing embryos transferred in infertility treatments to three or less, fencing swimming pools, home support for socially disadvantaged parents.
- Probable: early routine ultrasound, avoiding excessive alcohol intake in pregnancy, phototherapy for neonatal jaundice, vitamin K at birth to prevent brain hemorrhage, infant restraints in cars, child abuse prevention strategies, sudden infant death syndrome prevention strategies.
- Possible: mode of delivery for very preterm births including breech presentations, zinc, folate or fish oil to prevent intrauterine growth retardation (IUGR), methods of detecting IUGR, operative delivery for fetal distress, amnioinfusion for umbilical cord compression, rescue therapy for birth hypoxia–ischemia.
- Doubtful: electronic fetal monitoring for fetal distress – addition of fetal scalp sampling or ECG, bedrest for growth restriction, hospitalization for multiple pregnancies, multifetal pregnancy reduction for high order multiples, antenatal indometacin or thyrotropin-releasing hormone.

In spite of the proven or probable interventions available, the rate of cerebral palsy remains steady. Such interventions might not be enough. We may not understand all the steps in a complex causal pathway. There may be social factors, which influence people's decisions, which affect the outcome – access to a telephone, care of other children, independent transport, for instance. The balance between death and cerebral palsy may be irreducible. Even if it were possible to prevent the occurrence of cerebral palsy in children who entered labor as healthy, but who showed signs of intrauterine hypoxia–ischemia, to reduce by a quarter the 25% of cerebral palsy cases born preterm, and to prevent the 2% secondary to intrauterine infection, the total reduction in cerebral palsy cases would not exceed 20%. A preventative program might also increase survival rates of children with CP, thus offsetting any benefit.

CLINICAL FEATURES

Spastic diplegia

By the time diplegic children reach the age of 5 years or so they show spasticity in their legs more, or far more, than in their arms (Fig. 22.26).

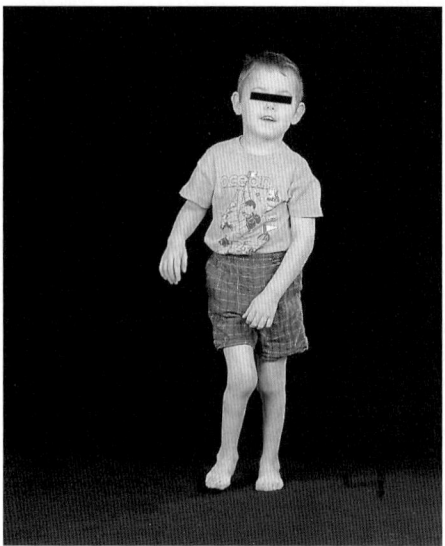

Fig. 22.26 Diplegic gait. Internal rotation with hip adduction.

If the signs are restricted to the legs, investigation of the spinal cord for a paraplegia should be undertaken, even though there is known to be brain damage from intracerebral bleeding, ischemia, meningitis or other conditions in infancy. Such spinal lesions as diastematomyelia, neurenteric or dermoid cysts, myelodysplasia, neurofibromata or vascular infarction may be found. The signs in the diplegic child's arms vary from mild spasticity to manual dyspraxia or dyskinesia, which may have emerged when the child was 3 or 4 years old.

Premature infants in the special care baby unit commonly show neurological abnormalities or ambiguities, which are hard to assess. They may show increased or decreased tone. Episodes are observed which may be seizures. The need for parenteral or nasojejunal feeding removes oral feeding behavior as an indicator of health. Ultrasound scans may show focal lesions of uncertain significance. Risk of cerebral palsy is known to be high for extremely low birth weight premature babies, though most premature babies grow up to be healthy children, free of neurological deficits. Parents and health professionals are bound to be concerned for each individual baby: 'is he/she going to be all right?' An explanation of attendant risk, in the light of neuroimaging findings, with regular review helps manage that uncertainty. Parents respect honesty.

Dystonia of prematurity is a form of extensor hypertonus emerging around 40 weeks' gestational age and reaching its peak by 4 months old. This causes much parental concern and makes affected children difficult to handle in the first 7 or 8 months. It is most marked when the infant is lying supine, with the neck extended, or when the child is suspended under the armpits. The arms become extended rigidly with internal rotation and fisting of the hands. The mouth may open widely, the legs become extended and stiff, the feet adopt an equinus posture with a spontaneous extension of the big toes and fanning of the other toes. Clonus is not seen. The back arches in extension, even opisthotonos, if the feet come in contact with a firm surface. When the head is turned to the side there is an obligatory asymmetrical neck reflex in the first few months. Attempting to position the child in a sitting position is unsuccessful, as the child remains stiff as a board. When the feet touch the floor, with the child suspended, rapid automatic walking is observed, with a degree of scissoring so that the feet tread on each other. The signs are most marked when the child is agitated, hungry, in discomfort or even at the beginning of feeding. However, when prone, especially when the neck is flexed, the child adopts a flexed posture. If a child has spastic cerebral palsy by this age, which is rare, posture does affect the degree of spasticity but turning the child into a prone position does not abolish spasticity or increased extensor tone.

Dystonia of prematurity, unless severe, resolves, spontaneously leaving no persistent motor signs. While it is present parents appreciate advice on handling and activities by a physiotherapist. In a small proportion of children the dystonia persists and may be a life-long condition. Prediction of outcome at 4–6 months is difficult. An explanation of probable outcome is helpful with physiotherapy advice. In children who turn out to have spastic cerebral palsy, the dystonia merges into spasticity, after a period of mixed rigidity and spasticity in the legs. The dystonia in the neck, trunk, arms and hands resolves leading to a spurt in development, especially hand function. Sitting is late, but is achieved. Spasticity may first be noted at the ankles where clonus can be elicited. It soon becomes evident in the hip adductors and the hamstrings. In some children the spasticity is not demonstrable at rest and is only observed during exertion.

Spastic quadriplegia

The children with spastic quadriplegia have a high risk of associated learning disability and epilepsy (Fig. 22.27). They may be hypotonic in early infancy but spasticity emerges in the early months of life. There is a continuing need to find suitable positioning and seating. Gastrostomy feeding is often indicated. Standing frames give experience of upright position and promote stronger bone growth. Hydrotherapy is beneficial. Medication for spasticity in cerebral palsy is disappointing. It is rare for baclofen or diazepam to be beneficial in doses which are free of causing unacceptable levels of drowsiness or vomiting. Botulinum toxin, in experienced hands, has a place in prevention of fixed deformities.

Ataxic cerebral palsy

In infancy, children who develop ataxic cerebral palsy show hypotonia and very delayed motor development (Fig. 22.28). Sitting is long delayed. Truncal ataxia predominates over limb dysmetria. Eventually they may cruise round furniture or walk with support for many months before walking independently. Even then they may be advised to use a walking aid. Hydrotherapy is much enjoyed by ataxic children.

ATAXIC DIPLEGIA

Children who grow up to demonstrate signs of ataxic diplegia do not go through a dystonic phase. On the contrary, they show very low tone in the trunk and limbs until signs of spasticity evolve, usually distally in

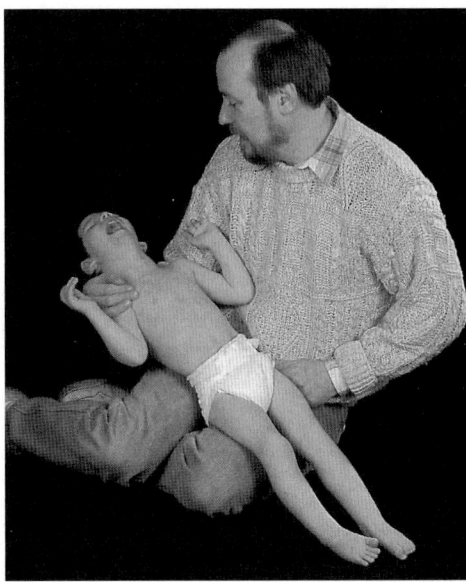

Fig. 22.27 Four limb cerebral palsy.

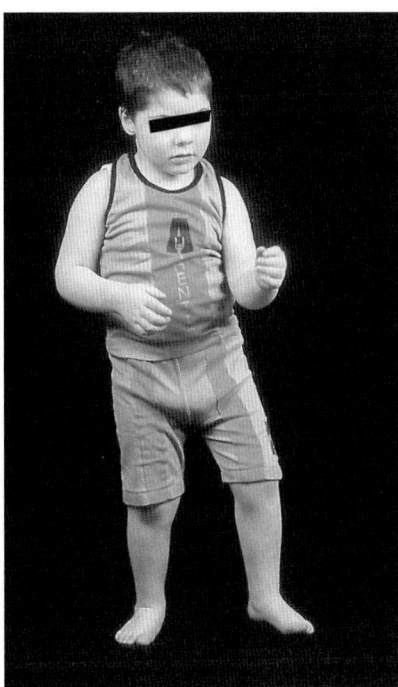

Fig. 22.28 Ataxic 3-year-old child showing broad-based gait and elevated arms.

their legs. Motor development is markedly delayed, usually more by the ataxia than the spasticity.

Autosomal recessive diplegia

Children who turn out to have genetic diplegias show normal tone in early infancy but begin to show signs of spasticity distally at about a year. It is important to remember that children who have a symmetrical diplegia or quadriplegia involving dystonia may have a dopa-responsive dystonia, especially where investigations are normal (see section on 'Movement disorders').

Differential diagnosis. At first it may be difficult to know whether the tightness at the ankles indicates Duchenne muscular dystrophy, metachromatic leukodystrophy or some other progressive disorder. These conditions have to be distinguished from hereditary spastic paraplegias, some of which are autosomal dominant though autosomal recessive forms also occur associated with loci mapping to chromosomes 8 (spg5), 15 (spg11) and 16 (spg7 which encodes for the protein paraplegin, apparently involved in mitochondrial function). In these disorders, which are of unknown pathogenesis, there is a progressive gait disturbance due to lower limb spasticity. They have hyperreflexia in their legs and extensor plantar responses. Ataxia, amyotrophy, neuropathy, extrapyramidal signs or pigmentation may be found also. In the dominant form there is an affected parent. In the recessive form more than one sibling is affected with or without parental consanguinity or there is an isolated patient with parental consanguinity.

Hemiplegia

Children present in the second half of the first year of life when pincer grasp, individual finger movements, bimanual activities and manipulation of objects are seen to be asymmetrical (Fig. 22.29). At first it may be attributed to the unaffected side being unusually dominant, an inappropriate conclusion so early in life. However it is evident that the affected hand tends to be fisted and there is poverty of movement in this arm and hand. If the child is able to sit unsupported, the lateral guarding reaction when the child is pushed to that side is absent or much less than on the unaffected side. The forward parachute reaction is asymmetrical. Hemiplegic children are a little late to pull to stand, to cruise

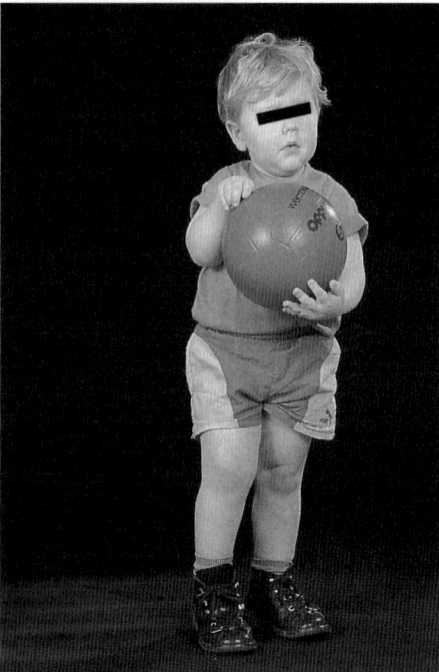

Fig. 22.29   Spastic hemiplegia, right-sided – hyperpronated.

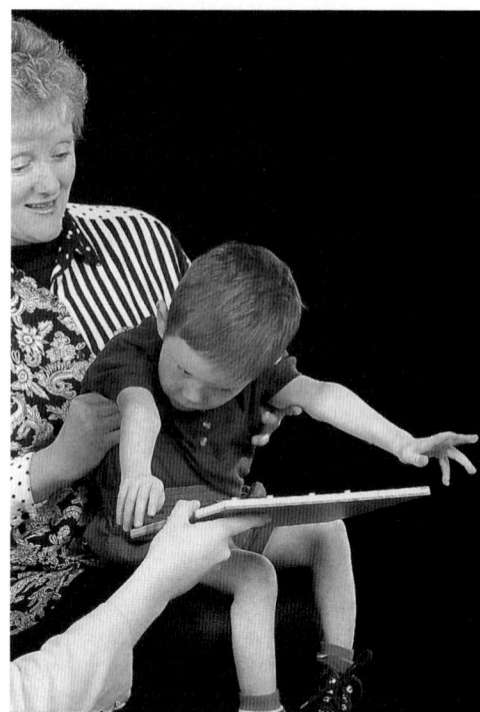

Fig. 22.30   A child with dyskinetic cerebral palsy, showing uncontrolled patterns of movement and flaccid trunk, while attempting to reach out.

around furniture and to walk independently, but not to a marked degree unless there is a comorbid global learning disability. A striking feature is that the child tends to go up on the toes of the affected foot. When walking begins, the heel tends to remain off the ground. As children grow older it is helpful to examine their outdoor shoes when they have been using them for some weeks. It is evident that there is a marked asymmetry with excessive wear at the toe and little or no wear at the heel compared with the unaffected side. As years pass there comes to be a clear asymmetry of growth between the limbs on the affected and unaffected sides, most evident in the hands and feet, in distinction from the symmetrical findings in children with acquired hemiplegia in later childhood.

Children with hemiplegia may have associated sensory loss on the affected side of the body and may also have a partial or complete hemianopia. As they grow older, some develop dyskinetic movements on the affected side. It may also become clear that there are mild signs of spasticity and increased reflexes on the supposedly unaffected side so that the condition is a markedly asymmetrical form of spastic quadriparesis. About a third of hemiplegic children have seizures and these are the first presentation in some of them. A surprising proportion of hemiplegic children have sufficient associated learning difficulties or other disabilities to attend special schools. In Salford, Manchester, in 1988, of 110 children with cerebral palsy, 27 had a hemiplegia of whom 17 attended special schools.[364]

Dyskinetic/dystonic cerebral palsy

Though pediatric neurologists with a regional practice will have a number of patients with dyskinetic/dystonic cerebral palsy, the condition arises infrequently in any local service, whether as a consequence of acute near-total intrapartum terminal hypoxia–ischemia or as an autosomal recessive disorder (Fig. 22.30). About 1:7000 children is affected. Only one in ten primary care physicians (general practitioners) will ever have such a child born into his or her practice in a working lifetime. Though families may expect their doctors to know about the condition, it is only through close liaison with therapy and specialist neurology services that knowledge and confidence will grow.

In infancy the children seem hypotonic with poor conjugate use of their eyes to follow people or objects. They have impassive facies, do not learn to speak, and have major feeding difficulties. Hand function is of little or no functional benefit. Dystonic posturing may make the child hard to handle. Commonly these children show emotional lability and

they are easily distressed but cannot easily demonstrate their intelligence. The involuntary choreiform or athetoid movements do not appear until the second year or subsequently. Parents may be convinced of their child's intelligence yet the standardized developmental assessments of ability yield results suggesting very low function.

As these children grow up they need expert advice on seating, feeding and communication particularly.[365] Saddle seating may be more secure and more suitable than conventional seating. Gastrostomy feeding may be required, at least for a time. There are a number of Advisory Centers for Education around Britain to give advice on aids to communication for personal and educational purposes.[366] Expert advice on physiotherapy,[367,368] hydrotherapy, horse riding[369] and other forms of exercise should be sought. Medication may be considered, only to be rejected.[370] It is exceptional for a child to benefit from drug therapy. A conceptual framework for reviewing outcomes in developmental disabilities has been proposed[371] but more research is needed.[372] As school leaving age approaches, there should be a multidisciplinary approach to transition planning and a college with the appropriate expertise should be sought. Expert careers advice is invaluable and suitable recreational opportunities should be investigated. There is justified concern for the decline in adult rehabilitation services over the past 30 years.[373–375]

Clinical progress

In early childhood the principal parental concern is to promote independent walking in children with diplegia or other forms of cerebral palsy. Facilitating hand function, feeding[376–380] and communication become increasingly important with time. Increasingly sophisticated technical options are available. However promotion of independence, recreation,[380,381] personal and social development is most important as preparation for adult life.[382]

MULTIDISCIPLINARY TEAMS AND CHILD DEVELOPMENT CENTERS

For parents of children with cerebral palsy, the discovery of the many associated potential problems can be daunting. There may be a multiplicity of appointments with different medical specialists, including dietitians, therapists, specialist nurses, orthoptists, audiometricians, medical social workers and diverse doctors. Coordination of investigation and treatment is best carried out through a child development team[383] based in a child development center[384,385] as recommended in the Court Report.[386] The nature of such teams and the facilities in these centers differ from place to place,[387] not least because of diversity of services from agencies other than health services. Making the services work in co-operation needs continuous attention as personnel and policies change frequently. These are among the keys to successful provision:

- good coordination of health, education and social services;
- clear lines of communication between primary care and specialist health services;
- shared single set of case notes for hospital and community health services;
- access to necessary expertise including seating, communication aids, orthotics, prosthetics, clinical psychology, dental services, feeding team;
- medical specialist services: vision, hearing, epilepsy service, orthopedics, psychiatry, genetics;
- close links with voluntary organizations;
- parental choice at all times;
- parent-held records;
- children's needs are paramount.

ASSOCIATED HEALTH PROBLEMS IN CEREBRAL PALSY

Feeding problems due to bulbar palsy, handling and seating difficulties, involuntary movements or posture and tone problems are a common first presentation. The children are prone to oral hypersensitivity and to bite on whatever is put in their mouths. Parents can be taught to desensitize the child's mouth before feeds. The reverse may be the case and the child's mouth may need stimulation during feeds. There may be aspiration of food with consequent respiratory symptoms. When this is chronic, the chest develops an increased anteroposterior diameter. Gastroesophageal regurgitation may occur leading to postprandial dyspepsia (heartburn) and vomiting. These symptoms may provoke crying or reflex syncope. Food thickeners and barrier treatment such as Gaviscon can be used as well as an upright position after meals. They may drool saliva. If this is persistent, they may benefit from hyoscine skin patches behind the ear or between the scapulae or from oral glycopyrrolate. Surgery on salivary glands or salivary ducts is not very successful in the long term.

Gastrostomy will be considered for those children with an unsafe swallow or whose intake is insufficient for growth, reflected in a markedly delayed bone age. A multidisciplinary team makes the assessment and simpler management strategies will be tried first. Assessment for gastrostomy includes a videofluoroscopy, by an experienced radiologist, with the child's speech and language therapist in attendance. The procedure is seen as mutilating, so parents need careful preparation and support. Subsequent satisfaction is usually good, with less coughing and choking; medication can be given more reliably and feeding time is improved, allowing the parent to spend more time doing other things including play, and with other children.[388] A dietitian will advise on the content of gastrostomy feeds. A common practice is to give a slow overnight infusion of feed by syringe pump, to reduce the volume that has to be given in the day. The cost–benefit of tube feeding has been questioned by Strauss et al[389] who demonstrated an increased mortality risk in tube-fed children (relative risk 2.1, with no increased risk in the most severely disabled children, but a doubled risk in those with less severe disabilities with increased risk of aspiration of vomit), but the lesson may be in the selection process and the appropriate use of fundoplication. There is a need for prospective studies[390] including comparison of the available gastrostomy tubes.

When reflux and vomiting are troublesome and persistent, and this can become more of a problem after gastrostomy, as feeding volume increases, *fundoplication* is considered. This is a major procedure and requires postoperative high dependency backup till breathing is safe.

The procedure – wrapping part of the fundus of the stomach around the lower part of the esophagus – is not an exact science. Sometimes it turns out to be too tight and swallowing becomes difficult, as is burping air. Sometimes it turns out to be too slack and makes little difference. So re-operation may be required. When it works well it makes a great difference to reflux and vomiting. There is, however, a significant risk of complications with gastrostomy and fundoplication.[391,392]

Constipation is a risk in all children who are inactive and if this is allowed to persist there is a risk of acquired megacolon, a lot of colicky pain after meals and soiling with overflow. Sometimes constipation can build up when the child is unwell. Pushing frequent fluids is wise.

The mainstays of treatment are:

- adequate, frequent fluid intake including fresh fruit juice especially during fever;
- varied, stimulating diet;
- communicative mealtimes – social occasions not just 'feeding time';
- some pureed fruit and fiber in the diet but not too much as it packs the colon;
- exercise including hydrotherapy;
- relaxed but consistent toileting;
- lactulose as a stool softener morning and evening mixed with a cordial;
- Senokot syrup in the morning.

Prune juice and syrup of figs are effective but are used less than they used to be, probably because children don't like the tastes. There is a range of unstandardized herbal preparations of cascara, frangula, rhubarb, senna, aloes, colycynth and jalap which should be avoided in children because of their unpredictable laxative effects. Osmotic laxatives such as magnesium hydroxide (milk of/cream of magnesia) or magnesium sulfate (Epsom Salts, Andrews Liver Salts) can be used in older children.

Judicious short term use of sodium picosulfate can help clear the bowel but is not appropriate in very young children.

Incontinence is persistent for children with severe cerebral palsy. It is also a problem, alongside enuresis, for many less severely affected children for longer than is seen in most children. Toileting routines should be attempted when the child is ready developmentally. Extra consideration is needed for time taken to go to the toilet, transfer from a wheelchair in some, unfastening and fastening clothes, for balancing on the toilet, with help from a rail if needed, and for wiping, which may be difficult. While parents and care staff will help young children, this is not appropriate from the onset of puberty when a toilet that washes, then dries, the youngster's bottom is a more dignified solution. For those who are not capable of a continence program there needs to be a regular supply of nappies of appropriate size.

Osteopenia[393] is a risk in immobile children with cerebral palsy, with consequent increased risk of fractures. This is not due to abnormalities of vitamin D or parathyroid hormone.[394] While enabling children to spend part of each day in a standing frame and promoting physical activity, e.g. with hydrotherapy, is likely to promote improved bone density, use of bisphosphonates for 12–18 months has been shown to increase bone density by 20–40%, with no apparent adverse effects.

A third of the children have a *global learning disability*, which may be moderate or severe. It may be thought that this is also true of children with dyskinetic cerebral palsy because there is so little that they can do; their eye movements may be randomn and communication is extremely difficult. Beware – some of these children are very intelligent but remain 'locked in' until technological means are found to enable them to control speech synthesizers, computers, environmental control systems and other technology. In the past, many such children and adults have languished, completely inappropriately, in provision for people with profound and multiple disabilities. A third of children have patchy or *specific learning difficulty*. The commonest specific difficulties are in language and communication, in visual perception or in mathematical tasks and calculation. There has been little reliable research into the communication difficulties of children with cerebral palsy[394–397] and the subject has been referred to only briefly in standard texts. Yule and Rutter[395] suggest that this is because few therapists work with children with physical disabilities. There is a substantial risk of hearing impairment in children with cerebral palsy, either from associated sensorineural loss or from secretory otitis media, which is very common in children with eustachian tube dysfunction in bulbar palsy. There has been a good deal of attention to communication before speech and to means of augmented communication (signing and symbol systems, information technology, speech synthesizers for instance) among practitioners. Doctors rely on advice from their speech and language therapy colleagues throughout. It is wise to beware early judgments on the communication potential of children with choreoathetoid (dyskinetic) cerebral palsy. So often they turn out to be much more capable than first thought. Perceptual difficulty may make it difficult for children to tell the time from a conventional clock, to understand maps and diagrams or to find their way about, including difficulty in avoiding obstacles with their wheelchairs.

Hearing impairment is very common in children with cerebral palsy, usually from fluctuating loss with secretory otitis media, but sometimes from sensorineural loss, or a combination of the two. Grommets can produce dramatic short term benefits but hearing aids may be the more effective long term solution, combined with expert learning support services.

Visual impairment is common in children with cerebral palsy, more than half of whom have visual problems for several reasons.[398] The condition causing the cerebral palsy such as congenital cytomegalovirus, toxoplasmosis or rubella may also have caused a cataract, colobomas or retinal lesions including pigmentary retinopathy. Retinopathy of prematurity is amenable to control by laser therapy or cryotherapy, but skilled ophthalmic examination of preterm infants' eyes has been available in recent years. The eyes may be too small (microphthalmia) or too big (buphthalmos or congenital glaucoma). The child may be shortsighted or longsighted. Cortical visual defects are common.

Epilepsy is common in children with cerebral palsy, affecting about a third overall.[399] Hadjipanayis et al[400] reported a prevalence of epilepsy of 41.8% in 323 patients with cerebral palsy in Athens, Greece. However the rate varies between studies, as the type of cerebral palsy in children in each study is different. The risk of epilepsy varies from rare, in pure ataxic cerebral palsy, to very high (up to 94% in some series but 71% would be more typical) in children with spastic quadriplegia and severe learning disability.[400] The prevalence of epilepsy in spastic or ataxic diplegia is 16–27%, but only 3% in encephalopathy of low birth weight (Little disease). In dystonic/dyskinetic cerebral palsy the prevalence is about a quarter and in hemiplegia between 30% and 50%.[400] Diagnosis of the condition is difficult enough in general[401,402] in children. This is more difficult in a child with cerebral palsy, who may have difficulty describing symptoms. It depends on careful observation and history taking while detection of side-effects requires constant vigilance: a child who lost her sitting balance (possible neurodegeneration?) got better when her phenytoin was stopped, another with a cachectic state (possible malignancy?) regained his weight when his carbamazepine was stopped. Vigabatrin may cause visual field defects which are difficult to detect in disabled children though there is a program to attempt to do this. Sodium valproate can lead to considerable weight gain. Always weigh costs versus benefits.

Psychiatric aspects

The commonest psychiatric reactions to having cerebral palsy are anxiety, depression and/or withdrawal. Other features include attention deficit hyperactivity disorder, tantrums, social naivety, passivity and autistic spectrum disorders which Nordin and Gillberg[403] found in 10.5% of children with cerebral palsy. The implications of the differences in neurobiological findings between children with cerebral palsy and those with learning disability or autism are not understood. Concentrations of neuropeptides and neurotrophins are raised in the blood of newborn infants who subsequently go on to develop severe learning disability and/or autism, but not in children with cerebral palsy.[404] Conversely altered secretion of androgens is a feature of children with cerebral palsy, but is not a feature of children with autism or learning disability.

Sleeping difficulties

It is very common for children with cerebral palsy to be difficult to settle at night, or to wake up unduly frequently during the night. For those with four-limb involvement or with severe spasticity in the legs the lack of activity in the day does not leave them tired at night. They may benefit from melatonin, 2 mg half an hour before a bedtime routine. Some require a higher dose of 4 mg.[405] If this does not help, it is worth trying 6 mg daily for a month. Of the other night sedatives, among the most reliable is chloral hydrate elixir. Though it tastes strongly and needs to be mixed with a palatable disguise, it does not suppress dreaming sleep and can be omitted without causing withdrawal symptoms. Some children with cerebral palsy cannot turn in bed and become uncomfortable unless supplied with a sheepskin, a ripple mattress, special cushion or need to be turned in bed on a regular basis. Antihistamine analogs such as alimemazine tartrate (Vallergan) can help on a one-off basis, but they may have a paradoxical effect of exciting the child or provoking seizures.

TREATMENTS FOR CEREBRAL PALSY
Treatment of spasticity

Parents and carers may seek treatment for spasticity with expectations that exceed clinical possibilities. The most important starting point is an understanding of the limitations of all forms of treatment, alongside the usually moderate gains that can be made. A spastic diplegic gait will always be recognizable as such but improved function, efficiency and comfort are all worthwhile. A child will be well advised to walk a little, without rushing, in as good a gait as possible, rather than walk as far or as fast as possible. Unrealistic expectations will burden the child, as well as the physician, with a sense of failure.

Dynamic spastic tone can be modified by ankle–foot orthoses, serial casting with progressive dorsiflexion of the ankle, medication or surgical procedures. The balance to be struck is between useful relaxation on the one hand and undesirable weakness or constitutional side-effects on the other. Scoliosis may be contained by wearing bracing or jackets. Children with ataxic or dyskinetic cerebral palsy may feel more secure in Lycra splinting but this has little part to play for spasticity.

Fixed contractures may be released by orthopedic operations, but these must be carefully selected so that the child does not consequently suffer any deterioration in functional level.

The aims for the child are to relieve pain and discomfort, improve function, facilitate care and contain contractures.[406] The authors' approach to therapy is summarized in Table 22.32.

Oral medication

Baclofen acts at the level of the neurones in the spinal cord, enhancing gamma-aminobutyric acid (GABA) activity as a GABA agonist, inhibiting some of the excess excitatory activity responsible for spastic tone. Dosage is built up gradually, according to effect and tolerance, to 2 mg/kg/day. Its effect will be global, rather than targeted, which may produce undesirable hypotonia of truncal muscles, adversely affecting sitting posture, for instance. It is essential that all treatments should be monitored in conjunction with physiotherapy assessments as well as the observations of the carers. This is very important for the child with four-limb spasticity in whom important side-effects may be overlooked, and who is especially susceptible to increasing polypharmacy. When there is doubt about benefit, then a planned withdrawal gradually (so as to avoid rebound spasticity, fits or hallucinations) will usually clarify its role.

Adverse effects on the child's alertness, diminished appetite, nausea or vomiting, and exacerbation of epilepsy should all be looked for. As for any treatment, there should be a general agreement between doctor and carer that only substantial, trouble free gains from treatment can justify its prolonged prescription.

Table 22.32 Schema for the treatment and management of cerebral palsy

Goals[371]
1. Facilitating care
2. !mproving function
3. Contaning contractures
4. Relieving pain and discomfort

Spasticity

Medication	Baclofen
	Tizanidine
	Benzodiazepines, esp. Valium
	Intramuscular – botulinum toxin
Surgery	Release of contractures, tendo-Achilles, hamstrings, hip adductors
	Scoliosis – spinal brace (operative fixation rarely?)
	Hip dislocaton
	– *prevention*: adductor tenotomy/obturator neurectomy, derotation osteotomy
	– *correction*: open reduction, resection of head of femur (Girdlestone procedure)
	Upper limb – hand surgery? Reasons for (hygiene)
Neurosurgery	Intrathecal baclofen
	Dorsal rhizotomy
Physical and occupational therapy	Stretching, splinting, seating, standing, walking aids
	Home and school, aids and adaptations
	Advice on handling and posture
Pediatrician	Attention to associated conditions that will *exacerbate* spasticity: pain (e.g. ear infection, pressure area, reflux esophagitis, constipation, upper airways obstruction. Or *compound* it, as with sleep disorder, seizures, failure to thrive
Athetosis and dyskinetic cerebral palsy	Medication most difficult, consider L-DOPA
	Valium and possibly oral baclofen for dystonia
	For children with later acquired disorder consider biotin and pyridoxine
	Physical/occupational therapy as above (? Lycra suits)
	Pediatrician as above
	Orthopedic surgery as above
	Neurosurgery? stereotactic basal ganglia stimulation
Ataxia	Supportive therapy only – walking frames/Lycra suits?

Dantrolene acts on calcium channels, reducing the power of muscle contraction. Relaxation may be at the cost of reduced function. Side-effects also include nausea, vomiting and diarrhea. Hepatotoxity has been reported.

Tizanidine is an alpha$_2$-adrenergic agent, which modifies excitatory transmitter activity. It has not been fully appraised for spastic cerebral palsy, in spite of manufacturers' claims that it may have a better side-effect profile for some patients compared with baclofen.

Tiagabine has not been effective in recent experience.[407]

Diazepam can be a very effective muscle relaxant, but its use is limited by systemic side-effects of drowsiness. However this is not inevitable, and when spastic tone is distressing, it is worth a trial. It can be very helpful for instance in seeing a child through a painful episode such as a fracture. Rebound spasticity can be severe following a prolonged period in plaster. Baclofen can also give relief at such times. Botulinum toxin (see below) may have a similar role.

Botulinum toxin

Botulinum toxin A (BTA) is a paralyzing agent derived from *Clostridium botulinum*. It causes muscle relaxation by chemically blocking acetylcholine release, with the loss of motor end plates. Its effect reverses over 3–6 months as affected nerve roots sprout forming new junctions. It is given intramuscularly, usually targeting lower limb muscle groups in spastic diplegic children. These include hip adductors, hamstrings, gastrocnemius and soleus, which all contribute to the classic crouched gait and scissoring typical of this group. Multiple site injections, selected after clinical and video assessment by a multidisciplinary team, are most effective. The team usually comprises at least a dedicated physiotherapist, an orthopedic surgeon and pediatric neurologist.

Three groups of patients may benefit: (i) ambulant children with a dynamic equinus throughout the gait cycle with knee flexion > 20 degrees or scissoring; (ii) children who are losing ability to get to standing or maintain standing; (iii) children of any functional category who are in pain or discomfort around the hip, or where adductor spasm seriously hampers care and hygiene.

The treatment is only effective for dynamic spasticity, especially in the young child, where therapeutic gains are greater and realistic aims to delay surgery beyond 8 years of age likely to be achieved by repeated injections. Toward adolescence many patients experience diminishing returns because of the added problems of growth. It is probably best considered as a possible treatment for windows of time in the child's life.[408] It must always be complemented by continuing physiotherapy and conventional containment of contractures, e.g. with orthoses.

The injections are painful, requiring sedation and local anesthetic cream for most children. Dose guidelines must be carefully followed, since it is a paralyzing agent. Systemic spread from an injection site can cause bladder incontinence, lethargy and laryngeal weakness temporarily in a few children, though in the main side-effects are not common.

Orthopedic surgery

The consensus in orthopedic intervention is for multilevel surgery delayed until the age of 8–11 years for the release of contractures at tendo-Achilles (TA), hamstrings and hip adductors. The skill is as much in selecting the operation that is right for the child as in performing it. An ill-chosen isolated release of the TAs may bring the foot out of equinus, but put the child into a worsened crouch at the hips and knees, speeding their progression to wheelchair dependence. Hamstring release may weaken hip extension, worsening the crouch position at the hip.

Hip subluxation can be contained by timely release of psoas and adductor muscles. The adducting hip is the one at risk of dislocation, but in the windswept posture the opposite abducting hip can also develop an abduction contracture, hampering seating. Femoral osteotomy can realign the femoral head into the acetabulum, correcting a persisting fetal alignment that lends to dislocation. In more severe cases the acetabulum may be refashioned as well. In extreme cases the femoral head may be resected (the Castle procedure) but sitting balance, if present, is likely to be lost.

Scoliosis is most common in non-ambulant four-limb spasticity. Early attention to seating with scoliosis support inserts is important, as is standing time in a frame, use of bracing or molded jackets. Spinal fixation is a major operation which may be selected for some patients with a curve of >40 degrees before the age of 15 years. However the general state of health of the child with respect to risks and likely change in quality of life postoperatively have all to be weighed thoughtfully.

Neurosurgery

Intrathecal baclofen delivered at very low doses through a pump driven by an implanted battery may be very effective for children with four-limb spasticity. The implant is positioned subcutaneously or subfascially in the abdomen or loin. A fine tube leads intrathecally to the mid-to-lower thoracic level, and there is a reservoir of baclofen that is replenished at intervals by injection. Complications include infection and meningitis, CSF leaks and wound infection. The system itself can become displaced or disconnected.

It has been used less hitherto in the UK for ambulant patients than in the USA. However it does have the advantage of an effective preoperative assessment by injecting a test dose at lumbar puncture. The response is measurable in a few hours.

Selective dorsal rhizotomy is a neurosurgical procedure by which selected lower nerve roots in the lumbar sacral distribution are partially deafferented. This reduces spasticity permanently. It is thought to work by reducing the afferent stimulation of alpha motor neurones, which already lack inhibition from the dysfunctional or damaged corticospinal tracts. There can be bladder dysfunction as a complication and significant muscle weakness that impairs function. Functional improvement has not been demonstrated in all studies and therefore it is a form of treatment that is still being assessed.

DISCLOSURE OF DIAGNOSIS OF CEREBRAL PALSY

As soon as it becomes clear that the child is developing signs of spastic diplegia or any other form of cerebral palsy, arrangements should be made for a senior doctor to discuss the findings with the parents. Guidelines on good practice have been published by the UK-based charity Scope[409] based on the recommendations of Cunningham et al[410] in relation to infants with Down syndrome, which is a life-long condition, diagnosable at birth. The reason for including this in the section on spastic diplegia is that there are many reasons for clinical uncertainty on the way to making this diagnosis. Yet there comes a time when it is possible to be reasonably confident. It is a way of describing how a child functions at present. In future it is possible for some children to grow out of this condition or other forms of cerebral palsy[411] so this, and other uncertainties, will be part of the discussion with parents. Important points are as follows:

- planned appointment as soon as feasible after diagnosis made;
- both parents present;
- with a relative, friend or professional (nurse, social worker, therapist) if parents wish;
- senior doctor with wide experience of developmental disabilities;
- trainee present if parents agree;
- quiet, comfortable room, free of interruption or disturbance;
- as much time available for discussion as parents find helpful;
- a full account of the condition and possible associated problems;
- details of further investigations or assessments;
- explanation of treatment plans and timetable;
- permission to notify the local education authority that the child may have special educational needs;
- information about help available from the social services department;
- details of local and national voluntary organizations who can help (photocopy the relevant pages of the Contact a Family Directory);
- write in the parent-held child health record;
- let parents have a copy of the clinic letter to the general practitioner;
- offer a home follow-up visit by a colleague to help the parents understand what they have been told;
- arrange a follow-up clinic visit and encourage parents to make a list of questions;
- assure parents of your willingness and that of your colleagues to help their child to find what he/she can do best and to make the most of that at each stage through childhood and adolescence;
- at all times show willingness to seek a second opinion.

LIFE EXPECTANCY

The life expectancy of children and adults with cerebral palsy is reduced but this is explained, almost entirely, by those with four-limb involvement lacking independent movement and self-care abilities. Strauss and Shavelle[412] reported findings on 24 768 individuals aged 15 or over and receiving services in California between January 1980 and December 1995. This work was extended, in a study period from 1986 to 1995, to a Californian population of 45 292 individuals of all ages with cerebral

palsy.[413] Detection of other conditions was poorer in people with cerebral palsy, so that mortality from breast cancer was three times that of the general population. The risk of brain tumors was raised dramatically, especially in children (standardized mortality ratio = 24) indicating an increased risk in those diagnosed as having cerebral palsy. There was a range of life expectancy of over 40 years in the adult study, according to the functional level. Some with the least independent function had a life expectancy of only 11 years. Similar findings have been reported in North East and South East Thames Regions in Britain,[414-416] in British Columbia, Canada,[417] and in Western Australia.[418]

In South East Thames, 79% of children with severe learning disability and cerebral palsy survived to a mean age of 16 years. This is higher than in an earlier study in Rochester, Minnesota over the period 1950–1976.[419] In the Australian study, half the children with profound and multiple learning disability with cerebral palsy (DQ < 20) lived to adult life. Of those with a DQ of 20–34, 76% survived to adult life, while 92% of those with higher ability did so. Those who reached 25 years had good subsequent life expectancy. There was no evidence in this study that advances in medical care and improvement in community awareness had improved the survival of people with cerebral palsy. It is premature to judge the impact on life expectancy of gastrostomy feeding, food supplements and the involvement of speech and language therapists, dietitians and others in feeding teams, tracheostomies for those prone to respiratory failure and the contemporary range of antiepileptic drugs. There is evidence of improved quality of life but, as yet, not of significant change in length of life. Comparison between the survival data from Western Australia and California was made by examination of both databases by Shavelle et al[420] and the differences were found to be slight if severity of learning disability was controlled for. The apparent disparity in survival was not due to differences in care, but because the Australian population included a higher proportion of mildly affected people and a lower proportion of people with severe or profound learning disability. This is the first published controlled comparison of survival in cerebral palsy between countries.

The interaction between cerebral palsy and learning disability in life expectancy has been reported to be an increasing problem (from 0.7 to about 0.9/1000 live births over the decade studied by Nicholson and Alberman[421]). Learning disability is, in itself, a risk factor for early death, especially from respiratory disease, which is three times commoner than in the general population.[422] Whereas 83% of the whole population live to be 65 years old or more, fewer than 50% of 2000 with an IQ < 70 and known to services in two London districts did so in this 8-year study. The risk of death before 50 was 58 times higher than in the population of England and Wales. Early death was associated with cerebral palsy, incontinence, problems of mobility and residence in hospital. Nonetheless, for children and adolescents with cerebral palsy and learning disability we must plan for their survival into adult life and advocate their case for transition into suitable health services when they leave pediatric care. More recently Hutton and Pharoah[423] reported a new finding that severe visual disability and lack of information on hearing (probably as a surrogate for severe impairment) had a significant association with reduced survival.

QUALITY OF LIFE AND COSTS OF CARING

In a review of 1365 published measures of quality of life only 5% were found to be applicable to children.[424] There are few published data on the views of children with disabilities on their quality of life and none of children with cerebral palsy and/or learning disability. Quality of life assessments of and by children with epilepsy have been reported.[425] Sociometric study of fifty-five 9- to 11-year-old children with hemiplegia in 54 mainstream schools has demonstrated increased risk of peer rejection, lack of friends and victimization.[426] As increasing inclusiveness is promoted for children with disabilities in mainstream schools there is a need to make provision for their social as well as physical and academic development. Fostering the social skills of children with disabilities may reduce the risk of social disadvantage.

The views of children with attention deficit hyperactive disorder (ADHD) concerning behavior disturbance, social competence and familial environment have been found to differ from those of their parents.[427] Children perceived themselves as equally competent and socially accepted as their peers, in contrast to their parents' ratings. Though parenting a preschool child with ADHD was found to be stressful it was not considered by parents or children to affect family functioning adversely. Parents of children with physical and/or learning disabilities have reported lower quality of life in all family members compared with parents of children without disabilities.[428,429] The substantial impact of severe disablement in a child on parental careers, family income and expenditure patterns has been demonstrated clearly in a study of nearly 500 children with disabilites and nearly 700 controls.[430] In that study, 67% of mothers of children with disabilities were unable to enter or keep paid employment after the birth of their child compared with 60–69% of mothers of children without disabilities who are able to do this.[431–433] In a study of time costs of caring for 16 children with severe disabilities, including cerebral palsy, compared with 31 children without disabilities, it was found that personal care time was significantly greater per waking hour throughout the day for the former.[434] Twelve of the 16 mothers of children with disabilities were not in paid employment. Twelve had little or no extended family support. Care needs did not decline with increasing age, preventing mothers working outside the home outwith school hours. (The same would be true of fathers when, as is now increasingly common, they act as main carers.) This is the only published study of time costs of caring for a child with a disability carried out entirely in the family home. Two previous studies were based on observation of institutional care[435,436] while that of Edebol-Tysk[437] was a study partly in an institution and partly at home.

Most parents do not regret the changed way of life consequent upon having a child with a disability but some find it a struggle. In a study of 110 children with cerebral palsy in Salford[364] 39% of the children attended mainstream schools. Of those attending special schools 22% had attended mainstream schools but the placement had broken down. Thirty-nine percent of those now in mainstream had been in a special school or nursery in the past. Of the children attending mainstream schools 88% were community ambulant compared with 17% in special schools. Two of the mainstream children were partially sighted compared with 11 who were partially sighted and 11 who were blind in special schools. Of the mainstream children 95% could feed themselves compared with 36% in special schools. Only 5% of those in mainstream school had current epilepsy compared with 52% of those in special schools. No mainstream child was bowel or bladder incontinent though help was needed for 17%/9% of the children for these functions. Fifty-three percent of the special school children were incontinent and an additional 18%/12% needed help for bladder or bowel function. Thus the children in special schools had more severe and complex disabilities than the mainstream children. Of the mainstream children 11% had a single parent compared with 35% of the special school children. Fifteen (14%) of these 110 children with cerebral palsy were on or had been on the child protection register compared with 1:500 in Salford children in general at that time. Four percent of mainstream children and 18% of special school children were in residential or foster care and two children had been adopted. In addition a further child had suffered a skull fracture, one had sustained extensive scalds in the bath, one had hypoxia–ischemiated as a result of having a large screw in his mouth and another had a sibling on the child protection register.

Knowing of the pressures experienced by families of children with disabilities should prompt services to go out of their way to be helpful, to be pre-emptive and to minimize the risks of dysfunction.[438]

MEDICOLEGAL ASPECTS

Despite immense changes in obstetric and pediatric practice since William Little[439] ascribed cerebral palsy to perinatal causes, and a major decline in neonatal death rate, the incidence of these disorders has remained relatively unchanged in resource rich countries at about 2:1000 children for the last 40 years.[440–442] The incidence in resource limited countries has been reported to more than twice this.[443]

The widespread lay belief that cerebral palsy is likely to be the consequence of brain damage (intrapartum hypoxia–ischemia) during birth has led to extensive litigation. Yet intrapartum causes only account for a small minority (about 10%),[444,445] and most affected children have suffered an unforeseen disaster rather than lack of care.[446] In an Oxford study comparing the relationship between quality of intrapartum care for 34 children with cerebral palsy compared with 377 controls,[447] only 2.9% of the cerebral palsy cases were considered to have experienced suboptimal care in labor compared with 14.5% of controls. None of the cerebral palsy cases had received suboptimal quality of care in response to fetal distress compared with 1.4% of controls. A change in practice toward no-fault compensation and a care package for children with cerebral palsy has been proposed. This would have the advantage of relative speed and would obviate the need to prove negligence in a protracted medicolegal process.

Diagnosis of cerebral palsy in early childhood is difficult[448] and often changes with time. Children may go through periods of transient motor abnormalities and may outgrow cerebral palsy in the same way as the motor signs abate after head injuries and acquired brain diseases.[411] Other conditions may resemble cerebral palsy.[449] Brain magnetic resonance imaging is helpful in distinguishing genetic-metabolic from acquired causes of extrapyramidal cerebral palsy.[450–453] In a very large American cohort most children considered to have definite cerebral palsy at 1 year had outgrown it by 7 years and very few of those considered to have probable or possible cerebral palsy had abnormal motor signs by this age.[411] In a study conducted in 1975 of children considered to show symptomatic hypoxia–ischemia only a quarter showed continuing motor signs in later childhood,[454] though there was an excess of children with learning difficulties.

Infants withstand 10 minutes of total intrapartum hypoxia–ischemia without long term consequences, but are very unlikely to survive more than 20 minutes of this. Of those who have suffered an intervening period of total hypoxia–ischemia, the effects are variable. The typical outcome is one of dyskinetic cerebral palsy, with or without seizures but with relative intellectual sparing or normal intelligence. MRI scans show lesions in the basal ganglia and/or thalamus in most affected children.[455] Only with very prolonged subtotal intrapartum hypoxia–ischemia is it likely that a child will suffer major learning difficulties[456,457] and only in association with severe cerebral palsy (as with sensorineural hearing loss). Children with known biomedical causes of learning disability can have low Apgar scores at birth without any hypoxia–ischemia.[458] The combination of low tone and severe learning disability in a child of school age is likely to be the result of a constitutional disorder, not acquired intrapartum damage.

In court, much may be made of cardiotocographic abnormalities but this is an unsatisfactory technique for preventing symptomatic hypoxia–ischemia.[459,460] The practice, during the last 40 years, of widespread continuous fetal heart monitoring has led to increased cesarean section rates, with associated maternal morbidity and mortality and no significant effect on perinatal morbidity or mortality,[461,462] though conflicting opinions have been expressed.[463] It has been of minimal benefit for low risk patients and its use in high risk patients has yet to be subjected to adequate evaluation. In the current medicolegal climate perhaps it never will be. If midwifery staffing is adequate, as it should be, intermittent fetal heart recording by Pinard stethoscope or hand-held ultrasound monitors is competent practice. This would not detect total hypoxia–ischemia due to placental separation during the second stage in a breech delivery but cesarean section is not an option in such circumstances and attempts at heroic emergency vaginal deliveries are likely to cause more harm than good. When staffing is inadequate there is a temptation to use cardiotocography as an electronic babysitter.

The greater number of premature infants who survive with cerebral palsy reflects a greater survival of such infants, most of whom survive in a healthy condition,[464] rather than an increased risk of cerebral palsy for such children. This justifies the enthusiasm for high quality neonatal care for premature infants. The changes in causes of cerebral palsy indicate a shift from the consequences of traumatic delivery of term infants many years ago to the higher proportion of very low birth weight survivors who would have died in time past. Overall the prevalence of cerebral palsy remains little changed.

The contribution of survivors of <1500 g birth weight largely accounts for the proportion of children with cerebral palsy who have acquired it postnatally increasing to 18% in the Mersey region between 1966 and 1977.[465] The expected proportion is about 10%.[466,467] In three series from New York, Chicago and Western Australia quoted by Stanley et al,[468] CNS infection accounted for over 60% of 856 cases of postnatal cerebral palsy. It is hoped that the introduction of immunization against measles, mumps, rubella, *Hemophilus influenzae*, pneumococcus and meningococcus C has reduced the ongoing risk of postnatal cerebral palsy. Other causes include accidental and non-accidental head injury, anoxia and cerebrovascular accidents.

TRANSITION TO ADULT SERVICES

As school leaving age approaches, there should be a multidisciplinary approach to transition planning and a college with the appropriate expertise should be sought.[469] Expert careers advice is invaluable and suitable recreational opportunities should be investigated. An adult specialist resource should be sought as a source of advice in future. Such services have been difficult to find in many places. Many adults with cerebral palsy and other disabling conditions are either not in touch with social services or specialist medical advice or are dissatisfied with the services received.[470] There is justified concern for the decline in adult rehabilitation services over the past 30 years[373] and the lack of coherent and sustained funding for academic rehabilitation research.[374]

DEGENERATIVE BRAIN DISORDERS

INTRODUCTION

The neurodegenerative disorders of childhood are a heterogeneous group of diseases that result in the progressive deterioration of neurological function with loss of speech, vision, hearing, locomotion, bulbar functions and cognitive abilities. They are often associated with seizures. They are rare with a prevalence of 0.6/1000 live births. Many are caused by specific genetic and/or biochemical defects but they can also be caused by infections and toxins with the cause of some remaining unknown.

They are important because:
1. Some of them are treatable and the earlier treatment is started the better the outcome.
2. Knowing and understanding the condition helps to predict and to plan the multidisciplinary management and ultimate terminal care needs.
3. Most have specific genetic implications with possible antenatal diagnosis.

CLINICAL APPROACH
History

A history of loss of skills helps distinguish the neurodegenerative from static, nonprogressive conditions. Usually, initial development is either normal or slightly delayed. Development then plateaus over a period of time with no acquisition of new skills followed by loss of previously acquired skills. The onset may be insidious but is sometimes acute sometimes in association with viral infections. Both may cause diagnostic difficulty. Regression may progress steadily at varying speeds or else spasmodically, with periods of progression followed by a plateauing of abilities prior to the next period of deterioration. Again, periods of deterioration may be triggered by intercurrent viral infections. Sometimes the presentation is with behavioral or psychiatric disturbances, or educational difficulties. Neurodegenerative conditions in early childhood often present with or include myoclonic or polymorphous seizures so that an epileptic encephalopathy, such as the Lennox–Gastaut syndrome may be suspected (see p. 858).

White or gray matter involvement

Some neurodegenerative conditions are localized to white or gray matter or may involve both. White matter involvement is characteristically associated with upper motor neurone signs, episodic hypertonia and difficulties in mobility. Gray matter involvement is particularly associated with intellectual and visual impairment and seizures.

Systemic involvement

The involvement of other organs is common. Physical examination should include a search for organomegaly and skeletal deformity. The retina should be examined carefully for pigmentation which might, for example, suggest a peroxisomal disorder or a mitochondrial cytopathy and for cherry-red spots due to abnormal perimacular deposition of storage material seen in a number of lysosomal storage disorders.

Family history

This, especially a history of consanguinity, may be important as most of these conditions, especially the neurometabolic, are autosomal recessive.

AGE-RELATED PRESENTATIONS

Neurodegenerative disorders (ND) can present at any age with obvious loss of skills, plateauing or delayed development with or without clinical clues.

Infancy (see also Table 22.33)

A loss of motor skills may not be appreciated in infancy. Regression at this age often presents with a loss of interest which may be visual or in nonverbal communication.[471] Hypothyroidism, the aminoacidopathies, and metabolic (organic) acidosis are the main conditions associated with regression without obvious clinical clues. Nonketotic hyperglycinemia and Menke syndrome with its characteristic twisted hair (see Ch. 26, p. 1124) often present with seizures. In this age group, irritability with extensor hypertonus can be a prominent presenting features of some conditions and may or may not be associated with organomegaly.

Table 22.33   Regression in infancy

With no obvious clue:
Hypothyroidism
Aminoacidopathies
Metabolic (organic) acidosis

With seizures:
Menke kinky syndrome
Nonketotic hyperglycinemia
Glucose transporter protein (Glut 1) deficiency
Serine biosynthesis disorders
Biotinidase deficiency
Carbohydrate deficient glycoprotein (CDG) syndromes

With irritability:
Krabbe
Infantile Gaucher
Tay–Sachs
Niemann–Pick
Glutaric aciduria type 1
Pelizaeus–Merzbacher
Infantile ceroid - lipofuscinosis (CLN 1)

The toddler age group (see also Table 22.34)

In the toddler, changes are seen in speech and behavior combined with motor difficulties.[471] In some conditions, there are specific, but often subtle features suggesting a specific diagnosis. For example, in Sanfilippo disease there are often soft dysmorphic features and a spleen may be palpable. In Moya Moya disease dementia and regression occur and HIV encephalopathy is usually characterized by failure to thrive with brain atrophy being prominent on neuroimaging. In others, specific neurological signs at presentation may suggests the diagnosis: peripheral neuropathy with ataxia and bulbar signs suggests metachromatic leukodystrophy; ataxia with ocular apraxia and conjunctival capillary dilation suggests ataxia telangiectasia; progressive cerebellar ataxia with mild dementia suggests juvenile Sandhoff disease; impairment of eye movement control and respiration with ataxia is characteristic of Leigh disease; and splenomegaly with a vertical gaze palsy suggests Niemann–Pick disease type C. The clinical manifestations of some conditions with autistic features such as Rett syndrome and a number of psychoses also start in this age group. Again, epilepsy can be the presenting feature.

The school-age child (see also Table 22.35)

In the school-age child regression is often manifested with a decline in school performance, including concentration and pencil skills. New learning is hindered because of poor memory and coordination is impaired.[471] A wide range of conditions can include epilepsy in this age group, although this is rarely the presenting problem (Table 22.35).

Table 22.34 Regression in toddlers

With neurological signs:
Metachromatic leukodystrophy
Juvenile Sandhoff
Ataxia telangiectasia
Leigh disease
Niemann–Pick type C

With autistic features:
Rett syndrome
Infantile Batten disease
Missed phenylketonuria
Biotinidase deficiency
Carbohydrate deficient glycoprotein (CDG) syndromes

With seizures:
Late infantile Batten disease (CLN 2)
Alper disease

Table 22.35 Regression in school age

With seizures as a prominent feature:
Juvenile Batten disease (CLN 3) (although seizures only prominent in later stages)
Lafora body disease
Sialidosis type 1
Myoclonic epilepsy with ragged red fibers
Juvenile Gaucher disease
Juvenile GM2 gangliosidosis

With seizures not a prominent feature:
Juvenile metachromatic leukodystrophy
Adrenoleukodystrophy
Subacute sclerosing panencephalitis
Wilson disease
Juvenile Huntington disease
Hallervorden–Spatz disease

CLASSIFICATION OF DEGENERATIVE BRAIN DISEASES

The neurodegenerative disorders can be classified in many different ways. One is shown below:

- lysosomal storage disease;
- sphingolipidoses e.g. GMI -, GM2-gangliosidosis, Krabbe disease, metachromic leucodystrophy, etc.;
- glycoproteinoses, e.g. mannosidosis, fucosidosis etc.;
- mucopolysaccharidoses;
- mucolipidoses;
- peroxisomal disorders, e.g adrenoleucodystrophy;
- organic acidurias, e.g. Canavan disease;
- trace metal metabolism e.g Wilson disease and Menke syndrome;
- neuronal ceroid lipofuscinoses;
- spinocerebellar degeneration, e.g. Friedreich ataxia, abetalipoproteinemia, olivopontocerebellar atrophy, ataxia telangiectasia etc.;
- basal ganglia degeneration, e.g. Hallervorden–Spatz disease and dystonia musculorum deformans;
- infections, e.g. subacute sclerosing panencephalitis, progressive multifocal leuco-encephalopathy, prion disease;
- miscellaneous, e.g. Pelizaeus–Merzbacher and Alexander disease.

SPECIFIC NEURODEGENERATIVE CONDITIONS

Detailed descriptions of all the neurodegenerative disorders for which there is a known biochemical defect are given in the chapter on metabolic disorders. There remain some conditions in which the presumed biochemical defect is unknown or the cause is due to some other mechanism, such as infection. These disorders will be considered here.

Rett syndrome

Rett syndrome (RS) was first described in 22 girls who, after normal development for 6 months, deteriorated in a devastating fashion. It affects females almost exclusively. Incidence figures vary widely but it probably affects about 1 in 10 000 females and possibly 1 in 100 000 males. Most cases (99.5%) are due to spontaneous mutations.

The diagnostic criteria for classic Rett syndrome are:[472]

- apparently normal prenatal and perinatal period;
- apparently normal development through at least the first 5–6 months of life;
- normal head circumference at birth;
- deceleration of the head growth (aged 3 months to 3 years);
- loss of acquired skills (aged 3 months to 3 years), including learned purposeful hand skills, acquired babble and/or learned words, and communicative abilities;
- appearance of obvious mental deficiency;
- appearance successively of intense hand stereotypies, including hand wringing and/or squeezing, hand washing and/or patting and/or rubbing, and hand mouthing and/or tongue pulling;
- gait abnormality among the ambulant girls, including gait apraxia and/or dyspraxia and jerky truncal ataxia and/or body dyspraxia;
- diagnosis tentative until the individual is aged 2–5 years.

The muscle tone is variable. Initially patients with RS patients are hypotonic. With progression of the disease spasticity and wasting develops. Some become wheelchair bound after 10 years, but they retain some functional ability and 60% of patients with RS continue to walk.

Other problems include breath holding and apnoea during wakefulness with normal breathing during sleep, epilepsy, oral-motor dysfunction with gut motility problems (e.g. constipation, gastroesophageal reflux [GER]), scoliosis, autonomic dysfunction (cold blue extremities), and somatic growth failure). During the regression period, individuals with RS demonstrate screaming episodes, sleep disturbances and poor social interactions.

Atypical cases with Rett syndrome (Rett syndrome variant) can be difficult to diagnose. The following criteria help:

- loss (partial or subtotal) of acquired fine finger skills in late infancy and/or early childhood;

- loss of acquired single words and/or phrases and/or nuanced babble;
- RS hand stereotypies, hands together or apart;
- early deviant communicative ability;
- deceleration of head growth of 2 standard deviations (2 sd), even when still within normal limits.

Currently, diagnosis of RS is made if the patient meets defined clinical criteria. The diagnosis is supported by a positive mutational analysis of MECP2. However, as many as 20% of females meeting the full clinical criteria for RS may have no identified mutation.[473] Mutations on the MECP2 gene are present in 85% of cases. Males with mutations on this gene show a spectrum of symptomatology, ranging from severe congenital encephalopathy, dystonia apraxia and retardation to psychiatric illness with mild mental retardation.[474]

Because no cure exists, treatment is palliative and supportive. A multidisciplinary approach to care for persons with RS is recommended.

The leukodystrophies

The leukodystrophies are disorders of cerebral white matter, either alone or combined with other CNS or peripheral nervous system problems. Many have known metabolic defects and are described in more detail in Chapter 28. There remain a few specific leukodystrophies not due to known metabolic defects and other unclassified leukodystrophies.

Pelizaeus–Merzbacher disease

This is usually an X-linked white matter myelination disorder. A mutation in the PLP gene is present in about 75% of cases. The clinical severity of PMD varies widely, primarily depending upon the precise nature of the causative mutation and probably, to a certain extent, upon other genetic and environmental influences.[475]

The presentation of classic PMD is of *infantile-onset* (typically within the first 2 months of life) nystagmus, titubation and weakness. Ataxia, cognitive delay, and spasticity then follow. Most children never walk. Most do acquire some degree of language skills, which may approach normal levels, but the speed of expressive language is usually slow giving impression of more severe degree of mental retardation than is present. These patients may survive to the sixth decade of life or longer.

More severely affected patients, those with the so-called *connatal PMD*, have nystagmus present from birth or at least in the first week or two of life, often have stridor and respiratory difficulty and hypotonia, and may even have seizures. These patients typically have limited language skills, never ambulate, and develop severe spasticity with little voluntary movement. These individuals usually die before the third decade of life.

Individuals with the least severe form of PMD, which merges with SPG2, present with childhood-onset spastic paraplegia, mild cognitive impairment, ataxia and athetosis. Survival to the sixth decade of life or later is characteristic. Typically, neurological signs progress but at a gradual rate with reported periods of relative stability. Generally, those who learn to walk begin to lose ambulatory abilities during adolescence.

PMD typically affects males, but female heterozygotes can be clinically affected, especially those who carry alleles that are relatively mild. As the defective oligodendrocytes die and are replaced by healthy oligodendrocytes in heterozygous females, neurological function improves. Females heterozygous for the less severe alleles of PLP1 that are not believed to cause oligodendrocyte cell death or apoptosis may develop a more progressive and nonremitting syndrome that usually begins during adulthood.

Some females with PMD (such as the original PMD family) probably have a clinical course much like that of affected males, in which the symptoms do not remit and may be the result of skewed X inactivation, i.e. the majority of oligodendrocytes have inactivated the normal X chromosome and insufficient healthy oligodendrocytes are available to myelinate the CNS effectively.[475]

Leukoencephalopathy with vanishing white matter disease

This is a group of autosomal recessive conditions with extensive MRI changes restricted to white matter. They may present with progressive spasticity and ataxia but often show step-wise progression following infections and minor head traumas, with a sudden onset of symptoms, followed by a period of stability and then further deterioration. van der Knapp et al[476] described families with MRI scan changes restricted to the white matter with cavitations in the frontal and/or temporal lobes. Affected patients had a relatively mild clinical course presenting with late spasticity, cerebellar signs and macrocephaly. A more rapid course with progressive diplegia and ataxia was reported in three siblings without cystic changes.[477] Yet other cases have been reported with onset in infancy or early childhood who have shown progressive ataxia and spasticity with exacerbations with infections and mild head trauma.[478]

VWM is caused by mutations in one of the five genes that are collectively called eIF2B, or eukaryotic initiation factor 2B. Changes in these genes reduce the function of eIF2B. This reduction in function becomes a particular problem during episodes of fever, infection or head traumas, and deterioration accelerates following such episodes.[479]

Alexander disease

Alexander disease is a rare disorder of the nervous system. It is considered one of the leukodystrophies. Most cases begin before age 2 years (the infantile form). Signs and symptoms of the infantile form typically include an enlarged brain and head (megalencephaly), seizures, stiffness in the arms and/or legs (spasticity), mental retardation and delayed physical development. Less frequently, onset occurs later in childhood (the juvenile form) or adulthood. Common problems in juvenile and adult forms of Alexander disease include speech abnormalities, swallowing difficulties and poor coordination (ataxia).

Alexander disease is characterized by abnormal protein deposits known as Rosenthal fibers, which are found in astroglial cells which support and nourish nerve cells in the brain and spinal cord. Mutations in the GFAP gene cause Alexander disease. This gene provides instructions for making a protein called glial fibrillary acidic protein. As a result, glial fibrillary acidic protein accumulates as a component of Rosenthal fibers and interferes with the normal activities of astroglial cells. It is not well understood how impaired astroglial cells contribute to the abnormal formation or maintenance of myelin.[480]

Alexander disease is considered an autosomal dominant disorder. However almost all cases result from new mutations. In some rare adult cases, a GFAP mutation may be passed to children of an affected parent.[481]

Cockayne syndrome

Cockayne syndrome (CS) includes the classic form (CKN1) and a more severe form with symptoms present at birth (CKN2). These are also termed CS types A and B, respectively. Patients present with delayed psychomotor development, poor feeding, photosensitive rashes and cataracts. All patients with CKN1 have mental retardation. and growth failure, which includes progressive microcephaly in most patients in the first year. Ambulant patients present with an unusual gait resulting from leg spasticity, ataxia, and contractures of the hips, knees and ankles. Muscle tone and reflexes are increased or decreased. Most patients have photodermatitis that leads to dry scaly skin. Patients develop an aged appearance. Pigmentary degeneration of the retina is one hallmark of this disorder, with cataracts and optic atrophy or optic disc pallor as frequent findings. These ophthalmologic changes are progressive. More than one half of patients with CKN1 have mild to severe sensorineural hearing loss. Many patients have moderate to severe dental caries; permanent teeth have short roots.

CKN1 is caused by a defect in the Cockayne syndrome type A gene (CSA or ERCC8) located on chromosome 5. Affected persons inherit two mutant genes, one from each parent. Cells carrying ERCC8 mutations are hypersensitive to UV light. They do not recover the ability to synthesize ribonucleic acid (RNA) after exposure to UV light. In addition, the cells cannot remove and degrade deoxyribonucleic acid (DNA) lesions from strands that have active transcription.[482]

Aicardi–Goutieres syndrome

Aicardi–Goutières syndrome is an autosomal recessive mimic of congenital infection presenting either in the immediate neonatal period with microcephaly, thrombocytopenia, anemia, deranged liver function, hepatosplenomegaly and seizures or within a few weeks or months of life with irritability, feeding difficulties, seizures and a loss of skills. Affected infants develop a spastic quadraparesis with dystonia and usually demonstrate severe psychomotor retardation. Periventricular or basal ganglia calcification is often present on CT and a fronto-temporal leukodystrophy with cystic formation is observed on MRI. Raised numbers of white cells are usually, but not always, present in the CSF and CSF interferon alpha, biopterin and neopterin levels are elevated. Distinctive 'chilblain-like' lesions can occur on the hands and feet. The disease results from mutations in any of four genes and molecular testing is available as a first-line investigation. The diagnosis should be considered in any child with features of congenital infection in the absence of corroborating serological data.[483]

Canavan disease

Canavan disease (CD) is a relatively rare, but always fatal, inherited, leukodystrophy. Presentation is in early infancy with variable symptoms; rapidly increasing head circumference, lack of head control, reduced visual responsiveness and abnormal muscle tone such as stiffness or floppiness. Children with Canavan disease cannot crawl, walk, sit or talk. Over time they may suffer seizures, become paralyzed, mentally retarded or blind and have trouble swallowing. Although hearing usually remains a functioning sense, deafness may also result. Most children do not live past age 10.

Canavan disease, like the more well-known Tay–Sachs disease, is one of a number of genetic disorders which affect Ashkenazi Jews at high frequency.

Canavan disease is autosomaly recessive inherited. It can be diagnosed antenatally by blood test that screens for the missing enzyme or for mutations in the gene that controls aspartoacylase. The ASPA gene is located on the short (p) arm of chromosome 17 between the end (terminus) of the arm and position 13.[484]

Progressive neuronal degeneration of childhood (PNDC, infantile poliodystrophy or Alper disease)

This term encompasses a group of diseases characterized by presentation in infancy or early childhood with neuronal degeneration with or without liver failure. The clinical picture is with hypotonia, fail to thrive, developmental delay, seizures and hepatic derangement. Epilepsia partialis continua is common, as are episodes of status epilepticus and often late hepatic failure develops with rapid progression to death. Sodium valproate can precipitate hepatic failure and some cases of 'valproate hepatotoxicity' in young children may have been PNDC.

The condition can be familial, usually autosomal recessive or sporadic. It has been associated with deficiencies of pyruvate carboxylase, pyruvate dehydrogenase and respiratory chain abnormalities. Many cases appear to be associated with mutations of the POLG1 gene which is a nuclear gene encoding the catalytic subunit of mitochondrial DNA polymerase. POLG1 is a major disease gene in mitochondrial disorders. Mutations of it can be associated with multiple deletions, depletion or point mutations of mitochondrial DNA (mtDNA). In turn, these different molecular phenotypes lead to an extremely heterogeneous spectrum of clinical outcomes, ranging from rapidly fatal hepatocerebral presentations, including Alper syndrome to adult-onset progressive ophthalmoplegia to juvenile ataxic syndromes with epilepsy.

Pantothenate kinase-associated neurodegeneration; Hallervorden–Spatz disease

This is a progressive neurodegenerative condition with characteristic accumulation of iron in the basal ganglia. The onset is in the first two decades of life with progressive dystonia, rigidity, choreoathetosis and cognitive deterioration. Other variable features are retinitis pigmentosa, optic atrophy, sensorineural deafness and acanthocytosis. Epilepsy is not prominent. The rate of progression is very variable and misdiagnosis as cerebral palsy is common. Neuro-imaging (MRI) demonstrate the characteristic basal ganglia 'tiger eye 'sign. Many patients have detectable mutations in PANK2, the gene encoding pantothenate kinase 2.[485] Iron chelation has not proven useful.

Spinocerebellar and peripheral nerve degenerations

These are primary neuronal degenerations, without metabolic markers. Their common features are their selective nature affecting one or only a few parts of the central or peripheral nervous system, their progressive nature though not necessarily fatal, and the likelihood of symmetrical involvement. With the rapid advances in neurogenetics, many of them now have a specific molecular DNA test. As knowledge of the different genotypes grows, it is evident that the same gene defect can lead to heterogeneous clinical features. This variable clinical picture with overlapping symptom and sign complexes has made classification difficult. The recognized conditions included in the group are summarized in Table 22.36. Particularly rapid advances have been made in the genetics of the spinocerebellar degenerations (which are considered elsewhere in this chapter) and in ataxia telangiectasia .

Neuroaxonal dystrophy

This is an autosomal recessive condition or conditions. The histopathological hallmark is the spheroid which is an axonal swelling formed by branched tubular structure and bundles of filament with mitochondria. Spheroids are present in peripheral nerves, especially presynaptically, but are also widespread throughout the CNS.

The infantile form starts between 6 months and 2 years of age with motor difficulties. The child is hypotonic but with pyramidal signs differentiating it from a neuromuscular condition. The condition progresses to severe dementia with spasticity and eventually decorticate rigidity. Nystagmus and optic atrophy commonly occur by the age of 3 years while seizures are a late feature. Death occurs by 5–10 years. Neuroimaging reveals cerebellar atrophy with, on MRI, increased signal on T2 in the cerebrum and cerebellum and sometimes basal ganglia calcification. EMG shows denervation with nerve conduction studies being normal. Visual evoked potentials disappear after a few months. The diagnosis is confirmed by the finding of spheroids on peripheral biopsy of skin, conjunctiva, nerves and/or muscle.

Rare cases of late onset (juvenile type) neuroaxonal dystrophy are reported. Onset is in late childhood with progressive myoclonic epilepsy and retinal degeneration. The diagnosis is by rectal or skin biopsies.[486]

No treatment or antenatal diagnosis is available.

Hereditary spastic paraparesis (HSP)

HSP is not a single disease entity, but rather a group of clinically and genetically diverse disorders that share the primary feature of progressive and generally severe lower extremity weakness and spasticity.

HSP is generally classified as uncomplicated or complicated. In uncomplicated HSP, symptoms are usually limited to gradual weakening in the legs; urinary bladder disturbance; and, sometimes, impaired sensation in the feet.

In complicated HSP, which is rare, additional symptoms may include peripheral neuropathy, epilepsy, ataxia, optic neuropathy, retinopathy, dementia, ichthyosis, mental retardation, deafness, or problems with speech, swallowing or breathing.[487]

The inheritance mode of HSP may be X-linked, autosomal dominant or autosomal recessive, with each type having several subtypes based on the location of the gene. The mode of inheritance cannot be used to predict severity of the disorder since symptoms can vary greatly within each type. Several genes have been located. There are ten types of dominantly inherited uncomplicated or complicated HSP, seven types of recessively inherited HSP and three types of X-linked HSP.[488]

The classic symptom of HSP is progressive difficulty in walking of variable severity. Some patients continue to be mobile while others eventually may require the use of a wheelchair. Patients usually have difficulty lifting their toes, which results in them dragging the toes when

Table 22.36 Spinocerebellar and peripheral nerve degenerations

Disorders	Genetics	Age at onset	Neurology and other clinical features
Dentatorubra rubro pallido luysian atrophy (DRPLA) (Ramsay–Hunt syndrome)	Familial (triplet repeat disorder)	Late childhood to adolescence	Myoclonic epilepsy; cerebellar ataxia
Friedreich ataxia	AR triplet repeat disorder (chromosome 9)	Mean 10.5 years (range 2–16 years)	Presenting: ataxia (limbs and trunk), scoliosis, tremor, cardiomyopathy (T inversion and LVH). Later: dysarthria, pyramidal signs with extensor plantars and diminished reflexes, proprioceptive loss, pes cavus, distal amyotrophy (distal wasting and weakness), optic atrophy and nystagmus, deafness, CCF or arrhythmias, gradually progressive diabetes mellitus; sudden cardiac death in the thirties
Familial spastic paraplegia	AR AD	11.5 years 18.5 years	Slow learning to walk; mild spastic paraplegia; stiff gait; scissoring of legs; slowly progressive (variable)
Progressive cerebellar ataxia	AR	Mean 9.4 years	Dysarthria, pyramidal signs, absent ankle jerks (others normal); sensory loss. Better prognosis than Friedreich ataxia
Familial spastic-ataxic syndrome	AR		Progressive insidious involvement with signs relative to cerebellum, corticospinal tract and occular signs. Death over 5–20 years
Olivopontocerebellar atrophy (OPCA) (Types I–V)	AD–OPCA (Types I, III, IV, V) AR–OPCA (Type II)		With retinal degeneration, progressive cerebellar ataxia; parkinsonian rigidity; resting tremor; impairment of speech
Ataxia telangiectasia (Louis–Barr syndrome)	AR (chromosome 11)		Progressive neurological deterioration with ocular and cutaneous telangiectasia. Early: cerebellar ataxia (often less than developmental progress). Later: decreased IgA, dysarthria; choreoathetosis; titubation. Sometimes progressive dementia. Telangiectasia of conjunctiva, pinnae, face, V of the neck, and flexures begins after 3 years; oculomotor dyspraxia, growth retardation; with wheelchair by 10–12 years; survivors show distal weakness, wasting, posterior column signs after 10 years; death before adulthood. Immunological: tonsils hypoplastic, abnormal IgM, thymic hypoplasia. Neoplasia: lymphomas, sarcomas, leukemia, Hodgkin, lymphosarcomas, ovarian and gastric tumors. Blood: lymphocytopenia. Endocrine: abnormal carbohydrate metabolism
Ataxia with occulomotor apraxia	AR. Two forms (Types 1 and 2) caused by mutations on the APTX and SETX genes respectively		Resemble ataxia telangiectasia but without the telangiectasia and the systemic features
Infantile neuroaxonaldystrophy	AR	6 months to 2 years	Loss of motor and mental milestones with regression; early visual involvement (ocular wobble); symmetrical pyramidal tract signs; marked hypotonia; anterior horn cell involvement (peripheral motor and sensory defect); dementia and decerebration
Multiple sclerosis in childhood		12–13 years	Death less than 10 years. Remitting course (1–2 episodes in childhood); optic/retrobulbar neuritis bilaterally (a quarter of childhood cases subsequently develop MS); gait disorder (with spasticity or ataxia)
Giant axonal neuropathy	AR	Early school years	Chronic peripheral mixed neuropathy; regression of gait, movement and IQ; fits; nystagmus; precocious puberty; pale, slightly reddish tightly curly hair

walking and catching them on stairs or on uneven sidewalks or curbs. In the later stages of the disease, patients experience difficulty flexing the thigh muscle to raise the leg when walking. A reduced sense of balance is noted. Some people also experience urinary problems.

The amount of spasticity experienced is variable depending on the circumstances. Many people notice that their muscles seem tighter when they are emotionally stressed or upset. Other factors that can affect spasticity are cold temperature, poor posture, high humidity and illness. The increasing stiffness in the legs is associated with frequent tripping, particularly when the patient is walking on uneven terrain.

Infectious progressive encephalitides

Some neurodegenerative conditions result from some slow viral infections. The main examples are: subacute sclerosing panencephalitis

(SSPE), progressive rubella panencephalitis, Lyme disease, HIV dementia and prion disease. Lyme disease and HIV dementia are considered elsewhere in this chapter and in the section on aseptic meningitis in this chapter and in the chapters on immunodeficiency and infections (see Chs 27 and 28). Here SSPE and prion disease will be considered.

Subacute sclerosing panencephalitis (SSPE)

SSPE is by far the most common of the chronic encephalitides. It most frequently follows measles infection in the first 2 years of life with an incidence of 1:1 000 000. It represents an altered host response to the virus. The interval between measles and the onset of SSPE is usually 5–7 years. The onset is often insidious with slow intellectual and bizarre behavior followed by the onset of intractable myoclonus. Occasionally unilateral symptoms and signs make early diagnosis difficult. Extrapyramidal and pyramidal features follow and the condition progresses to dementia. The speed of progression is variable, but more than half of patients have a rapid course.[489]

The EEG shows a characteristic pattern with so-called periodic complexes. The CSF shows evidence of intrathecal antimeasles antibody production. CT scan and MRI may be normal, especially early in the disease. Later, they may show variable cortical atrophy and ventricular dilation. Focal or multifocal white matter abnormalities may also be seen.

The prognosis is poor and the SSPE invariably results in profound disability or death. Rapidly evolving forms may lead to death in only a few months. A combination of intraventricular interferon and isoprinosine was reported to increase the rate of remission from 10% up to 45%. However late reoccurrence may happen after several years of remission.[490]

Prion diseases

Prions are infectious agents which affect only the CNS, are distinct from viruses and have very long incubation periods. The diseases caused by these agents were previously called the transmissible spongiform encephalitides and include scrapie in sheep, the human disease Kuru and Creutzfeldt–Jakob disease (CJD). Attempts to identify specific nucleic acid within highly purified preparations of prion were not successful.[491]

The major infectious component of prions is composed of a protein designated PrPSc. Cloning the prion protein gene resulted in the discovery of a point mutation for humans with familial CJD and established that prion diseases are genetic and infectious in humans.

Creutzfeldt–Jakob disease. Progressive dementia, loss of intellectual functions, sometimes with cerebellar and visual defects, are the main characteristics of CJD. The onset is usually in adults though there is a reported case in a 10-year-old. CJD is transmissible through growth hormone derived from human pituitary glands, through corneal transplants and by contaminated surgical instruments. The infectious agent is highly resistant to sterilization.[492]

New CJD variant. In the UK, there have been reports of a new variant of CJD occurring in adolescents and young adults. The characteristic features are personality changes, mental disturbance, dysesthesia and progressive dementia and ataxia. Myoclonus may be a feature. Affected young people often present with severe depression. A period of dysphoria follows accompanied by the onset of a florid, worsening ataxia. Dementia and an evolving spastic quadriparesis then follow with death occurring in 2 years or so. MRI shows high signal in the posterior thalamus. The place of tonsillar biopsy and specific CSF proteins in diagnosis is being defined. The histopathology is different from that of classic CJD.

INVESTIGATION OF DEGENERATIVE DISEASES

The clinical history, including the age of onset of the condition, together with specific clinical features referable to the nervous and other systems, may suggest a differential diagnosis. However, frequently specific features are lacking and in such cases 'screening' in relation to the age of onset can be useful. In all cases MRI is indicated.

In infancy, screening should include thyroid function tests (for hypothyroidism), urine and plasma amino acids (for aminoacidopathies), urine organic acids (for organic acidosis) and white cell enzymes (WCE) (for the neurolipidoses such as Niemann–Pick and Tay–Sachs diseases). EEG can sometimes be useful, for example revealing hypsarrhythmia, suggesting infantile spasms as a cause of apparent regression or a burst suppression pattern in nonketotic hyperglycinemia. Other investigations which may be useful include plasma copper (low in Menke syndrome), CSF with simultaneous blood and urine glycine (raised in nonketotic hyperglycinemia) and DNA studies such as for Pelizaeus–Merzbacher disease and mitochondrial cytopathies.

Screening in toddlers should include urine and plasma amino acids and urine organic acids. Metachromatic leukodystrophy (MLD) and the neurolipidoses can be detected from WCE. The diagnosis of Batten disease is undergoing a transformation. Previously neurophysiological studies along with skin and rectal biopsies (to detect neuronal inclusions) were required. However, nearly all cases of CLN 1, 2 and 3, can now be diagnosed using a combination of enzyme assays done on blood combined with molecular DNA studies. DNA studies now also assist in the diagnosis of Rett syndrome. Liver function tests and CSF and blood lactate levels can be helpful in Alper disease due to mitochondrial cytopathies.

In school-age children (Table 22.37) investigations should include WCE for juvenile metachromatic leukodystrophy, juvenile Gaucher disease and juvenile GM2 gangliosidosis; investigations (as above) for Batten disease; DNA for juvenile Huntington and in some cases of Hallervorden–Spatz diseases; muscle biopsy, EEG and DNA for mitochondrial cytopathies; very long chain fatty acids for adrenoleukodystrophy; EEG and CSF measles antibodies for SSPE; plasma ceruloplasmin and copper and urine copper for Wilson disease. Depending on the clinical picture, other investigations may need to be considered but the temptation to undertake all known tests should be resisted.

Table 22.37 Investigation for neurodegenerative conditions in school-age children

Blood
Liver function tests
Copper, ceruloplasmin
Lactate
Amino acids
Very long chain fatty acids
Immunoglobulins
Thyroid function tests
Autoantibodies, including antinuclear antibodies
White cell enzymes (targeted for conditions being considered)
Toxicology
Appropriate genetic tests, esp. DNA studies for specific disorders

Urine
Amino acids/organic acids
Renal epithelial metachromatic granules

CSF
Immunoglobulins
Electrophoresis
Cells (cytospin)
Measles IgG
Lactate
Neurotransmitters

Neurophysiology
EEG
Electroretinogram
Visual evoked potentials

Neuroimaging
CT scan
MRI

MANAGEMENT OF THE NEURODEGENERATIVE CONDITIONS

A very few neurodegenerative conditions have specific treatment. These include D-penicillamine for Wilson disease, specific diets and vitamins in some aminoacidopathies, pyridoxine and pyridoxal phosphate dependent seizures, folinic acid responsive seizures, biotinidase deficiency, glucose carrier protein deficiency (Glut 1 deficiency), serine biosynthesis disorders and creatine deficiency syndromes. The vast majority of the neurodegenerative disorders are untreatable, resulting in progressive neurodisability and death at variable ages. Having an accurate diagnosis is essential for appropriate genetic counseling. There is still much that can be offered to children and their families to tackle and ease the main difficulties facing the daily care and activities such as feeding and mobility, and to prevent or delay unwanted and inevitable complications such as bed sores and severe contractures.

Management can be arbitrarily divided into three stages: early, middle and late phases.

In the early phase the emphasis is likely to be on maintaining normal function, such as mobility, and normal activities, such as mainstream schooling, as long as is possible. Feeding difficulties often respond well to specific measures, as do associated medical problems such as seizures. In the middle phase as the child or young person becomes more dependent involvement of hospices and other shared care arrangements are often of immense value to the child and their family. Careful attention to nutrition will often help maintain health and general well-being, including mood. In the late phase mood disturbances including dysphoria and agitation can be problematic and often respond to medication. Opiates should not be considered as a last resort. Their judicious use may greatly enhance the quality of the child's life. Following death, if the diagnosis remains unclear, postmortem examination should be encouraged as its findings may be of great help in planning future pregnancies. Finally, families should be offered an opportunity to discuss unresolved issues at a suitable interval following the child's death.

NEUROMUSCULAR DISEASE

MODES OF PRESENTATION

In neuromuscular diseases the principal problem lies at the anterior horn cell (the spinal muscular atrophies), the peripheral nerve (the peripheral neuropathies), the neuromuscular junction (the myasthenic syndromes) or the skeletal muscle (the myopathies and muscular dystrophies). It used to be considered that the central nervous system was not involved. However, it often is. For example in Duchenne muscular dystrophy learning difficulties are common while the congenital muscular dystrophies are associated with a variety of structural brain disorders. Mitochondrial cytopathies often feature prominent muscle involvement but are of course multisystem disorders. Clinical evaluation can often be helpful in defining the likely site of involvement in neuromuscular disorders. Hence fasciculation, muscle atrophy and severely decreased or absent tendon reflexes are characteristic of anterior horn cell disease. In peripheral neuropathies absent tendon reflexes and muscle atrophy, but not fasciculation, are characteristic. Myasthenia is characterized by fatiguability. Tendon reflexes are usually normal or only slightly depressed. In the myopathies and muscular dystrophies the main finding is of weakness; tendon reflexes are usually preserved. Beyond such broad generalizations, the presentation of neuromuscular disorders shows considerable variation according to the age of the child.

Neonatal period

Pregnancy with a fetus with a neuromuscular condition may be complicated by polyhydramnios and reduced fetal movement.

Neuromuscular conditions must be suspected in infants who have arthrogryposis, are hypotonic, have feeding difficulties, respiratory problems or a need for respiratory support in the absence of any significant pulmonary pathology.

As any examination candidate knows conditions which may lead to a 'floppy infant' are legion. How does one distinguish infants who may have a neuromuscular condition? The traditional teaching, that these infants are weak in addition to being hypotonic, holds true. However, even if an infant is profoundly weak, without any antigravity limb movement, there are pitfalls to recognizing that the infant has a neuromuscular condition. An infant who unexpectedly fails to breathe after birth may be thought to have a hypoxic–ischemic encephalopathy and subsequent lack of movement may be attributed to the sequelae of this. Indeed, to confuse matters further, the infant may have had a degree of hypoxic–ischemic encephalopathy secondary to profound respiratory muscle weakness. Assessment of level of consciousness is difficult in neonates and is particularly difficult in an infant with ptosis and facial weakness.

Arthrogryposis may be caused by any condition resulting in restricted fetal movement. Neuromuscular disorders reported in patients with arthrogryposis include distal spinal muscular atrophy, neuropathy, congenital myopathy and congenital muscular dystrophy.

Feeding difficulties may be profound, with inability to suck and swallow and respiratory embarrassment on attempted feeding, or may mean feeds take longer than expected with weight gain less than ideal.

Conditions presenting in the neonatal period with limb weakness and respiratory and feeding difficulty include myotonic dystrophy and the congenital myopathies. The birth of an infant with congenital myotonic dystrophy is often the first presentation of this condition in the family. It is always useful to examine the mother of a weak neonate for ptosis, facial weakness and myotonia. The congenital myopathies, which are most likely to present with a need for respiratory support, are nemaline myopathy and myotubular myopathy. Ophthalmoplegia in a male infant is particularly suggestive of myotubular myopathy and there may be a history of neonatal death in other males in the family. Antenatal onset of spinal muscular atrophy is rare but severely affected neonates with deletions in the SMN1 gene are described.[493]

Congenital myasthenic syndromes must always be considered in neonates with feeding difficulty and episodes of respiratory distress or apnea.

Infancy and early childhood

Delayed motor development with age-appropriate cognitive abilities should prompt consideration of a neuromuscular condition. Global developmental delay may be the presenting feature in dystrophinopathies[494] and, in a boy with developmental delay, investigation should always include creatine kinase estimation. Episodic weakness or exacerbations of weakness during intercurrent illnesses suggest metabolic myopathy or congenital myasthenic syndrome.

Later childhood

The manifestations of limb muscle weakness include difficulty with or inability to run, abnormal gait, difficulty climbing stairs and rising from the floor (Fig. 22.31). Fatiguability should suggest a myasthenic disorder. Muscle pain or cramp on exertion and episodes of rhabdomyolysis are suggestive of metabolic myopathy.

Occasionally neuromuscular disease presents with 'abnormal liver function tests'. When creatine kinase is very elevated, other enzymes such as alanine transferase (ALT) may also be elevated, leading to the suspicion of liver disease. When ALT is elevated but other measures of liver function such as bilirubin and coagulation studies are normal, checking the creatine kinase level may reveal the true source of this enzyme and lead to appropriate investigations.

Toe-walking may be a manifestation of many conditions in childhood. Neuromuscular conditions, particularly dystrophinopathy, Emery–Dreifuss muscular dystrophy and Charcot–Marie–Tooth disease (CMT), must be considered in the differential diagnosis. Foot deformity is a frequent presenting feature of CMT and is also seen in distal spinal muscular dystrophy.

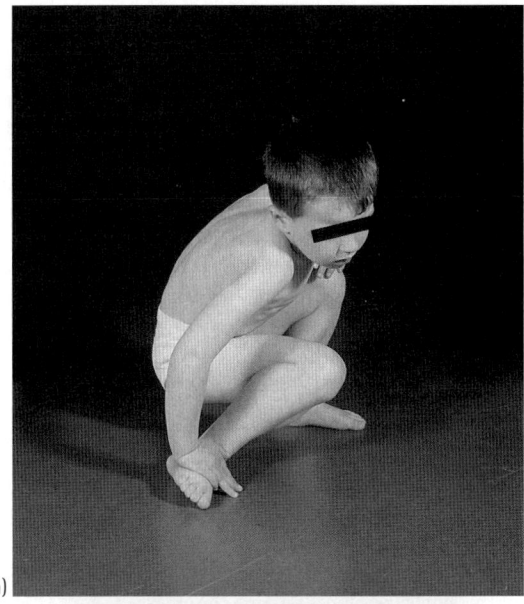

(a)

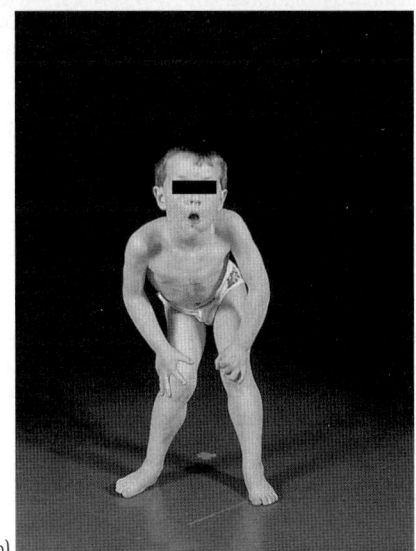

(b)

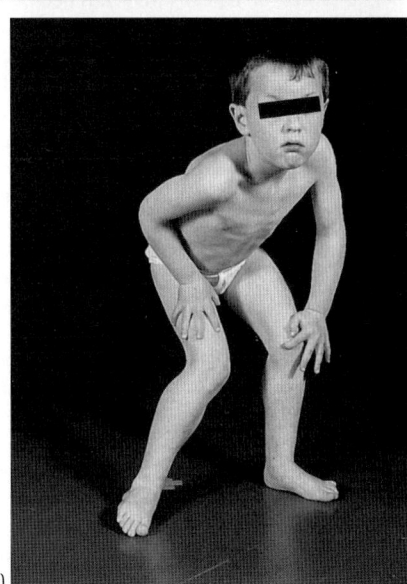

(c)

Fig. 22.31   A child with hip girdle weakness demonstrates a Gower maneuver: on rising from supine he turns prone then pushes himself up with his hands on his legs to the standing position.

INVESTIGATION

Appropriate investigation is only possible when preceded by comprehensive clinical assessment with particular attention to pattern of muscle weakness.

There are a few neuromuscular conditions in which specific and highly sensitive DNA tests are available (Table 22.38). These are myotonic dystrophy, spinal muscular atrophy and fascioscapulohumeral muscular dystrophy. DNA analysis is an appropriate first-line investigation for such conditions. Around 65% of boys with dystrophinopathy have a deletion in the dystrophin gene. DNA analysis for such a deletion is an appropriate early investigation to confirm the clinical diagnosis. If such a deletion is found opinion is divided as to whether muscle biopsy is indicated in order to determine with certainty whether the boy has Duchenne or Becker muscular dystrophy. In boys in whom initial DNA analysis is negative but a dystrophinopathy is confirmed on muscle biopsy further more detailed DNA analysis may detect other defects, such as point mutations. In a large number of other neuromuscular conditions DNA analysis can be helpful in confirming or further defining the diagnosis.

Muscle biopsy

Muscle biopsy may be by needle or with an open technique. Needle muscle biopsy is usually sufficient but may not yield enough muscle for biochemical enzyme analysis or comprehensive immunoblotting in limb girdle dystrophy.

Analysis of muscle biopsy may include:
- hematoxylin and eosin;
- fiber typing;
- immunohistochemistry;
- oxidative enzyme staining;
- immunoblotting;
- enzyme analysis;
- mitochondrial DNA analysis;
- electronmicroscopy.

Neurophysiology

Nerve conduction studies will usually confirm the presence of neuropathy and define whether this is of the demyelinating or axonal type.

EMG may show a clear myopathic or denervating pattern, however the picture is often mixed. Moreover, it is often normal even in confirmed myopathies.

Repetitive stimulation and single fiber EMG may be helpful in confirming a defect of neuromuscular transmission.

Biochemistry

Biochemical tests which may be useful in the investigation of neuromuscular disorders are shown in Table 22.39.

Muscle imaging

Muscle ultrasound can be valuable in detecting myopathies and muscular dystrophies, both of which are associated with increased

Table 22.38   DNA analysis in investigation of neuromuscular disease

DNA analysis for diagnosis	DNA helpful following diagnosis
Myotonic dystrophy	Charcot–Marie–Tooth 1
Spinal muscular atrophy	Limb girdle dystrophy
Facioscapulohumeral MD	Congenital muscular dystrophy
+/– dystrophinopathy	Congenital myopathies – nemaline, myotubular, minicore, central core
	Emery–Dreifuss MD
	Ion channel disorders
	Congenital myasthenic syndromes

Table 22.39 Biochemical investigations

Creatine kinase	Marked ↑ in most muscular dystrophies, may be mildly ↑ in neuropathic conditions Often normal in myopathies
Lactate	↑ May occur in mitochondrial myopathy
Carnitine/acylcarnitine profile	May be helpful in fatty acid oxidation defects
Glycolytic enzyme analysis	Useful in metabolic myopathy
Forearm ischemic exercise test	< Fivefold rise in lactate in glycogen storage defect < Fivefold rise in ammonia in adenylate deaminase deficiency

echogenicity of involved muscles. MRI can identify the pattern of muscle groups involved. Currently information is being gathered, largely in relation to the congenital myopathies, and it may ultimately become a useful clinical tool. The place of MR spectroscopy in helping to define the metabolic myopathies is still at the research stage.

MANAGEMENT

Accurate diagnosis is the first step in management and allows some estimation of the future course of the child's condition. Accurate diagnosis can also predict the need to be watchful for the development of particular complications such as respiratory insufficiency in minicore myopathy (see below). If a molecular genetic diagnosis can be made this allows accurate genetic counseling and antenatal testing.

To date, with the exception of some of the congenital myasthenic syndromes and metabolic myopathies, there is no specific treatment for inherited neuromuscular conditions.

The aims of management are therefore:
1. family support and education;
2. prevention and management of complications;
3. enhancing function;
4. palliation of symptoms.

Family support and education

Family support is vitally important, not only following diagnosis, but also in negotiating the various hurdles encountered by the family of a child with physical disability. Families now have access to a vast array of information about their child's condition but making sense of what all this means for an individual child can be challenging. Although there are principles for good practice, for example in disclosing a diagnosis, families vary and no single approach fits all so it is important support is tailored to an individual family's need with the aim of enabling them to achieve the best for their child.

Prevention and management of complications
Contractures

Contractures are inevitable in neuromuscular conditions when there is marked weakness. In some conditions there is a propensity to early contractures, for example in Emery–Dreifuss muscular dystrophy flexion contractures at the elbows and Achilles tendon contractures develop in the presence of only mild weakness.

Passive stretching of joints and splinting are the mainstays of contracture prevention. Physiotherapy entailing extensive exercises may be recommended, but there is no evidence that it is helpful and it is very difficult to comply with. Brief passive joint stretching is more likely to be tolerated by child and parents. Achilles tendon stretching can be carried out for a few minutes twice a day without major interruption of daily routine. A period of prone lying will stretch the hip flexors.

When there is useful muscle strength around a joint, splints which interfere with function are unlikely to be worn. In the prevention and management of Achilles tendon contractures, daytime ankle–foot orthoses (AFOs) will be helpful if there is marked ankle dorsiflexion weakness. If ankle dorsiflexion is not weak or there is a dynamic advantage from toe-walking, daytime AFOs will not be tolerated and night splints can be used. For example, in ambulant boys with dystrophinopathy daytime AFOs are unlikely to be tolerated so night splints are used; once ambulation is lost AFOs can also be used.

Surgery for release of contractures is of benefit in ambulant patients or may be needed prior to rehabilitation in knee–ankle–foot orthoses. Particular care is required in assessing the role of surgery in children with Achilles tendon contractures and weak hip flexors as tendon lengthening may cause a loss in ambulation.

Scoliosis

Bracing probably does not prevent progression of scoliosis in neuromuscular conditions; however it may facilitate seating in a child with marked truncal weakness.

Surgery is well established in the management of neuromuscular scoliosis. Posterior fusion is the procedure usually performed as respiratory compromise usually precludes an anterior approach.[495,496] More recently, rods which may be repeatedly extended have been useful in children who require surgery at a younger age and risk the development of secondary crankshaft deformity during the adolescent growth spurt. Careful attention must be paid to respiratory function in this group, so that completion of lengthening is performed while the child is still fit for surgery.

Respiratory management

Respiratory insufficiency is inevitable in the late stages of progressive neuromuscular conditions. In some conditions, however, respiratory muscles are selectively involved so respiratory insufficiency may occur when limb weakness is mild.

Weakness of inspiratory muscles restricts lung capacity. Weakness of inspiratory and expiratory muscles reduces the effectiveness of the cough. Bulbar dysfunction and aspiration will also contribute to respiratory compromise. The presence of a scoliosis or spinal rigidity will also complicate the picture.

Regular monitoring of forced vital capacity (FVC) is important in predicting the development of symptoms and should be performed at each clinic visit and before surgery is contemplated. When FVC is < 50% of predicted for height (arm span equates well with height in those unable to stand) there is a high risk of respiratory complications.

Assessment of bulbar function is important (Table 22.40) and the possibility of gastroesophageal reflux with aspiration also needs to be considered. If there is significant risk of aspiration because of bulbar weakness it may be necessary to limit oral intake, giving most of the nutritional requirements by nasogastric tube or gastrostomy.

Hemophilus influenzae vaccination is included in routine childhood immunizations. Pneumococcal vaccine and an annual flu vaccine should be offered to those at risk of respiratory problems. Chest physiotherapy is helpful during respiratory infections and when there are retained secretions. There is conflicting evidence about the relative efficacy of the various methods available. Cough assist devices may also be helpful in removing secretions. There is no strong evidence that respiratory muscle training is of benefit.

Table 22.40 Assessment of bulbar function

Questions in clinic	Any coughing or choking on eating or drinking? How long does it take to complete meals? What consistency of food can be managed?
Specialist assessment	Speech and language therapy assessment Videofluoroscopy of swallowing

Respiratory tract infections should be treated early and aggressively.

The first stage of respiratory failure is the development of nocturnal hypoventilation with oxygen desaturation during rapid eye movement (REM) sleep. Sleep is disturbed so the affected child wakes more frequently (this may be attributed to a need for turning), is not refreshed after the night's sleep and is tired during the day. Nocturnal hypoxemia with hypercapnia causes morning headache and a loss of appetite for breakfast. Left untreated, daytime hypoxemia and hypercapnia will ensue, with eventual cor pulmonale.

Nocturnal hypoventilation can be effectively managed with nocturnal non-invasive positive pressure ventilation (NIPPV). In boys with Duchenne muscular dystrophy this has been shown to prolong life and provide a quality of life equivalent to that of individuals with nonprogressive conditions receiving ventilatory support.[497,498]

Respiratory complications vary in different conditions. For example, in the dystrophinopathies and limb girdle dystrophies, respiratory muscle weakness will usually lead to nocturnal hypoventilation before there are significant bulbar problems. In spinal muscular atrophy, bulbar weakness often, but not invariably, contributes to recurrent respiratory tract infections before nocturnal hypoventilation occurs.

Cardiac complications

Ventricular dysfunction may be seen in many of the muscular dystrophies, in female dystrophinopathy carriers and in metabolic and congenital myopathies. Treatment for cardiac failure will relieve symptoms. Some children with dystrophinopathy with mild or even no skeletal muscle involvement may develop severe cardiomyopathy necessitating cardiac transplant.

Young people with some neuromuscular conditions have a propensity to develop cardiac dysrhythmias. Those with Emery–Dreifuss muscular dystrophy should have annual 24-hour ECG monitoring. Individuals with myotonic dystrophy are also predisposed to cardiac dysrhythmias.

Malnutrition

Children who have restricted mobility can easily gain weight excessively and the encouragement of healthy eating habits from the time of diagnosis is recommended. Bulbar weakness and secondary orthodontic problems may cause failure to thrive. Assessment of swallowing and dietary intake will indicate appropriate lines of management, which may be nutritional supplements, advice on consistency of food, or need for supplementary feeds via nasogastric tube or gastrostomy (Table 22.40).

Enhancing function

Prolonging mobility and standing. Prolongation of mobility and standing has been shown to delay the onset of scoliosis. Mobility may be prolonged with the use of ischial weightbearing long leg splints, knee–ankle–foot orthoses (KAFOs). These may be used in any neuromuscular condition. The use of a standing frame is of particular benefit in children with spinal muscular atrophy type II and in children with congenital myopathies and congenital muscular dystrophy.

Independent mobility. Electrically powered indoor–outdoor chairs (EPIOCs) allow children who have only very limited or no mobility to join others safely in the playground or elsewhere to partake in activities with their peers.

Education. Physical disability should not preclude education in mainstream school with access to the full curriculum. Adaptations may be needed. Use of information technology may be helpful: many children find a keyboard allows them to be more productive than they can be when writing. Many children with neuromuscular conditions also have learning needs which need to be addressed.

Adaptations and aids. Adaptations to the home and the use of environmental controls increase the independence of young people with neuromuscular conditions. Accessibility to public buildings and transport also allow a degree of independence.

Allowances

Individuals with physical disability and care needs may be entitled to financial help.

Palliative care

Most care in neuromuscular disease is palliative rather than curative. It is important that not only the physical but also the psychosocial and spiritual needs of the individual are met. Affected young people and their families should have an understanding of the benefits and burdens of treatment, be given an opportunity to express their views on those benefits and burdens and an assurance that there will be appropriate action in the light of those views.

In the progressive conditions, however, there comes a time when despite active management a terminal stage is reached, at which time alleviation of symptoms should be a priority (see Ch. 38).

MUSCULAR DYSTROPHIES

This group of conditions is characterized by the finding of dystrophic change on muscle biopsy: variation in fiber size, fiber splitting, necrotic fibers, excess of fatty and fibrous tissue. Classified originally according to clinical phenotype, these conditions can now frequently be defined at the level of the specific protein deficiency with immunohistochemistry and immunoblotting and at DNA level by mutation analysis.

Duchenne and Becker muscular dystrophy – dystrophinopathy

The dystrophinopathies are the most common form of muscular dystrophy seen in pediatric practice and have X-linked recessive inheritance. There is a wide spectrum of severity, boys with loss of ambulation before 13 years of age are considered to have Duchenne muscular dystrophy (DMD), those with preservation of ambulation beyond 16 years are considered to have the Becker variant. Boys losing ambulation between 13 and 16 years of age are said to have an intermediate type.

Dystrophin is a 427-kDa protein, which forms part of the cytoskeleton of the muscle cell plasma membrane. It consists of an N-terminal domain, which binds actin, a central rod domain, a cysteine-rich domain and a C-terminal globular domain. The N-terminal and rod domains bind to actin filaments with the greatest affinity at the N-terminal; the C-terminal domains bind to the transmembrane dystroglycan complex. The cysteine-rich domain, the beginning of the C-terminal globular domain and the N-terminal actin binding domain are very important for dystrophin function, with those deleted for this region having more severe phenotypes. The central rod domain is less important with deletions for much of this region resulting in mild phenotypes.

The dystrophin gene is located on the X chromosome and at 14 kb is the largest human gene cloned so far. Around 65% of males with dystrophinopathy are found to have a deletion of one or more exons of the gene, 5% have a duplication, the remainder have point mutations. Approximately one third of the mutations are new mutations. The clinical phenotype depends on the amount of functional dystrophin. Boys with the more severe Duchenne phenotype have absence of dystrophin, males with the milder Becker phenotype have partial dystrophin deficiency.[499–501] Clinical severity cannot be predicted by the size of the deletion or the region of the gene deleted.[502] The main factor that appears to determine clinical severity is whether there is disruption of the reading frame.[503] If the exons flanking the deletion share the same reading frame, protein translation can continue to produce a protein which, although it is missing amino acids, retains some biochemical function. If there is disruption to the reading frame no functional protein is produced.

With the identification of the gene and its protein product has come the realization that the clinical phenotype of dystrophinopathy is very wide indeed and includes asymptomatic cases with elevated creatine kinase (CK) only, cases with dilated cardiomyopathy and no skeletal muscle involvement and cases with elevated CK, cramps and myalgia.

Occasional female cases are seen, with a translocation involving the X chromosome.[504,505] Female carriers, heterozygous for a dystrophin gene mutation, occasionally exhibit overt muscle weakness, which can often be asymmetrical. Approximately 10% of isolated females, with a muscular dystrophy with high CK and proximal muscle weakness, can be shown to be manifesting carriers.[506,507] About 17% of female carriers have some demonstrable muscle weakness. Female carriers without muscle weakness may have cardiac involvement, with approximately 8% showing evidence of dilated cardiomyopathy.[508]

In a study of a cohort of 33 males born between 1953 and 1983, the mean age of diagnosis of DMD was 4.6 years, the median age of wheelchair dependency was 10 years and the median age of death 15 years.[509] Non-invasive ventilatory support can extend the length and quality of life considerably. The rate of learning disability is higher in the population with DMD than in the normal population. A meta-analysis of 1224 cases of DMD found a mean full scale IQ (FIQ) of 80.2. Of these children, 34.8% had a FIQ less than 70, of these 79.3% had mild (FIQ 50–70) learning difficulty, 19.3% moderate (FIQ 35–50), and 1.1% profound learning difficulty. In this study 6% of the children had FIQ > 110.[510]

Fatal rhabdomyolysis during anesthesia has been reported in a patient with BMD.[511] Smooth muscle involvement also occurs with acute gastric dilation and intestinal pseudo-obstruction.[512] Boland et al[509] found cardiac failure in 21% of males with DMD at a median age of 21.5 years.

The use of steroids in Duchenne muscular dystrophy

There is evidence from randomized controlled trials that corticosteroids produce a significant improvement in muscle strength and function in the short term (6–24 months).[513-516] The most effective dose of prednisolone appears to be 0.75 mg/kg/day. There appears to be an increase in muscle strength in the first 6 months of treatment followed by stabilization for up to 2 years and then decline in muscle strength which is slower than that in natural history controls. Other steroid regimens have been used. Deflazacort may produce less weight gain but cataract occurs more frequently. A regimen of intermittent prednisolone may produce some benefit but fewer unwanted effects.[517] There are no data from randomized controlled trials (RCTs) on long term effects; there is a suggestion from nonrandomized trials that there may be a benefit on respiratory and cardiac function in the longer term.[518,519] Significant unwanted effects include weight gain, behavior changes, vertebral fractures and cataract.

The exact mechanism by which corticosteroids produce an increase in strength in DMD is unknown. Potential mechanisms include: inhibition of muscle proteolysis; increase in myogenic repair; anti-inflammatory effect; stimulation of myoblast proliferation; and upregulation of utrophin.

Limb girdle dystrophy (LGMD)

This is a group of genetically heterogeneous conditions which have in common a syndrome of proximal limb weakness. Each condition can vary in severity from a severe Duchenne type phenotype to a mild phenotype. Even within a family there may be variation in severity between affected family members.

Classification of limb girdle dystrophies is now by mode of inheritance (autosomal dominant or recessive), protein deficiency and gene mutation. To date, the protein deficiency in three autosomal dominant and ten autosomal recessive LGMDs have been identified (Table 22.41). In addition, the gene loci for two more autosomal dominant LGMDs have been identified.

Facioscapulohumeral dystrophy

Facioscapulohumeral muscular dystrophy (FSHMD) is an autosomal dominant condition. The characteristic pattern is of facial weakness and weakness of scapular fixation, with winging of the scapulae and difficulty raising the arms. Weakness is frequently asymmetrical. Later there is weakness of biceps and triceps, truncal weakness and lower limb weakness, which usually starts distally, but proximal lower limb weakness is frequently present.

Table 22.41 Limb girdle muscular dystrophy

Inheritance	Classification	Gene product
Autosomal dominant	LGMD1A	myotilin
	LGMD1B	laminA/C
	LGMD1C	caveolin-3
Autosomal recessive	LGMD2A	calpain 3
	LGMD2B	dysferlin
	LGMD2C	γ-sarcoglycan
	LGMD2D	α-sarcoglycan
	LGMD2E	β-sarcoglycan
	LGMD2F	δ-sarcoglycan
	LGMD2G	telethonin
	LGMD2H	E3-ubiquitine ligase
	LGMD2I	fukutin-related protein
	LGMD2J	titin

In the severe infantile onset FSHMD there is marked facial weakness and a severe lumbar lordosis.

High frequency hearing loss is detected in most affected individuals. This is most likely to be clinically significant in the infantile onset FSHMD. The majority of affected individuals also have retinal telangiectasia on fluorescein angiography; only rarely does Coats syndrome, an exudative retinopathy with retinal detachment, occur. Cardiac involvement is rare and is most commonly manifest as dysrhythmia.

FSHMD is linked to 4q35. There is a deletion of an integral number of copies of a 3.3-kb DNA repeat. Affected individuals have 10 or fewer repeats, normal individuals 15 or more repeats.[520] No transcribed gene sequences are contained within this area. The proposed mechanism by which the deletion produces the condition is by position effect variegation, where the deletion may influence expression of distant genes.[521]

Emery–Dreifuss muscular dystrophy

Emery–Dreifuss muscular dystrophy (EDMD) is characterized by early contractures, particularly involving Achilles tendons, elbows and paraspinal muscles causing spinal rigidity, slowly progressive muscle weakness in a humeroperoneal distribution and cardiomyopathy with a propensity to dysrhythmias and a risk of sudden death.

EDMD is genetically heterogeneous. Two genes have been identified so far, the emerin gene on Xq28 and the laminA/C gene on 1q11–q13. The products of both these genes form part of the inner nuclear membrane. Emerin-deficient EDMD is inherited in an X-linked recessive fashion. Female carriers occasionally have cardiac conduction abnormalities and so warrant cardiology assessment. EDMD due to laminA/C deficiency may be inherited in an autosomal dominant or recessive fashion.

CONGENITAL MYOPATHIES

The congenital myopathies are a group of conditions that frequently, but not always, manifest in infancy with hypotonia and motor delay. Classification has traditionally been on the morphological appearance of muscle biopsies. It has long been recognized that the morphological appearances may not be specific and some changes may be seen in other conditions. With the elucidation of the genetic basis of some of these conditions it appears that the same morphological changes and clinical features may be seen in genetically heterogeneous conditions. Most notable to date, nemaline myopathy may be caused by defects in five different genes (Table 22.42). Determination of the genotype in a child with a congenital myopathy allows more informative genetic counseling and the possibility of antenatal diagnosis.

Most of these conditions are apparently nonprogressive, or only very slowly progressive, but important specific clinical features may occur, for example respiratory failure and paraspinal muscle contractures in minicore myopathy.

Table 22.42 The congenital myopathies

Congenital myopathy	Pathology	Important clinical features	Inheritance	Gene locus	Gene product
Myotubular	Central nuclei surrounded by clear area without myofibrils	Ophthalmoplegia, respiratory insufficiency in neonatal period, coagulopathy and hepatic dysfunction with subcapsular hemorrhages	XR	Xq28	MTM1 Myotubularin
Nemaline	Rod bodies derived from Z-band material	Respiratory insufficiency in neonatal period, occasional cardiomyopathy, selective diaphragmatic involvement with early respiratory insufficiency in milder cases	AD	1q21–q23	NEM1 α-tropomyosin
			AR	2q21.2–q22	NEM2 nebulin
			AD/AR	1q42.1	ACTA1 Alpha actin, skeletal muscle
			AD	9p13.2–p13.1	TPM2 β-tropomyosin
			AR	19q13.4	TNNT1 troponin T1
			AD	15q21–q24	?
Central core	Central areas of derangement of sarcomeres with absence of oxidative enzyme activity	Congenital hip dysplasia may occur, cardiomyopathy and respiratory insufficiency rare	AD	19q13.1	CCD Skeletal muscle ryanodine receptor
Minicore	Multiple small areas devoid of oxidative enzyme, type 1 fiber predominance	Contracture of paraspinal muscles with complicated scoliosis, early diaphragmatic involvement and respiratory insufficiency	?AR	?	

Myotubular myopathy and centronuclear myopathy

These terms may be used interchangeably or myotubular myopathy may be used for the severe X-linked early onset form and centronuclear myopathy used for sporadic, dominant or recessive cases. Muscle fibers, with centrally located nuclei with a surrounding halo devoid of myofilaments, resemble myotubes. In all types, ptosis and ophthalmoplegia are frequent features. Calf hypertrophy is described in late onset cases.

The X-linked form is due to mutation in the myotubularin (MTM1) gene. The gene product is a protein tyrosine phosphatase, which is required for muscle cell differentiation.[522] The severe X-linked early onset form is frequently associated with respiratory insufficiency and ventilator dependency. In a study of 55 males with confirmed MTM1 mutations Herman et al[523] found a survival rate at 1 year of age of 74%; 80% of these remained ventilator dependent. Care must be taken to distinguish this condition from congenital myotonic dystrophy. In the latter condition, examination of the mother may be helpful and DNA analysis will identify the CTG triplet repeat (see below).

Spherocytosis, gallstones, renal stones and a vitamin K-responsive coagulopathy are described[523] and it is prudent to assess coagulation prior to any operative procedures.

Later onset disease is usually only very slowly progressive. Cardiomyopathy is rare but has been reported as the presenting feature. Mutations in the dynamin2 gene have recently been found to cause a dominant centronuclear myopathy.[524] In females, care must be taken to exclude manifesting carrier status for the X-linked variety.

Nemaline myopathy

Nemaline myopathy is defined by the presence of nemaline rods in muscle fibers. These rods contain Z disc material. Intranuclear rods, which are identical to cytoplasmic rods, may be seen and may indicate an unfavorable prognosis.[525]

Various clinical phenotypes are seen. In the severe congenital form, there are no spontaneous movements or respiration. In the typical congenital type, onset is in infancy or early childhood with weakness predominantly affecting neck flexors, facial, bulbar and respiratory muscles. The course is slowly progressive but respiratory insufficiency may occur. Onset in later childhood or adult life may also occur. Nemaline myopathy has also been reported in the fetal akinesia sequence.[526]

Mutations in five genes: alpha-tropomyosin (TPM3),[527] nebulin (NEB), alpha-actin (ACTA1),[528] beta-tropomyosin (TPM2)[529] and troponin T1 (TNNT1)[530] have been found in nemaline myopathy. Autosomal dominant and autosomal recessive inheritance has been found in families with TPM3 and ACTA1 mutations. All TPM2 mutations have been autosomal dominant and all NEB and TNNT1 mutations autosomal recessive.

Genotype and mode of inheritance cannot be predicted from the clinical severity. Neonatal presentation has been seen with recessive mutations in NEB and TPM3 and dominant mutations in ACTA1. In the group with adult onset only dominant mutations have been found.

Central core disease (CCD)

The characteristic histological feature of CCD is the presence of central cores devoid of oxidative enzyme activity in type 1 muscle fibers (Fig. 22.32). In addition there is type 1 fiber predominance.

Inheritance may be autosomal dominant or recessive. Mutations in the ryanodine receptor gene (RYR1) have been identified in a few patients with CCD.[531,532] Mutations in this gene have also been found in families with susceptibility to malignant hyperthermia and these two conditions may coexist within a few patients and families.

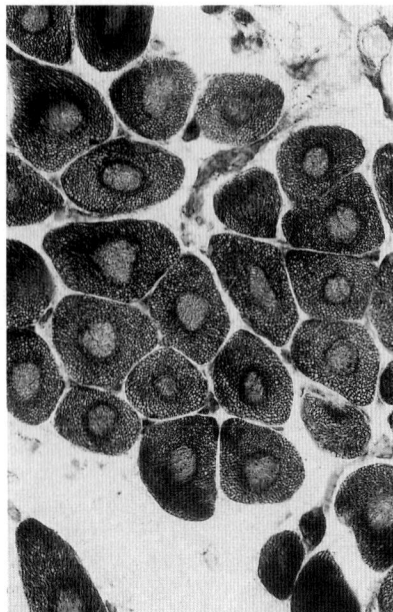

Fig. 22.32   Central core disease: the cores show absence of staining with NADH.

CCD is usually nonprogressive or only very slowly progressive even in the severe cases described.[533] Presentation is usually with hypotonia and delayed motor development in infancy. Congenital hip dislocation, contractures, scoliosis or foot deformity may occur.[534] Cardiac involvement and respiratory insufficiency do not usually occur.

Minicore myopathy (multiminicore disease)

Minicore myopathy is defined by the presence of small cores, which do not extend through the full fiber length but are histochemically and ultrastructurally similar to central cores. They are not confined to type 1 fibers.

Mutations of the selenoprotein N gene (SEPN1) have been found in individuals with recessively inherited minicore myopathy.[535]

Presentation is most frequently with hypotonia and delayed motor development. Muscle weakness is most marked in axial muscles and proximal limbs. Ophthalmoplegia is described. The weakness is static or very slowly progressive. Scoliosis, cardiomyopathy and respiratory insufficiency may occur in ambulatory patients.[536,537]

Other congenital myopathies

Other congenital myopathies occur more rarely. Desmin-related myopathies are clinically and genetically heterogeneous. Some types are associated with cardiomyopathy, others with respiratory insufficiency. Actin-related myopathy, a congenital myopathy with an excess of thin myofilaments, has been described in a small number of severely affected infants and has been associated with mutations in the ACTA1 gene.

CONGENITAL MUSCULAR DYSTROPHY

The congenital muscular dystrophies are a group of genetically heterogeneous conditions. The clinical features which they have in common are muscle weakness and hypotonia, which is present from birth or the first few months of life, contractures, which occur early or may be congenital, raised or normal CK levels and dystrophic changes on muscle biopsy. All are autosomal recessive and a number of gene defects have been identified to date. Some of the defective proteins responsible for congenital muscular dystrophy (CMD) interact with components of the extracellular matrix. Several congenital muscular dystrophies have been found to be due to mutations in glycosyltransferase genes responsible for the post-translational glycosylation of α-dystroglycan.

Important clinical features, which may help define a specific diagnosis, include whether intellect is normal or there is associated learning difficulty, and the presence of muscle hypertrophy or distal joint laxity. Brain MRI may be normal or may show the presence of abnormalities such as white matter changes, neuronal migration disorders, cerebellar or brainstem abnormalities. There may also be associated eye abnormalities such as myopia, glaucoma, cataract and retinal dysplasia.

Congenital muscular dystrophy without mental retardation
Primary laminin-α2 (merosin) deficiency

This is the most common form of CMD and accounts for 50% of CMD cases in the Caucasian population.[538] Severe muscle weakness involves the face, trunk and limbs symmetrically and is present from birth. CK is markedly elevated. Feeding and respiratory difficulties are common. Some improvement in muscle strength is usually seen so that independent sitting is achieved. Only very few children with complete laminin-α2 deficiency are able to stand or walk a few steps. Muscle strength tends to remain fairly stable through childhood.

All patients have white matter changes on brain imaging[539] (Fig. 22.33). Structural abnormalities such as occipital agyria and cerebellar hypoplasia have also been reported.[540] Most children are of normal intelligence unless there is gross occipital agyria. Epilepsy occurs in up to 30% of affected children.[540] A demyelinating neuropathy also occurs in this condition.[541]

Patients with partial laminin-α2 deficiency may have a clinical phenotype ranging from early onset of weakness and hypotonia to adult onset of limb girdle weakness.

Laminin-α2 is expressed in skin basement membrane and in the trophoblast. Immunofluorescence of fetal trophoblast may be used along with haplotype analysis or mutation analysis for antenatal diagnosis.

Secondary laminin-α2 (merosin) deficiency

Several families with an abnormality of laminin-α2 staining, but not linked to the LAMA-2 gene on chromosome 6q2, have been described. Mutations in a fukutin-related protein gene (FKRP) on chromosome 19q13.3 have been found in a number of families.[542] The clinical features are onset in the first weeks of life, severe weakness and wasting

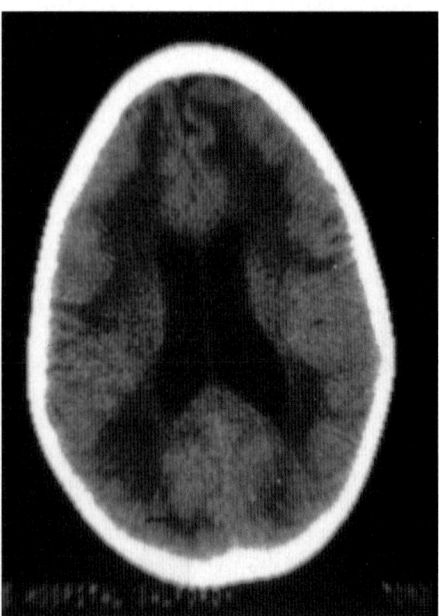

Fig. 22.33   CT scan in laminin-α2 deficiency showing extensive white matter changes.

of the shoulder girdle muscles, hypertrophy and weakness of leg muscles with inability to walk and respiratory failure in the second decade. Mutations in this gene are also described in children with limb girdle dystrophies of varying severity.

Ullrich syndrome

Recently mutations in the collagen VI genes COL6A1, COL6A2 and COL6A3 have been demonstrated in this condition.[543] The characteristic clinical features are proximal contractures and marked distal joint laxity. Intelligence is normal.

Rigid spine syndrome

Spinal rigidity is a feature of many myopathies. A group of children with early onset spinal rigidity, axial and proximal muscle weakness and severe respiratory failure have been described and classified as having a type of congenital muscular dystrophy (RSMD). In some of these families mutations have been found in the selenoprotein N gene (SEPN1).[544]

Congenital muscular dystrophy with mental retardation

Fukuyama congenital muscular dystrophy (FCMD)

This condition is essentially only seen in the Japanese population or patients of Japanese descent. Muscle weakness and learning difficulty are usually severe. Seizures occur in around 60%. Over 80% have high myopia, 60% glaucoma and 90% retinal dysplasia. The MRI brain scan shows abnormal signal in periventricular white matter in addition to neuronal migration defects.

Mutations in the fukutin gene on chromosome 9q3 are responsible for the condition.

Muscle eye brain disease (MEB)

Most children with MEB are severely affected. Brain MRI shows neuronal migration defects in addition to partial absence of the septum pellucidum, corpus callosum dysplasia, hydrocephalus, pontine and cerebellar hypoplasia and periventricular white matter changes. Eye abnormalities are severe with severe myopia and glaucoma. Most patients have severe visual handicap.

Mutations in the O-mannose β-1,2-N-acetylglucosaminyltransferase gene (POMGNT1) have been found in this condition.[545]

Walker–Warburg syndrome

In this condition there is almost complete lissencephaly (absence of cortical sulcation), microphthalmia with persistence of hyaloid vasculature and retinal detachment in combination with a muscular dystrophy. Other features may include encephalocele, ocular colobomas, cataract, genital abnormality and cleft lip and palate.[546]

Mutations in the O-mannosyltransferase 1 gene (POMT1) have been described.[547]

MYOTONIC DYSTROPHY

Myotonic dystrophy is a autosomal dominantly inherited condition in which there is a combination of a progressive myotonic myopathy and multiorgan involvement. There are two distinct types defined by their underlying molecular genetic cause.

DM1 (Steinert)

Muscle weakness predominantly affects facial muscles, levator palpebrae, neck flexion and distal limb muscles. Muscle weakness is commonly more extensive and often involves the diaphragm and intercostal muscles. Myotonia is unusual before the age of 6 years. Smooth muscle involvement causes dysphagia, which may be life threatening, and bowel dysfunction. Cardiac conduction defects and tachyarrhythmias are common and may occur when neuromuscular involvement is mild.[548] Central nervous system involvement causes learning difficulty in children and somnolence and lethargy in older individuals. Endocrine

disturbances include subfertility and in females there is a high rate of fetal loss.[549]

DM1 is a trinucleotide repeat disorder with an expansion of CTG repeats. There is a relationship between the size of DNA expansion and clinical severity[550] with those presenting with the condition in adult life having a DNA expansion band size between 0.25 and 3.5 kb, whereas about one in three children presenting in the newborn period will have DNA band expanded above 5 kb. Germ line instability accounts for the tendency of the mutation to expand in subsequent generations. Diminution may occur but is much less frequent. Expansion of the mutation accounts for the anticipation recognized clinically in this condition before its genetic basis was elucidated.

Congenital myotonic dystrophy is characterized by marked muscle weakness and hypotonia from birth (Fig. 22.34). Affected neonates have feeding difficulty with reduced reflexes and may have respiratory insufficiency. Mechanical ventilation may be required and the need for this is associated with a high mortality. Affected babies have a characteristic facial muscle posture with an open mouth and a tent-shaped or inverted V-shaped upper lip. Foot deformity and hip dislocation are occasionally seen. The finding of a large head with ventricular dilation in association with talipes on an antenatal ultrasound scan should prompt consideration of this diagnosis. All have learning difficulties with a wide spread of ability, some mild, some severe though few are able to obtain employment in adult life.[551]

With few exceptions congenital myotonic dystrophy is maternally transmitted.[552,553] Two thirds of the affected mothers have minimal or no symptoms of their own disease at the time of delivery.

Children with congenital myotonic dystrophy have a 25% chance of death before 18 months and a 50% chance of survival into the mid-thirties.[551] Life expectancy for adults is shortened, with a mean of about 60 years for men and women. Death usually results from respiratory insufficiency or cardiac arrhythmias. About half those with adult onset disease become wheelchair users. A higher proportion of those with childhood onset disease will use a wheelchair for mobility.

As childhood progresses, and particularly through adolescence, treatment for myotonia can be considered. Phenytoin and procainamide have been used successfully.

Type 2 (PROMM)

Features are similar to but less severe than type 1, the social and cognitive difficulties seen in DM1 are mild or absent. Anticipation does

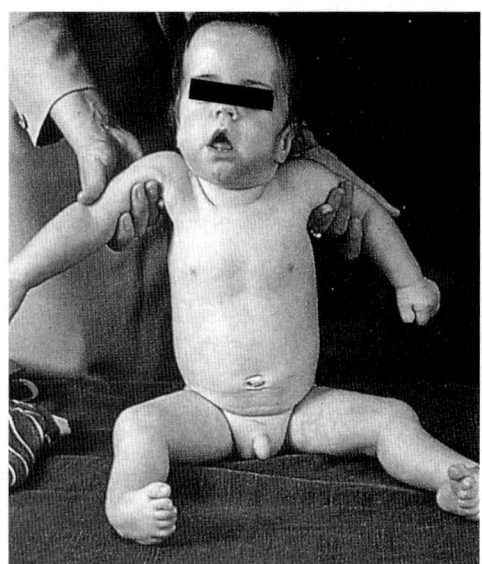

Fig. 22.34   Congenital myotonic dystrophy in a 1-year-old child with facial weakness, foot deformity and developmental delay.

not occur so no severely affected children are described. The condition is due to a repeat expansion (CCTG)n in the zinc finger protein 9 gene (ZNF9).[554]

ION CHANNEL MUSCLE DISEASES

This group of disorders is caused by abnormalities of membrane excitation caused by specific mutations in genes coding for various ion channels in the muscle fiber membrane.

Myotonic disorders
Chloride channel myotonias

Point mutations, deletions or an insertion in the skeletal muscle chloride channel gene (CLCN1) on chromosome 7q35 cause Thomsen myotonia congenita (dominant inheritance) and Becker myotonia congenita (recessive generalized myotonia).[555]

In Thomsen myotonia congenita myotonic stiffness is usually present from early childhood and causes toe-walking and clumsiness. The myotonia is worse after a period of rest and improves with repetition of movement. The myotonic stiffness is sometimes painful. Muscle hypertrophy is frequently seen. Tightness of the tendo-Achilles often occurs. Tapping a muscle produces an indentation for a few seconds (percussion myotonia). Lid lag and/or blephrospasm may be present. More recently it has been recognized that there may be considerable variation in the age of onset and severity of symptoms both between and within families. Some individuals may be minimally affected with only lid lag or electrical myotonia on EMG. Males tend to be more severely affected than females.

The recessive form is more common with an incidence of about 1 in 23 000 to 50 000. The clinical features are very similar to the dominant type, but they often appear after the age of 10 years and the myotonic stiffness is generally more severe. There is usually generalized muscle hypertrophy. On initiating movement there is muscle weakness but after a few contractions muscle strength becomes normal.

Should treatment be necessary, the myotonic stiffness responds well to drugs that reduce the increased excitability of the cell membrane by interfering with the sodium channel and these include local anesthetics, antifibrillar and antiarrhythmic drugs with mexiletine being the drug of choice.

Sodium channel myotonias and paramyotonia

Mutations in the skeletal muscle sodium channel (SCN4A) on chromosome 17q23, lead to a variety of dominantly inherited conditions including paramyotonia congenita with or without hyperkalemic periodic paralysis.

In paramyotonia congenita the myotonia appears with exercise and increases with continued exercise. It is exacerbated by cold and is most obvious in the muscles of the face, neck and distal upper extremities. The myotonic stiffness may be painful. Myotonia may be very difficult to detect on clinical examination unless movements are repeated, e.g repeated forceful closure of the eyes may elicit eyelid paramoyotonia. Symptoms may vary between individuals with the same mutation.[556,557] Many individuals with an SCN4A mutation will have episodes of weakness in addition to the myotonic stiffness, these are usually brief and are exacerbated by cold and by rest after exercise.

SCN4A mutations may also cause myotonia fluctuans in which the myotonic stiffness fluctuates in severity. It is not associated with episodes of weakness and may be exacerbated by rest after exercise but not by cold. Mutations may also lead to myotonia permanens with severe myotonia particularly affecting muscles of the neck, shoulder and chest which may at times lead to impairment of ventilation with hypoxia and loss of consciousness with the possibility of a misdiagnosis of epilepsy.

Sodium channel myotonic stiffness may be exacerbated by oral potassium. It is often responsive to acetazolamide. If this is not effective mexiletine or tocainamide may be.

Periodic paralyses
Hypokalemic periodic paralysis

Dominant point mutations in the muscle calcium channel dihydropyridine gene, CACNL1A3, on chromosome 1q31–q32 lead to hypokalemic periodic paralysis.[558] More rarely this can be caused by mutations in the skeletal muscle sodium channel gene (SCN4A)[559] or the potassium channel gene (KCNE3).[560]

With an estimated incidence of 1 in 100 000 this is the most common of the periodic paralyses. Maximum weakness usually develops during the night and early hours of the morning and attacks are often provoked by high dietary intake of sodium or carbohydrate especially late at night and in association with alcohol. Weakness affects the legs more than the arms and begins proximally. Previous exercise increases the likelihood of an attack and muscles which have previously been exercised may show the greatest weakness. There may be a sinus bradycardia during an attack. During episodes the potassium decreases (not always below normal) and there is urinary retention of sodium, potassium, chloride and water. Attacks are initially infrequent but increase in frequency and may be daily. In the fourth and fifth decades attacks become less frequent again but patients often have some fixed weakness after many years of attacks.

Management is by adjustment of lifestyle to avoid provoking factors. Attacks of weakness can be treated with potassium. Acetazolamide or dichlophenamide may be helpful in preventing attacks.

Hyperkalemic periodic paralysis

This is a dominantly inherited condition caused by mutations in the skeletal muscle sodium channel gene (SCN4A). It may present with or without paramyotonia or myotonia (see above). Attacks usually begin before the age of 10, are of shorter duration and more frequent than the attacks in hypokalemic periodic paralysis. The episodes are triggered by rest and they are often provoked by previous exercise. Potassium loading often precipitates an episode, and these are worsened by cold, stress, glucocorticoids or pregnancy. Some episodes are heralded by paresthesia or a sensation of muscle tension.

During an episode the sodium channels open and sodium moves into muscle cells causing a fall in serum sodium of between 3 and 9 mmol/L. Water follows the sodium causing hemoconcentration and an increase in the serum potassium. This in turn leads to potassium excretion in the urine, which may itself curtail the attack. Preventative therapy consists of frequent meals, rich in carbohydrate, a low potassium diet and the avoidance of fast and strenuous work and exposure to cold. The prompt intake of a thiazide diuretic or acetazolamide or the inhalation of a beta-adrenergic agent can curtail episodes in some people. Continuous use of these diuretics is not recommended.

Andersen syndrome

This condition is the triad of periodic paralysis, prolonged QT with ventricular dysrythmias and dysmorphic features. The dysmorphic features include low set ears, retrognathia or micrognathia, short stature and clinodactyly but may not be very striking. There may be a mild degree of fixed muscle weakness. Episodes of weakness may occur with normal, low or high serum potassium. Inheritance is autosomal dominant and mutations have been demonstrated in a potassium channel gene (KIR2.1).[561]

THE INFLAMMATORY MYOPATHIES
Juvenile dermatomyositis (see also Ch. 29)

The estimated incidence of juvenile dermatomyositis in the UK and Ireland is 1.9 per million aged under 16 years.[562] The median age of onset in this study was 6.8 years with five girls affected to each boy. The cause remains unknown. There is an association with HLA-B8/DR3 but the adult association with malignancy is not seen in children. It is a systemic vasculopathy associated primarily with inflammation of skin and muscle. About 10% of children with dermatomyositis test positive for myositis-associated antibody (MSA) (compared to about 50%

of adults), and 60% are positive for antinuclear antibodies. The MSA is most commonly directed against Mi-2 (in adults it is most often toward one of the tRNA synthetases). About 50% of children have circulating evidence of endothelial damage, while others have different indicators of disease activity such as elevated neopterin, or increased circulating B cells with peripheral lymphopenia.[563] Heterogeneity of this sort may well be associated with differing outcomes and in time define more specific approaches to therapy.

Presentation

The onset is usually insidious with slowly increasing proximal muscle weakness. Affected muscles are stiff, sore and tender and occasionally indurated. Nonpitting edema or thickening of the overlying skin may be seen. Bulbar muscles may be involved and occasionally weakness is so severe that respiratory failure ensues.

The skin lesions often have a characteristic violaceous (heliotrope) hue best seen on the eyelids (Fig. 22.35). The skin over the extensor surfaces of joints often becomes erythematous, atrophic and scaly, capillary loops may be prominent in the nail beds. Pigmentation may appear in these areas in time. A papular or pustular eruption may appear in the same position in oriental children.[564] A malar butterfly rash may appear similar to that seen in systemic lupus erythematosus. Calcification of subcutaneous tissues may occur.

There may be gastrointestinal involvement with functional large or small bowel symptoms or bleeding, arthropathy, fever, pulmonary disease, iritis and very occasionally seizures.

Diagnosis

High levels of muscle enzymes usually mirror muscle inflammation. Biopsy shows an inflammatory infiltration with muscle fiber necrosis and macrophage activity. Real diagnostic difficulty only arises when the rash is not evident. The differential diagnosis then includes conditions that may give insidious weakness including postinfectious polyneuropathy, metabolic and endocrine myopathies, myasthenia gravis or acute infectious myopathies.

Treatment

Many children will respond well to corticosteroid treatment. A starting dose of prednisolone 1 mg/kg/day is used, tapering off over 6–12 months. Further immunosuppression may be required and azathioprine is a valuable agent in a dose of 2.5 mg/kg/day. Low dose ciclosporin may also be used starting at 4 mg/kg/day.

A number of centers have reported that intravenous immunoglobulin therapy has allowed the dose of steroid to be reduced in resistant cases.[565] Intravenous methylprednisolone and methotrexate may prove to be effective in children with severe dermatomyositis – defined as those with associated dysphagia and severe vasculitis.[566] Great care must be taken with the supportive care of those children with bulbar involvement. Oral feeding should be suspended when dysphagia is present and serial measurements of forced expiratory volume made. Ventilatory support may be required.

Outcome

The outlook with modern immunosuppressant therapy is generally good. Before steroids up to 40% died, usually from bulbar and respiratory involvement. Tabarki et al[567] followed 36 children for a mean of 4.9 years. Twenty-eight of the children (78%) were well without functional impairment; five had inactive disease but with functional impairment and three had retained their active disease. Fifteen children developed dystrophic calcifications, which in five affected function. There is no satisfactory treatment for calcinosis, though aluminum hydroxide[568] and alendronate[569] have both been reported to bring benefit. Excision might be considered where functional impairment is significant. The best indicators of a good outcome were early treatment and a low creatine kinase level at diagnosis.

Acute infectious myositis
Viral myositis

This may occur in association with Coxsackie, echo and influenza viral infections. The presentation is of acute, distressing muscle aches, which are often symmetrical, and most commonly affects the thighs. There may be associated weakness. Occasionally it is very focal, affecting only one group of muscles. Viral invasion of muscle has not been demonstrated, but biopsy does show muscle cell necrosis and an inflammatory cell infiltrate. The creatine kinase may not be raised, although it usually is. Treatment is symptomatic and the condition is self-limiting and benign.

Pyogenic myositis

The commonest cause is *Staphylococcus aureus*. It is usually secondary to a penetrating injury, although in the tropics it may result from spreading infection from a superficial wound. There is intense local pain, swelling and loss of function. Treatment is with antibiotics and drainage as appropriate.

Parasitic myositis

Infestation with *Trichinella spiralis* results from the ingestion of undercooked, infested pork. Fever and myalgia are the commonest presentations. There may be periorbital edema, if periorbital muscles are involved or even dysphagia where bulbar muscles are involved. The calves, forearms or paraspinal muscles may be painful. Treatment is with thiabendazole 25–50 mg/kg/day or with mebendazole 100–200 mg twice daily and steroids. Mebendazole may have fewer unwanted effects.[570] Recovery is usually complete. In heavy infections of cysticercosis muscle may be affected.

Rarer forms of myositis
Congenital or infantile myositis

This was described by Shevell et al[571] and more recently by Vajsar et al.[572] Hypotonia and weakness are marked. Ventilatory support has often been required. The diagnosis is by muscle biopsy. Some cases are steroid responsive but the pathophysiology is poorly understood.

Inclusion body myositis

This is exceptional in childhood and presents as a chronic myositis simulating a dystrophy. The biopsy shows sarcoplasmic vacuoles containing basophilic and eosinophilic inclusions. The cause is unknown and treatment is usually ineffective.

METABOLIC MYOPATHY (see also Ch. 26)

Metabolic myopathies are the result of genetic defects of energy production, which may affect muscle alone or may also affect other high energy dependent tissues. The defect may be in glycogen or fatty acid metabolism or in mitochondrial oxidative phosphorylation.

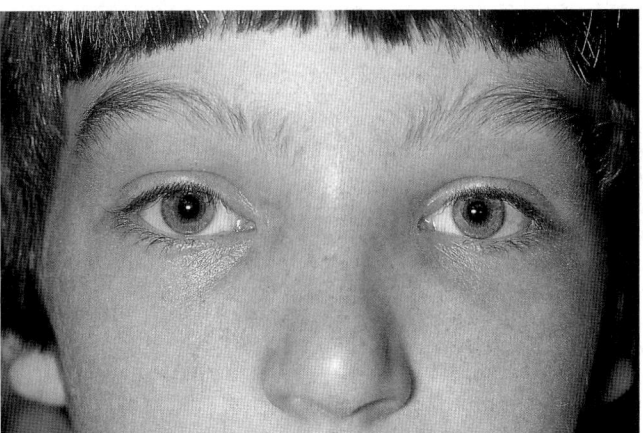

Fig. 22.35   Dermatomyositis: heliotrope rash around eyes.

Presentation may be with progressive weakness, recurrent symptoms of exercise intolerance, reversible weakness and myoglobinuria or both. Neonates and infants frequently present with severe multisystem disorders. In recent years advances in the understanding of the biochemical and genetic basis for many of these disorders has lead to new diagnostic tests. Nonetheless a specific enzyme abnormality could be detected in only 24% in a series of children with recurrent myoglobinuria.[573]

The glycogenoses

These defects of glycogen metabolism are rare and only those with prominent muscle involvement are included in Table 22.43. Recognition of Pompe disease (see Ch. 29, p. 1112) is now important because of the availability of enzyme replacement therapy.

Defects of mitochondrial fatty acid oxidation

Beta-oxidation results in the sequential cleavage of two carbon atoms from fatty acids and provides an important energy source during times of fasting and metabolic stress. Clinical features of muscle involvement include recurrent rhabdomyolysis and/or weakness and muscle pain provoked by prolonged exercise, which may occur some time after the exercise. Rhabdomyolosis may also occur during intercurrent infection. Proximal weakness without pain or rhabdomyolysis may also occur. Cardiomyopathy frequently occurs with dysrhythmia and/or progressive cardiac failure. Pigmentary retinopathy and peripheral neuropathy may also be seen. The most common presentation of this group of conditions in childhood is with hypoketotic hypoglycemia. These are all autosomal recessive conditions.

Diagnosis requires a high level of suspicion. It is essential to obtain urine and blood samples during the acute episode as biochemical abnormalities may not be present when the patient is well. Initial investigations should include urine organic acids, CK, lactate, carnitine and acylcarnitine profiles. Mutational analysis is available for the common mutations found in medium chain acyl-CoA dehydrogenase (MCAD) and long chain 3-hydroxyacyl-CoA dehydrogenase (LHCAD) deficiency. Specific enzyme analysis can be performed for many of these conditions on cultured fibroblasts. Table 22.44 lists the features of muscle involvement in some defects of beta-oxidation.

Defects of oxidative phosphorylation (OXPHOS)

Oxidative phosphorylation occurs in the mitochondria. Mitochondrial DNA encodes for only 13 subunits of the OXPHOS enzymes with more than 70 nuclear encoded subunits.

Isolated muscle involvement is unusual in this group of conditions in childhood. In a population-based study of OXPHOS disorders in childhood in Sweden eight out of 32 patients had myopathy, six infantile mitochondrial myopathy with cytochrome oxidase (COX) deficiency and two myopathy.[574]

A defect of OXPHOS is suggested by high plasma lactate and the finding of ragged red fibers or COX-deficient fibers on muscle biopsy. Electron microscopy of muscle biopsy may show structurally abnormal mitochondria with paracrystalline inclusions. OXPHOS enzyme analysis can be performed on muscle.

THE MYASTHENIC SYNDROMES
Myasthenia gravis

This is an autoimmune disorder, which is heterogeneous with respect to age at onset, ophthalmic changes and distribution of muscle weakness.

The annual incidence is between 0.25 and 2 people per 100 000. Although there has been an increase in the incidence in the over forties the incidence in childhood appears to be static. Boys and girls are equally affected in the first decade although the incidence in adolescence rises in girls with a ratio of three girls to two boys.

In most young people, myasthenia gravis is caused by autoantibodies specific for the human nicotinic acetylcholine receptor (AChR), which is concentrated at the postsynaptic region of the neuromuscular junction. These antibodies cause impaired neuromuscular transmission and muscle weakness.

There appears to be an immunogenetic predisposition to the development of idiopathic myasthenia gravis. Those with early onset myasthenia gravis have different HLA associations from those with late onset myasthenia gravis. Those with onset in childhood and adolescence also have an increased frequency of other autoimmune diseases. Monozygotic twins are at increased frequency of concordance and some families have more than one member affected. In Chinese and Japanese populations up to 30% present in early childhood, many with ocular myasthenia only. They show an association with HLA-BW46. This suggests that a particular environmental agent could be important. In Caucasians, about 60% of those with early onset myasthenia gravis are HLAB8 and DR3 positive.

Myasthenia gravis is associated with 30–60% of thymomas and about 10% of affected people of all ages have a thymoma.

Clinical features

The onset may be insidious or sudden. A common presentation is with ptosis and diplopia due to weakness of the extraocular and levator palpebrae muscles. This may or may not then spread to involve proximal limb and bulbar muscles. Respiratory muscles may also be involved. The weakness is variable and commonly progresses as the day goes on. This may lead a child to have difficulty with chewing and swallowing at the time of the evening meal. The weakness can remain localized to one group of muscles for many years, commonly the eye muscles. In some the weakness may only be obvious with tests of fatigue, for example, sustained upward gaze or repetitive shoulder abduction. Tendon reflexes are normal and there is no sensory impairment.

Table 22.43 Glycogen storage diseases with muscle involvement

Enzyme defect	Clinical features		Inheritance
Acid maltase (Pompe disease)	Infantile	Hypotonia, weakness, cardiomegaly, hepatomegaly, respiratory and feeding difficulty, death usually before 2 years	AR
	Juvenile	Muscle weakness proximal > distal, selective respiratory muscle involvement	
	Adult	Slowly progressive myopathy, one third present with respiratory failure	
Myophosphorylase (McArdle disease)	Muscle pain, weakness, stiffness during slight-moderate exertion, 'second wind' phenomenon, ↑ CK		AR
Phosphofructokinase (Tarui disease)	Exercise intolerance, hemolysis		AR
Phosphoglycerate kinase	Exercise intolerance, muscle cramps, myoglobinuria, CNS involvement, learning difficulty, epilepsy		XR
Debranching enzyme deficiency	Protuberant abdomen, muscle aching, progressive weakness		AR

Table 22.44 Defects of beta-oxidation of fatty acids

	Clinical features
Primary carnitine deficiency	Progressive muscle weakness, cardiomyopathy, hypoglycemia in some
Carnitine palmitoyl transferase II deficiency	Recurrent myalgia, rhabdomyolysis induced by fasting or prolonged exercise
Very long chain acyl-CoA dehydrogenase deficiency	Exercise-induced myalgia and rhabdomyolysis (presentation most often with hypoglycemia)
Medium chain acyl-CoA dehydrogenase deficiency	Rarely muscle pain, lipid storage myopathy, rhabdomyolysis
Short chain acyl-CoA dehydrogenase deficiency	Slowly progressive proximal lipid storage myopathy, secondary carnitine deficiency
Riboflavin responsive multiple acyl-CoA dehydrogenase deficiency	Muscle pain, proximal weakness, improvement with riboflavin
Long chain 3-hydroxyacyl-CoA dehydrogenase deficiency and mitochondrial trifunctional protein deficiency	Proximal myopathy, rhabdomyolysis, peripheral neuropathy, pigmentary neuropathy

If symptoms and signs remain confined to the eyes (ocular myasthenia) for longer than 2 years, the risk of subsequent development of generalized myasthenia gravis is low. Titers of antibodies to AChR are lowest in ocular myasthenia, although if the disease does become generalized the antibody titers tend to become positive.

Hoch and colleagues[575] showed that a high proportion of people without antibodies to AChR have antibodies to a muscle-specific receptor tyrosine kinase, MuSK.

Antibodies in myasthenia gravis lead to a functional loss of acetylcholine receptors at the neuromuscular junction by complement-dependent lysis of the postsynaptic membrane; cross-linking AChRs on the surface of the membrane lead to an increase in the rate of internalization and degradation of AChR and also direct inhibition of AChR function.

The importance of the recently discovered presence of MuSK antibodies in AChR negative myasthenia gravis has yet to be defined. MuSK is an essential component of the developing neuromuscular junction and MuSK antibodies might cause complement-mediated damage to the neuromuscular junction.

The thymus gland is probably necessary for the deletion of autoreactive T cells and has an important role in the pathogenesis of myasthenia gravis, even without the presence of a thymoma. In most children and adolescents the thymus is typically enlarged and contains many germinal centers with T and B cell areas very similar to those seen in lymph nodes. B cells obtained from the thymus spontaneously synthesize anti-AChR and thymic T cells are clonally restricted. A few T cells cloned from the thymus have proved specific for AChR epitopes. It seems probable that thymoma epithelium sensitizes T cells to these AChR epitopes and that T cells leave the thymus and initiate antibodies against AChR and other muscle antigens.

Investigations

AChR antibodies are positive in 85% of young people with generalized disease. When present this finding is diagnostic. Peripheral neurophysiology shows an increased decrement (greater than 10%) of the evoked compound muscle action potential in response to repetitive supramaximal stimulation.

Edrophonium (Tensilon) is a short acting anticholinesterase. When this is given intravenously there is a rapid (usually within 2 minutes), but often short lived (less than 5 minutes) improvement in strength (Fig. 22.36). Interpretation can be difficult, however. It must be remembered there is a small risk of inducing a cholinergic crisis with respiratory arrest.

Once the diagnosis is made, CT or MRI of the mediastinum should be carried out to exclude an associated thymoma. Thyroid function and thyroid antibodies should be measured because of the association with other autoimmune disease.

In childhood and adolescence, where ocular myasthenia is relatively common, the main diagnostic dilemma is distinguishing it from mitochondrial cytopathy. It must be remembered that 50% of those with ocular myasthenia are AChR antibody negative. For those with generalized myasthenia who are also antibody negative the difficulty is differentiating their problem from other neuromuscular disorders and other disorders of the neuromuscular junction. If the onset of bulbar myasthenia is sudden, a brainstem stroke also enters the differential diagnosis.

Treatment

The first-line management is with oral anticholinesterase drugs such as pyridostigmine. The dose should be titrated carefully with the response, remembering that too high a dosage can lead to a cholinergic crisis. Children under 20 kg should receive a dose of 30 mg initially. Those over about 20 kg should have 60 mg initially. The dosage can then slowly be increased in increments of 15–30 mg daily until maximum improvement is obtained. Total daily requirements are usually in the range of 30–360 mg. The effect of the drug usually wears off within 3–4 hours and the timing of the doses needs to be made accordingly. Unwanted gastrointestinal effects may occur, in particular abdominal pain and diarrhea. These may be countered with the use of propantheline. In generalized myasthenia gravis immunosuppression is indicated. Alternate day prednisolone is generally used, starting with a low dose, which is gradually increased (high doses may exacerbate myasthenia). On remission, the dose is gradually reduced. Azathioprine may have a steroid-sparing effect. In severely affected young people, plasma exchange or intravenous immunoglobulins can bring temporary improvement. These are useful strategies if the person involved poses an anesthetic risk prior to thymectomy.

Thymectomy is usually performed in children or adolescents who are AChR antibody positive with generalized myasthenia. Evidence from retrospective uncontrolled studies suggests benefit.[576] Thymectomy is rarely carried out for ocular myasthenia and for those who are AChR antibody negative. It nonetheless demands careful consideration where the symptoms prove to be anticholinesterase resistant.

Other neuromuscular junction disorders

The Lambert–Eaton syndrome

This is caused by antibodies to voltage gated calcium channels on the presynaptic nerve terminals of the motor nerve. Peripheral neurophysiology reveals a small compound muscle action potential at rest and an increase in the amplitude of the action potential after maximal voluntary contraction. Antibodies to voltage gated calcium channels can be detected in most. 3,4-Diaminopyridine prolongs the motor nerve action potential thus increasing neurotransmitter release. It can be effective when used in combination with the anticholinesterases.

Acquired neuromyotonia

This is caused by antibodies to the voltage gated potassium channels present on motor nerve terminals. Most patients present with muscle twitches (fasciculations and myokymia) and cramps. The condition may

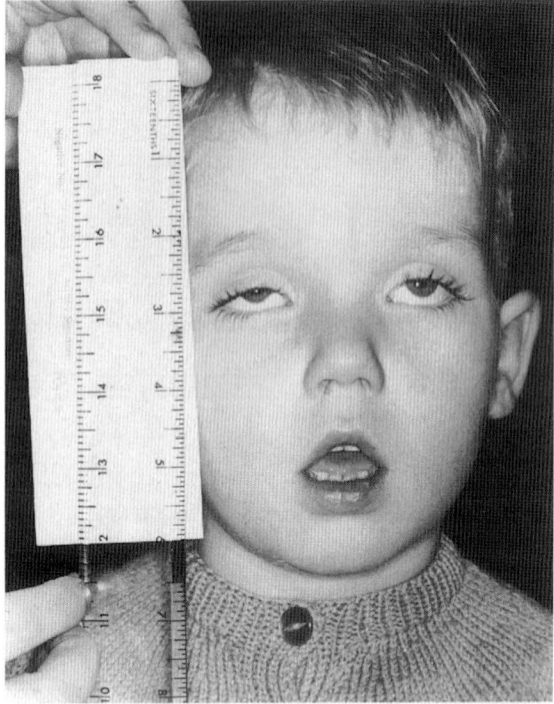

(a)

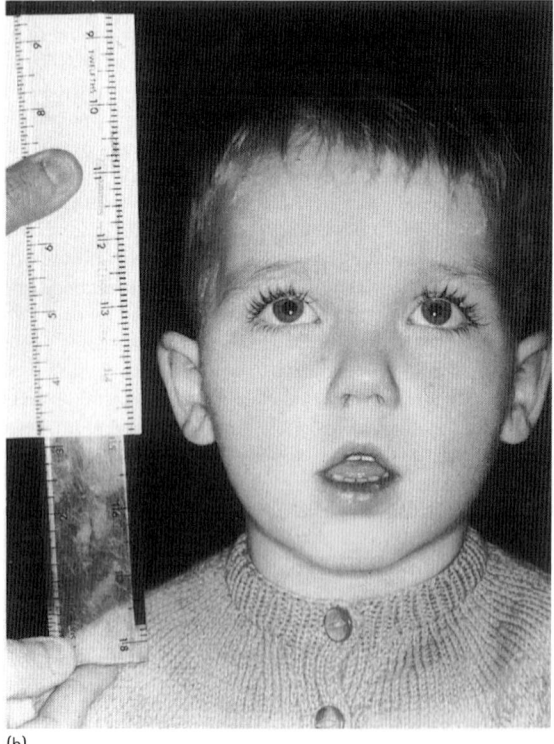

(b)

Fig. 22.36 Myasthenia gravis: (a) before and (b) after intravenous edrophonium.

be present alongside neuropathies or those with myasthenia gravis (particularly in the presence of a thymoma). Muscle weakness is often the major complaint. Membrane stabilizers such as carbamazepine may improve symptoms.

Congenital myasthenic syndromes

The congenital myasthenic syndromes are a group of genetic disorders of neuromuscular transmission. Fatiguable muscle weakness occurs and in some, progressive weakness and wasting may occur. They are

rare conditions but notable because respiratory crises may occur, especially in childhood, and some will benefit from treatment with anticholinesterases. The defect may be presynaptic, synaptic or postsynaptic. Gene mutations responsible for a number of these conditions have now been identified.

In childhood, presentation is usually with feeding difficulty, episodic respiratory difficulty, motor delay, facial weakness, impaired eye movements and fatiguable ptosis. With the exception of slow-channel syndrome, inheritance of these conditions is autosomal recessive.

Confirmation of the diagnosis may be difficult. A trial of an anticholinesterase may lead to improvement in muscle strength and help confirm clinical suspicion but some conditions will not respond to anticholinesterases or may even be worsened. Neurophysiology may be helpful especially if a decrement of more than 10% in compound muscle action potential occurs on repetitive stimulation or increased jitter is found on single fiber EMG. Cytochemical and morphological analysis of the neuromuscular junction is confined to centers with a research interest in this group of conditions. Increasingly the underlying genetic defect will be used in diagnosis and classification Table 22.45.

SPINAL MUSCULAR ATROPHY

Spinal muscular atrophy (SMA) is the result of anterior horn cell disease. The spinal muscular atropies are clinically and genetically heterogeneous. By far the most common type of SMA is proximal SMA caused by deletions in the SMN1 gene. Other types of SMA are very much rarer.

Proximal SMA

Spinal muscular atrophy (SMA) is the second most frequent lethal gene disorder in Caucasians after cystic fibrosis. Prevalence is 1/10 000. SMA is inherited in an autosomal recessive fashion; carrier frequency is estimated to be 1/40–1/60. The majority of cases are due to deletions within the SMN1 gene, the telomeric copy of the survival motor neurone gene on chromosome 5q12.2-q13.3. This area on the short arm of chromosome 5 is complicated with an inverted duplication containing the SMN, neuronal apoptosis inhibitor protein (NAIP) and P44 genes.[577] The SMN1 gene is the causative gene in SMA. The telomeric copy (SMN1) and the centromeric copy (SMN2) of the SMN gene differ by seven base pairs, which results in a splicing difference. There is evidence in transgenic mice that increasing the number of copies of the SMN2 gene ameliorates the severity of the disease. In humans some mutations in SMAII and SMAIII patients may be gene conversions with SMN1 being replaced by SMN2.[578] There is some correlation between SMN protein levels and disease severity.

In proximal SMA, weakness is more severe in the legs than the arms and is more marked proximally than distally. Intercostal muscles are affected with diaphragmatic sparing. Clinically there is a wide spectrum in the severity of SMA. Classification is clinical and based on age of onset and motor function. Life span however depends on respiratory and bulbar function. Within a type there is also a range of severity such that Dubowitz suggested classification should be on a decimal scale, type 1.0 to 1.9 and so on.[579]

Onset may be prenatal, with profound weakness, including facial weakness, contractures and respiratory failure in the neonatal period. Onset within the first 2 months of life is associated with early death. A few infants with SMA type I will have more prolonged survival. Infants with SMA type I are alert with normal facial expression; there is tongue fasciculation, and the limbs are profoundly weak (Fig. 22.37). Often the forearms are contracted in pronation leading to the classic 'jug handle' posture. Bulbar problems with aspiration and the need for tube feeding are invariable. Death is from respiratory causes.

Children at the more severe end of SMA type II may develop respiratory compromise early and will benefit from aggressive management of respiratory complications including the use of NIPPV. The majority of children with type II SMA can be expected to survive beyond childhood. Children with SMA have a hand tremor, polyminimyoclonus, which is very characteristic.

Table 22.45 The classification of the congenital myasthenic syndromes

		Clinical features	Response to anticholinesterase	Inheritance	Gene defect
Presynaptic	Congenital myasthenic syndrome with episodic apnea	Onset in neonatal period. Episodic severe respiratory and bulbar weakness causing apnea, may be provoked by fever, infection or excitement. Facial weakness. Fatiguable ptosis. No eye movement impairment	+	AR	Choline acetyltransferase (CHAT)
Synaptic	End plate acetylcholinesterase (AChE) deficiency	Childhood onset. Fatiguable generalized weakness. Slowly progressive (deterioration)	−	AR	ColQ mutations (ColQ polypeptide binds AchE tetramers)
Postsynaptic	Acetylcholine receptor (AChR) deficiency	Early onset. Feeding difficulty. Ptosis. Impaired eye movements. Motor delay	+ 3,4-Diaminopyridine may also be useful	AR	AChR ε, β or δ subunit mutations
	Fast channel syndrome	Similar to AChR deficiency	−	AR	AChR ε, α or δ subunit mutations
	Slow channel syndrome	Onset variable. Weakness of scapular muscles and finger extensors. Slowly progressive	− Quinidine is beneficial	AD	AChR ε, α, β or δ subunit mutations
	Congenital myasthenic syndrome with rapsyn deficiency	Onset variable, at birth may be associated with arthrogryposis or facial malformation, apnea may occur especially in febrile illnesses. Later onset may mimic antibody negative myasthenia gravis	+ 3,4 Diaminopyridine may produce further benefit	AR	RAPSN mutations

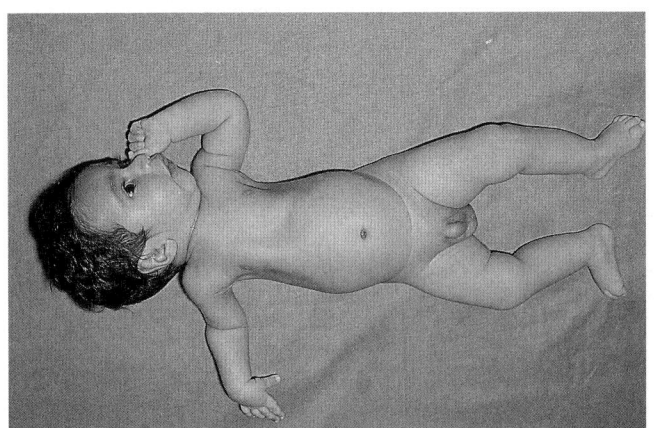

Fig. 22.37 SMA type 1: alert infant with severe limb and intercostals muscle weakness.

Individuals with SMA type III walk with a waddling gait and increased lumbar lordosis. Life expectancy is not affected Table 22.46.

Spinal muscular atrophy with respiratory distress (SMARD)

The presentation of this condition is usually with respiratory distress due to diaphragmatic paralysis; often there is eventration of the diaphragm. Limb weakness is more marked in the upper limbs and distally.

SMARD is genetically heterogeneous. Inheritance is autosomal recessive, mutations in the immunoglobulin mu-binding protein2 have been found in patients with the condition.[580]

Pontocerebellar hypoplasia type 1 (PCH 1)

This condition is characterized by neonatal onset, congenital contractures, ventilatory insufficiency and early death.[581] There is neurophysiological and histopathological evidence of anterior horn cell disease. Hypoplasia of the brainstem and cerebellum is seen on brain imaging. Linkage to the SMN1 gene has been excluded.[582] No gene locus has yet been identified.

Table 22.46 SMA; clinical spectrum

Type	Age of onset	Motor skills	Life expectancy
I Werdnig–Hoffmann	<6 months	Never sits alone	80% die by 1 year
II Intermediate	6–18 months	Sits alone, unable to walk	Variable
III Kugelberg–Welander	>18 months	Walks more than 4 steps alone	Normal

Spinal muscular atrophy, congenital benign with contractures

A number of families have been described with lower limb deformity present at birth and complete sparing of the upper limbs.[583] Motor and sensory nerve conduction is normal with giant motor units present on EMG. The condition is nonprogressive and inheritance is autosomal dominant. The gene locus is on chromosome 12q23-q24.[584]

THE INHERITED NEUROPATHIES

Introduction

Tooth, in 1886, described five cases with predominantly distal limb weakness and wasting, later referred to as peroneal muscular atrophy, suggesting that the primary pathology was in nerve.[585] In the same year Charcot and Marie described five further cases of peroneal muscular atrophy.[586] Despite their conclusion that the primary pathology was probably in the spinal cord, their names along with that of Tooth became eponymously associated with inherited neuropathies. Over the past decade, rapid progress has been made in defining the mutant genes causing this heterogeneous group of conditions. The nomenclature used has therefore also been in a state of flux with neurologists tending to use the term hereditary motor sensory neuropathy (HMSN) while in the genetic literature the term Charcot–Marie–Tooth (CMT) is more commonly found. The population prevalence of hereditary peripheral neuropathies is approximately 1 in 2500.

CMT is classified as type 1, demyelinating with a median nerve motor conduction velocity of less than 38 ms, or type 2, axonal with normal nerve conduction velocity.

The genes and proteins involved

CMT 1A is the most common form of CMT1, accounting for 70% of cases, and is caused by a 1.5-Mb duplication of chromosome 17p11.2.[587] The gene involved is peripheral myelin protein 22 (PMP22). Deletions in this gene can also occasionally cause CMT 1A, although they are usually responsible for hereditary neuropathy with liability to pressure palsies (HNPP).[588] HNPP usually presents in adult life. Autosomal dominant point mutations in the human myelin protein 0 (P_0) gene on chromosome 1q22-q23 lead to CMT 1B and occasionally the axonal neuropathy CMT 2 phenotype.[589]

Mutations in the early growth response 2 gene (EGR2) on chromosome 10 can cause either a dominant or recessive inherited demyelinating neuropathy.[590]

Point mutations in the Connexin 32 gene (CX32) cause X-linked CMT.[591]

The myelin proteins PMP22, P_0 and CX32 all play a part in the maintenance of myelin integrity. P_0 is an abundant myelin protein accounting for 50% of peripheral myelin protein. It transverses the Schwann cell membrane once and contributes the homophilic linkages between adjacent myelin lamellae thus bonding together the concentric myelin wraps.

PMP22 accounts for only 2–5% of peripheral myelin protein. Its role is unknown, though it is thought to play a part in cellular growth.

Connexin 32 is a gap junction protein. It mediates the formation of intracellular gap junctions between the folds of Schwann cell cytoplasm, particularly in the paranodal regions. These act as a channel for the transport of electrolyes and metabolites between the myelin wraps of an individual cell, the flow extending to the axon.

Phenotypes

CMT 1 refers to autosomal dominant demyelinating CMT. Most affected people present in childhood or adolescence with a slowly progressive distal wasting and weakness, associated with evolving areflexia, distal sensory loss and pes cavus. Affected people show evidence of demyelination and remyelination with onion bulb formation and Schwann cell proliferation on nerve biopsy.

Affected males with X-linked CMT arising from point mutations in the CX32 gene present in a way indistinguishable from those with CMT 1. Carrier females are mildly affected.

Dejerine–Sottas disease and congenital hypomyelinating neuropathy (CHN) represent a more severe phenotype. They present in the first 10 years of life with extremely slow motor conduction velocities. Point mutations in PMP22, P_0 and EGR2 can exist in either the heterozygous or the homozygous state, meaning these conditions may be either dominant or recessive.

To date five genes have been identified in families with autosomal recessive demyelinating neuropathies (referred to as HMSN type 1 autosomal recessive or CMT 4).

Autosomal dominant CMT 2 carries the same phenotype as CMT 1 though symptoms tend to develop later, in less severe form with preserved reflexes. Three loci and nine genes are described. An X-lined form of CMT 2 has been described in association with deafness and mental retardation.[592]

The clinical approach

Most children presenting with CMT present with motor difficulties of some sort. There may be an earlier history of motor developmental delay and hypotonia, or the story may be of slowly increasing unsteadiness, falling off in performance in games at school, or increasing tightness in the tendo-Achilles with the emergence of pes cavus making shoe fitting ever more difficult. Sensory symptoms tend to be mild and late.

More severe forms, particularly those with recessive inheritance, may present with what appears to be a cerebellar ataxia with a scanning dysarthria. This means when children are investigated for ataxia the possibility of CMT should be considered.

The common clinical picture is that of a pattern of wasting and weakness of the calves and small muscles of the feet, pes cavus, hammer toes and broadening of the forefoot appearing later (Fig. 22.38). Weakness and wasting of intrinsic hand muscles is also frequently present (Fig. 22.39). The tendo-Achilles tends to be tight. In the forms of CMT

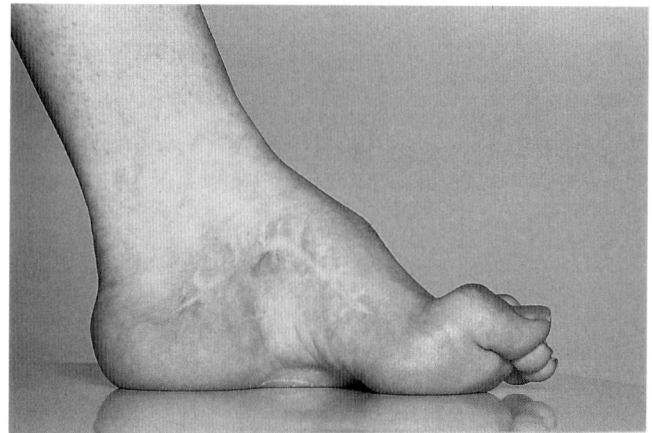

Fig. 22.38   CMT: pes cavis and clawing of toes.

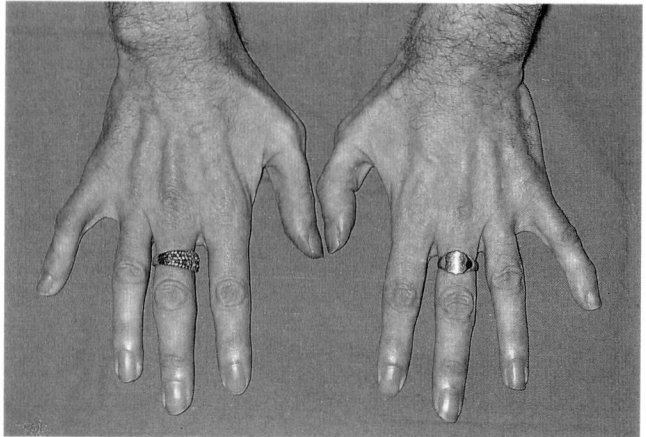

Fig. 22.39   CMT: wasting of intrinsic hand muscles.

with a faster rate of progression, bilateral foot drop may emerge. These forms tend to have an earlier loss of tendon reflexes with the emergence of sensory symptoms and signs.

The first investigation is peripheral neurophysiology. In most children, assessment of the motor nerve conduction velocities will help define whether this is a demyelinating or axonal neuropathy. Where the neuropathy is demyelinating a common duplication in the PMP22 gene can be sought. This will account for almost 70% of children in the CMT 1 group.

Clearly the family history is a useful adjunct in reaching a diagnosis and in this way the CMT may be classified as dominant, recessive or in the absence of male to male transmission probably X-linked. In a typical small family, however, this is often impossible.

Many laboratories also offer screening for PMP22, P_0 and CX32 point mutations though the other rarer genes mentioned have only been identified in interested research laboratories.

In a child or adolescent with clinical and neurophysiological CMT 1, where there is no evidence of male to male transmission, no chromosome 17 duplication and nothing to suggest Dejerine–Sottas disease or congenital hypomyelinating neuropathy, screening should be carried for CX32 mutations. If negative, mutations in P_0 and PMP22 should then be screened, followed lastly by ERG2, if available. In the very small number of remaining demyelinating cases, especially the more severe ones

with a suggestion of recessive transmission, the MTMR2 and periaxin genes should be screened where possible.

In the axonal form of CMT screening for mutations in the known genes is not yet widely available. If there is no male to male transmission, and especially if the index case is female, CX32 should be screened first. If this is negative, P_0 should be screened next. If these are both negative the rarer genes might then be sought.

Hereditary sensory and autonomic neuropathies (HSAN)

Hereditary sensory neuropathies are rare, accounting for 3% of hereditary neuropathies in the European population.[593] In this group of disorders there is loss of one or several modalities of sensation with less prominent clinical involvement of motor and autonomic function. Prominent features in presentation therefore are a conspicuous alteration of pain sensation related to the preferential progressive atrophy of small myelinated (delta) and usually the unmyelinated (C) nerve fibers.

Affected children may well therefore cause concern with painless burns, fractures, indolent ulcers and self-mutilation in infancy. Repeated injury may lead to an incorrect diagnosis of non-accidental injury.[594]

The HSANs are clinically and genetically heterogeneous; Table 22.47 gives the characteristics of the main types.

Table 22.47 The current classification of HSAN

Type	Clinical features	Inheritance	Gene
I	Onset after first decade Lack of pain sensation, reduced sweating especially over distal lower limbs Mild-moderate lower limb weakness Hyporeflexia Abnormal sensory conduction, motor conduction normal	AD	SPTLC1 (serine palmitoyl transferase long chain base subunit 1)
II	Early onset Fungiform papillae absent from tongue Repeated trauma, ulcers, infected sores on hands and feet Diminished pain, temperature and touch sensation No weakness Reflexes absent or decreased Absent sensory nerve action potentials, normal motor nerve conduction velocities	AR	Unknown
III Riley–Day	Feeding difficulty from birth Absence of tears Abnormal temperature control Postural hypotension Emotional ability Absent fungiform papillae from tongue Absent corneal reflexes Relative indifference to pain Absent flare to intradermal histamine Reflexes decreased or absent Motor nerve conduction velocities slightly slow Sensory conduction normal	AR	IKBKAP (inhibitor of kappa light polypeptide gene enhancer in B cell, kinase complex-associated protein)
IV	Anhydrosis with recurrent fevers Painless injury and self-mutilation Learning difficulty frequent Reflexes preserved	AR	Receptor tyrosine kinase for nerve growth factor TRKA
V	Early onset Painless injuries of extremities No weakness Normal reflexes Normal motor and sensory conduction	Uncertain, presumed AR	Unknown

DECREASED CONSCIOUSNESS AND COMA (INCLUDING HYPOXIC–ISCHEMIC, TOXIC AND METABOLIC ENCEPHALOPATHIES)

The approach to the child with decreased conscious level should be systematic. There are many potential causes and many specific treatments need to be considered. Reduced conscious level may be difficult to detect in infants and in all children may be obscured by the other features at presentation.

Initially it may not be apparent that the child has a primary neurological problem. For example, a high fever or abnormal cardiac or respiratory signs may distract the clinician. Conversely, reduced conscious level is most commonly caused by problems outside the CNS, e.g. hypoxia of primary respiratory or cardiac origin. Treatment of these will often improve CNS function and conscious level. In the emergency situation, the approach recommended in the APLS (Advanced Pediatric Life Support) manual[595] should be followed. These follow the ABC (Airway, Breathing, Circulation) principles of resuscitation. This systematic approach will address problems in other organ systems that are affecting the CNS. For example, in a child with meningococcal septicemia, reduced conscious level may be prominent at presentation but securing an adequate airway, optimizing oxygenation and treating shock will improve CNS function.

CLINICAL ASSESSMENT

The main causes of decreased conscious level are shown in Table 22.48. The initial history should concentrate on detecting these and, for example, a history of recent trauma, previous seizures or potential drug ingestion will guide appropriate investigations and may suggest specific treatments.

Symptoms of raised intracranial pressure (ICP) include poor feeding, vomiting, irritability, lethargy and seizures. Signs include a full fontanel (in babies), scalp vein distension, macrocephaly, bradycardia, hypertension, abnormal respiratory patterns, and focal neurological deficits including false localizing signs, particularly sixth nerve palsies.

Clinical examination should be thorough. General examination should seek signs suggestive of the causes in Table 22.48, e.g. the rash of meningococcal disease. In school-age children the conscious level should be assessed using the Glasgow Coma Score (GCS) (Table 22.49). In the preschool child the verbal response component of the GCS is unreliable and modified coma scores have been proposed (Table 22.49). In the intubated child modifications to the GCS use grimace rather than vocalization. While in adults the GCS is well validated and scores have been shown to have prognostic significance, this is not yet the case in children. However, a coma score of 8 or less should generally prompt intubation, as the child is unlikely to be able to protect the airway adequately. The coma score is a useful tool for the ongoing assessment of the encephalopathic child, in order to detect improvement or deterioration in the child's condition.

It is important to complete and document a neurological examination early in the assessment of the unconscious child. Management of the child may include ventilation, sedation and muscle paralysis, which are likely to interfere with later assessments. Particular attention should be paid to pupil size and reactivity. Pinpoint pupils may be a sign of poisoning, particularly with opiates and barbiturates. Small reactive pupils are a feature of medullary lesions and mid-size, nonreactive pupils of midbrain lesions. Fixed dilated pupils are an ominous sign, often indicating terminal coning, but can also occur temporarily, after severe hypoxia and as a consequence of hypothermia, seizure activity and occasionally after the administration of certain drugs, notably barbiturates such as thiopental. Metabolic conditions can cause all these types of pupillary abnormality. A unilateral dilated pupil may indicate incipient herniation, causing dysfunction of the third cranial nerve. This is particularly likely to occur with ipsilateral space-occupying lesions, such as extradural hematomas.

Table 22.48 Important causes of acute encephalopathy

Infectious and parainfectious encephalopathies
Meningitis (mainly bacterial, rarely fungal, protozoal and viral)
Cortical thrombophlebitis
Cerebral abscess and empyema
Primary viral encephalitis
Postinfectious encephalitis
Acute disseminated encephalomyelitis
Cerebral malaria
Severe systemic infections, including septicemia

Hypoxic ischemic encephalopathies
Perinatal asphyxia
Severe pulmonary disease
Carbon monoxide poisoning
Methemoglobinemia
Severe anemia
Status epilepticus
Near-miss sudden infant death syndrome
Postcardiac arrest
Cardiac bypass surgery
Near drowning
Cardiac arrhythmias
Congestive cardiac failure
Hypotension
Disseminated intravascular coagulation
Hypoglycemia
Anesthetic accidents
Vitamin or cofactor deficiencies (B_{12}, B_6, folate, etc.)

Trauma
Accidental
Non-accidental

Exogenous toxins
Drugs: antihistamines, anticholinergics, antidepressants, hypnotics and sedatives, analgesics, antiepileptics, anti-inflammatory, antimetabolites, antibiotics, etc.
Illicit substances: alcohol, solvents, cannabis, cocaine, amfetamines, opiates
Environmental toxins: carbon monoxide, phosphates, DDT, iron, lead, pesticides, heavy metals, insect and snake venoms, plants, etc.
Hypothermia
Heat stroke

Endogenous agents
Water intoxication
Electrolyte imbalances, esp. hypo- and hypernatremia
Acidosis and alkalosis
Scalds
Endocrine disorders: diabetes mellitus, hypoglycemia, hypo- and hyperthyroidism, hypo- and hyperparathyroidism, hypopituitarism, hypoadrenalism
Organ failure: hepatic, renal, pancreas
Hypertension
Inborn errors of metabolism: aminoacidopathies, organicacidurias, urea cycle defects, fatty acid oxidation defects, mitochondrial disorders, carnitine deficiency, porphyria

Cerebrovascular disease
Hemorrhagic stroke
Ischemic stroke

Epileptic seizure related
Postictal
Nonconvulsive status epilepticus
Postconvulsive status epilepticus

Table 22.49 Glasgow Coma Scale and Children's Coma Scale (modified Glasgow Coma Scale)

Eyes	Score	Best motor response	Score	Best verbal response		Score
Glasgow Coma Scale						
Open		*To verbal command*				
Spontaneously	4	Obeys	6	Orientated and converses		5
To verbal command	3	*To painful stimulus*		Disoriented and converses		4
To pain	2	Localizes pain	5	Inappropriate words		3
No response	1	Flexion – withdrawal	4	Incomprehensible sounds		2
		Flexion abnormal	3	No response		1
		Extension	2			
		No response	1			
Children's Coma Scale						
Spontaneous	4	Spontaneous (obeys verbal command)	6	Smiles, orientated to sound, follows objects, interacts		5
Reaction to speech	3	Localizes pain	5	*Crying*	*Interacts*	
Reaction to pain	2	Withdraws in response to pain	4	Consolable	Inappropriate	4
No response	1	Abnormal flexion in response to pain (decorticate posture)	3	Inconsistently consolable	Moaning	3
		Abnormal extension in response to pain (decerebrate posture)	2	Inconsolable	Irritable restless	2
		No response	1	No response	No response	1

GCS total 3–15; CCS total 3–15.

The fundi should be examined for signs of metabolic disease, retinal hemorrhage and papilledema. Absence of papilledema does not rule out raised ICP and does not indicate that it is necessarily safe to do a lumbar puncture. Voluntary and reflex eye movements should be assessed, facial weakness and asymmetry looked for and bulbar muscle functions tested. When oculocephalic reflexes are preserved (doll's eye movements) the eyes are able to maintain fixation when the head is moved side to side or up and down. When these are lost the eyes move with the head. Oculovestibular reflexes (caloric responses) are usually tested as part of brainstem death tests and require the eardrum to be intact. Deviation of the eyes toward a cold water stimulus and away from a warm water stimulus occurs.

The child's body posture and any abnormal movements should be noted. The presence of decorticate (arms flexed, legs extended) or decerebrate (arms and legs extended) postures are particularly significant. Tone, power, reflexes and plantar responses in the limbs should be documented and interpreted in the light of recently administered drugs such as neuromuscular blockers.

INVESTIGATIONS

During the primary assessment and resuscitation blood should be taken for FBC, U&E, calcium, blood cultures and blood glucose. Specific treatments such as glucose for hypoglycemia, antibiotics for meningococcal septicemia and calcium for seizures caused by hypocalcemia may be indicated. Further investigations which will aid the supportive care of the child include arterial blood gases, coagulation screen and urine and plasma osmolality (Table 22.50).

Subsequently, further investigations may be indicated for specific conditions. These may include a toxicology screen, blood alcohol level, specific drug levels (such as anticonvulsants), plasma ammonia and lactate levels and liver function tests. Urine for amino and organic acids and porphyrins should be collected. An early CT scan is usually indicated unless a cause for the child's condition is apparent. Lumbar puncture should usually be deferred at least until the results of this are known.[596,597] An X-ray skeletal survey may be useful at this point if non-accidental injury is suspected. Children who are hypoglycemic should have blood and urine collected while hypoglycemic or immediately thereafter for later metabolic investigations. Laboratory advice should be sought on the samples required and their subsequent handling and storage.

CONTINUING MANAGEMENT

The continuing management of the child with reduced conscious level is directed at maintaining homeostasis and at detecting and treating the underlying cause. Maintenance of cerebral perfusion pressure (CPP), cerebral blood flow (CBF) and normal cerebral metabolism are important. Raised ICP should be detected and treated. However, CPP is also affected by systemic factors such as hypotension. Children in coma require repeated reassessment and skilled neurological nursing usually on an intensive care or high dependency unit. Specific therapy for certain causes of encephalopathy, such as hemodialysis for removal of drugs after overdose, may be required.

Table 22.50 Useful investigations in coma

Basic hematological and biochemical investigations, including glucose, Ca, PO_4, Alk P and LFTs
Markers of inflammation, including ESR and CRP
Blood and urine osmolality
Blood clotting studies
Bacteriological and virological studies including cultures, serology, PCRs, Mantoux, etc.
Neuroimaging:
Ultrasound, CT, MRI
Blood gases
Plasma ammonia
Plasma lactate
Urine toxicology
Blood toxicology – alcohol, lead and specific toxins where indicated
Blood anticonvulsant levels
Urine metabolic screen
Urine amino and organic acids
CSF examination including lactate and glycine if indicated
TFTs and other endocrine investigations if indicated
Blood and urinary porphyrins
Skeletal survey
EEG

The physiology of intracranial pressure, cerebral perfusion pressure and cerebral blood flow

Intracranial pressure

Raised ICP can arise by a number of different mechanisms. The commonest causes are intracranial space-occupying lesions, CNS infections, hydrocephalus, intracranial hemorrhage, metabolic disease (with cerebral edema), meningeal inflammation (reducing CSF resorption) and dural sinus thrombosis (raising venous pressure) are the commonest. A rise in ICP may lead to secondary brain shifts with herniation of brain contents. A critical reduction in perfusion to the brain may result, leading to disability or death.

Cerebral edema has several pathological types. Both focal and generalized cerebral edema can cause raised ICP and decreased consciousness. Focal cerebral edema may be associated with localized brain dysfunction and focal neurological signs. Generalized cerebral edema may be associated with false localizing signs. Vasogenic edema results from changes in capillary permeability and occurs with CNS infections, head trauma and in encephalopathies due to toxins, hypertension and seizures. Osmotic edema is seen in hyponatremia, diabetic ketoacidosis and excessive fluid resuscitation. Cytotoxic edema is secondary to intracellular energy failure and occurs with hypoxic-ischemic insults, status epilepticus and severe infection. Hydrocephalus may result in transependymal resorption of CSF and periventricular interstitial edema. Finally, loss of cerebral autoregulation as occurs with systemic hypertension and in hypercapnia results in hydrostatic edema.

In children under 12–18 months the open sutures enable the skull volume to increase and large intracranial masses may accumulate without rapid or large rises in ICP. After 2 years of age the cranial cavity behaves more like the adult with a fixed volume. The development of cerebral edema as a normal response of the central nervous system to injury causes an increase in the volume of the brain. With the volume of the skull cavity fixed there will inevitably be either diminution in the total volume of CSF spaces and/or diminution of the pool of venous blood within the skull. As ICP increases there will be an increased resistance to inflow of arterial blood and thus a fall in the cerebral perfusion pressure. Cerebral perfusion pressure (CPP) equals the mean systemic blood pressure (SBP) minus the mean ICP. A fall in CPP leads to a fall in the CBF and if this is below 20 ml/100 g of tissue per min, brain ischemia will develop. Brain ischemia further increases the formation of cerebral edema leading to a further rise in ICP. If CBF falls below 10 mL/100 g per min electrical dysfunction of the neurones and loss of intracellular ion homeostasis occurs.

Generalized rises of ICP will first cause transtentorial and eventually transforaminal herniation. Unilateral increases in ICP, for example secondary to hematoma, will cause ipsilateral uncal herniation and compression of the third nerve against the free border of the tentorium with ipsilateral pupillary dilation secondary to loss of parasympathetic constrictor tone to the ciliary muscles. Uncontrolled further herniation will cause, in addition, contralateral third nerve palsy. At the same time the brainstem is shifted downward to the foramen magnum, which impairs the blood supply to the brainstem from the perforating branches of the basilar artery and results in brainstem ischemia. The signs of cingulate gyrus herniation, tentorial herniation and foramen magnum coning are given in (Table 22.51).

Monitoring ICP can be useful in head trauma, certain metabolic encephalopathies and in intracranial infection. There is little evidence of benefit in Reye syndrome, hepatic encephalopathy or hypoxic–ischemic injury (such as postcardiac arrest). A number of techniques have been described for monitoring ICP.[598] All depend on the principle, which is generally but not invariably correct, that the pressure within the cranium is the same in all departments. The preferred technique will depend on whether ventricular dilation is present or whether the ventricles are small and shifted as a result of the brain swelling. In the child with cerebral edema it is possible to monitor the ICP continuously by the use of a subdural or subarachnoid Teflon catheter. In infants this can be placed percutaneously through the anterior fontanel. Ventricular transducers record either the

Table 22.51   Clinical features of brain herniation

Tentorial
Sunsetting
Dilated pupils
VIth nerve palsy
Cortical blindness
Hemiplegia
Extensor motor pattern (decerebrate)
Coma
Respiratory irregularity
Systemic hypertension
Tonic seizures

Cingulate gyrus herniation
Diplegia or hemiplegia
Visual symptoms

Foramen magnum cone
Cardiorespiratory arrest
Bulbar palsy
Neck stiffness
Hypotonia
Stridor
Spinal flexion
Hypotension
Hyperthermia

ventricular pressure, or if not in the ventricle, the brain parenchymal pressure. Cerebral intraparenchymal devices are also available. The normal ICP in adults is 0–15 mmHg (0–2 kPa). In the newborn, older infants and toddlers the upper limits are 3.5 mmHg, 5.5 mmHg and 6.5 mmHg respectively.[599]

Brief rises in ICP may occur during coughing, straining and crying, as well as other physiological activities that increase the central venous pressure. Sustained elevations or intermittent rises in pressure in the form of pressure waves may also occur and may require treatment. An increase in the ICP may come about as a result of increasing the brain, blood or CSF contents of the skull. The increase in ICP that results from a given increment in volume depends on the ICP–volume status. As the ICP increases small changes in volume may result in significant changes in pressure.

Cerebral perfusion pressure

With increasing ICP there is an increase in the cerebral venous pressure. This remains about 3 mmHg below the ICP so that cerebral circulation continues. The cerebral perfusion pressure is the difference between the mean systemic arterial pressure (MAP) and the ICP, i.e. CPP = MAP − ICP.

The relationship between ICP and cerebral perfusion pressure is complex. Raised ICP may be caused by an increase in CBF or it may be the limiting factor producing a reduction in CBF. In encephalopathies the brain is frequently pale and devoid of blood flow as a result of raised ICP producing ischemia. The normal cerebral perfusion pressure is 60–70 mmHg. There is a progressive fall in brain perfusion with decreasing CPP down to a CPP of 40 mmHg. Below this ischemic infarction may result.

Cerebral blood flow

During acute encephalopathy there are changes in general and regional cerebral blood flow (CBF). Cerebral autoregulation is the maintenance of cerebral blood flow by alteration of the cerebral blood volume in response to large changes (increases or decreases) in the systemic perfusion pressure. Cerebral autoregulation is often impaired (globally or regionally) with encephalopathy so that CBF is related directly to systemic arterial pressure. Excessive blood flow (luxury perfusion) is sometimes seen after hypoxic–ischemic injury. It is possible using the Fick

glucose. Acid fast bacilli are rarely seen but culture may be positive in up to 50%. The use of PCR for mycobacterium DNA on blood and CSF has aided rapid diagnosis but false positives are seen. Further consideration is given to this illness under aseptic meningitis below.

CEREBRAL ABSCESS AND SUBDURAL EMPYEMA

Cerebral abscesses can result from hematogenous spread of infection, often in association with congenital heart disease, local spread of infection from sinusitis or mastoiditis or arise as a complication of meningitis. *Streptococcus*, *Staphylococcus* and anaerobic organisms are the most common causes, but many other organisms have been reported. Abscesses are usually located in the cerebral hemispheres and present with encephalopathy, seizures and sepsis. CT with contrast is usually diagnostic, often showing enhancement of the abscess cavity with intense surrounding edema.

Intravenous antibiotics are the main treatment although surgical drainage may be needed. A prolonged course of 4–6 weeks is often needed with progress monitored by serial scans. Mortality is around 10% with 30% of survivors developing epilepsy.

Subdural empyemas are essentially abscesses lying in the subdural space. Their presentation is similar to that of cerebral abscesses in general. Surgical evacuation is usually necessary combined with prolonged antibiotic treatment.

ACUTE DISSEMINATED ENCEPHALOMYELITIS (ADEM)

This acute patchy demyelination, occurring in the central nervous system, is thought to be an abnormal immunological response to infection. It may be considered a special form of postinfectious encephalitis. After an interval, following the precipitating viral infection, the child develops focal neurological signs, headache, mild encephalopathy and occasionally seizures. The focal neurological deficits depend on the sites of demyelination and may follow any pattern. There may be fluctuation or progression of signs in the days after presentation. CT scanning in the acute phase may be normal. MR scanning is usually diagnostic. The spinal cord may be involved. CSF examination characteristically shows a mild pleocytosis, usually lymphocytic, a normal or mildly raised CSF protein level and a normal glucose level. Oligoclonal bands may be present in some patients. Investigations looking for evidence of the precipitating infection often prove negative.

A good response is usually seen to steroids although it is unclear if the final outcome is influenced by such treatment. A 3- to 5-day course of intravenous methyl prednisolone is often given. More than 90% of children with ADEM make a full recovery from the initial episode, although this may take many months. Relapses are occasionally described.

MULTIPLE SCLEROSIS

Clinically it is not possible to distinguish between ADEM and the first attack of demyelination due to multiple sclerosis. Long term follow-up studies have suggested that as many as 10% of patients with ADEM later develop multiple sclerosis and 2.7% of adults with MS had onset before 16 years of age, but it is rare under the age of 10 years. Clinical features include the relapsing remitting course. Visual and sensory symptoms are prominent as in adults. Seizures occur more commonly than in adults. Optic neuritis is characterized by a sudden reduction in monocular or binocular vision. A large central scotoma and papillitis are usually found on ocular examination. Though often considered a principal feature of multiple sclerosis in adults, few children with optic neuritis go on to develop multiple sclerosis.

Diagnosis of multiple sclerosis depends principally on the clinical picture combined with the results of MRI. CSF examination and visually evoked responses remain useful adjuvant investigations. High dose steroid treatment is effective for acute relapses but the use of beta-interferon remains controversial.

CHRONIC INFLAMMATORY AND INFECTIOUS MENINGOENCEPHALOPATHIES

Aseptic meningitis

Not all children with CNS sepsis present with acute encephalopathy. The onset may be insidious, diagnostically confusing, and if appropriate therapy is not initiated significant disability may result. Thus, the child with subacute or chronic meningitis who fails to respond to adequate antibiotic therapy presents the pediatrician with a worrying and perplexing problem. Most of these children will present with fever, nuchal rigidity and headache, probably after an insidious prodromal illness of general malaise and anorexia. The CSF initially may show pleocytosis changing to lymphocytosis within a few hours or a day or two. Antibiotic therapy for at least 48 hours is appropriate until cultures are shown to be negative, along with supportive therapy with fluids, analgesia and antipyretics.

As for acute encephalopathy a variety of viruses are potentially implicated. The enteroviruses account for 80% of all cases of aseptic meningitis in American studies. The UK picture is similar in infancy, but the mumps virus is a more common pathogen in the 1- to 9-year-old age group. This may change with the advent of mumps, measles, and rubella vaccination. Other common causes of aseptic meningitis include herpes simplex, adenovirus, measles, cytomegalovirus, rubella, varicella, Epstein–Barr, influenza, parainfluenza and rotavirus. The Epstein–Barr and Coxsackie virus in particular may run a subacute or chronic course. A rash may accompany the illness, which can be specific. Febrile convulsions may occur. Generally, younger children are irritable and resent handling, while older children complain of myalgia, photophobia and retrobulbar pain with evidence of nuchal rigidity in only about 50%.

It is generally accepted that after 12 hours of illness, almost all (97%) of the cellular response in CSF will be lymphocytic and that antibiotics can be withheld if the child seems otherwise well. CSF glucose may be low in up to 20% and CSF protein may be increased in up to 50%. Laboratory tests for bacteria will be negative but should be complemented by specific viral culture of CSF and other sites, including throat, feces and urine, as well as the measurement of serum viral-antibody titers. Raised alpha-interferon levels usually indicate a viral meningoencephalitic illness, but slightly raised levels may also occur in bacterial infection. Viral identification can shorten antibiotic courses and reduce time spent in hospital.

After 48 hours of treatment the main alternative diagnoses to consider with a sterile polymorphic or pleocytic CSF are partially treated bacterial or tuberculous meningitis (TBM). Partially treated meningitis is particularly likely if there is a history of a course of oral antibiotics given for an intercurrent infection. This treatment may render microbacterial techniques unreliable, and it is reasonable at this stage to stop all antibiotics in order to clarify the situation. If deterioration ensues, antibiotic therapy may be reinstituted.

Tuberculous meningitis

Tuberculosis (TB) of the CNS occurs in all ethnic groups; diagnosis and treatment are difficult. Late diagnosis carries an associated high morbidity and mortality. The incidence of TB of the CNS is increasing in part as a result of the acquired immunodeficiency syndrome becoming more common. In children, TB of the CNS is often a complication of primary infection with or without miliary spread. TB of the CNS should be considered in any child with a subacute history of fever, headache, seizures, vomiting, behavioral change or impairment of consciousness. Respiratory symptoms may or may not be present. It is important to note that tuberculous meningitis (TBM) results from Rich's focus produced in an intensive inflammatory response, particularly at the base of the brain. There is an associated vasculitis, which may result in convulsions, cranial nerve palsies, dyskinesia, hemiparesis or signs of a mild radiculopathy.

The CSF sugar is typically low, but may be normal in up to 10% of patients. When the ratio of blood to CSF sugar is greater than 2:1 in the presence of a lymphocytic meningitis, TBM must be given very serious consideration. The Mantoux test may remain negative for some weeks due to anergy following primary exposure; the combination of lobar consolidation on a chest X-ray and aseptic meningitis is a particularly strong indication for antituberculous therapy. The decision to treat is rather easier when the X-ray shows classic miliary mottling, or examination of the fundi reveals choroidal tubercles.

Neuroimaging with MRI or CT with contrast may be helpful in diagnosis; tuberculomas may not be evident on an unenhanced scan. Lumbar puncture may be negative for culture of acid-fast bacilli, this diagnosis being made only on ventricular drainage. Acid-fast bacilli have to be searched for carefully in CSF specimens. The use of the polymerase chain reaction to detect antigen or metabolic products of tubercle bacilli can be misleading, with a one in ten false positive rate.

Treatment of tuberculous meningitis involves administration for at least a year of two antituberculous therapeutic agents that penetrate the blood–brain barrier and tuberculomas. Isoniazid and rifampicin are the mainstay of continued treatment during this period. Initially, four drugs are required, usually rifampicin, isoniazid, pyrazinamide and ethambutol. Steroids are of value when there is progressive neurological disorder or deteriorating consciousness, once appropriate antituberculous chemotherapy is begun. Further detail on treatment is given in Chapter 29.

Other causes

When a child with lymphocytic CSF does not improve as expected, a full reappraisal of the history and findings is appropriate, and thoughts on differential diagnosis should be broadened. Possibilities are rarer bacteria (see below), an immune paresis with opportunistic infection, a fistula, autoimmune disease or toxins.

Five percent of all children with acute lymphoblastic leukemia have CNS disease at presentation. The CNS is the most common site for relapse. Usually, associated signs of bone marrow failure (anemia, thrombocytopenia, recurrent infection) will aid diagnosis. Rarely, primary CNS lymphoma may present in this way. It is essential that bone marrow investigation is performed before the use of steroids.

In an immunocompromised or severely debilitated child, fungal infection, including candida and cryptococcus, may spread to the CNS from specific skin or oral lesions. Stains for fungi, swabs, cultures, antibody titers and urine microscopy should identify the cause. When the degree of debility is severe, and particularly when there is marked and rapid wasting of muscles, it may be justified to administer a course of amphotericin. In immunocompromised children, in addition to severe illnesses caused by the common agents, opportunistic pathogens may cause an encephalopathy.

Neurological manifestations of nervous system infection with *Borrelia burgdorferi* (a spirochete) are protean. It is a multisystem disorder, known also as Lyme disease, affecting the skin, joints, nervous system and cardiovascular system. *Borrelia* inhabits the gut of the *Ixodes* tic. The tic is widespread throughout the UK but found in greater numbers in woodland.

Man is infected by the bite of a tic producing (in most cases) a slowly enlarging patch of erythema (erythema chronicum migrans). A nonspecific flu-like illness may occur at this stage. These symptoms may be followed by cranial poly- or mononeuropathies, aseptic meningitis, transverse myelitis, postinfectious polyneuritis and encephalitis. A history of skin lesion or a tic bite is not always obtained.[615] Diagnosis is difficult, and serological studies may not be positive at the time of neurological presentation. Specific IgM is the most valuable serological test and intrathecal synthesis of specific antibodies which immunoblot the spirochetal antigen may also (in due course) be helpful diagnostically. Treatment in childhood is usually with penicillin or erythromycin. Nervous system disease must be treated aggressively as chronic encephalopathy may ensue. There is increasing evidence[616,617] in neuroborreliosis that intravenous cephalosporins are superior to penicillin, because of the latter's relatively poor CNS penetration.

The protozoon *Toxoplasma gondii* may cause meningitis in immunosuppressed children. It is usually accompanied by lymphadenopathy. The histology of an affected node may give the diagnosis, as may the presence in the serum of specific IgM. Treatment with sulphonamides, pyrimethamine or spiramycin is effective.

Leptospirosis results from contact with infected animal urine (mainly rats), usually in contaminated water or from farm machinery. After an incubation period of 10 days, the illness typically produces a high fever, sweating, headaches, conjunctival suffusion, muscle tenderness and pain with meningitis. Cardiac or renal failure may occur, with spontaneous improvement after 3 weeks. Diagnosis is based on cultured blood and urine and rising antibody titers after the first week. Penicillin, erythromycin and tetracycline are the treatment options, along with supportive therapy, though the immune-mediated effects of the illness may not be affected. Tetracyclines are contraindicated in renal failure and, depending on the severity of the illness, are contraindicated in children. Usually high doses are given for 10 days. Cerebral malaria may need to be considered in those who have recently traveled abroad.

Mycoplasma pneumoniae is reported to cause CNS disease in 7% of those admitted to hospital with associated upper or lower respiratory tract illness. A meningoencephalitis, which may be severe, is the commonest result, but polyneuropathy or transverse myelitis may also occur.

Neurobrucellosis may also cause meningoencephalitis. It is usually contracted from animals known to harbor the organism, or from the ingestion of unpasteurized milk products. Sweating, abdominal pain, fever, hepatosplenomegaly and arthritis commonly accompany the illness. Axonal polyneuropathy has been reported. *Brucella melitensis* may be isolated from CSF and there may be rising antibody titers. Regimens advocated include (either alone or in combination) co-trimoxazole, rifampicin or streptomycin. In chronic brucellosis suppression of intracellular infection may be attempted in the hope that the host's immunity will eventually eliminate or contain infection. Regimens advocated include protracted courses of the antibiotics used in acute brucellosis. Tetracyclines are useful but obviously cannot be used in children unless there is no alternative. Most children make a full recovery.

Kawasaki disease or mucocutaneous lymph node syndrome is a relatively uncommon disorder. It predominates in the under-fives and, although the etiology is uncertain, infective agents have been implicated in its etiology. Presentation is with persistent fever, characteristic skin rashes, with desquamation of the extremities, mucosal and buccal involvement and lymphadenopathy. It may be associated with aseptic meningitis though rarely as an isolated feature. The association of aseptic meningitis with an autoimmune vasculitis is dealt with in Chapter 29.

Aseptic meningitis may follow the administration of certain drugs. These include OKT3 (in renal transplantation), immunoglobulin (in idiopathic thrombocytopenic purpura and Kawasaki disease), isoniazid, sulfamethiazole, co-trimoxazole and azathioprine. A cellular response has also been reported in lead poisoning, although meningism is rare and reduced conscious level common.

It must also be remembered that migraine at times leads to a cellular response in the CSF, particularly in complicated migraine. If the hemiplegia is fleeting, the child's presentation at hospital may be with headache and the picture of an aseptic meningitis. Migraine may also present with fever, neck stiffness and aseptic meningitis. Although uncommon, recognition of this syndrome should help to avoid unnecessary invasive investigations.

The clinician needs to be aware that aseptic meningitis may well be the presenting feature of a number of less common but important conditions specified here. While the diagnosis is being investigated, due attention should be paid to the child's parents, who will also be feeling worried and perplexed. Adequate time needs to be allocated to inform them of investigation and treatment strategy at each stage, in order to maintain their confidence at a time when the medical team themselves may be feeling unsure.

Recurrent or chronic meningitis

Recurrent meningitis may result from anatomical abnormalities of the inner ear or cranioverterbal axis. The causes are acquired (following trauma) or congenital, immunodeficiency or distant untreated foci of infection.

In any child with recurrent meningitis, a communication between the CNS and the exterior must be assiduously sought. Congenital abnormalities of the inner ear leading to fistulae may present with recurrent meningitis. Otoscopy is usually normal, and diagnosis requires expert neuroradiological and possibly radioisotope investigation. CSF fistulae may also result from trauma or infection. Recurrent meningitis (often with unusual organisms for age) may result from infection via a midline dermal fistula (often referred to as a sinus), usually associated with spina bifida occulta. The fistula can occur at any point in the midline, though the natal cleft is the commonest site. There may be associated cord tethering, intraspinal dermoid, lipoma or cyst or diastematomyelia.

The second commonest site for a fistula is the occiput, and there may be associated cerebellar or brainstem signs of hydrocephalus. Infection of a dermoid cyst and proximal end of a neurodermal sinus may result in intraspinal abscess rather than meningitis.

Any neurodermal sinus that ends above the sacrum should be dealt with neurosurgically. Surgical results are poorer when definitive treatment is delayed until after the occurrence of meningitis.

Other infectious encephalopathies

Chronic encephalitides include subacute sclerosing panencephalitis (SSPE), progressive rubella panencephalitis and HIV encephalopathy. SSPE is an exceptionally rare disease caused by direct invasion by the measles virus of the CNS and usually first manifests some years after the initial measles illness, which has often occurred within the first 2 years of life. It has been described after measles immunization. An initial stage marked by intellectual and behavioral changes is followed by repetitive involuntary movements, resembling myoclonus. Dementia and early death follow inexorably. Diagnosis is by the detection of an oligoclonal CSF pattern and raised measles antibody titers in the CSF. SSPE is covered in detail in the section on neurodegenerative conditions (see p. 903). There is no specific treatment. HIV encephalopathy is dealt with in detail elsewhere (see Ch. 27, see pp. 1269).

ACUTE PARAPARESIS OR QUADRAPARESIS

It may be difficult to determine if an unwell child has actual muscle weakness. Many children present with nonspecific symptoms of irritability, lethargy and pallor. Some conditions with acute weakness are commonly associated with encephalopathy and this may be the predominant feature at presentation. Children with abnormal gait, limp or refusing to walk may present to orthopedic or trauma clinics, or be suspected of 'putting it on'. Failure to consider a neurological cause for nonspecific presentations is a common reason for delay in diagnosis of treatable conditions such as Guillain–Barré syndrome and acute myelopathy.

Initial assessment of any acutely ill child should concentrate on the ABC principles of resuscitation especially where there is co-existing encephalopathy. Neurological assessment should determine the pattern of weakness so that it can be classified according to the likely site of the lesion. The pattern of weakness will generally be that of hemiplegia, quadriplegia, paraplegia or asymmetrical variants of these. Further information from the pattern of tendon reflexes, sensory signs and symptoms of bladder and/or bowel involvement are important. Although not always clear after the initial neurological examination, it should be possible to determine whether the weakness is due to a lesion in the brain, spinal cord, anterior horn cell, peripheral nerve, neuromuscular junction or muscle. Points on history taking which aid the diagnosis are dealt with in the relevant sections below.

Children with weakness due to upper motor neurone lesions present initially with a flaccid limb weakness and loss of reflexes. Typical upper motor neurone signs of increased tone and brisk reflexes may not be present for several days or weeks.

There are a number of conditions that present with acute weakness where specific treatment is available and improves long term outcome. Diagnosis of these and early referral to specialist advice is important. Guillain–Barré syndrome, acute myelopathy due to cord compression and myasthenia gravis are important examples. In the child with an acute hemorrhagic or ischemic stroke, neurological and neurosurgical advice should be sought immediately. Children with acute stroke often have associated cerebral edema and raised ICP.

In children who present with an acute hemiparesis the differential diagnosis includes hemorrhagic and ischemic stroke, brain tumor, extradural or subdural hematoma, focal central nervous system infection (encephalitis or abscess), hemiplegic migraine, mitochondrial encephalomyopathy, lactic acidosis and stroke-like episodes (MELAS), acute demyelination and Todd paresis secondary to an epileptic seizure.

The differential diagnosis in children with paraplegia or quadriplegia includes Guillain–Barré syndrome, acute dermatomyositis, myasthenia gravis, acute peripheral neuropathy other than Guillain–Barré syndrome, CNS infection such as poliomyelitis or spinal cord abscess, acute transverse myelitis, spinal cord compression from tumor, abscess or hematoma and multifocal cerebral cortical dysfunction (although in the latter an encephalopathy is often prominent).

In paraparesis the weakness is confined to the lower limbs. A quadriparesis affects all four limbs. In the acute situation these are usually caused by lesions of the spinal cord, although anterior horn cell disease such as poliomyelitis and polio-like illnesses due to enteroviruses, lesions of the cauda equina or peripheral nerves, such as in Guillain–Barré syndrome, also need to be considered. Vascular lesions of the cord such as anterior spinal artery infarction and spinal arteriovenous malformations may need excluding. A very acute onset of dermatomyositis may present in a similar way. A raised CPK, heliotrope rash, muscle tenderness and irritability are useful diagnostic clues. Acute periodic paralysis should also be considered in the differential diagnosis. Vertebral osteomyelitis or discitis can present with lower limb weakness.

The main clinical distinction to be made is usually between spinal cord compression and Guillain–Barré syndrome. The onset of spinal cord dysfunction may be very acute, such as in transverse myelitis, or slowly progressive. A history of bony dysplasias or storage disorders such as a mucopolysaccharidosis suggest spinal cord compression. Guillain–Barré syndrome can have a very acute onset and differentiating it in the early phase of the illness can be difficult. Both disorders will show a flaccid, relatively symmetrical weakness of the lower limbs and trunk (depending on the site and extent and of the lesion). Autonomic dysfunction may be seen in both with skin changes, sweating and pulse and blood pressure instability. Cardiovascular instability can be life threatening. There may be dysfunction of bladder and bowel in both disorders although it is more consistently present in spinal cord lesions. Sensory signs with loss of pain, light touch, temperature discrimination and proprioceptive loss are commonly seen in spinal cord lesions. A sensory level may be apparent. Although sensory symptoms are present in Guillain–Barré syndrome, sensory signs are usually absent.

SPINAL CORD COMPRESSION

In children in whom spinal cord compression is slow in onset a history of progressive weakness and spasticity on examination may be seen. If the posterior columns are involved a loss of proprioception is expected. More extensive compression involving spinothalamic tracts will impair pain and temperature sensation. Corticospinal tract involvement leads to weakness, spasticity, hyperreflexia and extensor plantar response. Symptoms related to spinal route compression are unusual in childhood but may be seen in children with bony abnormalities or neurofibromatosis. Voluntary control over the bladder may be affected with difficulty in initiating micturition. Constipation may be seen.

TRANSVERSE MYELITIS

This is an inflammatory lesion of the spinal cord thought to be immune-mediated. Pathologically changes are similar to acute disseminated encephalomyelitis (ADEM) and similar preceding illnesses have been implicated. Direct viral infection of the spinal cord is unusual, but needs to be considered, and treatment with aciclovir may be necessary until herpes simplex virus infection is excluded. Borrelia infection may present in this way.

Transverse myelitis often presents over a matter of hours or days with symptoms and signs of acute spinal cord dysfunction, both sensory and motor. In 80%, the level is thoracic. Segmental edema of the spinal cord is seen on MRI imaging, although this may not be clear in the acute phase. An intraspinal tumor may be difficult to exclude on initial imaging.

There is no treatment that is of proven benefit. Steroids and intravenous immunoglobulin have been given to patients, but no systematic trials support their use. Investigation of blood and CSF for evidence of viral infection is often undertaken but rarely reveals a specific cause.

Clinical management follows the same lines as acute cord compression. Recovery from transverse myelitis may continue for 2 or 3 years. Return of sensation, motor function and finally bladder function often occurs sequentially. The prognosis, however, is difficult to predict. Approximately 20% of children have little or no recovery of function. Others recover fully.

PROGRESSIVE MYELOPATHY

Children who develop slowly progressive compression of the spinal cord may present diagnostic difficulties. Initial symptoms are usually a subtle stiffening of the legs followed by increasing difficulty caused by weakness of hip flexion and ankle dorsiflexion. Pyramidal weakness with hyperreflexia may then become apparent. Initial sensory involvement may cause paresthesiae below the level of the lesion, or if spinal thalamic pathways are involved, unpleasant and painful limb sensations.

Conditions that predispose to progressive myelopathy, particularly cervical myelopathy, include Down syndrome, the mucopolysaccharidoses and other storage disorders, bony dysplasias such as spondylometaphyseal dysplasia and, in children with CNS malformations, particularly, hindbrain malformations. It is important in boys to consider the peroxisomal disorder adrenomyelopathy, which is a form of adrenoleukodystrophy.

Children with spinal cord developmental disorders may develop progressive myelopathy due to lesions in the lumbar spinal cord or cauda equina. A small number of these may be due to the effect of tethering of the spinal cord and neurosurgical release of this may be useful. Tethering of the cord may lead to damage from traction as the cord cannot ascend with growth of the spinal column. The child may present with weakness in one leg or with bladder or bowel problems. Progressive neurological deterioration is an indication for surgery. If prophylactic untethering is not undertaken then careful neurological follow-up is mandatory, especially at peak growth periods. With modern MRI scanning it is now possible to diagnose the condition with more accuracy and criteria for operation should become clearer.

An important cause of tethering is a bony or fibrocartilaginous spur, which arises from a vertebral body and passes between the halves of a bifid cord – diastematomyelia. In some cases this fixes the cord and results in increasing traction with growth. In other cases the cord divides well above the spur and passes around the diastematomyelia in two separate dural canals – diplomyelia.

Damage from tethering or compression may cause spastic paraplegia. More frequently, however, the child presents with distal weakness of the foot with clawing of the toes and equinovarus posture and weakness of the peronei. Dribbling incontinence of urine may be an early feature and there may be sensory loss in the sacral territory, loss of ankle jerk and anal reflexes and trophic changes in the feet.

The presence of a cutaneous lipoma or lipomeningocele may penetrate in dumb-bell fashion into the spinal canal. It may cause an increase in pressure within the canal. Treatment of the lipoma can be difficult, as the cord itself, as well as nerve roots, may be enmeshed in fatty tissue.

GUILLAIN–BARRÉ SYNDROME

This is a form of acute or subacute polyneuropathy seen at all ages. Several variants are described including acute inflammatory demyelinating polyneuropathy, acute motor axonal neuropathy and Miller–Fisher syndrome. All have an immunological basis.

The clinical presentation in Guillain–Barré syndrome is with progressive motor weakness of more than one limb, and areflexia, of varying degree. The weakness should not be still progressing 4 weeks into the illness and should be relatively symmetrical. Most patients report a prodromal upper respiratory or gastrointestinal illness in the 4 weeks prior to the onset of weakness. Pain and paresthesia, without sensory signs, is a common feature at presentation. Autonomic symptoms, such as constipation, urinary retention and vasomotor disturbances, may occur. Although lower limb weakness is the usual presentation, it may be generalized and proximal or distal. Facial and bulbar weakness occurs in around a quarter of children. Abnormal eye movements, meningeal irritation and papilledema (rarely) may be present, making distinction from a primary cerebral problem difficult. Deep tendon reflexes are lost in most children early in the illness, but this is variable.

The most serious complication of Guillain–Barré syndrome is respiratory failure and ventilation is required in around 10% of cases. A rapid onset, cranial nerve involvement and high CSF protein are associated with the need for ventilation.[618] Monitoring of respiratory function through peak flow or formal forced vital capacity measurements (which may be difficult in the preschool child) is essential.

The maximum weakness is often present for several days before improvement starts. Recovery may take several months, but is complete in the majority of children. In 25% or so of children, mild long term problems such as foot drop or hand weakness is found. Mortality is 2–5%, usually related to respiratory failure. Features influencing prognosis include severity of distal weakness and length of time from maximal weakness to onset of recovery.

The CSF protein level is raised in almost all children with Guillain–Barré syndrome. The cell count should be > 10 cells/mm³. However, the protein may be normal during the first week of the illness. Nerve conduction studies characteristically show a patchy conduction block consistent with demyelination. They also may be normal in the first week of the illness. Investigation for the preceding infection may be useful. Many cases are associated with *Campylobacter jejuni* infection. This in turn may be associated with antiganglioside antibodies.

Treatment in Guillain–Barré syndrome is mainly symptomatic and supportive. Particular attention must be paid to symptoms and signs suggesting respiratory failure and autonomic instability. Regular measurement of respiratory function and consideration of elective ventilation are vital. Bulbar dysfunction may require nasogastric feeding. Chest and limb physiotherapy are helpful.

Specific treatment is now by the use of intravenous immunoglobulin (IVIG) or plasmapheresis. Studies have shown these to be equally effective.[619] The former is considerably easier to administer. IVIG in a dose of 2 g/kg split over 5 days is the conventional regimen although single dose regimens and regimens given over 3 days are also described. Treatment is usually given when the patient is non-ambulant or appears to be losing the ability to walk. Steroids are not beneficial. Symptomatic treatment for pain and paresthesia may be needed.

TRAUMATIC (ACCIDENTAL AND NON-ACCIDENTAL) BRAIN AND SPINAL CORD INJURY AND NEUROREHABILITATION

EPIDEMIOLOGY

Traumatic brain injury (TBI) is the commonest cause of acquired brain injury in children, and it is the commonest cause of accidental death in children. Severity is scored according to the Glasgow Coma Scale (GCS)

(Table 22.49). Five percent are severe (GCS ≤ 8) and another 5–10% are moderately severe (GCS 9–12). In severe TBI the male to female ratio is 2.75:1. Around 4 per 1000 children per year aged 15 years or under are admitted to hospital in the UK with TBI. The majority are minor head injuries but 5.6 per 100 000 per year are admitted to intensive care (ICU).[620] They are more likely to be socially deprived and pedestrian injuries are common in those requiring admission to ICU with a summer peak in the UK. The mortality rate is highest in pedestrian TBI, and the overall mortality rate for all severe TBI from the scene of trauma through ICU is 20–30%. Environmental as well as health care factors have a bearing on incidence and outcome, such as access to, and provision of, health care facilities, socioeconomic status of the child's family, the local environment (city or rural) and the amount of preventive legislation.[621]

It is probable that published figures for both incidence and mortality of head injury are an underestimate of the true figures. Though mortality is reducing with modern assessment and management (Fig. 22.40), there is still a major role for preventative measures such as compulsory seat belts, rear-facing baby car seats, speed control by cameras and traffic-calming measures, cycle helmets and modification of children's playgrounds with a forgiving surface such as forest bark and rails on slides. Most injuries result from falls or road traffic accidents, with the child as pedestrian, although the causes of head injury vary with the age of the child (Fig. 22.41).

The Royal College of Pediatrics and Child Health have published guidelines on the acute management of head injury in children.[622]

MECHANISMS OF BRAIN INJURY

Trauma can cause primary (or immediate) brain injury and secondary (or delayed) head injury.

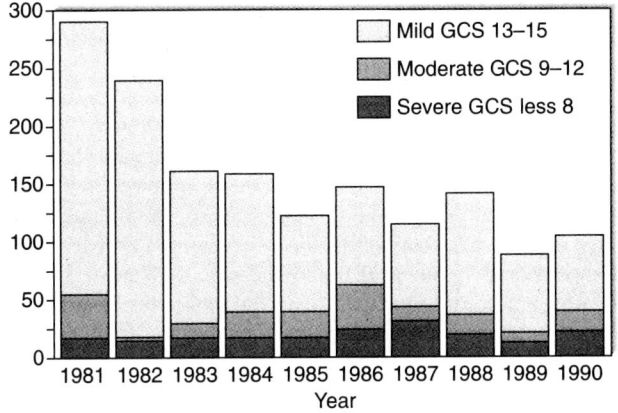

Fig. 22.40   Head injury in children under 16 years over a 10-year period. GCS, Glasgow Coma Score.

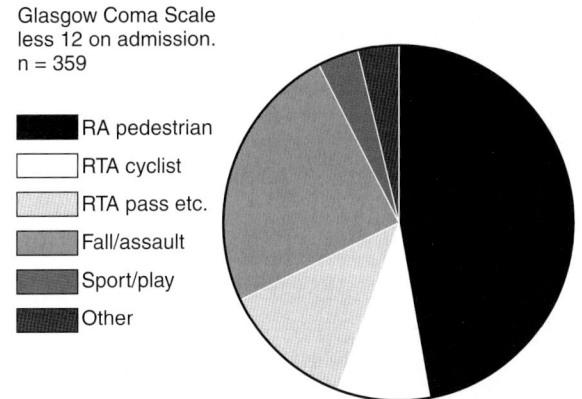

Fig. 22.41   Causes of accidental head injury in children under 16 years.

Primary brain injury

A high velocity, high energy impact over a small area will cause depressed or complex skull fractures and penetrating trauma. Knives, scissor blades and screwdrivers can penetrate the vault of the skull. Gunshot wounds are rare in the UK. Accidental penetrating injuries through the orbit or nose with sticks, pencils and toys occur. Objects in the mouth may penetrate the tonsillar fossa and cause carotid artery injury. There may be a delay of a day or more before the onset of neurological signs, as a dissecting aneurysm forms. Cavernous sinus thrombosis or caroticocavernous fistulae can result from intracranial injuries to the carotid artery. Blows, car accidents and falls commonly cause low velocity impacts and often lead to linear skull fractures. At the time of injury, linear or rotational forces of acceleration or deceleration cause deformation of the skull and its contents. The commonest primary brain injuries seen are due to shearing or contusion.

Shearing injury occurs when the brain moves, often with a rotational component, at the time of impact. The exact cascade from diffuse axonal injury to cerebral oedema is not yet fully understood, but children are more susceptible than adults to diffuse cerebral oedema. Secondary brain injury may ensue from this with compromise of cerebral perfusion. Inflammation, oxidative injury and iron-induced damage may provide therapeutic targets.[623] Primary contusions are best demonstrated on MRI. Deeper lesions correlate with poorer functional outcome at discharge, whereas initial GCS is more predictive of outcome at 12 months.[624]. The frontal lobes are commonly affected, even in the absence of focal lesions on MRI.[625] Volumetric MRI studies indicate reduced cerebral volume after TBI. Serial imaging implicates a degenerative process, with evidence of hemosiderin deposits as well as volume loss.[626] Contusion is often seen on the side of the brain opposite to to the site of impact (contra coup injury), thought to be due to the brain abutting on bony prominences especially in the frontal and temporal lobes. Compression injuries and lacerations of the brain are occasionally seen.

Collections of blood intraparenchymally, in the subarachnoid space, subdural or extradural spaces will add to cerebral irritation and increase intracranial pressure, diminishing cerebral blood flow.

Regional cerebral blood flow varies within a contused area compared with the surrounding brain, being reduced in the contusion.[627] Also cerebral vascular reactivity varies over time.[628] Such findings have consequences for targeting therapy. Ischemic change occurs in three phases.[629] The first is one of depressed metabolism with increased extracellular K^+ and intracellular Ca^{2+}. The second phase is one of energy failure and anoxic depolarization with loss of normal electrochemical gradients across the neuronal cell wall for different ions and concomitant release of neurotransmitters.[630] The third phase is neurodegenerative, which may take hours or days. The effectiveness of reperfusion and recovery processes will influence the final outcome.

Secondary brain injury

Much of the focus in the management of head injury has been on the prevention of secondary brain injury. It is assumed that primary brain injury is established by the time the child is seen at hospital. The clinical scenario of the child who 'talks and dies' is well known and although not all of these deaths are preventable, a number are.[621]

Associated thoracic, abdominal and pelvic injuries have the potential to cause additional brain injury through extracranial hypoxia and ischemia. Skilled resuscitation will minimize the impact of these on the brain. Status epilepticus will cause a further rise in intracranial pressure (ICP). Seizures require prompt recognition and management. Cerebral autoregulation of cerebral perfusion may be impaired in diffuse TBI. Raised ICP and status epilepticus need to be recognized and promptly treated. Cerebral autoregulation may be impaired. Diffuse cerebral edema may take 24 hours or more to reach its peak.

Intracranial hemorrhage (extradural hematoma, acute subdural hematoma, subarachnoid and intracerebral hemorrhage) needs prompt neurosurgical assessment and appropriate management. Extradural and subdural hemotmata may occur very soon after injury and may be evident on an initial CT scan. However they can accumulate over a period of hours or even minutes after admission. Repeat imaging is essential if GCS changes or neurological signs, such as focal weakness or pupillary asymmetry, appear. Subdural collections may take weeks to present clinically. Subarachnoid and intraventricular hemorrhage can lead to an acute or subacute hydrocephalus. Intraparenchymal hemorrhage with focal contusion may very occasionally require resective surgery to contain ICP. It is unusual, except very occasionally in infants, for the amount of blood loss intracranially to, by itself, cause shock and other sources of blood loss should be sought. Intracranial hemorrhages are usually seen in moderate or severe head injuries and rarely occur as an isolated injury.

MANAGEMENT OF ICP

The protocols most widely advocated for prevention of secondary injury depend on ICP monitoring and maintenance of cerebral perfusion pressure (CPP). Precise protocols vary between centers but all include attention to head-up neutral position in nursing and adequate sedation during ventilation. Significant rises in ICP which are sustained (over 5 minutes) may be managed with boluses of 20% mannitol or hypertonic saline. In adults there is evidence for a significantly greater and more sustained reduction of ICP with hypertonic saline.[631]

If these lines of management fail to contain ICP within accepted norms for the child's age other interventions which are still under clinical trial include moderate hypothermia and craniectomy. Outcome from TBI has been shown to relate to ICP and CPP. Younger children may tolerate a lower CPP. They also have a lower normal ICP than older children.[632] Moderate hypothermia may have more potential benefit for children than adults and trials so far show it to be safe.[633] In adults craniectomy has shown a significant increase in blood flow velocity and decrease in cerebrovascular resistance but no clear correlation with outcome yet.[634] A randomized controlled trial of early craniectomy after pediatric head trauma showed a clear benefit,[635] but a consensus on indications for such an invasive intervention has not yet been reached. There are consequences for the child in terms of a period of disfigurement and possible restrictions by education authorities on returning to school because of perceived vulnerability of the resected areas of the cranium. It may be several months before repair of the craniectomy can be effected.

Neuroimaging

The use of CT scanning has revolutionized the management of head injuries. CT scans are excellent for visualizing blood, bone and CSF. The main advantages are precise anatomical location of intracranial hematomas and accuracy in the diagnosis and differentiation of intracerebral, subdural and extradural hematomas.

Ultrasound may be useful in young children with an open anterior fontanel both for imaging and by utilizing Doppler for monitoring possible raised ICP and its subsequent response to treatment. There are great advantages in a portable, bedside and easily repeatable investigation with no radiation risk. The main disadvantages are the need for a 'window' through the skull through which to operate. MRI is mainly used to correlate neuroradiological abnormalities with functional disability in those children with residual neurological or neuropsychological deficits.[636]

Guidelines published on neuroimaging following head injury by the Royal College of Pediatrics and Child Health are shown in Figure 22.42.

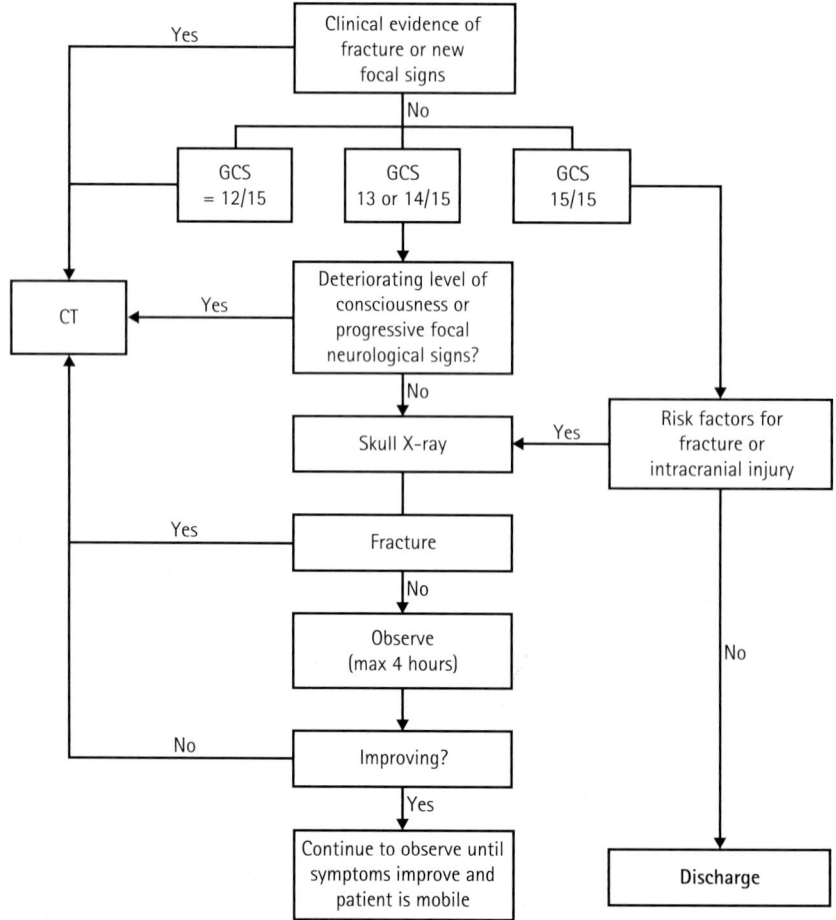

Fig. 22.42   Use of radiographic investigations in patients (> 5 years of age) with a head injury.

EARLY COMPLICATIONS OF TRAUMATIC BRAIN INJURY

Skull fractures

Forty percent of infants hospitalized with cranial trauma have skull fractures, but sequelae in the form of intracranial hematoma occur in only 8–22%. Leggate et al[637] showed that all infants, under 6 months of age, operated on for an extradural hematoma, had either a skull fracture or suture separation seen on X-ray. In a group of 40 infants with extradural hematomas, 90% had an abnormal X-ray. Most skull fractures are linear.

The skull in the neonate consists of poorly mineralized membranous bone. Linear fractures due to birth trauma occur but are rare in the compressive head injuries associated with traumatic deliveries, unless the baby is postmature. Under these circumstances, it offers little protection to the underlying brain, which is easily compressed in a ping-pong ball or Pond fracture. These may be associated with severe localized bruising and hemorrhage into the brain with minimal fracture.

Skull fractures do not heal by callus formation and so dating of the time of injury is difficult. If the edges are rounded and smooth, it is more than 2 weeks old. At autopsy, the margins are heaped, smooth and discolored with hemosiderin. A skull fracture normally heals in 2–3 months and has disappeared on X-ray by 6 months. In small infants the fracture site may not heal but form a growing skull fracture. This may present as a palpable, pulsating lump. Diagnosis is by X-ray. Management consists of closure of the underlying dural defect with natural or artificial membrane and closure of the bony defect either with an acrylic graft or a graft from the patient's own bone.

Most skull fractures are only medically significant if they:
- are depressed;
- go through the anterior fossa and cribriform plate, allowing CSF rhinorrhea and a risk of meningitis;
- go through the petrous temporal bone into the ear, allowing CSF otorrhea and a risk of meningitis;
- enter the sinuses or are across the skull base with brainstem injury.

Compound fractures, secondary to penetration injuries, may be obvious, or subtle (e.g. orbital trauma from an object such as a pencil or sharp pointed stick penetrating the medial aspect of the orbit, passing into the ethmoid sinus and through the cribriform plate into the intracranial cavity in its subfrontal compartment). Another common site for a penetrating injury is the temporal region. In all such cases, extensive preoperative investigation is required, including CT scanning and MRI angiography, prior to a thorough exploration of the penetrating tract with debridement of damaged brain and formal closure of the dura. The use of prophylactic antibiotics is controversial, but intravenous cefotaxime is often used.

Infection

Basal skull fractures may present with bilateral 'black eyes', or CSF leaks from the ear or nose. The eardrums should be examined routinely in all TBI to look for evidence of bleeding behind the tympanum, another sign of basal skull fracture. Prophylactic use of antibiotics in basal skull fracture is also controversial, but meningitis complicating such head injuries can be early or late with CSF leakage and must always be borne in mind. A persistently raised core temperature with raised peripheral white count and inflammatory markers signal possible meningitis. Lumbar puncture may be hazardous in acute TBI as peak oedema can be as late as 3–5 days in severe trauma. Repeat imaging and the clinical picture guide the decision whether to use antibiotics without LP. This is not infrequently the case unless ventricular CSF is available from a ventricular drain. A third generation cephalosporin (with metronidazole if anaerobic infection is possible as with penetrating wounds) given intravenously is the preferred choice.

Deafness

Fractures of the petrous temporal bone, with or without CSF otorrhea, can result in deafness and/or facial nerve palsy from direct cranial injury. Deafness can ensue with such events with only mild or moderate TBI. All such patients need formal audiology as part of head injury rehabilitation care, as do all children with severe TBI.

Diabetes insipidus

Diabetes insipidus may be seen following basal skull fractures and following any brain injury. Most cases are transient. Management consists of maintenance of the systemic blood pressure by adequate fluid replacement and desmopressin (DDAVP) to reduce the continuing urine output. In other cases, diabetes insipidus develops following profound and prolonged raised ICP. This is a poor prognostic indicator and is often accompanied by incipient brain death. Some children will survive with chronic diabetes insipidus following basal skull fracture and severe TBI. Patients in this situation should be assessed later for the possible development of panhypopituitarism.[638]

Extradural hematomas

An extradural hematoma consists of a collection of blood lying between the skull and the dura. It results either from torn dural veins or bleeding from meningeal arteries. Half of all cases occur in children under 2 years. The development of symptoms and signs may be rapid but, often in children, occur over several hours or days. Following a significant head injury, the child will become progressively drowsy with a deterioration in the GCS. Vomiting, focal weakness and ipsilateral third nerve palsy may be seen. A skull fracture is seen in only half of children. CT scan will show the hematoma. Neurosurgical evacuation is usually necessary although a few cases may be managed conservatively.

Subdural hematomas

These result from tearing of the bridging veins as they cross the subdural space. The hematoma lies between the dural and the arachnoid membranes. Subdural hematomas are conventionally classified as acute or chronic, although there is significant overlap. Subdural hematomas are nearly always caused as a result of trauma, with rotation between brain and dura. This causes shearing of bridging veins and is the likely mechanism in non-accidental injuries caused by shaking, with or without impact. Subdural hematomas are occasionally seen as a consequence of bleeding from penetrated vessels in depressed skull fractures[639] or in primary penetrating injuries, or in association with brain contusions with oozing from surface veins.

Acute subdural hematomas may be isolated or can be associated with brain contusion and/or skull fracture. The symptoms are those of raised ICP. Seizures are common. If there is no clear history of significant accidental trauma then the possibility of non-accidental injury should be considered. The management is that of raised ICP, with possible evacuation of the hematoma. Some thin hematomas with no evidence of midline brain shift or significantly raised ICP can be managed non-operatively. All should be discussed with a neurosurgical team. CT scan will show a high density, often unilateral, collection. If the scan is done some days after the injury, the collection may be isointense to brain and can be missed. After 2–4 weeks it becomes hypodense in comparison with brain tissue.[640] The collection usually lies over the convexity of the cerebral hemispheres, but may involve the posterior fossa, particularly in babies and infants. Underlying brain injuries may best be visualized with ultrasound and MRI.

Chronic subdural hematomas occur mainly in children under 1 year of age and may follow known trauma or may be apparently idiopathic. They may arise following instrumental delivery. Non-accidental injury must always be considered. The presentation may be with signs and symptoms of raised ICP, isolated macrocephaly, vomiting, failure to thrive or seizures. Chronic subdurals are usually bilateral lying over the frontoparietal regions. Though bleeding is probably responsible for initiating the process, why the hematoma organizes and becomes chronic is incompletely understood. A membrane surrounds the clot and fluid is probably absorbed across it by osmosis. The collection acts as a space-occupying lesion. There may be associated hydrocephalus, although the role of subarachnoid blood should then be considered.

The most appropriate management of chronic subdural hematomas is not straightforward. If the collection is evacuated, it will often reform within 24 hours or so, since a gap between brain and skull is formed by the chronic nature of the lesion allowing fluid to collect again. Tapping is usually reserved for treatment of symptoms of raised ICP rather than done routinely. In some children, placement of a subdural–peritoneal shunt may be required if accumulation of fluid continues.

Chronic subdural hematomas on CT scan appear as extra-axial collections of fluid iso- or hypointense to brain tissue. Depending on whether there has been associated damage to the brain, brain atrophy may be seen. MRI scanning may be helpful in determining the age of the collections.

The prognosis for subdural hematomas depends on the underlying cause and any associated brain injury from raised ICP or direct trauma. There is a mortality (mainly from acute subdural hematomas) of up to 3%. At follow-up 57–80% of survivors have normal development.

Intraparenchymal hemorrhage

Most intraparenchymal hemorrhages are associated with edema or contusion and are small in size, although often multiple. They are usually seen in the white matter, brainstem, cortex and corpus callosum. Operative treatment is rarely needed. Management is of the raised ICP, which almost always accompanies intraparenchymal hemorrhages. Intracerebellar hemorrhage is rare but may present with acute cerebellar signs, raised ICP, bilateral sixth nerve palsies or acute hydrocephalus.

Hydrocephalus

This may occur early in the period after head injury, in association with subarachnoid or intraventricular hemorrhage or localized brain edema. It may also be seen in the weeks or months following injury resulting in prolonged coma. It can be difficult, in some cases, to distinguish between hydrocephalus and postinjury cerebral atrophy with ventricular dilation. Pressure monitoring may be required. Treatment is by ventriculoperitoneal shunt or third ventriculostomy.

Seizures

In the conscious or nonparalyzed child, seizures will usually be clinically obvious. In an unconscious or paralyzed, ventilated child there may be clinical signs of seizures such as changes in systemic blood pressure or ICP, accompanied by tachycardia with or without pupillary dilation. Similar signs can also be seen during the recovery period after head injury as a non-epileptic phenomenon and are termed brainstem release symptoms. Immediate control of the seizure may be effectively obtained with lorazepam (0.1 mg/kg) given intravenously or diazepam (0.5 mg/kg) given rectally. Continuing treatment consists of intravenous phenytoin (18 mg/kg) or phenobarbital (15–20 mg/kg) and thereafter by maintaining blood levels in the therapeutic range. Resistant seizures may require control with a thiopental or midazolam infusion.

In the acute phase of injury antiepileptic drugs can be used to treat observed seizures. However EEG monitoring has shown that electrical seizures may still be recorded in spite of apparently protective levels of medication.[641] There is no evidence that continuation of treatment after the acute phase is protective against late seizures. With increasing awareness of potentially adverse effects of anticonvulsants on neurodevelopmental pathways such as the promotion of apoptosis, prophylactic treatment is not recommended.

OUTCOME

The prognosis for a head-injured child is related to the severity of the initial impairment of consciousness. Modern imaging techniques and easy access to neurosurgical units have diminished the mortality of treatable lesions such as acute extradural hematomas. The mortality of extradural hematoma in the pre-CT scan era was between 10% and 30% but is now reduced to almost zero. Overall most series of severely head-injured patients show a combined mortality and morbidity of approximately 30%. About 10% will die, 5% at the accident scene and 5% in the first few days. Details concerning the long term morbidity of head injuries is given in the section, in this chapter, on rehabilitation

TRAUMATIC SPINAL INJURY

Trauma is the commonest cause of acute spinal injury in children. However children comprise 1–10% of all spinal injury patients. They are relatively protected, compared with adults, by their greater ligamentous laxity and differing anatomy. However they can sustain serious spinal cord injury without radiological abnormality (SCIWORA). This comprised 6% of pediatric spinal injuries in a recent study from Baltimore.[642] Motor vehicle accident is the commonest cause in infants. Birth injury and non-accidental injury are other possible causes but their incidence is unclear. Falls are commonest in the 2–9 year olds, and sports injuries in the 10–14 year olds. The overall mortality rate is around 4%, attributable mainly to associated injuries especially TBI.

Spinal protection should govern the physical handling and management of all unconscious children with injury. The ABC of critical care must always apply to spinal injury with or without coma. Examination may reveal tenderness, swelling, bruising, or a palpable defect along the spinous processes.[643] Acute and severe spinal cord compression may cause spinal shock. There is complete flaccid paralysis, loss of reflexes and retention of urine and feces. Autonomic involvement may be severe and life threatening. In spinal shock there is both a direct effect on nerve conduction by the compressing lesion and also an indirect effect due to compromise of the vascular supply to the cord leading to ischemia and edema below the site of compression. MRI can reveal soft tissue, ligamentous or disc injury.[644] Cervical cord lesions may lead to respiratory and diaphragmatic muscle weakness requiring ventilation. Surgical decompression may reverse paralysis and MR scanning is urgent in this context. Intravenous dexamethasone is of proven benefit.

In the medium term, respiratory insufficiency, temperature control, bowel and bladder function and skin integrity may need weeks and months of expert medical and nursing management. These complex needs are best met in a spinal unit. Long term problems include possible paralysis with spastic elements, a neurogenic bowel and bladder, ventilator dependency and pressure sores. Overall the prognosis is better for children than adults.[645] Severe high grade injuries tend to be at the atlanto-occipital level with early death and complete cord involvement. Cervical dislocation carries a poor prognosis. However recovery for other categories can proceed over a prolonged postinjury period of 1 year at least.

REHABILITATION OF TRAUMATIC BRAIN INJURY
Long term sequelae
Physical

Physical neurological deficits often appear the most serious initially. Occasionally a severe physical deficit may remain with long term dependency. More often, sometimes several weeks or days from the injury, an accelerated phase of recovery is seen, leading to independent walking and restoration of fine motor skills for self-care. Fine motor deficits tend to be more prevalent than gross motor 12 months into recovery.[646] Where there has been basal ganglia injury there can be a delayed onset of choreoathetosis, which is difficult to treat. Early onset visual impairment and extrapyramidal signs often settle over the early weeks though visual perceptual difficulties may persist for longer. Otherwise measurable improvement in physical recovery may be detectable over 2 years or more.

Problems with feeding and swallowing, and protection of the airways may be pseudobulbar or dyspraxic in origin. Delayed return of language and articulation difficulties can be expected in this situation. A tracheostomy may be required to enable the child to be weaned from the ventilator, but was required in the long term in only 1 out of 82 children in the North West of England brain injury rehabilitation study.[646]

Risk of epilepsy

Seizures following TBI are classified as early in the first week, and thereafter they are classified as late. A Finnish study[647] showed that children of 7 years or under were more likely to have early seizures than adolescents or adults. Overall early fits with depressed skull fracture related to the origin of late post-traumatic seizures. Risk factors for late seizures include persisting neurological deficit, linear skull fracture and a persisting lesion on imaging. Late seizures did relate to a worse functional outcome in this study, and in the North West of England brain injury rehabilitation study[646] the need for anticonvulsants at 12 months from discharge correlated with a worse cognitive and behavioral outcome. In the Finnish study there was no correlation between late seizures and severity of brain injury scores without focal lesions. Barlow et al in Edinburgh concluded that the severity of early post-traumatic seizures related to the severity of the primary brain injury and the neurodevelopmental outcome.[648]

A large study of 4541 children and adults with TBI of varying severity showed an overall standardized incidence ratio for late epilepsy of 3.1. This ranged from 1.5 for mild head injury, 2.9 for moderate head injury to 17.0 for severe brain injury. Significant risk factors for late seizures in this study included cerebral contusion with subdural hematoma, skull fracture, loss of consciousness or amnesia for > 24 hours and an age > 65 years.[649]

Language, behavior and cognition

These have overlapping consequences for return to the family environment, to education and to society at large. Long term disorders are common, having far-reaching effects beyond childhood into adult prospects for family life and success in the workplace. Behavioral change has been reported by mothers of brain-injured children and young men 13 years after injury. Significantly those mothers were more likely to suffer from depression.[650]

Language

Language involvement is obvious in a mute or grossly dysphasic child but lesser degrees will be missed unless a planned assessment approach is adhered to. This is important because impairments of more complex higher language processing will disable information processing. This has consequences for education and social integration, compounding behavioral disorder. Language deficits detected by speech therapy assessment into the second year of recovery are associated with long term problems in written expressive language.

Early speech difficulties range from mutism, through dyspraxia to dysarthria and related swallowing difficulties.[651] Word-finding problems are common, as is lack of organization of thoughts, leading to expressive limitations that can be frustrating for the child with consequent behavioral reactions. The use of language can become concrete, alongside inappropriate social interactions such as impulsiveness, a tendency to tactless outspokenness and untimely interruption.

Behavior

The emotional and behavioral characteristics of frontal lobe dysfunction are most frequently associated with TBI. Executive functioning is usually affected, influencing cognitive as well as social performance. Commonly agreed aspects of executive function include the initiation, choosing and planning of tasks, 'seeing ahead', shifting thoughts and attention to find solutions, retaining information actively in working memory, monitoring one's own behavior and attaining social discernment. These aspects have been reviewed in detail by Levin and Hanten.[652] Normal executive function allows individuals to recognize when a problem-solving strategy is failing, moving them on to another logical approach. In executive dysfunction the individual is distractable/haphazard in the approach to problem solving and may return to failed strategies.

Prefrontal and frontotemporal damage may lead to typical psychiatric symptoms of mood swings, impulsivity, attention deficit, disinhibition, aggressive reactions and agitation. Other features may include over-talkativeness, repetition and obsession with ideas that, in extreme cases, may lose touch with reality. This can be associated with extreme restlessness, making the child difficult to contain. Over-familiarity and lack of normal social inhibition frequently disenchants friends and teachers who regard the child as rude and disruptive. The child's social set of friends may change on return to school as they may attract more dysfunctional children, leading them into trouble or delinquency. Frontal lobe dysfunction is found in about two thirds of severely brain injured children.[646]

Family functioning is affected.[653] In the home environment, parents experience the effects of the cognitive and emotional changes in terms of the child's impulsivity, flaring tempers, lack of motivation and poor judgment. The stress is multifactorial for a parent trying to steer between safe containment on the one hand, and encouragement toward independence on the other. Siblings are affected and family happiness may be seriously diminished.

Though the concept of plasticity of the immature brain may apply to aspects of severe brain injury recovery, there is a lack of evidence for the popular concept that the young recover better. In one study of 118 head-injured children under 12 years, children injured under the age of 5 years with left hemisphere injury had the poorest cognitive scores.[654] Frontal lobe damage at such an age may not become fully apparent in its social consequences until adolescence when frontal lobe development accelerates.

Cognition

Recent learning may be lost in severe head injury and the processes of new learning affected. Problems reside with attention, encoding information into memory, and retrieval of information when needed. Some brain-injured children exhibit many features of attention deficit hyperactivity disorder but slowing of information processing speed appears to be specific to TBI. Classroom learning will be hindered also by the distractions in that environment. Studying or revising for examinations becomes difficult and stressful, increasing the cycle of behavioral dysfunction with anxiety, poor self-esteem and possibly depression. Protracted post injury headache patterns and fatigue are likely to worsen in an unsupported school situation.

It usually takes between 6 and 9 months for behavioral and cognitive consequences to be recognized. By this time, the child may seem to his/her teachers to be the same person physically as before the injury. The outcome, without planned re-entry to education, is usually criticism of behavior and 'lack of effort', leading to failure or even exclusion from school. In secondary years, leading to important exam years, the timetable may be overwhelming for the severely or moderately head-injured teenager. A reduction in timetable can allow achievement to progress in time to consolidate that aspect of recovery, especially into the second year. Otherwise the child may 'drop out' of educational opportunities altogether, with all the associated adverse consequences for adult life.

The effects of language deficits on learning have been discussed above. Dominant hemisphere injury may hinder sequencing abilities important to spelling and mathematical concepts. Additionally, frontal lobe deficits in executive functioning interfere with the logistical approach to problem solving. Visual–perceptual deficits as well as fine motor problems will impair the accurate and speedy recording of work. It is easy to conceive how such deficits will be compounded by frontal lobe dysfunction.

Detailed psychometric testing, as well as clinical psychological support for the child and family is essential but the timing is crucial, as tests done too soon will be too pessimistic in an evolving recovery.

PREDICTION OF OUTCOME

The GCS 72 hours after injury was found to correlate with survival and degree of disability of the child at discharge in a study by Michaud et al.[655] The quality of eye movements has also been shown to relate to outcome. Children may recover from ventilation and sedation initially with purposive movements, which are then lost in a phase of brainstem release mechanisms of extensor posturing, sweating and sympathetic instability. This may take a number of weeks to subside before more encouraging physical signs emerge. It is important to be alongside the child to assess the early examination in the recovery phase. Jaffe et al[656] found a correlation between the GCS in the emergency admission room and later cognitive impairment. Post-traumatic amnesia (PTA) lasting for more than 7 days is also associated with greater cognitive and psychiatric deficits. PTA parallels neurosurgical severity of injury scores in this way.

Intracranial pressure measurements above 20mmHg appear to correlate adversely with survival rather than quality of outcome in Michaud's study of TBI. In Minns' study of medical brain injury, cerebral perfusion maintained above 40mmHg predicted a better quality of survival.[657] However there are age-related norms for ICP and cerebral perfusion pressure.[632]

Mention has already been made of the relationship between the depth of MR scan lesions and the severity of head injury.[624] Single photon emission tomography (SPECT) has a stronger relationship with neuropsychological outcome than MR findings.[658] Functional MR is likely to be more informative still, but limited in its availability at this time.

BRAIN INJURY REHABILITATION
In the intensive care unit (ICU)
In a severe brain injury this is a time of invasive procedures and intensive monitoring, such as the evacuation of extradural collections, exploration of depressed fractures and insertion of intracranial pressure monitoring systems. Many disciplines may be involved in the circumstances of multiple injury. The records quickly bear witness to important multidisciplinary interventions. However it is very important to find time to document a full pediatric history and examination. It is very occasionally the case that the 'head injury' may not be the cause of the child's loss of consciousness. The history also allows the pediatric neurologist to get to know the child and family, which may be important to the clinical care of the child in ICU, and will most certainly be of prime importance in supporting and providing for the child and family in the recovery phase. For those children who do not survive, this getting to know stage is of no less importance for later counseling.

The neurological examination is important in interpreting possible seizures and abnormal patterns of posture and movement. Purposeful movements recorded when sedation is first lifted may be overwhelmed by a phase of brainstem reflexes with increased extensor tone and excessive sympathetic drive. This is reflected in periods of hypertension, excessive sweating with notable sodium losses and blotchy flushing of the skin. Most often the original picture of purposeful patterns of movement will reappear with a resumed recovery, though uncertainties may reign over a period of weeks.

The family needs preparation and explanation of the stages ahead. These stages will entail adjustments to new environments such as a high dependency ward, a children's ward, and eventually the care of the pediatric teams in the child's district of residence. It is advantageous to the child and family to coordinate the continuing care of various surgical specialties in a neurorehabilitation setting.

The rehabilitation ward
After the ICU, multidisciplinary care is essential allowing all participants to meet on a regular basis to share information and observations. This needs to be facilitated by a nominated member of that team to whom the family and various specialties can refer usually on a weekly basis. When the child is well enough it is important to include them according to age and awareness, and sometimes siblings can join in to the mutual benefit of the child and his/her sibling. In the UK the consultant community pediatrician (CCP) for the child's district should be informed at an early stage. A visit by the CCP and relevant district therapy representative enhances the early provision of services, and some will be assisted by a

period of stay in their district hospital to allow all members of the child development center (CDC) team to plan continuation of rehabilitation.

Those involved will include a combination or all of the following.

The child and family
The family supply information about the child before the injury. This is important on a clinical and developmental level, and is important to the understanding of the child's personality, likes and dislikes. Parents need to express their concerns and receive support and understanding at a time which is inevitably fraught. They will be most aware of subtle changes in their child and provide one of the few constant factors in this situation. Parents need to have their confidence restored by being involved in their child's care, after the experience of ICU, when they handed over that role to others. They need to learn about the likely recovery pattern clinically, and the recovery pathway practically and temporally. There will be many items important to them and the child, like returning to favorite activities, advice on degrees of freedom and supervision, and how they will get back to their school and friendships. There must be a point of contact made clear before discharge.

The child and family will need to be encouraged to engage with changing teams of carers in the moves from ICU to the ward, on to district level and finally home. Teams in these different situations need to be mutually supportive and share information. However, no matter how much information is handed over, each service has to be allowed space and opportunity to get to know the child and create their own relationship with the child and family. Each team must use their own skills and initiative to assess changing needs in an evolving recovery. The need for team meetings carries on through all stages of recovery, including pre-discharge planning meetings with community services and in the early months/years of return to education. Specialist head injury liaison nurses play a valuable role.

Pediatrician/pediatric neurologist
Regular examination, integration of advice from other specialties and facilitation of team meetings constitute the main elements of care. The importance of pediatric input at every stage has been discussed above, especially to communicate with the child and family.

Nursing staff
Nurses spend most time with the child and family. They will be next to the parents in their perception of the child's recovery, physically and psychologically. Parents tend to share their anxiety or frustration first with them, and in this way the nurses can alert appropriate team members to address those problems. They are in a position of advocacy for the child and family, and are able to look ahead at the practical challenges of living at home.

Physical therapists
Physiotherapy and occupational therapy need a distraction-free working area and access to equipment. Therapy may be passive in the bed-bound patient, to limit contractures and provide chest care. As awareness improves they will work through elements of postural control. Early therapy may be limited by a confused pattern of recovery in the child who resists interaction. Such a pattern is often followed by fluctuating lucidity interspersed with intense tiredness and the need to sleep. All the team then need to plan their interventions so as to take advantage of the more wakeful times without overwhelming the child.

Equipment that can be important at this time includes tilt tables enabling a gradual readjustment to the upright posture as well as stretching tight Achilles tendons; wheelchair; walking aids; orthoses to help contain positional deformities; access to pool therapy and gymnasium areas.

Therapists work to restore independence to the child for personal and everyday needs. Occupational therapists contribute to the assessment of the child in the preparation for return to school, including implications of fine motor and perceptual deficits. Keyboard skills may need to be introduced to enhance the recording of work. Fine motor control and sitting position may also be crucial to an appraisal of feeding, which overlaps with the speech therapist's and nurses' roles.

In the community, the therapists need to plan ahead with colleagues for the return home, including housing implications and school placement. They will visit and assess those environments to give advice for adaptations and supervision. Initial school timetables can depend to some extent on the outcome of these assessments.

Speech therapy

Where there is bulbar and brainstem dysfunction affecting mouth opening and safe swallowing, the speech therapist may first have a role in desensitization programs to overcome reflex patterns before tastes or feeds are offered. They may contribute to assessments of tongue, lip and palate movements when airway protection is uncertain. Augmentive communication (the use of communication aids) is very important to children who have lost speech centrally with aphasia or dyspraxia, or peripherally with bulbar weakness. Awareness and degrees of understanding return in advance of expressive language, leading to frustration for the child who cannot speak. Where there has been base of skull fracture, the possibility of deafness must be examined.

Examination of higher functioning complex language performance is extremely important as a more likely long-lasting disability, especially when detected into the second year of recovery. Deficits have consequences for cognitive performance in the long term. Social language tends to return to a degree that may mask higher deficits. Semantic-pragmatic difficulties may be perceived alongside frontal lobe dysfunction as subtle personality change by family and friends.

Teaching

A hospital-based teaching facility is an essential component of rehabilitation, concerned with assessing and facilitating remediation of learning difficulties consequent upon brain injury. The teacher needs to be involved at an early stage of ward recovery, even when the patient is still drowsy or confused. This assists in planning assessments according to the pattern of recovery. Fundamental elements of learning are worked through so as not to take anything for granted in terms of basic perceptual skills. Dedicated teaching areas with mainstream curriculum facilities are essential, and it is important to be aware that the availability of teaching in hospital for children with acquired disability such as traumatic brain injury is a statutory right of the child in many countries such as the UK.[659]

Parental permission should be obtained early to allow the hospital teacher to contact the child's mainstream school to obtain background information on pre-injury ability and attainment, and to inform the child's school about the likely degree of recovery and persisting difficulties when the child returns to education. The school's special educational needs coordinator should be encouraged to visit and should be involved in discharge planning meetings.

In the UK the school health service, including community pediatric nurses, will support teachers as they get to know the child during home teaching and as reintegration into school takes place. The community pediatrician will liase with the Educational Psychology Service, which will be notified well before discharge.

Educational psychology involvement needs to be more flexible than the standard approach in the UK of a statement of special educational needs,the legal instrument for ensuring the provision of appropriate support for the child. In the 6 months that assessment and provision usually takes, the child with brain injury is likely to have changed, usually improved, in their abilities. A modification of the child's school timetable or a reduction in the proposed number of state examination subjects, including a reassessment of aims for post 16 years, is essential for children entering years 10 and 11 of mainstream school.

Clinical psychology and psychiatry

The clinical psychologist provides an essential understanding of the emotional, behavioral and psychometric consequences of the injury. This involves an inclusive approach to the family, including siblings. The consequences of frontal lobe dysfunction can be modified by a behavioral approach, and the clinical psychologist can engage directly with education in the formulation of a return to school. The psychologist's input into team meetings very often provides support to the team as well.

Psychiatry and psychology roles overlap, since social disinhibition is a specific psychiatric feature characteristic of traumatic brain injury. Occasionally the marked restlessness and aggressive mood swings that accompany the early confused phase of recovery merit treatment with medication such as methylphenidate or risperidone.

Social services

The learning support limb of the social services team can provide important practical support to families on discharge where safe containment of the child is an issue. They also have a role, with community occupational therapy advice, in assessing housing needs, including access (steps and stairs, corridors and doorways, toilet and bathing facilities, seating) and financial budgeting for adaptations in the home in the event of persisting physical deficits.

Discharge planning

The success of this depends on early involvement of the district community team of CCP and therapists. In fact it is likely that the severely injured child will need a period of time in their district hospital under the care of the CCP to enable all of this team to get to know the child and embark on their own problem solving approach. The North West rehabilitation study[646] showed that this enhances discharge provision of need compared to those children who have no CCP visit or district stay.

While the child is an inpatient, it is essential that the family, including the child whenever possible, should participate in weekly rehabilitation meetings where progress reports can be shared and plans adjusted accordingly. Caregivers need to understand the program that will take over well before discharge. Restrictions on activities need to be considered in a practical way that does not stifle the child's independence nor expose them to physical risk. This situation must be revisited and the family helped to adjust as recovery continues.

Children injured in their early years may not reveal the full consequences of frontal lobe dysfunction until adolescence, when frontal lobe development occurs. It is advisable therefore to follow all these children throughout their school years, with good liaison between Community Child Health, Social Services and Education. A proportion will need support into adulthood. There can be long term effects on employment prospects, social integration and prospects for a family life.

Outcome measures and standards of service provision

Outcome and standards of care are linked, one influencing the other. Standards of care should be part of the clinical process, and the outcomes should allow comparison. Disability outcome scores may attempt to incorporate the adequacy of provision of need, but generally this is confounded by the influence of medical factors that may not lend themselves to therapeutic correction. It is difficult to show the outcome benefit of, for instance, physiotherapy, occupational therapy, speech therapy or even surgical intervention such as intracranial pressure monitoring on the basis of disability scores. This is the problem when considering impairments consequent upon irreversible aspects of neurological injury. The King's Outcome Scale for Childhood Head Injury (KOSCHI) is a modification of the Glasgow Coma Scale for children.[660] Outcome is expanded descriptively under categories 1–5 as follows:

1. Death.
2. Vegetative.
3a and b. Severe disability.
4a and b. Moderate disability.
5a and b. Good recovery.

Interobserver reliability is less good for categories 3, 4 and 5, than 1 and 2. More studies are needed on the ways that effective help can be delivered to children with deficits and to their carers.[661] This demands an agreed assessment of need, provision of care, assessment of progress, and quality of life scores that take account of the adaptive competence of the child and their environment. Adult studies have shown that patients self-report a greater recovery than do their relatives or clinicians. Patients focus on residual physical deficits, whereas carers are more aware of cognitive and behavioral change.[662] This may partly reflect the lack of insight accompanying frontal lobe dysfunction. Relatives' questionnaires show a large degree of consistency over time.[663] In children, the Pediatric Quality of Life Inventory promises to be a useful tool, with versions developed for infants and toddlers, as well as self-reported (child) forms for children aged 5 and older.[664]

Setting standards according to unmet needs requires an approach to care that serves a spectrum of disorders needing rehabilitation and identifies environmental and personal factors, which may act as barriers or facilitators toward a successful outcome. It allows monitoring according to met and unmet needs. Key outcomes such as family adjustment, psychosocial adjustment, re-entry to education, the attainment of life skills progressing to employment and later family life all identify the essential members of a rehabilitation team. Standards of care start with the resourcing of these services, according to the phase of recovery, not only in pediatric hospitals but also locally with community pediatric services, educational services and transitionally into adult services as well.

NON-ACCIDENTAL HEAD INJURY (see also Ch. 6)

Child abuse has an incidence of 6/1000 of the childhood population.[665] However, less than 10% of all physically abused children will have a significant head injury, with brain involvement. In these children, approximately 75% also have bruises, 20% have burns, 40% have fractures and intracranial damage is seen in 40%. All socioeconomic groups are involved and 60–90% of abusers were themselves abused as children. Children born prematurely, children with learning difficulties and those with cerebral palsy are especially vulnerable. The outlook for children who survive non-accidental head injury is worse than following accidental injury. Neurological sequelae were reported in 30% of survivors with 57% having an IQ below 80.[666]

Neurological presentation of child abuse

The neurological presentation is not specific and may not immediately suggest abuse. The history may be vague. The child may present as an acute encephalopathy. Meningitis, encephalitis or metabolic disease may be suspected, rather than poisoning or shaking. Some children may present with repeated episodes of encephalopathy. Fabrication of symptoms, especially seizures (fictitious epilepsy), is a form of child abuse in Munchausen by proxy (Meadows syndrome). Seizure or status epilepticus is a possible presentation of non-accidental head injury; they are usually accompanied by encephalopathy. Attempts at suffocation may present as odd turns, seizures, apneic attacks, cyanotic attacks, rigidity or coma. It may be perpetrated in hospital as well as at home.[667]

The abused child may present with a traumatic head injury with scalp bruising, swelling, lacerations, skull fracture and neurological signs and symptoms. Injuries remote from the head may cause seizures and coma (e.g. burns, encephalopathy). In shaking injury, there may be no evidence of trauma to the head unless there has been an associated impact. The commonest presentation is as an unwell child who is irritable or excessively quiet, refusing feeds and vomiting. The infant is often hypothermic, pale and shocked with low blood pressure and tachycardia suggesting sepsis, hypoglycemia or intussusception. There may be seizures, tonic extensor spasms, breathing difficulties and cyanotic attacks.[668] A history of an attempted resuscitation is often given. It may be contended that the child was shaken because he/she was found gravely ill rather than this being the cause of the illness. Studies have shown that the force required to produce shaking injury in an infant is such that 'no reasonable parent would apply such force' (American Academy of Pediatrics). Rib fractures and retinal hemorrhages are commonly associated and are extremely rare after cardiopulmonary resuscitation.[669,670]

Skull fractures

Most accidental fractures are simple linear fractures, usually parietal and over the vertex or coming from the coronal suture. If the fracture line branches, crosses suture lines, is bilateral, stellate, multiple with separate fractures, more than 50 mm wide at presentation or expands as a growing fracture, then non-accidental fracture is more likely. A depressed fracture, especially of the occipital bone in a child under 3 years, is suggestive of abuse. Any of these features merits a full skeletal survey.[671]

A history that the infant fell from a couch or suffered some similar trauma is often obtained. Of 330 children under 2 years of age who were witnessed falling from couches, cots, etc., skull fractures occurred in only three and a subdural hematoma in only one. Fewer than 10% had evidence of concussion.[672]

Shaking whiplash injuries

The injury most characteristic of non-accidental head injury is the whiplash shaking injury. The full picture, originally described by Caffey,[673] consists of a subdural hematoma, massive cerebral edema, hemorrhagic retinopathy, fractured ribs and metaphyseal injury. These may occur in any combination. Often there is no skull fracture, bruising of the scalp, scalp edema or other evidence of direct head trauma. However, when present, these features suggest direct impact. This may be due to the head banging against a hard surface during the shaking, or the child may be thrown or dropped on the floor after the shaking or may be hit against a wall. The manner in which shaking injuries are caused have been admitted to by a number of perpetrators.[668,674,675]

The commonest age for shaking injury is 5 months. In children under 2 years of age 64% of head injuries and 95% of severe head injuries are due to abuse.[676] Of 100 children studied in a carefully controlled prospective study,[677] 24% of head injuries were presumed inflicted and these carried a higher mortality and risk of permanent brain damage than true accidental injuries. Many children die from their injuries.

The child may be shaken by the shoulders and upper arms, causing spiral humeral fractures or periosteal avulsion. Humeral fractures in very young children, excluding supracondylar fractures, were all found to be due to child abuse.[678] Alternatively the smaller child may be held by the rib cage, which is often severely squeezed, leaving finger-mark bruising and fractured ribs and causing a high central venous pressure which may contribute to the retinopathy. Rib fractures are very rarely caused in young infants by falls, coughing or birth injury; even very vigorous cardiac massage and resuscitation do not normally fracture ribs.[669] Concurrent injuries to the cervical spine with spinal epidural hemorrhage and bruising of the cervicomedullary junction are probably underestimated; they were found in five of six fatal cases of whiplash shaking injury by Hadley et al.[679]

Pathophysiology of brain injury from shaking

Shaking causes the brain to swirl first in one direction and then the reverse. The brain and skull start and stop rotating at different times causing tearing of bridging veins. Gray matter is firmer than white matter and they move at different velocities causing small tears that can best be demonstrated on ultrasound imaging.[680] The tentorium anchors the brainstem and the midbrain acts as a pivot upon which the cerebral hemispheres can rotate. This may cause a primary brainstem injury with concussion.

In child abuse, tears in the white matter of the orbital, first and second frontal convolutions and temporal lobe are common. Shaking may cause slit-like cavities in white matter and the ependyma may be torn so that necrotic brain extrudes into the ventricles.[681] Shearing injuries occur in the white matter of the hemispheres, particularly the corpus callosum, superior cerebellar peduncle and in the midbrain. Lesions in the latter may be unilateral or bilateral but are usually asymmetrical and often multiple. Although CT is the initial imaging method of choice, in cases of suspected non-accidental injury, MRI should also be obtained and serial imaging performed. This greatly helps in dating injuries, particularly subdural hematomas.[682] In shaking injuries combined with impact, cerebral edema is often very severe but may take some hours to appear after the injury. The cause of the edema is probably multifactorial.[683]

Retinal hemorrhages are most characteristic of non-accidental shaking injuries with chest compression. In Duhaime's series nine out of 10 children with retinal hemorrhage had been subjected to physical abuse; the one other case was a fatal high speed impact injury in a car.[677] Retinopathy can occur without subdural hemorrhage or cerebral edema but is seen in 50–70% of subdural hematomas. The bleeding involves all retinal layers and is also preretinal, extending into the vitreous or backwards, i.e. subretinal, to cause retinal detachment. Severe visual defects are common in survivors.

Subdural hematomas in the first 2 years of life are more commonly acute and due to child abuse than birth injury or accidental injury. Interhemispheric hematomas are particularly likely to be the result of being shaken. Most fatal non-accidental head injuries and many of those with persisting handicap have subdural hematomas (Fig. 22.43). Seventy-five percent of subdural hematomas are bilateral, 90% are supratentorial and 10% infratentorial. Eighty percent of interhemi-

spheric subdural hematomas, caused by non-accidental injury, have an associated retinopathy.

Arteriovenous malformations can bleed into the subdural space and hemorrhagic diatheses can cause spontaneous subdural bleeding, but this is rare without trauma. Scurvy, Menke disease, osteogenesis imperfecta, coagulopathies, thrombocytopenia and glutaric aciduria must also be included in the differential diagnosis.

The majority of small acute subdural hematomas, without mass effect, will resolve spontaneously. Larger or persisting hematomas can be treated by aspiration through the fontanel or drained via burr hole. This may, in addition to relieving symptoms, also be of medicolegal significance. The hematoma may re-accumulate. If it becomes chronic, a subduroperitoneal shunt may be required.

CHILDHOOD STROKE SYNDROMES

Stroke is defined by the World Health Organization as 'a clinical syndrome typified by rapidly developing signs of focal or global disturbance of cerebral functions, lasting more than 24 hours or leading to death, with no apparent causes other than of vascular origin'. Although in adults acute presentation with focal neurological signs such as hemiparesis is likely to have a vascular basis, the range of underlying pathologies is much wider in childhood and etiology will *not* be vascular in up to a third.[684] Childhood stroke has an annual incidence of 3–8/100 000 children, with equal proportions being ischemic and hemorrhagic. Stroke is one of the top 10 causes of childhood death in the USA;[685] contrary to common belief the majority of survivors have residual neurological impairments. Here we will focus on the acute evaluation and management of arterial ischemic stroke (AIS), sinovenous thrombosis (SVT) and nontraumatic intraparenchymal hemorrhage (IPH) in children beyond the neonatal period.

In the child presenting with acute hemiparesis distinction between the above pathologies, and nonvascular disorders such as tumor or demyelination, will require brain imaging. CT readily identifies intracranial hemorrhage and over 80% of cases of SVT. CT is commonly normal in the first 24 hours following infarction and either repeat CT or MRI will be required (Fig. 22.44). Cranial ultrasound is relatively sensitive in identifying intracranial hemorrhage in the newborn but is less reliable at excluding focal ischemia. Diagnoses such as Todd paresis or hemiplegic migraine should only be made after exclusion of vascular pathology by neuroimaging. Many children with transient focal symptoms are subsequently shown to have cerebral infarction on imaging.

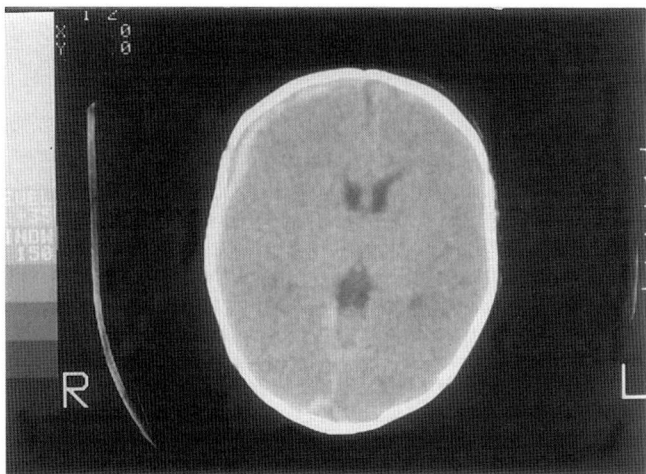

Fig. 22.43   Acute subdural hemorrhage over right hemisphere with hemispheric swelling and poor gray–white differentiation and some shift of midline.

ARTERIAL ISCHEMIC STROKE

Arterial ischemic stroke (AIS) is an acute focal neurological deficit secondary to cerebral infarction in an arterial distribution. As the

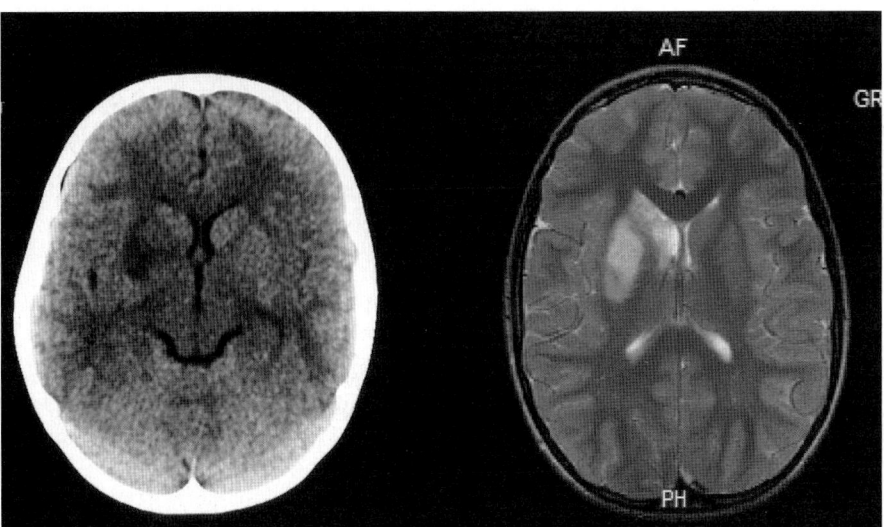

Fig. 22.44   CT scan (left) and axial T2-weighted MRI scan (right) of right basal ganglia infarction in childhood. Although the lesion is evident as a focal area of low density in the right lentiform nucleus, it is more easily identified on the MRI scan. In addition, MRI will identify abnormalities earlier than CT and permit concurrent examination of the cerebral circulation.

territory of the middle cerebral artery is most commonly affected, clinical presentation is usually with acute hemiparesis. Neonates may present with seizures and minimal focal symptoms or signs. Seizures occur at presentation in around 20% of older children. Large infarcts associated with mass effect, particularly in the posterior fossa, may present with coma. Early recognition of impaired consciousness and neurosurgical referral for cerebral decompression can be life saving. Posterior circulation stroke accounts for around 15% of all cases; there is a striking male preponderance. Recent data which suggests that posterior circulation arteriopathy may be a feature of stroke related to Fabry disease (see Ch. 26, p. 1104) may partially account for this male preponderance.[686] Half of cases of posterior circulation stroke in childhood are caused by vertebral artery dissection.

The evaluation of the child with AIS should include identification of risk factors, especially those which may influence clinical management. Half of children with AIS have a prior diagnosis, such as sickle cell disease (SCD) or congenital cardiac disease. The history should include enquiry about antecedent trauma, previous chickenpox (relevant if within the previous 12 months), associated medical conditions and family history of thrombosis or premature vascular disease. Clinical examination should include evaluation of vital signs, conscious level, neurological and cardiovascular examination, including blood pressure and peripheral pulses. A proposed algorithm for investigation is summarized in Figure 22.45.

Abnormalities of the cerebral circulation are identified in 80% of children with AIS; although these are commonly intracranial, arterial dissection affects the cervical arteries, thus the arterial circulation should be imaged from the aortic arch to the circle of Willis. This is most efficiently achieved using magnetic resonance angiography (MRA). Ultrasound of the carotid arteries can be a useful method of identifying dissection. Catheter cerebral angiography (CCA) is the gold standard for vascular imaging but is usually reserved for cases where MRA is nondiagnostic or there is potential pathology in smaller arteries that those visualized using MRA, for example in suspected cerebral vasculitis. CCA should also be considered in posterior circulation stroke as MRA is less sensitive for pathology in this area. Stenosis of the terminal internal carotid or proximal anterior and/or middle cerebral arteries is often transient ('transient cerebral arteriopathy' – TCA). TCA is thought to be due to transient arterial inflammation and is often related to antecedent chickenpox infection.

Moyamoya, endemic in Japan but also seen elsewhere, is a rare but potentially treatable arteriopathy (Fig. 22.46). This commonly bilateral disorder comprises occlusive disease of the terminal internal carotid arteries with basal ganglia collaterals, commonly described as a 'puff of smoke'. Most cases are idiopathic although there is a long list of associated conditions including Down syndrome, cranial irradiation, SCD and neurofibromatosis. Around 20% of affected children have abnormalities of other large arteries, for example renal artery stenosis. Affected children are at high risk of recurrent stroke as well as of intracranial hemorrhage. Vascular bypass procedures appear to reduce the risk of recurrent AIS.[687]

There are two major clinical guidelines for the management of childhood AIS. These are summarized in Table 22.55. Supporting the airway and circulation are essential components of the acute management of

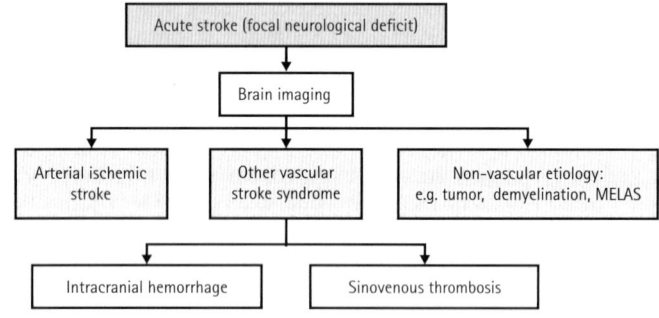

- **History:** ?prior diagnosis ?previous chickenpox ?head trauma
- **Examination:** neurocutaneous signs
- **Look for risk factors** which will change acute management:
  1. Echocardiogram and ECG
  2. Vascular imaging of neck and circle of Willis to look for dissection with MRA
  3. Evaluate for sepsis; exclude SCD, active coagulopathy, anemia and hypoxia
  4. Screen for thrombophilia
- **Targetted additional evaluation** in selected patients, e.g.
  - evaluate for vasculitis if inflammatory markers raised or multisystem involvement
  - CCA in posterior circulation stroke if MRA not diagnostic
  - screen for Fabry disease in males with posterior circulation AIS

Fig. 22.45 Algorithm for investigation of childhood arterial ischemic stroke. Thrombophilia screening should be undertaken following advice from a hematologist; specific tests undertaken will vary according to the local prevalence of genetic thrombophilia. Evaluation for vasculitis should include measurement of inflammatory markers (ESR, CRP), CSF examination for cells and protein, autoimmune and coagulation profile, and assessment for other organ involvement, e.g. urine dipstick and blood pressure measurement. Catheter angiography, including selective visceral angiography, may need to be considered, Assessment for Fabry disease involves measurement of alpha galactosidase A. ECG, electrocardiogram; MELAS, mitochondrial emcephalomyelitis, lactic acidosis and stroke like episodes; SCD, sickle cell disease; MRA, magnetic resonance angiography; CCA, catheter cerebral angiogram; AIS, arterial ischemic stroke.

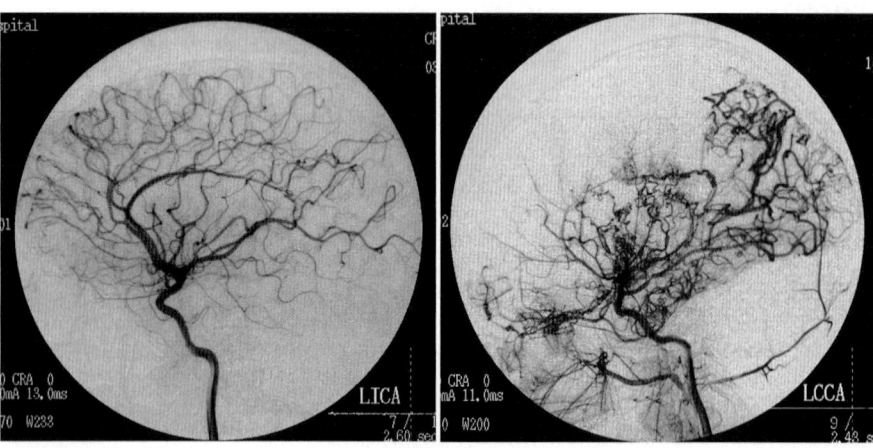

Fig. 22.46 Catheter cerebral angiogram (lateral view). **Left:** Normal anatomy of the left internal carotid artery and its branches. **Right:** (Common carotid artery injection) features of moyamoya, including occlusion of the terminal left internal carotid artery and profuse lenticulostriate collaterals.

Table 22.55 Summary of acute and longer term treatment recommendations from the two current [UK] clinical guidelines for management of acute childhood arterial ischemic stroke (AIS)

	RCP Guideline[a]	'Chest' guideline,[a,b]
Acute treatment of AIS[a]		
SCD	Exchange transfusion, target HbS < 30%	As RCP; iv hydration
All others	Aspirin 1–5 mg/kg/day	Anticoagulate for 5–7 days
Secondary prevention in AIS[a]		
SCD	Blood transfusion, HbS < 30%; consider BMT	Long-term transfusion
Dissection	Anticoagulate for up to 6 months	Anticoagulate 3–6 months
Cardioembolic	Consider anticoagulation depending on other clinical factors	Anticoagulate 3–6 months
Moyamoya	Evaluate for surgical revascularization	–
Other arteriopathy	Aspirin 1–3 mg/kg/day	Aspirin 2–5 mg/kg/day (after cessation of anticoagulation)
Recurrence on aspirin	Anticoagulate	–

RCP, Royal College of Physicians.
[a] http://www.rcplondon.ac.uk/pubs/books/childstroke.
[b] Monagle et al.[690]

AIS. Derangements in homeostasis, such as fever or hypoxia, should be corrected and infection should be treated. Specific treatment will be directed by the underlying risk factors but can be summarized as (i) exchange transfusion for patients with SCD (ii) anticoagulation for cardioembolic stroke and extracranial dissection and (iii) low dose aspirin in the rest. Childhood AIS recurs in up to 30% of children; this is related to moyamoya, multiple risk factors and some prothrombotic states such as protein C deficiency. Recurrence affects over 60% of children with SCD in whom regular blood transfusion is used to maintain HbS% < 30% and hemoglobin > 10 g/dl. Secondary prevention is also summarized in Table 22.55.

SINOVENOUS THROMBOSIS (SVT)

Thrombosis of the cerebral venous system may affect either the venous sinuses or the cortical veins. The latter is more difficult to identify as clinical features may be subtle and the normal anatomy is highly variable. Clinical presentation of SVT is with symptoms and signs of raised intracranial pressure (headache, vomiting, papilloedema) or with signs related to focal venous infarction (hemiparesis, seizures). It is impossible to distinguish between arterial and venous thrombosis on clinical grounds and a high index of suspicion is needed to make the correct diagnosis. Over 80% of SVT is identified on CT;[688] as with AIS, venous infarction may not be apparent if the CT is done within 24 hours. Venous infarction is often hemorrhagic and needs to be distinguished from primary intracranial hemorrhage. The venous sinuses can be imaged using MR venography or CT venography if CT is uninformative.

Up to 90% of children with SVT have one or more identifiable predisposing factors. These include infection of the head and neck, for example, sinusitis and otitis media. Many also have a prothrombotic disorder.

Other risk factors for SVT include dehydration, chemotherapy (especially L-asparaginase) and nephrotic syndrome (due to loss of anticoagulant proteins). Once the diagnosis is made, current guidelines recommend anticoagulation for 3–6 months.[689] The presence of hemorrhage is not a complete contraindication to anticoagulation but decisions regarding the risks (mainly bleeding) and benefits (preventing extension of the thrombosis) should be assessed on a case by case basis. Thrombolysis (systemic or local) is also sometimes used but the evidence supporting this is anecdotal. As with AIS supportive treatment with adequate hydration and treatment of sepsis is crucial. Up to two thirds of children with SVT have long term sequelae; this is more likely if there has been venous infarction or seizures in the acute period.

NONTRAUMATIC INTRAPARENCHYMAL HEMORRHAGE (IPH)

The clinical presentation of IPH may be indistinguishable from other stroke syndromes. However, coma and seizures are more common compared with AIS. Mortality is around 10%. IPH is a neurosurgical emergency and patients should be referred to a neurosurgical center as soon as the diagnosis is made. Subsequent evaluation will be directed toward identification of the underlying etiology which may be vascular (arteriovenous malformation (AVM), arterial aneurysm (AA) or cavernoma, or nonvascular (e.g. hemophilia or hemorrhage into a tumor).

AVMs represent abnormal communications between arterial and veins without an intervening capillary network. Clinical presentation is as a consequence of hemorrhage or local effects of the abnormal vessels (e.g. focal seizures, hemiparesis). The lifetime risk of hemorrhage related to AVM can be expressed using the formula (100 − (age in years)) expressed as a percentage; thus the lifetime risk of hemorrhage in a child is greater than in an adult, justifying a more aggressive treatment approach in childhood. Potential treatment options include surgical excision, endovascular occlusion or stereotactic radiosurgery. AA (dilation of the arterial wall) is a less common cause of IPH; it may be secondary to genetic conditions such as Ehlers–Danlos syndrome (especially type IV, the vascular type) or may be acquired (e.g. secondary to infection or trauma). Treatment is surgical or endovascular occlusion. Cavernomas are clusters of abnormally dilated blood vessels lined with endothelial tissue, without intervening neural tissue. There is no arteriovenous shunting and blood flow is slow. Cavernomas may be multiple and are inherited in an autosomal dominant manner in some families. They are not evident on CCA due to the slow flow but are usually identified on MRI. Treatment is usually by surgical excision.

In the child presenting with IPH, clinical status will strongly influence the immediate investigations and management. If the patient's clinical state mandates urgent evacuation of the hematoma, the child may have an abbreviated CCA in the operating theatre so that any associated AVM can be excised at the same time. If patients do not require urgent surgery evaluation options include CTA, MRI, MRA and CCA, according to the clinical context and likely underlying pathology. Patients should be also be evaluated for neurocutaneous disorders (e.g. PHACE (posterior fossa malformation, hemangioma, arterial, cardiac and eye anomalies) or Osler–Weber–Rendu syndromes) and have a routine coagulation screen. If no vascular or structural etiology is identified coagulation studies should be extended with advice from a hematologist.

VEIN OF GALEN MALFORMATION

Although rare, vein of Galen malformation (VGM) is a potentially treatable vascular malformation that may present to the pediatrician. It represents abnormal persistence of the median prosencephalic vein, a normal embryological structure. The net result is abnormal arteriovenous shunting. In the neonate this results in high output cardiac failure, often with multi-organ involvement. In older children venous hypertension can present as acute white matter ischemia ('melting brain syndrome'), with seizures and acute focal deficits, or more insidiously as macrocephaly. Hemorrhage is rare but is occasionally seen in adults. The advent of endovascular treatment (where glue injected via a micro-catheter is used to occlude the abnormal communications between arteries and veins) has revolutionized the outlook and may be curative. However, it is a high risk intervention and many children will have sustained irreversible cerebral injury prior to treatment. Once the diagnosis is made prompt referral should be made to a center with appropriate neurovascular expertise.

SPEECH AND LANGUAGE DELAY AND DISORDERS

INTRODUCTION

Children have inbuilt capacities to communicate by words, sounds, gestures and music.[691] Even neonates when awake and not hungry will show interest in a face and will mimic a facial expression. From early infancy, children will enjoy making reciprocal noises when alert and comfortable. Babble, which is the same throughout the world, emerges any time after 6 months and subsides by about 15 months. Children with severe hearing impairment babble normally, but fall silent thereafter. The function of babble is to engage adults in conversation. The nature of the words the child learns to speak depends on the adult language they hear. Later, the accent they use depends on that of their peers. There are inbuilt capacities to infer language rules to save time in learning. Sometimes these will lead a child to say words they have never heard from anyone else – 'I goed to my gran's', 'I got some chocolate mices' – for instance. The alternative – learning all language by listening and copying – would take far too long.

Delay refers to a normal pattern of speech and language acquisition but at a later age than most children. It may be specific in a child whose development is otherwise age appropriate. It may be associated with other specific delays, e.g. in motor development.[692] In children with global moderate learning disability the usual pattern of speech and language development is one of delay. Disorder refers to a pattern of development that is not seen in general. Speech examples include dysarthria or dyspraxia. Language disorders include word finding difficulty, receptive or expressive dysphasia or the excessively literal 'concrete thinking' of autistic children.

The age of uttering first words is variable, from well before the first birthday, to long after the second, in children who turn out to be university graduates, never mind mainstream schoolchildren. It is not related to social class, but there may be a family history of late talking and a higher proportion of boys are late to talk. By the age of 2 years, all but 6% of children have uttered their first words.[693] By the age of 3 years all but 4% can utter appropriate three-word phrases (Fig. 22.47).[694] Extension

of language into phrases and sentences is related to social class and is predictive of subsequent academic progress. Of children not yet talking in phrases at 3 years, 30% have walked before 1 year and 40% walked between 12 and 16 months but 30% walked after 16 months. Early talking in phrases and sentences predicts a good academic performance. Late talking in sentences, but early walking (before 12 months) predicts a good outcome, but with an increased risk of literacy difficulties (dyslexia). Late talking in sentences and walking after 16 months predicts limited academic performance and an increased likelihood of a need for learning support or special education.

Two thirds of children[695] have:
- first words between 9 months and 1 year;
- first phrases between 17 months and 2 years;
- and are intelligible to strangers at 2 years.

Children seem much more intelligible to those who hear them speak regularly – siblings and mothers particularly – than to professionals or strangers. By 3 years 9 months Morley reported that only 6% had incomplete sentences, but that 11% were unintelligible to strangers and 10% to health visitors, who reported 5% as unintelligible at 4 years 9 months and 0.7% as unintelligible at 6 years 6 months. The improvements were the consequence of maturation rather than treatment. In the National Child Development Study,[696] reduced intelligibility at 7 years was reported for 14% of children by doctors (but only for 1.4% was the problem marked). Teachers reported reduced intelligibility in 11% of the same children (marked in 2.6%). Phonological difficulties such as omissions, substitutions and reversals are common and are seen in early written work also.

PRESENTATION OF SPEECH AND LANGUAGE DISORDERS

When children have difficulty understanding speech they may be thought to be disobedient or deaf. When they have difficulty expressing themselves in speech they may become aggressive or frustrated and may have tantrums or behave destructively. Attempts to attract the attention of others by tapping them or pulling on their sleeves may be interpreted as aggressive behavior. In children who are late to talk, evidence of good comprehension is reassuring. Pure expressive dysphasia is rare and it is more likely that the child is simply showing a variant of normal development and will be fine shortly. Autistic children usually show signs of being remote from the first weeks of life, but a fifth show promising early development then regress. In girls, this should prompt consideration of Rett syndrome.[697] However Rett syndrome only affects 1 girl in 20 000 and the usual diagnosis is idiopathic autism or acquired aphasia. In boys, it is likely to be diagnosed as idiopathic autism. Some consideration may be given to fragile X, in that some children who appear odd, very withdrawn and uncommunicative in groups may have this condition, even though in individual consultation the child's communication is not autistic. Children who have communication problems, including those who are deaf, may be thought to be hyperactive until the problem is diagnosed.

PATHOLOGICAL SPEECH AND LANGUAGE DELAY AND DISORDER

There may be a known pathological cause for speech and/or language difficulties (Table 22.56). The child may have a *global learning disability*, due to a chromosomal abnormality, or other demonstrable medical cause. The child may have a suprabulbar palsy, due to *cerebral palsy*. There may be a bulbar palsy, due to a *neuromuscular disorder*. The mean verbal quotient of boys with Duchenne muscular dystrophy is 80 with a distribution from profound communication difficulty and autism to superior intelligence, compatible with university education. In the mouth there may be structural malformations such as *cleft palate* or *micrognathia* (moderate in Down syndrome and severe in Pierre Robin syndrome). One child in 500 has bilateral severe *sensorineural hearing loss*, which explains lack of early speech and language. *Central auditory*

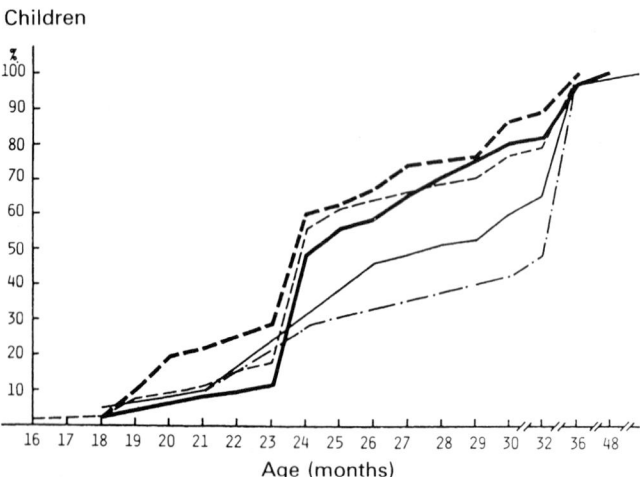

Children

Fig. 22.47 Onset of four-word sentences. Term boys, — ; term girls, –– ; preterm boys — and girls –– without cerebral palsy; boys and girls with cerebral palsy, —·—.[620]

Table 22.56 Investigation of children with speech and language delay/disorder

Hearing
Chromosomes especially for sex chromosome abnormalities, e.g. XXX, XXY, fragile X
Amino acid chromatogram, e.g. phenylketonuria
Creatine kinase in boys
EEG, e.g. in acquired aphasia
CT scan, e.g. in tuberous sclerosis or with partial complex seizures
MRI scan in congenital suprabulbar palsy

inattention[698] describes a condition in which the child behaves as if deaf although the ears can be demonstrated to hear normally by physiological tests. It is analogous to developmental visual inattention and, as with that condition, may resolve spontaneously.

Semantic and pragmatic language disorders are seen in children with *autism/autistic spectrum disorders*, which it is considered result from a developmental brain disorder. The condition known as *selective mutism* is a very persistent condition, often continuing into adult life, with a probable biological cause. Congenital suprabulbar palsy[699–701] may be associated with bilateral parasagittal areas of cortical dysplasia or with an abnormality of chromosome 22. Around the age of 3–9 years some children who have seizures, not necessarily severe ones, may lose their receptive language skills, either acutely or progressively over time, with acquired epileptic aphasia.[702–705] This condition has no known cause and can occur in children. About a third of all cases have not had seizures, but show left hemisphere seizure discharge on EEG.[706] The type with acute onset has a better prognosis for recovery. Cerebrovascular accidents, head injury, accidental or abusive, meningoencephalitis and encephalitis are causes of acquired pathological speech and language disorders (Table 22.57).

AUTISM AND AUTISTIC SPECTRUM DISORDERS
(see also Ch 34)

Autism, Asperger syndrome, high functioning autism, autistic spectrum disorders, atypical autism and pervasive developmental disorders are discussed elsewhere from a child psychiatric perspective (see Ch. 34). Here they are considered within the context of speech, language and communication disorder, which is a core feature of the autistic syndrome. Autistic behavior has long been regarded by pediatricians and pediatric neurologists as a familiar feature of children who have had

Table 22.57 The causes of pathological speech and language delay/disorder

Neurological
Global learning disability (mental retardation)
Cerebral palsy
Autism
Developmental dysphasia
Selective mutism
Congenital suprabulbar palsy
Acquired epileptic aphasia
Acquired brain injury

Neuromuscular
Duchenne muscular dystrophy
Dystrophia myotonica
Congenital bulbar palsy (nuclear agenesis)

Local structural
Malformations: tongue, lips, palate, teeth

Sensory
Bilateral sensorineural hearing loss
Deafblindness
Severe visual impairment

Mixed

infantile spasms which were idiopathic or associated with tuberous sclerosis.[707] It is also seen as a symptom in some children with idiopathic learning disability and/or in some children with epilepsy. This triad causes confusion for parents in the sense that they ask 'what is wrong with my child – is it learning disability, autism or epilepsy?'

For the pediatrician, all of these are symptoms of an underlying biological disorder of brain development, to be diagnosed medically if possible as the cause of the child's condition. To give autism, learning disability or epilepsy as 'the diagnosis' risks closing minds to the need to continue to search for the cause. However, in spite of much excellent work on the subject,[708–713] it remains the case that an underlying medical cause is still unknown for most autistic children. There is an excess in males, which is still present when boys with fragile X are excluded. The concordance for autism in monozygotic twins is 36–89% in published studies. Concordance in dizygotic twins is up to 30% and there is a substantial excess of autism (about 3%) and heterogeneous developmental language disorders in non-autistic twins and siblings of autistic children.

There has been a growing acknowledgment among pediatricians that children with autistic behavior present particular challenges to their families, their teachers and all who come in contact with them. It has implications for teaching methods, for speech and language therapy and for behavioral management. The voluntary organizations for families of autistic children have published very helpful and informative literature for parents and professionals. They put parents in touch with each other and provide innovative, appropriate local and national services for autistic people. For such reasons, pediatricians have become increasingly willing to diagnose children as having an autistic disorder, to discuss this with families and colleagues and to seek help from child mental health services. Many children who would have been considered to be 'loners', dyspraxic, eccentric or to have a schizoid personality disorder, in the past, are now being recognized as having autistic features. This increasing identification has contributed to the apparent increase in the prevalence of autistic children in recent years. The Medical Research Council in Britain has published an extensive Autism Review[714] on the Internet.

Childhood autism is characterized by the following developmental features:
- communication difficulties;
- problems with social interaction;
- behavioral problems including stereotopies and obsessional interests;
- onset in the first 3 years.

The communication difficulties in higher functioning autistic children, or children with Asperger syndrome, are described as a semantic/pragmatic disorder.[715] By this is meant that children use words without understanding their meaning and in an inappropriate context. It is a sophisticated form of echolalia. Some such children can pick up and repeat long passages of filmscore in appropriate accents. They may come out with apparently grown-up language, in a variety of settings, throughout the day but, if pressed, cannot explain their utterances. Their speech is monotonous in tone (a disorder of prosody). They do not understand similes or metaphors, and have a very concrete, literal understanding of words and objects. They do not understand or engage in symbolic play where one object can represent something else, e.g. a box representing a boat or a pencil representing a rocket. Their visual learning may be well be ahead of their auditory learning and they may be hyperlexic (much better at the mechanics of reading than at reading comprehension). The use of visual prompts may be helpful in structuring their learning and other activities.

A key component of their problems with social interaction is a lack of empathy, analogous to color blindness, in that it cannot be taught. This inability to know how others are feeling or to predict how others would be likely to feel in response to the autistic child's remarks or behavior leads to much conflict and confusion. Autistic children will regard the responses of others as bullying, persecution and utterly unjust. The children will involve themselves in activities along with other children, but not in a collaborative manner. Their highly developed sense of rules may

- Discuss the findings with the parents who may bring a grandparent, friend or professional.
- Inform the local education authority.
- Contribute to the interdisciplinary process of considering the appropriate form of education.
- Review progress at regular intervals – discuss findings with teachers, therapists and parents.

Speech and language therapists have a key role as consultants and advisers of parents, teachers, doctors and others in regular contact with children affected by speech and language delay and disorder. They are the experts, in collaboration with clinical psychologists, teachers and parents, in working out the way children's minds are working, in the way they are understanding and using language, including context and syntax and in the state of their phonological development. However the 'treatment' is not in the therapy sessions but in the day to day communication between adults and children, the anticipation and avoidance of frustration and the way the children are encouraged to succeed. Progress reassessment and revision of goals by therapists guide those who are in daily contact in helping the children. Sometimes parents complain that it seems they are being expected to adopt a treatment role but they should not be expected to spend too much time grappling with the limits of the child's ability. Rather they will be helping their children to consolidate on their abilities, finding out what their children do best and helping them to make the most of these.

Augmented communication

There are many ways of augmenting spoken language in everyday life. Gestures and other forms of body language are part of our repertoire. Actors develop these to a subtle and remarkable extent. For children whose speech is lacking or incomprehensible, systems involving

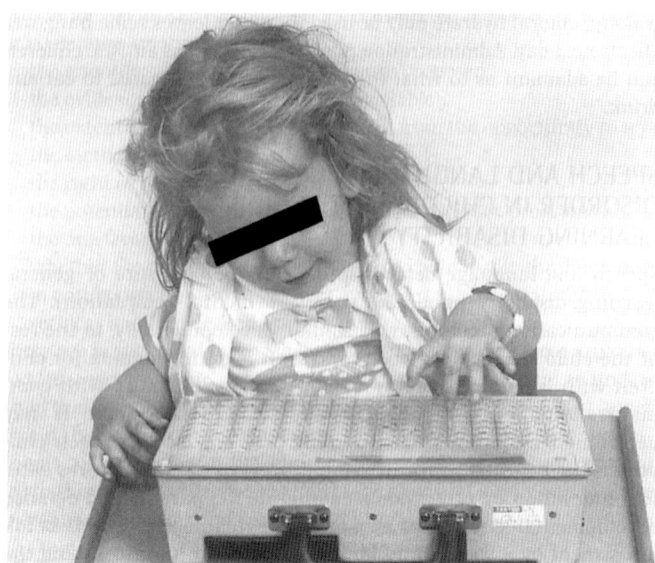

Fig. 22.48   Augmentative communication with Reybus Introtalker (pictograms) being used by an anarthric child with severe mixed cerebral palsy.

gestures or symbols can be beneficial. Instead of being reactive, the child can become proactive for the first time. There are specialist centers for augmentative communication, with expertise in signing, symbol and switching methods. The local speech and language therapy service will have a specialist expert who can advise on the best source of help (Fig. 22.48).

REFERENCES (* Level 1 Evidence)

The neurological consultation

1. Cunningham C, Newton R. A question sheet to encourage written consultation question. Qual Health Care 2000; 9:42–46.
2. Viswanathan V, Bridges SJ, et al. Childhood headaches: discrete entities or continuum? Dev Med Child Neurol 1998; 40:544–550.
3. Silva PA. Epidemiology, longitudinal course and some associated factors: an update in language developments and disorders. In: Yule W, Rutter M, eds. Clinics in developmental medicine. Oxford: MacKeith Press; 1987:101/102:12–15.
4. Lees J, Urwin S. Children with language disorders. London: Whurr Publishers; 1997.
5. Levene MI. The asphyxiated new born infant. In: Levene MI, Chervenak FA, Whittle M, eds. Fetal neonatal neurology and neurosurgery. London: Churchill Livingstone; 2001.487–498.
6. Alvarez LA, Maytal J, Shinnar S. Idiopathic external hydrocephalus: natural history and relationship to benign familial macrocephaly. Pediatrics 1986; 77:901–907.
7. Wallace GB, Newton RW. Gowers' sign revisited. Arch Dis Child 1989; 64:1317–1319.

Giving the news of disablity

8. Cunningham CC, Morgan PA, McGucken RB. Down's syndrome: is dissatisfaction with disclosure of diagnosis inevitable?. Dev Med Child Neurol 1984; 26:33–39.
9. Lingham S, Newton RW. Giving the news of disability – paediatric practice guideline. London: Royal College of Paediatrics and Child Health; 1996.
10. Nelson KB, Ellenberg JH. Children who outgrow cerebral palsy. Paediatrics 1982; 69:529–536.

11. Cunningham CC, Newton R, et al. Epilepsy – giving the diagnosis. A survey of British Paediatric Neurologists. Seizure 2002; 11:500–511.
12. Houston EC, Cunningham CC, et al. The information needs and understanding of 5 to 10 year old children with epilepsy, asthma or diabetes. Seizure 2000; 9:340–343.

Development of the human brain

13. Huttenlocher PR, Dabholkar AS. Regional differences in synaptogenesis in human cerebral cortex. J Comp Neurol 1997; 387:167–178.
14. Hittmair K, Wimberger D, Rand T, et al. MR assessment of brain maturation: comparison of sequences. Am J Neuroradiol 1994; 15:425–433.
15. Klingberg T, Vadya CJ, Gabrieli JDE, et al. Myelination and organisation of the frontal white matter in children: a diffusion tensor MRI study. Neuro Report 1999; 10:2817–2821.
16. Barkovich AJ, Kuzniecky RI, Dobyns WB, et al. A classification scheme for malformations of cortical development. Neuropediatrics 1996; 27:59–63.
17. van der Knapp MS, Valk J. Classification of congenital abnormalities of the CNS. Am J Neuroradiol 1988; 9:315–326.
18. Sarnat HB, Flores-Sarnat L. A new classification of malformations of the nervous system: an integration of morphological and molecular genetic criteria as patterns of genetic expression. Eur J Paediatr Neurol 2001; 5:57–64.
19. Hudgins RJ, Edwards MSB, Goldstein R, et al. Natural history of foetal ventriculomegaly. Pediatrics 1988; 82:692–697.
20. Gupta JK, Bryce FC, Lilford RJ. Management of apparently isolated foetal ventriculomegaly. Obstet Gynecol Surv 1994; 49:716–721.

21. Pilu G, Falco P, Gabrielli S, et al. The clinical significance of foetal isolated cerebral borderline ventriculomegaly: report of 31 cases and review of the literature. Ultrasound. Obstet Gynecol 1999; 14:320–326.
22. Ouahba J, Luton D, Vuillard E, et al. Prenatal isolated mild ventriculomegaly: outcome in 167 cases. Br J Obstet Gynaecol 2006; 113:1072–1079.
23. Serlo W, Kirkinen P, et al. Prognostic signs in foetal hydrocephalus. Childs Nerv Syst 1986; 2:93–97.
24. Chervenak FA, Duncan C, Ment LR, et al. Outcome of foetal ventriculomegaly. Lancet 1984; 2:179–181.
25. Adzick NS, Harrison MR. Foetal surgical therapy. Lancet 1994; 343:897–902.

Neural tube defects

26. van Allen MI, Kalousek DK, Chernoff GF, et al. Evidence of multi-site closure of the neural tube in humans. Am J Med Genet 1993; 47:723–743.
27. Cuckle H, Wald N. The impact of screening for neural tube defects in England and Wales. Prenat Diagn 1987; 7:91–99.
*28. Medical Research Council Vitamin Study Group. Prevention of neural tube defects: results of the Medical Research Council vitamin study. Lancet 1991; 238:131–133.
29. Meuli M, Meuli-Sommen C, Hutchins GM, et al. In utero surgery rescues neurological function at birth in sheep with spina bifida. Nat Med 1995; 1:342–347.
30. Bowman RM, McLone DG, Grant JA, et al. Spina bifida outcome: a 25 year prospective. Pediatr Neurosurg 2001; 34:114–120.
31. McDonnell GV, McCann JP. Issues of medical management in adults with spina bifida. Child Nerv Syst 2000; 16:222–227.

32. Rintoul N, Sutton LN, Hubbard AM, et al. A new look at myelomeningoceles; functional level, vertebral level, shunting and the implications for fetal intervention. Pediatrics 2002; 109:409–413.

33. Pit-ten Cate IM, Kennedy C, Stevenson J. Disability and quality of life in spina bifida and hydrocephalus. Dev Med Child Neurol 2002; 44:317–322.

34. Bruner JP, Tulipan N, Paschall RL, et al. Foetal surgery for myelomeningocele and the incidence of shunt dependent hydrocephalus. JAMA 1999; 282:1819–1825.

35. Bruner JP, Tulipan N, Reed G, et al. Intrauterine repair of spina bifida: preoperative predictors of shunt-dependent hydrocephalus. Am J Obstet Gynecol 2004; 190:1305–1312.

36. Minns RA. The management of children with spina bifida. In: Gordon N, McKinlay I, eds. Neurologically handicapped children. Oxford: Blackwell; 1986.

37. Johnston LB, Borzyskowski M. Bladder dysfunction and neurological disability at presentation in closed spinal bifida. Arch Dis Child 1998; 79:33–38.

Hydrocephalus

38. Cheung CS, Myrinthopolous NC. Factors affecting risks of congenital malformations. Report from the Collaborative Perinatal Project. Birth Defects 1975; 11:1–22.

39. Blackburn BL, Fineman RM. Epidemiology of congenital hydrocephalus in Utah, 1940 to 1979: report of an aetrogenically related epidemic. Am J Med Genet 1994; 52:123–129.

40. Fernell E, Hagberg G, Hagberg B. Infantile hydrocephalus epidemiology. An indicator of enhanced survival. Arch Dis Child Fetal Neonatal Ed 1994; 70:F123–F128.

41. Minns RA, Brown JK, Engelman HM. CSF production rate: real time estimation. Z Kinderchir 1987; 42(suppl I):36–40.

42. Kirkpatrick M, Engelman HA, Minns RA. Symptoms and signs of progressive hydrocephalus. Arch Dis Child 1989; 64:124–128.

43. Leggate JRS, Baxter P, Minns RA. Role of a separate subcutaneous cerebrospinal fluid reservoir in the management of hydrocephalus. Br J Neurosurg 1988; 2:327–337.

44. Minns RA, Engelman HM, Sterling H. A cerebrospinal fluid pressure in pyogenic meningitis. Arch Dis Child 1989; 64:814–820.

45. Minns RA, Merrick MV. Cerebral perfusion pressure and net cerebral mean transit time in childhood hydrocephalus. J Paediatr Neurosci 1989; 5:69–77.

46. Minns RA, Goh D, et al. A volume–blood flow relationship derived from CSF compartment challenge as an index of progression of infantile hydrocephalus. In: Proceedings of the International Symposium on Hydrocephalus, Japan, November 1990.

47. Chumas Tyagia, Livingston J. Hydrocephalus – what's new?. Arch Dis Child Fetal Neonatal Ed 2001; 85:F149–F154.

48. Jallo GI, Kothbauer KF, Abbot IR. Endoscopic third ventriculostomy. Neurosurg Focus 2005; 19(6):E11.

49. Schroeder HW, Niendorf WR, Gaab MR. Complications of endoscopic third ventriculostomy. J Neurosurg 2002; 96:1032–1040.

*50. Anonymous. Randomised trial of early tapping in neonatal haemorrhagic ventricular dilatation. Ventriculomegaly Trial Group. Arch Dis Child 1990; 65:3–10.

51. Tortorolo G, Luciano R, et al. Intraventricular hemorrhage: past, present and future, focusing on classification, pathogenesis and prevention. Child Nerv Syst 1999; 15:652–661.

52. Fulmer BB, Grabb PA, et al. Neonatal ventriculo subgaleal shunts. Neurosurgery 2000; 47:80–83.

*53. Kennedy CR, Ayers S, Campbell MJ, et al. Randomised, controlled trial of acetazolamide and furosemide. In posthemorrhagic ventricular dilation in infancy: follow-up at 1 year. Pediatrics 2001; 108:597–607.

54. Brydon HL, Bayston R, Hayward R, et al. The effect of protein and blood cells on the flow pressure characteristics of shunts. Neurosurgery 1996; 38:498–504.

55. Brydon HL, Hayward R, Harkness W, et al. Does the cerebrospinal fluid protein concentration increase the risk of shunt complications? Br J Neurosurg 1996; 10:267–273.

56. Gaston H. Does the spina bifida clinic need an ophthalmologist?. Z Kinderchir 1985; 40(suppl 11):45–50.

The neurocutaneous diseases

57. Gutmann DH, Aylsworth A, Carey JC, et al. The diagnostic evaluation and multi-disciplinary management of neurofibromatosis I and neurofibromatosis II. JAMA 1997; 278:51–57.

58. Evans DJR, Birch JM, Ramsden RT. Paediatric presentation of type 2 neurofibromatosis. Arch Dis Child 1999; 81:496–499.

59. Roach ES, DiMario FJ, Candt RS, et al. Tuberose Sclerosis Consensus Conference: Recommendations for diagnostic evaluation. National Tuberose Sclerosis Association. J Child Neurol 1999; 14: 401–407.

Seizures, epilepsy and other paroxysmal disorders

60. Steinlein OK, Mulley JC, et al. A missense mutation in the neuronal nicotinic acetylcholine receptor alpha 4 subunit is associated with autosomal dominant nocturnal frontal lobe epilepsy. Nat Genet 1995; 11:201–203.

61. Biervert C, Schroeder BC, et al. A potassium channel mutation in neonatal human epilepsy. Science 1998; 279(5349):403–406.

62. Singh NA, Charlier C, et al. A novel potassium channel gene, KCNQ2, is mutated in an inherited epilepsy of newborns. Nat Genet 1998; 18:25–29.

63. Claes L, Del-Favero J, et al. De novo mutations in the sodium-channel gene SCN1A cause severe myoclonic epilepsy of infancy. Am J Hum Genet 2001; 68:1327–1332.

64. Macdonald RL. Cellular effects of antiepileptic drugs. In: Pedley TAm, ed. Epilepsy: a comprehensive textbook. Philadelphia: Lippincott-Raven; 1997: 1383–1391.

65. Sander JW, Shorvon SD. Epidemiology of the epilepsies [erratum appears in J Neurol Neurosurg Psychiatry 1997; 62:679]. J Neurol Neurosurg Psychiatry 1996; 61:433–443.

*66. Kotsopoulos IA, van Merode T, Kessels FGH, et al. Systematic review and meta-analysis of incidence studies of epilepsy and unprovoked seizures. Epilepsia 2002; 43:1402–1409.

*67. Wallace H, Shorvon S, et al. Age-specific incidence and prevalence rates of treated epilepsy in an unselected population of 2 052 922 and age-specific fertility rates of women with epilepsy. Lancet 1998; 352(9145):1970–1973.

68. Forsgren L. Incidence and prevalence. In: Wallace SJ, Farrell K, eds. Epilepsy in children. London: Arnold; 2004:21–25.

*69. Kurtz Z, Tookey P, et al. Epilepsy in young people: 23 year follow up of the British National Child Development Study. BMJ 1998; 316(7128):339–342.

*70. Heaney DC, MacDonald BK, Everitt A, et al. Socioeconomic variation in incidence of epilepsy: prospective community based study in south east England. BMJ 2002; 325:1013–1016.

*71. Hesdorffer DC, Tian H, Anand K, et al. Socioeconomic status is a risk factor for epilepsy in Icelandic adults but not in children. Epilepsia 2005; 46:1297–1303.

72. Reading R, Haynes R, Beach R. Deprivation and incidence of epilepsy in children. Seizure 2006; 15:190–193.

*73. Eriksson KJ, Koivikko MJ. Prevalence, classification, and severity of epilepsy and epileptic syndromes in children. Epilepsia 1997; 38:1275–1282.

74. Berg AT, Shinnar S, et al. Newly diagnosed epilepsy in children: presentation at diagnosis. Epilepsia 1999; 40:445–452.

*75. Shinnar S, O'Dell C, et al. Distribution of epilepsy syndromes in a cohort of children prospectively monitored from the time of their first unprovoked seizure. Epilepsia 1999; 40:1378–1383.

*76. Oka E, Ohtsuka Y, Yoshinaga H, et al. Prevalence of childhood epilepsy and distribution of epileptic syndromes: a population-based survey in Okayama, Japan. Epilepsia 2006; 47:626–630.

*77. Shinnar S, Berg AT, et al. Predictors of multiple seizures in a cohort of children prospectively followed from the time of their first unprovoked seizure [see comments]. Ann Neurol 2000; 48(2):140–147.

*78. Berg AT, Levy SR, et al. Predictors of intractable epilepsy in childhood: a case-control study. Epilepsia 1996; 37:24–30.

*79. Hauser E, Freilinger M, et al. Prognosis of childhood epilepsy in newly referred patients. J Child Neurol 1996; 11:201–204.

*80. Casetta I, Granieri E, et al. Early predictors of intractability in childhood epilepsy: a community-based case-control study in Copparo, Italy. Acta Neurol Scand 1999; 99:329–333.

81. Duchowny M. Seizure recurrence in childhood epilepsy: the future ain't what it used to be [letter comment]. Ann Neurol 2000; 48:137–139.

*82. Arts WF, Geerts AT, et al. The early prognosis of epilepsy in childhood: the prediction of a poor outcome. The Dutch study of epilepsy in childhood. Epilepsia 1999; 40:726–734.

83. Berg AT, Shinnar S, et al. Defining early seizure outcomes in pediatric epilepsy: the good, the bad and the in-between. Epilepsy Res 2001; 43:75–84.

*84. Cockerell OC, Johnson AL, et al. Prognosis of epilepsy: a review and further analysis of the first nine years of the British National General Practice Study of Epilepsy, a prospective population-based study. Epilepsia 1997; 38:31–46.

*85. Sillanpaa M, Jalava M, et al. Long-term prognosis of seizures with onset in childhood. N Engl J Med 1998; 338:1715–1722.

*86. Sillanpää M, Schmidt D. Natural history of treated childhood-onset epilepsy: prospective, long-term population-based study. Brain 2006; 129:617–624.

*87. Wakamoto H, Nagao H, et al. Long-term medical, educational, and social prognoses of childhood-onset epilepsy: a population-based study in a rural district of Japan. Brain Dev 2000; 22(4):246–255.

88. Ficker DM. Sudden unexplained death and injury in epilepsy. Epilepsia 2000; 41(suppl 2):S7–S12.

*89. Ficker DM, So EL, et al. Population-based study of the incidence of sudden unexplained death in epilepsy. Neurology 1998; 51:1270–1274.

90. O'Donoghue M, Sander JW. Does early antiepileptic drug treatment alter the prognosis for remission of the epilepsies?. J R Soc Med 1996; 89:245–248.

91. Shinnar S, Berg AT. Does antiepileptic drug therapy prevent the development of chronic epilepsy?. Epilepsia 1996; 37:701–708.

92. Walczak TS, Jayakar P. Interictal EEG. In : Pedley TA, ed. Epilepsy: a comprehensive textbook. Philadelphia: Lippincott-Raven; 1997:831–848.

93. Goodin DS, Aminoff MJ. Does the interictal EEG have a role in the diagnosis of epilepsy? Lancet 1984; 1:(8381):837–839.

94. Schmidt D. The influence of antiepileptic drugs on the electroencephalogram: a review of controlled clinical studies. Electroencephalogr Clin Neurophysiol Suppl 1982; 36:453–466.

95. Sperling MR, Clancy RR, Ictal EEG. In: Pedley TA, ed. Epilepsy: a comprehensive textbook. Philadelphia: Lippincott-Raven; 1997:849–885.

96. Verrotti A, Pizzella V, Trotta D, et al. Magnetoencephalography in pediatric neurology and in epileptic syndromes. Pediatr Neurol 2003; 28:253–261.

97. Raybaud C, Guye M, et al. Neuroimaging of epilepsy in children. Magn Reson Imaging Clin N Am 2001; 9:121–147,viii.

98. Ruggieri PM, Najm IM. MR imaging in epilepsy. Neurol Clin 2001; 19:477–489.

99. Berkovic SF, Newton MR. Single photon emission computed tomography. In: Pedley TA, ed. Epilepsy: a comprehensive textbook. Philadelphia: Lippincott-Raven; 1997:969–975.

100. Henry TR. Positron emission tomography. In: Pedley TA, ed. Epilepsy: a comprehensive textbook. Philadelphia: Lippincott-Raven; 1997:947–968.

*101. Devous MD Sr, Thisted RA, et al. SPECT brain imaging in epilepsy: a meta-analysis. J Nucl Med 1998; 39:285–293.

102. Robinson RO, Ferrie CD, et al. Positron emission tomography and the central nervous system. Arch Dis Child 1999; 81:263–270.

103. Lawson JA, O'Brien TJ, et al. Evaluation of SPECT in the assessment and treatment of intractable childhood epilepsy. Neurology 2000; 55:1391–1393.

104. Gutierrez-Delicado E, Serratosa JM. Genetics of the epilepsies. Curr Opin Neurol 2004; 17:147–153.

105. Robinson R, Gardiner M. Molecular basis of Mendelian idiopathic epilepsies. Ann Med 2004; 36:89–97.

106. MacLeod S, Mallik A, Tolmie JL, et al. Electro-clinical phenotypes of chromosome disorders associated with epilepsy in the absence of dysmorphism. Brain Dev 2005; 27:118–124.

107. Guerrini R, Fillipi T. Neuronal migration disorders, genetics and epileptogenesis. J Child Neurol 2005; 20:287–299.

108. Suri M. The phenotypic spectrum of ARX mutations. Dev Med Child Neurol 2005; 47:133–137.

109. Kato M, Dobyns WB. X-linked lissencephaly with abnormal genitalia as a tangential migration disorder causing intractable epilepsy: proposal for a new term, "interneuronopathy". J Child Neurol 2005; 20:392–397.

110. Commission. Proposal for revised clinical and electroencephalographic classification of epileptic seizures. From the Commission on Classification and Terminology of the International League Against Epilepsy. Epilepsia 1981; 22:489–501.

111. Commission. Proposal for revised classification of epilepsies and epileptic syndromes. Commission on Classification and Terminology of the International League Against Epilepsy. Epilepsia 1989; 30:389–399.

112. Blume W, Luders H, et al. Glossary of descriptive terminology for ictal semiology: report of the ILAE task force on classification and terminology. Epilepsia 2001; 42:1212–1218.

113. Engel J Jr. A proposed diagnostic scheme for people with epileptic seizures and with epilepsy: report of the ILAE Task Force on Classification and Terminology. Epilepsia 2001; 42:796–803.

114. Treiman DM. Generalized convulsive status epilepticus in the adult. Epilepsia 1993; 34(suppl 1): S2–S11.

115. Livingston J. Status epilepticus. In: Wallace SJ, Farrell K, eds. Epilepsy in children. London: Arnold; 2004:290–303.

116. Roger J, Bureau M, et al. Epileptic syndromes in infancy, childhood and adolescence. London: John Libbey; 2002.

117. Engel J, Pedley TA. Epilepsy: a comprehensive textbook. Philadelphia: Lippincott-Raven; 1998.

118. Panayiotopoulos CP. The epilepsies: seizures, syndromes and management. London: Bladon; 2005.

119. Mizrahi EM, Kellaway P. Characterization and classification of neonatal seizures. Neurology 1987; 37:1837–1844.

120. Plouin P. Benign familial neonatal convulsions and benign idiopathic neonatal convulsions. In: Pedley TA, ed. Epilepsy: a comprehensive textbook. Philadelphia: Lippincott-Raven; 1997:2247–2255.

121. Auvin S, Pandit F, De Bellecize J, et al. Benign myoclonic epilepsy in infants: electroclinical features and long-term follow up of 34 patients. Epilepsia 2006; 47:387–393.

122. Berkovic SF, Heron SE, Giordano L, et al. Benign familial neonatal-infantile seizures: characterization of a new sodium channelopathy. Ann Neurol 2004; 55:550–557.

123. Szepetowski P, Rochette J, Berquin P, et al. Familial infantile convulsions and paroxysmal choreoathetosis: a new neurological syndrome linked to the pericentric region of human chromosome 16. Am J Hum Genet 1997; 61:889–898.

124. Vigevano F, Fusco L, et al. The idiopathic form of West Syndrome. Epilepsia 1993; 34:743–746.

125. Koo B. Vigabatrin in the treatment of infantile spasms. Pediatr Neurol 1999; 20:106–110.

126. Riikonen RS. Steroids or vigabatrin in the treatment of infantile spasms? Pediatr Neurol 2000; 23:403–408.

127. Chiron C, Dulac O, et al. Therapeutic trial of vigabatrin in refractory infantile spasms. J Child Neurol Suppl 1991; 2:S52–S59.

128. Appleton RE, Peters AC, et al. Randomised, placebo-controlled study of vigabatrin as first-line treatment of infantile spasms. Epilepsia 1999; 40:1627–1633.

*129. Lux AL, Edwards SW, Hancock E, et al. The United Kingdom Infantile Spasms Study comparing vigabatrin with prednisolone or tetracosactide at 14 days: a multicentre, randomised controlled trial. Lancet 2004; 364:1773–1778.

*130. Lux AL, Edwards SW, Hancock E, et al. The United Kingdom Infantile Spasms Study (UKISS) comparing hormone treatment with vigabatrin on developmental and epilepsy outcomes to age 14 months: a multicentre randomised trial. Lancet Neurol 2005; 4:712–717.

131. Wong M, Trevathan E. Infantile spasms. Pediatr Neurol 2001; 24:89–98.

132. Hancock E, Osborne JP. Vigabatrin in the treatment of infantile spasms in tuberous sclerosis: literature review. J Child Neurol 1999; 14:71–74.

133. Eisermann MM, DeLaRaillere A, Dellatolas G, et al. Infantile spasms in Down syndrome – effects of delayed anticonvulsive treatment. Epilepsy Res 2003; 55:21–27.

134. Dravet C, Bureau M, Oguni H, et al. Severe myoclonic epilepsy in infancy (Dravet syndrome). In: Roger JM, Bureau M, Dravet C, et al, eds. Epileptic syndromes in infancy, childhood and adolescence. London: John Libbey; 2002:81–103.

135. Scheffer IE. Severe infantile epilepsies: molecular genetics challenge clinical classification. Brain 2003; 126:513–514.

136. Berkovic SF, Harkin L, McMahon JM, et al. De-novo mutations of the sodium channel gene SCN1A in alleged vaccine encephalopathy: a retrospective study. Lancet Neurol 2006; 5:488–492.

137. Guerrini R, Dravet C, et al. Lamotrigine and seizure aggravation in severe myoclonic epilepsy. Epilepsia 1998; 39:508–512.

*138. Chiron C, Marchand MC, Tran A, et al. Stiripentol in severe myoclonic epilepsy in infancy: a randomised placebo-controlled syndrome-dedicated trial. STICLO study group. Lancet 2000; 356:1638–1642.

139. Guerrini R, Dravet C. Severe epileptic encephalopathies of infancy, other than West syndrome. In: Pedley TA, ed. Epilepsy: a comprehensive textbook. Philadelphia: Lippincott-Raven; 1997:2285–2302.

140. Duncan JS, Panayiotopoulos CP. Typical absences and related epileptic syndromes. London: Churchill Communications; 1995.

141. Aicardi J. Myoclonic-astatic epilepsy. In: Wallace SJ, Farrell K, eds. Epilepsy in Children. London: Arnold; 2004.163–168.

142. Tassinari CA, Bureau M, Thoma P, et al. Epilepsy with myoclonic absences. In: Roger J, Bureau M, Dravet C, eds. Epileptic syndromes in infancy, childhood and adolescence. London: John Libbey; 1992:151–160.

143. Singh R, Scheffer IE, et al. Generalized epilepsy with febrile seizures plus: a common childhood-onset genetic epilepsy syndrome. Ann Neurol 1999; 45:75–81.

144. Parker AP, Agathonikou A, et al. Inappropriate use of carbamazepine and vigabatrin in typical absence seizures. Dev Med Child Neurol 1998; 40:517–519.

145. Panayiotopoulos CP. Benign childhood partial seizures and related epileptic syndromes. London: John Libbey; 1999.

146. Ferrie CD, Grunewald RA. Panayiotopoulos syndrome: a common and benign childhood epilepsy. Lancet 2001; 357(9259):821–823.

147. Ferrie C, Caraballo R, Covanis A, et al. Panayiotopoulos syndrome: a consensus view. Dev Med Child Neurol 2006; 48:236–240.

148. Panayiotopoulos CP. Elementary visual hallucinations in migraine and epilepsy. J Neurol Neurosurg Psychiatry 1994; 57:1371–1374.

149. Berkovic SF, McIntosh A, et al. Familial temporal lobe epilepsy: a common disorder identified in twins. Ann Neurol 1996; 40:227–235.

150. Scheffer IE, Phillips HA, et al. Familial partial epilepsy with variable foci: a new partial epilepsy syndrome with suggestion of linkage to chromosome 2. Ann Neurol 1998; 44:890–899.

151. Gayatri NA, Livingston JH. Aggravation of epilepsy by anti-epileptic drugs. Dev Med Child Neurol 2006; 48:394–398.

152. Elger CE. Semeiology of temporal lobe seizures. In: Oxbury JM, Polkey CE, Duchowny M, eds. Intractable focal epilepsy. London: WB Saunders; 2000:63–68.

153. Avanzini G, Beaumanoir A, et al. Limbic seizures in children. London: John Libbey; 2001.

154. Bartolomei F, Chuvel P. Seizure symptoms and cerebral localization: frontal lobe and rolandic seizures. In: Oxbury JM, Polkey CE, Duchowny M, eds. Intractable focal epilepsy. London: WB Saunders; 2000.55–62.

155. Gobbi G, Bouquet F, et al. Coeliac disease, epilepsy, and cerebral calcifications. The Italian Working Group on Coeliac Disease and Epilepsy. Lancet 1992; 340(8817):439–443.

156. Hart Y, Andermann F. Rasmussen syndrome. In: Oxbury JM, Polkey CE, Duchowny M, eds. Intractable focal epilepsy. London: WB Saunders; 2001:233–248.

157. Aicardi J, Chevrie JJ. Atypical benign partial epilepsy of childhood. Dev Med Child Neurol 1982; 24:281–292.

158. Doose H, Hahn A, et al. Atypical benign partial epilepsy of childhood or pseudo-Lennox syndrome. Part II: family study. Neuropediatrics 2001; 32:9–13.

*159. Anonymous. Efficacy of felbamate in childhood epileptic encephalopathy (Lennox–Gastaut syndrome). The felbamate study group in Lennox–Gastaut syndrome. N Engl J Med 1993; 328:29–33.

160. Motte J, Trevathan E, et al. Lamotrigine for generalized seizures associated with the Lennox–Gastaut

syndrome. Lamictal Lennox–Gastaut Study Group. N Engl J Med 1997; 337:1807–1812.

*161. Sachdeo RC, Glauser TA, et al. A double-blind, randomized trial of topiramate in Lennox–Gastaut syndrome. Topiramate YL Study Group. Neurology 1999; 52:1882–1887.

*162. Hancock E, Cross H. Treatment of Lennox–Gastaut syndrome. Cochrane Database Syst Rev 2006; 3.

163. Ben-Menachem E, Hellstrom K, et al. Evaluation of refractory epilepsy treated with vagus nerve stimulation for up to 5 years [see comments]. Neurology 1999; 52:1265–1267.

164. Irwin K, Birch V, et al. Multiple subpial transection in Landau–Kleffner syndrome. Dev Med Child Neurol 2001; 43:248–252.

165. Robinson RO, Baird G, et al. Landau–Kleffner syndrome: course and correlates with outcome. Dev Med Child Neurol 2001; 43:243–247.

166. Deonna T. Cognitive and behavioral manifestations of epilepsy in children. In: Wallace SJ, Farrell K, eds. Epilepsy in children. London: Arnold; 2004:250–256.

*167. Verity CM, Butler NR, et al. Febrile convulsions in a national cohort followed up from birth. II – Medical history and intellectual ability at 5 years of age. BMJ (Clin Res Ed) 1985; 290(6478):1311–1315.

168. Wallace SJ. Febrile seizures. In: Wallace SJ, Farrell K, eds. Epilepsy in children. London: Arnold; 2004:123–130.

169. Barlow WE, Davis RL, et al. The risk of seizures after receipt of whole-cell pertussis or measles, mumps, and rubella vaccine. N Engl J Med 2001; 345:656–661.

*170. Offringa M, Moyer VA. Evidence based paediatrics: evidence based management of seizures associated with fever. BMJ 2001; 323:1111–1114.

171. Allen JE, Ferrie CD, et al. Recovery of consciousness following epileptic seizures in children. Arch Dis Child 2007; 92:39–42.

172. Knudsen FU. Febrile seizures: treatment and prognosis. Epilepsia 2000; 41:2–9.

173. Baumann RJ, Duffner PK. Treatment of children with simple febrile seizures: the AAP practice parameter. American Academy of Pediatrics. Pediatr Neurol 2000; 23:11–17.

*174. Scott RC, Besag FM, et al. Buccal midazolam and rectal diazepam for treatment of prolonged seizures in childhood and adolescence: a randomised trial [see comments]. Lancet 1999; 353(9153):623–626.

*175. Lahat E, Goldman M, et al. Comparison of intranasal midazolam with intravenous diazepam for treating febrile seizures in children: prospective randomised study. BMJ 2000; 321(7253):83–86.

*176. McIntyre J, Robertson S, Norris E, et al. Safety and efficacy of buccal midazolam versus rectal diazepam for emergency treatment of seizures in children: a randomised controlled trial. Lancet 2005; 366:205–210.

*177. Annegers JF, Hauser WA, et al. Factors prognostic of unprovoked seizures after febrile convulsions. N Engl J Med 1987; 316:493–498.

*178. Verity CM, Greenwood R, et al. Long-term intellectual and behavioral outcomes of children with febrile convulsions. N Engl J Med 1998; 338:1723–1728.

*179. Annegers JF, Grabow JD, et al. Seizures after head trauma: a population study. Neurology 1980; 30(7 Pt 1):683–689.

180. Hahn YS, Fuchs S, et al. Factors influencing posttraumatic seizures in children. Neurosurgery 1988; 22:864–867.

181. Chandler C. Posttraumatic seizures and posttraumatic epilepsy. In: Oxbury JM, Polkey CE, Duchowny M, eds. Intractable focal epilepsy. London: WB Saunders; 2000.185–193.

182. Shahwan A, Farrell, Deanty N. Progressive myoclonic epilepsies: a review of genetic and therapeutic aspects. Lancet Neurol 2005; 4:239–248.

183. Minassian BA, Ianzano L, et al. Identification of new and common mutations in the EPM2A gene in Lafora disease. Neurology 2000; 54:488–490.

184. Lehesjoki AE, Koskiniemi M. Progressive myoclonus epilepsy of Unverricht–Lundborg type. Epilepsia 1999; 40(suppl 3):23–28.

185. Mole S, Gardiner M. Molecular genetics of the neuronal ceroid lipofuscinoses. Epilepsia 1999; 40(suppl 3):29–32.

186. Lelloch-Tabiana A, Boddaetr N, Bourgeois M, et al. Angiocentir neuroepithelial tumor (ANET): a new epilepsy-related clinicopathological entity with distinctive MEI. Brain Pathol 2005; 15:281–286.

187. Galvan-Manso M, Campistol J, et al. Analysis of the characteristics of epilepsy in 37 patients with the molecular diagnosis of Angelman syndrome. Epileptic Dis 2005; 7:19–25.

188. Huppke P, Held M, et al. The spectrum of phenotypes in females with Rett syndrome. Brain Dev 2003; 25:346–351.

189. Garcia-Alvarez M, Nordli DR, et al. Inherited metabolic disorders. In: Pedley TA, ed. Epilepsy: a comprehensive textbook. Philadelphia: Lippincott-Raven; 1997:2547–2562.

190. Baxter P. Pyridoxine-dependent and pyridoxine-responsive seizures. Dev Med Child Neurol 2001; 43:416–420.

191. Carlsson M, Hagberg G, Olsson I. Clinical and aetiological aspects of epilepsy in children with cerebral palsy. Dev Med Child Neurol 2003; 45:371–376.

192. Austin JK, de Boer HM. Disruptions in social functioning and services facilitating adjustment for the child and adult. In: Pedley TA, ed. Epilepsy: a comprehensive textbook. Philadelphia: Lippincott-Raven; 1997:2191–2201.

193. Timmings P. Toxicity of antiepileptic drugs. In: Pedley TA, ed. Epilepsy: a comprehensive textbook. Philadelphia: Lippincott-Raven; 1997:1165–1173.

194. Kasteleijn-Nolst Trenite D, de Saint-Martin A. Cognitive aspects. In: Wallace SJ, Farrell K, eds. Epilepsy in children. London: Arnold; 2004:443–446.

195. Appleton RE. Guideline may help in prescribing vigabatrin. BMJ 1998; 317(7168):1322.

196. Perucca E. Pharmacokinetics. In: Pedley TA, ed. Epilepsy: a comprehensive textbook. Philadelphia: Lippincott-Raven; 1997:1131–1153.

197. Aicardi J. Epilepsy and other seizure disorders. In: Aicardi J, ed. Diseases of the nervous system in childhood. London: Mac Keith Press; 1998:575–637.

198. Gilman JT. Drug treatment: children. In: Oxbury JM, Polkey CE, Duchowny M, eds. Intractable focal epilepsy. London: WB Saunders; 2000:491–504.

*199. Mattson RH, Cramer JA, et al. A comparison of valproate with carbamazepine for the treatment of complex partial seizures and secondarily generalized tonic–clonic seizures in adults. The Department of Veterans Affairs Epilepsy Cooperative Study No 264 Group. N Engl J Med 1992; 327:765–771.

*200. Verity CM, Hosking G, et al. A multicentre comparative trial of sodium valproate and carbamazepine in paediatric epilepsy. The Paediatric EPITEG Collaborative Group. Dev Med Child Neurol 1995; 37:97–108.

*201. Marson AG, Williamson PR, et al. Carbamazepine versus valproate monotherapy for epilepsy. Cochrane Database Syst Rev 2002

202. Marson AG, Al-Kharusi AM, Alwaidh M, et al. The SANAD study of effectiveness of valproate, lamotrigine or topiramate for generalised and unclassifiable epilepsy: an unblinded randomised controlled trial. Lancet 2007; 369:1016–1026.

203. Marson AG, Al-Kharusi AM, Alwaidh M, et al. The SANAD study of effectiveness of carbamazepine, gabapentin, lamotrigine, oxcarbazepine, or topiramate

for treatment of partial epilepsy: an unblinded randomised controlled trial. Lancet 2007; 369:1000–1015.

204. Camfield C, Camfield P, et al. Asymptomatic children with epilepsy: little benefit from screening for anticonvulsant-induced liver, blood, or renal damage. Neurology 1986; 36:838–841.

*205. Sirven JL, Sperling M, et al. Early versus late antiepileptic drug withdrawal for people with epilepsy in remission. Cochrane Database Syst Rev 2002; 1.

*206. Berg AT, Shinnar S. Relapse following discontinuation of antiepileptic drugs: a meta-analysis. Neurology 1994; 44:601–608.

*207. Verrotti A, Morresi S, et al. Discontinuation of anticonvulsant therapy in children with partial epilepsy. Neurology 2000; 55:1393–1395.

*208. Chadwick D. Does withdrawal of different antiepileptic drugs have different effects on seizure recurrence? Further results from the MRC Antiepileptic Drug Withdrawal Study. Brain 1999; 122(Pt 3):441–448.

*209. Ranganathan LN, Ramaratnam S. Rapid versus slow withdrawal of antiepileptic drugs. Cochrane Database Syst Rev 2006; 2.

210. Matricardi M, Brinciotti M, et al. Outcome after discontinuation of antiepileptic drug therapy in children with epilepsy. Epilepsia 1989; 30:582–589.

211. Bouma PAD, Peters ACB, Brower OF. Long term course of childhood epilepsy following relapse after antiepileptic drug withdrawal. J Neurol Neurosurg Psych 2002; 72:507–510.

212. Camfield PR, Camfield CS, et al. If a first antiepileptic drug fails to control a child's epilepsy, what are the chances of success with the next drug? J Pediatr 1997; 131:821–824.

213. Nicolson A, Appleton RE, et al. The relationship between treatment with valproate, lamotrigine, and topiramate and the prognosis of the idiopathic generalised epilepsies. J Neurol Neurosurg Psych 2004; 75:75–79.

*214. Castillo S, Schmidt DB, et al. Oxcarbazepine add-on for drug-resistant partial epilepsy. Cochrane Database Syst Rev 2002; 1.

*215. Chaisewikul R, Privitera MD, et al. Levetiracetam add-on for drug-resistant localization related (partial) epilepsy. Cochrane Database Syst Rev 2002; 1.

*216. Jette NE, Marson AG, et al. Topiramate add-on for drug-resistant partial epilepsy. Cochrane Database Syst Rev 2002; 1.

*217. Levy R. Lamotrigine add-on for drug-resistant partial epilepsy. Cochrane Database Syst Rev 2002; 1.

*218. Marson AG, Kadir ZA, et al. Gabapentin add-on for drug resistant partial epilepsy. Cochrane Database Syst Rev 2002; 1.

*219. Ramaratnam S, Marson AG, et al. Lamotrigine add-on for drug-resistant partial epilepsy. Cochrane Database Syst Rev 2002; 1.

220. Aicardi J, Shorvon S. Intractable epilepsy. In Pedley TA, ed. Epilepsy: a Comprehensive textbook. Philadelphia: Lippincott-Raven; 1997:1325–1331.

221. Freeman J, Pierangelo V, Lanzi G, Tagliabue A, Perucca E. The ketogenic diet: from molecular mechanisms to clinical effects. Epilepsy Res 2006; 68:145–180.

222. Kossoff EH, McGrogan JR, Bluml RM, et al. A modified Atkins diet is effective for the treatment of intractable pediatric epilepsy. Epilepsia 2006; CD1001911

*223. Privitera MD, Wely TE, et al. Vagus nerve stimulation for partial seizures. Cochrane Database Syst Rev 2002; 1.

224. Parker AP, Polkey CE, et al. Vagal nerve stimulation in epileptic encephalopathies. Pediatrics 1999; 103(4 Pt 1):778–782.

225. Polkey CE. Temporal lobe resections. In: Oxbury JM, Polkey CE, Duchowny M, eds. Intractable focal epilepsy. London: WB Saunders; 2000:667–695.

226. Silfvenius H. Extratemporal cortical excisions for epilepsy. In: Oxbury JM, Polkey CE, Duchowny M, eds. Intractable focal epilepsy. London: WB Saunders; 2000:697–714.

227. Tuite GF, Polkey CE, et al. Hemispherectomy. In: Oxbury JM, Polkey CE, Duchowny M, eds. Intractable focal epilepsy. London: WB Saunders; 2000:715–733.

228. Anonymous. Stopping status epilepticus. Drug Ther Bull 1996; 34:73–75.

229. Scott RC, Surtees RAH, Neville BGR. Status epilepticus: pathophysiology, epidemiology, and outcomes. Arch Dis Child 1998; 79:73–77.

230. Shorvon S. Status epilepticus: its clinical features and treatment in adults and children. Cambridge: Cambridge University Press; 1994.

231. Knudsen FU. Rectal administration of diazepam in solution in the acute treatment of convulsions in infants and children. Arch Dis Child 1979; 54:855–857.

232. DeLorenzo RJ, Pellock JM, et al. Epidemiology of status epilepticus. J Clin Neurophysiol 1995; 12:316–325.

233. Shinnar S, Berg AT, Moshe SL, et al. The risk of seizure recurrence after a first unprovoked afebrile seizure in childhood: an extended follow-up. Pediatrics 1996; 98:216–225.

234. Maytal J, Shinnar S, et al. Low morbidity and mortality of status epilepticus in children. Pediatrics 1989; 83:323–331.

235. The Status Epilepticus Working Party. The treatment of convulsive status epilepticus in children. Arch Dis Child 2000; 83:415–419.

236. Lal Koul R, Aithala GR, Chacko A, et al. Continuous midazolam infusion as treatment of status epilepticus. Arch Dis Child 1997; 76:445–448.

237. Kofke WA, Young RSK, Davis P, et al. Isoflurane for refractory status epilepticus: a clinical series. Anesthesiology 1989; 71:653–659.

238. Tasker RC. Emergency treatment of acute seizures and status epilepticus. Arch Dis Child 1998; 79:78–83.

239. Stephenson JBP. Fits and faints. Oxford: Mac Keith Press; 1990.

240. Horrocks IA, Nechay A, et al. Anoxic-epileptic seizures: observational study of epileptic seizures induced by syncopes. Arch Dis Child 2005; 90:1283–1287.

241. McLeod KA, Wilson N, et al. Cardiac pacing for severe childhood neurally mediated syncope with reflex anoxic seizures. Heart 1999; 82:721–725.

242. Zaidi A, Clough P, et al. Misdiagnosis of epilepsy: many seizure-like attacks have a cardiovascular cause. J Am Coll Cardiol 2000; 36:181–184.

243. McClure RJ, Davis PM, et al. Epidemiology of Munchausen syndrome by proxy, non-accidental poisoning, and non-accidental suffocation. Arch Dis Child 1996; 75:57–61.

244. Fernandez-Alvarez E, Aicardi J. Movement disorders in children. London: Mac Keith Press; 2001.

245. Surtees R. Inherited ion channel disorders. Eur J Pediatr 2000; 159(suppl 3):S199–S203.

246. Jen J, Kim GW, Baloh RW. Clinical spectrum of episodic ataxia type 2. Neurology 2004; 62:17–22.

247. Bakker ML, van Dijk G, et al. Startle syndromes. Lancet Neurol 2006; 5:513–524.

248. Fertleman CR, Rees M, Parker KA, et al. Identification of the gene underlying an inherited disorder of pain sensation. Presented at the 54th Annual Meeting of the American Society of Human Genetics. October 30, 2004. Bethesda, Maryland, USA.

249. Stores G. Recognition and management of narcolepsy. Arch Dis Child 1999; 81:519–524.

250. MacLeod S, Ferrie C, Zuberi SM. Symptoms of narcolepsy in children misinterpreted as epilepsy. Epileptic Dis 2005; 7:13–17.

251. Lemon MD, Strain JD, Farver DK. Sodium oxybate for cataplexy. Ann Pharmacol 2006; 40:433–440.

252. Dauvilliers Y, Carlander B, Rivier F, et al. Successful management of cataplexy with intravenous immunoglobulins at narcolepsy onset. Ann Neurol 2004; 56:905–908.

253. Chen DK, So YT, Fisher RS. Therapeutics and technology assessement subcommittee of the American Academy of Neurology. Use of serum prolactin in diagnosing epileptic seizures: report of the Therapeutics and Technology Assessement Subcommittee of the American Academy of Neurology. Neurology 2005; 65:668–675.

254. Mikati MA, Kramer U, et al. Alternating hemiplegia of childhood: clinical manifestations and long-term outcome. Pediatr Neurol 2000; 23:134–141.

255. Shorvon SD. The epidemiology and treatment of chronic and refractory epilepsy. Epilepsia 1996; 37(suppl 2):S1–S3.

Headache and migraine

*256. Bille B. A 40-year follow-up of school children with migraine. Cephalalgia 1995; 17:488–491.

*257. Abu-Arafeh I, Russell G. Prevalence and causes of headache in schoolchildren. BMJ 1994; 309:765–769.

258. Pothmann R, v. Frankenberg SV, Mueller B, et al. Epidemiology of headache in children and adolescents: evidence of high prevalence of migraine among girls under 10. Int J Behavior Med 1994; 1:76–89.

259. Mortimer MJ, Kay J, Jaron A. Childhood migraine in general practice: clinical features and characteristics. Cephalalgia 1992; 12:238–243.

260. Sillanpää M, Anttila P. Increasing prevalence of headache in 7-year-old schoolchildren. Headache 1996; 36:466–470.

261. Chambers CT, Reid GJ, McGrath PJ, et al. Self-administration of over-the-counter medication for pain among adolescents. Arch Pediatr Adolescent Med 1997; 151:449–455.

262. Dengler R, Roberts H. Adolescents' use of prescribed drugs and over-the-counter preparations. J Public Health Med 1996; 18:437–442.

263. Simon HK, Weinkle DA. Over-the-counter medications. Do parents give what they intend to give?. Arch Pediatr Adolescent Med 1977; 151:654–656.

264. Lewis DW, Qureshi FA. Acute headache in the pediatric emergency department. Headache 2000; 40:200–203.

265. van der Wouden JC, van der Pas P, Bruijnzeels MA, et al. Headache in children in Dutch general practice. Cephalalgia 1999; 19:147–150.

266. Abu-Arafeh I, MacLeod S. Serious neurological disorders in children with chronic headache. Arch Dis Child 2005; 90:937–940.

*267. Headache Classification Committee of the International Headache Society. Proposed classification and diagnostic criteria for headache disorders, cranial neuralgias, and facial pain. Cephalalgia 1988; 8:9–96.

*268. Headache Classification Subcommittee of the International Headache Society. The International Classification of Headache Disorders, second edition. Cephalalgia 2004; 24(suppl 1):1–160.

269. Viswanathen V, Bridges S, Whitehouse W, et al. Childhood headaches: discrete entities or continuum?. Dev Med Child Neurol 1998; 40:544–550.

270. Blumenthal HJ, Rapoport AM. The clinical spectrum of migraine. Med Clin North Am 2001; 85:897–909.

271. Abu-Arafeh I, Callaghan M. Headache clinics for children. In: Childhood headache, clinics in developmental medicine. London: Mac Keith Press/ Cambridge University Press; 2002:175–184.

*272. Russell MB, Iselius L, Olesen J. Migraine without aura and migraine with aura are inherited disorders. Cephalalgia 1996; 16:305–309.

*273. Gervil M, Ulrich V, Kyvik KO, et al. Migraine without aura: a population-based twin study. Ann Neurol 1999; 46:606–611.

*274. Ulrich V, Gervil M, Kyvik KO, et al. Evidence of a genetic factor in migraine with aura: a population-based Danish twin study. Ann Neurol 1999; 45:242–246.

*275. Ophoff RA, Terwindt GM, Vergouwe MN. Familial hemiplegic migraine and episodic ataxia type-2 are caused by mutation in Ca++ channel gene CACNLA4. Cell Tissue Res 1996; 87:543–552.

276. Sanchez del Rio M, Moskowitz M. The trigeminal system. In: Olesen J, Tfelt-Hansen P, Welch KMA, eds. The headaches. Philadelphia: Lippincott Williams and Wilkins; 2000:141–149.

277. Golden GS. The Alice-In-Wonderland syndrome in juvenile migraine. Pediatrics 1979; 65:517–519.

278. Bickerstaff ER. Basilar artery migraine. Lancet 1961; 1:15–17.

*279. Lewis D, Ashwal S, Hershey A, et al. Practice parameter: pharmacological treatment of migraine headache in children and adolescents; Report of the American Academy of Neurology Quality Standards Subcommittee and the Practice Committee of the Child Neurology Society. Neurology 2004; 63:2215–2224.

*280. Damen L, Bruijn JK, Verhagen AP, et al. Symptomatic treatment of migraine in children: a systematic review of medication trials. Pediatrics 2005; 116:295–302.

*281. Hämäläinen ML, Hoppu K, Valkeila E, et al. Ibuprofen or acetaminophen for the acute treatment of migraine in children – a double-blind, randomized, placebo-controlled, crossover study. Neurology 1997; 48:103–107.

*282. Winner P, Rothner AD, Saper J, et al. A randomized, double-blind, placebo-controlled study of sumatriptan nasal spray in the treatment of acute migraine in adolescents. Pediatrics 2000; 106:989–997.

*283. Ahonen K, Hamalainen ML, Rantala H, et al. Nasal sumatriptan is effective in treatment of migraine attacks in children: a randomized trial. Neurology 2004; 23:(62):883–887.

*284. Hämäläinen ML, Hoppu K, Santavuori P. Sumatriptan for migraine attacks in children: a randomized placebo-controlled study. Do children with migraine respond to oral sumatriptan differently from adults? Neurology 1997; 48:1100–1103.

285. Linder SL. Subcutaneous sumatriptan in the clinical setting – the first 50 consecutive patients with acute migraine in a pediatric neurology office practice. Headache 1996; 36:419–422.

*286. Ludvigsson J. Propranolol used in prophylaxis of migraine in children. Acta Neurol Scand 1974; 50:109–115.

287. Forsythe WI, Gillies D, Sills MA. Propranolol (Inderal) in the treatment of childhood migraine. Dev Med Child Neurol 1984; 26:737–741.

*288. Winner P, Pearlman EM, Linder SL, et al. Topiramate for migraine prevention in children: a randomized, double-blind, placebo-controlled trial. Headache 2005; 45:1304–1312.

*289. Symon DN, Russell G. Double blind placebo controlled trial of pizotifen syrup in the treatment of abdominal migraine. Arch Dis Child 1995; 72:48–50.

*290. Gillies D, Sills M, Forsythe I. Pizotifen (Sanomigran) in childhood migraine. A double-blind controlled trial. Eur Neurol 1986; 25:32–35.

*291. Sorge F, De Simone R, Marano E, et al. Flunarizine in prophylaxis of childhood migraine. A double-blind, placebo-controlled, crossover study. Cephalalgia 1988; 8:1–6.

292. Caruso JM, Brown WD, Exil G, et al. The efficacy of divalproex sodium in the prophylactic

treatment of children with migraine. Headache 2000; 40:672–676.

293. Hershey AD, Powers SW, Bentti AL, et al. Effectiveness of amitriptyline in the prophylactic management of childhood headaches. Headache 2000; 40:539–549.

294. Sorge F, Barone P, Steardo L, et al. Amitriptyline as a prophylactic for migraine in children. Acta Neurol Napoli 1982; 4:362–367.

295. Sillanpää M. Changes in the prevalence of migraine and other headaches during the first seven school years. Headache 1983; 23:15–19.

296. Bille B. Migraine in childhood and its prognosis. Cephalalgia 1981; 1:71–75.

297. Bille B. Migraine in childhood: a 30 years follow-up. In: Lanzi G, Balottin U, Cernibori A, eds. Headache in children and adolescents. Amsterdam: Elsevier Science Publishers; 1989:19–26.

298. Verret S, Steele JC. Alternating hemiplegia in childhood: A report of eight patients with complicated migraine beginning in infancy. Pediatr 1971; 47:675–680.

299. Mikati MA, Kramer U, Zupane ML, et al. Alternating hemiplegia of childhood: clinical manifestation and long-term outcome. Pediatr Neurol 2000; 23:134–141.

300. Deonna T, Martin D. Benign paroxysmal torticollis in infancy. Arch Dis Child 1981; 56:956–959.

301. Kimura S, Nezu A. Electromyographic study in an infant with benign paroxysmal torticollis. Pediatr Neurol 1998; 19:236–238.

302. Watson P, Steele JC. Paroxysmal dysequilibrium in the migraine syndrome of childhood. Arch Otolaryngol 1974; 99:177–179.

*303. Abu-Arafeh I, Russell G. Paroxysmal vertigo as a migraine equivalent in children: a population-based study. Cephalalgia 1995; 15:22–25.

304. Fischer AJ. Histamine in the treatment of vertigo. Acta oto-laryngologica 1991; (suppl 479): 24–28.

*305. Abu-Arafeh I, Russell G. Prevalence and clinical features of abdominal migraine compared with those of migraine headache. Arch Dis Child 1995; 72:413–417.

*306. Dignan F, Abu-Arafeh I, Russell G. The prognosis of childhood abdominal migraine. Arch Dis Child 2001; 84:415–418.

307. Worawattanakul M, Rhoads JM, Lichtman SN, et al. Abdominal migraine: prophylactic treatment and follow-up. J Pediatr Gastroenterol Nut 1999; 28:37–40.

*308. Abu-Arafeh I, Russell G. Cyclical vomiting syndrome in children: a population-based study. J Pediatr Gastroenterol Nut 1995; 21:454–458.

*309. Dignan F, Symon DN, Abu-Arafeh I, et al. The prognosis of cyclical vomiting syndrome. Arch Dis Child 2001; 84:55–57.

310. Abu-Arafeh I. Chronic tension type headache in children and adolescents. Cephalalgia 2001; 21:830–836.

311. Terzano MG, Manzoni GC, Maione R. Cluster headache in one year old infant?. Headache 1981; 21:255–256.

312. Maytal J, Lipton RB, Solomon S, et al. Childhood onset cluster headaches. Headache 1992; 32(6):275–279.

313. Goadsby PJ, Edvinsson L. Human in vivo evidence for trigeminovascular activation in cluster headache. Brain 1994; 117:427–434.

314. McNabb S, Whitehouse W. Cluster headache-like disorder in childhood. Arch Dis Child 1999; 81:511–512.

315. Lanzi G, Balottin U, Borgatti R, et al. Late post-traumatic headache in pediatric age. Cephalalgia 1985; 5:211–215.

316. Callaghan M, Abu-Arafeh I. Chronic posttraumatic headache in children and adolescents. Dev Med Child Neurol 2001; 43:819–822.

*317. The Childhood Brain Tumor Consortium. The epidemiology of headache among children with brain tumor. Headache in children with brain tumors. J Neuroncol 1991; 10:31–46.

318. Vazquez-Barquero A, Ibanez FJ, Herrera S, et al. Isolated headache as the presenting clinical manifestation of intracranial tumors: a prospective study. Cephalalgia 1994; 14:270–272.

319. Rossi LN, Vassella F. Headache in children with brain tumors. Childs Nerv Syst 1989; 5:307–309.

320. Edgeworth J, Bullock P, Bailey A, et al. Why are brain tumours still being missed? Arch Dis Child 1996; 74:148–151.

321. Wilne SH, Ferris RC, et al. The presenting features of brain tumours: a review of 200 cases, Arch Dis Child 2006; 91:502–506.

322. Soler D, Cox T, Bullock P, et al. Diagnosis and management of benign intracranial hypertension. Arch Dis Child 1998; 78:89–94.

323. Salman MS, Kirkham FJ, MacGregor DL. Idiopathic 'benign' intracranial hypertension: case series and review. J Child Neurol. 2001; 16:465–470.

Disorders of movement

324. Towen BC, Sporrel T. Soft signs and MBD. Dev Med Child Neurol 1979; 21:528–530.

325. Zhou B, Bae SK, Malone AC, et al. hGFRalpha-4: a new member of the GDNF receptor family and a candidate for NBIA. Pediatr Neurol 2001; 25:156–161.

326. Fenichel GM. Movement disorders. In: Fenichel GM, ed. Clinical pediatric neurology, 4th edn. Philadelphia: WB Saunders; 2001.281–299.

*327. Bressman SB, Sabatti C, Raymond D, et al. The DYT1 phenotype and guidelines for diagnostic testing. Neurology 2000; 54:1746–1753.

328. Swaiman KF. Movement disorders and disorders of the basal ganglia. In: Swaiman KF, Ashwall S, eds. Pediatric neurology. St Louis: Mosby; 1999, 3rd edn. 801–809.

329. Darvet C, Griaud N, Burean M. Benign myoclonus of early infancy. Neuropediatrics 1986; 17:33–38.

330. Di Capua M, Furio L, et al. Benign neonatal sleep myoclonus. Mov Disord 1993; 8:191–194.

331. Brown P. Cortical myoclonus. Curr Opin Neurol 1996; 9:314–316.

332. Kinsbourne M. Myoclonic encephalopathy of infancy. J Neurol Neurosurg Psychiatry 1962; 25:271–276.

333. Comings DE. Tourette syndrome and human behavior. Duarte, CA: Hope Press; 1990.

334. Fernandez-Alvarez E, Aicardi J, eds. APA Diagnostic and Statistical Manual of Mental Disorders, 4th eds. Washington DC: American Psychiatric Association; 1994. In: Fernandery-Aevareg E, Aicardi J, eds. Tic disorders in movement disorders in children. London: Mackeith press for the International Child Neurology Association; 2001.

335. Robertson MM. Tourette syndrome, associated conditions and the complexities of treatment. Brain 2000; 123:425–462.

336. Swedo SE. Paediatric autoimmune neuropsychiatric disorders associated with streptococcal infections, clinical description of the first fifty cases. Am J Psychiatry 1998; 155:264–271.

337. Vanasse M, Bedard P, Andermann F. Shuddering attacks in children and early manifestation of essential tremor. Neurology 1976; 6:1027–1030.

338. Morrison PJ. The spinocerebellar ataxias: molecular progress and newly recognized paediatric phenotypes. Eur J Paediatr Neurol 2000; 4:9–15.

Cerebral palsy

339. Bax M, Goldstein M, Rosenbaum P, et al. Executive Committee for the Definition of Cerebral Palsy. Proposed definition and classification of cerebral palsy, April 2005. Dev Med Child Neurol 2005; 47:571–576.

340. Carr LJ, Reddy SK, Stevens S, et al. Definition and classification of cerebral palsy. Dev Med Child Neurol 2005; 47:508–510.

341. Hagberg B, Hagberg G. Dyskinetic and dystonic cerebral palsy and birth. Acta Paediatr 1992; 81:93–94.

342. Neville B. The Worster–Drought syndrome: a severe test of paediatric neurodisability services? Dev Med Child Neurol 1997; 39:982–984.

343. Palisano R, Rosenbaum P, Walter S, et al. Development and reliability of a system to classify gross motor function in children with cerebral palsy. Dev Med Child Neurol 1997; 39:214–223.

344. Palisano RJ, Cameron D, Rosenbaum PL, et al. Stability of the gross motor function system. Dev Med Child Neurol 2006; 48:424–428.

345. Himmelman K, Beckung E, et al. Gross and fine motor function and accompanying impairments in cerebral palsy. Dev Med Child Neurol 2006; 48:417–423.

346. Dobson F, Morris ME, Baker R, et al. Clinician agreement on gait patterns in children with spastic hemiplegia. Dev Med Child Neurol 2006; 48:429–435.

347. Barry MJ, VanSwearingen JM, Albright AL. Reliability and responsiveness of the Barry–Albright dystonia scale. Dev Med Child Neurol 1999; 41:404–411.

348. Hughes I, Newton R. Genetic aspects of cerebral palsy. Dev Med Child Neurol 1992; 34:80–86.

349. Kuzniecky R, Andermann F, Guerrini R. Congenital bilateral peri-Sylvian syndrome: study of 31 patients. The CBPS Multicentre Collaborative Study. Lancet 1993; 341:608–612.

350. Felix JF, Badawi N, Kurinczuk JJ, et al. Birth defects in children with newborn encephalopathy. Dev Med Child Neurol 2000; 42:803–808.

351. Volpe JJ. Brain injury in the premature infant: Is it preventable?. Paediatr Res 1990; 27(suppl):S28–S33.

352. Veelken N, Hagberg B, et al. Diplegic cerebral palsy in Swedish term and pre-term children – differences in reduced optimality, relations to neurology and pathogenetic factors. Neuropediatrics 1983; 14:20–28.

353. Rezaie P, Dean A. Periventricular leukomalacia, inflammation and white matter injury in the developing nervous system. Neuropathology 2002; 22:106–132.

354. Krägeloh-Mann I, Hagberg B, Petersen D, et al. Bilateral spastic cerebral palsy. Pathogenetic aspects from MRI. Neuropediatrics 1992; 23:46–48.

355. Brown JK, Lin JP, Minns RA. Causes of congenital hemiplegic cerebral palsy. In: Campbell AJM, MacIntosh N, eds. Forfar & Arneil's textbook of pediatrics. 5th edn, Edinburgh: Churchill Livingstone; 1998: 741.

356. Wiklund LM, Uverbrandt P, Flodmark O. Computed tomography as an adjunct to aetiology analysis of hemiplegic cerebral palsy. 1. Children born pre-term. 2. Children born at term. Neuropediatrics 1991; 22:50–56,121–128.

357. Okumura A, Hayakawa F, Kato T, et al. MRI findings in patients with spastic cerebral palsy. 1. Correlation with gestational age at birth. 2. Correlation with type of cerebral palsy. Dev Med Child Neurol 1997; 39:363–368.369–372.

358. Lebeer J. How much brain does a mind need? Scientific, clinical, and educational implications of ecological plasticity. Dev Med Child Neurol 1998; 40:352–357.

359. Pharoah POD, Cooke T, Cooke RWI. Hypothesis for the aetiology of spastic cerebral palsy – the vanishing twin. Dev Med Child Neurol 1997; 39:292–296.

360. Blickstein I. Reflections on the hypothesis for the aetiology of spastic cerebral palsy caused by the vanishing twin syndrome. Dev Med Child Neurol 1998; 40:358.

361. Association of Clinical Cytogenetists Working Party on Chorionic Villi in Prenatal Diagnosis. Cytogenetic analysis of chorionic villi for prenatal diagnosis: an ACC collaborative study of UK data. Prenat Diagn 1994; 14:363–379.

362. Stanley FJ, Blair E, Alberman E. Causal pathways to the cerebral palsies: a new aetiological model. In: Stanley F, Blair E, Alberman E, eds. Cerebral palsies: epidemiology and causal pathways. London: Mac Keith Press/Cambridge University Press; 2000.

363. Hill AB, Hill ID. Statistical evidence and indifference. In: Hill AB, Hill ID, eds. Bradford Hill's principles of medical statistics, 12th edn. London: Edward Arnold; 1991:272–276.

364. McKinlay IA, Ismail H. Health services for children with neurodevelopmental disabilities. In: Petridou E, Nakou S, eds. Children and families with special needs: the right to hope. Athens: European Society for Social Pediatrics; 1991.

365. Almost D, Rosenbaum P. The effectiveness of speech intervention for phonological disorders: a randomised controlled trial. Dev Med Child Neurol 1998; 40:319–325.

366. Ko MLB, McConachie H, Jolleff N. Outcome of recommendations for augmentative communication in children. Child Care Health Dev 1998; 24:195–205.

367. McKinlay IA. Physical therapies for cerebral palsies. In: Jukes AM, ed. Baclofen: spasticity and cerebral pathology. Northampton: Cambridge Medical Publications; 1978:4–6.

368. McKinlay I. Autism: the paediatric neurologist's tale. Br J Disord Commun 1989; 24:201–207.

369. Sterba JA, Rogers BT, et al. Horseback riding in children with cerebral palsy: effect on gross motor function. Dev Med Child Neurol 2002; 44:302–308.

370. McKinlay I, Hyde E, Gordon N. Baclofen: a team approach to drug evaluation of spasticity in childhood. In: Boyle IT, Johnston RV, Forbes CD, eds. Baclofen: a broader spectrum of activity. Scott Med J. 1979;S26–S28.

371. Butler C, Chambers H, Goldstein M, et al. Evaluating research and developmental disabilities: a conceptual framework for reviewing treatment outcomes. Dev Med Child Neurol 1999; 41:55–59.

372. Sussman M. Why don't we know more about what we are doing? Dev Med Child Neurol 2001; 43:507.

373. Dyson R. Shortage of therapists: radical solutions will be needed. BMJ 1990; 300:4.

374. Grahame R. Decline of rehabilitation services and its impact on disability benefits. J R Soc Med. 2002; 95:114–117.

375. Chamberlain MA. Advances in rehabilitation: an overview and an odyssey. Clin Med 2003; 3:62–67.

376. Mizuno K, Ueda A. Neonatal feeding performance as a predictor of neurodevelopmental outcome at 18 months. Dev Med Child Neurol 2005; 47:299–304.

377. Blasco PA. Management of drooling: 10 years after the Consortium on Drooling, 1990. Dev Med Child Neurol 2002; 44:778–781.

378. Cass H, Wallis C, Ryan M, et al. Assessing pulmonary consequences of dysphagia in children with neurological disabilities: when to intervene? Dev Med Child Neurol 47:347–352.

379. Gisel E. Gastrostomy feeding: too much of a good thing? Dev Med Child Neurol 2006; 48:869.

380. Sullivan PB, Alder N, Bachlet AME, et al. Gastrostomy feeding: too much of a good thing? Dev Med Child Neurol 2006; 48:877–882.

381. Potter CR, Unnithan VB. Interpretation and implementation of oxygen uptake kinetics studies in children with cerebral palsy. Dev Med Child Neurol 2005; 47:353–357.

382. Varni JW, Burwinkle TM, Berrin SJ, et al. The PedsQL in pediatric cerebral palsy: reliability, validity and sensitivity of the generic core scales and cerebral palsy module. Dev Med Child Neurol 2006; 48:442–449.

383. Robards MF. Running a team for disabled children and their families. London: Mac Keith Press/Cambridge University Press; 1995.

384. Bax MCO, Whitmore K. District handicapped teams in England, 1983–8. Arch Dis Child 1991; 66:656–664.

385. Bax MCO, Whitmore K. District handicapped teams in England 1983–8. Arch Dis Child 1991; 66:1103 (letter).

386. Court Report: Fit for the future. Report of a Committee on Child Health Services. Cmnd.6684. London: HMSO; 1976: vol 1.

387. Bax MCO, Whitmore K. District handicapped teams: structure, function and relationships. Report to DHSS London, Community Paediatric Research Unit, Westminster Children's Hospital; 1985.

388. Tawfik R, Dickson A, et al. Care givers perceptions following gastrostomy in severely disabled children with feeding problems. Dev Med Child Neurol 1997; 39:746–751.

389. Strauss D, Kastner T, et al. Tube feeding and mortality in children with severe disabilities and mental retardation. Pediatrics 1997; 99:358–362.

390. Sullivan PB. Is tube feeding in disabled children associated with excess mortality? J Pediatr Gastroenterol Nutr 1998; 27:240–241.

391. Kuttiyanawala MA. Gastrostomy complications in infants and children. Ann R Coll Surg Engl 1998; 80:240–243.

392. Khattak IU. Percutaneous endoscopic gastrostomy in paediatric practice. Complications and outcome. J Pediatr Surg 1998; 33:67–72.

393. Shaw NJ, White CP, et al. Osteopenia in cerebral palsy. Arch Dis Child 1994; 71:235–238.

394. Lassman FM, Fisch RO, Vetter DK, La Bens ES. Early correlates of speech, language and hearing: the collaborative perinatal project of the National Institute of Neurological and Communicative Disorders and Stroke. Littleton, Massachusetts: PSG Publishing; 1980:140–144,220–225.

395. Yule W, Rutter M. Language development and disorders. Oxford: Mac Keith Press; 1987: 20–21,357–358.

396. Haynes C, Nidoo S. Children with specific speech and language impairment. Oxford: Mac Keith Press; 1991:202–203.

397. Lees J, Urwin S. Children with language disorders. London: Whurr Publishers; 1991:197–202, 211–212.

398. Fielder AR, Best AB, Bax MCO. The management of visual impairment in childhood. London: Mac Keith Press/Cambridge University Press; 1993:32–33.

399. Wallace SJ. Epilepsy in cerebral palsy. Dev Med Child Neurol 2001; 43:713–717.

400. Hadjipanayis A, Hadjichristodoulou C, Youroukos S. Epilepsy in patients with cerebral palsy. Dev Med Child Neurol 1997; 39:659–663.

401. Clinical Standards Advisory Group. Services for people who have epilepsy. London: Department of Health; 2000.

402. Chadwick C, Smith D. The mis-diagnosis of epilepsy. BMJ 2002; 324:495–496.

403. Nordin V, Gillberg C. Autism spectrum disorders in children with physical or mental disability or both. 1: Clinical and epidemiological aspects. Dev Med Child Neurol 1996; 38:297–313.

404. Nelson KB, Jarether JK, Croen LA, et al. Neuropeptides and neurotrophins in neonatal blood of children with autism or mental retardation. Ann Neurol 2001; 49:597–606.

405. Jan JE, Espezel H, Appleton RE. The treatment of sleep disorders with melatonin. Dev Med Child Neurol 1994; 36:97–107.

406. Neville B, Albright AL. The management of spasticity associated with the cerebral palsies in children and adolscents. Secaucus, NJ: Churchill Communications; 2000.

407. Chu M-L, Sala DA. The use of Tiagabine in pediatric spasticity management. Dev Med Child Neurol 2006; 48:456–459.

408. Carr LJ, Cosgrove AP, Gringras P, Neville BG. Position paper on the use of botulinum toxin in cerebral palsy. UK Botulinum Toxin and Cerebral Palsy Working Party. Arch Dis Child 1998; 79:271–273.

409. Scope. Right from the start. London: Scope; 1994.

410. Cunningham CC, Morgan PA, McGucken RB. Down's syndrome: is dissatisfaction with disclosure of diagnosis inevitable?. Dev Med Child Neurol 1984; 26:33–39.

411. Nelson KB, Ellenberg JH. Children who outgrew cerebral palsy. Paediatrics 1982; 69:529–536.

412. Strauss D, Shavelle R. Life expectancy of adults with cerebral palsy. Dev Med Child Neurol 1998; 40:369–375.

413. Strauss D, Cable W, Shavelle R. Causes of excess mortality in cerebral palsy. Dev Med Child Neurol 1999; 41:580–585.

414. Williams K, Alberman E. Survival in cerebral palsy: the role of severity and diagnostic labels. Dev Med Child Neurol 1998; 40:376–379.

415. Evans PM, Alberman E. Certified cause of death in children and young adults with cerebral palsy. Arch Dis Child 1990; 65:325–329.

416. Evans PM, Evans SJW, Alberman E. Cerebral palsy: why we must plan for survival. Arch Dis Child 1990; 65:1329–1333.

417. Crichton JU, Mackinnon M, White CP. The life expectancy of persons with cerebral palsy. Dev Med Child Neurol 1995; 37:567–576,1032–1033 (letters).

418. Blair E, Watson L, Badawi N, Stanley FJ. Life expectancy among people with cerebral palsy in Western Australia. Dev Med Child Neurol 2001; 43:508–515.

419. Kudrjavcev T, Schoemberg BS, et al. Cerebral palsy: survival rates, associated handicaps and distribution by clinical sub-type (Rochester MN, 1950–1976). Neurology 1985; 35:900–903.

420. Shavelle RM, Strauss VJ, Day SM. Comparison of survival in cerebral palsy between countries. Dev Med Child Neurol 2001; 43:574.

421. Nicholson A, Alberman E. Cerebral palsy – an increasing contributor to severe mental retardation? Arch Dis Child 1992; 67:150–155.

422. Hollins S, Attard MT, Fraunhofer N, et al. Mortality in people with learning disability: risk causes, and death certification findings in London. Dev Med Child Neurol 1998; 40:50–56.

423. Hutton JL, Pharoah POD. Effects of cognitive, motor and sensory disabilities on survival in cerebral palsy. Arch Dis Child 2002; 86:84–90.

424. McLaughlin JF, Bjornson KF. Quality of life and developmental disabilities. Dev Med Child Neurol 1998; 40:435.

425. Ronen GM, Rosenbaum P, et al. Health-related quality of life in childhood epilepsy: the results of children's participation in identifying the components. Dev Med Child Neurol 1999; 41:554–559.

426. Yude C, Goodman R. Peer problems of 9–11 year old children with hemiplegia in mainstream schools Can these be predicted? Dev Med Child Neurol 1999; 41:4–8.

427. De Wolfe NA, Byrne JM, Bawden HN. ADHD in pre-school children: parent rated psycho-social correlates. Dev Med Child Neurol 2000; 42:825–830.

428. Andrew FW, Withey SB. Social indicators of well-being. London: Plenum Press; 1976.

429. Bode H, Weidner K, Stork M. Quality of life in families with children with disabilities. Dev Med Child Neurol 2000; 42:354.

430. Baldwin S. The costs of caring families with disabled children. London: Routledge & Keegan Paul; 1985.

431. Kew S. The cost of handicap. Health Social Serv J 1973; 14:860–861.

432. Baldwin S. Disabled children. Counting the costs. London: The Disability Alliance; 1977.

433. Lawton D. The family fund database. York UK: University of York; 1996.

434. Curran AL, Sharples PM, White C, Knapp M. Time costs of caring for children with severe disabilities compared with caring for children without disabilities. Dev Med Child Neurol 2001; 43:529–533.

435. Hagberg B, Edebol-Tysk K, Edstrom B. The basic care needs of profoundly mentally retarded children with multiple handicaps. Dev Med Child Neurol 1988; 30:287–293.

436. Barabas G, Matthews W, Zumoff P. Care-load for children and young adults with severe cerebral palsy. Dev Med Child Neurol 1992; 34:979–984.

437. Edebol-Tysk K. Evaluation of care-load for individuals with spastic tetraplegia. Dev Med Child Neurol 1989; 31:737–745.

438. Sloper T, Beresford B. Families with disabled children: social and economic needs are high but remain largely unmet. BMJ 2006; 333:928–929.

439. Little WJ. On the influence of abnormal parturition, labour, premature birth and asphyxia neonatorum on the mental and physical condition of the child especially in relation to deformities. Trans Obstet Soc Lond 1862; 3:293–344 (reprinted Cerebral Palsy Bull 1958; 1:5–36)

440. Stanley FJ, Blair E, Alberman E. How common are the cerebral palsies?. In: Stanley F, Blair E, Alberman E, eds. Cerebral palsies: epidemiology and causal pathways. London: Mac Keith Press/Cambridge University Press; 2000:22–39.

441. Blair E. Trends in cerebral palsy prevalence in Northern Ireland, 1981–1997. Dev Med Child Neurol 2006; 48:405.

442. Dolk H, Parkes J, Hill N. Trends in the prevalence of cerebral palsy in Northern Ireland, 1981–1997. Dev Med Child Neurol 2006; 48:406–412.

443. Serdaroglu A, Cansu A, Ozkan S, Tezcan S. Prevalence of cerebral palsy in Turkish children between the ages of 2 and 16 years. Dev Med Child Neurol 2006; 48:413–416.

444. Pschirrer ER, Yeomans ER. Does asphyxia cause cerebral palsy? Semin Perinatol 2000; 24:215–220.

445. Blair EM, Stanley FJ. Intra-partum asphyxia: a rare cause of cerebral palsy. Paediatrics 1988; 133:955.

446. Bakketeig LS. Only a minor part of cerebral palsies cases begin in labour: but still room for controversial child birth issues in court. BMJ 1999; 319:1016–1017.

447. Niswander KR. In: Stanley FJ, Chalmers I, eds. Cerebral palsy, intrapartum care and a shot in the foot. Lancet. 1989:1251–1252.

448. Baxter P, Rosenbloom L. CP or not CP? Dev Med Child Neurol 2005; 47:507.

449. Gupta R, Appleton RE. Cerebral palsy: not always what it seems. Arch Dis Child 2001; 85:3556–3560.

450. Hoon AH, Reinhardt EM, Kelley RI, et al. Brain magnetic resonance imaging and suspected extrapyramidal cerebral palsy: observations in distinguishing genetic–metabolic from acquired causes. J Pediatr 1997; 131:240–245.

451. Nelson KB. Neonatal encephalopathy: etiology and outcome. Dev Med Child Neurol 2005; 47:292.

452. Badawi N, Felix JF, Kurinczuk JF, et al. Cerebral palsy following term newborn encephalopathy: a population-based study. Dev Med Child Neurol 2005; 47:293–298.

453. Bax M, Tydeman C, Flodmark O. Clinical and MRI correlates of cerebral palsy: the European cerebral palsy study. JAMA 2006; 296:1602–1608.

454. Brown JK. Infants damaged during birth: perinatal asphyxia. In: Hull D, ed. Recent advances in paediatrics. Edinburgh: Churchill Livingstone; 1976:57–88.

455. Pasternak JF, Gorey MT. The syndrome of acute near-total intrauterine asphyxia in the term infant. Paediatr Neurol 1998; 18:391–398.

456. Nelson KB, Ellenberg JH. Antecedents of cerebral palsy. Multivariate analysis of risk. N Engl J Med 1986; 315:81–86.

457. Yeargin-Allsopp M, Murphy CC, Cordero JF. Reported biomedical causes and associated medical conditions for mental retardation among 10 year old children: Metropolitan Atlanta, 1985–1987. Dev Med Child Neurol 1997; 39:142–149.

458. Low JA, Muir DW, Pater EA, Karchmar EJ. The association of intrapartum asphyxia in the mature fetus with newborn behaviour. Am J Obstet Gynecol 1990; 163:1131–1135.

*459. Neilson JP, Levene MI. The Cochrane Collaboration: progress in perinatal medicine. Arch Dis Child 1997; 77F:176–177.

460. Umstad MP, Permezel M, Pepperell RJ. Litigation and intra-partum cardiotocograph. Br J Obstet Gynaecol 1995; 102:89–91.

461. Savage LW. The rise in caesarean section: anxiety or science? In: Chard T, Richards MPM, eds. Obstetrics in the 1990s: current controversies. London: Mac Keith Press; 1992:167–191.

462. Smith JH. Is continuous intra-partum foetal monitoring necessary? In: Chard T, Richards MPM, eds. Obstetrics in the 1990s: current controversies. London: Mac Keith Press; 1992:192–201.

463. Edington PT, Sibanda J, Beard RW. Influence on clinical practice of routine intra-partum foetal monitoring. BMJ 1975; 3:341–343.

464. Forfar JO, Hume R, McPhial FM, et al. Low birth weight: a 10 year outcome study of the continuum of reproductive casualty. Dev Med Child Neurol 1994; 36:1037–1048.

465. Pharoah POD, Cooke T, Cooke RWI, Rosenbloom L. Birth weight specific trends in cerebral palsy. Arch Dis Child 1990; 65:602–606.

466. Stanley FJ, Alberman E. Birth weight, gestational age and the cerebral palsies. In: Stanley FJ, Alberman E, eds. The epidemiology of the cerebral palsies. Spastics International Medical Publications. Oxford: Blackwell; 1984:57–68.

467. Pharoah POD, Cooke T, Rosenbloom I, Cooke RWI. Trends in birth prevalence of cerebral palsy. Arch Dis Child 1987; 62:379–383.

468. Stanley FJ, Blair E, Alberman E. Postneonatally acquired cerebral palsy: incidence and antecedents. In: Stanley FJ, Blair E, Alberman E, eds. Cerebral palsies: epidemiology and causal pathways. London: Mac Keith Press/Cambridge University Press; 2000:124–137.

469. Michelsen SI, Uldall P, Kejs AMT, Madsen M. Education and employment prospects in cerebral palsy. Dev Med Child Neurol 2005; 47:511–517.

470. Thomas A, Bax M, Coombes K, et al. The health and social needs of physically handicapped young adults: are they being met by the statutory services?. Dev Med Child Neurol 1985; 27:(suppl 50):1–20.

Degenerative brain disorders

471. Stephenson JBP, King MD. Regression. In: Handbook of neurological investigations in children. London: Wright; 1989:209–222.

472. Armstrong DD. Review of Rett syndrome. J Neuropathol Exp Neurol 1997; 56:843–849.

473. Dayer AG, Bottani A, Bouchardy I, et al. MECP2 mutant allele in a boy with Rett syndrome and his unaffected heterozygous mother. Brain Dev 2007; 29:47–50.

474. Moog U, Smeets EE, van Roozendaal KE, et al. Neurodevelopmental disorders in males related to the gene causing Rett syndrome in females (MECP2). Eur J Paediatr Neurol 2003; 7:5–12.

475. Garbern J, Krajewski KM, Hobson GM. PLP1-related disorders. Geneclinics. 2004. http://www.geneclinics.org

476. van der Knapp MS, Lyter PR, et al. Leukoencephalopathy with swelling and a discrepantly mild clinical course in eight children. Ann Neurol 1995; 37:324–334.

477. Hanefeld F, Holzbach U, Kruse B, et al. Diffuse white matter disease in children: an encephalopathy with unique features on magnetic resonance imaging and proton magnetic resonance spectroscopy. Neuropediatrics 1993; 24:244–248.

478. van der Knapp MS, Gabreels FJM, et al. A new leukoencephalopathy with vanishing white matter. Neurology 1997; 48:845–855.

479. Leegwater PA, Vermeulen G, Konst AA, et al. Subunits of the translation initiation factor eIF2B are mutant in leukoencephalopathy with vanishing white matter. Nat Genet 2001; 29:383–388.

480. Rodrinquez D, Gauthier F, Britini E, et al. Infantile Alexander disease: spectrum of GFAP mutations and genotype–phenotype correlation. Am J Hum Genet 2001; 69:1134–1140.

481. Messing A, Goldman JE, Johnson AB, et al. Alexander disease: new insights from genetics. J Neuropathol Exp Neurol 2001; 60:563–573.

482. Cao H, Williams C, Carter M, et al. CKN1 (MIM 216400): mutations in Cockayne syndrome type A and a new common polymorphism. J Hum Genet 2004; 49:61–63.

483. Aicardi J, Crow YJ. Aicardi–Goutieres syndrome. In: GeneReviews. 2005. Online. Available at:http://www.genetests.org.

484. Bennett MJ, Gibson KM, Sherwood WG, et al. Reliable prenatal diagnosis of Canavan disease (aspartoacylase deficiency): comparison of enzymatic and metabolite analysis. J Inherit Metab Dis 1993; 16:831–836.

485. Hayflick SJ, Hartman M, et al. Brain MRI in neurodegeneration with and without PANK2. Am J Neuroradiol 2006; 27:1230–1233.

486. Dorfman LJ, Pedley TA, et al. Juvenile neuroaxonal dystrophy: clinical, electro-physiological and pathological features. Ann Neurol 1978; 3:419–428.

487. Appleton RE, Farrell K. 'Pure' and 'complicated' forms of hereditary spastic paraplegia presenting in childhood. Dev Med Child Neurol. 1991; 33:304–312.

488. Fink JK, Heiman-Patterson T, Bird T, et al. Hereditary spastic paraplegia: advances in genetic research. Hereditary Spastic Paraplegia Working Group. Neurology 1996; 46:1507–1514.

489. Asber DM. Slow viral infections. In: Behrman RE, Kliegman R, Nelson WE, Vaughan VC, eds. Nelson textbook of pediatrics. Philadelphia: WB Saunders; 1996:1723–1728.

490. Anlar B, Gucuyener K, Imir T, et al. Cimitedine as an immuno-modulator in subacute sclerosing panencephalitis: a double blind, placebo controlled study. Pediatr Infect Dis J 1993; (12):578–581.

491. Meyer N, Rosenbaum V, et al. Search for putative scrapie genome in purified prion fraction reveals a paucity of nucleic acids. J Gen Virol 1991; 72:37–49.

492. Levin M, Walter S. Infections of the nervous system. In: Brett E, ed. Paediatric neurology. London: Churchill Livingstone; 1998:621–690.

Neuromuscular disease

493. MacLeod MJ, Taylor JE, Lunt PW, et al. Prenatal onset of spinal muscular atrophy. Eur J Paediatr Neurol 1999; 2:65–72.

494. Essex C, Roper H. Lesson of the week: late presentation of Duchenne's muscular dystrophy as global developmental delay. BMJ 2001; 323:37–38.

495. Westerlund LE, Gill SS, Jarasz TS, et al. Posterior only unit rod instrumentation for neuromuscular scoliosis. Spine 2001; 26:1984–1989.

496. Hopf CG, Eysel P. One stage versus two-stage spinal fusion in neuromuscular scoliosis. J Pediatr Orthop B 2000; 9:234–243.

497. Simonds AK. Nasal ventilation in progressive neuromuscular disease: experience in adults and adolescents. Monaldi Arch Chest Dis 2000; 55:237–241.

498. Simonds AK, Ward S, Heather S, et al. Outcome of paediatric domiciliary mask ventilation in neuromuscular and skeletal disease. Eur Respir J 2000; 16:476–481.

*499. Arahata K, Ishiura S, Ishiguro T, et al. Immunostaining of skeletal and cardiac muscle surface membrane with antibody against Duchenne muscular dystrophy peptide. Nature 1988; 333:861–863.

*500. Bonilla E, Samitt C, Miranda A, et al. Duchenne muscular dystrophy: deficiency of dystrophin at the muscle cell surface. Cell 1988; 54:447–452.

501. Hoffmann EP, Fischbeck KH, Brown RH, et al. Characterisation of dystrophin in muscle biopsy specimens from patients with Duchenne's or Becker's muscular dystrophy. N Engl J Med 1988; 318:1363–1368.

502. Koenig M, Beggs AH, Moyer M, et al. The molecular basis for Duchenne versus Becker muscular dystrophy: correlation of severity with type of deletion. Am J Hum Genet 1998; 45:498–506.

503. Monaco AP, Bertelson CJ, Leichti-Gallati S, et al. An explanation for the phenotypic differences between patients bearing partial deletions of the DMD locus. Genomics 1988; 2:90–95.

504. Greenstein RM, Reardon MP, Chan TS. An X-autosome translocation in a girl with Duchenne muscular dystrophy – evidence for DMD gene localisation. Pediatr Res 1977; 11:457.(abstract)

505. Verellen-Doumoulin C, Freund M, De Mayer R, et al. Expression of an X-linked muscular dystrophy in a female due to translocation involving Xq21 and non-random inactivation of the normal X chromosome. Hum Genet 1984; 67:115–119.

506. Arikawa E, Hoffmann EP, Kairdo M, et al. The frequency of patients having dystrophin abnormalities in a limb girdle patient population. Neurology 1991; 41:1491–1496.

507. Hoffmann EP, Arahata K, Minetti C, et al. Dystrophinopathy in isolated cases of myopathy in females. Neurology 1992; 42:967–975.

508. Hoogerwaard EM, Bakker E, Ippel PF, et al. Signs and symptoms of Duchenne muscular dystrophy and Becker muscular dystrophy among carriers in the Netherlands: a cohort study. Lancet 1999; 353:2116–2119.

509. Boland BJ, Silbert PL, Groove RV, et al. Skeletal, cardiac and smooth muscle failure in DMD. Pediatr Neurol 1996; 14:7–12.

*510. Cotton S, Voudoria NJ, Greenwood KM. Intelligence and Duchenne muscular dystrophy: full-scale, verbal and performance intelligence quotients. Dev Med Child Neurol 2001; 43:497–501.

511. Bush A, Dubowitz V. Fatal rhabdomyolysis complicating general anaesthesia in a child with BMD. Neuromuscul Disord 1991; 1:201–204.

512. Barohn RJ, Levine EJ, Olson JO, et al. Gastric hypomotility in Duchenne muscular dystrophy. N Engl J Med 1988; 319:15–18.

513. Griggs RC, Moxley RT, Mendell JR, et al. Prednisone in Duchenne dystrophy: a randomized controlled trial defining the course and dose response. Clinical Investigation of Duchenne Dystrophy Group. Arch Neurol 1991; 48:383–388.

514. Mendell JR, Moxley RT, Griggs RC, et al. Randomised double-blind six-month trial of prednisone in Duchenne's muscular dystrophy. N Engl J Med 1989; 320:1592–1597.

515. Backmann E, Henriksson KG. Low dose prednisolone treatment in Duchenne and Becker muscular dystrophy. Neuromuscul Disord 1995; 5:133–241.

516. Manzur AY, Kuntzer T, Pike M, et al. Glucocorticosteroids for Duchenne muscular dystrophy. Cochrane Rev 2004; (2):CD 003725.

517. Sansome A, Royston P, Dubowitz V. Steroids in Duchenne muscular dystrophy; pilot study of a new low dose schedule. Neuromuscul Disord 1993; 3:567–569.

518. Biggar WD, Gringas M, Fehlings DL, et al. Deflazacort treatment of Duchenne muscular dystrophy. J Pediatr 2001; 138:45–50.

519. Silversides CK, Webb GD, Harris VA, et al. Effects of deflazacort on left ventricular function in patients with Duchenne muscular dystrophy. Am J Cardiol 2003; 91:769–772.

520. van Deutekom JCT, Wijmenga C, van Tienhoven EA, et al. FSHD associated DNA rearrangements are due to large deletions of integral copies of a 32kb tandemly repeated unit. Hum Mol Genet 1993; 2:2037–2042.

521. Winokur ST, Bengtsson U, Feddersen J, et al. DNA rearrangement associated with facioscapulo-humeral muscular dystrophy involves a hetero-chromatin-associated repetitive element: implications for a role of chromatin structure in the pathogenesis of the disease. Chromosome Res 1994; 2:225–234.

522. Taylor GS, Maehama T, Dixon JE. Myotubularin, a protein tyrosine phosphatase mutated in myotubular myopathy, dephosphorylases the lipid second messenger phosphatidylinositol 3-phosphate. Proc Natl Acad Sci USA 2000; 97:8910–8915.

523. Herman G, Finegold M, Zhao W, et al. Medical complications in long-term survivors with X-linked myotubular myopathy. J Pediatr 1999; 134:206–214.

*524. Bitoun M, Maugenre S, Jeannet PY, et al. Mutations in dynamin 2 cause dominant centronuclear myopathy. Nat Genet 2005; 37:1207–1209.

525. Goebel HH, Warlo I. Nemaline myopathy with intranuclear rods – intranuclear rod myopathy. Neuromuscul Disord 1997; 7:13–19.

526. Lammens M, Moerman P, Fryns JP, et al. Fetal akinesis sequence caused by nemaline myopathy. Neuropediatrics 1997; 2:116–119.

*527. Laing NG, Wilton SD, Akkari PA, et al. A mutation in the alpha-tropomyosin gene TPM3 associated with autosomal dominant nemaline myopathy NEM1. Nat Genet 1995; 9:75–79.

*528. Nowak KJ, Wattanasirichaigoon D, Goebel HH. Mutations in the skeletal muscle alpha-actin gene in patients with actin myopathy and nemaline myopathy. Nat Genet 1999; 23:208–212.

529. Donner K, Ollikainen M, Ridanpää M, et al. Mutations in the β-tropomyosin (TPM2) gene – a rare cause of nemaline myopathy. Neuromuscul Disord 2002; 12:151–158.

530. Johnston JJ, Kelley RI, Crawford TO, et al. A novel nemaline myopathy in the Amish caused by a mutation in troponin T1. Am J Hum Genet 2000; 67:814–821.

531. Quane KA, Healy JM, Keating KE, et al. Mutations in the ryanodine receptor gene in central core disease and malignant hyperthermia. Nat Genet 1993; 5:51–55.

532. Jungbluth H, Müller CR, Halliger-Keller B, et al. Autosomal recessive inheritance of RYR1 mutations in a congenital myopathy with cores. Neurology 2002; 59:284–287.

533. Manzur AY, Sewry CA, Ziprin J, et al. A severe clinical and pathological variant of central core disease with possible autosomal recessive inheritance. Neuromuscul Disord 1998; 8:467–473.

534. Nagai T, Tsuchiya Y, Maruyama A, et al. Scoliosis associated with central core disease. Brain Dev 1994; 16:150–152.

535. Ferreiro A, Quijano-Roy S, Pichereau C, et al. Mutations of the selenoprotein N gene, which is implicated in rigid spine muscular dystrophy, cause the classical phenotype of multiminicore disease: reassessing the nosology of early-onset myopathies. Am J Hum Genet 2002; 71:739–749.

536. Jungbluth H, Sewry C, Brown SC, et al. Minicore myopathy in children: a clinical and histopathological study of 19 cases. Neuromuscul Disord 2000; 10:262–273.

537. Rowe PW, Eagle M, Pollitt C, et al. Multicore myopathy: respiratory failure and paraspinal muscle contractures are important complications. Dev Med Child Neurol 2000; 42:340–343.

538. Dubowitz V. Workshop report: the 41st ENMC sponsored workshop on congenital muscular dystrophy. Neuromuscul Disord 1996; 6:295–306.

539. van der Knaap M, Smit LM, et al. Magnetic resonance imaging in classification of congenital muscular dystrophies with brain abnormalities. Ann Neurol 1997; 42:50–59.

540. Philpot J, Cowan F, Pennock J, et al. Merosin deficient congenital muscular dystrophy: the spectrum of brain involvement on magnetic resonance imaging. Neuromuscul Disord 1999; 9:81–85.

541. Shorer Z, Philpot J, Muntoni F, et al. Demyelinating peripheral neuropathy in merosin-deficient congenital muscular dystrophy. J Child Neurol 1995; 10:472–475.

*542. Brockington M, Blake DJ, Prandini P. Mutations in the fukutin related protein gene (FKRP) cause a form of congenital muscular dystrophy with secondary laminin-α2 deficiency and abnormal glycosylation of α-dystroglycan. Am J Hum Genet 2001; 69:1198–1209.

*543. Camacho Vanegas O, Bertini E, Zhang RZ, et al. Ullrich scleroatonic muscular dystrophy is caused by recessive mutations on collagen type VI. Proc Natl Acad Sci USA 2001; 98:7516–7521.

544. Moghadaszadeh B, Petit N, Jaillard C, et al. Mutations in the SEPN1 gene cause congenital muscular dystrophy with spinal rigidity and restrictive respiratory syndrome. Nat Genet 2001; 21:17–18.

545. Yoshida A, Koyayashi K, Manya H, et al. Muscular dystrophy and neuronal migration disorder caused by mutations in a glycosyltransferase POMGnT1. Dev Cell 2001; 1:717–724.

546. Dobyns WB, Pagon RA, Armstrong D, et al. Diagnostic criteria for Walker Warburg syndrome. Am J Med Genet 1998; 32:195–210.

547. Beltran Valero De Bernabe D, Currier S, Steinbrecher A, et al. Mutations in the O-mannosyltransferase gene POMT1 give rise to the severe neuronal migration disorder Walker–Warburg syndrome. Am J Hum Genet 2002; 71:10.

548. Phillips MF, Harper PS. Cardiac disease in myotonic dystrophy. Cardiovasc Res 1997; 33:13–22.

549. O'Brien T, Harper PS. Reproductive problems and neonatal loss in women with myotonic dystrophy. Clin Genet 1984; 23:366–369.

550. Harley HG, Brook JD, Rundle SA, et al. Expansion of an unstable DNA region and phenotypic variation in myotonic dystrophy. Nature 1992; 6:545–546.

551. Reardon W, Newcombe R, Fenton I, et al. The natural history of congenital myotonic dystrophy: mortality and long term clinical aspects. Arch Dis Child 1993; 68:177–181.

552. Bergoffen J, Kant J, Sladky J, et al. Paternal transmission of congenital myotonic dystrophy. J Med Genet 1994; 31:518–520.

553. Ohya K, Tachi N, Chiba S, et al. Congenital myotonic dystrophy transmitted from an asymptotic father. Neurology 1994; 44:1958–1960.

554. Liquori CL, Ricker K, Moseley ML, et al. Myotonic dystrophy type 2 caused by a CCTG expansion in intron 1 of ZNF9. Science 2001; 293:864–867.

555. Koch M, Steinmeyer K, Lorenz C, et al. The skeletal muscle chloride channel in dominant and recessive human myotonia. Science 1992; 257:797–800.

556. Lehmann-Horn F, Jurkat-Rott K. Voltage gated ion channels and hereditary disease (review). Physiol Rev 1999; 79:1317–1372.

557. Plassart E, Reboul J, Rime CS, et al. Mutations in the muscle sodium channel gene (SCN4A) in 13 French families with hyperkalaemic periodic paralysis and paramyotonia: phenotype to genotype correlation and demonstration of the predominance of two mutations. Eur J Hum Genet 1994; 2: 110–124.

558. Ptacek LJ, Tawill R, Grigos RC, et al. Dihydropyridine receptor mutations cause hypokalemic periodic paralysis. Cell 1994; 78:1021–1027.

559. Bulman DE, Scoggan KA, van Oene MD, et al. A novel sodium channel mutation in a family with hypokalaemic periodic paralysis. Neurology 1999; 53:1932–1936.

560. Abbott GW, Butler MH, Bendahhou S, et al. MIRP2 forms potassium channels in skeletal muscle with Kv3.4 and is associated with periodic paralysis. Cell 2001; 104:217–231.

561. Plaster NM, Tawil R, Tristani-Firouzi, et al. Mutations in Kir2.1 cause the developmental and episodic electrical phenotypes of Andersen's syndrome. Cell 2001; 105:511–519.

562. Symmons DPM, Sills JA, Davis SM. The incidence of juvenile dermatomyositis: results from a nationwide study. Br J Rheumatol 1995; 34:732–736.

563. Pachman LM. An update on juvenile dermatomyositis. Curr Opin Rheumatol 1995; 7:437–441.

564. Lister RK, Cooper ES, Paige DG. Papules and pustules of the elbows and knees: an uncommon clinical sign of dermatomyositis in oriental children. Pediatr Dermatol 2000; 17:37–40.

565. Al-Mayouf SM, Laxer RM, Schneider R, et al. Intravenous immunoglobulin therapy for juvenile dermatomyositis: efficacy and safety. J Rheumatol 2000; 27:2498–2503.

566. Al-Mayouf S, Al-Mazyed AA, Bahbri S. Efficacy of early treatment of severe juvenile dermatomyositis with intravenous methylprednisolone and methotrexate. Clin Rheumatol 2000; 19:138–141.

567. Tabarki B, Ponsot G, Prieur A-M, et al. Childhood dermatomyositis: clinical course of 36 patients treated with low doses of corticosteroids. Eur J Paediatr Neurol 1998; 2:205–211.

568. Aihara Y, Mori M, Ibe M, et al. A case of juvenile dermatomyositis with calcinosis universalis – remarkable improvement with aluminium hydroxide therapy. Ryumachi 1994; 34:879–884.

569. Mukamel M, Horev G, Mimouni M. New insight into calcinosis of juvenile dermatomyositis. J Pediatr 2001; 138:763–766.

570. Watt G, Saisorn S, Jongsakul K, et al. Blinded, placebo-controlled trial of antiparasitic drugs for trichinosis myositis. J Infect Dis 2000; 182:371–374.

571. Shevell M, Rosenblatt B, Silver K, et al. Congenital inflammatory myopathy. Neurology 1990; 40:1111–1114.

572. Vajsar J, Jay V, Babyn P. Infantile myositis in the newborn period. Brain Dev 1996; 18:415–419.

573. Tein I, DiMauro S, DeVivo D. Recurrent childhood myoglobinuria. Adv Pediatr 1990; 37: 77–117.

574. Darin N, Oldfors A, Moslemi A-R, et al. The incidence of mitochondrial encephalomyopathies in childhood: clinical features and morphological, biochemical and DNA studies. Ann Neurol 2001; 49:377–383.

575. Hoch W, McConvill J, Melms A, et al. Autoantibodies to the receptor tyrosine kinase MuSK in patients with myasthenia gravis without acetylcholine receptor antibodies. Nat Med 2001; 7:365–368.

576. Gronseth GS, Barohn RJ. Practice parameter: thymectomy for autoimmune myasthenia gravis (an evidenced based review): Report of the Quality Standards Subcommittee of the American Academy of Neurology. Neurology 2000; 55:7–15.

577. Lefebvre S, Burglen L, Reboullet S. Identification and characterisation of a spinal muscular atrophy determining gene. Cell 1995; 80:155–165.

578. Campbell L, Potter A, Ignatius J, et al. Genomic variation and gene conversion in spinal muscular atrophy: implications for disease process and clinical phenotype. Am J Hum Genet 1997; 61:40–50.

579. Dubowitz V. Chaos in the classification of SMA: a possible resolution. Neuromuscul Disord 1995; 5:3–5.

*580. Grohmann K, Scheulke M, Diers A, et al. Mutations in the gene encoding the immunoglobulin mu-binding protein 2 cause spinal muscular atrophy with respiratory distress type 1. Nat Genet 2001; 29:75–77.

581. Goutières F, Aicardi J, Farkas E. Anterior horn cell disease associated with pontocerebellar hypoplasia in infants. J Neurol Neurosurg Psychiatry 1977; 40:370–378.

582. Muntoni F, Goodwin F, Sewry C. Clinical spectrum and diagnostic difficulties of infantile pontocerebellar hypoplasia type 1. Neuropediatrics 1999; 30:243–248.

583. Frijns CJM, Van Deutekom J, Frants RR, et al. Dominant congenital benign spinal muscular atrophy. Muscle Nerve 1994; 17:192–197.

584. van der Vleuten AJW, van Ravenswaaij-Arts CMA, Frijns CJM. Localisation of the gene for a dominant congenital spinal muscular atrophy predominantly affecting the lower limbs to chromosome 12q23–q24. Eur J Hum Genet 1998; 6:376–387.

585. Tooth HH. The peroneal type of muscular atrophy. London: HK Lewis; 1886.

586. Charcot JM, Marie P. Su rune forme particuliére d'atrophie musculaire progressive souvent familiale, debutante par les pieds et les jambes, et atteignant plus tard les mains. Rev Med Fr 1886; 6:97–138.

587. Timmerman V, Nelis E, Van Hul K, et al. The peripheral myelin protein gene PMP-22 is contained within the Charcot–Marie–Tooth disease 1A duplication. Nat Genet 1992; 1:171–175.

588. Nicholson GA, Valentijn LJ, Cherryson AK, et al. A frame shift in the PMP 22 gene in hereditary neuropathy with liability to pressure palsy. Nat Genet 1994; 6:263–266.

589. Hayasaka K, Himoro M, Sato W, et al. CMT neuropathy type 1B is associated with mutations of myelin P0 gene. Nat Genet 1993; 5:31–34.

590. Warner LE, Mancias P, Butler IJ, et al. Mutations in the early growth response 2 (EGR2) gene are associated with hereditary myelinopathies. Nat Genet 1998; 18:382–384.

591. Bergoffen J, Scherer SS, Wang S, et al. Connexin mutations in X-linked Charcot–Marie–Tooth disease. Science 1993; 262:2039–2042.

592. Priest JM, Fischbeck KH, Nouri N, et al. A locus for axonal motor-sensory neuropathy with deafness and mental retardation maps to Xq24–26. Genomics 1995; 29:406–412.

593. Hagberg B, Lyan G. Pooled European series of hereditary peripheral neuropathies in infancy and childhood. Neuropediatrics 1981; 12:9–17.

594. Makari GS, Carroll JE, Burton EM. Hereditary sensory neuropathy manifesting as possible child abuse. Pediatrics 1994; 93:842–844.

Decreased consciousness and coma (including hypoxic–ischemic, toxic and metabolic encephalopathies)

595. Advanced Life Support Group. Advanced paediatric life support. The practical approach. 3rd edn. London: BMJ Books; 2001.

596. Addy DP. When not to do a lumbar puncture. Arch Dis Child 1987; 62:873.

597. Archer BD. Computed tomography before lumbar puncture in acute meningitis: a review of the risks and benefits. CMAJ 1993; 148:961–965.

598. Leggate JRS, Minns RA. Intracranial pressure monitoring – current methods. In: Minns RA, ed. Problems of intracranial pressure in childhood. Clinics in developmental medicine nos 113–114. London: Mac Keith Press; 1991:123–140.

599. Minns RA, Merrick MV. Cerebral perfusion pressure and net cerebral mean transit time in childhood hydrocephalus. J Pediatr Neurosci 1989; 5:69–77.

*600. Schierhout G, Roberts I. Anti-epileptic drugs for preventing seizures following acute traumatic brain injury. Cochrane Rev 2001: CD000173.

*601. Alderson P, Roberts I. Corticosteroids for acute traumatic brain injury. Cochrane Rev 2000; (2):CD000196.

*602. Roberts I, Schierhout G, Alderson P. Absence of evidence for the effectiveness of five interventions routinely used in the intensive care management of severe head injury: a systematic review. J Neurol Neurosurg Psychiatry 1998; 55:729–733 (review).

603. Schaad UB, Lips U, Grehm HM, et al. Dexamethasone treatment for bacterial meningitis in children. Lancet 1993; 342:457–461.

*604. Roberts I, Schierhout G, Wakai A. Mannitol for acute traumatic brain injury. Cochrane Rev 2003: CD001049.

605. Tomlin PI, Clarke MA, et al. Rehabilitation in severe head injury in children: outcome and provision of care. Dev Med Child Neurol 2002; 44:828–837.

606. Shaw KN, Briede CA. Submersion injuries: drowning and near drowning. Emerg Med Clin North Am 1989; 7:355–370.

607. Ashwal S, Schneider S, Tomasi L, et al. Prognostic implications of hyperglycaemia and reduced cerebral blood flow in children with near drowning. Neurology 1990; 40:820–823.

608. Hawkins M, Harrison J, Charters P. Severe carbon monoxide poisoning: outcome after hyperbaric oxygen therapy. Br J Anaesth 2000; 84:584–586.

609. Antoon AY, Volpe JJ, Crawford JD. Burn encephalopathy in children. Pediatrics 1972; 50:609–616.

Infectious and inflammatory disorders of the CNS

610. Baraff LJ, Lee SI, Schiger DL. Outcome of bacterial meningitis in children: a meta analysis. Pediatr Infect Dis J 1993; 12:389–394.

611. Schaad UB, Lips U, Grehm HM, et al. Dexamethasone treatment for bacterial meningitis in children. Lancet 1993; 342:457–461.

612. Trinka E, Dubeau F, Andermann F, et al. Clinical findings, imaging characteristics and outcome in catastrophic post-encephalitic epilepsy. Epileptic Disord 2000; 2:153–162.

613. Ito Y, Kimura H, Yabuta Y, et al. Exacerbation of herpes simplex encephalitis after successful treatment with acyclovir. Clin Infect Dis 2000; 30:185–187.

614. Schmutzhard E. Viral infections of the CNS with special emphasis on herpes simplex infections. J Neurol 2001; 248:469–477 (review).

615. Bingham PM, Galetta SL, Arhreya B, et al. Neurologic manifestations in children with Lyme disease. Pediatrics 1995; 96:1053–1056.

616. Li M, Masuzawa T, Wang J, et al. In-vitro and in-vivo antibiotic susceptibilities of Lyme disease *Borrelia* isolated in China. J Infect Chemother 2000; 6:65–67.

617. Klempner MS, Hu LT, Evans J, et al. Two controlled trials of antibiotic treatment in patients with persistent symptoms and a history of Lyme disease. N Engl J Med 2001; 345:85–92.

Acute para- or quadraparsis

618. Rantala H, Uhari M, Cherry JD, et al. Risk factors for respiratory failure in children with Guillain–Barré syndrome. Pediatr Neurol 1995; 13:289–292.

619. van Der Meche FGA, Schmitz PIM The Dutch Guillain–Barré study group. N Engl J Med 1992; 326:1123–1129.

Traumatic (accidental and non-accidental) brain and spinal cord injury and neurorehabilitation

620. Parslow RC, Morris KP, Tasker RC, et al. Epidemiology of traumatic brain injury in children receiving intensive care in the UK. Arch Dis Child 2005; 90:1182–1187.

621. Sharples PM, Storey A, Aynsley-Green A, et al. Avoidable factors contributing to death of children with head injury. BMJ 1990; 300:87–91.

622. Royal College of Paediatrics and Child Health. Guidelines for good practice: early management of patients with a head injury. London: RCPCH; 2001.

623. Potts MB, Koh SE, Whetstone WD, et al. Traumatic injury to the immature brain: inflammation, oxidative injury and iron-mediated damage as potential therapeutic targets. NeuroRx 2006; 3:143–153.

624. Grados MA, Slomine BS, et al. Depth of lesion model in children and adolescents with moderate to severe traumatic brain injury: use of SPGR MRI to predict severity and outcome. J Neurol Neurosurg Psychiatry 2001; 70:350–358.

625. Berryhill P, Lilly MA, et al. Frontal lobe changes after severe diffuse closed head injury in children: a volumetric study of magnetic resonance imaging. Neurosurgery 1995; 37:392–399.

626. Levin HS, Benavidez DA, Verger-Maestre K, et al. Reduction of corpus callosum after severe traumatic brain injury in children. Neurology 2000; 54:647–653.

627. Hoelper BM, Reinhert MM, et al. RCBF in haemorrhagic, non-haemorrhagic and mixed contusions after severe head injury and its effect on perilesional cerebralblood flow. Acta Neurochir Suppl 2000; 76:21–25.

628. Jackson SA, Piper I, et al. Assessment of the variation in cerebrovascular reactivity in head injured patients. Acta Neurochir Suppl 2000; 76:445–449.

629. Tasker RC. Pharmacological advance in the treatment of acute brain injury. Arch Dis Child 1999; 81:90–95.

630. Gopinath SP, Valadka AB, et al. Extracellular glutamate and aspartate in head injured patients. Acta Neurochir Suppl 2000; 76:437–438.

631. Battison C, Andrews PJ, Graham C, et al. Randomised controlled trial on the effect of a 20% mannitol solution and a 7.5% saline/6% dextran solution on increased intracranial pressure after brain injury. Crit Care Med 2005; 33:196–202; discussion 257–258.

632. Chambers IR, Jones PA, Minns RA, et al. Which paediatric head injured patients might benefit from decompression? Thresholds of intracranial pressure and cerebral perfusion pressure in the first six hours. Acta Neurichir Suppl 2005; 95:21–23.

633. Adelson PD, Ragheb J, Muizelaar JP, et al. Phase II clinical trial of moderate hypothermia after severe traumatic brain injury in children. Neurosurgery 2005; 56:740–754.

634. Bor-Seng-Shu E, Hirsch R, Teixeira MJ, et al. Cerebral hemodynamic changes gauged by transcranial Doppler ultrasonography in patients with post-traumatic brain swelling treated by surgical decompression. J Neurosurg 2006; 104:93–100.

635. Taylor A, Butt W, Rosenfield J, et al. A randomized trial of very early decompressive craniectomy in children with traumatic brain injury and sustained intracranial hypertension. Child Nerv Syst 2001; 17:154–162.

636. Levin HS, Eugenio GA, Eisenberg HM, et al. Magnetic resonance imaging after closed head injury in children. Neurosurgery 1989; 24:223–227.

637. Leggate JRS, Lopez-Ramos N, Genitori L, et al. Extradural haematoma in infants. Br J Neurosurg 1989; 3:533–540.

638. Edwards OM, Clark JD. Post-traumatic hypopituitarism. Six cases and a review of the literature. Medicine (Baltimore) 1986; 65:281–290.

639. Choux M, Lena G, Genitori L. Intracranial haematomas. In: Raimondi AJ, Choux M, di Rocco C, eds. Head injuries in the newborn and infant. Heidelberg: Springer-Verlag; 1986:203–216.

640. Faerber EN. Intracranial tumours. In: Faerber EN, ed. CNS magnetic resonance imaging in infants and children. Clinics in developmental medicine, no.134 London: Mac Keith Press; 1995:165–172.

641. Vespa PM, Nuwer MR, et al. Increased incidence and impact of non-convulsive and convulsive seizures after traumatic brain injury as detected by continuous electro-encephalographic monitoring. J Neurosurg 1999; 91:750–760.

642. Cirak B, Ziegfield S, Knight VM, et al. Spinal injuries in children. J Pediatr Surg 2004; 39:607–612.

643. Vialle LR, Vialle E. Pediatric spine injuries. Injury 2005; 36:B102–B112.

644. McCall T, Fassett D, Brockmeyer D. Cervical spine trauma in children: a review. Neurosurg. Focus 2006; 20:(2):E5.

645. Wang MY, Hoh DJ, Leary SP, et al. High rates of neurological improvement following severe pediatric spinal cord injury. Spine 2004; 29: 1493–1497; discussion E266.

646. Tomlin PI, Clarke MA, et al. Rehabilitation in severe head injury in children: outcome and provision of care. Dev Med Child Neurol 2002; 44:828–837.

647. Asikainen I, Kaste M, Sara S. Early and late post-traumatic seizures in traumatic brain injury rehabilitation patients: brain injury factors causing late seizures and influence of seizures on long-term outcome. Epilepsia 1999; 40:584–589.

648. Barlow KM, Spowart JJ, Minns RA. Early posttraumatic seizures in non-accidental head injury: relation to outcome. Dev Med Child Neurol 2000; 42:591–594.

649. Annegers JF, Hauser WA, et al. A population based study of seizures after traumatic brain injuries. N Engl J Med 1998; 338:20–24.

650. Kinsella G, Packer S, Olver J. Maternal reporting of behaviour following very severe blunt head injury. J Neurol Neurosurg Psychiatry 1991; 54:422–426.

651. Massagli TL, Jaffe KM. Pediatric traumatic brain injury: prognosis and rehabilitation. Pediatr Ann 1994; 23:29–36.

652. Levin HS, Hanten G. Executive functions after traumatic brain injury in children. Pediatr. Neurol 2005; 33:79–93.

653. Rivara JMB. Family functioning following pediatric traumatic brain injury. Pediatr Ann 1994; 23:38–44.

654. Chadwick O, Rutter M, et al. Intellectual performance and reading skills after localised head injury in childhood. J Child Psychol Psychiatry 1981; 22:117–139.

655. Michaud LJ, Rivara GP, et al. Predictors of survival and severity of disability after severe brain injury in children. Neurosurgery 1992; 31:254–264.

656. Jaffe KM, Fay GC, et al. Severity of pediatric traumatic brain injury and early neurobehavioural outcome. Arch Phys Med Rehabil 1992; 73:540–547.

657. Minns RA. Intracranial pressure monitoring. Arch Dis Child 1984; 59:486–488.

658. Goldenberg G, Oder W, et al. Cerebral correlates of disturbed executive function and memory in survivors of severe closed head injury. J Neurol Neurosurg Psychiatry 1992; 55:362–368.

659. Department for Education and Skills. Special Educational Needs Code of Practice: SEN Toolkit, Section 7: Writing a Statement of Special Educational Needs; Section 12: The role of Health Professionals. Annesley, Nottinghamshire, UK: DfES Publications; 2001.

660. Couchman M, Rossiter L, et al. A practical outcome scale for paediatric head injury. Arch Dis Child 2001; 84:120–124.

661. Helders PJ, Engelbert RH, et al. Paediatric rehabilitation. Disabil Rehabil 2001; 23:497–500.

662. Powell JM, Machamer JE, et al. Self-report of extent of recovery and barriers to recovery after traumatic brain injury: a longitudinal study. Arch Phys Med Rehabil 2001; 82:1025–1030.

663. Hellawell DJ, Signorini DF, Pentland B. Reliability of the relative's questionnaire for assessment of outcome after brain injury. Disabil Rehabil 2000; 22:446–450.

664. McCarthy ML, Mackenzie EJ, Dennis R, et al. The Pediatric Quality of Life Inventory: an evaluation of its reliability and validity for children with traumatic brain injury. Arch Phys Med Rehabil 2005; 86:1901–1909.

665. Barlow KM, Minns RA. Annual incidence of shaken impact syndrome in young children. Lancet 2000; 356(9241):1571–1572.

666. Elmer E, Gregg GS. Developmental characteristics of abused children. Pediatrics 1967; 40:596–602.

667. Southall DP, Stebbens VA, Rees SV. Apnoeic episodes induced by smothering: two cases identified by covert video surveillance. BMJ 1987; 294:1637–1641.

668. Duhaime AC, Gennarelli TA, Thibault LE, et al. The shaken baby syndrome. J Neurosurg 1987; 66:409–415.

669. Feldman KW, Brewer DK. Child abuse, cardiopulmonary resuscitation and rib fractures. Pediatrics 1984; 73:339–342.

670. Odom A, Christ E, Kerr N, et al. Prevalence of retinal hemorrhages in pediatric patients after in-hospital cardiopulmonary resuscitation: a prospective study. Pediatrics 1997; 99:E3.

671. Carty H. Skeletal manifestations of child abuse. Bone 1989; 6:3–7.

672. Kravitz H, Driesen G, Gomberg R, et al. Accidental falls from elevated surfaces in infants from birth to 1 year of age. Pediatrics 1969; 44:869–876.

673. Caffey J. The whiplash shaken infant syndrome, 2nd edn. Pediatrics 1974; 54:396–403.

674. Kleinman PK, Blackbourne BD, Marks SC, et al. Radiological contributions to the investigation and prosecution of cases of fatal infant abuse. N Engl J Med 1989; 320:507–511.

675. Aoki N, Masuzawa H. Subdural haematomas in abused children: report of six cases from Japan. Neurosurgery 1986; 18:475–477.

676. Billmire ME, Myers PA. Serious head injury in infants: accident or abuse? Pediatrics 1985; 75:340–342.

677. Duhaime AC, Alario AJ, Lewander WJ, et al. Head injury in very young children: mechanisms, injury types and ophthalmological findings in 100 hospitalized patients younger than 2 years of age. Pediatrics 1992; 90:179–185.

678. Thomas SA, Rosenfield NS, Leventhal JM, et al. Long bone fractures in young children: distinguishing accidental injuries from child abuse. Pediatrics 1991; 88:471–476.

679. Hadley MN, Sonntag VKH, Rekate HL, et al. The infant whiplash-shake injury syndrome: a clinical and pathological study. Neurosurgery 1989; 24:536–540.

680. Jaspan T, Narborough G, Punt JAG, et al. Cerebral contusional tears as a marker of child abuse – detection by cranial sonography. Pediatr Radiol 1992; 22:237–245.

681. Rorke LB. Neuropathology of homicidal head injury in infants. Childs Nerv Syst 1990; 6:295.(abstract)

682. Barlow KM, Gibson RJ, McPhillips M, et al. Magnetic resonance imaging in acute non-accidental head injury. Acta Paediatr 1999; 88:734–740.

683. Barlow KM, Minns RA. The relation between intracranial pressure and outcome in non-accidental head injury. Dev Med Child Neurol 1999; 41:220–225.

Childhood stroke syndromes

684. Ganesan V, et al. Investigation of risk factors in children with arterial ischemic stroke. Ann Neurol 2003; 53:167–173.

685. Fullerton HJ, et al. Deaths from stroke in US children, 1979 to 1998. Neurology 2002; 59:34–39.

686. Rolfs A, et al. Prevalence of Fabry disease in patients with cryptogenic stroke: a prospective study. Lancet 2005; 366:(9499):1794–1796.

687. Fung LW, Thompson D, Ganesan V. Revascularisation surgery for paediatric moyamoya: a review of the literature. Childs Nerv Syst 2005; 21:358–364.

688. deVeber G, et al. Cerebral sinovenous thrombosis in children. N Engl J Med 2001; 345:417–423.

*689. Stam J, de Bruijn S, deVeber G. Anticoagulation for cerebral sinus thrombosis. Stroke 2003; 34:1054–1055.

690. Monagle P, et al. Antithrombotic therapy in children: the Seventh ACCP Conference on Antithrombotic and Thrombolytic Therapy. Chest 2004; 126(3 suppl):645S–687S.

SPEECH AND LANGUAGE DELAY AND DISORDERS

691. Bishop DBM. How does the brain learn language? Insights from a study of children with and without language impairment. Dev Med Child Neurol 2000; 42:133–142.

692. Owen SE, McKinlay IA. Motor difficulties in children with developmental disorders and speech and language. Child Care Health Dev 1997; 23:315–325.

693. Davie R, Butler N, Goldstein H. From birth to 7: A report of a National Child Development Study. London: Longman; 1972.

694. Fundudis TI, Kolvin I, Garside RF. Speech retarded and deaf children, their psychological development. London: Academic Press; 1997.

695. Morley ME. The development and disorders of speech in childhood. 2nd edn. Edinburgh: E & S Livingstone; 1965.

696. Largo RH, Molinari L, Comenale Pinto L, et al. Language development of term and preterm children during the first five years of life. Dev Med Child Neurol 1986; 28:33–35.

697. Hagberg B. Rett syndrome – clinical and biological aspects. London: Mac Keith Press, Cambridge University Press; 1993.

698. Gordon N. The concept of central deafness. In: Renfrew C, Murphy K, eds. The child who does not talk. Clinics in Developmental Medicine 13. London: William Heinemann; 1964.

699. Worster-Drought C. Congenital suprabulbar paresis. J Laryngol Otol 1956; 70:453–463.

700. Kuzniecky R, Andermann F, Gurerrini R. Congenital bilateral peri-sylvian syndrome: study of 31 patients. The CBPS Multicentre Collaborative Study. Lancet 1993; 341:608–612.

701. Gordon NS. Worster–Drought and congenital bilateral peri-sylvian syndromes. Dev Med Child Neurol 2002; 44:201–204.

702. Landau WM, Kleffner FR. A syndrome of acquired aphasia with convulsive disorder in children. Neurology 1957; 7:523–530.

703. Lees J, Urwin S. Acquired childhood aphasia. In: Children with language disorders. London: Whurr Publishers; 1991.179–210.

704. Mantovani JF. Autistic regression and Landau–Kleffner syndrome: progress or confusion?. Dev Med Child Neurol 2000; 42:349–353.

705. van Slyke PA. Classroom instruction for children with Llandau–Kleffner syndrome. Child Lang Teaching Ther 2002; 18:23–42.

706. Deonna T, Beaumanoir A, Gaillard P, et al. Acquired asphyxia in childhood with seizure disorder. A heterogeneous syndrome. Neuropediatriä 1977; 8:263–273.

707. Ferguson AP, McKinlay IA, Hunt A. Care of adolescents with severe learning disability from tuberose sclerosis. Dev Med Child Neurol 2002; 44:256–262.

708. McKinlay IA. Autism: the paediatric neurologists tale. Br J Disord Commun 1989; 24:201–207.

709. Gillberg C, Coleman M. The biology of the autistic syndromes. Oxford: Mac Keith Press; 1992.

710. O'Brien G, Yule W. Why behavioural phenotypes/methodological issues in behavioural phenotypes research. In: O'Brien G, Yule W, eds. Behavioural phenotypes. London: Mac Keith Press, Cambridge University Press; 1995.1–23,35–44

711. Gillberg C, Coleman M. Autism and medical disorders: a review of the literature. Dev Med Child Neurol 1996; 38:191–202.

712. Rutter M. Autism: two-way interplay between research and clinical work. J Child Psychol Psychiatry 1999; 40:169–188.

713. Lauritsen M, Mors O, Mortensen PV, et al. Infantile autism and associated autosomal chromosomal abnormalities. A registered based study and a literature survey. J Child Psychol Psychiatry 1999; 40:335–345.

714. Medical Research Council. Review of autism research: epidemiology and causes. 2001 www.rcac.uk

715. Bishop DBM. Autism, Asperger's syndrome, and semantic-pragmatic disorders. Where are the boundaries? Br J Disord Commun 1989; 24:107–121.

716. Johnson E, Hastings RP. Facilitating factors and barriers to the implementation of intensive home based behavioural intervention for young children with autism. Child Care Health Dev 2002; 28:123–129.

717. British Paediatric Association. Services for children and adolescents with learning disability (mental handicap): report of a BPA Working Party. 1994. London: Royal College of Paediatrics & Child Health.

718. Thompson NP, Montgomery SM, Wakefield AJ, et al. Is measles vaccination a risk factor for inflammatory bowel disease? Lancet 1995; 345:1071–1074.

719. Wakefield AJ, Murch SH, Linnel AAJ, et al. Ileal-lymphoid-nodular hyperplasia, non-specific colitis and pervasive developmental disorder in children. Lancet 1998; 351:637–641.

720. Smith A, McCann R, McKinlay I. Second dose of MMR vaccine: health professionals level of confidence in the vaccine and attitudes towards the second dose. Commun Dis Public Health 2001; 4:273–277.

721. Taylor B, Miller E, Lingam R, et al. Measles, mumps and rubella vaccination and bowel problems or developmental regression in children with autism: population study. BMJ 2002; 324:393–396.

722. Legge B. Can't eat, won't eat. London: Jessica Kingsley; 2002.

723. Gordon NS. Stuttering: incidence and causes. Dev Med Child Neurol 2002; 44:278–281.

724. Martin JAM. Hearing loss and hearing behaviour. In: Rutter M, Martin JAM, eds. The child with delayed speech. Clinics in Developmental Medicine 43: Spastic International Medical Publications. London: William Heinemann; 1972:83–94.

725. Lassman FM, Fisch RO, Vetter DK, et al. Early correlates of speech, language, and hearing loss. Littleton, MA: PSG Publishing; 1980.

726. Chalmers D, Stewart I, Silver P, et al. Otitis media with effusion in children – the Duneden study. Oxford: Mac Keith Press; 1989.

727. Maw AR. Glue ear in childhood: a prospective study of otitis media with effusion. London: Mac Keith Press/Cambridge University Press; 1995.

23

Disorders of the blood and bone marrow

Paula Bolton-Maggs, Angela Thomas

Many different factors, including environment, diet and illness can affect the blood picture, so that 'abnormalities' of the blood count are relatively common in childhood. Children have more reactive bone marrow than adults resulting in more impressive changes with relatively smaller stimuli. Infection commonly results in a mild or moderate degree of anemia and particularly produces elevation of the platelet count. The more serious hematological disorders will form the focus of this chapter. Hematological laboratory parameters in children must be assessed against normal ranges for age as these may be significantly different from adults. A table of normal ranges is given in Appendix 1. Developmental hemopoiesis is covered in Chapter 12. Normal ranges for hematological values in the neonatal period, including coagulation factors, are given in Appendix 1.

HEMATOLOGICAL ASSESSMENT IN CHILDHOOD

Hematological disorders present with nonspecific symptoms. Anemia may be profound before a child has any symptoms – pallor is eventually noted in an otherwise well child. Children with severe anemia may have respiratory distress and be misdiagnosed.[1] Children with leukocyte abnormalities may present with infection; thrombocytopenia is often asymptomatic until the count is profoundly low (less than 10×10^9/L). Demonstration of anemia, or a reduction of any one of the cell lines, is not a diagnosis in itself. Once an abnormality has been identified the next step is to establish the cause, which will determine the course of action. The quality of the blood sample from a child is important. Traumatic or lengthy venepuncture or difficult capillary collection often results in activation and partial coagulation, and visual inspection may miss small clots in a sample. The commonest cause of a low platelet count is a poorly collected sample which can also result in a falsely low white cell count or low hemoglobin.

ANEMIA

APPROACH TO ANEMIA

Anemia is a sign, not a diagnosis. The diagnosis may be clear from the history and examination together with the result of the blood count.

1. Is the child anemic? Results must be assessed against normal ranges for age. Many hospitals only quote adult normal ranges; this may lead to a mistaken diagnosis of anemia in a child, as the normal range is lower.
2. What are the characteristics of the red cells? The red cell indices and smear appearances may suggest potential diagnoses and initial investigations (Fig. 23.1 and Table 23.1).
3. What is the pathophysiological mechanism of the anemia? This requires synthesis of the clinical and laboratory findings, and consideration of the mechanisms shown in Figure 23.2.

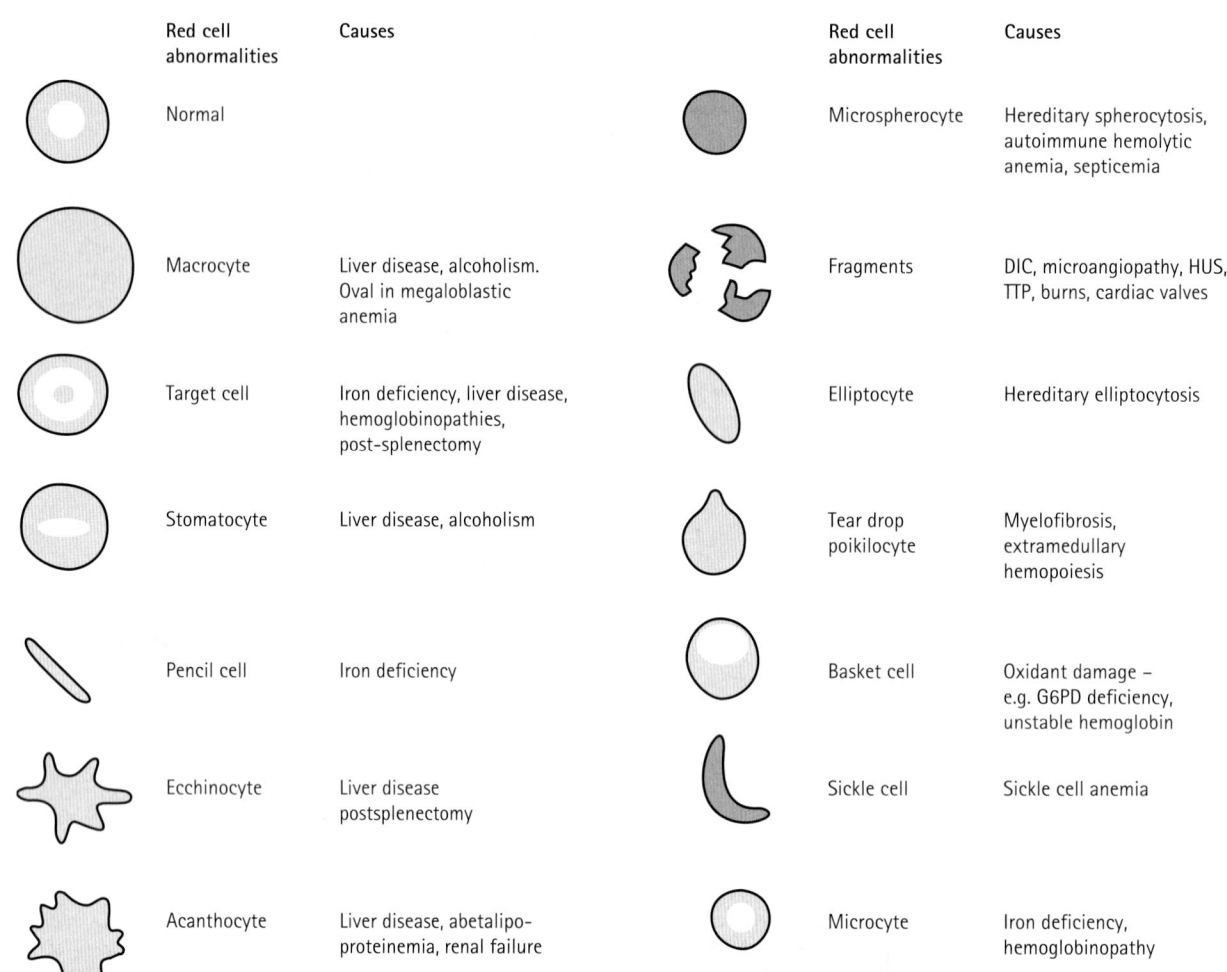

Fig. 23.1   Morphological appearance of red blood cells in different anemias. DIC, disseminated intravascular coagulation; G6PD, glucose-6-phosphate dehydrogenase; HUS, hemolytic uremic syndrome; TTP, thrombotic thrombocytopenic purpura. (From Hoffbrand et al 2001[36] with permission.)

Table 23.1   Morphological diagnosis of anemia

Red cell appearances	Hypochromic microcytic		Normochromic normocytic		Macrocytic	
Discriminatory test	Serum ferritin		Reticulocyte count		B_{12}/folate assay bone marrow examination	
Result	Reduced	Normal or increased	Reduced	Normal or increased	Megaloblastic	Non-megaloblastic
Possible diagnoses	Iron deficiency	Thalassemia Hemoglobinopathy Sideroblastic anemia	Bone marrow hypoplasia Red cell aplasia	Hemolysis Blood loss Secondary anemia	Deficiency of B_{12}/folate Abnormality of B_{12}/folate metabolism	Liver disease Thyroid disease Congenital dyserythropoietic anemia

DEFICIENCY ANEMIAS

Iron deficiency anemia is very important and common in childhood. Iron deficiency without anemia is significant because iron is also required for normal development of the central nervous system. Deficiencies of other hematinics are rare.

IRON DEFICIENCY

Etiology

In contrast to adults where the diagnosis of iron deficiency prompts a search for a source of blood loss, the commonest cause of iron deficiency in children is an inappropriate diet; blood loss is uncommon. Iron deficiency occurs from 6 months of age onwards when the child's total body mass is expanding in the face of an inadequate iron intake (Fig. 23.3).

Studies show that 10–18% of Caucasian children, and 17–31% of children of ethnic minorities, have iron deficiency with hemoglobin levels of less than 1 g/dl. Many other infants will be iron deficient (serum ferritin <12 µg/L) without anemia. Iron is required for the developing brain (see below) as well as for red cell production, so that it is important that iron deficiency, even without anemia, is corrected. Many infants and young children admitted to hospital for other reasons have blood tests which indicate iron deficiency as an incidental finding. This opportunity to correct iron deficiency (by a combination of therapy and dietary re-education) should not be missed. Routine prophylactic supplementation

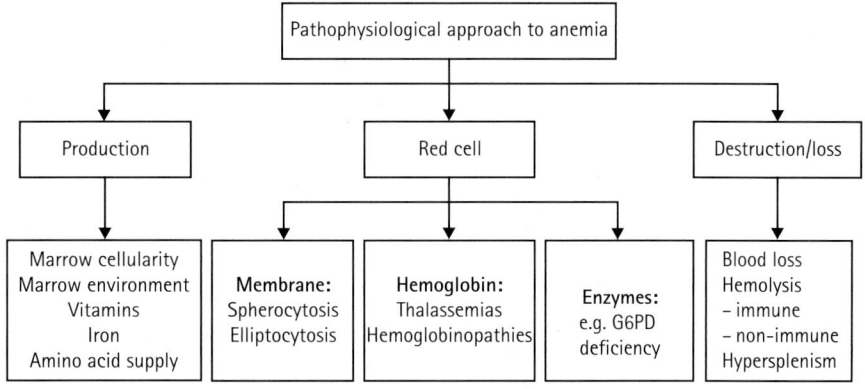

Fig. 23.2   Pathophysiological approach to anemia. G6PD, glucose-6-phosphate dehydrogenase.

of diets with iron may not necessarily be beneficial. Two randomized clinical trials have reported different results; in Nepal no difference in mortality was found,[2] but in a similar study of children in East Africa in a population with high rates of malaria there was an increase in hospital admissions and death in the treated group, possibly related to an increase in infection.[3] The inflammatory response, which leads to restriction of iron availability to erythroid precursors in infection,[4] may have a protective effect by reducing iron availability to micro-organisms. A Cambodian study of weekly iron and folate supplementation resulted in a decrease in the prevalence of anemia in children aged 5–11 years in two schools from 62% to 11%, and from 57% to 26%.[5] In resource-limited countries iron supplementation is only one part of necessary changes in child nutrition and health.

Diagnosis

Iron deficiency may present with pallor – the hemoglobin level can be extremely low (3–5 g/dl) without symptoms. Pica (the persistent compulsive ingestion of food or nonfood substances, for example soil, stones, chalk, sand, foam rubber and carpet) is an insufficiently recognized symptom. Usually these cravings cease with correction of the iron deficiency. Other signs (such as koilonychia or angular cheilitis) are very rare. Iron deficiency causes serial changes in the blood before anemia develops (Figure 23.3). Serum ferritin is reduced and eventually a microcytic, hypochromic anemia results. Usually the MCV (mean cell volume) and MCH (mean cell hemoglobin) fall before the hemoglobin, but the changes can occur together. The MCHC (mean cell hemoglobin concentration) is less useful because it is often normal in the face of hypochromia. (The value is calculated from the PCV and Hb and may be falsely elevated due to trapped plasma in the hematocrit where there are abnormal red cells.)

Iron deficiency is suspected when:

1. The hemoglobin is normal but the MCV and MCH are slightly reduced (the most important differential diagnosis is from thalassemia traits).
2. The hemoglobin is reduced with low MCV and MCH (Fig. 23.4). Reductions in MCV and MCH are usually proportional to the reduced hemoglobin level, e.g. with Hb of 3–4 g/dl, the MCV and MCH will be markedly low, e.g. 50 and 18 respectively.

When the diagnosis is unclear it should be confirmed by measurement of ferritin (reduced) or zinc protoporphyrin (raised). A low ferritin is diagnostic of iron deficiency. (Ferritin is an acute phase reactant and will be elevated in acute inflammatory states and liver disease. A normal ferritin does not absolutely rule out iron deficiency.) Measurement of the serum iron and iron binding capacity (transferrin saturation) adds little to the diagnosis in straightforward cases. The serum iron level on its own is unreliable having significant diurnal variation. It may be helpful to request these additional tests in children with chronic disease and in those with suspected iron overload.

Differential diagnosis

Other causes of a hypochromic microcytic blood picture are:

1. Anemia of chronic disease or 'anemia of inflammation' (modification of iron regulation by the inflammatory response).
2. Thalassemia traits – these require quantitation of hemoglobins A2 and F, and not simply hemoglobin electrophoresis. Thalassemias are not excluded by normal results and further tests (genetic analysis) may be required. The advice of a hematologist should be sought.
3. Sideroblastic anemias (see below).

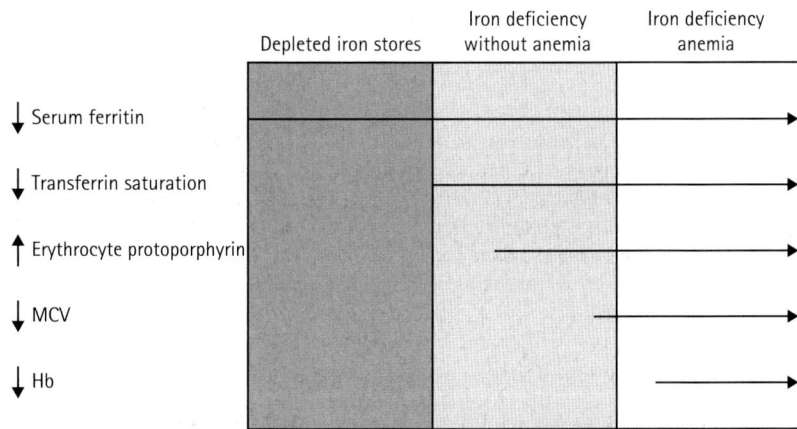

Fig. 23.3   Three stages of iron depletion based on results of laboratory tests. Hb, hemoglobin; MCV, mean cell volume. (From Nathan & Oski 1992[124] with permission.)

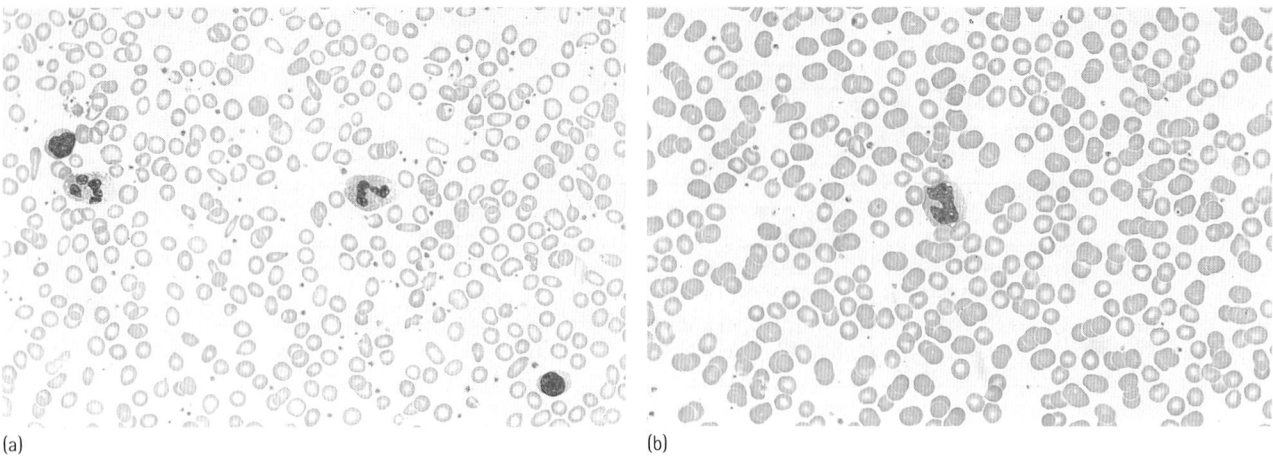

(a)   (b)

Fig. 23.4   Peripheral blood appearances in severe hypochromic iron deficiency with (a) microcytic red cells compared with (b) a normal film (same magnification).

Iron deficiency and neuropsychological effects

Animal experiments have clearly shown that early iron deficiency irreversibly affects brain iron content and distribution, leading to neurotransmitter and behavioral alterations. Anemia due to iron deficiency is significantly associated with poorer scores in developmental testing when compared with controls, particularly in coordination and spatial orientation skills. Some trials have shown definite benefit in treating the iron deficiency, but have suggested that not all the neurological deficit is reversed. Treating the hemoglobin level without replenishing the iron stores is probably insufficient. Further trials are needed, looking at long term school performance, academic achievements and career patterns in relation to iron deficiency in infancy, but would be very difficult to do. Prevention of iron deficiency is much better than attempts to reverse damage done. This topic has been reviewed[6,7] and the impact of iron therapy on psychomotor development and cognitive function in children under the age of 3 years has been considered in a Cochrane review.[8] Another more recent systematic review concluded that iron supplementation improved mental development.[9]

Nutritional aspects and diet

Iron requirements are relatively high in infancy and early childhood because of rapid growth (Fig. 23.5). Stores laid down in pregnancy are depleted after 6 months of age so it is important to establish a good intake of iron early in weaning. Preterm infants have lower iron stores at birth and may become iron deficient as early as 3 months of age.

Dietary iron occurs in two forms – heme and nonheme. Heme iron (in meat, fish and poultry) is well absorbed and its bioavailability is not affected by other dietary factors. Non-heme iron is less well absorbed and its bioavailability is affected by dietary factors because of the way it is bound in foods. It is present in beans, pulses, peanut butter, green leafy vegetables, dried fruit and fortified breakfast cereals. Absorption is enhanced by vitamin C and proteins, but is inhibited by a number of constituents of food and drink, for example tannins (in tea and legumes), phytates (in unrefined cereals), phosphates (in eggs), oxalates (in rhubarb, spinach) and polyphenols (in spinach, coffee). The main causes of iron deficiency are delayed weaning, use of cows' milk before 1 year as a main drink, excessive intake of milk and other drinks in older children, a diet low in iron-rich foods, poor intake of vitamin C and increased intake of foods which inhibit iron absorption. Primary care support and education should be aimed towards establishing good weaning practices and continued good eating patterns in later childhood.

Therapy

Choice of preparation

The daily iron requirement for full-term infants is 1 mg/kg/day (maximum total daily dose 15 mg) starting no later than 4 months of age until 3 years of age. Between 4 and 10 years, the requirement is 10 mg/day and above 11 years and through adolescence, 18 mg/day. The treatment dose for iron deficiency is 3 mg iron/kg body weight/day up to a maximum of 180 mg daily.

When a child fails to respond to iron therapy, the commonest reason is failure of adherence. Although many preparations may be prescribed three times a day, better adherence may be achieved with a single daily dose or twice daily dosing. Iron is available as iron salts and iron chelates.

1. **Iron salts** (e.g. sulphate, fumarate, gluconate and glycine sulphate), *ferrous sulphate*. Although ferrous sulphate is optimal for adults, the liquid is no longer recommended as it is not commercially available, and tastes terrible. Other preparations are available either as tablets, e.g. *ferrous sulphate*, *ferrous gluconate* or liquids such as *ferrous fumarate* and *ferrous glycine sulphate* 141 mg (equivalent to 25 mg Fe) in 5 ml.

2. **Iron chelates** (sodium iron edetate, and polysaccharide iron complex). Chelates have major advantages in paediatric practice – they do not stain the teeth and sodium iron edetate can be mixed with milk or juice without altering absorption. In general there are fewer gastrointestinal side-effects, and they are sugar-free. Perhaps most importantly, the child usually likes them.

- From birth to 4 months total body iron remains stable
- In the next 8 months there is a considerably increased requirement
  - rapid growth
  - increasing blood volume

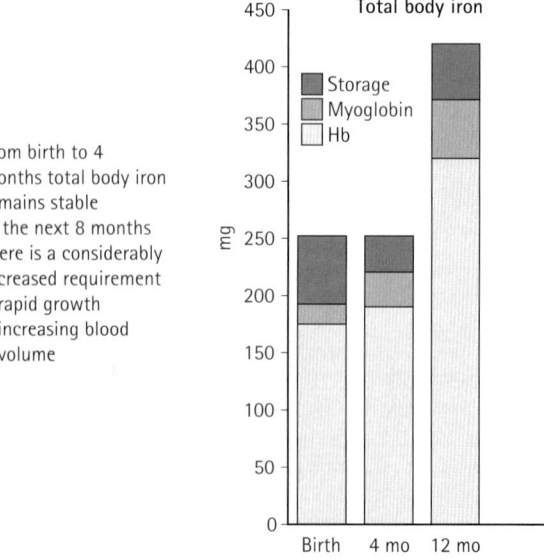

Fig. 23.5   Changes in body iron during infancy. (From Nathan & Oski 1992[124] with permission.)

Response to treatment

There is no difference in response between the types of iron medication providing sufficient iron is given. However severe the anemia, there is no advantage in giving iron parenterally. The hemoglobin increases by about 1 g/dl per week if adherence is good. Failure to respond is nearly always due to failure of adherence. If the hemoglobin is repeatedly less than 8 g/dl, a short admission to hospital may be considered in order to monitor adherence and reinforce dietary education. In severe iron deficiency anemia (Hb < 6.0 g/dl), the hemoglobin should be checked within 2 weeks to ensure that the child is responding (adhering). In very severe iron deficiency (e.g. Hb of 3 g/dl), early monitoring (e.g. within 3–4 days) will show an increase in the RDW (red cell distribution width) on the automated count, and the appearance of some polychromasia on the film. Then the monitoring interval can be extended. Children with severe iron deficiency will need a minimum of 3 months' iron therapy, often considerably more. The ferritin can be used to monitor treatment once the anemia and abnormal indices (hypochromia and microcytosis) have been corrected. In older children, the question of occult intestinal blood loss should be considered.

Conditions that may be associated with iron deficiency – lead poisoning

Although lead toxicity is thought to lead to anemia, severe lead toxicity, manifested by serious neurological effects, can occur without anemia. Coincidental iron deficiency is more likely to cause anemia; lead poisoning and iron deficiency are likely to occur in the same population. Lead poisoning and its management has been reviewed in detail.[10] Typically there is punctate basophilia on the blood film.

Anemias that can be confused with iron deficiency – the sideroblastic anemias and thalassemia traits (see later)

Sideroblastic anemias are rare, and in childhood usually congenital and may exhibit X-linked inheritance. The red cells are usually hypochromic and microcytic. The ferritin is normal or raised, and the anemia is characterized by erythroid hyperplasia and the presence of abnormal iron staining (ringed sideroblasts) in the bone marrow. Some drugs can also induce sideroblastic change, but this is rare in children.

Sideroblastic anemia (sometimes transient) may be the presenting feature of Pearson syndrome, a serious multisystem disease due to mitochondrial DNA deletions usually with pancreatic insufficiency, neurological involvement and a tendency to episodes of lactic acidosis. Liver failure may occur and the syndrome is usually lethal early in life.[11]

FOLATE DEFICIENCY

Etiology

Megaloblastic anemia is very rare indeed in children but when it does occur it is most commonly due to folate deficiency. Unlike iron, folate stores are relatively labile and in constant need of replenishment. Folates are required for nucleic acid synthesis and 1-carbon unit transfer in all cells of the body, particularly growing tissues (Fig. 23.6). Breast milk from a folate-replete mother contains about 25 μg/L of folate and provides enough folate for the normally developing child. However, if preterm babies are not supplemented with oral folate about a third will develop low serum folate levels by 6 weeks of age and 10% will develop megaloblastic anemia by 8 weeks of age when the hepatic stores have been depleted. Heating of milk results in a 40% loss of folate and reheating of pasteurized milk causes an 80% loss. In short, all babies are in a precarious state of folate balance during the first weeks of life. Rapid growth, fever, infection, diarrhea or hemolysis all increase folate requirements and may further deplete the stores to the level of clinical deficiency.

Folate is absorbed in the upper jejunum by an active transport mechanism that is impaired in malabsorption states, particularly celiac syndrome. In these disorders, the deficiency does not usually

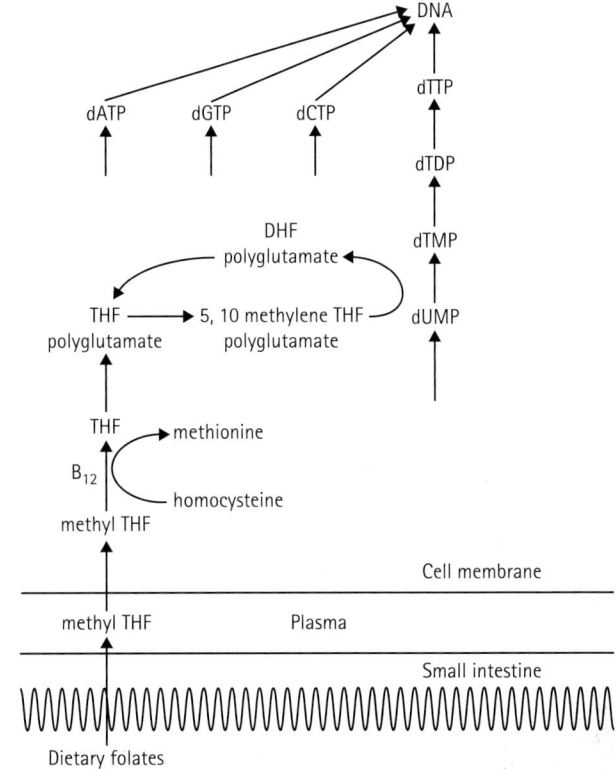

Fig. 23.6 Role of vitamin B_{12} and folate in DNA synthesis. Dietary folates are converted to methyltetrahydrofolate (methyl THF) by the small intestine. Inside marrow and other cells, methyl THF transfers a methyl group to homocysteine to form methionine. Vitamin B_{12} (B_{12}) is needed for this reaction. The THF formed is conjugated to the polyglutamate form possibly after formulation. 5,10-methylene THF polyglutamate is coenzyme for thymidylate synthetase, responsible for the methylation of the pyrimidine deoxyuridine monophosphate (dUMP). The folate coenzyme is oxidized to dihydrofolate (DHF) polyglutamate which is recycled to the fully reduced (THF) form by the enzyme dihydrofolate reductase (DHFR). dTMP is phosphorylated to thymidine triphosphate (dTTP). This is polymerized with the other three deoxyribonucleoside triphosphates, dA (deoxyadenosine) TP, dG (deoxyguanosine) TP, and dC (deoxycytidine) TP to form DNA. (From Hoffbrand 1983[125] with permission.)

produce a frank megaloblastic anemia. Other malabsorptive disorders such as tropical sprue, Crohn disease, multiple diverticula of the small intestine and blind loop syndrome will frequently produce folate deficiency.

Increased requirements for folate and subsequent deficiency occur in chronic hemolytic anemias, but deficiency is unusual as most children consume in excess of the necessary daily recommended intake, however deficiency may be common in poor socioeconomic groups.[12] Although regular folate therapy is recommended in chronic hemolytic states there is little evidence that this is always needed, and a double-blind controlled trial of folate therapy in sickle cell disease led the authors to conclude that this policy needs critical review.[13] Various drugs are associated with deficiency of folate, e.g. phenytoin, barbiturates, methotrexate, pentamidine and trimethoprim. Maternal folate deficiency predisposes to neural tube defects and possibly to other congenital abnormalities including Down syndrome. Congenital deficiencies of several enzymes in the folate pathway are described.[14]

Clinical features and diagnosis

The presentation, like many hematological disorders, is nonspecific. Folate deficiency will produce macrocytosis (which can be masked by associated iron deficiency in conditions with malabsorption); more severe forms will be associated with leucopenia and thrombocytopenia.

Hypersegmented neutrophils on the blood film is an important clue. Serum and red cell folate levels should be requested to confirm the diagnosis.

Treatment

Treatment is straightforward with oral folic acid in a dose of 1–5 mg daily and should be continued for several months. Where demand for the folate remains high (e.g. in chronic hemolytic anemias) lifelong supplementation may sometimes be required. There is often a dramatic clinical response within a few days with a reticulocytosis by the end of a week.

VITAMIN B12 DEFICIENCY

Vitamin B12 deficiency is very rare indeed in childhood. The infant usually has an insidious onset of pallor, lethargy and anorexia, often with neurological symptoms. With the popularity of vegetarianism, maternal dietary deficiency may produce profound deficiency in infancy with neurological sequelae and is currently the commonest cause of infantile B12 deficiency.[14] It may occur in older children as part of a more generalized gastrointestinal disease with malabsorption. B12 deficiency has been reported in infants whose mothers have undergone gastric bypass procedures for obesity,[15] and those whose mothers are in the early stages of traditional pernicious anemia.[16] B12 deficiency occurs in early infancy due to congenital defects in the absorption or metabolic pathway. Recent advances in the molecular and genetic mechanisms are reviewed by Whitehead.[14] The diagnosis should be considered in any infant who develops pancytopenia with megaloblastic anemia in the first 3 years of life. Methylmalonic aciduria with homocystinuria is associated with vitamin B12 deficiency. Diagnosis is very important but treatment with B12 does not necessarily reverse the neurological defects.[14]

Diagnosis

The blood picture is indistinguishable from folate deficiency – there is often a pancytopenia with macrocytosis. The serum vitamin B12 level will be low (less than 100 µg/ml) except in the deficiency of transcobalamin (TC) II. This latter finding occurs because the assay measures mainly vitamin B12 bound to TCI. The serum folate level will be high or normal and the red cell folate misleadingly low. These infants are difficult to investigate and should be referred to specialists for further workup.

Treatment

The usual dose of vitamin B12 (as hydroxocobalamin) for children is 100 µg, given intramuscularly, three times a week until the hemoglobin is normal, followed by 100 µg monthly thereafter. Some disorders may be successfully treated with oral B12 therapy.[17] The neurological defects may take longer to recover. In TCII deficiency very large doses are required.

OTHER CAUSES OF MEGALOBLASTIC ANEMIA

Some very rare metabolic disorders are associated with megaloblastic anemia such as orotic aciduria, Lesch–Nyhan syndrome, and thiamine responsive congenital dyserythropoietic anemia Type I.

APLASTIC ANEMIAS

Bone marrow failure usually presents with pancytopenia that may be moderate or severe, or initially there may only be a single lineage affected with evolution to full aplasia over months or years. Aplastic anemia may be idiopathic (70–80%) or secondary to a constitutional abnormality. Table 23.2 lists agents that may be associated with aplastic anemia. In many cases it is not possible to be certain about their etiologic role. Withdrawal may lead to improvement in the pancytopenia. Marrow aplasia is diagnosed by bone marrow examination, including trephine biopsy (Fig. 23.7). Whatever the underlying cause, severe aplasia (70%), defined as pancytopenia with neutrophils $< 0.5 \times 10^9$/L, platelets $< 10 \times 10^9$/L and reticulocytes $< 1\%$, with documented bone

Table 23.2 Agents associated with aplastic anemia. (After Alter and Potter 1978[123])

Drugs	Insecticides
Acetazolamide	Chlordane
Amodiaquine	DDT
Arsenicals	Gamma benzene hexachloride
Barbiturates	Parathione
Chloramphenicol	
Chlordiazepoxide	
Cimetidine	**Radiation**
Colchicine	Trinitrotoluene
Hydantoins	
Meprobamate	
Phenothiazines	**Solvents**
Phenylbutazone	Benzene
Pyrimethamine	Carbon tetrachloride
Quinacrine	Stoddart's solvent
Quinidine, quinine	Glues
Streptomycin	Toluene
Sulfonamides	
Thiazides	
Thiocyanate	
Thiouracils	

marrow hypocellularity, is associated with a high mortality from infection or bleeding. Good supportive care is essential, and early hemopoietic stem cell transplantation (HSCT) from an HLA-matched sibling donor is the optimal definitive treatment. These children should be referred to a specialist service early. If a sibling donor is not available the most appropriate treatment is intensive immunosuppression using antilymphocyte globulin combined with ciclosporin. Immunosuppression produces a response in over two-thirds of patients but over a long period of follow-up many patients develop myelodysplasia or leukemia suggesting ongoing clonal stem cell disorder.[18] An international group have published guidelines on the management of aplastic anemia.[19]

CONSTITUTIONAL APLASTIC ANEMIAS

Inherited bone marrow failure syndromes are important and are responsible for about 25% of children with aplastic anemia. Patients with these disorders have a genetic propensity for bone marrow failure presenting at birth or developing later.[20]

Fanconi's anemia (FA)

This rare and heterogeneous disorder can present from birth to 48 years of age although 75% present between 3 and 14 years of age. The median age at diagnosis is 7 years. The most common presentation is with pancytopenia, single lineage defects (particularly thrombocytopenia) or malignancy (particularly leukemia). Half have typical physical findings especially short stature, hyperpigmentation, café-au-lait spots, microsomy, microcephaly, thumb, ear, genital and renal anomalies, and developmental disability. FA is inherited as an autosomal recessive with a prevalence of 1–5 per million and a heterozygote frequency of about 1 in 300.[21,22]

Children may present with single lineage failure, particularly thrombocytopenia. Other clues are macrocytosis and fetal characteristics of red cells (raised HbF and an increased expression of i antigen). Chromosome fragility is the hallmark of this disorder, readily seen in metaphase spread from blood lymphocytes stimulated with suitable agents. FA subtyping is important because the complications and outlook vary.[21]

Treatment of FA is difficult – the median survival from diagnosis reported in the international registry (764 subjects) is 24 years.[23] Allogeneic HSCT may be curative for bone marrow failure with a 75% 2-year survival with sibling donors, but only a 33% 3-year survival with matched unrelated donors.[24] Patients with FA do not tolerate irradiation therapy well and modified conditioning is required. As with all cases of

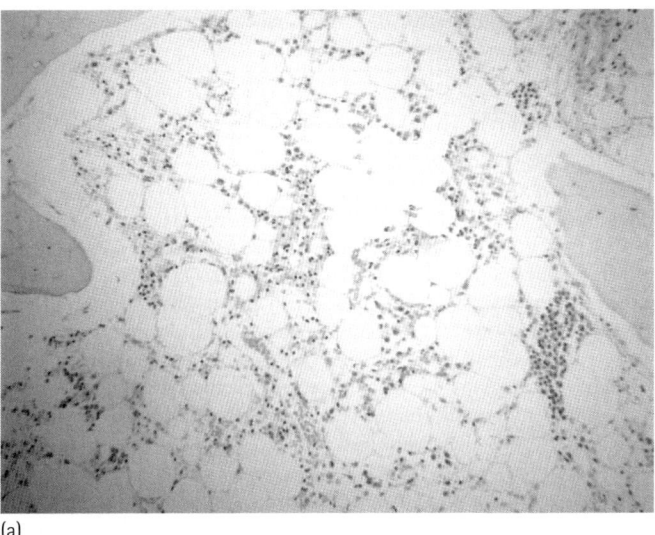

(a)

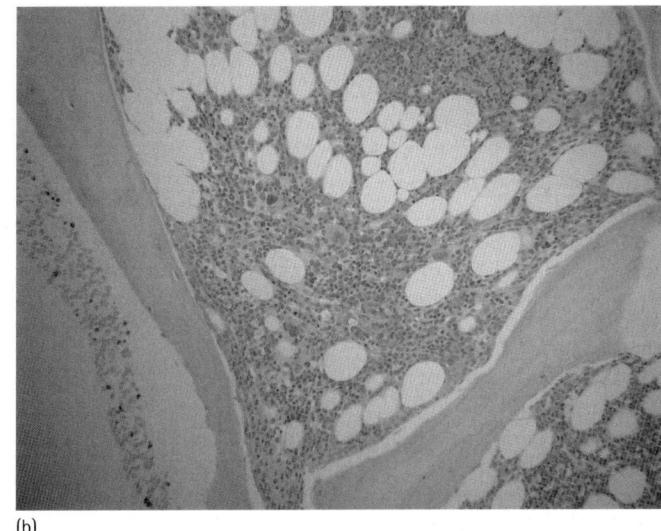

(b)

Fig. 23.7   The appearances of (a) aplastic bone marrow with (b) a normal marrow for comparison (trephine biopsy).

pancytopenia, good supportive care with red cell and platelet transfusion and antibiotics is essential until more specific therapy can be instituted. Androgens have been used for many years with some success in FA.

More than 20% of FA patients develop a malignancy, the risk increasing with age, 60% hematological. Androgens may well exacerbate a genetic risk for liver tumors. The risk of malignancy persists after HSCT and may be increased by irradiation.[22] Significant advances in the genetics, pathology and management have been reviewed.[21,25] At least 11 separate genes are identified; some of these are also found in a wide variety of other cancers with mechanisms related to defects in DNA repair and cell cycle check points. Some individuals with FA have given birth to children, genetic in utero testing is possible for some cases, and gene therapy may become a reality in the future.

Dyskeratosis congenita

Ectodermal dysplasia and X-linked recessive inheritance characterize this disorder. Skin manifestations begin during the first decade and progress. Features include reticulated hyperpigmentation of the face, neck and shoulders; dystrophic nails; mucous membrane leukoplakia; epiphora; hyperhidrotic palms and soles; poikiloderma; thin sparse hair; early loss of teeth; esophageal strictures and dysphagia; subnormal intelligence and hypogenitalia. Fifty six percent of cases develop hematological manifestations, usually after the dermatological problems at a mean age of 17 years. There may be single cell deficiencies or pancytopenia and the bone marrow may show hypercellularity, at the onset, with progressive loss of cellularity. Macrocytosis and elevated HbF levels are found. In reported series, the overall death rate is about 33% at 20 years, with 45% death rate in those with pancytopenia. Thirteen percent of cases develop malignancy. Treatment is the same as for other constitutional aplastic anemias and HSCT has been carried out successfully, although the dermatological and malignant sequelae will probably not be affected. Two genes encoding components of the telomerase are mutated in some but not all families. This disorder has been reviewed by Dokal.[26,27]

Shwachman–Diamond syndrome (SDS)

Children with SDS develop pancreatic insufficiency with variable blood abnormalities (most commonly neutropenia in > 80%) usually detected in infancy, often with skeletal abnormalities and additional immune dysfunction (consider in the differential diagnosis of cystic fibrosis). Anemia or thrombocytopenia can occur, and pancytopenia supervenes in many.[28] Multidisciplinary supportive care with aggressive management of infections, and pancreatic enzyme replacement with a high calorie diet are key therapies. The SBDS gene was identified in 2002 and is located at 7q11 encoding a protein implicated in

RNA metabolism.[29,30] There is a high risk of transformation (often with a myelodysplastic phase) to myeloid leukemia with a poor prognosis, so patients should have regular bone marrow examination. The median survival is 35 years with death from infection, bleeding and leukemia. Some patients have been successfully treated with HSCT. This disorder must be distinguished from **Pearson's syndrome** where affected children have pancreatic insufficiency and vacuolation of marrow precursors in association with congenital sideroblastic anemia (which may show spontaneous recovery).

Congenital amegakaryocytic thrombocytopenia (CAT)

Severe thrombocytopenia in infancy leads to purpura and bleeding within a few months. Megakaryocytes are absent in the bone marrow and there is a genetic defect in the thrombopoietin receptor.[31] About half the children have additional congenital abnormalities, particularly cardiac or neurological. Bleeding is treated with platelet transfusions, but these children need urgent referral for HSCT. Amegakaryocytic thrombocytopenia with radioulnar synostosis is a defined syndrome with mutations in the *HOXA11* gene.[32]

PURE RED CELL APLASIA (PRCA)

PRCA in childhood is caused by transient erythroblastopenia or constitutional red cell aplasia.

Transient erythroblastopenia of childhood (TEC) is an important cause of transient red cell aplasia, causing unexplained, sometimes severe, anemia in young children and toddlers.[33] The cause is unknown and may be related to infection, but parvovirus B19, implicated in aplastic crises in hemolytic states, is not the cause. Diamond–Blackfan syndrome or anemia (DBA) – constitutional and congenital red cell aplasia – presents usually at an earlier age, in the first year of life; 95% of cases by 2 years of age with occasional cases occurring up to 6 years. Diagnosis of either of these is made by the presence of anemia with reticulocytopenia and very few marrow erythroid precursors. TEC recovers within days or weeks, DBA does not. Children with TEC may need transfusion to tide them over, but usually do not.

DBA is a heterogeneous disorder with an incidence of 4–7 per million live births. There is a familial incidence of about 45%. About 50% of children have other physical abnormalities, particularly craniofacial or thumb. About 25% of patients have a mutation in the DBA1 gene, *RPS 19*, which codes for a ribosomal protein. Some children with DBA respond to steroids (> 70%), but many remain steroid dependent (45%) and others require life-long regular transfusion therapy (39%) with iron chelation with subcutaneous desferrioxamine. An international registry has revealed an unexpectedly high incidence of treatment-associated mortality from infection, and confirmed an increased risk of malignancy.[34] Some patients have been successfully treated with HSCT.

HEMOLYTIC ANEMIAS

GENERAL FEATURES

Hemolysis is defined by an increased rate of red cell destruction with a shortening of the normal life span of the cell from the normal 120 days to as little as a few days in severe hemolysis. The marrow can increase erythrocyte production six- or eight-fold so mild degrees of hemolysis are not associated with anemia. Mild hemolysis may be almost undetectable with no clinical clues; severe hemolysis can lead to a rapid and profound fall in hemoglobin, and be life threatening. The hemoglobin level is a balance between increased red cell destruction and ability of the bone marrow to compensate. Hemolysis is suspected when polychromatic cells are seen on the blood film (reticulocytes); further diagnostic and confirmatory tests are then indicated. A simplified diagnostic classification of causes is shown in Figure 23.8.[35] Hemolysis is usually associated with raised blood unconjugated bilirubin. Generally, hemolytic states are divided into those with spherocytes and those without, where the morphology may be normal, or characteristic of the underlying disorder. Hemolysis can be caused by inherited or acquired disorders. Diagnosis of the cause of the hemolysis is made according to the family history; clinical features and red cell morphology that together will indicate what further laboratory tests are required. Marrow examination is generally unnecessary.

The child with hemolysis may be pale with fluctuating jaundice (usually mild) and splenomegaly. Pigment gallstones may complicate the disorder – hemolytic anemia should always be excluded in a child with stones. Aplastic crises may occur, usually precipitated by parvovirus infection or rarely by folate deficiency, both of which are characterized by 'switching off' of erythropoiesis. This leads to reticulocytopenia and anemia. Parvovirus infection typically produces severe anemia sometimes requiring transfusion, and a modest thrombocytopenia and leucopenia. Folate deficiency is uncommon.

HEREDITARY HEMOLYTIC ANEMIAS
Membrane defects
Hereditary spherocytosis (HS)

HS is the commonest hereditary hemolytic anemia in north Europeans, caused by a variety of different genetic defects in the red cell skeletal proteins, ankyrin, spectrin, band 3 or protein 4.2 (Fig. 23.9).[36] It is dominantly inherited in 75% of families. There may be variable expression – investigation of other family members may identify asymptomatic individuals with a milder phenotype. The blood film shows the typical features – multiple small dense cells termed microspherocytes. The marrow produces normally shaped biconcave cells and progressive loss of membrane results in the spherical shape (Fig. 23.10). In an individual with spherocytes and no other affected family members autoimmune hemolysis must be excluded by a negative direct antiglobulin test. The child may or may not have jaundice and anemia, but splenomegaly is usual. (This is not associated with an increased risk of rupture, and these children should lead a normal active life.) Laboratory diagnosis is usually straightforward and the osmotic fragility test is not necessary for confirmation.[37] For difficult cases there are better investigations (membrane protein analysis).

Individuals with HS are usefully classified as mild moderate or severe by their baseline hemoglobin, reticulocyte count and bilirubin level. This classification, which should be made when the individual is well, helps to indicate those in whom splenectomy is beneficial – generally those with severe and moderate disease.[38] Individuals with severe disease should probably receive folate supplements although the evidence for this is limited.[37]

Splenectomy cures all the clinical manifestations of HS by removing the site of destruction of the abnormal red cells, but is associated

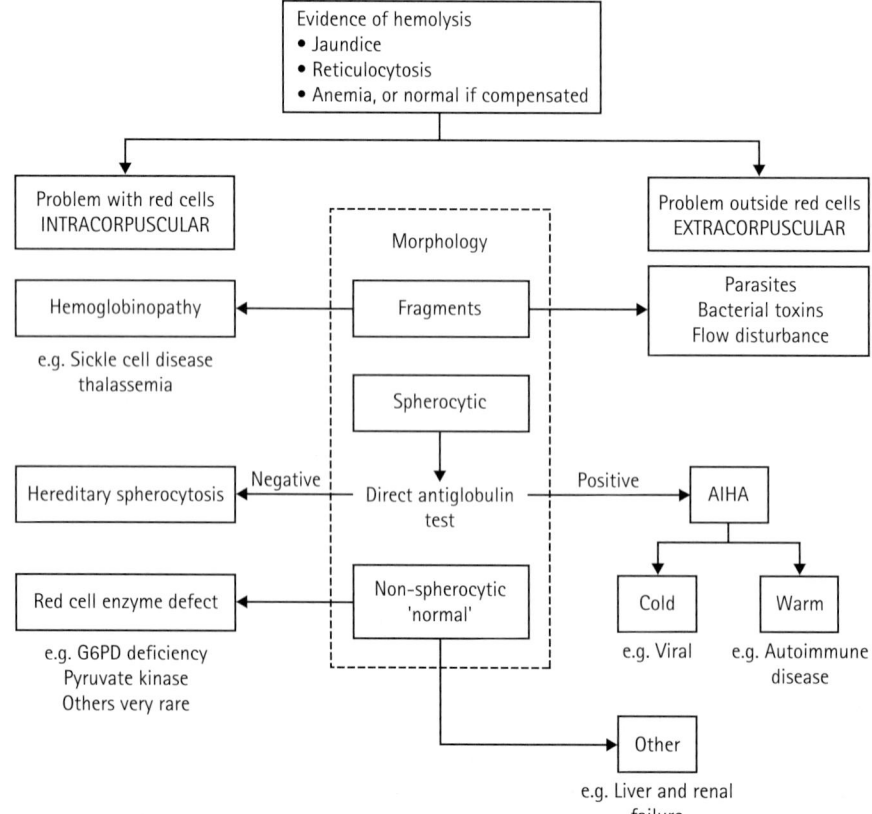

Fig. 23.8 A diagnostic approach to hemolytic anemia. AIHA, autoimmune hemolytic anemia; G6PD, glucose-6-dehydrogenase. (From Lissauer & Clayden 2001[35] with permission.)

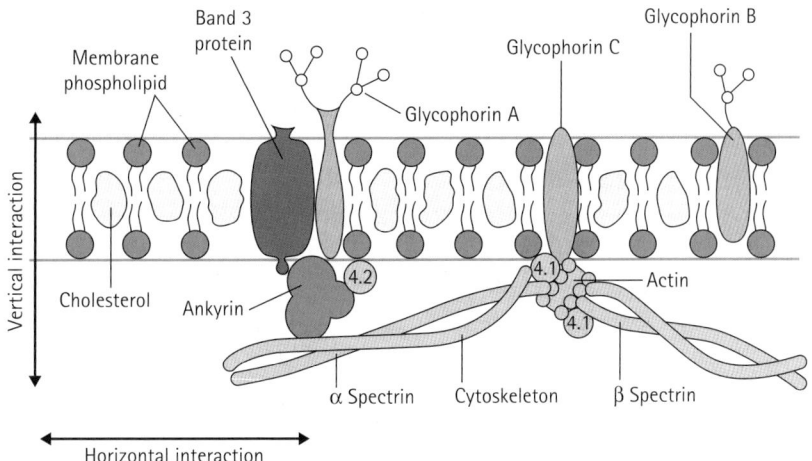

Fig. 23.9 Schematic structure of the red cell membrane. Some of the penetrating and integral proteins carry carbohydrate antigens; other antigens are attached directly to the lipid layer. (From Hoffbrand et al 2001[36] with permission.)

with a lifelong risk of overwhelming sepsis particularly with encapsulated organisms (*Pneumococcus*). It should be avoided in all but the most severe cases, during the first 10 years of life, when the risk of postsplenectomy sepsis is highest. There are guidelines for the management of splenectomized individuals, and in families with HS there may be others who have had splenectomy in the past, who need information about their increased risks of infection.[39] Patients should be immunized with pneumococcal, hemophilus and meningococcal vaccines before splenectomy and warned of their increased risk of infection with malaria. Antibiotic prophylaxis should be given on a long term basis but adherence may be poor. Patients should be issued with a medical card indicating they have had a splenectomy and warned about the importance of early reporting of symptoms of infection. Children with HS may develop gallstones in the first decade of life. This is an indication for both cholecystectomy and splenectomy at the same time. Following splenectomy the individual usually has a normal hemoglobin and near-normal red cell lifespan. Annual follow up may serve to remind the individual about the postsplenectomy risks. Immunity to pneumococcus and hemophilus may wane with time, and survey of antibody levels to these agents may provide a more evidence-based foundation for repeat immunizations. There is currently no consensus in this area.[37]

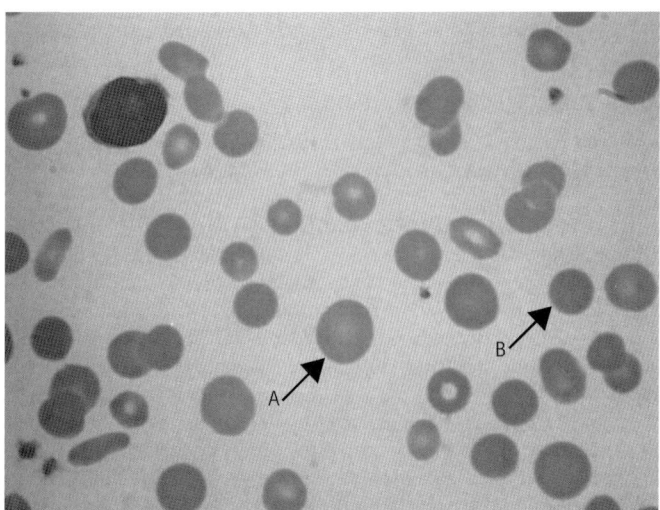

Fig. 23.10 Peripheral blood appearance in spherocytosis with spherocytes and polychromasia. A, polychromatic cell; B, microspherocyte.

Hereditary elliptocytosis (HE)

This common disorder is usually inherited as an autosomal dominant trait, usually diagnosed as an incidental finding when the blood count is performed for some other reason, but rare homozygous variants have been described in whom chronic severe hemolysis occurs. In the rare severe homozygous cases splenectomy usually provides symptomatic improvement.

Other less common membrane disorders are reviewed elsewhere.[40]

Red cell enzyme defects

Figure 23.11 shows the pathways of glucose metabolism and energy production in the red cell. Although defects of almost all the separate enzymes have been described, most are very rare and have been reviewed.[41,42] They are generally associated with a nonspherocytic blood picture, with no helpful morphological features of the red cells (apart from one or two exceptions). Deficiencies of almost all of the enzymes involved in the Embden–Meyerhof pathway and hexose monophosphate shunt can be associated with significant hemolysis. Some of these are chronic with exacerbations by intercurrent illnesses such as viral infections, others are clinically silent, most of the time, with sudden hemolytic episodes which bring the patient to medical attention. Most hospitals will be able to diagnose the two commonest deficiencies; analysis of the others requires specialist investigation only available in a few centers.

Glucose-6-phosphate dehydrogenase (G6PD) deficiency

This is the commonest cause of hemolysis worldwide, and is caused by a number of different mutations in the gene, which is on the X chromosome. These produce different phenotypes; most are associated with episodic hemolysis, the blood picture being normal at other times. A few variants are associated with chronic hemolysis. G6PD maintains glutathione in its reduced state and so is one of the vital mechanisms for protecting red cell membranes from oxidant stress. Oxidative stress induced by drugs, chemicals (Table 23.3) or an intercurrent infection can produce hemolysis. The different mutants of G6PD occur in different racial groups with differences in clinical severity. The racial incidence varies greatly from extreme rarity in northern Europeans through 1–35% in different Mediterranean races, up to 10% in African Negroes. Deficiency leads to various clinical presentations; neonatal jaundice is more common in oriental male babies, especially in the presence of infections or acidosis or if oxidant drugs are given to the mother in late pregnancy or to the neonate. Infections and diabetic ketoacidosis can precipitate hemolysis at all ages. Favism (eating broad beans) produces severe hemolysis, and is commonest in Mediterraneans and in the Middle East, although it does occur in Orientals and Europeans. Rare cases of chronic hemolysis in northern European races have also been described.

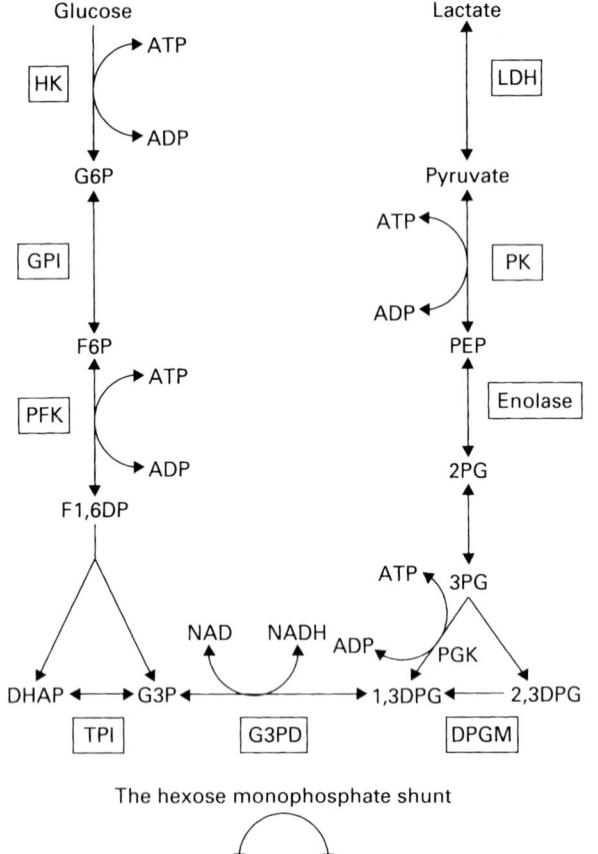

The hexose monophosphate shunt

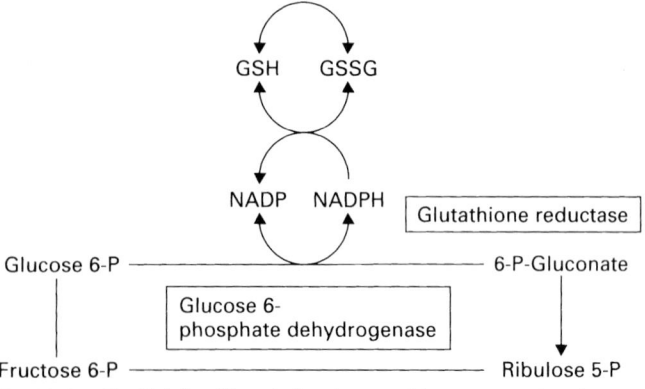

Fig. 23.11 The Embden–Meyerhof pathway and hexose monophosphate shunt. Enzymes: HK, hexokinase; GPI, glucose phosphate isomerase; PFK, phosphofructokinase; TPI, triose phosphate isomerase; G3PD, glucose 3-phosphate dehydrogenase; PGK, phosphoglycerate kinase; DPGM, 2,3-diphosphoglycerate mutase; PK, pyruvate kinase; LDH, lactate dehydrogenase. Intermediates: G6P, glucose 6-P; F6P, fructose 6-P; F1,6DP = fructose 1,6 di-P; 3PG, 3-P glycerate; 1,3DPG, 1,3-diphosphoglycerate; G3P, glyceraldehyde 3-P; PEP, phosphoenolpyruvate; DHAP, dihydroxyacetone P.

Hemolytic crises vary in severity and degree. Favism is associated with the most explosive course and intravascular hemolysis. A typical sign is the dramatic darkening of the urine with hemoglobin and urobilinogen to produce so-called 'Coca-Cola' urine. This may lead to renal dysfunction (sometimes severe). Diagnosis depends on an enzyme assay but reticulocytes nearly always have higher levels of all red cell enzymes so the test is best done when the child (usually male) has recovered from the acute episode.

Neonatal jaundice may require exchange transfusion. At other times all that is necessary is to be aware of the problem in appropriate ethnic groups and to avoid the precipitating factors. Patients should be informed of the hazards and supplied with written information about which foods and drugs to avoid.

Table 23.3 Drugs and chemicals associated with hemolysis in G6pd deficient subjects

Group	Drugs
Antimalarials	Primaquine, pamaquine, quinacrine, quinine
Sulfonamides	Sulfapyridine, sulfisoxazole, salicylazosulfapyridine
Nitrofurans	Nitrofuranatoin, furaltadone
Analgesics and related compounds	Acetylsalicylic acid, para-aminosalicylic acid
Miscellaneous	Synthetic water-soluble vitamin K analogs, chloramphenicol, phenylhydrazine, naphthalene, aniline dyes, nalidixic acid

Pyruvate kinase (PK) deficiency

PK deficiency is the commonest cause of nonspherocytic hemolysis in Northern Europe. It is autosomal recessively inherited and produces chronic hemolysis with varying grades of severity in different individuals. Neonatal jaundice occurs and infection can also precipitate more severe hemolysis. Parvovirus infection can, as in other hemolytic states, produce a dramatic aplastic crisis. Splenomegaly is usually present. Drugs do not precipitate crises.

The blood film in PK deficiency does not have any specific diagnostic features, although irregularly contracted cells are seen, especially after splenectomy. Diagnosis depends on measurement of the enzyme level, which must be carefully corrected for high reticulocyte count. Unfortunately some poorly functioning variants of PK can produce normal assay results; this can be sorted out by specialist measurement of the intermediate products of the Embden–Meyerhof pathway in order to demonstrate a block at the appropriate point.

Because of its position in the energy pathway, PK deficiency causes a rise in 2,3-DPG levels and thus a shift to the right in the oxygen dissociation curve and a consequent improvement in oxygen availability. For this reason, patients with PK deficiency can tolerate very low hemoglobin levels (and conversely hexokinase-deficient patients may require blood transfusion at relatively high hemoglobin levels). Thus, it is very important not to transfuse PK-deficient patients unless they are clinically unwell, failing to thrive or are otherwise genuinely symptomatic. Many patients are transfused unnecessarily on the basis of a perfectly acceptable hemoglobin level of about 5–6 g/dl. Severely affected patients may require intermittent transfusions when decompensated by infections, and occasionally patients require regular transfusions with iron chelation. In these children, splenectomy usually produces a beneficial reduction or abolition of the need for blood transfusion and should be considered in severe cases.

ACQUIRED HEMOLYTIC ANEMIAS

Acquired hemolysis in childhood is relatively uncommon but can be severe; it is important to make the correct diagnosis.

Autoimmune hemolytic anemias (AIHA)

The development of hemolysis caused by autoantibodies to red cell antigens is uncommon and can occur as a complication of some viral infections, as part of a larger dysregulation of immune function, either in autoimmune diseases such as systemic lupus erythematosis, or in some forms of immune deficiency. Autoimmune hemolysis is suspected when the child has anemia with a reticulocytosis sometimes with jaundice, and splenomegaly. The blood film usually shows spherocytes, and the condition is differentiated from HS by a positive direct antiglobulin test due to antibodies (IgG) or complement (in IgM-associated AIHA) attached to the red cells. After viral infections the antibody is usually IgM, and reactive in tests at room temperature ('cold') rather than at 37°C which is typical of IgG ('warm') antibodies. Infectious mononucleosis, CMV and mycoplasma are infections most commonly implicated in 'cold' autoimmune hemolysis (caused by antibodies to the i/I red cell antigens). These antibodies cause intravascular red cell destruction and may present with brown urine (hemoglobinuria) which is not usually seen in IgG-induced hemolysis where the red cells are destroyed predominantly in the spleen. Another type causing sudden onset of hemoglobinuria is paroxysmal cold hemoglobinuria caused by an unusual type of red cell antibody, a complement-fixing IgG which attaches to the red cells in the cold and lyses the cells in the warm – the Donath Landsteiner antibody. Treatment is rarely required, the hemolysis being short lived and resolving with the infection. It is prudent to keep the child warm; occasionally transfusion and steroids may be required. Hemolysis occurring as part of a wider autoimmune process can be chronic and difficult to manage; steroid therapy is often beneficial, transfusion is often difficult and best avoided because the antibodies react with all donor blood. Warm AIHA (rarely in childhood) can also be caused by drugs.

Immune hemolysis caused by maternal antibodies is discussed in detail elsewhere (see Ch. 12). AIHA may occur with immune thrombocytopenic purpura, when it is known as Evans syndrome. This is a potentially serious disorder with a chronic course and may require HSCT.[43]

Microangiopathic hemolytic anemia (MAHA)

Red cell fragmentation on the blood film (schistocytes – Fig. 23.12) is the pathognomonic feature, associated with reticulocytosis. This may be associated with thrombocytopenia, depending upon the underlying cause (Table 23.4). The red cells are damaged by fibrin strands deposited in small blood vessels and consumption of platelets within the resultant microthrombi, or by trauma passing through a damaged heart valve or other cardiac abnormality. A variety of causes are recognized, particularly hemolytic uremic syndrome (HUS) described more fully elsewhere (see Ch. 18). MAHA may be the first signal of a problem with a replaced heart valve. Disseminated intravascular coagulation from any cause may be associated with MAHA.

Other causes of hemolysis
Hypersplenism

Splenic enlargement, from any cause, such as portal hypertension, leishmaniasis and storage disorders, may produce a shortening of red cell survival due to excessive sequestration in the expanded reticuloendothelial system. The anemia is mild and usually associated with mild leucopenia and thrombocytopenia.

Infections

Malaria is an infection in which micro-organisms are present within red cells at the time of hemolysis. Mild hemolysis may occur with many

Table 23.4 Causes of red cell fragmentation syndromes

Microangiopathic
Hemolytic uremic syndrome
Thrombotic thrombocytopenic purpura
Meningococcal sepsis
Disseminated intravascular coagulation
Cardiac valves or arterial grafts
March hemoglobinuria
Infections – malaria, clostridia
Chemical and physical – burns
Liver and renal disease

other infectious processes. Septicemia, particularly due to clostridial organisms, may produce an acute hemolytic process usually as part of a consumptive coagulopathy. *Bartonella* infection is another documented cause of hemolysis (see Ch. 28).

DISORDERS OF HEMOGLOBIN SYNTHESIS

HEMOGLOBINOPATHIES AND THALASSEMIA
Etiology

Hemoglobin is the essential pigment that makes blood red, and carries oxygen to the tissues. There are several different normal hemoglobins specific for different ages; hemoglobin is made up of two pairs of globin chains, each containing a heme group which can bind oxygen (Fig. 23.13[44]). Some hemoglobins are only evident during early stages of gestation; later in fetal life the predominant hemoglobin is HbF (alpha-2gamma2). After birth, when the oxygen affinity does not need to be so high HbA (alpha2beta2) gradually replaces this, the switch starting at about 32 weeks gestation. Normal blood also contains a small amount of HbA2 (alpha2delta2) (Table 23.5). Various hemoglobin disorders result in clinically significant effects. There may be a qualitative or quantitative defect. The most common are discussed here, but there are many others.

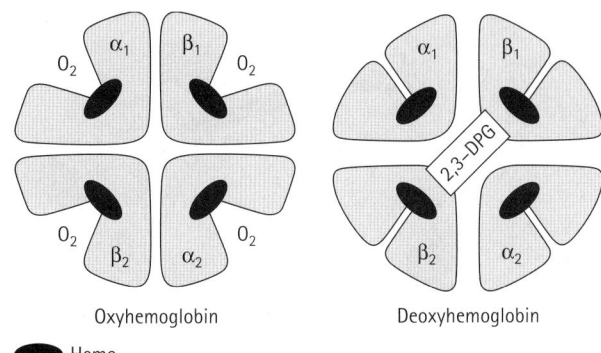

Oxyhemoglobin   Deoxyhemoglobin

● Heme

Fig. 23.13 The oxygenated and deoxygenated hemoglobin molecule. Alpha, beta globin chains of normal adult hemoglobin (hemoglobin A); 2,3-DPG, 2,3 diphosphoglycerate. (From Hoffbrand & Pettit 1993[44] with permission.)

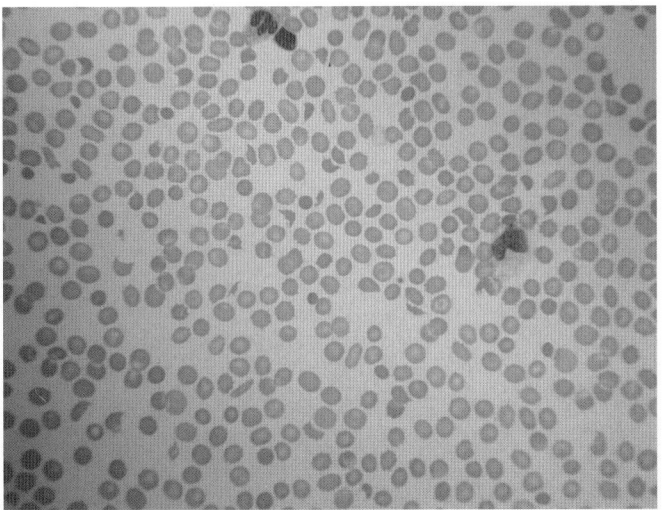

Fig. 23.12 Red cell appearances in red cell fragmentation syndromes.

Table 23.5 The types and quantities of different hemoglobins in infancy and adulthood

Type of Hb	HbA	HbF	HbA$_2$
Notation	α2β2	α2γ2	α2δ2
Normal % at birth	20	80	1
Normal % in older children	98	1	2

The sickling disorders

The most important structural hemoglobin disorder is due to a single amino acid change affecting the solubility of hemoglobin. Sickle hemoglobin results from a point mutation at position 6 of the beta chain (adenine to thymine) resulting in an amino acid change of glutamic acid to valine. Sickle hemoglobin forms crystals at low oxygen tension; these polymerise into long strands. The sickle gene has occurred from at least four separate mutation events, and is most common across the tropical zones (Fig. 23.14[44]). The high frequency of the gene in these areas may be related to some protection against malaria conferred by heterozygosity for the sickle cell gene. The clinical outcome depends upon whether the sickle gene is inherited from one or both parents, (sickle cell trait AS, or sickle cell disease, SS) and whether it is inherited with another hemoglobin disorder which modifies the effects (hemoglobin C, alpha thalassemia, beta thalassemia). It is important to make the correct diagnosis. Most screening tests detect the presence of sickle hemoglobin without quantification, and no information about other possible abnormalities. Full diagnosis requires analysis of the full blood count with red cell indices, hemoglobin electrophoresis with quantification of S and other hemoglobins. The affected individual then requires adequate information and counselling about the genetic implications, even if clinically mild or insignificant. A national screening program for sickling disorders and thalassemia has been rolled out across the UK between 2003 and 2005 (www-phm.umdcs.ac.uk/haemscreening/). In the USA, 49 states have mandatory newborn screening and the resultant education and clinical management has resulted in decreased morbidity and mortality.[45]

Sickle cell trait

Sickle cell trait (AS) is not a disease; affected individuals have less than 50% HbS, normal hemoglobin indices and no adverse clinical sequelae, unless exposed to severe hypoxic conditions. They should be treated as normal and reassured, but given appropriate genetic advice. No special precautions are required for anesthesia or other medical interventions in these individuals.

Sickle cell disease

Sickle cell disease denotes all genotypes containing at least one sickle gene in which HbS makes up at least 50% hemoglobin. Homozygous SS is one of these and is a very variable disorder, but affected individuals are prone to a number of serious complications which need careful management. The red cells have reduced survival, and this chronic hemolytic anemia (Hb 6–9 g/dl) leads to marrow expansion and typical bossing of the skull. Growth is often less than anticipated. Some individuals have a relatively trouble-free life; others have many vaso-occlusive crises. The relatively insoluble HbS precipitates into crystals distorting the red cell shape (sickle cells)(Fig. 23.15[35]) leading to microvascular sludging and infarction of surrounding tissues producing ischemic pain. In the infant the first sign may be dactylitis. In older children the long bones are more commonly affected. These attacks may be precipitated by a variety of external events of which the most important is probably intercurrent infection. Sickling episodes can be life threatening, particularly if the lungs are involved, and are usually very painful. Early and adequate pain relief is an important component of the management which also includes a diligent search for infection, and good hydration; sickle cell disease usually produces a urinary concentrating defect. Sickling causes necrosis in bones – while the changes may be reversible, avascular necrosis of the femoral or humoral heads leads to early and severe disability. In early life the child typically has an enlarged spleen but with defective function; this gradually infarcts (autosplenectomy) increasing the risk of overwhelming pneumococcal sepsis.[46] Prophylactic penicillin is protective and should be started early in life by 3 months of age. Pneumococcal vaccine should be given (in the UK with the heptavalent conjugate vaccine three doses in infants 2–6 months of age and a fourth dose in the second year of life[39]). Such children need open access to an experienced team preferably in an established hemoglobinopathy center. Hospitals in areas with few such patients should ensure that appropriate management protocols are available. Other serious complications of sickle cell disease are aplastic crises, most commonly associated with parvovirus B19 (as with all types of hemolysis), and rare sequestration crises in which there is sudden and dramatic pooling of blood in the

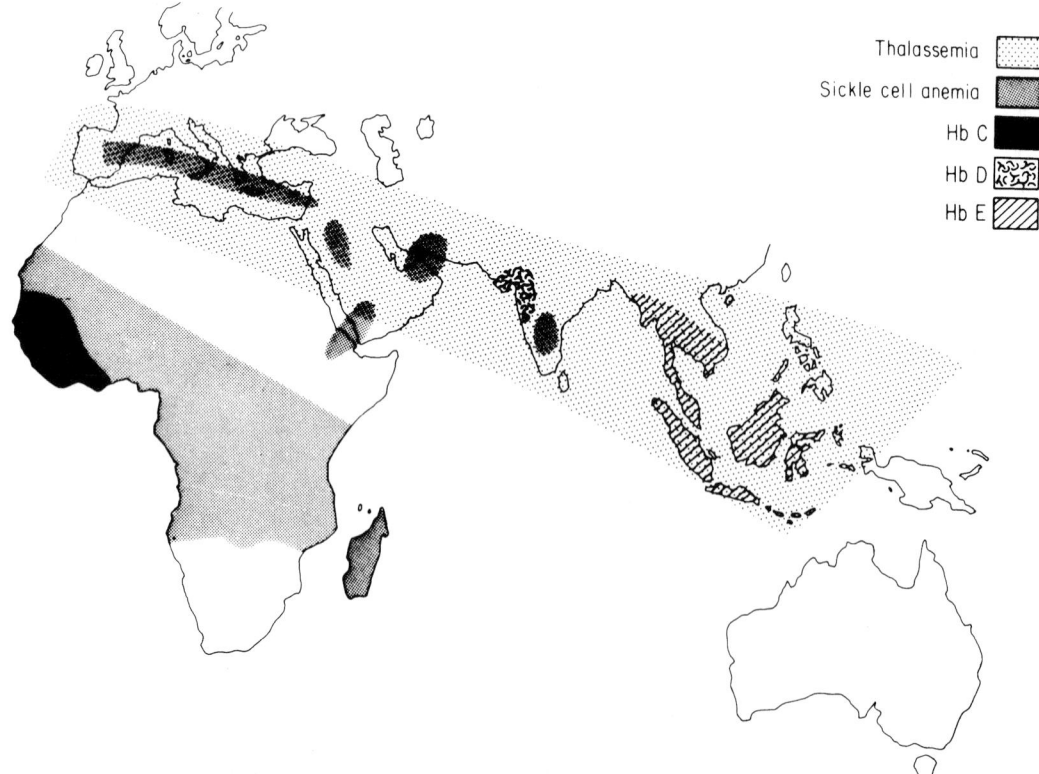

Fig. 23.14 The geographical distribution of the thalassemias and more common inherited structural hemoglobin abnormalities. (From Hoffbrand & Pettit 1993[44] with permission.)

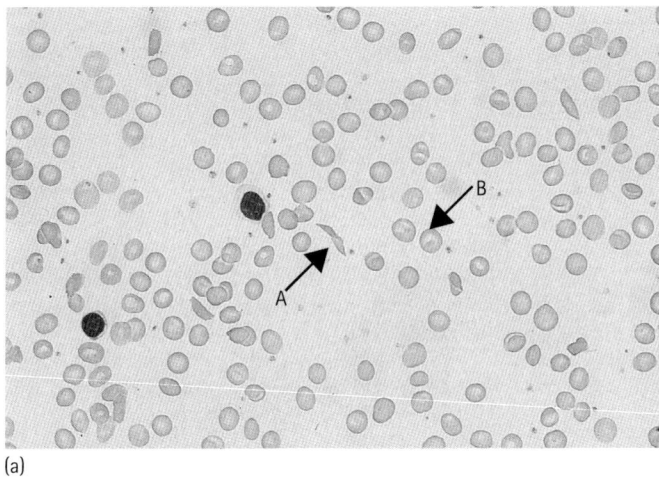

(a)

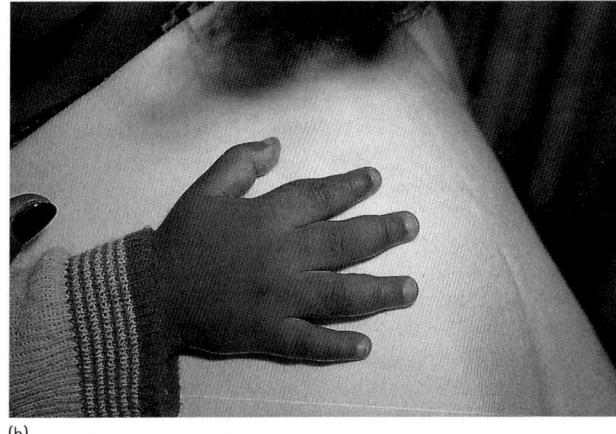

(b)

Fig. 23.15 (a) Peripheral blood appearance in homozygous sickle cell disease with target cells, polychromasia and distorted red cells (A, sickle cell; B target cell). (b) Swelling of the fingers from dactylitis, a common mode of presentation of sickle cell disease in late infancy. (From Lissauer & Clayden 2001[35] with permission.)

spleen or liver; the child presents with very rapidly falling hemoglobin. Splenic sequestration is an indication for splenectomy. Other important complications occur – chronic hemolysis predisposes to the development of gallstones; vascular occlusion can result in stroke, priapism and leg ulcers and retinal vaso-occlusion leads to proliferative retinopathy. Stroke has the highest incidence between 2 and 5 years and a cumulative incidence of 11% by 20 years of age. High risk patients can be identified by transcranial Doppler ultrasound scans (which detect high flow through stenotic segments of the cerebral arteries). This screening should be carried out annually from age 2–3 years because a first stroke can be prevented by blood transfusions (90% reduction), and following a stroke, chronic transfusion therapy reduces the risk of recurrence.[47,48] Stroke is more common in HbSS and HbS/beta[0] thalassemia compared to the other sickle disorders.

Management in sickle cell disease is supportive; blood transfusion is required only under some circumstances but not simply to raise the Hb level. Recent trials have demonstrated that increasing the proportion of HbF with hydroxyurea therapy reduces sickling episodes,[49] particularly acute chest syndrome.[50] Chronic lung complications including pulmonary hypertension are increasingly recognized as an important cause of morbidity and mortality both in the sickling disorders and other hereditary hemolytic anemias.[45,51] HSCT may be curative.[45] Transplantation from an HLA-matched sibling achieves 80–85% disease free survival, and US families with affected children are encouraged to consider umbilical cord blood collection from subsequent unaffected siblings.

Sickle cell variants

HbS can be inherited with HbC, each parent being heterozygous. The child with SC disease has a higher Hb than SS individuals, usually has fewer painful crises, but is nevertheless more prone to avascular necrosis, and to neovascularization of the eyes; these children should have regular ophthalmic review. When HbS is inherited with beta thalassemia the disorder may be less severe, but this depends upon the type of beta thalassemia (Table 23.6). For further information the reader is referred to Serjeant.[52]

Thalassemia syndromes

Thalassemias are a large and heterogeneous group of red cell disorders resulting from impaired or absent synthesis of globin chains. The different globin chains are coded for on either chromosome 16 (alpha-like) or 11 (beta, delta and gamma chains) shown in Figure 23.16a.[44] If alpha chains are affected alpha thalassemia results, if beta chains, beta thalassemia. The clinical effects depend upon both the type and extent of gene mutations and upon whether inherited from one or both parents (thalassemia trait or a more serious disorder). Large gene deletions

Table 23.6 The sickle syndromes – variable clinical severity

Most severe	Homozygous SS, HbS/β[0] thalassemia (β globin mutation with no β globin chain produced)
Intermediate	Hb SC disease
Least severe	HbS/β thalassemia (some β chains produced)
Severity also reduced by:	High HbF level Coincidental inheritance of α thalassemia genes

on chromosome 11 may affect more than one globin gene producing more complex gamma delta thalassemia. Some disorders which affect only HbF (gamma chain mutations) may produce only transient disorders (e.g. hemolytic anemia due to unstable gamma chains) in the neonatal period that disappear as the HbF is replaced by HbA. The racial and geographic origin of the patient will help point towards the most likely hemoglobin abnormalities and will help guide investigations. The pathology of the thalassemias is related to globin chain imbalance; a reduction of one chain leads to an excess of the other; this disturbs red cell production leading to anemia and other consequences of ineffective erythropoiesis.

Alpha thalassemias

Because alpha globin chains are part of fetal hemoglobin, disorders affecting alpha chains may be evident at or before birth, depending upon the severity. There are four alpha globin genes; the clinical phenotype depends upon the number of genes affected (Fig. 23.16b).[44] The most severe form, where all four alpha genes are deleted, is incompatible with life and leads to hydrops fetalis (Fig. 23.16c).[44] The milder forms may lead to a mild hemolytic anemia due to globin chain imbalance. The red cells contain tetramers of beta globin, HbH, which tends to precipitate out and may be visualized on the blood film with special stains. The mildest forms of alpha thalassemia manifest red cells with reduced MCV and MCH. The alpha thalassemia genes are particularly common in Asia, but mild genotypes are also common in Africa, where they may modify the clinical severity of sickle cell disease.

Beta thalassemias

The beta thalassemias occur mainly in countries bordering the Mediterranean but are also important in Asia. In some of the Mediterranean countries the heterozygote rate is as high as 20%; antenatal

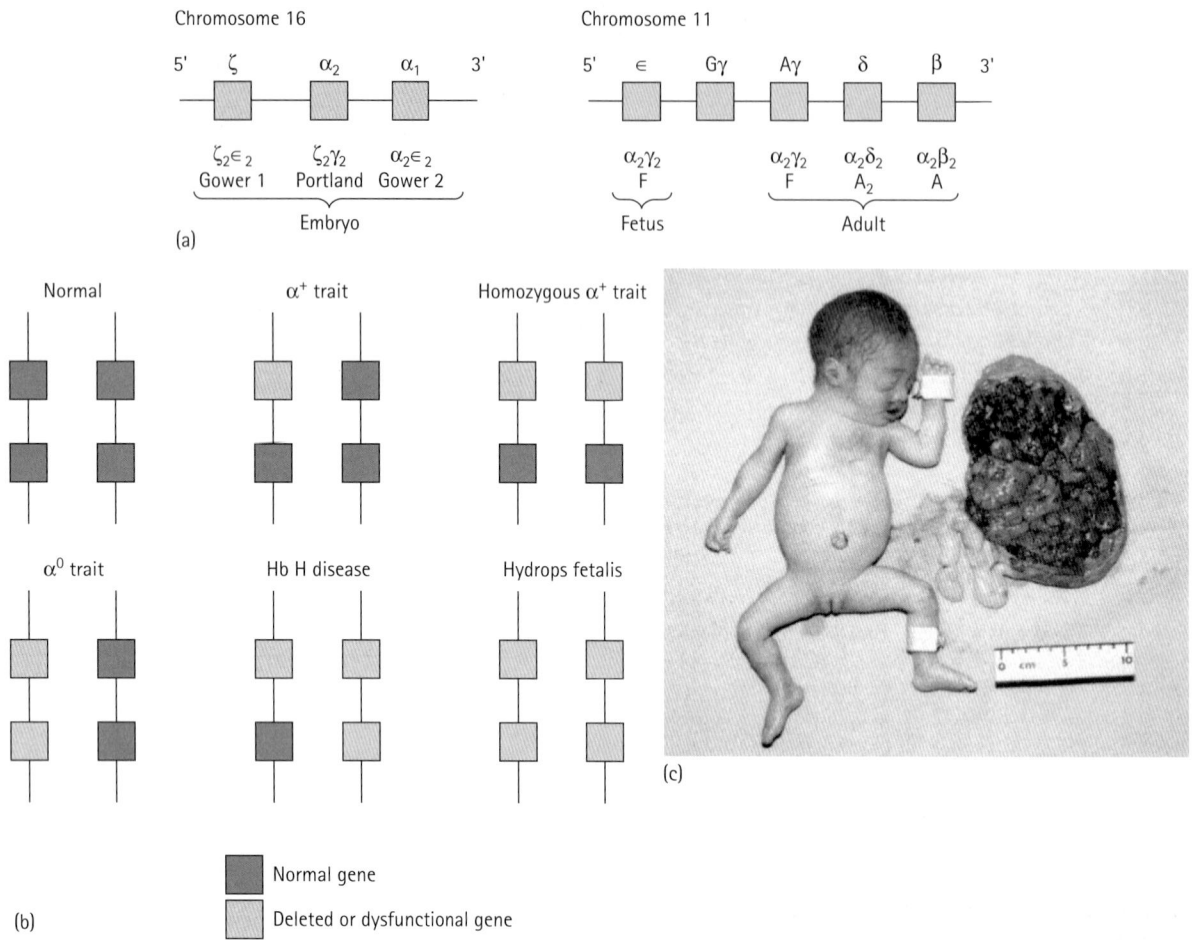

Fig. 23.16 (a) Globin gene clusters on chromosomes 11 and 16. (b) The genetics of alpha thalassemia. (c) Alpha thalassemia hydrops fetalis, the result of deletions of all four alpha globin genes. (From Hoffbrand & Pettit 1993[44] with permission.)

screening programmes have been particularly important in reducing the birth rate of severely affected homozygous infants. Individual mutations are common in different populations which enables screening by mutation detection. While the heterozygote state, beta thalassemia trait, is usually without symptoms or serious sequelae, the homozygous state results in beta thalassemia major – the child is unable to make HbA and usually presents with progressive anemia towards the end of the first year of life.

The pathogenesis of the clinical manifestations of beta thalassemia major is shown in Figure 23.17. Untreated, a child develops severe anemia with growth retardation, hepatosplenomegaly (extramedullary hemopoiesis), failure to thrive and skeletal abnormalities due to marrow hyperplasia. The bones are thin and prone to fracture. In addition to typical maxillary bone expansion which gives rise to the thalassemic facies, the skull X-ray has typical 'hair-on-end' appearance due to medullary expansion (Fig. 23.18a) and there is a typical peripheral blood picture (Fig. 23.18b). Children with beta thalassemia major require regular transfusions of red cells to maintain adequate hemoglobin levels, to promote normal growth and development, and suppress the erythroid hyperplasia and skeletal manifestations. Before embarking on regular transfusion the child should receive hepatitis B vaccine, the red cells should be more fully phenotyped to enable transfusion with blood additionally matched for some of the other red cell antigens. This is particularly important where the child is of a different ethnic group in order to reduce the risk of sensitization against the other red cell antigens. Repeated transfusions lead to iron overload, which is inevitable and must be treated with an iron chelator to remove the excess. The standard chelator is desferrioxamine (DFO) usually given by subcutaneous

infusion over several hours daily for maximal effect. Iron loading results in tissue damage to endocrine glands (parathyroids, pancreas, failure to progress through puberty), skin discoloration, but most seriously can lead to heart failure and dysrythmias. Death results from cardiac complications in inadequately chelated patients, often before the end of the second decade. Adherence is a major issue for many children, especially in teenage years. DFO itself has side-effects and the dose regimen must be carefully calculated. Children should be monitored regularly for ear and eye toxicity. There is good evidence that iron overload, as measured by high ferritin levels and liver biopsy, is clearly related to mortality. Oral iron chelation with deferiprone has been effective, particularly for cardiac iron loading, but carries concerns about toxicity.[53–56] A new oral agent, deferasirox, is as effective as DFO and represents a significant advance.[57] Further research is needed; all these agents have a place and the choice must be individualized.[58] The transfusion requirements (transfusion of packed red cells exceeding 180–200 ml/kg/year) will often indicate when removal of the enlarged spleen (which acts as a reservoir) may be of benefit. Patients often benefit from contact with other affected individuals and patient support groups.

Some individuals who are homozygous for a thalassemia gene show a clinically less severe course (thalassemia intermedia). These individuals may not be transfusion dependent but can show other complications of 'homozygous' beta thalassemia, such as skeletal deformity, to a varying degree. Management may be difficult and such children should be referred to specialists.

HSCT is potentially curative in thalassemia major.[59] Risk factors for a poor outcome were hepatomegaly, liver fibrosis and quality of iron

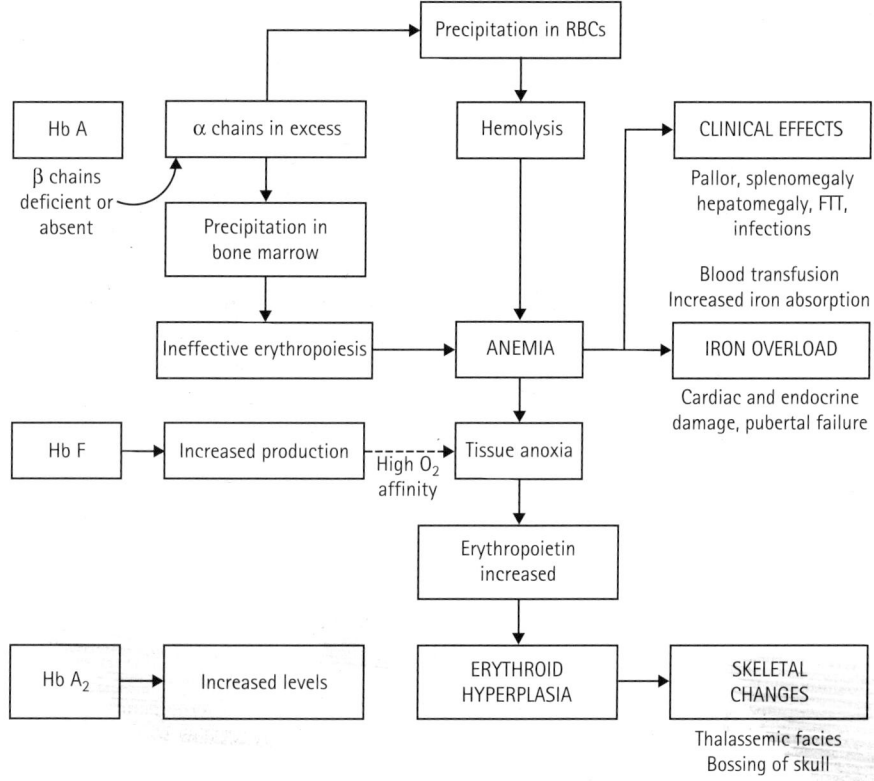

Fig. 23.17 The pathogenesis of beta thalassemia major. FTT, failure to thrive; RBCs, red blood cells.

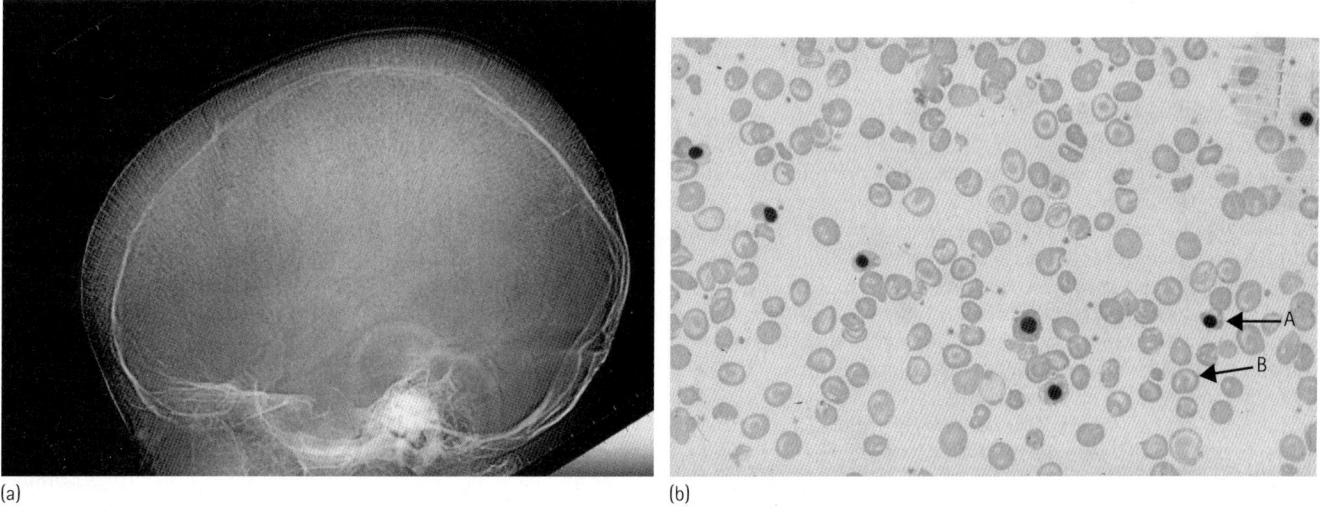

(a)   (b)

Fig. 23.18 Beta thalassemia major. (a) Skull X-ray showing 'hair on end' appearance caused by marrow hyperplasia and expansion. (b) Peripheral blood (postsplenectomy) showing target cells, nucleated red cells, red cell fragments and hypochromia. A, nucleated red cell; B, target cell.

chelation treatment. In 'Class I' patients who lacked any risk factors the overall survival was 96% at 10–11 years with an event-free survival of 92%, whereas 'Class III' patients with all three risk factors had an overall survival of 76% with an event-free survival of 53% at 10–11 years because of increased transplant-related morbidity and mortality. HSCT should be undertaken in young children before there has been significant transfusion iron overload.[60–62] Cord blood from a sibling can also be used.[63,64] Unrelated donor transplant may also be successful.[65] Another approach is preimplantation genetic diagnosis enabling selection of an unaffected fetus, or a fetus which is HLA compatible with an affected sibling with a view to HSCT,[66] but this raises important ethical considerations.

Rare hemoglobin disorders
Unstable hemoglobins
A variety of mutations are described which lead to destabilization of the structure of the globin complex. Some produce congenital Heinz body hemolytic anemia. (Heinz bodies are red cell inclusions visualized by staining with methyl violet). Affected individuals may have significant clinical manifestations or none; variants affecting the beta chains tend to be worse than the alpha chain variants. Children may present with chronic hemolytic anemia or with a more sudden event such as aplastic crisis due to parvovirus or an exacerbation of hemolysis triggered by an infection. Others can produce a picture very similar to thalassemia. Some hemoglobin variants exhibit increased oxygen affinity (leading to polycythemia),

decreased oxygen affinity, or oxidization of heme iron to the ferric state (resulting in methemoglobinemia). These are reviewed by Kulozik.[67]

SECONDARY ANEMIAS

The normal bone marrow produces 10^{11} red cells daily – disease processes readily affect this activity. Children often develop anemia as a consequence of some other illness. Even a transient infection may cause a significant fall in hemoglobin, but this will recover rapidly when the infection clears. More chronic illness is often complicated by 'anemia of inflammation' due to erythropoietin resistance and iron-restricted erythropoiesis.[4] The inflammatory cytokine interleukin 6 up-regulates production of the iron-regulatory hormone, hepcidin. Hepcidin inhibits iron release from macrophages and probably from hepatocytes, resulting in hypoferremia but normal or elevated ferritin. Hepcidin binds to the sole iron export channel from cells, ferroportin, leading to its loss from cell membranes. The anemia may be mild and normochromic or severe and microcytic. Chronic inflammatory disorders are commonly associated with this. Patients may become genuinely iron deficient because of poor diet or blood loss from the gut (possibly due to nonsteroidal anti-inflammatory drugs). Rheumatoid arthritis is particularly complex because the patients may also develop marrow hypoplasia due to drugs, e.g. gold. Patients with connective tissue disorders such as SLE can develop autoimmune hemolysis. Other diseases associated with anemia are acute and chronic renal failure, and some endocrine disorders, particularly hypothyroidism.

DRUGS

Drugs must always be considered as a cause of blood dyscrasias; there are several different potential mechanisms such as blood loss (aspirin and other nonsteroidal anti-inflammatory agents), development of immune phenomena or marrow suppression.

NEUTROPENIA

The time taken to develop from a stem cell to a mature neutrophil is only 24 hours. However, the mature neutrophil may then spend up to 10 days in marrow storage before release when it then circulates in the peripheral blood for only 6–10 hours. A proportion is 'marginated' along the endothelium and is not counted in the full blood count, so reliance on the peripheral blood neutrophil count alone to determine risk of bacterial sepsis can be misleading. The neutrophil reserve (marrow storage pool) is about 13 times the number in the blood. The most important functions of the neutrophils are to phagocytose and kill bacteria. Disorders of neutrophil function are considered in Chapter 27.

The neutrophil count tends to be lower in children, particularly infants, than in adults, and there are racial variations – black races have absolute neutrophil counts that are 0.2 to 0.6×10^9/L lower than Caucasians. If blood is left to stand for several hours before being analysed, the neutrophil count will be falsely low. Neutropenia is defined as a reduction of the absolute neutrophil count below the normal for age, and is divided according to severity, giving some indication of the likely clinical consequences, although this is heavily dependent upon the cause.

- Mild: 1.0 to 1.5×10^9/L (adjust for the first 6 months of life) – usually no clinical problems.
- Moderate: 0.5 to 1.0×10^9/L – clinical problems more common.
- Severe: less than 0.5×10^9/L – risk of life threatening sepsis, especially if neutropenia is prolonged beyond a few days.

Fortunately severe neutropenia in childhood is rare. Intercurrent viral infection is the commonest reason for mild neutropenia (neutropenia occurring during the first 24–48 h and persisting for up to 6 days). If this is the likely cause, then there is no need to repeat the blood count when the child recovers just to see if the count is back to normal. It is more important to be guided by the clinical picture.

NEUTROPENIAS SECONDARY TO MARROW FAILURE OR INFILTRATION

In children with marrow failure or infiltration the risk of serious sepsis is logarithmically increased at neutrophil counts of less than 0.1×10^9/L. In this group a responsible organism is identified in infections in all cases with persistent neutropenia for more than 12 weeks.[68] Endogenous organisms (i.e. part of the resident flora) result in the high risk of serious septicemia. Pathogenic organisms (such as *Pseudomonas*, *Klebsiella* and *Proteus* species) often replace normal less pathogenic flora in many patients with serious underlying disorders such as malignancy. *Staphylococcus aureus* and Gram negative bacilli translocate from the gastrointestinal tract when mucosal defences are breached, for example by the disease or chemotherapy. Neutrophils are normally responsible for some of the clinical features of acute inflammation such as redness, pus and swelling. Such features are therefore often minimal or absent in severe neutropenia. Because of this, and the speed with which sepsis can be fatal, any child with severe neutropenia who develops a significant fever (e.g. one reading over $39°C$ or two over $38°C$ half an hour apart) should be admitted to hospital, have blood and other relevant cultures sent, and be started on broad spectrum parenteral antibiotics while the culture results are awaited. Patients with chronic severe neutropenia should either have open access to a familiar ward, or carry a letter detailing the importance of blood culture as an initial investigation followed by admission for parenteral antibiotics if they attend the general practitioner or hospital emergency room with a fever. As most infections are caused by the child's own resident flora, the addition of protective isolation is not of any proven benefit. It is more important to screen regularly (surveillance throat and rectal swabs) for colonization by the more pathogenic Gram negative organisms (*Klebsiella* and *Pseudomonas* species which confer a higher risk of serious septicemia) and to use selective nonabsorbable antibiotics for gut decontamination. Good hygiene (including mouth and dental care) and prophylaxis against *Candida* are also beneficial. Salads may be significantly contaminated with *Pseudomonas* and other Gram negative organisms and are best avoided.

In other children with neutropenia where there is normal marrow reserve (see below) there is a reduced risk of serious sepsis despite the low count.

AUTOIMMUNE NEUTROPENIA

Autoimmune neutropenia is probably the commonest cause of persistent neutropenia in childhood occurring in perhaps 1 in 100 000 children per annum. Fortunately it is rarely associated with severe sepsis and usually resolves spontaneously after a variable period of time. Typically the child of either sex is aged between 5 and 24 months at presentation. A useful review[69] described 240 children aged 5–15 months at diagnosis. Ninety percent had benign infections and 95% recovered spontaneously within 7–24 months. Bone marrow examination may show maturation arrest with lack of the more mature precursors, or some myeloid hyperplasia, or can be normal. Antineutrophil antibodies can be demonstrated in the serum, which is helpful in confirming the diagnosis. Until the clinical pattern is clear, fever should be managed carefully with appropriate cultures and parenteral antibiotics while excluding a significant infection. When the diagnosis is clear, these children can be managed conservatively and the parents should be encouraged to continue with normal living. Fevers and other infections can be managed in the same way as any other non-neutropenic child. In the rare case with severe infection (usually the younger child) neutrophils can be temporarily increased by steroids or intravenous immunoglobulin but G-CSF (granulocyte-colony stimulating factor) is the treatment of choice for severe infection or to cover surgery.

SEVERE CONGENITAL NEUTROPENIAS

These disorders are rare, but very important to recognise because of the potential seriousness and need for aggressive management. The important difference from autoimmune neutropenia is that these children are likely to present with septicemia or other severe bacterial infections that can lead to early death if not appropriately managed. As neutropenia can occur as a secondary feature in the course of severe sepsis (particularly in neonates and in the presence of endotoxemia), the nature of such a disorder is often not clear at initial presentation. Any child with severe sepsis in whom neutropenia persists should be investigated with bone marrow examination.

Kostmann described 24 cases of severe neutropenia (neutrophils $< 0.2 \times 10^9$/L) in a consanguineous Swedish family in 1956. About 200 similar cases have been described in the literature, but 'Kostmann syndrome' is now recognized to be a heterogeneous group of congenital neutropenias[70] – some children have been shown to have mutations in the G-CSF receptor gene. Presentation is usually before 6 months of age with severe pyogenic infections – half present in the first month of life – and the outlook was poor before the advent of HSCT and the use of G-CSF. The bone marrow shows maturation arrest. Such children should be referred to a pediatric hematologist and most do well on daily injections of G-CSF. They should also receive mouth care and antibiotic prophylaxis. Data from an international registry has confirmed an increased risk of developing acute leukemia, but it is not clear whether this is related to the underlying disorder or to the therapy with G-CSF.[71]

Reticular dysgenesis is another form of severe neutropenia described in Chapter 25.

Cyclical neutropenia is a very rare disorder where there is a nadir of the neutrophil count usually every 21 days to below 0.2×10^9/L. During the neutropenia the child may have mouth ulcers, gingivitis, malaise and fever, and other evidence of bacterial sepsis. There is often some asymptomatic cycling of other blood parameters. Diagnosis requires attention to detail, and twice weekly blood counts for 6 weeks. The bone marrow can show either hypoplasia or maturation arrest of the myeloid series. The condition may improve with age. G-CSF therapy, timed to prevent the neutropenic phase, can give good relief. These patients have no clear evidence of an increased risk of hematological malignancy. It is important to establish whether the neutropenia is associated with any other congenital abnormalities. Neutropenia is well-recognized in about two thirds of cases of Shwachman–Diamond syndrome (see above). Neutropenia may also be seen in other congenital immune deficiency states, such as antibody deficiency.

ACQUIRED NEUTROPENIA

This is most commonly due to intercurrent viral infection or secondary to drug ingestion. The neutrophil count may fall to less than 0.2×10^9/L in an idiosyncratic and unpredictable way; any drug associated with the onset of neutropenia must be considered suspect. In the face of unexplained neutropenia it is advisable to stop the drug. Many different mechanisms have been implicated and there is no convenient diagnostic test.

EOSINOPHILIA

Eosinophilia is arbitrarily defined at a level of greater than 0.5×10^9/L. The commonest cause is the presence of allergic disease, especially atopy – asthma or eczema. Parasitic diseases such as hookworm, ascariasis, tapeworm and schistosomiasis should be sought when eosinophilia persists. A good history of overseas travel is essential. There are other causes that are listed elsewhere.[72]

DISORDERS OF HEMOSTASIS

The normal hemostatic mechanism depends upon the integrity of the vessel wall, and in particular the endothelial cells, the presence of normal numbers and function of platelets, and a normal coagulation mechanism. When an injury occurs these components act in concert to prevent excessive bleeding. The blood vessel wall contracts, the endothelium becomes procoagulant and platelets and coagulation factors are activated resulting in a platelet plug stabilized by fibrin. Several other homeostatic mechanisms come into play – activation of the natural anticoagulant and fibrinolytic systems limit the extent of fibrin formation and maintains the patency of the vessels. Clinical problems with bruising or bleeding can be caused by abnormalities of any part of the hemostatic mechanism or with the connective tissues.

Differentiation of bleeding disorders from non-accidental injury may be difficult. Investigation of a bruised child is mandatory in all cases where the bruising is unexplained or implausible. The history (particularly a detailed family history of any other bleeding tendency – menorrhagia, bleeding after surgery and dental extractions) and examination play an important part in their differentiation. Screening investigations should aim to identify the commonest disorders and those associated with significant bleeding. A blood count including a platelet count, and a coagulation screen – prothrombin time (PT), activated partial thromboplastin time (APTT) and fibrinogen level should be performed. Measurement of plasma factor VIII and IX level is recommended, as significant deficiencies can occur with a near normal coagulation screen. Von Willebrand factor (vWf) antigen and activity should be measured, because von Willebrand disease (vWd) is the commonest inherited bleeding disorder and the coagulation screen is usually normal. Interpretation of these investigations, if abnormal, may need the advice of a hematologist. The demonstration of a bleeding diathesis does not exclude non-accidental injury and these children may be at greater risk of harm from such injury due to their bleeding disorder.

PLATELET DISORDERS
Thrombocytopenic purpuras

Thrombocytopenia is common. A poorly taken blood sample is often responsible – if the low platelet count is unexpected it may need repeating to ensure that it was not a spurious result. Thrombocytopenia is often secondary to infection; sick neonates usually have low platelet counts, and the count may drop in a variety of viral infections, either due to mild and temporary marrow suppression, or occasionally by an autoimmune mechanism.

Symptoms are related to the degree of thrombocytopenia, and if the function is normal, there are very few symptoms until the count is less than 10×10^9/L (Table 23.7a). A raised platelet count is common in children and is nearly always 'reactive' (Table 23.7b). The causes of thrombocytopenia are divided into those with normal or increased numbers of megakaryocytes in the marrow (thrombocytopenia caused by increased peripheral destruction) and those with reduced or absent megakaryocytes (failure of production) (Table 23.8a). Thrombocytopenia in children is commonly caused by increased destruction. The hemostatic defect is mainly due to failure of formation of an adequate platelet 'plug' at the site of endothelial damage. Coagulation screening tests will be normal.

Table 23.7a   Clinical presentation of thrombocytopenia (normal range = 150–450 × 10⁹/L)

Platelet count × 10⁹/L	Symtoms
50–100	Bleeding only produced by trauma or surgery. Often no symptoms at all
30–50	Bruising with minor trauma
10–30	Spontaneous bruising and dependant purpura. Menorrhagia, epistaxis
< 10	Spontaneous bruising and purpura. Mucosal bleeding. At risk for more serious bleeding, e.g. from the gastrointestinal tract or in the central nervous system, depending upon cause of thrombocytopenia (much more likely in circumstances with reduced production than increased destruction)

Table 23.7b Causes of a raised platelet count (thrombocytosis)

In children nearly always reactive or secondary:
Infection
Iron deficiency
Postoperative
Inflammation
Malignancy
Hemorrhage
Primary disease of the marrow is very rare

Table 23.8a Causes of thrombocytopenia

Decreased production:
Congenital – rare
Acquired
Increased destruction:
Immune (common)
Nonimmune
Disseminated intravascular coagulation
Hemolytic uremic syndrome and its variants
Hypersplenism

Table 23.8b Causes of immune thrombocytopenia

Idiopathic autoimmune (ITP or AITP):
Acute (80–90% in children)
Chronic (i.e. >6 months' duration)
Alloantibodies:
Neonatal (NAIT)
Post-transfusion purpura
Drug-induced
Disease-associated (e.g. systemic lupus erythematosus, immunodeficiency and some infections)

Differential diagnosis

A careful clinical history and examination will point to the cause, bearing in mind the incidence of the different disorders.

Congenital thrombocytopenias are very rare and so are often missed. The time of onset of symptoms should be carefully defined, because patients with congenital disorders will have a life-long history. There may be a family history but many of these disorders are inherited recessively. Consanguinity of parents will increase the risk, so that disorders such as Bernard–Soulier syndrome are commoner in populations where cousin marriage is common.

Bernard–Soulier syndrome is caused by a deficiency of platelet glycoprotein 1b, resulting in thrombocytopenia (typically 30–40 × 10^9/L) and defective function so that the bleeding manifestations (bruising, mucous membrane bleeding) occur at a higher platelet count than expected. The blood film shows giant platelets.

Wiskott–Aldrich syndrome is an X-linked disorder that classically leads to severe thrombocytopenia with small platelets associated with eczema; it is associated with immune defects and a significant risk of transformation to malignancy. Mild forms are recognized and not all patients have eczema at the time of presentation with bleeding; some have very severe bleeding symptoms and have been cured by HSCT.

Clearly the implications of a diagnosis of one of these disorders are quite different from immune thrombocytopenias (see below). Other inherited thrombocytopenias are associated with various physical abnormalities, and are reviewed by various authors.[73–76] The children have a lifelong bleeding tendency that can be very difficult to manage, and need expert management in a specialist center.

Thrombocytopenia may be the presenting feature of a more sinister disorder, such as idiopathic aplastic anemia, or one of the constitutional marrow failure syndromes (see above). Limping or bone pain, with lymphadenopathy or splenomegaly, suggests leukemia, but it is rare for this to present without other abnormalities in the blood count. If these diagnoses are suspected a bone marrow examination will help (to rule out aplasia or malignancy) and other tests of platelet function, with analysis of platelet surface molecules, may be required to exclude the congenital disorders. Careful examination of a peripheral smear by an experienced hematologist in possession of the full clinical history is essential.

Coagulation screening tests are not usually indicated unless there is a possibility of consumptive coagulopathy (e.g. in association with suspected sepsis) or hypersplenism that may be associated with hepatic dysfunction. Generally, in a well child with purpura alone, the coagulation screen is normal and unnecessary. Purpura is not a symptom of a coagulation factor defect. In a child with thrombocytopenia and a hemangioma, even if very small, a coagulation profile is essential as this may indicate *Kasabach–Merritt syndrome* with a potentially serious consumption coagulopathy. This combination is fortunately rare, but may be very difficult to manage, with life threatening bleeding.[77]

Idiopathic thrombocytopenic purpura (ITP)

Immune thrombocytopenia can be caused by a variety of different mechanisms (Table 23.8b) but ITP is the most common. Despite this, it is not a common condition; the incidence is about the same as acute leukemia, 1 in 25 000. ITP is caused by antibody production against platelet antigens, switched on as an inappropriate immune response to a trivial viral

infection or immunization. There are well-recognized associations with varicella, MMR vaccine and with infectious mononucleosis.

The clinical onset is usually abrupt with presentation within 24–48 hours. Although the platelet count is dramatically decreased (80% less than 20 × 10^9/L), the typical child, of either sex aged 1–10 years, will have predominantly, or exclusively, cutaneous symptoms and signs often, with florid purpura and easy bruising. Mucosal bleeding is less common, with epistaxis occurring in 20%, usually not severe. Severe bleeding symptoms such as torrential nose bleeds, hematemesis, melena, menorrhagia or frank hematuria are uncommon, occurring in about 4%.[78] Intracranial hemorrhage is rare and not as high as the 1–3% often quoted. The incidence is much closer to 1 in 500 or 1 in 1000, is not confined to early in the course of the disorder, is not necessarily fatal and may be caused by an additional underlying abnormality or provoked by an injury.[79] The outlook in childhood ITP is very good; most children will fully recover within a short time – sometimes even within a few days, and mostly within 6 weeks.

There is no diagnostic test; other disorders have to be considered and excluded as appropriate. Bone marrow aspiration is not required, unless there is doubt about the diagnosis, as it can only exclude other disorders and show a picture that is consistent with increased peripheral destruction (an increase of megakaryocytes in an otherwise normal marrow).

The management of this disorder is controversial because many doctors fear that a very low platelet count carries a high risk of serious or life threatening bleeding. The evidence does not support this. Surveys from Germany[80] and the UK illustrate the safety of a 'no treatment' policy based on mild clinical presentation rather than the platelet count.[81] New standardized parameters are required for the assessment of these children which take into account symptoms as well as the platelet count.[82,83] A clinical classification or 'bleeding index' is shown in Table 23.9. When treatment is required for bleeding symptoms the choice is between oral steroids in high doses (e.g. 1–2 mg/kg/day for 2 weeks; 4 mg/kg/day for 4 days), or intravenous immunoglobulin (IVIG). If a child is treated for a low platelet count alone, it becomes difficult to withdraw steroids as the count drops when the steroid dose is lowered. Prolonged treatment with high dose steroids is toxic and dangerous. IVIG is a blood product (from pooled plasma donations), so may carry a risk of infection (hepatitis C has been transmitted in the past); it has a high frequency of side-effects (fever, headache, malaise) and has to be given by intravenous infusion. It is usually given as 1 g/kg daily for 1 or 2 doses; 800 mg/kg as a single dose may be sufficient. It is indicated in the child with significant bleeding

Table 23.9 Clinical bleeding assessment in children with immune thrombocytopenic purpura – irrespective of platelet count

Bleeding category	Clinical description
Asymptomatic	No symptoms. Low platelet count found incidentally
Mild	Cutaneous features only; purpura and bruising; occasional mucosal lesion; trivial nosebleeds. No interference with normal living
Moderate	More troublesome bleeding including menorrhagia, more severe nosebleeds, moderate interference with daily living
Severe	Bleeding requiring hospital admission and/or blood transfusion. Gastrointestinal bleeding; torrential nosebleeds. Serious life-threatening bleeding such as intracranial hemorrhage

(less than 4% of children) as it raises the platelet count faster than oral steroids. Many other agents have been used for the very rare child with serious hemorrhage who is refractory to steroids and IVIG. These complex cases should be referred to a specialist.

About 15% children do not remit within 6 months, which is defined as 'chronic' ITP. These children are still likely to remit (60% over 10 years) so that management can continue to be expectant.[84] Chronic ITP is more common in children over 10 years of age, and females. These children may develop other features of autoimmune diseases and may be screened for these on an annual basis (antinuclear factor, anti-double stranded DNA, lupus anticoagulants, anticardiolipin antibodies). In the absence of symptoms the finding of other autoantibodies may not alter the management, but will be a useful forewarning of possible trouble to come.

Splenectomy may be considered for children with severe bleeding problems, preferably more than 6 months from diagnosis. The child's lifestyle may be taken into consideration, but about 25% will not remit despite splenectomy and the longer the splenectomized individuals are followed, the higher the relapse rate with no evidence of a plateau. Splenectomy is associated with a life-long increased risk of infection (see above).

Thrombocytopenia secondary to infection
Mild thrombocytopenia of the order of $50–100 \times 10^9$/L is common following recent infection in young children, sometimes accompanied by splenomegaly; both resolve within a week or two. The infection may be a simple upper respiratory tract infection but is sometimes due to glandular fever, cytomegalovirus or toxoplasmosis. Many of the more serious infections (particularly meningococcal disease) produce consumptive coagulopathy. Thrombocytopenia is common in HIV infection, and may be the presenting feature in adults.

Drug-induced thrombocytopenia
Drugs such as alkylating agents and antimetabolites used in leukemia treatment regularly produce dose-dependent general marrow suppression. The other main type of drug-induced thrombocytopenia is that produced by immunological mechanisms, usually of the drug–hapten variety. This has been shown in adults to occur with sedormid, quinidine, quinine, sulfamethazine, antazoline and other drugs. Anti-epileptic medication can rarely produce marrow toxicity with both thrombocytopenia and leucopenia.

Disorders of platelet function
Inherited disorders of platelet function are rare; there are many more common acquired conditions in which moderate platelet dysfunction can play a role. Platelet disorders typically lead to mucosal bleeding, prolonged bleeding from superficial cuts, bruising and purpura. The extent of bleeding is related to the severity of the disorder.

Acquired
The main causes of acquired platelet dysfunction are indicated in Table 23.10. Many drugs cause some platelet dysfunction. Aspirin causes inhibition of prostaglandin synthetase and impaired thromboxane A2 synthesis. There is a failure of the release reaction and aggregation with adrenalin and adenosine diphosphate (ADP). A single small dose can have an effect for the lifespan of the platelet, 7–10 days. Other nonsteroidal anti-inflammatory drugs cause variable interference with platelet function. Heparin and intravenous antibiotics may become important in the seriously ill patient with multiorgan failure in intensive care. Uremia and liver dysfunction may be contributory. Myeloproliferative disorders are extremely rare in childhood. Although in adults a high platelet count may indicate a marrow disorder, in children a raised platelet count is common, and nearly always reactive. It is a marker of inflammation and challenge in a nonspecific manner similar to the erythrocyte sedimentation rate, and does not need further investigation or repeated measurement.

Hereditary
Glanzmann thrombasthenia is a serious bleeding disorder that usually presents early in life with bruising and mucous membrane bleeding. As with other autosomal recessive disorders cases are commonest in families with consanguineous partnerships. The platelet membrane lacks the IIb/IIIa receptor complex that is critical for normal platelet function. The platelet count is normal, laboratory testing shows that the platelets fail to aggregate with any of the usual agonists. Serious bleeding episodes require treatment with platelet transfusions, but these carry a risk of alloantibody stimulation, and so should be used very judiciously. Patients may need HSCT. Recent experience suggests that recombinant activated factor VII may be a useful agent for hemostasis, but the high cost precludes use except in severe bleeding episodes.

Platelets are complex organelles with several types of granule that are important for function. There are a number of inherited platelet storage pool diseases resulting in defective platelet function that produce usually only a mild bleeding tendency. The investigation of these in children is unsatisfactory, and specialist advice should be sought. The association with tyrosinase-positive albinism is called *Hermansky–Pudlak syndrome* and the bleeding problems are usually mild.

COAGULATION DISORDERS

Normal blood coagulation has been described as a 'cascade', where a series of enzymes are activated sequentially, each step adding magnification to the process, leading to the formation of a fibrin clot. In recent years this theory has been revised and it is now more helpful to visualise the relevant factors being brought into proximity with one another on cell surfaces which are crucial to normal coagulation[85,86] (Fig. 23.19a).

Table 23.10 Causes of acquired platelet dysfunction

1. Drugs:
   Inhibition of cyclo-oxygenase, e.g. aspirin and other nonsteroidal anti-inflammatory agents
   Elevation of cyclic AMP levels:
      Inhibitors of phosphodiesterase – dipyridamole
      Activators of adenyl cyclase
   Antibiotics – penicillins and cephalosporins
   Heparin
   Alcohol
2. Uremia
3. Disseminated intravascular coagulation
4. Primary marrow disorders
   Acute leukemias
   Myeloproliferative disorders (very rare in children)
5. Cardiac bypass surgery

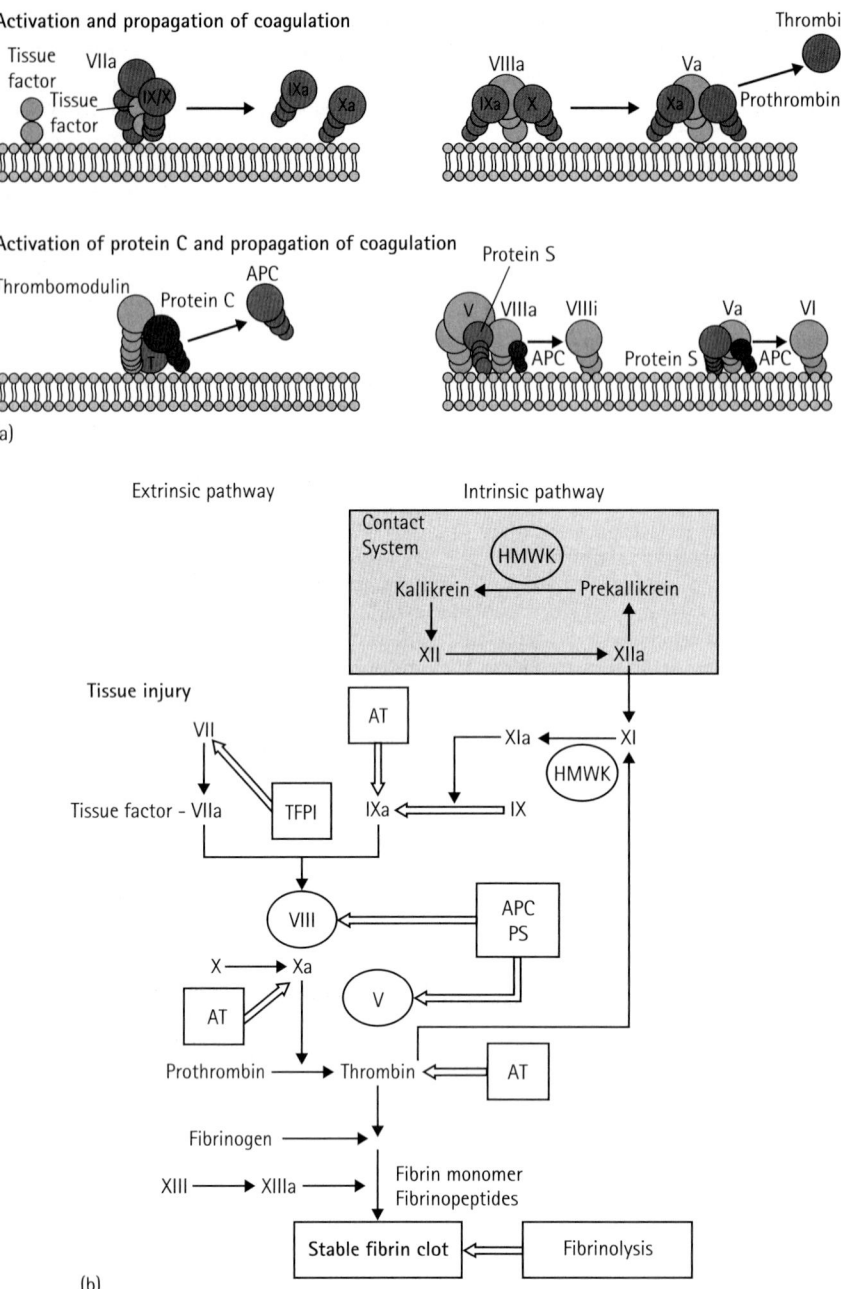

Fig. 23.19 Coagulation pathways. (a) Schematic models illustrating some of the phospholipid-bound reactions that are involved in the activation and regulation of coagulation. Factor VIIa binds to tissue factor and activates factors IX and X. Factors IXa and Xa together with factors VIIIa and Va, respectively, form the tenase and prothrombinase complexes that activate factor X and prothrombin, respectively. Thrombin-mediated activation of factor XI, factor V and factor VIII, which gives positive feedback amplification of the system, is not shown. Thrombomodulin is present on endothelial cells. Thrombin generated in the vicinity of intact endothelial cells binds to thrombomodulin and efficiently activates protein C. Activated protein C (APC) and protein S form a complex to the plasma membrane of endothelial cells and possibly also on other cells. This complex inactivates factors Va and VIIIa, which results in downregulation of the coagulation system. The degradation of factor VIIIa by APC is stimulated by protein S and by factor V, which in this context functions as an anticoagulant protein. (From Dahlback 2000[85] with permission.) (b) Schematic representation of the coagulation pathways. The physiological activation of coagulation occurs via the extrinsic system, after activation of tissue factor VII. The end result of activation is the production of a stable fibrin clot. Open shafted arrow, inhibitory action. Inhibitors: APC, activated protein C; AT, antithrombin; PS, protein S; TFPI, tissue factor pathway inhibitor. Tint box outlines the contact system; factors in this box affect the laboratory tests but do not play a significant role in hemostasis. Ovals indicate cofactors; HMWK, high molecular weight kininogen. (From Lissauer & Clayden 2001[35] with permission.)

Coagulation screening tests give important indications of where a coagulation problem lies, but do not take into account many other important physiological systems which add to the balance of hemostasis and thrombosis. In addition to the coagulation factors that contribute to the formation of the fibrin clot, the naturally occurring anticoagulants, antithrombin, protein C and its cofactor protein S, and tissue factor pathway inhibitor are important in preventing excessive coagulation

activation. Other so-called coagulation factors, such as factor XII, whose deficiency may produce an abnormal screening test, have no physiological role in coagulation; a defect is not associated with a bleeding disorder. Some of these interactions are shown in Figure 23.19b. Although the hemophilias are the best characterized of the inherited coagulation disorders, the rare ones have taught us much about normal hemostasis. The physiological pathway for a fibrin clot is the stimulation of tissue factor – factor VII. Infants with complete deficiency of either factor VII or factor X are particularly at risk of intracranial hemorrhage in the first week of life (also a major risk for the same reason in vitamin K deficiency), in contrast to severe factor VIII or IX deficiency where this complication is much less common.

Coagulation tests do not give any information about the fibrinolytic system, complement activation, the activity of the endothelial cell (a very important regulator of hemostasis) or of the other cell systems which may be implicated, such as monocytes and neutrophils where tissue factor expression can vary; up-regulation can produce a thrombotic milieu. At present there are no satisfactory routine ways of examining these other homeostatic mechanisms.

HEREDITARY COAGULATION DEFECTS

The three most common serious defects are due to deficiency of factors VIIIC and IXC and von Willebrand factor. The other disorders are autosomally inherited and either very rare (e.g. factor VII and X deficiencies, afibrinogenemia) or they produce less severe bleeding problems (factor XI deficiency). Inheritance patterns and incidence are detailed in Table 23.11.

Hemophilia A and B

Hemophilia A occurs with an incidence of 1 in 10 000 births, and is thought to be of similar incidence in all the populations of the world. Factor IX deficiency, hemophilia B, is about 5 times less common, but all the clinical manifestations are as for hemophilia A, and both are inherited as X-linked disorders. The degree of factor VIII or IX deficiency varies in different families, but remains constant within kindreds. They are divided clinically into mild, moderate and severe on the basis of the factor level, which predicts bleeding (Table 23.12). Boys with severe hemophilia often present at 12–18 months of age with joint bleeds when they begin to walk, or with mucosal bleeding from the mouth as a result of a fall. Bleeding is typically not severe but rather a constant ooze, or may stop temporarily with a friable clot, which is easily dislodged, leading to further bleeding. These infants may also have easy bruising leading to the suspicion of non-accidental injury. Children with moderate hemophilia will mostly have been diagnosed by the age of 5 years, but those with mild hemophilia may only be diagnosed much later (even in adulthood) when they present with bleeding after dental extraction or other challenges. The hallmark of severe hemophilia is recurrent bleeding into joints and muscles starting in infancy (Fig. 23.20). If inadequately treated, these result in progressive joint deformity and a severe destructive arthropathy (Fig. 23.21). Muscle bleeds can result in permanent damage due to fibrosis and contractures. Relatively minor trauma can also lead to life threatening bleeding. Bleeding initially appears relatively mild, but is persistent and can last for weeks if no treatment is available;

Table 23.12 Hemophilia A and B – level of clotting factor related to clinical features

Level of clotting factor (% of normal)	Clinical features
<1%	Severe disease Spontaneous bleeding into joints and muscles
1–5%	Moderate disease Bleeding after trauma Occasional spontaneous bleeding
5–40%	Mild disease Bleeding after trauma

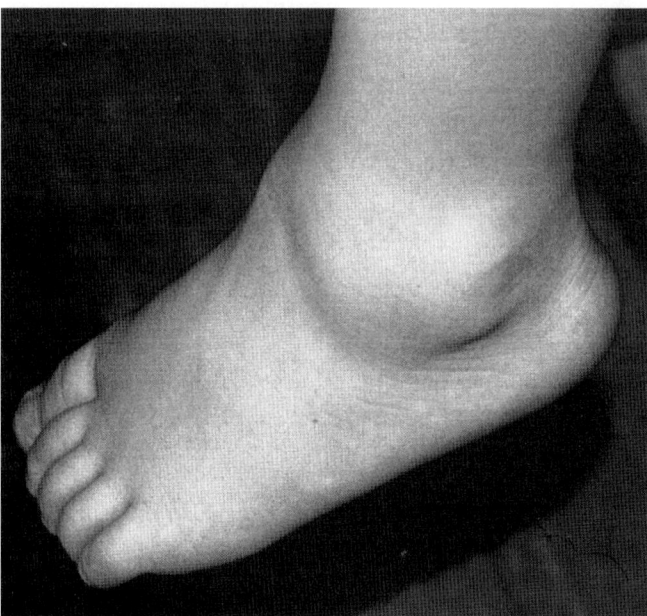

Fig. 23.20 Acute ankle hemarthrosis in a child with severe hemophilia A.

for example a child with a bitten tongue may bleed intermittently for 3 weeks leading to severe anemia necessitating blood transfusion as well as correct replacement therapy. Children with all grades of severity are at risk of bleeding after surgery, particularly in areas of increased fibrinolysis such as the mouth (dental extractions) and genitourinary tract (circumcision). Surgery should never be performed in a hemophiliac without appropriate replacement therapy.

Table 23.11 Hemorrhagic disorders

Deficient factor	Site of production	Synonym	Inheritance	Approximate incidence
VIIIC	Liver	Hemophilia A	X-linked	1:10 000 males
IXC	Liver	Hemophilia B, Christmas	X-linked	1:150 000
vWF	Endothelial cell and platelets	von Willebrand	Autosomal	1:30 000
XIC	Liver	PTA	Autosomal	Approximately 8% Ashkenazi Jews are heterozygous
XC	Liver	Stuart Prower	Autosomal recessive	1:100 000
VIIC	Liver	Proconvertin	Autosomal recessive	1:500 000
I	Liver	Fibrinogen	Autosomal recessive	1:1 000 000
IIC	Liver	Prothrombin	Autosomal recessive	1:2 000 000
XIII	Liver or platelets	Fibrin stabilizer	Autosomal recessive	1:2 000 000

C, coagulant activity; PTA, plasma thromboplastin antecedent; vWF, von Willebrand factor.

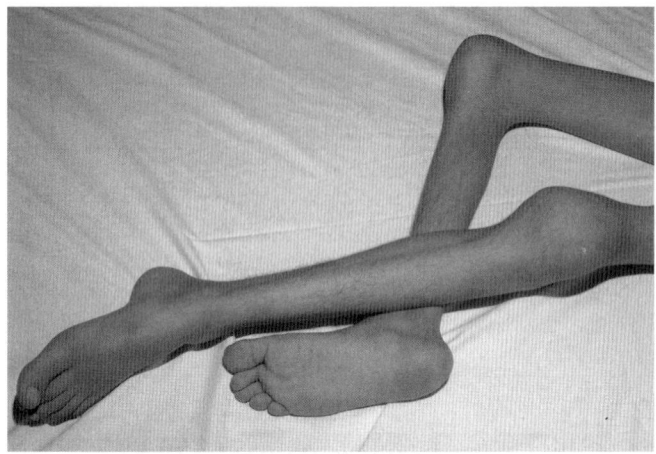

(a)

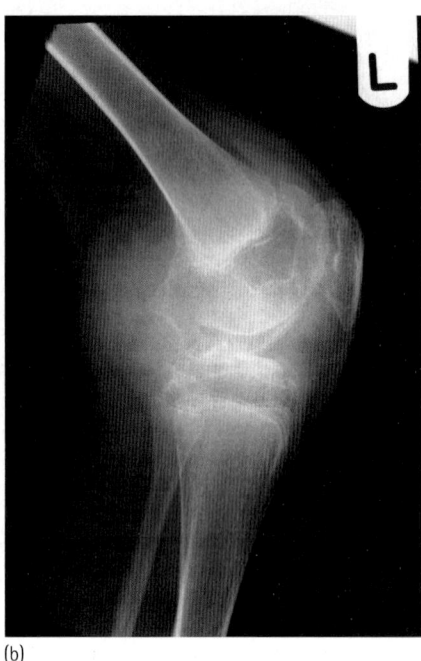

(b)

Fig. 23.21 (a) Severe hemophilia in an adolescent showing fixed flexion of right knee, marked arthropathy of left knee and muscle wasting. (b) Radiological appearance of left knee.

Diagnosis

Severe hemophilia can be diagnosed at birth in an infant with a known family history as the factor VIIIC level at birth is at normal adult levels. The initial screening test will show a markedly prolonged APTT. This will not distinguish between factor VIIIC and IXC – the appropriate factor assay must be performed. Severe hemophilia B can also be diagnosed at birth, but milder forms may not be reliably diagnosed within the first 6 months as the factor IX level only reaches adult levels later. The quality of the blood sample for coagulation testing and factor assays is crucial. Traumatic samples may contain tissue factor causing activation of the coagulation pathways and give an inaccurate and falsely normal results.

Genetics and counseling

About a third of hemophiliacs have no known family history and these individuals either represent new mutations or transmission via asymptomatic women over many generations. About a third of female carriers have low factor VIIIC (or IXC) levels because in each cell one X chromosome is inactivated (the Lyon hypothesis). On average, the factor level in carriers is half normal, but in some it is low enough to cause bleeding symptoms after trauma or surgery (effectively mild hemophilia). The relevant female relatives of any hemophiliac should have factor assays performed. A normal level will not exclude carrier status, which can generally be detected by mutation analysis of the index patient in the kindred and testing possible carriers for the known mutation. Genetic diagnosis should not be performed without consent from the possible carrier and should be delayed until the girl is old enough to understand and give informed consent. About 500 different mutations have been reported for the factor VIIIC gene, and more than 700 for the factor IX gene. It is very important to identify which women are at risk of giving birth to a severely affected boy. Parents need the opportunity to consider this, and appropriate management plans need to be in place for delivery. Most hemophiliac babies are born by normal vaginal delivery, but instrumentation should be avoided, and male infants tested at birth. It is possible to undertake antenatal testing in consultation with the appropriate services.

Management

Hemophilia is a potentially serious and life-long disorder. Families can be taught to manage this very well indeed, but this requires considerable investment of time and support best provided by specialist centers (hemophilia centers). In addition to information and training families are often helped by being put in touch with one another, and with support organizations (hemophilia societies). Families need to learn how to live with the disorder. Fortunately with current treatment options in resource-rich countries, there need to be few restrictions on activity. Contact sports should be avoided, but sport is generally beneficial; children should be encouraged to be fit, but regular soccer football is likely to lead to damaged ankle joints in the long-term. The important principal is to give replacement therapy for bleeding episodes. Treatment can be given on demand for bleeds in severe and moderate hemophilia. A concentrate of factor VIIIC is used (or factor IXC in factor IX deficiency), either plasma-derived or genetically engineered (recombinant). Fresh frozen plasma contains factor VIIIC and IXC but an unacceptably large volume would be required for an adequate factor increase. Cryoprecipitate is effective in hemophilia A (but not hemophilia B) but is not virally inactivated and is less convenient because of the volume required. Plasma-derived factor concentrates have been available in resource rich countries since the 1970s and have changed the lives of severe hemophiliacs, providing early and adequate treatment of joint bleeds preventing severe joint deformity in many young men. Unfortunately the early products transmitted both hepatitis C and HIV infection with tragic consequences. More than 1000 of the total 5000 people with hemophilia A in the UK were infected with HIV between 1979 and 1985, and more than 3000 people have been infected with hepatitis C. Viral inactivation steps introduced in the 1980s have prevented virus transmission (HIV and HCV) since 1986–87. In many countries recombinant products are the treatment of choice, but at a high cost. The half-life of factor VIII in the circulation is only 8–12 hours, and is less in small children. Doses need to be given twice or three times daily for surgery, where the aim is to keep the factor VIIIC level above 50 iu/dl. Minor bleeding episodes respond rapidly to a single dose of 20–25 iu/kg; more severe bleeds may need higher initial doses and repeat doses over a few days. Factor IXC needs to be given in higher dosage as the recovery is less (40–50 iu/kg), but less frequently as the half-life is longer.

Current treatment of severe hemophilia aims to prevent joint damage by giving prophylactic therapy. Factor VIIIC is given three times a week, or on alternate days, at a dose sufficient to prevent the trough level falling below 2 iu/dl, effectively converting severe to moderate hemophilia which is far less likely to be complicated by recurrent joint and muscle bleeds. Experience has shown benefit in serial cohorts monitored over decades.[87] Additional data from an orthopaedic outcomes study (data collected from 21 centers world-wide) demonstrated that those patients with more than 45 weeks of regular prophylaxis per year had better joint function at 6-year follow-up than those treated 'on demand'. Total factor VIII usage per annum also correlated with outcomes; in general, more treatment was better.[88] Prophylaxis is optimal therapy for young hemophiliacs, generally with a regimen of alternate day (or 25 iu/kg three times a week) therapy in hemophilia A, and twice weekly (40 iu/kg) injections for hemophilia B, starting in the first or second year of life. Prophylaxis is divided into: primary – started before the age of 2 years or after the first joint bleed and secondary – either as continuous therapy starting after the age of 2, or after two or more joint bleeds. Secondary prophylaxis can also be periodic treatment given to settle a series of repeated bleeds. The benefit of prophylaxis has been confirmed by a controlled trial in the USA,[89] and other studies are underway in Canada and Italy. Several questions remain, in particular, should prophylaxis be started in the first year of life before there are any joint bleeds? (Not all individuals with very low factor levels have repeated joint bleeds.) Venous access is usually very difficult in the young child – perhaps dosing weekly with escalation with age as veins become more accessible may be as effective. Central venous lines have advantages but are complicated by infection and thrombosis. Swedish and other smaller uncontrolled studies clearly demonstrate improvement in quality of life – reduced days off school and greater satisfaction among the families – but other families have found it very hard to persist with the regular injections for a variety of reasons. The availability and cost of factor concentrates is a major issue even in resource rich countries. Even within the European Network of 20 hemophilia centers (16 countries) the proportion of severe hemophiliac children on continuous prophylaxis varies from 15–100%.[90]

Mild hemophilia A (but not hemophilia B) can often be treated with parenteral high dose desmopressin (0.3 µg/kg i.v. or s.c.). This stimulates release of factor VIIIC from storage sites and can increase the level threefold within 1–2 hours of the end of the infusion. This is usually appropriate for minor procedures such as tooth extraction. Desmopressin is an antidiuretic hormone analogue, with potential fluid retention, which must be watched, and the risk of fits due to cerebral oedema is increased in small infants. Desmopressin is not usually given to infants less than 2 years of age. Major procedures can also be managed in this way, although the response declines after several days (tachyphylaxis).

Von Willebrand disease (vWd)

Von Willebrand disease (vWd) is the commonest inherited bleeding disorder with a prevalence of 1 in 100 to 1 in 1000. Mild forms (the commonest) are not usually detected by a 'routine coagulation screen' as the factor VIIIC and APTT are often normal and speficic assays of the von Willebrand factor are required (vWf – assays measure immunologically available protein or activity), often on more than a single occasion. The bleeding time is not usually helpful. It is the least sensitive diagnostic test in mild vWd. The defect is in the von Willebrand factor with secondary effects on factor VIIIC, normally protected from degradation in the circulation by binding to vWf. Von Willebrand factor has an important role binding platelets to the vessel wall with activity mediated through the glycoprotein 1b receptor on the platelets. Symptoms are those of 'platelet-type' bleeding – bruising, mucous membrane bleeding including epistaxis and menorrhagia in women. This is an important and often overlooked symptom. People with mild forms of vWd are likely to bleed excessively after surgery. vWf is a large molecule and can have both quantitative or qualitative defects. Von Willebrand disease has many subtypes; full workup should be performed in a hemophilia center with adequate diagnostic facilities. It is generally a mild disorder inherited autosomally with variable expression in different family members. The level of vWf is also affected by factors outside the vW gene, particularly blood group. A good family history is essential and the implications of the diagnosis explained carefully to other members of the family. Severe vWd is uncommon, usually occurring when each parent has a vWf defect which may be asymptomatic or expressed as mild vWd. Individuals with severe vWd may experience joint bleeds similar to severe hemophilia. Mucous membrane bleeding in mild vWd is often helped by antifibrinolytic drugs. Surgery can often be managed with parenteral desmopressin, but severe forms of vWd require factor replacement using a plasma-derived intermediate purity factor VIIIC concentrate containing vWf, or a vWf concentrate. Management of the different subtypes can vary; in particular there are some variants in which desmopressin is contraindicated so these patients should always be managed with appropriate hematological advice. Cryoprecipitate should no longer be used as concentrates are safer and usually effective.

Other hereditary bleeding disorders

Congenital deficiencies of all the other coagulation factors have been described, but are rare. A coagulation screen will indicate where the defect lies (but is normal in FXIII deficiency), and which further tests and assays are required. Bleeding symptoms should always be investigated. Families with all types of bleeding disorders are often misdiagnosed initially as non-accidental injury as, sadly, this is more common. Specific factor concentrates are available for some of the severe homozygous disorders (factor VII; factor X is contained in plasma-derived factor IX concentrates). Factor XI deficiency is clinically mild even in severe deficiency and more common amongst Jewish people (with a carrier rate of 8%). Factor XIII is the fibrin-stabilizing factor (normal coagulation screen) and in deficiency typically produces delayed hemorrhage 24–36 hours after injury, with delayed wound healing and sometimes scarring. Bleeding from the umbilical stump and delayed separation of the cord also occur. Specific assays define the diagnosis of all of these disorders.[91]

ACQUIRED COAGULATION DEFECTS

Although the congenital coagulation deficiencies are important, in clinical practice the acquired causes are much more common, and are usual in the sick child.

Deficiency of vitamin K-dependent coagulation factors

Factors II, VII, IX and X, synthesized in the liver, require vitamin K-dependent addition of gamma-carboxyl group to make a functional protein. Deficiency can cause a very serious bleeding disorder with a risk of intracranial hemorrhage. Vitamin K is fat soluble and obtained from green vegetables and bacterial synthesis in the gut. Vitamin K-dependent factors are low at birth and fall further in breast-fed infants in the first few days of life. Premature and ill babies are prone to deficiency and should always be supplemented. Classic hemorrhagic disease of the newborn is rarely seen in resource rich countries, partly because of universal prophylaxis but also due to general good standards of living. Later presentation of vitamin K deficiency can occur in infants with malabsorption and should be screened for in children with celiac disease, cystic fibrosis and other long-term gastrointestinal disorders including obstructive jaundice, pancreatic and small bowel disease. Prophylaxis can be achieved with 5 mg vitamin K orally daily. The prothrombin time is very sensitive to factor VII deficiency and is a useful screening test; the APTT will also be long. Parenteral vitamin K produces a rapid shortening of the prothrombin time, within 2–4 hours, but serious bleeding must be treated immediately with concentrates containing factors II, VII, IX and C or with fresh frozen plasma (preferably pathogen inactivated). Oral supplements can be used where absorption is likely to be normal.

Liver disease

Liver disease can produce a variety of complex alterations in hemostasis. Acute hepatocellular failure produces a rapidly progressive failure of coagulation factor synthesis detected initially as marked prolongation of the PT (effect on factor VII) and reduction in fibrinogen. Chronic disease produces variable effects often associated with thrombocytopenia. Liver dysfunction can lead to disruption of fibrinogen synthesis with abnormal forms but these do not predict bleeding. It also affects the fibrinolytic system and can be prothrombotic because of failure of clearance of activated coagulation proteins.

Consumptive coagulopathy – disseminated intravascular coagulation (DIC)

Blood coagulation is kept in sensitive balance with other homeostatic pathways, anticoagulant, pro-inflammatory, fibrinolytic. Under many conditions these are disturbed resulting in profound clinical derangements. Normal coagulation is triggered by tissue factor activation. Tissue factor expression is increased by diverse agents and endothelial damage leading to a pro-coagulant state. The endothelial cell has a key role as gatekeeper, regulating not only blood flow but the pro- versus anticoagulant properties. Any condition causing endothelial disturbance (shock from any cause) and sepsis can lead to activation of coagulation with consumption of platelets and coagulation factors producing disseminated intravascular coagulation. Microvascular thrombosis leads to end-organ dysfunction; consumption of factors and triggering of fibrinolysis lead to a bleeding diathesis. The condition varies from subclinical, detectable by testing only, to an acute florid hemorrhagic state. There are no diagnostic laboratory tests, rather a constellation of abnormalities associated with the appropriate clinical circumstances lead to the diagnosis. The commonest triggers in pediatric practice are infections, particularly Gram negative sepsis and meningococcal infection, and vascular injury (trauma, burns). Neonates with shock are particularly vulnerable, resulting in profound hypofibrinogenemia, very long coagulation screening tests and thrombocytopenia. The picture may be rapidly evolving, and repeated monitoring is essential in the acute situation. The key principal in management is to treat the underlying cause – remove the trigger; the bleeding child will need replacement therapy with blood products dictated by the laboratory tests (cryoprecipitate for a low fibrinogen, platelet transfusions for severe thrombocytopenia, and possibly plasma as well). Recently it is appreciated that the natural anticoagulants, protein C and S, and antithrombin, are usually consumed in addition; there may be a role for replacement of these, particularly in severe sepsis with protein C deficiency[92] particularly in relation to meningococcal disease.[93]

THROMBOSIS IN CHILDREN

Thrombosis is rare in children; the incidence of venous thrombosis is 0.6 per 100,000 of the Dutch population under 14 years of age, compared to 20.2 in those aged 15–24 years, 37 in those aged 25–39 years and 74 in those aged 40–54 years. Nevertheless, sick children are at risk, particularly those with central venous lines[94] and thrombotic events occur in neonates often related to the use of central lines. The incidence of thrombotic events after trauma in children is negligible under the age of 13 years and this group do not need thromboprophylaxis.[95] In addition to such acquired causes, there is increasing interest in a number of inherited risk factors that predispose to thrombosis in adults. A mutation in the factor V gene (factor V Leiden) which makes activated factor V resistant to inactivation is particularly common in Northern Europeans (2–7% of the population); protein C, protein S and antithrombin deficiency also increase the risk in heterozygotes, but screening for these in asymptomatic offspring of an adult with thrombosis is not justified. Such genetic screening should only be performed with appropriate consent. A study of Swedish children and adolescents presenting with a first thromboembolic event found acquired risk factors in 81% (commonly central lines) but 64% of those studied were found also to have heritable risk factors, and 20% had two or more.[96] Long-term studies show a significant incidence of postphlebitic syndrome and recurrent events. Infants with severe protein C deficiency have a severe thrombotic phenotype that usually presents at or shortly after birth with intracerebral thrombosis, blindness and typical microvascular thrombosis of the skin (Fig. 23.22). Diagnosis is urgent as the infant may be treated with protein C concentrate. Severe protein S deficiency may produce a similar picture. Homozygous antithrombin deficiency has not been reported; it is probably incompatible with life. Anticoagulant therapy is appropriate for many of these children, and appropriate protocols are now available, but should be supervised by a suitably trained person.

LEUKEMIA

INCIDENCE

Leukemia is the commonest malignancy of childhood accounting for approximately 35% of the total. Acute lymphoblastic leukemia (ALL)

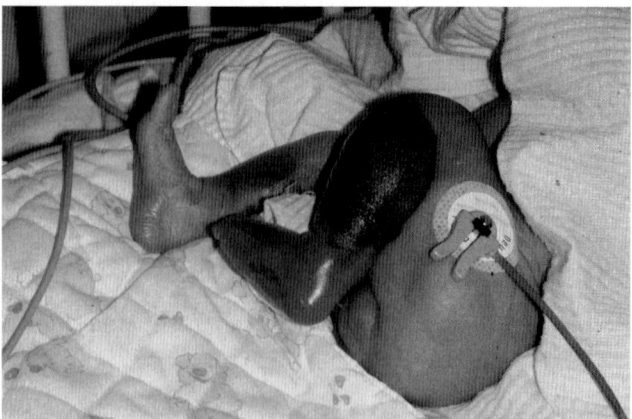

Fig. 23.22   Infant with severe congenital protein C deficiency. Microvascular thrombosis of the skin.

is much commoner than acute myeloid leukemia (AML) representing 80–85% of all leukemias in this age group. The incidence of leukemia is not constant throughout the world and this can partly be explained by genetic and environmental differences. In Western countries, the incidence is approximately 4/100 000 children up to the age of 15 years,[97] with boys having an incidence 1.2 higher than girls.

CLASSIFICATION OF LEUKEMIA

Distinction between the different types and subtypes of leukemia is essential for optimizing treatment and predicting outcome of disease. Leukemias are classified firstly into acute or chronic forms, indicating the speed of progression of the disease without treatment. Chronic leukemia in children is very rare and is confined to chronic myeloid leukemia (CML). CML accounts for between 2% and 5% of all childhood leukemias and presents as one of two forms: chronic granulocytic leukemia (CGL), which is identical to the adult type CGL, or juvenile CML (JCML), recently renamed juvenile myelomonocytic leukemia (JMML), which is a form of myelodysplasia. CGL, JMML and other forms of myelodysplasia carry a risk of progression to acute leukemia.

Cases of acute leukemia can be classified on the basis of morphology, cytochemistry, immunophenotype or cytogenetic abnormality, or by combinations of these characteristics. Ideal classifications of acute leukemias do not yet exist and so information from all these sources must be used together (Table 23.13).

Morphologically, the acute leukemias are divided into ALL and AML. The classification most widely used now was first described by the French–American–British (FAB) group in 1976[98] subsequently expanded, modified and clarified over the years. Pediatric myelodysplasia is recognized as a distinct entity with a prognostic scoring system. Classification of all these disorders requires examination of both peripheral blood and bone marrow films with differential counts performed on both. Cytochemical staining can help distinguish lymphoid from myeloid leukemia and also assign the two different leukemias to specific subtypes. However, it has mostly been superseded by immunophenotyping.

Immunological typing of leukemic cells utilizes immunoenzymatic and immunofluorescent techniques employing a panel of antibodies which recognize particular blast cell-surface or cytoplasmic antigens. Immunophenotyping is particularly useful in ALL and in classifying certain types of AML (M0 and M7) where the blasts are not easily classifiable morphologically. It will also help identify the occasional biphenotypic acute leukemias where there is expression of the specific markers from both lymphoid and myeloid lines. In ALL, it confirms the diagnosis and separates cases into leukemias of T cell and B cell lineage. Further separation into categories reflecting

Table 23.13 The leukemias and myelodysplastic syndromes. (After Bennett et al 1976, 1982[98,100] Emanuel 1999,[99] Passmore et al 1995,[101] Bain 1999[122])

Main group	Subtypes		Chromosomal associations
Acute lymphoblastic leukemia	Early B-precursor Common Pre-B Null	immunophenotype	t(12;21), t(1;19), t(4;11) t(12;21), high hyperdiploidy
	T		t(10;14)
	B		t(8;14); t(8;22), t(2,8)
	L1	morphological	t(12;21), high hyperploidy
	L2		t(12;21), high hyperdiploidy
	L3		t(8;14), t(8;22), t(2;8)
Acute myeloblastic leukemia	M0 undifferentiated		
	M1 without maturation		
	M2 with granulocytic maturation		t(8;21)
	M3 promyelocytic		t(15;17)
	M4 myelomonocytic		
	M4Eo myelomonocytic with eosinophils		inv(16) or t(16;16)
	M5 monocytic/monoblastic		11q23
	M6 erythroleukemia		
	M7 megakaryoblastic		t(1;22)
Myelodysplasia	RA refractory anemia		
	RARS refractory anemia with ringed sideroblasts		
	RAEB refractory anemia with excess blasts (5–20%)		
	RAEBT refractory anemia with excess blasts in transformation (20–30%)		
	JMML juvenile myelomonocytic leukemia		Monosomy 7, never bcr/abl+
	Imo 7 infantile monosomy 7		Monosomy 7
	EOS eosinophilia		

the stage of maturation at which the abnormal clone expanded is possible, particularly for the B cell leukemias where precursor B cell leukemias (null, pre-B and common) are distinguishable from mature B cell leukemia. These categories show some correlation with cytogenetic subsets. It is important to identify mature B cell leukemia which is also identifiable morphologically (FAB L3), and cytogenetically [t(8; 14)] (Table 23.13), because this is treated with chemotherapy designed for B cell non-Hodgkin lymphoma, not standard ALL therapy.

The mainstay of AML classification is morphological characteristics seen on both an ordinary, stained bone marrow aspirate film and those after specific cytochemical staining. Sometimes monoclonal antibody staining is required for precise classification as in megakaryoblastic leukemia (M7). The FAB classification is based on identifying the predominant cell type and the degree of differentiation of the cells. Certain types have characteristic laboratory or clinical features such as disseminated intravascular coagulation [promyelocytic leukemia (M3)], gum hyperplasia, skin rash and raised lysozyme levels [monoblastic leukemia (M5)] and osteosclerosis and Down syndrome with M7. Certain cytogenetic abnormalities are also associated with specific morphological types and can be important prognostic indicators. These include t(15;17) in M3 and inv(16) in myelomonocytic leukemia with eosinophils (M4Eo), both associated with a good prognosis in children.

The myelodysplastic syndromes (MDS) are rare in childhood and represent between 1% and 9% of all pediatric hematological malignancies.[102] They are often associated with other conditions such as Down syndrome, cardiac abnormalities, neurofibromatosis type 1 and congenital bone marrow disorders. These include FA and SDS which may progress to acute leukemia. Classification by the FAB group[100] is not ideal in childhood as this does not accommodate JMML or infantile monosomy 7, a myelodys-

plastic condition occurring in young infants which shares many characteristics with JMML. In addition, MDS occurring in association with the congenital bone marrow disorders may not be classifiable, as the bone marrow is often hypoplastic, whereas in adult MDS this occurs in only 10% of cases.

Refractory anemia (RA), anemia with myelodysplastic features, with or without a few ringed sideroblasts, is rare and must be distinguished from the congenital dyserythropoietic anemias (see Ch. 12) and megaloblastic anemia (see above). Refractory anemia with ringed sideroblasts (RARS) is exceptionally rare in childhood and must be distinguished from a mitochondrial cytopathy such as Pearson's syndrome (see above). RA and RARS can only be diagnosed with confidence in the presence of clonal cytogenetic abnormalities, but both carry a much better prognosis than other MDS in adults. The distinction between the other types of myelodysplasia, such as refractory anemia with excess blasts (RAEB) or refractory anemia with excess blasts in transformation (RAEBT) and AML depends on the percentage of blasts in the bone marrow. Review of treatment of this group of children shows that it is appropriate for them to be treated as for AML.[103] The FAB classification has been expanded and a scoring system developed taking into consideration the level of hemoglobin F, platelet count and complexity of karyotype.[101] A favorable score gives a 5-year survival of approximately 60% with all of those with an unfavorable score being dead within 4 years of diagnosis.

CLINICAL TRIALS

It is well recognized that the increased intensity of treatment has improved prognosis in general for leukemia. However, within a particular regimen, it is possible to increase intensity for those at highest risk while decreasing intensity for those with the best prognosis, thus reducing both early and late toxicity. Classification of leukemias morphologically, immunologically and cytogenetically along with certain clinical features has enabled stratification of children into different risk groups within a given type of leukemia, making it possible to give risk-adapted therapy. Many groups have developed different treatment regimens over the past 30 years, building on experience and introducing new drugs or methods of delivery in a controlled way to enable the true effect of any change to be determined. In the UK, >90% of children with acute leukemia are treated within clinical trials. This enables reliable comparisons between treatments and advances to be made. By standardizing risk categories internationally, it is also possible to compare results from trials conducted in the USA or other parts of Europe, for example.

PRESENTATION

Acute myeloblastic leukemia has a steady incidence throughout childhood although the monoblastic/monocytic types tend to occur relatively more often in infancy. Acute lymphoblastic leukemia is most common between the ages of 2 and 5 years with an increased incidence in boys. Rare cases of congenital leukemia do occur and these are usually but not exclusively malignancies of early B cells. JMML and monosomy 7 tend to occur in infants.

The diagnosis of acute leukemia usually starts from a clinical suspicion. Only very occasionally is it discovered serendipitously when a blood count is done for another reason. The clinical presentation is, for the most part, determined by the degree of bone marrow failure, but other features, secondary to the infiltration of different organs, may give specific signs and symptoms.

General symptoms and signs

The majority of children will give a short history of fewer than 4 weeks, although a prodrome of a few months is also seen. General symptoms include lethargy, loss of appetite and exhaustion. Bone marrow failure results in anemia, neutropenia and thrombocytopenia.

Anemia

This occurs in most cases but the fall in hemoglobin is gradual and can be very well tolerated initially. The low hemoglobin causes some of the commoner symptoms and signs such as pallor, lethargy, anorexia and breathlessness. Cardiac failure is uncommon even at very low levels of hemoglobin, but tachycardia and flow murmurs are common.

Infection

Susceptibility to infection may be apparent for some time before presentation and some patients may have a serious infection at diagnosis. Pyrexia at presentation may be due to the disease process itself, but since many children are neutropenic, and all are immunosuppressed, the child should be treated for infection with broad-spectrum intravenous antibiotics.

Hemorrhage

This is a frequent presenting feature and can be catastrophic. This is still the commonest cause of the rare deaths, which occur during the first few hours in hospital, and there is a strong association with leukostasis secondary to very high blast counts in the peripheral blood. Most bleeding episodes are milder and secondary to thrombocytopenia. Thrombocytopenia leads to petechiae and other hemorrhagic manifestations, especially mucosal bleeding and easy bruising. Bleeding may also be due to hepatic dysfunction and disseminated intravascular coagulation, the latter particularly with acute promyelocytic leukemia (M3).

Bone and joint involvement

Orthopedic surgeons, rheumatologists and accident and emergency staff frequently see children with bone pain and/or arthralgia and accompanying limp or failure to walk. Up to two thirds of children with

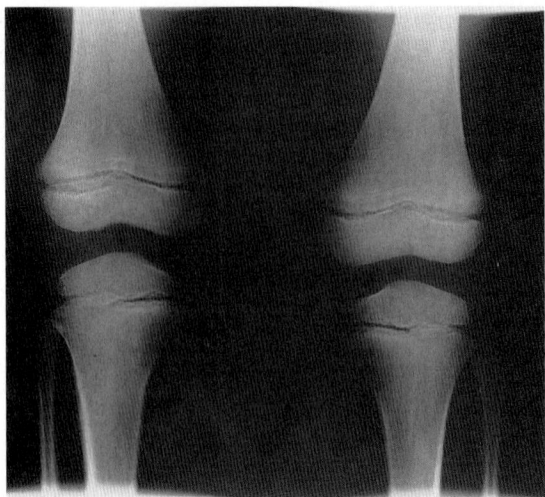

Fig. 23.23 Lymphoblastic leukemia. Knees showing generalized osteoporosis with transverse radiolucent bands across long bone metaphyses adjacent to metaphyseal bone ends, found in malignant infiltration of bone marrow.

ALL present with bone pain and therefore a full blood count should be checked in children with such symptoms. Examination for hepatosplenomegaly and lymphadenopathy may also help to identify the true diagnosis. Roentgenograms of these children will show changes in at least half, the most frequent of which are transverse radiolucent lines at the metaphyses (Fig. 23.23) and osteopenia sometimes with vertebral collapse. In acute megakaryoblastic leukemia (M7) and other types of leukemia, osteosclerosis can occasionally occur. Bone pain responds rapidly to antileukemic therapy although there may be some exacerbation when treatment starts. Another childhood malignancy, neuroblastoma, may also present with bone pain and anemia with or without thrombocytopenia. However, abnormal cells are rarely seen on the blood film, although the bone marrow may be virtually replaced by malignant cells. Immunophenotyping may be helpful and specific tests for neuroblastoma such as urinary catecholamines should be performed.

Hepatosplenomegaly, lymphadenopathy and other organ enlargement

Splenomegaly is present in up to 80% of children with acute leukemia and is particularly marked in CGL and JMML. The enlargement is smooth, firm and nontender unless it is chronically enlarged as in CGL when infarction can cause pain and tenderness. Hepatosplenomegaly is present in up to 60% of patients and the kidneys are palpable only occasionally, although abdominal ultrasound will reveal nonpalpable renal enlargement quite often in ALL and acute monoblastic leukemia (M5). Ovarian and testicular enlargement are rarely found at diagnosis but regular examination of the testes throughout follow-up, both on and off treatment, is essential as relapse at this site is quite common. Mediastinal enlargement, seen on chest roentgenogram, is almost exclusive to those with T cell ALL and can cause superior vena cava obstruction (Fig. 23.24). Abdominal masses of leukemia/lymphoma tissue not related to the liver and spleen typically occur in B-ALL cases. Infiltration of the sinuses may also occur (Fig. 23.25).

Gum hypertrophy occurs with all types of leukemia but is particularly common with M4 and M5 types (Fig. 23.26). Skin infiltration with leukemia is rare but does occur in the neonatal variety, when it is seen as bluish papules, and can also be seen in M4 and M5 (Fig. 23.27). JMML is associated with a nonspecific skin rash, especially on the face.

Meningeal leukemia

Children with ALL virtually all have presymptomatic meningeal leukemia at the time of diagnosis as shown by the inevitability of relapse in

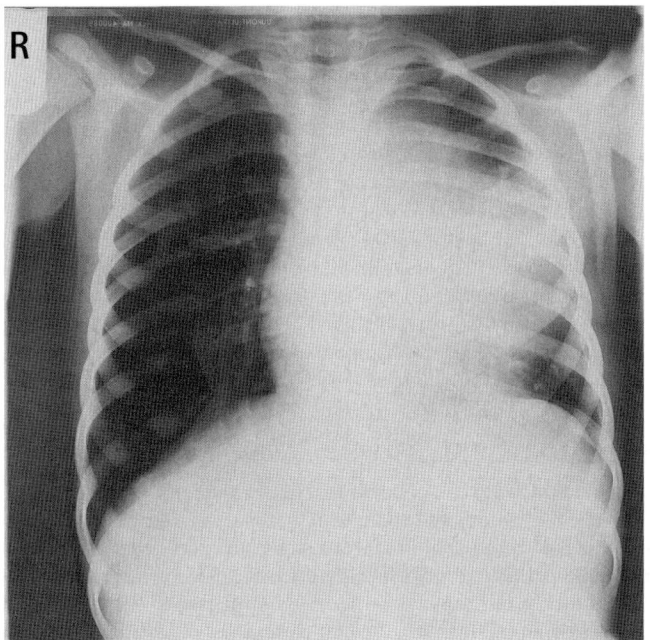

Fig. 23.24 Chest X-ray appearances in acute T cell leukemia with mediastinal widening and hilar lymphadenopathy causing superior vena cava obstruction.

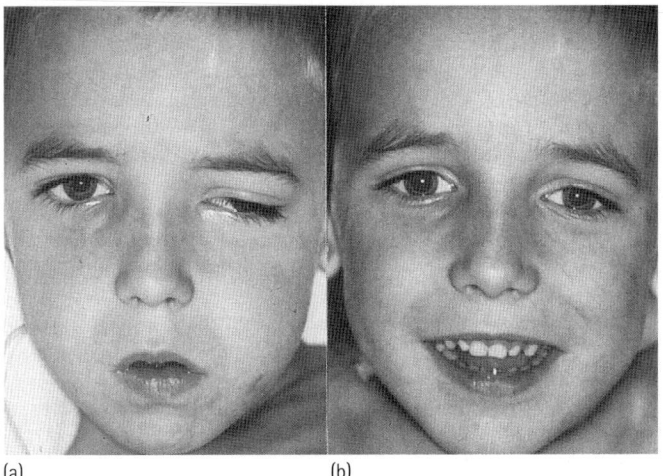

(a)   (b)

Fig. 23.25 Acute B cell leukemia causing (a) sinus infiltration and 3rd nerve palsy at presentation. (b) After 3 days of therapy.

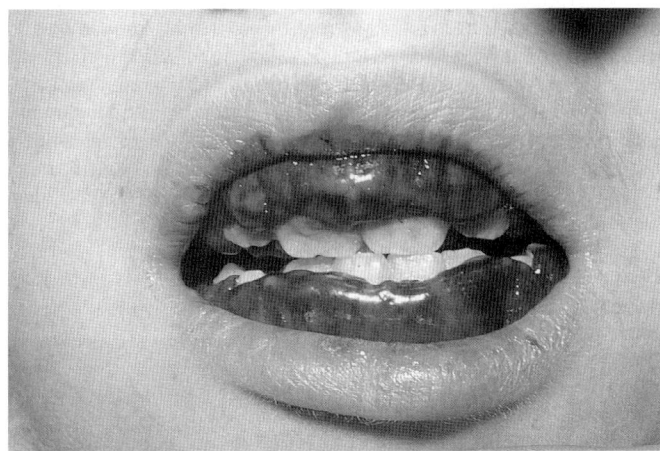

Fig. 23.26 Acute monocytic leukemia causing gum infiltration.

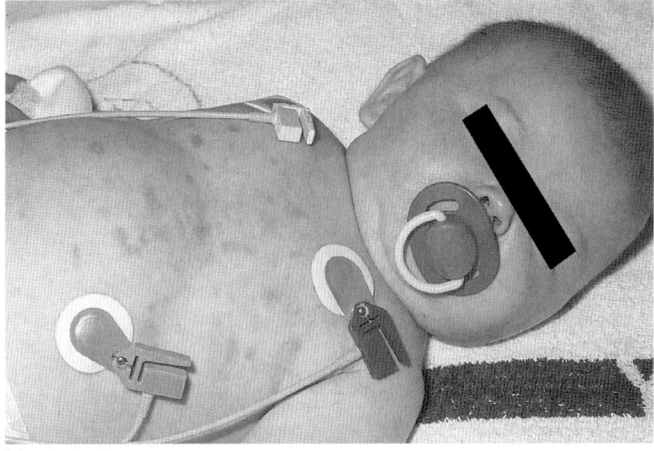

(a)

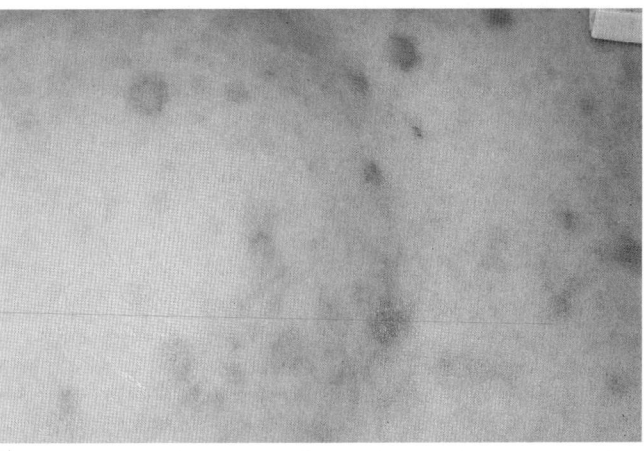

(b)

Fig. 23.27 Skin infiltration in an infant with acute monocytic leukemia.

those who do not receive CNS-directed therapy. However, a proportion present with blast cells in the CNS, which are often asymptomatic, but can give rise to diffuse or focal neurological signs. The commonest time to present is once treatment has stopped and such a relapse is frequently associated with the symptoms of raised intracranial pressure such as vomiting and severe headaches. Papilledema may be seen and cranial nerve palsies especially of the VIth nerve are common.

Tumor lysis syndrome

Children with hyperleukocytosis and/or a high leukemia burden secondary to massive organ infiltration, may develop metabolic abnormalities such as hyperkalemia, hyperphosphatemia and hypocalcemia. This is a particular hazard in B-ALL. Hyperuricemia to a varying degree is a common finding at presentation but can be very marked. When treatment is started there is further lysis of the leukemic cells so the metabolic abnormalities may worsen and can lead to renal failure and death. A forced diuresis, a uric acid lowering agent and careful steroid-based cytoreductive treatment may avoid this complication. Renal dialysis, leukopheresis and/or exchange transfusion may be required in severe cases.

DIAGNOSIS

It is essential before starting treatment for leukemia that the diagnosis has been made with certainty. Clinical examination and morphological review of well-stained blood and bone marrow films remain the most important parameters for diagnosis. If the bone marrow aspirate is inadequate, a repeat sample with a bone marrow trephine (biopsy) is mandatory. Other diagnostic techniques such as immunophenotyping are complementary but cannot alone be used to make the diagnosis.[104]

In young children, a relatively high proportion of lymphocytes both in the blood and bone marrow will express more immature markers, especially if there is a reactive lymphocytosis secondary to an infection for example. Aplastic anemia may also be mistaken for leukemia, as the bone marrow aspirate is often difficult and again may contain a high proportion of early B cells. If there is any doubt, supportive treatment and repeat sampling is essential.

MORPHOLOGY

The most constant finding at presentation of leukemia is an abnormality in the peripheral blood with 99% of children presenting either with circulating blasts and/or thrombocytopenia, 90% with anemia and 67% with neutropenia. Acute leukemia is diagnosed from the bone marrow sample if at least 30% of the total nucleated cells are blasts. Cytochemical stains are sometimes prepared to help distinguish between ALL and AML. Criteria for the classification of the acute leukemias have been described above.

The presence of CNS disease is assessed from cytospin preparations of cerebrospinal fluid (CSF). The CSF is considered to be positive if > 5 cells/mm^3 with recognizable blast cells are present. Immunophenotyping may be helpful in equivocal cases, as well as cytogenetic analysis, if enough material can be obtained. It is important to determine whether there is involvement with leukemia or not since these patients usually receive more intensive intrathecal chemotherapy and, if over the age of 2 years, cranial irradiation.

In CGL the most consistent finding in the peripheral blood is a leukocytosis, predominantly of mature neutrophils and their precursors (myelocytes and promyelocytes). Eosinophilia and basophilia are commonly present and the white cell count is usually $>100 \times 10^9$/L at diagnosis. Anemia is usual and platelets are often normal or slightly raised. The bone marrow is markedly hypercellular due to hyperplasia of the granulocyte series. In its chronic phase, blasts constitute < 5% of nucleated cells but increase in the accelerated phase and blast crisis. Cytogenetic analysis shows the Philadelphia chromosome t(9;22) in 90% of patients and the bcr/abl fusion gene can be detected in a proportion of Ph-negative patients.

JMML usually presents with thrombocytopenia and a dysplastic blood film with abnormal monocytes and blast cells. The marrow can be relatively uninformative but associated features include a reversion to a fetal type of hemopoiesis with a high hemoglobin F and the 'i' red cell antigen, and sometimes monosomy 7.

Immunophenotyping

It must be remembered that immunophenotyping is complementary to morphological diagnosis and does not replace it; mistakes in diagnosis can be made if this technique is relied upon in isolation. Immunophenotyping is particularly useful in cases of acute leukemia that are not obviously myeloid, so that a positive diagnosis of ALL can be made and cases of M0 and M7 AML identified. A panel of monoclonal antibodies is used which combines both highly specific and highly sensitive antibodies. Additional antibodies are required for conformation of erythroid leukemia (M6) and M7. Specific antibodies include cytoplasmic (cy) CD22 for B lineage, cy CD3 for T lineage and antimyeloperoxidase (MPO) for myeloid lineage. Sensitive antibodies include CD19, expressed on B cells, CD7 on T cells and CD13/33 on myeloid cells but all may be expressed on cells of other lineage. This aberrant antigen expression is a feature of both ALL and AML and does not mean that the leukemia is biphenotypic. This description is reserved for those leukemias where the more specific antigens (e.g. CD22, CD3, MPO) of more than one lineage are expressed. The prognosis of such leukemias is related to the accompanying cytogenetic abnormalities and many are associated with the Philadelphia chromosome.

Chromosomal analysis

Cytogenetic analysis is carried out by microscopic analysis of cells in metaphase when suitably stained. This technique can be supplemented by fluorescent in situ hybridization (FISH). Molecular cytogenetic analysis, where the DNA from the abnormal cells is analyzed using Southern blotting, or polymerase chain reaction (PCR) for example, can be used to establish clonality and also used for detection of minimal residual disease (MRD) to help direct therapy (see later). While some cytogenetic abnormalities identify subtypes of leukemia in a highly specific way, other chromosomal abnormalities occur in both acute and chronic leukemias, ALL and AML and also MDS. Specific cytogenetic abnormalities include t(15;17) in M3, inv(16) in M4Eo and t(8;14) in mature B cell ALL. Other cytogenetic abnormalities such as the Philadelphia chromosome, t(9;22) and monosomy 7 can arise in a variety of leukemias and MDS. It is becoming clear that in both AML and ALL cytogenetic analysis plays a crucial role in assignment of patients to different risk groups, allowing risk directed therapy.[105-107]

PROGNOSTIC INDICATORS

Type and intensity of treatment in ALL are the most important determinants of prognosis and changes in therapy may alter the significance of other risk factors.[108,109] Prognostic factors are used to stratify children into different risk groups allowing intensification of therapy in those at highest risk of relapse while decreasing intensity in those in the best prognostic group. In AML, the two parameters of greatest prognostic significance are the karyotype of the malignant cells and response to therapy.

Demographics

In ALL, age, sex and presenting white cell count have a significant influence on outcome. The US National Cancer Institute (NCI) set internationally agreed criteria for risk classification based on these parameters.[110] Standard risk patients are aged between 1 and 9 years with a presenting white cell count of $<50 \times 10^9$/L, while high risk patients are aged ≥ 10 years or have a presenting white cell count of $\geq 50 \times 10^9$/L. Approximately 75% of patients with B lineage leukemia are standard risk, while 75% of patients with T lineage leukemia are in the high risk category. Boys have a worse prognosis than girls even after adjusting for age and white cell count. CNS disease at diagnosis is not of prognostic significance.

Morphology

The original morphological classification in ALL is less important than originally thought[111] but has enabled identification of mature B cell leukemias with a specific morphology (L3).

In AML, morphology is closely associated with karyotype which does correlate with outcome.

Chromosomes

Karyotype has now been included in the NCI risk stratification, (see above). Bcr/abl, hypodiploidy (< 45 chromosomes), or, if 12–24 months old, an MLL gene rearrangement carries the worst prognosis. The MLL gene rearrangement has a particularly poor prognosis if associated with the translocation t(4;11) but additional chromosomal abnormalities do not affect prognosis.[106] Recent work has shown that those with 42–45 chromosomes overall have standard rather than high risk[105] and that not all those with a high hyperdiploid karyotype, that is > 50 chromosomes per cell, do well as was initially described.[107,112] This demonstrates the importance of continued refinement of chromosomal classification.

In AML, favorable karyotypes are those with t(8;21), t(15;17) seen with the M3 subtype and inv(16) seen with M4Eo.

Response to treatment

Analysis of the United Kingdom Medical Research Council trials for ALL (UKALL), 1980–2002, has consistently shown a relationship between time to respond to treatment and outcome.[112,113] The ALL97 trial included three risk groups taking both response to treatment and karyotype into consideration. The standard risk group (60–65% of children) is as previously defined by NCI criteria; the intermediate risk group (20% of children) has the same parameters as the previous high-risk group. A new high-risk group (10–12% of children) includes all children irrespective of initial risk group, who have a slow early response to treatment (assessed on bone marrow samples at day 15 for standard risk patients and day 8 for intermediate risk patients) or who have an unfavorable karyotype (see above).

In AML, complete remission (CR), that is < 5% leukemic cells in the bone marrow after the first course of chemotherapy, confers the best prognosis, while partial remission (PR), that is 5–20% leukemic cells, is only slightly worse. Patients with resistant disease (RD), defined as > 20% leukemic cells in the bone marrow after the first course of chemotherapy, have a very poor outlook. There is a correlation between karyotype and bone marrow status, however karyotype carries the greater prognostic weight. Good risk patients are therefore defined as those with a favorable karyotype regardless of their bone marrow status after course 1. Standard risk patients include all those who have no favorable karyotype and do not have RD after course 1. The poor risk group includes all those with RD after course 1 except those with a favorable karyotype.

Minimal residual disease (MRD)

It is hoped that MRD, as a more sensitive measure of response to treatment, will allow a much more accurate stratification of relapse risk than the prognostic indicators described above. MRD detected prior to bone marrow transplant predicts relapse post-transplant and would allow pretransplant intensification.[114] Improved techniques for detection of MRD and long term prospective study of large, comparable cohorts of patients has shown that clearance of MRD is an independent prognostic factor in childhood ALL.[115] This has opened the way for clinical application of MRD measurement in the management of ALL and this is incorporated into the current UK ALL trial (see below).

In AML, studies on the use of MRD measurement and drug resistance are underway.

TREATMENT

The treatment of acute leukemia requires both the eradication of the leukemic clone, so that normal bone marrow function may be restored, and supportive care during the period of bone marrow failure, both secondary to the disease itself and to the treatment. AML and ALL are both treated with a combination of chemotherapeutic drugs, with or without radiotherapy, but the pattern of treatment is quite different. In AML, the treatment is concentrated in four or five intensive blocks over a period of 6 months or so whereas in ALL, the treatment begins with an induction block, then intensification blocks followed by a period of maintenance for up to 2 years in girls and 3 years in boys.

Supportive care

Intensive chemotherapy requires expert supportive care best given in a limited number of centers familiar with the treatment of leukemia in children. A multidisciplinary team including nurses, physiotherapists, pharmacists and social workers delivers all aspects of hospital treatment and care of the child at home. In the UK most children are treated within United Kingdom Children's Cancer and Leukemia Group (UKCCLG) centers. Results from such centers are superior to ad hoc therapy elsewhere. In many cases care is shared to some extent with pediatricians in hospitals closer to the patients' homes.

Acute lymphoblastic leukemia

The dramatic increase in survival rates from ALL has been achieved by carefully planned progressive randomized trials.[116] Most regimens for ALL are based on the schema in Figure 23.28 and the drugs used are variations of these. With this type of treatment over 97% of patients achieve a remission within the first 4 weeks. Following this, additional blocks of intensification are required, including drugs not used in the first phase, to eradicate resistant leukemic clones. CNS-directed treatment is given during this phase. For those with CNS disease, intrathecal (i.t.) methotrexate and cranial irradiation are given, but this is not required if the CSF is negative for leukemic cells. In those with a negative CSF and a peripheral white cell count < 50×10^9/L, a long course of i.t. methotrexate is effective and for those with counts ≥ 50×10^9/L high dose i.v. methotrexate is used in addition to i.t. methotrexate.[112,117,118]

The UKALL XI study (1990–97) failed to show benefit when compared to the previous study, UKALL X, with an event-free survival (EFS) at 8 years of 61%.[109] Overall survival (OS) at 8 years was significantly better however, 81% versus 74%, owing to improved management of relapse. Although patients may be salvaged with further treatment, it is at the price of greater toxicity. To address the lower EFS, the next Medical Research Council (MRC) trial, MRC ALL 97/99, used the NCI criteria assigning patients to three different risk categories increasing the intensity of induction therapy and intensification blocks with increasing risk. Once completed, maintenance therapy (daily thiopurine, weekly oral methotrexate and monthly pulses of vincristine with 5 days of steroid) continued for a total treatment period of just over 2 years for girls and 3 years for boys. Dexamethasone was compared with prednisolone and 6-mercaptopurine with 6-thioguanine in a randomized way. Patients with high risk factors such as bcr/abl, hypodiploidy or t(4;11) were considered for allogeneic HSCT during first remission of disease.

Early results (trial closed in June 2002) are encouraging showing an 81% EFS at 5 years.[119] Five-year EFS was significantly better for those on dexamethasone compared with prednisolone, 84% versus 76%, with a decrease in both CNS and non-CNS relapse; 6-thioguanine has been replaced by 6-mercaptopurine in both the intensification and maintenance phases of treatment due to association with veno-occlusive disease.[120,121] The current UKALL 2003 trial is designed to see whether treatment can be reduced without compromising efficacy in MRD-defined low risk groups and whether postremission intensification can improve outcome in MRD-defined high risk groups.

Relapsed ALL

The commonest type of relapse occurs in the bone marrow following cessation of therapy. Most occur in the first year after stopping therapy with a diminishing risk thereafter. Further investigation may reveal disease in other sites, particularly the CNS or testicles or both. Relapse at other sites such as the ovary, eye, tonsils and skin is very rare. All relapses require intensive chemotherapy with CNS-directed therapy and appropriate local therapy. The intensity of treatment prior to relapse appears to influence the chance of success of further treatment. The usual treatment plan includes the standard four-drug induction therapy and subsequent intensification with different drugs in high dosage in an attempt to eradicate the residual resistant disease. For those in a high risk group (predominantly patients with early relapse, fewer than 6 months off treatment) once in remission, allogeneic HSCT from a

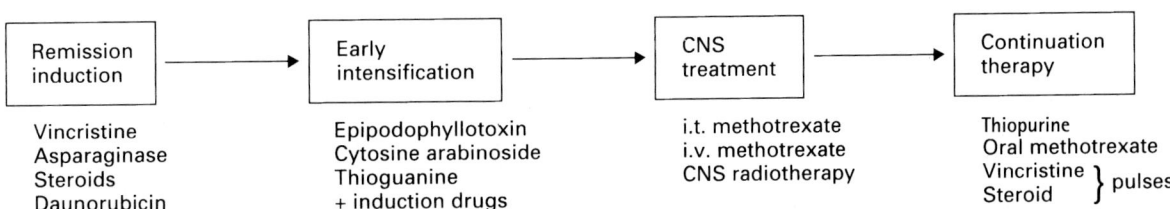

Fig. 23.28 Scheme for treatment of acute lymphoblastic leukemia. Drugs listed are only examples of those which can be used.

related or unrelated donor is indicated. A retrospective analysis of children on the UKALL R2 (R for relapse) protocol shows an OS of 56% and EFS of 47%. Duration of first remission and immunophenotype but not sites of relapse were predictive of survival. When stratified according to the Berlin-Frankfurt-Münster criteria, the OS and EFS were as follows: for standard risk 92% and 92%, intermediate risk 64% and 51%, and high risk group 14% and 15%. Those with very early isolated CNS relapse (<18 months from diagnosis) had a significantly worse outcome and are now being classified as high rather than intermediate risk. The current UKALL R3 trial is looking to improve outcome in the intermediate risk group by examining whether MRD at the end of induction is a suitable criterion on which to decide whether to proceed with chemotherapy or HSCT.

CNS relapse is the commonest site after bone marrow relapse and should be regarded as a local manifestation of systemic disease. Thus treatment should include intensive systemic therapy as well as local therapy, which is cranial or craniospinal irradiation. With this type of therapy, about one half of patients achieve a long-term remission (> 5 years) unless relapse is very early (see above).

Testicular relapse is the third likely site of relapse but can be treated with a good chance of success, especially if isolated. With intensive systemic therapy, CNS-directed therapy and testicular irradiation, there is a > 70% chance of cure.

AML

Therapy in AML includes remission induction, CNS-directed therapy and postremission therapy. However, in contrast to ALL, treatment is given in intensive blocks over a shorter duration. This, along with improved supportive care, has resulted in a significant increase in survival over the past 15 years. The MRC AML trial, AML 12, was based on risk-directed therapy, taking account of karyotype and response to treatment (see above). In the good and standard risk groups, chemotherapy alone was recommended, with randomization of four courses versus five, whereas in the poor risk group, transplantation was considered if there was a matched sibling donor. Preliminary analysis suggests there is no survival advantage for five courses over four.

The AML 12 trial (including adults and children) resulted in a 5-year OS of 66% and EFS of 56%. Specific therapy for different subtypes of leukemia is not given except in the case of M3 which responds to all-trans retinoic acid (ATRA) in conjunction with the standard chemotherapy. CNS-directed therapy is given as three courses of triple i.t. therapy. If CNS disease is present, an extended course of i.t. therapy is given with cranial irradiation at the end of treatment for those > 2 years of age. The current AML 15 trial tests the feasibility of reducing anthracycline dosage by comparing with high dose ara-C and whether targeted chemotherapy offers an advantage.

HSCT

The principle of HSCT is the provision of a source of hemopoietic stem cells to repopulate the bone marrow after conditioning therapy has destroyed the patient's own bone marrow cells. The sources of hemopoietic stem cells include bone marrow, peripheral blood and cord blood.

Allogeneic stem cells may be obtained either from an HLA-identical sibling, a partially matched relation or unrelated donor. The most data currently available are from transplants with matched sibling donors, although increasing experience is being gained with unrelated donor transplantation.

Preparative or conditioning therapy in leukemia is designed to eradicate residual leukemia and immunosuppress sufficiently to prevent graft rejection. Preparative regimens include high dose chemotherapy, with or without total body irradiation (TBI). The morbidity of HSCT, both early and late, is considerable and there is a significant mortality associated with the procedure. It is essential that the use and effectiveness of HSCT in the treatment of leukemia be carefully monitored in controlled trials to ensure that the benefits outweigh the morbidity and mortality.

Late sequelae of leukemia therapy

About 30 years ago very few children recovered from leukemia; now more than half survive. Currently around one in a thousand adolescents is a survivor of malignant disease in childhood, many of whom will have been treated in an era of less intensive therapy. Recognition of the long term effects of therapy and their impact upon quality of life is of increasing importance in the management of leukemia. Risk stratification is used to try to identify those who will be cured with less intensive therapy thus reducing toxicity and to target the more intensive therapy at those at greatest risk of relapse. Both chemotherapy and irradiation have long-term effects, but irradiation can be particularly toxic leading to growth retardation, cataracts, hypothyroidism, infertility and other endocrine function disturbances. Chemotherapy can result in cardiotoxicity, predominantly from anthracycline use. The neuropsychologic effects of TBI and different modes of CNS-directed therapy are unknown.

The risk of developing a second malignancy after successful treatment of leukemia is low with an estimated cumulative risk of around 2.5% at 15 years. The majority of tumors develop in the radiation field and exposure to radiotherapy appears to have a continuous risk of a second neoplasm.

It is essential that long term survivors of childhood malignancy are carefully followed up and late effects recorded so that appropriate modifications to therapy can be made for current and future generations of patients.

REFERENCES (*Level 1 Evidence)

1. Hetzel TM, Losek JD. Unrecognized severe anemia in children presenting with respiratory distress. Am J Emerg Med 1998; 16:386–389.
*2. Tielsch JM, Khatry SK, Stoltzfus RJ, et al. Effect of routine prophylactic supplementation with iron and folic acid on preschool child mortality in southern Nepal: community-based, cluster-randomized, placebo-controlled trial. Lancet 2006; 367:144–152.
*3. Sazawal S, Black RE, Ramsan M, et al. Effects of routine prophylactic supplementation with iron and folic acid on admission to hospital and mortality in preschool children in a high malaria transmission setting: community-based, randomized, placebo-controlled trial. Lancet 2006; 367:133–143.
4. Ganz T. Molecular pathogenesis of anemia of chronic disease. Pediatr Blood Cancer 2006; 46:554–557.

5. Longfils P, Heang UK, Soeng H, et al. Weekly iron and folic acid supplementation as a tool to reduce anemia among primary school children in Cambodia. Nutr Rev 2005; 63:(12 Pt 2):S139–S145.
6. Walter T. Effect of iron-deficiency anemia on cognitive skills in infancy and childhood. Baillières Clin Haematol 1994; 7:815–827.
*7. Grantham-McGregor S, Ani C. A review of studies on the effect of iron deficiency on cognitive development in children. J Nutr 2001; 131:(2S-2): 649S–666S; discussion 666S–668S.
*8. Logan S, Martins S, Gilbert R. Iron therapy for improving psychomotor development and cognitive function in children under the age of three with iron deficiency anemia (Cochrane Review). Cochrane Database Syst Rev 2001; 2:CD001444.
*9. Sachdev H, Gera T, Nestel P. Effect of iron supplementation on mental and motor development

in children: systematic review of randomized controlled trials. Public Health Nutr 2005; 8:117–132.
10. Piomelli S. Lead poisoning. In: Nathan DG, Orkin SH, eds. Hematology of infancy and childhood, 5th edn. Philadelphia: WB Saunders: edn. 1998.480–496.
11. Knerr I, Metzler M, Niemeyer CM, et al. Hematologic features and clinical course of an infant with Pearson syndrome caused by a novel deletion of mitochondrial DNA. J Pediatr Hematol Oncol 2003; 25:948–951.
12. Garcia-Casal MN, Osorio C, Landaeta M, et al. High prevalence of folic acid and vitamin B_{12} deficiencies in infants, children, adolescents and pregnant women in Venezuela. Eur J Clin Nutr 2005; 59:1064–1070.
*13. Rabb LM, Grandison Y, Mason K, et al. A trial of folate supplementation in children with homozygous sickle cell disease. Br J Haematol 1983; 54:589–594.

14. Whitehead MV. Acquired and inherited disorders of cobalamin and folate in children. Br J Haematol 2006; 134:125–136.

15. Grange DK, Finlay JL. Nutritional vitamin B_{12} deficiency in a breastfed infant following maternal gastric bypass. Pediatr Hematol Oncol 1994; 11:311–318.

16. Monagle PT, Tauro GP. Infantile megaloblastosis secondary to maternal vitamin B_{12} deficiency. Clin Lab Haematol 1997; 19:23–25.

17. Altay C, Cetin M. Oral treatment in selective vitamin B_{12} malabsorption. J Pediatr Hematol Oncol 1997; 19:245–246.

18. Ball SE. The modern management of severe aplastic anemia. Br J Haematol 2000; 110:41–53.

19. Schrezenmeier H, Bacigalupo A, Aglietta M, et al. Guidelines for the treatment of aplastic anemia. Consensus document of a group of international experts. In: Schrezenmeier H, Bacigalupo A, eds. Aplastic anemia. Cambridge: Cambridge University Press; 2000.308.

20. Alter BP. Aplastic anemia, pediatric aspects. Oncologist 1996; 1:361–366.

21. Taniguchi T, D'Andrea AD. Molecular pathogenesis of Fanconi anemia: recent progress. Blood 2006; 107:4223–4233.

22. Tischkowitz M, Dokal I. Fanconi anemia and leukaemia – clinical and molecular aspects. Br J Haematol 2004; 126:176–191.

23. Kutler DI, Singh B, Satagopan J, et al. A 20-year perspective on the International Fanconi Anemia Registry (IFAR). Blood 2003; 101:1249–1256.

*24. Guardiola P, Pasquini R, Dokal I, et al. Outcome of 69 allogeneic stem cell transplantations for Fanconi anemia using HLA-matched unrelated donors: a study on behalf of the European Group for Blood and Marrow Transplantation. Blood 2000; 95:422–429.

25. Dokal I. Severe aplastic anemia including Fanconi's anemia and dyskeratosis congenita. Curr Opin Hematol 1996; 3:453–460.

26. Dokal I. Dyskeratosis congenita in all its forms. Br J Haematol 2000; 110:768–779.

27. Dokal I, Vulliamy T. Dyskeratosis congenita: its link to telomerase and aplastic anaemia. Blood Rev 2003; 17:217–225.

28. Smith OP, Hann IM, Chessells JM, et al. Haematological abnormalities in Shwachman–Diamond syndrome. Br J Haematol 1996; 94:279–284.

29. Dror Y. Shwachman–Diamond syndrome. Pediatr Blood Cancer 2005; 45:892–901.

30. Hall GW, Dale P, Dodge JA. Shwachman–Diamond syndrome: UK perspective. Arch Dis Child 2006; 91:521–524.

31. van den Oudenrijn S, Bruin M, Folman CC, et al. Mutations in the thrombopoietin receptor, Mpl, in children with congenital amegakaryocytic thrombocytopenia. Br J Haematol 2000; 110:441–448.

32. Thompson AA, Woodruff K, Feig SA, et al. Congenital thrombocytopenia and radio-ulnar synostosis: a new familial syndrome. Br J Haematol 2001; 113:866–870.

33. Farhi DC, Luebbers EL, Rosenthal NS. Bone marrow biopsy findings in childhood anemia: prevalence of transient erythroblastopenia of childhood. Arch Pathol Lab Med 1998; 122:638–641.

34. Lipton JM, Atsidaftos E, Zyskind I, et al. Improving clinical care and elucidating the pathophysiology of Diamond–Blackfan anemia: an update from the Diamond–Blackfan Anemia Registry. Pediatr Blood Cancer 2006; 46:558–564.

35. Lissauer T, Clayden G. Illustrated textbook of paediatrics. In: 2nd edn. Edinburgh: Mosby; 2001.301.

36. Hoffbrand AV, Pettit JE, Moss PAH. Essential haematology, 4th edn. Oxford: Blackwell Science; 2001.

37. Bolton-Maggs PH, Stevens RF, Dodd NJ, et al. Guidelines for the diagnosis and management of hereditary spherocytosis. Br J Haematol 2004; 126:455–474.

38. Agre P, Asimos A, Casella JF, et al. Inheritance pattern and clinical response to splenectomy as a reflection of erythrocyte spectrin deficiency in hereditary spherocytosis. N Engl J Med 1986; 315:1579–1583.

39. Guidelines for the prevention and treatment of infection in patients with an absent or dysfunctional spleen: Working party of the British Committee for Standards in Haematology Clinical Haematology Task force. BMJ 1996; 312:430–434.

40. Mentzer WC, Lubin BH. Red cell membrane abnormalities. In: Lilleyman JS, Hann IM, Blanchette VS, eds. Pediatric hematology, 2nd edn. London: Churchill Livingstone; 1999.257–283.

41. Jacobasch G. Biochemical and genetic basis of red cell enzyme deficiencies. Baillières Best Pract Res Clin Hematol 2000; 13:1–20.

42. Beutler E, Luzzatto L. Hemolytic anemia. Semin Hematol 1999; 36:(4 Suppl 7):38–47.

43. Norton A, Roberts I. Management of Evans syndrome. Br J Haematol 2006; 132:125–137.

44. Hoffbrand AV, Pettit JE. Essential haematology, 3rd edn. Oxford: Blackwell; 1993.

45. Thompson AA. Advances in the management of sickle cell disease. Pediatr Blood Cancer 2006; 46:533–539.

46. Overturf GD. Infections and immunizations of children with sickle cell disease. Adv Pediatr Infect Dis 1999; 14:191–218.

*47. Adams RJ. Lessons from the Stroke Prevention Trial in Sickle Cell Anemia (STOP) study. J Child Neurol 2000; 15:344–349.

*48. Adams RJ, McKie VC, Hsu L, et al. Prevention of a first stroke by transfusions in children with sickle cell anemia and abnormal results on transcranial Doppler ultrasonography. N Engl J Med 1998; 339:5–11.

*49. Davies S, Olujohungbe A. Hydroxyurea for sickle cell disease (Cochrane Review). Cochrane Database Syst Rev 2001; 2:CD002202.

*50. Charache S, Terrin ML, Moore RD, et al. Effect of hydroxyurea on the frequency of painful crises in sickle cell anemia. Investigators of the Multicenter Study of Hydroxyurea in Sickle Cell Anemia. N Engl J Med 1995; 332:1317–1322.

*51. Ataga KI, Moore CG, Jones S, et al. Pulmonary hypertension in patients with sickle cell disease: a longitudinal study. Br J Haematol 2006; 134:109–115.

52. Serjeant G. Sickle cell disease. In: Lilleyman JS, Hann I, Blanchette VS, eds. Pediatric hematology, 2nd edn. London: Churchill Livingstone; 1999.219–230.

53. Olivieri NF. The beta thalassemias. N Engl J Med 1999; 341:99–109.

54. Olivieri N. Thalassaemia: clinical management. Baillières Clin Hematol 1998; 11:147–162.

*55. Olivieri NF, Brittenham GM, McLaren CE, et al. Long-term safety and effectiveness of iron-chelation therapy with deferiprone for thalassemia major. N Engl J Med 1998; 339:417–423.

56. Hoffbrand AV, Cohen A, Hershko C. Role of deferiprone in chelation therapy for transfusional iron overload. Blood 2003; 102:17–24.

57. Cappellini MD, Cohen A, Piga A, et al. A phase 3 study of deferasirox (ICL670), a once-daily oral iron chelator, in patients with beta thalassemia. Blood 2006; 107:3455–3462.

58. Neufeld EJ. Oral chelators deferasirox and deferiprone for transfusional iron overload in thalassemia major: new data, new questions. Blood 2006; 107:3436–3441.

59. Mentzer WC. Bone marrow transplantation for hemoglobinopathies. Curr Opin Hematol 2000; 7:95–100.

60. Lucarelli G. Bone marrow transplantation for thalassaemia. J Intern Med Suppl 1997; 740:49–52.

61. Lucarelli G, Galimberti M, Giardini C, et al. Bone marrow transplantation in thalassemia. The experience of Pesaro. Ann NY Acad Sci 1998; 850:270–275.

62. Lucarelli G, Clift RA, Galimberti M, et al. Bone marrow transplantation in adult thalassemic patients. Blood 1999; 93:1164–1167.

63. Walters MC, Quirolo L, Trachtenberg ET, et al. Sibling donor cord blood transplantation for thalassemia major: experience of the sibling donor cord blood program. Ann NY Acad Sci 2005; 1054:206–213.

64. Miniero R, Rocha V, Saracco P, et al. Cord blood transplantation (CBT) in hemoglobinopathies. Eurocord. Bone Marrow Transplant 1998; 22: (suppl 1): S78–S79.

65. Hongeng S, Pakakasama S, Chuansumrit A, et al. Outcomes of transplantation with related- and unrelated-donor stem cells in children with severe thalassemia. Biol Blood Marrow Transplant 2006; 12:683–687.

66. Kuliev A, Rechitsky S, Verlinsky O, et al. Preimplantation diagnosis and HLA typing for hemoglobin disorders. Reprod Biomed Online 2005; 11:362–370.

67. Kulozik AE. Hemoglobin variants and the rarer hemoglobin disorders. In: Lilleyman JS, Hann I, Blanchette VS, eds. Pediatric hematology, 2nd edn.London: Churchill Livingstone; 1999.231–256.

68. Bodey GP, Buckley M, Sathe YS, et al. Quantitative relationships between circulating leukocytes and infection in patients with acute leukemia. Ann Intern Med 1966; 64:328–340.

69. Bux J, Behrens G, Jaeger G, et al. Diagnosis and clinical course of autoimmune neutropenia in infancy: analysis of 240 cases. Blood 1998; 91:181–186.

70. Zeidler C, Schwinzer B, Welte K. Congenital neutropenias. Rev Clin Exp Hematol 2003; 7:72–83.

71. Rosenberg PS, Alter BP, Bolyard AA, et al. The incidence of leukemia and mortality from sepsis in patients with severe congenital neutropenia receiving long term G-CSF therapy. Blood 2006; 107:4628–4635.

72. Dinauer MC. Th phagocyte system and disorders of granulopoiesis and granulocyte function. In: Nathan DG, Orkin SH, eds. Hematology of infancy and childhood. Philadelphia: WB Saunders; 1998.922.

73. Balduini CL, Cattaneo M, Fabris F, et al. Inherited thrombocytopenias: a proposed diagnostic algorithm from the Italian Gruppo di Studio delle Piastrine. Haematologica 2003; 88:582–592.

74. Cattaneo M. Inherited platelet-based bleeding disorders. J Thromb Haemost 2003; 1:1628–1636.

75. Drachman JG. Inherited thrombocytopenia: when a low platelet count does not mean ITP. Blood 2004; 103:390–398.

76. Kunishima S, Saito H. Congenital macro-thrombocytopenias. Blood Rev 2006; 20:111–121.

77. Hall GW. Kasabach–Merritt syndrome: pathogenesis and management. Br J Haematol 2001; 112:851–862.

78. Bolton-Maggs PH, Moon I. Assessment of UK practice for management of acute childhood idiopathic thrombocytopenic purpura against published guidelines. Lancet 1997; 350:620–623.

79. Lilleyman JS. Intracranial hemorrhage in chronic childhood ITP [editorial]. Pediatr Hematol Oncol 1997; 14:iii–v.

80. Dickerhoff R, von Ruecker A. The clinical course of immune thrombocytopenic purpura in 55 consecutive children who did not receive intravenous immunoglobulin or sustained prednisone. J Pediatr 2000; 137:629–632.

81. Bolton-Maggs PH, Dickerhoff R, Vora AJ. The nontreatment of childhood ITP (or "the art of medicine consists of amusing the patient until nature cures the disease"). Semin Thromb Hemost 2001; 27:269–275.

82. Buchanan GR, Adix L. Grading of hemorrhage in children with idiopathic thrombocytopenic purpura. J Pediatr 2002; 141:683–688.

83. Buchanan GR. Bleeding signs in children with idiopathic thrombocytopenic purpura. J Pediatr Hematol Oncol 2003; 25:(suppl 1):S42–S46.

84. Lilleyman JS. Management of childhood idiopathic thrombocytopenic purpura. Br J Haematol 1999; 105:871–875.

85. Dahlback B. Blood coagulation. Lancet 2000; 355:1627–1632.

86. Hoffman M. Remodeling the blood coagulation cascade. J Thromb Thrombolysis 2003; 16:17–20.

87. Ljung RC. Prophylactic treatment in Sweden – overtreatment or optimal model? Haemophilia 1998; 4:409–412.

88. Aledort LM, Haschmeyer RH, Pettersson H. A longitudinal study of orthopaedic outcomes for severe factor-VIII-deficient hemophiliacs. The Orthopaedic Outcome Study Group. J Intern Med 1994; 236:391–399.

*89. Manco-Johnson MJ, Abshire TC, Brown D, et al. Initial results of a randomized, prospective trial of prophylaxis to prevent joint disease in young children with Factor VIII (FVIII) deficiency. ASH Annual Meeting Abstracts 2005; 106:3.

90. Ljung R, Aronis-Vournas S, Kurnik-Auberger K, et al. Treatment of children with haemophilia in Europe: a survey of 20 centers in 16 countries. Haemophilia 2000; 6:619–624.

91. Bolton-Maggs PH, Perry DJ, Chalmers EA, et al. The rare coagulation disorders – review with guidelines for management from the United Kingdom Haemophilia Center Doctors' Organization. Haemophilia 2004; 10:593–628.

*92. Bernard GR, Vincent JL, Laterre PF, et al. Efficacy and safety of recombinant human activated protein C for severe sepsis. N Engl J Med 2001; 344:699–709.

*93. de Kleijn ED, de Groot R, Hack CE, et al. Activation of protein C following infusion of protein C concentrate in children with severe meningococcal sepsis and purpura fulminans: a randomized, double-blinded, placebo-controlled, dose-finding study. Crit Care Med 2003; 31:1839–1847.

94. Andrew M, David M, Adams M, et al. Venous thromboembolic complications (VTE) in children: first analyses of the Canadian Registry of VTE. Blood 1994; 83:1251–1257.

95. Azu MC, McCormack JE, Scriven RJ, et al. Venous thromboembolic events in pediatric trauma patients: is prophylaxis necessary? J Trauma 2005; 59:1345–1349.

96. Rask O, Berntorp E, Ljung R. Risk factors for venous thrombosis in Swedish children and adolescents. Acta Paediatr 2005; 94:717–722.

97. Parkin DM, Stiller CA, Draper GJ, et al. The international incidence of childhood cancer. Int J Cancer 1988; 42:511–520.

98. Bennett JM, Catovsky D, Daniel MT, et al. Proposals for the classification of the acute leukaemias. French–American–British (FAB) co-operative group. Br J Haematol 1976; 33:451–458.

99. Emanuel PD. Myelodysplasia and myeloproliferative disorders in childhood: an update. Br J Haematol 1999; 105:852–863.

*100. Bennett JM, Catovsky D, Daniel MT, et al. Proposals for the classification of the myelodysplastic syndromes. Br J Haematol 1982; 51:189–199.

*101. Passmore SJ, Hann IM, Stiller CA, et al. Pediatric myelodysplasia: a study of 68 children and a new prognostic scoring system. Blood 1995; 85:1742–1750.

102. Chessells JM. Myelodysplastic syndromes. In: Lilleyman JS, Hann I, Blanchette VS, eds. Pediatric hematology; 1999.83–101.

103. Webb DK, Passmore SJ, Hann I, et al. Results of treatment of children with refractory anemia with excess blasts (RAEB) and RAEB in transformation (RAEBt) in Great Britain 1990–99. Br J Haematol 2002; 117:33–39.

104. Chessells JM. Pitfalls in the diagnosis of childhood leukaemia. Annotation. Br J Haematol 2001; 114:506–511.

105. Harrison CJ, Moorman AV, Broadfield ZL, et al. Three distinct subgroups of hypodiploidy in acute lymphoblastic leukaemia. Br J Haematol 2004; 125:552–559.

106. Moorman AV, Raimondi SC, Pui CH, et al. No prognostic effect of additional chromosomal abnormalities in children with acute lymphoblastic leukemia and 11q23 abnormalities. Leukemia 2005; 19:557–563.

*107. Moorman AV, Richards SM, Martineau M, et al. Outcome heterogeneity in childhood high-hyperdiploid acute lymphoblastic leukemia. Blood 2003; 102:2756–2762.

*108. Hann I, Vora AJ, Richards S, et al. Benefit of intensified treatments for all children with acute lymphoblastic leukaemia: results from MRC UKALL XI and MRC ALL97 randomized trials. UK Medical Research Council's Working Party on Childhood Leukaemia. Leukemia 2000; 14:356–363.

*109. Chessells JM, Harrison G, Richards SM, et al. Failure of a new protocol to improve treatment results in paediatric lymphoblastic leukaemia: lessons from the UK Medical Research Council trials UKALL X and UKALL XI. Br J Haematol 2002; 118:445–455.

110. Smith M, Arthur D, Camitta B, et al. Uniform approach to risk classification and treatment assignment for children with acute lymphoblastic leukemia. J Clin Oncol 1996; 14:18–24.

*111. Lilleyman JS, Hann IM, Stevens RF, et al. Cytomorphology of childhood lymphoblastic leukaemia: a prospective study of 2000 patients. United Kingdom Medical Research Council's Working Party on Childhood Leukaemia. Br J Haematol 1992; 81:52–57.

*112. Eden OB, Harrison G, Richards S, et al. Long-term follow-up of the United Kingdom Medical Research Council protocols for childhood acute lymphoblastic leukaemia, 1980–1997. Medical Research Council Childhood Leukaemia Working Party. Leukemia 2000; 14:2307–2320.

*113. Roy A, Bradburn M, Moorman AV, et al. Early response to induction is predictive of survival in childhood Philadelphia positive acute lymphoblastic leukaemia: results of the Medical Research Council ALL 97 Trial. Br J Haematol 2005; 129:35–44.

114. Goulden N, Oakhill A, Steward C. Practical application of minimal residual disease assessment in childhood acute lymphoblastic leukaemia annotation. Br J Haematol 2001; 112:275–281.

115. Coustan-Smith E, Sancho J, Hancock ML, et al. Clinical importance of minimal residual disease in childhood acute lymphoblastic leukemia. Blood 2000; 96:2691–2696.

*116. Schrappe M, Camitta B, Pui CH, et al. Long-term results of large prospective trials in childhood acute lymphoblastic leukemia. Leukemia 2000; 14:2193–2194.

*117. Clarke M, Gaynon P, Hann I, et al. CNS-directed therapy for childhood acute lymphoblastic leukemia: Childhood ALL Collaborative Group overview of 43 randomized trials. J Clin Oncol 2003; 21:1798–1809.

*118. Hill F, Richards S, Gibson BE, et al. Successful treatment without cranial radiotherapy of children receiving intensified chemotherapy for acute lymphoblastic leukaemia: results of the risk-stratified randomized central nervous system treatment trial MRC UKALL XI (ISRC TN 16757172). Br J Haematol 2004; 124:33–46.

*119. Mitchell CD, Richards SM, Kinsey SE, et al. Benefit of dexamethasone compared with prednisolone for childhood acute lymphoblastic leukaemia: results of the UK Medical Research Council ALL97 randomized trial. Br J Haematol 2005; 129:734–745.

120. Ravikumara M, Hill F, Wilson DC, et al. 6-thioguanine-related chronic hepatotoxicity and variceal hemorrhage in children treated for acute lymphoblastic leukaemia: a dual-center experience. J Pediatr Gastroenterol Nutr 2006; 42:535–538.

121. Stoneham S, Lennard L, Coen P, et al. Veno-occlusive disease in patients receiving thiopurines during maintenance therapy for childhood acute lymphoblastic leukaemia. Br J Haematol 2003; 123:100–102.

122. Bain BJ. Acute leukemia: immunophenotyping, cytogenetics and molecular genetics – the MIC and MIC-M classifications. In: Bain BJ, ed. Leukemia diagnosis. Oxford: Blackwell Science; 1999.53–112.

123. Alter BP, Potter NU. Classification and aetiology of the aplastic anemias. Clin Haematol 1978; 7:431–466.

124. Nathan DG, Oski FA. Hematology of infancy and childhood. 4th edn. London: WB Saunders; 1992.

125. Hoffbrand AV. Pernicious anemia. Scot Med J 1983; 28:218–227.

24

Oncology

Guy Makin, Stefan Meyer

INCIDENCE AND PREVALENCE

The cumulative incidence rate for cancer in children less than 15 years in the UK from 1981 to 1990 was 1774 per million with an age-standardized rate of 122.1 per million for England and Wales and 1806 and 124.9 per million for Scotland.[1,2] This means that of the 10 million children in the UK approximately 1200 (1 in every 8000) are diagnosed with cancer every year, which equates to 1 child in every 600 developing a malignancy before their fifteenth birthday.[3] Relative and absolute incidence figures for individual tumor types are shown in Tables 24.1 and 24.2 (derived from Parkin et al[3]). The total incidence of childhood tumors is constant around the world, with cumulative incidences (0–15 years) in the range of 1–2.5 per 1000 and age-standardized rates between 70 and 160 per million.[3] There are marked variations in the incidence of particular types of childhood cancer between countries and geographical areas. These variations may be caused by other diseases masking cancer and variable diagnostic and reporting methods, as well as genuine variations in incidence due to differences in a variety of genetic and environmental factors.

It is essential to have comprehensive population-based registration of all cancers in a particular region or country before firm conclusions about such variations can be drawn. This requires a universal agreement on tumor classification.[4] The standard system used is the international classification of childhood cancer developed in collaboration with the International Society of Pediatric Oncology based on the Birch and Marsden scheme.[5,6] Whereas most malignancies in the adult population are carcinomas, childhood malignancies are much more diverse and classified histologically or molecularly rather than by primary site.

Acute leukemia is the commonest individual childhood malignancy in the UK and accounts for 30% of malignant disease. Acute lymphoblastic leukemia (ALL) accounts for 80–85% of cases. A childhood peak between 2–6 years of age in ALL is seen in resource rich countries. Acute myeloid leukemia (AML) shows less variation except for apparently high rates among indigenous Pacific Island populations. Genetic variations alone, or in combination with environmental factors, may explain the high rates of certain malignancies. Infectious environmental factors undoubtedly explain the high incidence of B cell lymphomas in equatorial Africa and variations in overall and subset types of Hodgkin disease around

991

Table 24.1   Crude relative incidence figures for childhood cancers and relative percentage for ages 0–15 years. (Data derived and modified from Parkin et al 1998[3])

Tumor type	England and Wales		Nigeria Ibadan		India Madras	
	M/F	Rel %	M/F	Rel %	M/F	Rel %
Leukemia	1.2	32.6	2.1	12.0	1.7	29.4
ALL	1.3	26.1	2.8	3.9	1.7	22.1
ANLL	1.0	5.3	3.0	1.0	1.7	5.3
Lymphomas	2.4	10.0	2.3	39.7	2.8	23.0
Hodgkin	2.2	4.3	8.0	4.7	3.1	10.3
Non-Hodgkin	2.5	4.9	1.8	2.9	2.6	8.4
Burkitt	3.2	0.4	2.0	26.6	1.5	0.5
Unspecified	1.9	0.2	2.5	5.5	2.4	3.8
Brain and spinal neoplasms	1.2	22.5	1.3	15.9	1.7	10.4
Neuroblastoma (and other sympathetic nervous system)	1.1	7.0	–	0.3	1.0	2.4
Retinoblastoma	1.2	2.7	1.5	9.7	1.0	9.4
Renal	0.9	5.8	0.7	6.5	1.0	4.5
Wilms	0.9	5.7	0.6	6.3	1.0	4.5
Hepatic	1.4	0.9	1.0	1.6	2.7	1.0
Hepatoblastoma	1.4	0.7	–	0.8	2.5	0.6
Malignant bone	0.9	4.8	1.8	2.9	1.2	4.8
Osteosarcoma	0.9	2.5	2.0	0.8	1.3	1.9
Ewing sarcoma	1.0	2.1	–	–	0.6	2.0
Soft tissue sarcoma	1.2	6.8	1.4	7.6	1.5	5.6
Rhabdomyo-sarcoma	1.2	4.3	1.0	5.2	1.5	3.1
Germ cell and gonadal	0.9	3.5	–	0.5	0.3	3.0
Carcinomas and epithelial	0.8	3.0	3.5	2.3	1.3	3.6

M/F ratio, male to female ratio; ALL, acute lymphoblastic leukemia; ANLL, acute nonlymphoblastic leukemia.

Table 24.2   Age-standardized incidence rates per million children for ages 0–15 by sex. (Data derived from Parkin et al 1998[3])

Tumor type	England and Wales		USA, SEER			
			White		Black	
	M	F	M	F	M	F
All tumors	130.8	113.1	160.7	139.3	116.3	119.6
Leukemias	43.7	37.7	50.8	42.8	30.9	27.9
Lymphomas	15.3	6.8	19.9	10.2	13.0	8.1
Hodgkin	6.2	2.9	7.1	5.2	5.4	3.2
Non-Hodgkin	7.8	3.4	7.6	3.5	5.5	3.7
Burkitt	0.7	0.2	4.1	0.7	0.9	0.3
Brain and spinal	28.7	25.1	34.0	29.5	27.6	27.1
Neuroblastoma	9.4	9.2	13.3	12.2	8.9	10.4
Retinoblastoma	4.0	3.5	4.8	5.0	5.6	5.1
Renal	7.2	8.1	10.0	10.1	8.3	10.9
Wilms	7.1	8.1	9.9	10.0	7.4	10.3
Hepatic	1.3	1.0	2.3	2.3	2.2	1.6
Hepatoblastoma	1.0	0.8	1.9	2.1	1.7	1.4
Bone	4.8	5.4	6.6	6.3	2.9	5.0
Osteosarcoma	2.4	2.8	3.4	3.2	2.6	4.1
Ewing sarcoma	2.2	2.3	2.7	2.6	0.3	0.3
Soft tissue sarcoma	8.9	7.7	10.9	9.1	11.2	11.5
Rhabdomyosar-coma	5.8	4.9	6.4	4.3	5.8	4.7
Germ cell/gonadal	4.1	4.3	3.5	5.1	1.8	7.8
Carcinomas	2.8	3.6	3.5	5.9	3.2	2.6
Other and unspecified	0.5	0.3	0.6	0.5	–	1.3

F, female; M, male.

CAUSATION, TREATMENT AND SURVIVAL – GENERAL POINTS

Table 24.3 gives 5-year actuarial survival showing significant improvement for the majority of cancers until 2002. Prognostic factors for each tumor type are discussed in the individual sections but some general factors are important. Improvement from 10% to 70% overall survival and 60% long term cure for all childhood cancers over the last 35 years has been achieved by the use of multi-agent chemotherapy along with radiotherapy and surgery for local tumor control. This complex treatment is delivered in specialized centers with a multidisciplinary team approach, as acute toxicity often requires intensive nursing support and a comprehensive blood transfusion service. Worldwide this treatment is only available to less than 20% of all children. One of the great challenges for the future is to extend the availability of such care throughout the world.[14]

Pediatric oncology has vigorously embraced the approach of randomized controlled trials and more recently the use of overview analyses.[15] The success of this approach is shown by the increase in survival rates for childhood leukemia at specialized centers from 77% in the years 1980–1984 to 89% in the period 1990–1994.[16] Five-year survival rose from 67% to 81% over this time. Entry of patients into therapeutic trials showed an even greater difference with 5-year survival figures of 64% for those treated off protocol in 1980–1984 compared with 70% when treated on a trial, while for the later time period (1990–1994) the figures were 68% and 84%. These figures translate into an increased annual survival of over 50 patients in the 1990s who would have died of their disease in the 1980s. Centralization of care has also been demonstrated to improve survival for acute non-lymphoblastic leukemia, non-Hodgkin lymphoma, nephroblastoma, osteosarcoma, Ewing sarcoma and rhabdomyosarcoma.[17] The effect of trial entry includes an increased emphasis on protocol compliance,

the world. Other variations such as the low incidence of Ewing sarcoma seen in West Africa and among Afro-Caribbean Americans have not yet been explained. Similarly, the reason for sex differences in incidence and survival seen for many tumors are not understood (Table 24.2).

The incidence of cancer in childhood is increasing. Significant linear increases in precursor B ALL (average annual increase 0.7%) and Hodgkin disease (1.2% average annual rise) have been reported in the North West of England over the 45-year time period 1954–1998.[7–9] CNS tumors and extracranial solid tumors appear to have an annual increase in incidence of approximately 1%. These increases are not solely attributable to changes in diagnostic or reporting practice and at present lack a biological explanation.[7–10]

The prevalence of childhood cancer patients in the general population is rising dramatically. This is to a large extent the result of improved survival. Table 24.3 shows the survival trends for individual tumor types over the last two decades (data derived from the UKCCSG scientific report compiled by C Stiller[11]). Approximately 1 in 900 individuals aged 20 years are now cancer survivors. Long term effects of their cancer and its treatment now present a significant public health concern. However, despite successful treatment in many cases, childhood cancer still constitutes the second commonest cause of death after accidents for those aged 5–14 years. After the first month of life cancer accounts for 1 in 10 of all childhood deaths.[12,13]

Table 24.3 Five-year actuarial survival percentage of patients treated in United Kingdom Children's Cancer Study Group Centers 1977–1999 by period of diagnosis. (Data derived from United Kingdom Children's Cancer Study Group Scientific Report 2002, compiled by Stiller CA, personal communication)

Tumor type	77–84	85–89	90–94	95–99	X^2(1df) for trend
ALL	63	72	80	82	246.3***
ANLL	21	42	52	62	132.3***
Hodgkin disease	90	93	94	91	4.43*
Non-Hodgkin disease	60	76	76	83	61.5***
Ependymoma	42	45	54	69	14.6***
Low grade astrocytoma	81	84	89	93	19.3***
High grade astrocytoma	38	27	19	20	(7.34)**
PNET (inc medulloblastoma)	52	46	45	56	0.59
Neuroblastoma	37	39	50	58	82.6***
Retinoblastoma					
Bilateral	94	91	91	96	3.65
Unilateral	89	93	97	98	6.72**
Wilms	81	84	81	89	5.63*
Hepatoblastoma	37	41	68	69	23.9
Osteosarcoma	44	56	55	58	8.81**
Ewing sarcoma	40	55	65	74	30.5***
Rhabdomyosarcoma	56	60	63	65	12.6***
Germ cell					
CNS	48	59	63	82	8.62**
Non-CNS, nongonadal	47	82	80	80	15.0***
Gonadal malignant	87	96	97	97	12.3**

*p < 0.05; **p < 0.01; ***p < 0.001.
If X^2 in ( ) = negative trend (decreasing survival) which appears to be as a result of increased referral to centers of high risk patients who do not survive long enough to receive adjuvant therapy.
ALL, acute lymphoblastic leukemia; ANLL, acute nonlymphoblastic leukemia; PNET, primitive neuroectodermal tumor.

more consistent supportive care, audit and sharing of toxicity data and international exchange of information. Adoption of the 'best' therapy from other reported trial groups has become a feature of modern oncology therapy.[18] Further improvement is likely to result from more extensive collaborative efforts on an international level to reach meaningful patient numbers in addition to a better understanding of the biology of the individual malignancy.

ETIOLOGY

Little is yet known about the cause of most childhood cancers. Single environmental factors, e.g. smoking, which play a significant part in adult malignant disease, have not been identified for childhood malignancies (see below). Genomic damage that leads to malignant transformation takes time to develop, which explains the rising incidence of cancer with age in the general population, where cancer is a common disease. In childhood malignancies it is likely that genetic factors play a more important role in the etiology. A strong genetic basis for some childhood malignancies can be inferred from the observation of a high incidence of malignancies in certain genetic syndromes (Tables 24.4 and 24.5). These account for a minority of childhood cancers. However, susceptibility to childhood malignancies associated with genetic variation, which could affect handling of environmental factors or genomic damage, might account for a greater proportion of childhood cancers. The UK-wide National Case Control Study was established in 1991 in order to determine the role of exposure of parental germ cells, or children, to ionizing radiation, extremely low frequency electromagnetic fields or chemicals in the causation of childhood cancer.[19] Overall, a picture is emerging that the role of these environmental factors in the causation of childhood cancers is very limited. However, there is emerging evidence that abnormal responses to one or more common infections may play a role in the etiology of hematological and solid malignancies. This hypothesis suggests that there might be a paucity of exposure to infections in infancy and subsequent exposure shortly before the onset of cancer symptoms. However, even if common environmental factors like infections play a role for the initiation or progression of malignant diseases in children, genetic factors, which determine the host response at a given time in life will be important.

INHERITED PREDISPOSITION TO CHILDHOOD CANCER

The proportion of childhood tumors which are truly hereditary is estimated to be less than 5%, but might be higher.[20] Germline mutations may be inherited from parents (e.g. the retinoblastoma gene in familial retinoblastoma or the p53 gene in Li–Fraumeni syndrome). New genetic rearrangements and mutations may also arise within the oocyte or sperm prior to fertilization (e.g. in Down syndrome where there is a significantly increased risk of developing leukemia). Some tumors, for example nephroblastoma, are associated with more than one genetic syndrome.[21] Other cancers cluster in families, and predisposing genes are not all yet fully defined.

Constitutional chromosomal disorders

These disorders are usually characterized by a specific phenotype and associated with increased risk of malignancy. Altered chromosome number (aneuploidy) or structural rearrangements can be detected by routine karyotyping. The most common abnormality is constitutional trisomy 21, Down syndrome. These children have a nearly 20-fold increased risk of developing leukemia (1 in 100 compared with the general population of 1 in 2000 by the age of 10 years).[22,23] Interestingly many constitutionally normal childhood ALL patients have trisomy 21 in the leukemic cells, but the relevant genetic changes involved have not yet been fully elucidated. Both ALL (60%) and AML (40%) occur in Down syndrome but with many more AML cases in young children (under 2 years) than in the overall childhood leukemic population. A high percentage of such patients have acute megakaryocytic leukemia (M7) which is very responsive to therapy. Provided toxicity can be controlled Down patients fare as well as if not better than non-Down patients.[24] Further studies are now underway to explore why excess material of chromosome 21 not only plays a role in the development of leukemia but also seems to lead to excess toxicity with chemotherapy.

Numerical or structural sex chromosome abnormalities are also associated with an increased risk of malignancy. The extra X chromosome material seen in Klinefelter syndrome is associated not only with an increased risk of breast carcinoma but also with acute leukemia, lymphoma and extra gonadal germ cell tumors. Sex chromosome aneuploidy is associated with retinoblastoma in the conditions where there is excess of Y chromosome material. In 45 X0 Turner syndrome, there is increased risk of malignant transformation of rudimentary gonad tissue, but also increased risk of neuroblastoma, Wilms tumor and other malignancies.[20]

Detailed analysis of some chromosomal abnormalities has led to the identification of important genes involved in tumorgenesis in children. For example, chromosomal analysis of children with WAGR syndrome (consisting of Wilms tumor, aniridia, genital abnormalities and mental retardation) led the initial identification of the WT1 gene on 11p13, as a number of children with these abnormalities were found to have a deletion at 11p13. A small percentage (1–3%) of Wilms tumor patients were identified as having aniridia, often with a degree of developmental delay and genital abnormalities including hypospadias.[25,26] Subsequently disruption of this locus was also found in the

Table 24.4 Familial autosomal dominant disorders associated with childhood malignancy

Syndrome	OMIM	Locus	Gene	Associated childhood malignacy
Familial retinoblastoma	180200	13q14	RB1	Retinoblastoma Osteosacoma
Familial Wilms tumor	601363	17q12–21	FWT1	Wilms tumor
Familial Wilms tumor 2	605982	19q13	FWT2	Wilms tumor
Li–Fraumeni Syndrome	151623	17p13 22q12 22q11	TP53 CHK2 SNF5	Adrenocortical carcinomas Soft tissue sarcoma Osteosarcoma, CNS tumors
Hered!tery nonpolyposis colon cancer	114500	2p22–21 3p21 7p22	MSH2 MLH1 PMS2	Glioma
Famililal adenomatous poypopsis	175100	5q21	APC	
Gorlin syndrome	109400	9q31	PTCH	Medulloblastoma
Neurofibromatosis type 1	162200	17q11	NF1	Astrocytoma, JMML, AML, ALL, rhabdomyosarcoma
Neurofibromitosis type 2	101000	22q12	NF2	Menigioma
Multiple café au lait spots	114030	2p22 3p21	MSH2 MLH1	ALL, NHL, glioma
Multiple endocrine neoplasia type 2	171400			
Multiple endocrine neoplasia type 2B	162300	10q11	RET	Medullary thyroid carcinoma

OMIM, Online (database of) Mendelian Inheritance in Man.

Table 24.5 Disorders with immunodeficiency or chromosomal instability predisposing to childhood malignancy. (Adapted from Stiller[18])

Clinical syndrome	OMIM	Inheritance	Locus	Gene	Associated malignancies
Ataxia telangiectasia	208900	AR	11q22	ATM	Lymphoma, Leukemia
Wiscott–Aldrich syndrome	30100	X-linked	Xp11	WAS	NHL
Bloom syndrome	210900	AR	15q26	BLMN	Variable
Common variable immunodeficiency	240500	Various	Various	Various	Lymphoma
X-linked agammaglobulinemia	300300	X-linked	Xq13	BTK	Lymphoma
IgA deficiency	137100	AD	6p21	IGAD	Lymphoma
Severe combined immunodeficiency	300400	X-linked	Xq13	IGAD1	Lymphoma
X-linked lymphoproliferative disease (Duncan disease)	208240	X-linked	Xq25	Various	Lymphoma
Nijmegen breakage syndrome	251260	AR	8q21	NBS1	NHL, medulloblastoma RMS
Fanconi anemia	227650	AR and X-linked	Multiple	FANCA,B,C, D1/BRCA2, D2,E,F,G,I,J,K,L,M	AML, liver tumors, brain tumors, Wilms
Diamond–Blackfan anemia	205900	AD	19q13.2, 8p23.3-p22	RPS19 (in <50%) other	AML, osteosarcoma
Shwachman–Diamond syndrome	260400	AR	7q11	SBDS	MDS, AML

XR, X-linked recessive; AR, autosomal recessive; AD, autosomal dominant
OMIM, Online (database of) Mendelian Inheritance in Man.

Denys–Drash syndrome (characterized by severe urogenital abnormalities and Wilms tumor). However, there are other families reported with apparent dominant inheritance of Wilms tumor that do not have mutations at 11p13, and Wilms tumor has been reported in many genetic syndromes.[21] This implies that disruption of genes encoding for proteins involved in a variety of cellular functions can contribute to the genesis of this tumor. This includes two syndromes involving tissue overgrowth, Beckwith–Wiedemann (intrauterine and postnatal overgrowth, organomegaly, macroglossia and linear ear creases linked with nephroblastoma and hepatoblastoma) and hemihypertrophy (asymmetrical overgrowth of one side of the body, or face alone, linked with Wilms tumor). The risk in both conditions is high enough to warrant regular abdominal ultrasonography in patients recognized to have such overgrowth. The genetics of these syndromes are complex and can involve other mechanisms of genetic changes, such as imprinting. The insulin-like growth factor 2 gene (IGF2), which is normally a maternally imprinted gene but expressed from the paternal copy, is the gene involved in Beckwith–Wiedemann syndrome.[26] In many pediatric tumors the normal delicate balance of proliferation, differentiation and programmed cell death, apoptosis, is disturbed by the inappropriate activation of genes that promote proliferation, and inappropriate suppression of pathways which normally prevent proliferation. A complex picture is emerging that not only points at genetic changes affecting DNA structure, but also changes involving expression, transcription and indeed post-translational modification of encoded proteins (see below).

Single gene disorders

Table 24.4 shows some of the disorders predisposing to childhood tumors, inherited in an autosomal dominant fashion through several generations. There may be individuals with the same genetic mutation who have no or minimal overt manifestations of the malignant phenotype. The characteristics of these autosomal dominant cancer family syndromes are that:

1. inheritance can be from either father or mother;
2. multiple generations are most likely to be involved;
3. onset of the cancer will be at an earlier age compared with sporadic cases of the same cancer;
4. there are more likely to be multiple rather than single tumors;
5. there may be a clustering of increased risk of one or several different types of tumor within the family.

Retinoblastoma is the most carefully documented genetically determined tumor of childhood. In 1971 Knudson proposed that bilateral retinoblastoma was the familial form of this condition and patients had already acquired a germline mutation. His two-hit hypothesis proposed that such patients only required one further somatic cell hit for the tumor to develop whereas sporadic retinoblastoma, which occurs at an older age, requires at least two somatic mutations in the same cell for the tumor to develop. The affected gene, Rb1, is located on chromosome 13q14.1–14.2 and the normal function of the Rb1 gene product is to negatively regulate cell division (tumor suppression). Loss of this function gives rise to tumor development. Since in the inherited form all cells of the body contain the first mutation, tumors can arise not only in the retina but theoretically anywhere else. These other tumors do occur especially in the pineal gland, bone and soft tissue (particularly in response to irradiation), and skin as melanoma. In the nonhereditary form only retinal tumors develop. In the inherited form the second event may include loss of the whole chromosome 13, deletions and gene conversion. The complexity of genetic changes and phenotypic findings however is exemplified by the fact that about 15% of unilateral retinoblastoma are of the inherited type, which is not completely explained. There may also be no family history, either because the mutation has arisen de novo in the affected child or because there may be a mild form of the tumor in parents (known as a retinoma) which has spontaneously regressed. This sometimes can be identified by careful examination of the retina. Life-long follow-up of patients with inherited retinoblastoma shows them to progressively develop other malignancies over their lifetime including osteosarcoma and malignant melanoma as well as, in later life, carcinomas.[27] Another tumor suppressor gene involved in pediatric and familial cancers is the TP53 gene located at 17q12–13. Li and Fraumeni detected an increased incidence of breast cancer in mothers of young children with soft tissue sarcoma.[28] Considerable clustering of cancers including sarcomas, breast carcinoma, leukemias, brain tumors and adrenocortical carcinomas is seen in these families.[29,30] Malkin et al reported germline point mutations in the TP53 gene in a large number of such families.[31] However in some families with such a pattern of increased incidence of malignancy no p53 mutations have been found, suggesting that other genes within the same or interacting cellular pathways e.g. cell cycle control, can also be involved. The relationship between specific mutations within the gene and the malignant phenotype might also apply to other cancer genes. It is estimated that about 3% of osteosarcomas, 5% of rhabdomyosarcomas and probably all adrenocortical carcinomas are associated with germline TP53 mutations.[32]

Adenomatous polyposis coli and Gardner syndrome are characterized by the development of multiple colonic polyps in childhood and adolescence with progression to colon carcinoma in the second and third decade of life.[33,34] Individuals affected by these conditions also have an increased risk of other gastrointestinal and liver malignancies (including childhood hepatoblastoma). The syndrome involves the APC gene on 5q21. Molecular diagnostic testing of at-risk individuals, regular colonoscopy and surgical intervention can be life-saving in young patients. Another familial condition, hereditary non-polyposis colon cancer syndrome (HNPCC), involves right-sided colon tumors arising as early as the second decade of life. Such tumors can arise as a result of mutations in the mismatch repair gene hMSH2.[35] Many genes are for the maintainance of DNA integrity and mutations of these genes appear to prime cells for mutagenesis.[36] Turcot syndrome, in which familial clustering of brain tumors in childhood and polyposis/colon cancer is found, has been shown to involve mutations of the APC gene in some families and of mismatch repair genes in others (hMLH1 and hPMS2).

There are at least three forms of the multiple endocrine neoplasia (MEN) syndrome, all inherited in an autosomal dominant fashion. MEN2A can affect children (medullary thyroid carcinoma, pheochromocytoma), MEN2B (also includes ganglioneuromas of the gut and skeletal abnormalities) can even affect infants. The gene involved in MEN2A is the proto-oncogene RET (receptor tyrosine kinase gene) located on chromosome 10q11.2.[37] Neurofibromatosis type 1 which affects 1 in 2500 of the population is described elsewhere in the text. The NF1 gene (17q11.2) has been identified for over a decade. Its product, neurofibromin, acts as a transcriptional modulator during development of nerve and muscle. Mutations are associated with a range of benign and malignant neoplasms as well as the characteristic stigmata of the syndrome. NF2, which is much rarer, is related to a separate gene on chromosome 22 and is characterized by café-au-lait spots, bilateral vestibular schwannomas, neurofibromas and meningiomas and rarely presents in adolescence.

Other phakomatoses including tuberous sclerosis (TS) and von Hippel–Lindau disease (VHL) are associated with a range of benign and malignant neoplasms. In tuberous sclerosis these are mostly giant cell astrocytomas, but also other other tumors have been described; in VHL renal cysts and carcinomas, pheochromocytomas, cerebellar hemangioblastomas and retinal angiomas have been described. The nevoid basal cell carcinoma syndrome (Gorlin) is characterized by an association of early onset basal cell skin lesions and medulloblastomas.

Disorders which are recessively inherited appear to be less frequently or obviously associated with cancer early in life (Table 24.5). Some of that rarity may relate to failure to recognize the recessive disorder, without obvious family history and overt signs of disease at the time of cancer diagnosis. There are however some notable exceptions in childhood which predominantly involve genes involved in maintenance of DNA integrity and the DNA damage response, disruption of which leads to increased DNA fragility (spontaneous or in response to exogenous compounds such as irradiation or toxic chemicals) and in some cases immunodeficiency.

Xeroderma pigmentosum is characterized by eye and skin sensitivity progressing to basal and squamous cell carcinomas, melanomas and tip of tongue carcinomas. These lesions are all in sun-exposed areas but internal malignancies may occur. Some children show neurological deterioration. Mutations can occur in several genes and result in a defect in nucleotide excision repair.[38] There are related disorders, trichothiodystrophy and Cockayne syndrome. Ataxia telangiectasia (AT) presents in childhood with progressive truncal and subsequent limb ataxia, choreoathetosis and ocular motor apraxia. Telangiectasiae usually start in the conjunctivae in the first 5 years of life. However, many patients are missed until they present with leukemia and/or lymphomas.[39] Thirteen percent of UK-registered cases of AT have leukemia or lymphoma. There is associated deficiency of IgA and IgG$_2$ leading to sinopulmonary infections. It would appear that AT heterozygotes (1–2% of the population) are at much greater risk of developing breast cancer than the general population, possibly due to increased sensitivity to environmental DNA damage such as ionizing iradiation. The DNA of homozygotes is highly sensitive to damage from radiation and chemicals.[40,41] The AT gene on chromosome 11q22–33 encodes for a protein with kinase activity and signal transduction function.[42] Loss of AT results in a failure of normal cell cycle control. Nijmegen breakage syndrome (NBS) is a disorder with overlapping clinical features with AT such as immunodeficiency, but also marked microcephaly without teleangiectasia, which is also associated with non-Hodgkin lymphoma, but also brain tumors and soft tissue sarcoma.[43,44] The inherited disease Fanconi anemia (FA) shares some clinical feature of related disorders AT and NBS1 such as microcephaly and café au lait skin pigmentations. Characteristically there is hypersensitivity to DNA damaging agents, such as mitomycin C and other cross-linkers. FA patients can exhibit complex congenital abnormalities, but can also appear entirely normal. They are at extreme risk of progressive marrow failure and acute myeloid leukemia, but also brain tumors and Wilms tumor in addition to squamous cell carcinoma. There are at least 12 genes that can be mutated in FA, which are both autosomal and X-chromosomal. Most FA patients carry mutations in the FANCA gene (60%), followed by FANCC and FANCG (both approximately 15%).[45] The other genes appear less commonly mutated in FA patients, but might be extremely important in familial cancer syndromes, as patients of the rare Fanconi-D1 group carry mutations in the BRCA2 gene.[46,47] Heterozygous BRCA2 mutation carriers are at very high risk of developing breast, ovarian and pancreatic cancer, and it is quite possible that heterozygous carrier status of mutations and also other genes encoding for proteins involved in maintenance of DNA integrity play a significant role in cancer in the general population.

Genetically determined immunodeficiency

Where immune competence is impaired by inherited defects such as AT and NBS1 there is a high risk of leukemia and lymphoma development[48] (Table 24.6). Similarly, other forms of inherited and acquired immunodeficiency secondary to chemotherapy, intensive immunosuppression and infection predispose to malignancy, especially of lymphoid tissue (see below under lymphomas). With the increased burden of clinical AIDS resulting from HIV infection, especially in the resource rich world, and the more sophisticated use of immunosuppressant therapy this problem is growing.

GENETIC SUSCEPTIBILITY

The concept that some individuals may be more susceptible to develop genetic changes leading to malignancy is currently the subject of detailed investigations. Inappropriate maintenance of DNA integrity in response to ultraviolet light is seen in xeroderma pigmentosa (XP), in response to irradiation in ataxia telangiectasia and to cross-linking chemicals in Fanconi anemia (FA). For other cancer predisposing syndromes, immunodeficiency is a common clinical feature, while epidemiological data also point to a role for infectious agents. Additional factors might arise from differences in metabolizing enzymes, which might play a role especially in early development. For most sporadic childhood tumors we now suspect a combination of environmental factors with an inherent aberrant response, probably genetically determined, at a vulnerable point during development, to be at the root cause of the malignancy.

Most progress has been made in our understanding of infant and childhood ALL. Evidence from identical twins and retrospective analysis of neonatal blood spots has identified that for some, if not all such leukemias, initiation of the first genetic changes occurs before birth.[49,50] Genetic rearrangements involving the MLL gene, which are present in the majority of infant leukemias, appear adequate for development of overt leukemia. However, for precursor B cell ALL (peak age 2–6 years) additional postnatal genetic events are required. Carriage of the commonest leukemia-associated gene rearrangement TEL-AML1 (a cryptic translocation involving chromosomes 12 and 21) has been found in a frequency as high as 1–2% in normal cord blood.[51] Genetic epidemiological studies have found that the risk of developing infant MLL-associated leukemia is increased in pregnancies where the mother carries a low functioning polymorphic variant of the metabolizing NQ01 gene.[52] This protein plays a role for detoxification of quinone-containing substances which include both naturally occurring and synthetic topoisomerase 2 inhibitors.[53,54] Topoisomerase inhibitors can cause DNA breaks to be inappropriately relegated and may lead to genetic rearrangements. Dietary bioflavonoids can induce MLL cleavage and may contribute to infant acute leukemia.[55] Low function of the methylene tetrahydrofolate reductase (MTHFR) appears to confer protection against infant leukemia and precursor B cell ALL with hyperdiploidy. Low function MTHFR leads to greater available folate and increased DNA stability.[56] There has been some evidence that dietary supplementation with folate early in pregnancy may afford some protection against the development

Table 24.6 Recessive, sporadic and X-linked syndromes associated with childhood cancer

Syndrome	OMIM	Inheritance	Locus	Gene	Associated malignancy
Xeroderma pigmentosum	278720	AR	19q13 and others	ERCC2 and others	Skin cancer, melanoma
Rothmund–Thompson syndrome	268400	AR	8q24	REQL4	Osteosarcoma
WAGR syndrome	194072	Sporadic	11p13	WT1	Wilms tumor
Denys–Drash syndrome	194080	Sporadic	11p13	WT1	Wilms tumor
Beckwith–Wiedemann syndrome	130650	Sporadic/AD	11p15	Complex	Wilms tumor, hepatoblastoma, neuroblastoma, pancreatoblastoma
Costello syndrome	218040	AD	11p15.5	HRAS	Rhabdomyosarcoma, bladder carcionoma
Simpson–Golabi–Behmel syndrome	312870	X-linked	Xq26	GPC3	Wilms tumor
Perlman syndrome	267000	AR?	?11p	?	Wilms tumor
Sotos syndrome	117050	Sporadic	5q35	NSD1	Variable
Tuberous sclerosis	191100	AD	9q34 16p13	TSC1 TSC2	Subependymal giant cell astrocytoma
Tyrosinemia	276700	AR	15q23–25	FAH	Hepatocellular carcinoma

OMIM, Online (database of) Mendelian Inheritance in Man.

of childhood ALL.[57] In a similar fashion variations in genes encoding for other metabolizing enzymes have been investigated. In all of these instances dietary factors interact with the ability to metabolize/detoxify and appear to increase or decrease the risk of DNA damage. It is possible that other genetically determined factors, e.g. polymorphic variation within the more than 150 genes involved in DNA repair or genetic variants in genes that handle xenobiotics or other environmental factors as discussed below, may play a part in carcinogenesis in children.

In precursor B cell ALL abnormal response to infection may play a part in the later events or proliferation of the malignant clone. There is evidence that HLA class II alleles might influence risk.[58] Supportive evidence for a role of environmental, possibly infectious, agents in causation of childhood cancer comes from epidemiological studies detecting a rising incidence, onset seasonality and space–time clustering in leukemia, some lymphomas and solid tumors.[7,8,59,60]

ENVIRONMENTAL FACTORS
Ionizing radiation
Prenatal exposure
Stewart et al first reported an approximately 1.5-fold increase in childhood cancer for those fetuses exposed to X-rays performed on the maternal abdomen and pelvis during the first trimester of pregnancy.[61] There appeared to be a dose–risk relationship. Some but not all subsequent studies have confirmed an apparent increased risk associated with intrauterine X-ray exposure. In a series of studies on 1599 children born to mothers exposed to the Hiroshima and Nagasaki atomic bombs, those who received doses above the threshold of 10–20 cSv showed evidence of small head size, mental retardation and seizures.[62] Yoshimoto et al reported a 38% increase in cancer, with no dose threshold for those exposed in utero to atomic bomb irradiation, a similar rate to those exposed in the first decade of life in Japan.[63] In recent times there has been an interest in the concept of preconception effects particularly from radiation to the paternal germline.[64]

Postnatal exposure
Children who were within 1 kilometre of the epicenter of the Hiroshima bomb experienced an excess of acute and chronic myelogenous leukemia and acute lymphoblastic leukemia 3–10 years after the exposure. Young people surviving the atomic bomb have still developed thyroid and other adult cancers even decades after the event.

Therapeutic (low dose) external irradiation delivered to the scalp for tinea capitis or to the thymus have both been associated with significant increases in leukemia, brain tumors and thyroid carcinoma.[65,66] Dosages to the infant thyroid as low as 0.2 cGy have been reported in association with the development of carcinoma 12–17 years later. Speculation about the effects of radionucleotide ingestion from fallout has mostly centered on military personnel observing nuclear tests, although there has been a reported excess of childhood leukemia in Utah following exposure to fallout from atmospheric nuclear detonations.[67]

An increased risk of childhood malignancy, specifically leukemia, has been reported around nuclear reprocessing plants in the UK and elsewhere.[68–71] Studies of known environmental nuclide levels, routes of access and associated exposure to chemicals have failed so far to explain this risk. However, population mixing, and abnormal infection response might also account as a possible etiological factors in these communities.[72] The UK National Case Control Study has failed to show any relationship between household radon or gamma irradiation and the incidence of childhood malignancy.[73–75] However, irradiation (and chemotherapy) as treatment for a primary malignancy carries a definitive risk for development of a second tumor (see section 'Specific late effects', p. 1000).

There may be a life-long risk for children who receive extensive diagnostic X-rays with radiation dosages in excess of 10 cSv, in terms of developing breast and prostate cancer and leukemia in later life. Since such procedures cannot often be avoided clinicians need to be careful in their choice of procedure and avoid repetitive scanning wherever

possible (a CT scan of the head and body gives an effective body radiation dose of 0.1 cSv, while for a plain chest X-ray the dose is 0.008 cSv).

It is clearly important to remember that some children (e.g. with germline mutations of the Rb1, ATM, NBS1, FA genes or nevoid basal cell carcinoma genes) are particularly sensitive to ionizing irradiation, and that they may not be recognized as carrying the risk at the time of X-ray exposure. On the other hand, current exposure to radiation with diagnostic X-rays is extremely small compared with historical data.

Ultraviolet radiation
The fastest rising cancer incidence in the UK is for skin malignancy resulting from increased sunlight exposure on sunshine holidays and sunbed usage. The risk begins in childhood with unprotected and excessive sun exposure although the actual incidence of skin cancer in childhood is low.[76] Preventative measures are effective and population education needs to be enhanced (use of hats, clothing, sunscreens and avoidance of prolonged and/or repeated exposure to sun in childhood). The pediatrician has a key role in such education. Patients with xeroderma, Gorlin syndrome and albinism are at dramatically increased risk. The risk of developing melanoma appears to be increased if the sun exposure is obtained in conjunction with repeated exposure to chlorinated water in open air swimming pools. Some byproducts of chlorination are clearly mutagenic.[77]

Electricity and electromagnetic fields
Wertheimer and Leeper[78] reported an excess of childhood cancer in those exposed to excess electromagnetic fields derived from household electrical wiring. Subsequent studies where actual magnetic field measurements have been recorded have not consistently supported this observation. In the UK the large National Case Control Study has found no evidence to support such a relationship,[79] although the percentage of UK houses found to have high levels of exposure (greater than 0.4 micro-Tessler) was very small. By contrast, a Swedish study relating proximity to power lines and generated magnetic fields showed an apparent dose relationship with leukemia but not with all cancers, brain tumors or lymphomas.[80] Overall analysis does suggest the differences in study design might explain the conflicting results but for the vast majority of UK homes there appears to be no risk from generated electromagnetic fields nor from adjacency to power lines.

Drugs
Prenatal
Diethylstilbestrol is the only established transplacental carcinogen and exposure is associated with clear cell carcinoma of the vagina and cervix in female offspring as well as genital anomalies in both sexes.[81] Maternal phenytoin has been associated with increased incidence of neural crest tumors, and maternal alcohol with adrenal, neural crest and liver tumors and teratomas.[82] There may be a long latent period, e.g. the vaginal tumors did not occur until the children exposed to stilbestral before 20 weeks of gestation were aged 14–23 years.

Postnatal exposure
Intensive immunosuppression (e.g. in solid organ transplantation) is associated with a 20- to 40-fold increased risk of developing lymphoma with a short latent period. Modern intensive cancer therapy carries an increased risk of inducing secondary leukemia (mostly acute myeloid leukemia) and other neoplasms (e.g. brain). Chronic malnutrition, by inducing immune paralysis, coupled with chronic infective antigenic stimulation may be important in the induction of B cell neoplasias in tropical Africa.

There is an increased risk of developing AML for those treated with alkylating agents for other tumors (at the rate of 5–10% over the 10 years following exposure).[83] The most common alkylating agent used, cyclophosphamide, which can induce hemorrhagic cystitis, has also been incriminated as causative of bladder cancer. The exact risk for children treated with cyclophosphamide for either cancer or renal problems has not been adequately quantified but the avoidance of combined irradiation and alkylating agents especially when the bladder is involved appears wise. The increasing use of the highly effective cytotoxics, the topoisomerase 2 inhibitors (epipodophyllotoxins and anthracyclines) has been associated with a rise in early onset (median 30 months) therapeutically induced acute myeloid leukemia. The risk appears to be dose and schedule dependent.[84] For both alkylators and topoisomerase 2 inhibitors concurrent use of other cytotoxics and irradiation may increase the risk, although a genetic component is also likely to play an important role in these treatment related malignancies.

Long term use of androgens and other anabolic steroids has been associated with the development of hepatomas. Barbiturates used frequently and in high dosage in early infancy have also been incriminated in brain tumor formation, and phenytoin with lymphoma, but definitive evidence does not exist.

Golding et al reported that neonates receiving intramuscular vitamin K prophylaxis had an increased risk of developing leukemia.[85] Subsequent studies and more recent pooled analysis of the six major case control studies including that of Golding et al has found no convincing evidence to support the link.[86] The studies however have shown up major variations in clinical practice which need addressing. The risks of hemorrhage in the newborn appear to far outweigh any other risks of vitamin K prophylaxis.

Chemicals

Table 24.7 shows some of the parental occupations or exposures which have been incriminated in childhood tumor formation.[87] The exposure may be maternal or paternal, e.g. solvent exposure in the aircraft industry may act on the male germ cells which is then transmitted to the fetus. Although close exposure to asbestos mines in childhood was associated with the development in later life of mesotheliomas in the South African population, the rare mesotheliomas of childhood do not appear to be related to asbestos exposure. What has proved very difficult regarding chemicals, unlike with radiation, has been the ability to assess evidence of real exposure and its extent, plus to quantify risks.

There is conflicting evidence regarding parental smoking and alcohol consumption with regard to childhood cancer. Recently some association between smoking and particular subtypes of AML (M_1/M_2) has been suggested for young adults.

Viruses

Although infectious agents have been repeatedly associated with childhood leukemia and cancer no definite evidence has emerged to link any specific viral agent known to cause intrauterine infection with oncogenesis. However, mainly epidemiological data support a promoting role of infection in childhood leukemogenesis while repeated searches for viral genomic inclusion in ALL patients have proved negative.[88–90]

Table 24.7 Possible parental occupations associated with childhood malignancy

Occupation	Exposure	Tumor type
Petroleum industry	Petroleum	CNS
Lead industry	Hydrocarbons, lead	Wilms (lead)
Aircraft manufacturer	Organic solvents	CNS
Painting		Leukemia, ?hepatoblastoma (paints/pigments)
Paper/pulp mill workers, printing industries	Organic solvents	CNS, leukemia (sawdust)
Farming	Pesticides	CNS, leukemia, Wilms
Metal industries	Heavy metal solvents	Brain, leukemia (metal dust), lymphoma (foundries)

Postnatal exposure to Epstein–Barr virus (EBV) is associated with B cell lymphoid malignancies (Burkitt lymphoma and leukemia) in malarial areas of Africa where they comprise up to 50% of all childhood tumors. African Burkitt lymphoma occurs almost exclusively in areas of endemic malaria with early exposure to EBV (almost the whole population has been exposed by the age of 3 years). Most of the tumors in endemic areas show evidence of inclusion of viral DNA and the most consistently detectable antigen is the EBV surface capsid antigen. Infection early in life is thought to increase the size of certain pre B and B cell populations and maintains them in a proliferative state making them more likely to undergo genetic change. Alternatively EBV may induce an immortal cell clone with genetic transformation already present. Repeated infection, in particular with malaria (itself a T cell suppressor and B cell mitogen), and malnutrition lead to a major degree of T cell immunosuppression and B cell hyperplasia. It is not entirely clear whether the initial infection or subsequent events lead to the very characteristic translocation of DNA from chromosome 8 into the immunoglobulin coding sites on chromosomes 14, 2 or 22. The role of other cofactors, such as plant extracts, in promoting proliferation has not yet been fully evaluated. Outside equatorial Africa where exposure to EBV is usually much later, B cell tumors, especially extensive abdominal lymphomas, have been shown to contain viral antigen but in a lower percentage of cases. There are other differences between the endemic and sporadic cases but the same genetic translocation may be found in both forms. EBV has also been associated with nasopharyngeal carcinoma in nonmalarial areas and rare familial cases of both Burkitt lymphoma and nasopharyngeal carcinoma have been observed in tropical Africa.

EBV has also been linked to Hodgkin disease (HD).[91] In children and young adults it has been postulated that HD represents an abnormal outcome of delayed exposure to a common infectious agent. EBV is found in Hodgkin–Reed–Sternberg cells in a significant percentage of young cases, especially in boys and those with mixed cellularity subtype. What is not yet clear is whether the EBV is causative, contributory or a bystander in young people with altered immune responses.[92,93] Immune response genes may play a critical role in susceptibility to Hodgkin disease.[94]

Post transplantation and following severe immunosuppression for other conditions an EBV-driven lymphoproliferative disorder is increasingly observed (see lymphoma section).

Retroviruses alter the growth and differentiation of cells from various hemopoietic lineages. There is a clear relationship between infection with the retrovirus HTLV1 and a form of adult T cell leukemia and lymphoma,[95] and, although there has been recent speculation about in utero transmission, no childhood case has yet been reported. HIV infection, presumably as a result of its profound effect on helper T cells, predisposes to the development of a particularly virulent lymphoma in young adults. An increasing incidence of Kaposi sarcoma has been reported in African children.

Hepatitis B infection has long been associated with hepatocellular carcinoma. The mechanism of oncogenesis and the role of added effects resulting from other toxins such as aflatoxins still requires clarification.[96] Although some viruses may cause tumors by direct genetic transformation, some clearly induce host responses but the majority so far identified appear to function by oncogene activation. This can lead to interference with cell cycle control (e.g. HPV, E6, E7), or immortalization (EBV) or persistent activation of, for example, NFκB pathway with upregulation of the cytotoxic cascade (e.g. HTLV1 and Tax, or EBV and LMP-1) or promotional effects (mitogen exposure leads directly to proliferation, e.g. HTLV1–Tax gene leading to viral replication, HbV and HcV).

Other factors

There are other factors that are difficult to categorize in genetic or environmental causes that have been investigated in the context of childhood cancer. The observed association of inguinal hernias in children with Ewing sarcoma as well as other studies that found an increased incidence of isolated congenital abnormalities without defined syndromic association could point to environmental as well as genetic causes, but again might reflect gene–environment interaction.[97] Several case reports of malignancies occurring in children conceived by assisted reproduction technology (ART) give rise to concern about the neoplastic risk in ART. Several large national studies have failed to show an increased risk, but these studies will need to continue with the use of more sophisticated techniques in ART.[98,99]

EPIDEMIOLOGICAL CONCLUSIONS

Unlike in adults we have so far failed to identify significant connections between environmental factors and the majority of childhood cancers. Strong predisposition as part of a genetic syndrome accounts for the minority of cases but increasingly it is recognized that genetic susceptibility may play a significant part in a large number of tumors by altering response to or repair of damage caused by exogenous factors including viruses, chemicals, irradiation, etc. Initiation of the genetic damage, accumulation of a full malignant phenotype and ultimately proliferation of a premalignant clone require an accumulation of contributory factors. Each childhood tumor is likely to have a different combination of such factors in its etiology.

GENERAL PRINCIPLES OF DIAGNOSIS

A complete history and thorough clinical examination will suggest a diagnosis in most childhood malignancies. Histology is usually needed to confirm the diagnosis. Radiology is necessary to determine disease extent, and specific tumor markers (eg alpha fetoprotein in germ cell tumors) and baseline renal, liver and bone profiles are essential. Full blood count and coagulation profile are also needed, and it is useful to check the patient's antibody status to varicella and measles at diagnosis.

PATHOLOGY

Liaison with the pathologist about the clinical picture is crucial to successful diagnosis and a regular multidisciplinary review meeting bringing together radiology, clinical findings and histopathology should be standard practice. Morphology on H&E section is complemented by immunohistochemistry, cytogenetics, and DNA studies for specific gene abnormalities. Parental consent should be sought for tumor and constitutional DNA storage (from lymphocytes) for future study. Central review of pathology is mandatory for patients on clinical trials and has enabled audit and consistency of diagnosis.

RADIOLOGY

Specific radiological investigations will be discussed under each tumor heading but some general principles are important. Plain radiographs may be very suggestive of a specific diagnosis, e.g. suprarenal calcification in neuroblastoma, but are never diagnostic. As far as possible investigations should be rapid, noninvasive and avoid the need for general anaesthetic. Ultrasound examination is very useful as a first line, as sedation is rarely needed. Spiral CT scanners and MRI technology enable very precise tumor delineation. MRI is especially helpful for brain, spinal and liver tumors, while CT is particularly good for the detection of small chest metastases. Positron emission tomography (PET) scanning is increasingly available and offers an excellent means for monitoring residual disease.[100]

BIOCHEMICAL MARKERS

A few tumors secrete specific markers which can assist in diagnosis and in monitoring the response to treatment. Re-emergence of markers frequently precedes clinical relapse. Examples are urinary catecholamine excretion in neuroblastoma (total catecholamines, VMA and HVA); serum alpha-fetoprotein (AFP) in hepatoblastoma and teratomas; and human chorionic gonadotrophin (HCG) in some germ cell tumors.

CYTOGENETICS

Banding techniques and in situ hybridization studies have revolutionized routine karyotyping and tumor cytogenetics respectively. As more cytogenetic abnormalities are identified in tumors more specific probes have become available to detect translocations, deletions and amplifications of DNA. It is essential to combine tumor studies with analysis of nontumor DNA to exclude constitutional defects.

BONE MARROW EXAMINATION

Most childhood tumors are highly malignant and likely to be disseminated at presentation, with many (e.g. neuroblastoma, lymphoma, rhabdomyosarcoma, Ewing sarcoma, retinoblastoma) potentially metastasizing to the bone marrow. To exclude infiltration two aspirates and two trephines from different sites are considered a minimum requirement. The posterior iliac crest is the preferred site for bone marrow sampling in children.

PRINCIPLES OF THERAPY

The ultimate aim of therapy for childhood cancer is control of disease with minimum short and long term toxicity to normal tissue. Childhood tumors are generally extremely sensitive to cytotoxic agents in comparison with the common epithelial malignancies of adulthood. Most types of tumor will require multimodality therapy; surgery and/or radiotherapy for local tumor control, and chemotherapy for distant metastases, either macro or micro). The specific combination of therapies, and the schedule in which they are combined is tumor specific and is discussed in the relevant section.

As a general principle chemo- and radiotherapy are most effective against dividing cells; traditionally this has been felt to be the reason for their effectiveness against rapidly dividing tumor cells and for their toxicity to bone marrow and gut. In recent years the role of programmed cell death (apoptosis) both in tumor development, and as a mode of tumor cell response to treatment, has been increasingly appreciated. In normal tissue proliferation decreases the threshold for apoptosis so that cells can only proliferate in the presence of appropriate survival signals (growth factors, cytokines). This acts as a failsafe mechanism to ensure that cells can only proliferate in the right place and at the right time.[101] Tumor cells have acquired a relative resistance to this mechanism of engaging apoptosis so that they can proliferate without such signals, and evasion of apoptosis is felt to be a hallmark of cancer.[102] However tumor cells are 'primed' to undergo apoptosis if it can be triggered by an alternative route and there is an increasing focus on the modulation of apoptosis as an area for future development of more directed anticancer therapy.[103]

Hypoxia (a reduction of tissue oxygen to 1% or less) is a universal feature of tumors as a consequence of poorly organized tumor-derived new blood vessels. Hypoxia has profound effects on tumor cell response to radio- and chemotherapy, and has been correlated with poor prognosis in adult tumors.[104] Evidence is now emerging that hypoxia may also be an important contributor to tumor resistance in pediatric tumors.[105–107]

TUMOR CELL RESISTANCE

There are a number of mechanisms that prevent tumors being killed by drugs.[108]

Primary resistance

Extrinsic resistance occurs when inadequate drug reaches the tumor cell. This can arise from poor bioavailability, enhanced metabolism or excretion, or from inbuilt barriers to drug penetration such as the blood–brain barrier. There may be limited drug penetration into very large tumors or it may be that the concentration needed to kill the tumor produces excessive host toxicity and therefore cannot be used. In ALL therapy studies have shown that poor patient compliance as well as variable drug metabolism contribute to worse prognosis.[109]

Intrinsic resistance is a consequence of molecular abnormalities in the tumor cell that prevent cell death after cytotoxic damage. Primary resistance of this type is not prominent in pediatric tumors but is a common feature of adult epithelial malignancies, especially where the tumor supressor gene p53 is mutated.

Secondary resistance

This is more common in pediatric tumors. Relapse follows a good initial response to treatment or after finishing chemotherapy. Resistance may be against a single drug or against a range of cytotoxic agents with different mechanisms of action. To reduce acquired drug resistance it is common practice to deliver dose-intensive multiagent regimens alternating between drugs with different toxicities. A number of mechanisms for the development of tumor cell resistance have been described.

1. *Drug transport*: Decreased tumor cellular drug uptake and increased drug efflux have both been described as contributing to drug resistance. Polymorphisms in the reduced folate carrier resulting in decreased cellular methotrexate levels are associated with poorer outcome in acute lymphoblastic lymphoma[110]. Many cytotoxics are targets of drug efflux proteins, including p-glycoprotein (P-gp) and multidrug resistance protein (MDR/MRP). However while P-gp expression may be increased at relapse in childhood leukemia[111] there is minimal evidence for prognostic significance in other settings.[112]
2. *Drug target*: Amplification of the gene encoding the enzyme dihydrofolate reductase, the target for the widely used cytotoxic agent methotrexate, is associated with methotrexate resistance and has been reported in patients with ALL at relapse.[113]
3. *Drug inactivation*: Platinum drugs can be inactivated by glutathione-*S*-transferase (GST) mediated conjugation to glutathione. High levels of both glutathione and GST can be found in platinum-resistant tumor cells and tumor levels of GST correlate with survival in adult head and neck cancer.[114]
4. *DNA repair*: A number of cellular mechanisms exist to repair DNA damage induced by cytotoxic agents. Platinum compounds form DNA adducts and these are removed by nucleotide excision repair. This is a complex process involving many proteins, high levels of one of which, ERCC1, correlate with poor response to platinum.[115] Mismatch repair seems also to be important for response to platinum compounds and loss of mismatch repair has been reported in cisplatin-resistant ovarian tumors.[116]

At present our increased understanding of mechanisms of tumor drug resistance has not translated into therapeutic strategies to overcome them. However it is likely that with the next generation of rational therapeutics that many of the problems seen with resistance to conventional cytotoxic agents will become less important.

SURGERY AND IRRADIATION

Many pediatric tumors require definitive local control for long term cure. Local control requires either surgical excision with wide margins of normal tissue, or where this is impractical or technically impossible, then local radiotherapy. There are also many situations in which local radiotherapy is needed after surgical resection, either because of poor margins of normal tissue in the resected tumor, or because of evidence of microscopic local spread in the resected sample. The timing of such therapy needs to be carefully considered so as to disrupt ongoing treatment as little as possible.

The main limitation of irradiation is its effect on normal tissues. Modern megavoltage therapy has a sharper beam edge, better depth of penetration and can give a more even dose distribution thus avoiding damage to skin and overlying tissues when administered to deep organs. When therapy is planned, careful clinical and radiological assessment of the tumor is undertaken so that radiation fields can be calculated to minimize the radiation dose to normal tissue. New radiation technology is facilitating much more focused therapy with sharp cutoff to minimize damage to surrounding normal tissues. When irradiation is

included with chemotherapy in treatment protocols there is a potential for additive toxicity as well as efficacy. In the short term, radiation recall especially with actinonycin, can be troubling. In the long term the combination of alkylating agents and irradiation leads to an increased risk of the development of secondary neoplasms.

MONITORING TUMOR RESPONSE

Standardization of tumor response criteria is essential to facilitate comparison of treatment protocols. What constitutes each category of response is not always easy in any specific tumor.

1. *Complete regression* (CR): complete macroscopic regression of all apparent tumor.
2. *Partial regression* (PR): more than 50% reduction, but less than 100% of any single measurable lesion without any new lesions appearing or growth of other identifiable lesions. This category is sometimes split into good partial response and poor partial response.
3. *Stable disease*: no change in any tumor as defined by less than 50% reduction of any single measurable lesion without any new lesions appearing.
4. *Progressive disease*: enlargement of at least one measurable lesion and/or the development of new lesions while on therapy.

SPECIFIC EFFECTS OF TREATMENT

Ionizing irradiation

Ionizing irradiation may kill or severely damage a cell. Sublethal cell damage, particularly to normal tissue surrounding a tumor, can cause tissue aging, malformation, growth impairment or induce carcinogenesis. Irradiation is generally given in daily fractions to facilitate normal cell recovery. As cells in the periphery of the tumor mass are killed, more centrally placed and hypoxic cells will undergo a reoxygenation process and will become susceptible to therapy, particularly if there is an interval between radiation exposures.

Multiple fractions of radiation produce the same effect as a single large dose, but are better tolerated and more efficacious for most tumors. Tolerance curves can be produced for normal and malignant tissues. It is sometimes possible to calculate split course therapy during the intervals of which normal tissues can repair and some tumor cells will be recruited into the proliferative phase where they will be more susceptible to therapy.

Chemotherapy

Table 24.8 shows some adverse drug effects. Most agents produce alopecia and varying degrees of myelosuppression and some gastrointestinal upset. Patients worry about the nausea and vomiting, physicians about infection risks and hemorrhage.

Hematological toxicity

The degree and duration of neutropenia increases the risk of sepsis. It is essential that patients and parents are aware of the need to urgently seek medical attention should they become febrile or unwell. Regular monitoring of counts and careful education of parents as to the risks are essential.[117]

Neutropenia and infection

Neutropenia leads to a significant risk of bacterial and fungal sepsis when the total neutrophil count is less than 1.0×10^9/L. Skin and gastrointestinal flora can rapidly produce septicemia. The commonest isolated organisms are Gram-positives especially *Staphylococcus aureus* and coagulase negative staphlocococci, but the gravest threat to life comes from Gram-negative organisms including *Escherichia coli*, *Klebsiella* and *Pseudomonas*.[118]

Meticulous hand washing techniques by all staff can reduce nosocomial infection including colonization with some pathogens.[119,120] All rectal procedures should be prohibited during neutropenia unless absolutely unavoidable.

Table 24.8 Specific drug toxicity effects of some commonly used chemotherapeutic agents

Drug	Myelo-suppression	Immuno-suppression	Tissue irritant	Nausea + vomiting	Cystitis	Nephrotoxicity	Cardiotoxicity	Neuropathic	Ototoxicity	Pulmonary	Hepatotoxicity
Anthracyclines (adriamycin + daunomycin)	++	+	+++	++	-	-	+++	-	-	-	Radiation recall effect
Actinomycin	++	+	+++	++	-	-	-	-	-	-	Radiation recall effect + VOD
Bleomycin	-	+/-	+	+/-	-	-	-	-	-	++	-
Alkylating agents											
Cyclophosphamide	++	++	+	++	++	+	+ (high dose)	+ (IADH)	-	+	-
Ifosfamide	++	++	+	++	+++	++	?++	++ (> in adults)	-	+	-
(Nitrosoureas, e.g. CCNU)	+++ (cumulative)	++		++	-	++ (cumulative)	-	+ (rare)	-	++	-
Nonclassical alkylating											
Cisplatinum	+	+	+/-	+++	-	+++	-	++	+++ (cumulative)	-	-
Dacarbazine DTIC	+	+/-	+ (+ pain)	++	-	-	-	-	-	-	++ (+ VOD)
Antimetabolites											
Methotrexate oral, i.v., i.m., i.t.	++	++	-	Mucositis ++	-	++ (high dose)	-	++ (high dose) (chronic i.m.)	-	++ (high dose systemic) +	++ (acute/chronic)
6-mercaptopurine oral + i.v.	+	+	-	Rarely	-	-	-	-	-	-	+
Cytosine i.v./i.m.	++	++	-	++ (diarrhea)	-	-	-	Cerebellar (high dose)	-	-	-
Vinca alkaloids											
Vincristine	+/-	++	+++	-	-	-	-	+++ (+ IADH)	+++	-	-
Vinblastine	++	++	+++	+/-	-	-	-	+/-	-	-	-
Epipodophyllotoxins											
Etoposide	++	+	+	+/- Mucositis	-	-	+/- (hypotension)	+ (mild peripheral)	-	-	+ (enzymes)
Steroids	-	+++	High dose pain	-	-	-	-	-	-	-	-
Asparaginase	++	++	-	-	-	-	-	Encephalopathy	-	-	++

In addition epipodophyllotoxins, asparaginases, bleomycin and rarely cytosine + cisplatinum are associated with acute life threatening hypersensitivity reactions.
+-+++ denotes varying degree of toxicity.
- denotes no recorded toxicity of type.
VOD, veno-occlusive disease.

Any child who is neutropenic and febrile should rapidly receive broad spectrum antibiotics. Clinical signs of infection without fever necessitate a similar response.[121] The antibiotic regimen chosen should reflect local sensitivity profiles but must cover both Gram-negative and Gram-positive organisms (e.g. an aminoglycoside and a carbapenem). With more use of broad spectrum antibiotics fungal infection rates have increased. Failure of resolution of pyrexia after 96 hours of i.v. antibiotics or if there is clinical deterioration is an indication for systemic antifungal therapy. Fungal infections are particularly problematic in patients with prolonged neutropenia (> 10 days). There is no indication for prophylactic antiviral agents in the absence of clinical evidence of viral disease and no evidence for the routine use of granulocyte transfusions. Whilst granulocyte colony stimulating factor can reduce the duration of neutropenia there is no evidence of effectiveness in reducing duration of neutropenic fever. Current guidelines advise against its routine use.[121] There is no consensus on the use of prophylactic antibiotics in neutropenic patients.

Localizing signs are often absent in the face of profound neutropenia, but initial evaluation of these patients should include a thorough examination. Bacterial cultures should be taken from blood and any superficial lesion. Fungal and viral cultures plus serology should be performed if there is poor response. Chest X-ray is indicated in the presence of respiratory symptoms or lack of resolution of fever. Persistent fever indicates the need for further imaging to look for evidence of fungal infection. However in nearly two thirds of patients no initial focus of infection is identified. It is important that all medical and nursing staff are aware that these patients can become very ill very rapidly and it is essential that they are regularly monitored. Early intervention with aggressive fluid resuscitation and inotropic and ventilatory support can be life saving.

Immunosuppression

Both chemotherapy and radiotherapy can induce lymphopenia and impaired T and B cell function. Viral infections may not be adequately cleared and common viruses may be excreted for months. Varicella and, increasingly, measles pose major risks. Varicella infection formerly carried a high mortality but zoster immune globulin (ZIG) given prophylactically within 96 hours of contact is effective at preventing primary infection.[122] Varicella infection (either primary or shingles) can be effectively managed with aciclovir 5–10 mg/kg i.v. 8-hourly for at least 5 days followed by at least 2 weeks of oral therapy to prevent recrudescence.[123,124] Immunosuppressed patients contracting measles and developing either immune encephalitis or giant cell pneumonitis have a near 100% mortality.[125] Prevention of measles in these patients is best achieved by high community uptake of measles vaccination and avoidance of close contact with cases. Although immunization programs have reduced measles prevalence, only uptake rates in excess of 90% will make epidemics a feature of the past.

Pneumocystis carinii pneumonitis may occur during periods of profound lymphopenia. It presents with intractable fever and tachypnea often with no clinically detectable chest signs despite florid radiographic changes. It can be effectively prevented by the use of prophylactic co-trimoxazole.[126] Treatment of the pneumonitis requires a higher dose (trimethoprim 20 mg/kg/day and sulfamethoxazole 100 mg/kg/day given in two divided doses daily). About 80% of patients respond, with some doing so only on the addition of steroids.[127] Nebulized pentamidine can be used in those hypersensitive to sulfonamides but has had disappointing results in leukemic patients. Cytomegalovirus may coexist with pneumocystis and can produce a similar pneumonitis. Ideally broncho-alveolar lavage should be performed to confirm the diagnosis, certainly if there is poor response to therapy. Disease infiltration, fungi and drug reactions can all mimic *Pneumocystis carinii* pneumonitis.

Live vaccines, including measles and polio, must be avoided during therapy but it is recommended that the normal schedule of childhood immunization should otherwise be followed. Patients should receive single booster doses of all vaccines that they have previously received 6 months after finishing chemotherapy, and 12 months after bone marrow transplant.[128]

Blood product support

Children have more efficient platelets and good blood vessel wall support when compared with adults and only tend to bleed overtly at very low platelet counts (< 10 × 10⁹/L) except in the presence of severe infection. There is little evidence in favor of prophylactic platelets given at specific levels but most units will transfuse platelets once the count is < 10 × 10⁹/L in well patients. In those who are febrile and neutropenic it is usual to keep platelet counts > 20 × 10⁹/L. If invasive high risk procedures, such as lumbar punctures, are to be carried out, it is advisable to keep counts above 50 × 10⁹/L for 24 hours.[129] Frequent platelet transfusion can lead to antibody development with poor increases in platelet number. There is even less evidence for the use of prophylactic red cell transfusions but again most units have a hemoglobin limit at which they will transfuse patients regardless of symptoms; this is usually in the order of 8 g/dl.[130] The CMV immune status should be assessed for all patients at diagnosis and only CMV-negative donors used for those with no immunity. There is a significant risk of transfusion related graft versus host disease in patients with profoundly compromised cell mediated immunity. In oncological practice this includes all patients with Hodgkin disease, bone marrow transplant recipients and any patient who has received fludaribine. To minimize this risk, these patients should receive irradiated blood products at all times.

Local tissue toxicity

Many cytotoxics will cause tissue damage if they extravasate (e.g. vincristine and anthracyclines). Use of central lines has decreased the risk. For both central and peripheral lines, only experienced fully trained staff should give cytotoxics and correct line placement should always be checked prior to injection (good blood flow back, easy flushing with saline and no pain).

Nausea and vomiting

Many cytotoxics can produce profound nausea and vomiting. Symptom control has been greatly enhanced by use of the 5-HT₃ receptor antagonists. In the majority of patients vomiting can be controlled by regular ondansetron starting before chemotherapy.[131] The addition of i.v. dexamethasone is helpful in children receiving highly emetogenic regimens.[132] Metoclopramide and cyclizine can be used effectively with less emetogenic regimens and may also be useful in older patients with vomiting that is refractory to ondansetron and dexamethasone. Nabilone and levopromazine (nozinan) have also been effective in this setting.[133] Initial bad experiences with chemotherapy may induce anticipatory vomiting especially in teenagers, for which oral benzodiazepines (lorazepam) 12 hours prior to therapy can be effective. Lorazepam can also increase the effectiveness of dexamethasone.[134] Delayed vomiting can be a problem particularly with cisplatin but should also alert the physician to the possibilities of infection, hepatotoxicity or ongoing anxiety and psychological problems.

Mucositis

Methotrexate, the anthracyclines and actinomycin all induce mucositis which is frequently complicated by secondary candida infection. There is some evidence that ice chips can prevent mucositis but none of the other currently used prophylactic agents are effective.[135] There is evidence that prophylactic antifungal agents can reduce the clinical signs of oral candidiasis.[136] Mucositis can be extremely painful and intravenous opiate analgesia should be used at an early stage.

Bowel dysfunction

Myelo-ablative therapy regimens, high dose cytosine and irinotecan can all produce profound watery diarrhoea which can lead to significant (> 10% of body weight) weight loss for which parenteral nutrition is required. In the absence of diarrhoea such weight loss is usually due to tumor cachexia and loss of appetite is an indication for enteric feeding.

The vinca alkaloids can produce severe constipation and ileus. This autonomic neuropathy may be complicated by enterocolitis, bowel wall edema and even intussusception. Regular use of bowel softeners (e.g. lactulose) may decrease the risk but when established it may need more aggressive management. Prevention by attention to fluid intake, maximizing activity, avoidance of excess narcotics and stool softeners is preferable.

Renal toxicity

Cisplatin causes progressive tubular and glomerular deterioration with increasing cumulative dosage and occasionally acute tubular necrosis. Vigorous hydration (saline and mannitol) can protect to some degree. Concomitant diuretics and aminoglycoside antibiotics should be avoided. Hydration should be continued for 24 hours after cisplatin. Glomerular function should be monitored regularly and no further cisplatin should normally be given if the GFR falls below 60 ml/min/1.73 m^2. Profound tubular leakage of magnesium and calcium can produce weakness and tetany and require careful replacement. Methotrexate and melphelan can cause further nephrotoxicity in the face of renal impairment, delaying their own clearance and worsening myelosuppression.

Cyclophosphamide and ifosfamide can both cause hemorrhagic cystitis. Regular voiding and hydration for 24 hours after administration are essential. The metabolites can be inactivated by concomitant 2-mercaptoethane sulfonate sodium (Mesna).[137]

The alkylators and vincristine can have an antidiuretic hormone effect with resultant fluid overload and dilutional hyponatremia, sometimes resulting in seizures. Urinary flow must be maintained, if necessary with diuretics. Ifosfamide also can produce long-lasting renal tubular defects with hypophosphatemia, clinical rickets and reduction in glomerular filtration rate with cumulative dosage.

The nephrotoxicity of the commonly used antifungal agent amphotericin is an additive problem for these patients. Renal tubular damage can render them dependant upon electrolyte supplementation for prolonged periods. These problems can be largely avoided by the use of the liposomal formulations of this drug.[117]

Cardiotoxicity

The anthracyclines produce cardiotoxicity. Acute toxicity with arrhythmias, conduction defects and fall in left ventricular output is relatively rare, transient and does not absolutely prevent future use of the drugs. Late cardiomyopathy is related to cumulative dosage with the incidence of congestive cardiac failure increasing steeply beyond 450 mg/m^2 of doxorubicin. Echocardiography and endomyocardial biopsies have, however, demonstrated functional abnormalities at much lower cumulative dosages.[138] Dose rate and infusion time both affect toxicity.[139] Studies have reported echocardiographic changes in children who have received only 200–250 mg/m^2 of doxorubicin.[140] Up to 5% of patients will develop anthracycline-induced clinical heart failure 15 years after treatment, and those receiving more than 300 mg/m^2 are at highest risk.[141] Careful monitoring of ventricular function is mandatory when using these agents.

Neurotoxicity

Vincristine can produce peripheral neuropathy (ranging from loss of ankle jerks during therapy, through foot drop (5%), wrist drop (2%) to slapping gait and paresthesia of extremities), and rarely convulsions and encephalopathy.[142] The central effects may be complicated by an antidiuretic hormone effect with dilutional hyponatremia and seizures. The neuropathy can be very painful and is effectively treated with either amitriptyline[143] or gabapentin.[144] Encephalopathy has been recorded with leukemic induction therapy of weekly vincristine. However, such patients receive concomitant l-asparaginase and intrathecal methotrexate both of which can induce seizures and encephalopathic features.

CNS-directed therapy in leukemia can cause a leukoencephalopathy, most commonly if intrathecal or systemic methotrexate is administered after cranial irradiation. The least toxic modality is continuing intrathecal methotrexate alone (see below); ifosfamide produces an encephalopathy more commonly in adults than children.[145]

Ototoxicity

Platinum analogues, especially cisplatin, cause progressive high frequency hearing loss with increasing cumulative dosage. Tinnitus and, especially if combined with cranial irradiation, rapid deterioration of hearing can occur.[146]

Hepatotoxicity

Oral methotrexate can induce a cirrhotic state and mercaptopurine can cause cholestatic jaundice. High dose methotrexate can induce florid hepatic disturbance with mucositis and severe myelosuppression (more likely if combined with other drugs cleared by the liver). Actinomycin and anthracyclines should be avoided if possible for the first 4–6 weeks following abdominal (liver encroachment) irradiation. These and busulphan/cyclophosphamide conditioning for transplantation have been associated with veno-occlusive disease (VOD). This condition presents with hepatomegaly, ascites, encephalopathy and thrombocytopenia 5–10 days after actinomycin treatment.[147] An incidence of 1.2% has been reported for this condition in patients treated on the IRS IV protocol,[148] and as high as 8% for children treated for Wilms tumor.[149] There is no effective treatment and it can be associated with multi-organ failure and death. A strong case can be made for the avoidance of actinomycin in patients who have even a mild episode of VOD.

Biochemical disturbance

Rapid tumor cell breakdown, either after treatment or spontaneously, can result in tumor lysis syndrome, seen most commonly in T and B cell lymphoblastic disorders. Hyperkalemia, hyperphosphatemia, and consequent hypocalcemia, hyperuricemia, and urate nephropathy are seen. The risks can be reduced by gradual introduction of chemotherapy, often with a steroid pre-phase, hyperhydration (125 ml/m^2/h), allopurinol (10 mg/kg/day in divided doses) and careful urinary alkalinization with bicarbonate. In patients at greatest risk of tumor lysis syndrome recombinant urate oxidase (rasburicase) is highly effective at preventing its development.[150]

Acute psychological effects

Painful procedures and toxic therapy can become intolerable for the child unless kept to a minimum. The family need to make the child realize the absolute need for such treatment and must expect and tolerate the natural reaction to it and show that they care for their child as a special individual. The pediatric oncologist must support and help the whole family. The parents must know and understand the diagnosis and the effect of treatment if the child is to come through emotionally intact. The initial shock at the diagnosis precludes 'real' hearing and, subsequently, phases of anger at the apparent injustice are often misdirected at the staff.[151] Excess optimism or pessimism must be avoided but if treatment is offered and accepted, some feeling of hope must be conveyed. Involvement in nursing their child often provides a sense of purpose for parents. As they come to terms with the shock of diagnosis, parents frequently ask more searching questions which must be answered truthfully. If more than one member of staff explains matters, it is essential to stress that words used may be different but the meaning is the same. The caring team must be coordinated, and unit meetings are essential for this purpose. There are a few genuine circumstances where the extent of disease or nature of tumor diagnosis precludes cure. For such a child where there is no realistic treatment option and if parents agree, support for the whole family is even more important. Parents must realize that they are always told the truth, 'good' means good and the converse is true about any bad news. Parents may wish their child to be protected from the facts of the disease and diagnosis, but for the majority of children this is a mistake. Children are usually much more resilient than adults and provided appropriate words are used, and they have confidence in the person conveying the problem, they can cope admirably with even the worst of news. Time is necessary to build up confidence for the child and parents, and if such time is not spent at the beginning, management will become fraught with problems. Secrets about the disease within the family, especially keeping facts from siblings, is also unwise. When trust has developed, even if treatment fails and the patient becomes terminal, the team can usually support the patient and family through the final illness more adequately.

For teenagers the news of cancer and its necessary treatment can be particularly hard as it inevitably requires compliance with and dependence upon those from who they are striving to emotionally separate. They require great understanding and sometimes even a little support in their rebellion.

The involvement of a dedicated child psychiatrist in the team who can help staff to understand family interactions and can guide both staff and family through specific crises has proved very useful in many oncology centers. It may be that help is required by specific families where stress has become too great or where previous psychopathology is present. Cancer does not select specific families but affects the spectrum of the population independent of intelligence, insight and behavior.

LONG TERM SEQUELAE

There are many potential long term sequelae of childhood cancer survivors and these are summarized in Table 24.9.

Late recurrence

Hawkins[152] followed up over 11 000, 3-year cancer survivors, for at least 10 further years (Table 24.10). Overall 75% of late deaths were due to either treatment or recurrence of primary disease. No excess late deaths were seen in patients treated for non-Hodgkin lymphoma and nongenetic retinoblastoma, and were very rare in children treated for

Table 24.9 Potential long term sequelae of childhood cancer

Late recurrence of primary cancer
Second malignancy
Impairment of normal growth
Endocrine dysfunction
Infertility
Educational and psychological dysfunction
Other organ toxicity, e.g. cardiac, pulmonary
Impairment of normal life, e.g. obtaining work, insurance, being allowed to adopt children

Table 24.10 Long term survivors in childhood cancer. (Data derived from Hawkins 1989[152])

Tumor type	% of survivors at 3 years still alive at +10 years	Excess deaths (per n survivors at + 10 years)
Acute lymphoblastic leukemia	60	1 in 100
Hodgkin disease	74	< 1 in 100
Non-Hodgkin lymphoma	85	None
Neuroblastoma	89	< 1 in 200
Nephroblastoma	94	< 1 in 200
Retinoblastoma		
Genetic	93	1 in 200
Nongenetic	100	None

nephroblastoma and neuroblastoma. Late excess deaths in ALL were due to recurrent leukemia, which has been seen more than 10 years from diagnosis. Excess deaths in patients with genetic retinoblastoma and Hodgkin disease were due to second tumors rather than recurrence of primary disease.

Second tumors

The incidence of second tumors has been reported as 8% at 20 years from diagnosis (15 times higher than the general population at this age range).[153] It is inevitable that this incidence reflects therapeutic strategies of the past, and not those which we currently employ. Whilst survival overall may be better than twenty years ago, and thus the number of treated patients at risk for second tumors may be increasing, it is also possible that the reduction in the use of some treatment modalities, such as craniospinal irradiation for ALL, may reduce the risk of second tumors. Patients with 'genetic' retinoblastoma and Hodgkin disease were most likely to develop second tumors and the risk factors were identified as genetic susceptibility (with an Rb1 gene mutation up to 30% of patients will develop a second tumor[27]) and the combination of irradiation with alkylating agents in Hodgkin disease.[153,154] Other genetic disorders predisposing to multiple malignancies in childhood include Li–Fraumeni syndrome, neurofibromatosis type 1 and Gorlin syndrome. Two thirds of all the second solid tumors occurred within radiation fields (30% being soft tissue or bony sarcomas). These tumors have a long latency with a median time to diagnosis of 10–15 years. Total dosage greater than 30 Gy, old-style orthovoltage treatment and young age at treatment all increased the risk.[83,155] Secondary leukemia was associated in a dose dependant fashion with previous treatment with alkylating agents.[83] Secondary acute nonlymphoblastic leukemia with a shorter latency period (median 30 months) than with alkylating agents (median 5–7 years) has been increasingly described in patients exposed to topoisomerase 2 inhibitors such as etoposide. The risk appears to be total dose and schedule dependent.[84,156] The risk of developing second tumors after treatment for acute lymphoblastic leukemia appears to be relatively low at 2.5–3% at 15–20 years from diagnosis and the commonest tumors seen are gliomas and meningiomas in cranial irradiation fields.[157,158] The risk continues to increase with time from treatment well beyond 20 years.[159]

Growth impairment

Direct radiation damage to the hypothalamic–pituitary axis from cranial irradiation impairs growth hormone secretion and in higher dose also gonadotrophic and adrenocorticotrophic hormone secretion.[160] Precocious puberty can occur in children receiving cranial irradiation and young age at treatment increases the risk. Puberty may be both premature and foreshortened, further reducing final height and giving less time during which growth hormone replacement can be delivered. Growth hormone may need to be given in combination with gonadotrophin releasing hormone (GnRH) to attempt to arrest pubertal maturation. Growth hormone replacement may be less effective in gaining height for such patients than it is in idiopathic growth hormone deficiency. Growth hormone therapy appears totally safe to administer to patients with previous malignancies provided at least 1 year (but normally 2 years) have elapsed from treatment, and the patient is in full remission. To date there has been no convincing evidence of tumor reactivation or induction of second malignancies by growth hormone.[161]

The use of more intensive chemotherapy with cranial irradiation for childhood leukemia appears to increase the risk of growth impairment and there is increased likelihood of body disproportion with short spines in children treated with craniospinal irradiation and chemotherapy.[162,163] These children also have altered body composition with central obesity, hyperleptinemia[164] and reduced bone mineral density.[165] It is essential that all children who receive irradiation and intensive chemotherapy should be regularly assessed for linear growth, pubertal status and weight on a long term basis until they have reached maturity.

Thyroid dysfunction

Radiation damage results in a rise in thyroid stimulating hormone (TSH) and then hypothyroidism. This follows total body, craniospinal and local neck irradiation. Low doses (100 cGy) may be sufficient. Thyroid adenomas and carcinomas have been reported.[166] Persistent TSH elevation on follow-up requires replacement even in the absence of clinical or biochemical hypothyroidism.

Gonadal dysfunction and infertility

The germinal epithelium of the testis, from which the spermatozoa develop, is exquisitely sensitive to radiation and to cytotoxic drugs. Radiation doses as low as 1.2 Gy can result in permanent azoospermia.[167] The effects of cytotoxic agents are more variable but alkylating agents are particularly associated with poor sperm counts,[168] and procarbazine-containing regimens for Hodgkin disease can induce azoospermia in up to 97% of patients.[169] The gonadotoxicity of many chemotherapy regimens remains undefined and thus it is probably wise to recommend sperm banking for all post-pubertal boys, unless they are receiving a regimen which has been shown not to be gonadotoxic. Leydig cell function is far less sensitive than spermatogenesis, so many of these patients will develop normal secondary sexual characteristics and undergo a normal puberty.[168] Female gonadal dysfunction after treatment is much harder to predict than in males. Ovarian damage is related to both radiation and cytotoxic therapy, and to age at therapy; so that the younger the girl the more likely it is that she will recover ovarian function with time after treatment.[168] However procarbazine-containing regimens are still likely to impair female fertility; half of all pre-pubertal girls treated with 6 cycles of ChLVPP had elevated FSH, and 60% of these developed symptomatic ovarian failure requiring hormone replacement.[169] Irradiation decreases uterine volume, blood flow and endometrial thickness, and these changes are not usually reversible with androgen replacement. It is thus important to consider not just ovarian function when evaluating female fertility.[170] At present there are no nonexperimetal techniques for the preservation of female fertility, but it is likely that these will become available reasonably soon.

Gonadal function is also affected by hypothalamic-pituitary damage from radiation and it is thus important to monitor FSH and LH levels in patients who have received cranial radiotherapy.[168] It is valuable to have an endocrinologist involved in the long term follow-up and management of childhood cancer survivors.

Educational and psychosocial effects

Time lost from nursery and schooling at critical stages of learning may impair educational achievement. This may result from illness, sequelae of treatment and parental anxiety about allowing the child to mix in 'society'. CNS directed radiation therapy for leukemia and CNS tumors produces long standing neuropsychological sequelae including cognitive dysfunction, short term memory impairment and difficulties in problem solving. Young age at the time of treatment (especially under 3 years) increases the risk of damage.[171] The combined effect of cranial irradiation in leukemia patients on both growth and educational achievement has led to alternative CNS directed strategies being utilized. Such approaches are effective in controlling CNS disease but are not totally without effect on neuropsychological functioning.[172]

The incidence of long term overt psychological and psychiatric problems appears remarkably low among cancer survivors. However, many patients, particularly those who have received cranial irradiation, appear to be 'loners' with low self-esteem, working but in undemanding jobs and are much less likely than their peers to be in long term relationships. Child–parent relationships and life-long family coping does seem to influence psychological outcome. The impact of 'waiting for a relapse' is too much for some families to cope with.[173] Nevertheless the vast majority of childhood cancer patients complete normal education and have higher rates of employment than their matched peers.[174] Some face outdated prejudice from employers, some insurance and pension schemes (excessive weighting of premiums long term) and have difficulty in being considered as adoptees when rendered infertile by treatment.

Cardiorespiratory

Acute cardiac effects after anthracycline drugs have been described above, but the extent of the long term effects on endocardial muscle remains controversial. There are reports of sudden death after strenuous exercise or during pregnancy, and deteriorating cardiac function only rescued by cardiac transplantation in others. Total anthracycline doses in excess of 200 mg/m^2 have been associated with long term echocardiographic changes but it is not clear how many progress to overt cardiac disease.[175]

Sixty-five per cent of 5-year leukemia survivors in one study showed one or more defects of low vital capacity, total lung capacity, residual volume or transfer factor[176] but very few were symptomatic. These features represent impairment of lung growth during the first 5–6 years of life. This may be of significance, especially among smokers, later in life. Amongst solid tumor survivors chest wall growth impairment, restriction defects and/or fibrosis are more frequently identified, especially where the lungs have been irradiated.[177,178]

Conclusions on sequelae

Without intensive treatment most children with cancer died 30–40 years ago. Now approximately 70% survive long term and most have good quality of life. Some sequelae such as gonadal failure and infertility may be an acceptable, if regrettable, price for cure but second tumors and late cardiac deaths are not. It is essential that all childhood cancer patients are followed for life so that lessons can be learnt and therapy modified where appropriate without any loss of efficacy.

CENTRAL NERVOUS SYSTEM TUMORS

Central nervous system tumors as a group are the commonest solid tumors of childhood, accounting for about 25% of all pediatric malignant disease.[179] Recognized etiologic factors are shown in Table 24.11, and Table 24.12 shows the incidence of different childhood brain tumors. The primary CNS tumors of childhood are a highly disparate group; application of the revised WHO classification is probably the best approach to their categorization.[180] The vast majority of childhood CNS tumors arise from neuroepithelial tissues (the principle exceptions are intracranial germ cell tumors and craniopharyngioma). The WHO classification divides neuroepithelial tumors into: 1) glial (which includes all gliomas, ependymomas and choroid plexus tumors); 2) neuronal; 3) mixed neuronal-glial; 4) embryonal (which includes primitive neuroectodermal tumor (PNET)) and 5) pineal cell tumors. With modern immunohistochemistry and molecular biological methods it is possible

Table 24.11 Etiological factors for CNS tumors

Heritable syndromes
    Neurofibromatosis (visual pathway tumors + gliomas)
    Tuberous sclerosis (glial ependymomas)
    Von Hippel–Lindau (cerebellar + retinal + pheochromocytomas)

Familial clustering without identifiable genetic factor (various tumors including pinealomas)

Familial with autosomal dominant inheritance: astrocytoma

Retinoblastoma and pinealoblastoma (13q-)

Rhabdoid renal tumors and primitive neuroectodermal tumors of brain

Monosomy 22: meningiomas + acoustic neuromas

Ionizing irradiation: after low dose scalp irradiation and possible dental investigations

Immunodeficiency (intracerebral lymphomas) especially:
    a. Postrenal transplantation
    b. Wiskott–Aldrich
    c. Ataxia telangiectasia

Parental exposure to organic compounds such as nitrosamines and polycyclic hydrocarbons

Table 24.12 Relative incidence of CNS neoplasms in childhood (1981–1990) with male/female ratio of each group of tumors. (Data from Parkin et al 1998[3])

Tumor type	%	M/F ratio
Astrocytoma	38.3	1.1
Primitive neuro-ectodermal tumors	21.2	1.7
Ependymoma	10.8	1.4
Other gliomas	15.2	1.1
Other specified	8.6	1.1
Unspecified	5.9	0.9

to accurately identify the cells within CNS tumors. Commonly used neuronal antibodies such as glial fibrillary acidic protein (GFAP) and neurofilament protein (NFP) are coupled with non-neuronal markers such as smooth muscle actin (SMA), epithelial membrane antigen (EMA), keratin, vimentin, desmin and AFP to assign a diagnosis.

SYMPTOMS AND SIGNS

The presenting symptoms and signs of brain tumors in childhood depend more on the site than on type of tumor. Neurological features are due to infiltration, compression of neuronal structures or raised intracranial pressure (ICP) secondary to obstruction of CSF pathways. Raised ICP presents early in the majority of the infratentorial tumors with the classic triad of morning headache, vomiting and visual disturbance. There may be more vague symptoms of tiredness, deteriorating school performance, personality change and nonlocalized headache for a variable period before this. Headaches in young children should always be taken seriously and investigated. Infants may present with irritability, loss of appetite and developmental delay or regression. Infants under 2 years may develop an increase in the occipitofrontal circumference (OFC) with springing of the sutures as intracranial pressure increases and in babies the 'setting sun' sign may be seen. Fundi are frequently pale with just the early signs of papilledema. Fundal examination can be very difficult and sedation and pupillary dilatation may be appropriate. Developmental assessment should be part of the full examination. Specific signs depend on the site of the tumor.

Infratentorial lesions

Raised ICP and disturbance of balance (truncal and extremity) and specific cranial nerve dysfunction are the cardinal signs of the well-established tumor. Midline medulloblastomas may present only with raised intracranial pressure and truncal unsteadiness and without localizing features while cerebellar hemisphere lesions may present early with lateralizing features. It is, however, usually not possible to distinguish between astrocytoma and medulloblastoma clinically. VI nerve palsy may be a false localizing sign arising from raised intracranial pressure. When present bilaterally and especially when in combination with 5th, 7th or 9th nerve palsies, brainstem involvement is likely. Head tilt is frequently seen together with cochlear nerve palsy and vertical or horizontal diplopia when cerebellar tonsillar herniation occurs.

Supratentorial lesions

Both the site and the size of the tumor determine the presenting signs. With these lesions nonspecific headaches, seizures of all types and long tract signs may predominate. Raised ICP may be the first sign of tumors in relatively silent areas of the cortex (frontal, parietal or occipital) and the tumor may be very large. Raised pressure may be an early feature in small third ventricular lesions. Visual field defects may help to localize tumors. In primitive neuroectodermal tumors dissemination throughout the CNS via the cerebrospinal fluid may lead to symptoms and signs far removed from the primary lesion with consequent diagnostic confusion. Careful documentation of all signs and symptoms in the order that they appear is important.

DIAGNOSIS

Widespread availability of MR scanning has revolutionized the diagnosis of pediatric brain tumors. CT is useful for rapid identification of hydrocephalus and mass effect but MR is far better at defining tumor anatomy and extent.[181] Positron emission tomography (PET) may prove useful in detecting variations in metabolism between residual tumor and normal brain, and MR spectroscopy may also prove useful in noninvasive diagnosis.[182] For PNETs, exclusion of spinal deposits by MR scanning is essential.

GENERAL PRINCIPLES OF TREATMENT

Surgery

Preoperative steroids to reduce edema, external decompression of hydrocephalus and new scanning techniques have facilitated more complete surgical removal of visible tumor without increased morbidity. Extent of excision is a determinant of outcome for many tumor types.[183,184] Midline posterior fossa tumors more frequently require long term ventriculoperitoneal shunting. There is no evidence that this increases the likelihood of extracerebral metastases. Operative mortality for most tumors has been reduced to under 1%, although morbidity may be as high as 20%.

Radiotherapy[185]

Fields and volumes treated should be limited to minimize normal tissue damage. High grade astrocytomas do require whole brain irradiation and ependymomas, PNETs and some germ cell tumors, craniospinal irradiation. Although local areas can tolerate total dosages as high as 50–55 Gy, whole brain dosages over 35 Gy are associated with significant sequelae. Fraction size, number of fractions and duration of treatment all influence toxicity.

Acute radiation side-effects include headache, vomiting, skin erythema, alopecia and otitis externa. Lymphopenia is universal and may persist for 6 months. Profound myelosuppression may follow spinal irradiation and make subsequent chemotherapy difficult to deliver. Five to ten weeks after cranial irradiation 'somnolence syndrome' can occur (profound sleepiness and mild pyrexia) owing to a temporary disturbance of myelination. A similar effect on the spine produces Lhermitte sign (shooting arm pains).

Chemotherapy

The vulnerability of the developing CNS to radiation-induced damage, coupled with the poor survival for many types of tumor has resulted in considerable interest in the role of chemotherapy. The blood–brain barrier limits access to the brain of most drugs. At the margins of tumors, the tight capillary endothelial junctions persist, while neoplastic neovascularity makes the core of tumors more accessible. Lipid solubility, molecular size, protein binding and plasma concentration all determine the ability of a drug to penetrate the CNS. Lipophilic drugs (e.g. nitrosoureas) will penetrate tumor margins and water-soluble agents (e.g. cisplatinum) the core. The initial goal of many of the early studies of chemotherapy for CNS tumors was to delay or avoid radiotherapy especially in the very young. A large number of such 'baby brain' studies have now been reported with varying degrees of success,[186] and such a strategy is now routinely adopted for most infants. The use of multiagent chemotherapy with curative intent is variable between tumor types and for most randomized prospective trials are only just beginning to be done to determine the role of chemotherapy in a multimodality treatment plan.

GLIAL TUMORS

ASTROCYTOMAS

Astrocytomas are by far the commonest pediatric brain tumor and the majority are low grade. Low grade and high grade astrocytomas are very different and are best considered as separate tumor types.

Low grade glioma (LGG)

This group contains a number of histologically different types of astrocyte or oligodendrocyte derived tumor, but all are WHO grade I or II.[180]

Between 30% and 40% of all pediatric primary CNS tumors are low grade gliomas. The commonest site is the cerebellar hemispheres (35%), and then the cerebral hemispheres (20%), hypothalamus (12%), thalamus (12%), brainstem (12%), spinal cord (4%) and optic nerve (3%). One third of children are less than 5 years at diagnosis[187] and the median age of presentation is around 7 years. The male to female ratio is approximately 1:1. Between 5% and 15% of patients with NF-1 will develop LGG of optic tract or hypothalamus.[188] Subependymal giant cell astrocytomas are seen in up to 15% of patients with tuberous sclerosis,[189] and LGG is also seen in patients with Li–Fraumeni syndrome.

Presentation

This is dependent upon the tumor site. Posterior fossa tumors tend to present relatively early with signs of raised intracranial pressure; morning headache and vomiting, and with cerebellar signs such as ataxia. Supratentorial tumors may also present with signs of raised ICP but they are more likely to have seizures or motor symptoms. Optic tract tumors cause visual disturbance which can be difficult to detect in younger children, and hypothalamic tumors usually present with endocrinopathy. The presentation of spinal tumors is often insidious in onset with weakness, pain, sensory change, change in gait and eventually sphincter dysfunction.

Diagnosis

Low grade gliomas are hypo- or iso-dense on MRI on T1 and hyperdense on T2. They may be solid or cystic and usually enhance with gadolinium. Histologically the juvenile pilocytic astrocytoma and the fibrillary astrocytoma are the commonest variants. The most frequent cytogenetic abnormality is gain of chromosome 7 and 8.[190] NF-1 is associated with optic tract gliomas, and up to a third of patients with these tumors may have NF-1.[191] Low grade gliomas are not usually metatstatic and transformation to high grade tumors is rare.

Management

The guiding principle for the management of these tumors is to achieve local control without inflicting major morbidity on the patient. The approach is thus dependent on the site of the tumor and the age of the patient. Cerebral hemisphere and cerebellar tumors can usually be fully resected without major morbidity; in series up to 90% of patients achieved gross total resection.[187] These patients have extremely good survival with most series giving 90–100%. Progression free survival (PFS) is significantly worse for patients with residual disease. Although there are no randomized trials comparing radiotherapy with no treatment for these patients local radiotherapy for patients with gross residual disease in cerebral hemispheres or cerebellum has been traditionally given. There is however no evidence that it improves survival. Optic and hypothalamic tumors cannot usually be resected. For these patients radiotherapy is effective in controlling symptoms and disease progression.[192] The devastating late effects of radiotherapy on younger children have lead to considerable interest in the use of chemotherapy for these patients with vincristine and carboplatin in various schedules being increasingly accepted as standard therapy. The success of such a strategy has been variable, some series report excellent PFS for younger children, while in others the PFS is worse in the younger age group.[193,194] The current SIOP strategy for low grade gliomas includes all low grade (WHO I–II) tumors anywhere in the CNS, except diffuse intrinsic pontine gliomas. The strategy is complex and takes into account extent of surgery, age, and presence of NF 1. The fundamental principle is to resect the tumor if possible. Patients with completely resected tumors are observed and only treated if they relapse or progress. Patients with incompletely resected or inoperable tumors are observed and treated according to progression of disease or severity of neurological symptoms; for example a patient with optic glioma with severe visual disturbance such that their eyesight is threatened. These patients receive radiotherapy only if older than 8 years, or chemotherapy with vincristine and carboplatin for 16 months if younger than 8. All children with NF1 receive chemo- rather than radiotherapy. For children less than 8 years without NF1 the study is evaluating the effectiveness of adding etoposide to the induction chemotherapy.

High Grade Glioma (HGG)

These are WHO grade III–IV tumors and account for 7–11% of childhood brain tumors. Although the outlook is slightly better than for adults the overall survival remains extremely poor. Some may develop from previous LGG, and they are also seen after radiotherapy, and in the same tumor predisposing conditions as LGG.

Presentation

Most HGG are thalamic or in the cerebral hemispheres and as such tend to present with seizures, motor symptoms or raised ICP.

Diagnosis

HGG are usually infiltrative lesions and MRI will show an area of edema surrounding the tumor itself, which is often of heterogenous density and variable enhancement after gadolinium (Fig. 24.1). Metastatic

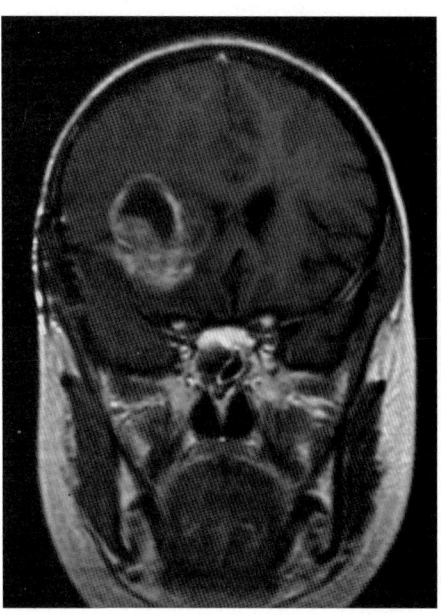
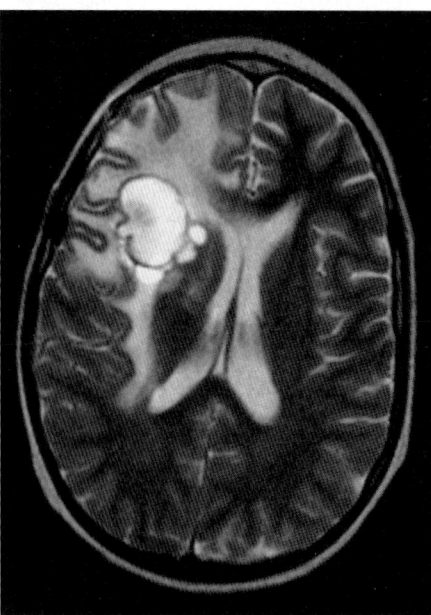

(a)   (b)

Fig. 24.1 (a) T1-weighted coronal MR scan post gadolinium showing a high grade glioma of the right frontoparietal lobe, with cystic and solid components. (b) T2-weighted axial MR scan showing the same tumor with extensive signal change in the right frontoparietal lobe around the solid/cystic tumor.

disease and extensive local spread along neuronal pathways are both common. Histologically these are less differentiated, more cellular and pleomorphic tumors than LGG.

Management

The mainstay of the treatment of HGG is extensive surgical resection and radiotherapy. Extensive resection does seem to improve survival for both anaplastic astrocytoma and glioblastoma.[195] Several randomized studies in adults have shown a significant benefit with radiotherapy, and there is evidence that doses up to 60 Gy improve survival compared to lower doses.[196] Given the poor outcome for these patients much work has been produced on the use of chemotherapy. Combinations of CCNU, vincristine and prednisolone have long been used in the US with evidence of improved survival in comparison to radiotherapy alone.[197] Intensification of chemotherapy has been tried by a number of groups and the combination of ifosfamide, etoposide, methotrexate, cisplatin and cytarabine preradiotherapy produced a highly significant survival benefit in comparison to radiotherapy followed by the European standard regimen procarbazine, CCNU and vincristine (PCV).[198] The current UK and French study for these patients is evaluating the use of the combination of cisplatin and temozolamide, which appeared promising in phase I studies.[199]

BRAINSTEM TUMORS

Brainstem tumors collectively account for 10–15% of childhood CNS malignancies. The median age at presentation is between 5 and 10 years and there is no sex difference. Seventy-five per cent occur in the pons and the rest in the medulla and midbrain. About 50% are low grade gliomas, 35–40% are high grade astrocytomas, and 10% are ependymomas and PNETs.

Presentation

Brainstem tumors can be considered in two groups, favorable and unfavorable. The favorable tumors are focal intrinsic, dorsal exophytic and cervicomedullary junction. These are usually pilocytic astrocytomas. Focal intrinsic tumors are usually found in the medulla and the midbrain. They are slow growing and present with either CSF obstruction or cranial nerve deficits according to site. Dorsal exophytic tumors arise from the floor of the fourth ventricle and do not usually invade the brainstem. Again they usually present with symptoms of CSF obstruction, and lesions of the IX–XII cranial nerves. Cervicomedullary junction tumors arise from the top of the spinal cord and grow up through the foramen magnum to compress the medulla. They usually present with lesions of IX-XII cranial nerves. Unfavorable brainstem tumors are diffuse intrinsic pontine tumors, PNETs and atypical teratoid/rhabdoid tumors. Diffuse intrinsic pontine gliomas account for 70% of brainstem tumors. These tumors present with a very short history of multiple bilateral cranial nerve defects.

Diagnosis

MRI is the imaging modality of choice for patients with a suspected brainstem lesion. All the tumor types described above appear hypodense on T1-weighted images and hyperintense on T2-weighted images. Low grade gliomas usually enhance briskly after gadolinium, whist intrinsic pontine tumors enhance poorly (Fig. 24.2).

Management

For cervicomedullary junction tumors complete resection can be achieved in the majority of patients with excellent long term control.[200] For dorsal exophytic tumors it is always necessary to leave a layer of tumor on the floor of the fourth ventricle. However again most of these patients do well.[201] Resection of focal intrinsic tumors is difficult and should only be attempted on easily accessible tumors with the imaging characteristics of pilocytic astrocytomas. For diffuse pontine glioma the clinical and radiological appearances are so characteristic that even biopsy is unnecessary, and may worsen the patient's neurological

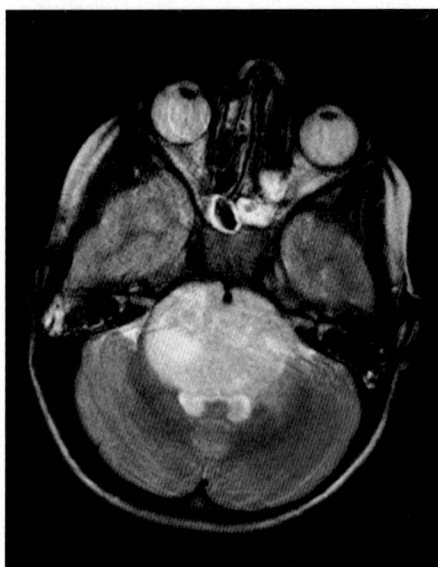

Fig. 24.2   T2-weighted axial MR scan showing a diffuse intrinsic pontine glioma.

condition.[202] Radiotherapy is indicated for favorable tumor types that cannot be safely surgically resected, or where there is progression after resection. 54 Gy delivered in 30 fractions results in tumor control in most patients.[203] Radiotherapy, again with 54 Gy in 30 fractions is indicated for patients with diffuse pontine tumors and will rapidly improve symptoms in most patients. However survival is extremely poor (20% at 2 years).[204] Hyperfractionated therapy (total dose up to 72 Gy) has proved disappointing.[205] To date no clear benefit has been shown from chemotherapy in either favorable or unfavorable brainstem tumors.[206]

EPENDYMOMA

These arise from the lining of the ventricular system and central canal of the spinal cord (75% in the posterior fossa, 25% in the cord). Half the cases occur before the age of 5. There is considerable variation in anaplasia, pleomorphism and differentiation. The *subependymoma* is often silent and found coincidentally at autopsy. Spinal subarachnoid space involvement is much more likely with infratentorial tumors (20–30%) than with the supratentorial tumors (3–8%). High grade ependymomas may disseminate within the CNS through the CSF but systemic spread is rare.

Presentation

Raised intracranial pressure is common in all posterior fossa tumors. There may be some cerebellar dysfunction. Local cranial nerve deficits are more commonly seen than in medulloblastoma because of local infiltration and invasion of the floor of the fourth ventricle and brainstem. Supratentorial ependymomas more commonly present with seizures and long tract signs. The duration of the history depends on the site and the grade of the tumor.

Diagnosis

CT scans will show a hyperdense and contrast-enhancing tumor with hydrocephalus; MR scanning will delineate tumor relations and spinal CSF metastases (Fig. 24.3). CSF examination is needed operatively.

Prognostic features

Spinal cord and especially myxopapillary cauda equina tumors fare better but otherwise site is not of prognostic significance. It is unclear for ependymomas whether histology (anaplasia) or degree of resection are of significance.[207] Young age (<5 years) and brainstem invasion do adversely affect outcome.

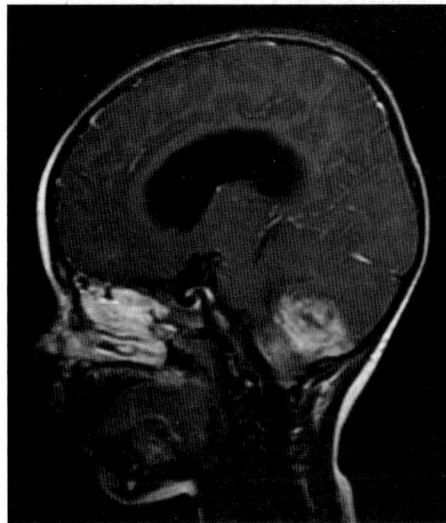

Fig. 24.3 T1-weighted sagittal MR scan post gadolinium showing a posterior fossa ependymoma.

Management

Attempts at primary total resection are indicated and usually possible for supratentorial tumors, less so in the posterior fossa where brainstem infiltration increases perioperative morbidity (5–10%). With surgery alone 5-year survival is 15–20%. For supratentorial tumors extended local field irradiation to a total dose of 50–55 Gy and for posterior fossa lesions a field to extend down to C3–4 are indicated. Most relapses are local but 10–15% have subarachnoid spread. This may be greater in posterior fossa and anaplastic tumors; for them, craniospinal irradiation has been recommended. For low grade tumors, surgery and extended field radiotherapy yield 50% 5-year survival. Intramedullary spinal cord tumors may be cured by complete microsurgical resection. Chemotherapy has not been shown to significantly improve survival.[208] The current SIOP study gives vincristine, cyclophosphamide and etoposide to patients with residual disease after surgery, before radiotherapy.

CHOROID PLEXUS NEOPLASMS

These are extremely rare tumors accounting for only about 0.5% of all childhood CNS tumors. Most occur before 2 years of age. Most occur in the lateral ventricles and are intraventricular papillomas which secrete CSF. About 15% are slow-growing carcinomas which can reach huge dimensions and can metastasize.

Presentation

This is usually with raised intracranial pressure and hydrocephalus (they can produce CSF up to four times the normal rate) owing to ventricular obstruction with or without hemorrhage. CT scan will show hydrocephalus and an isodense to hyperdense intraventricular tumor with contrast enhancement and often with calcification, MRI will show where the fronds of the tumor extend into the ventricles.

Management

Surgery is the treatment of choice but there is a high mortality and morbidity. For papillomas, curative complete resection appears to be possible in between 75 and 100%. Shunting may be necessary to relieve persistent hydrocephalus. For the papillomas there is no need for further therapy. For carcinomas degree of surgical resection seems to be a prognostic factor.[209] Radiotherapy seems to improve survival[210] and there are some reports of a role for chemotherapy.

EMBRYONAL TUMORS

MEDULLOBLASTOMA (PNET OF CEREBELLUM)

This is a midline PNET usually arising from the cerebellar vermis in the roof of the fourth ventricle. All PNETs tend to seed within the CSF, and up to 35% of medulloblastomas may have metastatic disease at presentation. The peak age incidence is 5 years. There is a male preponderance.

Presentation

Obstruction of the fourth ventricle leads to raised intracranial pressure, progressive ataxia of the lower limbs, diplopia, and 5th, 7th and other cranial nerve deficits. Long tract signs appear rather later. Nuchal rigidity and/or head tilt suggests cerebellar tonsillar herniation and necessity for rapid relief. The differential diagnosis includes cerebellar astrocytoma, ependymoma, brainstem glioma, and infectious encephalitis (although the last is usually of more acute onset). CT scan shows a solid homogeneous, iso- or hyperdense lesion which is enhanced by contrast but these features are not unique to medulloblastoma (Fig. 24.4a). An MR scan may more easily differentiate a medulloblastoma from the other tumors by clearly showing the site of origin (Fig. 24.4b).[211] Lumbar CSF examination should *not* be performed before surgery.

Prognostic features

Young children (under 3) have a poorer prognosis than older children and are generally considered unsuitable for craniospinal radiotherapy because of the profound neurodevelopmental sequelae. Meningeal enhancement on MR of brain or spine is sufficient evidence of metastatic disease (Chang stage M2/3) and is associated with worse prognosis. The presence of isolated tumor cells in the CSF (Chang stage M1) is now accepted to confer a poorer prognosis.[212] The prognostic significance of gross total resection is disputed with some studies showing a survival advantage[212] and others not (HIT 91). The commonest genetic abnormality in medulloblastoma is deletion of 17p, seen in 40–50% of tumors although the prognostic significance of this finding is debated.[213] High expression of ErbB2 and ErbB4 are associated with more aggressive tumors and worse prognosis.[214] MYC oncogene amplification is seen in only 6% of medulloblastomas but is associated with worse outcome.[215]

Pathology

This is a highly cellular soft and friable tumor full of small round undifferentiated cells with hyperchromatic nuclei and abundant mitoses. There can be variable glial or neuroblast differentiation which may be of prognostic significance.

Management

Complete macroscopic resection is achievable in about 50% of cases. These tumors are the most radiosensitive of the primary CNS childhood tumors and radiotherapy is required to the whole neuraxis (36 Gy) with at least 50 Gy to the posterior fossa. Three-year survival figures of up to 60% have been reported for surgical resection followed by craniospinal irradiation.[216] Medulloblastoma has been shown to be chemosensitive in relapse schedules and in vitro. Although early multicenter trials (SIOP I, II) were unable to confirm the survival advantage seen with adjuvant chemotherapy in single-center trials, SIOP PNET 3 showed a significant increase in event free survival (EFS) for patients treated with etoposide, vincristine, cyclophosphamide and carboplatin as opposed to those receiving radiotherapy alone (3-year EFS 78% vs. 65%).[217] Excellent results have also been reported using cisplatin, vincristine and CCNU (Packer chemotherapy)[218,219] and this combination is now the recommended treatment in most studies. These patients have high morbidity from whole CNS irradiation (intellectual impairment and growth) and as a result there has been an impetus toward reducing doses of craniospinal radiation. The current SIOP study for nonmetastatic patients compares reduced dose conventional radiotherapy with hyperfractionated radiotherapy (HFRT) with both groups receiving Packer chemotherapy. In contrast the UK strategy for patients with metastatic disease is to use hyperfractionated accelerated radiotherapy (HART) to deliver a

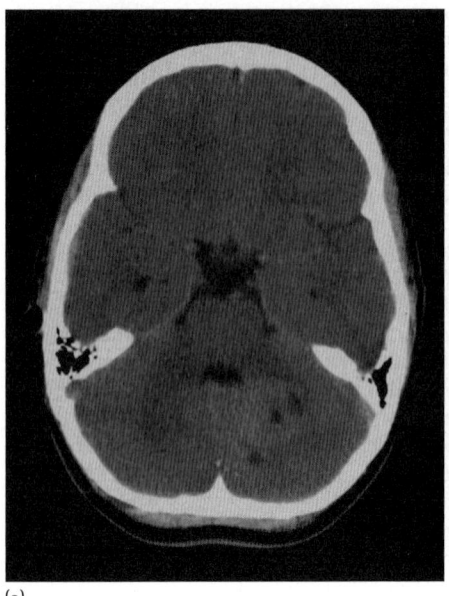
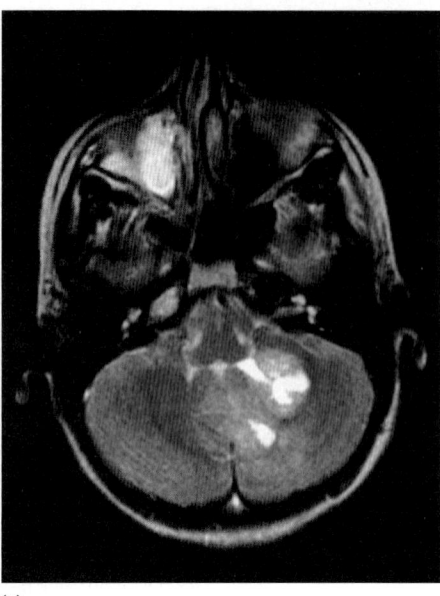

(a)   (b)

Fig. 24.4   (a) Noncontrast CT image of a left-sided medulloblastoma. (b) T2-weighted axial MR scan of the same tumor.

craniospainal dose of 40 Gy, with a total primary dose of 60 Gy to try to improve survival without worsening neurological sequelae.

SUPRATENTORIAL PNETs

Eighty per cent of these tumors occur within the cerebral hemispheres and the remaining 20% in the midline, especially the pineal gland. Historically they have been treated in the same way as medulloblastoma, but there is now evidence that the nonpineal tumors have a significantly worse prognosis with 5-year PFS of 41% compared to 71% for pineal tumors and 78% for medulloblastoma.[220]

Presentation

This is usually with raised intracranial pressure, seizures and motor signs. The time from symptom onset to diagnosis may be quite long (up to 10 months).

Management

Despite adequate surgery, conventional chemotherapy and craniospinal radiotherapy the majority of nonpineal stPNETs recur locally (71% in German studies and 72% in SIOP PNET 3). The current UK strategy is to combine early HART with Packer chemotherapy.

PINEAL TUMORS

Most pineal tumors are germ cell tumors, seen much more commonly in boys and girls in the second decade of life. 20–40% are pineal parenchymal tumors (pinealoblastomas or pinealocytomas) and occur in the first 10 years and more frequently in girls.

Pinealoblastomas are best categorized as PNETs, often showing some differentiation resembling retinoblastoma. Pinealocytomas are generally more differentiated. Pineal tumors spread locally and pinealoblastomas and germinomas may disseminate, but teratomas tend to remain localized.

Presentation

Raised intracranial pressure from third ventricular outflow obstruction is the most common presenting feature. Other signs will depend on the site and the degree of extension of the tumor. The classic presentation of a pineal tumor is with failure of upward gaze (Parinaud syndrome) and pupils that react to accommodation but not to light. Imaging will identify the lesion but not differentiate the type since both teratomas

and parenchymal tumors tend to have irregular mixed density mass lesions with calcification but with a fairly uniform contrast enhancement. CSF examination is needed following decompression particularly in pinealoblastoma and germinoma.

Management

Biopsy is recommended to clarify the diagnosis. It is associated with a high morbidity (though low mortality), with frequent impairment of vision. In well-circumscribed teratomas, excision may be possible but for the rest, where local infiltration is quite common, biopsy with some debulking and relief of hydrocephalus is all that can be achieved with surgery. The primary treatment for the majority is radiotherapy with whole brain irradiation in the region of 35–45 Gy and a boost of 10–15 Gy to the tumor area for germ cell tumors and pinealoblastomas. There is controversy as to who actually needs spinal irradiation. It should probably be judged by the presence or absence of cells in the CSF and MR appearances but some recommend routine whole neuraxis radiation in pinealoblastoma. There is no blood–brain barrier in the pineal region and drugs such as vinblastine, bleomycin, cisplatinum and VP16 have all been shown to have some efficacy in pineal tumors.

INTRACRANIAL GERM CELL TUMORS

These account for about 3% of childhood CNS tumors in the UK. They are most common in the second decade of life. Virtually all are either pineal or suprasellar in location. Up to 20% will present with concurrent primary tumors, and up to 15% will have CSF metastases at diagnosis. The majority of intracranial germ cell tumors are germinomas, the remainder are mature and immature teratomas and the secreting tumors; yolk sac tumors, choriocarcinoma and embryonal carcinoma.

Presentation

The features of pineal tumors are described above. Suprasellar tumors usually present with raised ICP and endocrinopathy, ranging from isolated diabetes insipidus to panhypopituitarism. Visual field deficits related to chiasmal compression are also seen, and some will present with signs of hypothalamic compression, including anorexia. MR imaging of brain and spinal cord are needed because of the risk of CSF seeding. Germinomas are usually relatively homogenous and isodense to brain, with bright enhancement after gadolinium (Fig. 24.5). Teratomas usually contain calcification and are more heterogenous in

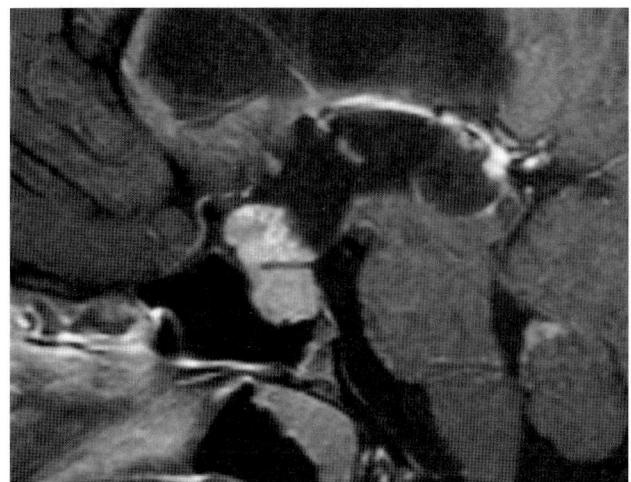

Fig. 24.5 T1-weighted sagittal MR scan showing a suprasellar intracranial germ cell tumor with CSF metastases.

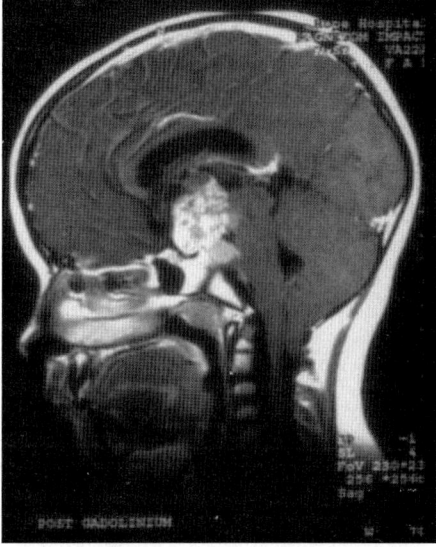

Fig. 24.6 T1-weighted sagittal MR scan post gadolinium showing the typical location and appearance of a craniopharyngioma.

signal intensity. Serum AFP and βHCG should be obtained before surgery and CSF should be examined for tumor cells and levels of AFP and βHCG either pre- or perioperatively. Tissue diagnosis is not mandatory for tumors with elevated serum or CSF markers.

Management

Germinomas are radiosensitive and extensive surgical resection should not be attempted. Craniospinal radiotherapy results in greater than 90% survival in the most recent SIOP germ cell study. Mature teratomas need surgical resection for cure and 93% 10-year survival can be expected, while immature teratomas fare less well, with 75% 10-year survival.[221] In SIOP CNS GCT 96 secreting tumors received four courses of cisplatin, ifosfamide and etoposide, followed by focal or craniospinal radiation. Survival for both groups was around 70%.[222]

CRANIOPHARYNGIOMA

Two thirds of these tumors occur before the age of 20 with a median age of 8 years. There is no sex difference. Craniopharyngioma arises either in the pituitary stalk or from the floor of the third ventricle. They may be solid, mixed or cystic with or without calcification. Although they are frequently well differentiated and benign histologically their close association with the hypothalamus, pituitary and optic chiasm makes their management challenging.

Presentation

The usual presentation of these patients is with the combination of visual failure (secondary to compression of the optic chiasm), endocrinopathy (especially growth failure) and raised ICP (due to obstruction of the third ventricle). Classic diabetes insipidus is relatively rare, seen in only 15%.

Diagnosis

CT scanning will show a cystic low density lesion with contrast enhancement and often considerable calcification. The MR scan may define the solid and cystic components of this tumor better and identify the surrounding anatomy (Fig. 24.6).

Management[223]

For this low grade tumor with visual and neuropsychological disturbances the efficacy of treatment is often difficult to evaluate. With preoperative steroids to reduce pressure and vasopressin to control diabetes insipidus, morbidity and mortality have decreased. Seventy-five to eighty per cent of tumors can be completely removed with recurrence rates of 20–25% (most in the first 2 years). Morbidity is high with secondary

bleeding and local tissue damage. Periodic CT or MR scanning plus endocrine follow-up are essential. If scans show no disease and no calcification postsurgery there is a 70% 10-year event-free survival. If there is residual tumor or calcification, radiotherapy (50–55 Gy local field) is required. Many now recommend subtotal resection and radiotherapy rather than radical surgery.[224] Intracystic radiocolloid injection has been used successfully in recurrent cystic lesions. No role has yet been established for chemotherapy.

LYMPHOMAS

Lymphoid malignancies in childhood arise from malignant transformation of lymphoid precursor cells at various stages of maturation. Lymphomas make up the third commonest group of childhood cancers. They are classified into Hodgkin's lymphoma or Hodgkin disease (HD) and Non-Hodgkin lymphoma (NHL) according to the WHO updated REAL (revised European-American Lymphoma) classification. This classification takes into account clinical and morphological as well as genetic and immunophenotypic features.[225]

The strong associations with congenital and acquired immunodeficiencies for NHL and to a lesser extent HD as well as the high incidence in geographical areas with high incidence of malaria and early EBV infection suggests a role for viral infections in the pathogenesis of these malignancies.[226,227] However, primary evidence of viral involvement in oncogenesis in other parts of the world is rare, and the precise role of EBV and other viruses is still unclear.

NON-HODGKIN LYMPHOMA

Childhood non-Hodgkin lymphomas represent a heterogeneous group of high grade malignancies of immature T or B cell precursors. NHL in the pediatric age group can be divided into Burkitt, precursor B- and T cell lymphoblastic lymphomas, large B cell lymphomas and anaplastic large cell lymphomas. The characteristics that are important for the biology and the diagnosis of NHL are listed in Table 24.13. Typical nonrandom chromosomal rearrangements have been identified in Burkitt lymphoma, where the oncogene *c-myc* is translocated adjacent to the gene coding for heavy chain immunoglobulin, which leads to overactivation of *c-myc*, which is thought to play a crucial role in pathogenesis and malignant proliferation. Anaplastic large cell lymphoma (ALCL) carries a characteristic translocation between 2p23 and 5q35 that leads to activation of the ALK tyrosine kinase

Table 24.13   Common childhood non-Hodgkin lymphoma characteristics and frequency

	Burkitt	Precursor T/B lymphoblastic	Large B-cell	Anaplastic large cell
Stage of development	Germinal center	Immature	Germinal center	Mature T-cell
Immunophenotype	CD20+ CD79a+ S Ig+	TdT B-lineage T-lineage CD19+CD7+ CD79a+CD2+ S Ig-CD3+	CD20+ CD79+a	CD30+
Cytogenetics/molecular biology	t(8;14)(q24;q32) or variant resulting in transcriptional deregulation of c-MYK	No specific abnormalities	Occasional t(8;14)(q24;q32) der(3)(q27) resulting in deregulation of bcl6	t(2;5)(p23;q35) or variant Activation of NPM/ALKtyrosin kinase receptor
Frequency (UK)	45%	25%	5%	20%

receptor. Advances in the understanding of the cellular biology has contributed to clinical management of children with NHL, as these findings have not only made an important contribution to accurate diagnosis but have also been found to have prognostic implications. The uncommon ALCL without ALK expression appear to have a much worse prognosis.[228] There are promising data that also could lead to novel therapeutic strategies targeting deregulated genes, such as ALK in ALCL.[229]

Presentation

The scope for presentation is wide and depends upon the site of the primary lymphoid mass and the presence of features of disseminated disease such as fatigue, pain and anemia.[230,231]

Abdominal primary

The abdomen is the most common primary site. In Europe B cell lymphomas normally present as a diffuse abdominal tumor often involving the omentum and mesentery with infiltration into kidney, liver and spleen and ascites (Fig. 24.7). Frequently the bone marrow and central nervous system are also involved. Sometimes there are localized tumors of the bowel wall especially in the terminal ileum (thought to arise in Peyer's patches). These masses may lead to intussusception or bleeding and sometimes to perforation of the bowel. These tumors can resemble appendicitis or an appendix mass since they often present with a right iliac fossa mass and pain.

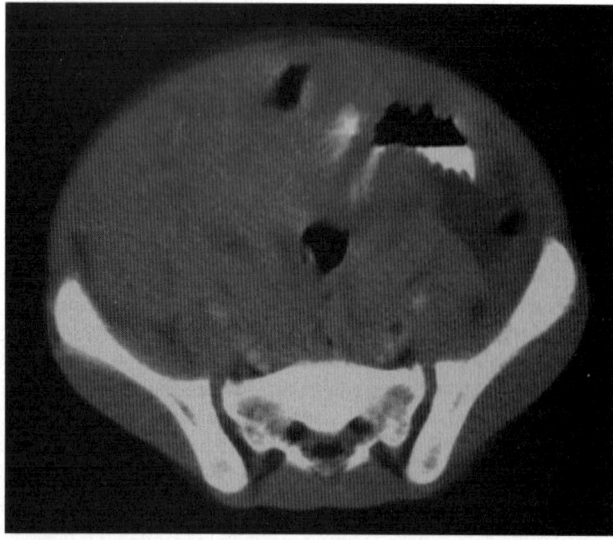

Fig. 24.7   Contrast-enhanced CT image of the pelvis showing the typical appearance of a diffuse abdominal B cell non-Hodgkin lymphoma.

Mediastinal primary

In the UK approximately 20% of children with NHL present with a mediastinal mass with or without pleural effusions. Most T lymphoblastic lymphoma present in this way. There may be signs of superior vena caval obstruction, dysphagia, dyspnea and pericardial effusion. There may be associated neck and axillary lymphadenopathy. Hepatospenomegaly and bone marrow involvement (present in more than 50% of cases) and central nervous system disease are common in these patients. These patients are at high risk of developing airway obstruction with general anesthesia.

Other sites

In Europe jaw or neck masses are unusual, but in Africa this is the usual presentation. Fifty percent of African patients with jaw primaries also have abdominal disease but marrow disease is unusual.[232] Lymphoid swellings can occur anywhere but most commonly in the head and neck including Waldeyer's ring and the facial bones. Other sites of origin include the pharynx (usually B cell origin) and primary tumors of bone, skin, thyroid, testis (usually lymphoblastic), orbit, eyelid, kidney and epidural space have all been described. Bone lymphomas may be localized or disseminated and may be associated with hypercalcemia.

Anaplastic large cell lymphomas have additional distinct clinical features and can present with painful lymphadenopathy, skin involvement and a systemic inflammatory response with widely fluctuating fever.

Central nervous system involvement

Primary intracranial lymphomas are rare although more frequent with postorgan transplantation and other forms of immunosuppression or immunodeficiency. However secondary CNS involvement is common in advanced lymphoblastic and Burkitt lymphoma. When present there are the characteristic features of headache, vomiting, papilledema, cranial nerve dysfunction and seizures.

Diagnosis

A full history and examination usually gives a clue to the type of lymphoma and the extent of dissemination. All patients require a preliminary chest radiograph for assessment of the mediastinum. This must be performed prior to any anesthetic procedure. Imaging of lymphoid masses is best carried out by MRI particularly for tumors of the head and neck. Ultrasonography is the quickest and most efficient way to define liver, spleen and kidney involvement and extent of abdominal primaries without requiring sedation or anesthesia in young children. Either MRI or CT scanning can follow. All patients require bone marrow examination. The specimens should be examined cytogenetically and immunophennotyped as well as routine cytomorphology. All patients require examination of cerebrospinal fluid provided that there is no clinical evidence of raised intracranial pressure. If this is present then a CT or MRI scan should be carried out before lumbar puncture to exclude any focal deposit. Sometimes the diagnosis can be made on cytological examination of pleural fluid or bone marrow. In the presence of any accessible localized disease excision biopsy should be carried out. If there is truly isolated mediastinal disease with no involvement of bone marrow or CSF, material will need to be obtained preferably by percutaneous needle or mediastinoscopy. For abdominal primaries diagnosis should be attempted by cytological examination of ascitic fluid or by percutaneous needle biopsy. Unless there is an acute abdominal emergency (such as gastrointrastinal obstruction or intussusception) laparotomy should be avoided wherever possible to avoid sequelae of prolonged ileus and even ruptured abdominal wounds. Tumor material needs to be submitted for routine histological diagnosis, immunophenotyping and cytogenetics. Clinical patterns of presentation, histology, cytomorphology, immunophenotype and cytogenetics usually facilitate very precise definition of the tumor. Initial blood tests should include a full blood count, liver and renal function tests and an electrolyte profile to monitor for tumor lysis. Lactate dehydrogenase (LDH) serum levels which are thought to be prognostic, especially in B cell disease, should be assessed pretreatment.[231]

Staging

Table 24.14 shows the most commonly used staging system for childhood NHL.[233] All primary mediastinal tumors and diffuse abdominal tumors are at least Stage III. The spread in NHL, unlike Hodgkin disease, is not orderly and contiguous from node to node. There is no place for routine staging laparotomy in NHL nor for lymphangiography. To what extent PET (positron emission tomography) is useful in staging and management of childhood NHL is currently under evaluation.

Management

Many patients with lymphomas present with poor nutrition, concomitant infection and metabolic problems resulting from spontaneous tumor lysis. These require attention and, if possible, correction before

Table 24.14   St Jude modified staging system for non-Hodgkin lymphoma

Stage		Approximate frequency by stage seen in UK
I	Single tumor (extranodal) or single anatomic area (nodal) (not mediastinum or abdomen)	5%
II	Single tumor (extranodal) with regional node involvement. Primary gastrointestinal tumor with or without involvement of associated mesenteric nodes only On the same side of diaphragm: a. two or more nodal areas b. two single (extranodal) tumors with or without regional node involvement	20%
III	On both sides of the diaphragm: a. two single tumors extranodal b. two or more nodal areas. All primary intrathoracic tumors (mediastinal, pleural, thymic); all extensive primary intra-abdominal disease; all primary paraspinal or epidural tumors regardless of other sites	50%
IV	Any of the above with initial CNS* or bone marrow involvement† (<25%)	25%

* CNS disease = unequivocal blasts > 5/mm³ in a cytocentrifugal cerebrospinal fluid specimen ± neurologic deficits, e.g. cranial nerve palsies ± intracranial nodal deposits
† Arbitrary cutoff of 25% to distinguish leukemia from lymphoma. This may not be useful for all, e.g. in B cell NHL no difference in outcome between Stage III and IV disease up to 70% bone marrow infiltration

intensive therapy can be delivered. Prophylactic use of allopurinol or urate oxidase and more recently rasburicase has reduced the risks of therapeutic tumor lysis.[234,235]

Except for the diagnostic biopsy there is no routine role for surgery in childhood NHL. Radiotherapy can be helpful to control local disease and may be warranted in emergency situations such as spinal cord compression, and for the management of mediastinal masses. Chemotherapy is the preferred modality of treatment since all tumors have the potential to disseminate. Considerable improvement in survival from childhood NHL has been achieved with combination therapy, which has evolved over many national and international multicenter trials treating large numbers of patients.

In general chemotherapy in pediatric NHL is subtype specific. While B cell disease appears to be responsive to pulsed intensive treatment, T cell lymphomas and precursor B cell disease appears to benefit from prolonged and continuous treatment similar to that used in the treatment of lymphoblastic leukemia. Anaplastic large cell lymphoma is treated in Europe as an own identity with a more 'B cell like' approach.

Localized lymphomas (Stage I and II)

Localized NHL is best treated with short course therapy of not more than 6 months' duration. For Stage I and abdominal Stage II disease there is no need for CNS directed therapy.[236] Over 80% event free survival can be achieved with short course pulsed therapy for low stage B cell lymphoma. Some groups have attempted to reduce the risk of late cardiotoxicity by limiting or omitting anthracyclines and reducing the risks of infertility or second tumor development by reducing anthracycline and alkylator dosages. Patte et al reported high cure rates with only two pulses of cyclophosphamide-based chemotherapy and Reiter et al very successfully treated Stage I and IIa B cell lymphomas using only three courses.[236–238] The only exceptions are localized lymphoblastic tumors which appear to require more intensive and sustained therapy similar to that used for advanced lymphoblastic leukemia and lymphoma.[239]

Advanced stage B cell lymphomas

The best results are those reported by the SFOP and BFM groups.[236–238] Both groups used initial low dose cytoreductive therapy (cyclophosphamide, vincristine and prednisolone) in order to reduce tumor bulk before a more intensive induction regimen. The LMB protocol consists of high dose methotrexate, fractionated high dose cyclophosphamide, vincristine, prednisolone and doxorubicin followed by a consolidation phase using continuous infusion cytosine arabinoside. CNS-directed therapy is with high dose methotrexate and intrathecal therapy but not irradiation except for those with Stage IV disease involving the CNS at diagnosis. Event free survival has progressively improved over the last 20 years with therapy modified in duration and intensity. In recent times there has been a multinational protocol stratifying disease by stage attempting to reduce intensity and subsequent toxicity for lower risk patients and giving very intensive therapy for those with the highest risk, in particular those with bone marrow involvement of greater than 70% and those with CNS disease at diagnosis. The initial response to the cytoreductive therapy has also proven to be a significant prognostic indicator. Application of such therapy even in the most advanced disease now carries with it over 80% chance of 5-year event free survival.[238]

Advanced stage non-B cell lymphoma

Since the mid-1970s patients with lymphoblastic lymphoma usually of T cell origin (but with a small percentage having precursor B cell disease) have been treated with leukemia type therapy.[237,239] The BFM Group have shown somewhat superior results because of their very sustained induction, consolidation and maintenance therapy similar to that used for acute lymphoblastic leukemia. With such intensive treatment there seems to be very little difference in survival between Stage III and IV disease. The most significant adverse prognostic feature appears to be failure to respond early (as defined by the BFM Group for acute lymphoblastic leukemia). Such slow responders may benefit from early intensification. The BFM 90 protocol has transformed the previously observed pattern of ongoing relapses out beyond 4 years, to early relapses and virtually no late relapses.[239] A European wide international protocol is now in use.

Anaplastic large cell lymphoma

Multi-agent chemotherapy as trialed by the SFOP and BFM groups results in an over 80% event free survival, with skin involvement and splenomegaly forming the most adverse features.[240,241] The duration of therapy is determined by stage and consists of short pulsed intensive treatment. As with T lymphoblastic leukemia there has been creation of a European Intergroup of investigators to create a trial using a prephase with vincristine, cyclophosphamide, and dexamethasone followed by a multi-agent BFM type regimen (ifosfamide, etoposide, cytosine arabinoside, dexamethasone and intrathecal therapy).

Immunosuppression/immunodeficiency related lymphoproliferative disease (LPD)

There are increasing reports of patients developing what is thought to be an EBV driven lymphoproliferation of B cell phenotype following severe immunosuppression, especially after organ transplantation. The recognized strategy for dealing with them has first been to reduce immunosuppressive therapy. There is a clear correlation between the incidence of LPD and the severity of immunosuppression. It is not always possible to reduce immunosuppression in the post-transplant situation, and most appear to require some chemotherapy. Some respond to the use of cytoreductive therapy with cyclophosphamide, vincristine, and steroids. Some tumors require intensive B cell lymphoma type therapy. Numbers have been too small in the past to address some of the questions in clinical trials, but this might change with increasingly important international collaborations. Use of targeted anti-B cell monoclonal antibodies[242] and the production of cytotoxic T lymphocytes against EBV-infected cells have been reported.[243]

Alternative strategies

Bone marrow transplantation has limited use in modern day therapy for NHL and should be reserved for those who have partial remission after intensive therapy, or those who relapse early but respond on re-induction with second line therapy. Specific targeted monoclonal antibody therapy has been used in adult high grade lymphomas but not systematically in children. Relapse in childhood NHL is still associated with a high mortality.

HODGKIN DISEASE

Hodgkin's lymphoma or Hodgkin disease (HD) arises from malignant transformation of germinal center derived B-lineage precursors.[244] HD is characterized by the presence of giant multinuclear Hodgkin's and Reed–Sternberg cells, which are the malignant cells in this lymphoma. HD has a peak incidence in teenagers and is uncommon in children under five and rare in children under two. As for NHL, infection, in particular by EBV, is thought to contribute to the etiology. The Epstein–Barr virus genome has been detected in Reed–Sternberg cells in a significant percentage (at least 60%) of young cases especially boys and those with mixed cellularity subtype.[91–93,245] Although no typical recurrent nonrandom cytogenetic changes have been identified in HD, recurrently observed gains of material on chromosome 2p, which are found in approximately 50% of HD, point to deregulation of the REL gene, which is a putative oncogenic transcription factor in the pathogenesis of HD.[246,247]

Classification

According to the WHO classification HD can be subdivided into four subtypes.[225]

1. *Lymphocyte predominance*: Reed–Sternberg cells may be quite scarce, fibrosis is rarely seen and the prognosis is very good.
2. *Mixed cellularity*: Reed–Sternberg cells are usually profuse (5–15 per high power field) often with fine fibrosis and focal necrosis.
3. *Lymphocyte depletion*: large abnormal mononuclear cells are often seen as well as Reed–Sternberg cells with few lymphocytes. Fibrosis

and necrosis are common and often quite diffuse. This form is rarer in children.

4. *Nodular sclerosis*: lacunar cells are a characteristic finding with a thickened capsule and bands which divide the tissue into nodules. This histology is especially common in lower cervical, supraclavicular and mediastinal HD of childhood.

The prognosis appears to be related to the proportion of lymphocytes present in types 1–3. Mixed cellularity is seen much more commonly in younger patients and in those from developing countries. Overall in the UK and Northern Europe nodular sclerosing and mixed cellularity types are seen in roughly equal proportions.

There is some correlation between patterns of presentation and histopathology with mixed cellularity and lymphocyte depleted forms usually presenting with more disseminated disease and nodular sclerosis classically presenting with mediastinal disease in adolescence. Lymphocyte predominant disease almost always presents with focal nodal disease characteristically in the neck or groin. Hodgkin disease generally follows an orderly pattern of spread from node to contiguous node. When the spleen is involved, infiltration usually starts as a small nodule. Liver infiltration is usually focal.

Clinical presentation

In childhood most patients present with painless swelling of the cervical or supraclavicular nodes, which can feel firm or rubbery on palpation. Two thirds of children have mediastinal involvement, which may be found coincidentally on chest radiograph but may compromise the airway and cause respiratory distress (Fig. 24.8a). Involvement of the pleura or pericardium with effusions may worsen the chest symptoms. Axillary or inguinal node involvement is less common. The groin is involved in less than 5% of childhood cases. Hepatic and splenic involvement indicates advanced disease (Fig. 24.8b). Approximately 30% of young patients have nonspecific features of tiredness and anorexia but very specific symptoms of fever, weight loss (more than 10%) and night sweating. Other unspecific symptoms are generalized pruritus and unexplained pain on taking alcohol. These are designated as B symptoms and carry a worse prognosis and are therefore part of pretreatment staging.

Diagnosis

Differential diagnosis includes infective causes of lymphadenopathy (e.g. infectious mononucleosis, atypical TB, and other viruses) and non-Hodgkin lymphoma particularly in lymphocyte-predominant disease. Usually NHL has a more rapid onset and rapid tumor growth. Diagnostic investigations which are essential include:

1. Clinical assessment for any node or organ enlargement and documentation of any symptoms.
2. Standard posteroanterior (PA) and lateral chest radiograph. It is important to document the extent of a mediastinal mass since its dimensions determine whether the patient may require subsequent radiotherapy (Fig. 24.8a).
3. CT scan of chest, neck and abdomen to define precise dimensions and extent of disease. Although MR scanning may be better for neck masses, CT is more commonly used enabling scanning from neck through to the abdomen (Fig. 24.8b,c).
4. Node biopsy to confirm diagnosis, subtype and to carry out molecular and EBV screening studies.
5. Bone marrow aspirates and trephine biopsy to exclude infiltration in patients with advanced disease and those with B symptoms.

In the past laparotomy and splenectomy have been part of the management of HD, but now the procedures are safely avoided wherever possible because of the risk of overwhelming sepsis associated with splenectomy. Table 24.15 shows the staging system most commonly used throughout the world.

Management

Hodgkin disease is very responsive to treatment, in particular to radiotherapy, but universal use of radiotherapy was associated with

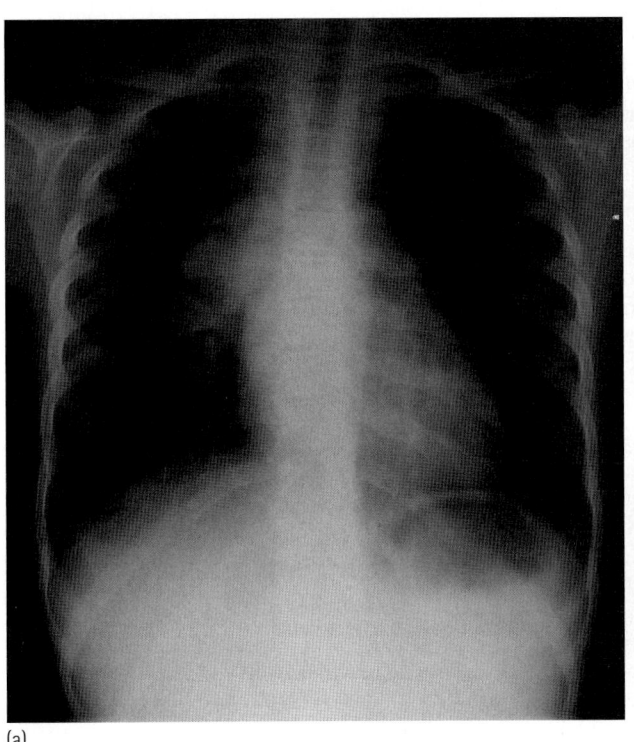

(a)

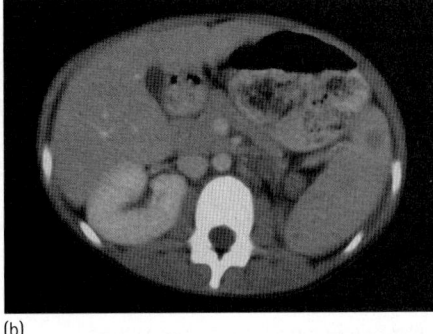

(b)

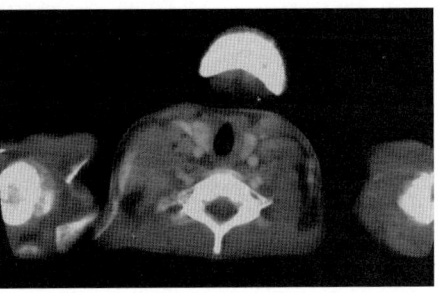

(c)

Fig. 24.8 (a) PA chest radiograph showing right-sided hilar lymphadenopathy in Hodgkin disease. (b) Contrast-enhanced CT image of the abdomen showing the typical appearance of Hodgkin disease in the spleen. (c) Contrast-enhanced CT of the neck showing bilateral cervical lympadenopathy in Hodgkin disease.

unacceptable local tissue growth problems in earlier trials. Combined modality therapy was adopted to minimize the toxicity of both radiation and chemotherapy but optimize cure. Newer evidence accrued that the combination of alkylating agents such as procarbazine and radiation increased the risk of some late toxicity, especially second tumor formation and infertility.[248,249] As a consequence modern therapy has contained radiotherapy in a dose range of 20–35 Gy only for those with localized Stage IA disease where an involved field was included. Since such tumors are primarily in the neck there still is the consequence of developing hypothyroidism.[250] Chemotherapy is now used for all stages including low stage disease. Positron emission tomography (PET) has become very important in assessing response to initial therapy in pediatric HD.[251] In lymphocyte predominant HD the approach today is surgery and resection only if the tumor is operable (mainly Stage IA and IIA). More extensive disease of this histology, which has an excellent prognosis, is treated with low intensity chemotherapy consisting of prednisolone, vinblastine and low dose cyclophosphamide. Response is assessed with PET scanning. For patients with Stage II and IIIA HD the aim of therapy is to achieve cure with least long term sequelae. The current

aim is to minimize the potential toxicity of alkylating agents and etoposide, which include infertility and second malignancies. The current approach in the UK has adapted the experiences from the GPOH trials and now uses two courses of OEPA chemotherapy consisting of prednisolone, vincristine, adriamycin and etoposide for patients with Stage I and IIA disease. If re-assessment with PET after the two courses indicates no active disease it is safe to give no further treatment.[252] Patients with Stage IIB, IIIA receive an additional two cycles of COPP (procarbazine, cyclophosphamide, vincristine, procarbazine and prednisolone) chemotherapy, if PET scanning after induction indicates no active disease. If the tumor is PET-positive after the initial OEPA involved field radiotherapy (IFRT) is delivered to sites of disease. Patients with Stage IIIB and IV disease require more therapy and receive four courses of COPP with IFRT if there is evidence of PET-positive residual disease after initial courses of OEPA, and without radiation if PET scanning indicates the absence of active disease. The responsiveness of HD to treatment has made it difficult now to run randomized trials with low stage Hodgkin disease, which has a 5-year event free survival greater than 95%. In Stage IV patients results have been less favorable (in the region of 50–60% 5-year survival in the past). Relapsed and progressive HD is still a problem, and no uniform strategy for second line treatment exists. In the UK EPIC chemotherapy, consisting of etoposide, prednisolone, ifosphamide and cisplatin is currently used for refractory or relapsed disease, which can be followed by high dose chemotherapy and stem cell rescue in high risk patients. A similar approach was reported by the GPOH, which conferred over 60% overall survival after relapse of HD, however early relapse after initial treatment and progressive disease remain difficult to cure.[253,254]

NEUROBLASTOMA

Although most frequently presenting as a large abdominal mass, this tumor is metastatic in 70% of patients at diagnosis. The commonest primary sites are the adrenal gland 40%, other abdominal sites 25%, chest 15%, pelvis 5% and neck 5%. The thorax is more frequently involved in those under 1 year. Neuroblastoma arises from primordial neural crest cells which form part of the sympathetic and rarely the parasympathetic nervous system. 1 in 250 neonates dying of other causes are found to have small foci of adrenal neuroblasts but disease

Table 24.15 Ann Arbor staging system for Hodgkin disease

Stage I	Involvement of a single lymph node region (I) or of a single extralymphatic organ or site (I_E)
Stage II	Involvement of two or more lymph node regions on the same side of the diaphragm (II) or localized involvement of an extralymphatic organ or site and one or more lymph node regions on the same side of the diaphragm (II_E)
Stage III	Involvement of lymph node regions on both sides of the diaphragm (III) which may be accompanied by involvement of the spleen (III_S) or localized involvement of extralymphatic organ or site (III_E) or both (III_{SE}).
Stage IV	Diffuse or disseminated involvement of one or more extralymphatic organs or tissues with or without associated lymph node involvement

+B, presence of fever, night sweats or weight loss > 10% in previous 6 months; +A, none of above

occurs only in 1 in 10 000 live births. These foci may represent tumors in situ or may be a reflection of a normal stage of adrenal development which regresses in health but persists in malignancy. Spontaneous regression of malignant neuroblastoma to benign ganglioneuroma has been recorded even in infants with quite widespread disease (see below).

Epidemiology and etiology

Neuroblastoma occurs slightly more frequently in boys and occasional familial clusterings have been reported. Genetic rearrangement involving the short arm of chromosome 1 has been described and it is possible that up to 20–25% of cases may be heritable. Geographical variations may reflect genuine genetic or environmental factors or may be a reflection of low detection rates. Neuroblastoma occurs with increased frequency in Beckwith–Wiedemann syndrome, neurofibromatosis, nesidioblastosis and in fetal phenytoin syndrome.

Presentation

The features of neuroblastoma are protean because of early dissemination and origin anywhere along the sympathetic chain. Superficial or abdominal lesions usually present as a mass, while pelvic or thoracic lesions often present with obstruction of bowel, bladder or airway. The classic presentation of Stage 4 disease is with an abdominal mass with the features of marrow infiltration including anemia, bruising, fever, lethargy and irritability. Anemia is present in approximately 90% of cases even in the absence of marrow infiltration. Bony disease gives characteristic deep-seated intractable pain in one or more limbs and often causes a limp. Proptosis with periorbital bruising is a characteristic but rare feature of Stage 4 disease due to infiltration either within the orbit or in the sphenoid bone. Local extension through an intervertebral foramen can produce cord compression at any level in some 5% of patients. These patients may need urgent treatment, either with radiotherapy, laminectomy or chemotherapy. Full neurological recovery can be expected in 50% of these patients, but recovery is unlikely if the presenting motor defect is severe.[255] Approximately 1–2% of tumors produce vasoactive intestinal peptide which produces intractable diarrhea associated with hypokalemia. Most (90%) tumors secrete catecholamines usually homovanillic acid (HVA) and vanillylmandelic acid (VMA), and although blood levels may be very high they do not normally cause hypertension. Hypertension does occur but is usually renovascular. Skin metastases present as nontender bluish, mobile subcutaneous nodules ('blueberry muffin') and are characteristically seen in Stage 4S disease.

A syndrome of opsoclonus/myoclonus in which the patient has acute cerebellar and truncal ataxia with rapid eye movements may be seen (dancing eye syndrome). CNS disease is rare although increasingly described as length of survival improves.

Investigations

The diagnosis must be confirmed and extent of disease evaluated.

Biopsy

All should have histological confirmation from the most easily accessible tumor deposit. In addition to histology fresh tumor material is needed for molecular diagnostics. Deletions of the short arm of chromosome 1 are found in 70–80% of near diploid cells and can assist in differentiation from other small round cell tumors. DNA content overall is of prognostic significance (pseudodiploidy is associated with advanced disease and poorer survival). MYCN amplification is associated with advanced disease and poor prognosis. Consequently, tumor cytogenetics, ploidy and MYCN amplification studies are all required. Histologically, neuroblastoma consists of small blue round cells with fibrillary bundles, hemorrhage, necrosis, calcification and attempts at rosette formation. Maturation to ganglion cells with fibrils may be diffuse (ganglioneuroma) or patchy (ganglioneuroblastoma). Table 24.16 shows ways in which small round cell tumors of childhood may be distinguished.

Bone marrow

Multiple site aspirates and trephines are necessary to exclude involvement since it is the commonest metastatic site. When present, infiltration may be very heavy and mimic ALL or show patchy clumps or rosettes (Fig. 24.9a).

Diagnostic imaging

CT, MR and ultrasound scans can all be used to define primary tumor extent (Fig. 24.9b). It is essential to have three-dimensional assessment of tumor size to document response accurately. MR is optimal to determine any spinal extension (Fig. 24.9c). Iodine-123 metaiodobenzylguanine (MIBG) scanning is needed to determine the extent of metatstatic disease (Fig. 24.9d). If negative a technetium bone scan is needed to exclude bone metastases.

Urinary catecholamines

Between 85% and 95% of patients have detectable excess in their urine and the total levels of catecholamines and VMA and HVA can be used to monitor tumor response. Catecholamines should ideally be measured on 24-hour specimens but can be done on spot specimens in younger children.

Blood tests

In addition to the usual baseline investigations it is usual to measure lactate dehydrogenase (LDH), ferritin and neuron specific enolase (NSE) in patients with neuroblastoma.

Biology

The molecular biology of neuroblastoma has been extensively studied. It is well established that amplification of the proto-oncogene MYCN is associated with higher stage tumors and a worse prognosis.[256] Deletion of the short arm of chromosome 1 (1p deletion), with its loss of a putative tumor suppressor gene is similarly associated with more advanced disease and disease progression.[257,258] Gain of the long arm of chromosome 17 (17q gain) is also a powerful negative prognostic factor.[259] Expression of the high affinity nerve growth factor (NGF) receptor, TrkA, and to a lesser extent the low affinity NGF receptor (LNGFR/p75), correlates with good outcome.[260,261] Expression of TrκB, the receptor for brain derived neurotrophic factor (BDNF), correlates with MYCN amplification and poor prognosis[262] while expression of TrkC, the receptor for neurotrophin 3 (NT-3), is associated with good outcome.[263] These correlations suggest a difference in differentiation state between those tumors with a favorable prognosis and those which do badly. On the basis of these markers patients can be divided into three prognostic groups (Table 24.17). The first group consists of those whose tumors have a hyperdiploid or triploid karyotype, without MYCN amplification or 1p deletion and high expression of TrkA. These tend to be infants, less than 1 year of age, with Stage 1, 2, or 4s tumors who have an excellent prognosis. The second group contains those whose tumors have a diploid or tetraploid karyotype, no MYCN amplification, but deletion of 1p and low expression of TrkA. This group tends to contain children over the age of 1 year with Stage 3 and 4 disease who respond initially to chemotherapy but often relapse. They have an intermediate prognosis with 25–50% 5-year survival. The third group have tumors with diploid or tetraploid karyotypes, amplified MYCN, deletion of 1p, and absence of TrkA. These children have an appalling prognosis with a 5-year survival of 5%.[261]

Staging

Brodeur et al[264] published an international neuroblastoma staging system (INSS) (Table 24.18) which has been widely adopted. Standardization has enabled comparison of treatment results which was difficult in the past. All previous criteria were based on clinical, radiological and bone marrow examination but now staging includes the division of Stage 2 into those with and without lymph node involvement which alters prognosis and may indicate the need for a change in therapy. The overall distribution by stage is approximately 10–15% Stage 1, 8–10% Stage 2,

Table 24.16 Useful markers in the differentiation of small round cell tumors of childhood

Tumor	Tdt	Cytoplasmic immunoglobulin	Markers now identified immunologically					Intermediate filament proteins			
			Actin	Myosin	Neuron-specific enolase	S100 protein	Desmin	Vimentin	Neurofilament	Cytokeratins
Rhabdomyosarcoma	-	-	+	+ (if differentiated type)	+/- (rare)	+/-	+	+	-	+/-
Neuroblastoma	-	-	-	-	+	+	-	-	+	-
Askin tumor	-	-	-	-	+	-/+	-	+/-	?	+/-
Peripheral PNET	-	-	-/+	-	+	+	-/+	+/-	+/-	+/-
Ewing sarcoma 'typical'	-	-	-	-	- (+) (occasional)	- (+)*	-	+	-	+/-
Non-Hodgkin lymphoma	+T -B	In B cell	-	-	-	-	-	+	-	-
ALL	+ (95%)	In pre-B (10–15%)	-	-	-	-	-	-	-	-

This battery of markers should be combined with specific antibodies to detect surface antigens, e.g. UJ13A for neuroectodermally derived cells or UJ181A from fetal brain cell origin.
(+)*, occasional in Ewing sarcoma. ALL, acute lymphoblastic leukemia; PNET, primitive neuroectodermal tumor; Tdt, terminal deoxynucleotidy transferase.

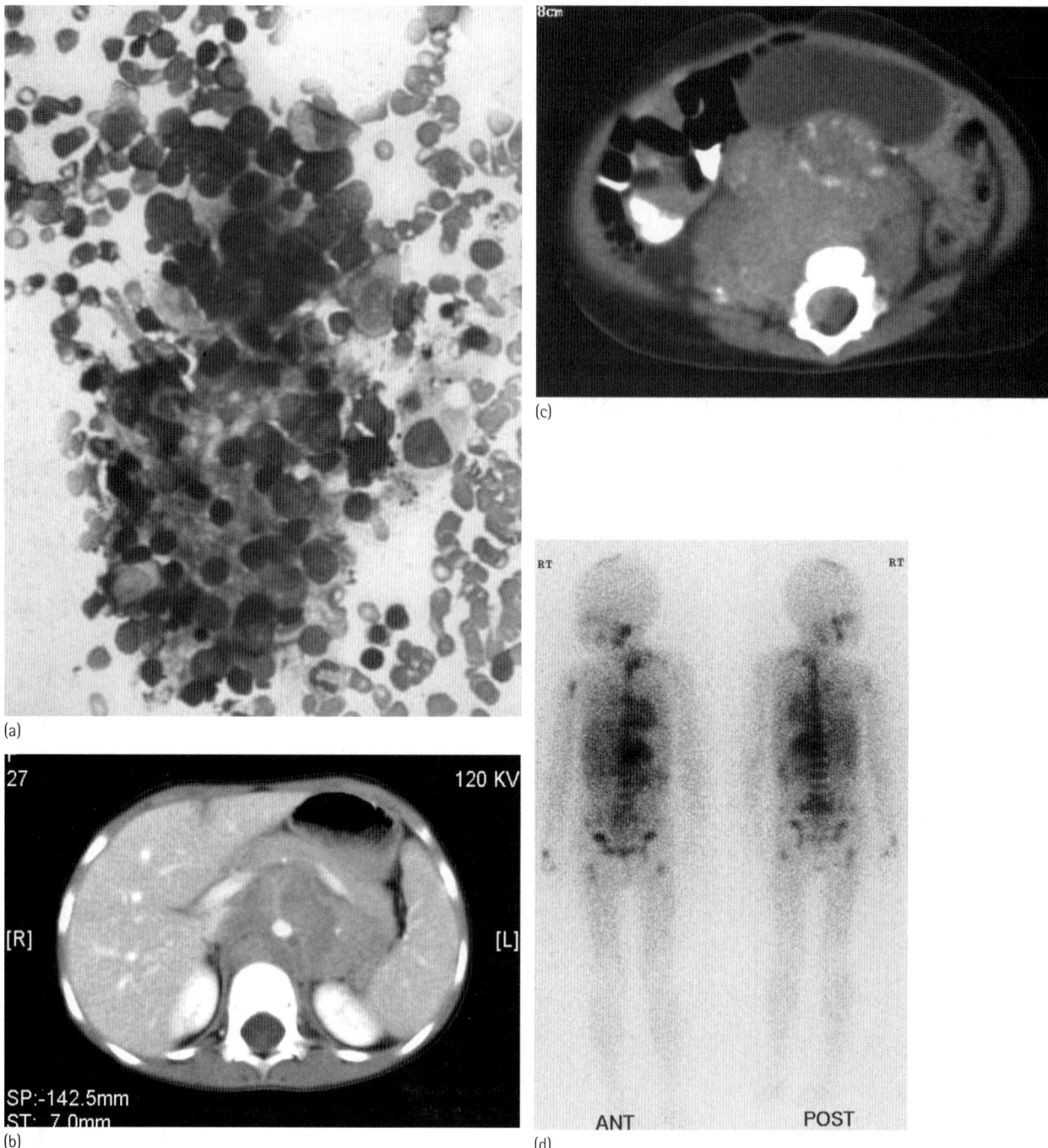

Fig. 24.9 (a) Bone marrow aspirate showing a clump of neuroblastoma cells. (b) Contrast-enhanced CT image of abdominal neuroblastoma – note the encased blood vessels displaced anteriorly. (c) Contrast-enhanced CT image of abdominal neuroblastoma – note the calcification anteriorly in the tumor and the intraspinal component. (d) MIBG scan of a patient with Stage 4 neuroblastoma. Note the uptake in the abdominal primary tumor and the extensive bony uptake.

Table 24.17 Prognostic features in neuroblastoma

Good	Intermediate	Adverse
Age < 1 year	Age > 1 year	Age > 1 year
INSS stage 1, 2, 4S	INSS stage 3, 4	INSS stage 3, 4
Single copy MYCN	Single copy MYCN	Amplified MYCN
Intact chromosome 1p	Deleted 1p	Deleted 1p
No gain of 17q	Gain of 17q	Gain of 17q
Hyperdiploid	Diploid/tetraploid	Diploid/tetraploid
High TrkA	Low TrkA	Low TrkA

15–20% Stage 3 and 60% Stage 4. In those under 1 year almost 30% have Stage 1 disease. Nearly 40% of infants (1 year) affected have localized disease compared with 20% of older children. Stage 4S (Stage 1 or 2 with dissemination limited to liver, skin and/or bone marrow) is almost exclusively seen in infants. Table 24.17 shows recognized prognostic features.

Management
Low risk group
(INSS Stage 1, 2 and 3, Stage 4 without bone, lung, pleural, or CNS metastases in infants, and INSS Stage 4S disease, without MYCN amplification.)

Table 24.18 International staging system for neuroblastoma

Stage 1	Localized tumor confined to the area of origin, complete gross excision, with or without microscopic residual disease, identifiable ipsilateral and contralateral lymph nodes negative microscopically
Stage 2A	Unilateral tumor with incomplete gross excision, identifiable ipsilateral and contralateral lymph nodes negative microscopically
Stage 2B	Unilateral tumor with complete or incomplete gross excision, with positive ipsilateral regional lymph nodes, identifiable contralateral lymph nodes negative microscopically
Stage 3	Tumor infiltrating across the midline with or without regional lymph node involvement; or unilateral tumor with contralateral regional lymph node involvement; or midline tumor with bilateral regional lymph node involvement
Stage 4	Dissemination of tumor to distant lymph node, bone, bone marrow, liver and/or other organs (except as defined in 4S)
Stage 4S	Localized primary tumor as defined for stages 1 and 2 but with dissemination limited to liver, skin and/or bone marrow

Surgery only is recommended for Stage 1 and 2 disease (99% and 98% overall survival respectively) and for resectable Stage 3 disease in infants, in the absence of MYCN amplification. Chemotherapy is reserved for any recurrence and may be needed in 10% of Stage 1 patients and 20% of Stage 2.[265] Unresectable Stage 2 or 3 disease in infants in the absence of MYCN amplification can be managed with short non-intensive combination chemotherapy based on cyclophosphamide/vincristine (CO), etoposide/carboplatin (VP-CARBO) and cycophosphamide/doxorubicin/vincristine (CADO). A subset of Stage 2 patients with a poorer prognosis can be identified by MYCN amplification and age over 2 years.[266] These patients merit aggressive chemotherapy and should be regarded as high risk. Stage 4S disease is associated with spontaneous regression and good overall survival. However a group of infants who present at less than 2 months of age tend to have rapidly enlarging abdominal disease (either an abdominal primary or metastases in the liver) and a poorer prognosis. Whilst most patients with 4S neuroblastoma do not need treatment this group merit early combination chemotherapy[267,268] with VP-CARBO and CADO. A small group of infants with Stage 4 disease without bony metastases and without MYCN amplification, who would be categorized as 4S but for the presence of a large usually abdominal primary can also be treated with a similar expectant strategy and will regress spontaneously.

Intermediate risk group
(Unresectable INSS Stage 2 and 3 without MYCN amplification and infants with Stage 4 with bone, lung, pleural, or CNS disease, but without MYCN amplification.)

This group of patients is relatively small, only 15% of cases of neuroblastoma are Stage 3, and 15% of these will be high risk due to MYCN amplification. Combination chemotherapy alternating VP-CARBO and CADO is recommended with surgical resection of any remaining tumor.

High risk group
(Any child with INSS Stage 2 or 3 with MYCN amplification, infants with Stage 4 or 4S disease with MYCN amplification, Stage 4 disease over the age of 1.)

Infants with disease above Stage 1 with amplification of MYCN do not do well in the absence of intensive therapy. Current European guidelines for this group of patients include chemotherapy with VP-CARBO and CADO followed by radiotherapy to the tumor site and myeloablative therapy with autologous bone marrow transplantation (ABMT).

Children over the age of 1 year with Stage 4 disease constitute 40–50% of all patients with neuroblastoma. Without intensive chemotherapy the survival for this group of patients is < 5%. With intensive induction chemotherapy, high dose myeloablative therapy with stem cell transplantation and maintenance therapy with 13-cis retinoic acid the survival for this group has improved dramatically, but remains stubbornly stuck at around 30%.[269] Many different induction regimens have been utilized for high risk neuroblastoma; most involve cisplatin/carboplatin in combination with cyclophosphamide, etoposide and vincristine. In the US doxorubicin has usually been included. No schedule has been convincingly shown to be superior, although the best European results to date have been with the Rapid COJEC schedule (vincristine/cisplatin alternating with vincristine/carboplatin/ etoposide and vincristine/cyclophosphamide/ etoposide every 10 days for eight cycles) on ENSG 5 (5-year overall survival, 39.6%). The current European cooperative trial uses Rapid COJEC as induction therapy, followed by surgical resection of the primary tumor, ABMT with either busulfan/melphalan or carboplatin/etoposide/melphalan as myeloablative therapy, 21 Gy of radiotherapy to the primary site, and 6 monthly cycles of 13-cis-retinoic acid. The use of immunological approaches including anti-G2 ganglioside antibodies and/or interferon are now under investigation as adjuvant therapy.

Since neuroblastoma is radiosensitive, a place for total body irradiation or targeted radiotherapy with MIBG in the above plan has been suggested. The optimal timing of such therapy remains unclear.

Screening
Since the prognosis for localized disease is good and that for advanced disease is so very poor and there is a readily obtainable marker for disease (urinary catecholamines) attempts have been made to carry out urinary screening of infants. Studies of screening in Japan and Canada have convincingly shown that it fails to detect Stage 4 disease in children over 1 year, and merely increases the number of previously asymptomatic and presumably spontaneously resolving cases detected.[270-274] Mass screening for neuroblastoma with urinary catecholamines thus cannot currently be recommended.

NEPHROBLASTOMA (WILMS TUMOR)
The incidence of Wilms tumor is approximately 1 in 10 000 live births with a very slight female preponderance (Tables 24.1, 24.2). The complex genetic picture is covered in the etiology section and Table 24.4. About 1% of patients have a family history of such tumors and it is possible that all bilateral (5% of all cases) and up to 20% of unilateral forms might be predominantly genetic in origin.

Presentation
Presentation is usually with an abdominal mass in a well child, often found coincidentally on routine examination. Fever is present in about 25%, hematuria in 25%, abdominal pain in 40% and hypertension in 5–10% of patients. It is important to examine specifically for aniridia, hemi-hypertrophy and genitourinary tract abnormalities.

Investigations
Ultrasound examination will define the mass and enable assessment of the contralateral kidney and patency of the inferior vena cava. Cross-sectional imaging with CT usually provides convincing evidence of the renal origin of the tumor, with the remaining renal parenchyma spread around the tumor (the so-called 'claw sign') as well as visualizing the contralateral kidney (Fig. 24.10a). Chest CT is needed to exclude pulmonary metastases (the usual site for Wilms tumor metastatses) (Fig. 24.10b). If histology reveals a clear cell sarcoma then isotope bone scan is needed to exclude bone metastases, and if the histology is of a rhabdoid tumor then CT of brain is needed to exclude intracranial metastases.

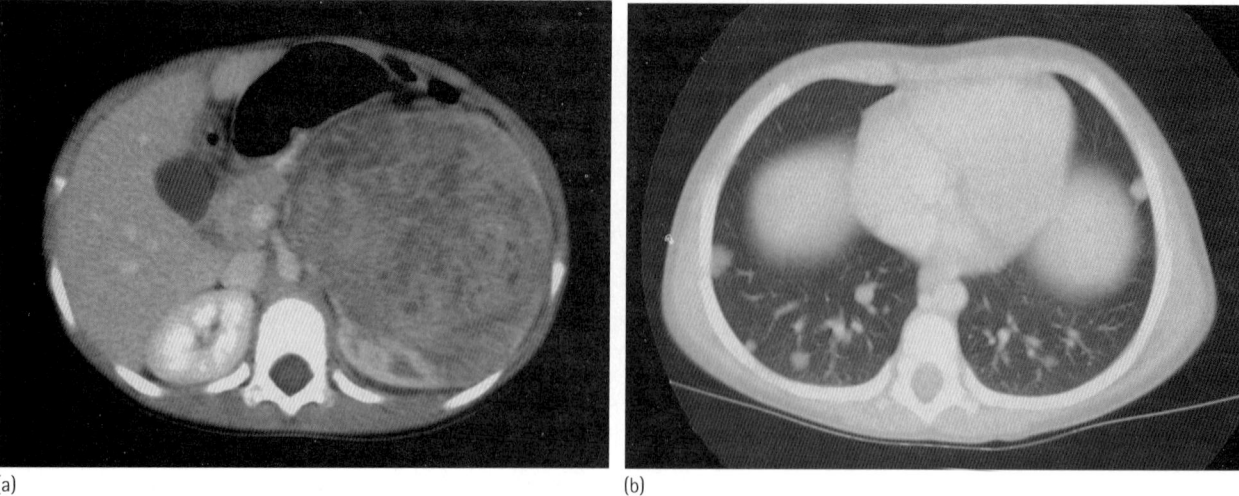

(a)   (b)

Fig. 24.10   (a) Contrast-enhanced CT of abdomen showing the typical appearance of an intrinsic renal tumor stretching the renal parenchyma around it (the 'claw sign'). (b) CT of thorax showing multiple pulmonary metastases of Wilm tumor.

Histology

The current SIOP working classification of renal tumors defines low, intermediate and high risk groups. Mesoblastic nephroma (see below) is classified as low risk, while clear cell sarcoma and rhabdoid tumors are considered high risk. The risk classification of Wilms tumor varies according to whether the patient has received chemotherapy before nephrectomy. The SIOP approach to Wilms tumor treatment with pre-nephrectomy chemotherapy for all patients means that the diagnostic needle biopsy is really only to confirm the diagnosis of Wilms tumor and the risk classification and tumor stage are defined by the post-chemotherapy nephrectomy specimen. In post-chemotherapy nephrectomy specimens only cystic partially differentiated nephroblastoma (CPDN) or completely necrotic tumors are classified as low risk. Blastemal type and diffuse anaplasia are classified as high risk, while all other histological types constitute intermediate risk.

Clear cell sarcoma comprises 5% of childhood renal tumors. It is always unilateral and is usually seen between 2 and 3 years of age. The most useful diagnostic feature is a trabecular pattern of blood vessels, and the clear cytoplasm is only present in a minority of tumors. Rhabdoid tumors comprise just 2% of childhood renal tumors, and have a poor prognosis. Eighty percent of patients are younger than 2 years. These patients often have hypercalcemia. Histologically the tumor cells have large eccentric nuclei with prominent eosinophilic nucleoli and are vimentin and cytokeratin positive. Wilms tumor with diffuse anaplasia, clear cell sarcoma and rhabdoid tumors account for more than 50% of deaths from renal tumors.[274]

Prognosis

Stage and tumor histology (see Table 24.19 and above) influence outcome.[275] In the second UK Wilms tumor study (UKW2) 32% of patients were Stage I, 14% were Stage II, 29% Stage III, 15% Stage IV and 5% Stage VI. In this study 4-year overall survival was 94% for Stage I, 91% for Stage II, 84% for Stage III, 75% for Stage IV and 78% for Stage V.[276]

Management

The aims of therapy are to cure without excessive toxicity in Stage I to III and improve long term disease control in Stage IV disease. The International Society of Pediatric Oncology Studies have shown that pre-operative chemotherapy reduces the risk of tumor rupture, down-stages tumors and consequently reduces the numbers requiring flank irradiation.[277,278] As a result the current European practice is for all children over the age of 6 months to have pre-operative chemotherapy after needle biopsy confirmation of diagnosis. SIOP studies have also shown that for selected subgroups therapy can be

Table 24.19   Staging system for nephroblastoma

Stage I	Tumor limited to one kidney and totally excised. The renal capsule intact with no rupture pre- or during surgery. No residual tumor is apparent beyond the margins of excision. Tumor may have been biopsied
Stage II	Tumor extension beyond the kidney but totally excised. The extension is regional referring to renal vessels outside kidney, infiltrated or containing thrombus. There may be penetration through the capsule to the outer surface and into the perirenal soft tissue. Biopsy may have been performed with local flank spillage. No residual tumor beyond margins of excision
Stage III	Residual nonhematogenous tumor confined to abdomen. Any one or more of the following may be present: 1. Extension beyond surgical margins micro- or macroscopically 2. Diffuse peritoneal contamination by spread or spillage 3. Involved nodes (renal hilar nodes previously) 4. Tumor not fully resectable because of local infiltration into vital organs, e.g. liver
Stage IV	Blood-borne metastases, e.g. lung, liver, bone and/or brain
Stage V	Bilateral kidney tumors initially or subsequently

reduced without compromising cure.[279] Primary nephrectomy is only recommended for children less than 6 months of age with localized intrarenal tumors.

Pre-operative chemotherapy

For localized tumors vincristine weekly for 4 doses with actinomycin in weeks 1 and 3, followed by nephrectomy in week 5.

For metastatic tumors vincristine weekly for 6 doses with actinomycin weeks 1, 3 and 5 and doxorubicin in weeks 1 and 5, followed by nephrectomy in week 6.

Postoperative chemotherapy

This is determined by the combination of local stage and histological classification at nephrectomy for localized disease, and by this and the response of pulmonary metastases for those with metastatic disease. Stage I tumors are limited to the kidney, without involvement of the vessels of the renal sinus, and are completely resected. Stage II tumors extend beyond the kidney, infiltrate the renal sinus or adjacent organs or vena cava, but have been completely resected. Stage III tumors extend beyond the resection margins or involve abdominal lymph nodes, including post-chemotherapy changes in resected lymph nodes.

Localized tumors

Histological low risk, Stage I tumors do not need any further treatment. Stage II and III tumors receive 27 weeks of vincristine (20 doses) and actinomycin (9 doses)(AV-2). Intermediate risk, Stage I tumors receive 4 doses of vincristine and 1 of actinomycin (AV-1). Intermediate risk Stage II and III patients are randomized between actinomycin, vincristine and doxorubicin (AVD) and AV-2. Stage III patients receive local flank radiotherapy. High risk patients with Stage I disease receive AVD, Stage II and III patients receive the high risk strategy described below and local radiotherapy.

Metastatic tumors

Patients with complete radiological clearance of their pulmonary metastases prenephrectomy receive AVD with flank radiotherapy if they have local Stage III disease, unless they have histological high risk disease at nephrectomy. Patients with persistent metastases that cannot be surgically removed receive the high risk strategy with flank radiotherapy for local Stage III tumors and pulmonary radiation. Patients with high risk tumors of any stage receive the high risk strategy, etoposide and carboplatin alternating with cyclophosphamide and doxorubicin for 34 weeks with flank radiotherapy for Stage II and II tumors and pulmonary radiotherapy for all.

Specific late effects

Long term renal problems are uncommon in Wilms tumor patients these days. The small group of patients with Denys–Drash syndrome are at risk of nephritis in the remaining kidney. Flank radiation fields including the full vertebral width have reduced bony anomalies and lower dosages have reduced abdominal wall muscle atrophy. An acute veno-occlusive syndrome is occasionally seen when right-sided flank irradiation is combined with actinomycin D or adriamycin (both should be avoided for 6 weeks postradiation). Lung irradiation for residual pulmonary metastases can cause an acute pneumonitis, fibrosis and impairment of lung function.[177] Meadows et al[153] described 24 second tumors among Wilms tumor patients, with 22/24 having received radiotherapy and 10/24 chemotherapy and radiotherapy. As with Hodgkin disease, increasingly attempts are made to avoid radiation combined with chemotherapy wherever possible, hence the use of presurgical chemotherapy to reduce tumor rupture and the subsequent need for radiotherapy.

MESOBLASTIC NEPHROMA

This tumor forms only a small percentage of childhood renal tumors but it is the commonest in the neonatal period with a mean age at diagnosis of 3–4 months. It is a quite distinct entity from Wilms tumor. The kidney may be large with no pseudocapsule. Hemorrhage, cysts and necrosis are rare but the tumor may appear to infiltrate into the normal kidney and into the perinephric connective tissue. The mass is most commonly felt coincidentally at the time of an examination for other reasons. Occasionally there is hematuria, hypertension secondary to a rise in renin and even congestive cardiac failure. Babies with this tumor can have increased risk of preterm delivery due to polyhydramnios. Prenatal diagnosis has been made using ultrasound. The differential diagnosis is between hydronephrosis and multicystic kidney. Ultrasound can distinguish between these but cannot distinguish a nephroma from nephroblastoma. The treatment of choice is nephrectomy; recurrence is rare and usually only in children presenting beyond 3 months of life. Adjuvant treatment is only required for recurrent disease or significant but rare renal rupture or if the patient is older than 3 months with marked cellular mitosis on histology.

SOFT TISSUE SARCOMAS (STS)[280]

Sarcomas can arise from primitive mesenchymal cells anywhere in the body. They are the sixth most common form of childhood cancer.

RHABDOMYOSARCOMA (RMS)

The vast majority (75%) of soft tissue sarcomas are rhabdomyosarcomas. Bladder and vaginal rhabdomyosarcomas are more common in the young and are most often embryonal or botryoid in type. Truncal and extremity lesions are more common in older patients and are more likely to have alveolar histology.

Specific etiologic factors

Most cases of RMS are sporadic and of unknown etiology. However STS in children is associated with a significant increase in risk of breast cancer in their mothers due to germline mutations of the p53 tumor suppressor gene on chromosome 17.[28,281] RMS has also been associated with the nevoid basal cell carcinoma syndrome (Gorlin) which results from a germline mutation of the human homologue of the Drosophila segment polarity gene, patched (ptc).[282,283] The protein product of ptc is a membrane receptor that is involved in the regulation of sonic hedgehog (shh) and wnt-1 signaling. Shh and wnt-1 are very important in the induction of embryonal myogenesis, via expression of the developmental transcription factors Pax-3 and Pax-7.[284] Chromosomal translocations involving either Pax-3 (t(2;13)) or Pax-7 (t(1;13)) and the Forkhead (FKHR) transcription factor are seen commonly in alveolar RMS.[285] Thus a model is beginning to emerge in which abnormalities in the ptc/shh/Pax signaling pathway contribute to the development of RMS.[286]

Clinical presentation

Rhabdomyosarcomas can arise at any site in the body as mass lesions. They are usually nontender and the presentation depends on the site of the tumor.

Head and neck (40% of all rhabdomyosarcomas)

About 10% of tumors arise in the orbit producing proptosis and ophthalmoplegia. These are usually small, localized tumors with good prognosis (Fig. 24.11). Parameningeal tumors (about 20%) arise from the nasopharynx, paranasal sinuses, middle ear, mastoid and pterygopalatine fossa, producing nasal airway and ear symptoms often with purulent or bloody discharge. There is a high risk of cranial nerve or meningeal involvement and raised intracranial pressure may be the presenting feature. Other head and neck sites including scalp, face, oral mucosa, oropharynx, larynx and neck do not carry the same risk of CNS spread and present as mass lesions; they tend to be of low stage and nonmetastatic.

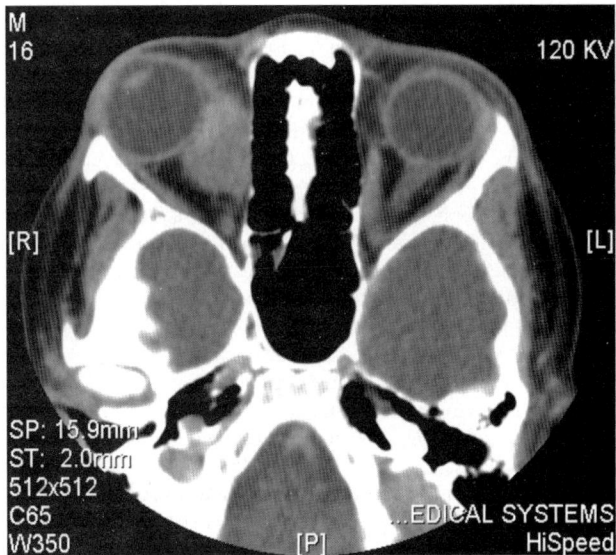

Fig. 24.11 Contrast-enhanced CT of orbit showing a rhabdomyosarcoma of the medial rectus muscle.

Genitourinary tract (20%)

These usually arise in the bladder and prostate (12%) presenting as a polypoid mass inside the bladder leading to hematuria, urinary obstruction or even extrusion of the tumor into the urethra in females. They tend to be localized. Prostatic tumors lead to bladder outlet obstruction. Constipation may arise from obstruction of the rectum. Bladder tumors tend to occur in younger patients. Prostatic tumors have a higher risk of dissemination. Vaginal and uterine rhabdomyosarcomas make up 2% of the total. Most are botryoid (grape-like) and present with a mucosal or bloody discharge. Paratesticular tumors make up about 6% of the total and usually present as painless swellings in the scrotum or inguinal canal. The genitourinary tract tumors tend to have embryonal histology.

Extremity lesions (20%)

The majority have alveolar histology. Nodal and metatstatic involvement is common.

Truncal (10%)

On the trunk the mass may reach massive proportions before diagnosis. Local recurrence and distant spread is more likely than lymphatic or nodal involvement.

Other sites (10%)

Intrathoracic and retroperitoneal tumors may reach large dimensions before diagnosis. Intrathoracic primaries may present with airway obstruction or other respiratory symptoms and abdominal tumors with gastrointestinal obstruction. Perineal lesions are rare but can present like an abscess or a polyp. They often have alveolar histology and nodal spread.

Diagnosis

Careful assessment of primary tumor extent and regional node involvement (clinical and radiological) is required as a baseline. A truly localized lesion should have a full excision biopsy attempted but most will have diagnostic biopsy. In parameningeal sites, investigations should include full CNS visualization by CT or MR plus CSF examination if there is no evidence of an intracerebral mass lesion. CT scan of the chest and isotope bone scan to exclude lung and bone metastases are needed. Bilateral marrow trephines and aspirates are required to exclude marrow involvement.

Histological classification

Traditionally several forms of rhabdomyosarcoma were recognized.[287] Differences in classification of these tumors existed between North American and European pathologists and an attempt to produce a unifying classification based upon prognostic categories (International Classification of RMS) has been proposed.[288] This divides these tumors into three groups:

1. *Superior prognosis*: This consists of the botryoid and spindle cell subtypes of embryonal RMS. Both of these variants are uncommon, botryoid accounting for 6% of STS and spindle cell 3%. However both have an excellent prognosis; 95% 5-year overall survival (OS) for botryoid and 88% for spindle cell reported in the second Intergroup study (IRS II). Botryoid lesions are usually found at sites that allow growth into a cavity, normally in the genitourinary tract. They tend to have a distinctive macroscopic 'bunch of grapes' appearance, and microscopically a subepithelial layer of condensed tumor cells. Spindle cell RMS is of low cellularity and is almost exclusively formed of spindle-shaped cells. These tumors are normally paratesticular in site.

2. *Intermediate prognosis*: This group contains embryonal RMS. Histologically these consist of blastemal mesenchymal cells which tend to differentiate into cross-striated muscle cells. Considerable cytologic variation can exist. These tumors tend to be found in children less than the age of 10 years and in sites including head and neck, pelvis and retroperitoneum. In IRS II these patients accounted for 49% of STS and had a 66% 5-year OS.

3. *Poor prognosis*: This group contains alveolar RMS and the undifferentiated sarcomas. Alveolar RMS features a connective tissue stroma lined with tumor cells giving rise to the so-called alveolar pattern. This may not be present throughout the tumor, but any amount of alveolar tumor even within a predominantly embryonal RMS carries a worse prognosis and the tumor should be regarded as alveolar. Alveolar RMS tends to present in older patients in association with skeletal muscle, usually involving the extremities or the trunk. Undifferentiated sarcomas are usually diffuse and contain primitive mesenchymal cells which are negative for the antigenic markers of RMS. In IRS II, 31% of tumors were alveolar and 10% undifferentiated sarcoma; alveolar RMS had a 5-year OS of 54% and undifferentiated sarcoma 40%.

Although rhabdomyosarcoma is the commonest STS of childhood, other tumors including extraosseous Ewing sarcoma, fibrosarcoma and peripheral primitive neuroectodermal tumors may need to be considered in the differential. Identification on light and electron microscopy of cross-striations will facilitate a specific diagnosis. Immunocytochemistry as outlined in Table 24.16 has enabled easier differentiation of rhabdomyosarcoma from other tumors.[289] Desmin is the most useful marker but caution is required for its interpretation. Multiple monoclonal antibodies may help to confirm the diagnosis. It is the pattern of positivity rather than any single marker which determines the diagnosis.

Staging

The system used by the Intergroup collaborators (IRS) is the most widely accepted (Table 24.20) but attempts are now being made to adapt the TNM system[290] and relate it to site and extent of disease. A new grouping system is being tested in most recent trials.

Prognostic variables

RMS is a heterogenous condition and several prognostic factors have been identified, in addition to the histological groupings described above. Both pre-operative stage and postsurgical extent of disease are important. For those with localized tumors, complete excision (Group I) yields better survival than those with microscopic residual tumor or regional extension (Group II). Even poorer survival is seen for those with macroscopic (Group III) residual tumor and the worst for those with metastatic disease (Group IV). In IRS III 5-year OS for Group I disease was 93%, while for Group IV disease it was only 30%.[291] The site of the primary influences the lag time between first symptoms and diagnosis, the likelihood of metastatic spread and the possibility of surgical excision, and is also related to histological type. Orbital tumors had a 5-year OS of 95% in IRS III, while 5-year OS for parameningeal tumors was only 70%, a difference that was still seen in IRS IV.[292] In all trials to date, alveolar histology confers a worse prognosis than embryonal (see above). Tumor size

Table 24.20 Intergroup rhabdomyosarcoma study clinical grouping system

Clinical group	Definition
I	A. Localized, completely resected, confined to site of origin
	B. Localized, completely resected, infiltrated beyond site of origin
II	A. Localized, grossly resected, microscopic residual
	B. Regional disease, involved lymph nodes, completely resected
	C. Regional disease, involved lymph nodes, grossly resected with microscopic residual
III	A. Local or regional grossly visible disease after biopsy only
	B. Grossly visible disease after >50% resection of primary tumor
IV	Distant metastases present at diagnosis

(< 5 cm) and patient age (< 10 years) are also important prognostic features. Some data also exist to suggest that different molecular abnormalities may confer different prognoses. Event free survival among a group of patients with alveolar RMS having the Pax7-FKHR gene fusion was significantly better than for a group containing the Pax3-FKHR translocation.[293] Rate of response to treatment and achievement of complete response also closely predict for outcome.

Management

The outcome of treatment for RMS has improved steadily over the last 30 years. Overall survival was only 25% in 1970 but was 70% by 1991. This improvement in outcome has been achieved through cooperative studies; Intergroup Rhabdomyosarcoma Study Group (IRSG) in North America, and the SIOP Malignant Mesenchymal Tumor (MMT) studies in Europe. The major differences between these two groups' strategies lie in the intensity of initial therapy and the use of radiotherapy. IRSG studies tend to give radiotherapy earlier and to a greater proportion of patients than MMT studies with the result that although overall survival is not significantly different, event free survival is better in IRS studies.[292] The focus in the current European collaborative study (EpSSG RMS 2005) is on increasingly sophisticated risk group stratification.[294]

Low risk

A. This contains nonalveolar, localized tumors ≤ 5 cm in maximum diameter in patients < 10 years of age in any site which have been fully resected (IRS Group I). These patients receive vincristine and actinomycin alone for 22 weeks, a strategy that has been effective in all previous European studies, with a 5-year EFS in these patients of > 90%.[295]

Standard risk

This contains three subgroups of patients all with nonalveolar, localized tumors:

B. Fully resected (IRS I) tumors that were > 5 cm or in patients ≥ 10 years. This is effectively an upstaging of older patients who seem to do worse.[296] These patients receive 4 cycles of IVA and then 5 of VA.

C. This contains those patients with micro- or macroscopic residual disease (IRS II/III) after surgery for localized tumors in special sites (orbit, nonparameningeal head and neck, nonbladder/prostate genitourinary tract). This group contains most of the patients who have not received radiotherapy in MMT studies. IRS IV treated these patients with VA and radiotherapy with very good results.[292] The aim of the EpSSG study is to reduce chemotherapy for this group, so they receive 4 cycles of IVA and 5 of VA, and to use response to 3 cycles of IVA to determine need for radiotherapy.

D. Localized, ≤ 5 cm, non-alveolar tumors with residual disease in all other sites in patients < 10 years. These patients receive 9 cycles of IVA and local radiotherapy with or without surgery.

High risk

This again contains three subgroups:

E. Those patients with localized, non-alveolar tumors with residual disease in other sites who either have tumors > 5 cm or are ≥ 10 years.

F. Non-alveolar, ≤ 5 cm tumors in any site with nodal disease in patients < 10 years.

G. Localized alveolar tumors of any size, in any site, in any age of patient. All three of these subgroups will be randomized between 9 cycles of IVA and 4 cycles of IVA with doxorubicin followed by 5 cycles of IVA (IVADo). Those patients in CR at the end of 9 cycles are randomized between stopping and 24 weeks of vinorelbine and cyclophosphamide.[297,298]

Very high risk

Those patients with alveolar disease with nodal spread. These patients have a very poor prognosis in previous European studies with survival comparable to that for metastatic disease. They will thus be treated with the intensive IVADo and vinorelbine/cyclophosphamide arm.

Metastatic disease

In IRS III the survival for patients with metastatic disease was only 30%[291] and in MMT 89 was only 29%. Both groups have used the up-front window study as a means of evaluating the effectiveness of novel agents. In the IRS IV study single agents found to be effective when used alone were subsequently incorporated into the continuation chemotherapy regimen. Topotecan was shown to be highly effective in the treatment of newly diagnosed metastatic RMS[299] and IRS V is using a similar approach with irinotecan. However despite the activity of topotecan the overall survival for patients receiving the topotecan-based regimen was still only 20% at 3 years.[300] MMT 98 used the up-front window approach described above and followed this with a six drug regimen of IVA and carboplatin, epirubicin and etoposide, the combination having been previously shown to be effective in this setting,[301] followed by 9 cycles of maintenance chemotherapy with VAC. However MMT 98 also defined a high risk group of patients older than 10 years or those with bone or bone marrow disease who were treated with high dose sequential monotherapy (cyclophosphamide, etoposide, carboplatin) and nine courses of VAC as maintenance. Pooled analysis of the results from five up-front IRS window studies suggests that future strategies for metastatic RMS should include ifosfamide, etoposide, doxorubicin and topotecan/irinotecan.[302]

OSTEOSARCOMA

The age-standardized incidence of osteosarcoma in Europe is 5.5 per million for boys and girls aged 0–14 years. However it is commoner in the second decade of life when the incidence rises to 19.3 per million for boys and 10.7 per million for girls aged 14–19 years. Between 51% and 55% of bone tumors in children are osteosarcomas.[303]

Etiology

The peak age incidence is at the time of maximum bone growth and osteosarcoma usually occurs at the metaphyses of rapidly growing long bones (distal femur, proximal tibia, proximal humerus). It has a slightly younger peak age for girls, corresponding to earlier onset of puberty. These features all point toward malignant transformation of rapidly proliferating bone forming cells. The question then is whether transformation is a spontaneous event or induced by other environmental factors. Trauma frequently draws attention to the tumor but is almost certainly not causative. About 3% of all osteosarcomas are secondary to therapeutic irradiation. Latency between initial treatment and onset of a secondary osteosarcoma can be 10–15 years. Osteochondromas and chronic osteomyelitis can predispose to tumor formation. There is a strong association with retinoblastoma and 50% of the second tumors in heritable retinoblastoma are osteosarcomas. The same chromosome 13 defect has been demonstrated in both tumors. It has been speculated that rapidly proliferating bone forming cells may be particularly susceptible to mitotic errors and lead to loss of heterozygosity at the Rb locus. A number of other familial clusterings have also been described, including in families with demonstrated p53 germline mutations. Many osteosarcomas show somatic rearrangements of p53.

Presentation

Most osteosarcomas present as a mass. Symptom duration is usually about 2–3 months. A more delayed presentation is commoner in periosteal sarcomas when symptoms may be present for many months or even years. Distal femur (33–35%), proximal tibia (15%), proximal humerus (9–10%), mid-femur (5%) and proximal femur (4–5%) are the commonest sites. Axial flat bones can be affected, especially in the pelvis, and constitute 15–20% of all tumors. These sites tend to occur in older patients. Up to 20% of patients have metastases at diagnosis, most commonly in the lungs. Occasionally multifocal osteosarcoma is seen and this carries a very poor prognosis.

agents in osteosarcoma are cisplatinum, doxorubicin and methotrexate. Ifosfamide has been shown to be a promising agent with greater than 20% single drug efficacy in relapsed patients and is often used in combination with etoposide. The amount of tumor necrosis after presurgical therapy relates to outcome with those with < 10% viable tumor having 75% 5-year survival compared to 45% for poor responders.[306] The current collaborative European and North American trial (EURAMOS 1) compares cisplatin, doxorubicin and methotrexate (MAP) with MAP and ifosfamide and etoposide (MAPIE) in those with poor response to pre-surgery chemotherapy, and MAP with MAP and pegylated interferon α_{2b} for good responders. Importantly this study includes patients with axial primary tumors, primary metastatic disease, and those with secondary tumors who may all have comparable survival to those with localized extremity tumors, with complete surgical excision.[308,309]

Modern surgical practice avoids amputation if possible. However this is not always the case and it is probably best discussed as an option at the time of diagnosis. Both endoprosthetic replacement and amputation can have very good functional outcomes, but high quality physiotherapy is important in achieving the maximum function after surgery.[310]

Previously patients relapsing with pulmonary metastases have been salvaged with the use of second line intensive therapy, e.g. using ifosfamide and etoposide plus high dose methotrexate when they have initially received just cisplatinum and doxorubicin followed by thoracotomies to remove metastases. With these aggressive approaches to pulmonary metastases 30–40% of such patients may be alive 5 years from the time of relapse. The therapy for such patients who have already received all of these agents before relapse remains to be clarified.

EWING SARCOMA

This is the second most common malignant bone tumor of childhood with a peak age at 10–15 years. Worldwide variations are seen in Tables 24.1 and 22.2 with a low risk especially among black Americans and the Chinese. Ewing, Askin and peripheral neuroectodermal tumors are all included in this group. These tumors consist of small round blue cells and more than 95% show re-arrangements of chromosome 22, usually an 11;22 translocation resulting in an EWS-FLI1 fusion oncogene.[311]

Presentation

The commonest presentation is with a painful swelling of an affected bone and adjacent soft tissue. Around 20–25% of patients will have metastatic disease at presentation and tiredness, anorexia, weight loss and fever can be expected. Radiological appearances and the presence of fever may lead to the diagnosis of osteomyelitis and delay appropriate therapy (Fig. 24.13a). The most common sites are the pelvis, proximal humerus and femur but any bone can be involved. The axial skeleton is more frequently involved than with osteosarcoma. In long bones, metaphyseal and diaphyseal sites are the rule. Rib primaries often present with pleural effusions and respiratory difficulties. Sacral tumors may present with sacral nerve compression and either limb or bladder signs and symptoms.

Diagnosis

The differential diagnosis includes osteomyelitis, arthritis, traumatic injury to bone, osteosarcoma, neuroblastoma, lymphomas and even leukemia. MR imaging is required to determine the local extent of tumor within bone and soft tissue (Fig. 24.13b). CT is necessary to exclude pulmonary metastases and bone scan to exclude bony metastases (Fig. 24.13c,d). At biopsy

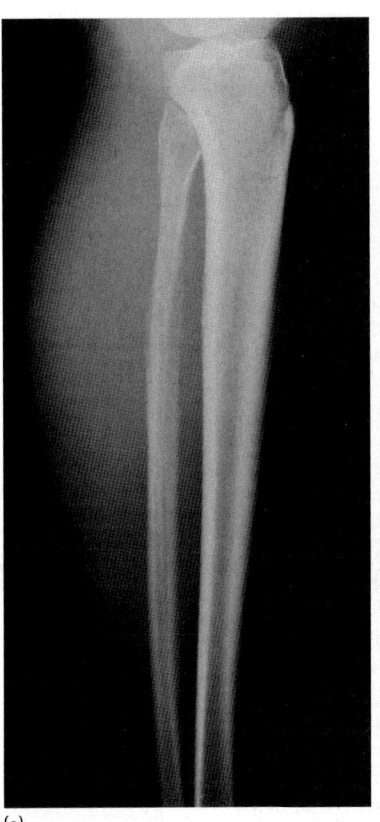 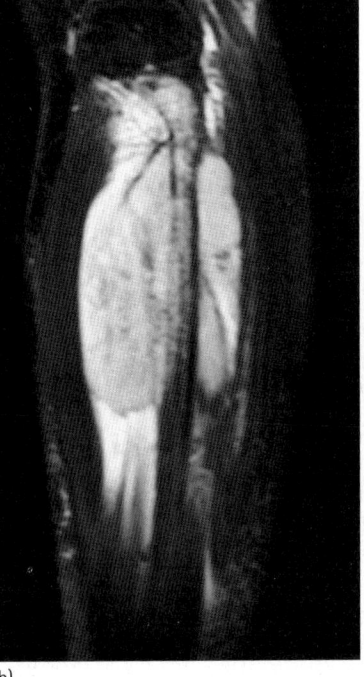 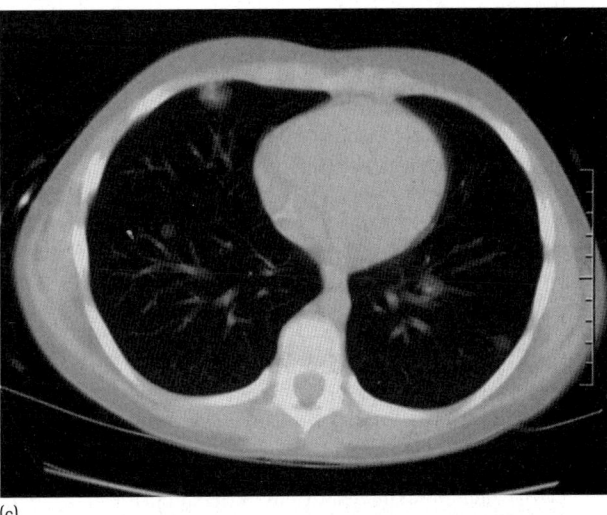

(a) (b) (c)

Fig. 24.13 (a) Plain radiograph of the leg showing a Ewing sarcoma of the proximal fibula. Note the 'moth-eaten' appearance of the upper fibula, extensive periosteal reaction and associated soft tissue swelling. (b) T2-weighted sagittal MR scan of the leg in Ewing sarcoma showing an extensive soft tissue component surrounding the fibula and signal change affecting the upper half of the fibula. Contrast this with relatively discrete changes on plain radiography. (c) CT of chest showing pulmonary metastases of Ewing sarcoma.

(Continued)

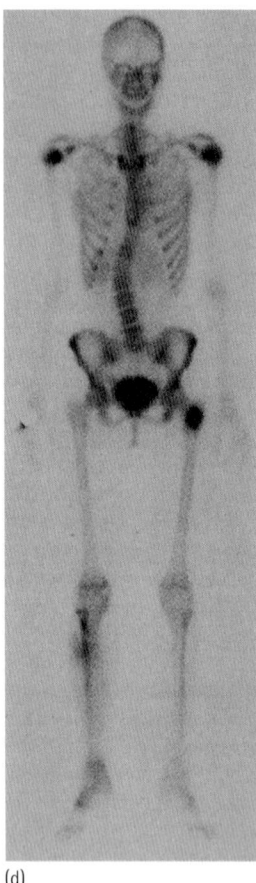

(d)

Fig. 24.13 Continued   (d) Technetium isotope bone scan showing extensive bony metastases in Ewing sarcoma.

adequate material must be obtained. Incision for biopsy must be in a place where if further definitive surgery is to take place the scar can be excised, as with osteosarcoma. Diagnostic biopsy is best performed in a supraregional unit specializing in bone tumors. Two bone marrow aspirations and trephines from different sites should be performed to exclude marrow infiltration.

Pathology

Typical Ewing sarcoma consists of sheets of small round cells with minimal stroma. These cells are usually strongly vimentin positive and negative for neural markers, although in PNET NSE and S100 are often positive. Most Ewing sarcomas and PNETs will be strongly positive for MIC2. Identification of the EWS-FLI1 translocation by FISH is often useful in confirming the diagnosis.

Prognostic features

Metastatic disease at presentation is the strongest adverse prognostic feature in Ewing sarcoma. In CESS 81–EICESS 92 the 10-year disease free survival for patients with localized disease was 55%, for those with pulmonary metastases alone 30% and for those with bone or bone marrow metastases only 18%.[312] The structural type of EWS-FlI1 fusion transcript has also been reported to be an independent prognostic factor, patients with the type 1 transcript having a better prognosis than those without.[313] Tumor volume greater than 200 ml is associated with worse outcome in patients with localized disease.[314] The histological response to chemotherapy correlated with prognosis in both the French EW88 and CESS 86 studies.[314,315] Pelvic and spinal tumors are usually bigger at presentation and less amenable to surgical resection than distal limb tumors and thus tend to have a worse prognosis.

Management
Chemotherapy

The role of chemotherapy in Ewing sarcoma is both to treat systemic disease and to shrink local tumor to allow for easier or less mutilating surgery.

Chemotherapy based on vincristine, cyclophosphamide and doxorubicin has been effective and replacement of cyclophosphamide with ifosfamide resulted in an improvement in 5-year overall survival from 44% to 62% in UK studies,[316] and was associated with improved outcome in CESS 86.[314] Further intensification with ifosfamide and etoposide in CCG/POG studies resulted in improved overall survival for localized, but not metastatic, disease.[317,318] To improve survival for patients with primary metatstatic disease further dose intensification and up-front windows studies of new agents have been tried. Whilst topotecan alone did not seem to be active, the combination of topotecan and cyclophosphamide is promising.[319] Myeloablative theray with peripheral blood stem cell support does not seem to improve survival for this group of patients.[320] The current European study (Euro-Ewing 99) gives six courses of vincristine, ifosfamide, doxorubiciɴ and etoposide (VIDE) before local therapy, and then maintenance therapy with vincristine, actinomycin and cyclophosphamide (VAC) or vincristine, actinomycin and ifosfamide (VAI) for patients with localized disease and good histological response to VIDE. Patients with poor response to VIDE or pulmonary metastases at diagnosis are randomized between VAI and MAT with PBSC support. Patients with nonpulmonary metastatic disease are eligible for an up-front windows study of irinotecan and receive MAT with PBSC support after local therapy.

Surgery

Definitive local therapy to achieve complete clearance of tumor is required for Ewing sarcoma. The increasing sophistication of prosthetic surgery means that this can now be achieved in many patients without amputation. However the primary consideration in deciding upon surgical approach remains the need to achieve good margins of tumor clearance. Evidence from EICESS 92 suggests that a more aggressive surgical approach, and even the use of pre-operative radiotherapy to improve operability, have a significant effect on both overall survival and on local recurrence rates. In EICESS 92 75% of German patients received surgery compared to 51% of UK patients, and 45% received pre-operative radiotherapy compared to 3% of UK patients. Overall survival for these groups was 66% versus 54% and local recurrence rates were 7% versus 21%.[321]

Radiotherapy

Whilst surgery should be considered the primary mode of local control in Ewing sarcoma there will be many patients, particularly those with pelvic or other axial tumors, for whom this is not possible. In the EICESS 92 study even in the German patient group 25% of patients had inoperable tumors. Whilst Ewing sarcoma is radiosensitive the EICESS 92 patients receiving radiotherapy alone as local therapy had the worst overall survival[321] and the same differential survival has been seen in POG studies.[322] Despite this radiotherapy is effective for local control; in the POG 8346 study local control rates were 88% for patients receiving surgery with or without radiotherapy, but still 65% for those receiving radiotherapy alone, and among patients receiving appropriate treatment volumes the local control rate was 80%.[322] The majority of treatment failures with this disease are systemic rather than local.

GERM CELL TUMORS

These tumors are derived from primordial germ cells and arise within the gonads and at a number of other midline sites in the sacrococcygeal, retroperitoneal, mediastinal, neck or pineal regions. Malignant germ cell tumors account for 3% of all childhood cancers. A number of structural chromosomal changes have been detected in germ cell tumors, most consistently an isochrome 12p, in about 80% of patients with testicular lesions.[323] Klinefelter syndrome is strongly associated with mediastinal tumors (20% of males so affected). 46XY gonadal dysgenesis is frequently complicated by germ cell tumors.

TERATOMAS

These are tumors with tissue arising from all three germinal layers, with a lack of organization and variable maturation. They may be solid or cystic and are most often found in the sacrococcygeal region. Teratomas can contain three types of tissue; mature, with well-differentiated tissues; immature, with embryonic components; and malignant with disorganized embryonic tissue and malignant germ cell elements.

GERMINOMA[324]

The commonest sites for these tumors in childhood are the ovary (dysgerminoma), anterior mediastinum and pineal region (Fig. 24.14). Ten percent of all ovarian and 15% of all germ cell tumors are germinomas and they are the commonest in undescended testicles (seminoma). There is a characteristic histological appearance of large round cells, vesicular nuclei and clear eosinophilic cytoplasm. Serum levels of AFP and HCG levels are not elevated in pure germinoma.

EMBRYONAL CARCINOMA

This is a poorly differentiated tumor usually with an epithelial appearance. Apparent pathological maturation to teratoma has been noted after chemotherapy. These tumors stain markedly for AFP and HCG. In pediatric practice it is rare to see pure embryonal carcinoma, but it may be found as a component of other germ cell tumors. In young males, the commonest site is the testis.

YOLK SAC TUMOR

This tumor occurring alone or in combination with teratoma is the most common malignant germ cell tumor in childhood. The sacrococcygeal region is the usual site in infancy but later the ovary and testes are more frequently affected, although it can occur elsewhere. The tumors are often soft and friable with a papillary, reticular or a solid pattern.

CHORIOCARCINOMA

This highly malignant tumor is rare in childhood and arises from nongestational extraplacental tissue. The commonest sites are the mediastinum, ovary and pineal region. βHCG but not AFP is markedly elevated in serum. Histology shows large round cells with vesicular nuclei (cytotrophoblasts) and large, usually vacuolated, cells which form syncytia (syncytiotrophoblasts). Hemorrhage and necrosis are common.

GONADOBLASTOMA

This tumor is most frequently found in dysgenetic gonads. Thirty percent of patients with gonadal dysgenesis develop gonadoblastoma (bilateral in 40% of cases). Local invasion is seen within the gonads but if elements of germinoma are present it is more likely to spread. AFP and HCG are not produced by this tumor.

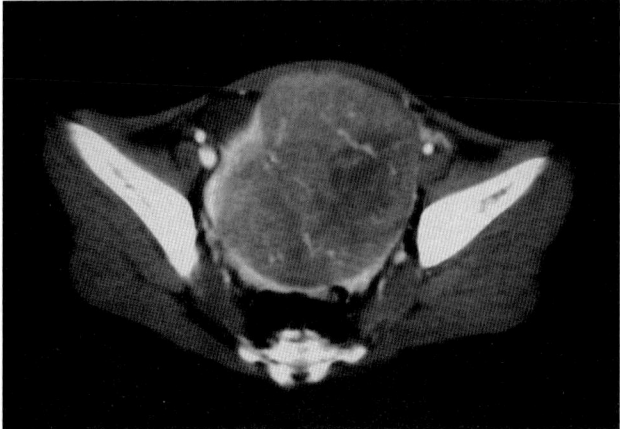

Fig. 24.14 Contrast-enhanced CT of pelvis showing a large ovarian dysgerminoma.

POLYEMBRYOMA

This is a rare tumor of the ovary or anterior mediastinum. Both AFP and HCG are elevated. The tumor contains elements resembling small embryos.

Biochemical markers

Three markers may help with diagnosis and monitoring of therapy.

Alpha-fetoprotein

Alpha-fetoprotein (AFP) production from the yolk sac is maximal at about 12–15 weeks of gestation. Normal adult blood levels are not reached until 6–12 months postpartum. Tumors arising from the pluripotential germ cells of the yolk sac secrete AFP with the exception of pure dysgerminoma, pure choriocarcinoma, mature teratomas and gonadoblastoma. Monitoring of serum levels can be useful, especially for evidence of resistant or recurrent disease. Staining of tumor for AFP is a useful diagnostic tool.

Beta-human chorionic gonadotrophin

This glycoprotein is produced by specialized placental cells so that tumor with trophoblastic elements (choriocarcinoma and hydatidiform moles) have high levels. The half-life is extremely short (45 minutes) so rapid normalization occurs with tumor kill.

Lactate dehydrogenase isoenzyme 1

Elevation of this isoenzyme is seen in tumor derived from the yolk sac. It can be used to monitor response to therapy.

SACROCOCCYGEAL TERATOMAS

The incidence is 1 in 35 000 live births with 65% being benign, 30% malignant and 5–10% having an immature appearance. Approximately 40% of all germ cell tumors occur in this area. There is a marked female sex preponderance (70%). The mode of presentation will depend on the precise site of the tumor:

1. The buttocks with a minimal presacral component. This is the commonest site in the newborn (186 out of 398 in one series[325]).
2. External but with a significant intrapelvic component (138 out of 398).
3. External but with most of the mass intrapelvic and extending into the abdomen (35 out of 398). This is the group most likely to be malignant de novo.
4. Entirely presacral with no external component or significant pelvic extension (39 out of 398). These are more difficult to detect and may lead to constipation, urinary frequency or lower limb weakness from sacral nerve compression.

Diagnosis

The early detection and surgical removal of even a benign tumor is necessary because of the risk of subsequent malignant change. If the diagnosis is made before 2 months of age the chance of malignancy is low (10% in boys and 7% in girls). After 2 months, the risk of malignancy is over 60% in boys and 45–50% in girls. The estimation of AFP and HCG levels is mandatory. CT or MRI scanning will delineate the tumor extent, and determine the presence of any intraspinal component. Pulmonary metastases must be excluded.

MEDIASTINAL TERATOMAS

These almost always arise in the anterior superior mediastinum along the urogenital ridge which extends from C6 to L4. They are sometimes found coincidentally on chest X-ray or they may present with airway obstruction, cough, wheeze and dyspnea. Many histological types have been reported, ranging from pure teratoma to embryonal carcinoma and yolk sac tumor. Radiological appearances are of a rounded mass often with calcification. Sometimes teeth may be identified in a mature teratoma. Cross-sectional imaging is essential to determine tumor extent. AFP, HCG levels and urinary catecholamines should be measured. It is important to exclude other diagnoses because, for a mediastinal teratoma, complete surgical excision is necessary for cure whereas in other tumors (especially lymphomas) chemotherapy is the treatment of choice.

ABDOMINAL GERM CELL TUMOR

Most arise in the retroperitoneum but they can occur within the gastrointestinal tract, omentum or liver. In the stomach they may present as obstruction or hemorrhage and in the liver as a mass or jaundice. The retroperitoneum is the third commonest site after the sacrococcygeal and mediastinal regions in those under 2 years. Pressure from the mass causes pain, constipation or urinary difficulties. Cross-sectional imaging and measurement of urinary catecholamines and serum AFP levels will aid diagnosis.

INTRACRANIAL TERATOMAS

These account for about 6% of germ cell tumors. Most arise in the pineal region but they can also arise in the suprasellar and infrasellar regions, more frequently leading to CSF pathway obstruction at third ventricular level. A wide variety of histological types including germinomas, embryonal carcinoma and pure teratoma are reported and it is important to distinguish between them since the treatment will be different. For teratoma, surgical excision is the treatment of choice; for embryonal carcinoma, which is more likely to be highly malignant, intensive chemotherapy and radiotherapy will be needed.

Other sites for extragonadal germ cell tumors are the oral cavity, the pharynx, the orbit and the neck, collectively making up about 6% of germ cell tumors. These are mostly found at birth and are of benign histology though they can cause death from airway obstruction. Vaginal tumors, mostly of the endodermal sinus tumor type, usually present with bloody discharge.

GONADAL TUMORS
Ovarian tumor

These account for about 30% of all germ cell tumors; 65% are benign teratomas, 5% are immature teratomas and about 30% are malignant. In children epithelial carcinoma of the ovary is rare. Most malignant ovarian germ cell tumors occur around the time of puberty. Presentation is usually with acute or chronic pain associated with nausea and vomiting. There may be fever. These tumors are not infrequently misdiagnosed as appendicitis and found at laparotomy. The mass may be large with omental seeding before presentation. If βHCG secretion is marked, pregnancy may be misdiagnosed. The tumor can spread locally to the adnexae, throughout the abdomen (with ascites), to nodes or via the blood. Cross-sectional imaging is needed to define site and extent of tumor (Fig. 24.14). Pulmonary metastases should be excluded. AFP levels will be elevated if the tumor contains yolk sac elements or immature teratoma and βHCG if it is an embryonal carcinoma or choriocarcinoma.

Testicular tumors[326]

These comprise about 7% of all germ cell tumors and about 70% of all testicular tumors in childhood. Eighty percent are malignant and nearly 20% are pure teratomas. The most common malignant tumor is yolk sac tumor. The presentation is with a slowly growing painless testicular mass, with or without accompanying hydrocele (25%) and/or inguinal hernia (20%). These tumors may be misdiagnosed as either epididymitis or hydrocele. If the testis is undescended the risk of malignancy is 20–40 times greater. The risk of malignant change is also higher in the contralateral descended testis in a patient with unilateral cryptorchidism. Ultrasound of the testis with CT scanning of abdomen, pelvis and chest, and measurement of AFP and HCG levels will help diagnosis and staging.

MANAGEMENT
Benign germ cell tumors

The optimal treatment for mature teratomas is complete surgical excision. In the UKCCSG study 123 of 125 patients with mature or immature germ cell tumors had primary surgical resection and 114 of these needed no further treatment.[327] Six of these patients developed yolk sac recurrence which was successfully treated with combination chemotherapy. The AFP should be followed long term to identify any recurrence. External sacrococcygeal tumors require a transacral approach but if the pelvis is involved an abdominal combined approach is needed. Removal of the coccyx is essential if recurrence is to be avoided. Spillage from cysts must be avoided and the surgeon should ensure that there is no intraspinal extension of the tumor.

Immature germ cell tumors

Controversy exists about the ideal treatment of immature teratomas. For localized but immature forms, most authorities still recommend surgery and follow-up, as the diagnosis is often only made after tumor removal. The UK and US practice is to treat recurrence with chemotherapy if it arises; the POG experience in 68 children receiving surgery alone was of three recurrences, all salvaged with chemotherapy[328] and a 3-year disease free survival of 96.7%; the UK experience is of four recurrences out of 41 patients, three salvaged with chemotherapy.[327]

Malignant germ cell tumor

Einhorn et al[329] showed that cisplatinum, bleomycin and vinblastine (BVP) were superior to all previous chemotherapy for malignant ovarian and testicular germ cell tumors. More recently the UKCCSG has demonstrated that pulsed carboplatin, etoposide and bleomycin (JEB) is as effective and less toxic for all malignant extracranial nongonadal tumors. Five-year event free survival was 87% and overall survival 91% in GCII with JEB as compared with 46% and 63% respectively with the previous regimen (GCI). Rates of renal toxicity and deafness in children treated on GCI were 20% and 35% respectively, while on GCII they were 0% and 10%.[330] The current UK GCIII study attempts to use a risk group strategy to reduce the chemotherapy exposure for many of these patients.[331] All those with gonadal Stage 1 tumors are considered low risk and need no therapy beyond surgical resection. Stage 4 tumors, other than those of the testes in children < 5 years and pure germinomas, thoracic tumors (other than Stage 1), and tumors with AFP ≥ 10 000kU/l (except Stage 1 tumors and testicular tumors in children < 5 years) are considered high risk and receive 6 cycles of JEB. All other tumors are considered intermediate risk and receive 4 courses of JEB. For relapsing adult patients cisplatin and ifosfamide have been effective[332] and high dose chemotherapy with autologous bone marrow rescue have also been used successfully but there are few published pediatric data.[333]

RETINOBLASTOMA[334]

This malignant embryonal tumor occurs predominantly in the first 2 years of life (75% are diagnosed before 3 years). Its relative incidence varies considerably around the world (see Table 24.1). The increase in Africa and India is of nongenetic retinoblastoma and strongly suggests an environmental factor may be involved in etiology. The age-standardized incidence rate in the UK is 7.5 per million children which amounts to between 40 and 50 new cases diagnosed per annum in the UK. There is no obvious sex difference in incidence. There is a family history in about 10% of cases, the remaining 90% appearing sporadic. However 20–30% of all tumors are bilateral and clearly 'genetic' (even if there is no family history) and about 10–12% of unilateral cases are also inherited. This means that overall about 40% are genetic or 'heritable' from an affected, surviving parent, from a non-affected carrier parent or as the result of a new mutation in the patient. Sixty percent are 'nonhereditary' and result from spontaneous somatic cell mutations within retinal cells. They are always unilateral and have no family history. Knudson[335] proposed that in the 'genetic' form the first mutation occurred prezygotically, while a second somatic event triggered the tumor in the retina or elsewhere in the body.

In nongenetic tumors both events occur within the retinal cells. Carriers of the retinoblastoma gene (13q14) mutation can develop single or multiple retinal tumors and/or neoplasms at other sites. Indeed germline Rb mutations have been implicated in the development of osteosarcoma, small cell lung carcinoma, bladder and breast carcinoma and various soft tissue sarcomas. Abnormalities of the p53 gene often occur concurrently with the inactivation of the retinoblastoma susceptibility gene.[336] The retinoblastoma gene encodes for a 928 amino acid protein, which is a nuclear phosphoprotein with DNA-binding activity, that plays a critical role in cell cycle regulation. Very accurate genetic counseling is possible from the mode of presentation, family history and search for evidence of the Rb gene mutation in the parents. Any child of a surviving parent who had retinoblastoma has a 50% chance of developing a tumor. If normal parents have one affected child, the next one has a 1% risk if the first child had unilateral disease and 6% if it was bilateral. As with all tumor suppressor genes, sequencing has demonstrated heterozygous point mutations along the 27 exons of the Rb gene. Prenatal and postnatal prediction using such sequencing of this large gene, although cumbersome at present, clearly enables even more accuracy in terms of risk assessment.

Despite much research we do not know what causes the initial germline mutation in genetic retinoblastoma but such mutations may arise merely as a result of spontaneous mutations at a 'background' mutation rate.[337] New mutations appear to more frequently derive from the paternal allele, i.e. arise during spermatogenesis.[338,339] About 5% of retinoblastoma patients carry a constitutional deletion on the long arm of chromosome 13.[337] Sporadic nonhereditary retinoblastoma risk factors include older maternal and paternal age and paternal employment in the 'metal' industries.[340]

Presentation

Nowadays most children are identified with the tumor still intraocular. The commonest presenting feature is leukocoria or loss of the red reflex. The tumor shows as a creamy to pinkish mass through the iris. Strabismus is common if the tumor arises in the macula. Occasionally, patients may show inflammatory changes or even a fixed pupil. A common reason for delay in diagnosis is a mistaken diagnosis of uveitis or endophthalmitis. The tumor is not painful unless there is secondary glaucoma or inflammation. If the involvement is unilateral the child will probably not complain of visual loss. Most often parents note the eye abnormality and seek help. A full ophthalmological examination under general anesthetic is required. Ultrasonography, CT and MR scanning have enabled better visualization of the tumor. Bone marrow aspiration and lumbar puncture should also be performed under general anesthetic to exclude dissemination. Hemorrhage and calcification are quite common and pieces of tumor may break off and seed either into the vitreous or elsewhere on to the retina. External layer disruption can lead to choroid involvement and a greater risk of blood-borne metastases. The iris may be pushed forward by a mass effect or the trabecular network infiltrated leading to glaucoma. Spread can occur along the optic nerve to invade the brain and CSF. Blood-borne spread commonly goes to bone and brain. Lymphatic spread to the preauricular and submandibular nodes is rare. A staging system based on size of tumor, site of tumor on the retina, extension to involve the choroid, optic nerve or vitreous and presence/absence of metastases is now employed.

Management

All patients require treatment in highly specialized multidisciplinary centers. For those patients with unilateral nongenetic tumors near 100% cure is possible by enucleation.

There is clear benefit of adjuvant chemotherapy for patients with deep choroidal or optic nerve infiltration.[341] Limited dosage JOE (carboplatin, vincristine and etoposide) has been used successfully with the least toxicity and lowest rate of secondary tumors to date, from any chemotherapy regimen. The UK approach is to give 4 cycles of JOE post enucleation to those patients with deep choroidal invasion and 6 cycles with intrathecal therapy, and local radiotherapy to those with involvement of the cut end of the optic nerve at enucleation. For those with small

unilateral lesions (less than 4 disk diameters) cryotherapy and photocoagulation offer an alternative to enucleation, but very careful expert follow-up is required to ensure that the tumor is sterilized.[342] For 'genetic' disease, enucleation in unilateral disease, and the worse eye in bilateral disease, is usually performed. With the high risk of tumors developing in the other eye with such genetic tumors, if not already present, radiotherapy and/or chemotherapy is used as well to try to conserve some vision in both eyes. Careful attention must be paid to scheduling and total dosage.[343] Even with bilateral disease, event free survival at 5 years can be 90% unless there is orbital or CNS invasion, but with germline Rb carriage it would appear that the development of secondary neoplasia is a very high risk over the ensuing 30–40 years.[27] All planned combined modality therapy should attempt to minimize the risk by avoiding for example combinations of irradiation and alkylators and careful attention to the dose and scheduling of drugs such as the topoisomerase 2 inhibitors.

LIVER TUMORS

Presentation

Hepatoblastoma

This tumor usually presents as an abdominal mass in a child under 2 years. Weight loss, anorexia, vomiting and pain can be seen but symptoms are less prominent than in hepatocellular carcinoma. Occasionally the tumor ruptures and presents as an acute abdomen. Abdominal distention with an enlarged liver is the most common finding. Jaundice is rare but the patient may be anemic.

Hepatocellular carcinoma (HCC)

These tumors usually present as painful right-sided abdominal masses, often with features of underlying liver disease. Splenomegaly with finger clubbing and spider nevi is often seen. Nausea, vomiting, fever, weight loss and anorexia are more common than in hepatoblastoma. These tumors may also rupture. Jaundice is reported in up to 25% of cases. There may also be associated thrombocytosis and polycythemia due to raised erythropoietin and probably thrombopoietin levels.

Diagnosis

Ultrasound examination will define the liver mass, up to 10% of which may show calcification, and the inferior vena cava, hepatic and portal veins. Hepatoblastoma and HCC are deeply infiltrative and may be multicentric. MR scanning is superior to CT for definition of tumor margins. Hepatoblastoma occurs most commonly in the right lobe of the liver. Cooperation between radiologist and surgeon is likely to result in more reliable anatomical information (Fig. 24.15). CT of chest is needed to exclude pulmonary metastases. Blood tests should include a full blood

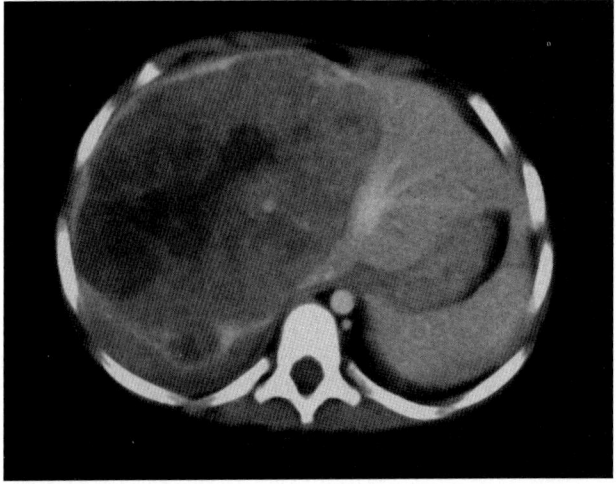

Fig. 24.15 Contrast-enhanced CT of abdomen showing a hepatoblastoma arising from the right lobe of the liver.

count. Mild normochromic normocytic anemia is quite common but, particularly in HCC, increased erythropoietin production may lead to polycythemia. The platelets may be elevated in excess of $1000 \times 10^9/L$ in childhood liver tumors. The most useful marker is AFP, produced exclusively in the liver in postnatal life. AFP is raised in about two thirds of patients with hepatoblastoma and in about 50% of patients with HCC and is useful for monitoring the course of the disease. Failure to fall along the usual gradient or a late rise suggests persistent or recurrent disease, often prior to any clinical evidence of relapse. Liver function should be evaluated and monitoring of calcium, phosphate and alkaline phosphatase levels are necessary particularly if there is any significant osteopenia. Hepatitis B serology is often positive in hepatocellular carcinoma but rarely in hepatoblastoma.

Staging and histology

Staging in Europe is based on the relationship between the tumor and the anatomy of the liver (the PRETEXT classification). Surgical resection is crucial for cure of hepatoblastoma and HCC, and this staging system aims to predict the anatomy of the healthy liver that will remain after resection and describes the number (out of four) of sections of the liver involved. The presence of tumor beyond the liver, either local spread to vena cava and/or portal vein or distant pulmonary metastases is sufficient to categorize the disease as high risk. Biopsy is usually necessary, although in children between 6 months and 3 years with a raised AFP it is not mandatory. Hepatoblastoma most often metastasizes to lungs and nodes at the porta hepatis and rarely to bone. HCC similarly metastasizes to the lungs, nodes and later to bone.

Management

Hepatoblastoma

Hepatoblastoma requires total surgical excision for cure. Preoperative chemotherapy, with doxorubicin and cisplatin, produces tumor shrinkage and increases the number of patients whose tumors can be fully resected. Between 80% and 100% of hepatoblastomas are chemoresponsive, and 67–80% will be resectable after this treatment.[344] In the first SIOP liver tumor trial, SIOPEL-1, all patients received pre-operative chemotherapy regardless of initial resectability. The 3-year overall survival in this trial was 79%.[345] The presence of pulmonary metastases at diagnosis has been consistently found to be an adverse prognostic factor.[346] SIOPEL-1 also identified tumor affecting all four liver sections, extrahepatic tumor and multifocal tumor as poor prognostic factors. In the current SIOP trial (SIOPEL-3) this group of patients are regarded as high risk and receive an intensive chemotherapy regimen alternating cisplatin with carboplatin/doxorubicin (SuperPLADO). This regimen was piloted in SIOPEL-2 and produced a 67% resection rate and a 3-year overall survival of 53%.[347] The remaining patients are standard risk and receive either cisplatin as a single agent or cisplatin/doxorubicin, as cisplatin single agent therapy was effective for standard risk patients in SIOPEL-2, with a 97% resection rate and a 3-year overall survival of 91%. In SIOPEL-1 10 patients had liver transplantation because of unresectable disease, all but 1 of these patients were alive without evidence of disease at median 3-year follow up. The presence of pulmonary metastases at diagnosis is not a contraindication to transplantation, providing that these are no longer visible at the time of surgery; 4 of the successfully transplanted patients in SIOPEL-1 had pulmonary metastases at diagnosis.

Hepatocellular carcinoma

In the SIOPEL-1 study, pre-operative therapy (cisplatin, doxorubicin) was given to 40 patients of whom 12 had complete resection, and 2 incomplete. Seven of these patients were alive without disease at 10- to 46-month follow-up while 22 were still unresectable. Overall survival for these patients on SIOPEL-1 was 28% at 5 years, the presence of metastases and the PRETEXT stage were both predictive of survival. In SIOPEL-2 these patients received SuperPLADO but there was no improvement in survival. In the American Pediatric Intergroup Study there were 46 patients with HCC. Seventeen percent had Stage 1 disease (complete

resection with clear margins) and for these patients the survival was 88%. Survival for the whole patient group was 19% and, as in SIOPEL-1, no patients with metastatic disease survived.[348] In the current HCC specific study SIOPEL-5 those patients with localized respectable tumors will undergo primary surgery. Those patients with unresectable, extra-hepatic or metastatic tumors receive PLADO in combination with thalidomide as an anti-angiogenic agent pre-operatively, surgery if possible, and then 12 months of metronomic therapy with cyclophosphamide and thalidomide. In multifocal nonresectable HCC in childhood, liver transplantation may also have a place; two patients were transplanted on SIOPEL-1, both were alive and disease free at 40 and 55 months follow up.

LANGERHANS CELL HISTIOCYTOSES

Histiocytoses are a heterogeneous group of uncommon proliferative diseases involving bone marrow derived immature histiocytic cells, which can have more reactive than malignant features. The classification of histiocytic disorders by the Writing Group of the Histiocyte Society includes hematological malignancies and hemophagocytic lymphohistiocytosis (HLH), which are discussed elsewhere in this book.[349] Relevant in the context of pediatric oncology are dendritic cell related class 1 disorders as these manifest mainly as nonhematopoietic organ dysfunction (see below) and are treated with antineoplastic agents (Table 24.21).

To understand Langerhans Cell Histiocytosis (LCH) it is useful to look at the development of the histiocyte. The hematopoetic bone marrow stem cell develops into committed granulocyte and macrophage precursors, which divide and differentiate producing myelocytes and monocytes. When these migrate into the peripheral circulation they undergo terminal differentiation into macrophages and histiocytes in many tissues determined by the local microenvironment, e.g. Kupffer cells in the liver and Langerhans cells (LCs) in the skin, which are involved in antigen-processing or antigen presentation to the circulating T cells. All of the antigen-presenting cells, and in particular LCs, have a strong affinity for class 2 antigens which the T4 or helper T cells recognize. LCs contain

Table 24.21   Classification of histiocytosis syndromes in children

Class I	Class II	Class III
Langerhans' cell histiocytosis	1. Primary hemophagocytic lymphohistiocytosis (FHLH ± family history)	Malignant histiocytic disorders: 1. Acute monocytic leukemia 2. Malignant histiocytosis 3. True histiocytic lymphoma
I Single bone	2. Secondary HLH (infection, malignancy, etc.)	
II Multiple bone	3. Other mononuclear phagocytosis (not Langerhans' cell)	
IIIA Bone + soft tissue		
IIIB Soft tissue only	4. Sinus histiocytosis + massive lymphadenopathy (Rosai–Dorfman)	
	5. Juvenile xanthogranuloma	
(Birbeck granules CD1A antigen positive S100 morphology)	6. Reticulocytoma	

structured organelles called Birbeck granules (these are rod-like structures with central striations and a terminal vesical expansion which looks like a tennis racket under electron microscopy) and express the CD1a surface antigen. Normal LCs make up not more than 2% of all epidermal cells and play in important role in immunosurveillance.

In LCH the normal LCs are stimulated to proliferate and accumulate in affected tissues with a variable mixture of other cells to form granulomas with locally destructive behavior, which interfere with normal organ function. Although features of clonality have been described in LCH it is regarded as reactive rather than malignant.[350] This atypical immunological response is thought to be triggered by a pathological response to infection, but no infectious agent has been identified as responsible.

Clinical features and staging

The generic name 'Langerhans cell histiocytosis' is used to encompass historical terms like eosinophilic granuloma, Hand–Schuller–Christian triad and Letterer–Siwe disease, which were descriptions of different stages of LCH (Table 24.21). Pathological staging includes breakdown of bony lesions into those with or without contiguous soft tissue involvement and/or involvement of immediately adjacent lymph nodes. Stage I is a single lytic bone lesion; Stage II are multiple lytic bone lesions, which were formerly called eosinophilic granulomata. Bone lesions most commonly affect the skull, long bones and, vertebrae, where these lesions can lead to vertebral collapse, mandible or maxilla and can lead to gingival disease with even loss of teeth. Bone scans may identify such lesions but sometimes they can be missed but picked up preferentially by plainX-rays (Fig. 24.16a,b). Magnetic resonance imaging has identified lesions not seen either by X-rays or bone scans. Almost every bone in the body has at sometime been reported to show such lytic lesions. The skull is involved in nearly 50% of cases. Stage IIIA, bone plus soft tissue lesions, is often associated with diabetes insipidus if the pituitary is involved or proptosis of the orbit (previously termed Hand–Schuller–Christian triad); Stage IIIB, soft tissue only, is the disseminated form previously termed Letterer–Siwe disease. The absence of bone disease carries worse prognostic implications.[351] Stage IIIB typically

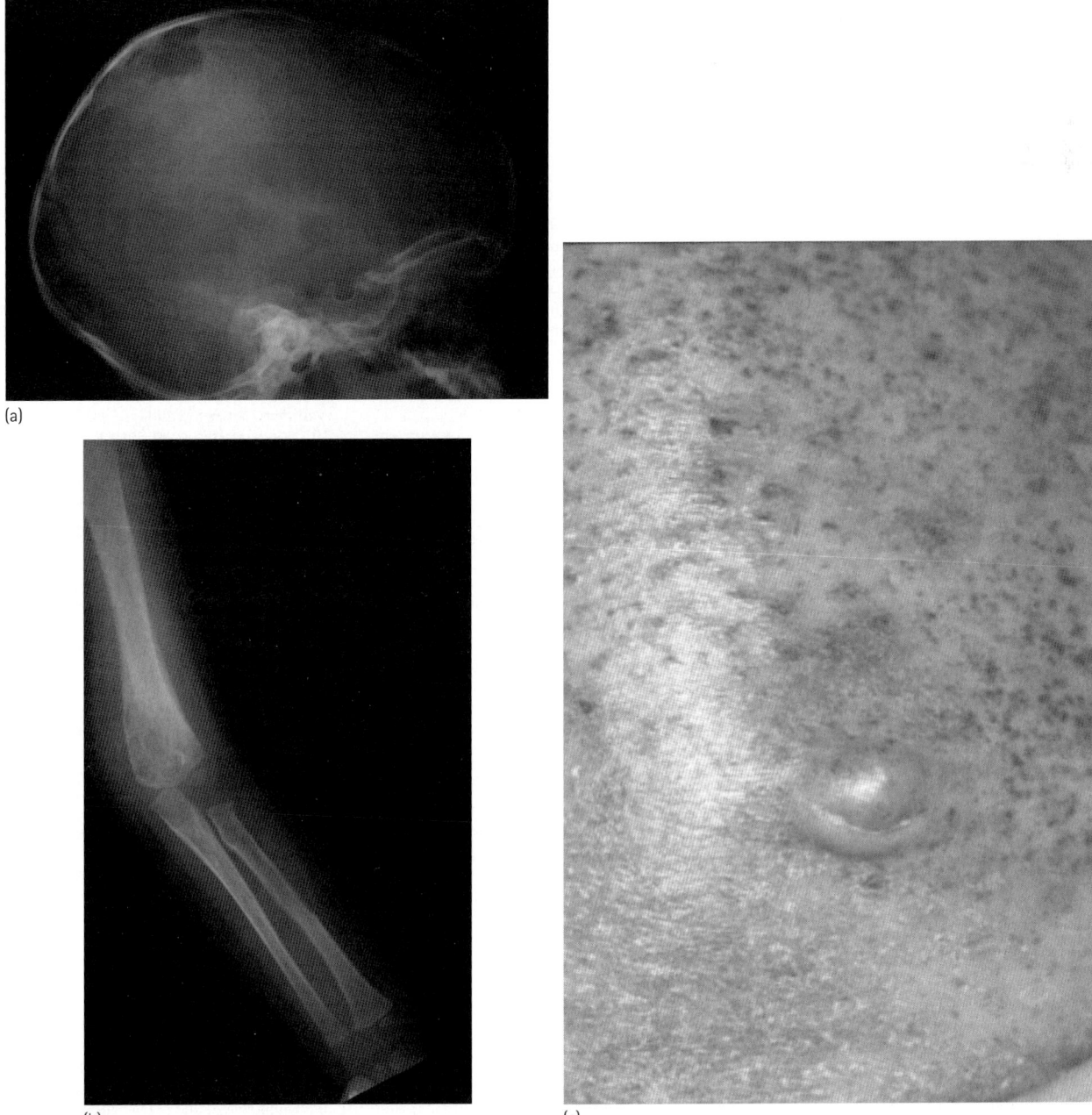

(a)

(b)

(c)

Fig. 24.16 Lateral plain radiograph of the skull showing the typical lytic lesions of Langerhans cell histiocytosis. (b) Plain radiograph of the elbow showing a destructive lesion of LCH. (c) Skin rash in LCH.

affects young infants and although overall LCH has a low mortality, those aged under 6 months with disseminated soft tissue disease have a mortality of 50–60%. They often have failure to thrive, lymphadenopathy, hepatosplenomegaly, anemia and pancytopenia with red to purple skin lesions, a high incidence of seborrheic dermatitis and multiple organ involvement. A wide range of skin lesions have been identified, ranging from patterns similar to seborrhoeic dermatitis through nodular lesions, bronzing of the skin, and xanthomatous lesions (Fig. 24.16c). Skin involvement carries adverse prognostic features.[351] Over 70% of all patients with LCH have bone lesions, while 30–45% have skin and mucous membrane involvement, 25–30% pulmonary involvement, 25–30% hepatosplenomegaly, 30% lymphadenopathy and 30% hemopoietic disorders. The pituitary is involved in about 15–20% of cases. CNS involvement and protein losing enteropathy are less common. CNS involvement is rare apart from pituitary disease but can present with space occupying lesions and neurological dysfunction and is an unfavorable feature. These patients usually have multisystem disease and a high mortality.[352,353] Definitive diagnosis of LCH depends on the characteristic pathological appearances with Birbeck granules and CD1a antigen positivity in the cells on biopsy specimen from skin, lymph node, bone or soft tissue.

Management

For Stage I and II bone disease excision biopsy or curettage for diagnosis with the intra-lesional injection of steroids is the treatment of choice.[354] Local low dosage irradiation has been used for deposits which cannot easily be treated by curettage but require treatment. For more advanced disease systemic chemotherapy with prednisolone, vinblastine and etoposide has been subjected to evaluation by clinical trails.[355,356] For the approximately 15% patients with extensive dysfunction particularly of liver, lung or hemopoietic system, more aggressive chemotherapy has been used including the use of moderate dose systemic methotrexate and cytosine arabinoside in addition to prednisolone, mercaptopurine and vinblastine.[355,356] Response to initial chemotherapy appears to be of prognostic significance.[357] In the Japanese trial from 1996 poor responders were allocated much more intensive treatment including anthracyclines, cytosine arabinoside, methotrexate and cyclophosphamide, which resulted in improved overall survival.[358] The role of high dose therapy including etoposide, cyclophosphamide and busulfan prior to allogeneic marrow transplantation or alternatively antithymocyte globulin, prednisolone and ciclosporin where there is no donor for high risk patients has not been established, but such treatment as used for hemophagocytic lymphohistiocytosis (HLH) could be an option for high risk patients.[359] Recent pilot data from France which addressed the role of 2-chlorodeoxyadenosine in combination with cytosine arabinoside have shown promising response rates but also treatment related mortality from bone marrow suppression.[360] The small patient numbers with relapsing and severe multisystem LCH necessitate continuing international collaboration in order to further improve the outlook of children affected by this disorder, which carries considerable long term morbidity in survivors.[361]

REFERENCES (* Level I evidence)

*1. Stiller CA, Allen M, Bayne A, et al. UK national registry of childhood tumors England and Wales (1981–1990) in International Incidence of Childhood Cancer Vol II IARC. Scientific Publications 1998; 144:365–367.

*2. Sharp L, Gould A, Harris V, et al. UK Scottish Cancer Registry 1981–90 in International Incidence of Childhood Cancer Vol II IARC. Scientific Publications 1998; 144:369–371.

*3. Parkin DM, Kramarova E, Draper GJ, et al, eds. International Incidence of Childhood Cancer Vol II IARC. Lyon: Scientific Publications; 1998:144.

*4. Steliarova-Foucher E, Stiller C, Kaatsch P. Geographical patterns and time trends of cancer incidence and survival among children and adolescents in Europe since the 1970s (the ACCIS project): an epidemiological study. Lancet 2004; 364:2097–2105.

*5. Kramarova E, Stiller CA, Ferlay J, et al, eds. The international classification of childhood cancer. IARC Technical Report No 29. Lyon: IARC; 1996.

6. Birch JM, Marsden HB. A classification scheme for childhood cancers. Int J Cancer 1987; 40:620–624.

*7. McNally RJQ, Birch JM, Taylor GM, et al. Temporal increases in the incidence of childhood peak precursor B cell ALL seen in North West England. Lancet 2000; 356:485–486.

*8. McNally RJQ, Cairns DP, Eden OB, et al. Examination of temporal trends in the incidence of childhood leukemia and lymphoma provides etiological clues. Leukemia 2001; 15:1612–1618.

*9. McNally RJQ, Kelsey AM, Cairns DP, et al. Temporal increases in the incidence of solid tumors seen in North West England 1954–98 are likely to be real. Cancer 2001; 927:1967–1976.

*10. Dreifaldt AC, Carlberg M, Hardell L. Increasing incidence rates of childhood malignant diseases in Sweden during the period 1960–1998. Eur J Cancer 2004; 40:1351–1360.

11. Stiller CA. Personal communication. From UKCCSG Annual Scientific Report; 2002.

12. Botting B, Crawley J. Trends and patterns in childhood mortality and morbidity. In: The health of our children decennial supplement OPCS series DS no 1995; 11:62–81.

*13. Coebergh JW, Capocaccia R, Gatta G, et al. Childhood cancer survival in Europe, 1978–1992: the EUROCARE study. Eur J Cancer 2001; 37:671–672.

14. Pizer B, Eden T. The treatment of childhood cancer. In: Southall D, Coulter B, Ronald C, et al, eds. International child health care – a practical manual for hospitals worldwide. London: BMJ Books; 2002:302–313.

15. Simone JV. History of the treatment of childhood ALL: a paradigm for cancer cure. Best Pract Res Clin Hematol 2006; 19:353–359.

16. Stiller CA, Eatock EM. Patterns of care and survival for children with acute lymphoblastic leukemia diagnosed between 1980 and 1994. Arch Dis Child 1999; 81:202–208.

*17. Stiller CA. Centralization of treatment and survival rates for cancer. Arch Dis Child 1988; 63:23–30.

18. Pritchard J, Stiller CA, Lennox EL. Overtreatment of children with Wilms tumor outside pediatric oncology centers. BMJ 1989; 299:835–836.

19. UK Children's Cancer Study Investigators. The United Kingdom Childhood Cancer Study: objectives, materials and methods. Br J Cancer 2000; 825:1073–1102.

20. Stiller CA. Epidemiology and genetics of childhood cancer. Oncogene 2004; 23:6429–6444.

21. Scott RH, Stiller CA, Walker L, et al. Syndromes and constitutional chromosomal abnormalities associated with Wilms tumor. J Med Genet 2006; 43:705–715.

22. Stiller CA, Kinnier-Wilson LM. Down syndrome and leukemia. Lancet 1981; 2:1343.

23. Zipursky A, Thorner P, de Harven E, et al. Myelodysplasia and acute megakaryoblastic leukemia in Down syndrome. Leukemia Res 1994; 18:163.

24. Rao A, Hills RK, Stiller C, et al. Treatment for myeloid leukemia of Down syndrome: population-based experience in the UK and results from the Medical Research Council AML 10 and AML 12 trials. Br J Hematol 2006; 132:576–583.

25. Miller RW, Fraumeni JF, Manning M. Association of Wilms tumor with aniridia, hemihypertrophy, and other congenital malformations. N Engl J Med 1964; 270:922–927.

26. Call KM, Glaser J, Ho CY, et al. Isolation and characterisation of a zinc finger polypeptide gene at the human chromosome II. Wilms tumor locus. Cell 1990; 60:509.

*27. Draper GJ, Sanders BM, Kingston JE. Second primary neoplasms in patients with retinoblastoma. Br J Cancer 1986; 53:661.

*28. Li FP, Fraumeni JF. Soft tissue sarcoma, breast cancer and other neoplasms. A familial syndrome. Ann Intern Med 1969; 71:747–752.

*29. Garber JE, Goldstein AM, Kantor AF, et al. Follow-up study of twenty four families with Li–Fraumeni syndrome. Cancer Res 1991; 51:6094–6097.

30. Birch JM, Hartley AL, Blair V, et al. Cancer in the families of children with soft tissue sarcoma. Cancer 1990; 66:2239–2248.

*31. Malkin D, Li FP, Strong LC, et al. Germline p53 mutations in a familial syndrome of breast cancer, sarcomas and other neoplasms. Science 1990; 250:1233–1238.

32. Birch JM, Aliston RD, McNally RJQ, et al. Relative frequency and morphology of cancers in carriers of germline TP53 mutations. Oncogene 2001; 20:4621–4628.

33. Dukes CE. The hereditary factor in polyposis intestini, or multiple adenomata. Cancer Rev 1930; 5:241.

*34. Gardner EJ. Follow-up study of a family group exhibiting dominant inheritance for a syndrome including intestinal polyps, osteomas, fibromas and epidermal cysts. Am J Hum Genet 1992; 14:376.

35. Fishel R, Lescoe MK, Rao MRS, et al. The human mutator gene homologue MSH2 and its association with hereditary nonpolyposis colon cancer. Cell 1993; 75:1027.

36. Wood RD, Mitchell M, Lindahl T. Human DNA repair genes. Mutat Res 2005; 577:275–283.

*37. Mulligan L, Kwok J, Healey C, et al. Germline mutations of the RET proto-oncogene in multiple endocrine neoplasia type 2A. Nature 1993; 363:458.

38. Wood R. Seven genes for three diseases. Nature 1991; 350:190.

39. Woods C, Taylor AM. Ataxia telangiectasis in the British Isles: the clinical and laboratory features of 70 affected individuals. Q J Med 1992; 298:169.

40. Taylor AMR, Metcalfe JA, Thick J, et al. Leukemia and lymphoma in ataxia-telangiectasia. Blood 1996; 87:423–438.

41. Stankovic T, Kidd AM, Sutcliffe A, et al. ATM mutations and phenotypes in ataxia-telangiectasia

families in the British Isles: expression of mutant ATM and the risk of leukemia, lymphoma, and breast cancer. Am J Hum Genet 1998; 62:334–345.

42. Savitsky K, Bar-Shira A, Gilad S, et al. A single ataxia telangiectasia gene with a product similar to Pl-3 kinase. Science 1995; 268:1749.

43. Digweed M, Sperling K. Nijmegen breakage syndrome: clinical manifestation of defective response to DNA double-strand breaks. DNA Repair (Amst) 2004; 3:1207–1217.

44. Meyer S, Kingston H, Taylor AM, et al. Rhabdomyosarcoma in Nijmegen breakage syndrome: strong association with perianal primary site. Cancer Genet Cytogenet 2004; 154:169–174.

45. Taniguchi T, D'Andrea AD. Molecular pathogenesis of Fanconi anemia: recent progress. Blood 2006; 107:4223–4233.

46. Howlett NG, Taniguchi T, Olson S, et al. Biallelic inactivation of BRCA2 in Fanconi anemia. Science 2002; 297:606–609.

47. Wagner JE, Tolar J, Levran O, et al. Germline mutations in BRCA2: shared genetic susceptibility to breast cancer, early onset leukemia and Fanconi anemia. Blood 2004; 103:3226–3229.

48. Gatti RA, Good RA. Occurrence of malignancy in immunodeficient disease. Cancer 1971; 28:89–98.

*49. Gale KB, Ford AM, Repp R, et al. Backtracking leukemias to birth: identification of clonotypic gene fusion sequences in neonatal blood spots. Proc Natl Acad Sci USA 1997; 94:13950–13954.

*50. Wiemels JL, Cazaniga G, Daniotti M, et al. Prenatal origin of acute lymphoblastic leukemia in children. Lancet 1999; 354:1499–1503.

51. Greaves MF. Childhood leukemia. BMJ 2002; 324:283–287.

52. Wiemels JL, Pagnamenta A, Taylor GM, et al. (and UK Childhood Cancer Study Investigators). Lack of function NAD(P)H: quinone oxidoreductase alleles are selectively associated with pediatric leukemias that have MLL fusions. Cancer Res 1999; 59:4095–4099.

53. Ross JA. Dietary flavonoids and the MLL gene: a pathway to infant leukemia? Proc Natl Acad Sci USA 2000; 97:4411–4412.

54. Alexander FE, Patheal SL, Biondi A, et al. Transplacental chemical exposure and risk of infant leukemia with MLL gene fusion. Cancer Res 2001; 61:2542–2546.

55. Strick R, Strissel PL, Borgers S, et al. Bioflavonoids do induce MLL cleavage and may contribute to infant leukemia. Proc Natl Acad Sci USA 2000; 97:4790–4795.

56. Wiemels JL, Smith RN, Taylor GM, et al. Methylene tetrahydrofolate reductase (MTHFR) polymorphisms and risk of molecularly defined subtypes of childhood acute leukemia. Proc Natl Acad Sci USA 2001; 98:4004–4009.

*57. Thompson JR, Fitzgerald P, Willoughby MLN, et al. Maternal folate supplementation in pregnancy and protection against common acute lymphoblastic leukemia in childhood: a case control study. Lancet 2001; 358:1935–1940.

58. Taylor GM, Dearden S, Payne N, et al. Evidence that an HLA-DQA1-DQB1 haplotype influences susceptibility to childhood common acute lymphoblastic leukemia in boys provides further support for an infection related etiology. Br J Cancer 1998; 785:561–565.

*59. Westerbeck RMC, Blair V, Eden OB, et al. Seasonal variations in the onset of childhood leukemia and lymphoma. Br J Cancer 1998; 781:119–124.

60. Birch JM, Alexander FE, Blair V, et al. Space time clustering patterns in childhood leukemia support a role for infection. Br J Cancer 2000; 829:1495–1509.

61. Stewart A, Webb J, Giles D, et al. Malignant disease in childhood and diagnostic radiation in utero. Lancet 1956; ii:447.

62. Miller RW, Mulvihill JJ. Small head size after atomic irradiation. Teratology 1976; 14:355–357.

63. Yoshimoto Y, Kato H, Sihull WJ. Risk of cancer among in utero children exposed to A-bomb radiation 1950–84. Lancet 1988; ii:665.

*64. Gardner MJ, Snee MP, Hall AJ, et al. Results of a case control study of leukemias and lymphoma among young people near Sellafield nuclear plant in West Cumbria. BMJ 1990; 300:423–429.

65. Modan B, Ron E, Verner A. Thyroid cancer following scalp irradiation. Radiology 1977; 123:741–744.

*66. Upton AC, Albert RE, Burns FJ, et al. Radiation carcinogenesis. New York: Elsevier; 1986.

*67. Lyon JL, Klauber MR, Gardner JW, et al. Childhood leukemias associated with fallout from nuclear testing. N Engl J Med 1979; 300:397–402.

68. Black D. New evidence on childhood leukemia and nuclear establishments. BMJ 1987; 294:591–592.

*69. Committee on Medical Aspects of Radiation in the Environment (COMARE). 1986/1988 Bobrow M (Chairman) HMSO Report 1 (West Cumbria 1986), HMSO Report 2 (Dounreay, 1988). London: HMSO.

*70. Committee on Medical Aspects of Radiation in the Environment (COMARE) 4th Report. The incidence of cancer and leukemia in young people in the vicinity of the Sellafield site, West Cumbria. London: HMSO; 1996.

*71. Heasman MA, Urquhart JD, Black RJ, et al. Leukemia in young persons in Scotland. A study of its geographical distribution and relationship to nuclear installations. Health Bull 1987; 45:147–151.

72. Kinlen LJ, Clarke K, Hudson C. Evidence from population mixing in British new towns 1946–85 of an infective basis for childhood leukemia. Lancet 1990; 336:577–582.

73. Greaves MF. Speculations on the cause of childhood acute lymphoblastic leukemia. Leukemia 1988; 1:120–125.

74. UK Childood Cancer Study Investigators. The United Kingdom childhood cancer study of exposure to domestic sources of ionising radiation: 1: radon gas. Br J Cancer 2002; 86:1721–1726.

75. UK Childood Cancer Study Investigators. The United Kingdom childhood cancer study of exposure to domestic sources of ionising radiation: 2: gamma radiation. Br J Cancer 2002; 86:1727–1731.

*76. Holman CDJ, Armstrong BK, Heenan PJ. Relationship of cutaneous melanoma to individual sunlight exposure habits. J Natl Cancer Inst 1986; 76:403.

77. Meier JR. Genotoxic activity of organic chemicals in drinking water. Mutat Res 1988; 196:211.

*78. Wertheimer N, Leeper E. Electrical wiring configurations and childhood cancer. Am J Epidemiol 1979; 109:273.

79. UK Children's Cancer Study Investigators. Exposure to power frequency magnetic fields and the risk of childhood cancer. Lancet 1999; 354:1925–1931.

*80. Feychting M, Ahlbom A. Magnetic fields and cancer in children residing near Swedish high-voltage power lines. Am J Epidemiol 1993; 138:467.

81. Melnick S, Cole P, Anderson D, et al. Rates and risks of diethylstilbestrol related clear cell adenocarcinoma of the vagina and cervix. An update. N Engl J Med 1987; 316:514–516.

82. MacKinney AA, Booker HE. Diphenylhydantoin effects on human lymphocytes in vitro and in vivo. An hypothesis to explain some drug reactions. Arch Intern Med 1972; 129:988–992.

83. Tucker MA, Meadows AT, Boice JD, et al. Leukemia after therapy with alkylating agents for childhood cancer. J Natl Cancer Inst 1987; 78:459–464.

84. Ng A, Taylor GM, Eden OB. Treatment related leukemia – a clinical and scientific challenge. Cancer Treat Rev 2000; 265:377–391.

*85. Golding J, Paterson M, Kinlen LJ. Factors associated with child cancer in a national cohort study. Br J Cancer 1990; 62:304–308.

*86. Roman E, Fear NT, Ansell P, et al. Vitamin K and childhood cancer: analysis of individual patient data from six case-control studies. Br J Cancer 2002; 86:63–69.

87. Kwa SL, Fine LJ. The association between parental occupation and childhood malignancy. J Occup Med 1980; 22:792–794.

88. McNally RJ, Eden TO. An infectious aetiology for childhood acute leukemia: a review of the evidence. Br J Hematol 2004; 127:243–263.

89. MacKenzie J, Perry J, Ford AM, et al. JC and BK versus sequences are not detectable in leukemia samples from children with common acute lymphoblastic leukemia. Br J Cancer 1999; 81:898–899.

90. MacKenzie J, Gallagher A, Clayton RA, et al. Screening for herpes virus genomes in common acute lymphoblastic leukemia. Leukemia 2001; 15:415–421.

*91. Jarrett RF, Gallagher A, Jones DB, et al. Detection of Epstein-Barr virus genomes in Hodgkin disease: relation to age. J Clin Pathol 1991; 44:844–848.

92. Mueller NE, Grufferman S. The epidemiology of Hodgkin disease. In: Mauch PM, Armitage JO, Diehl V, et al, eds. Hodgkin disease. Philadelphia: Lippincott Williams & Wilkins; 1999. ch. 5

93. Flavell KJ, Murray PG. Hodgkin disease and the Epstein-Barr virus. J Clin Path/Molec Pathol 2000; 53:262–269.

*94. Taylor GM, Gokhale DA, Crowther D, et al. Further investigation of the role of HLA-DPB1 in adult Hodgkin disease suggests an influence on susceptibility to different Hodgkin disease subtypes. Br J Cancer 1999; 80:1405–1411.

*95. Yoshida M, Miyoshi I, Hinuma Y. Isolation and characterisation of retrovirus from cell lines of human adult T cell leukemia and its implication in the disease. Proc Natl Acad Sci USA 1982; 79:2031–2035.

96. Kremsdorf D, Soussan P, Paterlini-Brechot P, et al. Hepatitis B virus-related hepatocellular carcinoma: paradigms for viral-related human carcinogenesis. Oncogene 2006; 25:3823–3833.

97. Valery PC, Holly EA, Sleigh AC, et al. Hernias and Ewing's sarcoma family of tumors: a pooled analysis and meta-analysis. Lancet Oncol 2005; 6:485–490.

98. Bruinsma F, Venn A, Lancaster P, et al. Incidence of cancer in children born after in-vitro fertilization. Hum Reprod 2000; 15:604–607.

99. Klip H, Burger CW, de Kraker J, et al. OMEGA-project group. Risk of cancer in the offspring of women who underwent ovarian stimulation for IVF. Hum Reprod 2001; 16:2451–2458.

100. Kushner BH, Yeung HWD, Larson SM, et al. Extending positron emission tomography scan utility to high risk neuroblastoma: fluorine-18 fluorodeoxyglucose positron emission tomography as sole imaging modality in follow-up of patients. J Clin Oncol 2001; 19:3397–3405.

101. Pelengaris S, Khan M, Evan GI. Suppression of Myc-induced apoptosis in beta cells exposes multiple oncogenic properties of Myc and triggers carcinogenic progression. Cell 2002; 109:321–334.

102. Hanahan D, Weinberg RA. The hallmarks of cancer. Cell 2000; 100:57–70.

103. Makin GWJ, Dive C. Recent advances in the understanding of apoptosis: new therapeutic opportunities in cancer chemotherapy. Trends Molec Med 2003; 9:251–256.

104. Brown JM, Wilson WR. Exploiting tumor hypoxia in cancer treatment. Nature Revs Cancer 2004; 4:437–447.

105. Das B, Yeger H, Tsuchida R, et al. A hypoxia-driven vascular endothelial growth factor/Flt1 autocrine loop interacts with hypoxia-inducible factor-1 through mitogen-activated protein kinase/extracellular signal-regulated kinase 1/2 pathway in neuroblastoma. Cancer Res 2005; 65:7267–7275.

106. Kilic M, Kasperczyk H, Fulda S, et al. Role of hypoxia inducible factor-1 alpha in modulation

of apoptosis resistance. Oncogene 2006; E-pub 16 October DOI 10.1038/sj.onc.1210008

107. Hussein D, Estlin EJ, Dive C, et al. Chronic hypoxia promotes hypoxia-inducible factor-1α-dependent resistance to etoposide and vincristine in neuroblastoma cells. Mol Cancer Ther 2006; 5:2241–2250.

108. Longley DB, Johnson PG. Molecular mechanisms of drug resistance. J Pathol 2005; 205:275–292.

*109. Davies HA, Lennard L, Lilleyman JS. Variable mercaptopurine metabolism in children with leukemia: a problem of noncompliance? BMJ 1993; 306:1239–1240.

*110. Laverdiere C, Chiasson S, Costea I, et al. Polymorphism G80A in the reduced folate carrier gene and its relationship to methotrexate plasma levels and outcome of childhood acute lymphoblastic leukemia. Blood 2002; 100:3832–3834.

*111. Ivy SP, Olshefski RS, Taylor BJ, et al. Correlation of P-glycoprotein expression and function in childhood acute leukemia: a children's cancer group study. Blood 1996; 88:309–318.

112. den Boer ML, Pieters R, Kazemier KM, et al. Relationship between major vault protein/lung resistance protein, multidrug resistance-associated protein, P-glycoprotein expression, and drug resistance in childhood leukemia. Blood 1998; 91:2092–2098.

113. Goker E, Waltham M, Kheradpour A, et al. Amplification of the dihydrofolate reductase gene is a mechanism of acquired resistance to methotrexate in patients with acute lymphoblastic leukemia and is correlated with p53 gene mutations. Blood 1996; 86:677–684.

114. Shiga H, Heath EI, Rasmussen AA, et al. Prognostic value of p53, glutathione-S-transferase Pi, and thymidylate synthase for neoadjuvant cisplatin-based chemotherapy in head and neck cancer. Clin Cancer Res 1999; 5:4097–4104.

115. Lord RV, Brabender J, Gandara A, et al. Low ERCC1 expression correlates with prolonged survival after cisplatin plus gemcitabine chemotherapy in non-small cell lung cancer. Clin Cancer Res 2002; 8:2286–2291.

116. Watanabe Y, Koi M, Hemmi H, et al. A change in microsatellite instability caused by cisplatin-based chemotherapy of ovarian cancer. Br J Cancer 2001; 85:1064–1069.

*117. Prentice HG, Hann IM, Herbrecht R. A randomized comparison of liposomal versus conventional amphotericin B for the treatment of pyrexia of unknown origin in neutropenic patients. Br J Hematol 1997; 98:711–718.

118. Pizzo PA. Fever in immunocompromised patients. N Engl J Med 1999; 341:893–900.

*119. Boyce JM, Pittet D. Guideline for hand hygiene in health-care settings recommendations of the Healthcare Infection Control Practices Advisory Committee and the HICPAC/SHEA/APIC/IDSA Hand Hygiene Task Force. Infect Control Hosp Epidemiol 2002; 23:(suppl):S3–S40.

*120. Girou E, Loyeau S, Legrand P, et al. Efficacy of handrubbing with alcohol based solution versus standard handwashing with antiseptic soap randomised clinical trial. BMJ 2002; 325:362–366.

*121. Hughes WT, Armstrong D, Bodey GP, et al. Guidelines for the use of antimicrobial agents in neutropenic patients with cancer. Clin Infect Dis 2002; 34:730–751.

122. Brunell PA, Ross A, Miller LH, et al. Prevention of varicella by Zoster immune globulin. N Engl J Med 1969; 280:1191–1194.

*123. Prober DG, Kirk LE, Keeney RE. Acyclovir therapy of chickenpox in immunosuppressed children: a collaborative study. J Pediatr 1982; 101:622–625.

*124. Carcao MD, Lau RC, Gupta A, et al. Sequential use of intravenous and oral acyclovir in the therapy of varicella in immunocompromised children. Pediatr Infect Dis J 1998; 17:626–631.

*125. Gray M, Hann IM, Glass S, et al. Mortality and morbidity caused by measles in children with malignant disease. BMJ 1987; 295:19–22.

*126. Hughes WT, Rivera GK, Schell MJ, et al. Successful intermittent chemoprophylaxis for Pneumocystis carinii pneumonitis. N Engl J Med 1997; 316:1627–1632.

*127. Darbyshire P, Eden OB, Jameson B, et al. Pneumonitis in lymphoblastic leukemia in childhood. Eur J Paediatr Hematol Oncol 1985; 2:141–147.

128. Royal College of Paediatrics and Child Health. Immunisation of the immunocompromised child; Best practice statement. London: Royal College of Paediatrics and Child Health; 2002.

*129. Stanworth SJ, Hyde C, Heddle N, et al. Prophylactic platelet transfusion for hemorrhage after chemotherapy and stem cell transplantation. Cochrane Database Syst Rev 2004; Oct 18:(4):CD004269.

130. Ruggiero A, Ricardi R. Interventions for anemia in pediatric cancer patients. Med Pediatr Oncol 2002; 39:451–454.

*131. Jurgens H, McQuade B. Ondansetron as prophylaxis for chemotherapy and radiotherapy-induced emesis in children. Oncology 1992; 49:279–285.

*132. Alvarez O, Freeman A, Bedros A, et al. Randomized double-blind crossover ondansetron-dexamethasone versus ondansetron-placebo study for the treatment of chemotherapy-induced nausea and vomiting in pediatric patients with malignancies. J Pediatr Hematol Oncol 1995; 17:145–150.

133. Dupuis LL, Nathan PC. Options for the prevention and management of acute chemotherapy-induced nausea and vomiting in children. Paediatr Drugs 1993; 5:597–613.

134. Van Hoff J, Olszewski D. Lorazepam for the control of chemotherapy-related nausea and vomiting in children. J Pediatr 1988; 113:146–149.

*135. Worthington HV, Clarkson JE, Eden OB. Interventions for preventing oral mucositis for patients with cancer receiving chemotherapy. Cochrane Database Syst Rev 2004; Apr 19:(2):CD000978.

*136. Worthington HV, Clarkson JE, Eden O. Interventions for preventing oral candidiasis for patients with cancer receiving treatment. Cochrane Database Syst Rev 2004; Oct 18:(4):CD003807.

*137. Hows JM, Mehta A, Ward L, et al. Comparison of mesna with forced diuresis to prevent cyclophosphamide induced haemorrhagic cystitis in marrow transplantation: a prospective randomised study. Br J Cancer 1984; 50:753–756.

*138. Hausdorf G, Morf G, Beron G, et al. Long term doxorubicin cardiotoxicity in childhood: noninvasive evaluation of the contractile state and diastolic filling. Br Heart J 1988; 60:309–315.

*139. Bielack SS, Erttman R, Winkler K, et al. Doxorubicin: effect of different schedules on toxicity and antitumor efficiency. Eur J Cancer Clin Oncol 19889; 25:873–882.

*140. Lipshultz SE, Colan SD, Gelber RD, et al. Late cardiac effects of doxorubicin therapy for ALL in childhood. N Engl J Med 1991; 324:808–815.

*141. Kremer LCM, van Dalen EC, Offringa M, et al. Anthracycline-induced clinical heart failure in a cohort of 607 children: long term follow-up study. J Clin Oncol 2001; 19:191–196.

142. Weiss HD, Walker MD, Wiernik PH. Neurotoxicity of commonly used antineoplastic agents. N Engl J Med 1975; 291:75–127.

*143. McQuay HJ, Tramer M, Nye BA, et al. A systematic review of antidepressants in neuropathic pain. Pain 1996; 68:217–227.

*144. Caraceni A, Zecca E, Bonnezzi R, et al. Gabapentin for neuropathic cancer pain: a randomized controlled trial from the Gabapentin Cancer Pain Study Group. J Clin Oncol 2004; 22:2909–2917.

145. Pratt CB, Green AA, Horowitz ME, et al. Central nervous system toxicity following the treatment of pediatric patients with ifosfamide/mesna. J Clin Oncol 1986; 4:1253–1261.

146. Brock PR, Pritchard J, Bellman SC, et al. Ototoxicity of high-dose cisplatinum in children. Med Ped Oncol 1987; 16:368–369.

147. D'Antiga L, Baker A, Pritchard J, et al. Veno-occlusive disease with multi-organ involvement following actinomycin-D. Eur J Cancer 2001; 37:1141–1148.

148. Ortega JA, Donaldson SS, Ivy SP, et al. Veno-occlusive disease of the liver after chemotherapy with vincristine, actinomycin D, and cyclophosphamide for the treatment of rhabdomyosarcoma. Cancer 1997; 79:2435–2439.

149. Bisogno G, de Kraker J, Weirich A, et al. Veno-occlusive disease of the liver in children treated for Wilms tumor. Med Ped Oncol 1997; 29:245–251.

*150. Goldman SC, Holcenberg J, Finklestein JZ, et al. A randomised comparison between rasburicase and allopurinol in children with lymphoma or leukemia at high risk for tumor lysis. Blood 2001; 97:2998–3003.

151. Eden OB, Black I, Mackinlay GA, et al. Communication with parents of children with cancer. Palliat Med 1994; 8:105–114.

*152. Hawkins MM. Long term survival and cure after childhood cancer. Arch Dis Child 1989; 64:798–807.

*153. Meadows AT, Baum E, Fossati-Bellani F, et al. Second malignant neoplasms in children: an update from the Late Effects Study Group. J Clin Oncol 1985; 3:532–538.

*154. Meadows AT. Risk factors for second malignant neoplasms: report from the Late Effects Study Group. Bull Cancer 1988; 75:125–130.

155. Tucker MA, D'Angio GJ, Boice JD, et al. Bone sarcomas linked to radiotherapy and chemotherapy in children. N Engl J Med 1987; 317:588–593.

156. Pui C, Behm SG, Raimondi SC, et al. Second acute myeloid leukemia in children treated for acute lymphoid leukemia. N Engl J Med 1989; 321:136–142.

157. Nygaard R, Garwicz S, Haldorsen T, et al. Second malignant neoplasms in patients treated for childhood leukemia. A population based cohort study from the Nordic countries. Acta Pediatr Scand 1991; 80:1220–1228.

*158. Neglia JP, Meadows AT, Robison LL, et al. Second neoplasms after acute lymphoblastic leukemia. N Engl J Med 1991; 325:1330–1336.

*159. Relling MV, Rubnitz JE, Rivera GK, et al. High incidence of second brain tumors after radiotherapy and antimetabolites. Lancet 1999; 354:34–40.

160. Shalet SM, Clayton PE, Price DA. Growth and pituitary function in children treated for brain tumors or acute lymphoblastic leukemia. Hormone Res 1988; 30:53–61.

161. Ogilvy-Stuart AL, Ryder WD, Gattamaneni HR, et al. Growth hormone and tumor recurrence. BMJ 1992; 304:1601–1605.

*162. Kirk JA, Raghupathy P, Stevens MM, et al. Growth failure and growth hormone deficiency after treatment for acute lymphoblastic leukemia. Lancet 1987; 1:1990–1993.

*163. Davies HA, Didcock E, Didi M, et al. Disproportionate short stature after cranial irradiation and combination chemotherapy for leukemia. Arch Dis Child 1994; 70:472–475.

164. Brennan BMD, Rahim A, Blum WF, et al. Hyperleptinanemia in young adults following cranial irradiation in childhood: growth hormone deficiency or leptin insensitivity. Clin Endocrinol 1999; 50:163–169.

*165. Brennan BMD, Rahim A, Adams JA, et al. Reduced bone mineral density in young adults following cure of acute lymphoblastic leukaemia in childhood. Br J Cancer 1999; 79:1850–1863.

166. Bessho F, Ohta K, Akunuma A. Dosimetry of radiation scattered to thyroid gland from prophylactic

cranial irradiation for childhood leukemia. Pediatr Hematol Oncol 1994; 11:47–53.

167. Howell SJ, Shalet SM. Spermatogenesis after cancer treatment: damage and recovery. J Natl Cancer Inst Monographs 2005; 34:12–17.

168. Relander T, Cavallin-Stahl E, Garwicz S, et al. Gonadal and sexual function in men treated for childhood cancer. Med Pediatr Oncol 2000; 35:52–63.

*169. Clark ST, Radford JA, Crowther D, et al. Gonadal function following chemotherapy for Hodgkin disease: a comparative study of MVPP and a seven drug regime. J Clin Oncol 1995; 13:134–139.

170. Critchley HO, Wallace WH, Shalet SM, et al. Abdominal irradiation in childhood: the potential for pregnancy. Br J Obstet Gynaecol 1992; 99:393–394.

*171. Kun LE, Mulhearn RK, Crisco JJ. Quality of life of children treated for brain tumors: intellectual, emotional and academic function. J Neurosurg 1986; 58:1–6.

*172. Hill FGH, Vargha-Khadem F, Gibson B, et al. UKALL XI randomized trial of stratified CNS treatment and prospective neuropsychological assessment in childhood ALL. Blood 2000; 9:466.

173. Meadows AT, McKee L, Kazak AE. Psychosocial status of young adult survivors of childhood cancer: a survey. Med Pediatr Oncol 1989; 17:466–470.

174. Malpas JS. Cancer: The consequences of cure. Clin Radiol 1988; 39:166–172.

175. Steinherz LJ, Steinherz PG, Tan CT, et al. Cardiac toxicity 4–20 years after completing anthracycline therapy. JAMA 1991; 266:1672–1677.

*176. Shaw NJ, Tweeddale PM, Eden OB. Pulmonary function in childhood leukemia survivors. Med Pediatr Oncol 1989; 17:149–154.

*177. Shaw NJ, Eden OB, Jenney MEM, et al. Pulmonary function in survivors of Wilms tumor. Pediatr Hematol Oncol 1991; 82:131–137.

*178. Attard-Montalto SP, Kingston JE, Eden OB, et al. Late follow-up of lung function after whole lung irradiation for Wilms tumor. Br J Radiol 1992; 66:1114–1118.

179. Estlin E, Lowis S. Clinics in Developmental Medicine 166. London: MacKeith Press; 2005.

180. Kleihues P, Louis DN, Scheithauer W, et al. The WHO classification of tumors of the nervous system. J Neuropathol Exp Neurol 2002; 61:215–225.

181. Packer RJ, Zimmerman RA, Bilanuik LT. Magnetic resonance imaging in the evaluation of treatment related central nervous system damage. Cancer 1986; 58:635–640.

182. Brunelle F. Noninvasive diagnosis of brain tumors in children. Childs Nerv Syst 2000; 16:731–734.

*183. Campbell JW, Pollack IF, Martinez AJ, et al. High grade astrocytomas in children: radiologically complete resection is associated with an excellent long term prognosis. Neurosurgery 1996; 38:258.

*184. Tait DM, Thornton-Jones H, Bloom HJG, et al. Adjuvant chemotherapy for medulloblastoma: the first multicenter controlled trial of the International Society of Pediatric Oncology (SIOP1). Eur J Cancer 1990; 26:464.

185. Habrand J-L, De Crevoisier R. Radiation in the management of childhood brain tumors. Childs Nerv Syst 2001; 17:121–133.

186. Kellie SJ. Chemotherapy of central nervous system tumors in infants. Childs Nerv Syst 1999; 15:592–612.

187. Gajjar A, Sanford RA, Heideman R, et al. Low grade astrocytoma: a decade of experience at St Jude Children's Research Hospital. J Clin Oncol 1997; 15:2792–2799.

188. Vinchon M, Soto-Ares G, Ruchoux MM, et al. Cerebellar gliomas in childen with NF-1: pathology and surgery. Child Nerv Syst 2000; 16:417–420.

189. Jozwiak S, Schwartz RA, Janniger CK, et al. Usefulness of diagnostic criteria of tuberous sclerosis complex in pediatric patients. J Child Neurol 2000; 15:652–659.

190. Cokgor I, Friedmann AH, Friedmann HS. Gliomas. Eur J Cancer 1998; 34:1910–1915.

191. Janss AJ, Grundy R, Cnaan A, et al. Optic pathway and hypothalamic/chiasmatic gliomas in children younger than 5 years with a 6-year follow-up. Cancer 1995; 75:1051–1059.

192. Tao ML, Barnes PD, Billett AL, et al. Childhood optic chiasm gliomas: radiographic response following radiotherapy and long-term clinical outcome. Int J Radiat Oncol Biol Phys 1997; 39:579–587.

193. Packer RJ, Ater J, Allen J, et al. Carboplatin and vincristine chemotherapy for children with newly diagnosed progressive low-grade gliomas. J Neurosurg 1997; 86:747–754.

*194. Laithier V, Grill J, LeDeley MC, et al. Progression-free survival in children with optic pathway tumors: dependence on age and the quality of the response to chemotherapy – results of the first French prospective study for the French Society of Pediatric Oncology. J Clin Oncol 2003; 21:4572–4578.

*195. Wisoff JH, Boyett JM, Berger MS, et al. Current neurosurgical management and the impact of the extent of resection in the treatment of malignant gliomas of childhood: a report of the Children's Cancer Group trial no. CCG-945. J Neurosurg 1998; 89:52–59.

196. Garden AS, Maor MH, Yung WK, et al. Outcome and patterns of failure following limited-volume irradiation for malignant astrocytomas. Radiother Oncol 1991; 20:99–110.

*197. Sposto R, Ertel IJ, Jenkin RD, et al. The effectiveness of chemotherapy for treatment of high grade astrocytoma in children: results of a randomized trial. A report from the Children's Cancer Study Group. J Neurooncol 1989; 7:165–177.

198. Wolff JE, Gnekow AK, Kortmann RD, et al. Preradiation chemotherapy for pediatric patients with high-grade glioma. Cancer 2002; 94:264–271.

199. Geoerger B, Vassal G, Doz F, et al. Dose finding and O$_6$-alkylguanine-DNA alkyltransferase study of cisplatin combined with temozolomide in pediatric solid malignancies. Br J Cancer 2005; 93:529–537.

200. Epstein F, Wisoff J. Intra-axial tumors of the cervicomedullary junction. J Neurosurg 1987; 67:483–487.

201. Khatib ZA, Heideman RL, Kovnar EH, et al. Predominance of pilocytic histology in dorsally exophytic brainstem tumors. Pediatr Neurosurg 1994; 20:2–10.

202. Hood TW, Gebarski SS, McKeever PE, et al. Stereotaxic biopsy of intrinsic lesions of the brainstem. J Neurosurg 1986; 65:172–176.

203. Farmer JP, Montes JL, Freeman CR, et al. Brainstem gliomas. A 10-year institutional review. Pediatr Neurosurg 2001; 34:206–214.

*204. Kaplan AM, Albright AL, Zimmerman RA, et al. Brainstem gliomas in children: a Children's Cancer Study Group review of 119 cases. Pediatr Neurosurg 1996; 24:185–192.

*205. Packer RJ, Boyett JM, Zimmerman RA, et al. Outcome of children with brainstem gliomas after treatment with 7800cGy of hyperfractionated radiotherapy: a Children's Cancer Study Group Phase I/II trial. Cancer 1994; 74:1827–1834.

*206. Jenkin RDJ, Boesel C, Ertel I, et al. Brainstem tumors in childhood: a prospective randomized trial of irradiation with or without CCNU, VCR and prednisone. A report of the Children's Cancer Study Group. J Neurosurg 1987; 66:227–233.

207. Bouffet E, Perilongo G, Canete A, et al. Intracranial ependymomas in children: a critical review of prognostic factors and a plea for cooperation. Med Pediatr Oncol 1998; 30:319–329.

*208. Evans AE, Anderson JR, Lefkowitz-Boudreaux IB, et al. Adjuvant chemotherapy of posterior fossa ependymoma: craniospinal irradiation with or without adjuvant CCNU, vincristine and prednisolone: a Children's Cancer Study Group Study. Med Pediatr Oncol 1996; 27:8–14.

209. Berger C, Thiesse P, Lellouch-Tubiana A, et al. Choroid plexus carcinomas in childhood: clinical features and prognostic factors. Neurosurgery 1998; 42:470–475.

210. Wolff JE, Sajedi M, Coppes MJ, et al. Radiation therapy and survival in choroid plexus carcinoma. Lancet 1999; 353:2126.

211. Packer RJ, Zimmerman RA, Bilanuik LT. Magnetic resonance imaging in the evaluation of treatment related central nervous system damage. Cancer 1986; 58:635–640.

*212. Zeltzer PM, Boyett JM, Finlay JL, et al. Metastasis stage, adjuvant treatment, and residual tumor are prognostic factors for medulloblastoma in children: conclusions from the Children's Cancer Group 921 randomized phase III study. J Clin Oncol 1999; 17:832–845.

213. Biegel JA, Janss AJ, Raffel C, et al. Prognostic significance of chromosome 17p deletions in childhood primitive neuroectodermal tumors (medulloblastomas) of the central nervous system. Clin Cancer Res 1997; 3:473–478.

214. Gilbertson RJ, Perry RH, Kelly PJ, et al. Prognostic significance of HER2 and HER4 coexpression in childhood medulloblastoma. Cancer Res 1997; 57:3272–3280.

215. Scheurlen WG, Schwabe GC, Joos S, et al. Molecular analysis of childhood primitive neuro-ectodermal tumors defines markers associated with poor outcome. J Clin Oncol 1998; 16:2478–2485.

*216. Tait DM, Thornton-Jones H, Bloom HJG, et al. Adjuvant chemotherapy for medulloblastoma: the first multicenter controlled trial of the International Society of Pediatric Oncology (SIOP1). Eur J Cancer 1990; 26:464.

*217. Taylor RE, Bailey CC, Lucraft H, et al. Results of a randomized study of pre-radiotherapy chemotherapy (carboplatin, vincristine, cyclophosphamide, etoposide) with radiotherapy alone in Chang Stage M0/M1 medulloblastoma (SIOP/UKCCSG PNET 3). Med Pediatr Oncol 2001; 37:191.

*218. Packer RJ, Goldwein J, Nicholson HS, et al. Treatment of children with medulloblastoma with reduced dose craniospinal radiation therapy and adjuvant chemotherapy: a Children's Cancer Study Groups Study. J Clin Oncol 1999; 17:2127–2136.

*219. Kortman RJ, Kuhl J, Timmerman B, et al. Postoperative neo-adjuvant chemotherapy before radiotherapy as compared to immediate radiotherapy followed by maintenance chemotherapy in the treatment of medulloblastoma of childhood: results of the German HIT '91 study. Int J Radiat Oncol Biol Phys 2000; 46:269–279.

*220. Pizer BL, Weston CL, Robinson KJ, et al. Analysis of patients with supratentorial primitive neuroectodermal tumors entered into the SIOP/UKCCSG PNET 3 study. Eur J Cancer 2006; 42:1120–1128.

221. Matsutani M, Sano K, Takakura K, et al. Primary intracranial germ cell tumors: a clinical analysis of 153 histologically verified cases. J Neurosurg 1997; 86:446–455.

222. Nicholson JC. Interim guidelines for the treatment of intracranial germ cell tumors. UK: CCSG Germ Cell Tumor Working Group; 2006.

*223. Amendola BE, Gebarski SS, Bermudez AG. Analysis of treatment results in craniopharyngioma. J Clin Oncol 1985; 3:252–258.

*224. Habrand J-L, Ganry O, Couanet D, et al. The role of radiation therapy in the management of craniopharyngioma: a 25-year experience and review of the literature. Int J Radiat Oncol Biol Phys 1999; 44:255–263.

225. Harris NL, Jaffe ES, Diebold J, et al. World Health Organization classification of neoplastic diseases of the hematopoietic and lymphoid tissues: report of the Clinical Advisory Committee meeting – Airlie House, Virginia, November 1997. J Clin Oncol 1999; 17:3835–3849.

226. Sandlund JT, Downing JR, Crist WM. Non-Hodgkin's lymphoma in childhood. N Engl J Med 1996; 334:1238–1248.

227. Gutierrez MI, Bhatia K, Barriga F, et al. Molecular epidemiology of Burkitt lymphoma from South America: difference in breakpoint location and EBV association from tumors in other world regions. Blood 1992; 79:3261–3266.

228. ten Berge RL, Oudejans JJ, Ossenkoppele GJ, et al. ALK-negative systemic anaplastic large cell lymphoma: differential diagnostic and prognostic aspects – a review. J Pathol 2003; 200:4–15.

229. Piva R, Chiarle R, Manazza AD, et al. Ablation of oncogenic ALK is a viable therapeutic approach for anaplastic large-cell lymphomas. Blood 2006; 107:689–697.

230. Magrath IT. Malignant non-Hodgkin lymphomas in children. Hematol Oncol Clin North Am 1987; 1:577–602.

231. Perkins SL. Work-up and diagnosis of pediatric non-Hodgkin's lymphomas. Pediatr Dev Pathol 2000; 3:374–390.

232. Burkitt D. A sarcoma involving the jaws in African children. Br J Surg 1958; 46:218–223.

233. Murphy SB. Classification. Staging and end results of treatment of childhood non Hodgkin's lymphoma: dissimilarities from lymphomas in adults. Semin Oncol 1980; 7:332–339.

*234. Patte C, Philip T, Rodany C, et al. High survival rate in advanced stage B cell lymphomas and leukemias without CNS involvement with short intensive polychemotherapy. Results from the French Pediatric Oncology Society of a randomized trial of 216 children. J Clin Oncol 1991; 9:123–132.

235. Goldman SC, Holcenberg JS, Finklestein JZ, et al. A randomized comparison between rasburicase and allopurinol in children with lymphoma or leukemia at high risk for tumor lysis. Blood 2001; 97:2998–3003.

*236. Patte C, Auperin A, Michon J, et al. The Societe Francaise d'Oncologie Pediatrique LMB89 protocol: highly effective multiagent chemotherapy tailored to the tumor burden and initial response in 561 unselected children with B cell lymphomas and L3 leukemia. Blood 2001; 97:3370–3379.

*237. Reiter A, Schrappe M, Parawaresch R, et al. Non Hodgkin's lymphoma of childhood and adolescence: results of a treatment stratified for biologic subtypes and stage. A report of the BFM group. J Clin Oncol 1995; 13:359–372.

238. Reiter A, Schrappe M, Tiemann M, et al. Improved treatment results in childhood B cell neoplasms with tailored intensification of therapy: a report of the Berlin–Frankfurt–Munster Group Trial NHL-BFM 90. Blood 1999; 94:3294–3306.

*239. Reiter A, Schrappe M, Ludwig WD, et al. Intensive ALL-type therapy without local radiotherapy provides a 90% event-free survival for children with T cell lymphoblastic lymphoma: a BFM group report. Blood 2000; 95:416–421.

*240. Brugieres L, Deley MC, Pacquement H, et al. CD30(+) anaplastic large-cell lymphoma in children: analysis of 82 patients enrolled in two consecutive studies of the French Society of Pediatric Oncology. Blood 1998; 92:3591–3598.

*241. Seidemann K, Tiemann M, Schrappe M, et al. Short-pulse B-non-Hodgkin lymphoma-type chemotherapy is efficacious treatment for pediatric anaplastic large cell lymphoma: a report of the Berlin–Frankfurt–Munster Group Trial NHL-BFM 90. Blood 2001; 97:3699–3706.

242. Fischer A, Blanche S, Le Bidois J, et al. Anti B cell monoclonal antibodies in the treatment of severe B cell lymphoproliferative syndrome following bone marrow and organ transplantation. N Engl J Med 1991; 324:1451–1456.

243. Papadopoulos BE, Ladanyi M, Emmanuel D, et al. Infusions of donor leucocytes to treat EBV associated lymphoproliferative disorders after allogeneic bone marrow transplantation. N Engl J Med 1994; 330:1185–1191.

244. Re D, Kuppers R, Diehl V. Molecular pathogenesis of Hodgkin's lymphoma. J Clin Oncol 2005; 23:6379–6386.

245. Weiss L, Movahed LA, Warnke RA, et al. Detection of Epstein–Barr viral genomes in Reed–Sternberg cells of Hodgkin disease. N Engl J Med 1989; 320:502–506.

246. Barth TF, Martin-Subero JI, Joos S, et al. Gains of 2p involving the REL locus correlate with nuclear c-Rel protein accumulation in neoplastic cells of classical Hodgkin lymphoma. Blood 2003; 101:3681–3686.

247. Martin-Subero JI, Gesk S, Harder L, et al. Recurrent involvement of the REL and BCL11A loci in classical Hodgkin lymphoma. Blood 2002; 99:1474–1477.

248. Bhatia S, Yasui Y, Robison LL, et al. High risk of subsequent neoplasms continues with extended follow-up of childhood Hodgkin's disease: report from the Late Effects Study Group. J Clin Oncol 2003; 21:4386–4394.

249. Ben Arush MW, Solt I, Lightman A, et al. Male gonadal function in survivors of childhood Hodgkin and non-Hodgkin lymphoma. Pediatr Hematol Oncol 2000; 17:239–245.

250. Sklar C, Whitton J, Mertens A, et al. Abnormalities of the thyroid in survivors of Hodgkin's disease: data from the Childhood Cancer Survivor Study. J Clin Endocrinol Metab 2000; 85:3227–3232.

251. Korholz D, Kluge R, Wickmann L, et al. Importance of F18-fluorodeoxy-D-2-glucose positron emission tomography (FDG-PET) for staging and therapy control of Hodgkin's lymphoma in childhood and adolescence – consequences for the GPOH-HD 2003 protocol. Onkologie 2003; 26:489–493.

252. Dorffel W, Luders H, Ruhl U, et al. Preliminary results of the multicenter trial GPOH-HD 95 for the treatment of Hodgkin's disease in children and adolescents: analysis and outlook. Klin Padiatr 2003; 215:139–145.

253. Schellong G, Dorffel W, Claviez A, et al. Salvage therapy of progressive and recurrent Hodgkin's disease: results from a multicenter study of the pediatric DAL/GPOH-HD study group. J Clin Oncol 2005; 23:6181–6189.

254. Stoneham S, Ashley S, Pinkerton CR, et al. Outcome after autologous hemopoietic stem cell transplantation in relapsed or refractory childhood Hodgkin disease. J Pediatr Hematol Oncol 2004; 26:740–745.

255. De Bernandi B, Pianca C, Pistamiglio P, et al. Neuroblastoma with symptomatic spinal cord compression at diagnosis: treatment and results with 76 cases. J Clin Oncol 2001; 19:183–190.

*256. Brodeur GM, Seeger RC, Schwab M, et al. Amplification of N-Myc in untreated human neuroblastoma correlates with advanced disease stage. Science 1984; 224:112–114.

*257. Caron H, Van Sluis P, De Kraker J, et al. Allelic loss of chromosome 1p as a predictor of unfavorable outcome in patients with neuroblastoma. N Engl J Med 1996; 334:225–230.

*258. Maris JM, Weiss MJ, Guo C, et al. Loss of heterozygosity at 1p36 independently predicts for disease progression but not decreased overall survival probability in neuroblastoma patients: a Children's Cancer Group Study. J Clin Oncol 2000; 18:1888–1899.

*259. Bown N, Cotterill S, Lastowska M. Gain of chromosome arm 17q and adverse outcome in patients with neuroblastoma. N Engl J Med 1999; 340:1954–1961.

*260. Nakagawara A, Arima M, Azar CG, et al. Inverse relationship between Trk expression and N-Myc amplification in human neuroblastoma. Cancer Res 1992; 52:1364–1368.

*261. Nakagawara A, Arimanakagawara M, Scavarda NJ, et al. Association between high levels of expression of the Trk gene and favorable outcome in human neuroblastoma. N Engl J Med 1993; 328:847–854.

262. Nakagawara A, Azar CG, Scavarda NJ, et al. Expression and function of Trk-B and BDNF in human neuroblastomas. Mol Cell Biol 1994; 14:759–767.

263. Yamashiro DJ, Liu XG, Lee CP, et al. Expression and function of Trk-C in favorable human neuroblastomas. Eur J Cancer 1997; 33:2054–2057.

264. Brodeur GM, Seeger RC, Barrett A, et al. International criteria for diagnosis, staging and response to treatment in patients with neuroblastoma. J Clin Oncol 1988; 6:1874–1881.

*265. Perez CA, Matthay KK, Atkinson JB, et al. Biologic variables in the outcome of stages I and II neuroblastoma treated with surgery as primary therapy: a Children's Cancer Group Study. J Clin Oncol 2000; 18:18–26.

*266. Rubie H, Hartmann O, Michon J, et al. N-Myc gene amplification is a major prognostic factor in localized neuroblastoma: results of the French NBL 90 study. J Clin Oncol 1997; 15:1171–1182.

*267. Nickerson HJ, Matthay KK, Seeger RC, et al. Favorable biology and outcome of Stage IV-S neuroblastoma with supportive care or minimal therapy: a Children's Cancer Group Study. J Clin Oncol 2000; 18:477–486.

*268. Katzenstein HM, Bowman LC, Brodeur GM, et al. Prognostic significance of age, MYCN oncogene amplification tumor cell ploidy, and histology in 110 infants with stage DS neuroblastoma: the Pediatric Oncology group experience – a Pediatric Oncology Group Study. J Clin Oncol 1998; 16:2007–2017.

*269. Matthay KK, Villablanca JG, Seeger RC, et al. Treatment of high-risk neuroblastoma with intensive chemotherapy, radiotherapy, autologous bone marrow transplantation, and 13-cis-retinoic acid. N Engl J Med 1999; 341:1165–1173.

270. Bessho F, Hashizume K, Nakajo T, et al. Mass screening of infants with neuroblastoma without a decrease of cases in older children. J Pediatr 1991; 119:237–241.

271. Sawada T, Kidowaki T, Sakamoto I, et al. Neuroblastoma: mass screening for early detection and its prognosis. Cancer 1984; 53:2731–2735.

*272. Woods WG, Tuchman M, Robison LL, et al. A polulation-based study of the usefulness of screening for neuroblastoma. Lancet 1996; 348:1682–1687.

273. Yamamoto K, Hanada R, Kikuchi A, et al. Spontaneous regression of localized neuroblastoma detected by mass screening. J Clin Oncol 1998; 16:1265–1269.

274. Beckwith JB. Pathological aspects of renal tumors in childhood. In: Broecker BH, Klein FA (eds). Pediatric tumors of the genitourinary tract. New York: Alan Liss; 1988.25–48.

275. Breslow NE, Beckwith JB. Epidemiological features of Wilms tumor. Results of the National Wilms Tumor Study. J Nat Cancer Inst 1982; 68:429.

*276. Mitchell C, Jones PM, Kelsey A, et al. The treatment of Wilms tumor: results of the United Kingdom Children's cancer study group (UKCCSG) second Wilms tumor study. Br J Cancer 2000; 83:602–608.

*277. Tournade MF, Com-Nougue C, Voute PA, et al. Results of the Sixth International Society of Pediatric Oncology Wilms Tumor Trial and Study: a risk-adapted therapeutic approach in Wilms tumor. J Clin Oncol 1993; 11:1014–1123.

*278. Tournade MF, Com-Nougue C, de Kraker J, et al. and International Society of Pediatric Oncology Nephroblastoma Trial and Study Committee. Optimal duration of pre-operative therapy in unilateral and nonmetastatic Wilms tumor in children older than 6 months: results of the Ninth International Society of Pediatric Oncology Wilms Tumor Trial and Study. J Clin Oncol 2001; 19:488–500.

*279. de Kraker J, Graf N, van Tinteren H, et al. Reduction of postoperative chemotherapy in children with Stage I intermediate-risk and anaplastic Wilms tumor (SIOP 93–01 trial): a randomised controlled trial. Lancet 2004; 364:1229–1235.

280. Arndt CAS, Crist WM. Common musculoskel et al. tumors of childhood and adolescence. N Engl J Med 1999; 341:342–352.

281. Birch JM, Hartley AL, Marsden HB, et al. Excess risk of breast cancer in the mothers of children with soft tissue sarcomas. Br J Cancer 1984; 49:325–331.

282. Hahn H, Wicking C, Zaphiropoulos PG, et al. Mutations of the human homolog of Drosophila patched gene in the nevoid basal cell carcinoma syndrome. Cell 1996; 85:841–851.

283. Hahn H, Wojnowski L, Zimmer AM, et al. Rhabdomyosarcomas and radiation hypersensitivity in a mouse model of Gorlin syndrome. Nature Med 1998; 4:619–622.

284. Zahn S, Helman LJ. Glimpsing the cause of rhabdomyosarcoma. Nature Med 1998; 4:559–560.

285. Barr FG. Gene fusions involving PAX and FOX family members in alveolar rhabdomyosarcoma. Oncogene 2001; 20:5736–5746.

286. Anderson J, Gordon A, Pritchard-Jones K, et al. Genes, chromosomes, and rhabdomyosarcoma. Genes Chromosomes Cancer 1999; 26:275–285.

287. Marsden HB. The pathology of soft tissue sarcomas. In: D'Angio GJ, Evans AE, eds. Bone tumors and soft tissue sarcomas. London: Edward Arnold; 1985:4–46.

288. Newton WA, Gehan EA, Webber BL, et al. Classification of rhabdomyosarcomas and related sarcomas. Pathologic aspects and proposals for a new classification – an Intergroup Rhabdomyosarcoma Study. Cancer 1995; 76:1073–1085.

289. Kemshead JT. Monoclonal antibodies. Their use in the diagnosis and therapy of pediatric and adult tumors derived from the neuroectoderm. In: Baldwin RW, ed. Monoclonal antibodies for cancer detection and therapy. London: Academic Press; 1985.281.

290. Lawrence W, Gehan EA, Hays DM, et al. Prognostic significance of staging factors of the UICC staging system in childhood rhabdomyosarcoma. A report from the Intergroup Rhabdomyosarcoma Study IRSII. J Clin Oncol 1987; 5:46–54.

*291. Crist W, Gehan EA, Ragab AH, et al. The Third Intergroup Rhabdomyosarcoma Study. J Clin Oncol 1995; 13:610–630.

*292. Crist WM, Anderson JR, Meza JL, et al. Intergroup Rhabdomyosarcoma Study-IV: results for patients with nonmetastatic disease. J Clin Oncol 2001; 19:3091–3102.

293. Kelly KM, Womer RB, Sorensen PHB, et al. Common and variant gene fusions predict distinct clinical phenotypes in rhabdomyosarcoma. J Clin Oncol 1997; 15:1831–1836.

*294. Meza JL, Anderson J, Pappo AS, et al. Children's Oncology Group. Analysis of prognostic factors in patients with nonmetastatic rhabdomyosarcoma treated on intergroup rhabdomyosarcoma studies III and IV: the Children's Oncology Group. J Clin Oncol 2006; 24:3844–3851.

*295. Ferrari A, Bisogno G, Casanova M, et al. Paratesticular rhabdomyosarcoma: report from the Italian and German Cooperative Group. J Clin Oncol 2002; 20:449–455.

*296. Stewart RJ, Martelli H, Oberlin O, et al. International Society of Pediatric Oncology. Treatment of children with nonmetastatic paratesticular rhabdomyosarcoma: results of the Malignant Mesenchymal Tumors studies (MMT 84 and MMT 89) of the International Society of Pediatric Oncology. J Clin Oncol 2003; 21:793–798.

297. Casanova M, Ferrari A, Spreafico F, et al. Vinorelbine in previously treated advanced childhood sarcomas: evidence of activity in rhabdomyosarcoma. Cancer 2002; 94:3263–3268.

298. Casanova M, Ferrari A, Bisogno G, et al. Vinorelbine and low-dose cyclophosphamide in the treatment of pediatric sarcomas: pilot study for the upcoming European Rhabdomyosarcoma Protocol. Cancer 2004; 101:1664–1671.

*299. Pappo AS, Lyden E, Breneman J, et al. Up-front window trial of topotecan in previously untreated children and adolescents with metastatic rhabdomyosarcoma: an Intergroup Rhabdomyosarcoma Study. J Clin Oncol 2001; 19:213–219.

*300. Walterhouse DO, Lyden ER, Breitfeld PP, et al. Efficacy of topotecan and cyclophosphamide given in a phase II window trial in children with newly diagnosed metastatic rhabdomyosarcoma: a Children's Oncology Group study. J Clin Oncol 2004; 22:1398–1403.

*301. Frascella E, Pritchard-Jones K, Modak S, et al. Response of previously untreated metastatic rhabdomyosarcoma to combination chemotherapy with carboplatin, epirubicin and vincristine. Eur J Cancer 1996; 5:821–825.

*302. Soft Tissue Sarcoma Committee of the Children's Oncology Group; Lager JJ, Lyden ER, Anderson JR, et al. Pooled analysis of phase II window studies in children with contemporary high-risk metastatic rhabdomyosarcoma: a report from the Soft Tissue Sarcoma Committee of the Children's Oncology Group. J Clin Oncol 2006; 24:3415–3422.

303. Stiller CA, Bielack SS, Jundt G, et al. Bone tumors in European children and adolescents, 1978–1997. Report from the Automated Childhood Cancer Information System project. Eur J Cancer 2006; 42:2124–2135.

304. Dahlen D, Unni K. Osteosarcoma of bone and its important recognisable varieties. Am J Surg Pathol 1977; 1:61–72.

305. Enneking WF, Spanier SS, Goodman MA. Current concept reviews: the surgical staging of musculo-skeletal sarcoma. J Bone Joint Surg 1980; 62:1027–1030.

*306. Bielack SS, Kempf-Bielack B, Delling G, et al. Prognostic factors in high-grade osteosarcoma of the extremities or trunk: an analysis of 1702 patients treated on neoadjuvant cooperative osteosarcoma study group protocols. J Clin Oncol 2002; 20:776–790.

307. Grimer RJ, Bielack S, Flege S, et al. European MusculoSkeletal Oncology Society. Periosteal osteosarcoma – a European review of outcome. Eur J Cancer 2005; 41:2806–2811.

*308. Bielack SS, Kempf-Bielack B, Heise U, et al. Combined modality treatment for osteosarcoma occurring as a second malignant disease. Cooperative German-Austrian-Swiss Osteosarcoma Study Group. J Clin Oncol 1999; 17:1164.

*309. Kager L, Zoubek A, Potschger U, et al. Cooperative German-Austrian-Swiss Osteosarcoma Study Group. Primary metastatic osteosarcoma: presentation and outcome of patients treated on neoadjuvant Cooperative Osteosarcoma Study Group protocols. J Clin Oncol 2003; 21:2011–2018.

310. Grimer RJ. Surgical options for children with osteosarcoma. Lancet Oncol 2005; 6:85–92.

311. Delattre O, Zucman J, Melot T, et al. The Ewing family of tumors – a subgroup of small-round-cell tumors defined by specific chimeric transcripts. N Engl J Med 1994; 331:294–299.

*312. Paulussen M, Ahrens S, Braun-Munzinger G, et al. EICESS 92 (European Intergroup Cooperative Ewing's Sarcoma Study) – preliminary results. Klin Padiatr 1999; 21:276–283.

*313. de Alava E, Kawai A, Healey JH, et al. EWS–FLI1 fusion transcript structure is an independent determinant of prognosis in Ewing's sarcoma. J Clin Oncol 1998; 16:1248–1255.

*314. Paulussen M, Ahrens S, Dunst J, et al. Localized Ewing tumor of bone: final results of the cooperative Ewing's Sarcoma Study CESS 86. J Clin Oncol 2001; 19:1818–1829.

*315. Oberlin O, Deley MC, Bui BN, et al. Prognostic factors in localized Ewing's tumors and peripheral neuroectodermal tumors: the third study of the French Society of Pediatric Oncology (EW88 study). Br J Cancer 2001; 85:1646–1654.

*316. Craft A, Cotterill S, Malcolm A, et al. Ifosfamide-containing chemotherapy in Ewing's sarcoma: The Second United Kingdom Children's Cancer Study Group and the Medical Research Council Ewing's Tumor Study. J Clin Oncol 1998; 16:3628–3633.

*317. Grier HE, Krailo MD, Tarbell NJ, et al. Addition of ifosfamide and etoposide to standard chemotherapy for Ewing's sarcoma and primitive neuroectodermal tumor of bone. N Engl J Med 2003; 348:694–701.

*318. Miser JS, Krailo MD, Tarbell NJ, et al. Treatment of metastatic Ewing's sarcoma or primitive neuroectodermal tumor of bone: evaluation of combination ifosfamide and etoposide – a Children's Cancer Group and Pediatric Oncology Group study. J Clin Oncol 2004; 22:2873–2876.

*319. Bernstein ML, Devidas M, Lafreniere D, et al. Children's Cancer Group Phase II Study 9457; Children's Oncology Group. Intensive therapy with growth factor support for patients with Ewing tumor metastatic at diagnosis: Pediatric Oncology Group/ Children's Cancer Group Phase II Study 9457 – a report from the Children's Oncology Group. J Clin Oncol 2006; 24:152–159.

*320. Meyers PA, Krailo MD, Ladanyi M, et al. High-dose melphalan, etoposide, total-body irradiation, and autologous stem-cell reconstitution as consolidation therapy for high-risk Ewing's sarcoma does not improve prognosis. J Clin Oncol 2001; 19:2812–2820.

*321. Whelan J, McTiernan A, Weston C, et al. Consequences of different approaches to local treatment of Ewing sarcoma within an international randomized controlled trial: analysis of EICESS-92. J Clin Oncol (ASCO Annual Meeting Proceedings Part 1) 2006; 24:(18S):9533.

322. Donaldson SS, Torrey M, Link MP, et al. A multidisciplinary study investigating radiotherapy in Ewing's sarcoma: end results of POG #8346. Pediatric Oncology Group. Int J Radiat Oncol Biol Phys 1998; 42:125–135.

323. Horwich A, Huddart R, Dearnely D. Markers and management of germ-cell tumors of the testes. Lancet 1998; 352:1535–1538.

324. Dehner LP. Gonadal and extragonadal germ cell neoplasia of childhood. Hum Pathol 1983; 14:493–511.

325. Altman RP, Randolph JG, Lilly JR. Sacrococcygeal teratomas. J Pediatr Surg 1974; 9:389–398.

326. Bosl GJ, Motzer RJ. Testicular germ cell cancer. N Engl J Med 1997; 337:242–253.

*327. Mann JR, Raafat F, Robinson K, et al. Mature and immature extracranial teratomas in children: the UK Children's Cancer Study Group's experience. In: Jones I, Appleyard P, Harnden P, Joffe JK, eds. Germ cell tumors. . London: John Libbey; 1998:237–246.

*328. Cushing B, Giller R, Cohen L, et al. Surgery alone is effective treatment of resected immature teratoma in children: a pediatric intergroup report. Med Pediatr Oncol 1996; 27:221.

329. Einhorn LH, Williams SD, Troner M, et al. The role of maintenance therapy in disseminated testicular cancer. N Engl J Med 1981; 305:727–731.

*330. Mann JR, Raafat F, Robinson K, et al. UKCCSG's germ cell tumor GCT studies: improving outcome for children with malignant extra-cranial nongonadal tumors. Carboplatinum, etoposide and bleomycin are effective and less toxic than previous regimes. Med Pediat Oncol 1998; 30:217–227.

331. Baranzelli MC, Kramar A, Bouffet E, et al. Prognostic factors in children with localized malignant nonseminomatous germ cell tumors. J Clin Oncol 1999; 17:1212–1219.

332. McCaffrey JA, Mazumdar M, Bajorin DF, et al. Ifosfamide- and cisplatin-containing chemotherapy as first-line salvage therapy in germ cell tumors: response and survival. J Clin Oncol 1999; 15:2559–2563.

*333. Siefert W, Beyer J, Strohscheer I, et al. High-dose treatment with carboplatin, etoposide, and ifosfamide followed by autologous stem-cell transplantation in relapsed or refractory germ cell cancer: a phase I/II study. J Clin Oncol 1994; 12:1223–1231.

334. Doz F, Brisse H, Stoppa-Lyonnet D, et al. Retinoblastoma. In: Pinkerton CR, Plowman PN, Pieters R, eds. Pediatric oncology, 3rd edn. London: Arnold: 2004:323–338.

335. Knudson AG. Mutation and cancer: statistical study of retinoblastoma. Proc Natl Acad Sci USA 1971; 68:820–823.

336. Stratton MR, Moss S, Warren W, et al. Mutation of the p53 gene in soft tissue sarcomas: association with abnormalities of the RB1 gene. Oncogene 1990; 5:1297–1301.

337. Knudson AG, Meadows AT, Nichols WW, et al. Chromosomal deletion and retinoblastoma. N Engl J Med 1976; s295:1120–1123.

*338. Dryja TP, Mukai S, Petersen R, et al. Parental origin of mutations of the retinoblastoma gene. Nature 1989; 339:556–558.

339. Zhu XP, Dunn JM, Phillips RA, et al. Preferential germline mutation of the paternal allele in retinoblastoma. Nature 1989; 340:312–313.

*340. Bunin GR, Petrakova A, Meadows AJ, et al. Occupations of parents of children with retinoblastoma: a report from the Children's Cancer Study Group. Cancer Res 1990; 50:7129–7133.

341. Honavar SG, Singh AD, Shields CL, et al. Postenucleation adjuvant therapy in high-risk retinoblastoma. Arch Ophthalmol 2002; 20: 923–931.

342. Shields CL, Mashayekhi A, Cater J, et al. Chemoreduction for retinoblastoma. Analysis of tumor control and risks for recurrence in 457 tumors. Am J Ophthalmol 2004; 138:329–337.

343. Kingston JE, Hungerford JL, Madreperna SA, et al. Results of combined chemotherapy and radiotherapy for advanced intraocular retinoblastoma. Arch Ophthalmol 1996; 114:1339–1343.

*344. Douglas EC, Green AA, Wrenn E, et al. Effective cisplatin based chemotherapy in the treatment of hepatoblastoma. Med Pediatr Oncol 1985; 13:187–190.

*345. Plaschkes J, Perilongo G, Shafford E, et al. Pre-operative chemotherapy – cisplatin (PLA) and doxorubicin (DO) PLADO for the treatment of hepatoblastoma and hepatocellular carcinoma: results after two years follow-up. Med Pediatr Oncol 1996; 27:256.

*346. Perilongo G, Brown J, Shafford E, et al. Hepatoblastoma presenting with lung metastases. Treatment results of the first cooperative, prospective study of the International Society of Pediatric Oncology on childhood liver tumors. Cancer 2000; 89:1845–1853.

347. Perilongo G, Shafford E, Maibach R, et al. Risk-adapted treatment for childhood hepatoblastoma: final report of the second study of the International Society of Pediatric Oncology-SIOPEL 2. Eur J Cancer 2004; 40:411–421.

348. Katzenstein HM, Krailo MD, Malogolowkin MH, et al. Hepatocellular carcinoma in children and adolescents: results from the Pediatric Oncology Group and the Children's Cancer Group intergroup study. J Clin Oncol 2002; 20:2789–2797.

349. Chu T, D'Angio GJ, Favara B, et al. Classification of histiocytosis syndromes in children – from the Writing Group of the Histiocyte Society. Lancet 1987; i:208–209.

350. Willman CL, Busque L, Griffith BB, et al. Langerhans cell histiocytosis (histiocytosis X) – a clonal proliferative disease. N Engl J Med 1994; 331:154–160.

*351. Broadbent V. Favorable prognostic features in histiocytosis X: bone involvement and absence of skin disease. Arch Dis Child 1986; 61:1219–1221.

352. Arico M, Egeler RM. Clinical aspects of Langerhans' cell histiocytosis. Hematol Oncol Clin North Am 1998; 12:247–258.

353. Grois NG, Favara BE, Mostleck GH, et al. Central nervous system disease Langerhans' cell histiocytosis. Hematol Oncol Clin North Am 1998; 12:287–305.

354. Titgemeyer C, Grois N, Minkov M, et al. Pattern and course of single-system disease in Langerhans cell histiocytosis data from the DAL-HX 83- and 90-study. Med Pediatr Oncol 2001; 37:108–114.

*355. Ladisch S, Gadner H, Arico M, et al. LCH-1: a randomized trial of etoposide versus vinblastine in disseminated Langerhans' cell histiocytosis. Med Pediatr Oncol 1994; 23:107–110.

*356. Gadner H, Grois N, Arico M, et al. A randomized trial of treatment for multisystem Langerhans'cell histiocytosis. J Pediatr 2001; 138:728–734.

*357. Mittheisz E, Seidl R, Prayer D, et al. Response to initial treatment of multisystem Langerhans cell histiocytosis: an important prognostic indicator. Med Pediatr Oncol 2002; 39:581–585.

*358. Morimoto A, Ikushima S, Kinugawa N, et al. Improved outcome in the treatment of pediatric multifocal Langerhans cell histiocytosis: results from the Japan Langerhans Cell Histiocytosis Study Group-96 protocol study. Cancer 2006; 107:613–619.

359. Henter J, Arico M, Egeler RM, et al. HLH-94: a treatment protocol for hemophagocytic lymphohistiocytosis. Med Pediatr Oncol 1997; 28:342–347.

360. Bernard F, Thomas C, Bertrand Y, et al. Multi-center pilot study of 2-chlorodeoxyadenosine and cytosine arabinoside combined chemotherapy in refractory Langerhans cell histiocytosis with hematological dysfunction. Eur J Cancer 2005; 41:2682–2689.

361. Minkov M, Steiner M, Prosch H, et al. Central nervous system-related permanent consequences in patients with Langerhans cell histiocytosis. Pediatr Blood Cancer 2006; Feb 8 [Epub ahead of print].

25

Gynecological diseases

Anne S Garden

INTRODUCTION

The awareness of gynecological problems in children and adolescents has increased in recent years. Some children's hospitals have dedicated gynecological and multidisciplinary clinics but the majority of girls and teenagers seen are still seen by general practitioners, pediatricians or gynecologists with no particular expertise.

There is a need for such a service. Gynecologists do not always appreciate that girls are not miniature women but have specific anatomy and physiology, and psychology. Pediatricians often feel inadequate dealing with sexual and hormonal problems. A report that 30% of males and 26% of females under the age of 16 are sexually active[1] is not always remembered in pediatric practice. Additionally, while all our patients deserve to be treated with sensitivity, this is especially true for girls with gynecological problems. A painful, inappropriate examination may cause fears and phobias in young girls that stay with them during their teenage years – and even into adulthood, with unfortunate effects on their future reproductive health.

PHYSIOLOGY

Prior to birth, high levels of estrogens produced by the placenta inhibit gonadotrophin release from the fetal pituitary. Following delivery and the loss of maternal estrogens a transient rise in neonatal gonadotrophin levels may result in neonatal ovarian activity. Such activity, however, is short-lived and both gonadotrophin and estrogen levels drop within a short time of delivery and remain so throughout childhood until just before puberty.

The high levels of circulating estrogens may cause secretion of milk from the neonatal breast and a white vaginal discharge to be present. The loss of the estrogens after delivery may result in a vaginal bleed due to breakdown of the endometrium.

The high levels of circulating estrogens affect the appearance of the neonatal genitalia. The labia majora and minora are large and rounded and the hymen appears edematous. These changes disappear with the loss of maternal hormones – the labia majora becoming flattened, the labia minora thin and attenuated and the hymen less prominent. The hymenal changes are often the last to regress with the result that for the first year of life the hymen can appear quite prominent; the appearance of the external genitalia then remain unchanged until puberty.

Gonadotrophin-releasing hormone begins to be released in a pulsatile fashion between the ages of 6 and 9 years, initially during sleep. This results in release of gonadotrophins, initially luteinizing hormone (LH) but later also follicle-stimulating hormone (FSH) from the pituitary. As the duration of gonadotrophin release becomes prolonged, the ovary responds with the production of estrogens.

Estrogen production, along with adrenal androgen production, causes the physical changes of pubertal development that were classically described by Tanner and his colleagues in the 1960s and 1970s. The first sign of puberty is the appearance of the subareolar breast bud at the mean age of 10.8 years (range 8.8–12.8 years). Pubic hair growth occurs approximately 6 months later, although in approximately one third of girls it occurs before breast development.[2] Thereafter, pubertal development proceeds in a recognized sequence of events – increase in growth velocity, pubic and axillary hair development to Tanner Stage 4, breast development to Tanner stage 3–4, menstruation.[3] The median age of menarche in British teenagers is 13 years[4] with little geographic, social or ethnic variation. In the UK 95% will reach menarche by the age of 15 and one in eight while still in primary school.

PROBLEMS AT BIRTH

DISORDERS OF SEXUAL DIFFERENTIATION

The diagnosis, investigation and management of girls with disorders of sexual differentiation (DSD) have been dealt with in Chapter 15. Surgical correction of the genital abnormalities has traditionally been performed soon after birth, with the belief that it is important to correct the appearance of the genitalia as soon as possible – and certainly before the girl reached her adolescent years. More recently clinicians have been questioning this management. Delaying corrective surgery until later years allows the girl to be involved in the decision-making. Additionally, the growth of the structures and the estrogenization of the tissues make the surgery easier, allowing, for instance, better dissection of the neural bundle during clitoridectomy, thus preserving function. Recent articles showing poor sexual function in later life in women who had surgery performed in childhood have strengthened the argument that corrective surgery should be delayed until adolescence.[5,6]

HYDROCOLPOS

Hydrocolpos presents at birth with a bulging membrane visible at the introitus, less commonly as an abdominal mass rising out of the pelvis. It is caused by the failure of breakdown of the membrane at the junction of the Mullerian duct and the urogenital sinus, allowing the collection of fluid. Treatment is by excision of the membrane. Failure to recognize that an abdominal/pelvic mass may be due to hydrocolpos may have serious consequences. In the only published series, 35% of neonates died after an unnecessary laparotomy for hydrocolpos.[7] Although the paper is old it emphasizes the importance of making the correct diagnosis.

PROBLEMS IN EARLY CHILDHOOD

VULVOVAGINITIS

Vulvovaginitis is without doubt the commonest condition seen at a pediatric gynecology clinic – and has almost always been misdiagnosed and mismanaged before being referred.

Vulvovaginitis occurs because the anatomy and physiology of the genitalia of the prepubescent girl do not provide the resistance to bacterial infections found in the adult woman. In the pre-pubescent girl, the labia minora are thin and attenuated. The changes in vaginal secretion that occur at puberty, under the influence of estrogen (acidic vaginal secretions and the presence of Doderlein's bacilli), and which help prevent infection, are not present. This results in the girl being prone to bacterial infection. The common age of presentation, between the ages of 3 and 8, may be due to the girl being more responsible for her own personal hygiene at this age. The common organisms involved are fecal flora and nasopharyngeal organisms (*Haemophilus influenzae* and Group A beta-hemolytic streptococci),[8] although the significance of these organisms is uncertain because of the lack of information about normal vaginal flora in pre-pubertal girls.[9] Other organisms, particularly *Candida*, are much less common.

Girls with vulvovaginitis present with symptoms of vaginal irritation or pain, which can be severe and vaginal discharge, which can be profuse and often described as 'green' or 'brown'. Dysuria may also be present and the girl may well have been investigated for urinary tract infection before the correct diagnosis is made. Examination shows the labia to be inflamed and often excoriated. Careful inspection should also be undertaken to exclude dermatological conditions.

The differential diagnosis of vulvovaginitis includes other conditions that cause vulvar irritation or vaginal discharge that are mentioned later.

Management is usually limited to treatment for the relief of symptoms. The role of investigation is a vexed one. It is impossible to take an uncontaminated high vaginal swab in a young girl without a general anesthetic and no attempt should be made to do so. An introital swab may be helpful but interpretation may be difficult because of the presence of contaminants. The use of antibiotics in response to a specific swab result is limited as subsequent attacks are likely to be due to different organisms. Antibiotics should only be used if a pure growth of a pathogen is identified.[9]

The mainstay of treatment should be advice regarding personal hygiene and clothing. The use of an emollient cream such as E45 or Sudocrem may relieve symptoms and provide a barrier, especially to relieve pain on micturition. There is no place for antifungal therapy unless a *proven* candidal infection is present.

It is essential to explain to the mother why the condition has occurred along with reassurance that it will improve as the girl approaches puberty. It is also important to stress that the girl will not have any long-term gynecological consequences.

BLOODSTAINED VAGINAL DISCHARGE

Bloodstained vaginal discharge is relatively uncommon. It may be due to infection but a foreign body or tumor must be excluded.

Foreign bodies in the vagina in this age group are not unusual, resulting from the normal practice of girls exploring their own bodies. Examination under anesthesia is mandatory. Imaging with ultrasound or X-rays will not pick up foreign bodies such as pieces of toilet paper or sponge. In any case, general anesthesia will be required for removal.

Genital rhabdomyosarcoma is an unusual tumor that may present with bloodstained discharge. It is dealt with more fully later.

VULVAR IRRITATION

Other common causes of vulvar irritation in this age group are:
- dermatological conditions;
- threadworms;
- nonspecific vulvitis.

Dermatological conditions

Any dermatological condition such as eczema or psoriasis may occur on the vulva just as in any other part of the body.

A dermatological condition that is not uncommon in prepubertal girls is lichen sclerosus. This condition may occur anywhere on the body but is found on the vulva at the extremes of reproductive life – in the prepubertal girl and the postmenopausal woman. The etiology is unknown, although genetic susceptibility and an autoimmune basis have both been suggested.[10] It presents with extreme irritation. Examination shows characteristic appearances of shiny white ('pearly white') macules or papules that may coalesce into larger plaques. There are often associated hemorrhagic areas that may appear as bruising. Ulcerated areas may also be present (Fig. 25.1). To the unaware, the condition may be suggestive of sexual abuse[11] and it has been suggested that lichen sclerosus is more common in girls who have been sexually abused.[12]

Treatment depends on the severity of the symptoms. If the irritation is severe, treatment is with high-potency steroids, most commonly clobetasol propionate 0.05%. In less severe cases or when the disease is asymptomatic, an emollient cream is all that is required. As the condition may also involve the perianal skin ('figure of eight appearance'), constipation is often a feature and laxative therapy may also be required. Most girls have complete remission of symptoms after 2 or 3 months[13] and the condition usually resolves completely before puberty. There is no risk of malignancy with lichen sclerosus in this age group, unlike that debated in the postmenopausal group, and it may be worth emphasizing that to parents, who in this age of the Internet may be alarmed by the information they find there.

Threadworms

Threadworms (*Enterobius vermicularis*) are common in this age group and although the most common presentation is with anal irritation, vulvar irritation may also be present or may be the only presenting symptom. Diagnosis is by a Sellotape test, the tape being applied to the perianal region overnight, removed in the morning and fixed to a glass slide. Examination of the slide will reveal ova and adult worms. Treatment is with mebendazole 100 mg as a single dose to all members of the family over the age of 2 years.

Nonspecific vulvitis

Nonspecific vulvitis is common but difficult to treat. Common precipitating factors are washing powder, fabric conditioners and bubble bath. Treatment is by identifying and removing the cause.

OTHER VULVAR DISORDERS

Vulvar warts

Vulvar or perianal warts (Fig. 25.2) present the dilemma of whether or not they are indicative of sexual abuse. They may well have been transferred quite innocently from the hands of a parent or childminder, or the child herself, and the situation requires sensitive handling. It has been suggested that DNA typing of the virus may be helpful but this is debatable except in cases of child abuse, where a matching to genital warts

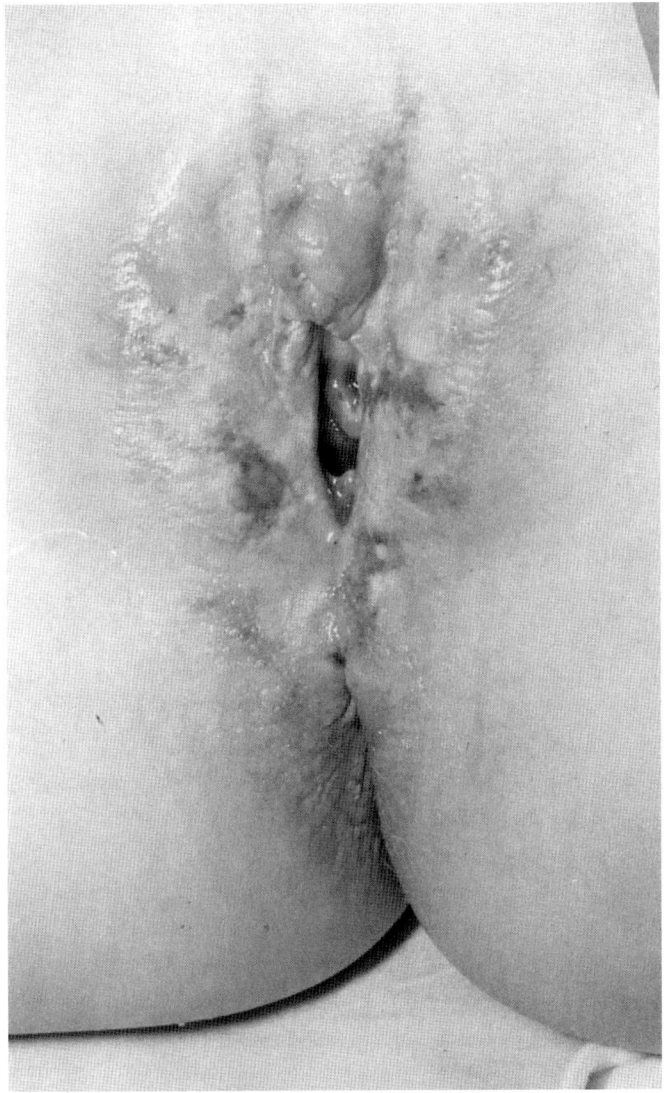

Fig. 25.1 Lichen sclerosus on the vulva of a prepubertal girl showing the classical appearances of pearly white areas with hemorrhage and ulceration.

from the alleged abuser will provide confirmation. Warts on the hymen are always significant.

Treatment is by cautery under general anesthesia or, in the older girl, by using podophyllin, taking care not to damage the surrounding skin.

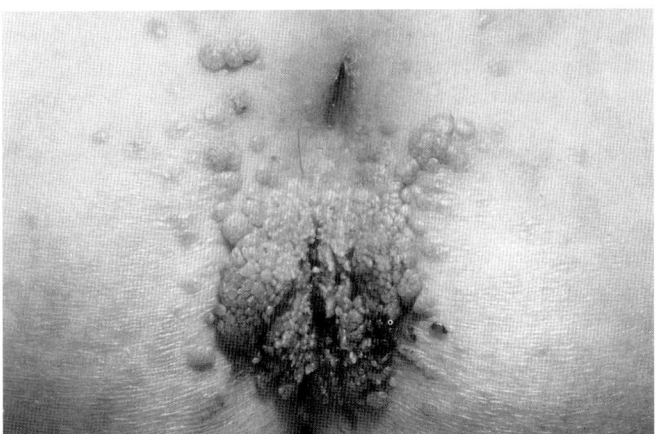

Fig. 25.2 Perianal warts in a young girl (reproduced by kind permission of Edward Arnold).

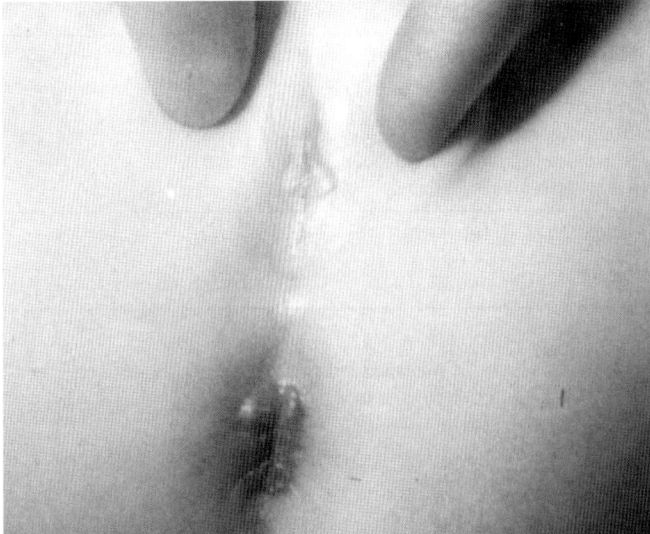

Fig. 25.3 Labial adhesions in a child of 18 months. Note the completely flat appearance of the perineum.

LABIAL ADHESIONS

Labial adhesions are seen most commonly in girls under the age of 3 years and are thought to be secondary to chronic irritation. It is important to make the correct diagnosis. The child is commonly brought up by parents, who are panic-stricken, having been told that their child has a congenital abnormality that will require major reconstructive surgery.

The difference between labial adhesions and congenital absence of the vagina is quite straightforward. In a girl with labial adhesions, the perineum is quite flat, with the fused labia preventing visualization of the urethra, clitoris or hymen (Fig. 25.3). The line of the fused labia can often be clearly seen. In a girl with congenital absence of the vagina, separation of the labia shows clearly the introital structures.

Labial adhesions are usually asymptomatic, a chance finding by the mother or a health worker. Occasionally, the presentation may be that of incontinence, urine being trapped behind the adhesion when the girl is squatting on the toilet but being expelled when she stands up.

Treatment, if required, is with estrogen cream. There is debate that treatment should be restricted to those girls who are symptomatic as the condition is a self-limiting one and resolves spontaneously as the child becomes older. There is no place for surgical separation.

The debate as to whether labial adhesions are diagnostic of, or more common in, girls who have been sexually abused is unresolved.

PROBLEMS OF PUBERTY

PRIMARY AMENORRHEA

Amenorrhea is considered as 'primary' when the girl has never menstruated and 'secondary' if she has not had a period for 6 months or more. Primary amenorrhea is usually subdivided into two groups – girls who have no pubertal development in whom the problem is most likely due to a hormonal cause and girls who have normal pubertal development in whom the cause is most likely an anatomical one. The causes of primary amenorrhea are shown in Table 25.1.

It is standard practice to advise investigation of girls with primary amenorrhea without pubertal development by the age of 14 and girls with normal pubertal development by the age of 16. It is equally important to remember that pubertal development is a continuum and that a break in the continuum is as significant as arbitrary cut-offs of age.

Primary amenorrhea without sexual development
Constitutional delay

Girls with constitutional delay may have a family history of the condition. Investigations show low estrogen and low gonadotrophin levels.

Table 25.1   Causes of primary amenorrhea

Without pubertal development
Constitutional delay
Chronic systemic disease
Absent ovarian function
Hypothalamic pituitary dysfunction
(Polycystic ovarian syndrome)

With pubertal development
Absent uterus
(Absent or imperforate vagina)

Bone age is delayed compared to chronological age. Reassurance is all that is required although girls in whom puberty is significantly delayed should be considered for induction of puberty.

Chronic systemic disease

Chronic diseases such as poorly controlled diabetes or hypothyroidism are not usually a diagnostic problem. Estrogen and gonadotrophin levels are low. Puberty follows control of the disease.

Absent ovarian function

Absent ovarian function may be due to primary or premature ovarian failure or to gonadal dysgenesis. The characteristic findings on investigation are high follicle-stimulating hormone (FSH) and luteinizing hormone (LH) levels and low estrogen. Ovarian failure may also present as secondary amenorrhea depending on the stage of development at which the failure occurred. It is a devastating diagnosis to have to give any woman of reproductive years but worse for an adolescent girl and it requires sensitive handling.

The most common identified cause of premature ovarian failure in modern practice is subsequent to chemotherapy or irradiation for childhood or adolescent malignancy. Recent advances in techniques of ovarian tissue cryopreservation suggest that it may be possible in the future to preserve fertility in some patients whose gonadal function is threatened by premature menopause, or by treatments such as radiotherapy, chemotherapy or surgical castration.[14] While most cases are idiopathic, identified causes of ovarian failure in this age group are autoimmune, chromosomal (e.g. 46XXX, fragile X), metabolic (e.g. galactosemia).

Gonadal dysgenesis most commonly is associated with a 45X or variant karyotype (Turner syndrome) but may also be found in girls with a 46XY karyotype (Swyer syndrome or pure gonadal dysgenesis). Turner syndrome is found in 1:2000 to 1:3000 of the female population. It is characterized by short stature and ovarian failure, the ovaries being only streaks of tissue (streak ovaries). However, only approximately 50% of girls with Turner syndrome have the 45X karyotype on lymphocyte culture, the remainder being due to abnormal X chromosomes or mosaic karyotypes. Because of this, the phenotype varies greatly, but the main additional features include web neck, shield chest with wide-spaced nipples and wide carrying angle (Fig. 25.4). Delay in the diagnosis is often due to the failure to appreciate the variation in phenotype.

Hypothalamic pituitary dysfunction

Hypothalamic or pituitary disorders, such as craniopharyngiomas, hydrocephaly or Kallmann syndrome may result in primary amenorrhea.

Treatment

Treatment involves hormone replacement in such a way as to mimic the normal physiological response of the ovary. Obviously in girls with constitutional delay or those with chronic illness, development may proceed normally given time. However, while waiting for spontaneous development, adolescents may experience psychological stress or even bullying at school so induction of puberty should be considered and discussed.

Estrogen replacement should begin around the age of 10 or 11, unless it is wished to delay it for the administration of growth hormone

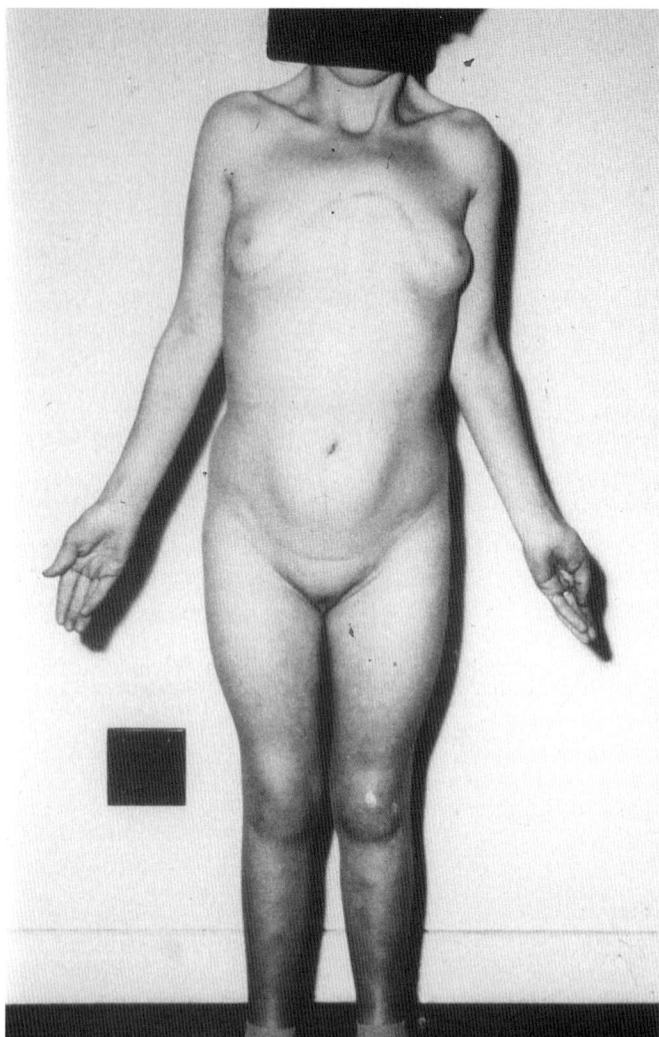

Fig. 25.4   Classical appearance of a girl with Turner syndrome showing web neck, wide-spaced nipples and wide carrying angle. Mosaic conditions are common so that a wide variation in phenotype is seen.

in girls with Turner syndrome. The initial dose should be 1 mcg ethinyl estradiol increasing every 6 months to 2 mcg, 5 mcg and 10 mcg. After this period of time a cyclical preparation of estrogen and progestogen should be introduced, either in the form of the combined oral contraceptive or, preferably, hormone replacement therapy. Girls on long-term oestrogen replacement should be monitored for dosage and compliance to reduce the long-term risks of estrogen lack such as osteoporosis.

Primary amenorrhea with sexual development

Primary amenorrhea with normal development is usually due to an anatomical cause, either absence of the uterus (or more correctly the endometrium) or absence or blockage of the vagina, which more correctly causes cryptomenorrhea.

Absence of the uterus

Failure of development of the Mullerian duct causing congenital absence of the uterus may be found in Rokitansky–Kuster–Hauser syndrome or as part of complete androgen insensitivity syndrome (CAIS).

Rokitansky–Kuster–Hauser syndrome. Girls with this condition are phenotypically normal, with a 46XX karyotype and normal ovaries. Associated renal tract abnormalities are found in 40% of patients and vertebral column abnormalities such as hemivertebrae or fused vertebrae in 12%. The degree of failure of development (Fig. 25.5) varies from total absence of Mullerian duct structures to varying degrees of uterine

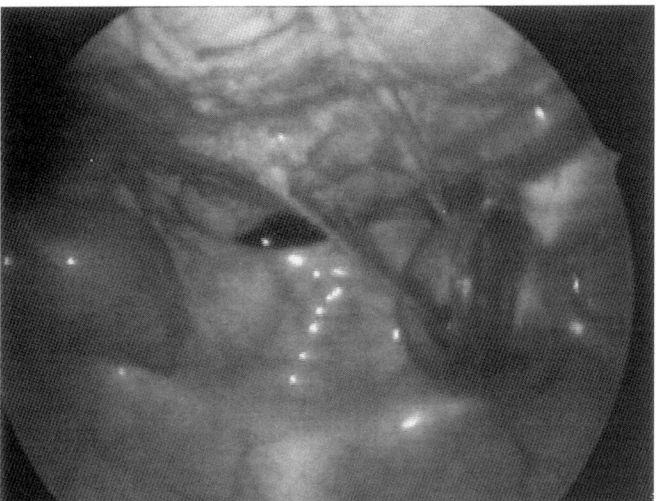

Fig. 25.5 Rudimentary uterine horns in a girl with Rokitansky–Kuster–Hauser syndrome (adhesions surrounding the left horn).

horn development, very occasionally including endometrium within a small blind uterine horn causing cryptomenorrhea. It is not necessary to remove the rudimentary uterine horn unless there is cryptomenorrhea. Vaginal reconstruction with dilators or surgically is required.

Complete androgen insensitivity syndrome (CAIS). Girls with CAIS have a 46XY karyotype. They are often slightly taller than average, have good breast development and sparse pubic and axillary hair. The condition arises as a result of the cells of the mesonephric duct and genital tubercle failing to respond to circulating androgens with the resulting failure of development of male external genitalia. The condition is an X-linked disorder and a history of a sister or aunt with the condition may be obtained.

Treatment is by removal of the testes because of the 5% risk of malignancy[15] and vaginal reconstruction. Long-term estrogen replacement is required to protect against osteoporosis.

Girls with CAIS and their families require sensitive management, particularly in regard to their sexual identity.[16]

Cryptomenorrhea

Cryptomenorrhea or 'hidden menstruation' presents with amenorrhea in the presence of increasingly severe cyclical lower abdominal pain. The common blockage occurs at the lower end of the vagina, but higher lesions may occur.

In severe cases, the girl may present with acute urinary retention due to blockage of the urethra by the vaginal mass. Examination of the abdomen reveals a mass arising out of the pelvis, the size being dependent on the duration of menstruation. With a low blockage, examination shows the classical bulging blue membrane at the introitus on separation of the labia (Fig. 25.6). Treatment is by cruciate incision of the membrane.

More rarely, cryptomenorrhea may occur in the presence of menstruation when there is a blockage of a duplex genital tract, in which case presentation is with severe dysmenorrhea.

PROBLEMS OF ADOLESCENCE

HEAVY PERIODS

A complaint of heavy periods is the commonest reason for seeing a teenager at a gynecological clinic. It is essential when seeing these patients that an accurate history is taken. In practice, it is difficult to assess a girl's menstrual loss objectively in the absence of evidence such as anemia. Information about cycle length and duration is subjective and rarely helpful, although the use of a menstrual diary or a pictorial chart[17] may help. A history of how her periods affect activities such as attendance at school, having to get up at night to change sanitary protection or

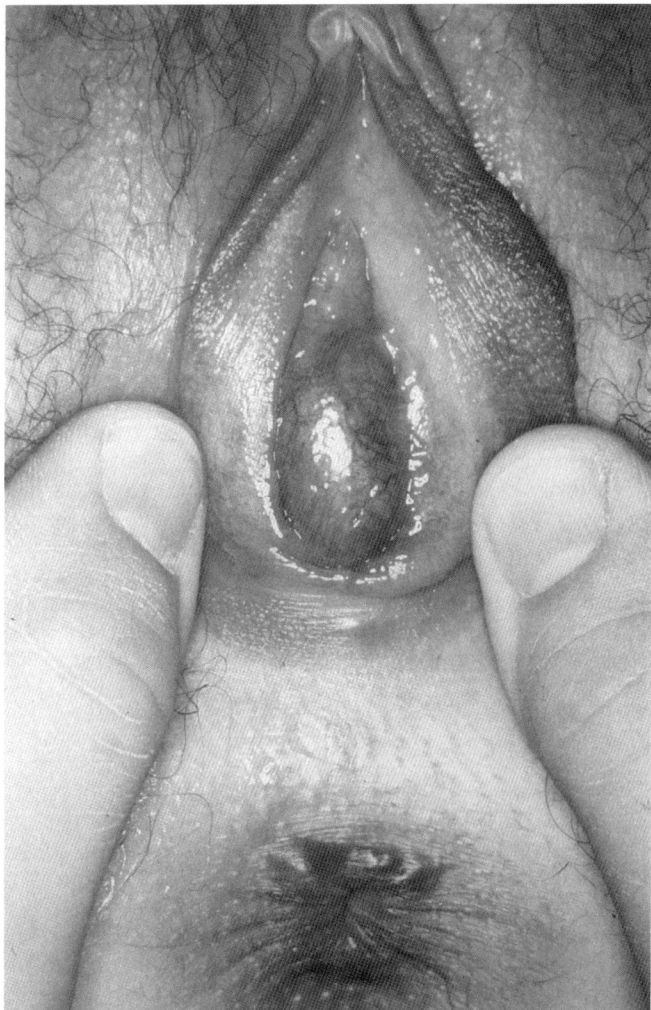

Fig. 25.6 Bulging membrane at the introitus of an adolescent with cryptomenorrhea due to a low transverse vaginal septum.

nightwear may be more helpful. However, a study in adult women with a complaint of heavy periods that showed that in 68% the blood loss was less than 80 ml and in 42% it was less than 50 ml[18] illustrates the difficulty in making an accurate assessment of the problem through history. It is essential however that an objective assessment is made as acceptance that a problem exists may affect a girl's perception of her menstruation into adulthood.

Pathophysiology

Girls with heavy, irregular periods are unlikely to be ovulating. Whereas in their early twenties, 95% of women are having ovulatory cycles, regular ovulation only occurs in 15% of girls in the first year after menarche.[19] In the absence of progesterone produced as a result of ovulation, the endometrium continues to proliferate under the action of unopposed estrogen until the endometrium breaks down irregularly with resultant extremely heavy loss. Girls with regular heavy periods are more likely to be ovulating and the mechanism for the heavy loss is thought to be due to increased endometrial fibrinolysis[20] and an alteration in prostaglandin balance.[21]

Management

There is no place for bimanual vaginal or rectal examination of these girls. It is unlikely that there will be any pelvic pathology causing these symptoms and such an examination is only likely to cause distress and deter them from attending future gynecological examination. If it is essential that an assessment is made of the pelvic organs, then pelvic ultrasound should be performed.

Full blood count should be performed. Thyroid function should only be assessed if there are features in the history or examination suggestive of thyroid dysfunction.[22] There is no indication in this age group for hysteroscopy or dilatation and curettage.

Girls who are not anemic and whose periods are not disrupting their school or personal life require reassurance only. Girls with heavy regular periods should be treated with tranexamic acid 1 g 6 hourly and mefenamic acid 500 mg 8 hourly.[23] Tranexamic acid has been shown to reduce menstrual flow by 54% and mefenamic acid to reduce menstrual flow by 20%.

In girls with irregular periods, treatment should be with cyclical progestogens, such as dydrogesterone, norethisterone or medroxyprogesterone, or the combined oral contraceptive pill. Treatment should continue for 6–12 months in the first instance before stopping, with the information that the medication is not curing anything, merely controlling symptoms until ovulatory cycles occur. Treatment should therefore be continued in the long term until the symptoms have settled.

Concerns about giving the combined oral contraceptive pill to adolescents are largely unfounded. The most commonly expressed are premature closure of epiphyses, which is unfounded as a girl producing enough estrogen to have heavy periods will already have closed epiphyses, and an increased risk of developing breast cancer. The risk of the latter has been defined by the Collaborative Group on Hormonal Factors in Breast Cancer[24] as being 0.5 excess cancers per 100 000 women when used in the ages 16–19.

PAINFUL PERIODS

Dysmenorrhea affects 60% of adolescents – 14% of them having symptoms severe enough to cause them to miss school.[25] Dysmenorrhea occurs in ovulatory cycles and is caused by increased levels of prostaglandins being released by the menstrual endometrium. The pain starts with the onset of menstruation, or just before, and lasts 24–48 h. It may be accompanied by nausea, vomiting, diarrhea, backache and pain in the thighs. Treatment is with one of the prostaglandin synthetase inhibitors, usually mefenamic acid 500 mg 8 hourly.[26] Although good-quality trials are lacking,[27] the combined oral contraceptive pill is the treatment of choice for those girls who fail to respond to the prostaglandin synthetase inhibitors and has the added advantage of reducing menstrual flow and providing contraception.

In girls who fail to respond to the combined oral contraceptive pill, underlying pathology should be excluded. The commonest underlying cause is endometriosis (Fig. 25.7), found in approximately 40% of adolescent girls investigated.[28] Treatment is with the combined oral contraceptive pill, progestogens, danazol and gonadotrophin-releasing hormone (GnRH) agonists, the choice being made principally on the basis of the side effects as they are equally effective in relieving pain.[29]

Loss of bone mass is the main limiting side effect of the use of GnRH agonists but has been shown to be reversible in adolescents.[30] GnRH agonists may be used with add-back estrogen/progestogen to prevent bone loss without apparent loss of effective therapy.[31]

The other condition that should be considered in girls who fail to respond to the combined oral contraceptive pill is cryptomenorrhea in a patient with a duplex system. Ultrasound examination in such girls may show an 'ovarian cyst', which is, of course, the blind uterine horn filled with menstrual blood. Depending on the level of the blockage, treatment is either by removing the vaginal septum blocking the uterus or removing the uterine horn. Endometriosis is often additionally present. Imaging of the renal tract should be performed as 47% of girls with Mullerian duct abnormalities have renal tract anomalies.[32]

SECONDARY AMENORRHEA

Secondary amenorrhea is defined as the cessation of periods for 6 months or more. The main causes are listed in Table 25.2.

Polycystic ovarian disease

Polycystic ovarian syndrome (PCO) presents with irregular periods or secondary amenorrhea and is associated with obesity, hirsutism, acne and anovulation. Endocrinologically it is characterized by LH hypersecretion and insulin resistance, and a finding of an LH:FSH ratio of greater than three with slightly raised testosterone levels and low sex hormone-binding globulin (SHBG). Ultrasound examination reveals a slightly enlarged ovary with hyperechoic stroma and 10 or more follicles of no greater than 10 mm around the circumference (Fig. 25.8). These ultrasound appearances are found in up to one third of women and diagnosis should not be made on these appearances alone.

Treatment should emphasize the importance of weight loss through exercise and diet[33] as this reduces insulin resistance and is associated with improved regularity of menstruation, hirsutism and ovulation. It is also important as women with PCO have an increased risk of developing diabetes mellitus, or having a stroke or a transient ischemic attack.[34] Treatment otherwise is aimed at controlling the symptoms. In the case of secondary amenorrhea or irregular periods, this is achieved with the

Table 25.2   Causes of secondary amenorrhea

Pregnancy
Premature ovarian failure
Polycystic ovary syndrome
Pituitary disorders
Hypothalamic disorders

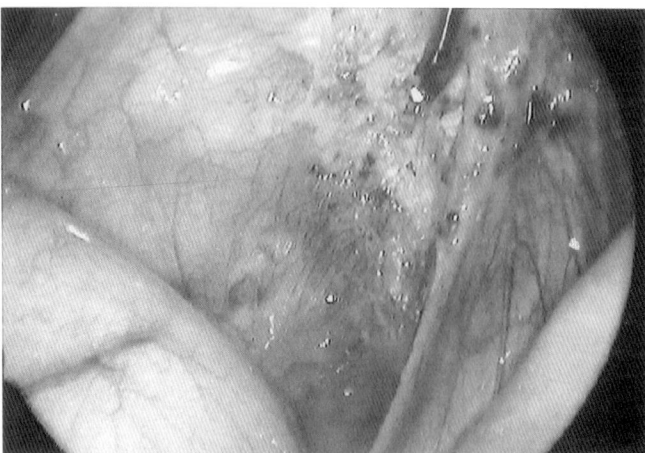

Fig. 25.7   Extensive endometriosis involving the right uterosacral ligament and pouch of Douglas in an adolescent girl.

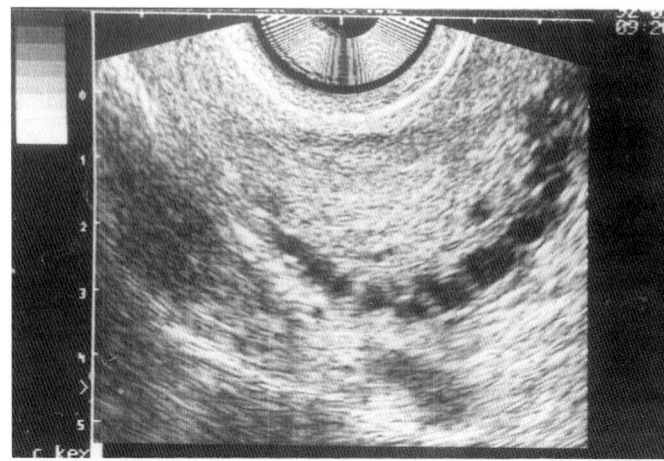

Fig. 25.8   Ultrasound appearances of polycystic ovarian syndrome.

combined oral contraceptive pill. Metformin has been shown to reduce hyperinsulinemia and hyperandrogenemia[35] although there is no literature about the safety of long-term use in young women.[36]

Pituitary disorders

Pituitary disorders as a cause of secondary amenorrhea in adolescents are very rare.

Hypothalamic disorders

Girls who have a low body mass index (BMI) due to dieting, anorexia nervosa or excessive exercising will have amenorrhea secondary to hypothalamic dysfunction and low levels of gonadotrophin. Investigation reveals low levels of FSH, LH and estrogen. Menstrual cycles will normally resume when, or just after, the girl achieves normal weight. Management in the meantime, however, can be difficult as such girls often refuse replacement hormones as they fear putting on weight.

HIRSUTISM AND VIRILISM

Hirsutism is defined as the presence of excessive hair in a female in a distribution that is characteristic of an adult male. It is an extremely embarrassing and distressing condition for a teenager. Causes include ovarian disorders, adrenal disorders, drugs and hypothyroidism; polycystic ovarian syndrome is the most common.

Examination should include careful recording of the extent of the abnormal hair growth as a baseline prior to treatment. Initial investigation is by hormone profile including FSH, LH, testosterone, SHBG, 17alphahydroxyprogesterone and the specific adrenal androgen dehydroepiandrosterone sulfate (DHEAS). Cortisol levels and thyroid function tests should also be assessed.

Treatment should be started as soon as possible as terminal hair growth can be difficult to stop once stimulated. Cosmetic treatments such as waxing, laser therapy or electrolysis should be used. Specific treatment depends on the cause. Ovarian or adrenal androgen-secreting tumors should be removed. Late-onset congenital adrenal hyperplasia is treated with dexamethasone.

Hirsutism due to polycystic ovarian syndrome is treated with the antiandrogen cyproterone acetate in conjunction with estrogen. Low-dose cyproterone acetate may be given in the form of the combined oral contraceptive Dianette (Schering). Higher doses may be given.

Spironolactone and finasteride have also been used for the treatment of hirsutism although neither is licensed for the treatment of hyperandrogenism.

FEMALE GENITAL MUTILATION

Female genital mutilation is a complex issue that raises concerns about competing cultural backgrounds, autonomy, health education and sexuality. It is practiced in many cultures but most widely in northern Africa and in the Arab peninsula. The age at which it is performed varies with culture but most commonly around the ages of 7–9.

Immigration figures show that the number of women from communities that traditionally practice female genital mutilation is rising in the UK.[37] Girls from cultures where it is the practice for the procedure to be performed but who live in Britain probably have the operation performed in the country of their family.

Four main types are recognized:
1. **Circumcision.** This is the least extensive and involves cutting of the prepuce of the hood of the clitoris. In some countries this is known as 'Sunna'.
2. **Excision.** This involves removal of the clitoris and all or part of the labia minora with the remainder of the labia minora being stitched together, leaving a small opening to allow urine and menstrual blood to be passed (Fig. 25.9).
3. **Infibulation.** This is the most extensive. It involves removal of the clitoris, labia minora and a substantial part of the medial aspect

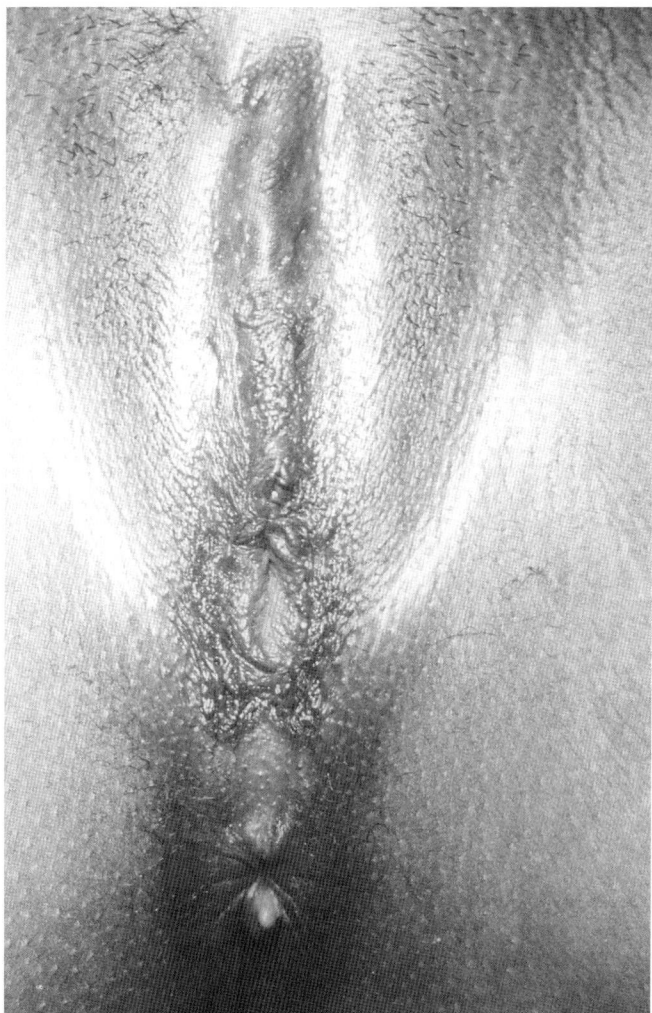

Fig. 25.9 Appearance of the external genitalia in an adolescent girl who has had excision of the genitalia (reproduced by kind permission of Edward Arnold).

of the labia majora. The remainder of the labia majora are then pinned together to leave a small opening.
4. **Intermediate.** This involves removal of the clitoris and varying amounts of the labia minora and majora.

The most common problems likely to be seen by pediatricians in girls who have had circumcision performed are recurrent urinary tract infection and dysmenorrhea.

In Britain, female genital mutilation is illegal (Prohibition of Female Circumcision Act 1985); it is regarded as a form of abuse[38] and raises child protection issues. It differs from other forms of abuse in that it may be done with the best intentions for the future welfare of the child, there is no possibility of its repetition during childhood and it is approved by sections of the communities in which it is practiced.

GYNECOLOGICAL TUMORS

Gynecological tumors are rare in childhood and adolescence – and malignant tumors particularly so. The commonest are ovarian lesions with tumors of the vagina and cervix being the next most common. Late presentation is a major problem, partly due in the case of ovarian lesions to the nonspecific presenting symptoms, and partly due to the rarity of the tumors resulting in a low index of suspicion. The main presenting symptoms are nonspecific lower abdominal pain, occasionally with vomiting. Vaginal bleeding may be the presenting symptom in estrogen-secreting tumors.

BENIGN OVARIAN TUMORS

Follicular cysts are the most common, frequently being found incidentally as part of an ultrasound examination. Management for lesions less than 5 cm is simply by follow-up ultrasound examination to ensure that the cysts resolve. Larger cysts should be aspirated, either under ultrasound control or laparoscopically. If surgical removal is required, care should be taken to preserve as much of the normal ovarian tissue as possible.

Teratomas are the most common neoplasm. They arise from totipotential primordial cells and may contain tissue derived from all three tissue layers. The predominant tissue is usually ectodermal – i.e. sebum and hair – earning the common term 'dermoid cyst'. Treatment is by surgical removal, with conservation of as much ovarian tissue as possible, and close examination of the other ovary as 10–15% of these tumors are bilateral.

MALIGNANT OVARIAN TUMORS

Dysgerminomas are the most common malignant ovarian tumor in childhood and adolescence; 60% of these tumors are found in females under the age of 20. They are bilateral in 10–15% of cases. As they are usually of low malignant potential unilateral oophorectomy may be carried out, unless the girl has a Y chromosome – or part of one – in her karyotype, when bilateral oophorectomy should be performed.

Other malignant tumors of the ovary such as immature teratomas, endodermal sinus tumors, embryonal carcinoma, mixed germ-cell tumors and granulosa cell tumors are less common.

OTHER MALIGNANT TUMORS

Genital rhabdomyosarcoma (previously known as sarcoma botryoides) is the most common genital tract neoplasm in children under the age of 16. The tumor occurs most commonly in the vagina, less commonly in the cervix and uterus. Vaginal lesions occur most commonly in girls under the age of 2 years, with lesions of the cervix and vagina being found most commonly in older girls and young adults.

The tumor presents with vaginal bleeding and bloodstained discharge and such symptoms should always be assessed by examination under anesthesia and should include cystoscopy and proctoscopy. Treatment is with multimodal regimes using triple chemotherapy (vincristine, actinomycin D and cyclophosphamide), with or without radiotherapy. The use of this regime has reduced the need for surgical resection from 100% in the initial Intergroup Rhabdomyosarcoma Study Group (IRSG) to only 13% in the most recent study.[39]

TEENAGE PREGNANCY

The problems associated with teenage pregnancy are those associated with social deprivation rather than specifically related to young maternal age. The incidence of teenage pregnancies varies between countries and within countries. The Guttmacher Institute recently reported trend data on adolescent birth rates for 46 countries over the period 1970–1995. Lowest rates were reported from the Netherlands (12/1000 adolescents/year) with the highest among resource rich countries being the Russian Federation (> 100/1000 adolescents/year). Japan and most western European countries had rates of < 40/1000 adolescents/year.[40] Within the Netherlands, four times as many pregnant teenagers had non-Dutch ethnicity compared to all pregnant women.[41] Psychosocial problems, and the consumption of alcohol, cigarettes, marijuana, heroin and solvents are higher among pregnant teenagers than in the general teenage population.[42] Pregnant teenagers with higher levels of education are more likely to undergo termination of pregnancy than continue with the pregnancy.[43] There is some evidence that, in some areas, the difference in teenage pregnancy rates between more affluent and more deprived areas has widened over the last 2 decades.[44]

Antenatal problems reported in pregnant teenagers include pregnancy-induced hypertension, anemia,[45] premature labor and low birth weight,[46] although some of these are also associated with social factors such as smoking and deprivation. There are no specific intrapartum problems faced by pregnant teenagers, high rates of spontaneous delivery with low rates of prolonged labor and cesarean section being consistently reported.[46] While no differences have been reported in outcome of first teenage pregnancy, a second teenage pregnancy is associated with three times the average risk of stillbirth.[47]

REFERENCES (* Level 1 evidence)

1. Wellings K, Nanchahal K, MacDowall W, et al. Sexual behaviour in Britain: early heterosexual experience. Lancet 2001; 358:1843–1850.
2. Tanner JM. Foetus into man, 2nd edn. Ware: Castlemead Publications; 1989:58–74.
3. Marshall WA, Tanner JM. Variation in the pattern of pubertal changes in girls. Arch Dis Child 1969; 44:944–954.
4. Whincup PH, Gilg JA, Odoki K, et al. Age of menarche in contemporary British teenagers: survey of girls born between 1982 and 1986. BMJ 2001; 322:1095–1096.
5. Alizai NK, Thomas DF, Lilford R, et al. Feminizing genitoplasty for congenital adrenal hyperplasia: what happens at puberty. J Urol 1999; 161:1592–1593.
6. Minto CL, Liao L-M, Woodhouse C, et al. The effect of clitoral surgery in individuals who have intersex conditions with ambiguous genitalia. Lancet 2003; 361:1252–1257.
7. Gravier L. Hydrocolpos. J Ped Surg 1969; 4:563–568.
8. Pearce AN, Hart CA. Vulvovaginitis: causes and management. Arch Dis Child 1992; 67:509–512.
9. Joishy M, Ashtekar CS, Jain A, et al. Do we need to treat vulvovaginitis in prepubertal girls? BMJ 2005; 330:186–188.
10. Powell J, Wojarowska F, Winsey S, et al. Lichen sclerosus premenarche: autoimmunity and immunogenetics. Br J Dermatol 2000; 142:481–484.

11. Muhlendahl KE. Suspected sexual abuse in a 10 year old girl. Lancet 1996; 348:30.
12. Warrington SA, de San Lazaro C. Lichen sclerosus et atrophicus and sexual abuse. Arch Dis Child 1996; 75:512–516.
13. Fischer G, Rogers M. Treatment of childhood vulvar lichen sclerosus with potent topical steroid. Pediatr Dermatol 1997; 14:235–238.
14. Donnez J, Martinez-Madrid B, Jadoul P, et al. Human Reprod Update 2006; 12:519–535.
15. Verp MS, Simpson JL. Abnormal sexual differentiation and neoplasia. Cancer Genet Cytogenet 1987; 25:191–218.
16. Goodall J. Helping a girl to understand her testicular feminisation. Lancet 1991; 337:33–35.
17. Higham JM, O'Brien PMS, Shaw RW. Assessment of menstrual loss using a pictorial chart. Br J Obstet Gynaecol 1990; 97:734–749.
18. Cameron IT. Dysfunctional uterine bleeding. Baillière's Clin Obstet Gynaecol 1989; 3:315–337.
19. Apter D, Vihko R. Hormonal patterns of adolescent cycles. J Clin Endocrinol Metab 1978; 47:944–954.
20. Dokery CJ, Sheppard B, Daly L, et al. The fibrinolytic enzyme system in normal menstruation and excessive uterine bleeding and the effect of tranexamic acid. Obstet Gynecol Reprod Biol 1987; 24:309–318.
21. Smith SK, Abel MH, Kelly RW, et al. Prostaglandin synthesis in the endometrium of women with ovular

dysfunctional bleeding. Br J Obstet Gynaecol 1981; 88:434–442.
22. Prentice A. Medical management of menorrhagia. BMJ 1999; 319:1343–1345.
*23. Bonnar J, Sheppard BL. Treatment of menorrhagia during menstruation: randomised controlled trial of ethamsylate, mefenamic acid and tranexamic acid. BMJ 1996; 313:579–582.
*24. Collaborative Group on Hormonal Factors in Breast Cancer. Breast cancer and hormonal contraceptives. collaborative re-analysis of individual data on 53297 women with breast cancer and 100239 women without breast cancer from 54 epidemiological studies. Lancet 1996; 347:1713–1727.
25. Klein JR, Litt IF. Epidemiology of adolescent dysmenorrhoea. Pediatrics 1981; 68:661–664.
*26. Marjoribanks J, Proctor ML, Farquhar C. Nonsteroidal anti-inflammatory drugs for primary dysmenorrhoea. Cochrane Database Syst Rev 2003; 4:CD001751.
*27. Proctor ML, Roberts H, Farquhar C. Combined oral contraceptive pill (OCP) as treatment for primary dysmenorrhoea. Cochrane Database Syst Rev 2001; 2:CD002120.
28. Vercellini P, Fedele L, Arcaini L. Laparoscopy in the diagnosis of pelvic pain in adolescent women. J Reprod Med 1989; 34:156–160.
*29. Royal College of Obstetricians and Gynaecologists. The investigation and management of endometriosis. RCOG Guideline No. 24. London: RCOG; 2000.

30. Fogelman I. Gonadotropin releasing hormone agonists and the skeleton. Fertil Steril 1992; 57:715–724.

31. Surrey ES. Steroidal and nonsteroidal 'add-back' therapy: extending safety and efficacy of gonadotrophin-releasing hormone agonists in the gynaecologic patient. Fertil Steril 1995; 64:673–685.

32. Fore SR, Hammond CB, Parker RT, et al. Urologic and skeletal anomalies in patients with congenital absence of the vagina. Obstet Gynecol 1975; 46:410–416.

33. Pasquali R, Casimirri F. The impact of obesity on hyperandrogenism and polycystic ovary syndrome in premenopausal women. Clin Endocrinol 1993; 39:1–16.

34. Wild S, Pierpoint T, McKeigue P, et al. Cardiovascular disease in women with polycystic ovary syndrome at long-term follow-up: a retrospective cohort study. Clin Endocrinol 2000; 52:595–600.

*35. Moghetti P, Castello R, Negri C, et al. Metformin effects on clinical features, endocrine and metabolic profiles, and insulin sensitivity in polycystic ovary syndrome: a randomized, double-blind, placebo-controlled 6-month trial, followed by open, long-term clinical evaluation. J Clin Endocrinol Metab 2000; 85:139–146.

*36. Lord JM, Flight IHK, Norman RJ. Meformin in polycystic ovary syndrome: systemic review and meta-analysis. BMJ 2003; 327:951–955.

37. Forward (Foundation for Women's Health, Research and Development). Newsletter. November 1998.

38. Black JA, Debelle GD. Female genital mutilation in Britain. BMJ 1995; 310:1590–1594.

39. Andrassy RJ, Weiner ES, Raney RB, et al. Conservative surgical management of vaginal rhabdomyosarcomas: a 25 year review from the Intergroup Rhabdomyosarcoma Study III. J Pediatr Surg 1999; 34:731–734.

40. Singh S, Darroch JE. Adolescent pregnancy and childbearing levels and trends in developed countries. Fam Plann Perspect 2000; 32:14–23.

41. Van Enke WJ, Gorissen WH, van Enk A. Teenage pregnancy and ethnicity in the Netherlands: frequency and obstetric outcome. Eur J Contracept Reprod Health Care 2000; 5:77–84.

42. Quinlivan JA, Petersen RW, Gurrin LC. Adolescent pregnancy: psychopathology missed. Aust N Z J Psych 1999; 33:864–868.

43. Henderson LR. A survey of teenage pregnant women and their male partners in the Grampian region. Br J Fam Plann 1999; 25:90–92.

44. McLeod A. Changing patterns of teenage pregnancy: population based study of small areas. BMJ 2001; 323:199–203.

45. Konje JC, Palmer A, Watson A, et al. Early teenage pregnancies in Hull. Br J Obstet Gynaecol 1992; 99:969–973.

46. Van Eyk N, Allen LM, Sermer M, et al. Obstetric outcomes of adolescent pregnancies. J Pediatr Adolesc Gynecol 2000; 13:96.

47. Smith GC, Pell JP. Teenage pregnancy and risk of adverse perinatal outcomes associated with first and second birth: population based retrospective cohort study. BMJ 2001; 323:476.

26

Inborn errors of metabolism: biochemical genetics

Edited by Neil R M Buist and Robert D Steiner

"Nature is no where accustomed more openly to display her secret mysteries than in cases where she shows traces of her workings apart from the beaten path; nor is there any better way to advance the proper practice of medicine than to give our minds to the discovery of the usual law of nature, by careful investigation of cases of rarer forms of disease. For it has been found in almost all things that what they contain of useful or applicable, is hardly perceived unless we are deprived of them, or they become deranged in some way." (William Harvey 1642: letter to John Vlackveld)

INTRODUCTION

THE EVIDENCE BASE

Randomized, controlled, clinical trials are the basis of evidence-based medicine. However, for rare disorders, there are so few subjects, even with multicenter studies, that they are very difficult or impossible to conduct. In addition, wide clinical and genetic heterogeneity can render the generalizing results of such trials invalid. For rare diseases, treatment is often based on anecdote, empiric data and theory that can lead to a perception of treatment efficacy, as happened with the use of Lorenzo's oil for adrenoleukodystrophy and supplemental cholesterol for Smith–Lemli–Opitz syndrome. Recent successful trials of enzyme replacement therapy for several lysosomal storage diseases have been funded by the pharmaceutical industry without which they would have been difficult, if not impossible, to perform.

USEFUL REFERENCES

The major reference on biochemical genetics is the four-volume textbook edited by Scriver et al.[1] Additional sources for clinicians are Nyhan et al,[2] Gilbert-Barness and Barness[3] and Fernandes et al.[4] Other useful texts are by Holton,[5] Blau and Blaskovics,[6] Hommes,[7] Lyon et al[8] and Clarke.[9]

On-line Mendelian Inheritance In Man (OMIM), accessed through Pubmed on the Internet (http://www3.ncbi.nlm.nih.gov/omim/), provides invaluable information about all known human genetic conditions. Other sites include http://www.genetests.org, which is a listing of laboratories providing specific DNA tests, and links to Genereviews which provides online chapters on many inborn errors of metabolism (IEM). Other good sites are http://www.kumc.edu/gec/geneinfo.html, 'Children Living with Inherited Metabolic Disease' (http://www.climb.org.uk/) and the National Organization for Rare Disorders (NORD), New Fairfield, CT, USA (http://www.rarediseases.org/).

BIOCHEMICAL AND GENETIC CONSIDERATIONS

For 80 years after the term 'inborn errors of metabolism' was coined,[10] metabolic disorders were viewed as mostly involving amino acids. The field now includes over 600 disorders in almost every metabolic pathway and including defects of subcellular organelles, membrane structure and function, and disorders of protein processing, ion channeling, signal transduction, etc. The boundaries between environmental, genetic and metabolic conditions, never very clear, have increasingly merged. Over 400 conditions are discussed in this chapter; others, such as the metabolic endocrinopathies (Ch. 15), genetic defects of digestion and absorption (Ch. 19) and the metabolic defects of erythrocytes and leukocytes (Ch. 23) are discussed elsewhere.

Biochemical considerations

Expression of an enzyme activity usually represents the sum of the effect of two alleles. In Figure 26.1 the contribution of each allele (0–50%) and the total enzyme activity as a percentage are shown. The mother (I-2) is heterozygous for an allele producing a nonfunctional protein and I-1 is heterozygous for a mild mutation. Individuals such as I-3, who is a compound heterozygote with 11% of residual function, might be totally asymptomatic, be mildly affected or may only exhibit problems when the enzyme is stressed. Such heterogeneity results in 0–100% of normal activity, giving rise to severe or mild cases of a disorder even within a single pedigree.

Readers should always be mindful of the artificial nature of enzyme assays that usually involve highly unphysiological conditions, including high substrate levels and the use of artificial substrates. Some mutant enzymes require high in vivo levels of substrates to work adequately, as seen in some vitamin-dependent diseases. Occasionally healthy people have no activity against an artificial substrate in vitro. Conversely, it is possible to have normal in vitro activity but none in vivo. Similarly, in immunological assays, the epitope of the antibody may not involve the active site of the enzyme; immunological cross-reactivity can therefore be present even though a mutant protein is functionally defective.

Many enzymes exist in different forms in different tissues. Such *isoenzymes* may share some subunits while others are under separate genetic control. It is thus possible for a defect to occur in one tissue while normal activity is present in others. This must be remembered when leukocytes or surrogate tissues are used to diagnose an enzyme defect that is suspected to exist in other organs. A further confounding fact is that some isozymes derive from a single gene but are matured to different forms in different tissues; in an unusual form of acute intermittent porphyria, the erythrocyte isoform is normal but the enzyme is deficient in liver.

The potential consequences of an enzyme deficiency are illustrated in Figure 26.2. In phenylketonuria (PKU), for example, the metabolic

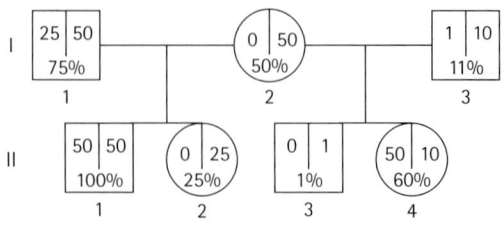

Fig. 26.1 Hypothetical pedigree showing the contribution of different mutant alleles to the total activity of an enzyme that is indicated as a percentage of the normal. Each normal allele contributes 50% of total normal function as seen in II-1. The index case II-3 has only 1% of normal activity. Case I-3 and even case II-2 might, under some circumstances, show evidence of the defect.

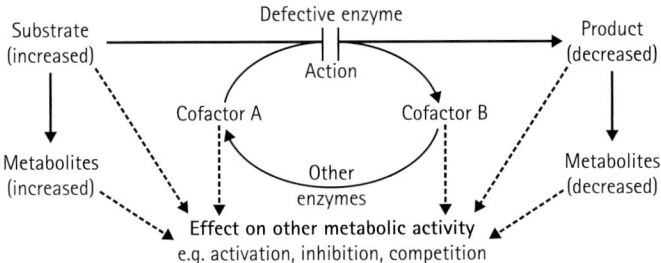

Fig. 26.2 Theoretical consequences of an enzyme deficiency.

derangements include inhibition of amino acid transport into brain cells, diminished synthesis of myelin and aromatic amines and inhibition of pyruvate metabolism, but it is not known how the brain damage is actually caused. Phenotypic variations even within a single family are presumed to be due to different environmental exposures or to inherited differences in the other metabolic steps that are affected by the biochemical upset (*epigenetics*). Genotype–phenotype correlations are proving to be very difficult to predict.[11]

Genetic considerations

The rapid advances fostered by the Human Genome Project have radically changed the specialty of genetics and are ever more impinging upon all branches of medicine. While some disorders are caused by one or only a few mutations, most are caused by many, sometimes numbering over 1000. New genes and new mutations make it almost obligatory to check the Internet before consulting on almost any genetic condition.

Some mutations are common in certain populations and rare in others, often due to founder effects or closed populations, but the high incidences of Tay–Sachs, Gaucher disease and mild congenital adrenal hyperplasia in Ashkenazim, which are caused by several different mutations, raise questions not only of founder effects but also of selective advantages.

Most heterozygotes can be identified if a specific test can be devised. For example, carriers of maple syrup urine disease have normal plasma amino acid levels and amino acid tolerance tests, but reduced enzyme activity in leukocytes. On the other hand, 80% of carriers for PKU can be identified by the phenylalanine:tyrosine ratio in fasting plasma or a phenylalanine tolerance test, though DNA analysis is now preferred. However, even in vitro enzyme assays may not clearly differentiate between carriers and affected or normal subjects. If available, DNA analysis is the optimum way to detect heterozygotes.

When a known metabolic disease is associated with other unrelated problems such as dysmorphic features, consideration should always be given either to the possibility of a micodeletion syndrome (e.g. glycerol kinase; see p. 1070), incest or the possibility of two conditions coexisting.

Most metabolic defects are recessively inherited. In this chapter, the genetics of each condition will not necessarily be discussed unless they vary from this pattern. Gene loci are not routinely provided in this chapter; they can be found on OMIM.

CLINICAL CONSIDERATIONS

Incidences

At least 1–2% of individuals have a pathogenic metabolic disorder of which most, such as hyperuricemia and the hyperlipidemias, are of minor clinical importance in childhood. Almost all of the conditions in this chapter are rare (~1 in 100 000–250 000); many are extremely rare (1 in 10^6–10^7). However, if there are 1000 diseases each with an incidence of only one in a million, 1 in 1000 people will have one of them and for *each* of these conditions, 1 in 500 is a carrier! This rarity constitutes a major diagnostic stumbling block for clinicians.[12–15]

Some of the commonest reasons for referral to a metabolic clinic are:

- disorders detected by expanded newborn screening;
- suspected or confirmed lactic acidosis;
- suspected or confirmed metabolic neurological disorders; including nonspecific developmental delay;
- metabolic bone diseases such as nutritional or hereditary rickets;
- failure to thrive;
- hypercholesterolemia;
- suspected porphyria;
- visceromegaly.

Clinical features

Metabolic disorders should always be considered when patients present with puzzling or unexplained problems, whether of growth, development or specific organ pathology. They can disrupt the function of any organ and may present at any age to specialists in any clinical discipline. Review of Tables 26.7, 26.10, 26.11, 26.26 and 26.28, which list common symptoms in various classes of disease, show the enormous diversity of presentations. Superb diagnostic algorithms are given in Chapter 66 of Scriver et al.[1]

Metabolic screening

Because the symptoms of metabolic disorders mimic nongenetic disease, some kind of 'metabolic screen' is frequently done on blood and/or urine of potential cases in the hope that an abnormality may assist in the diagnosis. This screening is different from the newborn screen and varies in different centers but may include rather insensitive tests for sugars, mucopolysaccharides, amino acids and a variety of other compounds. Quantitative assay of plasma amino acids, carnitine derivatives and urine organic acids are increasingly available and used for screening.[16] Such screening of 'at risk' children reveals an IEM in about 10% of cases.[17,18] It must always be remembered that many disorders are not associated with abnormal metabolite levels and thus cannot be detected by such assays. In most centers, the cost of such testing is less than that of a computed tomography (CT) or magnetic resonance imaging (MRI) scan. Increased number and availability of specific metabolic tests is improving the possibility of accurate diagnosis (Table 26.1).[19]

Large-scale metabolic screening in subjects with neurodevelopmental delay has led to the discovery of many new defects; most are rare. When an unusual defect is associated with clinical symptoms it is tempting to assume that they are causally related; however, this is often not the case. Amino acid disorders once thought to cause neurodevelopmental delay but now considered benign include cystathioninuria, methionine adenosyl transferase deficiency, some hyperlysinemias, saccharopinuria, 2-ketoadipic aciduria, sarcosinemia, hyperprolinemia, hydroxyprolinemia, histidinemia, carnosinemia, urocanic aciduria and beta-aminoisobutyricaciduria.

Routine newborn metabolic screening (including tandem mass spectrometry [MS/MS]) has entered a new phase with as many as 40 different conditions being detectable. Interpretation of the results requires considerable biochemical knowledge and is outside the scope of this chapter (see Appendix 1). It remains to be seen how radically expanded screening will alter our understanding of these diseases and reveal as yet unknown biological diversity.

THERAPEUTIC CONSIDERATIONS

Roughly 12% of metabolic diseases are markedly ameliorated by therapy; in about 50% treatment is partially effective, but treatment has little effect in the remainder.[20] For most, the approach is still to try and induce activity, as in the vitamin-responsive conditions, or to counteract the biochemical disturbance by diet or drug therapy. However, even total correction of a biochemical defect may not improve the symptoms (see Fig. 26.2). For example, in the Lesch–Nyhan syndrome, the blood urate is easily controlled with allopurinol, but the neurological symptoms are unchanged.

Table 26.1 Specialized investigations used in biochemical genetics

Test	Disorders detected
Blood	
Carnitine	Defects of amino, organic and fatty acid metabolism
Acyl-carnitines	Defects of amino, organic and fatty acid metabolism
Amino acids	All the aminoacidopathies
Very long chain fatty acids	Screening for peroxisomal defects
Plasmalogens	Screening for peroxisomal defects
Fatty acids	Several disorders, including the Smith–Lemli–Opitz syndrome
White blood cells/skin lysosomal enzymes	Lysosomal storage diseases
Transferrin (isoelectric focusing)	Congenital disorders of glycosylation
Creatine	Defects of creatine synthesis
Total homocysteine	Defects of folate and clotting abnormalities
Biotinidase	Biotinidase deficiency
Prolactin	Used to assess neurotransmitter dysfunction
Urine	
Organic acids	This is a primary test for many different disorders
Sulfate	For defects of trans-sulfuration and sulfite oxidase deficiency
Glycine conjugates	For derivatives of many organic and amino acids
Purines and pyrimidines	Several defects in these pathways
Pterins	Cofactors for synthesis of several neurotransmitters
Creatine	Low in defects of creatine synthesis
Guanidinoacetic acid	Abnormal in defects of creatine synthesis
Glycosaminoglycans	Mucopolysaccharidoses
Oligosaccharides	Oligosaccharidoses
Cerebrospinal fluid	
Neurotransmitters (biogenic amines)	Several synthetic defects
Pterins	Cofactors for synthesis of several neurotransmitters
γ-Aminobutyric acid	Specific defect
S-Adenosyl methionine	Defect of methionine metabolism
Folate	Several defects
Amino acids	Nonketotic hyperglycinemia (with simultaneous blood)

Adapted from Buist et al.[19]

Transplantation of bone marrow, liver, kidney, as well as stem cells offers the possibility of 'cure' for a variety of disorders. Increasingly, enzyme replacement therapy is being deployed, especially for lysosomal storage disorders, since problems of delivery of stable, active enzyme to the appropriate organelle are being solved. However, these treatments are very costly; enzyme replacement for Gaucher disease is dramatically effective but can cost more than £100 000/year. Similar therapy for other lysosomal disorders costs even more.[21]

Substrate inhibitors as used in tyrosinemia type I, if available, can be very effective. Chaperones are a class of proteins that are essential for the proper tertiary folding of proteins. Studies on chaperone treatment, especially for lysosomal storage diseases, are being initiated to improve the structural configuration of mutant enzymes.

DISORDERS OF AMINO ACID METABOLISM

GENERAL CONSIDERATIONS

Of the disorders of amino acid metabolism, defects of catabolism represent the largest group, but abnormalities also exist in amino acid biosynthesis and transport. The clinical manifestations vary widely and involve many different organs. Systemic manifestations are common because of the presence of high levels of circulating small molecules, many of which are toxic to different tissues.

Pyridoxine dependent transamination of an amino acid to the corresponding keto acid is an early step in amino acid catabolism. Therefore, the accumulation of abnormal organic acids and systemic acidosis are the primary biochemical manifestation of many disorders of amino acid metabolism. Collectively, these conditions are a subgroup of the 'organic acidemias'. This has important implications for the diagnosis of these disorders. While many can be diagnosed by quantitative analysis of plasma amino acids, examination of urine organic acids is often the single most valuable diagnostic test. The more distal the enzyme deficiency lies in the degradation pathway, the more likely plasma amino acid levels will be normal and urine organic acid analysis abnormal. Usually, if one of these disorders is suspected, both plasma amino acids and urine organic acids should be analyzed.

The nutritional characteristics of proteins and amino acids are discussed in Chapter 16. Hydrolysis of protein to oligopeptides and free amino acids in the gut is controlled by enzymes that may be defective as a result of a hereditary disorder (Ch. 19).

Figure 26.3 shows the possible metabolic fate of plasma amino acids that are normally maintained within narrow limits, although they are affected by nutrition, systemic diseases and hormones. Insulin and glucagon usually lower the plasma levels; conversely, many amino acids stimulate the release of insulin and other hormones. In obesity and early in fasting, the branched chain amino acids may be elevated. In starvation the essential amino acids are low and the non-essential amino acids may be elevated, although alanine, a major gluconeogenic substrate, is usually low. In sepsis, stress, renal failure and liver disease, there may be considerable changes, liver disease often causing marked elevation of methionine, phenylalanine and tyrosine. In early life, high protein intake and immature regulatory systems may cause major elevations of many amino acids. The level of most free amino acids in intracellular fluid is about 10 times higher than in plasma.

In PKU, the blood phenylalanine concentration may be 20–60 times normal. Conversely, a rise of alanine of only 10–20% above normal may be the first indication of serious lactic acidosis or hyperammonemia.

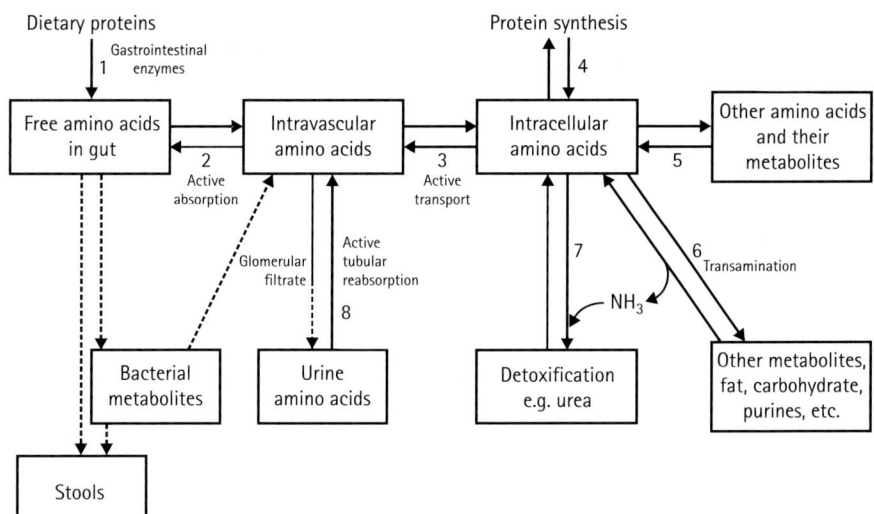

Dietary proteins

Protein synthesis

Fig. 26.3 Potential metabolic fate of amino acids. Numbers represent processes requiring active metabolism where congenital defects could occur. Dotted lines represent processes independent of metabolic activity.

In some conditions, such as argininosuccinic aciduria and nonketotic hyperglycinemia, the amino acid is excreted readily in the urine and blood levels may be only mildly abnormal, although in both these conditions the levels are markedly increased in the cerebrospinal fluid (CSF).

The quantity of amino acids in normal urine can vary over 10-fold and depends greatly upon age and nutrition; the levels are higher in infants. Values expressed per unit volume are worthless and even when calculated per milligram creatinine or per square meter, may be misleading. The predominant amino acids in urine (% of total in parentheses) are glycine (20–25%), taurine (5–15%), histidine (10–20%) and glutamine (7–10%). Normally, renal tubular reabsorption is nearly 100%, notable exceptions being histidine and glycine. In early infancy, amino acids may be reabsorbed poorly, adult rates being reached by 3–6 months. Normal urine contains many metabolites arising from the diet, drugs or bacterial action in the gut; these compounds often pose diagnostic problems since many are detected on amino acid or organic acid analyses. Increased urinary excretion is termed *aminoaciduria*; it can be due to increased filtration from raised plasma levels or defective reabsorption by the renal tubular cells. Amino acids are transported across cell membranes in specific groups. Excess of a single amino acid may saturate the renal absorption mechanism for others that share the same transport site and cause a competitive aminoaciduria.

DESIGNING AN AMINO ACID RESTRICTED DIET

When dietary restriction of amino acids is required to treat aminoacidopathies, certain basic nutritional principles apply. These include:

1. The basal nutritional requirements of the patients are similar if not identical to those of normal infants. This includes the need for enough of the restricted amino acid(s) to allow for normal growth and development.
2. The diet must be adequate in every respect, nutritionally, acceptability and palatability for the patient.
3. It is critical to recognize the catabolic effects of even minor illness or emotional upset upon normal metabolic homeostasis.
4. A normal diet provides only about 25% of the daily amino acid pool; the remainder comes from endogenous turnover; illness can increase catabolism many fold. For each gram of protein catabolized for energy (~4 calories), 65 000 mcg of ammonia is generated.
5. Unlike in normal people, deficiency of any essential nutrient (such as phenylalanine in PKU), causes increased catabolism that will *raise* the blood level of the limiting amino acid. This is particularly difficult in maple syrup urine disease since all three of the

branched chain amino acids (leucine, isoleucine and valine) must be present in adequate amounts.

6. Diet therapy is very challenging and requires detailed knowledge of the food options available, their nutritional compositions and limitations and how they can be optimally combined.
7. With few exceptions, the amino acid profile of most foods is relatively similar, e.g. all proteins, animal or vegetable, contain about 4–5% phenylalanine; what is different is the actual protein content.
8. The essential principle is to reduce natural protein sources as far as necessary while maintaining the energy intake as high as possible. With this as a base, additional medical foods and normal low-protein, high-energy foods are added to develop a complete intake.
9. Special low-protein, high-energy foods are becoming more available and should be freely used in designing these diets.
10. It is hard to overemphasize the effect of these diets upon patients as well as their families. Every effort must be made to make the diet as 'normal' and as varied as possible.

PHENYLALANINE–TYROSINE GROUP
Phenylketonuria and hyperphenylalaninemia

The term phenylketonuria (PKU) was coined in 1930 to describe patients with severe neurodevelopmental delay and high blood phenylalanine levels. It is now clear that it represents only one end of a spectrum of hyperphenylalaninemia (HPA) in which 30–40% of infants, detected by newborn screening, never develop high enough blood phenylalanine levels to cause brain damage. Such clinical heterogeneity is now apparent for virtually all IEMs but for the PKU/HPA spectrum, the central debate is over what level of phenylalanine requires treatment, what the treatment goals should be, and what constitutes PKU and what HPA. All are recessively inherited disorders. In all of them, phenylalanine cannot be converted to tyrosine. Blood phenylalanine is elevated and, when high, phenylpyruvic acid is excreted in the urine.

Clinical findings

Almost all classic, untreated PKU patients exhibit severe brain damage with an IQ < 30 because persistently elevated phenylalanine is toxic to the central nervous system (CNS). This damage begins to become irreversible within 3–6 weeks of birth and therefore early screening and treatment are important. Phenylketonuric infants appear normal at birth, but some show nonspecific feeding problems. In the early months, vomiting, irritability, an eczematoid rash, developmental slowing and a mousy, musty odor, derived from phenylacetic acid (the same metabolite that is frequent in chronically incontinent patients), usually emerge.

General physical development is usually normal. Over 90% of untreated patients are fair haired, fair skinned and blue eyed, but dark skin, hair or irises do not exclude the diagnosis. Peripheral neurological findings are usually not prominent, but one third have minimal upper motor neuron signs. Seizures occur in about 25%, predominantly in the most severely retarded. Electroencephalographic (EEG) abnormalities can be seen in approximately 80% and brain CT or MRI scan may reveal cortical atrophy and white matter abnormalities.

Behavioral problems, including restlessness, aggression, learning difficulties and sleep disturbances, are common in patients treated early in life but in whom the restriction diet was later discontinued.

Diagnosis and screening

Phenylalanine is converted to tyrosine by hepatic phenylalanine hydroxylase (PAH). In the absence of PAH, tyrosine becomes an essential amino acid, and phenylalanine is diverted to other pathways producing phenylpyruvic acid and phenylacetic acid, which are normally only present in trace amounts. Untreated patients with classic PKU usually have plasma concentrations over 1200 mcM ([20 mg/dl]; normal ~60 mcM, [~1 mg/dl]). Throughout infancy, levels as high as 3600 mcM (60 mg/dl) can be seen.

Where newborn screening is available, PKU should always be diagnosed in the neonatal period (see Ch. 12). Initial abnormal screening results require urgent quantitation of plasma phenylalanine and tyrosine. Transient HPA can take as long as 2 months to resolve, and even in mild HPA, the plasma phenylalanine can be very high in the first weeks of life. In classic PKU the plasma phenylalanine generally rises over 1–2 weeks to levels well over 1200 mcM; the concentration of tyrosine is low.

About 1–2% of patients with HPA do not have a defect in PAH, but in synthesis or recycling of the cofactor tetrahydrobiopterin (see below). Every infant with persistently raised blood phenylalanine should be tested for this group of disorders since treatment and prognosis of these disorders is radically different (see p. 1120).

HPA occurs in 1 in 10000–20000 persons but is more frequent in some countries such as Ireland. The carrier frequency in most populations is ~1–2%. Over 500 mutations have been defined, but none accounts for a majority of patients (http://www.pahdb.mcgill.ca/). Carrier detection and prenatal diagnosis are possible with molecular genetic methods.

Treatment (also see above)

Clinical manifestations of classic PKU can be completely prevented by early and continued restriction of dietary phenylalanine to maintain blood levels at 120–360 mmol/L (2–6 mg/dl) in infancy and childhood; values up to 600–750 mmol/L (10–12 mg/dl) are often unavoidable in adolescence and adulthood.

Infants generally require ~60–80 mg/kg/d phenylalanine but the phenylalanine tolerance must be individually established and falls to ~7–15 mg/kg by 5 years. The blood levels should be tightly monitored (two to three times weekly for 2–3 months, falling to once a week by 3–4 years). Breast milk is relatively low in phenylalanine and breastfeeding should be encouraged, usually supplemented with a phenylalanine-free formula as needed. Over-restriction of phenylalanine results in tissue breakdown, *increasing* levels of phenylalanine and, if prolonged, growth problems, seizures, mental retardation and death are reported sequelae.

There is still debate about when treatment of HPA is indicated. We believe treatment should be started for blood levels over 360–500 mcM (6–8 mg/dl) or if phenylalanine metabolites are detected in the urine.

It was formerly common to discontinue dietary restriction of phenylalanine by school age but it is now clear that this leads to IQ loss and behavioral disturbances.[22] The diet is now recommended to be continued for life at least for classic cases. Even severely affected adult PKU patients who were not treated in childhood usually benefit from phenylalanine restriction in terms of psychiatric manifestations of the disease.

It is now clear that blood phenylalanine levels in many cases of HPA, particularly those running at < 1000 μmol/L, can be substantially reduced or even normalized by treatment with tetrahydrobiopterin. While this drug is not yet widely available, it offers the possibility that for as many as 50% of cases, the diet can be relaxed or even stopped.[23] In addition, recent studies on the use of large neutral amino acids (NeoPhe, Prekulab, Korsor, Denmark) 0.5–1.0 g/kg/d have shown that, by competitive inhibition of absorption of phenylalanine, they too can reduce the blood levels by as much as 50%.[24]

Maternal phenylketonuria

High phenylalanine levels are exquisitely toxic to the developing fetal brain and thus offspring of mothers with HPA can be severely damaged. All offspring are obligatory heterozygotes and ~1 in 100 are homozygotes.[25] The miscarriage rate is high and affected children have prenatal microcephaly typically with severe, mental retardation and sometimes congenital heart defects. This outcome can be prevented if the maternal phenylalanine levels are maintained in the range 0.15–0.25 mmol/L from conception. Table 26.2 indicates the risk of damage to the fetus depending on maternal phenylalanine levels.

Defects in the synthesis or recycling of biopterin (malignant PKU) (see also p. 1120)

Tetrahydrobiopterin (BH_4) is an essential cofactor for phenylalanine, tyrosine and tryptophan hydroxylases. At least five defects in the synthesis or recycling of BH_4 are the cause of ~1% of HPA diagnosed by newborn screening. If, however, the true nature of the defect is not recognized, and treatment is limited to dietary restriction of phenylalanine, patients show severe and progressive neurological symptoms in spite of normal phenylalanine levels.[26] All these defects result in deficient conversion of phenylalanine to tyrosine, even though the PAH apoenzyme itself is normal. Severe neurological disease may occur with only mild hyperphenylalaninemia, suggesting that BH_4 levels may be relatively more adequate for phenylalanine hydroxylation than for that of tryptophan or tyrosine. Affected patients have marked hypotonia, parkinsonism, as well as spasticity and dystonic posturing. Some have seizures, myoclonus and EEG abnormalities. Drooling is common. The delay in psychomotor development is usually profound.

Testing for these defects by blood and urine biopterin profiling should be done routinely in all patients with hyperphenylalaninemia, because early treatment is vital. CSF neurotransmitter and biopterin levels and phenylalanine loading tests are often useful in diagnostic confirmation. The diagnosis of specific enzyme deficiency can be confirmed in many cases in cultured fibroblasts.

The treatment for this group of patients consists of administration of biogenic amine precursors, such as 5-hydroxytryptophan (5-HT) and L-dopa that do not require hydroxylation. Carbidopa is a necessary adjunct to prevent decarboxylation of these precursors before they reach the CNS. BH_4 is used in patients with synthesis defects, but if not sufficient by itself it should be supplemented by phenylalanine restriction. In order to optimize the drug dosages, monitoring of neurotransmitter levels in CSF is often indicated. Unfortunately, however, even early

Table 26.2 Maternal phenylalaninemia: percentage risk of damage to fetus according to maternal phenylalanine level

	Blood phenylalanine (mmol/L)		
	> 1.25	0.65–1.2	< 0.625
Spontaneous abortion	24	22	8
Mental retardation	92	53	21
Microcephaly	73	57	24
Congenital heart disease	12	11	0
Low birth weight	40	52	13

and aggressive therapy does not always prevent neurological deterioration and eventual death.

Inherited isolated deficiency of tyrosine hydroxylase causes severe parkinsonism in infancy. It and other disorders affecting aromatic acid neurotransmitters are discussed on p. 1120.

Tyrosinemia

The tyrosinemias are a group of disorders in which tyrosine is elevated (Fig. 26.4). The commonest, most often seen in premature infants, is transient tyrosinemia of the newborn resulting from delayed maturation of tyrosine-metabolizing enzymes. Tyrosinemia can also occur in scurvy and many forms of liver disease.

Hepatorenal tyrosinemia (hereditary tyrosinemia type 1)

Clinical features. The liver and kidney are the primary organs affected in this disorder. Symptoms may begin early in infancy with an acute rapid course to demise, or they may progress more chronically. Most patients present with failure to thrive and liver dysfunction. Untreated, the liver disease is progressive, causing cirrhosis and liver failure. Renal tubular damage results in the Fanconi syndrome with tubular acidosis and rickets. Neurodevelopmental delay is not a feature. Surviving patients have a high risk for hepatocarcinoma.

Diagnosis

This disease is caused by deficiency of fumarylacetoacetate hydrolase, the last enzyme in tyrosine catabolism. Biochemical alterations include elevated plasma concentrations of tyrosine and methionine and the excretion of tyrosyl compounds in the urine. The presence of succinylacetone in urine is diagnostic. Highly elevated blood concentrations of alpha-fetoprotein (AFP) are seen, even before the elevation in tyrosine

(note that AFP can be falsely high in infants). Hypoglycemia may occur, and coagulation defects are common.

Mutation analysis can be used for prenatal diagnosis and carrier detection. Hepatorenal tyrosinemia is common in the Canadian province of Quebec, where a single founder mutation is responsible for most cases.

Treatment

The liver failure and renal Fanconi syndrome of hepatorenal tyrosinemia can be effectively treated with 2(2-nitro-4-trifluoromethylbenzoyl)-1,3 cyclohexanedione (NTBC) which blocks tyrosine metabolism by inhibiting its second step (Fig. 26.4), thus preventing the accumulation of toxic metabolites. NTBC raises blood tyrosine levels and thus needs to be combined with a dietary restriction of phenylalanine and tyrosine. The prognosis of patients with this disease has vastly improved with this new therapy.[27,28]

Oculocutaneous tyrosinemia (tyrosinemia type 2)

Tyrosine aminotransferase is deficient in oculocutaneous tyrosinemia. The characteristic features of this disease are corneal ulcers or dendritic keratitis early in life and erythematous papular or keratotic lesions on the palms and soles. About 50% of patients display mental retardation, but this may be due in part to ascertainment bias or gene deletions. Tyrosine itself is not toxic and the liver and kidney are unaffected. Plasma concentrations of tyrosine are higher than in other forms of tyrosinemia, and the urine contains large amounts of tyrosine metabolites generated by other transaminases. The lesions on the palms and soles and in the eyes relate directly to the accumulation and crystallization of tyrosine. Both respond rapidly to treatment with diets low in tyrosine.

Tyrosinemia type 3

The second step in tyrosine catabolism is catalyzed by 4-hydroxyphenylpyruvate dioxygenase. Several patients lacking this enzyme have been identified and all suffer from mild psychomotor retardation, but no other organ systems are involved. Plasma tyrosine levels are elevated, but usually not to levels that cause corneal ulcers or hyperkeratosis. Treatment consists of a low tyrosine diet.

Alkaptonuria

Garrod's suggestion that the disorder results from absence in the liver of the enzyme that catalyzes the oxidation of homogentisic acid (Fig. 26.4) gave rise to the one-gene, one-enzyme hypothesis, the notion of IEM and the field of biochemical genetics.[10]

Alkaptonuria results from defective activity of the enzyme homogentisic acid dioxygenase. Blood tyrosine is not elevated and the disorder is characterized by the excretion of homogentisic acid in urine. Urine appears normal when fresh but on standing, and particularly after alkalinization, homogentisic acid is oxidized forming a dark brown or black pigment. This can be seen in diapers (nappies) and should permit the condition to be recognized in infancy, but the diagnosis is usually first made in adulthood during routine urinalysis or during investigation of arthritis. Alkaptonuria is usually asymptomatic in childhood. After the third decade, deposition of brownish or bluish pigment is seen, particularly in the ears and sclerae, and is extensive in fibrous tissues. This is referred to as ochronosis. It leads to progressive arthritis, produces symptoms resembling rheumatoid arthritis or osteoarthritis, with limitation of motion; complete ankylosis is common with a characteristic appearance on X-ray. NTBC should also be useful.

SULFUR-CONTAINING AMINO ACIDS (Fig. 26.5)

Methionine plays an important role in methylation reactions. Some is resynthesized from homocysteine by two separate pathways, one of which interdigitates with folate metabolism, the 1-carbon pool and with vitamin B_{12}. Some defects of folate or vitamin B_{12} metabolism can therefore cause accumulation of homocysteine. The disulfides, homocystine and cystine, are formed from two molecules of homocysteine and cysteine, respectively. In proteins, two molecules of cysteine condense to form

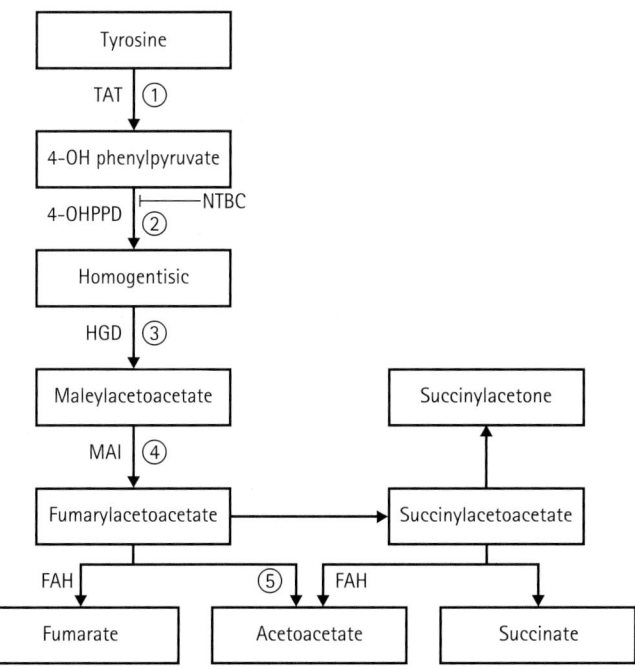

1= Tyrosinemia type II-> corneal ulcers, hyperkeratosis
2= Tyrosinemia type III-> mental retardation
3= Alkaptonuria-> ochronosis, black urine
4= Maleylacetoacetate isomerase deficiency->
     phenotype?
5= Tyrosinemia type I-> liver failure, renal damage

Fig. 26.4 The tyrosine catabolic pathway. The enzymes for each reaction are given on the left, the disease corresponding to its deficiency on the right. TAT, tyrosine aminotransferase; HPD, 4-PH phenylpyruvate dioxygenase; HGD, homogentisic acid dioxygenase; MAI, maleylacetoacetate isomerase; FAH, fumarylacetoacetate hydrolase.

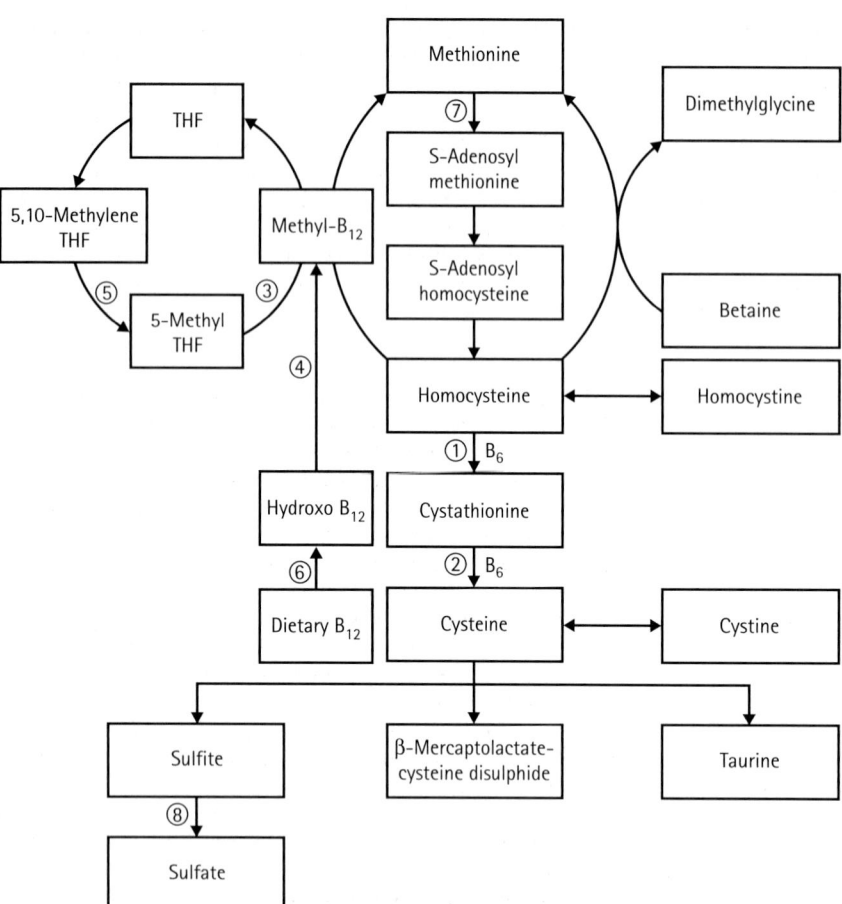

Fig. 26.5   Metabolism of the sulfur-containing amino acids. 1, Cystathionine synthase (homocystinuria); 2, cystathioninase (cystathioninuria); 3, 5-methyltetrahydrofolate-homocysteine methyl transferase; 4, cobalamin-activating system (homocystinuria and methylmalonic aciduria); 5, 5,10-methylenetetrahydrofolate reductase (homocystinuria); 6, gut absorption and reduction of vitamin B$_{12}$ (homocystinuria and methylmalonic aciduria); 7, methionine adenosyltransferase (hypermethioninemia); 8, sulfite oxidase (sulfite oxidase deficiency). THF, tetrahydrofolic acid.

disulfide bonds that help to maintain the three-dimensional shape of the protein. Homocystine is not present in protein. Cystinosis is discussed on p. 1112 and in Chapter 18 (p. 550). Breast milk contains the sulfur-containing amino acid taurine which is also present in high levels in muscle, leukocytes and other tissues; it is frequently excreted in large quantities as a result of liver disease, a high protein intake, leukemia or endogenous protein catabolism. No primary defect of taurine metabolism is known and its role in metabolism is unclear.

Homocystinuria

The term homocystinuria is sometimes used to indicate one specific form of the disease caused by defective activity of the enzyme cystathionine beta-synthetase (CBS). However, several other enzyme defects can also cause elevated homocysteine, including defects of folate and B$_{12}$ metabolism. Therefore, homocystinuria refers to a heterogeneous group of disorders. Plasma methionine, cystine and B$_{12}$ levels, as well as urine organic acids, should be measured in all patients with elevated plasma homocystine. Biosynthesis of the sulfur amino acid cysteine involves the demethylation of methionine to homocysteine, followed by its reaction with serine to form cystathionine. This latter step is catalyzed by the pyridoxine-requiring enzyme cystathionine beta-synthetase.

Homocystinuria due to cystathionine beta-synthetase deficiency

Clinical findings

This autosomal recessive defect is the most common cause of homocystinuria. The most characteristic feature of this disorder is subluxation of the ocular lens. Most patients have a marfanoid habitus, with skeletal abnormalities similar to those seen in Marfan syndrome. In homocystinuria, however, the joints tend to be limited in mobility rather than hypermobile. There is also lenticular subluxation in both conditions; however,

in Marfan syndrome the lens is usually displaced upwards, whereas in homocystinuria it is displaced downwards and medially. Additional features include developmental delay, osteopenia and predisposition for thrombosis. Presentation is usually in the first decade with the exception of thromboembolism that may occur at any age. Homocystinuria is one of the few amino acid disorders in which manifestations tend to progress in adulthood, because many clinical manifestations result from thrombotic complications. Classic tests of clotting function are normal, but elevated homocystine levels cause increased platelet adhesiveness.

Diagnosis

Homocystine is not normally detected in the usual assays of amino acids in body fluids. In CBS deficiency, elevated homocystine can be detected in both urine and blood. Levels of methionine are usually also elevated and levels of cystine are reduced. Because homocystine is unstable, testing should be done on fresh urine and measurement of blood total homocystine is also essential. Because homocystinuria can be caused by several genetic defects, it is important to confirm the diagnosis of CBS deficiency by DNA mutation analysis or enzyme assay. DNA based diagnosis can theoretically be used for prenatal detection.

Treatment

Since CBS is a pyridoxine-dependent enzyme, some activity may be restored by pharmacological doses of pyridoxine. Seven days of 100–500 mg/d should always be tried to determine any degree of vitamin responsiveness. (Prolonged high doses can be associated with peripheral neuropathy.) If the homocystine levels normalize, no additional therapy may be needed. Those who do not respond should be treated with a low-methionine diet supplemented with L-cystine. All patients should probably receive high doses (5 mg)/day of folic acid. In addition, the compound betaine may be used to aid in the reconversion of homocysteine to methionine.[29,30] Medications to reduce platelet adhesiveness can be prescribed, but do not abolish all thromboembolic events.

Oral contraceptives may be contraindicated in women due to the increased risk of thrombosis.

Other causes of homocystinuria

The second most important cause of homocystinuria is *N5,10-methylenetetrahydrofolate reductase (MTHFR) deficiency* which is involved in the recycling of homocysteine to methionine. It is associated with low rather than high plasma methionine levels. Neurological features and a clotting propensity predominate this rare condition but eye and skeletal involvement are lacking. The specific enzyme diagnosis can be made on cultured skin fibroblasts. For treatment, no pyridoxine is given and methionine may be supplemented rather than restricted in the diet. Folate administration may also be beneficial.

A mild form of MTHFR deficiency associated with a thermolabile variant of the MTHFR gene is found in 5–7% of people. It can be easily diagnosed by DNA mutation analysis. Homozygous individuals are prone to develop thromboembolic and arteriosclerotic disease and there is a minor degree of hyperhomocysteinemia. In addition to screening for individuals at risk for atherosclerosis who might benefit from administration of folate, B_6 and/or B_{12}, measurement of blood free and total homocysteine levels can detect true inborn errors of sulfur amino acid metabolism in those who have very high levels, and is a valuable test for monitoring response to therapy.

Methylcobalamin is required for resynthesis of methionine from homocystine and defects in the vitamin B_{12} pathway can cause varying mixes of megaloblastic anemia, homocystinuria and/or methylmalonic aciduria. At least eight different complementation groups that involve vitamin B_{12} metabolism are known (see Fig. 26.43). There may be more since not all cases appear to have a demonstrable defect. These conditions are often associated with neurological deficits and have a guarded prognosis. For this reason it is important that every patient with homocystinuria has a urine organic acid analysis to assay for the presence of methylmalonic acid. If a vitamin B_{12} synthetic defect is found, B_{12} injections (usually hydroxycobalamin) are used in addition to the usual treatments for homocystinuria.

Sulfite oxidase and molybdenum cofactor deficiency

The terminal step in the oxidative degradation of cysteine, the conversion of sulfite to sulfate, is catalyzed by the molybdenum-containing enzyme sulfite oxidase. Severe neurological diseases are associated with deficiency of the oxidase or the cofactor. Molybdenum cofactor deficiency is discussed on p. 1123 and 1126.

Clinical findings

Most patients present with neonatal neurological disease including severe hypotonia, seizures and myoclonic spasms. Symptoms are progressive and usually lead to early death. Patients with milder forms of the disease have progressive cerebral palsy and choreiform movements. Infantile hemiplegia has been reported and lens dislocation is frequent even in neonates.

Diagnosis and treatment

Deficiency of sulfite results in increased amounts of sulfite, thiosulfate and S-sulfocysteine in the urine. These compounds require special analyses for their detection. Sulfite oxidase deficiency can be caused by a defect in the gene for this protein or by defects in the synthesis of the molybdenum cofactor required for its function. In molybdenum cofactor deficiency the serum uric acid is very low and urinary hypoxanthine and xanthine are markedly elevated. Prenatal diagnosis is available. Ophthalmologic examination is indicated in all suspected cases.

Currently, no effective therapy is available.

Other disorders of S-containing amino acids

Cystathioninuria, an inborn error of amino acid metabolism in which there is a deficiency of the activity of cystathionase, was first reported in two adults with mental deficiency. Subsequently, however, cystathioninuria has been found in a number of individuals with no clinical signs and is currently considered a benign variant.

Persistent hypermethioninemia occurs in *methionine adenosyl transferase deficiency* which, in most cases, appears to be benign.

Transient neonatal hypermethioninemia occurs in a small number of infants, most of whom are receiving a high protein intake. Although there are no known toxic sequelae, modest protein restriction seems warranted in view of the toxicity of methionine in laboratory animals. It is also frequent in tyrosinemia type 1 and in hepatocellular damage.

A defect of *S-adenosylhomocysteine hydrolase* causes hypermethioninemia and is associated with developmental delay and a severe destructive myopathy accompanied by high plasma creatine kinase.[31]

DISORDERS OF THE GAMMA-GLUTAMYL CYCLE

The synthesis and recycling of the sulfur-containing tripeptide glutathione involves a series of six enzymatic reactions termed the gamma-glutamyl cycle (Fig. 26.6). Six disorders causing disease are known; pyroglutamic aciduria is discussed below.

Pyroglutamic aciduria (5-oxoprolinuria)

Pyroglutamic aciduria, or 5-oxoprolinuria, is caused by autosomal recessive deficiency of glutathione synthetase. Pyroglutamic acid is 2-pyrrolidone-5-carboxylic acid, a condensation product of glutamic acid or glutamine. It can be readily detected by urine organic acid analysis. Acquired, nongenetic pyroglutamic aciduria is due to glutathione depletion, most often caused by acetaminophen.

In the newborn, marked nonketotic acidosis without accompanying coma and massive hemolysis are usual and may recur. The disease is often characterized later by neurological symptoms, including spasticity, ataxia and mental retardation. Therapeutic attempts have been aimed at increasing cellular glutathione concentrations and antioxidant activity. However, this does not eliminate neurological problems in severely affected patients. Drugs such as acetaminophen that require glutathione for detoxification should be avoided.

Treatment involves providing antioxidants, vitamin E, vitamin C and Bicitra or bicarbonate in large enough amounts to control the acidosis. The prognosis is variable. Mild cases may have a normal outcome; severe cases may be partially helped by therapy.

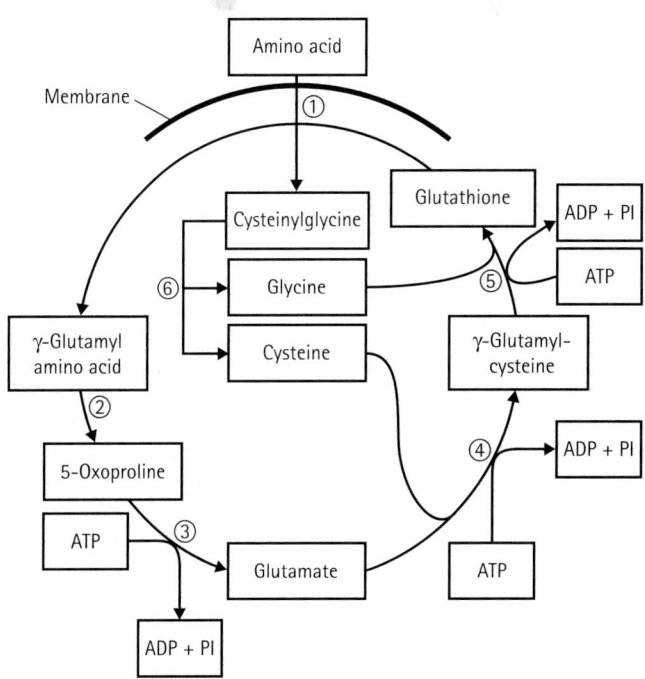

Fig. 26.6 γ-Glutamyl cycle. 1, γ-Glutamyl transpeptidase; 2, γ-glutamyl cyclotransferase; 3, 5-oxoprolinase; 4, γ-glutamyl-cysteine synthase; 5, glutathione synthase; 6, peptidase.

DISORDERS ASSOCIATED WITH HYPERAMMONEMIA

Most diets contain excess amino acids, the nitrogen of which is mostly excreted as urea. The enzymes of the urea cycle are active before birth. The first three steps of the pathway are mitochondrial so the full cycle requires the transport of ornithine into and the transport of citrulline out of mitochondria. Arginine is an important regulator of the cycle since it induces N-acetylglutamate synthetase. N-acetylglutamate, in turn, activates carbamyl phosphate synthetase.

The urea cycle is only complete in the liver where urea is synthesized. Defects at all steps of the urea cycle have been described, the common feature of which is hyperammonemia, although it may not occur in argininemia. Some of the enzymes are present in other tissues where the enzymes must have other roles. In severe liver damage, hyperammonemia is sometimes found and may contribute to the cerebral symptoms of liver failure.

Clinical features

The clinical features of the different disorders associated with hyperammonemia are similar and therefore will be discussed as a group. Patients with severe defects in the urea cycle present in the newborn period with coma and acute metabolic crisis. Postnatal catabolic events and protein intake contribute to the metabolic derangement. In infancy, the symptoms include episodes of poor feeding, vomiting, failure to thrive, lethargy, irritability or other neurological symptoms, all of which are aggravated by any metabolic stress or formula changes that increase protein intake, and may be alleviated by reducing the protein content of the diet. Respiratory alkalosis is not uncommon.

Most babies with hyperammonemia are initially thought to be septic and therefore ammonia measurements are essential in any infant with suspected sepsis, especially if accompanied by lethargy or CNS depression. Elevated blood ammonia levels can cause an increased respiratory rate resulting in some degree of respiratory alkalosis. In older children with, presumably, less severe mutations, symptoms often develop for the first time during weaning. Food intolerance or distaste for protein may be evident; some have failure to thrive, developmental or neurological problems with seizures, migraine, ataxia and abnormal EEG. Even adults may present with new onset of hyperammonemic symptoms, particularly during times of high catabolic stress such as the postpartum period, dieting or during intercurrent illnesses such as infections, dehydration, surgery or chemotherapy.

Transient neonatal hyperammonemia

Hyperammonemia is sometimes seen in infants receiving intravenous alimentation. In these cases it may be due to an inappropriately high nitrogen intake. Other infants with profound, but transient, hyperammonemia have mostly been preterm; respiratory distress is usual. Rapid development of neurological damage with apnea, loss of reflexes and coma ensues within 12–48h of birth. Ammonia levels may be as high as 5000 µmol/L. Liver function tests and plasma amino acids, including glutamine, may be normal. If the condition is treated early and vigorously the babies rapidly improve, the protein tolerance becomes normal, liver enzyme assays show no abnormality and the prognosis is excellent. The cause is unknown but rapid protein catabolism, mitochondrial dysfunction, maternal carnitine deficiency and/or portocaval shunting may play a role.

Enzyme defects of the urea cycle (Fig. 26.7)

With the exception of ornithine transcarbamylase deficiency which is X-linked, all these disorders are autosomal recessive traits. All have both severe (neonatal) forms and milder, later onset forms that may not even present until adulthood.

N-Acetylglutamate synthetase deficiency (step 1)

This disorder usually presents in the first weeks of life. N-Acetylglutamate does not participate directly in the urea cycle, but is an allosteric activator of carbamyl phosphate synthetase (CPS). Thus, the absence of this compound results in secondary CPS deficiency. Several acyl-CoA derivatives of organic acids such as methylmalonyl-CoA, propionyl-CoA or valproyl-CoA can inhibit N-acetylglutamate synthesis, which explains the profound hyperammonemia that can occur in the 'ketotic hyperglycinemias' and valproic acid toxicity.

Treatment of this disease differs from that for the other urea cycle disorders[32] in that carbamylglutamate, which is structurally similar to N-acetylglutamate, can stimulate CPS activity. Arginine (1 mmol/kg/d) and carbamylglutamate (1.7 mmol/kg/d) are effective in controlling hyperammonemia.[33,34]

Carbamyl phosphate synthetase I deficiency (step 2)

This enzyme is mitochondrial and provides carbamyl phosphate for the synthesis of urea. Deficiency (step 2) usually presents with severe neonatal hyperammonemia, although later onset is possible. Prenatal detection is possible. CPS II is a separate cytoplasmic enzyme involved in the synthesis of pyrimidines (p. 1123).

Ornithine transcarbamylase deficiency (step 3)

This is the most common urea cycle defect; the only one inherited as an X-linked trait. Most affected males present as newborns in severe hyperammonemic crisis. About 20–30% are less severely affected and some have normal mental development and almost normal tolerance for protein, except during stress. Some female carriers are totally asymptomatic, others have mild aversion or intolerance to protein and some have recurrent hyperammonemic crises, e.g. during dieting, that can be fatal. Plasma amino acids are never grossly distorted; citrulline is low,

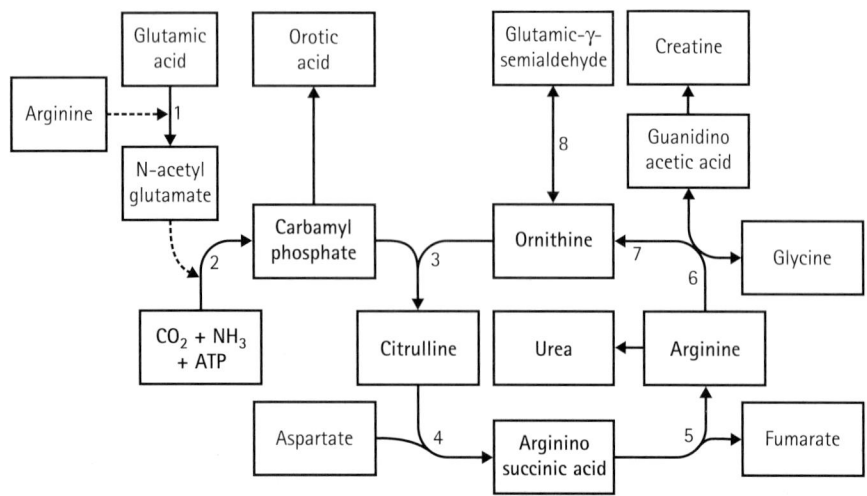

Fig. 26.7 Urea cycle. 1, N-acetylglutamate synthase; 2, carbamyl phosphate synthase; 3, ornithine transcarbamylase; 4, argininosuccinate synthase; 5, argininosuccinate lyase; 6, arginase; 7, ornithine uptake into mitochondria; 8, ornithine ketoacid aminotransferase.

ornithine is normal but glutamine, alanine and sometimes lysine are increased in blood and sometimes in urine; during stress, orotic acid is usually increased in the urine. The combination of the clinical presentation, elevated urine orotic acid, normal urine organic acids and blood amino acids showing only elevated glutamine and alanine is diagnostic.

The enzyme can be assayed in liver or duodenal mucosa but not in fibroblasts. Enzyme activity from multiple liver biopsies from a female carrier may vary widely, representing different degrees of inactivation of the mutant X chromosome in different areas. Most carriers can be detected by increased urine orotic acid from 0 to 8 and 8 to 16 h after a provocative challenge of allopurinol (100 mg/kg p.o.) either alone or together with 1.0 g protein/kg or L-alanine 0.5 g/kg p.o. DNA analysis, when possible, is best for prenatal diagnosis and carrier detection since, when informative, it obviates the need for liver biopsy

Citrullinemia (step 4)

Citrullinemia is caused by argininosuccinate synthetase deficiency. The presentation varies greatly from death in the neonatal period to being asymptomatic. Many patients who have suffered severe hyperammonemia become mentally retarded. Hepatic function is occasionally impaired. The etiology of this hepatocellular dysfunction is unknown. Plasma and urine citrulline levels are markedly elevated, even between crises. The enzyme can be assayed in fibroblasts; prenatal diagnosis is possible.

Argininosuccinic aciduria (step 5)

Argininosuccinic aciduria is caused by deficiency of argininosuccinic acid lyase. Death in infancy is not rare and even mild cases tend to have developmental delay, even when they have never had prolonged coma or overt hyperammonemia. Trichorrhexis nodosa, an abnormal fragility of the hair, is found in some cases. Hepatocellular dysfunction and hepatic enlargement are common findings. Plasma citrulline is elevated, but to a much lesser degree than in citrullinemia. This, along with the presence of argininosuccinic acid and its anhydrides in plasma, urine and CSF, are diagnostic. The enzyme defect can be shown in several tissues, including red blood cells. Prenatal diagnosis is available. Large supplements of arginine are added to the normal treatment since urinary argininosuccinic acid provides a major pathway for waste nitrogen disposal.

Argininemia (step 6)

Argininemia is caused by arginase I deficiency; it has a different presentation from the other urea cycle disorders in that profound hyperammonemia is unusual. This disease usually presents with increasingly severe pyramidal tract signs starting within the first 2 years of life. It may mimic cerebral palsy. The plasma arginine is markedly raised. The urinary amino acid pattern may be similar to that seen in cystinuria, caused by arginine saturating the group reabsorptive site in the proximal renal tubules. Alternatively, urine amino acids may be normal or there may be a generalized aminoaciduria. Deficient arginase activity can be shown in the red blood cells of both patients and heterozygotes.

Hyperammonemia–hyperinsulinism

This autosomal dominant disorder is caused by specific mutations in the glutamate dehydrogenase (GLUD1) gene. Glutamate dehydrogenase enzyme activity in pancreatic beta cells is allosterically regulated by intracellular leucine levels. Thus, it acts as sensor that couples insulin secretion to amino acid levels just as glucokinase links glucose levels to insulin production. In the liver GLUD1 activity negatively modulates the urea cycle and hence ammonia metabolism. The mutations that cause hyperammonemia–insulinism result in constitutive activation of GLUD1, independent of intracellular amino acid levels. This results in simultaneous hyperinsulinism (beta cell) and hyperammonemia (hepatocyte).

Clinically, the hyperinsulinism is more significant and can present as severe (usually leucine sensitive) hypoglycemia in infancy. The hyperammonemia is typically mild with levels elevated only 3–5-fold.

Hyperammonemic crises are very rare. Treatment includes inhibition of insulin release with drugs such as diazoxide and avoidance of fasting; pancreatectomy, which reveals nesidioblastosis, may be necessary. The hyperammonemia is usually mild enough not to require specific therapy. Diagnosis is confirmed by molecular analysis. (see also Ch. 15)

Citrullinemia, type II (citrin deficiency)

Both neonatal and adult forms of type II citrullinemia are becoming increasingly recognized. Neonatal cases typically present with severe cholestasis and hepatic dysfunction. Plasma levels of citrulline, methionine and galactose are markedly elevated and often detected by newborn screening but hyperammonemia is not typical. Most patients respond to a low-protein, lactose-free diet with improved hepatic function.

The adult-onset form is characterized mainly by psychiatric symptoms and/or delayed development. Hyperammonemia is frequent. Drowsiness and coma occur and several patients have died from cerebral edema during these neurological episodes.

This disorder is caused by mutations in a transporter responsible for shuttling aspartate and glutamate across the mitochondrial membrane. Citrin deficiency is associated with decreased hepatic activity of argininosuccinate synthetase deficiency and thus causes elevated blood citrulline levels. The disease is most common in Japan and may be rare elsewhere. Arginine supplementation and ammonia scavenger therapy are thought to be beneficial.

Lysinuric protein intolerance

This condition is caused by a defect in the uptake of arginine and other amino acids in several tissues. The result is deficiency of urea cycle substrates in the liver (see p. 1067).

Hyperornithinemias
Hyperornithinemia with hyperammonemia and homocitrullinuria

Two distinct disorders of elevated plasma ornithine levels exist, but only the hyperornithinemia with hyperammonemia and homocitrullinuria (HHH) syndrome has associated hyperammonemia. Most reported patients have a history of developmental delay and older patients tend to have spasticity. Symptoms may develop at any age. Excretion of ornithine, polyamines, orotic acid and glutamine may be increased. The primary defect is in the mitochondrial uptake of ornithine. Large, bizarre mitochondria may be present in the liver. Oral ornithine supplements have been reported to be beneficial. Homocitrulline can also be formed during pasteurization of milk and, if ingested, is excreted in the urine.

Gyrate atrophy of the retina

Hyperornithinemia in the absence of hyperammonemia also occurs in gyrate atrophy of the choroid and retina, caused by deficiency of ornithine k aminotransferase. The disease presents in adults with a characteristic retinopathy, subcapsular cataract and progressive loss of peripheral vision leading to blindness by middle age. In children, small discrete circular patches of degeneration may be seen in the periphery of the retina; later these coalesce to form a characteristic lobular appearance that gives rise to the name. The electroretinogram (ERG) dark adaptation is abnormal. Plasma and CSF ornithine levels are markedly elevated. The enzyme is deficient in several tissues, including cultured skin fibroblasts. Heterozygotes may be detected by oral ornithine loading tests (100 mg/kg) or by enzyme assay. Abnormal inclusions have been reported in muscle and bizarre, elongated mitochondria are present in liver. Direct toxicity of ornithine and low proline, lysine or creatine have all been suggested as a cause of the retinal damage.

Pharmacological doses of vitamin B_6, the cofactor of the mutant enzyme, may improve the biochemical and ERG findings in some cases. Ornithine is not contained in protein and hence cannot be restricted in the diet. Instead, long term arginine restriction may result in improved visual function but such treatment is very hard to maintain.

Secondary hyperammonemias

Other causes of hyperammonemia include:

- liver disease (Ch. 19);
- Reye syndrome (Chs 19 and 22);
- the ketotic hyperglycinemias (p. 1065);
- methylmalonic aciduria (p. 1065);
- propionic aciduria (p. 1065);
- 3-ketothiolase deficiency (p. 1071);
- 3-hydroxy-3-methylglutaric aciduria (p. 1070);
- familial lysinuric protein intolerance (p. 1067);
- neonatal glutaric aciduria type II (p. 1070 and Ch. 12);
- defects of fatty acid oxidation (p. 1068);
- valproic acid toxicity;
- ureterostomy;
- shock and after surgery.

Diagnostic approaches

Blood ammonia should be routinely assayed in any acutely sick child with neurological findings and in patients with mild, episodic symptoms. Hyperammonemia may be present in the fasting state but is sometimes induced only by a protein load. Hyperammonemia up to 2–3 times the normal limit is sometimes seen in severely ill infants, especially those with impaired hepatic function. In contrast, the ammonia levels in patients with primary hyperammonemia may exceed 1000 μmol/L.

Great care must be taken in handling samples and in the assays – erroneously high values are common. When hyperammonemia is confirmed, immediate assay of blood amino acids and urine organic acids is indicated. Raised levels of glutamine and alanine reflect increased transamination and should always suggest this possibility. Defect at steps 3–6 of the urea cycle (see Fig. 26.7) may cause orotic aciduria due to diversion of carbamyl phosphate to the overproduction of pyrimidines.

An algorithm for the work-up of hyperammonemia is provided in Figure 26.8.[35]

Treatment[36,37]

Every effort must be made to minimize catabolism for energy needs. Management of acute, severe hyperammonemic crises includes the following steps:

1. Maximal hydration p.o. or i.v. to enhance renal excretion.
2. Maximum tolerable nonprotein caloric intake p.o. or i.v. Central venous access may be necessary to administer high concentrations and quantities of glucose (D20–D30); often an insulin drip is added to enhance amino acid synthesis and to control hyperglycemia.
3. Hemodialysis is the most effective method to remove ammonia rapidly and should be considered in any comatose hyperammonemic patient. Dialysis should not be delayed to await the effects of alternate pathway drugs (see below). Peritoneal dialysis is less effective.
4. Administer i.v. ammonia scavenging drugs. For sodium benzoate and sodium phenylacetate, usually given together, the loading dose of each is 250 mg/kg (or 5.5 g/m²) given in 25–30 ml/kg of 10% dextrose solution over 90 min. The maintenance dose is 250 mg/kg/d (or 5.5 g/m²/d) for each drug given as a 24 h infusion. Great care in dosing, administration and monitoring is essential.
5. Administer L-arginine-HCl i.v. The loading dose is 600 mg/kg (or 12 g/m²) given along with the sodium benzoate and sodium phenylacetate. The maintenance dose is 250 mg/kg/d (or 5.5 g/m²/d). The HCl derivative can produce serious acidosis.

The doses stated above are for acute hyperammonemia without a known enzyme defect. Arginine is very effective in reducing blood ammonia in citrullinemia and argininosuccinic aciduria and the high dose is aimed at these disorders. In patients with known CPS or ornithine transcarbamylase (OTC) deficiency, a lower dose is used for loading (200 mg/kg or 4 g/m²) and maintenance (200 mg/kg/d or 4 g/m²/d). In argininemia, neither arginine nor the ammonia scavenging drugs are indicated.

Maintenance therapy[37–39]

After the acute crisis, dietary protein is cautiously introduced at 0.5–0.75 g/kg/d and increased as tolerated. A mix of essential amino acids may be added. The protein intake is increased to the minimum daily requirement as tolerated. The ammonia scavenging drugs are gradually switched from i.v. to p.o. For chronic oral therapy sodium phenylbutyrate is preferred.[40] The dose is 450–600 mg/kg/d if the patient weighs < 20 kg and 10–13 g/m²/d in larger patients. Arginine is used in patients with citrullinemia or argininosuccinic aciduria at 400–600 mg/kg/d (10–13 g/m²/d). For CPS and OTC deficiency oral L-citrulline is preferred and is given at a dose of 170 mg/kg/d (3.3 g/m²/d).

Liver transplantation has been successful in correcting the metabolic disease and preventing hyperammonemic brain damage in many patients.[41]

GLYCINE

Nonketotic hyperglycinemia

Clinical findings

Nonketotic hyperglycinemia (NKH) usually presents with intractable seizures in the neonatal period. Hypotonia, lethargy, hyperreflexia, hiccupping and myoclonic jerks are frequent. Many patients require assisted ventilation and death is a common outcome. The EEG shows a typical burst–suppression pattern. Most patients who survive have profound mental retardation.

Rarer forms of NKH include an infantile form in which there is a symptom-free interval and apparently normal development for several months. Patients then present with seizures with various degrees of mental retardation. In an even milder form, patients present in childhood with mild mental retardation and episodes of delirium, chorea and vertical gaze palsy during febrile illness. There is a late-onset form that presents in childhood with progressive spastic diplegia and optic atrophy, but intellectual function may be preserved and seizures are not common. Rare infants have presented with symptoms and laboratory tests consistent with classic NKH, but then had complete, spontaneous reversal of both hyperglycinemia and neurological problems.

Diagnosis

Glycine levels are usually elevated in all body fluids including blood, urine and CSF. However, the blood levels may be normal, although they are always elevated in the CNS and an abnormal ratio of CSF: blood glycine is considered diagnostic except in the presence of valproate which can interfere with this ratio. Urine glycine is virtually always markedly elevated but should not be relied upon since physiological hyperglycinuria is common in neonates. Atypical cases, and cases where prenatal diagnosis may later be requested, may necessitate liver biopsy for enzyme analysis and/or mutation analysis.

The basic defect is in the glycine cleavage system that catalyzes the conversion of glycine to CO_2 and hydroxymethyltetrahydrofolic acid. The enzyme is multimeric with four distinct protein components designated P, H, T and L. Mutations in the P and T genes have been found with the P protein being most commonly affected. Prenatal diagnosis can be performed by biochemical analysis of chorionic villus sample biopsies.

Treatment

There has been modest success in treatment, particularly in late-onset cases. Sodium benzoate combines with glycine to form hippurate which is readily excreted; large doses may reduce CSF glycine and decrease seizures. Glycine is a neurotransmitter and anticonvulsants that block the N-methyl-D-aspartate (NMDA) receptor may be beneficial. Dextromethorphan has resulted in some improved outcome.[42,43] Similarly, imipramine has had some beneficial effects. For infants with classic severe neonatal NKH, consideration should be given towards allowing the lethal form to take its natural course.

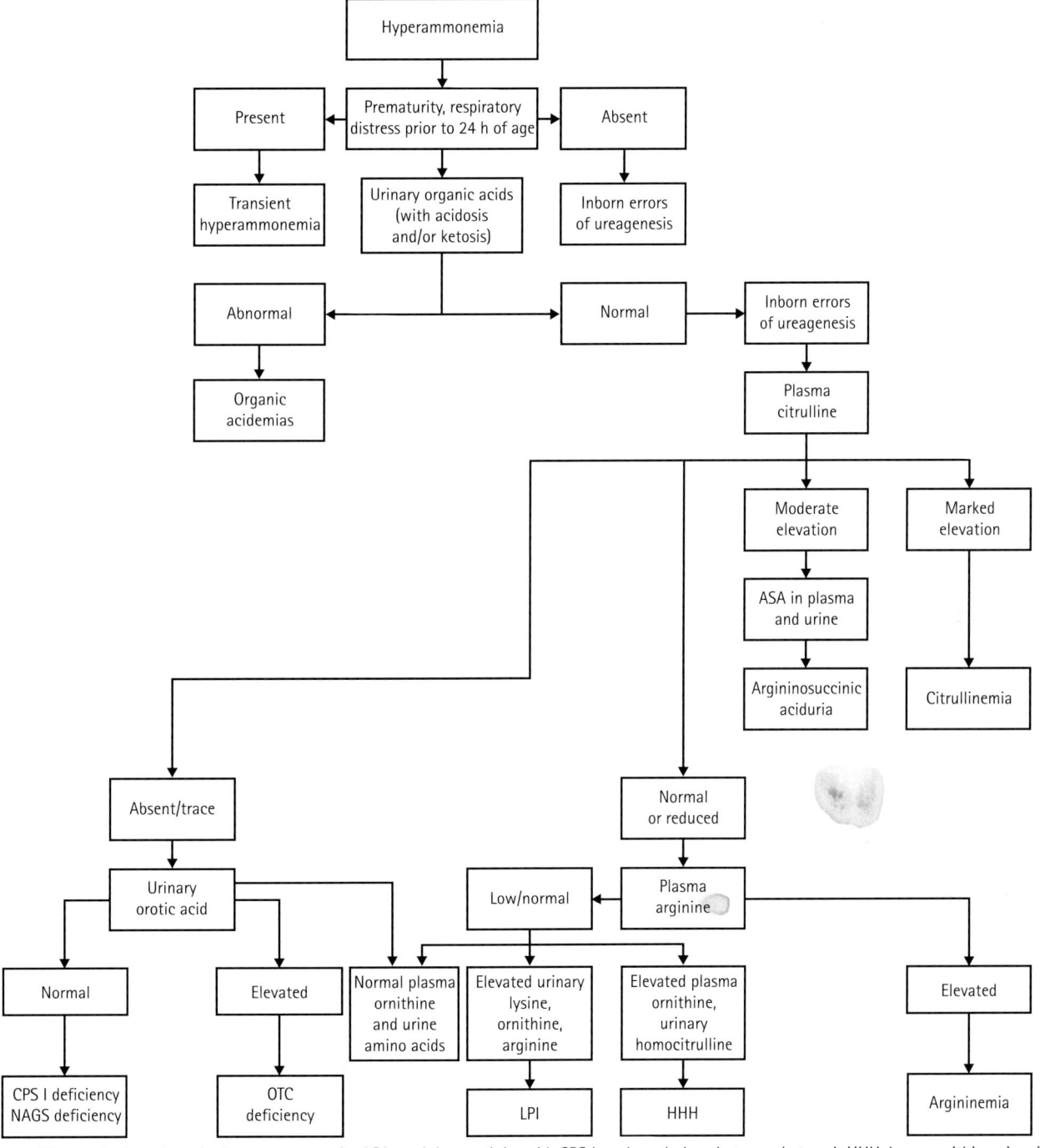

Fig. 26.8 Diagnostic flow chart for hyperammonemia. ASA, argininosuccinic acid; CPS I, carbamyl phosphate synthetase I; HHH, hyperornithinemia with hyperammonemia and homocitrullinuria; LPI, lysinuric protein intolerance; NAGS, N-acetylglutamate synthetase deficiency; OTC, ornithine transcarbamylase.

Hyperoxaluria (oxalosis)

Clinical findings

In primary hyperoxaluria large amounts of oxalate are excreted in the urine, leading to calcium oxalate lithiasis and nephrocalcinosis and massive extrarenal deposits of oxalate (oxalosis). Two distinct types are known with type 1 generally being more severe than type 2. Renal failure is common and first signs or symptoms are often before age 5 years (see Ch. 18).

Diagnosis

Primary hyperoxaluria type 1 is caused by deficiency of the hepatic enzyme alanine:glyoxylate aminotransferase and type 2 by D-glycerate/

glyoxylate reductase. In addition to hyperoxaluria, there is additional excretion of glycolic acid in type I and of L-glycerate in type 2.

Oxalic acid is a dicarboxylic acid that forms a calcium salt of very low solubility. Oxalate in the urine is clearly of endogenous origin, and glycine is a precursor. Patients with hyperoxaluria may excrete 30 times as much oxalate as normal. Genes for both types have been identified; prenatal diagnosis is available.

Treatment

This is aimed at reducing the intake of oxalate and calcium as far as possible with only minimal intake of vitamin C. The urine should be alkalinized and the volume should be kept as high as possible. Some type 1 patients respond to oral pyridoxine (200–500 mg/d), possibly by increasing conversion of glyoxylate to glycine. However, dietary and pharmacological treatment is often ineffective in the long term. Combined hepatorenal transplantation is usually successful,[44] but renal transplantation alone is not because systemically generated oxalate is deposited in the transplanted kidney.

Creatine deficiency

Two autosomal recessive diseases affect the biosynthesis of creatine from glycine and arginine via the intermediate metabolite guanidinoacetate. The deficient enzymes are arginine:glycine amidinotransferase (AGAT) and guanidinoacetate methyltransferase (GAMT). The resulting lack of phosphocreatine is most damaging to the CNS and is associated with major neurological problems including hypotonia, developmental delay, progressive movement disorder and seizures. A third, X-linked disorder associated with creatine deficiency is caused by mutations in a creatine transporter (SLC6A8). The clinical symptoms consist of developmental delay and hypotonia.

Diagnosis and treatment

The diagnosis of AGAT and GAMT deficiency is made by measuring creatine, creatinine and guanidinoacetate in blood or urine. Creatine is very low in both disorders. Guanidinoacetate is low in AGAT and elevated in GAMT deficiency. Plasma and urine creatinine levels may be low but normal levels do not rule out the diagnosis. Importantly, treatment with creatine monohydrate has been reported to reverse neurological symptoms.[45,46] Disease-causing mutations have been found in both types.

In the transporter defect, plasma creatine levels are not decreased and the diagnosis is made by measuring phosphocreatine levels in brain using proton magnetic resonance spectroscopy (MRS). The urinary creatine:creatinine ratio is high and supplementation with creatine is not clinically beneficial. The diagnosis is confirmed by mutation analysis.

Sarcosinemia

Sarcosine is formed from dimethylglycine, which may be a product of betaine or choline. It is not normally detectable in blood or urine although sarcosinuria may occur after the ingestion of lobster and some other foods. Sarcosine dehydrogenase deficiency has been found in individuals with short stature and mental retardation, but a causal relationship is unclear.

LYSINE, HYDROXYLYSINE AND TRYPTOPHAN

Glutaric aciduria type I is caused by a defect in the catabolic pathway of lysine, hydroxylysine and tryptophan. Alpha-ketoadipic acid, the common product of all three amino acids, is oxidatively decarboxylated to form glutaryl-CoA in a reaction catalyzed by alpha-ketoadipic acid dehydrogenase. Glutaryl-CoA dehydrogenase, the enzyme deficient in glutaric aciduria type I, is a mitochondrial flavin adenine dinucleotide (FAD)-dependent enzyme, which converts glutaryl-CoA to crotonyl-CoA.

Glutaric aciduria type II is a very different disease with deficiency in the activity of many acyl-CoA dehydrogenases. It is also known as multiple acyl-CoA dehydrogenase deficiency (MADD; see p. 1070).

Glutaric aciduria type 1 (GA₁)

Clinical findings

Glutaric aciduria type I is usually asymptomatic for some months after birth. Symptoms usually develop during an intercurrent illness with lethargy followed by the sudden onset of severe extrapyramidal neurological signs, after which the patient is left with dystonia and choreoathetosis. Mild macrocephaly may be found in early infancy. Metabolic stress such as intercurrent infections can trigger ketosis, acidosis, liver dysfunction, vomiting and acute neurological symptoms such as seizures and coma. The biochemical reason for the sudden emergence of catastrophic CNS damage is not known. The neurological deficits can probably be prevented if the disorder is effectively treated before the first metabolic crisis.

Diagnosis

This disorder is readily detected by expanded newborn screening. The cardinal characteristic is massive glutaric aciduria together with increased 3-hydroxyglutaric acid (see Appendix 1). Prenatal diagnosis can be performed on cultured amniocytes and by DNA based diagnosis.

Treatment

Therapy consists of protein restriction, especially lysine and tryptophan. In addition L-carnitine (100–300 mg/kg/d) and often riboflavin (100 mg/d) are used, starting at the time of diagnosis. Some success has been reported with the use of anticonvulsants that stimulate gamma-aminobutyric acid (GABA) receptors. Early treatment can significantly improve or prevent the neurological outcome. Aggressive management of intercurrent illness is critical. Young children with GA1 should be hospitalized and receive i.v. glucose (D10W at twice maintenance) and i.v. L-carnitine (150–300 mg/kg/d) very early in any situation that could result in metabolic decompensation, including febrile illnesses, decreased food intake, vomiting and diarrhea.

Other disorders of lysine metabolism

Deficiency of the bifunctional protein alpha-aminoadipic semialdehyde synthase causes familial hyperlysinemia. The clinical significance of this enzyme deficiency is controversial. Psychomotor retardation has been reported in many but not all affected individuals.

Individuals who lack 2-ketoadipic acid dehydrogenase excrete large amounts of 2-ketoadipic acid and 2-hydroxyadipic acid in their urine. The disorder is termed 2-ketoadipic acidemia. Although there are some case reports of neurological disease in this condition, other patients have been clinically normal.

Hydroxylysinemia has been found in several mentally retarded patients. The amino acid comes solely from collagen, where lysine is hydroxylated after incorporation into protocollagen. However, collagen metabolism was normal and the disorder was due to a defect in the metabolism of free hydroxylysine. An X-linked disorder in lysine hydroxylation is found in Ehlers–Danlos syndrome type VI (see Ch. 29, p. 1398).

Hyperprolinemia, hydroxyprolinemia and prolidase deficiency

Hyperprolinemia and hydroxyprolinemia are defects of the imino acids. Three distinct metabolic defects have been identified: proline oxidase is deficient in type I hyperprolinemia; 1-pyrroline-5-carboxylate dehydrogenase is deficient in type II hyperprolinemia; and hydroxyproline oxidase is deficient in hydroxyprolinemia. Although some patients with hyperprolinemia type II have been normal into adult life, it may be responsible for seizures in some patients.

Prolidase is an enzyme that cleaves X-pro linkages. Deficiency is associated with developmental delay, minor dysmorphic features and recalcitrant skin lesions that appear anywhere on the body from infancy to adult life. Massive amounts of many X-pro dipeptides are found in the urine. There is no specific treatment.

BRANCHED CHAIN AMINO ACIDS

Defects in the degradation of the branched chain amino acids valine, leucine and isoleucine result in the accumulation of organic acid intermediates (Fig. 26.9). High levels of leucine are toxic, particularly to the CNS. These diseases are most readily detected by analysis of urine organic acids and in many cases there is a characteristic odor. There are many different enzymes involved in this pathway, all of which are autosomal recessive traits.

Several of the disorders of branched chain amino acid metabolism are associated with elevated plasma glycine levels and/or hyperammonemia. These disorders were historically termed 'ketotic hyperglycinemias'. They are discussed as a group in this section.

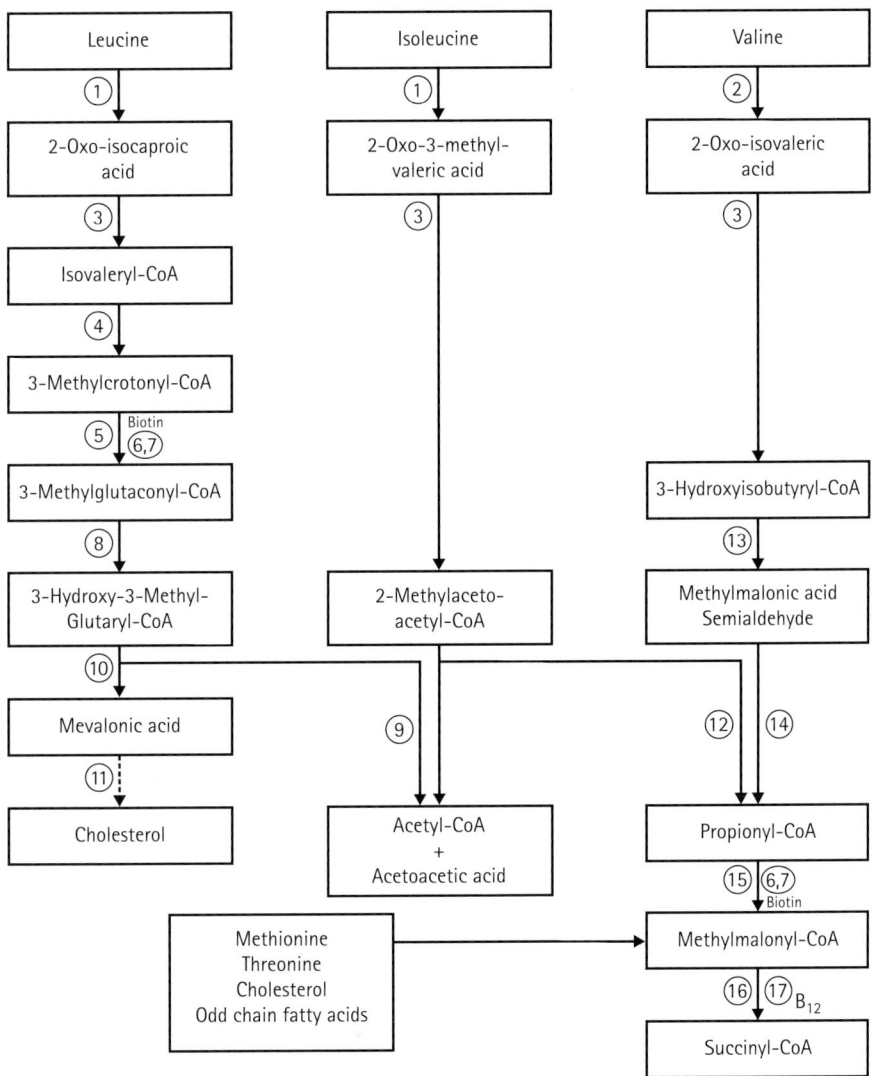

Fig. 26.9 Branched chain amino acid metabolism: numbers indicate known metabolic errors. 1, Leucine aminotransferase; 2, valine aminotransferase; 3, branched chain keto acid decarboxylase (maple syrup urine disease); 4, isovaleryl-CoA dehydrogenase; 5, 3-methylcrotonyl-CoA carboxylase; 6, biotinidase; 7, holocarboxylase synthetase; 8, 3-methylglutaconyl-CoA hydrolase; 9, 3-hydroxy-3-methylglutaryl-CoA lyase; 10, 3-hydroxy-3-methylglutaryl-CoA reductase; 11, mevalonate kinase; 12, 2-methylacetoacetyl-CoA thiolase (β-ketothiolase); 13, 3-hydroxyisobutyryl-CoA deacylase; 14, methylmalonic semialdehyde dehydrogenase; 15, propionyl-CoA carboxylase; 16, methylmalonyl-CoA mutase; 17, cobalamin defects.

AMINO ACID RELATED ORGANIC ACIDEMIAS

Many of the disorders of branched chain amino acids present with acidosis that is sometimes severe; they are an important subgroup of the organic acidemias. Diagnostic and therapeutic approaches to metabolic acidosis will be discussed first, followed by the description of individual disorders. Table 26.3 lists disorders associated with metabolic acidosis.

Diagnostic approaches (see also lactic acidosis, p. 1080)

Unexplained metabolic acidosis, with or without ketosis, should always suggest the possibility of an organic acidemia and demands urgent evaluation. The blood pH may be normal or low, and an anion gap or base deficit is to be expected. In some disorders, hypoglycemia is frequent and hyperammonemia or lactic acidosis reflect disturbed mitochondrial function. Hyperuricemia can be caused by inhibition of renal tubular secretion of uric acid by other organic acids. In the 'ketotic hyperglycinemia' syndromes (methylmalonic acidemia, propionic acidemia, isovaleric acidemia and 2-methyl-3-hydroxybutyric aciduria) the blood glycine is often raised; an elevated plasma glycine:alanine ratio is more consistent. In contrast, in lactic acidosis, hyperalaninemia reflects increased transamination of pyruvate. The urine pH is low and the Acetest (Ames), Ketostix (Ames) or dinitrophenylhydrazine tests may be abnormal depending upon which metabolites are being excreted. Diagnosis can usually be made by identification of the organic acid pattern, or their glycine and carnitine conjugates, in blood or urine and can be confirmed by specific enzyme assays (see also Appendix 1).

In milder cases, the diagnosis may be easily missed unless samples are obtained during an acidotic episode. Provocative tests with precursor amino acids have proved fatal and should not be used. *Blood and urine samples for metabolite identification should be taken from any child with unexplained acidosis.*

A number of organic acids may occur in the urine of sick, ketotic or acidotic children without IEM, presumably reflecting secondary metabolic disturbances. Lactate can reflect poor tissue perfusion. The *dicarboxylic acids* adipic, suberic and sebacic acids, 3-hydroxyisobutyric acid, 2-methyl-3-hydroxybutyric acid and 3-hydroxyisovaleric acid, as well as the ketone bodies, can all accumulate when lipolysis is increased, making it difficult to distinguish between primary or secondary effects on fatty acid breakdown (see also p. 1067). Many of these disorders are detected by expanded newborn screening (see Ch. 10).

Treatment

Since dehydration is associated with endogenous protein catabolism, it must be avoided; a urine output of 150–200 ml/kg/d or more, if tolerated, may help in the elimination of the metabolites. Although sodium bicarbonate is not a mainstay of therapy, and does not treat the cause of acidosis, it may be required along with definitive therapy to help correct the base deficit. Before the abnormal metabolites are identified, protein and fat should be restricted with as many calories from carbohydrate as can be tolerated, i.v. or p.o. If carbohydrate aggravates a lactic acidosis, the defect may be in pyruvate dehydrogenase (see Fig. 26.17) for which protein and fat are given and glucose

Table 26.3 Disorders associated with metabolic acidosis and/or organic aciduria. The major metabolite excreted is indicated either by the name of the disorder or by the compounds in parentheses (see also Table 26.8 and 9)

Branched chain amino acid disorders
Maple syrup urine disease (branched chain keto acids)
Methylmalonic acidemia
Propionic acid acidemia
Isovaleric acidemia
3-Methylcrotonylglycinuria
3-Methylglutaconic aciduria
3-Hydroxy-3-methylglutaryl-CoA lyase deficiency
Mevalonic acidemia
2-Methylacetoacetyl-CoA thiolase deficiency
3-Ketothiolase deficiency (3-hydroxybutyrate)
3-Hydroxyisobutyryl-CoA deacylase deficiency
Methylmalonic semialdehyde dehydrogenase deficiency
(3-hydroxypropionate)

Other disorders
2-Ketoadipic aciduria
Glutaric aciduria types I and II
Crotonic acidemia
5-Oxoprolinuria
Succinic semialdehyde dehydrogenase deficiency (4-hydroxybutyrate)
Succinyl-CoA:3-ketoacid CoA transferase deficiency
Threonine sensitive acidosis
2-Hydroxyglutaric aciduria
Barth syndrome (3-methylglutaconic acid)
Fanconi syndrome
The tyrosinemias (tyrosyluria) (succinyl acetone)
Renal tubular acidosis
Lactic/pyruvic acidosis
Multiple carboxylase and biotinidase deficiencies
Mitochondrial disorders
Krebs cycle disorders
Fructose 1,6-diphosphatase deficiency (lactate)
Glycogen storage disease type 1 (lactate)
Ketoacidosis as in diabetes mellitus
Carnitine depletion
Disorders of fatty acid catabolism
Disorders of ketone body utilization

Other disorders in which pathological organic aciduria can occur
Urea cycle disorders (orotic acid)
Canavan disease (N-acetylaspartate)
Phenylketonuria (phenylpyruvate)

Other acquired causes of acidosis
Poisoning: salicyclate, methanol, benzyl alcohol, antifreeze, etc
Ethanol
Starvation
Dehydration
Diarrhea
Reye syndrome

is minimized. Once the abnormal metabolites are identified, their precursors are restricted in the diet to the limits of metabolic tolerance. Calories are then supplied from all other available sources. Thus in maple syrup urine disease, all three branched chain amino acids are restricted, whereas in isovaleric acidemia only leucine needs to be controlled. Before the diagnosis is established, large doses of vitamin B_{12} (1–2 mg), pyridoxine (150–500 mg), thiamin (200–500 mg), folic acid (10–20 mg), biotin (10–20 mg), nicotinamide (100–500 mg) and riboflavin (100–500 mg) should be given in case the disorder is vitamin responsive. Once the definitive diagnosis is known, those unlikely to be useful can be stopped.

Abnormal quantities of any CoA derivative combines with carnitine to make acylcarnitine derivatives that are then excreted. This frequently causes profound carnitine depletion that in turn aggravates the metabolic acidosis and may induce muscle weakness, hypoglycemia,

hepatocellular damage and cardiomyopathy. Initial treatment should include L-carnitine 100–300 mg/kg/d in divided doses.

In extreme cases, hemodialysis or continuous extra corporal hemoperfusion should be used; peritoneal dialysis is less effective. A glucose/insulin drip may help to reverse endogenous protein catabolism. Once the crisis is over, a diet appropriate to the particular disorder is cautiously re-introduced over several days.

Maple syrup urine disease

In maple syrup urine disease (MSUD; branched chain ketoaciduria), major cerebral symptoms typically appear early in the newborn period, and the urine has an odor reminiscent of maple syrup. The branched chain amino acids – leucine, isoleucine and valine – are present in high concentration in the blood and urine, and the ketoacid analogues are found in the urine. The catabolic pathway is initiated by a transamination reaction to the respective ketoacids. The defect in MSUD is in the next step, namely oxidative decarboxylation of the ketoacids to their CoA derivatives. This is catalyzed by a mitochondrial multienzyme complex similar to pyruvate dehydrogenase and alpha-ketoglutarate dehydrogenase. For this reason autosomal recessive mutations in four different genes can cause MSUD. Patients have been identified with defects in the E1alpha, E1beta, E2 and E3 subunits of the complex. The E3 subunit is shared by all three complexes and defects in this gene cause simultaneous deficiency of all three dehydrogenases. MSUD is rare in most populations with an incidence of ~1:150 000.

Clinical findings

Infants with MSUD appear well at birth. Typically, symptoms begin after 3–5 d and progress rapidly. Early manifestations include feeding difficulty, irregular respirations and progressive CNS depression. Severe hypoglycemia may occur. Characteristically these patients develop convulsions, opisthotonos and generalized muscular rigidity with or without intermittent flaccidity. Death usually occurs within a few weeks after decerebrate rigidity develops. Cortical atrophy may be seen on CT or MRI, and the myelin is usually hypodense. This is consistent with defective myelinization as has been observed at autopsy. "A characteristic odor of maple syrup, caramel or fenugreek is present in urine sweat and cerumen. A similar odor is sometimes reported in normal infant's diapers"

Milder forms of the disease due to different mutations occur. There is an intermittent form with repeated episodes of ataxia and lethargy progressing to coma, but without neurodevelopmental sequelae. Episodes are usually precipitated by infection or anesthesia.

Diagnosis

Any traces of odor should be sought in all infants with such a presentation. Increased quantities of leucine, isoleucine and valine, and their keto acids are found in the plasma and urine. The presence of an abnormal amino acid, alloisoleucine, is diagnostic for MSUD.

Treatment

Treatment demands a diet with strict control of leucine which is acutely neurotoxic. Isoleucine and valine are normally restricted as well but they are not actually neurotoxic and, since all three are essential nutrients, they are sometimes *added* back to the diet to reduce the possibility that deficiency of one of them may be contributing to poor biochemical control (see p. 1064). With care, the plasma amino acids can be maintained near normal limits but this must be continued for life. A normal IQ may be achieved in those treated early and well. In a severe crisis, special intravenous solutions of amino acids can be used. Rare patients have a thiamine responsive form of MSUD and therefore this vitamin should be tried in all cases.

KETOTIC HYPERGLYCINEMIAS

Secondary elevation of plasma glycine is found in some defects of branched chain amino acid metabolism, particularly in propionic acidemia, methylmalonic acidemia and 3-ketothiolase deficiency. Because these conditions are also associated with ketoacidosis, they were originally termed the ketotic hyperglycinemias in contrast to nonketotic hyperglycinemia (see above). Urine organic acids should be analyzed in any patient with elevated plasma glycine.

Propionic acidemia
Clinical findings
This disease is characterized by recurrent episodes of lethargy, coma and metabolic acidosis with severe ketosis, similar to those observed in diabetic coma. There may be symptomatic hyperammonemia due to secondary inhibition of the urea cycle. Neutropenia, thrombocytopenia and osteoporosis severe enough to lead to pathological fracture may occur. Mental retardation, seizures and cerebral palsy are common in older patients, with the basal ganglia often involved. Symptoms begin within 24 h after birth, with vomiting, lethargy, acidosis and ketonuria. Death can occur with intractable acidosis. Surviving patients are susceptible to metabolic strokes, cardiomyopathy, progressive renal dysfunction and recurrent pancreatitis, any of which may prove fatal. The cause of these later complications is not known.

Diagnosis
The defect is in the enzyme propionyl CoA carboxylase, a multimeric enzyme with non-identical alpha and beta subunits; it catalyzes the formation of methylmalonyl CoA from propionyl CoA (see Fig. 26.9). Mutations in both genes have been identified.

Propionyl CoA is formed in the catabolism of several precursors (valine, isoleucine, methionine and threonine, odd-chain fatty acids and cholesterol, which creates a memorable mnemonic, 'VOMIT'). Propionic acidemia is most readily diagnosed by organic acid analysis of the urine for methylcitrate, 3-OH propionate, propionyl-glycine and others. Elevated quantities of glycine in the blood and urine may be suggestive. Patients frequently have an abnormal plasma carnitine profile with low free carnitine levels and an elevated fraction of short chain acyl-CoA carnitine. The defect can be demonstrated in leukocytes and in cultured fibroblasts: prenatal diagnosis is possible using molecular techniques as well as analysis of amniotic fluid for abnormal metabolites.

Treatment
Restricting the intake of the precursor amino acids reduces the frequency and severity of attacks of ketosis and acidosis (see p. 1070). Treatment with L-carnitine serves to reduce toxic quantities of propionyl CoA as well as reversing secondary deficiency of carnitine.[47] With bone marrow suppression, intercurrent illness and infection readily occur and must be treated vigorously with large amounts of glucose, fluids and electrolyte, often including sodium bicarbonate and L-carnitine. The acidosis or hyperammonemia can be life threatening and dialysis may be needed during acute decompensation. Patients diagnosed early in infancy and raised according to these principles clearly have improved survival and a more favorable developmental outcome. However, even when treated from birth, and in the absence of any known metabolic decompensation, the outcome can be very poor. Milder cases are sometimes not even detected until adult life. Liver transplantation has been used in this disorder, but has not been completely curative and in particular has not prevented neurological deterioration.

Methylmalonic acidemias
The methylmalonic acidemias are a genetically heterogeneous family of disorders in which methylmalonic acid accumulates in body fluids. The most severe disorders have a primary defect in the same pathway as propionic acidemia (see above) and the same compounds are toxic. Methylmalonic acid is normally formed from methylmalonyl-CoA, which is a product of the propionyl-CoA carboxylase reaction (see Fig. 26.9). Methylmalonyl-CoA mutase, a dimer of identical subunits, converts

methylmalonyl-CoA to succinyl-CoA, which can then be metabolized through the citric acid cycle. The mutase enzyme requires a vitamin B_{12} coenzyme, deoxyadenosylcobalamin (AdoCbl).

Impaired methylmalonyl CoA mutase activity can also be caused by several primary defects in vitamin B_{12} metabolism (styled Cbl A-G), all of which are autosomal recessive (see p. 1079 and Fig. 26.43). These defects affect the transport or synthesis of both methylcobalamin (MeCbl) and AdoCbl and thus can cause both abnormalities in both pathways at the same time. These patients tend to have lower plasma levels of methylmalonic acid than those with mutase mutations; they may not become ketotic and may also have megaloblastic anemia. High plasma homocysteine levels may be present.

Clinical findings
The clinical manifestations, complications and outcome of the severe forms are similar to those of propionic acidemia, patients usually presenting in the first weeks after birth. Hyperammonemia, hypoglycemia and ketosis are prominent. Growth retardation may be striking. Convulsions and abnormalities of the EEG have been observed. Failure to thrive may be extreme and death can occur in early infancy. However, later presentations, including serendipitous diagnosis in adults, have been reported. The cobalamin defects are somewhat different.

Diagnosis
Methylmalonic acid is elevated in plasma or urine, where it is normally present only in trace quantities. The urine also contains methylcitrate and plasma glycine may be elevated. Because plasma homocysteine levels may be elevated with defects in B_{12} metabolism, this compound should be measured in every patient with methylmalonic acidemia. Blood concentrations of vitamin B_{12} are normal, except when B_{12} deficiency is the cause of elevated methylmalonic acid. The activity of methylmalonyl CoA mutase is defective in leukocytes, cultured fibroblasts and amniotic fluid cells.

Several of the involved genes have been cloned and some mutations identified. In order to provide accurate prognostic information and genetic counseling, the exact cause of the methylmalonic acidemia needs to be determined, if feasible.

Treatment
The treatment for patients defective in the mutase structural gene is similar to that of propionic acidemia. It includes L-carnitine supplementation as well as dietary protein restriction.[48] Liver transplantation has been shown to be partially beneficial.

Some patients with Cbl defects are responsive to injection of high doses of specific isoforms of vitamin B_{12}. Those that do not respond may require specialized pharmacological and dietary management to control the elevated plasma homocysteine.

Isovaleric acidemia
Isovaleryl-CoA is the product of the branched chain decarboxylation of the ketoacid analogue of leucine that normally converts isovaleryl-CoA to 3-methylcrotonyl-CoA. Isovaleryl-CoA dehydrogenase is deficient in this disorder.

Clinical findings
Isovaleric acidemia normally presents within days of birth with lethargy, vomiting, coma, acidosis, ketosis and symptomatic hyperammonemia. The most distinguishing feature is a characteristic pungent odor, reminiscent of sweaty feet, which is that of isovaleric acid. Many patients die within a few weeks after birth.

In infants who survive the initial attack but remain untreated, there are recurrent episodes of vomiting, acidosis and ataxia, progressing to lethargy and coma. Acute episodes often occur with infections or after surgery. The odor is more likely to be appreciated during an episode of acute illness, but it may be absent. Mental retardation can be seen, especially among those diagnosed late, but normal IQ and good health are not uncommon. Patients with isovaleric acidemia also may have leukopenia, thrombocytopenia and anemia.

Diagnosis

During acute episodes, concentrations of isovaleric acid in the serum and urine may be enormous. Increased urinary isovalerylglycine is the most reliable biochemical indicator, and this compound is easily identified in routine organic acid analysis.

Treatment

Acute episodes are treated by vigorous use of parenteral fluids that contain glucose and electrolytes. The acidosis may require sodium bicarbonate. Hemodialysis or peritoneal dialysis may be indicated to treat hyperammonemia and/or acidosis. Long term treatment requires restricting the dietary intake of protein until the amount of leucine ingested is that necessary for growth. The conjugation of isovaleric acid with glycine (250 mg/kg/d) permits the possibility of adjunctive treatment with exogenous glycine. Additionally L-carnitine 100–200 mg/kg/d is administered.[49] If treatment is begun early, the prognosis is good.

OTHER BRANCHED CHAIN ORGANIC ACIDURIAS

3-Methylcrotonylglycinuria, due to isolated deficiency of 3-methylcrotonyl-CoA carboxylase, is similar to isovaleric acidemia except there may be an odor similar to cats' urine. 3-Methylcrotonylglycine and 3-hydroxyisovaleric acid are excreted in large amounts in the urine but are not elevated in blood. A trial of biotin (10–20 mg/d) is indicated because most cases who excrete these metabolites have multiple carboxylase deficiency. Most of these cases are asymptomatic.

A defect of *3-methylglutaconyl-CoA hydratase* (step 8, see Fig. 26.9) causes excretion of 3-methylglutaconic acid and 3-methylglutaric acid. The usual symptoms are progressive neurological deterioration in infancy, *without obvious metabolic acidosis*. However, hypoglycemia, metabolic acidosis and cardiomyopathy have also been reported although these could have been due to carnitine depletion. Other patients with 3-methylglutaconic aciduria but normal enzyme studies have presented with various symptoms of neurological deterioration, including choreoathetosis, spasticity, optic atrophy, tapetoretinal degeneration and nerve deafness. Metabolic acidosis may be absent or marked and most such cases die. Some cases are associated with defects of the respiratory chain but in most, the primary enzyme defect is not known. Barth syndrome is discussed on p. 1098.

2-Methylbutyryl-CoA dehydrogenase deficiency is a defect of isoleucine metabolism. The presentation includes neurological symptoms in the newborn period along with mild acidosis and hypoglycemia. Most cases are asymptomatic. The abnormal metabolites included 2-methylbutyrylglycine and 2-methylbutyrylcarnitine.

The last step in leucine catabolism, *3-hydroxy-3-methylglutaryl-CoA lyase*, commits leucine to ketogenesis and is discussed on p. 1070.

MULTIPLE CARBOXYLASE AND BIOTINIDASE DEFICIENCIES

Biotin is an essential cofactor for many carboxylases, including several involved in branched chain amino acid metabolism. For this reason perturbations of its association with these enzymes affect multiple different carboxylases. There are two distinct causes of multiple carboxylase deficiency. One is a deficiency of holocarboxylase synthetase and the other a deficiency of biotinidase. Holocarboxylase synthase catalyzes the association of biotin with the various carboxylases to form functional holoenzymes. Defects in this protein usually cause a severe, neonatal form of the disease. Biotinidase is involved in recycling of the vitamin and deficiency is usually clinically milder.

Clinical findings

Neonatal and infantile forms of the disease are distinguished. The former generally presents with life threatening acidotic illness in the newborn period, like that of propionic acidemia. Symptoms include severe ketosis, acidosis, dehydration and coma. Death can occur unless vigorous treatment is instituted. Patients who survive the first days of life have alopecia totalis and an impressive red, scaly total body eruption. The infantile form presents later with periorificial dermatitis resembling acrodermatitis enteropathica, partial alopecia and neurological abnormalities such as ataxia, delayed mental development and convulsions. These patients too may develop life threatening acidotic episodes. Immunodeficiency may be found in either form of the disease and may involve T- and B-cell function. Mild deficiency of biotinidase may be asymptomatic.

Diagnosis and treatment

Urine organic acid analysis is characteristic with excretion of 3-methylcrotonylglycine, 3-hydroxyisovaleric, methylcitric, 3-hydroxypropionic and lactic acids. Tiglylglycine may also be found. The two forms of the disease can be distinguished by mutation analysis or by enzyme measurement in cultured fibroblasts.

Newborn screening for biotinidase deficiency is employed in several programs because the disorder is readily treated and sequelae can be completely avoided. The incidence of complete deficiency is ~1 in 100 000.

Both genes for holocarboxylase synthetase and biotinidase have been identified. Two alleles for biotinidase account for ~50% of all mutations. Holocarboxylase synthetase deficiency is rarer than biotinidase deficiency and there are also two mutations that are more frequent. Prenatal diagnosis and successful prenatal treatment of affected fetuses has been reported.

All cases of biotinidase deficiency and most patients with multiple carboxylase deficiency are responsive to exogenous biotin.[50] Doses of 10 mg/d are usually sufficient to reverse all of the findings, but some patients require more. Carnitine may be a useful adjunct to therapy.

AMINO ACID TRANSPORT DISORDERS

In the kidney and gut, amino acids are actively transported across cell membranes in five major groups (Table 26.4). In addition, there are other separate, but minor, transport systems.

Disorders of both group-specific and individual amino acid transport systems exist. In tissues other than the kidney and gut there are similar, but not identical, active transport processes, but only in lysinuric protein intolerance is any other tissue known to be involved. Renal transport defects result in specific patterns of aminoaciduria, when, if anything, the plasma levels of the same amino acids are lower than normal. Plasma elevation of a single amino acid usually causes a single aminoaciduria, as in PKU, but a single amino acid may saturate the transport mechanism for all the others in the group, causing a group aminoaciduria. For example, in hyperglycinemia, the imino acids (group 2) may also be excreted.

Inherited defects of four group transport systems are known but they probably do not affect all cells. For example, the two types of iminoglycinuria imply that several genes must be required for amino acid transport in different tissues. *Dicarboxylic aminoaciduria* is a benign trait.

Cystinuria (see also Ch. 18)

Although the disorder bears the name of only one amino acid, cystinuria is a disorder of transport of cystine and all of the dibasic amino acids – cysteine, ornithine, lysine and arginine ('COLA'). The defect is in the SLC7A9 gene, which encodes a subunit of a family of amino acid transporters expressed in kidney, liver, small intestine and placenta. The condition is mainly important because cystine is very insoluble in normal urine and patients tend to develop renal calculi at any age. About 1–5% of patients with renal stones have cystinuria. Cystine crystals, which are flat and hexagonal, may be found in the urine. The diagnosis is based upon the nitroprusside test, amino acid chromatography or stone analysis. The aim of treatment is to keep urine cystine levels in the range of maximum solubility (approx. 0.1 mmol/mmol creatinine). It consists of maintaining a urine flow of 2–3 L/m²/24 h or more; 25%

Table 26.4   Group systems of amino acid transport in kidney and gut and their disorders

Group	Disorder
1. a. Cystine, lysine, ornithine, arginine b. Lysine, ornithine, arginine	Cystinuria type I, II and III Dibasic aminoaciduria: • Lysinuric protein intolerance • Without protein intolerance
2. Glycine, proline, hydroxyproline	Iminoglycinuria
3. β-Amino acids, taurine	None known
4. Aspartic and glutamic acid	Dicarboxylic aminoaciduria
5. Neutral amino acids (e.g. glycine, alanine, valine, leucine, isoleucine, serine, threonine, cysteine, cystine, phenylalanine, tyrosine, methionine, histidine, tryptophan)	Hartnup disease

of the fluid intake should be taken during the night. Maximum alkalization of the urine to around pH 7.5 is important, since the solubility of cystine decreases markedly below that.

Isolated cystinuria, isolated dibasic aminoaciduria (lysine, ornithine, arginine) and isolated lysinuria have been reported, showing that partial transport defects within the group can also occur.

Lysinuric protein intolerance
Clinical features
In this disorder, most common in Finland, symptoms of hyperammonemia become evident following weaning, when food intolerance, diarrhea, vomiting, hypotonia, hepatosplenomegaly, sparse hair, osteoporosis and marked failure to thrive develop. Interstitial pulmonary fibrosis is a late feature and may prove lethal. Mental development may be normal.

Diagnosis and treatment
There is a defect in the renal, liver and intestinal transport of lysine, arginine and ornithine, resulting in increased excretion in the urine and low levels in plasma. Cysteine transport is normal. The hyperammonemia is explained by deficient transport of urea cycle substrates into liver cells. In addition to other treatment for hyperammonemia, supplementation with citrulline (2–10 g/d) is very beneficial.

Iminoglycinuria
Free imino acids are normally present in urine in the first 6 months but they fall to very low levels thereafter. A defect of proline, hydroxyproline and glycine transport appears to be benign. Gastrointestinal transport may be either normal or defective. Hyperglycinuria is usually marked but glycine normally varies within wide limits, accounting for up to 25% of the urinary amino acids. It is common in iminoglycinuria heterozygotes, the ketotic and nonketotic hyperglycinemias and in valproate therapy. Glycinuria with glucosuria can occur either alone or with vitamin D-resistant rickets, although the reason for this is not known.

Hartnup disease
Hartnup disease is caused by defective transport in the kidney, and usually the gut, of amino acids in group 5 (see Table 26.4). The only constant feature is a characteristic aminoaciduria. The symptoms, if they occur, are those of pellagra caused by malabsorption of tryptophan. They include photodermatitis, ataxia, psychiatric changes and mental deterioration, but these are usually intermittent and are only precipitated during protein deprivation or periods of stress. Symptoms usually lessen with age. Patients on a normal protein or niacin-supplemented diet are symptomless. Deficiency of the other amino acids causes no problem. Treatment with oral nicotinic acid (25 mg/d) is effective.

Other amino acid transport defects
Methionine malabsorption in gut and kidney has been associated with mental retardation, convulsions, diarrhea and white hair. 2-Hydroxybutyric acid produced by gut bacteria has a peculiar, beer-like body odor that gives rise to the name oast-house syndrome. No treatment is known.

The blue diaper (nappy) syndrome is a rare isolated defect in gut absorption of tryptophan; gut bacteria degrade tryptophan to indoles that are then absorbed, metabolized in the liver and excreted in the urine as the blue pigment indican. The defect may be associated with mental retardation, hypercalcemia and nephrocalcinosis.

MISCELLANEOUS AMINO ACID DISORDERS

A number of patients with *carnosinemia* have been reported. Most have had abnormalities of the CNS, but others with the same defect are completely normal, so this defect is probably benign.

Histidinemia is a disorder in which large amounts of histidine are found in blood, urine and CSF. Deficiency of histidase (histidine-ammonia-lyase) has been demonstrated by direct assay of the enzyme in skin. More than half of these patients have had speech, mental and growth retardation; however, prospective studies have shown conclusively that histidinemia does not cause disease.

Histidine is normally converted by histidase to urocanic acid, which is ultimately metabolized to glutamic acid. Rare case reports have associated urocanase with severe mental retardation and neurological deterioration.

FATTY ACID OXIDATION DISORDERS (Fig. 26.10)
(in aggregate ~1 in 10,000–20,000)

GENERAL CONSIDERATIONS

After birth, fatty acids are the major fuel for cardiac and skeletal muscle, both at rest and during aerobic exercise. Following release from circulating or stored triglycerides by lipoprotein lipase (step 1), free fatty acids are bound to albumin in the plasma. After diffusing across the cell membrane, the long chain fatty acids, primarily palmitic and oleic acids, are converted to fatty acyl-CoA esters by an acyl-CoA synthase (step 3). Neither this step nor the transport systems into mitochondria seems to be required for medium or short chain fatty acids but these are usually minor metabolic pathways.

Transport into mitochondria requires L-carnitine, which is both endogenously produced and also comes from animal sources in the diet. Carnitine palmitoyl transferase (CPT)-I (step 4) forms fatty acyl-carnitine conjugates that are transported into the mitochondria by a translocase (step 5). Once inside the matrix, the reaction is reversed by CPT-II and free carnitine and long chain fatty acyl-CoA are reformed (step 6).

Fatty acid beta-oxidation occurs in a repeating four-reaction cycle, each 'spiral' of the cycle releasing one molecule of acetyl-CoA (steps 7–12). The first reaction is performed by one of four acyl-CoA dehydrogenases, the choice of enzyme dependent upon the structure and chain length of the fatty acid substrate. Straight chain C_{12-18} fatty acids are metabolized by very long chain acyl-CoA dehydrogenase (VLCAD), which is bound to the inner mitochondrial membrane. Long chain branched or desaturated fatty acids are probably substrates for long chain acyl-CoA dehydrogenase (LCAD), an enzyme within the mitochondrial matrix. Shortened fatty acids become substrates for either medium chain (C_{6-12}) or short chain (C_{4-6}) acyl-CoA dehydrogenases (MCAD or SCAD). All these reactions provide reducing equivalents and are coupled directly through electron transfer flavoprotein (ETF) and ETF:coenzyme Q (CoQ) oxidoreductase (ETF:QO) (steps 13–15) to CoQ of the electron transport chain. Three further enzymes (steps 10–12) complete one cycle leaving a fatty acyl-CoA two carbons shorter for further beta-oxidation.

For long chain fatty acids, steps 10–12 are all catalyzed by a single membrane bound enzyme complex called the trifunctional protein. For

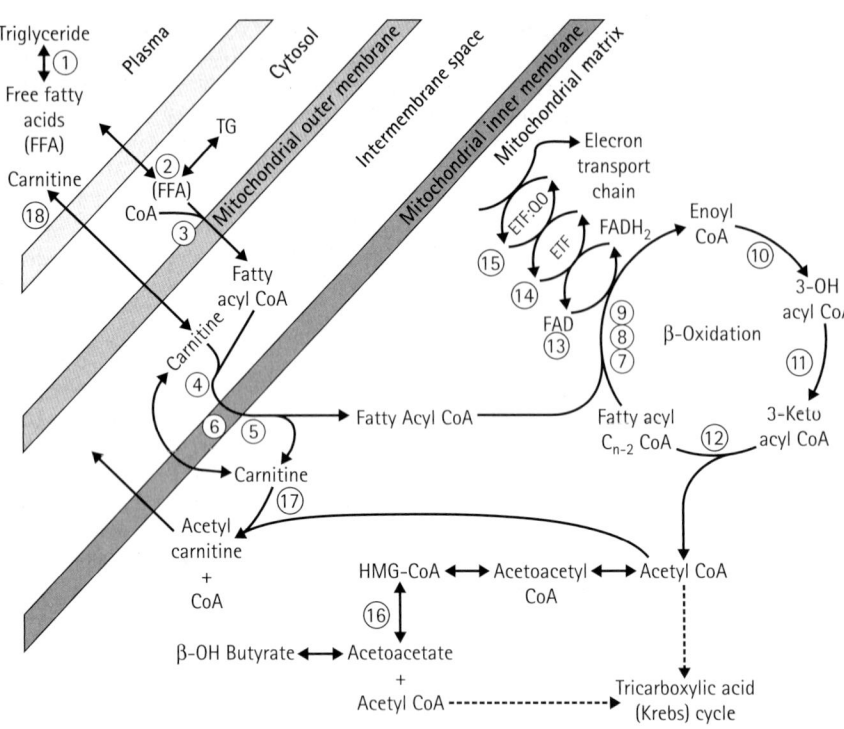

Fig. 26.10 Steps involved in fatty acid oxidation. 1, Lipoprotein lipase;* 2, fatty acid binding protein; 3, fatty acyl-CoA synthase; 4, carnitine palmitoyl transferase I (CPT-I);* 5, carnitine palmitoyl transferase II (CPT-II);* 6, fatty acyl carnitine translocase;* 7, long chain acyl CoA dehydrogenase (LCAD);* 8, medium chain acyl CoA dehydrogenase (MCAD);* 9, short chain acyl CoA dehydrogenase (SCAD);* 10, enoyl-CoA hydratase; 11, 3-hydroxyacyl-CoA dehydrogenase;* 12, thiolase; 13, flavin adenine dinucleotide (FAD);* 14, electron transfer flavoprotein (ETF);* 15, ETF: coenzyme Q oxidoreductase (ETF: QO);* 16, 3-hydroxy, 3-methylglutaryl CoA lyase (HMGCoA);* 17, carnitine acetyl transferase;* 18, carnitine transport. * Defects identified (see text).

shorter fatty acids, three distinct mitochondrial matrix proteins are required. Reducing equivalents generated in step 11 (3-hydroxyacyl-CoA dehydrogenase) are coupled to complex I of the electron transport chain. Fatty acid oxidation in the liver produces the ketone bodies, acetoacetate and beta-hydroxybutyrate, which, under homeostatic conditions, are recycled to fatty acids for use in other tissues, although they can be directly metabolized by the brain for energy during prolonged fasting. In liver and muscle, acetyl-CoA generated through fatty acid oxidation is a substrate for the citric acid cycle, sparing glycogen and preventing glucose depletion.

Transition from the continuous supply of glucose in fetal life to a mixed fuel system after birth requires efficient beta-oxidation, which is not usually stressed by the normal frequent feeding schedules of newborn infants. It is often only when breast milk let-down is insufficient, when the time between feeding increases, or during a catabolic illness, that these disorders tend to cause symptoms.

When beta-oxidation is increased or disrupted, the dicarboxylic acids adipic (C_6), suberic (C_8) and sebacic (C_{10}) are produced by omega-oxidation of the excess intermediates. Thus they are seen in fasting and in ketoacidosis from any cause, as well as in the disorders of fatty acid catabolism or ketone utilization.

Isolated deficiencies of most of the enzymes involved in fatty acid oxidation have been described, and collectively these disorders appear to be relatively common. All are inherited in an autosomal recessive pattern, and specific gene defects have been identified for most of the disorders.

The role of carnitine is discussed below.

Clinical features

Disorders of fatty acid metabolism commonly present with one of three phenotypes:

1. sudden infant death;
2. hypoketotic hypoglycemia in association with recurrent vomiting and hepatic encephalopathy;
3. recurrent rhabdomyolysis and myoglobinuria.

The expected phenotypes associated with the known disorders of fatty acid oxidation are presented in Table 26.5. Sudden infant death due to occult hypoglycemia often occurs in the setting of fasting or intercurrent illness, but sudden death may also occur in nonfasting neonates (particularly in infants with long chain fatty acid metabolism

defects such as VLCAD deficiency) due to cardiac arrhythmia or cardiomyopathy.

More commonly, disorders of fatty acid metabolism cause episodes of lethargy with nausea and vomiting, hypoketotic hypoglycemia, progressive somnolence and hepatic encephalopathy. As many as one third of the initial episodes may be fatal, the diagnosis not being established unless appropriate perimortem metabolic studies are performed.[51] Some children may have recurrent episodes of decompensation prior to diagnosis and may exhibit muscle weakness, hypotonia and developmental delay. Dysmorphic features and cardiomyopathy may occur in some of the disorders and CNS symptoms, when they occur, may be life threatening. Fatty acid metabolism defects may also

Table 26.5 Clinical presentations of fatty acid oxidation disorders

Enzyme deficiency	Hepatic	Myopathic
Carnitine transporter		X
Carnitine palmitoyl transferase (CPT)-I	X	Rarely
Carnitine acyltranslocase	X	
CPT-II	X	X
VLCAD	X	X
MCAD	X	
SCAD	X	
LCHAD/MTP	X	X
SCHAD	X	X
Ketolytic defects	X	

Hepatic presentation – recurrent Reye-like syndrome, hypoglycemia, acidosis; myopathic presentation – hypotonia, recurrent rhabdomyolysis.
LCHAD, long chain 3-hydroxyacyl-CoA dehydrogenase; MCAD, medium chain acyl-CoA dehydrogenase; MTP, microsomal triglyceride transfer protein; SCAD, short chain acyl-CoA dehydrogenase; SCHAD, short chain 3-hydroxyacyl-CoA dehydrogenase; VLCAD, very long chain acyl-CoA dehydrogenase.

present as exercise intolerance and recurrent episodes of rhabdomyolysis and myoglobinuria, often with initial onset during adolescence or adulthood. It is now clear from newborn screening that asymptomatic adults are not uncommon.

Diagnosis

Hypoketotic hypoglycemia is discussed below. Fatty acid oxidation defects should be sought by studies of urine organic acids and plasma carnitine status in patients with encephalopathy, myopathy, cardiomyopathy, unexplained liver disease or hypoglycemia. These patterns may be diagnostic at all times or only abnormal during metabolic stress. Plasma acylcarnitine or urine acylglycine profiles should also be assessed.

Histologically, microvesicular fat in the liver and myocytes are characteristic of carnitine depletion. Enzyme assays can usually be done on peripheral blood lymphocytes or cultured skin fibroblasts. Some of the defects, such as MCAD or LCHAD deficiency, are associated with common, specific disease-causing mutations. However, negative findings on specific mutation analysis does not rule out these disorders.

Treatment

Optimal therapy for disorders of fatty acid oxidation is generally based upon anecdotal experience. Avoidance of fasting and the ready provision of nonfat calories during stress, either orally or parenterally, are critical. L-Carnitine (50–300 mg/kg/d orally or 50–100 mg/kg/d i.v.) is given to reverse deficiency and to enhance urinary excretion of toxic acyl-CoA intermediates as carnitine conjugates,[52] but no controlled trials of carnitine supplementation have been published to prove its clinical efficacy. The safety and efficacy of L-carnitine therapy in disorders of long chain fatty acid metabolism remain anecdotal. Carnitine supplementation in acute carnitine deficiency syndromes, such as cardiomyopathy secondary to a defect in the cellular carnitine transporter, can be life saving.[53]

For defects in long chain fatty acid oxidation, dietary long chain fat restriction under the guidance of an experienced nutritionist may be useful, and medium chain triglyceride (MCT) oil is an effective alternative fuel source.[54] Specific nutritional deficiencies, including essential fatty acid deficiency (associated with hair loss, eczema and poor growth), fat soluble vitamin deficiency, vitamin B_{12} and iron deficiency, may complicate extreme dietary fat restriction (total energy from fat < 20% of total energy intake); these parameters must be carefully and repeatedly monitored during such dietary therapy.

SPECIFIC DISORDERS

Defects in the carnitine cycle

Carnitine derives mostly from the diet and partly from endogenous synthesis. It can be depleted in liver or kidney disease, malnutrition and malabsorption. Low blood levels are usual in premature and neonatal infants and in pregnancy, in which lowered values are probably physiologically normal.

Marked depletion occurs either from renal loss (e.g. Fanconi syndrome – see Ch. 18, p. 550) or increased utilization (e.g. the organic acidemias or valproate therapy). The latter occurs because carnitine accepts any acyl-CoA ester and the resulting acylcarnitine is then excreted. In removing the toxic acyl-CoA esters, the carnitine is lost. In addition, acylcarnitines inhibit the renal reabsorption of free carnitine, aggravating the depletion. In such cases, free carnitine levels are reduced but the acylcarnitine (bound) values are high. It is important to assay both fractions in plasma; an acyl:free ratio above 0.5 is abnormal. All the disorders of carnitine metabolism can be detected by newborn screening (see Appendix 1) and those with liver damage may develop hyperammonemia.

Carnitine transporter deficiency ('primary carnitine deficiency')

No primary defect of carnitine synthesis is currently known. The term 'primary deficiency' is reserved for a defect in the uptake of carnitine into cells. Such defects may be pancellular or tissue specific in myocytes, renal tubular cells or, rarely, hepatocytes. Renal tubular losses produce very low plasma values and very high urine levels, resulting in systemic deficiency involving all tissues. Muscle depletion presents with hypotonia or weakness; cardiac depletion causes acute or chronic cardiomyopathy and hepatocellular depletion can cause hepatic steatosis or fulminant Reye syndrome, any of which can be precipitated during stress or minor starvation. In other cases, the plasma levels may be normal but the involved tissues are deficient. L-Carnitine (250–350 mg/kg/d) should be used as replacement therapy.[53]

Carnitine palmitoyl transferase deficiency I and II
(steps 4 and 5) (~1:500 000)

Deficiency of the liver isoform of CPT-I causes symptomatic fasting hypoketotic hypoglycemia and occasionally hepatocellular damage. Recurrent rhabdomyolysis is the hallmark of deficiency of muscle CPT-I deficiency. In either form, total and free plasma carnitine are characteristically elevated; this observation is unique among all known fatty acid oxidation defects and is otherwise seen only with carnitine supplementation, renal insufficiency or cardiac muscle damage.

In CPT-II deficiency, an infantile form presents with severe hypoglycemia, myopathy and cardiomyopathy leading to death. Plasma carnitine is low with elevated acylcarnitines. A milder form presents with lipid myopathy, recurrent rhabdomyolysis and myoglobinuria in young adults.

Carnitine/acylcarnitine translocase deficiency is clinically similar to infantile CPT-II deficiency.

Treatment of these disorders is frequent intake of dextrose or sugary snacks to diminish the need for fat during exercise or stress.

Medium chain acyl–CoA dehydrogenase deficiency (MCADD) (step 8) (1:10–20 000)
Clinical features

This is the most common defect in fatty acid oxidation. The typical acute presentation includes fasting- or illness-induced hypoketotic hypoglycemia, often associated with metabolic acidosis and hepatocellular dysfunction that can progress to full-blown Reye syndrome. Chronically, cardiomyopathy and/or signs of muscle carnitine depletion such as fatigue, lethargy, weakness or hypotonia can also occur. As with all disorders of fuel-related pathways, these problems are produced or aggravated by poor nutrition or the stress of even a minor illness, and may be recurrent.

The most severe presentation is of sudden death in the first days or months of life, presumably due to occult hypoglycemia. These cases may be mislabeled as sudden infant death syndrome (SIDS), especially if a detailed postmortem examination including metabolic testing is not performed.[55] The risk of sudden infant death can be prevented through avoidance of prolonged fasting, making medium chain acyl-CoA dehydrogenase deficiency an ideal candidate for newborn screening (see Ch. 4), although death can occur soon after birth before screening results are available.

Some individuals with MCADD may never become symptomatic, presumably because they never develop carnitine depletion under sufficient stress or because they carry mutations with relatively mild physiological effects. It is important to note however that the initial presentation of MCADD may occur in adolescence or even adulthood.

Diagnosis

Characteristic medium chain fatty acid metabolites, acylglycine and acylcarnitine conjugates, are present in urine or blood. Fatty acid metabolites are often detected by urine organic acid analysis, especially during acute crises, but may be normal between episodes. Analysis of acylcarnitine conjugates is more sensitive and is often diagnostic even between clinical episodes. Newborn screening using tandem mass spectrometry is now being increasingly used.

Of patients presenting clinically, 80–90% are homozygous for an A985G mutation in the MCAD gene, but the frequency of this mutation is lower in cases detected by newborn screening, suggesting that other mutations may be associated with mild or subclinical disease.[56] Whether phenotype can be accurately predicted from genotype is still under evaluation.

Defects of long chain fatty acid oxidation

A trifunctional enzyme comprises *long-chain 3-hydroxy-acyl-CoA dehydrogenase (LCHAD)*, enoyl-CoA hydratase and thiolase activities, the so-called trifunctional protein (TFP). LCHAD deficiency (step 11) appears to be the second most common fatty acid oxidation defect and is frequently caused by homozygosity for a G1528C mutation in the TFP alpha subunit gene. Cases with other mutations in either the alpha or beta TFP subunit genes often exhibit deficiency of all three enzymatic activities; this may alter both the pattern of diagnostic metabolites and the clinical presentation. Long chain hydroxy acids may be detectable by urine organic acid analysis during acute metabolic crises, but as in MCADD, analysis to detect long chain 3-hydroxylated carnitine esters is often more sensitive.

In LCHAD/TFP deficiency and in *very long chain acyl-CoA dehydrogenase deficiency (VLCADD)* (step 7), the clinical features are often similar to, but more severe than, MCADD. Older patients may develop late-onset cardiomyopathy or myopathy with recurrent myoglobinuria, and patients are generally carnitine deficient. Pigmentary retinopathy and vision loss during childhood is a complication specific to LCHAD/TFP deficiency. In addition to fasting avoidance and ingestion of a fat-restricted diet, treatment with dietary MCT oil and L-carnitine may be beneficial.[54] Acute fatty liver of pregnancy or the 'HELLP' syndrome occurs in many women who carry LCHAD deficient fetuses;[57] the pathophysiological mechanism of this complication is currently unknown.

Defects of short chain fatty acid oxidation

These include defects of *short chain acyl-CoA dehydrogenase (SCADD)* (step 9), *short chain 3-hydroxyacyl-CoA dehydrogenase (SCHAD)*[58] and *malonyl-CoA decarboxylase*. These disorders tend to cause failure to thrive, recurrent vomiting with or without hypoglycemia and/or ketosis, hypotonia, marked developmental delay, seizures and early demise. The urine organic acid profiles tend to suggest the site of the defects but confirmation requires detailed studies in fibroblasts or other tissues.

Many individuals with clinical symptoms and biochemical evidence of SCADD have inherited variations in the SCAD gene that are also common in the normal population. In one study, 69% of 133 patients with biochemical findings of SCADD were either homozygous for a single mutation or were compound heterozygous for two different SCAD polymorphisms (G625C or C511T); yet 14% of the general population also carry these polymorphisms.[59] So, the exact pathophysiological relationship between the presence of these polymorphisms and clinical disease is not clear. All of these disorders are detectable by expanded newborn screening (see Appendix 1).

Glycerol kinase deficiency

Glycerol derives from hydrolysis of fats and, reversibly, from glycolysis, making it available for gluconeogenesis. Glycerol kinase deficiency causes recurrent attacks of a Reye-like syndrome with vomiting, acidemia, CNS depression and hypotonia that are precipitated by a high fat intake or fasting. Milder cases are found by chance with pseudohypertriglyceridemia on routine multichannel blood testing. It also can be part of an X chromosome microdeletion syndrome that can include Duchenne muscular dystrophy, retinopathy and adrenal hypoplasia, which usually dominates the clinical picture; note that glycerol in urine may derive from body lotions or suppositories. Frequent high carbohydrate feeding with mild fat restriction is indicated.

Glycerol intolerance is a different condition associated with recurrent hypoglycemia and Reye-like attacks that may actually be a manifestation of fructose-1, 6-diphosphatase deficiency.[60]

Multiple acyl-CoA dehydrogenase deficiency

This comprises several different disorders that are all associated with a defect in the entry of electrons into the electron transport chain (see Fig. 26.19). All affect the handling of reducing equivalents generated from the catabolism of several amino acids and by numerous different acyl-CoA dehydrogenases, hence the name multiple acyl-CoA dehydrogenase deficiency. Defects of transport, processing or binding of FAD (Fig. 26.10) (step 13), ETF (step 14) or the ETF:QO (step 15) are all possible. Three forms are generally recognized with clinical overlap between groups and genetic heterogeneity within each group.

The severe form (MAD:S), also called *glutaric aciduria type II*, is often lethal in the newborn period, secondary to profound acidosis, hypoglycemia, coma and multiple organ system involvement. A subgroup of these patients exhibits dysmorphic facial and other features, characteristic subependymal brain cysts, dysmyelination of brain and polycystic kidneys. Milder cases lack dysmorphism but usually exhibit severe failure to thrive, hypotonia, cardiomyopathy and liver damage. An unusual 'acrid' odor and the 'sweaty feet' odor of isovaleric acid are often described. The biochemical profile on urine organic acid analysis is generally diagnostic, with accumulation of ethylmalonic, glutaric, 2-hydroxyglutaric, adipic, suberic and sebacic acids, isovaleryl, isobutyryl- and 2-methylbutyryl-glycines, with sarcosine often detected by urine amino acid screen.

A milder form of the disorder termed MAD:M (sometimes called *ethylmalonic-adipic aciduria*) may not present until adulthood; the presentation being similar to other acyl-CoA dehydrogenase deficiencies. The urine organic acid profile is simpler than in MAD:S, usually containing only ethylmalonic, adipic and methylsuccinic acids and hexanoyl and butyrylglycines. Dicarboxylic acids are abundant and sometimes disappear following riboflavin supplementation, giving rise to the original term riboflavin-responsive dicarboxylic aciduria. A similar metabolite pattern may also be seen in isolated SCADD and is often detected by newborn screening (Ch. 4).

Defects of both ETF and ETF:QO dehydrogenase have been found in both forms of MAD. Generally, the severity of the enzyme deficiency correlates with the severity or type of disorder. Some of these patients improve on riboflavin (100–300 mg/d) and carnitine (100–200 mg/kg/d).[61]

Disorders of ketone metabolism
3-Hydroxy-3-methylglutaric aciduria

The last steps of leucine catabolism are mitochondrial *3-hydroxy-3-methylglutaryl-CoA synthase* and *lyase* which are essential to the formation of the ketone bodies acetoacetyl-CoA and acetyl-CoA. Defective function of these enzymes is characterized by *hypoketotic hypoglycemia* as well as metabolic acidosis. The disease is particularly likely to be mistaken for Reye syndrome (Ch. 22, p. 875).

In the cytosol, *3-hydroxy-3-methylglutaryl-CoA synthase* reverses this reaction and *3-hydroxy-3-methylglutaryl-CoA reductase*, the enzyme inhibited by statin drugs, is the next and rate-limiting step in cholesterol synthesis (see p. 1090).

Clinical findings

Patients deficient in the mitochondrial synthase or the lyase have acute episodes of life threatening illness in early infancy, often with persistent vomiting as the first symptom. Coma and dehydration may lead to apnea and death. Seizures, hepatomegaly, elevated liver enzymes, metabolic acidosis, hypoglycemia and hyperammonemia can occur. Acute episodes, reminiscent of Reye syndrome, are likely to follow an acute infectious illness and may be followed by mental retardation, neurological abnormalities and cerebral atrophy.

Diagnosis

Concentrations of glucose may be strikingly low, but ketonuria is absent, and this distinguishes these patients from most others with organic acidemias. Liver function tests may be abnormal at times of acute illness. The organic aciduria is characteristic; in addition to large quantities of 3-hydroxy-3-methylglutaric acid, the urine contains 3-methylglutaconic acid, 3-methylglutaric acid and 3-hydroxyisovaleric acid. During illness, the urine may also contain large amounts of lactic acid.

Treatment. Parents should be alerted to the need for early, vigorous management of the acute crises, especially when the oral route is compromised by fasting or anorexia. Long term management depends on the avoidance of fasting and hypoglycemia. A high carbohydrate diet is useful, and the intake of both fat (ketone precursors) and protein should be limited. L-Carnitine has limited usefulness, because 3-hydroxy-3-methylglutaric acid does not form carnitine conjugates.

Defects of ketone utilization
3-Ketothiolase deficiency
Defects of ketone utilization cause facile hyperketosis; they include deficiencies of *succinyl-CoA:3-ketoacid-CoA transferase, 2-methylaceto-acetyl-CoA thiolase* or of several different enzymes with *3-ketothiolase* activity (step 12). *Mitochondrial acetoacetyl-CoA thiolase* is an enzyme in the isoleucine pathway that converts 2-methylacetoacetyl-CoA to propionyl-CoA and acetyl-CoA.

All can present with severe neonatal acidosis, intermittent episodes of ketoacidosis with lethargy and coma, or may be asymptomatic. Developmental delay and episodes of diarrhea may occur. Mitochondrial acetoacetyl-CoA thiolase is associated with progressive neurological deterioration, neuropathy and an extrapyramidal movement disorder. Hypoglycemia, ketotic hyperglycinemia and hyperammonemia are reported.

The urine contains 2-methyl-3-hydroxybutyric acid, tiglylglycine, 2-methylacetoacetic acid and other organic acids and butanone. Acetoacetic and beta-hydroxybutyric acids can be greatly elevated, and the differential diagnosis must include acquired ketotic hypoglycemia (see below), as well as salicylism. Lactic acidosis with abnormal lactate:pyruvate ratios and increased ketone body levels are usual. Continued elevation of diagnostic metabolites between ketotic episodes strongly suggests the diagnosis. The enzyme defect can be demonstrated in cultured skin fibroblasts.

Treatment for these disorders is again based primarily upon avoidance of fasting.

Hypoglycemia as a presenting feature of metabolic disorders
Hypoglycemia is often considered the purview of endocrinologists since changing rates of glucose consumption are balanced by intricate hormonal controls and the coordinated release of fuels from glycogen, fat or protein. Metabolic causes should never be forgotten; often, hepatomegaly or acidosis suggests a metabolic diagnosis but evaluation of hypoglycemia may require extensive metabolic testing. The half-life of metabolic fuels in the plasma is about 100 secs, so, as with hormone assays, tests for high or low levels of ketones, free fatty acids, amino acids, carnitine and its conjugates, and possibly glycerol *must be obtained during hypoglycemia (< 2.2 mmol/L [40 mg/dl]) and before any treatment has been given.* Urine organic acids and acylcarnitine analyses can be diagnostic. Hyper- or hypo-ketosis is often not recognized because quantitative assays are not readily available. If these tests are not diagnostic, then starvation/fasting stress tests can be used to recreate an acute hypoglycemic episode but should only be performed in hospital with full emergency support and expert consultation available.[62]

Hypoglycemia with ketosis and/or acidosis
Ketotic hypoglycemia occurs frequently in small undergrown infants and children. Most cases are due to poor growth, poor nutrition with inadequate and/or infrequent feeding, but symptoms can sometimes occur even in apparently healthy, well fed infants. Lack of glycogen stores and of muscle protein for gluconeogenesis necessitates increased lipolysis. As a result, fatty acid intermediates and ketones readily accumulate in patterns that mimic hereditary defects of fuel homeostasis. In nutritional deprivation or hormonal problems, plasma alanine and lactate are low and there is no response to intramuscular glucagon. The differential diagnosis includes glycogen storage disorders and defects of ketone utilization, pyruvate, the citric acid cycle and organic acid metabolism.

Hypoketotic hypoglycemia
Hypoglycemia with inappropriately low levels of blood ketones suggests a defect of fatty acid oxidation or of ketone production; it is also typical in hyperinsulinism. Quantitation of serum free fatty acids during a hypoglycemic episode assists with the differential diagnosis; free fatty acid levels are suppressed in hyperinsulinism while they are elevated in fatty acid oxidation disorders.

DISORDERS OF CARBOHYDRATE METABOLISM

The hereditary disorders of digestion and absorption, including *lactase, sucrose-isomaltase, trehalase* and *glucose–galactose malabsorption* are addressed in Chapter 19 (p. 621).

In the kidneys, renal glycosuria is caused by a defect in glucose reabsorption. Pentosuria is a benign condition, most common in Jewish people due to deficient *l-xylulose reductase* activity; xylulose is excreted in the urine where it reacts with Benedict's solution or Clinitest to give a false positive test for glucose.

DEFECTS OF GLYCOLYSIS (FIG. 26.11)
In erythrocytes
Severe defects of glycolysis in erythrocytes are usually associated with hemolytic anemia (Ch. 23). Such conditions include defects of *glucose-6-phosphate dehydrogenase, hexokinase* (step 2), *glucosephosphate isomerase* (step 4), *phosphofructokinase* (step 5), *aldolase triose phosphate isomerase (TPI)* (step 7), *phosphoglycerate kinase (PGK)* (step 9), *diphosphoglycerate mutase* (step 10), *pyruvate kinase* (step 12) and *lactate dehydrogenase.* In contrast, deficiency of either *2,3-diphosphoglycerate (DPG) mutase* or *diphosphoglycerate phosphatase* causes mild erythrocytosis. Hemolysis can also be caused by defects of glutathione metabolism (see p. 1057) and certain steps in purine and pyrimidine metabolism (see p. 1122) and *adenosine triphosphatase.* Another red cell enzymopathy is a deficiency of *6-phosphogluconate dehydrogenase* in the pentose monophosphate shunt. Finally, *cytochrome b_5 reductase* deficiency is often associated with methemoglobinemia and developmental delay.

In the nervous system
Several of these disorders also cause neurological or muscular disease. Severe TPI deficiency is associated with severe, progressive neurological disease with both upper and lower motor neurone damage. The intellect is relatively well preserved but there is a tendency to sudden death and increased susceptibility to infection. Severe PGK deficiency can cause developmental delay and attacks of behavioral and emotional abnormalities, movement disorders including hemiplegia and even coma that develop during hemolytic crises. *Glutathione reductase* deficiency can also cause a variety of neurological abnormalities, including myelopathy. About 15% of cases with cytochrome b_5 reductase deficiency have severe progressive neurological deterioration with microcephaly, athetosis and hypertonia in addition to methemoglobinemia. In all of these disorders, management of these neurological symptoms is unsatisfactory but should include avoidance of oxidant drugs.

In muscle – the metabolic myopathies (see also p. 1088)
There is a large and growing number of metabolic myopathies, almost all of which involve energy metabolism. Since several are glycolytic disorders, the whole group is summarized here (Table 26.6).

Clinical features
The usual symptoms are muscle weakness, lack of endurance and post-exercise muscle pain or cramps. Infants are often hypotonic. Muscle wasting, when present, is often due to disuse rather than to the intrinsic muscle disease. Disorders associated with lactic acidosis are characterized by exercise-induced dyspnea. In glycolytic or fatty acid defects, excessive exercise leads to severe cramping and rhabdomyolysis with increased serum creatine phosphokinase (CPK) levels and recurrent myoglobinuria that can cause severe renal damage. These diseases may

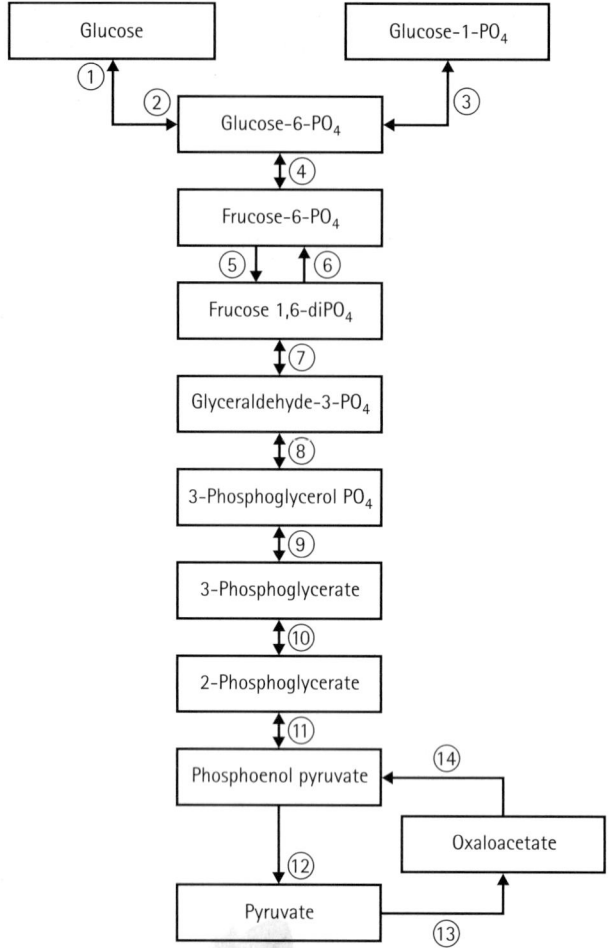

Fig. 26.11 Embden–Meyerhof glycolytic pathway. 1, Hexokinase; 2, glucose-6-phosphatase; 3, phosphoglucomutase; 4, phosphohexose isomerase; 5, phosphofructokinase; 6, fructose-1,6-bisphosphatase; 7, triose phosphate isomerase; 8, glyceraldehyde-3-phosphate dehydrogenase; 9, phosphoglycerate kinase, 10, phosphoglyceromutase; 11, enolase; 12, pyruvate kinase; 13, pyruvate carboxylase; 14, phosphoenolpyruvate carboxykinase.

Table 26.6 Metabolic myopathies

Glycogen storage diseases (GSDs)
  Acid maltase deficiency (GSD type II)
  Glycogen debrancher deficiency (III)
  Glycogen brancher deficiency (IV)
  Phosphorylase deficiency (V)

Glycolytic defects
  Phosphofructokinase
  Phosphoglycerate kinase
  Phosphoglycerate mutase
  Glucosephosphate isomerase
  Lactate dehydrogenase
  Lactate transporter

Fatty acid oxidation disorders
  Long chain fatty acid oxidation disorders
  (VLCAD, LCHAD/TFP deficiency)
  Carnitine palmitoyl transferase deficiency
  Secondary carnitine depletion

Purine disorders
  Myoadenylate deaminase deficiency

Mitochondrial defects
  Defects in respiratory chain complexes I–IV
  Luft syndrome (complex V – ATPase deficiency)
  Krebs cycle defects
  Adenine nucleotide translocase defect
  Pyruvate dehydrogenase deficiency
  Defect in the malate–aspartate shuttle

Others
  Ion channelopathies
  Periodic paralyses (hypo- or hyper-kalemic)
  Malignant hyperthermia

LCHAD, long chain 3-hydroxyacyl-CoA dehydrogenase; TFP, trifunctional protein; VLCAD, very long chain acyl-CoA dehydrogenase.

Metabolic screening with plasma amino acid analysis, plasma carnitine levels, plasma acylcarnitine profile and urine organic acid analysis may also yield the diagnosis.

Blood lactate and ammonia, inosine and hypoxanthine (from the purine nucleotide cycle) normally rise after exercise but in many metabolic myopathies this is not so. A semi-ischemic forearm exercise test may provide useful information. In some of the glycogen storage diseases and mitochondrial defects, the lactate rises very fast and limits the duration of the test. In glycogenolytic defects, lactate and ammonia should rise abnormally and in glycolytic lesions, ammonia and purines rise but the lactate does not; in myoadenylate deaminase deficiency, the ammonia, inosine and hypoxanthine do not rise normally.

The test is carried out as follows: a blood pressure cuff is inflated above systolic pressure. A handgrip is formed and opened every second for 1 min. Prior to and for eight 1 min intervals after starting the exercise, venous blood is collected for assay of lactate, ammonia and hypoxanthine. Other physiological measurements of muscle function including electromyography (EMG), or treadmill exercise test, may assist with the diagnosis and help assess exercise tolerance but should be done with caution in these patients.

Before a muscle biopsy is performed, it is essential to plan for the tests that might be required, including histochemistry, electron microscopy, isolation of mitochondria, biochemical analyses, immunohistochemistry and DNA studies, because processing of the tissue varies for different studies and in different laboratories. For example, immediate flash freezing is essential for glycogen quantitation, enzyme assays require fresh tissue or flash freezing while preparation for histochemistry and electron microscopy varies upon the laboratory. Glycogen content is often increased in the glycogen storage diseases, the glycolytic defects and frequently in electron transport defects. The lipid content is usually increased in the lipid disorders and often in electron transport

be aggravated by fasting or a high fat diet and tend to present in adolescence or later. Curiously, the disorders of the electron transport chain, which may occur at any age, are rarely associated with myoglobinuria, perhaps because the dyspnea from lactic acidosis is so marked that exercise capacity is too limited to result in much muscle cell damage.

Myoadenylate deaminase is an enzyme of the purine pathway (p. 1123). Deficiency is found by histochemical staining in 1–2% of muscle biopsies. It is frequently asymptomatic but can cause a variety of muscular symptoms.

Diagnosis

Nonspecific complaints of muscle weakness, lack of endurance or muscle cramps are very common and only 10–20% of such cases prove to have a real muscle disorder. Real cases are often not detected or evaluated for years or until a crisis such as rhabdomyolysis develops. The differential diagnosis includes both cardiovascular and respiratory disease as well as a psychogenic disorder. The key to the diagnosis is in the history and consideration of its veracity regarding the symptoms and their effects upon daily life. Physical signs including muscle wasting or hypertrophy and muscle weakness are supportive of the diagnosis, but their absence does not preclude a metabolic defect. Elevation of serum CPK levels and myoglobinuria indicate ongoing rhabdomyolysis; blood electrolyte abnormalities or lactic acidosis may suggest specific defects.

chain defects. Muscle biopsy for mitochondrial disease is discussed on p. 1088.

In some research laboratories, intracellular levels of ATP, phosphocreatine and phosphate are measured in vivo by ^{31}P-NMR spectroscopy; this technique may be used to detect defects of energy generation and to monitor the effects of treatment

Treatment

This is usually restricted to limiting exercise which should be stopped before symptoms are provoked. Mild aerobic exercise can be encouraged[63] but rigorous training may be dangerous. In glycolytic and fatty acid disorders, 'carbo loading' may be useful and continuous intake of glucose during exercise is helpful; fasting and high fat diets should be avoided, especially before exercise. Anecdotal reports suggest that carnitine therapy (50–100 mg/kg/d) may help prevent rhabdomyolysis in certain fatty acid oxidation defects such as VLCAD deficiency. Dietary supplementation with MCT oil provides a fuel source that bypasses the block in long chain fatty acid oxidation disorders and may also improve exercise intolerance.[64]

DEFECTS IN GALACTOSE METABOLISM

The main source of dietary galactose is lactose (glucose–galactose disaccharide), the predominant carbohydrate in milk and most milk-based infant formulae, in which it provides a considerable amount of energy. Galactose is metabolized for energy mainly in the liver, but must first be converted to glucose. Other tissues, such as erythrocytes, can metabolize galactose too, which provides a means to screen for galactose problems in the newborn. The metabolic pathway of galactose is depicted in Figure 26.12. Three metabolic errors are known.

Galactose-1-phosphate uridyltransferase deficiency (galactosemia) (step 2)

Clinical features

Infants with severe transferase deficiency become sick soon after beginning to ingest milk. The severity of the presentation depends on the quantity of milk ingested (breast milk contains more lactose than milk-based formulae) and the presence of residual transferase activity in liver. Severe cases mimic sepsis and many do develop Gram negative (especially *Escherichia coli*) or beta-streptococcal sepsis. Prior to the availability of newborn screening and in areas where newborn screening for galactosemia is not routine, many transferase-deficient infants die from sepsis and/or liver failure without the diagnosis being entertained, with the true cause of the infant's death not being revealed until the disease recurs in a subsequent sibling.

Typically, transferase-deficient infants present within a few days after birth with vomiting, diarrhea, failure to thrive and persistent jaundice. Hepatosplenomegaly, progressive liver dysfunction, hypoglycemia, anemia, coagulopathy with purpura and deficient clotting factors, and the biochemical findings of the renal Fanconi syndrome (see Ch. 18, p. 550) are typical. Cataracts may be evident at birth or appear

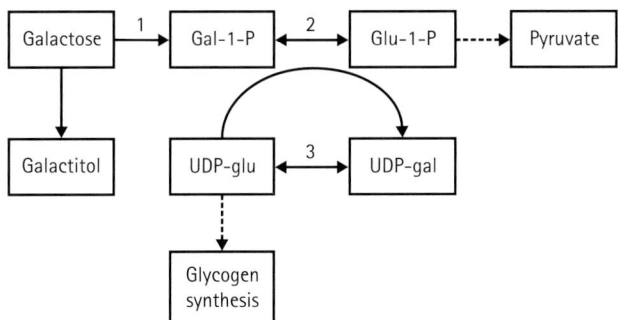

Fig. 26.12 Galactose metabolism. 1, galactokinase; 2, galactose 1-phosphate uridyltransferase; 3, uridine diphosphate galactose 4-apimerose.

soon after. Edema, ascites, malnutrition, cachexia and septicemia usually presage a fatal outcome from hepatic failure within a few weeks if the condition is not treated. Mental retardation and behavioral abnormalities develop in the absence of treatment if the disease has a more protracted course. When residual enzyme activity is present, or with poor control, the course is less catastrophic, with failure to thrive and cataracts being the major features.

The acute abnormalities are rapidly corrected by complete elimination of galactose from the diet.[65] With treatment, the cataracts and even the cirrhosis reverse. However, long term complications are frequent, regardless of how early or how well the infant is treated. Overall, there is a slight reduction in intelligence and visual perceptual skills; 50% have dyspraxic speech, and hypergonadotrophic hypogonadism with ovarian failure and often sterility occurs in approximately 80% of females. The causes of these late complications are unknown but probably prenatal.[65] Testicular function is unaffected.

Diagnosis

The simplest screening test is examination of the urine for reducing sugars (Clinitest) performed 24–36 h *after* the start of lactose-containing feeds. This test, however, is neither completely sensitive nor specific. If the infant is feeding poorly, there may be no galactose in the urine. In addition, other reducing substances, such as antibiotics, may cause a false positive Clinitest reaction. It must be noted that dipstick tests for 'sugar' in urine specifically detect glucose and do not react with galactose.

Newborn screening tests (see Ch. 4) for blood galactose, galactose metabolites or erythrocyte transferase enzyme activity (Beutler test) are in wide use, but often the results are only available after symptoms have already developed. The metabolite galactose-1-phosphate (gal-1-P) is markedly elevated even in cord blood, enabling early detection in high-risk infants. Vomiting or the use of nonlactose formulae may obscure the diagnosis and blood transfusion or exchange transfusion negate the erythrocyte assays for gal-1-P and the enzyme. Clinical suspicion, even without supporting lab results, is enough reason to initiate treatment and for quantitative assays of erythrocyte galactose metabolites, enzyme assays or mutation analysis. Galactose tolerance tests should never be undertaken if the diagnosis is suspected.

The most obvious histological changes occur in the liver. There is fatty infiltration, fibrosis, bile duct proliferation and pseudoacinar arrangement of hepatic cells. The renal changes consist of widening of the proximal tubules and alterations of the tubular epithelium.

Transferase activity can be assayed in erythrocytes, cultured fibroblasts and chorionic villi.

Variants

There are many variants with lesser deficiencies of enzyme activity. The commonest is the Duarte mutation; 1 in 25 people are carriers and they have about 75% of normal enzyme activity. Duarte homozygotes have about 50% and Duarte/classical compound heterozygotes (who carry one Duarte and one galactosemia allele) have about 10–25% activity. Such cases often, but not invariably, have elevated blood gal-1-P and are often detected by routine newborn screening. If they drink lactose-containing formula or breast milk, gal-1-P remains high for months but gradually falls to normal as lactose becomes a smaller portion of total energy intake.

There is no evidence that the gal-1-P or other galactose metabolites are toxic in these cases or that there is any risk for any of the long or short term complications of classical galactosemia, and opinion is divided as to whether galactose restriction should be recommended. Some authorities recommend nonlactose formula for the first year; others allow partial breast-feeding, while still others allow lactose intake to continue unrestricted. Often, clinical practice in this matter seems to be guided by medicolegal concerns.

Several other known mutations cause partial transferase deficiency and are associated either with mild galactosemia or are entirely asymptomatic. A specific mutation common to blacks is associated with complete transferase deficiency in erythrocytes but 10% normal activity in the liver and intestine and a mild phenotype.

Treatment

In infants with the full-blown disease (i.e. complete transferase deficiency), elimination of dietary galactose corrects all of the acute problems within a few days if treatment is begun soon enough to prevent irreversible complications. Soy milk (which contains galactose but in a nonbioavailable form) or synthetic formulae, which do not contain lactose, are used. On the diet, weight gain ensues, residual liver damage is rare and usually the cataracts resolve.[64]

Without question, the diet should be strictly followed for the first several years. It is less clear how important strict galactose restriction is for older children. Some authorities believe that the diet requires life-long meticulous attention to detail, but the occurrence of long term complications from galactosemia, including speech dyspraxia, tremor, ataxia and seizures, does not correlate with dietary galactose exposure.[66] Once solid foods are introduced, it becomes more difficult to offer a truly galactose-free diet. Many foods contain unlabeled lactose and even many fruits and vegetables contain galactose largely in the form of complex saccharides (fiber) that, for the most part, are not bioavailable; the overall contribution of galactose from these sources is unknown. In general, the list of foods to be avoided includes dairy products, some breads, sausage and candies which contain lactose, and other food products that list whey, casein or caseinates, or milk solids as ingredients. Also, some medications may contain lactose. Such diets are very restrictive and can lead to eating disorders and serious parental anxiety.

With the evidence that individuals with galactosemia synthesize significant quantities of galactose metabolites (see below), other authorities now believe that, after childhood, obsessive adherence is unnecessary and small quantities of galactose are safe, although deliberate and continuous high exposure is clearly contraindicated. Adults can tolerate small quantities of galactose without acute symptoms or obvious biochemical abnormalities; the long term safety of this is not known and some restrictions are clearly needed until further studies have been performed. Some children on a relaxed regimen show deteriorating school performance and behavior problems. Life-long galactose restriction remains the standard of care.

Because cataracts may be present at birth, cord blood gal-1-P is often markedly elevated and because gal-1-P may also be increased in the mother's blood, prenatal restriction of galactose has been attempted. However, this seems to have no effect upon the long term outcome.[67] Heterozygote offspring of properly treated homozygous mothers appear to be completely normal.

Self-intoxication

About 12–24 mg/kg/d galactose is synthesized by these patients;[68] some galactose is essential for the synthesis of galactolipids and galactoproteins. Moreover, lactose is synthesized normally in the milk of a lactating galactosemic mother. It is not surprising that, even with the use of strict galactose-free diets or parenteral nutrition, gal-1-P remains elevated in the blood of classical galactosemics. Galactose ingestion certainly raises the erythrocyte gal-1-P further and this test is still used to monitor diet compliance; in view of the dual sources, elevated values may be misinterpreted.

Galactitol from free galactose is the likely cause of cataracts. The cause of the acute and long term complications is not known; they have been attributed to gal-1-P toxicity but, by inference from the variants, this seems unlikely. It appears likely that they are largely determined prenatally.

Galactokinase deficiency

As soon as galactose is consumed by individuals with galactokinase deficiency, it accumulates in the blood and urine; some is reduced to the polyol galactitol that causes cataracts because of osmotic swelling and disruption of lens fibers. Gal-1-P and UDP-galactose (UDP-gal) levels are normal and cataract is the only clinical abnormality directly related to the enzyme defect. Fetuses of affected females may also develop cataracts, as may heterozygotes in later life. A galactose-free diet is indicated and should be continued for life. Early treatment prevents cataracts or

arrests their further increase. A similar diet has been proposed for heterozygotes but no long term studies have been reported. Prenatal diagnosis is possible

Uridine diphosphate galactose-4-epimerase deficiency

This disorder occurs in two forms: one confined only to erythrocytes, the second being generalized, affecting the liver as well. The former is completely symptomless and needs no treatment. Generalized epimerase deficiency is clinically similar to transferase deficiency and galactose, gal-1-P and UDP-gal increase after galactose consumption. Dietary galactose restriction is followed by a drop of all three metabolites in the blood. UDP-gal is a critical substrate for the production of sphingolipids for the brain and dietary intake of approximately 1.5–2 g galactose/d is thought to be necessary to meet the requirement of UDP-gal while simultaneously preventing gal-1-P accumulation.

DEFECTS IN FRUCTOSE METABOLISM (FIG. 26.13)

The main dietary sources of fructose are fruits, fruit juices, vegetables, potatoes, honey and all products that contain sucrose (fructose–glucose). Sorbitol, an artificial sweetener, is oxidized by the enzyme sorbitol dehydrogenase to fructose.

Fructose-1-phosphate aldolase deficiency (hereditary fructose intolerance) (step 2)

There are three aldolase isozymes, A, B and C, each with specific properties and tissue localization. In this condition, aldolase B is deficient; it is localized in liver, intestine and kidneys and normally cleaves fructose-1-phosphate (F-1-P) and fructose-1,6-diphosphate (F-1,6-P) into two trioses. These trioses are then substrates either for glycolysis or for

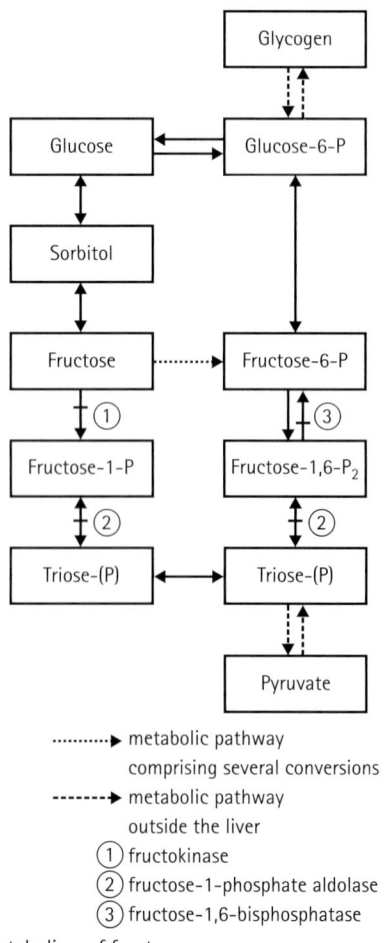

Fig. 26.13   Metabolism of fructose.

gluconeogenesis. In hereditary fructose intolerance, F-1-P accumulates as soon as the patient ingests fructose; it is very toxic and it inhibits several enzymes of glycogenolysis and gluconeogenesis, causing rapid and profound hypoglycemia. Furthermore, the intracellular supply of phosphate is sequestered as F-1-P which prevents the regeneration of ATP from ADP. Under these conditions, ADP is dephosphorylated to AMP and then further metabolized to uric acid.

Clinical features

Symptoms develop at the very first introduction of fruit or fructose containing infant formula (some soy formulae contain fructose), or when honey is misused as a pacifier. This usually occurs during weaning, since breast milk and most infant formulae do not contain fructose. Acute symptoms include vomiting, diaphoresis, tremor, lethargy, convulsions and other manifestations associated with hypoglycemia. Chronic exposure to fructose leads to progressive liver damage with anorexia, failure to thrive, jaundice, hepatomegaly, splenomegaly, ascites, edema and hemorrhage. Aversion to sweets develops early in life and, by avoiding sweetened foods, most patients, if they survive infancy, unknowingly protect themselves from the toxic effects of fructose. Occasionally the condition is only diagnosed in adult life. Remarkably, the teeth often remain free of caries.

Diagnosis

Fructosemia is easy to diagnose if the feeding history is carefully obtained. Metabolic abnormalities following acute fructose ingestion include hypoglycemia, hypophosphatemia, hyperuricemia and hypermagnesemia. Chronic ingestion is associated with all the manifestations of renal Fanconi syndrome (see Ch. 18) and markedly abnormal liver function tests often with increased levels of some amino acids such as tyrosine and methionine. Absence of these findings in a patient with fructose avoidance behavior does not eliminate the diagnosis. Liver biopsy, during acute or chronic fructose ingestion, shows extensive abnormalities, including focal areas of necrosis, fatty degeneration, proliferation of bile ducts, formation of pseudoacini and ultimately biliary cirrhosis.

The presence of a reducing sugar in urine following fructose ingestion is an important clue. When the diagnosis is suspected but not proven, DNA analysis can be definitive. More than 80% of individuals of European descent with hereditary fructose intolerance can be identified by DNA analysis for a small set of common mutations.[69] However, most laboratories only test for specific mutations.

In this disease, a fructose tolerance test can be dangerous and even fatal. If it is deemed absolutely necessary, the test should be executed in hospital with full medical support available, under the guidance of a metabolic specialist and only when the patient is clinically stable. A positive test is signaled by a rise of at least 50% in serum uric acid and a drop of 40–50% in the serum glucose and phosphate. In unclear cases, enzymatic assay of a liver biopsy may be necessary.

Treatment

All dietary sources of fructose must be strictly eliminated; this includes fruits, fruit juices, vegetables, potatoes, honey and all products that contain sucrose (fructose–glucose) or sorbitol. This diet prevents all abnormalities and restores liver and kidney function to normal, except in cases of severe liver failure. The effects of the treatment are influenced by the age of the patient, the amount and duration of fructose ingestion and the residual aldolase B activity. Young infants are most susceptible to life threatening fructose toxicity. In older children, even small amounts of fructose can elicit symptoms, and continued exposure to small amounts, although insufficient to cause acute symptoms, may cause growth retardation. Successful treatment requires detailed knowledge of the fructose content of all foods.

Fructose-1,6-diphosphatase deficiency (step 3)

This enzyme is one of the unidirectional enzymes in the pathway of gluconeogenesis and is also important for the conversion of fructose into glucose. Fasting, fructose ingestion or metabolic stress lead to hypoglycemia and increased protein and fat catabolism, resulting in the accumulation of lactate, pyruvate, alanine, ketone bodies and glycerol.

Clinical features

The symptoms of this disorder are similar to those of fructosemia or type 1 glycogen storage disease. They may develop in the neonatal period or later, provoked by insufficient food intake. Dietary sugar ingestion is usually not the inciting event precipitating metabolic crisis, as these patients are not nearly as sensitive to fructose as are those with hereditary fructose intolerance. Fulminating lactic acidosis and hypoglycemia can lead to hyperventilation, hypotonia, hepatomegaly, nausea, vomiting, lethargy and convulsions. Liver and kidney function may deteriorate and the course may be either severe and rapidly fatal or episodic, being exacerbated during acute metabolic stress. Hepatomegaly is often present.

Diagnosis

Hypoglycemia and lactic acidosis together with or without evidence of liver dysfunction demand metabolic investigation. Characteristically, glycerol and glycerol-3-phosphate accumulate during hypoglycemia and are excreted in the urine. These metabolites derive from excessive proteolysis and fatty acid oxidation that increase to compensate for the lack of glucose. The lactic acidosis can be profound and recalcitrant to therapy. Liver histology may show fatty degeneration and fibrosis and the renal Fanconi syndrome may be apparent. All these are reminiscent of type 1 glycogen storage disease. A fasting test might elicit the above symptoms. Fasting fructose or glycerol stress tests are not without risk, and should be avoided in most cases. Definitive diagnosis requires enzyme assay of leukocytes or liver biopsy tissue but the leukocyte assay is fraught with difficulties.

Treatment

Treatment consists of frequent meals and the restriction, but not total elimination, of fructose, sucrose and sorbitol intake. Prolonged fasting must be avoided and early and aggressive treatment with i.v. glucose and bicarbonate may be necessary during infections.

Other disorders of fructose metabolism

In *fructokinase* deficiency (essential fructosuria) (step 1), fructose metabolism is blocked in the liver, intestine and kidney, and fructose levels in blood and urine rise if the patient consumes fructose. The condition is benign. Fructose malabsorption is reasonably common and is associated with fermentative diarrhea following quite modest fructose ingestion.

A defect of *aldolase A*, detectable in fibroblasts, is associated with nonspherocytic hemolytic anemia; some cases have had microcephaly and dysmorphic features.

DEFECTS IN GLYCOGEN METABOLISM: GLYCOGEN STORAGE DISORDERS AND ALLIED DISEASES

Several inherited enzyme defects interfere with the metabolism of glycogen. Defects in glycogen synthesis severely limit glycogen storage and are associated with postprandial hyperglycemia followed by rebound fasting hypoglycemia. Defects in degradation often raise the glycogen content of the organ in which the enzyme is normally localized, causing local tissue dysfunction. Glycogen is a giant polysaccharide that is stored mainly in liver and muscle. Around 90% of the glucose molecules are linked in straight chains through alpha-1,4 bonds; about 8% are linked through alpha-1,6 bonds that form branching points. The usual glycogen concentration of the liver is 5–7 g/100 g wet weight and in muscle < 2 g/100 g wet weight, these concentrations being influenced by factors such as the nutritional status, the pre- or post-prandial condition of the patient and hormones. Therefore, quantitative glycogen analyses on tissue biopsies, while often done, may be difficult to interpret.

The major function of glycogen in liver is to provide reserve glucose for export to other organs, mainly the brain. In contrast, muscle glycogen is only used as a fuel for ATP synthesis during muscle contraction. It follows that a glycogen storage disorder (GSD) involving the liver is usually characterized by fasting hypoglycemia, whereas the muscle defects are characterized by myopathy.

For the synthesis of glycogen (Fig. 26.14), glucose is phosphorylated to glucose-6-phosphate, then converted to glucose-1-phosphate. The enzyme glycogen synthase (enzyme 1) then catalyzes the polymerization of glucose-1-phosphate molecules into straight chain glycogen. Branching enzyme (enzyme 2) adds glucose-1-phosphate in alpha-1,6 linkages to form branch points.

In the initial step of glycogenolysis, whether in liver or muscle, a phosphorylase cleaves glucose-1-phosphate molecules from the alpha-1,4 linkages of the outer chains. Liver phosphorylase (enzyme 3) is distinct from muscle phosphorylase (enzyme 4). The activity of both enzymes is influenced by hormones, mainly glucagon, insulin and epiniphrine (adrenaline). Phosphorylase activity ceases as it nears a branch point; further degradation of the glucose polymer and removal of the branch point is mediated by debranching enzyme (enzyme 5). The product of glycogenolysis, glucose-1-phosphate, is converted to glucose-6-phosphate. In the liver, glucose-6-phosphate is predominantly dephosphorylated to glucose by glucose-6-phosphatase (enzyme 6). In muscle, glucose-6-phosphate is consumed as a substrate for glycolysis and ATP production.

This main pathway of glycogen degradation by phosphorylation and dephosphorylation in the cytoplasm is different from that in lysosomes. Pompe disease (GSD II), a lysosomal GSD, results from deficiency of lysosomal alpha-1,4-glucosidase. The severity of this disorder illustrates the importance of lysosome-mediated glycogen degradation (see p. 1112).

Traditionally, the GSDs have been classified numerically or by eponym. However, different numbers have been assigned to the same enzymatic defect and the specific enzyme nosology is now preferable (Table 26.7). For historical reasons, all three systems are used in this chapter.

Two defects of glycogen synthesis are known, glycogen synthase (enzyme 1) deficiency and branching enzyme (enzyme 2) deficiency. The

Table 26.7 Glycogen storage diseases, classification

Type	Deficient enzyme	Tissue involved	Main clinical findings
IA	Glucose-6-phosphatase	Liver, kidney	Hepatomegaly, hypoglycemia, lactic acidosis
IB	Glucose-6-phosphatase-related transport	Liver, leukocytes	Same as IA + immunological abnormalities
IC			Same as IA
ID			Same as IA
II	Acid α-glucosidase (lysosomal)	Generalized	Infant form: cardiorespiratory failure. Later forms: myopathy
III	Debranching enzyme	Liver, muscle, heart	Hepatomegaly, hypoglycemia, myopathy
IV	Branching enzyme	Liver	Hepatosplenomegaly, cirrhosis
V	Phosphorylase	Muscle	Myopathy, exercise intolerance
VI	Phosphorylase system	Liver (muscle)	Hepatomegaly (myopathy)
VII	Phosphofructokinase and other defects of glycolysis	Muscle (erythrocytes)	Myopathy, exercise intolerance (hemolysis)
0	Glycogen synthase	Liver	Hypoglycemia

disorders of glycogenolysis can generally be separated into two groups, hepatic dysfunction and hypoglycemia or skeletal myopathy, depending upon the normal location of the missing enzyme.

Glycogen synthase deficiency (GSD type 0)
Clinical features
This defect is usually grouped with the GSDs since it involves the same metabolic pathway. Failure to synthesize glycogen results in rapid and profound hyperglycemia after even quite modest meals. This is followed by a rapid and profound fall of the blood glucose when postprandial events normally turn to glycogenolysis to maintain blood glucose. Facile ketosis and postprandial hyperlactacidemia can be seen. The liver is not enlarged and its glycogen content is low.

Diagnosis and treatment
The enzyme defect can only be demonstrated in the liver. Mutation analysis may also be helpful. The differential diagnosis can include Munchausen-by-proxy (see Ch. 5, p. 50) from occult insulin administration.

Treatment consists of small, frequent protein-rich meals and regular uncooked cornstarch feedings to prevent hypoglycemia and ketosis.

Branching enzyme deficiency (GSD type IV)
Clinical features
The main features of this disorder are marked hepatomegaly with progressive cirrhosis, splenomegaly, muscle hypotonia and weakness, hypo- or areflexia, retarded motor milestones, growth retardation and normal mental development. Death usually occurs in the first years of life, although liver transplant may prolong survival, and milder forms exist. Rarely, milder variants with myopathy are observed in adults and cardiomyopathy with heart failure may be the only presentation.

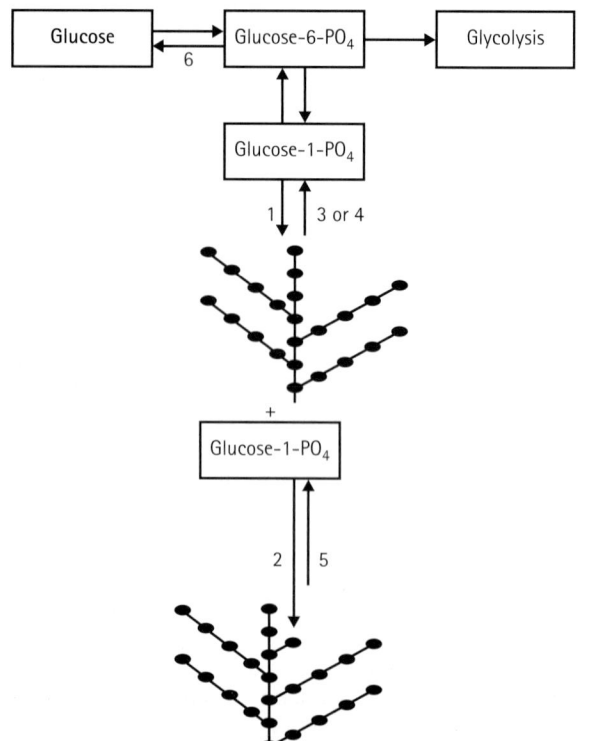

Fig. 26.14 Glycogen metabolism. 1, glycogen synthase; 2, branching enzyme; 3, liver phosphorylase; 4, muscle phosphorylase; 5, debranching enzyme; 6, glucose-6-phosphatase.

Diagnosis and treatment

The metabolic derangements are hypoglycemia, usually mild, increased transaminases and decreased clotting factors. The enzyme defect causes insufficient branching of the glycogen molecule and its prolonged inner and outer chains give it the appearance and properties of amylopectin. Apparently this abnormal glycogen is difficult to mobilize. It acts as a foreign body and glucose release from it is hampered. In contrast to the liver, muscle histology is usually normal in spite of absent enzyme activity in that tissue. The enzyme defect is expressed in many tissues including fibroblasts; antenatal diagnosis is feasible.

Treatment is symptomatic and consists of frequent high carbohydrate feedings and, eventually, gastric drip feeding. This treatment, however, does not prevent liver failure. Liver transplantation has been successful but does not address the myopathy.

Glucose-6-phosphatase deficiency (GSD type IA, von Gierke disease)

Clinical features

The most conspicuous clinical findings are a protruding abdomen because of marked hepatomegaly, hypotrophic muscles, truncal obesity, a rounded 'doll face' and short stature (Fig. 26.15). Because glucose-6-phosphatase activity is required for both glycogenolysis and gluconeogenesis, severe symptomatic hypoglycemia is frequent, often occurring during the night or after even short periods of reduced caloric intake. Even minor delays or reduction of carbohydrate intake may provoke hypoglycemic attacks that are accompanied by lactic acidosis. The liver may be enlarged at birth; its size increases gradually and it may achieve a total span of 15–20 cm. Initially, the liver is smooth with a normal consistency, but by 10–20 years age, it becomes firmer and nodular due to the development of benign adenomas. Cirrhosis, however, does not typically develop. Severe hypertriglyceridemia is caused by poor glycemic control and can be associated with acute pancreatitis. The spleen is normal in size, but the kidneys are moderately enlarged. Easy bruising, epistaxis and even frank hemorrhage after surgery or other event, may be troublesome due to impaired platelet function. Linear growth is retarded but truncal obesity is obvious; both are improved through judicious treatment. Cerebral function is usually normal so long as hypoglycemic damage is prevented. Left untreated, associated hyperuricemia frequently causes gout.

Because of effective therapy preventing fatal hypoglycemia, the life expectancy of these individuals has greatly improved, and consequently some late-onset complications have emerged. Rarely, hepatic adenomas become malignant, hyperuricemia and gout are now rare, but progressive focal glomerular sclerosis is a serious risk and can lead to renal failure. Anemia and osteopenia are also late-onset problems.

Metabolic derangements

Failure to dephosphorylate glucose-6-phosphate means that glucose production from both glycogenolysis and gluconeogenesis is blocked. However, the Embden–Meyerhof glycolytic pathway (see Fig. 26.11) is intact and during fasting is intensified under hormonal stimulation. This increases lactate production that can serve as a fuel to the brain. However, chronic lactic acidemia is usual and probably contributes to the retarded growth and osteoporosis. Excess acetyl-CoA is also produced and is converted into fatty acids and cholesterol; this probably underlies the hypertriglyceridemia, hypercholesterolemia and hyperprebetalipoproteinemia seen in most of these patients. Some of the excess glucose-6-phosphate is channeled via the pentose monophosphate shunt to urate, thus explaining the hyperuricemia, which can be severe.

Diagnosis

In the past, oral glucose tolerance tests were employed as a diagnostic aid. During this test, in GSD I patients, the blood lactate *decreases* from an initially high level to (near) normal. This is the opposite from the normal response. Oral glucose tolerance tests, fasting and other stress tests, however, can be hazardous. Assay of glucose-6-phosphatase activity in liver confirms the diagnosis and delineates the different forms of this syndrome (see below). In the liver, fat accumulation often exceeds that of glycogen; this does not contradict the biochemical diagnosis. DNA mutational analysis is becoming increasingly available. Antenatal diagnosis can only be done on fetal liver tissue or by DNA studies.

Treatment

Acute hypoglycemia should be treated with glucose 0.25 g/kg in 50–100 ml water orally or by intravenous bolus infusion; importantly, this should be followed immediately by an intravenous drip providing twice the normal glucose requirement (see below). Lactic acidosis usually resolves without the need for sodium bicarbonate since glucose administration suppresses lactate overproduction. Oral nutrition is reintroduced as soon as possible.

For maintenance, a high carbohydrate diet with 60–65% of the total energy as carbohydrates, 10% as protein and 20–25% as fat is used. Both lactose and sucrose intake should probably be restricted since neither galactose nor fructose can be converted to glucose because of the enzyme defect. Low-lactose, sucrose-free formulae are preferable if breast milk is not available. Maltose or dextrins can be added to give a total 65% of energy as carbohydrate. Feedings should be administered at 2–3 h intervals around the clock before the age of 3 months, followed by a wider spacing from 3–6 months onwards. Gastric drip feeding at night is introduced as early as possible using carbohydrate derived from glucose, maltose or glucose polymers to provide a constant supply of carbohydrate at 7–9 mg/kg/min for infants, 5–6 mg/kg/min for 1–6-year-olds and 4 mg/kg/min for older children. This treatment improves the clinical condition, decreases the liver size, suppresses the bleeding tendency and promotes growth. Since disconnection of the tubing or pump malfunction in the GSD I patient receiving enteral feedings can be fatal, good equipment and alarm systems are crucial.

Most older patients prefer to use uncooked cornstarch as a slow-release form of carbohydrate which becomes the mainstay of therapy. Because of its thick consistency, even mixed in water, it cannot easily be given via a gastric or nasogastric tube but can be given orally, between or together with meals, and normalizes the blood sugar for several hours (Fig. 26.16); with close supervision, care and good parents, it can also

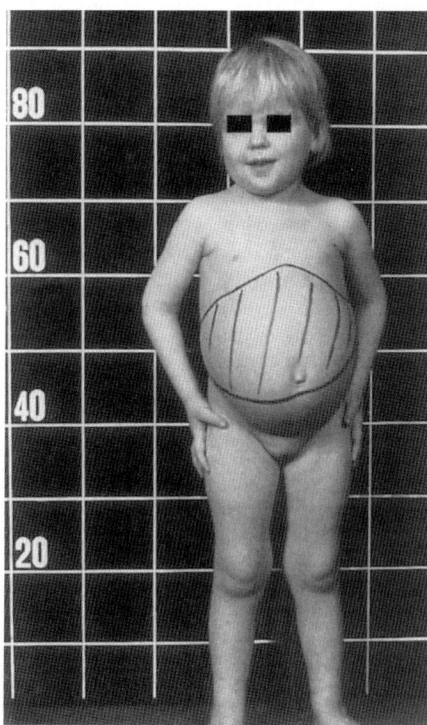

Fig. 26.15 Typical features of a patient with glucose-6-phosphatase deficiency.

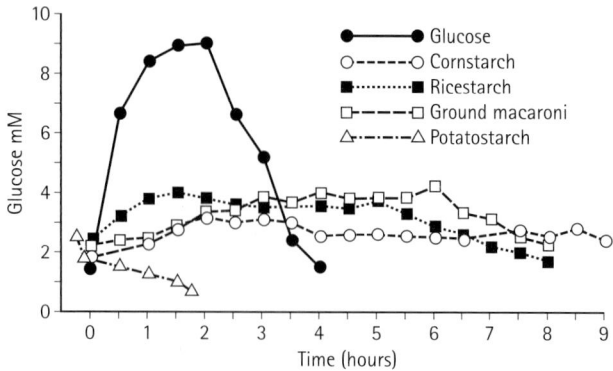

Fig. 26.16 Blood glucose curves of a patient with glucose-6-phosphatase deficiency after the ingestion of glucose or various uncooked starches, 2 g/kg body weight each.

be used in infants, although prior to about 1 year of age infants may not produce sufficient amylase to metabolize the cornstarch effectively. Early introduction of cornstarch may, however, induce earlier production of amylase. Even optimum treatment may not correct the hypoglycemia, lactic acidosis and hyperlipidemia completely and some patients continue to grow poorly. Captopril is being evaluated for treating the renal disease; osteoporosis requires a generous calcium and vitamin D intake and periodic assessment of bone density. Hyperuricemia is treated with allopurinol. Liver transplantation has been successful.

Glucose-6-phosphate translocase deficiencies (GSD types IB and IC)

These are defects of translocases located on the luminal wall of the endoplasmic reticulum that normally allow entry of glucose-6-phosphate (GSD type IB) and exit of phosphate (GSD type IC). Both defects render glucose-6-phosphatase functionally inactive. A defect of glucose translocase has not yet been described.

The clinical and metabolic symptoms and treatment of GSD IB are not discernibly different from GSD IA except for a grave propensity to immunological abnormalities. There is neutropenia and defective neutrophil and monocyte function; bacterial infections are frequent and may be fatal. Inflammatory bowel disease akin to Crohn disease and myelogenous leukemia are added potential complications. The prognosis of translocase deficiency traditionally was worse than that of type IA because of the increased risk of metabolic derangements due to the frequent infections, but the introduction of granulocyte macrophage-stimulating factor (GM-CSF) as a treatment has improved the prognosis tremendously (see Ch. 27).

Translocase 1 defect (GSD type IB) accounts for 12–15% of the total cases of glucose-6-phosphatase deficiency; type IC is extremely rare.

Debranching enzyme deficiency (GSD type III, 'limit dextrinosis')

During glycogenolysis, this enzyme normally prunes the alpha-1,6 linkage branch points as the straight, alpha-1,4 links are being broken down by phosphorylase. When this does not happen, glycogen degradation stops at the branch points, leaving 'limit dextrin'. This abnormal glycogen may behave as a foreign body and elicit high transaminase levels, recurrent jaundice, fibrosis and even cirrhosis. Gluconeogenesis, however, is unimpeded and this drains glucogenic amino acids from muscle protein, presumably contributing to poor growth and muscle wasting. This also explains the observation that GSD III patients are not as prone to severe hypoglycemia as GSD I patients.

Clinical features

Two forms exist; one is confined to liver but the more common one involves the muscles as well. In younger children the liver symptoms predominate and are very similar to GSD type IA with hypoglycemia

in the neonatal period or later or during decreased food intake or metabolic stress. The liver is markedly enlarged and extremely high transaminases are common; the spleen and kidneys are not affected. Hypotonia, truncal obesity and a doll face develop and the patient may show retarded growth which gradually catches up later. Motor development is slow but mental development is usually normal. The liver has a normal consistency, but rarely cirrhosis may develop. Surprisingly, for unknown reasons, the liver size often returns to normal at or before puberty.

In the myopathic form, which has probably been underdiagnosed in the past, there is increasing muscle weakness and a slowly progressive distal muscle wasting, starting in childhood or later. It may be accompanied by cardiomyopathy with left ventricular hypertrophy and electrocardiogram (ECG) abnormalities. These developments warrant close supervision of muscle function and regular ECG in all patients.

Diagnosis

Conspicuous findings during fasting are ketosis (not lactic acidosis), hyperlipidemia (mainly hypercholesterolemia) and hypoglycemia. An oral galactose tolerance test elicits a normal increase of blood glucose and an abnormal increase of blood lactate. A fasting glucagon test is characterized by an abnormally flat glucose response but such stress tests can be dangerous in GSD.

The liver pathology shows an increase of reticulin fibers between hepatocytes and of fibrous tissue in portal tracts. In the myopathic form, the muscles show myofibrillary destruction and degeneration of the neuromuscular junctions. Enzyme assay in liver or muscle is required to confirm the diagnosis.

Treatment and prognosis

Treatment of the hepatic form is similar to that of GSD I except that restriction of galactose and fructose is not necessary as both can be converted normally into glucose. Although gastric drip-feeding is not a prerequisite for glucose homeostasis at a later age, this treatment and extra protein may be useful in delaying or improving the myopathy. Thus, the diet for both forms of the disease should contain approximately 55–60% energy as carbohydrates, particularly starch, 15–20% energy as protein and 20–25% energy as fat, predominantly polyunsaturated; uncooked cornstarch is also often used. The late development of myopathy and cardiomyopathy remains a concern.

Liver phosphorylase and liver phosphorylase b kinase deficiencies (GSD type VI)

Phosphorylase b kinase is required to convert phosphorylase b (inactive) to the activated form and the kinase itself is regulated by another (cyclic AMP-dependent) kinase, the whole system being stimulated by hormones, particularly glucagon. The clinical heterogeneity of phosphorylase b kinase deficiency is due to the fact that it consists of four different subunits at least one of which is coded on the X chromosome. These two defects are discussed together because their clinical features and metabolic derangements are similar.

Clinical features

In early childhood, pronounced hepatomegaly, without splenomegaly, and a protuberant abdomen due to muscle hypotonia are the most striking features; the liver enlargement resolves slowly and usually disappears by puberty. Equally, the muscle hypotonia and weakness, which initially cause slow motor development, also tend to improve. Growth and puberty are often delayed. Mental development is normal. There are exceptions to this usually mild course, particularly in phosphorylase b kinase deficiency, of which many variants exist. Rare cases have had combinations of hepatic symptoms and myopathy, fatal cardiomyopathy and even myopathy without hepatic symptoms. The X-linked form of phosphorylase b kinase deficiency is the most common and mildest form, and can present with isolated hepatomegaly in children.

Diagnosis

A tentative diagnosis is based on the pronounced hepatomegaly in contrast to the mild clinical and metabolic findings. Mild fasting hypoglycemia may develop; elevated serum transaminases, hypercholesterolemia and a marked tendency to fasting ketosis are evident at a young age, but normalize completely by puberty.

An oral galactose test is abnormal as blood lactate increases excessively. Contrary to expectation, glucagon tests are not of much help as the increase of blood glucose is variable. Fasting or stress tests may be dangerous. Kinase defects can theoretically be detected in blood cells but assay of liver or muscle or DNA studies may be required in some cases.

Treatment

Treatment of this self-limiting disease is not necessary except for prevention of hypoglycemia, which may require uncooked cornstarch. Use of polyunsaturated fat suppresses hypercholesterolemia. Severe forms of phosphorylase b kinase deficiency may be refractory to dietary treatment, and liver transplantation may be indicated for severe cases with liver failure.

Muscle phosphorylase deficiency (GSD type V, McArdle syndrome)

Clinical features

This disorder is characterized by increasing intolerance for strenuous exercise. During early childhood no symptoms occur except easy fatiguability. In adults, strenuous muscle activity is accompanied by severe cramps and may be followed by rhabdomyolysis, which can precipitate anuria and renal failure. In middle life, the fatigue increases and muscle wasting and weakness predominate. The serum CPK may be permanently or intermittently elevated.

Diagnosis

In myophosphorylase deficiency, ischemic exercise testing shows that lactic acid production is blocked and release of ammonia and the purine nucleotide cycle compounds is exaggerated. The ensuing myogenic hyperuricemia is one of the characteristic features of defects of muscle glycogenolysis. The normal increase in lactate is also absent in other glycolytic defects in muscle, such as phosphofructokinase deficiency.

Phosphorylase activity must be assayed in muscle; liver phosphorylase is presumably normal, as is glucose homeostasis. DNA mutation analysis can be useful as there are several common mutations.

Treatment

Treatment is symptomatic and consists of the avoidance of strenuous exercise. 'Carbo loading' and a high protein diet are of some help and glucose should always be taken during exercise. Strenuous exercise is always a risk. Carefully monitored exercise training has been shown to improve muscle function.[63]

Muscle phosphofructokinase deficiency (GSD type VII)

Clinical features

The three clinical and metabolic characteristics of this rare disorder are myopathy, increased hemolysis and gout. The myopathy is similar to GSD type V and manifests itself in childhood by weakness, limitation of vigorous activity and exercise-induced cramps, accompanied by myoglobinuria and raised CPK. As in muscle phosphorylase deficiency, there is no rise of venous lactate after exercise and ammonia, inosine, hypoxanthine and urate are produced in excess. Continued myogenic hyperuricemia explains the gout. The block in glycolysis may be partly compensated by increased fatty acid oxidation. Different isoenzymes of phosphofructokinase exist in various tissues. The absence of the M-subunit in erythrocytes results in hemolytic anemia (see Ch. 23, p. 967).

Treatment

Provision of extra glucose does not bypass the enzyme defect and is therefore of no help. This is different from muscle phosphorylase defi-

ciency in which glucose enters the glycolytic pathway 'downstream' from the enzyme defect. A high protein diet and prevention of excessive activity are the only measures.

Lysosomal alpha-1,4-glucosidase deficiency (GSD type II, Pompe disease)

Deficiency of this enzyme, also called acid maltase deficiency, leads to a generalized GSD. However, this defect is not in the regular cascade of glycogenolysis and is not associated with defects of circulating fuels (see p. 1112).

DISORDERS OF PYRUVATE METABOLISM AND THE KREBS CYCLE, AND LACTIC ACIDEMIA

Glycolytic (see p. 1072), gluconeogenic, ketone and fatty acid (see p. 1067) pathways all feed into the Krebs cycle (Fig. 26.17) for aerobic metabolism. Pyruvate, derived from glycolysis or glucogenic amino acids, is converted to acetyl-CoA via the unidirectional pyruvate dehydrogenase complex (PDHC). Pyruvate is in equilibrium with lactate and the normal lactate:pyruvate ratio is about 20:1, being dependent upon the NAD:NADH ratio and the availability of oxygen for aerobic metabolism. If pyruvate oxidation is compromised, lactate accumulates, resulting in lactic acidosis. When this central furnace is disrupted, other precursor fuels such as organic acids also accumulate and can be detected in body fluids.

All the disorders of pyruvate metabolism are associated with neurological damage, usually of a severe onset any time after birth. Developmental and motor delay, seizures, pyramidal and/or basal ganglion signs are usually severe and present major problems.

Pyruvate dehydrogenase complex

Defects in this three-enzyme complex are the most common of the pyruvate disorders. The first component, E1, is the thiamine-dependent *dehydrogenase*. It has two subunits one of which is coded for on the X-chromosome. Female carriers of this defect may be almost as severely affected as males. Severe cases may show mild mid-facial hypoplasia,

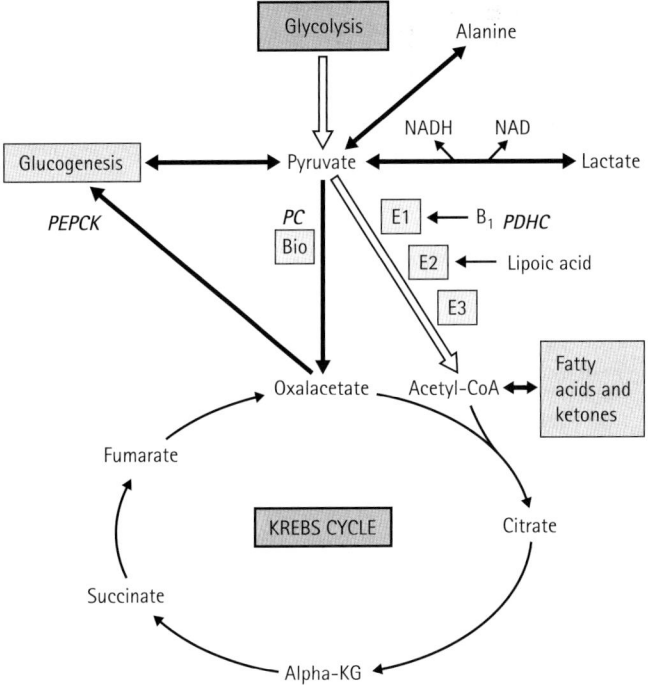

Fig. 26.17 Metabolic pathways involving lactate and pyruvate. PEPCK: phosphoenolpyruvate carboxykinase; PDHC: pyruvate dehydrogenase complex; PC: pyruvate carboxylase; Bio; biotin; B1: thiamine; E1,E2,E3: Separate complexes of PDHC; Alpha-KG: Alpha-ketoglutarate.

evidence of prenatal effects of the block. Apart from the severe neonatal forms, milder mutations can present with later onset of cerebellar signs with ataxia being prominent and proportionally less developmental delay. These signs are exacerbated by carbohydrate ingestion that can induce coma.

The other two components are *dihydrolipoamide acyltransferase* and *dihydrolipoamide dehydrogenase* (E2 and E3). These two involve lipoic acid and are common to other dehydrogenases, including branched chain aminoacid dehydrogenase and, if defective, involve additional metabolic systems. Deficiency usually causes very serious neurological damage.

Pyruvate carboxylase and phosphoenolpyruvate carboxykinase

These enzymes are both involved in recycling pyruvate to glucogenesis and defects can provoke hypoglycemia. Both can present with severe neonatal crises or with a more indolent course. Pyruvate carboxylase (PC) requires biotin and is thus involved in multiple carboxylase deficiency (p. 1066).

Diagnosis can be done on fibroblasts. Treatment is supportive with avoidance of hypoglycemia.

DEFECTS OF THE KREBS CYCLE

These include *alpha-keto acid dehydrogenase, fumarase* and *succinic dehydrogenase* (complex II of the respiratory chain, see below) deficiencies. All are associated with severe neurological disease and poor prognosis.

LACTIC ACIDEMIA

Diagnosis and treatment

Transient and acquired lactic acidemia is not an infrequent finding in any seriously ill child and may be caused by a number of conditions (Table 26.8). A struggling child, use of tourniquets during blood draw, poor tissue perfusion secondary to sepsis, cardiac or pulmonary disease, severe anemia, seizures, liver failure, toxins and IEM can all lead to an abnormal accumulation of L-lactate. Ischemia of tissues including brain and various brain defects, including cerebral atrophy, agenesis of the corpus callosum and brainstem, and deep gray matter abnormalities can also cause persistent lactic acidosis.

When acquired causes are not evident, primary (hereditary) lactic acidemia must be sought. However, it is often difficult to determine whether it is primary or secondary to conditions in a very sick child who does not have an IEM; indeed, these two possibilities are not mutually exclusive. Lactic acidosis may be fulminating or minimal. There may be facile ketosis and abnormal organic aciduria.

Initial laboratory investigations include serial measurements of blood (if feasible, arterial), lactate and, if possible, pyruvate. In general, a blood lactate:pyruvate ratio > 20 suggests a respiratory chain disorder; below that, a block proximal to the respiratory chain (e.g. pyruvate

dehydrogenase deficiency) is more likely. While the lactate:pyruvate ratio reflects the redox state in *the cytoplasm*, the plasma beta-hydroxybutyrate:acetoacetate ratio reflects the intramitochondrial redox state; a ratio > 1 suggests mitochondrial dysfunction. However, in most centers, *quantitative* assays for pyruvate, and the ketone bodies are unavailable or notoriously unreliable. Plasma alanine, which is transaminated pyruvate, is normally maintained in narrow limits and when elevated, often reflects an elevated pyruvate or a distorted redox state. Elevated CSF lactate may be present in some patients with normal blood lactate.

In general, acquired lactic acidemia corrects relatively quickly after the underlying cause is treated but primary causes tend to persist. This is a generalization because even in proven primary disorders the lactic acidemia may be transient. Every effort should be made to find the cause of the lactic acidosis, including echocardiography, brain MRI (preferably with spectroscopy as MRS can quantitate brain lactate) and appropriate metabolic investigations (Table 26.9). Confirmation of a suspected abnormality may be provided by measuring lactate and pyruvate levels in cultured fibroblasts. Precise diagnosis requires assays of leukocytes or fibroblasts and is only available in a few centers. Prenatal diagnosis is very tricky.

In most cases, the primary cause of the acidosis is not clear at the outset; thus it is necessary to make some empiric decisions. The acidosis may require large doses of bicarbonate for an extended period. PDHC may respond to a strict ketogenic diet; however, PC and phosphoenolpyruvate carboxykinase (PEPCK) deficiencies can become dramatically worse with it. Most other causes do not respond to such diets. In EI cases, thiamine up to 750 mg/d for an adult can be beneficial. Dichloroacetate is used to maintain the E1 in active form and it has had some limited success.[70]

D-Lactic acidemia

D-Lactate is not made by humans. D-Lactic acidemia is caused by intestinal bacterial overgrowth, usually associated with short bowel and blind loop syndromes, and may cause intermittent neurological symptoms, including dizziness, ataxia and disorientation. D-lactic acidemia is one

Table 26.8 Differential diagnosis of elevated blood lactate

Acquired causes
Poor peripheral perfusion
Sepsis/shock
Cardiorespiratory dysfunction
Spurious elevation/lab error
Tight tourniquet/difficult blood draw

Inborn errors of metabolism
Disorders of pyruvate metabolism and the Krebs cycle
Disorders of glucogeogenesis
Glycogen storage diseases
Disorders of fatty acid oxidation
Disorders of mitochondrial function
Disorders of organic acid metabolism
Disorders of biotin metabolism

Table 26.9 Evaluation of lactic acidemia

History	Traumatic delivery, infectious contacts, toxin/drug ingestion, family history of metabolic disease
Physical examination	Cardiac hemodynamic state, capillary refill,* ?hepatomegaly
Bedside tests	Blood pressure, pulse oximetry*
Other studies	Chest X-ray, ECG, echocardiography, EEG, head imaging
Laboratory tests	Routine – complete blood count with differential, glucose, electrolytes, liver enzymes, blood urea nitrogen, creatinine, blood gases, serial lactate/pyruvate measurements, blood cultures (urine and CSF cultures if indicated), toxicology screen
Special tests	Metabolic studies – quantitative plasma amino acids, ammonia level, acylcarnitine profile, urine organic acids Assay of enzyme activities in WBC or fibroblasts Muscle exercise testing Muscle biopsy for histochemistry, electron microscopic, immunological and biochemical studies 31P NMR spectroscopy DNA studies on muscle, WBC, fibroblasts, liver, etc

*Decreased cardiac function (e.g. secondary to cardiomyopathy) may be present in patients with apparently normal perfusion, blood pressure and cardiac examination.

cause of unexplained acidosis because the D dimer is not detected by standard lactate assays but is seen on organic acid analysis; it requires a specific method. It is easily treated by a course of oral antibiotics.

MITOCHONDRIAL DISEASE

Mitochondria contain a special DNA (mtDNA) that replicates continuously and is highly pleomorphic with differences between individuals and even greater differences between populations. This makes it useful for forensic and anthropological studies. mtDNA is double-stranded and circular, being 16 569 base pairs long. It encodes 13 subunits of the respiratory chain, 22 transfer RNAs (tRNAs) and two ribosomal RNAs (rRNAs) (Fig. 26.18). Mitochondria contain ~1000 structural proteins and enzymes, including the tricarboxylic acid and fatty acid oxidation cycles, part of the urea cycle and numerous others, all of which are encoded by nuclear genes, being imported into the mitochondrial matrix after initial cytoplasmic synthesis.

The term mitochondrial disease is limited to disorders of the respiratory (electron transport ETC) chain with resultant decreased production of adenosine triphosphate (ATP). Disorders of other intramitochondrial enzymes are not classified as mitochondrial diseases.

Each mitochondrion contains between 2 and 10 copies of mtDNA, and each cell contains a few to 1000 mitochondria, depending on its energy requirements. With rare exceptions, mtDNA is inherited entirely from the ovum and mitochondria are distributed randomly to daughter cells during embryogenesis. If an mtDNA mutation arises in a cell, both mutant and normal mtDNA molecules will coexist in that cell, a condition known as *heteroplasmy*. At all subsequent cell divisions, a mix of mutant and normal mtDNAs are then transmitted randomly to daughter cells, so that the proportion of normal to mutant DNA in each cell is determined stochastically. Even without functional or environmental pressure, with repeated cellular division, the proportions of the two tend to drift towards either completely normal or completely mutant in a given cell line (*replicative segregation*).

The term *threshold effect* refers to the expression of an abnormal phenotype only when the percentage of mitochondria harboring mutant mtDNA exceeds the proportion of normal mitochondria needed for the energy demands of the tissue. In general, there is a greater likelihood of tissue dysfunction if a high percentage of abnormal mitochondria is present.[71] In most maternally inherited disorders, heteroplasmy is common although *homoplasmic* disorders also exist. The clinical phenotype and potential disease expression ultimately depends on the severity of the mutation, the percentage of affected mitochondria and the energy requirements of the involved tissues (Table 26.10).

Mitochondrial disorders have an overall incidence of approximately 1 in 8500 children and are therefore more common than phenylketonuria or myotonic dystrophy.[72] They may occur sporadically or be inherited in a Mendelian (autosomal recessive, autosomal dominant, X-linked) fashion. Defects of mtDNA are inherited by maternal inheritance (see below). Mitochondrial disorders have been recently reviewed.[73]

THE RESPIRATORY CHAIN

The mitochondrial respiratory (electron transport) chain (Fig. 26.19) produces the majority of energy through the process of oxidative phosphorylation (OXPHOS), in which the reduction of oxygen to water is coupled to the production of the high energy compound ATP. Because of the critical role mitochondria play in generating cellular energy, mitochondrial disorders can cause dysfunction of any organ system, although the high energy needs of the neuromuscular system make it the most vulnerable.

The respiratory chain consists of four inner mitochondrial membrane multi-subunit protein complexes (complexes I–IV) that transport electrons down an electrochemical gradient using a variety of electron carriers, including iron–sulfur clusters, cytochromes and coenzyme Q_{10}, and an ATPase (complex V). Electron transport between the complexes is coupled to the extrusion of protons across the inner mitochondrial membrane by proton pump components of the respiratory chain.

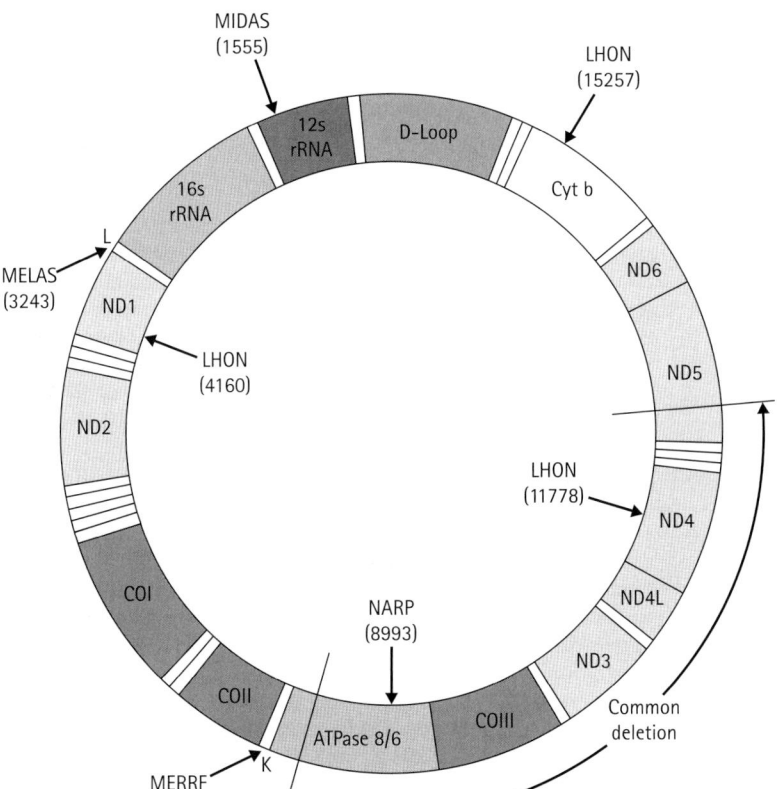

Fig. 26.18 Mitochondrial genome. Human mtDNA is a double-stranded, circular genome of 16 569 base pairs that encodes 13 OXPHOS subunits, 22 tRNAs, and two rRNAs. The locations of common pathogenic mutations are shown, with the base pair positions given in parentheses. Different disease phenotypes may occur with the same mutation. For example, mutations at position 3243 have been reported in MELAS, PEO, cardiomyopathy and MIDD and 8344 mutations are associated with MERRF, deafness and cardiomyopathy, and PEO with myoclonus. On the other hand, different mutations may cause a similar clinical presentation (e.g. LHON). The common deletion is associated with KSS, PEO and PS. ATPase 8/6, complex V subunits; COIII, complex IV subunits; Cyt b, cytochrome b (complex III subunit); K, lysine tRNA; KSS, Kearnes–Sayre syndrome; L, leucine tRNA; LHON, Leber hereditary optic neuropathy; MELAS, mitochondrial encephalomyopathy, lactic acidosis and stroke-like episodes; MERRF, myoclonic epilepsy with ragged-red fibers; MIDAS, maternally inherited deafness with aminoglycoside sensitivity; MIDD, maternally inherited diabetes and deafness; NARP, neurogenic weakness, ataxia and retinitis pigmentosa; ND1-6, complex I subunits (7); PEO, progressive external ophthalmoplegia; PS, Pearson marrow–pancreas syndrome. White bars indicate position of mitochondrial tRNAs.

Table 26.10   Presenting clinical symptoms and signs in mitochondrial respiratory chain disorders

Brain and muscle	Hypotonia/hypertonia Weakness Seizures Stroke-like episodes Ataxia Exercise tolerance	Leigh syndrome, Alpers syndrome Recurrent myoglobinuria Peripheral neuropathy Spinal muscular atrophy-like Elevated CSF protein
Eye	Cataracts Pigmentary retinopathy Optic atrophy	Progressive external ophthalmoplegia Ptosis Diplopia
Ear	Sensorineural deafness Aminoglycoside-induced ototoxicity	
Heart	Cardiomyopathy Cardiac conduction defects	
Gastrointestinal tract	Hepatic dysfunction/failure Exocrine pancreatic dysfunction Villous atrophy Gastroenteritis-like illness Failure to thrive	Cyclic vomiting Chronic diarrhea Valproate-induced liver failure
Bone marrow	Pancytopenia Megaloblastic anemia Sideroblastic anemia	
Kidney	Renal failure Fanconi syndrome Nephrotic syndrome	Renal tubular acidosis Vitamin D-unresponsive rickets Tubulointerstitial nephritis
Endocrine system	Diabetes mellitus Short stature Hypoparathyroidism	Hypothyroidism Adrenocorticotrophin deficiency Infertility
Skin	Rashes Mottled pigmentation	Trichothiodystrophy Ichthyosis
Dysmorphology	Dysmorphic features	

ATP is synthesized by complex V from adenosine diphosphate (ADP) and inorganic phosphate using energy from the flow of protons back into the mitochondrial matrix from the intermembrane space (Fig. 26.19). This process converts physicochemical energy into a biomedical source of energy.

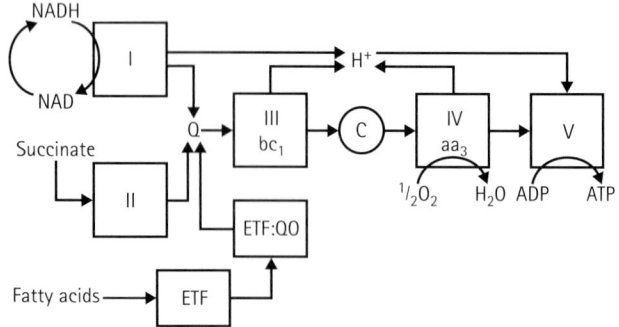

Fig. 26.19   The respiratory chain is embedded in the inner mitochondrial membrane and consists of five multisubunit enzymes (complexes I–V). Complex I, (NADH Co Q oxidoreductase); complex II, succinate Co Q oxidoreductase; complex III, ubiquinol cytochrome c reductase; complex IV, cytochrome c oxidase; complex V, ATP synthase; Q, coenzyme Q; C, cytochrome c; ETF, electron transfer flavoprotein; ETF:QO, electron transfer flavoprotein oxidoreductase. Electrons generated by complexes I, III and IV create the proton gradient that drives ATP synthesis. Their transport (using transition metal compounds, flavins and coenzyme Q_{10}) is coupled to proton extrusion across the inner mitochondrial membrane by complexes I, III and IV. Protons then re-enter the mitochondrial matrix through complex V and ATP is synthesized from ADP and inorganic phosphate. NADH (via complex I) and FADH2 (via complex II or coenzyme Q_{10}) donate electrons to the respiratory chain.

Dysfunction of the ETC causes decreased ATP production, as well as increased production of reactive oxygen and free radicals that can further impair respiratory chain function and exacerbate the already diminished energy production. These changes subsequently activate the mitochondrial membrane permeability transition pore, resulting in egress of apoptotic factors and cell death. All these factors play a role in the pathogenesis of these disorders.[74] They are also postulated to explain the progressive emergence of mutant mtDNA in several adult-onset diseases.

mtDNA codes for 7 of the 43 subunits in complex I, 0 of 4 in complex II, 1 of 11 in complex III, 3 of 13 in complex IV and 2 of 14 in complex V. Nuclear DNA encodes the remaining subunits as well as all the other proteins responsible for the assembly and maintenance of the respiratory chain, ribosomal proteins and enzymes responsible for mtDNA replication. The respiratory chain is thus formed and maintained by the coordinated interaction of two genomes.

CLINICAL FEATURES

Mitochondrial diseases are typically multisystem disorders that affect virtually any tissue or organ system and they may present with a broad array of symptoms and signs: myopathy, neurological symptoms and cardiomyopathy being the most common. With the capricious nature of mtDNA distribution during meiosis and cell replication, it should not surprise clinicians to find unusual combinations of tissue involvement in these cases. Once a family is recognized, it is usual to find members with apparently unrelated diseases (see below) and others who possess the mutant mtDNA but who are totally normal. Progressive dysfunction of seemingly unrelated organ systems may indeed provide the first clue to the presence of underlying mitochondrial disease.[75] While several classic clinical syndromes have been described (Table 26.11),[76,77] there is considerable overlap in their presentations. Mitochondrial disease can

Table 26.11   Clinical features of mitochondrial encephalopathies*

Tissue	Signs and symptoms	KSS	MERRF	MELAS	MILS	NARP
CNS	Seizures	−	+	+	+	−
	Ataxia	+	+	+	±	+
	Myoclonus	−	+	±	−	−
	Psychomotor retardation	−	−	−	+	−
	Psychomotor regression	+	±	+	−	−
	Hemiparesis/hemianopia	−	−	+	−	−
	Cortical blindness	−	−	+	−	−
	Migraine-like headaches	−	−	+	−	−
	Dystonia	−	−	+	+	−
	Peripheral weakness	±	±	±	−	+
Muscle	Weakness	+	+	+	+	+
	Ophthalmoplegia	+	−	±	−	−
	Ptosis	+	−	±	−	−
Eye	Pigmentary retinopathy	+	−	−	±	+
	Optic atrophy	−	−	−	±	±
Endocrine	Diabetes mellitus	±	−	±	−	−
	Short stature	+	+	+	−	−
	Hypoparathyroidism	±	−	−	−	−
Heart	Conduction block	+	−	±	−	−
	Cardiomyopathy	±	±	±	±	−
Gastrointestinal	Intestinal pseudo-obstruction	−	−	±	−	−
ENT	Sensorineural hearing loss	−	+	+	−	±
Kidney	Fanconi syndrome	±	−	±	−	−
Skin	Lipomas	−	+	−	−	−
Genetics	Sporadic	+	−	−	−	−
	Maternal	−	+	+	+	+

*Boxes highlight the typical clinical features of each syndrome except for MILS, which is defined by neuroradiological findings.
CNS, central nervous system; ENT, ear, nose, and throat; KSS, Kearns–Sayre syndrome; MELAS mitochondrial encephalomyopathy, lactic acidosis and stroke-like episodes; MERRF, myoclonus epilepsy with ragged red fibers; MILS, maternally inherited Leigh syndrome; NARP, neuropathy, ataxia and retinitis pigmentosa; PNS, peripheral nervous system.
Adapted from DiMauro et al:[76]

present at any age, prenatal to adulthood.[75] The disorders are listed in Table 26.12.

Leigh syndrome and Alpers syndrome

The terms Leigh syndrome (subacute necrotizing encephalomyelopathy) and Alpers syndrome are clinical descriptions that do not imply a specific biochemical cause. Leigh syndrome is a severe neurological disorder characterized by pyramidal and extrapyramidal symptoms, brainstem dysfunction and a progressive course that typically presents in children aged 1–5 years. Onset is usually gradual hypotonia, weakness, ataxia, tremor, optic atrophy, ophthalmoplegia, retinitis pigmentosa and respiratory abnormalities. Bilateral basal ganglia lesions are a common neuroradiological finding. Symmetric necrotic lesions in the thalami, brainstem and posterior columns of the spinal cord are pathological features. Patients usually do not have ragged-red fibers on histochemistry of muscle. Leigh syndrome is heterogeneous and may be caused by mtDNA, autosomal recessive and X-linked disorders. The most common are in nuclear genes coding for various subunits of complex I and II and in SURF I and II, proteins that are required for assembly of complex IV. The usual mtDNA mutations are mtATP6 (complex V; maternally inherited Leigh syndrome [MILS], see Table 26.9) and in several mitochondrial tRNAs. Leigh syndrome can also be seen in pyruvate dehydrogenase deficiency, an X-linked disorder (see p. 1079).

Alpers syndrome (progressive infantile poliodystrophy) is a comparable neurodegenerative disorder with onset in infancy and death in early childhood in which liver disease is characteristic. Patients have lactic acidemia and a variety of symptoms, including myoclonic epilepsy, ataxia, hypo- or hyper-tonia and abnormal respirations. Alpers syndrome primarily affects the cerebral cortex and cerebellum, with lesser involvement of the basal ganglia and brainstem. Both respiratory chain and tricarboxylic acid cycle defects have been found in this disorder. Alpers syndrome is primarily caused by mutations in the gene coding for mtDNA polymerase (POLG), an enzyme essential for mtDNA replication and repair.[78] A mutation in mtDNA-encoded cytochrome c oxidase II gene may cause a similar clinical picture.[79]

Mitochondrial myopathy

Stable or progressive hypotonia, muscle weakness and poor exercise tolerance with dyspnea are common features in mitochondrial disorders of muscle; myalgia and myoglobinuria are much less frequent. The severity ranges from fatal infantile myopathy to milder presentation in later childhood or adulthood. Although severe lactic acidosis and multiorgan system failure may accompany severe infantile forms of mitochondrial myopathy, there is one form in which complete, spontaneous remission occurs during the first years of life.[80]

Histologically, there are usually subsarcolemmal aggregates of mitochondria that, on staining with Gomori trichrome, give what is termed a ragged-red fiber picture (RRF). On electron microscopy, the mitochondria are large and misshapen with inclusions. Numerous mtDNA (especially involving mitochondrial tRNAs) and nuclear DNA (nDNA) mutations (e.g. mtDNA depletion syndrome) have been associated with myopathy.

Cardiomyopathy

Respiratory chain dysfunction is also a cause of cardiomyopathy from birth through adult life. This is usually concentric and hypertrophic but dilated forms are not uncommon. Heart pathology usually shows fibroelastosis, interstitial fibrosis and abnormal mitochondria. Cardiac

Table 26.12 Classification of mitochondrial respiratory chain disorders

Defects of mitochondrial DNA (maternal inheritance)
Point mutations
    MELAS, MERRF, LHON, NARP, MIDAS
Single deletions
    KSS, CPEO, PS
Duplications or duplications/deletions
    KSS

Defects of nuclear DNA (Mendelian inheritance)
Respiratory chain subunit disorders
    Complex I deficiency: NDUFV1, NDUFS1, NDUFS2, NDUFS4, NDUFS7,
    NDUFS8 mutations
    Complex II deficiency: Fp subunit of succinate dehydrogenase
Disorders of intergenomic communication
    Respiratory chain subunit stability/assembly: SURF-1, SCO1, SCO2,
    COX10 mutations
    mtDNA replication: mtDNA depletion syndrome, multiple mtDNA
    deletions (autosomal dominant and recessive types), thymidine
    phosphorylase deficiency (MNGIE)
Defective oxidative phosphorylation coupling
    Luft disease
Mitochondrial substrate pores/translocase defects
    ANT deficiency
    VDAC deficiency
    Malate/aspartate shuttle deficiency
Defects of mitochondrial protein importation
    Chaperonins: hsp60, parplegin (SPG7 mutations), Mohr–Tranebjaerg
    syndrome (DPP1 mutations)
Defects of intramitochondrial metal homeostasis
    Freidreich ataxia (frataxin mutations)
    X-linked sideroblastic anemia and ataxia (ABC7 mutations)
    Wilson disease (ATP7B mutations)
Other nuclear genome defects
    Barth syndrome (G4.5/taffazin mutations)
    Cartilage-hair hypoplasia (RNase MRP mutations)
Other neurodegenerative disorders
    Alzheimer disease
    Parkinson disease
    Huntington disease
    Amyotrophic lateral sclerosis

ANT, adenine nucleotide translocator; CPEO, chronic progressive external ophthalmoplegia; KSS, Kearns–Sayre syndrome; LHON, Leber hereditary optic neuropathy; MELAS, mitochondrial encephalomyopathy, lactic acidosis and stroke-like episodes; MERRF, myoclonic epilepsy and ragged-red fibers; MIDAS, maternally inherited deafness with aminoglycoside sensitivity; MNGIE, myoneurogastrointestinal disorder and encephalopathy; NARP, neurogenic weakness, ataxia, and retinitis pigmentosa; PS, Pearson marrow–pancreas syndrome; VDAC, voltage-dependent anion channel.

conduction defects are relatively common. The cardiomyopathy may be isolated or associated with other organ involvement.

A number of respiratory chain defects (especially complex I and complex IV deficiencies), mtDNA point mutations and deletions have been associated with cardiomyopathy.[81,82] Mutations of nDNA that affect the function of the respiratory chain may cause cardiomyopathy in addition to causing neurological impairment (e.g. mutations in the SCO2 or frataxin genes). The X-linked Barth syndrome is an important cause of dilated cardiomyopathy in boys (see p. 1098).

Hepatic disease

Severe early-onset liver failure is associated with a mitochondrial depletion syndrome caused by a defect in *deoxyguanosine kinase*. Both infantile and more indolent hepatic disease also have been associated with various defects of the respiratory chain, often affecting multiple complexes. Other organs can also be involved. Histopathology is nonspecific, often showing steatosis, fibrosis and cholestasis. General

depletion of mtDNA and mtDNA rearrangements have been found in some of these patients.

Renal disease

Renal tubules depend on oxidative metabolism, so it is not surprising that kidney involvement is relatively common in mitochondrial disease. Proximal renal tubular dysfunction, manifesting as the *renal Fanconi syndrome*, is most frequently encountered, but the nephrotic syndrome, focal segmental glomerulonephrosis and chronic interstitial nephropathy have also been reported (see Ch. 18). The Fanconi syndrome (see also p. 550) may be extreme or partial with only mild aminoaciduria or renal tubular acidosis. It can present at any age. Kidney involvement is often associated with disease in other organ systems.

Endocrine disease

Diabetes mellitus, hypoparathyroidism, growth failure secondary to IgF1 deficiency, hypothyroidism, hypothalamic dysfunction and adrenocorticotrophic hormone (ACTH) deficiency may occur in children with mitochondrial disease, particularly in Kearns–Sayre syndrome (KSS). These are often associated with other features including sensorineural hearing loss, cardiomyopathy, myopathy, renal tubular defects and neuropsychiatric disease (e.g. Maternally inherited diabetes and deafness MIDD). Various mtDNA point mutations, including the A3243G tRNA mutation associated with MELAS syndrome, and mtDNA rearrangements have been associated with diabetes. Patients may present as neonates with ketosis, prominent hyperglycemia and lactic acidosis or in later childhood or adulthood.

Pearson marrow–pancreas syndrome is characterized by exocrine, and sometimes endocrine, pancreatic dysfunction and refractory sideroblastic anemia with variable neutropenia and thrombocytopenia, and is caused by a large mtDNA deletion.

Wolfram syndrome is characterized by diabetes insipidus, diabetes mellitus, optic atrophy and deafness (DIDMOAD) (see also p. 112). Wolfram syndrome in many cases is an autosomal recessive condition caused by mutations in the WFS1 gene which codes for a protein that localizes to the endoplasmic reticulum and is likely involved in membrane trafficking, protein processing and/or calcium homeostasis, but has also been described in patients with mtDNA point mutations and deletions.[83]

Mitochondrial encephalopathy, lactic acidosis and stroke-like episodes (MELAS)

Mitochondrial encephalopathy, lactic acidosis and stroke-like episodes (MELAS) classically presents with stroke-like episodes and focal neurological deficits (which may be transient), headache, emesis, lactic acidosis, myopathy with abnormal muscle morphology; symptoms occur by age 15 years in 80%. Short stature, seizures, developmental regression, pigmentary retinopathy, deafness, diabetes mellitus and cardiomyopathy are variably present. A heteroplasmic A3243G tRNALeu(UUR) mtDNA mutation is the most common cause. This same mutation has been associated with mitochondrial epilepsy and ragged red fibers (MERFF), progressive external ophthalmoplegia (PEO), MIDD and autistic spectrum disorders.[84] Multiple white matter lesions and basal ganglia calcification are common.

Muscle histochemistry shows cytochrome c oxidase (COX)-positive RRF and strong succinate dehydrogenase reactivity in blood vessels most of the time. Although biochemical studies may be normal, complex I deficiency or partial combined deficiencies of complexes I, II and IV have been described.

Mitochondrial epilepsy and ragged-red fibers (MERRF)

Mitochondrial epilepsy and ragged-red fibers (MERRF) is characterized by myoclonic epilepsy, myopathy and progressive cerebellar ataxia. Deafness is common, and optic atrophy, peripheral neuropathy and heart block may occur. Symptoms usually emerge in the second or third decade.

Mild to moderate elevations of lactate and creatine kinase may be present. On histochemistry, the muscle shows prominent COX-negative RRF and, most often, complex I and IV deficiencies. The most common mutation is A8344G in the mtDNA tRNALys gene, although other mtDNA point mutations may result in a similar phenotype.

Leber hereditary optic neuropathy

Leber hereditary optic neuropathy (LHON) is one of the most common causes of blindness in young men (1 in 10 000–50 000). Although most patients show only sudden or subacute vision loss due to degeneration of the optic nerve, non-ophthalmological features also occur and can include encephalomyopathy, deafness, ataxia, a multiple sclerosis-like illness and cardiac conduction defects. The male:female ratio is about 3:1 but the reason for this is not understood. A G11778A mutation in the ND1 subunit of complex I causes > 60% of cases, but ~20 different mutations in mtDNA are known. These mutations are usually homoplasmic, in contrast to the heteroplasmy in most mitochondrial disorders. It should be recognized that homoplasmy can also be found in *unaffected* members of a known pedigree. This disorder should not be confused with Leber hereditary amaurosis.

Neurogenic weakness ataxia and retinitis pigmentosa (NARP)

The disorder NARP is characterized by proximal neurogenic weakness, pigmentary retinopathy, seizures, ataxia, sensory neuropathy and developmental delay. Mutations in mtDNA (T8993G and T8993C) cause dysfunction of the ATPase 6 subunit of complex V. Leigh syndrome is often present when the mutant mtDNA load is particularly high (> 90%). Imaging may show cerebral or cerebellar atrophy, in addition to features of Leigh syndrome. Biochemical findings on muscle biopsy may be normal and RRF or COX-negative fibers are usually absent.

Kearns–Sayre syndrome, chronic progressive external ophthalmoplegia and Pearson syndrome

Large single deletions or duplications of mtDNA are most often sporadic, with patients having only a single type of abnormal mtDNA, theoretically arising from clonal expansion of a chance rearrangement event in oogenesis or early embryogenesis. Human oocytes contain approximately 100 000 mtDNA molecules, but only about 1000 are passed on to the fetus. If a defective mtDNA molecule passes through this 'bottleneck', transmission to the fetus may result in mitochondrial disease.[85] Kearns–Sayre syndrome (KSS), chronic progressive external ophthalmoplegia (CPEO) and Pearson syndrome can be associated with sporadic mtDNA duplications/deletions.

Patients with KSS present in childhood with variable combinations of CPEO, pigmentary retinopathy, endocrinopathy, ataxia, proximal myopathy, areflexia, sensorineural deafness, stroke-like episodes, bulbar symptoms, heart block, CSF protein > 1g/L (100 mg/dl) and lactic acidosis. Up to 60% of muscle fibers are COX negative, with RRF in 5–20%. Nearly all patients have a large mtDNA deletion; one that encompasses 4.9 kb from nucleotide 8482 to 13459 is present in ~40% of cases. This 'common deletion' is also associated with isolated PEO or Pearson syndrome.

PEO consists of ptosis, external ophthalmoplegia and proximal weakness; the autonomic innervation of the eye is not affected. Life span may be normal. The muscle pathological features are similar to KSS.

Pearson syndrome presents in early infancy with a refractory sideroblastic anemia, variable neutropenia and thrombocytopenia, and exocrine pancreatic dysfunction. Diabetes mellitus, liver dysfunction and renal tubular dysfunction may also occur. The 'common deletion' is present in 90% of total blood or bone marrow mtDNA, but may be quite low in muscle or fibroblasts. Muscle histology and biochemistry are often normal. The initial refractory anemia resolves in patients surviving infancy, but these children may progress to KSS, with subsequent accumulation of deleted mtDNA species in muscle and lessening of the mutant mtDNA in blood.[86]

Mitochondrial DNA depletion syndromes

This term encompasses a number of autosomal recessive conditions in which the concentration of mtDNA is decreased or nearly absent.[87] Deficiency of mitochondrial *DNA polymerase gamma*, encoded by POLG1, causes Alpers syndrome, epilepsy and fulminant hepatic failure associated with mtDNA depletion.[88] Mitochondria do not contain enzymes for de novo deoxyribonucleoside-5′-triphosphate (dNTP) synthesis and thus rely on salvage pathways, including thymidine kinase and deoxyguanosine kinase for mtDNA replication.

Profound mtDNA depletion may occur in patients with a severe myopathy, lactic acidemia and elevated creatine kinase levels (900–4000 IU/L) who had reduced activity of *mitochondrial thymidine kinase*.[89] Marked elevation of creatine kinase is otherwise rare in mitochondrial disorders and, therefore, serves as a diagnostic clue.

A significant depletion of mtDNA occurs in children with early progressive liver failure and neurological abnormalities secondary to a single nucleotide deletion in the mitochondrial *deoxyguanosine kinase (dGK)* gene.[90] Severe infantile liver disease associated with mtDNA depletion may also be caused by mutations in MPV17, which codes for a mitochondrial inner membrane protein.[91] Mutations in MPV17 also cause *Navajo neurohepatopathy*, a condition characterized by hepatopathy, peripheral neuropathy, corneal anesthesia, failure to thrive and leukoencephalopathy.[92]

Mutations in SUCLA2, a gene that encodes *succinyl-CoA synthetase*, cause early infantile-onset encephalomyopathy and mtDNA depletion.[93] Autosomal recessive POLG1 mutations also cause mtDNA depletion and variable clinical phenotypes, including Alpers syndrome.

Although the majority of cases of mtDNA depletion have autosomal recessive inheritance, the X-linked *mental retardation, epileptic seizures, hypogonadism and hypogenitalism, microcephaly, obesity (MEHMO) syndrome* has been associated with a decreased amount of mtDNA.[94]

Mutations in OPA1, a gene that encodes a dynamin-related protein with GTPase activity that is targeted at mitochondria, cause a common form of autosomal dominant optic atrophy characterized by progressive loss of visual acuity in childhood and mtDNA depletion.[95–97] Some HIV patients treated with nucleoside reverse transcriptase inhibitors have mtDNA depletion and subsequent organ toxicity, possibly secondary to inhibition of DNA polymerase gamma by this class of drug.[98]

Myoneurogastrointestinal disorder and encephalopathy (MNGIE)

This disorder is characterized by a chronic intestinal pseudo-obstruction, ophthalmoplegia, peripheral neuropathy with 'stocking/glove' sensory loss and myopathy. Deafness is common and developmental regression with white matter disease may be present. Histologically, RRF, a partial COX deficiency and neurogenic changes are seen on muscle histology.[99]

MNGIE is most often caused by mutations in the nuclear gene ECGF1, which encodes thymidine phosphorylase, and is inherited in an autosomal recessive fashion; however, in some cases, mtDNA depletion, multiple mtDNA deletions and a single base pair deletion in the mitochondrial tRNA[Thr] gene have been reported.

Luft hypermetabolic syndrome

This rare disorder is associated with defective OXPHOS coupling. Patients develop symptoms in childhood consisting of myopathy and euthyroid hypermetabolism, with increased body temperature, sweating, respiratory rate and heart rate. Skeletal muscle OXPHOS is uncoupled with dissipation of the electrochemical gradient generated by the respiratory chain and decreased ATP production.[100]

Coenzyme Q_{10} deficiency

Coenzyme Q_{10} is essential to the function of the electron transport chain. Defective synthesis results in loss of coupling and a wide range of typical mitochondrial symptoms in differing combinations. Activities of the individual complexes are normal but when linked together in the assay, are shown to be defective.

Treatment with coenzyme Q_{10} in doses up to 300 mg/d are helpful especially in this disorder but also often in other forms of mitochondrial disease

Other clinical features

Additional manifestations of mitochondrial disease are prenatal effects, including intrauterine growth retardation, hydranencephaly, polyhydramnios, microcephaly, facial dysmorpism and abnormalities of fetal tone and movement.[101,102] In addition, gastrointestinal illness (cyclic vomiting, chronic diarrhea, exocrine pancreatic dysfunction, intestinal pseudo-obstruction, failure to thrive), as well as dermatological findings (mottled pigmentation) can occur.[81,103]

CLASSIFICATION (Table 26.12)

Because the components of the respiratory chain are coded by both the nuclear and mitochondrial genomes, familial cases of mitochondrial disorders may show either maternal or Mendelian inheritance. Sporadic cases also occur as a result of new mutations, presumably in the oocyte or early after fertilization.

Defects of the mitochondrial genome
Point mutations

Many benign mtDNA polymorphisms are known; they are used in anthropologic studies. Over 100 pathogenic mtDNA point mutations have been described. MELAS, MERRF, LHON and NARP have each been associated with several specific point mutations.[77] Conversely, the same mtDNA mutations can lead to different findings in different patients. *Maternally inherited deafness with aminoglycoside sensitivity (MIDAS)* is caused by an A to G transition at base pair 1555 in the mitochondrial 12S ribosomal subunit gene.

Multiple deletions, duplications or duplications/deletions

Other major rearrangements of mtDNA include duplications, most commonly present in the context of duplications/deletions, and multiple deletions. While *single* mtDNA deletions may exhibit maternal inheritance and can be associated with various phenotypes, including KSS, *multiple* deletions of mtDNA exhibit Mendelian inheritance and are caused by defective signaling between the nuclear and mitochondrial genomes, with resultant defective mtDNA replication (see below).

Nuclear genome defects

Defects of nDNA that result in abnormal mitochondrial respiratory chain function are inherited in a Mendelian fashion and may be responsible for the majority of cases of mitochondrial disease. They can cause dysfunction of specific respiratory chain subunits; intergenomic communication between nuclear and mitochondrial genomes, oxidation/phosphorylation coupling; substrate pores or translocases; mitochondrial protein importation; or intramitochondrial metal homeostasis.[76,77]

Defects in nuclear genes of respiratory chain subunits

Defects in respiratory chain subunits encoded by nDNA are inherited in an autosomal recessive manner. The first reported defect was a mutation in the flavoprotein (Fp) subunit gene of succinate dehydrogenase (complex II) in Leigh syndrome.[104] Succinate dehydrogenase mutations have been associated with familial pheochromocytoma and paraganglionoma, highlighting an interesting link between mitochondrial dysfunction and hereditary cancer.[105,106]

Mutations in 10 nuclear genes coding for complex I have been described; these cause brain and brainstem pathology, especially Leigh syndrome or leukoencephalopathy. Mutations in complex I subunit genes NDUFS2 and NDUFV2 cause hypertrophic cardiomyopathy and encephalomyopathy.[82,107]

Defects in intergenomic communication

Certain nDNA mutations result in either aberrant subunit biogenesis/maintenance or mtDNA replicative errors. Mutations in NDUFS6 cause defective assembly or stability of complex I, resulting in a lethal neonatal encephalomyopathy.[108] Mutations in BSCIL, an assembly gene for complex III, result in encephalopathy, renal tubulopathy and liver disease.[109] Similarly, nuclear mutations have been detected in a number of genes coding for assembly factors for COX (complex IV). Patients with COX deficiency secondary to mutations of SURF-1, which is important in the assembly of stability of complex IV, develop Leigh syndrome.[110,111] Impaired mitochondrial copper metabolism, and subsequent defective COX activity, occurs in mutations affecting the SCO1 and SCO2 genes, with patients having early-onset encephalopathy and either liver disease or hypertrophic cardiomyopathy, respectively.[112,113] COX10 codes for heme A:farensyltransferase, an inner mitochondrial membrane protein important in the biogenesis of COX; deficiency has been reported in siblings who have died with progressive neurological deterioration and proximal renal tubulopathy.[114] Nuclear defects involved in the biosynthesis of complex V have also been reported. Clinical features include severe neonatal disease with lactic acidosis, hypotonia or hypertonia, seizures, contractures, cardiomegaly and hepatomegaly.[115,116]

Because nDNA codes for enzymes involved in mtDNA transcription, translation and replication, defects in intergenomic communication may cause qualitative or quantitative alterations of mtDNA. Although all the genes responsible have not yet been identified, multiple mtDNA deletions (cf. single sporadic deletions) and depletion in the amount of mtDNA are inherited in a Mendelian fashion.[87] Autosomal recessive and autosomal dominant forms of PEO are associated with multiple deletions of mtDNA. POLG1 encodes mitochondrial DNA polymerase gamma; mutations in this gene are a relatively common cause of autosomal dominant and autosomal recessive PEO.[117] POLG1 mutations are also associated with a wide array of overlapping clinical features, including severe encephalomyopathy, ataxia, myalgia and liver failure.[118] PEO may also be caused by mutations in POLG2, the gene encoding the p55 accessory subunit of polymerase gamma.[119] Mutations in ANT1 (encodes the heart and muscle-specific isoform of the mitochondrial adenine nucleotide transporter) and C10orf0002 (encodes Twinkle, a mtDNA helicase) are less common causes of autosomal dominant PEO.[121,122]

Defects in mitochondrial substrate pores or translocases

All the molecules required for OXPHOS reactions, including ATP, ADP, phosphate and other ions, must cross the inner and outer mitochondrial membranes through protein channels. Dysfunction of the *adenine nucleotide* translocator (ANT) by voltage-dependent anion channel (VDAC), or the *malate-aspartate shuttle* may cause classic symptoms and signs of mitochondrial disease.

The ANT transports ADP and ATP across the inner mitochondrial membrane; a defect of this system has been reported in a patient with myopathy and lactic acidosis.[122] (Mutations in ANT1 have also been associated with autosomal dominant PEO.) VDAC (also called porin) is an outer mitochondrial membrane transporter that opens differentially for anions, cations and certain uncharged molecules at different transmembrane voltages. VDAC deficiency was documented in a dysmorphic infant with hypothalamic hypothyroidism and psychomotor retardation.[123] Investigation of a young adult with exercise-induced myalgia documented a defect in the inner mitochondrial membrane malate–aspartate shuttle.[124]

Defects in importation of mitochondrial proteins

Proteins that are destined for import into mitochondria contain a leader sequence that acts as a targeting signal. They are then translocated into the mitochondrial matrix by import machinery consisting of chaperonins and *translocases of the outer and inner mitochondrial membranes (Tom and Tim complexes)*. The mitochondrial matrix chaperonin heat shock protein 60 (hsp60) ensures proper folding of the imported proteins.

Defective hsp60 synthesis was associated with decreased activities of multiple mitochondrial enzymes in a patient who died aged 2 d, after presenting with dysmorphic features, hypotonia and severe lactic acidosis.[125] A defect in *paraplegin*, a ubiquitous inner mitochondrial membrane protein with proteolytic and chaperonin activities, was found in patients with hereditary spastic paraplegia (HSP) in which progressive weakness and spasticity of the lower limbs occur; other features, including developmental delay, optic atrophy, retinitis pigmentosa, deafness, ataxia and ichthyosis, may be present. Muscle biopsies from two patients with HSP showed RRF, a finding consistent with impaired OXPHOS.[126]

Finally, the X-linked neurodegenerative disorder *Mohr-Tranebjaerg syndrome* (DFN-1/MTS) is caused by mutations in the gene coding for the deafness/dystonia peptide (DDP), a protein which bears strong resemblance to the Tim subclass of mitochondrial transmembrane carrier proteins.[127] Mutations in the DDP1 gene cause decreased levels of the inner mitochondrial membrane Tim23 complex, which is required for mitochondrial import of proteins responsible for the translocation, assembly and integrity of the OXPHOS system. Patients with MTS have dystonia, spasticity, developmental delay and progressive sensorineural hearing loss.

Defects in intramitochondrial metal homeostasis

The neurodegenerative disorders Friedreich ataxia, X-linked sideroblastic anemia and ataxia (XLAS/A), and Wilson disease are associated with aberrant intramitochondrial metal homeostasis, which may secondarily cause dysfunction of the respiratory chain.[128] Friedrich ataxia (see Ch. 29) is caused by an expansion of a GAA triplet repeat in the gene frataxin that codes for a mitochondrial protein involved in iron homeostasis. The result is an intramitochondrial accumulation of free iron, which impairs oxidative metabolism, possibly by interfering with the normal production of heme and iron–sulfur clusters.[129]

Iron homeostasis is also altered in XLSA/A, a disorder characterized by nonprogressive cerebellar ataxia and mild anemia starting in infancy or early childhood. The mitochondrial inner membrane iron transporter ABC7 is defective in XLSA/A.[130]

In Wilson disease (see p. 1125) a modified, cleaved, form of the mutant protein is found in mitochondria.[131] The mutation results in intramitochondrial copper overload, mtDNA deletions and abnormal respiratory chain function. Mutations in SCO1 and SCO2, nuclear genes that play a role in mitochondrial copper delivery, have been found in patients with COX deficiency.

Other nuclear genome defects

Barth syndrome (3-methylglutaconic aciduria type II) is discussed on p. 1098.

Other neurodegenerative disorders

Diminishing respiratory chain function and increasing clones of mutant mtDNA occur as we age and are thought to play a role on the development of several neurodegenerative disorders with onset in adulthood, including Alzheimer disease, Parkinson disease, Huntington disease and amyotrophic lateral sclerosis.[132-134] In this context, the roles of aging, damage from free radicals, external toxins and genetics are still not understood.

GENETIC COUNSELING (see also Ch. 14)

A meticulous pedigree is essential to evaluating any patient with suspected mitochondrial disease; it may reveal Mendelian (dominant, recessive or occasionally X-linked) or maternal inheritance [matrilineal] with family members having variable phenotypes). A family history of hearing loss, vision problems, muscle weakness, behavior abnormalities, migraines, diabetes mellitus and other endocrine disease, or short stature, transmitted only by females, should always be sought.

Single mutations in mtDNA are transmitted matrilinearly. Both single and large deletions in mtDNA are usually sporadic with little or no risk of recurrence, but more complex deletion/duplications of mtDNA may be inherited (possibly ~5% transmission to offspring, but little data exist to support this figure). Multiple mtDNA mutations may be inherited in an autosomal dominant or autosomal recessive manner. Genetic counseling is more straightforward in cases of nDNA mutations; affected relatives tend to have similar features and classic Mendelian inheritance can be more readily understood by the family.

Most children with mitochondrial disease are diagnosed clinically or by the finding of decreased activity in one or more of the respiratory chain complexes and do not have a specific mutation identified. In these cases, it is difficult to provide accurate recurrence risk estimates, unless a particular mode of inheritance is suggested by the pedigree. Because of the inherent characteristics of mitochondrial biology (heteroplasmy, replicative segregation, threshold effect), genetic counseling is particularly challenging. Moreover, even if maternal inheritance seems likely on the basis of family history, it may not be possible to predict the expression of disease in current or future children. In a given family with mtDNA disease, future offspring may be more, similarly or less affected than the proband. Empiric recurrence risks have been estimated for some of the more common mtDNA disorders based on maternal blood mutation loads.[71] The blood percentage of abnormal mtDNA in MELAS and MERRF does *not* correlate well with expression of clinical features, but there appears to be relatively good correlation with mutant load and outcome in NARP. Nevertheless, while counseling is relatively straightforward in NARP with either a very high or very low percentage of mutant mtDNA, difficulty is encountered in less clear-cut patients with intermediate mutant loads.[135]

Prenatal diagnosis of mtDNA disorders has been attempted by mutation analysis on amniocytes or chorionic villi. However, the mutant load in these tissues does not necessarily predict the distribution or percentage of mutant mtDNA in other tissues after birth. It has been suggested that mutant loads < 30% or > 90% may predict a low or high probability, respectively, of having a child with clinical disease, although this information must still be treated with caution.[71]

Molecular prenatal genetic diagnosis of oocytes, oocyte cytoplasmic transfer to dilute mutant mtDNA and transfer of an unfertilized oocyte nucleus into an enucleated donor oocyte (followed by in vitro fertilization and reimplantation) are experimental techniques that may offer female carriers of an mtDNA mutation reproductive options in the near future.

CLINICAL EVALUATION OF SUSPECTED MITOCHONDRIAL DISEASE

Lactic acidosis is discussed on p. 1080 and the organic acidurias on p. 1066. Urine organic acid analysis may be normal, or show variable elevations of lactate, pyruvate, ketone bodies, tricarboxylic acid cycle intermediates or other organic acids, including ethylmalonic, malic, fumaric, 3-methylglutaconic, 2-ethylhydracrylic, 2-methylsuccinic and glutaric acids.[136] Orotic acid, from the urea cycle, and dicarboxylic acids, from compromised fatty acid oxidation, may also be present. All these reflect distorted intramitochondrial homeostasis secondary to primary respiratory chain dysfunction.[137] Generalized aminoaciduria is present in the renal Fanconi syndrome (see Ch. 18, p. 550).

Because elevations of specific acylcarnitines are characteristic of fatty acid oxidation disorders, a plasma acylcarnitine profile may help to differentiate a fatty acid oxidation disorder from a defect in the respiratory chain (see Appendix 1). Plasma carnitine can be low due to increased excretion of conjugates or to poor nutrition. Highly elevated creatine kinase levels are unusual, but have been reported in the mtDNA depletion syndrome.

Periodic screening tests to monitor ophthalmological, hearing, cardiac, liver and renal function are an essential part of the evaluation of these patients. In patients with neurological symptoms, brain MRI is routinely performed and EEG may be indicated. Positron emission tomography (PET), single photon emission computed tomography

(SPECT) and proton MRS have also been used to study blood flow, lactate, oxygen and glucose metabolism in brain and muscle. Deep gray matter signal abnormalities on MRI and abnormal lactate elevation on proton MRS are relatively common.[138]

Muscle biopsy

Muscle tissue for histology, histochemical staining, ultrastructural morphology and biochemical analysis may be needed to diagnose a respiratory chain disorder.[76] It is essential that processing of the tissues be discussed with the referral laboratories *before* any biopsy is done since samples are processed differently depending on what tests might be required; this is especially true for biochemical testing.

Histologically, the modified Gomori trichrome stain detects abnormal red-staining subsarcolemmal collections of mitochondria that give rise to the term RRF and are considered to be a classic feature of mitochondrial disease. However, these are often not present in children and therefore, their absence does *not* exclude the consideration of mitochondrial disease. Conversely, RRF and ultrastructurally abnormal mitochondria, reflecting oxidative stress, may be present in other conditions, including overtraining, inflammatory myopathies, myotonic dystrophy and Duchenne muscular dystrophy.[76] Histochemical staining for succinate dehydrogenase (SDH) and COX activities is also routine. SDH staining is a sensitive indicator of mitochondrial proliferation. COX staining is particularly useful in distinguishing mtDNA defects, which show a differential mosaic staining pattern with some fibers staining COX positive and others COX negative. In nuclear defects that affect COX activity, fibers are uniformly COX negative.[76] In addition, COX-positive RRF are seen in MELAS. Other nonspecific histopathological findings of respiratory chain disorders include accumulation of glycogen and/or lipid, fiber-type variation, or neurogenic changes.[139] In some cases, muscle histology may appear entirely normal. Abnormal mitochondria, often with paracrystalline inclusions or alteration in shape and size, or an increased number of mitochondria may be apparent by electron microscopy, but such changes are nonspecific.

Muscle is the best surrogate tissue for quantitation of respiratory chain function using spectrophotometric or polarographic techniques, because of its higher oxidative enzyme activities. However, some defects are only expressed in an affected tissue, in which case that tissue must be tested to find the biochemical defect.[75] Biochemical analyses may reveal isolated respiratory chain deficiencies, indicating a new somatic mutation in a specific mtDNA respiratory chain subunit gene or a nuclear defect, or combined partial complex deficiencies suggestive of a mtDNA tRNA mutation. The absence of a biochemical defect does not exclude a diagnosis of mitochondrial disease, and may be seen, for example, in some cases of mtDNA mutations affecting mitochondrial tRNAs. Some laboratories use monoclonal antibodies that recognize different respiratory chain subunits to perform immunohistochemical and/or Western blotting analyses on skin fibroblasts or biopsy specimens.[140,141]

When mitochondrial disease is suspected, some experts prefer to start by searching for mutations in blood since tests for several common point mutations and deletions of mtDNA are available. However, these are limited and if none is found, a mitochondrial disorder is not excluded. Furthermore, the mutation may simply not be present in a high enough concentration to be detected in the assayed tissue. While many mtDNA point mutations and some deletions or duplications can be detected in blood, multiple mtDNA deletions or complex rearrangements may require analysis of a muscle specimen. Overall, mtDNA deletions have been found in approximately 12% (11% single, 1% multiple) of patients with documented respiratory chain dysfunction and mitochondrial tRNA mutations in 16%, while the remainder are undiagnosed at the molecular level (possibly reflecting the presence of rare mtDNA or nDNA mutations that are not usually screened for).[142] In cases where a nuclear gene is suspected, further investigations may be available in specialized laboratories. On the Internet, Genetests (http://www.genetests.org) is a reliable search tool.

THERAPY

There is no proven specific therapy for most respiratory chain disorders although some successes have been reported. Almost all approaches attempt to capitalize upon compounds that are known to facilitate or to interdigitate with the respiratory chain. These include various combinations of L-carnitine, ascorbate, tocopherol, succinate, riboflavin, menadione, nicotinamide, thiamine, creatine, idebenone and coenzyme Q_{10} (Table 26.13).[72] However, it is difficult to assess the efficacy of any therapy given the genetic heterogeneity and broad clinical spectra of these diseases. Riboflavin may stabilize or improve features in some cases of complex I deficiency[143] and rarely, menadione can act as an electron acceptor. In some patients, especially those with a primary deficiency of coenzyme Q_{10} in muscle,[144-146] coenzyme Q_{10} decreases blood lactate levels and may improve oxygen utilization and clinical symptoms. Vitamin E and coenzyme Q_{10} have improved cardiac and skeletal muscle bioenergetics in Friedreich ataxia.[147] Succinate, if given

Table 26.13   Vitamin, cofactor and drug therapy of mitochondrial disease

Medication	Mechanism	Dose
Ubiquinone (coenzyme Q_{10})	Bypass of complex I Antioxidant	5 mg/kg/d 30–250 mg/d in adults
Idebenone	Bypass of complex I Antioxidant	90–270 mg/d in adults
Carnitine	Corrects secondary Deficiency	50–100 mg/kg/d Up to 3 g/d in adults
Dichloroacetate	Stimulates PDH activity	15–200 mg/kg/d
Succinate	Directly donates electrons to complex II	1–6 g/d
Thiamin (vitamin B_1)	PDH cofactor Stimulates NADH production	15–30 mg/kg/d 500–1000 mg/d in adults
Riboflavin (vitamin B_2)	Cofactor for complex I and II and ETF after conversion to FAD	10–15 mg/kg/d 500–1000 mg/d in adults
Nicotinamide	Increase NAD, NADH pool	20 mg/kg/d 100–1000 mg/d in adults
Ascorbic acid (vitamin C)	Antioxidant Bypass complex III when given with K_1 or K_3	25–100 mg/kg/d Up to 6 g/d in adults
Menadione (vitamin K_3)	Antioxidant Bypass complex III when given with ascorbate	40–80 mg/d
Creatine	Increases muscle phosphocreatine	Up to 10 g/d in adults
Pantothenic acid	Increases CoA synthesis	15 mg/kg/d
A-Tocopherol (vitamin E)	Antioxidant	15 mg/kg/d (22 IU/kg/d)
Lipoic acid	Antioxidant	15 mg/kg/d

These vitamins and cofactors are typically given together in various combinations. For example, coenzyme Q_{10}, vitamin C, vitamin E and lipoic acid are often used simultaneously for antioxidant action, because together their cooperative action is more effective in free radical defense than if given singly. Vitamin K3 should not be given unless there is conclusive evidence of a complex III deficiency. K3 shunts electrons from complex I to complex IV in the presence of vitamin C, effectively bypassing complex III. This has the potential to decrease ATP production in patients without complex III deficiency. ETF, electron transfer flavoprotein; FAD, flavin adenine dinucleotide; FMP, flavin monophosphate; NAD, nicotine adenine dinucleotide (oxidized); NADH, nicotine adenine dinucleotide (reduced); PDH, pyruvate dehydrogenase complex.

in quantities as a potential fuel, may be beneficial in patients with complex I deficiency, because of its ability to donate electrons directly to complex II.

Dichloroacetate (DCA) stimulates pyruvate dehydrogenase (p.1080) activity and causes a decrease in blood lactate, improved brain oxidative metabolism on MRS, and amelioration of clinical symptoms in some patients with mitochondrial disease.[148,149] However, a controlled clinical trial using DCA to treat a variety of causes of lactic acidemia, including mitochondrial disorders, showed that the medication was well tolerated and blunted the postprandial increase in circulating lactate, but did not improve neurological or other measures of clinical outcome.[70] A trial of DCA in MELAS patients was terminated early because it was found to cause peripheral neuropathy.[150] On the other hand, L-arginine (a precursor of creatine) appears to improve endothelial function and has potential for treatment in MELAS.[151] Patients with mitochondrial disease may have uridine deficiency and supplementation with triacetyluridine has resulted in improved strength, growth and renal tubular function in some patients.

OXPHOS disorders may cause hyperglycemia due to difficulty in oxidative metabolism of a large glucose load; in which case, a diabetic diet may be of value. In patients with secondary impairment of beta-oxidation of fatty acids, a low fat diet should be tried.

When mtDNA mutations in muscle are heteroplasmic, a novel therapeutic approach has been proposed by which exercise-induced muscle damage could result in altering the proportions of normal and mutant mtDNA as the tissue repairs. This is called *gene shifting*.[152] Resistance exercise training that induces muscle damage has the potential to stimulate dormant myoblast satellite cells to fuse with regenerating myofibers. In theory, myoblasts with normal mtDNA (and energy production) would be at a selective advantage and more likely to undergo such fusion as has been shown in a patient undergoing such exercise training. Spontaneous improvement, with a decrease in the proportion of mutant mtDNA in muscle, has been observed in a patient with a mtDNA point mutation, giving further support to the theoretical possibility of this approach.[153] Aerobic exercise appears to increase oxidative capacity in patients with mtDNA mutations, possibly by inducing mitochondrial proliferation. It is not clear, however, why production of the normal mtDNA might exceed that of the mutant and the long term outcome of such training is unknown.[154]

Experiments in gene therapy for respiratory chain disorders include complementation by cytosolic synthesis of mitochondrial proteins containing an appropriate targeting sequence, with subsequent translocation into mitochondria; direct mitochondrial transfection with an entire normal mitochondrial genome or polymerase chain reaction (PCR)-generated fragments of complementing DNA;[155] and sequence specific oligonucleotide or peptide–nucleotide conjugate targeting of mutant mtDNA.[156]

DISORDERS OF LIPID, LIPOPROTEIN AND BILE ACID METABOLISM

Disorders of lipid and lipoprotein metabolism are important and common in pediatrics, frequently with a genetic basis. Detection of dyslipidemia or early onset of cardiovascular disease in a closely related adult is an indication for young relatives also to be tested. Treatment of affected children with lipid-lowering medication may be warranted in some situations. Although atherosclerotic vascular disease is almost non-existent in children, homozygous familial hypercholesterolemia may cause myocardial infarction (MI) and death before age 20 years, and other forms of severe hyperlipidemia may cause MI in the third or fourth decade. Severe hypertriglyceridemia is also associated with increased risk of pancreatitis, a potentially life threatening complication. In addition to familial disorders, hyperlipidemia is an important complication of other metabolic disorders such as diabetes, obesity and the use of some medications. Finally, identification of secondary hyperlipidemia may indicate an underlying condition, such as hypothyroidism.

Basic biochemistry

The primary lipids in plasma are triglycerides, cholesterol and phospholipids. Other lipids that occur in small amounts in plasma include free fatty acids, mono- and di-glycerides, steroid hormones (e.g. testosterone, estradiol, cortisol), sterol-derived vitamins (e.g. vitamin D), terpenes (e.g. vitamins A, E and K) and sterols other than cholesterol (e.g. desmosterol, 7-dehydrocholesterol). Because of their innate insolubility in aqueous media, lipids are transported in plasma as a constituent of lipoproteins or bound to plasma carrier proteins.

Triglycerides and fatty acids

Triglycerides, which are composed of three fatty acid molecules covalently bound to a glycerol molecule, are synthesized in the liver from acetate or fatty acids and in the intestinal mucosa from absorbed dietary fat. Triglycerides are secreted into plasma in lipoproteins via the endogenous and exogenous pathways (Fig. 26.20). Free fatty acids (non-esterified) are normally present in plasma in small amounts, primarily bound to albumin, and have a short half-life of 4–8 min, but the majority of fatty acids in plasma occur in the form of triglycerides and to a lesser extent in phospholipids and cholesteryl esters in lipoproteins. Release of free fatty acids and glycerol from adipose tissue triglyceride stores normally is increased during exercise, stress and fasting as a consequence of increased activity of hormone sensitive lipase. Increased release of free fatty acids in patients with uncontrolled diabetes occurs as a result of the loss of insulin-mediated inhibition of phosphorylative activation of hormone-sensitive lipase. A sustained increase in delivery of free fatty acids and/or glucose to the liver, as occurs in uncontrolled diabetes, greatly stimulates hepatic synthesis of triglycerides, leading to hypertriglyceridemia. Relative deficiency of lipoprotein lipase in uncontrolled diabetes contributes to hypertriglyceridemia by delaying triglyceride lipolysis. During hydrolysis of triglycerides, mono- and di-glycerides are generated as intermediate products.

Fatty acids are classified on the basis of chain length and degree of saturation. Short chain fatty acids contain 2–6 carbon atoms, medium chain fatty acids contain 8–10 carbon atoms and long chain fatty acids contain > 12 carbon atoms. Very long chain fatty acids normally are a minor component of the fatty acid pool, but these molecules accumulate in patients with peroxisomal disorders (see p. 1113). Saturated fatty acids (e.g. stearic acid, C18:0) contain no double bonds, whereas mono-unsaturated fatty acids (e.g. oleic acid, C18:1ω9) contain a single double bond and polyunsaturated fatty acids (e.g. linoleic acid, C18:3ω6) contain two or more double bonds. Unsaturated fatty acids are further subclassified into four classes, ω3 (e.g. linolenic acid), ω6 (e.g. linoleic acid), ω7 (e.g. palmitoleic acid) and ω9 (e.g. oleic acid), on the basis of

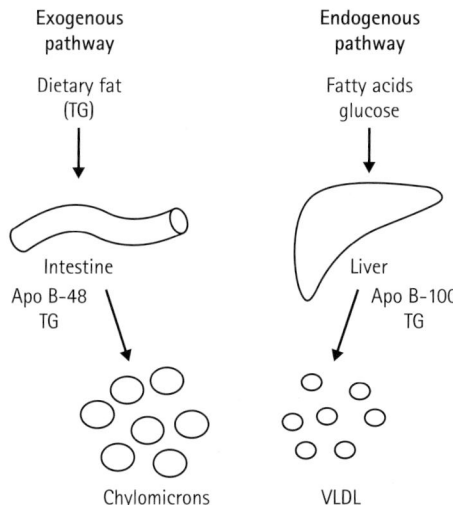

Fig. 26.20 Exogenous and endogenous sources of plasma triglycerides. TG, triglyceride; VLDL, very low density lipoprotein.

the position of the first double bond from the methylene end of the molecule. The ω3 fatty acids found in marine oils and fish, such as eicosapentanoic acid (EPA, C20:5ω3) and docosahexanoic acid (DHA, C22:6ω3), have potent triglyceride-lowering effects when given in sufficient doses, may modulate immunity and platelet function, may have additional cardioprotective effects, and also may have a role in pre- and post-natal development of the brain and retina.

Cholesterol

Cholesterol is synthesized from acetate by the liver and intestinal mucosa and released into plasma in lipoproteins. Other cell types also have the capacity to synthesize cholesterol in response to local cellular requirements, but most of this does not appear in plasma. All cholesterol in the brain is synthesized within the CNS. Current evidence suggests that a large proportion of cholesterol in high-density lipoprotein (HDL) particles may be derived by receptor-mediated efflux from peripheral tissues. Although the majority of cholesterol in the body is synthesized endogenously, dietary cholesterol nonetheless influences the plasma cholesterol concentration by modulating hepatic secretion and uptake of cholesterol via transcriptional regulation of key enzymes and receptors. Delivery of dietary cholesterol to the liver inhibits proteolytic activation of sterol regulatory element binding protein-2 (SREBP-2), which is an agonist for the SRE in the regulatory sequence of the low density lipoprotein (LDL) receptor gene and other genes. Hence, increased intake of dietary cholesterol decreases hepatic expression of the LDL receptor, thereby contributing to hypercholesterolemia. Under normal conditions, about 40–50% of dietary cholesterol is absorbed. Cholesterol biosynthesis is regulated in the liver by the rate-limiting enzyme, 3-hydroxy-3-methylglutaryl coenzyme A reductase (HMG-CoA reductase), which is the inhibitory target of 'statin' cholesterol lowering medications. A large amount of cholesterol and cholesterol derived bile acids circulate in the enterohepatic circulation, a pathway that consists of hepatic secretion of bile acids and cholesterol into the intestinal lumen via the bile duct followed by reabsorption of a portion of bile acids and cholesterol distally. The majority of cholesterol in plasma and tissues is esterified with a single fatty acid molecule to form cholesteryl esters.

Phospholipids

The plasma phospholipids are primarily derived from hepatic and intestinal synthesis, but can be synthesized by many body tissues. Phospholipids are acylglycerols that contain phosphoric acid esterified to the C_3-hydroxyl group. The four major classes of phospholipids are phosphatidyl choline (lecithin), phosphatidyl serine, phosphatidyl ethanolamine and phosphatidyl inositol. As a consequence of their polar structure, three of the four phospholipid classes form bilayers in aqueous media and are a critical component of cell membranes and the surface coat of lipoproteins. Phosphatidyl ethanolamine also is incorporated into cell membranes, but in isolation it has a tendency to form hexagonal complexes. As a consequence of the localization of phospholipids in the surface coat of lipoproteins, the phospholipid content of lipoprotein particles (expressed as a percentage of total weight) tends to be inversely proportional to particle size.

Lipoproteins

The three main lipids, triglycerides, phospholipids and cholesterol, are transported in plasma as constituents of various lipoproteins that can be characterized on the basis of lipid composition, protein composition, particle size and density, nuclear magnetic resonance (NMR) spectroscopy and electrophoretic mobility. The various lipoprotein particles also differ in their origin and metabolic fate. The characteristics of the six major lipoprotein classes are shown in Table 26.14. The lipoprotein classes are sometimes subfractionated on the basis of density (e.g. HDL2a, HDL2b, HDL3; LDL1, LDL2, LDL3) or size (e.g. LDL pattern A [large] and B [small]), but subfractionation is unnecessary for most clinical situations. The protein moieties of lipoproteins, which are referred to as apoproteins (Table 26.15), contribute to the structure and metabolic fate of various lipoprotein particles. HDL particles also can be subfractionated into particles containing apo A-I without A-II [HDL(A-I)] and particles containing apo A-I and A-II [HDL(A-I/A-II)]. HDL(A-I) particles may be more cardioprotective than HDL(A-I/A-II) particles.

LIPOPROTEIN METABOLISM

Chylomicrons

Chylomicrons are synthesized by enterocytes in the small intestine and secreted into the thoracic duct in response to absorption of dietary fat. Dietary lipids undergo hydrolysis in the intestinal lumen, allowing absorption of the resulting fatty acids and glycerol by enterocytes. Fatty acids with a chain length of <10–12 carbon atoms tend to be absorbed into the portal circulation, whereas other fatty acids are utilized by the intestinal mucosal cells for synthesis of chylomicrons. Enterocytes use hydrolyzed lipid products as substrates for synthesis of triglycerides, cholesteryl esters and phospholipids, which are combined with a single apo B-48 molecule, apoproteins A-I, A-II, A-IV and some apo C-II and E to form chylomicrons. Chylomicrons are slowly released into the circulation via the thoracic duct, normally resulting in a peak plasma triglyceride concentration 4–6 h after fat ingestion and return to baseline after 8–10 h. After release into the plasma, chylomicrons are

Table 26.14   Characteristics of plasma lipoproteins

Lipoprotein	Electrophoretic mobility	Density (g/ml)	Size (Å)	Lipid composition (% of total weight)*	Major apoproteins	Origin
Chylomicrons	Alpha$_2$	0.95	800–5000	2% P, 7% PL, 2% FC, 5% CE, *84% TG*	B-48, C-I, C-II, C-III, E	Intestine
VLDL	Pre-beta	0.95–1.006	300–800	8% P, 19% PL, 7% FC, 13% CE, *53% TG*	B-100, C-I, C-II, C-III, E	Liver
IDL	Low pre-beta (broad beta)	1.006–1.019	250–350	19% P, 19% PL, 9% FC, *29% CE*, 23% TG	B-100, E	VLDL, chylomicrons
LDL	Beta	1.019–1.063	200–250	21% P, 22% PL, 8% FC, *37% CE*, 11% TG	B-100	VLDL, liver
Lipoprotein(a)	Sinking pre-beta	1.06–1.08	200–300	33% P, 22% PL, 9% FC, *33% CE*, 3% TG	B-100, apo(a)	Liver
HDL	Alpha$_1$	1.063–1.21	75–100	*50% P*, 23% PL, 4% FC, 18% CE, 4% TG	A-I (70–75% of protein) A-II, (A-IV, D, CI-III, E)	Liver, peripheral tissues, intestine

*Dominant lipid in each protein is in italics.
CE, cholesteryl ester; FC, free cholesterol; HDL, high density lipoprotein; IDL, intermediate density lipoprotein; LDL, low density lipoprotein; P, protein; PL, phospholipid; TG, triglyceride; VLDL, very low density lipoprotein.

Table 26.15   Major plasma apoproteins

Apoprotein	Origin	Molecular weight	Metabolic function
A-I (apolipoprotein I)	Liver, intestine	28 000	Activates LCAT; ligand for ABC-A1 receptor, ABCG1, SR-B1, cubulin/megalin
A-II	Liver, intestine	17 500	May facilitate activation of hepatic lipase, may inhibit LCAT
A-IV	Intestine, liver	44 500	May facilitate LPL activation; activates LCAT, affects HDL assembly and metabolism
A-V	Liver		May be important determinant of plasma triglyceride concentrations
Apo(a)	Liver	Variable: 400–800 000	Covalently bound to apo B-100 in Lp(a) via sulfhydryl linkage; may adversely influence fibrinolysis and lipid deposition at sites of arterial injury
B-48	Intestine	264 000	Structural protein in chylomicrons. Truncated version of apo B-100
B-100	Liver	550 000	Structural protein in LDL and VLDL, binds to LDL receptor; essential for synthesis and secretion of VLDL
C-I	Liver, adrenal	7000	Cofactor for LCAT, inhibits CETP
C-II	Liver, (intestine)	9000	Cofactor for LPL
C-III	Liver	9000	Inhibits LPL activation, cofactor for sphingomyelinase, may activate LCAT
C-IV	Liver	16 000	Associated mostly with VLDL, some in HDL. Probably involved in triglyceride metabolism
D	Adrenal, kidney, pancreas, placenta, brain, intestine, spleen, testes	29 000	May facilitate interlipoprotein and intercell lipid transfer, involved in brain lipid metabolism, activates LCAT. Carried in HDL
E (E2, E3, E4)	Liver, (intestine), CNS, peripheral tissues, macrophages	34 000	Binds to LDL and apo E receptors, facilitates hepatic uptake of VLDL and chylomicron remnants. Dominant apoprotein in brain
F	Liver	33 000	Lipid transfer inhibitor protein (LTIP), inhibits CETP, associated with LDL
H (β2-glycoprotein I)	Liver	43 000	Component of HDL and chylomicrons, may facilitate LPL activation
J (clusterin)	Liver, other?	70 000	Binds to megalin (LRP2); found in amyloid, may be involved in neurodegenerative disorders, found in all human fluids including CSF
M (protein G3a)	Liver, kidney	26 000	Member of lipocalin protein superfamily. Associates with HDL, but also VLDL and LDL. Binds to megalin (LRP2).
Transfer proteins	Liver	Variable	Transfer of lipids between lipoproteins

CETP, cholesteryl ester transfer protein; HDL, high density lipoprotein; LCAT, lecithin–cholesterol acyltransferase; LDL, low density lipoprotein; LPL, lipoprotein lipase; SR-B1, scavenger receptor-B1; VLDL, very low density lipoprotein.

rapidly remodeled and catabolized with a half-life < 15 min. Transfer of apo C and E from HDL to chylomicrons facilitates the hydrolysis of chylomicron triglycerides by lipoprotein lipase (LPL) and subsequent hepatic uptake of triglyceride-depleted chylomicron remnants via the LDL receptor-related protein (LRP), apo E receptor and proteoglycan-mediated uptake pathways. During chylomicron degradation, fatty acids released by LPL in peripheral tissues can be utilized for energy or storage as triglycerides in adipose tissue. Apoproteins A-I and A-II and phospholipids are transferred to HDL during chylomicron catabolism.

Very low density lipoprotein

Very low density lipoprotein (VLDL) particles are primarily secreted by the liver, although there is evidence for intestinal secretion of VLDL. The rate of synthesis of VLDL is dependent on hormonal factors (such as insulin), time of day, diet, amount of adiposity (particularly visceral fat mass), and availability of substrate for triglyceride synthesis. Apo B-100 synthesis is essential for VLDL synthesis and secretion. During the initial steps of VLDL synthesis, apo B-100 is required on the endoplasmic reticulum to facilitate the aggregation of triglyceride and other lipids

to form VLDL particles. Thus, lack of apo B-100, or the presence of truncation mutations in apo B-100, can suppress VLDL secretion. The metabolic pathways for VLDL particles in plasma are similar to those of chylomicrons, but VLDL particles also are remodeled by hepatic lipase and typically have a much longer half-life in plasma of 6–12 h. In addition, VLDL particles are sequentially metabolized to become intermediate density lipoprotein (IDL) particles and subsequently LDL particles. VLDL remnants can be taken up by hepatic LDL, apo E and LRP receptors. The important role of apo E in hepatic clearance of VLDL from plasma is illustrated by the marked accumulation of VLDL and chylomicron remnants in patients with type III hyperlipidemia resulting from increased VLDL secretion in the context of homozygosity for apo E2, a defective ligand for the apo E receptor and LRP.

Low density lipoprotein

The majority of LDL particles in plasma derives from intravascular catabolism and remodeling of VLDL particles. To a lesser extent, de novo synthesis of LDL does occur in the liver. Unlike chylomicrons and VLDL particles that can sequentially deliver fatty acids and other lipids to various tissues during catabolism, LDL particles primarily deliver cholesterol, which occurs via whole particle uptake by the LDL receptor or alternative pathways. Modified LDL particles may be taken up by scavenger receptors or oxidized LDL receptors. Transfer of cholesteryl esters from HDL to LDL is mediated in part by cholesteryl ester transfer protein (CETP) in the process of reverse cholesterol transport. Modification of LDL by LPL and hepatic lipase (HL) influences the size and density of LDL particles, as well as their atherogenicity. Small dense LDL (pattern B) is more atherogenic than buoyant LDL (pattern A). The normal half-life of LDL particles in plasma is 3–4 d. Although peripheral tissues can catabolize LDL particles, and steroidogenic endocrine tissues (e.g. adrenal) take up proportionally large amounts of LDL per amount of tissue, the liver is the major site of LDL removal from plasma. Decreased numbers of functional LDL receptors in the liver resulting from genetic defects (e.g. familial hypercholesterolemia), hypothyroidism or aging, lead to hypercholesterolemia due to accumulation of LDL particles in plasma. The liver is a key regulator of plasma LDL cholesterol concentrations.

High density lipoprotein and reverse cholesterol transport

HDL particles are believed to be the primary mediators of reverse cholesterol transport, the process whereby cholesterol is removed from peripheral tissues and delivered to the liver for disposal. Studies of Tangier disease (see below) have greatly advanced our understanding of the genesis and metabolism of HDL particles. In Tangier disease, the absence of functional ABCA1 receptors results in dramatic reductions in the formation of HDL particles and a very low plasma HDL cholesterol concentration. This observation suggests that the acquisition of free cholesterol from peripheral tissues by apo A-I via the ABCA1 transporter is a major source of HDL cholesterol in plasma. Apo E-rich HDL is the dominant lipoprotein in the brain.

Most free cholesterol in nascent HDL particles is normally esterified in plasma by lecithin–cholesterol acyltransferase (LCAT) to form cholesteryl esters. Sequestration of additional cholesterol by HDL via SRB1 and ABCG1, and further remodeling in plasma, results in larger mature HDL particles, typically in the HDL2 subfraction. CETP mediates the transfer of cholesteryl ester from HDL to VLDL and LDL for subsequent delivery to the liver via the LDL, apo E and LRP receptors. HDL also can selectively deliver cholesterol directly to the liver via the scavenger receptor class B, type 1 (SR-B1), without uptake of the whole HDL particle. Cubulin is an additional HDL receptor that may mediate uptake of free apo A-I in the renal tubule. Megalin, a member of the LDL receptor family, also binds apo A-I and may mediate catabolism of HDL. After delivery of cholesterol to the liver at the terminus of the reverse cholesterol transport pathway, a portion of the cholesterol is utilized for bile acid synthesis by the rate-limiting enzyme CYP7A1 under the regulatory control of heterodimers of the nuclear retinoid X receptor (RXR) and farnesoid X (bile acid) receptor (FXR). Cholesterol and bile acids are secreted into the bile for subsequent excretion of a portion of the enterohepatic circulatory pool of cholesterol and bile acids in the feces. Additional cardioprotective effects of HDL may be related to antioxidant (related in part to paraoxonase) and anti-inflammatory properties.

Exercise, weight loss, alcohol intake, estrogen and phenytoin can increase plasma HDL cholesterol concentrations, but not all mechanisms for HDL cholesterol elevation are beneficial. Among lipid-lowering medications, niacin and fibrates have the greatest HDL cholesterol-raising efficacy. Torcetrapib, an experimental CETP inhibitor, substantially increases the plasma HDL cholesterol concentration, but this drug has been withdrawn due to excess mortality. Puberty in males (testosterone), weight gain, type 2 diabetes, hypertriglyceridemia, cigarette smoking and a low fat diet can be associated with decreases in plasma HDL cholesterol. It is important to realize that the cardioprotective benefits from HDL are probably more dependent on the flux of cholesterol from peripheral tissues to the liver for disposal than on the absolute HDL cholesterol sponcentrations. For example, increased removal of HDL cholesterol from plasma by overexpression of hepatic SR-B1 receptors in experimental animals lowers the plasma HDL cholesterol concentration, but reduces the risk of atherosclerosis. Conversely, deficiency of

CETP in humans increases the plasma HDL cholesterol concentration to 3.8–5.1 mmol/L (150–200 mg/dl) by blocking transfer of cholesteryl esters from HDL to VLDL and LDL, but this condition can be associated with increased risk for atherosclerosis if the LDL cholesterol concentration also is high. Thus, the relationship between risk for atherosclerosis and increases or decreases in plasma HDL cholesterol needs to be interpreted with an understanding of the potential effects of such changes on reverse cholesterol transport.

Lipoprotein(a)

Lipoprotein(a) [Lp(a)] probably is formed in plasma as a consequence of the covalent cysteine–cysteine disulfide linkage of circulating apo(a) to the C-terminal region of apo B-100 in LDL particles. More than 95% of apo(a) in plasma is found in Lp(a). The liver is the predominant site of apo(a) synthesis. Plasma concentrations of Lp(a) vary 100-fold in the general population, largely due to genetic factors resulting in > 70–80% heritability of plasma Lp(a) concentrations. Genetically mediated apo(a) size polymorphisms are an important determinant of the Lp(a) concentration, as reflected by the inverse association between the apo(a) size and the plasma Lp(a) concentration. Additional factors that can increase plasma Lp(a) concentrations are renal insufficiency, menopause and dietary intake of trans fatty acids. Factors that may decrease plasma Lp(a) concentrations are postmenopausal estrogen replacement, treatment with niacin, anabolic steroids and LDL apheresis (a process that removes apo B-containing particles from plasma). High plasma concentrations of Lp(a) are associated with increased risk for cardiovascular disease, but the atherogenicity of Lp(a) may require the presence of elevated plasma concentrations of LDL cholesterol. Reducing the LDL cholesterol concentration below ~2.0 mmol/L (80 mg/dl) may abrogate the atherogenicity of elevated Lp(a). The normal physiological function of Lp(a) is unclear, but it may be involved in the delivery of cholesterol and other lipids to sites of vascular injury. A deficiency syndrome is unknown, even among individuals with very low concentrations of Lp(a). The presence in apo(a) of multiple kringle-4 repeats with homology to plasminogen may contribute to alterations in fibrinolysis.

Enzymes and transfer proteins involved in lipoprotein metabolism

A variety of enzymes and transfer proteins serve important roles in lipoprotein metabolism (Table 26.16). Beginning in the small bowel, pancreatic lipase hydrolyzes dietary fats to release glycerol and triglycerides that are absorbed by enterocytes. Within the enterocyte, microsomal triglyceride transfer protein (MTP) is involved in the formation of chylomicrons. MTP also is involved in formation of VLDL particles in the liver. Three additional enzymes are involved in intravascular metabolism of lipoproteins.

LPL and HL are bound by heparan sulfate to the vascular endothelium, where they are involved in hydrolysis of triglycerides (and phospholipids by hepatic lipase) in triglyceride-rich lipoproteins, remodeling of lipoproteins (LDL, remnants and HDL), and hepatic uptake of remnant lipoproteins. Heterozygous deficiency of LPL may be a subgroup of the familial disorder, familial combined hyperlipidemia, which is discussed below. Endothelial lipase is primarily a phospholipase that may be involved in HDL metabolism, placental lipid metabolism and release of fatty acids from phospholipids for energy utilization.

Cholesterol ester transport protein (CETP) and phospholipid transfer protein (PLTP) are involved in the bidirectional transfer of lipids between lipoproteins. CETP is secreted by the liver and circulates in plasma mainly bound to HDL. It plays an important role in reverse cholesterol transport by facilitating the transfer of cholesteryl esters from cholesterol replete HDL particles to VLDL and LDL for subsequent delivery to the liver for disposal. CETP deficiency results in very high plasma HDL cholesterol concentrations, but may increase risk for atherosclerosis due to the block in reverse cholesterol transport. PLTP is involved in the transfer of surface phospholipids from shrinking triglyceride-rich lipoprotein particles during their catabolism.

Table 26.16 Enzymes and transfer proteins involved in lipoprotein metabolism

Enzyme	Function
Pancreatic lipase	Hydrolysis of dietary fat in intestinal lumen
Hormone-sensitive lipase	Hydrolysis of triglycerides in adipose cells to release free fatty acids
Lipoprotein lipase	Hydrolysis of triglycerides in circulating VLDL and chylomicrons to release free fatty acids to peripheral tissues; uptake of triglyceride-rich lipoproteins
Hepatic lipase	Hydrolysis of triglycerides and phospholipids in VLDL and VLDL remnants, uptake of remnant lipoproteins, facilitation of SR-BI-mediated uptake of HDL cholesteryl esters by liver
Endothelial lipase	Hydrolysis of lipoprotein phospholipids, involved in HDL metabolism
Lecithin cholesterol acyltransferase (LCAT)	Catalyzes transfer of position 2 fatty acids from phosphatidyl choline to cholesterol in HDL to form cholesteryl esters
Acyl cholesterol acyltransferase (ACAT)	Catalyzes esterification of cholesterol to form cholesteryl esters in intracellular pools
Transfer proteins Cholesteryl ester transfer protein (CETP)	Facilitates transfer of cholesteryl esters from HDL to VLDL and LDL
Phospholipid transfer protein (PLTP)	Facilitates transfer of phospholipids from triglyceride-rich lipoproteins to HDL, may facilitate recycling of HDL back to discoidal particles

HDL, high density lipoprotein; LDL, low density lipoprotein; SR-B1, scavenger receptor-B1; VLDL, very low density lipoprotein.

Lipoprotein receptors

The number of recognized lipoprotein receptors has been expanding rapidly during recent years. These receptors are important for the metabolism and uptake of lipoproteins by various tissues (Table 26.17). The classic genetic disorder caused by defective lipoprotein receptors is familial hypercholesterolemia, which most commonly is a consequence of a variety of types of mutations in the LDL receptor. It is anticipated that a myriad of genetic disorders related to mutations in lipoprotein receptors, lipolytic enzymes and transfer proteins have yet to be identified.

HYPERLIPIDEMIA

The hyperlipidemias have traditionally been classified descriptively as Fredrickson types I–V on the basis of the type of lipoprotein particle that is increased in plasma (Table 26.18). Although the classification of hyperlipidemia as types I–V is still occasionally used, it rarely adds information that is not already apparent from the fasting lipid profile. In addition, problems arise because multiple disorders can result in the same lipoprotein phenotype. For example, both the genetic disorder familial hypercholesterolemia and hypothyroidism can be associated with type IIa hyperlipidemia. Moreover, a single disorder may cause several patterns of hyperlipidemia in different individuals, and in a single individual over time. The Fredrickson classification does not accommodate important disorders such as hypoalphalipoproteinemia (low HDL cholesterol), elevated Lp(a) or qualitative changes in lipoprotein particles such as small dense LDL. The one exception to these limitations is the diagnosis of type III hyperlipidemia, which refers to a specific genetically mediated metabolic disorder that is described in more detail below.

The hyperlipidemias can be subdivided into primary (hereditary) hyperlipidemias (Table 26.19), and secondary hyperlipidemias resulting from acquired (often reversible) metabolic conditions (Table 26.20). The best 'classification scheme' involves identifying the precise genetic and/or metabolic defect in an individual patient, although currently this is often not possible.

PRIMARY HYPERLIPIDEMIAS
Familial hypercholesterolemia

Familial hypercholesterolemia (FH) occurs in ~1 in 500 people and is classically an autosomal dominant disorder of the LDL receptor, resulting in an absent or functionally defective receptor protein; hundreds of mutations are known. Defects have been identified in transcription, post-translation modification, translocation to the plasma membrane, LDL binding, localization to clathrin coated pits, internalization and degradation. Individuals heterozygous for such LDL receptor defects typically have about half-normal levels of LDL-receptor expression in the liver and twice-normal plasma LDL-cholesterol concentrations. Other dominant causes of FH include defects in apo B that diminish LDL receptor binding (familial defective apo B) and heterozygous gain of function defects in PCSK9, a gene that encodes NARC1, an LDL receptor ligand that promotes degradation of the LDL receptor after internalization from the plasma membrane. Autosomal recessive familial hypercholesterolemia (ARH) is caused by homozygous defects in ARH-1, an adapter-like protein that modulates internalization of LDL–LDL receptor complexes from clathrin coated pits.

Severe hypercholesterolemia in FH greatly increases the risk for atherosclerotic vascular disease, with about 50% of untreated males and females developing myocardial infarction by the ages of 50 and 60 years, respectively. The lifetime risk for myocardial infarction is > 85% in untreated patients. In accordance with the concept that atherosclerosis is a generalized process that can affect multiple arterial trees, the risk for stroke and peripheral vascular disease also is increased in patients with this disorder, although myocardial infarction is the most common. In some families, other atherogenic factors, such as increased Lp(a), may accentuate the risk for vascular disease, resulting in earlier clinical expression of cardiovascular disease as early as the third decade. Homozygous familial hypercholesterolemia is associated with LDL cholesterol levels > 12.8–18 mmol/L (500–700 mg/dl) and myocardial infarction and death in childhood without very aggressive treatment.

Clinical findings and treatment

The primary physical manifestations of heterozygous FH are early corneal arcus and tendon xanthomas, which are not always present and may not develop until the fifth or sixth decade. Children with homozygous FH commonly develop tendon and tuberous xanthomas in early childhood. Treatment for homozygous FH requires aggressive pharmacological therapy, often in combination with LDL apheresis, which should be provided in collaboration with a lipid disorders clinic. Liver transplantation has been used successfully in some patients to alleviate the severe hypercholesterolemia, but this aggressive intervention is itself associated with complications. It is possible that targeted gene therapy for delivery of normal LDL receptors to the liver may become feasible at some point in the future.

Treatment is discussed on p. 1100.

Familial defective apo B

This autosomal dominant disorder is a subtype of FH in which a defect in apo B-100 prevents binding of LDL to normal LDL receptors. The most common mutation is a glutamine to arginine point mutation at amino acid 3500, but other mutations have been described.

Polygenic hypercholesterolemia

This is a heterogeneous group of prevalent disorders that clearly have a familial component, presumably resulting from interactions between two or more genes. Polygenic hypercholesterolemia is probably the most common primary hyperlipidemia. The genetic basis for such disorders is unknown, but is an area of intense interest.

Table 26.17   Lipoprotein receptors

Receptor (R)	Family	Ligand(s)	Function(s)
LDL-R	LDL-receptor	Apo B-100, E	Uptake of LDL, IDL and VLDL remnants
VLDL-R	LDL-receptor	Apo B-100, E, reelin	VLDL uptake
Apo E-R2	LDL-receptor	Apo E, reelin	Uptake of apo E-containing lipoproteins
MEGF7	LDL-receptor		
LDL-R related protein (LRP orLRP-1)	LDL-receptor	Apo E, LPL, PAI-1, tPA, lactoferrin, others	Uptake of VLDL and chylomicron remnants. Multiple LRP subtypes exist; some are not involved in lipoprotein metabolism
LRP1B	LDL-receptor	Comparable to LRP	Comparable to LRP
Megalin (LRP-2)	LDL-receptor	Apo E, HDL	Endocytic uptake of retinoids and steroids
Scavenger receptor, class A, types I and II (SRA-I, SRA-II)	Scavenger receptor, class A	Acetylated LDL, oxidized LDL, polyanionic molecules, others	Uptake of modified lipoproteins, and apoptotic and senescent cells by macrophages
CD36	Scavenger receptor, class B	Oxidized LDL, acetylated LDL, others	Uptake of oxidized LDL
SR-BI	Scavenger receptor, class B	LDL, HDL, acetylated LDL, oxidized LDL	Uptake of modified lipoproteins, selective uptake of HDL cholesteryl ester by liver, transfer of cholesterol from peripheral cells to HDL and other lipoproteins
SR-BII	Scavenger receptor, class B	Modified lipoproteins	SR-BI splice variant
Lectin-like oxidized LDL receptor-1 (LOX-1)	C-type lectin-like protein super family	Oxidized LDL	Uptake of oxidized LDL
ATP binding cassette subfamily A, member 1 (ABCA1)	ABC transporter	Apo A-I	Peripheral HDL receptor, mediates formation of nascent HDL from tissue derived cholesterol and apo A-I, modulates uptake of sterols in small intestine
ATP binding cassette subfamily G, member 1 (ABCG1)	ABC transporter		Facilitates transfer of cholesterol from peripheral cells to HDL and other lipoproteins
Cubulin		Apo A-I, intrinsic factor-vitamin B_{12} complexes	Uptake of apo A-I in renal tubule

HDL, high density lipoprotein, IDL, intermediate density lipoprotein; LPL, lipoprotein lipase; LRP, LDL receptor-related protein; PAI, Plasminogen activator inhibitor; SR, scavenger receptor; tPA, tissue plasminogen activator; VLDL, very low density lipoprotein.

Table 26.18   Descriptive classification of hyperlipidemia on the basis of lipoprotein accumulation

Type	Lipoprotein abnormality	Possible etiologies	Lipid values
I	↑Chylomicrons	LPL deficiency, apo C-II deficiency	↑↑TG. Total cholesterol is 4–7% of TG level
IIa	↑LDL	Familial hypercholesterolemia, hypothyroidism	↑Total cholesterol and LDL-cholesterol
IIb	↑LDL and VLDL	Familial combined hyperlipidemia, type 2 diabetes	↑Total cholesterol, LDL- and VLDL-cholesterol and TG
III	↑Remnants (IDL)	Homozygosity for mutant apo E2 + disorder of lipoprotein overproduction	↑↑IDL and remnants, ↑total cholesterol (TG
IV	↑VLDL	Type 2 diabetes, familial combined hyperlipidemia, ethanol	↑TG (< 1000 mg/dl), 11.2 mmol/L ↑Total and VLDL cholesterol
V	↑VLDL and chylomicrons	Type 2 diabetes, ethanol, high fat diet	↑↑TG (> 1000 mg/dl), 11.2 mmol/L total cholesterol. 7–10% of TG level

IDL, intermediate density lipoprotein; LDL, low density lipoprotein; LPL, lipoprotein lipase; TG, triglyceride; VLDL, very low density lipoprotein.

Table 26.19 Primary hyperlipidemias and lipoprotein deficiencies

Disorder	Prevalence	Inheritance	Lipoprotein pattern	Genetic cause
Hyperlipidemias				
LPL deficiency	1 in 10^6	Recessive	Type I	LPL mutation resulting in absent or defective protein
Apo C-II deficiency	Rare	Recessive	Type I	Apo C-II deficiency
Familial hypercholesterolemia (heterozygous)	1 in 500	Dominant	IIa/IIb	Defective LDL receptor; hundreds of mutations. Homozygotes occur in 1:10^6
Familial defective apo B	1 in 700–1000	Dominant	IIa/IIb	Glutamine < arginine 3500 in apo B-100 causes defective binding to LDL receptor. Phenotype similar to familial hypercholesterolemia
PCSK9 polymorphisms	Variable	Dominant	↑ or ↓ LDL cholesterol	PCSK9 gene encodes a protein that promotes degradation of the LDL receptor. Gain of function or loss of function mutations modulate hepatic LDL receptor activity
Polygenic hypercholesterolemia	1 in 100?	Polygenic	IIa/IIb	Unknown
Familial combined hyperlipidemia	1 in 100–200	Dominant	IIa/IIb, IV, V	Associated with increased apo B secretion. Single defects in a variety of genes may cause a common phenotype. Polymorphisms in upstream transcription factor-1 (USF1) may be a key underlying defect.
Familial hypertriglyceridemia	1 in 200–500	Dominant	IV/V	Unknown
Type III hyperlipidemia	1 in 5000–10000	Usually recessive	III	Homozygosity for mutant apo E2 is permissive, but not sufficient
(Broad-beta disease, dysbetalipoproteinemia)				Requires concurrent disorder of increased lipoprotein secretion Prevalence of E2/E2 homozygotes is about 1 in 100; most do not have hyperlipidemia. Rare dominant mutations occur
Sitosterolemia	≈40–60 cases reported	Recessive	IIa	Mutations in ABCG5 and G8 sterol transporters
Cerebrotendinous xanthomatosis (CTX)	≈150 cases reported	Recessive	IIa/IIb	Defect in 27-hydroxylase blocks bile acid synthesis
Lipoprotein deficiencies				
Tangier disease	< 100 cases reported	Recessive	Very low HDL-C	Defect in ABCA1 (HDL receptor)
Abetalipoproteinemia	Rare	Recessive	Cholesterol 20–30 mg/dl 0.5–0.75 mmol/L	Absence of apo B-100 with decreased or absent apo B-48; MTP mutations
Hypobetalipoproteinemia	1 in 1000–2000	Dominant	LDL-C 20–40 mg/dl 0.5–1.0 mmol/L	Apo B truncations
Chylomicron retention disease	Rare	Recessive	Low cholesterol, TG	Inability to synthesize or secrete chylomicrons
Familial hypoalphalipoproteinemia	> 1 in 100–200	Dominant	HDL-C 30 mg/dl 0.75 mmol/L	Apo A-I mutations, heterozygous ABCA1 mutations
Fish eye disease	Rare	Recessive	–	Defect in LCAT activity
LCAT deficiency	Rare	Recessive	–	Absence of LCAT activity

HDL, high density lipoprotein; LCAT, lecithin-cholesterol acyltransferase; LDL, low density lipoprotein; LPL, lipoprotein lipase; MTP, microsomal triglyceride transfer protein; TG, triglyceride.

Familial combined hyperlipidemia

Familial combined hyperlipidemia is genetically heterogeneous with a common phenotype characterized by hepatic overproduction of apo B-100 and accumulation in plasma of apo B-100-containing lipoproteins (VLDL, IDL and LDL). This disorder has a prevalence of 1–2% and may account for up to 20% of premature coronary heart disease.

The resulting hyperlipidemia is variable among affected family members and can vary over time in a given individual. The lipoprotein abnormalities often consist of increased plasma apo B in association with increased plasma concentrations of triglycerides (in VLDL) or LDL-cholesterol, or both. The plasma HDL cholesterol concentration often is reduced and the LDL particles often are characterized as small

Table 26.20   Secondary dyslipidemias

Category	Condition	Lipoprotein abnormality
Dietary	Excess saturated fat/cholesterol	↑cholesterol, ↑LDL-C, ↑TG from fat intake in susceptible patients
	Very low fat	↓LDL-C, ↓HDL-C, possible ↑ TG
	Excess calories	↑TG, ↓HDL-C
Endocrine	Diabetes	↑TG if uncontrolled; abnormal lipoprotein composition in type 2
	Insulin resistance	↑TG
	Hypothyroidism	↑total cholesterol, ↑LDL-C, ↑TG
	Obesity	TG overproduction
	Cushing syndrome	↑TG, possible ↑LDL-C
	Lipodystrophy	↑TG
	Acromegaly	↑TG
Drugs	Alcohol	↑TG
	Thiazide diuretics	↑LDL-C, ↑TG
	Beta-adrenergic blockers	↑TG, ↓HDL-C
	Glucocorticoids	↑TG, possible ↑LDL-C
	Oral estrogen/tamoxifen	↑TG
		↑TG
	Retinoic acid derivatives	↑Total cholesterol, ↑LDL-C
	Ciclosporin	↑TG (↑total cholesterol, ↑ LDL-C)
	Protease inhibitors	
Other	Renal failure/nephrotic syndrome	↑Total cholesterol, ↑LDL-C, ↑ TG, ↑lipoprotein(a)
	Cholestatic liver disease	↑↑Total cholesterol, ↑lipoprotein X
	Lupus, myeloma, autoimmune disease	↑TG
	Some glycogen storage diseases	↑TG, ↑LDL-C

HDL, high density lipoprotein; LDL, low density lipoprotein; TG, triglyceride.

and dense (e.g. pattern B), which are more atherogenic than buoyant larger LDL particles. Patients with this disorder develop premature myocardial infarction, stroke and peripheral vascular disease in mid-adulthood. It has been suggested that the hyperlipidemia phenotype of familial combined hyperlipidemia may not be fully expressed until young adulthood, but hyperlipidemia may emerge in childhood. Heterozygous LPL deficiency appears to be one subtype of this disorder. The genetic basis for familial combined hyperlipidemia may be related to upstream transcription factor-1 (USF1), a ubiquitous basic-helix-loop-helix leucine zipper transcription factor that modulates expression of at least 13 genes involved in lipid and glucose metabolism. The results of recent studies suggest that polymorphisms in USF1 may be the key defect that confers susceptibility to familial combined hyperlipidemia.

Familial hypertriglyceridemia

This disorder may be a subtype of familial combined hyperlipidemia, although the phenotype is one of hypertriglyceridemia with triglyceride concentrations usually < 11.2 mmol/L (1000 mg/dl). Older studies suggested this condition may be benign, other than the increased risk for pancreatitis during exacerbation of hypertriglyceridemia (triglycerides > 16.8–22.4 mmol/L [1500–2000 mg/dl]). The absence of coronary artery disease in a family with an autosomal dominant pattern of inheritance of hypertriglyceridemia suggests the diagnosis, but the possibility of increased risk for coronary artery disease should not be excluded. The genetic basis for this disorder is uncertain.

Type III hyperlipidemia

Type III hyperlipidemia, also known as broad beta disease or familial dysbetalipoproteinemia, is associated with homozygosity for the abnormal apoprotein E2 that is a poor ligand for triglyceride-rich lipoprotein receptors in the liver. Rare autosomal dominant forms of this disorder have been identified. Surprisingly, apo E2/E2 homozygosity is seen in about 1% of the general population, but the prevalence of type III hyperlipidemia is only 1 in 5000–10 000. Thus, only 1–2% of individuals with the homozygous genetic abnormality in apo E develop type III hyperlipidemia. Under normal conditions, the apo E2/E2 mutation alone is insufficient to cause hyperlipidemia, since alternative pathways exist for clearance of small amounts of triglyceride-rich lipoprotein remnants. However, in the setting of overproduction of triglyceride-rich lipoproteins, which occurs in hypothyroidism, obesity, high fat diet consumption, menopause, uncontrolled diabetes, familial combined hyperlipidemia, and other conditions, the clearance pathways become saturated, thereby resulting in the accumulation of atherogenic VLDL and chylomicron remnants.

Clinical findings

Palmar xanthomas (yellowish deposits in palmar creases) are said to be pathognomonic, but often are not present. Tuberoeruptive xanthomas also occur, but resolve over months during effective lipid lowering therapy. Patients with this disorder are susceptible to diffuse premature atherosclerosis.

Treatment

Treatment is directed to alleviation of factors causing lipoprotein overproduction. A low fat diet, regular exercise, and avoidance of obesity are key lifestyle interventions. Alcohol exacerbates the dyslipidemia. Fibrates are the first line drug therapy, but statins, niacin and fish oil also are helpful.

Lipoprotein lipase and apo C-II deficiency

LPL deficiency is a rare condition detectable at birth that is thought to occur with a frequency of about 1 in 10^6. Causes of LPL deficiency can include homozygous deficiency of functional enzyme, absence of the cofactor apo C-II and dominant inheritance of a lipase inhibitor.

Clinical findings

The clinical manifestations of recurrent pancreatitis and eruptive xanthomas may not be recognized until late infancy or childhood, but the severity of hypertriglyceridemia and its complications are related to dietary fat intake. Other symptoms may include abdominal pain in the absence of pancreatitis, dyspnea and mild cognitive dysfunction. Plasma triglyceride concentrations may be > 33.7–112 mmol/L (3000–10 000 mg/dl; lower in young children) in association with moderately increased plasma cholesterol concentrations. Lipemia retinalis often is visible when the triglyceride concentration is > 44.9–56 mmol/L (4000–5000 mg/dl), but it is much easier to examine the blood ex vivo after separation of plasma or serum from blood cells by centrifugation or standing. The plasma typically appears turbid when the triglyceride concentration exceeds 5.6–6.7 mmol/L (500–600 mg/dl). Plasma with a triglyceride concentration of 11.2 mmol/L (1000 mg/dl) has the appearance of skimmed milk. Plasma with a triglyceride concentration > 22.4–33.7 mmol/L (2000–3000 mg/dl) (2–3% fat) appears creamy, whereas levels > 33.7–67.4 mmol/L (5000–6000 mg/dl) (5–6% fat) will have the appearance of whipping cream.

Treatment

Initial treatment for severe hypertriglyceridemia requires a very low fat diet containing no more than a few grams of dietary fat daily. Children with overt pancreatitis require hospitalization for intravenous hydration and cessation of oral intake. In stable children, the fat intake may be increased to 5–10 g/d or higher as tolerated. Medium chain triglycerides, which are absorbed into the portal circulation and do not contribute to chylomicron formation, may be used to improve the palatability of the low-fat diet. Older children may succumb to the high fat dietary habits of their peers, but the development of abdominal pain helps to attenuate such behavior. Pharmacological therapy is generally unhelpful.

Wolman disease and cholesterol–ester storage disease (lysosomal acid lipase deficiency)

This lysosomal enzyme hydrolyses esterified cholesterol back to the free form. This step is required for feedback inhibition of new cholesterol synthesis. Its absence results in excess cholesterol production.

Wolman disease is most severe with xanthomatous deposits in many tissues resulting in hepatosplenomegaly, steatorrhea, failure to thrive and death in infancy. In cholesterol-ester storage disease (CESD) xanthomas are much less evident but this is one cause of hypercholesterolemia and should be aggressively treated. The disorders are allelic.

Phytosterolemia/sitosterolemia

This is a rare autosomal recessive disorder that is associated with tendon xanthomas, premature atherosclerosis and occasionally hemolytic anemia. It can present as 'pseudohomozygous familial hypercholesterolemia' with LDL-C > 12.8 mmol/L (500 mg/dl) in childhood, and xanthomas occasionally on the buttocks. Affected patients typically are very sensitive to diet-induced hypercholesterolemia due to enhanced intestinal absorption of cholesterol, as well as plant sterols. Sitosterol and other plant sterols, which are normally present in minimal amounts in plasma, accumulate in plasma of affected individuals. The disease is caused by defects in ABC-G5 or ABC-G8, two sterol transporters that normally export nonspecifically absorbed sitosterol and other plant sterols from the intestinal mucosa back into the intestinal lumen.

The diagnosis can be established by identifying increased levels of plasma sitosterol, or possibly by genetic testing. A low cholesterol diet in combination with bile acid-binding agents is helpful. Avoidance of dietary plant sterols is difficult, but affected individuals should avoid using over-the-counter cholesterol-lowering margarines containing sitosterol or sitostanol esters (Benecol and Take Control margarines in the USA). A selective inhibitor of cholesterol absorption, ezetimibe, is efficacious in these patients and can also lower LDL-C in conditions other than sitosterolemia.

OTHER GENETIC AND METABOLIC DISORDERS AFFECTING LIPID METABOLISM

Generalized lipodystrophy

There are several distinct genetic forms; some may be evident at birth (Berardinelli–Seip congenital lipodystrophy), others develop in childhood or adult life (Lawrence syndrome). Patients with generalized lipodystrophy have minimal amounts of body fat (subcutaneous and visceral). The congenital form of this disorder is often familial whereas the acquired form is commonly sporadic. Familial generalized lipodystrophy is primarily caused by mutations in the seipin gene (type 2 lipodystrophy) and AGPAT 2 (1-acylglycerol-3-phosphate O-acyltransferase 2 [lysophosphatidic acid acyltransferase, beta]) (type I lipodystrophy). Children with generalized lipodystrophy tend to be tall, have advanced bone age, and have the appearance of increased muscle bulk. Insulin resistance and subsequent development of type 2 diabetes and hypertriglyceridemia are common. Treatment consists primarily of correction of the metabolic abnormalities, but leptin may be efficacious for hyperglycemia and hypertriglyceridemia in some subtypes of lipodystrophy.

Partial lipodystrophy

Partial lipodystrophy consists of several overlapping phenotypes. Some may be due to recessive mutations in zinc metalloproteinase Ste-24 homolog (ZMPSTE-24) (type B lipodystrophy), recessive mutations in lamin A/C (type A lipodystrophy), dominant mutations in lamin A/C (Dunnigan type) or lamin A alone, lamin B2 (acquired) or defects in PPAR-gamma, but many cases seem to be sporadic. Typically there is progressive symmetrical loss of subcutaneous body fat, most commonly from the face, with progressive involvement of the arms, trunk and hips.

Other variations can involve loss of fat in the extremities (Kobberling type), preservation of subcutaneous fat in the face or patchy lipoatrophy. The age of onset varies from 5 to young adult life. Girls are affected much more frequently than boys. Insulin resistance is common and can be severe, resulting in very high insulin requirements and possibly increased responsiveness to insulin-sensitizing thiazoladinediones in those who develop type 2 diabetes. Hypertriglyceridemia can be a consequence of insulin resistance and/or hyperglycemia.

The use of highly active antiretroviral therapy (HAART) for human immunodeficiency virus (HIV) infections (see Ch. 27) is commonly associated with lipodystrophy, insulin resistance and dyslipidemia, all of which contribute to increased risk for atherosclerosis in patients with HIV. Abnormal fat distribution is seen in some of the carbohydrate deficiency syndromes.

Tangier disease

Tangier disease, a rare autosomal recessive disorder, is characterized by the near absence of plasma HDL cholesterol, very low plasma concentrations of apo A-I, and pathognomonic orange–yellow tonsillar enlargement, lymphadenopathy and splenomegaly. The physical findings are a consequence of the accumulation of cholesteryl esters in the reticuloendothelial system. Premature atherosclerosis may occur in individuals with sufficient amounts of LDL cholesterol in plasma. The genetic basis was once thought to be due to primary deficiency of HDL, but defects in the ABCA1 transporter protein are now known to be the cause. In Tangier disease, apo A-I is unable to sequester cholesterol from peripheral cells due to impaired interaction with the defective or absent ABCA1 protein, resulting in a dramatic reduction in formation of HDL particles and increased degradation of apo A-I. Typically, the LDL cholesterol concentration is low, which diminishes the risk of cardiovascular disease, but premature atherosclerosis occurs in individuals with the highest LDL cholesterol concentrations.

Familial hypoalphalipoproteinemia

Familial hypoalphalipoproteinemia is typically a consequence of heterozygous defects in ABCA1 (resulting in decreased formation of HDL and increased degradation of apo A-I) or apo A-I. Affected subjects have low concentrations of plasma HDL cholesterol (<0.9 mmol [11 35 mg/dl]) and increased risk of atherosclerosis. Uncommon forms of low HDL cholesterol may result from accelerated reverse cholesterol transport, which may lower the plasma HDL cholesterol without increasing the risk of atherosclerosis.

Abetalipoproteinemia

Abetalipoproteinemia is characterized by nearly complete absence of LDL in plasma. It is caused by autosomal recessive defects in microsomal triglyceride transfer protein (MTP) or homozygous truncation defects in apo B.

The net result of the defect is deficient assembly of chylomicrons, resulting in failure to absorb fat and fat-soluble nutrients from the gut, and inability to form VLDL in the liver, resulting in defective transport of vitamin E to peripheral tissues. Fat malabsorption causes steatorrhea and consequent growth failure with deficiency of several nutrients. The malabsorption can be so marked that night blindness (vitamin A deficiency), rickets (vitamin D deficiency) and neurological disease (ataxia, peripheral neuropathy; vitamin E deficiency) may occur in childhood. Pigmentary degeneration of the retina also occurs. Abnormal red cell membranes lead to acanthocytosis and anemia.

Diagnosis and treatment

The plasma cholesterol concentration is usually below 1.2 mmol/L (45 mg/dl). It may be possible to confirm the defect by DNA studies.

Treatment involves the monitored use of a low fat diet that is supplemented with high doses of essential fatty acids and fat-soluble vitamins, especially high-dose vitamin E to prevent neurological disease. Many of the complications are related to vitamin E deficiency. Heterozygotes may have normal or low plasma lipids.

Hypobetalipoproteinemia

Hypobetalipoproteinemia is an uncommon disorder characterized by a low plasma concentration of LDL cholesterol < 1.3 mmol/L (50 mg/dl). It typically is a consequence of heterozygous truncation mutations in apo B, resulting in the absence of apo B-100, or heterozygous defects in MTP. Apo B-100 is required for formation of VLDL particles, which are subsequently metabolized to become LDL particles. The disorder is associated with protection against atherosclerosis.

Lecithin:cholesterol transferase deficiency and fish eye disease

Familial lethicin:cholesterol transferase (LCAT) deficiency (complete) and fish eye disease (partial LCAT deficiency) are caused by autosomal recessive mutations in LCAT. Normally, 95% of LCAT in plasma is associated with HDL particles (alpha-LCAT) and the rest is associated with VLDL and LDL (beta-LCAT). LCAT is required for synthesis of esterified cholesterol and lysolecithin. In 'classical' deficiency, LCAT activity on HDL and VLDL/LDL is nearly absent, which results in corneal opacities and progressive renal disease. If the deficiency is less severe, sometimes associated with deficiency of LCAT only in HDL particles, the eye findings are present (fish eyes) but there is no renal disease. Most cases are diagnosed in adulthood.

The diagnosis is made by finding low levels of HDL-C, severely reduced LCAT activity in plasma or by DNA studies. The ratio of free:total cholesterol in plasma may be elevated. Treatment is with a low fat diet and statins.

Cerebrotendinous xanthomatosis

The primary abnormality in this disease is the accumulation in plasma of cholestanol resulting from homozygous deficiency of the mitochondrial enzyme sterol 27-hydroxylase, a key enzyme involved in hepatic bile acid synthesis and cholesterol oxidation (see Table 26.19). It is a rare disorder characterized by development of xanthomas in tendons, the lungs and brain in the setting of low or normal plasma cholesterol concentrations. Affected patients may also develop progressive cerebellar ataxia, dementia, spinal cord paresis, diminished intelligence and cataracts. Diarrhea may be frequent in infants and young children. Dementia, ataxia, tendon xanthoma and cataracts may become apparent between the ages of 10 and 18 years, but milder cases may not be identified until later in adulthood.

Treatment with chenodeoxycholic acid has beneficial effects on plasma cholestanol levels, but it may take years to diminish levels of cholestanol in the brain. Sometimes statins are added, but must be used with caution. Early initiation of treatment is advised.

Barth syndrome

Barth syndrome is an X-linked disorder associated with cardiomyopathy, biventricular hypertrophy, systemic myopathy, neutropenia and growth failure associated with increased tissue lipid deposition. Plasma cholesterol and carnitine are reduced and levels of urinary 3-methylglutaconic and 3-methylglutaric acids are increased. Barth syndrome is caused by mutations in the tafazzin gene (TAZ1, G4.5). Mutation analysis can be diagnostic. Urine organic acids should be evaluated in all children with cardiomyopathy. Treatment with carnitine and possibly additional cholesterol have been proposed. Advanced cases may require cardiac transplantation.

DISORDERS OF CHOLESTEROL SYNTHESIS

Mevalonate kinase deficiency

Mevalonate is the product of HMG-CoA reductase, the rate-limiting enzyme for cholesterol and isoprenoid synthesis. Deficiency of mevalonate kinase, a peroxisomal enzyme, may be associated with developmental delay, dysmorphic features, cataracts, cerebellar atrophy hepatosplenomegaly, lymphadenopathy, anemia, diarrhea, malabsorption and early death. Recurrent crises with fever, lymphadenopathy, arthralgia, edema and a morbilliform rash are reported. A milder vari-

ant causes the autoinflammatory hyper IgD/periodic fever syndrome without other manifestations.

Mevalonic acid is massively increased in blood and urine. Plasma cholesterol is normal. No specific treatment is known, but gene therapy is a theoretical possibility.

Smith–Lemli–Opitz syndrome

This condition is the most prevalent genetic disorder of cholesterol synthesis; it occurs in ~1 in 30 000 births. The genetic basis for this syndrome is homozygous deficiency of 7-dehydrocholesterol-delta^7-reductase, an enzyme that catalyzes the final step in cholesterol synthesis.

Clinical findings

It is characterized by dysmorphic features with characteristic facies, micrognathia, microcephaly, high forehead, a short anteverted nose, low-set ears, cleft palate, syn- and/or poly-dactyly (particularly second and third toes), mental retardation and growth failure (Fig. 26.21). Male infants have hypospadias or more severe feminization of the external genitalia. Frequent additional features are cleft palate, hepatocellular

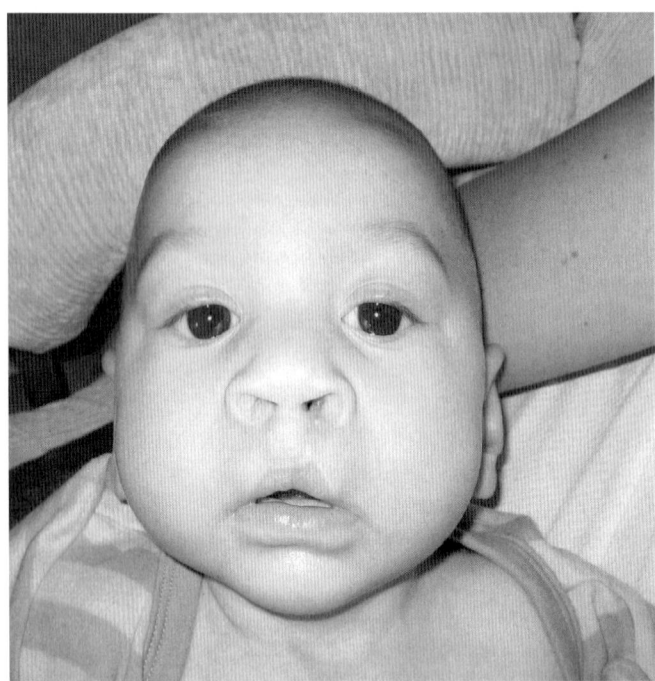

(a)

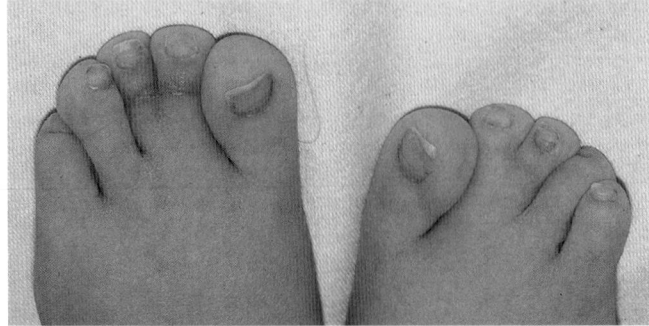

(b)

Fig 26.21   Smith–Lemli–Opitz syndrome. (a) Face showing typical features; note the microcephaly, arched eyebrows, upturned nares, 'cod fish' mouth, micrognathia and cleft palate (not infrequent). These features with hypotonia, developmental delay and ambiguous genitalia are very suggestive. (b) Syndactyly of second and third toes.

damage, heart malformations, renal and cerebellar hypoplasia. Severely affected individuals may die at birth or in infancy, but survival into later adulthood is common in milder cases.

Diagnosis and treatment

Plasma cholesterol concentrations are usually low, but an elevated 7-dehydrocholesterol concentration establishes the diagnosis. Brain development is presumably impaired due the lack of availability of cholesterol, but toxicity of cholesterol precursors cannot be excluded. Increased dietary intake of cholesterol in egg yolk, sometimes with bile acid supplementation to enhance intestinal cholesterol absorption, increases plasma cholesterol and decreases the 7-dehydrocholesterol concentration, but does not improve outcomes. Plasma cholesterol does not cross the blood–brain barrier, so exogenous cholesterol cannot ameliorate cholesterol deficiency in the brain. Strategies to diminish prenatal complications will require initiation of treatment early in gestation and methods of delivering cholesterol to the brain.

Other defects in cholesterol synthesis

A number of other genetic disorders associated with enzymatic defects in cholesterol synthesis have been identified. Most are characterized by severe developmental anomalies, including brain malformation and mental retardation. They include X-linked dominant chondrodyslasia punctata (CDPX2 or 'Conradi–Hunermann syndrome') caused by 3-beta-hydroxysteroid delta⁸,delta⁷-isomerase deficiency and X-linked dominant CHILD syndrome (congenital hemidysplasia with ichthyosiform erythroderma and limb defects) caused by mutation of a gene coding for 3-beta-hydroxysterol dehydrogenase. A defect of 4-alpha-methylsterol-4-demylase is also associated with developmental delay, cataracts and severe, generalized psoriatiform dermatitis. Desmosterolosis and lathosterolosis are caused, respectively, by 3-beta-hydroxysterol delta²⁴-reductase and 3-beta-hydroxysteroid-delta⁵-desaturase (sterol C5-desaturase) deficiency. They are identified by analysis of plasma sterols.

DEFECTS IN BILE ACID METABOLISM

The bile acids, cholic and chenodeoxycholic acids, are synthesized in a complicated process that involves peroxisomes, mitochondria, the endoplasmic reticulum and the cytosol. They are essential for normal absorption of fats from the gut and undergo considerable recycling and reuse. At least 10 inherited synthetic diseases have been identified; they fall into two main categories:

1. disorders affecting specific enzymes of the bile acid synthetic pathway (Table 26.21);
2. disorders in which bile acid metabolism is secondarily altered as a consequence of abnormal peroxisomal function. Enzymatic defects usually result in accumulation of synthetic intermediates.

These disorders all cause progressive familial intrahepatic cholestasis presumably the consequence of bile acid intermediate accumulation. In some cases this leads to cirrhosis and liver failure.

These defects cannot be readily differentiated clinically from other causes of aggressive liver disease with biliary obstruction, except by sophisticated mass spectrometry analysis of urine and/or serum bile acids.

Early treatment with chenodeoxycholic or cholic acid may be very effective and can be continued for years. Liver transplantation is required in advanced cases.

Progressive familial intrahepatic cholestasis (PFIC)

This term comprises a heterogeneous group of autosomal recessive disorders caused by defects in the transport of bile acids and associated with early-onset cholestasis and the development of hepatic fibrosis, cirrhosis and end-stage liver disease before adulthood. Progressive familial intrahepatic cholestasis type 1 PFIC1 is severe and usually lethal in the first decade of life. Symptoms include early onset of loose, foul-smelling stools, jaundice, hepatosplenomegaly and impaired growth. Extreme pruritus without jaundice has been described in the last trimester of pregnancies carrying affected infants. PFIC1 was

Table 26.21   Inherited disorders of bile acid synthesis: Enzyme defects and phenotype

Enzyme defect	Gene	Biochemical phenotype	Clinical symptoms
Affecting the sterol ring			
7-Dehydrocholesterol reductase	DHCR7	↓Cholesterol ↓PBA	↓Growth, mental retardation, rare neonatal cholestasis
Cholesterol 7β-hydroxylase	CYP7A1	↑LDL- and liver cholesterol ↓↓PBA	No liver disease, hyperlipidemia, premature vascular disease, gallstone disease
Oxysterol 7β-hydroxylase	CYP7B1	↑Oxysterols ↓PBA, ↑BIA	Neonatal liver failure, cholestasis, cirrhosis (-)
3β-hydroxy-β5-C27-steroid oxidoreductase (C27 3βHSD)	HSD3B7	↓PBA, ↑BIA	Neonatal liver failure, fat-soluble vitamin deficiency, steatorrhea (+)
β4–3-Oxosteroid 5β-reductase (5βRD)	AKR1D1	↑BIA	Neonatal liver failure, cholestasis, jaundice (+)
Affecting the side chain			
Sterol 27-hydroxylase	CYP27A1	↓PBA ↑Bile alcohols ↑Cholesterol	Cerebrotendinous xanthomatosis (CTX), CNS neuropathy (slow progression)
2-Methylacyl-CoA racemase	AMACR	↑(*R*) BIA ↑Pristanic acid	Adult-onset sensory motor neuropathy, neonatal hepatitis, fat-soluble vitamin deficiency (+)
D-Bifunctional protein	EHHAD17	↑BIA ↑Pristanic acid ↓PBA	Neurological deficiencies, minimal liver failure
25-Hydroxylase pathway*	?	↑Bile alcohols	Neonatal (giant cell) hepatitis, cirrhosis
Bile acid CoA:amino acid N-acyltransferase (BAAT)	?	↓Conjugated PBA	Minimal/transient liver disease, fat-soluble vitamin deficiency

*Enzyme defect has not been identified.
BAI, bile acid synthetic intermediates; LDL, low density lipoprotein; PBA, primary bile acids (cholic and chenodeoxycholic acids); (*R*), bile acid *R* enantiomers; + or –, response to bile acid treatment.

first described in the old order Amish, and is also known as Byler disease. It results from mutations in the ATP8B1 gene.[157] Mutations in the same gene are also found in benign recurrent intrahepatic cholestasis (BRIC1), which is characterized by recurrent episodes of cholestatic jaundice with elevation of serum bile acids that spontaneously resolves after a period of weeks to months. Mutations of ABCB11, which encodes a liver-specific ATP-binding cassette transporter gene, can also result in similar severe (PFIC2) and benign (BRIC2) forms of intrahepatic cholestasis. A further form (PF1C3) results from mutations in ABCB4, which encodes a multidrug resistant P-glycoprotein (MDR3); it is unique among the three types of PFIC, showing high serum gamma-glutamyltransferase levels, portal inflammation and ductular proliferation in an early stage.

SECONDARY HYPERLIPIDEMIA

Secondary hyperlipidemia is the most common form of hyperlipidemia and can exacerbate primary hyperlipidemias. Excess intake of dietary saturated fat and cholesterol is the most common cause of secondary hyperlipidemia which is prevalent in Western populations; diabetes and hypothyroidism also are common causes. Additional types of secondary hyperlipidemia are described in Table 26.20.

TREATMENT OF HYPERLIPIDEMIA

The cornerstone of treatment for all forms of hyperlipidemia is lifestyle modification consisting of regular physical activity, healthy diet and avoidance of excess body weight and smoking. A healthy diet typically is based on complex carbohydrates with increased amounts of fruits and vegetables, increased dietary fiber and reduced intake of saturated and total fat and cholesterol. Although controversy still prevails regarding the optimal dietary composition, such a diet helps to minimize body weight, is replete with essential vitamins and phytochemicals, and helps to minimize most forms of hyperlipidemia. A low fat, low cholesterol diet, such as the American Heart Association Step 1 diet, is generally safe in children, but more restrictive diets in children should not be prescribed without supervision of a dietitian and/or pediatric health care provider.

Drug therapy for treatment of hyperlipidemia is usually reserved for young adults unless there are compelling reasons for initiation of treatment in childhood. Concerns about possible unforeseen toxicity of lipid-lowering medications in growing children, the typically long delay in the onset of clinically significant vascular disease, and the imperfect association of hyperlipidemia in childhood with hyperlipidemia in adulthood, support the avoidance of drug therapy in children. Important exceptions need to be considered, however.

Untreated homozygous familial hypercholesterolemia usually results in death from myocardial infarction in childhood. Thus, aggressive drug and nondrug therapy (often including LDL apheresis) is essential in affected children. Among children with heterozygous familial hypercholesterolemia (or other severe conditions) associated with a very early onset of cardiovascular events in relatives (e.g. before age 30), it often is advisable to initiate some form of drug treatment during childhood to prevent the accumulation of a heavy burden of atherosclerosis prior to adulthood.

Bile acid-binding agents are believed to have the lowest risk for toxicity because they are not absorbed systemically, and they are approved for use in children, but such agents alone may lack efficacy. Several studies of children with heterozygous familial hypercholesterolemia showed no evidence of toxicity after 1–2 years of treatment with several statins. Additional studies have demonstrated normalization of accelerated progression of carotid intima-media thickening by long term treatment with statins in children with heterozygous familial hypercholesterolemia. The results of such studies have suggested that it may be appropriate to initiate lipid lowering drug therapy at the age of 8–10 years in affected children. It may be acceptable to treat with a low or moderate dose of a 'statin' in combination with a bile acid-binding agent and a healthy lifestyle, but the long term safety and benefit of such an intervention remain unproven. Ezetimibe, an inhibitor of cholesterol absorption, can reduce the plasma LDL cholesterol concentration by 16–20% and may be useful in treatment of children, but experience in children is limited. Drugs available for treatment of hyperlipidemia are outlined in Table 26.22. In the USA, the FDA has approved lovastatin, fluvastatin, simvastatin, pravastatin and atorvastatin for use in boys and postpubertal girls ≥10 years (8 years

Table 26.22   Drugs for treatment of hyperlipidemia*

Indication	Possible drugs
Elevated LDL cholesterol	'Statins' (lovastatin, simvastatin, pravastatin, fluvastatin, atorvastatin, fosuvastatin) Niacin Lovastatin + niacin (Advicor) Bile acid sequestrants (colestyramine, colestipol, colesevelam) Cholesterol absorption inhibitors (ezetimibe)
Hypertriglyceridemia (not type I)	Fibrates (gemfibrozil, clofibrate, fenofibrate) Niacin Fish oil (>6 g/d in adults). Omacor (3–4 g/d) is distilled fish oil (>80% EPA + DHA)
Type I hypertriglyceridemia (chylomicronemia)	Drugs not helpful. Treatment is very low fat diet
Combined hyperlipidemia (LDL cholesterol and triglycerides)	'Statins' Niacin Fibrates Lovastatin + niacin (Advicor)
Type III hyperlipidemia	Fibrates Statins Niacin Fish oil Oral estrogen in estrogen-deficient women may help (raises triglycerides in other conditions)
Low HDL cholesterol	Niacin (most efficacious agent) Fibrates 'Statins' (less efficacious than niacin and fibrates) CETP inhibitors (experimental); torcetrapib (withdrawn in late 2006) – caused increased mortality
Elevated lipoprotein(a)	Niacin (clinical benefit unproven)

CETP, cholesteryl ester transferase protein; DHA, docosahexanoic acid; EPA, eicosapentanoic acid; HDL, high density lipoprotein; LDL, low density lipoprotein;
*Most of these interventions have not been tested adequately for safety and efficacy in children.

for pravastatin) with heterozygous familial hypercholesterolemia. All of these statins and rosuvastatin are approved for treatment of homozygous familial hypercholesterolemia.

LYSOSOMAL STORAGE DISEASES

GENERAL CONSIDERATIONS

Lysosomes are cytoplasmic organelles containing hydrolytic enzymes that digest a wide range of macromolecules, thus acting as waste disposal units. The majority of lysosomal storage diseases (LSDs) arise from defects in sugar hydrolases in the acidic intralysosomal environment. In common with all other intraorganelle proteins, lysosomal hydrolases are synthesized on ribosomes and then glycosylated in the Golgi, receiving specific mannose side chains that function as recognition sites for targeting and uptake into lysosomes. Deficiency of a lysosomal enzyme leads to intralysosomal accumulation of the undegraded substrates, in the tissues where they are normally metabolized. As the stored materials accumulate within the affected cells, they lead to increasingly impaired function of the involved organs. Table 26.23 summarizes these disorders.

There are over 40 recognized LSDs.[1] Classification can be confusing. Eponyms as well as numbering systems and alphabetical designations have accumulated haphazardly as new conditions have emerged. The LSDs include glycolipidoses, mucopolysaccharidoses, glycogenoses, oligosaccharide and glycoprotein disorders, defects of entry of enzymes or egress of products into or out of lysosomes, and the neuronal ceroid lipofuscinoses. Apart from cystinosis, accumulated substrates have a common structure – carbohydrate attached to a protein or a lipid. Figure 26.22 illustrates the biochemical pathways implicated in many of these disorders.

Incidence and genetics

Individually, LSDs are rare with incidences ranging from about 1 in 50000 to just a few known cases. Some affect up to 10000 patients worldwide; the overall incidence for LSDs is estimated at 1 in 7000 to 1 in 10000 births.[158,159] Some, particularly Tay–Sachs and Gaucher disease, are much more frequent in specific populations (these two being frequent in Ashkenazim). All, with the exceptions of Hunter syndrome, Fabry disease and sialuria, are inherited as autosomal recessive traits. Most of the disorders present in childhood but almost all have late-onset variants that may not emerge until adult life. With few exceptions, genotype–phenotype correlations are not well understood and should rarely be used for counseling.

Clinical features

Storage diseases characteristically have three clinical phases. In the first, which may last from weeks to decades, clinical findings are absent or occult. This is followed by emerging evidence of tissue involvement that can be relatively acute or evolve over years. Finally, the involved tissues begin to lose function.

LSDs should be considered in: developmental delay, especially with loss of milestones or loss of fine motor control; coarsening of facial features; hepatosplenomegaly; leukodystrophy; ophthalmological abnormalities especially corneal clouding; characteristic radiological skeletal changes; angiokeratomas; and hydrops fetalis.

Diagnosis

Diagnostic evaluation of LSDs can be complex, and assistance of a specialist in clinical biochemical genetics is critical since testing involves a progressive cascade of biochemical and genetic testing. Mucopolysaccharides (MPS, now known as glycosaminoglycans [GAGs]) and oligosaccharides can be screened, identified and quantitated in urine. Specific enzyme assays for almost all the disorders are available but often only in special centers. Some enzymes can be measured in serum, while others require leukocytes or cultured skin fibroblasts. Occasionally, high enzyme activities erroneously appear to rule out disease and falsely low activities can be due to vagaries of testing

and enzyme behavior (e.g. Tay–Sachs variants and pseudodeficiencies in metachromatic leukodystrophy and others). Carrier testing is usually feasible but overlap between carrier and normal values can be confusing; mutation analysis, if available, is preferable.

When considering the possible diagnosis of an LSD, it may be appropriate to start with simple urine screening tests for GAGs and/ or oligosaccharides. If a specific disorder is suspected, then appropriate enzyme assay is indicated. If the diagnosis remains obscure, electron microscopic study of fibroblasts from skin, conjunctival or rectal biopsy, or even leukocytes may reveal lysosomal inclusions that then lead to further analyses. Virtually all of these disorders are amenable to prenatal diagnosis using chorionic villus samples or cultured amniocytes.

Treatment

There is currently no cure for any of these disorders. Where specific therapies are in use or under trial, these are discussed under the individual disorders. Genetic counseling and family support are always required.

Great care must be taken when considering surgery or anesthesia in patients with LSDs since uncontrolled neck movements can pose a grave risk of atlanto-occipital dislocation. Airway narrowing from tissue infiltration, possible cardiopulmonary disease, and the need to position and stabilize the neck during induction make anesthesia high risk in many LSDs.

SPHINGOLIPIDOSES

In sphingolipids, sphingosine is linked through its amino group to a variety of fatty acids containing 16–26 carbon atoms. Ceramide is a C-18 sphingosine linked to a fatty acid and therefore, is a long chain aminoalcohol base attached to carboxylic acid (Fig. 26.23). Esterification through the hydroxyl group on the first carbon of ceramide is the basis for synthesis of many lipid compounds. Ceramide with sialyl-oligosaccharides yields gangliosides, with phosphorylcholine it yields sphingomyelins, and with monosaccharides or oligosaccharides it yields neutral glycolipids. The degradative pathway for higher gangliosides to sphingosine is depicted in Figure 26.22.

Although the sphingolipidoses are closely related chemically, their phenotype varies considerably depending on the role of the individual metabolites or their precursors in different tissues. For example, glucocerebroside, which accumulates in Gaucher disease, derives from peripheral cells which are particularly rich in membrane glycolipids. Gangliosides, on the other hand, are concentrated in neuronal membranes, thereby involving the gray matter of the brain.

Tay–Sachs and Sandhoff diseases: the GM$_2$-gangliosidoses

Both disorders result in a progressive neurodegenerative disorder caused by deficiency of N-acetyl glucosaminidase (beta-hexosaminidase) and accumulation of ganglioside GM$_2$. Hexosaminidase exists in two forms: hex a is a heterodimer and has two alpha and beta subunits; hex b has four beta subunits; both isozymes cleave terminal sugars from GM$_2$. Defects in the alpha subunit cause hex a deficiency (Tay–Sachs disease [TSD]); defects in the beta subunit cause hex a and b deficiency (Sandhoff disease). Gangliosides are glycosphingolipids consisting of ceramide and an oligosaccharide side chain with sialic acid residues.

An activator protein facilitates the binding of GM$_2$-ganglioside to hex a; deficiency of the activator can also cause TSD.

Clinical features

Classic infantile TSD is characterized by the gradual onset of progressive weakness, hypotonia, poor head control, decreasing attentiveness followed by paralysis, dementia, blindness and seizures in early infancy. Although some motor skills may be achieved, most affected children never sit alone or crawl. An exaggerated startle response is characteristic, indicating brainstem involvement. By 6–10 months, upper and

Table 26.23 Classification of the lysosomal storage diseases

Sphingolipidoses			Mucolipidoses		
GM$_2$-gangliosidosis			Mucolipidosis II (I-cell disease)	I*	N-acetyl-glucosamine-I-phosphotransferase
Tay–Sachs	I,J,A	Hexosaminidase A (alpha chain)	Mucolipidosis III	J*	N-acetyl-glucosamine phosphotransferase
Sandhoff	I,J,A	Hexosaminidase A and B (beta chain)			
Gaucher disease	I,J,A	Glucocerebrosidase	Other lysosomal disorders		
Fabry disease	J→A	Alpha-galactosidase A	Pompe syndrome (glycogenolysis II)	I,J,A	Alpha-D-glucosidase (acid maltase)
Niemann–Pick disease type A, B	I,J,A	Sphingomyelinase	GM$_1$-gangliosidosis	I,J,A*	Beta-galactosidase
Niemann–Pick type C	J→A	Defect in cholesterol esterification	Aspartylglucosaminuria	J*	Aspartylglucosaminidase
Metachromatic leukodystrophy	I,J,A	Arylsulfatase A	Fucosidosis	I,J*	Alpha-fucosidase
MLD with 'normal' enzyme	J	Arylsulfatase A activator protein	Alpha-mannosidosis	I,J*	Alpha-mannosidase
Multiple sulfatase deficiency	I,J*	Multiple sulfatases	Beta-mannosidosis	J*	Beta-mannosidase
Krabbe disease	I,J,A	Galactocerebrosidase	Schindler disease	I,J*	Alpha-N-acetylgalactosaminidase
Farber syndrome	I	Acid ceramidase			
Mucopolysaccharidoses			Disorders involving sialic acid		
Hurler syndrome (MPS I H)	I,J*	Alpha-L-iduronidase	Sialidosis type I	J,A*	Neuraminidase
Hurler–Scheie (MPS I H-S)	J	Alpha-l-iduronidase	Sialidosis type II (Mucolipidosis I)	I,J*	Neuraminidase
Scheie syndrome (MPS I S)	J*	Alpha-L-iduronidase	Galactosialidosis	I,J*	Neuraminidase and beta-galactosidase
Hunter syndrome (MPS II)	I,J,A*	Iduronate sulfatase	Mucolipidosis IV	I*	Mucolipin 1
Sanfilippo syndrome			Infantile sialic acid storage disease, Salla disease	I,J,A*	Sialic acid egress from lysosomes
MPS III			Sialuria	I,J,A	Impaired feedback on synthesis of sialic acid
MPS IIIA	J*	Heparan-N-sulfatase			
MPS IIIB	J*	Alpha-N-acetyl glucosaminidase			
MPS IIIC	J*	Acetyl-CoA; alpha acetylglucosaminide acetyl-transferase			
MPS IIID	J*	N-acetyl-glucosamine-6-sulfatase			
Morquio syndrome (MPS IV)					
MPS IV-A	J*	N-acetyl-galactosamine-6-sulfatase			
MPS IV-B	J*	Beta-galactosidase			
Maroteaux–Lamy syndrome (MPS VI)	I,J,A*	Arylsulfatase B			
Sly syndrome (MPS VII)	I,J*	Beta-glucuronidase			
MPS IX	I,J	Hyaluronidase			

* Conditions that usually have a 'Hurler-like' storage phenotype.
I, infantile: symptoms or diagnosis usual within infancy; J, juvenile: symptoms or diagnosis usual within childhood; A, adolescents or adult: symptoms or diagnosis usually during or after adolescence.

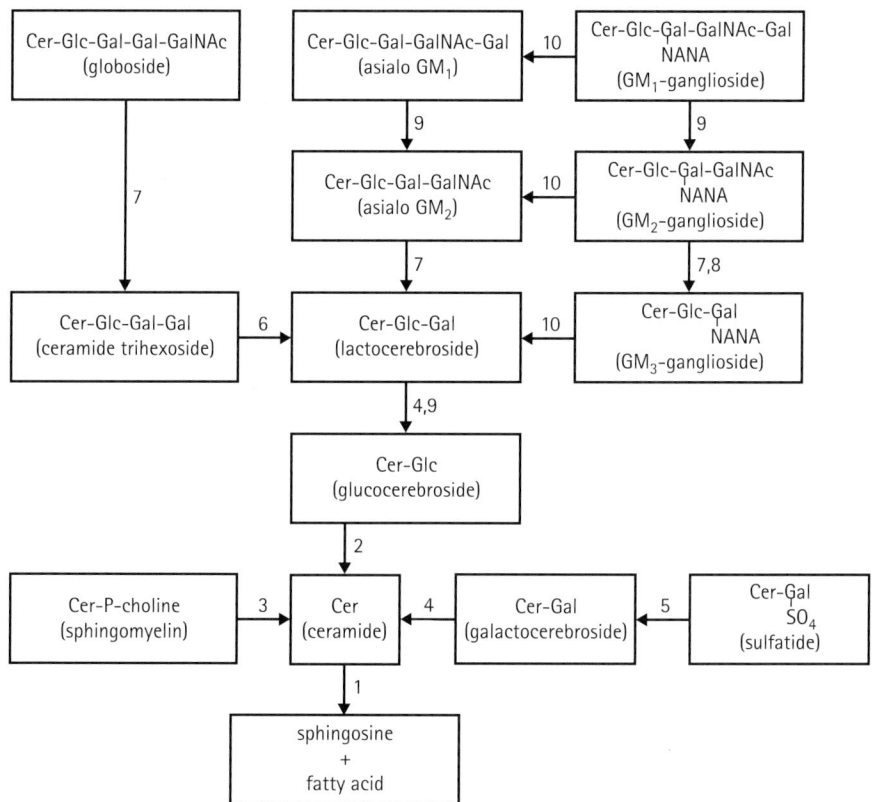

Fig. 26.22 Schematic representation of ganglioside and sphingolipid degradation, showing enzyme steps and metabolic blocks. 1, Ceramidase (Farber); 2, α–glucosidase (Gaucher); 3, sphingomylinase (Niemann–Pick); 4, galactocerebrosidase (Krabbe); 5, arylsulfatase A (metachromatic leukodystrophy); 6, α–galactosidase (Fabry); 7, total hexosaminidase (Sandhoff); 8, hexosaminidase A (Tay–Sachs); 9, β–galactosidase (GM$_1$-gangliosidosis); 10, α–neuraminidase (sialidosis).

Fig. 26.23 Structure of a typical ceramide.

lower neurone involvement is obvious and seizures and macrocephaly become evident. Ophthalmological examination reveals 'cherry red spots' at the maculae – a gray–white halo of lipid-laden cells that creates the appearance of a central red spot (Fig. 26.24). They were once considered diagnostic of TSD, but can be found in other GM$_2$-gangliosidoses and variably in GM$_1$-gangliosidosis, Niemann–Pick disease, Farber disease and sialidosis. Continued deterioration leads to complete unresponsiveness, blindness, deafness and spasticity with decerebrate posture and death by 3–5 years.

Variants of TSD include juvenile, adult and b$_1$ (normal activity with artificial substrate) variants and activator protein defect. Late-onset juvenile hex a deficiency usually presents between 2 and 10 years with ataxia, progressive spasticity, dementia and increasing seizures. Most patients die as teenagers. Adult forms present somewhat later and are often misdiagnosed as multiple sclerosis.

Infantile Sandhoff disease is similar to infantile TSD but with the combined hex a and b deficiency, there is more extraneural involvement with mild visceromegaly and occasional foamy histiocytes in bone marrow or vacuolated lymphocytes in blood. Minor bony changes may also be present. There is no ethnic predilection. Juvenile and adult forms are similar to their counterparts of TSD with delayed onset, slower progress and longer survival.

Activator protein deficiency is clinically and histologically identical to TSD except that hexosaminidase activities are normal when measured by conventional methods.

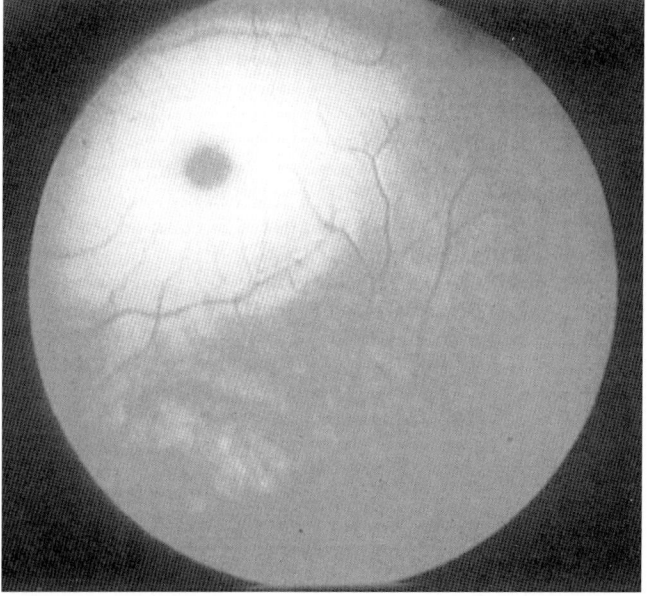

Fig. 26.24 Tay–Sachs disease. A cherry-red spot is seen at the posterior pole due to the presence of ganglioside in the ganglion cells of the macula. There are no ganglion cells at the fovea which presents as a red spot but the surrounding area appears white or milky in color.

Diagnosis

Enzyme assays using artificial substrates are done in serum, leukocytes or tissues. In TSD, hex a is reduced but hex b activity is normal; Sandhoff disease shows both hex a and b deficiency. Serum assays can give erroneous results especially in pregnancy, with liver disease and with certain medications including oral contraceptives; in these circumstances, the assay must be done in leukocytes. Sophisticated assays are needed to identify unusual variants. Urine oligosaccharides are normal in TSD but in Sandhoff, oligosacchariduria can be seen.

Enzymatic prenatal diagnosis for TSD is available but molecular testing is optimal, although > 70 mutations for TSD are described.

Population screening for Tay–Sachs disease. Prior to population screening, TSD incidence was about 1 in 3500 Ashkenazim but only about 1 in 300 000 non-Ashkenazim; it was also common in French Canadians. There are common mutations in Ashkenazi Jews, so that mutational analysis is sometimes used for screening. Since about 1 in 27 Ashkenazim is a heterozygote (~1 in 160 in non-Jews), widespread screening for heterozygotes is now common practice in selected populations. In the international TSD prevention program, > 1 million people have been tested, resulting in a dramatic decrease in TSD in Jewish infants. Since 1970, screening has reduced the incidence from approximately 60/year to 3–5/year in Jews in the USA.

Treatment
Supportive care is the only treatment option at present. Platt et al evaluated a potential strategy for treatment based on N-butyldeoxynojirimycin (formerly OGT-918, now miglustat), an inhibitor of glycosphingolipid biosynthesis. TSD mice treated with this agent had no accumulation of GM$_2$ in the brain.[160] Clinical trials with miglustat in later-onset forms are in progress. Animal studies of bone marrow transplant showed some encouraging preliminary results,[161] but this was ineffective in a child also treated with miglustat.[162]

Gaucher disease
Clinical features
Gaucher disease is the most prevalent of the LSDs. Three types have been described (Table 26.24). Type 1 is by far the most frequent. Common signs include splenomegaly (typically 4–70 times normal) often with hypersplenism and bone marrow crowding leading to thrombocytopenia and/or anemia with easy bruising or bleeding, especially menorrhagia and nosebleeds. Less extreme hepatomegaly (1.5–10 times normal) is usual; bony infiltration leads to avascular necrosis of the hip and disseminated damage elsewhere, and bone pain can lead to a misdiagnosis of trauma or infection and, with the bleeding tendency, to consideration of malignancy. Growth retardation and delayed puberty are common in children. There are no neurological problems in type 1. Rarely, pulmonary hypertension, infiltrative lung disease, portal hypertension, and renal involvement are seen.

Type 2 presents in infancy with opisthotonus, visceromegaly, strabismus, severe neurological dysfunction with spasticity, failure to thrive and cachexia leading to early death (Fig. 26.25). Type 3 is characterized by visceral enlargement which may be massive, and slowly progressive neurological dysfunction. Age at presentation for type 3

is later than type 2, and progression is slower. The presentation, however, is variable, and some patients with type 3 do not have massive organomegaly.

Gaucher disease is panethnic with an incidence of about 1 in 1000 in Ashkenazim in whom it is much more common than in the general population.

Diagnosis
Often typical 'Gaucher cells' are the initial finding in bone marrow or liver. Diagnosis is confirmed by enzyme activity in leukocytes or by mutation analysis. There are well-established genotype–phenotype correlations, so mutation analysis can be used, with some caution, to predict prognosis. High levels of acid phosphatase, chitotriosidase, and angiotensin converting enzyme in blood and/or increased levels of glucocerebroside in tissues are also found but are not considered diagnostic.

Treatment
In the past, supportive care was limited to blood transfusions, splenectomy and androgen therapy. Treatment for skeletal complications included pain management for bone crises and orthopedic management of bone lesions. Bone marrow transplantation is now superceded.[163]

Enzyme replacement therapy (ERT) has become the treatment of choice.[164] Response to therapy is shown in Figure 26.26. It partially or completely reverses the hepatomegaly and the bone marrow abnormalities, and can probably prevent bone crises and avascular necrosis of the hips if begun early enough. However, established skeletal changes may require 2–3 years to improve.

Virtually all children with symptomatic Gaucher disease, even those with isolated splenomegaly, should be considered for treatment with ERT since presentation in childhood indicates moderate to severe disease. Asymptomatic adults are sometimes not treated with ERT because treatment requires intravenous infusions every 2 weeks, and is extremely expensive.[21,165] Substrate reduction therapy with miglustat, as discussed above for TSD, may also prove helpful[166] and is now approved in several countries.

Fabry disease
Fabry disease is caused by decreased alpha-galactosidase a activity, with intralysosomal accumulation of globotriasylceramide (GB-3) (also known as CTH, ceramide trihexosamide or GL-3). The frequency is estimated at 1 in 40 000–117 000 births with no apparent ethnic predisposition. Most families have a unique mutation. Although Fabry disease is inherited as an X-linked trait, most female heterozygotes, though not often symptomatic in childhood, eventually develop signs, symptoms and complications of the disease, though this often occurs more slowly and later than in men.

Table 26.24 Clinical types of Gaucher disease

Clinical features	Type 1	Type 2	Type 3
Age at onset of signs/symptoms	Any	Infancy	Childhood
Splenomegaly	Mild to extreme	Moderate	Mild to extreme
Hepatomegaly	Mild to extreme	Moderate	Mild to extreme
Skeletal disease/bony crises	Absent to severe	Absent	Moderate to severe
Primary central nervous system disease	Absent	Significant	Mild to significant, increasing with age
Life span	Normal with enzyme replacement therapy	~2 years	2–60 years
Ethnicity	Panethnic	Panethnic	Panethnic
Demographic group	Ashkenazi Jewish		Norrbottnian
Frequency	~1 in 60 000–200 000 (~1 in 500–1000 Ashkenazim)	< 1 in 100 000	< 1 in 50 000

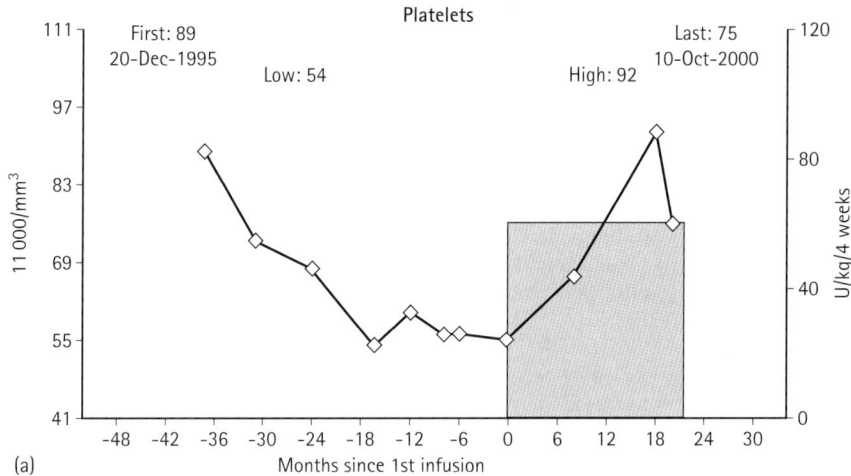

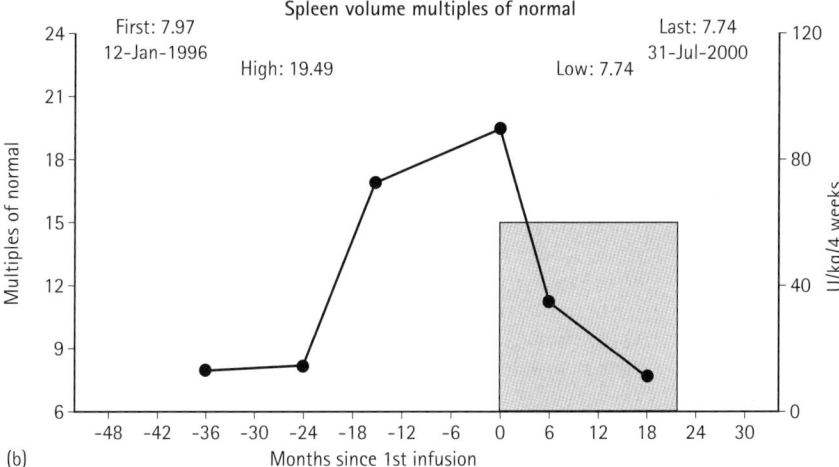

Fig. 26.26 Response of (a) platelet count and (b) spleen volume to enzyme replacement therapy in a patient with Gaucher disease. Shaded area indicates the period of enzyme replacement therapy.

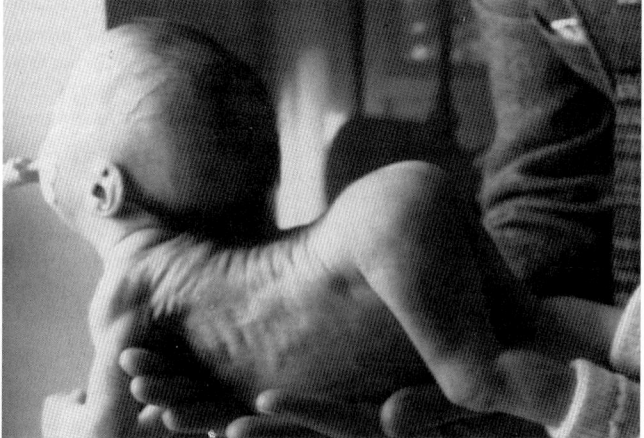

Fig 26.25 Severe opisthotonus in a 3-month-old infant with type II Gaucher disease.

Clinical features

Males typically present in childhood with peripheral neuropathy, the most striking feature being attacks of acroparesthesia characterized by intense pain in the hands and feet; over time the neuropathy worsens causing impaired temperature and vibratory perception. Suspicion of psychiatric disease often delays the diagnosis for years. Renal damage, evidenced by increasing proteinuria, occurs typically in adulthood, fol-lowed years later by renal dysfunction and renal failure. Without treat-ment, renal failure is usually fatal in males typically in their fourth or fifth decade.

Other major sites of involvement are the skin, heart and nervous system. Angiokeratomas are clusters of dark, nonblanching, petechi-oid punctate lesions that are usually present in the 'bathing trunk' area, and especially the umbilicus or scrotum. Hypertrophic cardiomyopathy is the most common cardiac manifestation. Autonomic nervous system involvement is characterized by dysautonomia, decreased vessel com-pliance and hypo/anhydrosis. Abdominal pain is not uncommon and gastrointestinal dysfunction can result in pain, diarrhea and mesenteric infarction. CNS involvement may cause transient ischemic attacks and stroke, especially in older men. The corneae have whorl-like opacities and tortuous retinal vessels which can occlude. Constitutional difficul-ties may include fatigue, depression and an impaired quality of life. Cases due to milder mutations can present with cardiomyopathy in adulthood but few, if any, other problems.

Diagnosis

Decreased activity of alpha-galactosidase a in serum, leukocytes or other tissue is diagnostic. In urine, crystalline glycosphingolipids show bire-fringence under polarization microscopy (so called 'maltese crosses'). Histologically, lysosomal inclusions are present in almost all cell types, including the skin and glomeruli.

The corneal changes are virtually pathognomic, can be seen by slit lamp examination, and may be a useful adjunctive test for females who, even when affected, often have normal enzyme activity levels. DNA mutation analysis is the definitive diagnostic test in females.

Treatment

Analgesics are usually required, and phenytoin, neurontin, carbamazepine or narcotics were often used for pain before ERT was developed. Renal dialysis or transplant are used for renal failure but the disorder progresses in other tissues. ERT given by intravenous infusion has revolutionized the treatment of this disorder.[167,168,169]

Niemann–Pick disease types a and b

Clinical features

The common feature of these disorders is accumulation of sphingomyelin due to a defect of sphingomyelinase. Typically, type a patients present in infancy with marked hepatosplenomegaly, failure to thrive and relentlessly progressive psychomotor regression; about 50% have Jewish ancestry. Lymphadenopathy is also often present. Neurological regression leads to hypotonia and weakness with feeding difficulties. A macular cherry red spot is seen in about 50% of cases, and corneal clouding and retinal abnormalities can be seen. Xanthomas and a yellow–brown discoloration of the skin may be observed. Hypersplenism can be aggressive with widespread infiltration of foam cells. Most patients die before 2 years.

Type b is a chronic non-neuronopathic disorder with variable onset from early childhood to adult life. All patients have marked hepatosplenomegaly usually with hypersplenism. Patients may suffer general malaise and there may be a delay in sexual development. Lung infiltration may become prominent and lead to respiratory difficulties and cardiopulmonary failure. There is generally no bone or neurological involvement and cherry red spots are rarely found. Most affected children survive into adulthood.

Diagnosis and treatment

Deficient enzyme activity in leukocytes or cultured fibroblasts is diagnostic, the values being very low in type a but there is up to 15% residual activity in type b. Characteristic foam cells (or 'sea-blue histiocytes') can be seen in bone marrow, liver and spleen, but they are not diagnostic.

Only supportive care is currently available. Liver transplantation has been used in the severe non-neuropathic cases. ERT is in early clinical trials for type b but is unlikely to be effective for type a.

Niemann–Pick type c

Niemann–Pick type c (NPC) is entirely different from types a and b and is caused by one of two non-allelic defects: NPC1 codes for a large endosomal glycoprotein and NPC2 codes for a lysosomal cholesterol binding protein. It is known by several other names including juvenile dystonic lipidosis, neurovisceral storage disease with vertical supranuclear ophthalmoplegia and sea-blue histiocytosis. NPC is characterized by defective cholesterol esterification.

Clinical features

Onset may vary from infancy to late adult life; findings include intellectual impairment and impaired fine motor movements and behavioral problems, progressive ataxia, dementia, dysarthria, dystonia and tremors, seizures, cataplexy and mild hepatosplenomegaly. Supranuclear ophthalmoplegia with impairment of upward gaze is almost invariable. A history of neonatal hepatitis, sometimes with cholestasis, is often reported and rare cases develop liver failure. With time, the disease progresses to bulbar palsy and encephalopathy but patients seem to maintain a cheerful demeanor though they gradually lose contact with the environment. There is generally no cherry red spot. Death typically occurs after one to three decades of deterioration, though early-onset cases often die in early childhood.

Diagnosis

Many cases are misdiagnosed for years as multiple sclerosis, Parkinson disease, Leigh syndrome or other neurological conditions, although the vertical ophthalmoplegia is highly suggestive. Foamy histiocytes that stain an unusual sea-blue color are usually found in many tissues. These are similar to those seen in Niemann–Pick types a and b, Wolman disease and cholesterol ester storage disease. Skin, nerve and conjunctival biopsies usually show a variety of inclusions. Unesterified cholesterol and secondarily, sphingomyelin, phospholipids and glycolipids are stored in excess in the liver, spleen and other organs. Sphingomyelinase activity may be low, but this is not the primary defect. Cultured fibroblasts show a disorder of cholesterol processing and accumulation of unesterified cholesterol in lysosomes. There is a characteristic pattern of filipin-cholesterol staining in cultured fibroblasts (filipin stains unesterified cholesterol). These approaches are used for the definitive diagnosis, though mutational analysis is becoming more widely available. Prenatal diagnostic testing is offered in a few centers.

Treatment

Substrate reduction therapy with miglustat is in clinical trials, but results are not yet available. Allopregnanolone may soon be tested in clinical trials. For now, treatment remains supportive.

Metachromatic leukodystrophy

Three arylsulfatases are designated as a, b and c. Metachromatic leukodystrophy is caused by deficiency of arylsulfatase a; the b enzyme is deficient in Maroteaux–Lamy syndrome (MPS VI) and arylsulfatase c in steroid sulfatase deficiency. All three, as well as iduronate sulfatase, heparan N-sulfatase and N-acetyl-galactosamine-6-sulfatase, are involved in multiple sulfatase deficiency.

Deficiency of arylsulphatase a leads to accumulation of lipid in neurones. Since sulfatide is a major constituent of myelin, progressive demyelination occurs, leading to a characteristic leukodystrophy. The most common forms are late infantile and juvenile.

Clinical features

In the late infantile type, onset is usually between 1 and 2 years of age with learning difficulties and incoordination, and gradually increasing signs of deteriorating psychomotor function with signs of cortical, cerebellar and peripheral nerve involvement. Increasing speech difficulties with dysarthria, ataxia and optic atrophy accompany marked mental and motor regression and within a few years the children are decerebrate, rarely surviving beyond 8 years.

The juvenile form usually presents before 6 years, but may be delayed past puberty. Subtle behavioral difficulties and declining school performance accompany or precede increasing signs of cortical and cerebellar dysfunction. Clumsiness progresses to ataxia, spasticity and increasingly obvious deterioration. The course is variable but most patients die by about 20 years of age.

An adult-onset form is rare but may emerge at any age, starting with behavioral or personality changes that may include paranoia, dementia or psychosis. Neurodegenerative signs and peripheral neuropathy become progressively more obvious. Most succumb after a prolonged course.

A defect of the enzyme activator, saposin b, results in a disease that is clinically indistinguishable from the usual cases except that the activity of arylsulfatase a is totally normal when initially assayed.

Diagnosis

Symmetrical attenuation of white matter, most prominent in the parietal and occipital regions, is seen on brain MRI. Peripheral neuropathy causes decreased nerve conduction velocity and raised protein levels in CSF. Peripheral nerve biopsy shows segmental demyelination with metachromatic material within Schwann cells and histiocytes.

Diagnosis requires enzyme assay in leukocytes or cultured fibroblasts. Diagnosis of the activator protein deficiency form requires special assays in cultured fibroblasts. Urine sulfatide excretion measurement may occasionally be helpful in diagnosing atypical cases.

The standard enzyme assay uses artificial substrates: values < 10% of control occur in all types of metachromatic leukodystrophy; however, 2.5% of healthy individuals have 'pseudodeficiency' due to a mutant enzyme with in vitro activity as little as ~20% of normal; these cases require mutational analysis. Because disease-causing and pseudodeficient genes can coexist, prenatal diagnosis should always test the parents as well as the proband. Special care is required if using chorionic villus tissue due to the presence of high steroid sulfatase activity.

Treatment

Treatment is supportive; bone marrow transplantation has its detractors and advocates since there is some evidence of slowing or halting of the neurodegenerative process in select cases.[170]

Other sulfatase deficiencies

Multiple sulfatase deficiency affects several sulfatases (see above) and thus exhibits similarities with other LSDs, particularly the mucopolysaccharidoses. Thus, coarse features, stiff joints, hepatosplenomegaly and short stature are standard findings, along with the findings of metachromatic leukodystrophy.

Arylsulfatase c (steroid sulfatase) deficiency causes X-linked ichthyosis and reduced activity in the placenta that often results in delayed onset of labor. The gene is located on the Xp22.3-pter region and escapes X-inactivation.

Krabbe disease

Clinical features

Krabbe disease is caused by deficiency of galactocerebrosidase (galactocerebroside beta-galactosidase or galactosylceramidase). It is a rapidly progressive, invariably fatal disease. Most patients present between 3 and 6 months with pronounced irritability and increased sensitivity to stimulation. An exaggerated startle response may be seen, similar to TSD. Progressive psychomotor retardation soon becomes obvious with increasing hyperactivity often accompanied by tonic spasms and spasticity but with clear evidence also of peripheral neuropathy. There is usually no retinal degeneration nor cherry red spot; however, optic atrophy leads to blindness. Seizures become more frequent and patients rapidly deteriorate, most dying by 2 years of age. There is no visceromegaly and microcephaly is usual but not invariable.

Rare late infantile, juvenile and adult forms occur. They are similar to the infantile form but with a more protracted course. The earlier the onset, the more aggressive is the neurological deterioration; later variants may present with loss of vision and hemiparesis.

Diagnosis and treatment

This requires specific enzyme assay in leukocytes or cultured fibroblasts. Leukodystrophy is apparent on brain MRI and most patients have delayed nerve conduction velocity. CSF protein levels are usually raised in infants but may be normal in older patients.

Supportive treatment is often all that is available. Bone marrow or umbilical cord blood transplantation in patients with only minimal neurological involvement has shown some efficacy.[171,172]

Farber disease

This disorder, caused by ceramidase deficiency, leads to lipogranulomatosis deposits in various tissues. It presents in infancy with painful subcutaneous swellings around joints and bony prominences. Lymphadenopathy and heart and lung involvement are usual and the brain is also variously involved; cherry-red spots may be present. Laryngeal involvement leads to a characteristic hoarse cry with both breathing and feeding difficulties that usually cause death in the first 2 years. Some variants have little tissue involvement and no brain damage. The differential diagnosis includes juvenile rheumatoid arthritis, histiocytosis and hyperphosphatemic tumoral calcinosis. Enzyme assay is available; no treatment is known.

MUCOPOLYSACCHARIDOSES

Mucopolysaccharides (MPS), now usually called glycosaminoglycans (GAGs), are complex sugar/protein compounds that require at least 10 enzymes for their degradation. Deficiency of any of these enzymes leads

to accumulation of GAGs in tissues and their excretion in the urine. The GAGs include dermatan sulfate, heparan sulfate, keratan sulfate and chondroitin sulfate, and characteristic excretion patterns help to differentiate these disorders. Because lysosomal hydrolases are linkage specific, alpha-L-iduronidase cleaves terminal alpha-L-iduronide from both dermatan sulfate and heparan sulfate, resulting in accumulation of both compounds in Hurler syndrome (Fig. 26.27). These disorders are classified by the enzyme deficiency and type of GAG excreted. They are numbered I to IX but some numbers have been dropped as allelic disorders have been recognized, e.g. the designations MPS V and VIII are no longer used.

As in most LSDs, there is an initial period of normalcy followed by a chronic and progressive course, generally characterized by coarse facial features, hepatosplenomegaly, corneal clouding, skeletal abnormalities, cardiac valvular disease, stiff joints and later, cardiomyopathy. The Sanfilippo syndromes primarily exhibit developmental regression with little or no dysmorphism.

The radiographic features of these disorders are referred to as 'dysostosis multiplex'. The earliest findings are in the spine where defective ossification distorts the vertebral bodies giving rise to 'beaking' starting in T12 and L1; this extends to other vertebrae, resulting in a worsening gibbus (Fig. 26.28). There are obvious changes in the long bones, hands, ribs and clavicle (Fig. 26.29); the basilar portions of the ilia are hypoplastic with flaring of the iliac wings. Coxa valga and dysplasia of the capital femoral epiphyses can vary from minimal to severe. Macrocephaly is usual with thickening of the calvarium most apparent over the occiput. The sella becomes J- or shoe-shaped and the optic foramina are enlarged. In addition, cardiomegaly is progressive and increased pulmonary markings are frequent.

Several forms of MPS have prominent CNS involvement and developmental regression. Hydrocephalus, blindness, hearing loss, carpal tunnel syndrome, obstructive airway disease, persistent rhinorrhea, recurrent upper respiratory infections and otitis media, inguinal and umbilical hernias, hirsutism and thick hair, and spinal cord compression are variably present, all being due to accumulation of GAGs in the affected tissues.

Diagnosis

There are several simple urine screening tests; however, they are relatively insensitive and nonspecific so that GAG quantitation and identification is preferred. Definitive diagnosis requires enzyme analysis either in leukocytes or cultured skin fibroblasts. Thus far, mutational analysis has not proven very useful in diagnosis nor in providing genotype–phenotype correlations. Hunter syndrome is an X-linked recessive trait

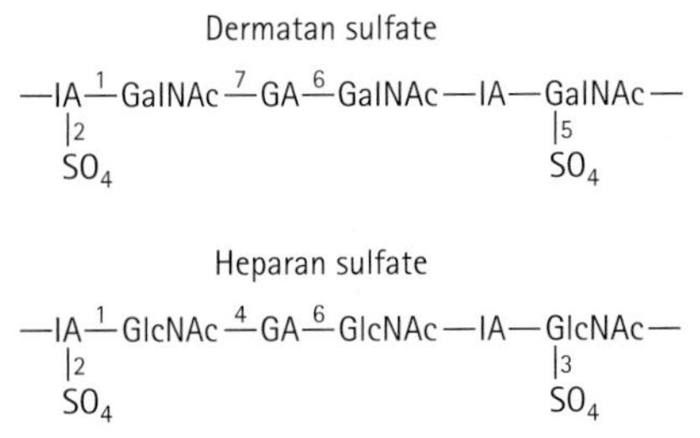

Dermatan sulfate

$$-IA\overset{1}{-}GalNAc\overset{7}{-}GA\overset{6}{-}GalNAc-IA-GalNAc-$$
$$|2|5$$
$$SO_4SO_4$$

Heparan sulfate

$$-IA\overset{1}{-}GlcNAc\overset{4}{-}GA\overset{6}{-}GlcNAc-IA-GlcNAc-$$
$$|2|3$$
$$SO_4SO_4$$

	MPS
1. α-L-iduronidase	I
2. Iduronate sulfatase	II
3. Heparin-N-sulfatase	III-A
4. N-acetyl-α-glucosaminidase	III-B
5. Galactosamine-4-sulfatase (arylsulfatase B)	VI
6. β-glucuronidase	VII
7. N-acetyl-β galactosaminidase	IV

Fig. 26.27 Portions of polysaccharide chains of dermatan and heparan sulfate and nature of the defects in the various mucopolysaccharidoses.

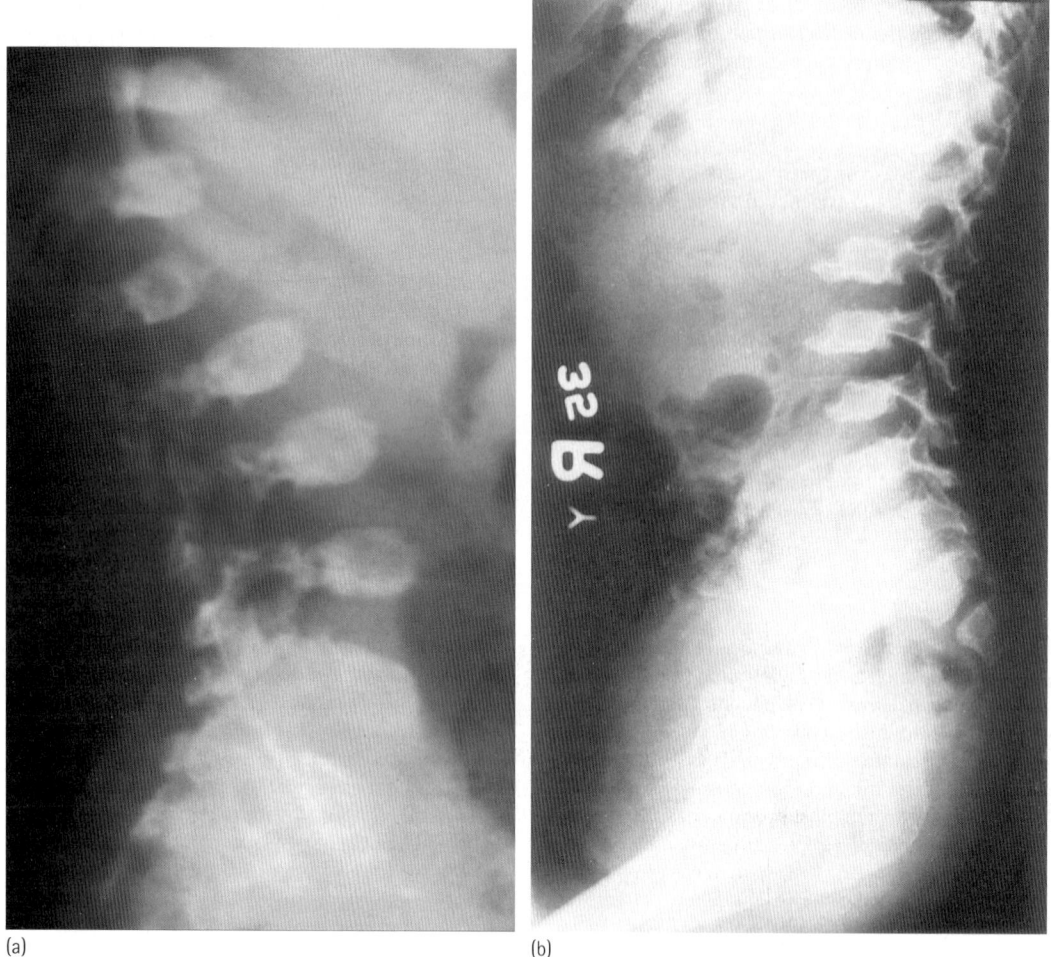

(a)   (b)

Fig. 26.28   (a) Lateral view of the spine showing early changes in a 3-year-old child with Hurler syndrome and (b) late changes in the spine of a patient with Morquio syndrome.

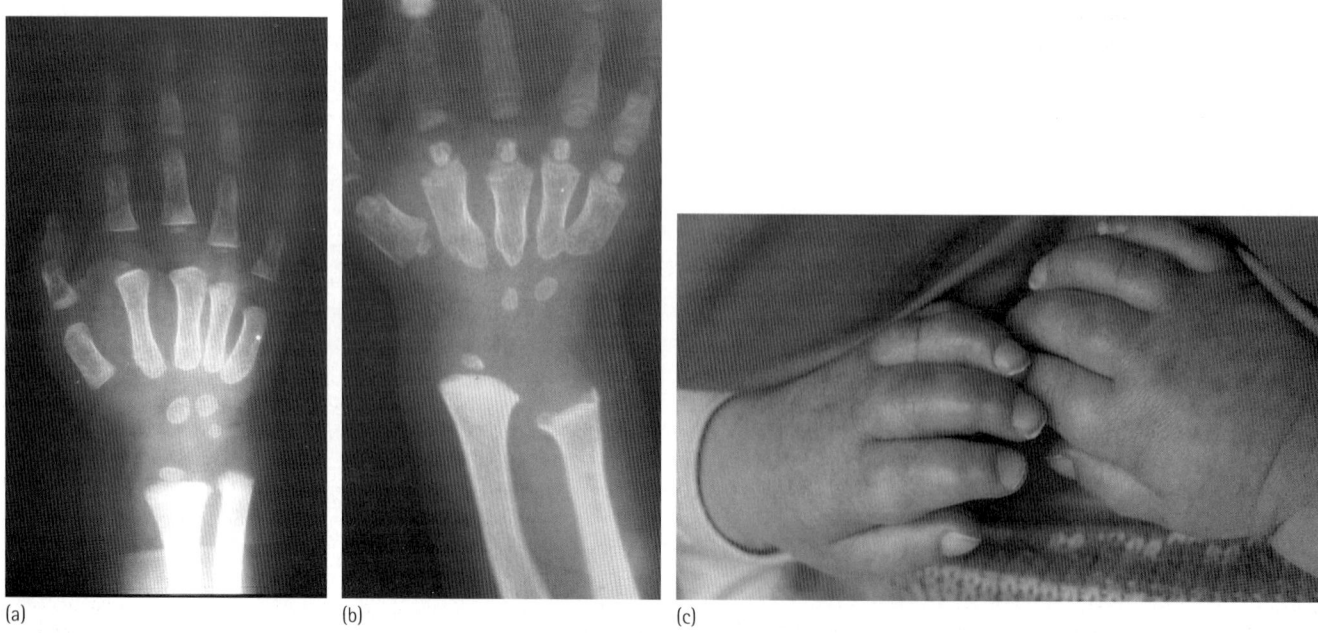

(a)   (b)   (c)

Fig. 26.29   Dysostosis multiplex: (a,b) Hand X-rays of two 3-year-old children with mild and more severe bony changes; (c) the claw hands of Hurler syndrome.

but all the others are autosomal recessive traits. Prenatal diagnosis is available for most MPS but is not always easily available. Carrier testing is possible, but is not always conclusive.

Treatment

Surgery poses great risk for these patients since airway narrowing from tissue infiltration, possible cardiopulmonary disease, and manipulation of the neck, which may be unstable in MPS disorders, during induction make anesthesia high risk.[173-177]

ERT is now available for MPS I, MPS II and MPS VI. Unfortunately, ERT does not address the neurological complications, so it may not prevent death in severe cases. Bone marrow or cord blood stem cell transplantation has shown some efficacy, especially for MPS I.[174,176] Other than this, supportive care is all that is available.

MPS I – Hurler, Hurler–Scheie (I/V) and Scheie (V) syndromes

These conditions, earlier thought to be different disorders, are allelic and caused by different mutations of the gene encoding alpha-L-iduronidase, leading to severe and milder forms of the same disease. The accumulating GAGs are heparan and dermatan sulfates.

Clinical features

The frequency of MPS I – Hurler syndrome is around 1 in 100 000. These patients are usually diagnosed at 1–2 years of age, and typically have a life expectancy of 6–10 years. Major clinical manifestations include cardiomyopathy, hepatosplenomegaly, skeletal deformity, developmental regression, corneal clouding, hearing loss, rhinorhea and dysostosis multiplex.

The frequency of MPS I – Hurler–Scheie syndrome is around 1 in 115 000. The clinical findings are similar to Hurler syndrome with the exception that there is no CNS involvement. Patients are often diagnosed at age 2–5 years, with death occurring in the late 20s without treatment.

The least severe form is Scheie syndrome which occurs in about 1 in 500 000. It is characterized by joint stiffness with tendon compression syndromes, glaucoma and variable aortic valve disease. There is normal growth and no CNS involvement, and life expectancy can be normal. The differential diagnosis includes acquired polyarthropathies and the multiple epiphyseal dysplasias.

Hunter MPS II

Hunter syndrome is caused by a deficiency of iduronate sulfatase, with storage of dermatan and heparan sulfate. The presentation is very similar to MPS I except that the corneae never become cloudy and a pebbly skin lesion, usually most apparent over the scapulae ('peau d'orange'), is common. Severely affected children usually die in the second decade. Mild cases can have normal intelligence, short stature and survival into the sixth decade.

Diagnosis and treatment

Increased levels of the GAGs dermatan and heparan sulfate in urine are suggestive. Measurement of iduronate sulfatase in leukocytes or cultured fibroblasts is diagnostic.

Neither bone marrow nor cord blood stem cell transplant has been successful but ERT is beneficial.

Sanfilippo syndrome MPS III A, B, C and D

Symptoms in all forms include the subtle onset of developmental regression, extreme hyperactivity and behavioral difficulties including aggressive behavior, mild hepatosplenomegaly and, frequently, very mild dysostosis. Coarsening of facial features in these disorders may be minimal or absent, making clinical recognition difficult. Life span is into the second to third decade. Sanfilippo A is a result of heparan N-sulfatase deficiency; MPS III B is caused by a deficiency of alpha-N-acetylglucosaminidase. MPS III C is a result of deficient acetyl-CoA: alpha-glucosaminide acetyltransferase and MPS III D is caused by N-acetylglucosamine 6-sulfatase deficiency.

Diagnosis and treatment

The absence of dysmorphic features, subtle onset and psychiatric problems often delay the diagnosis for years. All forms are characterized by increased excretion of heparan sulfate but this may not be marked, so a normal urine screen does *not* rule out the diagnosis. Enzyme analysis in leukocytes or cultured fibroblasts is necessary.

Neither bone marrow nor cord blood stem cell transplant has been successful.

Morquio syndrome A and B (MPS IV)

Morquio A is caused by deficiency of N-acetyl-galactosamina-6-sulfatase, Morquio B by deficient beta-galactosidase – the same enzyme deficiency that causes GM₁-gangliosidosis. Morquio A and B are clinically identical; both have less severe forms; atlantoaxial subluxation can occur.

Presentation is usually at 18–24 months with gait problems from genu valgum, coxa valga, kyphosis and growth failure. The trunk and neck are short and the facies are broad, but without the coarseness of MPS I. In the upper limbs, especially the hands, there is joint laxity rather than contractures. By 6 years, the corneae are typically cloudy, and there is progressive spinal and chest deformity with lumbar lordosis and dorsal kyphosis (see Fig. 26.28b). Contractures of the knees and hips produce a jockey-like stance and the fingers are short and hypermobile with ulnar deviation. Cardiac valvular lesions may occur. Intelligence is usually normal. An enamel dysplasia occurs that is not seen in other LSDs. Survival well into adulthood is usual, females seeming to fare better than males. A common and critical problem is odontoid hypoplasia with subluxation of C1 on C2. Myelopathy may occur acutely or insidiously, being precipitated by even minor trauma including flexion of the neck as during anesthesia. Mechanically induced pulmonary insufficiency and valvular heart disease are eventually fatal.

Diagnosis and treatment

The diagnosis is made with specific enzyme assays. The accumulated GAGs are keratan sulfate and chondroitin 6-sulfate. In early childhood MPS IV is similar to other MPSs, and a number of skeletal dysplasias with platyspondyly are easily confused, but, in them, corneal clouding and keratansulfaturia are absent.

Myelopathy may benefit from early treatment by surgical fusion of the spine or other orthopedic procedures, but the decision on whether to operate should be carefully considered by experts. Bracing alone is rarely satisfactory.

Maroteaux–Lamy syndrome (MPS VI)

Maroteaux–Lamy syndrome results from deficiency of N-acetylgalactosamine-4-sulfatase (arylsulfatase B). Dermatan sulfate is excreted in excess. Mild and severe forms of the disorder are seen. MPS VI is usually diagnosed between 6 and 24 months. Signs include short stature, dysostosis multiplex, stiff joints, corneal clouding and normal intelligence. Eventually, cardiac valvular disease occurs and myelopathy is common. In the severe forms, life expectancy without treatment is into the second decade.

Diagnosis and treatment

Diagnosis is by assay of arylsulfatase B in leukocytes or cultured fibroblasts. Increased urinary dermatan sulfate is suggestive.

Bone marrow or cord blood stem cell transplant were formerly used but clinical trials have now confirmed efficacy of ERT.[177,178]

Other mucopolysaccharide disorders (MPS VII and IX)

Sly syndrome (MPS VII) is rare and caused by beta-glucuronidase deficiency, with resultant excretion of dermatan sulfate, heparan sulfate and chondroitin 6-sulfate. Severe cases may have hydrops fetalis. Major clinical manifestations include dysostosis multiplex and hepatosplenomegaly with a wide variation in severity. Diagnosis is by enzyme analysis in serum, leukocytes or cultured fibroblasts. No specific therapy is available.

Hyaluronidase deficiency (MPS IX) with transient bilateral nodular soft tissue masses and painful generalized edema has been reported. The patient had mildly dysmorphic features, acquired short stature, normal joint movement and intelligence. Pelvic radiographs revealed multiple intra-articular soft tissue masses and acetabular erosions.

MUCOLIPIDOSES [I-CELL DISEASE (ML II) AND PSEUDO-HURLER POLYDYSTROPHY (ML III)]

These two conditions are allelic and caused by a defect of N-acetyl-glucosamine-1-phosphotransferase which normally attaches phosphate to a polymannose side chain on the precursor proenzymes in the Golgi. This destroys the uptake-recognition site on the enzymes and results in several of them showing elevated levels in serum, having altered electrophoretic patterns and multiple intralysosomal enzyme deficiencies. This accounts for a heterogeneous accumulation of intralysosomal storage material. The gross cytoplasmic inclusions seen in cultured fibroblasts gave rise to the name 'inclusion (I) cell disease'.

ML II and ML III are similar to severe and mild Hurler syndrome, respectively, except that corneal clouding never develops. In ML II, the features may even be detectable at birth. ML III is milder and is often diagnosed as polyarticular arthropathy for years before the true cause is recognized. Clinical and radiological appearances are shown in Figures 26.30.

Diagnosis and treatment

Diagnosis is suspected based on the clinical findings associated with elevated levels of several lysosomal enzymes in serum. Assay of the specific enzyme defect is available in a few centers. Mutation analysis should become available soon. No specific therapy is available.

OLIGOSACCHARIDOSES AND GLYCOPROTEINOSES

The glycoproteinoses are rare disorders in which different enzyme deficiencies result in accumulation of oligosaccharides that are excreted

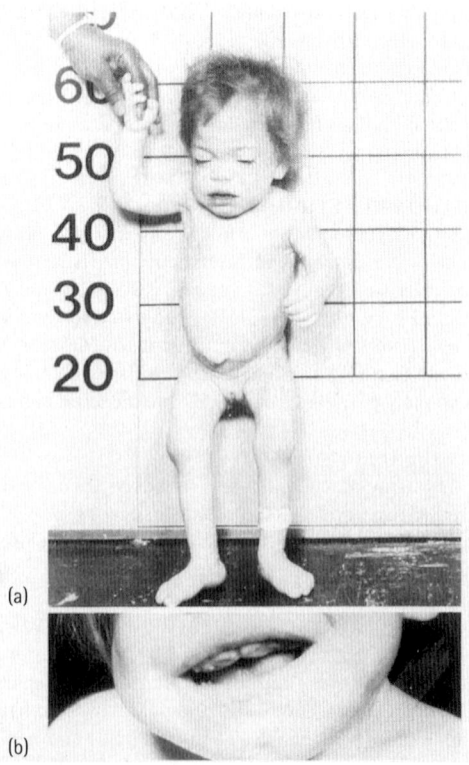

Fig. 26.30   Mucolipidosis II (I-cell disease) in an 18-month-old girl. (a) Facies and habitus, (b) gum hypertrophy.

in urine; some have ethnic predilections. The clinical presentations are often similar to a mild MPS but with no increased excretion of GAGs. Two typical oligosaccharide chains are shown in Figure 26.31. As with all untreated LSDs, once the conditions manifest, they follow a steady downhill course. No specific treatment is available.

GM₁-gangliosidosis (beta-galactosidase deficiency)

Early-, severe- and later-onset forms are described; they involve the same enzyme as MPS IV B and galactosialidosis (combined with neuraminidase deficiency).

Clinical features

Infantile GM_1-gangliosidosis (type I) is the commonest form. It presents in infancy and mimics a severe Hurler phenotype with increasing psychomotor retardation and failure to thrive. Dysostosis and hepatosplenomegaly are prominent and cardiomyopathy may develop. About 50% have a macular cherry red spot and by 1 year, blindness and seizures are usual. Continued deterioration results in death by 2 years of age.

In juvenile GM_1-gangliosidosis, development starts to slow around 1 year, progressing to seizures, abnormal movements and progressive decline, leading to death between 3 and 10 years of age. Skeletal changes, hepatomegaly and cherry red spots are usually absent. Adult GM_1-gangliosidosis presents in the second or third decade; it is the rarest form but is more frequent in Japan. Symptoms include slowly progressive dystonia, spinocerebellar degeneration and increasing cognitive deficits. Dysmorphic features, visceromegaly, cherry red spots and seizures are absent.

Diagnosis and treatment

Beta-galactosidase is deficient in all tissues and may be assayed in leukocytes. Lymphocytes often show a characteristic vacuolation. Low levels of keratan sulfate may be excreted; more often there is a characteristic oligosacchariduria that includes a specific octasaccharide. At autopsy, many tissues contain large histiocytes ballooned with GM_1-ganglioside.

No specific therapy is available.

Aspartylglucosaminuria
Clinical features

Most cases have originated from Finland, where a consistent phenotype, reminiscent of the MPSs, is found. They present between 1 and 5 years of age with coarse features and loose, sagging skin, often with prominent acne. Angiokeratomas are common and connective tissue involvement leads to joint laxity. Growth is usually poor, often with mild dysostosis. There is generally no significant hepatosplenomegaly but recurrent respiratory infections, urinary tract infections, hernia, clubfoot or planovalgus deformity, corneal opacities and strabismus are frequent. Mental deterioration and bizarre behavior become evident between 6 and 15 years with death 20–30 years later from pulmonary disease.

Diagnosis and treatment

Deficient aspartylglucosaminidase activity can be demonstrated in leukocytes or fibroblasts. Most patients have vacuolated lymphocytes, lymphopenia and increased urinary levels of glycoasparagines that may be detected on amino acid analysis.

No specific treatment is available.

Fucosidosis

A severe form with onset between 3 and 18 months and a milder form are described; both are rare. Both are similar to the MPS phenotype with skeletal abnormalities, coarse facial features, growth retardation, hepatosplenomegaly, cardiomegaly and mental retardation. Early-onset cases are severely delayed and never achieve normal milestones. Milder patients have angiokeratomas identical to Fabry disease.

Deficient enzyme activity in leukocytes is diagnostic. Vacuolated lymphocytes are found. Oligosaccharide analysis of urine is helpful. No specific treatment is available.

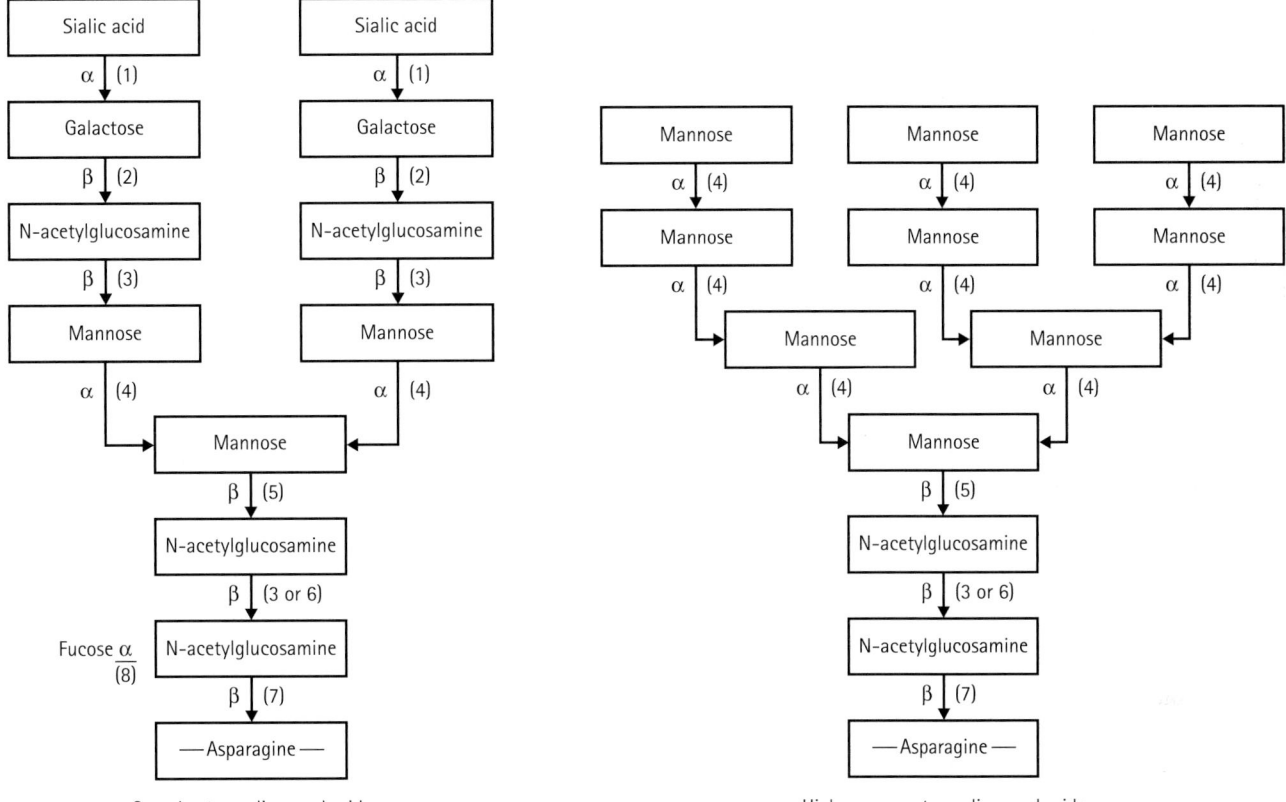

Fig. 26.31 Structures of two typical oligosaccharide chains as found on glycoproteins. Alpha and beta linkages are indicated and the specific degradative enzyme steps are numbered as follows: 1, α-neuraminidase; 2, β-galactosidase; 3, β-hexosaminidase; 4, α-mannosidase; 5, β-mannosidase; 6, endo-β-hexosaminidase; 7, aspartylglucosaminidase; 8, α-fucosidase.

Alpha-mannosidosis

Two phenotypes are described; both are rare. Type I presents in infancy and type II between 1 and 4 years of age. The clinical features are very similar and include mildly coarse MPS-like facies, marked mental retardation, recurrent infections, impaired speech, hearing loss, corneal clouding, hepatosplenomegaly and dysostosis. There may also be marked hyperplasia of the gingiva.

Vacuolated lymphocytes are generally present in peripheral blood and bone marrow. Several mannose-rich oligosaccharides are found in urine. The enzyme is measurable in leukocytes. No specific treatment is available.

Beta-mannosidosis

The few reported severe cases have had seizures, quadriplegia and rapid decline to death. Symptoms have included mental retardation, angiokeratoma, feeding difficulties, recurrent infections, speech difficulties and hearing loss. The enzyme can be measured in leukocytes. Vacuolated lymphocytes are not present and the major storage substance is an oligosaccharide. No specific therapy is available.

Schindler disease

This rare disorder is due to deficiency of alpha-N-acetylgalactosaminidase. Type I is an infantile-onset neuroaxonal dystrophy with rapid deterioration starting about 1 year and leading to pancerebral damage, blindness and myoclonic seizures. There is no visceromegaly or any peripheral storage cells. Type II develops later, even in midlife. Angiokeratoma corporis diffusum, lymphedema and mild, progressive cerebral involvement are reported; inclusions may be seen in leukocytes and dystrophic axons in rectal biopsies. Urinary oligosaccharides are abnormal. The enzyme assay can be performed in leukocytes.

SIALIDOSES

The sialic acids are a family of compounds derived from neuraminic acid. Neuraminidase deficiency occurs in several forms.

Clinical features

In type I (cherry red spot–myoclonus syndrome), debilitating myoclonic seizures and movement disorders develop, usually in the second decade and are accompanied by progressive visual loss associated with macular cherry red spots. Nystagmus, ataxia and seizures may occur. Intelligence is usually preserved until late, and visceromegaly and dysostosis are mild or absent.

The phenotype of type II (previously called mucolipidosis type I) is of a severe MPS disorder presenting in infancy or even as fetal hydrops. The phenotype is with dysostosis, hepatosplenomegaly and developmental delay. Survival depends upon the severity of the symptoms.

Galactosialidosis is very similar to type II sialidosis. An early infantile form is characterized by coarse facies, macrocephaly, growth disturbance, hepatosplenomegaly, fetal hydrops, ascites, kidney and heart involvement, angiokeratomata, telangiectasia, seizures, myoclonus, ataxia, pyramidal tract signs, progressive neurological deterioration, cherry red spots, corneal and lens opacity, hearing loss and dysostosis multiplex. Late infantile cases are less severe with slower progression. A late juvenile form, most common in Japan; develops more insidiously with survival into adult life.

Diagnosis and treatment

In types I and II, deficient alpha-neuraminidase activity can be shown in cultured fibroblasts. In galactosialidosis, combined deficiency of neuraminidase and beta-galactosidase is caused by the primary defect of an intralysosomal protein that protects these enzymes from degradation. In all three disorders, foam cells may be seen in bone marrow.

Vacuolation is rare in lymphocytes in type I but present in type II and can be prominent in other cells. The urine contains several sialylated oligosaccharides.

No specific therapy is available.

Mucolipidosis IV

This is a rare disorder that typically presents in infancy or early childhood, with psychomotor retardation that becomes evident by 2–3 years of age. There is corneal clouding and retinal degeneration but no facial dysmorphism, visceromegaly or skeletal changes. Survival is usually well into the third decade. Later-onset, milder cases are known. More than 80% of patients have been Ashkenazi Jews in whom the carrier frequency is ~1 in 100 (giving a frequency of ~1 in 40 000). There is no cellular metachromasia or mucopolysacchariduria, although gangliosides, MPS, lamellar membrane structures and amorphous, periodic-acid Schiff (PAS)-positive cytoplasmic inclusions can be seen in many tissues, including conjunctiva, and even in conjunctival swabs. The defect is in a protein (mucolipin) the function of which is unknown. Plasma gastrin levels are elevated for unknown reasons. Two mutations account for 95% of disease alleles in Ashkenazim so that molecular testing can be diagnostic. No specific therapy is available.

Infantile sialic acid storage disease, Salla disease and sialuria

Clinical features

Four clinical entities present with intracellular accumulation and urinary excretion of sialic acid; all are rare.

1. Infantile sialic acid storage disease (ISSD) and Salla disease are probably allelic, caused by mutations in a lysosomal membrane transport protein.
2. Sialuria is an error of impaired feedback inhibition in the synthesis of sialic acid.
3. Sialidosis is due to deficiency of lysosomal neuraminidase leading to storage of sialyloligosaccharides, or bound sialic acid.
4. Galactosialidosis is due to deficiency of a 32 kDa protective protein; affected patients also excrete sialyloligosaccharides in urine.

ISSD presents with a severe 'Hurler' phenotype. Growth retardation is common but there may only be mild dysostosis. Some patients have had punctate calcification of the epiphyses similar to Zellweger syndrome. There is also marked hypopigmentation with pale wispy hair. Corneae are usually clear but optic atrophy is common. Failure to thrive leads to death in the first years of life.

In Salla disease, symptoms emerge in the first year or two of life and include ataxia, athetosis and pyramidal signs. Many patients are exotrophic and later, most develop mild 'storage' facies. There is usually no corneal clouding and the fundi are normal. Most patients have a very low IQ. Growth retardation is usual, but apart from a somewhat thickened calvarium, the radiological picture is usually normal. Most patients live for decades.

Sialuria presents with developmental delay, visceromegaly and coarse facies. There is massive excretion of free sialic acid in urine but no lysosomal storage. It is caused by overproduction of sialic acid due to a failure in negative feedback control on uridine diphosphate N-acetyl-glucosamine-2-epimerase.

Galactosialidosis and sialidosis are described above.

Diagnosis and treatment

In ISSD and Salla disease there are prominent lysosomal vacuoles in lymphocytes and free sialic acid levels are markedly increased in urine, leukocytes and fibroblasts. Urinary oligosaccharides are abnormal. In sialuria, the cells contain sialic acid in the cytosol. Prenatal diagnosis is possible for all conditions; sialic acid is markedly raised in amniotic fluid in ISSD but not in Salla disease. Chorionic villus cells are vacuolated. No specific therapy is available.

OTHER LYSOSOMAL DISEASES

Lysosomal alpha-1,4-glucosidase deficiency (GSD type II, Pompe disease)

This condition is caused by lysosomal alpha-1,4-glucosidase (acid maltase) deficiency, with an incidence of 1 in 40 000–100 000. Acid maltase catalyzes the cleavage of alpha-1,6 and alpha-1,4 linkages in glycogen and therefore completely hydrolyzes glycogen. It is present in all tissues. Infantile, juvenile and adult forms are known. The clinical presentation of infantile Pompe disease is a result of massive glycogen deposition in the heart and skeletal muscle. Previously it has been classified as a glycogen storage disorder (see p. 1076).

Clinical features

Infantile Pompe disease is characterized by the rapid onset in the first months of life of profound muscle hypotonia, weakness, hyporeflexia, macroglossia, massive cardiomyopathy and variable hepatomegaly. The infant is usually alert and the cognitive development is normal. The clinical course is downhill and, without treatment, cardiopulmonary failure or pneumonia lead to death by around 1 year.

Childhood or adult forms are less severe and progress more slowly. The heart is not usually affected in late-onset Pompe disease but motor milestones are delayed and weakness of limb girdle and truncal muscles mimics chronic myopathies, especially the limb girdle muscular dystrophies. Involvement of respiratory muscles ultimately causes ventilatory insufficiency with death often between the second and fourth decade.

Diagnosis

The diagnosis can be suspected from the characteristic ECG that shows huge QRS complexes, left or biventricular hypertrophy and shortened PR interval. Muscle biopsy reveals glycogen freely dispersed in the cytoplasm and vacuoles that stain for glycogen (PAS positive) and acid phosphatase. Increased glycogen content is usually found, and electron micrographs showing intralysosomal accumulation of glycogen are also highly suggestive, though not diagnostic.

The enzyme can theoretically be assayed in leukocytes but that assay is fraught with difficulties and assay in muscle and/or fibroblasts is often preferred. A new and reliable assay in blood has been developed but should only be done in experienced laboratories. In the infantile form, glycogen-laden lysosomes are present in all organs except the kidneys and the cerebral cortex, being particularly abundant in anterior horn cells and motor nuclei of the brainstem. In the adult disorder, glycogen storage may be absent in heart, brain and liver, and varies greatly in different muscles (note this can cause difficulties with diagnostic testing). A second enzyme, neutral maltase, is produced by the kidneys and is also present in the leukocytes and must be differentiated during enzyme analysis. Antenatal diagnosis is possible.

Treatment

Recent trials of intravenous recombinant alpha-glucosidase infusions have been promising,[179-185] particularly for the myopathic forms, and ERT is now approved for use both in the USA and Europe.[184] Extensive supportive care is required.[185]

Cystinosis

Cystinosis (see also Ch. 18, p. 550) Cystinosis occurs in approximately 1 in 60 000 births. It is a disorder in which there is intralysosomal storage of cystine in many tissues, secondary to deficient egress from the lysosomes. It is the most common cause of a chronic renal Fanconi syndrome in childhood (see p. 550).

Clinical features

Infantile cystinosis presents in infancy with tremendous water and salt craving (ketchup and pickle juice!), food refusal and failure to thrive, vomiting, lethargy, polyuria, irritability, anorexia and signs of progressive renal tubular and glomerular damage that can lead to death in the first decade. Growth failure is usually severe and rickets may be prominent. The skin is pale and the hair becomes blonde due to inhibition of melanin formation; photophobia is common due to a crystal keratopathy and a characteristic retinopathy. Later, progressive damage of the thyroid gland causes hypothyroidism, proximal myopathy, and sometimes, cerebral lesions.

Milder variants present in childhood or adolescence with slower progression of retinopathy and renal disease; there is also an adult form in which there is no renal damage, although cystine crystals are still present in the cornea.

Diagnosis

The symptoms, blonde hair and blood values are so striking that the diagnosis should suggest itself. The biochemical features of the severe form are those of the renal Fanconi syndrome with renal tubular acidosis, hyponatremia, hypokalemia, hypouricemia, hypophosphatemia, hypocalcemia and raised alkaline phosphatase. In the urine polyuria, glycosuria, proteinuria and aminoaciduria are prominent. Plasma amino acids, including cystine, are normal or low. The diagnosis can be confirmed by the demonstration of refractile corneal crystals seen on slit lamp examination (they can also be seen in other tissues) and by measurement of intracellular cystine levels in leukocytes or cultured skin fibroblasts (up to 100 times normal); levels in heterozygotes are typically 5–10 times normal. Histological examination shows severe damage of the proximal renal tubules. Cystinotic cells take up 35S-cysteine at about twice the normal rate but accumulate the disulfide, cystine, in greatly increased amounts.

Treatment

There is no cure. Therapy is directed towards correction of the fluid and electrolyte imbalances, acidosis, rickets and hypothyroidism. Dietary restriction of cystine and methionine, and also penicillamine, are ineffective. Cysteamine or phosphocysteamine are the drugs of choice since they deplete intracellular cystine; they must be given every 6 h and the dose monitored by regular assay of leukocyte cystine. They are used as eye drops to control cystine levels in the cornea and thus to mitigate the photophobia. These drugs delay or prevent renal failure and other systemic consequences. Transplanted kidneys do not express the cystinotic defect and have the same prognosis as any renal transplant. The biochemical defect, however, continues in other tissues and long term complications, including myopathy and CNS damage, are now recognized.

Neuronal ceroid lipofuscinosis
Genetics

Lipofuscin is an autofluorescent complex of lipid and protein that can be detected in lysosomes by electron microscopy. The neuronal ceroid lipofuscinoses (NCLs) are a group of disorders that collectively are probably the most common causes of progressive neurodegeneration in childhood. Infantile (Santavuori–Haltia), late infantile (Jansky–Bielschowsky), juvenile (Batten, Spielmeyer–Vogt), and adult (Kufs)-onset forms represent the 'classic' clinical presentations but as many as 20% of cases are 'atypical', and a Finnish variant, Gypsy/Indian early-juvenile variant, Turkish variant and Northern epilepsy are additional well defined variants described in specific populations. Seven different gene loci are currently known. It is important to recognize that identical clinical variants can be caused by different protein/enzyme/gene defects (Table 26.25).

Clinical features

All forms of NCL develop signs of neurological impairment that may be rapid or slow, followed by seizures, often myoclonic, and overt deterioration, involving all brain functions, and that leads inevitably to death. Retinal degeneration is prominent in virtually all forms of NCL; the younger the onset, the more rapid the progression. Infants may die within a year or two, but juvenile cases may survive for 10–20 years. In the juvenile form, the first symptom is either rapid loss of vision over a few months or the sudden onset of seizures. Cerebral atrophy is often apparent by brain MRI even before the onset of symptoms. In adults, initial symptoms include psychiatric disorders, myoclonic seizures and signs of pyramidal involvement. In most NCLs, there is a characteristic pigmentary retinopathy; it is notably absent in at least one form of late infantile NCL reported from Finland. There is no dysmorphism or visceromegaly.

Diagnosis

The history of rapid loss of sight and neurodegeneration, especially when brain imaging reveals only atrophy, is highly suggestive. Early changes can be seen in visual evoked responses, ERG and MRI of the brain. Diagnosis formerly was based on detection of characteristic 'curvilinear' and fingerprint inclusions by electron microscopic examination of lysosomes of conjunctiva, rectum, leukocytes or skin. Experts differ, depending upon their experience, as to which tissue is optimal for finding the inclusions. In the juvenile form, leukocytes often show inclusions; however, in some NCLs, the inclusions are sparse or absent in leukocytes. The deposits are distinctive but with subtle differences in each subtype; rare cases show a granular appearance. In the late infantile and juvenile forms, the lipofuscin contains large amounts of subunit c of ATP synthase; in the infantile form this is absent but the deposits are rich in sphingolipid activator protein. The reason for the incorporation of these products is unknown. Activity of the enzymes defective in several forms of NCL can now be measured in blood. In addition, mutation analysis for many of the types of NCL is available. Prenatal diagnosis can often be achieved through a combination of microscopic and/or biochemical and genetic studies.

Treatment

There is no proven treatment for any of the NCLs although cysteamine is under investigation as a potential treatment in the infantile forms. A gene therapy trial for late infantile NCL and a trial of purified human fetal neural stem cells are underway for infantile and late infantile NCL.

PEROXISOMAL DISORDERS

GENERAL CONSIDERATIONS

Peroxisomes are single membrane-bound organelles found in most eukaryotic cells. They are responsible for a variety of metabolic functions. Biosynthetic activities include synthesis of plasmalogens, which are important components of cell membranes and myelin, cholesterol, bile acids, glyoxylate and docosahexanoic acid (DHA). Additionally, two aminotransferases involved in gluconeogenesis are located in liver peroxisomes. Catabolic functions include H_2O_2-based cellular respiration, glutaryl-CoA, purine and pipecolic acid catabolism, alpha-oxidation of branched chain fatty acids (phytanic acid) and beta-oxidation of very long chain fatty acids (VLCFAs) which have more than a 22-carbon chain.[186,187]

Table 26.25 Types and features of neuronal ceroid lipofuscinosis

Clinical types	Frequency (% of total)	Age of onset (years)	Usual gene defect	Other reported genes
Infantile	~16	0–3	CLN1	
Late infantile	~50	2–8	CLN2	CLN 1,3,5,6,7
Juvenile	~30	4–10	CLN3	CLN1,2 (5–8?)
Adult	~2	11–55	CLN4	

From Zhong, 2000. Genereviews.

Peroxisomal disorders can be classified into two categories: disorders of biogenesis (PBDs), which are associated with a general loss of peroxisomal function, and disorders associated with single enzyme deficiencies.

DISORDERS OF PEROXISOME BIOGENESIS

Zellweger syndrome, neonatal adrenoleukodystrophy and infantile Refsum disease

There are at least 12 different complementation groups that account for three distinct but overlapping diseases. All three disorders show dysmorphic features and all share some common clinical and biochemical abnormalities.

Clinical features

These three conditions all result from defects in peroxisome assembly.[186] Their overall incidence is approximately 1 in 50 000. They share clinical and biochemical features and represent a spectrum of disease severity. Microscopically, the peroxisomes may be absent or in the form of 'peroxisome ghosts', remnant membrane structures that lack normal matrix enzymes. Rhizomelic chondrodysplasia punctata (RCDP) is considered a partial PBD and is considered separately below.

Zellweger syndrome (cerebrohepatorenal syndrome) is the most severe phenotype and is characterized by marked neonatal hypotonia, seizures, psychomotor retardation, feeding difficulties, hepatomegaly, renal cysts, sensorineural deafness and developmental brain abnormalities, such as polymicrogyria, heterotopias and agenesis of the corpus callosum. Ocular abnormalities include corneal clouding, cataracts, glaucoma, nystagmus and pigmentary retinopathy. There is characteristic craniofacial dysmorphism that includes a high forehead, large fontanelles, midface hypoplasia, shallow orbital ridges, hypertelorism with upslanting palpebral fissures and epicanthal folds, posteriorly rotated ears with abnormal helices, anteverted nares, and micrognathia (Fig. 26.32). There is often radiographic stippling of epiphyses, most prominent in the knee and hip. Prolonged neonatal jaundice and liver disease are frequent. Death usually occurs within the first year.[187–189] Individuals with prolonged survival (> 1 year) are at increased risk for hyperoxaluria, nephrocalcinosis and subsequent nephropathy.[190] Histologically peroxisomes are absent from the liver and kidneys.

Infants with neonatal adrenoleukodystrophy (NALD) and infantile Refsum disease (IRD) show milder phenotypes. In NALD, there are similar but less pronounced dysmorphic features than seen in Zellweger syndrome and renal cysts, cataracts and epiphyseal stippling are absent. Patients with NALD may initially show relatively normal development, but this is followed by regression. While survival may extend into the teen years, such children typically exhibit severe neurodevelopmental delay, with sensorineural hearing loss and blindness due to pigmentary retinopathy.[186,189] In the brain, demyelination is frequent as are neuronal migration abnormalities. NALD is also characterized by adrenal dysfunction, as well as liver disease. Of note, NALD is a completely separate entity from X-linked adrenoleukodystrophy (see below).

Dysmorphic features in IRD are more subtle but include fairly marked mid-facial hypoplasia (Fig. 26.33). The main features of IRD include severe sensorineural deafness, pigmentary retinopathy, failure to thrive, hypotonia, absent limb reflexes and psychomotor retardation. Neuronal migration abnormalities are present but there is no overt demyelination, as seen in NALD. Occasionally infants with IRD present with bleeding due to a vitamin K-responsive coagulopathy. Non-infantile Refsum disease is discussed below.

Rhizomelic chondrodysplasia punctata

Three different genetic defects are known to cause this disorder. It has a distinct clinical presentation and is associated with defects in only two peroxisomal metabolic functions: plasmalogen biosynthesis and branched chain fatty acid oxidation.[186] The most striking difference between rhizomelic chondrodysplasia punctata (RCDP) and the Zellweger spectrum disorders is the presence of major skeletal abnormalities which include rhizomelia (shortening of the proximal limbs), short stature, coronal clefts of vertebrae, metaphyseal splaying, kyphoscoliosis and joint contractures; calcific stippling is present but disappears within the first year of life. As with the other PBDs, there is also characteristic facial dysmorphism, cataracts, sensorineural deafness, psychomotor retardation and feeding difficulty with severe failure to thrive (Fig. 26.34). The majority of children with RCDP die before 2 years of age. However, milder cases are now recognized, characterized by congenital cataracts and chondrodysplasia, with or without rhizomelia.[191]

Type I RCDP is associated with a peroxisomal receptor defect (PTS2) and deficiency of at least three peroxisomal enzymes. Types 2 and 3 are each associated with single enzyme defects, dihydroxyacetone phosphate acyltransferase (DHAPAT) and alkyl-DHAP synthase, respectively.

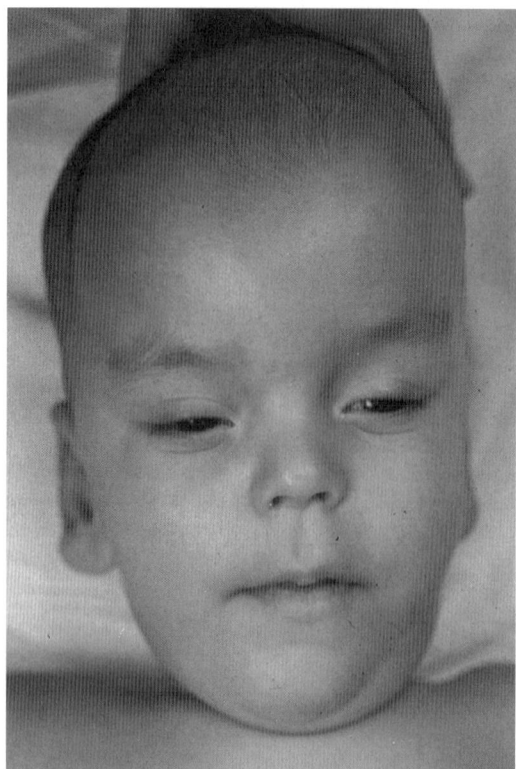

Fig 26.32   Facies of Zellweger syndrome with a high forehead, anteverted nares, micrognathia and hypertelorism.

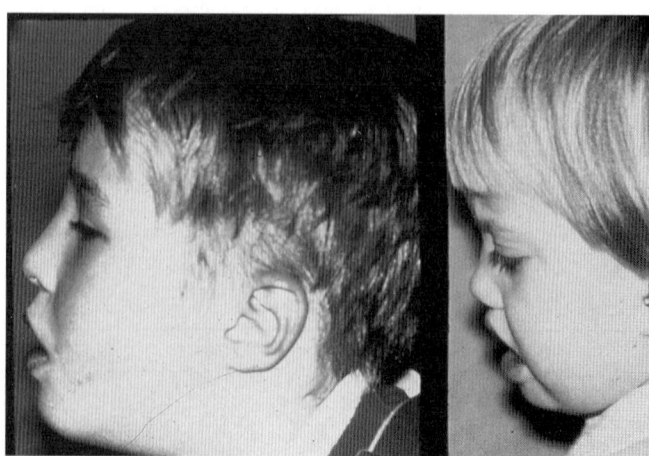

Fig 26.33   Side view of two children with infantile Refsum disease, showing the marked similarity and mid-facial hypoplasia.

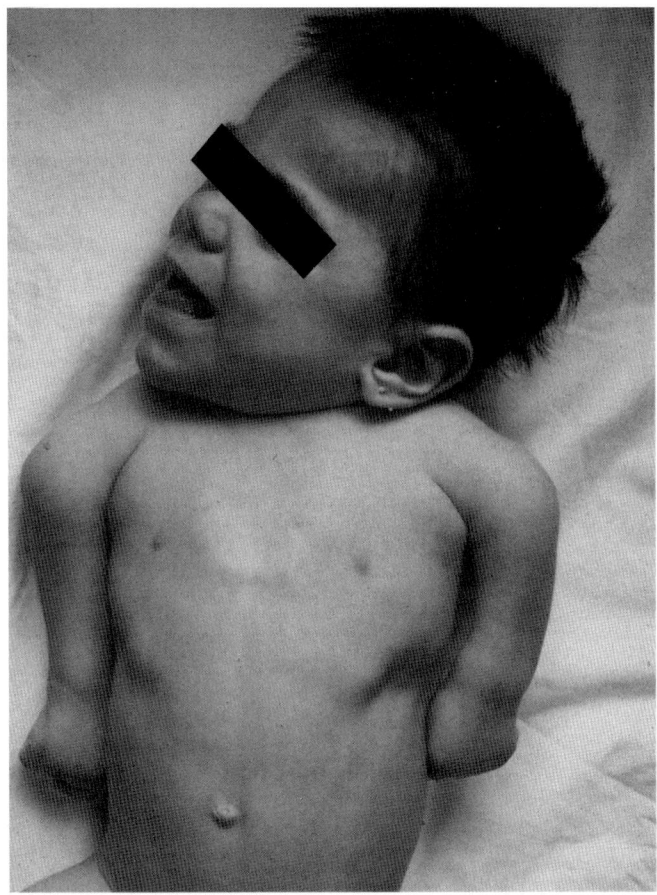

Fig 26.34   Rhizomelic chondrystrophia punctata in a 4-year-old.

Biochemical features

In varying degrees, all three disorders of peroxisome biogenesis share the same biochemical abnormalities: elevations of plasma VLCFAs, phytanic and pipecolic acids, and decreased plasmalogen and DHA (Table 26.26). In RCDP, the findings are similar except the VLCFAs are normal.

Molecular genetics

To date, pathogenic mutations are known in 12 PEX genes that encode peroxisomal membrane proteins, targeting signals and receptors required for peroxisome assembly and protein importation.[192] Approximately 65% of these patients have mutations in PEX1. A complete lack of PEX1 protein is associated with the Zellweger phenotype, while residual amounts are found in patients with NALD and IRD.[193] Correlations between clinical and biochemical phenotype and genotype are gradually emerging.[188,194] RCDP type 1 is associated with mutations in PEX7.[191]

Diagnosis

These disorders should always be considered in infants with both nerve deafness and visual deficit, particularly when associated with hypotonia and psychomotor retardation and/or characteristic dysmorphic features.

The best screening test is measurement of plasma VLCFAs, which are increased in all three disorders but not in RCDP. Additional assays of plasma phytanic acid, pipecolic acid, plasmalogen, bile acid intermediates and essential fatty acids may also be useful in characterizing the diagnosis, but abnormalities of phytanic acid and plasmalogen may be age dependent.[186] Definitive diagnosis may require enzymatic studies in cultured fibroblasts, particularly to differentiate a generalized PBD from a single enzyme defect, or in the characterization of RCDP. Molecular genetic testing is currently available for PEX1, PXMP3 (PEX2), PEX3, PEX5, PEX6, PEX7, PEX10 and PEX12.[189,191,193]

Therapy

The underlying etiology of clinical features of the PBDs is not known and their treatment remains largely supportive and symptomatic. Coagulation abnormalities may require treatment with vitamin K; adrenal insufficiency may require steroid treatment; liver dysfunction may improve with oral bile acid treatment;[195] and hyperoxaluria may require increased fluid intake and oral citrate to prevent nephrolithiasis.[188,190]

As individuals with milder phenotypes are surviving longer, there is active research into possible primary treatment. Because patients with PBDs have low levels of DHA, an important component of brain and retina, oral administration of its ethyl ester has been studied. While controlled trials are lacking, an open label study of 20 patients with PBDs receiving DHA ethyl ester 100–500 mg/d reported normalization of DHA levels in plasma and erythrocytes, decrease in plasma VLCFAs, improvement in liver function, improved vision in 50%, and MRI findings suggesting improvement in myelination.[196] Sodium 4-phenylbutyrate has been shown to increase peroxisome numbers and functions in normal fibroblasts but no trials are yet reported.[197]

DISORDERS ASSOCIATED WITH ISOLATED ENZYME DEFICIENCIES

Numerous enzymatic reactions are localized to peroxisomes and pathogenic disorders involving five metabolic pathways are currently recognized: fatty acid beta-oxidation, phytanic acid alpha-oxidation, etherphospholipid synthesis, glyoxylate detoxification, and possibly isoprenoid synthesis. Table 26.27 summarizes the clinical and screening biochemical abnormalities associated with the best characterized disorders in this group. The two most common disorders, X-linked adrenoleukodystrophy (X-ALD) and Refsum disease, are discussed below.

X-linked adrenoleukodystrophy

X-ALD is caused by a defect in the gene ABCD1 that codes for ALDP, a peroxisomal membrane adenosine triphosphate (ATP)-binding cassette transporter, and is associated with increased levels of VLCFAs in blood and tissues.

Table 26.26   Biochemical abnormalities in selected peroxisomal disorders

	Plasma VLCFA	Plasma phytanic acid	RBC plasmalogens
Peroxisome biogenesis disorders: Zellweger syndrome, adrenomyeloneuropathy, infantile Refsum disease, neonatal adrenoleukodystrophy	Increased	Increased	Increased
Rhizomelic chondrodysplasia punctata	Normal	Increased (type I) Normal (types 2 and 3)	Decreased
X-linked adrenoleukodystrophy/adrenomyeloneuropathy	Increased	Normal	Normal
Refsum disease (classical)	Normal	Increased	Normal

RBC, red blood cell; VLCFA, very long chain fatty acids.

Table 26.27   Peroxisomal disorders due to single enzyme deficiencies

Metabolic pathway	Disorder	Clinical phenotype	Best screening test
Fatty acid beta-oxidation	X-ALD/AMN	Progressive neurodegeneration, adrenal insufficiency, myeloneuropathy	Increased VLCFA
	Acyl-CoA oxidase deficiency Thiolase deficiency Bifunctional protein deficiency	NALD-like	Increased VLCFA
	2-Methylacyl-CoA racemase deficiency	Late-onset neuropathy	
Phytanic acid oxidation	Refsum disease	Retinitis pigmentosa, cerebellar ataxia, polyneuropathy	Increased phytanic acid
Etherphospholipid synthesis	DHAPAT synthase deficiency Alkyl DHAP synthase deficiency	RCDP	Decreased RBC plasmalogen
Isoprenoid synthesis	Mevalonate kinase deficiency	Dysmorphic features, hepatosplenomegaly, hypotonia, cerebral atrophy, failure to thrive	Increased urinary mevalonic acid
Glyoxylate detoxification	Hyperoxaluria type 1	Recurrent nephrolithiasis and nephrocalcinosis	Increased urinary oxalic, glyoxylic and glycolic acids

AMN, adrenomyeloneuropathy; DHAP, dihydroxyacetone phosphate; DHAPAT, DHAP acyltransferase; NALD, neonatal adrenoleukodystrophy; RCDP, rhizomelic chondrodysplasia punctata; VLCFA, very long chain fatty acids; X-ALD, X-linked adrenoleukodystrophy.

Clinical features

This disease (once known as Schilder disease) occurs in 1 in 20 000–50 000 males. There are several distinct phenotypes, all of which can be seen within the same family. In childhood-onset cerebral X-ALD, which accounts for approximately 35% of cases, development is entirely normal prior to the onset, typically between 4 and 8 years. School difficulty, behavioral disturbances and vision impairment are the most frequent initial symptoms.[198] These are followed by progressive neurological deterioration with seizures, nystagmus, vision and hearing impairments, behavior and memory problems. As the disease progresses, dementia, blindness and quadriplegia develop, and death ensues. Adrenal insufficiency is present in at least 90%.[198] This rapidly progressive cerebral form is associated with an inflammatory, demyelinating leukodystrophy.

The second phenotype, adrenomyeloneuropathy (AMN), accounts for 35–40% of cases and presents either with Addison disease or with signs of myelopathy with progressive polyneuropathy and bladder dysfunction in the second or third decade of life. Less common phenotypes include adults with adrenal insufficiency but without neurological abnormalities, and adults who develop cerebral symptoms without evidence of myelopathy. Neurological abnormalities occur in approximately 15% of heterozygous females and are commonly misdiagnosed as multiple sclerosis. It should be noted that some patients never develop neurological abnormalities.

Diagnosis

The diagnosis of X-ALD in males can be made by the detection of elevated plasma VLCFAs. Plasma VLCFA should be measured in all males who develop Addison disease. Plasma VLCFA is normal in 15% of heterozygous females, therefore DNA analysis is required for reliable diagnosis and carrier testing.[199] Approximately 85% of patients with the childhood form have characteristic abnormalities on brain MRI consisting of symmetrical areas of increased signal in the parieto-occipital region on T2-weighted imaging.[198]

Over 400 different mutations have been identified; DNA mutation analysis is available.[199] There appears to be no genotype–phenotype correlation associated with mutations within the X-ALD gene and the basis of the unpredictable intrafamilial phenotypic variability is unknown.

Therapy

Stem cell (bone marrow or cord blood) transplantation, if performed at the very earliest sign of CNS symptoms, has been shown to stabilize the progression of cerebral X-ALD. In a recent 5–10 year follow-up study of 12 patients with childhood-onset cerebral X-ALD who had undergone bone marrow transplantation early in the course of the disease, there was MRI evidence for stabilization or even reversal of demyelination.[200] Eight of the 12 children were functioning normally in school with no additional support. At this time, transplantation prior to the onset of any neurological signs or symptoms is not recommended since a fair proportion of affected males do not develop neurological symptoms, even without treatment.

Diet therapy with 'Lorenzo's oil' (a 4:1 mixture of glyceryl trioleate and glyceryl trierucate) has been shown to normalize plasma concentrations of VLCFA in patients with X-ALD, but lack of well-controlled clinical studies has limited conclusions regarding clinical efficacy.[199] Single-arm clinical trials have shown little effect of Lorenzo's oil in changing the course of cerebral or myelopathic X-ALD among symptomatic individuals.[201] However, in a recent single-arm study in 89 asymptomatic boys with normal baseline brain MRI findings, Moser et al reported that 74% remained free of neurological symptoms with normal MRI results over the mean study period of 6.9 years.[202] This compares with the authors' estimation that at least 35% of untreated X-ALD patents become symptomatic by age 10 years. Adverse effects include thrombocytopenia and elevated liver enzymes.

New therapeutic approaches are based on the observations of an improved ability of cultured fibroblasts to metabolize VLCFAs in the presence of lovastatin and 4-phenylbutyrate. Two small studies on the efficacy of lovastatin/simvastatin have failed to show clinical or biochemical benefit.[203,204] There are currently no published randomized controlled trials.

Refsum disease
Clinical features

Refsum disease is an autosomal recessive disorder with cardinal manifestations that include retinitis pigmentosa, cerebellar ataxia and polyneuropathy.[205] The age of onset is very variable; 40% of patients develop symptoms prior to 10 years of age and up to 75% by age 20.[205] The onset is usually insidious and often begins with night blindness. Sensory–motor polyneuropathy typically begins in the distal lower extremities and, if untreated, progresses to involve the upper extremities and trunk. Ataxia and cerebellar dysfunction usually become evident later than the retinal degeneration and polyneuropathy. Additional clinical features can include sensorineural hearing loss, anosmia, ichthyosis and skeletal manifestations (epiphyseal dysplasia, shortening or elongation of the third or fourth metatarsals, hammer toes). Cardiac conduction abnormalities and cardiomyopathy are a frequent cause of sudden death in untreated patients.

Refsum disease is caused by a deficiency of phytanoyl-coenzyme A (CoA) hydroxylase, an enzyme in alpha-oxidation that catalyzes an essential step in phytanic acid degradation. Deficiency of this enzyme results in the accumulation of phytanic acid, with plasma levels usually > 200 μmol/L.[206] Mutations in PHYH account for over 90% of cases; mutations in PEX7, which encodes the PTS2 receptor, account for fewer than 10% of cases. Molecular testing is available for confirmatory testing, prenatal diagnosis and carrier testing.[206]

Therapy

Phytanic acid enters the food chain from plants so therapy focuses on diets low in phytanic acid. Aggressive dietary intervention results in stabilization or improvement in the peripheral neuropathy, auditory and visual deficits.[205] Fasting and rapid weight loss, which result in the release of phytanic acid-containing lipids, should be avoided. Plasmapheresis or lipid apheresis can be used to reduce plasma phytanic acid rapidly in the management of acute arrhythmias or severe weakness, and may have a role in maintenance therapy.[206]

OTHER GENETIC DISORDERS OF PEROXISOMES

Other peroxisomal disorders include mevalonate kinase deficiency (see p. 1098), oxalosis type I (see p. 1061), at least four other disorders of fatty acid oxidation, two defects in etherphospholipid synthesis and an ill-defined defect of hyperpipecolic acidemia.

CONGENITAL DISORDERS OF GLYCOSYLATION

GENERAL CONSIDERATIONS

Glycosylation of proteins and lipids is a multienzyme process that adds carbohydrate side chains, known as glycans, which confer special characteristics to lipids and to proteins or classes of proteins. For protein glycoconjugates, this attachment is either through asparagine residues (N-glycosylation) or serine/threonine residues (O-glycosylation).[207] In spite of the fact that over 25 enzyme defects are now known, two broad clinical categories of congenital disorders of glycosylation (CDG) are recognized although the clinical spectrum of these disorders is still emerging. In type I CDGs, defects of N-glycosylation result from malfunction of cytosolic or endoplasmic reticulum enzymes involved in oligosaccharide assembly or the attachment of oligosaccharides to proteins.[208,209] In type II CDGs the abnormalities involve the endoplasmic reticulum and Golgi.[210,211]

To date, at least 12 different CDG I and six CDG II disorders have been reported (Tables 26.28 and 26.29; Fig. 26.35).

CONGENITAL DISORDERS OF GLYCOSYLATION TYPE I

CDG type Ia

The first CDG to be described was type Ia, which is panethnic and the most common entity. The defect is in phosphomannomutase which blocks conversion of mannose-6-phosphate to mannose-1-phosphate.[208,212] It is a multisystem disease affecting the central and peripheral nervous system, as well as the gastrointestinal tract, liver, fat, muscles, skeleton, heart, kidney, gonads and hematoimmunological system.[213–218] Not all forms of CDG are dysmorphic and some are being found with hypoglycemia or thromoembolic disease as a presenting feature.

Once observed, it can be seen that the facies are remarkably similar and mildly dysmorphic (Figs 26.36 and 26.37). Cardinal manifestations include psychomotor retardation, micro- or macro-cephaly, strabismus, roving eye movements, pigmentary retinopathy, hypotonia, hyporeflexia, ataxia, muscular dystrophy and epilepsy. In some cases, stroke-like episodes are often associated with febrile illness, transient lethargy, coma, hemiparesis, hemiplegia and vision loss, without neuroradiological evidence for thrombosis or hemorrhage. The neurological symptoms are stable; cerebellar hypoplasia is almost invariable and approximately 20% of cases die in the first year. Cardiomyopathy or pericarditis is not uncommon. Inverted nipples may be present, and in the early months, unusual fat pads may be seen, especially supra-iliac/pubically (see Fig. 26.36c) but also on the trunk and extremities.[208] Females never enter puberty.

The defect in glycosylation involves transferrin and many other proteins, including most hormone and lipid-binding proteins (thyroid, sex hormones, apo B and cholesterol binding); other findings are increased arylsulfatase activity and Factor XI. Phosphomannomutase activity may be determined in leukocytes and fibroblasts (although occasionally affected patients manifest intermediate activities) and mutation analysis is available. There is no specific treatment.[217,219–221]

CDG type Ib

In CDG type Ib phosphomannose isomerase deficiency blocks conversion of fructose-6-phosphate to mannose-6-phosphate. It is characterized by gastrointestinal illness (recurrent diarrhea, vomiting, liver dysfunction, coagulopathy and hypoglycemia) without prominent neurological symptoms.[223–225] The diagnosis is critical since this disorder responds to oral mannose supplementation (4 × 150 mg/kg/d) with correction of clinical and biochemical abnormalities.[222]

Table 26.28 Clinical features of congenital disorders of glycosylation

Neurological	Hypotonia, developmental delay, hypo/areflexia, ataxia, seizures, stroke-like episodes, peripheral neuropathy, microcephaly, cerebellar hypoplasia, demyelination, epilepsy, demyelinating polyneuropathy
Ophthalmological	Strabismus, abnormal eye movements, optic atrophy, nystagmus, retinitis pigmentosa, iris or retinal colobomata, cortical blindness, corneal dystrophy
Gastrointestinal	Protein-losing enteropathy, failure to thrive, cyclic vomiting, hepatic dysfunction, liver fibrosis, intestinal villus atrophy, hypoalbuminemia, low protein C, protein S, antithrombin III, increased aspartate aminotransferase
Hematological	Coagulopathy, thrombosis, thrombocytopenia, thrombocytosis, decreased Factor XI
Cardiac	Pericardial effusion, cardiomyopathy
Endocrinological	Hyperinsulinemic hypoglycemia, hypothyroidism, hypogonadism, hypoplastic genitalia
Renal	Nephrotic syndrome, renal tubular defects, hyperechogenic kidneys
Immunological	Recurrent infections, hypogammaglobulinemia
Orthopedic	Scoliosis, contractures, osteopenia, thoracic scoliosis
Other	Cholinesterase and pseudocholinesterase deficiency
	Craniofacial dysmorphy, inverted nipples, unusual fat distribution

Table 26.29   Congenital disorders of glycosylation types I and II

Disorder	Enzymatic or protein defect	Gene
CDG Ia	Phosphomannomutase	PMM2
CDG Ib	Phosphomannose isomerase	PMI
CDG Ic	Dolichol-P-Man:Man5GlcNAc-PP-dolicholmannosyltransferase	ALG6
CDG Id	Dolichol-P-Man:Man5GlcNAc-PP-dolicholmanosyltransferase	ALG3
CDG Ie	Dolichol-P-mannose synthase	DPM1
CDG If	LEC35 protein	LEC25MPDU1
CDG Ig	Dolichol-P-Man:Man7GlcNAc-PP-dolicholmannosyltransferase	ALG12
CDG Ih	Dolichol-P-glucose:Glc-1-Man-9-GlcNAc-PP-dolichyl-alpha-3-glucosyl transferase	ALG8
CDG Ii	GDP-Man:Man1GlcNAc$_2$-PP-dolichol mannosyltransferase	ALG2
CDG Ij	UDP-GlcNAc:dolichyl-phosphate-N-acetylglucosamine phosphotransferase	DPAGT1
CDG Ik	Beta-1,4-mannosyltransferase	ALG1
CDG IL	Alpha-1,2-mannosyltransferase	ALG9
CDG IIa	N-acetylglucosaminyltransferase II	MGAT2
CDG IIb	Glucosidase I	GSI
CDG IIc	GDP-fucosetransporter-1	FUCT1
CDG IId	Beta-1,4-galactosyltransferase	B4GALT1
CDG IIe	Oligomeric Golgi complex-7	COG7
CDG IIf	Cytidinemonophosphate (CMP)-sialic acid transporter	SLC35A1

CDG, congenital disorders of glycosylation; Glc, glucose; GlcNAc, N-acetylglucosamine; Man, mannose; P, phosphate; PP, pyrophosphate; GDP, guanosine diphosphate; UDP, uridine diphosphate.

Other forms of CDG type I

Severe neurological impairment is the most striking finding in most other forms of CDG type I (Table 26.28).[226] Although such patients (CDG types Ib–II) have different biochemical defects (Table 26.29), the transferrin isoelectric focusing (IEF) pattern is similar to that of CDG type Ia.[209,212,223] Clinically, CDG type Ic (glucosyltransferase I deficiency) is similar to type Ia in terms of axial hypotonia and seizures, but with milder psychomotor retardation, strabismus and absence of cerebellar hypoplasia or retinitis pigmentosa.[227] Patients with type Id (mannosyltransferase VI deficiency)

present with profound psychomotor retardation, hypoplasia of the corpus callosum, epilepsy, microcephaly, optic atrophy and colobomas.[228] CDG type Ie (dolichol-phosphate mannose synthase deficiency) manifests profound psychomotor retardation, epilepsy, hypotonia, failure to thrive, mild dysmorphic features and a mildly increased serum creatine kinase activity.[229] In CDG type If (lec 35 deficiency) the phenotype is of severe psychomotor retardation, epilepsy, poor vision and ichthyosiform skin anomalies, variably associated with dwarfism, hypotonia, contractures and feeding difficulties.[209,230] CDG Ig (mannosyltransferase

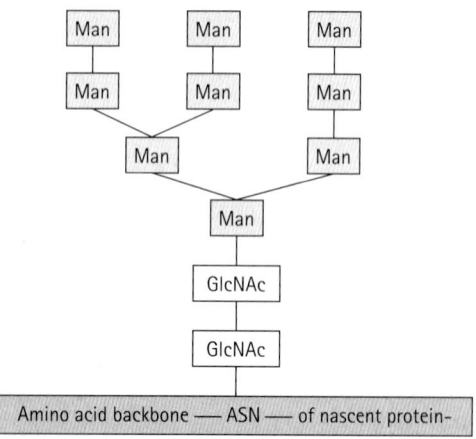

Fig 26.35   Metabolic scheme of a typical N-linked carbohydrate side chain built upon asparagine (ASN). This represents one form of a mature side chain. The linkages between the sugars vary and other sugars including N-acetylgalactosamine, galactose and sialic acid are commonly present. The side chain is built step by step and additional sugars are added and then later pruned. GlcNAc, N-acetylglucosamine; Man, mannose.

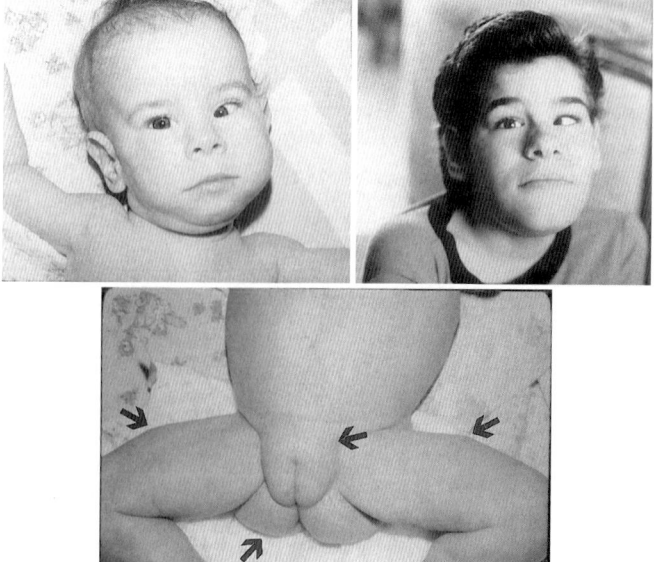

Fig. 26.36   Congential disorder of glycosylation (CDG) syndrome. (a) Facies at 15 months. (b) Facies at 16 years. (c) Pelvic area at 18 months showing the fat pads.

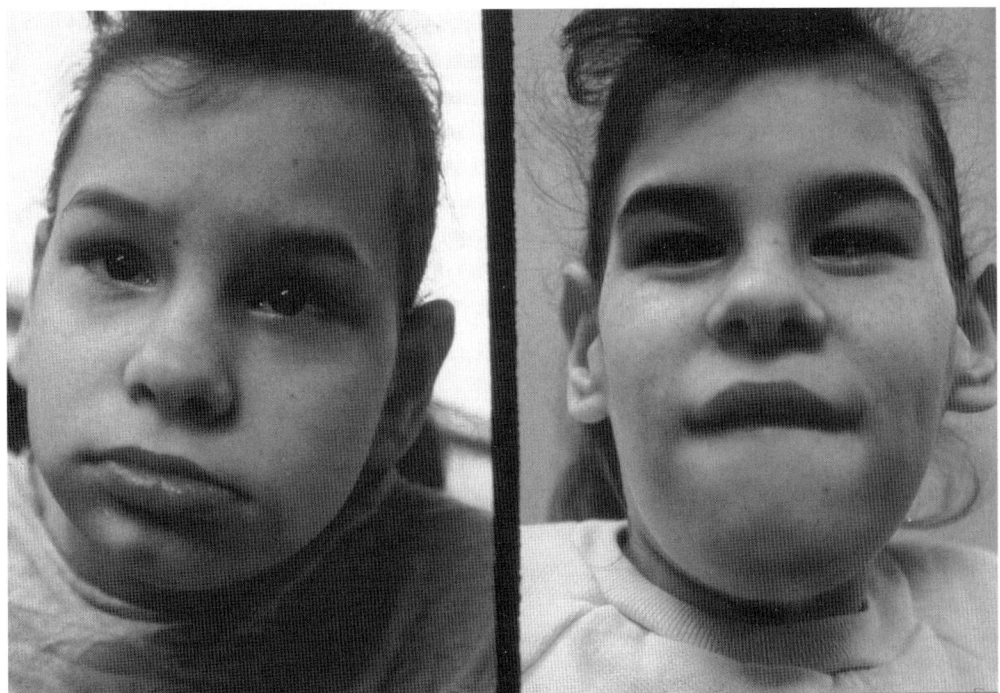

Fig 26.37 Two siblings aged 15 and 17 years with congenital disorder of glycosylation (CDG) type Ia.

VIII deficiency) manifests a clinical phenotype of generalized hypotonia, facial dysmorphism, severe psychomotor retardation, feeding difficulties and progressive microcephaly.[231] CDG Ih mimics the non-neural phenotype of the Ib disorder with protein-losing enteropathy, moderate hepatomegaly and severe hypoalbuminemia.[232]

The phenotype of CDG type Ii includes psychomotor retardation, hyperreflexia, retarded myelination, infantile spasms and bilateral iris coloboma associated with unilateral cataract.[233] CDG type Ij is a disorder associated with infantile spasms, esotropia, severe hypotonia, microcephaly, micrognathia and psychomotor retardation.[234] CDG Ik presents with intractable seizures, generalized hypotonia, blindness and liver dysfunction,[235] whereas the type IL disorder features severe microcephaly, axial hypotonia, seizures, hepatomegaly and psychomotor retardation.[236]

CONGENITAL DISORDERS OF GLYCOSYLATION TYPE II

Type IIa CDG (N-acetylglucosaminyl-transferase II deficiency) presents with developmental retardation, stereotypical behavior, craniofacial dysmorphism, epilepsy and mild liver damage with increased serum transaminases.[237-239] CDG type IIb (glucosidase I deficiency) manifests dysmorphic features, severe hypotonia and epilepsy, and is associated with an unusual urine tetrasaccharide.[240,241] The phenotype of CDG IIc (GDP-fucose transporter deficiency) includes a severe neurological syndrome, retarded growth, craniofacial dysmorphism and recurrent infections (e.g. leukocyte adhesion deficiency syndrome II).[210,211,242] CDG type IId (beta-1,4-galactosyltransferase deficiency) manifests psychomotor retardation associated with a Dandy–Walker malformation and myopathic features.[243,244] CDG type IIe manifests multiple defects associated with a defect in COG 7 (conserved oligomeric Golgi complex, subunit 7), involved in shuttling various glycoproteins from the ER to the Golgi.[210,211,245] The defect results in both N- and O-linked glycosylation defects. The findings included dysmorphic features, neurological findings and cholestatic liver disease. CDG IIf is a disorder of CMP sialic acid transport across the Golgi membrane, and manifests primarily hematological findings (microthrombocytopenia with hemorrhage, and neutropenia leading to opportunistic infections).[210,211,246]

DIAGNOSIS OF THE CONGENITAL DISORDERS OF GLYCOSYLATION SYNDROMES

These disorders are multifaceted and not well recognized by most clinicians. The primary screening tool is assessment of the glycosylation pattern of serum transferrin using IEF or other methods.[225,247,248] Typically, increased asialo- and disialo-transferrin and decreased tetrasialo- and pentasialo-transferrin suggests a type I, whereas elevated tri- and disialotransferrin patterns with decreased tetrasialotransferrin species suggest a type II disorder. Although transferrin is the surrogate protein for these analyses, many other transport proteins are also affected. Rare cases of both types I and II have been identified with normal transferrin patterns.

Transferrin IEF should be used freely as an initial diagnostic tool in evaluating patients with dysmorphism, developmental delay and evidence of multisystem involvement. Enzymatic confirmation is available in special centers.

CONGENITAL DISORDERS OF LIPID GLYCOSYLATION

A disorder of ganglioside synthesis, GM₃ synthase deficiency (lactosylceramide alpha-2,3-sialyltransferase deficiency) represents the first defect in lipid glycosylation.[249] Clinical features in the single old order Amish pedigree included early onset of irritability and poor feeding, seizures, profound developmental regression and diffuse brain atrophy. The plasma contained decreased quantities of GM₃ ganglioside and increased lactosylceramide associated with deficient GM₃ synthase activity.

DISORDERS OF NEUROTRANSMITTER METABOLISM

BACKGROUND – METABOLISM AND FUNCTION OF BIOGENIC AMINES

Biogenic amines include the catecholamines (dopamine, epinephrine [adrenaline] and norepinephrine [noradrenaline]) and serotonin, which are derived from hydroxylation of tyrosine and tryptophan by their respective hydroxylases (Figs 26.38 and 26.39).[250,251] Both enzymes

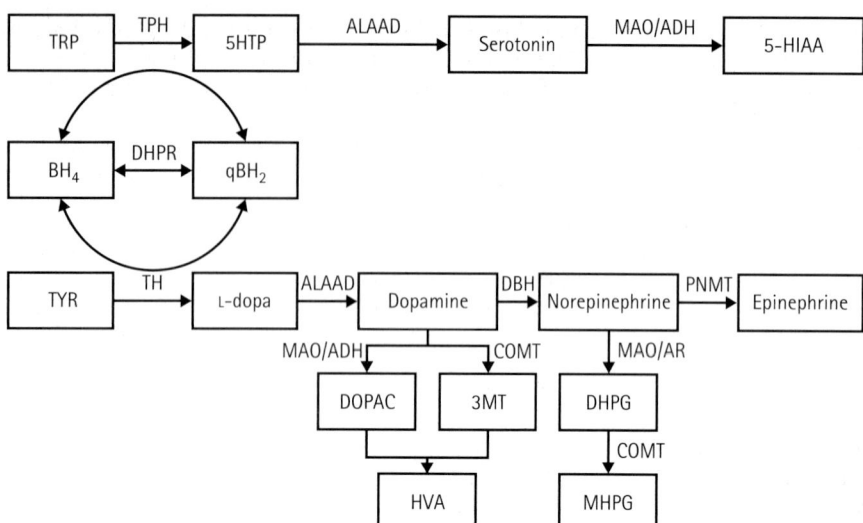

Fig. 26.38 Schematic diagram of catecholamine and serotonin metabolism. Not all steps are shown. TRP, tryptophan; TPH, tryptophan hydroxylase; 5HTP, 5-hydroxytryptophan; ALAAD, aromatic L-amino acid decarboxylase; MAO, monamine oxidase; ADH, aldehyde dehydrogenase; 5-HIAA, 5-hydroxyindoleacetic acid; BH$_4$, tetrahydrobiopterin; qBH$_2$, quinoid dihydrobiopterin; DHPR, dihydropteridine reductase; TYR, tyrosine; TH, tyrosine hydroxylase; L-dopa, L-3,4-dihydroxyphenylalanine; COMT, catechol-O-methyltransferase; DOPAC, dihydroxyphenylacetic acid; 3MT, 3-methoxytyramine; HVA, homovanillic acid; DBH, dopamine beta-hydroxylase; AR, aldehyde reductase; DHPG, dihydroxyphenylglycol; MHPG, 3-methoxy-4-hydroxyphenylglycol; PNMT, phenylethanolamine-N-methyltransferase.

utilize tetrahydrobiopterin (BH$_4$; see p. 1054), a product of guanosine 5 -triphosphate (GTP) metabolism, as a cofactor. The products of the hydroxylation reactions, 3,4-dihydroxy-L-phenylalanine (L-dopa) and 5-hydroxytryptophan, are further metabolized to active neurotransmitters (dopamine and serotonin) via decarboxylation catalyzed by aromatic L-aminoacid decarboxylase (AADC), a pyridoxine-dependent reaction. Dopamine is further metabolized to norepinephrine (noradrenaline) in noradrenergic neurons in a reaction catalyzed by dopamine beta-hydroxylase. Serotonin is converted to melatonin in the pineal gland.

Catechol O-methyltransferase (COMT) and monoamine oxidase (MAO) catalyze the breakdown of dopamine, serotonin and norepinephrine (noradrenaline) to homovanillic acid (HVA), 5-hydroxyindoleacetic acid (5-HIAA) and 3-methoxy-4-hydroxyphenylglycol (MHPG), respectively (Fig. 26.38). The latter are the primary metabolites quantitated in human CSF on the presumption that CSF correctly reflects

brain neurotransmitter metabolism. The biogenic amines control a host of critical processes, including (but not limited to) psychomotor function, memory, appetite, mood, sleep, vascular tone and body temperature.[250-252] Thus, defects in the metabolism of neurotransmitters are expected to have severe, multisystem manifestations.

Recent studies have shown abnormal numbers of 5-hydroxytryptophan neurons and receptors in the brainstems of sudden infant death syndrome (SIDS) victims; the significance is not yet clear.[253]

DEFECTS OF BIOGENIC AMINE SYNTHESIS

Defects of biogenic amine synthesis include deficiencies of tyrosine hydroxylase (TH) and aromatic aminoacid decarboxylase (ALAAD) (Fig. 26.38). Because BH$_4$ is a critical cofactor for tryptophan hydroxylase and TH (as well as phenylalanine hydroxylase, see p. 1054), defects of enzymes in its synthetic pathway can also cause pathologically low levels of biogenic amines (Fig. 26.39). These include guanine triphosphate cyclohydrolase I (GTPCH), 6-pyruvoyl tetrahydrobiopterin synthase (PTPS), sepiapterin reductase (SR), pterin carbinolamine reductase (PCD) and dihydropterin reductase (DHPR). While most of these disorders are also inherited in an autosomal recessive manner, autosomal dominant GTPCH deficiency (also called Segawa disease, dystonia with diurnal fluctuation, or dopa-responsive dystonia) is the most common disorder of biogenic amine metabolism.

Clinical features

Deficiency of *tyrosine hydroxylase* causes impaired synthesis of dopamine, which in turn leads to deficiencies in the other catecholamines. It manifests with parkinsonism, oculogyric crises, ptosis, miosis, postural hypotension, truncal hypotonia and irritability.[254,255] CNS catecholamine levels (dopamine, norepinephrine [noradrenaline] and epinephrine [adrenaline], as well as HVA and MHPG) are decreased, while serotonin metabolism (5-HIAA) remains unaffected. BH$_4$ and neopterin levels are normal, enabling distinction between TH deficiency and the disorders of BH$_4$ synthesis described below.[256]

Deficiency of *aromatic aminoacid decarboxylase* causes symptoms similar to TH deficiency.[257] A neonatal presentation has been reported with early feeding difficulties, hypotonia and autonomic dysfunction.[258] Other clinical features are limb and orofacial dystonia, athetosis and an overall paucity of voluntary movement. Dysautonomic features include diaphoresis, temperature instability, nasal congestion, ptosis, pupillary changes, hypotension and bradyarrhythmias.[259] Dysautonomia related to impaired catecholamine synthesis may underlie paroxysmal events in these patients, including apneic spells and sudden cardiorespiratory arrest.

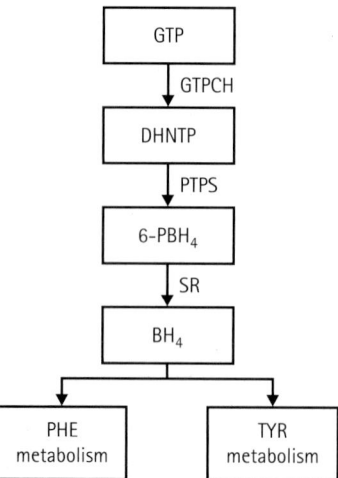

Fig. 26.39 Generation of tetrahydrobiopterin from guanosine triphosphate. Not all steps are shown. GTP, guanosine triphosphate; DHNTP, dihydroneopterin triphosphate; PTPS, 6-pyruvoyltetrahydrobiopterin synthase; 6-PBH$_4$, 6-pyruvoyltetrahydrobiopterin; SR, sepiapterin reductase; PHE, phenylalanine; TYR, tyrosine. Tetrahydrobiopterin serves as bound cofactor in phenylalanine and tyrosine hydroxylase reactions, the first committed steps in the metabolism of both amino acids. Regeneration of tetrahydrobiopterin from quinoid dihydrobiopterin requires the action of pterin-4a-carbinolamine dehydratase (PCD), which is not shown.

Metabolically, ALAAD deficiency results in central and peripheral deficiency of catecholamines, serotonin, HVA, MHPG and 5-HIAA. In addition, the CSF profile shows high L-dopa, 5-OH-tryptophan and 3-OH-methyldopa, OMD (an L-dopa metabolite), and normal pterin levels.[250] Neither TH or ALAAD deficiency demonstrates hyperphenylalaninemia.

Segawa syndrome is due to autosomal dominant guanosine triphosphate cyclohydrolase deficiency (GTPCH). It presents with dystonia and parkinsonism, with resting tremor, spasticity, postural instability and oculogyric crises with normal cognition. There tends to be a diurnal fluctuation of symptoms, with worsening in the evenings and improvement following sleep.[250] Both the dystonia and tremor may have a prominent postural component. Isolated toe gait, female predominance and presentation with only prominent postural tremor in adulthood have all been described.[260] Adults have a striking incidence of major depression and obsessive-compulsive disorder, as well as sleep disorders including insomnia, excessive daytime somnolence and frequent parasomnias characterized as nightmares.[261] Thus, an expanded phenotype with psychopathology appears to be present in this disorder.

The defects in BH$_4$ metabolism are important since they are detectable by newborn screening, can cause the 'malignant PKU' syndrome and are treated differently from PKU (see p. 1054). They include autosomal recessive synthetic steps of *GTPCH, 6-pyruvoyltetrahydropterin synthase (PTPS)*, and *sepiapterin reductase (SR)* and the recycling enzyme *dihydropteridine reductase (DHPR)*. Untreated, they all present with progressive psychomotor retardation, dystonia, seizures, choreoathetosis, temperature instability, hypersalivation, microcephaly and irritability. Patients with SR deficiency also manifest dystonic posturing with diurnal variation, oculogyric crises, tremor, hypersomnolence, oculomotor apraxia and weakness.[250,262]

An early defect in this pathway, pterin-4a-carbinolamine dehydratase, may not manifest significant clinical abnormalities, other than transient alterations in tone.

DEFECTS OF MONOAMINE DEGRADATION
Clinical features
Orthostatic hypotension is the hallmark of *dopamine beta-hydroxylase (DBH) deficiency*, which results in decreased norepinephrine (noradrenaline) production from dopamine.[263] The disease has generally been diagnosed in adults, with retrospective case histories suggesting a neonatal period associated with ptosis, hypothermia, hypoglycemia and hypotension.[250] A normal variant of undetectable DBH levels associated with normal norepinephrine and epinephrine (adrenaline) concentrations has been identified in 4% of the population.[264]

Catabolism of serotonin and catecholamines requires the actions of *monoamine oxidase A or B (MAO-A and MAO-B)*.[265] A point mutation in the MAO-A gene on the X chromosome has been associated with borderline mental deficits and aggressive behavior.[250] Conversely, several males with X chromosome deletions, including the MAO-A and MAO-B genes, manifested severe retardation, while males with an unusual deletion involving a portion of the MAO-B gene (but with an intact MAO-A gene) had normal mental capacity. To date, no specific isolated abnormality of the MAO-B gene has been reported.

Diagnosis
In general, CSF is required for measurement of biogenic amines and metabolites but is available in only a few specialty laboratories. Collection of CSF requires special considerations, including a rostro-caudal gradient of metabolite levels, and oxidation of BH$_4$ and neurotransmitter metabolites that occurs without immediate freezing or via contamination with blood.[266] Thus, a specific protocol with orderly collection of predefined volumes and rapid handling on dry ice is essential so that the values can be compared to reference ranges established with the same collection criteria.

TH deficiency results in low levels of catecholamines and related metabolites; ALAAD deficiency results in similar decreases accompanied by low CSF serotonin concentrations. Neurotransmitter precursors (5-hydroxytryptophan, levodopa and OMD) also accumulate in ALAAD deficiency. Urine organic acid testing may show elevation of vanillactic acid, representing a potential clue during metabolic screening.[267]

The disorders PTPS, DHPR, PCD and recessive GTPCH deficiencies are usually detected by newborn screening since BH$_4$ is required for phenylalanine hydroxylase activity. Blood phenylalanine levels are normal in autosomal dominant GTPCH deficiency (Segawa disease) and SR deficiency, as well as TH and ALAAD deficiencies. Further evaluation for these disorders requires accurate quantification of CSF pterins, HVA and 5-HIAA. In many cases, loading with phenylalanine and tetrahydrobiopterin followed by measurement of phenylalanine and tyrosine can provide important diagnostic information (see also p. 1054).[250,268] Prenatal diagnosis of TH deficiency by mutation analysis has been reported.[257]

Measurement of urinary biopterin further helps to distinguish these disorders, with decreased biopterin in PTPS deficiency and elevated in DHPR deficiency (versus normal in PKU); it is mandatory in any infant detected by newborn screening to have an elevated phenylalanine.

In DBH deficiency, CSF shows low levels of MHPG with accumulation of HVA, while patients with MAO-A deficiency manifest increased biogenic amine and O-methylated metabolites. The most sensitive index of MAO-A activity is MHPG, the major norepinephrine (noradrenaline) metabolite.[269]

Treatment
Treatment for the monoamine synthesis disorders and MAO/COMT include substitution with neurotransmitter precursors (dopa, 5-HTP) and BH$_4$. Autosomal recessively inherited GTPCH-1 deficiency and PTPS deficiency should be treated with BH$_4$. Dietary phenylalanine restriction is beneficial in DHPR and PCD deficiencies, but may also require tyrosine supplementation.[270,271] Folinic acid supplementation in DHPR deficiency restores methyltetrahydrofolate and prevents progressive calcification of the basal ganglia and subcortical white matter.[250,269] Dietary supplementation of long chain polyunsaturated fatty acids may have therapeutic relevance in those disorders with hyperphenylalaninemia.[272] Patients with BH$_4$ synthesis disorders may deteriorate if given folate antagonists such as methotrexate, which interfere with a salvage pathway through which BH$_2$ is converted into BH$_4$ via dihydrofolate reductase. Use of dihydroxyphenylserine (which may be decarboxylated to norepinephrine [noradrenaline]) is aimed at correction of norepinephrine (noradrenaline) deficiency in DBH deficiency.[250]

Patients with Segawa disease and SR, ALAAD and TH deficiency all show improvement often with L-dopa combined with carbidopa; the latter is a peripheral dopa-decarboxylase inhibitor.[269,273] A diagnostic trial of L-dopa for dystonia can be clinically helpful and, if positive, should be followed by more definitive testing.[274]

Segawa disease is the most amenable to treatment.[258,275] It should be initiated with levodopa 1 mg/kg/d, with gradual titration usually to 4–5 mg/kg/d based on efficacy or adverse effects.[274] Some authorities recommend up to 20 mg/kg/d, but this is isolated L-dopa without carbidopa.[260] The diagnoses should be considered in atypical presentations, such as spastic diplegia, asymmetric limb dystonia or even writer's cramp. The genetic penetrance is incomplete and phenotypic variation can be highly variable even within the same family.[276] Contraindications to L-dopa therapy include psychosis, narrow-angle glaucoma and melanoma.[275] L-Dopa should be used with caution in hypotension and asthma, and with antihypertensive agents. Reduced benefit may occur if combined with dopamine receptor blockers, e.g. neuroleptics. Adverse effects are frequent and dyskinesias are reported in 20% of patients with Segawa disease, although they respond to reduction in dose.[277] Trihexyphenidyl may also be tried. Tetrahydrobiopterin may be helpful but is rarely used. The dopamine synthesis line appears far more involved than the serotoninergic line; hence, serotonin reuptake inhibitors are not standard therapy.

Results of treatment of ALAAD deficiency are variable. Several agents have been tried in a small number of patients. As described above, standard initial treatment is L-dopa 1 mg/kg/d with doses tailored to results.[269] TH deficiency is a progressive and often lethal disorder, which can be improved by L-dopa. A combination of low-dose L-dopa (3 mg/kg/d divided in six doses) with selegiline (5 mg/d in a single dose) has been reported as beneficial; hypersensitivity to L-dopa has been described.[273,278] As with all cases of parkinsonism and basal ganglion dysfunction, treatment must be individually tailored, making use of emerging medications and adapting to changing presentations.

Succinic semialdehyde dehydrogenase deficiency

Succinic semialdehyde dehydrogenase (SSADH) deficiency is a disorder in the catabolism of the neurotransmitter GABA. GABA is transaminated to form succinic semialdehyde, which is then reduced by SSADH to succinate. In the presence of a block at this step, succinic semialdehyde is reduced to gamma-hydroxybutyric acid that accumulates in the urine, serum and CSF.

Patients with this disease have variable degrees of ataxia and hypotonia, convulsions and mild psychomotor retardation. Gamma-hydroxybutyric aciduria is an interesting model disorder of metabolism because the basic defect leads to the accumulation of a compound of known neuropharmacological activity. Gamma-hydroxybutyric acid was originally developed as an analogue of GABA that could readily cross the blood–brain barrier and be used as an intravenous anesthetic. It is currently employed for treatment of cataplexy associated with narcolepsy.

The gene is known and many mutations have been found. Prenatal diagnosis is available. Treatment is supportive and employs standard anticonvulsant drugs. Recent work with a murine model of SSADH deficiency suggests that treatment with taurine and/or antagonists of the GABA-B receptor may be of benefit.[279]

GABA-transaminase deficiency

Deficiency of GABA transaminase has been reported associated with progressive neurological deterioration, leukodystrophy and hypotonia resulting in eventual death. CSF levels of GABA and homocarnosine were highly elevated.

Riley–Day syndrome, familial dysautonomia

This disease, long thought to be due to a defect of neurotransmitter metabolism, is actually one of the hereditary sensory and autonomic neuropathies (type 3 HSAN3). It occurs mostly in Ashkenazim and is associated with varying signs of autonomic dysfunction, alacrima, vasomotor instability, cardiac dysfunction and variable peripheral neuropathy; abnormal tongue papillae were once thought to be pathognomonic.

DISORDERS OF PURINE METABOLISM

For clinicians, the best known purine is uric acid which, however, is only the end product of a complex synthetic and catabolic pathway in which at least 14 metabolic disorders are known (Fig. 26.40). In these disorders, the most common symptoms are those of gout or nephrolithiasis; however, since purines are bases for DNA and RNA synthesis and other compounds, some disorders present with hematologial, neurological, musculoskeletal or immunological problems.[280]

HYPERURICEMIA

Hypoxanthine-guanine phosphoribosyl transferase deficiency

This enzyme is coded on the X chromosome. Mild deficiency is extremely common and results in hyperuricemia that frequently leads to gout. Gout is caused by precipitation of uric acid in and around joints, very often the big toe, which leads to extremely painful arthritis (podagra). Renal involvement can lead to uric acid nephrolithiasis and progressive renal damage. Hyperuricemia can be asymptomatic for many years.

Hyperuricemia can be caused by several mechanisms including dehydration, a high meat diet, increased absorption and reduced renal excretion. In the kidney, uric acid is filtered and then reabsorbed in the proximal tubules before being re-excreted. Re-excretion occurs in a system that also transports other organic acids; thus, in ketoacidosis, hyperuricemia is frequent as a result of competitive inhibition at that site. Increased production, due to faulty feedback inhibition, occurs in several of the inherited disorders discussed in this section and also in glycogen storage disease type I (see p. 1077). It is also commonly seen during the early stages of chemotherapy for malignancy.

Lesch–Nyhan syndrome
Clinical features

This condition is caused by severe deficiency of hypoxanthine-guanine phosphoribosyl transferase (HGPRT).[281,282] The first sign may be a pink discoloration of the diapers (nappies) due to large amounts of urate crystals that presage nephrolithiasis. The condition is characterized by severe choreoathetosis that emerges in the first months of life; it is so severe that most patients never walk. Dysarthria is extreme and this, together with the neurological picture, leads many to believe that these patients are mentally retarded which is not necessarily the case. The most distressing aspect is an extraordinary degree of self-mutila-

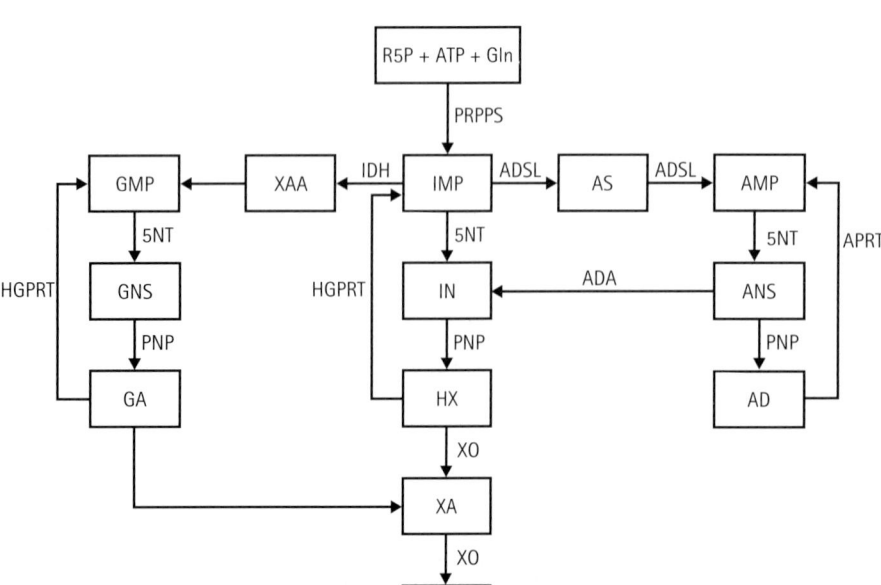

Fig. 26.40 Schematic overview of purine metabolism (not all steps are shown). R5P, ribose-5-phosphate; Gln, glutamine; PRPPS, phosphoribosylpyrophosphate synthetase; IMP, inosine monophosphate; 5NT, 5 -nucleotidase; IN, inosine; HX, hypoxanthine; XO, xanthine oxidase; XA, xanthine; UA, uric acid; ADSL, adenylosuccinate lyase; AS, adenylosuccinate; AMP, adenosine monophosphate; ANS, adenosine; PNP, purine nucleoside phosphorylase; AD, adenine; APRT, adenine phosphoribosyl transferase; ADA, adenosine deaminase; IDH, IMP dehydrogenase; XAA, xanthylic acid; GMP, guanosine monophosphate; GNS, guanosine; GA, guanine; HGPRT, hypoxanthine guanine phosphoribosyl transferase.

tion that manifests with biting, hitting, kicking or head banging that the patients are unable to control. It is so bad that most patients beg to be restrained in their wheelchairs or beds. Dental prostheses or even total edentulation may be required to prevent damage of oral tissues and other sites. The basis of the neurological damage is not known.

Diagnosis

The clinical diagnosis is often delayed but is based upon the classical presentation associated with hyperuricemia that, however, may only be marginally abnormal. DNA diagnosis is possible but most families exhibit private mutations of the gene.[283-287]

Treatment

Allopurinol must be used to control the uric acid levels but results in accumulation of xanthine that is also lithogenic so metabolite levels should be monitored. It does nothing for the neurological problems that can only be marginally helped by the standard drugs used for movement disorders. Education is very challenging but often rewarding. It is important to recognize the emotional state of the patients (and their families), especially during adolescence. Antidepressants, anxiolytics and extensive counseling are required for this condition.

OTHER DISORDERS OF PURINES

For the remaining disorders of purine metabolism, the phenotype is predominantly neurological with renal abnormalities, but may also involve the musculoskeletal system.

Adenine phosphoribosyl transferase (APRT) deficiency causes marked urolithiasis with all of its complications due to the insolubility of 2,8-dihydroxyadenine.[288,289] In *phosphoribosyl pyrophosphate (PRPP) synthetase superactivity*, hearing loss, developmental delay, ataxia, dysmorphism, gout and uric acid lithiasis are variable.[289] *Adenylosuccinate lyase (ADSL)* deficiency presents with psychomotor retardation, hypotonia, epilepsy, autism and occasionally cerebellar hypoplasia.[290-293] ADSL-deficient patients accumulate succinylaminoimidazole carboxamide riboside (SAICAR) which may be identified colorimetrically using a spot test of urine.[293]

Xanthine oxidase/dehydrogenase, combined xanthine oxidase/sulfite oxidase, xanthine dehydrogenase/aldehyde oxidase and *molybdenum cofactor deficiencies* (see pp. 1056 and 1126) variably manifest psychomotor retardation, intractable seizures, features of hypoxic ischemic encephalopathy, lens dissociation and xanthine lithiasis, often leading to renal failure.[294-299] Hypouricaemia is characteristic of all these conditions. Increased hypoxanthine may serve as a benzodiazepine agonist at the $GABA_A$ receptor complex, perhaps contributing to neurological sequelae.[300] Hypouricaemia is also seen in starvation and from renal loss in the renal Fanconi syndrome, such as cystinosis.

Adenosine deaminase (ADA) deficiency presents with severe combined immunodeficiency (see Ch. 27, p. 1150) and lymphopenia,[301-304] potentially related to lymphocyte toxicity induced by accumulated ADA substrates, adenosine and 2'-deoxyadenosine.[305] Recent studies have revealed that the ADA gene is responsive to tumor suppressor elements linked to the p53 family.[306] *Purine nucleoside phosphorylase (PNP)* deficiency manifests isolated T-cell deficiency, developmental delays, lymphopenia and dysplastic marrow morphology.[307-309] Patients with both disorders are subject to unrelenting infection.

The remaining defects of purine metabolism are heterogeneous. *Myoadenylate deaminase deficiency (MDA)* is discussed on p. 1072.[310-312] Deficiency of *thiopurine methyltransferase (TPMT)*, which converts thioinosine monophosphate (IMP) to methylthio-IMP, does not manifest as 'disease' until intervention with thiopurine which may be used in chemotherapy, thus making TPMT deficiency a 'pharmacogenetic' disorder.[313-315]

Diagnosis and treatment

For most of these disorders, the initial suspicion comes from the clinical presentation backed up by plasma uric acid levels. Measurement

of uric acid:creatinine ratio in urine may be helpful, but is very variable. Adequate, age related control ranges for uric acid are needed, and dietary intake of purines varies considerably between populations; purine analogues are found in many foods including all flesh, chocolate and caffeine. Disorders featuring accumulation of insoluble purine bases (e.g. xanthine, 2,8-dihydroxyadenine) should be included in the differential of urolithiasis.

In all forms of hyperuricemia, treatment with allopurinol controls the blood levels but does not address the underlying causes. Colchicine, or rarely aspirin, is also used during acute podagra crises.[280]

Severe combined immune deficiency in ADA deficiency makes it one of the prototypic disorders amenable to bone marrow transplantation, enzyme replacement therapy employing polyethylene glycol (PEG)-associated ADA or erythrocyte-encapsulated ADA, in addition to gene therapy.[302,316] Limited reports have suggested clinical efficacy of ribose intervention for ADSL deficiency.

DISORDERS OF PYRIMIDINE METABOLISM

Clinical features

Pyrimidines, like purines, are essential for DNA and RNA synthesis. Disorders of pyrimidine metabolism (Fig. 26.41) manifest significant

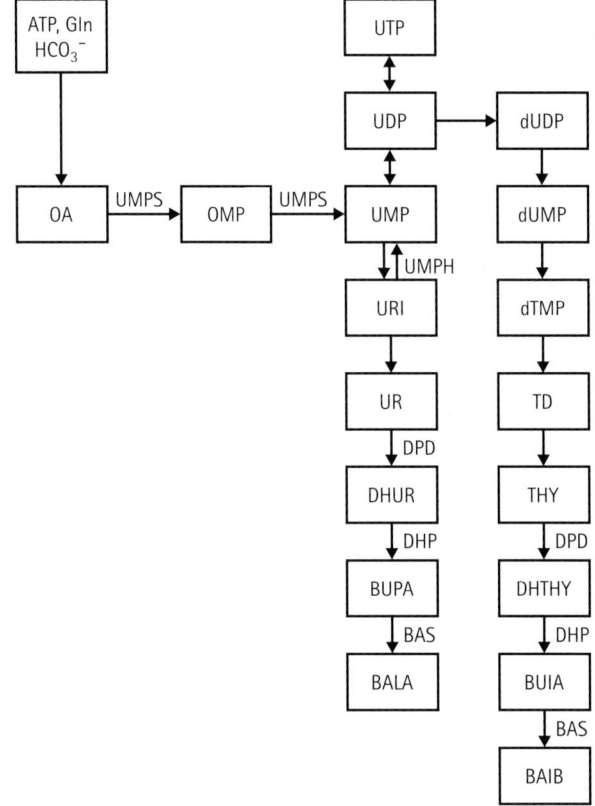

Fig. 26.41 Schematic diagram of pyrimidine catabolism (not all steps are shown). Gln, glutamine; OA, orotic acid; UMPS, uridine monophosphate synthetase; OMP, orotidine monophosphate; UMP, uridine monophosphate; UDP, uridine diphosphate; UTP, uridine triphosphate; dUDP, deoxyuridine diphosphate; dUMP, deoxyuridine monophosphate; UMPH, uridine monophosphate hydrolase; URI, uridine; dTMP, deoxythymidine monophosphate; UR, uracil; TD, thymidine; DPD, dihydropyrimidine dehydrogenase; THY, thymine; DHUR, dihydrouracil; DHP, dihydropyrimidinase (dihydropyrimidine amidohydrolase); DHTHY, dihydrothymine; BUPA, beta-ureidopropionic acid; BUIA, beta-ureidoisobutyric acid; BAS, beta-alanine synthase; BALA, beta-alanine; BAIB, beta-aminoisobutyric acid.

phenotypic/genotypic heterogeneity. Three disorders affect metabolism of uridine monophosphate (UMP), including *UMP synthetase (UMPS) deficiency*, *UMP hydrolase 1 (UMPH 1) deficiency* and *UMP hydrolase (UMPH) superactivity*.[280,289,301]

UMPS deficiency, sometimes known as hereditary *orotic aciduria*, causes megaloblastic anemia and T-cell immunodeficiency, failure to thrive, orotic acid crystalluria associated with renal orotic acid accumulation and intractable diarrhea. UMPH 1-deficient patients display a characteristic nonspherocytic hemolytic anemia with basophilic stippling, while those with UMPH superactivity manifest developmental delays, seizures, hyperactivity and recurrent infection.

In *dihydropyrimidine dehydrogenase (DPD)* deficiency[317] there is a variable phenotype including psychomotor retardation, seizures, microcephaly, feeding difficulties, autistic features and hypertonia.[318,319] DPD deficiency is a 'pharmacogenetic' disease, since treatment with 5-fluorouracil (5-FU) in patients with DPD deficiency can lead to severe 5-FU toxicity.[320,321] Neurological dysfunction in *dihydropyrimidine amidohydrolase (DHP)* deficiency includes microcephaly, psychomotor retardation, spastic quadriplegia and seizures. Both DPD and DHP deficiencies have 'thymine/uraciluria', with accumulation of dihydrothymine and dihydrouracil in DHP deficiency.[317,320]

Beta-ureidopropionase (beta-alanine synthase; BAS) deficiency is a rare neurological disorder, manifesting optic atrophy, dystonia, convulsions and severe mental retardation associated with excretion of beta-ureidopropionate and beta-ureidoisobutyrate.[322-325] The latter may be detected by NMR analysis.

Thymidine phosphorylase (TP) deficiency is an autosomal recessive disorder that causes a mitochondrial syndrome known as MNGIE (mitochondrial neuropathy, gastrointestinal encephalomyopathy; see p. 1085), in which gastrointestinal symptoms are found along with demyelinating polyneuropathy and leukoencephalopthy.[326-330]

Diagnosis and treatment

Several specialist laboratories now offer extended screening for purine and pyrimidine disorders employing HPLC, capillary electrophoretic and/or tandem mass spectrometric screening protocols.[331-334] For the disorders described above, DPD deficiency is detectable by employing a recently devised [2-^{13}C] uracil breath test.[335,336]

Few of the above disorders are treatable beyond palliative measures. However, uridine treatment of UMPS deficiency reverses the biochemical and clinical abnormalities.

DISORDERS OF METAL METABOLISM

(Calcium and magnesium metabolism and the nutritional aspects of trace metals are discussed in Chapter 16.)

Metals function via association with proteins in a way similar to vitamins. They are required for a variety of functions, including electron transfer, oxygen binding and structural support. Inherited disorders that result in either deficiency or overload can have severe consequences.

COPPER

An adult body contains approximately 100 mg of copper. Copper is capable of functioning in electron transfer reactions (a so called redox active metal) and is required for the activity of many critical enzymes in a wide variety of metabolic pathways (Table 26.30). Consequently, copper deficiency has numerous effects on metabolism. Copper excess also has significant clinical consequences, which result from the ability of copper to transfer electrons to oxygen and generate toxic oxygen free radicals.

In serum, over 90% of copper is bound to ceruloplasmin (see below). The circulating pool of available copper is believed to be bound to histidine and other amino acids. Copper homeostasis is maintained via a balance between copper absorption from the gut and loss via biliary excretion. The two most common inherited disorders of copper

Table 26.30 Copper-dependent enzymes and their function

Enzyme	Function
Cytochrome c oxidase	Electron transport
Tyrosinase	Melanin biosynthesis
Peptidylglycine α-amidating Monooxygenase	Activation of neuropeptides (gastrin, vasoactive intestinal peptide, melanocyte stimulating hormone, thyrotrophin releasing hormone, cholecystokinin, vasopressin, corticotrophin releasing hormone and calcitonin)
Dopamine β-hydroxylase	Catecholamine biosynthesis
Lysyl oxidase	Collagen cross-linking
Cu-Zn superoxide dismutase	Protection from oxidative stress
Ceruloplasmin	Iron metabolism

metabolism affect either the absorptive (Menkes disease) or excretory (Wilson disease) phases of copper homeostasis.[337]

Menkes disease

Menkes disease (~1 in 250 000) is an X-linked disorder resulting from mutations in a gene (ATP7A) that encodes an ATP-dependent copper transporter that is expressed in nearly all tissues except the liver. The Menkes protein is required for the absorption of copper from the gut and the placenta. Lack of this protein results in accumulation of high levels of copper in enterocytes and the placenta due to an inability to release copper absorbed from the gut or maternal blood, respectively, resulting in profound systemic copper deficiency. ATP7A also functions in the transport of copper across the blood–brain barrier.

Clinical features

Menkes disease results in severe developmental delay and failure to thrive. Drowsiness, lethargy, hypotonia, hypothermia and feeding difficulties are often evident within a few days of birth, and low birth weight is common.[338] The skin is pale, soft and doughy. The most characteristic feature is the hair, which is sparse and depigmented, with a corkscrew-like microscopic appearance (pili torti) and a texture reminiscent of steel wool, leading to the term 'Menkes kinky hair syndrome' (Fig. 26.42). Seizures are common. Death occurs commonly in the first decade.

The clinical features are caused by the loss of function of copper-dependent enzymes (Table 26.30). Tyrosinase deficiency results in hypopigmentation of the skin and hair. Peptidylglycine alpha-amidating monooxygenase (PAM) deficiency leads to a broad spectrum of neuroendocrine derangements. Abnormalities of collagen cross-linking due to lysyl oxidase deficiency cause osteoporosis, flared metaphyses and fractures, which may suggest battering; Wormian bones are also common. Arteries are often tortuous and may rupture, which can lead to subdural hematomas. The ureters and the bladder wall are weakened and dilated. Deficiency of cytochrome oxidase and dopamine beta-hydroxylase results in CNS degeneration, characterized by abnormalities of myelin, and cerebral and cerebellar atrophy.

Heterozygous females have normal levels of copper, ceruloplasmin and catecholamines. Patches of pili torti are present in approximately 50% of obligate carriers; their absence does not exclude carrier status.

A well characterized variant of Menkes disease, associated with milder mutations in the ATP7A gene, is the *occipital horn syndrome*, also known as X-linked cutis laxa (see Ch. 29, p. 1397). This is a disorder of connective tissues characterized by lax skin and joints, bladder diverticula, inguinal hernias and arterial tortuosity. Ossification within the tendons that attach the trapezius and sternocleidomastoid muscles to the skull give rise to the pathognomonic occipital horns, which can be felt by palpation and demonstrated radiographically. As in Menkes, these abnormalities are caused by deficient activity of lysyl oxidase. Dopamine beta-hydroxylase activity is also sometimes affected, leading to symptoms of autonomic dysfunction, such as orthostatic hypotension.

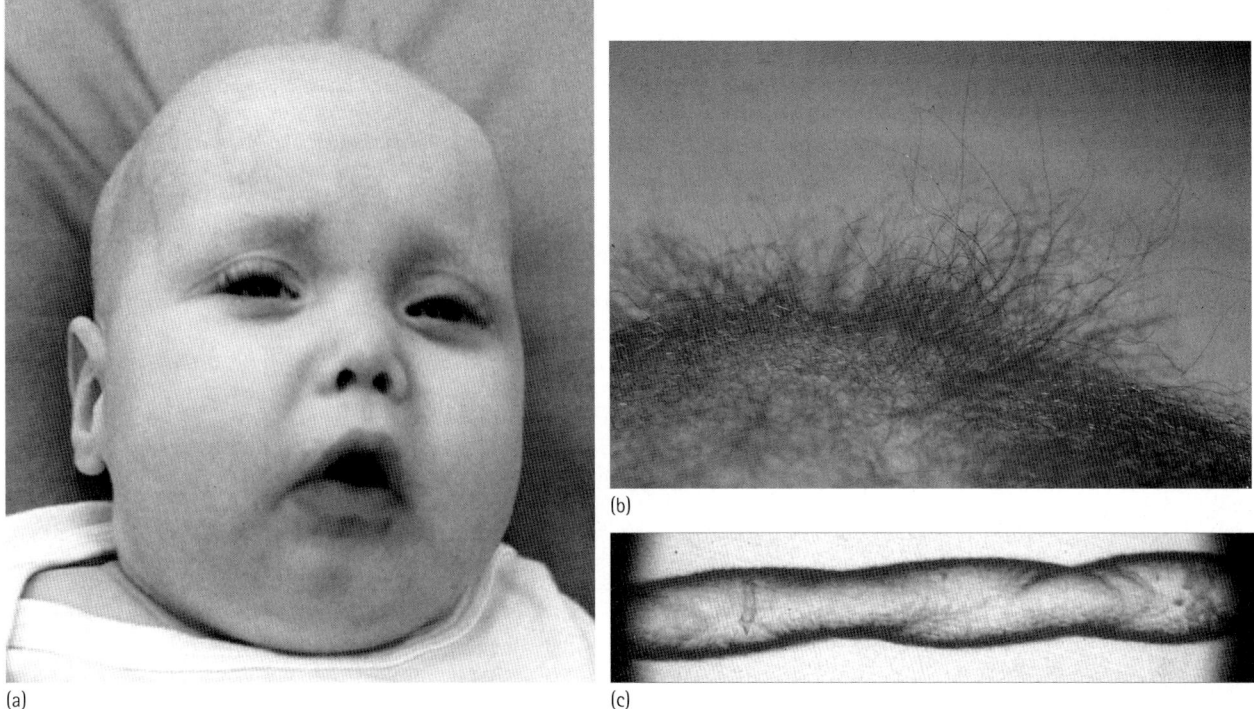

Fig. 26.42   (a) Features and (b,c) typical hair of Menkes syndrome.

Diagnosis

The clinical picture is so striking that a presumptive diagnosis should be easy. Usually, the serum copper and ceruloplasmin are low, but these can be low even in healthy infants. Abnormalities of catecholamine levels in serum, CSF and urine, secondary to dopamine beta-hydroxylase deficiency, are more consistent; in neonates, plasma levels of these neurotransmitters are the preferred diagnostic tool.[339] Radioactive copper uptake by cultured fibroblasts is increased and can also be used for diagnosis. Because of the large number of mutations that have been identified in the gene, molecular diagnosis is not readily available.

Treatment

Since copper absorption from the gut is defective, oral copper supplementation is ineffective. In contrast, parenteral administration of copper–histidine can rapidly normalize serum levels of copper and ceruloplasmin. However, most of the enzymes that require copper are intracellular, and it is difficult to evaluate the adequacy of treatment effectively, particularly in the brain. When begun prior to the onset of severe neurological symptoms, copper–histidine may improve neurological outcome and decrease seizure activity, but since significant connective tissue problems persist, this therapy should be considered experimental.[340] A single unsuccessful attempt at in utero copper treatment has also been reported.[341]

Wilson disease

Wilson disease is an autosomal recessive disorder caused by mutations in the ATP7B gene, which codes for a different copper transporting ATPase that is homologous to ATP7A. Lack of either results in a defect of intracellular copper transport. The differences between Menkes and Wilson diseases are a result of the different tissue distributions of the two proteins; Wilson primarily affecting the liver, whereas the Menkes gene is expressed in nonhepatic tissues. The Wilson protein is required for the export of copper from hepatocytes into the bile and also for transport of copper into the Golgi apparatus for ceruloplasmin synthesis.

Clinical features

Wilson disease, also known as hepatolenticular degeneration, primarily affects the liver and the nervous system, particularly the basal ganglia. Patients may present at any time from early childhood to the fifth decade. Children most commonly present with liver disease, which usually becomes evident in the first or second decade. Hepatosplenomegaly, jaundice and symptoms of hepatitis are the most common findings; acute hepatic failure can occur. Hemolytic anemia is not uncommon.

After adolescence, the disease more commonly presents with neurological symptoms. The first signs of CNS involvement, which can occur even in the absence of hepatic damage, include deterioration of school performance and changes in mood and behavior. Concomitantly or subsequently, findings of basal ganglia damage develop. Progressive extrapyramidal signs, including rigidity, dysarthria, dysphagia, drooling and intellectual deterioration may mimic Parkinson disease. Psychiatric symptoms ranging from mania to depression, paranoia or anxiety can also be encountered. Occasionally, flapping tremor, schizophrenic behavior or the renal Fanconi syndrome may be the presenting feature. A brown or green ring around the corneal limbus in the eye – the Kayser–Fleischer ring – is caused by copper deposited in Descemet's membrane but may not be present in the first decade.

Diagnosis

Wilson disease should be considered in any child with unexplained liver disease, neurological dysfunction or hemolytic anemia. Plasma copper and ceruloplasmin are usually, but not invariably, low, but this is not specific for Wilson disease, being seen in other liver diseases. The best diagnostic test is determination of 24 h urine copper excretion, which is elevated (>100 mcg/24 h; normal = 20–50 mcg/24 h) in nearly all symptomatic patients. Presymptomatic patients and carriers can have intermediate levels of copper excretion (50–100 mcg/24 h), and may require a liver biopsy and direct measurement of copper content for definitive diagnosis. A Kayser–Fleischer ring is best identified by slit lamp examination and is nearly always present in patients with neurological and psychiatric symptoms. It is rarely present in children, particularly in the absence of neurological symptoms. Though singly not 100%

effective for diagnosis, the combination of 24 h urine copper excretion, ceruloplasmin level and a slit lamp examination is unlikely to miss a real case.[342] The large number of disease-causing mutations makes DNA diagnosis impractical at present.

Treatment

D-Penicillamine was the drug of choice for many years; it is now superseded. In children with minimal liver dysfunction, zinc acetate, combined with a diet limited in high copper containing foods (shellfish, chocolate) is highly effective. Oral zinc induces metallothionein expression in enterocytes, which binds to copper and blocks its absorption. This affects the absorption of both dietary copper and that secreted into the gastrointestinal tract. Overtreatment can cause copper deficiency, which manifests with hypochromic, microcytic anemia. Significant liver disease should be treated with trientine (Syprine), a copper chelator, in addition to zinc.[343] For patients with neurological or psychiatric symptoms, a recently developed chelator, tetrathiomolybdate, is effective in halting and in many cases reversing symptoms.[344] Currently, this agent is available as an investigational new drug. Patients with significant liver and/or neurological disease should be referred to a center with extensive experience in the treatment of Wilson disease. Liver transplantation is indicated for progressive hepatic insufficiency and in fulminant hepatic failure. Liver transplant results in complete correction of copper homeostasis and reversal of most neurological dysfunction.

Aceruloplasminemia

Aceruloplasminemia is a rare autosomal recessive disorder affecting the ceruloplasmin gene.[345] Ceruloplasmin is a copper-containing ferroxidase that is required for the mobilization of iron from reticuloendothelial cells. It is also expressed in astrocytes, where it functions in iron metabolism. Accumulation of iron in the pancreas, basal ganglia and retina are responsible for the primary symptoms, which usually develop in the fourth decade of life. Clinical features include an extrapyramidal movement disorder, diabetes mellitus and retinal degeneration. Excess iron is also seen in the liver. Plasma copper is low secondary to the ceruloplasmin deficiency. The abnormalities of iron metabolism result in a mild anemia and decreased serum iron level. No specific treatment is known.

IRON

The nutritional aspects of iron metabolism are discussed in Chapter 16.

Maintenance of normal iron homeostasis depends of the ability to regulate the rate of iron absorption from the gut in response to total body iron stores. The major iron transport protein of the plasma is transferrin. After birth, transferrin is about 65% saturated with iron, this value falling to a norm of 20–30% as iron stores are used. Transferrin saturation decreases in iron deficiency, and increases in the presence of iron overload. Adult total body iron content is about 3–4 g, of which 40–60% is in hemoglobin, 10–20% is in myoglobin and tissue enzymes, and 10–40% is stored as ferritin. Newborn infants have total body iron levels of about 250–400 mg.

Hereditary hemochromatosis

Hemochromatosis results when too much dietary iron is absorbed. It can be acquired, but hereditary hemochromatosis is one of the most common genetic disorders of Caucasians, with an incidence of 3–5 in 1000. However, the penetrance of clinical symptoms is low, with estimates ranging from 1% to 50%.[346,347] The most common form results from mutations in the HFE gene and it is inherited as an autosomal recessive condition. The total body iron levels are 5–10 times normal (15–40 g). Only a few milligrams of excess iron are absorbed each day, usually resulting in a delay of symptoms until adulthood. Rare forms can present during the second or third decade, and it may be identified in children serendipitously during routine lab testing of iron status. Clinical onset is delayed in females as a result of menstrual blood loss.

Clinical features

The most common symptoms in adults are fatigue, arthralgia, loss of libido and impotency. Associated findings include hepatomegaly leading to cirrhosis and sometimes hepatocellular carcinoma, increased skin pigmentation, diabetes mellitus (an old name for this condition was 'bronzed diabetes'), abdominal pain and cardiomyopathy. The first symptoms in juvenile-onset forms are commonly hypogonadotrophic hypogonadism and heart failure. All of the tissue damage is from excess accumulation of iron, which is believed to be due to iron-catalyzed generation of toxic oxygen radicals.

Diagnosis

Biochemical measures of iron status must be used for diagnosis. A persistent elevation of the fasting transferrin saturation (>45% for one year) identifies 98% of affected patients.[348] The transferrin saturation is elevated even when the level of ferritin and total body iron stores are normal, allowing for diagnosis prior to the onset of symptoms.

Treatment

Decisions regarding initiation of treatment should be based upon measures of total body iron load and symptoms. Most patients with an elevated transferrin saturation and normal ferritin do not require therapy, but should be re-evaluated yearly. When the ferritin is elevated (≥200 mcg/L in pre-menopausal women, ≥300 mcg/L in men and post-menopausal women), or in the presence of liver disease, therapy should be started.

The iron can be readily mobilized, allowing for treatment via repeated phlebotomy (500 ml of blood contains 200–250 mg of iron). Therapy is monitored by monitoring the serum ferritin, which should be maintained in the low normal range. When treatment is begun before significant tissue damage occurs (cirrhosis, diabetes mellitus), the prognosis is excellent. However, much of the damage that occurs in hemochromatosis is irreversible, emphasizing the need for early diagnosis and treatment. Because of the high incidence and excellent response to early therapy, population screening for hereditary hemochromatosis has been considered.

Neonatal hemochromatosis

Neonatal hemochromatosis is a rare cause of neonatal liver failure that results from the accumulation of excess iron in utero. The liver demonstrates cirrhosis, fatty infiltration and bile duct proliferation with hemosiderin deposits. The pancreas, adrenals, thyroid and myocardium may also be affected. The cause is uncertain, but maternal immunization against a fetal antigen has been proposed,[349,350] and is leading to attempts at immunotherapy. Elevated iron has also been seen in the liver of neonates with viral infections (cytomegalovirus, echovirus), neonatal lupus and inherited disorders of bile acid synthesis. There is no specific therapy, though liver transplant has been successfully employed.

ZINC

Zinc is an essential element that plays both catalytic and structural roles in many proteins. Zinc deficiency is rare in the absence of generalized malnutrition (see Ch. 16), or malabsorption. Acrodermatitis enteropathica (see also Ch. 30, p. 1458)) is an inherited disorder associated with severe zinc deficiency due to mutations of the SLC39A4 gene, which encodes an intestinal zinc transporter.[351] Typical symptoms include diarrhea, acrodermatitis, alopecia and failure to thrive. Infants present shortly after weaning from breast milk or in the first weeks of life in formula fed infants. The symptoms respond rapidly to oral zinc sulfate supplementation. Hereditary hyperzincemia is benign.

MOLYBDENUM (see also p. 1057 and p. 1123)

Molybdenum is required for the function of three oxidases, xanthine, sulfite and aldehyde oxidase. The functional complex of molybdenum is called the *molybdenum cofactor*, and consists of a single metal atom in complex with a pterin. Mutations in three genes (MOCS1 and 2, and GPHN) can cause molybdenum cofactor deficiency; all result in severe progressive neurological deterioration, seizures, dislocated lenses and early death. Serum uric acid is very low and the urine contains xanthine, hypoxanthine, sulfite and thiosulfate.

Diagnosis can be made on the basis of low serum uric acid, an abnormal urinary purine profile and an elevation of urine sulfite, which can be detected by special dipstick in fresh urine. A more stable marker is urine S-sulphocysteine, which is the preferred metabolite for diagnosis. No successful treatment has been reported. The genes for all three proteins are known and prenatal diagnosis is possible.

PORPHYRIAS

The porphyrias are a heterogeneous group of disorders resulting from inherited or acquired abnormalities in heme biosynthesis.[352] Symptoms associated with these disorders result primarily from the accumulation of heme precursors, as opposed to heme deficiency. The tissues with the highest rates of heme biosynthesis are the liver and the erythroid bone marrow, leading to the frequent classification of porphyria as either hepatic or erythropoietic. An alternative classification is based upon the nature of the clinical symptoms. Acute porphyrias are characterized by symptom-free periods alternating with episodic attacks. Non-acute or cutaneous porphyrias are more chronic conditions.

Heme is biosynthesized in eight sequential steps, the first and last three occurring in mitochondria. The initial and rate-limiting enzyme is delta-aminolevulinic acid synthase (ALAS), which catalyzes the first committed step in the pathway. This enzyme is subject to feedback inhibition by heme. Deficiency at any subsequent step of the pathway results in decreased heme production, loss of the normal feedback inhibition and thus increased synthesis of the early, symptom-producing intermediates.

The cytochrome P450 enzymes involved in metabolite and drug metabolism in the liver require large amounts of heme. Drugs such as phenobarbital that induce P450 enzymes, lead to an increased rate of heme production by stimulating ALAS production (see Table 26.31). In the acute forms of porphyria, a rapid rise of heme precursors then precipitates symptoms. In contrast, the cutaneous porphyrias are primarily the result of the chronic accumulation of photosensitizing intermediates of heme biosynthesis in the skin. The specific symptoms in individual patients vary widely in all types of porphyria, depending on the nature of their specific mutation(s). Since an absolute block in heme biosynthesis would be lethal, all patients have some residual enzyme activity.

ACUTE PORPHYRIAS

Acute intermittent porphyria (AIP) is the most common of the acute porphyrias in the UK (1 in 10 000–20 000); it results from a 50% reduction in hydroxymethylbilane synthase (formerly known as porphobilinogen deaminase) activity. It is an autosomal dominant disorder, as are the two other common forms of acute porphyria, variegate porphyria and hereditary coproporphyria, resulting from mutations in the *protoporphyrinogen oxidase* and *coproporphyrinogen oxidase* genes, respectively.

Table 26.31 Drugs and toxins which may aggravate acute porphyries (the list is not exhaustive)

Barbiturates	Oral contraceptives
Chloroquine	Pentazocine
Erythromycin	Phenytoin
Estrogens	Primidone
Ethanol	Sulfonamides
Griseofulvin	Theophylline
Ketamine	Trimethadione
Meprobamate	Valproic acid

Though rare in the general population, variegate porphyria has a prevalence of 1 in 3000 in Afrikaners. A very rare form of acute porphyria, *aminolevulinic acid dehydratase* deficiency porphyria, is an autosomal recessive condition. In spite of the genetic basis, a family history of acute porphyria is frequently negative. Only 10–20% of patients who inherit the gene for AIP ever develop symptoms, and symptoms almost never occur before the onset of puberty.

Clinical features

The most common symptom of acute porphyria is attacks of severe abdominal pain, typically constant and poorly localized, and often associated with nausea, vomiting and constipation. Tachycardia is the second most common symptom. Dark urine, motor neuropathy and psychiatric symptoms, including depression, anxiety, hallucinations and paranoia, are also frequently observed. In severe cases, muscle weakness can lead to paralysis and respiratory compromise. Peripheral neuropathy may result in sensory changes and urinary retention. The symptoms of acute porphyrias are believed to result primarily from the effects of ALA and porphobilinogen (PBG) on the nervous system. Heme deficiency and free radical damage may also be involved. Significantly, the symptoms of acute porphyrias are not associated with an inflammatory response, thus fever, leukocytosis and raised erythrocyte sedimentation rate are not typical.

Both endogenous and exogenous agents can trigger the onset of symptoms, the common feature being their induction of liver cytochrome P450s and increased liver heme biosynthesis. Precipitating factors include prescription and illicit drugs, fasting, smoking, starvation, alcohol and stress. The cyclical hormonal changes associated with menstruation as well as oral contraceptives can also precipitate attacks, resulting in a higher incidence of symptoms in females. Drugs that have been associated with symptoms are listed in Table 26.31. (A more complete listing is available at http://www.drugs-porphyria.com/.)

Patients with variegate porphyria and hereditary coproporphyria have neuroviseral symptoms similar to, but generally milder than, those seen in AIP. In addition, variegate porphyria (and occasionally hereditary coproporphyria) can cause cutaneous photosensitivity and skin lesions similar to those seen in the non-acute porphyrias (see below). Aminolevulinic acid dehydratase deficiency porphyria is highly variable in regards to both age of onset and severity. This variability likely results from heterogeneity in regards to the amount of residual enzyme activity in individual patients. In general the symptoms resemble those of AIP.

Diagnosis

Symptoms of acute porphyria before puberty are extremely rare; therefore, more common causes of acute abdominal symptoms must first be excluded. In adults, the symptoms are often attributed to psychosomatic disease or dysfunctional family dynamics. Any history of affected relatives must be carefully evaluated. Photosensitive skin lesions in addition to the neuroviseral symptoms are highly suggestive of variegate porphyria and may be seen in hereditary coproporphyria. With the exception of aminolevulinic acid dehydratase deficiency, all other acute porphyrias result in marked elevations of urine porphobilinogen (PBG) during an acute attack. Levels of urine ALA are also elevated to a lesser degree. Initial testing can be done on a single urine specimen, but requires special handling to avoid sample degradation and referral to an experienced laboratory. Normal levels of ALA and PBG on a spot urine sample taken during an acute episode effectively rule out the diagnosis of acute porphyria. In the presence of skin lesions total plasma porphyrins and fecal porphyrins should also be measured.

Between episodes of AIP, urinary levels of PBG are often normal but can remain elevated and can be quantitated in a 24 h urine sample. Specific enzyme testing is essential to confirm the diagnosis. DNA testing is available for most of the porphyrias, and can be used as an alternative to enzymatic testing in the evaluation of asymptomatic family members. Minor elevations of porphyrins can be seen in a variety of disorders, including constipation and lead poisoning, and care must be taken to interpret the values correctly. Many patients with chronic pain syndromes are erroneously labeled as porphyrics and often develop narcotic dependency.

Treatment

Measures to reduce the increased heme synthesis in the liver include elimination of any drugs that may have contributed, infusion of heme and i.v. fluids containing glucose. Infusion of a 10% glucose solution and correction of any electrolyte imbalances should begin immediately. Heme arginate (Normosang, Leiras) (3 mg/kg i.v. in a single daily dose) is given to inhibit the endogenous production of heme and decrease the production of ALA and PBG. Nausea and vomiting can be treated with chlorpromazine or other phenothiazines. Pain should be managed aggressively, using narcotics if required. Symptoms usually resolve in several days, so long term treatment with narcotics should not be necessary. Propranolol can be used for tachycardia and hypertension. Long term management includes the avoidance of precipitating drugs and a high carbohydrate diet (60–70% of total calories). Regular infusions of heme arginate may also be effective.

CHRONIC (NON-ACUTE) PORPHYRIAS

The non-acute porphyrias usually present in childhood and symptoms are chronic rather than episodic. Their primary symptom is skin damage, which results from photosensitivity caused by the accumulation of porphyrins in the skin. In contrast to the acute porphyrias the cutaneous forms of porphyria are exacerbated by exposure to ultraviolet (UV) light.

Congenital erythropoietic porphyria (HEP)

This is a rare autosomal recessive porphyria, associated with reduced uroporphyrinogen III synthase activity. The first sign is often red tinted discoloration of urine, which fluoresces in the diaper (nappy). Accumulation of porphyrins in red cell membranes results in hemolytic anemia, which can cause severe in utero anemia and hydrops fetalis. Chronic anemia and splenomegaly are characteristic features in older patients. Accumulation of porphyrins in the skin results in blistering and friability following exposure to UV light. Abnormalities of pigmentation, hypertrichosis and thickening of the skin occur with repeated damage. Recurrent skin infections can lead to loss of digits and scarring of the eyelids, nose and ears. Deposition of porphyrins in the teeth results in red discoloration (erythrodontia). The porphyrins that accumulate in congenital erythropoietic porphyria (CEP) are fluorescent, and can be seen by long wave illumination of the teeth, red blood cells and urine. The severe symptoms in this disorder often lead to premature death.

Porphyria cutanea tarda

There are two forms of porphyria cutanea tarda (PCT); type I is acquired and accounts for 80%, type II is inherited. Combined, they are the most common form of porphyria. Both result from decreased activity of liver uroporphyrinogen decarboxylase (UROD). Type I is the result of the sensitivity of UROD to a variety of insults including alcohol, hepatitis C, HIV infection, estrogens and smoking. Iron overload in hemochromatosis is a common precipitant. Type II is due to a mutation in the UROD gene. Patients with type II disease have a 50% reduction in UROD activity; its inheritance is autosomal dominant. The primary manifestation of PCT is photosensitivity, which results in somewhat milder symptoms than those of CEP. Mild elevations of liver enzymes are also characteristic. Patients with a homozygous deficiency of UROD have a more severe form of PCT called hepatoerythropoietic porphyria (HEP), which is similar to CEP.

Erythropoietic protoporphyria

This is the most common inherited form of cutaneous porphyria. Erythropoietic protoporphyria (EPP) results from a reduction in ferrochelatase activity, and is an autosomal dominant disorder. Ferrochelatase

catalyzes the final step of heme biosynthesis, the addition of Fe^{2+} to protoporphyrin. The cutaneous manifestations of EPP include burning, itching, erythema and swelling. Chronic sun exposure and skin damage can lead to scarring, though this is usually less severe than in CEP and HEP. Occasional patients develop severe liver dysfunction secondary to porphyrin accumulation. A mild hypochromic anemia may be present, but hemolysis is uncommon.[353]

Diagnosis

In contrast to the acute porphyrias, most of the porphyrins that accumulate in the non-acute porphyrias are not highly water-soluble and therefore are not primarily excreted in the urine. Initial screening of patients suspected of having a cutaneous porphyria can be done by analysis of total plasma porphyrins. Subsequent analysis of stool, urine and red blood cells may be required for specific disease identification.

Treatment

Because of the role of sun and UV exposure in the pathophysiology, their avoidance is essential. Special protective clothing and high sun protection factor (SPF) sunscreen lotions should be routinely utilized. Oral beta-carotene and cysteine may result in improved sun tolerance, particularly in EPP.[354] As in the acute porphyrias, avoidance of drugs that induce heme synthesis is also important. In CEP repeated blood transfusion to suppress bone marrow heme production is effective but chelation therapy is then essential to avoid iron overload. Because of the sensitivity of UROD to iron, phlebotomy to lower liver iron levels is beneficial in all types of PCT. Low dose chloroquine treatment is also beneficial in PCT. The liver dysfunction in EPP may be improved by a combination of oral bile acid supplementation to facilitate porphyrin excretion and cholestyramine to inhibit their reabsorption.

Liver transplantation has been performed in EPP where it has been shown that porphyrins accumulate in the transplanted liver allograft, indicating that the erythroid bone marrow is the main source of porphyrins in this disorder.[355] Bone marrow transplantation in an animal model of EPP resulted in a marked drop in tissue porphyrin levels, indicating that this approach may be helpful in EPP patients. Successful gene therapy for the photosensitivity in EPP has also been reported in the mouse. Several patients with CEP have been treated successfully by bone marrow transplant.[356,357] Gene therapy for this disorder is currently being developed.[358]

DISORDERS OF BILIRUBIN

The pathophysiology and differential diagnosis of jaundice are discussed elsewhere (see Ch. 19) and only genetic abnormalities of bilirubin and bile acid metabolism are considered here.

UNCONJUGATED HYPERBILIRUBINEMIA

Crigler–Najjar syndrome

The severe form (type I) of Crigler–Najjar syndrome results from a lack of hepatocyte uridine diphosphate-bilirubin glucuronosyl transferase (bilirubin-UGT) activity. Patients present as neonates with severe unconjugated hyperbilirubinemia (360–850 μmol/L [21–50 mg/dl]). Kernicterus rapidly develops unless repeated exchange transfusions or plasmapheresis and continuous phototherapy are instituted. Affected patients are always at risk of kernicterus, even as adults, if therapy is interrupted. Heterozygotes have normal bilirubin levels but may have impaired glucuronidation of other substrates. Diagnosis is based on the exclusion of other causes of hyperbilirubinemia, normal liver histology, lack of bilirubin conjugates and absent enzyme activity.

Treatment with enzyme-inducing agents such as phenobarbital is ineffective; however, phototherapy and plasmapheresis can be used to lower unconjugated bilirubin levels. Liver transplantation is curative, and preliminary studies suggest that partial transplantation may also be effective.[359] Infusion of isolated hepatocytes and gene therapy approaches are also being investigated.[360]

The type II form is allelic, caused by less severe mutations in the UGTIAI gene. Patients usually present with jaundice in infancy but this may be delayed until childhood or later. The serum bilirubin may be intermittently raised to 80–360 μmol/L (5–21 mg/dl), but falls with phenobarbital and other bilirubin-UGT inducing agents. Kernicterus is rare. Relatives may give a history of a similar pattern of jaundice. Molecular testing is available for both types I and II.

Gilbert syndrome

Gilbert syndrome (~1 in 1000) is characterized by a mild, chronic and variable unconjugated hyperbilirubinemia (~50 μmol/L [3 mg/dl]) that may be exacerbated by intercurrent infection, fasting, exertion and excessive alcohol intake. Hepatic morphology is normal and kernicterus does not occur. Males are more commonly affected than females, which likely reflects differences in rates of bilirubin production.[361] The disorder is benign but if skin pigmentation is distressing, phenobarbital reduces the bilirubin level. It is usually inherited as an autosomal recessive condition caused by a sequence variation in the promoter region of the UGT1A1 gene but autosomal dominant inheritance is also described. Compound heterozygosity for a severe UGT1A1 mutation and the promoter mutation seen in Gilbert patients results in an intermediate phenotype. Molecular testing is available.

PREDOMINANTLY CONJUGATED HYPERBILIRUBINEMIA
Dubin–Johnson syndrome

This is an autosomal recessive condition caused by a defect in the transport of conjugated bilirubin and other low molecular weight organic anions from hepatocytes into bile. The disorder results from mutations in a gene that encodes a canalicular multispecific organic anion transporter (cMOAT, also known as MRP2). Patients usually present during adolescence with mild conjugated hyperbilirubinemia (30–80 μmol/L [2–5 mg/dl]), though levels can reach 340 μmol/L (20 mg/dl), particularly during intercurrent illness, pregnancy or with oral contraceptives. Prolonged cholestatic jaundice may occur during infancy, but this usually resolves until the teen years.[362] The bromsulfthalein secretion test gives a characteristic rebound picture. Stools may be acholic and the urine dark; patients may complain of generalized weakness, anorexia, nausea and vague upper abdominal pain. The liver may be enlarged and tender. Serum transaminases, alkaline phosphatase and bile salts are normal. Total urinary coproporphyrinogen is normal or slightly increased but the ratio of coproporphyrinogen I:coproporphyrinogen III is markedly elevated, and can be used to make the diagnosis. Histologically, the liver demonstrates accumulation of a black pigment in lysosomes, but is otherwise normal. Long term follow-up studies show no evidence for chronic liver damage and suggest a benign course.[363]

Rotor disease

Rotor disease is characterized by cholestatic jaundice, but in contrast to Dubin–Johnson syndrome there is no hepatic pigmentation. Bromsulfthalein clearance from the plasma is prolonged, but without the rebound phenomenon seen in Dubin–Johnson syndrome. The two disorders can also be distinguished by urinary coproporphyrinogen levels, which are markedly increased in Rotor disease, but have a normal ratio of coproporphyrinogen I to coproporphyrinogen III. Inheritance is likely autosomal recessive, though the molecular basis is still unknown.

HEREDITARY DISORDERS OF VITAMIN METABOLISM

No genetic disorders affecting vitamins A or C are known. *Familial hypercarotinemia* is usually benign but plasma vitamin A levels should be measured. Most disorders of vitamin metabolism are discussed elsewhere but are summarized here for consistency.

In *thiamine responsive megaloblastic anemia with deafness and diabetes mellitus (TRADD)* the anemia is marked; MCVs well over 100 are seen. The diabetes and profound nerve deafness develop in childhood.

Thiamine 10–20 mg/d is enough to restore normal red cells but does not reverse the diabetes or deafness; these latter may be preventable by presymptomatic thiamine therapy.

Pyridoxine dependent seizures are discussed on p. 863 and *biotinidase* deficiency on p. 1066.

Lipoic acid is sometimes used in treating pyruvate dehydrogenase deficiency (see p. 1079).

There are five known defects of *folate* metabolism. Methylene-H4 folate reductase and methyl-H4 folate homocysteine methyltransferase are both in the recycling pathway to methionine (see p. 1056). Another defect is in the histidine pathway (see p. 1067) and hereditary malabsorption, which causes megaloblastic anemia, is also known. Several others defects have been proposed but are not proven.

Folinic acid responsive seizures are part of a severe nondysmorphic neurodevelopmental condition. The CSF contains an unknown compound that is characteristic of the condition.[364] The dose is between 10 and 40 mg/d; folic acid is ineffective.

For *vitamin B$_{12}$*, hereditary lack of intrinsic factor, of ileal absorption and the plasma transport proteins transcobalamin I and II are just the early aspects of a cascade of defects (Fig. 26.43). Vitamin B$_{12}$ is known to be involved with only two pathways, namely in homocystine (see p. 1056) and methylmalonic acid metabolism (see p. 1065). At least nine defects are known (Cbl A–I). Those that interfere with methyl B$_{12}$ functions affect homocysteine metabolism, cause serious brain damage and are usually associated with megaloblastic anemia. Those that affect mutase activity all cause methylmalonic aciduria. Thus some cause a combined defect of both pathways. It should be noted that plasma B$_{12}$ levels are low in the absorptive defects but normal in the remainder. Plasma methylmalonic acid is a sensitive indicator of B$_{12}$ deficiency and is usually abnormal in newborn infants whose mothers are B$_{12}$ deficient.

Disorders of *vitamin D* metabolism include defects of both the 1-alpha-hydroxylase and 25-hydroxylases (D-dependent rickets type I). Both are associated with severe rickets that responds to therapy with 1,25-dihydroxyvitamin D3. A defect of the vitamin D receptor (D-dependent rickets type II) is far more serious; the rickets resists almost all therapy and most patients have total alopecia, those who do not have hair loss exhibit a different D-binding protein defect. Vitamin D resistant rickets is discussed in Chapter 15, p. 478–527.

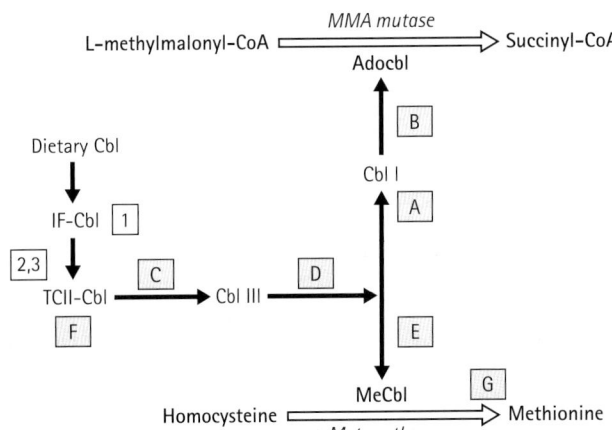

Fig 26.43 Vitamin B$_{12}$ metabolism. 1, denotes intrinsic factor deficiency; 2, defective absorption (in the distal ileum); 3, transcobalamin I and II deficiencies. Defect A results from failure of reduction of the cobalt from 2$^+$ to 1$^+$ in mitochondria. B results from failure of adenosyltransferase to synthesize adenosyl-B12. C and D are due to failures in the reduction of the central cobalt from 3$^+$ to 2$^+$ after efflux from the lysosomes. E is due to a defect in a reductase required to keep Cbl in a functional state. F is due to a failure to transport Cbl across the lysosomal membrane. G is due to a defect in methionine synthase.

A disorder of *vitamin E* metabolism is associated with progressive cerebellar dysfunction (similar to that seen in abetalipoproteinemia); it responds to increased doses of the vitamin.

MISCELLANEOUS INBORN ERRORS OF METABOLISM

Cerebral glucose transporter (GLUT 1) deficiency

There are several distinct glucose transporters. GLUT 1 is required for the transport of glucose into the CNS. Deficiency manifests as an autosomal dominant; it results in low CNS and CSF glucose *in the presence of normal blood glucose levels*. The result is severe and early onset of seizures and progressive brain damage. A high ketone diet, given to encourage brain metabolism of ketones, is beneficial. Well over 100 proteins have been identified in plasma. Many exhibit considerable genetic variation that is usually without functional significance. Selected disorders are discussed below.

Alkaline phosphatase

Alkaline phosphatase comprises a family of at least four gene products that are normally bound to plasma membranes and accept a number of substrates such as phosphoethanolamine, pyrophosphate and pyridoxal-5'-phosphate. One isoenzyme is isolated to the intestine, a second to placenta, a third to germ cells. The fourth, which is present in most tissues and is called tissue nonspecific alkaline phosphatase (TNSALP), undergoes post-translational modification in almost all tissues producing liver, kidney, bone, leukocyte, etc isoenzymes that can be recognized electrophoretically. Alkaline phosphatase in plasma probably has no metabolic role; normally, in children, it derives largely from osteoblastic activity in bone, particularly during growth spurts. It can also reflect tissue damage in various organs, particularly the bile duct epithelium.

Hypophosphatasia

This condition is due to absence or defective function of tissue nonspecific alkaline phosphatase (TNSALP). As with most disorders, there are severe and mild variants and both autosomal recessive and dominant inheritance are encountered. The principal presentations are of bone and/or dental abnormalities that may occur together or independently.

Clinical features

The most severely affected cases can be detected prenatally by X-ray and these infants usually die prenatally or soon after birth. The skull and skeleton may be so unmineralized as to be almost invisible on X-ray. Shortening, bowing and rachitic changes of the bones are usual and undermineralization may seem reminiscent of osteogenesis imperfecta, although the radiological features are distinct. Thoracic dystrophy causes severe neonatal asphyxia; the differential diagnosis therefore includes Jeune asphyxiating thoracic dystrophy. This form is found in ~1 in 2500 Mennonite infants.

In less severely affected infants, failure to thrive, vomiting, hypotonia and constipation usually develop in the first year; they are related to hypercalcemia which is a usual feature of the condition and may be severe enough to cause nephrocalcinosis. The fontanelle is widely open and often tense. The skull may be misshapen and the face asymmetrical. In the skull, osteoporosis or copper-beaten skull is evident and may be associated with delayed bone growth. Bony deformities consist of shortening of long bones, bowing, thickening of the wrists, shortening of the digits, lordosis and a Harrison's sulcus; the metaphyses show characteristic translucencies in the growth plates. There may be premature loss of primary teeth, especially the incisors; there is no compensatory early eruption of permanent teeth.

In older children and in the dominant forms, the presentation can be more variable with little more than premature loss of primary teeth without periodontal disease, but with abnormal alveolar attrition and enlarged pulp chambers and root canals. Permanent teeth can also be involved. The condition may be first recognized in adults and presents with calcium nephrolithiasis. In such cases, osteoporosis and fractures are frequent,

pseudofractures can be seen on X-ray and some have the deformities of previous 'rickets'. Dental abnormalities may be the only finding.

Hypercalcemia is frequent in the infantile forms and can be life threatening when older patients are immobilized, as for orthopedic treatment. The hypercalcemia develops from failure of synthesis of apatite crystals in bone.

Diagnosis and treatment

In the most severe cases, all TNSALP isozyme activities are virtually absent. In milder cases, the activity is present but diminished, a finding that becomes increasingly hard to evaluate in adults since normal values are lower than in childhood. In severe but not in mild cases, phosphoethanolamine is increased in the urine and pyridoxal-5'-phosphate is markedly increased in the blood. The latter test is less available but seems to be a better discriminant; both are most abnormal in the most severe cases. Prenatal diagnosis is tricky; ultrasound studies may help and analysis of TNSALP in an experienced laboratory is critical.

Pseudohypophosphatasia was reported in a family with the findings of hypophosphatasia but normal enzyme levels. Low values for TNSALP may occur in a number of conditions including malnutrition, hypothyroidism, zinc deficiency and glucocorticoid therapy.

There is no effective treatment; craniostenosis and limb deformity may require surgery.

Hyperphosphatasia

The normal plasma alkaline phosphatase varies considerably throughout life and normal ranges are not clearly defined. Elevated values, derived from osteoblasts, occur in any condition with increased bone turnover, such as rickets, fractures, osteogenic sarcoma, osteolytic malignancies or juvenile Paget disease. The liver isozyme of ALP is increased whenever bile duct epithelium is damaged, as in obstructive jaundice.

Familial hyperphosphatasia, usually involving liver ALP, is usually benign, but may be associated with bone disease (e.g. juvenile Paget), and association with mental retardation, seizures and neurological damage is reported in several families.

Transient hyperphosphatasemia of infancy is not uncommon; it involves the bone and liver forms and can occur following a minor viral prodrome and is often detected during routine blood tests. The plasma level can easily reach well over 2000 IU/L but this only lasts for a few weeks; no other laboratory tests are abnormal. The etiology is unknown and no treatment is indicated.[365]

Carbonic anhydrase II deficiency

This is a rare autosomal recessive trait that causes osteopetrosis, mixed proximal and distal renal tubular acidosis and developmental delay with cerebral calcifications; growth failure and dental malocclusion occur frequently. The osteopetrosis in this condition is usually less severe than in the classic disorder and patients may be asymptomatic for months or years after birth, but eventually fractures, failure to thrive or developmental delay bring the patient to attention.

Treatment for this disorder is symptomatic, whereas bone marrow transplantation is beneficial in 'classic', severe osteopetrosis. Prenatal diagnosis is not currently available.

Transport proteins

In *congenital analbuminemia* plasma albumin is missing and the substances in plasma that are normally bound to it, such as calcium, are reduced. However, the unbound (active) fractions of these compounds in the plasma are normal and mild edema may be the only finding. The reason for the lack of gross edema is unclear. Heterozygotes have normal levels. Occasionally, electrophoretic variants of albumin are found in healthy people. Hypoalbuminemia due to malnutrition, hepatocellular disease and protein-losing enteropathy are discussed inch 19.

Congenital deficiency of hormone-binding proteins are discussed inch 15. Normal serum contains 0.3–2 g/L of haptoglobin, which binds to free hemoglobin in plasma. There are several common genetic variants and even total deficiency seems to be benign.

REFERENCES

1. Scriver CR, Beaudet AL, Valle D, et al, eds. The metabolic and molecular bases of inherited disease, 8th edn. New York: McGraw Hill; 2001.

2. Nyhan WL, Barshop B, Ozand PT. Atlas of metabolic diseases, 2nd edn. London: Chapman & Hall; 2005.

3. Gilbert-Barness E, Barness L. Metabolic diseases. Natick, MA: Eaton Publishing; 2000.

4. Fernandes J, Saudubray J-M, van den Berghe G, eds. Inborn metabolic diseases: diagnosis and treatment. 3rd edn. Berlin: Springer-Verlag; 2000.

5. Holton JB, ed. 2nd edn. The inherited metabolic diseases. Edinburgh: Churchill Livingstone; 1994.

6. Blau N, Blaskovics M, eds. 2nd ed The physician's guide to the laboratory diagnosis of inherited metabolic diseases. London: Chapman & Hall; 2002.

7. Blau N, Hoffmann GF, Leonard J, et al. eds. Physician's guide to the treatment and follow-up of metabolic diseases. Springer-Verlag Berlin, Heidelberg New York, 2006 (ISBN-13 978-3-540-22954-4).

8. Lyon G, Adams RD, Kolodny EH. Neurology of hereditary metabolic diseases of children. New York: McGraw-Hill; 1996.

9. Clarke JTR. A clinical guide for inherited metabolic diseases. Cambridge: Cambridge University Press; 2000.

10. Garrod AE. The incidence of alkaptonuria: a study in chemical individuality. Lancet 1902; 2:1616.

11. Iper JS. Genetic complexity in single gene diseases. BMJ 1996; 312:196–197.

12. Dionisi-Vici C, Rizzo C, Burlina AB, et al. Inborn errors of metabolism in the Italian pediatric population: a national retrospective survey. J Pediatr 2002; 140:321–327.

13. Applegarth DA, Toone JR, Lowry RB. Incidence of inborn errors of metabolism in British Columbia, 1969–1996. Pediatrics 2000; 105:e10.

14. Baird PA, Anderson TW, Newcombe HB, et al. Genetic disorders in children and young adults: a population study. Am J Hum Genet 1988; 42:677–693.

15. Lee PJ, Cook P. Frequency of metabolic disorders; more than one needle in the haystack. Arch Dis Child 2006; 91:896–899.

16. Fitzpatrick D. Inborn errors of metabolism in the newborn: clinical presentation and investigation. J R Coll Physicians Edin 2006; 36:147–151.

17. Gu XF, Han LS, Ye J, et al. Outcome study of tandem mass-spectrometry on clinical selective screening in Chinese patients. J Inherit Metab Dis 2006; 29(suppl 1) p17.

18. Usha D. Screening of high-risk neonates and children using GC/MS in India. J Inherit metab Dis 2006; 29(suppl 1) p17.

19. Buist NRM, Dulac NO, Bottiglieri T, et al. Metabolic evaluation of infantile epilepsy: recommendations of the Amalfi group. 2002. J Child Neurol 2002; 102(suppl 3):3S98.

20. Treacy E, Childs B, Scriver CR. Response to treatment in hereditary metabolic disease. 1993 Survey and 10-year comparison. Am J Hum Genet 1995; 56:359–367.

21. Beutler E. Lysosomal storage diseases: natural history and ethical and economic aspects. Mol Genet Metab 2006; 88:208–215.

22. Smith I, Lobascher ME, Stevenson JE, et al. Effect of stopping low-phenylalanine diet on intellectual progress of children with phenylketonuria. BMJ 1978; 2:723–726.

23. Matalon R, Michals-Matalon K, Koch R, et al. Response of patients with phenylketonuria in the US to tetrahydrobiopterin. Mol Genet Metab 2005; 86(suppl 1):S17.

24. Matalon R, Michals-Matalon K, Bhatia G, et al. Large neutral amino acids in the treatment of phenylketonuria (PKU). J Inherit Metab Dis 2006; 29:732–738.

25. Hanley WB, Clarke JT, Schoonheyt W. Maternal phenylketonuria (PKU) – a review. Clin Biochem 1987; 20:149–156.

26. Hyland K, Arnold LA, Trugman JM. Defects of biopterin metabolism and biogenic amine biosynthesis: clinical diagnostic and therapeutic aspects. Adv Neurol 1998; 78:301–308.

27. Lindstedt S, Holme E, Lock EA, et al. Treatment of hereditary tyrosinaemia type I by inhibition of 4-hydroxyphenylpyruvate dioxygenase. Lancet 1992; 340:813–817.

28. Holme E, Lindstedt S. Tyrosinaemia type I and NTBC (2-(2-nitro-4-trifluoromethylbenzoyl)-1,3-cyclohexanedione). J Inherit Metab Dis 1999; 22:665–666.

29. Sakura N, Ono H, Nomura S, et al. Betaine dose and treatment intervals in therapy for homocystinuria due to 5,10-methylenetetrahydrofolate reductase deficiency. J Inherit Metab Dis 1998; 21:84–85.

30. Walter JH, Wraith JE, White FJ, et al. Strategies for the treatment of cystathionine beta-synthase deficiency: the experience of the Willink Biochemical Genetics Unit over the past 30 years. Eur J Pediatr 1998; 157(suppl 2):S71–S76.

31. Baric I, Fumic K, Glenn B, et al. S-adenosylhomocysteine hydrolase deficiency in a human: a genetic disorder of methionine metabolism. Proc Natl Acad Sci U S A 2004; 101:4234.

32. Anon. Consensus statement from a conference for the management of patients with urea cycle disorders. J Pediatr 2001; 138:S6–S10.

33. Guffon N, Vianey-Saban C, Bourgeois J, et al. A new neonatal case of N-acetyl glutamate synthase deficiency treated by carbamylglutamate. J Inherit Metab Dis 1995; 18:61–65.

34. Hinnie J, Colombo JP, Wermuth B, et al. N-acetylglutamate synthetase deficiency responding to carbamylglutamate. J Inherit Metab Dis 1997; 20:839–840.

35. Steiner RD, Cederbaum SD. Laboratory evaluation of urea cycle disorders. J Pediatr 2001; 138:S56–S60. discussion S60–61

36. Brusilow SW, Danney M, Waber LJ, et al. Treatment of episodic hyperammonemia in children with inborn errors of urea synthesis. N Engl J Med 1984; 310:1630–1634.

37. Batshaw ML, MacArthur RB, Tuchman M. Alternative pathway therapy for urea cycle disorders: twenty years later. J Pediatr 2001; 138:S46–S54.

38. Brusilow SW. Phenylacetylglutamine may replace urea as a vehicle for waste nitrogen excretion. Pediatr Res 1991; 29:147–150.

39. Widhalm K, Koch S, Scheibenreiter S, et al. Long-term follow-up of 12 patients with the late-onset variant of argininosuccinic acid lyase deficiency: no impairment of intellectual and psychomotor development during therapy. Pediatrics 1992; 89:1182–1184.

40. Burlina AB, Ogier H, Korall H, et al. Long-term treatment with sodium phenylbutyrate in ornithine transcarbamylase-deficient patients. Mol Genet Metab 2001; 72:351–355.

41. Saudubray JM, Touati G, Delonlay P, et al. Liver transplantation in urea cycle disorders. Eur J Pediatr 1999; 158(suppl 2):S55–S59.

42. Hamosh A, Maher JF, Bellus GA, et al. Long-term use of high-dose benzoate and dextromethorphan for the treatment of nonketotic hyperglycinemia. J Pediatr 1998; 132:709–713.

43. Wiltshire EJ, Poplawski NK, Harrison JR, et al. Treatment of late-onset nonketotic hyperglycinaemia: effectiveness of imipramine and benzoate. J Inherit Metab Dis 2000; 23:15–21.

44. Saborio P, Scheinman JI. Transplantation for primary hyperoxaluria in the United States. Kidney Int 1999; 56:1094–1100.

45. Stockler S, Holzbach U, Hanefeld F, et al. Creatine deficiency in the brain: a new, treatable inborn error of metabolism. Pediatr Res 1994; 36:409–413.

46. Stockler S, Hanefeld F, Frahm J. Creatine replacement therapy in guanidinoacetate methyltransferase deficiency, a novel inborn error of metabolism. Lancet 1996; 348:789–790.

47. Roe CR, Millington DS, Maltby DA, et al. L-Carnitine enhances excretion of propionyl coenzyme A as propionylcarnitine in propionic acidemia. J Clin Invest 1984; 73:1785–1788.

48. van der Meer SB, Poggi F, Spada M, et al. Clinical outcome of long-term management of patients with vitamin B12 unresponsive methylmalonic acidemia. J Pediatr 1994; 125:903–908.

49. Roe CR, Millington DS, Maltby DA, et al. L-Carnitine therapy in isovaleric academia. J Clin Invest 1984; 74:2290–2295.

50. Moslinger D, Stockler-Ipsiroglu S, Scheibenreiter S, et al. Clinical and neuropsychological outcome in 33 patients with biotinidase deficiency ascertained by nationwide newborn screening and family studies in Austria. Eur J Pediatr 2001; 160:277–282.

51. Wilcox R, Steiner RD. Metabolic disease and sudden unexpected death. J Pediatr 2003; 142:357.

52. Rinaldo P, Schmidt-Sommerfeld E, Posca AP, et al. Effect of treatment with glycine and L-carnitine in medium-chain acyl-coenzyme A dehydrogenase deficiency. J Pediatr 1993; 122:580–584.

53. Pierpont ME, Breningstall GN, Stanley CA, et al. Familial carnitine transporter defect: a treatable cause of cardiomyopathy in children. Am Heart J 2000; 139:S96–S106.

54. Gillingham M, Van Calcar S, Ney D, et al. Dietary management of long-chain 3-hydroxyacyl-CoA dehydrogenase deficiency (LCHADD). A case report and survey. J Inherit Metab Dis 1999; 22:123–131.

55. Wang SS, Fernhoff PM, Khoury MJ. Is the G985A allelic variant of medium-chain acyl-CoA dehydrogenase a risk factor for sudden infant death syndrome? A pooled analysis. Pediatrics 2000; 105:1175–1176.

56. Andresen BS, Dobrowolski SF, O'Reilly L, et al. Medium-chain acyl-CoA dehydrogenase (MCAD) mutations identified by MS/MS-based prospective screening of newborns differ from those observed in patients with clinical symptoms: identification and characterization of a new, prevalent mutation that results in mild MCAD deficiency. Am J Hum Genet 2001; 68:1408–1418.

57. Ibdah JA, Bennett MJ, Rinaldo P, et al. A fetal fatty-acid oxidation disorder as a cause of liver disease in pregnant women. N Engl J Med 1999; 340:1723–1731.

58. Bennett MJ, Weinberger MJ, Kobori JA, et al. Mitochondrial short-chain L-3-hydroxyacyl-coenzyme A dehydrogenase deficiency: a new defect of fatty acid oxidation. Pediatr Res 1996; 39:185–188.

59. Corydon MJ, Vockley J, Rinaldo P, et al. Role of common gene variations in the molecular pathogenesis of short-chain acyl-CoA dehydrogenase deficiency. Pediatr Res 2001; 49:18–23.

60. Beatty ME, Zhang YH, McCabe ER, et al. Fructose-1,6-diphosphatase deficiency and glyceroluria: one possible etiology for GIS. Mol Genet Metab 2000; 69:338–340.

61. Mooy PD, Przyrembel H, Giesberts MA, et al. Glutaric aciduria type II: treatment with riboflavine, carnitine and insulin. Eur J Pediatr 1984; 143:92–95.

62. Saudubray JM, Charpentier C. Clinical phenotypes: diagnosis/algorithms. In: Scriver CR, Beaudet AL, Sly WS, et al, eds. The metabolic and molecular bases of inherited disease, 8th edn. New York: McGraw-Hill; 2001.1327–1403.

63. Haller RG, Wyrick P, Taivasslo T, et al. Aerobic conditioning: an effective therapy in McArdle's disease. Ann Neurol 2006; 59:922–928.

64. Gillingham MB, Scott B, Elliott D, et al. Metabolic control during exercise with and without medium-chain triglycerides (MCT) in children with long-chain 3-hydroxy acyl-CoA dehydrogenase (LCHAD) or trifunctional protein (TFP) deficiency. Mol Genet Metab 2006; 89:58–63.

65. Waggoner DD, Buist NR, Donnell GN. Long-term prognosis in galactosaemia: results of a survey of 350 cases. J Inherit Metab Dis 1990; 13:802–818.

66. Kaufman FR, McBridechang C, Manis FR, et al. Cognitive functioning, neurologic status and brain imaging in classical galactosemia. Eur J Pediatr 1995; 154:S2–S5.

67. Irons M, Levy HL, Pueschel S, et al. Accumulation of galactose-1-phosphate in the galactosemic fetus despite maternal milk avoidance. J Pediatr 1985; 107:261–263.

68. Berry GT, Nissim I, Lin Z, et al. Endogenous synthesis of galactose in normal men and patients with hereditary galactosaemia. Lancet 1995; 346:1073–1074.

69. Tolan DR, Brooks CC. Molecular analysis of common aldolase B alleles for hereditary fructose intolerance in North Americans. Biochem Med Metab Biol 1992; 48:19–25.

70. Stacpoole PW, Kerr DS, Barnes C, et al. Controlled clinical trial of dichloroacetate for treatment of congenital lactic acidosis in children. Pediatrics 2006; 117:1519–1531.

71. Thorburn DR, Dahl H-HM. Mitochondrial disorders: genetics, counseling, prenatal diagnosis and reproductive options. Am J Med Genet 2001; 106:102–114.

72. Chinnery PF, Turnbull DM. Epidemiology and treatment of mitochondrial disorders. Am J Med Genet. 2001; 106:94–101.

73. Schapira AH. Mitochondrial disease. Lancet 2006; 368:70–82.

74. Wallace DC. Mouse models of mitochondrial disease. Am J Med Genet 2001; 106:71–93.

75. Munnich A, Rustin P. Clinical spectrum and diagnosis of mitochondrial disorders. Am J Med Genet 2001; 106:4–17.

76. DiMauro S, Bonilla E, De Vivo D. Does the patient have a mitochondrial encephalomyopathy? J Child Neurol 1999; 14(suppl 1):S23–S35.

77. DiMauro S, Schon E. Mitochondrial DNA mutations in human disease. Am J Med Genet 2001; 106:18–26.

78. Naviaux RK, Nguyen KV. POLG mutations associated with Alpers syndrome and mitochondrial DNA depletion. Ann Neurol 2004; 55:706–712.

79. Uusimaa J, Finnilä S, Vainionpää L, et al. A mutation in mitochondrial DNA-encoded cytochrome c oxidase II gene in a child with Alpers–Huttnelocher-like diseases. Pediatrics 2003; 111:e262–e268.

80. DiMauro S, Nicholson JF, Hays AP, et al. Benign infantile mitochondrial myopathy due to reversible cytochrome c oxidase deficiency. Ann Neurol 1983; 14:226–229.

81. Böhm M, Pronicka E, Karczmarewicz E, et al. Retrospective, multicentric study of 180 children with cytochrome c oxidase deficiency. Pediatr Res 2006; 59:21–26.

82. Janssen RJ, Nijtmans LG, van den Heuvel LP, et al. Mitochondrial complex I: structure, function and pathology. J Inherit Metab Dis 2006; 29: 499–515.

83. Bespalova IN, van Camp G, Bom SJH, et al. Mutations in the Wolfram syndrome 1 gene (WFS1) are a common cause of low frequency sensorineural hearing loss. Hum Mol Genet 2001; 10:2501–2508.

84. Pons R, Andreu AL, Checcarelli N, et al. Mitochondrial DNA abnormalities and autistic spectrum disorders. J Pediatr 2004; 144:81–85.

85. Poulton J, Macaulay V, Marchington DR. Mitochondrial genetics '98: is the bottleneck cracked?. Am J Hum Genet 1998; 62:752–757.

86. Larsson NG, Holme E, Kristiansson B, et al. Progressive increase of the mutated mitochondrial DNA fraction in Kearns–Sayre syndrome. Pediatr Res 1990; 28:131–136.

87. Suomalainen A, Kaukonen J. Diseases caused by nuclear genes affecting mtDNA stability. Am J Med Genet 2001; 106:53–61.

88. Naviaux RK, Nyhan W, Barshop B, et al. Mitochondrial polymerase gamma deficiency and mtDNA depletion in a child with Alpers' syndrome. Ann Neurol 1999; 45:54–58.

89. Saada A, Shaag A, Mandel H, et al. Mutant mitochondrial thymidine kinase in mitochondrial DNA depletion myopathy. Nat Genet 2001; 29:332–344.

90. Mandel H, Szargel R, Labay V, et al. The deoxyguanosine kinase gene is mutated in individuals with depleted hepatocerebral mitochondrial DNA. Nat Genet 2001; 29:337–341.

91. Spinazzola A, Viscomi C, Fernandez-Vizarra E, et al. MPV17 encodes an inner mitochondrial membrane protein and is mutated in infantile hepatic mitochondrial DNA depletion. Nat Genet 2006; 38:570–575.

92. Karadimas CL, Vu TH, Holve SA, et al. Navajo neurohepathopathy is caused by a mutation in the MPV17 gene. Am J Hum Genet 2006; 79:544–548.

93. Elpeleg O, Miller C, Hershkovitz E, et al. Deficiency of the ADP-forming succinyl-CoA synthetase activity is associated with encephalomyopathy and mitochondrial DNA depletion. Am J Hum Genet 2005; 76:1081–1086.

94. Leshinsky-Silver E, Naviaux RK, Zinger A, et al. MEHMO (mental retardation, epileptic seizures, hypogenitalism, microcephaly, obesity): a new X-linked mitochondrial DNA depletion syndrome. Mitochondrion 2001; 1:95–96.

95. Alexander C, Votruba M, Pesch UEA, et al. OPA1, encoding a dynamin-related GTPase, is mutated in autosomal dominant optic atrophy linked to chromosome 3q28. Nat Genet 2000; 26:211–215.

96. Delettre C, Lenaers G, Griffoin J-M, et al. Nuclear gene OPA1, encoding a mitochondrial dynamin-related protein, is mutated in dominant optic atrophy. Nat Genet 2000; 26:207–210.

97. Kim JY, Hwang JM, Ko HS, et al. Mitochondrial DNA content is decreased in autosomal dominant optic atrophy. Neurology 2005; 64:966–972.

98. White AJ. Mitochondrial toxicity and HIV therapy. Sex Transm Infect 2001; 77:158–173.

99. Hirano M, Vu TH. Defects of intergenomic communication: where do we stand?. Brain Pathol 2000; 10:451–461.

100. DiMauro S, Bonilla E, Lee CP, et al. Luft's disease. Further biochemical and ultrastructural studies of skeletal muscle in the second case. J Neurol Sci 1976; 27:217–232.

101. Castro-Gago M, Alonso A, Pintos-Mart'nez E, et al. Congenital hydranencephalic-hydrocephalic syndrome associated with mitochondrial dysfunction. J Child Neurol 1999; 14:131–135.

102. Von Kleist-Retzow JC, Cormier-Daire V, Viot G, et al. Antenatal manifestations of mitochondrial respiratory chain deficiency. J Pediatr 2003; 143:208–212.

103. Garcia-Cazorla A, De Lonlay P, Nassogne MC, et al. Long-term follow-up of neonatal mitochondrial cytopathies: a study of 57 patients. Pediatrics 2005; 116:1170–1177.

104. Bourgeron T, Rustin P, Chretien D, et al. Mutation of a nuclear succinate dehydrogenase gene results in mitochondrial respiratory chain deficiency. Nat Genet 1995; 11:144–148.

105. Baysal BE, Ferrell RE, Willett-Brozick JE, et al. Mutations in SDHD, a mitochondrial complex II gene, in hereditary paraganglioma. Science 2000; 287:848–851.

106. Astuti D, Latif F, Dallol A, et al. Gene mutations in the succinate dehydrogenase subunit SDHB cause susceptibility to familial pheochromocytoma and to familial paraganglioma. Am J Hum Genet 2001; 69:49–54.

107. Triepels RH, Van den Heuvel LP, Trijbels JM, et al. Respiratory chain complex I deficiency. Am J Med Genet 2001; 106:37–45.

108. Kirby DM, Salemi R, Sugiana C, et al. NDUFS6 mutations are a novel cause of lethal neonatal mitochondrial complex I deficiency. J Clin Invest 2004; 114:837–845.

109. De Lonlay P, Valnot I, Barrientos A, et al. A mutant mitochondrial respiratory chain assembly protein causes complex III deficiency in patients with tubulopathy, encephalopathy and liver failure. Nat Genet 2001; 29:57–60.

110. Tiranti V, Hoertnagel K, Carrozzo R, et al. Mutations of SURF-1 in Leigh disease associated with cytochrome c oxidase deficiency. Am J Hum Genet 1998; 63:1609–1621.

111. Zhu Z, Yao J, Johns T, et al. SURF1, encoding a factor involved in the biogenesis of cytochrome c oxidase, is mutated in Leigh syndrome. Nat Genet 1998; 20:337–343.

112. Papadopoulou LC, Sue CM, Davidson MM, et al. Fatal infantile cardioencephalomyopathy with COX deficiency and mutations in SCO2, a COX assembly gene. Nat Genet 1999; 23:333–337.

113. Valnot I, Osmond S, Gigarel N, et al. Mutations of the SCO1 gene in mitochondrial cytochrome c oxidase (COX) deficiency with neonatal-onset hepatic failure and encephalopathy. Am J Hum Genet 2000; 67:1104–1109.

114. Valnot I, von Kleist-Retzow JC, Barrientos A, et al. A mutation in the human heme A: faresyltransferase gene (COX10) causes cytochrome c oxidase deficiency. Hum Mol Genet 2000; 9:1245–1249.

115. Houstek J, Klement P, Floryk D, et al. A novel deficiency of mitochondrial ATPase of nuclear origin. Hum Mol Genet 1999; 8:1967–1974.

116. De Meirleir L, Seneca S, Lissens W, et al. Respiratory chain complex V deficiency due to a mutation in the assembly gene ATP12. J Med Genet 2004; 41:120–124.

117. Van Goethem G, Dermaut B, Löfgren A, et al. Mutation of POLG is associated with progressive external ophthalmoplegia characterized by mtDNA deletions. Nat Genet 2001; 28:211–212.

118. Horvath R, Hudson G, Ferraro G, et al. Phenotypic spectrum associated with mutations of the mitochondrial polymerase γ gene. Brain 2006; 129:1674–1684.

119. Longley MJ, Clark S, Man CYW, et al. Mutant POLG2 disrupts DNA polymerase γ subunits and causes progressive external ophthalmoplegia. Am J Hum Genet 2006; 78:1026–1034.

120. Kaukonen J, Juselius JK, Tiranti V, et al. Role of adenine nucleotide translocator 1 in mtDNA maintenance. Science 2000; 289:782–785.

121. Spelbrink JN, Li F-Y, Tiranti V, et al. Human mitochondrial DNA deletions associated with mutations in the gene encoding Twinkle, a phage T7 gene 4-like protein localized in mitochondria. Nat Genet 2001; 28:223–231.

122. Bakker HD, Scholte HR, van den Bogert C, et al. Deficiency of the adenine nucleotide translocator in muscle of a patient with myopathy and lactic acidosis: a new mitochondrial defect. Pediatr Res 1993; 33:412–417.

123. Huizing M, Ruitenbeek W, Thinnes FP, et al. Deficiency of the voltage-dependent anion channel: a novel cause of mitochondriopathy. Pediatr Res 1996; 39:760–765.

124. Hayes DJ, Taylor DJ, Bore PJ, et al. An unusual metabolic myopathy: a malate–aspartate shuttle defect. J Neurol Sci 1987; 82:27–39.

125. Huckriede A, Agsteribbe E. Decreased synthesis and inefficient mitochondrial import of hsp60 in a patient with a mitochondrial encephalomyopathy. Biochim Biophys Acta 1994; 1227:200–206.

126. Casari G, De Fusco M, Ciarmatori S, et al. Spastic paraplegia and OXPHOS impairment caused by mutations in paraplegin, a nuclear-encoded mitochondrial metalloprotease. Cell 1998; 93:973–983.

127. Rothbauer U, Hofmann S, Muhlenbein N, et al. Role of the deafness dystonia peptide 1 (DDP1) in import of human Tim23 into the inner membrane of mitochondria. J Biol Chem 2001; 276:37327–37334.

128. Orth M, Schapira AHV. Mitochondria and degenerative disorders. Am J Med Genet 2001; 106:27–36.

129. Tan G, Chen L-S, Lonnerdal B, et al. Frataxin expression rescues mitochondrial dysfunctions in FRDA cells. Hum Mol Genet 2001; 19:2099–2107.

130. Allikmets R, Rashkind WH, Hutchinson A, et al. Mutation of a putative mitochondrial iron transporter gene (ABC7) in X-linked sideroblastic anemia and ataxia (XLSA/A). Hum Mol Genet 1999; 8:743–749.

131. Lutsenko S, Cooper MJ. Localization of the Wilson's disease protein product to mitochondria. Proc Natl Acad Sci U S A 1998; 95:6004–6009.

132. Beal MF. Mitochondrial dysfunction in neurodegenerative diseases. Biochim Biophys Acta 1998; 1366:211–223.

133. Schapira AHV. Mitochondrial dysfunction in neurodegenerative disorders. Biochim Biophys Acta 1998; 1366:225–233.

134. Comi GP, Bordoni A, Salani S, et al. Cytochrome c oxidase subunit I microdeletion in a patient with motor neuron disease. Ann Neurol 1998; 43:110–116.

135. Enns GM, Bai RK, Beck AE, et al. Molecular-clinical correlations in a family with variable tissue mitochondrial DNA T8993G mutant load. Mol Genet Metab 2006; 88:364–371.

136. Shoffner JM. Oxidative phosphorylation disease diagnosis. Sem Neurol 1999; 19:341–351.

137. Enns GM, Bennett MJ, Hoppel C, et al. Mitochondrial respiratory chain complex I deficiency presenting with clinical and biochemical features of long-chain 3-hydroxyacyl-CoA dehydrogenase (LCHAD) deficiency. J Pediatr 2000; 136:251–254.

138. Dinopoulos A, Cecil KM, Schapiro MB, et al. Brain MRI and proton MRS findings in infants and children with respiratory chain defects. Neuropediatr 2005; 36:290–301.

139. Enns GM, Hoppel CL, DeArmond S, et al. The relationship of mitochondrial dysfunction to the pathogenesis of fiber type abnormalities in skeletal muscle. Clin Genet 2005; 68:337–348.

140. Capaldi RA, Murray J, Byrne L, et al. Immunological approaches to the characterization and diagnosis of mitochondrial disease. Mitochondrion 2004; 4:417–426.

141. De Paepe B, Smet J, Leroy JG, et al. Diagnostic value of immunostaining in cultured skin fibroblasts from patients with oxidative phosphorylation defects. Pediatr Res 2006; 59:2–6.

142. Jaksch M, Kleinle S, Scharfe C, et al. Frequency of mitochondrial transfer RNA mutations and deletions in 225 patients presenting with respiratory chain deficiencies. J Med Genet 2001; 28:665–673.

143. Bugiani M, Lamantea E, Invernizzi F, et al. Effects of riboflavin in children with complex II deficiency. Brain Dev 2006; 28:576–581.

144. Chan A, Reichmann H, Kögel A, et al. Metabolic changes in patients with mitochondrial myopathies and effects of coenzyme Q10 therapy. J Neurol 1998; 245:681–685.

145. Abe K, Matsuo Y, Kadekawa J, et al. Effect of coenzyme Q10 in patients with mitochondrial myopathy, encephalopathy, lactic acidosis, and stroke-like episodes (MELAS): evaluation by noninvasive tissue oximetry. J Neurol Sci 1999; 162:65–68.

146. Musumeci O, Naini A, Slonim AE, et al. Familial cerebellar ataxia with muscle coenzyme Q10 deficiency. Neurology 2001; 56:849–855.

147. Hart PE, Lodi R, Rajagopalan B, et al. Antioxidant treatment of patients with Friedreich ataxia. Arch Neurol 2005; 62:621–626.

148. De Stefano N, Matthews PM, Ford B, et al. Short-term dichloroacetate treatment improves indices of cerebral metabolism in patients with mitochondrial disorders. Neurology 1995; 45:1193–1198.

149. Saitoh S, Momoi MY, Yamagata T, et al. Effects of dichloroacetate in three patients with MELAS. Neurology 1998; 50:531–534.

150. Kaufmann P, Engelstad K, Wei Y, et al. Dichloroacetate causes toxic neuropathy in MELAS: a randomized, controlled clinical trial. Neurology 2006; 66:325–330.

151. Koga Y, Akita Y, Junko N, et al. Endothelial dysfunction in MELAS improved by L-arginine supplementation. Neurology 2006; 66:1766–1769.

152. Taivassalo T, Fu K, Johns T, et al. Gene shifting: a novel therapy for mitochondrial myopathy. Hum Mol Genet 1999; 8:1047–1052.

153. Kawakami Y, Sakuta R, Hashimoto K, et al. Mitochondrial myopathy with progressive decrease in mitochondrial tRNALeu(UUR) mutant genomes. Ann Neurol 1994; 35:370–373.

154. Taivassalo T, Shoubridge EA, Chen J, et al. Aerobic conditioning in patients with mitochondrial myopathies: physiological, biochemical, and genetic effects. Ann Neurol 2001; 50:133–141.

155. Khan SM, Bennett Jr JP. Development of mitochondrial gene replacement therapy. J Bioenerg Biomembr 2004; 36:387–393.

156. Collombet J-M, Coutelle C. Towards gene therapy of mitochondrial disorders. Mol Med Today 1998; 4:31–38.

157. Bull LN, van Eijk MJ, Pawlikowska L, et al. A gene encoding a P-type ATPase mutated in two forms of hereditary cholestasis. Nat Genet 1998; 18:219–224.

158. Applegarth DA, Toone JR, Lowry RB. Incidence of inborn errors of metabolism in British Columbia, 1969–1996. Pediatrics 2000; 105:e10.

159. Meikle PJ, Hopwood JJ, Clague AE, et al. Prevalence of lysosomal storage disorders. JAMA 1999; 28:249–254.

160. Platt FM, Reinkensmeier G, Dwek RA, et al. Extensive glycosphingolipid depletion in the liver and lymphoid organs of mice treated with N-butyldeoxynojirimycin. J Biol Chem 1997; 272:19365–19372.

161. Norflus F, Tifft CJ, McDonald MP, et al. Bone marrow transplantation prolongs life span and ameliorates neurologic manifestations in Sandhoff disease mice. J Clin Invest 1998; 101:1881–1888.

162. Jacobs JF, Willemsen MA, Groot-Loonen JJ, et al. Allogeneic BMT followed by substrate reduction therapy in a child with subacute Tay–Sachs disease. Bone Marrow Transplant 2005; 36:925–936.

163. Ringden O, Groth CG, Erikson A, et al. Ten years' experience of bone marrow transplantation for Gaucher disease. Transplantation 1995; 59:864–870.

164. Barton NW, Brady RO, Dambrosia JM, et al. Replacement therapy for inherited enzyme deficiency—macrophage-targeted glucocerebrosidase for Gaucher's disease. N Engl J Med 1991; 324:1464–1470.

165. Charrow J, Esplin JA, Gribble TJ, et al. Gaucher disease: recommendations on diagnosis, evaluation, and monitoring. Arch Intern Med 1998; 158:1754–1760.

166. Cox T, Lachmann R, Hollak C, et al. Novel oral treatment of Gaucher's disease with N-butyldeoxynoj-irimycin (OGT 918) to decrease substrate biosynthesis. Lancet 2000; 355:1481–1485.

167. Schiffmann R, Kopp JB, Austin 3rd HA, et al. Enzyme replacement therapy in Fabry disease: a randomized controlled trial. JAMA 2001; 285:2743–2749.

168. Wilcox WR, Banikazemi M, Guffon N, et al. International Fabry Disease Study Group. Long-term safety and efficacy of enzyme replacement therapy for Fabry disease. Am J Hum Genet 2004; 75:65–74.

169. Eng CM, Guffon N, Wilcox WR, et al. Safety and efficacy of recombinant human-galactosidase A replacement therapy in Fabry's disease. N Engl J Med 2001; 345:9–16.

170. Krivit W, Shapiro E, Kennedy W, et al. Treatment of late infantile metachromatic leukodystrophy by bone marrow transplantation. N Engl J Med 1990; 322:28–32.

171. Krivit W, Shapiro EG, Peters C, et al. Hematopoietic stem-cell transplantation in globoid-cell leukodystrophy. N Engl J Med 1998; 338:1119–1126.

172. Escolar ML, Poe MD, Provenzale JM, et al. Transplantation of umbilical-cord blood in babies with infantile Krabbe's disease. N Engl J Med 2005; 352:2069–2081.

173. Kakkis ED, Muenzer J, Tiller GE, et al. Enzyme-replacement therapy in mucopolysaccharidosis I. N Engl J Med 2001; 344:182–188.

174. Krivit W. Allogeneic stem cell transplantation for the treatment of lysosomal and peroxisomal metabolic diseases. Springer Semin Immunopathol 2004; 26:119–132.

175. Wraith JE, Clarke LA, Beck M, et al. Enzyme replacement therapy for mucopolysaccharidosis I: a randomized, double-blinded, placebo-controlled, multinational study of recombinant human alpha-L-iduronidase (laronidase). J Pediatr 2004; 144:581–588.

176. Muenzer J, Wraith JE, Beck M, et al. A phase II/III clinical study of enzyme replacement therapy with idursulfase in mucopolysaccharidosis II (Hunter syndrome). Genet Med 2006; 8:465–473.

177. Harmatz P, Giugliani R, Schwartz I, et al. VI Phase 3 Study Group. Enzyme replacement therapy for mucopolysaccharidosis VI: a phase 3, randomized, double-blind, placebo-controlled, multinational study of recombinant human N-acetylgalactosamine 4-sulfatase (recombinant human arylsulfatase B or rhASB) and follow-on, open-label extension study. Pediatrics 2006; 148:533–539.

178. Harmatz P, Whitley C, Belan K, et al. A phase I/II double blind two dose group study of rhASB enzyme replacement therapy in patients with MPS VI (Maroteaux–Lamy syndrome). Am J Hum Genet 2001; 69(suppl):674, A2896.

179. Van den Hout H, Reuser AJ, Vulto AG, et al. Recombinant human alpha-glucosidase from rabbit milk in Pompe patients. Lancet 2000; 356:397–398.

180. Amalfitano A, Bengur AR, Morse RP, et al. Recombinant human acid alpha-glucosidase enzyme therapy for infantile glycogen storage disease type II: results of a phase I/II clinical trial. Genet Med 2001; 3:132–138.

181. Kishnani PS, Nicolino M, Voit T, et al. Chinese hamster ovary cell-derived recombinant human acid alpha-glucosidase in infantile-onset Pompe disease. J Pediatr 2006 July; 149(1):89–97.

182. Kishnani PS, Hwu WL, Mandel H, et al. Infantile-onset Pompe Disease Natural History Study Group. A retrospective, multinational, multicenter study on the natural history of infantile-onset Pompe disease. J Pediatr 2006 May; 148(5):671–676.

183. Winkel LP, Hagemans ML, van Doorn PA, et al. The natural course of non-classic Pompe's disease; a review of 225 published cases. J Neurol 2005 Aug; 252(8):875–884.

184. Kishnani PS, Corzo D, Nicolino M, et al. Recombinant human acid (alpha)-glucosidase. Major

clinical benefits in infantile-onset Pompe disease. Neurology 2007; 68:99–109.

185. Kishnani PS, Steiner RD, Bali D, et al. Pompe disease diagnosis and management guideline. Genet Med 2006; 8:267–288.

186. Gould SJ, Raymond GV, Valle D. The peroxisome biogenesis disorders. In: Scriver CR, Beaudet AL, Sly WS, et al, eds. The metabolic and molecular basis of inherited disease, 8th edn. New York: McGraw-Hill; 2001.2287–2324.

187. Suzuki Y, Shimozawa N, Imamura A, et al. Clinical, biochemical and genetic aspects and neuronal migration in peroxisome biogenesis disorders. J Inherit Metab Dis 2001; 24:151–165.

188. McKusick VA, eds. Online Mendelian Inheritance in Man. 2001. http://www3.ncbi.nlm.nih.gov/Omim/ed

189. Steinberg SJ, Raymond GV, Braverman NE, et al. Peroxisome biogenesis disorders, Zellweger spectrum. In: Gene reviews at Gene Tests: Medical Genetics Information Resource. Available at: http://www.genetests.org

190. Van Woerden CS, Groothoff JW, Wijburg FA, et al. High incidence of hyperoxaluria in generalized peroxisomal disorders. Mol Genet Metab 2006; 88:346–350.

191. Braverman NE, Moser AB, Steinberg SJ. Rhizomelic chondrodysplasia punctata type 1. In: Gene Reviews at Gene Tests: Medical Genetics Information Resource. Available at: http://www.genetests.org.

192. Brown L-A, Baker A. Peroxisome biogenesis and the role of protein import. J Cell Mol Med 2003; 7:388–400.

193. Walter C, Gootjes J, Mooijer PA, et al. Disorders of peroxisome biogenesis due to mutations in PEX1: phenotypes and PEX1 protein levels. Am J Hum Genet 2002; 69:35–48.

194. Steinberg S, Chen L, Wei L, et al. The PEX gene screen: molecular diagnosis of peroxisome biogenesis disorders in the Zellweger syndrome spectrum. Mol Genet Metab 2004; 83:252–263.

195. Kohji M, Akihiko D, Yasuhiko Y, et al. Oral bile acid treatment in two Japanese patients with Zellweger syndrome. J Pediatr Gastroenterol Nutr 2002; 35:227–230.

196. Martinez M. Restoring the DHA levels in the brains of Zellweger patients. J Mol Neurosci 2001; 16:309–316.

197. Wei H, Kemp S, McGuinness MC, et al. Pharmacological induction of peroxisomes in peroxisome biogenesis disorders. Ann Neurol 2000; 47:286–296.

198. Moser HW, Smith KD, Watkins PA, et al. X-linked adrenoleukodystrophy. In: Scriver CR, Beaudet AL, Sly WS, et al, eds. The metabolic and molecular basis of inherited disease, 8th edn. New York: McGraw-Hill; 2001.3257–3293.

199. Moser HW, Moser AB, Steinberg SJ. X-linked adrenoleukodystrophy. In: Gene Reviews at Gene Tests: Medical Genetics Information Resource. Available at: http://www.genetests.org.

200. Shapiro E, Krivit W, Lockman L, et al. Long-term beneficial effect of bone marrow transplantation of childhood-onset cerebral X-linked adrenoleukodystrophy. Lancet 2000; 356:713–718.

201. Van Geel BM, Assies J, Haverkort EB, et al. Progression of abnormalities in adrenomyeloneuropathy and neurologically asymptomatic X-linked adrenoleukodystrophy despite treatment with 'Lorenzo's oil'. J Neurol Neurosurg Psychiatry 1999; 67:290–299.

202. Moser HW, Raymond GV, Lu S-E, et al. Follow-up of 89 asymptomatic patients with adrenoleukodystrophy treated with Lorenzo's oil. Arch Neurol 2005; 62:1073–1080.

203. Pai GS, Khan M, Barbosa E, et al. Lovastatin for X-linked adrenoleukodystrophy: clinical and biochemical observations in 12 patients. Mol Genet Metab 2000; 69:312–322.

204. Verrips A, Michel AAP, Wilemsen MD, et al. Simvastatin and plasma very-long-chain fatty acids in X-linked adrenoleukodystrophy. Ann Neurol 2000; 47:552–553.

205. Wanders RJA, Jacobs C, Skjeldal OH. Refsum disease. In: Scriver CR, Beaudet AL, Sly WS, et al, eds. The metabolic and molecular basis of inherited disease, 8th edn. New York: McGraw-Hill; 2001.3303–3321.

206. Wanders RJA, Waterham HR, Leroy BP. Refsum disease. In: Gene Reviews at Gene Tests: Medical Genetics Information Resource. Available at: http://www.genetests.org.

207. Jaeken J, Carchon H. Congenital disorders of glycosylation: a booming chapter of pediatrics. Curr Opin Pediatr 2004; 16:434–439.

208. Freeze HH. Disorders in protein glycosylation and potential therapy: tip of the iceberg? J Pediatr 1998; 133:593–600.

209. Jaeken J, Carchon H. Congenital disorders of glycosylation: the rapidly growing tip of the iceberg. Curr Opin Neurol 2001; 14:811–815.

210. Eklund EA, Freeze HH. The congenital disorders of glycosylation: a multifaceted group of syndromes. NeuroRx 2006; 3:254–263.

211. Sparks SE. Inherited disorders of glycosylation. Mol Genet Metab 2006; 87:1–7.

212. Jaeken J, Matthijs G. Congenital disorders of glycosylation. Annu Rev Genomics Hum Genet 2001; 2:129–151.

213. Blennow G, Jaeken J, Wiklund LM. Neurological findings in the carbohydrate-deficient glycoprotein syndrome. Acta Paediatr Scand 1991; 375(suppl):14–20.

214. Jaeken J, Hagberg B, Stromme P. Clinical presentation and natural course of the carbohydrate-deficient glycoprotein syndrome. Acta Paediatr Scand 1991; 375(suppl):6–13.

215. Barone R, Pavone L, Fiumara A, et al. Developmental patterns and neuropsychological assessment in patients with carbohydrate-deficient glycoconjugate syndrome type IA (phosphomannomutase deficiency). Brain Develop 1999; 21:260–263.

216. van Ommem CH, Peters M, Barth PG, et al. Carbohydrate-deficient glycoprotein syndrome type 1a: a variant phenotype with borderline cognitive dysfunction, cerebellar hypoplasia, and coagulation disturbances. J Pediatr 2000; 136:400–403.

217. Grünewald S, Schollen E, van Schaftingen E, et al. High residual activity of PMM2 in fibroblasts: possible pitfall in the diagnosis of CDG-Ia (phosphomannomutase deficiency). Am J Hum Genet 2001; 68:347–354.

218. Schoffer KL, O'sullivan JD, McGill J. Congenital disorder of glycosylation type Ia presenting as early-onset cerebellar ataxia in an adult. Mov Disord 2006; 21:869–872.

219. Charlwood J, Clayton P, Keir G, et al. Prenatal diagnosis of the carbohydrate-deficiency glycoprotein syndrome type 1A (CDG1A) by a combination of enzymology and genetic linkage analysis after amniocentesis or chorionic villus sampling. Prenat Diagn 1998; 18:693–699.

220. Mayatepek E, Schröder M, Kohlmüller D, et al. Continuous mannose infusion in carbohydrate-deficient glycoprotein syndrome type I. Acta Paediatr 1997; 86:1138–1140.

221. Kjaergaard S, Kristiansson B, Stibler H, et al. Failure of short-term mannose therapy of patients with carbohydrate-deficient glycoprotein syndrome type IA. Acta Paediatr 1998; 87:884–888.

222. Niehues R, Hasilik M, Alton G, et al. Carbohydrate-deficient glycoprotein syndrome type Ib: phosphomannose isomerase deficiency and mannose therapy. J Clin Invest 1998; 101:1414–1420.

223. Babovic-Vuksanovic D, Patterson MC, Schwenk WF, et al. Severe hypoglycemia as a presenting symptom of carbohydrate-deficient glycoprotein syndrome. J Pediatr 1999; 135:775–781.

224. de Lonlay P, Cuer M, Vuillaumier-Barrot S, et al. Hyperinsulinemic hypoglycemia as a presenting sign in phosphomannose isomerase deficiency: a new manifestation of carbohydrate-deficient glycoprotein syndrome treatable with mannose. J Pediatr 1999; 135:179–183.

225. Damen G, de Klerk H, Huijmans J. Gastrointestinal and other clinical manifestations in 17 children with congenital disorders of glycosylation type Ia, Ib, and Ic. J Pediatr Gastroenterol Nutr 2004; 38:282–287.

226. de Lonlay P, Seta N, Barrot S, et al. A broad spectrum of clinical presentations in congenital disorders of glycosylation I: a series of 26 cases. J Med Genet 2001; 38:14–19.

227. Kahook MY, Mandava N, Bateman JB, et al. Glycosylation type Ic disorder: idiopathic intracranial hypertension and retinal degeneration. Br J Ophthalmol 2006; 90:115–116.

228. Schollen E, Grunewald S, Keldermans L, et al. CDG-Id caused by homozygosity for an ALG3 mutation due to segmental maternal isodisomy UPD3 (q21.3-qter). Eur J Med Genet 2005; 48:153–158.

229. Garcia-Silva MT, Matthijs G, Schollen E, et al. Congenital disorder of glycosylation (CDG) type Ie. A new patient. J Inherit Metab Dis 2004; 27:591–600.

230. Schenk B, Imbach T, Frank CG, et al. MPDU1 mutations underlie a novel human congenital disorder of glycosylation, designated type If. J Clin Invest 2001; 108:1687–1695.

231. Grubenmann CE, Frank CG, Kjaergaard S, et al. ALG12 mannosyltransferase defect in congenital disorder of glycosylation type 1g. Hum Mol Genet 2002; 11:2331–2339.

232. Eklund EA, Sun L, Westphal V, et al. Congenital disorder of glycosylation (CDG)-Ih patient with a severe hepato-intestinal phenotype and evolving central nervous system pathology. J Pediatr 2005; 147:847–850.

233. Thiel C, Schwarz M, Peng J, et al. A new type of congenital disorder of glycosylation (CDG-Ii) provides new insights into the early steps of dolichol-linked oligosaccharide biosynthesis. J Biol Chem 2003; 278:22498–22505.

234. Wu X, Rush JS, Karaoglu D, et al. Deficiency of UDP-GlcNAc: Dolichol phosphate-N-acetylglucosamine-1 phosphate transferase (DPAGT1) causes a novel congenital disorder of Glycosylation Type Ij. Hum Mutat 2003; 22:144–150.

235. Kranz C, Denecke J, Lehle L, et al. Congenital disorder of glycosylation type type Ik (CDG-Ik): a defect of mannosyltransferase I. Am J Hum Genet 2004; 74:545–551.

236. Weinstein M, Schollen E, Matthijs G, et al. CDG-IL: an infant with a novel mutation in the ALG9 gene and additional phenotypic features. Am J Med Genet 2005; 136:194–197.

237. Jaeken J, Schachter H, Carchon H, et al. Carbohydrate deficient glycoprotein syndrome type II: a deficiency in Golgi localised N-acetyl-glucosaminyltransferase II. Arch Dis Child 1994; 71:123–127.

238. Cornier-Daire V, Amiel J, Vuillaumier-Barrot S, et al. Congenital disorders of glycosylation IIa cause growth retardation, mental retardation, and facial dysmorphism. J Med Genet 2000; 37:875–877.

239. Van Geet C, Jaeken J, Freson K, et al. Congenital disorders of glycosylation type Ia and IIa are associated with different primary haemostatic complications. J Inherit Metab Dis 2001; 24:477–492.

240. De Praeter CM, Gerwig GJ, Bause E, et al. A novel disorder caused by defective biosynthesis of N-linked oligosaccharides due to glucosidase I deficiency. Am J Hum Genet 2000; 66:1744–1756.

241. Volker C, De Praeter CM, Hardt B, et al. Processing of N-linked carbohydrate chains in a patient with glucosidase I deficiency (CDG type IIb). Glycobiology 2002; 12:473–483.

242. Etzioni A, Sturla L, Antonellis A, et al. Leukocyte adhesion deficiency (LAD) type II/carbohydrate deficient glycoprotein (CDG) IIc founder effect and genotype/phenotype correlation. Am J Med Genet 2002; 110:131–135.

243. Foulquier F, Vasile E, Schollen E, et al. Conserved oligomeric Golgi complex subunit 1 deficiency reveals a previously uncharacterized congenital disorder of glycosylation type II. Proc Natl Acad Sci U S A 2006; 103:3764–3769.

244. Steet R, Kornfeld S. COG-7-deficient human fibroblasts exhibit altered recycling of golgi proteins. Mol Biol Cell 2006; 17:2312–2321.

245. Wopereis S, Morava E, Grunewald S, et al. Patients with unsolved congenital disorders of glycosylation type II can be subdivided in six distinct biochemical groups. Glycobiology 2005; 15:1312–1319.

246. Martinez-Duncker I, Dupre T, Piller V, et al. Genetic complementation reveals a novel human congenital disorder of glycosylation of type II, due to inactivation of the Golgi CMP-sialic acid transporter. Blood 2005; 105:2671–2676.

247. Valmu L, Kalkkinen N, Husa A, et al. Differential susceptibility of transferrin glycoforms to chymotrypsin: a proteomics approach to the detection of carbohydrate-deficient transferring. Biochemistry 2005; 44:16007–16013.

248. Zamfir A, Peter-Katalinic J. Glycoscreening by on-line sheathless capillary electrophoresis/electrospray ionization-quadrupole time of flight-tandem mass spectrometry. Electrophoresis 2001; 22:2448–2457.

249. Simpson MA, Cross H, Proukakis C, et al. Infantile-onset symptomatic epilepsy syndrome caused by a homozygous loss-of-function mutation of GM3 synthase. Nat Genet 2004; 36:1225–1229.

250. Blau N, Thony B, Cotton RGH, et al. Disorders of tetrahydrobiopterin and related biogenic amines. In: Scriver CR, Beaudet AL, Sly WS, et al, eds. The molecular and metabolic bases of inherited disease, 8th edn. New York: McGraw-Hill; 2001:1725–1776.

251. Bonafe L, Blau N, Burlina AP, et al. Treatable neurotransmitter deficiency in mild phenylketonuria. Neurology 2001; 57:908–911.

252. Rajput AH. The protective role of levodopa in the human substantia nigra. Adv Neurol 2001; 86:327–336.

253. Paterson DS, Trachtenberg FL, Thompson EC, et al. Multiple serotonineric brainstem abnormalities in sudden infant death syndrome. J Am Med Assoc 2006; 296:2124–2132.

254. Eells JB, Rives JE, Yeung SK, et al. In vitro regulated expression of tyrosine hydroxylase in ventral midbrain neurons from Nurr1-null mouse pups. J Neurosci Res 2001; 64:322–330.

255. Hoffman GF, Assmann B, Brautigam C, et al. Tyrosine hydroxylase deficiency causes progressive encephalopathy and dopa-nonresponsive dystonia. Ann Neurol 2003; 54:S56–S65.

256. Bonafe L, Thony B, Leimbacher W, et al. Diagnosis of dopa-responsive dystonia and other tetrahydrobiopterin disorders by the study of biopterin metabolism in fibroblasts. Clin Chem 2001; 47:477–485.

257. Moller LB, Romstad A, Paulsen M, et al. Pre- and postnatal diagnosis of tyrosine hydroxylase deficiency. Prenat Diagn 2005; 25:671–675.

258. Pons R, Ford B, Chriboga CA, et al. Aromatic L-amino acid decarboxylase deficiency: Clinical features, treatment and prognosis. Neurology 2004; 62:1058–1065.

259. Swoboda KJ, Saul JP, McKenna CE, et al. Aromatic L-aminoacid decarboxylase deficiency: Overview of clinical features and outcomes. Ann Neurol 2003; 54:S49–S55.

260. Segawa M, Nomura Y, Nichiyama N. Autosomal dominant guanosine triphosphate cyclohydrolase

I deficiency (Segawa disease). Ann Neurol 2003; 54:S32–S45.

261. Van Hove JLK, Steyaert J, Matthijs G, et al. Expanded motor and psychiatric phenotype in autosomal dominant Segawa syndrome due to GTP cyclohydrolase deficiency. J Neurol Neurosurg Psychiatry 2006; 77:18–23.

262. Bonafe L, Thony B, Penzien JM, et al. Mutations in the sepiapterin reductase gene cause a novel tetrahydrobiopterin-dependent monoamine-neurotransmitter deficiency without hyperphenylalaninemia. Am J Hum Genet 2001; 69:269–277.

263. Cryan JF, Dalvi A, Jin SH, et al. Use of dopamine-beta-hydroxylase-deficient mice to determine the role of norepinephrine in the mechanism of action of antidepressant drugs. J Pharmacol Exp Ther 2001; 298:651–657.

264. Denium J, Steenbergen-Spanjers GCH, Jansen M, et al. DBH gene variants that cause low plasma dopamine beta hydrozylase with or without a severe orthostatic syndrome. J Med Genet 2004; 41:e38.

265. Salichon N, Gaspar P, Upton AL, et al. Excessive activation of serotonin (5-HT) 1B receptors disrupts the formation of sensory maps in monoamine oxidase A and 5-HT transporter knock-out mice. J Neurosci 2001; 21:884–896.

266. Hyland K. The lumbar puncture for diagnosis of pediatric neurotransmitter diseases. Ann Neurol 2003; 54:S13–S17.

267. Abdenur JE, Abeling N, Specola N, et al. Aromatic L-aminoacid decarboxylase deficiency: unusual neonatal presentation and additional findings in organic acid analysis. Mol Genet Metab 2006; 87:48–53.

268. Bandmann O, Goertz M, Zschocke J, et al. The phenylalanine loading test in the differential diagnosis of dystonia. Neurology 2003; 60:700–702.

269. Swoboda KJ, Hyland K. Diagnosis and treatment of neurotransmitter-related disorders. Neurol Clin 2002; 20:1143–1161.

270. van Sponsen FJ, van Rijn M, Bekhof J, et al. Phenylketonuria: tyrosine supplementation in phenylalanine-restricted diets. Am J Clin Nutr 2001; 73:153–157.

271. Kalsner LR, Rohr FJ, Strauss KA, et al. Tyrosine supplementation in phenylketonuria: diurnal blood tyrosine levels and presumptive brain influx of tyrosine and other large neutral amino acids. J Pediatr 2001; 139:421–427.

272. Agostoni C, Scaglioni S, Bonvissuto M, et al. Biochemical effects of supplemented long-chain polyunsaturated fatty acids in hyperphenylalaninemia. Prostaglandins Leukot Essent Fatty Acids 2001; 64:111–115.

273. Haussler M, Hoffmann GF, Wevers RA. L-dopa and selegiline for tyrosine hydroxylase deficiency. J Pediatr 2001; 138:451.

274. Brandmann O, Wood NW. Dopa responsive dystonia – The story so far. Neuropediatrics 2002; 33:1–5.

275. Mink JW. Dopa-responsive dystonia in children. Curr Treat Opt Neurol 2003; 5:279–282.

276. Uncini A, De Angelis MV, Di Fulvio P, et al. Wide expressivity variation and high but no gender-related penetrance in two dopa-responsive dystonia families with a novel GCH-I mutation. Mov Disord 2004; 19:1139–1145.

277. Hwang WJ, Calne DB, Tsui JK, et al. The long-term response to levodopa in dopa-responsive dystonia. Parkinsonism Relat Disord 2001; 8:1–5.

278. Dionisi-Vici C, Hoffmann GF, Leuzzi V, et al. Tyrosine hydroxylase deficiency with severe clinical course: clinical and biochemical investigations and optimization of therapy. J Pediatr 2000; 136:560–562.

279. Pearl PL, Capp PK, Novotny EJ, et al. Inherited disorders of neurotransmitters in children and adults. Clin Biochem 2005; 38:1051–1058.

280. Simmonds HA. Purine and pyrimidine disorders. In: Blau N, Duran M, Blaskovics ME, eds. Physician's guide to the laboratory diagnosis of metabolic diseases. London: Chapman & Hall; 1996.341–357.

281. Jinnah HA, Visser JE, Harris JC, et al. Delineation of the motor disorder of Lesch–Nyhan disease. Brain 2006; 129:1201–1217.

282. Schretlen DJ, Ward J, Meyer SM, et al. Behavioral aspects of Lesch–Nyhan disease and its variants. Dev Med Child Neurol 2005; 47:673–677.

283. Becker MA. Hyperuricemia and gout. In: Scriver CR, Beaudet AL, Sly WS, et al, eds. The molecular and metabolic bases of inherited disease, 8th edn. New York: McGraw-Hill; 2001.2513–2536.

284. Jinnah HA, Friedmann T. Lesch–Nyhan disease and its variants. In: Scriver CR, Beaudet AL, Sly WS, et al, eds. The molecular and metabolic bases of inherited disease, 8th edn. New York: McGraw-Hill; 2001:2537–2570.

285. Hall S, Oliver C, Murphy G. Self-injurious behaviour in young children with Lesch–Nyhan syndrome. Dev Med Child Neurol 2001; 43:745–749.

286. Allen SM, Rice SN. Risperidone antagonism of self-mutilation in a Lesch–Nyhan patient. Prog Neuropsychopharmacol Biol Psychiatry 1996; 20:793–800.

287. Cossu A, Micheli V, Jacomelli G, et al. Kelley–Seegmiller syndrome in a patient with complete hypoxanthine-guanine phosphoribosyltransferase deficiency. Clin Exp Rheumatol 2002; 20:851–853.

288. Sahota AS, Tischfield JA, Kamatani N, et al. Adenine phosphoribosyltransferase deficiency and 2,8-dihydroxyadenine lithiasis. In: Scriver CR, Beaudet AL, Sly WS, et al, eds. The molecular and metabolic bases of inherited disease, 8th edn. New York: McGraw-Hill; 2001:2571–2584.

289. Nyhan WL. Disorders of purine and pyrimidine metabolism. Mol Genet Metab 2005; 86:25–33.

290. Van den Berghe G, Jaeken J. Adenylosuccinate lyase deficiency. In: Scriver CR, Beaudet AL, Sly WS, et al, eds. The molecular and metabolic bases of inherited disease, 8th edn. New York: McGraw-Hill; 2001.2653–2662.

291. Ciardo F, Salerno C, Curatolo P. Neurologic aspects of adenylosuccinate lyase deficiency. J Child Neurol 2001; 16:301–308.

292. Edery P, Chabrier S, Ceballos-Picot I, et al. Intrafamilial variability in the phenotypic expression of adenylosuccinate lyase deficiency: a report on three patients. Am J Med Genet A 2003; 120:185–190.

293. Castro M, Perez-Cerda C, Merinero B, et al. Screening for adenylosuccinate lyase deficiency: clinical, biochemical and molecular findings in four patients. Neuropediatrics 2002; 33:186–189.

294. Raivio KO, Saksela M, Lapatto R. Xanthine oxidoreductases – role in human pathophysiology and in hereditary xanthinuria. In: Scriver CR, Beaudet AL, Sly WS, et al, eds. The molecular and metabolic bases of inherited disease, 8th edn. New York: McGraw-Hill; 2001; 2639–2652.

295. Gille L, Staniek K, Nohl H. Effects of tocopheryl quinone on the heart: model experiments with xanthine oxidase, heart mitochondria, and isolated perfused rat hearts. Free Radic Biol Med 2001; 30:865–876.

296. Ichida K, Matsumura T, Sakuma R, et al. Mutation of human molybdenum cofactor sulfurase gene is responsible for classical xanthinuria type II. Biochem Biophys Res Commun 2001; 282:1194–1200.

297. Ohtsubo T, Rovira II, Starost MF, et al. Xanthine oxidoreductase is an endogenous regulator of cyclooxygenase-2. Circ Res 2004; 95:1118–1124.

298. Hobson EE, Thomas S, Crafton PM, et al. Isolated sulphite oxidase deficiency mimics the features of hypoxic ischaemic encephalopathy. Eur J Pediatr 2005; 164:655–659.

299. Sass JO, Kishikawa M, Puttinger R, et al. Hypohomocysteinaemia and highly increased proportion of S-sulfonated plasma transthyretin in

molybdenum cofactor deficiency. J Inherit Metab Dis 2003; 26:80–82.

300. Deutsch SI, Long KD, Rosse RB, et al. Hypothesized deficiency of guanine-based purines may contribute to abnormalities of neurodevelopment, neuromodulation, and neurotransmission in Lesch–Nyhan syndrome. Clin Neuropharmacol 2005; 28:28–37.

301. Chiarelli LR, Bianchi P, Fermo E, et al. Functional analysis of pyrimidine 5′-nucleotidase mutants causing nonspherocytic hemolytic anemia. Blood 2005; 105:3340–3345.

302. Hershfield MS, Mitchell BS. Immunodeficiency diseases caused by adenosine deaminase deficiency and purine nucleoside phosphorylase deficiency. In: Scriver CR, Beaudet AL, Sly WS, et al, eds. The molecular and metabolic bases of inherited disease, 8th edn. New York: McGraw-Hill; 2001:2585–2626.

303. Hershfield MS. Genotype is an important determinant of phenotype in adenosine deaminase deficiency. Curr Opin Immunol 2003; 15:571–577.

304. Apasov SG, Blackburn MR, Kellems RE, et al. Adenosine deaminase deficiency increases thymic apoptosis and causes defective T cell receptor signaling. J Clin Invest 2001; 108:131–141.

305. Blackburn MR, Kellems RE. Adenosine deaminase deficiency: metabolic basis of immune deficiency and pulmonary inflammation. Adv Immunol 2005; 86:1–41.

306. Tullo A, Mastropasqua G, Bourdon JC, et al. Adenosine deaminase, a key enzyme in DNA precursors control, is a new p73 target. Oncogene 2003; 22:8738–8748.

307. Grunebaum E, Zhang J, Roifman CM. Novel mutations and hot-spots in patients with purine nucleoside phosphorylase deficiency. Nucleosides Nucleotides Nucleic Acids 2004; 23:1411–1415.

308. Myers LA, Hershfield MS, Neale WT, et al. Purine nucleoside phosphorylase deficiency (PNP-def) presenting with lymphopenia and developmental delay: successful correction with umbilical cord blood transplantation. J Pediatr 2004; 145:710–712.

309. Dror Y, Grunebaum E, Hitzler J, et al. Purine nucleoside phosphorylase deficiency associated with a dysplastic marrow morphology. Pediatr Res 2004; 55:472–477.

310. Sabine RL, Holmes EW. Myoadenylate deaminase deficiency. In: Scriver CR, Beaudet AL, Sly WS, et al, eds. The molecular and metabolic bases of inherited disease, 8th edn. New York: McGraw-Hill; 2001:2627–2638.

311. Sabbatini AR, Toscano A, Aguennouz M, et al. Immunohistochemical analysis of human skeletal muscle AMP deaminase deficiency. Evidence of a correlation between the muscle HPRG content and the level of the residual AMP deaminase activity. J Muscle Res Cell Motil 2006; 27:83–92.

312. Scola RH, Iwamoto FM, Camargo CH, et al. Myotonia congenita and myoadenylate deaminase deficiency: case report. Arq Neuropsiquiatr 2003; 61:262–264.

313. Evans WE, Hon YY, Bomgaars L, et al. Preponderance of thiopurine S-methyltransferase deficiency and heterozygosity among patients intolerant to mercaptopurine or azathioprine. J Clin Oncol 2001; 19:2293–2301.

314. Frohman EM, Havrdova E, Levinson B, et al. Azathioprine myelosuppression in multiple sclerosis: characterizing thiopurine methyltransferase polymorphisms. Mult Scler 2006; 12:108–111.

315. Evans WE. Pharmacogenetics of thiopurine S-methyltransferase and thiopurine therapy. Ther Drug Monit 2004; 26:186–191.

316. Carbonaro DA, Jin X, Petersen D, et al. In vivo transduction by intravenous injection of a lentiviral vector expressing human ADA into neonatal ADA gene knockout mice: A novel form of enzyme replacement therapy for ADA deficiency. Mol Ther 2006; 13:1110–1120.

317. Webster DR, Becroft DMO, van Gennip AH, et al. Hereditary orotic aciduria and other disorders of pyrimidine metabolism. In: Scriver CR, Beaudet AL, Sly WS, et al, eds. The molecular and metabolic bases of inherited disease, 8th edn. New York: McGraw-Hill; 2001.2663–2704.

318. Yu J, McLeod HL, Ezzeldin HH, et al. Methylation of the DPYD promoter and dihydropyrimidine dehydrogenase deficiency. Clin Cancer Res 2006; 12:3864.

319. Ezzeldin HH, Lee AM, Mattison LK, et al. Methylation of the DPYD promoter: an alternative mechanism for dihydropyrimidine dehydrogenase deficiency in cancer patients. Clin Cancer Res 2005; 11:8699–8705.

320. Kuhara T, Ohdoi C, Ohse M. Simple gas chromatographic-mass spectrometric procedure for diagnosing pyrimidine degradation defects for prevention of severe anticancer side effects. J Chromatogr B Biomed Sci Appl 2001; 758:61–74.

321. Altundag O, Altundag K, Silay K, et al. Gender differences in the dihydropyrimidine dehydrogenase expression may contribute to higher toxicity in women treated with 5-fluoroacil therapy. Med Hypoth 2005; 65:1196.

322. Moolenaar SH, Gohlich-Ratmann G, Engelke UF, et al. Beta-ureidopropionase deficiency: a novel inborn error of metabolism discovered using NMR spectroscopy on urine. Magn Reson Med 2001; 46:1014–1017.

323. Assmann B, Gohlich G, Baethmann M, et al. Clinical findings and a therapeutic trial in the first patient with beta-ureidopropionase deficiency. Neuropediatrics 2006; 37:20–25.

324. van Kuilenburg AB, Meinsma R, Beke E, et al. Beta-ureidopropionase deficiency: an inborn error of pyrimidine degradation associated with neurological abnormalities. Hum Mol Genet 2004; 13:2793–2801.

325. Assmann BE, Van Kuilenburg AM, Distekmaier F, et al. Beta-ureidopropionase deficiency presenting with febrile status epilepticus. Epilepsia 2006; 47:215–217.

326. Nishino I, Spinazzola A, Hirano M. MNGIE: from nuclear DNA to mitochondrial DNA. Neuromuscl Disord 2001; 11:7–10.

327. Hirano M, Marti R, Spinazzola A, et al. Thymidine phosphorylase deficiency causes MNGIE: an autosomal recessive mitochondrial disorder. Nucleosides Nucleotides Nucleic Acids 2004; 23:1217–1225.

328. la Marca G, Malvagia S, Casetta B, et al. Pre- and post-dialysis quantitative dosage of thymidine in urine and plasma of a MNGIE patient by using HPLC-ESI-MS/MS. J Mass Spectrom 2006; 41:586–592.

329. Bedlack RS, Vu T, Hammans S, et al. MNGIE neuropathy: five cases mimicking chronic inflammatory demyelinating polyneuropathy. Muscle Nerve 2004; 29:364–368.

330. Labauge P, Durant R, Castelnovo G, et al. MNGIE: diarrhea and leukoencephalopathy. Neurology 2002; 58:1862.

331. Hartmann S, Okun JG, Schmidt C, et al. Comprehensive detection of disorders of purine and pyrimidine metabolism by HPLC with electrospray ionization tandem mass spectrometry. Clin Chem 2006; 52:1127–1137.

332. Czarnecka J, Cieslak M, Michal K. Application of solid phase extraction and high-performance liquid chromatography to qualitative and quantitative analysis of nucleotides and nucleosides in human cerebrospinal fluid. J Chromatogr B Analyt Technol Biomed Life Sci 2005; 822:85–90.

333. Adam T, Lochman P, Friedecky D. Screening method for inherited disorders of purine and pyrimidine metabolism by capillary electrophoresis with reversed electroosmotic flow. J Chromatogr B Analyt Technol Biomed Life Sci 2002; 767:333–340.

334. Friedecky D, Adam T, Bartak P. Capillary electrophoresis for detection of inherited disorders of purine and pyrimidine metabolism: a selective approach. Electrophoresis 2002; 23:565–571.

335. Mattison LK, Fourie J, Hirao Y, et al. The Uracil breath test in the assessment of dihydropyrimidine dehydrogenase activity: pharmacokinetic relationship between expired $^{13}CO_2$ and plasma [2-^{13}C]dihydrouracil. Clin Cancer Res 2006; 12:549–555.

336. Mattison LK, Ezzeldin H, Carpenter M, et al. Rapid identification of dihydropyrimidine dehydrogenase deficiency by using a novel 2-^{13}C-uracil breath test. Clin Cancer Res 2004; 10:2652–2658.

337. Culotta VC, Gitlin JD. Disorders of copper metabolism. In: Scriver CR, Beaudet AL, Sly WS, et al, eds. The molecular and metabolic bases of inherited disease, 8th edn. New York: McGraw-Hill; 2001.3105–3126.

338. Kaler SG. Menkes disease. Adv Pediatr 1994; 41:263–304.

339. Kaler SG, Gahl WA, Berry SA, Holmes CS, et al. Predictive value of plasma catecholamine levels in neonatal detection of Menkes disease. J Inherit Metab Dis 1993; 16:907–908.

340. Tumer Z, Horn N, Tonnesen T, et al. Early copper-histidine treatment for Menkes disease. Nat Genet 1996; 12:11–13.

341. Kaler SG, Buist NR, Holmes CS, et al. Early copper therapy in classic Menkes disease patients with a novel splicing mutation. Ann Neurol 1995; 38:921–928.

342. Gow PJ, Smallwood RA, Angus PW, et al. Diagnosis of Wilson's disease: an experience over three decades. Gut 2000; 46:415–419.

343. Askari FK, Greenson J, Dick RD, et al. Treatment of Wilson's disease with zinc. XVIII. Initial treatment of the hepatic decompensation presentation with trientine and zinc. J Lab Clin Med 2003; 142:385–390.

344. Brewer GJ, Askari F, Lorincz MT, et al. Treatment of Wilson disease with ammonium tetrathiomolybdate: IV. Comparison of tetrathiomolybdate and trientine in a double-blind study of treatment of the neurologic presentation of Wilson disease. Arch Neurol 2006; 63:521–527.

345. Gitlin JD. Aceruloplasminemia. Pediatr Res 1998; 44:271–276.

346. Beutler E, Felitti VJ, Koziol JA, et al. Penetrance of 845G − > A (C282Y) HFE hereditary haemochromatosis mutation in the USA. Lancet 2002; 359:211–218.

347. Bulaj ZJ, Ajioka RS, Phillips JD, et al. Disease-related conditions in relatives of patients with hemochromatosis. N Engl J Med 2000; 343:1529–1535.

348. Powell LW, George DK, McDonnell SM, et al. Diagnosis of hemochromatosis. Ann Intern Med 1998; 129:925–931.

349. Schoenlebe J, Buyon JP, Zitelli BJ, et al. Neonatal hemochromatosis associated with maternal autoantibodies against Ro/SS-A and La/SS-B ribonucleoproteins. Am J Dis Child 1993; 147:1072–1075.

350. Whitington PF, Hibbard JU. High-dose immunoglobulin during pregnancy for recurrent neonatal haemochromatosis. Lancet 2004; 364:1690–1698.

351. Wang K, Zhou B, Kuo YM, et al. A novel member of a zinc transporter family is defective in acrodermatitis enteropathica. Am J Hum Genet 2002; 71:66–73.

352. Anderson KE, Sassa S, Bishop DF, et al. Disorders of heme biosynthesis; X-linked sideroblastic anemia and the porphyrias. In: Scriver CR, Beaudet AL, Sly WS, et al, eds. The molecular and

metabolic bases of inherited disease, 8th edn. New York: McGraw-Hill; 2001.2961–3062.

353. Gross U, Hoffmann GF, Doss MO. Erythropoietic and hepatic porphyrias. J Inherit Metab Dis 2000; 23:641–661.

354. Murphy GM (for the British Photo-dermatology Group). The cutaneous porphyrias: a review. Br J Dermatol 1999; 140:573–581.

355. de Torres I, Demetris AJ, Randhawa PS. Recurrent hepatic allograft injury in erythropoietic porphyria. Transplantation 1996; 61:1412–1433.

356. Zix-Kieffer I, Langer B, Eyer D, et al. Successful cord blood stem cell transplantation for congenital erythropoietic porphyria (Gunther's disease). Bone Marrow Transplant 1996; 18:217–220.

357. Tezcan I, Xu W, Gurgey A, et al. Congenital erythropoietic porphyria successfully treated by allogeneic bone marrow transplantation. Blood 1998; 92:4053–4058.

358. Pawliuk R, Bachelot T, Wise RJ, et al. Long-term cure of the photosensitivity of murine erythropoietic protoporphyria by preselective gene therapy. Nat Med 1999; 5:768–773.

359. Rela M, Muiesan P, Vilca-Melendez H, et al. Auxiliary partial orthotopic liver transplantation for Crigler-Najjar syndrome type I. Ann Surg 1999; 229:565–569.

360. Seppen J, Bakker C, de Jong B, et al. Adeno-associated virus vector serotypes mediate sustained correction of bilirubin UDP glucuronosyltransferase deficiency in rats. Mol Ther 2006; 13:1085–1092.

361. Schmid R. Gilbert's syndrome – a legitimate genetic anomaly. N Engl J Med 1995; 333:1217–1218.

362. Lee JH, Chen HL, Ni YH, et al. Neonatal Dubin–Johnson syndrome: long-term follow-up and MRP2 mutations study. Pediatr Res 2006; 59:584–589.

363. Machida I, Wakusawa S, Sanae F, et al. Mutational analysis of the MRP2 gene and long-term follow-up of Dubin-Johnson syndrome in Japan. J Gastroenterol 2005; 40:366–370.

364. Hyland K, Arnold LA. Value of lumbar puncture in the diagnosis of infantile epilepsy and folinic acid responsive seizures. J Child Neurol 2002; 17(suppl 3):3S48–3S55. discussion 3S56

365. Wolf PL. The significance of transiet hyperphosphatasemia of infancy and childhood to the clinician and clinical pathologist. Arch Pathol Lab Med 1995; 119:774–775.

Appendix 1

Metabolic diseases and their associated abnormalities[1-3]

Results from expanded newborn screening using tandem mass spectrometry (MS/MS) to show the different metabolic diseases and the usual abnormal acyl-carnitines associated with them.

The designation 'C3, C5, etc' denotes the chain length of the metabolites detected. The amino acids are not listed since they are recognized by their own names.

Normal values and reference values vary in different programs and are therefore not provided here.

	Acylcarnitines by MS/MS
Organic acid disorders	
Propionic acidemia	C3
Methylmalonic acidemia	C3,
Malonic acidemia	C3DC
Isobutyryl-CoA dehydrogenase deficiency	C4
Isovaleric acidemia	C5
2-Methylbutyrul-CoA dehydrogenase deficiency	C5
3-Methylcrotonyl-CoA carboxylase deficiency	C5-OH
3-Methylglutaconic aciduria	C5-OH
3-Hydroxy-3-methylglutaric aciduria	C5-OH, C6DC
Holocarboxylase synthetase and biotinidase deficiencies	C5-OH and/or C3
2-Methyl-3-hydroxybutyric aciduria	C5-OH, C5:1
β-Ketothiolase deficiency	C5:1 and/or C5-OH
Glutaric academia type 1 (GAI)	C5DC
Fatty acid oxidation disorders	
Carnitine uptake defect/carnitine transport defect	C0 (low free carnitine)
Short chain acyl-CoA dehydrogenase deficiency (SCAD)	C4
Medium/short chain L-3-hydroxyacyl-CoA dehydrogenase deficiency	C4-OH
Glutaric acidemia type II (multiple acyl-CoA dehydrogenase deficiency [MADD, GAII])	C4–C18 saturated and unsaturated species, C14:1
Medium chain ketoacyl-CoA thiolase deficiency (MCAT)	C8, C8-OH and C10-OH
Medium chain acyl-CoA dehydrogenase deficiency (MCADD)	C6–10, C10:1
2,4-Dienoyl-CoA reductase deficiency	C10:2
Very long chain acyl-CoA dehydrogenase deficiency (VLCAD)	C14, C14:1, C14:2, C16, C16:1, C14:1/C12:1
Carnitine palmitoyltransferase I deficiency (CPT IA)	C0/C16, C0/C18, C0/(C16+C18)
Carnitine palmitoyltransferase II deficiency (CPT II)	C16 (high), C18, C18:1, C0 (low)
Carnitine acylcarnitine translocase deficiency (CACT)	C16, C18:1 (high)
Long chain L-3-hydroxyacyl-CoA dehydrogenase deficiency (LCHAD)	C16-OH and/or C18:1-OH, C16:1,C18-OH
Trifunctional protein deficiency (TFP)	C16-OH and/or C18:1-OH

REFERENCES

1. Zytkovicz TH, Fitzgerald EF, Marsden D, et al. Tandem mass spectrometric analysis for amino, organic, and fatty acid disorders in newborn dried blood spots: a two year summary from the New England Newborn Screening Program. Clin Chem 2001; 47:1945–1955.

2. Sweetman L, Millington DS, Therrell BL, et al. Naming and counting disorders (conditions) included in newborn screening panels. Pediatrics 2006; 117(suppl):S308–S314.

3. Northwest Regional Newborn Screening Program. Oregon State Health Department. Portland, OR, USA.

27

Immunodeficiency

Andrew J Cant, E Graham Davies,Catherine Cale, Andrew R Gennery

INTRODUCTION

'Immunity' describes the immune system response to a given antigenic challenge in a useful (protective) sense. The main role of the immune system is to repel invasion by microorganisms. Abnormalities in this system may increase susceptibility to infection as well as other non-infective problems such as allergy and autoimmunity. Our increased understanding of the immune mechanisms used in handling microbes has led to a better understanding of both primary and secondary immunodeficiency.[1] Conversely, much has been learned of the intricacies of immune function from studying patients with immunodeficiency.

THE IMMUNE SYSTEM

The immune system protects the host from infectious or dangerous microbes in the environment and has evolved to contain or eliminate pathogens in a complex variety of ways. Key to this is the ability to distinguish between host and pathogen. Many of the mechanisms used, as with many of the defense processes, are found in a range of organisms including invertebrates and plants. The more complex parts of the immune system (such as T and B lymphocytes, the key players in adaptive immunity) have evolved to work in tandem with these aspects of recognition systems and innate immunity.

The initial host defense against infection involves innate factors. Physical and chemical barriers play an important role in pathogen exclusion by direct antimicrobial effects or prevention of microbial attachment. Physical barriers such as epithelial surfaces and mucous membranes provide the first line of defense, augmented by hair and cilia in conjunction with respiratory tract mucus secretions, stomach acids and other mucous membrane secretions. Commensal intestinal and skin flora produce locally acting antibiotics, excluding potential pathogens. The importance of such defenses is clearly demonstrated when they are significantly breached, e.g. bacterial sepsis following severe burns or repeated bacterial infection causing bronchiectasis in immotile bronchial cilia syndrome or cystic fibrosis (see Ch. 20). Although the role these barriers play in the initial defense is critical they will not be considered further in this chapter.

COMPONENTS OF THE IMMUNE SYSTEM

The main organs of the immune system are the bone marrow, thymus, spleen and lymph nodes. The immune system is not predominantly organ based, and all parts of the body have a local immune system, for example Peyer's patches in the gut. The cells of the immune system are derived from pluripotent stem cells which originate in utero from fetal liver and bone marrow. Immune cells signal to each other and the rest of the body via cell surface molecules and soluble messengers. The latter are termed cytokines, chemokines or interleukins, depending on their exact function. The more important cytokines and their main effects are listed in Table 27.1. Many of these proteins have multiple and overlapping effects and are important in the innate and adaptive immune systems. Cytokines interact with their ligands (or receptors) on the surface of target cells. Receptors are frequently composed of more than one protein chain, one of which is common to a group of receptors and one defines the exact specificity of the receptor. An example is the gamma chain of the interleukin (IL)-2 receptor which is shared with the receptors for IL-4, -7, -9, -15 and -21. Mutations in the gene for this chain result in X-linked severe combined immunodeficiency (SCID) (p. 1154).

Functional lymphocyte subsets are identified by their surface antigens. Particular antigens [defined by recognition by a specific monoclonal antibody and termed the cluster of differentiation (CD) number] are used to define cell type (e.g. T or B lymphocyte) or their state of differentiation or activation (e.g. naive or memory cell). The more important surface antigens recognized by different CD antibodies are listed in Table 27.2. The functional roles of many of these surface antigens have been established.

INNATE AND ADAPTIVE IMMUNITY

Pathogens that breach barrier defenses encounter two fundamentally different, but closely linked, types of response (Fig. 27.1): innate then adaptive components of the immune system. Innate immune responses employ a limited number of receptors specific for conserved microbial structures but are highly effective and include neutrophil and mononuclear phagocytes as well as humoral factors such as complement. This response is immediate but limited in scope.

The adaptive immune system is distinguished by the specificity of its response and ability to generate immunological memory. This results in an initial delay in immune response, when innate immune responses are critical, but leads to more rapid and enhanced responses upon subsequent antigen exposure.

Innate and adaptive mechanisms are interdependent and many adaptive immune mechanisms exert their effects using the innate elements. Innate function is often greatly potentiated by factors produced by the adaptive immune response.

INNATE IMMUNE MECHANISMS

Humoral innate immune mechanisms
Complement

One of the most important humoral defenses is the complement system, of which the central component (Fig. 27.2) is C3b, the active product of cleavage of the C3 molecule. Antigen bound C3b acts as a powerful opsonin by interacting with neutrophil and monocyte C3b receptors. C3 is cleaved by one of three pathways. The classical (antibody-dependent) pathway requires specific antibody – antigen interaction. In the alternative pathway, microbial products, such as polysaccharides and endotoxin, directly activate another cascade of reactions involving serum protein factors B and D to form an alternative C3 convertase which is stabilized by factor P (properdin). In the lectin pathway, mannose binding lectin binds to bacterial sugars and interacts with serine proteases MASP1 and 2 to cleave C4. The lectin pathway is of crucial importance early in an infection prior to the production of specific antibodies and in young children.[2]

The fixing of C3b to the surface of a microorganism becomes self-amplifying, since C3b itself forms a component of the enzyme responsible for C3 cleavage. This is strictly controlled by a number of soluble and cell surface regulatory proteins. The later complement components C5–C9 produce a membrane-attack complex which can lyse cell membranes, a mechanism particularly important in the handling of systemic neisserial infections.

As well as lysis and opsonization, the complement reactions generate pharmacologically and chemotactically active by-products, such as the cleavage products C3a and C5a, for which there are cell surface receptors.

Cell surface complement receptors bind complement components and any associated cells or organisms, resulting in activation of other parts of the immune system. Complement receptor 1 (CR1, CD35, Table 27.2) is found on neutrophils, monocytes, erythrocytes, B lymphocytes and glomerular epithelial cells. It recognizes C3b- and C4b-coated particles and facilitates phagocytosis. Erythrocyte CR1 helps clear circulating immune complexes. CR2 (CD21), found predominantly on B lymphocytes and recognizing C3d, the main C3b breakdown product, is believed to modulate activity of these cells. It is the receptor for Epstein–Barr virus (EBV). CR3 (CD11b/CD18) on phagocytic cells and on natural killer (NK) cells recognizes inactivated C3b (C3bi) and is important in phagocytosis. CR4 (CD11c/CD18) weakly binds C3bi. CR3 and CR4 are members of a family of adhesion molecules, the leukocyte integrins, also involved in intracellular adhesion.

Other acute phase reactants

Serum levels of this diverse group of proteins, including clotting factors, amyloid proteins and C-reactive protein (CRP), rise rapidly at the onset of acute inflammatory responses. Their precise biological role is poorly characterized. CRP has some immunomodulating effects and acts as a nonspecific opsonin for bacterial phagocytosis.

Table 27.1   Principal cytokines

Cytokine	Other (previous) names	Produced by	Main actions
IL-1		Monocytes	Proinflammatory; fever; T cell activation
IL-2	T cell growth factor	T cells	T (mainly T_H1), NK cell activation/proliferation
IL-3	Multicolony stimulating factor	T cells	Proliferation of bone marrow progenitor cells
IL-4	B cell stimulating factor	T cells (T_H2)	T_H2 cell growth factor; B cell isotype switching especially to IgE
IL-5		T cells	T_H2 cytokine; activation and proliferation of eosinophils (and B cells)
IL-6		T, B cells monocytes	General cell growth and differentiation factor
IL-7	Lymphopoietin I	Bone marrow and thymic stroma	General cell growth factor
IL-8		T cells, monocytes, PMN	PMN activation, chemotaxis and adhesion
IL-9		T cells	T cell, mast cell growth and differentiation
IL-10	Cytokine synthesis inhibitory factor	T cells (T_H2) monocytes, mast cells	Inhibits T_H1 cytokine production
IL-11		Stromal cells	Growth factor similar in actions to IL-6
IL-12	NK stimulating factor	B cells, monocytes	Increases T and NK cell cytotoxicity; T_H1 growth and differentiation factor
IL-13		T cells (T_H2)	B cell isotype switching similar to IL-4
IL-14	High mol wt B cell growth factor	T, B cells	B cell growth and differentiation
IL-15		Stromal cells, monocytes	Similar actions to IL-2 (utilizes same receptor)
IFN α and β		Leukocytes-α Fibroblasts-β	Antiviral, antiproliferative Increased MHC expression, increased cytotoxic activity
IFN γ	Macrophage activating factor	T cells (T_H1) NK cells	Macrophage activation, increased MHC expression, T_H1 effects
TNF α	Cachectin	Monocytes	Proinflammatory
TNF β	Lymphotoxin	T cells	Proinflammatory
GM CSF		Leukocytes	Increased myelopoiesis, increased cytokine production by macrophages, proinflammatory
G CSF		Leukocytes	Increased granulopoiesis, activates PMN, reduces inflammatory cytokine production
M CSF		Monocytes, T, B cells	Increased monocyte growth and differentiation, increased cytokine production
TGF β		Platelets, monocytes	Suppresses inflammation and cell proliferation

IL, interleukin; IFN, interferon; TNF, tumor necrosis factor; CSF, colony stimulating factor; GM granulocyte macrophage; G, granulocyte; M, monocyte; TGF, transforming growth factor; PMN, polymorphonuclear cells; T_H1/T_H2, T helper cells.

Interferon

Alpha- and beta-interferons are proteins produced by virally infected cells. They render other cells immune to virus infection by producing an antiviral state. Interferons increase NK cell activity, increase human leukocyte antigen (HLA) class I antigen expression on cells, and decrease cell growth including that of tumor cells. Interferon (IFN) gamma, although it has some antiviral effect, is primarily a cytokine which upregulates immune responses, particularly by enhancing intracellular killing of microorganisms such as mycobacteria.

Iron-binding proteins

Many bacteria require iron for growth, and decreasing its availability is one mechanism of defense used by the host. An avid iron-binding protein, lactoferrin, present in human milk, reduces the growth of Escherichia coli. The reduction of serum iron which occurs during infections increases the bacteriostatic effect of serum.

Cellular innate immune mechanisms
Adhesion molecules

These molecules and ligands help cell-to-cell association, essential for normal immune and inflammatory responses. Found on all cells of the immune system and on vascular endothelium, their expression is tightly controlled during inflammatory responses by cytokines such as the interleukins, tumor necrosis factor (TNF) alpha and IFN-gamma. Two groups of adhesion molecules (the selectins and integrins) are crucial for the migration of immune cells out of the bloodstream to areas of inflammation.

Interaction between the selectins and their ligands results in the transient endothelial interactions of 'rolling' and margination which occur early in inflammatory reactions. Beta-2 integrins are subsequently upregulated, and their expression is responsible for the firm tethering of neutrophils to the endothelium and their subsequent egress from the circulation. Integrin expression is greatly upregulated by the proinflammatory cytokines such as TNF-alpha or IL-1 beta.

Effector cells

Phagocytic cells include neutrophils and monocyte/macrophages. Bacterial phagocytosis requires migration of neutrophils to the site of infection (chemotaxis). Products of the acute inflammatory response, including cleaved complement fragments (e.g. C5a), act as chemo-attractants in this process. Chemotaxis is followed by adherence to the bacterium and ingestion (phagocytosis). This is aided by opsonization, particularly by immunoglobulin G (IgG) and complement (C3b), which bind to bacteria and also phagocyte cell surface receptors Fc gamma and CR1/3 respectively, but also C-reactive protein and soluble forms of fibronectin. Following phagocytosis, lysosomes rapidly fuse with the bacterium-containing phagosome exposing the bacterium to lysosomal enzymes (e.g. myeloperoxidase) which are involved in killing and digestion. The process is accompanied by the generation of hydrogen peroxide, superoxide and hydroxyl radicals which aid bacterial killing. Neutrophil numbers and function are enhanced by the inflammatory response.

Monocytes and macrophages ingest and kill extracellular bacteria in a similar fashion to neutrophils but more slowly and less efficiently.

Table 27.2   Leukocyte antigens

Designation	Main cellular expression	Properties/function
T cells		
CD1	Thymocytes. Langerhans' cells	Unknown
CD2	Mature T cells	Sheep erythrocyte (E Rosette) receptor; LFA-3 ligand
CD3	Pan T cell marker	Part of T cell receptor complex
CD4	Helper/inducer T cells	MHC class II receptor; HIV receptor
CD5	Mature T cells. B cell subset (B1)	Unknown
CD8	Cytotoxic/suppressor T cells	MHC class I receptor
CD25	Activated T cells	IL-2α receptor
CD28	T cells	CD80 receptor; T cell activation
CD38	Thymocytes Activated cells	Unknown
CD71	Activated T cells Thymocytes	Transferrin receptor
B cells		
CD19	Pre B and B cells	Unknown
CD20	Pre B and B cells	Unknown
CD21	B cells	Complement receptor (CR) 2 EBV receptor
CD22	Pre B and B cells	Unknown
CD23	B cells	Low affinity IgE receptor
CD40	B cells	Ig isotype switching
Surface immunoglobulin	B cells	Antigen receptor
Monocytes		
CD14	Monocytes	Receptor for lipopolysaccharide
NK cells		
CD16	NK, monocytes	Fc γ receptor III
CD56	PMN, NK and some T cells	Unknown
General		
CD11a	Leukocytes	Cell adhesion ICAM-I receptor
CD11b	NK cells, MΦ, PMN	CR3
CD11c	NK cells, MΦ, PMN	CR4
CD15	PMN	Lewis X antigen
CD18	Leukocytes	β_2 integrin associated with CD11 antigens
CD34	BM progenitor cells	L selectin ligand
CD35	Monocytes, PMN, B cells	CR1
CD43	All leukocytes	Sialophorin
CD45	All leukocytes	Tyrosine phosphatase. T cell activation. Variable isoforms – see text
CD58	All leukocytes	LFA-3; CD2 ligand
CD80	Activated B and T mono	CD28 receptor
HLA class I	All leukocytes	Antigen presentation
HLA class II	B, monocytes, activated T cells	Antigen presentation

CD, cluster of differentiation; LFA, lymphocyte function-related antigen; MHC, major histocompatibility complex; HIV, human immunodeficiency virus; IL = interleukin; EBV, Epstein–Barr virus; NK, natural killer cells; PMN = polymorphonuclear cells; ICAM, intercellular adhesion molecule; MΦ = macrophage; BM, bone marrow; HLA, human leukocyte antigen.

However, they are important in defenses against intracellular micro-organisms, including bacteria such as *Mycobacterium tuberculosis* and *Listeria monocytogenes*. Such pathogens are recognized directly by the cell surface mannose/fucose receptor interacting with microbial carbohydrate moieties such as mannose, or are opsonized and bound to Fc gamma or CR1/3 receptors. Monocytes are also cytotoxic against infected host cells or malignant cells. Macrophage activity is greatly enhanced by cytokines, particularly IFN-gamma, produced by T lymphocytes as part of the specific cell-mediated immune response.

NK cells are part of the non-T, non-B cell lymphoid population and recognize and kill tumor and virus-infected cells. They have surface receptors for the Fc fragment of IgG and, when 'armed' with specific IgG against a target cell antigen, kill by a process called antibody-dependent cellular cytotoxicity (ADCC). They also have killer-activating and killer-inhibitory receptors. Killer-activating receptors recognize a number of different cell surface molecules and, when engaged, issue a 'kill'

message, normally over-ridden by the killer-inhibitory receptors engaging major histocompatibility complex (MHC) I molecules. Loss of MHC I expression due to viral cell infection or malignancy removes the inhibitory control, resulting in cytotoxic cell killing.

ADAPTIVE IMMUNE MECHANISMS

Adaptive responses are orchestrated by T and B lymphocytes, whose receptors are highly specific for the antigens presented to them. Receptor diversity is generated during B and T lymphocyte development by random recombination of different genetic elements. Binding of antigen to receptor leads to the generation of antigen specific effector immune mechanisms, such as antibody production or the generation of cytotoxic T lymphocytes. This process converts a naive T or B lymphocyte to an effector T lymphocyte or plasma cell respectively. As part of this process, memory T and B lymphocytes are also generated.

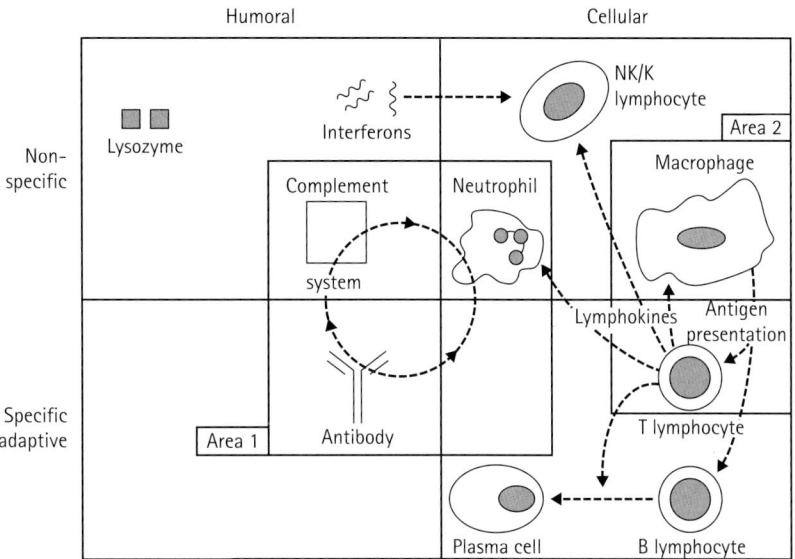

Fig. 27.1   Functional compartments of the immune system illustrating some of the more important interactions (dotted arrows). Area 1 is mainly involved in handling pyogenic bacteria. Area 2 is mainly involved with intracellular pathogens.

Antigen presenting cells (APCs) (e.g. specialized cells of the macrophage lineage called dendritic cells and also B lymphocytes) present antigens to T lymphocytes. APCs take up antigens, degrade them to small peptide fragments and express them on the cell surface in association with the MHC molecules.[3] The T lymphocyte receptor (T cell receptor, TCR) will only recognize the peptide in association with a self MHC molecule. Some MHC polymorphisms provoke better responses than others to specific antigens, explaining part of the genetic variability in immune responsiveness. CD4 positive helper T lymphocytes respond to antigen bound within the groove of class II MHC molecules (HLA DR) whilst

CD8 positive cytotoxic T lymphocytes respond to antigen bound to class I (HLA AB) molecules. Other receptor ligand interactions between the APC and T lymphocyte, including adhesion molecules, are important for maximizing T lymphocyte stimulation and are essential for the initial stimulation of naive cells.

When presented, antigen sits in a groove in the MHC molecule where it can interact with a complementary groove in the TCR (Fig. 27.3). Some antigens (superantigens) crosslink the presenting cell MHC molecule with other nonvariable parts of the TCR chains, resulting in stimulation of large numbers of T lymphocytes in an antigen nonspecific way. This causes immune mediated inflammatory diseases such as toxic shock syndrome. Superantigens are usually microbial products such as exotoxins.

There are two arms of the specific immune system – antibody mediated and cell mediated.

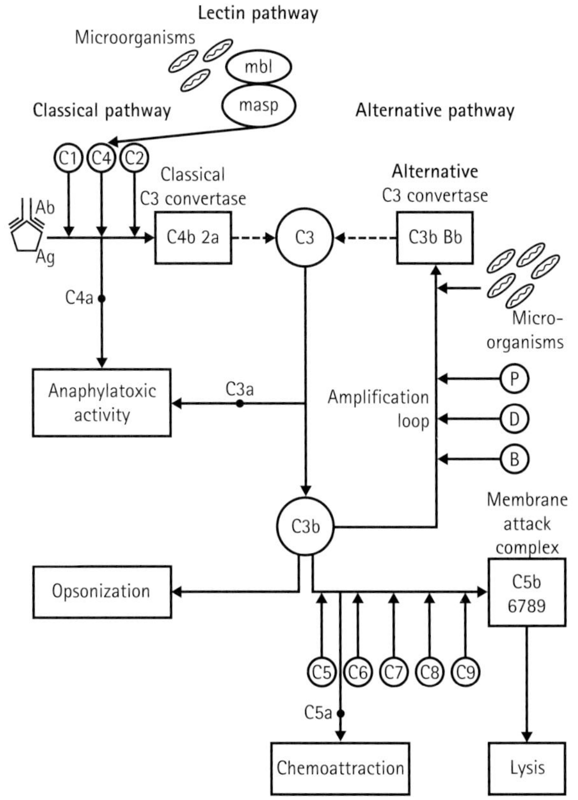

Antibodies

These are immunoglobulins produced by B lymphocytes and their effector cells, plasma cells, in response to exposure to specific antigens, e.g. during infection or after vaccination. Sometimes, specific antibodies may be present in the serum without prior exposure to the relevant

Fig. 27.2   The main features of the classical, alternative and lectin pathways of the complement system. Inactive cleavage and breakdown products are not shown.

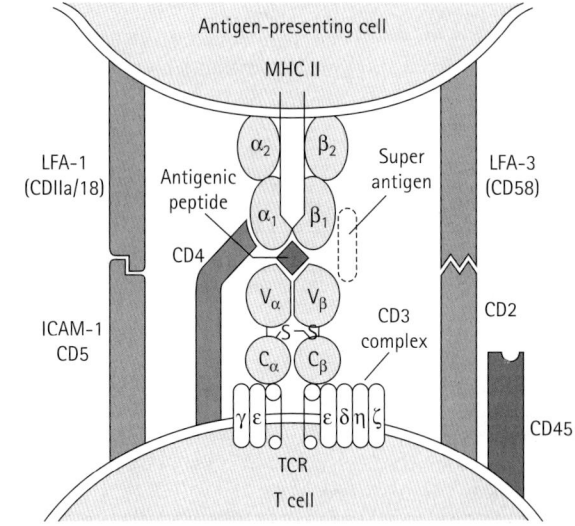

Fig. 27.3   Antigen presentation.

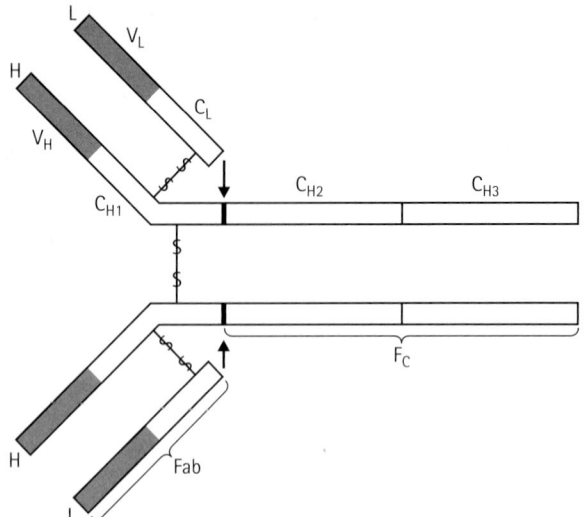

Fig. 27.4 Basic structure of an antibody molecule. Heavy (H) and light (L) chains comprise variable regions (V_H and V_L) – shown by solid bars – and constant regions (C_H and C_L) open bars. Constant region domains (C_{H1}, C_{H2} and C_{H3}) are shown. Arrows indicate the site of pepsin-mediated cleavage to give Fc and Fab fragments.

antigen – so-called 'natural' antibodies, resulting from cross-reactivity between antigens, particularly nonprotein (polysaccharide) antigens.

The basic structure of the immunoglobulin molecule is shown in Figure 27.4. The variable region has a unique amino acid sequence, giving the antibody its unique specificity which ensures that there is an antibody complementary to every antigen that could be constructed. There are five main classes of immunoglobulin, each with its own structure and functions (Tables 27.3 and 27.4).

Immunoglobulin class or isotype is determined by the heavy chain. During B lymphocyte development, rearrangement of genes coding for the variable and constant parts of the immunoglobulin chain occurs (Fig. 27.5). One each of the V, D and J heavy chain genes is rearranged to lie adjacent to the relevant heavy chain constant region gene, so that transcription produces a single protein with a constant and a variable portion. Approximately 10^{16} different receptors are generated. A similar process occurs during T cell development. Further rearrangement to bring a particular variable gene combination to lie adjacent to a different heavy chain constant region gene allows the B lymphocyte to switch to another antibody class (isotype) with the same antigen specificity. A mu chain is always produced first; class switching to other isotypes occurs later. Specific antibody diversity is created by the large number of possible combinations of variable region genes which can be selected and is increased further by a very high mutation rate in V genes and the effect of the enzyme deoxynucleotidyltransferase (TdT) during the rearrangement process. A similar but slightly less complex process takes place with light chains, of which there are two types – kappa and lambda.

IgM

This is the first antibody class produced in primary immune responses. For most antigens, there is a subsequent switching to other classes but for some, e.g. responses to the lipopolysaccharides of Gram negative bacilli, IgM remains the predominant class. Its large pentameric structure confines it to the intravascular space where it fixes complement.

IgG

This is the main class of antibody produced in secondary immune responses. Functions include opsonization, complement fixation leading to C3 opsonization and complement mediated lysis, neutralization of toxins or viruses, and participation in antibody dependent cellular cytotoxicity. Though there is considerable overlap, the four subclasses of IgG tend to have different functions. In adults, antibodies to bacterial polysaccharides are predominantly of IgG2 subclass, but in children significant amounts are found in the IgG1 subclass. Responses to protein antigens are mainly in the IgG1 and IgG3 subclasses. The role of IgG4 is, as yet, unclear.

IgA

This is the main antibody in secretions, where it forms a dimeric molecule consisting of two IgA subunits joined by a J chain and associated with a protective secretory piece synthesized by epithelial cells. In addition to protecting mucous membranes and the gastrointestinal tract from infection, IgA may have a role in limiting food antigen uptake from the gut. Serum IgA is mainly in monomeric form, though dimeric and trimeric forms are also found.

IgD

This is mainly a surface molecule on the membrane of B lymphocytes which regulates B lymphocyte differentiation and maturation. Small amounts found free in plasma are not thought to have any biological role.

Table 27.4 Properties of IgG subclasses

	G1	G2	G3	G4
Mol wt ($\times 10^{-3}$)	150	150	165	150
% of total IgG (adults)	70	20	7	3
Biological half-life (days)	23	23	9	23
Complement-fixing ability	++	+	++	−
Fc receptor binding				
Monocytes	++	+/−	++	+/−
Neutrophils	++	+	+	+
Lymphocytes	+	+/−	+	+/−

Table 27.3 Properties of serum immunoglobulins

	IgG	IgM	IgA	IgD	IgE
Heavy chain	γ	μ	α	δ	ε
Light chain	κ/λ	κ/λ	κ/λ	κ/λ	κ/λ
Mol wt ($\times 10^{-3}$)	150	900	160–320	180	200
Polymeric status	Monomer	Pentamer	Monomer or dimer*	Monomer	Monomer
Sedimentation coefficient (Svedberg units)	6.7	19	7	7	8
Mean adult serum concentration (g/L)	12	1.5	3	0.03	0.001
Biological half-life (days)	23	5	7	2.8	2.3
Placental transfer	+	−	−	−	−

*Trimeric IgA may also occur. Secretory IgA is in dimeric form.

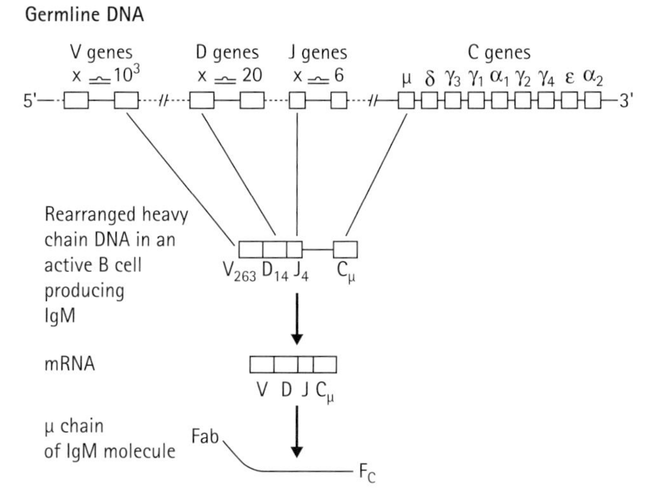

Germline DNA

Fig. 27.5 Immunoglobulin heavy chain gene arrangements on chromosome 14 in germline configuration and showing an example of a rearrangement using V gene number 263, D_{14} and J_4 to produce a unique antigen binding site. In this example, the variable genes (V, D and J) have been combined with a μ constant region heavy chain gene (Cμ) to produce a complete μ chain of an IgM molecule.

IgE

Mast cells and basophils have receptors for the Fc part of this molecule. Antigen binding may cause degranulation of the cells, triggering an immediate hypersensitivity response. Such reactions are often harmful rather than beneficial, but evolved as a mechanism for removing parasites.

Antibody production

Antibodies are produced by B (bone marrow derived) lymphocytes. Naive B lymphocytes have membrane antibody which acts as a receptor for antigen. Initial stages of B cell development are antigen independent, but the final stages of B lymphocyte differentiation require stimulation with the appropriate antigen leading (after final class switching) to maturation into plasma cells. The full process requires the cooperation of antigen specific T helper (CD4 positive) lymphocytes. Isotype switching from IgM production to the other antibody classes is critically dependent on T/B lymphocyte interaction via the CD40 antigen on B lymphocytes and its ligand expressed on activated T lymphocytes (CD40L, CD154). The responses to some antigens, e.g. bacterial polysaccharides, can result in limited antibody production without T lymphocyte help. There is no immunological memory generated in such responses.

Cell-mediated immunity

T (thymus-derived) lymphocytes predominate in immune responses to intracellular microbes and regulate immune responses by secreting cytokines and growth factors.

T lymphocytes are generated from bone marrow derived stem cells, but acquire functional capabilities during thymic maturation. Here the cells undergo a series of developmental stages including gene rearrangement to generate diversity in the variable domains of the TCR. They also become 'educated' with regard to self/nonself recognition so that self-reactive clones are deleted and only clones recognizing antigen in the context of self MHC are preserved.

The TCR, although not an immunoglobulin molecule, has a similar arrangement of constant and variable parts and the generation of diverse specificity is achieved along similar lines to the generation of antibody diversity in B lymphocytes. The TCR is a heterodimeric molecule with each chain having a constant and variable portion. The majority (> 90%) of mature circulating T lymphocytes express alpha and beta

chains, the remainder are gamma and delta. Diversity is acquired in a method similar to that of the immunoglobulin molecule. A number of genes [artemis, recombinase activating genes 1 and 2 (RAG1, 2), DNA ligase 4, cernunnos-XLF] are critical for this gene rearrangement, and mutations in these genes lead to T− B− SCID (p. 1155).

During thymic maturation T lymphocytes also acquire important functional surface molecules. CD3 is constitutively expressed on T lymphocytes and is closely associated with the TCR (Fig. 27.3). Initially both CD4 and CD8 are expressed on the same cells, but only one of the molecules is retained. Most gamma delta T lymphocytes do not express CD4 or CD8. Their precise function is unclear, but they seem to play a role in mucosal defense and gut antigen clearance and tolerance.

The primary effector cell in the adaptive response is the CD4+ T helper lymphocyte (Fig. 27.6). Once activated by antigen presentation these cells develop in one of two ways: the T_H1 route with production of IL-2 and IFN-gamma whose main role is in stimulating macrophage function and cell-mediated immunity but also has effects on B lymphocytes including antibody class switching, particularly to IgG2. T_H2 cells on the other hand produce predominantly IL-4 and IL-10 which promote antibody responses and class switching, particularly towards IgG1, IgG4 and IgE. Allergic responses and those against parasites are of T_H2 type. Responses to an antigen may follow a T_H1 or T_H2 route depending on a complex set of circumstances. Once established these responses are self-amplifying in that production of IFN-gamma or IL-4 promotes T_H1 and T_H2 responses respectively and inhibits the other.

The functions of T lymphocytes can be summarized as:

1. help and regulation of antibody production by B lymphocytes;
2. cytokine production which stimulates and regulates other nonspecific immune effector cells;
3. secretion of growth and differentiation factors, e.g. colony-stimulating factors, B lymphocyte growth factors;
4. T lymphocyte-mediated specific cytotoxicity, e.g. against virus-infected cells or against foreign tissues.

Signal transduction

Once T and B lymphocytes have engaged antigen via their specific receptors they must activate to generate the next step in the immune response. Cell surface receptors that have a signaling function are either transmembrane proteins or part of a complex of protein that contains intracellular signaling elements (Fig. 27.7). Both T and B lymphocyte receptor complexes have proteins with cytosolic tails containing immunoreceptor tyrosin-based activation motifs (ITAMs) that can be phosphorylated. After antigen binding, B and T lymphocyte receptors cluster on

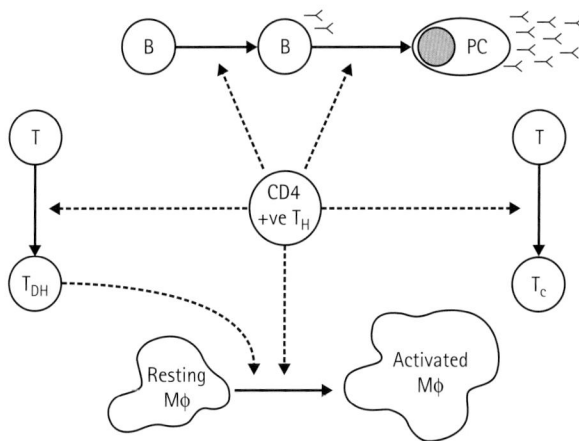

Fig. 27.6 Central role of CD4+ve T helper (T_H) cell in immune responses. T_C, cytotoxic T cell; T_{DH}, delayed hypersensitivity T cell; Mφ, macrophage; B, B cell; PC, plasma cell.

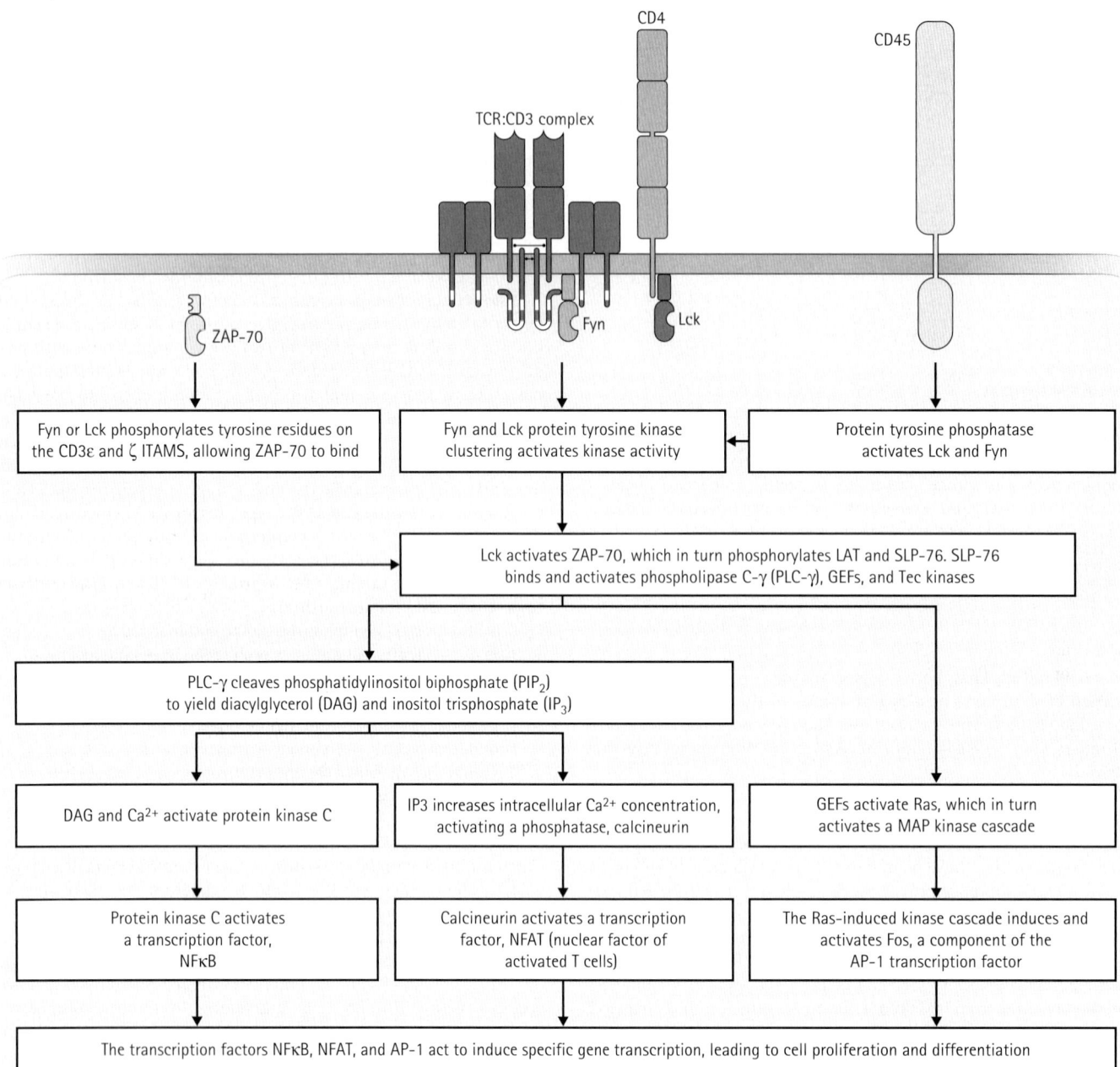

Fig. 27.7 Intracellular signaling pathways are induced following antigen-presenting cell/T cell receptor interaction. The T cell receptor (TCR) complex associates with Fyn, and the co-receptor (CD4/CD8) with Lck. Antigen/MHC binding to the TCR brings together the CD4 or CD8 co-receptor, TCR and CD45. The CD45 protein tyrosine phosphatase activates Fyn/Lck which in turn activate zeta chain associated protein (ZAP)-70. ZAP-70 activation signals through three separate pathways to activate three transcription factors, NFκB, NFAT and AP-1. These act on T cell genes in the nucleus to initiate gene transcription leading to T cell differentiation and proliferation. (Adapted from Janeway et al 2005[4] with permission.)

the surface of the lymphocyte which leads to the formation of a supramolecular adhesion complex (SMAC) in which the antigen receptors are co-localized with other cell surface signaling and adhesion molecules. This association between the APC and the T lymphocyte is termed the immunological synapse. Once clustered, the intracellular portions of antigen receptors associate with tyrosine kinases, in particular the Src family. This results in tyrosine phosphorylation of ITAMs in the receptor complex, and a cascade of intracellular proteins is activated. These include SH2 domain containing proteins, and small G proteins which transmit the signal to the nucleus after converting bound GTP to GDP. Antigen receptor signaling is enhanced by co-receptors that bind the same ligand; these include CD19, CD21 and CD81 for B lymphocytes.

THE DEVELOPMENT OF THE IMMUNE SYSTEM

PRENATAL DEVELOPMENT

T and B lymphocyte development commences very early in the gestation of the human fetus. Cells capable of responding in mixed lymphocyte culture or to the mitogen, phytohemagglutinin (PHA), and recognizable NK cells are present in the fetal liver from 6 weeks. T and B lymphocyte precursors are identifiable from 7–8 weeks and T lymphocyte precursors colonize the rudimentary thymus from the 9th week. By the second trimester, circulating lymphocytes with mature T lymphocyte surface markers including CD3, CD4 and CD8 are identifiable. Absence of these markers can be used for the antenatal diagnosis of SCID by fetal blood sampling (p. 1154). B lymphocyte precursors also originate in the fetal liver, and mature in the bone marrow in mammals. Surface B lymphocyte markers, including surface immunoglobulin, can be detected by the second trimester, although at low levels.

Although the cellular elements of the specific immune system are present from early in gestation, their ability to respond to antigens, especially by making immunoglobulin, is limited until the time of birth.

The elements of the innate immune system also develop early in fetal life. Neutrophil precursors can be identified in the yolk sac. Mature neutrophils appear in the circulation in the second trimester but numbers are low until the onset of labor. C3 has been detected from 6 weeks of gestation. The serum levels of complement components, which are produced mainly by the fetal liver, rise slowly throughout fetal life.

THE IMMUNE SYSTEM IN THE NEWBORN

The newborn immune system exhibits a physiological immunodeficiency[5,6] in full-term and preterm infants, but is more exaggerated in the premature and particularly marked in sick or stressed preterm infants. This accounts for the increased susceptibility to infection of the newborn, whether overwhelming group B streptococcal sepsis, or disseminated herpes simplex infection. Placentally transferred IgG partially offsets the deficiency. However, transfer of significant amounts of immunoglobulin (Fig. 27.8)[7] is a late event in gestation, and so preterm infants have significantly reduced levels; those at the limits of viability (23–24 weeks) have extremely low levels. The protective effect of maternal immunoglobulin depends on the mother having IgG antibody to the appropriate antigens and, in group B streptococcal sepsis, lack of maternal-type specific antibody to the relevant bacterial polysaccharides is a major risk factor. The newborn infant shows poor antibody responses, especially to T-independent antigens, poor ability to switch immunoglobulin isotypes and poor maturation of antibody affinity. These poor responses are a function of intrinsic B and T lymphocyte and APC immaturity. T lymphocyte responses are poor in neonates largely because of the high proportion of naive T lymphocytes which are more difficult to stimulate.

T lymphocyte surface marker expression differs between neonates and adults. There is a high CD4:CD8 ratio, a high expression of the thymocyte antigen CD38 and low numbers of cells expressing the gamma delta TCR. There is also a high proportion of B lymphocytes expressing the CD5 antigen (B1 cells). Expression of crucial signaling molecules such as CD40L is also reduced. These differences resolve over the early months of life as a result of antigen exposure. Neonatal T lymphocytes have usually less than 10% of the CD45RO (memory) isoform and predominant expression of the CD45RA (virgin, naive) isoform. These proportions gradually reverse during childhood. Exposure to intrauterine infection may alter these neonatal patterns towards a more mature picture.

The overall balance of neonatal T lymphocyte responsiveness is tilted towards T_H2 rather T_H1 response. This may contribute to the susceptibility to intracellular bacterial pathogens, such as *Listeria monocytogenes* or *Salmonella* species, since defenses to these pathogens rely on a T_H1 pattern response.

Nonspecific immune mechanisms are also immature at birth. Neutrophil bone marrow reserves are easily exhausted leading to neutropenia; chemotaxis and cell deformability may be reduced compared to values in adults or older children.[8] In contrast to the situation at other ages, neutrophil numbers and function have a tendency to deteriorate in the presence of infection or other stress.[9] Complement factor levels and function in a full-term infant are at approximately two thirds of the adult level, and often below one half in preterm babies. Alternative pathway factors are at relatively lower levels than classical pathway levels. The precise significance of these findings in predisposing to neonatal sepsis is not clear.

Low immunoglobulin and complement levels are directly proportional to gestational age. Depressed T lymphocyte function may occur in babies who have suffered severe intrauterine growth restriction. The latter has been demonstrated up to < 5 years of age, though the clinical significance of such findings is unclear.[10] The placental transfer of immunoglobulin in situations of severe intrauterine growth restriction is probably also compromised, though not all studies have confirmed this.[11]

POSTNATAL DEVELOPMENT

Following birth the neonate is exposed to a wide variety of antigenic stimuli which trigger immunological maturation regardless of gestational age. Immunoglobulin production and specific antibody responses commence soon after birth. Initially, mostly IgM is produced, but gradually IgG responses develop and by 2 months of age infants are able to produce good IgG antibody responses to protein vaccines, such as tetanus toxoid. During this period, maternal IgG levels fall due to catabolism,

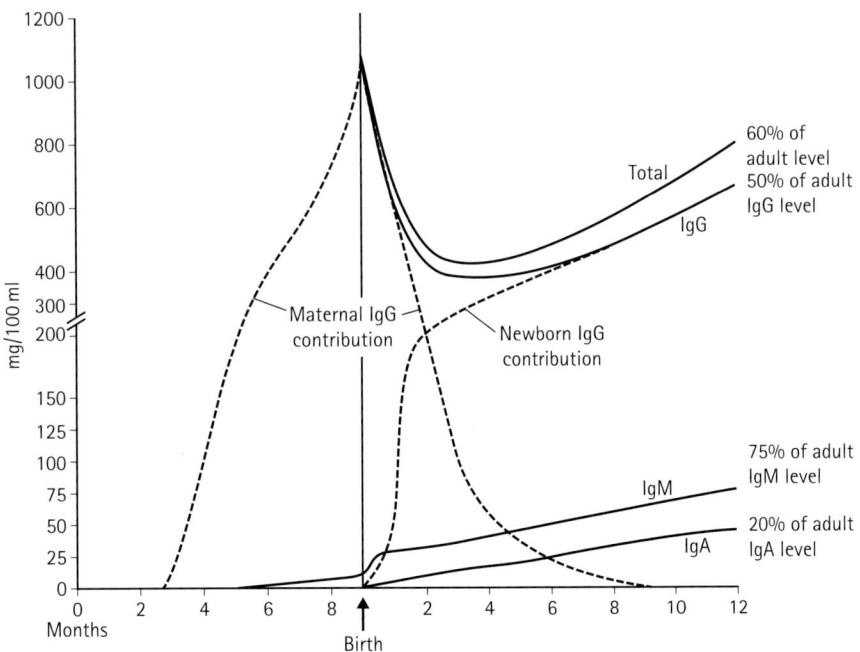

Fig. 27.8   Immunoglobulin levels in fetal life and in the first year postnatally. (From Miller & Steihm 1983[7] with permission.)

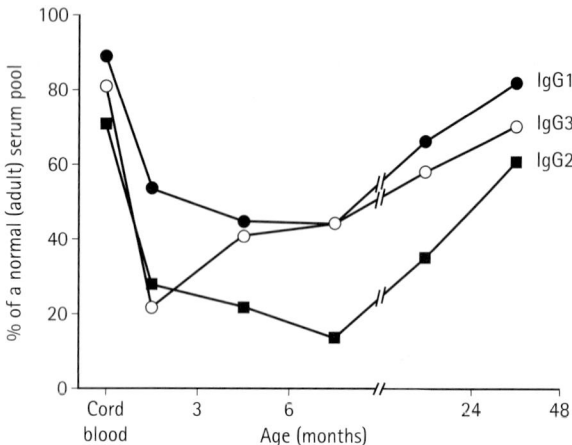

Fig. 27.9 Mean levels of IgG subclasses 1–3 in early life. Note the exaggerated fall and slow rise of IgG2 levels compared to IgG1 and IgG3. (Drawn from the data of Oxelius 1979[12].)

and a physiological nadir in IgG level occurs at 3–6 months of age before the infant's production picks up (Fig. 27.8). Thereafter isotype levels rise at different rates: adult levels of IgM are achieved by 4–5 years, and IgG by 7–8 years, whilst serum IgA levels (and secretory IgA) rise only very slowly, not achieving adult values until teenage years.

The pattern of maturation of IgG subclass levels also varies. IgG2 shows a prolonged physiological trough compared to IgG1 and IgG3 (Fig. 27.9).[12] Though antibody responses to most protein antigens mature early, responses to many polysaccharide antigens do not. Most antipolysaccharide IgG antibody in adults is found in the G2 subclass, while in young children the G1 subclass contains these. There is a high degree of susceptibility to polysaccharide-encapsulated organisms such as pneumococcus in young children, and a lack of responsiveness of children under the age of 18–24 months to pure polysaccharide vaccines, such as the polysaccharide pneumococcal vaccine. Conjugation of the polysaccharide to a protein or peptide facilitates early responsiveness to both components as demonstrated by the high efficacy of *Haemophilus influenzae* type B (Hib) and the new pneumococcal conjugate vaccines.[13]

T lymphocyte immunity appears to mature rapidly in the early weeks of life following antigen exposure. T lymphocyte expression of CD40 ligand improves, as does cytokine production with the T_H2/T_H1 balance shifting towards T_H1. However, the differences in T lymphocyte numbers and CD4:CD8 ratios between children and adults, and the unreliable responses of children to delayed hypersensitivity skin test antigens, such as *Candida* antigen, does suggest that maturation and development of the cell-mediated immune system continues through early childhood. Subtle immaturities in cell-mediated immunity probably account for the increased susceptibility of young children to tuberculosis (TB), and of young infants to invasive salmonellosis and listeriosis.

IMMUNODEFICIENCY DISORDERS: GENERAL PRINCIPLES

CLASSIFICATION AND GENETICS

Immunodeficiency may be due to a primary (inherited) or secondary (acquired) defect. The WHO working party on immunodeficiency[14] has classified the primary disorders, and the main categories are listed in Tables 27.5A,B.[14] Figure 27.10[1] and Table 27.6 show the relative frequencies of the various disorders. The overall incidence of any significant immunodeficiency disorder (excluding selective IgA deficiency) has been estimated at 1 in 10000.

Many of the primary disorders have a genetic basis.[14] Identification of the responsible gene(s) has been achieved in an increasing number of conditions. Chromosomal aberrations may be found in some immunodeficiency disorders. Deletions of heavy chain constant region genes have been described in a minority of patients with immunoglobulin class or subclass deficiencies, while deletions on chromosome 18 (in some cases of IgA deficiency) and on chromosome 22 (most cases of DiGeorge syndrome) have also been recorded. Immunodeficiency is often a feature of chromosomal breakage/repair disorders, such as ataxia telangiectasia.

The molecular basis of many of the primary immunodeficiency disorders has been elucidated. Usually several different mutations in the relevant gene have been described. Occasionally mutations at certain points are associated with partial forms of disease, presumably because of some residual function of the protein concerned. Recognition of the molecular pathways involved enhances understanding of the immune response, and identification and clarification of precise molecular mechanisms enable focused treatment of primary immune deficiencies, e.g. X-linked hyper-IgM used to be considered an antibody deficiency, although immunoglobulin replacement does not prevent liver disease secondary to *Cryptosporidium parvum* infection. Recognition of the primary T lymphocyte defect has led to curative hemopoietic stem cell transplant (HSCT) in selected patients. Identification of the genes involved enables genetic diagnosis (including antenatal diagnosis) and involves a number of techniques including restriction fragment length polymorphism (RFLP) and single strand conformational polymorphism (SSCP) analysis.

DIAGNOSIS AND INVESTIGATION OF IMMUNODEFICIENCY

A careful history and examination will help determine which children should be investigated further and the nature and extent of investigations, and should precede any laboratory tests.

Table 27.5A Primary immunodeficiencies – predominantly antibody deficiency (Adapted from Notarangelo et al 2006[14])

Immunodeficiency	Defect	Inheritance
X-linked agammaglobulinemia	Btk protein	XL
Autosomal recessive hyper-IgM syndromes	AID, CD40, UNG	AR
Common variable immunodeficiency	Unknown – some closely linked to C4 gene	Varied (occasionally AR or AD)
Ig heavy chain deletions	Deletion at Ig heavy chain locus (14q32)	AR
Ig kappa chain deletion	Mutation in Igκ chain locus (2p11)	AR
Selective IgA deficiency	Unknown – some closely linked to C4 gene	Varied (occasionally AR or AD)
IgG subclass deficiency (± IgA deficiency)	Unknown	Unknown
Antibody deficiency with normal immunoglobulin levels	Unknown	Unknown
Transient hypogammaglobulinemia of infancy	Unknown	Unknown

AD, autosomal dominant; AR, autosomal recessive; XL, X-linked.

Table 27.5B Combined immunodeficiencies (Adapted from Notarangelo et al 2006[14])

Immunodeficiency	Defect	Inheritance
CD40 ligand deficiency (X - linked hyper-IgM syndrome)	CD40 ligand	XL
Wiskott–Aldrich syndrome (WAS)	WAS protein	XL
X-linked lymphoproliferative disease	SLAM-associated protein	XL
DiGeorge anomaly defect chromosomal deletion (usually 22q11.2)	Developmental field	Sporadic (some AD)
Cartilage–hair hypoplasia	RMRP gene	AR
Ataxia telangiectasia	ATM protein	AR
Nijmegen breakage syndrome	NBS1 (nibrin) gene	AR
Ataxia telangiectasia-like syndrome	Mre11	AR
DNA Ligase 4 deficiency	LIG4	AR

AD, autosomal dominant; AR, autosomal recessive; XL, X-linked.

Table 27.5C Defects of phagocytic function (Adapted from Notarangelo et al 2006[14])

Immunodeficiency	Defect	Inheritance
XL chronic granulomatous disease	Killing defect gp91phox	XL
AR chronic granulomatous disease	Killing defect gp22phox, gp47phox, gp67phox	AR
Leukocyte adhesion deficiency type I	β integrin (CD18)	AR
Leukocyte adhesion deficiency type II	CD15	AR
Neutrophil G6PD deficiency	Neutrophil G6PD	XL
Myeloperoxidase deficiency	Myeloperoxidase	AR
AR severe congenital neutropenia	Elastase	AR
Chediak–Higashi syndrome	Lyst gene	AR
Griscelli syndrome	Rab27a gene	AR
Primary hemophagocytosis	Perforin	AR
	MUNC13–4	AR
	Syntaxin 11	AR
XL severe congenital neutropenia	WAS activating mutation	XL
Mycobactericidal defect	IFN γ receptor 1 deficiency	AR
	IFN γ receptor 2 deficiency	AR
	IL-12 receptor deficiency	AR
	IL-12 deficiency	AR

AR, autosomal recessive; G6PD, glucose-6-phosphate dehydrogenase; WAS, Wiskott–Aldrich syndrome; XL, X-linked.

HISTORY

Pregnancy and birth history may provide information regarding possible congenital infection, intrauterine growth retardation or prematurity, all of which are associated with immune defects. Delayed separation of the umbilical cord, in the absence of local infection, may suggest a neutrophil defect. Most children will present with an infective problem. The

Table 27.5D Complement deficiencies (Adapted from Notarangelo et al 2006[14])

Component	Inheritance	Main clinical associations
C1q	AR	SLE, MPGN, pyogenic infections
C1r*	AR	SLE
C1s*	AR	SLE
C4	AR	SLE
C2	AR	SLE, MPGN, HSP, pyogenic infections
C3	AR	Severe pyogenic infections
C5	AR	Neisserial infections, SLE
C6	AR	Neisserial infections, SLE
C7	AR	Neisserial infections, SLE
C8	AR	Neisserial infections, SLE
C9	AR	Neisserial infections (less marked than for C5–8 deficiency)
Factor D	AR	Neisserial infections
Properdin	XL	Neisserial infections
C1 esterase inhibitor	AD	Hereditary angioedema
Factor H	AR	Hemolytic uremic syndrome, MPGN
Factor I	AR	Pyogenic infections
MBP deficiency	AR	Pyogenic infections, usually asymptomatic
MASP2 deficiency	AR	SLE, pyogenic infections

AD, autosomal dominant; AR, autosomal recessive; HSP, Henoch–Schönlein purpura; MPGN, membranoproliferative glomerulonephritis; SLE, systemic lupus erythematosus; XL, X-linked; MBP, mannose-binding protein; MASP2, mannose-binding protein-associated serine protease 2. *NB* SLE is the most common immune complex disorder in complement deficiencies.
* C1r and C1s deficiency usually occur together.

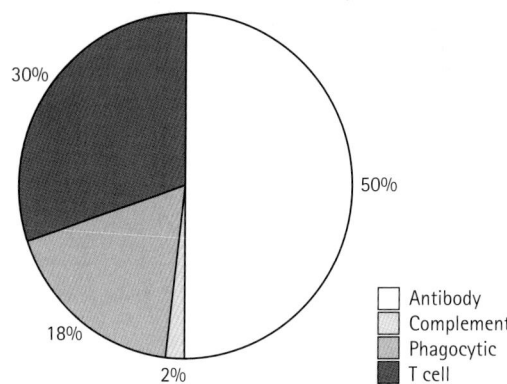

Fig. 27.10 Relative distribution of primary immunodeficiencies, based on combined experience from Japan, Switzerland and USA, excluding cases of asymptomatic selective IgA deficiency. The T cell deficiency group includes patients with combined cell-mediated and antibody deficiencies.

Table 27.6 Incidence of some primary immunodeficiencies

Immunodeficiency	Incidence
Severe combined immunodeficiency	1 in 66 000
DiGeorge syndrome	1 in 4 000
Common variable immunodeficiency	1 in 50 000
Chronic granulomatous disease	1 in 181 000
Selective IgA deficiency	1 in 500
X-linked agammaglobulinemia	1 in 250 000

age of onset of infections, their site, proven or suspected organisms and time to recovery with conventional treatments are all important considerations. An immunodeficient child is likely to have more infections which take longer to resolve or have an atypical course compared to other children. The type of organism involved, including the occurrence of atypical infections, should direct further investigations (Table 27.7). The occurrence of frequent upper respiratory tract infections (URTI) alone in a young child is not indicative of an underlying immune defect unless associated with frequent bacterial infections. There are a few studies on the frequency of URTI, but clinical experience suggests that up to eight URTI per year is normal in the preschool years. When evaluating the number of infections, other factors such as parental smoking, attendance at daycare and anatomical problems should be considered. Infections with common organisms may run an atypical course in that they are unusually severe, e.g. hemorrhagic chickenpox, or they fail to respond to standard treatments, e.g. a bacterial pneumonia which fails to respond to appropriate antibiotic therapy. Alternatively, infections may be caused by uncommon (atypical) organisms which are in themselves highly suggestive of immunodeficiency, e.g. *Pneumocystis carinii* pneumonia.

The history should include inquiries about related problems associated with immunodeficiency disorders. Failure to thrive is common, and may be associated with diarrhea due to chronic or recurrent infection or autoimmune enteropathy. Evidence of end-organ damage, such as a cough productive of sputum consistent with bronchiectasis, should also be sought. Allergic/atopic problems are common and may be unusually severe. Autoimmune and malignant diseases, though not common, have an increased incidence. Taking a careful family history may reveal other children with unusual or fatal infectious complications in keeping with an autosomal recessive or X-linked pattern of inheritance. A history of consanguinity should be sought. Some tactful inquiries to ascertain whether the parents have any risk factors for infection with the human immunodeficiency virus should be made as infection with this virus is often a differential diagnosis. In some disorders, e.g. IgA deficiency, there may be a family history of collagen vascular or other immune mediated disease. Older relatives who are carriers of or who are affected by milder variants of primary immune defects may have autoimmune manifestations [e.g. mouth ulcers and systemic lupus-erythematosus variant in chronic granulomatous disease, (CGD)] or

have a history of malignant disease [lymphoma in X-linked lymphoproliferative disease, XLP, or Wiskott–Aldrich syndrome, (WAS)].

EXAMINATION

General physical examination should be directed towards potential sites of infection, including the throat, ears and sinuses and examination of the oral cavity and napkin area for candidiasis. The presence or absence of lymphoid tissue should be noted, as should cutaneous problems consistent with an immune defect. In more severe antibody states such as X-linked agammaglobulinemia, there is a lack of tonsils and lymphoid tissues. Signs of end-organ damage from infections, such as clubbing and respiratory abnormalities, must be sought. Some diseases may have specific physical signs, such as oculocutaneous albinism in Chediak–Higashi syndrome, typical facies and/or cleft palate in DiGeorge syndrome, telangiectasia or neurological abnormalities in ataxia telangiectasia, and disproportionate short stature in some forms of combined immunodeficiency (see cartilage–hair hypoplasia, p. 1160).

DIAGNOSTIC IMAGING

Radiological evaluation, directed by findings from history and examination, may be useful. The exception is in DNA repair defects (see below) where the effects of exposure to ionizing radiation may be harmful, and X-ray and computerized tomography (CT) evaluation should be limited as much as possible. Magnetic resonance imaging (MRI) and ultrasound are safe alternatives.

Evidence of bony abnormalities may support a diagnosis of adenosine deaminase deficiency, Shwachman–Diamond syndrome or other dysplasias associated with immune defects. Dilatation of the common bile duct may be suggestive of sclerosing cholangitis, associated with a number of combined immunodeficiencies especially CD40 ligand deficiency.[15] Careful review of chest radiographs may suggest bronchiectasis, and should prompt high resolution CT imaging. Although thymic absence on anterior posterior and lateral chest radiographs is consistent with a combined immune defect in infants and young children, thymic atrophy may also occur in response to stress (e.g. infection) and this finding is not diagnostic.

LABORATORY INVESTIGATION

Two main questions need to be addressed: which children to investigate, and how extensively to investigate selected children. The following should trigger investigation: family history consistent with immune deficiency, single infection with an unusual/opportunistic organism, single infection which is atypically severe, has an atypical course or occurs at an atypical age, recurrent minor bacterial infections [e.g. otitis media > two per year despite appropriate ear, nose and throat (ENT) management, resulting in significant school absence], or more than one episode of serious bacterial infection.

Laboratory investigations can be directed to a certain extent by the organism causing infection (Table 27.7) and the age of the child.

The laboratory investigations range from those readily available in all centers, to highly specialized tests performed in a few research centers. Only a small proportion of children presenting with recurrent infections require complex investigation; most can be adequately investigated using a few relatively straightforward tests.

Hematology

Much can be learnt from a full blood count and blood film examination. Modern analyzers rapidly perform a white count and differential. Neutropenia is readily detected. If cyclical neutropenia is suspected, twice weekly counts should be performed for 8 weeks as the nadir may be brief and easily missed. Bone marrow aspiration should be considered in neutropenic children to distinguish between failure of production and increased peripheral destruction, and to exclude a myelodysplastic or

Table 27.7 Examples of association between infecting organisms and most likely type of immune defect

Organism	Candidate immune defect
Pneumococcus, Haemophilus influenzae	Antibody, complement
Staphylococcus	Neutrophil
Meningococcus	Complement
Gram negative bacteria	Neutrophil
Salmonella	Type 1 cytokine defects, cell-mediated
Cryptosporidium	Cell-mediated
Giardia lamblia	Antibody, cell-mediated*
Mycoplasma spp.	Antibody
Candida albicans	Cell-mediated, neutrophil, monocyte
Aspergillus spp.	Neutrophil
Herpes viruses (e.g. CMV)	Cell-mediated
Enteroviruses	Antibody, cell-mediated
Other viruses (e.g. measles)	Cell-mediated
Mycobacteria (typical and typical)	Type 1 cytokine defects
Bacille Calmette–Guérin (BCG)	Cell-mediated, type 1 cytokine defects

* particularly patients with HIV.

malignant process. Neutrophilia in the absence of overt infection suggests a neutrophil adhesion defect or functional problem (e.g. CGD). Lymphopenia, using appropriate age related ranges (see Appendix), is highly suggestive of a combined immunodeficiency of primary or secondary etiology,[16] although SCID can occur in the presence of a normal lymphocyte count. Nucleated red cells in infants and abnormal leukocyte morphology in sick children may render a manual differential necessary. Abnormal leukocyte granules are characteristic of Chediak–Higashi syndrome. Platelet volume is universally low in Wiskott–Aldrich syndrome, and is a rapid and very reliable diagnostic pointer.[17]

TESTS OF INNATE IMMUNITY
Complement
C3 and C4 can be routinely measured in pathology departments using nephelometry (see below); reference ranges for C3 are well defined. However, null alleles for C4 are present at a relatively high frequency in the population so that the significance of an isolated low C4 in an individual with recurrent infections is less certain. Furthermore, normal levels of C3 and C4 do not exclude deficiencies of other complement components. It is therefore better to assess the functional integrity of the complement pathway using assays which test the ability of patient serum to lyse sensitized erythrocytes. All assays measure the intactness of one activation pathway plus the final common effector pathway (formation of the membrane attack complex). The species of erythrocyte used in the assay and chelation of magnesium and/or calcium determines whether components of the classical pathway (CH50/CH100 or THC) or alternative pathway (AP50) are assayed. Deficiency in any one component will result in a failure of lysis. However the most common reason for failure of lysis is active infection, with consumption of complement components, or degradation of complement components if the sample is not separated and frozen within 2 h of venesection. If repeat testing shows a persistent abnormality, evaluation of individual complement components should be performed.

Assays for the activity of the lectin pathway are not widely available, although assay of serum concentrations of mannose binding lectin by enzyme linked immunosorbent assay (ELISA) is available in some centers. Polymorphic variants within the MBL gene affect serum concentrations of the protein.[18]

Neutrophil function tests
Neutrophil function has three main components: chemotaxis, phagocytosis and activation of the respiratory burst. Neutrophil function tests are difficult as neutrophils rapidly activate upon venesection and also die quickly. Historically, a wide range of neutrophil function tests have been performed, although their validity is questionable. This particularly applies to assays of neutrophil chemotaxis.

Chemiluminescence
This test evaluates the opsonizing capacity of patient serum, the ability of neutrophils and monocytes to phagocytose and activation of the respiratory burst. The use of autologous or third party serum can be used to distinguish defects in opsonization from defects in the respiratory burst. Phagocytosis of organisms by neutrophils and monocytes results in the activation of the respiratory burst and the production of oxygen free radicals. These react with oxidizable substances on microbes, such as unsaturated lipids, nucleic acids and peptides, to form unstable intermediates. When these intermediates return to their original state, light energy is emitted. This chemiluminescence is readily measured with a spectrophotometer or chemiluminometer. Such assays are being superseded by flow cytometric assays (see below).

Nitroblue tetrazolium reduction test
Nitroblue tetrazolium (NBT) is a yellow dye readily taken up by phagocytes and, upon stimulation [for example with phorbol myristate acetate (PMA)], is reduced to the purple dye formazan by the oxidative burst. In normal individuals, at least 95% of neutrophils should contain a purple deposit in stimulated cells. In CGD, less than 1% of neutrophils reduce NBT.

Carrier mothers of the X-linked disease can be detected by this method; they show an intermediate level of NBT reduction (20–80%) (Fig. 27.11). In experienced hands, this is a rapid and sensitive test for CGD.

Flow cytometric assays of neutrophil function
Phagocytosis
Fluorescently labeled organisms or inert agents can be used to assess the phagocytic ability of neutrophils. This assay is still primarily a research tool, but has the advantage of being able to study the phagocytic capability of the neutrophil to different organisms, and may help define the defect in undefined immunodeficiencies. Comparison of phagocytosis with autologous and control serum can be used to assess opsonization.

Oxidative burst
Neutrophils take up dihydrorhodamine, and activation of the respiratory burst by preincubation with PMA or other stimuli results in fluorescence within cells, which can be assessed using the flow cytometer. As with an NBT, carriers for CGD can also be detected.

Enzyme assays
Neutrophil killing defects may also occur in deficiency states of myeloperoxidase and glucose-6-phosphate dehydrogenase (G6PD), which can be assayed separately.

TESTS OF ADAPTIVE IMMUNITY
Test of humoral immunity
Immunoglobulins
IgG is the predominant circulating immunoglobulin. Smaller amounts of IgA, IgM, IgD and IgE are found in serum. A reduced or absent gamma globulin portion may be seen in serum electrophoresis in significant hypogammaglobulinemia. IgG, A and M are routinely quantified by nephelometry. This technique involves mixing of a known quantity of antibody to the test protein (in this case IgG, A or M) with serum containing an unknown quantity of the protein. Immune complexes form which will scatter light, the amount of light scattered being proportional to the quantity of protein within the sample. Results must be evaluated with reference to age-specific normal ranges, as production of all five classes of immunoglobulin is low at birth and gradually matures over the first 5 years of life. Immunoglobulin can be lost through the gut or urinary tract. Thus, low Ig levels can only be attributed to a production defect if gut or renal losses have been excluded and the serum albumin is within the normal range. A number of catabolic states, such as myotonic dystrophy, can also lower total immunoglobulin levels.

IgE is measured using a variety of techniques, including ELISA and automated solid-phase ELISAs. Measurement of IgE is indicated if hyper-IgE syndrome is included in the differential diagnosis.

IgD is present in the serum in very low concentrations. It may be nonspecifically increased as a part of multiple inflammatory reactions, but is not used as part of the routine assessment of immune deficiency. IgD is not routinely measured unless a periodic fever syndrome is suspected (see Ch. 28).

IgG subclasses
IgG subclasses are commonly measured by nephelometry or radial immunodiffusion. Results should be interpreted in the light of age-specific normal ranges. The utility of measuring IgG subclasses in children under 2 years of age, or if the total IgG is low, is debatable. In addition, approximately 10% of the normal population have undetectable IgG4, and normal ranges should be adjusted to reflect this.

Measures of in vivo antibody responses
The ability of the immune system to produce functional antibody is more important than the amount of circulating antibody. Functional tests of IgG production rely on measuring antibody titers to antigens to which the child is known to have been exposed either naturally or by vaccination. Responses to protein antigens such as tetanus, diphtheria and the conjugated Hib vaccine are widely available. However, although normal ranges

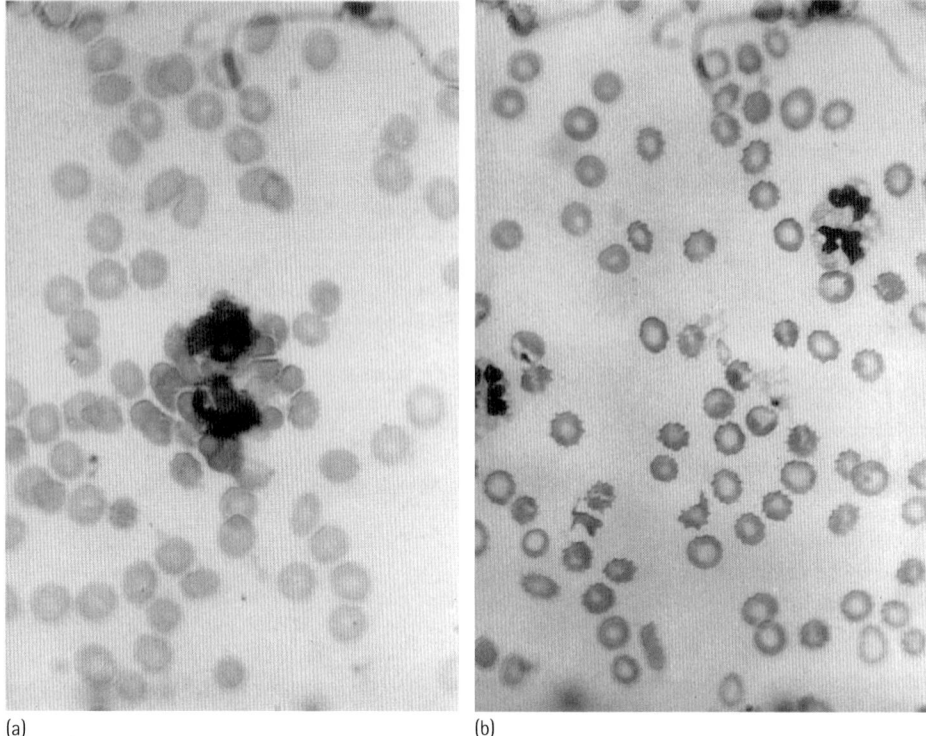

(a)   (b)

Fig. 27.11 Slide nitroblue tetrazolium (NBT) reduction test. (a) Normal subject. Neutrophils have taken up and reduced NBT to form a dense brown/black deposit. (b) Patient with chronic granulomatous disease. None of the cells has produced the deposit due to failure to reduce the NBT.

for antibody titers exist these are not well validated for antigens other than Hib, and may not be a true reflection of immunological memory. If antibody titers are low, booster vaccinations should be given to assess the memory response. In children over 2 years of age, administration of 23 serovalent polysaccharide vaccine (Pneumovax®) is useful to assess the ability to respond to carbohydrate antigens. Loss of this response may be the first sign of an evolving immunodeficiency in patients with common variable immunodeficiency or WAS. However, with the introduction of heptavalent conjugated pneumococcal vaccine into the national immunization program, assessment of pneumococcal polysaccharide antibodies is difficult as the Pneumovax® assay result is not possible to interpret if the child has received conjugate pneumococcal vaccine. Assessment of antibody responses to common respiratory viral pathogens and varicella zoster may provide useful additional information, although negative tests in the absence of microbiologically proven disease are difficult to interpret.

The optimal test of in vivo antibody production is assessment of IgM and IgG responses and rate of clearance to a novel antigen whose clearance is dependent on opsonization by a specific antibody. The harmless bacteriophage φX174 can be administered intravenously for this purpose, but this investigation is rarely used in current practice.[19,20]

Cell–mediated immunity

Humoral and cell-mediated immunity do not exist in isolation. Cell-mediated defects are likely to result in a degree of humoral immunodeficiency as the latter is dependent on the former for help in making an antibody response with memory.

Quantification of cell numbers

Cell-mediated immunity can be assessed by measuring the number and function of cells. Lymphocytes can be enumerated using flow cytometry, which uses fluid dynamics to separate cells into a single cell stream, passing through beams of laser light to scatter the light with a pattern determined by their size and granularity. The scattered light is detected by photon multiplier tubes. The different light scatter properties of cells enable populations of neutrophils, monocytes and lympho-cytes to be differentiated. Lymphocytes can be characterized further by

cell surface markers, tagged with monoclonal antibodies, whose fluorescent labels are excited by incident light beams (Fig. 27.12, Table 27.8). The number of cells staining with a particular monoclonal antibody can be expressed as a percentage of the lymphocyte pool or as an absolute number. Proportions of different lymphocytes and absolute numbers vary with age, and reference should be made to published age-related normal ranges.[21,22] Approximately 60–80% of circulating lymphocytes are T lymphocytes, with 10–20% B lymphocytes and 5–15% NK cells.

Functional tests of cell-mediated immunity

In vitro lymphocyte proliferation assays. When lymphocytes encounter antigen in vivo, they upregulate activation markers and proliferate, without which an effective immune response cannot occur. This can be mimicked in vitro by culturing lymphocytes for a defined time period with appropriate stimuli and using the incorporation of tritiated thymidine or a nonradioactive marker such as bromodeoxyuridine into the DNA of dividing cells as a surrogate measure of cell proliferation. A range of stimuli can be used. Plant lectins, e.g. PHA and concavalin A, act as potent T lymphocyte mitogens and cause high levels of proliferation in normal cells. A more physiological assessment of proliferative capacity can be obtained using a monoclonal antibody to the T lymphocyte surface protein, CD3, which results in direct receptor stimulation, or by using a recall antigen such as tetanus. Proliferation tests of in vitro B lymphocyte function, e.g. using pokeweed mitogen and EBV, are rarely indicated in modern clinical practice. The results of responses to recall antigens need to be interpreted in the light of previous exposure, which reduces their clinical utility in children. Mixed lymphocyte cultures (MLC) are a modification of lymphocyte proliferation assays where the stimulating cells are irradiated lymphocytes from an HLA disparate donor. MLC responses may be useful in assessing the suitability of donors prior to HSCT.

Other measures of lymphocyte function. As well as dividing upon stimulation, T lymphocytes produce a range of cytokines (e.g. IFN-gamma, IL-2) and express activation markers on their surface (e.g. CD69, CD25, MHC II). The latter may be detected after only a few hours of incubation with an appropriate stimulus. Neither of these assays provides the same

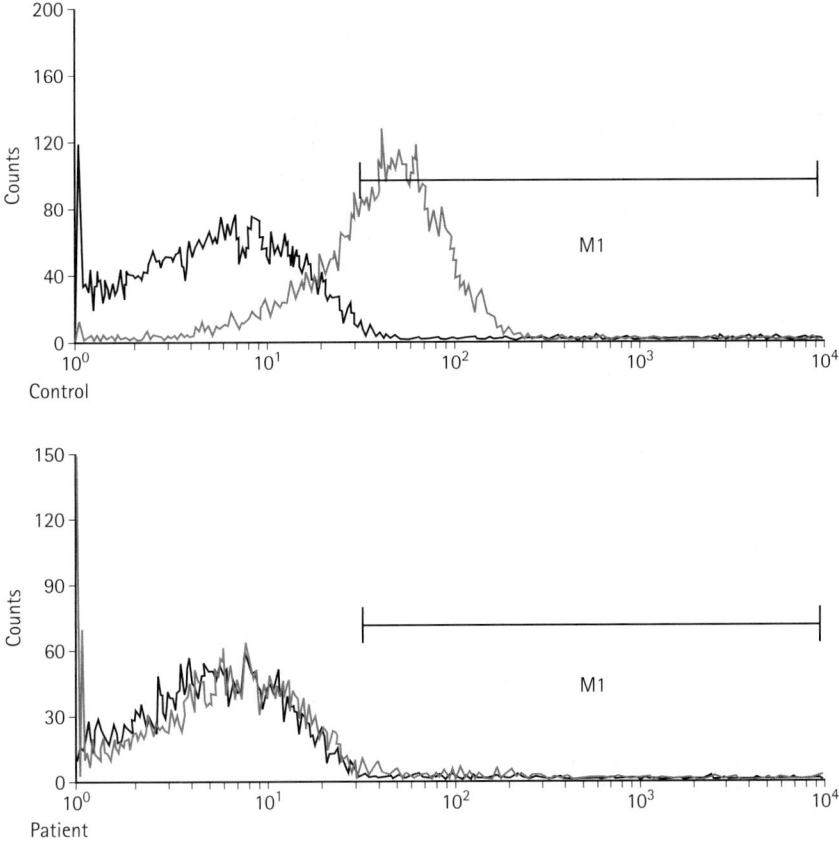

Fig. 27.12 Flow cytometric lymphocyte assay. Both plots show isotype control and staining for common gamma chain using flow cytometry. The control has normal levels of expression, represented by a shift in the histogram peak. Surface expression is lacking in the patient, enabling rapid molecular diagnosis of gamma chain deficient SCID.

information as that given by formal proliferation assays. Rare immune defects have been described with aberrant cytokine production, and cytokine assays may be useful in this context.

In vivo tests: delayed hypersensitivity skin tests. Delayed hypersensitivity skin tests can be performed using a number of common antigens, including those derived from candida, streptococcus, mumps and tetanus toxoid. Induration at the site is indicative of an intact cell-mediated immune response to the test antigen and makes it unlikely that the patient has a significant cell-mediated immune defect. Responses are dependent on established memory. Corticosteroids and some intercurrent viral infections may abrogate the response, which limits their clinical utility in children. They may, however, be useful in circumstances where in vitro lymphocyte proliferation assays are not readily available.

Definition of molecular defects

Protein assays. The genetic basis of an increasing number of immunodeficiencies is well defined; many occur because a surface or cytoplasmic signaling protein is absent or defective. In most cases a defect in the gene

coding for the protein results in either no protein expression, expression of low amounts, or expression of abnormally sized protein. These abnormalities can be detected using a combination of Western blotting (Fig. 27.13) and flow cytometry.[23] These are highly specialized investigations available in a limited number of centers.

Table 27.8 Common markers used to identify cell types

Cell type	Detected with fluorescent monoclonal light antibody to
All T lymphocytes	CD3
T helper cells	CD4
Cytotoxic T lymphocytes	CD8
B lymphocytes	CD19 or CD20
Natural killer cells	CD16 and CD56 or CD57
Memory T lymphocytes	CD45RO
Naive T lymphocytes	CD45RA

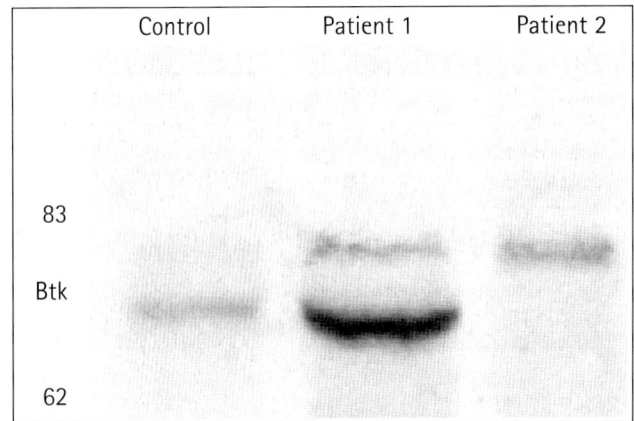

Fig. 27.13 Western blotting for btk protein, defective in X-linked agammaglobulinemia. Protein lysates are made from mononuclear cell extracts from peripheral blood. Btk is concentrated by immunoprecipitation with a btk specific antibody. Immunoprecipitates are then subjected to electrophoresis, which separates the proteins on the basis of size. Gels are incubated with a second anti-btk antibody to allow specific detection. Btk is seen in the control and patient 1, who lacked B cells but did not have X-linked agammaglobulinemia. Patient 2 lacked btk expression, and a mutation in btk was later defined.

Genetics. In the presence of an appropriate history or abnormal protein expression, genetic analysis may be undertaken. Genes can be screened using SSCP analysis or direct sequencing of genes. However, not all genetic differences between individuals result in clinical problems. Significant numbers of polymorphisms exist within the human genome which may have no clinical effects.

Carrier testing. Appropriate genetic counseling should be offered to all families. Once mutations have been defined, parents can be tested for carrier status. In a number of conditions nongenetic tests may be useful in determining carrier status. These include the NBT, in which intermediate numbers of neutrophils will reduce NBT in mothers who carry the mutation for X-linked CGD, and intermediate levels of adenosine deaminase (ADA) in carriers of ADA deficiency. Females randomly inactivate one of their X chromosomes in all cells. If a gene that is critical for the development of a particular cell lineage is carried on the X chromosome, this will result in apparent nonrandom X inactivation as cells where the good gene is inactivated will fail to develop. Detection of nonrandom X activation was historically a powerful tool for carrier detection, but as the X-linked immune deficiencies have now had their genetic basis defined, the need to rely on nonrandom X inactivation in the mother for carrier detection has been largely superseded. Carrier testing of siblings raises a number of ethical issues, and children should usually reach the age of informed consent before any tests are undertaken (see Ch. 10).

Antenatal diagnosis. Appropriate counseling by an individual conversant with the outcome of immunodeficiencies in the modern era should be undertaken before antenatal diagnosis is undertaken. Due to the small risk of miscarriage, screening should only be offered to mothers in whom the result would determine whether the mother would terminate the pregnancy. The gestation at which antenatal diagnosis can be undertaken is influenced by the nature of the immunodeficiency. Defined mutations can be screened for on CVS at 10–12 weeks' gestation. Fetal blood sampling at 18–20 weeks can be used where there is a clear phenotype, e.g. absent T lymphocytes, absent respiratory burst.

DISORDERS OF CELL-MEDIATED IMMUNITY: COMBINED IMMUNODEFICIENCIES

SEVERE COMBINED IMMUNODEFICIENCY (SCID)

Failure to develop normal T lymphocytes leads to lymphocyte-mediated immunodeficiency. T lymphocytes are also critical for the maturation and function of B lymphocytes and so the more severe T lymphocyte deficiencies are nearly always accompanied by defective antibody responses resulting in a combined (lymphocyte-mediated and humoral) deficiency. In other combined immunodeficiencies single gene defects affect both B and T lymphocyte development. The severity of the humoral deficiency varies from a subtle defect of specific antibody response to complete hypogammaglobulinemia. Thus, it is unusual to find a significant primary T lymphocyte deficiency syndrome accompanied by normal humoral immune function. Combined immunodeficiency results from a large number of disorders with X-linked or autosomal recessive inheritance.[24] The molecular basis of many combined immunodeficiencies has now been elucidated (Table 27.9). The most severe phenotype, SCID, is associated with a profound T lymphopenia and panhypogammaglobulinemia with early death from infection. Whilst the usual clinical features of this group of diseases are well characterized, atypical presentations and 'leaky' forms with an attenuated phenotype are increasingly recognized. Circulating T lymphocyte numbers are usually low or absent but may be normal. In the classic SCID presentation, lymphocyte responses to mitogen are absent, but may be present in attenuated forms where immunoglobulin may also be produced. However, tests of antigen-specific T lymphocyte proliferation and antibody production are defective and there is cutaneous anergy. Patients usually have a limited diversity of T lymphocyte receptor and immunoglobulin gene rearrangements. Diagnosis may be more difficult in atypical patients. Identifying the molecular defect in specific patients with combined immunodeficiency or SCID is important for prognosis, treatment, genetic counseling and increasing our knowledge about these rare diseases. When identified, the name of the underlying molecular defect should be used.

General features of severe combined immunodeficiency

The presenting clinical features are characterized by early onset, persistent respiratory tract or gut infection and failure to thrive.[25] Affected babies appear well at birth but within the first few months of life fail to clear infection and fall progressively away from their birth centile. Chronic diarrhea and failure to thrive are due to persistent and sometimes multiple gastrointestinal viral infections, often with associated food intolerance. Persistent respiratory tract infections with respiratory syncytial virus or parainfluenza viruses are common, with failure to clear virus accompanying persistent bronchiolitic-like signs. An insidiously progressive persistent respiratory infection with radio-

Table 27.9 Classification of severe combined immunodeficiency

Syndrome	T lymphocytes	B lymphocytes	NK lymphocytes	Inheritance
Reticular dysgenesis	−	−	−	AR
ADA deficiency	−	−	−	AR
RAG1, 2 deficiency	−	−	+	AR
Artemis deficiency (RS*)	−	−	+	AR
CgC deficiency	−	+	−	XL
JAK-3 deficiency	−	+	−	AR
IL-7Rα deficiency	−	+	+	AR
ZAP-70 kinase deficiency	CD4+	+	+	AR
MHC II deficiency	CD8+	+	+	AR
p56lck deficiency	CD8+	+	+	AR
IL-2/IL15Rb	CD8+	+	−	AR
Idiopathic CD4 lymphopenia	CD8+	+	+	AR
CD45 deficiency	+	+	+	AR
WHN gene deficiency	+	+	+	AR
Omenn syndrome	+	−	+	AR
Nonhost T lymphocytes (MFE or transfusion GvHD)	+	+/−	+/−	

ADA, adenosine deaminase; AR, autosomal recessive; CgC, common interleukin gamma chain; GvHD, graft versus host disease; IL-7Rα, interleukin 7 receptor alpha; JAK-3, janus-associated kinase 3; MFE, maternofetal engraftment; RAG, recombination activating genes; WHN, winged-helix-nude; XL, X-linked; ZAP-70, zeta-associated kinase-70.
* RS, radiosensitive.

logical evidence of interstitial pneumonitis should raise the suspicion of *Pneumocystis carinii* infection, often a co-pathogen with respiratory viruses. Other presentations include prolonged otitis media and invasive bacterial infections, particularly staphylococcal or pseudomonas septicemia and pneumonia, which may respond poorly to appropriate treatment. Severe invasive fungal infection is rare, but often fatal. Extensive, persistent superficial candidiasis is more common. Occasionally babies present with disseminated BCG or vaccine-strain poliomyelitis virus. Children presenting within the first 6 months or so of life are more likely to have SCID or a severe T lymphocyte defect.

Non-infectious manifestations mainly result from graft versus host disease (GvHD) caused by the inability to reject foreign lymphocytes acquired either from the mother in utero or from un-irradiated blood transfusion. Engraftment of transplacentally acquired maternal lymphocytes (maternofetal GvHD, MFGvHD) sometimes, but not always provokes GvHD, typically with a mild reticular skin rash with or without slightly deranged liver function tests. Its role in the gastrointestinal symptoms is not known. Fatal GvHD can follow transfusion with non-irradiated blood or with white lymphocyte or platelet concentrates. In these cases the skin rash is more severe and lymphadenopathy and hepatosplenomegaly may be present; here cases may be clinically indistinguishable from Omenn syndrome (see below), but identification of maternal cells by karyotype or DNA fingerprinting will distinguish MFGvHD from Omenn syndrome. EBV infection may lead to uncontrolled B lymphoproliferative disorders, similar to that seen in solid organ transplant recipients.

Examination usually reveals a wasted child (Fig. 27.14) who has dropped through the growth centiles, with evidence of candidiasis and other infections. Skin rashes may be indicative of infection or GvHD. There is no clinically detectable lymphoid tissue. There may be hepatomegaly.

Investigations show severe lymphopenia from birth; in infancy a normal lymphocyte count is $> 2.7 \times 10^9$/L, and if the normal adult lower limit of 1.0×10^9/L is quoted, the lymphopenia will be missed. Lymphocyte phenotyping shows severely depleted T lymphocyte numbers; B lymphocytes and NK cells may be present, or absent. Occasional variants show unusual patterns of mature T lymphocyte markers; in such cases maternal engraftment should be excluded. Mitogen responses, MLC reaction, and in vitro antigen specific responses are usually absent. Immunoglobulin estimations show low levels of IgG, IgA and IgM but may be misleading as residual maternal IgG may give a falsely reassuring result and it can be difficult to distinguish IgA and IgM levels in SCID from the low levels seen in normal infants; furthermore some SCID infants make IgM, but this is not functionally active. Isohemagglutinins are a useful measure of in vitro IgM production and absence is significant. If SCID is suspected, lymphocyte phenotyping is more reliable than immunoglobulin estimation. Chest radiographs show an absent thymus, and hyperinflation and/or interstitial pneumonia, if infection is present. Typical cupping and flaring

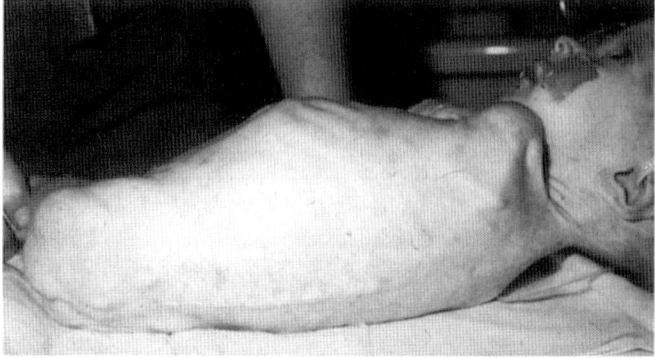

Fig. 27.14 Wasting in a child with severe combined immunodeficiency (SCID).

of the costochondral junction is also evident in patients with ADA deficient SCID.

In children who die, postmortem examination reveals severely depleted lymphoid tissue, with nodes and thymus showing no lymphoid lymphocytes and absent Hassall's corpuscles in the latter. Plasma lymphocytes are absent.

Without treatment, patients die from infection by about 12 months of age. Currently, the only curative treatment is hemopoietic stem cell transplantation (HSCT), although clinical gene therapy trials for common gamma chain deficiency and ADA deficiency are in progress. Supportive interim treatments include antibiotic prophylaxis with co-trimoxazole as antipneumocystis treatment, antifungal prophylaxis and immunoglobulin replacement. Live vaccines should be avoided. The diagnosis of SCID is a pediatric emergency, and suspected cases should be urgently referred to a designated treatment center for further assessment and treatment.

TYPES OF SEVERE COMBINED AND COMBINED IMMUNODEFICIENCIES
T negative B positive SCID
Common gamma chain deficiency (X-linked SCID)
The most common form of SCID is characterized by severe lymphopenia, absence of mature T and NK lymphocytes, but normal numbers of circulating B lymphocytes. It is caused by a deficiency of the gamma chain common to the IL-2, -4, -7, -9, -15 and -21 receptors. The easiest form of SCID to treat, the first successful gene therapy was performed for this condition. Carriers show nonrandom skewed X inactivation of T lymphocytes.

JAK-3 deficiency
This autosomal recessive form of SCID is phenotypically identical to the X-linked common gamma chain deficiency. It is due to mutations in the gene encoding Janus-associated-kinase 3, a protein which binds to the intracellular tail of the common gamma chain, and through which signals are transduced following cytokine binding.

IL-7R alpha deficiency
This autosomal recessive form of SCID is characterized by a T− B+ NK+ phenotype, and is due to mutations in the gene encoding the IL-7R alpha.

T negative B negative SCID
Four forms of this autosomal recessive disorder have been described. Phenotypically they are identical, with absent T and B lymphocytes, but normal numbers of NK lymphocytes present. The first form is due to defects in the recombinase activating genes (RAG) which are necessary for the development of diverse T and B lymphocyte antigen receptors. In the second form cells cannot repair DNA normally following radiation damage and patients' fibroblasts show in vitro radiosensitivity. The defect is in the artemis gene, which is necessary for rejoining DNA following TCR and B cell receptor (BCR) recombination. Two other DNA repair defects, DNA ligase 4 deficiency and cernunnos-XLF, can also present with a T− B− NK+ phenotype, sometimes associated with microcephaly. Whilst treatable by HSCT, results are not as good as in the T− B+ form of SCID. 'Leaky' RAG and artemis defects have been shown in some patients with Omenn syndrome.

Omenn syndrome
Omenn syndrome is characterized by a generalized erythematous rash, often with scaling and erythroderma, lymphadenopathy, hepatosplenomegaly, increased serum IgE levels with a marked eosinophilia and combined immunodeficiency.[26] Children usually present in early infancy but atypical forms may present towards the end of the first year of life, with the clinical features described, as well as diarrhea, failure to thrive and persistent infection. There are normally high numbers of oligoclonal activated poorly functional T lymphocytes of the T_H2 phenotype but few if any B lymphocytes and low levels of immunoglobulin. The syndrome has

been called a 'leaky' form of SCID in that small numbers of very abnormal T lymphocytes 'leak' past the block in T lymphocyte development. The underlying defect, at least in some cases, is a mutation in the RAG or artemis genes. Other cases with defects in IL-7R alpha are described.

In some families, one affected individual has presented with T− B− NK+ SCID whilst another has presented with Omenn syndrome. The clinical picture may resemble SCID with maternofetal engraftment, when maternal T lymphocytes crossing the placenta cause a GvHD-like reaction in an immunocompromised patient. Molecular genetic studies to identify the origin of the dermal infiltrative T lymphocytes can differentiate the two disorders. Activated oligoclonal lymphocytes in skin seemingly provoke Langerhans' cells to migrate to lymph nodes, liver and spleen where lymphoid tissue architecture is severely disrupted. It has been suggested that IFN-gamma may ameliorate the clinical symptoms, but HSCT is the only curative treatment.

Reticular dysgenesis
This rare form of SCID, inherited as an autosomal recessive trait, is characterized by defective lymphoid and myeloid differentiation. Bone marrow examination confirms the absence of myeloid precursors. Platelets and erythrocytes are formed normally. There is some evidence that this is not a discrete entity, but due to other forms of SCID, complicated by severe maternal engraftment and bone marrow GvHD.[27] The absence of the innate cellular elements of the immune system makes the immunodeficiency even more severe than in other forms of SCID. Clinical presentation often occurs earlier, as does the inevitable fatal outcome if immune reconstitution cannot be achieved.

Lymphocyte metabolism defects
ADA deficiency
This variety of SCID is due to a single gene defect which results in absence of the purine metabolic pathway enzyme, ADA.[28] Although the enzyme is expressed widely throughout the body, accumulation of adenosine and 2 -deoxyadenosine in immature lymphocytes is particularly damaging resulting in cell death. Patients typically present earlier than with other forms of SCID, with very low numbers of T, B and NK lymphocytes. Skeletal abnormalities (cupping deformities of the ends of the ribs, as well as abnormalities of the transverse vertebral processes and the scapulae) are reported in up to 50% of cases and can be correlated with histological changes.[29] Neurodevelopmental problems may also occur in some patients.[30]

Partial forms of ADA deficiency are associated with a milder immunodeficiency. Occasional cases of ADA deficiency have been described where, inexplicably, immune function is normal. The diagnosis is confirmed by finding very low erythrocyte ADA activity and high levels of deoxyadenosine triphosphate in the urine. First trimester antenatal diagnosis can be made by assaying ADA activity in chorionic villus sampling. Treatment is by HSCT or by use of replacement polyethylene glycol-coupled ADA (PEG-ADA). Over several weeks immune function improves considerably, and although not to full normality, often to a degree sufficient to keep the child free of infections and thriving. PEG-ADA has been used on a long term basis in those without a suitable donor. The disadvantages of this include the enormous cost, the continuing dependence on intensive medical input and concerns that the beneficial effects will not be maintained in the long term. Patients can develop antibodies against the bovine ADA but to date in most cases these have not been of great clinical significance.[31] Gene therapy is being offered for some patients with this condition.

Purine nucleoside phosphorylase (PNP) deficiency
Deficiency of the purine metabolic pathway enzyme, PNP, which results in combined immunodeficiency, is initially less severe than ADA deficiency though there is progression with age. It is an autosomal recessive condition, the gene for which is found on chromosome 9. The metabolites deoxyguanosine and deoxyguanosine triphosphate are particularly toxic for thymocytes resulting in a T lymphocyte deficiency with relatively preserved B lymphocyte function.[32]

The onset of symptoms is usually later than in ADA deficiency, and can be delayed for several years though most cases present in infancy with recurrent and severe infections, particularly with viruses and fungi, diarrhea and failure to thrive. There is a marked tendency to autoimmune disease, especially hemolytic anemia which can progress to red cell aplasia and a predisposition to GvHD following non-irradiated blood transfusion. Skeletal abnormalities do not occur, but neurodevelopmental problems are found in over half of all patients, particularly spastic paresis, disequilibrium and ataxia. There may also be more general neurodevelopmental and behavioral problems. In one series 20% of patients presented primarily with neurological disorder.[33]

Laboratory tests show a progressive fall in T lymphocyte numbers and function with time, poor in vitro mitogen responses and negative delayed hypersensitivity skin tests. Immunoglobulin levels and antibody responses are initially normal but in the late stages levels fall. Serum uric acid levels are very low. The diagnosis is confirmed by demonstrating absent PNP activity in erythrocytes or fibroblasts and deoxyinosine and deoxyguanosine in the urine. Asymptomatic forms of the deficiency have not been reported. Prenatal diagnosis can be made by enzyme activity assays on chorionic villus samples.

The prognosis without corrective treatment is poor with most cases dying in early childhood. The risk of development of malignancy is high. Treatment with HSCT is therefore indicated as early as possible. If successful this corrects the immunodeficiency but its effect on the neurological disease is uncertain. Enzyme replacement therapy with fresh irradiated red blood cells and other biochemical manipulations have not met with sustained success.

Other combined immunodeficiencies
Other rare immunodeficiencies have been described in only a few patients to date, with defects in other surface and signaling molecules (Table 27.10). It is likely that these will become increasingly recognized as more laboratories are able to offer diagnostic testing. Other atypical or unusual presentations may be due to defects in molecules already described, or to as yet unidentified molecules or mutations.

ZAP-70 kinase defect (CD8 deficiency)
Defective signal transduction in T lymphocytes results from this autosomal recessive condition.[34] The defective kinase is important in T lymphocyte activation via the CD3/TCR complex. There is a marked effect on CD8+ lymphocyte development, resulting in a profound CD8+ lymphopenia which is the hallmark of this condition. Though CD4 lymphocytes are present in normal numbers, they are nonfunctional.

Idiopathic CD4 lymphocytopenia
A marked depression in the CD4 positive lymphocyte count characterizes this condition. Most reports have been on adult patients, but it can be seen in children. It is best regarded as a primary immunodeficiency disorder[35] as strenuous efforts to look for a retroviral cause have proved negative and the epidemiology of the condition does not fit with a viral infection. Affected individuals may be highly susceptible to opportunistic infections. The nature of the defect is poorly understood. There may well be a number of different causes.

Table 27.10 Other forms of severe combined immunodeficiency

Defect	Phenotype
IL-2Rβ/IL-15Rβ deficiency	T^{LOW} B+ NK−
CD45 deficiency	T^{LOW} B+ NK^{LOW}
IL-2Rα deficiency	T^{LOW} B+ NK+
CD3γ deficiency	T^{LOW} B+ NK+
CD3δ deficiency	T− B+ NK+
CD3ε deficiency	T^{LOW} B+ NK+

Immunoglobulin levels and antibody responses may be normal. The natural history of this condition is not well understood. The CD4 cell count remains stable for a prolonged period in most patients rather than progressively declining as in HIV infection. Prophylaxis against *Pneumocystis carinii* infection should be given. HSCT has been successfully performed.

MHC ANTIGEN DEFICIENCY

MHC CLASS II DEFICIENCY

Major histocompatibility complex (MHC) class II antigens (HLA DR, DP, DQ) are expressed on a limited repertoire of cells and present antigen to CD4+ T lymphocytes, which, following an appropriate second signal, activate T helper lymphocytes specific for that antigen and initiate an effective immune response. Expression of MHC II in the thymus is essential for positive selection of CD4+ T lymphocytes, and lack of MHC II expression, previously described as a variant of the 'bare lymphocyte syndrome', results in a profound susceptibility to viral, bacterial, fungal and protozoal infections.[3]

The disease is rare and is inherited in an autosomal recessive manner. The MHC II genes are normal and MHC II deficiency results from mutations in several different genes which code for a complex of regulatory factors controlling transcription of MHC II genes. The genes involved include MHC2TA, RFX5 and RFXAP.[36] The clinical and laboratory variability does not correlate with genotype.

The clinical picture resembles SCID, although often infections develop slightly later. Intestinal and hepatic complications due to cryptosporidial infections are more common than in other immune defects. Neurological manifestations due to a range of viral infections are also well described. Coxsackie virus, adenovirus and poliovirus were the most frequently reported causes of meningoencephalitis.

The laboratory phenotype is variable, but most patients have CD4 lymphopenia and hypogammaglobulinemia, with normal lymphocyte proliferation responses. The diagnosis can be confirmed flow cytometrically by showing absent or significantly reduced levels of class II molecules, e.g. DR, on cells that constitutively express class II (B lymphocytes and monocytes).

Affected children require treatment with replacement immunoglobulin, co-trimoxazole and antifungal prophylaxis pending HSCT, which is the definitive treatment although this has had limited success in comparison to other types of SCID.[37]

MHC CLASS I DEFICIENCY

Although described before MHC II deficiency, SCID due to abnormal expression of the A, B and C components of the MHC I complex is much less common. MHC I is required for development of CD8 positive T lymphocytes, and affected children have low numbers of these cells. Mitogen responses are frequently normal. The genetic basis for the disease is mutations in TAP1 or 2.[38] These proteins are required for transport of antigen from the cytoplasm into the endoplasmic reticulum where they associate with MHC I. If the assembly of the antigen/MHC I complex cannot be completed due to antigenic lack, then the MHC is destroyed in the cytoplasm.

Clinically this disease has a milder phenotype than MHC II deficiency with symptoms often not beginning until late childhood. Recurrent respiratory tract infections leading to bronchiectasis and sinus problems are common. Gastrointestinal disease is rare. Unusual skin lesions thought to be due to vasculitis have been reported in a few patients.

Diagnosis is confirmed by showing absent HLA class I expression in peripheral blood. Treatment is directed towards prevention/limitation of lung disease with judicious use of antibiotics (directed by sputum cultures), physiotherapy and bronchodilators as required. Prophylactic continuous antibiotics are of unproven benefit, but may be helpful. The majority of cases do not require replacement immunoglobulin therapy or bone marrow transplantation.

COMBINED IMMUNODEFICIENCY FORMING PART OF OTHER SYNDROMES

DiGEORGE ANOMALY

This condition results from abnormal cephalic neural crest cell migration into the third and fourth pharyngeal arches in early embryological development. A microdeletion at chromosome 22q11.2 is present in 90% of cases whilst others are associated with other chromosomal anomalies, including 10p−. The 22q microdeletion is also found in velocardiofacial or Shprintzen syndrome, as well as some cases of Opitz G/BBB, a syndrome which should now be considered as a part of the same spectrum. In a few families with the DiGeorge phenotype, mutations have been identified in Tbx1, a gene within the 22q11 deleted region. Tbx1 is required for the development of the pharyngeal arches, which are important for the development of the thymus and parathyroid glands. DiGeorge anomaly is sporadic in occurrence, though familial cases, some associated with 22q chromosomal deletions, have been reported with a prevalence of 1 in 3000–4000 live births. The syndrome is extremely heterogeneous: partial forms are more common than the complete phenotype. Whilst it is classically recognized by the triad of congenital heart defects, immunodeficiency secondary to thymic hypoplasia and hypocalcemia secondary to parathyroid gland hypoplasia, an expanded phenotype is increasingly recognized with dysmorphic facies [low set, abnormally formed ears, hypertelorism and antimongoloid slant, micrognathia, short philtrum to the upper lip and high arched palate; (Fig. 27.15)], palatal abnormalities (cleft palate, velopharyngeal insufficiency), autoimmune phenomena, learning difficulties (particularly speech delay), renal anomalies, neuropsychiatric disorders and short stature. Conotruncal heart defects are classically associated with the syndrome, but other defects are seen including tetralogy of Fallot, septal defects, pulmonary atresia and aberrant subclavian vessels (see Ch. 21). Some patients have normal cardiac anatomy.

Severe T lymphocyte immunodeficiency presenting with a SCID phenotype of profound lymphopenia and poor lymphocyte proliferation is rare (< 1.5% of cases). Humoral immunodeficiency is more common, presenting with recurrent sinopulmonary infection, which may improve with time. Occasionally significant lung damage may occur due to repeated infection. Autoimmune features are increasingly recognized, including juvenile chronic arthritis, autoimmune thyroiditis and autoimmune cytopenias. The long term immunological outlook is not well defined.

All children diagnosed with 22q11.2 deletion should have an immunological evaluation including lymphocyte subset analysis, T lymphocyte proliferative responses, immunoglobulin levels and specific antibody responses to vaccination antigens. Laboratory findings may show severe T lymphocyte depletion with poor mitogen responses or relatively normal findings. Previously considered a T lymphocyte defect, recent studies have shown that antibody responses, particularly to polysaccharide antigens, may be impaired. Immunoglobulin levels may be normal but hypogammaglobulinemia may develop, and minor humoral abnormalities are common. Chest radiographs show absence of a thymic shadow.

In the severe phenotype, the cardiac problems are the main prognostic determinant. Blood products should be irradiated if T lymphocyte mitogen responses are poor. Patients with severe immunodeficiency have been successfully treated with fetal thymus implants. In the partial phenotype with normal T lymphocyte function, the usual infant vaccination schedule can be followed and it is safe to give live vaccines such as measles, mumps, rubella vaccine or varicella zoster vaccine as long as the CD4 count exceeds 400/mm³ and there are normal T lymphocyte mitogen responses. Demonstration of good antibody responses to tetanus and Hib vaccination gives further reassurance that live vaccines can be safely administered.[39] Prophylactic antibiotics and occasionally intravenous immunoglobulin can be helpful, particularly for young children with recurrent infection due to humoral deficiency.

Some infants with CHARGE syndrome (coloboma; heart anomaly; atresia, choanal; retardation of mental and somatic development;

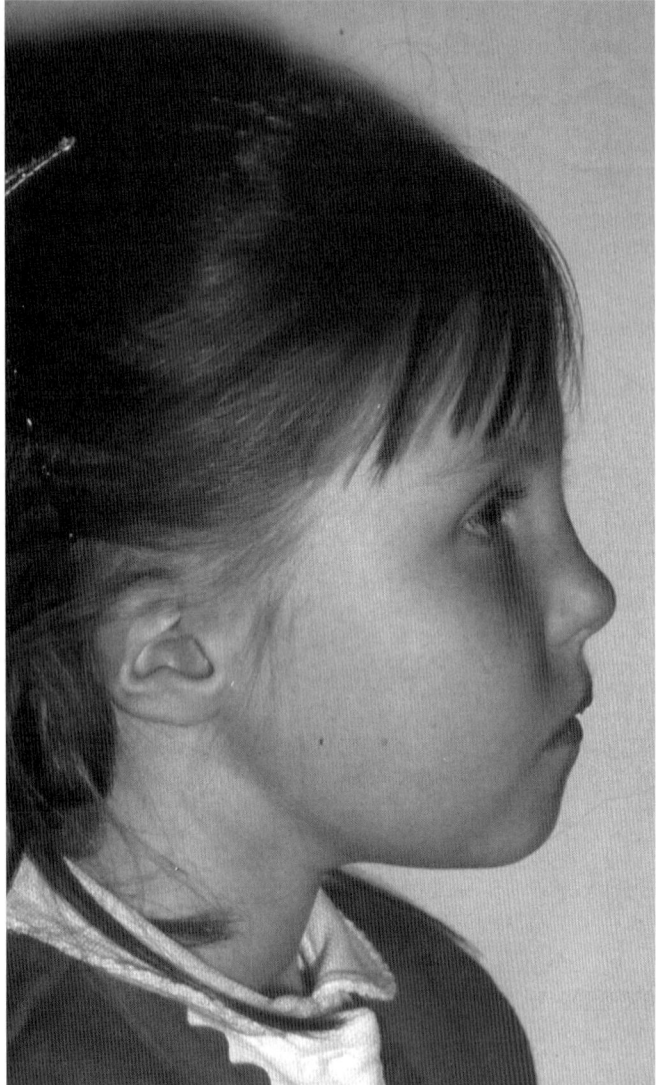

Fig. 27.15 Facies of a child with DiGeorge syndrome. (Reproduced with permission of the Bubble Foundation and the family.)

microphallus; ear abnormalities and/or deafness) due to a defect in the CHD7 gene can also present with severe immunodeficiency.[40] Treatment is the same as that for severe immunodeficiency in DiGeorge syndrome.

WISKOTT–ALDRICH SYNDROME (WAS)

Immunodeficiency, thrombocytopenia, eczema and an increased risk of autoimmune disorders and malignancy characterize this X-linked recessive condition. The gene codes for a novel 501 amino acid protein, the Wiskott–Aldrich syndrome protein (WASP), only found in bone marrow derived cells. Mutations in the same gene are found in patients with X-linked thrombocytopenia (XLT) and X-linked severe congenital neutropenia.

Clinical features

The classic features of thrombocytopenia, recurrent infections and eczema vary in severity and in some patients the eczema is surprisingly mild. The condition usually presents in early life with bruising, petechiae and bleeding: thrombocytopenia and bleeding episodes may require platelet transfusions. In XLT, thrombocytopenia with small platelet volume is the only symptom, perhaps with mild eczema. In WAS, bacterial and/or viral infections of the upper and lower respiratory tract are common and opportunistic infection, such as *Pneumocystis carinii*, may occur. Herpes viruses, including herpes simplex and varicella zoster

virus, are poorly handled and may cause severe and recurrent disease. Impetigo, cellulitis and skin abscesses are common; molluscum contagiosum and viral warts may be very extensive. Infection exacerbates the bleeding tendency, and early death may result from bleeding. With increasing age, infective problems replace bleeding as the major cause of death. Immunization with polysaccharide vaccines is ineffective and can cause severe, even fatal, reactions. The median survival is between 3 and 15 years. Autoimmunity, particularly autoimmune hemolytic anemia and vasculitis, and lymphoreticular malignancy become more common with increasing age and in many cases are related to abnormal persistence of EBV infection.[41] Scoring systems have been used to distinguish the milder phenotype of XLT from classic WAS. Heterozygous female carriers are clinically normal and demonstrate random X inactivation in all hemopoietic cells.

Laboratory tests

Thrombocytopenia with an abnormally small mean platelet volume (mean platelet volume < 5 fl) is pathognomonic. The severity of immunodeficiency is variable, but affects cellular and humoral responses. T lymphopenia is progressive with depressed responses to mitogens and antigens and negative delayed hypersensitivity skin tests. Serum immunoglobulins show a characteristic pattern with a very low IgM, normal IgG and raised IgA and IgE. Antibody responses to tetanus, *Haemophilus influenzae* type B and pneumococcus are often low, as are isohemagglutinin titers. The direct Coombs test is frequently positive, with or without a hemolytic anemia. In vivo neutrophil and monocyte chemotaxis is impaired. Electron microscopy shows greatly reduced numbers of microvilli on lymphocytes and platelets due to failure of the normal binding of actin bundles which is critical to the organization of the cytoskeleton. Lymphoid and myeloid cell lines are all affected so that phagocytes migrate poorly to sites of inflammation and do not put out normal filopodia, dendritic cells do not present antigen effectively, lymphocytes do not signal to each other normally and platelets form imperfectly from megakaryocytes.[42] WASP has a number of unique domains, suggesting multiple functions, which may explain the complex phenotype of a single gene mutation. Mis-sense mutations in exons 1–3 which lead to normal or truncated sized protein result in the milder phenotype of XLT, whereas most other mutations result in the classic WAS phenotype.

Treatment

Acute bleeding episodes may be controlled by platelet transfusions (irradiated to prevent GvHD). Splenectomy and systemic steroids should be avoided if possible as they will increase the risk of infection. Topical steroids are required for the eczema. Immunoglobulin replacement, with or without prophylactic antibiotics, reduces bacterial sinopulmonary infections and in high dose may help treat autoimmune phenomena.

With only these supportive measures the prognosis remains poor. Immunological and hematological reconstitution can be achieved by HSCT, and despite a higher risk of EBV-driven lymphoproliferative disorders 5-year survival is 87% after HLA identical sibling donor HSCT and 71% after unrelated donor HSCT.[43] Partial chimerism may lead to the presence of autoimmune features, but the risk of lymphoid malignancy should be diminished.

X-LINKED HYPER-IgM SYNDROME (CD40 LIGAND DEFICIENCY)

X-linked hyper-IgM syndrome is a T lymphocyte immunodeficiency due to a defect in the gene encoding for the CD40 ligand glycopeptide (CD154) expressed on activated T lymphocytes. CD40L binds to CD40, expressed on B lymphocytes and monocyte/macrophage derived cells. Lack of binding prevents immunoglobulin isotype switching from IgM to IgA, IgG and IgE as well as activation of Kupffer cells and pulmonary macrophages. Lack of IgA and IgG results in a similar clinical picture to X-linked agammaglobulinemia (XLA) with sinopulmonary and invasive

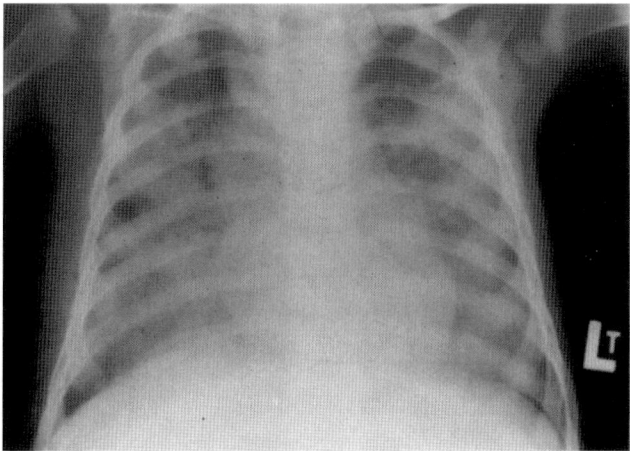

Fig. 27.16   Chest radiograph of a 6-month-old boy, presenting with *Pneumocystis carinii* pneumonia. The underlying immune deficiency was found to be CD40 ligand deficiency.

bacterial infection but in contrast to XLA, opportunistic infections also occur; failure of T lymphocytes to activate pulmonary macrophages results in *Pneumocystis carinii* pneumonia (Figs 27.16 and 27.17) whilst ineffective Kupffer cell function allows repeated infections of bowel, pancreas and biliary tree with *Cryptosporidium parvum* and similar organisms leading to sclerosing cholangitis, cirrhosis, pancreatitis and hepatic malignancy which becomes clinically apparent in the second or third decade. Neutropenia with oral ulceration is common, and when combined with low or absent IgA and IgG and normal or raised IgM should suggest the diagnosis. Fatal CMV infection or enteroviral meningoencephalitis can occur. Autoimmune phenomena are relatively common and include hemolytic anemias, thrombocytopenia, hypothyroidism, arthritis and liver disorders.[15]

Patients should receive co-trimoxazole as *Pneumocystis carinii* pneumonia prophylaxis and high doses of immunoglobulin replacement therapy are often required. With adequate replacement the rising IgM levels may normalize. The neutropenia sometimes responds to granulocyte colony stimulating factor (G-CSF) and immunoglobulin replacement. All drinking water should be boiled. Azithromycin prophylaxis may lessen the risks of *Cryptosporidium parvum* infection. Despite conventional treatment, many patients do not survive beyond the second decade of life, but a few patients with a common variable immunodeficiency-like clinical course are relatively well in middle life. HSCT is increasingly recommended for this condition[44] and combined HSC and liver transplantation has been successful.

X-LINKED LYMPHOPROLIFERATIVE DISEASE

An X-linked immunodeficiency associated with fulminant fatal EBV-driven infectious mononucleosis was first recognized in the Duncan kindred.[45] There are three common clinical presentations: fulminant infectious mononucleosis (58%), dysgammaglobulinemia, often evolving to common variable immunodeficiency (CVID) (31%) and EBV-driven B lymphocyte lymphoma, usually extranodal, and affecting the gastrointestinal tract or central nervous system (20%). Less commonly patients present with vasculitis, aplastic anemia, hemophagocytic lymphohistiocytosis or pulmonary lymphomatoid granulomatosis.[46] The prognosis is poor with 45–96% mortality, depending on the clinical presentation, and registry data indicate no survivors after 40 years of age. Most patients are well until infected with EBV, although other viruses may act as triggers. The gene responsible for the disease, SH2D1A in the Xq25 region of the X chromosome, was identified in 1998.[47] The gene encodes a small protein, signaling lymphocyte activation molecule (SLAM) associated protein (SAP), which appears critical for T lymphocyte and NK cell control of EBV-infected B lymphocytes but why this causes the clinical features is not yet understood.

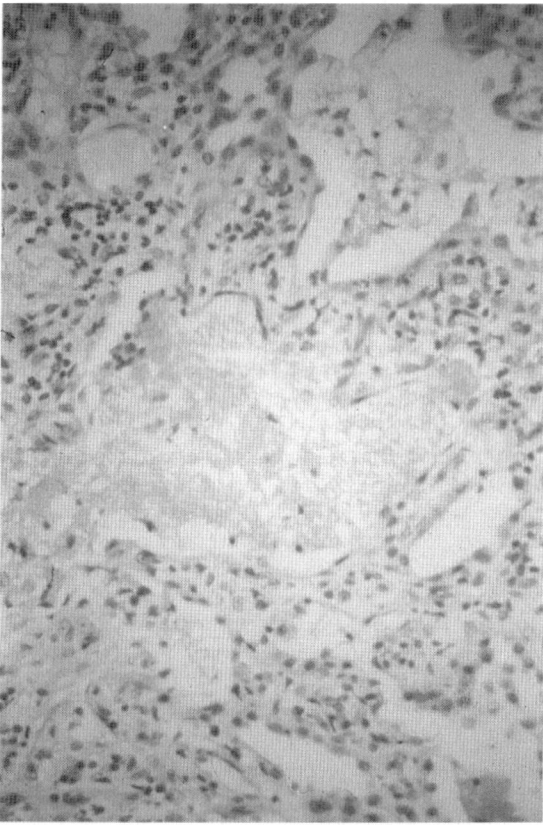

(a)

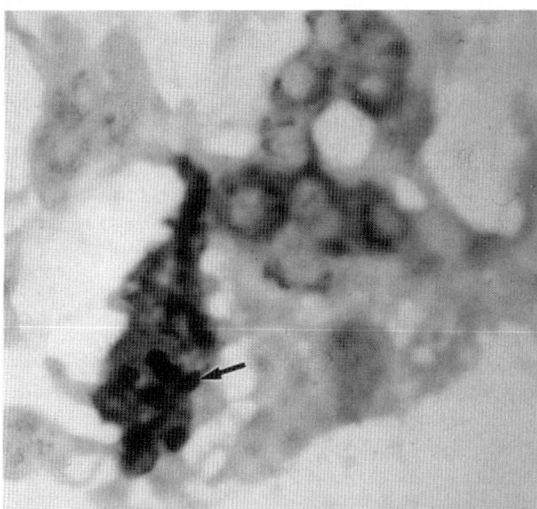

(b)

Fig. 27.17   Lung histology following open lung biopsy in the patient whose chest radiograph is shown in Figure 27.16. (a) Hematoxylin and eosin stain showing marked inflammatory infiltrate. (b) Grocott methenamine stain showing *Pneumocystis* organisms (arrowed).

Confirmation of the diagnosis involves demonstrating EBV genome in blood by PCR, together with the immune defects outlined above and an abnormal serological response to the virus with absent antibody response to EB nuclear antigen. Mothers of affected boys also have abnormal EBV serology, with persisting very high titers against viral capsid antigen. Whilst the majority of cases appear to be triggered by EBV infection, EBV negative clinical cases have been described.[48] Protein analysis reveals absent or abnormal SAP protein in many cases, although a gene mutation is not apparent in up to 40% of patients, raising the possibility of mutations in intrinsic elements or other control proteins. Regular treatment with immunoglobulin replacement as passive immunization against EBV is recommended in affected patients, particularly if hypogammaglobulinemia is present. Hemophagocytic lymphohistiocytic episodes may be treated with immunosuppression with ciclosporin. Correction of the disorder by HSCT has been achieved and is the only curative treatment. Other family members may be diagnosed from the index case and should be offered HSCT.

IMMUNODEFICIENCY AND SHORT-LIMBED DWARFISM

T and B lymphocyte function abnormalities are seen in a number of osteochondrodysplasias, including Shwachman syndrome, where there is neutropenia and pancreatic insufficiency, and Schimke immuno-osseous dysplasia which features radiographic changes of spondyloepiphyseal dysplasia, nephrotic syndrome and cellular immunodeficiency. Other short-limbed dwarfisms associated with immunodeficiency are less clearly delineated.

Cartilage–hair hypoplasia is the most well described variant, inherited in an autosomal recessive manner, and mutations in the RMRP gene, which encodes mitochondrial RNA-processing endoribonuclease RNA, have been described. Severe short-limbed short stature (−11.8 SD to −2.1 SD) with radiographic appearances of metaphyseal and spondyloepiphyseal dysplasia is always present, accompanied by sparse light hair in most patients. Severe anemia and Hirschsprung disease are well recognized associations, as are malignancies, notably lymphoma and skin carcinoma. The immunodeficiency is surprisingly variable; most have T lymphopenia and impaired in vitro mitogen proliferative responses, but only half suffer recurrent infection.[49] However, some have IgA and/or IgG subclass deficiencies with frequent ear infections. Patients are excessively vulnerable to viral infections, particularly varicella zoster, EBV and other human herpes virus infections and the risk of infective death is 300 times greater than normal.[50] Severely affected patients should be assessed for HSCT, which has been successful in correcting the immunodeficiency.

DNA REPAIR DEFECTS AND IMMUNODEFICIENCY

Recognition of a wide array of foreign antigens requires a huge number of genetically diverse lymphocytes, each bearing a unique receptor. These are created by rearranging the variable (V), diversity (D) and joining (J) gene segments that code for T or B lymphocyte receptor genes (VDJ recombination). This is initiated by introducing DNA double strand breaks between the gene segments, and then rejoining the rearranged segments using the cells' ubiquitous DNA repair machinery. Without the ability to repair DNA damage, cells may apoptose or undergo malignant proliferation and so individuals with defective DNA repair mechanisms have a predisposition to neurodegeneration, developmental anomalies and cancer as well as defective immunity. The mechanisms are complex with scope for many single gene defects to give rise to distinct clinical entities.[51]

Ataxia telangiectasia (AT)

This multisystem autosomal recessive disorder, the best known of the DNA repair disorders, is characterized by progressive cerebellar ataxia, oculocutaneous telangiectases, variable immunodeficiency and an increased risk of lymphoid malignancy and is associated with chromosomal instability and cellular radiosensitivity. Diagnosis, in the absence of a family history, is usually by a pediatric neurologist on the basis of gait anomalies. Before telangiectases appear it may be difficult to distinguish from other ataxia syndromes (see also Ch. 22). Ataxia and cerebellar signs are always present and usually appear in the second year, but may be delayed. Neurological degeneration is progressive, resulting in severe disability by late childhood. Mental function is usually preserved though retardation has been described. Telangiectases appear later, usually between 2 and 8 years of age, first on the bulbar conjunctivae (Fig. 27.18) but later elsewhere, particularly on the nose, the ears, and in the antecubital and popliteal fossae. Other cutaneous manifestations include patches of hypo- or hyperpigmentation, cutaneous atrophy and atopic dermatitis.

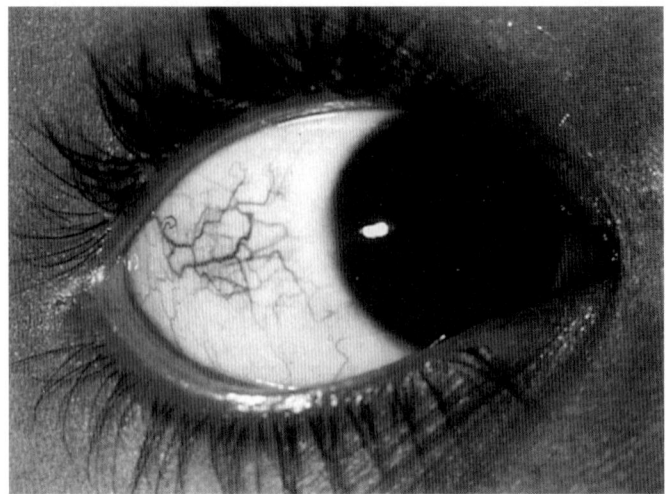

Fig. 27.18 Ataxia telangiectasia.

Gonadal atrophy occurs in both sexes, and growth failure is also prominent in the later stages. Cellular and humoral immunodeficiency affects 60–80% of cases but clinical manifestations are extremely variable. Recurrent sinopulmonary infection is common and may lead to bronchiectasis and clubbing. Recurrent pulmonary infection may be exacerbated by aspiration, common as the disease progresses. Lymphoreticular malignancies and, unusually for immunodeficiency, carcinomas, occur with increased frequency. Radiosensitivity means that treatment with radiotherapy is toxic and often lethal. Irrespective of the development of malignancy, survival beyond early adult life is unusual. Heterozygosity for the AT gene mutation confers an increased risk of developing breast cancer.

Laboratory features

Immunological findings are extremely variable. Low or absent levels of IgA, IgE, IgG, IgG2 and IgG4 subclasses are frequently found and antibody responses are particularly poor to polysaccharide and viral antigens. IgM may be raised and autoantibodies are sometimes found. Cellular immunodeficiency is characterized by defective thymic development and lymphopenia, predominantly of CD4+ T lymphocytes with an increase in the number of T lymphocytes bearing the gamma/delta receptor. Decreased mitogen and antigen responses can be demonstrated due to defective cytoplasmic to nuclear signaling. A raised alpha-fetoprotein (abnormal in 90%) supports the diagnosis, as does evidence of increased chromosome breakage on exposure to ionizing radiation. Patients are efficient at V(D)J rejoining, but have a high incidence of translocations at the sites of the T lymphocyte receptor and immunoglobulin heavy chain genes (chromosome 7:14 translocations). The ATM gene on chromosome 11q22.23 codes for a phosphatidyl kinase involved in meiotic recombination and cell cycle control.[52] The protein detects DNA damage and signals to proteins involved in DNA repair and cell cycle control;[53] it is absent or inactive in AT patients.

Treatment

Prophylactic antibiotics or immunoglobulin replacement can reduce the morbidity of sinopulmonary infection in some patients. As the immunodeficiency is often progressive, the need for such treatment should be reviewed intermittently.

Nijmegen breakage syndrome

Nijmegen breakage syndrome (NBS), an autosomal recessive disorder, is characterized by microcephaly with mild to moderate mental retardation, 'bird-like' facies, immunodeficiency, predisposition to malignancy, radiation sensitivity and chromosomal instability. Bacterial sinopulmonary infection is common. Hypogammaglobulinemia is the most common immunological abnormality and a third of patients make no immunoglobulin. A CD4+ T lymphopenia with diminished T lymphocyte proliferative responses is also found.[54] Alpha-fetoprotein levels are normal. Patients have an increase in chromosome 7:14 translocations on karyotype analysis. Mutations in the gene encoding nibrin cause NBS.[55] Nibrin is a component of a protein complex which is part of the ATM signal transduction cascade. Treatment with antibiotic prophylaxis or immunoglobulin replacement can be helpful, and patients should be monitored carefully for development of lymphoid malignancy. In rare cases HSCT may have a role in improving immunodeficiency, although the long term effects on malignancy are not known.

Ataxia-telangiectasia-like disorder
Patients with similar features to AT patients but with no mutation in the ATM gene have been described. In some, mutations have been found in the Mre11 protein, part of the complex with which nibrin associates and which is one of the complexes downstream from ATM. Some patients are microcephalic.

Other disorders associated with DNA repair (artemis, DNA ligase IV, cernunnos-XLF) have been described in the section on SCID. Patients with artemis and DNA ligase IV deficiency can present with CID. Microcephaly has been described in some of these patients.

Bloom syndrome
This rare autosomal recessive disorder is associated with increased sister chromatid exchange, severe growth failure, increased malignancy and immunodeficiency. Affected individuals may develop facial telangiectases and facial photosensitivity. Recurrent bacterial sinopulmonary infections associated with hypogammaglobulinemia, most often low IgM, are the most common clinical manifestation of immunodeficiency, and may lead to bronchiectasis. The Bloom protein, mutated in the disease, unwinds the DNA helix. The mechanism of the immunodeficiency is unclear.

Fanconi anemia (see also Ch. 23)
Progressive bone marrow failure leading to pancytopenia is the main problem in this condition. There may also be skeletal malformations. Immunodeficiency can occur, and selective IgA deficiency and T lymphocyte abnormalities have been recorded. At least 11 genes are implicated in the disorder, encoding for proteins which form a complex involved in sensing crosslinking DNA damage and facilitating repair.[56] A subgroup of patients with defects in the FAND2 gene show similarity to patients with NBS and fibroblasts exhibit sensitivity to ionizing radiation as well as DNA crosslinking agents.

Xeroderma pigmentosa
Immune deficiency, predominantly involving NK cells, may occur but is not a prominent feature. The mechanism of the immunodeficiency is unclear.

DEFECTS ASSOCIATED WITH OTHER SYNDROMES
Immunodeficiency, centromeric instability, facial anomalies (ICF) syndrome
Immunodeficiency, centromeric instability, facial anomalies syndrome is an autosomal recessive disorder in which there are characteristic structural abnormalities in chromosomes 1, 9 and 16 in lymphocytes. Affected children develop severe recurrent infections and have immunoglobulin deficiency, often with agammaglobulinemia but with normal T and B lymphocyte numbers.[57] T lymphocyte immunity is not normal and *Pneumocystis carinii* infection, severe viral warts and cutaneous fungal infection are described. The differential diagnosis is CVID. Mental retardation may occur but there is no increased risk of malignancy. Mutations in the DNMT3B gene have been identified in some patients, leading to hypomethylation of their DNA. The immunodeficiency may be due to lymphogenesis-associated gene dysregulation caused by indirect effects on gene expression that interfere with normal lymphocyte signaling, maturation and migration. HSCT has corrected the immunodeficiency in some patients who are able to discontinue immunoglobulin replacement.

OTHER IMMUNODEFICIENCIES
A number of syndromes have been described which include primary immunodeficiency as part of the phenotype. In some, the syndrome is well described, and in a few the underlying molecular defect has recently been elucidated. Most lack clear definition.

Hoyeraal–Hreidarsson syndrome
This X-linked disorder is characterized by microcephaly, cerebellar hypoplasia, aplastic anemia and growth retardation. A progressive combined immunodeficiency with hypogammaglobulinemia and lymphopenia is a well recognized association. Mutations in the dyskeratosis congenita gene (DKC1) have been found in some patients.

Netherton syndrome
This triad of generalized infantile erythroderma, diarrhea and failure to thrive may be associated with variable immunodeficiency including mild lymphopenia. The clinical features are similar to those seen in Omenn syndrome and SCID with maternofetal engraftment. Distinguishing these entities is important as the other conditions are treated by HSCT, whereas Netherton syndrome is not. Hair shaft abnormalities are diagnostic (bamboo hairs), and mutations in the serine protease inhibitor (PI) gene SPINK5 have been described.

DISORDERS OF IMMUNE REGULATION

AUTOIMMUNE LYMPHOPROLIFERATIVE SYNDROME (ALPS)
Apoptosis, or programmed cell death, downregulates immune responses once an infection has been countered. Defects in this process lead to marked autoimmune and lymphoproliferative features which characterize ALPS.[58] Apoptosis can be induced by a number of pathways; one of the most important is initiated through a cell surface molecule, Fas (CD95). Ligation of Fas initiates a cascade of intracellular reactions culminating in apoptosis induced by proteolytic enzymes including caspases. Mutations in several molecules in this cascade result in molecularly distinct but clinically similar forms of ALPS (Table 27.11).

Most of the cases described have been heterozygotes though a few homozygous cases are also reported. The variability of clinical severity and the occurrence of asymptomatic individuals make estimation of the incidence of this condition very difficult.

Clinical features
Many cases present in early childhood, often co-incident with the first encounter of human herpes virus infection (CMV, EBV, HHV6), but adult presentation is also described. Asymptomatic cases may occur in the families of symptomatic individuals. Autoimmune disease most commonly affects the hemopoietic system causing hemolytic anemia or thrombocytopenia but the CNS, kidney and skin can be involved. Lymphoproliferation often results in characteristically massive lymphadenopathy in the anterior triangle of the neck, together with splenomegaly in nearly all cases and hepatomegaly in some. Fever is a common feature. Lymphoreticular malignancy (Hodgkin and non-Hodgkin) is reported with increased frequency but has probably been overdiagnosed because the histological picture of proliferation resembles malignancy:

Table 27.11 Different molecule types of ALPS

Type	Molecule affected
Ia	Fas (CD95)
Ib	Fas ligand
II	Caspase 10
III	Caspase 8
IV	Unknown

clonality studies distinguish the two.[59] Homozygous Fas deficiency has a more severe clinical phenotype, sometimes with prenatal onset resulting in hydrops.

Laboratory features

Affected individuals usually have high lymphocyte counts and normal or high immunoglobin levels. Autoantibodies are usually present; the direct Coombs test is often positive. A universal feature is the occurrence of circulating CD3 positive T lymphocytes expressing the alpha/beta receptor but not expressing CD4 or CD8 (so-called 'double negative T lymphocytes') and usually constituting 5–20% of the total CD3 cell count. Many of these cells also express HLA DR (normally only expressed on activated T lymphocytes). CD95 is not normally constitutively expressed on lymphocytes but is after activation with mitogens, and failure of this expression can be demonstrated in type 1a ALPS after appropriate cellular activation. Apoptotic assays involving artificial ligation of CD95 with an antibody and then measurement of cell death can be used to confirm an ALPS defect. Mutation analysis of Fas, Fas L and the appropriate caspase genes will confirm the precise molecular diagnosis.

Treatment and prognosis

Autoimmune phenomena usually respond to treatment but there is a tendency for recurrence or the emergence of new autoimmune problems. Splenectomy for the control of hematological problems should be avoided if possible since there are reports of severe infective complications following this. However it may prove unavoidable, in which case penicillin prophylaxis should be given. The immune dysregulation can often be 'reset' with a course of rituximab in combination with a 6 month course of high dose intravenous immunoglobulin (IVIG) (2 mg/kg fortnightly) and steroids (initially 2 mg/kg/day prednisolone, tapering with response). Malignant disease is treated along standard lines but at the moment there are insufficient data to determine whether the response to treatment differs from non-ALPS patients. HSCT has been successful in patients with homozygous Fas deficiency but currently not enough is known of the long term prognosis to justify elective HSCT in (milder) heterozygous cases, especially as some patients improve with age.

CHRONIC MUCOCUTANEOUS CANDIDIASIS

Chronic mucocutaneous candidiasis (CMC) describes a group of disorders characterized by chronic infection of skin, nails and mucous membranes by organisms of the genus *Candida*, most commonly *Candida albicans*. Recurrent and persistent candida of the mouth, napkin area, skin and nails is the hallmark of this condition, but the severity varies considerably and invasive disease almost never occurs. Failure of usually effective antifungal drugs to clear candida distinguishes CMC from other conditions that predispose to candida such as secondary immunodeficiency, steroid treatment or systemic antibiotics. Candidiasis is usually first noticed early in infancy and in severe cases gross esophageal involvement causes dysphagia, gastroesophageal reflux and failure to thrive whilst skin lesions may be extremely disfiguring and distressing (Fig. 27.19). As a patient becomes older, candida may become less severe. Nail dystrophy and dental enamel hypoplasia are associated.

In some patients there is an associated endocrinopathy (hypoparathyroidism, Addison disease, pernicious anemia, hypothyroidism, diabetes mellitus) which suggests that CMC is part of autoimmune polyendocrinopathy, candidiasis, ectodermal dystrophy (APECED), inherited in an autosomal recessive manner. In some of these, a defect in the AIRE (AutoImmune REgulator) gene has been identified. This codes for a protein expressed in thymus that is critical for the deletion of autoreactive T lymphocytes. A minority of patients suffer from invasive bacterial sepsis, opportunistic infection, autoimmune hemolytic anemia, malabsorption and chronic active hepatitis. Bronchiectasis and restrictive lung disease can occur.[60]

The underlying non-autoimmune immunodeficiency is poorly defined and variable. There may be diminished T lymphocyte

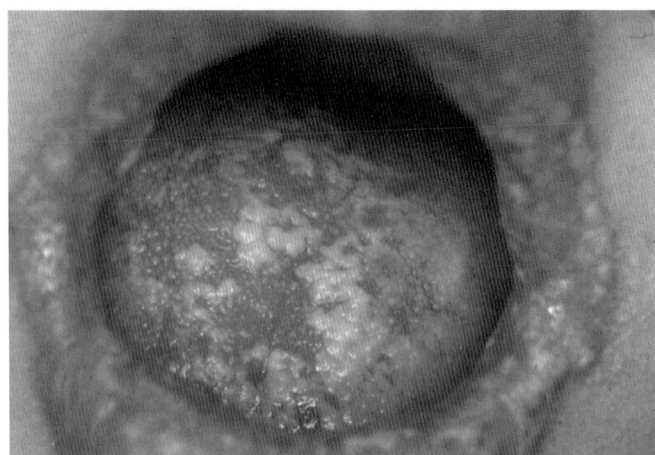

Fig. 27.19   Chronic mucocutaneous candidiasis. (Reproduced with permission of the Bubble Foundation.)

proliferation and cytokine production in response to candida antigens with impaired antibody production to polysaccharide antigens, and sometimes IgG2 subclass deficiency.[61]

Treatment with azole antifungals such as fluconazole can be very effective, even in severe cases, but often does not completely eradicate infection, or infection recurs on stopping treatment. Continuous treatment is necessary in severe cases.

THE IMMUNE DYSREGULATION, POLYENDOCRINOPATHY, ENTEROPATHY, X-LINKED (IPEX) SYNDROME

The IPEX syndrome is characterized by infantile ichthyosiform dermatitis, protracted diarrhea, insulin dependent diabetes mellitus and thyroiditis; other autoimmune features may be apparent, particularly autoimmune cytopenia. Gut biopsies show autoimmune enteropathy. Mutations in the FOXP3 gene have been described in some affected patients. FOXP3-expressing T lymphocytes are regulatory T cells with a role in preventing autoimmunity. HSCT is the only curative treatment, and short term results are encouraging. Whilst the initial response is often dramatic, with rapid resolution of diarrhea and the disappearance of autoantibodies, the long term prognosis following HSCT is unknown.

DEFECTS OF ANTIBODY PRODUCTION

X-LINKED AGAMMAGLOBULINEMIA (XLA, BRUTON DISEASE)

First described by Bruton in 1952,[62] this X-linked condition is due to an intrinsic defect in the normal differentiation of B lymphocytes beyond the pre-B lymphocyte stage. The defective gene encodes a cytoplasmic enzyme, Bruton tyrosine kinase (btk). Affected boys classically show a complete failure to produce immunoglobulins and antibody responses, but cell-mediated immunity is normal. Milder phenotypes have been found although it has not proved possible to correlate severity with the many different mutations that have been found.

Clinical features

Typically, recurrent pyogenic infections commence in the latter half of the first year of life, after maternal IgG levels have declined. The diagnosis is often made surprisingly late; in one series, the average age at diagnosis was 3.5 years without, and 2.5 years with, a positive family history.[63] The situation may not have improved since then as a more recent audit of all forms of immunoglobulin deficiency in adults and children in the UK found an average delay of 6.26 years between onset of symptoms and diagnosis.[64]

Table 27.12 Presenting features in 96 patients with X-linked agammaglobulinemia (From Lederman & Winkelstein 1985[63])

Presenting feature	%
Ear, nose and throat infections (otitis media)	75 (59)
Lower respiratory tract infections (pneumonia)	65 (56)
Gastrointestinal infections (diarrhea)	35 (32)
Pyoderma	28
Arthritis (septic)	20 (8)
CNS infections (meningitis)	16 (10)
Septicemia	10
Neutropenia	10
Positive family history	26
Others: Failure to thrive; fever of uncertain origin; complications of immunization; osteomyelitis and dermatomyositis	< 5% each

Diagnoses and figures in brackets indicate the predominant type of infection in each system and its overall incidence in the 96 patients.

Table 27.13 Comparison of X-linked agammaglobulinemia (XLA) and common variable immune deficiency (CVID)

	XLA	CVID
Inheritance	X-linked	Mostly unknown (some may be AR or AD)
Age of onset	Infancy	Any age
Immunological defect	Antibody	Antibody ± cell-mediated
Immunoglobulin classes	All decreased	One (usually IgM) or more often preserved
B cell numbers	Absent	Usually present
T cell numbers and function	Normal	Normal or decreased
Pyogenic infections	Yes	Yes
Opportunistic infections	Very rare	Yes
Autoimmune phenomena	Very rare	Yes
Chronic gastrointestinal problems	Rare	Common

AD, autosomal dominant; AR, autosomal recessive.

Sinopulmonary infections are most common, but gastroenteritis, pyoderma, arthritis, meningitis and osteomyelitis may be presenting features (Table 27.12).[63] Common gastrointestinal pathogens include *Campylobacter jejuni* and *Giardia lamblia*.[65] Chronic conjunctivitis caused by *Pseudomonas* species may also occur. Recovery from viral infections is normal with the notable exception of those caused by enteroviruses (especially echoviruses) which can cause a chronic meningoencephalitis or dermatomyositis-like picture. Vaccine-associated paralytic poliomyelitis has been reported with live vaccine. Pathogens in which cell-mediated immunity is thought to be important are not usually a problem, though occasional cases of *Pneumocystis carinii* infection have been reported. Other complications include a nonpurulent arthritis affecting predominantly large joints. In some cases this has been shown to be due to mycoplasma infection. Neutropenia, alopecia totalis and amyloidosis are infrequent complications.

Laboratory findings

Once maternal IgG has declined, the usual pattern is absence or severe depletion of all serum immunoglobulin classes. It is not possible to demonstrate any antibody response to vaccines or to bacteriophage ΦX174. Circulating lymphocyte markers show a normal number of T lymphocytes, but absence of B lymphocytes. Bone marrow aspirate shows pre-B lymphocytes (containing cytoplasmic mu chains). Lymph nodes show absent follicles and germinal centers. Plasma cells cannot be demonstrated at any site. An associated neutropenia is found in some cases. Confirmation of the diagnosis can be made rapidly in over 90% of cases by demonstrating absence of the btk protein in cell lysates.[66] The finding of absent or abnormal btk in boys with partial antibody deficiency means that the condition should be considered in the presence of any form of antibody deficiency in boys, particularly if circulating B lymphocyte numbers are low. Foremost in the differential diagnosis of XLA is CVID. Table 27.13 lists some of the important differences between the two.

The mainstay of treatment is immunoglobulin replacement therapy (p. 1172). Infections may still occur, especially giardiasis and chronic conjunctivitis. Chronic lung damage and sinus disease may also progress on treatment and for this reason vigorous and early antibiotic therapy should be used for respiratory tract infections. If the problems are recurrent despite increased doses of immunoglobulin, continuous prophylactic antibiotics may be required. A large series of patients treated before IVIG was available revealed a high incidence of chronic lung disease (75% of those over 20 years) even with treatment with intramuscular immunoglobulin, and 17% of patients had died with a mean age of 16.9 years. With the widespread use of IVIG, lung disease seems less common and a recent sizable retrospective study[67] found that the patients developing progressive lung and sinus disease while on treatment tended to be those with damage sustained before immunoglobulin therapy was commenced. These data emphasize the importance of early diagnosis and treatment for this condition. The same study also found that maintaining patients at higher IgG levels reduced the risk of lung disease but not of sinus problems.

RELATED VARIANTS

X-linked agammaglobulinemia and sensorineural hearing loss

Three unrelated boys with XLA have been described with mutation confirmed XLA and progressive sensorineural hearing loss.[68] They all had large deletions in the terminal part of the btk gene which were believed to involve a contiguous gene coding the deafness, dystonia protein, DDP. Mutations in the latter gene have been associated with the Tranebjaerg syndrome of deafness, dystonia and mental retardation. At the time of reporting the patients did not exhibit the other features.

Hypogammaglobulinemia with growth hormone deficiency

Very rarely hypogammaglobulinemia with low/absent B lymphocytes consistent with XLA has been described associated with isolated growth hormone deficiency. In the first case described no btk mutation was identified. In subsequent cases mutations in btk have been identified but the same mutations have also been found in boys without growth hormone deficiency. The relationship between the two conditions therefore remains enigmatic.

AUTOSOMAL RECESSIVE FORMS OF AGAMMAGLOBULINEMIA

When hypogammaglobulinemia is found in girls or when a patient's parents are consanguineous, autosomal recessive genetic defects affecting B lymphocyte differentiation should be considered. Mutations have been described so far in genes coding for: mu heavy chain, Ig-alpha (part of the signal transduction complex of the B lymphocyte antigen receptor), lambda$_{5/14.1}$ light chain, BLNK (B lymphocyte linker protein). These proteins are required for early B lymphocyte development from pro-B lymphocyte to pre-B lymphocyte stage. Unlike XLA, pre-B lymphocytes are therefore not detectable in marrow samples. Other families have also been described in whom the molecular defect is yet to be identified. In all cases the defect is B lymphocyte specific. The number of cases described is too small to draw firm conclusions but the clinical picture would seem to be similar to XLA, although patients with mu heavy chain deficiency may have more serious life-threatening infections than those with XLA with an earlier onset of symptoms.[69]

IMMUNOGLOBULIN DEFICIENCY WITH TRANSCOBALAMIN II DEFICIENCY

Hypogammaglobulinemia due to a failure of terminal (antigen driven) B lymphocyte differentiation can result from congenital absence of one of the vitamin B_{12} carrier proteins, transcobalamin II. There is associated pernicious anemia. Parenteral high dose vitamin B_{12} corrects the immunological defect.

COMMON VARIABLE IMMUNE DEFICIENCY

CVID is a poorly defined entity characterized by the presence of quantitative or qualitative hypogammaglobulinemia. The incidence is between 1:10000 and 1:100000 of the population and although the onset of symptoms is typically seen within the second or third decade of life it is increasingly being diagnosed in childhood.

Familial inheritance is seen in up to 25% of cases, but the variability of phenotype both within and between families suggests a polygenic inheritance. Selective IgA deficiency appears to be one end of the spectrum of this disease.[70] Autoimmune diseases such as rheumatoid arthritis also have an increased incidence in these kindreds. As with all patients with humoral immune defects, patients with CVID present with recurrent sinopulmonary and gastrointestinal infections. They are particularly susceptible to *Giardia lamblia*. They are also at risk from enteroviral infections, causing choriomeningitis in particular, and arthritis may result from chronic mycoplasma infection. Other clinical manifestations exemplify the inherent immune deregulation with an increased incidence of autoimmune disease, particularly autoimmune hemolytic anemia, thrombocytopenia and neutropenia. Nonmalignant granulomatous lymphadenopathy, hepatosplenomegaly and involvement of the gastrointestinal tract is a frequent finding in a subgroup of patients,[71] and clinical differentiation from malignancy may be difficult although histologically lesions resemble those seen in sarcoidosis. These granulomata are normally sensitive to steroid treatment. Patients with CVID also have a significantly increased risk of lymphoreticular and gastrointestinal malignancies.

Laboratory findings

Hypogammaglobulinemia is the hallmark of these patients. This may vary from a failure of specific vaccine responses to panhypogammaglobulinemia. B lymphocyte numbers are frequently normal. A significant proportion of patients have T lymphocyte abnormalities, in particular a reversed CD4/8 ratio and a generalized lymphopenia.[72] Such abnormalities at presentation should prompt a search for other defined immune defects. As the molecular basis of other immune deficiencies is being defined, it is clear that a number of patients with CVID have milder phenotypes of other immunodeficiencies such as X-linked agammaglobulinemia, CD40 ligand deficiency or X-linked lymphoproliferative disease.[73,74] Additionally, defects in ICOS, TACI, BAFF-R and CD19 have been described in a few individuals, but for the majority of cases the genetic basis is unknown.

Treatment

The aim of treatment is prevention of further infections and consequent end-organ damage such as bronchiectasis. Mild phenotypes may require only prophylactic antibiotics. Significant degrees of hypogammaglobulinemia should be treated with immunoglobulin replacement therapy. If patients have significantly abnormal cell-mediated immunity, they should be given prophylactic co-trimoxazole. Granulomatous lesions and autoimmune phenomena may respond to treatment with steroids.

IgA DEFICIENCY

Studies on healthy blood donors have shown that 1 in 600–700 Caucasians have no demonstrable serum IgA. Deficiency of serum IgA is usually associated with a lack of salivary IgA. The clinical significance of low IgA in isolation is unclear as the majority of affected individuals are asymptomatic. However, in populations of patients with chronic lung disease and autoimmune diseases there is an increased incidence of IgA deficiency. As the majority of patients with IgA deficiency are well, the pathophysiology of disease in these individuals is probably multifactorial; other contributory elements may include IgG subclass deficiency and reduced levels of mannan-binding lectin. Selective IgA deficiency is part of the spectrum of CVID; both may be present in the same family and rarely patients with IgA deficiency progress to CVID. In an infant, low IgA may be the last manifestation of transient hypogammaglobulinemia to resolve. Acquired IgA deficiency (usually reversible) may occur as a result of drug therapies (e.g. penicillamine, phenytoin, sodium valproate, captopril). It has also been described in congenital infections and after hepatitis C infection.

Assessment of patients with IgA deficiency

If it is an incidental finding without a history of recurrent infections, an isolated low IgA is unlikely to be of clinical significance. If recurrent infections are present, further investigation should be undertaken, including assessment of IgG subclasses and specific vaccination responses. IgG subclass deficiencies occur in approximately 15% of cases. True IgA absence should be differentiated from low levels, which are common in childhood, by performing an Ouchterlony test, which will detect IgA in those patients with low levels.

Symptoms

Infective. Recurrent sinopulmonary infections are the commonest symptoms in young children. Middle ear infections can be troublesome, and recurrent lower respiratory tract infections may result in lung damage. In the majority of children the frequency and severity of infections improve with age, regardless of the IgA level. Gastrointestinal infections, in particular with *Giardia lamblia*, have an increased incidence.

Autoimmunity. There is a strong correlation between autoimmune disease of all types and IgA deficiency,[75] whether or not the latter is associated with infections. Mechanisms are poorly understood, but may include abnormalities in antigen handling.

Gastrointestinal disease. The increased incidence of gastrointestinal infection has been discussed above. There is also an increase in celiac disease in IgA deficiency, which may give a false negative test if the diagnosis of celiac disease is based on the presence of IgA antigliadin and endomysial antibodies.

Malignancy. There are multiple reports of lymphomas and gastric malignancies in patients with IgA deficiency, although the true incidence of this problem has not been well defined.

Treatment

Patients with significant symptoms may respond to prophylactic antibacterial treatment, particularly over the winter. Very occasionally patients may require replacement immunoglobulin therapy. If they have a total IgA deficiency, they may have anti-IgA antibodies, which can result in severe anaphylactoid reactions if given IgA-containing preparations (including IVIG or blood). The risks can be minimized by choosing an immunoglobulin preparation with the lowest IgA content.

IgG SUBCLASS DEFICIENCY

Many individuals with isolated subclass deficiencies are completely healthy. Immunoglobulin subclass deficiency is more likely to be associated with infection in patients who make poor specific antibody responses, particularly to polysaccharide antigens. The utility of IgG subclass measurement is therefore questioned by some authorities and assessment of results should occur in the context of clinical features and specific antibody responses.[76]

Criteria for diagnosis should include a normal total IgG with a subnormal level of one or more IgG subclasses.[14] As IgG1 is the predominant IgG subclass, low levels of IgG1 will result in low total IgG, and this should be defined as CVID. Although deletions of the corresponding gamma genes have been demonstrated in a few cases, a majority of patients suffer from a regulatory dysfunction, and the deficiencies are most often relative rather than absolute.[77]

IgG3 is the most common subclass deficiency in adults, with IgG2 predominating in children. IgG4 levels vary widely in normal individuals, with up to a fifth of the population having very low levels. The clinical significance of selective IgG1 deficiency is difficult to assess. IgG subclass deficiencies may be associated with IgA deficiency, be a part of the spectrum of the immune defect in combined or T lymphocyte immunodeficiency such as AT, or be an early manifestation of CVID.

Recurrent sinopulmonary infections are the usual clinical presentation of a significant subclass defect. Most children can be effectively treated with prophylactic antibiotics, such as co-trimoxazole or a macrolide, over the winter months. Hearing loss and lung damage should be monitored. Very occasionally children may require treatment with replacement immunoglobulin.

SELECTIVE ANTIBODY DEFICIENCY WITH NORMAL IMMUNOGLOBULINS

A small number of individuals have normal immunoglobulin levels, but fail to respond to specific antigens. The most frequent defect is a failure to respond to polysaccharide antigens (e.g. the polysaccharide pneumococcal vaccine, Pneumovax®). The majority of individuals are normal, and clearly have other immune mechanisms that can compensate for this defect. A number, however, have recurrent sinopulmonary infections.

Lack of polysaccharide responses may also be seen in Wiskott–Aldrich syndrome, be normal in the first 2 years of life, or be an early manifestation of CVID. Children over the age of 3 years who are found to lack pneumococcal responses should be followed up until it is clear that they are not developing an immune defect.

DISORDERS OF PHAGOCYTIC CELLS

CHRONIC GRANULOMATOUS DISEASE

Chronic granulomatous disease (CGD) is an inherited defect of the phagocyte nicotinamide adenine dinucleotide phosphate (NADPH) oxidase enzyme complex which generates superoxide and other reactive oxygen species that are toxic to organisms ingested into phagosomes. The commonest X-linked gene defect, accounting for up to 60% of cases, is in the major membrane component gp91phox. Defects in the cytoplasmic components p67phox and p47phox are inherited in an autosomal recessive pattern, as are mutations in the second membrane component p22phox, the latter being very rare.

The disease has protean clinical manifestations, but the hallmark is acute, and potentially fatal, bacterial or fungal infection.[78] A subgroup of patients with some residual enzyme function may not present until adult life. A common manifestation is acute suppurative lymphadenitis in the neck, axilla or groin. Other frequent pyogenic infections include liver abscesses, osteomyelitis, arthritis, pneumonia, skin sepsis and perianal abscesses. Pathogens such as *Staphylococcus aureus*, *Burkholderia cepacia*, *Aspergillus* species and *Serratia marcescens* are common because they are catalase positive: this enzyme destroys any hydrogen peroxide produced by the organism within the phagosome. Infections with catalase negative organisms, such as *Streptococcus pneumoniae*, are rare. Fungal infection often manifests as pneumonia, but disseminated infection is frequently seen, with osteomyelitis and hepatic involvement. Once established, fungal infection is hard to treat and frequently fatal.

The occurrence of non-infectious granulomatous complications is increasingly recognized. These include inflammatory bowel disease, restrictive lung defects, genitourinary obstruction and cutaneous granulomata. Many children have colitis, which may be subclinical, manifested only as a persistent iron deficiency anemia and which histologically may be mistaken for Crohn disease. These non-infective manifestations respond well to corticosteroid treatment.[79] Female carriers of the X-linked form may have a number of manifestations including skin abscesses and an increased incidence of autoimmune diseases and mouth ulcers.

Diagnosis is suggested by failure of reduction of nitroblue tetrazolium or dihydrorhodamine by neutrophils (see diagnosis section). In the X-linked form, mothers may have intermediate levels of dye reduction.

Treatment

The use of prophylactic antibiotics, in particular co-trimoxazole which is concentrated in neutrophils, has significantly reduced morbidity and mortality from bacterial infections in this disease. Children should also receive oral prophylactic antifungal agents such as itraconazole or voriconazole which help reduce the incidence of fatal fungal disease in these patients.[79]

Infections or unexplained fevers should be treated aggressively. IFN-gamma is a useful adjunctive treatment in severe bacterial or fungal infections, and in Europe is mainly used for prophylaxis only after documented failure of oral antibacterial and antifungal agents.[80] White cell infusions may be used as adjunctive therapy in severe infection. Registry data suggest that the outlook in early childhood has improved considerably in recent years,[81] but considerable morbidity and mortality occurs and consideration should be given to HSCT when a suitable donor is available.[82] Clinical gene therapy trials are in progress.

ENZYMATIC DEFICIENCIES RESULTING IN NEUTROPHIL KILLING DEFECTS

Myeloperoxidase (MPO) deficiency is the commonest inherited disorder of neutrophils. Almost half of those affected have a complete deficiency, the rest have structural or functional defects in the enzyme. MPO is the primary component of azurophilic (primary) granules. The majority of patients with MPO deficiency are asymptomatic, a notable exception being diabetic patients with MPO deficiency, who appear to have a particular susceptibility to candidiasis.

Other enzyme defects are less common and include glutathione synthetase deficiency, pyruvate kinase deficiency and complete neutrophil G6PD deficiency (note: in the common red cell G6PD deficiency there is sufficient enzyme present in neutrophils for normal killing to occur). The phenotypes may be very mild, with variable numbers of bacterial infections. G6PD deficiency will result in an abnormal NBT test; otherwise the diagnosis is established by measurement of specific enzyme levels.

NEUTROPHIL-SPECIFIC GRANULE DEFICIENCY

This rare disorder is characterized by recurrent skin and lung infections with staphylococci and enteric bacteria. The diagnosis can be confirmed by electron microscopy of patient neutrophils, which show reduced or absent primary granules. Specific stains will also demonstrate lack of the proteins that constitute the granules, including lactoferrin and vitamin B_{12} binding protein. Proteins that reside in azurophilic (primary) granules, such as lysozyme and myeloperoxidase, are present. Neutrophils also show abnormalities in migration and nuclear morphology. Mice lacking the transcription factor CCAAT/enhancer binding protein have a similar phenotype, and patients with mutations in this gene have been reported.[83]

The clinical course of patients is variable. Treatment options include prompt institution of antibiotic therapy for infections and prophylactic antibiotic treatment. HSCT should be considered in patients with a severe phenotype

OTHER NEUTROPHIL DISORDERS

Neutropenia

This includes cyclical neutropenia and severe congenital neutropenia, which are covered in Chapter 23.

Shwachman–Diamond syndrome

This rare autosomal recessive disorder is characterized by exocrine pancreatic insufficiency, skeletal abnormalities, bone marrow dysfunction and recurrent infections. Neutropenia occurs in all patients, whilst 10–25% of patients also have pancytopenia. There is an increased incidence of malignancy. The genetic defect has recently been identified. HSCT may be indicated in some patients.

HEMOPHAGOCYTIC SYNDROMES

Chediak–Higashi syndrome

Chediak–Higashi syndrome (CHS) is a rare autosomal recessive disease with partial oculocutaneous albinism, recurrent bacterial infections and the development of an accelerated lymphocyte and macrophage activation syndrome [similar to that seen in hemophagocytic lymphohistiocytosis (HLH) and X-linked lymphoproliferative disease (XLP)] in approximately 85% of patients, which is usually fatal. Variable neurological manifestations are also recognized. Characteristic giant lysosomal granules are seen in the cytoplasm of all cells containing these organelles, and are easily detected on a peripheral blood film. A characteristic pattern of hair pigment can be seen by light microscopy. The gene for this disease (Lyst) codes for a regulator of lysosomal transport;[84] proteins normally transported through lysosomes enter these organelles but cannot exit, with subsequent lysosomal hypertrophy. In melanocytes this is thought to result in abnormalities of melanin transport and consequent albinism. In neutrophils degranulation of lysosomes cannot occur, with failure of release of bactericidal proteins into the phagosome and defective intracellular killing. The impaired NK cell function is not fully elucidated, whilst monocyte function is probably impaired because giant lysosomes interfere with intracellular motility systems leading to abnormal processing of MHC II in endosomes, and thus defective antigen presentation. The activation syndrome may result from failure to transport inhibitory molecules such as CTLA4 to the surface of leukocytes, with consequent failure of negative feedback mechanisms after T lymphocyte and macrophage activation. Common pathogens in CHS include *Staphylococcus aureus*, streptococci and pneumococci. Hemophagocytosis may be triggered by viral infection, particularly human herpes virus infection.

Treatment

Prophylactic co-trimoxazole should be given to prevent bacterial infection. The accelerated phase cannot be predicted, and patients should be closely monitored, particularly if febrile. Symptoms, signs, laboratory and clinical findings and diagnosis and treatment of the accelerated phase are as for HLH (see below). The only definitive treatment for the hematological problems is HSCT. This should be considered early if there is a matched sibling donor. Successful HSCT will not prevent late onset neurological sequelae however.

Griscelli syndrome

Individuals with Griscelli syndrome resemble those with CHS in that they have variable hypopigmentation of the skin. The hair is characteristically silvery grey from birth, and recurrent pyogenic infections associated with absent delayed type cutaneous hypersensitivity and impaired natural killer cell function should suggest the diagnosis. Hypogammaglobulinemia can be seen as a secondary phenomenon. In contrast to CHS, large lysosomal granules are not seen and examination of hair by electron microscopy shows large clumps of pigment, with the accumulation of mature melanosomes in melanocytes. This provides a rapid diagnostic test. Three distinct types of Griscelli syndrome have been identified, but only patients with mutations in Rab27a have an accelerated phase.[85]

Hemophagocytic lymphohistiocytosis (familial)

Hemophagocytic lymphohistiocytosis (HLH) may be primary (familial) or secondary to a viral infection or an immune deficiency (e.g. Griscelli syndrome, CHS and XLP) or other immune dysregulation (macrophage activation syndrome in juvenile arthritides). The primary form is universally fatal without treatment. Patients present with high swinging fevers, hepatosplenomegaly and pancytopenia, and may appear septic. Laboratory findings include an acute phase response, elevated ferritin and elevated fasting triglycerides. Examination of bone marrow, cerebrospinal fluid, pleural effusions or ascitic fluid may demonstrate hemophagocytosis. This may be very difficult to find, and repeated sampling may be required. Diagnosis of familial HLH should be suspected in an infant with an appropriate clinical picture.[86] Older children are more likely to have secondary HLH.

Of patients with familial HLH, 20–30% will have a mutation in perforin and a similar proportion in munc13–4. Mutations in syntaxin 11 have also been identified, particularly in Turkish families.[87] A group of patients remains in whom the genetic defect remains to be identified. The exact pathophysiology of the disease has not been elucidated, but it is thought that all the identified molecules have a regulatory role, and absence leads to dysregulated immune activation.[88]

Treatment with a combination of chemotherapeutic agents, steroids, and monoclonal antibodies that deplete lymphocytes may induce remission, but HSCT is required for cure.

LEUKOCYTE ADHESION DISORDERS

To counter infection in tissues, leukocytes egress from the circulation toward sites of inflammation as described earlier in this chapter (p. 1141). Inherited defects in some of the cell surface molecules responsible for the process have been recognized.

Leukocyte adhesion deficiency type 1

Deficiency of the 95 kd beta chain (CD18), common to the beta-2 integrin family of cell surface adhesive molecules, leads to a profound immunodeficiency affecting the function of neutrophils, monocytes and certain lymphocytes, including T and NK cytotoxic cells.[89] Inheritance is autosomal recessive. Chemotaxis, adherence and phagocytosis are markedly depressed. Different mutations result in phenotypes of variable severity depending on the number of surface molecules that can be expressed. Occasional patients have also been described whose cells express normal levels of CD18 but have a mutation affecting the function of the molecule. This can be demonstrated by showing failure of expression of an activation epitope on the molecule. Although these molecules are involved in the lymphocyte interactions necessary for specific immune responses, these responses are preserved. Even the impaired lymphocyte cytotoxicity, which can be demonstrated very clearly in the laboratory, is of uncertain clinical significance. The clinical picture is almost entirely explained by the way in which leukocytes are attracted to areas of infection and can become fixed to the vessel walls at sites of inflammation in the usual way but cannot pass out into the tissues. This leads to blockage of small vessels and rapidly expanding necrotic lesions without pus. The beta-2 integrin family is also involved in the platelet function molecule Gp 2b3a, and patients with a combined leukocyte and platelet defect have been found.[90]

Individuals affected by the most severe phenotype (< 1% expression) present in the first weeks of life with delayed umbilical cord separation (the cord fails to shrink down and may not separate until 3–4 weeks of age), together with rapidly progressive erosive perianal ulcers. Delayed umbilical cord separation does not seem to occur in patients with some expression of the molecule (usually in the range 2–10% of normal expression). In all forms there is excessive susceptibility to bacterial and fungal infections. Gingivitis and periodontitis are common and more deep seated infections of bone, respiratory and gastrointestinal tracts are often seen. Non-infective inflammatory lesions, particularly affecting the skin and resembling pyoderma gangrenosum, can occur in the partial forms of the deficiency and are often responsive to steroids.

Investigations almost invariably show a circulating neutrophilia (because of failure of the cells to migrate out of the circulation) and a profound neutrophil chemotactic defect. Diagnosis is confirmed by demonstrating the absence of the cell surface markers recognized by the anti-CD11/CD18 monoclonal antibodies.

In the severe form, early death from infection is the rule unless a successful HSCT can be performed. In the partial forms supportive and expectant management is pursued in the first instance but HSCT may become necessary.

Leukocyte adhesion deficiency (LAD) type II

In this extremely rare disorder a defect of fucose metabolism results in a failure of fucosylation to generate sialyl lewis x (CD15s) and other ligand molecules to which the selectin molecules bind. This results in a failure of the 'rolling' type weak adhesion of leukocytes to endothelium which slows down the circulating leukocytes before beta-2 integrin binding can occur. There is a neutrophilia, and neutrophil chemotaxis and migration from the circulation is severely impaired. There is no deficiency in specific immune responses. As in LAD I deficiency, patients have a neutrophilia and suffer repeated bacterial infections and periodontal disease. Delayed umbilical cord separation is, however, not seen. Other features peculiar to LAD II include mental retardation, short stature and the Bombay (hh) blood phenotype.[91]

CYTOKINE DEFECTS

Type 1 cytokine defects

Defects in the IL-12 dependent IFN-gamma pathway have been described in patients affected by persistent severe, invasive or intractable mycobacterial infections with bone and soft tissue abscesses complicated by persistent discharging sinuses. Implicated pathogens are usually BCG or poorly pathogenic environmental nontuberculous mycobacteria and are often fatal.[92] Invasive non-typhi salmonella infections have been described, and may be successfully treated with antibiotics. There may also be increased susceptibility to viral infection including human herpes viruses, respiratory viruses including respiratory syncytial virus and parainfluenza type 3. Infections result from a failure of upregulation of macrophage killing. The clinical picture depends on the precise molecular defect that is present. Defects have been described in a number of constituents of the IL-12/IFN-gamma pathway, including complete or partial IFN-gamma-R1 deficiency, IL-12p40 subunit deficiency, and complete IL-12bn1 deficiency. The outcome of patients with complete IFN-gamma-R1 deficiency is poor, but HSCT has been successfully attempted.

HYPER-IgE SYNDROME

This complex disorder is characterized by extreme elevation of the serum IgE level (usually in the range 2000–40000 units/L), chronic dermatitis and repeated lung and skin infections.[93] The predominant organism is staphylococcus, although infections with other organisms and secondary fungal infections may occur. The total IgE levels may fall in adulthood, sometimes to the normal range. Autosomal dominant and autosomal recessive forms occur: the former (Job syndrome) is characterized by the formation of pneumatoceles and multiple systemic problems, including coarse facies, delayed loss of primary dentition and a variety of skeletal abnormalities including an increased fracture rate and joint hypermobility.[94]

While the immunological features can be explained as the consequence of a T cell regulatory defect, the other features are not easily explained. Abnormal bone and connective tissue turnover as a consequence of abnormal cytokine profiles has been postulated as a possible way of tying all the features together. The mode of inheritance is thought to be autosomal dominant with incomplete penetrance. The gene for the disorder has not been identified but studies on the autosomal dominant cases have found linkage to the proximal part of chromosome 4q.[95]

The autosomal recessive form was more recently described.[96] Although these children have skin and lung infections and very high IgE, they do not develop pneumatoceles or have any of the soft tissue or skeletal markers of the autosomal dominant form.

The mainstay of treatment is long term antistaphylococcal antibiotic prophylaxis, usually with flucloxacillin. HSCT failed to correct the IgE levels in the one patient in whom it was reported as being attempted despite successful engraftment of donor myeloid and lymphoid cells.[97] Subsequent follow-up has demonstrated less frequent and severe infections.

ANHYDROTIC ECTODERMAL DYSPLASIA, INCONTINENTIA PIGMENTI AND DEFECTS IN THE NEMO GENE, AND RELATED DISORDERS

X-linked anhydrotic ectodermal dysplasia has been associated with immunodeficiency. Patients present with sparse scalp hair, conical teeth and absent sweat glands. Some suffer from recurrent sinopulmonary infection, often with encapsulated organisms, and have poor antibody responses to polysaccharide antigens, or frank hypogammaglobulinemia. Incontinentia pigmenti is a rare X-linked dominant condition characterized by developmental abnormalities in skin, hair, teeth and the central nervous system. Previously thought lethal in male fetuses, rare male infants with a progressive combined immunodeficiency have been described.

Hypofunctional mutations in the NEMO gene encoding a protein required to activate the transcription factor NF-kappaB have been described in male patients with both X-linked anhydrotic ectodermal dysplasia and incontinentia pigmenti, suggesting that these conditions represent variants of the same disorder.[98]

Similar presentations have been described in patients found to have defects in I-kappa-B-alpha, with recurrent Gram positive and Gram negative bacterial infections and raised IgM. Other rare patients with similar bacterial infections but no ectodermal dysplasia have been described with IRAK-4 deficiency.

COMPLEMENT DISORDERS

PRIMARY INHERITED DEFICIENCIES

The main inherited deficiencies of complement components are listed in Table 27.5D (p. 1149). Severe disease is inherited in an autosomal recessive manner with absolute deficiency of a complement component due to gene defects in both alleles. However, heterozygosity results in approximately half normal levels of the protein which can sometimes be clinically important. A number of clinical patterns can occur depending upon which factor is deficient.

Autoimmune disease

A predisposition to autoimmune disease, particularly systemic lupus erythematosus and the other immune complex disorders, is a feature of most of the complement deficiency syndromes. Deficiency of C1q carries a very high risk with over 90% of patients in one series developing either systemic lupus erythematosus (SLE) or discoid LE.[99] Evidence, based on the finding that null alleles for a number of complement components (notably C2 and C4) occur with greater frequency in patients with autoimmune diseases such as SLE, suggests that heterozygosity for deficiency is also a risk factor. In general, the course of these diseases is similar to that in patients without complement deficiency.

Pyogenic infections

Recurrent pyogenic infections are a feature of complement deficiencies. Organisms such as streptococci and *Haemophilus influenzae* are the main problem as opsonization/binding of antibody and complement to bacteria is critical for their elimination. C3 deficiency is the most severe. Deficiency of the classical pathway components C1q and C2 and of factor D in the alternative pathway also predisposes to infection and the first two also carry a predisposition to autoimmune phenomena. Deficiencies of the alternative pathway control proteins, factors H or I lead to uncontrolled consumption of C3 resulting in increased susceptibility to pyogenic infections.

Neisserial infections

Deficiency of one of the later complement components, C5–C9 (leading to failure of membrane lysis), or of the control factor properdin (the only deficiency inherited in an X-linked manner) leads to a specific deficiency in handling neisserial species (*Neisseria meningitidis* and *N. gonorrhoeae*) but not to a generalized increase in susceptibility to pyogenic infections. There is a predominance of disease caused by rare serogroups of meningococci (W135, X, Y and Z) in these patients. In a Dutch study[100] complement deficiency (most commonly late components or properdin) was found in 33% of survivors of meningococcal disease due to rare serogroups compared to 2, 0 and 7% in patients who suffered Group A, B and C disease respectively. The disease is said to run a milder course in these patients. Recurrent attacks of meningococcal septicemia/meningitis and severe invasive gonococcal disease are also associated with late complement deficiencies in factors 6–9. Late complement deficiencies are more common in individuals from the Middle East and Japan; C9 deficiency in Japan affects up to 0.1% of the population.[101] Screening for deficiencies should be undertaken in patients and their immediate families where there has been recurrent meningococcal disease due to common serogroups or single episodes caused by a rare serogroup. In the UK, screening children with single episodes of meningococcal disease due to common serotypes is unlikely to reveal a complement defect.[102]

Hereditary angioedema

Deficiency of the control protein, C1 esterase inhibitor (C1INH), leads to spontaneous episodes of localized edema (angioedema) without urticaria due to excessive release of proinflammatory breakdown products of complement. C1INH is also a negative regulator of the kallikrein pathway and edema may be due to the increased release of kinins. These occur spontaneously anywhere in the body but those affecting the upper airway are most serious and can be life threatening. Precipitating factors can include local trauma (including surgical procedures, endoscopy and dental work), exposure to extreme cold and emotional stress. Intra-abdominal swelling can occur causing pain and swelling which can be misdiagnosed as a surgical condition. There is a high incidence of SLE and related diseases. C4 levels are also persistently low due to excessive consumption (which occurs even between attacks) although C3 levels are normal. In most cases C1INH assay shows very low levels or absent protein but in approximately 15% of cases the protein is present but functionally defective. The condition is inherited in an autosomal dominant fashion. Episodes of visible swelling do not usually occur until the second decade of life, but younger children suffer from attacks of abdominal pain. Infusions of purified C1INH are effective in terminating attacks and should be used for all attacks affecting the head and neck and for intra-abdominal attacks which are running a protracted course. The concentrate should also be given prophylactically to cover surgical and dental procedures. For prevention of attacks, the treatment of choice after puberty is one of the 'retarded' androgenic steroids, such as danazol. In prepubertal children prophylactic use of tranexamic acid, a fibrinolytic agent which inhibits plasmin formation, is recommended. This raises functional C1INH levels sufficiently to prevent attacks and is relatively free of virilizing side-effects. Monitoring of liver function tests should be performed with long term usage.

SECONDARY COMPLEMENT DEFICIENCIES

Many immunopathological diseases can result in excessive complement activation and consumption. In SLE and other immune complex diseases, low levels of C3 and the early classical pathway components can occur. In acute nephritis, C3 levels are acutely depressed, while in membrano-proliferative glomerulonephritis a more persistent depression of C3 levels occurs due to the presence of an autoantibody – C3 nephritic factor – directed against C3bBb, the alternative pathway C3 convertase. This autoantibody can also be associated with the condition partial lipodystrophy, with or without membranoproliferative glomerulonephritis. An increased susceptibility to pyogenic infections occurs when C3 levels are reduced below approximately 10%. Gram negative sepsis, acute pancreatitis and acute vasculitis can all be associated with complement consumption.

INTERACTION OF ANTIBODY AND COMPLEMENT DEFICIENCIES

Deficiency of the early classical pathway complement components has been shown to be associated with poor antibody responses, presumably because of some immunoregulatory role of the complement factors. Later components are not implicated.

Alternative pathway opsonization is less efficient in the absence of specific antibody to bacterial surfaces. There is evidence that antibody may 'neutralize' surface molecules, such as sialic acid, which otherwise inhibit alternative pathway activation.

MANNAN–BINDING LECTIN (MBL) DEFICIENCY

MBL provides another antibody independent mechanism for opsonization of microorganisms by binding to mannose residues common on the surface of a number of different microorganisms.[103] Several allelic variants of the molecule are found and appear to be common findings in different populations. The variant affecting codon 54 is found in up to 20% of Caucasians while a variant at codon 57 has a frequency of 20–30% in West Africans.

The variant alleles affect the stability of MBL protein structure and so result in low serum levels of MBL in the heterozygous state and extremely low levels in those who are homozygous. Two promoter region polymorphisms also cause low levels of MBL.[104] It has been suggested that the persistence of such high frequencies of MBL deficiency in humans occurs because low levels may protect against certain parasitic infections.[2] Individuals with low levels have an increased incidence of bacterial infections, particularly in early childhood before the ability to make high affinity antibodies is fully developed. They also have an increased incidence of autoimmune disease.[105] The true significance of MBL deficiency is much debated and may only be important when other 'minor' immunodeficiencies coexist, or in early childhood, when other immune pathways are not fully developed.

DEFICIENCIES OF C3 RECEPTORS

The distribution and function of cell surface receptors for C3b and its derivatives have been described (p. 1140). Specific clinical syndromes have been attributed to deficiencies of some of these receptors. A dominantly inherited CR1 deficiency is associated with SLE and other immune complex disorders, presumably related to failure of the immune complex clearing function of this molecule.

Deficient expression of the CR3 receptor occurs as part of the leukocyte adhesion deficiency type I syndrome (p. 1166) since it is a member of the beta integrin family affected in this disorder though what contribution this makes to the overall clinical picture in that condition is unclear.

PAROXYSMAL NOCTURNAL HEMOGLOBINURIA

The membrane bound complement regulatory proteins DAF (CD55) and CD59 prevent the activation of complement on host cells. They are part of a family of proteins which are attached to the cell surface by a glycophosphatidylinositol anchor. A clonal defect in stem cells can result in abnormal expression which increases the susceptibility of cells, especially red blood cells, to complement mediated lysis. This can result in paroxysmal nocturnal hemoglobinuria.

MANAGEMENT OF COMPLEMENT DEFICIENCIES

Apart from C1 esterase inhibitor there are no specific replacement factor preparations. Fresh plasma infusions have been used prophylactically or can be reserved for the treatment of serious episodes of infection. Life-long prophylactic penicillin and meningococcal vaccination are advised in those complement deficiencies resulting in susceptibility to neisserial infections. A polyvalent vaccine (A, C, W135 and Y) should be given. Prophylactic co-trimoxazole can be used in deficiencies which result in an increased susceptibility to a wider range of organisms. Clinical monitoring may allow earlier diagnosis and treatment of autoimmune disorders should they emerge.

SECONDARY IMMUNODEFICIENCY

Secondary immunodeficiencies are more common than primary disorders and are easily overlooked. Increasing success in treating cancer and transplantation mean that more and more children receive immunosuppressive drugs (Table 27.14). Children with autoimmune disease also receive immunosuppressive treatment, and newly available biological agents, e.g. etanercept, are associated with infection. Viral infections also depress immune function and specific aspects of immunity may be lost in other conditions, e.g. immunoglobulin deficiency secondary to protein-losing states, or complement consumption states. The causes of more generalized, and sometimes less well-defined, secondary immunodeficiency are discussed here.

INFECTION-INDUCED IMMUNODEFICIENCY

Many different infections have been shown to depress immunity. This is seen most commonly after viral infection[106] but chronic infection with

Table 27.14 Some causes of secondary immunodeficiency

Drugs
Corticosteroids
Cytotoxic drugs
Specific immunosuppressive, e.g. cyclosporin A (ciclosporin), antilymphocyte globulin
Miscellaneous, e.g. phenytoin

Radiation

Malnutrition

Protein-losing states
Nephrotic syndrome
Gastrointestinal disease (especially intestinal lymphangiectasia)
Burns

Excessive immunoglobulin catabolism
Myotonic dystrophy
Metabolic disturbance
Inherited – galactosemia
– glycogen storage disease
Acquired – uremia
– diabetes mellitus

Infections
Viruses – human immunodeficiency virus
– cytomegalovirus, Epstein–Barr virus
Bacteria – overwhelming infections
Protozoa – e.g. malaria

Immune complex disorders, e.g. systemic lupus erythematosus

Hyposplenism
Congenital asplenia
Sickle cell anemia
Splenectomy

Malignancy, esp. lymphoid

Histiocytic disorders
Langerhans' cell histiocytosis
Hemophagocytic lymphohistiocytosis

Miscellaneous
Sarcoidosis
Surgery and anesthesia

other organisms can have similar effects. Examples include the depressed antibody responses in malaria infected children which correlate with the parasite load, or the T lymphocyte depression that complicates advanced mycobacterial disease and which may be due to the immunosuppressive effects of specific mycobacterial cell wall products.

Acute viral infection
Decreased numbers of circulating lymphocytes associated with markedly reduced T lymphocyte proliferative responses and cutaneous anergy are a 'normal' reaction to a wide variety of common acute viral infections. This was first recognized in measles infection by Von Pirquet in 1908. It has also occurred after live viral vaccines, including measles and oral polio. In some cases, it is due to direct infection of lymphocytes and/or macrophages. In others, there is an alteration in immunoregulation, most marked in acute infectious mononucleosis due to EBV infection in which there is B and T lymphocyte proliferation and a reversal of the normal helper:suppressor T lymphocyte ratios. Influenza and measles virus infections also have nonspecific depressive effects on neutrophil and monocyte function. The clinical importance of these observations is not always certain but in resource limited countries they probably account for the very high incidence of secondary bacterial infection after measles and the fatal downward spiral of infection and malnutrition that is commonly seen after measles.

Chronic viral infectizon
Congenital viral infection (and toxoplasmosis) results in an immune depression with specific failure of T lymphocyte reactivity, or tolerance, to the relevant agent and in some cases a more generalized depression of antibody responses and even hypogammaglobulinemia, sometimes of a pattern which mimics the hyper-IgM syndrome. Congenital cytomegalovirus and rubella infections can result in prolonged excretion of these viruses for several years. Other chronic viral infections, e.g. subacute sclerosing panencephalitis or persistent EBV infection, are associated with an ill-defined immune suppression, possibly partly due to an element of pre-existing immune incompetence. Hepatitis C virus infection is associated with acquired IgA deficiency.[107]

IMMUNODEFICIENCY DUE TO DRUGS AND RADIATION
Specific immunosuppressive agents
Antibodies to human lymphocytes (antilymphocyte globulin) or specific T lymphocyte subpopulations are used to treat idiopathic aplastic anemia, GvHD and graft rejection. They induce prolonged, profound lymphopenia and depress primary antibody and delayed hypersensitivity responses. B lymphocyte monoclonal antibodies have been used in the treatment of B lymphoproliferative disease in transplant patients with some success but deplete the B lymphocyte population for many months and can lead to hypogammaglobulinemia.

The newer biologic monoclonal antibody agents such as etanercept (soluble TNF-alpha receptor), infliximab (anti-TNF-alpha), basiliximab (anti IL-2R-alpha), and others are increasingly used in transplantation settings, and to treat inflammatory disorders such as juvenile idiopathic arthritis and Crohn disease. Their use is associated with an increased infection risk, particularly tuberculosis associated with the use of TNF-alpha blockade.

Ciclosporin and tacrolimus are reversible calcineurin antagonists used in organ and bone marrow transplantation, affecting predominantly T lymphocytes, but also B lymphocytes and other cell types. They inhibit antigen processing as well as diminishing IL-1 and IL-2 production, and IL-2 receptor expression.

Corticosteroid drugs are less specific, but potent, immunosuppressive drugs.[108] The degree of immunosuppression induced is related to the dose and length of treatment course and probably varies between individuals. An equivalent dose of prednisolone 2 mg/kg/day for more than a week, or 1 mg/kg/day for greater than a month is generally considered immunosuppressive. Lymphopenia results from a diminution of recirculation of long-lived T lymphocytes. Cytotoxic function, mitogenic responses and delayed hypersensitivity responses are all depressed. With high dose treatment for prolonged periods antibody responses, especially primary responses, also become impaired. Corticosteroids also affect recirculating monocytes and polymorphs, and microbicidal ability is depressed.

Cytotoxic drugs used in the treatment of leukemia and solid tumors have major immunosuppressive side-effects. Cyclophosphamide particularly affects B lymphocyte function and antibody production, but T lymphopenia (especially of CD4+ T lymphocytes) also occurs.

Azathioprine, mycophenolate mofetil and 6-mercaptopurine suppress antibody production, particularly primary responses. T lymphocyte functions including delayed hypersensitivity responses are also depressed.

Methotrexate has potent anti-inflammatory activity and may also suppress antibody responses in higher doses.

Radiation therapy, particularly total body or total lymphoid irradiation, has profound and long-lasting effects on lymphocyte-mediated immune function and on antibody responses.

The most severe immunosuppressed states occur during HSCT for malignant disease. In these cases, a combination of radiotherapy and chemotherapy is often used.

Clinical effects

The immunosuppressed child is susceptible to opportunistic infection, especially fungal infections and *Pneumocystis carinii* pneumonia (see Figs 27.16, 27.17). After HSCT, there is a recognized pattern of susceptibility to different pathogens, depending on the elapsed time since the procedure (Fig. 27.20). In the absence of neutropenia, susceptibility to pyogenic infections is less of a problem. 'Live' vaccines should be avoided, as should contact with cases of measles and chickenpox. Postexposure prophylaxis should be given when inadvertent exposure to these viruses occurs. Co-trimoxazole is effective as prophylaxis against *Pneumocystis carinii* pneumonia.

Other drugs

A variety of miscellaneous drugs may cause immunosuppression as part of their side-effect profile. The effects of phenytoin and other agents on IgA production are discussed in the section on IgA deficiency. Moderate or severe depression of neutrophil counts is a side-effect of a large number of drugs including antibiotics such as sulfonamides and flucloxacillin and results in a susceptibility to bacterial disease.

MALNUTRITION

Nutritional status, infection and immunity are closely linked, and nutritional deficiency can have profound effects on all aspects of the immune system. The most profound and wide-ranging effects are seen in protein/

Table 27.15 Main immunological effects of severe malnutrition

Cell-mediated immunity
T cell lymphopenia
Reduced CD4 cell numbers
Reduced CD4:CD8 ratio
Reduced delayed hypersensitivity responses
Reduced proliferative T cell responses to mitogens and antigens
Reduced lymphokine production

Antibody production
Polyclonal hypergammaglobulinemia
Decreased IgA in secretions
Increased serum IgE
Defective antibody responses
Reduced antibody affinity
Depressed function of antigen-presenting cells

Nonspecific immune system
Depressed neutrophil bactericidal capability
Depressed levels of complement factors, especially C3

calorie deficiency (Table 27.15), with changes in lymphocyte number and function, antibody production and quality, complement synthesis and phagocytosis.[109] There is increased susceptibility to TB, measles, *Pneumocystis carinii* as well as staphylococcal pneumonia, and Gram negative sepsis.

Specific nutritional deficiencies also affect immune function. Zinc deficiency in autosomal recessive acrodermatitis enteropathica or secondary to nutritional deficiency causes thymic atrophy, T lymphopenia, anergy, impaired cytotoxicity and decreased immunoglobulin production. Many immunological effects of zinc deficiency may be related to the critical role of zinc in intracellular zinc-finger-dependent transcription factors, and in DNA synthesis and lymphocyte proliferation. Treatment with zinc supplements reverses most effects. Iron deficiency, even without anemia, has subtle effects on T lymphocyte and phagocytic lymphocyte function. The clinical importance of this is not clear. Some studies have shown an increased frequency of infections which reverses with iron therapy, but others have not confirmed this. Vitamin A deficiency is associated with depressed T lymphocyte and humoral responses, and a dominant T_H2 pattern of response. In populations at risk from malnutrition, vitamin A supplementation improves antibody responses to vaccines. In similar populations treatment with vitamin A during measles infection reduces mortality and has been shown to reverse some of the induced abnormalities in lymphocyte numbers and function.

VACCINATION OF THE CHILD WITH A POTENTIALLY IMPAIRED IMMUNE RESPONSE

Immunocompromised children are often more in need of the protection vaccination can offer because of their greater risk from infection, and yet are less likely to be vaccinated because of concerns about the underlying immunodeficiency. In general, live vaccine should be avoided in children with malignancy who are being treated with or have received chemotherapy within 6 months. Booster vaccines may be appropriate after completion of treatment. Children who have undergone HSCT should be reimmunized 12–18 months post HSCT, providing immunosuppression has been stopped for 6 months or more and they do not have GvHD. Measles, mumps and rubella (MMR) vaccine should be given 6 months after commencement of the vaccination schedule. Vaccinations should be up to date before transplantation in those receiving solid organ transplants. As they remain on life-long immunosuppression following transplantation, live vaccines should be avoided. HIV infected children should receive killed polio vaccine, but MMR seems safe to give. Children with primary immunodeficiency should be immunized. Those with lymphocyte-mediated immunodeficiency should not receive live vaccines; in all other forms

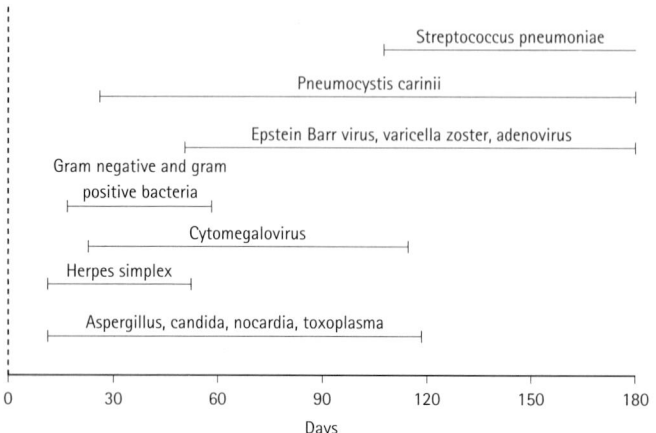

Streptococcus pneumoniae
Pneumocystis carinii
Epstein Barr virus, varicella zoster, adenovirus
Gram negative and gram positive bacteria
Cytomegalovirus
Herpes simplex
Aspergillus, candida, nocardia, toxoplasma

0   30   60   90   120   150   180
Days

Fig. 27.20 Timeline showing periods of maximal risk for various infectious complications after bone marrow transplantation with immunosuppression/marrow ablation. (Courtesy of the Bubble Foundation).

of immunodeficiency live vaccine can safely be administered, except BCG in patients with CGD. Children on pharmacological doses of steroids (an equivalent dose of prednisolone 2 mg/kg/day for > 1 week, or 1 mg/kg/day for > 1 month) or other immunosuppressive therapy should not be given live vaccines. Conjugate pneumococcal vaccine should be given to children with asplenia, hyposplenism or nephrotic syndrome, although from late 2006 it is part of the routine UK primary vaccination schedule. Zoster-specific immunoglobulin should be given to those with significant immunosuppression who are chickenpox contacts and non-immune. Children receiving immunoglobulin replacement should not be vaccinated, as protective antibody is present in the immunoglobulin given.[110]

HYPOSPLENISM

Congenital asplenia, splenectomy and sickle cell disease are the major causes of hyposplenism in childhood. Finding Howell–Jolly bodies on a blood film or absence of a spleen on ultrasound are helpful when it is unclear whether the spleen is absent. Patients are at risk of pyogenic infection including pneumonia, septicemia or meningitis with polysaccharide encapsulated bacteria such as *Streptococcus pneumoniae* or *Neisseria meningitidis*. The absolute risk of infection of 0.42% per year is significant when viewed over a lifetime, and the risk is four times higher in young children with congenital asplenia where other aspects of immunity are less well developed. Young asplenic children also suffer infection with a greater range of pathogens including *Haemophilus influenzae* and Gram negative organisms. The immunodeficiency is multifactorial and probably largely functional. Factors thought to contribute include failure of clearance of opsonized bacteria in the spleen, lack of the B lymphocyte reservoir function, and low activity of the alternative pathway of complement. Defective alternative pathway complement activity was found in 10% of splenectomized and 16% of sickle cell patients. In older patients, IgG antibody responses to pneumococcal vaccine are similar to normal individuals although low serum IgM levels have been reported. Antipolysaccharide IgG levels decay more quickly.[111]

As pneumococcal infection is the most common severe infection, prophylaxis with penicillin is used in the UK, but alternative treatment may be necessary where penicillin-resistant pneumococci are common. In children below 4 years of age, the risks from other infections mean a broader spectrum antibiotic such as amoxicillin (or co-trimoxazole) is recommended. Vaccination with conjugated pneumococcal, *Haemophilus influenzae* type B and meningococcus C vaccines may diminish the risk but does not remove the need to give penicillin. Immunization should be performed prior to elective splenectomy. Antipneumococcal antibody levels should be measured annually, and patients revaccinated if levels are low.[112]

Much, but not all, of the increased susceptibility to infection in sickle cell disease stems from the hyposplenism which develops as the spleen is infarcted. In addition, sickle cell patients have impaired reticuloendothelial clearing capacity (due to chronic hemolysis) and focal tissue ischemia (as a result of sickling). As well as being susceptible to pneumococcus, these patients are also prone to Gram negative sepsis, including salmonella osteomyelitis. The risk of these problems is less in the variant form, hemoglobin S, hemoglobin C disease, but is still higher than background so prophylactic measures are still indicated.

TREATMENT OF IMMUNODEFICIENCY

SUPPORTIVE CARE

Children with immunodeficiency disorders often require the full spectrum of pediatric care. Particular attention needs to be paid to nutritional status and the management of dietary intolerances secondary to the gastrointestinal problems which frequently occur. Supporting the emotional needs of the family is also very important. Prevention and treatment of infections is the mainstay of supportive care.

GENERAL MEASURES FOR PREVENTION OF INFECTIONS

Newborns suspected of having a severe immunodeficiency disorder should be protected using isolation techniques, including limitation of the numbers of persons involved with care; individuals with respiratory or gastrointestinal symptoms of infection should avoid contact. Breast-feeding should be encouraged. Wherever the child is managed the importance of strict hand washing procedures cannot be overemphasized. If HSCT with conditioning chemotherapy is embarked upon (see below), isolation in facilities with positive pressure filtered air supply is necessary, mainly to reduce the risk of aspergillosis and droplet borne viral infections.

SPECIFIC MEASURES FOR PREVENTION OF INFECTIONS

Co-trimoxazole as prophylaxis against *Pneumocystis carinii* should be given for defects involving cell-mediated immunity mechanisms. For *Pneumocystis carinii* pneumonia prophylaxis only, co-trimoxazole need only be given on 2 or 3 days a week. If this is not tolerated, alternatives include dapsone or atovaquone. Inhaled pentamidine can be used in older children. Injectable pentamidine should not be used prophylactically because of the potential side-effects and possible reduced efficacy. Co-trimoxazole probably also reduces the incidence of pyogenic infections in these patients and those with phagocytic or humoral immune deficiencies and for this purpose it is usually given daily (dose 30 mg/kg/day in one or two doses). In circumstances of poor nutrition, increased bone marrow turnover and in all cases after HSCT, weekly folinic acid supplements are given to lessen the risk of bone marrow depression without compromising the antimicrobial efficacy. Antifungal prophylaxis should be used in combined immunodeficiencies or phagocytic cell defects. In chronic granulomatous disease and other conditions where the risk of aspergillus infection is high, itraconazole is preferred. Otherwise fluconazole or non-absorbed agents such as nystatin are used.

Where the immune deficiency predisposes to infection with relatively few organisms, prophylaxis with a narrow spectrum antibiotic can be used, e.g. penicillin prophylaxis for the terminal complement deficiencies where only neisserial infection is a risk. Prophylactic antibiotics are most commonly used for patients with relatively minor humoral deficiencies such as symptomatic IgA deficiency. There is no scientific basis for the choice of antibiotic in these circumstances because of the great difficulty in performing a trial looking at efficacy. Co-trimoxazole has been widely used but concerns over potential side-effects have led to the use of other agents such as azithromycin which, because of its long half-life, can be given on 3 days out of every 14 and provides continuous prophylaxis against sinopulmonary bacterial infections. This is attractive, but less is known of its effects when given over many years. Cefixime is a further alternative given as a single daily dose. Antiviral prophylaxis with aciclovir is used in patients with cell-mediated immunodeficiency and previous herpes simplex infection. It is also used in the context of HSCT to prevent herpes simplex and CMV reactivation.

Immunizations may be used judiciously if sufficient immune function is judged to be present to give an antibody response. 'Live' vaccines are contraindicated in combined immunodeficiencies and in the more severe antibody deficiency states. Passive immunization is the basis of immunoglobulin replacement therapy (see below) and specific hyperimmune globulins are available for postexposure prophylaxis in patients with primary or secondary immunodeficiency exposed to chickenpox or hepatitis B. For measles exposure, standard immunoglobulin is used. The role of immunoglobulins with high titers of anti-respiratory syncytial virus (RSV) or of monoclonal anti-RSV antibodies in protecting against RSV in children with primary immunodeficiencies during the winter season has not been evaluated and is unlikely to be formally investigated because of the rarity of these conditions. They may have a role in SCID patients before and during transplant, particularly as common cold symptoms in carers may be caused by this virus.

The prevention of complications of recurrent infections is most important. Evidence of middle ear disease which might lead to deafness should be sought and treated. Chronic lung disease leading to bronchiectasis is a serious complication, particularly of antibody deficiency states. Regular physiotherapy with sputum cultures to direct appropriate antibiotic therapy and monitoring of pulmonary status are useful. Breakthrough infections threatening organ damage despite prophylactic antibiotics may be an indication for starting immunoglobulin therapy even if the tests show relatively minor abnormalities of humoral immunity. Serial measurements of lung function tests and judicious use of high resolution CT (HRCT) scanning may detect early damage or progression of existing damage. HRCT scans are relatively contraindicated in disorders associated with increased radiosensitivity such as ataxia telangiectasia.

TREATMENT OF INFECTIONS

A policy of vigorous and early antimicrobial treatment of infections should be observed. Unusual agents may cause infection, and broader spectrum antimicrobial cover may therefore be needed. In neutrophil disorders it is important to cover *Pseudomonas* and other Gram negative bacilli. Early treatment of an infection may be life saving, but its initiation should not detract from full attempts at identification of the causative agent. Invasive diagnostic procedures, such as bronchoalveolar lavage or, if this fails to produce a diagnosis, open lung biopsy, will facilitate precise and optimal therapy. The mainstay of treatment for systemic fungal infection remains amphotericin B, mostly used in its liposomal form to reduce toxicity and enable larger doses to be given. New agents increasingly used for treating invasive aspergillosis include voriconazole and caspofungin.

Antivirals such as the broad spectrum agent, ribavirin, and the anticytomegalovirus agents, ganciclovir and foscarnet, are particularly useful in the immunocompromised infant. Newer antivirals include cidofovir for resistant CMV, adenovirus and severe molluscum contagiosum and pleconaril for enteroviral infections. The role of zanamivir in immunocompromised children with influenza has not been assessed.

BLOOD PRODUCT SUPPORT

Blood product infusions may be necessary in some disorders. In combined deficiencies and in patients undergoing heavy immunosuppression (as for HSCT), all such products except intravenous immunoglobulin and fresh frozen plasma may contain viable leukocytes and should be irradiated with 2000–3000 rad to prevent possible GvHD. In those with no evidence of previous exposure to CMV, blood products should be obtained from CMV-antibody-negative donors. White cell infusions have a role in specific situations such as adjunctive therapy in poorly responding infections in patients with CGD and other neutrophil function disorders particularly if they are harvested from G-CSF primed donors.

SUPPORT FOR FAMILIES AND PATIENTS

Patient support organizations which are established in most resource rich countries are very helpful in providing information and advice and in helping families to meet others with the same (rare) diagnoses. In the UK the organization is the Primary Immunodeficiency Association (PIA) (http://www.pia.org.uk/). Further information may be generally available on the Web but families should be warned that sometimes this is produced without reference to expert advice. Other specific diseases may have their own organizations.

REPLACEMENT IMMUNOGLOBULIN THERAPY

This is the mainstay of treatment for the more severe antibody states and various combined immunodeficiencies. The need for immunoglobulin must be evaluated on an individual patient basis. Absolute indications include quantitative defects (IgG less than the 95th percentile for age or less than 3 g/L in an older child) and qualitative defects (failure of response to booster vaccinations). Other indications include failure of

antibiotic prophylaxis in a child with quantitatively minor Ig abnormalities (e.g. IgA and IgG subclass deficiency) and risk of end-organ damage (e.g. bronchiectasis) in a child with any degree of antibody deficiency. As immunoglobulin is a blood product, and there is a limited supply, new and existing uses should be carefully evaluated.

Risks of replacement therapy

Replacement immunoglobulin must contain the full range of protective antibodies in order to provide effective prophylaxis against infections. Unlike coagulation factors where the invariant protein needed can be made using molecular techniques, a polyclonal product cannot be generated by recombinant technology and human plasma has to be used as a source. To ensure that immunoglobulin contains the full spectrum of protective antibody, preparations are made from pooled (5–100 000 donors) plasma donations, which increases the risk of transmission of an infectious agent.[113] Pools are screened for known agents (e.g. hepatitis B and C) and the process of cold ethanol precipitation, universally used for the fractionation of plasma, effectively kills some viruses, including HIV. New intravenous and subcutaneous products must include a further viral inactivation step such as pasteurization or nanofiltration before they are licensed. The risk of transmission of variant Creutzfeldt – Jakob disease (vCJD) is theoretical and not quantifiable using modern techniques, but plasma is no longer sourced from the UK in an effort to minimize the risk. Taken together, these precautions have reduced the risk of infection to a very low level. Patients should be evaluated by PCR for hepatitis B and C prior to commencement of therapy, and require regular monitoring of immunoglobulin levels and liver function tests. Any elevation in liver function tests should prompt re-evaluation of their hepatitis status. Batch numbers of all products administered must be recorded to facilitate patient tracing if there is a problem with an individual batch. Switching between different preparations should be avoided unless there are good clinical reasons.

Mode of administration

The efficacy of replacement immunoglobulin therapy was established in the 1950s using i.m. preparations. However, this is painful and only limited volumes can be given so that adequate serum levels of IgG were rarely achieved. Improvements in manufacturing techniques in the 1980s meant IMIG was superseded by IVIG preparations. Large volumes of the latter could be given, achieving better symptom control and trough IgG levels well within the normal range. Doses are in the range of 0.3–0.5 g/kg/3 weeks, infused over 2–3 h. Immediate reactions to IVIG are more common than to the i.m. preparation and include nausea, vomiting, flushing, rigors and occasionally hypertension. These can normally be controlled by slowing the infusion rate. Rarely, anaphylactoid reactions occur, particularly in IgA-deficient patients who may have anti-IgA antibodies.[114] Patients with known anti-IgA antibodies should be given a preparation with a low IgA content. In the 1990s subcutaneous (s.c.) administration of immunoglobulin was shown to be efficacious in adults with far fewer side-effects, other than local reactions, and specific products are now licensed for use in children. Advantages include lack of need for venous access and ease of training parents for home therapy. However, given that only a limited volume can be given in one site, frequency of administration is normally increased, and SCIg should be given weekly.

REPLACEMENT THERAPY FOR COMBINED DEFICIENCIES

REPLACEMENT OF THYMUS FUNCTION

Fetal thymus and/or fetal liver (as a source of stem cells) transplants have been used for SCID with some limited success. Delayed immune reconstitution, severe infection, GvHD and lack of availability of fetal tissues together with significant improvement in HSCT techniques have led to these procedures being abandoned. However, fetal thymus transplantation appears to be effective in patients with severe DiGeorge anomaly who have normal hemopoietic stem cells but who lack the thymic machinery to undergo

T lymphocyte receptor gene rearrangement. Thymic transplant in these patients is still being evaluated, but early results look promising.[115]

HEMOPOIETIC STEM CELL TRANSPLANTATION

Virtually all primary T lymphocyte and phagocyte immunodeficiency disorders are potentially correctable by HSCT.[116] Patients with immediately life-threatening conditions, mainly SCID, are treated by HSCT. Improving results from HSCT, together with an increasing understanding of the basis of the immunodeficiencies, and international registry data on their long term outcome have led to more conditions such as Wiskott–Aldrich syndrome, CD40L deficiency and CGD being treated by HSCT (Table 27.16).

Early attempts at HSCT using poorly matched donors were largely unsuccessful and so only transplants using HLA matched sibling donors were performed, an approach available only to about 20% of patients. Since the early 1980s, techniques have been developed to allow parent-to-child (haploidentical) grafts, by removing mature T lymphocytes that would otherwise cause fatal GvHD. These have become the most common HSCT procedure for patients with SCID.[117,118] Matched unrelated donor transplants are being increasingly used, particularly for non-SCID immunodeficiencies. Overall results are improving, probably due to a combination of factors (Table 27.17).

Table 27.16 Primary immunodeficiency disorders which have been treated with bone marrow transplantation

Lymphocyte disorders
Severe combined immunodeficiency
(including adenosine deaminase deficiency)
Wiskott–Aldrich syndrome
Omenn syndrome
Major histocompatibility antigen
class II deficiency
DiGeorge syndrome
Purine nucleoside phosphorylase deficiency
Cartilage–hair hypoplasia syndrome
X-linked lymphoproliferative disease
Hyper-IgM syndrome (CD40 ligand deficiency)
Mucocutaneous candidiasis
Immunodeficiency with partial albinism (Griscelli syndrome)

Phagocytic cell disorders
Chronic granulomatous disease
Leukocyte adhesion defect type I
Congenital agranulocytosis
Chediak–Higashi syndrome
Familial hemophagocytic lymphohistiocytosis
IL-12-dependent interferon-gamma pathway defects
Hyper-IgE syndrome

Table 27.17 Factors associated with improvement in results of HSCT in primary immunodeficiency

- Use of new stem cell sources (peripherally mobilized blood stem cells, umbilical cord blood stem cells)
- Development of low toxicity (reduced intensity) conditioning chemotherapy
- Improved HLA matching with high resolution molecular DNA techniques
- Improved early detection of viral infection by PCR enabling preemptive treatment
- Development of new antiviral and antifungal agents
- Development of new immunosuppressive agents to treat GvHD, e.g. infliximab
- Early use of aggressive supportive care including intensive care

Complications of HSCT

The five main complications of HSCT are toxicity from conditioning agents, graft failure, graft rejection, GvHD, and infection which may be pre-existing due to immunodeficiency or be acquired after HSCT. Rejection is less likely following transplantation with replete rather than T lymphocyte depleted marrow, but the risk of GvHD after replete marrow is greater. Graft rejection is unusual in SCID, but more likely in the NK+ phenotypes, or if clinically evident maternofetal engraftment is present. Myeloablation with chemotherapy helps reduce the chance of rejection and may result in better engraftment quality. The risk of infectious complications is greatest in T lymphocyte depleted grafts where there is a prolonged period before functioning immunity develops.

GvHD primarily affects skin, gut and liver causing an erythematous maculopapular papular rash, watery diarrhea and jaundice. Diagnosis is clinical, but should usually be confirmed by biopsy of the affected organ. GvHD is rarely fatal but the associated severe acute inflammatory changes may be life threatening. The process itself causes further immunosuppression and bone marrow depression, which may cause delay or failure of graft maturation which, in turn, increases the risk from infection. Cyclosporin A (ciclosporin) is generally given as prophylaxis against GvHD with or without methotrexate. Corticosteroids and intravenous immunoglobulin are also sometimes used as GvHD prophylaxis, the latter also reducing the risk of infection. Acute GvHD is treated with immunosuppressive agents including high dose steroids, mycophenolate mofetil and increasingly biologic agents such as infliximab and basiliximab. In extreme cases antithymocyte globulin may be needed, which further increases the infection risk. Chronic, ongoing GvHD is rarely a problem following HSCT for immunodeficiency. Recalcitrant GvHD may respond to extracorporeal phototherapy.

Infection after transplantation is discussed above (see secondary immunodeficiencies and Fig. 27.20).

Matched related donor HSCT

Usually only sibling donors are matched, but when parents are consanguineous, other family members may be a full match. For severe combined immunodeficiency, HLA-matched grafts are relatively straightforward. Prior immunosuppression ('conditioning') is not usually required or can be minimal. GvHD can occur but is usually mild and self-limiting and prophylaxis is not usually given. Full and long-lasting immune reconstitution is usually achieved though in some cases B lymphocyte engraftment and therefore reconstitution of humoral immunity does not occur, necessitating continuing immunoglobulin therapy. In recent years, the success rate in the European experience has been of the order of 90%.[116] Failure is usually related to the pre-existing condition of the child, rather than the technique.

Matched transplants for other conditions (where a residual immune system is capable of graft rejection) have a lower success rate, at least in part because of the need to give conditioning treatment, with the consequent risks of lung and liver toxicity and infection. Nevertheless, encouraging results have been reported[116] with overall survival of 81% since 1995. The use of lower intensity chemotherapy conditioning regimens has enabled sick patients with pre-existing lung and liver damage to undergo successful treatment.[119]

Mismatched bone marrow transplantation

By removing all T lymphocyte lineage cells (back to the prethymic stage) from harvested bone marrow, GvHD can be prevented even in an HLA-mismatched situation. At first, T lymphocytes were removed by their propensity to bind to plant lectins, but now specific monoclonal antibodies are used that either remove T lymphocytes or positively select HSC in a semiautomated system. The resulting T lymphocyte-depleted, stem cell-enriched marrow will reconstitute T lymphocyte immunity by producing precursor T lymphocytes which are 'educated' into a state of tolerance towards the foreign HLA haplotype in the recipient thymus. The fact that there is half matching of human leukocyte antigen allows most immune functions to proceed normally.

However, successful mismatched bone marrow transplants are not as easily achieved as matched ones. Even in SCID, the T lymphocyte depleted bone marrow can be rejected (or fail to take), and to prevent this conditioning therapy (marrow ablation) is often needed. Development of immune function is often slow (120 days before the appearance of T lymphocytes versus 42 days following matched antigen HSCT), and full immune reconstitution will take months. B lymphocyte function (antibody responses) is generally good following fully conditioned HSC transplantation,[120] although polysaccharide responses may remain poor. Failure to remove all the T lymphocytes can result in severe GvHD, which may require the use of immunosuppressive drugs. On the other hand absolute deficiency of T lymphocytes inhibits engraftment. The adding back of small numbers of T lymphocytes has been attempted to overcome this problem but it increases the risk of GvHD. Clinical trials are in progress investigating the co-infusion of mesenchymal stem cells, which may facilitate engraftment and modulate GvHD. The prolonged period of immunodeficiency greatly increases the risk of opportunistic infections. In this group of transplants the use of high technology isolation facilities (such as laminar air flow) improves the outcome.

Despite these problems, refinements of the technique over recent years have resulted in continuing improvement in results, with success rates for SCID of around 78% for T lymphocyte depleted grafts, and > 90% for matched sibling donors.[116] Success is dependent on type of SCID, with better results for B+ SCID than the B− phenotype.[117] Age at presentation also influences outcome, with very good results for those transplanted in the neonatal period, before they have contracted infections.[121]

The problems and risks of mismatched bone marrow transplantation have meant that it has been used less for non-SCID conditions. Nevertheless results are improving[116] with 47% survival in the post-1995 period in Europe.

Matched unrelated donor bone marrow transplantation

For many years there have been national and international registries of tissue typed volunteers willing to donate bone marrow, allowing the option of using phenotypically matched unrelated donors. There is considerable experience of this approach in the hematological field. Early results in SCID suggested that using mismatched haploidentical donors gave better results. However, with the increased sophistication of tissue typing techniques this may no longer be the case and unrelated donors are increasingly being used with similar results to those following mismatched bone marrow transplantation.

Storage of screened umbilical cord donations is also performed. Advantages to using cord blood include high stem cell dose, no risk to the donor, less GvHD and 'instant' availability of a suitable unit. This is particularly important in treating infants with SCID where the delay involved in identifying, screening and harvesting an unrelated donor may mean new or worsening infection, decreasing the chance of successful transplantation. Relatively low stem cell dose/kg is less of a problem than for adult transplantation, particularly for infants with SCID. Immune reconstitution appears to be as good as for other stem cell sources.[122]

Transplantation technique

This is relatively straightforward for donor and recipient. Under general anesthesia marrow is harvested by multiple punctures along the posterior iliac crest. If it is to be given unfractionated it is passed through a coarse filter to remove bone particles, the nucleated cells are counted and if necessary the volume adjusted. T lymphocyte depletion, if required, is done under strict aseptic conditions (details of this are beyond the scope of this chapter). Another approach which avoids the need for bone marrow harvest is the technique of peripheral stem cell harvest which is increasingly being used and is under evaluation. Umbilical cord blood is harvested at time of delivery, and in families with known immunodeficiencies, directed cord donation is possible, targeted for potential future affected family members.

OTHER REPLACEMENT THERAPIES

Enzyme replacement

Some reconstitution of immunological function can be achieved by administering replacement enzyme in ADA deficiency. Purified bovine ADA is conjugated with polyethylene glycol (PEG-ADA) and given by intramuscular injection. In the severe SCID phenotype this can significantly improve immune function, but regular treatment is needed and the long term outcome is not known. If a suitable donor is available, HSCT seems the best treatment. However PEG-ADA may be useful in partial forms of the condition. Its role as an adjunct to transplantation is unclear.

Cytokines

Several cytokines and growth factors are available in recombinant synthetic form. Their widespread use in immunodeficiency disorders awaits evaluation. IFN-gamma and IL-2 have been useful in improving cell-mediated immune function in deficiencies where their production was demonstrably absent.[123] Growth factors such as G-CSF or granulocyte–macrophage colony stimulating factor may be of benefit in phagocytic series defects. The use of IFN-gamma in chronic granulomatous disease has been discussed under the description of this disorder.

Somatic gene therapy

This has been attempted in adenosine deaminase deficiency using ADA transfected CD34 positive autologous cells, with improvement in immunological and clinical parameters.[124] Successful gene therapy has also been performed for common gamma chain deficiency.[125] Although early results were encouraging, leukemia has subsequently occurred in some cases.[126] It is not yet clear how widespread this risk is, and it may be confined to specific disorders. Preclinical gene therapy trials for RAG deficiency in animal models have demonstrated a malignancy risk. A number of other conditions may be amenable to gene therapy. Clinical trials are currently planned for selected patients with X-linked chronic granulomatous disease or Wiskott–Aldrich syndrome who have no suitable donor. At present HSCT remains the treatment of choice for all but a handful of patients.

REFERENCES (* Level 1 evidence)

1. Steihm RE, Ochs HD, Winkelstein JA, eds. Immunological disorders in infants and children, 5th edn. Philadelphia: WB Saunders; 2005.
2. Turner MW. The role of mannose-binding lectin in health and disease. Mol Immunol 2003; 40:423–429.
3. Klein C, Lisowska-Grospierre B, LeDeist F, et al. Major histocompatibility complex class II deficiency: clinical manifestations, immunologic features, and outcome. J Pediatr 1993; 123:921–928.
4. Janeway CA, Travers P, Walport M, et al. Immunobiology. 6th edn. Garland Publishing; 2005.
5. Burgio GR, Hanson LA, Ugazio AG, eds. Immunology of the neonate. Berlin: Springer-Verlag; 1987.

6. Marshall-Clarke S, Reen D, Tasker L, et al. Neonatal immunity: how well has it grown up? Immunol Today 2000; 21:35–41.
7. Miller ME, Steihm ER. Immunology and resistance to infection. In: Remington JS, Klein JO, eds. Infectious diseases of the fetus and newborn infant. Philadelphia: Saunders; 1983.
8. Hill HR. Biochemical, structural and functional abnormalities of polymorphonuclear leukocytes in the neonate. Pediatr Res 1987; 22:375–382.
9. Cairo MS. Neonatal neutrophil host defence: prospects for immunologic enhancement during neonatal sepsis. Am J Dis Child 1989; 143:40–46.
10. Ferguson AG. Prolonged impairment of cellular immunity in children with intrauterine growth retardation. J Pediatr 1978; 93:52–56.

11. Shapiro R, Beatty DW, Woods DL, et al. Serum complement and immunoglobulin values in small for gestational age infants. J Pediatr 1981; 99:139–142.
12. Oxelius VA. IgG subclass levels in infancy and childhood. Acta Pediatr Scand 1979; 68:23–27.
13. Choo S, Seymour L, Morris R, et al. Immunogenicity and reactogenicity of a pneumococcal conjugate vaccine administered combined with a haemophilus influenzae type B conjugate vaccine in United Kingdom infants. Pediatr Infect Dis J 2000; 19:854–862.
14. Notarangelo L, Casanova JL, Conley ME, et al. International Union of Immunological Societies Primary Immunodeficiency Diseases Classification Committee. Primary immunodeficiency diseases: an update from the International Union of Immunological

Societies Primary Immunodeficiency Diseases Classification Committee Meeting in Budapest, 2005. J Allergy Clin Immunol 2006; 117:883–896.

15. Levy J, Espanol-Boren T, Thomas C, et al. Clinical spectrum of X-linked hyper-IgM syndrome. J Pediatr 1997; 131:47–54.

16. Hague RA, Rassam S, Morgan G, et al. Early diagnosis of severe combined immune deficiency syndrome. Arch Dis Child 1994; 70:260–263.

17. Ochs HD, Slichter SJ, Harker LA, et al. The Wiskott–Aldrich syndrome: studies of lymphocytes, granulocytes and platelets. Blood 1980; 55:243–252.

18. Gadjeva M, Thiel S, Jensenius JC. The mannan-binding-lectin pathway of the innate immune response. Curr Opin Immunol 2001; 13:74–78.

19. Pyun KH, Ochs HD, Wedgewood RJ, et al. Human antibody responses to bacteriophage FX174: sequential induction of IgM and IgG subclass antibody. Clin Immunol Immunopathol 1989; 51:252–263.

20. Ochs HD, Davis SD, Wedgewood JR. Immunologic responses to bacteriophage fX174 in immunodeficiency diseases. J Clin Invest 1971; 50:2559.

21. Comans–Bitter WM, de Groot R, van den Beemd R, et al. Immunophenotyping of blood lymphocytes in childhood. Reference values for lymphocyte subpopulations. J Pediatr 1997; 130:388–393.

22. Berrington JE, Barge D, Fenton AC, et al. Lymphocyte subsets in term and significantly preterm UK infants in the first year of life analysed by single platform flow cytometry. Clin Exp Immunol 2005; 140:289–292.

23. Gilmour KC, Cranston T, Loughlin S, et al. Rapid protein-based assays for the diagnosis of T− B+ severe combined immunodeficiency. Br J Haematol 2001; 112:671–676.

24. Fischer A, Le Deist F, Hacein-Bey-Abina S, et al. Severe combined immunodeficiency. A model disease for molecular immunology and therapy. Immunol Rev 2005; 203:98–109.

25. Fischer A. Severe combined immunodeficiencies (SCID). Clin Exp Immunol 2000; 122:143–149.

26. Notarangelo LD, Villa A, Schwarz K. RAG and RAG defects. Curr Opin Immunol 1999; 11:435–442.

27. Muller SM, Ege M, Pottharst A, et al. Transplacentally acquired maternal T lymphocytes in severe combined immunodeficiency: a study of 121 patients. Blood 2001; 98:1847–1851.

28. Hirschhorn R, Vauter GF, Kirkpatrick JA Jr, et al. Adenosine deaminase deficiency frequency and comparative pathology in autosomally recessive severe combined immunodeficiency. Clin Immunol Immunopathol 1979; 14:107–120.

29. Cederbaum SD, Kaitila I, Rimoin DL, et al. The chondro-osseous dysplasia of adenosine deaminase deficiency with severe combined immunodeficiency. J Pediatr 1976; 89:737–742.

30. Rogers M, Lwin R, Fairbanks L, et al. Cognitive and behavioral abnormalities in adenosine deaminase deficient severe combined deficiency. J Pediatr 2001; 139:44–50.

31. Hershfield MS. Immunodeficiency caused by adenosine deaminase deficiency. Immunol Allerg Clin North Am 2000; 20:161–175.

32. Cohen A, Grunebaum E, Arpaia E, et al. Immunodeficiency caused by purine nucleoside phosphorylase deficiency. Immunol Allerg Clin North Am 2000; 20:143–159.

33. Soutar RL, Day RE. Dysequilibrium/ataxic diplegia with immunodeficiency. Arch Dis Child 1991; 66:982–983.

34. Elder ME, Hope TJ, Parslow TG, et al. Severe combined immunodeficiency with absence of peripheral blood CD8+ T cells due to ZAP-70 deficiency. Cell Immunol 1995; 165:110–117.

35. Piketty C, Weiss L, Kazatchkine M. Idiopathic CD4 lymphocytopenia. Presse Med 1994; 23:1374–1375.

36. Masternak K, Muhlethaler-Mottet A, Villard J, et al. Molecular genetics of the bare lymphocyte syndrome. Rev Immunogenet 2000; 2:267–282.

37. Renella R, Picard C, Neven B, et al. Human leucocyte antigen-identical haematopoietic stem cell transplantation in major histocompatibility complex class II immunodeficiency: reduced survival correlates with an increased incidence of acute graft-versus-host disease and pre-existing viral infections. Br J Haematol 2006; 134:510–516.

38. de la Salle H, Hanau D, Fricker D, et al. Homozygous human TAP peptide transporter mutation in HLA class I deficiency. Science 1994; 265:237–241.

39. Driscoll DA, Sullivan KE. DiGeorge syndrome: a chromosome 22q11.2 deletion syndrome. In: Ochs HD, Smith CIE, Puck JM, eds. Primary immunodeficiency diseases; a molecular and genetic approach, Oxford: Oxford University Press; 2007:485–495.

40. Theodoropoulos DS, Theodoropoulos GA. Immune deficiency and hearing loss in CHARGE Association. Pediatrics 2003; 111:711–712.

41. Nonoyama S, Ochs HD. Characterization of the Wiskott–Aldrich syndrome protein and its role in the disease. Curr Opin Immunol 1998; 10:407–412.

42. Thrasher AJ, Kinnon C. The Wiskott–Aldrich syndrome. Clin Exp Immunol 2000; 120:2–9.

43. Filipovich AH, Stone JV, Tomany SC, et al. Impact of donor type on outcome of bone marrow transplantation for Wiskott–Aldrich syndrome: collaborative study of the International Bone Marrow Transplant Registry and the National Marrow Donor Program. Blood 2001; 97:1598–1603.

44. Gennery AR, Khawaja K, Veys P, et al. Treatment of CD40 ligand deficiency by hematopoietic stem cell transplantation: a survey of the European experience, 1993–2002. Blood 2004; 103:1152–1157.

45. Purtilo DT, Cassel CK, Yang JPS, et al. X-linked recessive progressive combined variable immunodeficiency (Duncan's disease). Lancet 1975; I:935–940.

46. Morra M, Howie D, Simarro Grande M, et al. X-linked lymphoproliferative disease: a progressive immunodeficiency. Annu Rev Immunol 2001; 19:657–682.

47. Coffey AJ, Brooksbank RA, Brandau O, et al. Host response to EBV infection in X-linked lymphoproliferative disease results from mutations in an SH2-domain encoding gene. Nat Genet 1998; 20:129–135.

48. Sumegi J, Huang D, Lanyi A, et al. Correlation of mutations of the SH2D1A gene and Epstein–Barr virus infection with clinical phenotype and outcome in X-linked lymphoproliferative disease. Blood 2000; 96:3118–3125.

49. Makitie O, Kaitla I, Savilahti E. Susceptibility to infections and in vitro immune functions in cartilage-hair hypoplasia. Eur J Pediatr 1998; 157:816–820.

50. Makitie O, Kaitla I. Cartilage–hair hypoplasia – clinical manifestations in 108 Finnish patients. Eur J Pediatr 1998; 152:211–217.

51. Gennery AR. Primary immunodeficiency syndromes associated with defective DNA double-strand break repair. Br Med Bull 2006; 77–78:71–85.

52. Savitsky K, Bar-Shira A, Gilad S, et al. A single ataxia telangiectasia gene with a product similar to PI-3 kinase. Science 1995; 268:1749–1753.

53. Chun HH, Gatti RA. Ataxia-telangiectasia, an evolving phenotype. DNA Repair (Amst) 2004; 3:1187–1196.

54. Hiel JA, Weemaes CM, van den Heuvel LP, et al. Nijmegen breakage syndrome. Arch Dis Child 2000; 82:400–406.

55. Varon R, Vissinga C, Platzer M, et al. Nibrin, a novel DNA double-strand break repair protein is mutated in Nijmegen breakage syndrome. Cell 1998; 93:467–476.

56. Dokal I. Fanconi's anaemia and related bone marrow failure syndromes. Br Med Bull 2006; 77–78:37–53.

57. Ehrlich M. The ICF syndrome, a DNA methyltransferase 3B deficiency and immunodeficiency disease. Clin Immunol 2003; 109:17–28.

58. Worth A, Thrasher AJ, Gaspar HB. Autoimmune lymphoproliferative syndrome: molecular basis of disease and clinical phenotype. Br J Haematol 2006; 133:124–140.

59. Straus SE, Jaffe ES, Puck JM, et al. The development of lymphomas in families with autoimmune lymphoproliferative syndrome with germline Fas mutation defective apoptosis. Blood 2001; 98:194–200.

60. Kirkpatrick CH. Chronic mucocutaneous candidiasis. Pediatr Infect Dis J 2001; 20:197–206.

61. Lilic D, Calvert JE, Cant AJ, et al. Chronic mucocutaneous candidiasis. II. Class and subclass of specific antibody responses in vivo and in vitro. Clin Exp Immunol 1996; 105:213–219.

62. Bruton OC. Agammaglobulinaemia. Pediatrics 1952; 9:722–727.

63. Lederman HM, Winkelstein JA. X-linked agammaglobulinaemia: an analysis of 96 patients. Medicine 1985; 64:145–156.

64. Spickett GP, Chapel HM. Report on the audit of patients with primary antibody deficiency in the United Kingdom 1993–1996. London: NHS Management Executive; 1998.

65. Hermaszweski RA, Webster ADB. Primary hypogammaglobulinaemia: a survey of clinical manifestations and complications. Q J Med 1993; 86:31–42.

66. Gaspar HB, Lester T, Levinsky RJ, et al. Bruton's tyrosine kinase expression and activity in X-linked agammaglobulinaemia (XLA). Clin Exp Immunol 1998; 111:334–338.

67. Quartier P, Debre M, De Blic J, et al. Early and prolonged intravenous immunoglobulin replacement therapy in childhood agammaglobulinaemia: a retrospective survey of 31 patients. J Pediatr 1999; 134:589–596.

68. Richter D, Conley ME, Rorher J, et al. A contiguous deletion syndrome of X-linked agammaglobulinaemia and sensori-neural deafness. Pediatr Allerg Immunol 2001; 12:107–111.

69. Grunebaum E. Agammaglobulinaemia caused by defects other than btk. Immunol Allerg Clin North Am 2001; 21:45–63.

70. Vorechovsky I, Cullen M, Carrington M, et al. Fine mapping of IGAD1 in IgA deficiency and common variable immunodeficiency: identification and characterization of haplotypes shared by affected members of 101 multiple-case families. J Immunol 2000; 164:4408–4416.

71. Knight AK, Cunningham-Rundles C. Inflammatory and autoimmune complications of common variable immune deficiency. Autoimmun Rev 2006; 5:156–159.

72. Cunningham-Rundles C, Bodian C. Common variable immunodeficiency: clinical and immunological features of 248 patients. Clin Immunol 1999; 92:34–48.

73. Gilmour KC, Cranston T, Jones A, et al. Diagnosis of X-linked lymphoproliferative disease by analysis of SLAM-associated protein expression. Eur J Immunol 2000; 30:1691–1697.

74. Kanegane H, Tsukada S, Iwata T, et al. Detection of Bruton's tyrosine kinase mutations in hypogammaglobulinaemic males registered as common variable immunodeficiency (CVID) in the Japanese Immunodeficiency Registry. Clin Exp Immunol 2000; 120:512–517.

75. Etzioni A. Immune deficiency and autoimmunity. Autoimmun Rev 2003; 2:364–369.

76. Shackleford PG. IgG subclasses: importance in pediatric practice. Pediatr Rev 1993; 14:291–296.

77. Pan Q, Hammarstrom L. Molecular basis of IgG subclass deficiency. Immunol Rev 2000; 178:99–110.

78. Rosenzweig SD, Holland SM. Phagocyte immunodeficiencies and their infections. J Allergy Clin Immunol 2004; 113:620–626.

79. Cale CM, Jones AM, Goldblatt D. Follow up of patients with chronic granulomatous disease diagnosed since 1990. Clin Exp Immunol 2000; 120:351–355.

80. Fischer A, Segal AW, Seger R, et al. The management of chronic granulomatous disease. Eur J Pediatr 1993; 152:896–899.

81. Winkelstein JA, Marino MC, Johnston RB Jr, et al. Chronic granulomatous disease. Report on a national registry of 368 patients. Medicine (Baltimore) 2000; 79:155–169.

82. Seger RA, Gungor T, Belohradsky BH, et al. Treatment of chronic granulomatous disease with myeloablative conditioning and an unmodified hemopoietic allograft: a survey of the European experience, 1985–2000. Blood 2002; 100:4344–4350.

83. Lekstrom-Himes JA, Dorman SE, Kopar P, et al. Neutrophil-specific granule deficiency results from a novel mutation with loss of function of the transcription factor CCAAT/enhancer binding protein. J Exp Med 1999; 189:1847–1852.

84. Barbosa MDFS, Barrat FJ, Tchernev VT, et al. Identification of mutations in two major mRNA isoforms of the Chediak–Higashi syndrome gene in human and mouse. Hum Mol Genetics 1997; 6:1091–1098.

85. Menasche G, Feldmann J, Fischer A, et al. Primary hemophagocytic syndromes point to a direct link between lymphocyte cytotoxicity and homeostasis. Immunol Rev 2005; 203:165–179.

86. Henter JI, Horne A, Arico M, et al. HLH-2004: Diagnostic and therapeutic guidelines for hemophagocytic lymphohistiocytosis. Pediatr Blood Cancer 2006; 48:124–131.

87. zur Stadt U, Schmidt S, Kasper B, et al. Linkage of familial hemophagocytic lymphohistiocytosis (FHL) type-4 to chromosome 6q24 and identification of mutations in syntaxin11. Hum Mol Genet 2005; 14:827–834.

88. Stepp SE, Dufourcq-Lagelouse R, Le Deist F, et al. Perforin gene defects in familial hemophagocytic lymphohistiocytosis. Science 1999; 286:1957–1959.

89. Crowley CA, Curnutte JT, Rosin RE, et al. An inherited abnormality of neutrophil adhesion: its genetic transmission and its association with a missing protein. N Engl J Med 1980; 302:1163–1168.

90. Inwald D, Davies EG, Klein NJ. Demystified... adhesion molecule deficiencies. Mol Pathol 2001; 54:1–7.

91. Etzioni A, Frydman M, Pollack S, et al. Recurrent severe infections caused by a novel leukocyte adhesion deficiency. N Engl J Med 1992; 327:1789–1792.

92. Mansouri D, Adimi P, Mirsaeidi M, et al. Inherited disorders of the IL-12-IFN-gamma axis in patients with disseminated BCG infection. Eur J Pediatr 2005; 164:753–757.

93. Buckley RH. The hyper-IgE syndrome. Clin Rev Allergy Immunol 2001; 20:139–154.

94. Grimbacher B, Holland SM, Gallin JI, et al. Hyper-IgE syndrome with recurrent infections – an autosomal dominant multisystem disorder. N Engl Med 1999; 340:692–702.

95. Grimbacher B, Holland SM, Puck JM. Hyper-IgE syndromes. Immunol Rev 2005; 203:244–250.

96. Renner ED, Puck JM, Holland SM, et al. Autosomal recessive hyperimmunoglobulin E syndrome: a distinct disease entity. J Pediatr 2004; 144:93–99.

97. Gennery AR, Flood TJ, Abinun M, et al. Bone marrow transplantation does not correct the hyper IgE syndrome. Bone Marrow Transplant 2000; 25:1303–1305.

98. Doffinger R, Smahi A, Bessia C, et al. X-linked anhidrotic ectodermal dysplasia with immunodeficiency is caused by impaired NF-kappaB signalling. Nat Genet 2001; 27:277–285.

99. Bowness P, Davies KA, Norsworthy PJ, et al. Hereditary C1q deficiency and systemic lupus erythematosus. Q J Med 1994; 87:455–464.

100. Fijen CAP, Kuijper EJ, Bulte MT, et al. Assessment of complement deficiency in patients with meningococcal disease in the Netherlands. Clin Infect Dis 1999; 28:98–105.

101. Tedesco F, Nürnberger W, Perissutti S. Inherited deficiencies of the terminal complement components. Int Rev Immunol 1993; 10:51–64.

102. Hoare S, El-Shazali O, Clark JE, et al. Investigation for complement deficiency following meningococcal disease. Arch Dis Child 2002; 86:215–217.

103. Thiel S, Frederiksen PD, Jensenius JC. Clinical manifestations of mannan-binding lectin deficiency. Mol Immunol 2006; 43:86–96.

104. Madsen HO, Garred P, Thiel S, et al. Interplay between promotor and structural gene variants control basal serum level of mannan-binding protein. J Immunol 1995; 155:3013–3020.

105. Davies EJ, Snowden H, Hillarby MC, et al. Mannose binding gene polymorphisms in systemic lupus erythematosus. Arthritis Rheum 1995; 38:110–114.

106. Lamelin J-P, Lenoir GM. Immunodeficiency secondary to viral infection. In: Chandra RK, ed. Primary and secondary immunodeficiency disorders. Edinburgh: Churchill Livingstone; 1983.204–218.

107. Ilan Y, Shouval D, Ashur Y, et al. IgA deficiency associated with chronic hepatitis C virus infection. Arch Intern Med 1993; 153:1588–1592.

108. Mukwaya G. Immunosuppressive effects and infections associated with corticosteroid therapy. Pediatr Infect Dis J 1988; 7:499–504.

109. Chandra RK. Nutrition and the immune system: an introduction. Am J Clin Nutr 1997; 66:460S–463S.

110. Skinner R, Cant A, Davies G, et al. Immunisation of the immunocompromised child. Best Practice Statement. London: Royal College of Paediatrics and Child Health; 2002.

111. Spickett GP, Bullimore J, Wallis J, et al. Northern Region asplenia register – analysis of first two years. J Clin Pathol 1999; 52:424–429.

112. Cavill I, for the Working Party of the British Committee for Standards in Haematology Clinical Haematology Task Force. Guidelines for the prevention and treatment of infection in patients with an absent or dysfunctional spleen. BMJ 1996; 312:430–434.

113. Chapel HM. Safety and availability of immunoglobulin replacement therapy in relation to potentially transmissible agents. Clin Exp Immunol 1999; 118:(suppl):29–34.

114. Misbah SA, Chapel HM. Adverse effects of intravenous immunoglobulin. Drug Saf 1993; 9:254–262.

115. Markert ML, Alexieff MJ, Li J, et al. Postnatal thymus transplantation with immunosuppression as treatment for DiGeorge syndrome. Blood 2004; 104:2574–2581.

116. Antoine C, Muller S, Cant A, et al. European Group for Blood and Marrow Transplantation; European Society for Immunodeficiency. Long-term survival and transplantation of haemopoietic stem cells for immunodeficiencies: report of the European experience 1968–99. Lancet 2003; 361:553–560.

117. Bertrand Y, Landais P, Friedrich W, et al. Influence of severe combined immunodeficiency phenotype on the outcome of HLA non-identical, T-cell-depleted bone marrow transplantation. J Pediatr 1999; 134:740–748.

118. Buckley RH, Schiff SE, Schiff RI, et al. Hematopoietic stem-cell transplantation for the treatment of severe combined immunodeficiency. N Engl J Med 1999; 340:508–516.

119. Rao K, Amrolia PJ, Jones A, et al. Improved survival after unrelated donor bone marrow transplantation in children with primary immuno-deficiency using a reduced-intensity conditioning regimen. Blood 2005; 105:879–885.

120. Gennery AR, Dickinson AM, Brigham K, et al. CAMPATH-1M T-cell depleted BMT for SCID: long-term follow-up of 19 children treated 1987–98 in a single centre. Cytotherapy 2001; 3:221–232.

121. Kane LC, Gennery AR, Crooks BNA, et al. Neonatal bone marrow transplantation for severe combined immunodeficiency. Arch Dis Child (Fetal Neonatal Ed) 2001; 85:F110–F113.

122. Bhattacharya A, Slatter MA, Chapman CE, et al. Single centre experience of umbilical cord stem cell transplantation for primary immunodeficiency. Bone Marrow Transplant 2005; 36:295–299.

123. Cunningham-Rundles C, Kazbay K, Zhou Z, et al. Immunologic effects of low-dose polyethylene glycol-conjugated recombinant human interleukin-2 in common variable immunodeficiency. J Interferon Cytokine Res 1995; 15:269–276.

124. Aiuti A, Slavin S, Aker M, et al. Correction of ADA-SCID by stem cell gene therapy combined with nonmyeloablative conditioning. Science 2002; 296:2410–2413.

125. Cavazzana-Calvo M, Hacein-Bey S, de Saint Basile G, et al. Gene therapy of human severe combined immunodeficiency (SCID)-xl disease. Science 2000; 288:669–672.

126. Hacein-Bey-Abina S, Von Kalle C, Schmidt M, et al. LMO2-associated clonal T cell proliferation in two patients after gene therapy for SCID-X1. Science 2003; 302:415–419.

28

Infections

Edited by David Isaacs, Kim Mulholland

MORTALITY AND MORBIDITY IN INFECTIOUS DISEASE

THE GLOBAL PERSPECTIVE

Worldwide, infections are responsible for the majority of deaths and loss of good health in children. In 2005, infectious diseases were estimated to have caused about 6.7 million of a total of 10.1 million deaths among the estimated global child population of under-5-year-olds of 616.2 million.[1,2] These deaths occurred disproportionately in resource limited countries, where it is also estimated that five groups of infections caused the death of more than 7 million children: acute respiratory infections (ARIs); diarrheal diseases; congenital infections including human immunodeficiency virus (HIV) and hepatitis B; malaria; and vaccine-preventable diseases including measles.[1,2] Although there has been improvement worldwide in the all cause under-5 child mortality rate from 1990 to 2005 (from 95 to 76 per thousand) there is little reason to believe the proportion of deaths attributable to infection has changed much over this time, except that the numbers of children dying as a result of HIV have considerably increased.[2,3] This and other factors means that there has been far less improvement in under-5 mortality in sub-Saharan Africa where the decline between 1990 and 2005 has been only from 188 to 169 per thousand. Indeed there are countries most heavily affected by HIV such as Botswana and South Africa where HIV has reversed previous trends with the estimated under-5 mortality rising from 58 to 120 per thousand and 60 to 68 per thousand respectively.[2] The relationship between infection, malnutrition and socially determined factors such as wars and orphanhood is subtle but important, as poor nutrition, poverty and social dislocation greatly multiply the impact of infections. To a considerable extent this explains why infections are so much more important as a cause of death and disability in resource limited compared to resource rich countries.[4] The rising incidence of HIV infection in resource limited countries has added another multiplier and these relations are shown schematically in Figure 28.1, contrasting sub-Saharan Africa with South Asia in the early years of the new millenium.[2,3]

Malnutrition underlies a substantial proportion of the deaths from diarrheal diseases, respiratory infections, measles and malaria, while HIV is of particular importance in sub-Saharan Africa and some parts of Asia.[2,3] In contrast, in Western Europe and other resource rich countries, malnutrition plays little role as a cofactor for the effects of infection, except in children with serious constitutional diseases such as malignancies or congenital immunodeficiencies. However, a growing population of immunocompromised children (very low birth weight babies, children with congenital immunodeficiencies or HIV infection and children on powerful immunocompromising therapies) represents an increasingly important source of deaths due to infections, often with organisms that are usually innocuous for immunocompetent children. It has been estimated that infections are responsible for around 17% (37 000) of 214 000 deaths under 5 years old that take place among 78 million children annually in resource rich countries.[1,2] Proportionately, the burden of infections is far higher in primary care. In England and Wales, infectious diseases are responsible for 40% of all new episodes of illness presenting to general practitioners with annual rates of around 730 episodes per 1000 population. Rates are even higher for infants (children before their first birthday).[5] Mortality statistics and data on acute consultations need to be supplemented by estimates of the burden of disability (morbidity) and to allow for the varying implications of the disability or death of an individual at different ages. This can be done by use of a measure such as disability adjusted life years (DALYs).[1,6] Combining estimates of chronic disability and mortality statistics, this measure calculates the likely numbers of healthy years of life lost because of specific diseases and conditions and, by 'weighting', an allowance is made for the different significance of ill-health and mortality among infants, elderly persons and adults providing for dependants. Estimates of the burden of disease experienced (Table 28.1 and Figure 28.1)[1] further emphasize the importance of infectious disease in resource limited

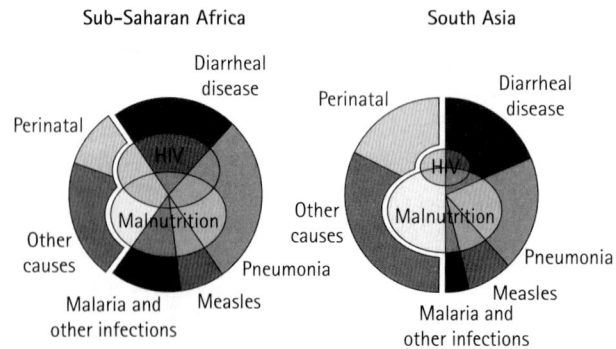

Fig. 28.1 Principal causes of death in children under age 5, sub-Saharan Africa and South Asia, circa 2000.

Table 28.1 Estimated distribution of burden of disease (combined mortality and chronic morbidity) in children in resource limited countries – 1990. (Source World Bank 1993[1])

	Total DALYs lost (million)	
	Age under 5 years	Age 5–14 years
Perinatal conditions	13.5	Nil
Communicable disease	63.3	33.9
Congenital STDs (HIV and syphilis)	(2.0%)	(4.0%)
Diarrheal diseases	(32%)	(15%)
Tuberculosis	(1.0%)	(11%)
Other vaccine-preventable disease	(20%)	(18%)
Malaria	(8%)	(9%)
Intestinal helminths	Nil	(27%)
Respiratory infections	(35%)	(16%)
Noncommunicable disorder	20.8	16.9
Injuries	6.2	9.7
Total	103.8	60.5

countries and the particular contribution to mortality in children under age 5 played by respiratory disease, diarrheal disease, the five vaccine-preventable diseases (diphtheria, measles, pertussis, polio and tetanus), and in older children by tuberculosis and intestinal helminths.[1]

HIV AND AIDS

Since the 1990s there has been an inexorable rise in the global importance of HIV. In 2006, the United Nations AIDS program and WHO estimated that 39.5 million persons worldwide were infected with HIV, of whom 2.3 million were children under the age of 15, and 530 000 children became infected with HIV.[2,3] The majority of childhood infections occur through mother-to-child transmission, with a smaller number from unscreened blood transfusions in resource limited settings. The distribution of deaths varies dramatically by global region, with the highest numbers and rates in sub-Saharan Africa where the rates have reversed previous improving trends in child mortality rates (Figs. 28.2 and 28.3). HIV rarely kills children directly, but by lowering the child's immunocompetence it leaves the infected child increasingly vulnerable to other infections. In addition, HIV infection affects children by making them lose their parents to HIV prematurely and it is estimated that 15.2 million children (under age 18) were living having lost one or more parents to HIV.[3] Since the appreciation that the risk of mother-to-child transmission of HIV infection can be reduced to under 2%, screening for HIV infection has resulted in a fall in early AIDS cases in France, Italy, Spain and the UK, the countries most affected in Western Europe (Fig. 28.4).[7] The fall in early pediatric AIDS has taken place despite rising levels of HIV infection in mothers in the UK, notably in London, but also in the rest of the UK (Fig. 28.5).[8]

THE UK

Infections remain an important cause of death in UK children. Conventional death registration data indicate that in 2005 infections (including infections of the central nervous and respiratory systems) were the main cause of death in 127 children in England and Wales (Table 28.2). The figure rises to 199 if sudden infant death syndrome is included. This represents a considerable change over time. In 1995 there were 193 deaths where infections were the main cause, with the figure including SIDS being 537.

Recent trends in a number of important infections in the UK are shown in Figures 28.4–28.14. Trends in vertically acquired HIV

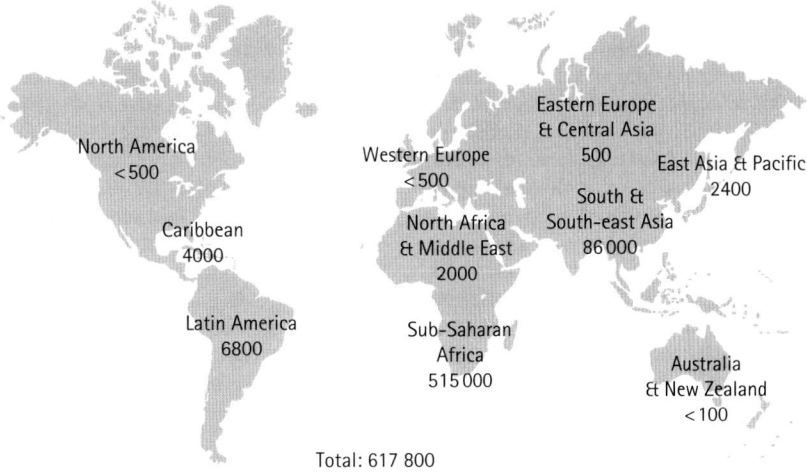

Fig. 28.2   New HIV infections in children globally and by region in 2001.
Source: Joint United Nations Programme on HIV–AIDS (UNAIDS).

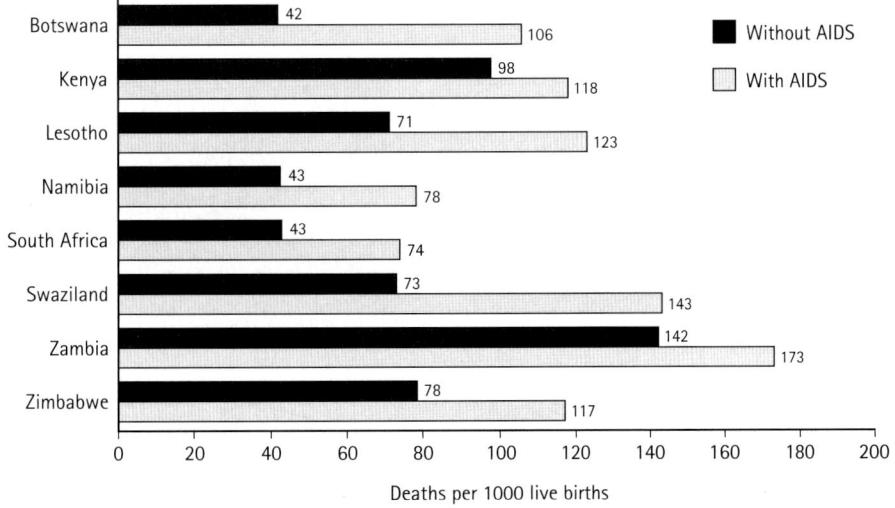

Sources: UNICEF (2005); United Nations Population Division, World Population Prospects: The 2004 Revision, database

Fig. 28.3   Estimated impact of HIV and AIDS on under-5 mortality rates 2002–2005.
Source: Joint United Nations Programme on HIV–AIDS (UNAIDS).

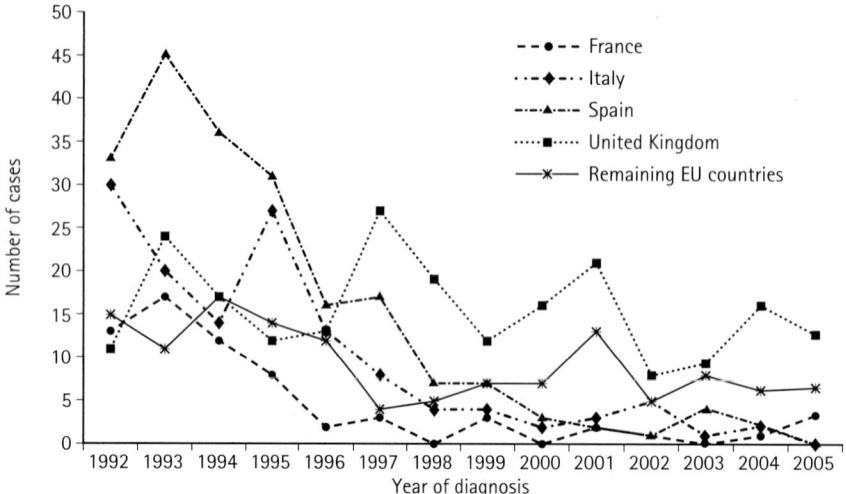

Fig. 28.4   Mother-to-child HIV transmission in European countries. AIDS cases in children aged less than 1 year at diagnosis. 2002–2005.
Source: EuroHIV European Centre for the Epidemiological Monitoring of AIDS.

infection (Figs 28.4 and 28.5) have already been mentioned.[7,8] The introduction of immunization against *Haemophilus influenzae* type b (Hib) in 1992 led to a dramatic decline in invasive infections attributed to this organism (Fig. 28.6). However, a booster dose of Hib was added when it became clear that primary immunization alone was insufficient and numbers began to rise again after 2000 (Fig. 28.6).[9] There has been heightened awareness of meningococcal infections as the most important single cause of septicemic and meningitic infections in immunocompetent children. The introduction of a conjugate vaccine against type C meningococcal infections has resulted in a fall in cases attributed to this infection in the earliest targeted groups, the under-1-year-olds and teenagers (Fig. 28.7).[10] Immunization was highly effective in reducing the incidence of measles in the 1970s (Fig. 28.8). However, measles vaccination coverage is incomplete. Sero-epidemiological investigations in England in the early 1990s indicated a growing number of susceptible (antibody negative) older children and hence an increasing risk of a substantial measles epidemic in school age children, with its inevitable morbidity and mortality, and more recently there have been significant

outbreaks.[11,12] To pre-empt further larger epidemics a UK-wide initiative immunized 8 million schoolchildren (90% of those eligible) in 1994. Transmission of indigenous measles was almost entirely interrupted and confirmed notifications fell dramatically. Hence the risk of an epidemic was averted, at least temporarily.[12] Subsequent declines in measles, mumps and rubella (MMR) vaccination following unwarranted parental concern over the safety of vaccine left more children underprotected (Fig. 28.9) and substantial outbreaks of measles followed in the late 1990s and early 2000s.[13,14] Trends in whooping cough (pertussis) in the late 1980s and early 1990s, following the collapse of professional and public confidence in pertussis vaccine, had provided earlier evidence of what can happen if myths about immunization are allowed to prevail over science (Fig. 28.10).[15,16] The rate of diphtheria and poliomyelitis declined dramatically in the UK following the introduction of immunization in the 1940s and 1950s rather as it did for *Haemophilus* in the 1990s. In contrast, control of another illness for which there is a vaccine, tuberculosis,[17] has been less successful with an overall rise in notifications in the 1990s, which particularly reflects trends in London

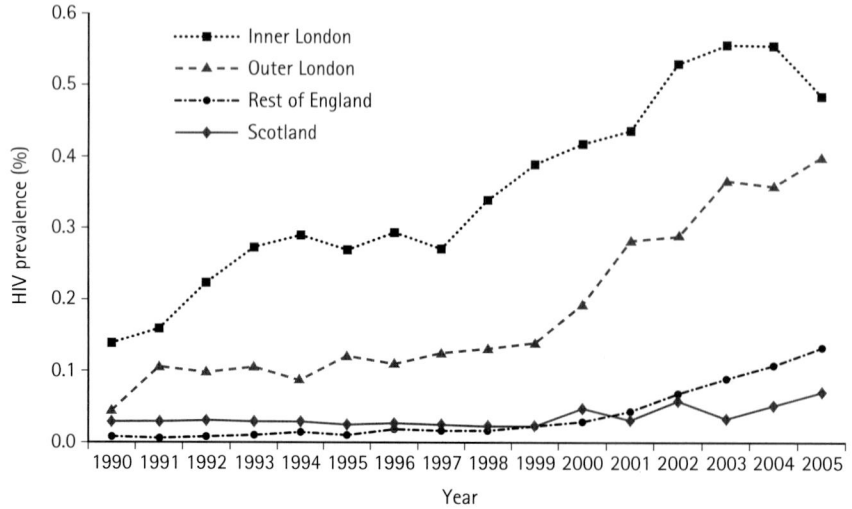

Fig. 28.5   Trends in prevalence of HIV infection in pregnant women in the UK by area of residence 1990–2005.
Source: UK Unlinked Anonymous HIV Monitoring Programme – Health Protection Agency, University College London Institute of Child Health, Health Protection, Scotland.

Table 28.2 Deaths due to infections in children aged 14 years and under; England and Wales 1990–2005. (Source of original data: Office of National Statistics)

ICD-9 code	ICD-10 code		1990	1991	1992	1993	1994	1995	1996	1997
001–009	A00–A09	Intestinal infectious disease	18	20	12	23	22	28	17	35
036	A39	Meningococcal infection	108	110	87	102	85	107	112	100
038	A40–A41	Septicemia	24	21	26	28	33	50	44	39
030–041*	A30–A49*	Other bacterial infection*	13	10	10	12	9	9	11	8
042–044	B20–B24	HIV	0	0	0	6	8	4	11	5
052	B01	Chickenpox	3	5	3	6	3	2	7	2
055	B05	Measles	1	0	1	0	0	0	0	0
042–079*	A80–B34	Other viral diseases*	31	24	16	24	27	26	22	23
001–139	A00–B99	All infectious and parasitic disease	212	199	170	227	203	250	240	230
320–322	G00–G03	Meningitis	52	59	53	49	19	28	32	36
323	G04–G05	Encephalitis	9	8	3	4	10	7	2	8
466–469	J20–J22	Acute bronchitis and bronchiolitis	59	65	31	44	38	27	34	34
480–486	J10–J18	Pneumonia	135	127	83	137	124	104	115	129
487	J10–J11	Influenza	4	3	0	2	2	4	2	2
798–799	R95–R99	SIDS	1090	927	466	431	421	371	394	384
All cause mortality		All cause	4491	4264	3495	3386	3167	3023	2973	2970
Population	Population denominator		9 529 400	9 659 000	9 777 400	9 866 500	9 913 900	9 921 300	9 921 800	9 956 900

ICD-9 code	ICD-10 code		1998	1999	2000	2001	2002	2003	2004	2005
001–009	A00–A09	Intestinal infectious disease	44	45	40	4	3	3	7	10
036	A39	Meningococcal infection	86	84	69	85	49	59	33	46
038	A40–A41	Septicemia	38	48	46	20	19	23	27	16
030–041*	A30–A49*	Other bacterial infection*	16	18	8	42	40	27	44	31
042–044	B20–B24	HIV	5	1	1	8	2	4	3	1
052	B01	Chickenpox	6	3	2	2	1	2	7	2
055	B05	Measles	0	1	0	0	1	0	0	0
042–079*	A80–B34	Other viral diseases*	23	15	20	16	18	31	20	17
001–139	A00–B99	All infectious and parasitic disease	232	238	201	187	144	155	150	135
320–322	G00–G03	Meningitis	43	35	35	32	29	40	29	29
323	G04–G05	Encephalitis	7	5	1	2	7	5	11	6
466–469	J20–J22	Acute bronchitis and bronchiolitis	34	32	22	33	19	16	24	14
480–486	J10–J18	Pneumonia	125	122	87	63	69	73	53	73
487	J10–J11	Influenza	6	8	3	5	5	16	1	15
798–799	R95–R99	SIDS	310	300	271	95	81	101	104	95
All cause mortality		All cause	2826	2767	2495	2523	2377	2407	2248	2242
Population	Population denominator		9 970 100	9 972 500	9 905 500	9 970 100	9 972 500	9 685 352	9 637 426	9 589 141

*Contains other totals not shown above.

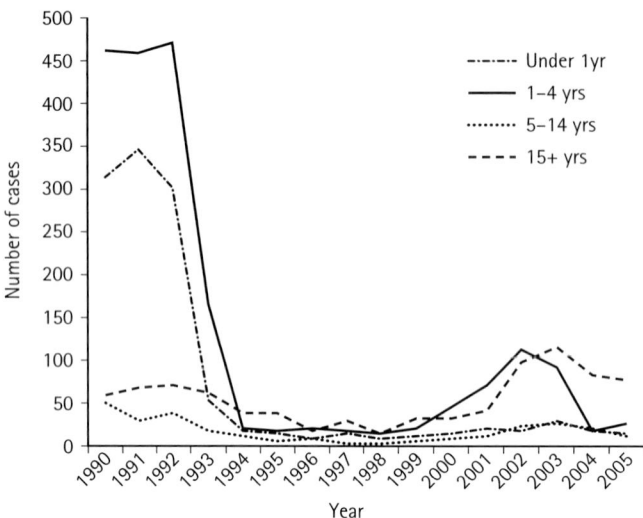

Fig. 28.6 Invasive Hib infections by age group, 1990–2005. Supplied by the Health Protection Agency Centre for Infections and relying on laboratory reporting, reporting by clinicians, genitourinary medicine (GUM) clinic returns (KC60) (gonorrhea), tuberculosis notifications, COVER Vaccination coverage statistics, reports through the Royal College of General Practitioners Research Unit (influenza).

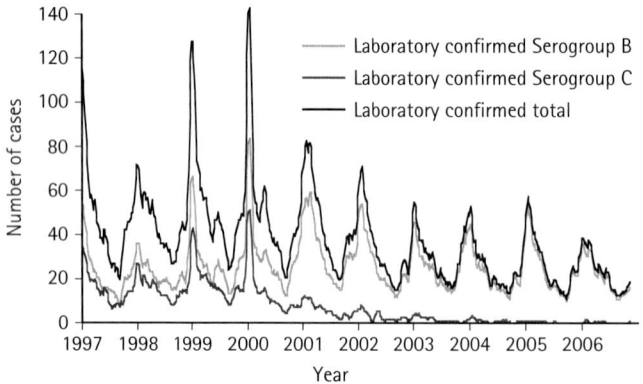

Fig. 28.7 Laboratory confirmed cases of meningococcal disease. England & Wales Five Weekly Moving Averages: 1997–2006. Supplied by the Health Protection Agency Centre for Infections and relying on laboratory reporting, reporting by clinicians, genitourinary medicine (GUM) clinic returns (KC60) (gonorrhea), tuberculosis notifications, COVER Vaccination coverage statistics, reports through the Royal College of General Practitioners Research Unit (influenza).

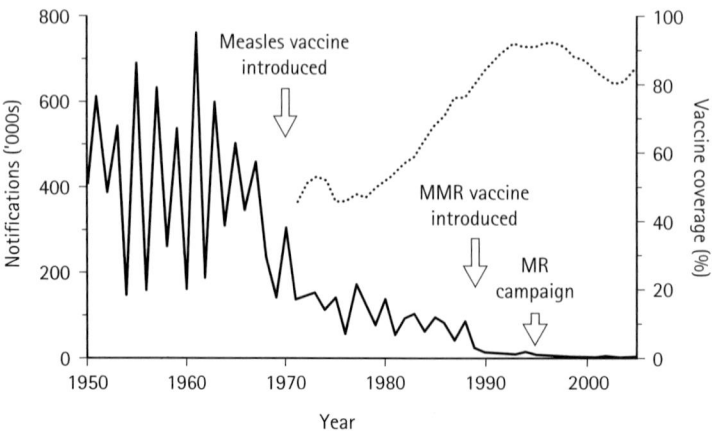

Fig. 28.8 Annual measles notification and vaccine coverage in England and Wales 1950–2005. Supplied by the Health Protection Agency Centre for Infections and relying on laboratory reporting, reporting by clinicians, genitourinary medicine (GUM) clinic returns (KC60) (gonorrhea), tuberculosis notifications, COVER Vaccination coverage statistics, reports through the Royal College of General Practitioners Research Unit (influenza).

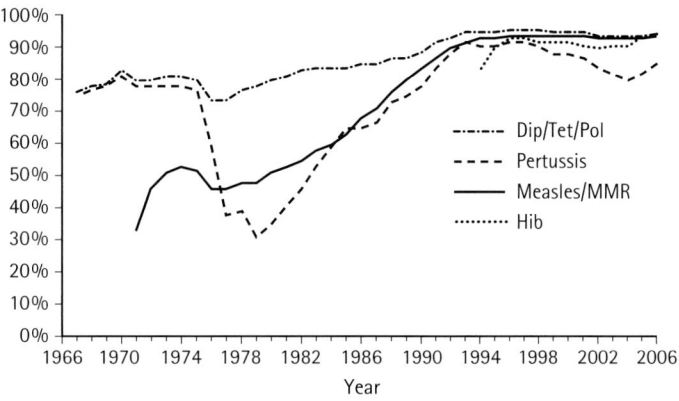

Fig. 28.9   Two year vaccine coverage in England and Wales 1966–2005/6. Supplied by the Health Protection Agency Centre for Infections and relying on laboratory reporting, reporting by clinicians, genitourinary medicine (GUM) clinic returns (KC60) (gonorrhea), tuberculosis notifications, COVER Vaccination coverage statistics, reports through the Royal College of General Practitioners Research Unit (influenza).

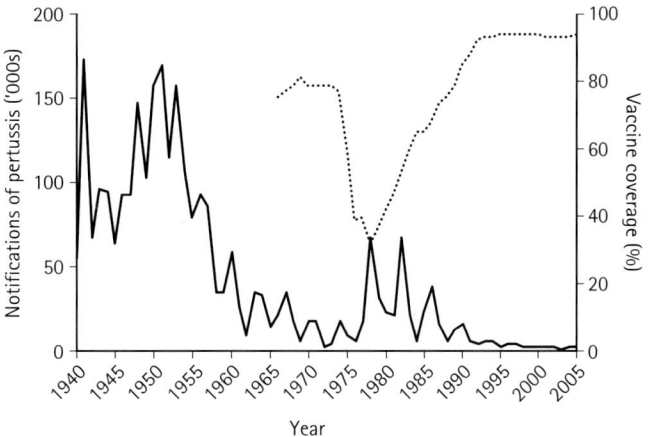

Fig. 28.10   Whooping cough cases and vaccine coverage in England and Wales 1940–2005. Supplied by the Health Protection Agency Centre for Infections and relying on laboratory reporting, reporting by clinicians, genitourinary medicine (GUM) clinic returns (KC60) (gonorrhea), tuberculosis notifications, COVER Vaccination coverage statistics, reports through the Royal College of General Practitioners Research Unit (influenza).

and imported cases (Fig. 28.11). Influenza epidemics occur every winter though they vary in their severity and the proportion of infections that occur among children (Fig. 28.12). Food poisoning has become the commonest notifiable infection in children. Sharply increasing trends in notified numbers of cases of food poisoning in the 1980s and 1990s were mirrored by trends in national laboratory reporting of salmonellosis. Since 1997, however, salmonella reports have declined while reports of *Campylobacter* spp. have risen (Fig. 28.13). Though numbers are far less than for campylobacter or salmonella, the emergence of *Escherichia coli* O157 since the 1980s is of concern because of the severe disease and specific renal pathology that often follows this infection. Not all countries see this subtype of verocytotoxigenic *E. coli* (VTEC): in Australia for example the predominant subtype is *E. coli* O111.[18]

Sexually transmitted diseases are now appreciated to be a substantial problem among adolescents in the UK. Rates of gonorrhea rose by over 50% between 1995 and 2000 (Fig. 28.14) with the highest percentage rise among adolescents.[19] The highest incidences of gonorrhea and chlamydia seen among genitourinary medicine clinic attenders are in females aged 16–19 years.[8,19] After intensive campaigns the rates of gonorrhea are now declining.[8] Chlamydia is the more important, because of its widespread distribution and serious sequelae of pelvic inflammatory disease, infertility and ectopic pregnancies. It is clear that the chlamydia infections seen in genitourinary medicine clinics are only

a fraction of those prevalent in the teenage population and campaigns in the UK are now aiming to control this infection through opportunistic screening in primary care.[20]

General practitioner (GP) reporting provides the least-selected surveillance data in the UK on the nature and burden of infectious disease in children in the community, particularly on conditions such as chickenpox or influenza that are unlikely to be investigated microbiologically or to lead to hospital admission. These data show that respiratory tract infections (mainly upper tract infections) account for over 80% of new GP consultations for infectious diseases in children.[5]

EMERGING AND RE-EMERGING INFECTIONS

In the 1960s and 1970s it was often stated that improving social conditions and medical treatments were leading to a relentless decline in the importance of infectious diseases. Emerging and re-emerging infections such as HIV and tuberculosis (Figs. 28.1 and 28.11), high profile nosocomial outbreaks of legionnaires' disease and food poisoning in the UK, and most recently the appearance of severe acute respiratory syndrome (SARS) and highly pathogenic avian influenza (H5N1) have changed medical opinion. In addition, the deliberate release of organisms such as anthrax in the USA has brought a new threat to health from infections.[21] It is now realized that infections remain important threats to the health

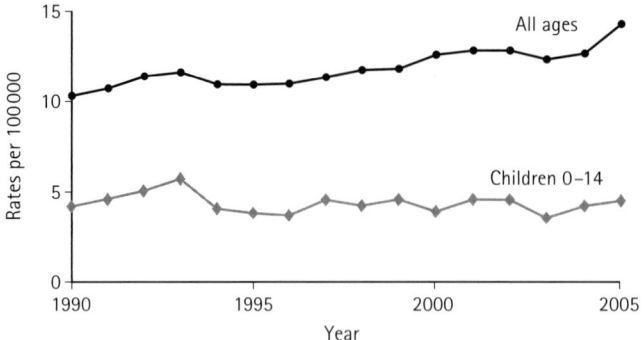

Fig. 28.11 Tuberculosis notification rates per 100 000 population in England and Wales 1993–2005. Supplied by the Health Protection Agency Centre for Infections and relying on laboratory reporting, reporting by clinicians, genitourinary medicine (GUM) clinic returns (KC60) (gonorrhea), tuberculosis notifications, COVER Vaccination coverage statistics, reports through the Royal College of General Practitioners Research Unit (influenza).

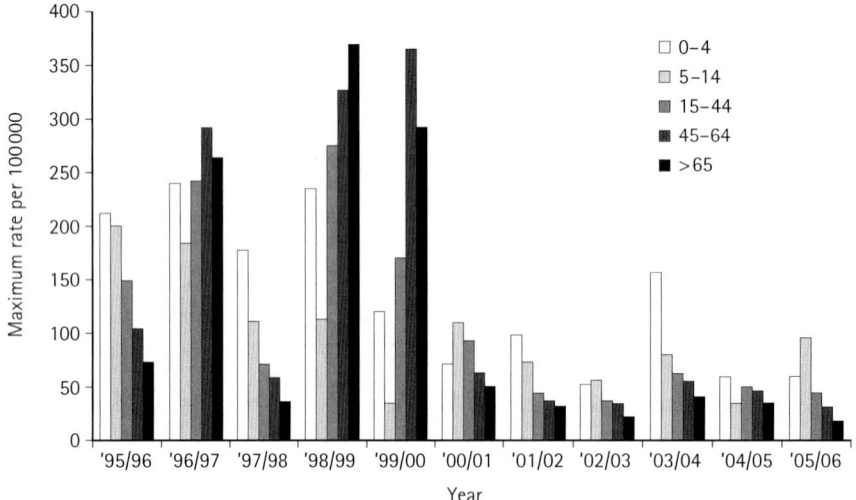

Fig. 28.12 Rates of influenza reports 1990–2006 by age group (RCGP). Supplied by the Health Protection Agency Centre for Infections and relying on laboratory reporting, reporting by clinicians, genitourinary medicine (GUM) clinic returns (KC60) (gonorrhea), tuberculosis notifications, COVER Vaccination coverage statistics, reports through the Royal College of General Practitioners Research Unit (influenza).

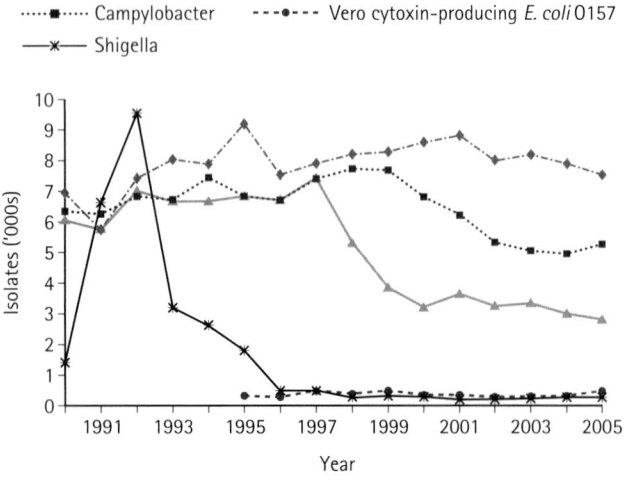

Fig. 28.13 Laboratory reporting of selected gastrointestinal pathogens in England and Wales 1977–2005. Supplied by the Health Protection Agency Centre for Infections and relying on laboratory reporting, reporting by clinicians, genitourinary medicine (GUM) clinic returns (KC60) (gonorrhea), tuberculosis notifications, COVER Vaccination coverage statistics, reports through the Royal College of General Practitioners Research Unit (influenza).

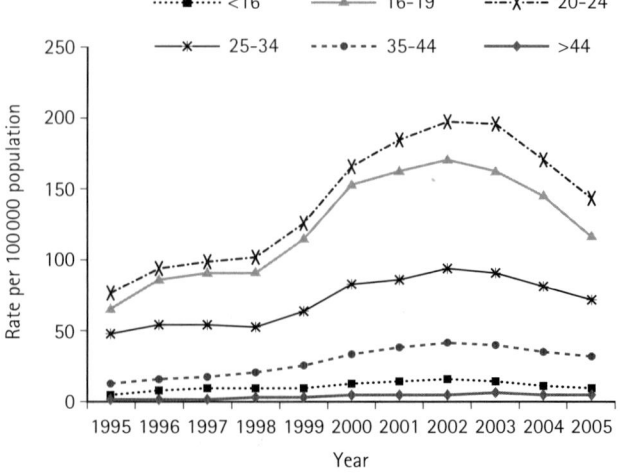

Fig. 28.14 Rates of uncomplicated gonorrhea seen in genitourinary medicine clinics by age group in the UK 1995–2005.

of children and adults in every country. Following a lead from the United States Centers for Disease Control and Prevention (CDC), in 1995 the World Health Organization established a Division of Emerging Viral and Bacterial Disease Surveillance and Control (www.who.int/emc/index.html). Some countries and regional bodies (for example the European Union and WHO's Western Pacific Region) have been establishing or strengthening infrastructures to detect and respond to emerging or re-emerging infections and in 2005 the International Health Regulations were radically revised so that they would detect any new threat. The new regulations require all governments to strengthen surveillance and to report any potential previous public health emergency of international concern (the previous regulations only required countries to report cases of cholera, plague and yellow fever).[22] Some emerging infections are new or involve newly recognized pathogens (Table 28.3),[23] examples being human herpesvirus types 6 and 7, variant Creutzfeldt–Jakob disease, and *Clostridium difficile* O27.[24] Other infections derive from animal infections that have only latterly come to affect humans, such as HIV, Lassa fever, avian influenza virus type A/H5N1 and SARS. Yet a third group is established infections whose incidence, pathogenicity or antimicrobial resistance has recently increased, for example dengue fever, methicillin resistant *Staphylococcus aureus* infection (MRSA) and tuberculosis (both drug susceptible and multiply resistant *Mycobacterium tuberculosis*).

Table 28.3 New and emerging infections – new and newly recognized agents identified since 1973. (Source: European Centre for Disease Prevention and Control)

Year of report	Agent	Disease
1973	Rotavirus	Major cause of infantile diarrhea worldwide
1975	Parvovirus B19	Fifth disease; aplastic crisis in hemolytic anemia
1976	*Cryptosporidium parvum*	Acute enterocolitis
1977	Ebola virus	Ebola hemorrhagic fever
1977	*Legionella pneumophila*	Legionnaires' disease
1977	Hantaan virus	Hemorrhagic fever with renal syndrome (HFRS)
1977	*Campylobacter* sp.	Enteric pathogens distributed globally
1980	Human T cell lymphotropic virus-I (HTLV I)	T cell lymphoma leukemia
1981	*Staphylococcus* toxin	Toxic shock syndrome associated with tampon use
1982	*Escherichia coli* O157:H7	Hemorrhagic colitis; hemolytic uremic syndrome
1982	HTLV II	Hairy cell leukemia
1982	*Borrelia burgdorferi*	Lyme disease
1983	HIV	HIV disease including AIDS
1983	*Helicobacter pylori*	Peptic ulcers
1988	Human herpesvirus-6 (HHV-6)	Roseola infantum and encephalitis
1989	*Ehrlichia chaffeensis*	Human ehrlichiosis
1989	Hepatitis C	Parenterally transmitted non-A, non-B hepatitis
1990	Human herpesvirus-7 (HHV-7)	Roseola infantum and encephalitis
1991	Guanarito virus	Venezuelan hemorrhagic fever
1992	*Vibrio cholerae* O139	New strain associated with epidemic cholera
1992	*Bartonella* (=*Rochalimaea*) *henselae*	Cat-scratch disease; bacillary angiomatosis
1993	Sin nombre hantavirus	Hantavirus pulmonary syndrome
1994	Sabiá virus	Brazilian hemorrhagic fever
1994	Hendra virus infection	Severe respiratory illness, neurologic syndrome
1995	Human herpesvirus-8 (HHV-8)	Kaposi sarcoma
1997	Bovine spongiform encephalopathy (BSE) agent (a prion)	New variant Creutzfeldt–Jakob disease
1997	Influenza A, H5N1	Severe respiratory illness
1999	Nipah virus, West Nile virus in USA	West Nile fever, meningitis, encephalitis, acute flaccid paralysis
2001	Human metapneumovirus (hMPV)	From asymptomatic infection to severe bronchiolitis
2003	SARS coronavirus (SARS CoV)	Severe acute respiratory syndrome (SARS)
2003 (USA)	Monkeypox virus (previously seen in Africa from 1970s)	Similar to smallpox, but usually milder
2004	Simian foamy retroviruses	No evidence of pathology
2005	Human retroviruses, HTLV3 and HTLV4	Immunodeficiency?
Islands in the Indian Ocean 2006	Chikungunya virus (previously first described in Tanzania in 1956)	Joint pains which may or may not be accompanied by muscle pain, high fever, conjunctivitis, and a rash.
Past decade	Emergence of: multidrug resistant organisms (MDROs), including methicillin resistant *Staphylococcus aureus* (MRSA), vancomycin resistant enterococci (VRE) and certain Gram negative bacilli (GNB) including those producing extended spectrum beta-lactamases (ESBLs)	Sepsis, pneumonia, surgical infection, ventilator-associated pneumonia (VAP), etc.
	Clostridium difficile type O27	
	Extended spectrum drug resistant *M. tuberculosis* (XDR-Tb)	
	Drug resistant *Streptococcus pneumoniae* (DRSP)	Meningitis, pneumonia, sepsis

Of particular importance to children are HIV, diphtheria, pertussis, *E. coli* O157 causing hemolytic uremic syndrome (HUS) and avian influenza (A/H5N1), and sexually transmitted infections in adolescents.

The reasons for emergence and re-emergence are almost as varied as the organisms themselves (Table 28.4).[25] Failure of public health programs can be an important cause. Diphtheria reappeared in the 1990s as an epidemic in Russia because of a collapse in vaccine production and the emergence of mistaken reasons among the public and professionals for refusing immunization. A similar phenomenon affecting pertussis occurred in the UK in the 1970s and 1980s from the mistaken impression that the vaccine was more dangerous than the disease (see Fig. 28.10).[15,26] Both *E. coli* O157 and various salmonellas have been spread efficiently through industrialized production and distribution of foods.[27] An outbreak of HUS due to contaminated commercial hamburgers occurred in the USA in 1993[28] and in 1995 an outbreak of gastrointestinal disease in children due to *S. agoma* in north London was traced to defective production in a factory in Israel. Changes in behavior can result in disease emergence. International trends towards earlier menarche and sexual debut are causing younger females to be exposed to STDs with a consequent rise in pelvic inflammatory disease, ectopic pregnancy and secondary infertility.[20,29]

EFFECTIVE INTERVENTIONS

In 1990, at a World Summit for Children, government leaders including that of the UK committed their administrations to 27 goals to improve the health and lives of children. There have been some major achievements towards these goals and subsequent aspirational targets such as the Millenium Goals.[2] More than 60 countries have reached their national goals of reducing mortality rates of children < 5 years by a third or more. Polio has been eradicated in more than 175 countries and deaths from diarrheal illnesses have been more than halved.[2]

Interventions designed to prevent or treat infections may be assessed by measuring their resulting health gain as healthy years of life and comparing their costs relative to other interventions. Thus it is possible to come up with 'best buys' for countries, and this has been undertaken for resource limited countries by the World Bank using the 'DALY' measure.[1,6] Interventions targeted against acute respiratory infections, diarrheal disease, malaria and the six vaccine-preventable diseases represent four of the six top interventions for health gain in children under age 5, and five out of six of those targeted at children aged 5–14 years[30] (Tables 28.5 and 28.6). While new technologies and developments are necessary, greater health gains can come from the application of established interventions of proven effectiveness such as the early detection and treatment of acute respiratory infections, and the use of oral rehydration therapy (ORT) for gastrointestinal infections.[30] Immunization represents a success story. By 1990, the Expanded Program of Immunization (EPI) reached a goal of immunizing 80% of children in most countries with an estimated benefit of 3 million lives saved in 1995. A particular priority has been polio immunization. The EPI, supported by Rotary International, had, by 1995, eliminated wild polio from 145 countries, including all of the Americas.[30] However, the 80% target remains unachieved in sub-Saharan Africa where overall immunization rates are static and there have been outbreaks extending out of West Africa into

Table 28.4   Factors in infectious disease emergence and re-emergence relevant to child and adolescent health (Adapted from Morse 1995[25])

Factor	Example of specific factors	Examples of disease (more than one factor may be driving the emergence of an infection)
Ecological changes including: those due to economic development and land use, distribution of animal populations and climate changes	Agriculture: dams, changes in water ecosystems; deforestation/reforestation; flood/drought; famine; changes in animal distribution; climate changes	Schistosomiasis (dams); Rift Valley fever (dams, irrigation); Argentine hemorrhagic fever (agriculture); West Nile virus (bird movement), highly pathogenic avian influenza Hantaan–Korean hemorrhagic fever (agriculture); hantavirus pulmonary syndrome, southwestern US, 1993 (weather anomalies)
Human demographics, behavior	Societal changes and events: population growth and migration (movement from rural areas to cities); practices of keeping animals and contact with wild animals, war or civil conflict; urban decay; sexual behavior; intravenous drug use; preference for 'fast foods'; use of high-density facilities	Introduction of HIV; spread of dengue; spread of HIV and other sexually transmitted diseases, appearance of zoonoses [highly pathogenic avian influenza (H5N1), SARS (corona virus)], meningococcal disease, cholera, increases in food poisoning (*Salmonella enteritidis*)
International travel and commerce	Worldwide movement of goods and people; air travel	'Airport' malaria; dissemination of mosquito vectors; rat-borne hantavirusues; antibiotic-resistant gonorrhea; introduction of cholera into South America; dissemination of O139 *V. cholerae*
Technology and industry	Globalization of food supplies; changes in food processing and packaging; organ or tissue transplantation; drugs causing immunosuppression; widespread use of antibiotics	Hemolytic uremic syndrome (*E. coli* contamination of hamburger meat), *S. agoma* in kosher snacks; transfusion-associated hepatitis (hepatitis B, C), opportunistic infections in immunosuppressed patients, Creutzfeldt–Jakob disease from contaminated batches of human growth hormone (medical technology)
Microbial adaptation and change	Microbial evolution, response to selection in environment	Antibiotic-resistant bacteria (multiply resistant *M. tuberculosis*), 'antigenic drift' in influenza virus; zidovudine-resistant HIV
Breakdown in public health measures	Curtailment or reduction in prevention programs; inadequate sanitation and vector control measures, immunization myths	Whooping cough in the UK, resurgence of tuberculosis in the US; cholera in refugee camps in Africa; resurgence of diphtheria in the countries of the former Soviet Union

Table 28.5 Main cause of disease burden in children in demographically developing countries in 1990 and the cost-effectiveness of the interventions available for their control. (Adapted from Morse[25])

Disease and injuries	Number of DALYs lost* millions (% total)	Main intervention	Cost-effectiveness ($ per DALY)
Respiratory infections	98 (14.8)[†]	Integrated management of the sick child	30–100
Perinatal morbidity and mortality	96 (14.6)	a. Prenatal and delivery care	30–100
		b. Family planning	20–150
Diarrheal disease	92 (14.0)	Integrated management of the sick child	30–100
Childhood cluster (diseases preventable through immunization)	65 (10.0)	Expanded Program on Immunization (EPI) EPI-plus[†]	12–30
Congenital malformation	35 (5.4)	Surgical operations	High (unknown)
Malaria	31 (4.7)	Integrated management of the sick child	30–100
Intestinal helminths	17 (2.5)	School health program	20–34
Protein-energy malnutrition	12 (1.8)	Integrated management of the sick child	30–100
Vitamin A deficiency	12 (1.8)	EPI-plus[†]	12–30
Iodine deficiency	9 (1.4)	Iodine supplementation	19–37
Subtotal	467 (71.0)	–	–
Total DALYs lost	660 (100)	–	–

*DALYs lost (for specific diseases and the total) are taken from the 1993 World Development Report (World Bank 1993[1]).
[†]EPI-plus includes the six vaccines of the Expanded Program on Immunization (EPI), plus the vaccine against hepatitis B and vitamin A supplementation.

Table 28.6 The global balance sheet – child health 1990–2000. (Source WHO 2001[22])

Goal	Gains	Unfinished business
Infant and under-5 mortality (U5MR): reduction by one third in infant mortality and U5MR	More than 60 countries achieved the goal of U5MR At the global level, U5MR declined by 14%	U5MR rates increased in 14 countries (nine of them in sub-Saharan Africa) and were unchanged in 11 others Serious disparities remain in U5MR within countries: by income level, urban vs. rural, and among minority groups
Polio: *global eradication* by 2000	More than 175 countries are polio free	Polio is still endemic in 20 countries
Routine immunization: *maintenance of a high level of immunization coverage*	Sustained routine immunization coverage at 75% [three doses of combined diphtheria/pertussis/tetanus vaccine (DPT3)]	Less than 50% of children under 1 yr of age in sub-Saharan Africa are immunized against DPT3
Measles: *reduction by 95% in measles deaths and 90% in measles cases by 1995 as a major step in global eradication in the longer run*	Worldwide reported measles incidence has declined by nearly two thirds between 1990 and 1999	In more than 15 countries, measles vaccination coverage is less than 50%
Neonatal tetanus: *elimination* by 1995	104 of 161 resource limited countries have achieved the goal Deaths caused by neonatal tetanus declined by 50% between 1990 and 2000	27 countries (18 in Africa) account for 90% of all remaining neonatal tetanus
Deaths due to diarrhea: *reduce them by 50%*	This goal was achieved globally, according to World Health Organization (WHO) estimates	Diarrhea remains one of the major causes of death among children
Acute respiratory infections (ARIs): *reduction of ARI deaths by one third in children under 5*	ARI case management has improved at health center level The effectiveness of *Haemophilus influenzae* type b and pneumococcus vaccines is established	ARI remains one of the greatest causes of death among children Vertical, single-focus ARI programs seem to have had little global impact

other parts of Africa. Because of economic or social reasons there are at least some war-torn countries where polio elimination looks difficult or impossible. The infection is also proving hard to eradicate in India.[31,32] This makes the goal of global polio elimination, and its prize of release of resources currently committed to polio immunization, look difficult.[2]

SURVEILLANCE TO INFORM PUBLIC HEALTH ACTION

Given adequate resources and will, many infectious diseases can be prevented or contained, but eradication of all infection-related morbidity

and mortality is unachievable as many microorganisms have extensive animal and environmental reservoirs. Interventions can prevent infections or ameliorate the effects of disease. Knowledge as to which interventions are effective must be combined with timely surveillance data on the epidemiology of infection and susceptibility so as to allow rational decisions to be made on resource allocation for public health action. Equally, surveillance provides the basis for health protection, for example in detecting and directing action on deliberate release of biological agents.[21]

Data for surveillance of the commoner infectious diseases in the UK are derived from mortality statistics, disease notifications and laboratory reporting although in recent years enhanced surveillance to answer specific public health questions has become far more important (Table 28.7).[7-14,19,24,33] An infection may be made statutorily notifiable in the UK, either because there is a need for rapid information for effective local control or for the purpose of monitoring national immunization programs. Often taken for granted, these systems are among

Table 28.7 Infectious disease morbidity and mortality: principal sources of data in the UK

Data source	Collected by	Type of information
Mortality data	OPCS, GRS, DHSS	Death entries from medical practitioners
Statutory notifications	OPCS, LGAs, SHHD, DH	Currently (1995) list of 39 IDs; selected because need for rapid local information for control, or to monitor national immunization program; clinical diagnoses
Laboratory reports	CfI and HPA from routine and specialist laboratories	Wide range of microbiologically confirmed infections
General practitioners	Computerized reporting by GPs including the RCGP from weekly returns from 40 practices	Wide range of infectious diseases presenting in general practice; clinical diagnoses
NHS Direct	Daily outputs from NHS Direct systems	Wide range of infectious diseases presenting as syndromes through the NHS Direct centers
Computerized hospital discharge data	ONS and SHHD from individual hospitals and health boards	All diagnoses categorized by ICD code; combination of clinical and microbiological
Enhanced surveillance systems	From many sources to CfI, HPS, CDSC-PHS (Wales), CDSC NI	A wide variety of conditions answering specific questions: e.g. levels of MRSA in hospitals, rates of completion of treatment courses by those with tuberculosis, performance of antenatal screening for HIV
Consultant pediatricians	British Paediatric Surveillance Unit	Changing 'menu' of rare infections and infection-related disorders; specified case definitions
Consultant clinicians (genitourinary medicine)	HPA Centre for Infections	HIV and AIDS cases including detailed demographic data
Public health specialists	HPA Centre for Infections	Significant outbreaks and incidents

CDSC-PHS (Wales), Communicable Disease Surveillance Centre of the Public Health Service, Wales; CDSC NI, Communicable Disease Surveillance Centre (Northern Ireland); CfI, Health Protection Agency Centre for Infections; DH, Department of Health; DHSS, Department of Health and Social Security, Northern Ireland; GRS, General Registrar's Office for Scotland; HA, health authority; HB, health board; HPS, Health Protection Scotland; ID, infectious disease; LGA, local government authority; ONS, Office for National Statistics; OPCS, Office of Population Censuses and Surveys; PHLS, Public Health Laboratory Service; RCGP, Royal College of General Practitioners; SHHD Scottish Home and Health Department.

the best in the world. Routine reporting is supplemented by special or enhanced surveillance systems for rare and/or more important infections such as HIV and congenital rubella syndrome. An example of this is active reporting by clinicians through the British Paediatric Surveillance Unit (BPSU) of the Royal College of Paediatrics and Child Health (RCPCH), whereby researchers combine reports from RCPCH members with data from other systems to give optimal coverage.[33] Other innovative mechanisms are using primary care mechanisms through general practice or NHS Direct. Surveillance of infectious disease mortality and morbidity in England and Wales is undertaken by the Office for National Statistics (ONS) and by the Centre for Infections and Local and Regional Services of the Health Protection Agency (HPA) and the Public Health Service-Wales. In Scotland this function is performed by Health Protection Scotland though public health policy is coordinated by national departments of health and enacted by local specialists in public health medicine. In Wales it is performed by the Communicable Diseases Surveillance Centre (CDSC) of the Public Health Service Wales and in Northern Ireland by CDSC (Northern Ireland). The HPA and ONS collaborate closely to obtain, analyze and interpret data from several sources which often overlap, but which are also complementary allowing validation of reports (Table 28.7). From these national reporting centers data and information are routinely reported to the European Centre for Disease Prevention and Control and the World Health Organization. The legal basis of these reporting mechanisms is established under the European Union Legislation and the new (2005) International Health Regulations.[22,34]

ACKNOWLEDGMENTS

In the preparation of this section the assistance is gratefully acknowledged of a large number of colleagues in the European Centre for Disease Prevention and Control; the United Nations Special Program on AIDS; the European HIV Centre (EUROHIV) at INVS, Paris; the Office for National Statistics; the Registrar General's Office, Scotland; the Department of Health and Social Security, Northern Ireland; the Centre for Infections of the Health Protection Agency; the Royal College of General Practitioners Research Unit; Health Protection Scotland; the Communicable Disease Surveillance Centre of the Public Health Service, Wales; and the Communicable Disease Surveillance Centre (Northern Ireland).

CLINICAL PROBLEMS

THE CHILD WITH FEVER

The most useful temperature measurement is the core or central temperature which has a normal range in young adults of 36.4–36.9 °C, and fluctuation around these values of up to 0.4 °C. Infants have a rectal temperature above 37 °C which falls by about 0.8 °C during sleep and rises before waking.[35] There is a circadian rhythm in childhood with the highest temperature at 6 P.M. The peripheral temperature is normally 0.5 °C lower than that recorded centrally.[36] What is regarded as fever varies. Studies of infants define fever as a central temperature of greater than 38 °C. Antipyretic agents have the same effect on fever of either bacterial or viral origin and the response should not be used as a distinguishing feature. There are a number of different devices available for temperature measurement. Electronic probes are widely used in hospital for oral (central), axillary (peripheral) or rectal (central) sites. Tympanic membrane thermometers are moderately accurate providing they are inserted correctly but are not recommended in young infants. Other methods using strips or chemical dots are of variable accuracy. Mercury thermometers, sometimes regarded as the 'gold standard', are not recommended because of the risks from broken glass and the toxic effects of the metal.

Although a central temperature reading is of value in the sick child, and measurement of the temperature difference between core and periphery is of particular value in the shocked patient, for most purposes a peripheral reading is adequate.

The commonest cause of fever in childhood is viral infection, usually resolving within a week of onset. Persistence of fever demands thorough investigation; the term pyrexia or fever of unknown origin (PUO, FUO) is normally applied when fever has been present for 14 days.

FEVER IN THE NEWBORN

Fever during the neonatal period may be the presenting sign of bacterial infection. If investigation is delayed until other signs occur, such as lethargy, anorexia or apnea, infection may be far advanced before treatment is started. It is generally accepted that any febrile newborn should have cultures of blood, cerebrospinal fluid (CSF) and urine taken, and then should be started on empirical antibiotics.[37] Other investigations such as a peripheral white blood count (WBC), serum C-reactive protein (CRP) and serum procalcitonin (PCT) may indicate the likelihood of bacterial infection.[38] If an infant is tachypneic then a chest X-ray (CXR) should be performed.

Infections presenting within 48 h of birth are likely to have resulted from maternal transmission with bacteria such as group B streptococcus (GBS, *Streptococcus agalactiae*), *S. pneumoniae* and *Escherichia coli*. Later infections in the neonatal period are more likely to be nosocomial, and are more common in the preterm infant undergoing intensive care. Typical organisms are *Staphylococcus aureus* and *S. epidermidis*. However, maternally acquired infections with organisms such as GBS, and those acquired in the community, are also seen later in the neonatal period.

Viral infections, either congenital or acquired, may also be associated with fever. Babies who acquire herpes simplex virus (HSV) infection from their mothers at birth may present after 2–7 days with fever and nonspecific signs of sepsis, and HSV should be considered in the differential diagnosis. Clinical features may include skin, eye or mouth lesions, pneumonitis, hepatitis, encephalitis and disseminated intravascular coagulopathy (DIC). Other viruses that commonly present with fever in the neonatal period include enteroviruses, influenza and respiratory syncytial virus.

FEVER DURING INFANCY AND CHILDHOOD

The commonest cause of fever in this group is viral infection, which tends to be short lived. The challenge for the pediatrician is to determine whether the fever is the result of a viral or bacterial infection. In a series of 292 infants < 2 months old admitted to hospital with a history of fever, 19 (6.5%) were described as having serious bacterial infection (SBI), although 5 of the 19 were afebrile at the time of admission.[39] In a prospective study of children 3–36 months of age, pathogenic bacteria were isolated in blood culture from 60/519 (12%) with a fever greater than 39.5 °C (method of temperature measurement not described). The risk of bacterial infection was found to be higher among infants with an elevated white blood count.[40] In the young infant the signs of SBI are relatively nonspecific and it is generally accepted that children < 3 months old require hospital admission. The strategy described by Baraff et al is widely accepted.[41]

The infant is assessed as toxic or nontoxic based on level of activity, responsiveness, feeding and peripheral perfusion. Toxic infants need to be evaluated urgently for bacteremia or meningitis and started on antibiotics. Nontoxic infants should have blood cultures and lumbar puncture and can be classified as low risk if they have normal CSF and urinalysis, and a WBC between 5 and 15 000/mm³. The well looking infant in the high risk group should also be started on antibiotics. A CXR should be performed in the presence of abnormal respiratory signs.

Guidance on many aspects of fever in the infant and child is published by the National Institute for Clinical Excellence.[42]

The typical signs of viral upper respiratory infection include coryza, inflamed tympanic membranes, tonsillitis and fever. Bacterial tonsillitis and otitis media are difficult to differentiate from viral causes.

A good history and thorough examination are essential if a speedy diagnosis is to be achieved. Direct questions should be asked about the following:

1. previous immunizations;
2. family members with fever;
3. travel abroad;
4. consumption of unpasteurized milk (to exclude listeriosis, brucellosis), or raw eggs (*Salmonella* spp.);
5. history of congenital heart disease;
6. symptoms of this illness (abdominal pain, urinary frequency and dysuria);
7. signs noticed, e.g. rash, joint swelling.

Examination should take note of rash, lymphadenopathy, hepato- and splenomegaly, chest signs, heart murmurs, abdominal masses and tenderness. The bones and joints should be assessed for swelling and tenderness.

When fever has been persistent – over a week for instance – and no cause has been found, serious consideration should be given to hospital admission to confirm pyrexia and to initiate investigations. The physical signs and investigations required to exclude conditions producing FUO or PUO are given in Table 28.8.

However, certain basic investigations should be performed, of which urine and blood culture are arguably the most important.

FEVER AND NEUTROPENIA

The neutropenic child with fever is in a similar clinical situation to the neonate with fever, in that there is no time to wait for culture results. Antibiotics should be started after blood cultures have been taken. The antibiotics chosen must cover infections due to staphylococci and Gram negative enteric bacilli. Neutropenic children are also at risk of fungal infection, and empirical antifungal therapy is indicated if fever persists despite antibiotics and negative cultures.

THE CHILD WITH A RASH

In some cases a rash will be diagnostic, and in others the diagnosis will only be reached in conjunction with the history and appropriate investigations. Failure to recognize certain rashes could cost the life of a child, as in meningococcal infection or varicella in an immunocompromised child.

If an infectious cause is suspected, certain information should be obtained by history: prior infectious disease and/or rashes; recent contact with infectious disease; prior immunization; foreign travel; prodromal illness; fever.

In the general examination, note should be taken of the child's general state, the temperature, appearance of conjunctivae, ears and throat. Careful auscultation of the chest should be performed; all groups of lymph glands as well as liver and spleen should be examined.

Once this has been done, interest should return to the rash, which should be described carefully (e.g. hemorrhagic, macular, papular):

1. macules – flat and impalpable;
2. papules – circumscribed, elevated lesions;
3. vesicles – circumscribed, elevated, filled with clear fluid, and normally less than 0.5 cm in diameter;
4. pustules – elevated lesions containing a purulent exudate;
5. petechiae and other hemorrhagic spots – cannot be blanched by compression and may be flat or raised; the term purpura usually refers to the larger lesions with a diameter greater than 0.5 cm.

The distribution may be an important clue to certain infections, and it may be relevant whether or not the rash is itchy.

INFECTIOUS RASHES IN THE NEWBORN

Rashes are common in the neonatal period. Neonatal urticaria, or erythema toxicum, is characterized by a mixture of erythematous macules and white or yellow papules that usually develop over the first few

Table 28.8   Causes of pyrexia of unknown origin

Disease	Signs	Investigations
Bacterial		
Brucellosis	Lymphadenopathy, splenomegaly	Antibody titers
Bacterial endocarditis	Murmur, splinter hemorrhages	Blood culture × 3, *Brucella*, *Coxiella* titers
Leptospirosis	Hematuria, jaundice, conjunctivitis	Blood culture, serology
Osteomyelitis	Bone swelling, tenderness, redness, immobility	Blood culture, bone aspirate culture, bone radioisotope scan
Pelvic abscess	Abdominal tenderness, tender mass rectally	Leukocytosis on full blood count
Pyelonephritis	Loin tenderness	Urine microscopy and culture
Tuberculosis	Pneumonia, meningitis	Tuberculin test, culture gastric washings ± cerebrospinal fluid, chest X-ray
Typhoid fever	Abdominal tenderness, rose spots, splenomegaly	Blood culture
Septic arthritis	Swelling, tenderness, immobility at single joint	Joint aspirate culture
Psittacosis	Chest crackles, tachypnea	Chest X-ray, serology
Listeriosis	Arthritis, meningism	Blood culture, cerebrospinal fluid culture
Virus		
Cytomegalic inclusion disease	Lymphadenopathy, hepatosplenomegaly	Urine culture, etc., blood and urine PCR
Human immunodeficiency virus	Lymphadenopathy, failure to thrive, chronic infection, e.g. candida	T4/T8 lymphocyte ratio, HIV antibody, HIV PCR
Infectious mononucleosis	Tonsillitis, hepatosplenomegaly	Paul–Bunnell/Monospot, Epstein–Barr viral antibody
Hepatitis	Icterus, hepatomegaly	Hepatitis A, hepatitis B serology, hepatitis B and C PCR
Parasite		
Malaria	Splenomegaly, hepatomegaly, encephalopathy	Thick or thin blood film
Toxoplasmosis	Cervical, supraclavicular lymphadenopathy	Smear from biopsy specimen, serology
Miscellaneous		
Crohn's disease	Abdominal tenderness and mass	GI endoscopy or barium study of GI tract. Exclude *Yersinia* and *Campylobacter* infection
Diabetes insipidus	Polyuria, polydipsia	Dilute urine following water deprivation
Juvenile rheumatoid arthritis		
1. Systemic	Fever, characteristic maculopapular rash, lethargy, arthritis, pericardial effusion	No diagnostic test
2. Monoarticular/polyarticular	Fever not a consistent sign	
Kawasaki disease	Cervical lymphadenopathy, bilateral conjunctival injection, red, fissured lips and tongue, maculopapular rash, swelling and desquamation of hands and feet	No diagnostic test
Malignancy	Includes anemia, lymphadenopathy, splenomegaly, abdominal mass, bone pain	Full blood count, blood film, lymph node biopsy, bone marrow trephine, vanillylmandelic acid
Leukemia		
Lymphoma		
Neuroblastoma		
Factitious fever (Munchausen by proxy)	Pyrexia only recorded by parent	None

days and may persist until the end of the second week. Staphylococcal infection of the newborn may be difficult to distinguish from neonatal urticaria. Although erythematous lesions are seen with staphylococcal infection, pustules and vesicles predominate. When there is uncertainty as to the diagnosis, a Gram stain of vesicle fluid should be performed. Plentiful polymorphs as well as Gram positive cocci should be seen in the presence of staphylococcal infection; eosinophils predominate in neonatal urticaria.

Vesicles are also seen in neonatal varicella and herpes simplex virus (HSV) infection. In the former, a history of maternal varicella will be elicited. In the latter, however, a history of past or current genital herpes is obtained in only a quarter of cases. The vesicles of HSV tend to be larger and less opaque than those of staphylococcal infection. Urgent treatment of neonatal HSV is essential. Rapid diagnosis can be achieved by rapid viral identification tests such as immunofluorescence on vesicle fluid or by electron microscopy if available. PCR of vesicle fluid, if available in a timely way, can also be diagnostic.

Other rashes associated with infection may be petechial or purpuric as a result of thrombocytopenia, as seen in congenital cytomegalovirus (CMV) or congenital rubella infections. In such cases the rash is usually just one of several clinical features of congenital infection.

INFECTIOUS RASHES IN INFANCY AND CHILDHOOD

These will be described under descriptive headings.

Vesicular rashes
Varicella

Lesions normally appear without a prodromal illness, and progress rapidly (within a few hours) from papules to vesicles surrounded by an erythematous base. Crops of vesicles appear over 3 days, predominantly on the trunk and proximal limbs. Vesicles may also develop on mucous membranes.

Herpes zoster

Lesions similar to those seen in varicella infection may develop over specific dermatomes or cranial nerves. Although the immunosuppressed are at increased risk from zoster, this condition is also seen in normal children.

Herpes simplex virus (HSV)

HSV infection in childhood may be primary, usually associated with gingivostomatitis, may be secondary (reactivation) as with cold sores and other recurrent herpetic lesions, or may occur as eczema herpeticum, a spreading vesicular rash in association with eczema (caused by HSV but sometimes confusingly called Kaposi's varicelliform eruption). Pyrexia is followed by the appearance of crops of vesicles on the eczematous skin, which may occur over several days. Rapid diagnosis, e.g. with immunofluorescence, and treatment with antivirals is essential because untreated severe infection may be fatal.

Hand, foot and mouth
This is caused by enteroviruses, the commonest being Coxsackie virus type 16, and occurs in epidemics. It is associated with a papular–vesicular eruption of the mouth, hands, feet and sometimes buttocks.

Impetigo
This condition usually presents as a red macule and then becomes vesicular. The small vesicles burst to leave a honey-colored crust. Both streptococcal and staphylococcal impetigo occur most commonly around the mouth.

Molluscum contagiosum
This is caused by a pox virus. Flesh-colored papules with a central dimple are firm initially, but become softer and more waxy with time. Lesions are 2–5 mm in size and may occur anywhere. Molluscum is more severe in HIV infection.

Maculopapular rashes
Measles
Measles rash is blotchy, red or pink in color, raised in places, and starts behind the ears and on the face, spreading downwards. The lesions tend to become confluent on the upper part of the body and remain more discrete lower down. The rash fades, usually after 2–3 days. The skin becomes brown and although desquamation occurs this is not usually seen on the hands and feet, as it is in scarlet fever.

Rubella
Rubella results in a pink rash which progresses caudally. The lesions are normally discrete and the rash develops more quickly and disappears earlier than in measles. Desquamation is not a characteristic.

Scarlet fever
The eruption is dark red and punctiform. The rash tends to be most prominent on the neck and in the major skinfolds. A distinctive feature is circumoral pallor as a result of the rash sparing the area around the mouth. Desquamation of the hands and feet is common after 1–2 weeks. True scarlet fever is associated with inflammation of the tongue (white and red strawberry tongue). Scarlatina refers to the rash, which may occur alone in milder streptococcal infection and is often short lived.

Kawasaki disease
Although several features are required for the diagnosis of this condition, which is of unknown etiology, the rash may be confused with that of scarlet fever. Discrete red maculopapules are seen on the feet, around the knees and in the axillary and inguinal skin creases. Desquamation of the hands and feet is a common feature (Fig. 28.15).

Erythema infectiosum or fifth disease
Infection caused by parvovirus B19 is associated with a rash which develops in two stages. The cheeks appear red and flushed, giving rise to a 'slapped cheek' appearance. A maculopapular rash develops 1–2 weeks later, predominantly over the arms and legs which, as it fades, appears lace-like.

Roseola infantum
The main cause is human herpes virus 6 (HHV-6). Roseola infantum is characterized by a widespread morbilliform (measles-like) rash, seen in its most florid form on the trunk. The lesions tend to be discrete. As the rash appears the fever, which is normally present over the previous

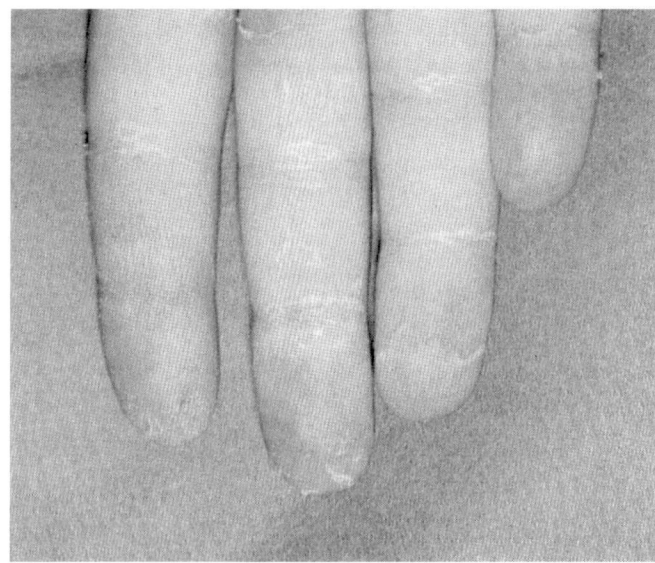

Fig. 28.15 Kawasaki disease: finger desquamation starting at the tips.

4 days, resolves and the child looks well (in contrast to measles, in which the child is febrile and unwell when the rash appears).

Viral infections
Many viral infections, particularly those associated with the enteroviruses, may cause maculopapular rashes.

Petechial and purpuric rashes
Meningococcal infection
The first sign of meningococcal septicemia may be a petechial or purpuric rash anywhere on the body and often localized (Fig. 28.16). On occasions these lesions may be preceded by or accompany a maculopapular rash which may blanch (Fig. 28.17). The petechiae will not blanch, and although it is conventional to make a microbiological diagnosis on blood culture and PCR, bacteria can often be seen on Gram stain and cultured on scrapings of the skin lesions.

Meningococcal petechiae can be confused with those seen on the face around the eyes following events that result in a transient rise in venous pressure such as vomiting. Rarely petechial rashes are associated with septicemia caused by other bacteria, such as *S. pneumoniae*, *S. aureus* and *Haemophilus influenzae* type b.

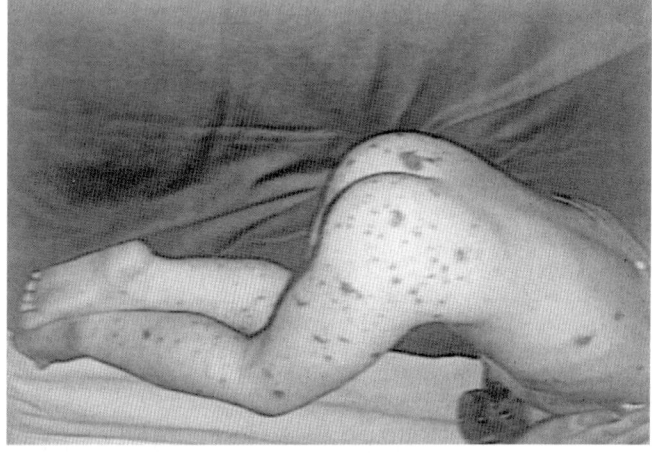

Fig. 28.16 Purpuric rash of meningococcemia.
(Courtesy of Department of Medical Illustration, University of Aberdeen.)

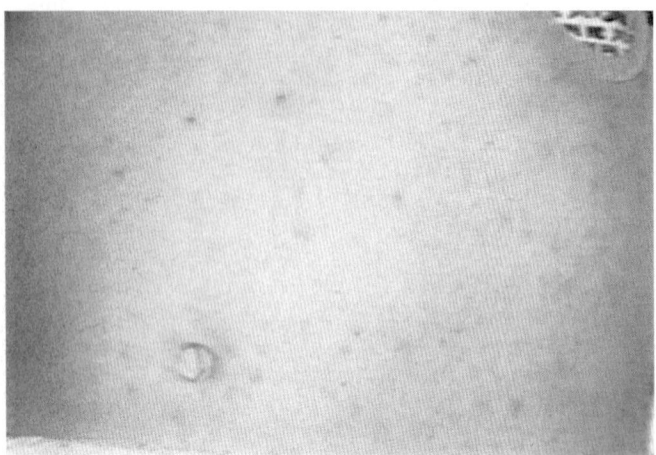

Fig. 28.17 Maculopapular/morbilliform rash of early meningococcemia. (Courtesy of Department of Medical Illustration, University of Aberdeen.)

Henoch–Schönlein purpura

This condition often follows an upper respiratory tract infection but no single infective agent has been implicated. Hemorrhagic macules and papules develop on the buttocks and extensor surfaces of the limbs, particularly the knees and ankles. The lesions come in crops and fade over a few days leaving a brown pigmentation.

Idiopathic thrombocytopenic purpura (ITP)

A purpuric rash sometimes associated with frank bleeding is seen in this condition. Even post-infective cases are often referred to as ITP, and rubella infection is considered to be the commonest infectious cause.

Leukemia

Children with leukemia may present with a hemorrhagic rash as a result of thrombocytopenia but in addition, the pallor of severe anemia will usually be obvious.

FEVER AND INCREASED RESPIRATORY RATE

The combination of fever and rapid breathing is a common and important pediatric presentation. While the differential diagnosis is vast (Table 28.9), a serious underlying condition must always be considered, in particular sepsis (bacteremia or septicemia) and bacterial pneumonia.

Table 28.9 Differential diagnosis of the child with fever and increased respiratory rate

Serious infections
  Bacteremia/septicemia
  Bacterial pneumonia (with or without parapneumonic effusion)
  Other focal bacterial infections (including meningitis, osteomyelitis, septic arthritis)
Less serious infections
  Viral or *Mycoplasma* bronchopneumonia
Mild infections
  Viral upper respiratory tract infection (URTI)
  Viral bronchitis
  Viral exanthema
Fever and increased respiratory rate with upper airways obstruction (stridor)
  Viral laryngotracheobronchitis (viral 'croup')
Fever and increased respiratory rate with lower airways obstruction (wheeze)
  Acute viral bronchiolitis (usually due to RSV)
  Asthma triggered by intercurrent viral upper respiratory tract infection

Fortunately, these serious conditions are uncommon and most infants and young children presenting with fever and increased respiratory rate simply have a relatively minor viral upper respiratory tract infection. In this situation, the respiratory rate is only mildly elevated and not associated with any other obvious signs of increased work of breathing (such as intercostal and/or subcostal retractions).

Both the level of the fever and the degree of tachypnea are key indicators of a serious versus minor infection: the higher the level, the greater the likelihood of a serious bacterial infection. In addition, infants and young children with serious infections will have other features, both on history and physical examination, which will assist with the diagnosis. These include signs of marked increased work of breathing, and 'grunting' respirations with extensive bacterial pneumonia. Further, infants and young children with serious bacterial infections will look ill, with signs such as pallor, cyanosis, apathy and altered level of consciousness. On the other hand infants and young children with a viral acute respiratory infection will have a history and physical evidence of a viral/coryzal illness with mild fever, clear rhinorrhea, conjunctival injection, redness of the tympanic membranes, sore throat and dry cough.

Clearly, the source or focus of infection must be thoroughly sought, both when taking the history and when performing the physical examination, in children presenting with this combination of symptoms. Recent contact with other children suffering from a viral infection (including one of the viral exanthemata) is vital information. Symptoms of a viral upper respiratory tract infection, or symptoms which localize the inflammation to a specific area of the respiratory tract, need to be elicited. This includes: a barking cough and inspiratory stridor indicating viral laryngotracheobronchitis (croup); coryzal symptoms plus acute history of significant cough (acute viral bronchitis); coryzal symptoms with acute wheeze, cough and shortness of breath (acute viral bronchiolitis in infants; acute asthma in older children).

A major symptom and sign to look for in children with fever and tachypnea is wheezing. In infants this is most likely to be due to acute viral bronchiolitis (usually due to respiratory syncytial virus), and in older children to an episode of acute bronchospasm (asthma) triggered by an intercurrent viral respiratory tract infection. In both these situations wheeze will be present, either audible with the ear or with a stethoscope. Generally, there will also be hyperinflation of the thoracic cage, tachypnea and other signs of increased work of respiration. In infants with acute viral bronchiolitis, diffuse inspiratory crackles are generally audible throughout the chest plus the loud expiratory, musical wheezing.

Infants and children with viral or *Mycoplasma* bronchopneumonia generally have other coryzal symptoms and signs in the ear, nose and throat plus a marked cough, which is often the major complaint. By contrast bacterial pneumonia presents with high fever, 'grunting' respirations and tachypnea, but no cough, particularly in the early phases of the illness.

The infant and young children with bacterial sepsis will generally have high fever (over 38.5 °C), rapid respiratory rate and rapid pulse and will look ill. On close inspection some of these children may have localized features of serious infection such as meningitis, osteomyelitis, septic arthritis or endocarditis. Infants with a bacterial urinary tract infection will have very few localizing symptoms or signs apart from fever and mild elevation of respiratory rate.

In summary, there is a large differential diagnosis of the infant or young child presenting with a combination of fever and increased respiratory rate. This can range from a severe life-threatening illness to a trivial head cold. The latter is far more likely, and most will have only mildly elevated temperature and respiratory rate plus other symptoms and signs to indicate an intercurrent viral upper respiratory tract syndrome. On the other hand, a markedly elevated temperature and respiratory rate in a very sick child indicates a serious infection, particularly bacteremia/septicemia or bacterial pneumonia.

When in doubt, further investigations and/or a further period of observation are essential. These may include CXR, blood cultures, lumbar puncture and blood or urine for bacterial antigen testing.

In obviously sick infants and children, or those in whom a serious underlying bacterial infection is likely, appropriate antibiotics should be given while waiting for the results of the above testing.

COUGH AND FEVER

The presence of cough signifies irritation or stimulation of cough receptors in the upper or lower airways. This is most commonly secondary to inflammation from a viral infection of the upper or lower airways and will be accompanied by mild fever. Cough is also a feature of bronchial asthma, which is also often accompanied by fever, since the commonest trigger for an acute exacerbation in young children is an intercurrent viral upper respiratory tract infection.

Thus the combination of fever and cough suggests an infection somewhere in the respiratory tract and this is far more likely to be due to a virus rather than bacteria. Diffuse, mild inflammation is typical of viral infection, while focal, severe inflammation is typical of bacterial infection in the respiratory tract. Indeed, one of the major distinguishing features between streptococcal pharyngitis and a viral upper respiratory tract infection is the absence of cough and coryzal symptoms in streptococcal throat infections.

To determine the likely cause of cough and fever requires a comprehensive history and physical examination. Laboratory investigations may occasionally be required to further elucidate the cause.

If there is a past history of bronchial asthma, the fever and cough are almost certainly due to episodic asthma or 'wheezing associated respiratory infection' (WARI). If there is a past history of chronic bronchitis (frequent episodes of protracted cough with intercurrent viral acute respiratory infections) then it should be obvious from the history that the child is having a further episode of acute viral bronchitis.

Fever and cough due to an upper respiratory tract infection should be readily distinguishable by the coryzal symptoms of rhinorrhea, conjunctival injection and a dry cough but no increased work of breathing and no wheeze. While the child with viral laryngotracheobronchitis will have signs of a coryzal illness, the striking features will be the barking, 'croupy' quality of the cough and probable inspiratory stridor, particularly when the child is upset. When severe this inspiratory stridor will be associated with increased work of breathing (chest wall retractions, tracheal tug). Acute viral bronchitis is characterized by troublesome dry or wet cough in association with an acute respiratory infection. On auscultation there may be scattered coarse crackles (due to excessive airway secretions), which should clear following active coughing. Acute viral bronchiolitis is characterized by coryzal symptoms plus hyperinflation of the chest, loud wheezing, inspiratory crackles throughout both lung fields, and varying degrees of respiratory difficulty in addition to fever and cough. Viral and *Mycoplasma* bronchopneumonia will be characterized by coryzal symptoms, marked cough, increased work of breathing and widespread, scattered, inspiratory crackles.

A less common but important cause of cough and fever is foreign body inhalation, e.g. nuts and peanuts. Initially this is a dry cough, often with wheeze and difficulty breathing. If retained, the cough becomes loose and productive of purulent sputum. A child with a loose, productive cough and fever could also be suffering from chronic suppurative lung disease – bronchiectasis or chronic bronchitis. Most of these children will have some underlying problem (e.g. cystic fibrosis or immune deficiency).

In summary, fever and cough signify some inflammatory process in the airways. This can range from a relatively uncomplicated viral upper respiratory tract infection due to rhinovirus through to viral or *Mycoplasma* bronchopneumonia (Table 28.10). A major differential to consider is whether the fever and cough are due to an exacerbation of asthma in the child with underlying episodic asthma.

RHINITIS

Rhinitis implies inflammation of the nasal 'mucosa', and in children this is most commonly due to a viral upper respiratory tract infection. The

Table 28.10 Causes of cough and fever

Acute respiratory tract infections
  Viral upper respiratory tract infection (URTI)
  Acute viral bronchitis
  Acute viral laryngotracheobronchitis (viral croup)
  Acute viral bronchiolitis (infants)
  Acute viral bronchopneumonia
  Mycoplasma (bronchitis and bronchopneumonia)
Asthma syndromes
  Classical bronchial asthma
  Wheezing associated respiratory infection (WARI)
Less common causes
  Foreign body inhalation
  Suppurative lung disease (chronic bronchitis/bronchiectasis)

inflammation normally results in a combination of rhinorrhea and nasal obstruction. Sneezing is commonly associated with these symptoms.

The major differential diagnosis of rhinitis secondary to a viral upper respiratory tract infection is allergic rhinitis. In children allergic rhinitis is generally perennial rather than seasonal and is characterized by its persistence for weeks or months rather than the short term nasal symptoms of an acute viral infection. The symptoms of allergic rhinitis have a typical diurnal pattern (classically worse in the mornings) and there is absence of fever and other signs suggesting a viral upper respiratory tract infection. Nasal itch and sneezing are common as are clear rhinorrhea and nasal obstruction. There is often an associated allergic conjunctivitis which can simulate a viral rhino-conjunctivitis. The child with allergic rhinitis generally has other signs of clinical atopy, particularly atopic eczema or bronchial asthma.

Vasomotor rhinitis is uncommon in young children and typically causes sudden onset (and sudden cessation) of clear rhinorrhea – often for only hours – but with recurrent episodes.

Other rarer causes of rhinitis include:
- Foreign body – particularly small parts of toys and polystyrene beads. Causes unilateral nasal symptoms.
- Unusual infections (e.g. nasal diphtheria).

The distinction between acute viral rhinitis secondary to a viral infection and acute sinusitis is subtle and arbitrary. Most definitions base the distinction on duration of symptoms. Conventionally, acute sinusitis is the appropriate diagnosis if the nasal discharge is severe and persists for more than 10 days. These symptoms would generally be associated with cough and possibly bad breath.

Chronic sinusitis is arbitrarily defined as a persistent, mucopurulent nasal discharge for over 30 days. This is most commonly seen in children with underlying abnormalities of mucus, mucociliary clearance or immune function (e.g. cystic fibrosis, primary ciliary dyskinesia, agammaglobulinemia).

Drug therapy for rhinitis associated with a viral upper respiratory tract infection is generally not required. However, in small infants the nasal obstruction and rhinorrhea may interfere with feeding and saline drops followed by suctioning of the drops ('nasal lavage') may be helpful, particularly immediately prior to feeds. Acute sinusitis is generally viral although secondary bacterial infection may occur. While there is some uncertainty as to whether or not antibiotics are indicated in this situation, there is little doubt that the color of the nasal discharge changes promptly with administration of antibiotics, but such treatment is best reserved for those who are more severely affected by the symptoms. Chronic sinusitis should be treated with antibiotics and prolonged courses (three weeks) may be necessary.

Perennial allergic rhinitis in children warrants treatment, particularly if the symptoms are severe. The most effective treatment is regular nasal topical corticosteroid (e.g. budesonide nasal spray).

In summary, while there are many possible causes for rhinitis (Table 28.11), most commonly it is the result of either a respiratory virus or allergic rhinitis.

Table 28.11   Causes of rhinitis

Common
    Viral upper respiratory tract infection (acute viral nasopharyngitis
    – most commonly due to rhinovirus)
    Perennial allergic rhinitis
Uncommon
    Acute viral or bacterial sinusitis
    Vasomotor rhinitis
Rare
    Retained foreign body
    Uncommon infections (e.g. nasal diphtheria)

NOISY BREATHING

Audible noises of respiration are common in children. Clarification of the type of noise is critical with respect to identifying the most likely underlying cause. In general, noisy breathing signifies some obstruction to airflow, and the specific type of noise – especially which phase of respiration – can greatly assist in determining the anatomic site of the airflow obstruction.

The types of noises identifiable are listed below in Table 28.12, together with the phase of respiration in which they are most audible, and the usual anatomic site for the noise.

An important principle is: the noise is predominantly inspiratory when the obstruction is outside the thoracic cage (upper airways), and predominantly expiratory when the obstruction is inside the thorax (lower airways).

If a child has the noise when being examined then there is no difficulty determining its features. However, when the noise is from history alone this can create difficulties with respect to the terminology used by parents. In such instances, mimicking these noises will often assist with the accurate diagnosis. Alternatively, asking the parents to obtain tape recordings will enable clear identification of the type of noise.

There will generally be associated symptoms and signs with these noises, which will assist clinically in determining the exact site and

cause for the obstruction. For example, a child with acute onset inspiratory stridor and a barking cough in association with an URTI has acute viral 'croup' (laryngotracheobronchitis). On the other hand, a child with grunting respirations and high fever who looks toxic and unwell is probably suffering from acute (bacterial) pneumonia.

The causes of obstruction are numerous and are summarized in Table 28.13.

In summary, the child presenting with the problem of noisy breathing requires a comprehensive history and examination to determine the exact nature of the noise and to determine whether there are any associated symptoms or signs. By accurately determining the nature of the noisy breathing, the likely anatomical site of the obstruction can usually be determined, and this will greatly assist with the final diagnosis.

SUSPECTED MENINGITIS

Over the last five years, notified cases of bacterial meningitis have fallen to less than 1500 cases a year in England and Wales (Table 28.14). The mortality from these infections has also declined in recent years, but there is evidence that the long term consequences of meningitis are considerable, particularly when the disease occurs early in life.

ETIOLOGY AND PATHOPHYSIOLOGY OF BACTERIAL MENINGITIS

The commonest route of meningeal infection is from the bloodstream, so the spectrum of pathogens causing meningitis is similar to that seen in bacteremia and sepsis. The introduction of the *Haemophilus influenzae* type b (Hib) polysaccharide-conjugate vaccine into the UK vaccination program has had a dramatic effect.[43] The incidence of Hib meningitis has dropped from around 2500 cases per year to 44 per year, with *Neisseria meningitidis* now the commonest cause of community acquired bacterial meningitis in the UK, followed by *Streptococcus pneumoniae*. The relative importance of these pathogens varies considerably with age (Table 28.14) and the nature of the immunization programs in operation. In the neonatal period, group B streptococcus is the prominent meningeal pathogen, followed by Gram negative bacilli, *S. pneumoniae* and *Listeria monocytogenes*. In children older than 3 months and in young adults, the most frequent cause of bacterial meningitis is *N. meningitidis* followed by *S. pneumoniae*. Infants between 1 and 3 months old are susceptible to *N. meningitidis* and *S. pneumoniae*, as well as the neonatal pathogens. The propensity of neonates to get meningitis is in part due to their immunological immaturity. Older children with congenital or acquired deficiencies in complement, immunoglobulin production, lymphocytes, neutrophils or splenic function are at increased risk from meningitis, sometimes due to atypical pathogens. A rare but serious form of bacterial meningitis is caused by *Mycobacterium tuberculosis*. This organism can affect patients of all ages and should be considered in any atypical presentation of meningitis, particularly patients presenting with an insidious illness.[44]

Table 28.12   Types of identifiable noises

Noise	Inspiration	Expiration	Site of obstruction
Snuffliness	+ +	±	Nasal
Snoring	+ +	±	Oronasopharynx
Stridor	+ + +		Extrathoracic trachea (subglottis/larynx)
Rattliness	+ +		Central tracheobronchial tree (trachea)
Wheeze		+ +	Small and medium sized intrathoracic airways
Grunting		+ + +	Alveoli

Table 28.13   Causes of obstruction

	Causes of noise	
	Acute	Persistent
Snuffliness	Viral upper respiratory tract infection	Perennial allergic rhinitis
Snoring	Acute tonsillitis/upper respiratory tract infection	Chronic enlargement of tonsils and adenoids
Stridor	Viral croup	Congenital subglottic stenosis or other fixed upper airway malformations
Rattle	Acute viral bronchitis	Cerebral palsy/CNS disorders ('sputum retention')
Wheeze	Asthma	Chronic small airways obstruction (e.g. cystic fibrosis)
Grunt	Acute bacterial (lobar) pneumonia Hyaline membrane disease (neonate)	Chronic interstitial lung disease (e.g. pulmonary fibrosis)

Table 28.14 Statutory notifications of meningitis cases in 2000 and 2005 (data from Health Protection Agency)

	Year	Age group				
		1–11 months	1–4 years	5–9 years	10–14 years	15–24 years
Haemophilus influenzae	2005	11	15	3	2	3
	2000	5	10	1	1	2
Neisseria meningitidis	2005	163	121	42	26	92
	2000	231	220	105	86	219
Streptococcus pneumoniae	2005	63	32	10	7	5
	2000	53	27	4	9	14

While meningitis often occurs in the context of systemic infections, it can also follow bacterial invasion from a contiguous focus of infection, such as the mastoids or paranasal sinuses, or from osteomyelitis of the skull. Skull fractures, craniospinal dermal sinuses, neurenteric or dermoid cysts, occult intranasal encephaloceles, or transethmoid meningoceles are also potential portals of entry for pathogens into the subarachnoid space.[45] The possibility of a cranial defect should be considered in children with recurrent meningitis. Neurosurgical procedures and the presence of ventriculoperitoneal shunts also provide routes for meningeal infection. In such cases, *Staphylococcus aureus* and coagulase negative staphylococci are more likely pathogens.

Bacterial invasion of the cerebrospinal fluid (CSF) is followed by an outpouring of inflammatory cells which cross the blood–brain barrier and enter the CSF. Inflammatory cytokines such as tumor necrosis factor and interleukins 1, 6 and 8 are central to the inflammatory response. These mediators increase adhesion molecule expression on endothelial cells and leukocytes, which act in concert to facilitate the migration of cells into the CSF. Antibodies to adhesion molecules limit leukocyte migration and the consequences of meningeal infection.[46] The meninges become inflamed, swollen and covered by fibrino-purulent exudate. The thickest exudate is usually at the base of the brain. This leads to obstruction of the exit foramina of the fourth ventricle or the subarachnoid basal cisterns, restricting the CSF circulation to produce hydrocephalus. The ependymal lining of the cerebral ventricles may also be a site of intense inflammation (ventriculitis), causing ventricular enlargement and subsequent subependymal gliosis. A combination of cerebral vasculitis, thrombosis, cerebral edema and raised intracranial pressure leads to globally reduced cerebral blood flow and focal ischemia. This results in neuronal injury and cerebral damage, manifest clinically as coma, seizures and focal neurological signs.

CLINICAL FEATURES

The fully developed clinical picture of acute meningitis in children is sufficiently characteristic to be recognized without difficulty. More than 80% of children will have fever, vomiting, severe headache and signs of meningeal irritation. However, in the early stages of disease, and in young children, the symptoms and signs are often nonspecific. Fever may be absent in up to 30% of individuals, and 20–30% do not have signs of meningism at presentation. Previous antibiotic therapy may also mask the significance of the presenting illness.[47]

Older children will often complain of headache or pain at the back of the neck, nausea and photophobia. The physical signs of meningeal irritation are neck stiffness and a positive Kernig test, which reflect inflammation of nerve roots of the spinal canal and adjacent sensory nerves. The most comfortable position for the patient is to lie with an extended neck and flexed hips and knees to reduce tension on the nerves emanating from the spinal cord. Neck stiffness can be detected by placing a palm of the hand on the supine child's occiput. Any attempt at flexing the child's neck will result in the lifting of the whole trunk. Kernig's sign is elicited with the child supine. The hip and knee joints are bent 90 degrees and then an attempt is made to extend the knee fully. In the presence of meningitis, there is resistance and severe pain as the sciatic nerve is stretched. A positive Brudzinski sign is involuntary muscular contraction causing leg flexion upon passive flexion of the neck, but this is a less reliable sign of meningitis. Additional evidence of neurological involvement includes convulsions, which occur in 30% of children within 3 days of presentation, cranial nerve palsies (particularly III, IV, VI, and VII), delirium, drowsiness and coma.

In infants and toddlers, the symptoms are often those of a generalized illness. Irritability, lethargy, convulsions, refusal of feeds, vomiting, a high pitched cry and a bulging fontanelle should all alert the physician to the presence of meningitis. The 'typical' features of meningitis may be absent or difficult to interpret or elicit. When present they are often indicative of advanced disease.

Neisseria meningitidis is the commonest cause of bacterial meningitis in the UK (Table 28.14). More than 50% of patients infected with this organism will have a petechial rash, so a vigilant search for petechiae should be made in any child with features suggesting a diagnosis of meningitis. The whole skin surface should be carefully examined, since there may initially be only one or two petechiae. However it is also important to note that initially the rash of *N. meningitidis* may be maculopapular or urticarial in nature, and so an atypical rash should not be taken as evidence to exclude the diagnosis. In all age groups, the clinical manifestations of bacteremia and sepsis may be the earliest evidence of infection (see section on sepsis and meningococcal infection). If the condition can be picked up at this stage and treated appropriately, meningitis can be prevented.

DIAGNOSIS

If meningitis is suspected, the diagnosis should be confirmed by lumbar puncture and examination of CSF. Over the last 10 years, there has been a move away from performing diagnostic lumbar punctures (LP) in patients presenting with suspected meningitis, since it is frequently argued that an LP will not affect patient management and may be hazardous. However, an LP offers immediate confirmation of the diagnosis and allows appropriate treatment to be started, which may be particularly important in neonates and immunocompromised patients in whom the differential diagnosis is wide. Identifying the etiological agent and its antibiotic sensitivities may be crucial to administering the most appropriate antibiotics and providing important prognostic information.[47]

There are, however, specific and clear contraindications to LP in patients with meningitis.[48] These are:

1. signs of raised intracranial pressure with changing level of consciousness, focal neurological signs or severe mental impairment;
2. cardiovascular compromise with impaired peripheral perfusion or hypotension;
3. respiratory compromise with tachypnea, an abnormal breathing pattern or hypoxia;
4. thrombocytopenia or a coagulopathy.

An LP should also be avoided if it will result in a significant delay in treatment. The association between LP and cerebellar tonsillar herniation has not been shown to be causal, and has not been reported in the absence of the specific contraindications listed above.

Lumbar puncture should be performed in the third to fourth lumbar space using a needle with a stylet, since use of a needle alone has been associated with the development of implantation dermoid cysts. CSF should be collected for microscopy and culture, bacterial and viral polymerase chain reaction (PCR), latex agglutination tests for bacterial antigens, protein and glucose. Blood cultures may also identify the etiological agent if an LP is not performed or fails to establish the cause of meningitis.

Analysis of the CSF leukocyte count, glucose and protein can usually establish a positive diagnosis of meningitis, but normal results do not necessarily exclude meningitis. The absence of cells may indicate very early meningitis before the migration of leukocytes into the CSF. Very high white cell counts of up to 20 000/mm³ can be observed in bacterial meningitis, although the number of cells is usually less than 3000/mm³. There is a broad association between a predominance of polymorphonuclear leukocytes in the CSF and bacterial meningitis. However, lymphocytes may predominate in early or partially treated bacterial meningitis, in tuberculous meningitis and in neonates. In bacterial meningitis, CSF glucose is usually low with a CSF:blood ratio of less than 0.5, and protein is frequently raised to more than 0.4 g/L. Numerous studies have now shown that even after the administration of intravenous antibiotics, the diagnostic cellular and biochemical changes in the CSF may persist for at least 48 h. In the context of a negative Gram stain and CSF culture, the presence of bacterial antigens and PCR tests may prove invaluable for establishing a diagnosis of bacterial meningitis.

THE USE OF CT SCANS

Following the clinical diagnosis of bacterial meningitis, it has become common practice to arrange a computerized tomographic (CT) brain scan to exclude raised intracranial pressure prior to undertaking a lumbar puncture. This approach has three important drawbacks. First, raised intracranial pressure (ICP) is very common amongst children with meningitis and clinically significant raised ICP cannot be ruled out by brain CT. Second, it is hazardous to transport patients to a CT scanner before they have been adequately stabilized. Third, the inevitable delay in undertaking the CT scan requires that empirical antibiotics be given while awaiting the procedure, therefore impairing the diagnostic yield from a subsequent LP. Patients presenting with clinical signs of raised ICP are the minority, and these children should not undergo LP, regardless of their CT findings. CT scans can exclude lesions requiring neurosurgical intervention and identify conditions such as cerebral abscess or hydrocephalus requiring shunting. The diagnostic yield from a CT scan in children is, however, low and should not be allowed to compromise the procedures required for diagnosis and to initiate appropriate treatment.[47]

ANTIBIOTICS

Except in cases where the patient is well and the diagnosis very uncertain, antibiotics should be administered empirically while awaiting the result of the LP. The selection of the optimal antibiotic for the treatment of bacterial meningitis should be based on the following criteria: the spectrum of pathogens known to cause meningitis in different age groups (Table 28.14); the changing pattern of antimicrobial resistance;[49,50] the pharmacological properties of the antibiotics available and the results of therapeutic trials. In infants up to 3 months of age, a combination of ampicillin and cefotaxime is a logical choice, as cefotaxime provides cover for both neonatal and infant pathogens, and ampicillin is effective against Listeria monocytogenes. For the same reason, ampicillin should be included as part of empirical therapy for immunocompromised patients. Penicillin-resistant meningococci are emerging worldwide, as are chloramphenicol-resistant strains, but these have not yet resulted in treatment failures. Fortunately, almost all strains in the UK remain sensitive to the third generation cephalosporins.

In the USA and some countries in Europe including Spain, France and Romania, more than 25% of pneumococcal isolates are resistant to penicillin and this proportion exceeds 50% in South Africa. Penicillin-insensitive strains of pneumococci are more likely to be resistant to third generation cephalosporins, and there have been documented cases of microbiological failure in the treatment of pneumococcal meningitis with third generation cephalosporins. In the UK, the level of penicillin resistance is stable at less than 5%.[50] In most UK cases, penicillin resistance is low level and cephalosporin resistance is rare and so a third generation cephalosporin (cefotaxime or ceftriaxone) is adequate for most community acquired meningitis in children over 3 months. The routine use of vancomycin for community acquired meningitis is not justified in the UK at the present time. However, vancomycin should be added to the treatment regimen for any patient coming from an area where high levels of penicillin resistance are endemic. The addition of rifampicin to vancomycin or the administration of vancomycin intraventricularly has been recommended by some authorities.[51]

THE ROLE OF CORTICOSTEROIDS

It is now widely accepted that much of the cerebral damage which occurs in bacterial meningitis is not caused by the invading organism itself but by the host mediated inflammatory response.[52] While a number of adjunctive anti-inflammatory agents have been suggested, only corticosteroids have been extensively tested in clinical trials. Several studies have shown some improvement in morbidity (deafness or neurological deficit), although these studies were largely conducted in children with Haemophilus influenzae type b meningitis, and this approach requires administration of corticosteroids either before antibiotic administration or at the same time.[53] Fewer data are available in children with pneumococcal and meningococcal meningitis. However, a recent systematic review of 18 studies in children and adults supports the use of steroid administration as a means of reducing the mortality and morbidity associated with meningitis.[54] These data imply that, at least at the present time, concerns that limiting meningeal inflammation could actually delay sterilization of the CSF by agents such as vancomycin, since these antibiotics cross the blood–brain barrier poorly, have not been substantiated.

NEUROLOGICAL AND FLUID MANAGEMENT

Hyponatremia is frequently observed in patients with bacterial meningitis. While this is associated with elevated serum antidiuretic hormone (ADH), possibly suggesting inappropriate ADH secretion (SIADH), more recent studies indicate that SIADH is overdiagnosed and the patients are hypovolemic.[55] Treatment of suspected SIADH with fluid restriction could potentially compromise circulating volume and therefore cerebral blood flow. Circulatory shock should be treated aggressively, significant dehydration corrected carefully, fluid balance monitored frequently and maintenance fluids given with care.

Patients presenting with clinical signs of raised ICP require very careful fluid balance monitoring to help maintain adequate cerebral blood flow. Intubation and mechanical ventilation should be instituted early to facilitate oxygenation, allow adequate sedation and permit normalization of $PaCO_2$. Such patients should be nursed head up and central venous catheters should not be placed in the neck. Intravenous mannitol may be useful for managing acute changes in intracranial pressure, and anticonvulsants for control of fits.[47]

COMPLICATIONS

Convulsions occur in 20–30% of children, usually within 72 h of presentation. The onset of late or persistent fits is associated with a poor prognosis. Subdural collections of fluid are common, particularly during infancy. They are usually sterile and rarely require aspiration unless there is evidence of increasing ICP, the presence of focal neurological signs, convulsions or persistent fever due to subdural empyema. Cerebral abscesses are rare outside the neonatal period. More frequent causes of persistent fever include intercurrent viral infection, ongoing inflammation and drug fever. In the absence of a definitive microbiological etiology, the combination of persistent fever and poor clinical condition may indicate that the meningitis is due to organisms resistant to the prescribed antibiotic therapy. A repeat LP should then be performed.

The commonest long term complication of meningitis is sensorineural deafness. This appears to develop early in the course of the disease and may occur in spite of early recognition and appropriate treatment. All children should undergo audiological assessment after recovery from infection. The overall rate of permanent deafness following meningitis may be less than 5% but is higher in cases of pneumococcal meningitis than in meningococcal infections. However, reversible hearing loss is seen in many more children, with reports of up to a third of children showing some impairment during the early phase of infection. In a study of morbidity after an episode of meningitis in infancy, almost a fifth of patients had some degree of disability.[56] This figure is higher if subtle defects are included, such as behavioral problems, middle ear disease and squints. Morbidity was highest following neonatal meningitis and also after meningitis caused by S. pneumoniae, group B streptococcus and atypical pathogens.

PREVENTION

Conjugate vaccines against H. influenzae type b (Hib), N. meningitidis group C and S. pneumoniae are now routinely given in the UK as part of the primary course of immunization and as a booster in the second year of life. An effective vaccine against N. meningitidis group B is not yet available.

When a child presents with meningococcal or Hib meningitis, other family members and close contacts are at increased risk of infection. Rifampicin (rifampin) is currently recommended for contacts of meningococcal disease (four doses of 10 mg/kg per dose 12 hourly) and H. influenzae type b (20 mg/kg per dose daily for 4 days). Decisions on who should receive prophylaxis can be difficult, and advice should be sought from the Consultant in Communicable Disease Control.

SEPTIC SHOCK

Despite the vast array of potential pathogens, the human host is remarkably resistant to life-threatening infection. Most pathogens are restricted by host defenses to their primary sites of invasion, with minimal clinical consequences. These first line defense mechanisms successfully intercept invading organisms in the majority of cases. On occasion, however, microbial invasion of the bloodstream can and does occur, even in apparently immunocompetent children, with potentially devastating consequences. The sequence of events following successful entry of microbes or microbial products to the circulation is complex, and depends both upon the virulent properties of the offending microorganism and the host response. Initial microbial invasion may be clinically silent and indeed may resolve without antimicrobial therapy. If, however, bacterial proliferation ensues, a systemic response is initiated in the host. This is referred to as the systemic inflammatory response syndrome (SIRS) and is defined by the presence of abnormalities in two or more of the following: temperature, heart rate, respiratory rate and white blood count, of which one must be temperature or white count. SIRS can follow any severe insult including infection, trauma, major surgery, burns or pancreatitis, but when SIRS occurs in the context of infection, the patient is described as septic.

The term severe sepsis can be used to describe a state characterized by hypoperfusion, hypotension and organ dysfunction, while the term septic shock is restricted to patients with persistent hypotension despite adequate fluid resuscitation and/or hypoperfusion even following adequate inotrope or pressor support.[57] In practice it can be difficult to divide patients neatly into these defined states, but the use of these terms serves to highlight the sequential nature of the events associated with microbial invasion, and will help in the evaluation of future clinical trials in septic patients.

MICROBIAL ETIOLOGY OF SEPSIS

In view of the multitude of potential pathogens with the capacity to cause disease, it is perhaps surprising that a very limited range of microorganisms is responsible for invasive infections in healthy children beyond the neonatal period. Three organisms predominate: Streptococcus pneumoniae, Neisseria meningitidis and Haemophilus influenzae type b.

The incidence of sepsis due to vaccine preventable organisms has been drastically reduced in countries with appropriate vaccination programs. However, even in these countries, otherwise healthy children who are not yet fully vaccinated, children in whom the vaccine has not provided adequate cover (vaccine failures), and children with infections caused by N. meningitidis group B continue to present with severe and life-threatening infections. Rarer causes of sepsis in healthy children include Staphylococcus aureus, group A, C and G streptococci and Salmonella spp., and these may be associated with wound and skin infections or a history of diarrhea respectively. In vulnerable patient groups other pathogens are implicated. In neonates, group B Streptococcus, Escherichia coli, other Gram negative bacteria, and Listeria monocytogenes are the usual causes of sepsis. In immunocompromised patients, Gram negative organisms such as Pseudomonas aeruginosa, and fungi may be responsible. Any patient with an indwelling catheter is particularly at risk of sepsis from coagulase negative staphylococci and enterococci as well as methicillin resistant Staphylococcus aureus (MRSA). With all of these organisms, the onset of bacteremia is a crucial event in the pathogenesis of sepsis, but invasion of the bloodstream is not necessary for bacteria to induce features of septic shock. Enterotoxins from staphylococci and streptococci are potent stimulators of T cell proliferation and activation, and can produce toxic shock syndromes even in patients with an apparently localized focus of infection. Some viruses, including herpes viruses, enteroviruses and adenoviruses, can produce diseases which may be indistinguishable clinically from bacterial sepsis, particularly in neonates and infants.

PATHOPHYSIOLOGY OF SEPSIS

Over the last three decades it has emerged that it is the host response to microbial invasion which is predominantly responsible for the clinical features of sepsis and septic shock. Lipopolysaccharides (LPS) from Gram negative bacteria, and a variety of other microbial products have the capacity to stimulate the production of mediators from many cells within the human host. Tumor necrosis factor, interleukin 1 and interleukin 6 are just a few of the many inflammatory mediators reported to be present at high levels in septic patients. It has now been established that families of pattern recognition receptors exist which are able to transduce cellular signals in response to microorganisms, including bacteria. One important family, the human Toll-like receptors (hTLR), consists of at least ten proteins, with hTLR4 acting as the principal mediator of LPS signaling, while other members of the family, such as hTLR1, hTLR2 and hTLR6, can mediate signals induced by lipoproteins of mycobacteria and Gram positive bacterial peptidoglycans. The cytokines and inflammatory mediators produced in response to microbial stimuli activate neutrophils, endothelial cells and monocytes and influence the function of vital organs, including the heart, liver, brain and kidneys. The net effect of excessive inflammatory activity is to cause the constellation of pathophysiological events seen in patients with sepsis and septic shock.

PRO- VERSUS ANTI-INFLAMMATORY MECHANISMS IN SEPSIS

The proinflammatory mediators produced in response to microbial invasion prime and activate cells to fight infection. However, the host also responds to proinflammatory stimuli by producing antagonists, known collectively as anti-inflammatory mediators. Interleukin 10 and soluble cytokine receptors or antagonists such as interleukin 1 receptor antagonist occur naturally and act to limit the effects of proinflammatory cytokines. The balance between pro- and anti-inflammatory mediators is probably more critical than the levels of either alone. Patients who survive the initial inflammatory insult, but who still require assisted ventilation and intravenous support, have high levels of anti-inflammatory mediators. These patients are resistant to further proinflammatory stimulation and may be more susceptible to nosocomial infections. Such patients may actually benefit from immune stimulation[58] to provoke the production of more inflammatory mediators, and the balance of pro- and anti-inflammation may prove crucial in therapeutic interventions. In the future, a clear characterization of the inflammatory status of septic patients may therefore be essential before adjuvant therapy is instituted (see below).

CLINICAL PRESENTATION AND DIAGNOSIS

The symptoms and signs of the initial phase of bacteremia are dependent upon the age and pre-existing health of the patient and the duration of the illness, as well as the causative organism. Bacteremia, with little inflammatory response, can be very difficult to diagnose clinically because of the overlap in clinical presentation with common viral illnesses. A number of clinical parameters have been examined to try to estimate the probability of bacterial rather than viral infection: children with a bacteremic illness are more likely to have a fever $> 39\,^{\circ}C$ and a white blood cell count (WBC) $> 15 \times 10^9/L$ or $< 2.5 \times 10^9/L$. However, the specificity and sensitivity of these parameters for diagnosing bacteremia is low and does not greatly add to the physician's general assessment of the child's condition.[59] Therefore frequent reassessment of the patient may be necessary if impending severe sepsis is to be recognized at an early stage. Nonspecific signs, including lethargy, irritability, hypotonia, poor feeding, nausea and vomiting, may be the earliest features of impending severe sepsis. Fever is not invariably present and hypothermia may also occur, particularly in neonates and infants. Cardiovascular involvement with tachycardia or bradycardia, inadequate peripheral perfusion, prolonged capillary refill, cold extremities, peripheral edema, decreased urine output and evidence of shock may all be manifest as the systemic response to bacterial invasion progresses. Respiratory, gastrointestinal and neurological derangement may indicate systemic disease or involvement of these specific organs in the infectious process. A petechial rash may be indicative of meningococcal disease, and in staphylococcal and streptococcal toxin-mediated shock, erythroderma, conjunctival and mucosal erythema and edema are usually present.

In all patients with suspected sepsis, blood cultures should be taken. The success of this procedure is dependent upon adequate blood inoculation of the culture media. If only a small volume of blood is available for culture, this should be added to the aerobic bottle, as few of the causative organisms will be anaerobes. Samples from potential sources of infection should be collected where appropriate. These include indwelling catheters, urine microscopy and culture, diagnostic radiology and aspiration for intra-abdominal sepsis, and lower respiratory tract secretions in ventilated patients, preferably by bronchoalveolar lavage. A lumbar puncture should be considered in patients with suspected meningeal involvement but is contraindicated in the presence of shock, coagulopathy, reduced conscious level or focal neurological signs. Samples can also be analyzed by molecular microbiological techniques for bacteria, fungi and viruses, although these investigations are not always routinely available. In patients with suspected toxic shock syndrome, analysis of staphylococcal and streptococcal isolates for the presence of toxin production and of V beta T cell receptor repertoires may be instructive. WBCs, high or low, and markers of inflammation including C-reactive protein (CRP), procalcitonin and proinflammatory cytokine levels may be useful. However, none of these investigations is specific or diagnostic. Coagulation studies, hemoglobin, urea and electrolytes, glucose and liver function tests should be performed to help inform further management and guide fluid and electrolyte replacement and general support.

MANAGEMENT OF SEPSIS
Recognition

Most cases of sepsis begin with the invasion of the bloodstream by a limited number of microbes. As the organisms multiply, often logarithmically, the host response intensifies and the condition of the patient deteriorates. The chances of a favorable outcome are greatly enhanced by initiating treatment at the earliest possible stage, so the most important aspect of sepsis management is the earliest possible recognition of the condition. In view of the diagnostic difficulties described above, it is imperative that otherwise healthy children presenting with nonspecific features are observed carefully. Even if a health care professional considers the risk of impending sepsis to be low and the patient well enough to be at home, a detailed plan of management should be discussed with the family. The parents or guardians should have a clear understanding of the clinical features to observe and what actions to take if there is deterioration or failure to improve and a plan agreed for the clinician to review the child's condition. In patients at increased risk of bacteremia, such as neonates, immunocompromised children and children with neutropenia or sickle cell disease, there should be a low threshold for initiating antimicrobial therapy.

Antimicrobial therapy

The choice of antibiotics is dependent upon the most likely pathogens and the particular antibiotic resistance patterns of the community or hospital. In otherwise healthy children without an obvious source, a third generation cephalosporin such as cefotaxime or ceftriaxone is appropriate. The emergence of antibiotic resistance precludes penicillin as adequate initial therapy. In more vulnerable populations, other considerations apply. For example, in neonates, a third generation cephalosporin is frequently used together with ampicillin to treat *Listeria monocytogenes*, sometimes with the addition of an aminoglycoside for additional Gram negative bacterial cover.

Immunocompromised patients are vulnerable to infection with a wider spectrum of pathogens. Children with B cell and antibody deficiencies or with reduced or absent splenic function are at increased risk from encapsulated bacterial infections. Neutropenic patients are particularly susceptible to staphylococcal and Gram negative bacteria including pseudomonal infections. A combination of an antipseudomonal penicillin (e.g. piptazobactam) with an aminoglycoside (e.g. gentamicin) is usually prescribed for this population. However, a glycopeptide (e.g. vancomycin) and antifungal therapy may be required if initial therapy fails to control the infection. Patients with sickle cell disease are at risk of salmonella septicemia and may require treatment with ciprofloxacin. In patients with staphylococcal toxic shock syndrome, treatment with antistaphylococcal therapy is advisable, even though the total number of bacteria may be small. These are general guidelines, and advice about local antimicrobial prescribing policies should always be sought.

Subsequent management

The details of the emergency treatment of shock are covered in Chapter 36. Children will usually require transfer to a pediatric intensive care unit. Hypovolemia is invariably present due to fluid maldistribution, which occurs as a result of the release of vasoactive mediators by host inflammatory and endothelial cells. The loss of circulating volume is compounded by a loss of intravascular proteins and fluid due to endothelial dysfunction (capillary leak). Continuous monitoring of central venous pressure and urine output is required to guide fluid replacement. Large volumes of plasma or blood are normally required, and mechanical ventilation may be necessary to manage capillary leakage of fluid into the lungs.[60] The net effect of the host response to infection frequently leads to myocardial depression, necessitating the use of inotropic support. Severe peripheral vasodilatation compounds hypotension, and vasopressors may be required. Dysregulation of the coagulation and thrombotic pathways leads to widespread microvascular thrombosis and consumption of clotting factors. Treatment of disseminated intravascular coagulation (DIC) is largely symptomatic, with administration of fresh frozen plasma and platelets if bleeding occurs. While administration of antibiotics will prevent further bacterial proliferation, the concentration of microbial components such as LPS and outer membrane proteins may persist for some time. These will continue to cause inflammation and further deterioration in the patient's condition. Continuous reassessment and adjustment of supportive therapy is therefore required to optimize further management.

Adjuvant therapy

The recognition that much of the pathology seen in sepsis is due to host-derived mediators has led to the development of numerous antagonists to offending bacterial and host components. Initial attempts to reduce the inflammatory response in sepsis used steroids. However, high doses of methylprednisolone were found to be detrimental in sepsis, and as a result routine use of high dose steroids in sepsis was abandoned. More recent data have shown that physiological doses of glucocorticoids may shorten the duration of shock and improve survival rates.[61] More selective agents have been developed, including antagonists of tumor necrosis factor, interleukin 1, platelet activating factor and endotoxin. None of these has proved to be beneficial in large clinical trials. However, it is too early to discard these new forms of treatment, since a clearer understanding of the sequence of events in sepsis may identify subgroups of patients who might benefit from these interventions.

The use of high doses of intravenous immunoglobulin may be beneficial in toxic shock syndromes and may be useful in other septic populations.[62] There is also evidence that administration of activated protein C (APC) can reduce mortality in adults with sepsis-induced organ failure.[63] This suggests that downstream inflammatory pathways, such as the protein C anticoagulation pathway, critical in thrombosis and hemostasis, may present potential targets for future interventions. However, in a trial of APC in children, no beneficial effect was observed. Perhaps the most important recent development in critical illness concerns the modulation of endocrine pathways. The administration of growth hormone to critically ill adults was found to significantly increase mortality, whilst low doses of steroids and tight glycemic control appear to be advantageous.[64] The role of the endocrine axis in children with sepsis is still unclear but is currently under investigation.

CONGENITAL AND NEONATAL INFECTIONS

SPECIFIC INFECTIONS
Congenital rubella

The association between rubella infection during pregnancy and congenital cataracts in the newborn was first made by an Australian ophthalmologist, Norman Gregg, in 1941.[65] The introduction of effective rubella vaccination programs has made congenital rubella syndrome (CRS) an uncommon disorder in resource rich countries such as the UK. Falling vaccine coverage and immigration of nonvaccinated women was the likely cause of a small resurgence in the number of reported cases of CRS over the period 1996–2000.[66,67]

Both the risk of fetal infection and the risk of sequelae vary with the gestation when maternal infection occurs. Transmission of the virus to the fetus occurs in 90% in the first 11 weeks, 50% from 11 to 20 weeks' gestation, 37% from 20 to 35 weeks, and 100% during the last month of pregnancy.[68] However, the risk of serious sequelae to the fetus after confirmed maternal rubella infection is greatest in early pregnancy, being 90% if infected <11 weeks, 30% at 12–20 weeks and none thereafter, aside from some mild growth retardation.[68] The majority of infants with congenital rubella disease result from primary maternal rubella infection, although maternal reinfection may rarely result in an infant with anomalies.[69]

Clinical manifestation

The common manifestations of congenital rubella infection are shown in Table 28.15. Important clinical manifestations are disorders of the eye (microphthalmia, cataract, congenital glaucoma, retinitis), congenital

Table 28.15 Clinical features of rubella, cytomegalovirus and toxoplasmosis

	Cytomegalovirus	Rubella	Toxoplasmosis
CNS			
Hydrocephaly	+	–	+++
Microcephaly	+	+++	–
Calcification	+++	+	++
Deafness	++	+++	++
Encephalitis	–	–	+
Eyes			
Microphthalmia	+	+	+++
Cataracts	–	++	+
Chorioretinitis*	+	+	+++
Intrauterine growth retardation	+	+++	+
Cardiac lesion	–	++	+
Purpuric rash	++	+++	–
Pneumonia	+++	++	++
Hepatosplenomegaly	++	+++	++++
Lymphadenopathy	–	–	+
Bony lesion	+	+++	–

*The choroidoretinitis caused by *Toxoplasma gondii* and *Treponema pallidum* has been confused with the Aicardi syndrome, in which the lesions are always bilateral, rarely peripheral, and lack pigments, in contrast to that due to these two organisms.
Infecting organisms are listed alphabetically and not in order of likelihood.

heart disease (patent ductus arteriosus, peripheral pulmonary artery stenosis), and neurological sequelae (mental retardation, behavioral disorders, meningoencephalitis, convulsions). There may also be intrauterine growth retardation, microcephaly, thrombocytopenia, hepatosplenomegaly, purpuric skin lesions, pneumonitis and linear bone lesions. Only 68% of infected infants show signs at birth and up to 20% of these may die in infancy. A number of manifestations, however, present much later in life. These include hearing loss 87%, congenital heart disease 46–60%, mental or psychomotor retardation 30–50%, cataract or glaucoma 30–40%, diabetes mellitus and thyroid dysfunction.

Diagnosis

Virus isolation, either from nasopharyngeal washing, urine or cerebrospinal fluid (CSF) is the most direct method of diagnosis, but may take many weeks. A positive rubella-specific immunoglobulin M (IgM) in a neonate and/or the detection of rubella RNA in urine or nasopharyngeal secretions by polymerase chain reaction (PCR) usually indicates recent postnatal or congenital infection, although false positive results do occur. A number of sensitive immunoassays are available for the detection of rubella-specific IgG. Rising or persistently stable levels of IgG from the newborn period to beyond 9 months of age confirm perinatal or congenital infection.

Management

There is no specific treatment for rubella infection. In countries where routine rubella vaccination has been used, the infection rate has been considerably reduced. Seronegative women of childbearing age should be offered vaccination either after a pregnancy test or immediately postpartum. Rubella immunization of 13-year-old girls, which started in the UK in 1970, reduced the incidence considerably and the use of the measles, mumps and rubella (MMR) vaccine in the UK from 1988 has made congenital rubella rare.[66] Most new reports of congenital rubella in the UK are of infants born to mothers who were themselves born abroad and came to the UK after the age of schoolgirl immunization. In 2004, the World Health Organization adopted a strategy to improve global control of rubella and CRS by 2010 by increasing vaccination coverage of women of childbearing age using the combined measles–rubella vaccine, and by improving surveillance for CRS.[70,71]

Cytomegalovirus (CMV)

Cytomegalovirus (CMV) infection is the most common congenital infection in Europe with a prevalence of 3–4 per 1000 births. CMV is a member of the herpes virus family and, as such, establishes a latent infection after the initial infection and reactivates, especially under states of altered cellular immunity. It is ubiquitous in the community, although not highly infectious. It may be transmitted transplacentally or through genital secretions, saliva, breast milk or blood transfusion.

About 50% of women of childbearing age in the UK remain susceptible to CMV infection and 1% of those susceptible at the beginning of pregnancy will have a primary infection during pregnancy. Like rubella, the greatest risk of fetal damage occurs after primary maternal infection. In about 50% of primary infections of the mother, the fetus will be infected, but only 10% of these infants will display symptoms at birth or through childhood. After a recurrent maternal CMV infection, there is a low risk of transmission to the infant ($\leq 1\%$), with an equally low risk of sequelae.[72] However, some cases of infants with severe, symptomatic congenital CMV disease due to either maternal reinfection with a new CMV strain or reactivation of latent CMV infection during pregnancy have been reported.[73] Unlike rubella, fetal damage may follow primary infection or recurrent infection at any stage of pregnancy.

Clinical manifestations

The majority of infants with congenital CMV infection are asymptomatic. When symptomatic, the main clinical features are as shown in Table 28.16. The risk of neurological sequelae and intrauterine growth retardation in the fetus is greatest after infection in the first 20 weeks of pregnancy, but infants of mothers with pre-existing immunity to CMV can have clinical sequelae.[74] Such effects include microcephaly, chorioretinitis, mental retardation, sensorineural hearing loss and intracerebral periventricular calcification. Infection in the second half of pregnancy usually results in visceral disease such as hepatitis, purpura, hyperbilirubinemia and thrombocytopenia. Other effects include dental abnormalities and inguinal hernias. Pneumonitis is a common feature of postnatally acquired CMV infection, especially in the premature infant, but rarely follows true congenital infection. Those infants who have symptoms in the newborn period nearly always have subsequent handicap. The presence of microcephaly at birth is the strongest predictor of poor cognitive outcome in later life.[75] Of the infected infants who are asymptomatic at birth, up to 10% will have CMV-related problems by 3 years of age, the most common problem being sensorineural hearing loss.[76,77] High CMV viral blood load (10^4 viral DNA copies per 10^5 poly-morphonuclear leukocytes) in the newborn has recently been identified as a strong predictor for adverse long term clinical sequelae.[78]

Perinatal CMV infection

Many infants acquire CMV infection through breast-feeding or by contact with other infected secretions in the first weeks of life or, in hospitalized babies, through blood products. This usually results in an asymptomatic infection. The exception is premature infants, especially those with extremely low birth weight, or infants with cellular immunodeficiency in whom CMV infection may result in pneumonitis, hepatitis, thrombocytopenia, neutropenia and, uncommonly, gastroenteritis. In general, postnatal CMV infection does not result in long term sequelae, with the possible exception of babies less than 2000 g.[79]

Diagnosis

Diagnosis is based on isolation of the virus in throat washings or urine or by detection of CMV DNA in these specimens by PCR. Cultures must be obtained within the first 3 weeks of life to distinguish congenital CMV infection from perinatally acquired infection. Demonstration of CMV-specific IgM antibody in neonatal serum is also suggestive of congenital infection, but it can only be detected in about 70% of infected newborns. Later in infancy, in the absence of clinical signs suggestive of congenital infection, laboratory methods alone will not make the distinction between CMV acquired during intrauterine life and postnatal infection. Retrospective diagnosis of congenital CMV infection can be made by detection of CMV DNA in dried blood on the filter paper from newborn screening cards.

Treatment and prevention

Ganciclovir therapy may be used to treat some congenitally infected infants with life-threatening CMV-related organ disease or retinitis involving the macula. Work is in progress towards production of a vaccine. Intravenous ganciclovir has also been used in a series of small clinical trials to try to reduce the risk and extent of central nervous system damage after symptomatic congenital CMV infection.[80,81] However, no firm conclusions about the efficacy of this treatment could be drawn due to the small sample sizes, and until more efficacy data are available it is not routinely recommended. Some groups nevertheless recommend ganciclovir therapy for infants with signs of disseminated disease without severe hearing loss [≥ 100 dB by brainstem auditory evoked response (BAER)] due to the high risk of late progression,[82] and others prescribe prolonged therapy with oral valaganciclovir.[83] However, there is a lack of clinical trial data to support these opinions.

Table 28.16   Lesions that may be caused by prenatally acquired viral infections

Pathogen	Clinical sequelae
1. Coxsackie virus	Abortion, mild febrile disease, rash, meningitis, hepatitis, gastroenteritis, myocarditis, congenital heart disease and neurological deficits
2. Cytomegalovirus	Microcephaly, hydrocephaly, microphthalmia, retinopathy, cerebral calcification, deafness, psychomotor retardation, anemia, thrombocytopenia, hepatosplenomegaly, jaundice and encephalopathy
3. ECHO virus	Same as coxsackie virus
4. Hepatitis B virus	Low birth weight, asymptomatic hepatitis carrier, acute hepatitis, chronic hepatitis
5. Herpes simplex virus	Abortion, microcephaly, cerebral calcification, retinopathy, encephalitis, multiple organ involvement
6. Human immunodeficiency virus	Abortion, hydro/microcephaly, limb deformities, intrauterine growth retardation, failure to thrive, rash, hepatosplenomegaly, pneumonia
7. Influenza virus	Abortion
8. Measles virus	Abortion, congenital measles
9. Polio virus	Abortion, congenital poliomyelitis with paralysis
10. Rubella virus	Abortion, microcephaly, cataract, microphthalmia, congenital heart disease, deafness, low birth weight, hepatosplenomegaly, petechiae, osteitis
11. Vaccinia virus	Abortion, congenital vaccinia
12. Varicella-zoster virus	Abortion, limb, cerebral and skin malformation
	Stillbirth, low birth weight, chorioretinitis, congenital chickenpox, or disseminated neonatal varicella or zoster
13. Variola virus	Abortion, congenital variola

In alphabetical order and not in order of frequency or seriousness.

CMV is spread by intimate contact with infected secretions. Pregnant caregivers and hospital personnel should employ careful hand washing after exposure to the secretions of a CMV-infected infant. Passive immunotherapy with CMV hyperimmune globulin of women with primary CMV infection during early pregnancy has been shown in an open labeled phase I trial to be safe and possibly effective at reducing transmission to and sequelae in the offspring.[84] Results have yet to be confirmed in a randomized clinical trial.

Varicella-zoster (chickenpox)
Congenital infection
Maternal varicella-zoster infection during the first 20 weeks of pregnancy may result in spontaneous abortion or fetal death in utero, or in an embryopathy characterized by dermatomal skin scarring and limb hypoplasia. There may also be disorders of the central nervous system (microcephaly, cortical atrophy) and eyes (cataracts, chorioretinitis), of the gastrointestinal tract and of the genitourinary tract. It is hypothesized that the damage results from in utero reactivation of varicella-zoster virus (VZV) or disseminated fetal infection.

Maternal infection in the second half of pregnancy may result in an asymptomatic primary fetal infection followed by herpes zoster in the first years of life in about 1% of exposed infants. A large prospective study from the UK and Germany of the effects of maternal VZV infection in pregnancy estimated the overall risk of embryopathy during the first 20 weeks of pregnancy to be 1%, with the highest risk of transmission of 2% being in the period 13–20 weeks.[85] Occasional cases resulting from maternal infection at 23 weeks have been reported.[86] Administration of varicella-zoster immunoglobulin (V-ZIG) to the mother may modify the course of chickenpox, but it has not been shown to alter the risk of transmission to the fetus.[87]

Perinatal infection
Maternal varicella that occurs in the period 5 days before delivery to 2 days after delivery may result in life-threatening, disseminated VZV infection in the infant due to transplacental passage of the virus in the absence of maternal antibody. If the onset of maternal infection is more than 7 days prior to delivery, there is usually sufficient passive transfer of antibody, unless the infant is less than 28 weeks' gestation. Administration of V-ZIG to the infant has been shown to prevent or modify the course of the illness in most cases. However, as a significant number of infants will develop systemic VZV despite the administration of V-ZIG,[88] all infants with perinatal VZV exposure should be monitored closely for systemic disease, with prompt initiation of intravenous aciclovir should vesicles appear. Hospitalized infants with chickenpox should be placed in respiratory and contact isolation until the lesions have crusted, but breast-feeding can continue.

Herpes simplex virus (HSV)
Neonatal HSV infection carries a high mortality if untreated. The incidence of disease ranges from 1:2500 live births in some parts of the USA[89] to 1:60000 live births in the UK.[90] In the past, up to 75% of cases of neonatal infection were due to HSV type 2 and the rest due to type 1. More recently, the proportion of cases due to neonatal HSV-1 infection is increasing in the UK and elsewhere around the world, possibly due to an increase in genital HSV-1 disease.[90] The infection is acquired from passage through an infected birth canal in 85% of cases, and is postnatally acquired from the oral lesions of an infected caregiver in 10–15% of cases. A true congenital syndrome is seen in < 5% of cases. The greatest risk for transmission (about 50%) is from a primary maternal infection when there has been insufficient time for seroconversion and transplacental transfer of antibody.[91] If a woman with a recurrent infection is shedding virus at delivery, the risk may be 5% or less. Cesarean delivery is not completely effective in preventing transmission to the infant.

Clinical manifestations
Neonatal HSV disease may manifest as lesions localized to the skin, eye or mouth (SEM), as encephalitis, as pneumonitis or as a disseminated multiorgan infection with or without central nervous system involvement.

The age of presentation varies with the category of disease. In general, neonatal HSV disease usually presents in the first 3 weeks of life, but it may manifest at any time from day 1 to 4 weeks of life. About 50% of cases now present as SEM disease, possibly due to better awareness of the condition. The typical vesicular, ulcerative lesion usually occurs on the presenting part. Up to 70% of SEM disease will spread to the central nervous system or elsewhere without treatment, but is rarely fatal. Infants with SEM disease have 10% long term morbidity, with higher rates seen if there are frequent cutaneous recurrences in early life.

The disseminated form typically commences at about 1 week of age with a shock-like syndrome in the absence of positive bacterial cultures with thrombocytopenia, disseminated intravascular coagulation, hepatitis, jaundice, and sometimes encephalitis and seizures. Skin lesions appear in 50% of these cases. Disseminated HSV infection may also present as an interstitial pneumonitis, usually presenting about day 3 of life. The mortality in this group is as high as 50% even with treatment, and over half of the survivors are left with long term sequelae (mental retardation, blindness, seizures, learning defects). The third group presents with central nervous system symptoms such as poor feeding, apnea, lethargy and seizures without visceral involvement, typically in the second to third week of life. It has been hypothesized that this group represents reactivation of an earlier asymptomatic infection. They have a 15% mortality, with severe long term central nervous system effects seen in 65%.[92]

Congenital infection
Intrauterine HSV infection may manifest as the presence of vesicles or scarring at birth, chorioretinitis, microphthalmia, microcephaly, hydranencephaly or cerebral atrophy on CT scan in the first week of life, organ calcification or organomegaly. The majority of reported cases are due to HSV-2. There is a high rate of early neonatal death and long term central nervous system sequelae.

Diagnosis
If neonatal HSV disease is suspected, viral swabs of skin vesicles, eyes, nasopharynx and rectum should be sent for HSV culture and immunofluorescence or HSV PCR, CSF collected for routine examination, HSV PCR and culture, blood sent for liver function tests, platelet count and coagulation screen, and empirical therapy with systemic intravenous aciclovir promptly commenced. A chest radiograph may be indicated if respiratory distress is present. Imaging of the head by ultrasound or CT scan should be performed. Serologic assays are usually not helpful in the acute diagnosis of neonatal HSV disease.

Treatment and prevention
Mothers with primary lesions should be delivered electively by Cesarean section while mothers with recurrent lesions, if they have a negative culture and do not have lesions or prodrome of infection, may be delivered vaginally. The use of invasive fetal monitoring and vacuum delivery should be avoided where possible in women with known genital HSV disease. Some suggest that the infant should be screened for infection by surface viral swabs at 48 h of life.

Aciclovir 60 mg/kg/d in three divided doses given intravenously should be commenced as soon as neonatal HSV disease is suspected. Many suggest it should be commenced empirically in the offspring of women with known primary genital HSV infection due to the high attack rate. The duration of therapy is 14 days for SEM disease and 21 days for all other categories or where a lumbar puncture could not be performed.[93] Topical therapy may be given in addition to systemic therapy for HSV eye disease under the direction of an ophthalmologist. The prognostic significance of persistence of HSV DNA at the end of therapy is currently under evaluation.

Prevention of neonatal HSV disease demands a vaccine to prevent maternal infection and/or reactivation. Recently a recombinant HSV type 2 glycoprotein subunit vaccine has been shown to be partly effective at reducing the risk of infection and development of clinical disease in women without prior immunity to HSV types 1 or 2.[94] Its efficacy is currently being evaluated in HSV-1 seronegative girls prior to the onset of sexual activity.[95] Other prevention strategies include the use of an oral antiviral in late pregnancy in women with primary HSV infection during pregnancy or in HSV-seropositive women with frequent clinical recurrences in the genital area.[96]

The shock-like syndrome associated with the disseminated form of neonatal HSV disease has been associated with signaling through Toll-like receptor (TLR)-2,[97] raising the possibility that future therapeutic strategies for this condition may target TLR signaling pathways.

PARASITIC INFECTIONS

Toxoplasmosis

Toxoplasmosis is a worldwide disease. In the UK between 20 and 40% of the population have been infected with this protozoan by adult life. The incidence of congenital toxoplasmosis in Europe is 1–10 in 10 000 newborns.[98,99]

Congenital toxoplasmosis infection usually occurs as a result of placental infection after a primary infection in a pregnant woman. Parasites form small focal lesions in the placenta, proliferate and are released as active forms into the fetal bloodstream. Rare cases of fetal transmission have been reported after preconception maternal infection in immunocompetent women,[100] presumably due to myometrial infection. It is generally accepted that women who bear a congenitally infected child do not have infected children in subsequent pregnancies, probably owing to persistence of immunity after the primary infection. Exceptions to this rule do occur, and it is suggested that the persistence of *Toxoplasma gondii* as cysts in the myometrium with liberation of active forms during pregnancy is one of the main infectious causes of repeated abortion in women. Congenital toxoplasmosis has been reported following reactivation in women with HIV infection, although it is a rare event as shown by a European Collaborative Study.[101]

The risk of transmission and the clinical outcome after maternal toxoplasmosis infection vary with the trimester of pregnancy. Recently, up-to-date risk estimates of maternal transmission of toxoplasmosis during pregnancy have come from a large study of women with confirmed infection who were referred to a toxoplasmosis reference laboratory in France.[98] Infection in early pregnancy carried a low risk of transmission; this rose to 6% by 13 weeks, thereafter rising sharply to 40% at 26 weeks, and 72% at 36 weeks. If a fetus is infected, the risk of developing clinical signs (and the severity of disease) is greatest the earlier in pregnancy the infection occurs, falling from 61% at 13 weeks, to 25% at 26 weeks, to 9% at 36 weeks.[98]

Clinical manifestations

Infection of the fetus with virulent strains early in pregnancy may produce fetal death and abortion; still later, severe fetal damage or stillbirth; and later still, a liveborn infant with stigmata of congenital toxoplasmosis. However, up to 70% of infants with congenital toxoplasmosis are asymptomatic at birth. The most common single presenting feature is chorioretinitis and both eyes are involved in 40% of cases. Other important clinical features are given in Table 28.15. They include hydrocephalus, intracranial calcification, hepatosplenomegaly, jaundice, thrombocytopenia and a maculopapular rash. Clinical sequelae of congenital infection, including visual disturbance, seizures and mental retardation, may not manifest until later in life. A recent long term follow-up study of visual sequelae from congenital toxoplasmosis infection has confirmed that late onset retinal lesions and relapse in existing visual lesions can occur many years after birth. The prognosis for patients with central nervous system involvement must be extremely guarded.

Diagnosis

This is usually based on *Toxoplasma* IgM and/or *Toxoplasma* IgA antibody test. The sensitivity of the IgM-ISAGA test is probably the highest. Persistently elevated *Toxoplasma* IgG beyond 12 months of life, and detection of *Toxoplasma* DNA by PCR in the placenta, neonatal blood or CSF may also be used to make the diagnosis. In the infant with suspected congenital toxoplasmosis, ophthalmological examination, hearing assessment and central nervous system examination and imaging should also be performed.

Treatment

Infants diagnosed with symptomatic or asymptomatic congenital toxoplasmosis infection should be treated to reduce the incidence of long term sequelae such as chorioretinitis. Two synergistic antimicrobials, either sulfadimidine or sulfadiazine together with pyrimethamine, are used in various combinations. Prolonged treatment for up 12 months is required to reduce the risk of late reactivation in the eye.[102] Corticosteroids should be used in the presence of chorioretinitis or raised CSF protein. Many advise treatment of pregnant women with primary toxoplasmosis. A recent systematic review suggests that there are still insufficient data on whether this treatment is effective in preventing neonatal infection.[103]

Pregnant women should be educated to avoid ingestion of *Toxoplasma* cysts by adequate cooking of meat, washing of garden produce, and washing hands after contact with soil.

ENTEROVIRUSES (NON-POLIO)

Intrauterine, perinatal and postnatal transmission of enteroviruses [coxsackie viruses group A and B, enteric cytopathogenic human orphan (ECHO) viruses, enteroviruses 68–71] has been documented, although there are no data available on the risks of transmission to the fetus or of sequelae should this occur. While maternal enterovirus infection during pregnancy has not been conclusively proven to cause an embryopathy, there have been links between some specific maternal enteroviral infections and anomalies in the infant (coxsackie B virus infection with urogenital anomalies, coxsackie B3 and B4 viruses with cardiac anomalies, coxsackie A9 with digestive anomalies).

Perinatal enteroviral infections generally cause asymptomatic infection or mild, nonspecific illness, particularly if the baby acquires infection 'horizontally' from other babies. However, if a woman is infected just before or after delivery, severe disease may develop in the 'vertically' infected newborn, in the first week after birth. The mother may present with severe abdominal pain mimicking abruption, or with respiratory or gastrointestinal symptoms. The baby may present with one or more of the following: a sepsis-like syndrome [fever or hypothermia, anorexia, vomiting, lethargy, disseminated intravascular coagulation (DIC)], gastrointestinal (vomiting, diarrhea, fulminant hepatitis, pancreatitis), neurological (aseptic meningitis, encephalitis or paralysis), respiratory (pneumonitis, pharyngitis, laryngotracheobronchitis), skin or mucosal manifestations (erythematous, maculopapular rash, herpangina, hemorrhagic conjunctivitis) or cardiac disease (myocarditis, pericarditis). Some specific enteroviruses are associated with particular syndromes (see Enteroviruses). Severe ECHO virus infections are more likely to cause hepatitis with massive hepatic necrosis, DIC and death, while coxsackie viruses are more likely to cause myocarditis and meningitis. Neonatal outbreaks of enterovirus 71 (EV 71) have recently been associated with neurological manifestations such as encephalitis, Guillain–Barré syndrome and neurogenic pulmonary edema.[104,105]

Diagnosis

Enteroviruses may be cultured from the nasopharynx, throat swab or feces. Serology is rarely helpful due to poor sensitivity. Detection of enterovirus nucleic acid in the CSF by PCR can be useful in the diagnosis of enteroviral meningitis.

Treatment

The antiviral agent pleconaril has been shown to have in vitro activity against a number of enteroviruses, but not EV 71.[106] In a small case series, treatment of severe neonatal enterovirus infection with oral pleconaril was associated with both virological and clinical improvement, but the sample size was too small to determine if this outcome was significant. Intravenous immunoglobulin has also been used to treat life-threatening disease, but its efficacy is unproven for this use.

HOSPITAL INFECTION CONTROL

Nosocomial infections are defined as infections acquired by hospitalized patients which were not present or incubating at the time of their hospital admission.[107] Infection control developed as a formal discipline during the 1950s and 1960s primarily as a response to nosocomial staphylococcal infections. Today infection control, enhanced by the application of epidemiological methods and the use of statistical analysis, has a major role in identifying and analyzing adverse outcomes in the health care setting. The central role of an infection control program is to reduce the risk of nosocomial infection with resulting protection of patients, health care workers, students and visitors.

All hospitals should have in place a multidisciplinary infection control committee with members who are interested and knowledgeable in infection and infection control and represent areas of the hospital where infection is either a potential problem or are involved in controlling these infections. The infection control committee must have the delegated authority of the hospital executive to efficiently and tactfully implement actions to control infection. It is recommended that the committee should consist of a medical microbiologist, medical virologist, infection control practitioner and an infectious disease physician and, in addition, personnel from medical and nursing and administration as well as pharmacy, operating theaters, housekeeping, engineering and maintenance. Ideally the chair of the committee should have expertise in hospital epidemiology and infection control.

Nosocomial infections are predominantly transmitted via contact, primarily by the contaminated hands of health care workers who have touched a colonized patient or something in the patient's environment. Hand washing with soap and water remains the single most important method in the prevention of nosocomial infections, but numerous studies have shown that hand washing compliance by health care workers is poor and often less than 50%. To improve the situation, there has been a recent increase in use of alcohol-based hand antiseptics. The application of these alcohol-based hand antiseptics, a process called hand hygiene, kills bacteria (except *Clostridium difficile*) very rapidly. Hand hygiene takes much less time than traditional hand washing and is gentler on the skin of the hands than repeated use of soap and water. In addition, hand lotions and moisturizers should be available to health care workers to decrease skin irritation which may result from frequent hand washing and hand hygiene.[108]

Isolation of patients is done to prevent the spread of microorganisms from infected or colonized patients to other patients or health care workers, thus interrupting transmission. The current isolation guidelines are based on our understanding of the mechanisms of disease transmission. There is essentially a two-tiered approach to isolation. The first is the use of **standard precautions**, the basis of infection control, which applies to all patients. The second approach is **transmission-based precautions**, contact, droplet and aerosol, which apply to patients with documented or suspected infections (see Table 28.17).

Standard precautions involve hand washing before patient contact and after leaving the patient's environment. In addition, personal protective equipment, masks, gowns, gloves and eye protection, provides a barrier to reduce the opportunities for transmission of infectious agents if there is contact with body fluids. A fluid resistant gown or apron made with impervious material, fluid repellent mask or face shield and protective eyeware should be worn when performing any procedure where there is the likelihood of splashing or spreading of blood or other body substances.[109] Gloves are worn as a barrier to protect the health care worker's hands from contamination and prevent the transfer of microorganisms. The type of gloves selected should be appropriate to the type of risk of the procedure. Sterile gloves are worn if the procedure involves contact with tissues that would be sterile under normal circumstances. Medical examination gloves, which are clean but not sterile, are used in all procedures that may involve direct skin or mucous membrane contact with blood or fluids capable of transmitting blood-borne pathogens. General purpose gloves are used for housekeeping activities and cleaning instruments. The gloves must be changed and discarded as soon as they are torn or punctured, after contact with an individual is completed and before care is

Table 28.17   Isolation and types of precautions

Isolation precautions	Requirements	Examples of infections
Standard	Hand washing before and after patient contact Personal protective equipment (PPE): Gloves, gown and mask should be worn by staff when touching or handling blood or body substances Hands must be washed before attending patients and after removal of gloves	All patients require standard precautions
Contact	Standard precautions plus: Single room if possible and cohorting of patients with like illness if possible	Respiratory syncytial virus Rotavirus Impetigo Herpes zoster (shingles) Hepatitis A Methicillin-resistant *S. aureus* (MRSA) Extended-spectrum beta-lactamase (ESBL) positive Enterobacteriaceae Carbapenem-resistant *Acinetobacter baumannii*
Droplet	Contact precautions plus: Use of a mask if within 1 meter of the patient The room door must remain closed	Influenza virus Adenovirus *N. meningitidis* (invasive) *B. pertussis*
Airborne	Droplet precautions plus: Single negative pressure room with 6–12 air changes per hour	Measles Chickenpox Tuberculosis

provided to another individual or when performing separate procedures on the same patient where there is a risk of transmitting infection from one part of the body to the other. It should be emphasized that hands must be washed and cleaned after the removal and disposal of gloves.

Health care workers are susceptible to infectious diseases and may therefore be infected by, or transmit infection to, patients. It is therefore strongly recommended that health care workers working in clinical areas be protected against those infectious diseases where vaccination is possible. It is recommended that health care workers be vaccinated against diphtheria, tetanus, pertussis, measles, mumps, rubella, varicella, influenza and hepatitis B.[109] Other vaccinations such as meningococcal, typhoid and hepatitis A virus vaccines may be indicated in special circumstances.[110]

The potential transmission of blood-borne diseases is greatest where a needle, scalpel blade or other sharp instrument is used. All health care workers are responsible for the management and disposal of the sharps they have used and should take care to ensure they are disposed of in a safe manner. Particular care should be taken in removing disposable scalpel blades from scalpel handles. In addition, needles should not be removed from disposable syringes and should not be purposefully bent or broken. Needles should not be re-sheathed after use, if possible. All sharps should be disposed of immediately after use into a sharps container which is puncture resistant and waterproof.[111]

It is generally agreed that antimicrobial resistance is driven by antibiotic use, and excessive and unnecessary use of antimicrobials can be expected to increase the prevalence of resistant microorganisms. Infection of patients with multiresistant organisms leads to increased morbidity and mortality as well as increased financial costs. All health care institutions need to develop policies for the control of antimicrobial use by developing guidelines and authorization for their use in specific situations. Advice from the medical microbiologist or infectious diseases physician may assist general clinicians in more appropriate selection of antimicrobial agents.[112]

Routine surveillance for selected pathogens may be a method to assess the efficacy of infection control policy and procedures and determine if an outbreak occurs. A nosocomial infection outbreak may be described as an epidemic, or an increase above normal of the expected level of an infection in the clinical setting. The main goal of managing an outbreak is to prevent a further increase in the incidence of health care associated infection by identifying factors which may have contributed to the outbreak. This also allows for the development and implementation of measures to prevent future outbreaks. General management of an outbreak involves first determining a case definition and, second, confirming an increase in cases by the infectious agent above the background rate. It is then necessary to collect information regarding cases as descriptive epidemiology to determine if there are any recognized modes of transmission.[113] Implementation of appropriate infection control measures as described in Table 28.17 should be undertaken to contain the outbreak.

Managing infection control in a pediatric hospital presents some unique challenges. Young children usually have poor personal hygiene and require significant adult supervision to ensure this practice. They are also mobile and quite impulsive and may require isolation to prevent contact spread of infecting organisms to other patients. Isolation of small children can often distress them and it is essential to provide adequate supervision for their safety and suitable age-related activities to relieve their distress.

BACTERIAL INFECTIONS

THE USE OF THE BACTERIOLOGY LABORATORY BY THE PEDIATRICIAN

A proficient and well managed microbiology laboratory is essential for any health care institution.[114] Pivotal to the function of the microbiology laboratory is excellent communication between the physician and the laboratory personnel. After considering the clinical and epidemiological circumstances of the patient infection, the physician must collect appropriate samples for culture. Ideally specimens should be obtained directly from the site of infection before commencement of antibiotic therapy. However, this may not always be possible in patients who are critically ill, when antimicrobial therapy may need to start immediately. It is critical that all specimens submitted to the laboratory be correctly collected, labeled and transported as well as being of sufficient quality and quantity for adequate microbiological testing. They should be submitted promptly to the laboratory along with all relevant clinical and epidemiological data to assist the laboratory in selection of appropriate testing protocols.

DIRECT MICROSCOPY

Gram stain is one of the most useful and rapid diagnostic tests offered by the microbiology laboratory. It can be performed on exudates, tissue smears, fluids and aspirates to detect bacteria and fungal elements. In addition to bacteria, the presence and type of inflammatory cells is also detected. Information about bacterial morphology, i.e. cocci or rods, and the staining appearance, Gram positive or Gram negative, can give important preliminary information about the possible genus of the infecting microorganism and thus guide empiric antimicrobial therapy. If infection with mycobacteria or *Nocardia* spp. is suspected, the acid-fast or modified acid-fast stains respectively can be performed to detect these microorganisms.

BLOODSTREAM INFECTIONS

Blood cultures are among the most important specimens processed by the microbiology laboratory. Bloodstream infections can be considered to be transient, intermittent or continuous, and diagnosis of a bloodstream infection is very important in managing sick patients.

An example of transient bacteremia is that which occurs following cleaning one's teeth; transient bacteremia is rarely of clinical significance. An intermittent bacteremia occurs in patients who have serious bacterial infections such as pneumonia, urinary tract infections or osteomyelitis, where organisms may be isolated from the bloodstream but this is not uniformly the case. Continuous bacteremia occurs in patients who have infection within the vascular space and this includes patients with bacterial endocarditis or septic thrombophlebitis.

Because diagnosis of a bloodstream infection may be critical for patient care, it is essential that these specimens are collected correctly. Optimal collection of a blood culture starts with proper skin preparation. The skin must first be cleaned with 70% alcohol followed by tincture of iodine for 1 min or alternatively povidone–iodine for 2 min. It is important to allow these disinfectants to dry as killing bacteria takes time. Alcohol should not be used as a second antiseptic agent when an iodophor is used as it may inactivate these compounds. It is also recommended to clean the septum of the blood culture bottle with 70% alcohol and allow this to dry before injecting blood. The blood must be injected without changing needles.

It is important to take the volume of blood which is recommended for the blood culture system being used. Optimal blood volume enhances recovery of agents as blood is an important component of the culture media itself. The maximum amount of blood that can be taken from a child will depend on the weight and the clinical status of the child and it is usual for 1–3 ml to be obtained from a child younger than 6 years, whereas the neonate may only be able to afford 0.5–1 ml. When collecting blood cultures from children it is advisable to use a pediatric blood culture system which is optimized to function with much smaller volumes than adult blood culture systems. Addition of extra blood can often lead to a false positive signal due to blood cell metabolism, as modern automatic blood culture systems detect carbon dioxide production, and additional blood does not enhance bacterial detection. Blood culture media also contain an anticoagulant, sodium polyanethole sulfonate (SPS), which in addition to its anticoagulant action has an anticomplement and antiphagocytic effect that prevents intracellular killing of microorganisms by neutrophils following injection of the blood into the culture bottle and thus enhances sensitivity. However, SPS may inhibit recovery of organisms such as *Neisseria gonorrhoeae*, *Neisseria meningitidis*, *Gardnerella vaginalis*, *Streptobacillus moniliformis* and *Peptostreptococcus anaerobius*. Ideally blood cultures should be obtained before the start of antibiotic therapy to prevent inhibition of microorganism growth.

More recently, bacteremias have been associated with the increased use of indwelling intravenous catheters for a variety of vascular access needs.[115] Where the use of indwelling catheters is common, institutions have seen an increase in organisms such as coagulase negative staphylococci, corynebacteria, bacilli, yeasts and a variety of uncommon but opportunistic Gram negative rods. When collecting blood cultures through an indwelling catheter, it is strongly recommended that blood cultures are collected simultaneously from a peripheral noncannulated site, to determine if a positive culture represents true bacteremia or infection of the central venous line. While it is recommended not to take blood cultures through central venous lines, this practice is usually quite common because of the ease of drawing blood through these catheters with little discomfort to the patient. Identification of a contaminated catheter may result in treating patients with antibiotics for a period of time, possibly preventing more serious systemic infection and also obviating the need to remove the catheter.

Blood cultures are usually incubated for 5–7 days before being declared negative. The length of culture may be extended in specific situations, for example when fastidious organisms are anticipated as in subacute bacterial endocarditis or in prolonged fever of unknown origin.

URINARY TRACT INFECTIONS

The commonest site of clinically significant bacterial infection in infants and children is the urinary tract. Urinary tract infections may occur within the renal parenchyma, in the tubules or pelvis, or at any point along the ureters, urinary bladder or urethra. Studies relating clinical infection to the number of bacteria in a voided urine specimen demonstrated that at least 100 000 variable bacteria on culture per milliliter of urine correlated strongly with infection in the upper urinary tract. Most urinary tract pathogens grow easily and quickly and include *Escherichia* spp., *Klebsiella* spp., *Enterobacter* spp., *Proteus* spp., *Pseudomonas* spp., *Enterococcus* spp. and *Staphylococcus* spp. Bacteria that are generally considered contaminants and disregarded include lactobacilli, diphtheroids, non-enterococcal alpha-hemolytic streptococci and coagulase negative staphylococci, other than *Staphylococcus saprophyticus* which is a common cause of urinary tract infection in pubertal girls and young women.

Yeasts, particularly *Candida* spp., may cause urinary tract infections. Determination of true urinary tract infection due to the yeast is more complex than with bacteria as there is no correlation with colony number and formal diagnosis may require an invasively obtained specimen, e.g. catheterization of the bladder, to avoid genital colonization which may contaminate the culture. Urine specimen may on occasions be used to detect *Mycobacteria* spp. and leptospira.

In addition to culture information, with identification of the bacterium and provision of antibiotic sensitivity results, the cell count per high power field is also helpful in determining the significance of results. The presence of a high white blood cell count, greater than 100 per high power field, indicates the presence of a significant inflammatory reaction occurring within the upper urinary tract. Where there is sterile pyuria, consideration must be given to whether the patient has already received an antibiotic rendering the sample sterile or whether there is some other non-infectious inflammatory lesion of the upper urinary tract. Some laboratories will also test the urine to see if it contains antibacterial activity, indicating the presence of antibiotic in the urine and thus warning the clinician of possible false negative results.

The presence of greater than 10 epithelial cells per high power field in the urine specimen is indication of significant contamination from the terminal urethra or vulva, so culture results need to be interpreted with great caution. Collection of the urine specimen should be done so as to minimize possible contamination by external colonizing bacteria in the urogenital tract. Suprapubic bladder aspiration of urine is the procedure least likely to result in contaminated urine. Alternatively, urine obtained by insertion of a catheter through the urethra into the bladder, collection of the urine specimen and removal of the catheter is also much less likely to be contaminated than voided specimens. If a voided specimen is to be collected, careful cleaning of the urethral meatus with sterile water in both males and females is strongly recommended prior to collection of a mid-stream urine specimen. It is desirable to ask the patient to void a small volume first (about 5 ml) and then collect the next urine passed, a mid-stream urine specimen. The initial voiding helps clean any colonizing bacteria from the terminal urethra prior to collection of the specimen for culture.

RESPIRATORY TRACT INFECTION

Respiratory tract infections can be divided into upper respiratory and lower respiratory. Common upper respiratory tract specimens include throat swabs and nasopharyngeal swabs or aspirates. Aspirates from sinuses or the middle ear are submitted only occasionally, because they are difficult to collect and empiric therapy without culture is usually effective. Throat swabs are cultured only for group A streptococci (*Streptococcus pyogenes*) unless there is a specific request to look for other agents.[116] Group C and group G beta-hemolytic streptococci can also cause throat infection, but there is no association with rheumatic fever or acute post-streptococcal glomerulonephritis. If diphtheria (*Corynebacterium diphtheriae*) or whooping cough (*Bordetella pertussis*) is suspected, the laboratory should be contacted so that the specimens are collected in the correct way and cultured on appropriate media for detection of these organisms.

Expectorated sputum is the most common specimen for diagnosis of lower respiratory tract infections (primarily pneumonia). In addition to sputum culture, more invasive methods for collection of specimens from the lower respiratory tract include bronchial washes, bronchial brushes, transbronchial biopsy and bronchoalveolar lavage. In difficult and serious clinical situations a surgical open lung biopsy may be indicated.[117]

Microbiology laboratories routinely use screening microscopy guidelines to reject sputum specimens of poor quality and thereby minimize unnecessary and potentially misleading culture results. The quality of the specimen is assessed by the number of squamous epithelial cells present per high power field with numbers exceeding 25 per low power field indicating that the specimen is heavily contaminated with saliva (oropharyngeal contamination) and unlikely to produce reliable results. The presence of polymorphonuclear leukocytes indicates a sputum specimen usually of apparent good quality. These criteria are not suitable and have not been validated for rejection of specimens where *Legionella* spp., fungi or *Mycobacteria* spp. are being cultured. The range of microorganisms that can cause lower respiratory tract infections is very diverse and it is important to provide an appropriate history to the laboratory so that testing can be targeted to the most relevant causes. Lower respiratory tract infection may be community acquired or nosocomial and other relevant clinical information including the type of infiltration seen on chest X-ray, the immunological status of the patient, any underlying diseases such as cystic fibrosis, a history of exposure to tuberculosis or travel, occupational or other exposures may be very helpful to the laboratory in identifying the causative organism.

CENTRAL NERVOUS SYSTEM INFECTION

Cerebrospinal fluid (CSF) must be transported to the laboratory promptly, because fastidious organisms such as *Neisseria meningitidis* may become nonviable if the specimen cools. In addition, cells in the specimen begin to degenerate and are difficult to identify morphologically in specimens greater than 6 h old.

It is customary to collect at least three tubes of CSF to send to the laboratory and it is important that a sufficient quantity is collected for all testing that is requested. In addition to culture, all CSF specimens are examined for cell count including red cells and white cells, with the white cells differentiated into polymorph lymphocytes and monocytes, as well as determining the biochemical parameters of protein and glucose concentration.[118]

Gram stains must be performed on all spinal fluids and any microorganism seen immediately reported to the responsible clinician as this may be of critical assistance in managing the patient and optimizing antibacterial coverage. Bacterial antigen tests for *Neisseria meningitidis*, *Streptococcus pneumoniae*, *Haemophilus influenzae* type b, group B streptococcus (*Streptococcus agalactiae*) and *Escherichia coli* are not routinely performed by many laboratories as the sensitivity of these tests does not exceed that of Gram stains. More recently, polymerase chain reaction (PCR) testing for *Neisseria meningitidis* and *Streptococcus pneumoniae* has become available, and these tests have been particularly helpful in the early management of cases of acute bacterial meningitis, especially when antibiotics have been given before taking cultures.[119] However, culture remains essential as the infecting organism can be tested for antibiotic susceptibility to guide therapy.

In addition to bacterial cultures, cultures for mycobacteria and fungi may also be indicated in specific clinical situations. However, cultures for both these types of organisms require reasonable volumes of CSF, at least 2 ml per sample and preferably 5–10 ml.

DIARRHEAL DISEASES

Acute diarrhea can be caused by a broad range of microorganisms including bacteria, viruses and parasites. Ideally stool specimens are preferred to rectal swabs and should be transported to the laboratory promptly. Most laboratories will reject a stool specimen which is not diarrheal, i.e. the specimen must take up the shape of the container, unless one is specifically looking for *Salmonella* spp. carriage. Most laboratories routinely culture for *Salmonella*, *Shigella* and *Campylobacter*. In addition, white and red cells are often looked for by direct microscopy as an indication of colitis. It is important to provide a good history to complement the specimen, such as any history of travel, ingestion of seafood or recent antibiotic therapy, and it is necessary to inform the laboratory if the clinician is looking for *Vibrio* spp., *Aeromonas* spp., *Plesiomonas* spp., *Yersinia* spp. or enterohemorrhagic *Escherichia coli*, as specific techniques in the laboratory will be needed to detect these organisms.[120] Parasites can be a common cause of diarrhea in young children, including *Cryptosporidium* and *Giardia*, and microscopy or antigen detection is required to detect these.

GENITAL TRACT INFECTIONS

Genital specimens are usually collected on pediatric patients when looking for evidence of sexually transmitted disease following alleged sexual assault and child abuse. The genital tract contains many nosocomial organisms including coagulase negative staphylococci, lactobacilli, corynebacteria, streptococci, anaerobes and yeasts. Some genital tract infections not associated with sexually transmitted disease may be caused by endogenous bacteria, for example *Gardnerella vaginalis* or group B streptococci or rarely *Staphylococcus aureus*.

The common sexually transmitted diseases which need investigation are *Neisseria gonorrhoeae*, *Chlamydia trachomatis* and *Treponema pallidum* (syphilis). Both gonorrhea and chlamydia can be confirmed by culture. It is important to ensure that the cultures are collected with the correct type of swabs, as both organisms are extremely fastidious and the method of specimen collection and transport to the laboratory are critical. More recently, detection of these microorganisms using PCR on first void urine specimen has proved both sensitive and specific as well as having increased patient acceptance. It should be noted that PCR for gonorrhea should not be performed on any other specimen other than the urogenital specimens as there is a high rate of false positive results if eye or throat specimens are collected, due to cross-reaction with nonpathogenic nosocomial *Neisseria* spp. It is important to have culture evidence if at all possible as antibiotic susceptibility testing can be done for gonorrhea and these results are more reliable if legal proceedings arise from the case. Syphilis can be detected by dark field examination of exudate from any ulcerative lesion, but is more commonly diagnosed serologically.

ANTIMICROBIAL SUSCEPTIBILITY TESTING

Antimicrobial susceptibility testing is advisable for presumed pathogens where response to antimicrobial agents is not predicted from identification alone. It is becoming increasingly needed with dissemination of resistance genes amongst bacteria. The aim of antimicrobial susceptibility testing is to demonstrate that in vitro growth inhibition of an infecting microorganism by a specific antimicrobial agent correlates with clinical response to that agent. Most testing is performed to detect the minimal inhibitory concentration (MIC), which is the lowest concentration of a specific antimicrobial agent that prevents visible growth of the test organism. Minimal bacterial concentration (MBC) is the lowest concentration of a specific antimicrobial agent that kills most (greater than 99.9%) of the inoculum of the organism and is rarely performed except under specialized circumstances. The more common and non-fastidious organisms can be tested. There need to be adequate data substantiating the clinical response of a species, and a minimal inhibitory concentration (MIC) for that agent, to provide interpretive data. There are many organisms for which these data are not available, examples being *Bacillus* species other than *Bacillus anthracis*, *Corynebacterium* spp. and many fastidious or unusual species, e.g. *Eikenella*, *Capnocytophaga*, *Leuconostoc*. It is also important to know that there are some specific organism–antimicrobial agent combinations where results are not reported because in vitro data are often misleading.

PRINCIPLES OF ANTIMICROBIAL THERAPY

Antimicrobial therapy is indicated when there is clinical or culture evidence of an infection and the use of an antimicrobial agent would be expected to significantly shorten the duration of illness or lower the incidence of complications. However, not all bacterial infections need specific antimicrobial treatment, including minor skin infections and some gastrointestinal infections, e.g. *Salmonella* spp., where host defense mechanisms usually effect cure.

INITIAL MICROBIOLOGICAL EVALUATION

Patients in whom an infectious illness is suspected should always be investigated to establish a microbiological diagnosis as this will aid ongoing therapeutic decisions. Initial microscopic examination of a Gram stained specimen from a sterile site often shows excellent correlation with the cause of the infection. However, if the specimen must pass through an area which is normally colonized with commensal bacteria, such as wound cultures or the mouth with sputum specimens, then the Gram stain should be evaluated carefully. In these situations, the bacterial culture report should be interpreted cautiously and contamination with commensal bacterial flora and the pathogenic potential of the isolated organism carefully considered. With sputum specimens, the presence of many polymorphs compared to epithelial cells on Gram stain and microscopy can be used to quality control the specimen, with predominance of polymorphs supporting purulent sputum while predominance of epithelial cells indicates heavy salivary contamination and probable invalid and contaminated culture results.

When there are clinical signs suggestive of a systemic infection, blood cultures should always be collected. Positive cultures from normally sterile fluid such as blood, CSF, pleural and synovial fluid should always be considered accurate, unless there is strong evidence to suggest otherwise. Bacteria such as *Neisseria meningitidis* and *Streptococcus pneumoniae* growing on cultures from sterile sites are never contaminants and the *Enterobacteriaceae* are rarely contaminants. However, when normal skin flora, such as alpha-hemolytic streptococci, *Propionibacterium acnes* or coagulase negative staphylococci are isolated, their significance and the clinical picture must be carefully reviewed to decide whether the isolated bacteria are indeed pathogens.

CHOICE OF ANTIBACTERIAL AGENT

The optimal antibiotic for treating a bacterial infection is one with action against the infecting agents, the narrowest possible spectrum of antibacterial activity, the fewest side-effects and the lowest toxicity.

The microbiology laboratory reports bacteria as susceptible or resistant to a particular antibacterial agent, depending on the amount of antibiotic that corresponds to achievable serum concentrations with standard dosage and schedule. Many infections occur at sites other than the bloodstream where there may be issues of antibiotic penetration (e.g. the CSF) or activity (e.g. aminoglycoside activity is decreased in pus). The antibiotic should be administered in a dose, at a dose interval and by a route that achieves an antibacterial level at the site of infection at least equal to, or preferably several times higher than, the level of that agent required to inhibit bacterial growth in vitro.

The choice of an empiric antibiotic agent for a suspected or proven infection is based upon (1) the site(s) of infection, (2) those bacteria that are most likely to cause that particular infection, (3) the bacteria presumptively identified by Gram stain of a specimen from the infected site, (4) the predicted susceptibility of the organism to the antibiotic, (5) the pharmacological properties of the antibiotic, and (6) the cost.

TREATMENT WITH MORE THAN ONE ANTIBIOTIC

The indications for using more than one antibiotic in the treatment of an infection are: (1) to treat infection due to more than one microorganism if they are not susceptible to the same drug; (2) to treat empirically a life-threatening infection where the causative bacterium is unknown and broad spectrum coverage of potential infecting bacteria must be achieved immediately; (3) to treat difficult organisms or infections for which synergy of an agent has been demonstrated or is postulated, e.g. enterococcal endocarditis; (4) to prevent the emergence of resistance during treatment.

DURATION OF ANTIMICROBIAL THERAPY

The appropriate duration of an antibacterial treatment course is defined as the shortest period necessary to prevent bacteriological or clinical relapse, i.e. produce a cure. The duration of treatment for a bacterial infection depends on the site and extent of the infection, the bacterium and the host response. The duration of treatment for cure has been reliably established for some infections, e.g. streptococcal pharyngitis, but it has not been established for many others. Response to therapy in patients with infections is best monitored clinically rather than bacteriologically. Repeat cultures are usually unnecessary and not helpful in the patient who has a good clinical response.

FAILURE OF ANTIMICROBIAL THERAPY

Failure of antibiotic therapy is defined as detection of bacteria beyond the expected time of clearance, usually accompanied by clinical failure of response to therapy. It is self-evident that antibiotics cannot be expected to cure a nonbacterial disease. If there is a failure of therapy with antibiotic therapy then details of the regimen should be examined, such as the susceptibility of the bacterium, dosage, route of administration, dosage interval and penetration into the site of infection. When there is an abscess, drainage is often far more effective than antibiotic treatment in resolving the infection. Common reasons for antibiotic treatment failure are: (1) failure of the patient to take medication as directed; (2) deficiency in host defense mechanisms including poor nutritional status; (3) inability to clear respiratory or other secretions; and (4) poor penetration of the antibiotic to the site of infection, e.g. poor tissue perfusion. The development of antibiotic resistance by an initially susceptible bacterium during treatment occurs but is uncommon.

ANTIBACTERIAL PROPHYLAXIS

Antibiotic prophylaxis is the use of an antibacterial agent to prevent infection and is most efficacious when attempting to prevent infection for a relatively brief period. The administration of antibiotics to prevent postoperative wound infection is now well established. The risk of contamination of the wound occurs at the beginning of the operation, so if prophylaxis is to be effective the antibiotic must be administered immediately prior to the operation to maintain high effective blood and tissue levels throughout the procedure. The use of prophylactic antibiotics has resulted in a significant decrease in the incidence of infections in procedures involving areas that are heavily contaminated with bacteria, such as the head and neck, and in gynecological and colonic surgery. Factors that predispose to contamination in surgery are long operations and the placement of prosthetic devices. Preventing infection of a prosthesis can be achieved with a short duration of therapy, up to 12 h. However, in specific situations such as cardiac surgery or placement of orthopaedic prostheses, prophylactic antibiotics are frequently continued for 2 days.

CLINICAL PHARMACOLOGY OF ANTIMICROBIAL AGENTS
Absorption

Many antimicrobial agents are well absorbed after oral administration while others are very poorly absorbed, e.g. vancomycin and aminoglycosides are very rapidly degraded in the intestinal tract so they must be administered parenterally to treat systemic infections. With few exceptions, oral administration of antibiotics results in lower serum concentrations of antibiotics than when using identical parenteral dosing, exceptions being metronidazole and chloramphenicol.

Serum concentrations achieved by the usual oral doses of agents such as ampicillin, first generation cephalosporins and tetracycline are generally not high enough to inhibit Gram negative enteric bacteria susceptible to these drugs. However, they may be used in urinary tract infection, because they are concentrated in the urine. In hospitalized patients with severe infection, antimicrobial therapy is generally administered parenterally to ensure adequate levels.

Distribution

After administration and absorption, antimicrobial agents are bound to plasma proteins to varying degrees. The time of serum decline relates to excretion and inactivation and is measured as serum half-life, i.e. the time required for a 50% decrease in serum concentration, which is a measure of the duration of the pharmacological effect. Serum half-life is an important determinant of a dosage schedule, in both normal patients and those in whom the half-life is prolonged because of decreased drug excretion or metabolism.

The initial rise in serum concentration after drug administration is followed by a decrease as the drug is distributed to body tissues. The tissue concentration of antibiotic depends on the degree of protein binding, the concentration gradient from serum to tissue, and the drug diffusibility. Most antibiotics penetrate well into pleural, peritoneal, pericardial and synovial fluid. Penetration into brain, CSF, eye and placenta is more variable. In general, penetration of antibiotics into body compartments increases with the presence of inflammation, e.g. penicillin penetrates into the CSF much more easily in an inflammatory state.[121]

Inactivation and excretion

There are several mechanisms of excretion and inactivation of antimicrobial agents, which include excretion by the bowel, removal by the kidney, inactivation by the liver, or inactivation by other unknown means. Antimicrobial agents may be inactivated by more than one mechanism.

Renal excretion is the major means of clearance of most antimicrobials, exceptions being chloramphenicol, erythromycin, clindamycin, doxycycline, ceftazidime and metronidazole. Renal failure results in accumulation of antimicrobials normally excreted by the kidney and dosage changes are essential for such agents as aminoglycosides and glycopeptides which have a low therapeutic-to-toxicity ratio and a single means of excretion or inactivation.

MECHANISM OF RESISTANCE

Bacteria acquire resistance to antibiotics most commonly by one of three main mechanisms:

1. Inability to reach the site of action due to decreased cell wall permeability or increased action of efflux pumps. Examples of this type of mechanism occur in *Pseudomonas* spp. and *Enterobacteriaceae* as a mechanism of resistance to aminoglycosides.
2. Alteration in the antimicrobial target. An example is alteration in the penicillin-binding protein 2 in staphylococci to PBP-2a encoded by the mec A gene, which renders all beta-lactam antibiotics, including the penicillinase-resistant penicillins, inactive, i.e. MRSA.[122]
3. Production of an enzyme that inactivates the antibiotic. Examples are beta-lactamases, which cleave the beta-lactam ring and render these antibiotics inactive.[123] Beta-lactamases have co-evolved with the increased use of beta-lactam antibiotics over the last 50 years, and are a major mechanism of defense by Gram negative bacteria against beta-lactam antibiotics. The introduction of penicillin saw a very rapid increase in prevalence of beta-lactamase production by staphylococci which inactivate penicillin but not penicillinase-resistant penicillins (see below) which are stable and therefore remain active.[122] Beta-lactamases have spread to organisms which previously did not have them, including *Haemophilus influenzae* and *Neisseria gonorrhoeae*.

Hundreds of beta-lactamases have been described and can be assigned to one of four groups, A to D. Class A beta-lactamases are usually plasmid-mediated and can spread easily between bacteria of different genera. They occur commonly in *E. coli* and other *Enterobacteriaceae*. More recently, mutants have emerged with an 'extended spectrum', which can attack not only penicillins but many of the first, second and third generation cephalosporins, called extended-spectrum beta-lactamases or ESBLs.[124-126] The class A beta-lactamases can be inhibited by beta-lactamase inhibitors such as clavulanic acid (see below). On the other hand, class C beta-lactamases, which have a broader spectrum than class A enzymes and mediate resistance to penicillins and most cephalosporins, are chromosomal, intrinsically produce a beta-lactamase, and are confined to specific bacterial species such as *Enterobacter* spp., *Serratia marcescens*, *Citrobacter freundii*, *Acinetobacter* spp., *Aeromonas* spp., indole positive *Proteus* spp. and *Morganella morganii*, often referred to as the ESCAAPM group. The class C beta-lactamases cannot be inhibited by clavulanic acid. Both class A and class C beta-lactamases inactivate penicillins and cephalosporins but do not inactivate carbapenems. However, more recently, metallobeta-lactamases, which are usually class B and inactivate all beta-lactams including carbapenems, have become more prevalent by spreading on plasmids among Gram negative bacteria.[123]

Aminoglycosides, which are very potent bactericidal antibiotics with a broad range of activity especially against Gram negative bacteria, can induce enzymes which catalyze phosphorylation, acetylation or adenylation of this class of antibiotics causing covalent modifications leading to poor ribosomal binding resulting in high-level resistance to these agents.[127]

CLASSES OF ANTIMICROBIAL AGENTS

Beta-lactams

The antimicrobial agents of most value in treating infants and children are the beta-lactams, including penicillins, cephalosporins, monobactams and carbapenems, which have in common a beta-lactam ring.

The bacterial targets of beta-lactam antibiotics are penicillin binding proteins (PBPs), which are vital for bacterial cell division, shape and structural integrity. The exact mechanism of action of beta-lactams remains elusive. Recent evidence suggests it is a complex process involving both inhibition of cell wall synthesis and activation of endogenous autolytic systems. Their action is usually bactericidal. Some bacteria have a deficiency in this system of autolytic enzymes that results in inhibition but not killing of the bacteria by the beta-lactam. This phenomenon is called tolerance and is demonstrated, in vitro, by a minimal inhibitory concentration (MIC) in the susceptible range but a minimal bacterial concentration (MBC):MIC ratio of 32 or greater.

The nature of the bactericidal activity of beta-lactam has been described as time-dependent killing. The important determinant of bactericidal activity for beta-lactams is the length of time during the dosing interval that the concentration of the antibiotic exceeds the MIC of the infecting microorganism. Bactericidal activity is thought to be greatest when the concentration of the beta-lactam antibiotic at the site of infection is 4–10 times greater than the MIC of the infecting microorganism. The rapidity and extent of bacterial killing are not increased when concentrations exceed this ratio.

Resistance to beta-lactam antibiotics is either by production of a beta-lactamase or by alterations in the PBPs.

Penicillin

The penicillins can be classified into four groups based on their antimicrobial activity. There are some overlaps in activity. The four groups are the natural penicillins, the amino-penicillins, the penicillinase-resistant penicillins and the extended-spectrum penicillins. The mechanism by which most bacteria have acquired resistance to penicillins G is beta-lactamase production. Resistance to penicillin by *Streptococcus pyogenes* (group A streptococcus) and *Streptococcus agalactiae* (group B streptococcus) has not emerged. Resistance caused by altered PBPs occurs less commonly, but the increasing resistance of *Streptococcus pneumoniae* to penicillin is a result of altered PBPs.

1. *Aqueous penicillin G* produces high peak concentrations of antibacterial activity in the serum within 30 min of administration. The drug is rapidly excreted by the kidneys resulting in low serum concentrations within 2–4 h. When treating severe disease such as meningitis, pneumonia or endocarditis, penicillin G should be administered usually every 4 h until the infection has been cured.

2. *Procaine penicillin G* given intramuscularly produces serum levels of approximately 10–30% of those of aqueous penicillin, but the activity persists in serum for as long as 4 h. IM procaine penicillin is very painful and can cause injection site abscesses. It is only recommended for short term treatment of children with mild to moderate disease when IV access cannot be achieved.

3. *Benzathine penicillin G* is given intramuscularly as a depot preparation that provides for low continuous concentrations approximately 1–2% of those achieved by the aqueous penicillin G. Penicillin is detectable in the serum for 3 weeks or more following injection. Benzathine penicillin G can be used for the treatment of group A streptococcal pharyngitis, impetigo or prophylaxis of streptococcal infections in children who have rheumatic carditis, although pain at the injection site is a major deterrent to the use of this antibiotic.

4. *Phenoxymethylpenicillin* (oral penicillin or penicillin V) is well absorbed from the gastrointestinal tract with peak concentrations in serum approximately 40% of that of the same dose of aqueous penicillin G. Oral penicillin is satisfactory for treating mild to moderate infections with susceptible organisms.

All penicillins are excreted by both glomerular filtration and tubular secretion. Concomitant use of probenecid, a drug that blocks tubular secretion of organic acids, can produce higher peaks and more sustained serum concentrations resulting in greater antimicrobial activity. Dosages and dosing intervals will need adjustment when penicillins are administered to persons with decreased renal function.

Penicillinase-resistant penicillin

Penicillinase-resistant penicillins are the drug of choice for the initial management of patients with suspected staphylococcal disease, as most strains of *S. aureus* produce a beta-lactamase, penicillinase. Common penicillinase-resistant penicillins are cloxacillin, dicloxacillin, flucloxacillin, oxacillin and nafcillin. These agents are active against streptococci and can be used for treatment of infections commonly caused by both staphylococci and streptococci, e.g. impetigo. However, as these agents are less active than penicillin G against streptococci, penicillin G should be used if streptococci alone are isolated from culture. It should be noted that penicillinase-resistant penicillins have no activity against Gram negative bacteria or enterococci.

Disease caused by methicillin-resistant *Staphylococcus aureus* (MRSA) was reported shortly after the introduction of methicillin in the 1960s. Methicillin resistance is caused by alterations in PBP-2 rather than by production of a beta-lactamase, so MRSA is resistant to all currently available beta-lactam agents including penicillins, cephalosporins and carbapenems.

Coagulase-negative staphylococci, most commonly *Staphylococcus epidermidis*, a skin commensal, may be a pathogen in neonates or cause infections of prosthetic devices such as heart valves, CSF shunts and intravenous lines. Many strains of coagulase-negative staphylococci produce beta-lactamase and have altered PBPs making them methicillin resistant. Vancomycin is the drug of choice for diseases known to be caused by MRSA or methicillin-resistant *Staphylococcus epidermidis* (MRSE).

Amino-penicillin

The amino-penicillins include ampicillin and amoxicillin which have extended activity compared with penicillin, with activity against some Gram negative organisms, including *H. influenzae*, *E. coli*, *Proteus mirabilis*, *Salmonella* spp. and *Shigella* spp. The amino-penicillins can also retain activity against penicillin-susceptible Gram positive bacteria. Amino-penicillins are the drug of choice for treatment of infections caused by *Listeria monocytogenes* and the enterococci. These drugs are used frequently in the treatment of susceptible pathogens causing (1) lower respiratory tract infection, (2) acute otitis media, (3) urinary tract infections, and (4) acute diarrheal disease when therapy is indicated. It should be noted that amoxicillin is significantly less effective than ampicillin for the treatment of shigellosis. Ampicillin is associated more frequently with diarrhea than amoxicillin.

Extended-spectrum penicillins

Extended-spectrum penicillins are semisynthetic derivatives of ampicillin and have better activity against Gram negative bacteria because of high affinity for PBPs and greater penetration to the Gram negative outer membrane. The carboxypenicillins include carbenicillin and ticarcillin while the ureidopencillins include piperacillin and mezlocillin. These extended-spectrum penicillins have activity against *Pseudomonas aeruginosa* but are significantly less active against Gram positive cocci than ampicillin.

Extended-spectrum penicillins (often combined with an aminoglycoside) have been used for the treatment of intra-abdominal and upper urinary tract infections as well as for sepsis in neutropenic patients. They are only available as parenteral formulations.

Beta-lactamase inhibitor/beta-lactam combinations

Beta-lactamase inhibitors, such as clavulanic acid, sulbactam and tazobactam, are compounds that have weak intrinsic antibacterial activity but bind irreversibly to many beta-lactamases rendering the beta-lactamases inactive. Beta-lactamase inhibitors are combined in a fixed ratio with a beta-lactam antibiotic, e.g. amoxicillin/clavulanic acid or piperacillin/tazobactam. The spectrum of activity of the combination is determined primarily by the spectrum of activity of the beta-lactam. The main indication for use of these combination antimicrobial agents is the treatment of infections caused by susceptible beta-lactamase producing pathogens.

Ampicillin/sulbactam or amoxicillin/clavulanic acid can be used to treat beta-lactamase producing strands of *Staphylococcus aureus* (but not methicillin-resistant *Staphylococcus aureus*), *Haemophilus influenzae*, *Moraxella catarrhalis*, *Neisseria gonorrhoeae*, *Escherichia coli*, some *Proteus* spp., *Klebsiella* spp. and some anaerobic bacteria including *Bacteroides fragilis*.

Adverse effects and allergies of penicillins

The penicillins have very little dose-related toxicity. Adverse reactions include electrolyte disturbance of sodium and potassium, gastrointestinal problems with diarrhea, and hematological changes with hemolysis, neutropenia or platelet dysfunction. Drug-induced hepatitis can occur determined by elevated aspartate aminotransferase (AST), neurological abnormalities are rare and include seizures, while renal problems can occur with interstitial nephritis.

Allergy, however, is an important factor and can occur quite frequently with penicillin compounds.[128] The penicillin are haptens, low molecular weight compounds too small to induce an immune response but which bind to host proteins and are highly immunogenic. The four types of immune-mediated reactions that can occur after the administration of penicillins are: (1) immediate hypersensitivity (IgE mediated); (2) cytotoxic antibody reactions; (3) immune complex reactions (Arthus reactions); and (4) delayed cell-mediated hypersensitivity. It is estimated that serious immediate reactions will occur in 2 of every 10 000 cases and fatal reactions in 1 in 100 000 treatment cases of penicillin administration. Identifying patients who will have a significant reaction to penicillin remains difficult. At present, physicians must rely on the patient's history of reactions after administration of penicillin to identify those likely to be allergic and avoid administration of penicillin in these patients for anything other than very serious infections, e.g. endocarditis, where desensitization may be necessary. All penicillins are cross-reactive with regards to sensitization, and allergy to one implies sensitization to all, although this cross-sensitivity is less than 100%.

Cephalosporins

The cephalosporins have a very broad range of activity which includes Gram positive, Gram negative and anaerobic bacteria. Cephalosporins are categorized as first, second, third and fourth generation depending on their pattern of in vitro activity. Cephalosporins have no activity against enterococci or methicillin-resistant staphylococci.

First generation cephalosporins. The first generation cephalosporins are effective against Gram positive cocci including beta-lactamase producing *Staphylococcus aureus*. They have variable activity against Gram negative enteric bacilli, such as *Escherichia coli*, *Proteus mirabilis* and *Klebsiella* species, with minimal if any activity against *Haemophilus influenzae* and *Moraxella catarrhalis* and are inadequate against penicillin-sensitive *Streptococcus pneumoniae*. They should therefore not be used for treatment for respiratory tract infection.

Second generation cephalosporins. The second generation cephalosporins in common use are cefuroxime and cefaclor. When compared with the first generation cephalosporins, second generation cephalosporins have similar or somewhat less activity against Gram positive cocci with better activity against *Haemophilus influenzae*, *Moraxella catarrhalis*, *Neisseria meningitidis* and *Neisseria gonorrhoeae* and some members of the *Enterobacteriaceae*.

Third generation cephalosporins. The common parenteral third generation cephalosporins used in children are cefotaxime, ceftriaxone and ceftazidime. There are oral third generation cephalosporins and cefixime is the most commonly used. Third generation cephalosporins are very potent against Gram negative and enteric bacteria and have excellent activity against *Haemophilus influenzae*, *Moraxella catarrhalis*, *Neisseria gonorrhoeae* and *Neisseria meningitidis*, group A streptococci and penicillin-susceptible pneumococci. They have relatively poor activity against staphylococci. Ceftazidime is the only third generation cephalosporin used in children with activity against *Pseudomonas aeruginosa*. The increasing prevalence of extended-spectrum beta-lactamases (ESBL) in the *Enterobacteriaceae* is increasing the prevalence of resistance to these agents. The parenteral third generation cephalosporins achieve high levels in the serum and adequate concentration in CSF.

Fourth generation cephalosporins. The fourth generation cephalosporin, cefepime, exhibits very rapid entry into the bacterial cell and stability against a range of beta-lactamases as well as increased binding affinity to multiple PBPs. These factors explain cefepime's expanded spectrum of activity and improved efficacy against Gram negative pathogens compared with third generation cephalosporins.[129]

Adverse reactions. The safety profile of cephalosporins is similar to penicillins with hypersensitivity reactions being the most frequent.

Monobactams

Aztreonam is the prototype monobactam. It has aerobic Gram negative antibacterial activity similar to that of ceftazidime but has no significant Gram positive activity.

Carbapenems

The carbapenem class of antimicrobial agents exhibits the broadest spectrum of activity of all beta-lactam antibiotics. They include imipenem-cilastatin and meropenem and have activity against most clinically significant Gram positive and Gram negative pathogens including anaerobic organisms.

The glycopeptides

The glycopeptides, vancomycin and teicoplanin, exhibit time-dependent bactericidal activity against most clinically significant Gram positive bacteria except that they are only bacteriostatic for enterococci. The glycopeptides interfere with the development of the peptidoglycan cell wall at a site of action distinct from that of beta-lactams, so there is no cross-resistance or competitive inhibition between these drug classes.

Vancomycin is not metabolized significantly and is excreted by glomerular filtration. In patients with severe renal failure the half-life may extend 7 or more days, and furthermore vancomycin is not removed effectively by either peritoneal or hemodialysis. The dosing interval needs to be adjusted when using vancomycin in patients with impaired renal function.[130]

Adverse effects. Ototoxicity and nephrotoxicity have been considered serious adverse effects of vancomycin therapy in the past, but these serious events are much less frequent than previously thought. Infusion-related side-effects are the most common side-effect seen with vancomycin with the rapid onset of a widespread erythematous rash. This can usually be managed by slowing the infusion rate or premedicating the patient with antihistamines.

Aminoglycosides

The aminoglycosides, gentamicin, tobramycin and amikacin, demonstrate rapid concentration-dependent bactericidal activity with a post-antibiotic effect, i.e. killing of bacteria continues in the absence of any detectable serum antibiotic.[131] The higher the peak concentration of the aminoglycoside, the longer the duration of the post-antibiotic effect. The mechanism of the bactericidal action is binding to the bacterial ribosome and interfering with bacterial protein synthesis by inducing translational errors. The uptake of aminoglycosides by bacteria can be facilitated by concomitant therapy with a cell wall-active antibiotic such as vancomycin or a beta-lactam. Aminoglycosides have activity against a range of facultative aerobic bacteria, but their activity is reduced in infections at sites with reduced oxygen tension, e.g. abscesses. Anaerobic bacteria and fermentative bacteria such as streptococci are inherently resistant to aminoglycosides. Aminoglycosides penetrate the blood–brain barrier very poorly in the absence of inflammation and thus are not very successful in the treatment of Gram negative meningitis. Aminoglycosides are not metabolized after parenteral administration and are excreted unchanged in the kidney by glomerular filtration.

Resistance to aminoglycosides can evolve in a number of ways: (1) alteration in the bacterial target affecting binding; (2) decreased cell permeability making it more difficult for the drug to reach the ribosomal target; and (3) breakdown of the drug by bacterial enzymes.

The major use of aminoglycosides in children is for serious infections caused by Gram negative enteric infections, neonatal sepsis, sepsis in a child with immunodeficiency, especially neutropenia, abdominal and systemic infections associated with fecal contamination of the peritoneum, and complicated urinary tract infections.

Adverse effects. All aminoglycosides can damage the proximal renal tubules, the cochlea, the vestibular apparatus or a combination of these, and rarely can cause neuromuscular blockade. To avoid toxicity and ensure therapeutic levels, the concentration of aminoglycoside in serum should be monitored in all patients.

Macrolides

The macrolides, erythromycin, clarithromycin and azithromycin, have similar antibacterial spectra, mechanism of action and mechanism of resistance but they differ in their pharmacokinetic characteristics. They all bind reversibly to the 23S component of the 50S ribosomal subunit and inhibit protein synthesis. The macrolides are bacteriostatic but clarithromycin and azithromycin are bactericidal against *Streptococcus pyogenes, Streptococcus pneumoniae* and *Haemophilus influenzae*.

The newer macrolides have a spectrum of activity similar to that of erythromycin, but clarithromycin has greater activity against *Moraxella catarrhalis, Haemophilus influenzae, Mycoplasma pneumoniae, Chlamydophila pneumoniae, Chlamydia trachomatis, Legionella pneumophila, Ureaplasma urealyticum* and *Neisseria gonorrhoeae*. Clarithromycin also has activity against organisms that are resistant to erythromycin, including *Toxoplasma gondii, Mycobacterium leprae, Mycobacterium chelonae* and *Mycobacterium avium-intracellulare* (MAC).

Azithromycin is effective in vitro against a diverse group of microorganisms including *Bordetella pertussis, Legionella pneumophila, Corynebacterium diphtheriae*, spirochetes including *Treponema pallidum*, the mycoplasmas (except *M. hominis*), chlamydiae, and aerobic and anaerobic Gram positive cocci.[132] Azithromycin is highly active against *Campylobacter jejuni*. When compared with erythromycin, azithromycin has less activity against Gram positive bacteria and greater activity

against Gram negative bacteria including some *Enterobacteriaceae* such as *Shigella* and *Salmonella* species.

Adverse effects These include local gastrointestinal irritation with nausea, vomiting and abdominal pain. Cholestatic hepatitis occurs rarely but is a serious reaction requiring cessation of therapy. Erythromycin has been associated with infantile hypertrophic pyloric stenosis.

Miscellaneous antibacterial agents
Clindamycin

Clindamycin is a semisynthetic derivative of lincomycin and has much better oral absorption and greater antimicrobial activity. It has action against Gram positive bacteria as well as Gram positive and Gram negative anaerobes including *B. fragilis*. Clindamycin penetrates well into most tissues including bone but has poor penetration into the CNS. It is inactivated in the liver and excreted in bile with very little renal excretion. It is useful in the treatment of staphylococcal infections in penicillin-allergic individuals and MRSA.

Adverse effects. Clindamycin can often cause diarrhea and less commonly the more serious *Clostridium difficile* associated pseudomembranous colitis. The occurrence of pseudomembranous colitis is a strong indication to cease this agent. Clindamycin is also associated with allergic reactions and rashes and rarely causes erythema multiforme and anaphylaxis.

Trimethoprim–sulfamethoxazole (co-trimoxazole)

Trimethoprim is active against many Gram positive and Gram negative bacteria, except *Pseudomonas aeruginosa*. Trimethoprim is often combined with sulfamethoxazole because the two drugs act synergistically. The drug is widely distributed in tissues including the CNS, and a significant amount is excreted unchanged in the urine giving high concentrations which makes it useful for treating urinary tract infections. Trimethoprim–sulfamethoxazole also has activity against *Haemophilus influenzae* and *Pneumocystis carinii*.

Adverse effects. The most common side-effects are nausea, vomiting, diarrhea and hypersensitivity reactions. Prolonged administration may be associated with a megaloblastic bone marrow or leukopenia; thrombocytopenia and anemia may also occur.

A discussion of the mechanisms of action, clinical indications and modes of resistance of antiviral agents and antifungal agents is beyond the scope of this chapter. The reader is referred to other publications for this information.[133–135]

Management of infections is complex. The clinician needs a good understanding of infectious clinical syndromes, likely pathogens, antimicrobial resistance patterns, and knowledge of antimicrobial agents, their spectrum of activity, penetration to the site of likely infection and possible adverse effects, to effectively and safely treat common childhood illnesses.

BACTERIAL INFECTIONS: BOTULISM

The name botulism derives from the Latin *botulus* for sausage, and was coined following an outbreak in Germany in 1793 in which 13 people who shared a large sausage became ill and 6 died.

Classical botulism is a paralytic disease caused by ingestion or absorption of one or more preformed neurotoxins produced by the soil organism, *Clostridium botulinum*. Cases occur singly or in small clusters following consumption of home-canned or prepared foods in which the heat-resistant spores of *C. botulinum* have germinated under anaerobic conditions. Canned or bottled foods, especially soil-contaminated vegetables, smoked fish and continental sausage, are classic food vehicles. High temperatures are required to inactivate spores. If toxin production does occur, poisoning can be avoided by adequate cooking or reheating of the food, because the toxin is inactivated by moderate heat. Raw fish or fish products are also potential sources of botulinum toxin.

Infant botulism is a different condition from the botulism due to preformed toxin. Infant botulism results from multiplication of *C. botulinum* in the baby's intestine, and causes an indolent presentation. The median age of onset is 2 months, with a range of less than 3 weeks to

12 months.[136-138] Infant botulism is more common in babies living in rural areas or on a farm: in Australia cases occur when it is hot, dry and windy and spores may blow into the baby's mouth or into the water supply.[136] There is a particular association with babies whose pacifiers were dipped in honey, although only 11 of 68 US babies reported with infant botulism had honey exposure.[137,138] Corn syrup ingestion (20 of the 68 babies) and breast-feeding were other risk factors. Breast milk is thought to generate favorable conditions for germination of spores.

CLINICAL FEATURES AND DIAGNOSIS

Classic botulism

Typically, after an interval of 12–36 h, patients present acutely with malaise, nausea, vomiting, dizziness, weakness and dry mouth. After hours or days cranial nerve palsies develop, causing ptosis, blurred vision, diplopia, dysphagia and dysarthria. Paralysis may progress over a period of hours or days to involve many muscle groups and the patient may require respiratory support. Recovery occurs over weeks to months.

Infantile botulism

This is characterized by an insidious onset of severe, progressive hypotonia, poor suck, constipation and bilateral ptosis. The pupils are often dilated and there may also be pooling of oral secretions, reduced facial movements and ophthalmoplegia. The gag reflex is often weak. Peripheral tendon reflexes are normal or diminished, but not usually absent. Paralysis may progress to involve the respiratory muscles and the infant may require respiratory support.[138]

The differential diagnosis includes spinal muscular atrophy (absent reflexes, fasciculations), myotonic dystrophy [myotonia, electromyogram (EMG) pattern], wild-type or vaccine-associated paralytic poliomyelitis (asymmetric paralysis, CSF pleocytosis) and Guillain–Barré syndrome (ascending paralysis, raised CSF protein). The EMG in infant botulism shows denervation. The diagnosis is primarily based on clinical findings and EMG, and can be supported by detecting *C. botulinum* toxin in stools (by PCR or animal inoculation) and/or by growing *C. botulinum* from stool culture. An association between infant botulism and sudden infant death syndrome (SIDS) has been proposed but is unproven.

TREATMENT

Infant botulism is managed by protecting the airway and using artificial ventilation if required. Babies who require artificial ventilation recover after 3–4 weeks. With proper supportive care the outcome is excellent, with complete recovery the rule.

Tracheostomy prolongs hospitalization.[138] Nasogastric tube feeds are usually well tolerated. Antibiotics such as penicillin do not speed recovery and gentamicin may exacerbate neuromuscular problems. Antibiotics are only indicated for complications such as pneumonia. Botulism antitoxin, harvested from hyperimmune adults (hBIG) and available only to investigators in the USA, halves the mean time to resolution of symptoms in infant botulism.[139,140] Equine antitoxin made in horses (eBIG) has long been used in the treatment of adult botulism but has not been shown to be effective in infant botulism.[141] A new intravenous botulinum immunoglobulin, produced in the USA, reduced the duration of mechanical ventilation and hospitalization significantly in infant botulism.[142]

In older children, circulating toxin needs to be neutralized with antitoxin, in the form of botulinum immune globulin, as soon as possible. This has no effect on bound toxin but it is always indicated as toxin may circulate for days. The remainder of the care is supportive of respiration, as for infant botulism.

BACTERIAL INFECTIONS: BRUCELLOSIS; UNDULANT FEVER

Brucellosis is usually caused by one of three organisms: *Brucella abortus*, *Brucella melitensis* or *Brucella suis*. All three are primarily diseases of domesticated animals (cattle, goats and pigs, respectively). The clinical picture ranges from clinically asymptomatic infection via acute brucellosis (with septicemic manifestations) to chronic brucellosis.

EPIDEMIOLOGY

Human brucellosis is mostly a disease of those who come into contact with infected animals in rural areas. Spread of infection from animal to animal occurs readily and the resulting illness is often chronic with long term excretion of the organism. Infection is transmitted to humans by infected milk or milk products and, less frequently, by direct contact or entry through skin. Person-to-person spread rarely occurs. Elimination of brucellosis in animal populations (by vaccination or slaughter policies) will eliminate new infections in humans. World Health Organization sources estimate that there are 500 000 cases worldwide each year (childhood infections accounting for less than 10% of cases). In the UK there are about 20 patients each year, most with disease caused by imported *B. melitensis* infection or laboratory accident. The low incidence of brucellosis in children which results from milk-borne infection is unexpected and some have suggested that environmental exposure may be more relevant.

PATHOLOGY

Acute brucellosis is a septicemic illness, with seeding of organisms in the body, which may become apparent immediately or later after the systemic features have resolved. There is widespread reticuloendothelial system hyperplasia and focal manifestations may occur in many organs, particularly in the liver or spleen. Chronic brucellosis may follow acute brucellosis or begin insidiously. In chronic brucellosis the organisms usually remain intracellularly where they are relatively protected against host defenses and antibiotics.

B. melitensis often produces more invasive manifestations and debility than *B. abortus*, an important point to realize when generalizing about brucellosis. Those with low gastric acid levels are thought to be at particular risk of infection.

CLINICAL FEATURES

The incubation period of acute brucellosis is from a few days to a month.

With acute brucellosis symptoms develop rapidly with high fever, rigors, arthralgia and profuse sweating: patients often feel much more ill than signs suggest but recovery follows in most. Fever has no particular pattern. Weight loss and secondary anemia may develop. If the patient does not recover then a state of chronic brucellosis ensues with vague irritability, malaise, fatigue, musculoskeletal aches and pains, headaches and depression. Fever may be intermittent, occurring every few weeks – hence the name 'undulant fever'.

Although chronic brucellosis is rarely life threatening the morbidity may be significant.

With both acute and chronic brucellosis suggestive signs may be prominent or absent, constituting a pyrexia of unknown origin. There may be hepatomegaly, splenomegaly or lymph node enlargement. Particularly with *B. melitensis* infection lymph nodes may suppurate and osteomyelitis or arthritis may develop.

Other rare, but potentially life-threatening manifestations include meningitis, endocarditis, peritonitis and encephalitis.

DIAGNOSIS AND DIFFERENTIAL DIAGNOSIS

Clinical diagnosis may be easy in areas where animal infection is endemic. In non-endemic areas clinical diagnosis may be difficult unless it is realized that patients have visited endemic areas or ingested milk products from endemic areas.

In acute brucellosis blood cultures may be positive, but the organisms are difficult to culture and cultures may take up to 2 weeks to become positive. Agglutination tests to detect IgM and IgG antibodies may be helpful but may be positive in asymptomatically infected patients in endemic areas. Nevertheless increasing titers are almost certainly diagnostic. Agglutination titers of greater than 1:160 in a patient with appropriate clinical features are very suggestive.

In chronic brucellosis blood cultures are rarely positive and bone marrow culture or, less often, liver or splenic biopsy culture may be necessary. If there is renal involvement urine cultures may be positive. Biopsy shows noncaseating granulomas.

If available, the presence of *Brucella*-specific IgM is diagnostic of acute brucellosis or of chronic brucellosis in an acute relapse, whilst *Brucella*-specific IgG indicates infection at some stage. Lymphocytosis with neutropenia may be found.

The differential diagnosis of acute brucellosis includes malaria, salmonellosis (including typhoid fever), tuberculosis, tularemia, rheumatic fever, infective endocarditis, Q fever, leptospirosis and non-infective conditions. If malaise and debility predominate, depression enters the differential diagnosis, as well as being a complication in its own right.

TREATMENT[143]

In acute brucellosis antibiotic treatment probably shortens the illness and reduces the risk of progression to chronic brucellosis. Opinions differ as to the optimal treatment: comparison of treatment results of *B. abortus* and *B. melitensis* infection is not necessarily valid. Most studies of children with brucellosis deal with children with *B. melitensis* infection. Regimens advocated include (either alone or in combination) co-trimoxazole, rifampicin or streptomycin. In chronic brucellosis suppression of intracellular infection may be attempted in the hope that the host's immunity will eventually eliminate or contain infection. Regimens advocated include protracted courses of the antibiotics used in acute brucellosis. Tetracyclines are useful but obviously cannot be used in children unless there is no alternative.

Single agent treatment carries a relapse rate of 5–40%, thought to be caused by inadequate killing rather than development of resistance.

Antipyretics, analgesics and antidepressant treatment may be indicated. Vaccination of humans with the live attenuated organisms used in animals is not practicable and would certainly make subsequent interpretation of serological tests very difficult.

BACTERIAL INFECTIONS: CHOLERA

Cholera is an acute bacterial enteric disease characterized in its severe form by sudden onset, profuse, painless, watery stools, occasional vomiting, and, in untreated cases, rapid dehydration, acidosis, hypoglycemia and circulatory collapse. Cholera is caused by infection with toxin-producing strains of *Vibrio cholerae*: 01 (includes two biotypes – classical and El Tor) and 0139 (non-01). The clinical picture is similar, because the organisms elaborate a similar enterotoxin that is critical in the pathogenesis. In any single epidemic, one particular biotype tends to be dominant.

EPIDEMIOLOGY

From the nineteenth century, pandemic cholera has spread repeatedly from the Gangetic delta of India to most of the world. Since 1961, *V. cholerae* of the El Tor biotype has spread through most of Asia into Eastern Europe, Africa and Latin America, assuming a worldwide distribution in resource limited countries. Sporadic imported cases occur among returning travelers or immigrants to high-income countries. Humans are the main reservoir of infection, but other environmental reservoirs such as small crustaceans exist in brackish water or estuaries. Outbreaks occur as a result of ingestion of infected water due to poor sanitation and hygiene and occasionally as a result of ingestion of infected food, especially shellfish.

The arrival of cholera in a region may be heralded by an epidemic of severe disease among all age groups: the presentation of large numbers of adults (as well as children) with severe dehydrating diarrhea should alert to the possibility of a cholera epidemic. The initial outbreak may be explosive due to the short incubation period (1–5 days) and the ease of fecal–oral transmission in areas where standards of environmental sanitation and personal hygiene are low. Cholera may then become endemic, causing disease mainly in young children of less than 5 years. This is particularly likely with the El Tor biotype, which has a longer carrier period (up to 2–4 weeks) than classical, a longer viability in water and a higher infection:case ratio. El Tor cholera has largely replaced classical cholera as the major pathogen of public health importance worldwide. *V. cholerae* 0139 has been a cause of severe outbreaks in the Bay of Bengal region since 1992.

ORGANISM AND PATHOPHYSIOLOGY

V. cholerae are Gram negative curved rods measuring $1.5–3.0\,\mu m \times 0.5\,\mu m$. In culture, they may assume other forms such as spiral shapes. They possess somatic (O) antigens and flagellar (H) antigens that may be used to distinguish serological strains such as Ogawa, Inaba and Hikojima. In hanging-drop preparations, they are highly motile. Diarrhea is mediated via an enterotoxin that consists of A and B subunits. The B subunit binds the toxin to surface receptors on the enterocyte and activates arachidonic acid metabolism. Once binding has occurred, the A subunit activates the enzyme adenylate cyclase to produce cyclic adenosine monophosphate (cAMP) which inhibits the absorption of sodium chloride and water. cAMP also stimulates secretion of sodium chloride and bicarbonate from the crypt epithelial cells. The excessive intestinal secretions accumulate in the intestinal lumen and are then expelled in the diarrheal stools. The severity of disease depends on the size of the infecting dose, and the organism is easily destroyed by gastric acid. Most patients with cholera are infected with large inocula of the organism or have relative achlorhydria. Breast-feeding is protective.

The electrolyte content of stools of patients with adult cholera, cholera in children and diarrhea due to other organisms is summarized in Table 28.18. Generally, stool osmolarity in pediatric cholera is isotonic with plasma. The stool sodium content of children with cholera is intermediate (~ 100 millimoles/litre) between that found in childhood diarrhea due to other organisms such as rotavirus (~ 30 mmol/L) or *Shigella* (~ 60 mmol/L) and that found in adult cholera (130–150 mmol/L). Stool potassium is higher in pediatric cholera (~ 30 mmol/L) compared to adult cholera (~ 15 mmol/L) and bicarbonate losses (~ 45 mmol/L) are also high. Cholera does not invade the gut mucosa, but colicky abdominal pain and ileus can occur due to electrolyte disturbances such as hypokalemia and hypocalcemia with acidosis.

CLINICAL FEATURES

The majority of infections with *V. cholerae* are asymptomatic or mild and clinically indistinguishable from other causes of acute watery diarrhea. The typical presentation of severe disease is of acute frequent diarrhea with copious, odorless, virtually colorless (described as 'rice-water') stools. Vomiting is common but fever is unusual. A similar presentation can occur in infants with rotavirus gastroenteritis. In older age groups, the presentation of acute diarrhea among a family group may be confused with food poisoning but severe vomiting which precedes diarrhea and marked abdominal pain are characteristics of food poisoning that are unusual with cholera.

Table 28.18 Relative electrolyte constituents of stools

	Sodium	Potassium	Chloride	Bicarbonate
Cholera in adults	+++	+	+++	+++
Cholera in children	++	++	++	++
Noncholera infantile diarrhea	+	++	+	+

The main clinical features of cholera are those due to severe water and electrolyte loss. Dehydration is commonly isotonic or hypotonic with typical sunken eyes, reduced skin turgor, thirst and dry mucous membranes. Hypovolemic shock may occur within hours of onset. Hypoglycemia is not uncommon and, along with acidosis and hypovolemic shock, leads to deterioration in level of consciousness and occasional convulsions. Hypokalemia and hypocalcemia may also develop and cause colicky abdominal pain, paralytic ileus, muscle cramps and arrhythmias. In severe untreated cases, death may occur within a few hours, and the case-fatality rate may exceed 50%. With proper treatment, the mortality is < 1%.

DIAGNOSIS

Infection with *V. cholerae* is confirmed microbiologically by culture of stools or rectal swabs. Isolates should be serogrouped, and tested for toxin production and antibiotic susceptibility. If laboratory facilities are not nearby, specimens should be transported in special medium such as Cary-Blair transport medium.[144] Traditional culture techniques usually take over 48 h to complete. For clinical purposes, a quick, presumptive diagnosis can be made by dark field or phase microscopic examination of wet preparation showing the vibrios moving like 'shooting stars' and inhibited by serotype-specific antiserum. Rapid dipstick tests that could be used by non-laboratory trained health workers show promise.[145] Earlier confirmation of a cholera outbreak could reduce the case-fatality rate, usually highest at the beginning of an outbreak, and lead to earlier implementation of infection control measures.

MANAGEMENT

The basis of therapy is replacement of water and electrolyte losses from the stool. In cases with no dehydration or mild dehydration, oral solutions will suffice but ongoing review is important. The World Health Organization oral rehydration solution (WHO-ORS) was developed for cholera management and the electrolyte content is appropriate replacement for the above mentioned stool losses. Absorption is dependent on the glucose-facilitated membrane transport of sodium. Other more complex substrates with a lower osmolality such as in cereal-based ORS (e.g. rice-based) are more effective at reducing fluid losses in children with acute watery diarrhea.[146] Stool sodium content is higher in cholera than in noncholera diarrhea, yet a meta-analysis[147] concluded that reduced osmolarity ORS (sodium 75 mEq/L, glucose 75 mmol/L, osmolarity 245 mmol/L) is safe and at least as effective as WHO-ORS (sodium 90 mEq/L, glucose 111 mmol/L, osmolarity 311 mmol/L). The WHO now recommends low osmolarity ORS and zinc supplementation for all children with acute watery diarrhea.[148]

Patients with moderate dehydration have a fluid deficit of between 5 and 10% with decreased skin turgor, thirst, sunken eyes and tachycardia but an intact sensorium. Rehydration and maintenance may be oral or intravenous. Those with severe dehydration, with fluid deficits of more than 10%, will show all the above signs together with peripheral cyanosis, drowsiness or coma, and weak or absent peripheral pulses. Such patients require rapid rehydration with intravenous (or intraosseous) fluids. Ringer's lactate is the most appropriate, widely available intravenous fluid for rehydration but normal saline can also be used. Provision must be made for ongoing stool losses and frequent review of fluid management is essential. Electrolytes and blood sugar should be assessed at intervals to guide ongoing therapy. Potassium will need to be added (at least 20 mmol/L) if normal saline is used during the maintenance phase.

Antibiotics can shorten the duration of diarrhea, reduce fluid losses and requirements and reduce vibrio excretion. Alternatives include doxycycline, erythromycin, azithromycin or ciprofloxacin. Antibiotic-resistant strains are increasingly common, and treatment protocols should be guided by in vitro susceptibility testing. Chemoprophylaxis for contacts has never succeeded in markedly limiting spread but is justified for close household contacts of an index case or if the outbreak is in a closed group, e.g. aboard ship. Mass chemoprophylaxis of whole communities is never indicated and encourages antibiotic resistance.

CONTROL AND PREVENTION

During an outbreak, a coordinated response is important.[144] An emergency treatment center should be established that is accessible to the community and appropriately supplied and staffed. Standardized treatment regimens and frequent review are essential for effective therapy. Early case-finding and management of household contacts should be organized. Educate the population at risk concerning the need to seek appropriate treatment without delay. Initiate a thorough investigation designed to find the vehicle and circumstances of transmission (time, place, persons). Support with laboratory examination of implicated water or food sources and sewage, and plan control measures accordingly. It may be necessary to educate the community by dissemination of important, factual information relating to water safety, food preparation and human waste disposal, and to obtain public support for control activities. Adopt emergency measures to ensure a safe water supply. Chlorinate public water supplies and chlorinate or boil water used for drinking, cooking and washing dishes and food containers. Provide appropriate safe facilities for sewage disposal.

Cholera will ultimately be brought under control only when water supplies, sanitation and hygienic practices attain such a level that fecal–oral transmission of *V. cholerae* becomes an improbable event. Active immunization with a cheap, oral killed whole-cell vaccine that provides a moderate level of protection is gaining recognition as an effective control strategy.[149,150] Indirect herd protection to nonvaccinated neighbors improves effectiveness[151] and the vaccine may provide protection for 3–5 years.[152]

BACTERIAL INFECTIONS: DIPHTHERIA

Diphtheria is an acute infectious disease caused by exotoxin-producing *Corynebacterium diphtheriae*. Although local disease at the primary site of infection, usually the respiratory tract, may be severe, the most significant clinical manifestations are often those at distant sites following systemic absorption and dissemination of the extremely potent diphtheria toxin. Having been one of the leading causes of pediatric mortality in Europe and the USA in the early twentieth century, a combination of improved social welfare and the introduction of mass immunization programs resulted in a dramatic decline in the incidence of diphtheria in resource rich countries by the 1980s (Table 28.19). However, a major resurgence occurred in the newly independent states of the former Soviet Union during the 1990s,[153] emphasizing the potential for rapid re-emergence of the disease in situations where overcrowding, lack of basic infrastructure, natural disasters and/or social unrest disrupt immunization programs and increase exposure to the organism.[154] Nowadays, diphtheria is encountered most frequently among children in South and Southeast Asia, where it remains endemic. Worldwide, more than 5000 deaths from the disease were reported in 2002.[155] Imported cases continue to occur in Europe, particularly among inadequately vaccinated travelers to or from the Indian subcontinent.[156–158]

Table 28.19 Diphtheria – England and Wales

	Cases	Deaths
1920	69 481	5648
1930	74 043	3497
1940	44 281	2480
1950	962	49
1960	49	5
1970	22	3
1980	5	0

BACTERIOLOGY AND PATHOGENESIS

Corynebacterium diphtheriae is a nonmotile unencapsulated nonsporu-lating Gram positive bacillus. It grows readily on ordinary nutrient agar but is more easily identified by early growth on the nutritionally inad-equate Loeffler's medium or on blood tellurite agar, on which growth of other throat organisms is inhibited. Conventionally, three biotypes (gravis, intermedius and mitis) are recognized on the basis of differ-ences in colonial morphology, fermentation reactions and hemolytic potential. Toxin production, the major virulence factor of *C. diphtheriae*, depends on the presence of a lysogenic phage carrying the tox structural gene and is not related to biotype. Highly toxic strains may carry two or three tox+ genes inserted into the genome. Strains lacking the phage do not produce toxin, although conversion to toxigenicity by transfer of a tox+phage can occur. An immunoprecipitation assay was tradi-tionally used to demonstrate toxigenicity of individual strains, but both PCR for the gene and rapid enzyme immunoassays for the toxin are now available.[159-161]

In the absence of toxin production, *C. diphtheriae* is not particularly invasive, usually remaining in the superficial layers of the respiratory mucosa and inducing only a mild inflammatory reaction. The toxin, a 58 kDa polypeptide, consists of two fragments; fragment B binds to spe-cific receptors on susceptible cells allowing fragment A to enter the cell and catalyze the inactivation of elongation factor 2, thereby inhibit-ing protein synthesis and leading to cell death.[162] At the site of infec-tion, local toxin production induces tissue necrosis and the formation of a dense, necrotic mass of fibrin, leukocytes, dead epithelial cells and organisms, closely adherent to the underlying mucosa (Fig. 28.18). Attempts to remove this 'pseudomembrane' often result in bleeding from the edematous submucosal layers. Systemically absorbed toxin can affect all organs in the body, but the major clinical consequences gener-ally involve the heart, kidneys and nervous system. Renal involvement is seen in persons with massive toxin absorption, most of whom die within the first week of illness. In contrast there is often a latent period before cardiac and neurological complications become apparent. The sever-ity of these late complications usually reflects the severity of the initial infection and the extent of the membrane.

Reports of endocarditis and osteomyelitis caused by invasive non-toxigenic strains indicate that other virulence factors may exist.[163,164] A related microorganism, *Corynebacterium ulcerans*, is also able to pro-duce diphtheria toxin and has occasionally been isolated from patients with otherwise classical diphtheria, as well as from individuals with milder symptoms.[165,166]

CLINICAL MANIFESTATIONS
Acute disease

The incubation period is typically between 2 and 5 days. The clinical manifestations depend on the site of the primary infection, the immu-nization status of the host, and the degree to which systemic absorption of toxin has occurred. The disease is conveniently classified into several clinical phenotypes according to the site of primary infection.

Nasal diphtheria is characterized by a serosanguinous or seropu-rulent nasal discharge associated with a subtle membrane inside the nostrils, and sometimes excoriation of the external nares and upper lip.

If the infection is limited to the anterior nares, the acute illness is often mild, absorption of toxin is limited and systemic complications rare.

Faucial diphtheria is usually a more severe presentation. Anorexia, malaise, sore throat and low grade fever are followed after one or two days by the development of membrane, typically on one or both tonsils, extending variously up to the uvula and soft palate, or down to the lar-ynx and trachea and compromising the patency of the airway. Local soft tissue edema and lymphadenitis give rise to the 'bull-neck' appearance seen in severe cases (Fig. 28.19). The extent of the membrane corre-lates with the severity of the bull-neck, the degree of airway obstruc-tion and the signs of acute systemic toxicity. In very severe cases massive toxin absorption occurs resulting in cardiac and respiratory collapse, renal failure and death within a few days. However, with appropriate treatment and good supportive care the membrane sloughs off after 5–7 days and the patient recovers from the local infection, although remaining at risk of the delayed toxin-mediated problems.

Laryngeal involvement generally represents downward extension of the membrane from the pharynx and is correspondingly severe. In some cases the membrane extends to involve the whole of the tracheo-bronchial tree and death is virtually inevitable. Occasionally, however, isolated laryngeal disease occurs and the membrane is limited to the lar-ynx alone; hoarseness, a brassy cough, and rapidly progressive stridor and respiratory distress develop after a short prodromal illness. Relief of the airway obstruction by emergency tracheostomy provides dramatic relief and late complications are unusual as absorption of toxin tends to be limited in such cases.

Cutaneous, ocular, aural and genital diphtheria may all occur, but are rarely associated with significant toxin-mediated disease. The indolent ulcers of cutaneous diphtheria are common in the trop-ics and may serve as a reservoir for the organism, whilst at the same time inducing good immunity in the host. Cutaneous diphtheria is also seen among alcoholics, the indigent and the homeless in resource rich countries.[167,168]

Late complications

Characteristically cardiac complications become evident during the sec-ond, or occasionally third, weeks of illness and are often insidious in onset. ECG abnormalities such as subtle ST–T wave changes, increased rates of ectopy and/or first-degree heart block are detectable in many patients, but clinical dysfunction is apparent in only 10–25%.[169-171] In these patients, the initial ECG abnormalities tend to progress to more complex conduction abnormalities, notably complete heart block, as clinical myocarditis develops. Findings at this stage include profound bradycardia, diminished heart sounds, a gallop rhythm, and varying degrees of congestive failure. A hypotensive low output state is a very poor prognostic sign, usually associated with major conduction distur-bances, and suggests extensive myocardial damage. Ventricular and supraventricular tachyarrhythmias may also occur and are often fatal.

Neurological complications occur in around 10–20% of patients overall. Bulbar involvement is sometimes seen during the first or second week, although minor dysfunction can be difficult to identify in children during the acute stage. In general neurological symptoms are identified later, usually arising between the third and eighth weeks of illness. In some cases there may be a biphasic course with initial partial recovery

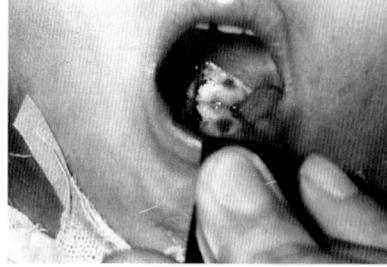

Fig. 28.18 Typical 'pseudomembrane' in a child with faucial diphtheria.

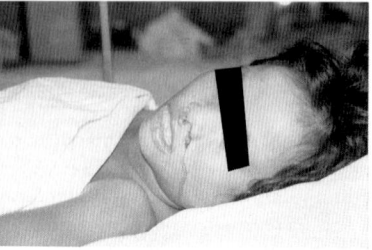

Fig. 28.19 Severe diphtheria showing brawny erythematous swelling of the neck (bull-neck) and serosanguinous nasal discharge.

from early bulbar symptoms, followed by late secondary deterioration with bulbar and peripheral manifestations.[172] The early symptoms are likely due to local effects of toxin on the nerve endings in bulbar muscles, while the later effects reflect systemic absorption and dispersion of the toxin. The neurological manifestations are typically bilateral and motor rather than sensory, and electrophysiological studies indicate an underlying demyelinating process. Difficulty in swallowing with nasal regurgitation due to palatal paralysis is often the first symptom, followed by ocular and other cranial nerve palsies, and later a peripheral polyneuropathy similar to but usually more severe than Guillain–Barré syndrome.[173] If diaphragmatic or respiratory muscle paralysis occurs, the course may be severe and prolonged.

DIAGNOSIS

The diagnosis of diphtheria should be made on the basis of clinical findings, without waiting for laboratory confirmation, since any delay in treatment may have serious consequences. Definitive diagnosis relies upon isolation of the organism; swabs should be obtained urgently and the microbiology service informed of the possibility of diphtheria so that appropriate cultures can be set up and tests for toxigenicity performed.

Differential diagnoses include infectious mononucleosis, herpetic tonsillitis, Vincent's angina, streptococcal pharyngitis and blood dyscrasias. In resource rich countries where diphtheria is a rarity it may easily be missed, and a high index of suspicion is required, particularly in patients without adequate immunization cover and in those who have recently visited an area endemic for diphtheria.

MANAGEMENT

Neutralization of free toxin with diphtheria antitoxin is the most important aspect of management. The antitoxin is only effective before the toxin enters cells so prompt administration is critical. Empirical dosage recommendations are given in Table 28.20.[174] As the antiserum is raised in horses, after preliminary sensitivity testing with 0.1 ml of a 1:1000 dilution of antitoxin, a single dose should be given to try to avoid sensitization. Facilities for resuscitation must be available, even in the absence of a reaction to the test dose.

Antibiotic therapy should be given to eliminate the organism and prevent spread, with penicillin probably the antibiotic of choice. Erythromycin may be more effective at preventing carriage but some resistant clinical isolates have been identified.[175] Parenteral treatment (benzylpenicillin 25000–50000 units/kg/d, or erythromycin 40–50 mg/kg/d for those with a history of penicillin allergy) should be started immediately, changing to oral therapy as the patient improves. Treatment should be continued for 10–14 days and the patient should be barrier nursed until eradication of the organism has been confirmed by culture of appropriate swabs. The disease is notifiable and all suspected cases should be reported immediately to the relevant authority so that measures can be taken to minimize the likelihood of spread.

Good supportive care is also critical. Emergency tracheostomy may be lifesaving in children with severe airway obstruction. However, endotracheal intubation should be avoided unless absolutely necessary in case part of the membrane becomes dislodged and obstructs the lower airways. Ventilatory support is not usually required except in those with extensive pulmonary involvement or those with respiratory failure due to neurological dysfunction. A short course of corticosteroids is often given to patients with 'bull-neck' or upper airway obstruction in order to reduce local edema.

Patients recovering from moderate to severe local disease should be kept on strict bed rest for a minimum of 2 weeks until cardiac involvement has been excluded. Careful clinical examination and regular ECG and echocardiographic monitoring allow early detection of conduction disturbances and impending myocarditis.[176] Patients who develop mild to moderate cardiac failure but maintain normal blood pressure can usually be managed successfully with bed rest, oxygen, diuretics and ACE inhibitors. However, recovery may take many weeks and occasional patients are left with permanent conduction abnormalities. Steroids have not been shown to be of benefit for treatment or prevention of myocarditis, although the number of patients involved in formal research studies has been limited.[177]

The prognosis for patients developing severe conduction disturbances depends largely on the severity of the overall myocardial involvement. Profound bradyarrhythmias are usually associated with major heart muscle disease; if a low output state with hypotension and renal compromise develops, the response to cardiac pacing and/or inotropic agents is poor and the outlook is bleak.[178] Cardiac pacing may be helpful in those with significant conduction abnormalities in whom a reasonable stroke volume is maintained.[179] However, in some such cases the conduction disturbance resolves without intervention after a few days.

Later still, patients with severe neurological involvement may require assisted ventilation and nutritional support for prolonged periods, together with physiotherapy, treatment for nosocomial infections as they arise, and eventually rehabilitation.

PROGNOSIS

Before the introduction of antitoxin, antibiotics and routine immunization, the prognosis was grave, with mortality rates of 30–50%. Currently mortality rates of around 5–10% are usual,[180] with the majority of deaths in those with overwhelming disease at presentation or those who develop myocarditis. If antitoxin is administered within the first 72 h severe disease and death are rare.

PREVENTION

Humans are the only known reservoir for *C. diphtheriae*. The principal modes of spread are by respiratory droplets from acute cases or asymptomatic carriers, or by direct contact with infected skin lesions. Immunization with diphtheria toxoid (formalin inactivated toxin) is very effective at protecting against the effects of the toxin, but does not prevent infection with the organism. Before the vaccine era diphtheria was predominantly a disease of the young and most people acquired natural life-long immunity through repeated exposure to the organism during childhood. Vaccine induced immunity wanes gradually over time, however, and during the recent resurgence of diphtheria in the former Soviet Union many adults acquired the disease and mortality was high in this group.[181]

The standard schedule for routine immunization should include a minimum of 3 doses of the triple vaccine (DTP) early in the first year of life, with a DTP booster at school entry, and a further booster at school

Table 28.20 Dosage of antitoxin recommended for various types of diphtheria

Type of diphtheria	Dosage (units)	Route
Nasal	10000–20000	Intramuscular
Tonsillar	15000–25000	Intramuscular or intravenous
Pharyngeal or laryngeal	20000–40000	Intramuscular or intravenous
Combined types or delayed diagnosis	40000–60000	Intravenous
Severe diphtheria, e.g. with extensive membrane and/or severe edema (bull-neck diphtheria)	40000–100000	Intravenous or part intravenous and part intramuscular

leaving using the low dose adult vaccine (usually as Td). Supplementary boosters should be given to high-risk groups including health care workers, travelers to endemic areas, alcoholics and the homeless, and periodic boosters for the general population may become routine in the future. Patients suffering from diphtheria should receive active immunization after recovery, since clinical disease may not induce adequate antitoxin levels.

BACTERIAL INFECTIONS: *ESCHERICHIA COLI*

Escherichia coli was first described by Theodore Escherich in 1885. It is a Gram negative, non-spore-forming, fimbriate bacillus which is motile by means of flagella (Fig. 28.20). Although *E. coli* is responsible for the vast majority of human infections there are four other species in the genus, *E. blattae*, *E. vulneris*, *E. fergusonii* and *E. hermannii*. *E. blattae* is an intestinal commensal of cockroaches and does not cause human infection, but the other three have been described as rare opportunists. In contrast *E. coli* is a major pathogen, both primary (Table 28.21) and opportunist. It is also the major aerobic Gram negative rod found in the human (and other animals) gastrointestinal tract at a concentration of approximately 10^8 colony forming units (cfu) per gram. It can be found in soil and water, but this is invariably a result of fecal contamination.

The complete genome sequences of both *E. coli* K12 (a nonpathogenic laboratory strain) and *E. coli* O157 are available.[182,183] *E. coli* K12 encodes some 4405 genes on a large circular chromosome of 4639 kilobase pairs. *E. coli* O157, which causes hemorrhagic colitis and hemolytic uremic syndrome (HUS), has a larger genome with 1387 new genes encoded in clusters or islands not found in *E. coli* K12. *E. coli* K12 and *E. coli* O157 share a common backbone but diverged some 4.5 million years ago.[184] Most of the differences result from acquisition of islands of genes. These islands encode pathogenicity determinants (pathogenicity islands),

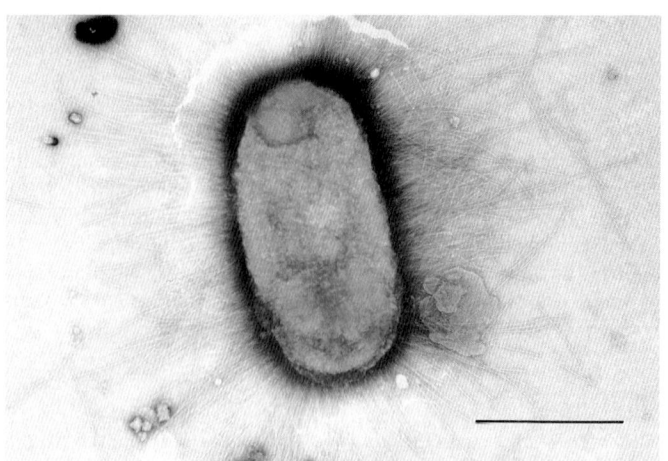

Fig. 28.20   Negative stain electron micrograph of *Escherichia coli* showing numerous fimbriae.

metabolic functions (metabolic islands) and several pro-phages (bacterial viruses whose genome has been incorporated into the bacterial chromosome). Other pathogenic *E. coli* such as enteropathogenic *E. coli* (EPEC), uropathogenic P-fimbriate *E. coli* (PFEC) and the neonatal pathogen *E. coli* K1 also encode different pathogenicity islands in their genomes.

EPIDEMIOLOGY

E. coli is subdivided into a large number of serotypes based on O- or somatic (on lipopolysaccharide on the outer membrane of the bacterium) antigens, H- or flagellar antigens and K- or capsular antigens. There are

Table 28.21   *Escherichia coli* as a primary pathogen

	Serogroups	Pathogenicity determinants	Infection sites	Disease associations
Gastrointestinal tract				
Enterotoxigenic *E. coli* (ETEC)	O6, O8, O5, O20, O25, O128, O139, O148, O153, O159	CFA (pili), heat labile (LT) and heat stable (ST) toxins	Small bowel	Secretory diarrhea in travelers and children in resource limited countries
Enteroinvasive *E. coli* (EIEC)	O28, O29, O124, O136, O143	*Ipa* pathogenicity island on plasmid *ial*, adhesin	Large bowel	Mild dysentery in children in resource limited countries
Enteropathogenic *E. coli* (EPEC)	O55, O86, O111, O119, O125, O126, O127, O128, O142	Locus of enterocyte effacement pathogenicity island (LEE), *tir, eae*	Small and large bowel	Acute and chronic diarrhea in neonates and infants in resource limited countries
Enterohemorrhagic *E. coli* (EHEC)	O26, O111, O128, O157	*eae*A, *eae*B, shigatoxins 1 & 2	Large bowel	Hemorrhagic colitis, hemolytic uremic syndrome, encephalopathy
Enteroaggregative *E. coli* (EaggEC)	O44, O111, O121 but most are nongroupable	Adhesin, EAST-1	Small and large bowel	Acute and chronic diarrhea in children and travelers
Diffuse adhering *E. coli* (DAEC)	O75 but most are nongroupable	Adhesins	Unknown	Perhaps a cause of diarrheal disease
Urinary tract				
P-fimbriate *E. coli* (PFEC)	O1, O2, O3, K1	P-fimbriae (adhesions) encoded on a pathogenicity island	Urinary tract, septicemia	Cystitis, pyelonephritis
S-fimbriate *E. coli* (SFEC)	O1, O2, O3	S-fimbriae (adhesins)	Urinary tract, septicemia	Cystitis, pyelonephritis
Neonatal meningitis and bacteremia				
E. coli K1	O1, O2, O3, K1	K1 capsule plus pathogenicity island function unclear	Urinary tract, meninges, septicemia	Urinary tract infection, meningitis, septicemia

167 different O-serogroups and at least 82 K-antigens.[185] Serogrouping is of importance not just for epidemiological purposes but also delineation of pathogenicity. However, a number of molecular biological techniques provide more accurate epidemiological and pathogenicity related markers. These include techniques for whole genome analysis such as pulsed field gel electrophoresis (PFGE) of macrorestricted chromosomal DNA,[186] analysis of housekeeping genes (multilocus sequence testing; MLST) or of insertion sequence distribution (eubacterial repetitive intergenic consensus sequences; ERICS). E. coli can also be divided into four main phylogenetic groups by analysis of two genes (chuA, yjaA) and an anonymous DNA fragment.[187] Most virulent extra-intestinal strains belong to group B2 and to a lesser extent group D, whereas most commensal strains are in group A.

E. coli is part of the normal flora of most mammalian species. For example. E. coli O157 is excreted asymptomatically by cattle but can be transferred to humans as a 'food-poisoning' to cause hemorrhagic colitis, HUS and encephalopathy. The uropathogenic PFEC and the neonatal pathogen E. coli K1 colonize the gastrointestinal tract[188] thence reaching their infective sites by ascending the urinary tract and by hematogenous spread respectively. In addition the commensal E. coli that do not possess defined pathogenicity determinants are important opportunist pathogens, for example after gastrointestinal surgery or in patients with indwelling urinary catheters. Finally the commensal E. coli are an important reservoir of antibiotic resistance genes that can be transferred to more pathogenic bacteria.[189]

Enteropathogens

Enterotoxigenic E. coli (ETEC) are solely human pathogens, although similar bacteria can cause diarrheal disease in domestic animals. They cause up to 25% of cases of diarrheal disease in children in resource limited countries and are a major cause of traveler's diarrhea (c. 80% of cases). Infection is usually acquired via food or water contaminated with human excreta. The infective dose is high (c. 10^7 cfu). Enteroinvasive E. coli (EIEC) are a minor cause of diarrheal disease, in most surveys being responsible for less than 5% of cases in children in the tropics. Enteropathogenic E. coli (EPEC) were responsible for epidemics of infantile diarrhea in the UK and the USA in the 1940s and 1950s but are now found predominantly in neonates and infants in resource limited countries (in one study causing 11% of cases of infantile diarrhea). The infective dose is low (< 10^4 cfu) so direct person-to-person spread is also possible.

Enterohemorrhagic E. coli (EHEC) are most often acquired as food poisoning, but since the infective dose is low (< 10^2 cfu), person-to-person spread in households and hospitals has been described. Enteroaggregative E. coli (EaggEC) are the most recently described group and are responsible for cases of acute and chronic diarrhea in children and traveler's diarrhea. They are particularly associated with chronic diarrhea in children in resource limited countries. The infective dose is unknown. It is still unclear what role diffuse adhering E. coli (DAEC) play in diarrheal disease and little is known of their epidemiology.

Uropathogens

Most E. coli causing urinary tract infection fall into serogroups O1, O2, O4, O6 and O75, have thick capsules and express adhesins. Of particular importance are PFEC which bind to the P-blood group receptor. They colonize the intestine and, in females, the vagina, perineum and anterior urethra. From there they ascend to produce cystitis and pyelonephritis.

Neonatal sepsis

E. coli K1 is responsible for 40% of the cases of neonatal bacteremia and 75% of the cases of neonatal meningitis that are due to E. coli. The incidence rate of E. coli neonatal meningitis in the USA is 1 case per 1000 live births. Infection is acquired from mother-to-baby at birth or baby-to-baby and staff-to-baby in neonatal intensive care units. Approximately 50% of women of childbearing age have intestinal carriage of E. coli K1 and 70% of neonates born to carrier mothers will acquire carriage. The colonization to disease ratio is approximately 200–300 to 1.

PATHOGENESIS

Enteropathogens

ETEC cause a non-inflammatory, secretory, small intestinal diarrhea. To do this they must colonize the upper small intestine by adhering to enterocytes using fimbriae (protein spikes) termed colonization factor antigens (CFA) in human ETECs. In addition they secrete one or both of heat labile (LT) and heat stable (ST) toxins. The LTs (I and II) are subunit toxins. They consist of five (toxophore) B subunits that carry and bind the toxin to ganglioside receptors on the enterocyte surface and one A (toxin) subunit. The A subunit is activated by cleavage to A1 which activates adenosine diphosphate (ADP) ribosylation of a regulatory subunit of adenyl cyclase. This results in activation of adenyl cyclase and raised intra-enterocyte concentrations of cyclic adenosine monophosphate (AMP). This results in fluid and electrolyte secretion into the small intestinal lumen, and thus a voluminous watery diarrhea. LTI is very similar to cholera toxin. ST (a and b) are smaller (16–18 amino acids) and activate guanylate cyclase by mimicking guanylin, the endogenous modulator of cyclic guanosine monophosphate (GMP) signaling. How raised intracellular cyclic GMP levels induce diarrhea is unclear. EIEC cause colitis and an inflammatory diarrhea. They have similarity with Shigella spp. in that similar pathogenicity genes (on a pathogenicity island) are encoded as large plasmids in both genera. They attach to and invade colonic enterocytes (Fig. 28.21). They can then migrate laterally from colonocyte to colonocyte. How this causes colonocyte death, loss of mucous membrane integrity and an inflammatory response is unclear, but the initial stages might involve induction of colonocyte apoptosis.

EPEC produce specific ultrastructural lesions on the enterocyte surface, termed attaching effacement, in which there is very close intimate attachment of the bacteria to the enterocyte surface with local loss of the microvilli (brush border) (Fig. 28.22). Although this lesion can be detected throughout the gastrointestinal tract it is the effect on the small intestine that is most important. EPEC initially adhere to the enterocyte surface by means of bundle forming pili. This then activates a chromosomal pathogenicity island called the locus of enterocyte effacement (LEE) which assembles a type III secretion system. Through this, the bacterium injects effector molecules into the enterocyte. One is Tir (transferable intimin receptor) which inserts into the enterocyte membrane and acts as a receptor for a molecule (intimin) on the bacterial surface thus promoting intimate attachment of the bacterium to the enterocyte. Other effectors cause damage to the microfilaments of the terminal web causing loss of the microvilli (termed effacement). This causes a great loss of surface area for absorption and of the brush border disaccharidases sucrase, maltase and lactase, and leads to malabsorption and an osmotic diarrhea.

EHEC such as E. coli O157 have a pathogenicity island very similar to the EPEC LEE but their attaching effacement is confined to the

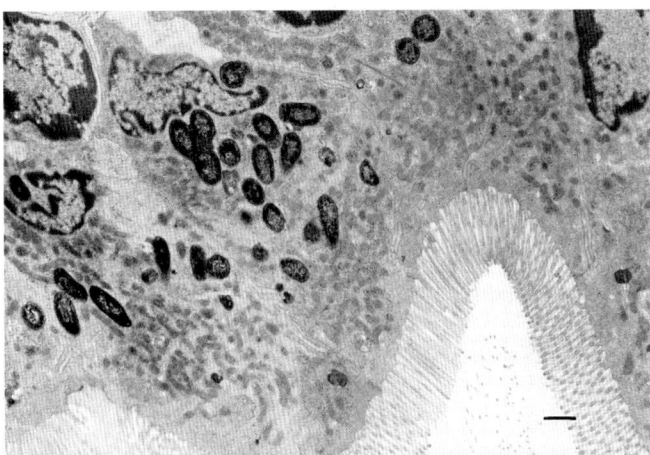

Fig. 28.21 Thin section electron micrograph of colonic enterocytes with numerous enteroinvasive *Escherichia coli* in the cytoplasm.

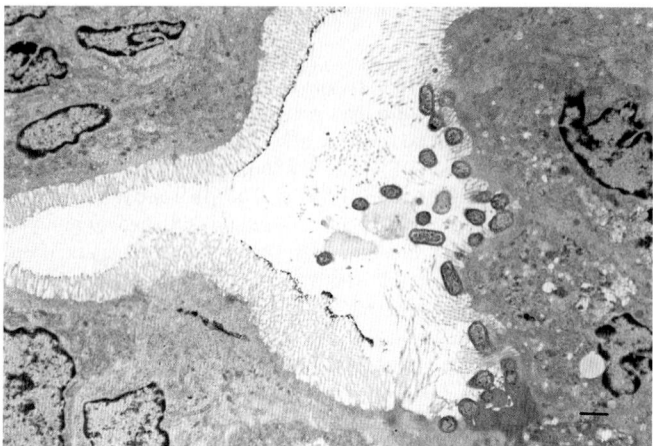

Fig. 28.22   Thin section electron micrograph showing enteropathogenic *Escherichia coli* closely adherent to duodenal enterocytes with loss of microvilli (attaching effacement).

terminal ileum and colon. In addition they elaborate Shiga toxins (ST) 1 and/or 2 (previously known as verocytoxins). These are subunit toxins with five B (toxophore) units and one A (toxin) unit. The B units carry, protect, and bind the A subunit to the enterocyte utilizing a globoside glycolipid receptor. The A subunit inhibits protein synthesis and is one of the most potent toxins known. ST-1 is identical to Shiga toxin and both it and ST-2 are encoded on promiscuous bacteriophages. This means that these toxin genes are widely distributed in enteric bacteria, but in order to produce disease, *E. coli* must have both LEE and ST. ST kills colonocytes causing hemorrhagic colitis. If ST enters the circulation it binds to receptors on endothelial cells, in particular in the renal vasculature. This causes fibrin deposition, cell swelling and narrowing of the lumen of the vessel, and results in a microangiopathic hemolytic uremia or HUS.

EaggEC are so called because they produce a 'stacked brick' appearance when adherent to cells in culture and each other. They adhere to both small and large intestinal mucosa by means of plasmid-encoded fimbriae (AAF/I, AAF/II). They elaborate toxins including EaggEC heat stable toxin-1 (EAST-1) which resembles ETEC ST and a plasmid encoded toxin (Pet) which induces mucin release, exfoliation of cells and crypt abscesses. Recently it has been shown that a novel flagellin from EaggEC induces the release of the inflammatory chemokine IL-8 from intestinal epithelial cells.

PFEC have two pathogenicity islands in their genome which encode expression of fimbriae with a receptor binding molecule at their tip which recognizes the P-blood group antigen. This is a glycolipid with terminal digalactose residues and is expressed on most tissues including the epithelium of the urinary tract. Thus the bacteria are able to adhere and resist the flushing action of urine. How they induce inflammation is less clear but probably involves induction of cytokine and chemokine release.

E. coli K1 produces a thick capsule that allows it to evade the killing effects of neutrophils and complement. It, like the group B meningococcal capsule, is a homopolymer of N-acetyl neuraminic acid which is a self-antigen being expressed on neuronal tissue in particular. Further pathogenicity determinants are gradually being uncovered.

CLINICAL FEATURES

The clinical features associated with enteropathic *E. coli* are outlined in Table 28.21. For a more detailed description of this and of urinary tract infections and neonatal sepsis, see the appropriate sections.

DIAGNOSIS AND DIFFERENTIAL DIAGNOSIS
Enteropathogens

For definitive diagnosis, *E. coli* must be isolated from fecal samples. Although O-serogrouping was the method originally used to describe the different pathogenic types it is of little value except in outbreaks. For specific diagnosis, the pathogenicity genes or their products must be detected. This is most conveniently done by polymerase chain reaction (PCR) and a number of multiplex PCR systems have been described although none is commercially available.

Uropathogens and neonatal sepsis

Standard microbiological procedures are used to isolate *E. coli* from urine, blood or CSF. It is possible to demonstrate PFEC or *E. coli* K1 using specific antisera, although this is not entirely necessary.

TREATMENT, PROGNOSIS AND PREVENTION
Enteropathogens

In general, diarrheal disease should be managed by assessment of dehydration and appropriate rehydration. Antimicrobial therapy is not normally indicated and in some cases, for example with *E. coli* O157, might be harmful. However, some infections with EPEC and EaggEC can produce persistent diarrhea and in such cases antimicrobial chemotherapy directed by in vitro sensitivity testing is appropriate.

The prognosis is good with full recovery without antibiotic therapy in most cases. There are no vaccines currently available, so good hygiene and recognition of risk are the mainstay of infection prevention both in hospital and the community.

Uropathogens

For uncomplicated infections, short course (3–5 days) antimicrobial chemotherapy will suffice. If complicated by pyelonephritis or septicemia, longer duration of treatment will be needed. For prognosis, prevention and follow-up, see the appropriate section on urinary tract infection.

Neonatal sepsis

For pre-emptive, empiric therapy, see the section on neonatal sepsis. This will need to be modified in the light of the local antimicrobial susceptibility patterns. No vaccine is available, especially since the K1 capsule is a self-antigen.

BACTERIAL INFECTIONS: *HAEMOPHILUS INFLUENZAE*

GENERAL FEATURES AND EPIDEMIOLOGY

Haemophilus influenzae was first reported by Pfeiffer in 1892. A small Gram negative bacterium, it may be encapsulated or non-encapsulated (nontypable). In 1931 Pitmann[190] described six antigenically distinct capsular types, designated a to f. The possession of the capsule is an important virulence determinant and it is *H. influenzae* of capsular serotype b (Hib) that stands out as the most virulent strain, responsible for the great majority of invasive *Haemophilus* infections. Prior to the widespread use of effective vaccines against Hib, it was the major cause of bacterial meningitis and the predominant cause of epiglottitis in young children. In the Oxford region between 1985 and 1990 for example, the incidence of all invasive Hib disease was 36 cases/100 000 children < 5 years old.[191] Table 28.22 summarizes several characteristics relating to carriage and pathogenicity.

H. influenzae is among the bacteria normally found in the human pharynx and also colonizes the mucosae of the conjunctiva and genital tracts. Spread from one individual to another occurs by airborne droplets or by direct transfer of secretions. Exposure begins during or immediately after birth so that from infancy onwards, carriage of one or more strains for periods lasting from days to months is common. The presence of *H. influenzae* in cultures obtained from the upper (but not the lower) respiratory tract is therefore a common and normal finding. In about 3–5% of individuals, the organisms are encapsulated, most often with the serotype b antigen (in an unvaccinated population). Following widespread vaccination, however, carriage of type b strains has declined. In general, carriers of *H. influenzae*, whether colonized

Table 28.22   Carriage and pathogenicity of *Haemophilus influenzae*

Strains	Common upper respiratory tract carriage rates	Principal manifestation of pathogenicity
Non-encapsulated (nontypable)	50–80%	Exacerbations of chronic bronchitis, otitis media, sinusitis, conjunctivitis, lower respiratory tract infections Bacteremic infections rare
Encapsulated, type	2–4% b (pre-vaccine)	Meningitis, epiglottitis, pneumonia and empyema, septic arthritis, cellulitis, osteomyelitis, pericarditis, bacteremia
Encapsulated, types a and c through f	1–2%	Rarely incriminated as pathogens. May cause bacteremia and meningitis

with encapsulated or nontypable organisms, remain healthy, but occasionally disease occurs. Two contrasting patterns of *H. influenzae* disease can be identified. The more serious in its consequences is invasive infections such as meningitis, septic arthritis, epiglottitis and cellulitis; these infections typically occur in young children, are associated with bacteremia and are caused by encapsulated type b strains. The second category includes less serious, but numerically more common infections that occur as a result of contiguous spread of *H. influenzae* within the respiratory tract. *H. influenzae* is a common cause of otitis media (accounting for 23% of bacteria isolated by tympanocentesis),[192] sinusitis, conjunctivitis and lower respiratory tract infection. These infections are usually, but not invariably, caused by nontypable strains. These generalizations are not hard and fast; nontypable strains are a cause of neonatal sepsis, as well as sepsis and meningitis in infants and children.[193] They are a common cause of severe, acute lower respiratory tract infections (often accompanied by bacteremia) among young children living in resource limited countries[194] and are responsible for about 50% of all *H. influenzae* causing invasive disease in adults.[195] Epiglottitis, however, appears to be a syndrome associated overwhelmingly with serotype b. Brazilian purpuric fever is a rare disease caused by a nontypable *H. influenzae*, biotype *aegyptius*. This occurs in young children who present initially with a conjunctivitis and go on to develop a serious, potentially fatal form of septicemia which can mimic meningococcemia.

PATHOGENESIS

The host and microbial determinants of colonization by *H. influenzae* are poorly understood. In animal experiments infection is potentiated by viruses such as influenza. Adhesins facilitate attachment to mucus and to human epithelial cells and there are cell wall components that inhibit the normal ciliary function of respiratory tract epithelium. The primacy of type b capsule as a crucial factor in the pathogenesis of invasive disease has been well established. Lipopolysaccharide is also important in facilitating bloodstream survival and blood–brain barrier damage in experimental infections. In rat and primate models of *H. influenzae* type b meningitis, organisms were found to invade the submucosa of the nasopharynx and to reach the meninges as a result of bacteremia rather than by direct penetration of contiguous structures such as the cribriform plate or the inner ear. The occurrence of meningitis correlated strikingly with the duration and intensity of bacteremia; experimental manipulation of the host factors that decrease the efficiency of intravascular clearance (e.g. splenectomy) increased the incidence of meningitis.[196]

IMMUNITY

Among the host factors governing susceptibility to invasive type b infection, the role of serum antibodies to polyribosyl-ribitol phosphate (PRP), the type b capsular antigen, has been shown to be critical. Serum anti-PRP antibodies in conjunction with complement-mediated bactericidal and opsonic activity mediate protective immunity against systemic infections in humans. The sera of newborns and young infants (up until about 3 months old) generally have sufficient amounts of passively acquired antibody to afford protection. Thereafter, the natural decline of these maternally derived antibodies is followed by a period lasting until the age of 2–4 years when the levels of antibody are inadequate to provide protection. The delay in the acquisition of serum anti-PRP antibodies is characteristic of children less than 2 years old and is a major reason for the high attack rates of *H. influenzae* b invasive disease in early infancy. Although some infants may be exposed to type b *H. influenzae* through nasopharyngeal carriage, the antigenic stimulus for these antibodies may also be different commensal bacteria or ingested foods, which immunize through their cross-reacting antigens.

In an infant rat colonization model, anti-PRP antibodies given intranasally are able to prevent nasopharyngeal colonization by Hib. The same effect is seen when these antibodies are given intraperitoneally and a minimum effective serum level can be defined.[197] If it is assumed that anti-PRP antibodies function in a similar manner on the oropharyngeal mucosa of human children, both serum-derived IgG and locally produced IgA may reduce Hib carriage and thereby protect against invasive disease. A clinical study has correlated protection against carriage of *H. influenzae* b in infants with vaccine-induced serum anti-PRP IgG antibodies of greater than or equal to 5 mcg/ml.[198]

CLINICAL FEATURES

Meningitis is the most serious manifestation of invasive infection due to *H. influenzae* b. Antecedent symptoms of upper respiratory infection are common. The most common signs are fever and altered behavior – including poor feeding, vomiting, irritability and drowsiness. Thus, none of these clinical features distinguishes the child with *H. influenzae* meningitis from several other infectious diseases or other forms of meningitis. In particular, young infants have few specific signs; nuchal rigidity and a bulging fontanelle are typical, but often absent, early in the course of established meningeal infection. Seizures, cranial nerve involvement and coma may develop as the disease progresses and the effects of raised intracranial pressure, cerebral edema and vasculitis prevail. Subdural effusions are common but these very rarely require specific management and are usually sterile. Overall mortality for *H. influenzae* meningitis is less than 5% in resource rich countries but significantly higher, ranging from 22 to 40%, in resource limited countries. Sequelae occur in 15–30% of those who survive; the commonest complication is sensorineural deafness.

Acute respiratory obstruction caused by involvement of the supraglottic tissue by *H. influenzae* b (epiglottitis) is a potentially lethal disease of characteristically rapid onset. Typically, the child is aged 2–7 years and presents with sore throat, fever, dyspnea and dysphagia (causing pharyngeal pooling and then oral drooling of secretions). The child is restless and anxious and often adopts a characteristic posture in which the neck is extended and the chin is protruded in order to minimize airway obstruction. Abrupt deterioration leading to death within a few hours may occur if adequate treatment is not provided. The characteristic findings are supralaryngeal. The epiglottis is red and swollen and resembles a red cherry at the base of the tongue. Although an abrupt death is usually the result of acute airway obstruction, sudden collapse may result from less well defined mechanisms associated with acute toxemia. It should be emphasized that examination of the pharynx of a child in whom acute epiglottitis is suspected should only be attempted under conditions in which the airway can be secured immediately, otherwise the examination may precipitate respiratory arrest.

Invasive disease due to non-type-b encapsulated and nontypable *H. influenzae* is rarer but may present in a similar fashion. Presentation may also be similar in the rare group of children who develop invasive disease with *H. influenzae* b despite vaccination, 'vaccine failures'. In both groups, predisposing host factors such as immunodeficiency should be sought.[193,199]

Confirmation of the clinical impression of invasive *H. influenzae* infection depends upon cultures of normally sterile fluids (e.g. CSF, blood, pleural or synovial fluid). Positive nasopharyngeal cultures are not helpful since carriage is common among healthy persons. Needle aspiration of the middle ear (tympanocentesis), sinuses, the margins of an area of cellulitis or lung may occasionally prove helpful in selected cases, especially in a very sick child in whom no diagnosis has been established. Whenever practical, the results of Gram stain should be sought immediately; in up to 70% of cases of meningitis, CSF smears show the typical pleomorphic, Gram negative coccobacilli. Detection of capsular antigen in serum, CSF or concentrated urine by immunoassay (e.g. latex agglutination) may be useful, especially in children who have received prior antibiotic treatment. This test should be interpreted with caution, however, in those who have recently received Hib vaccine, as a false positive result is possible.

TREATMENT

Severe infections due to *H. influenzae* should be treated with parenteral third generation cephalosporins, for example cefotaxime or ceftriaxone. Ampicillin resistance has emerged among both encapsulated and nontypable strains (in the range of 10–30% for European and USA strains). Resistance is almost always mediated by beta-lactamases. This has particular relevance to the antibiotic management of less severe infections, such as otitis media and sinusitis. Although ampicillin/amoxicillin remains the antibiotic of choice, others such as amoxicillin–clavulanate or macrolides have become alternative first- and second-line choices.

The use of dexamethasone as adjunctive therapy in Hib meningitis can result in a reduction in sensorineural deafness.[200] Early administration, close to or even prior to the first dose of antibiotic, is preferable. Elective intubation and antibiotics are usually mandatory in cases of epiglottitis.

PREVENTION

Active immunization

The first generation of vaccines against Hib consisted of the purified type b polysaccharide. A trial in 1974 in Finland demonstrated efficacy in children older than 18 months of age but not in younger infants.[201] This led to the development of a second generation of vaccines in which the immunogenicity of PRP is enhanced by covalent linkage of the capsular polysaccharide or oligosaccharides to protein to form conjugate vaccines. Conjugate vaccines elicit significantly enhanced antibody responses when compared to PRP and, in contrast to the latter, are found to prime for a secondary antibody response. Clinical trials and national surveillance have confirmed their efficacy in infancy.[202] An unexpected outcome has been a reduction in Hib colonization of the upper respiratory tract and this has contributed to the near elimination of Hib disease in countries where immunization has become routine. Unfortunately, on a global scale too few countries have had the resources to use this vaccine for routine immunization. Experience from The Gambia[203] and Kenya[204] suggests that a dramatic effect on disease rates can be expected when vaccination is eventually implemented in all resource limited countries.

Children and adults who have an increased risk of invasive disease, e.g. those without spleens or with malignancy, should also receive *H. influenzae* b conjugate vaccines. These vaccines are safe and, in general, protective antibody responses are seen.

The burden of disease due to nontypable *H. influenzae* strains is also recognized and its prevention through vaccination is desirable. A recent study with an 11-valent pneumococcal polysaccharide–protein conjugate vaccine, in which the protein is protein D, a highly conserved cell surface lipoprotein of *H. influenzae*, has, for the first time, demonstrated efficacy against otitis media due to *H. influenzae*.[205]

Chemoprophylaxis

Young unimmunized or partially immunized children living in the same household as a case of invasive *H. influenzae* b disease are likely to be at significantly increased risk of secondary disease. In the pre-vaccine era secondary attack rates in household contacts were estimated to be 2–4% and in 'day-care centers' up to 1.3%. It is plausible that antibiotic prophylaxis could decrease this secondary attack rate. Rifampicin (20 mg/kg, maximum dose 600 mg/d), given orally once daily for 4 days, is effective in eradicating nasopharyngeal carriage. Treatment of household contacts (children and adults) where there are susceptible children less than 4 years old should be considered, as should treatment of such children in nurseries who are contacts of a case. The course of Hib vaccines should also be completed. The index case should also receive rifampicin prior to discharge unless he or she has been treated with a third generation cephalosporin.

BACTERIAL INFECTIONS: LEPROSY

EPIDEMIOLOGY

Worldwide, 4 million individuals have or are disabled by leprosy. The incidence, however, remains stable at around 450 000 new cases annually with high rates of childhood cases. India dominates the global picture with 67% of the global caseload. Few childhood cases are seen in Europe and North America, but in India childhood cases comprise at least 17% of the new case detection. In the UK, all new leprosy cases acquired their infection abroad. Average incubation times of 2–5 years and 8–12 years have been calculated for tuberculoid and lepromatous cases respectively. Age, sex, household contact and BCG vaccination are important determinants of leprosy risk. Leprosy incidence reaches a peak at age 10–11 years, and equal numbers of male and female cases are seen until puberty, after which there is an excess of male cases. Improved socioeconomic conditions, extended schooling and good housing reduce the risk of leprosy. HIV infection is not a risk factor for leprosy but may worsen leprosy nerve damage, and leprosy has been reported presenting as an immune reconstitution syndrome in adults treated for HIV.

MICROBIOLOGY AND PATHOLOGY

Leprosy is caused by *Mycobacterium leprae*, an acid-fast, intracellular organism that has the longest doubling time of all known bacteria (12 days) and cannot be cultivated on artificial media. *M. leprae* is a hardy organism, retaining viability for 5 months drying in the shade. The optimum temperature for growth is 27–30 °C, which corresponds with the clinical observation of maximal *M. leprae* growth at cool superficial sites (skin, nasal mucosa and peripheral nerves). The *M. leprae* 3.27 Mb genome has been sequenced. Less than half the genome contains functional genes: 165 genes are unique to *M. leprae*, but functions can be attributed to only 29. *M. leprae* has lost many genes for carbon catabolism and many carbon sources (e.g. acetate and galactose) are unavailable to it. The genome sequence is opening new possibilities for understanding the biological uniqueness of *M. leprae*.

Untreated lepromatous patients sneeze organisms into the environment. In Indonesia and Ethiopia, *M. leprae* DNA has been detected in nasal swabs in up to 5% of the population. After entry via the nose, *M. leprae* is inhaled, multiplies on the inferior turbinates and then has a brief bacteremic phase before binding to Schwann cells and macrophages. The skin is unimportant in leprosy transmission. Bacilli are not excreted by the skin and are rarely found in the epidermis. Untreated lepromatous leprosy mothers excrete *M. leprae* in their breast milk, but treatment renders the bacteria nonviable.

PATHOLOGY

There are four important aspects to the pathogenesis of leprosy: bacterial load, the host immune response, the nerve damage and immune-mediated reactions. Schwann cells and skin macrophages are infected early with granuloma formation. In established infection the host immune response determines not only the histological picture but also the clinical features of disease and the prognosis. The Ridley–Jopling spectrum describes the range of responses with tuberculoid and lepromatous poles. At the tuberculoid (TT) pole there is well-expressed cell-mediated immunity and delayed hypersensitivity control of bacillary multiplication, with formation of epithelioid cell granulomas. In the lepromatous (LL) form there is cellular anergy towards *M. leprae*, with abundant bacillary multiplication and unactivated macrophages. Between these two poles is a continuum, varying from the patient with moderate cell-mediated immunity (borderline tuberculoid, BT) through borderline (BB) to the patient with little cellular response, borderline lepromatous (BL).

Nerve damage occurs in small dermal nerves in skin lesions and peripheral nerve trunks. Acute immune-mediated reactions are serious complications because they cause nerve damage. Reversal reactions (type 1) are episodes of delayed hypersensitivity occurring at sites of localization of *M. leprae* antigens. Erythema nodosum leprosum (ENL) (type 2) reactions are due to immune complex deposition.

CLINICAL FEATURES

Patients commonly present with skin lesions, weakness or numbness due to a peripheral nerve lesion, or a burn or ulcer in an anesthetic hand or foot. Borderline patients may present with nerve pain, sudden palsy, multiple new skin lesions or pain in the eye. Childhood cases are frequently detected in school surveys or as household contacts of adult leprosy patients. In an Indian study based on a survey area, 30% of cases had a household contact with leprosy, usually a parent or grandparent.[206]

Cardinal signs
- Typical skin lesions, which are anesthetic at the tuberculoid end of the spectrum
- Thickened peripheral nerves
- Acid-fast bacilli on skin smears or biopsy.

Presenting symptoms
Early lesions
Indeterminate lesions are slightly hypopigmented or erythematous macules, a few centimeters in diameter, with poorly defined margins. Hair growth and nerve function are unimpaired. The indeterminate phase may last for months or years before resolving or developing into one of the determinate types of leprosy.

Skin
The commonest skin lesions are macules or plaques; more rarely papules and nodules are seen.

Anesthesia
Anesthesia may occur in skin lesions when dermal nerves are involved or in the distribution of a large peripheral nerve. In skin lesions, the small dermal sensory and autonomic nerve fibers supplying dermal and subcutaneous structures are damaged causing local sensory loss and loss of sweating within that area.

Peripheral neuropathy
Peripheral nerve trunks are vulnerable at sites where they are superficial or are in fibro-osseous tunnels. Damage to peripheral nerve trunks produces characteristic signs with dermatomal sensory loss and dysfunction of muscles supplied by that peripheral nerve. The sites of predilection for peripheral nerve involvement are ulnar (at the elbow), median (at the wrist), radial, radial cutaneous (at the wrist), common peroneal (at the knee), posterior tibial and sural nerves (at the ankle), facial nerve (on the zygomatic arch), and great auricular in the posterior triangle of the neck.

The leprosy spectrum
Classifying patients according to the Ridley–Jopling scale is clinically useful. Table 28.23 gives the skin and nerve features of disease across the spectrum. There is also a simpler field classification of paucibacillary/ multibacillary (Table 28.24) which guides the length of treatment. BB disease is unstable, and BT leprosy may be associated with rapid, severe nerve damage. BL patients are at risk of both reversal and ENL reactions.

LL has an insidious onset. The earliest lesions are ill defined with shiny erythematous macules. Gradually the skin becomes infiltrated and thickened and nodules develop; facial skin thickening causes the characteristic leonine facies. Dermal nerves are destroyed and sensory loss develops in a glove and stocking distribution. Sweating is lost. Damage to peripheral nerves is symmetrical and occurs late in disease. Testicular atrophy results from diffuse infiltration and the acute orchitis that occurs with ENL reactions.

Most studies in childhood report all types of leprosy; incidence rates and proportion of lepromatous cases increase with age. Few children present under the age of 5 years.

Eye
Eye damage results from both nerve damage and bacillary invasion. Lagophthalmos results from paresis of the orbicularis oculi due to involvement of the facial (7th) nerve. Damage to the ophthalmic branch of the trigeminal (5th) nerve causes anesthesia of the cornea putting it at risk of ulceration. Invasion of the iris and ciliary body makes them extremely susceptible to reactions.

DIAGNOSIS
Leprosy should be considered as a possible diagnosis in anyone with peripheral nerve or skin lesions who has lived in a leprosy endemic area. The diagnosis is clinical and based on finding a cardinal sign of leprosy, supported by the finding of acid-fast bacilli on slit skin smears. Where resources permit, histological examination of a skin or nerve biopsy

Table 28.23 Major clinical features of the disease spectrum in leprosy

Classification	TT	BT	BB	BL	LL
Skin					
Infiltrated lesions	Defined plaques Healing centers	Irregular plaques Partially raised edges	Polymorphic Punched out centers	Papules, nodules	Diffuse thickening
Macular lesions	Single, small	Several, any size	Multiple, all sizes Geographic	Innumerable, small	Innumerable, confluent
Nerve					
Peripheral nerve	Solitary, enlarged nerves	Several nerves Asymmetrical	Many nerves Asymmetrical	Late neural thickening Asymmetrical anesthesia and paresis	Slow, symmetrical loss Glove and stocking anesthesia
Microbiology					
Bacterial index (0–6)	0–1	0–2	2–3	1–4	4–6

BB, borderline; BL, borderline lepromatous; BT, borderline tuberculoid; LL, lepromatous leprosy; TT, tuberculoid.

Table 28.24 Modified WHO recommended multidrug therapy regimens

Type of leprosy	Drug treatment		Duration of treatment
	Monthly supervised	Daily self-administered	
Paucibacillary	Rifampicin 450 mg (or 10 mg/kg)	Dapsone 50 mg (or 1 mg/kg)	6 months
Multibacillary (MB)	Rifampicin 450 mg (or 10 mg/kg) Clofazimine 150 mg (or 3 mg/kg)	Clofazimine 50 mg (or 1.5 mg/kg) alternate days Dapsone 50 mg (or 1 mg/kg)	24 months
Paucibacillary single lesion	Rifampicin 450 mg, ofloxacin 200 mg, minocycline 50 mg (supplied in a single blister pack)		Single dose

WHO classification for field use when slit skin smears are not available:
• paucibacillary single lesion leprosy (one skin lesion);
• paucibacillary (2–5 skin lesions);
• multibacillary (more than five skin lesions).
In this field classification WHO recommends treatment of MB patients for 12 months only.

is ideal for accurate classification. Serological and polymerase chain reaction based diagnostic tests are not yet clinically useful.

Skin examination
The whole body should be inspected in a good light, otherwise lesions may be missed, particularly on the buttocks in borderline disease. Skin lesions should be tested for anesthesia.

Neurological examination
The peripheral nerves should be palpated systematically looking for enlargement and tenderness. Nerve function should be assessed by testing the small muscles of the hands and feet. Sensation on the hands and feet can be assessed and monitored using Semmes Weinsteinmonofilaments. These are now widely used in leprosy and diabetic clinics.

Slit skin smears
These should be undertaken from suspect lesions and standard sites (earlobes, arms and buttocks). Slit skin smears should be read by experienced technicians.

Outside leprosy endemic areas doctors frequently fail to consider the diagnosis of leprosy. Diagnosis had been delayed in over 80% of new patients seen between 1995 and 1999 at The Hospital for Tropical Diseases, London.[207] Patients had been misdiagnosed by dermatologists, neurologists, orthopedic surgeons and rheumatologists. A common problem was failure to consider leprosy as a cause of peripheral neuropathy in patients from leprosy endemic countries. These delays had serious consequences for patients, with over half of them having nerve damage and disability.

DIFFERENTIAL DIAGNOSIS
Skin
The variety of leprosy skin lesions means that many skin conditions need to be included in the differential diagnosis. In suspected tuberculoid lesions the presence of lesional anesthesia is crucial in differentiating leprosy from fungal infections, vitiligo, vitamin A deficiency and eczema. Single facial patches in children may be difficult to test for anesthesia and one may have to observe a lesion over some months. In lepromatous disease the presence of acid-fast bacilli in smears differentiates leprosy nodules from onchocerciasis and post kala-azar dermal leishmaniasis.

Nerves
Peripheral nerve thickening is rarely seen except in leprosy. Hereditary sensory motor neuropathy type III is also associated with palpable peripheral nerve hypertrophy.

TREATMENT
The treatment of leprosy has six main components: chemotherapy, monitoring and treating nerve damage, management of reactions and neuritis, patient education, prevention of disability and social and psychological support.

Chemotherapy
All children with leprosy should be given an appropriate multidrug combination. The first line anti-leprosy drugs are rifampicin, dapsone and clofazimine. Table 28.24 shows the drug combinations, doses and duration of treatment.

Rifampicin
Rifampicin is a potent bactericidal drug for *M. leprae*. Because *M. leprae* resistance to rifampicin can develop as a one-step process, rifampicin should always be given in combination with other anti-leprotics. Parents and children should be warned that their urine, sweat and tears will be red for 48 h after taking rifampicin.

Dapsone (DDS)
Dapsone (4,4-diaminodiphenylsulfone) is only weakly bactericidal. It commonly causes mild hemolysis but rarely anemia. Glucose-6-phosphate dehydrogenase deficiency is rarely a problem.

Clofazimine
Clofazimine has a weakly bactericidal action. It also has an anti-inflammatory effect, which has reduced the incidence of ENL reactions. Skin discoloration is the most troublesome side-effect, ranging from red to purple-black. The pigmentation usually fades slowly after stopping clofazimine. Clofazimine also produces a characteristic ichthyosis on the shins and forearms.

More than 14 million patients have been treated successfully with multiple drug treatment (MDT). Clinical improvement is rapid, toxicity rare, and duration of treatment is shortened. Monthly supervision of the rifampicin component has been crucial to success. The three drugs used for MDT are donated by Novartis free of charge for distribution in blister packs (pediatric and adult). At the end of 6 months' treatment of borderline disease there may still be signs of inflammation, which should not be mistaken for active infection. The distinction between relapse and reaction may be difficult. WHO studies have reported a cumulative relapse rate of 1.07% for paucibacillary leprosy and 0.77% for multibacillary leprosy at 9 years after completion of MDT. *M. leprae* is such a slow-growing organism that relapse only occurs after many years. Patients with a high initial bacterial load may be at greater risk of relapse and so require treatment until skin-smear negative.

Short course chemotherapy regimens have been tested for pauci-bacillary (PB) leprosy using either rifampicin in weekly doses or single dose chemotherapy using a combination of currently used drugs. So far all of these regimens have had higher relapse rates than the current WHO PB regimen. The fluoroquinolones (pefloxacin and ofloxacin) and the macrolide minocycline are all highly active against *M. leprae*, but because of cost are rarely used in field programs. A single dose of triple drug combination (rifampicin, ofloxacin and minocycline) has been tested in India for patients with single skin lesions and produced marked clinical improvement at 18 months in 52% of patients. Although the study had major flaws, and single dose treatment is less effective than the conventional 6-month treatment for PB leprosy, it is an operationally attractive field regimen.

Monitoring and treating nerve damage

Nerve damage may occur before diagnosis, or during and after MDT. It may occur during a reaction or without overt signs of nerve inflammation (silent neuropathy). About 30% of newly diagnosed patients have nerve damage and at least 25% of multibacillary patients develop nerve damage during treatment. Children are at the same risk as adults of developing nerve damage and having reactions. Monitoring sensation and muscle power in a child's hands, feet and eyes should be part of the routine follow-up so that new nerve damage is detected early. Any new damage should be treated with a course of oral steroids, starting with prednisolone 0.5 mg/kg/d and reducing by 0.1 mg/d each month. Response rates vary depending on the severity of initial damage, but even when promptly treated, nerve damage will only improve in 60% of cases.

Management of reactions and neuritis

Reversal (type 1) reactions

Reversal reactions manifest clinically with erythema and edema of skin lesions and tender, painful peripheral nerves. Loss of nerve function may be dramatic and foot drop can occur overnight. Awareness of the early symptoms of reversal reactions by both patient and physician is important, because, if left untreated, severe nerve damage may develop. The peak time for reversal reactions is in the first 2 months of treatment. The treatment of reactions is aimed at controlling acute inflammation, easing pain, reversing nerve damage and reassuring the patient. MDT should be continued. If there is any evidence of neuritis (nerve tenderness, new anesthesia and/or motor loss) corticosteroid treatment should be started using the regimen given above.

Erythema nodosum leprosum type 2 (ENL) reactions

This complication affects only BL and LL patients and presents with crops of small, pink, tender skin lesions on the face and the extensor surfaces of the limbs. In a cohort study from Hyderabad, India, 31% of children with BL/LL disease developed ENL.[208] The patient is usually unwell with malaise and fever. Other accompanying signs are acute iritis and episcleritis, lymphadenitis, orchitis, bone pain, dactylitis, arthritis and proteinuria. This is a difficult condition to treat and frequently requires treatment with high dose steroids (1 mg/kg daily, tapered down rapidly) or thalidomide. Since ENL frequently recurs, steroid dependency can easily develop. Thalidomide (5 mg/kg daily) is superior to steroids in controlling ENL and is the drug of choice for young men with severe ENL. Unfortunately thalidomide is unavailable in several leprosy endemic countries despite its undoubted value. Clofazimine has a useful anti-inflammatory effect in ENL and can be used at 3 mg/kg daily for several months.[209] Acute iridocyclitis is treated with 4-hourly instillation of 1% hydrocortisone eye drops and 1% atropine drops twice daily.

Neuritis

Silent neuritis should be treated similarly to reversal reaction (see above). In the Hyderabad study 24% children developed neuritis.[208]

Patient education

Patients and their parents deserve a clear explanation of the etiology, diagnosis and prognosis of leprosy. It should be emphasized that the infection is curable provided that they comply with the antibiotic regimen. It is important to stress that deformity is not an inevitable disease endpoint. It may be helpful to ask parents and older patients about their views of leprosy as there are many myths about leprosy, which can be dispelled. Lepromatous patients become non-infectious within 72 h of starting antibiotics. Patients and their families should be encouraged to lead a normal life and be reassured that family activities such as eating together, sharing baths and bed linen pose no risks to other family members. It should be emphasized that leprosy is not transmitted sexually nor is it hereditary.

Prevention of disability

It is vital in preventing disability to create patient self-awareness so that damage is minimized. In a study from south India, 33% of children presenting to a referral center had visible deformities.[210] The child with an anesthetic hand or foot needs to understand the importance of daily self-care, especially protection when doing potentially dangerous tasks and regular inspection for trauma. For each patient it is helpful to identify potentially dangerous situations, such as cooking, radiators and hot food. Soaking dry hands and feet followed by rubbing with oil keeps the skin moist and supple.

An anesthetic foot needs the protection of an appropriate shoe. For anesthesia alone, a well-fitting 'trainer' with a firm sole and shock-absorbing inner will provide adequate protection. Once there is deformity, such as clawing, special shoes must be made to ensure protection of pressure points and even weight distribution.

Children should be taught to work out why an injury occurred so that the risk can be avoided in future. Plantar ulceration occurs secondary to increased pressure over bony prominences. Ulceration is treated by rest. In leprosy, ulcers heal if they are protected from weightbearing. No weightbearing is permitted until the ulcer has healed. Appropriate footwear should be provided to prevent recurrence.

Physiotherapy exercises should be taught to maximize function of weak muscles and prevent contractures. Contractures of hands and feet, foot drop, lagophthalmos, entropion and ectropion are amenable to surgery.

Social, psychological and economic rehabilitation

The social and cultural backgrounds of the patient determine the nature of many of the problems that may be encountered. The family may have difficulty in coming to terms with leprosy. The community may reject the patient. Education, confidence from family, friends and doctor, and plastic surgery to correct stigmatizing deformity all have a role to play.

PROPHYLAXIS

In non-endemic areas it is very unusual to see leprosy in contacts of leprosy patients. The last case of secondary transmission in the UK was reported in 1923. Household contacts of new patients should be examined for clinical signs of leprosy and advised to report any new skin lesions promptly and to tell their physicians that they have had contact with a known case of leprosy. In the UK, BCG vaccination is given to contacts under the age of 12; chemoprophylaxis is reserved for children under 10 years who are household contacts of lepromatous cases. They are given prophylaxis with rifampicin 15 mg/kg body weight given monthly for 6 months.[211] BCG gives variable protection, ranging from 80% in Uganda to 20% in Burma. In trials in Malawi and Venezuela, adding killed *M. leprae* to BCG did not enhance protection.

BACTERIAL INFECTIONS: LEPTOSPIROSIS

Leptospirosis is a worldwide zoonosis transmitted to humans by infected urine of a wide range of domestic and wild animals: often the causative spirochetes are excreted asymptomatically for long periods of time.

Adults usually acquire infection because of occupational exposure: children may acquire infection by playing in areas contaminated with animal urine or by playing with the animals themselves.

PATHOLOGY

In the UK and USA the common serotypes of the genus *Leptospira* include *Leptospira icterohaemorrhagiae* (commonly acquired from rat's urine*)*, *Leptospira canicola* (commonly acquired from dog's urine), *Leptospira pomona* (commonly acquired from pig's urine), *Leptospira hebdomadis* and *L. ballum*. Correlation of named serotypes with specific syndromes is impossible because of the variability of illness produced by each serotype.

Leptospires gain entry to humans via ingestion, mucous membranes, skin abrasions or the conjunctivae. After entry, the organisms affect capillary epithelium and may cause capillary damage, hypoxia and hemorrhage into various organs. Liver damage may cause jaundice (although hemolysis may also play a part), renal damage may cause renal failure, central nervous system damage meningitis and encephalitis, and skeletal muscle involvement muscle pain. Blood clotting parameters are often not disordered enough to account for the hemorrhagic tendency. Illnesses may be biphasic with initial symptoms caused by leptospiremia and later symptoms by host immune responses.

CLINICAL FEATURES

The incubation period is probably from a few days to just under 3 weeks.

The clinical manifestations range through asymptomatic infection to multisystem disease. With clinical disease there is usually an abrupt onset of fever with several possible accompaniments:
1. muscular pains;
2. marked constitutional upset and hemorrhagic manifestations;
3. nephritic features usually without associated hypertension;
4. jaundice with or without hemorrhages;
5. jaundice with leukocytosis or a raised erythrocyte sedimentation rate (leukocytosis and a raised sedimentation rate are unusual in viral hepatitis);
6. meningitis with injected or hemorrhagic conjunctivae, or a lymphocytic meningitis with normal biochemical parameters: this syndrome is typically associated with *L. canicola* infection;
7. persistent fever lasting up to 3 or 4 weeks, perhaps without other signs;
8. jaundice with nephritis – Weil syndrome, usually caused by *L. icterohaemorrhagiae* infection in which renal failure is a common cause of death (in contrast most patients with viral hepatitis have a low or normal blood urea and present with gradual-onset malaise and fever which usually remits once jaundice is apparent).

DIAGNOSIS AND DIFFERENTIAL DIAGNOSIS

Blood cultures may be positive in early illness, but some *Leptospira* resist standard culture and the diagnosis has to be confirmed by dark ground microscopy or by serology. Usually reactive antibody becomes detectable after the first week of illness. Agglutination and complement fixation tests are often used. If there is a meningitic clinical picture the CSF is usually lymphocytic; the CSF biochemistry is often normal and CSF culture may be positive. Urine culture or dark ground microscopy may be positive once infection is established, and may remain positive for several weeks.

The differential diagnosis is very wide: if a zoonosis is suspected, Q fever and brucellosis are major contenders.

TREATMENT

Eradication of noncommercial animals (such as rats) or reducing potential exposure to animal urine is ideal. *Leptospira* are sensitive to penicillin, tetracyclines (which are contraindicated in renal failure and which, depending on the severity of illness, are contraindicated in children) and erythromycin. Usually high doses are given for 10 days. Early treatment is essential as antibiotics will do little to alleviate the immune-mediated elements of the illness. Isolation of patients is unnecessary as person-to-person spread is unlikely. Despite serious dysfunction of infected organs in acute illness, recovery is usually complete in survivors.

LYME DISEASE

Lyme disease is a seasonal non-occupational bacterial zoonosis which is distributed throughout the temperate zones of the world.[212] It was first recognized in 1975 because of a geographic clustering of children with arthritis in Lyme, Connecticut.[213] It is now recognized that the causative agent is an arthropod-borne spirochete called *Borrelia burgdorferi* which is transmitted by the hard tick *Ixodes dammini* or related ixodid ticks depending on the geographical distribution, e.g. *Ixodes ricinus* is predominant in Europe.[214] The tick, which has a wide range of hosts (deer, cattle, sheep, mice, squirrels, dogs), appears to prefer the white-footed mouse and white-tailed deer. Birds are now also recognized as reservoirs.

The anatomical location of tick bites appears important. Patients bitten on the head and neck had significantly more neurological manifestations, perhaps explaining the higher frequency of neuroborreliosis among children compared with adults.[215]

The illness is a multisystem disorder, which consists of a prodromal febrile illness with the characteristic rash of erythema chronicum migrans (ECM) and associated symptoms. Without antibiotic treatment a substantial number of patients will go on to cardiac, neurological and rheumatological sequelae. However, progression from early to late stage is not inevitable, even in the absence of antibiotic treatment. 'Incomplete' cases with minimal or absent rash can occur, and patients may have aseptic meningitis, facial palsy, carditis or arthritis as the first sign of disease.

ETIOLOGY AND VECTOR

In 1982 a previously unrecognized spirochete was isolated from *I. dammini* ticks that had been collected from Shelter Island, New York. This discovery was followed in 1983 by the successful culture of the spirochete named *B. burgdorferi* from patients with Lyme disease.

The main vector species are *I. ricinus* in Europe and the *I. scapularis* group in North America.[216] The life cycle of the tick consists of larval, nymphal and adult stages. The larvae and nymphs primarily feed on rodents such as the white-footed mouse, the natural reservoir for *I. dammini*. The adults usually feed on large mammals like deer, sheep and horses. Furthermore, the growth of the vector population is promoted by deer and fails to occur in their absence. The nymphal stage, whose peak questing period is May through July, is primarily responsible for transmission of disease. As these immature ticks feed aggressively on more animal species they facilitate rapid transmission of the organisms and often escape detection by the human host because they remain very small, even after a feed.

EPIDEMIOLOGY

Lyme disease is the most common vector-borne disease among children with more cases in children than in adults. However, there is substantial regional variation in the incidence of Lyme disease although most cases appear to occur during the summer months. The estimated incidence in the USA in 1992 was 3.9 per 100 000 population with Connecticut having the highest incidence (53.6/100 000). These figures are undoubtedly underestimates as only a small proportion of cases are reported. In the UK, for example, the incidence of Lyme disease is not well documented although experience suggests that serious disease is not common. Children between the ages of 5 and 10 years appear to be at highest risk in endemic areas.

PATHOGENESIS

In early Lyme disease the spirochete is injected into the bloodstream or skin through tick saliva. It may also be deposited in fecal material on the skin, and from there the organism may invade the skin or blood. Following an incubation period of 3–32 days the organism migrates outwards in the skin to produce the classical immune-mediated lesion of ECM. It may also spread to the lymphatics or disseminate in the blood or organs such as the brain, heart or joints or to other sites to produce the secondary lesions of late stage disease. The propensity to produce damage of a specific target organ appears to be determined by a number of factors including genospecies of *Borrelia* isolate as well as host factors such as human leukocyte antigen (HLA) phenotype. For example, *B. afzelii* is more common in patients with mainly dermatological manifestations, whereas *B. garinii* is more often associated with neurological complications. Furthermore, arthritis, which is a more common presentation of early or late Lyme disease in Europe as opposed to ECM in North America, is more commonly seen in patients with HLA-DR4 and -DR2.[217] There is also some evidence that patients with severe and prolonged illness, especially neurological or joint disease, have an increased frequency of the B cell alloantigen HLA-DR2.[218]

CLINICAL CHARACTERISTICS

Like other spirochetal infections the illness can occur in distinct stages which may overlap or occur alone without recalling earlier features.

Early manifestations[219]

Up to one third of patients remember a tick bite which often leaves a nonspecific small red macule or papule. About 1 week later this area expands to the pathognomonic warm, painless, erythematous, annular lesion called ECM which reaches a maximum diameter of 15 cm (larger areas up to 70 cm have been reported) and usually has a bright red outer border. In the largest community-based prospective study reported in children, 89% of those studied presented with a single or multiple lesions of ECM.[220]

This lesion, which resolves within 4 weeks without therapy, can occur at any site although the thigh, groin and axilla are particularly common. Concomitant signs and symptoms include high fever (particularly in children), malaise, regional lymphadenopathy, meningism, myalgia and migratory arthralgias. Most of the early clinical features are characteristically intermittent and fluctuating during a period of several weeks, before spontaneous resolution occurs. About 10% of patients have features suggestive of anicteric hepatitis. Cellulitis secondary to an infected insect bite is a common misdiagnosis.

Two uncommon skin lesions, acrodermatitis chronica atrophicans and lymphadenosis benigna cutis, which are rare both in children and in North America, are regarded as specific late skin manifestations in Lyme disease.[221]

Late manifestations

These manifestations occur some weeks to months after the initial infection and the clinical features are dependent on the organ affected and the severity of damage.

In about 10–40% of patients, frank *neurological abnormalities* usually occur weeks to months after infection. The classical triad of early neurological disease includes a lymphocytic meningitis, cranial neuropathy and radiculoneuritis. Neuroborreliosis in children most commonly presents as mild encephalopathy, lymphocytic meningitis and cranial neuropathy.[222] Radiculopathy, particularly in European children, and peripheral neuropathy, both of which occur late in the disease, are rare in children. Typically patients develop a fluctuating lymphocytic meningitis about 4 weeks after the onset of ECM often with superimposed cranial (especially facial) neuritis. Patients will have a CSF lymphocytic pleocytosis. Other less common neurological complications include ataxia, spastic paraparesis due to an acute myelitis, hemiparesis, optic neuritis, hydrocephalus, Guillain–Barré syndrome and a pseudotumor cerebri-like syndrome.

Cardiac disease, which is relatively uncommon in children, occurs roughly 5 weeks after the tick bite. The disease spectrum includes myopericarditis, cardiomegaly, left ventricular dysfunction and especially fluctuating degrees of atrioventricular block, which may progress to complete heart block. The latter may require temporary pacing. The duration of cardiac involvement is usually brief (3 days to 6 weeks) and self-limiting. The clinical features show similarities to rheumatic fever although valvular involvement has not been reported.

Arthritis is a common late sequela of Lyme disease occurring in up to 60% of patients within a few weeks to 2 years after the onset of illness; 20–40% of patients do not remember having ECM. The spectrum of Lyme arthritis ranges from subjective joint pains which are often migratory, to intermittent attacks of arthritis to chronic erosive disease (10%).[223] The commonest pattern of joint involvement is an acute asymmetric mono- or oligoarticular arthritis primarily affecting the large joints. Most commonly (> 90%) involved is the knee joint and the child typically presents with subacute effusion of the knee. The attacks of arthritis typically last for a few weeks to months and recur intermittently over several years. Fatigue is the commonest associated non-articular symptom, whereas fever or other systemic symptoms are unusual.

Numerous other rare manifestations have been associated with Lyme disease. These include ophthalmic complications (conjunctivitis, episcleritis, photophobia, uveitis), hepatitis, hepatosplenomegaly and testicular swelling. There is no clear evidence that *B. burgdorferi* causes congenital disease, although the existence of this rare syndrome cannot be ruled out.[224] Furthermore, transmission of Lyme disease in breast milk has not been documented.

DIAGNOSIS

The diagnosis is not always easy, given that symptoms may be nonspecific and serology may be misleading.[225] The hallmark for confirming the diagnosis is to obtain appropriate fluid or tissue for culture. Such tests are unlikely to be of value in everyday clinical practice and future diagnostic tests such as polymerase chain reaction (PCR) have not yet been adequately tested. Therefore, the diagnostic tests used most frequently are serological and detect antibodies against *B. burgdorferi*. The most commonly used of these tests, which is now widely available as a pre-packed commercial kit, is the enzyme linked immunosorbent assay (ELISA). Unfortunately, this test yields many false positive reactions with other spirochetal infections, connective tissue diseases and certain viral infections.[224] There is also cross-reactivity with antigens of spirochetes belonging to the normal flora. The immunoblotting technique currently offers the best means of validating a positive or equivocal ELISA in a patient with a low likelihood of Lyme, although this test is not widely available and its proper interpretation is as yet unclear.[226]

Currently the diagnosis of early Lyme disease, especially in the presence of skin lesions, is made on clinical and epidemiological grounds since serology (*B. burgdorferi* IgM) does not usually become positive until 3–6 weeks after the onset of the erythema migrans. Also, the antibody response may be aborted in patients with early Lyme who are treated promptly with an effective antimicrobial agent. The specific IgG antibody rises slowly and may not reach a level of diagnostic significance in early disease. It usually peaks months or years later, often when arthritis is present, and can persist for many years despite adequate treatment or cure. Furthermore, a substantial proportion of people who become infected by *B. burgdorferi* never have a clinical illness but have positive serology. Serological testing is not necessary for diagnosing typical ECM but is helpful in untreated atypical skin lesions, patients with acute meningitis, neuropathies and arthritis due to Lyme. The negative and positive predictive values of currently available serological tests are very much dependent on the pretest likelihood that a patient has Lyme disease. For example, a patient with ECM who lives in an endemic area has a very high probability of having Lyme even if the serological test is negative. Conversely, a patient with vague nonspecific symptoms with a positive test is unlikely to have Lyme despite positive serology. Therefore, serological tests should not be used on patients with nonspecific symptoms but clinicians should order serological tests for Lyme disease in selected groups such as those with clinical findings suggestive of Lyme or in highly prevalent areas so that the predictive value of the test is high.[224]

Notably the predictive value of positive serology in patients with erythema chronicum migrans as a single manifestation of Lyme disease is low.[227]

Patients reported to have Lyme disease who did not meet the United States Centers for Disease Control and Prevention (CDC) case definitions had increased symptoms and worsening quality of life indices, the implication being that such patients did not have Lyme disease.[228] A consensus paper noted that the risks of intravenous antibiotics in patients with nonspecific complaints outweighed potential benefits.[229]

The differential diagnosis is wide but includes other tick-borne diseases including ehrlichiosis and babesiosis.

TREATMENT

Since no clinical trials of treatment have been performed in children the recommendations for treatment have been extrapolated from adult studies.[230,231] Doxycycline 2.5 mg/kg (max 100 mg) orally, 12-hourly for 14–21 days is the oral antibiotic of choice for children 8 years or older. For younger children, amoxicillin 25 mg/kg orally, 12-hourly for 14–21 days, is recommended. Ceftriaxone 75–100 mg/kg, IM, once daily is recommended for persistent or recurrent arthritis and either ceftriaxone or benzylpenicillin 50 000 U/kg IV, 4-hourly for carditis, meningitis or encephalitis. Lyme disease will respond well to antibiotic therapy if treated early, shortening the duration of illness and reducing the incidence of complications. The long term prognosis for this group as well as those treated for late Lyme disease is excellent.

PREVENTION

Acquisition of Lyme borreliosis can be reduced by simple practical methods such as wearing long trousers, tucking trousers into socks, wearing boots, promptly removing any attached ticks and impregnating clothes with DEET or permethrin. A vaccine is currently under development.

BACTERIAL INFECTIONS: MENINGOCOCCEMIA

Despite the recent introduction of an effective vaccine against group C organisms in the UK, *Neisseria meningitidis* is still the most frequent cause of septicemia in childhood, and affects otherwise healthy children of all ages after the neonatal period. In the UK, there are over 1200 microbiologically confirmed cases a year (Statutory Notifications of Infections Diseases 1995–2006)[232] and probably double that number diagnosed on clinical grounds alone. About 50% will have meningitis. In the last decade, wider public awareness, better diagnosis and intensive care have improved the outcome, but mortality is still between 5 and 10%.

N. meningitidis is a Gram negative diplococcus which is surrounded by an outer polysaccharide capsule, an outer membrane and an underlying peptidoglycan layer. Pili or fimbriae extend through the capsule and are thought to play a role in the attachment to epithelial cells within the nasopharynx. Between 2 and 10% of the general population are colonized, but carriage rates may be much higher in outbreaks. The precise relationship between carriage and invasive disease remains unclear. Spread is predominantly by respiratory droplets from close contacts.

In Western Europe, the group B organism is still the most commonly isolated strain but is closely followed by group C organisms. In the UK, the introduction of a group C conjugate vaccine has reduced the rate of group C infections in the younger age group dramatically. Group A organisms have been responsible for large epidemics, particularly in sub-Saharan Africa, and another serogroup, W135, has caused a number of infections in pilgrims returning from the Hajj.

In spite of high colonization rates, only a relatively small number of colonized individuals develop invasive disease. Progression from nasal carriage to bacteremia is thought to be influenced by both bacterial and host factors. Certain bacterial properties, such as the presence of a capsule, pili and lipopolysaccharide (LPS) structure are known to be associated with invasive disease. There are also some data to indicate that smoking, respiratory tract infections and mucosal injury may aid colonization. However, the most important host factor predisposing individuals to this infection is the presence of defects within the complement cascade. Deficiencies of terminal complement components C5–C9, properdin and mannose-binding lectin all lead to an increased incidence of disease, and sometimes recurrent disease.

Having gained access to the circulation, bacterial components including LPS cause a host inflammatory response with the release of pro-inflammatory mediators such as tumor necrosis factor, IL-1, IL-6 and IL-8. These cytokines influence a number of cellular and noncellular functions including neutrophil, monocyte and endothelial cell activation, thrombotic and hemostatic pathway imbalance and complement activation. In addition, the organism can bind to vascular endothelial cells inducing adhesion molecule expression, with consequent leukocyte attachment and migration. Uninterrupted, this intense inflammatory process leads to tissue injury and ultimately to multiple organ failure and death.[233]

CLINICAL FINDINGS

There are two major clinical presentations of meningococcal disease: meningitis and septicemia. A proportion of patients will have evidence of sepsis and meningitis. Once in the bloodstream, however, *N. meningitidis* can localize to other sites including joints, bones, eyes and heart. Most deaths occur in the predominantly septicemic form of the disease. The presence of meningitis is a good prognostic indicator, and may indicate that host defenses have contained the infection long enough for the bacteria to invade the blood–brain barrier. Sepsis commonly presents with nonspecific symptoms of fever, vomiting, abdominal pain and muscle aches. These patients may also have a characteristic rash, which can occur anywhere and may be purpuric or morbilliform (Fig. 28.17). The extent of the inflammatory response will influence other signs of sepsis or septic shock. In the early stages, fever, tachycardia and tachypnea may be present with the rash. Later, signs of shock develop, with poor peripheral perfusion, hypotension and oliguria. These are generally accompanied by an extensive purpuric rash and evidence of disseminated intravascular coagulopathy (DIC) (Fig. 28.16). Recent evidence indicates that polymorphisms within the cytokine and hemostatic/thrombotic pathways can influence the severity of this disease. Hemorrhage into internal organs may occur. Classically, this involves the adrenal glands in the Waterhouse–Friderichsen syndrome. In those who recover, skin necrosis or vascular occlusion may cause the loss of an extremity, though most small lesions heal with minimal scarring.

The predominantly meningitic form of the disease presents with symptoms and signs of meningitis with fever, vomiting, headache and neck stiffness. Patients with meningitis may develop convulsions, focal neurological signs, a depressed level of consciousness, coma and death due to raised intracranial pressure (see Suspected meningitis). As the organism gains access to the central nervous system (CNS) from the blood, the petechial rash may be present and helpful in the diagnosis.

Arthritis, pericarditis and pleural effusions may occur as autoimmune phenomena 5–10 days after the acute infection. This is due to immune complex formation and is self-limiting, although a large pericardial effusion may cause cardiac tamponade. A rare chronic form of meningococcal sepsis can occur and is characterized by anorexia, weight loss, fever, arthralgia or arthritis and skin rash; erythema nodosum or bacterial endocarditis may also occur.

In the differential diagnosis, other bacterial and viral infections which cause purpura must be considered. Anaphylactoid purpura and idiopathic thrombocytopenic purpura may cause similar purpuric rashes. A morbilliform rash may be confused with a drug eruption or a number of viral infections including measles. Subacute or chronic meningococcemia presents a greater challenge. The differential diagnosis includes the many causes of arthritis and fever in children. However, a petechial rash in a febrile child should be considered as suggestive of meningococcal disease until proved otherwise.

LABORATORY INVESTIGATION

The diagnosis is established by recovery of *N. meningitidis* from the blood, petechial lesions or the CSF, but lumbar puncture is contraindicated in the presence of shock, coagulopathy, reduced conscious level or focal neurological signs. The practice of giving penicillin before hospital admission to patients in whom meningococcal infection is suspected, which has saved lives, has also decreased successful culture of the organism. In these situations, meningococcal DNA may still be detected by polymerase chain reaction (PCR) in blood and CSF. Serology may confirm the clinical diagnosis retrospectively. The complete blood count may show a polymorphonuclear leukocytosis. Neutropenia is invariably present in severe disease, however, and indicates a poor prognosis (see below). There is usually also evidence of DIC with thrombocytopenia, a coagulopathy and intravascular fibrin and thrombosis within dermal vessels. The importance of platelets and neutrophils in this disease is highlighted in a number of studies, which show that reduced circulating numbers of both cell types is correlated with a worse outcome.

TREATMENT

The most important aspect of meningococcal disease management is recognition. Recent work has shown that the classical signs of meningococcal disease with rash and meningism occur relatively late, 13–22 h after onset of illness. Early signs of disease include leg pains, cold hands and feet and pallor or mottling.[234] It is essential for the disease to be recognized early because, as with other forms of bacterial sepsis, bacterial load is critical, with higher bacterial concentrations leading to a more severe inflammatory response and organ dysfunction.[235] In patients with little capacity to limit bacterial growth within blood, a single bacterium may proliferate to more than a million organisms in under 8 h. Most deaths occur in patients with a bacterial load of more than a million organisms/ml. Early intervention with antibiotics will rapidly arrest bacterial growth and reduce levels of circulating LPS and other bacterial components. A third generation cephalosporin, such as cefotaxime or ceftriaxone, has become the standard therapy for the initial treatment of suspected meningococcal disease. Once the organism is isolated and sensitivity determined, penicillin can be used in the majority of cases. It is recommended that family doctors who see a patient with suspected meningococcal infection in the home give a dose of intramuscular penicillin immediately. Some recent data suggest that this course of action is associated with a higher mortality, but this is probably because primary care physicians administer penicillin to the sickest children.

In shocked children, vigorous resuscitation is required. Volume expansion with plasma and/or 4.5% albumin (20 ml/kg and repeat as required) is the crucial first step. Emergency transfer to the regional intensive care unit is usually advisable as inotropic and vasopressor agents, artificial ventilation and hematological support are frequently required (see section on sepsis). In very severe disease, extracorporeal membrane oxygenation may be life saving.

New therapies, which alter the immune response or inflammatory cascade, are under investigation at present, but no such agents have been shown to be effective to date. However, as in other forms of sepsis (see section on sepsis), corticosteroids, endotoxin and inflammatory modulation, activated protein C administration and endocrine manipulation may prove beneficial in the future.

PROPHYLAXIS

Prophylaxis against invasive disease should be given to the family and close contacts of the patient. Rifampicin, given in 4 doses over 2 days, has been shown to be effective in clearing the organism. A single injection of ceftriaxone, or an oral dose of ciprofloxacin, are appropriate alternatives.

In the UK, a conjugate meningococcal C vaccine has now been introduced with evidence of a marked decline in this organism in vaccinated individuals. Polysaccharide vaccines are available for *N. meningitidis* groups A, C, Y and W135 for patients traveling to endemic areas. Trials continue on vaccines against *N. meningitidis* group B.

PROGNOSIS

The mortality from acute meningococcemia remains high at between 5 and 10%, most deaths occurring in patients with very high bacterial loads. Early recognition is the key to improved outcome. Survivors may suffer extensive tissue injury, sometimes requiring amputation and/or skin grafting. A number of prognostic scores have been developed, the most frequently quoted being the Glasgow meningococcal septicemia prognostic score. This is predominantly based upon clinical parameters such as blood pressure and coma, but as supportive care has improved, this score may no longer accurately identify patients at greatest risk of mortality. Other scores have now been developed which revolve around hematological parameters, and a simple score based on the product of the initial platelet and neutrophil count has been shown to be a better prognostic guide to mortality. This score may help to identify those patients at whom novel therapeutic agents should be targeted.[236]

BACTERIAL INFECTIONS: *MYCOBACTERIUM TUBERCULOSIS*

In technically advanced countries, morbidity and mortality from tuberculosis have declined progressively over the decades. This is associated with improved living conditions and medical care, particularly case finding and chemotherapy. However, it is still an important problem, especially in immigrant and minority groups. In some resource limited countries, the case rate has hardly changed and any decline is offset by an increase in population.

The majority of children infected by *M. tuberculosis* are asymptomatic. However, in a small number, especially young children, the disease is serious or fatal, due to meningitis or disseminated disease, and survivors may be left with sequelae such as cerebral palsy, mental retardation or chronic lung or bone and joint disease.

MICROBIOLOGY

The 'tubercle bacillus' was first described by Robert Koch in 1882 and is now called *Mycobacterium tuberculosis*. Mycobacteria derive their name from their mold-like appearance on culture. One of their unique characteristics is a highly complex, lipid-rich cell wall which protects the bacillus from digestion by the lysosomal enzymes of macrophages and which, when stained, resists decolorization by acid alcohol. Like *Mycobacterium leprae*, but different from other mycobacteria, *M. tuberculosis* is an obligate parasite with total dependence on the living host.

The two major species of mycobacteria infecting man are *M. tuberculosis* and *M. bovis*. *M. bovis* differs from the other types in its resistance to pyrazinamide. *M. tuberculosis* is aerophilic but *M. bovis* is micro-aerophilic (prefers reduced oxygen tension). Within the host, mycobacteria may lie dormant for many years.

M. tuberculosis is cultured on Lowenstein–Jensen medium and is slow growing, taking an average time of 21 days, and occasionally 1–2 months or longer. Growth of *M. tuberculosis* may be detected in 7–10 days using liquid culture media, e.g. the BACTEC radiometric or Roche biphasic systems.

There are two major methods for direct identification in specimens: Ziehl–Neelsen stain and fluorescence microscopy with auramine–rhodamine stain. The latter is the more rapid, more sensitive and more specific.

A number of serological tests have been developed using purified protein derivatives of *M. tuberculosis* in enzyme linked immunosorbent assay (ELISA) or solid-phase radioimmunoassays. However, many lack sensitivity and specificity, especially for culture-negative cases, and thus are not used for routine laboratory diagnosis.[237] Tests for antigen in CSF are useful, but not routinely available. Gene probes can identify mycobacteria rapidly once they have grown in culture. In adults, nucleic acid amplification (NAA) has sensitivity >90% and specificity 98% for smear positive respiratory specimens, but only 50–70% sensitivity for smear negative specimens.[238] Sensitivity for nonrespiratory specimens, particularly CSF, is lower than for respiratory specimens. This is partly due to inhibitors especially in pleural, ascitic and CSF specimens. There are few studies in children and they are limited by numbers of confirmed or probable cases of tuberculosis.[239,240] Sensitivities for polymerase chain reaction (PCR) in gastric aspirates in children with confirmed or clinical pulmonary tuberculosis vary from 40 to 80% and generally are higher than culture. Sensitivity is increased by testing multiple samples. Specificity is reported to be 94–100%, although PCR may be positive in a third of children with tuberculous infection only. Sensitivities are no higher in bronchoalveolar lavage (BAL) than in gastric aspirates. PCR can differentiate between *M. tuberculosis* and environmental mycobacteria and PCR methods are available to detect rifampicin resistance. DNA fingerprinting is a valuable tool in studying transmission of tuberculosis.

EPIDEMIOLOGY

In studies of tuberculosis, differentiation has to be made between tuberculous infection (as evidenced by a positive tuberculin test) and disease. In tuberculous disease there is clinical, radiological or bacteriological evidence of infection. The great majority of infected people remain asymptomatic. In England and Wales in 1949–1950, a national survey showed that nearly half of 14-year-old children were tuberculin positive. Today, less than 1% of 11–13-year-old children are tuberculin positive at routine school examination.

Three quarters of tuberculosis cases occur in resource limited countries where 0.2–1% of the population are expectorating the tubercle bacillus. A rise in case rates in adults and children has been observed in countries with a high prevalence of HIV infection, especially sub-Saharan Africa.[241]

In technically advanced countries, with a low prevalence of smear positive cases, the infection rate in children will be low and the majority of adults with tuberculosis will have endogenous reactivation. Conversely, in resource limited countries, the high prevalence of smear positive cases will result in a significant proportion of children and young adults developing primary tuberculosis, and exogenous reinfection in older adults will be common. Children under 14 years may comprise up to 20% of case load in the Indian subcontinent, 39% in South Africa and 5% in the United States.[241,242]

National surveys for England and Wales for the periods 1978–1979, 1983, 1988, 1993 and 1998 found 747 (estimate based on 6 month survey), 452, 308, 408 and 364 newly notified children under 15 years respectively.[243] In 1998, rates (per 100 000) for children were highest for black African (70.6) and Indian subcontinent (23.1) compared to black Caribbean (9.0) and white (1.1) groups. Although rates for the Chinese group were high (82.1), cases were low (14).

The decline in the incidence of tuberculosis began in Europe before the introduction of BCG and chemotherapy. In the decade 1979–1988 there was an average reduction in notification rates in England of 7.2% per year. However, since 1988 there has been a 21% rise in notifications, with the highest increase in the London area. In the 1998 survey, 49% of children with tuberculosis were resident in London, 44% of whom were born abroad, compared to 10% resident elsewhere.[243] There has also been a rise in notifications in parts of Europe and the USA. Factors associated with the rise in notifications in the USA since 1987 include HIV infection, homelessness, immigration and decline in resources for tuberculosis control. The increase is focal, mainly confined to inner cities, and 80% of childhood cases are in minority ethnic groups. Multidrug resistance is a major problem. However, with increased support for tuberculosis control, the rise in cases has reversed. In the period 1993–2003 the incidence decreased by 44%.[244]

Most cases of tuberculosis are caused by *M. tuberculosis*. *M. bovis*, which was an important cause of tuberculosis of the gastrointestinal tract, lymph nodes and bones, has virtually disappeared from technically advanced countries through eradication of tuberculosis in cattle and pasteurization of milk. In the UK before 1950, *M. bovis* was the cause of 33% of childhood and 10% of adult extrapulmonary disease.

However, there has been a recent increase in tuberculosis in cattle which is considered to be related to infection in badgers.[245] *M. bovis* infection is also an uncommon cause of tuberculosis in resource limited countries, except in communities where large amounts of raw milk are consumed, when it commonly presents with cervical adenitis. In the UK, it is still isolated from reactivated lesions in approximately 1% of adults.[245] *M. bovis* is resistant to pyrazinamide.

PATHOLOGY

The pathology of tuberculosis has been described by Miller.[246] The first response to the presence of the tubercle bacilli at the point of entry and in the regional nodes is a serous exudate. Neutrophils accumulate, then macrophages which ingest the bacilli and may be transformed into epithelioid cells, which contain more effective digestive enzymes in their lysosomes. Fusion of either macrophages or epithelioid cells forms characteristic multinucleate giant cells. Death of cells in the center of the tubercle (granuloma) results in caseation necrosis. Lymphocytes form a zone around the tubercle and are particularly apparent during the second month of infection, which coincides with the development of tuberculin sensitivity. Healing takes place with the deposition of collagen fibrils by fibroblasts, which wall off the caseous area from healthy tissue. After 12 months or more, calcification may be seen, which remains for years but may be completely reabsorbed. It usually has a stippled appearance. Alternatively, healing may not occur, or the tubercle-containing dormant bacilli may reactivate after months or years. Extensive necrosis with caseation and liquefaction may develop. Liquefaction allows bacilli to survive, inhibits macrophage and lymphocyte function because of lack of oxygen, and prevents drug penetration. Activity and healing of the lesion may occur concurrently.

IMMUNOLOGY

The main defense against infection by the tubercle bacillus is cell mediated. The role of B cells is unclear.

Tubercle bacilli are readily ingested, but are not killed by macrophages, in which they multiply. Toxic substances and other properties in the lipid-thick cell wall protect the bacillus against lysosomal enzymes. CD4 T lymphocytes (T helper cells), when sensitized by tubercle bacilli, produce cytokines which activate macrophages and CD8 cytotoxic T lymphocytes (CTL). CTLs lyse cells containing mycobacteria and enable macrophages to kill their ingested bacilli. The positive effect of T helper cells may be countered by suppressor activity. In advanced disease or in the presence of a large bacterial load these suppressor effects may predominate, which may explain the anergy commonly seen in these children.

Defense against tuberculosis has two major components: (1) cell-mediated immunity (CMI) controls the infection by activating macrophages which enables them to kill ingested mycobacteria, and (2) delayed type hypersensitivity (DTH) is active when the bacillary antigens reach high levels.[247] DTH is responsible for the tissue damage and caseation necrosis characteristic of post-primary tuberculous disease. There is no correlation between the degree of hypersensitivity and resistance to tuberculosis. The balance between hypersensitivity and resistance will influence the manifestation of tuberculosis, i.e. the former will be associated with clinical and radiological signs of the disease, whereas with the latter there will be a paucity of signs. Improved knowledge of T helper cells has enhanced understanding of the above mechanisms.[248] Three types of T helper cells are recognized: T_H0 (naive cells), T_H1 and T_H2. T_H0 cells differentiate into T_H1 cells or T_H2 cells. T_H1 lymphocytes secrete IL-2, interferon-gamma (IFN-gamma) and lymphotoxin-alpha and stimulate type 1 immunity, which is pro-inflammatory and characterized by phagocytic activity and DTH. IFN-gamma and lymphotoxin-alpha promote secretion of pro-inflammatory cytokines such as tumor necrosis factor-alpha (TNF-alpha). T_H2 cells secrete interleukins such as IL-4 and IL-5, which promote eosinophils and IgE and stimulate a more allergic type 2 immune response. The immunological reactions to tuberculosis are not as clearcut in humans as in mice (in which most experimental work has been undertaken), nor as in leprosy. It would seem, however, that in humans a type 1 response is important in protective inflammation and mounting a DTH response, and a switch to a type 2 response is associated with the period of healing and granuloma organization. High or prolonged type 1 activity may result in excessive DTH reactions and tissue destruction, associated with raised IFN-gamma and TNF-alpha levels. Conversely, failure to control infection, as in immunocompromised patients, is associated with increased type 2 activity. It is suggested that, in humans, excessive tissue destruction may relate to mixed T_H1/T_H2 response whereby a factor produced by type 2 cells makes tissues very sensitive to TNF-alpha.[249] Other important factors include transforming growth factor beta (TGF-beta) produced by mononuclear phagocytes, which may have negative effects on T_H1 activity and 1,25 $(OH)_2$ vitamin D_3 which appears important for action of macrophages in controlling intracellular mycobacterial replication.

A number of primary factors influence the outcome of the immune response, including the number of inhaled bacilli, their virulence and the immune response by the host. These are affected by secondary factors, e.g. age of the patient, infections such as measles, malnutrition, malignancy and immunodeficiency states. Children under 5 years and adolescents (especially females) are at higher risk of developing tuberculous disease.

PATHOGENESIS

The first infection by tubercle bacillus occurs most commonly by inhalation through the lungs, less often by ingestion through the alimentary tract (tonsils and ileum), and rarely by infection of an open wound on the skin. Infection of the mouth, skin and eyes may result from exposure to a dental surgeon with pulmonary tuberculosis. Enlargement of the regional lymph nodes provides an indication of the site of primary focus.

Primary infection

The primary focus in the lung is usually single and situated just under the pleura (Ghon focus) in a well-ventilated part of the lung. Bacilli multiply at the primary focus and in the regional lymph nodes. The primary focus and nodes form the primary complex. In most cases there is hematogenous and lymphatic dissemination throughout the body and to other parts of the lungs. Certain organs favor survival of the bacilli and these may later be affected by disease, e.g. apical and subapical regions of the lungs (Simon focus), where there is a higher oxygen tension, renal parenchyma, epiphyseal lines of bones, cerebral cortex and regional nodes. At about 4–8 weeks, acquired immunity develops and usually contains the infection; sensitivity to tuberculoprotein develops simultaneously. Bacilli stop multiplying and, in the great majority of cases, die or remain dormant indefinitely within the healing tubercle or macrophages. Tubercles, especially if large and apical or subapical, may reactivate at any time in life, if the balance between the organism and the host defense is upset.

In children, the primary focus in the lung is usually small or invisible on chest X-ray, but the regional nodes are enlarged and prominent. In contrast, regional nodes are usually not prominent in primary infection in adults.

The initial infection is usually asymptomatic. Occasionally a short period of fever and malaise may have been noted. Erythema nodosum may appear within a few weeks of the primary infection, coinciding with tuberculin conversion. It is an allergic hypersensitivity reaction, which may be associated with high levels of circulating immune complexes. Phlyctenular conjunctivitis is another, though rare, manifestation of hypersensitivity.

If the infecting load of bacilli is large or the host defense inadequate there may be (Fig. 28.23):

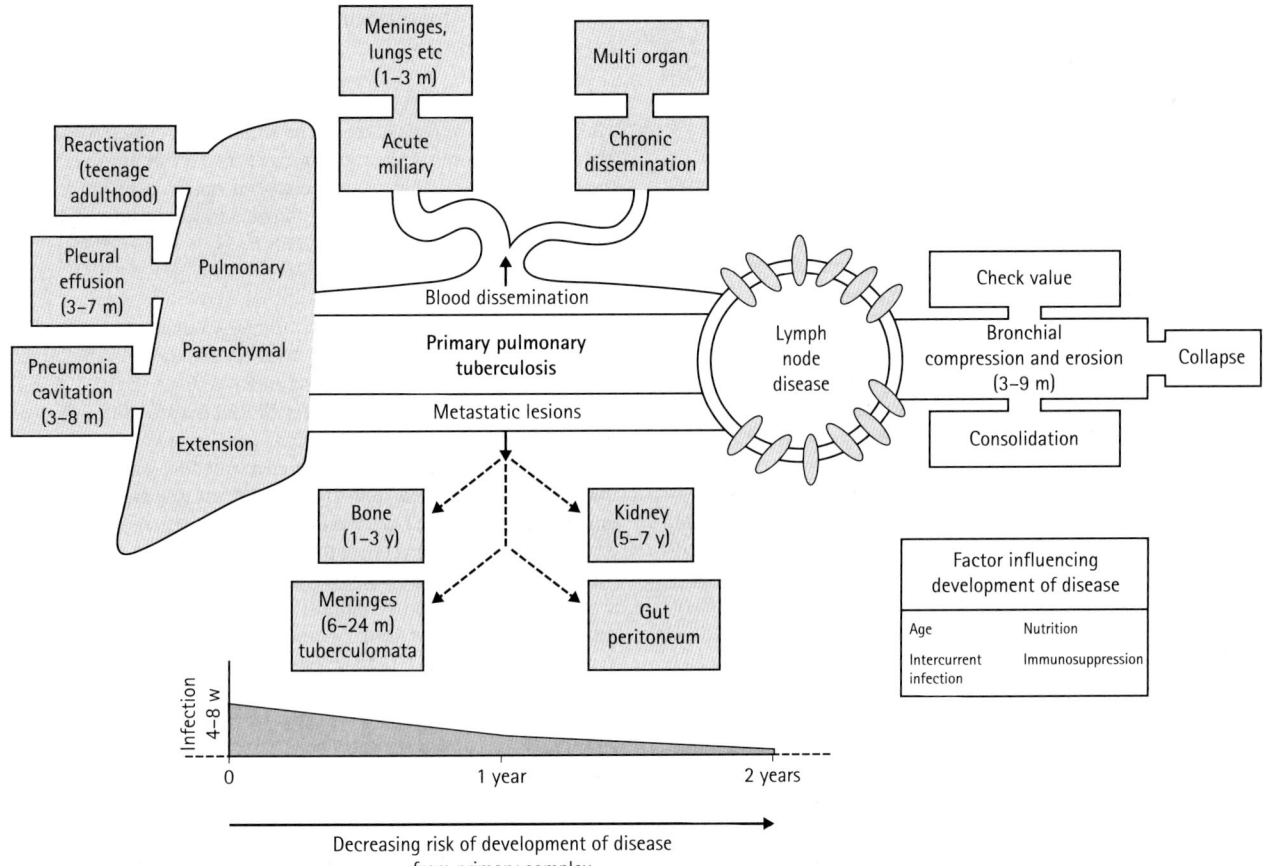

Fig. 28.23 Complications of primary pulmonary tuberculosis. Approximate interval between establishment of primary complex and development of complications in parentheses.

1. extension of the lung focus;
2. softening of the regional nodes;
3. extension of foci in other parts of the body;
4. hematogenous spread with dissemination of bacilli throughout the body (miliary tuberculosis), or chronic low grade dissemination (cryptogenic tuberculosis).

In a newly infected person the risk of developing tuberculous disease is highest in the first 2 years following a primary infection (especially in the first year). The risk is greater in infants and young children and those with malnutrition or immunosuppression. Infants have a risk of 40% or more of developing disease compared with 5% for adults. Pulmonary disease, miliary tuberculosis and meningitis are usually manifest within 1 year of infection, especially in young children, whereas bone disease presents later (within 3 years), and renal disease usually much later (over 5–7 years).

Post-primary tuberculosis

Post-primary tuberculosis occurs when a person who has previously had tuberculosis develops active disease. Post-primary tuberculosis can develop from endogenous reactivation of a primary lesion, from exogenous reinfection or both. Though sometimes termed 'adult'-type pulmonary tuberculosis, it may be seen in children.[246] It is characterized by strong resistance, which keeps the disease localized to the affected organ, and an active hypersensitivity state, which results in extensive tissue destruction and necrosis. The tubercle bacillus may have reached the area through blood spread following primary infection or via the airways in exogenous reinfection. For the latter, as the apices are not well ventilated, multiple exposure will usually be necessary.[250] It affects particularly the apical regions of the lungs, where the oxygen tension is higher. There is widespread caseation necrosis, liquefaction with cavity formation and healing by fibrosis.

TUBERCULIN SENSITIVITY

The intradermal tuberculin test using old tuberculin was described by Charles Mantoux in 1908. A positive response results in induration within 72 h, associated with migration of activated lymphocytes and macrophages to the site of injection.

Purified protein derivative (PPD)-S 5 IU is the standard strength in many countries. PPD RT 23 Statens Serum Institute (SSI), Copenhagen is administered at a strength of 2 tuberculin units (TU). Induration of ≥6 mm with RT 23 is regarded as positive. Because the active principle of RT 23 adheres to glass walls of containers, Tween 80 is added to reduce absorption. This multiplies the strength by a factor of 4–5. Weaker and stronger products are available. In phlyctenular conjunctivitis or tuberculosis of the eye it is suggested to use a weaker strength initially as a stronger solution may result in a severe eye reaction. Stronger solutions, e.g. 10 TU, are rarely indicated as they may give false positive reactions with environmental mycobacterial infections.

Technique of tuberculin test

The skin is cleaned and dried, and the injection given *intradermally* into the upper third of the flexor surface of the forearm (Mantoux test) with a 1 ml syringe and a small needle (short bevel gauge 25–26) producing a wheal of at least 5 mm (see BCG technique). The result should be read at 48–72 h, but a valid result may be obtained at up to 96 h. In strongly tuberculin positive subjects, a wheal may appear within 24 h. Rarely, lymphangitis or a systemic reaction may develop following the tuberculin test. If necrosis and ulceration develop, local hydrocortisone ointment may relieve the discomfort.

Interpretation

The transverse diameter of induration is measured. In older children and adults, an indurated wheal of 5 mm or less is regarded as negative, 6–9 mm is likely to be associated with infection by environmental mycobacteria, and 10 mm or greater is indicative of infection by *M. tuberculosis*, unless the person has received BCG recently. In infants and young children with clinical evidence suggestive of tuberculosis, those with malnutrition or immunosuppression or in close contact with a case, an intermediate reaction of 6–9 mm should be considered positive. After BCG, the tuberculin response is usually less than 15 mm. A tuberculin reaction of 15 mm or greater in any child is suggestive of sensitivity to *M. tuberculosis*. Where there is doubt about interpretation of the tuberculin reaction, an IFN-gamma assay should be undertaken.

A negative or weak response in the presence of tuberculosis may occur in the following conditions: 6–10 weeks after onset of infection, but before tuberculin sensitivity has developed; malnutrition; miliary or overwhelming tuberculosis; nonrespiratory disease, especially tuberculous meningitis; tuberculosis in infants less than 6 weeks of age; recent viral infections such as measles and glandular fever, or whooping cough; recent immunization (within 6 weeks) against measles, mumps and rubella; immunosuppressive diseases including HIV, malignancy, and other debilitating diseases; and current treatment with immunosuppressive agents (including corticosteroids). In resource limited countries the tuberculin test is often negative in children with tuberculosis, probably owing to immunosuppression due to malnutrition, HIV infection and/or overwhelming disease.

When the tuberculin test is negative in children with tuberculosis due to malnutrition, overwhelming infection or other causes, if it is repeated some months after treatment when the general condition of the patient has improved, it will usually be positive. However, a small proportion of children with culture-proven tuberculosis (perhaps 5%) are consistently negative, despite the absence of adverse factors such as malnutrition, overwhelming tuberculosis or other infections.[251] In children infected by *M. tuberculosis* (and those given BCG), tuberculin sensitivity may revert to negative over some years, particularly in those in whom there was not a strong initial reaction or who have had prompt treatment. This does not necessarily imply that they are not protected from reinfection. Repeated administration of tuberculin in subjects sensitized by BCG or tuberculosis may enhance tuberculin sensitivity (booster phenomenon).

Multiple puncture techniques

Multiple puncture tests such as the Heaf test are used to screen large numbers of children. Other tests include the Tine and Imotest. The Heaf test is the most reliable, but all doubtful reactions following multiple puncture techniques should be confirmed by a Mantoux test. The Heaf test was discontinued in the UK in 2005.

Interferon-gamma assays

IFN-gamma assays are based on antigens encoded by genes located within the region of difference 1 (RD1) of the *M. tuberculosis* genome, e.g. early secretory antigenic target 6 (ESAT6) and culture filtrate protein 10 (CFP10). Neither ESAT6 nor CFP10 is present in BCG strains or in most environmental mycobacteria.

Presently there are two commercial IFN-gamma assays, the QuantiFERON-TB Gold and T SPOT-TB assays. Both measure IFN-gamma released from T cells sensitized when they are exposed to ESAT6 and/or CFP10. The former is an ELISA and the latter an enzyme-linked immunospot (ELISPOT) assay. IFN-gamma assays have similar or higher sensitivity than the tuberculin test.[252] A study in South African children which included those with HIV infection and severe malnutrition found that the ELISPOT had a higher sensitivity than the tuberculin test.[253]

The main advantage of IFN-gamma assays over the tuberculin test is the higher specificity due to lack of cross-reactivity with BCG and environmental mycobacteria and likely higher sensitivity in children with HIV infection and malnutrition.

BCG VACCINATION

BCG vaccine is an attenuated bovine strain of mycobacteria introduced by Calmette and Guérin in France in 1921 and originally given orally. It was first used in Sweden in 1927 and in England in 1948.

After intradermal injection of BCG, there is dissemination of small numbers of bacilli to internal organs, particularly the liver and lungs, where granulomata develop. BCG sensitizes individuals so that when they are infected by *M. tuberculosis* multiplication of bacteria is curtailed and a granuloma develops quickly which walls off the infection. Systemic hematogenous dissemination is reduced, as also is secondary infection of the lung either from local extension of lesions or seeding from the blood. BCG vaccination does not prevent tuberculous infection; it particularly reduces the risk of meningitis and disseminated disease (and death), and, to a lesser extent, pulmonary disease.

Indications

In the UK, BCG vaccination is recommended for the following groups:[254]
1. all neonates and infants (0–12 months) living in areas where the incidence of tuberculosis is greater than 40 per 100 000;
2. neonates, infants and children under 16 years with a parent or grandparent born in a country with an incidence of tuberculosis greater than 40 per 100 000;
3. previously unvaccinated new immigrants aged under 35 years who were born in, or lived for more than 3 months in a country with an incidence of tuberculosis greater than 40 per 100 000;
4. contacts of those with respiratory tuberculosis;
5. individuals at occupational risk aged under 35 years including health care workers and laboratory staff who are likely to have contact with patients, clinical materials or derived isolates, veterinary and other staff who handle animal species susceptible to tuberculosis, and staff working directly with prisoners, in care homes for the elderly, or in hostels or facilities for the homeless or refugees;
6. individuals aged under 35 years intending to live or work with local people for more than 1 month in a country with an incidence of tuberculosis greater than 40 per 100 000.

Contraindications

BCG vaccination is contraindicated in patients with immunosuppressive disorders or malignancy, those receiving corticosteroids or immunosuppressive treatment, and in generalized infective conditions. If eczema exists, vaccination should be given in an area free from skin lesions. An interval of 3 weeks should be allowed between administration of BCG vaccine and other live vaccines, with the exception of oral polio vaccine. BCG vaccination is not given to tuberculin positive subjects

The recommendations for BCG vaccination of infants born to mothers infected by HIV vary according to the prevalence of tuberculosis. In industrialized countries, BCG is contraindicated in infants suspected of HIV infection. In countries where both HIV infection and tuberculosis are endemic, routine BCG immunization of newborns is recommended. However, in resource limited countries where neonatal BCG is routine, a small proportion of recipients with perinatal HIV infection or congenital immunodeficiency syndromes will develop distant or disseminated disease with a high mortality.[255,256]

Technique

BCG is given to subjects whose tuberculin reaction is < 6 mm. Re-vaccination is unnecessary for people with a definite BCG scar, even if the tuberculin test is negative. A pre-vaccination tuberculin test is not required in children < 6 years old unless they have stayed > 1 month in a country with an incidence of tuberculosis > 40 per 100 000 or had contact with a person with tuberculosis.

BCG vaccine is injected intradermally, usually into the left upper arm at the insertion of the deltoid muscle: 0.1 ml is given with a 1 ml syringe and a short bevelled needle gauge 25–26 (as per Mantoux test). It is advised that neonates and infants < 12 months are given 0.05 ml because of the increased risk of local lymphadenopathy. Proper technique is essential. The needle should be inserted, bevel upwards, into the superficial layers of the dermis (almost parallel with the surface) for about 3 mm and a wheal of at least 5–7 mm produced. If resistance is not felt during injecting, the needle has been inserted too far (or the fluid has leaked externally) and it should be withdrawn. Injecting the vaccine subcutaneously may result in an abscess or large ulcer. Normally a small papule develops at the site of vaccination within 2–6 weeks. Sometimes it may ulcerate and discharge but it usually heals after about 2–3 months, leaving a small scar (for management see Complications).

Accelerated BCG reaction

If BCG vaccine is given to persons infected by tuberculosis or who have received BCG previously, an accelerated reaction may result: a papule appears within 24–48 h, a pustule by 5–7 days, and a scab by 2 weeks. In malnourished children with tuberculosis, the tuberculin test is often negative, but there may be an accelerated reaction to BCG which could potentially be used as a diagnostic test for tuberculosis. A papule of 5 mm or more appearing by the third day is regarded as positive. BCG is considered to be equivalent to 20–50 TU PPD. Because of the risk that a malnourished child has HIV infection, this practice is now not recommended.

Complications

If > 1% of recipients develop an adverse local reaction to BCG, this usually indicates incorrect dosage or bad technique. The commonest complication is the development of a local abscess or large ulcer. Unless there is superinfection with a pyogenic organism, the abscess is non-tender and the child afebrile. Swelling of local lymph nodes with or without sinus formation is more likely in young infants. These complications usually result from an inadvertent subcutaneous injection.

Nonfluctuant enlarged nodes should be left untreated. Abscesses should be aspirated. If repeated aspiration of fluctuant nodes does not result in resolution they may be excised. Discharging ulcers should be cleaned with an antiseptic two or three times a day, left uncovered as much as possible, and, when necessary, a non-adherent dressing should be used. For ulcers that do not respond to these methods, isoniazid 6 mg/kg/d for 6 weeks usually results in healing. Hypertrophic or keloid scars may develop at the site of vaccination, especially if given at sites other than insertion of the deltoid. Excision is not always successful. Local injection of triamcinolone at monthly intervals for 3–4 doses may result in atrophy.

Other rare complications of BCG vaccination include anaphylactic reactions, satellite lesions, bone lesions, meningitis or overwhelming infection. The latter usually occurs in immunodeficient infants (see above under Contraindications and HIV infection).[257] Focal lesions such as osteitis may occur in apparently immunocompetent infants and in some cases have been associated with increased potency of the vaccine.[258] Osteitis may develop 6–9 months to some years after vaccination. In HIV-infected infants, enlarged lymph nodes (usually ipsilateral to BCG injection) with sinus formation may develop months to years after the vaccination has apparently healed, coinciding with the onset of immunosuppression or administration of antiretroviral therapy.[256]

Efficacy

The effectiveness of BCG in preventing tuberculosis, particularly meningitis and disseminated disease, has been demonstrated in a number of prospective trials and case control studies.[259-261] It also provides some protection against leprosy and Buruli ulcer. Protection persists for up to 10 years. However, results of studies vary between different communities and are influenced by factors such as the prevalence of and exposure to tuberculosis, distance from the equator, the prevalence of environmental mycobacteria, the administration and potency of the vaccine, and the age and nutritional status of the population.[262]

Schoolchildren in the UK vaccinated at around 13 years have demonstrated a consistent level of protection of about 75%, persisting for 15 years.[263]

Two controlled trials of BCG in the newborn, one in North American Indians living in Saskatchewan, the other in Chicago, have shown 75–80% protection, and some case control studies have also demonstrated over 70% protection.[259,261]

In the northern hemisphere, BCG continues to provide substantial protection against tuberculosis overall and up to 80% for meningitis and disseminated disease.

Tuberculin sensitivity after BCG vaccination

When the technique and potency of vaccine is adequate, most vaccinated infants will have a scar and > 90% will be tuberculin positive (≥ 6 mm). Low grade tuberculin sensitivity will remain in most children for at least 5–12 years.[264,265] Preterm infants and those with severe intrauterine growth retardation may have a reduced response to BCG vaccination, possibly due to impaired cell-mediated immunity. Scars are less likely to persist in infants vaccinated in the neonatal period.

In resource limited countries, tuberculin sensitivity following neonatal BCG wanes considerably over the first few years. After 2–3 years most children will be tuberculin negative or have low sensitivity.[266] Thus neonatal BCG should not affect the interpretation of the tuberculin test in these areas. In children recently vaccinated with BCG, who are in contact with a smear positive case of tuberculosis, a Mantoux reaction of ≥ 15 mm should be interpreted as likely infection by *M. tuberculosis*. Repeat BCG vaccination is associated with larger tuberculin reactions. An IFN-gamma assay should help in identifying a false positive tuberculin test.

New vaccines

Vaccines are required which are more effective in preventing exogenous reinfection, especially in adolescents and adults, in people already infected by environmental mycobacteria and in those who have received conventional BCG. Candidate vaccines include live attenuated vaccines comprising BCG or *M. tuberculosis* subunit vaccines and fusion proteins formulated in various adjuvants.[267] Phase 1 trials have been completed for some and phase 2 trials are in progress or planned.

PREVENTION AND CONTACT TRACING

In the UK today, the majority of children in whom tuberculosis is diagnosed are detected through contact tracing of smear positive cases of tuberculosis. Children with primary tuberculosis (as opposed to adolescents with cavitary disease) and patients with nonrespiratory tuberculosis are rarely infectious. However, children with tuberculosis and their visitors should be segregated from the rest of the ward until family and visitors have been screened. Smear positive adults who receive drug regimens which include rifampicin usually have a negative sputum culture within 2 weeks.

Procedures for control and prevention of tuberculosis in the UK have been outlined.[268] When a case of tuberculosis is diagnosed, household contacts should be screened. Children and young adults should have a tuberculin test and, when positive, a chest X-ray. Older adults and those who have received BCG vaccination should have a chest X-ray. If the tuberculin test is negative, it should be repeated after 6 weeks as the first test may have been done too early in the course of infection. Tuberculin negative subjects should be offered BCG. Tuberculin positive subjects with a normal chest X-ray should be given chemoprophylaxis (see below).

Young children are usually infected in the home. For older children it may be necessary to search outside the home, e.g. staff at school, a swimming pool attendant or a youth leader. In tuberculosis of the face or gums, the possibility of infection by a dentist should be considered.

Chemoprophylaxis and follow–up of contacts

This section outlines the recommendations for chemoprophylaxis of contacts of a known case of tuberculosis.

Chemoprophylaxis is indicated for tuberculin positive children (≥ 10 mm) or those with a positive IFN-gamma assay with a normal chest X-ray, who have not had BCG. It should be considered in those with ≥ 15 mm who have received BCG. Guidelines for children < 2 years in close contact with smear positive pulmonary disease are as follows:

1. *No prior BCG*: give chemoprophylaxis irrespective of tuberculin test. Repeat tuberculin test after 6 weeks: if negative, stop chemoprophylaxis and give BCG; if positive (and chest X-ray excludes disease) give full chemoprophylaxis.
2. *Prior BCG*: if tuberculin test is strongly positive (≥ 15 mm) give chemoprophylaxis. If tuberculin test is weak (≤ 10 mm), repeat in 6 weeks. If there is no change, no further action is required. If size of reaction increases (and chest X-ray excludes disease), give full chemoprophylaxis. Routine follow-up chest X-rays are only required for those who are eligible for, but did not receive, chemoprophylaxis.

For chemoprophylaxis, isoniazid (INH) plus rifampicin (RIF) should be given for 3 months, or INH only 6 mg/kg/d should be given for 6 months. In young infants exposed to smear positive patients, or in contacts at any age when the source is suspected to harbor INH-resistant *M. tuberculosis*, RIF may be added to INH and the combination given for 4–6 months. If INH resistance is confirmed, RIF alone may be given for 6 months.[268,269]

CLINICAL FORMS OF TUBERCULOSIS

The commonest presentation of tuberculosis is respiratory disease, followed by involvement of lymph nodes.[243] In resource limited countries, extrapulmonary disease accounts for 35–40% of tuberculosis, compared to around 20% in the USA.[241] It is important to remember that tuberculosis can infect virtually any part of the body. Figure. 28.23 shows an outline and a time scale of some of the complications of primary tuberculosis.

Intrathoracic tuberculosis

Primary pulmonary tuberculosis

The primary complex consists of a focal lesion usually 1–2 cm in diameter which may be found in any part of the lung, and enlarged hilar nodes or, in heavier infections, paratracheal nodes. Lymph node enlargement is particularly prominent in infants and young children (Figs. 28.24b and 28.25a). The primary complex is usually asymptomatic and discovered during contact tracing or a routine tuberculin test. Often the primary focus has resolved or is not visible and the diagnosis is based on enlarged regional nodes. Calcification of the focus and, more often, the nodes may occur after about 12 months, generally within 2–3 years of the infection, and remains an indication of previous infection. Calcification usually indicates healing of the tuberculous process, but healing and progression of the disease may continue concurrently. In many cases the calcium slowly resolves leaving clear lung fields, which explains the common finding in adults where the tuberculin test is positive and the chest X-ray normal.

In older children and adolescents, the lung component is more prominent and commonly presents as an enlarging upper lobe infiltrate and cavitation, usually without lymph node enlargement, and is indistinguishable from postprimary tuberculosis. Pleural effusion is more common at this age.

Progression of primary tuberculosis

Progression of primary tuberculosis may result from extension of the pulmonary focus (progressive primary tuberculosis) or, more commonly, softening of regional lymph nodes. Extension of the pulmonary focus may cause bronchopneumonia or rupture into the pleura resulting in pleural effusion. Tuberculous empyema may result from rupture of caseous material into the pleural space, which may be complicated by pneumothorax (pyopneumothorax). Evacuation of caseous material into a bronchus may result in the appearance of a cavity. Cavities in primary pulmonary tuberculosis are not uncommon in malnourished and debilitated infants with progressive primary tuberculosis (Fig. 28.24b).

Complications from enlargement or softening of regional nodes have a variety of manifestations. The bronchus may be compressed externally; more likely, the wall is eroded and caseous material either partly or completely blocks the lumen (endobronchial tuberculosis); or rupture

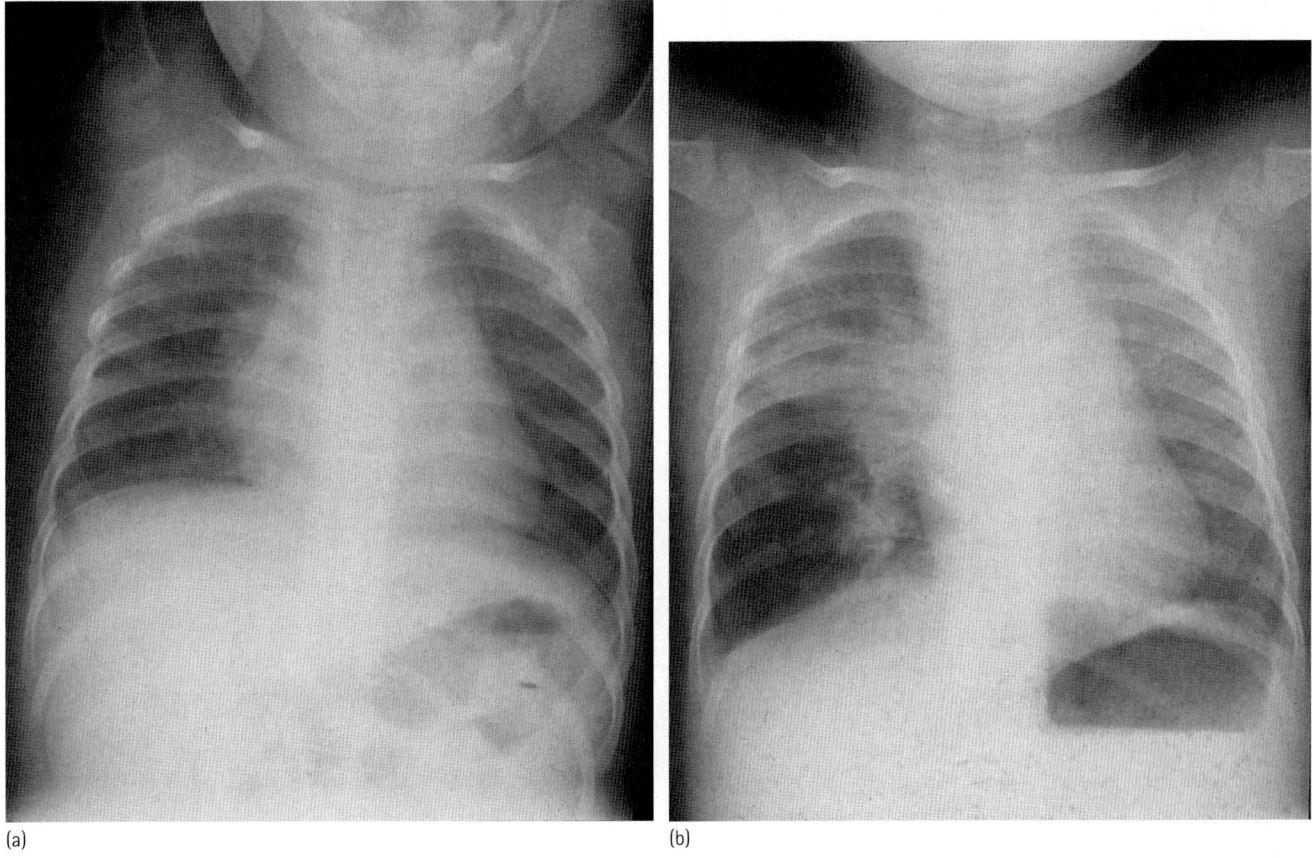

(a)   (b)

Fig. 28.24   (a) A 2½-year-old asymptomatic girl with a strongly positive tuberculin test was in contact with a smear positive case of tuberculosis. Chest X-ray shows a nonspecific opacity in the right upper zone. (b) She was put on chemoprophylaxis with isoniazid plus rifampicin but did not comply with treatment. Chest X-ray taken 2 months later shows an enlarged right mediastinal node with compression of the trachea, collapse/consolidation in all three zones of the right lung, a cavity in the upper lobe and hyperinflation of the right lower lobe. She now had symptoms – cough, stridor and wheeze. This case demonstrates progression of untreated primary tuberculosis.

of the wall results in bronchopneumonia. Partial obstruction may result in a ball-valve effect with lobar emphysema (Fig. 28.24b). This is often transient, because either the bronchus blocks completely or the material is coughed up with clearing of the obstruction.[270] More commonly, there is *segmental* collapse with or without consolidation. Rupture of caseous material into the bronchus may result in a predominantly allergic response with exudation, or, if there are a large number of bacteria present, a progressive tuberculous bronchopneumonia. The former may be associated with marked changes on chest X-ray but which clear spontaneously, whereas the latter, which is more often seen in debilitated children, may prove fatal if not treated. Spread of infected material into both main bronchi may result in bilateral bronchopneumonia.

Rarely, a caseous node may rupture into the trachea, resulting in bilateral obstructive emphysema or asphyxia, into the esophagus resulting in a fistula or the development of an esophageal pouch, or into the pericardium. Other complications from enlarged nodes include superior vena cava obstruction and recurrent laryngeal or phrenic nerve compression.

There may be nonspecific symptoms of irregular fever, anorexia and weight loss. In severe or long-standing cases, the child may be severely wasted. Compression of the bronchi may result in a spasmodic cough simulating whooping cough. When there is obstructive emphysema, the symptoms may be mistaken for asthma, though clinical examination will usually demonstrate signs of mediastinal shift. In long-standing cases, the child may present with clubbing of the fingers and bronchiectasis.

Adolescent tuberculosis

In adolescents, infection is usually in the upper lobes or the superior segments of the lower lobes, and is usually confined to the lungs with no hematogenous spread. In some cases it results from reactivation of a former primary lesion (post-primary tuberculosis) and, though usually associated with adults, this may occur in children and adolescents (Fig. 28.25a, b). Evidence of a previous primary pulmonary complex may be detected.[270] In other cases it is a primary exogenous infection. Common symptoms include a productive cough, especially in the morning, and there may be hemoptysis, fever, night sweats, malaise and weight loss.

Chest X-ray may show a variety of lesions including nodular or patchy shadows, cavities and various stages of healing with fibrosis and calcification. Both lungs may be affected and there may be a pleural effusion.

Diagnosis

The diagnosis of primary pulmonary tuberculosis is based on a positive tuberculin test (10 mm) and/or a positive IFN-gamma assay and enlarged nodes on chest X-ray with or without a pulmonary infiltrate. History of contact provides strong support. Enlarged lymph nodes may not be easily demonstrated; a lateral chest X-ray may be helpful. Persistent pulmonary infiltrate(s) in the presence of a positive tuberculin test is highly suggestive of tuberculosis.

Chest X-ray usually shows enlarged nodes with opacities more often in the right than left lung, due to collapse and/or consolidation. Bilateral disease may be seen in 25% of cases. In progressive disease, cavities may be seen. Lymph nodes may be detected on CT scan in children with normal chest X-rays.[271] The tuberculin test may be negative in debilitated children. This is a common problem in resource limited countries where, in the absence of facilities for mycobacterial culture, the diagnosis is often based on the response to a trial of chemotherapy.

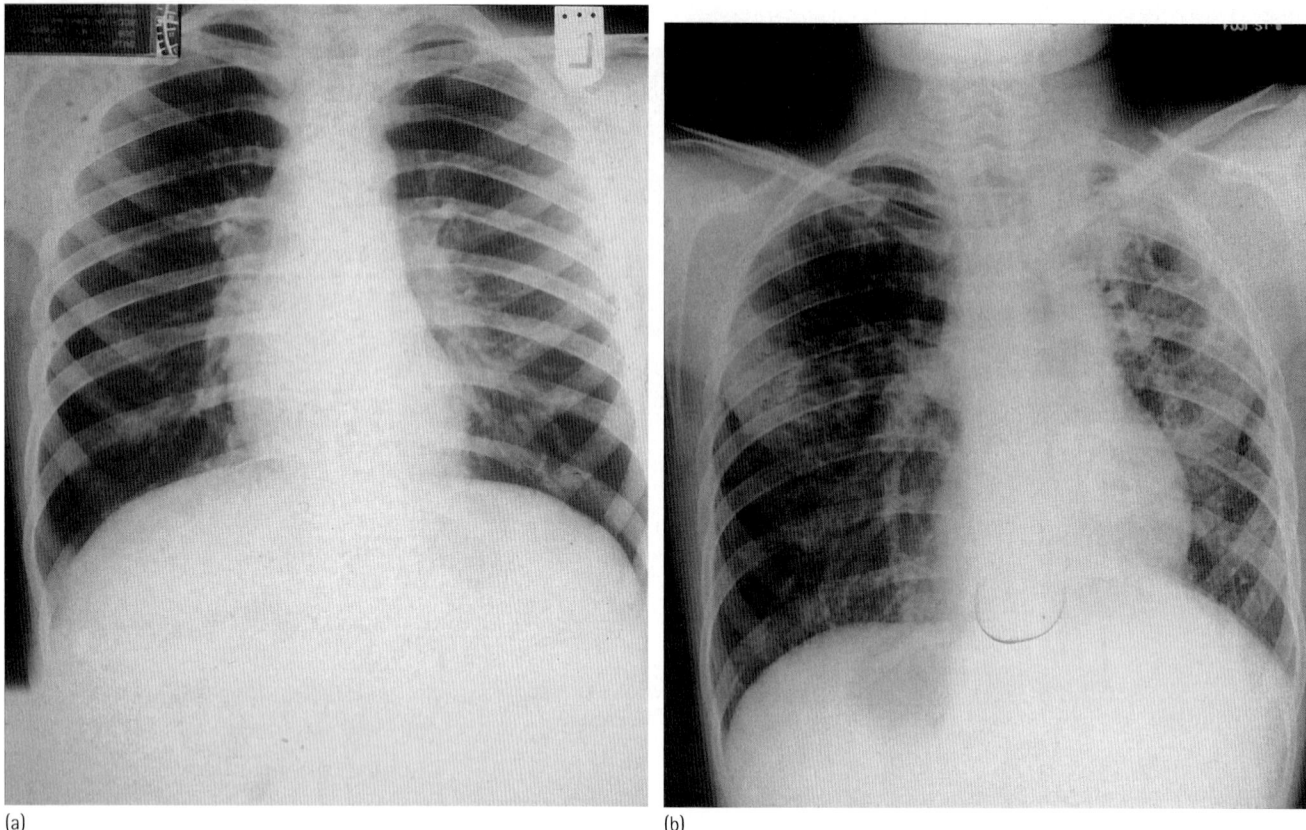

(a)   (b)

Fig. 28.25 (a) An 8-year-old boy was in contact with his grandmother who had smear-positive tuberculosis. His tuberculin test was negative. Although the chest X-ray shows an enlarged right hilar node it was regarded as normal and he did not receive chemoprophylaxis. He was given BCG and developed an accelerated reaction to it. (b) Four years later he presented with a cough for 6 months, dyspnea and weight loss. Chest X-ray shows loss of volume of the right lung with multiple cavities and fibrosis in the right upper lobe and a cavity in the left apex and left mid zone and a miliary pattern. Sputum smear was strongly positive for acid-fast bacilli. This is an example of post-primary tuberculosis. (Fig. 28.25b Reproduced with permission from the *Journal of Medical Microbiology* 1996; 44:7, Fig 1.)

In older children with post-primary or adult type tuberculosis, diagnosis is made by smear and culture of sputum. For younger children, if sensitivities of the contact are not available or diagnosis is unclear, three early morning gastric aspirations should be undertaken while the child is recumbent and has been fasted overnight. If the gastric aspirate (usually 5–10 ml) is very small or the tube is blocked, sterile water (< 20 ml) may be injected and after a few minutes aspirated. If there is delay in transporting the specimen to the laboratory, the acid should be neutralized (pH 7.0) by adding approximately 3 ml of sodium bicarbonate (100 mg/ml). Smear is seldom positive on gastric aspirates in industrialized countries and in some cases it may be due to environmental mycobacteria. However, in resource limited countries where the infective load of *M. tuberculosis* may be high, 10–15% of patients may have a positive smear. Culture is positive in no more than 30–50% of cases.[272] It is more likely to be positive in infants (75%) and those with extensive parenchymal disease.[273] However, it may be positive in children with only enlarged intrathoracic nodes and rarely in those with normal chest X-ray. Gastric aspiration undertaken in an ambulatory clinic has generally lower sensitivity for culture than when taken in the early morning.

Alternative methods to obtain sputum include induced sputum, laryngeal swab and nasopharyngeal aspirate.[274] Laryngeal swabs or nasopharyngeal aspirates are useful for ambulatory clinics and when gastric aspiration is not possible.[275-277] Induced sputum is increasingly used for diagnosis of tuberculosis and may be undertaken in infants, or in adolescents without productive sputum.[278,279] Culture of respiratory secretions obtained through induced sputum, laryngeal swab or nasopharyngeal aspirate is less sensitive (25–30%) than gastric aspirate (30–50%).[276-279] Bronchoscopy is no more sensitive for culture

of *M. tuberculosis* than gastric aspiration.[280,281] If diagnosis is important for management, biopsy of enlarged lymph nodes should be considered.

The blood count usually shows a normal white cell count. A raised ESR is associated with activity of the disease but otherwise has no diagnostic value.

A *pleural effusion* is due to an allergic response to the mycobacteria and thus the tuberculin test is usually strongly positive, except in very debilitated children. If large, or required for diagnostic purposes, it should be aspirated. The fluid is usually clear and straw-colored, but may be opalescent if there is a high cell count. Lymphocytes will be seen on microscopy, but early in the disease neutrophils may also be present. The protein content will be raised, > 40 g/L, and the glucose low, < 1.7 mmol/L. Mycobacteria are often not detected on direct smear, but in about half the cases they may be cultured, especially if a large volume of fluid is centrifuged. Mycobacteria are more likely to be cultured from an empyema. Pleural biopsy may also be taken for histology.

Management

Uncomplicated primary infection usually heals without treatment. The main purpose of chemotherapy is to prevent hematogenous spread and progression of disease, which is more likely in young, debilitated or malnourished children. Segmental collapse may occur despite chemotherapy, but tuberculous bronchopneumonia or pleural effusion is usually prevented. Radiological changes resolve slowly and 50% of children may still have evidence of the primary complex after 18 months. Lymph nodes may enlarge during chemotherapy, but there is usually no necessity to prolong therapy because of this.

Standard three-drug chemotherapy is isoniazid (INH), rifampicin (RIF) and pyrazinamide (PZA) for 2 months followed by INH and RIF for 4 months. Ethambutol (EMB) is added if drug resistance is suspected or burden of infection is high. If PZA is not given, INH + RIF should be given for 9 months. For alternative regimens see section on Chemotherapy. For hilar lymphadenopathy alone a three-drug regimen followed by INH + RIF for just 2 months or INH + RIF for 6 months may be adequate.[282]

Bronchial obstruction. Incomplete bronchial obstruction with air trapping and the development of *obstructive emphysema* may respond to corticosteroids (see Management). However, the transient nature of this lesion should be remembered, i.e. it may resolve or the bronchus may become completely obstructed. Complete obstruction will result in absorption collapse, and bronchoscopy should be performed to exclude other pathology, such as foreign body, and to suck out as much of the caseous material in the bronchial lumen as possible. Unfortunately, the obstruction may be difficult to visualize, especially in young infants.

Pleural effusion. The infective load in pleural effusion is low and responds quickly to treatment. The addition of corticosteroids may enhance the absorption of fluid but long term benefit regarding reduction of pleural thickening and adhesions has not been demonstrated.[283] In the presence of empyema, surgical drainage may be required.

Pericarditis

M. tuberculosis may reach the pericardium by lymphatic extension from mediastinal lymph nodes, direct extension from caseous lung tissue or lymph nodes, or from hematogenous spread. It is more common in resource limited countries.[284] A loud pericardial rub may be heard in dry pericarditis. Occasionally, there is a large effusion, which may cause tamponade. An effusion will be detected by echocardiography. Pericardial aspirate is often blood-stained, and polymorphonuclear leukocytes may be seen in the early stages, after which lymphocytes predominate. *M. tuberculosis* may be cultured in over half the cases, and in up to 75% using double strength Kirchner culture medium. Diagnosis may also be made by culture and histology of a pericardial biopsy. Constrictive pericarditis may ensue in spite of treatment.

Standard antituberculous treatment is given. Open drainage may prevent subsequent requirement for pericardial aspiration. Corticosteroids may enhance the rate of improvement and reduce the requirement for aspiration, but seem not to reduce the need for pericardectomy.[285,286]

Extrathoracic tuberculosis

Nonrespiratory disease usually results from hematogenous spread. Virtually any organ may be affected. Some of the common types are described below. Tuberculosis may also affect the larynx, middle ear and mastoid bones. Middle ear disease may be associated with HIV infection. Virtually any part of the eye may be infected and tuberculosis should be remembered as a cause of an orbital mass. Tuberculosis of the skin may result from primary inoculation, from hematogenous dissemination, or from a cold abscess in an underlying structure.

Lymph node tuberculosis

Superficial lymph node tuberculosis commonly occurs in the cervical or supraclavicular, and, less often, the axillary or inguinal regions. As in primary tuberculosis of the lungs, the regional nodes enlarge in response to a focus. Less commonly, enlargement of a number of superficial lymph nodes results from hematogenous spread. The focus may be the tonsils, gums, lungs or elsewhere. In cervical adenitis, the commonest focus is the upper lung fields. Enlarged axillary or inguinal nodes may be due to disseminated disease or infection of the skin. In the UK, in the majority of cases of white children with histological evidence of mycobacterial infection of the cervical glands, it is associated with environmental mycobacteria such as *M. avium-intracellulare*. *M. tuberculosis* is more common in immigrant children.

Initially the nodes are discrete, mobile and non-tender, later becoming matted together. Without treatment, softening of nodes usually develops within 6 months of infection, and nodes may discharge forming a sinus or track along the fascial planes. Swelling and softening may occur in up to a third of patients during treatment or even years after the node is calcified and apparently healed. This phenomenon of paradoxical enlargement may be due to hypersensitivity to tuberculoprotein, released at intervals from the lesion, and does not usually indicate active infection.

The tuberculin test is usually positive and a chest X-ray should be taken to exclude pulmonary tuberculosis. Calcification within the node may be detected radiologically. Ultrasound or MRI is helpful in confirming that the lesion is a lymph node and in detection of caseous necrosis. Fine needle aspiration for smear and culture, or preferably excision biopsy, will usually confirm the diagnosis. All specimens, either from biopsy or aspiration, should be cultured as it is important to ascertain whether the infection is caused by *M. tuberculosis* or environmental mycobacteria. However, culture may be positive in only two thirds of cases. The main differential diagnosis is from a cervical pyogenic abscess. Local viral or streptococcal infection of the tonsils may cause enlargement of existing tuberculous nodes. Other differential diagnoses include glandular fever, HIV infection, cat-scratch disease, malignancy or an infected branchial or thyroglossal cyst and, in HIV endemic regions of sub-Saharan Africa, Kaposi sarcoma.

Treatment with standard chemotherapy is adequate. If softening of the node occurs, it may be aspirated. If excision is necessary, the primary node should be removed intact, or, if not feasible, as much of the caseous material as possible.[246] Cold abscesses are frequently of the 'collar stud' variety, and will recur if the abscess in the deep fascia is not adequately drained.

Disseminated tuberculosis

Hematogenous dissemination of small numbers of bacilli probably occurs in the majority of children with primary uncomplicated tuberculosis. In resource limited countries, a liver biopsy for an unconnected disease may show tuberculous granulomata in children not known to have had tuberculosis. These rarely become symptomatic. Massive hematogenous spread is referred to as acute miliary tuberculosis and if untreated is usually rapidly fatal. It may be associated with caseous necrosis involving a blood vessel or inadequate immunological response to the infection. It may be found at autopsy without being evident on chest X-ray. A more chronic form, cryptogenic disseminated, also occurs. In both forms, disease may develop in virtually any organ of the body.

Acute miliary tuberculosis. Acute miliary tuberculosis (miliary means 'millet seed') is most common in young children and usually occurs within a year of the primary infection. The most important complication is meningitis. The onset is usually insidious. Presenting signs include pyrexia, dyspnea, anemia, hepatosplenomegaly and lymphadenopathy.[287] Anorexia and weight loss are common and variable degrees of malnutrition will be evident depending on the length of the illness. The lungs show a 'snowstorm' picture on chest X-ray. Rarely, respiratory failure with adult respiratory distress syndrome may develop. Choroid tubercles are pathognomonic of the disease. Cutaneous lesions include macules, papules, purpura and papulonecrotic tuberculides.

Except in the early stages, the diagnosis will usually be evident from a chest X-ray. Miliary disease may be detected on CT scan when the chest X-ray is normal. There may also be lobar infiltrates and hilar lymphadenopathy. The tuberculin test may be weak or negative in the early stages or if the child has severe debility. A lumbar puncture is essential in all cases to exclude meningitis. Bacteriological confirmation will be obtained in the majority of children, particularly from culture of gastric contents, and also CSF and urine. In difficult cases the diagnosis is sometimes made on liver, lung or marrow biopsy.

Acute miliary disease usually responds promptly to chemotherapy. Most deaths are related to meningitis and/or late diagnosis. A short course of corticosteroids will speed the resolution of symptoms, especially if there is alveolar capillary block. Standard chemotherapy is adequate. Prolonged (9 months) therapy may be required in complicated cases or meningitis.

Chronic disseminated (cryptic) tuberculosis. In chronic disseminated tuberculosis, small numbers of bacilli seed the bloodstream at intervals and produce metastatic foci in organs throughout the body. Apart from the lung lesions, there is usually generalized lymphadenopathy and often hepatosplenomegaly, and involvement of the pleural, pericardial and peritoneal cavities, bones and kidneys may occur. There may be multiple bone involvement with dactylitis or involvement of the skin with papulonecrotic tuberculides. In some cases the chest X-ray is normal and the primary site is unknown. A variety of hematological abnormalities may be seen, e.g. pancytopenia, or leukemoid reactions, which suggest leukemia or a lymphoma. The tuberculin test may be negative. Bone marrow biopsy may show necrotic foci with little cellular reaction but teeming with mycobacteria.

Treatment is similar to that of acute miliary disease. Corticosteroids may be of benefit in debilitated children.

Tuberculosis of the central nervous system

Tuberculosis of the central nervous system may have a variety of manifestations.[288] There may be generalized inflammation affecting brain and spinal cord; less commonly, single or multiple tuberculomata enlarge and present as an intracranial space-occupying lesion or rarely tuberculous disease may be confined to the spine.

Tuberculous meningitis. Tuberculous meningitis is most common in children under 5 years of age, often occurring within 6 months and usually within 2 years of primary infection, but it may occur at any age. It results from rupture of one or more tubercles (Rich focus) into the subarachnoid space. The tubercle(s) is commonly situated in the sub-cortex of the brain, and less often in the meninges or spinal cord. Characteristically, the severe inflammatory response results in a thick gelatinous exudate and adhesions around the base of the brain with hydrocephalus and spinal block. Involvement of cranial nerves may result in single or multiple palsies. Arteritis may cause thrombosis and infarction of nervous tissue with permanent damage. Occasionally there is little exudate and the illness is termed *serous meningitis*. Spontaneous recovery without treatment has been described in some of the latter cases.

Symptoms develop over some weeks and may be grouped into stages, which give a guide to prognosis. Initially, the symptoms are nonspecific and include irritability, malaise, anorexia, vomiting, constipation and low grade fever. Unless the child is a contact of tuberculosis or there is a high index of suspicion, the diagnosis is rarely made at this stage. Within a few weeks specific features in addition to the above become apparent: there is headache, disorientation, meningism, focal neurological signs, such as cranial nerve palsy, hemiplegia or visual defect, and seizures may develop. In young infants the fontanelle may be distended. Fundoscopy may demonstrate choroid tubercles, especially when there is miliary disease, papilledema or the development of optic atrophy. The third and often terminal stage is manifest by coma, a posture of decerebrate rigidity, dilated pupils, and the child is usually wasted.

Diagnosis. The diagnosis is based on CSF findings with or without a positive tuberculin test. There may be radiological evidence of pulmonary disease, or clinical evidence of disease elsewhere in the body. The tuberculin test may be negative in over a third of cases, especially in the advanced stages when there is wasting.

The CSF is clear, unless there is a high cell count, when it may appear turbid. The cell count is usually less than 500/mm³ and mainly lymphocytic, except in the very early stages when neutrophils may predominate. Neutrophils may also increase after commencement of chemotherapy. The protein is usually raised (0.8–4 g/L) and in spinal block may be > 10 g/L, and the CSF is xanthochromic. The glucose is usually low. However, it should be remembered that the first lumbar puncture may be normal, that the cell count, protein and glucose levels may fluctuate from day to day, and that the cell count and protein may be lower in ventricular than in spinal fluid.[289] The chance of detecting tubercle bacilli microscopically is higher if a large amount of CSF is obtained and centrifuged; the success rate claimed varies from 30 to 90% depending on the volume of CSF and the care taken in examining the fluid. Brain

imaging will be abnormal in 75–100% of cases; usually there is hydrocephalus, parenchymal disease and basilar meningitis. Tuberculomata may be detected on initial brain scans or appear later. If raised intracranial pressure is suspected, CSF should be taken off slowly with a fine needle or from the ventricles. The CSF should always be cultured for mycobacteria, but is positive in less than half the cases. It may be possible to detect tubercle bacilli after chemotherapy has commenced. Occasionally, tuberculous meningitis may be complicated by pyogenic meningitis. Studies of tuberculous meningitis, mainly in adults, have demonstrated sensitivities and specificities for PCR in CSF ranging from 33 to 100% and 88 to 100%, respectively, and generally higher sensitivity than culture.[238]

Spinal tuberculosis. Spinal tuberculosis is usually secondary to downward extension of the tuberculous process, and usually occurs during treatment of tuberculous meningitis. There is pain and stiffness in the spine at the level of the lesion and symptoms are related to involvement of the spine or nerve roots. The CSF protein is high and there is evidence of a spinal block, which can be confirmed by MRI scan or a myelogram.

Rarely, diffuse tuberculous spinal subarachnoiditis may occur as a result of extension of a primary focus in the spine. It presents as a subacute, transverse or ascending myelitis with upper and lower motor neurone signs and may be mistaken for other causes of cord compression and polyneuritis.

Tuberculoma. A tuberculoma is a tuberculous focus, which enlarges within brain tissue. It may be single or multiple. It may give rise to signs of raised intracranial pressure or a hemiplegia, or cranial nerve palsy if in the brainstem. A skull X-ray may show calcification. CT scan usually shows a hypodense mass and ring enhancement with contrast. MRI scan is more sensitive for detecting tuberculomas, infarcts and spinal lesions. Tuberculomas may expand weeks to months after commencing treatment for meningitis or pulmonary tuberculosis and result in raised intracranial pressure sometimes requiring surgical decompression.[290,291] This phenomenon of paradoxical enlargement may be a hypersensitivity response (as in cervical lymphadenitis).

Management. The key to success in treating tuberculous meningitis is early diagnosis and immediate treatment. If there is doubt, antituberculous chemotherapy should be commenced, along with conventional antimicrobials for bacterial meningitis if necessary.

Optimal chemotherapy is a combination of drugs with good penetration into the CSF and low toxicity. Standard chemotherapy is INH (15–20 mg/kg) and RIF (15–20 mg/kg) given for 9–12 months, with the addition of PZA (40 mg/kg) for the first 2 months of treatment. If drug resistance is suspected, ethionamide or protionamide 20 mg/kg, or ethambutol (EMB) [or streptomycin (SM)] should be added. A 6-month course may be adequate in most cases.[292,293]

A study of 99 children in Cape Town, of whom 96% had stage II or III, treated for 6 months with INH 20 mg/kg, RIF 20 mg/kg, PZA 40 mg/kg and ethionamide 20 mg/kg, had a satisfactory outcome, with only one probable relapse.[293]

Drugs cross the blood–brain barrier more readily in the first 2–3 months of the disease when the meninges are inflamed. INH and PZA achieve high levels in the CSF, even when meninges are not inflamed. Ethionamide has adequate, RIF and EMB moderate to poor, and SM poor penetration across the meninges.[294–296] Ethionamide is useful for isoniazid-resistant *M. tuberculosis*. In children who are vomiting, INH, RIF and SM can be given parenterally and other drugs by nasogastric tube. Controlled trials on the value of corticosteroids in tuberculous meningitis have demonstrated benefit especially in stage II and III disease.[295,297–299] The rationale is based on their ability to reduce the inflammatory exudate and thus prevent the development of adhesions which result in internal hydrocephalus and basilar arachnoiditis. In South Africa, 141 children with stage II–III disease were randomized to receive prednisolone 4 mg/kg or placebo for 1 month.[298] The prednisolone treated group had a reduced mortality in stage III, a better cognitive function in survivors and a reduction in size of existing, and development of new, tuberculomas. Dexamethasone 0.6 mg/kg/day or prednisolone 4 mg/kg/day may be given for 2–3 weeks then tailed off over 2–3 months. A higher dose of corticosteroids was used in the South African study because of theoretical concerns about interaction with rifampicin, but others have used a more conventional dose of prednisolone to equal effect.

Serial brain imaging will detect cerebral edema and the presence or development of hydrocephalus or tuberculomas. In the presence of cerebral edema, controlled ventilation (with monitoring of intracranial pressure if necessary) may be indicated. Obstructive hydrocephalus is common and is not always clinically evident. If it is symptomatic, it should be treated by a ventriculo-peritoneal shunt. In the initial stages, before the drugs have controlled the infection, the shunt may be exteriorized.

Spinal arachnoiditis with a CSF block may develop during treatment. If not improved by corticosteroids, release of pressure by surgery may be necessary.

Tuberculomas are treated on similar lines to meningitis. Most of the small and medium-sized lesions resolve completely with chemotherapy. Rarely, large lesions and those not responding to chemotherapy may require excision. Enlargement during treatment of pulmonary or tuberculous meningitis can cause raised intracranial pressure or cranial nerve palsies. Corticosteroids should be tried and, failing this, a ventriculo-peritoneal shunt may be necessary. Most patients with unresolved tuberculomas have been given prolonged antituberculous therapy, e.g. 12–18 months or more. In some cases of meningitis, a second course of corticosteroids may be indicated for treatment of tuberculomas.

Prognosis. The prognosis for meningitis is related to age of the child (young children have a worse prognosis) and the stage of the disease at which therapy is commenced. The stages have been classified as follows:

Stage I: consciousness undisturbed; no, or only mild and focal, neurological signs.

Stage II: consciousness disturbed, but patient not comatosed or delirious. Mild or moderate neurological signs, such as paraparesis, hemiparesis, and cranial nerve palsies, may be present.

Stage III: patient comatose or delirious with mild, moderate or severe neurological signs.

In a study of 199 children in Hong Kong, complete recovery occurred as follows: stage I 96%, stage II 78% and stage III 21%. Of children in stage III, 17% died as opposed to 1% in stage II.[300] Resolution of neurological disability may continue for many months after commencement of therapy.

Abdominal tuberculosis

Abdominal tuberculosis usually results from swallowed sputum or *M. bovis*-infected milk, but may be associated with extension from thoracic nodes or hematogenous dissemination, or may be an extension of pelvic tuberculosis post menarche. The primary focus is usually in the terminal ileum. Symptoms of disease in children are usually due to enlargement or softening of regional mesenteric nodes and/or involvement of the peritoneum. In adults with cavitatory pulmonary disease, there may be a chronic enteritis and fistulo in ano resembling Crohn's disease or other inflammatory bowel disease.

Common symptoms are abdominal pain, fever, weight loss and abdominal swelling or there may be symptoms of intestinal obstruction. Enlarged mesenteric lymph nodes or a mass associated with adhesions of the omentum and intestines may be palpated, usually on the right side of the abdomen.

Peritonitis may be the dominant condition and is often unassociated with demonstrable pulmonary disease. It may result from extension of a mesenteric node or hematogenous spread. In the latter situation, rarely there may be a polyserositis with involvement of the pleura and pericardium. The ascitic fluid has a predominance of lymphocytes and a protein concentration above 25 g/L (usually lower than in a tuberculous pleural exudate). Mycobacteria are not often identified and the culture may be positive in only a quarter of cases.

Diagnosis is made on the basis of a positive tuberculin test, peritoneal aspiration and bacteriological and histological examination of specimens obtained by laparoscopy, endoscopy, or at laparotomy.

Ultrasonography and CT scan are useful for diagnosis and guidance for needle aspiration. Calcification may be detected on abdominal X-ray.

Treatment is by standard chemotherapy.

Tuberculosis of bones and joints

Tuberculosis of bones and joints results from hematogenous spread, usually affecting a single or a few joints within 6–36 months of primary infection. The spine is affected in over half the cases (Pott disease), followed by the knee, hip and ankle. In chronic disseminated tuberculosis, multiple large or small joints may be affected, with or without associated abscesses, or there may be dactylitis of one or both hands. Sometimes punched out cystic lesions are seen with few inflammatory changes affecting surrounding tissue. Lesions confined to the skull may resemble eosinophilic granuloma of bone, or, if associated with miliary disease, the systemic form of Langerhans' cell histiocytosis.

Infection usually starts in the well-vascularized metaphyses near the epiphyseal line of long bones, or, less commonly, in the synovium of the joint. Typically there is minimal periosteal reaction or new bone formation. Progression of the disease may result in destruction of the joint, and/or abscess or sinus formation. The cold abscess may track a considerable distance from the primary focus. For example, a cold abscess from the cervical vertebrae may present as a retropharyngeal mass or, from the lumbar vertebrae, as a psoas abscess pointing in the groin.

Treatment is standard 6-month chemotherapy. However, if evacuation of necrotic sequestrum and abscesses is not adequate, drug penetration might be impaired and a longer course (9–12 months) necessary.[301] Ambulatory chemotherapy without surgery has been found the most satisfactory treatment for spinal disease in resource limited countries. Acute cord compression may respond to chemotherapy alone, but if the necessary technical expertise is available, early spinal decompression is the treatment of choice. A bone graft may be necessary in cases of extensive destruction of vertebrae or weightbearing bones, such as the neck of the femur.

Genitourinary tuberculosis

Tuberculosis of the kidneys is uncommon in children as it usually presents 5–7 years or more after the primary infection, although it may occur sooner. The first symptom is dysuria and typically there is a sterile pyuria with or without red cells. There may not be any symptoms and even in advanced disease there may be very few leukocytes in the urine. Culture of urine for mycobacteria is usually positive.

Glomerulonephritis with immune complex disease complicating miliary tuberculosis has been described, and may be found to be more common if actively sought.[302]

Tuberculous epididymitis is seen in young boys and epididymo-orchitis in older boys.[246] The development of a cold abscess may be the first manifestation of disease. In girls, tuberculosis of the uterus or Fallopian tubes occurs after the onset of puberty and may be complicated by peritonitis.

Tuberculosis of the kidneys and genital tracts should be treated by standard chemotherapy.

Management during pregnancy and of the newborn

Active tuberculosis during pregnancy is associated with infection of the placenta in approximately half the cases; congenital tuberculosis is rare. The main considerations are of the mother during pregnancy and management of the infant at birth.

The only commonly used drug absolutely contraindicated during pregnancy is SM because of its ototoxic effect on the fetus. INH and RIF are given for 6 months and PZA is added during the first 2 months of treatment. Pyridoxine supplements should be given with INH because of increased requirements during pregnancy.

At birth, if the mother has completed treatment or has inactive disease, the infant is given BCG. If she has active disease and/or is receiving treatment, the infant is given INH 6 mg/kg/d for 3 months and is then given a tuberculin test (and a chest X-ray if necessary). If these are negative INH may be stopped (presuming the mother is not infectious) and BCG given. If respiratory symptoms develop a chest X-ray should be taken. Where it is doubtful that the mother will comply with treatment, BCG may be given at birth and the infant also given INH for 3–6 months. The extent to which INH may interfere with BCG vaccination is not clear, but is probably small.[303] It is not necessary to use isoniazid-resistant BCG.

If the tuberculin test is positive (> 5 mm), full investigation for tuberculosis should be undertaken. If no clinical or bacteriological evidence of disease is detected, INH should be continued for a total of 6 months. If disease is detected, full treatment as for congenital infection should be given.

Unless the mother has multidrug resistant tuberculosis she should not be separated from her child and should continue breast-feeding, once both are on appropriate chemotherapy. Small amounts of antituberculous drugs are excreted in breast milk, but they are not harmful to the infant. Consideration should be given to testing mother and infant for HIV infection.

Perinatal tuberculosis

Perinatal tuberculosis is uncommon, although increasing numbers are reported in areas where HIV/tuberculosis coinfection of women has risen.[304] Whether the infection is contracted before birth (congenital) or in the neonatal period is probably only of epidemiological significance. There are three possible routes for congenital infection:

1. transplacental, when the primary infection will be in the liver, or it may possibly bypass the liver through the ductus venosus and be detected in the lungs;
2. aspiration of infected amniotic fluid or infected material in the genital tract, when the lungs will be infected;
3. ingestion, when presumably the liver will be infected.

Symptoms of congenital infection may occur from birth up to 2 months of age with the majority presenting within 2–5 weeks. In neonatal infection, onset of symptoms is later (1–2 months). Common clinical features are respiratory distress, fever, hepatosplenomegaly, lymphadenopathy, poor feeding, and failure to thrive. There may also be skin lesions, ear discharge, jaundice and, in late diagnosed cases, meningitis. The tuberculin test is usually negative but may become positive 6 weeks or more after birth. An IFN-gamma assay may help in assessing whether the baby is infected. Chest X-ray may show bronchopneumonia, sometimes resembling staphylococcal pneumonia, or miliary changes but may not be abnormal in the early stages. Mycobacteria are often isolated from gastric aspirates, tracheal aspirates or ear discharge. The diagnosis may also be made from CSF, or liver, lung or lymph node biopsy. PCR should be undertaken on all specimens. Placental histology or endometrial curettage may confirm a prenatal source of infection. The mortality is high in overwhelming or late-diagnosed cases and preterm infants. Other bacterial or viral infections may be superimposed.

Treatment is with standard chemotherapy. If drug resistance is suspected, SM or kanamycin should be added for the first 2 months and then replaced by ethambutol. Duration of chemotherapy should be 9 months. There are no studies on the efficacy of chemotherapy for the newborn.

HIV infection

In industrial countries, tuberculosis/HIV coinfection is not a major problem.[305] In sub-Saharan Africa, in contrast, there has been a marked increase in frequency of children treated for respiratory tuberculosis since the mid-1980s, and 60–70% of cases may be HIV seropositive. Because of confounding factors, including the high prevalence of HIV infection in mothers and of tuberculosis in the household, difficulty in confirming both HIV infection in infants and tuberculosis generally, and confusion with HIV-related pulmonary disease, the true incidence of tuberculosis/HIV coinfection is unknown.[306] What is clear is that in HIV-infected children not receiving antiretroviral therapy the cure rate for tuberculosis is reduced, there is a higher rate of both relapse and reinfection, and mortality is increased.[306–308] For most cases there is no difference in the radiological features between HIV-infected and non-infected children with tuberculosis, except possibly a tendency for increased frequency of disseminated disease in the more immunosuppressed. Coinfection with systemic environmental mycobacteria is also a feature in the latter group. In children presenting with tuberculosis and HIV-related pulmonary disease with bilateral reticulo-nodular changes, hilar lymphadenopathy and finger clubbing, the diagnosis of tuberculosis has to depend on methods other than radiology such as contact history, tuberculin test and culture of *M. tuberculosis*. Although the tuberculin test is often negative, it should always be undertaken as it is positive in a proportion of HIV-infected children.

Because of reports of slow eradication of *M. tuberculosis* and/or relapse, at least 9 months of chemotherapy is advised.[308] For HIV-infected children with a positive tuberculin test and no evidence of tuberculosis, 12 months of INH chemoprophylaxis is advised.[309] In HIV-endemic areas, SM should be avoided because of risks from unsterilized needles. Thiacetazone may cause severe skin reactions in HIV-infected children and is contraindicated.

The interaction of rifampicin with non-nucleoside reverse transcriptase inhibitors, nevirapine and efavirenz, and with protease inhibitors is a problem. Also an immune reconstitution inflammatory syndrome may occur, usually within 6 weeks of commencing antiretroviral therapy, comprising fever, lymphadenopathy and worsening of the chest X-ray.

General principles of chemotherapy

A 6 month short-course therapy is standard for respiratory and most nonrespiratory disease.[268,282,310,311] There are still differences of opinion regarding dosage of drugs, especially INH, and the management of meningitis, bone or joint disease, HIV infection and drug resistance. Duration of therapy need not exceed 1 year, except in unusual circumstances such as drug resistance or noncompliance. Intermittent therapy is useful where compliance may be in doubt and is cheaper, although probably only of practical value in areas where supervision is possible. Drugs are usually given twice- or thrice-weekly. Directly observed therapy (DOT) is indicated where there is poor compliance.[312]

Different drugs are effective (in order of efficacy) in:

1. killing actively dividing bacilli, e.g. in open cavities – INH, RIF, SM;
2. killing dormant, intermittently or nondividing bacilli, e.g. in closed caseous lesions – RIF, INH; or within macrophages – PZA, RIF, INH;
3. suppressing drug-resistant mutants – INH, RIF.

PZA is particularly active against bacteria inhibited by an acid environment (e.g. within macrophages and in areas of acute inflammation). Killing actively dividing bacilli and clearing the sputum of live infective bacilli can be accomplished rapidly but for cure or 'sterilization' a prolonged course of treatment is necessary to eradicate dormant and intracellular bacilli. Failure to do this may result in relapse. Mycobacteria may survive for years in a dormant state when metabolism is inhibited by low oxygen tension or low pH.

The most commonly used drugs are bactericidal, e.g. INH (the most potent), RIF, PZA, SM. INH can kill up to 90% of the bacillary population during the first few days of chemotherapy. Bacteriostatic drugs may be used along with bactericidal drugs to prevent emergence of resistance to the bactericidal drugs, e.g. EMB (bactericidal in large doses), ethionamide, thiacetazone and p-aminosalicylic acid (PAS).

The *standard regimen*, used for most types of tuberculosis, is INH + RIF for 6 months, with addition of PZA for the first 2 months. EMB is advised as a fourth drug for the first 2 months if drug resistance is a possibility or there is a high burden of organisms. A longer duration of 9–12 months is advised for some types of disease as indicated in the respective sections. Other schedules are shown in Table 28.25. Caution is advised for EMB in children < 5 years old, because they are too young to report symptoms of optic neuritis, although it is unlikely that problems would arise at a dose of 15 mg/kg.[269] Visual testing should be undertaken where possible. In Table 28.26, the drug dosage and common side-effects are shown. The doses for INH (6 mg/kg) and RIF are minimal and they should be rounded up rather than down. Higher doses, 15–20 mg/kg, are advised for serious forms of tuberculosis such

Table 28.25 Drug regimens

Regimen	Duration
Standard daily	
HRZ(E)[a]: 2 months, then HR: 4 months	6 months
HR: 9 months	9 months
HRZ: 2 months, then HR: 2 months	4 months[b]
Intermittent thrice weekly	
HRZ: 2 months, then HR thrice weekly: 4 months	6 months
Alternative less potent daily:[c]	
HRZ(E): 2 months, then HE: 6 months	8 months

[a] Add E if drug resistance is suspected or burden of organisms is high.
[b] For hilar lymphadenopathy alone.
[c] Resource limited countries.
H, isoniazid; R, rifampicin; Z, pyrazinamide; E, ethambutol.

as meningitis. Adverse reactions are reported in approximately 1–2% of patients.[313] They are less common in children and usually apparent within 6–8 weeks of starting treatment. Peripheral neuropathy as a complication of INH is rare in children. Slow acetylators are at increased risk and pyridoxine will prevent it. Pyridoxine 10 mg is indicated only for children on meat- or milk-deficient diets, breast-feeding infants, malnourished children, and during pregnancy. Higher doses may interfere with the activity of INH.

The main complication is hepatic toxicity.[314] Transient elevation of transaminases occurs in 7–17% of children taking INH, is dose-related and is more likely if RIF is also given. There are case reports of hepatocellular toxicity and death from INH therapy in children.[313] There is no need to monitor serum transaminases unless there is pre-existing liver disease or high doses of these drugs are administered, e.g. in meningitis. Parents should be asked to report persistent nausea, vomiting, malaise and especially jaundice. Children who are rapid acetylators do not have an increased risk of hepatitis when exposed to INH.

Cutaneous reactions, if mild, may not require cessation of treatment, but generalized hypersensitivity will. If toxicity occurs, all drugs should be stopped and reintroduced sequentially in the order INH, RIF and PZA in a small dose (approximately a quarter of the full dose) the first day, increasing to full dose over the next 2–3 days.[314]

Corticosteroids reduce the host's inflammatory response, which may contribute to tissue damage. However, there is only strong evidence of benefit in tuberculous meningitis, although they are sometimes used with less evidence in spinal block, obstruction of bronchi by lymph nodes, miliary disease with alveolar capillary block, pleural effusion and pericarditis.[315] Prednisolone 1.5–2 mg/kg/d is given for 2 weeks and gradually tailed off over 6 weeks. Higher doses are given by some for meningitis.[298]

In children, knowledge of drug resistance is usually obtained from culture and sensitivity of the contact. If drug resistance is suspected or is likely, four bactericidal drugs, e.g. INH, RIF, PZA and EMB, should be given. If possible, SM should be avoided because of the trauma of daily injections. In drug resistance, at *least two drugs* to which the mycobacteria are susceptible should be given. For INH resistance RIF, PZA and EMB are given for a 9–12 month course. For multiple drug resistance, e.g. to INH, RIF and SM, four or more drugs are required initially and treatment should continue for 12–24 months.[269,310] Depending on sensitivities, PZA and EMB are given with three or more second line drugs, e.g. ethionamide, ciprofloxacin, cycloserine or parenterally administered drugs, e.g. kanamycin, amikacin or capreomycin. DOT should be considered.

Patients should be seen monthly for the first 2–3 months to make sure of compliance and to monitor any problems with drugs. Chest X-ray should be repeated at 1–2 months, at the end of therapy, and 3 or more months later. Resolution of pulmonary infiltrates may take over a year and lymphadenopathy (intra- or extra-thoracic) 2–3 years. If adequate chemotherapy has been given, there is no need to prolong treatment; if

relapse occurs or the patient stops treatment for a period, the same standard drug regimen should be given, preferably for 9 months' duration. If in doubt about activity of a pulmonary lesion, gastric aspirates or sputum should be obtained for microscopy and culture. Chest X-rays should be repeated every 6–12 months after cessation of therapy until stable.

Children with primary tuberculosis are rarely infectious and sputum is usually non-infectious after 2–3 weeks of chemotherapy and so they may return to school after this period.

BACTERIAL INFECTIONS: MYCOBACTERIA – ENVIRONMENTAL

Mycobacteria may be divided into those associated with tuberculosis and leprosy and those causing disease associated with the environment, also referred to as nontuberculous, or atypical mycobacteria. The former (including *Mycobacterium leprae*) are highly infectious and are passed from person to person. Environmental mycobacteria, of which there are over 50 species, exist principally as harmless saprophytes in water, soil and vegetation, and also as pathogens in animals such as birds, reptiles and fish. Person-to-person transmission is extremely rare. Environmental mycobacteria generally prefer warm climates and the geographical distribution of the different species is quite variable. Water (fresh or salt) is probably a major vector, e.g. drinking, washing or aquatic sports, or by inhalation of aerosols.[316] The main portals of entry are probably through the skin or mucosa, and by inhalation or ingestion.

DIAGNOSIS

Environmental mycobacteria may be detected as commensals in sputum or gastric aspirates, swabs from wounds or abscesses, or in inadequately sterilized sputum pots. More definite proof of their pathogenicity is obtained when they are derived from a closed lesion, e.g. by aspiration or resection, or the same strain of mycobacteria is repeatedly isolated. Differentiation between mycobacteria is by their cultural characteristics or by PCR. Histologically, it is usually not possible to differentiate lesions from the granulomata of tuberculosis, although nontuberculous infection is more likely to show 'nonspecific' inflammation with less prominent caseation. Variable numbers of acid-fast bacilli may be seen.

There may be a moderate reaction to the tuberculin test (purified protein derivative, PPD-S), approximately 3–25 mm, or no reaction.[317] Differential intradermal tests with antigens prepared from specific environmental mycobacteria, e.g. *Mycobacterium avium*, *M. intracellulare*, *M. malmoense*, *M. scrofulaceum* or *M. kansasii*, are more likely to produce a larger reaction than that with PPD-S.

The commonest clinical problem due to infection by environmental mycobacteria in children is cervical adenitis. Other conditions include cutaneous infections, rarely pulmonary or otolaryngeal disease, osteitis, disseminated disease and meningitis.[318,319] In adolescents and adults, infection in the presence of pre-existing pulmonary disease (including cystic fibrosis) is the commonest association.

LYMPHADENITIS

There appears to be a relative if not an absolute increase in incidence of lymphadenitis due to environmental mycobacteria in areas of the world where tuberculosis is now rare, which may be partly due to decline in neonatal BCG vaccination.[320] However, it also occurs in resource limited countries but is under-reported due to lack of facilities to identify environmental mycobacteria.[321] A defect in the type 1 cytokine pathway could be a factor in some cases.[322] Disease usually presents in children aged between 1 and 5 years, and is usually unilateral and cervical. The submandibular group of nodes is most often infected, followed by tonsillar, pre-auricular and anterior cervical groups. Infection of axillary, inguinal and epitrochlear nodes has been described. The area of entry is rarely identified, although occasionally a lesion on the tonsil

Table 28.26 · Recommended drugs for tuberculosis

Drug	Daily dose			Thrice weekly dose			Side-effects
	Children	Adolescents		Children	Adolescents		
		<50 kg	>50 kg		<50 kg	>50 kg	
Isoniazid (INH)	6 mg/kg p.o., i.m., i.v. 15–20 mg/kg (meningitis)	300 mg	300 mg	15 mg/kg (max 900 mg)	15 mg/kg	Max 900 mg	Hepatic enzyme elevation, hepatitis, peripheral neuropathy, hypersensitivity
Rifampicin (RIF)	10 mg/kg p.o., i.v. 15–20 mg/kg (meningitis)	450 mg	600 mg	15 mg/kg (max 600 mg)	15 mg/kg	Max 900 mg	Orange discoloration of secretions and urine (also contact lens), nausea, vomiting, hepatitis, febrile reactions, thrombocytopenia
Pyrazinamide (PZA)	30–35 mg/kg p.o. 40 mg/kg (meningitis)	1.5 g	2.0 g	50 mg/kg	2.0 g	2.5 g	Hepatotoxicity, hyperuricemia, arthralgia, gastrointestinal upset, skin rash
Ethambutol (EMB)	15–20 mg/kg p.o.*	15 mg/kg (max 2.5 g)	15 mg/kg (max 2.5 g)	30 mg/kg	30 mg/kg	Max 2.5 g	Optic neuritis, skin rash
Streptomycin (SM)	15–20 mg/kg i.m.	750 mg	1.0 g	15–20 mg/kg	750 mg	1.0 g	Ototoxicity, nephrotoxicity
Thiacetazone	4 mg/kg p.o.	150 mg	150 mg	Not recommended	Not recommended	Not recommended	Gastrointestinal disturbance, vertigo, visual disturbance, hepatitis, agranulocytosis, exfoliative dermatitis in HIV infection
Ethionamide/ protionamide	15–20 mg/kg p.o. (divided doses)	750 mg	1.0 g	Not recommended	Not recommended	Not recommended	Gastrointestinal disturbance, hepatotoxicity, allergic reactions

*In children <5 years old, give 15 mg/kg.

or buccal mucosa is seen. Enlargement of pre-auricular nodes suggests that the eye might be a portal of entry in some cases. Enlargement of nodes occurs over weeks to months. The overlying skin becomes erythematous or purple prior to discharge of the abscess, but is not usually warm unless secondarily infected. It is commonly mistaken for a pyogenic cervical abscess. A sinus may develop and later calcification may occur. Some nodes probably settle spontaneously. Infection by environmental mycobacteria should be considered when a submandibular or pre-auricular node enlarges in a young child from a background of low tuberculous endemicity, in the presence of a normal chest X-ray and a negative or low grade sensitivity to PPD.

The treatment of choice is excision biopsy of the primary group of involved nodes.[317,318,323] Often the lesion is incised when mistaken for a cervical abscess, or it has discharged spontaneously. In these circumstances, as much necrotic material as possible should be removed and later, if necessary, the primary node excised. Fine needle aspiration is helpful for diagnosis, but mycobacterial culture or PCR is required for confirmation.

Chemotherapy is not usually indicated as the disease is local and the usual mycobacteria causing disease, e.g. *M. avium* complex (MAC) and *M. malmoense*, are commonly resistant to standard tuberculosis chemotherapy. However, if surgery is difficult, e.g. involvement of the parotid gland or closeness of the lesion to the facial nerve, limited incision and curettage may be undertaken and, if healing is slow, antimycobacterial therapy commenced. A suggested drug regimen is azithromycin (10 mg/kg) or clarithromycin plus rifabutin (6 mg/kg) daily for 6 months.[317] Occasionally, longer or repeat treatment is required. Azithromycin has the advantage of once daily treatment and high tissue concentration. There are no controlled trials on the value of single versus combined drugs or duration of therapy. Recurrence of disease in another site sometimes occurs and should be treated as usual.

OTOLARYNGEAL DISEASE

Chronic infection of the middle ear associated with tympanotomy tubes and chronic mastoiditis due to colonization by, particularly, rapidly growing mycobacteria, e.g. *Mycobacterium abscessus* and *Mycobacterium chelonei*, has been described. Debridement with removal of all diseased tissue and in the case of chronic mastoiditis securing maximum ventilation of the cavity is essential. Chemotherapy with appropriate drugs is given for 6 months. Treatment for *M. abscessus* and *M. chelonei* includes parenteral therapy with amikacin and cefoxitin or imipenem for a few weeks, followed by oral clarithromycin and/or ciprofloxacin, depending on sensitivities.[319,324]

SOFT TISSUE INFECTION

The most common soft tissue infections are 'swimming pool granuloma' and 'fish tank granuloma', both caused by *M. marinum*. Local abscesses may follow infection by *M. fortuitum* or *M. chelonei* at injection sites, trauma or surgery, and often present 3–4 weeks after infection, although the incubation period may be much longer in deep infections. Regional nodes are not usually enlarged. Mycobacteria can usually be detected in the lesions. Management comprises debridement of diseased tissue, with chemotherapy reserved for extensive or deep-seated disease.

'Swimming pool granuloma' commonly affects children bathing in infected water on areas of abrasion such as the knees or elbows. Papules, which may ulcerate, appear on the affected areas; scab formation follows. Spontaneous healing occurs within a few months. If drug therapy is required, a single agent such as co-trimoxazole, clarithromycin, ciprofloxacin, or, for more severe infections, dual therapy with rifampicin plus ethambutol, is given for 3–6 months.

Buruli ulcer derives its name from a district in northern Uganda and is known as Bairnsdale ulcer in Australia where the causative agent (*M. ulcerans*) was originally identified. *M. ulcerans* produces a potent toxin, mycolactone.[325] It occurs in localized places in a number of tropical rain forest areas around swamps and river banks. It is transmitted through minor skin injury after contact with water, soil or vegetation contaminated probably by water bugs.[325] It starts as a subcutaneous nodule, often on a leg or arm, ulcerates and gradually progresses to a large ulcer with deep, undermined edges. Satellite nodules or ulcers may be present. Perhaps a third of small lesions heal spontaneously. Diagnosis is by detection of acid-fast bacilli, culture, histology and PCR (98–100% sensitivity).[325] Treatment of large ulcers requires wide excision, cleansing with antiseptic such as 0.5% silver nitrate, and immediate skin grafting. Application of heat to maintain the temperature of the ulcer above 40 °C, which inhibits growth of *M. ulcerans*, may be successful, though not practical in resource limited countries. Chemotherapy is given along with surgery to assist healing. A suggested regimen is rifampicin plus streptomycin for at least 2 months. BCG may give some protection.

PULMONARY DISEASE

Pulmonary disease due to environmental mycobacteria is rare in immunocompetent children. It presents similarly to pulmonary tuberculosis: primary complex, bronchial obstruction, bronchopneumonia or primary progressive disease.[326] The majority of cases are caused by MAC, less often by *M. kansasii* and, in some cases, by other mycobacteria such as *M. fortuitum*. Obstruction of a bronchus should be resected either at bronchoscopy or thoracotomy. Prolonged chemotherapy may be required.

In about 13% of patients with cystic fibrosis, environmental mycobacteria may be recovered from respiratory tract specimens.[327] The decision to treat with chemotherapy depends on a number of indications including: recovery of mycobacteria on serial specimens, reduction in lung function not responding to standard management, changes on chest X-ray compatible with superinfection, and response to chemotherapy for mycobacteria. Choice of chemotherapy depends on species of mycobacteria. Drugs may need to be continued for up to 2 years.[328]

DISSEMINATED AND EXTRAPULMONARY DISEASE

Disseminated disease is usually associated with severe immunological defects, congenital or AIDS. When bone disease occurs, it is usually disseminated osteomyelitis, but can rarely be multifocal osteomyelitis without an apparent underlying immunodeficiency. Infection of the meninges may also occur. A variety of inherited defects in the IL-12 dependent gamma interferon (IFN-gamma) output pathway are recognized, which increase susceptibility to mycobacteria (especially environmental mycobacteria and BCG) and to Salmonella.[329] Some patients respond to IFN-gamma therapy.

In HIV infection, disseminated disease due to MAC is usually seen in older children with a low CD4 count and advanced disease. Trials are in progress regarding optimal chemotherapy. A suggested regimen is clarithromycin, ethambutol and rifabutin.[330] Other drugs include clofazimine, rifampicin, ciprofloxacin or amikacin.[324,328]

DRUG THERAPY

Drugs appropriate for environmental mycobacteria are outlined in Table 28.27. In vitro drug sensitivities may not predict clinical response. Duration of treatment and synergy between drug combinations are important factors. In general, neither isoniazid nor pyrazinamide is useful for environmental mycobacteria. Experience with many of the newer drugs is limited in children and it is important to be aware of side-effects, particularly when used in combination, e.g. plasma levels of rifabutin may be increased by clarithromycin and fluconazole with a risk of uveitis.

PERTUSSIS (WHOOPING COUGH)

Although theoretically vaccine-preventable, pertussis continues to be a significant health problem throughout the world. There are a number of reasons for this including:

Table 28.27 Suggested antimicrobials for treating environmental mycobacterial infection

Organism	Drugs
M. avium-intracellulare and M. scrofulaceum (MAIS complex) M. malmoense	Azithromycin/clarithromycin, rifabutin/ rifampicin, ethambutol, ciprofloxacin, clofazimine, amikacin
M. kansasii	Rifampicin, ethambutol, ciprofloxacin, clarithromycin
M. marinum	Rifampicin, ethambutol, clarithromycin, TMP-SMZ, ciprofloxacin
M. fortuitum M. chelonei M. abscessus	Amikacin, cefoxitin, clofazimine, clarithromycin, ciprofloxacin, imipenem

TMP-SMZ, trimethoprim–sulfamethoxazole.

- Immunization rates are low in some countries.
- The vaccine is not 100% effective and the immunity is transient.
- Because of potential adverse effects of the vaccine in older children and adults, booster vaccinations have rarely been given beyond the age of 5–6 years, although this is changing.
- Because of the transient nature of the immunity, many adults are non-immune and are now the major source of infection, particularly to pre-vaccinated or incompletely vaccinated infants.
- Because of perceived major adverse events from pertussis vaccine, many parents and medical practitioners are wary about giving this vaccine. Further, they will often give an incomplete course of pertussis vaccination if there have been any (even minor) adverse events from earlier vaccinations.
- Infants are born with no passive immunity to pertussis. The non-immune status of neonates means they are highly vulnerable to this disease until vaccination is complete (generally at 6 months). Unfortunately, this is also the age group where the disease is most deadly.

PATHOGENESIS

Pertussis is a bacterial infection due to a Gram negative coccobacillus, *Bordetella pertussis*. Although this organism is sensitive to antibiotics (particularly macrolides), once the paroxysmal cough is established, antibiotics have little or no effect on the clinical course of the illness, except to render that patient non-infectious to others. Thus, recognition and treatment of index patients to prevent further spread is an important public health measure.

It is ideal if pertussis is diagnosed *before* the development of the paroxysmal coughing phase, as antibiotics in this initial stage of the illness can reduce the severity of the clinical illness. Although recognition in the pre-paroxysmal phase is difficult, diagnosis of index cases and treatment of any household contacts with any respiratory symptoms (particularly young children) with the appropriate antibiotics is warranted. Indeed, in a young unimmunized infant (less than 6 months), contact with a known pertussis case is an absolute indication for immediate prophylactic antibiotics.

SPREAD

Droplet or aerosol spread is usual, and indirect spread (e.g. via fomites) is unlikely. The disease is highly infectious and over 80% of unvaccinated household contacts of a known case will develop the clinical illness.

CLINICAL FEATURES

There are several distinct phases of this illness (see Table 28.28). The initial early 'catarrhal' phase consists of upper respiratory tract symptoms and a nonspecific dry cough. This phase lasts for 7–10 days and is abruptly followed by the paroxysmal cough phase. During the early paroxysmal phase, there are violent spasms of uncontrollable cough with facial flushing. These spasms of cough can persist for several minutes and are classically followed by an inspiratory 'whoop'. Infants often vomit and may develop apnea and cyanosis with these coughing spasms, and a 'whoop' is often absent in this age group. This phase of the illness can persist for up to 3 months.

Between coughing spasms, children are strikingly well. Thus, pertussis is generally diagnosed on the basis of the history, unless a spasm is directly observed. The number of spasms per day is highly variable and generally peaks within the first 2–3 weeks of the illness, before a very gradual reduction in the frequency and severity of spasms.

In adolescents and adults the disease is highly modified, presumably reflecting their partial immune status. Thus, any adult with a troublesome cough which has persisted for 2–3 weeks should be suspected of having whooping cough. Epidemiological studies have repeatedly shown that adults are the major reservoir of *B. pertussis* infection, particularly of young unvaccinated or incompletely vaccinated infants.

CASE DEFINITION

The current World Health Organization case definition is as follows: *B. pertussis infection* should be suspected if there is severe cough for greater than or equal to *2 weeks* (i.e. 'probable' pertussis). If *one* of the following are present *in addition* to the above, the child should be notified and treated:

- Prolonged cough followed by apnea or cyanosis, and in the older child paroxysm followed by vomiting, inspiratory whoop or the presence of subconjunctival hemorrhages;
- exposure to suspected case in the previous 3 weeks;
- epidemic whooping cough in the area;
- a lymphocytosis of 15 000/mm³ or greater.

LABORATORY DIAGNOSIS

Confirmation of the diagnosis is an issue. While a positive culture is the gold standard, this lacks sensitivity and false negatives are common. Standardization of other laboratory methods, including PCR and serology, is required to firmly establish their role in diagnosis. Detection of *B. pertussis* by culture or PCR is used for infants and young children who do not mount a good serological response, while serology is more useful in older children and adults. The USA Centers for Disease Control suggest the following as a guide:

- during the first 7 weeks of the cough: culture and PCR;
- cough for 3–4 weeks: PCR and serology;
- cough for more than 4 weeks: serology only.

Table 28.28 Natural history of pertussis

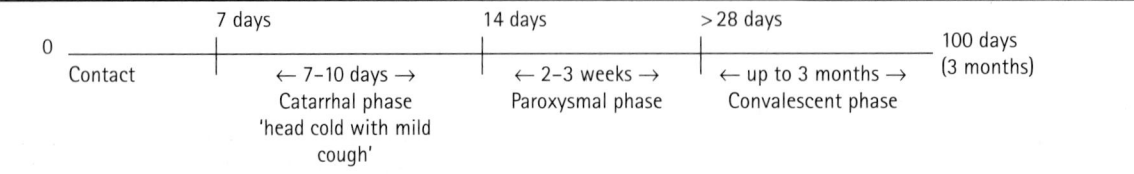

EPIDEMIOLOGY

The disease is endemic in most resource rich countries despite widespread immunization programs. In addition to the endemic cases, there are frequent epidemic peaks, which classically occur every 2–5 years. The endemic nature of this disease presumably reflects the large reservoir of adults who develop a modified illness and infect infants and young children. The true incidence of pertussis is difficult to determine because of the problems with accurate clinical diagnosis, the low sensitivity of microbiology, and uncertainty concerning PCR and serological testing methods. As well as lack of recognition, there is almost certainly under-reporting of the condition in resource rich countries.

MORTALITY/MORBIDITY

The estimated annual burden of disease, as reported by the World Health Organization, is 200 million–400 million infections worldwide, causing 200 000–300 000 deaths.

The quoted mortality in resource rich countries for this disease is approximately 0.3%, and is slightly higher in infants < 6 months old (0.5%). Major complications resulting in prolonged morbidity include hypoxic encephalopathy and subsequent brain damage. Most of the morbidity and virtually all of the mortality is in infants < 6 months of age.

VACCINATION

Until recently, the standard vaccine used was a whole cell pertussis vaccine, which unfortunately had a reputation for being both relatively ineffective and potentially harmful. As a consequence, vaccination rates for pertussis often fluctuated and most countries observed major increases in the rates of pertussis when vaccine uptake fell or was low.

Because of the widespread perception of a poor risk:benefit ratio with pertussis vaccine, complete coverage of children < 5 years of age fell to < 50% in the UK in the late 1980s, and was associated with major epidemics.

The introduction of acellular vaccines, with high quality studies showing excellent effectiveness and low adverse event rates, has dramatically altered the situation.[331] Most resource rich countries have replaced whole cell vaccine with acellular vaccine, with increased coverage of complete vaccination in young children. However, to control B. pertussis infection will require repeated booster vaccinations in adolescents and adults. The introduction of the acellular vaccine, which can be safely given to adolescents and adults, means that eradication is now a real prospect.

VACCINE EFFICACY

The published data on vaccine effectiveness have been quite variable. For the whole cell vaccine efficacy varied from approximately 35 to 98%. While the whole cell vaccine offered protection against more severe disease, it did not confer long term immunity. Recent studies show that the efficacy of the acellular vaccine has ranged from 85 to 90%, with a much lower incidence of adverse events.

TREATMENT

In the paroxysmal phase, antibiotics are indicated to prevent the spread of infection. However antibiotics have little or no impact on the child's coughing illness. Although the usual antibiotic is erythromycin for 7–10 days, newer macrolides (e.g. azithromycin) are equally effective and better tolerated.

In young infants with severe and frequent spasms, admission to hospital and close observation is essential. Treatment revolves around experienced, high quality pediatric nursing care. This includes: avoidance of provoking spasms; close observation and treatment of spasms (with oxygen if necessary); minimal handling; and for uncontrollable life-threatening spasms – endotracheal intubation and mechanical ventilation.

BACTERIAL INFECTIONS: *PNEUMOCOCCUS*

Pneumococcus (*Streptococcus pneumoniae*) is a common cause of serious disease in children, particularly otitis media, pneumonia and meningitis. It is also a frequent cause of occult bacteremia.[332] *S. pneumoniae* are Gram positive oval cocci. They cause beta hemolysis (a green zone around the colony) on blood agar, and occur in pairs (diplococci) or short chains. Pneumococci can be characterized serologically by the capsular polysaccharides or by molecular biological techniques. More than 90 pneumococcal serotypes have been characterized but only a small number are responsible for the majority of serious, invasive infection.

EPIDEMIOLOGY

Approximately 50% of healthy children and 8% of adults[333] carry *S. pneumoniae* in the upper respiratory tract and it is thought that spread is mainly by healthy carriers although patient-to-patient and patient-to-doctor transfer has been documented. Children under 2 years have the highest rate of carriage, but why some infants develop disease whereas others remain unaffected is unknown. In resource limited countries, a high proportion of lower respiratory infection in young children is due to *S. pneumoniae*, and pneumococcal meningitis is associated with a high mortality (30–35%). Globally, *S. pneumoniae* is thought to cause over 1 million deaths in children under the age of 5 years.[334] The 'pneumonia season' in late winter and early spring has been attributed to indoor crowding and damage to respiratory mucosal defenses by recent virus infections.

From the nasopharynx, *S. pneumoniae* may reach the lungs or through impaired respiratory mucosa spread to the middle ear or meninges. Bacteremic spread to a variety of sites may occur, notably the joints.[335]

Antibiotics have reduced the severity and mortality of pneumococcal disease but have had little influence on disease incidence. Despite timely administration of appropriate antimicrobial therapy, infants with pneumococcal meningitis remain at considerable risk from neurological sequelae and the pneumococcus is more likely to cause permanent deafness than either the meningococcus or *Haemophilus influenzae*. Recurrent pneumococcal meningitis is occasionally seen when CSF leakage complicates skull fracture. Children with an absent or nonfunctioning spleen, impaired antibody production and HIV infection are at particular risk of serious pneumococcal infection.

DIAGNOSIS

In pneumococcal pneumonia there is usually tachypnea with grunting, inspiratory retractions, nasal flaring and cyanosis, but physical examination of the chest may be unhelpful and the radiological changes surprisingly few in the early stages of illness. Blood and CSF cultures are helpful in diagnosis. In bacteremic disease, the white blood cell count is often elevated to over 20×10^9/L. Recovery of the pneumococcus from the upper respiratory tract is unhelpful because of the frequency of the carrier state. Pneumococcal antigen detection in CSF, pleural fluid, serum and urine may be useful for rapid diagnosis, especially in children who have received antibiotics prior to culture.

TREATMENT

A worrying trend is the increasing antimicrobial resistance among *S. pneumoniae* worldwide.[336] There is regional variation in the incidence of resistant organisms and risk factors include recent antimicrobial use. Penicillin remains the drug of choice for infections with penicillin-sensitive organisms and high drug levels may overcome drug resistance if they exceed the minimum inhibitory concentration (MIC) of the organism. It may not be possible, however, to achieve adequate CSF levels, and pneumococcal meningitis due to resistant organisms should not be treated with penicillin. Multiply drug resistant pneumococci can also be resistant to ceftriaxone and cefotaxime so, whilst awaiting sensitivity results, vancomycin use is recommended (usually in combination with ceftriaxone) if there is a strong clinical suspicion of multiply resistant organisms.

PREVENTION

Pneumococcal vaccine

Although pneumococcal vaccines have been available for many years they have had, until recently, limited efficacy in children under 2 years and their use was therefore targeted towards older children with risk factors such as splenectomy.

The older pneumococcal polysaccharide vaccines (PPV) are manufactured using 23 (23-valent) pneumococcal serotypes, do not stimulate T cells, do not induce a boostable memory response and are ineffective in children under 2 years of age.[337]

The pneumococcal conjugate vaccine (PCV) is manufactured by conjugating carrier proteins to capsular polysaccharides from the seven (7 or hepta-valent) or nine (9-valent) commonest pneumococcal serotypes responsible for 80% of invasive disease. These vaccines are T cell dependent and thus are immunogenic in infancy and induce memory so that the immunological response is boostable.[337]

A pivotal, randomized controlled trial of heptavalent PCV in more than 18000 children given from 2 months of age showed 97.4% protection against invasive pneumococcal disease.[338]

PCV was introduced for routine use in infants and toddlers in the USA in 2000 and since then significant reductions in invasive pneumococcal disease have been seen in vaccinated children.[339–342] Hospitalization rates for all-cause pneumonia in children less than 2 years (the target population) have declined by 39%[343] but the introduction of the vaccine has also been linked with reduced invasive pneumococcal disease in young infants and adults suggesting changes in pneumococcal carriage rates, transmission and herd immunity.[339,344,345] The vaccine also appears effective in children with chronic diseases[342] including HIV infection.[340,346]

PCV was introduced into the UK childhood immunization program in the autumn of 2006 and offered to children age 2, 4 and 13 months (http://www.immunisation.nhs.uk).

PPV is recommended as an additional strategy for children aged 2 years or older in whom pneumococcal infection is likely to be more common and/or dangerous:

- asplenia or severe dysfunction of the spleen, e.g. homozygous sickle cell disease and celiac syndrome;
- chronic renal disease or nephrotic syndrome;
- immunodeficiency or immunosuppression from disease or treatment (including HIV infection;)
- chronic heart, lung or liver disease;
- diabetes mellitus;
- cochlear implants
- history of invasive pneumococcal disease
- presence of CSF shunt or other condition with risk of CSF leak

Note: Where possible, the vaccine should be given 4–6 weeks (but at least 2 weeks) *before* splenectomy and *before* courses of chemotherapy, together with advice about the risk of pneumococcal infection. If this is not possible, as for splenectomy following trauma, the vaccine should be given as soon as possible after recovery and before discharge from hospital. If not given before chemotherapy and/or radiotherapy its use should be delayed for at least 6 months after completion of treatment.

Chemoprophylaxis

An alternative for children with functional or anatomical asplenia, for those receiving immunosuppressive therapy, or for infants under 2 years, is to give them continuous antibiotic prophylaxis, e.g. phenoxymethyl penicillin.[347]

EDUCATION

Patients at risk (or their parents) need to be educated about the risks and the importance of seeking medical help at the onset of illness.

A MedicAlert bracelet should be used. A patient card and information sheet for asplenic or hyposplenic patients is available from: Department of Health, PO Box 410, Wetherby LS23 7LL.

BACTERIAL INFECTIONS: *PSEUDOMONAS*

PSEUDOMONAS AERUGINOSA

Pseudomonas aeruginosa is an important nosocomial pathogen with innate resistance to many antimicrobial agents and disinfectants. The bacterium grows readily in moist environments including ventilator and incubator humidification systems. Known to pediatricians as a cause of life-limiting respiratory infection in cystic fibrosis, *P. aeruginosa* can infect virtually any part of the body. Infection is usually associated with congenital or acquired immunodeficiency, prematurity, neutropenia or white cell dysfunction, malignant disease and its treatment, transplantation, prolonged instrumentation of body cavities (e.g. tracheostomy, ventricular drainage, bladder catheterization, venous catheterization, peritoneal dialysis) and following puncture wounds. *P. aeruginosa* infections are generally restricted to immunocompromised patients, but severe infections may occur in healthy children and require prompt diagnosis and treatment. The most important *P. aeruginosa* infections in pediatric patients include:

Septicemia

P. aeruginosa is an important cause of septicemia in oncology and neonatal units. However, anti-pseudomonas activity is not usually included in antibiotic protocols to cover presumed sepsis in children with no previous medical disorders. Even when appropriate antibiotic therapy is given, mortality is high. The characteristic necrotic skin lesion, known as ecthyma gangrenosum, is a typical feature of *P. aeruginosa* septicemia and may be useful in diagnosis.

Meningitis

P. aeruginosa meningitis is seen mainly in premature babies and in patients with ventricular drainage catheters or those undergoing intrathecal therapy. It calls for immediate intravenous therapy with a suitable antibiotic, guided by the results of antibiotic sensitivities.

Ear infection

P. aeruginosa is commonly cultured from chronically infected ears (otitis externa) and mastoids, particularly in regular swimmers (swimmers' ear). Occasionally an aggressive and painful infection is produced which is difficult to eradicate and may require surgery.

Eye infections

P. aeruginosa is an important cause of pediatric keratitis following corneal trauma, or secondary to immunosuppression or prematurity. The response to apparently appropriate systemic and topical antibiotic therapy is often disappointing and keratoplasty may be necessary. *P. aeruginosa* also causes orbital cellulitis.

Urinary tract infection

Urinary tract infection usually follows long term catheterization, but also occurs when chronic infection has impaired local tissue viability. The organism is a common commensal under the prepuce, and this should be suspected as the source of unexpected *Pseudomonas* bacteriuria.

Respiratory infections

P. aeruginosa pneumonia occurs in the presence of the predisposing factors outlined earlier or following prolonged treatment of other bronchopulmonary infections. Chronic airway infections with mucoid variants of *P. aeruginosa* and repeated debilitating exacerbations are a major cause of morbidity and mortality in individuals with cystic fibrosis.

Osteomyelitis

Pseudomonas osteomyelitis is particularly associated with penetrating injuries to the foot through sports shoes such as from stepping on a nail ('sneaker osteomyelitis'). In this setting or when osteomyelitis fails to respond to antibiotic therapy directed against *Staphylococcus aureus*, *Pseudomonas* should be considered. It is not always possible to isolate the organism from blood cultures, and antibiotic therapy may have to be broadened blindly.

Skin infections

Pseudomonas skin infections are seen where the skin of the foot has become macerated from prolonged immersion or the wearing of rubber footwear. Ecthyma gangrenosum, an aggressive skin infection usually arising in children with one of the predisposing factors already mentioned, produces necrotic ulcerative lesions involving particularly the anogenital and axillary areas, and can be rapidly fatal.[348]

Management of *Pseudomonas aeruginosa* infections

Treatment of *P. aeruginosa* infections can be difficult if not diagnosed early. The choice of antibiotic therapy should depend on the laboratory sensitivity of the isolate.[349] Many strains are sensitive to broad spectrum penicillins such as ticarcillin, aminoglycosides such as gentamicin, and anti-pseudomonal beta-lactams such as ceftazidime, all of which must be given parentally and usually in combination. Safety concerns over the use of quinolones in pediatric patients have reduced, and agents such as ciprofloxacin can be given orally.

BURKHOLDERIA (PSEUDOMONAS) CEPACIA COMPLEX

Pseudomonas cepacia, now classified as a group of closely related species known as the *Burkholderia cepacia* complex, are important pulmonary and transmissible pathogens in children with cystic fibrosis or chronic granulomatous disease.[350] Outbreaks of nosocomial infection in intensive care units can also occur and usually be traced to contaminated solutions, including disinfectants. In individuals with cystic fibrosis, the *B. cepacia* complex can be aggressive pathogens producing a rapidly fatal necrotizing pneumonia, known as 'cepacia syndrome'.

B. cepacia complex species are intrinsically resistant to many antibiotics but may be sensitive to antibiotic combinations containing two or three agents. Of the newer antibiotics, meropenem is the most active agent.

BURKHOLDERIA (PSEUDOMONAS) PSEUDOMALLEI

Burkholderia pseudomallei causes melioidosis, is spread mainly by contaminated monsoon waters and is endemic in tropical areas of southeast Asia and Australia. Pediatric pneumonia is an important feature of melioidosis, but it may also present with multiple metastatic abscesses and 'imitate' other infections. Melioidosis has a high mortality and responds better to intravenous ceftazidime than to conventional therapy with tetracyclines and chloramphenicol.[351]

OTHER *PSEUDOMONAS* SPECIES

Numerous species of *Pseudomonas* (e.g. *P. fluorescens* and *P. putida*), some renamed (e.g. *Stenotrophomonas maltophilia* and *Ralstonia pickettii*), are recovered from time to time from clinical microbiology specimens, particularly from immunocompromised or otherwise vulnerable patients.

PREVENTION OF NOSOCOMIAL *PSEUDOMONAS* INFECTIONS

In the management of *Pseudomonas* infections, prevention is easier than cure. Thorough drying (and preferably sterilizing) of equipment after cleaning, and scrupulous attention to the manufacturer's instructions for the storage and use of antiseptic solutions are important in curtailing outbreaks of nosocomial infection.

BACTERIAL INFECTIONS: RELAPSING FEVER

Relapsing fever is a disease caused by *Borrelia* species. It is characterized by sudden onset of fever with recurrent episodes of fever. There are two types of relapsing fever (RF): epidemic or louse-borne relapsing fever (LBRF) and endemic or tick-borne relapsing fever (TBRF).

EPIDEMIOLOGY

Relapsing fever has a worldwide distribution, though epidemic RF is prevalent in East Africa, particularly Ethiopia and the Sudan. LBRF epidemics usually follow massive movement of people or disasters such as famine, flooding and earthquake.[352,353] Disaster situations cause overcrowding and lapses in personal and domestic hygiene. The seasonality of TBRF infection varies depending on the behavior of the ticks, whereas LBRF peaks in the rainy season, when people tend to crowd. RF affects both sexes equally in children. Infants account for less than 5% of cases.[354]

ETIOLOGY

LBRF is caused by *B. recurrentis*, while TBRF is caused by various *Borrelia* species in different areas, including *B. duttoni* (East Africa), *B. hispanica* (Spain), *B. persica* (Asia), *B. hermsii* and *B. turicatae* (North America).

PATHOGENESIS

LBRF is transmitted from person to person by body lice. Man is the only reservoir for *B. recurrentis*. The lice prefer normal body temperature to higher temperatures, so lice leave febrile patients and infect afebrile ones.[355] Lice acquire *Borrelia* while feeding on the blood of an infected person. The ingested *Borrelia* enter the mid-gut of the louse. From the mid-gut, the *Borrelia* penetrate the gut wall, enter the hemolymph, and multiply in the body cavity. They do not reach the salivary glands or the ovaries. Human beings are infected when the infected lice are crushed on the skin and *Borrelia* enter the human body through the skin abrasions or intact skin. The louse can remain infective throughout its life span.

Ticks of the genus *Ornithodoros* are important vectors for the transmission of TBRF. Ticks inhabit rodent burrows, earthen floors and crevices of houses. Ticks get infected while feeding on infected animals, especially rodents. Within a few days the spirochetes enter the salivary glands, coxal glands, central ganglion and Malpighian tubules. Infected ticks transmit *Borrelia* to human beings through bites. An infected tick can transmit *Borrelia* to its offspring, which can also transmit to human beings.

In both types of RF spirochetemia occurs and the spirochetes can be detected in the blood of the patient. The characteristic recurrence of symptoms in RF is due to antigenic changes that result in new clones, and during relapse new antibodies are formed. An important clinical characteristic of RF is a Jarisch–Herxheimer (JHR) reaction following destruction of the spirochetes in the course of the disease or treatment. The cause is unclear, although JHR is associated with raised levels of tumor necrosis factor alpha (TNF-alpha), IL-6 and IL-8.[356,357]

CLINICAL FEATURES

The incubation period for both LBRF and TBRF is about 7 days, range 4–18 days. The clinical manifestations may be indistinguishable from the common tropical febrile illnesses such as malaria, typhus fever and typhoid fever. Concomitant infection with typhus is not uncommon in LBRF as both are transmitted by lice.

The onset of RF is characterized by sudden onset of high grade fever, shaking chills, dry cough, abdominal pain and headache accompanied by joint pain, back pain, neck pain and myalgia. Some patients have neck stiffness. Hepatomegaly with hepatic tenderness is common and about a third of patients have splenomegaly. Jaundice with dark-colored urine is occasionally seen, with or without hepatic abnormalities. Hemorrhagic manifestations can include petechial rash, epistaxis and/or hematuria. Neurological abnormalities in TBRF include peripheral neuritis and focal neurological deficits, while patients with severe RF of either type may develop confusion and altered consciousness. Severe cases may develop pneumonia and myocarditis. Myocarditis is usually the cause of death in RF, especially during JHR.

In untreated cases, symptoms disappear in about a week, but tend to recur after 7 or more days. With each relapse the symptoms are milder and shorter in duration. In LBRF the usual number of relapses is 1–2, but for TBRF it is 3 or more.

JHR occurs within a few hours of starting antibiotics in about a third of children and severity varies.[358] JHR has two phases: the chill phase and the flush phase.[359] The chill phase, which begins about an hour after administration of an antibiotic and lasts for 10–30 minutes, causes a rise in heart rate, arterial blood pressure and breathing rate, rigors and anxiety. This is followed by the flush phase, in which the temperature and arterial blood pressure drop and the patient becomes diaphoretic and may become shocked.

DIAGNOSIS

Diagnosis is based on the identification of *Borrelia* in blood films taken during the febrile period and stained with Wright or Giemsa stains. Detection of spirochetes can be enhanced by staining fixed smears with acridine orange and by dark-field or phase-contrast microscopy of wet-mount preparations. *Borrelia* can be cultivated by inoculation of rodents or in artificial medium. The role of serology in the diagnosis of RF is not well established. The leukocyte count may be normal or elevated, but is low in JHR. The platelet count is often low. Urinalysis often reveals increased leukocytes, red blood cells (RBC) and RBC casts. Blood urea nitrogen is elevated until patients are rehydrated and urine output is increased. Liver transaminases and bilirubin levels may be elevated. Cerebrospinal fluid analysis may reveal pleocytosis in a few patients, but CSF culture is negative.[358]

TREATMENT

The aim of treatment is to clear spirochetes from blood and tissues and to prevent or control JHR. A wide range of antibiotics is effective. A single dose of an antibiotic often clears the organism from the blood, but it is recommended to continue antibiotics for a couple of days to prevent relapses. Fast destruction of the spirochetes with antibiotics such as tetracycline increases the severity of JHR. Hence, it is recommended to start treatment with less intense destruction of the organisms by using penicillin followed by tetracycline for LBRF. A single dose of benzylpenicillin 400 000 units is given intramuscularly, followed by tetracycline 50 mg/kg/d in 4 divided doses for 2 days for children > 8 years old. Erythromycin or chloramphenicol is an alternative for children less than 9 years old, for whom tetracycline is contraindicated. Penicillin does not eradicate spirochetes from the blood in some patients,[354,360] probably due to poor penetration of penicillin across the blood–brain barrier to clear spirochetes persisting in the cerebral vessels. For TBRF, a 7–10 day course of penicillin is recommended.

It is important to be vigilant for the occurrence of JHR by monitoring vital signs. Keep an IV line open with normal saline to combat shock in case it occurs during JHR. Meptazinol has been claimed to be effective in diminishing the JHR.[361] Recent studies have shown that JHR is associated with increased levels of TNF-alpha, IL-6 and IL-8; when anti-TNFalpha-Fab was given 30 minutes before penicillin, plasma levels of IL-6 and IL-8 were reduced and the incidence of JHR decreased.[356,357] However, the place of antibodies against TNF-alpha in the treatment of JHR has not been well established.

PREVENTION

The most important measure is avoidance of lice and ticks. Improvement in personal and domestic hygiene is an important step to prevent breeding of vectors. Insecticides should be used to delouse the body, clothing and dwellings. In epidemics early case identification and treatment will decrease the size of the human reservoir in LBRF.

PROGNOSIS

In adults, the case fatality rate of LBRF is 3–4% among treated patients[359] and may be as high as 40% among the untreated.[361] In TBRF, the case fatality rate in children admitted to hospital is 8.8% in Tanzania.[362] Among hospital admitted children with LBRF, the case fatality rate is < 2%.[354,358] In LBRF, death is associated with adulthood, delay in consultation and presence of vomiting.[363,364]

BACTERIAL INFECTIONS: SALMONELLOSIS

Salmonellosis is caused by nontyphoidal salmonellae (NTS) which are important causes of infection and disease in children worldwide. A relatively large dose (more than 10^5 colony-forming units) of *Salmonella* is usually required to cause infection. Neonates and young infants are at particular risk of infection because of relative achlorhydria and frequent milk feeds that increase gastric pH and because of lack of acquired immunity.

There are important differences between resource rich and resource limited countries regarding epidemiology and clinical presentation of salmonellosis.[365] In industrialized countries, NTS infection is usually food-borne, causing acute gastroenteritis, but extraintestinal disease is rare.[366] In the UK, most reported cases of food poisoning are due to *Salmonella*. These outbreaks are associated with infections contracted abroad and with infected food, especially from poultry, cattle and pigs. Infection may occur from unhygienic handling or inadequate cooking of food, especially of infected frozen meat that has not been allowed to thaw fully or of refrigerated eggs. Intensive farming methods with the addition of antibiotics to feeds have increased the frequency of infected food and added to the growing problem of multidrug resistant *Salmonella*. Intrafamilial spread and spread through institutions is common, and outbreaks at restaurants, parties and picnics are frequently reported. Pet reptiles are also occasional household sources of infection.

In resource limited countries NTS are also an important cause of invasive extraintestinal disease, particularly in tropical Africa during the rainy season.[367] Intensive rearing of food animals is uncommon in this context, but many children live in crowded conditions with poor sanitation and contaminated water sources. Human-to-human infection by chronic carriers and water-borne salmonellosis in sewage are more likely methods of spread in the community. Nosocomial infection is also relatively common.

PATHOGENESIS

The sites of invasion by salmonellae are usually the ileum and/or the colon. The bacilli can penetrate the mucosa to the lamina propria of the ileum without producing obvious damage to cells and invoke a mainly neutrophil response (as opposed to *S. typhi* which produces a monocytic response). Infection of the ileum results in a watery diarrhea, secretory in nature. Less commonly, invasion of the colon may produce a dysentery-type illness.

Under certain conditions there may be bloodstream invasion, resulting in septicemia or focal infection such as meningitis, osteomyelitis, septic arthritis or empyema. Risk factors for invasive disease include young age, malnutrition, and immunodeficiency including HIV infection. In tropical Africa, an association of invasive NTS disease with malaria and anemia has been reported. Conditions such as hypochlorhydria, hemoglobinopathies especially sickle cell disease, schistosomiasis and malignancy also increase risk of invasive disease.

In sickle cell disease, infarction of the gut may allow salmonellae access to the bloodstream, from where they may invade infarcted areas of bone resulting in osteomyelitis. Also, the impaired opsonization and phagocytic activity in sickle cell disease exacerbates the infection. People with schistosomiasis may harbor salmonellae within the worm or perhaps the granuloma, which protects them from the body's immune system. There may be prolonged or intermittent fever with joint pains and malaise. Treatment should include appropriate chemotherapy for schistosomiasis and *Salmonella*.

CLINICAL FEATURES

The incubation period of *Salmonella* enteritis is 12–48 h. Symptoms in essentially healthy individuals include nausea, vomiting, abdominal pains and diarrhea. In mild cases there may only be diarrhea. The diarrhea may be secretory in nature, with frequent high volume, watery stools resulting in hypotonic dehydration. Alternatively, the presence of blood and mucus may indicate colitis. In severe cases, toxic megacolon and perforation can occur.[367] Fever is common and occasionally there may be an enteric fever-type illness. A reactive arthritis may occur and is associated with HLA-B27 histocompatibility antigens. Symptoms usually settle after 5–7 days but loose stools may continue for several weeks.

In infants < 1 year old, especially neonates and infants < 3 months, septicemia with metastatic infections can occur. In systemic salmonellosis, gastrointestinal symptoms may not be prominent and the infection may be diagnosed only by blood culture. Serious consequences of blood invasion in young infants are meningitis, osteomyelitis and failure to thrive. In older infants and children, bacteremia is usually associated with fever or toxemia, but infants < 3 months old may be afebrile.

Studies in sub-Saharan African children have shown that invasive NTS disease is also common in children > 1 year old and is associated with a high mortality.[367,368] The presentation is often a nonspecific febrile illness or with cough, dyspnea or diarrhea. Associated clinical features are anemia, hepatosplenomegaly, malnutrition and malaria parasitemia. Other common presentations of extraintestinal disease include meningitis and septic arthritis.[367] Mortality is reported as 25% for NTS bacteremia and over 50% for NTS meningitis. In contrast, *Salmonella typhi* is the commonest blood isolate in under-5s in the Indian subcontinent, while NTS is relatively uncommon.[369]

DIAGNOSIS

Salmonella culture is more likely from feces than from a rectal swab. In suspected cases, repeat culture may be necessary as excretion of the organisms may be intermittent. Leukocytes are often seen, and red blood cells and mucus may be present. In *Salmonella* colitis, endoscopy may demonstrate a swollen edematous mucosa with mucus and areas of hemorrhage suggesting ulcerative colitis.

In invasive disease, blood, CSF, urine culture and culture of metastatic lesions such as bone will confirm the diagnosis. Blood culture is advised in infants < 3 months of age and immunocompromised children with *Salmonella*-positive stools, irrespective of whether or not there are symptoms of bacteremia. NTS are not fastidious organisms and are usually readily cultured.

MANAGEMENT

In cases of secretory diarrhea, rehydration and fluid maintenance alone may be necessary. Antibiotics are not indicated for otherwise healthy children with acute NTS gastroenteritis because they do not alter the course of the disease but may prolong excretion in stools and encourage development of multidrug resistance.[370,371] Resistance of NTS to antibiotics relates to their ability to acquire drug resistance from other bacteria in the gut through plasmids and transposons.

Antibiotics are indicated for children with invasive disease. Current preferred first choice is a third generation cephalosporin, cefotaxime or ceftriaxone, or one of the fluoroquinolones, e.g. ciprofloxacin, but multidrug resistance is increasingly common.[366] Treatment for NTS bacteremia should be given for at least 7 days, but longer courses are required for meningitis, osteomyelitis or for children with HIV/AIDS who are at

particular risk of relapse after cessation of antibiotics. The advantages of fluoroquinolones are excellent efficacy and tissue penetration with either parenteral or oral administration, and eradication of intestinal carriage.

Antibiotics are indicated in suspected *Salmonella* enteritis, pending blood culture results, for infants < 3 months of age (particularly febrile infants and neonates), and for immunocompromised children.[372] In prolonged illness, with failure to thrive or in immunocompromised children, intravenous feeding should also be considered before significant weight loss has occurred.

Persistent excretion of *Salmonella* may occur for weeks or some months, especially in young infants. No action is necessary, except for advice regarding hygiene, e.g. when changing nappies and washing the hands of young children. No restriction of activities is necessary, if stools are normal.

TYPHOID FEVER

In England and Wales, from 1996 to 2006, there were on average 182 reports of *S. typhi*, 177 of *S. paratyphi* A, and 22 reports of *S. paratyphi* B infection per annum, over two thirds of which were contracted abroad, particularly in the Indian subcontinent.[373] *S. paratyphi* C was rare. There has been a recent increase in *S. paratyphi* A consistent with the increase reported in parts of Asia.[374,375] In many resource limited countries, where hygiene and sanitation are poor, typhoid fever is endemic and constitutes a major health problem.[374] It is considered that up to 80% of infections are mild or subclinical and thus hospital statistics grossly underestimate the prevalence. The classical features of typhoid fever are mainly found in school-age children and young adults. When *S. typhi* is isolated from young children the presentation is often atypical.[376]

S. typhi only infects humans. Subjects are infectious during the acute phase of the disease and when chronic infection of the biliary system, especially the gallbladder, occurs, persistent excretion of the bacteria in feces results. In patients with structural abnormalities of the urinary tract, such as those resulting from *Schistosoma haematobium* infection, there may be prolonged excretion of *S. typhi*.

Epidemiology

In technically advanced countries, typhoid fever is usually caused by contamination of food by a carrier. *S. typhi* can survive for long periods in food and can withstand freezing and drying. Outbreaks may occur from infected milk and ice cream, and in institutions a wide variety of foods have been infected when a carrier is involved with preparation. Oysters and shellfish cultivated in contaminated sewage may be infected. In resource limited countries, flies and insects may transmit infection and a contaminated water supply may be the source of an outbreak. Contaminated ice may also be a cause. The infective dose is much smaller than in nontyphoidal salmonellosis.

Pathogenesis and pathology

After ingestion, the bacilli invade mainly the upper bowel, with minimal inflammation, and pass to the local lymphatics where they are taken up by macrophages. Their easy access through the bowel may be explained by the ability of *S. typhi* to invade the gut without stimulating an acute inflammatory response or recruitment of neutrophils. If the macrophages have not been sensitized by a previous infection they are unable to kill the bacteria, which are then transported within the macrophages to the thoracic duct and thus to the reticuloendothelial system where the uncontained bacilli proliferate in the bone marrow, lymphoid tissue, liver and spleen. At this stage, marrow and blood culture will be positive. The degree of infection depends on the dose and virulence of the organism, the protective effects of gastric juice, and the host's immune response.

Proliferation of bacilli, which is enhanced by bile, continues in the bile ducts and especially the gallbladder, from where large loads of bacteria pass into the gut and may be cultured from a duodenal aspirate. The organisms are taken up by macrophages in Peyer's patches, particularly those in the ileum. By now, the macrophages have been activated by sensitized lymphocytes and an inflammatory reaction takes place. This results in swelling, necrosis and ulceration of Peyer's patches, which in most cases heal uneventfully. However, erosion of blood vessels may cause intestinal hemorrhage, and extension of the necrosis through the bowel wall may result in perforation. At this stage, which is usually 2–3 weeks after the initial infection, most of the bacteria are intracellular and so blood culture is less often positive, but continuous proliferation in the gallbladder results in shedding of large numbers of bacilli into the gut and stool culture becomes positive. Infection of urine reflects the bacteremia, and a quarter to one third of patients may excrete S. typhi during the illness.

Within the body, reaction to the infection continues. Many tissues are affected including the liver, spleen, kidney, heart and lungs. Typhoid nodules, which are foci of macrophages and lymphocytes, can be detected in a number of organs. Cloudy swelling of the liver and kidney occurs and the enlarged spleen is packed with proliferating cells in the sinusoids and pulp. Toxemia is the most likely cause of organ dysfunction, as signs of inflammation are patchy, and is also probably responsible for the mental confusion. Glomerulonephritis and renal failure may occur and are, in some cases, due to immune complex disease.

Rarely, local suppurative infections may develop in bone, joints, lung, kidney and meninges. S. typhi osteomyelitis is commonly associated with sickle cell disease.

Clinical features

The incubation period is around 10–14 days and shorter in those receiving a high infecting dose of the organism. During the first week of illness there are vague influenza-like symptoms, namely fever, malaise, aches and pains and headache. Persistence of fever for over a week should alert one to the diagnosis. At this stage, common symptoms are headache, drowsiness, anorexia, vomiting, abdominal pain, diarrhea and cough; constipation may be a symptom in older children. On examination the temperature is often 39–40 °C and may have a 'swinging' septicemic pattern. Occasionally, the temperature may be normal in moribund children and rise after resuscitation. Signs of toxemia and confusion are common. The respiration rate is often raised and nonlocalized wheeze and crackles may be heard in the chest. The pulse rate is raised and may be weak in late-diagnosed cases. A bradycardia relative to the level of temperature, seen in some adults, is usually not present in young children. Signs of heart failure may be present, especially if there is anemia and/or myocarditis. The abdomen is mild to moderately distended with vague nonlocalized tenderness. The spleen is enlarged in 20–30% of cases and the liver in a similar proportion. Rates of hepatosplenomegaly vary geographically and according to the duration of the disease. Meningism may be detected. Rose spots, which are pink macules that fade on pressure, may be seen, especially on the trunk. S. typhi may be cultured from them. They may appear in successive crops lasting 2–3 days. They have rarely been reported in children with dark skin.

In uncomplicated cases, treatment results in symptomatic improvement within 2 days and the temperature is usually normal within the week. The physical signs resolve in 2–4 weeks but the child may not regain full strength for 1–2 months.

S. typhi infection during pregnancy may cause abortion. Though transplacental infection occurs, perinatal infection is commonly due to infection during parturition.

In infants and young children, infection by S. typhi may present as a rapid septicemic-type illness with respiratory signs, seizures and meningism. Conversely, presentation may be milder in some infants compared to older children.[376]

In resource limited countries, the presence of nutritional anemia and malnutrition and diseases such as malaria, tuberculosis, sickle cell disease, schistosomiasis and leishmaniasis may complicate the diagnosis. In these diseases, splenomegaly is a common feature. The tendency to anemia in typhoid, which is commonly due to marrow depression, may be exacerbated by the above diseases, and also by glucose-6-phosphate dehydrogenase deficiency and the thalassemias.

The association between Salmonella infections and sickle cell disease and schistosomiasis is described in the section Salmonellosis.

Complications

Perforation of the gut is one of the major complications. It appears to be less common in young children. It is most common in the second to third week of the illness but may occur at any time. If it is observed in hospital, it is often associated with sudden deterioration, hypotension, tachycardia and abdominal rigidity. Sometimes perforation is less dramatic and presents more as an ileus. Occasionally, air is detected under the diaphragm in a child who is not particularly sick. Presumably, the perforation, being small, has sealed off spontaneously. Intestinal hemorrhage may accompany or occur independently of perforation. Other complications include pneumonia, myocarditis, heart failure, glomerulonephritis, renal failure, hepatitis, focal or generalized central nervous system disorders and meningitis. The association between septic osteitis and sickle cell disease has already been mentioned.

Diagnosis

Blood culture is positive in 70–80% of cases in the first 7–10 days of the illness and in about half this number in the following 2–3 weeks and may still be positive after some weeks of illness. However, prior antibiotics may affect sensitivity, as may the volume of blood taken. For schoolchildren 10–15 ml, and for preschool children 2–4 ml are required to achieve optimal isolation rates.[374] Culture of marrow is more often positive than blood, and both may remain positive despite previous or current antibiotic therapy. Early on, stool culture may be positive in 50% of cases and later in the disease in over 70%. Urine culture may be positive in 25–30% of cases. Thus, the combination of blood, stool and urine cultures should diagnose most untreated cases. Leukocytes, predominantly mononuclear, are usually detected in the stool and there is often some proteinuria.

In resource limited countries where routine blood cultures may not be available the Widal test is commonly relied upon for diagnosis; however, it lacks sensitivity and specificity.[374,375] A high titer of O antibody (> 1:160) or four-fold rise in titer in a child in a non-endemic area who has not had a recent typhoid vaccination (within 1 year) is highly suggestive of typhoid fever. In endemic areas, H antibodies may be raised from previous infections and vaccination also results in a sustained raised H titer. Also, in endemic areas an anamnestic response of O antibody to nontyphoid illnesses may necessitate having a higher diagnostic level during the first week of illness. Conversely, O antibodies may fail to develop and, if present, fail to rise in confirmed typhoid fever. In tropical countries, immunosuppression by malaria may be a factor. Persistence of Vi antibodies may be used as evidence of carrier status, but they may be raised (> 1:5) in only 70% of cases. A number of rapid diagnostic tests are being evaluated. These include tests to detect IgM antibodies against specific S. typhi antigens, e.g. Typhidot-M®, Tubex®, a dipstick test and nested PCR.[374,375]

Anemia is common and the white cell count is usually normal or low. There may be neutrophilia in young infants or when bowel perforation or a pyogenic abscess is present. There is usually a decrease in eosinophil count. Thrombocytopenia may be detected, especially in severe cases. The serum bilirubin is usually normal unless there is a hemolytic anemia, but serum transaminases are often raised. Hyponatremia is common.

Management

Correction and maintenance of fluid and electrolyte balance is important. Blood transfusion may be necessary. Care regarding overhydration is necessary in the presence of anemia, heart failure, nephritis and/or renal failure.

When the organism is known to be sensitive there is little to choose between chloramphenicol, co-trimoxazole and amoxicillin. Unfortunately, because of multidrug resistance (MDR) alternatives are usually required such as fluoroquinolones (ciprofloxacin or ofloxacin), third generation cephalosporins (ceftriaxone or cefotaxime) and for uncomplicated cases, azithromycin.[374,375,377] However, there are increasing reports of *S. typhi* with reduced susceptibility to fluoroquinolones but fortunately full resistance and resistance to cephalosporins is still rare. Nalidixic acid resistance is commonly used as a marker for resistance to fluoroquinolones but some organisms with reduced susceptibility to fluoroquinolones may be susceptible to nalidixic acid.[378] Also, presumably because of less use of first line drugs in Asia there has been a recent rise in reports of *S. typhi* with sensitivity to chloramphenicol.[374,375] In sub-Saharan Africa, where resistance is generally lower, in many areas chloramphenicol remains the standard drug.

In industrialized countries where most cases of typhoid fever have been contracted abroad, until full sensitivity results are available it should be presumed that *S. typhi* will be multidrug resistant and some cases will have reduced susceptibility to fluoroquinolones. Ceftriaxone 60–80 mg/kg once daily for 7–14 days or until 3 days after defervescence is effective. Fluoroquinolones have the advantage of better tissue penetration, oral administration and eradication of the carrier stage. Relapse rates may be lower than with third generation cephalosporins. If sensitive, ciprofloxacin 25 mg/kg/d intravenously, followed by 30 mg/kg/d orally, is given for 7–14 days. Fluoroquinolones are not licensed for routine use in children, owing to concerns regarding arthropathic effects on weight-bearing joints in juvenile animals. However, short courses of fluoroquinolones appear safe.[379] For MDR isolates with reduced susceptibility to fluoroquinolones, azithromycin (10 mg/kg/d) given for 7–10 days is an alternative.[377] Cefixime (20 mg/kg/d) is also used but may not be effective in treating MDR.[374] In areas where chloramphenicol is still sensitive it is given in a dose of 50–75 mg/kg/d. Therapy needs to be continued for a minimum of 14 days; 21 days significantly reduces the relapse rate. When fever subsides the dose may be reduced to 30 mg/kg.

Corticosteroids may be beneficial in severe cases. A controlled trial of dexamethasone, 3 mg/kg followed by 1 mg/kg every 6 h for 48 h in severely ill patients, produced a significant reduction in mortality.[379] Perforation should be managed surgically, after full resuscitation with correction of electrolyte and fluid imbalance, and blood transfusion if necessary.[380] Procedures will vary according to circumstances and include simple oversewing of the perforation, or resection, especially in those with multiple perforations. Additional antibiotics to cover Gram negative organisms and anaerobes such as gentamicin and metronidazole should be given.

For clearance of infection, three consecutive stools should be cultured at weekly intervals after chemotherapy ceases. With adequate chemotherapy relapse is uncommon. Children may return to school when symptom free; stools do not have to be culture negative. Preschool children and children unable to practice normal hygiene may need to be excluded until clear of infection. Carriage of *S. typhi* for over 3 months indicates that the child may have become a chronic carrier, but this is uncommon in children. It may be associated with defective cell-mediated immunity to *Salmonella*. Ciprofloxacin or another fluoroquinolone should be given for relapse or chronic carriage.

Prognosis

In the pre-antibiotic era, the mortality rate for typhoid fever for all ages was around 7–20% and in technically advanced countries is now <0.5%. In resource limited countries, the overall mortality in children shows marked geographical variation. This may depend on age and stage of disease on admission, prior administration of antimicrobials, bacterial resistance and management.

Prevention

Care should be taken in the handling of stools of infected children and attention paid to hygiene, particularly hand washing. Supervision of young and handicapped children is important.

There are two vaccines available for general use: parenteral Vi capsular polysaccharide and oral live attenuated vaccines which use the Ty21a strain. They provide approximately 50–70% protection.[381] A single dose of Vi polysaccharide vaccine is given by intramuscular injection and side-effects are usually only local and mild. There may be

a suboptimal response in children under 2 years (vaccination is not recommended under 12 months). A booster dose is required about every 3 years. The Ty21a vaccine is given for three to four doses on alternate days. At present it is not recommended for children under 6 years. In unexposed children, reinforcement courses need to be given every year and every 3 years where there is repeated exposure.

The development of a Vi conjugate vaccine has the potential for mass immunization of infants and children in low income countries.[382]

PARATYPHOID FEVER

Paratyphoid fever, due to *S. paratyphi*, is similar to typhoid fever, but is usually milder with a shorter period of fever and a lower frequency of complications and mortality. The incubation period is often shorter and diarrhea is more common. However, in neonates and young infants complications and mortality may be high. It should be managed along the same lines as typhoid fever.

BACTERIAL INFECTIONS: *SHIGELLA* (BACILLARY DYSENTERY)

Shigella is a global infection that is notorious for disseminating rapidly in settings where there is crowding, inadequate sanitation and insufficient supply of clean water. The spectrum of symptoms ranges from mild watery diarrhea to fulminant bacillary dysentery, characterized by bloody stools, fever, prostration, cramps and tenesmus. The bacillus was first described by Kiyoshi Shiga in Japan in 1898. The organism he described was *Shigella dysenteriae* type 1, also known as the *Shiga bacillus*, the most virulent of all the shigellae.

Shigellae are nonmotile, Gram negative, non-lactose-fermenting rods belonging to the family Enterobacteriaceae. The genus *Shigella* is subdivided into four groups, or species: *Shigella dysenteriae* (12 serotypes), *Shigella flexneri* (15 serotypes and subtypes), *Shigella boydii* (18 serotypes) and *Shigella sonnei* (a single serotype). The most common serogroup of *Shigella* circulating in a community appears to be related to the level of industrialization. *S. flexneri* predominates in resource limited countries (~60% of isolates), with *S. sonnei* being the next most common (~15%).[383] In industrialized countries, *S. sonnei* is the most common serogroup (~77%).[383]

EPIDEMIOLOGY

The major mode of transmission is by fecal–oral contact, and a low infectious inoculum (as few as 10 organisms) renders *Shigella* highly contagious for humans, the only natural host. Persons symptomatic with diarrhea are primarily responsible for transmission. The majority of infections are due to endemic shigellosis which primarily affects children 1–4 years of age. Endemic strains of *Shigella* cause approximately 10% of all diarrheal episodes in resource limited countries and contribute disproportionately compared to other enteric pathogens to adverse outcomes such as persistent diarrhea, malnutrition, and even death. In contrast, *Shigella* causes fewer than 5% of diarrhea episodes among young children in industrialized countries where it generally has a benign outcome. *Shigella* is an important etiologic agent of diarrhea among residents of industrialized countries (including military personnel) who travel to less developed regions of the world and tends to produce a more disabling illness than other etiologic agents.

Outbreaks of shigellosis occur in settings where suboptimal hygiene allows fecal–oral transmission, such as children attending day care and persons residing in custodial institutions. Outbreaks in the child care setting often result in high attack rates (33–73%) and secondary cases in many families. Outbreaks which involve contaminated food and water in addition to direct contact can be quite extensive, involving thousands of people over a brief period of time. When feces are improperly disposed of, flies may transmit infection. In such settings, the simple introduction of fly-traps can effectively diminish the incidence of shigellosis.

One serotype of *S. dysenteriae* (type 1) is uniquely capable of pandemic spread. During the twentieth century, pandemics of *S. dysenteriae* type 1 appeared in Central America, south and south-east Asia and sub-Saharan Africa, primarily affecting populations in areas of political upheaval and natural disaster. Typically these strains are resistant to multiple antibiotics and induce high attack rates and case fatality in all age groups. A tragic example of the potential for devastation occurred among Rwandan refugees who fled into Zaire in 1994. During the first month alone, approximately 20 000 persons died from dysentery caused by a strain of *S. dysenteriae* type 1 that was resistant to all of the commonly used antibiotics.[184]

PATHOGENESIS AND PATHOLOGY

After oral inoculation, *Shigella* passes to the terminal ileum and colon where it invades and proliferates within enterocytes, produces cell death, incites an inflammatory reaction and induces intestinal fluid secretion. The ensuing cellular destruction and inflammation result in mucosal ulceration and microabscesses. Two *Shigella* enterotoxins (ShETs), designated ShET1 and ShET2, have been incriminated as mediators of the watery diarrhea seen early in the course and may possess other virulence properties. *S. dysenteriae* 1 uniquely produces the highly potent cytotoxin called Shiga toxin which has been implicated in hemolytic uremic syndrome (HUS). The Shiga toxin produced by *S. dysenteriae* 1 has genetic and functional homologies to the Shiga toxins produced by the enterohemorrhagic *Escherichia coli*, and both can cause HUS.

IMMUNITY

Exposure to wild-type *Shigella* infection confers immunity, at least to the same serotype. This immunity is associated with serum antibody recognizing the O-antigen of the lipopolysaccharide moiety. Cross-protection among *S. flexneri* serotypes and subtypes seems to occur, but there is no evidence to date that immunity is shared among *Shigella* species. Mucosal immunity is also important, as illustrated by the protective effect of breast-feeding on the severity of shigellosis in infants from endemic areas[385] and of passively transferred oral immunoglobulin in preventing experimental shigellosis in subjects.[386] Infection also induces cell-mediated immune responses, but their contribution to clinical protection has not been elucidated.

CLINICAL FEATURES

Shigellosis typically evolves through several phases. The incubation period is 1–4 days, but may be as long as 8 days with *S. dysenteriae*. First there is fever and other constitutional symptoms such as headache, malaise, anorexia and occasionally vomiting, followed in several hours by watery diarrhea. In a minority of cases, there is progression within hours to days to frank dysentery with frequent small stools containing blood and mucus, accompanied by lower abdominal cramps and rectal tenesmus. A variety of unusual but important extraintestinal manifestations may occur, including seizures (usually fever-associated), encephalopathy and metastatic infections such as meningitis, arthritis, and splenic abscess, infection of the vagina with bloody discharge, corneal infection and urinary tract infection. Hematologic complications include leukemoid reaction and HUS (following *S. dysenteriae* 1).

Most episodes of shigellosis in otherwise healthy persons are self-limited and resolve within 5–7 days without sequelae. Acute life-threatening complications are largely confined to infants and children from resource limited countries, particularly those with underlying malnutrition. Dehydration, electrolyte imbalance and hypoglycemia are the most common metabolic derangements and are associated with a poor outcome. Intestinal complications include toxic megacolon, rectal prolapse from tenesmus, and intestinal perforation. Sepsis is rare and seen mostly when there is malnutrition or immunodeficiency. Persistent diarrhea and malnutrition are the major long term sequelae resulting, at least in part, from a protein-losing enteropathy that follows *Shigella*-induced intestinal damage. An uncommon late sequel seen primarily in adults is reactive inflammatory arthritis, alone or as part of a constellation of arthritis, conjunctivitis and urethritis known as Reiter syndrome. Persons with HLA-B27 haplotype are predisposed, accounting for about half of the cases.

DIAGNOSIS

The diagnosis should be suspected in patients with dysentery, febrile diarrhea or close contacts of patients with such symptoms. These symptoms in a child 1–4 years old should trigger the highest suspicion. If the patient presents with fever and diarrhea without macroscopic blood in the stools, the diagnosis of *Shigella* infection may be suggested by the presence of large numbers of leukocytes in the stool. Stool microscopy is also useful for distinguishing enteroinvasive bacterial infection from amebic dysentery or enterohemorrhagic *Escherichia coli* (EHEC). Moreover, EHEC and amebic dysentery are less likely to cause fever, and EHEC typically produces voluminous bloody stools rather than dysentery. On the other hand, bacterial pathogens such as nontyphoidal *Salmonella*, *Campylobacter jejuni*, *Yersinia enterocolitica* and enteroinvasive *E. coli* can cause bloody stools or dysentery accompanied by fecal leukocytes, as can a heavy *Trichuris trichiura* or *Schistosoma mansoni* infection.

Definitive diagnosis of *Shigella* infection is made by culturing the organism from a fresh stool specimen or rectal swab. Areas of fecal mucus are optimal for sampling. *Shigella* survives poorly in stool samples that are left in ambient temperature; therefore, if the sample cannot be promptly plated onto solid media, it should be inoculated into appropriate transport media and refrigerated. Culture of two or more stool specimens before initiation of antibiotic therapy increases the yield. Blood culture should be undertaken in toxic patients, young infants and those who are immunocompromised.

MANAGEMENT

Careful attention to the patient's fluid and electrolyte balance with correction of deficits and replacement of ongoing losses is a central feature of management. Agents that suppress intestinal motility, such as diphenoxylate, loperamide and opium-containing preparations, should not be given to children, debilitated or immunocompromised patients with known or suspected shigellosis, or to patients infected with antibiotic-resistant strains or with *S. dysenteriae* as they may increase the severity of dysentery by delaying clearance of the organism.

Many controlled clinical trials of patients with shigellosis have demonstrated that appropriate antibiotics significantly decrease the duration of fever, diarrhea, intestinal protein loss, and excretion of the pathogen. Most patients in these studies were infected with either *S. flexneri* or *S. dysenteriae*. The advantages of treating *S. sonnei*, which is usually self-limited, are less clear. Treatment is recommended for patients with severe disease, dysentery or underlying immunosuppression and should be administered empirically while awaiting culture and antibiotic susceptibility results. The major indication for treatment in mild disease is to decrease excretion and eliminate the potential for transmission. For susceptible strains, ampicillin, trimethoprim–sulfamethoxazole, nalidixic acid and pivmecillinam are good choices. Amoxicillin is less effective, presumably because of its rapid absorption and low fecal concentrations. For cases in which susceptibility is unknown or there is resistance to first line agents, a fluoroquinolone (such as ciprofloxacin), azithromycin or parenteral ceftriaxone can be used. The efficacy of ceftriaxone has been attributed to excretion of its active form in the bile; despite in vitro susceptibility, other cephalosporins such as oral cefixime and parenteral cefamandole are inconsistently effective, perhaps due to their lack of intracellular activity. Treatment can be administered orally except in seriously ill patients and is generally given for 5 days.

PREVENTION

Interruption of transmission by individual hygienic behavior such as hand washing is effective in interrupting outbreaks. Segregation of ill persons is useful in settings where hygienic practices are difficult to enforce, such as outbreaks occurring in institutions for the mentally handicapped. Antibiotics should not be used to prevent transmission.

Oral live attenuated vaccines and parenteral O-polysaccharide conjugate vaccines have been developed that show promise in early clinical trials, but as yet no effective vaccine is in use.[387] A polyvalent vaccine will be required to cover the *Shigella* serotypes of clinical and epidemiologic importance.

BACTERIAL INFECTIONS: *STAPHYLOCOCCUS*

Staphylococci are Gram positive cocci and include the coagulase positive *Staphylococcus aureus* which is responsible for most of the clinical problems. Coagulase negative staphylococci (CNS) include *Staphylococcus saprophyticus*, a cause of urinary tract infection, and *Staphylococcus epidermidis*, a skin commensal, which has become an increasing problem with the use of intravascular and other implantable devices.

STAPHYLOCOCCUS AUREUS

Staphylococci are relatively resistant to heat and drying, enabling them to survive for some months on a variety of surfaces or in dust. Their pathogenicity depends on various cell wall components, enzymes and toxins. Toxic shock syndrome toxin-1 (TSST-1), for example, is associated with toxic shock, exfoliative toxins A and B (ETA and B) with scalded skin syndrome,[388] and Panton–Valentine leukocidin (PVL) with abscesses and necrotizing pneumonia.[389] The production of beta-lactamases (penicillinases and cephalosporinases) is of particular clinical relevance, as these enzymes effectively inactivate beta-lactam antibiotics, and agents such as flucloxacillin or clavulanate-potentiated amoxicillin are required to overcome this.

Asymptomatic carriage of *S. aureus* is common, and the organisms can be found in the anterior nares and less often on the skin, particularly the perineum and axillae. This can be a problem in hospitals, where staff and patients can become carriers of resistant staphylococci, and can have serious consequences in obstetric units, burns units and surgical wards. Immunocompromised patients on broad spectrum antibiotics are particularly at risk. Since the 1960s, the prevalence of methicillin resistant strains of *S. aureus* (MRSA) and epidemic MRSA (EMRSA) has increased both in hospital and in the community. Local hospital infection control strategies vary in terms of patient isolation, barrier nursing and 'decontamination programs' with detergent baths and topical use of mupirocin (pseudomonic acid) to the anterior nares. Serious infection can occur with MRSA, and although strains are generally sensitive to vancomycin and teicoplanin, there are now occasional reports of vancomycin-resistant *S. aureus* (VRSA)[390] and vancomycin-intermediate *S. aureus* (VISA).

Bacteremia and septicemia

Septicemia and bacteremia with *S. aureus* is generally associated with a focus of infection such as osteitis, pneumonia or a severe skin infection and can be associated with intravascular devices such as intravenous cannulae, central lines and prosthetic heart valves. Severe systemic upset with fever is common, and weight loss and anemia can occur with prolonged illness. Staphylococcal bacteremia can progress to endocarditis with risk of damage to previously normal heart valves.

Toxic shock syndrome can be associated with tampon use or with other foci of infection, particularly where the skin integrity is compromised by trauma, surgical wounds, burns, chickenpox, eczema, etc. Symptoms include fever, headache, diarrhea, myalgia and confusion. Clinical features include pyrexia, hypotension, a widespread erythematous rash, particularly on the hands and soles (which later desquamate) and mucosal involvement with conjunctivitis and red, inflamed lips. It is a multisystem disease with frequent renal impairment, hepatitis or thrombocytopenia.

Successful treatment depends on rapid institution of antistaphylococcal therapy and general supportive measures, including surgical drainage or removal of tampon, as indicated (Table 28.29). Eradication of staphylococci from indwelling devices such as central lines is unlikely with antibiotic therapy alone and removal of the infected device is usually required. Staphylococci are generally penicillin resistant and suitable antimicrobial agents include flucloxacillin, second generation cephalosporins, rifampicin and fusidic acid. Clindamycin or erythromycin may be useful in combination with fusidic acid, particularly if there is a history of penicillin allergy or to treat suspected or proven community acquired MRSA infection. Aminoglycosides, such as gentamicin, have antistaphylococcal action and can be used in combination with other antistaphylococcal agents. Vancomycin or teicoplanin is prescribed for more resistant organisms. Usually 2 weeks of therapy is sufficient for uncomplicated bacteremia.

Skin infection

Intact skin is a powerful barrier against staphylococcal infection and most skin infection is fairly minor resulting in boils, pustules, furunculosis, carbuncles, styes, paronychia and impetigo. Topical therapy with mupirocin or fusidic acid ointment should suffice for the treatment of impetigo. Large abscess formation may require surgical drainage. Children who are prone to recurrent minor staphylococcal skin infections should be investigated for possible nasal carriage as they may benefit from a course of mupirocin applied to the anterior nares, and if necessary other family members may also be treated. In children with recurrent staphylococcal skin infection, consideration should be given to screening for neutrophil abnormalities, although the vast majority of these children are immunologically normal.

Table 28.29 Antimicrobial therapy for *Staphylococcus aureus* infection

Parenteral				
Flucloxacillin or cloxacillin	i.v. or i.m.	1 month to > 12 years	12.5 mg/kg	6-hourly
Fusidic acid	i.v. only	1 month–12 years	6–7 mg/kg	8-hourly
		12 years	500 mg	Diethanolamine fusidate
Vancomycin (infusion over 60 min, monitor levels)	i.v. only	>1 month	15 mg/kg/d	
Oral				
Flucloxacillin		1 month–1 year	62.5 mg	6-hourly
		1–4 years	125 mg	6-hourly
		5–12 years	250 mg	6-hourly
		> 12 years	500 mg	6-hourly
Fusidic acid		1 month–1 year	12.5 mg/kg	8-hourly
		1–4 years	250 mg	8-hourly
		5–12 years	250–500 mg*	8-hourly
		> 12 years	500 mg*	8-hourly

*As sodium salt.

Cellulitis, a more deep-seated, spreading infection of the skin is an indication for systemic antimicrobial therapy. Orbital cellulitis carries risks of cavernous sinus infection and should be treated promptly with high dose intravenous antibiotics.

The scalded skin syndrome is discussed in Chapter 30.

Gastrointestinal infection

Food poisoning

Foodstuffs such as cooked meat products, cream, custard and pastry can be a source of staphylococcal food poisoning. The organism may be isolated from the food handlers involved, and often the food is found to have been undercooked and then refrigerated. Symptoms caused by the enterotoxin (which is heat stable) occur 2–5 h after consumption and result in an acute onset of sweating, abdominal pain, diarrhea and vomiting. The symptoms rarely last longer than a few hours but occasionally supportive therapy with intravenous fluids is required. Antibiotics are not helpful.

Pneumonia, osteitis, meningitis

These staphylococcal infections are discussed in Chapter 12.

STAPHYLOCOCCUS EPIDERMIDIS

With the increasing use of invasive procedures, this skin commensal has become an important pathogen, particularly in the neonate and in the presence of indwelling catheters and shunts. Children with ventriculoatrial shunts may have bacteremia, and ventriculoperitoneal shunts can lead to peritonitis. In this situation, eradication of infection with antimicrobial therapy may not be possible and relapse is common. Replacement of the infected device or catheter is, therefore, usually required.

Particularly in hospital acquired infection, resistance to many antimicrobial agents is common. Resistance to vancomycin is rare, though, despite its widespread use in this setting.

BACTERIAL INFECTIONS: STREPTOCOCCUS AND ENTEROCOCCUS

The large family of streptococci can be responsible for a variety of diseases and sequelae. Streptococci are Gram positive cocci, which tend to form chains. There are several classification systems based on serological or molecular biological techniques. A more traditional classification is based on the degree of hemolysis surrounding a colony on blood agar. Hemolysis can be complete (beta hemolysis), partial (alpha hemolysis) or absent (gamma hemolysis).

The beta hemolytic streptococci are responsible for most of the streptococcal disease in humans and are among the most common bacterial infections of childhood. Streptococci belonging to the other two groups are mainly commensals of the pharynx or gastrointestinal tract and tend to be less virulent pathogens.

THE BETA HEMOLYTIC STREPTOCOCCI

Beta hemolytic streptococci can be further classified into Lancefield groups depending on the serological characterization of the polysaccharide layer of the cell wall. Most human disease is caused by Lancefield group A streptococci (GAS), which include *Streptococcus pyogenes*. GAS can be further categorized into subtypes.

Beta hemolytic streptococci can produce disease by direct tissue invasion or by toxin production. Some strains have a hyaluronic acid capsule which is non-antigenic and has an inhibitory effect on phagocytosis. The cell wall is a complex structure built upon a peptidoglycan matrix. There are a variety of antigenic determinants, including the protein M antigen, which confer further resistance to phagocytosis and may act as a superantigen. Streptococci lacking this antigen are generally avirulent. The T antigens are useful for epidemiological tracing. The polysaccharide layer determines the Lancefield group. Lipoteichoic acid is a further cell wall component, which influences membrane affinity and adherence to epithelial cells. Virulence also depends on the production of toxins. Several strains can produce the streptococcal pyrogenic exotoxins (SPE) A, B and C, previously known as erythrogenic toxins, which act as a superantigen triggering the rash of scarlet fever and the syndrome of streptococcal toxic shock syndrome. The two streptolysins O and S are responsible for the hemolytic action of streptococci and the estimation of the antistreptolysin O (or ASO) titer can be useful in diagnosing streptococcal infection. Persisting high ASO titers are seen, for example, in rheumatic fever. Other extracellular products, which are possibly involved in spread of infection and the pyogenic process, include DNases, hyaluronidases and streptokinase.

Epidemiology

GAS are principally carried in the pharynx and asymptomatic carriage occurs in 15–20% of children. Infection is spread by direct contact or droplet spread and outbreaks may occur particularly in dormitory-type accommodation in winter months. Food- or water-borne outbreaks have been reported. There have been changing patterns in streptococcal disease worldwide. Scarlet fever, for example, is less of a clinical concern than previously, although over the last few decades[391] there has been an increase in more severe invasive forms of disease such as necrotizing fasciitis.

Immunity

In view of the antigenic variety of the streptococcal strains, repeated streptococcal infection is possible. A child who has suffered from scarlet fever and developed immunity to the SPEs should be protected against further attacks of the syndrome.

Clinical features

The usual focus for GAS infection is the throat, and infection generally presents with symptoms and signs of acute tonsillitis. In children up to the age of 5 years the illness may be less specific. The incubation period is 2–4 days and the child usually complains of a sore throat and headache, is febrile and may have cervical lymphadenopathy. The pharynx may appear mildly inflamed or a more severe form of exudative pharyngitis may be present. Clinical discrimination from viral infection is not usually possible and uncomplicated carriage is always a possibility when streptococci are isolated from the throat swab. Classically, after 10 days of illness, a rise in the ASO titer will be apparent. Tonsillitis, otitis media, mastoiditis, sinusitis and the much rarer GAS pneumonia, impetigo or pyoderma, empyema, meningitis and septicemia are described elsewhere. Scarlet fever and erysipelas are unique to streptococcal infection.

Scarlet fever

Scarlet fever is caused by infection with an SPE producing strain of GAS. The usual portal of entry is via the pharynx and the syndrome classically follows acute streptococcal tonsillitis. However, the streptococci may gain access via broken skin following pyoderma, minor cuts, burns, surgical wounds or chickenpox infection.

Clinical features

The incubation period is usually 2–4 days and the illness may be of variable severity with sudden onset fever, headache, vomiting, sore throat and refusal to eat. In the past, severe illness was more common and delirium a frequent feature. The erythematous rash appears some 2 or 3 days after the onset of illness and classically is first seen in the axillae and groins with blanching on pressure (Figs 28.26 and 28.27). Within 24 h the rash spreads to the trunk and limbs. The face may be flushed and circumoral pallor is a common feature. Pastia's sign – linear petechiae in the flexures – may be helpful diagnostically. After a week or so, desquamation usually occurs starting on the face, then the trunk and limbs. Initially the tongue appears swollen with a yellowish white coating and prominent papillae. This is known as the 'white strawberry' tongue, which later becomes the 'red strawberry' tongue as the coating disappears.

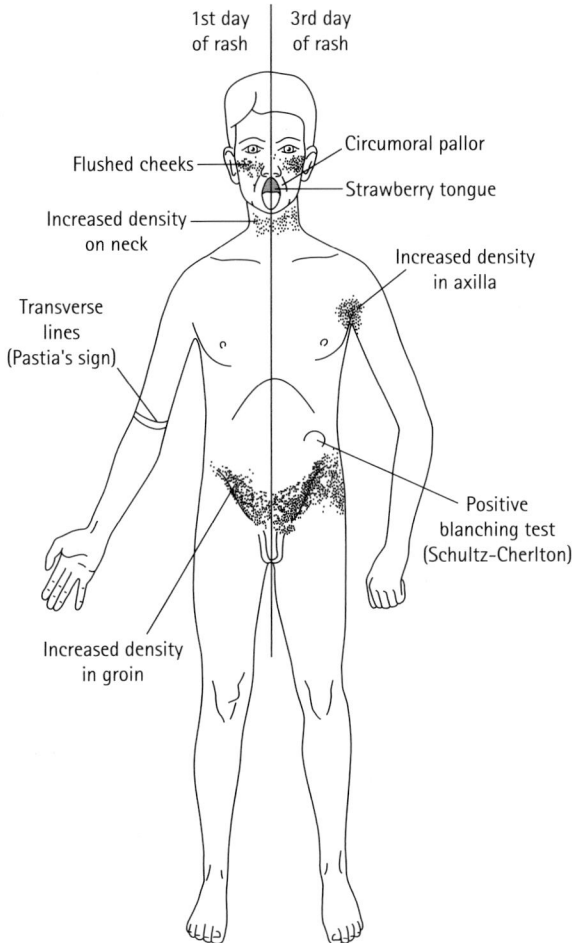

Fig. 28.26   The distribution and the development of rash in scarlet fever.

Untreated, the illness runs its course within 10 days or less. A high fever and tachycardia are common.

Albuminuria is a common finding and a polymorphonuclear leukocytosis is usual.

Since the availability of antibiotic therapy, serious complications are rare. Immediate complications include cervical lymphadenitis with more rarely abscess formation necessitating surgical drainage. Acute otitis media may develop and without treatment further complications including mastoiditis, meningitis or cerebral abscess may ensue. Involvement of the paranasal sinuses can lead to suppurative sinusitis. Other recognized local complications include peritonsillar cellulitis or abscess formation, laryngitis and retropharyngeal abscess.

Rarely, bacteremic spread can lead to metastatic foci of infection, and bronchopneumonia is a further complication, which may lead to empyema or suppurative pericarditis.

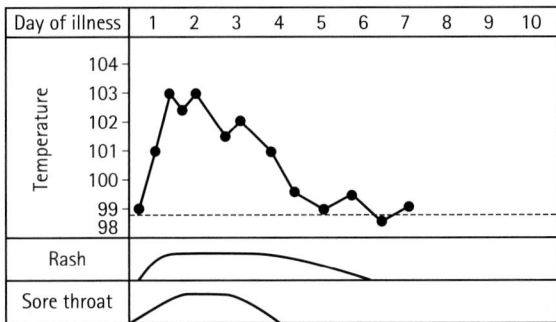

Fig. 28.27   The development of scarlet fever.

The later complications, occurring about 2–3 weeks after the onset of illness, include rheumatic fever, acute glomerulonephritis and erythema nodosum. Early antibiotic therapy should prevent such complications.

Differential diagnosis

Where acute tonsillitis is present the diagnosis is usually straightforward. With milder or subclinical pharyngitis the diagnosis may be less apparent and confused with other exanthemata. Measles is recognized by the prodromal catarrhal symptoms, diarrhea, conjunctivitis, the presence of Koplik spots and the different character and distribution of the rash. In rubella, the diffuse rash contrasting with the mild illness and the presence of predominantly occipital cervical lymphadenopathy are distinguishing features. Generalized lymphadenopathy with splenomegaly is often present in infectious mononucleosis; the blood film examination may reveal atypical mononuclear cells and Epstein–Barr virus (EBV) serology is positive. Other viral exanthemata run a shorter course and usually have leukopenia rather than polymorphonuclear leukocytosis.

Kawasaki syndrome may be difficult to differentiate. The rash, oral and peripheral changes are similar. The cervical lymphadenopathy of Kawasaki syndrome may be characteristically unilateral and matted, and the episcleritis with limbal sparing of Kawasaki syndrome is not usually seen in scarlet fever. In clinical practice, failure of a child with suspected scarlet fever to respond to antibiotics should arouse suspicion of Kawasaki syndrome.

A very similar rash may be seen with staphylococcal toxic shock syndrome but there is often an obvious focus of staphylococcal infection and the rash tends to be more severe on the palms and soles.

Drug rashes, particularly following antibiotic usage, can be scarlatiniform (scarlet fever-like). The other features of disease are not usually present, however, and the rash fades with the cessation of therapy.

Prevention and treatment

The main aim of antimicrobial therapy is to eradicate the infection and thereby prevent the sequelae of local suppurative disease or later rheumatic fever and post-streptococcal glomerulonephritis (Table 28.30). Penicillin is the drug of choice for the treatment of GAS. In severe cases intravenous or intramuscular administration of benzylpenicillin may be required initially. In milder cases, oral phenoxymethylpenicillin for 10 days is usually sufficient. Erythromycin is a suitable alternative in cases of penicillin allergy. Ampicillin and amoxicillin should be avoided, as if mistakenly given in infectious mononucleosis they can cause a severe rash and constitutional upset.

It is unusual to get multiple cases of scarlet fever in a family, although uncomplicated streptococcal throat infection may develop in other children.

Erysipelas

Erysipelas is a skin infection caused by any of the GAS, which can enter the skin through trivial wounds or abrasions. Children of all ages are susceptible and recurrent attacks often involving the same site can occur. Children with congenital lymphedema appear to be more at risk.

Clinical features

The illness may present with fever, malaise, vomiting and anorexia or the symptoms may be confined to the affected skin or occasionally the mucous membranes. A small erythematous patch may develop into a much larger area of affected skin, which becomes red, hot, painful, indurated and well demarcated by a raised edge. In infants, the periumbilical region is a common site, whereas in older children the extremities or the face are sites of predilection and both cheeks may be involved in a butterfly type of distribution. Facial erysipelas must be differentiated from the violaceous cellulitis caused by *Haemophilus influenzae* type b infection or the slapped cheek appearance of parvovirus B19 infection. Resolution of erysipelas starts centrally and may be followed by desquamation.

Table 28.30 Antimicrobial therapy for *Streptococcus pyogenes* infection

Parenteral				
Benzylpenicillin	i.m.	1–12 months	15 mg/kg	6-hourly
		1–4 years	150 mg	6-hourly
		5–12 years	300–600 mg	6-hourly
		>12 years	600 mg–1.2 g	6-hourly
	i.v.	All ages	25–50 mg/kg	4–6-hourly
Erythromycin	i.v. only	1 month–12 years	8–12 mg/kg	6-hourly
Oral				
Phenoxymethylpenicillin		<1 year	62.5 mg	6-hourly
		1–4 years	125 mg	6-hourly
		5–12 years	250 mg	6-hourly
		>12 years	500 mg	6-hourly
Erythromycin		1 month–1 year	125 mg	6-hourly
		2–8 years	250 mg	6-hourly
		>8 years	500 mg	6-hourly

Blood cultures are frequently negative but after 10 days of illness there may be a rise in the ASO titer.

Erysipelas responds quickly to penicillin or erythromycin. It may be difficult to differentiate erysipelas from other soft tissue infection such as cellulitis, the more deep-seated infection caused mainly by staphylococcal infection, and in cases where doubt exists, antistaphylococcal antimicrobial therapy should also be prescribed, e.g. flucloxacillin.

Streptococcal pyoderma

Although most impetiginous lesions are caused by staphylococcal infection, localized purulent streptococcal infection of the skin (streptococcal impetigo or pyoderma) may result from secondary infection of wounds or burns. In children, particularly in the age range 2–5 years and living in tropical or subtropical climates, it mainly involves the lower limbs and may follow intradermal inoculation of streptococci by minor trauma or insect bites. Multiple lesions are common and begin as small papules, becoming vesicular with surrounding erythema. Pustule formation occurs and the lesions then enlarge and break down with formation of thick crusts. Systemic upset is not common but regional lymphadenitis is usually present. Ten days of penicillin therapy is advised although there appears much less risk of rheumatic fever with this type of infection.

Lymphangitis, characterized by red, linear streaks leading to the enlarged regional lymph nodes, may follow very minor skin infection or inoculation with streptococci. It may accompany cellulitis.

Streptococcus agalactiae (group B streptococcus)

Streptococcus agalactiae, or group B streptococcus (GBS), is a beta hemolytic streptococcus belonging to Lancefield group B, and is a major cause of neonatal infections, both early and late.

VIRIDANS GROUP STREPTOCOCCI

Viridans streptococci are usually alpha hemolytic but can be nonhemolytic. They are generally oropharyngeal commensals, and include *Streptococcus mutans, S. salivarius, S. sanguis* and *S. mitis* groups and three streptococci formerly known as the *Streptococcus milleri* group (*S. anginosus, S. constellatus* and *S. intermedius*). Even minor dental procedures can be complicated by a transient bacteremia, which is of no clinical consequence except for children with cardiac disease, either congenital heart disease, such as patent ductus arteriosus or bicuspid aortic valves, or acquired, such as rheumatic heart disease. Infective endocarditis is a risk in such cases. Regular dental care with additional antibiotic prophylaxis for dental procedures is advised for children who have a history of rheumatic fever or congenital heart disease.

ENTEROCOCCI

Enterococci are commensals of the intestinal tract. They can cause urinary tract infection, particularly in cases of structural urinary tract abnormality or neurological dysfunction of the bladder such as in children with lumbar or sacral myelomeningocele. *Enterococcus faecalis* and *E. faecium* are the major pathogens of the 18 types of enterococci seen in humans. *E. faecalis* can cause infective endocarditis and has emerged as a major cause of bacteremia in hospitalized patients. Enterococci are often penicillin resistant, and determination of the antibiotic sensitivity is important. In endocarditis, combinations of antimicrobial chemotherapy are advised, such as the synergistic combination of amoxicillin and an aminoglycoside such as gentamicin. Vancomycin is an alternative, but this treatment is threatened by the emergence of vancomycin resistant enterococci (VRE). Fortunately, few of these isolates appear clinically relevant and the organisms are often no longer evident after cessation of vancomycin or removal of infected lines and devices. There are concerns that VRE may cause more clinical problems in the future and drugs with activity against vancomycin resistant *Enterococcus faecium* include linezolid and quinupristin/dalfopristin.[392]

BACTERIAL INFECTIONS: TETANUS

Despite the availability of an effective active vaccination since 1923, tetanus remains a major health problem in resource limited countries and is still encountered in resource rich countries. At least 1 million cases require hospital treatment worldwide each year and there are approximately 400 000 deaths.[393] There are approximately 800 000 tetanus deaths each year, of which approximately 400 000 are due to neonatal tetanus.[393] Approximately 12–15 cases are reported per year in the UK and between 40 and 60 cases per year in the USA.[393]

ETIOLOGY

Tetanus is caused by a toxin released following infection with *Clostridium tetani*, a Gram positive, spore forming, obligate anaerobic bacillus. Tetanus typically follows deep penetrating wounds where anaerobic bacterial growth is facilitated. The most common portals of infection are wounds on the lower limbs, postpartum or postabortion infections of the uterus, nonsterile intramuscular injections and compound fractures. Minor trauma can lead to disease and in up to 30% of cases no portal of entry is apparent.[393]

EPIDEMIOLOGY AND PATHOGENESIS

Clostridium tetani is a ubiquitous inhabitant of the intestinal tract of many animals and commonly found in soil. The toxin binds to gangliosides on peripheral nerves, and the toxin is internalized. It is then moved by retrograde axonal transport to the central nervous system. The toxin prevents release of the inhibitory neurotransmitter (GABA) into the synaptic cleft. The alpha motor neurones are therefore under no inhibitory control and undergo sustained excitatory discharge causing the characteristic motor spasms of tetanus.

PREVENTION

Tetanus toxoid is produced by formaldehyde treatment of the toxin, its immunogenicity improved by absorption with aluminum hydroxide.[394] In the UK and USA it is administered to children between 2 and 6 months old (3 doses at 4–8 week intervals) with boosters at 15 months in the USA and at 4 years. A further dose is recommended in both the USA and UK within 5–10 years. In order to maintain adequate levels of protection, five additional booster doses should be administered to ensure life-long protection.[394] Minor reactions to the tetanus toxoid are estimated to be 1 in 50000 injections. Severe reactions such as the Guillain–Barré syndrome and acute relapsing polyneuropathy are rare. Neonatal tetanus can be prevented by immunization of women during pregnancy.[395] Two or three doses of absorbed toxin should be given with the last dose at least one month prior to delivery. There is no evidence of congenital anomalies associated with tetanus toxin administered during pregnancy.[395] Maternal HIV and also malaria infection may limit the transfer of protective maternal antibodies. Passive immunization with human or equine tetanus immunoglobulin shortens the course and may reduce the severity of tetanus. The equine form, widely available throughout resource limited countries, has a higher incidence of anaphylactic reactions. In established cases, patients should receive 500–1000 IU/kg of equine antitoxin or 5000–8000 IU of human antitetanus immunoglobulin intravenously or intramuscularly. For prophylaxis 1500–3000 IU equine or 250–500 IU human antitetanus immunoglobulin should be given. Passive immunization should be administered as soon as possible after the injury; once the toxin is bound and internalized it will have no effect. In addition to passive immunization, active vaccination needs to be administered to all patients.

CLINICAL FEATURES

The incubation period (the time from inoculation to the first symptom) can be as short as 48 h or as long as many months after inoculation with *Clostridium tetani*. The period of onset is the time between the first symptom and the start of spasms. These periods are important in determining the prognosis: the shorter the incubation period or period of onset, the more severe the disease. Trismus (lockjaw), the inability to open the mouth fully owing to rigidity of the masseters, is often the first symptom. Generalized tetanus is the most common form of the disease, and presents with pain, headache, stiffness, rigidity, opisthotonus and spasms which can lead to laryngeal obstruction. These may be induced by minor stimuli such as noise or touch, or by simple medical and nursing procedures such as intravenous and intramuscular injections, suction or catheterization. The spasms are excruciatingly painful and may be uncontrollable leading to respiratory arrest and death. Spasms are most prominent in the first 2 weeks; autonomic disturbance usually starts some days after spasms and reaches a peak during the second week of the disease. Rigidity may last beyond the duration of both spasms and autonomic disturbance. Severe rigidity and muscle spasm necessitates paralysis for prolonged periods in severe tetanus.

DIAGNOSIS AND DIFFERENTIAL DIAGNOSIS

The diagnosis is a clinical one, relatively easy to make in areas where tetanus is seen frequently, but often delayed in resource rich countries where cases are less common. The differential includes tetany, strychnine poisoning, drug induced dystonic reactions, rabies and orofacial infection. In neonates the differential diagnosis includes hypocalcemia, hypoglycemia, meningitis and meningoencephalitis, and seizures.

TREATMENT

In patients with a deep wound, thorough debridement and toilet are critical to reduce the anaerobic conditions that the bacteria thrive in. Common complications in tetanus are those of prolonged periods in intensive care. Secondary infections are a frequent complication, most commonly associated with the lower respiratory tract, urinary catheterization and wound sepsis. Gram negative organisms, particularly *Klebsiella* and *Pseudomonas*, are common. Meticulous mouth care, chest physiotherapy and regular tracheal suction are essential to prevent atelectasis, lobar collapse and pneumonia, particularly as salivation and bronchial secretions are greatly increased in severe tetanus. Adequate sedation is mandatory before such interventions in patients at risk of uncontrolled spasms or autonomic disturbance and the balance between physiotherapy and sedation may be difficult to achieve. Energy demands in tetanus may be very high due to muscular contractions, excessive sweating and sepsis.

SPECIFIC TREATMENT

Penicillin is the standard antibiotic therapy for tetanus. The dose is 100000–200000 IU/kg/d intramuscularly or intravenously for 7–10 days. Metronidazole is a safe and effective alternative. Autonomic disturbance with sustained labile hypertension, tachycardia, vasoconstriction and sweating is common in severe cases. Profound bradycardia and hypotension may occur and may be recurrent or preterminal events. Diazepam has a wide margin of safety and a rapid onset of action, and is a sedative, an anticonvulsant and a muscle relaxant. However, it has a long cumulative half-life. Invariably, in the doses required to achieve adequate control of spasms, respiratory depression, coma and medullary depression are common. Magnesium sulfate has been used to reduce autonomic disturbance and help to control spasms.[396] There is very little information on follow-up of patients after tetanus; enuresis, mental retardation and growth delay have all been reported after neonatal tetanus.

PROGNOSIS

The prognosis in tetanus remains serious despite the best available treatment. Globally the mortality rate in neonatal infection is approximately 60%.[397] Older children and adults have a mortality rate of 10–30% depending on the availability of basic intensive care facilities.[393]

BACTERIAL INFECTIONS: TULAREMIA

ETIOLOGY

This disease derives its name from Tulare, a county in California, where it was first discovered amongst ground squirrels by McCoy in 1911. It is caused by a small, intracellular, nonmotile Gram negative coccobacillus, *Francisella tularensis*, that commonly causes disease in wild animals such as rabbits, hares, squirrels, foxes, rats and deer. There are four subspecies of the organism that are serologically identical but differ in biochemical properties and virulence.[398] *F. tularensis* subsp. *tularensis* represents over 90% of the isolates from North America and is highly virulent in man and rabbits.[399] It is usually recovered from rodents and arthropods. *F. tularensis* subsp. *holartica*, the type most commonly found in Europe and Asia, is less virulent in man and rabbits.[400] It is usually isolated from aquatic animals. The other two subspecies have only rarely been associated with disease in humans.

EPIDEMIOLOGY

The organism can be isolated from a wide variety of wild mammals, from domestic animals such as sheep, cattle and cats, and from the arthropods that bite these animals such as ticks, fleas and deer flies. Human infection occurs after a bite from an infected arthropod, by contact with an infected animal, by ingestion of a diseased animal or contaminated water, or by inhalation of infected secretions. Humans are highly susceptible to the organism, with fewer than 50 organisms required for infection. Tularemia occurs throughout the northern hemisphere, with large outbreaks reported in North America, the southern part of the former Soviet Republic, and northern Scandinavia. In the eastern part of the continental USA it occurs mostly in winter, related to the rabbit hunting season, whereas in the states west of the Mississippi River it occurs in summer when there is a preponderance of ticks. Human case-to-case contact has not been documented, though care must be taken in dressing discharging wounds. Tularemia is extremely infectious for laboratory workers, who must take exceptional care in the handling of infected material or cultures. Its high attack rate and virulence after inhalation has caused its frequent citation as a possible agent for bioterrorism.[401]

PATHOLOGY

There is a local lesion at the portal of entry and, at times, disseminated lesions throughout the body. Entry is usually through the skin, but may be via the conjunctiva, the respiratory tract or rarely the gastrointestinal tract. Dissemination occurs via the lymphatics or blood, and lesions may be found in the regional lymph nodes and in many other parts of the body. The local lesion is a painful, erythematous papule often with central ulceration and regional lymph node enlargement. The lesions are granulomatous, much like the lesions of miliary tuberculosis, but the center of the lesions is often necrotic and consists of polymorphonuclear leukocytes.

CLINICAL FEATURES

The incubation period ranges from 1 to 21 days but most cases occur 3–5 days after exposure. The severity of the disease depends on the route of entry, the subspecies involved, and the host's immune response. Children usually show more constitutional upset and less respiratory involvement than adults. Most frequently there is an abrupt onset of high fever, headache and malaise with or without regional adenopathy, chest X-ray changes, vomiting, and a cutaneous lesion at the site of entry. Sterile pyuria is also common. Rarely there may be pericarditis, osteomyelitis, meningitis, splenic abscesses or thrombophlebitis. Before antibiotics, reported mortality ranged from 7 to 30%. Six clinical syndromes have been described which occur according to the portal of entry. Most common is the *ulceroglandular syndrome* characterized by a primary painful maculopapular lesion at the point of skin entry with subsequent ulceration and slow healing. This is associated with painful, acutely inflamed regional lymph nodes that may ulcerate and proceed to abscess formation. Other forms of the disease include *typhoidal* tularemia, with high fever and hepatosplenomegaly, *pulmonary* tularemia, with pneumonia, pleuritis and hilar adenopathy, *ocular* tularemia, in which the eyelids become edematous and painful, *oropharyngeal* tularemia, in which the tonsils are covered by a pseudomembrane, and a *glandular* form in which no portal of entry can be identified.[402]

DIAGNOSIS

The circumstances of the disease onset, especially a history of bite or scratch or exposure to wild animals, should readily suggest the diagnosis in endemic areas. There is a significant risk to laboratory personnel when handling specimens so the laboratory should be informed if tularemia is suspected. Serology is the usual means of establishing the diagnosis: a four-fold or greater rise in serum agglutination titer to *F. tularensis* is evident after the second week of illness. Nonspecific, low titer cross-reactions may occur to *Brucella*, *Proteus* and *Yersinia* species. The organism can be cultured from infected sites on special media or by rodent inoculation, but this should be attempted only by personnel vaccinated against the organism.

PCR-based methods may be used to distinguish subspecies,[398] but are not routinely available.

The differential diagnosis depends on the presentation, but includes causes of skin lesions with regional adenopathy such as cat-scratch disease, causes of prolonged fever including brucellosis and salmonellosis (especially typhoid), and causes of atypical pneumonia.

TREATMENT

Streptomycin is the historical drug of choice for treatment of severe tularemia. However, as it is not widely available, gentamicin is an effective alternative although treatment failures have been reported.[403] Chloramphenicol should be added for tularemic meningitis. Options for outpatient therapy of older children include tetracyclines or the quinolones, although relapses have been reported after completion of therapy with both drugs.[404] Treatment is usually for 6–10 days, the duration depending on the severity of the illness.

PREVENTION

In endemic areas, opportunities for arthropod bites should be minimized by wearing protective clothing and regular tick inspections. Prevention also involves avoidance of contact with infected or potentially infected animals and insect vectors, adequate cooking of potentially infected meat and the boiling of water from springs and streams.

In the USA, a live attenuated vaccine is available for those repeatedly exposed to the organism such as laboratory technicians.[405]

BACTERIAL INFECTIONS: YERSINIOSIS AND PLAGUE

YERSINIOSIS[406,407]

Yersiniosis is caused by two species of enteric bacteria, *Yersinia enterocolitica* and *Yersinia pseudotuberculosis*. A wide spectrum of clinical manifestations occurs, including acute watery diarrhea, mesenteric adenitis, extraintestinal infection and bacteremia. Postinfectious sequelae such as arthritis or erythema nodosum are also common.

Microbiology and pathogenesis

Yersinia spp. are facultative anaerobic Gram negative coccobacilli which grow well on bile containing media. There are three human pathogens within the genus, *Y. pseudotuberculosis*, *Y. enterocolitica* and *Y. pestis*. Over 50 serogroups of *Y. enterocolitica* have been described. *Yersinia* infections occur through invasion of the gastrointestinal tract via a membrane protein, invasin, which binds to a cell surface ligand. Multiplication may occur within intestinal epithelial cells and Peyer's patches, with the potential for systemic spread.

Epidemiology

Yersinia enterocolitica infection occurs globally but is most common in temperate regions. Yersiniosis is a zoonotic infection but usually causes food-borne illnesses. The organism can be found in the gastrointestinal tract of a number of domestic and livestock animals. Infection of humans usually occurs after eating or drinking contaminated food or water; incompletely cooked pork is a major risk factor.[408] Infection may also occur by person-to-person or direct animal-to-person contact. Most infections are sporadic but a number of specific outbreaks due to contaminated food or water have occurred. Infants and young children are more susceptible to infection with *Y. enterocolitica* than adults.

Infection with *Y. pseudotuberculosis* is less common, apart from in Japan. Infection results from contact with both sylvatic and domestic animals and a number of birds. It usually affects patients aged between 5 and 20 years.

CLINICAL FEATURES[409]

The incubation period for acute yersiniosis is 3–7 days. *Y. enterocolitica* infection most commonly presents as acute gastroenteritis in young children with diarrhea, fever and abdominal pain, clinically indistinguishable from *Salmonella* or *Campylobacter* infection. Stools contain mucus, leukocytes and red blood cells. Patients may be symptomatic for up to 3 weeks and remain infectious over this period, due to shedding of organisms in the feces. Rare complications include diffuse ulceration of the small intestine and colon, perforation, intussusception and toxic megacolon.

Y. enterocolitica infection in older children most commonly causes mesenteric adenitis and terminal ileitis; this is also the most common manifestation of *Y. pseudotuberculosis* infection. The presentation mimics appendicitis. Diarrhea is unusual and the infection is usually self-limiting. Ultrasound and/or CT may help by demonstrating a normal appendix and enlarged mesenteric nodes. The differential diagnosis includes acute appendicitis or terminal ileal disease such as Crohn's or tuberculosis.

Y. enterocolitica bacteremia is rare and usually occurs in patients with other chronic medical conditions or immunosuppression. There is also a strong association with iron overload syndromes. Case fatality rates for *Y. enterocolitica* bacteremia range from 7.5 to 25%, but may reach 50% in patients with iron overload. Focal *Y. enterocolitica* infection can occur as a complication of bacteremia or occasionally in the absence of detectable bacteremia. *Y. pseudotuberculosis* bacteremia is much less common, but is also associated with chronic illness. Case fatality rates are extremely high in the immunocompromised population. In Japan, *Y. pseudotuberculosis* infection has been associated with renal failure in young children.

Secondary, immunologically mediated, postinfective complications may occur in up to 30% of patients following *Yersinia* infection. A reactive asymmetrical large joint polyarthropathy or erythema nodosum are the most common manifestations, occurring 1–2 weeks after the acute presentation. There is a strong association with the possession of HLA B27. Reiter syndrome, glomerulonephritis and myocarditis have also been described. Synovial fluid culture is normally sterile. Joint symptoms of reactive polyarthritis may last for several months.

Diagnosis

Definitive diagnosis of yersiniosis is by culture of the organism from stool, lymph nodes or blood. Isolation from stool may be optimized by using cold enrichment or cefsulodin–Irgasan–novobiocin (CIN) agar. High titers of *Yersinia* antibodies in a previously healthy individual are suggestive of infection but four-fold rises in titer are rarely found. Interpretation of serology is also complicated by low titers following yersiniosis in infants or immunocompromised patients, a high background prevalence of positive serology in some populations and cross-reactivity with *Brucella*, *Rickettsia* and *Salmonella* spp. Cultures are often negative by the time of appearance of postinfective symptoms.

Y. pseudotuberculosis may be found in sterile site samples, but is rarely isolated from stool. Serology is often the only mode of diagnosis available; antigens cross-react with those of *Y. enterocolitica*.

Treatment

Antimicrobial treatment does not shorten the course or severity of enterocolitis and is not indicated in uncomplicated cases. Localized infection, systemic disease or enterocolitis in an immunocompromised patient should be treated. *Y. enterocolitica* is resistant to most penicillins and first generation cephalosporins: amoxicillin–clavulanate combinations are also unsuitable due to variable minimum inhibitory concentrations. Aminoglycosides, chloramphenicol, tetracycline, co-trimoxazole and fluoroquinolones have been most effective in clinical practice: third generation cephalosporins may also be effective.[410] *Y. pseudotuberculosis* is sensitive to ampicillin and cephalosporins in addition to the drugs already discussed.

PLAGUE[411,412]

Epidemiology and pathogenesis

Plague is a zoonosis caused by *Yersinia pestis*. It occurs globally; approximately 2000 cases of plague are reported annually. Over 90% of cases occur in Africa, with current epidemics in the Democratic Republic of Congo and Madagascar; major active foci also exist in other parts of Africa, the Western USA, China and south-east Asia. Mammals, particularly rodents, act as host reservoirs. Fleas feed upon diseased hosts and organisms multiply within the midgut of the flea before being transmitted to humans or other mammals when the flea bites and regurgitates a blood meal. Human infection can also be acquired from direct contact with wild rodents or their predators (including cats), and person-to-person spread can occasionally occur in epidemics. Most human plague cases currently occur in rural settings with transmission from wild animals; epidemics in human settlements occur when domestic rat species become infected. Plague is a potential bioterrorism agent and this has led to an increased interest in the disease.

Clinical features

There are three main clinical forms of plague. *Bubonic* plague is most common. Bacteria multiply in regional lymph nodes following a flea bite, culminating 2–8 days later in systemic symptoms, fever, headache and malaise. Regional lymph nodes enlarge and become extremely tender with swelling and inflammation around the nodes: the bubo. Occasionally, pustules, eschars or papules occur at the site of flea bites. Most individuals develop a transient secondary bacteremia: in some this leads to septicemic or pneumonic plague.

Patients with *septicemic* plague present with Gram negative septicemic shock and may develop complications such as renal failure or DIC. Septicemic plague occasionally occurs in the absence of buboes; this presentation is more common in children.

Pneumonic plague is usually a complication of bacteremia and presents with cough, fever and hemoptysis: the chest X-ray may show bronchopneumonia, consolidation or cavitation. Large numbers of bacteria may be exhaled with the potential for respiratory spread to cause primary pneumonic plague.

Diagnosis

The patient's symptoms and an appropriate exposure history may lead to a clinical diagnosis of plague. Leukocytosis is common and liver function tests may be abnormal. *Yersinia pestis* may be demonstrated on smears from blood, bubo fluid or CSF: fluorescent antibody techniques increase the sensitivity. Definitive diagnosis depends upon culture of the organism, which grows readily on standard media. A rapid diagnostic test that detects plague antigens in blood has been developed and has helped considerably in field conditions, allowing confirmation of diagnosis within 15 minutes.[412] Serological tests are useful in retrospective diagnosis of plague.

Treatment

Case fatality rates may reach 30–50% in untreated plague. Streptomycin is the traditional drug of choice; gentamicin or doxycycline has been shown to be equally effective, with response rates of around 95%.[413] Seven days' therapy is required to prevent relapse: clinical improvement normally occurs within 3 days. Fluoroquinolones may also be effective, particularly for the rare strains with high level multidrug resistance, although clinical experience is limited. Ciprofloxacin is also indicated as prophylaxis for contacts of pneumonic plague.

Prevention

Plague vaccines are only usually administered to individuals at high risk in laboratories or field control teams: their efficacy against pneumonic plague is limited and frequent boosting is necessary. A number of new vaccines are being developed. Public education, reducing flea bites and rodent exposure, and avoidance of sick or dead animals are all measures that can help avoid infection.

INFECTIONS DUE TO VIRUSES AND ALLIED ORGANISMS

USE OF THE VIROLOGY LABORATORY BY THE CLINICIAN

VIROLOGY SPECIMEN COLLECTION AND TRANSPORT

When virus infection is suspected, it is important for the pediatrician to take a careful medical history and perform a thorough medical examination of the patient to decide the most likely viral pathogens causing an infection. The possible diagnoses should be discussed with the clinical virologist, so that appropriate specimens are collected and laboratory tests ordered. It is important to collect specimens for viruses as early as possible in the illness after the onset of symptom. Swabs and tissue specimens for viral culture should be placed in viral transport media, i.e. buffered media containing protein and antibiotics. The presence of antibiotics in viral transport media makes these specimens unsuitable for bacterial or fungal cultures. Separate swabs and specimens need to be collected if bacterial or fungal cultures are also required. Liquid samples such as CSF, bronchoalveolar lavage fluid or urine can be sent in clean sterile containers without transport media. Blood for virological tests should be sent in a tube containing an anticoagulant. Both heparin and EDTA are suitable for specimens for viral culture or antigen detection, but citrate should not be used. Heparin should not be used if polymerase chain reaction (PCR) testing of blood is to be performed, as it inhibits the reaction. All specimens for virological testing should be kept cold on ice after collection and during transport. Transport to the laboratory should be prompt and if there is a delay in transport the specimen should be frozen, preferably at $-70\,°C$ rather than $-20\,°C$, as this temperature often reduces virus viability. Most swabs are suitable for collection of specimens, e.g. cotton, Dacron, polyester and rayon, but calcium alginate may inactivate some viruses and inhibit PCR reactions. Swabs should have a metal or plastic shaft, as wood shafts can be toxic to cell cultures.

METHODS OF VIRUS DETECTION

There are five approaches to virus identification:
1. Sending patient material for direct examination by electron microscope.
2. Culturing body fluid or tissue for viruses.
3. Detecting viral antigen in clinical specimens.
4. Using PCR and nucleic acid probes to detect genomic material.
5. Identifying postinfection antiviral antibody by serological methods.

LABORATORY DIAGNOSIS OF VIRAL INFECTION

Respiratory viruses

Historically, cell culture techniques have allowed the detection of a wide range of viral pathogens which cause respiratory infections and also detect dual or mixed infections. However, traditional cell culture techniques are usually slow and often do not provide a diagnosis until the patient is recovering or has been discharged from hospital.

To enhance the clinical utility of viral diagnosis in respiratory infections, most laboratories now use virus specific fluorescent antibodies for direct identification of viruses in cells collected from the respiratory tract via nasopharyngeal aspirates, swabbing or bronchoalveolar lavages. There are now commercially available tools with monoclonal antibodies which are run simultaneously and can detect respiratory syncytial virus (RSV), influenza A, influenza B, parainfluenza viruses 1–3 and the adenovirus group. In addition these antibodies can be used to detect viruses in culture and decrease the culture time from 10–14 days to 3–5 days, thus improving the clinical utility of this test.[414] More recently molecular diagnosis using polymerase reverse transcription and polymerase chain reaction (RT-PCR) has increased the sensitivity of detection, but at a significantly increased cost.[415]

Rapid identification of respiratory viruses is important in health care, because it permits timely and appropriate cohorting (isolation) of patients to prevent nosocomial spread of disease and allows for prompt and appropriate clinical management, i.e. stopping unnecessary antibiotic therapy and commencing specific antiviral therapy for influenza or RSV if indicated.

Childhood exanthems

It is unusual to require laboratory diagnosis of common childhood exanthems such as measles, mumps and rubella and chickenpox, unless there is very severe or atypical disease.[416] Viral culture may be performed in these situations, but serological testing is used more commonly, with detection of IgM being most commonly performed by enzyme linked immunosorbent assay (ELISA) or immunofluorescence (IF) assay.

Enterovirus infection

Enteroviruses, now with more than 101 recognized members, are a common cause of many clinical syndromes including mild febrile illness, upper respiratory tract infections, viral pneumonia, exanthems, enanthems, myocarditis, pericarditis, aseptic meningitis, encephalitis and acute flaccid paralysis. Enterovirus infections are more prevalent in summer and early autumn in temperate climates, but can occur all year round. Enteroviruses are transmitted by the fecal–oral route; they replicate in the gastrointestinal tract, where they rarely cause gastrointestinal symptoms, but can cause diseases in other tissues or organs throughout the body.[417] During the acute illness, enteroviruses are excreted from the oropharynx for several days and continue to be excreted in the feces for several weeks. Most enteroviruses can be grown in tissue culture and usually take 4–8 days to detect. However, more recently PCR detection of enteroviruses has enabled more rapid diagnosis of enterovirus meningitis and encephalitis.

Gastrointestinal infection

Most viruses which cause diarrheal illnesses are not detectable by cell culture. Historically, viral gastrointestinal pathogens have been detected using electron microscopy, which is still used today. More commonly rotavirus, adenovirus or norovirus antigens are detected by immunological methods using ELISA, membrane enzyme immunoassay or latex agglutination. Potentially, PCR technology could be used to detect these viruses, but is not routinely available at present.

Arboviruses

Arboviruses (arthropod-borne viruses) include the alphaviruses and flaviviruses. These viruses are all transmitted by the bite of a hematophagous arthropod which transmits the virus to humans. As these viruses are transmitted by arthropods they occur seasonally, i.e. in the warm weather when arthropods are much more active and also are limited to specific geographic regions consistent with the distribution of the transmitting arthropod. Arboviruses are responsible for a significant amount of viral disease globally, e.g. dengue, yellow fever, Japanese encephalitis and West Nile virus.[418] Arbovirus infections may be asymptomatic. Clinical illnesses include mild febrile illness, acute hepatitis, viral arthritis, rash, hemorrhagic shock and encephalitis. Diagnosis of arbovirus infection is commonly performed by serology, commonly using ELISA technology to detect IgG and IgM antibodies.

Herpesviruses

The herpesviruses are a very large and diverse group of DNA viruses, of which eight have been recognized as the cause of infections in humans. Herpes simplex virus (HSV) types 1 and 2, cytomegalovirus (CMV), and varicella zoster virus (VZV) can be cultured from most sites by conventional cell culture or culture fluorescence. However, human herpes virus 6 (HHV-6), and HHV-7, HHV-8[419] and Epstein–Barr virus (EBV) cannot be cultivated. Diagnosis of central nervous system infections by HSV, CMV or VZV is now commonly done using PCR. Viral culture, while slower, can be performed. HSV and VZV can be detected in scrapings from vesicular skin lesions, using immunofluorescent antibody staining or PCR detection of a cell smear taken from the base of the vesicle. These assays are quite sensitive and specific.

Diagnosis of CMV infection in organ donors or recipients, neonates and pregnant women is usually performed using serology. Detection of IgM antibodies in the absence of IgG antibodies indicates acute infection in neonates and pregnant women while the presence of IgG antibodies indicates past infection in organ donors and recipients. The isolation of CMV from the urine and saliva of neonates in the first week of life is diagnostic of congenital CMV infection.

CMV infection and reactivation can cause significant disease in immunosuppressed patients, such as solid organ recipients, bone marrow transplant recipients, patients receiving chemotherapy and HIV positive patients. Culture for CMV alone is not adequate in these situations, as CMV shedding is quite frequent in immunosuppressed patients without the development of disease. The diagnosis of CMV disease in immunosuppressed patients is achieved by the detection of CMV in a biopsy of the affected organ. Detection of CMV in biopsy tissues can be achieved using histological evidence of CMV inclusions, evidence of CMV antigen, usually detected by immunoperoxidase antibody staining of tissue sections, or detection of CMV by culture or PCR. As tissue biopsies are very invasive, the detection of CMV viral load in blood as a surrogate marker for CMV disease or as an indicator for risk of development of CMV disease has become the standard of care. The usual method for detecting CMV in blood is a CMV antigenemia assay in infected leukocytes, using monoclonal antibody to the CMV late protein, pp65. By using a fluorescent label, CMV-infected cells can be counted using a microscope and the number per high power field determined, giving a relatively quantitative result. These assays can also be used to monitor the efficacy of CMV antiviral therapy in the prevention and treatment of CMV disease. More recently, detection of CMV DNA in blood using a quantitative PCR assay has been used.[420] Qualitative CMV PCR detection is adequate for the diagnosis of CMV retinitis by detection of CMV in aqueous or vitreous humor.

Serological methods are used for the diagnosis of primary EBV infection, whereas molecular methods are used to diagnose EBV-associated lymphoma of the brain and post-transplant lymphoproliferative disease. Diagnosis of acute EBV infection is performed with an EBV viral capsid antigen (VCA) IgM ELISA assay. Past infection of EBV can be determined by detecting IgG antibodies to VCA or Epstein–Barr virus nuclear antigen (EBNA). VCA IgG appears within one week of acute infection while EBNA IgG appears 1–2 months after acute infection. Quantitation of EBV DNA in serum can be used to monitor patients at risk for EBV associated lymphoproliferation; however, currently there are no established threshold levels of EBV DNA which indicate risk of disease.[421] These assays are most useful when run as serial assays to determine increases or decreases in EBV viral load in response to alterations in immunosuppression.

Hepatitis viruses

The hepatitis viruses are a group of unrelated DNA and RNA viruses that cause liver disease as the major clinical manifestation. Diagnosis of these infections is usually with serological techniques. More recently, quantitation of hepatitis B virus DNA and hepatitis C virus RNA has been developed to aid in monitoring antiviral therapeutic responses.

Human immunodeficiency virus infection

Human immunodeficiency virus (HIV) infection in infants greater than 18 months of age is confirmed with a positive HIV antibody test. The diagnosis of vertical HIV infection in an infant less than 18 months is achieved by culture of HIV or detection of HIV DNA in blood. Both these assays have a sensitivity of approximately 80% and are the current 'gold standard'. More recently, detection of HIV RNA (viral load assays) has been used. If using this assay, one has to be careful of the possibility of false positive results. Using these methods, greater than 90% of vertically infected HIV infants will be identified by 6 months of age.

Polyomaviruses

The human polyomaviruses, BK virus and JC virus, infect the majority of the population but remain latent in the kidneys after primary infec-tion. Reactivation can occur when there is T cell immunodeficiency. BK viruria in bone marrow transplant patients is associated with hemorrhagic cystitis. JC virus causes progressive multifocal leukoencephalopathy (PML), seen primarily in AIDS patients.

Detection of BK virus can be achieved by cytologic examination of exfoliated urinary epithelial cells or by PCR detection of BK virus DNA in the urine or blood. JC virus is detected by PCR detection of DNA in CSF.[422] Alternatively, a brain biopsy of a patient suspected of PML may indicate histopathological changes consistent with the diagnosis of PML.

New viruses

More recently, newly discovered respiratory viruses have caused significant illness globally. In 2001, human metapneumovirus was discovered as a cause of bronchiolitis in infants and young children, clinically indistinguishable from that caused by RSV.[423] In 2003, the agent of severe acute respiratory syndrome (SARS), a coronavirus, was associated with a global outbreak of respiratory illness associated with high mortality.[424] There are ongoing concerns regarding pandemic avian influenza virus (H5) which has been spreading around the world both in avian populations and to a much lesser extent in humans since it was first recognized in Hong Kong in 1977. All three of these agents can be identified using molecular technology and PCR assays.

ANTIVIRAL SUSCEPTIBILITY TESTING

Antiviral therapy is now available for the management of many viral infections, including HIV, HSV-1 and 2, CMV, VZV, influenza A and B, RSV, hepatitis B virus and hepatitis C virus. It is anticipated that resistant viruses will invariably occur and increase in prevalence with increased use of antiviral agents. Antiviral resistance is defined as a decrease in susceptibility to an antiviral agent established by in vitro testing and confirmed by genetic analysis of the viral genome and biochemical analysis of the altered enzyme. Clinical failure of antiviral therapy may not always be due to antiviral resistance and consideration must be given to the patient's immunological status, the pharmacokinetic properties of the drug in a given patient, and patient compliance. Antiviral resistance is more likely to occur with long term or recurrent administration of intermittent or suboptimal therapy.

Laboratory assays to detect the viral susceptibility to an agent can be either phenotypic or genotypic assays. Phenotypic assays require growth of the virus in vitro in the presence of the drug and establishment of the concentration of antiviral agent resulting in 50% and 90% inhibition of growth. These assays have not been standardized or correlated with therapeutic success, as they have for antibacterial susceptibility testing, and are not routinely available.

On the other hand, genotypic assays which detect genetic mutations known to confer antiviral resistance are more widely available, especially in the management of HIV infected patients and the selection of anti-HIV therapeutic agents. The major limitation of genotypic assays is that they can only detect resistance caused by known mutations and will not detect new resistance mechanisms.

HIV INFECTION

EPIDEMIOLOGY

The first cases of pediatric acquired immune deficiency syndrome (AIDS) were described in 1982 and the causative agent, HIV, was first isolated in 1983. Since then, a large amount has been learnt about the disease and for resource-rich countries and even increasingly in resource-limited settings, antiretroviral therapies (ART) have had a major impact in reducing morbidity and mortality in HIV infected adults[425] and children,[426] as well as dramatically reducing transmission from mother to child.[427,428] However, the global HIV epidemic has continued, with an estimated 40 million people living with HIV worldwide in 2006 (Fig. 28.28). Whilst the global prevalence (proportion of the population living with HIV) appears to have plateaued, the total number of people

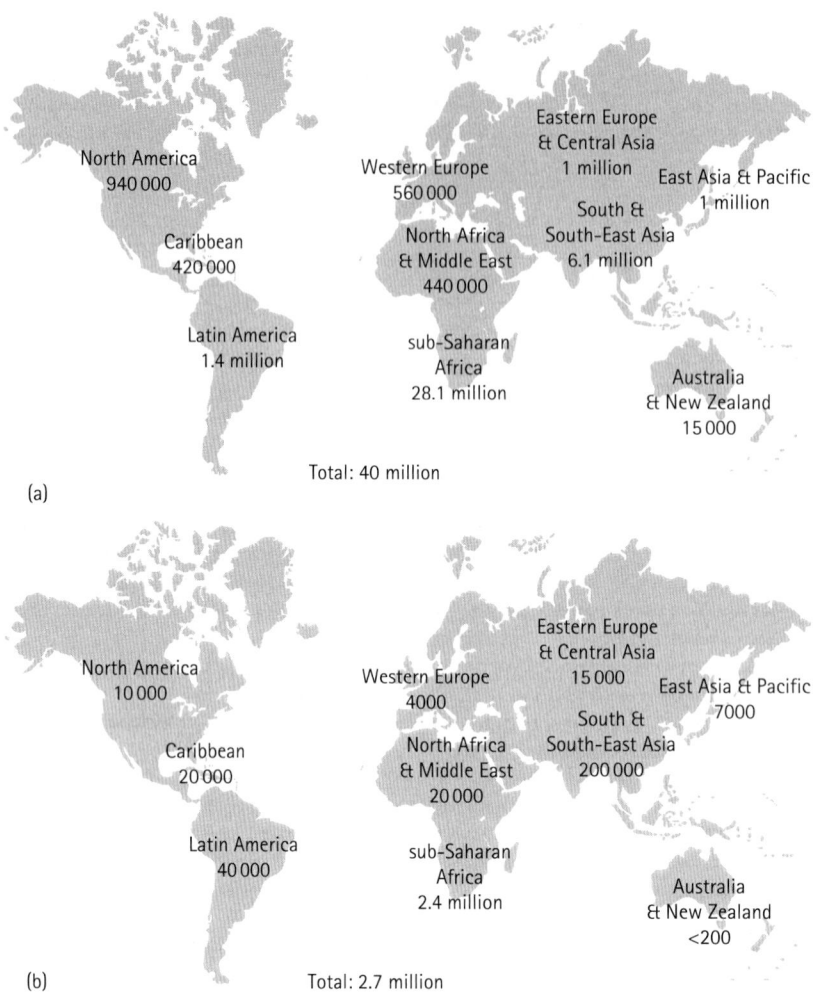

Fig. 28.28   (a) Adults and children estimated to be living with HIV/AIDS as of end 2001. (b) Children (< 15 years) estimated to be living with HIV/AIDS as of end 2001.

infected continues to rise with population growth and prolonged life expectancy from ART. About 95% of people infected with HIV live in resource-limited settings, with Africa continuing to bear the brunt of the epidemic (approximately 65% of global HIV infections), although incidence rates appear to have peaked in several African countries, and may even be falling in some countries (e.g. Kenya). Women are disproportionately affected by HIV, and HIV seroprevalence is over 20% among pregnant women in many sub-Saharan African countries. Because over 95% of pediatric infections are acquired from mother to child, this has major implications for HIV infection in children. In Africa, where almost 90% of the world's infected children live, HIV has reversed gains in child survival and has lowered life expectancy. In addition, large numbers of children have been orphaned. By the end of 2006, UNAIDS estimated that there were over 12 million children under 18 years of age in Africa who had lost their mother or both parents to AIDS,[429] placing enormous strains on communities already devastated by the social and economic impact of so many young adults prematurely dying.

The global HIV epidemic continues to grow outside Africa. Over half of the world's population lives in the Asia/Pacific region and in 2006 an estimated 8.3 million people were infected with HIV. Two thirds live in India, which now has the largest number of HIV infected persons of any single country.[429] Seroprevalence rates in pregnant women are over 1% in many states. The epidemic in Eastern Europe and Central Asia has seen a twenty-fold increase in the number of people living with HIV in under a decade; estimated at 1.5 million in 2006, the majority live in the Russian Federation and the Ukraine, where adult prevalence rates are above 1%. While intravenous drug use is a major risk factor, increasing reports of new sexually transmitted infections suggest HIV is spreading into the general population.[429] Increasing availability of surveillance data from China provides estimates that at least 650000 people are living with HIV, with highest prevalence rates seen in injecting drug users and sex workers.

Even in Western countries, prevention efforts appear to be stalling. Available information indicates that the number of newly infected people is no lower in 2006 compared with previous years, with 720000 adults and children estimated to have acquired HIV in Western and Central Europe and 1.2 million in North America.[429] Overall HIV prevalence has risen in both regions, because ART is resulting in HIV infected individuals living longer, and also likely as a result of more people coming forward for testing (including in particular, pregnant women). Thousands of infections are still occurring through unsafe sex between men, where complacency may be attributed to the fact that in the age of ART, HIV is seen as a treatable if not curable disease. However, it is also true that transmission rates of HIV are likely to be lower from persons on highly active ART (HAART) who will have lower plasma concentrations of the virus.[430] In the USA, there remain an estimated 25% of persons with HIV who have not been diagnosed, this proportion being higher in black African populations where HIV is now the leading cause of death in African American women aged between 25 and 34 years.[429] The proportion of persons with undiagnosed HIV is higher (around one third) in the UK. These persons are more likely to transmit HIV to their sexual partners as they are less likely to use barrier contraception and are not on HAART and therefore have higher levels of plasma viremia.

It is estimated that around 43% of transmission occurs around the time of seroconversion and thus generally before the infected person knows he or she has HIV infection.

By the end of 2006 there were an estimated 2.3 million children < 15 years old living with HIV infection worldwide, of whom 540 000 were newly infected and 360 000 died during 2006 alone; 87% live in sub-Saharan Africa.[429] Although contributing less than 1% of children infected with HIV worldwide, there are currently around 11 000 children living with HIV in North America and about 4000 in Western and central Europe, of whom over 1100 live in the UK and Ireland (www.chipscohort.org).[429] With dramatic decreases in transmission rates from mother to child in resource rich countries, new pediatric infections amongst babies usually occur only in countries where antenatal screening is not comprehensive and/or interventions to reduce mother-to-child transmission (MTCT) are not widely offered. Recent cases of MTCT in UK have been reported in infants of women with a negative HIV antibody test in early pregnancy who subsequently seroconvert during pregnancy or breast-feeding.[431] It is not surprising that pediatric infections in many countries of the north are increasingly in migrants from countries with a high prevalence of HIV infection. In the UK, over 75% of seropositive newborns are delivered to mothers born in sub-Saharan Africa, and whereas prior to 2000 approximately one third of HIV infected children were themselves born overseas, this proportion increased to around two thirds after 2003.[432] Similar patterns are being observed in many countries in Europe.[433]

Romania has the largest number of HIV infected children in Europe.[429] The majority belong to a cohort of children who were uniquely infected with HIV through contaminated blood products and needles in the late 1980s. Although many have died, there remain a considerable number of these children who are now teenagers in Romania. Maternal seroprevalence in Romania is about 0.3% in cities such as Costansa, on the Black Sea.

Surveillance for pediatric HIV infection

Unlinked anonymous monitoring of HIV through testing dried blood spots (Guthrie cards) collected on all newborns in many countries for metabolic screening, or antenatal bloods, can provide an unbiased estimate of the prevalence of HIV infection among women having live babies. This is a useful method of providing information about the extent of heterosexually acquired HIV infection in a population, particularly if monitoring is undertaken longitudinally. This might be done continuously or, if resources are scarce, it can be done intermittently (e.g. for 3 months each year). It is possible, while preserving full anonymity, to retain demographic information (e.g. mother's country of birth) which can then determine HIV seroprevalence among particular groups within a community as was done in North London, showing low HIV prevalence among women coming from Asian communities in

1998.[434] Data from anonymous serosurveys have also been combined with non-named confidential register data on HIV in pregnancy in order to provide an indication of the proportion of pregnancies being identified before or during pregnancy.[435] This can be a useful way to audit antenatal testing policy and provide local feedback to care providers (see below).

HIV antibody testing of Guthrie cards is being undertaken in the UK and covers approximately 70% of live births. In 2004, the HIV antenatal seroprevalence was 0.44% in Greater London and 0.11% in the rest of England, but women of sub-Saharan origin had a rate of 2.2%, over 30 times the rate of 0.07% in women born in the UK[436] (Fig. 28.29). Maternal seroprevalence rates in England and Scotland have risen from 0.16% in 2000 to 0.27% in 2004,[436] and this rise may in part reflect an increasing desire for HIV infected women on HAART and clinically well to have children, in the knowledge that the risk of MTCT with appropriate intervention is very low. In London in 2004, three quarters of seropositive newborns were delivered to mothers born in sub-Saharan Africa, and similar patterns are being observed in European countries such as France and Belgium. In Scotland, Ireland and southern Europe a higher proportion of seropositive children are still born to women with injecting drug use (IDU) as a risk factor, but here too the proportion of women acquiring HIV from heterosexual transmission is increasing.

Of 1441 children reported to the National Study of HIV in Pregnancy and Childhood (NSHPC) by June 2006, over 1300 are currently known to be living with HIV in the UK and Ireland. Over two thirds reside in London and were born to women who acquired HIV in sub-Saharan Africa. With dispersal of refugees to other cities in the UK, this is changing. Similarly, whereas the majority of HIV infected children in Scotland and Ireland are still white children born to mothers with IDU as a risk factor for acquiring HIV, this is changing and increasing numbers of mothers of more recently diagnosed HIV infected children acquired the disease through heterosexual contact, often abroad. Follow-up of infected children is being coordinated, along with follow-up of children in Europe participating in clinical trials [Paediatric European Network for Treatment of AIDS (PENTA)], through the Collaborative HIV in Paediatric Study (CHIPS) cohort which has over 1100 children in follow-up from over 40 centers and is coordinated through the MRC Clinical Trials Unit in London in collaboration with the Institute of Child Health (ICH) (www.chipscohort.ac.uk, www.pentatrials.org).[432]

With the advent of HAART, children with HIV are living longer and the average age of the cohort of infected children in the UK and Ireland is now around 8.5 years, with 12% being 15 years of age or older, and over 100 having transferred to adult clinics.[432] As children with HIV survive into adolescence they face many similar issues to other young people with chronic disease such as delayed growth, development and puberty and adherence to and the long term side-effects of drug therapy. However, these young people have the additional issues

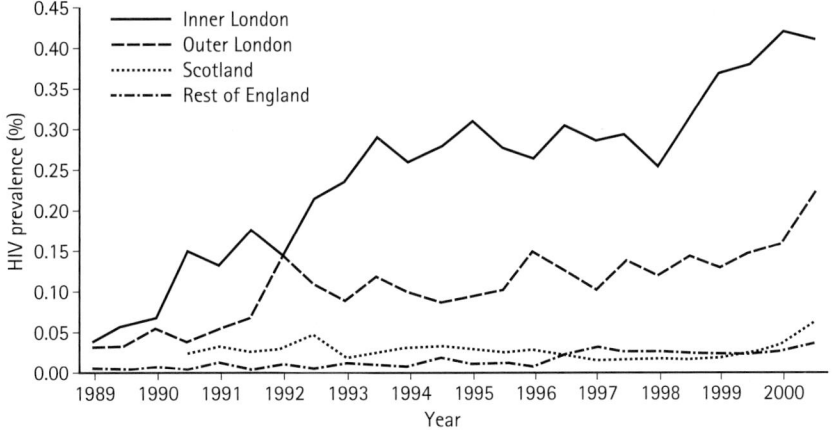

Fig. 28.29 Trends in prevalence of HIV infection in pregnant women by area of residence: 1989–2000.

of negotiating adolescence with a stigmatizing sexually transmissible disease. Many will also have lost a parent or will have to care for a sick family member. The complex medical, psychological and social needs of these young people require multidisciplinary team involvement with close liaison with adult colleagues when transitioning young people to adult services.[437]

MOTHER-TO-CHILD TRANSMISSION OF HIV

Mother-to-child transmission (MTCT) of HIV can occur during pregnancy, labor or breast-feeding.[438] In the absence of breast-feeding, approximately two thirds of transmission occurs around the time of delivery. In Europe and the USA, the rate of MTCT in the absence of breast-feeding prior to the advent of interventions was around 15–20%, compared with around 30–40% in Africa. Most of this difference is due to breast-feeding, which accounts for about one third of transmission in Africa.[439] Factors independently affecting the rate of transmission include the mother's clinical status, HIV viral load and CD4 cell count, particularly at the time of delivery, prematurity, factors around delivery such as duration of rupture of membranes and mode of delivery[438,440] (Table 28.31).

In the last 10 years, rates of MTCT in resource rich countries have fallen dramatically to 2% or less with strategies including use of antiretroviral therapy, elective Cesarean section (CS) and refraining from breast-feeding.[427,441] Unfortunately in most resource limited settings, despite increased availability of at least some interventions to reduce MTCT, only about 10% of women are diagnosed in pregnancy and therefore have access to such interventions.[429]

Antiretroviral therapy to reduce MTCT

In 1995, the first placebo-controlled trial (the ACTG 076 trial) of zidovudine (ZDV) monotherapy, given to the mother antenatally from a median of 26 weeks by continuous intravenous infusion during labor, and then orally to the infant from birth for 6 weeks, resulted in a 67% reduction in MTCT in non-breast-feeding US and French HIV infected women compared with placebo.[442] This trial was followed by non-randomized studies to document the effect of ZDV monotherapy on MTCT in the clinical setting[427,441,443] and of non-randomized studies of double[444] and triple antiretroviral therapy. The results showed that ZDV was highly effective in reducing MTCT and, compared with historical controls, the use of double therapy was superior to monotherapy.[444] With triple therapy, MTCT rates below 1% are achievable among women with undetectable HIV viral load at delivery.[445] Cohort studies have documented reductions in MTCT over calendar time with increasing use of triple HAART in pregnancy (Fig. 28.30).[428]

The importance of low maternal plasma HIV viral load around the time of delivery in reducing the risk of MTCT has been demonstrated in subsequent trials.[446] However, it is not the only important factor and it is clear that ART reduces MTCT both by decreasing maternal viral load and by providing pre- and post-exposure prophylaxis to the infant. In an individual patient meta-analysis of women with low HIV RNA of < 10 000 copies/ml, the transmission rate was reduced from 10% to

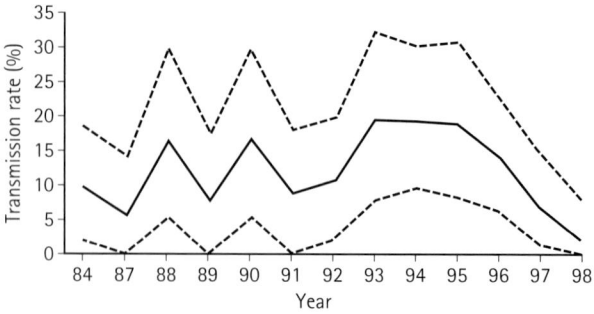

Fig. 28.30 Estimated vertical transmission rate (95% CI) in UK over time in non-breast-feeding women.
(From Duong et al 1999[428])

only 1% by the use of ZDV alone, which has only a minimal effect on maternal viral load (reduction by only about 0.3 log copies/ml).[447] This suggests that post-exposure prophylaxis to the fetus is also important, a factor borne out by the large impact on transmission of giving long acting nevirapine (NVP) to women during labor and to the baby.[448] Even if a woman has not received ART during pregnancy or delivery, ART given to the baby as soon as possible after birth is likely to have an effect on transmission. Guidelines for giving ART to pregnant women to reduce MTCT are available and are regularly updated.[449,450]

Trials have been conducted comparing different components of the ACTG 076 regimen and also evaluating other antiretroviral drugs. Most have taken place in resource-limited settings where an important goal was also to refine, simplify and reduce the costs of the initial ZDV regimen used in the ACTG 076 trial. A trial of ZDV monotherapy in non-breast-feeding women in Thailand showed that a 50% reduction of MTCT was possible by giving ZDV from 36 weeks' gestation, oral ZDV during labor and for 2 weeks to the baby.[451] However, another trial from Thailand emphasized that starting ART at 28 weeks added benefit compared with starting at 36 weeks,[452] suggesting that some in utero transmission may be prevented by ART. It is also true that if starting ART is left until 36 weeks, some women will go into premature labor having received minimal or no pre-labor ART.

Intrapartum ART alone does not appear to be useful[453] if given without postpartum prophylaxis to the baby. In HIVNET 012 undertaken in Uganda, a single 200 mg oral dose of NVP, given to the mother in labor, followed by a single oral dose of 2 mg/kg to the infant at 48 h (total cost US$4), led to a 40% reduction in MTCT at 16 weeks compared with intrapartum and neonatal (for 1 week) oral ZDV.[448] Follow-up to 18 months has shown continued efficacy of around 40% despite breast-feeding for an average of 9 months. However, probably due to its long plasma half-life,[454] nevirapine resistance rates of up to 75% in mothers and 46% in infants after single dose exposure have been reported.[455,456] As ART becomes increasingly available worldwide the therapeutic implications of NVP resistance for mothers and infants infected despite NVP are of increasing concern.[457,458] Methods to reduce rates of nevirapine resistance include the use of short course combination therapy to protect the nevirapine 'tail'. In the Treatment Option Study (TOPS) significantly reduced rates of NVP resistance were seen in women who received either 4 or 7 days of Combivir with single dose nevirapine (SD-NVP) when compared to women who received SD-NVP alone.[459,460] In a study from Malawi, infants who received SD-NVP plus AZT had lower rates of NVP resistance at 6–8 weeks of age than infants who received SD-NVP or mothers who had peripartum SD-NVP alone. Similar rates of MTCT were seen in all groups.[461] For those women who develop NVP resistance there are some data suggesting that these mutations fade over time. Women who had received peripartum SD-NVP had higher rates of virological failure when commencing subsequent NVP-based HAART than women who had received a placebo but only if they started HAART within 6 months of delivery.[462] Whether archived NVP mutations will continue to impact on the longer term response to subsequent

Table 28.31 Factors associated with mother-to-child transmission (MTCT) of HIV

- Without interventions, the rate of MTCT was 15–20% in Europe, and 25–40% in Africa
- Most MTCT occurs around the time of delivery
- Increased risk is associated with:
  - late stage maternal disease
  - high maternal plasma viremia
  - prolonged rupture of membranes
  - invasive obstetric procedures
  - prematurity
  - breast-feeding

NNRTI-based regimens requires further follow-up. The balance between preventing transmission of HIV to infants whilst minimizing impact on maternal health and future HAART options is a complex issue requiring continuing research, during which time NVP continues to have a role in the prevention of MTCT in resource poor settings.

Reducing MTCT in well resourced settings

Whilst randomized controlled trials of HAART are lacking, in a European cohort HAART was associated with a fall in transmission from 11.5% to 1.2%, with a greater reduction (0.25% versus 1.92% respectively) if started prior to pregnancy compared to during pregnancy.[463] Prior to 2004, women commencing HAART in pregnancy would typically receive NVP with two nucleoside reverse transcriptase inhibitors (NRTIs), often ZDV and 3TC. Following reports of fatal fulminant hepatitis in pregnant women with good CD4 counts receiving NVP-based HAART, nevirapine is no longer recommended for pregnant women with good CD4 counts (> 250 cell/uL) who are taking ART for the prevention of MTCT. Alternate regimens based on a protease inhibitor are used. NVP monotherapy is not recommended because of concerns about the development of resistance to all non-nucleoside reverse transcriptase inhibitor (NNRTI) drugs.

Problems with ART to reduce MTCT

Maternal pre-eclampsia and premature labor

Advances in the development of pharmaceutical interventions to reduce HIV MTCT are not without complications. Analysis of a Spanish cohort of HIV positive women delivering between 1985 and 2003 showed a marked reduction in MTCT but an increased risk of fetal death or pre-eclampsia with any form of HAART taken pre-pregnancy.[464] A European study found an increased risk of prematurity associated with combination therapy commenced before the pregnancy (OR 2.6, 95% CI 1.43–4.75),[465] but a US cohort reported similar rates of prematurity of 17% but no significant difference between mothers who had received ART and those who had not.[466] It is speculated that immune reconstitution due to ART may play a part in adverse pregnancy outcome.

Neonatal toxicity

In a French study of ZDV + 3TC, concerns were first raised about a possible link between mitochondrial dysfunction in HIV uninfected children and perinatal exposure to NRTIs.[467] This complication is also known to occur rarely in HIV infected individuals taking NRTIs. Retrospective analysis of other large cohort data failed to reveal other definitive cases.[468] Neonatal anemia, and neutropenia have been reported in uninfected infants perinatally exposed to NRTIs, but they rarely require transfusion and respond to discontinuing the NRTIs, although a small negative effect on hematopoiesis has been seen up to 18 months of age.[469] Although concerns about the potential carcinogenicity and reproductive effects of ART as well as mitochondrial toxicity remain, current evidence suggests that the benefit of ART in dramatically reducing MTCT far outweighs potential harm. Many countries are now setting up long term surveillance to follow all children born to HIV infected mothers, whether exposed or not to ARTs in utero. In the UK, the CHART study, the National Study of HIV in Pregnancy conducted at the ICH, assesses the long term health and development of ART-exposed children.

Effect of mode of delivery on MTCT

Several cohort studies have shown that factors around delivery contribute importantly to MTCT. In a meta-analysis of 15 large studies, including more than 5000 mother–child pairs from the USA and Europe, it was estimated that each hour longer in labor with ruptured membranes was associated with a 2% increase in the risk of MTCT.[470] A meta-analysis of these studies, a randomized European trial, and a European controlled trial, showed that among more than 8000 women the risk of transmission was 50% lower for babies delivered by elective CS prior to membrane rupture, compared with vaginal or emergency CS delivery.[471,472] Subsequent cohorts have shown that reduction of MTCT to around 2% is possible with ZDV, elective CS delivery and with not breast-feeding.[428,442] The question of how much additional reduction to transmission may occur if elective CS delivery is undertaken in women on HAART with undetectable HIV RNA viral load around the time of delivery is unclear[473] and is unlikely to be answered from controlled trials. However, as the risk is very low, most guidelines suggest that the women can undergo a normal vaginal delivery in this situation, but that membranes should not be ruptured prematurely, and invasive interventions during labor or delivery (e.g. use of scalp electrodes and instrumental delivery) should be avoided.[449,450] Increasingly, women on HAART with undetectable plasma viral loads are choosing vaginal delivery. This may be of particular importance for women returning to areas of the world where elective CS is not readily available for subsequent pregnancies.

Breast-feeding

HIV can be transmitted through breast milk.[474,475] Most transmission appears to occur early, and factors including HIV viral content in colostrum, immaturity of the infant gastrointestinal tract in the neonatal period, and the contribution of breast and nipple complications (e.g. mastitis and bleeding nipples which may increase the amount of virus in breast milk) all play a role. Breast milk transmission continues, however, throughout the duration of breast-feeding, posing extremely difficult dilemmas for policy in parts of the world where alternatives to breast-feeding are expensive, unsafe and culturally unacceptable, but where HIV prevalence is high.[476]

The current recommendation is that infants should continue to be breast-fed where infectious diseases and malnutrition are the main cause of infant mortality, because artificial feeding substantially increases the risk of illness and death.[476] Evidence suggests that mixed feeding is associated with a higher risk of transmission and therefore it has been recommended that women in these areas exclusively breast-feed for 4–6 months (which is anyway advocated for all women) and then wean as quickly as possible. After this time, the benefits of breast-feeding may be outweighed by the risk of HIV infection.[477] This strategy is likely to be more feasible than exclusive formula feeding, which in many settings is likely to increase infant mortality from other infections, to be socially unacceptable and unaffordable and risk a 'spill-over effect' on non-HIV infected mothers. Where infants of HIV infected mothers can be ensured uninterrupted access to nutritionally adequate, safely prepared breast milk substitutes, they are at less risk of illness and death from non-HIV related illness and their mothers should be encouraged not to breast-feed. Hopefully, larger prospective studies will help clarify the effects of exclusive breast-feeding followed by early weaning after short course anti-retroviral therapy on HIV transmission rates, and the morbidity and mortality of HIV infected and uninfected babies. The risk of transmission through breast-feeding in mothers with an undetectable plasma viral load on suppressive HAART is being assessed in studies in Africa.[478]

Other interventions to reduce MTCT

Other interventions that have been explored to reduce MTCT include trials of cleansing the birth canal and vitamin A supplementation during pregnancy. The rationale for the former is that the maximum risk of exposure appears to be around the time of delivery and, therefore, cleaning with chlorhexidine might reduce vertical transmission. However, clinical trials have failed to show significant reduction of MTCT with this approach.[479]

Observational studies suggested that low vitamin A levels were associated with increased MTCT.[480] Randomized trials have, however, failed to show a significant impact of supplementation with vitamin A on prevention of MTCT.[481]

ANTENATAL TESTING

In resource rich countries

The case for offering antenatal HIV testing is overwhelming. A recommendation that HIV testing should be offered to all women in pregnancy has been successfully implemented in most well resourced countries. In the UK, the universal offer of HIV testing during the antenatal period was endorsed in 1999 after an economic analysis showed that a universal offer policy was cost effective throughout the UK provided that a high uptake of testing was achieved.[482]

Statistical analysis of unlinked anonymous seroprevalence data with reported infections suggests that in 2004, 90% of infected women living in the UK were diagnosed prior to delivery and were therefore able to take up interventions to reduce MTCT. In most European countries and in the USA, a marked decrease in infected babies reflects the high proportion of pregnant women receiving appropriate care to reduce MTCT. However, a few infants continue to present with severe *Pneumocystis jiroveci*, previously called *P. carinii* pneumonia (PCP), and cytomegalovirus (CMV) infection[483] as a result of perinatal transmission of HIV from mothers who are unaware of their own HIV infection or from mothers who have seroconverted in pregnancy or during breast-feeding.[431] Discussions are underway in the UK to determine whether a second HIV antibody test in the later stages of pregnancy would be feasible and cost effective in further reducing the risk of MTCT.

In resource limited countries

In low income countries, ART to prevent MTCT is only one strand of a much more complex mesh of issues surrounding the prevention of vertical transmission.[484] With the available tools and knowledge that we have already, there is a strong argument for putting resources into providing antenatal diagnosis and the appropriate perinatal interventions. This undoubtedly requires a huge input of resources into the development of sustainable infrastructures in situations where antenatal care may currently be rudimentary.

Understandably, concerns have been raised that, rather than putting scarce resources into a 'magic bullet' of ART to pregnant women, efforts should be concentrated on the more difficult issue of preventing women getting infected in the first place. In sub-Saharan Africa pilot projects offering antenatal screening and intervention have been established since 2001, but the scaling up of these services has been disappointing, with less than 10% of infected pregnant women in sub-Saharan Africa offered intervention to prevent MTCT in 2006.[429] Preventing HIV infection in women will require both behavioral and biomedical interventions such as microbicides, several of which are currently being evaluated in phase III trials.

ETIOLOGY AND PATHOGENESIS

HIV is a retrovirus. Transmission occurs through sexual intercourse, via infected blood and blood products and by transmission from mother to child. Many of the clinical features of HIV can be ascribed to profound immune suppression, because HIV infects cells of the immune system and ultimately destroys them. An understanding of the way it does this is helpful in interpreting tests used in monitoring the disease and helps explain the difficulties in developing a vaccine for HIV.

The virus predominantly infects a subset of the thymus-derived lymphocytes carrying the surface molecule CD4, which binds the glycoprotein on the envelope of HIV called gp120. CD4 is also present on many monocytes and macrophages and on Langerhans' cells of the skin and dendritic cells of many other tissues. HIV also requires co-receptors to enter cells. Two of these, termed CCR5 and CXCR4, are of particular importance. These co-receptors are members of a family of receptors, expressed on the cells of lymphocytes, dendritic cells and cells of the rectal, vaginal and cervical mucosa, that function as receptors for chemokines that orchestrate the migration and differentiation of leukocytes during immune responses. Virus strains able to infect primary macrophages (R5 tropic viruses) use CCR5 as a co-receptor and these are detected early in infection, suggesting they are important for transmission. Further evidence for this comes from studies showing that individuals homozygous for a 32 pair deletion of CCR5 show increased resistance to being infected by HIV.[485,486] Both R5 and strains infecting T cells use CXCR4 as a co-receptor (T or X4 viruses) and they arise during the course of infection.

CD8 cytotoxic lymphocytes (CTL) capable of killing HIV infected targets develop early in primary HIV infection and are very important in the initial control of viremia.[487,488] Among CD8 cells, rapid expansion of strong T cell responses to multiple viral epitopes has been shown to be associated with better control of viremia following primary infection in adults. CD8 T cells kill infected cells and produce CD8 T cell antiviral factor (CAF) which inhibits viral replication. The breadth and strength of the CTL responses are determined by the degree of CD4 specific helper response, which may be determined by the level of HIV viremia and by genetic host factors. In adults who fail to control viral load, CTL responses are narrower and less marked. Because HIV replication is very rapid and errors occur in reverse transcription, these mutants can evade CTL response (escape mutants), i.e. the viral epitope mutates to 'escape' control by the CTL. Children surviving with perinatally acquired HIV have been shown to have more robust HIV-1-specific CD8 responses than was previously thought, comparable in magnitude and breadth to those of adults[489] and, as in adult studies, infants and children with unsuppressed viral loads had poorer CTL responses.[490]

In infants in whom the immune system is immature, the viral load rises over the first weeks after primary infection around the time of birth, and stays high throughout infancy. It then falls in the absence of therapy over the next 3–5 years (Fig. 28.31)[491,492] to reach a 'set point' which is much later after primary infection than in adults (set point at about 6 months). Unlike adults, infants have a highly active thymus which may 'work' to replenish CD4 cells destroyed by the virus. While this may appear to be advantageous, recent work has suggested these new thymic cells may quickly become infected with HIV and possibly delay reduction in HIV viremia in children on ART.[493]

As viremia starts to decline in adults, HIV antibody production increases. Detection of HIV antibodies is the principal way of making the diagnosis in adults and older children, as antibodies persist usually until death.

Polyclonal activation of B cells also occurs, resulting in high immunoglobulin levels in most children commencing during infancy, although infants with rapid disease progression may rarely be hypogammaglobulinemic. This polyclonal increase in immunoglobulin is in many cases nonfunctional, while antigen-specific antibody production is reduced, resulting in increased susceptibility to bacterial infections.

There are reports of both adults and children being exposed to HIV and remaining uninfected; these individuals have detectable HIV-specific CTL. In addition, individuals with strong CTL responses may have delayed disease progression (long term nonprogressors); the latter has also been associated with certain HLA type 1 alleles.[494]

The CD4 cell plays a central role in orchestrating the immune system, and their destruction by HIV accounts for much of the immunosuppressive

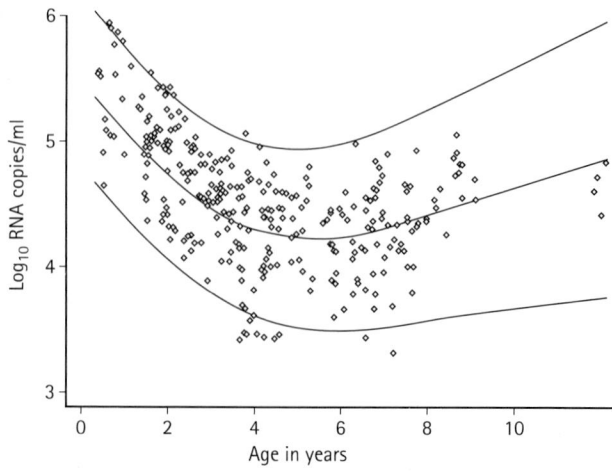

Fig. 28.31 Log_{10} HIV-1 RNA plotted against age in untreated HIV infected children (fitted line and 95% CI). (From Gibb et al 1998[492])

effect of the virus. Following fusion into CD4 and other cells, viral core material enters the host cell and the genetic material encoded in RNA is converted to DNA by reverse transcriptase. This DNA 'provirus' is then integrated into the host genome. HIV replicates at an enormous rate with > 10[6] particles being produced daily.[495] In addition, turnover of infected replicating CD4 cells is high, occurring approximately every 1.5 days. CD4 damage occurs both directly and through mechanisms resulting in apoptosis of infected cells. The exact role of both mechanisms is still debated. HIV in resting memory and long-lived cells both in the immune system and in other tissues remains latent for long periods of time and is largely responsible for persistence of the virus despite the ability of HAART to decrease virus to undetectable levels in plasma. In 1996, with the advent of HAART, there was great hope that the half-life of long-lived cells might be in the order of only a few years and that HIV eradication might be possible. Sadly this is not the case, and modeling exercises estimate the half-life of these long-lived infected cells to be around 70 years.[496] If HAART is stopped, even after plasma viral load has been undetectable for several years, HIV viral load rises again within 1–2 weeks, typically returning to the 'set point' seen prior to initiation of HAART. The virus also has a remarkable ability to mutate and develop resistance to antiretroviral drugs, as seen following single dose nevirapine exposure (see above). Mutant virus may remain in latent cells for many years but re-emerge if that drug is re-started in an individual.

Monitoring with CD4 and HIV RNA viral load

The most widely used markers for predicting disease progression in children, as in adults, are the CD4 cell count (or percentage) and viral load as measured by HIV-1 RNA in plasma.

Absolute CD4 counts are higher in young children than in adults and there is great within- and between-individual variability. CD4 percentages vary less with age, although they are still higher at very young ages as can be seen from percentile charts constructed from uninfected children born to HIV positive mothers (Fig. 28.32).[497] By around 4–5 years of age, the CD4 cell count number and range has fallen to nearer adult values. In children with HIV infection, as in adults, absolute lymphocyte counts and CD4 cell counts decrease with progression of the disease. Analyses of combined individual longitudinal data in untreated children prior to the advent of ART (HIV Paediatric Prognostic Markers Collaborative Study) have provided guidance for thresholds of CD4%, CD4 count and total lymphocyte counts (TLC) associated with a marked increase in disease progression at different ages.[498–500] These have formed the basis for new WHO guidelines[501]; clinicians can use a risk calculator (available on http://www.hppmcs.org/) to estimate risk of progression in an untreated child according to age and CD4% count or TLC level. Most pediatricians use CD4% up until the age of around 5 years when increasing account should be taken of the total CD4 count. Of particular note, in very young children, no marker is very good at predicting

disease progression. Whereas, in adults, a CD4 cell count below 200 cells/mm[3] is a useful predictor of risk of developing *Pneumocystis carinii* (*P. jiroveci*) pneumonia (PCP) and is therefore used to determine the time to start prophylaxis against this disease, during infancy even CD4 percentage is of limited predictive value.[502] After infancy, a CD4% greater than 25% is considered evidence of minimal immunosuppression, 15–25% moderate, and < 15% severe immunosuppression and these form the basis of the Centers for Disease Control (CDC) immunological classification of HIV in children.[503,504] The Revised WHO Clinical Staging and Immunological Classification of HIV/AIDS (2006) incorporates age-related immune classification from infancy through to adulthood.[501] Importantly, for the individual child the rate of fall of CD4% and at older ages of CD4 cell counts are of importance and should be taken into account when making decisions about when to start antiretroviral therapy. Further analyses of HPPMCS data are ongoing to try to define this more accurately.

Viral load as measured by plasma HIV RNA is an independent predictor of HIV progression in adults after the 'set point' has been reached. Several different assays are available in kit form with quality control (Roche, Chiron and NASBA). The Roche PCR version 1.5 and Chiron assays are widely used and include additional primers to ensure accuracy when measuring viral load in persons with different subtypes of HIV (e.g. subtype B is the most common virus subtype in white North Americans and Europeans but subtypes A, C and D are common in Africans). It is important to be aware that assay variability may be as high as 0.7 log and that results need to be interpreted on a log scale. Repeating results is advisable if treatment decisions are being taken based on viral load results; in general viral load is less predictive of disease progression than CD4% or count and used less to make decisions about starting therapy.[498] All assays are less precise at values above 750 000 copies/ml but all assays are more robust at low levels down to a cut-off of 50 copies/ml. In infants, HIV RNA is very high after infection around the time of birth and remains much higher (often 1 million copies/ml or more) than observed in adults for the first 2 years of life, gradually reducing by an average of about one log over the first 5 years of life in the absence of antiretroviral therapy (Fig. 28.33).[492,495]

LABORATORY DIAGNOSIS OF HIV

Enzyme linked immunosorbent assays (ELISA) for measuring HIV antibody are highly sensitive and specific for diagnosing HIV in adults and in children over 18 months of age. However, because of transplacental transfer of maternal antibody, all babies born to HIV infected women will have antibodies at birth which take a median of 10 months and a maximum of 18 months to clear. Other techniques, directed at viral components rather than the host immune response, are therefore required to diagnose HIV in young infants.

In Western countries, early diagnosis of HIV in infants has been improved significantly by polymerase chain reaction (PCR) techniques for detecting proviral DNA and RNA. Using these techniques, HIV infection can be definitively diagnosed in about 90% of infected infants by age 1 month and in virtually all by 3 months. HIV proviral DNA PCR is the preferred method for initial diagnosis. In a meta-analysis, 38% (90% CI = 29–46%) of infected children had positive PCR DNA tests by age 48 h, rapidly increasing in the second week with 93% of infected children (90% CI = 76–97%) testing positive by 2 weeks of age.[505]

HIV RNA tests may be more sensitive than DNA PCR for diagnosis, but limited data suggest lower specificity, immediately after birth. However, they may be alternatives if proviral DNA tests are not available and give additional information about the degree of viremia. Culture of HIV is time consuming and expensive and is no longer routinely undertaken. The detection of p24 antigen, both standard and immune-complex dissociated, although highly specific, is not as sensitive as DNA PCR. Nevertheless, detection of acid or heat dissociated p24 antigen by ELISA is considerably cheaper than PCR tests and is also technically less demanding, making it more promising as a diagnostic tool for resource limited settings; it is highly specific but less sensitive than proviral DNA.

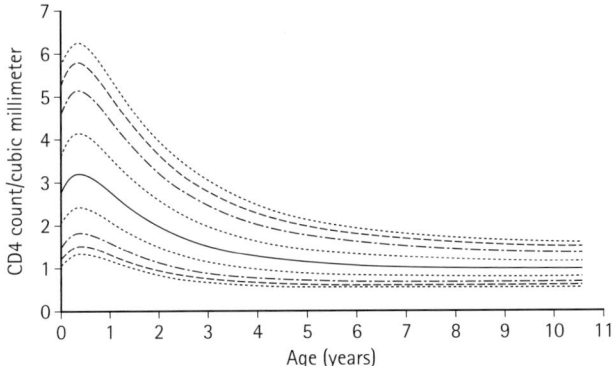

Fig. 28.32 CD4 lymphocyte counts in uninfected children by age: 3rd, 5th, 10th, 25th, 50th, 75th, 90th, 95th and 97th centiles. Created from data collected by the European Collaborative Study using the methods of Wade & Ades (1994).[497]

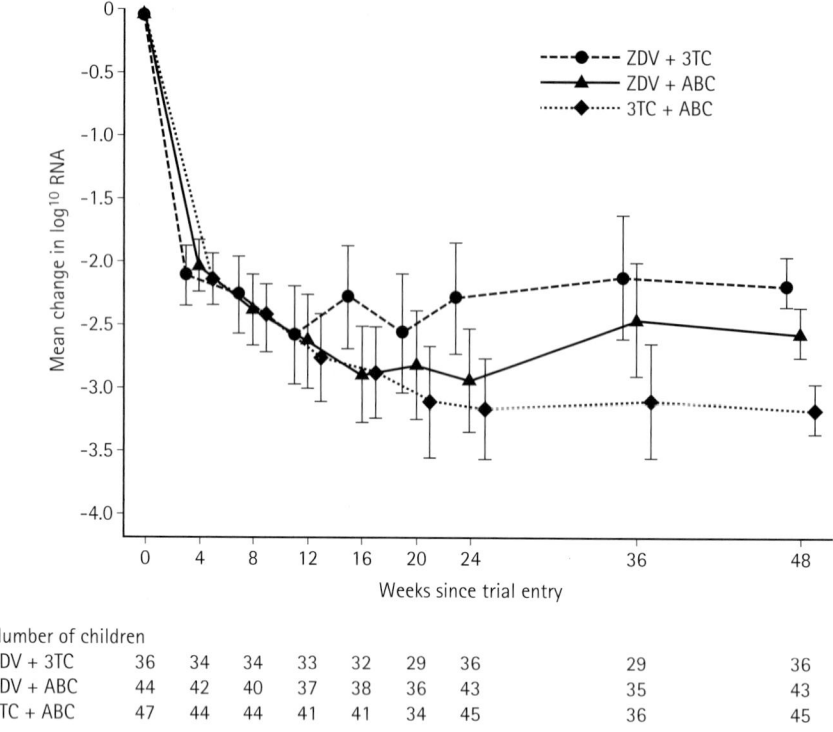

Fig. 28.33   Change in log[10] RNA after starting ART in the PENTA 5 trial. (From PENTA 2002[535])

Another laboratory clue that a child may have HIV infection is the presence of polyclonal hypergammaglobulinemia, which in the presence of CD4 lymphopenia should lead to a high suspicion of HIV infection.

In the last 5 years, there has been increased focus on developing cheaper ways of detecting early infection in infants. Although still outside the reach of most countries' budgets, early diagnosis using DNA PCR techniques is now available in many parts of South Africa and is being introduced into countries such as Uganda. Updated WHO guidelines recommend that treatment of symptomatic infants can start in the absence of a definitive diagnosis.[501] Early detection of infection among babies born to mothers who have received PMTCT is more problematic because, with reduced transmission rates, many babies have to be tested to detect a single infected baby. The issues of testing during breast-feeding also require attention; the WHO recommends that testing might be focused around timing of immunizations, and in women who wean at 6 months according to guidelines, after cessation of breast-feeding.[501] Debate continues about the best time to test if only one test per infant is available. However, unless it is undertaken early, it is clear that infected babies will die before there is time for diagnosis to occur.

CLINICAL ASPECTS IN WELL RESOURCED SETTINGS

HIV infected babies generally appear normal at birth, with birth weight in the normal range. Clinically one cannot usually detect any signs that a baby has HIV in the first days of life. Signs and symptoms develop over the first few weeks and most children have evidence of infection before 12 months of age. Anecdotally, axillary lymphadenopathy may be an early sign that a baby is infected. However, there is a wide spectrum and some infected children may not present to medical attention for several years, with a smaller number remaining asymptomatic into adolescence.

HIV can present with a spectrum of signs and symptoms in children. This is reflected in both the four-stage CDC classification[504] and more recently in the revised four-stage WHO classification system for children[501] (Table 28.32), and important differences between adults and children are summarized in Table 28.33. In the absence of antiretroviral

therapy or prophylaxis against PCP (see below), disease progression is faster than in adults, even in well resourced settings. Cohort studies reported in the early 1990s that 15–20% of children progressed to an AIDS-defining illness by 12 months of age.[506–508] Over half of this subset of perinatally infected children presented with PCP at around 3–6 months of age in the absence of using prophylactic co-trimoxazole. Data from prospective cohorts in Europe in the early 1990s reported overall survival rates in children on either no ART or only ZDV monotherapy of around 70% by 6 years and 50% by 9 years of age.[506–508]

Children with HIV infection frequently present with nonspecific signs and symptoms that are common in general pediatrics. The most usual clinical features associated with HIV infection include persistent generalized lymphadenopathy (particularly axillary), hepatosplenomegaly, chronic or recurrent diarrhea, prolonged or recurrent oral or diaper candidiasis, fever, recurrent otitis or sinusitis and chest infections. Children may also present with a picture of idiopathic thrombocytopenic purpura with no other signs and may be more prone to developing eczema, extensive molluscum, and recurrent allergic iritis and rhinitis. A typical and quite specific presentation is non-tender bilateral parotid enlargement, which may be associated with generalized cervical lymphadenopathy and X-ray appearances of lymphocytic interstitial pneumonitis (LIP) with hilar lymphadenopathy (see below). Such children often also have allergic rhinitis, tonsillar and/or adenoid enlargement and may present with sleep apnea. Herpes zoster (shingles) in childhood is uncommon and suggests a defect in cellular immunity justifying an HIV test in the absence of other explanations.

Persistent or recurrent oral candidiasis after the neonatal period, abnormal neurological signs, failure to thrive and poor growth in association with HIV are all indications of increasing immune deficiency and a poorer outcome. Conversely, thrombocytopenia does not indicate a poor prognosis and bilateral parotitis, lymphadenopathy and LIP (see below) are often associated with a relatively good prognosis. Details of the main AIDS (CDC stage C) presenting conditions are described below. Although the development of these conditions, along with immunological stage 3 disease, has been shown to be predictive of a poor outcome, the prognosis varies. For example, conditions such as recurrent

A number of factors need to be taken into account when starting ART in children (Table 28.35). Education of families, taking account of drugs other family members may be taking, as well as due care in choosing a regimen which the family can adhere to are important considerations. Considerable support is required to enable families to sustain high levels of adherence long term. Frequency of dosing has been a major development and once daily regimens are now feasible for children with well established once daily pharmacokinetics for drugs such as lamivudine and abacavir that were previously given twice daily.[550-552]

There is some evidence that adherence may be poorer among asymptomatic children who have never been ill. This disadvantage needs to be weighed against avoiding children becoming seriously ill before starting ART. Educating parents and carers about following CD4 and viral load as predictors of progression at monitoring visits is important to ensure that a consensus between health professionals and the family is achieved about the right time to start therapy. Viral load and CD4% can fluctuate, and at least two or three values should be obtained. Time spent on preparing and educating the family before commencing ART is always important. For children under 12 years the 'PENTA Calculator' (http://www.ctu.mrc.ac.uk/penta/) can be a useful tool in decision making and help parents and carers to further understand the risk of disease progression.

Older children presenting for the first time are a selected group who do not have rapid disease progression. For these children it is reasonable to monitor CD4 counts and only offer treatment if counts are declining steadily below 20% or counts are between 200 and 350 as in adults (Table 28.35).[501] There is no consensus level of viral load above which treatment should be started in children.

Which ART to start

When starting HAART, most prescribers would initiate triple therapy with two NRTI drugs and one PI or one NNRTI. Intensive induction with quadruple combination therapy, sparing at least one class of drugs, reducing to a maintenance regimen of three drugs when the plasma viral load is well maintained at undetectable levels is another possible option and has been used in infants with extremely high levels of plasma viremia in some centers. The PI drugs are difficult to formulate into palatable suspensions for children compared with the NRTIs and NNRTIs. No large randomized clinical trials in children or adults provide evidence to conclude that PI-containing or PI-sparing regimens have greater long term clinical efficacy. This question and when to switch therapy is being addressed in a randomized controlled trial of children in Europe and the US starting therapy randomized to either PI- or NNRTI-based HAART (PENPACT 1 trial; www.pentatrials.org).

Data from the UK and Ireland CHIPS cohort show that most children start HAART with a triple regimen and over time there has been a shift from a PI- to an NNRTI-based regimen.[426] NVP is the main NNRTI in young children, but efavirenz is increasingly being used in children over 3 years. The main PI was nelfinavir, but increasingly this is being replaced by ritonavir boosted lopinavir (Kaletra). NRTI fixed drug combination tablets are increasing being made available in adult doses to reduce pill burden and ease adherence, thereby potentially improving response to therapy. Combivir (ZDV+3TC), Trizivir (ZDV+3TC+ABC), Kivexa (3TC+ABC) and Truvada (TDF+FTC) are available, the latter two formulations administered once daily. However, no combination liquid formulations are available. Use of crushed whole or half tablets requires care as some pills (e.g. Combivir) have these drugs unevenly distributed through the tablet. Fixed drug combinations containing an NNRTI with

Table 28.35 WHO recommendations for initiating ART in HIV-infected infants and children according to clinical stage and availability of immunological markers[549]

WHO pediatric stage	Availability of CD4 cell measurements	Age-specific treatment recommendation	
		≤11 months	≥12 months
4	CD4	Treat all	
	No CD4		
3	CD4	Treat all	Treat all, CD4-guided in those children with TB, LIP, OHL, thrombocytopenia
	No CD4		Treat all[c]
2	CD4		CD4-guided
	No CD4		TLC-guided
1	CD4		CD4-guided
	No CD4		Do not treat

WHO age-specific recommendations for starting ART on immunological markers

Immunological marker	Age-specific recommendation to initiate ART			
	< 11 months	12–35 months	36–59 months	> 5 years
%CD4	< 25%	< 20%	< 15%	< 15%
CD4 count	< 1500 cells/mm³	< 750 cells/mm³	< 350 cells/mm³	< 200 cells/mm³

WHO TLC criteria for severe HIV immunodeficiency requiring initiation of ART; suggested for use in infants and children with clinical stage 2 and where CD4 measurement is not available

Immunological marker	Age-specific recommendation to initiate ART			
	< 11 months	12–35 months	36–59 months	> 5 years
TLC	< 4000 cells/mm³	< 3000 cells/mm³	< 2500 cells/mm³	< 2000 cells/mm³

What HAART to start?
Either: 2 NRTI + 1 PI (PI: NFV or lopinavir/r)
plus NRTI combinations: ZDV + ddI; ZDV + 3TC; ddI + d4T, d4T + 3TC; 3TC + ABC
Or: EFV + 2 NRTI (if over 3 years)
NVP + 2 NRTI (all ages)
Or: 3 NRTI: ZDV + 3TC + abacavir

two NRTIs are already available as generic formulations in resource limited countries, and a combined once daily pill of efavirenz, emtricitabine and tenofovir is available for adults and can be used for older adolescents in well resourced settings.

There is considerable inter- and intra-patient variation in drug levels achieved even when using standard ART doses for size. The role of therapeutic drug monitoring (TDM) has not been clearly defined in pediatrics but is frequently used in many centers. A randomized controlled trial assessing the impact of differing levels of TDM compared to no TDM (PENTA 14) was recently halted due to low levels of recruitment. TDM is definitely indicated where there is the possibility of drug interactions and can provide additional information regarding individual pharmacokinetics, absorption and adherence.

Adherence

It has become very clear from adult and pediatric studies that adherence is one of the principal determinants of both the degree and duration of virological suppression.[553] In one study, children whose caregivers reported no missed doses in the previous week were more likely to have an undetectable viral load (50% versus 24%).[554] The reasons for non-adherence are complex and multifactorial. Adherence is difficult to assess in the clinic. No pediatric intervention studies aimed at improving adherence have been conducted. Outpatient attendance and adherence are poorer in adolescents and young adults, increasing their risk of virological failure and the evolution of resistance.[555]

Changing therapy

Virological failure requires investigation into the potency of the regimen, including checking that the child is on the correct dose (which may be higher than the recommended dose in drug packet inserts)[548,550] and that the child has not outgrown their dose, checking for possible pharmacokinetic interactions with other drugs or food, and checking on adherence. These should all be done before switching therapy. A recent study demonstrated that children were frequently underdosed with antiretrovirals, a continuing issue for growing infants and children whose dosing is calculated on weight or surface area.[540] The level of viremia in children that should prompt a switch in therapy is the subject of an ongoing trial discussed above. Adult guidelines recommend switch consideration for sustained viral rebound, defined as two plasma viral loads at least one month apart > 400 copies/mm³, for patients whose viral loads have previously been undetectable.[528,529] Occasionally, despite virological failure, families and doctors may wish to continue the current regimen when the child is clinically and immunologically stable, and there is not an obvious easy palatable regimen to switch to. However this may lead to accumulation of resistance mutations and therefore fewer options for subsequent therapy. The choice of the new regimen will depend on the prior ART history, drug toxicity, availability of new drugs/formulations and adherence, and may be guided by resistance testing.

Resistance

Resistance testing is recommended for treatment of naive adults prior to initiation of HAART as transmitted resistance is well recognized and has also been reported in infants following mother-to-child transmission.[556] As the availability of ART increases worldwide, baseline resistance testing may be considered for children if there is any uncertainty regarding ART exposure either for the child directly or the mother prior to or during pregnancy or breast-feeding.[530] Resistance testing is increasingly routinely performed in children on HAART with virological failure, although virological or immunological benefit was not demonstrated in a recently published pediatric trial with long term follow-up[557] and results from short term adult studies are conflicting. Further validation of resistance testing is difficult as, like TDM, it has increasingly become part of standard care.

Toxicity

Children on HAART are now surviving into adult life, but as the length of exposure to HAART grows, the long term side-effects are becoming increasingly apparent. Lipodystrophy (LD) is defined as abnormality in lipid metabolism resulting in dyslipidemia (high lipids) and body changes characterized by truncal obesity alongside disfiguring loss of fat on the face and in the periphery. A European cross-sectional study reported fat redistribution in a quarter of children. Increased risk was associated with more advanced disease, female gender, use of protease inhibitors and of stavudine, which are similar risk factors to adults.[558,559] However, studies are hampered by the lack of a standard definition of LD in the growing child, and many reports are clearly subjective although efforts are being made to standardize assessments.[560] Hyperlipidemia is being increasingly reported but there is uncertainty as to the level of hyperlipidemia that should precipitate a treatment switch or addition of lipid lowering drugs. Insulin resistance resulting in hyperglycemia and occasionally exogenous insulin dependence is seen in adults and occasionally in pediatric cohorts and has been associated with length of time on PI-based HAART.[561] Adult cohorts have reported an increase in cardiovascular events when compared to the general population. HIV itself has a pro-inflammatory effect on the endothelium but coupled with the metabolic complications described above, concern is growing about the cardiovascular risk in adult life for children with perinatally acquired HIV infection.[562]

A high prevalence of bone demineralization has been reported in children in association with HIV infection and HAART, raising concerns of risk of progression to osteopenia and osteoporosis in early adult life. The optimum management strategy is currently unclear and requires further consideration.[563,564] Mitochondrial toxicity, at least in part due to the inhibition of DNA polymerase by nucleoside analogues, has rarely been associated with severe, even fatal, lactic acidosis in children on HAART.[565] Asymptomatic hyperlactatemia occurs more frequently but may be temporary and current evidence does not support routine lactate measurements for children on HAART.[566] Unexplained nausea, vomiting, fatigue and/or neurological deterioration in a child on HAART should prompt assessment of lactic acid status and consideration of mitochondrial toxicity.

As toxicity associated with long term continuous ART becomes more apparent, strategies to reduce ART exposure, including structured treatment interruptions (STI) and immune therapies, are being evaluated in children and adults. Recent trials of STIs in adults have been halted early due to an excess of clinical adverse events in patients off treatment, although overall absolute risk of events in the SMART trial was small.[543] Interim analysis of a pilot European pediatric trial (PENTA 11) was satisfactory. The argument prevailed that STI in children has a compelling rationale and may be safer because of a more active immune system; the trial is continuing, with a parallel trial also continuing in Botswana. The cost/benefit for children may be different to adults as they potentially face a lifetime of ART with its cumulative toxicities.

Prophylaxis against opportunistic infections
Co-trimoxazole prophylaxis for prevention of PCP
There is good evidence from randomized trials in adults with HIV that co-trimoxazole is very effective at preventing PCP and this is the drug of choice. Dapsone or inhaled pentamidine can be used in the event of hypersensitivity to co-trimoxazole but they are less efficacious. The evidence for efficacy of co-trimoxazole in preventing PCP in infants with HIV is indirect, and comes from studies showing decreased PCP after the introduction of guidelines recommending starting all babies on co-trimoxazole.[567,568]

The MTCT rates are now so low in Europe and the USA that, coupled with the ability to exclude HIV infection by 3 months of age, the need for PCP prophylaxis has decreased and can be restricted to babies born to mothers who do not take interventions in pregnancy to reduce MTCT, or have a high risk of MTCT (e.g. because of detectable HIV RNA viral load at delivery) or babies where the mother is reluctant for the baby to be tested early in life.[449] Prophylaxis can be stopped once it has been established that the baby is uninfected. Infected infants should continue prophylaxis throughout the first year of life, as CD4 counts are unreliable indicators of PCP risk. Thereafter, it is not unreasonable to stop prophylaxis unless the CD4 count is under 15%.

Guidelines for PCP prophylaxis in adults permit discontinuation of both primary and secondary PCP prophylaxis when the CD4 cell count is above 200 cells/μL for greater than 3 months in response to HAART. Although evidence is more limited in pediatric populations, most practitioners consider discontinuation of primary and secondary prophylaxis when the CD4 count has increased above 200 cells/μL or 15% on HAART,[568] and the majority of children on HAART in the UK are not on PCP prophylaxis. A prospective study in children over 2 years in the US supported the safe withdrawal of OI and PCP prophylaxis following immune reconstitution in response to HAART.[569] In all children, whether or not they are on HAART, guidelines recommend restarting co-trimoxazole when the CD4% falls below 15% or 200 cells/μL.

Prophylaxis against other infections

Co-trimoxazole has also been shown, in a large placebo controlled trial of Zambian HIV infected children aged 1–14 years (mean age 4.5 years), to reduce mortality by 43%.[513] The efficacy was maintained over a period of 18 months and occurred despite high background prevalence of *S. pneumoniae* and non-typhi *Salmonella* species with resistance to co-trimoxazole. The trial also showed a reduction in hospital admissions and use of antibiotics in the arm treated with active drug. Although most causes of death and hospital admissions were presumptive diagnoses, it appeared that reduction in bacterial lung infections was the most likely mode of action and PCP was not observed in nasopharyngeal aspirates.[534] Updated WHO guidelines recommend that all HIV infected children in resource limited settings continue to receive co-trimoxazole prophylaxis while awaiting HAART.[501] The question about continued benefit of co-trimoxazole prophylaxis in the presence of HAART requires further evaluation.

In well resourced countries, as a result of advances in antiretroviral therapy, there has been a shift in focus from diagnosing and managing opportunistic infections to restoring and maintaining cellular immunity with HAART and thereby preventing opportunistic infections.

HIV infected children who are contacts of individuals with open pulmonary TB should be carefully assessed, bearing in mind skin testing is frequently unhelpful because of anergy. If there is no evidence of infection, prophylactic isoniazid for 6 months, or isoniazid plus rifampicin for 3 months is recommended. Prophylaxis against *Mycobacterium avium-intracellulare* in children is not recommended because of adverse reactions and the potential for resistance and breakthrough on single agents such as rifabutin.

Primary prophylaxis against CMV is not recommended. With respect to secondary prophylaxis following CMV infection, infants who have had CMV usually reconstitute their immune systems very well, obviating the need for secondary prophylaxis.

For most other established opportunistic infections, such as cryptosporidiosis for which there were few useful therapeutic options, the best treatment is HAART, which should be started as soon as possible if a child presents initially with HIV infection and an acute opportunistic infection. Immune reconstitution disease, which may occur particularly in severely immunocompromised children, may make opportunistic infection symptoms worse initially. Some individuals with immune reconstitution disease may require steroids in addition to HAART and specific therapy for opportunistic infections.

Immunizations

Children with HIV infection should be immunized according to normal schedules with both live and killed vaccines. The exception is that BCG is not advised for children with HIV infection in low prevalence areas because of the risk of dissemination. However, it should be given in areas of high TB prevalence and this, in the author's view, should include babies born to African women in the UK who have a high rate of TB and may also return to Africa either to live or to visit. In line with current UK vaccination schedules, inactivated polio vaccine (IPV) is to be preferred to live oral polio vaccine because of theoretical concerns about paralytic poliomyelitis in contacts of children excreting live virus. Pneumococcal polysaccharide vaccine has been recommended for HIV

infected children over 2 years of age, but a trial of its use in adults with HIV in Africa showed no benefit. Conjugate pneumococcal vaccine should be given to children under 2, in line with national UK guidelines. Annual influenza vaccination is also recommended. All children with HIV should be screened for hepatitis A, B and C co-infection; hepatitis A and B vaccination should be offered to those who are susceptible to infection.

The efficacy of all vaccines is improved among children who have immune reconstitution following ART. Children immunized before starting ART in whom responses are inadequate should be revaccinated.

Passive immunization of symptomatic children with CD4% < 15% is recommended if they are in contact with varicella zoster virus (VZV) and are either VZV naive or have no detectable specific antibodies to VZV. Varicella zoster immunoglobulin (VZIG) ideally should be given within 72 h of contact. VZIG may prolong the incubation period to 28 days, so clinicians need to consider isolating these patients at clinic visits. Similarly, normal human immunoglobulin should be given for susceptible symptomatic children in contact with measles. The role of oral aciclovir in preventing VZV infection following contact has not yet been ascertained but it is used by some pediatricians.

Regular intravenous immunoglobulin infusions (400 mg/kg every 28 days) should only be given to children with recurrent bacterial infections despite good compliance with HAART and co-trimoxazole prophylaxis, or those with proven hypogammaglobulinemia. Higher doses may be useful in the management of thrombocytopenia (0.5–1.0 g/dose every day, for 3–5 days). However, in the era of HAART, the number of children requiring such therapy should be minimal.

Supportive care

Unlike most other severe chronic diseases of children, HIV simultaneously affects family members including the parents and other siblings. The parents' own health, their social isolation and feelings of guilt compound the difficulties of caring for a sick child. An effective well coordinated multidisciplinary team is required to address the changing needs of infected children and their caregivers. Continuity of care needs to be developed between inpatient and outpatient services, local referring hospitals and the community. Ideally adults and children should be treated in family based units.[570] All too often parents will ignore their own health needs because they put their children first.

The work of the multidisciplinary team has increasingly shifted towards ways of helping families achieve long term adherence to HAART. As children survive longer, meeting the needs of adolescents and planning transition to adult clinics is placing new demands on services. The decision as to who should be informed should be tailored individually. Families may need help in explaining the diagnosis to older children. This needs to be undertaken at the child's pace, and is frequently most effectively achieved in gradual steps. It is not mandatory to tell staff at schools, as universal precautions should be employed for all children with injuries. The risk of transmission from casual contacts in school or daycare settings is virtually zero. Ensuring that adolescents are well informed and responsible before they become sexually active is a priority and pediatric family clinics in London are setting up specific adolescent clinics with their adult colleagues. Peer support for adolescents is important to help young people with HIV come to terms and live with their disease.

The multidisciplinary team should include a dietician, as nutritional problems and growth faltering are not uncommon even in the era of HAART and particularly in children with chronic lung disease. Balanced supplements are sometimes required and enteral feeding through gastrostomy tubes may be necessary. Gastrostomy tubes have been used with success to allow unpalatable medicines to be given, particularly in children on multiple therapies such as in TB co-infection, those with neurological impairment, or in children who have failed first/second line therapy due to poor adherence. In addition, dietary and exercise advice is increasingly needed to prevent and treat obesity in HIV infected children on HAART.

Pain management is important in late stage disease. Complementary therapies frequently used in adults with late disease, such as aromatherapy, may be useful and require evaluation. With the continuing success of HAART, there are currently very few children in industrialized countries needing palliative or terminal care. However a small number of children and adolescents in Europe and more in the USA have multidrug resistant virus and urgently require novel therapies.

Prevention remains the top priority in managing HIV infection in children. Reducing national perinatal transmission rates to below 2% is an achievable target that can only be realized if HIV infected mothers can be identified prenatally and offered appropriate interventions. Antenatal detection rates in most European countries and the USA have reached high levels for several years and continued effort by health professionals, public health planners and community organizations is essential.

EXANTHEMATA

MEASLES (MORBILLI AND RUBEOLA)

Measles is a viral disease of high infectivity, which presents with an acute catarrhal illness, fever, and characteristic Koplik spots on the buccal mucous membranes followed by a distinctive maculopapular rash. There is a high incidence of serious complications of the respiratory and nervous systems. In large cities and towns, measles is most likely to occur in infants and preschool children, but in rural and less crowded urban areas the principal incidence is between the ages of 5 and 10 years. Measles is extremely rare under 3–4 months of age, because of protective maternal antibody, but authenticated cases have occurred.

In some countries measles outbreaks have shown a characteristic biennial periodicity but such a pattern is by no means universal and the introduction of active immunization has altered the natural epidemiology of the disease.

Mortality

In resource limited countries, where malnutrition is common, measles may have a mortality as high as 25% and produce serious complications.[571] Children are at increased risk of dying for a year after their measles due to impaired cellular immunity. Inhibition of macrophage production of interleukin-12, a cytokine important for driving cell mediated immunity, by binding of measles virus to CD46, a cellular protein that regulates complement, is thought to be partly responsible for this immunosuppression.[572] Measles can cause devastating outbreaks when the virus is introduced into naive populations such as on remote islands. Although the morbidity and mortality are lower in highly immunized, industrialized countries, outbreaks can still occur if a population of unimmunized children, usually preschool, is allowed to develop. In more exposed communities, measles is now comparatively mild and its morbidity and mortality lower, although occasional deaths still occur in the UK. Children who contract measles when in remission from acute leukemia or who have other conditions in which immunity is compromised are at particular risk.

Etiology

Measles virus is an RNA virus of the paramyxovirus family, genus *Morbillivirus*, and morphologically resembles the parainfluenza viruses. It is usually transmitted by droplet infection from the respiratory tract of a case before, or close to, the onset of the rash. Entry mainly occurs through the respiratory tract, but infection through the intact conjunctiva has been postulated. Clinically significant antigenic variation has not been described. An attack is usually followed by life-long immunity and there is little or no authenticated evidence of second attacks of measles except in individuals with severe immunological defects. Subclinical infection can probably occur but is rare.

Clinical features

Measles has an incubation period of 8–14 days. A mild illness may occur at the time of infection but most cases develop a prodromal illness some 3–5 days before the eruptive stage. The main features of this illness are pronounced catarrh, characterized by a constantly running nose, conjunctivitis and a harsh dry cough. Fever and irritability are usually present and there may be a fleeting scarlatiniform or morbilliform rash. Koplik spots, the most pathognomonic sign of measles, appear during this stage and are seen as small, grayish white lesions on the buccal mucosa close to the posterior molar teeth; they are usually quite numerous but may be scanty or occasionally cover the entire lining of the cheek. They can be difficult to demonstrate and the angle of the inspecting light is critical; having faded, they are replaced by a dry, matte appearance on the mucosa, which has a ground-glass-like surface.

The true rash of measles (Fig. 28.34)[573] starts behind the ears and along the hairline. Fever, which will have lessened at the end of the prodromal period, may now rise again to 39–40 °C (Fig. 28.35),[573] and the eruption spreads rapidly to involve the face. The lesions are maculopapular in character and of a dusky hue. Over the next two days the eruption spreads downwards and becomes generalized; marked confluence of the spots develops and this gives a blotchy appearance.

The extent and severity of the rash shows wide variation. In some, especially the younger cases, the eruption may be unusually sparse and modification by maternal antibody has been suggested. There is frequently some degree of hemorrhage or diapedesis into the rash giving it a purpuric quality and subsequent skin staining. This should not be confused with the rare, and usually fatal, hemorrhagic measles in which extensive bleeding occurs into the skin and from the mucous membranes. In the immunocompromised child, the rash occasionally does not develop.

Fading of the rash can be surprisingly rapid but it usually disappears quite slowly, beginning to fade on the third day in the order of

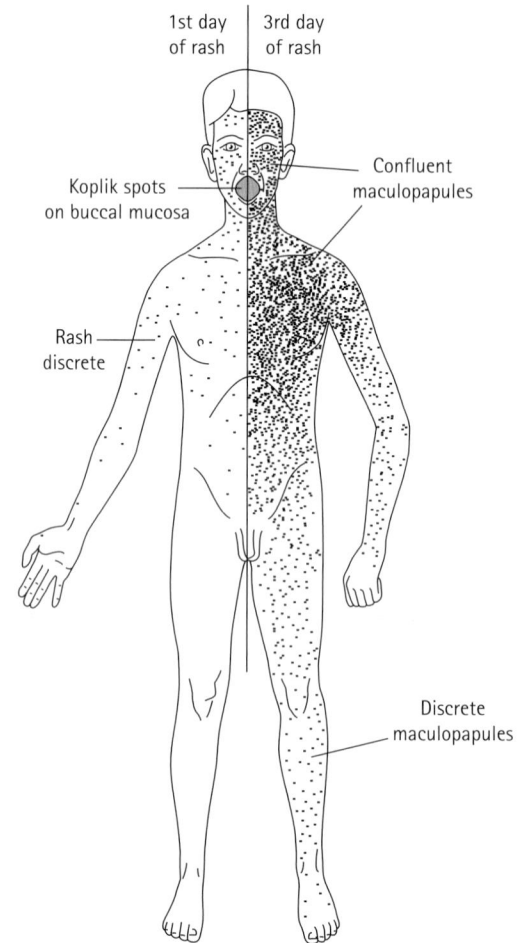

Fig. 28.34 The distribution and the development of rash in measles. (From Krugman & Ward 1968[573])

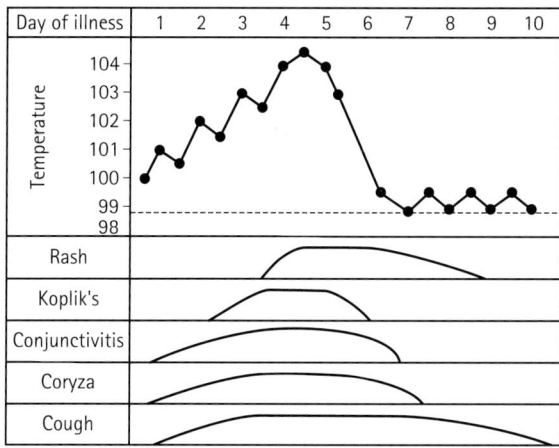

Fig. 28.35 The development of measles. (From Krugman & Ward 1968[573])

appearance; the rash may be largely gone from the face and upper trunk by the fourth day though persisting on the lower extremities. After a further 3–4 days a brownish staining appears, probably due to capillary hemorrhage and, on occasions, this staining can be very intense. In severe cases, a fine desquamation may occur at the site of the rash, but this does not usually involve the hands and feet like scarlet fever.

Complications
Respiratory
Measles virus always attacks the respiratory tract causing some degree of laryngotracheobronchitis. An element of bronchitis is universal and can be severe, extending even to bronchiolitis; the latter can be complicated by acute mediastinal emphysema. Croup may be prominent. Viral damage may denude the respiratory tract of its protective lining and allow the aspiration of bacteria. Bronchopneumonia may result and the severity will depend on the nature of the aspirated material. Staphylococcal pneumonia can be life threatening.

In a few instances measles virus involvement of the respiratory tract may spread to the lung parenchyma, giving rise to the condition known as giant cell pneumonia. This complication may be prolonged and is often fatal, and the illness may be accompanied by little or no rash. It is usually found in association with underlying disease such as HIV infection, leukemia, or other immune deficiency with impaired T cell function. In view of its atypical nature, this illness is often undiagnosed during life and the true diagnosis is made as a result of autopsy findings.

Ophthalmic
Some degree of conjunctivitis and keratitis occurs in every case of measles. It is typically exudative, nonpurulent and nonfollicular and can be characterized by Koplik spots. When pseudomembranes or corneal ulcers occur they are the result of secondary bacterial infection. Optic neuritis and retinitis are associated with measles encephalitis.

Ear
Involvement of the middle ear used to be commonplace and could result in suppurative otitis media, chronic perforation or mastoiditis. The lessening severity of measles and prompt antibiotic treatment has reduced the incidence of these complications to a low level.

Gastrointestinal tract
Severe oral inflammation due to secondary infection by bacteria, *Treponema vincentii*, or thrush can occur but cancrum oris is only likely to be seen where malnutrition is rife. Cancrum oris (noma) is a gangrenous form of stomatitis that commences with a dusky red spot on the inside and outside of the cheek. This rapidly spreads to form a sloughing gangrene of the gums and jaws and in extreme cases teeth

may be shed. The breath develops a peculiarly foul odor and death can supervene.

Gastroenteritis is common in measles in non-industrialized countries and can be prolonged; it probably results from direct viral involvement of the gut with or without superinfection with organisms such as *Cryptosporidium*. Appendicitis can occur in measles though abdominal pain is more commonly due to associated mesenteric adenitis.

Enlargement of the spleen is more frequently encountered in measles than is generally realized.

CNS
Measles, with its pronounced constitutional upset and high fever, is often complicated by febrile convulsions. These are most commonly encountered at the start of the eruptive stage and either settle spontaneously or in response to simple sedation; they should not be assumed to be indicative of encephalitis.

True postinfectious encephalomyelitis occurs in from 1 in 1000 to 1 in 5000 cases of measles and has a mortality of about 10% and leaves about 15% with neurological residua. It normally presents after 7–14 days, when the rash is subsiding, but can commence earlier in the disease and rarely even before the rash. Drowsiness, fits, a recrudescence of fever, focal neurological signs and progressive coma suggest that severe cerebral involvement is occurring. In some cases the process may arrest at this juncture and be followed by rapid improvement; in others there is a steady deterioration and death. Between these extremes there are patients in whom recovery is slow and permanent cerebral damage likely.

Rarely subacute sclerosing panencephalitis (SSPE) may complicate measles infection, though not apparently measles immunization. In SSPE, measles virus becomes latent in the cerebrum following primary infection and is then reactivated, usually 5–10 years later, by some unknown stimulus. An alternate hypothesis suggests that a partially immune individual is reinfected by measles which then provokes this unique form of encephalitis. It is more common in children in whom primary measles occurs before 1 year of age.

Others
Uncomplicated measles tends to produce leukopenia, and significant thrombocytopenia is occasionally encountered. Epistaxis is a common and occasionally troublesome feature.

There is a traditional but unconfirmed belief that measles may activate or predispose to tuberculosis. Diagnostic difficulty is provided by the fact that measles may suppress the Mantoux reaction for several weeks.

Diagnosis
Provided the medical attendant is consulted at its inception, measles can be diagnosed on clinical grounds with a fair degree of accuracy. Immunofluorescence can be used to detect measles virus antigen in respiratory secretions if rapid diagnosis is needed. Difficulties can arise when an opinion is required later in the disease.

Neutralizing, complement-fixing and hemagglutination-inhibiting antibodies to measles develop during the illness and appropriate serological tests can confirm their presence. Detection of measles IgM on a single specimen is the simplest method for diagnosis. Measles IgM can be detected from 3 days after the onset of the rash for about a month. Sensitivity rates, however, vary according to the type of assay used and the time after the onset of the rash, with the hemagglutination-inhibiting antibodies assay being the most sensitive and complement fixation the least (87% and 37% of cases, respectively, 3 days after the onset of the eruptive phase).[574] The demonstration of a significant rise (four-fold or greater) in antibody titer to measles virus confirms the clinical diagnosis. The hemagglutination-inhibition and complement fixation tests are usually employed, on account of the ease and rapidity with which they can be performed.

Measles virus can be isolated in primary tissue cultures of human kidney, human amnion or monkey kidney, and several other tissue culture systems have been used. The growth rate of measles virus in tissue culture is relatively slow and serological tests will often yield a positive result before the virus has been isolated and identified. During the late prodromal stage of the illness virus can be recovered from the nasopharynx, urine, conjunctival secretions and blood. By the second day of the rash, virus isolation becomes more difficult, though the urine may continue to contain virus for a further 2 days. In the immunocompromised child, there may be prolonged shedding of measles from the sites after the initial infection.[575]

In SSPE, measles antibody in high titer is demonstrable in the serum many years after a typical attack of measles. Antibody may also be detected in the CSF and the ratio of this antibody to that in the serum may be of diagnostic significance. Brain biopsy can confirm the diagnosis of SSPE where facilities for electron microscopy and immunofluorescence are available.

Differential diagnosis

Kawasaki disease can cause a morbilliform rash with fever, conjunctivitis and lymphadenopathy and can be quite difficult to distinguish clinically from measles. The milder illness of rubella with its pinker rash and selective involvement of the suboccipital glands is usually distinguishable. The rash of infectious mononucleosis can cause confusion but its other clinical and laboratory features usually lead to the correct interpretation. Enteroviral infections associated with a rash are usually more transient and lack the catarrhal involvement. Influenza virus infections, both A and B, can occasionally cause a morbilliform rash with respiratory symptoms and fever. In roseola infantum, the rash is very like measles, but as it appears the fever falls and the child is well, in contrast to measles. Scarlet fever and drug eruptions have readily distinguishing features.

Treatment

There are currently no antiviral agents available with demonstrated efficacy in vivo against measles virus. Ribavirin has been shown to inhibit measles virus replication in vitro, and there are anecdotal reports of its use either intravenously or by aerosol to treat severe pneumonitis or encephalitis in the immunocompromised child.[576] However, this treatment remains experimental in the absence of data from a randomized controlled trial.

Amongst the earliest complications that may require treatment are croup and febrile convulsions. These are managed symptomatically (see Chs 20 and 22).

Secondary bacterial infection, superimposed on viral damage to the respiratory tract, will require treatment. Staphylococcal pneumonia is the most feared complication, and if bacterial pneumonia is suspected antistaphylococcal antibiotics should be used. Prophylactic antibiotics are unnecessary, as confirmed by a recent systematic review on the subject.[577]

Mastoiditis should not occur if adequate treatment of otitis media is given early, but if it does occur surgical drainage is required. Any sign of secondary infection of the conjunctiva should be treated with appropriate antibiotics, and chloramphenicol eye ointment smeared on to the lids often proves efficacious.

It is rare for gastroenteritis to be so severe as to cause fluid and electrolyte depletion but where this occurs appropriate measures require to be taken. True appendicitis can present in the course of measles.

Postinfectious encephalitis requires intensive supportive treatment, including anticonvulsants for seizures. The use of corticosteroids remains controversial, but many clinicians feel such therapy warrants trial in severe cases whose progress is unsatisfactory.

Preventive measures
Quarantine
Because this disease is highly infectious and the maximum infectivity is before the rash appears, quarantine measures are frequently ineffective. However, any child who is suffering from a severe, debilitating disease should be protected from exposure whenever possible. In the hospital setting, appropriate quarantine measures should be in place for up to

4 days after the onset of the rash while the child is infectious via the respiratory route. The immunocompromised child with measles should be placed on respiratory isolation for the duration of the illness.

Passive immunization
Passive immunization has been used as post-exposure prophylaxis against measles for many years, although the evidence for it is sparse. Normal human immunoglobulin (gamma globulin) is used (0.2 ml/kg intramuscularly for normal children, 0.5 ml/kg for immunocompromised children, maximum dose 15 ml). The use of passive immunization is particularly important when immunocompromised children, for whom active immunization is contraindicated, are exposed to measles.

Active immunization
In the early years of measles vaccines, an inactivated measles vaccine was used which not only failed to protect against infection but resulted in the children developing severe, atypical illness with giant cell pneumonitis when exposed to wild-type virus.

Live, attenuated measles vaccines are highly protective and have very few side-effects. Where they have been used to immunize whole populations, acute measles, encephalitis and subacute sclerosing panencephalitis have virtually disappeared. In countries where immunization rates are relatively low, there are many cases of acute encephalitis, with several children each year dying or handicapped as a result.[578] Measles vaccine is readily inhibited by maternal antibody and may be ineffective if given before 1 year of age. If it is wished to protect a child exposed to measles who has no contraindications to immunization and is over 1 year old, then measles vaccine is preferable to passive immunization. Many countries now give measles vaccine in conjunction with mumps and rubella vaccines (MMR) in the second year of life, and a second dose may be given at school entry or at 12–14 years old. The only contraindication to measles vaccine is immune deficiency (including high dose but not low dose steroids). Anaphylactic egg allergy is no longer considered to be a contraindication.[579] HIV infection is not a contraindication unless the patient is severely immunocompromised; on the contrary, as they are at high risk from wild-type measles virus, every attempt should be made to immunize HIV positive children against measles. Measles continues to be a significant public health concern despite an effective vaccine. Recent outbreaks in countries such as the USA[580] and UK[581] where endemic infection was considered to be virtually eliminated have highlighted the need for sustained high vaccination coverage in areas where wild-type virus no longer circulates. There is also concern that infants, who are at greater risk of severe disease, are becoming susceptible to measles earlier in their first year due to declining levels of maternal antibody.[580]

RUBELLA (GERMAN MEASLES)

Postnatal rubella is characterized by its mild nature and relative freedom from complications. Some of the original accounts of the disease emanated from Germany and because of this and a certain similarity to measles, the name of German measles became a popular, if ill-conceived, descriptive title.

Etiology
Rubella virus is an RNA virus of the Togaviridae family. It was first cultured and identified as recently as 1962. Since then it has proved possible to grow it quite readily on suitable tissue cultures, a factor that has considerably enhanced our knowledge of the disease. Transmission is primarily through droplet spread of infected nasopharyngeal secretions from a few days before to up to 14 days after the onset of the rash.

Incidence
The true incidence of rubella is difficult to assess as infection is subclinical in a sizable proportion of cases. Even the clinical illness itself has no pathognomonic features, a point that is substantiated in surveys where rubella antibody levels correlate poorly with the history of previously

suspected infection. By early adult life as many as 90% of city dwellers may show serological evidence of previous rubella but the figure can be much lower in rural communities. Rubella is less common in preschool children than, for example, measles and in one survey less than 10% of children under 2 years showed evidence of previous infection, though this figure had risen to 25% between the ages of 2 and 5 years. By 12 years of age, 80% had antibody, suggesting the bulk of infection occurs between 6 and 12 years of age.

Clinical features

Rubella has an incubation period of 14–21 days, with an average of 17 days. In children it is rare to have a significant prodromal illness and the first indication of rubella infection is the appearance of a rash over the face (Fig. 28.36).[573] This soon spreads to cover the trunk and later the limbs. The basic lesions are fine, pink macules which, originally discrete, can soon coalesce over the face and trunk. The rash usually disappears within 2–3 days but may persist for as long as 5 days. Occasionally it has a duration measured in hours and in this instance can be readily missed. A biphasic type of rash, with complete regression in between, has been described and a small area of the eruption may persist on the medial aspect of the thighs after the main rash has subsided. Small purpuric spots sometimes appear on the soft palate but have no diagnostic significance, as other infections are associated with a similar enanthem.

Lymph node enlargement is an important feature of the disease. It may appear as much as a week before the rash, though usually just before, and may persist for some time after the eruption has faded. The cervical, postauricular and suboccipital glands are most commonly involved, can be tender and are sometimes unassociated with any rash.

In adolescents and adults, especially female, prodromal symptoms are more likely and include malaise, headache, stickiness of the eyes,

conjunctivitis and fever. In children the temperature rarely rises above 37.1–37.4°C but in adults it can attain 39.5–40.0°C (Fig. 28.37).[573]

The clinical stigmata of congenital rubella are described in Chapter 12.

Complications

In general, complications are unusual though a higher incidence is encountered in certain epidemics and some seem age or gender dependent.

Polyarthritis may be a sequel of rubella. It usually commences when the rash has subsided, is more common after florid eruptions and occurs in adults, especially women, rather than in children. The small joints of the hands and the wrist joints are most often involved but the large joints can also be attacked. The condition usually resolves within 2 weeks.

Postinfectious encephalitis, myelitis and polyradiculitis may follow an attack of rubella and have a similar pathology to these syndromes when they occur after other infections. However, in rubella they appear to have a better prognosis.

Thrombocytopenia is quite common in the course of the illness and may become clinically manifest as purpura. Epistaxis, hematuria and melena can also develop. Some cases of so-called 'idiopathic thrombocytopenic purpura' can be shown by laboratory tests to have resulted from subclinical rubella infection. Leukopenia is frequently found at the height of the illness and there may be an increase in plasma or Turk cells.

Diagnosis

Owing to the lack of pathognomonic features, one cannot rely on a clinical diagnosis of rubella and, whenever confirmation is important, laboratory tests (in the form of appropriate serological studies) should be used.

A serological diagnosis depends on the demonstration of a significant rise in antibody titer (four-fold or greater) when a sample of serum collected at the onset of the illness and a further sample taken 2–3 weeks later are compared.

Antibodies to rubella virus may be detected by hemagglutination-inhibition, neutralization, complement-fixation or radial hemolysis test. Nowadays, the hemagglutination test is generally preferred, owing to its reliability and the ease with which it can be performed.

Following infection both neutralizing and hemagglutination-inhibition antibodies persist, at a variable titer, for a long time whereas complement-fixation antibodies disappear more rapidly.

Virus may be recovered with relative ease from the nasopharynx during the last week of the incubation period and for up to 2 weeks thereafter. It is less readily isolated from the urine and blood. However, many laboratories do not offer viral culture for rubella.

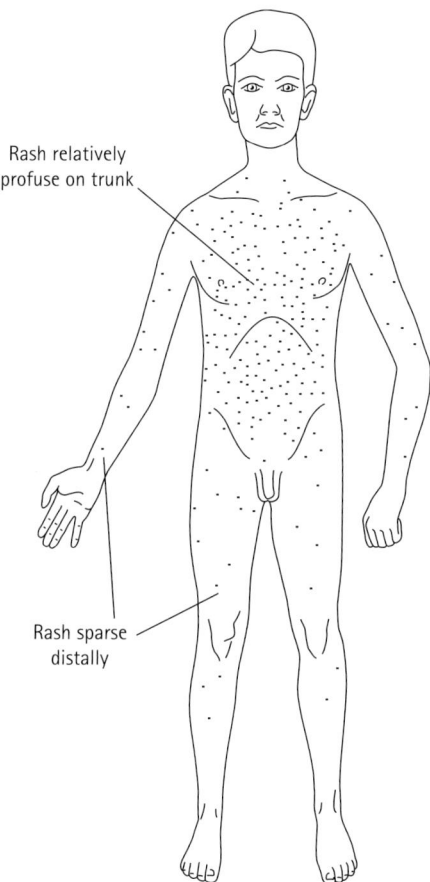

Fig. 28.36 The distribution and development of rash in rubella. (From Krugman & Ward 1968[573])

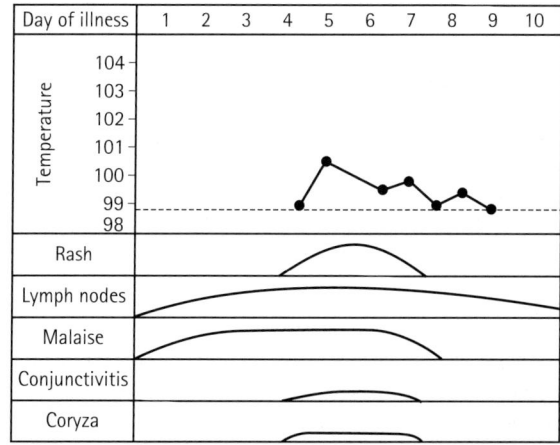

Fig. 28.37 The development of rubella. (From Krugman & Ward 1968[573])

Differential diagnosis

Rubella may be confused with many common exanthemata and other skin eruptions. Differentiation from measles, glandular fever and drug eruptions does not present great difficulty but scarlet fever can cause confusion. Enteroviral infections accompanied by a rash, especially those associated with ECHO virus infection, provide the greatest diagnostic challenge. The presence of the herald patch, the distribution over the trunk and the complete well-being of the patient help to distinguish pityriasis rosea.

Resort to laboratory tests is always desirable when doubt exists in regard to a suspicious rash in a pregnant woman or her contacts.

Treatment

There is no specific treatment for rubella. A rapid recovery is to be expected. Prodromal symptoms rarely cause trouble but analgesics may be needed when polyarthritis occurs. Neurological complications are managed along the usual lines for such conditions.

Prevention

As a general rule, preventive measures are unnecessary in view of the mild nature of the disease. However, the situation is quite different in the case of women in early pregnancy, and attempts to prevent rubella were traditionally made using intramuscular normal human immunoglobulin. Evaluation of this procedure proved difficult, but laboratory-confirmed cases of rubella occurred despite immunoglobulin. Attenuated live rubella vaccines are now widely used and in general stimulate reasonable antibody levels. Opinions differ as to how they are best employed. Some recommend they are given to girls around puberty and non-immune pregnant women postpartum (selective immunization) while others believe children of both sexes should be given the vaccine in early childhood, usually in conjunction with measles and mumps vaccine as MMR, in an attempt to reduce the pool of infection in the community (universal immunization). Although terminations of pregnancy are frequently performed on pregnant women who have been inadvertently immunized there have been no cases of congenital rubella syndrome caused by the vaccine.

ERYTHEMA INFECTIOSUM (FIFTH DISEASE, SLAPPED CHEEK DISEASE)

This disease may occur at any time of year, but outbreaks in primary school children are classically in the winter and spring. Joint involvement may occur. Children with shortened red cell survival can develop profound anemia (aplastic crises), including children with endemic malaria,[582] and sickle cell disease.[583] Infection during pregnancy can lead to hydrops fetalis.

Etiology

Erythema infectiosum is caused by parvovirus B19 (human parvovirus), a small, single-stranded DNA virus. Spread is by droplet infection, although as the virus can be seen in plasma during infections, it could be transmitted by blood products. Erythrocyte precursors are particularly susceptible to the virus, causing a mild fall in hemoglobin (of about 1 g/dl) in normal individuals but profound anemia in those whose red cell survival is already shortened.

Clinical features

B19 infection may be asymptomatic or may cause a mild febrile illness with rash. In children the first sign of infection is usually marked erythema of the cheeks or slapped cheek appearance often with relative circumoral pallor (Fig. 28.38). In volunteer studies, however, there is an initial febrile episode with headache, chills, myalgia and malaise associated with viremia and the rash appears about 7 days later (Fig. 28.39). Then 1–4 days after the slapped cheeks an itchy, erythematous, maculopapular rash develops on the trunk and limbs. As the rash on the limbs clears it leaves a lacy, reticular pattern. The rash may fluctuate over the next 1–3 weeks and a hot bath, for example, may lead to recrudescence of an evanescent rash.

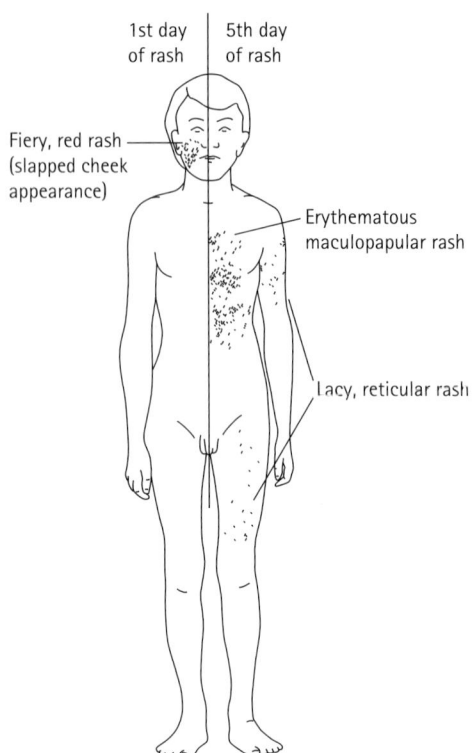

Fig. 28.38 The distribution and development of rash in erythema infectiosum (fifth disease).

Complications

Arthritis or arthralgia is more common in adults, but certainly can occur in children. It usually appears 1–6 days after the rash but there may be no history of rash at all. Arthritis is characteristically transient and asymmetrical, affecting wrists, knees, ankles, elbows and fingers, though it may persist for weeks or even months.

Children with a shortened red cell survival, such as those with sickle cell anemia, thalassemia major, hereditary spherocytosis or other hemolytic anemias, may have severe aplastic crises with hemoglobin levels falling as low as 1–2 g/dl and no reticulocytes.

Children with malignancy, particularly acute leukemia, or with HIV infection may develop prolonged anemia from chronic parvovirus B19 infection.

Infection during pregnancy can result in hydrops fetalis due to fetal anemia, which may be fatal, but no congenital syndrome has been described in babies of infected mothers who delivered at term.[584]

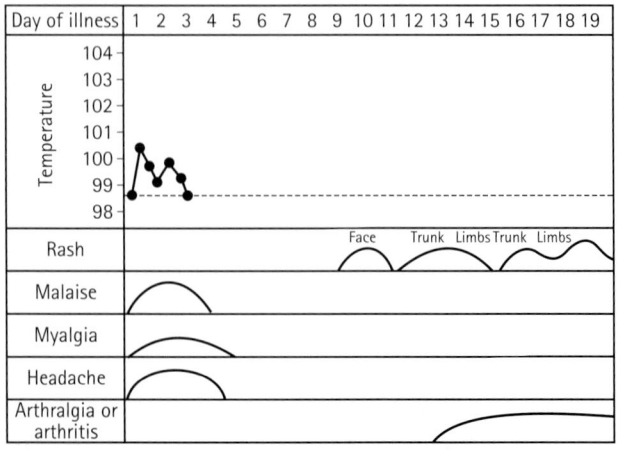

Fig. 28.39 The development of erythema infectiosum (fifth disease).

Encephalitis with or without neurological sequelae has rarely been reported after clinical erythema infectiosum, but it is not certain that this is a true complication of B19 infection.

Diagnosis

Erythema infectiosum may closely mimic rubella, and the two diseases can circulate concurrently. The slapped cheek appearance with circumoral pallor can be mistaken for scarlet fever.

The diagnosis can be made serologically by demonstrating parvovirus B19-specific IgM on an acute serum sample, although it is always better to get a paired sample in case there is a late rise in antibody. The virus can be detected by electron microscopy or PCR of plasma of patients with aplastic crises. This is particularly important in patients with sickle cell disease in whom severe anemia might be due to sequestration or pneumococcal sepsis. DNA probes and PCR have been used to detect the viral genome in stillbirths with hydrops fetalis and to demonstrate persisting antigen in children with leukemia and chronic anemia.

Treatment

There is no specific treatment. Isolation of patients is unnecessary since they are no longer infectious when the rash appears.

Arthritis may require salicylates or nonsteroidal anti-inflammatory agents. Children with aplastic crises may require blood transfusion until the red cell aplasia resolves spontaneously after 1–2 weeks.

ROSEOLA INFANTUM (SIXTH DISEASE, EXANTHEM SUBITUM, THREE DAY FEVER)

Roseola infantum is a common disease of infancy, characterized by fever and the appearance of an erythematous maculopapular rash as the fever defervesces. It may be confused with measles clinically. It is generally benign.

Etiology

Human herpesvirus 6 (HHV-6) is the main causative agent of roseola.[585,586] HHV-7 is responsible for most clinical cases of roseola infantum which are HHV-6 negative.[587] These double-stranded DNA viruses are members of the herpesvirus family, and as such, persist for the life of the host with frequent asymptomatic reactivation. There are two variant strains of HHV-6: type A and type B. Most of the primary infections in childhood are due to type B infection, and nearly 80% of children acquire HHV-6 by 2 years of age.[588] Primary HHV-6 infection is usually symptomatic and often results in presentation for medical evaluation.[588]

Clinical features

The illness starts abruptly with fever and some anorexia and irritability although in general the child appears relatively well. Mild cough, coryza, diarrhea and vomiting rarely occur. The pyrexia of 38.9–40.6 °C persists for 3–5 days, then falls precipitously as the rash appears (Fig. 28.40).[573] The rash is erythematous, with discrete macular or maculopapular

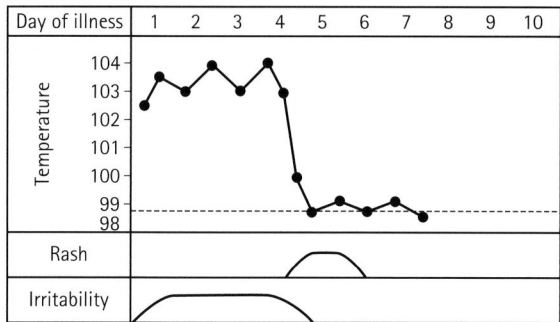

Fig. 28.40 The development of exanthem subitum. (From Krugman & Ward 1968[573])

lesions, and starts on the trunk and neck, sometimes spreading to the face and limbs. It lasts 1–2 days. Cervical lymphadenopathy is common and may sometimes be prominent: the suboccipital, posterior cervical and posterior auricular nodes are most commonly involved. There is no characteristic enanthem, although there may be pharyngitis, small exudative follicular tonsillar lesions, or small ulcers on the soft palate, tonsils and uvula.

For the first day or two of fever the white count is often elevated with a neutrophil leukocytosis, but then may fall as low as 3000/uL (3×10^9/L) predominantly lymphocytes with an absolute neutropenia.

A number of clinical syndromes (bone marrow suppression, pneumonia, hepatitis, encephalitis) have been associated with reactivation of HHV-6 in the immunocompromised, although a causal link has been difficult to prove.[586]

Complications

Convulsions may occur in association with roseola.[589] These are usually febrile convulsions but encephalitis has rarely been described, sometimes with severe residua such as hemiparesis or mental retardation. Rarely thrombocytopenic purpura may occur following roseola.[586]

Diagnosis

The diagnosis of roseola infantum is primarily clinical, although it can now be confirmed serologically. PCR assays to detect HHV-6 DNA are available, but cannot distinguish an acute infection from reactivation. The characteristic fever chart and discrete rash that does not become confluent distinguish roseola from other childhood exanthemata including measles. The rash may be confused with a drug rash if antibiotics have been given and a vaccine reaction may cause confusion if the illness comes on soon after immunization.

Treatment

There is no specific treatment. There are anecdotal reports of treatment of HHV-6 infection in immunocompromised children with ganciclovir, but there is no evidence to support efficacy from clinical trials. Antipyretics may lessen the risk of convulsions, but if these occur, encephalitis should be considered and the child treated appropriately.

HERPESVIRUSES

CHICKENPOX (VARICELLA)

Chickenpox is a common and highly infectious disease caused by varicella zoster virus (VZV). In general, chickenpox is relatively benign and has a virtually worldwide distribution. However, chickenpox is not endemic in some isolated areas and if introduced to such a community a more serious disease may occur. It can also prove severe and even fatal in neonates, when contracted by a patient on immunosuppressive drugs and rarely in previously healthy children and adults.[590]

Immunity following chickenpox is usually life-long and second primary attacks are rare. Like all herpesviruses, however, the virus can remain latent and recur years later, in the case of VZV, in the form of zoster (shingles).

Etiology

Chickenpox is transmitted from person to person by direct contact, droplet or airborne spread; infection can also arise through articles recently contaminated by an infected person. Viral entry is through the upper respiratory tract mucosa or via the conjunctiva. Infectivity is maximal during the prodromal period 1–2 days before the eruption of the rash and has completely waned by the time the eruption becomes crusted. In the immunocompromised, infectivity may continue after crusting has occurred if new lesions continue to develop.

The causative agent, VZV, is a large DNA herpesvirus. The virus is highly specific for humans and is very difficult to grow in culture in the laboratory.

Clinical features

Chickenpox is predominantly a disease of childhood and usually occurs between 2 and 8 years of age. Cases may occur in infancy. Peripartum intrauterine infection can lead to varicella neonatorum (see below) which, untreated, has a mortality up to 20%. Postnatal infection can cause classical chickenpox of a lesser severity occurring only in babies whose mothers have not had chickenpox.

Following an incubation period of 10–28 days, usually around 16 days, the disease starts with mild malaise and fever (Fig. 28.41).[573] In children prodromal symptoms may be absent and the illness begins with a rash. Older children and adults have more definite prodromata and symptoms include malaise, fever, headache, sore throat and backache.

The rash (Fig. 28.42)[573] commences as a crop of macules, which within hours pass through a papular stage to become vesicular; the vesicles persist

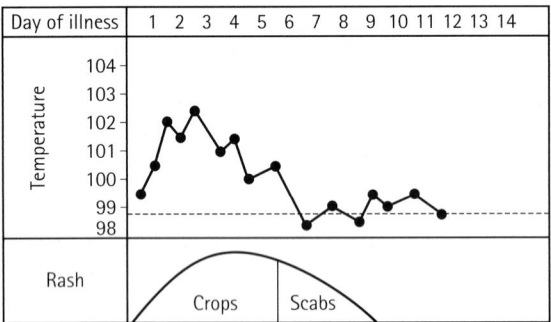

Fig. 28.41   The development of chickenpox. (From Krugman & Ward 1968[573])

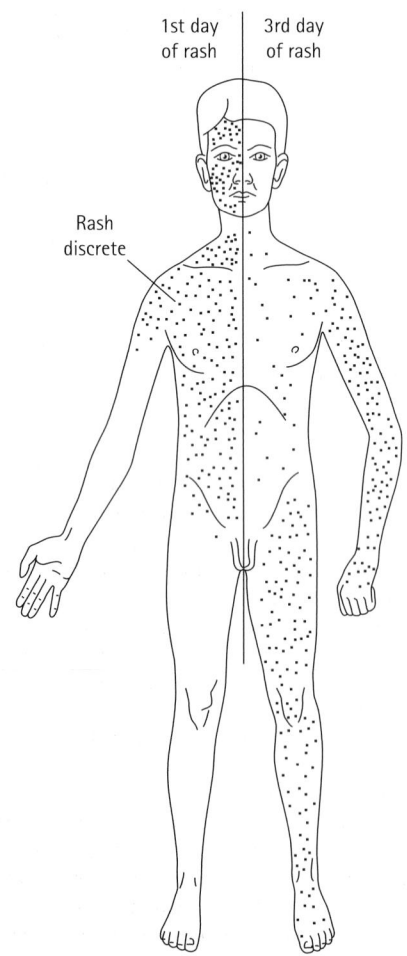

Fig. 28.42   The distribution of rash in chickenpox. (From Krugman & Ward 1968[573])

for 3–4 days, becoming pustular and finally forming a crust. The spots are superficial and the vesicles may be round, oval, elliptical or irregular in shape; they are often surrounded by a red areola. The rash is usually mild in children vaccinated against varicella with the Oka vaccine and may be atypical (maculopapular with few or no vesicles).[591]

Evolution of the rash occurs by a series of crops, and lesions at different stages may be seen. The trunk is principally involved but spots also appear over the face, scalp and the proximal parts of the limbs. Lesions tend to be more abundant on covered rather than exposed parts of the body.

In mild cases the entire eruption may consist of a few spots; less often, the rash is almost generalized, extending to the distal parts of the limbs including the soles and palms. By the time of vesiculation there is often an intense pruritus. In some patients crusts can be very tenacious and 2–3 weeks may elapse before their separation is complete.

An enanthem is usually found and presents as vesiculation over the palate, tongue or buccal mucous membranes; the conjunctivae and vagina may be similarly affected.

Hemorrhagic chickenpox

In this there is usually a marked constitutional disturbance and high fever. Extensive bleeding into the vesicles develops and the lesions become black; areas of ecchymosis can appear on otherwise uninvolved skin. Bleeding may occur from mucous membranes and present as hematuria or melena. Both children and adults may contract this form of chickenpox and it has been particularly reported in patients receiving corticosteroids or cytotoxic drugs suggesting the importance of cell mediated immunity as well as antibody in recovery from infection. It can be associated with profound thrombocytopenia (purpura fulminans) and is often fatal.

Varicella gangrenosa

This form of the disease usually results from severe secondary bacterial infection (usually due to group A streptococci) of the vesicles which may extend down to muscle. These lesions are slow to heal and can leave considerable scarring. Occasionally this form of varicella appears to start ab initio before any apparent secondary infection.

Varicella neonatorum

If the maternal rash appears less than 7 days before delivery or up to 2 days after delivery there is a risk that the baby will receive a large inoculum of virus without maternal antibody. Such babies are at very high risk of disseminated disease with death from pneumonitis, and should be protected at birth by giving zoster immune globulin (ZIG) (reviewed in Heuchan & Isaacs 2001[592]). Since this does not always protect them,[593] families of these infants should be informed of the risk of severe disease and early treatment with acycloguanosine (aciclovir) commenced promptly if symptoms develop. Babies whose mother's rash develops 7 days or more before or 3 days or more after delivery are at low risk. Postnatally acquired chickenpox is nearly always mild although if the mother has not had chickenpox the use of ZIG should be considered for a neonate exposed to the virus.

Varicella bullosa

Bullous varicella may occur in children, the lesions developing into large bullae with a positive Nikolsky sign. It is due to superinfection with a toxin-producing *Staphylococcus aureus*, and the prognosis for full recovery without scarring is excellent. Treatment is with antistaphylococcal antibiotics.

Complications

Sepsis

Secondary skin infection is the commonest complication. Abscesses may form locally or in regional lymph nodes. Cellulitis, erysipelas and scarlet fever can also develop. Bacteremic spread may give rise to pneumonia, osteomyelitis and septic arthritis. Common infecting organisms include group A streptococci and *S. aureus*.

Neurological

Postinfectious encephalitis can occur and usually starts as the rash reaches maturity. The most common manifestation is a pure cerebellar ataxia with an excellent prognosis. Complete recovery is virtually invariable, usually rapidly, though it may rarely take some weeks. Acute disseminated encephalomyelitis (ADEM) is a more sinister but rarer form of post varicella encephalitis with cerebral demyelination giving rise to long tract signs, cranial nerve lesions, convulsions, etc. Examination of the CSF may show a mild lymphocytic pleocytosis and slight elevation of the protein content. About 10% of cases of Reye syndrome occur secondary to chickenpox. Transverse myelitis, acute infantile hemiplegia and Guillain–Barré syndrome have been described complicating varicella.

Pneumonitis

Pneumonitis is usually seen in adults and immunocompromised children (and varicella neonatorum) and may present with acute respiratory distress or hemoptysis; diffuse nodular infiltration is seen on X-ray of the chest. The diagnosis is often obscure until the typical exanthem develops. Some cases die and, in those who recover, miliary calcification may be seen in the lung fields some years later.

In normal children, pneumonia complicating chickenpox is most likely to be bacterial, due to *S. pneumoniae*, group A streptococcus or occasionally *S. aureus*.

Others

Myocarditis, pericarditis, endocarditis, hepatitis and glomerulonephritis have rarely been reported. Appendicitis may also occur and can present before the eruptive phase; this sometimes leads to cross infection in pediatric surgical wards. Keratitis and conjunctivitis are rare and usually benign. Arthritis may mimic septic arthritis but the latter should always be excluded by examination of the joint fluid because septic arthritis can complicate chickenpox. If ampicillin is prescribed a drug eruption may occur as with EBV infection, probably as a result of drug–hapten interaction.

Congenital varicella

If the mother contracts chickenpox up to 20 weeks' gestation, there is about a 2% risk of the baby developing congenital varicella syndrome with cicatricial scarring of the limbs, cortical atrophy, hypoplasia of limbs, digital defects, retinitis or cataracts. Maternal chickenpox in the second 20 weeks of gestation may result in an inapparent primary infection in the fetus, and causes shingles in the first years of life in about 1% of exposed children.

Diagnosis

The clinical course of varicella and the nature of the rash are usually typical and a firm clinical diagnosis can be made. Rapid diagnosis can be by direct immunofluorescence (DFA) of cells scraped from the base of a vesicle and placed directly on a slide. DFA can also be performed on respiratory secretions obtained by nasopharyngeal aspirate or bronchoalveolar lavage for the diagnosis of infection in the immunocompromised.

VZV can be isolated from vesicle fluid collected during the first 3 or 4 days of the rash, but rarely from other sites. Tissue culture for varicella is not widely available. Detection of VZV DNA in body fluids or tissues by PCR is a sensitive technique that may be helpful in the diagnosis of VZV infection in the immunocompromised child.

A number of serological assays are available for diagnosis of past VZV infection that vary in their sensitivity. These have application in deciding if an exposed individual needs passive immunoprophylaxis. They can also be used to make a retrospective diagnosis of VZV infection if a significant rise in varicella IgG has occurred during the illness. In this setting, it is necessary to test two sera – an acute sample collected within a day or two of the onset of the illness and a convalescent sample collected 2 or 3 weeks later.

Differential diagnosis

Chickenpox can be confused with impetigo, scabies, dermatitis herpetiformis, eczema herpeticum or vaccinatum and erythema multiforme. In most of these the absence of the typical, centripetal distribution and cropping of varicella helps in the differentiation.

Treatment

General

No treatment is usually required and bed rest is probably unnecessary except in ill patients. Simple analgesics will control prodromal symptoms where these are troublesome. Aspirin should not be given because of the risk of Reye syndrome. Calamine lotion will normally soothe pruritus; if not, an antihistamine should be tried. If the enanthem is unusually severe careful oral toilet is needed and lesions on the conjunctiva should be protected from secondary infection. Treatment with aciclovir is indicated if infection develops in immunosuppressed cases, and in any patient with severe disease.

Sepsis

In convalescence, simple antiseptics should control superficial skin infection. More severe sepsis will require appropriate antibacterial chemotherapy, which should be guided by swabbing of the affected lesions and by cultures of the blood and of any pus. Flucloxacillin will adequately treat hemolytic streptococcal infection or staphylococcal infection until culture results are available.

Encephalitis

No specific treatment is available for the neurological complications and the usual supportive measures will be employed. Some clinicians favor the use of corticosteroids in severe cases despite the unhappy association of chickenpox with these drugs. It is argued that the encephalitis is of allergic origin and that by this stage of the illness there is sufficient antibody response to prevent further dissemination of the virus. In practice no serious untoward effects have been reported where steroids have been used in this condition although it is difficult to assess how much this therapy contributes to any recovery. Similarly the role of aciclovir in treating varicella encephalitis is unclear.

Others

Cases of severe varicella pneumonitis and profound thrombocytopenia have also been treated with aciclovir and corticosteroid drugs but an accurate evaluation of their benefit is impossible. Appendicitis should be treated surgically.

Prevention

The live attenuated Oka strain varicella vaccine is available in some countries for use in healthy children over 12 months of age or adults who have not had varicella. It has been shown to be highly effective (approximately 85% of children) in preventing clinical disease post exposure.[594] However, clinical disease in vaccinated persons is contagious and can sustain transmission, prompting the question of whether a two-dose regimen is required to prevent transmission during outbreaks. The Oka vaccine has been shown to be safe in solid organ transplant recipients post transplantation,[595] and in HIV infected children with CD4+ T cell counts ≥ 200 cells/μl (or 15%).[596]

The infectivity of chickenpox is such that the strictest isolation measures may fail to prevent its spread. In the community, it is usual practice to isolate a child from school or day care until the rash has become crusted. In the hospital setting, a child with active chickenpox should be quarantined in respiratory isolation while the rash remains vesicular.

Postexposure prophylaxis

In the case of patients who are receiving corticosteroid drugs or cytotoxic drugs, every effort should be made to prevent exposure to chickenpox and herpes zoster for reasons already described. If such exposure should occur then hyperimmune chickenpox gamma globulin (ZIG) has been shown to modify severity even if it does not always prevent the disease, and should be given. The use of ZIG in neonates has already been discussed. Chemoprophylaxis with aciclovir after exposure to VZV reduced the likelihood of clinical disease in a few small case control studies,[597-599] but has not been assessed in a properly evaluated randomized controlled trial and is not routinely advocated.[600] Postexposure immunization with the Oka VZV vaccine has been shown to protect against or modify chickenpox in nonrandomized cohort studies.[601] It is thought to be most effective if given within 5 days of exposure.

HERPES ZOSTER (ZOSTER: SHINGLES)

The clinical relationship between chickenpox and herpes zoster has long been recognized. The virus causing the two syndromes is identical, and is referred to as the varicella zoster virus (VZV). Non-immune persons may develop chickenpox when exposed to herpes zoster but the converse rarely occurs. The inoculation of children with virus obtained from zoster patients has resulted in clinical chickenpox which has then spread to other children as chickenpox.

Following an attack of varicella, the virus survives in a latent form in the sensory root ganglia of the cord and brain, a situation with similarities to latent infection by HSV. After an interval of many years, but sometimes earlier, the virus becomes activated by local precipitating factors or by some depression of protective immunological mechanisms. Virus then spreads along the sensory root in question; adjacent motor areas of the cord, or other parts of the cerebrum, may become involved. A degree of systemic spread can also occur which provokes a modified form of chickenpox. Such modification may result from the antigenic stimulus provided by the reactivated virus, and the very high antibody levels found early in the course of herpes zoster support this impression.

Patients who develop zoster are usually elderly, but the disease does occur in children and younger adults. In young children, pain is much less marked than in adults, and zoster is not suggestive of immune deficiency or malignancy. There is often a history of maternal varicella during pregnancy or early neonatal varicella: it is thought that varicella at a time of relatively poor immunity is more likely to result in childhood zoster. In a few instances, primary infection by VZV appears to provoke zoster rather than chickenpox; the explanation is not known. On occasion zoster may also occur simultaneously with a primary attack of chickenpox.

For reasons alluded to above, zoster is seen quite frequently in persons suffering from leukemia or other malignant disease and can follow radiotherapy.

Clinical features

Zoster may start with constitutional disturbance or progressive pain over a particular dermatome, although in children zoster may be pain free. Clusters of macules and papules appear on the skin overlying the dermatome, rarely crossing the midline. These soon vesiculate and the vesicles formed may be larger than in chickenpox and tend to coalesce. Extensive crusting follows, which slowly separates to expose a raw, ulcerated area. This will bleed readily and is susceptible to secondary infection. Healing is slow, vitiligo may develop after months or years and the involved skin is often anesthetic. Enlargement of the regional lymph nodes is very common.

Acute pain tends to subside as crusting sets in, but extreme irritation and neuralgia may persist for months and even years (post-herpetic neuralgia). In children the illness tends to be much milder, pain is mild or absent and recovery is considerably quicker.

Thoracic segments are most commonly involved in the community, but zoster of the trigeminal nerve, and usually of the ophthalmic division, is the commonest variety seen in hospital.

Geniculate herpes is of special interest and is frequently misdiagnosed; in this form of zoster, vesicles appear on the meatus and pinna of the ear. Pain may be experienced in the throat, in or behind the ear, and taste may be lost over the anterior two thirds of the tongue. Facial paralysis, sometimes permanent, may result. This condition is sometimes referred to as the *Ramsay Hunt* syndrome. A modified generalized rash over the trunk and face is seen in many cases provided examination is sufficiently diligent. Other features include involvement of the adjacent motor root with resultant paralysis, which can be permanent, and meningitis, encephalitis or myelitis can be encountered.

Occasionally zoster occurs without any accompanying rash, the so-called 'zoster sine herpete'.

Diagnosis

Prior to the appearance of the skin eruption diagnosis is difficult in children, in whom zoster is rather unexpected. Diagnoses such as pleurisy or fibrositis may be made but the difficulties are quickly resolved when the classical rash, along the line of a nerve, makes its appearance. If it is in a distribution that looks dermatomal, HSV infection may sometimes be mistaken for zoster. Laboratory tests are referred to in the section on chickenpox.

Treatment

The illness is usually mild in children and simple analgesics such as paracetamol will usually control pain. Relief may follow the application of a dusting powder of zinc oxide or the use of cold sprays.

Ophthalmic zoster requires special care because of the danger to the eyes. Topical or systemic antivirals may be needed for ophthalmic VZV. Consultation with an ophthalmologist is advisable.

In some instances, particularly severe zoster may show a dramatic response to treatment by corticosteroid drugs. However, their general use is not advised and they are best avoided in zoster affecting the eye and wherever any underlying immunological defect may be present. Aciclovir may be needed for immunocompromised children or those with severe zoster.

High doses of the live attenuated Oka vaccine (known as the 'zoster vaccine') have been shown to reduce disease incidence and severity in the elderly,[602] but the vaccine has not been evaluated for use in children or young adults.

Prognosis

This is usually good. Post-herpetic neuralgia is uncommon in children. Certain paralyses can prove permanent and impairment of vision has followed ophthalmic zoster. Such complications are more commonly found in adult cases.

HERPES SIMPLEX VIRUS

Primary infection by *Herpesvirus hominis* (HSV) usually occurs in early childhood and is generally subclinical. However, in a small percentage of children it may produce a variable clinical illness, the main features of which include localized vesiculation on some part of the body and a sharp constitutional reaction. Some children avoid infection altogether and may reach adolescence or adult life with no immunity to this virus. This is more likely to occur when they have been brought up in rural, as opposed to urban, areas and, as with many other viral infections, an attack in adult life can often be more severe.

An interesting feature of this virus is its ability to persist in a latent form once the primary infection, whether clinical or subclinical, has subsided. In some people, the virus becomes reactivated by certain nonspecific stimuli at various times in their lives and the resultant clinical manifestations tend to differ from those seen with primary infection. Reactivation of HSV with asymptomatic shedding or, less commonly, clinical disease is a common event after the initial infection.[603]

Etiology

HSV is a DNA virus surrounded by a membrane and is approximately 150–180 nm in diameter. There are two strains, HSV types 1 and 2. HSV type 2 primarily infects the genital tracts of adults, and infection in the pregnant woman near term can result in serious infection in the newborn infant. HSV type 1 is primarily oral, although type 2 can cause oral disease and type 1 can infect the genitalia.

Clinical features

A variety of different syndromes may result from primary infection by HSV beyond the neonatal period. Neonatal HSV disease is discussed in Chapter 12.

Acute herpetic gingivostomatitis (ulcerative stomatitis)

This, the commonest manifestation, commences with a sharp constitutional reaction with high fever, malaise, anorexia and irritability. The patient, usually a young child, has difficulty feeding due to pain in the mouth. Inspection, often hampered by severe discomfort, reveals marked swelling and inflammation of the gums which may bleed at the merest touch. Deeper inspection will reveal the typical shallow ulcers, white in color, on such sites as the tongue, palate, gums, buccal mucosa and tonsils. In mild cases, the ulcers are few; in more severe examples there may be a contiguous sheet of ulcers involving all the sites mentioned. Saliva tends to flow from the mouth and satellite lesions form down the chin or cheek where the child dribbles. Considerable swelling of the face and neck may accompany or even precede the appearance of lesions and cause diagnostic confusion. Mild cases subside rapidly but the worst may take up to 2 weeks before the local lesions disappear. Younger children may implant the virus onto other sites such as the sucked finger or perineal region, where vesiculation will develop. The isolation of HSV2 from an oropharyngeal lesion in a child prior to puberty should raise the question of sexual abuse.

Perineal herpes (acute herpetic vulvovaginitis)

This is a less common primary manifestation, though it may be underdiagnosed in view of confusion with severe napkin and other eruptions in the same area. It is diagnosed far more often in girls, though primary perineal herpes sometimes occurs in boys. Some degree of constitutional upset will again herald the infection, to be followed by painful vesiculation over the perineum, which may extend into the vagina in girls. Lesions close to the external urethral orifice may cause difficulties with micturition and regional adenitis may develop. The lesions usually subside without scarring despite the likelihood of secondary infection. Reactivation occurs over the buttocks, thighs or perineum.

Traumatic herpetic infection

The intact skin appears relatively resistant to this virus but primary infection may arise over the site of abrasions and burns. An interesting variety is the herpetic whitlow of the finger which is sometimes seen in nurses who contract the infection by virus entering such lesions as needle puncture wounds or the abrasions that can result from opening glass phials – lesions that are common on the nurse's hand. Here again there may be a marked constitutional upset and regional lymphadenitis.

Acute herpetic keratoconjunctivitis

Primary herpetic infection of the eye is a serious presentation of this infection though relatively rare. The majority of cases are due to HSV1, although HSV2 eye disease may occur as a consequence of neonatal infection. Normally only one eye is involved and cases present with constitutional upset and pain. Marked reddening and edema appear on the affected conjunctiva, the cornea becomes hazy and the eye will usually close. Vesicles appear around the lids and a purulent discharge often occurs. So long as the infection remains superficial the condition will usually subside without complications in 10–14 days. Deeper involvement may give rise to keratitis disciformis, hypopyon keratitis or iridocyclitis, all of which may be followed by scarring; however, these are more commonly encountered in recurrent herpetic infection. Recurrent herpetic keratitis has been shown to be an immune-mediated phenomenon.[604]

Kaposi varicelliform eruption (KVE) or eczema herpeticum

Children with eczema are prone to superinfection of the involved skin by a number of organisms including HSV. The disease starts with a particularly sharp constitutional upset and vesicles then appear on the skin and are most intense at the eczematous areas. An experienced observer may readily recognize the condition; more often the true diagnosis is unappreciated and extensive secondary infection accompanied by a marked serosanguinous discharge will develop. Further crops of vesicles may appear and the child's condition may deteriorate further. The most severe cases may be fatal without aciclovir therapy. In the remainder there is a slow recovery over a period of 3–4 weeks.

Primary herpetic meningoencephalitis

Previously considered an infrequent infection, modern virological techniques have shown that herpetic meningoencephalitis is more common than was believed. The signs of CNS involvement may appear shortly after a primary lesion at some other site but there is usually no clinical evidence to indicate the basic etiological agent. Cases may present as mild forms of aseptic meningitis or as a rapidly fatal form of encephalitis principally involving the temporal lobes. Recently, a genetic etiology for HSV encephalitis was demonstrated in two children with autosomal recessive deficiency in the intracellular protein UNC-93B, resulting in impaired cellular type I interferon responses.[605]

Clinical features: recurrent herpes

Exacerbations of latent HSV infection may be provoked by a variety of nonspecific stimuli which include upper respiratory infections, any febrile illness, gastrointestinal upsets, overexposure to sunlight and emotional upsets. Drugs and certain foods have also been incriminated.

Whatever the excitant, recurrent herpes presents as a crop of tiny vesicles which are sometimes painful and after a few days will dry up to form a scab. They may erupt on almost any part of the skin or on the mucous membranes of the mouth, conjunctivae or genitalia. The most usual site is on the skin around the nose and mouth (cold sores). Exacerbations tend to recur at the same site in any particular individual. Recurrent herpes gives rise to little or no constitutional upset or fever but the excitant, such as lobar pneumonia, may do so.

Diagnosis

The clinical features are often diagnostic in themselves but resort to laboratory aid is of help in certain instances. The procedures most commonly employed are:

1. growth of the virus in tissue culture;
2. demonstration of viral antigens in the material by a fluorescent antibody technique;
3. detection of HSV DNA in CSF or other bodily secretion or tissue by PCR.

Other procedures that may be employed are:

4. demonstration under the electron microscope of herpesvirus particles in material taken from a lesion;
5. antibody estimations on acute and convalescent serum samples to show specific IgM or a significant rise in IgG during a suspected primary infection;
6. histological evidence of intranuclear inclusions and giant cells.

Primary herpes

The oral lesions of primary herpetic gingivostomatitis may be confused with a variety of conditions such as thrush, tonsillitis, Vincent's stomatitis, agranulocytosis and leukemia. Careful clinical and laboratory studies readily differentiate most of these but herpangina, due to infection by coxsackie viruses group A, can cause genuine confusion; however, gingivitis does not normally accompany herpangina, but is common in herpetic infections. Virus studies may be needed in difficult cases. Herpetic vulvovaginitis is readily confused with ammoniacal dermatitis which has been secondarily infected. Impetigo of the vulva is usually accompanied by involvement elsewhere. Kaposi varicelliform eruption (eczema herpeticum) may be confused with bacterial superinfection of eczema, with eczema vaccinatum and occasionally with varicella. Herpetic meningoencephalitis is difficult to diagnose on clinical grounds; usually virological studies are required to make a conclusive diagnosis.

Recurrent herpes

Recurrent herpes produces a fairly precise diagnostic picture, but on occasion can resemble herpes zoster. The absence of pain, lack of a definable neurological distribution and differing nature of the vesicles should differentiate these conditions.

Treatment

As a rule, primary oral herpetic infections do not require other than supportive treatment. Children with severe gingivostomatitis may have feeding difficulties due to pain, and careful coaxing will be needed to ensure adequate hydration; cleansing of the mouth is also difficult on account of this pain. Irritating acidic fluids should be avoided and diet restricted to cold, bland drinks during the most acute phase. Superinfection by *Candida* may occur but this usually responds to treatment by the local application of nystatin suspension; secondary bacterial infection rarely warrants any antibiotic therapy though this may be required in herpetic vulvovaginitis. Intravenous aciclovir should be reserved for children requiring hospital admission for intravenous rehydration.

Eye involvement is best managed by an experienced ophthalmologist. Herpetic infections are amongst the few viral diseases in which highly successful treatment by antiviral agents has been reported; topical 5-iodo-2-deoxyuridine (IDU) or aciclovir are effective in herpetic eye infections.[606] Intravenous aciclovir is the treatment of choice for herpes simplex encephalitis, for KVE and for any manifestations of HSV disease in a neonate.

CYTOMEGALOVIRUS INFECTIONS

Cytomegalovirus (CMV) is a DNA virus of the herpesvirus group and as such, after the primary infection, causes latent infection with frequent subclinical reactivations for the life of the host. It is ubiquitous in the community, and in the immunocompetent host usually results in asymptomatic infection. CMV infection of the fetus and newborn (congenital and perinatal CMV infection) is discussed in Chapter 12. CMV can cause life-threatening disease in immunocompromised patients with HIV infection, or post solid organ or bone marrow transplantation, either after a primary infection or when a latent infection becomes reactivated.

Clinical features

In immunocompetent older children and adults, CMV infection is usually asymptomatic. On occasion, it may present with fever, cough, headaches and pains in the back and limbs. The clinical picture is one of infectious mononucleosis, with lymphadenopathy, hepatosplenomegaly and sometimes jaundice. Examination of the peripheral blood reveals the presence of atypical lymphocytes, and there is a varying degree of derangement in liver function tests. Hemolytic anemia can occur, and cold agglutinins, cryoglobulins and antinuclear factor may be present. Ampicillin may cause a rash as in EBV infection. CMV may produce a pneumonitis but this is usually seen in premature neonates with postnatally acquired infection or in children suffering from underlying diseases such as chronic hepatic disorders, leukemia and other malignancies.

A febrile illness with features suggesting infectious mononucleosis may also be encountered in patients who have recently undergone open heart surgery or organ transplantation and investigation of obscure postoperative illness in such cases should include tests for CMV infection. In patients with immune deficiency, particularly AIDS patients, CMV may cause pneumonitis, hepatitis, encephalitis or myelitis, severe retinitis and colitis. HIV infected children who acquire CMV during the first 4 years of life have been shown to have a more rapid progression to AIDS than those who remain CMV negative.[607] CMV is a frequent cause of hepatitis, pneumonitis or graft rejection in solid organ transplant recipients and is associated with increased rates of co-infection with other opportunistic pathogens in these individuals. The virus is usually acquired from the donor organ or blood products, although reactivation of latent host CMV may also occur.

Laboratory diagnosis

Histological lesions due to CMV infection are characterized by large cells containing intranuclear and cytoplasmic inclusion bodies. The inclusion-containing cells may be widely disseminated.

Rapid viral diagnosis using DNA probes or by early immunofluorescence testing of tissue cultures (so-called 'shell vial cultures') or detection of the CMV pp65 antigen in blood is particularly useful in the management of suspected CMV infection in immunocompromised patients.

A clinical diagnosis may be confirmed by:

1. isolation of the virus from urine, peripheral blood mononuclear cells, or other secretions;
2. demonstration of a significant rise in antibody titer during the illness;
3. the presence of typical histological lesions in a biopsy specimen, e.g. liver;
4. typical inclusion bodies in cell deposits of fresh urine.

With improved virological techniques, efforts should always be made to grow CMV when infection is suspected. Suitable specimens are fresh urine samples and saliva swabs but these specimens must be delivered to the laboratory with minimum delay as the virus easily loses its infectivity. Isolation of the agent is usually carried out in tissue cultures of human fibroblasts.

Quantification of the amount of CMV DNA or antigen in blood or other secretions to monitor recurrence and allow early pre-emptive therapy in the immunocompromised child is currently being evaluated.[608]

Differential diagnosis

CMV infections acquired in later life may mimic a variety of febrile states but infectious mononucleosis is the most likely condition to cause confusion. Where jaundice occurs, infectious hepatitis, serum hepatitis and leptospirosis require exclusion.

Prevention

Blood products from CMV antibody negative donors should always be given to preterm neonates and immunocompromised patients, particularly post-transplant or HIV infected patients. Alternatively, as the virus is cell associated, filtration or freezing of the donor blood to remove white cells also reduces the risk of acquired CMV infection.

Passive immunoprophylaxis of transplant patients with immunoglobulin is partially successful in reducing the risk of CMV infection. Seropositive CMV patients may reactivate when immunosuppressed, and interferon but not aciclovir reduces this risk.

Treatment

Ganciclovir, a derivative of aciclovir, has been successfully used to treat immunocompromised patients with CMV retinitis, enteritis and pneumonitis.[609] In adult patients, 70–80% cease excretion of CMV within a week, with the exception of marrow transplant patients with CMV pneumonitis, of whom somewhat fewer respond. However, relapse occurs in about half when ganciclovir is stopped, it causes significant marrow suppression, and the drug is incorporated into the host genome. Milder CMV disease can be treated with oral valganciclovir.

Foscarnet causes less marrow suppression, although transient renal impairment may occur. There are few controlled data on its use in CMV infections in childhood. Cidofovir is another antiviral agent with activity against CMV. Its main use is in CMV retinitis or prophylaxis in the organ transplant population.

Prophylaxis with oral antiviral agents in solid organ transplant recipients to prevent CMV disease has been recently demonstrated to be successful in a meta-analysis.[610]

Prognosis

Congenital CMV infection has a variable outcome. Normal individuals who contract CMV infection rarely suffer any sequelae, but in immunocompromised patients, blindness due to retinitis, graft rejection and death from pneumonitis, hepatitis and disseminated CMV infection or opportunistic infection may occur.

EPSTEIN–BARR VIRUS

EBV is the cause of infectious mononucleosis or glandular fever, a disease primarily of older children, adolescents and young adults. An almost identical syndrome can be caused by CMV and *Toxoplasma gondii* as well as EBV. An anginose form of glandular fever primarily affecting the tonsils is seen in younger children under 5 years of age. EBV is a DNA virus and like the other herpesviruses can persist in a latent state and reactivate. It has a worldwide distribution, is potentially oncogenic and has been linked with nasopharyngeal carcinoma, Burkitt lymphoma and other lymphomas, particularly in immunocompromised patients. It can also cause lymphoproliferative syndromes post transplant or in the HIV infected individual.

Etiology and epidemiology

Primary infection of the lymphoid tissue of the nasopharynx may be asymptomatic or may lead to symptomatic infection of lymph nodes. Humans are the only source of EBV, transmission is by the respiratory route and the virus is of low infectivity, usually requiring intimate oral contact. The 'kissing disease' refers to its spread among adolescents and young adults by this route. Epidemics are unusual. The virus persists in the nasopharynx and the uterine cervix. The virus primarily infects B lymphocytes but the atypical mononuclear cells seen in the blood film are activated T lymphocytes.

Clinical features

The anginose form of glandular fever is characterized by fever and sore throat with moderate or marked cervical lymphadenopathy. The tonsils are red and inflamed and there is often exudative folliculitis with white exudate. Other lymph nodes and spleen are rarely enlarged and the clinical picture is not readily distinguishable from acute streptococcal tonsillitis, except that EBV is more likely to cause palatal petechiae.

Glandular fever often starts insidiously with malaise, anorexia and fever, and sore throat is usually a prominent symptom. Occasionally the patient merely has malaise and fever for 1–3 weeks with chills and sweats (febrile form of infectious mononucleosis) and presents with pyrexia of unknown origin. Generally, however, there is marked enlargement of posterior and anterior cervical lymph nodes, and the suboccipital, postauricular, axillary, epitrochlear and inguinal nodes may also be enlarged (glandular form). The tonsils may be inflamed with exudate and rarely this can be sufficient to impair swallowing and even breathing. Splenomegaly is usual and hepatomegaly may also be present, sometimes with jaundice.

Skin eruptions occur in about 10–15% of cases. Most common is a widespread maculopapular rash but morbilliform, scarlatiniform, purpuric and urticarial rashes may occur. Ampicillin (or amoxicillin) causes a particularly florid, confluent maculopapular rash in EBV infection, and the ampicillin rash may be seen less commonly in conjunction with other herpesvirus infections, such as CMV and chickenpox.

In Duncan syndrome, or X-linked lymphoproliferative disease, affected males are unable to control EBV infection and develop generalized lymphadenopathy and hepatosplenomegaly which persists and is rapidly fatal. These patients usually have persistently high levels of IgG antibodies to the viral capsid antigen (VCA).

EBV may be responsible for the lymphoid interstitial pneumonitis that can occur in children with HIV infection, since the EBV genome has been demonstrated in lung biopsy specimens from these patients. It can also cause CNS and other lymphomas in patients with HIV infection.

Complications

Threatened obstruction of the airway may occur in the severe anginose variety, especially when there is secondary edema in the neck. Neurological complications include aseptic meningitis, cranial nerve palsies (including Bell's palsy), encephalomyelitis, transverse myelitis and Guillain–Barré syndrome. Cardiac involvement may present as myocarditis or as transient arrhythmias. Other complications include pneumonitis, orchitis, rupture of the spleen, hemolytic anemia, thrombocytopenic purpura and various ocular manifestations; hepatic involvement has been referred to previously. A prolonged illness with fatigue and relapses over many months has occasionally been described in children, in association

with raised EBV antibodies. Chronic EBV infection is not a common cause of the 'chronic fatigue syndrome' or myalgic encephalopathy (ME).

EBV is thought to be the cause of Burkitt lymphoma and of nasopharyngeal carcinoma, in both of which tumors the EBV genome can consistently be demonstrated.

Diagnosis

Five main points arise in the diagnosis of glandular fever: a suggestive clinical picture, typical changes in the peripheral blood, a positive heterophile antibody test, IgM antibody to EBV, and certain nonspecific changes in other laboratory tests.

Blood changes

Most important is the presence of large, atypical mononuclear cells which have an irregular nucleus, whose cytoplasm contains vacuoles, and which have characteristic pale staining of the cellular cytoplasm. Often there is a leukocytosis of $10–20 \times 10^9$ cells/L and sometimes the predominant cells are initially polymorphonuclear. However, atypical monocytes and lymphocytes soon appear, or may be present from the outset, and these can represent from 5 to 50% of the total leukocyte count. Other changes in the blood include occasional leukopenia and rare instances of profound thrombocytopenia and transient autoimmune hemolytic anemia.

Heterophile antibody test (Paul–Bunnell reaction)

There is massive B cell activation in acute EBV infection resulting in an outpouring of nonspecific antibodies. Sheep red cell agglutinins (heterophile antibodies) develop frequently by the second week of infectious mononucleosis, but occasionally not for 2 or 3 weeks, so an early negative test should be repeated.

Sheep red cell agglutinins are not specific for infectious mononucleosis and may occur in other conditions. However, by means of absorption tests using guinea pig kidney and ox erythrocytes the specificity of the test may be increased. The following are the salient features:

1. Antibodies present in infectious mononucleosis are not absorbed by guinea pig kidney but are absorbed by ox erythrocytes.
2. Antibodies found in normal serum are not absorbed by ox erythrocytes but they are absorbed by guinea pig kidney.
3. Antibodies found in serum sickness are absorbed by both guinea pig kidney and ox erythrocytes.

Agglutinins to horse erythrocytes may also be present in the serum of a patient suffering from infectious mononucleosis and in many laboratories a test based on the agglutination of horse erythrocytes is in use. This is the basis of the rapid slide test, the 'Monospot' test. This test may sometimes be negative early in the disease and if EBV is suspected should be repeated. The test is unreliable under 5 years of age, owing to false negative results.

EBV antibody tests

The presence of specific EBV anti-VCA IgM antibody indicates a recent or current infection, whereas the presence of IgG antibodies to the VCA or nuclear antigen (EBNA) merely indicates an infection with EBV some time in the past. Only a small proportion of affected patients show a rise in IgG to VCA, so the IgM test is preferred to show acute infection.

Nonspecific laboratory tests

In well over half the cases some derangement of liver function tests will be found. Most often there is a mild or moderate rise in the serum alanine aminotransferase (AAT) or glutamic pyruvate transaminase (SGPT) level but the alkaline phosphatase and serum bilirubin levels may also rise. Usually these changes are transient but in cases with clinical evidence of hepatic involvement the derangement in liver function tests is more marked.

On occasion, a false positive Wassermann reaction occurs in infectious mononucleosis. High antistreptolysin 'O' titers may be found, probably due to an anamnestic reaction.

The detection of EBV DNA by PCR or in situ hybridization in saliva or tissue of an immunocompromised child may indicate a lymphoproliferative syndrome.

Differential diagnosis

Infectious mononucleosis may be diagnosed too readily. Young children with mild fever and lymph node enlargement in the neck are more likely to have a respiratory viral infection.

Cases that present with fever and little else may be confused with influenza, brucellosis or typhoid; those with a sore throat need to be differentiated from streptococcal or other viral tonsillitis, diphtheria, agranulocytosis and leukemia. Glandular enlargement may be mistaken for toxoplasmosis, CMV infection or reticulosis, and the icteric form of the disease has to be distinguished from infectious hepatitis, leptospirosis and, occasionally, from obstructive liver disease.

The skin eruption of glandular fever has produced confusion with measles, rubella, secondary syphilis, Kawasaki disease and drug rashes.

Treatment

There is no specific treatment. Aciclovir has virtually no in vivo activity against EBV. The disease tends to be mild in children, but simple analgesics may be required to ease pain and gargles to soothe the sore throat. There is increasing evidence that antibiotics can do more harm than good, as toxic skin eruptions appear to follow their use, and ampicillin is especially incriminated in this direction. However, in cases where significant secondary infection is fully substantiated, antibiotics may need to be employed. Corticosteroids can have a dramatic, symptomatic effect but should be reserved for cases where edema of the airway is severe or where life-threatening complications such as thrombocytopenic purpura or severe neurological involvement are encountered. Reduction of immunosuppression or bone marrow transplantation may be of value in the management of EBV lymphoproliferative diseases.[611]

Prognosis

The prognosis is good and children recover more quickly than adults, though some cases run a protracted course and patients may take months to recover their full health. Death is rare and usually results from rupture of the spleen or severe neurological involvement. Recurrences in the immediate convalescent phase can occur but are usually short-lived.

VIRAL AND ALLIED INFECTIONS OF THE RESPIRATORY TRACT

Infections of the respiratory tract are frequent and ubiquitous. They are the most common cause of illness in almost any age group and have a predilection for the extremes of life. Agents that are capable of attacking one part or another of the respiratory tract include viruses, rickettsiae, mycoplasmas and fungi.

Respiratory infection frequently results from a combination of different organisms because, once the initial assault has damaged the defensive mechanisms within the air passages, secondary infection is readily superimposed. This often renders it difficult to prove the primary cause. Nevertheless, detailed studies on the etiology of acute respiratory tract infection indicate that up to 85% of such disease may be initiated by a virus.

In the ensuing account a description is given of the various viruses and allied organisms which play a significant role in the production of infective respiratory disease.

INFLUENZA

Influenza is an acute infectious disease of variable severity with an emphasis on general illness rather than on symptoms arising from the respiratory tract. It tends to occur in pandemic form every few years. In most instances the disease is a benign condition, but it may have a devastating effect in some normal children. Disease is often more severe with an increased mortality in immunosuppressed patients or those with chronic cardiorespiratory disease.

Etiology

Influenza viruses are RNA viruses of the orthomyxovirus family. There are three antigenic types: A, B and C. Infection by type C is relatively uncommon, results in mild or inapparent illness and does not produce epidemics. Type B virus produces significant illness, followed by reasonably effective immunity. Outbreaks or small epidemics may occur, especially in schoolchildren, but are often of a localized nature. Some variation in antigenicity of type B virus occurs and outbreaks appear sporadically at intervals of 3–6 years.

Most clinical, virological and epidemiological interest is focused upon type A viruses, as these produce the most noteworthy outbreaks or epidemics and, when major new variants emerge, pandemics. Pandemics have usually been identified by titles that reflect the suspected geographical origin, as in 'Asian flu' or 'Hong Kong flu'. The World Health Organization has devised a more definitive classification of influenza viruses which reflects the nature of mutation more precisely.[612] Influenza strains that cross the species barrier pose an increasing pandemic threat as shown by the recently identified avian influenza A strain (H5N1).[613]

Structurally, influenza viruses comprise a central core of ribonucleoprotein with a covering envelope. From this envelope spikes containing hemagglutinins project and between these spikes are mushroom-shaped protrusions composed of neuraminidase.

Each basic type of influenza (A, B or C) has its own distinctive ribonucleoprotein consisting of the S or soluble antigen. Protein antigens on the viral surface are related to hemagglutinins (the H antigens) and to neuraminidases (the N antigens). In the case of type A viruses minor changes may occur year by year, producing what is known as antigenic drift. However, at intervals usually exceeding a decade, major changes take place producing antigenic shift. The virtually new type A virus that emerges as a result of antigenic shift has thus acquired the potential to produce a pandemic.

Strain designation of influenza viruses is, therefore, based on the following points:

1. identification of the S antigen – that is, whether the virus is type A, B or C;
2. the host origin – when isolated initially from man, no specific identification is recorded but, if from an animal source, a suitable suffix is appended;
3. the geographical origin;
4. the strain number and the subtype of the hemagglutinin and neuraminidase identified;
5. the year of isolation.

Without an appreciation of the relatively complex antigenic structure and its variation, an understanding of the epidemiology of influenza is difficult.[614] Furthermore, effective vaccination requires using vaccines whose antigenic components accurately reflect the strain of influenza virus prevalent at the time of use.

Epidemiology

Man is the principal reservoir of infection and the disease is transmitted by direct contact, through droplet infection and by articles that have been freshly soiled with discharges from the nose or throat of infected persons. Infectivity appears to persist for 4–5 days after the clinical onset of the disease. Occasional cases originate from animals, e.g. pigs or chickens. In view of the high infectivity of influenza and the rapidity of modern travel, an epidemic can soon develop pandemic proportions. Human infection with avian influenza A strain (H5N1) was initially described in Vietnam, but the virus has now been isolated from individuals in most parts of the world.[613] It infects humans in contact with diseased birds and is associated with high mortality rates due to respiratory failure. At the current time, only low levels of human to human transmission of H5N1 have been shown to occur, but an increase in transmission efficiency via this route could result in a major world pandemic.

Pathogenesis

Influenza infection causes necrosis of ciliated respiratory epithelium and this commences in the nose and spreads downwards to the trachea and bronchi. Edema and leukocyte infiltration follow causing pharyngitis, tracheitis and bronchitis; in severe cases considerable exudation of blood and edema fluid may occur and enter the alveoli with resultant pneumonia.

Primary respiratory damage from influenza virus may in itself produce a severe illness, but secondary bacterial infection is more often the cause of fatal pneumonia; organisms such as *Staphylococcus aureus* and *Klebsiella pneumoniae* are particularly dangerous in this context.

Clinical features

The incubation period of influenza is short and ranges from 1 to 3 days. In children over 5 years of age there is a sudden onset of fever, headache and shivering, with pains in the limbs and back. Anorexia, listlessness and malaise may also be experienced and in some instances, particularly in children, nausea and vomiting may be unduly pronounced. Abdominal pain ('gastric flu') can be a prominent symptom. A dry, painful cough, discomfort in the throat, hoarseness and nasal discharge are usual.

The temperature may reach 39–40 °C, but apart from signs of pharyngitis, objective physical findings are few and in uncomplicated cases clinical and radiographic examination of the chest is usually clear. Leukopenia will be found in uncomplicated cases and the ESR becomes moderately elevated.

The illness usually runs a short course and is followed by rapid improvement. Some patients experience a period of mental and physical lethargy in convalescence but seriously complicated cases are rarely seen outside epidemics.

In younger children and infants influenza A typically causes high fever (over 39 °C) and upper respiratory tract infection with coryza, cough, irritability and pharyngitis. Otitis media, laryngotracheitis, bronchitis, bronchiolitis indistinguishable from that due to RSV, and pneumonia may all occur. Vomiting and diarrhea are frequent in infants. Febrile convulsions are frequent, as are fleeting erythematous rashes, which can be morbilliform. Despite these manifestations, a recent large scale epidemiological study in the USA confirmed that a significant burden of influenza disease in infants and young children goes unrecognized.[615] The risk of severe lower respiratory tract involvement is greater in immunocompromised children, and in children with neurological and neuromuscular disease.[616]

In neonates the picture is nonspecific, with apneic episodes, lethargy, poor feeding and impaired circulation. Outbreaks may occur in neonatal units.

Diagnosis

At epidemic times, a clinical diagnosis of influenza has a high likelihood of being correct, but such a diagnosis in a sporadic case can often be incorrect. Other respiratory viral infections and some quite unconnected diseases may present with a similar clinical picture and a specific diagnosis depends on definitive laboratory tests.

Virological confirmation of influenza can be established by serological studies or by demonstrating the presence of influenza virus. The latter can be isolated from pharyngeal swabs, nasal swabs or throat washing during the acute stage of the illness and can be grown in the amniotic cavity of chick embryos or in tissue cultures. Influenza may be isolated in monkey kidney tissue cultures. During epidemics, immunofluorescence using an antiserum to the epidemic strain to test nasopharyngeal secretions can be used for rapid diagnosis. Complement-fixation, neutralization and hemagglutination-inhibition tests are available for the serological study of antibody responses to infection with influenza. In all these tests it is desirable to show a significant (four-fold or greater) rise in antibody titer during the illness.

Complications

Viral complications such as myocarditis, polyneuritis, encephalitis and psychosis are rarely seen in childhood cases. Secondary bacterial infection of the respiratory tract is more likely and pneumonia, otitis media and purulent sinusitis may occur. Death can result from severe overwhelming infection by influenza virus itself, though a fatal outcome is more likely to result from secondary bacterial infection. Acute myositis may be severe, particularly affecting the calves, with a raised serum creatine phosphokinase (CPK). Reye syndrome has sometimes followed influenza infection.

Treatment

In mild cases this is essentially symptomatic. Bed rest is advisable and pain will be eased by simple analgesics such as paracetamol (acetaminophen). Troublesome cough may respond to codeine or similar preparations. Bacterial complications may require antibiotic treatment, whenever possible guided by appropriate laboratory studies. Amantadine and rimantadine have been successfully used to treat severe infection in immunocompromised children or those with underlying chronic illnesses. The neuraminidase inhibitors are a new class of antiviral agents that have been shown to be effective in the treatment of severe influenza in high risk patients.[617,618] Zanamivir is an inhaled preparation, and oseltamivir is an oral preparation. Their use in childhood disease is still under evaluation.

Prophylaxis

The extreme infectivity of influenza renders such measures as isolation and quarantine virtually ineffective. There is evidence that killed virus vaccine can significantly reduce the incidence of influenza, although the sudden emergence of a fresh influenza A mutant may render it impossible to produce the specific vaccine in time to influence an outbreak. Annual influenza vaccination should be considered for the child over 6 months with chronic pulmonary, circulatory or neuromuscular disorders, or with chronic renal disease or diabetes mellitus, or with immunosuppression (including HIV infection). Postexposure prophylaxis with amantadine or the neuraminidase inhibitors has been shown to be effective in preventing illness in adults and children.

In the USA, annual influenza vaccination is now recommended for all children aged 6–59 months, using either a trivalent inactivated influenza vaccine or a live attenuated vaccine.[619] Previously unvaccinated children under 9 years should receive two doses the first year.[619] In other countries, including the UK and Australia, annual influenza vaccination is recommended for children at high risk of severe influenza.

PARAINFLUENZA VIRUS INFECTIONS

The parainfluenza viruses are RNA viruses of the *Paramyxovirus* group. They are more closely related to mumps and Newcastle disease viruses than to influenza.

Four antigenic varieties, called 1, 2, 3 and 4, are recognized, although type 4 has no known role in causing disease in humans. Types 1, 2 and 3 have frequently been isolated from cases of acute laryngotracheobronchitis (croup), bronchitis, bronchiolitis and pneumonia in infants and children, and less often from rhinitis and pharyngitis. They are undoubtedly the commonest cause of acute laryngotracheobronchitis, in which other viruses such as influenza A, RSV and ECHO viruses play a lesser role.

Serological studies indicate that infection, especially with type 3, is common in preschool children. Type 3 infection is endemic and occurs at any time of the year. Type 1 infection tends to occur in summer or autumn outbreaks every second year while type 2 outbreaks are less predictable.

Laboratory diagnosis

Parainfluenza viruses can be isolated from nasal and pharyngeal swabs. The viruses are relatively labile so these swabs should be placed in virus transport medium and delivered to the laboratory with minimum delay. Antigen detection by immunofluorescence or ELISA is increasingly available. Serological diagnosis is rarely helpful, other than in epidemiological studies, because of heterotypic antibody rises among the three types and related viruses, particularly mumps.

Treatment

There is no specific treatment available. Symptomatic treatment of laryngotracheobronchitis with steroids or adrenaline (epinephrine) for severe airways obstruction may be indicated. Ribavirin has been used to suppress infection in immunocompromised hosts.

A live attenuated parainfluenza type 3 vaccine is currently in clinical trial in young infants.[620]

RESPIRATORY SYNCYTIAL VIRUS INFECTIONS

Respiratory syncytial virus (RSV), first identified in 1956, is now recognized to be amongst the most important agents causing respiratory infection in infants and young children worldwide. RSV is an RNA paramyxovirus. The virus grows well in many tissue cultures. In contrast to members of the myxovirus group, to which it shows some resemblance, RSV has no hemagglutinins so does not cause hemagglutination, but produces a fusion protein which causes in vitro and in vivo fusion of cells to form syncytia. Only two antigenic strains of RSV have been described.

Clinical features

RSV has been found in association with several clinical syndromes including mild upper respiratory tract infection, croup, bronchitis, bronchiolitis and pneumonia. Its principal association is with acute bronchiolitis in infants below 1 year of age. Epidemics of RSV infection occur annually in late autumn and winter in temperate climates. Outbreaks are mainly found in urban communities. In tropical climates there is not such a clear-cut annual epidemic. Nosocomial infections can be a major problem in hospitals.

Bronchiolitis is described elsewhere and although infection by influenza viruses, parainfluenza viruses, human metapneumovirus, mycoplasmas, adenoviruses and rhinoviruses may produce a similar picture, few clinical respiratory syndromes have so close an etiological association as bronchiolitis and RSV infection.

Neither maternal nor acquired antibody protects absolutely against RSV, so RSV can infect neonates. Reinfections throughout childhood are common, but successively milder. Preterm infants with symptomatic RSV bronchiolitis appear to have worse lung function at follow-up.[621] High RSV viral load is associated with more severe disease.[622] Toddler-age children may develop bronchitis or pneumonia, school-age children more commonly develop otitis media, while adults get a severe cold with sore throat. Infants with mutations in the Toll-like receptor 4 (TLR4) gene complex involved in the innate immune response to RSV are especially prone to severe disease.[623]

Laboratory diagnosis

The ideal specimen is a nasopharyngeal aspirate of mucus. Rapid viral diagnosis by immunofluorescence (or ELISA) has greatly aided the management of infants with bronchiolitis. The virus can be isolated successfully in various tissue culture systems, but as it is relatively unstable it is recommended that the specimen should be inoculated directly into the cultures without previous freezing. If the specimen has to be stored for a few hours it should be kept in virus transport medium at 4 °C.

Serology can be used in children over 6 months of age, usually by complement-fixation test on paired sera. Under this age there is often no IgG response.

Treatment

Treatment is primarily supportive with supplemental oxygen and/or fluids. Nebulized ribavirin may be indicated in proven severe RSV infection in infants at high risk, particularly those with pre-existing cardiopulmonary disease or immune deficiency.[624–626]

Prevention

Two agents have recently become available for the prevention of RSV in high risk infants (those born prematurely < 35 weeks' gestation, or those with underlying chronic lung disease, cardiac disease or immunosuppression). RSV intravenous immunoglobulin (RSV IVIG) from pooled donors is administered intravenously, and palizumab is a mouse monoclonal antibody to the RSV protein that is given intramuscularly. Both are given monthly during the RSV season and have been shown to significantly reduce the number of cases of hospitalized RSV bronchiolitis in at-risk groups,[627–629] but are expensive. The cost effectiveness of these agents in the UK has been questioned based on local data.[630]

HUMAN METAPNEUMOVIRUS

Human metapneumovirus (MPV) is an RNA virus that was discovered in 2001 in the respiratory isolates of young children.[631] It has been found to be a cause of respiratory illness in all age groups.[631–634] It is a member of the Paramyxoviridae family and has four major genotypes that fall into two antigenic subgroups (A and B). Humans are the only source of infection and transmission is thought to occur through contact with infected secretions. Infection occurs in yearly epidemics, peaking in late winter to spring.[632–634] Co-infection with other viral pathogens is common. Seroprevalence studies suggest that virtually all children have been exposed to MPV by the age of 5.[631]

Clinical features

The clinical features of MPV are similar to those of RSV.[630,631,633] It causes respiratory illnesses of both upper and lower respiratory tract, including bronchiolitis in infants and croup. Disease in normal hosts is usually mild, although MPV can occasionally cause severe pneumonitis. Preterm infants and children with underlying pulmonary or cardiac disorders or with immunodeficiency are at risk of severe disease from MPV, although RSV is a more common pathogen in this group.[635] Immunocompromised children may have persistent shedding of MPV.[636] Severe disease in children with HIV infection is usually associated with pneumococcal superinfection.[637] Like RSV, recurrent infections occur throughout life.

Laboratory diagnosis

There are currently no commercially available tests for the diagnosis of MPV. MPV can be isolated by culture of respiratory secretions, and MPV viral nucleic acid can be detected by RT-PCR in reference or research laboratories.[632,634]

Treatment

Treatment is supportive with supplemental oxygen and attention to hydration as required.

Prevention

Control of nosocomial MPV infection requires contact precautions, with particular attention to hand washing after contact with infected respiratory secretions.

ADENOVIRUSES

The first isolation of an adenovirus took place in 1953 from fragmented human adenoids grown in tissue culture, hence the name. Subsequently a number of different strains, chiefly types 1, 2, 5 and 6, were isolated from cultures of tonsils and adenoids. Outbreaks due to these agents have been encountered in children at boarding schools, at summer camps and amongst those attending communal swimming pools. Outbreaks in adults mainly involve military recruits. The nature of the clinical illness produced shows considerable variation and overlap but some relatively specific syndromes are included.

Adenoviruses are DNA viruses. They are relatively stable to changes in temperature and pH. They are widespread in nature and have been isolated from monkeys, pigs, dogs, birds and cattle, as well as from man. They may persist for weeks or even months in the upper respiratory tract.

Clinical features

Adenovirus infections are principally diseases of childhood, occurring mostly in children under 5 years old. Certain adenovirus types show a pronounced age association. Immunocompromised hosts are at risk of severe disease from adenovirus.[638]

Amongst syndromes recognized to be associated with adenoviral infection are the following:

Acute febrile pharyngitis

This syndrome has a high endemic rate in infants and young children and mainly results from infection by types 1, 2 and 5. It can also occur in epidemic form when type 3 is usually involved.

Pharyngoconjunctival fever (PCF)

Most commonly associated with infection by type 3, and less frequently with types 7A and 14, this syndrome can also follow infection by types 1, 2, 5 and 6. Epidemics occur in children, some associated with swimming pools. Symptoms include sore throat, headache, myalgia, eye discomfort, abdominal pain and back stiffness. Examination often reveals pharyngitis and unilateral or bilateral follicular conjunctivitis.

Acute respiratory disease (ARD)

Uncommon in children, ARD is usually found in military recruits. It is most commonly due to infection by types 4 and 7, less often by types 3 and 14. The main clinical features include pharyngitis, cough, hoarseness and chest pain.

Viral pneumonia in infants

Adenoviruses may cause severe pneumonia, and outbreaks have been reported in hospital nurseries. Types 3, 7 and 21 have caused the most severe, sometimes fatal, cases. Infection may disseminate (see below) or may result in bronchiolitis obliterans, bronchiectasis or unilateral hyperlucent lung. In immunocompetent infants hospitalized with severe adenovirus infection, disease severity correlates with serum LDH and oxygen saturation at admission.[639]

Ocular syndromes

Two specific ocular syndromes are associated with adenovirus infection. The first is called *epidemic keratoconjunctivitis* and is associated with type 8 infection; the second, *follicular conjunctivitis*, usually results from infection by type 3 and may expand into the fuller syndrome of pharyngoconjunctival fever.

Disseminated disease

Adenovirus types 7 and 21 are particularly prone to cause pneumonia and disseminate to involve the liver (hepatitis), heart (myocarditis or pericarditis) and CNS (meningitis or encephalitis). This is more likely in immunocompromised patients.

Gastroenteritis

Noncultivable enteric adenoviruses (types 40 and 41), seen on electron microscopy of feces, have been associated with gastroenteritis.[640]

Laboratory diagnosis

Adenoviruses can be grown in a wide range of tissue cultures. These viruses are relatively stable and can readily be isolated from throat swabs and feces. In respiratory disease, a pharyngeal swab should be sent to the laboratory in virus transport media. Growth may be slow, so cultures should be incubated for at least 3 weeks before being regarded as negative.

Serological evidence of infection is by detecting complement-fixing antibodies to adenoviruses in acute and convalescent serum samples. Antigen detection by immunoassays and detection of viral DNA by PCR in body fluids may aid in diagnosis of adenovirus infection in the immunocompromised.

Treatment

Treatment is largely supportive. The new antiviral agent, cidofovir, has been used with some success in the treatment of severe adenoviral infections in children post bone marrow transplantation.[641]

MUMPS (EPIDEMIC PAROTITIS)

To mump is an old English word meaning to mope. Mumps is an acute infectious disease characterized by nonsuppurative enlargement of the salivary glands, particularly the parotids. It results from infection by mumps virus, one of the myxoviruses, and is associated with an unusually diverse range of complications. Infection may be inapparent in as many as 30% of cases and the illness may present with a complication and no history of preceding salivary gland involvement.

Epidemiology and etiology

Mumps is an endemic disease of urban communities which occasionally occurs in epidemic proportions, especially in certain closed communities. Spread is by droplet infection or from recently contaminated articles and close contact is required. The relatively high incidence in adults bears witness to the comparatively low infectivity of the disease, though when mumps is introduced into a naive community, a serious and widespread outbreak may follow. There have been recent outbreaks of mumps in young adults in the UK.[642]

The responsible agent is an RNA virus. Man appears to be the only reservoir and the portal of entry is through the mouth or nose. Infectivity may extend from several days before the illness to several days after the first sign of salivary gland involvement. Virus has been isolated from the blood in the prodromal stage and from the urine up to 14 days after the commencement of clinical illness. It is not clear whether spread to the salivary glands occurs locally or through the bloodstream.

Clinical features

The main incidence occurs between 5 and 15 years of age; mumps is relatively uncommon in younger children and in adults over 30 years.

The incubation period is between 14 and 21 days and the illness may commence with malaise, fever, headache and anorexia; these prodromal symptoms may be absent. Salivary gland involvement commences 1–2 days later and the parotid glands are the most frequently affected. Pain develops around the ear and a swelling appears which extends forwards from the lobe of the ear, downwards over the angle of the jaw and backwards behind the pinna, which is usually pushed outwards. The swelling may be so trivial as to escape casual inspection or be very marked and exquisitely tender. Often only one parotid is involved initially, followed, in 75% of cases, by swelling of the other parotid 1–5 days later. Less often simultaneous and synchronous swelling of both parotids occurs.

Submandibular salivary gland involvement can easily be overlooked as the soft tissues under the jaw readily absorb such swelling, unless it is particularly marked, and it is often the concomitant swelling of the parotids that directs attention to it. Sublingual involvement is much less common but is extremely painful and can be seen readily beneath the upturned tongue.

In addition to salivary gland involvement, the orifice of Stensen's duct may be swollen and the mouth rather dry. Fever is present in the majority of cases, may reach 40 °C and persist for up to a week; in fact, cases without salivary gland involvement may present as examples of unexplained fever and recover without the true diagnosis being appreciated, though in others the later development of a typical pattern of complications may indicate mumps to be the cause.

There may be some degree of leukopenia in mumps though certain complications, such as meningitis and pancreatitis, may provoke a leukocytosis.

Complications

Complications are common and varied.

CNS

Aseptic meningitis is the commonest complication and may present before, coincidentally with, or after, the illness. The CSF will show a lymphocytic pleocytosis and the count may exceed 1000 cells/μl. The protein content may be moderately raised and the glucose level is usually normal. However, the latter is occasionally decreased in mumps meningitis and where no salivary gland enlargement occurs to indicate the diagnosis, confusion with tuberculous meningitis has occurred. Other less common complications include postinfectious encephalitis, myelitis and polyradiculitis. Although usually unilateral, bilateral nerve deafness, often complete, can also occur, as may transient facial paralysis. The virus is easily isolated from the CSF of patients with mumps meningitis, which is generally benign. The postinfectious encephalitis is, however, more severe; although complete recovery is usual, neurological sequelae and even death may occur. Virus can be grown from the CSF, but an immune-mediated mechanism is more likely to contribute to pathogenesis.

Orchitis

Orchitis may occur in 20% of postpubertal males and in younger children can occasionally occur in an undescended testicle. The involvement is usually unilateral but even after severe orchitis, sterility is rare, and males with orchitis should be firmly reassured of the good prognosis.

Pancreatitis

A significant degree of pancreatitis is rare and this complication is over-diagnosed. Salivary gland enlargement by itself raises the serum amylase level but when the pancreas is significantly involved intense pain will occur with rigidity of the abdominal wall and there is often a marked leukocytosis.

Other complications

These include oophoritis, mastitis, bartholinitis, myocarditis, hepatitis, thyroiditis and thrombocytopenic purpura. An occasional case of diabetes mellitus has also been reported following mumps.

Laboratory diagnosis

Viral confirmation of mumps depends on isolation of the virus or the demonstration of a significant rise in antibody titer during the illness.

Mumps virus can be cultured from saliva swabs and urine during the acute illness and from the CSF in cases complicated by meningitis.

Serological tests are readily available to demonstrate a significant rise in antibody titer during the illness and the complement-fixation test is most commonly employed. In this test, two specific antigens, soluble (S) and viral (V), are often used. In general, antibody to S antigen rises earlier in the illness than antibody to V antigen, but whereas S antibody may only persist for a few months, the V antibody is present for a very long period. Hemagglutination-inhibition and virus neutralization tests are also of help where available.

Differential diagnosis

In children, the differential diagnosis is more limited than in adults as in the latter one may encounter more diseases that involve the salivary glands. Conditions that cause lymph node enlargement produce most confusion but careful clinical examination should resolve the difficulty. Pyogenic submandibular abscesses and glandular fever can prove more perplexing and in these instances the blood picture and serum amylase estimations can be helpful. Suppurative parotitis may be considered where there is overlying inflammation and where pus can be expressed from the appropriate salivary duct. Recurrent parotitis is quite common in children. It is not due to repeated attacks of mumps. Sometimes an underlying allergic disorder, sialectasis or duct calculi may be found. Other conditions which may require exclusion are tumors, Mikulicz syndrome, uveoparotid fever in sarcoidosis, HIV infection, tuberculosis and dental conditions.

Treatment

There is no specific treatment. Pain may be relieved by simple analgesics and the application of heat to the glands can prove soothing. The mouth should be kept clean and a fluid diet is needed until swelling subsides. Neurological complications are managed along customary lines though the diagnostic lumbar puncture in mumps meningitis often produces dramatic relief of headache. In orchitis the testes should be supported and ice bags may ease the discomfort; there is no evidence that corticosteroid drugs, stilbestrol or incision of the tunica albuginea significantly alter the course of this complication.

Prognosis

This is generally good and a fatal outcome exceedingly rare, although permanent brain damage and deafness have been described. Sterility is most unlikely. One attack of mumps appears to provide life-long immunity.

Prevention

Injections of human anti-mumps immunoglobulin have been used prophylactically and appear beneficial if given sufficiently early in the incubation period. Live vaccines are safe and produce a good antibody response with long immunity though the duration has not been fully substantiated. They can be used to immunize contacts, and are incorporated into the MMR vaccine for routine immunization in many countries.

COXSACKIE AND ECHO VIRUS INFECTIONS

Respiratory illness in association with these enteroviruses is usually mild.

Certain coxsackie viruses produce specific respiratory syndromes. Some group A serotypes can cause herpangina and certain group B viruses are the agents responsible for causing pleurodynia (Bornholm disease). Agents from both groups of coxsackie viruses have been found in association with mild febrile respiratory disease and one strain, coxsackie A21 (Coe virus), has been recovered with particular frequency from outbreaks in young servicemen.

ECHO viruses are not usually regarded as respiratory pathogens, but they have been found in the throat or feces during upper respiratory disease. Amongst serotypes isolated in these circumstances are ECHO viruses types 6, 11, 19 and 20.

The laboratory diagnosis of infections due to coxsackie and ECHO viruses is described in the section specifically devoted to these agents.

RHINOVIRUS INFECTIONS

Rhinoviruses are the main cause of the common cold. There are many serologically distinct types. They belong to the large group of picornaviruses, meaning small RNA viruses, but unlike coxsackie and ECHO viruses they are acid labile at pH 3.

The common cold is probably the most ubiquitous infection in man and the illness tends to be more severe in children than in adults, with an acute catarrhal inflammation involving the nose, nasopharynx and accessory sinuses. The onset is usually abrupt and is accompanied by a copious watery discharge, which may later turn mucopurulent even in the absence of bacterial superinfection. Little or no fever occurs and constitutional symptoms are mild.

Apart from their ability to produce the common cold, rhinoviruses have been found in association with acute wheezing episodes in children and with pneumonia.[643]

Laboratory diagnosis

Nasopharyngeal aspirates in virus transport medium, nose swab or throat swab collected during the acute stage of the respiratory illness should be sent to the laboratory for the isolation of rhinoviruses. Serology is generally unhelpful. ELISA and PCR for rhinovirus have been developed but are not widely available.

CORONAVIRUSES AND SARS

Human coronaviruses (HCV) are probably almost as frequent a cause of colds and acute upper respiratory tract infections as rhinovirus infections.[644] Coronaviruses have also been associated with wheeze and pneumonia.[645] The exact frequency of HCV infections has been difficult to ascertain because coronaviruses are difficult to grow and can often only be isolated in tracheal organ cultures. The diagnosis can be made by ELISA on respiratory secretions or serologically by detecting antibody to one of the two main serotypes, 229E and OC-43. PCR is not widely available.

During 2002–2003, there was an acute outbreak of a severe atypical pneumonia, originally in China and Hong Kong, that did not respond to routine antimicrobial therapies.[646,647] The disease was labeled severe acute respiratory distress syndrome (or SARS). Commonly known viruses and bacteria were not isolated and eventually a novel coronavirus, SARS-CoV, was confirmed to be the causal agent.[648,649] The syndrome was characterized by fever of 38 °C or more, respiratory symptoms (cough, dyspnea), myalgia and marked infiltrates on chest X-ray which were often out of proportion to the degree of symptoms. Most patients did not experience upper respiratory tract symptoms. Gastrointestinal symptoms were present in 10% of patients. Severe disease was associated with deranged liver function enzymes, thrombocytopenia and leukopenia, and respiratory failure, and was associated with high mortality. Infected children < 12 years of age experienced only mild disease and rarely progressed to respiratory failure or death.[648,649]

Transmission of SARS-CoV is by contact with respiratory secretions, although urine, stool and blood can also be a source of infection. Infected individuals are most contagious during the second week of the illness. In the 2003 outbreak, high rates of human to human transmission were reported in exposed health care workers.[648,649] Routine diagnostic tests are not available for SARS-CoV, and the diagnosis is usually made by the combination of known exposure, clinical features and failure to isolate other pathogens. The virus is difficult to isolate in cell culture. Research laboratories have confirmed the infection by molecular techniques, serology or by immuno-electron microscopy. Although severe SARS has been treated with steroids, ribavirin and interferon alfa, there is no antiviral agent with proven efficacy against this virus.[648,649]

REOVIRUS INFECTIONS

In 1954, a new group of respiratory-entero or reovirus agents was recognized. It had originally been thought to belong to the ECHO virus group. Since then three distinct types (1, 2 and 3) have been serologically differentiated though they share a common complement-fixing antigen.

Following these preliminary investigations reoviruses have been isolated from many different animal hosts in widely separated areas. These viruses have also been recovered from rectal and throat swabs taken from children suffering from mild respiratory disease, diarrhea, and occasionally fatal pneumonia.

A recent seroprevalence study in the USA suggests that reovirus infections are common during early childhood.[650] However, the exact role of reoviruses in producing human disease is largely undetermined. The family Reoviridae also includes the rotaviruses, which are associated with gastroenteritis.

Laboratory diagnosis
Reoviruses can be isolated from pharyngeal swabs and nasal secretions, but are more commonly recovered from feces.

Acute and convalescent samples of serum are required for hemagglutination-inhibiting antibody titer estimations; a four-fold, or greater, rise in titer during the illness is evidence of infection with a reovirus.

Rotaviruses are difficult to culture and diagnosis depends on electron microscopic examination or ELISA tests on feces.

CHLAMYDOPHILA PSITTACI (PSITTACOSIS)

Psittacosis is a zoonosis contracted from birds or objects they have contaminated. It was originally considered that infection could only result from birds of the psittacine group (psittacosis) but it is now appreciated that infection may arise from many other birds, both wild and domesticated (ornithosis), and animals such as sheep and goats.

Chlamydophila (formerly Chlamydia) psittaci, the causative organism, is antigenically and genetically distinct from the genus Chlamydia in which it was previously grouped.[651] This obligate intracellular organism appears to occupy an intermediate position between viruses and rickettsiae and shows sensitivity only to certain antibiotics.

Clinical features
The presentation is usually with high fever, chills, headache, myalgia, chest pain, anorexia and fatigue. A dry cough may become productive and fine crackles may be heard. The pulse may be relatively slow. Contact with a sick bird is suggestive, but there may be no history of bird or animal contact. Chest radiography may show perihilar infiltrates, atelectasis or even consolidation. Children and adolescents seem less susceptible to psittacosis than adults. However, this may merely reflect the fact that less specific illness is produced in the young and the diagnosis may therefore be overlooked.

Laboratory diagnosis
A clinical diagnosis of psittacosis can be confirmed by serological tests. Treatment can suppress antibody responses. The estimation of complement-fixing antibodies in acute and convalescent samples of serum is a reliable and popular test which avoids the hazards involved in the isolation of a highly infectious agent but does not distinguish between other species of Chlamydia or Chlamydophila. The acute serum sample should be collected as early in the illness as possible and a convalescent sample taken about 2 weeks after the onset of the illness. It is often worthwhile examining a third sample of serum obtained after a further 2 weeks. A four-fold, or greater, rise in antibody titer during the illness is indicative of infection with a member of the psittacosis–lymphogranuloma venereum group of agents.

The psittacosis agent can be isolated from blood in the early stages of the illness and later from pleural fluid and infected tissues by reference laboratories where appropriate controls are enforced to prevent infection in personnel.

Sensitive immunoassays for C. psittaci are available in some reference laboratories.[652]

Prognosis
Spontaneous recovery is to be expected, but where the diagnosis is confirmed during the clinical illness, tetracycline (except in children less than 8 years old) or erythromycin may reduce symptoms and hasten convalescence.

CHLAMYDOPHILA PNEUMONIAE

C. pneumoniae is closely related to C. psittaci, and cross-reacts with it in complement-fixation serological tests. Infection can be subclinical or result in mild to moderate respiratory illnesses. The prodrome may include a sore throat, and there is often a protracted cough persisting up to 6 weeks with a biphasic course.[653] Serological surveys suggest it is a not uncommon cause of pneumonia in children, particularly in resource limited countries. Treatment is as for psittacosis.

CHLAMYDIA TRACHOMATIS

C. trachomatis, acquired by passage through an infected birth canal, can cause a pneumonitis usually at 3–11 weeks of age. There may be a history of maternal vaginal discharge and the infant may have had conjunctivitis. The infant is afebrile with a characteristic staccato cough. There are often crackles and wheezes on auscultation. About half the infants have otitis media with a pearly white tympanic membrane. The radiographic appearance is of diffuse pulmonary infiltrates with peribronchial thickening and focal consolidation. Definitive diagnosis is by culturing C. trachomatis or detecting antigen in a nasopharyngeal aspirate or conjunctival swab, or by detecting specific IgM by immunofluorescence. PCR and other nucleic amplification techniques can be used to detect C. trachomatis DNA in genital swabs or urine from the mother. They can also be used on conjunctival swabs from the infant, but the test has not proved sensitive when performed on infants' pharyngeal specimens. Presumptive evidence can be obtained by demonstrating characteristic inclusions on conjunctival scrapings if there is active conjunctivitis. Treatment of conjunctivitis is with erythromycin 40 mg/kg/d 6-hourly for 14 days. Parents should be alerted of the signs of infantile hypertrophic pyloric stenosis, which is associated with erythromycin use in infants < 6 weeks of age, although the link has not been proven to be causal.[653]

Chlamydia pneumonia can be treated with erythromycin as before or with azithromycin 20 mg/kg orally once daily for 3 days. The parents should also be treated.

MYCOPLASMA PNEUMONIAE

Mycoplasma pneumoniae is a common cause of atypical pneumonia in childhood but can also cause a variety of clinical syndromes. It is not a virus but a pleuropneumonia-like organism (PPLO) that lacks a cell wall and belongs to the distinctive genus of mycoplasmas.

Clinical features

M. pneumoniae may give rise to inapparent infection, mild upper respiratory tract infection, bronchitis, bronchiolitis, bronchopneumonia and bullous myringitis both in adults and children. Epidemics occur every 3–4 years. *M. pneumoniae* may have an etiological role in some cases of Stevens–Johnson syndrome and can also cause myocarditis, pericarditis, arthritis and encephalitis. When it causes pneumonia, the radiological appearance may be of bilateral, diffuse reticular infiltrates or of consolidation, including lobar consolidation. Small pleural effusions can occur.

Laboratory diagnosis

Isolation of *M. pneumoniae* from sputum, throat washings or pharyngeal swabs is possible, but the agent grows slowly.

For serological studies, acute and convalescent samples of serum should be collected. Various serological tests are available, but the complement-fixation test appears popular and reliable. A single high titer of IgG antibodies to *M. pneumoniae* on an acute serum sample may be helpful, since there is often a fairly long history of illness. Detection of *M. pneumoniae* IgM by immunofluorescence does not distinguish an acute infection from one in the recent past, as the antibody may persist for many months.

Cold agglutinins are present in the serum in many cases and may be useful in acute management, although their detection is not specific for *Mycoplasma* infection.

Treatment

Mild respiratory illnesses caused by *Mycoplasma* are usually self limiting and do not require treatment. Pneumonia caused by *M. pneumoniae*, where a diagnosis is made during the active stage of illness, can be treated with tetracycline (25–50 mg/kg/day) or doxycycline (2.5 mg/kg up to 100 mg twice daily) in children over 8 years old, or with erythromycin (30–50 mg/kg/day) or with one of the newer macrolides such as clarithromycin or azithromycin in younger children. There is no evidence that antimicrobial treatment alters the course of nonrespiratory forms of *Mycoplasma* disease.

VIRAL INFECTIONS OF THE CNS (INCLUDING MENINGITIS, ENCEPHALITIS, MYELITIS AND POLYNEURITIS)

See Chapter 22 (Infectious and inflammatory disorders of the CNS).

LYMPHOCYTIC CHORIOMENINGITIS

Lymphocytic choriomeningitis (LCM) virus was first recognized in 1934, and is classified as a member of the Arenavirus group. It occurs in mice.

Sporadic cases and small outbreaks of LCM aseptic meningitis in man have been reported in Europe and the USA, in circumscribed areas where infected mouse colonies have been shown to exist.[654] Although originally suspected to be a common cause of aseptic meningitis, it is now known to have a very small role except in these endemic areas.

Clinical features

The incubation period of LCM lies between 7 and 14 days. Any age group may contract the disease, if in contact with the relevant infected mouse colonies. The clinical picture and the abnormalities in the CSF are identical with those found in other types of viral meningitis and etiological diagnosis can only be made by laboratory studies. LCM can also cause mild respiratory illness and occasionally pneumonia. Orchitis, myopericarditis, arthritis or alopecia may rarely occur. The prognosis is usually excellent, although an occasional fatality has been reported in infants. No specific treatment is indicated. Control of infected mouse colonies should be undertaken by expert rodent exterminators.

Laboratory diagnosis

LCM virus can be isolated from blood in the initial febrile phase of the illness, and from CSF after the onset of meningitis. The virus can be propagated in young mice and in various tissue cultures.

Complement-fixing and neutralizing antibodies appear in the patient's serum following infection and a serological diagnosis can be made by demonstrating a significant rise in antibody titer during the illness. The antibodies tend to be produced rather late in the illness, so the convalescent serum sample for complement-fixing antibodies should be collected about the third week of the illness and that for neutralizing antibodies about 6 weeks after the onset of the disease.

RABIES (HYDROPHOBIA)

Rabies, the most feared of all zoonoses, has been a recognized disease of man since early times.[655] Spread to man may occur from a wide variety of warm-blooded animals which demonstrate variable susceptibility. Although this susceptibility is extremely high in such animals as foxes, jackals and wolves, it is only moderate in others including the dog. However, as man has a closer association with domestic animals, such as the dog, they provide a greater risk to him. In any particular geographical area, enzootic or epizootic infection may predominate in only one or two species of wild animal. In Central and South America the dominant animal is the vampire bat, in Russia the wolf, in North America the bat and skunk, and in Europe the fox.

Certain areas of the world are currently free of rabies including New Zealand, certain Pacific islands, parts of Scandinavia and the UK. In an attempt to retain this position, the movement of animals is governed by strict regulations including compulsory quarantine of animals, but such measures can be severely stretched. Enzootic rabies was eradicated from the UK in 1922, but fears exist that the current epizootic form amongst foxes in Europe, which has spread rapidly westwards over recent years, may result in the reintroduction of rabies.

Infection can follow the licking of abraded skin or mucosa by an infected animal as well as by a bite. Airborne infection from bats to man can also occur in caves where they are roosting. In most instances suspicion will arise that the animal concerned is rabid, especially where the furious form of the disease occurs. Should the less dramatic, dumb form occur, however, the true nature of the illness is not so readily suspected.

Clinical features

The incubation period may be as short as 10 days or as long as 7 years, but is usually between 1 and 3 months. Wounds on the hands, forearm and neck are especially dangerous and in them, or where there is extensive biting at any site, the incubation period may be shortened. Age may also be a factor, and cases in young children tend to have a shorter incubation period.

The onset of clinical illness is heralded by a prodromal period of 2–7 days. Indefinite sensory changes may be experienced at the site of the bite, together with such nonspecific features as slight fever, headache, malaise, nausea and sore throat. Paresis and paralysis then develop and the muscles of deglutition go into spasm at any attempt to swallow (hence the term hydrophobia). Increasing depression and anxiety become apparent and the patient may become very withdrawn.

The disease may now enter a stage of excitement (furious rabies) with alternating manic activity and calm. The patient will remain lucid but fearful and the spasms in the throat become more violent. Cranial nerve palsies may develop and generalized convulsions become frequent. Death follows in virtually every case, from either cardiac or respiratory arrest. Less often the picture is not so florid and a progressive ascending paralysis occurs, giving rise to the so-called 'dumb' form of the disease.

Clinical diagnosis
A classical case, following a significant bite, provides a clearly recognizable clinical picture. Otherwise, forms of viral encephalitis, bulbar poliomyelitis, hysteria and tetanus may produce similar features and cause diagnostic confusion. Encephalitis can occur following antirabies vaccination with the old vaccines and produce a similar picture to that of rabies itself, but this has not been recorded following the human diploid cell vaccine.

Laboratory diagnosis
Rabies virus is probably not a single antigenic species and four rabies-related viruses are recognized. These agents have a marked predilection for nervous tissue but multiply in other organs such as the salivary glands. Within the nervous system the main pathological process is an encephalomyelitis leading to the development of inclusion bodies, particularly within the hippocampus. These inclusions are known as Negri bodies.

During life, the laboratory diagnosis of rabies depends on testing such specimens as saliva, CSF and conjunctival secretions by animal inoculation and immunofluorescent techniques. Viral antigens may be detected in skin biopsies. The rapidly fatal outcome, and the confusion which serum or vaccine can introduce, may render serological tests unhelpful.

If the suspected animal is available, it should be sacrificed and the brain examined for rabies virus antigens by hybridization techniques.

After death, specimens of brain tissue should be inoculated intracerebrally into mice. The specimens should also be subjected to rabies immunofluorescent tests and examined for Negri bodies. These tests should yield results within 1–2 days. However, if they are inconclusive, the results of mouse inoculation must be awaited, and it may take up to 3 weeks to declare this test negative.

Treatment
The treatment of clinical rabies is largely symptomatic, but intensive supportive therapy including artificial ventilation has been employed and at least two cases of proven rabies have survived following such measures. Appropriate steps must be taken to avoid possible spread to the attendants and to the immediate environment.

Postexposure prophylaxis
Local treatment of the wound. This can prove highly beneficial and should not be overlooked or delayed. Ideally wounds should be thoroughly cleansed using a 20% soap solution and after washing any residual soap away with water, a 0.1% quaternary ammonium compound such as cetrimide should be applied. Alternatives include 40–70% alcohol or tincture and aqueous solutions of iodine. Should none of these agents be immediately available, extensive cleansing with clean water should be used as early as possible and the chemical agents employed when practicable. Primary suturing of the wounds should be avoided and human rabies immunoglobulin (HRIG) should be infiltrated into the tissue beneath the wound. If there is any suspicion of exposure to tetanus, tetanus prophylaxis should be instituted.
Special systemic treatment. The aim of prophylaxis by vaccination is to induce a rapid antibody response which may prevent clinical disease developing. The human diploid vaccines are safe and highly effective. The site and frequency of injections for postexposure prophylaxis will depend on the vaccine used. If the human diploid cell vaccine is used, vaccination should commence as soon as possible after the incident and injections should be given by deep subcutaneous or intramuscular injection on days 0, 3, 7, 14 and 28. As antibodies do not develop for some days, immunoprophylaxis with HRIG should be given intramuscularly as well as infiltrating the wound[656] of those not previously immunized,

ideally within 24 hours. Treatment may be discontinued if the suspect dog or cat remains healthy after observation for 5 days. Other animals may require longer observation.

Pre-exposure prophylaxis
Prophylaxis by the human diploid cell rabies vaccine may be used for those at high risk of contracting rabies, e.g. laboratory staff or veterinary staff in endemic areas. Immunization is not routinely recommended for those visiting endemic areas.

NEURODEGENERATIVE VIRUS DISEASES
Subacute sclerosing panencephalitis (SSPE)
See Chapter 22 (Infectious and inflammatory disorders of the CNS).

Rubella panencephalitis
See Chapter 22 (Infectious and inflammatory disorders of the CNS).

Progressive multifocal leukoencephalopathy
This disease is a demyelinating disease caused by infection of astrocytes and oligodendrocytes with one of two papovaviruses, JC virus or simian virus 40 (SV40). The more common of the two to cause disease, JC, is named after the initials of the first affected patient, a 38-year-old man with Hodgkin disease who developed progressive multifocal leukoencephalopathy.

All cases have been in patients who are immunosuppressed, e.g. post renal transplant, have a malignant lymphoproliferative disorder or have a chronic disease such as tuberculosis or sarcoidosis. All areas of the brain and spinal cord may be affected. The usual presentation is early dementia with confusion, impaired cerebration and labile affect. Focal weakness often progresses to hemiparesis and later to bilateral long tract signs. Blindness, aphasia and ataxia are usual, with death occurring in less than 6 months. Detection of JC viral nucleic acid in the CSF by PCR analysis may be helpful in making the diagnosis of progressive multifocal leukoencephalopathy, but the sensitivity of the assay varies widely between laboratories.

PRION DISEASES: TRANSMISSIBLE SPONGIFORM ENCEPHALOPATHIES
The transmissible spongiform encephalopathies (TSE) of man are a rare, neurodegenerative, fatal group of disorders in which there is progressive degeneration of neurones with demyelination and gliosis of gray matter, causing a spongiform appearance of the brain, and the accumulation of a rare protein or prion (proteinaceous infectious agent). Their existence was first postulated by Pruisner in his analysis of the pathogenesis of scrapie in sheep.[657] Prions are thought to cause neuronal dysfunction and pathology when an alpha helical protease-sensitive form of the prion converts to a protease-resistant protein form associated with a structural predominance of beta sheet. Human TSE disorders include Creutzfeldt–Jakob disease (CJD), variant-Creutzfeldt–Jakob disease (v-CJD), Gerstmann–Straussler–Scheinker disease, kuru and fatal familial insomnia.[658] They closely resemble two animal diseases, scrapie and transmissible mink encephalopathy.

Kuru was the first TSE to be identified over 40 years ago. It was initially thought to be caused by a slow virus. In kuru, the cerebellum is most affected, and the disease is characterized by a progressive ataxia with a shivering tremor (the word 'kuru' means shivering). The incubation period is up to 20 years. It was acquired by the women and children of the Fore tribe in New Guinea who ate the brains of dead kinsfolk.

CJD is a progressive dementia with varying neurological features. Myoclonus, ataxic tremor, spasticity and parkinsonian features have all been described. CJD is sometimes familial. Cases have occurred in children who received human growth hormone from human pituitary extracts unwittingly infected with the agent and through brain and eye surgery.

The TSE of most relevance to pediatricians is v-CJD. It was first identified in the UK in 1996,[659] and there is evidence to suggest it is linked to exposure to tissues from cattle infected with bovine spongiform encephalopathy (BSE),[660,661] although the route of infection and indeed much about the natural history of this disease remains unclear despite analysis of the dietary history of people with v-CJD.[662] There appears to be a genetic component to the disease, as all patients identified to date are homozygous for methionine at codon 129 of the 'PRNP' gene.[658] v-CJD is distinguished from CJD by a younger age at onset and some distinguishing clinical features such as a psychiatric presentation, altered pain sensation and the absence of the periodic electroencephalographic complexes seen in CJD. Neurological signs such as ataxia and myoclonus occur later in the illness than in CJD. Amyloid plaques and bilateral, increased thalamic densities may be seen on MRI.

Treatment

No specific treatment for prion diseases is available. Supportive therapy is indicated for the sequelae of the neurodegeneration.

INFECTIONS DUE TO ENTEROVIRUSES
Poliomyelitis (infantile paralysis, acute anterior poliomyelitis)

Poliomyelitis has been a disease of man for many centuries, but has become more virulent since the late nineteenth century.

In the great majority of infected people, poliomyelitis is a harmless subclinical event; nevertheless, severe epidemics can arise with remarkable rapidity and the mortality and morbidity that result demonstrate that the fear in which the disease is held is well founded.

Epidemiology

Man appears to be the main reservoir of polioviruses in nature, although the great apes can also develop poliomyelitis. In temperate climates, epidemics occur in summer months. The large epidemics of the early 1950s were associated with a higher attack rate and greater severity in older children and young adults in countries with a high standard of living. A possible explanation was that improved hygiene standards led to a diminished rate of subclinical infection in infancy. In countries where vaccination rates are low, poliomyelitis is still primarily a disease of infants and young children.

The Expanded Program of Immunization of the World Health Organization, having as one of its goals global eradication of polio, has led to a steady decline in the world incidence of poliomyelitis since 1973, and a 95% decline in cases worldwide.[663] Intense wild-type poliovirus activity is now limited to the Indian subcontinent and sub-Saharan Africa.[663] In the rest of the world there are rare cases of vaccine-associated paralytic poliomyelitis attributable to the oral poliovirus vaccine.

Etiology

There are three strains, polioviruses types 1, 2 and 3, which show little antigenic overlap. They are particularly small RNA viruses. Poliovirus type 1 has been associated with most of the major epidemics and shows the greatest propensity to cause paralytic forms of the disease, whereas type 2 causes sporadic cases or small outbreaks with a low incidence of paralysis; type 3 occupies an intermediate position. Clinical severity is increased by age and pregnancy. Excessive muscular activity in a recently infected person makes a paralytic form of the disease more probable as do intramuscular injections into the limbs and other minor, traumatic procedures. Recent tonsillectomy predisposes to bulbar poliomyelitis and corticosteroid drugs can have an adverse effect. Antibody is clearly important as there is a higher incidence in patients with antibody deficiency.

The disease is spread by direct contact with infected persons through pharyngeal secretions and feces. Infectivity is probably maximal early, and oral–oral spread may be more common than fecal–oral spread.

Rarely paralytic poliomyelitis may result from oral vaccine strains which revert to virulence.

Pathogenesis and pathology

Polioviruses enter the body via the oral route and multiply in the tonsillopharyngeal tissues and intestinal wall. The virus passes to regional lymph nodes. Infectivity of the pharyngeal secretions disappears rapidly, but there is continued excretion into the bowel and polioviruses can be isolated from the feces for weeks and sometimes months.

The viruses probably pass to the bloodstream from the infected lymph nodes and can be isolated from the blood on occasion. The mode of passage thereafter to the nervous system is not fully understood.

In man, the pathological lesions in the CNS are mainly found in the anterior horns of the spinal cord but the posterior horns and intermediate columns may be involved. The essential lesion is neuronal damage, and though some neurones will die, others may recover. Meningitis occurs, and in some cases there is an extensive encephalitis involving motor cells in the medulla and pons, the vestibular nuclei and the motor and premotor areas of the cerebral cortex. Sometimes the lesions are concentrated in the medulla with little damage at lower levels in the cord.

Clinical features

Poliomyelitis is highly infectious and has an incubation period of 1–3 weeks. Most people infected will have an inapparent illness, which can only be demonstrated by retrospective serological surveys or by examination of contacts in the course of an actual epidemic. Paralytic disease virtually only occurs in unimmunized children or adults, as the virus still circulates in the community.

The minor illness. People infected by polioviruses may respond with a mild, insignificant illness whose features may include fever, anorexia, headache, lassitude and gastroenteritic symptoms. The title of 'abortive poliomyelitis' was sometimes used to describe this condition, now more commonly referred to as the minor illness.

The major illness (nonparalytic or preparalytic poliomyelitis). The major illness may immediately follow the minor or there may be a short gap of apparent recovery. Occasionally the minor illness does not occur.

In the preparalytic stage of the major illness, the symptoms simulate those of aseptic meningitis with neck stiffness and a positive Kernig sign. The patient has headache, vomiting, malaise, fever, and may develop pain and stiffness in the neck and back. Patients may also complain of an aching pain and spasm in the limbs.

Lumbar puncture normally shows a mild CSF pleocytosis (either polymorphonuclear or lymphocytic) and slight to moderate elevation of the protein content.

A variable percentage of cases presenting with this picture will gradually improve over the ensuing 7–10 days and thereafter make an uninterrupted recovery (nonparalytic poliomyelitis). Others, unfortunately, proceed to paralysis, starting some 2–3 days later. Occasionally, paralysis comes on earlier or the preparalytic stage is absent.

Paralytic poliomyelitis. *Spinal paralysis.* The cervical and lumbar segments of the cord are most frequently involved and patchy, asymmetric paralysis in the limbs results. This may be trivial and can be confined to part of one muscle group when it is easily overlooked. Unilateral involvement of the dorsiflexors of the feet, of the quadriceps or of the deltoids is a common finding. The paralysis is of lower motor neurone type.

Spinal respiratory paralysis. This form is usually associated with rapid, severe limb paralysis, and neuronal damage may then extend through the central part of the cord. Paralysis of the abdominal muscles may show itself by a weak cough. Lower intercostal involvement may be symptomless to the patient at rest and only evident to the examiner. Eventually such signs as tachypnea, tachycardia, cyanosis, a rising blood pressure and mental confusion will become apparent. In some instances, the signs of increasing ventilatory failure are difficult to distinguish from those of bulbar involvement or encephalitis, which can be present simultaneously.

Bulbar poliomyelitis. This form may be seen with unusual frequency in some epidemics and can be associated with recent tonsillectomy. Difficulty in swallowing is the cardinal sign and the subject is unable to clear mucus and saliva from the throat. There is a reluctance on the part of the patient to breathe deeply, in case secretions become aspirated into the lung. Such symptoms arise from pharyngeal involvement and further spread may cause weakness of the flexors of the neck, facial paralysis, external ocular palsies and, occasionally, true laryngeal paralysis. Extension to the respiratory center, with totally irregular breathing and periods of apnea, has a grave prognosis and involvement of the circulatory center will result in circulatory collapse and an irregular, rapid pulse. Involvement of these vital centers is usually fatal.

Vaccine associated paralytic poliomyelitis (VAPP). The World Health Organization defines VAPP as 'acute flaccid paralysis in a vaccine recipient 7 to 30 days after receiving oral polio vaccine, with no sensory or cognitive loss and with paralysis still present 60 days after the onset of symptoms'.[664] It occurs in about one case in every 750 000 first doses distributed,[665] and has led to reintroduction of the inactivated Salk vaccine into the routine immunization schedule in many industrialized countries including the USA, the UK and Australia.

Laboratory diagnosis

Isolation of poliovirus from the patient is the method of choice. Polioviruses grow well in a variety of tissue cultures, and if specimens are collected early in the illness, successful virus isolation is not difficult. Virus may be recovered from throat swabs early and from the feces for several weeks after the onset. CSF should be cultured for polioviruses but, unlike coxsackie and ECHO viruses, these are found infrequently.

Acute and convalescent samples of serum should be obtained and tested for a significant rise in antibody titer during the illness; tests for both complement-fixing and neutralizing antibodies are available.

Differential diagnosis

Paralytic poliomyelitis may be confused with a variety of disorders including Guillain–Barré syndrome, botulism, localized paralysis following specific infections such as mumps or infectious mononucleosis, paralytic episodes in sickle cell disease, myasthenia gravis and familial periodic paralysis.

Particular forms of poliomyelitis can be specially confusing, such as isolated facial paralysis which may mimic Bell's palsy, and bulbar paralysis which can be mistaken for tetanus. Pseudoparalysis may be found in acute rheumatism, osteomyelitis, fractures, scurvy, congenital syphilis and hysteria.

A true poliomyelitis-like illness can follow infection by other enteroviruses such as coxsackie, ECHO viruses and enterovirus type 71. Wherever possible, the diagnosis of any case of clinical poliomyelitis should be supported by virus isolation and positive serological tests.

Complications, course and prognosis

Nonparalytic poliomyelitis. There are no complications of nonparalytic forms of poliomyelitis. However, unsuspected paralysis may be detected in cases of this type once they become mobilized and this is particularly seen in the back muscles, the strength of which is difficult to assess whilst the patient remains in bed.

Spinal paralytic poliomyelitis. Some recovery may occur in the first 4 weeks following paralysis. Improvement thereafter is much slower. In muscles where the neuronal supply has been severely affected, permanent paralysis with extremely rapid wasting will result.

Spinal respiratory paralysis. At the height of the illness in this group, various cardiac irregularities and even cardiac failure may occur, secondary to the respiratory complications or as a direct effect of the virus on the myocardium.

Major complications include pneumonia, hypertension, urinary retention and constipation. Renal calculi are not uncommon.

Bulbar poliomyelitis. This form of poliomyelitis is of great seriousness if it spreads to the vital centers in the medulla. However, in those cases without involvement of these centers there is remarkably full and quite rapid recovery of the cranial nerves. Involvement of the diaphragm may be permanent.

Late effects (post-polio syndrome). People with paralytic polio may develop new symptoms many years later, characterized by pain in muscles, weakness, fasciculation, breathlessness and problems with speech and swallowing. The mechanism is unknown.

Treatment

Spinal paralysis. The mainstay of therapy is physiotherapy, emphasizing passive movement, and hydrotherapy if available. Paralytic limbs should be supported and splinting may prevent contractures.

Patients may remain fecal excretors of poliovirus for several weeks and infection control precautions must be used.

In children, lack of growth in severely paralyzed limbs may lead to significant shortening, and skilled orthopedic advice is needed in such instances.

Spinal respiratory paralysis. Ventilatory support may be required and a constant watch for the incipient onset of respiratory insufficiency must be maintained. Late diagnosis may cause hypoxia and increased neuronal damage. Where respiratory paralysis is marked, ventilation is best achieved by the use of intermittent positive pressure ventilation combined with tracheostomy.

Bulbar poliomyelitis. Mild cases whose major defect is inability to swallow can often be managed conservatively with nasogastric tube feeding and suction of secretions. These patients often do well and undergo spontaneous recovery in 2–3 weeks. More severe cases require tracheostomy. Even in severe cases the prognosis is good and the tracheostomy can often be closed within a few weeks.

Prevention

Virtually all cases of paralytic poliomyelitis occur in children who have not been immunized. Poliomyelitis outbreaks are unlikely to occur in a community where a high level of protection by immunization is maintained. Active immunization can be produced by either killed virus vaccines (Salk type) or live attenuated virus vaccines (Sabin type). The former require to be given by injection and the latter by the oral route. A full primary course of either type involves three doses with a booster. In general, Sabin type vaccines result in higher humoral antibody levels, are easy and painless to administer and also produce local immunity in the gut. Children with immune deficiency are at increased risk of paralytic polio and should be immunized with the killed vaccine. Children with HIV infection can receive either live or killed vaccines, but if there is a relative at home with AIDS who might be infected by the vaccine virus, Salk (killed) vaccine should be given.

Non-polio enterovirus infections

The coxsackie and ECHO viruses, nonclassified enteroviruses and polioviruses are called enteroviruses and are classified with rhinoviruses into a larger group known as the picornaviruses (pico = small, RNA viruses). The agents in this group have a similarity in size, a similar nucleic acid core (RNA) and other common physical and chemical properties. Clinical and epidemiological studies show that the coxsackie and ECHO viruses are widely distributed in man and can cause a considerable variety of clinical syndromes. However, they have not demonstrated the same propensity to produce such large and serious epidemics as polioviruses.

Coxsackie virus infections

The existence of this group of viruses became apparent in 1948 when unidentifiable, filterable agents were isolated from the feces of two children in whom a clinical diagnosis of paralytic poliomyelitis had been suspected. These children resided in Coxsackie in New York State and the large group of similar viruses subsequently identified has been named after this town. At the present time there are approximately 30 different varieties of coxsackie viruses and these have been classified into two groups, known as A and B; 24 of the strains have been allocated to group A and the remaining 6 to group B.

Some, but not all, viruses of the coxsackie groups may be grown on suitable tissue cultures but all produce a characteristic histopathological effect when injected into suckling mice.

Coxsackie group A virus diseases

Relationship of group A viruses to disease. Viruses of this group may be isolated from a variable percentage of healthy individuals; as a result their isolation from a sick patient must not necessarily be construed as a diagnostic event.

Herpangina. This is one of the most clearly defined clinical syndromes caused by infection with coxsackie A viruses. It is most commonly seen in infants and children, though it can occur in adults. The onset is characterized by fever, anorexia and pain in the throat; other features include headache, abdominal pain and myalgia. Infection will normally derive from another human and the agent may be transmitted from nasal secretions as well as from the feces. The incubation period lies between 3 and 5 days and fecal infectivity may last for several weeks.

Local examination of the mouth will usually reveal hyperemia of the pharynx and characteristic papulovesicular lesions, approximately 1–2 mm in diameter and surrounded by an erythematous ring. Most commonly the lesions are present over the tonsillar pillars, soft palate and uvula, although the tongue may be involved. It is rare to find more than five to six lesions and these soon enlarge and form shallow ulcers. The illness will usually subside within a week and few complications are found in children. Second attacks may result from infection by different antigenic strains. The clinical picture is highly suggestive, but laboratory studies are required for full confirmation, and at least nine different group A viruses are known to produce this syndrome.

CNS involvement. Aseptic meningitis is the most common clinical manifestation and may result from infection by several different coxsackie A virus strains. As with other types of viral meningitis, young children are most likely to be involved and the incidence is rather higher in boys. There is no characteristic clinical picture that differentiates this from other causes of viral meningitis, although in a few instances one of the more specific syndromes associated with group A infection may be present simultaneously. On occasion non-polio enterovirus infection may be associated with paralytic disease that is clinically indistinguishable from poliomyelitis. Coxsackie virus A7 is the most frequently implicated, but other strains such as A9 have also been involved. Severe and fatal encephalitis has been described in a small number of cases of coxsackie A virus infection.

Hand, foot and mouth disease. Most cases of hand, foot and mouth disease are due to infection with coxsackie virus A16, but other coxsackie viruses (usually A5 and A10), ECHO viruses and enterovirus 71 have all caused cases or outbreaks.

Hand, foot and mouth disease usually presents with little or no constitutional upset. Reluctance to feed may be an early sign in babies. Examination of the mouth often shows mild ulceration of the tongue and pearly white vesicles, sometimes surrounded by a red halo, and further examination shows lesions on the palms and soles. The lesions are mainly found over the ventral surface of the fingers and toes and have a characteristic distribution along the sides of the feet. Some children also have a maculopapular rash over the buttocks which may extend on to the thighs and mimic Henoch–Schönlein purpura. Fever is rarely marked and there is little associated lymphadenopathy.

A fully developed case is extraordinarily characteristic and once seen is readily recognized thereafter. The mouth lesions can be confused with herpetic gingivostomatitis and herpangina as the peripheral lesions are painless and may be overlooked. An occasional case has been confused with scabies.

Outbreaks of this syndrome are usually small and tend to occur in the summer months. Subclinical infection of family contacts can be demonstrated by the isolation of viruses and the prognosis is excellent.

The association between HFM disease caused by enterovirus type 71 and brainstem encephalitis is described below.

Miscellaneous coxsackie A virus infections. Coxsackie A viruses have been isolated from children suffering from a febrile illness with a rash, from cases of pharyngitis and from cases of benign pericarditis. They have also been associated with mild undifferentiated respiratory tract infection, especially coxsackie A21 virus (previously known as Coe virus), with acute febrile lymphadenitis, gastroenteritis, tracheobronchitis and pleurodynia.

Laboratory diagnosis. The isolation of most coxsackie group A viruses is not difficult provided suitable specimens are sent to the laboratory. Suitable specimens include vesicle fluid, throat swabs, feces and CSF, depending on the clinical syndrome under investigation. Serological tests on acute and convalescent serum samples can be carried out, but owing to the large number of serotypes this is not a practical procedure unless an agent has been isolated. The coxsackie virus complement-fixation test frequently employed cross-reacts with all enteroviruses and is not very sensitive. Detection of viral RNA by PCR is now generally available and more sensitive than culture.

Coxsackie group B virus diseases

Bornholm disease or epidemic pleurodynia. This disease, first recognized clinically over a century ago, results from infection with certain group B coxsackie viruses. Children and young adults are usually involved and more severe cases occur in the latter.

After an incubation period of 2–4 days, the illness commences in a nonspecific manner with fever, malaise and headache. However, the characteristic pain will soon follow. This is principally experienced over the lower chest and may be associated with acute dyspnea. A clinical diagnosis of pleurisy can be made, even if no friction rub is audible and X-ray of the chest is clear. Pain may also be felt lower down the trunk and this may spread over the abdomen and simulate an acute surgical condition. Palpation over the affected muscles may reveal exquisite tenderness and this can have a band-like distribution suggestive of a neurological disorder or shingles.

In many instances the illness subsides within a few days but it may run a relapsing course and last for as long as 3–4 weeks. Several members of a family may be attacked in quick succession and show a wide variation in the severity.

Bornholm disease requires to be differentiated from pleurisy and pneumonia. Acute appendicitis and cholecystitis have been mimicked by an abdominal presentation but milder varieties, without significant pain, can be confused with influenza. In general, there is no significant leukocytosis and this may be helpful in the differentiation of pyogenic infection.

Outbreaks are small and often confined to family units. However, an epidemic can be more widespread and in these instances the correct clinical diagnosis may be made with reasonable accuracy. Nevertheless, full confirmation requires detailed virological assessment.

CNS involvement. All six group B coxsackie viruses can cause *aseptic meningitis*. The age incidence is similar to that encountered in aseptic meningitis due to other viruses. Clinical differentiation from other possible causes is impossible, although pleurodynia is an occasional accompaniment. Severe and fatal encephalitis has been described in only a small number of cases, as has mild paralytic disease.

Neonatal or infant coxsackie B virus myocarditis. Coxsackie viruses B1–5 can all cause myocarditis, but types B3 and B4 most frequently. The illness usually commences within the first 2 weeks of life though older babies have been involved. Most neonatal cases are probably caused by vertical spread from an infected mother, and a maternal history of respiratory or gastrointestinal illness is common. Nursery outbreaks can also occur.

Clinical features (see Ch. 21). The presentation can be abrupt or more insidious. Presenting symptoms include feeding difficulties, lethargy, fever, cyanosis, respiratory distress and shock. Cardiomegaly, tachycardia, hepatomegaly and electrocardiographic changes soon appear. Involvement may not be confined to the cardiovascular system. In up to one third of cases, there are central nervous signs such as convulsions, neck stiffness, and coma with CSF changes.

The prognosis is poor, and up to 75% of cases die in spite of intensive therapy. At autopsy an intense inflammatory infiltration and necrosis is found in the myocardium and changes may also be found in the liver, pancreas, suprarenal glands, bone marrow and CNS.

Differential diagnosis. Myocarditis is difficult to diagnose in a neonate. Most cases are initially considered to be some form of acute respiratory disorder (e.g. respiratory distress syndrome), other overwhelming infections or congenital heart disease.

Treatment. Infants with this condition require intensive nursing in hospital. Oxygen, diuretics and inotropes may be required. The heart is often very sensitive to digoxin and low doses may be needed if used.

Pericarditis and myocarditis due to coxsackie B viruses in older children. Acute pericarditis in older children and adults is a syndrome where the causative role of coxsackie B viruses (types B1–5) is well established. Less often, myocarditis may also occur in these age groups but, unlike infection in neonates, the prognosis is generally good. Clinical recovery is quite rapid and although the electrocardiographic changes can take some months to resolve, recovery seems complete and there is little evidence of any permanent cardiac damage. Rare cases of myocarditis are fulminant and fatal.

Miscellaneous coxsackie B virus infections. Group B coxsackie viruses can be associated with mild respiratory tract illness, febrile illness with an exanthem and orchitis. They are also reputed to cause endocardial fibroelastosis, the infection of the fetus occurring in utero.

Laboratory diagnosis. The six types of coxsackie group B viruses can be readily isolated in the laboratory either in tissue cultures or suckling mice. Virus can be grown from throat swabs, feces, CSF and in some cases from other organs, e.g. myocardium and testis. Acute and convalescent samples of serum should be sent to the laboratory so that, if present, a significant rise in antibody titer during the illness can be shown. Serological tests may be of special value if a coxsackie group B virus has been isolated as in this instance the sera need only be tested for an antibody rise against this specific isolate. In all cases it is advisable to try to isolate a virus from the patient as early in the illness as possible. Detection of viral RNA by PCR is available in many laboratories.

ECHO virus infections

Agents of this group are named after the initial letters of their original name, enteric cytopathogenic human orphan viruses. There are some 30 distinctive serotypes and their association with aseptic meningitis, encephalitis and paralytic diseases is well documented. They may also cause respiratory tract infections, gastroenteritis, myocarditis and exanthemata of a rather nonspecific character. Subclinical infection with this group is common. Infections may be sporadic or occur in moderate sized epidemics.

A number of different types of ECHO viruses have been associated with each of the various clinical syndromes that this group may cause and most types have been found in association with more than one syndrome. A few of the identified types have not, as yet, been found in association with obvious disease. In general, infection by this group of agents is relatively benign and, except in neonates, few fatalities have been described. They spread in a fashion similar to polioviruses and coxsackie viruses.

Clinical syndromes

A considerable number of different ECHO virus types can cause *aseptic meningitis*, which may be sporadic or in epidemics. In general, the prognosis is good and in many instances the cases are clinically indistinguishable from those produced by other viral infections. However, in some there is a rash and where this is seen in a reasonable proportion of cases in any outbreak of aseptic meningitis, it often indicates that an ECHO virus is responsible.

Sporadic cases of *poliomyelitis-like illness* with paralysis have been reported in association with confirmed ECHO virus infection. The paralysis is usually mild and reversible, but permanent residual paralysis can occur. Cases of *encephalitis* due to ECHO viruses have also been reported,

occasionally fatal. Children with antibody deficiency can get chronic ECHO virus encephalitis and/or myositis.

Mild upper respiratory illness has been found in association with a few ECHO viruses, particularly types 11, 19 and 20. ECHO viruses 5, 11, 14, 18, 19 and 20 have been associated with gastroenteritis in infants and young children.

ECHO viruses have been isolated in association with sporadic cases of pleurodynia, pericarditis and myocarditis. However, as these agents may be cultured from many otherwise healthy people their etiological relationship should not necessarily be assumed.

Where rashes do occur as a result of ECHO virus infection they tend to be of a fine, maculopapular character, have a widespread distribution and fade rapidly. Generally there is no classical distribution or typical enanthem, although lesions may be papular, arranged in lines and located peripherally, the so-called 'papular acro-located syndrome' (PALS).

Neonatal ECHO virus infection can disseminate and cause massive hepatic necrosis, disseminated intravascular coagulation, bleeding and usually death. Such severe cases are acquired vertically (from the mother) and a maternal history of peripartum illness with diarrhea or abdominal pain is common. Although nursery outbreaks may occur, most horizontally acquired or nosocomial cases are relatively mild, although occasionally complicated by meningitis and myocarditis.

Laboratory diagnosis

The ECHO viruses can be readily isolated in tissue culture, or enteroviral RNA can be detected by reverse-transcriptase PCR. Specimens usually required by the laboratory are CSF, throat swabs and feces depending on the clinical manifestations of the illness. Serology is not sufficiently sensitive to be useful clinically.

Enteroviruses types 68–71

In addition to the spectrum of symptoms outlined above, this group of enteroviruses is also associated with specific syndromes. Enterovirus type 70 has been isolated from patients with acute hemorrhagic conjunctivitis. Enterovirus type 71 (EV71) is associated with hand, foot and mouth syndrome. In Australia, Malaysia, Taiwan and Japan, outbreaks of EV71-associated hand, foot and mouth disease in children have been followed by severe neurological symptoms such as brainstem encephalitis often with neurogenic pulmonary edema, and by Guillain–Barré syndrome, acute transverse myelitis, cerebellar ataxia, opsomyoclonus, benign intracranial hypertension and febrile convulsions.

Treatment

No specific therapy is available. In a small, uncontrolled case series, the antiviral agent pleconaril was used in severe enteroviral infection in infants and immunocompromised children.[666] However, efficacy data from randomized controlled trials are as yet unavailable. Intravenous immunoglobulin and interferon have been used to treat chronic enteroviral infection in immunodeficient children. None of these agents is reportedly effective against EV71-associated disease.

VIRUSES AND THE GASTROINTESTINAL TRACT

Many viral agents may inhabit the intestinal tract without producing obvious clinical illness. As a result, when such agents are cultured in the presence of gastrointestinal symptoms, their etiological role is difficult to establish. Nevertheless epidemiological studies in the recent past seemed to indicate that some agents, such as certain ECHO viruses, may be involved in outbreaks of diarrhea in infants. The picture has, however, changed in the last few years as a wide variety of new viral agents has been discovered by electron microscopy of feces. Notable amongst these are *rotaviruses* and *noroviruses*, including *Norwalk virus*.

GASTROENTERITIS

Viruses associated with gastroenteritis include rotaviruses, noroviruses including Norwalk, caliciviruses, coronaviruses, astroviruses, adenoviruses, stool parvoviruses and enteroviruses. The role of rotaviruses and Norwalk virus is most clearly established, but other viruses can cause limited cases or outbreaks of infantile diarrhea.

Rotaviruses were initially found on electron microscopy of duodenal biopsies taken from children with diarrhea in Australia in 1973. Since then these agents have been found to be common worldwide and their presence may be detected by a variety of methods. Several different human types have been identified as well as many animal varieties. Species specificity appears incomplete.

Between 1 and 7 days after infection, but usually within 2 days, the affected child starts to vomit and develops a low grade fever. Watery diarrhea soon follows and, although mucus may be seen in the stools, blood is rarely present. The vomiting stops after 1–2 days, but diarrhea persists even if intravenous fluids are started with no oral intake. Nonspecific respiratory symptoms may occur and, although the illness terminates in about 5–7 days, virus may be found in the stool for up to 10 days.

The peak age of attack is between 6 and 24 months of age, mainly from 9 to 12 months. There is a slight male preponderance. Asymptomatic cases may be found in older members of the household. Neonatal infection occurs and has been associated with a clinical picture resembling necrotizing enterocolitis. However, neonatal infection is often subclinical, perhaps due to the presence of maternal antibody. It is suggested that breast-feeding can be protective.

Up to 50% of hospitalized cases of infantile gastroenteritis and a lower proportion of community cases are caused by rotaviruses.[667] Transmission is by the fecal–oral route. In temperate climates it is mainly a winter disease, although cases can occur throughout the year. Serological surveys show that up to 90% of children aged 3 years or over possess antibody to rotaviruses, and surveys in the adult population show figures of up to 70%.

Treatment of gastroenteritis due to rotavirus infection is along standard lines. Fatalities are rare in industrialized countries and usually in otherwise debilitated children. A variety of complications have been found but the role of rotaviruses in their production is not firmly established.

A tetravalent rotavirus vaccine was licensed in the USA in 1998 and introduced into the routine schedule. It was then voluntarily withdrawn from the market in 1999, due to a possible rare association with intussusception that was detected in post-licensing surveillance.[668] New rotavirus vaccines are safe and effective and have not been associated with intussusception.

The *Norwalk virus*, which was first discovered in 1972, and other caliciviruses are also known to produce gastroenteritis. Outbreaks have usually occurred in older children with secondary cases in adults, some involving schoolchildren and their teachers. These agents, first discovered in the USA and certain Far Eastern countries, are now found on a worldwide basis. After an incubation period of some 2 days the illness starts with nausea and vomiting. Diarrhea, abdominal cramps and fever follow in about half of those involved but symptoms usually abate within a day or so. Treatment is purely symptomatic.

Enteric adenoviruses are the second most important cause of viral diarrhea of infancy, in terms of hospitalization, and often cause prolonged diarrhea with or without vomiting. Astroviruses rarely result in hospital admission but can cause winter vomiting and may cause rare outbreaks in hospitals.

INTUSSUSCEPTION

Intussusception involves the invagination of a portion of the intestine into an adjacent portion. A study found *adenovirus infection* in 34% of Vietnamese and 40% of Australian children with intussusception, but no association with rotavirus, other enteric pathogens or oral polio vaccine.[669] It is thought that adenovirus infection causes inflammation of the Peyer's patches that acts as a focus for the intussusception. Adenoviruses have also been isolated from regional lymph glands in children with mesenteric adenitis and, as this condition is considered to be associated with the development of intussusception, the possible etiological role seems strengthened.

The association between intussusception and a live attenuated rotavirus vaccine, although not with wild-type rotavirus infection, is further evidence that intussusception may follow virus infections of the gastrointestinal tract.

OTHER CONDITIONS

Attempts to establish an association between viral infection and appendicitis have not proved very rewarding. Pancreatitis is a recognized complication of mumps and has occasionally been found in association with infection by coxsackie viruses.

LABORATORY DIAGNOSIS

In general, the main pathogens responsible for viral gastroenteritis, rotavirus, enteric adenoviruses, caliciviruses and astroviruses cannot be readily isolated by culture.[670] Although these agents may be demonstrated in stools by negative staining electron microscopy this has largely been replaced by enzyme immunoassays or PCR for rotavirus and enteric adenoviruses.

OCULAR DISEASES CAUSED BY VIRUSES AND ALLIED ORGANISMS

It is now recognized that viral and chlamydial infections of the eye constitute a larger proportion of ocular disease than was formerly appreciated. In part this stems from the enormous advances in viral technology but many ocular diseases are now recognized to have a viral basis because chemotherapy has cleared secondary bacterial infection and revealed the true, underlying viral pathogenesis.

In most instances viral infection of the eye presents as part of a systemic infection which may manifest itself by direct tissue invasion or indirectly through neural involvement, as in the viral encephalitides. Examples of viruses that may act this way are CMV and HSV in the congenitally infected or immunocompromised. However, some viral infections seem to involve the eye selectively, including certain adenoviral infections, trachoma, inclusion conjunctivitis and acute hemorrhagic conjunctivitis.

ADENOVIRUS INFECTIONS OF THE EYE

Two main ocular syndromes are associated with adenovirus infection – *pharyngoconjunctival fever* and *epidemic keratoconjunctivitis*.

Pharyngoconjunctival fever

Pharyngoconjunctival fever may result from infection by several types of adenoviruses, most commonly type 3. Clinically it may present as unilateral or bilateral follicular conjunctivitis, often with fever, pharyngitis and mild preauricular lymphadenopathy. The conjunctivitis shows follicular hypertrophy and a mild transient keratitis sometimes develops.

Children are most often affected and cases may occur sporadically or in epidemics, sometimes associated with swimming pools.

Epidemic keratoconjunctivitis

This disease presents as an acute keratoconjunctivitis with follicular hypertrophy of the conjunctiva and marked preauricular lymphadenopathy. A distinctive keratitis then develops and about a third of the cases have pseudomembranes.

Large epidemics may occur and adults are involved rather than children. Infection is usually due to adenovirus type 8 and spread may occur through ocular instruments, infected eye-droppers and contaminated solutions used in hospitals, first aid stations and surgeries. Complete recovery usually occurs but permanent impairment of vision can occasionally result.

Laboratory diagnosis

Ocular infection with an adenovirus can be confirmed by culture or PCR. Swabs or scrapings in virus transport medium should be sent to the laboratory for virus isolation. The adenoviruses are not difficult to grow.

TRACHOMA AND INCLUSION CONJUNCTIVITIS (see Ch. 12)

Chlamydia have properties intermediate between viruses and bacteria, and show sensitivity to certain antibiotics. *Chlamydia trachomatis* is the cause of trachoma, inclusion conjunctivitis, afebrile pneumonitis and lymphogranuloma venereum.

Trachoma

Trachoma is a specific form of keratoconjunctivitis that first involves the upper tarsal follicles. Later upper limbal changes appear followed by pannus formation and the development of Herbert's peripheral pits. The disease is mainly encountered in tropical areas where water is scarce. In such areas there is often a very high incidence. Permanent scarring and blindness may occur, especially where adequate facilities for treatment are not available.

All ages are affected, but the disease is especially common in children and is often associated with secondary infection. Theories to explain the spread have included person-to-person contact, infection through fomites and dissemination by flies.

Treatment

Among drugs which may be used are sulfonamides, tetracycline and less often erythromycin. Opinions differ as to the efficacy and mode of treatment. However, where topical therapy is conscientiously applied over a period of several weeks or even months, a good response can be anticipated. Some advocate supplementation by oral therapy.

Inclusion conjunctivitis

This condition is caused by certain strains of *Chlamydia trachomatis* that may reside in the genital tract and produce cervicitis or urethritis. There is a danger of spread to infants during their passage through the birth canal, resulting in inclusion blennorrhea. Older children and adults may contract inclusion conjunctivitis from swimming pools contaminated by urine or genital tract discharge.

Treatment of inclusion conjunctivitis is also by sulfonamides or topical broad spectrum antibiotics. However, the response is quicker than in trachoma and treatment need not be so prolonged. The prognosis is also better and permanent scarring does not occur. Neonates with inclusion conjunctivitis should be treated with oral erythromycin 10 mg/kg/dose 6-hourly for 14 days because of the risk of progression to afebrile pneumonitis.

Laboratory diagnosis

The agents are situated in the epithelial cells of the conjunctiva, and for successful culture epithelial scrapings or eye swabs in special transport medium should be sent to the laboratory. Cultural methods consist of inoculation of suitable tissue cultures and then, after incubation, examination under the microscope for typical inclusion bodies. Direct microscopy on Giemsa-stained smears may reveal typical inclusions. ELISA antigen detection tests and PCR that avoid the need for culture and give a rapid diagnosis are increasingly being used.

ENTEROVIRUS 70 (ACUTE HEMORRHAGIC CONJUNCTIVITIS)

This condition is caused by enterovirus type 70, which has been isolated from the conjunctiva of affected patients. Extensive outbreaks have been reported from Africa, Pakistan, India and South America. The disease appears to have an incubation period of about 24 hours and to be highly contagious in unhygienic and crowded conditions. The infection is of sudden onset with swelling, congestion, watering and pain in the eye. The most characteristic sign is subconjunctival hemorrhage of varying intensity, which may sometimes be accompanied by corneal keratitis. The disease is not influenced by antibiotics and symptoms usually subside within 1–2 weeks.

Laboratory diagnosis

Conjunctival scrapings or swabs should be sent to the laboratory where suitable tissue cultures can be used to isolate the causative agent.

VIRAL INFECTION OF THE LIVER

Acute inflammation of the liver may be caused by a number of viruses including hepatitis viruses A to E, CMV, adenoviruses, picornaviruses, HSV, EBV and the viruses of diseases such as yellow fever and rubella.

HEPATITIS A VIRUS INFECTION OR INFECTIOUS HEPATITIS (EPIDEMIC HEPATITIS, EPIDEMIC JAUNDICE OR CATARRHAL JAUNDICE)

This disease has an incubation period of 15–50 days (average 30 days) and is mainly found in young children. It is also quite common in older children and young adults but the attack rate declines with increasing age though a higher proportion of severe and complicated cases may be found in these older age groups. Pregnant women may contract a particularly severe form.

Infectious hepatitis occurs worldwide and epidemic periodicity varies greatly in different communities. The responsible agent, hepatitis A virus, is present in both blood and feces at the peak of the illness and persists in the feces for a relatively short time. Susceptible human volunteers have been fed filtered fecal extracts and virus could be found in the feces of those who developed jaundice from 14 to 26 days before the onset of icterus and for over a week thereafter. Furthermore, although at least two thirds of the recipients displayed no clinical evidence of hepatitis, subclinical evidence of infection was found on serial examination by appropriate liver function tests. This indicates a ratio of 1:2 for clinical, as opposed to subclinical, infection and this impression is further substantiated by epidemiological studies in naturally occurring epidemics.

Although infectious hepatitis is mainly transmitted by the fecal–oral route through contamination of food and water, transmission may also occur from blood, urine, nasopharyngeal secretions and saliva. Large epidemics usually occur in institutions and closed communities and, in some of these, infection of a communal water supply has been responsible. Prevention of waterborne outbreaks of this type is difficult, although carefully controlled super-chlorination may be effective. Outbreaks have also followed the ingestion of raw oysters and raw clams infected by sewage. Infection may also result from the use of imperfectly sterilized instruments, syringes and needles that have been contaminated by infected blood or blood products.

The diagnosis, differential diagnosis and detailed treatment of infectious hepatitis are referred to elsewhere (Ch. 19). Complement-fixation tests, immune-adherence hemagglutination, ELISA and radioimmunoassay can be used to detect specific IgM and IgG antibody to hepatitis A virus. The presence of specific IgM antibody indicates a recent infection with hepatitis A virus. In the majority of childhood cases the illness is mild and treatment need not extend beyond simple bed rest and a moderate period of convalescence.

Mortality amongst otherwise healthy, well-nourished individuals is as low as 0.1–0.2% but can rise to 2 or 3% in the poorly nourished. Death may either be early from fulminating hepatitis leading to acute hepatocellular failure or occur considerably later from chronic liver damage.

Prevention

Killed vaccines are safe and effective,[671] and indicated for older children and adults at long term risk. Human normal immunoglobulin is effective prophylaxis and should be given to adult and child contacts of index cases and to people traveling for short periods to areas with poor sanitation.

HEPATITIS B (SERUM HEPATITIS, AUSTRALIA ANTIGEN-POSITIVE HEPATITIS)

Hepatitis B is enormously important. Worldwide, there are about 200 million chronic carriers of hepatitis B virus (HBV), which is one of the most important causes of liver cirrhosis and hepatoma. HBV can be transmitted either vertically (mother to child) or horizontally (from an infectious contact). Infection is endemic in some parts of the world, notably South East Asia where carriage rates may exceed 15%. About half of all carriers will die liver-related deaths.

The incubation period is 60–160 days, much longer than hepatitis A. Virus antigen can be detected in the blood up to 3 months before jaundice occurs and often for many years after clinical recovery. The virus is mainly transmitted via infected blood and is highly infectious, far more so than HIV. Infected blood transfusions, needle sharing by intravenous drug abusers, tattooing and ritual scarification are all well-documented means of spread. The virus can be sexually transmitted and the incidence is high in many homosexual communities. Vertical spread is common and is thought to be mainly peripartum rather than transplacental, thus being largely preventable by intervention immediately after birth. Most vertically infected babies become chronic carriers. About a quarter to a third of asymptomatic HBV carriers remain infectious and go on to develop liver fibrosis[672] or carcinoma (hepatoma).[673,674] The virus is also found in breast milk, although breast-feeding has not been shown to be a clear risk factor for transmission. Clinical features of hepatitis B infection are discussed elsewhere.

Etiology

In 1965, geneticists investigating inherited variations in human plasma proteins discovered an unusual protein antigen in the serum of an Australian aborigine. This antigen, originally called Australia antigen (Au), and now hepatitis B surface antigen (HBs), was found to be associated with hepatitis of long incubation. On electron microscopy of serum three particles are identifiable. Dane particles, 42 nm in diameter, are complete virus comprising an inner core containing double-stranded HBV DNA within a core antigen (HBc) and surrounded by an outer coat of surface antigen (HBs). A further antigen, the e antigen, a component of the inner core, may also be seen (Fig. 28.43). The detection of e antigen in the absence of e antibody correlates with high infectivity. Subjects may be:

1. HBs antigen positive, with no e antigen or e antibody detected – these will be mainly chronic carriers;
2. HBe antigen positive, but e antibody negative – usually also HBs positive – are highly infectious: usually suggests recent, active infection, but can be chronic HBe Ag positive carriers;

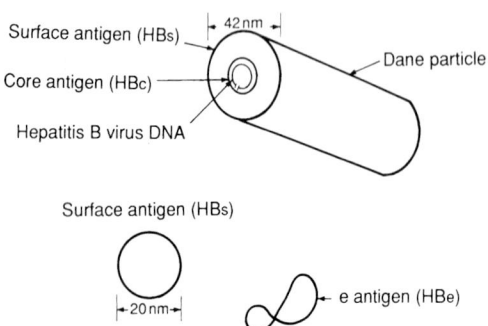

Fig. 28.43 Diagrammatic representation of electron microscopic appearance of hepatitis B virus.

3. HBe antibody positive – recovery phase, much less infectious.

Tests commonly used to detect the presence of HBV antigens and antibodies include hemagglutination tests and ELISA tests, which are often used to screen sera for surface antigen (HBs), and radioimmunoassays which are more sensitive.

Detection of HBs antibody indicates either recovery from acute HBV infection or a response to immunization. Presence of HBc IgM antibody indicates acute HBV infection, while HBc IgG antibody is detected following infection but not immunization (which uses only surface antigen).

Prevention

In many countries, blood or blood product donations are routinely screened for surface antigen (HBs) and antenatal screening of all pregnant women or those from high risk groups allows intervention to prevent vertical transmission. Great care should be taken when handling blood and excreta from HBV positive patients because of the high infectivity, although any person doing so should have been immunized.

Passive immunization with specific immunoglobulin is given for accidental contamination with infected blood, e.g. in the laboratory or from a syringe and needle from a drug abuser. It reduces vertical transmission if given to infected mothers in the first 72 h (ideally < 12 h) after birth.[675] There appears to be no additional benefit by giving further doses of HBV immunoglobulin beyond the newborn period.[675]

Recombinant DNA hepatitis B vaccines are now widely available. All health care personnel likely to come into contact with HBV positive patients (e.g. doctors, dentists, nurses, midwives, students, laboratory staff) should receive a course of three doses of the vaccine.

Babies of mothers who are in the above risk groups 1 (HBs positive) and 2 (HBe antigen positive) are at high risk of becoming chronic carriers without intervention. Indeed this will be the case in up to 90% of babies of HBe antigen positive mothers. Such babies should receive both passive HBV specific immunoglobulin and be actively immunized with hepatitis B vaccine, which provides additional protection against vertical transmission over HBV immunoglobulin alone.[675] Babies of mothers in group 3 (HBe antibody positive) are at lower risk but may rarely develop acute hepatitis, and there is a risk of later horizontal transmission from the mother or an infected sibling. They should therefore be immunized and many would feel they should also receive specific immunoglobulin.

Many countries are now advocating universal neonatal hepatitis B immunization.

Treatment

Pegylated interferon alpha and lamivudine have been used in the treatment of chronic hepatitis B disease in adults, and shown to be effective at reducing HBV viral load and inducing HbeAg seroconversion in some patients.[676,677] Lamivudine has been given to HBV infected women in the last weeks of pregnancy to reduce the risk of vertical transmission with variable success.[678] The use of these agents for the treatment of chronic HBV infection in children has also been reported in small case series,[679] but the efficacy of these therapies has not been fully evaluated.

HEPATITIS C (TRANSFUSION-ASSOCIATED NON-A, NON-B HEPATITIS)

Hepatitis C virus is a small single-stranded RNA virus that is a member of the flavivirus family. It is the cause of the great majority of transfusion-associated hepatitis.

The structure of hepatitis C virus (HCV) was determined by molecular biology techniques in 1988. There are multiple HCV genotypes and subtypes, each of which carries a different long term prognosis. Serological tests have been developed to screen blood products, and PCR testing for the presence of viral nucleic acid is widely available. The virus is extremely difficult to grow.

HCV has an incubation period of around 30–60 days. Transmission is mainly via blood transfusion or by needle sharing between intravenous drug abusers. Screening of donated blood for the presence of hepatitis C antibodies has greatly reduced the risk from blood transfusion. HCV is more resistant to inactivation than HBV or HIV, and blood products such as intravenous immunoglobulin have occasionally transmitted HCV despite viral inactivation steps.

Vertical transmission from mother to fetus occurs in about 5% of pregnancies, and is thought to occur antenatally or perinatally almost exclusively in the setting of high maternal viral load in the serum. Maternal co-infection with HIV is associated with a higher risk of transmission.[680] Other risk factors have been poorly defined. As yet unconfirmed associations include prolonged rupture of membranes, and invasive fetal monitoring[681] and female sex of the infant.[682] Elective Cesarean section does not confer protection from vertical transmission.[682] HCV RNA and antibody have been detected in breast milk,[683] although breast-feeding has not been shown to be associated with transmission to the infant by hepatitis C positive women.[684] Nevertheless, a theoretical risk remains and the decision of a hepatitis C positive woman whether to breast-feed should be made on an individual basis. The diagnosis of perinatally acquired HCV is usually based on the detection of HCV antibody and/or HCV RNA by PCR. The presence of maternal antibody makes interpretation of serological assays difficult in children less than 18 months. At 12 months, up to 10% of uninfected children remain HCV seropositive, but this figure has dropped to 0.1% by 18 months.[685] PCR for HCV RNA is sensitive over 1 month of age and is specific, but the test is expensive. Any positive PCR test should be repeated to exclude false positive results, and because of the possibility of viral clearance.[685]

Childhood HCV infection is largely asymptomatic,[686] but a high proportion of those infected with HCV become chronic carriers and may progress to cirrhosis. A large cohort study from Italy of HCV infected children has shown a shift in the dominant HCV genotype from genotypes 1 and 2, associated with poorer response to therapy and reduced viral clearance, to genotypes 3 and 4, with genotype 3 associated with a better prognosis.[687] Nevertheless, it is estimated that childhood HCV disease will have an important economic impact on direct medical costs in the next decade, as the burden of pediatric HCV infection increases.[688] Interferon alfa therapy alone or with ribavirin is effective in reducing viral replication in around 40% of adult chronic carriers, although half of these responders will relapse when interferon is stopped. Experience with the use of these agents in HCV infected children is increasing. Treatment may be considered for the child with severe hepatitis C induced liver disease, which should be managed by a pediatric hepatologist.[689]

Children with hepatitis C infection should be immunized against hepatitis A and hepatitis B to protect against further insults to the liver.

DELTA AGENT (HEPATITIS D)

The delta agent is a defective RNA virus which requires HBV for its own synthesis. This is one of the most important examples of viral co-infection described. The delta agent was detected by immunofluorescence studies of liver cell nuclei of chronic HBV carriers. Delta antigen and antibody are detected by radioimmunoassay or ELISA and have never been demonstrated other than in association with HBV. The delta agent is most prevalent in intravenous drug abusers in Italy and the Mediterranean but has been detected worldwide. It appears to be a risk factor for acute hepatitis in drug abusers. About half of HBs positive hemophiliacs in the USA and Italy have anti-delta antibodies.

HEPATITIS E (ENTERIC NON-A, NON-B HEPATITIS)

Hepatitis E is the enterically transmitted form of non-A, non-B hepatitis and is transmitted by the fecal–oral route. It is of major importance in resource limited countries as a cause of hepatitis due to waterborne epidemics, which mainly affect young adults, but rarely children. The mortality can be as high as 40% in pregnant women. The viral genome has been cloned and sequenced, and serological tests and PCR assays are available.

HEPATITIS G

This single-stranded RNA virus of the flavivirus family usually results in an asymptomatic infection. It can cause chronic infection, but rarely hepatitis. It has been documented in adults and children, especially those whose mothers are co-infected with HCV or HIV.[690] It can be diagnosed by detection of viral RNA by PCR.

HEPATITIS – THE ROLE OF OTHER VIRUSES

Other viral infections may involve the liver.

CMV is known to attack the liver in 85% of newborn infants suffering from cytomegalic inclusion disease; the same virus may also cause hepatitis when older children or adults contract the acquired form of the infection. *Infectious mononucleosis*, due to EBV, is frequently accompanied by some degree of liver involvement; most often this will reveal itself as a mild derangement of liver function tests though some cases will manifest obvious jaundice. Infection by *arboviruses* may cause a similar picture; yellow fever produces a more specific and severe form of hepatitis.

HSV infection of the newborn can manifest as severe and often fatal hepatitis.

Lastly, there are instances where transient liver involvement has been found in a variety of viral infections including ECHO viruses types 4 and 9, coxsackie viruses, adenoviruses and lymphocytic choriomeningitis virus. In most the involvement has been extremely mild with full recovery, although severe hepatitis may occur.

MISCELLANEOUS VIRAL INFECTIONS

ORF (CONTAGIOUS PUSTULAR DERMATITIS OF SHEEP, CONTAGIOUS ECTHYMA OF SHEEP)

This is a common and widespread viral infection of sheep and to a lesser extent of goats. In general infection is from animal to animal but virus can persist in the soil of affected pastures for several months. Lambs are most commonly involved and they develop a papulovesicular eruption on the mouth, lips and non-hair-bearing areas of the skin. Transmission to man is relatively rare and the main incidence is in springtime. The infection is most commonly encountered in shepherds, farm and abattoir workers. However, children can be infected owing to their liking for handling young lambs.

Orf virus is included amongst the poxviruses and has certain similarities to the virus of molluscum contagiosum. It can be grown with difficulty on tissue culture but is usually identified by electron microscopy. Scrapings from the base of the bullae are preferred to vesicle fluid in these studies.

Clinical features

Lesions, which are usually but not exclusively single, most commonly appear on the hand or forearm. Initially there is an area of infiltration presenting as brawny edema but this soon develops into a flaccid bulla. However, on puncture a rather clear serosanguinous fluid is obtained. There is little or no constitutional upset but the progression of the lesion is slow and may take 6–8 weeks before it finally heals. No specific treatment is available or required in view of the benign nature of the condition but it is wise to protect the lesion with dressings to counteract the possibility of secondary infection.

MOLLUSCUM CONTAGIOSUM

This viral disease (see also Ch. 30) is seen in children more often than in adults. The responsible agent is a DNA virus belonging to the pox group but serologically unrelated to vaccinia or variola; it is readily identified by electron microscopy of the curettings from a lesion or on the histological appearances of a biopsy. Transmission is by close contact but infectivity is low.

Clinical features

Molluscum contagiosum is unassociated with any constitutional upset and presents as a chronic viral infection of the epidermis. Lesions, which may be multiple, take the form of pinkish white or flesh-colored, dome-shaped nodules between 2 and 8 mm in diameter and most show a central depression or umbilication. They may appear on the face, arms, legs, buttocks, scalp or genitalia but sparing of the palms of the hands and the soles of the feet is a characteristic feature. Occasionally the margins of the eyelids are involved and chronic follicular conjunctivitis can supervene (Fig. 28.44). HIV infection may be associated with disseminated molluscum.

Treatment

The disease is benign and self-limiting. Treatment is advised only to prevent spread by autoinoculation or to others. Treatment is simple and consists of the removal of the lesions with a sharp curette. Other methods include electro- or cryocautery. The lesions will usually heal without scarring and recurrence is rare.

TRANSFUSION TRANSMITTED (TT) VIRUS

TT virus is a DNA virus that was first identified in 1997 in the serum of a patient with post-transfusion hepatitis of unknown etiology.[691] To date, there has been no disease association with this virus. It can be detected in the serum of 2% of healthy blood donors in the UK, and can be transmitted by transfusion, by fecal–oral spread and vertically.[692]

ARENA VIRUSES CAUSING HEMORRHAGIC FEVER

Lassa fever

Lassa fever was first reported from Lassa in Nigeria in 1969. The Lassa virus shows some morphological and antigenic similarities to lymphocytic choriomeningitis virus. It is one of the arenaviruses and it is widely distributed throughout West Africa. It is one of five African viruses (yellow fever, Lassa, Ebola, Marburg and Congo-Crimean) that cause hemorrhagic fever. The natural host is the rat *Mastomys natalensis*.

The virus is transmitted from person to person by close contact. It causes a diffuse serositis, hemorrhage and shock and is often fatal. Intravenous ribavirin reduces mortality from Lassa fever and is the treatment of choice. Additional treatment involves the use of plasma from a convalesced patient. For the adult 250–500 ml are used. Stocks of this are held in Nigeria, Sierra Leone, the London School of Hygiene and Tropical Medicine and the Communicable Disease Center, Atlanta, Georgia, USA. Strict isolation of patients is mandatory.

Marburg virus disease (green monkey disease, vervet monkey disease, Jo'burg virus disease)

Marburg virus disease was first recognized in Germany in 1967 in personnel who had handled a consignment of African green monkeys

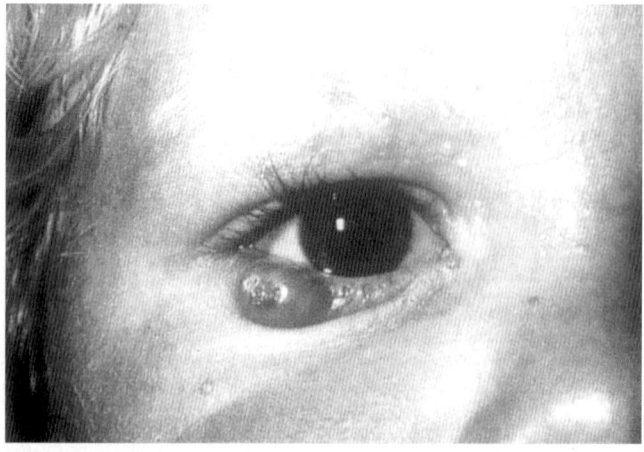

Fig. 28.44   Molluscum contagiosum.

(*Cercopithecus aethiops*) from Uganda. Outbreaks have occurred in Sudan and Zaire. The Marburg virus is long, rod shaped (rhabdovirus-like) and does not appear to possess antigenic affinity with other known viruses. Although the Marburg outbreak appeared to follow contact with African green monkeys, no similar infections have been recognized as a result of other contacts with these monkeys and such monkeys suffer 100% mortality if experimentally infected. Thus the natural host and possible vectors are unknown.

The disease is highly infectious and carries a high mortality: 7 of the 31 Marburg cases died. Secondary cases appear to have a better prognosis than primary cases. There is as yet no protective vaccine. Strict isolation and barrier nursing of patients is necessary.

Ebola virus disease

This disease is clinically indistinct from Marburg virus disease. The virus is morphologically identical to the Marburg virus, but antigenically distinct. The disease has been found in the Sudan and Zaire.

INFECTIONS DUE TO ARBOVIRUSES (TOGAVIRUSES)

The principal feature linking the viruses of this group is the fact that all are arthropod borne (hence the name) and well over 200 such agents have been recognized. Most viruses in this group are natural parasites of animals or birds and multiply in arthropod vectors, which are unharmed by the process. Infection in the human may take several forms; most commonly encephalitis of varying severity results. Other diseases produced include yellow fever, dengue and sandfly fever. Arboviruses may also result in mild influenza-like illness. Children are particularly susceptible to this group of diseases. The arboviruses are subdivided into a number of families: Bunyaviridae (sandfly fever virus, Hantaviruses), Togaviridae (western equine encephalitis virus, eastern equine encephalitis virus), Flaviviridae (yellow fever virus, dengue viruses, West Nile virus), Reoviridae and Rhabdoviridae. They may also be classified according to the clinical syndromes they produce.

Arboviruses group A

Some 20 arboviruses are included in this group, the best known being the viruses of eastern and western equine encephalitis, and more recently West Nile virus.[693] These present in humans as aseptic meningitis or meningoencephalitis of varying severity. Children tend to be more seriously affected and death may result. Those who survive the illness may have permanent mental retardation, deafness, epilepsy and paralysis. Mortality may vary with age and the responsible virus. On average, 5% of patients may die, but this figure is often considerably higher following infection by certain viruses, reaching 74% in eastern equine encephalitis.

Other viruses of this group produce a mild dengue-like illness and most have their animal reservoir in wild or domestic birds. Their arthropod vectors are culicine and anopheline mosquitoes.

Arboviruses group B

This, a larger group, can be divided into (1) *mosquito-borne* and (2) *tick-borne* sections. The best-known disease associated with the former is yellow fever. The latter are mainly associated with a variety of encephalitic illnesses.

Yellow fever (yellow jack)

Yellow fever has been a recognized clinical entity for over 300 years, and in 1881 Carlos Finlay suggested that *Aedes aegypti* spread the infection. This theory was substantiated by the classical studies of Walter Reed and his colleagues working on mosquitoes and yellow fever in Cuba.[694] Yellow fever occurs in parts of Africa, South America and central America, but not Asia. The last cases of infection acquired in the UK occurred in the latter part of the nineteenth century, when ships arrived carrying infected *A. aegypti*.

Disease may vary from a mild fever to a fulminant hepatitis with jaundice, hepatic necrosis, hemorrhage and shock. In the jungle it is predominantly an adult disease. Where infection occurs in an urban community, all ages and both sexes are equally affected.

There is no specific treatment.

Elimination of the responsible vector is of prime importance and infection has been eradicated from certain areas where this has been diligently performed. Vaccination with the 17 D attenuated strain of virus is compulsory for travel to endemic areas and immunity will usually last for up to 6 years. Complications of immunization are confined to an occasional case of benign encephalitis, usually encountered in young infants, and the vaccine is not recommended under 9 months of age if exposure to mosquitoes can be avoided.

Dengue fever

Dengue fever is mosquito-borne like yellow fever, is also caused by a virus from group B, and the same vector, *A. aegypti*, is involved. The disease is widespread and is mainly found in warm areas, including Australia, Greece, Japan, India, Malaysia and Hawaii. So far, four antigenic varieties, known as types 1, 2, 3 and 4 have been described.

Clinical features. There is an incubation period of 5–9 days. The illness starts with high fever, malaise, headache, pain in the eyes, backache and excruciatingly painful limbs (it is sometimes called breakbone fever). Between the third and fifth days, a maculopapular, scarlatiniform or petechial rash appears and lasts up to 4 days. Following this there is usually a rapid recovery. Occasionally, however, particularly in children, the disease progresses to a severe hemorrhagic form, dengue hemorrhagic shock syndrome (DHSS), which may be fatal (see Hemorrhagic fevers below). It is thought that DHSS follows prior sensitization with a different strain of dengue virus, and is an example of antibody-mediated enhancement of disease.

Control. Eradication of the vector is desirable. Dengue viruses are poor antigens, which has frustrated efforts to produce effective vaccines.

Hemorrhagic fevers

A number of virus infections may occur in a hemorrhagic form, e.g. Lassa fever, yellow fever and measles. The arboviruses, particularly the Chikungunya (group A) and dengue (group B) viruses, are also prone to cause hemorrhagic disease. Hemorrhagic fever due to the mosquito-borne Chikungunya virus has been reported in Africa, India and Thailand. In South East Asia, hemorrhagic fever due to dengue virus is transmitted by the bite of the *A. aegypti* mosquito which is common in urban areas.

The hemorrhagic fevers affect mainly children. Patients develop fever, erythematous or petechial rashes, hepatosplenomegaly and bleeding that may be mild or severe. The majority of patients recover, but some develop shock and die. Thrombocytopenia is common. In fatal cases there are gross effusions into the serous cavities, petechial hemorrhages on the surface of organs and bronchopneumonia. Treatment is symptomatic. In shocked cases, intravenous plasma should be administered, together with the usual measures for collapsed patients.

Hemorrhagic fever with renal syndrome

This name is used for several similar conditions including Korean hemorrhagic fever and nephropathica epidemica occurring in Scandinavia, central Europe, Russia, China, Japan and Korea.[695] At least two viruses, Hantaan (Hantavirus) and Puumala, transmitted by arboviruses from rodents, are implicated. The clinical manifestations are fever, shock, massive proteinuria followed by acute renal failure, and thrombocytopenia and bleeding with bruising, hematuria, hematemesis and melena. With supportive treatment, the mortality is low.

Tick-borne arbovirus infections

These including louping ill (a disease of sheep in Scotland and northern England; rarely aseptic meningitis can occur if man is infected by an infected tick), Russian spring–summer encephalitis (western and eastern forms), Omsk hemorrhagic fever and Kyasanur Forest fever. Illness associated with this group may range from aseptic meningitis to severe and even fatal encephalitis, although the prognosis is better than with

infection by group A strains. On occasion paralytic disease simulating poliomyelitis can occur and Omsk fever is usually characterized by bronchopneumonia and hemorrhage from various orifices.

Arboviruses group C and unclassified arboviruses

Group C, comprising seven viruses, is responsible for influenza-like illness in parts of South America. Amongst the unclassified infections, sandfly fever is perhaps the best documented illness.

Sandfly fever (phlebotomus fever, papataci fever)

This illness results from infection by one of the unclassified arboviruses. It is relatively common in countries bordering the Mediterranean and occurs in parts of Africa, Russia, India and China. The responsible vector *Phlebotomus papatasii*, often called sandfly, is extremely small and may pass through mosquito nets. Infection in these sandflies may be permanent, due to trans-ovarian infection, and no definite animal reservoir is known. Several different strains of virus have been isolated with established immunological variation.

Clinical features. The incubation period is 3–7 days. Onset is sudden and rigors may occur. Headache, pain behind the eyes, muscular aching and fever are typical features. Occasionally photophobia, neck and back stiffness occur and mimic meningitis. After 3 or 4 days there is an abrupt termination by crisis. Severe apprehension often accompanies this illness and acute depression may follow an attack for a short time. Leukopenia is common. A clinical diagnosis is readily made in endemic areas or during an outbreak.

There is no specific treatment and the prognosis is good. Control is confined to attempts at eradication of the vector in its breeding grounds.

RICKETTSIAL INFECTIONS

Rickettsial infection in man produces a number of different diseases, spread over a wide geographical area. The resultant illnesses have certain basic similarities and all but one are characterized by some form of skin eruption. Definitive clinical diagnosis can be difficult and confirmatory laboratory tests are desirable. A simple classification of rickettsial infection is shown in Table 28.36.

Rickettsiae have biophysical properties that place them in an intermediate position between viruses and bacteria and are small coccobacilli, usually less than half a micrometer in diameter, with rigid cell walls. They contain both RNA and DNA, but are obligate intracellular parasites and are sensitive to certain antibiotics.

LABORATORY TESTS

Procedures to isolate the causative organisms exist, but should only be undertaken by a laboratory well equipped to deal with the risks involved. In view of the hazards involved in isolation, serological methods of diagnosis are usually employed.

The Weil–Felix agglutination reaction, used for several years, depends on the fact that patients with certain rickettsial infections develop agglutinins in their serum during the illness which agglutinate some strains of Proteus organisms, namely OX 19, OX 2 and OXK. There are now a number of other serological assays available in specialist reference laboratories. If possible, paired sera should be examined in the Weil–Felix test, but agglutinins may appear as early as the fifth or sixth day after the onset of the fever and usually reach a peak during the second or third week. Detection of rickettsial DNA in the blood or tissue by PCR may allow the diagnosis to be made earlier in the illness.

TYPHUS FEVER (EPIDEMIC LOUSE-BORNE TYPHUS FEVER)

Historical writings suggest that typhus fever (classical or historic typhus) has been a scourge of humanity for many centuries. Typhus fever and war are inextricably linked. Although the responsible agent may be endemic in many parts of Europe, serious epidemics only arise

Table 28.36   Rickettsial diseases: causal agents, vectors, reservoirs and differential Weil–Felix reactions

	Disease	Causal rickettsiae	Principal vectors	Animal reservoir	Geographic occurrence
Typhus	Epidemic (louse-borne typhus)	R. prowazekii	Lice	Man	Worldwide
	Brill–Zinsser disease	R. prowazekii	–	Man	Worldwide
	Endemic murine (flea-borne) typhus	R. mooseri	Fleas	Rats	Worldwide
	Scrub typhus (mite-borne) (Tsutsugamushi fever)	R. tsutsugamushi	Mites	Small rodents	Japan, South East Asia, Pacific
Spotted fevers	Rocky Mountain spotted fever	R. rickettsii	Ticks	Small rodents	East and west USA
	Mediterranean fever (fièvre boutonneuse)	R. conorii	Ticks	Small rodents and dogs	Mediterranean, Caspian and Black Sea, Africa, South East Asia
Rickettsialpox		R. akari	Mites	House mice	USA, Russia, Korea
Q fever	Query fever	R. burnetii	Occasionally ticks	Cattle Sheep Goats Bandicoots	Worldwide

during times of war or in their aftermath, due entirely to the increased infestation by lice that occurs in these periods. Epidemics occur chiefly in winter when people are crowded together for warmth and shelter, enhancing chances of spread of the louse. Following the 1914–1918 war, it was estimated that 30 million cases of typhus occurred in Russia alone, and some 10% of these probably died. In the 1970s, large epidemics occurred in central Africa (Ruanda–Burundi).

The responsible organism is *Rickettsia prowazekii* and transmission is by the body louse *Pediculus corporis* or the head louse *Pediculus capitis*. The lice become infected by biting a human who is carrying the specific rickettsiae in the blood. Subsequent spread of the infection results from the infected feces of the lice rather than by an actual bite, and the irritation set up on the human body by the infestation results in the organisms being scratched into the skin. Infection may also result from the inhalation of louse feces in dust. At times fleas may act as a vector and also convey the infection through their feces.

Clinical features

The incubation period is 6–15 days. There are three main clinical phases – prodromal, invasive and eruptive.

Prodromal symptoms, not always present, include mild headache, lassitude, weakness and pyrexia. The invasive stage is characterized by a sharp rise in temperature, severe headache and generalized aching. Rigors may occur and the fever may reach 40–41 °C. The pulse is rapid, the blood pressure reduced and a variable degree of prostration develops. A wide variety of additional symptoms and signs may be encountered including suffusion of the conjunctivae, facial flushing, photophobia, deafness, tinnitus, vertigo and cough.

The characteristic rash arises about the fifth day of illness and the initial lesions, comprising pinkish red macules, appear on the trunk and soon spread to the limbs. Most cases show sparing of the face, palms and soles. In mild cases the rash may develop no further, but in the more severely ill the eruption becomes hemorrhagic or even purpuric. During this eruptive phase the mental state becomes dulled. Stupor, delirium and coma may follow. Hypotension also becomes more intense and oliguria with azotemia is common. Severe cases will die between the 9th and 18th day of illness. Those who recover slowly improve after 2 weeks, the mental recovery being more rapid than the physical. Typhus is usually accompanied by leukopenia and normochromic anemia.

Complications

Bronchopneumonia, otitis media, skin sepsis, arterial thrombosis and gangrene are all encountered. Less often there may be areas of skin necrosis and secondary infection of the salivary glands. Prolonged hypotension has a grave prognosis.

Differential diagnosis

Typhus may be readily considered and diagnosed at epidemic times, but sporadic cases can cause considerable confusion. Amongst diseases that may require differentiation are other rickettsial infections, typhoid fever, measles, malaria and meningococcal septicemia.

Treatment

In children, doxycycline 5 mg/kg/d 12 hourly (max 200 mg) or chloramphenicol 75–100 mg/kg/d (max 2 g) or tetracycline 50 mg/kg/d is used and should be continued until the temperature has settled for 48 h. Antibiotics should be re-instituted if there is clinical relapse.

Careful nursing and general supportive measures are required. A high protein diet is desirable and transfusion of blood or plasma may be needed. Electrolyte imbalance can readily occur and requires appropriate correction. Oxygen may be given for pulmonary complications and digoxin for cardiac failure.

Prognosis

The disease is rarely fatal in children, but about 10% of young adults and 60–70% of people over 50 may die.

Control

Killed vaccines prevent deaths, although not necessarily infection. Scrupulous hygiene is desirable and insecticides should be used to eliminate lice: DDT, lindane and malathion have proved effective.

BRILL–ZINSSER DISEASE (RECRUDESCENT TYPHUS)

This condition represents a recrudescence of epidemic louse-borne typhus that occurs years after the primary attack. It is usually mild and the illness is drastically modified. Skin rashes are usually absent and the prognosis is good. In view of its atypical clinical nature and the fact that a case may arise when no other typhus infection is occurring, diagnosis is difficult. Less markedly abnormal laboratory tests can also be misleading. However, if a diagnosis is made, treatment is along the lines employed for epidemic typhus. The real danger of Brill–Zinsser disease is to the community. If epidemiological factors are favorable, especially if the environment is heavily louse infested, an epidemic could arise from such a case.

MURINE TYPHUS (ENDEMIC FLEA-BORNE TYPHUS FEVER)

This disease is clinically similar to classical epidemic typhus but is milder and has a much lower fatality rate (2%); the management and treatment are also similar. The responsible agent is named *Rickettsia mooseri* and it is usually spread to man from its animal host by the rat flea (*Xenopsylla cheopis*).

Widely distributed throughout the world, the disease appears to be on the decline, probably owing to stricter control of rats. It is more common in summer when rats are more numerous and has a higher infection rate amongst persons in the food trade where rats may abound. Unlike lice, which die from *R. prowazekii*, the rat flea is not killed by the multiplication of *Rickettsia mooseri* in its tissue. Control depends on flea eradication and extermination of rats.

SCRUB TYPHUS (TSUTSUGAMUSHI FEVER)

This disease, known by many different names according to the locality where it occurs, is transmitted to man by the bite of the larvae of different species of chigger-like mites; best known of these are *Trombicula akamushi* and *Trombicula deliniensis*. The responsible agent is known as *Rickettsia tsutsugamushi* and the cycle of infection involves chiggermite and various wild rodents. Clinical features are again like those of other rickettsial infections though fairly mild. A diagnostic finding in some is a small necrotic ulcer or eschar where the responsible mite has attached itself to the skin and introduced the infection. The disease occurs in the south west Pacific and South East Asia between Japan, the Solomon Islands and Pakistan.

Treatment is with doxycycline 5 mg/kg/d 12 hourly (max 200 mg) or chloramphenicol 75–100 mg/kg/d (max 2 g) and the mortality is under 5%. Elimination of the disease is difficult and mite-infested areas are best avoided. Alternatively protective clothing, treated with a mite repellent, should be used. Vaccines have not proved effective in this condition.

ROCKY MOUNTAIN SPOTTED FEVER

This disease results from infection by *Rickettsia rickettsii* which is transmitted to man through a variety of ticks which are both the vector and the common reservoir for the responsible agent. Some rodents, dogs and sheep also act as additional but less prolific reservoirs. The clinical course has many similarities to classical typhus but the incubation period is often shorter (2–5 days in severe cases). Furthermore, the rash is usually more pronounced and frankly petechial. It can also be more widespread and may take some time to subside.

Complications, differential diagnosis, laboratory findings, treatment and management are all similar to epidemic typhus. Reported mortality rates have varied between 3 and 90% with an average, for all ages, of 20%. Despite its name, this disease is now much more common in the eastern than the western USA. In the western USA, adult males are most frequently attacked, whereas in the east children are most commonly affected.

Control is difficult owing to the disseminated nature of the vector in the wild, and where possible it is best to avoid tick-infested areas or to ensure that adequate protective clothing is worn.

TICK TYPHUS FEVERS (FIÈVRE BOUTONNEUSE)

There are three tick-borne spotted fevers caused by rickettsiae which share the same group-specific antigen as *Rickettsia rickettsii*, the cause of Rocky Mountain spotted fever, but have distinct type-specific antigens.

Rickettsia conorii causes fièvre boutonneuse, which is also called Mediterranean fever along the Mediterranean, Black and Caspian sea littorals; called Kenyan tick typhus and South African tickbite fever; and called Indian tick typhus in South East Asia. *Rickettsia australis* causes Queensland tick typhus in eastern Australia. *Rickettsia sibirica* causes Siberian tick typhus which occurs throughout central Asia.

The main animal reservoir is dogs. These tick typhus fevers are clinically similar. A small, indurated lesion, the tache noire, develops at the site of the tick bite, and central necrosis gives way to eschar formation. There is regional lymphadenopathy. The tick typhus fevers are much milder than Rocky Mountain spotted fever, with a mortality under 1%. Antibiotic treatment is as for the latter disease.

RICKETTSIALPOX

Due to *Rickettsia akari*, this disease is usually transmitted to man by a mite and the house mouse is the main animal reservoir. Epidemics tend to occur where mice and mites are found together, primarily in urban populations worldwide.

The illness is comparatively mild. The incubation period is 10–21 days. Fever is usual and a mild rash develops, most closely resembling adult chickenpox. Death is extremely rare. Doxycycline is the drug of choice.

Q FEVER (QUERY FEVER)

This disease results from infection by *Coxiella burnetii* and usually presents as an influenza-like illness with fever and headache, often followed by an atypical pneumonic illness. Unlike other rickettsial infections, Q fever is unaccompanied by a rash.

C. burnetii is an obligate intracellular parasite which is highly pleomorphic and contains both RNA and DNA. It is more resistant to chemical and physical agents than other pathogenic rickettsiae and is relatively sensitive to certain antibiotics.

The natural reservoir of *C. burnetii* is animals such as cattle, sheep and goats, as well as certain ticks, and the latter are probably involved in animal-to-animal spread. Infection in humans may arise from the handling of infected meat and placentae, the inhalation of infected dust in farmyards and the consumption of infected raw milk. Cases are most likely to be found in farm workers, slaughtermen and shepherds. Where milk is the vehicle of transmission, the disease may occur without any apparent occupational link and involve children.

Clinical features

Q fever is less commonly diagnosed in children than in adults because the illness produced in younger age groups is less severe and less intensively studied.

There is usually an incubation period of 2–3 weeks and the illness starts abruptly with fever, rigors, headache, malaise and weakness. In some instances the illness may terminate in approximately 1 week without any further progression, but in most diagnosed cases the patient goes on to develop a cough and chest pain. Physical signs may be absent or minimal, although the chest X-ray may show pneumonitis.

Severe cases may have symptoms for up to 3 weeks and radiological abnormalities can take a similar period to resolve. Inapparent infection can also occur. Occasionally Q fever presents with meningoencephalitis and diagnosis can be difficult.

Complications

Q fever, or rickettsial, endocarditis has only been seen in people with pre-existing valvular disease of the heart and the clinical presentation is with culture negative subacute bacterial endocarditis. Granulomatous hepatitis and bone granulomas have been described.

Laboratory diagnosis

C. burnetii can be isolated in laboratory animals or fertile hen's eggs. However, as it is a significant biohazard to laboratory workers, serological tests are preferred to confirm a clinical diagnosis, and a complement-fixation test or immunofluorescence is used on acute and convalescent sera. Detection of nucleic acid by PCR or hybridization techniques is also available.

Treatment

Prodromal symptoms require symptomatic treatment. Once the diagnosis is made, doxycycline (5 mg/kg/d up to 200 mg) or tetracycline (25 mg/kg/d) or chloramphenicol should be given in standard dosage for 2 weeks.. Therapy should not be withheld where the diagnosis is retrospective and the patient has recovered, because it is important to eradicate the infection and avoid the possibility of chronicity. Endocarditis has a grave prognosis.

PROTOZOAL INFECTIONS

AMEBIC INFECTIONS

Amebae are characterized by two forms – the motile, feeding trophozoite and the cyst. The cyst has a rigid wall, resistant to environmental conditions, which allows it to survive for variable periods without feeding. The major ameba of importance to man is *Entamoeba histolytica*, which is anaerobic and an obligate parasite of the gut. It has to be differentiated from other nonpathogenic gut amebae, e.g. *E. dispar*, *E. coli* and *E. hartmanni*. There are a number of free-living aerobic amebae which are found in the soil and feed on bacteria in muddy water. In dry conditions the cysts may be dispersed by wind. Species that are pathogenic to man and may cause meningoencephalitis are *Naegleria fowleri* and the opportunist *Acanthamoeba culbertsoni* and *Balamuthia mandrillaris*.

AMEBIASIS

Amebiasis is caused by *E. histolytica* and is transmitted by the fecal–oral route. Sources of infection include sewage contamination of water supplies, infection by food handlers and direct fecal contact from person to person, as may occur in mental institutions. Transmission by sexual contact, including oral and anal sex, also occurs. Rarely, amebic colitis or liver abscess may present within the neonatal period.

Infection occurs worldwide, with a high prevalence in resource limited countries where hygiene is poor.

E. histolytica cannot be differentiated by microscopy from the morphologically identical but nonpathogenic *E. dispar*. Methods required include stool antigen tests, culture characteristics, zymodeme analysis and molecular techniques, such as PCR.[696–698] *E. histolytica* trophozoites characteristically demonstrate active erythrophagocytosis. *E. dispar* is 9 times more prevalent than *E. histolytica* and is the most likely species when 'amebic cysts' are detected in stools of asymptomatic subjects in any part of the world. Up to 10% of asymptomatic carriers of *E. histolytica* develop invasive disease; the remainder clear the infection within a year.[696,698]

Why *E. histolytica* is activated to invade is not known. Malnutrition, pregnancy, ulcerative colitis, immunosuppression, corticosteroids and intercurrent infection by bacteria or parasites may be precipitating factors. Inflammatory bowel disease should not be treated with corticosteroids until amebiasis has been excluded.

The incidence of disease does not necessarily correlate with prevalence of infection. Invasive disease is reported particularly from South East Asia, Natal (South Africa), the west coast of Africa, Mexico and parts of South America. In the USA, infection is associated especially with children of Hispanic origin.

Pathogenesis and pathology

Infection occurs from ingestion of cysts, which, on digestion, release trophozoites in the intestine. The trophozoites feed on bacteria and fecal matter in the cecum and further down the colon. When they reach areas where the feces are more solid, they encyst and the cysts are passed in the stool. Trophozoites may be detected in the stool even if there is no intestinal hurry. The presence of either trophozoites or cysts in stool is not necessarily indicative of invasive disease. However, the presence of hematophagous trophozoites (containing ingested red blood cells) is usually suggestive of invasion. Invasion is accomplished by lytic enzymes secreted by the trophozoites which result in tissue necrosis and erosion of blood vessels, but with a surprising lack of inflammatory response. Initial lesions are small superficial erosions. With progression, they penetrate the muscularis mucosa and may expand to produce flask-shaped ulcers. Further extension may result in intestinal perforation, but more commonly the parasite is carried to the liver in the portal vein, and rarely to other organs such as the lung, heart or brain. The colonic lesions may vary from small pinhead erosions confined to the cecum and rectosigmoid to extensive, deep, confluent ulcers extending throughout the colon. It is probable that the majority of amebae

reaching the liver do not cause detectable disease. Possibly, an area of tissue necrosis is necessary for the disease to be established. As in the bowel, liver abscess is characterized by localized necrosis without much inflammatory response, unless there is secondary infection.

Clinical features

The major organs affected in invasive amebic disease are the colon, the liver and adjacent organs, such as the right lung, pericardium and rarely the skin or eye.

Intestinal amebiasis

Intestinal amebiasis has a wide spectrum of severity. It may occur within a few weeks of infection or be delayed several months. There may be mild, intermittent diarrhea with blood and mucus, usually with no systemic upset or fever. Severe, fulminating dysentery is associated with watery, blood-stained, mucoid stools resulting in dehydration, electrolyte disturbance and toxemia. Abdominal pain, tenesmus and tenderness may be present. Perforation, which is often multiple with slow leakage, and peritonitis may occur. Other complications include hemorrhage, ameboma, stricture, intussusception and rectal prolapse. Chronic or relapsing dysentery may occur unless the initial attack has been managed by adequate chemotherapy and nutritional support. Ameboma is a complication of previous amebic dysentery and presents as a tender mass in the cecum or colon.

Enlargement of the liver may occur without evidence of an abscess, presumably the result of toxic products transported in the portal vein from the diseased bowel.

Amebic liver abscess and related disorders

Amebic liver abscesses may be single or multiple and more often involve the right lobe. Multiple abscesses are common in young children (Fig. 28.45). The liver is tender and, if the abscess is situated anteriorly, a mass is commonly visible (Fig. 28.46). There is nearly always fever and usually anemia, leukocytosis and raised erythrocyte sedimentation rate

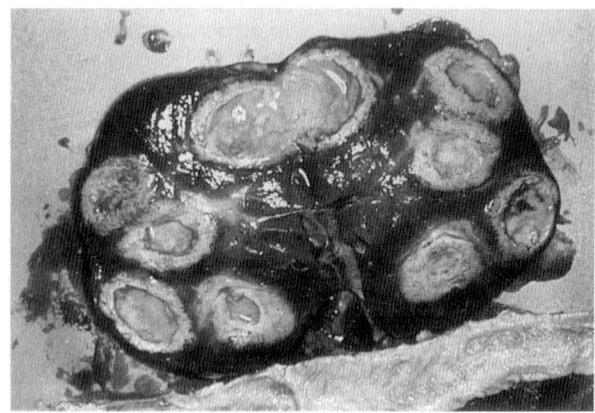

Fig. 28.45 Typical multiple amebic abscesses in the liver of an infant aged 8 months.

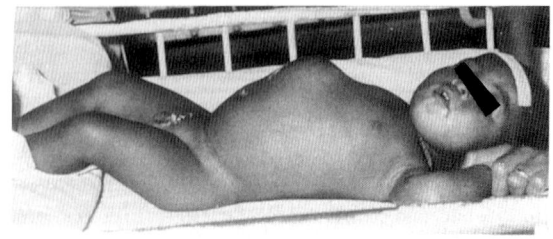

Fig. 28.46 An African infant of 10 months with a large amebic liver abscess presenting as a fluctuant mass in the epigastrium.

(ESR) and often also alkaline phosphatase. Jaundice is infrequent and serum transaminases are usually not raised. There is dysentery or a history of previous dysentery in only half the cases. In over two thirds of cases, elevation and immobility of the right diaphragm produces corresponding signs in the right lung.

Complications of amebic liver abscess include secondary bacterial infection, extension, or rupture into the peritoneal cavity, the pleural cavity and/or the lung. Involvement of the left lobe of the liver may result in a pericardial effusion or rupture into the pericardium. Rarely, there may be extension to abdominal organs including the stomach, gut or kidneys. Blood-borne spread may result in a brain or lung abscess.

Skin

Cutaneous amebiasis may be associated with rupture of a liver abscess, colostomy stoma or a laparotomy incision. In infants, amebic abscess of the perineum may result from direct contact with infected feces (Fig. 28.47).

Diagnosis

The diagnosis of amebic dysentery is based on the finding of motile, hematophagous E. histolytica trophozoites in feces. Red cells and bacteria but few leukocytes are usually present. Examination of a freshly passed warm stool (within 30 min of being passed) is important because, when the stool cools, the amebae stop moving and release the contained red cells in their vacuoles. Three or more stool examinations may be necessary and both direct and concentrated methods should be used. E. histolytica stool antigen test is more sensitive than microscopy and can differentiate E. histolytica from E. dispar. Endoscopy may demonstrate amebic ulcers, which are usually shallow, covered with a yellowish-gray exudate and contain numerous hematophagous trophozoites. Biopsy should be taken from the edge of the ulcer. The intervening mucosa is often relatively normal in appearance. Serum antibody titers to E. histolytica may be raised in two thirds of cases early in disease and in over 90% during convalescence.[697] In endemic areas, positive serology in young children suggests infection, but in older children does not distinguish between past and current infection.

The definitive diagnosis of amebic liver abscess is made by aspiration of bacteriologically sterile pus. The pus is usually gray-yellow at the first aspiration and only at subsequent aspirations takes on the pink or red-brown 'anchovy-paste' color. Amebae are seldom detected in necrotic material from the center of the abscess, but are more common in the walls of the cavity and thus are more likely to be detected in the last portions of the aspirate.

In most cases an ultrasound scan can localize and delineate the size of the abscess cavity. Ultrasound, CT and MRI have equal sensitivity in detecting amebic abscesses. Differential diagnosis includes pyogenic liver abscess, subphrenic abscess and hydatid disease. X-ray and screening may demonstrate a raised diaphragm with reduced movement and there may be an effusion or other signs of inflammation at the lung

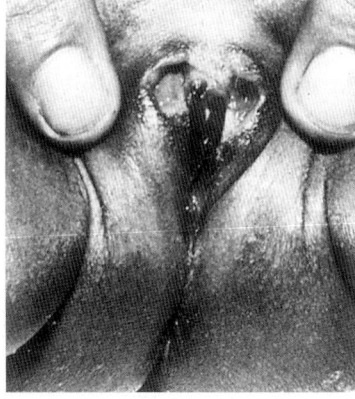

Fig. 28.47 Cutaneous amebiasis involving the vulva in an infant aged 5 months.

base. Usually there is a leukocytosis and a raised ESR. Antibody titers are usually high and may be detected in serum in over 95% of cases later on in disease.[697] ELISA has high sensitivity and specificity and usually becomes negative 6–12 months after response to treatment, whereas indirect hemagglutination titers may remain raised for many years. For unknown reasons, infection is only detected in the stool in about one third of cases, and usually only cysts are present.

Management

Chemotherapy of invasive amebiasis must include drugs which can eliminate amebae both from the tissues and the lumen of the bowel. Metronidazole and tinidazole (longer half-life) achieve both but are less effective as luminal amebicides.

For asymptomatic patients, and following invasive disease, the luminal amebicide diloxanide furoate is given, using 20 mg/kg/d in three divided doses for 10 days. Paromomycin 25–35 mg/kg/d in three divided doses for 7 days is an alternative. In endemic areas, older asymptomatic children are usually not treated, as reinfection is so common.

In symptomatic intestinal disease, metronidazole or tinidazole is recommended. Metronidazole 35–50 mg/kg/d in three divided doses orally is given for 7–10 days depending on the severity of the infection. Side-effects such as nausea and a metallic taste in the mouth may make compliance difficult. Alternatively, oral tinidazole 60 mg/kg is given as a single daily dose for 5 days. Both drugs may also be given intravenously. In severe colitis, correction of fluid and electrolyte imbalance is important, and gastric suction is necessary when there is ileus. Blood transfusion may be required. Broad spectrum antibiotics may be necessary if septicemia or other infection is suspected. Perforation of the bowel with leakage into the peritoneum may require surgery.

For liver abscess, metronidazole or tinidazole is usually effective and is given in doses similar to intestinal disease. Diloxanide furoate or paromomycin should be given to eradicate the bowel infection.

Indications for aspiration of the abscess include: suspected pyogenic abscess (particularly when there are multiple lesions), a palpable mass, a markedly raised diaphragm, failure of symptoms to remit after 72 h of drug therapy, and abscess in the left lobe. Aspiration, by relieving the pressure within the liver tissues, allows better drug penetration of the abscess. Surgical evacuation may be necessary for multiple or inaccessible abscesses, or when secondary infection has occurred. For needle aspiration, a wide-bore needle with a three-way tap should be used and the abscess cavity evacuated fully. Aspiration is usually through the right chest wall at the point of maximum tenderness, or through the abdomen if the abscess is superficial. Aspiration should be guided by ultrasound scan. If repeat aspiration is required, or in the case of drug resistance, percutaneous catheter drainage for 24–48 h may be undertaken.[699]

Resolution of the abscess cavity may take many months. Follow-up should be arranged to ensure complete eradication of infection, otherwise relapse may occur.

Intrathoracic and intraperitoneal rupture of amebic liver abscesses usually responds to standard anti-amebic chemotherapy.

As humans and primates are the only reservoirs of E. histolytica, eradication of disease is possible and vaccines are being developed with this aim.

NAEGLERIA AND ACANTHAMOEBA

Two distinct types of meningoencephalitis are caused by free-living amebae: primary amebic meningoencephalitis by Naegleria fowleri, and granulomatous amebic encephalitis usually by Acanthamoeba culbertsoni or Balamuthia mandrillaris.[700]

Primary amebic meningoencephalitis

This is an acute necrotizing meningoencephalitis caused by N. fowleri which gains access to the nasal cavities and results in direct invasion of the nervous system through the olfactory apparatus. There is usually a history of swimming under water or diving in warm fresh water or hot springs. Cysts transmitted in dust may colonize the nasal cavities of children. The cerebrospinal fluid (CSF) has changes similar to bacterial meningitis, viz. a predominant neutrophil count, often accompanied by red cells, a raised protein (usually > 1 g/L) and low glucose concentration. Careful search for trophozoites should be undertaken on fresh CSF. Nasal secretions or washings should also be examined for amebae.

The course of the disease is usually rapidly fulminating within 3–6 days. Intravenous and, if necessary, intraventricular (through a reservoir) amphotericin is the main treatment. In addition, parenteral fluconazole is usually given by the intravenous (and intrathecal) route and rifampicin orally. Duration of therapy is 8–10 days.

Granulomatous amebic encephalitis

This is a slowly progressive disease, occurring usually in immunocompromised individuals, although sometimes no immune defect can be demonstrated.[701] Infection by acanthamoeba may result from swallowing or inhaling cysts, or by direct skin or corneal contact. The CSF shows a lymphocytosis, a raised protein and low or normal glucose. Acanthamoeba may be detected in histological specimens. Sometimes the trophozoites may be detected by wet mount of CSF and subsequently cultured. Serology may also be of value.

Severe brain damage may have occurred by the time the diagnosis is made. Suggested drugs for treatment include polymyxin B, pentamidine isetionate, co-trimoxazole, ketoconazole and flucytosine.

Successful outcome is more likely in immunocompetent children.

Acanthamoeba keratitis

Most cases of acanthamoeba keratitis are associated with use of contact lenses, owing to a combination of abrasions of the cornea and contamination of the lens from washing in homemade solutions, especially fresh or tap water.[702]

Treatment is difficult and often requires keratoplasty. Local application of a combination of biocides, e.g. 0.02% polyhexamethylene biguanide plus 0.1% propamide isetionate and neomycin, is used. Local chlorhexidine may also be of value.[702] Corticosteroids are required to control inflammation. Only fresh, sterile, commercial solutions should be used to clean contact lenses.

Research on vaccines to prevent acanthamoeba keratitis is in progress.

BALANTIDIASIS

Balantidium coli is a parasite of pigs which may colonize the colon of man producing a disease similar to *E. histolytica*, but extracolonic disease does not occur. Treatment is with metronidazole or tetracycline for 8–10 days.

CRYPTOSPORIDIOSIS

Cryptosporidium spp. are second only to the enteric viruses in importance as causes of diarrheal disease in children. There are a number of different species of *Cryptosporidium*, some of which infect humans (Table 28.37). *C. muris* was first described by Tyzzer in 1907 as an asymptomatic infection of the gastric glands of mice. *C. parvum* was first described also by Tyzzer in 1912 in the intestines of mice. *C. meleagridis* was described as a cause of diarrhea in turkeys by Slavin in 1955 and since then the number of different *Cryptosporidium* species has expanded, contracted and then expanded again. It was first described as a human pathogen in 1976[703,704] and thought to be zoonotic. Interest in cryptosporidiosis increased, first because it was possible to diagnose infection by microscopic examination of stained fecal smears and second because of its association with AIDS.[705,706] It was originally thought of as a zoonotic infection, but person-to-person transmission was described in 1983[707] and it is clear that both anthroponotic and zoonotic transmission occur.

Originally *Cryptosporidium* was classified as a member of the subclass *Coccidiosina* in the phylum *Apicomplexa*. However, recent molecular

Table 28.37 *Cryptosporidium* species

	Major hosts	Minor hosts
C. hominis	Humans	Cattle, dugong, sheep
C. parvum	Cattle, sheep, goats, humans	Deer, mice, pigs
C. meleagridis	Turkeys, humans	Parrots
C. felis	Cats	Humans, cattle
C. canis	Dogs	Humans
C. wrairi	Guinea pigs	Humans
C. baileyi	Chickens, turkeys	Other birds, humans
C. muris	Rodents, Bactrian camels	Humans, rock hyrax, chamoix
C. andersoni	Cattle, Bactrian camels	Sheep
C. bovis	Cattle	
C. galli	Finches, chickens	
C. serpentis	Snakes, lizards	
C. saurophilum	Lizards	Snakes
C. molnari	Fish	

phylogenetic studies and the detection of extracellular stages have placed it closer to the Gregarines than Coccidia.[708]

Cryptosporidium spp. have a complex life cycle (Fig. 28.48) which can be simplified to (a) replication within the host and (b) the excreted infective form. The infective form is the oocyst, which is excreted in large numbers during acute infection (Fig. 28.49). It is highly resistant to disinfectants and is sufficiently small (c. 6 μm) to be able to pass through some water filtration units. The oocysts are infective as soon as they are excreted. Under the influence of gastric pH and duodenal enzymes, the oocyst excysts to release four sporozoites. These attach to and penetrate the enterocytes. Their location is just beneath the enterocyte membrane (Fig. 28.50) sometimes termed 'intracellular but extracytoplasmic'. It then undergoes cycles of asexual and sexual reproduction culminating in the production and excretion of the thick-walled oocysts. *C. hominis*

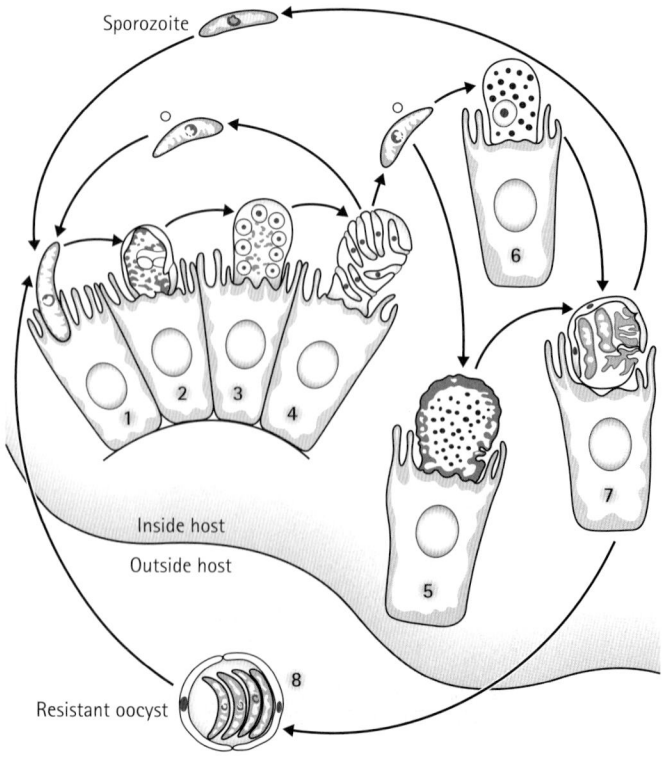

Fig. 28.48 The life cycle of *Cryptosporidium*.

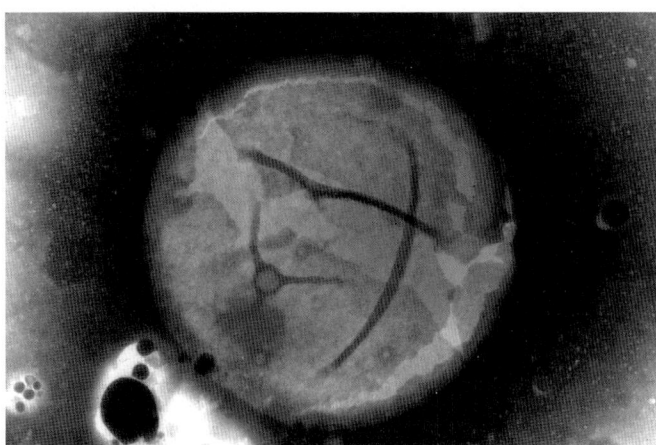

Fig. 28.49 An oocyst of *Cryptosporidium hominis*.

has a 9.2 megabase genome encoded on 8 chromosomes, the full sequence of which has recently become available.[709]

EPIDEMIOLOGY

Cryptosporidiosis has a worldwide distribution, being detected in every country where it has been sought. There are an estimated 250–500 million cases each year in Africa, Asia and Latin America.[710] It is an important cause of traveler's diarrhea and outbreaks can occur in crèches and day care centers. School visits to farms where children handle farm animals and then eat without washing their hands are another risk activity. In addition, *Cryptosporidium* can be acquired by the waterborne route. The largest such outbreak occurred in Milwaukee, USA, and affected 403 000 people.[711] It was related to a water treatment failure, although the fecal coliform count (the standard measure of water quality) was within normal limits.

Large numbers of oocysts are excreted during acute infection and the infective dose is low (30–300 oocysts), varying by *Cryptosporidium* species.[706] In some volunteer experiments one oocyst was able to initiate infection. Transmission of *C. hominis* is usually considered to occur by person-to-person transmission, directly or indirectly, and the other species by zoonotic transmission. However, *C. hominis* has been detected in cattle and *C. parvum* can be transmitted person to person. Most of the cases of cryptosporidiosis are due to *C. hominis* and *C. parvum* followed by *C. meleagridis*, *C. canis* and *C. felis*.[712–714] *C. muris* is rarely a cause of human disease.[712,715] In the UK and other temperate countries there is a distinct seasonality with peaks in spring and to a lesser extent in autumn.[705,710,716]

The impact of cryptosporidiosis is greatest in children, and prevalence rates are much higher in children in resource limited countries (5–19%) compared to industrialized (<4%) countries.[705] The highest prevalence (19%) was recorded among children in Gaza.[717] Although children have the highest prevalence of infection, cryptosporidiosis can occur at any age. The youngest recorded case was 3 days and the oldest 95 years old.[716] Patients immunocompromised by AIDS, immunosuppression, congenital immune deficiency or cytotoxic therapy are at risk of severe and prolonged cryptosporidiosis (see ref. 705).

PATHOLOGY AND PATHOGENESIS

Cryptosporidiosis is usually acquired by ingestion but there have been instances where it was acquired by the airborne route.[718] The shortest incubation period is presumed to be 3 days in a neonate who acquired infection intrapartum.[719] In a large study of Finnish travelers visiting Leningrad the mean incubation period was 7.2 ± 2.4 days with a median of 8 days.[720] Infection affects the small and large intestine in immunocompetent hosts but can spread along mucosal planes to the biliary tree, pancreas, liver, sinuses and lung in immunocompromised patients.

The mechanisms by which *Cryptosporidium* causes diarrhea are not entirely clear. Possible mechanisms include malabsorption and a local intestinal inflammatory response with increased production of prostaglandins and several cytokines.[721] In addition, *Cryptosporidium* delays apoptosis in infected cells but promotes it in adjacent enterocytes.[721] The histopathologic appearance of the intestine in cryptosporidiosis shows minimal inflammatory infiltrates with blunting of villi (Fig. 28.51). Electron microscopic examination of infected mucosa shows minimal damage to the brush border (Fig. 28.49).

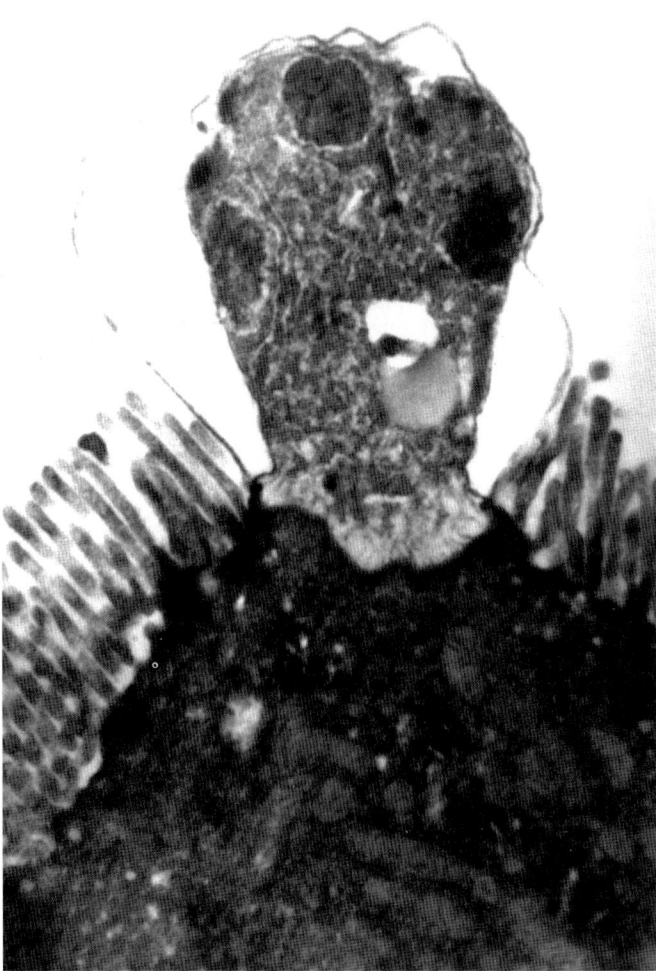

Fig. 28.50 A trophozoite of *Cryptosporidium hominis* just beneath the enterocyte membrane.

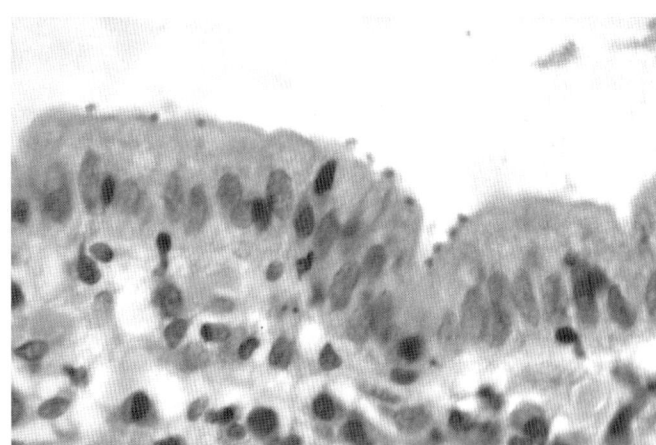

Fig. 28.51 Duodenal mucosal biopsy stained by hematoxylin and eosin showing villous blunting and cryptosporidia on the luminal surface.

CLINICAL FEATURES

The clinical features vary according to whether the patient is immuno-compromised or has an intact immune system.[705,710,716]

Immunocompetent children

The severity of disease varies across a spectrum from a short mild illness to one of prolonged watery diarrhea lasting over 6 months which has been mistakenly diagnosed as celiac disease. Anorexia (60–70% of cases), vomiting (50–75%), fever > 38 °C (25–50%) and abdominal pain (50–90%) are commonly described. The stool is watery (60–100% of cases), green (60–70%) and has a particularly offensive odor (80–100%). The stool frequently varies from 3 to 20 per day with 60–70% of children producing > 5 stools per day. The average duration of diarrhea is 12–14 days but with a wide range (5–60 days).[722,723] On average, patients excrete oocysts for 10–14 days after cessation of diarrhea.[724] In approximately one third of children the diarrhea is intermittent with bouts lasting for 2–3 days with 1–2 days quiescence until the next bout. Up to a third of children have respiratory tract symptoms,[723] which might be related to the presence of *Cryptosporidium* in a case of laryngotracheitis in a child in Papua New Guinea.[725]

Cryptosporidiosis is not a major cause of severe dehydration in well-nourished children,[705] but is in children from resource limited countries.[725] A major feature is loss of weight and failure to thrive, which occurred in 25% of children admitted to a Liverpool children's hospital.[723]

Immunocompromised patients

Although there is a spectrum of severity, cryptosporidiosis in immuno-compromised patients is much more likely to be severe and also less likely to be self-limiting. The diarrhea is often described as profuse, volu-minous and cholera-like. A stool frequency of up to 71 per day and a volume of 17 liters per day have been recorded in adults.[716] Another feature of cryptosporidiosis in immunocompromised patients is the occurrence of extraintestinal infection, which can involve the lung, sinuses, biliary tree or liver.

The immune deficits associated with severe cryptosporidiosis include B cell deficiency (hypo- or agammaglobulinemia, IgA deficiency), B and T cell deficiency (severe combined immunodeficiency, HIV/AIDS), immunosuppressive therapy (cytotoxic drugs, steroids, transplants), malnutrition, diabetes and measles.

DIAGNOSIS AND DIFFERENTIAL DIAGNOSIS

The first human cases of cryptosporidiosis were diagnosed by examination of duodenal biopsies.[703,704] However, it was soon realized that patients with cryptosporidiosis excrete sufficiently large numbers of oocysts for them to be detected by microscopic examination of stained fecal smears. Stains now include modified Ziehl–Neelsen, Kinyoun and Safranin methylene blue.[705] An auramine phenol method has greater sensitivity as on UV illumination the oocysts fluoresce apple-green against a dark background. Such tests are labor intensive, and detection of copro-antigens by commercially available enzyme immunoassay kits allows large numbers of samples to be processed rapidly.[726] However, their efficiency depends upon the quality of the antibody used, they may not detect all species of *Cryptosporidium*, and recently one test was recalled because of problems with false positives.

Genome detection by PCR amplification of the 18S rRNA gene is a sensitive diagnostic tool and coupled with restriction fragment length polymorphism (RFLP) analysis will provide assignment to species. However, it is not commercially available.

Finally serological diagnosis by detection of antibody is possible, which although valuable for population-based surveys of exposure is not useful for acute diagnosis.

TREATMENT

In most cases of infection in immunocompetent children only support-ive therapy is needed. The infection is self-limiting. This is not the case in immunocompromised patients and a large number of drugs (> 150) have been tried in the treatment of cryptosporidiosis. Paromomycin and spiramycin produce symptomatic improvement but no alterations in oocyst excretion. A new agent, nitazoxanide, has been licensed for treatment of cryptosporidiosis and in double-blind placebo-controlled trials shows great promise.[727] The only other intervention possible is to decrease the immune suppression by giving antiretroviral drugs in AIDS or stopping chemotherapy for malignancies.

CONTROL MEASURES

Great emphasis on personal hygiene is needed to limit person-to-person spread. In particular hand washing after toileting and nappy changing are very important. It is the mechanical effect of hand washing that is important as the thick-walled oocysts of *Cryptosporidium* are very resistant to most disinfectants and detergents. Prevention of waterborne disease is very difficult as evidenced by the Milwaukee experience.[711] The providers of potable water in the UK continuously screen the water to try to prevent infection. Boiling or freezing water should kill the oocysts. There is no vaccine to prevent cryptosporidiosis and as yet we still do not have a sound understanding of immunity to cryptosporidiosis.

PROGNOSIS

Except in immunocompromised or malnourished children, the prognosis is very good providing there is adequate nutrition during the recovery phase. However, one study from Guinea-Bissau indicated that crypto-sporidiosis in infancy was associated with a higher subsequent childhood mortality rate.[728]

GIARDIASIS

The enteric protozoan *Giardia* is a major cause of diarrheal disease of humans and other animals including dogs and cats. Although frequently referred to as *Giardia lamblia* in the medical literature, this has no taxonomic validity. *Giardia duodenalis* is the species affecting most mammals including humans, companion animals and food animals.[729] Other recognized species are *G. agilis* in amphibians, *G. muris* in rodents, and *G. psittaci* and *G. ardae* in birds. The vegetative form of *G. duodenalis* or trophozoite is a pear-shaped flagellate protozoan 12–15 μm long and 5–9 μm wide (Fig. 28.52). It has two nuclei and four symmetrically arranged flagella originating from basal bodies at the anterior poles of the nuclei. The concave

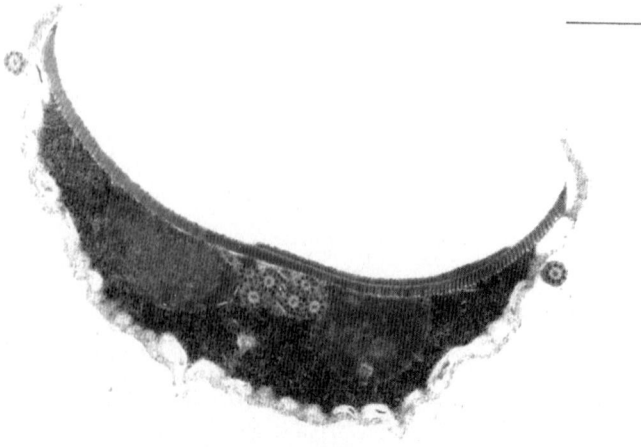

Fig. 28.52 Thin section electron micrograph of *Giardia duodenalis* showing the ventral disc and flagella in cross-sections.

ventral surface has a ventral disc composed of microtubules, which are used by the protozoan for attachment to intestinal cells. The trophozoites are unusual among eukaryotes in having only a few rudimentary intracellular organelles.[730] The infective form is the cyst which is excreted in feces. It can survive water chlorination and for months in cold fresh water. The cysts are quadric-nucleate, ovoid and 7–10 μm in length. The genome is small and consists of approximately 12 million base pairs on five chromosomes encoding an estimated 5000 genes.

EPIDEMIOLOGY

Giardiasis has a worldwide distribution and it is estimated that some 200 million people in Africa, Asia and Latin America have symptomatic infection and there are approximately 500 000 new cases each year.[731] It is an important cause of traveler's diarrhea and there is an increasing incidence of outbreaks in day care centers and crèches. Spread is fecal–oral, especially when hygiene is poor. Waterborne spread is increasingly important and, since a number of animal species can harbor G. duodenalis, a proportion of cases could be zoonotic.[732] Cyst concentrations excreted in feces are 150–20 000/g, but in contrast the infective dose is 10–100 cysts.

The impact of giardiasis is greatest in children. Prevalence rates are significantly higher in resource limited (20–30%) compared to resource rich (2–5%) countries. Recurrent and prolonged infections are not uncommon and some children may excrete cysts for long periods asymptomatically. Patients with hypo- or agammaglobulinemia are at particular risk of chronic giardiasis, but HIV and AIDS do not apparently increase the risk greatly.

Recently it has been shown that strains infecting humans can be subdivided on the basis of 18S rRNA gene sequences into two major groups. These are called assemblages A and B and there are clusters of genotypes within the two assemblages.[729] Not only are these subdivisions useful for epidemiologic purposes, but it also appears that assemblage A isolates tend to be associated with intermittent diarrhea and assemblage B with more severe, persistent diarrhea.[733]

PATHOLOGY AND PATHOGENESIS

Histologic changes in duodenal biopsies from cases of symptomatic giardiasis vary from entirely normal through partial, subtotal and total villous atrophy. Approximately 20–25% of patients will have normal villous architecture and < 10% subtotal villous atrophy.[734] On electron microscopic examination there can be shortening and disruption of microvilli even in biopsies appearing normal on light microscopy.

Following ingestion, cysts are excysted by the sequential exposure to low pH in the stomach and higher pH in the duodenum, which activates giardial proteases.[735] Interestingly, the newly excysted protozoa express different surface antigens (variant surface proteins, VSP) to those expressed by the trophozoite before it was encysted. The trophozoites then can be found free in the small intestinal lumen (here motility by flagella is important to prevent flushing out) and closely apposed to the enterocyte surface, often embedded in mucin. Most often their ventral surface is towards the enterocyte surface and it is thought that attachment is by the ventral disc; however, they also have a mannose-binding lectin on their surface. The trophozoites reproduce by binary fission and it is thought that bile salts stimulate growth. Trophozoites encyst in the small intestine when they are at high cell densities and this is stimulated by high bile salt concentrations, lipid metabolites and neutral pH. How diarrhea is induced is not entirely clear. Suggestions include the trophozoites acting as a mechanical barrier to prevent nutrient absorption (which is unlikely), structural and ultrastructural damage to enterocytes, and malabsorption. Recently it has been demonstrated that giardiasis is accompanied by disruption of inter-enterocytic tight junctions perhaps mediated by anexin-like alpha giardins.[736]

CLINICAL FEATURES

There are three clinical forms of giardiasis:
1. asymptomatic excretion of cysts;
2. acute diarrheal disease which is usually short and self-limited;
3. chronic diarrhea with malabsorption, weight loss and failure to thrive. The asymptomatic carrier state can occur in children or adults but whether carriage follows symptomatic infection or carriage occurs with no prior disease is unclear. There is no information on whether the asymptomatic carrier has subclinical enteropathy. However, it is clear that carriers can act as a reservoir of infection for others.

Acute giardiasis follows an incubation period of 3–20 days (mean 7 days) and the illness usually lasts 2–4 weeks, but may last as long as 7 weeks. Diarrhea (in over 90%) is the major feature and weight loss occurs in 60–70%. Other features are abdominal discomfort, flatulence, nausea and vomiting (in 30%). Approximately half the patients will have signs of steatorrhea. In patients with cystic fibrosis, giardiasis may worsen the malabsorption of fat and fat soluble vitamins.

A proportion of those with acute giardiasis (estimated to be about 30%) go on to develop chronic diarrhea, most often with steatorrhea. Weight loss can be great, with fat malabsorption in about 50%. In infants and young children this can cause failure to thrive. In some cases malabsorption of vitamins such as B_{12} or folate can lead to macrocytic anemia. Secondary lactase deficiency may occur and does not necessarily resolve with successful therapy.

DIAGNOSIS AND DIFFERENTIAL DIAGNOSIS

Giardiasis should be considered in cases of acute or chronic diarrhea. Specific diagnosis is by detection of the protozoon, its antigens or genome either in stool or duodenal fluid obtained by endoscopy, a nasoduodenal tube or a weighted nylon thread ('string-test'). Stool is the most appropriate specimen, but more invasive specimen collection is indicated when there is a high index of clinical suspicion yet stool samples are repeatedly negative. Although trophozoites are shed in the initial phase of acute diarrhea, giardiasis is most often confirmed by detection of cysts on microscopy of wet-mount or formalin–ethyl acetate concentrated stool samples. A single stool sample will detect giardiasis in 70% of cases and examination of three samples on separate days will detect it in 85%. The sensitivity of microscopy can be increased by using anti-Giardia fluorescent labeled antibody (direct immunofluorescence). In general, antigen detection by ELISA is more efficient and cost effective.[737] A number of commercial kits are available, including one that can simultaneously detect G. duodenalis, Entamoeba histolytica and Cryptosporidium parvum.[738] Diagnosis by genome detection, for example by PCR, is at present experimental.

TREATMENT

There is no evidence of benefit in treating asymptomatic infection. At least five classes of drugs – nitroimidazoles (metronidazole, tinidazole), benzimidazoles (albendazole), acridine dyes (mepacrine), nitrofurans (furazolidone) and nitazoxanide – are used for treating symptomatic giardiasis. A recent systematic review has concluded that drug treatment was associated with an improved cure rate (odds ratio 11.5; 98% confidence interval 2.3–58). Of the longer course regimens, metronidazole was the most effective (OR 2.4; 95% CI 1.2–4.4) with a smaller relapse rate. Tinidazole, which has a longer serum half-life than metronidazole, was best of the single dose regimens.[739] Unfortunately, there are few trials in children. The generally accepted regimen in children is metronidazole 15 mg/kg/d in three doses for 7–10 days. Mepacrine may be used as second line therapy (50 mg twice daily for children 1–5 years and 100 mg twice daily for children 5–10 years). Its use is limited by its bitter taste and induction of vomiting. In the USA, either metronidazole or furazolidone is preferred (tinidazole is not licensed for giardiasis). Furazolidone comes as a suspension, is given four times daily (6 mg/kg/d) for 7–10 days, and is less effective than metronidazole.

CONTROL MEASURES

In nurseries, crèches and child care centers, personal hygiene should be emphasized. Hand washing by staff and children should be stressed, especially after toileting and nappy changing. In outbreaks, attempts should be made to identify and treat all of those with symptomatic giardiasis. Those with symptomatic giardiasis should be excluded from work or nurseries until the diarrhea ceases. Although such infection control measures will decrease transmission, it must be remembered that routes other than direct person to person (e.g. waterborne, zoonotic) are possible. Recently, a vaccine has been licensed for the prevention of giardiasis in dogs and cats.[740] The vaccine, which is made from killed whole trophozoite preparations, proved highly effective. This could be of benefit to humans, firstly in decreasing an animal reservoir for zoonotic transfer and secondly by paving the way for a human vaccine.

PROGNOSIS

The prognosis is excellent, except in immunocompromised children, when relapse is common and treatment may need to be continued for prolonged periods. At the same time, attention must be paid to adequate nutrition and the treatment of concurrent infections.

LEISHMANIASIS

Leishmaniasis is caused by infection with a number of species of protozoan parasites of the genus *Leishmania*. It occurs in many parts of the world, including southern Europe, and is particularly problematic in Central and South America, the Middle East, South Asia, China and East Africa. An estimated 1–2 million new cases occur annually. Most forms of leishmaniasis are zoonoses with rodent or canine reservoirs of infection; man and other vertebrate hosts become infected by the bite of sandflies (genera *Phlebotomus* and *Lutzomyia*). Clinical syndromes are determined by the infecting species and range from self-limiting cutaneous lesions to potentially fatal visceral leishmaniasis.

LIFE CYCLE AND PARASITE BIOLOGY

Leishmania are transmitted by sandflies of the genus *Phlebotomus* in the Old World and *Lutzomyia* in the New World. Sandflies take in blood containing the aflagellate stage (amastigotes) from a hemorrhage made in the skin by their mouthparts. The amastigotes divide at least once before changing into the motile flagellate stage (promastigotes). These develop within the gut over 4–14 days and migrate forward to become inoculated when the sandfly attempts to take its next blood meal.[741] The intracellular stage in the vertebrate host (including man) is a small uninucleate ovoid body (2–5 µm long and 1–2 µm wide) containing a kinetoplast with a flagellar remnant and known as the amastigote (also referred to as the Leishman–Donovan body). The amastigote predominantly infects cells of the reticuloendothelial system and multiplies repeatedly by binary fission, eventually destroying the host cell.

Parasite biology

Two major subgenera of importance in human leishmaniasis can be distinguished by the site of development within the sandfly vector: *Leishmania* subgenus *Leishmania* (*L. donovani*, *L. mexicana*, *L. tropica* and *L. major*) and *Leishmania* subgenus *Viannia* (*L. braziliensis* complex).[742] Leishmania that infect man are morphologically similar apart from minor variations in size of amastigotes. However, isoenzyme profiles, DNA characterization, PCR, monoclonal antibody techniques and serotyping can all be used to distinguish species.[743] Culture of leishmania can be performed using specialized media. Some *Leishmania* species grow poorly in culture, and culture characteristics have been used to differentiate *L. braziliensis* which is slow growing from *L. mexicana*.

The important leishmania affecting man and the clinical syndromes that they cause are summarized in Table 28.38.

VISCERAL LEISHMANIASIS (KALA AZAR)

Visceral leishmaniasis (VL) is caused by leishmania of the *L. donovani* complex (*L. donovani*, *L. infantum* and *L. chagasi*).

Table 28.38 Summary of human leishmaniasis

Parasite	Geographical distribution	Animal reservoir	Disease
Visceral leishmaniasis (*Leishmania donovani* **complex**)			
L. donovani	India, Bangladesh, China	None	VL PKDL
	Kenya	(Dog)	VL PKDL
	Sudan and Ethiopia	Rodents	VL (CL) (MCL)
L. infantum	Mediterranean littoral, Central Asia, China	Canine sp.	VL (CL) VL CL
L. chagasi	Central and South America	Canine sp.	VL
Old World cutaneous leishmaniasis			
L. tropica	Middle East to India	(Dog)	CL (dry), LR
L. aethiopica	Ethiopia and Kenya	Rock hyrax	CL DCL
L. major	Africa, Middle East and Asia	Rodents	CL (wet)
American cutaneous leishmaniasis (*Leishmania mexicana* **complex**)			
L. mexicana	Mexico, Belize, Guatemala	Forest rodents	CL (DCL) Chiclero's ulcer
L. amazonensis	Brazil–Amazon basin	Forest rodents	CL DCL
American mucocutaneous leishmaniasis (*Leishmania braziliensis* **complex**)			
L. braziliensis	Brazil, Amazon forest, Peru, Ecuador, Bolivia, Venezuela, Colombia, Paraguay	Uncertain, forest animals	CL and MCL
L. guyanensis	North Amazon, Guyana	Sloth, lesser anteater	CL MCL
L. panamensis	Panama, Costa Rica	Sloth	CL (MCL)
L. peruviana	Western Andes	(Dog)	CL (Uta)

CL, cutaneous leishmaniasis; DCL, diffuse cutaneous leishmaniasis; LR, leishmania recidivans; MCL, mucocutaneous leishmaniasis; PKDL, post kala azar dermal leishmaniasis; VL, visceral leishmaniasis.

Epidemiology

L. donovani is endemic and epidemic in north-eastern India and Bangladesh, predominantly affecting young adults and children. Infection is confined to man and no animal reservoirs have been identified. The vector, *P. argentipes*, is peridomestic and readily feeds on man. The parasite is similar in East Africa, where the disease is widespread with endemic foci and occasional epidemics, particularly in association with population movements and land development. Children are predominantly affected. Rodents are reservoirs of disease in Sudan, but no animal reservoir has been identified in Kenya. Transmission is often seasonal due to fluctuations in sandfly populations.

L. infantum is widely distributed through the Mediterranean littoral, southern Europe, the Middle East, southern regions of the former USSR and China. In endemic areas, children under 5 are predominantly affected although infection may occur at any age in visitors or the immunosuppressed. The domestic dog is an important reservoir host; wild canines and foxes also act as reservoirs.

L. chagasi in South and Central America resembles *L. infantum* clinically and epidemiologically. Infection occurs in Amazonian Brazil, Bolivia, Paraguay, Argentina, Colombia and Venezuela. Children are predominantly affected and both domestic and wild canines and foxes are reservoir hosts.

Pathogenesis

After inoculation into the skin, the promastigotes convert to amastigotes in skin macrophages. These disseminate throughout the reticuloendothelial system and amastigote-laden macrophages are found in liver, spleen, bone marrow, lymphatic tissue and occasionally the skin. Progressive splenomegaly, hepatomegaly, anemia and thrombocytopenia result.

Clinical features

Subclinical or asymptomatic infection is common and protects against subsequent infection; clinical disease only occurs in 10–20% of infections. The clinical features of visceral leishmaniasis are similar throughout the world. A small cutaneous lesion may occur at the site of inoculation, but is usually not observed. After a variable incubation period (usually 4–6 months), symptoms develop. Classical clinical features are a triad of fever, splenomegaly and anemia. However, the spectrum of VL ranges from an acute febrile infection with anemia, pancytopenia and splenomegaly to a protracted illness slowly progressing over 2 or more years with severe anemia and massive splenomegaly. *L. infantum* infections are usually more acute than infection with *L. donovani* but acute forms of *L. donovani* occur, especially in children. *L. infantum* may also cause simple cutaneous leishmaniasis in adults in Southern Europe.

Fever is frequent, commonly remittent or intermittent, and may have a characteristic double diurnal periodicity. In very acute forms, fever is high, with prostration, toxemia and minimal splenomegaly. However, many patients remain active despite high fever and some patients with chronic infection may be afebrile for prolonged periods. Most patients develop progressive splenomegaly and hepatomegaly; in chronic infections, the spleen may be grossly enlarged, smooth and hard. Generalized or localized (often cervical) lymphadenopathy occurs in some geographical areas and may be present in the absence of hepatosplenomegaly or other features of visceral leishmaniasis.

Patients with chronic disease are pale and, especially in India, develop an earthy grey color with areas of hyperpigmentation (kala azar). In Africa a diminution in skin pigmentation is more typical. Chronic VL leads to progressive wasting, nutritional skin changes and hair changes similar to those observed in kwashiorkor. Pancytopenia with associated immunosuppression leads to secondary infections such as pneumonia, bronchitis, meningitis and tuberculosis. Episodes of diarrhea are common and may be due either to secondary infection or submucosal infiltration with leishmania-laden macrophages. Patients are rarely jaundiced but dependent edema and ascites occurs. Hemorrhagic features, especially recurrent epistaxis, are common; major or fatal hemorrhagic episodes may occur.

Visceral leishmaniasis and HIV

Visceral leishmaniasis is an important opportunistic infection in HIV, particularly in Southern Europe. Most cases occur in young adults but pediatric cases of co-infection have been reported. Both classical and atypical presentations with pulmonary, skin and gastrointestinal infection occur; fulminant infection without splenomegaly is also recognized. Leishmania serology is frequently negative, but parasites are usually easy to find in appropriate samples.

Laboratory findings

The hematological features of visceral leishmaniasis are classically moderate to severe normocytic, normochromic anemia with hemoglobin levels of 6–8 g/dl, accompanied by neutropenia and thrombocytopenia, commonly $80–100 \times 10^9$/L. Lymphocytes are usually in the normal range and circulating eosinophils reduced or absent from the peripheral blood. The serum albumin is reduced and there is a substantial elevation of immunoglobulins, predominantly IgG.

Diagnosis[744,745]

A parasitic diagnosis may be made by microscopy or culture of bone marrow or splenic aspirates. Splenic aspiration is more sensitive and reasonably safe in the absence of disturbed hemostasis or thrombocytopenia. Marrow aspiration is preferable in acute illness or in the presence of thrombocytopenia or disturbed hemostasis. Leishmania may also be identified by examination of the buffy coat and in lymph node and liver biopsy specimens. Smears are fixed in methanol and stained with Giemsa or Leishman that stain the cytoplasm of the amastigote blue, the nucleus pink or violet and the kinetoplast bright red. Culture is generally less sensitive than direct smear examination, but will detect some smear negative cases.

Anti-leishmania antibodies may be detected by a number of techniques, including IFAT, ELISA, and direct agglutination tests (DAT). ELISA and DAT techniques are highly sensitive and specific. High titers are associated with active disease and fall slowly after treatment. Rapid field diagnosis may be made by use of immuno-chromatographic strips which use recombinant antigens. PCR techniques can be used to detect leishmania DNA in peripheral blood and marrow with high sensitivity and specificity.

Differential diagnosis

Visceral leishmaniasis should be considered in the differential diagnosis of acute or chronic fever accompanied by hepatosplenomegaly and anemia, especially when there is a history of residence in an endemic area. Many other infections including malaria, especially *P. malariae* infection, typhoid, brucellosis, relapsing fever and tuberculosis (which may coexist with visceral leishmaniasis) should be considered. Splenomegaly must be differentiated from schistosomiasis, tropical splenomegaly syndrome and lymphoma or leukemia.

Treatment[744,745]

Pentavalent antimonial compounds remain the treatment of choice for most cases of visceral leishmaniasis. Two preparations are in common use: sodium stibogluconate containing 100 mg antimony (Sb) per ml (Pentostam) and methylglutamine antimonate containing 85 mg Sb per ml (Glucantime). Response rates are usually around 90%, but antimonial resistance, particularly in Bihar, India, is an increasing problem, and some regions report failure rates of up to 60%.

Sodium stibogluconate is administered by daily intravenous or intramuscular injection. The dose is 10–20 mg/kg Sb per day for 20–30 days. Children normally receive 20 mg/kg/d. Rapid extensive renal clearance occurs and dose adjustments should be made if renal function is poor. Common side-effects in adults include arthralgia, myalgia, biochemical and clinical pancreatitis, mild increase in liver enzymes and marrow suppression. The drug appears to be better tolerated by children.[746,747] Minor ECG changes are common; prolonged Q-T interval and dysrhythmias may occur in high dose regimens used for the treatment of antimony-resistant infections. Anaphylactic shock is a rare complication following administration. Sodium stibogluconate has been used in pregnancy without untoward effects on the fetus.

Amphotericin B. Both conventional and lipid formulations have been proven to be effective in various regimens lasting for between 10 and 40 days depending upon geographical location and the immune status of the patient. Standard amphotericin B is now the first line of therapy in some areas of India. Lipid formulations are better tolerated, have the theoretical advantage of being preferentially being taken up by macrophages and can be used in shorter courses of 10 days. They are currently the treatment of choice if expense does not preclude their use. Reported efficacy in children in Mediterranean VL is over 95%.[748]

Pentamidine. This may be effective, but resistance appears to develop rapidly and relapse is not uncommon. The main concern is toxicity, particularly the development of diabetes mellitus. The drug is now rarely used, except in areas of high resistance to antimonials or in patients who relapse.

Aminosidine (paromycin) is an aminoglycoside that has high efficacy and is well tolerated. It is administered intravenously or by intramuscular injection at a dose of 12–20 mg/kg/d for 3–4 weeks. Phase three trials with new formulations are currently underway.

Miltefosine is a new oral drug that is emerging as a very effective treatment option. It is given in a 4-week regimen at 2.5 mg/kg daily and is effective against antimony resistant strains. Cure rates are over 90% in children.[749,750]

Supportive and symptomatic treatment is important in addition to chemotherapy. Intercurrent bacterial infections are common and should be appropriately treated and attention paid to correcting nutritional status and vitamin deficiencies. Patients with hemorrhage should receive vitamin K. Blood transfusions are often required for the treatment of anemia in children.

Response to treatment
Fever normally subsides and patients start to feel better in the first week of treatment. Hemoglobin and white cell counts improve over 2–4 weeks while the splenomegaly reduces more gradually over subsequent weeks or months. Patients should be followed up for at least one year to detect relapse.

Relapse and nonresponsiveness
Relapse normally occurs within 6 months and relapse rates vary considerably depending upon the geographical location and the initial treatment regimen. Treatment of relapse is usually with prolonged courses of sodium stibogluconate, but depends upon geographical patterns of resistance. Pentamidine, aminosidine, amphotericin B and liposomal amphotericin have all been used successfully to treat relapse. Systemic interferon-gamma may be useful as an adjunctive therapy in resistant infections. HIV infected individuals are more likely to relapse and may need maintenance therapy.

Post kala azar dermal leishmaniasis
Post kala azar dermal leishmaniasis (PKDL) is most commonly seen in Indian visceral leishmaniasis (20%) and less often in African infections (1–5%). Following treatment of visceral disease, cutaneous lesions develop with symmetrical depigmented lesions especially on exposed surfaces. Lesions progress to become papular or nodular and mucosal surfaces may be involved with abundant leishmania (*L. donovani*) in lesions. Treatment with pentavalent antimonial compounds is effective although lesions also heal spontaneously.

CUTANEOUS LEISHMANIASIS
Epidemiology
L. tropica and *L. major* cause cutaneous leishmaniasis in the Middle East, Afghanistan, the southern Mediterranean, Sudan and sub-Saharan Africa. Clinical infection in endemic areas occurs mainly in children.

L. tropica has a human reservoir and transmission is mainly urban whereas *L. major* occurs in rural areas with rodent reservoirs.

L. mexicana and *L. braziliensis* cause cutaneous leishmaniasis in Central and South America. *L. mexicana* has a reservoir in forest rodents in Central and South America and particularly affects the pinna of the ear in forest workers, notably chicleros (chewing gum collectors). *L. braziliensis* has a reservoir in domestic animals and forest rodents. Cutaneous lesions may progress to mucocutaneous leishmaniasis (espundia).

Clinical features
Clinical features of cutaneous leishmaniasis are similar throughout the world with some slight differences between species. Typically, after an incubation period of several weeks, a localized, small, raised cutaneous nodule occurs, surrounded by a zone of erythema. The lesion grows slowly and central shallow ulceration may occur. Lesions remain raised above the level of normal skin; ulcers are shallow and do not have undermined edges. Lesions continue to progress for 6–24 months followed by spontaneous healing eventually leaving a slightly depressed papery scar. Satellite lesions may develop and regional lymphadenopathy is found in some forms. Lesions may be single or multiple and are more common on the face, hands, feet or limbs. *L. tropica* tends to cause single lesions lasting for 1–2 years with little tissue reaction and sometimes non-ulcerating lesions, whereas lesions in *L. major* are often multiple with a greater degree of ulceration and tissue reaction. Spontaneous healing occurs in 50% of lesions by 3 months in *L. major* or *L. mexicana*, 10 months in *L. tropica* and much longer in *L. braziliensis*.

Diffuse cutaneous leishmaniasis
In the Ethiopian highlands and western Kenya, *L. aethiopica* causes initial skin lesions similar to *L. tropica*. In very rare cases, leishmania disseminate throughout the skin to cause widespread, often symmetrical, lesions that resemble lepromatous leprosy. Similar syndromes occur in Central and South America due to infections with *L. mexicana* and *L. amazonensis*. A cell-mediated immune response to leishmania antigens is absent.

Leishmania recidivans
This is an unusual form of cutaneous leishmaniasis found in the Middle East and caused by *L. tropica*. The initial chronic skin lesion heals but then groups of lesions resembling lupus vulgaris occur around the healed scar. Leishmania amastigotes are difficult to find but the leishmanin skin test is strongly positive.

Mucocutaneous leishmaniasis
L. braziliensis complex infections cause single, often self-healing, primary lesions of the skin. However, in less than 10% of cases, subsequent metastatic spread to the oro-nasopharynx may occur (espundia). The time interval between initial infection and mucosal infection varies from a month to many years. The nasal septum is often involved initially causing symptoms of nasal stuffiness and epistaxis. Granulomatous lesions cause necrosis and destruction of cartilage and soft tissue and extend to involve the nose, mouth, tongue and soft palate. Lesions may ultimately involve the pharynx and larynx. Secondary infection is common and contributes to tissue destruction. Aspiration pneumonia occurs in the late stages and may be fatal.

Diagnosis of cutaneous leishmaniasis
The likelihood of finding parasites depends upon the infecting species and the stage of the lesion. Parasites are more numerous in early lesions and in *L. tropica* and diffuse cutaneous leishmaniasis. Aspirates and slit smear preparation from the raised margins of a lesion, dermal scrapings and biopsies are all useful. Care should be taken to reduce the chance of bacterial contamination of samples. Multiple sampling and a combination of techniques increase the chances of a successful diagnosis. Samples should be examined microscopically and cultured on appropriate media. Impression smears should be made from biopsy samples. Although histology is less sensitive in detecting parasites, it is useful in

excluding other causes of the lesion. Mucocutaneous disease is often difficult to diagnose due to the limited number of parasites. PCR may be helpful on lesion aspirates or biopsies and may distinguish between different species complexes. Species diagnosis may also be made on cultured parasites by isoenzyme analysis or other DNA diagnostic techniques.

The leishmanin skin test (a test of delayed hypersensitivity using leishmanial antigen) may become positive during the course of infection, but is now rarely used for diagnosis. Serodiagnostic tests are of limited value for the diagnosis of cutaneous disease but may be helpful for the diagnosis and follow-up of mucocutaneous disease.

Important differential diagnoses for cutaneous leishmaniasis include superficial mycoses such as sporotrichosis, cutaneous mycobacterial infections, yaws, syphilis, sarcoidosis and neoplasms. In mucosal disease, histoplasmosis, paracoccidioidomycosis and midline granuloma must also be considered.

Treatment[751]

Many cutaneous leishmaniasis lesions heal spontaneously without specific treatment. Local treatment should include cleansing and antibiotics to control secondary infection and covering to prevent secondary contact lesions. Local infiltration with antimonials is used in some areas for treatment of early non-inflamed lesions to accelerate healing.[752] This can be painful. Topical paromomycin may be effective in *L. major* infection; success rates in other species are variable.[744,745]

Oral agents such as allopurinol and imidazoles (ketoconazole, itraconazole) have been used for cutaneous leishmaniasis with variable and generally disappointing results. Miltefosine may be effective orally for American cutaneous leishmaniasis.[753]

In *L. braziliensis* areas where mucocutaneous leishmaniasis occurs, all leishmanial lesions must be treated with prolonged systemic pentavalent antimonials (20 mg/kg stibogluconate for 20 days) to prevent metastatic spread. The clinical response may be poorer in children under 5.[754] Systemic therapy is also indicated for multiple or potentially disfiguring lesions of any species; shorter, lower dose courses may be adequate for *L. major* or *L. tropica*. Established mucocutaneous disease is difficult to treat and may require prolonged courses of systemic antimony or amphotericin. Diffuse cutaneous leishmaniasis is resistant to pentavalent antimonials but may respond either to combinations of aminosidine and antimonials or to prolonged courses of pentamidine.

CONTROL OF LEISHMANIASIS

Control centers upon vector control and reduction in the reservoir host. In central Asia, the simultaneous use of rodenticide and insecticide in gerbil burrows has reduced markedly the incidence of *L. major* infection. Similarly, control of stray dog populations and residual insecticide spraying have reduced *L. infantum* infection in many areas. Effective control can be achieved by medical surveillance of the population at risk when man is the major host reservoir. Insecticide spraying of houses is useful for peridomestic vectors such as in Indian visceral leishmaniasis. Control remains problematic in the vast forested areas of the Americas; the use of insecticides in tropical rain forests is impractical and control of the extensive reservoir of infected wild animals equally impossible. A number of candidate vaccines have been developed but clinical trials have been disappointing in both cutaneous and visceral leishmaniasis. A number of studies suggest that treated or untreated bednets reduce the risk of visceral leishmaniasis.[755]

MALARIA

Malaria is a disease of humans caused by infection with one or more of four species of protozoa of the genus *Plasmodium* (*Plasmodium falciparum, Plasmodium vivax, Plasmodium malariae* and *Plasmodium ovale*). It is usually acquired through the bite of an infected female *Anopheles* mosquito, although it may also follow the transfer of infected blood as

in blood transfusion, or transplacentally or by the use of contaminated syringes. Worldwide some 45 *Anopheles* species effectively transmit malaria, although the identity, behavior and importance of local vectors vary widely with geographic location. The most effective vector is probably *Anopheles gambiae* – a mosquito that is widely distributed in tropical Africa. *P. falciparum* is the most pathogenic of the malaria parasites and infections with it must always be regarded as serious and potentially life threatening. The other three species tend to cause less serious illness, although on occasion a lethal nephrosis may complicate *P. malariae* infections.

THE PARASITE LIFE CYCLE

Malaria parasites undergo a complex stage of asexual development in the human host and a stage of sexual development (sporogony) which occurs partly in man and partly in the mosquito vector.[756]

Asexual development in man

This begins with the introduction of infective forms (sporozoites) in mosquito saliva during the biting act. Sporozoites circulate for less than 60 min, eventually gaining access to parenchymal liver cells either directly or after passage through Kupffer cells. The invasion process may entail specific ligand–receptor interaction. Once within the hepatocyte, the sporozoite initiates the exoerythrocytic (EE) phase of asexual development during which it grows and undergoes repeated nuclear fission (schizogony), eventually producing a cyst-like schizont filled with daughter parasites (merozoites). This phase usually proceeds without interruption and both the time taken to schizont maturity and the number of merozoites produced vary with the identity of the plasmodial species involved. *P. falciparum* completes its EE development fastest (about 5 days) and produces most merozoites per schizont (about 30 000). The other species are slower and less prolific, the respective values for *P. malariae*, for example, being about 15 days and about 15 000 merozoites. In two parasite species, *P. vivax* and *P. ovale*, some sporozoites initiate this uninterrupted EE stage of development but some do not. These latter, on entering hepatocytes produce small unicellular forms (hypnozoites) which persist without development for periods varying from several weeks to many months. Eventually the hypnozoites, activated by mechanisms as yet not known, resume growth and proceed to schizont maturation and merozoite liberation. Hypnozoites are currently widely believed to give rise to the relapsing parasitemias which characterize *P. ovale* and, particularly, *P. vivax* infections and which can occur even after drug treatment has effectively eliminated erythrocytic parasites. Hypnozoites do not develop in infections with *P. falciparum* and *P. malariae* and in these species recrudescence of parasitemia is generally considered to be due to persistent erythrocytic infection.

Merozoites liberated from EE schizonts are short lived and must find and enter a red blood cell within a few minutes. Within the erythrocyte each grows rapidly through ring form and uninucleate trophozoite stages eventually to form a schizont containing merozoites. On schizont rupture, the merozoites enter the bloodstream, attach to and penetrate fresh erythrocytes and again begin the cycle of erythrocytic asexual development. Attachment and penetration by merozoites are complex operations, which require specific ligand–receptor interactions. Erythrocyte invasion by *P. vivax* appears to require a ligand that is associated with Duffy blood group antigens, while attachment of *P. falciparum* merozoites to red cells requires one associated with sialic acid on the erythrocyte membrane. Age of the red cell also influences invasion by merozoites: *P. vivax* preferentially invades reticulocytes – a feature which tends to limit the density of parasitemia attained by this species – while *P. falciparum* can invade red cells of all ages.

The duration of the erythrocytic phase of asexual development and the merozoite yield per schizont vary with the plasmodial species. *P. malariae* has the longest cycle (72 h, i.e. quartan periodicity); the remaining species have cycles of about 48 h duration (i.e. tertian periodicity). *P. falciparum* has the greatest capacity to replicate and the merozoite yield of its schizonts is in the range 8–32. For the others the yields are 8–24 for *P. vivax*, 4–16 for *P. ovale* and 8 for *P. malariae*. The ability of *P. falciparum* to replicate rapidly in both the hepatic and erythrocytic phases of development partly accounts for the severity of the illness this species causes.

The time taken for parasites to become detectable in the peripheral blood following sporozoite inoculation is termed the prepatent period, while the time from infection to the onset of symptoms is termed the incubation period. While the two periods may be of equal duration, more usually the incubation period is about 2 days longer.

Late in its asexual erythrocytic cycle *P. falciparum* withdraws from the peripheral circulation and sequesters in deep vasculature. The phenomenon, which probably contributes importantly to the serious pathological effects that this *Plasmodium* causes, is effected by the binding of receptors on the surface of red cells infected with nearly mature parasites to ligands exposed on the surface of the endothelial cells lining deep blood vessels. Sequestration does not occur in the course of infections with the other plasmodial species that infect man.

Sexual development

In the course of blood stage schizogony in the human host some merozoites differentiate, by mechanisms which are not yet understood, to give rise to male and female sexual forms (gametocytes). In the case of *P. vivax*, gametocytes are formed early after the release of merozoites from the liver (before clinical symptoms), while *P. falciparum* gametocytes are generated after a number of erythrocytic cycles. Early treatment of fever with antimalarial drugs may therefore prevent gametocyte formation in *P. falciparum* but not in *P. vivax* infections. When mature, gametocytes circulate in the blood but do not undergo further development unless they are ingested by an anopheline mosquito during feeding. Once in the midgut of the mosquito, the female (macrogametocyte) escapes from the enclosing erythrocytic membrane and becomes a macrogamete. The male (microgametocyte) undergoes a process of exflagellation during which eight slender, uninucleate filaments (microgametes) are extruded and break free. Each microgamete seeks a macrogamete and, if successful, penetrates and fertilizes it. The two nuclei fuse and a zygote is formed. This is probably the only point in the life history of the parasite that genetic recombination occurs. The diploid zygote then undergoes meiosis and, as an ookinete, migrates to penetrate the epithelium of the mosquito midgut wall where it comes to rest on the external surface. There it rounds up, becomes an oocyst and begins a series of nuclear divisions. Oocyst maturity is reached after a period which is dependent on the identity of the plasmodial species and the ambient temperature to which the mosquito is exposed. It may be 1–4 weeks, or longer. At maturity the oocyst is filled with as many as 10 000 daughter parasites (sporozoites), each some 10–15 μm in length and feebly motile. The sporozoites escape at oocyst rupture and travel in the hemocelomic fluid to the salivary glands where they accumulate in the acinal cells to be discharged with saliva when the mosquito next feeds.

Infected humans constitute the only known source of mosquito infection for *P. falciparum*, *P. vivax* and *P. ovale*. For *P. malariae* some apes and monkeys may constitute reservoirs of infection in addition to humans.

EPIDEMIOLOGY

Despite widespread operations promoted by the World Health Organization between 1955 and 1975 with the aim of achieving global eradication, malaria remains probably the most prevalent, important, communicable disease throughout much of the tropical and subtropical world, the greatest burden of disease being in sub-Saharan Africa. Estimates of the world annual incidence of malarial illness have ranged from 200–450 million episodes[757] to over half a billion.[758] The much-quoted estimate of around 1 million malaria deaths annually in Africa, >75% of them in children, is supported by available evidence.[759] Over the past 25 years *P. falciparum* parasites have become increasingly resistant to chloroquine and other currently available antimalarial drugs.

This development appears to have been accompanied by an increase in malaria-attributed mortality in some endemic areas[760] and has required the development of new drug policies for malaria control and new regimens for chemoprophylaxis for travelers and other at-risk groups.

Many factors influence the epidemiology of malaria. Atmospheric temperature is important. For successful development in the mosquito vector, *P. vivax* requires a sustained temperature of at least 16 °C, while *P. falciparum* requires one of 20 °C. The geographical limits of *P. vivax* transmission are thus more widely set than those of *P. falciparum*. Other factors relate to the identity and biology of the *Plasmodium*, the identity and behavior of the vector, the social and economic customs of human populations and the topography and climate of the region. It follows, therefore, that the epidemiological pattern of the infection is not uniform but varies considerably between and within countries.

Where transmission occurs the measurement of endemicity has, in the past, relied on establishment of spleen rates and parasite positivity rates in ambulant children aged 2–9 years. Thus categories classified as hypo-, meso-, hyper- and holoendemic were characterized by both spleen and parasite rates of <10%, 11–50%, constantly >50% and constantly >75% respectively. In hyperendemic areas spleens in adults were frequently enlarged; in holoendemic areas they were not (this observation was attributed to the greater acquisition of immunity in holoendemic areas).

However, the widespread use of antimalarial drugs in areas where malaria is endemic has adversely affected these classical indices of endemicity and they are less useful today than formerly. This change has prompted the use of seroepidemiological techniques in the identification of malaria transmission and the measurement of its intensity. These techniques detect and quantify specific malaria antibody in serum and establish age-specific profiles for prevalence and titer. Briefly, profiles which show little change with age denote low transmission while profiles showing values which rise rapidly with age denote high transmission.[761]

Epidemiologically malaria presents in two extremes, one of which is stable and shows little change from one year to another, and the other which is unstable and may fluctuate violently in intensity at regular or irregular intervals. Stable malaria is most in evidence in areas where transmission rates are high; it is characterized by rates of mortality and morbidity which are high in infants and young children and which fall to low, even negligible, levels as age advances and effective immunity is acquired. Unstable malaria occurs where transmission rates remain low for periods of several years then suddenly increase greatly for climatic or other reasons; it is characterized by the occurrence of epidemics in which morbidity and mortality are conspicuous at all ages. Acquired immunity is not a feature of unstable malaria, save possibly at the end of a protracted epidemic period. Between the extremes of stability and instability, a range of intermediate epidemiological presentation occurs.

IMMUNITY

Malarial immunity may be innate, i.e. genetically determined, or acquired. Innate immunity may be due to a lack of ligands on the erythrocyte surface which bind to specific receptors on the merozoite surface at an essential stage in the invasion process, or to the presence of abnormal intramembranous erythrocytic components, which inhibit, but do not totally prevent, growth of the parasite within the red cell. An example of the former is the freedom from *P. vivax* infection that is apparent in people whose erythrocytes lack Duffy blood group antigens, while an example of the latter is the partial protection and survival advantage towards *P. falciparum* infections that heterozygosity for the sickle cell gene confers.[762]

Acquired immunity may be passive or active. Passive immunity due to the transplacental transfer of specific IgG malarial antibodies from mother to fetus probably accounts, at least in part, for the relative resistance to malaria that infants born in highly endemic areas show over the first few months of life. Acquired active immunity develops slowly in response to infection with malaria.[763] The first evidence is an ability to restrict the clinical effects of infection despite the persistence of high density parasitemia. This 'clinical' immunity is usually discernible in young children in highly endemic areas around the third to fourth year of life. Later, an ability to restrict parasite density develops and slowly strengthens throughout later childhood and adolescence to reach maximum expression in adult life. When fully developed, malarial immunity is species, strain and stage specific.

Acquired active immunity entails the collaboration of different cell populations, notably T cells, B cells and macrophages, during which specific and nonspecific humoral factors are elaborated which restrict parasite growth and replication.[764] Knowledge of how this complex response is assembled and controlled remains incomplete. T cells play a central role and their recognition of, and response to, defined malarial antigens are probably controlled by immune response (Ir) genes. Sensitized T cells respond to antigen by replication and the secretion of lymphokines which promote further T cell replication and diversification, induce replication of B cells with antibody production and activate macrophages.

Specific malarial antibodies belong to the immunoglobulin classes G, M and A. They function by agglutinating parasites and parasitized cells, inhibiting interactions between host cell surface ligands and parasite receptors, mediating cellular cytotoxicity and phagocytosis and inhibiting sequestration of mature asexual erythrocytic forms of *P. falciparum* in deep vasculature. Antibodies do not kill parasites directly through the activation of complement. Natural malaria infection induces synthesis of a wide range of antibodies directed against specific parasite antigens. Thus antibodies with specificity for the antigens of sporozoites, EE forms, asexual blood stages and sexual stages can be detected and titrated in the sera of residents of endemic areas.

The killing of parasites, which is probably carried out mainly by activated macrophages and cytotoxic T cells, involves release from the host cells of toxic oxygen derivatives and occurs principally in spleen and liver. However, other killing mechanisms exist. Interferon-gamma released by sensitized T cells has been observed to kill EE stages in hepatic cells, while tumor necrosis factor (TNF) liberated from macrophages stimulated with endotoxin has been reported to inhibit replication of both EE and erythrocytic stages of the parasite.

PATHOLOGY

The pathogenic sequences that develop in malaria are attributable to events that arise during the asexual erythrocytic stage of development of the parasite in man.

Anemia is common and is due partly to the rhythmic invasion and destruction of erythrocytes by parasites and partly to additional mechanisms, such as dyserythropoiesis and immune hemolysis following sensitization of nonparasitized red cells.[765] Bone marrow changes in dyserythropoiesis include erythroblast multinuclearity, karyorrhexis, incomplete and unequal nuclear division and cytoplasmic bridging. The marrow may contain large amounts of stainable iron and show evidence of phagocytosis of defective red cell precursors by macrophages. Whether these changes are initiated by toxic substances liberated by the parasite, or represent the nonspecific effects of macrophages rendered hyperactive by parasite antigens remains to be ascertained. The sensitization of uninfected red cells occurs commonly in malaria, often involves C3 and/or IgG and can be detected by the direct antiglobulin test (DAT) using specific antisera. DAT positivity of red cells, which is frequent in patients with falciparum malaria, has been found to be associated with enhanced blood destruction, but the association appears to be relatively uncommon.[765]

A characteristic feature of *P. falciparum* infections is the collection ('sequestration') of large numbers of late-stage parasites in the venules and capillaries of a variety of organs.[766] This results from the ability of this parasite, in the later stages of its development in the red cell, to display a number of proteins – known as *P. falciparum* erythrocyte membrane protein-1 (PfEMP-1) – on the red cell surface, by which the parasitized red cell attaches to host receptors on the microvascular endothelium.[767]

PfEMP-1 is a family of proteins encoded by recently identified highly variable var genes.[768] It is possible that sequestration is augmented by adhesion between parasitized erythrocytes, a phenomenon that can be demonstrated in vitro.[769] Sequestration is believed to be the mechanism underlying some of the clinical complications of *P. falciparum* infection, including the coma and convulsions of cerebral malaria. It is not known how sequestration may lead to tissue dysfunction: one possibility is that the huge number of actively metabolizing parasites consume oxygen and glucose at the expense of neighboring tissue, or produce toxic metabolites, including lactate, that may affect cellular function. Another possibility is that sequestration stimulates the release of host transmitters, such as nitric oxide, that may have a local effect on blood flow or on the conduction of nerve impulses. Host cytokines, too, are released and these may make endothelial cells more adhesive for the surface of parasitized red cells, thus augmenting sequestration.[770]

In some children with fatal cerebral malaria, histological changes include accumulations of platelets and microthrombi in cerebral and other microvessels.[771] CT scans of children surviving cerebral malaria with neurological sequelae show areas of brain infarction that may result from such vascular occlusions. Fortunately the majority of children and adults treated for cerebral malaria recover without neurological sequelae,[772] suggesting that microvascular occlusions from microthrombi are not a usual or major component of the pathology.

In children dying of encephalopathy with *P. falciparum* parasitemia, autopsies indicate that in a considerable proportion (about a quarter in one series[773]) the diagnosis may be a condition other than malaria, the parasitemia in these cases being incidental. This underlines the fact that, when a high proportion of a population is parasitemic, the diagnosis of severe malaria requires careful judgment and will sometimes be mistaken. This can result in failure to treat severe bacterial infection, often with fatal consequences.

Enlargement of the spleen and liver is common in acute and chronic infections and, on section, both organs are dark from the accumulation of malarial pigment (hemozoin). Evidence of phagocytosis of parasites, parasitized cells and hemozoin is usually present in the splenic pulp and in the sinusoidal macrophages and Kupffer cells of the liver.

In *P. falciparum* infections an acute diffuse glomerulonephritis may occur in which deposits of immunoglobulins, complement and malarial antigens are detectable in the mesangium and capillary loops. This is usually transient, but in non-immune adults with *P. falciparum* malaria it may lead to acute renal failure, usually characterized pathologically by acute tubular necrosis, from which recovery is usual if the patient can be sustained by supportive care and dialysis until renal function is restored. In *P. malariae* infections, however, a much more progressive and frequently lethal nephropathy may develop, again with evidence of antigen/antibody deposition. In children these lesions may progress despite antimalarial treatment to total glomerular sclerosis with secondary tubular atrophy. Clinically, the manifestations of a nephrotic syndrome develop with severe generalized edema and ascites accompanied by heavy proteinuria and hypoalbuminemia.

During pregnancy, *P. falciparum* may attain very high densities in the maternal placental blood and cause damage to the syncytiotrophoblast. Placental infection is associated with reduced infant birth weight and, in endemic areas, the association is most marked in first pregnancies. Occasionally, parasites cross the placenta, giving rise to congenital infection in the infant at or soon after birth. In endemic areas such infections seldom persist or cause disease in the neonate, but if the mother is a 'non-immune' individual, the baby may develop an illness with fever, anemia and jaundice.

Thrombocytopenia commonly occurs in *P. falciparum* infections for reasons that remain poorly understood. It usually occurs independently of changes in other measures of coagulation (prothrombin time, partial thromboplastin time) or to plasma fibrinogen concentrations and is usually unaccompanied by bleeding. Spontaneous bleeding may occur associated with disseminated intravascular coagulation (DIC), but this is an uncommon clinical feature of severe malaria in adults and is rare in children.

CHEMOPROPHYLAXIS

Large scale continuous chemoprophylaxis for children is not recommended in endemic areas, the main reason being that it is economically and logistically almost impossible to achieve over the long term on a national scale. It may be a useful measure, however, in focal high risk communities, such as refugees who have moved from a nonmalarious to an endemic area. Theoretical but unproven disadvantages of community-wide chemoprophylaxis include interference with the development of acquired immunity, enhancement of the development and spread of drug resistance and risk of toxicity from long term drug usage.

For individuals traveling from nonmalarious to malarious areas, however, chemoprophylaxis remains an important means of protection.

Drug prophylaxis should be seen as only one component of prevention. At least as important is sleeping under a permethrin-impregnated net (malaria-transmitting mosquitoes bite mainly in the middle of the night). Other measures can help: application of insect repellents [dimethylphthalate (DMP) or dimethyl-m-toluamide (DEET)] to exposed skin areas over periods of mosquito activity, the screening of houses and the use of knock-down insecticides in bedrooms before retiring.

Most prophylactic drugs should be taken for at least a week before travel (mainly in order to ensure acceptability) and for a month after exposure ends (to eliminate parasites that have developed in the liver in the intervening time).

Expatriates from a non-endemic country who intend to reside with their children for many years in a country with P. falciparum transmission must decide whether to take drug prophylaxis over the long term. The decision must be based on the extent of local risk, its seasonality, the local pattern of parasite resistance to various antimalarial drugs, and the availability of prompt health care. With screening and indoor residual spraying of the home and consistent use of insecticide-impregnated bednets, the risk may be low enough to avoid prophylaxis, provided that any fever is promptly diagnosed and treated. Expatriates may consider using chemoprophylaxis only during seasons of increased transmission or when visiting parts of the country where transmission is known to be high.

No prophylactic regimen, even if adhered to fully, guarantees protection against malaria absolutely. If a febrile illness develops during or up to 6 months after the period of exposure, malaria remains a possibility and should be investigated accordingly. Parents should be advised to ensure that physicians attending illness in children after return from endemic areas are aware of the need to exclude a diagnosis of malaria. Similarly, parents who live in endemic areas and are visited from time to time by children being educated in non-endemic areas should ensure that guardians and school authorities are alerted to the need to exclude malaria as a diagnosis in any illness developing in the repatriated child.

When contemplating the need for chemoprophylaxis in particular instances, the physician should ascertain the risk to which the child is or will be exposed, the duration of exposure, the pattern of drug resistance of malaria in the area to be visited, and possible drug toxicity. Useful information on disease incidence and drug resistance in the malarious countries of the world is to be found in the periodic reviews published by the World Health Organization in its Weekly Epidemiological Record.

Suggested chemoprophylactic regimens[774] (see also www.prodigy.nhs.uk/malaria_prophylaxis) are as follows:

1. Where only P. vivax malaria exists, prophylaxis should be by chloroquine proportional to an adult dose of 300 mg (two tablets) once weekly or by proguanil (Paludrine) proportional to an adult dose of 200 mg (two tablets) daily (see Table 28.39).
2. Where P. falciparum transmission occurs, options include:
   - Atovaquone–proguanil (Malarone), daily. This has the advantage of very little known toxicity and of attacking liver stage as well as blood stage parasites, so that it need be taken for only a week after exposure ends. Malarone is expensive.
   - Mefloquine (Lariam) once weekly. The weekly dosage is an advantage, but is easier to forget. Various side-effects are

Table 28.39 Age-related dosage of antimalarial drugs for chemoprophylaxis in children

Age	Fraction of adult dose
< 6 weeks	1/8
6 weeks–1 year	1/4
1–5 years	1/2
5–12 years	3/4
> 12 years	Adult dose

commonly reported, including insomnia and vivid dreams. Mefloquine should not be given to children who have a history of epilepsy or psychiatric disease.

Various prophylactic regimens used in the past are no longer recommended as prophylactics, although some of the component drugs remain important for treatment. Amodiaquine as a weekly prophylactic has been associated with occasional hepatic necrosis or neutropenia; weekly pyrimethamine–dapsone (Maloprim) with occasional agranulocytosis; and weekly sulfadoxine–pyrimethamine (SP, Fansidar) with Stevens–Johnson syndrome. Doxycycline, a useful prophylactic in adults, is contraindicated in children.

Continuous chemoprophylaxis is indicated for indigenous children in malarious areas who are homozygous for the sickle cell gene, because malaria may precipitate a crisis. Malaria increases viral load in adults with HIV infection,[775] but it is not yet known whether chemoprophylaxis against malaria will improve life expectancy in children with HIV infection or AIDS. Co-trimoxazole prophylaxis is beneficial in HIV infected children[776] and co-trimoxazole is an efficacious antimalarial drug, but it is not known whether or to what extent the benefit of co-trimoxazole is dependent on its antimalarial activity.

VACCINATION

A safe and effective vaccine for malaria is not yet available. Several candidate vaccines, making use of antigens from various combinations of sporozoite, erythrocytic and sexual stages of P. falciparum, are undergoing development or clinical trials. Promising results have been obtained among children in Mozambique in trials of the candidate vaccine RTS,S, a product consisting of sequences of the circumsporozoite protein of the P. falciparum merozoite linked to hepatitis B surface antigen and combined with the adjuvant ASO2.[777] In a double-blind randomized trial in children aged 1–5 years, the vaccine demonstrated 30% (95% CI 11%, 45%) protection against clinical malaria, 58% (16%, 81%) against severe malaria disease and 45% (31%, 56%) protection against P. falciparum infection, a benefit that was shown to persist over a subsequent year of observation.[778] Trials of this vaccine continue, with the aim of assessing its benefit when administered to young infants within existing standard EPI schedules.

CLINICAL FEATURES

The manifestations of malaria in an individual are determined by the infecting species of Plasmodium and the resistance or immunity of the host.

Each of the four species of parasite causing human malaria may produce a febrile illness with nonspecific symptoms including anorexia, malaise, headache, chills, rigors, sweating, irritability and failure to eat and drink. Symptoms begin about 10 days after the infective mosquito bite, but longer incubation periods are common, especially with the nonfalciparum malarias, and sometimes the first symptoms are not experienced until months or years after exposure. Diarrhea, vomiting and cough are common, but not severe, early symptoms. Febrile convulsions commonly complicate sudden rises of temperature in young children. The pattern of fever is irregular at first; the classical periodicity appears only if the illness is protracted and untreated, when P. malariae may cause quartan fever (72 h between spikes), P. vivax and

P. ovale tertian fever (48 h intervals) and *P. falciparum* subtertian fever (less than 48 h intervals). The liver and spleen may become palpable during the first few days of fever; the spleen may become enlarged during the course of a single episode, and may become very large after repeated or untreated infections.

Anemia develops, its degree being greatest in those with the heaviest or most protracted infections. Minor abnormalities of hepatic enzymes may be found, but jaundice is unusual even in severe falciparum malaria.

The most important distinction between species in their clinical effects is in the capacity of *P. falciparum* to cause, in susceptible individuals, a rapidly progressive severe ('complicated') disease, which may be fatal. Most of the many deaths from malaria every year are due to *P. falciparum* infections in young children living in endemic areas, the majority in sub-Saharan Africa.

In endemic areas the patient's first encounter with *P. falciparum* may be in utero. Parasitemia is common in pregnant women, and both placenta and cord blood may contain parasites at the time of delivery. Babies born to infected primigravid mothers may have a low birth weight but are otherwise unaffected. Parasitemia usually clears rapidly in the newborn, who remains relatively resistant to falciparum malaria for the first few months of life, probably because of a combination of maternal antimalarial antibodies and the fact that parasites grow less successfully in fetal than in adult hemoglobin. Occasionally (rarely in endemic areas) the newborn goes on to develop congenital malaria, features of which may include fever, failure to feed, anemia, jaundice and hepatosplenomegaly. Severe disease begins to affect children in endemic areas after the first few months of life, and for the next few years. During this time the majority of children are increasingly able to tolerate parasitemia with few or no symptoms, and malaria-related mortality decreases later in childhood.

In areas where there is little or no malaria transmission, children are susceptible to infection and severe disease at any age, and congenital malaria is sometimes seen.[779]

Acute *P. falciparum* infections

P. falciparum malaria usually presents as a febrile illness similar to that caused by other species of malaria. In a proportion of patients, however, complications develop which may threaten life. The most important manifestations of severe malaria in children are altered consciousness, labored breathing (due to acidosis) and severe anemia. These features may occur singly or in any combination.[780] A variety of metabolic complications may develop, resembling those that may complicate any severe systemic infection (reviewed in ref 781). Hypoglycemia may accompany any of the above syndromes and is associated with increased mortality, especially when the hypoglycemia is profound.[782] Some of the organ complications of falciparum malaria which are common in non-immune adults are uncommon in children. Renal failure, pulmonary edema and disseminated intravascular coagulation are less likely to develop in children, and are not present in most of those who die of falciparum malaria.

Cerebral malaria (CM)

When impaired consciousness in a child with falciparum malaria cannot be explained by the presence of hypoglycemia, seizures or a transient postictal state, and no other causative disease is present, the term 'cerebral malaria' is used.

Clinical measurements of the depth of coma are helpful in defining severity.[772]

CM develops rapidly. In the majority of children febrile symptoms precede coma by 2 days or less; in some the interval is only a few hours. Most patients have been feverish, irritable, listless and unable to eat or drink prior to losing consciousness. Convulsions are common and sometimes herald the onset of coma. In CM there is no postictal recovery of consciousness as occurs after a febrile convulsion. Other symptoms that may precede coma include vomiting and cough; minor looseness of stool may occur, but severe diarrhea is unusual.

The rectal temperature may exceed 40 °C, and is usually sustained during the first day or two of treatment. Occasionally a patient with CM may be afebrile when first examined, and rarely may remain so throughout the illness. Tachycardia is appropriate to the degree of fever, and the systolic blood pressure is normal in most patients. Dehydration is not clinically obvious, but vigorous fluid therapy in some patients leads to correction of acidosis and to improved tissue perfusion, suggesting that hypovolemia is commonly important. Respiration is rapid; in some patients breathing is stertorous, in others deep suggesting acidosis. About 5% of children with CM are jaundiced. The heart and lungs are normal on examination. The abdomen is soft; the liver may be moderately enlarged and the spleen may be palpable. In a minority of children with CM a shock-like state, with hypotension, cold peripheries and a wide core-to-skin temperature difference, may develop. Anemia is clinically apparent in some patients, and may develop during the course of illness in others.

The most striking clinical features are neurological. By definition the patient is unconscious and cannot be roused. Coma may be profound, the child being unable to withdraw from or localize a painful stimulus, and unable to moan or cry in response to pain. With less severe neurological impairment, motor and vocal responses to pain are retained but the patient is unable to watch or recognize familiar people. Corneal and pupillary reflexes are usually intact, but brainstem reflexes may be lost in the most severely ill. Retinal hemorrhages are common. Some of the most severely ill patients have papilledema.[783] Recently two further features have been identified that constitute a characteristic 'malarial retinopathy' not seen in other infections: these are areas of discrete retinal whitening, and a silver, orange or white appearance of some of the smaller vessels, usually in a patchy distribution.[784,785]

In some patients the motor picture suggests decerebration or decortication, with symmetrical rigidity or posturing of limbs, which may be sustained or repetitive. These may represent underlying seizure activity. It is not uncommon for patients to be opisthotonic. Focal asymmetrical twitching movements of the face or of a limb may be witnessed, sometimes (not invariably) proceeding to a generalized convulsion. If available, electroencephalography may reveal cerebral seizure activity in some cases in whom there is minimal or absent convulsive movement. Both overt and subtle seizures may occur in the absence of extremes of fever, and they cannot be regarded as febrile convulsions. The plantar reflexes may be abnormal. Abdominal reflexes are almost invariably absent.

The peripheral blood film reveals ring stages of *P. falciparum*. Occasionally parasites may be scanty, and rarely absent, in the blood film of a child with CM, perhaps as a result of the synchronous sequestration of mature parasites, and especially in a non-immune child; parasitemia is usually revealed with repeated examination at intervals of a few hours. In an endemic area, in a child with suspected CM who has scanty or moderate peripheral parasitemia, alternative diagnoses must be considered with particular care, as peripheral parasitemia may be an incidental finding in a child whose encephalopathy is due to something else. The likelihood that *P. falciparum* is the cause of a cerebral disease increases with the density of the parasitemia; it is not uncommon for up to 20% of red cells to be parasitized, and in some patients the figure exceeds 50%.

The packed cell volume may be normal or may be reduced; it usually falls further as the illness progresses. Life-threatening anemia may develop rapidly in patients with hyperparasitemia. Commonly the fall in hematocrit exceeds what would be predicted from the level of parasitemia. The peripheral white cell count is normal in the majority of patients but may be elevated in the very ill. The most severely affected patients are acidotic. There are minor abnormalities of hepatic enzymes, and the plasma creatinine may be mildly elevated. Plasma sodium, potassium, chloride, phosphate and calcium concentrations may show mild abnormalities but are commonly normal. Plasma and cerebrospinal fluid (CSF) lactate levels are abnormally raised in some patients, commonly in association with hypoglycemia. CSF opening pressure is raised in most patients, and fluctuates over time.[786] The mean and distribution of opening pressures were similar in a series of patients with fatal and nonfatal CM, and the pathogenetic importance of raised intracranial pressure remains uncertain.[787] The CSF is clear with normal cell counts and protein concentration.

A significant proportion of patients with CM are hypoglycemic when first admitted to hospital.[782,788] These patients do not differ from others in their duration of preceding illness, fasting or coma, or by any distinctive physical signs, but they tend to be younger and are more likely to be profoundly unconscious, to exhibit motor abnormalities and to have elevated levels of lactate and alanine in the plasma.

Even with optimal treatment, the mortality among children admitted to hospital with CM is 10–20%. The cause of death is not known, and in most cases cannot be attributed to renal, cardiac, pulmonary or hematological complications of malaria. Presenting features associated with an increased risk of death in children with CM include profound coma, age under 3 years, hypoglycemia, witnessed convulsions, motor abnormalities (hypertonicity, posturing), extreme hyperparasitemia (> 20% of red cells parasitized), acidosis, lactic acidemia and leukocytosis (> 15×10^9 white blood cells/L).[772]

In patients who survive CM, the duration of coma after the start of treatment ranges from a few hours to several days, the average duration being about 30 h. The change from deep coma to full consciousness may be dramatically rapid, and usually occurs before the temperature has fallen to normal and before parasitemia has cleared. The great majority of children who survive CM make a full neurological recovery; 5–10% of patients, however, suffer neurological sequelae, including hemiparesis, spasticity and cerebellar defects, from which a gradual recovery is made in some patients over the subsequent months. Risk factors for the development of sequelae are the same as those associated with mortality. Areas of intracerebral infarction have been demonstrated by computerized tomography in some children with neurological sequelae after CM.[789] Long term follow-up studies suggest that children recovering from CM are at increased risk of epilepsy in subsequent years, and that some may have cognitive and learning defects.[790]

Anemia

Anemia is a component of most episodes of malarial illness. In areas endemic for P. falciparum severe anemia (hemoglobin concentration < 5 g/dl) is an important clinical consequence of acute or recurrent malaria.[791]

The history of fever and associated symptoms may be similar to that of any malarial illness, but it is common for a child to present without such symptoms, or for anemia to be identified when a child is examined for an unrelated complaint. Some children with severe malarial anemia develop respiratory distress, which is usually due to acidosis resulting from impaired tissue perfusion and oxygenation.[792] Less commonly, breathlessness is due to cardiac failure, with enlarging liver, and a gallop rhythm on auscultation of the heart.

Peripheral blood films reveal parasitemia and a normochromic normocytic or, in chronic infections, hypochromic anemia. The reticulocyte count is inappropriately low. Unconjugated bilirubin may be increased in the plasma, free hemoglobin may be present in plasma and urine, and the plasma haptoglobin concentration is usually decreased or absent in the acute stage of the illness. The bone marrow shows normoblastic erythropoiesis with minimal dyserythropoiesis and increased myeloid precursors.[765] Unless other diseases are present, serum and red cell folate values are normal. Serum iron may be normal or moderately reduced, but there is usually normal or increased stainable iron in the bone marrow.

After the start of treatment for acute malaria, the hemoglobin level falls further in proportion to, or in excess of, the degree of parasitemia. In endemic areas, many children have a positive direct antiglobulin test. Reticulocytosis begins within a few days, and the hemoglobin level rises rapidly in convalescence.

Severe anemia recurs within a few weeks or months in an important proportion of children admitted to hospital for treatment of severe anemia. The role of malaria in this recurrence, and the potential for its prevention by antimalarial drugs, is under investigation.

Hyper-reactive malarial splenomegaly

Some children with protracted or frequent P. falciparum infection develop hyper-reactive malarial splenomegaly, a condition in which massive enlargement of the spleen is accompanied by raised serum IgM, high titers of antimalarial antibody, and hepatic sinusoidal lymphocytosis.[793] Splenomegaly resolves slowly with prolonged antimalarial treatment.

DIAGNOSIS AND DIFFERENTIAL DIAGNOSIS

Delayed diagnosis of P. falciparum malaria can have tragic consequences. In endemic areas it is a justifiable policy for all fevers without another obvious cause to be regarded as malarial and treated accordingly. In non-endemic areas a history of travel should alert the physician to the possibility of malaria, even if travel was many months or years ago. Malaria should be considered in puzzling clinical situations, even in individuals who have not traveled to an endemic area, as mosquitoes may transmit plasmodia after 'commuting' on an aeroplane ('airport malaria'), and parasites may be transmitted transplacentally or by needle-stick injury. Malaria should be considered in the differential diagnosis of all fevers accompanied by cerebral complications, acidosis or anemia, and in patients with fever who develop hypoglycemia, acute renal failure, disseminated intravascular coagulation or pulmonary edema.

The diagnosis of malaria depends on finding the parasite in the peripheral blood. Thick smears stained with Field's or Giemsa stain, and thin films stained with Leishman's, Giemsa or a modified Field's stain, allow identification of the species and density of malaria parasitemia. There have been occasional well-authenticated reports of fatal falciparum malaria in which blood films were repeatedly negative during life. Treatment should therefore not be withheld from a patient with an illness suggestive of malaria even if films are negative. In such patients blood films should be repeated at intervals during treatment, when parasitemia may be revealed. Serological methods of identifying malarial infection are valueless for individuals in endemic areas, and of limited use to the clinician seeing patients elsewhere. Serology identifies past or current infection, and may help towards diagnosis in a patient with recurrent fever in a non-endemic area in whom parasitemia cannot be found on repeated testing. Antigen-detecting test strips and DNA probes can identify parasitemia; these methods are valuable in clinical and epidemiological research, but have not become standard methods for use in clinical practice.

In high transmission areas where more than half of the child population may be parasitemic but apparently well at any given time, diagnosis of malaria as the cause of an illness must be speculative and will sometimes be wrong. In the comatose child, finding the distinctive ophthalmoscopic changes of malarial retinopathy (Fig. 28.53) strengthens the confidence with which the illness can be attributed to malaria. Other possible causes of the patient's clinical disease must also be considered.

A proportion of children with malaria have bacteremia, which may be either the principal or an additional cause of the child's illness.[794] Nontyphi bacteremia is particularly associated with malaria and severe anemia in infants and young children.

TREATMENT OF UNCOMPLICATED MALARIA

Most countries in endemic areas now have a national malaria control program with a stated policy of first line therapy for the treatment of presumed or proven malaria. In many areas it is a (necessary) part of national policy to base treatment on a presumptive diagnosis of malaria in the child with no obvious alternative explanation for fever. The correct drug, dosage and route are important. In general, antimalarial drugs should be given by mouth unless the patient is too ill to swallow. It is usual to prescribe additional symptomatic treatment, e.g. paracetamol, to reduce high fever, myalgia and headache.

In response to strong recommendations from WHO and funding bodies, countries are moving to adopt combination therapies as first line

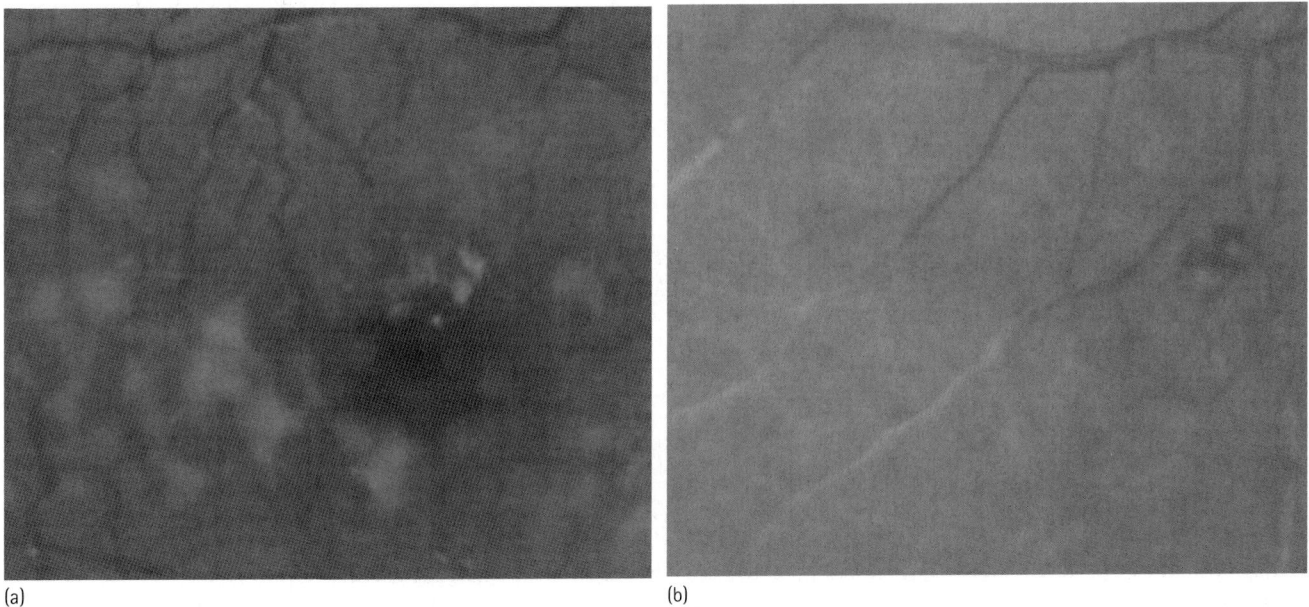

(a)   (b)

Fig. 28.53   Ophthalmoscopy in a child with cerebral malaria, showing (a) patchy retinal macular whitening, close to the fovea, (b) whitening of vessels, and two white-centered hemorrhages.

antiparasitic treatment in areas with a predominance of *P. falciparum* (i.e. most of sub-Saharan Africa). Artemisinin-containing combination therapies (ACTs) are preferred because of the rapid antiparasitic action of artemisinin drugs, their lack of toxicity, and the expectation that combination with another drug will prevent or delay the evolution of drug resistance to each component drug.[795]

Combination therapies that are being increasingly introduced include: artemether–lumefantrine (Coartem) – the only combination yet available (2006) for which the different components are co-formulated in the same tablet; amodiaquine plus artesunate; and amodiaquine plus sulfadoxine–pyrimethamine. The first of these must be given twice daily for three days, the others once daily for three days. Chlorproguanil–dapsone–artesunate (CDA) is a further option for which large scale field evaluations remain to be completed.

Policies usually include a second line therapy if the first line fails or is contraindicated in an individual. If a child vomits more than one attempted dosing by mouth, parenteral or rectal therapy with quinine or an artemisinin drug may be given.

Treatment of nonfalciparum malaria

Chloroquine is the treatment of choice for acute nonfalciparum malaria. Some *P. vivax* infections are chloroquine resistant, but since *P. vivax* does not progress to life-threatening disease, a trial of chloroquine is justified.

P. vivax and *P. ovale* malaria (unless acquired congenitally or by blood transfusion) may relapse if treatment does not include a drug to eliminate hepatic hypnozoites. Primaquine (0.25 mg/kg daily for 2 weeks) will achieve this, but is not worth giving in areas where reinfection is inevitable, and it should not be given to children under the age of 5 years. Primaquine causes severe hemolysis in patients with glucose-6-phosphate dehydrogenase deficiency; the red cell concentration of this enzyme should therefore be measured before the drug is given; if low, an alternative method of radical cure is weekly chloroquine for 6 months in prophylactic doses. Primaquine need not be given after malaria due to *P. falciparum* or *P. malariae*. Primaquine has the additional action of killing gametocytes of all species of malaria parasites; it therefore has the potential to reduce transmission and has occasionally been used for this purpose in areas of moderate endemicity, a function now more safely achieved using artemisinin drugs.

MANAGEMENT OF SEVERE (COMPLICATED) FALCIPARUM MALARIA

Malaria due to *P. falciparum* differs from disease due to other plasmodial species in that *P. falciparum* infections may progress to severe and complicated disease. In the patient with falciparum malaria treatment must therefore be undertaken urgently; complications must be foreseen, recognized and treated; and the antimalarial drugs must be carefully chosen and correctly and promptly administered. Most of the deaths in children admitted to hospital with severe malaria occur before specific antiparasitic drugs can be expected to affect the disease: supportive care during the early phase of management is therefore critically important.

Supportive measures
Hypoglycemia
This complication should be suspected in any child with impaired consciousness, convulsions or acidosis, whether at the time of admission or during the course of treatment. Glucose should be administered as 10% or 20% solution by slow intravenous injection (0.5 g/kg). (If only 50% glucose is available, it should be diluted two- to three-fold with normal saline before being infused over a few minutes.) The blood glucose concentration must be measured again at hourly intervals until the patient's condition improves.

Convulsions
Hypoglycemia and hyperpyrexia should be corrected. Prolonged seizures should be treated with the optimal available drug regimen: drugs which may be used include lorazepam, diazepam, paraldehyde, phenytoin or phenobarbital, using drugs in sequence if convulsions prove refractory.

Acidosis
Deep or labored breathing due to acidosis is a common presentation of severe malaria in children. Possible contributory (and often additive) causes are dehydration, severe anemia, shock, repeated convulsions and hypoglycemia, all of which should be looked for and corrected in the acidotic child (see below under Severe anemia).

Hyperpyrexia
Hyperpyrexia (rectal temperature > 39 °C) should be corrected by administration of oral or rectal paracetamol (15 mg/kg 4–6-hourly). Although important to reduce the risk of seizures in infants and for

symptomatic relief in the conscious child, antipyretic measures have not been demonstrated to affect the prognosis in severe malaria.[796]

Severe anemia

Because of the increasing risk of transmission of HIV by blood in parts of the world where malaria is endemic, blood transfusion should only be given if life-threatening anemia is present or can be predicted on the basis of the hematocrit and level of parasitemia on admission. Blood transfusion is particularly important for the child with severe anemia and respiratory distress.[797] Most children with severe malarial anemia who are breathless have acidosis rather than heart failure, and may be in urgent need of fluid volume replacement.[792]

Exchange transfusion has been advocated and successfully used for patients with hyperparasitemia, but no controlled trials have been done to prove the superiority of this measure. In countries with limited resources for blood transfusion and with high prevalence rates of HIV infection, exchange transfusion is not justifiable as a method for treating severe malaria.

Fluid therapy

This must be sufficient to correct hypovolemia, acidosis and oliguria. When a child has both volume depletion and encephalopathy, there is a therapeutic dilemma: infusion of isotonic electrolyte solution may correct hypovolemia but increase the risk of cerebral edema.[798] In this situation an infusion of albumin, plasma or other plasma expander may be safer (in the anemic child, whole blood will serve all of the needed functions). Current studies are in progress to provide appropriate guidelines. The usual precautions are important to avoid overhydration and the risk of pulmonary edema. Acute tubular necrosis is uncommon as a complication of P. falciparum malaria in children, but if it occurs peritoneal or hemodialysis may be required.

Antibiotics

Some children with severe malaria are bacteremic, the proportion differing between studies and sites. In a series in Kenya the overall rate of bacteremia among 421 children with malarial coma or severe anemia was 8.6% and mortality was three-fold higher in these patients than others, prompting the authors to recommend routine antibiotic treatment for patients with severe malaria.[794] Other studies have indicated a more specific association between severe malarial anemia (SMA) and nontyphoidal salmonella bacteremia, especially in infants and toddlers, suggesting that antibiotics should be considered in the management of SMA in very sick children and in those not responding to antimalarial and hematinic

therapy. Policies for antibiotic use in various severe malaria syndromes may best be decided on the basis of local experience.

In a child with malarial coma, it may be impossible on physical examination to exclude a diagnosis of bacterial meningitis. Since asymptomatic parasitemia is common in endemic areas, parasitemia in the febrile unconscious child cannot be assumed to be the cause of the disease. Some clinicians prefer to perform a lumbar puncture in these circumstances, to clarify the diagnosis. If lumbar puncture is deferred because of the child's clinical condition, antibiotics should be given to cover the possibility of bacterial meningitis.

There is no place for heparin, dexamethasone or dextran in the treatment of CM.[799]

Antimalarial drugs for severe malaria

For severe or complicated P. falciparum malaria, the antiparasitic treatment of choice depends on the context. Recent multicenter studies in South East Asia[800] have shown that intravenous artesunate is superior to quinine in the treatment of adults with severe malaria, but there were insufficient children in these studies to detect a comparable difference among children. Africa differs from South East Asia in two important respects relating to the treatment of severe malaria: (1) in Africa most patients are children, while in South East Asia most patients are adults; and (2) in Africa quinine resistance is unknown among P. falciparum isolates, while partial quinine resistance is well described in South East Asia. Studies are therefore under way to compare parenteral quinine with intravenous artesunate in African children with severe malaria.

Meanwhile, for children in Africa, parenteral quinine remains the drug therapy of choice for severe malaria. If quinine is unavailable, quinidine is an equally effective alternative. Appropriate schedules for treatment are given in Table 28.40.

Quinine may cause severe hypotension if given by rapid intravenous injection, so a dilute solution (1–2 mg/ml) must therefore be infused slowly (over 3 or more hours). If the intravenous route is problematic or impossible, quinine may be given by intramuscular injection in the same doses, the solution (diluted to contain 60 mg/ml) being divided and administered in two sites simultaneously. Parenteral quinine is known to stimulate the secretion of insulin from the pancreatic beta cells, but hypoglycemia in children being treated for malaria is usually due to the disease rather than to drug therapy.[782] If intramuscular quinine is used in the treatment of a comatose child, supplementary glucose must be given or the blood glucose level checked frequently.

Oral drugs should replace parenteral as soon as a patient can take them. If given as the only drug treatment, quinine must be continued

Table 28.40 Drug treatment of acute malaria. In this table the first regimen listed in each section is the treatment of choice

Diagnosis	If patient can take oral drugs	If patient unable to take oral drugs
Malaria due to P. vivax, ovale, malariae, and uncomplicated CQ-sensitive falciparum malaria	Oral CQ: 10 mg/kg first dose then 5 mg/kg after 6, 24 and 48 h Or: AQ, same doses	CQ: 10 mg/kg over 8 h in saline or 5% dextrose; then 5 mg/kg by similar infusions × 3 (total 25 mg/kg in 32 h) Or: CQ i.m. or s.c. 2.5 mg/kg 4-hourly to 10 doses. Substitute oral CQ when possible
Uncomplicated falciparum malaria of doubtful CQ sensitivity	S/P single dose (S: 25 mg/kg, P: 1.25 mg/kg) Or: oral AQ as above Or: oral MQ 15 mg/kg first dose, then 10 mg/kg after 8 h	As for complicated falciparum malaria
Severe or complicated falciparum malaria	QN: i.v., first dose* 16.7 mg/kg over 4 h in 5% dextrose, then 8.3 mg/kg over 2–4 h each, 8-hourly, until oral drug can be taken (viz. quinine 8.3 mg/kg 8-hourly) to complete 7-day course Or: QN i.m. 8.3 mg/kg 8-hourly as solution containing 60 mg/ml. Give supplementary glucose. Substitute oral quinine as soon as possible, 8.3 mg/kg 8-hourly to complete 7-day course Or: quinidine i.v. 7.5 mg/kg 8-hourly, each dose over 4 h in 5% dextrose, until oral treatment can be taken; this may be QN 8.3 mg/kg 8-hourly or quinidine 7.5 mg/kg 8-hourly. Total course 7 days	

*The first dose of i.v. quinine should be reduced to 8.3 mg/kg if the patient has received any quinine or mefloquine in the two preceding days.
CQ, chloroquine; AQ, amodiaquine; QN, quinine; MQ, mefloquine; S/P, sulfonamide–pyrimethamine combination, e.g. Fansidar. All doses of CQ, QN and quinidine refer to base, not salt (8.3 mg quinine base = 10 mg quinine dihydrochloride).

for at least 7 days. Alternatively, once oral treatment is resumed, quinine may be replaced by a locally efficacious oral combination therapy (as used for uncomplicated *P. falciparum* malaria).

MALARIA CONTROL

Since the epidemiology of malaria varies greatly between and even within countries, control measures which are effective in one area may prove ineffective in another. It is important, therefore, that national control programs be designed having regard to local epidemiological, social and economic circumstances.

There are currently four principal methods of malaria control relevant to the well-being of children in areas of intense transmission:

1. *Prompt recognition and treatment of both mild and severe disease* at all levels of the health service, with referral to a larger health facility when necessary. This requires appropriate diagnostic policies (often including presumptive diagnosis of fever as malarial), effective, safe and affordable treatment schedules, competent health staff, and health facilities that are accessible to the majority of people. Because health services are inevitably distant from the homes of many rural people, complementary strategies are needed, and several are being assessed. These include administration of antimalarial drugs for treatment or prevention by village health workers,[801] the training of shopkeepers in appropriate prescribing and dosages (most first line treatment for malaria in village communities is obtained from local grocery stores),[802] schemes to involve traditional healers in treatment or referral of patients with malaria, and making rectal artesunate available at village level for the early treatment of the convulsing or unconscious child.[803]

2. *The use of insecticide-treated nets (ITNs) or curtains.* Several controlled trials and a meta-analysis have demonstrated that sleeping under ITNs can reduce all-cause child mortality in communities.[804] Inevitably there is concern that such results depend on the presence of a scientific team, providing materials and encouraging their use. A study in Tanzania showed a 27% increase in child survival among ITN users in the context of a bednet program promoted by social marketing, i.e. without the involvement of an investigative team.[805] Impregnated nets and curtains therefore have a potentially important place in malaria control, which may depend on local culture and malaria transmission patterns. The need for annual re-impregnation of nets poses a challenge to sustainability; new methods (the 'permanet') may make re-impregnation unnecessary.

3. *Intermittent presumptive treatment (IPT).* Pregnant women, especially primigravidae, are at increased risk of malaria, and placental malaria is associated with low birth weight and increased infant mortality. Provision of two, three or more therapeutic doses of an antimalarial drug such as pyrimethamine–sulfadoxine (Fansidar) between the fourth and eighth months of pregnancy, irrespective of symptoms or parasitemia – intermittent presumptive treatment in pregnancy, or IPTp – reduces placental malaria and improves birth weights.[806] IPTp is now an instrument for control of malaria-induced morbidity in many endemic countries. *Intermittent presumptive therapy for infants (IPTi)* proved promising in an East African study, in which infants given a therapeutic dose of sulfadoxine–pyrimethamine at 2, 3 and 9 months of age, irrespective of fever or parasitemia, had fewer episodes of malaria and of severe anemia during the first year of life than controls.[807] Some (not all) subsequent studies have shown similar benefits, and multicenter trials of IPTi are in progress. Similar studies in older age groups of children (IPTc) are being considered.

4. *Indoor residual spraying (IRS)* – the spraying of the inside walls of dwellings with residual insecticide – was a mainstay of the malaria eradication campaigns in 1950–70, parts of which were spectacularly successful. But IRS encountered both political and vector resistance, was poorly sustained, and was never adequately achieved in Africa. IRS is now receiving renewed attention as novel methods and capacities are acquired, and it is being increasingly explored as a promising component of malaria control programs.

There is growing optimism that vaccination will, within the next few years, become a further weapon in the armamentarium available to fight malaria.

The success of any method or combination of methods of control is likely to be materially influenced by the degree to which the causes and consequences of malaria are appreciated by populations and by the willingness of communities to participate in, and even finance, specific operations.[799]

Meanwhile the international community is becoming more aware of the fact that tools for malaria control exist, and that their deployment needs expenditure on materials, infrastructure, health systems and staff development. Commitments of funding from major donors have increased in recent years and will need to be sustained if real progress is to be made.

TOXOPLASMOSIS

Toxoplasmosis is mainly of importance to pediatrics as a congenital infection (see p. 1202). Infection acquired after birth can cause choroidoretinitis or infectious mononucleosis and can cause significant disease in persons with underlying T cell immunodeficiencies. Occasionally, signs of congenital infection may not manifest until late in childhood or early adulthood.

The birth prevalence of congenital toxoplasmosis infection across Europe ranges from 1 to 10 per 10 000 newborns.[808] In the UK, only 10% of women show evidence of past infection with toxoplasmosis, whereas in France up to 55% of pregnant women show antibodies to toxoplasmosis on antenatal screening.

ETIOLOGY

The causative organism, *Toxoplasma gondii*, is, in its free active state, a small, crescentic protozoan, which is a strict intracellular parasite multiplying only within the cytoplasm of the nucleated host by binary fission or, probably more frequently, by internal budding (endodyogeny). The active form, responsible for acute infection, stimulates an immunological response by the host. At the same time, cyst forms of the parasite develop in any tissue, but chiefly in nervous tissue or striated muscle, and may persist for the life of the host.

PATHOGENESIS

T. gondii infects virtually all species of mammals and several species of birds. The cat family is the definitive host. Cats usually acquire the infection after eating infected rodents, birds or uncooked meat. After primary infection, they shed millions of oocysts in their feces for up to 14 days. Oocysts may remain viable in soil for many months, and are not found on the cat fur, thus explaining the failure to link cat exposure with the risk of human toxoplasmosis infection.[809]

Humans are most commonly infected after ingestion of tissue cysts in raw or poorly cooked meat, or by ingestion of soil, food or water contaminated with oocysts. Infection from meat has been shown to be responsible for up to two thirds of all new infections in pregnant women.[810] Traditionally pork, lamb, goat or game meats hold the highest risk for human infection, although undercooked beef has been shown to be a risk factor for toxoplasmosis seroconversion,[810] possibly due to combination with cheaper meats.[809] Congenital toxoplasmosis infection usually occurs as a result of placental infection after a primary infection in a pregnant woman. The risk of transmission and the clinical outcome after maternal toxoplasmosis infection vary with the trimester of pregnancy, with the first trimester having the lowest risk of transmission to the fetus but the highest risk of damage.

Transmission has also been rarely documented in children after blood or blood product transfusion, heart or bone marrow transplantation[811,812] and through infected breast milk.[813]

CLINICAL FEATURES

Acquired infection with *T. gondii* is uncommon in the UK in children under 5 years. Serological surveys suggest a peak acquisition of infection in early and mid teens. The disease is nearly always asymptomatic. The commonest manifestation, if clinical signs do occur, is lymphadenopathy, particularly of cervical nodes, which may be accompanied by no ill health, or may be accompanied by fever and prostration and resemble severe infectious mononucleosis. Muscle pain may also occur due, it is believed and occasionally confirmed, to infection of voluntary muscle. Acquired toxoplasmosis may also result in hepatosplenomegaly, lymphocytosis, and, rarely, pneumonitis, acute hepatitis, arthritis or cardiac arrhythmias (due to lesions in the region of the conducting system). The occurrence of cardiac failure due to toxoplasma infection of the myocardium is conjectural. Isolated visual disturbance due to toxoplasmosis retinitis in childhood used to be thought to be due to reactivation of an undiagnosed congenital infection, but is equally commonly due to acquired infection.[814]

Acquired toxoplasmosis infection has been documented in immunodeficient children with HIV infection, or post bone marrow or solid organ transplantation, but it occurs much less commonly than in adults. Toxoplasmosis in the immunocompromised child may manifest as encephalitis, pneumonitis or even a multiorgan systemic disease.

DIAGNOSIS AND DIFFERENTIAL DIAGNOSIS

Acquired toxoplasmosis should be considered in any case of unexplained lymphadenopathy, particularly when maximal in, or confined to, the cervical region, whether or not it is accompanied by pyrexia. Lymph node enlargement in acquired toxoplasmosis may persist for several months, leading to the consideration of lymphoma and tuberculous lymphadenopathy in the differential diagnosis.

In the immunocompromised child, it enters the differential diagnosis for neurological disease (encephalitis, meningoencephalitis, brain abscess), for interstitial pneumonitis, and for myocarditis.

Laboratory diagnosis

The most common laboratory aids to the diagnosis include serology, isolation of the organism, histology and the direct detection of *T. gondii* DNA in infected tissues or fluids by polymerase chain reaction (PCR). Other diagnostic methods used less commonly today include skin testing and the Sabin–Feldman dye test, which depends upon the inhibition by antibody-containing serum of methylene blue staining of laboratory cultures of *T. gondii*. The diagnosis of a congenital infection postnatally is discussed in Chapter 12.

Serological methods remain the most commonly used method for diagnosis. Acute infection in the older child or adult may be diagnosed by a four-fold rise in toxoplasma-specific IgG by indirect immunofluorescence, or enzyme immunoassay. Toxoplasma-specific IgM can be detected by 2 weeks post infection, and usually declines by 6 months, but at times may persist for months (and occasionally over a year) after the initial infection. Thus the detection of toxoplasma IgM may indicate either an acute or a recent past infection. Positive results should be confirmed by multiple tests in different laboratories, given a false positive rate of up to 2%. If timing of the infection is critical, as in the case of a pregnant woman, the presence of IgA and IgE antibodies to toxoplasmosis which decline more readily than IgM, and IgG avidity (high avidity suggests an infection >12 months prior) may be helpful in differentiating an acute infection from a past infection. However, some suggest that even current serological assays cannot predict the time of infection within the first year after infection (reviewed in Petersen et al[815]).

The detection of *T. gondii* DNA by PCR in amniotic fluid is now commonly used for the prenatal diagnosis of congenital toxoplasmosis.

Sensitivity rates of up to 90% have been reported, but there is a wide range in the quality of assays available, with false positive rates ranging from 0 to 10% reported in some laboratories (reviewed in Petersen et al[815]). Other applications of the assay are on cerebrospinal fluid, or peripheral white blood cells in the immunocompromised or congenitally infected infant.

Culture of *T. gondii* from lymph node biopsy material, amniotic fluid, placenta or, less often, other tissue fluids is possible, although generally less widely used than serological methods. The organism can be cultured in suitable laboratory animals, particularly mice, embryonated eggs and tissue cultures. The most reliable of these procedures is that of intraperitoneal inoculation of mice. Histological examination of biopsy material is also of value, limited chiefly by the availability of suitable material. Cysts can be identified readily, but vegetative forms are recognized with difficulty.

In the immunocompromised child, such as those with HIV infection, the ability to document seroconversion to toxoplasmosis is impaired. A diagnosis must be made by demonstrating the organism by PCR, culture or histology in infected tissues, or presumptively by characteristic findings on imaging that respond to an empirical trial of antiparasitic therapy.

Dermal hypersensitivity to injection of a suspension of killed toxoplasma is indicated by a delayed tuberculin type response. There is good correlation between a positive skin test and a positive dye test titer of 1:8 or more. The test may be negative in very recent infections and is used chiefly in epidemiological surveys in man.

TREATMENT AND PROGNOSIS

Treatment of acquired toxoplasmosis infection in childhood is usually only indicated for active ocular infection or severe disease in other organs.

Treatment of congenitally infected infants is discussed in Chapter 12. Antibiotics, other than spiramycin, have proved to be of little value in the treatment of acute toxoplasmosis. Sulfonamides have proved disappointing and sulfones too toxic in the doses required. The most effective form of chemotherapy is a combination of pyrimethamine and sulfadiazine for a total duration of 3–4 weeks. The hematological toxic effects of pyrimethamine, due to its antifolic acid action, can be prevented or reversed by folinic acid. Spiramycin, though less toxic than the pyrimethamine and sulfadiazine combination, is clearly less effective. An alternative is the use of a combination of trimethoprim and a sulfonamide, e.g. co-trimoxazole. Life-long suppressive therapy with these agents is indicated for HIV infected children after toxoplasmosis encephalitis.

In the pregnant woman, spiramycin may be given in early pregnancy for suspected primary toxoplasmosis to prevent transmission to the fetus, and after 17 weeks' gestation, pyrimethamine and sulfadiazine may be used for confirmed fetal infection to reduce the risk of transmission or complications in the child. However, a recent systematic review of randomized trials of antiparasitic treatment of toxoplasmosis in pregnancy concluded that there was still insufficient evidence available to determine whether such treatment has a positive effect on clinical outcomes or risk of transmission.[816]

Chemoprophylaxis to prevent reactivation of toxoplasmosis should be considered in the significantly immunosuppressed child with HIV infection or prior to heart transplantation.

TRYPANOSOMIASIS

AFRICAN TRYPANOSOMIASIS: SLEEPING SICKNESS

Human African trypanosomiasis (HAT) is caused by two 'subspecies' of *Trypanosoma brucei* which are transmitted by the bite of the tsetse fly. Sleeping sickness is widely distributed in 36 countries in sub-Saharan Africa. Approximately 18 000 cases are reported annually to the WHO, with an estimated total burden of 50–70 000.

T. b. gambiense occurs in west and central Africa and causes a disease which is slow in onset and progression (Gambian sleeping sickness). Infected humans provide long term sources of infection for the tsetse and the *T. b. gambiense* disease is largely an anthroponosis. Infection with *T. b. rhodesiense* occurs in east and south east Africa and causes an acute illness that is often lethal within a few months (Rhodesian sleeping sickness). It is a true zoonosis: infection is maintained within wild ungulate reservoirs. Both forms most commonly infect adults but any age may be affected; infection is 2–3 times more common in adults than children in *T. b. gambiense* endemic areas.[817]

Life cycle
In the tsetse fly, stumpy trypomastigotes ingested with the blood meal transform into slender midgut forms. These eventually reach the salivary gland and transform via epimastigotes to the infective metacyclic trypomastigote. After inoculation, the metacyclic trypomastigotes are converted into long slender forms in the subcutaneous tissue of the host. Blood forms are polymorphic with both slender and stumpy forms. The continual movement of the trypomastigote is activated by a flagellum and a fold of membrane which is lifted up by the motion of the flagellum – the 'undulating membrane'. Three 'subspecies' of *T. brucei* group exist; *T. b. brucei*, which is not infective to humans, cannot be distinguished morphologically from *T. b. rhodesiense* and *T. b. gambiense*. However, biochemical techniques, DNA analysis and isoenzyme characterization can distinguish different *T. brucei* populations. *T. b. rhodesiense* comprises two distinct zymodemes; the 'Zambezi' group in southern Africa and the 'Busoga' group in east Africa associated with more acute severe disease. *T. b. gambiense* is less variable.

Epidemiology
The reported number of infections has declined considerably over the last 6–7 years, because of improved surveillance and control measures in some regions. However, recent epidemics have occurred in areas such as DRC, Angola and Sudan, partly because of breakdown of control measures and population movement due to civil unrest. *T. b. gambiense* accounts for the vast majority of cases of trypanosomiasis.

T. b. gambiense is restricted to west and central Africa and is transmitted by 'palpalis group' tsetse (*Glossina palpalis, G. tachinoides* and *G. fuscipes*), which inhabit dense vegetation along rivers and in forests. Vectors feed on man at water collecting points and river crossings. The man–fly–man cycle of transmission may maintain the disease in the absence of an animal reservoir; infected individuals may be asymptomatically parasitemic for years. Although human parasites infect both wild and domestic animals, their epidemiological significance remains uncertain.

T. b. rhodesiense is usually transmitted by 'morsitans group' tsetse (*G. morsitans, G. pallidipes* and *G. swynnertoni*) in East African woodland savannah and lake shores. Most infection is sporadic such as in Tanzania when game hunters or honey gatherers are bitten by *G. morsitans* which transmit disease from the bushbuck host, or in south east Uganda and western Kenya where fishermen are bitten by *G. pallidipes* on lake shores. However, epidemics have occurred in western Kenya and in south eastern Uganda with infections occurring in both sexes and all age groups. The vector is *G. f. fuscipes*, a 'palpalis group' tsetse which invades *Lantana camora* thickets close to human habitation; domestic cows may play an important part in maintaining infection in such situations. Imported trypanosomiasis is also relatively rare, but an increased number of cases have been reported over the last 5 years in Europe and the USA as a result of exposure in game parks. Congenital infection with *T. b. rhodesiense* and *T. b. gambiense* does occur, but appears to be very rare.

Pathogenesis and pathology
Pathological processes are similar but vary in intensity between *T. b. gambiense* and *T. b. rhodesiense*. Parasites inoculated into the subcutaneous tissue multiply locally, forming a trypanosomal chancre, with edema and an infiltrate of polymorphonuclear leukocytes, lymphocytes and plasma cells. Parasites travel to regional lymph nodes where they continue to multiply and cause parasitemia 5–12 days after infection. Waves of parasitemia occur, each differing in its surface antigens (particularly variant surface glycoprotein) as the parasite attempts to avoid the host immune response.

Hyperplasia of the reticuloendothelial system, with lymph node and spleen enlargement, occurs as a response to infection; lymph nodes may subsequently become atrophic and fibrotic. Morular cells (Mott cells) are found; these are plasmacytes that may have an important role in the production of IgM. Blood parasites invade the central nervous system via the choroid plexus leading to the second stage of infection, a meningoencephalitis. A lymphocytic meningoencephalitis and focal vasculitis with perivascular infiltrates occurs particularly in the frontal lobes, pons and medulla. Parasites in the CNS are accompanied by changes in the cerebrospinal fluid with a raised protein concentration and the presence of mononuclear cells, particularly lymphocytes. Parasites can also be identified in the CSF.

The succession of variable antigens induces a profuse production of IgM antibody in the serum and it is also locally produced in the central nervous system by plasma cells and the morular cells. Immune complex damage (type III hypersensitivity) may cause less common lesions of the kidney, lungs, liver and heart. Expression of cell-mediated immunity, induction of cell-mediated immunity and expression of humoral immunity have been shown to be impaired in *T. b. gambiense* infections in man.

Clinical features
The trypanosomal chancre
The primary lesion (trypanosomal chancre) is a painful, erythematous and edematous swelling at the site of the bite that appears within 2 or 3 days. Skin vesicles and ulceration may develop and the chancre heals with residual scarring over 2–3 weeks. Chancres commonly occur in *T. b. rhodesiense* infection but are less common in *T. b. gambiense*. As the chancre develops, the regional lymph glands become enlarged and tender.

The hemolymphatic (first) stage
Waves of irregular remittent fever, in association with the waves of parasitemia, occur 5–12 days after the bite. This is most marked in *T. b. rhodesiense* infections; in *T. b. gambiense* the hemolymphatic stage may be mild, subclinical or asymptomatic. Febrile episodes, sometimes with rigors, are accompanied by malaise, headache, muscular tenderness, joint aches and weight loss. An annular erythematous rash (circinate erythema) may be visible, particularly on the trunk in the fair skinned. Generalized lymphadenopathy may develop, especially in *T. b. gambiense*. Winterbottom's sign, posterior cervical triangle lymphadenopathy, occurs in *T. b. gambiense* due to the predilection for *G. palpalis* to bite on the head. Edema may affect the ankles or feet or face, producing a dull expressionless facies. Irritability, insomnia and confusion may occur even in the early stage. The spleen and liver may enlarge. In the acute stage of *T. b. rhodesiense* infection, tachycardia is common; pleural or pericardial effusions may occur and myocarditis with arrhythmias or cardiac failure may lead to death.

Meningoencephalitic (second) stage
Meningoencephalitis is an inevitable consequence of untreated human African trypanosomiasis. In *T. b. gambiense*, it tends to occur after months or years while in *T. b. rhodesiense* it occurs early, often during the febrile illness, and progresses rapidly to a fatal outcome. Children develop meningoencephalitis more rapidly than adults. A wide variety of neurological signs occur. Behavioral changes and sleep disturbances are often the first signs; inappropriate diurnal somnolence with insomnia and agitation at night are common. Patients become apathetic, lacking in attention and may exhibit trance-like states. Behavior becomes inappropriate, aggressive or overtly paranoid. Nutritional deficiencies, intercurrent infections and progressive emaciation result. Generalized weakness, unsteadiness of gait, expressionless facies, slurred speech, tremors of the limbs, hyper-reflexia and delayed deep hyperalgesia all occur. In advanced disease, focal epileptic attacks, profound ataxia, choreoathetosis and psychotic changes may be followed by coma and death. There is little variation in symptoms or signs between adults and

children, apart from the incidence of malnutrition, which may be as high as 50–60% in children with second stage disease.[818]

Diagnosis[819]

Clinical diagnosis of African trypanosomiasis may be difficult. Although the presence of a chancre is pathognomonic, the hemolymphatic stage must be differentiated from a wide range of febrile illnesses including malaria. Differential diagnosis of second stage disease includes other causes of meningoencephalitis, particularly cryptococcal and tuberculous meningitis in the HIV infected, and psychiatric illness. Routine laboratory tests show a normal total white cell count, raised ESR, anemia, thrombocytopenia, low serum albumin and elevated serum IgM. Bilirubin and transaminases may be raised. Hematological abnormalities, including coagulopathy, are particularly prominent in acute *T. b. rhodesiense*. A parasitic diagnosis must be attempted in all suspected cases.

Parasitological diagnosis

In the early stages of *T. b. rhodesiense* infection, parasitological diagnosis is usually simple, as the concentration of trypanosomes in the blood or aspirates of trypanosomal chancres is high. Organisms can be seen by single or repeated microscopic examination of wet films or thick blood or aspirate fluid films stained with Field's stain or Giemsa. Blood film microscopy is less reliable in *T. b. gambiense*; repeated examination of blood films and concentration techniques are more often required. However, organisms are readily seen in fresh lymph node aspirates. Trypanosomes may also be identified in CSF, various effusions and marrow smears.

Concentration methods increase the sensitivity of microscopy; microhematocrit centrifugation and microscopic examination of the area above the buffy coat are commonly used. The quantitative buffy coat technique (QBC), where motile trypanosomes are stained with fluorescent acridine orange, tubes centrifuged and examined by fluorescent microscopy, is rapid and sensitive.[820] The miniature anion exchange centrifugation technique (MAEC[821]) involves passing a sample of blood through a DEAE-cellulose anion exchange column, which allows trypanosomes to pass into a collecting tube which is centrifuged and examined. This technique is sensitive but difficult in field conditions.

Once trypanosomiasis is diagnosed or suspected, the CSF must be examined, preferably within 15 min of lumbar puncture. Increase in cell count (more than 5 cells/mm³), protein elevation, CSF IgM or trypomastigotes in the centrifuged deposit indicate CNS involvement.

Immunodiagnosis

Immunodiagnostic tests include IFAT, ELISA, CFT and IgM estimation. IFAT is valuable in epidemiological investigation and screening of populations and suspects but provides only presumptive evidence of infection. A card agglutination test for trypanosomiasis (CATT) has been developed for the diagnosis of *T. b. gambiense*. The test provides a rapid field test for preliminary screening of populations in endemic areas. Positive serological tests require confirmatory parasitic diagnosis prior to treatment.[822] Antigen detection techniques (CIATT) have also been developed and appear to be sensitive and specific; they have potential for following the response to therapy.[823]

Treatment[824]

Treatment should be started as soon as possible after making a parasitological diagnosis although nutritional disturbances or intercurrent infection should first be treated in view of the toxicity of treatment. Routine use of antihelminth and antimalarial drugs is common. Examination of the CSF is mandatory to distinguish early stage from late stage disease as CNS involvement requires different, more toxic therapy. Lumbar puncture should not be performed until at least one dose of suramin (or pentamidine) has been given to clear parasites from the blood and prevent inoculation into the CSF at the time of LP.

Treatment of hemolymphatic trypanosomiasis

Suramin is effective in treatment of the hemolymphatic stage of both *T. b. rhodesiense* and *T. b. gambiense* disease and will rapidly clear the parasitemia in both early and late sleeping sickness. Pentamidine is the first line therapy for *T. b. gambiense* but is not effective in *T. b. rhodesiense*. Neither suramin nor pentamidine is effective in meningoencephalitis.

Suramin. Suramin is given intravenously with a test dose of 5 mg/kg on day 1 followed by 20 mg/kg on days 3, 7, 14 and 21. Fever, nausea, vomiting and urticaria are common side-effects: renal toxicity may occur.

Pentamidine. Pentamidine is usually given intramuscularly at doses of 4 mg/kg base daily or on alternate days for 7 days. Intravenous administration avoids local side-effects that include sterile abscesses, but requires close supervision. Side-effects include syncope and hypotension, vomiting and abdominal pain, especially in the first half hour after administration. Peripheral neuritis is a rare complication and severe hypoglycemic reactions may occur during the course of treatment. Adrenaline and glucose should be available when treatment with pentamidine is given.

Meningoencephalitic (late stage) trypanosomiasis

Melarsoprol. Melarsoprol (Mel B) is an arsenical compound which enters the CNS. Use is limited to late stage trypanosomiasis because of its toxicity. A variety of different treatment schedules have been used. In *T. b. rhodesiense* infection, melarsoprol is usually given in three or four courses, each course lasting three days and separated by a week, giving a total dose of 35–37.5 ml melarsoprol. Regimens which use lower doses initially and increase through four courses of treatment may be less toxic.

Many regimens have been advocated for treatment of *T. b. gambiense*. Recently, shortened 10-day regimens (2.2 mg/kg daily) have been used for *T. b. gambiense* with no loss of efficacy, and no increased relapse.[825,826]

Thrombophlebitis is a frequent complication of melarsoprol treatment; extravasation causes severe local reactions. The major side-effect is a *reactive arsenical encephalopathy* (RAE), which occurs in up to 5% of patients, usually after the third or fourth dose. The onset is usually sudden with neurological deterioration, confusion, convulsions and coma. It occurs more commonly in severe meningoencephalitis and is fatal in 10–50% of cases. In *T. b. gambiense* (but not *T. b. rhodesiense*) prophylactic prednisolone significantly reduces the incidence of RAE.[827] Other toxicity common with melarsoprol includes agranulocytosis, aplastic anemia, thrombocytopenia and peripheral neuropathy. Melarsoprol should not be given as initial therapy to parasitemic patients; it may cause a Jarisch–Herxheimer-like febrile reaction after the first injection. Treatment normally leads to a striking improvement in the mental and physical condition of patients with sleeping sickness, but there is increasing concern about rising relapse rates.

Eflornithine (difluoromethyl-ornithine, DFMO). This drug has been used for the treatment of both early and late stage *T. b. gambiense* with good results but is poorly effective in *T. b. rhodesiense*. The drug is given intravenously in a dose of 100 mg/kg 6-hourly for 14 days (4 g/m² for young children); oral preparations are being evaluated. Major side-effects are diarrhea and reversible marrow depression. Response rates vary from 73 to 97% with some geographical variability; shorter courses are less effective. Recent studies suggest that eflornithine may be more effective and safer than melarsoprol in some settings,[828,829] although efficacy may be reduced in those who are HIV positive.

Nifurtimox. (an oral agent) has occasionally been used in the treatment of *T. b. gambiense*. As a single agent it has high relapse rates, but when used in combination with a low dose 10-day course of melarsoprol, the combination regimen was superior to a standard melarsoprol regimen.[830]

Follow-up and relapse

Patients should be seen 3 months after treatment and followed up for 2 years to identify relapse which occurs in 5–20% of those treated, usually presenting as a chronic meningoencephalitis without a peripheral parasitemia. Follow-up should include routine lumbar puncture to identify a rising cell count or protein. Relapse in *T. b. gambiense* following treatment with suramin or pentamidine should be with melarsoprol; eflornithine can also be used in the treatment of relapse after melarsoprol therapy. Relapse in *T. b. rhodesiense* is usually treated with a second course of melarsoprol; nifurtimox may be effective, but more data are needed.

Control of sleeping sickness

There are two major components of control activities: detecting and treating human cases and vector control. Sleeping sickness caused by *T. b. rhodesiense* is usually detected at fixed medical units in rural areas when patients present with the symptoms of early parasitemia (passive surveillance). In *T. b. gambiense*, limited clinical symptoms in the early stage mean that active surveillance for infected individuals is necessary. Active surveillance may also be useful in *T. b. rhodesiense* epidemics. Blood film examination is used to screen for *T. b. rhodesiense*, but in *T. b. gambiense* CATT tests or gland aspiration are frequently used for initial population screening. Diagnoses should be confirmed parasitologically; serologically positive but parasite negative individuals should be followed at regular intervals. Community education may play a large part in encouraging early diagnosis and reducing the number of parasitemic individuals. There is no role for mass community prophylaxis: it may mask second stage infections and lead to resistance.[824]

Vector control measures used include destruction of tsetse habitats and insecticide spraying. Insecticide-impregnated (and/or odor-baited) traps have been very effective in reducing fly populations without the environmental problems associated with widespread application of insecticides.

AMERICAN TRYPANOSOMIASIS: CHAGAS' DISEASE

Chagas' disease is endemic throughout most countries of South and Central America. It is caused by *Trypanosoma cruzi*, which is transmitted to humans by triatomine bugs. Acute *T. cruzi* infection is usually benign; the major public health and socioeconomic significance of the disease arises from the chronic stages of the disease. Improved control has led to a reduction in disease: approximately 10 million are infected with an estimated 14 000 deaths annually.

Life cycle of *Trypanosoma cruzi*

The organism occurs in three distinct forms: amastigotes found in tissues of mammalian hosts, epimastigotes found in the digestive tract of the triatomine bug, and trypomastigotes found in mammalian blood. After ingestion by the vector, trypomastigotes change and multiply as epimastigotes and in the succeeding 2–4 weeks develop into metacyclic trypomastigotes in the gut of the bug. Infective forms, excreted with the feces, enter through an abrasion in the skin or through intact mucous membranes such as the conjunctiva. Within 1–2 weeks trypomastigotes circulate in the bloodstream. After an undetermined period, the trypomastigote invades tissue cells and is transformed into the amastigote.

Epidemiology

T. cruzi infect over 100 mammalian species; the commonest wild hosts are rodents and small marsupials. Many triatomine bugs are sylvatic and maintain infection among reservoir hosts. Three species have adapted to human dwellings: *Rhodnius prolixus*, *Triatoma infestans* and *Panstrongylus megistus*. Human infection usually occurs from transmission between man and domestic animals. There may be hundreds or thousands of bugs in a household due to factors such as poor housing, thatched roofs and lack of wall resurfacing. Up to 40–50% of bugs may be infected in some locations. Most transmission occurs rurally but peri-urban transmission is increasing as a result of the rapid urbanization occurring throughout much of South America.

Chagas' disease may also be acquired by blood transfusion, although widespread serological screening has decreased transmission considerably. Congenital disease is an important public health problem in rural areas of endemic transmission, occurring in up to 10% of seropositive women.

Pathogenesis

Parasites multiply at the site of entry which may lead to a chagoma, consisting of interstitial edema and focal inflammation. Parasites reach the blood but soon disseminate to enter cells, particularly histiocytes, neuroglia, smooth muscle, cardiac muscle and skeletal muscle cells. Amastigotes develop within cells to form pseudocysts. Pseudocyst rupture may lead to the development of acute inflammatory foci with tissue damage, such as the destruction of conducting tissue in the heart. A small proportion of individuals have acute complications, but in the vast majority the inflammatory reaction subsides and parasitemia and multiplication of parasites in the tissues is reduced by the immune response. Mechanisms of the chronic complications of Chagas' disease remain uncertain; tissue damage, neuronal loss and an autoimmune response are all likely to be important.[831]

Clinical features

Acute Chagas' disease

Acute Chagas' disease is usually an illness of children but can occur at any age. The acute phase of Chagas' disease is asymptomatic in over two thirds of affected infants and children. If symptomatic, the acute phase lasts for 1–3 months and resolves spontaneously. A chagoma may occur at the portal of entry. The skin over the chagoma becomes hard and may desquamate. Romaña's sign, unilateral eyelid edema and chemosis, is one of the classical syndromes associated with acute Chagas' disease, occurring when bug feces contaminate the conjunctiva.

One to two weeks later, a febrile reaction develops, often associated with headache and myalgia. Vomiting, diarrhea, lymphadenopathy, moderate hepatosplenomegaly and meningoencephalitis may all occur. Myocardial involvement, causing varying dysrhythmias to myocarditis and cardiac failure, may occur; these complications may occasionally be fatal. Meningoencephalitis in the very young has a bad prognosis. Leukocytosis and lymphocytosis accompany the parasitemia.

Following the acute phase, if untreated, low level infection may persist asymptomatically for many years (sometimes termed indeterminate phase). Between 15 and 40% of these patients will develop chronic Chagas' disease.

Chronic Chagas' disease

Chronic symptomatic disease is rarely a pediatric problem, usually occurring between the ages of 15 and 50 years. It is characterized by the reappearance of clinical disease 10–20 years after infection. In adults, classical manifestations are the development of a biventricular congestive cardiomyopathy or cardiac rhythm disturbances. Complete right bundle branch block with left bundle hemi-block is the most common abnormality; AV block, extrasystoles and Stokes–Adams attacks also frequently occur. Inflammatory changes and destruction of parasympathetic ganglion cells in muscle may also eventually lead to mega-esophagus and megacolon.

Congenital Chagas' disease

Congenital infection with *T. cruzi* occurs in between 2 and 10% of maternal infections. Infection is associated with abortion, stillbirth and severe illness or death in early infancy in a high proportion. Clinical features include cardiac problems, mega-esophagus, pneumonitis and meningoencephalitis. Transmission is also thought to occur through breast milk.

Chagas' disease in the immunocompromised

Chagas' disease in immunocompromised individuals is an increasing problem in South America due to HIV infection and the use of immunosuppressive drugs in transplant patients. Reactivation of latent *T. cruzi* infection or transplantation of an infected organ can cause the recurrence of parasitemia and the development of an intense myocarditis or severe neurological problems if careful monitoring and pre-emptive therapy is not used.[832]

Diagnosis

Parasitic diagnosis

A specific diagnosis, demonstrating *Trypanosoma cruzi* in the peripheral blood, is usually easy in the early acute illness. The parasite appears as a C- or S-shaped trypomastigote with a prominent kinetoplast in Romanowsky-stained thick or thin films. Centrifugation steps on separated red cells or lysed blood increase the sensitivity of microscopic examination. Culture requires specialized media and is difficult to perform outside a laboratory. Xenodiagnosis is a method for detecting sub-patent parasitemia in chronic infections (and occasionally in acute infection) by allowing triatomine bugs to feed on the individual patient: it is preferable to animal inoculation which is unreliable. Bugs are then dissected to look for gut infection after 20–40 days. PCR methods have published sensitivities of 60–100% when compared with serology; the technique may be more sensitive in children than in adults. It may also be particularly useful in the early detection of congenital infection.[833]

Serological diagnosis

An initial IgM response and life-long IgG response may be detected by a number of serological tests, including complement-fixation tests, indirect fluorescent antibody tests and enzyme-linked immunosorbent assays. Approximately 50% of individuals with positive serology will also be positive using xenodiagnosis, but there is a poor specificity with false positive tests from other parasitic infections, particularly leishmaniasis, and autoimmune disorders.

Following the response to therapy is difficult; xenodiagnosis may be negative in those with low parasite burdens and serological tests often remain positive after parasitological cure. PCR may be particularly useful in this situation.[834]

Treatment

Chemotherapy in Chagas' disease is problematic. Two drugs have been widely used: nifurtimox (8 mg/kg body weight daily for 60–90 days) and benznidazole (6–10 mg/kg body weight daily for 30 or 60 days). The latter is now more commonly used as it is better tolerated. Benznidazole side-effects are more common in adults than in children and occur in 4–30% of cases; hypersensitivity reactions cause rashes and fever, vomiting and peripheral neuropathy. Treatment in acute disease suppresses parasitemia, shortens the course of the acute illness and helps to prevent complications and deaths from acute myocarditis or meningoencephalitis. However, elimination of parasites and prevention of chronic illness only occurs in 50–70% of patients.

The value of treatment in the indeterminate and chronic phase is less certain; results of clinical trials vary both geographically and according to the stage of the infection. Standard recommendations have been that chemotherapy is of no benefit. However, increasing evidence and a Cochrane review suggests that treatment of patients with benznidazole in the indeterminate phase (chronic asymptomatic) leads to parasite clearance in around 60% of patients (measured by negative serology or xenodiagnosis) and reduces the proportion developing ECG changes or progressing to heart disease.[835,836]

Both allopurinol and itraconazole have been used for treatment of chronic disease with parasitological cure in 40–50% and normalization of ECG abnormalities in 36–48% of individuals; itraconazole appears to be superior in preventing the development of new ECG changes.[835,837,838] Further work is needed to evaluate the true value of chemotherapy in chronic disease. Heart failure is usually treated with vasodilators such as ACE inhibitors; digitalis may aggravate arrhythmias. Pacemakers are commonly implanted for heart block. A number of surgical procedures are used for mega-esophagus and megacolon. Treatment of symptomatic congenital infection is often unsatisfactory. Recent evidence suggests that routine screening of babies of seropositive mothers with treatment of positive infants is a safe and effective approach.[833,839]

Control

No vaccine exists for Chagas' disease. Major preventative efforts center upon control of transmission. Chagas' disease is predominantly a disease of poverty, which leads to poor quality housing and the inability to control domestic triatomine bugs. In recent years, control programs have been effective in countries in the southern cone of South America (Argentina, Brazil, Bolivia, Chile, Paraguay and Uruguay) with a reduction in incidence of between 60 and 99% from 1983–1997.[840]

Seroprevalence surveys are used to indicate areas and dwellings at risk, and pyrethroid insecticides are used for the spraying of housing and peri-domestic buildings; the use of fumigant canisters may also be useful. Community surveillance is then used to detect residual or new infections and further spraying performed. Housing improvements and health education help to promote sustainability. Programs to control blood transfusion transmission are based on routine serological testing and usually combine serological tests for HIV and hepatitis B as well as *T. cruzi*. If seropositive blood has to be used, the addition of gentian violet 24 h before is effective and safe in preventing transmission.

FUNGAL INFECTIONS

Fungi form a large and very diverse kingdom but only a small number are pathogenic for humans. Fungi are eukaryotes, that is, unlike bacteria, they have a nucleus and intracellular organelles. They also possess a cell wall composed of chitin. Infections are conveniently divided into superficial, subcutaneous and systemic or deep mycoses. In addition, an increasing number of opportunist fungi cause infection in immunocompromised children (Table 28.41).

Fungi can grow in a unicellular mode (yeasts) or a multicellular mode, when cells elongate and multiply to form long filaments called hyphae and collectively form a mycelium. Some fungi are dimorphic, existing as a yeast at one temperature but forming multicellular hyphae at another. Rather confusingly, some are given different names when in the different forms. Thus *Cryptococcus neoformans* is the name as a yeast and *Filobasidiella neoformans* is its hyphal form. *Actinomyces* and *Nocardia* spp. are not fungi but branching bacteria, but are more conveniently included in discussions of fungal disease (Table 28.42). Treatment of subcutaneous and systemic mycoses is most often by antifungals such as polyenes (e.g. amphotericin B) or imidazoles (e.g. ketoconazole) (Table 28.42). To prevent repetition, information on dosage, mode of administration and side-effects and toxicity is included at the end of the chapter.

ACTINOMYCOSIS

ETIOLOGY

Actinomycosis is an infection with a worldwide distribution that affects humans and other animals such as cattle and canines. *Actinomyces* spp. are Gram positive, non-spore-bearing, short or filamentous bacilli, which may exhibit true branching. Although *Actinomyces israelii* is the major pathogen, other species including *A. gerencserai*, *A. meyeri*, *A. naeslundii*, *A. odontolyticus*, *A. pyogenes*, *A. radicidentis* and *A. viscosus* do cause human infection. *Actinomyces* spp. can be found as commensals in the oral cavity, gastrointestinal tract and female genital tract.

PATHOGENESIS

Actinomyces spp. are incapable of invading normal tissues and thus require trauma to the mucous surface to initiate disease. This can result from mechanical (accidental or surgical) trauma, primary bacterial or viral infection or malignancy. In addition, this damage will produce injury that renders the tissue anaerobic which facilitates growth of the bacterium. Little is known of virulence determinants of *Actinomyces* spp. and, for example, toxins have not been detected. The commonest sites of actinomycosis are the cervicofacial region (60% of cases), abdomen (25%) and lungs (15%). In addition, *A. naeslundii* and *A. viscosus* are associated with periodontal disease and *A. radicidentis* with dental radiculitis. In actinomycosis there is a dense cellular infiltrate with abscess and sinus formation. The small yellow particles (sulfur granules) characteristic of actinomycosis occur especially with infection due to *A. israelii*.

CLINICAL FEATURES

Actinomycosis is uncommon in children but a case series has been reported.[841] Cervicofacial actinomycosis presents as an indurated swelling in the mandibular region. Subsequently one or more sinuses develop. Less commonly, the tongue, pharynx, lacrimal glands or bone can be affected. Regional lymph nodes tend not to be affected. Local spread to

Table 28.41 Medically important fungi

Superficial mycoses		
	Dermatophytes (tinea capitis, tinea cruris, tinea pedis, tinea unguium, endothrix, ringworm)	Epidermophyton floccosum Microsporum audouinii (M. gryseum, M. canis) Trichophyton rubrum (T. mentagrophytes, T. verrucosum, T. terrestre, T. violaceum, T. schoenleinii, T. tonsurans)
	Pityriasis versicolor	Malassezia (Pityrosporum) furfur
	Black piedra	Piedraia hortae
	Tinea nigra	Cladosporium werneckii
	Candidiasis (mucous membrane)	Candida albicans (C. tropicalis, C. parapsilosis)
Subcutaneous mycoses		
	Sporotrichosis	Sporothrix schenckii
	Chromomycosis	Phialophora verrucosa, Phialophora (Fonsecaea) pedrosoi, Cladosporium carrionii
	Mycetoma	Actinomadura madurae, Nocardia asteroides, N. brasiliensis, Streptomyces somaliensis
	Rhinosporidiosis	Rhinosporidium seeberi
	Zygomycosis	Basidiobolus haptosporus Conidiobolus coronatus
Systemic mycoses		
	Histoplasmosis	Histoplasma capsulatum
	Cryptococcosis	Cryptococcus neoformans
	Blastomycosis	Blastomyces dermatitidis
	Coccidioidomycosis	Coccidioides immitis
	Paracoccidioidomycosis	Paracoccidioides brasiliensis
	Penicilliosis	Penicillium marneffei
Opportunist pathogens		
	Aspergillosis	Aspergillus fumigatus
	Candidiasis	Candida albicans and other species
	Mucormycosis	Mucor spp.
	Pneumocystosis	Pneumocystis carinii

cause brain or spinal cord abscesses has been reported. In these cases there is usually a mixed bacterial population.

Thoracic actinomycosis can occur by aspiration of oral bacteria, hematogenous spread, or local spread from cervical or abdominal lesions. Thus the initial focus can be in the bronchial tree or lung parenchyma. Subsequently, multiple abscesses develop which form sinuses that traverse the chest wall. The main clinical features are chest pain, fever, productive cough and weight loss. Abdominal actinomycosis presents with fever, neutrophilia, chronic abdominal pain and an inflammatory mass. Sinus formation is uncommon. Most often abdominal actinomycosis follows a perforated appendix.[842] Pelvic actinomycosis occurs most often in association with intrauterine contraceptive devices (the coil) and is thus very uncommon in children. Disseminated actinomycosis is uncommon in pediatric practice but has been reported.[843]

DIAGNOSIS AND DIFFERENTIAL DIAGNOSIS

Cervicofacial actinomycosis is part of the differential diagnosis of an indurated swelling of the mandibular region, especially if there is sinus formation. Specific diagnosis is by bacteriological culture of aspirated pus, sinus discharge, biopsy tissue or fine needle aspirations, but care must be taken to avoid contamination by commensal bacteria. Cultures should be kept anaerobically at 35–37 °C for up to 14 days. More rapid diagnosis can be obtained by examination of crushed sulfur granules stained by Gram stain where filamentous, branching or beaded Gram positive bacteria will be seen. It must be distinguished from other chronic suppurative lesions of the cervical region including chronic pyogenic osteomyelitis and tuberculosis. Thoracic actinomycosis may be confused with other chronic lung infection, including bronchiectasis and pulmonary tuberculosis.[844] Culture of sputum, bronchial aspirates or biopsy material will confirm the diagnosis.

The mass of abdominal actinomycosis can mimic an appendix abscess, abdominal tuberculosis or intra-abdominal carcinoma.[843] Laparotomy with culture of pus or biopsy material is necessary to establish the diagnosis. Serologic diagnosis is unreliable.

TREATMENT AND PROGNOSIS

Benzyl penicillin is the treatment of choice. It is given in high doses, intravenously for 2 weeks at least, then orally for 6–8 months. This may be accompanied wherever possible with surgical drainage. For penicillin-allergic patients, tetracycline and perhaps ciprofloxacin can be tried. The prognosis is generally good, although thoracic actinomycosis may require even more prolonged and energetic treatment.

ASPERGILLOSIS

ETIOLOGY

Aspergillosis is a fungal infection with a worldwide distribution. There are over 90 Aspergillus species described and 19 have been associated with human disease. However, most infections are due to Aspergillus fumigatus, A. flavus and to a lesser extent A. niger. Aspergillus spp. are widely distributed in the environment and some cause infection in other animals. Aspergillus is a member of the Eumycetes (true fungi) and produces a mycelium with a fruiting body, the conidium, from which spores are released into the atmosphere. The spores can be found in air sampled anywhere on earth.

EPIDEMIOLOGY AND PATHOGENESIS

Most disease manifestations involve the lung. In general, community acquired disease tends to be non-invasive aspergillosis and hospital acquired disease either non-invasive or invasive aspergillosis. In addition,

Table 28.42   Subcutaneous and systemic mycoses

Disease	Causative organism	Geographical distribution	Predominant clinical features	Treatment
Actinomycosis	*Actinomyces israelii*	Worldwide	Abscesses and sinuses in face and neck, lungs, abdomen	Benzyl penicillin
Aspergillosis	*Aspergillus* spp.	Worldwide	Granulomata of lungs, skin or generalized, aspergilloma	Nystatin aerosol, i.v. amphotericin B or oral itraconazole or ketoconazole
North American blastomycosis	*Blastomyces dermatitidis*	North America	Granulomata of lungs or generalized	i.v. amphotericin B or oral itraconazole or ketoconazole
South American blastomycosis	*Paracoccidioides brasiliensis*	South America	Ulcerating granulomata of oropharynx, lungs or generalized	i.v. amphotericin B or oral itraconazole or ketoconazole
Candidiasis	*Candida* spp. usually *C. albicans*	Worldwide	Usually superficial infection. Systemic resembles septicemic illness	i.v. amphotericin B with or without 5-flucytosine or oral fluconazole i.v. caspofungin
Chromoblastomycosis	*Cladosporium werneckii* *Fonsecaea compacta* *F. pedrosoi* *Phialophora verrucosa* *Rhinocladiella aquaspersa*	Tropics	Nodular, verrucose, tumors, plaque or cicatricial lesions of skin and deeper tissues	Surgery and i.v. amphotericin B, with 5-flucytosine, itraconazole or ketoconazole but mixed results
Coccidioidomycosis (San Joaquin Valley fever)	*Coccidioides immitis*	North and South America	Influenza-like illness. Progressive pulmonary or central nervous system infection in minority	i.v. amphotericin B or 5-flucytosine or i.v. miconazole or oral itraconazole
Cryptococcosis (torulosis)	*Cryptococcus neoformans*	Worldwide	Chiefly central nervous system infection, meningoencephalitis, or focal lesion but can cause pneumonia	i.v. amphotericin B or oral fluconazole
Histoplasmosis	*Histoplasma capsulatum*	Central USA	Granulomata in lungs, or in miliary distribution	i.v. amphotericin B or oral itraconazole or fluconazole
Mycetoma (Madura foot, maduromycosis)	Actinomycetoma *Actinomadura madurae* *A. pellotieri* *Nocardia brasiliensis* *N. madurae* *Streptomyces somaliensis* Eumycetoma *Madurella grisea* *M. mycetomatis* *Pseudallescheria boydii*	Tropics	Localized chronic infection involving skin, subcutaneous tissue and bone (nodule, sinuses and discharge)	Surgery (removal of lesions, amputation). Actinomycetoma: dapsone plus streptomycin. Eumycetoma: griseofulvin or imidazoles plus penicillin (but poor results)
Mucormycosis	*Mincor* spp. *Absidia corymbifera* *Rhizomusco* spp. *Rhizopus* spp.	Worldwide	Rhinocerebral, rhino-orbital, cardiac involvement, pulmonary, gastrointestinal, skin and soft tissue, bone involvement	i.v. amphotericin
Nocardiosis	*Nocardia asteroides* or *N. brasiliensis*	Worldwide	Pulmonary suppuration, occasionally central nervous system infection	Sulfonamides
Penicilliosis	*Penicillium marneffei*	South East Asia	Generalized infection especially in immune compromised patients with skin, bone, liver, spleen and lung involvement	i.v. amphotericin and oral itraconazole
Pneumocystosis	*Pneumocystis carinii*	Worldwide	Acute or subacute pneumonia in children immunocompromised by HIV, malnutrition or cytotoxic drugs	Oral co-trimoxazole, nebulized pentamidine
Rhinosporidiosis	*Rhinosporidium seeberi*	India and Ceylon	Polypoid tumors of mucous membrane – nose, nasopharynx, conjunctival sac. Gelatinous lesions, bleeding easily. Diagnosis by microscopic examination of crushed fragments of polyp. Pulmonary and nasopalatal types with tissue destruction may occur in the patients subject to severe metabolic disturbance	Surgical removal
Sporotrichosis	*Sporothrix schenckii*	Worldwide	Subcutaneous nodule (usually on hands or feet) which enlarges and adheres to skin and breaks down to form chronic ulcer. Satellite nodules develop by lymphatic spread. Usually localized but may be widely disseminated. Diagnosis by culture of exudates or scrapings or antibody tests. Extracutaneous forms involving muscles, lungs eyes, CNS, urinary tract and wide dissemination may occur	For lymphangitic form, potassium iodide 30 mg/kg/d up to maximum tolerance. For disseminated form i.v. amphotericin B or oral itraconazole

mycotoxins such as aflatoxin may contaminate cereals, groundnuts and other foods. Aflatoxin is a potent carcinogen but its role in human disease remains to be clarified. The non-invasive manifestations of aspergillosis are extrinsic allergic alveolitis (EAA), allergic bronchopulmonary aspergillosis (ABPA) and aspergilloma. In the former two, disease results from an allergic response to *Aspergillus* spp., a type III hypersensitivity response in EAA and type I in ABPA. An aspergilloma is a fungal mycelial ball that develops in a pre-existing lung cavity. In each case, the fungus is acquired by inhalation. Invasive pulmonary aspergillosis occurs in those immunocompromised by radiation, steroids or chemotherapy, especially if there is neutropenia. An increase in numbers of cases is often preceded by building work in or near the hospital, which increases atmospheric contamination by aspergillus spores. Dissemination from invasive pulmonary aspergillosis can result in metastatic foci in most organs of the body.

CLINICAL FEATURES AND DIAGNOSIS

ABPA in pediatric practice is particularly associated with cystic fibrosis, but may also occur in asthma. It presents insidiously with worsening bronchospasm and less commonly low grade fever. Up to two thirds of patients expectorate brownish sputum, which contains aspergilli. Eight diagnostic criteria (aspergillus precipitins, aspergillus specific IgE, chest radiographic infiltrates, blood eosinophilia > 500/mm³, *A. fumigatus* skin test, total serum IgE > 1000 ng/ml, bronchiectasis, cough and wheeze) are widely used,[845] but must be applied regularly to be of benefit.[846]

Invasive pulmonary aspergillosis occurs most often in the setting of relapse of the underlying condition or post bone marrow transplant[847] and presents with unremitting fever, new pulmonary infiltrates, dyspnea and unproductive cough. These, together with hemoptysis and tachycardia, can mimic pulmonary embolus. Massive hemoptysis is rare. Radiographic changes are variable, but most often, patchy bronchopneumonic infiltrates or nodular densities are seen. After 2–3 weeks, cavitation may occur. Dissemination is clinically indistinguishable from bacterial septicemia in immunocompromised patients. The presentation of metastatic disease, which can occur almost anywhere, will depend on the site of infection. Specific diagnosis depends upon culture of aspergilli from the infective site but blood cultures are very rarely, if ever, positive. Since aspergilli are so frequently present in the environment it is also necessary to demonstrate tissue invasion by histologic examination.

TREATMENT, PROGNOSIS AND PREVENTION

Allergic bronchopulmonary aspergillosis requires early therapy with oral corticosteroids and addition of high dose inhaled steroids may be of benefit. Recurrence is common. The natural history of aspergillosis is variable but only a minority of children resolve spontaneously. If there is evidence of some pulmonary invasion from the aspergilloma, antifungal therapy with amphotericin B or oral itraconazole may be beneficial. Surgical removal is necessary, for example, if there is life-threatening hemoptysis; however, this does carry a risk of inoculating fungi into the field of surgery.

For invasive pulmonary or other aspergillosis, surgical drainage, debridement or resection is most important with antifungal therapy acting as an adjunct. Amphotericin B is the gold standard for therapy, and addition of 5-flucytosine might be of benefit. Itraconazole given orally is licensed for therapy but long term administration will be needed. The prognosis is generally poor but it is difficult to distinguish the relative contributions of the aspergillosis and the underlying condition.

BLASTOMYCOSIS

ETIOLOGY

Blastomyces dermatitidis is a dimorphic fungus. It exists as a yeast in human infection and when cultured at 37 °C, but in a mycelial form at room temperature or in the environment. Two serotypes and several genotypes have been described. *Paracoccidioides brasiliensis* is also dimorphic. In human lesions, it is found as a double-walled ovoid or round yeast 4–40 μm in diameter. In culture at 19–28 °C or in the environment it has a mycelial form. Isolates of *P. brasiliensis* vary greatly in their ability to cause disease.

EPIDEMIOLOGY AND PATHOGENESIS

Although sometimes referred to as North American blastomycosis, *B. dermatitidis* infection has been reported in North and South America, Europe, Africa and Asia. Within North America it has been reported from the mid-west and south east USA and parts of Canada. It appears that the environment along waterways is an important reservoir and infection is probably acquired by inhalation. Humans and other animals can be infected but person-to-person transmission does not occur and children are rarely infected. *P. brasiliensis* infection was originally called hyphoblastomycosis but is now known as South American blastomycosis, or, more correctly, paracoccidioidomycosis. It is limited to Central and South America from Mexico to Argentina but most cases (80%) are reported from Brazil. It is found in soil and is thought to be acquired by inhalation. It is rare in women, adolescents and children. Person-to-person transmission does not occur.

CLINICAL FEATURES

It is likely that most infections with *B. dermatitidis* are asymptomatic, but when clinically apparent can range from acute self-limiting pneumonia to disseminated infection. Occasionally, the acute pneumonia does not resolve and chronic pulmonary blastomycosis occurs, which is clinically indistinguishable from pulmonary tuberculosis or histoplasmosis. Cutaneous lesions are the most frequent manifestations of disseminated infection. These begin as subcutaneous nodules or papules. They then become ulcerated with raised irregular borders and a crusted center. Histologically these are granulomas.

P. brasiliensis causes a spectrum of disease ranging from acute pulmonary infection with or without mucocutaneous involvement to a progressive disseminated form with involvement of the mucocutaneous tissue, reticuloendothelial system and adrenals. It may also give a miliary appearance in the lung.

DIAGNOSIS AND DIFFERENTIAL DIAGNOSIS

Blastomycosis, although uncommon in children, should be suspected in patients from endemic areas with granulomatous and ulcerating lesions of the skin or mucous membranes, especially if it is of long duration or there is involvement of other organs. Acute pulmonary blastomycosis is difficult to diagnose clinically, as it presents as an influenza-like illness or with pleuritic pain. The chronic form is indistinguishable from tuberculosis, histoplasmosis or coccidioidomycosis. Specific diagnosis is by demonstrating the presence of *B. dermatitidis*, by culture of lesions or sputum, and for superficial lesions, biopsy stained by methenamine silver (the yeasts may not stain by hematoxylin and eosin).

Paracoccidioidomycosis has similar differential diagnoses to blastomycosis. Since children may present with an acute or subacute form with large numbers of yeast in the reticuloendothelial system and fungemia, specific diagnosis can also be aided by blood culture.

Treatment and Prognosis

Without treatment the mortality rate of blastomycosis is over 60%. Amphotericin B is the mainstay of therapy but higher doses are needed. Treatment should continue until symptoms resolve and continue for 3–4 months thereafter. Even with this, relapses occur in 10–20% of patients (up to 5 years later). Oral ketoconazole or, better still, itraconazole appears as effective as amphotericin B but there are no trials directly comparing the regimens. Treatment should continue for at least 6 months. Ketoconazole is effective in 85% of cases of paracoccidioidomycosis and relapse rates are low (0–11%) if therapy is continued for at least 6 months. Itraconazole appears superior to ketoconazole.

CANDIDIASIS

ETIOLOGY AND EPIDEMIOLOGY

There are almost 200 *Candida* species and they have a worldwide distribution. They exist in budding yeast, hyphal or pseudohyphal forms (Fig. 28.54). *Candida albicans* is the commonest species found both as a commensal, particularly in the mouth, rectum, vagina or on skin, and as a pathogen. The others are found less commonly as commensals but *C. glabrata* can be found in the mouth, rectum or vagina and *C. parapsilosis* and *C. tropicalis* on skin. Infections occur particularly in neonates and immunocompromised children, especially those with T cell defects.

PATHOGENESIS AND CLINICAL FEATURES

Different *Candida* spp. have differing virulence but *C. albicans* is the most competent pathogen. Virulence factors include adhesins, ability to switch from yeast to hyphal (invasive) forms, production of proteolytic enzymes, antigenic variability and host mimicry. In addition to these, however, there need to be breaches in the skin or mucosa, alterations in the normal flora (usually due to antibacterial therapy), or underlying conditions such as immune deficiency (congenital or acquired), diabetes mellitus or implanted devices.

Superficial candidiasis (thrush)

Oral thrush typically occurs in neonates. Adherent gray-white plaques on removal reveal a raw, red base. They are usually found on the tongue, gums or gingival mucosa but may extend into the esophagus or trachea, especially in HIV/AIDS. There may also be scaly, macular or vesicular, erythematous perianal lesions. In skin areas that are moist, occluded or irradiated, candidiasis can occur as intensely erythematous intertriginous lesions. These can be papular, plaque-like or confluent with surrounding satellite lesions. Commonly involved sites include the axillae, inguinal regions, perineum and digital web spaces. *Candida* spp. can also cause onychomycosis which, unlike that due to dermatophytes, is painful.

Chronic mucocutaneous candidiasis

This includes a heterogeneous group of patients with T cell deficits, some of which are highly specific to *Candida* spp. Most cases present in infancy or early childhood with oral thrush or perineal candidiasis which may become more widespread or just persist with localized lesions.

Deeper candidiasis

Candidal infection of deeper tissues and organs occurs rarely in otherwise healthy patients. Oral or esophageal candidiasis may be complicated by extension of infection to the intestine, typically with symptoms of diarrhea, abdominal pain and pruritus ani. The child may present with a celiac-like syndrome. In pulmonary candidiasis, the symptoms of fever and productive cough, sometimes with hemoptysis, are nonspecific. On radiological examination, patchy consolidation is seen, and cavitation may occur with infections of sufficient duration. Pulmonary candidiasis

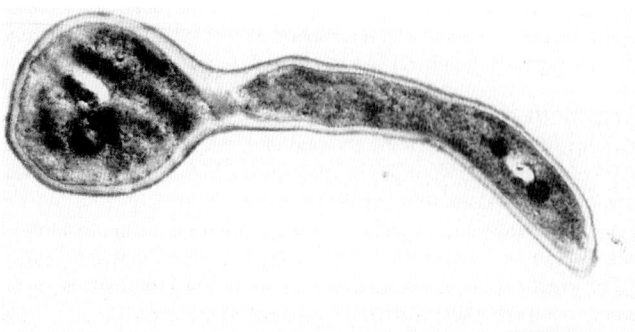

Fig. 28.54 A thin section electron micrograph of *Candida albicans* showing a pseudohypha (bar = 1 μm).

should be not diagnosed too readily on the evidence of culture of *Candida* from sputum, since the organism may be isolated in a proportion of healthy individuals, and particularly from hospital patients.

Disseminated *Candida* infection, although very uncommon in infancy and childhood, is thought to be increasing in frequency and has been reported in neonates, debilitated infants and children, particularly those treated with antibiotics or corticosteroids, or with diseases of the reticuloendothelial system, and in patients requiring prolonged intravenous therapy. Several *Candida* species have been isolated from such patients, whose clinical features are those of septicemia. Disseminated candidiasis, which may be confirmed by blood culture, should be suspected when a septicemic illness supervenes in premature neonates, debilitated infants, or children in the course of antibiotic therapy, especially in the presence of a portal of entry for the organism such as an indwelling intravenous cannula.

The isolation of *Candida* from a specimen of urine obtained by suprapubic aspiration is highly suggestive of disseminated infection but must be interpreted in the light of other clinical data. Urinary tract infections with *C. albicans* do occur, especially in neonates or in association with indwelling urinary catheters. In neonates infection can ascend to produce fungal balls in the renal pelvis. The appearance of papular lesions on the skin containing *Candida* has been noted in preterm infants under such circumstances.

Candida endocarditis, though rare, has been reported in childhood. Previously damaged heart valves are the site of localization of infection in a patient with disseminated *Candida* infection.

DIAGNOSIS AND DIFFERENTIAL DIAGNOSIS

Oral thrush can usually be diagnosed on observation of the typical lesion, which may be confused with deposits of milk. The latter can be scraped off without effort, revealing a normal mucosal surface. Candidal napkin rash may be confused with ammoniacal dermatitis, and, although it is common for the two lesions to coexist, the sharply demarcated edges of the former and its association with oral thrush should suggest the diagnosis. Confirmation of superficial candidiasis is readily made by the finding of typical pseudohyphae on microscopic examination and by culture of the organism from swabs from superficial lesions. Yeast cells are not significant in feces as they occur in 15% of normal children but hyphal forms occur only with invasion of mucous membranes and their presence can therefore be taken as an indication of enteric candidiasis.

The clinical and radiological features of pulmonary candidiasis can be confused with a number of subacute and chronic bacterial infections of the lungs. The presence of characteristic predisposing circumstances should suggest the diagnosis, especially if pulmonary cavitation is present. Laboratory confirmation is best made by repeated sputum culture, or preferably, by culture of tracheal or bronchial aspirates.

In disseminated candidiasis the organism can be isolated by blood or urine culture.

TREATMENT AND PROGNOSIS

Oral candidiasis is best treated by local application of antifungal agents. Preparations in common use are suspensions of nystatin (100 000 units/ml) and miconazole (2% in a gel). Gentian violet (1% aqueous solution) is by far the cheapest but it is messy, may produce excoriation of buccal mucosa, and generally fails to eradicate the fungus from the lower alimentary tract; it is now little used in Western countries. Nystatin and miconazole are probably equally effective. Nystatin is given in a dose of 1.0–2.0 ml dropped in the oral cavity 4 to 6 hourly for 7–10 days while miconazole gel is applied as 5.0 ml, two to four times each day. Apparent failure of such treatments is seldom, if ever, due to the presence of antibiotic-resistant species of *C. albicans*. While resistance to nystatin and amphotericin B by *Candida* species other than *C. albicans* can readily be induced in vitro, only a minor degree of diminished antibiotic sensitivity can be induced in *C. albicans*. A dose of 1 ml of nystatin by oral instillation 6 hourly may be inadequate; higher and more frequent doses should be employed if the infection appears to be unresponsive. In perianal forms or candidiasis of skin or nails, topical nystatin (100 000 units/g of ointment) or miconazole is effective. Oral therapy with either antibiotic is effective in candidal enteritis.

In the treatment of candidiasis of deeper structures and organs, oral nystatin therapy is not recommended, since absorption from the gastrointestinal tract is poor. Oral ketoconazole may be effective. In pulmonary candidiasis, nystatin may be administered by aerosol, e.g. 500 000 units in 15 ml distilled water. In systemic candidiasis and candidal endocarditis and probably in pulmonary candidiasis, the most effective treatment is the intravenous administration of amphotericin B. Recent reports have indicated that the liposomal amphotericin B (AmBisome) treatment is less toxic and at least equally effective.[848] Flucytosine has the advantages over amphotericin B of oral administration and lower toxicity. Many strains of *C. albicans* are resistant, however, and the drug cannot be administered parenterally to those patients too ill to take it by mouth. It should be reserved for those patients in whom amphotericin B has proved to be too toxic. Echinocandins such as caspofungin are also useful in treating such infections.

The prognosis of superficial candidiasis is excellent; that of candidal enteritis has to be guarded. Disseminated candidiasis carries a poor prognosis, largely related to the nature of the predisposing conditions. Meningeal candidiasis, however, may run a surprisingly mild course.

CHROMOBLASTOMYCOSIS

ETIOLOGY, EPIDEMIOLOGY AND PATHOGENESIS

This is the commonest infection by the dematiaceous or black pigmented fungi. A number of fungi including *Fonsecaea pedrosoi*, *F. compacta*, *Phialophora verrucosa*, *Cladosporium carrionii*, *Rhinocladiella aquaspersa* and, less commonly, *Exophiala jeanselmei* cause chromoblastomycosis. Although most common in the tropics, cases have been reported from more temperate regions such as Europe and the USA. The habitat of each of the fungi is soil, decomposing vegetation and woodland. Humans most often become infected by traumatic implantation of such material for example when walking barefoot. Person-to-person transmission has not been described.

CLINICAL FEATURES, DIAGNOSIS AND TREATMENT

Chromoblastomycosis usually begins as a small pink papule which enlarges to a nodule. Over time it evolves to a scaly, fissured pink brownish plaque which eventually becomes verrucose. Eventually thick, crusted, hyperkeratotic masses occur which are prone to secondary infection, leading eventually, after many years, to lymphatic blockage and elephantiasis. The differential diagnosis includes blastomycosis, lupus vulgaris, leishmaniasis and tertiary syphilis. Specific diagnosis is by histologic examination and isolation of the fungi, which requires up to 6 weeks incubation at both 25 and 37 °C. Treatment is difficult. For small lesions, wide surgical excision is possible. Itraconazole for 6–24 months is effective in above 60% of cases. Amputation may be required.

COCCIDIOIDOMYCOSIS

ETIOLOGY AND EPIDEMIOLOGY

Coccidioides immitis is a dimorphic fungus which exists as a mycelial saprophyte in soil but as an endosporulating spherule in the human lung. Infection is acquired by inhalation of arthroconidia from soil and is particularly prevalent in the San Joaquin Valley in California. Although most cases occur in and around this area, cases have been described in Central (Guatemala, Honduras) and South America (Venezuela, Colombia, Paraguay, Bolivia, Argentina). It may also occur when dust storms blow the arthroconidia into other areas.

PATHOGENESIS

Inhalation of arthroconidia results in a disease attack rate of about 40%. Once in the lungs the arthroconidia convert to the spherule-endospore phase within 3 days. This causes an initial influx of neutrophils and an inflammatory response which changes to a mononuclear cell infiltrate with granulomata once the spherule-endospore phase is well established. The spherules are too large (20–150 µm) to be ingested by neutrophils or even macrophages but they are important in defense presumably because they can engulf the released endospores (c. 2–5 µm). A brisk T_H1 (T helper type 1) response is needed for recovery from infection.

CLINICAL FEATURES

Most often coccidioidomycosis is a somewhat prolonged influenza-like illness, often with pneumonia, which follows an incubation period of 1–3 weeks. In 90%, recovery is complete; the remainder are left with pulmonary cavities and nodules.[849] Nonpulmonary features include fever, malaise, headache, arthralgia, myalgia and skin rashes. Approximately 25% of patients develop erythema nodosum 6–16 days after onset of symptoms. In about 1% of patients, there is dissemination with skin (subcutaneous abscesses), bone, meningeal and even miliary manifestations. Dissemination is particularly found in immune compromised patients including cardiac allograft recipients (5% of those in Arizona) and those with HIV/AIDS.

DIAGNOSIS AND DIFFERENTIAL DIAGNOSIS

Coccidioidomycosis should be suspected in children in or from endemic areas, especially if non-white, who develop an acute febrile illness. Primary pulmonary coccidioidomycosis especially with erythema nodosum can be confused with primary tuberculosis, and the postprimary nodular or cavitating disease with secondary tuberculosis. Diagnosis can be confirmed by culture of sputum, pus or blood (if disseminated), but the laboratory should be warned since this is a significant pathogen that will need special containment. The coccidioidin skin test (similar to tuberculosis) will become positive within 21 days of infection. Serologic tests such as complement-fixing titers are available and useful for confirmation of diagnosis.

TREATMENT AND PROGNOSIS

Primary coccidioidomycosis seldom requires more than symptomatic treatment. Amphotericin B, the most effective drug, should, in view of its toxicity, be reserved for severe primary or postprimary pulmonary disease. Intravenous amphotericin B therapy is, however, essential in disseminated coccidioidomycosis and, where there is infection of the central nervous system, may be given by intrathecal infection. Until recently, the only alternative form of therapy was intravenous miconazole but oral itraconazole has been shown to be of value and of relatively low toxicity.

The prognosis of primary coccidioidomycosis is excellent, while that of postprimary pulmonary disease is good. Disseminated coccidioidomycosis carries a poor prognosis, especially with meningeal infection, unless treated vigorously and at an early stage.

CRYPTOCOCCOSIS

ETIOLOGY AND EPIDEMIOLOGY

Cryptococcus neoformans exists as a yeast in mammalian infections and on artificial culture but in a mycelial form in the environment. *C. neoformans* has a worldwide distribution and there are two variants: *C. neoformans* var. *neoformans* and *C. neoformans* var. *gattii*. *C. neoformans* is subdivided into four serotypes (A–D). *C. neoformans* var. *neoformans* falls into serotypes A and D, and var. *gattii*, serotypes B and C. The former is associated with soil, especially that contaminated by pigeon droppings and causes infection in patients immunocompromised by HIV/AIDS, chemotherapy or steroid administration. The latter is associated with the tropics and has been isolated from debris around *Eucalyptus camaldulensis*, the Australian red river gum tree. It causes infection in immunocompetent individuals. Although infection occurs in all age groups, children are less often infected.

PATHOGENESIS AND CLINICAL FEATURES

Infection is acquired, it is thought, by inhalation of the fungus. Person-to-person transmission does not occur. Virulent strains of *C. neoformans* have a thick polysaccharide capsule (Fig. 28.55) that protects them from phagocytic killing by macrophages and neutrophils. In the lungs, they can cause pneumonia but this occurs in less than 15% of patients with cryptococcosis. Most often the organism passes through the lungs silently to infect at secondary sites. The major manifestation is chronic meningitis with headache, personality changes, dementia and focal neurologic signs. It can be entirely asymptomatic early in the infection and, especially in HIV/AIDS patients, neck stiffness and fever are not major presenting features (< 50% of cases). In approximately 15% of cases of cryptococcosis there is skin or bone involvement. The cutaneous manifestations can be acneiform, abscesses, ulcers, granulomas or plaques.

DIAGNOSIS AND DIFFERENTIAL DIAGNOSIS

Specific diagnosis depends on demonstrating the fungus or its capsular antigen in CSF, blood or other infective sites. However, it must be remembered that *C. neoformans* can be present in sputum in the absence of disease. In CSF the cellular response varies. In AIDS patients, the cell count is low (< 5/mm³) whereas in non-AIDS patients it ranges from 10 to 300/mm³, but in each case there is a prevalence of lymphocytes (> 80%). *C. neoformans* will stain violet on Gram stain (Gram positive), but the India ink stain is best for demonstration of the yeasts. This is a negative stain because the stain does not penetrate the yeast but shows it with its thick polysaccharide capsule against a black background. There are commercially available latex agglutination kits for detection of capsular antigen in CSF or serum. These can also be used to measure response to therapy. Finally *C. neoformans* can be cultured on suitable fungal culture medium. The differential diagnoses include other bacterial and viral causes of acute or chronic meningitis or meningoencephalitis, in particular tuberculous meningitis, and for the skin lesions molluscum contagiosum, penicilliosis and histoplasmosis, especially in AIDS patients.

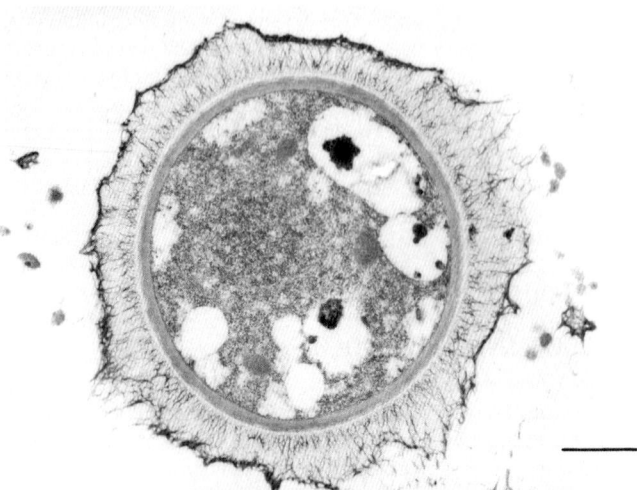

Fig. 28.55 A thin section electron micrograph of *Cryptococcus neoformans* showing its thick polysaccharide capsule (bar = 1 μm).

TREATMENT AND PROGNOSIS

For non-AIDS patients a combination of amphotericin B and 5-flucytosine for 6 weeks is curative in 75% of patients. In AIDS patients a number of regimens have been tried, principally because relapse is common after stopping therapy. Amphotericin B with or without 5-flucytosine for 2 weeks followed by 8 weeks of therapy with either fluconazole or itraconazole appears optimal in these cases. This is then followed by long term oral suppressive therapy with fluconazole. However, with the advent of combination antiretroviral therapy for HIV/AIDS the outlook is much better.[850] In addition to frequent relapse, obstructive hydrocephalus is a major complication of cryptococcal meningitis.

HISTOPLASMOSIS

ETIOLOGY AND EPIDEMIOLOGY

Histoplasma capsulatum is another dimorphic fungus which undergoes reversible morphologic variation according to the environment in which it is placed. Its normal habitat is soil, especially below where birds and bats have roosted. Here it exists in a mycelial form with hyphae bearing macroconidia (8–14 μm diameter) and microconidia (2–5 μm), which are the infective forms. At temperatures above 35 °C *H. capsulatum* grows as a yeast (2–3 × 3–4 μm) and this is the form found in human infections. Histoplasmosis is endemic in North America (especially the Ohio and Mississippi valleys) and Latin America, but cases have been reported from Europe and Asia. The taxonomy of *H. capsulatum* is currently under discussion. Three varieties are recognized: *H. capsulatum* var. *capsulatum*, *H. capsulatum* var. *duboisii* (which causes African histoplasmosis) and *H. capsulatum* var. *farciminosum* (which causes skin ulcers in horses and mules) but genetic analysis suggests *H. capsulatum* might harbor six species.[851] It is estimated that there are 200 000–500 000 cases each year worldwide. In endemic areas of the USA, it is estimated that 90% of the population have been exposed with frequent re-exposure.[852]

PATHOGENESIS AND CLINICAL FEATURES

Infection occurs when microconidia are inhaled. Most often this occurs when individuals disturb soil or dust containing microconidia, but they can travel for miles in the wind. In the lungs, the spores germinate to the yeast form, which elicits an influx of neutrophils, macrophages and lymphocytes and formation of granulomas. The yeasts are able to survive within macrophages,[853] and may persist for years within the reticuloendothelial system. Infection is more likely to progress, persist or disseminate if there is abnormal T cell function. Infection is also likely to disseminate in infants under 2 years,[854] but there is often an associated T cell defect. With exposure to a low infective dose, only 1% of patients develop clinical disease, but the rest have serologic evidence of infection. With a higher inoculum only 10–50% are asymptomatic. Most clinically expressed infections are self-limited and include acute pulmonary histoplasmosis, mediastinal lymph node enlargement, pericarditis and rheumatologic manifestations.

Approximately 80% of the symptomatic cases are of acute pulmonary histoplasmosis, which presents as a 'flu-like' illness with fever, chills, headache, myalgia and a nonproductive cough. This usually resolves within a few weeks. More diffuse pulmonary disease leading to respiratory insufficiency can occur with a higher infecting dose. The rheumatologic manifestations include erythema nodosum with arthralgia or frank arthritis, which can persist for months. Pericarditis occurs as an inflammatory complication of pulmonary disease. Chronic pulmonary histoplasmosis is very rare in children. It occurs mostly in middle-aged men with chronic obstructive airways disease. Disseminated histoplasmosis is a progressive illness with extrapulmonary spread of the fungus. It can occur following acute infection or years later. In infants it presents as fever, splenomegaly and/or hepatomegaly.[854] Subsequently, shock, liver or renal failure and central nervous system involvement can occur. Cutaneous or mucosal granulomas in children in endemic areas should also be considered as possible histoplasmosis.

DIAGNOSIS AND DIFFERENTIAL DIAGNOSIS

Diagnosis requires a high index of clinical suspicion in a child living in, or coming from, an endemic region. Specific diagnosis requires a battery of tests including histology, antigen and antibody detection and fungal culture of bone marrow, spleen, lymph node, liver or bronchoalveolar lavage samples.[854] The histoplasmin skin test is not useful, especially in those with T cell impairment and disseminated disease. The differential diagnosis includes pulmonary or miliary tuberculosis.

MYCETOMA[855]

Mycetoma is a chronic, subcutaneous granulomatous disease caused by either fungi (eumycetoma) or branching bacteria (actinomycetoma). It has a worldwide distribution and is endemic in a belt between latitudes 15°S and 30°N, which encompasses Senegal, Sudan, Somalia, Mexico, India and parts of Central and South America. In Sudan it is estimated that there are 300–400 new cases each year, mostly in males aged 20–40 years, but children may rarely be affected. The clinical triad of subcutaneous nodules, sinuses and discharge is suggestive. The differential diagnosis includes Kaposi's sarcoma, neurofibroma, malignant melanoma, syphilitic osteitis and bone tuberculosis, but specific diagnosis can be made by histologic examination. Culture is difficult and takes a long time. Surgical treatment is to remove all affected tissue, which can involve amputation of affected feet or hands. Actinomycetoma can be treated with dapsone and streptomycin for 1 month. Medical treatment of eumycetoma is much more difficult. Griseofulvin, ketoconazole or itraconazole have had mixed success but treatment must be continued for 1–10 years.

NOCARDIOSIS

ETIOLOGY AND EPIDEMIOLOGY

Nocardia spp. are Gram positive, acid alcohol fast, nonmotile, branching bacteria in the suborder *Corynebacterineae* that are closely related to the actinomycetes. There are 20 *Nocardia* spp. but most human infections are by *Nocardia asteroides* and less commonly by *N. farcinica* and *N. nova*. In tropical countries infection can also be by *N. brasiliensis* and *N. africana*.[856] *Nocardia* are environmental organisms living in soil and decaying vegetation. Person-to-person spread does not occur, and although *Nocardia* spp. can cause infections in animals they are not zoonotic. Primary infections do occur but most infections occur in immunocompromised individuals.

PATHOGENESIS AND CLINICAL FEATURES

Infection is acquired either by inhalation or direct inoculation into the skin. Characteristically *Nocardia* spp. produce abscesses and granulomas. Virulent strains of *N. asteroides* can evade phagocytic killing by inhibiting phagolysosome fusion or acidification of phagosomes.[857,858] Dissemination is much more likely to occur if there is some form of immune compromise and has been reported in HIV/AIDS when it may involve the skin, kidneys and adrenals. In 5% of patients it involves the central nervous system either as diffuse meningitis or abscesses.

Pulmonary infection is found in 75% of patients with nocardiosis, alone or in association with disseminated infection, and may produce no symptoms. In other patients malaise, cough, fever and dyspnea may develop. Hemoptysis is an uncommon symptom. Involvement of the central nervous system may result in the clinical features of meningoencephalitis, or, if the lesion is a single abscess, of a localized intracranial or intraspinous tumor. Primary cutaneous nocardiosis can present as cellulitis or as an abscess with or without lymphadenitis and can be mistaken for *Streptococcus pyogenes* or *Staphylococcus aureus* infections.[859] *Nocardia* spp. are also pathogens in mycetoma.

DIAGNOSIS AND DIFFERENTIAL DIAGNOSIS

There are no typical symptoms and signs, and the pulmonary form may readily be confused with other suppurative lung conditions. Radiological examination of the chest similarly provides no characteristic features, the most common being patchy infiltration perhaps with cavitation. Specific diagnosis depends upon laboratory help but unfortunately *Nocardia* spp. are difficult to recognize and identify in the routine diagnostic laboratory, compounded by the fact that they are slow growing.

TREATMENT AND PROGNOSIS

Prior to the advent of the sulfonamides, nocardial infection was usually fatal, and at present the outlook is poor, partly because of the nature of the predisposing conditions and partly because of delay in diagnosis.

The treatment of choice is prolonged administration of sulfonamides or co-trimoxazole. Treatment may be necessary for several months, and may be combined with surgery. It is recommended that sulfonamides be given in a dose adequate to maintain a blood level of not less than 10 mg/100 ml.

Treatment with antibiotics, including benzyl penicillin and chloramphenicol, has been reported to be successful on occasions and, as indicated by sensitivity of the organism in vitro, may be given in addition to sulfonamides.

PENICILLIOSIS

This is an emerging infection which is the third commonest opportunist infection in HIV infected patients in South East Asia.[860] Most cases are due to *Penicillium marneffei* but occasional cases of *P. chrysogenum* occur.[861]

Approximately 80% of patients with penicilliosis are immunocompromised. Penicilliosis can present as cutaneous or disseminated infection or both. The skin lesions are usually umbilicated papules resembling molluscum contagiosum. Disseminated disease usually presents as fever, weight loss and anemia. Specific diagnosis is by isolation of the fungus from skin, bone marrow or blood. Mild to moderate disease can be treated with itraconazole or ketoconazole but severe disease will require amphotericin B. There are no controlled trials of therapy.

SPOROTRICHOSIS[862]

Sporotrichosis is caused by the dimorphic fungus *Sporothrix schenckii*. It grows as a saprophyte in decaying vegetation and infection occurs following traumatic inoculation into the skin. Some cases have been transmitted by domestic cat scratch.[863] It has a worldwide distribution but, for example, is the commonest subcutaneous mycosis in Latin America. Infection is often related to occupation (e.g. farmers, florists, gardeners) and occurs most often in adults, although infections do occur in children.[864] The initial nodule at the inoculation site enlarges becoming red, pustular and ulcerating in turn. Extension occurs up the lymphatics to draining lymph nodes which themselves enlarge and drain to the skin. Spontaneous healing can occur but most often the lesions persist with gradual extension and scarring. Diagnosis depends upon demonstrating *S. schenckii* in lesions by immunohistochemistry or immunofluorescence. Fungal culture, however, provides the definitive diagnosis. There are no controlled trials of therapy, but oral itraconazole for 3–12 months has cure rates of 89–100%. Saturated potassium iodide (10 drops diluted in fruit juice three times daily) can be used in a resource poor setting but it is poorly tolerated. If disease is unresponsive to itraconazole, it might be necessary to use amphotericin B.

ANTIFUNGAL CHEMOTHERAPY[865]

Only a small number of antifungal drugs are available for treatment of systemic mycoses and there are very few controlled trials to demonstrate efficacy, none in children. Most of the antifungals act on the fungal cell membrane by either chelating ergosterol (polyenes) or inhibiting its synthesis (imidazoles, triazoles). 5-Flucytosine is a nucleoside analog that inhibits fungal transcription.

POLYENES

Nystatin is a microcrystalline suspension so should not be given parenterally. It is very effective in treating superficial infections due to sensitive fungi and resistance has developed very slowly if at all. Amphotericin B is active against a wide range of fungi in vitro including *Candida* spp., *C. neoformans*, *H. capsulatum* and *Aspergillus* spp. However, up to 40% of *P. marneffei* are resistant and the agents of chromoblastomycoses are usually resistant as are those causing eumycetoma.

For systemic mycoses, amphotericin B must be given intravenously by slow infusion but can also be given intrathecally, intraventricularly or intraperitoneally. The lyophilized powder must be reconstituted in 5% dextrose solution (not saline, which may cause it to precipitate) and is given as a slow infusion over 4–6 h at a concentration of 100 µg/ml. Usually treatment begins with a dose of 0.25 mg/kg/d with a gradual increase up to about 1 mg/kg/d as can be tolerated. A daily dose of 1.5 mg/kg/d should not be exceeded. For intrathecal use, doses of 0.1–0.5 mg or even 1 mg have been given to children according to weight and tolerance of the drug. Only 2–5% of the daily dose of amphotericin B is excreted in urine in the active form, and in experimental animals 20% is excreted in bile. The fate of the major part of the administered dose is unknown, but there are reports of detection of the drug in liver, spleen and kidney one year after cessation of therapy. There are no trials delineating duration of therapy, but treatment is usually given for 1–3 months depending upon the rate of clinical and laboratory improvement. Amphotericin B has a high toxicity profile. During a 4–6 h infusion, 50–90% of patients experience fever, chills, malaise, muscle and joint pains, nausea and vomiting. The major side-effect is nephrotoxicity: glomerular filtration rates fall by 40% in most patients and stabilize to 20–60% after multiple doses. Toxicity is manifest by increased blood urea and creatinine levels and the appearance of red cells, white cells and casts in the urine. If blood urea rises above 16.7 mmol/L or creatinine above 170 µmol/L treatment should be stopped until levels return to normal. Hematological side-effects occur in 75% of patients, most frequently a normochromic, normocytic anemia, and cardiac arrest, hepatotoxicity, neurotoxicity and allergic reactions do occur but are rare.

Encapsulating amphotericin B in liposomes (AmBisome, Abelcet) or in a colloidal dispersion (Amphocil) gives better tolerance and fewer side-effects in doses up to 3–5 mg/kg/d.

FLUCYTOSINE

5-Flucytosine is a fluorinated pyrimidine that was originally developed as an antineoplastic drug. Its mechanisms of action are, on conversion to 5-fluorouracil in the fungus, to act as an analog of uracil, inhibiting protein synthesis and to inhibit thymidylate synthetase and thus DNA synthesis. It has a narrow spectrum of activity but is usually active against *C. albicans* and *C. neoformans*. However, resistance even in these fungi can develop, so it is most often used in combination with amphotericin B. It is well absorbed orally and is usually given at 50–100 mg/kg/d in four divided doses in neonates and children. Although less toxic than amphotericin B, it can cause bone marrow suppression, cutaneous reactions (particularly in AIDS patients) and diarrhea. The risk of bone marrow suppression is greater with concomitant amphotericin B therapy and appears more likely in children. For these reasons, it is advisable to measure peak (2 h post oral or 30 min post intravenously) and trough (just prior to dose) serum levels twice weekly during therapy. Peak levels should not exceed 100 mg/L and the trough is around 25 mg/L.

IMIDAZOLES

Of the licensed imidazoles, clotrimazole is solely a topical agent, while ketoconazole can be given topically or orally and miconazole topically or intravenously. Miconazole has a broad range of antifungal activity in vitro but is less active against *Aspergillus* spp., *Hansenula* (now Pichia) *anomala* and *Mucor* spp. It is particularly useful for topical application in dermatophyte infections and in oral and cutaneous candidiasis. Intravenous miconazole should be considered in patients unable to tolerate amphotericin B and as an alternative to the latter drug in systemic infections with *Candida* resistant to flucytosine.

Recommended dosage for oral candidiasis is 5 ml of miconazole gel (20%) two to four times per day. For systemic infections, an ampoule containing 200 mg of miconazole should be diluted with 5% dextrose or physiological saline solution and administered by slow intravenous infusion three times daily. In children, the total daily dose is of the order of 40 mg/kg body weight.

Toxic effects are in general less frequent and less severe than those encountered with amphotericin B therapy. They include gastrointestinal, mental and liver enzyme disturbances. The poor water solubility of miconazole necessitates the use of a lipophilic solvent causing major problems with venous irritation and occlusion.

Ketoconazole has an even better antifungal spectrum of activity. It is a less toxic alternative to amphotericin B but does cause gastrointestinal problems (in 3–40%) and hepatocellular damage (most often in females over 40 years). Its use has been reported in systemic candidiasis, coccidioidomycosis and histoplasmosis. An appropriate dose is 3 mg/kg daily orally for a child and 200–400 mg once daily for an adult. Treatment should be maintained for 10 days, in the case of oral thrush, and for at least 1 month in the case of systemic infections. Less than 10% of either drug is excreted in urine, so they are of little use in urinary tract infections.

TRIAZOLES

The two major antifungals in this recently introduced class of drugs are fluconazole and itraconazole. Fluconazole has high bioavailability, and peak serum concentrations are similar by either the oral or intravenous routes. It is active against most *C. albicans* and *C. neoformans* but some other *Candida* spp. (e.g. *C. krusei*) are resistant. Its main clinical use is in treating cryptococcosis and candidiasis. In children over 4 weeks, recommended doses are 3 mg/kg/d for mucosal candidiasis, 6–12 mg/kg/d for systemic candidiasis or cryptococcosis and 3–12 mg/kg/d for prophylaxis in neutropenic children. Neonates aged 2–4 weeks should be given similar doses but every 2 days, and those aged 2 weeks and under every 3 days. Fluconazole is generally well tolerated with nausea, vomiting, abdominal pain and diarrhea in less than 5%. Asymptomatic elevation of hepatic aminotransferase enzymes occurred in 12% of children after 4 days of intravenous therapy.[866] About 80% of the drug is excreted by the renal route. Itraconazole has an even broader spectrum of activity being active against most *Candida* spp., *H. capsulatum*, *B. dermatitidis*, *C. immitis*, *P. braziliensis*, *P. marneffei*, *A. flavus* and *A. fumigatus*. It has an equally broad clinical use for infections by the above and in sporotrichosis, chromoblastomycosis and phaeochromomycosis. For the latter two, response depends on the infecting fungus. The dose is 2.5–5 mg/kg daily by the oral route. The duration of therapy depends upon the infection being treated. Itraconazole has a good safety profile but very little of the drug is excreted in urine.

ECHINOCANDINS

This novel class of antifungals includes caspofungin, micafungin and anidulafungin. They inhibit β(1,3)-D-glucan synthesis in the fungal cell wall. They are clinically effective in invasive candidiasis and candidemia but less effective in aspergillosis.[867] They have little or no activity against the rest of the fungi described here.

HELMINTH INFECTION

Helminth or worm infections occur worldwide, although in warmer, moister areas, especially where standards of hygiene are low, the range of species and prevalence tends to be greater and multiple infections are common. Because children tend to live more closely with nature and with their pets, many helminth infections are more common in children than in adults. Reviews listing the estimated prevalence of the variety of worm infections in humans worldwide indicate that a vast health problem exists. New and emerging helminth zoonoses continue to be identified.[868]

Many tentative prevalence figures are undoubtedly underestimates. One review[869] concluded that there are more trematodes infecting humans than any other group of animal parasites, over 75 species, mostly acquired from poorly prepared or cooked food.[870]

Helminth infections are by no means confined to tropical or resource limited countries and the increase in travel and of refugee movements in recent years has led to an increasing awareness in resource rich countries of the dangers of imported diseases.[871]

Helminth infections differ in most cases from those caused by viruses, bacteria or protozoa, in that the clinical effects exhibited by the host are mostly related to the worm load carried, and the latter in turn is usually related to the infective dose. The controversy regarding the possible adverse effects of helminth infections and the value of anthelmintic treatment on cognitive function and learning or educational ability remains unresolved, but the concept may well be valid.[872,873]

The common parasitic helminths infecting humans include the Nematoda (roundworms) and Platyhelminthes (flatworms) which comprises the Trematoda (flukes) and Cestoda (tapeworms). Less commonly humans may be infected with such worms as the Acanthocephala (thorny headed worms).[874]

The control of human helminth infections usually depends on a detailed knowledge of the epidemiology and life cycles of the species concerned – the aim being to break the cycle. The following principles are utilized, either alone or in combination, depending upon the species:

1. treatment of infected individuals, including mass treatment;
2. control of animal reservoirs where such exist;
3. hygiene, which includes education and provision of adequate and acceptable toilet facilities;
4. vector control where applicable;
5. the wearing of shoes where infection occurs from the soil through the skin;
6. instruction in food preparation and cooking;
7. immunization – a field which continues to be of great interest.

Of all the above, the most important method for the control of human helminthiases remains education combined with improved sanitation and personal hygiene. However, mass de-worming may play an important role in the control of some helminthiases and, in relation to immunization, Maizels et al[875] expressed the view that 'vaccines are the one major goal of the helminthological community'.

NEMATODES (ROUNDWORMS)

Nematodes are nonsegmented worms, round in transverse section with separate sexes. They possess both gut and body cavity (pseudocele). Species particularly important to humans include amongst others: *Ascaris lumbricoides, Toxocara canis, Enterobius vermicularis, Ancylostoma duodenale, Necator americanus, Trichuris trichiura, Strongyloides stercoralis, Trichinella spiralis, Onchocerca volvulus, Loa loa, Wuchereria bancrofti, Mansonella perstans, Mansonella ozzardi* and *Brugia malayi*.

ASCARIASIS

The intestinal roundworm *Ascaris lumbricoides* is cosmopolitan but variable in distribution, thriving in a moist climate, temperate or tropical, and especially under conditions of overcrowding. Ascariasis (like trichuriasis) tends to have a lower prevalence and worm load at higher altitudes.[876] The adult ascarids, male and female, live in the lumen of the small intestine, maintaining only an intermittent attachment to the mucosa. The gravid female lays an average of 200 000 eggs each day. Newly excreted eggs may remain dormant for a long period. If conditions are suitable they develop into an infective egg in about 2 weeks, in which condition they can remain viable for months or years until ingested.[877] The only hosts of these worms are humans, although cases of human infection with *A. suum*, the pig ascarid, have also been recorded. The life cycle of *A. lumbricoides* is depicted in Figure 28.56.

Clinical features

In 80% of cases the only manifestation of ascariasis is the asymptomatic passage of eggs and adult worms in the stool. Symptoms are related to three phases of the ascarid's life cycle:

1. invasion and migration of larvae;
2. presence of a large adult worm load;
3. migration of adult worms from their normal habitat.

To this one may add symptoms associated with the development of true allergy to the ascarid.[878]

Ascariasis is potentially serious and can contribute to a significant proportion of abdominal emergencies in children.[879]

Larval pneumonitis

The initial migration of larvae through the intestinal wall and via the portal circulation to the lungs may, in the case of heavy infection, or with repeated reinfections, cause a characteristic and often seasonal clinical picture.[880] The patient develops a dry spasmodic cough with intermittent wheezing and breathlessness, transient rhonchi and crackles in the lung fields; rarely, hemoptysis occurs. There may be malaise, with fever as high as 40 °C, discomfort over the liver, and urticarial rashes. Radiological examination of the chest reveals diffuse, mottled opacities, peribronchial infiltration or areas of pneumonitis. Marked eosinophilia is present. Symptoms and signs subside after 2 or 3 weeks and the eosinophilia generally diminishes to 3–5% of the total white cell count. Chronic lung disease occasionally results from repeated larval onslaughts. Severe pulmonary infiltration with asthma, eosinophilia and raised IgE levels can occur in children infected with *A. suum*.

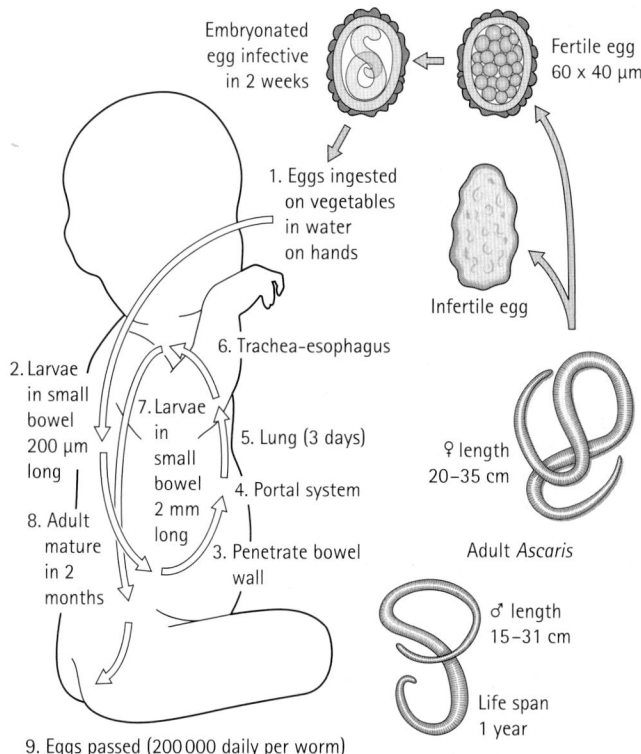

Fig. 28.56 Character and life cycle of *Ascaris lumbricoides*.

Worm load

Although some features of intestinal ascariasis are of an allergic nature, in the healthy child on a normal diet it is unlikely that the presence of a few ascarids will cause any significant disturbance.[880] A large worm load will, however, drain off a considerable proportion of a child's nutritional intake and in children can be associated with impaired lactose digestion and absorption.[879] Heavy infections are usually seen in underprivileged communities where nutrition is already inadequate. The combination of malnutrition, vitamin and iron deficiency, and the almost invariable presence of intestinal parasites of other types, makes the part played by ascarids difficult to assess. However, studies in Colombia have shown that steatorrhea and D-xylose malabsorption associated with heavy loads of *Ascaris* improved after de-worming. These children are ill, stunted and marasmic, with abdominal distention. Colicky abdominal pain is frequent. There may be low grade fever and a mass of worms can often be palpated abdominally. Toxins from ascarids may play a part in producing the chronic illness.

Intestinal complications associated with a heavy worm burden are frequently seen in hyperendemic areas.[881] A bolus of worms (usually both dead and living) may impact, particularly near the ileo-cecal junction (Fig. 28.57). A mass of ascarids may also precipitate temporary obstruction from spasm, cause inflammatory reactions and adhesions, or lead to volvulus or intussusception.

Migration of adult worms

Under certain circumstances, particularly with high fever, gastrointestinal upset or ineffectual anthelmintic therapy (e.g. the use of tetrachlorethylene for a concomitant hookworm infection), an ascarid may migrate from its normal habitat in the bowel and be vomited, or wriggle up the esophagus and emerge through the nose. Lodgment in the appendix or Meckel's diverticulum can result in obstruction and perforation. The common bile duct may be blocked by a roundworm, leading to severe upper abdominal pain, vomiting, tenderness and enlargement of the liver, a palpable gallbladder, and jaundice. Pancreatitis is a further complication. Other manifestations of the migrating ascarid include intestinal perforation with peritonitis, chronic peritonitis due to the presence of eggs, soft tissue or liver abscess, laryngeal impaction and even the passage of a worm per urethram. Ascarids can also penetrate perforations, suture lines and into drainage or suction tubes.

Roundworm sensitivity can produce a variety of allergic manifestations: nasal, pulmonary, dermal, or gastrointestinal.[880]

Diagnosis

Larval pneumonitis (Löffler syndrome) is generally suggested by the presence of eosinophilia, but other parasites can produce this syndrome (Table 28.43), and proof of diagnosis can only be obtained if a larva is identified in the sputum. Adult worms may later be passed in the stool or seen on radiological examination (Fig. 28.58) of the abdomen using barium. Diagnosis, however, rests almost wholly on finding eggs in the stools (Fig. 28.59), except in the event of early infection or a population of purely male worms. Serological and intracutaneous tests are available but as yet are of little practical value although they have been used in epidemiological surveys.[882]

Treatment

No treatment is known to remove migrating larvae, although some have claimed success using piperazine or pyrantel. The pneumonitis responds dramatically to prednisone.[880] Albendazole is a very valuable, broad spectrum anthelmintic with a wide activity against intestinal nematode species. It is generally well tolerated at doses recommended for these helminths and has, in fact, been designated as a 'WHO essential agent'. It is given at a dose of 400 mg as a single dose (200 mg for children < 10 kg).[877,880,883,884]

Two anthelmintics highly effective in ascariasis and with minimal side-effects are pyrantel embonate/pamoate (10–20 mg/kg, max. 750 mg) and mebendazole (100 mg 12-hourly for 3 days; children < 10 kg 50 mg 12-hourly for 3 days). Levamisole is also effective and

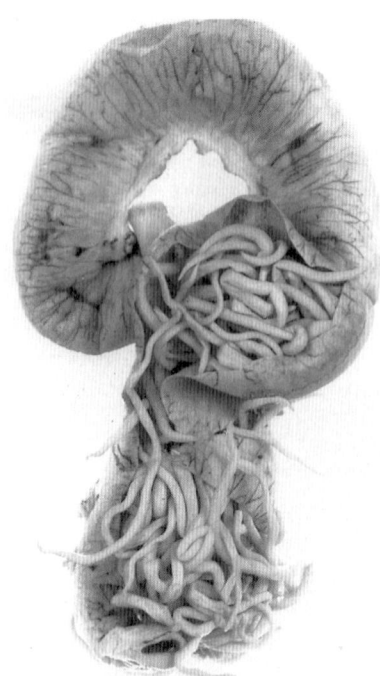

Fig. 28.57 Intestinal obstruction by *Ascaris lumbricoides* in a 14-year-old boy.

Table 28.43 Worms and fly larvae giving rise to pulmonary infiltrations, visceral larva migrans and cutaneous larva migrans

	Pulmonary infiltration with eosinophilia	Visceral larva migrans	Cutaneous larva migrans
Ancylostoma braziliense			×
Ancylostoma caninum			×
Ancylostoma duodenale	Rare		
Angiostrongylus cantonensis		×	
Anisakis species		×	
Ascaris lumbricoides	×	Rare	
Ascaris suum	×	×	
Capillaria hepatica		×	
Dirofilaria species	×	×	
Fly larvae			
Dermatobia species		×	
Gasterophilus species			×
Hypoderma species			×
Gnathostoma species		×	×
Necator americanus	Rare		'Ground itch'
Schistosoma species			'Swimmer's itch'
Strongyloides stercoralis	×	Rare	'Ground itch'
Toxocara canis	×	×	
Toxocara cati	Uncertain	Uncertain	
Uncinaria stenocephala			×

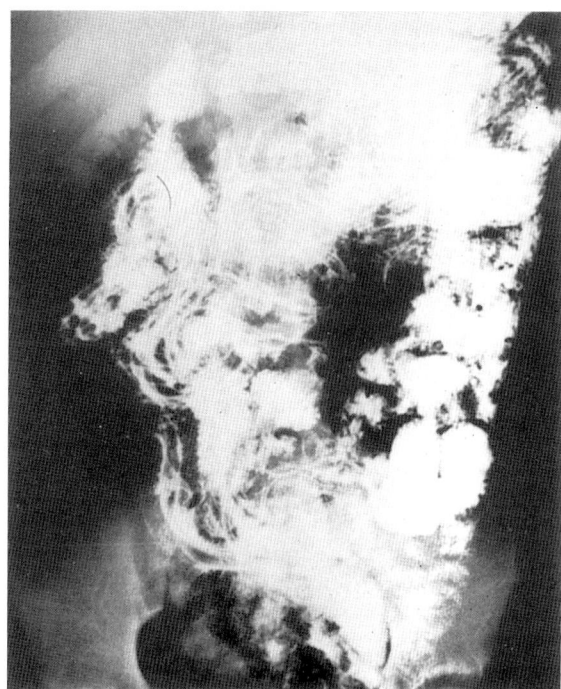

Fig. 28.58 *Ascaris lumbricoides.* Barium follow-through showing infestation in small bowel with worms coated with barium.

piperazine has been used with success in the past. Tiabendazole, although effective, is best avoided owing to its side-effects.[885,886]

Overall, albendazole seems to be the drug of choice for ascariasis but, while results can be achieved quickly with chemotherapy, they are

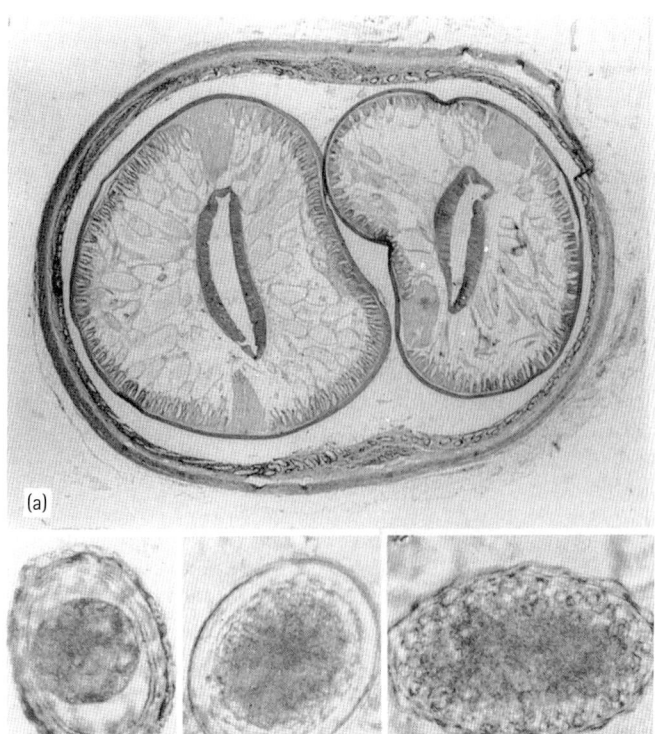

Fig. 28.59 (a) Pair of *Ascaris* in appendix (approx. × 10). (b) Fertilized egg of *Ascaris lumbricoides* (approx. × 600). (c) Decorticated fertilized egg of *A. lumbricoides* (approx. × 600). (d) Unfertilized egg of *A. lumbricoides* (approx. × 600).

only temporary in the absence of other control measures. Prevention of ascariasis depends on improving living conditions and the sanitary disposal of feces, on preventing contamination of drinking water and raw vegetables, and on education in hygiene. There is evidence too, to indicate that the mass delivery of anthelmintic treatment to children may be an important option in the control of geohelminth infections, including ascariasis. The 1993 World Development Report of the World Bank[887] includes mass de-worming in its 'essential package of health interventions' and school-based mass delivery is singled out as one of the most cost-effective measures – a concept supported by studies such as that of Guyatt.[888]

TOXOCARA CANIS AND VISCERAL LARVA MIGRANS

Toxocara canis is a close relative of *Ascaris*. Its natural hosts are the young dog and the fox, in which it undergoes a cycle essentially similar to *Ascaris* in humans (Fig. 28.60). The cycle in dogs is complicated by the development of immunity with expulsion of adult worms by the animals at about 6 months of age. In pregnant bitches, however, this immunity is lost and dormant larvae in the tissues are reactivated or reinfection occurs, resulting in the puppies being infected in utero and being born with worms. Children ingest infective eggs from dirt contaminated with dog feces or directly from the animals themselves, especially young puppies or lactating bitches.[889] The larvae, after penetrating the intestinal wall, are incapable of completing their pulmonary migration in an unnatural host and wander aimlessly, never to find their intestinal habitat. They pass through, or become encysted in liver, lungs, kidneys, heart, muscle, brain or eye, causing an intense local response from the tissue.

Clinical features

The child (most commonly 1–5 years of age) with visceral larva migrans (VLM) shows failure to thrive associated with pica (90% of cases), anemia (Hb < 9 g/dl in 45%), fever (80%) and enlargement of liver (65%) and spleen (45%). There is cough (80%), bronchospasm and wheezing (63%).[889] A single organ may bear the brunt of the infection so that pulmonary symptoms or neurological abnormalities due to brain involvement (convulsions, disturbances of consciousness, hemiparesis) may predominate. Intense and persistent eosinophilia lasting months or years and reaching levels as high as 80×10^9/L is characteristic and may be the only abnormality found. Serum globulin levels are raised, particularly IgM, IgG and IgE, and elevated titers of anti-A and anti-B isoagglutinins have been described in 39% of cases. Transient chest shadows are recorded in about 50% of cases and the CSF may show an eosinophilia where the CNS is involved. The infection usually runs a chronic, benign course of 18 months or so and generally the prognosis is good, although deaths have been reported.

Ocular manifestations of toxocariasis (ocular larva migrans, OLM) may be the only evidence of the disease. The age of maximal ocular involvement is higher than that of systemic involvement, the average age being about 7–8 years. Loss of sight in the affected eye generally results, and usually only one eye is involved. A diagnosis of ocular toxocariasis should be considered when there is inflammatory detachment of the retina or retinitis of the posterior pole in a child, especially in one with geophagic habits, who has contact with young dogs. The diagnosis can be confused with retinoblastoma, which may lead to the unnecessary surgical removal of an eye in a child with ocular toxocariasis.

It appears, therefore, that there are two toxocaral syndromes in humans:

1. larvae in the eye, presenting as granulomatous pseudotumors of the retina (OLM);
2. generalized toxocariasis with numerous larvae in the liver and other organs and associated with fever and eosinophilia (VLM).

Because ocular lesions are seldom found in the generalized forms, and because ocular disease is almost entirely confined to children, it has been postulated that ocular toxocariasis could be the manifestation of congenital infection of the child from an infected mother, in a similar fashion to the transplacental infection of puppies. This

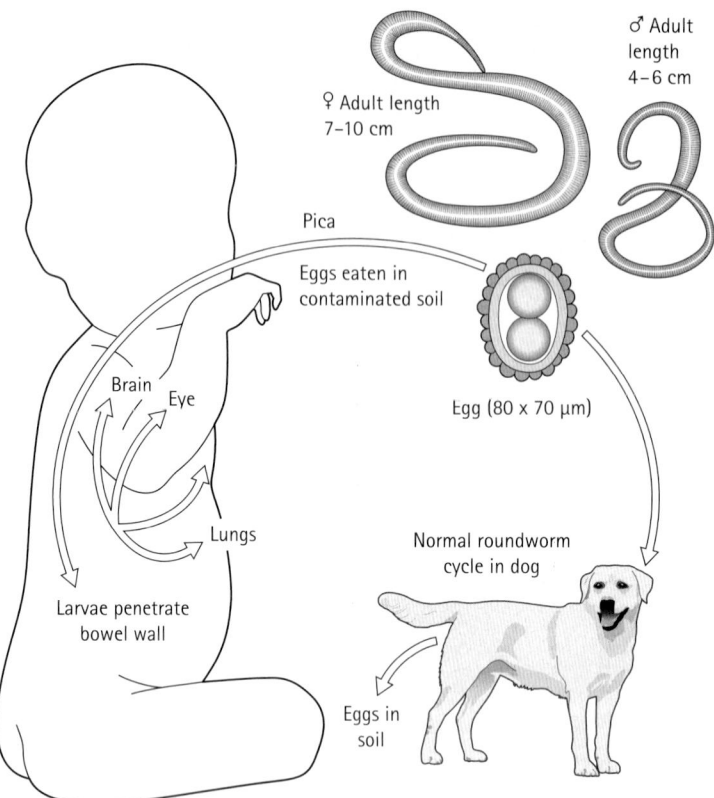

Fig. 28.60 Character and life cycle of *Toxocara canis*.

hypothesis, if true, would have important implications for expectant mothers. Similarly, contact with cats or cat litter might entail risk of fetus-damaging infection due to toxocariasis from *Toxocara cati* as well as toxoplasmosis.

It has been suggested that the eosinophilia so often seen in children suffering from lead poisoning resulting from pica may well be due to concurrent *Toxocara* infection. Physicians managing children with lead intoxication should be aware of this possibility and treat the toxocariasis concurrently.

A similar clinical syndrome can be caused in children by filarial parasites of animal origin and by larvae of other types[889] (Table 28.43). It still remains unclear whether *T. cati* (the cat roundworm) can be responsible for systemic larva migrans, and another dog ascarid, *Toxascaris leonina*, previously thought to be non-infective to humans, should be considered as a potential cause of visceral larva migrans.

Diagnosis

Acquisition of a puppy in the preceding year has proved to be a good suggestive indicator of *Toxocara* infection in symptomatic patients.[889] The diagnosis can only be established with certainty, however, by a biopsy (generally of the liver) or, undesirably and rather drastically, after enucleation of the eye. Skin tests and serological tests such as the indirect fluorescent antibody test and the *Toxocara* enzyme immunoassay (EIA) are available with the latter having a reported sensitivity of 78% and a specificity of 92%.[889,890] It is worth noting that 2–7% or more of symptomless adults and up to 23% of children with no symptoms may have detectable *Toxocara* antibodies.[889,891]

Fluorescein angiography, ultrasound and CT scans are also described as useful adjuncts to diagnosis.[890]

Treatment

Diethylcarbamazine (DEC) (2 mg/kg 8-hourly for 7–10 days) is reportedly effective.[883,890] An alternative regimen is up to 6 mg/kg in divided doses for 3 weeks.[889] Repeated courses may be necessary and if respiratory distress or myocardial involvement develops, corticosteroids may be life-saving.

Tiabendazole at a dose of 50 mg/kg per day for 3–5 days or 25 mg/kg for 1–4 weeks has also been recommended in the past and has been considered especially useful for early ocular cases where diethylcarbamazine should not be used, as the cellular response it elicits could aggravate visual problems. Corticosteroids are also important in controlling ocular lesions and should be given before the DEC is started.[890] Albendazole (400 mg 12-hourly for 3–5 days) has shown promise and flubendazole has also proved encouraging.[890,892]

Overall, however, the chemotherapy for toxocariasis remains unsatisfactory.

Prevention

While the dangers of infection from pets cannot be overstressed, this is a very emotive issue. Hungerford[893] stated: 'In our stress distorted society, pets...may be the critical factor in maintaining or restoring mental health or happiness to an only child, or to a psychotic, mentally distraught or lonely child or adult.'

The answer, therefore, is not destruction of pets, but regular and routine de-worming of dogs, especially puppies and pregnant bitches, with mebendazole, fenbendazole, piperazine or pyrantel pamoate. Also important is education to impress upon children and expectant mothers the need to wash their hands after handling pets and not to allow dogs to lick them on the face. Dogs and cats should also be prevented from defecating where children play (sandpits, etc.).

ENTEROBIUS VERMICULARIS (OXYURIASIS)

Enterobius vermicularis (threadworm, pinworm, seatworm) is common worldwide, but unlike most nematodes it is more prolific in temperate and cold climates. The incidence is highest in schoolchildren from 5 to 9 years with another peak at 30–49 years.[894] Boys and girls are equally affected. Enterobiasis is particularly common in highly populated districts, institutional groups, and among members of the same family. Incidences as high as 40–50% have been reported and in institutions such as mental hospitals, prevalence may reach 90–100%. The absence of a prolonged developmental stage outside humans (Fig. 28.61) favors reinfection and transmission from child to child. Hands are contaminated by scratching the perianal area where eggs are deposited, and by contact with soiled underclothing, nightclothing or bedding. Infection is also acquired by inhalation of egg-containing dust, which may be disseminated from bedclothing by shaking, or movements of the sleeper. At room temperature eggs survive for 2–3 weeks. Furthermore, retroinfection may occur when the eggs hatch on the perianal area and larvae find their way back through the anus into the intestinal tract.

The usual habitat of the threadworm of both sexes is the caecum and adjacent appendix, lower ileum, and colon. The worms are free in the intestinal lumen or lie with their heads attached to the mucosa. Gravid females migrate to the lower colon and rectum and crawl through the anus to deposit thousands of sticky eggs on the anal verge and perineum at night, usually dying thereafter. It is worth emphasizing that dogs and cats play no part in the transmission of enterobiasis to humans.

Clinical features

Threadworm infection is generally asymptomatic. The most common manifestation is anal pruritus due to migration of the worms and the presence of eggs. Restless sleep, nightmares, teeth grinding, and perhaps bed-wetting may result. In up to 20% of girls, vulval irritation and vaginal discharge are caused by threadworms and can persist for years[877] and night crying may be due to a threadworm in the vaginal introitus. Excoriation and pyogenic infection can follow from constant scratching.

It is most unlikely that threadworms play any significant part in causing the variety of symptoms commonly attributed to them. For example, threadworms are no more common in children with recurrent abdominal pain than in those without pain. Similarly, threadworms are found as often in normal appendices as in appendices showing acute or chronic inflammation, so that they are not considered to play any material role in the production of appendicitis, although appendiceal blockage resulting in a simulated chronic appendicitis may occur at times.[894]

Nail biting, nose picking, masturbation, convulsions, hyperkinesis and other behavior disturbances are also often erroneously ascribed to these parasites.

Very heavy infections can, however, result in catarrhal inflammation of the bowel from the attachment and irritation of worms, resulting in gastrointestinal disturbance. Intestinal obstruction has even been reported. Rarely, heavy infections have led to invasion of the bowel and appendiceal walls, peritoneum or viscera by larvae and immature worms. In their external migration gravid threadworms may occasionally crawl up the vagina into the uterus and Fallopian tubes or into the urethra and bladder depositing eggs in these sites with resulting low grade salpingitis, cystitis or urethritis, and cases are on record of worms penetrating the intestinal wall, probably through a pre-existing mucosal breach, to reach the peritoneal cavity.

Enterobiasis may be associated with infection by the protozoan flagellate, *Dientamoeba fragilis*, which is believed to be transmitted within the egg of the threadworm and may be a cause of diarrhea.[895]

Eosinophilia is usually absent in enterobiasis but may occur in up to 12% of cases.

Diagnosis

Often the first evidence of infection is the discovery of the adult worms in the feces, particularly after enemas, or on the perineum. Worms may be clearly visible on proctoscopy. The most widely used and effective method of obtaining eggs from the perianal region is the adhesive cellulose tape method. The adhesive side of a piece of transparent tape is applied to the anus and surrounding skin – either directly or wrapped round a test tube – and the tape then transferred adhesive side down to a glass slide. The adhering eggs are clearly visible under a microscope (Fig. 28.62a). The test is best performed in the morning before bathing or defecation, and in view of the irregular migrations of gravid worms at least three examinations should be made on consecutive days. Eggs are found in the stools in only 5–10% of cases, but five perianal swabs reveal eggs in 97% of infections.

Treatment

Drugs of choice for enterobiasis include mebendazole, albendazole and pyrantel embonate/pamoate. Mebendazole given in a single dose of 100 mg (one tablet) stat. is recorded as giving a cure rate of about 95% with no or very few side-effects.[877] Although some authorities advise that mebendazole should not be used in children < 2 years of age, others accept that a dose of 50 mg can be used for a child < 10 kg.[884] Albendazole is also reported as effective, at a dose of 400 mg orally (200 mg in children 10 kg or less).[896] Neither mebendazole nor albendazole should be used during pregnancy.[884]

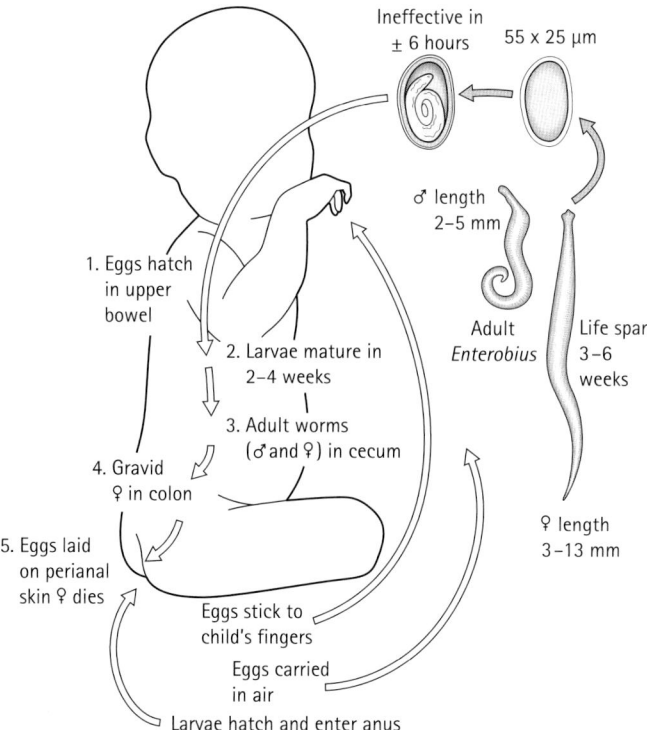

Fig. 28.61 Character and life cycle of *Enterobius vermicularis*.

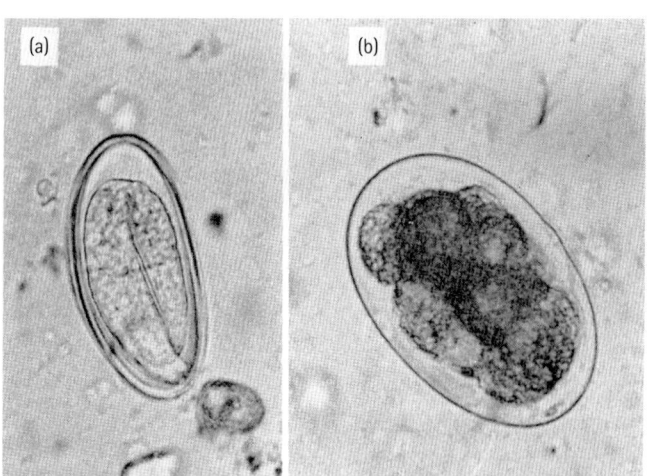

Fig. 28.62 (a) Fully developed egg of *Enterobius vermicularis* (approx. × 600). (b) Hookworm egg (approx. × 600).

Pyrantel 11 mg/kg is also very effective as a single dose treatment, giving cure rates greater than 90%. Side-effects are usually mild (e.g. nausea and vomiting), occurring in about 3% of cases.[877,886]

Piperazine citrate and pyrvinium pamoate are no longer in general use for enterobiasis, and tiabendazole, while efficacious, has unpleasant side-effects.

When a child is treated for enterobiasis, the whole family should be treated, and a second course should be given after 3 weeks. Unfortunately, reinfection is the rule rather than the exception. Intractable family infections can be controlled by the treatment of all family members with 100 mg (50 mg for children <10 kg) mebendazole a week for 12 weeks.

Prevention of recurrence is extremely difficult, particularly in crowded communities and in humid temperate climates, which facilitate prolonged survival of eggs. Personal cleanliness is essential and this includes cutting fingernails, regular hand washing before meals and after using the toilet, washing the anal area on rising, and regular changing of underclothing and bed linen.

HOOKWORM (ANCYLOSTOMIASIS)

Ancylostoma duodenale (Old World hookworm) and *Necator americanus* (tropical hookworm) are morphological variants, tropical hookworm being rather smaller with differences of fine morphology.

Hookworm occurs in most tropical and subtropical areas of the world, with *A. duodenale* distributed mainly around the Mediterranean littoral and *N. americanus* in south and central Africa and southern America. Both species are, however, widely distributed today in Asia as well as in most other tropical countries. In South East Asia and Brazil, *A. ceylanicum* infections of humans occur as well and *A. malayanum* is yet another species from humans.[877] Hookworm is one of the world's chief causes of anemia.

A. braziliense, one cause of cutaneous larva migrans (Table 28.43) and a natural parasite of dogs and cats, is widely distributed throughout tropical and subtropical areas, while the common dog hookworm *A. caninum* is also widely distributed, and *Uncinaria stenocephala* infects dogs in temperate regions. These latter two species can also cause cutaneous larva migrans in humans and it is claimed that in northern Queensland in Australia, *A. caninum* may be a cause of eosinophilic enteritis in humans as discussed by Smyth.[897]

The excreted egg, in favorable damp, shady conditions, hatches on the soil in about 2 days, releasing a rhabditiform larva which develops 8–10 days after hatching into the infective (filariform) larva. This larva penetrates the skin of the host, although *A. duodenale* is believed also to enter via the oral route with fecally contaminated food and water and may infect by the transmammary and transplacental routes from infected mother to child.[898] The life cycle in humans from larval penetration to oviposition lasts about 5 weeks (Fig. 28.63). The adult worm may survive within its host for 7 years or longer.

Adult worms are attached to the wall of the jejunum, or, less commonly, the duodenum, by their buccal capsules, sucking blood from their hosts. Each worm may suck up to 0.5 ml of blood per day; thus heavy worm loads may result in a loss of 100–150 ml/day. Significant damage is therefore produced by hookworms, but clinical manifestations depend on the host's general resistance, on the worm load, and on the child's dietary intake and iron reserves.

Clinical features
Larval invasion
Penetration of the skin, usually of the feet or buttocks, by the filariform larvae may produce, within minutes, a series of wheals, which soon develop into an itchy, papular and vesicular eruption ('ground/dew itch'). The rash may become ulcerative or pustular, but generally

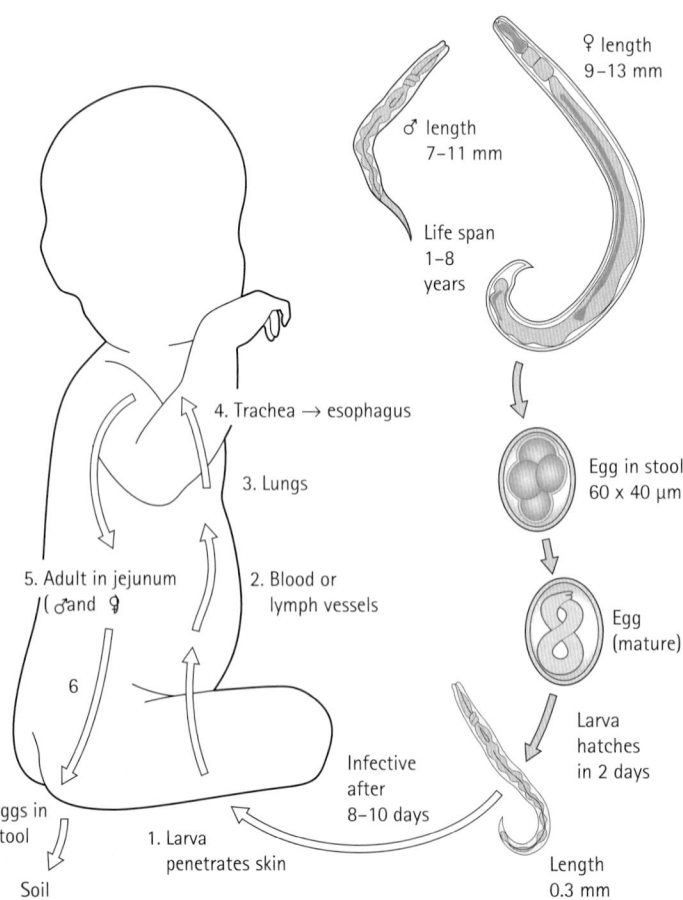

Fig. 28.63 Character and life cycle of hookworm.

subsides within 10 days and the larvae do not wander within the skin as in the case of cutaneous larva migrans (see below).

Migration through the lungs

After penetration of the skin, larvae reach the small intestine via the heart and lungs as in ascariasis.

Respiratory symptoms are unusual in children except in the case of heavy or repeated infections, particularly of *N. americanus*, when there may be cough, sore throat, bloody sputum and pulmonary changes on X-ray (Table 28.43).

Adult worms in the intestine

A distinction should be made between hookworm infection (where patients carry a subclinical worm load) and hookworm disease, which results from heavy worm loads and inadequate diet. Where heavy infections occur, symptoms develop 2–7 weeks after initial infection and consist of abdominal discomfort especially after meals, anorexia and sometimes nausea and vomiting. There may be intermittent diarrhea, general debility and undue tiredness. Once the adult worms are well established, there is little disturbance to the child, provided that the intake of iron, vitamins and protein keeps pace with the chronic blood loss produced by the parasites. When diet is inadequate and worm load heavy, severe hookworm disease results, characterized by profound iron deficiency anemia, hypoalbuminemic edema, cardiac failure and even death. It has been estimated that 100 worms will cause a daily loss of 4 mg of iron. A balanced diet easily compensates for this loss, but iron deficiency soon develops on a marginal dietary intake. Children with heavy hookworm infections are stunted, marasmic and anemic; their skin is dry and their face puffy. All aspects of development are retarded. An important concomitant which makes hookworm infection much more serious is sickle cell anemia.

A marked eosinophilia (40%) is characteristic of early hookworm infection. It reaches maximum intensity at about 3 months after initial infection and then diminishes gradually to levels of 5–20%. A partially effective protective immunity seems to develop in hookworm infection.[899,900]

Diagnosis

This depends on finding the eggs (Fig. 28.62b) in the feces, and an egg count should be performed if a causal relationship with a concomitant iron deficiency anemia is to be established. An egg count > 2000 eggs/g of feces is generally considered to be of clinical significance.

In old stool specimens rhabditiform larvae are occasionally found and can be distinguished from those of *Strongyloides* by the short buccal chamber and larger genital primordium of the latter.

Eggs similar to those of hookworms can be recovered from humans infected with *Trichostrongylus* spp., *Oesophagostomum* spp. and *Ternidens deminutus*. The eggs of the former species are more pointed than those of hookworm and the eggs of *T. deminutus* are significantly larger than those of the hookworm species. These infections can be treated as for hookworm.[901]

Treatment

Albendazole is reported to be effective against the migrating larval stages of the human hookworms, *A. duodenale* and *N. americanus*.[902] The avermectins (ivermectin) have shown promise against all stages of hookworm development, including migrating larvae.[877] Children with severe anemia, malnutrition or a heavy worm load should receive preliminary supportive treatment in the form of blood transfusion, high calorie and protein diet, vitamins and iron therapy before definitive treatment of the worms. A highly effective anthelmintic for hookworm infection is albendazole and at a single dose of 400 mg (200 mg for children 10 kg or less) it has also proved highly effective against a wide range of other intestinal helminths.[877,884] Albendazole is additionally reported to have ovicidal activity against hookworm, ascariasis and trichuriasis, making it especially valuable in integrated control programs for these infections.[902] Mebendazole also gives excellent cure rates for both species

of hookworm at a dose of 100 mg twice a day for 3 days or 50 mg for children 10 kg or less – and with few or no side-effects.

Pyrantel embonate/pamoate (11 mg/kg, max. 750 mg) is effective for *A. duodenale* given in a single dose regimen,[903] but for *N. americanus* needs to be given as a multiple dose treatment.

Other treatments for hookworm include phenylene diisothiocyanate and bephenium hydroxynaphthoate.

The preventive aspects of hookworm are complex and include education of the public into the mode of spread of the disease, provision and proper usage of latrines, improvement of diet, and, where the incidence is high, mass population treatment. The wearing of shoes will also help to prevent infection. Studies from Papua New Guinea by Quinell et al[903] suggest that host susceptibility differences may explain why different individuals are predisposed to heavy or light burdens. Interest continues regarding the possibility of vaccination against hookworm infection.[898,900,904]

CUTANEOUS LARVA MIGRANS (CREEPING ERUPTION, SAND WORM)
Clinical features

The larvae of the dog hookworms, *A. braziliense*, *A. caninum* and *U. stenocephala*, together with certain other parasites (Table 28.43), can produce in humans a long-lasting skin eruption which differs from that caused by 'human' hookworms. The larva, after penetrating the epidermis, is unable to enter the bloodstream or lymphatics and instead burrows just below the corium, traveling up to an inch a day. Papules mark the site of entry and advancing end of the larva and the tunneling causes slightly elevated, erythematous and serpiginous lines which itch intensely (Fig. 28.64). Vesicles may form along the course of the tunnels and scaling develops as the lesions age. The most common sites in children are the buttocks and the dorsum of the feet, but any area can be affected. The eruption generally disappears after 1–2 months, but may persist for 6 months or longer. The diagnosis is clinical.

Treatment

Topical tiabendazole 15% cream is the treatment of choice and can easily be made from the oral preparation by dissolving 500 mg tablets in a water base, if not commercially available. Ivermectin (children > 5 years) 200 µg/kg orally as a single dose, or albendazole 400 mg (200 mg for a child < 10 kg) orally, once daily for 3 days, is also effective.[884] Cryotherapy is unpleasant, ineffective and no longer used.

TRICHURIS TRICHIURA (TRICHOCEPHALIASIS, WHIPWORM)

The whipworm, so called for its thin anterior lash-like end (Fig. 28.65), is widely distributed, being most common in hot, damp environs. The adult nematode frequents the cecum but can occur in the appendix, colon or

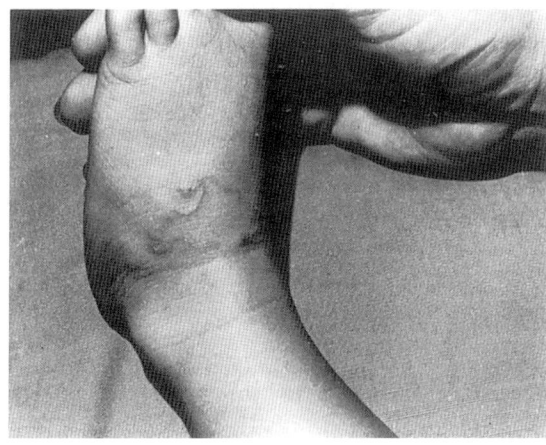

Fig. 28.64 Cutaneous larva migrans.

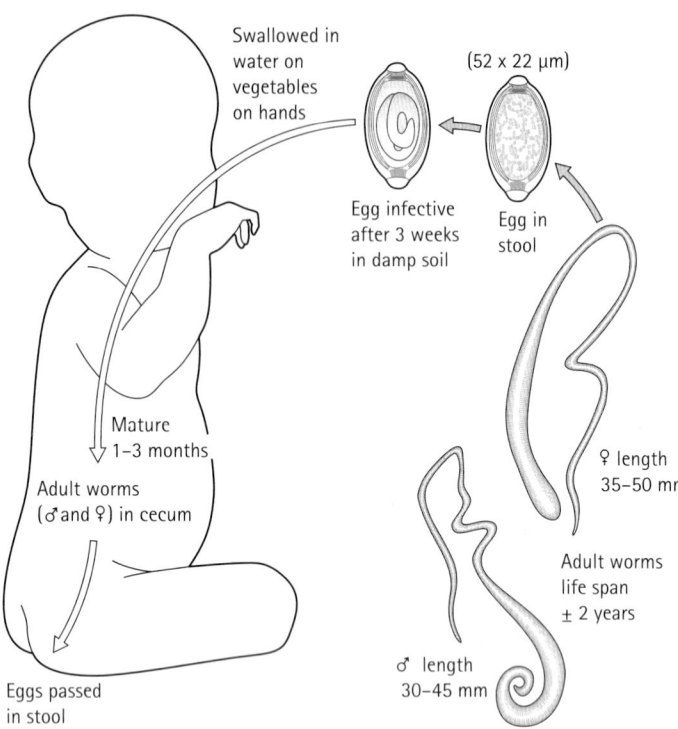

Swallowed in water on vegetables on hands

(52 x 22 μm)

Egg infective after 3 weeks in damp soil

Egg in stool

♀ length 35–50 mm

Mature 1–3 months

Adult worms (♂ and ♀) in cecum

Adult worms life span ± 2 years

♂ length 30–45 mm

Eggs passed in stool

Fig. 28.65 Character and life cycle of *Trichuris trichiura*.

terminal ileum, its thin anterior extremity threaded or embedded in the mucosa. Eggs pass out with the feces and mature on the soil in about 2–3 weeks. Children usually acquire whipworm by sucking fingers or objects contaminated with fecal-polluted soil containing infective eggs, but contaminated vegetables and fly-borne contamination of food are also important means of spread. Trichuriasis is by no means confined to the tropics[905] and may prove troublesome in mental institutions.

Trichuris vulpis, the dog whipworm, may occasionally infect humans.[891]

Clinical features

Whipworm infection is often asymptomatic but should not be underrated as a pathogen in humans.[905] Heavy worm loads may be responsible for intestinal symptoms including abdominal pain, which is most marked in the right iliac fossa simulating appendicitis, bloody diarrhea, tenesmus, and sometimes mild pyrexia. Heavy loads can lead to marked anemia, weight loss, and a picture closely resembling hookworm disease or amebic colitis. Clubbing of the fingers and toes is seen and is reversed with eradication of the infection. Rectal prolapse is a well-recognized complication. Trichuriasis often causes insidious disease and is frequently associated with growth retardation.[906]

Diagnosis

This is readily accomplished by finding the characteristic eggs (Fig. 28.66) in the stools. A barium enema may assist in diagnosis (Fig. 28.67).

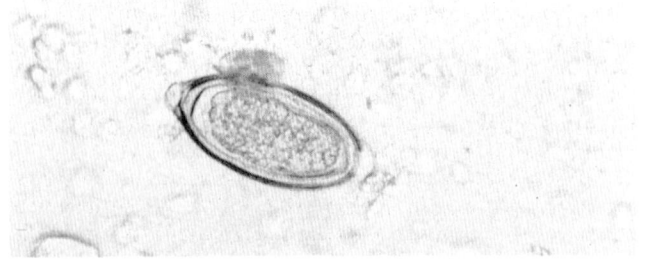

Fig. 28.66 Egg of *Trichuris trichiura* (approx. × 600).

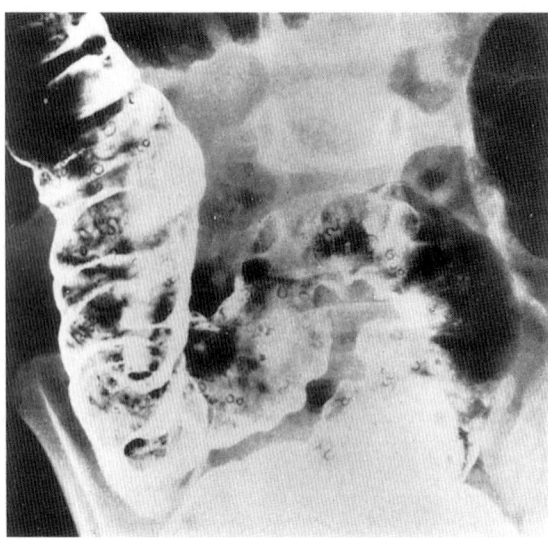

Fig. 28.67 *Trichuris trichiura*. Double contrast barium enema examination showing infestation and numerous small circular or sigmoid defects in barium coating of colon.

Treatment

Albendazole at a dose of 400 mg, or 200 mg for children 10 kg or less, given once, is the drug of choice,[884] but mebendazole can also be used at a dose of 100 mg (50 mg for a child 10 kg or less) 12-hourly for 3 days.[877] Difetarsone has been reported to be most useful in the treatment of whipworm, and oxantel pamoate is also reported to be effective.[877]

STRONGYLOIDES STERCORALIS (STRONGYLOIDIASIS)

Strongyloides stercoralis (sometimes termed 'threadworm' in the American literature) has a human cycle closely resembling hookworm, except that autoinfection is common and a free-living cycle can occur if external conditions are favorable (Fig. 28.68). Strongyloidiasis is most common in tropical or semitropical climates but may occur sporadically in temperate regions. The minute adult worms are to be found in the crypts of Lieberkuhn glands in the upper part of the small intestine, where they burrow into the mucosa.

In central Africa, *Strongyloides fülleborni* is often found in humans and a similar species is reported to cause 'swollen belly syndrome' in infants about 6 weeks of age in Papua New Guinea (PNG).[907] The species in PNG has been designated as *S. fülleborni Kellyi*, and infants as young as 18 days of age can become infected, possibly by transmammary infection, as may also occur with *S. fülleborni* in Africa.[908]

Clinical features

Skin penetration by filariform larvae may cause a transient prickling sensation, but following heavy infection there is a pruritic petechial rash with local edema. Internal and external autoinfection frequently occurs, especially in immunodeficient patients or patients on immunosuppressant drugs or corticosteroids, larvae in the feces entering through the rectal mucosa, anus or skin in the perianal region. This gives rise to an often recurring eruption resembling cutaneous larva migrans (termed larva currens) but of shorter duration. Generalized urticaria is sometimes seen as a result of hypersensitivity. Eosinophilia is common. Clinical manifestations of pulmonary migration of larvae are infrequent, but respiratory symptoms can occur and, rarely, chronic lung disease develops due to larvae maturing within the lung.

In chronic strongyloidiasis the presence of the adult worms in the intestine is often asymptomatic.[909] A heavy worm load causes epigastric pain, episodes of acute appendicitis,[896] bowel upset often with bloody diarrhea, iron deficiency anemia and debility. Infection can last 20 years or more, owing to constant internal and external autoinfection.[910]

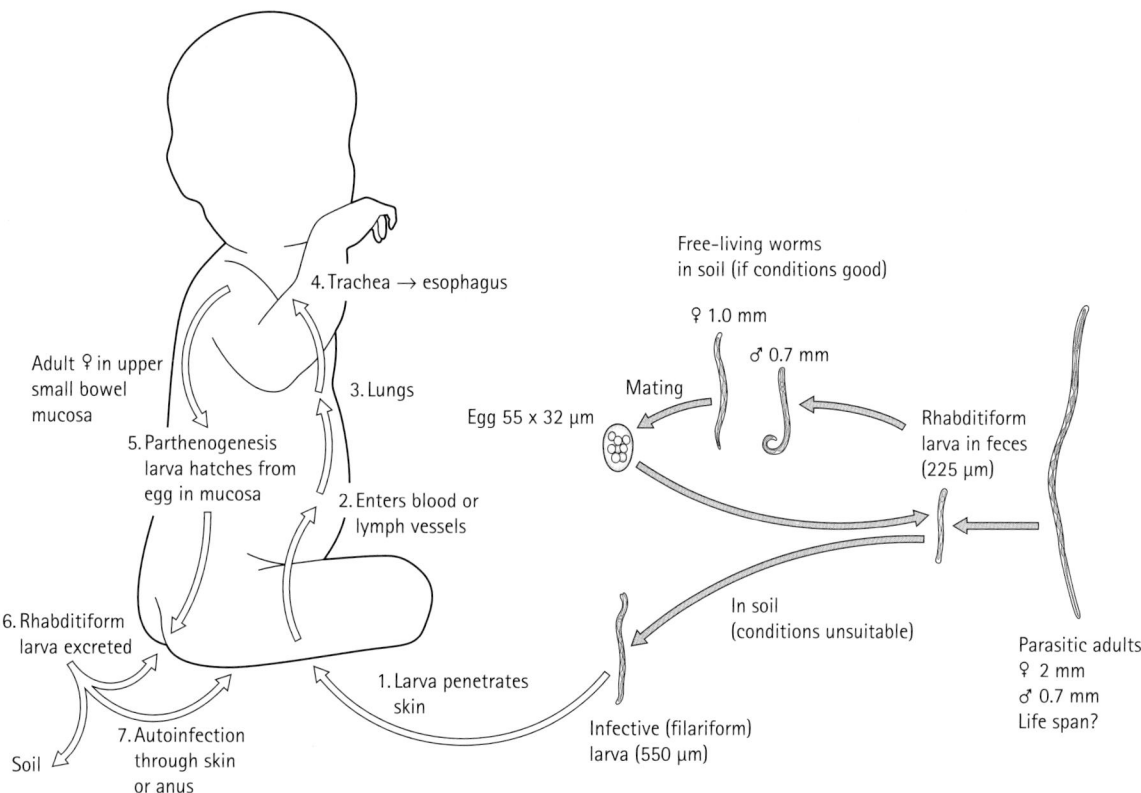

Fig. 28.68 Character and life cycle of *Strongyloides stercoralis*.

In immunocompromised patients, fatal infection can occur, but it is noteworthy that despite the HIV/AIDS pandemic in sub-Saharan Africa and elsewhere, *S. stercoralis* has not proved an important opportunistic pathogen, although an epidemiological association between strongyloidiasis and HTLV-1 has been reported.[901,909] *Strongyloides* hyperinfection syndrome may be complicated by Gram negative bacteremia in both immunocompromised and non-immunocompromised individuals and has a high mortality.[911,912]

Diagnosis

Considerable eosinophilia is usual and can be an important diagnostic indicator in some circumstances.[910] Diagnosis of *S. stercoralis* is established by demonstrating rhabditiform larvae (Fig. 28.69a) in fresh stools (repeat examinations may be necessary) or duodenal fluid. A useful method for diagnosing *S. stercoralis*, giardiasis, and other upper intestinal parasites is duodenal drainage or the use of the duodenal capsule (Enterotest), or 'string test'; a special pediatric size is available. The capsule, containing a length of thread and 3-ply nylon yarn, is swallowed while the protruding free end of thread is held at the mouth. The yarn within the capsule plays out, and within 3–4 h the line has almost invariably extended to the duodenum or jejunum. The gelatin capsule dissolves. The nylon yarn is then pulled back through the mouth and the adhering mucus examined for parasites.

Serological tests such as EIA are available in some countries, with sensitivities in the order of 80–90% and specificities of about 90%. These tests do not usually differentiate present from past infection and may cross-react with other nematode infections.[890]

In *S. fülleborni* infections, fully embryonated eggs (Fig. 28.69b) are passed in the feces. They are similar in appearance to hookworm eggs but much smaller, about 50 × 36 µm in size, are fully developed at time of passage[901] and hatch after about 2–3 h.

Treatment

Because of the dangers of autoinfection, especially in the immunocompromised, strongyloidiasis must always be treated when diagnosed.[913]

The treatment of choice for strongyloidiasis is now albendazole 400 mg 12-hourly, orally for 3 days (children 10 kg or less 200 mg), repeated after 7 days if the infection is disseminated.[884,902] Ivermectin 200 µg/kg orally each day as a single dose for 1–2 days can also be used

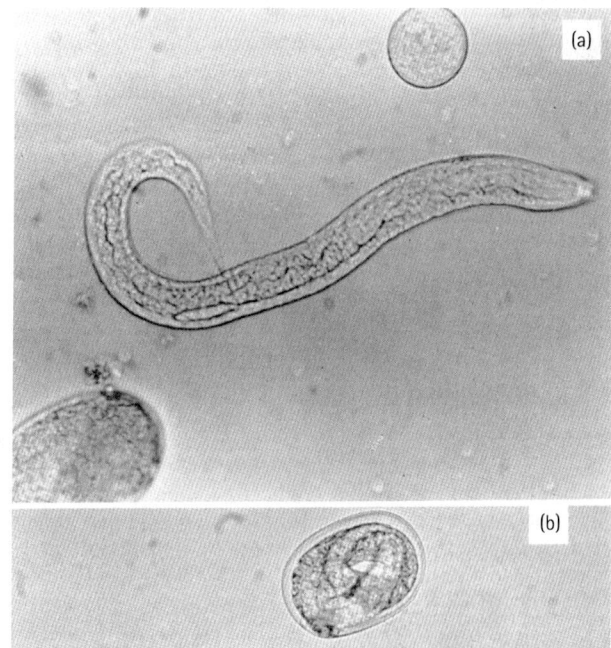

Fig. 28.69 (a) Rhabditiform larva of *Strongyloides stercoralis*. Note short buccal cavity and large genital primordium. Also in the field, an *Entamoeba* cyst and a hookworm egg (approx. × 600). (b) Egg of *Strongyloides fülleborni*. Note its small size. It contains a fully developed, motile larva when passed (approx. × 600).

for children > 5 years of age.[884,913,914] Tiabendazole, which is effective (25 mg/kg 12-hourly, orally, given morning and evening for 3 days up to a maximum total of 3 g daily), is an alternative, but can have unpleasant side-effects.[884,913]

ANGIOSTRONGYLIASIS

Angiostrongylus cantonensis is a natural parasite in the lungs of rats over much of the world, human infection being recorded from Indonesia, Papua New Guinea, Northern Australia, Africa, the Pacific, South East Asia, Cuba and Puerto Rico. The intermediate hosts are snails (such as the giant African land snail *Achatina fulica*) and slugs, which are eaten by the rodents. Humans become infected by eating certain edible snails or by accidental ingestion of small infected slugs on food plants or ingestion of paratenic (or 'carrier') hosts such as edible crustacea.[915]

In humans, larvae migrate to the brain causing eosinophilic meningitis, with neck stiffness, photophobia, pyrexia, decreased consciousness and vomiting.

The diagnosis can be suspected when large numbers of eosinophils are found in the CSF in patients with a history of eating snails or perhaps crustacea. Blood eosinophilia may also be present. Occasionally adults or larvae of *A. cantonensis* can also be detected. Surgical intervention may be necessary.[916] No effective specific treatment is presently available and may in any case be inadvisable as dead worms cause more clinical problems than live ones. However, mebendazole (100 mg 12-hourly for 5 days) together with corticosteroids (30–60 mg/day) is recommended for *A. cantonensis*.[890,913]

Other forms of angiostrongyliasis include an abdominal form caused by *A. costaricensis* in several Latin American countries. This species causes intestinal and liver lesions similar to those caused by *Toxocara*. It is usually diagnosed at surgery and has an epidemiology similar to *A. cantonensis*.[917] This species may require a higher dose of mebendazole than that recommended for *A. cantonensis*.[913]

HELMINTHOMA

Nodules in the bowel wall which contain the adult worms (helminthomas) can be caused by the nodular worms which belong to the genera *Oesophagostomum*, occurring naturally in simian and ruminant hosts, and the false hookworm, *Ternidens deminutus*, a natural parasite of nonhuman primates. These are known in Central Africa to cause human disease characterized, particularly in *Oesophagostomum*, by tumor-like granulomatous reactions in the wall of the colon.[918] *Ternidens* infections in humans have also been reported from Surinam and Thailand.[919,920] Eggs of these species are hookworm-like but those of *Ternidens* are larger in size.[901]

The drug treatment of choice for the expulsion of the adult worms is mebendazole (100 mg 12-hourly for 3 days). Albendazole is promising.[901,918]

ANISAKIASIS (ANISAKIDOSIS)

Anisakiasis in humans is caused by the larval stages of some 30 genera of anisakid nematodes, of which the most common are *Anisakis*, *Contracaecum*, *Terranova* and *Pseudoterranova*.[896,921] These helminths are intestinal parasites of a range of fish-eating vertebrates, including dolphins, and the larval stages of the worm are found in intermediate hosts such as small fish (e.g. mackerel, herring, salmon), squid or octopus.[922,923] Humans become infected when they eat raw or undercooked fish.

The ingested worms live in the human gastrointestinal tract or penetrate the tissues, giving rise to abscesses or eosinophilic granulomata.

Clinically the infection may be asymptomatic or mild with nausea, vomiting, epigastric pain and often an eosinophilia, which may exceed 40%. Rarely, death may result from peritonitis following perforation of the gut.[922]

While the infection has for many years been recognized in Japan, an increase has been noted in the USA owing to better diagnostic techniques.[923] Diagnosis is established at laparotomy, by X-ray or, most reliably, by endoscopy. Serological tests for diagnosis include the radioallergosorbent test (RAST) and counterimmunoelectrophoresis.

The most effective treatment, where possible, is removal of worms from the stomach by endoscopy. Prevention is best achieved by removing worms from fish prior to eating and by thorough cooking of fish. No effective anthelmintic treatment is presently available,[922] but Shorey et al[890] express the view that mebendazole might have some value, and albendazole at a dose of 400 mg 12-hourly for 21 days proved promising in one case.[921]

TRICHINOSIS

The genus *Trichinella* contains at least four species, the best known being *Trichinella spiralis*. This species has a cosmopolitan distribution, usually being transmitted to humans by eating inadequately cooked, infected pig meat, although outbreaks from other meat sources (e.g. horse meat) are recognized.[924,925] The disease may occur in outbreaks (Fig. 28.70). Trichinosis due to *T. spiralis* is rare in communities which shun pork and in those with vigilant agricultural control, but human disease, especially with other species (e.g. *T. pseudospiralis*, *T. nelsoni*, *T. britovi* or *T. nativa*), may follow eating the meat of other species of animal. Adult *T. spiralis* infect humans, pigs and rats, as well as other animals. Porcine infection usually results from the ingestion of either infected rats or garbage containing uncooked pork meat.

Clinical features

Human trichinosis is frequently mild or symptomless. Although symptoms may occur as early as 24 h following a pork meal, it is usually during the incubation period of 5–7 days or longer,[926] in which the ingested larvae mature into adults, that a clinical picture resembling food poisoning develops – nausea, vomiting, diarrhea and abdominal pain. This phase lasts about 5 days and is followed by signs and symptoms as the larvae enter the bloodstream and encyst in the muscle, a phase lasting a further 2–3 weeks. There is pyrexia, edema of the face and eyelids, splinter hemorrhages under the fingernails, tender lymphadenopathy and myalgia, often extreme. Cough may occur and in severe cases the illness may suggest encephalitis or myocarditis. Marked eosinophilia is usual. Final encystment of the larvae occurs only in voluntary muscles, particularly those of the diaphragm, throat, chest wall, extrinsic ocular apparatus and tongue, and patients may die of toxemia or myocarditis. The encysted larvae may live for many years.

Diagnosis

Diagnosis in the early stages can be made by finding worms in the feces, but in the later stages of the disease, diagnosis is established by muscle biopsy. Intracutaneous and fluorescent antibody tests, together with other serological procedures, are useful adjuncts.[890,926]

Treatment

Albendazole (400 mg for 3 days; 200 mg for children 10 kg or less) is the drug of choice. Mebendazole (200–400 mg daily for 3 days and then 400–500 mg for 10 days) is also recommended.[890,913]

There is evidence that tiabendazole (25 mg/kg per day 12-hourly for 5 days; max. 3 g daily) rapidly kills off migrating larvae and relieves the symptoms.[883] If taken early, the drug also kills larvae in the bowel but is not lethal to the adult worms. Corticosteroids, previously recommended for the treatment of trichinosis, should be restricted to critically ill cases,[916] and then only used in conjunction with anthelmintics.

PARACAPILLARIA PHILIPPINENSIS (CAPILLARIASIS)

It has long been known that the nematode *Capillaria hepatica* can cause a visceral larva migrans-like syndrome in people who have eaten meat (e.g. infected liver) or sand containing the eggs of the worm. Infected

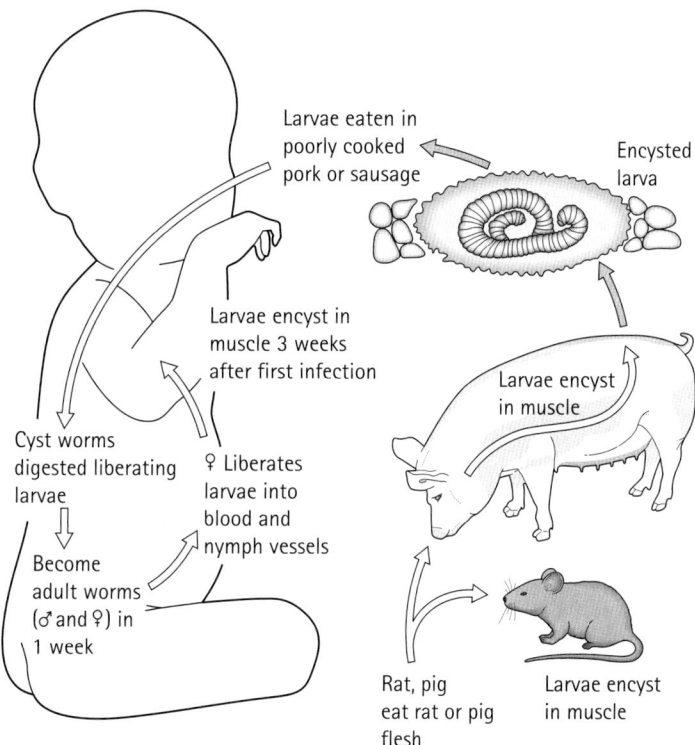

Fig. 28.70 Character and life cycle of *Trichinella spiralis*.

children exhibit such symptoms as fever, eosinophilia, abdominal pain and hepatomegaly, with large numbers of typical eggs being found in the liver on histological examination.

Another species of the genus, *Paracapillaria philippinensis*, has also been shown to be an important cause of epidemic diarrhea in humans in South East Asia and the Middle East. Clinical features in these cases include abdominal pain, malabsorption and diarrhea, which is often severe and not uncommonly fatal (35%) without medical care.[927]

P. philippinensis is a parasite of the small intestine, and is believed to be a zoonotic infection from birds and freshwater fish. Humans become infected by ingestion of eggs or infected raw fish, the usual intermediate host, and the host parasite load may increase as a result of autoinfection.[896]

Capillaria aerophila is found in the lungs of cats, and occasional human infections have been recorded.[890,896]

Diagnosis of capillariasis is based upon histology or finding eggs and larvae in feces. The eggs are like those of *Trichuris*, but the polar plugs are inset and the shells are striated or pitted. *C. hepatica* eggs can be found as spurious 'transit eggs' in feces of patients who have recently eaten infected liver.[928]

Tiabendazole has been used for treatment, but side-effects and relapses are common.[927] Mebendazole (200 mg 12-hourly for 20 days) and albendazole (400 mg daily for 10 days) are reported to be effective for the treatment of capillariasis.[896,913]

DRACUNCULOSIS (DRACONTIASIS)

Despite its bizarre mode of propagation, the guinea worm (*Dracunculus medinensis*) is widely distributed in equatorial Africa, the Middle East and India. However, with new international efforts to improve drinking water supplies, dracontiasis eradication may well be achievable.[929]

Clinical features

Children from the age of 2 years may be infected by drinking water containing *Cyclops*, a tiny crustacean which is infected with the larvae of *Dracunculus*. During the asymptomatic incubation period, lasting approximately 1 year, the guinea worm matures in retroperitoneal tissues. The male, having fertilized the female, apparently dies. The gravid female, often over 100 cm in length by 1.5 mm in width, then migrates

through the subcutaneous tissues to distal parts of the extremities, usually the lower limb, to form a large pruritic papule. This vesiculates, then bursts leaving a shallow ulcer. On immersion in water the worm's uterus prolapses through the ulcer releasing myriads of larvae. Occasionally adult worms may develop in ectopic sites.

Papule formation may be associated with a marked allergic reaction (vomiting, diarrhea, urticaria and bronchospasm).

Secondary infection of sinuses, subcutaneous cysts, sterile abscesses and periarticular fibrosis with joint deformity are recognized complications. Calcified worms may be discovered on radiological examination.

Treatment

The ancient technique of repeatedly stimulating the parturient worm with cold water, grasping the uterus which then protrudes, and then cautiously winding the worm round a stick an inch or two per day is still used. However, drug treatments recommended for dracontiasis include the use of niridazole (12.5 mg/kg 12-hourly for 7–10 days) and tiabendazole which has also been reported to be effective at a total dose of 25 mg/kg orally daily for 3 days.[883] Metronidazole is also claimed to be highly effective at an oral dose for children of 7.5 mg/kg (max. 250 mg) 8-hourly for 5–10 days.[883,885,913]

FILARIASIS

Filariasis is included among the diseases given priority by the United Nations Development Program/World Bank/WHO Special Program for Research and Training due to the huge number of people infected and the enormous burden of morbidity affecting whole communities in endemic regions.[930]

Humans are the primary hosts to several species of filariae, the adult worms living in the tissues. The adult female worms produce eggs which hatch to release pre-larval microfilariae. These are ingested by an appropriate blood-sucking arthropod vector, in which they undergo metamorphosis to form infective larvae. Important characteristics of the principal human filariae are shown in Table 28.44).

During the early stages of all filarial infections moderate to high eosinophilia is usual, but this gradually diminishes in those who have

Table 28.44 Types of filaria worms responsible for human disease

Type and distribution	Insect vector	Important features of microfilaria	Human adult worm location
Onchocerca volvulus, west, central and east Africa, Guatemala, Mexico, and Surinam	*Simulium* black flies	Do not occur in blood, but in skin as unsheathed intradermal microfilariae (microfilariae may penetrate eye)	Subcutaneous tissue
Mansonella perstans, tropical and subtropical areas mainly of Africa and South America	*Culicoides* midges	Occur in blood. Nonperiodic. Unsheathed. Nuclear column extends into tip of thick blunt tail	Mesenteric, perirenal and retroperitoneal tissues
Mansonella ozzardi, South America	*Culicoides* midges	Occur in blood. Nonperiodic. Nuclear column does NOT extend into tip of thin, pointed tail	Mesentery and serous body cavities
Wuchereria bancrofti, tropical and subtropical areas throughout the world	Many mosquitoes belonging to the genera *Culex, Acdes, Anopheles,* and *Mansonia*	Occur in blood. Nocturnal periodic. Sheathed. Nuclear column does NOT extend into tip of thin pointed tail	Lymphatic tissue
Brugia malayi, B. timori, East Indies and Southern Asia	Many mosquitoes belonging to the genera *Mansonia, Culex,* and *Anopheles*	Occur in blood. Nocturnal periodic. Sheathed. Nuclear column extends into tip of tail with single spaced nuclei in terminal bulb and subterminal swelling	Lymphatic tissue
Loa loa, west and central Africa	*Chrysops* flies	Occur in blood. Diurnal periodic. Sheathed. Nuclear column extends into tip of thick blunt tail	Subcutaneous tissue

been infected for long periods. Apart from *Onchocerca volvulus*, where microfilariae are found in skin snips, parasitological diagnosis is best achieved by using stained blood films or concentration techniques applied to peripheral blood. However, very promising and effective serological tests for the detection of circulating filarial antigen have been developed.

Onchocerca volvulus

Onchocerciasis is a filarial disease transmitted to humans by bites from black flies of the genus *Simulium*. It is characterized by subcutaneous nodules, containing adult worms of *O. volvulus*, by skin eruptions due to microfilariae, and by serious eye disease. The condition is only seen in Central Africa and in parts of South America (Table 28.44), especially along the banks of fast flowing rivers, in which the flies breed.

Clinical features

Adolescents are most commonly affected, but children down to 1 year of age may be afflicted. Signs of disease begin to appear after 4–18 months, and the commonest manifestation is the *Onchocerca* nodule. These subcutaneous fibrous nodules (onchocercomata), each containing one or more adult worms, vary from a few millimeters to about 3 cm in diameter and become fully developed within a year of exposure. In Africa, they tend to occur most commonly in the pelvic region, especially over the hips and on the buttocks, while in Latin America the head is more usually involved. Nodules do not generally give rise to much discomfort, but at times they may be painful, and secondary infection with abscess formation can occur. The number and size of nodules increases with intensity of infection.

Typical skin lesions (onchodermatitis) consist of an intensely itchy, papular dermatitis, with edema in the early stages, progressing to lichenification and atrophy ('lizard skin'). Large numbers of microfilariae are present in the skin, and involvement may be generalized or limited to one area of the body. Transient urticaria is often the only skin manifestation, and indeed the condition may be entirely asymptomatic despite the presence of microfilariae in the skin. General well-being is seldom disturbed.

Ocular lesions (river blindness), due to microfilariae penetrating the eyes, represent the most serious feature of onchocerciasis and are a frequent cause of blindness in endemic areas. They occur especially when the disease is present in the upper half of the body and are more common in South America. Children rarely show advanced ocular lesions,

but hyperemia of the conjunctiva and nummular keratitis may be seen in older children. Any part of the eye can be involved.

Diagnosis

Diagnosis is best established by demonstrating microfilariae in skin snips and the adult worms on nodule biopsy. Serological tests, including tests for antigen, are also available in onchocerciasis but there may be some cross-reaction with other filarial species (e.g. *Mansonella ozzardi*) in areas where they coexist.[931] Microfilariae are not uncommonly found in urine.

Treatment

Microfilariae are killed by diethylcarbamazine, but the drug is no longer considered justified for the treatment of onchocerciasis due to the common and often severe adverse reactions that it causes. Ivermectin is now accepted as the treatment of choice for onchocerciasis at a single dose of 150–200 µg/kg for both adults and children.[913,932–934] As it kills only the microfilariae but not the adult worms, treatment is long term and may need to be repeated every 3–6 months for 2–3 years.[890,935,936] It has been found, however, that adding doxycycline (100 mg daily for 6 weeks) to the ivermectin regimen significantly enhances microfilarial suppression by sterilizing female worms through depletion of the symbiotic *Wolbachia* bacteria.[937,938] The use of ivermectin for mass treatment has given hope for the effective control of this disease. Suramin is lethal to the adult worms but it may cause severe adverse reactions. Excision of nodules, especially those near the eyes, is sometimes recommended prior to chemotherapy, because of the danger of ocular involvement. Regular urine tests should be made as the drug is nephrotoxic. Amocarzine and albendazole are also being evaluated for efficacy in the treatment of onchocerciasis.[896]

Vector control requires the simultaneous application of control measures (spraying with appropriate insecticides) over whole river systems.

Loa loa

Loa loa is transmitted by flies of the genus *Chrysops*, which are infected by sucking human blood containing microfilariae. These are present in blood during the daytime, thus corresponding with the diurnal biting habits of most *Chrysops*. The disease is endemic in western and central Africa. Adult worms are found migrating through subcutaneous tissues, the male being some 3 cm and the female 6 cm in length. They may remain viable for as long as 30 years.

Clinical features

Symptoms of loiasis are usually trivial. The most characteristic manifestation is a recurrent, painless, puffy, pink swelling, often referred to as a calabar, or fugitive, swelling. This lesion marks the journey of the adult worm in the subcutis. It develops over a period of 3–4 h and may acquire a diameter of 10 cm or more, before subsiding in a few days. The upper extremities and eyelids are most often involved and on occasions the thin worm may be seen rapidly traversing the bulbar conjunctiva and sometimes accompanied by periorbital edema. The appearance of the calabar swelling is frequently associated with fever and malaise. Eosinophilia is present.

Some patients remain afilaremic, no microfilariae being found in the peripheral blood despite intensive investigation.[939]

Treatment

Diethylcarbamazine is used in the treatment of loiasis but can cause severe adverse reactions in people with microfilarial counts > 2000 mf/ml blood.[940] It is usually recommended that the drug be given in slowly increasing doses.[913]

Day 1: 50 mg (child 1 mg/kg) after food;
Day 2: 50 mg (child 1 mg/kg) 8-hourly;
Day 3: 100 mg (child 1–2 mg/kg) 8-hourly;
Days 4–21: 3 mg/kg 8-hourly.

In afilaremic patients, side-effects can be controlled by steroids and/or antihistamines. In patients with large numbers of microfilariae in their blood, meningoencephalitis may result from lysis of dead microfilariae and thus in these patients benefits of treatment must be weighed against the danger of the side-effects. In these people, steroids and antihistamines may not be effective in preventing side-effects.

Ivermectin (200 μg/kg stat repeated every 6–12 months) has been recommended[890] while mebendazole and albendazole have also been tried.[939]

Wuchereria bancrofti and Brugia malayi

Infections by *Wuchereria bancrofti*, *Brugia malayi* and *B. timori* (termed 'lymphatic filariasis') occur in the tropics and in some semitropical areas, being transmitted by various species of mosquito. The adult female and male worms (some 85 mm and 40 mm in length respectively) attain maturity in the lymphatic system about 1 year following entry to the body, after which time the nocturnal periodic sheathed microfilariae are demonstrable in peripheral blood between 10 pm and 2 am. Some Pacific strains of *W. bancrofti* are nonperiodic.

Clinical features

First infection may occur in children but the full clinical picture may take many years to develop. As with other filarial diseases, the early phases may be entirely asymptomatic or associated with florid allergic manifestations. The commonest manifestations of the mature filariae are acute and recurring lymphangitis. The affected lymph node, together with its afferent vessel, usually in the groin, is painful and tender. The lymphatic vessel becomes palpable and cord-like and is associated with a linear red streak in the overlying skin. This stage is often accompanied by pyrexia, malaise, nausea and headache. Dreyer et al[941] believe that acute attacks of lymphatic filariasis can be divided into a number of clearly defined clinical syndromes. The acute attacks, which subside after several days, have a variable periodicity of weeks or months, gradually becoming less severe, often with persistence of residual subcutaneous swelling. Recurrent funiculitis may occur and involvement of intra-abdominal lymph nodes may give rise to the clinical picture of peritonitis. Chylous ascites, chyluria, varicose groin nodes, hydrocele and elephantiasis are classical end results but as they arise from chronicity over many years, emphasis on this aspect is out of place in a pediatric context. Nevertheless, early manifestations of chronic disease may sometimes appear in the late years of childhood.

Work by Hightower et al[942] has suggested that children born to mothers infected with *W. bancrofti* are more susceptible to this infection than those born to uninfected mothers.

Tropical eosinophilia syndrome. In some patients, an abnormal response to *W. bancrofti* infection results in a clinical picture which reflects a specific allergic sensitization to filarial antigens, a condition known as tropical pulmonary eosinophilia or tropical eosinophilia syndrome. These patients present with cough, asthma-like symptoms, respiratory distress and eosinophil counts of 3000/mm³ or greater. X-ray of the lungs usually shows extensive changes. These patients often do not develop filaremia, hence the term 'occult filariasis'.

A similar condition can be caused by infection with *Brugia malayi* and perhaps by infection with nonhuman filariae.

Diagnosis

The clinical diagnosis of lymphatic filariasis based on symptoms can now be greatly aided by ultrasonography and lymphoscintigraphy.

The recovery of typical sheathed microfilariae in midnight blood slides and occasionally in urine will establish the diagnosis. Concentration techniques may need to be used to recover microfilariae from the blood.

In the case of tropical pulmonary eosinophilia, diagnosis is made clinically and confirmed by serology or rapid response to diethylcarbamazine.[943]

It is worth noting that visitors to endemic areas who contract lymphatic filariasis often do not develop a microfilaremia, which can make parasitological confirmation of the infection impossible. Thus the development of an EIA test (TropBio, Australia) to detect circulating filarial antigen has provided a major breakthrough in the diagnosis of lymphatic filariasis, the test for *W. bancrofti* being highly specific and very sensitive. Antigen-detecting tests, including DNA detection from blood spots, have also been developed for *B. malayi*, show great promise and are very cost-effective.[944-946]

Treatment

Diethylcarbamazine rapidly removes circulating microfilariae but large doses are required to kill adult worms. The dosage regimen for children utilizes increasing doses as for loiasis.[883,885,913] There is often an acute exacerbation during therapy, for which antihistamines should be given. Ivermectin, which has significantly fewer side-effects than diethylcarbamazine, is also very effective in the treatment of lymphatic filariasis. It kills microfilariae but not adult worms and the single oral dose of 150–200 μg/kg should be repeated at yearly intervals. Albendazole and doxycycline are also mentioned as showing promise.[938]

A single oral dose of ivermectin has been recommended for controlling lymphatic filariasis al[934,947] and the use of yearly or 6-monthly doses of ivermectin or the regular use of salt fortified with diethylcarbamazine has proved invaluable in the control of this condition in endemic regions. The control of lymphatic filariasis is a public health problem which is neither easy nor straightforward.[948] Even small areas omitted from a general filariasis vector control program due to, for example, difficult terrain, have the potential to disperse the infection.[949] As Molyneaux[950] says: 'environment remains a key determinant in changing patterns of vector-borne infections. Changes are rapid and vectors have the capacity to change equally rapidly, a capacity not matched by health systems'. He believes less time will be spent in future on developing new pesticides for insect vector control, and that the emphasis will be on genetic approaches to make insects less effective vectors.

Mansonella perstans and Mansonella ozzardi

Mansonella perstans has had many recent changes in its name[951] and is widely distributed in those tropical and subtropical areas which favor the habitat of the vector. The unsheathed microfilariae are transmitted by *Culicoides* midges from person to person, and the adult worms develop in the mesentery, perinephric and retroperitoneal tissues where they may survive for many years (Table 28.44).

Clinical features

This form of filariasis is often held to be harmless, but symptoms can be associated with infection, particularly in people visiting from non-endemic regions. Infection with these helminths may result in lethargy, arthralgia, urticaria and headache. Less frequently calabar-like swellings around the eye ('bung eye'), and pericardial or pleural effusions occur. Among indigenous inhabitants of endemic areas *M. perstans* is often asymptomatic.

The period from exposure to the appearance of nonperiodic microfilariae in the blood is unknown.

Diethylcarbamazine is ineffective in treatment of mansonellosis,[890,940] but trichlorophone has been used with success. Albendazole (400 mg bd for 30 days), mebendazole (100 mg 12-hourly for 30 days)[913] or a combination of mebendazole and levamisole have all been reported as effective.[940] The judicious use of corticosteroids is valuable in severe cases. Ivermectin (150 µg/kg stat p.o.) is reported to be effective in the treatment of *M. ozzardi* but not *M. perstans*.[890,940]

In rain forest areas of Central Africa, a related species, *M. streptocerca*, infects humans. Microfilariae of this species are unsheathed and have a curled tail with nuclei extending to the tip. The adult and microfilariae of this species are found in skin, and diagnosis is by skin snips as for *Onchocerca*. Symptoms include dermatitis, with macules and papules. Infection is more common in older people than in children.

M. ozzardi in South America is a species with many clinical similarities to *M. perstans*. In the past it has been considered a commensal, but studies have suggested that this parasite may also not be as harmless as is often believed (Table 28.44).

Dirofilaria immitis

The dog heartworm is a common filarial nematode infecting dogs in most tropical regions of the world including parts of the USA and northern Australia. It is transmitted by mosquitoes.

Occasional human cases are diagnosed during serological surveys or on biopsy for investigations of pulmonary 'coin' lesions found on X-ray.[897] Cases of pleural effusion, intraocular infection and eosinophilic meningitis are also caused by *D. immitis* in humans. Most cases of dirofilariasis are recorded in adults, but clinical infections are seen at times in children and Hungerford[893] believes that dirofilariasis is much more common in Australia than is believed at present.

As *D. immitis* infection in humans does not usually exhibit a filaremia, diagnosis is usually made on biopsy of a lung lesion or on removal of a worm from the eye. Skin tests or serological tests are unhelpful.

Other species of *Dirofilaria* are also recorded from humans, usually from subcutaneous tissue or from the conjunctival sac.

CESTODES (TAPEWORMS)

The cestodes are platyhelminths, which are dorso-ventrally flattened, have no gut or body cavity and are hermaphroditic. Adult tapeworms have a characteristic morphology with a scolex armed with suckers and sometimes hooks, an unsegmented neck region and a long segmented strobila.

Life cycles are complex, with the adult tapeworms living in the gastrointestinal tract of the vertebrate definitive hosts and larval stages occurring in a range of vertebrate or invertebrate intermediate host species. Larval forms vary from the free-living, ciliated coracidium larva and worm-like procercoid and plerocercoid (sparganum) larvae of the pseudophyllidean tapeworms (e.g. *Diphyllobothrium latum*) to the cysticercoid, cysticercus (bladderworm) or hydatid larvae of the cyclophyllidean tapeworms.

Humans can become infected with a range of cestode species and mostly harbor the adult tapeworm although human infection with larval cestodes includes sparganosis (*Spirometra* sp.), cysticercosis (*Taenia solium*) and hydatidosis (*Echinococcus granulosus*).

The main cestodes relevant to humans are *Taenia saginata*, *Taenia solium*, *Hymenolepis nana*, *H. diminuta*, *Dipylidium caninum*, *Diphyllobothrium latum*, *Echinococcus granulosus*, *E. multilocularis* and *Inermicapsifer madagascariensis*.

TAENIASIS

Taeniasis is caused by infection with adult *T. saginata* or *T. solium* (Table 28.45). In both these infections, the adult tapeworm is found in the

Table 28.45 Characteristics of *Taenia saginata* and *Taenia solium*

	Taenia saginata	Taenia solium
Parasite		
Scolex	4 suckers only	Crown of hooklets and 4 suckers
Length	5–20 m	3–15 m
Lateral branches of uterus	15 or more	8–13
Intermediate host	Cattle	Pig, but occasionally man
Final host	Man	Man

intestinal tract of humans – the only definitive host. The intermediate hosts harboring the larval stage (cysticercus) of the tapeworm are cattle in *T. saginata* (the beef tapeworm) and usually pigs in *T. solium* (the pork tapeworm). However, in the case of *T. solium*, in addition to pigs, a wide range of mammals, including humans, can harbor the cysticerci.

It has been suggested that in the Asia-Pacific region, other, but as yet incompletely defined, species of *Taenia* may infect humans.[952,953] One such species found in Indonesia, Taiwan and Korea morphologically resembles *T. saginata* but is acquired from pork and has been named *T. asiatica*.[870,896]

Infection with adult *Taenia* results from ingestion of infected meat and, as such, is not common in very young children.

Taenia saginata (the beef tapeworm)

The beef tapeworm is cosmopolitan, occurring in almost all countries where beef is eaten. It is especially common where local eating habits favor the consumption of raw or undercooked beef. The cysticerci in the beef can even survive salting and a moderate degree of drying.

The adult worm is harbored in the human intestine, attached by its scolex to the mucosa of the small intestine. It may reach 20–25 m in length and gravid proglottids (or segments), their uteri packed with eggs, break from the strobila singly or in chains of 2–5 segments, and either migrate actively out of the anus or pass out passively with the feces.

These proglottids crawl about on the ground releasing eggs, which are also liberated when the proglottid dies and disintegrates on pasture land. Eggs lying on the grass are ingested by grazing cattle (Fig. 28.71). The oncosphere (hexacanth) larva is released in the intestine, penetrates the intestinal wall using its six hooklets and is carried via the bloodstream to the heart and voluntary muscles, especially the tongue, shoulder

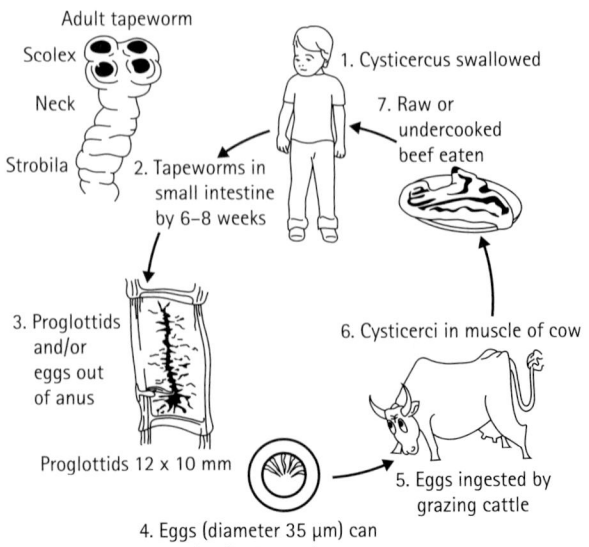

Fig. 28.71 Life cycle of *Taenia saginata*.

and masseter muscles. Here it loses its hooklets, develops an inverted scolex with suckers but no hooks and changes into a bladderworm (or cysticercus) larva, termed *Cysticercus bovis*, over about 3 months. These cysticerci are about 8 × 5 mm in size and meat infected with them is commonly termed 'measly' owing to its spotted appearance.

When ingested, the cysticercus evaginates the scolex and elongates into the adult stage. Humans eating such 'measly' beef raw or undercooked thus become infected with adult tapeworm. Gravid segments are shed about 3 months after infection.

Epidemics of 'measles' in cattle have not uncommonly resulted from cattle grazed on pastures fertilized with untreated effluent from sewage outlets. Such cattle become infectious about 3 months after ingestion of eggs.

Clinical features

In most cases infection with *T. saginata* is quite symptomless, the only feature being the intermittent passing of segments. In 5–50% of cases, eosinophilia may occur while abdominal pain, weight loss, malaise, an increase or decrease in appetite and such allergic features as urticaria and pruritus ani may be seen.

Adult tapeworms absorb digested food through their cuticles and thus they compete for food with the host and in this process food deprivation and digestive upset may occur.

Rarely, intestinal obstruction results and at times proglottids wander into the appendix and, impacting there, may cause obstructive appendicitis.

Diagnosis

Diagnosis is generally made when proglottids are seen in the stool. These can readily be identified by pressing them between two glass microslides and counting the number of uterine branches on each side of the central stem. In *T. saginata*, there are usually 15 or more primary uterine branches on each side.

In the cases where proglottids cannot be found, eggs (Fig. 28.72) may be detected in the feces or on anal tapes as used for *Enterobius*, a process which is more effective for recovery of *T. saginata* eggs than stool examination. Eggs of *T. saginata* and *T. solium* are identical.

Treatment

The treatment of choice for *T. saginata* infection is praziquantel as a single oral dose of 10–20 mg/kg.[883,884] Niclosamide is also effective, being usually given without purgation at a dose of 1 g (11–34 kg) or 1.5 g (34 kg and over), which should be chewed before swallowing.[883] The worm is passed in a partially digested state. Treatment can be followed, if desired, by a saline purge after 2 h.

Treated patients should be re-checked 3 months after treatment to assess cure. With modern anthelmintics it is not feasible to examine post-treatment stools for the scolex.

Prevention of *T. saginata* infection depends upon avoidance of consumption of raw or undercooked beef and hygienic disposal of human feces to prevent infection of cattle.[870] Freezing of meat (−10°C for 10 days) is also reported to be effective in killing cysticerci.

Taenia solium (the pork tapeworm)

T. solium is widely distributed, but less so than the beef tapeworm. It is common, however, in Africa, Asia, Latin America and parts of eastern Europe.

The life cycle of *T. solium* (Fig. 28.73) is similar to that of *T. saginata* but with some very important differences. In both species humans comprise the only definitive host and may harbor one or more tapeworms. In *T. solium* infections humans become infected with the adult tapeworm after eating raw or undercooked 'measly' pork containing cysticerci. The range of intermediate hosts of *T. solium* is wider than that of *T. saginata* and, besides pigs, can include the domestic dog. In fact, in areas where dogs form a significant part of human diet, they may serve as an important source of human *T. solium* infection. Humans too can become infected with cysticerci of *T. solium* (known as *Cysticercus cellulosae*) after ingestion of eggs, a condition termed cysticercosis.

The adult *T. solium* is, on average, a little shorter than *T. saginata*, reaching about 15 m in length. The scolex has both suckers and a double row of hooks. The cysticerci of both species are essentially similar, but again the invaginated scolex of *C. cellulosae* has hooks which are absent in *C. bovis*.

Clinical features

Taeniasis solium. Infection with the adult *T. solium* is much the same as with the adult *T. saginata* except that proglottids of the pork tapeworm are less mobile than those of the beef tapeworm and so such features as appendiceal blockage are more rare. Most cases are asymptomatic, but diarrhea and constipation have been recorded and a moderate eosinophilia may develop.

Cysticercosis. The greatest danger in infection with *T. solium* is the danger to others of infection with eggs via food or water (heteroinfection) and the danger to the patients themselves of autoinfection by external means (hand-to-mouth transfer of eggs) or internal means (vomiting up and re-swallowing of proglottids).

The clinical effects of cysticercosis are essentially dependent upon the number and sites of the cysticerci. Cysticerci can develop almost anywhere in the body: beneath the skin (subcutaneous cysticercosis); in the myocardium; in the muscles; within the eye or in the brain (cerebral cysticercosis or neurocysticercosis). If within the ventricles of the brain the cysticerci can become greatly enlarged resulting in a racemose cyst.

Usually cysticerci do not cause clinical symptoms until they die, swell and calcify – a process which occurs about 3 years or longer after infection. Whether or not they cause symptoms is also dependent upon their site. In the muscles, heart or beneath the skin they are relatively benign but within the eye they can cause retinal detachment, loss of vision and even blindness. If sited in the brain they may result

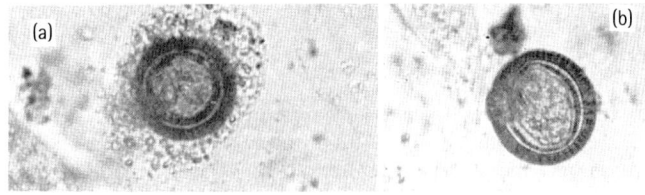

Fig. 28.72 Complete egg of *Taenia* sp., the embryophore being surrounded by the remains of the vitelline cell. (b) Other egg has lost all traces of the vitelline cell and consists only of the oncosphere larva surrounded by its thick, striated embryophore (approx. × 600).

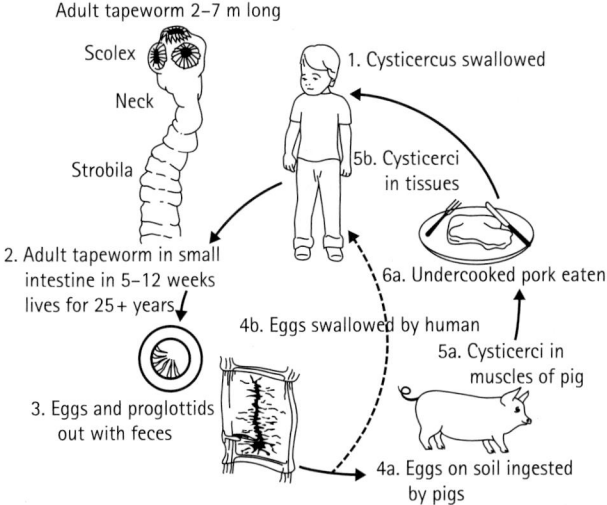

Adult tapeworm 2–7 m long
Scolex
Neck
Strobila
1. Cysticercus swallowed
5b. Cysticerci in tissues
2. Adult tapeworm in small intestine in 5–12 weeks lives for 25+ years
6a. Undercooked pork eaten
4b. Eggs swallowed by human
5a. Cysticerci in muscles of pig
3. Eggs and proglottids out with feces
4a. Eggs on soil ingested by pigs

Fig. 28.73 Life cycle of *Taenia solium*.

in neurological disorders, personality changes or epileptic convulsions. Neurocysticercosis is a common cause of epilepsy among Africans in southern Africa and, although more common in adults, it has even been recorded in children as young as 3 years of age.[954] Death can follow hydrocephalus resulting from blockage of the ventricular spaces.

Diagnosis

Taeniasis solium. Diagnosis of infection with adult *T. solium* is established by the finding of eggs (indistinguishable from those of *T. saginata*) in feces (Fig. 28.72) or by the passing of typical gravid proglottids. The proglottids of *T. solium* have fewer than 13 lateral uterine branches on each side and so can be differentiated from those of *T. saginata* although some degree of overlap may occur. (*Note:* gloves must be worn when examining proglottids for counting of the uterine branches, as eggs of *T. solium* are infective to humans.)

Cysticercosis. Cysticercosis can be diagnosed by palpation and biopsy of cysticerci if accessible and their microscopic examination after squashing between two glass microslides or after histological sectioning.

In patients in whom cysticercosis is clinically suspected confirmation can sometimes be obtained by radiology, where calcified cysticerci are visible as millet seed-shaped shadows in the muscles or small spotted areas on skull X-ray (Fig. 28.74a,b). X-rays are also useful in differentiating cerebral cysticercosis from CNS infection due to *Angiostrongylus, Gnathostoma* and *Paragonimus*.[955]

Eosinophils can at times be found in the CSF of patients with cerebral cysticercosis. About 25% of patients with cerebral cysticercosis will be found to harbor adult *T. solium* in their intestines or have a history of such infection.

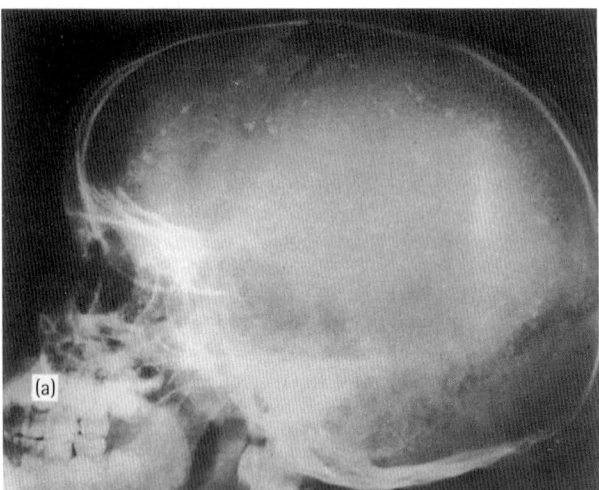

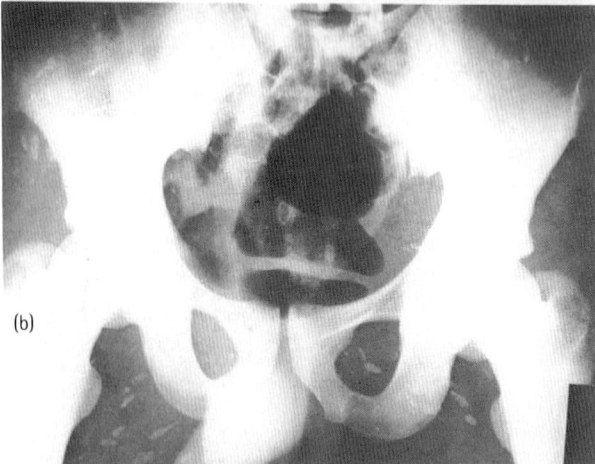

Fig. 28.74   (a) Cerebral cysticercosis. (b) Calcified cysticerci visible in the muscles in X-ray of pelvis.

Serological tests for blood or CSF are available for the diagnosis of cysticercosis.[955-957] In addition, tests have been developed to detect cysticercal antigen in CSF.

CT scans are of great value, not only for the diagnosis of cerebral cysticercosis, but also for an assessment of the length of infection and for post-treatment progress evaluation.[955,957,958]

Treatment

Treatment for *T. solium* is similar to that for *T. saginata*, with praziquantel or niclosamide being the drugs of choice.[913,959] Mepacrine, while effective, tends to cause nausea and vomiting and should thus be avoided because of the danger of regurgitation of proglottids into the stomach and re-swallowing them.

Cysticercosis. Albendazole (5 mg/kg 8-hourly for 8–15 days) is probably the treatment of choice for cysticercosis.[890] Although clinical studies have shown that praziquantel at a dose of 25–50 mg/kg/d in three divided doses for 14 days may be effective for the treatment of cysticercosis,[883,885,886,913,960] it is frequently associated with side-effects in neurocysticercosis and its use is not universally accepted in this situation.[883,961]

A number of authors have argued that the risks of cysticidal therapy in neurocysticercosis sometimes outweigh the benefits, and should be considered for each individual patient.[890,913,962] The simultaneous administration of steroids may help reduce inflammatory complications which can follow the death of the cysticerci after anthelmintic treatment.[896]

Surgical removal of cysticerci is seldom feasible, especially if the cysticerci are numerous and deep seated.

Anticonvulsants to control fits, steroids to control raised intracranial pressure and occasionally surgery to control hydrocephalus may be required for controlling the fits in neurocysticercosis.

Prevention of *T. solium* infection and cysticercosis is essentially the same as for *T. saginata*. Cysticerci can be destroyed during cooking by heating the meat to 50 °C.

Hymenolepis spp.

Two species of this genus of tapeworm infect humans, *Hymenolepis nana* (the dwarf tapeworm) and *H. diminuta* (the rat tapeworm). These are small tapeworms, reaching only 40 mm in length for *H. nana* and 40 cm in length for *H. diminuta*.

Hymenolepis nana

H. nana is harbored in the small intestine of the human (or sometimes rodent) host and the gravid proglottids disintegrate in the gut so that eggs pass out in the feces. When an egg is ingested by another person, it releases an oncosphere into the small intestine, and this burrows into a villus, forming a cysticercoid. It develops here before leaving the villus after about 14 days to grow into an adult tapeworm in the intestinal lumen (Fig. 28.75).

Because of its direct person-to-person mode of transmission, *H. nana* is a common tapeworm in resource limited countries and tends to be more common in children than in adults. In a survey in Zimbabwe, 18.7% of children were infected with *H. nana*, but only 3.8% of adults.[963]

Diagnosis is based on detecting characteristic *H. nana* eggs (Fig. 28.75). The treatment of choice is praziquantel or niclosamide as for taeniasis.[886,913] Praziquantel at a dose of 25 mg/kg has a cure rate of 98.5% and minimal side-effects.[964]

Hymenolepis diminuta

The rat tapeworm, *H. diminuta*, is common in many parts of the world in rats and mice. Its intermediate hosts are fleas and flour beetles. Children may become infected when they accidentally swallow the intermediate host – often with insect-infested meal or flour.

Diagnosis of *H. diminuta* infection is based on finding the eggs in feces. These eggs differ from those of *H. nana* in being larger, rounder, lemon yellow in color, and having a striated shell and no polar filaments.

Treatment is as for *H. nana*.

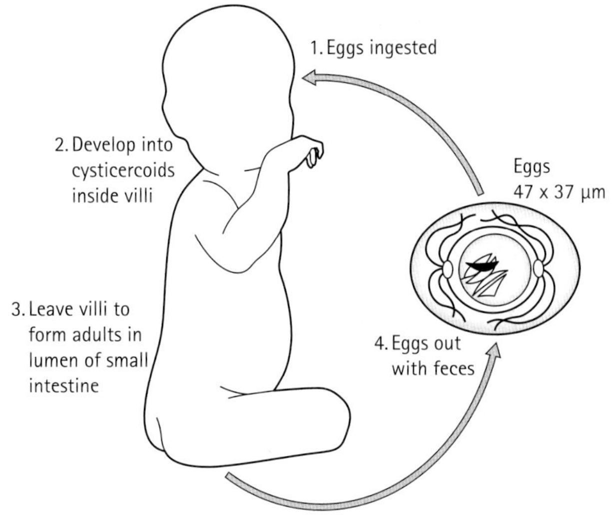

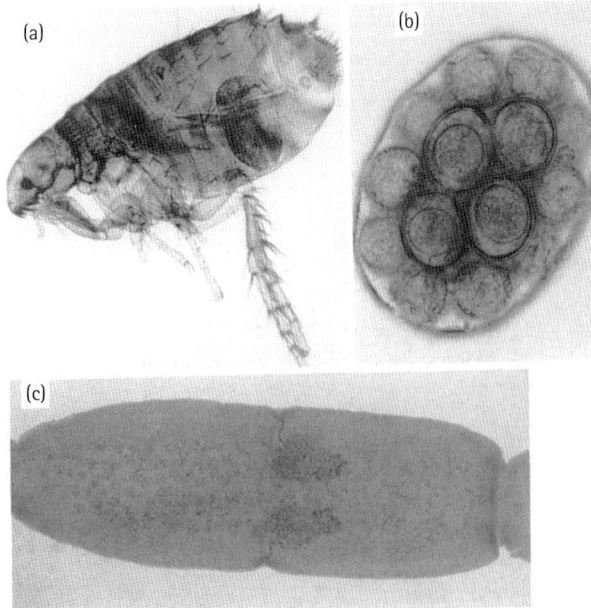

Fig. 28.75 Life cycle of *Hymenolepis nana*. Egg inset (approx. × 600).

Neither *H. nana* nor *H. diminuta* causes serious clinical effects, but abdominal pain, diarrhea, loss of appetite and eosinophilia may occur when loads are heavy. One problem with *H. nana* is a build-up of worm load as a result of external autoinfection by ingestion of eggs.

Dipylidium caninum

This tapeworm is worldwide, commonly infecting both dogs and cats. The intermediate hosts are fleas, such as the common dog and cat fleas (Fig. 28.76a), which contain the cysticercoids, and infection of the final host occurs when the flea is swallowed. Children can become infected when they accidentally swallow a flea or when they are licked on the mouth by a dog which has been 'fleaing' itself and has cysticercoids on the tongue.

Dipylidium caninum is a relatively small tapeworm (20 cm long) and usually causes little discomfort, although at times diarrhea, fever, restlessness and even convulsions have been recorded.

Diagnosis is made when actively motile proglottids with two genital pores (Fig. 28.76c) are found by the mother on nappies or when typical egg capsules (Fig. 28.76b) are found in the feces on microscopic examination.

Niclosamide is reported to be effective in treatment although in some cases repeated treatments with this drug have failed.[965] The recommended drug of choice is praziquantel at a single dose of 5–10 mg/kg.[965]

Diphyllobothrium latum

The adult fish tapeworm can reach 20 m or more in length. It is a common tapeworm of a variety of fish-eating mammals, including dogs and cats, in Scandinavia, the Baltic, South America, the Great Lakes of North America, parts of the Middle and Far East and Indonesia, while occasional cases are encountered in other parts such as Labrador and Australia.[896,959]

The scolex of this species has sucking grooves, and eggs are shed from the gravid proglottids to pass out with the feces.

When the eggs fall into water, a ciliated coracidium larva develops and is released through the operculum into the water. This is ingested by the microscopic crustacean, *Cyclops*, in which a procercoid larva is formed. When the *Cyclops* is eaten by a fish, the procercoid changes into a plerocercoid (sparganum) larva in the muscles of the fish. Finally the life cycle is completed when the fish is eaten by the mammalian definitive host (Fig. 28.77), which may include humans.

Clinical effects of heavy worm loads include diarrhea, abdominal pain, generalized weakness[959] and occasionally intestinal obstruction. *D. latum* is also recorded as causing a megaloblastic (macrocytic) anemia in susceptible patients who have a genetic predisposition and who are on a diet deficient in vitamin B_{12}, by competition with the host for this vitamin – especially when the worm is attached high up in the small intestine. Eosinophilia is not usually a feature of infection.

Diagnosis is based on finding typical operculate eggs in the feces (Fig. 28.78). Proglottids in the feces can be recognized by their centrally situated uterus and genital pore.

The recommended treatment is praziquantel 2.5–10 mg/kg orally as a single dose for people >4 years old. Niclosamide 1 g orally as a single dose for children 11–3 kg is an alternative.[890,913] Whichever anthelmintic is used, concurrent vitamin B_{12} should also be given if the patient is anemic.

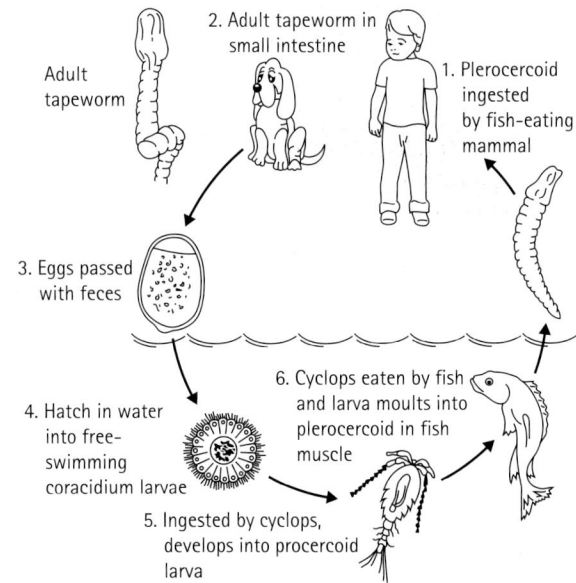

Fig. 28.77 Life cycle of *Diphyllobothrium latum*.

Fig. 28.76 (a) *Ctenocephalides* sp. – dog flea intermediate host of *Dipylidium caninum* (approx. × 50). (b) Egg capsule of *Dipylidium caninum* (approx × 600). (c) Stained gravid proglottid of *Dipylidium caninum*. Note characteristic double set of reproductive organs and twin genital pores (approx. × 20).

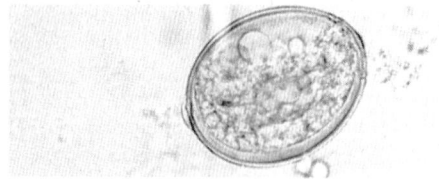

Fig. 28.78 Operculate egg of *Diphyllobothrium latum* (approx. × 600).

A common source of human infection is eating raw or smoked fish, so cooking fish is an important preventive measure.[870] Freezing fish (−10 °C for 15 min) is also effective in killing plerocercoids.

The plerocercoids of certain species belonging to the related genus, *Spirometra*, the adults of which inhabit the intestines of dogs, can infect humans and cause a condition called sparganosis. These elongated plerocercoid (sparganum) larvae can infect humans after ingestion of infected frogs or *Cyclops* with water (East Africa, North America) or by application of infected frog flesh to skin ulcers or eye wounds as poultices. Plerocercoids in the frog muscle migrate into the human flesh where they settle – a condition occurring in South East Asia.

These spargana can encyst in any tissues. Perhaps the commonest manifestations are nodules about 2 cm in size under the skin with painful surrounding edema. They can be detected radiologically as elongated shadows and can usually be removed surgically if accessible. One species of sparganum can bud and proliferate so spreading through the tissues.

ECHINOCOCCOSIS (HYDATID DISEASE)

Echinococcosis (hydatid disease) in humans is caused by the larval stage of *Echinococcus granulosus* and to a much lesser extent by *E. multilocularis*, *E. oligarthrus* or *E. vogeli*.

The life cycle of *E. granulosus* is shown in Figure 28.79. The small adult tapeworms (Fig. 28.80a) live in the intestine of the dog and related canids such as dingoes in Australia. After ingestion of the eggs by the intermediate hosts, which are usually sheep or sometimes cattle and in

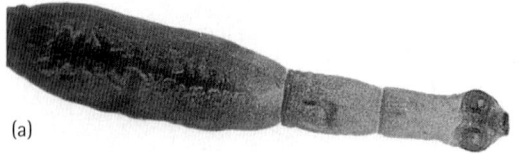

(a)

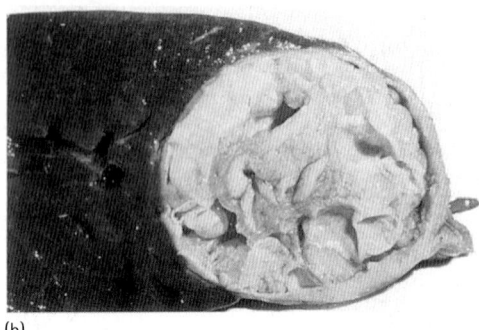

(b)

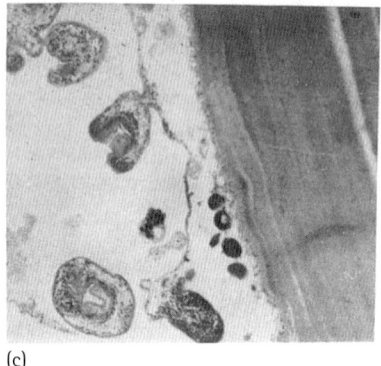

(c)

Fig. 28.80 (a) Adult *E. granulosus*. Note scolex and proglottids (approx. × 12). (b) Hydatid cyst in human liver. (c) Histological appearance of the wall of a pulmonary hydatid cyst.

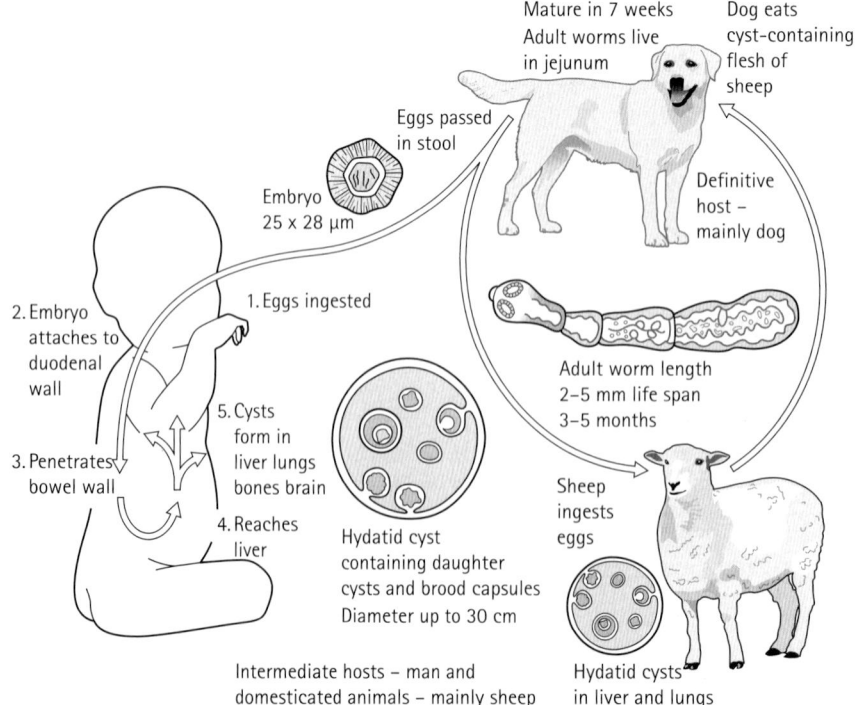

Fig. 28.79 Character and life cycle of *Echinococcus granulosus*.

Australia wallabies or other marsupials, the larval tapeworms develop into hydatid cysts in the viscera. Humans can also become infected when they ingest the tapeworm eggs, and children are particularly at risk because of their often intimate contact with dogs. They may pick up eggs contaminating the animal's coat or from the dog's tongue after being licked.

The infection is particularly common in rural sheep and cattle farming areas, especially where dogs are used for herding. It is widespread throughout Africa, Australasia, Asia, the Near East and South America and is also found in the Mediterranean, the USA and the UK.[871,966] *E. multilocularis* is widespread in the northern hemisphere, with human cases being common in parts of the former USSR, China, northern Japan, Alaska and central Europe, including possible spread into eastern Germany.[966-968] Cycles involving wild animals are also found in certain parts of the world.

In hydatidosis due to *E. multilocularis*, wolves, coyotes and foxes are the definitive hosts, and small field rodents serve as the natural intermediate hosts. Urban cycles involving the domestic cat and house mouse have been demonstrated.

The incidence of echinococcosis is decreasing in some areas owing to regular anthelmintic treatment of dogs and strict controls prohibiting the feeding of offal to dogs,[969] and global control has been mooted.[970]

Clinical features

Because development of cysts is slow, an infection acquired in childhood may only become clinically evident in adulthood, but manifestations of the disease in children are by no means uncommon.

The most frequent sites for cysts are the liver (Fig. 28.80b) and lungs (Fig. 28.80c). Spleen, peritoneum, kidneys, bone, orbital fossae, brain, heart and reproductive organs may also be invaded. In children, lung disease is reported to be the commonest form. Cysts sited in parenchymatous organs are large unilocular, well-circumscribed, fluid-filled structures in *E. granulosus* infections.

In bone, the parasite ramifies along bony canals, eroding bone and later involving the medullary cavity to form a large osseous cyst, which often results in spontaneous fracture. The much rarer *E. multilocularis* infection may produce complex, multilocular alveolar cysts with a gelatinous matrix and this alveolar hydatid disease has a 93% mortality within 10 years of diagnosis.[970]

Many cases of hydatid disease are silent. When symptoms occur they are usually those of a slow-growing tumor, with pressure on, or blockage to, the affected organ. Thus, recurrent pyrexia, paroxysmal cough, chest pain, hemoptysis and even expectoration of cyst fluid and membrane (should rupture occur into a bronchus) may occur as manifestations of pulmonary hydatidosis. Abdominal pain, vomiting, hepatomegaly and obstructive jaundice may indicate liver involvement. Intracranial localization can produce symptoms and signs indistinguishable from those of a tumor. Orbital cysts produce proptosis.

Sensitivity to cyst contents, resulting from slow leak of fluid, may develop with resulting allergic symptoms, notably urticaria. Severe anaphylaxis and even death can follow rupture of a cyst, while secondary metastatic cysts may develop in other parts of the body following such rupture.

Diagnosis

Diagnosis depends initially upon clinical awareness. A moderate eosinophilia is almost invariably present in childhood cases, except during febrile illnesses.

Often an X-ray provides the first indication of hydatid disease, especially in thoracic cases (Fig. 28.81). Ultrasound or CT scanning may be required to demonstrate the cystic nature of the lesion.[957] Serological tests may be helpful in confirming diagnosis. The historic Casoni skin test is no longer used because better serological tests are available, including the indirect hemagglutination test, a hydatid ELISA test and the improved immunoelectrophoresis, Arc 5 test and the double diffusion Arc 5 test.

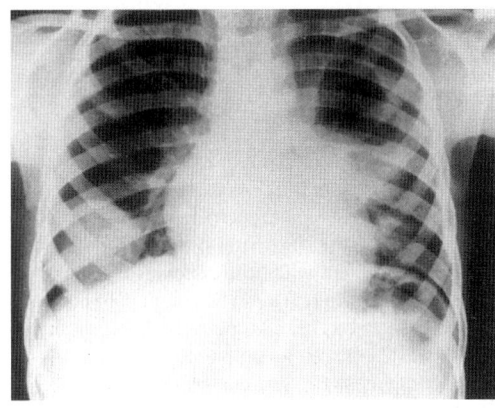

Fig. 28.81 Hydatid cysts in lung. Noncalcified cyst in right lung. Cyst in left lung has ruptured into a bronchus and contains fluid and air.

Pulmonary hydatids appear less serologically active than cysts in other parts of the body. After surgical removal of hydatid cysts, antibodies may be detectable in low titers for a while, but sooner or later disappear completely.

At times a cyst in the lung may rupture and diagnosis can then be made by finding hydatid sand or hooklets in the sputum. The latter are easily detected by using a standard Ziehl–Neelsen or auramine stain with UV microscopy, as they are intensely acid fast.

If hydatid cysts are suspected, diagnostic aspiration must *not* be attempted because of the danger of anaphylaxis and metastatic spread.

If children vomit what appear to be hydatid cysts, care should be taken to confirm their nature microscopically by the presence or absence of a germinal membrane (Fig. 28.80c), as gel cysts, closely resembling small hydatids, can easily mislead the unwary. These gel cysts may be vomited, by children up to 2 years, after ingestion of commercial fruit gels containing carrageenan.

Treatment

Treatment is surgical, if cysts are accessible, but due precautions must be observed to prevent release of hydatid fluid and to sterilize cysts prior to removal, using a scolicidal agent. Shorey et al[890] have summarized an approach to the treatment of uncomplicated hepatic hydatids using *p*uncture; *a*spiration of cyst contents; *i*ntroduction of a scolicidal agent such as alcohol or hypertonic saline; *r*e-aspiration of the solution – termed PAIR therapy.

Results of chemotherapy for hydatid cysts using mebendazole have been disappointing, but albendazole can be used as an adjunct to surgery or for the treatment of inoperable hydatids at a dose of 400 mg bd for 28 days, repeated as necessary or as 15 mg/kg/d in 2 doses (max 800 mg) for 28 days and repeated as necessary.[913,965] Albendazole can also be used in the treatment of infection with *E. multilocularis*, but treatment of multilocular hydatidosis remains largely surgical drainage.[958]

Prevention

While highly successful control programs have resulted in decreases in the prevalence of hydatid disease in Tasmania and New Zealand, elsewhere the disease remains common and may even be spreading.[871,966,970]

Dogs should not be allowed access to offal, to limit canine infection, and their regular treatment with an effective teniafuge such as praziquantel is indicated. In endemic areas this de-worming should be carried out every 2 months.

ANOPLOCEPHALID TAPEWORMS

This group of cestodes includes *I. madagascariensis*, *Raillietina* spp. (tapeworms of rodents with various arthropod intermediate hosts probably involved) and *Bertiella studeri* (a monkey cestode). Human infection with *I. madagascariensis* is particularly common in southern Africa but it has been sporadically reported also from a number of other tropical and subtropical areas. Outside Africa, the parasite seems to have dispensed with a need for a rodent reservoir.

These cestodes may reach 42 cm in length and their small, actively motile proglottids are shed in the stool and have the appearance of rice grains; they contain characteristic parenchymatous egg capsules.

I. madagascariensis most frequently involves children between the ages of 1 and 5 years, and while the infection is usually asymptomatic, anorexia, asthenia, anemia and abdominal pain have occasionally been attributed to it. It has been found to be the most common tapeworm affecting white children in Zimbabwe and more cases in African children are coming to light as awareness increases.[971,972]

Niclosamide is the treatment of choice for *I. madagascariensis*, one tablet (0.5 g) repeated in 1 h, while niclosamide or praziquantel is recommended for *Bertiella studeri*.[972]

TREMATODES (FLUKES)

Trematodes are parasitic helminths belonging to the class Platyhelminthes (flat worms). Trematodes are dorsoventrally flattened worms which have a gut, no body cavity and possess an oral and a ventral sucker. Most are hermaphrodite, except the schistosomes. The flukes have a complex life cycle involving various species of aquatic snail as intermediate hosts. Trematodes infecting humans include blood flukes (*Schistosoma*), liver flukes (*Fasciola, Clonorchis, Opisthorchis*), intestinal flukes (*Fasciolopsis, Heterophyes, Metagonimus*) and lung flukes (*Paragonimus*).

BLOOD FLUKE INFECTION (SCHISTOSOMIASIS OR BILHARZIASIS)

Schistosomiasis has been increasing as a hazard to humans through the construction of dams and the movement of human populations.

Adult blood flukes live in the veins of the final host. There are three main species which infect humans: *Schistosoma japonicum, S. mansoni* and *S. haematobium*[973] (Table 28.46). *S. japonicum* is a zoonotic species which frequents the superior mesenteric veins of humans and causes a more virulent and rapidly progressive illness than the other species, involving mainly the small and large intestine and liver. Adult *S. mansoni* worms live in the inferior mesenteric veins with resultant damage to the colon and liver while *S. haematobium* is found in the veins of the vesical plexus of humans, the disease thus predominantly affecting the urinary tract.

Other blood flukes less commonly recorded in humans include *S. intercalatum* (Central and West Africa), *S. mekongi* (Viet Nam), *S. malayensis* (Malaysia), *S. bovis* (in North Africa and Iraq) and *S. mattheei* (in southern Africa). The latter two are zoonotic species of cattle and sheep.

The life cycle of the human blood flukes is shown in Figure 28.82.

Pathogenesis and clinical features

Humans are usually infected by direct penetration of the cercariae through intact skin. The pathological changes in schistosomiasis are produced by cercariae, schistosomulae, adult worms and eggs – by their physical presence, by virtue of metabolic products or from the body's immune response to the infection. The severity of the disease depends primarily upon the number of parasites that can gain entry to the body and mature.

Despite the wealth of knowledge that has accumulated regarding the pathophysiology of schistosomiasis, the extent of ill health and mortality caused by this disease is still debatable.[974]

While large sections of a population may harbor the parasites, many individuals come to terms with the disease and suffer virtually no morbidity, owing to an interplay of factors such as immunological tolerance, worm load and rate of reinfection. The role of protective immunity in schistosomiasis continues to be a subject of debate.[975] Increased prevalence and intensity of infection in childhood lend credence at least to

Table 28.46 Geographical distribution of schistosomiasis (After Warren & Mahmoud 1975[973])

Species	Distribution				
	Africa	Middle East	Asia	South America	Caribbean
S. mansoni	Egypt Libya Sudan South of the Sahara Malagasy Republic	Yemen* Aden* Saudi Arabia*		Brazil Surinam Venezuela	Puerto Rico Dominican Republic* Guadeloupe Martinique St Lucia
S. japonicum			Malaysia*[1] China Japan Philippines Sulawesi* Thailand* Laos*[2] Kampuchea*[2] Vietnam[2]		
S. haematobium	Widespread including Malagasy Republic and Mauritius[†]	Lebanon Iran* Turkey Iraq Jordan Yemen Israel Saudi Arabia	India[†]		

*Very small focal areas.
[†]Focal distribution.
*Limited foci have been reported in Portugal in the past.
[1]Species known as *S. malayensis*.
[2]Species known as *S. mekongi*.

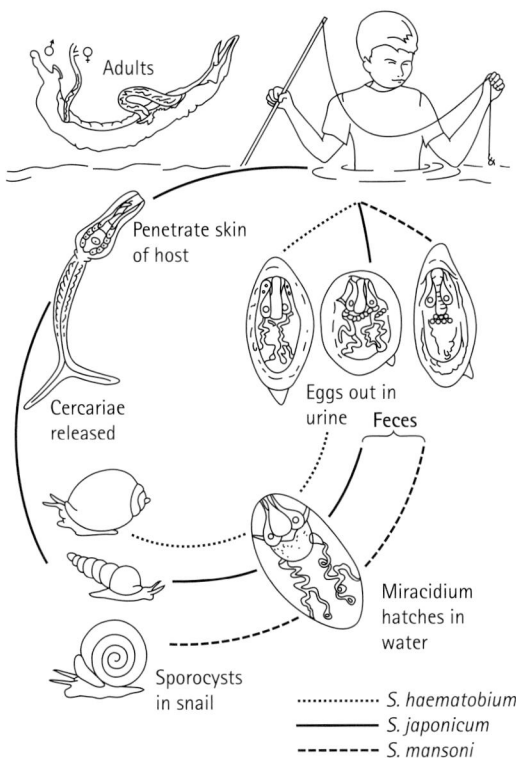

Fig. 28.82   Life cycle of schistosomes.

some protective immunity playing a part.[976] The immunity involved in schistosomiasis is complex,[975] being described as concomitant immunity, whereby the adult worms are not affected by the host's immune response to the infection, but newly invading cercariae are destroyed.[977–980]

The later stages of schistosomiasis generally take many years to develop so that the spectrum of clinical disease in children is narrowed. Nevertheless, such late manifestations as portal hypertension, calcification of the bladder and even vesical carcinoma are by no means rare in adolescents living in hyperendemic areas. A further difference in the disease as it affects children compared with adults is related to the caliber of blood vessels. Because of the smaller and more tenuous venous plexuses and collaterals, schistosomes are less able to migrate to sites far removed from their normal habitat in children than in older persons. The relative lack of immunity in young patients renders them more liable to severe systemic disturbance during the early stages of the disease. Determinants of infection in human communities are varied and involved.[981]

Clinical features can be related to the phase of parasitic invasion, and symptomatology is generally, but not always, proportionate to worm load. The pathogenesis of schistosomiasis is complex but it is essentially an immunological disease.[982–985]

Penetration of cercariae
At the time of penetration, within a few hours to a few days of exposure, a dermatitis termed swimmer's, or Kabure, itch may develop and last for 2–3 days. The condition is more common in non-indigenous inhabitants. It can also be caused by avian or mammalian schistosomes in countries where human schistosomiasis is unknown. For example it is quite common in Australia where it is sometimes termed 'pelican itch' and in the USA where it is known as 'seabather's eruption'. These latter cercariae, however, die while attempting to penetrate the skin. A prickly sensation is followed by intense itching and an urticarial, papular or occasionally vesicular rash appears, lasting from a few hours to several days.

Migratory/toxemic stage: the Katayama syndrome
Having passed through the skin, the cercariae lose their tails and the resulting schistosomulae enter the lymphatics, pass to the veins and

travel to the heart and hence to the lungs to circulate freely in the systemic circulation. Many die, but those that gain access to the portal system reach the liver where they mature into adult male and female worms. Rarely, worms mature in other ectopic sites such as veins of the brain and spinal cord. Coupling takes place in the liver and the male transports the female against the flow of blood to their sites of predilection where egg laying begins. The prepatent period in schistosomiasis (i.e. from infection to egg laying) is normally about 5–9 weeks.

During the migratory stage of the life cycle with a crescendo just prior to egg laying, the patient may develop an illness known as the Katayama syndrome due to antigenic challenge by the parasitic metabolites in the non-immune host. Malaise, pyrexia, liver tenderness and splenomegaly occur. Eosinophilia is constant. Urticaria, joint and muscle pains, cough, abdominal discomfort and diarrhea may also occur. Encephalopathy, myocarditis and anaphylactoid purpura are reported complications.[896]

Katayama syndrome is most common in *S. japonicum* infections, but can also occur when a previously uninfected individual is exposed to a heavy invasion by *S. mansoni* cercariae.

Early egg laying stage
Many eggs laid by female worms in the submucosal venules of the intestine or bladder pass through the tissues and are discharged in the feces (*S. japonicum* and *S. mansoni*) or urine (*S. haematobium*). This early egg laying stage may be associated with dysenteric symptoms or with dysuria, frequency and terminal hematuria.

Late egg laying stage – pathology of chronic schistosomiasis
Initially eggs pass through the tissues relatively easily but as infection progresses, marked tissue reaction occurs, eggs can no longer pass through the tissues so readily, and many are swept back by the flow of blood to be deposited elsewhere.

The morbidity of chronic schistosomiasis is mainly related to the presence of eggs,[985] which initially stimulate a granulomatous reaction characterized by a pseudotubercle, rich in eosinophils. This is followed by degeneration and calcification of the eggs with much reactive fibrosis. The principal pathological effects are as follows.

Genitourinary system. *S. haematobium* is the principal cause. The early bladder lesions usually occur on the trigone where deposition of phosphates round the egg deposits imparts a velvety appearance termed 'sandy patches'. Subsequent mucosal proliferation may produce multiple papillomata before ulceration, calcification (Fig. 28.83) and fibrosis lead to diminished bladder capacity. A similar process may involve the ureters, especially at their lower ends, leading to ureteric stricture and consequent hydronephrosis. This complication can also occur from vesical reflux

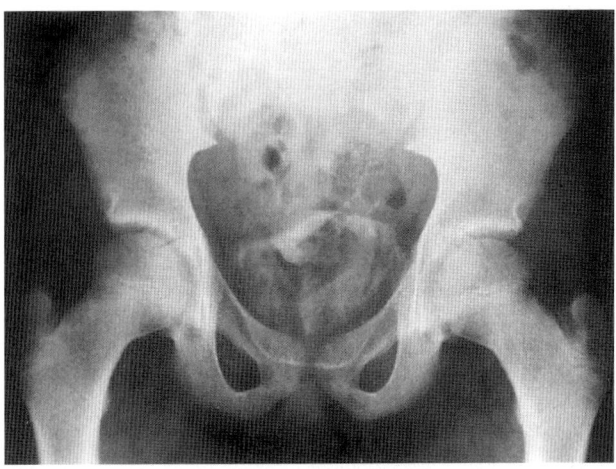

Fig. 28.83   X-ray showing bladder calcification due to schistosomiasis in a 10-year-old girl.

in the absence of overt ureteric involvement. Vesical or ureteric calculi may occur. An important long term complication is the predisposition of the bladder affected by schistosomiasis to develop carcinoma, usually of squamous cell type. The pathogenesis of bladder carcinoma in *S. haematobium* infection is complex and has still not been fully elucidated. While most common in adults, it is recognized to occur in adolescents. Genital lesions are usually diagnosed after puberty. These include epididymo-orchitis (often with associated secondary hydrocele), salpingo-oophoritis and chronic cervicitis. Large schistosomal granulomata (bilharziomas) consisting of masses of eggs enveloped in granulation tissue may involve the skin of the perineum and vulva. The lesions have a warty papillomatous appearance and when situated at the urethral meatus such a lesion is indistinguishable from a caruncle. Cutaneous schistosomiasis may rarely involve other parts of the body, and bilharzial granuloma of the conjunctiva has even been described in children.

An extended bacteremia with *Salmonella typhi* or *S. paratyphi* can occur, including a prolonged urinary carrier state, in concurrent *S. haematobium* infections.

Bacteriuria is generally considered to be more common in patients with *S. haematobium* than in uninfected controls.

Intestinal tract. Involvement of small bowel is usually only seen in *S. japonicum* infection but schistosomiasis of the colon may be due to both *S. japonicum* and *S. mansoni*. Eggs of *S. haematobium* may also be encountered in rectal snips taken from the lower part of the rectum. Mucosal involvement of the bowel gives rise to a similar appearance to that seen in the bladder with a velvety roughening of the mucosa. This may be associated with dysentery in the early egg laying phase of the disease, especially with *S. japonicum* infection. Gross lesions of the bowel are rare, but on occasions papillomata, granulomata, ulcers, stricture and fistulae occur. The appendix is frequently involved and signs of chronic appendicitis are common, although acute obstructive appendicitis consequent upon fibrosis is a rare complication.

Liver. Hepatic fibrosis may result from the presence of eggs of *S. mansoni* or *S. japonicum* with formation of granulomata and healing by fibrosis leading to thick tracts of periportal fibrous tissue traversing the liver in different directions. This 'pipe stem' fibrosis (Symmers' liver) gives the surface of the liver an irregular bosselated contour due to tethering of the capsule. In the later stage, eggs are scanty and may even be absent from biopsy material, in which the essential features are of preserved liver architecture associated with gross thickening of the portal tracts by collagenized bands of fibrous tissue. Kupffer cells usually contain schistosomal pigment. Liver involvement can lead to portal hypertension with ascites and splenomegaly, which is occasionally massive ('Egyptian splenomegaly'). Anemia is frequent and may be due to chronic hemorrhage from varices or to associated 'hypersplenism'. There is usually only mild impairment of liver function and thus the results of portal systemic shunting procedures usually give good results in selected cases. Splenectomy combined with lienorenal anastomosis is a helpful procedure if there is associated hypersplenism.

A relationship has been postulated between schistosome infection and carcinoma of the liver.

Cardiopulmonary systems. Lung involvement is usually the result of pulmonary embolization by eggs of *S. haematobium*. Though generally rare, it is reported with some frequency from Egypt. Two forms of lung disease occur:

1. a bronchopulmonary form, characterized by parenchymal egg granulomata: chronic bronchitis and bronchiectasis may result;
2. a cardiovascular form, due to occlusion of pulmonary arterioles by obliterative endarteritis, resulting in Ayerza's syndrome with cor pulmonale.

Nervous system. Eggs may lodge in any part of the CNS, generally seeded there by gravid females ectopically situated in nearby veins. Migrating schistosomulae may also be arrested in the nervous system if treatment is administered during the early migratory phase of the disease. However, neurological complications are unusual in schistosomiasis, cerebral involvement being best known with *S. japonicum* and spinal cord lesions with *S. mansoni* and *S. haematobium*.

Neuroschistosomiasis may well be more common than is currently recognized and is probably underdiagnosed according to Hughes and Biggs.[957]

It has been claimed that school performance can be adversely affected by chronic schistosomiasis.

In patients infected with *S. mansoni*, glomerulonephritis has been reported due to the deposition of immune complexes (IgM and IgG) in the kidney.

Laboratory diagnosis

Confirmation of the diagnosis of active schistosomiasis can only be obtained by finding typical viable eggs (Fig. 28.84a,b,c). Eggs can be recovered by examination of urinary deposit (*S. haematobium*) or from stool (all other species) by direct smear (including a Kato smear), sedimentation or water centrifugation.[986] Flotation techniques are not satisfactory and formol ether concentration kills the eggs with the result that no report can be made on egg viability as judged by miracidial activity or flame cell activity. Confirmation of viability of the egg is important to differentiate active disease from past infection.

Egg recovery is not easy and as many as 20% of infected persons may not pass eggs. Repeated examination of stool and urine specimens, the latter collected at midday, is essential. If urine or stools fail to reveal

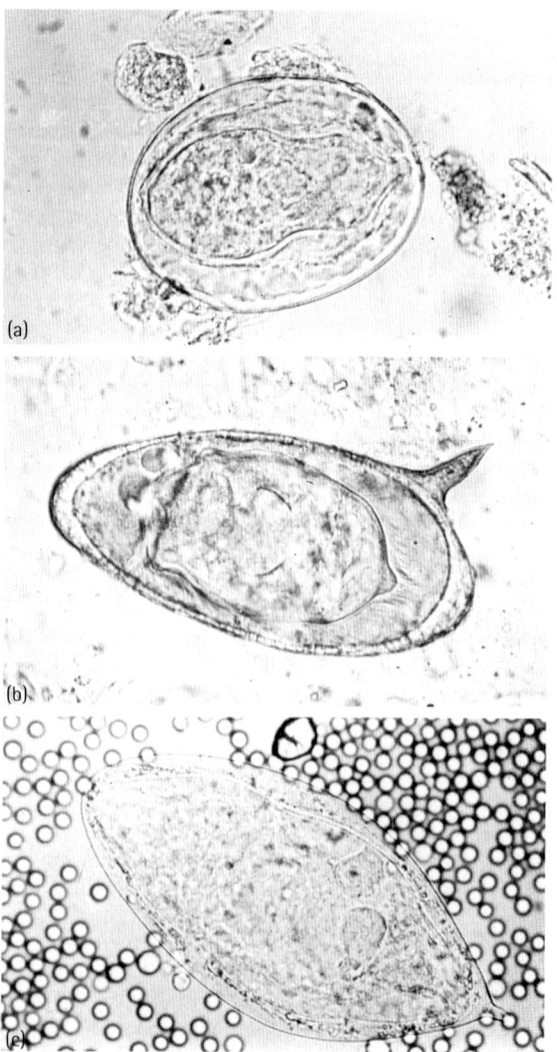

Fig. 28.84 (a) Egg of *Schistosoma japonicum* (approx. × 600). (b) Egg of *Schistosoma mansoni* (approx. × 600). (c) Egg of *Schistosoma haematobium* (approx. × 1000).

eggs, a rectal snip may prove rewarding in *S. japonicum, S. mansoni* and *S. haematobium* infections. In fact a single rectal snip gives more positives than three urines and stools. Cystoscopy may be indicated where urinary symptoms are present, the cystoscopic picture depending on the worm load.

A type I response skin test and various serological tests are available. These may be negative in early disease and positive results may indicate present or past infection, so a positive result is not, in itself, an indication for treatment. However, these tests often provide good negative screens to exclude a diagnosis of schistosomiasis and are particularly useful in screening returned travelers from endemic regions.

Treatment

The treatment of choice for all forms of schistosomiasis, and the only effective and safe treatment for *S. japonicum* infections, is praziquantel.[886,987-989] This drug is designated as a 'WHO essential agent', being extremely safe and highly effective when given as a single dose of 40 mg/kg (can be divided into two doses) for *S. haematobium* and *S. mansoni*[913,965,988,989] and at a dose of 60 mg/kg divided into three doses and given in a single day for *S. japonicum*.[884,885,965,990]

Of the other treatments available for schistosomiasis, metrifonate, an organophosphorus compound, appears to be less effective for treatment in cases of infection with *S. haematobium* than praziquantel.[989] It is not used for other species of schistosome. The dose used for children is 7.5 mg/kg per fortnight for a total of three doses.[885] Although side-effects are minimal, some have been recorded. The drug does depress cholinesterase levels and caution is needed in cases where patients may require some form of surgery necessitating the use of the muscle relaxant, suxamethonium. Oxamniquine is only effective against *S. mansoni* infections. The dose regimen is 10–20 mg/kg given as a single or divided doses over 1–2 days after food.[883,885,913,965,988,990] High cure rates and few side-effects are recorded.[886] This drug is useful for treating children orally at a rate of 20 mg/kg/d in 2 doses for 1 day.[913] Antischistosomal drugs such as the antimonials, niridazole and hycanthone have been superseded by the newer, more effective and safer compounds.

Prevention

As reinfection often follows successful treatment,[989] the control of schistosomiasis remains a priority. However, control is complex and generally employs a two-pronged attack on the life cycle of the fluke. The first is aimed at eliminating the snail population. Planned water systems for irrigation, which give a flow rate too high for survival of snails, are an ideal, but not always feasible method. Nontoxic molluscicides such as Frescon or Bayluscide have been found effective.

The experimental introduction of snail-eating predators and parasites has not had any lasting effect.

The second approach to control is aimed at preventing pollution of waterways by human excreta and involves public health education combined with provision of adequate and effective toilet facilities. In some control projects, mass treatment of infected humans has been used in conjunction with snail control. However, these aspects of prevention are ineffective in the case of *S. japonicum* which is extensively propagated by rodents. In *S. japonicum*, cercariae can be prevented from penetrating the skin by using topical applications of niclosamide or niclosamide-impregnated leggings.

Mass de-worming, repeated chemotherapy and the provision of safe water supplies through pump systems have all been proposed for the control of schistosomiasis.[991]

By 1988, schistosome vaccines were entering phase 1 trials[992] and research continues into the development of vaccines and chemoprophylaxis. The results to date appear to be encouraging, but there are concerns about the application of vaccine programs.[993-996]

OTHER TREMATODES

The life cycles of these flukes involve a variety of snail hosts with infective metacercariae settling on plants or aquatic invertebrates or vertebrates[870] (Table 28.47).

Liver fluke infection

The main trematode infections of the liver are fascioliasis, caused by the cattle and sheep liver flukes *Fasciola hepatica* (temperate regions) and *F. gigantica* (tropical Africa, Asia and Hawaii); clonorchiasis caused by *Clonorchis (Opisthorchis) sinensis* in the Far East; and opisthorchiasis, caused by *Opisthorchis felineus* in parts of Europe and Asia or *O. viverrini* in Thailand.

Clinical features

Infection with these flukes results when the metacercariae are ingested with aquatic plants (*Fasciola*) such as watercress to which the encysted metacercariae are attached, or in undercooked fish (*Clonorchis, Opisthorchis*).[870]

Symptoms of liver fluke infection depend largely upon the worm load and mild infections are often asymptomatic. Heavier infections tend to produce a triphasic response with an initial phase of invasion being accompanied by irregular fever and eosinophilia. Diarrhea and urticaria are common and there may be tender hepatomegaly. This phase lasts for about 4 weeks and is followed by an asymptomatic latent period

Table 28.47 Life cycles of intestinal and lung flukes

	Fascioliasis	Clonorchiasis	Opisthorchiasis	Fasciolopsiasis	Paragonimiasis
Adult fluke ↓	30 × 10 mm F. hepatica F. gigantica Liver	15 × 5 mm Cl. sinensis Liver	9 × 5 mm O. felineus O. viverrini Liver	50 × 15 mm F. buski Small intestine	12 × 6 mm Paragonimus spp. Lung
Egg ↓	Feces	Feces	Feces	Feces	Sputum/feces
Miracidium ↓	Free-swimming ↓	Ingested by snail ↓	Ingested by snail ↓	Free-swimming ↓	Free-swimming ↓
Snail ↓					
Cercariae ↓					
Metacercaria ↓	Water plants	Freshwater fish	Freshwater fish	Water plants (water chestnut)	Crabs and crayfish
Definitive host	Plant eater: sheep, cow human	Fish eater: dog, cat, pig, human	Fish eater: dog, human, seals	Water chestnut eater: pig, human	Crab/crayfish eater: dog, cat, human

usually lasting several months before the stage of obstructive jaundice occurs. Rarely the parasites of *F. hepatica* may settle in ectopic sites such as the pharynx after eating raw liver and mature there with resulting local reaction. Pharyngeal fascioliasis is known in the Middle East as *halzoun*. Individual worms may migrate into the liver parenchyma resulting in liver abscess formation. Eosinophilia is often present and the ESR is usually raised.

In Thailand, cholangiocarcinoma has been found to be associated with infection by *O. viverrini*.[997]

Local prevalences are often dependent upon social customs and dietary habits, and epidemic outbreaks of fascioliasis have been recorded.[997,998]

Diagnosis

The diagnosis is usually based upon the finding of typical operculate eggs in the feces (Fig. 28.85) although in some infected patients stools are consistently negative for eggs. The finding of eggs of *Fasciola* in the feces must be regarded with caution, as persons eating infected cattle or sheep liver can pass 'transit eggs' and this condition of spurious infection or false fascioliasis must be distinguished from true fascioliasis by the examination of repeat stool specimens.[928]

Treatment

On the whole, treatment of liver fluke infection remains unsatisfactory. For fascioliasis, treatment now consists of triclabendazole 12 mg/kg orally once daily for 1–2 days.[890,913,916] Bithionol 50 mg/kg orally in divided doses on alternate days for 2–3 weeks has been used,[965] and chloroquine, dehydroemetine and praziquantel have also been tried. Drug treatment of choice for clonorchiasis and opisthorchiasis is praziquantel 25–75 mg/kg/d in 3 doses for 1–2 days with albendazole (10 mg/kg for 7 d) as an alternative.[890,913,965]

Intestinal fluke infections

Many species of fluke infect the human intestinal tract[870,999] including the large intestinal fluke *Fasciolopsis buski* in parts of South East Asia, the small intestinal fluke *Heterophyes heterophyes*, in the Nile Delta and Far East, *Metagonimus yokogawai* in the Far East and eastern Europe and *Brachylaima* sp. in Australia.[1000]

Infection with these flukes results from ingesting metacercariae with aquatic vegetation (*F. buski*), with raw or undercooked fish (*H. heterophyes* and *M. yokogawai*) or by snail ingestion (*Brachylaima*). As in the case of liver fluke infection, a local high prevalence may be caused by local eating habits.[870,998]

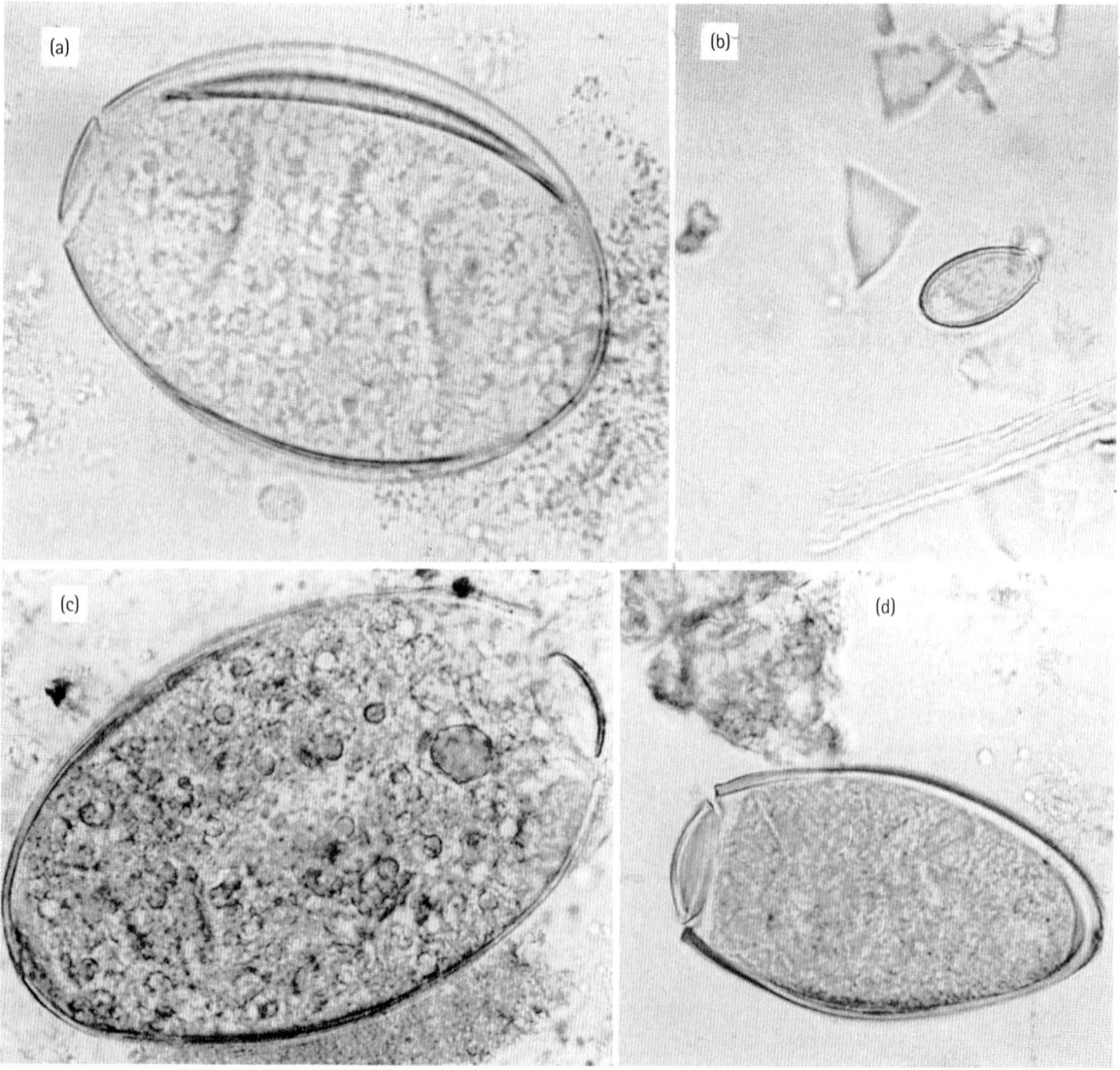

Fig. 28.85   Eggs of (a) *Fasciola hepatica* – ruptured to demonstrate operculum (approx. × 600); (b) *Opisthorchis sinensis* (approx. × 600); (c) *Fasciolopsis buski* – ruptured to demonstrate operculum (approx. × 600); (d) *Paragonimus westermani* (approx. × 600).

Symptoms of intestinal fluke infection may vary from a mild inflammatory reaction at the site of worm attachment in the small intestine to ulceration or abscess formation in the bowel wall, associated with severe bloody diarrhea.

Infections due to *F. buski* may result in vague abdominal symptoms, ascites and edema, probably as a result of protein-losing enteropathy and toxaemia.[999] An eosinophilia may be present, and iron deficiency anemia is common in fasciolopsiasis.

Diagnosis

As with liver fluke infection, diagnosis is made by finding typical operculate eggs in the feces of infected patients (Fig. 28.85).

Treatment

Intestinal fluke infections due to *F. buski*, *Heterophyes heterophyes* and *Metagonimus yokogawai* in children can be treated with praziquantel in a dose of 75 mg/kg in three doses for 1 day.[883,885,913,965] Niclosamide has also been used to treat intestinal fluke infections, while tetrachlorethylene has been described as an effective and cheap anthelmintic.[886,896]

Lung fluke infection

Human lung fluke infection is caused by 11 species of the genus *Paragonimus*. In the Far East, South East Asia and the Philippines, the species involved is *P. westermani* while in central and west Africa (and probably South Africa) the species is *P. africanus* or *P. uterobilateralis*. In the western hemisphere, *P. mexicanus* and *P. kellicotti* are the more common species.[896]

Infection occurs with the ingestion of the metacercariae in crabs and crayfish. Again local high prevalences are largely dependent upon dietary habits and culinary practices of preparing and cooking the crustacean intermediate hosts.[870,998] However, an interesting epidemic is on record which resulted from the use of crab juice as an antipyretic for children suffering from measles.

Symptoms of lung fluke infection are often suggestive of pulmonary tuberculosis, which may also often be present concurrently. The onset is insidious with cough and chest pain. Hemoptysis is usual, with copious blood-tinged sputum containing many eggs. Bronchiectasis and pulmonary fibrosis are late results, and finger clubbing is often present. An eosinophilia may occur and variable symptoms may result from flukes developing in ectopic sites, e.g. transverse myelitis and skin ulceration. In a small percentage of patients with paragonimiasis, the adult worms may settle in the CNS resulting in epilepsy, hemiplegia, visual impairment or an eosinophilic meningitis.[957]

Diagnosis

The diagnosis of paragonimiasis is established by finding the characteristic asymmetrical operculate eggs in sputum or feces (Fig. 28.85). X-rays, CT scans and serology may all prove useful.

Treatment

The drugs of choice are bithionol (or Bitin) at a dose of 30–40 mg/kg in divided doses given orally every other day for 10–15 days, or the newer derivative of bithionol, Bitin-S, given at a dosage regimen of 10–20 mg/kg every other day for 10–15 days. Praziquantel is very effective at a dose of 75 mg/kg/d in three doses for 2 days[883,885,886,913,965] and may be used in conjunction with corticosteroids if there is CNS involvement.[890]

Side-effects include diarrhea, nausea, vomiting and abdominal pain, but these are mild and soon subside.

ACANTHOCEPHALA

This group of helminths, the thorny-headed worms, are intestinal parasites of rats throughout the world. They are characterized by a proboscis covered with rows of recurved hooklets and have as their intermediate hosts insects such as cockroaches. The only species recorded from humans are *Moniliformis moniliformis* and *Macracanthorhynchus hirudinaceus*.

Humans, especially children, are occasionally infected after accidental ingestion of the intermediate host.[874] The worms live in the small intestine and diagnosis is made by passing adult worms or finding eggs in the feces. Spurious transit eggs can be passed by humans after eating of rodents as food.

Pyrantel pamoate and tiabendazole appear to be ineffectual, and mebendazole (Vermox) is the drug of choice, at a dose of 100 mg (one tablet) twice a day for 3 days.

FLIES, FLEAS, MITES AND LICE

MYIASIS

Myiasis is the infection by fly maggots of tissues of living animals, including humans. The larvae of a number of fly species may penetrate the skin of children or enter wound tissue.[1001] While the maggots of some myiasis-causing fly species only feed on dead and necrotic tissue (and even today are sometimes used in the medical treatment of wounds), the maggots of species such as the screw worm flies (*Callitroga americana* in the New World and *Chrysomyia bezziana* in the Old World) can be dangerous, as they extend their activities from necrotic to healthy tissue around the wounds.

Various clinical forms of myiasis are recognized: cutaneous (including wound infection), gastrointestinal, ocular, aural and urogenital. The clinical relevance varies according to the site and the species of fly involved, but infection of the sinuses and nasal cavities may be the most dangerous.[1002]

The tumbu, or putsi fly, *Cordylobia anthropophaga*, is found in tropical and subtropical Africa, and recently in Northern Europe.[1003] The large pale brown tumbu deposits her eggs on shady soil contaminated with urine, or damp clothing, where they hatch to release larvae in about 3 days. Laundry placed out to dry is an ideal site for oviposition, especially if laid out on grass or on the ground, so thorough ironing of clothes is desirable in endemic areas. The larvae penetrate intact skin where they grow rapidly, and unless removed, abandon the host and drop onto the ground in about 8 days to pupate.

Cutaneous lesions, which may be single or multiple, can occur on any part of the skin, particularly the waist, back (Fig. 28.86a) and feet. The characteristic lesion is a tender, large, furuncular swelling with a dark, central pore (Fig. 28.86b). Following application of petroleum jelly, the pore widens revealing movement of the posterior spiracles. The larva, about 0.5–1.0 cm in length, may then be squeezed out or grasped with forceps and extracted. Secondary infection of these lesions is rare.

In South America, the eggs and larvae of the tropical warble fly *Dermatobia hominis* may be transferred to the human skin by flies, mosquitoes or ticks and produce similar papular lesions.

Cutaneous myiasis is being increasingly recognized as an imported infection in many nontropical areas.[1003]

In areas of the world where sheep are farmed, the sheep nasal bot fly, *Oestrus ovis*, has been at times recorded as causing ophthalmomyiasis, a self-limiting but extremely painful condition.

Other larvae (e.g. those of *Gasterophilus*) may produce itching skin lesions related to the wanderings of the larvae, or tender short-lived subcutaneous cystic swellings. *G. intestinalis* can cause intestinal myiasis.

Maggots of some fly species tend to infest neglected wounds with excess necrotic tissue, even in hospital situations, and can be controlled by adequate wound toilet.

Myiasis may occur rarely in mucous membrane-lined orifices such as the mouth, anus and vagina, and in the eye. One species, *Auchmeromyia luteola*, lives in cracks and crevices of floors in Africa, coming out at night to suck blood from the sleeping human host.

TUNGIASIS

Tungiasis is infection with the jigger (or chigoe) flea, *Tunga penetrans*, originally endemic to South America, but now also endemic in central Africa and parts of India.

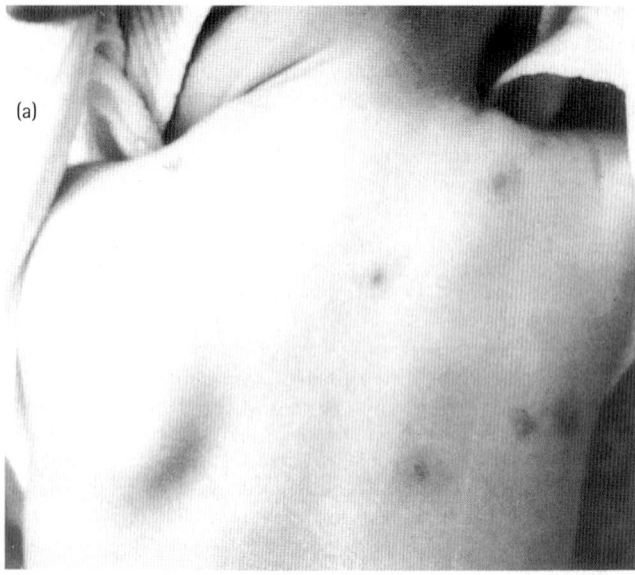

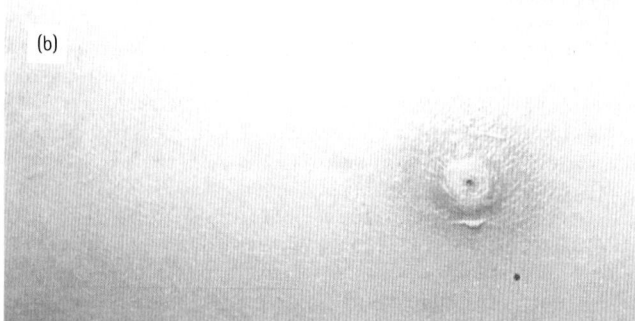

Fig. 28.86 (a) Child with multiple putsi lesions on back. (b) Lesion due to *Cordylobia anthropophaga* on leg to show characteristic appearance.

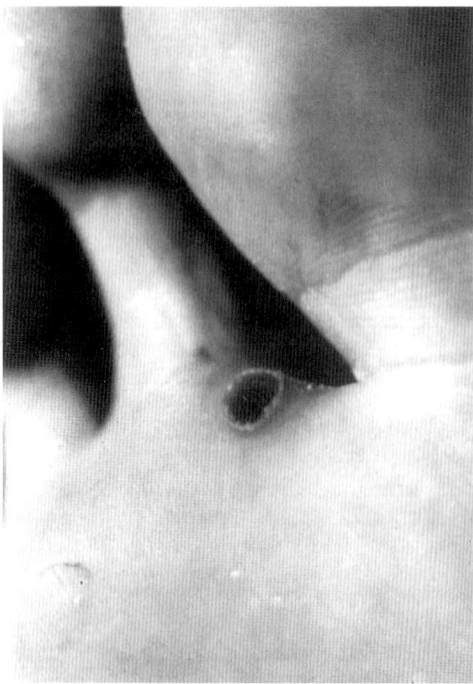

Fig. 28.87 Lesion due to jigger flea (*Tunga penetrans*). (Courtesy of Dr K. Ott)

The adult fleas live in soil or in the dust and cracks of earth floors of houses. After mating, the female flea penetrates the skin of the host (rodents, dogs, cats or humans) and develops in the epidermis under the stratum corneum, her abdomen swelling tremendously with developing eggs. The initial small lesion becomes inflamed and erythematous, developing into a pustule which may crust over or even form a suppurating ulcer if secondarily infected by bacteria. Lesions mostly occur on the feet, especially under the toenails or between the toes (Fig. 28.87). Itching, pain and even regional lymphadenopathy are common.

Eggs are expelled by the female flea, fall to the ground and form free-living larvae and pupae in the soil.

Diagnosis is made by finding the flea in the lesion and carefully removing it. In unsuspected cases, diagnosis may be made after biopsy of the lesion and finding the fragmented flea in the lesion.

Treatment consists of a careful removal of the flea, without rupturing it, using a sterile needle, followed by a cleaning of the wound with chloroform and a careful curetting of the affected area.

Jiggers are a potential source of tetanus in unimmunized children.

DEMODICIDOSIS

The hair follicle mite, *Demodex folliculorum* (Fig. 28.88), is one of the commonest parasites of the human skin, with infection rates of 25% or higher.

Human infection is probably acquired by direct person-to-person contact, often at a very young age (e.g. suckling babies infected from their mother). Human infection with other species of *Demodex* from animals has not been ruled out.

The mites live in the pilosebaceous glands and hair follicles especially of the face, scalp, external ear and breast. They are common in the eyelids and mites can often be found clinging to removed eyelashes.

Clinically the condition may be asymptomatic or infected hair follicles may result in the formation of 'blackheads' with crops of red papules appearing on the forehead. In heavy infestations, or in sensitized patients, dermatitis may follow, with scaling of the skin. Demodicidosis may be associated with HIV infection, causing an acute papulo-nodular rash, usually localized to the head and neck.[1004]

Diagnosis is established by finding the mites, often in sero-purulent fluid expressed from the lesions, or in biopsied specimens of skin in which mites can be found.

Treatment consists of good hygiene, soap and water together with sulfur ointment or gamma-benzene hexachloride if necessary.

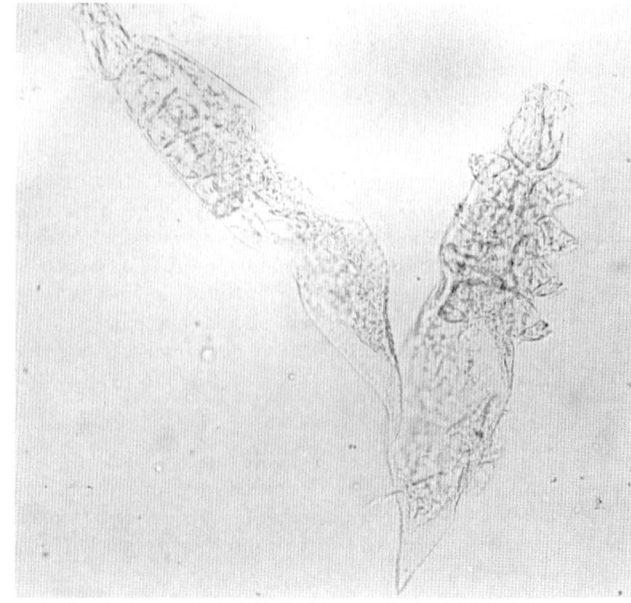

Fig. 28.88 *Demodex folliculorum* (approx. × 300).

SCABIES (see Ch. 30)

Scabies is a disease caused by the mite *Sarcoptes scabiei* (Fig. 28.89b). It occurs worldwide, especially in areas of crowding and in countries with a low standard of living. Scabies appears to sweep the world in cyclical pandemics.[1003,1005] It can afflict both rich and poor alike, and is more common in women and children.[1006] Most cases of human scabies are contracted from other infected humans, but occasionally animal strains of the scabies mite can infect humans.[1002]

The gravid female mites burrow into the horny layers of the skin, forming tunnels (Fig. 28.89c) in which the eggs are laid. The female mite lives for about one month, laying 2–3 eggs daily, which hatch in 3–4 days into six-legged larvae. These migrate to the surface and then burrow into the skin again and moult into eight-legged nymphs before becoming adults about 10 days after hatching. On average, each patient is infested with only 10–12 mites at any one time and much of the observed symptomatology is due to sensitization of the host to the mite and its products.[1007,1008]

CLINICAL FEATURES

Although the main sites infested can vary with the age of the patient, the commonest sites found to harbor mites include the hands (especially the sides of the fingers and the interdigital spaces), the finger webs, the wrists, the elbows, the feet, the penis and the scrotum, the buttocks and the axillae, with a lesser involvement of the body. The head and face is spared in most cases, except in infants.[1006,1009]

The feeding activities of the mites and host sensitization result in itching and the development of an extensive rash, which does not correlate with the predilection sites of the mites (Fig. 28.89a).

The characteristic lesions of scabies are the burrows in the skin, but there may also be pruritic papules, vesicles and pustules. Often there is eczematization and crusting of the lesions, especially when they are secondarily infected by bacteria. Scabies lesions can provide an entry site for infection with Group A beta hemolytic streptococci and thus glomerulonephritis may follow scabies.[1009]

Scabies may present in variable forms.[1006] In some healthy persons and in patients on corticosteroids, scabies may present with minimal signs and symptoms. In young children, vesicles rather than tunnels are often the rule, while in some patients the disease occurs in the nodular form. In mentally handicapped patients, debilitated patients and the immunosuppressed, extensive crusted or 'Norwegian scabies' is sometimes seen and in HIV infected individuals scabies can be particularly severe and persistent. In such cases the infestation is highly contagious and large numbers of mites can be found.

A common feature of scabies is the characteristic nocturnal itching, especially when the patient is warm in bed.

The infestation is transmitted by direct contact, including sexual contact. Fomites such as clothing and blankets generally play no part in the transmission of scabies.

DIAGNOSIS

Scabies is usually diagnosed clinically and should be considered in any patient presenting with an itchy rash covering the whole body but sparing the head and face.[1008,1010] In infants, scabies may present in an atypical form which can involve the face.[1006] Confirmation by the finding of mites is often difficult, even extensive lesions being associated with very few mites. Mites or their fecal pellets can sometimes be found in the tunnels after careful removal of the horny layers of skin. An improved method of obtaining mites is to scrape a suspect lesion and then float the mite out using mineral oil.

TREATMENT

The treatment of scabies involves the widespread application of topical preparations. Permethrin 5% cream or benzyl benzoate 25% emulsion are the treatments of choice.[1006,1008–1010] Full strength benzyl benzoate can cause an unpleasant stinging, so for children and sensitive adults it should be used diluted to half strength and in children under 2 years should be diluted with 3 parts water. Monosulfiram and crotamiton are possibly less effective, but the latter is said to have some antipruritic activity. Gamma-benzene hexachloride 1% has in the past proved to be cheap and effective,[1009] but is toxic if ingested. It should not be used in premature babies and should be used with care in pregnancy and in infants under 1 year of age.[1011] Children younger than 2 months can be treated with 5% sulfur cream daily for 2–3 days.[884,1006]

Resistance to both lindane and the pyrethroids (including permethrin) has been recorded and it may be difficult to distinguish resistance from incomplete treatment.[1009]

For adequate treatment and control, *all members of the family must be treated whether or not they exhibit symptoms*, or relapses and treatment failure will result.[1006] In conditions of overcrowding and poor hygiene, the regular use of monosulfiram soap prevents reinfection.

For mild scabies a single treatment should suffice but moderate or severe scabies might require re-treatment after 14 days. Symptoms may persist due to sensitization to treatment, and some patients have a 'parasitophobia' and see imaginary parasites; in these cases over-treatment must be avoided.

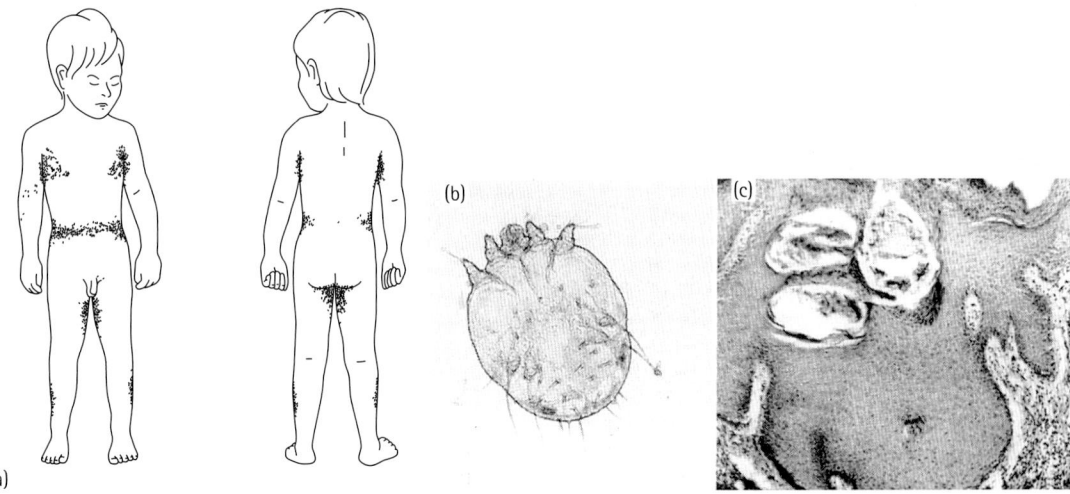

Fig. 28.89 (a) The distribution of the rash in scabies. (b) Adult *Sarcoptes scabiei* (approx. × 100). (c) Histological section of skin in scabies showing tunnels (approx. × 300).

Giving a child a hot bath before treatment for scabies commences is unnecessary.

Many animal parasitic mites (e.g. *Dermanyssus* and *Ornithonyssus* from rodents or birds and mange and cheyletid mites from dogs and cats) as well as many free-living and nonparasitic mites can attack humans and cause an extensive rash with a severe dermatitis and an itchy allergic reaction resulting in the formation of papules, vesicles and skin blotches. This condition can be very distressing and infestation usually derives from pets, animals nesting in roofs, straw and other packing materials.[1012]

The use of oral ivermectin (200 µg/kg orally as one dose for children > 5 years together with scabicides)[884,1006] may be required for the treatment of crusted scabies; toxicity can be a problem.[1008,1009] One review[1013] found no difference in clinical cure rates between crotamiton and lindane or benzyl benzoate and sulfur and concluded 'the evidence that permethrin is more effective than lindane is inconsistent. Lindane, permethrin and ivermectin appear to be associated with rare but serious drug reactions'. More research is needed on the safety and effectiveness of ivermectin and malathion compared to permethrin, on community management, and on different regimens and vehicles for topical treatment.

LOUSE INFESTATION

Humans can become infested with three types of lice: the head louse (*Pediculus humanus capitis*; Fig. 28.90); its morphologically identical, but behaviorally different variant, the body louse (*P. h. corporis*); and the crab or pubic louse, which forms a distinct species, *Pthirus pubis*. All three types are confined to humans worldwide and tend to be more prevalent in areas with poor living standards.[1014]

PEDICULUS HUMANUS CAPITIS (THE HEAD LOUSE)

P. h. capitis is worldwide in distribution. Its incidence is subject to unpredictable increases and decreases, with sporadic extensive pandemics. The prevalence varies from country to country and from year to year but may reach 60% or more of schoolchildren.[1007,1014]

Head lice tend to be confined to the scalp but are occasionally found on other hairy parts of the body. The insects live close to the scalp and feed on blood which they obtain with their sucking mouthparts. After mating, the female louse lays 6–8 eggs every 24 h. These eggs or 'nits' (Fig. 28.91) are glued tightly to the hairs close to the scalp and hatch in about 7 days into nymphs, which feed and pass through three instars before becoming adult in 10–11 days.[1014]

Head louse infestation is usually asymptomatic but heavy infestations may be manifested by scalp pruritus and, with secondary bacterial infection, by cervical gland enlargement.

Pediculosis capitis is found in people of all ages but is most common in children aged 3–13 years, and maximal at 6–9 years. Although not

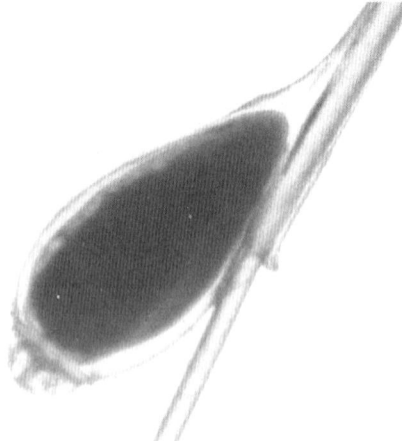

Fig. 28.91   Egg of crab louse (*Pthirus. pubis*) attached to hair (approx. × 60).

directly correlated to hair length, head lice are more common in girls than in boys. Both rich and poor alike are afflicted, but infestation is more frequent in low socioeconomic areas.

Diagnosis of pediculosis capitis is based on careful examination of the scalp for lice or their eggs. This is greatly facilitated using a hand lens. A more effective method for diagnosis involves treating dry hair with white conditioner, combing it with a fine tooth 'nit' comb, and examining the comb or, better still, the combings spread on a sheet of paper for nits.[1015,1016]

Head lice can only be controlled by regular inspection and treatment of infected cases *and all their family members*, whether or not lice or nits can be found in the latter. Dead nits remain tightly attached to the hairs and may have to be combed out with special fine toothed 'nit combs'.

In the past, DDT has been used for treatment, but its toxicity and resistance in the lice led to its replacement by gamma-benzene hexachloride (gamma BHC, gamma HCH; lindane). However, resistance is being recorded to HCH and this, plus its toxicity, has resulted in its being considered obsolete in many parts of the world.[1007,1017,1018] It is being replaced by safer preparations such as carbaryl, malathion and the synthetic pyrethroids such as permethrin. Of these, malathion (a 0.5% preparation in a spirit base) is the most widely used. It is twice as safe as HCH and has the added but variable advantage of possibly being residual for at least a month, through bonding to the hair. Additionally, malathion and carbaryl are reported to be ovicidal, killing both lice and nits, a feature absent in HCH which is not ovicidal. However, the concept of an inherent ovicidal efficacy for malathion and carbaryl has been challenged.[1019] Repeat treatments after a week or so might be advisable, irrespective of the insecticide used. Pyrethrins, especially those in a mousse formulation, may also be effectively used to treat head lice,[1014] with the third generation synthetic pyrethroids such as permethrin proving the most promising.[1017,1018] Permethrin, synergized pyrethrum and malathion are all effective in head louse treatment and the choice between them really depends on local resistance patterns.[1020] All these preparations are toxic to some extent and care should thus be exercised in their use, with particular care being taken to avoid accidental ingestion or contact with eyes. Shampoos and lotions are both available, but lotions are far superior.[1014,1021,1022] Developing resistance to head louse preparations may prove a problem, albeit a sometimes controversial one.[1014,1020,1023] Ivermectin may be considered for the treatment of more difficult cases.[1024]

The use of levamisole for pediculosis, although considered to be safe and economical by some,[1025] does not really seem a practical alternative to the more conventional methods of head louse control.

An alternative, non-insecticidal approach to the treatment of head lice involves applying hair conditioner to wet hair, then combing the hair thoroughly using a fine toothed comb to remove the lice and their eggs, a technique known as 'bug-busting' in the UK.

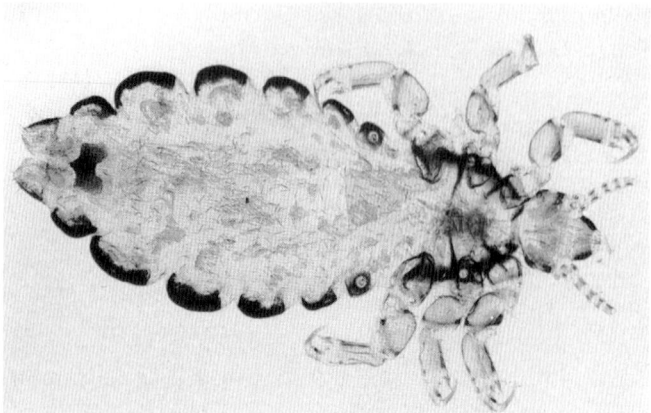

Fig. 28.90   Photomicrograph of adult *Pediculus humanus capitis* – the head louse (approx. × 50).

This does need dedication to ensure that the process is effectively carried out and results of its efficacy compared to insecticidal treatment vary.[1026–1028]

In the control of head lice, sterilization of clothing, bedding, combs, etc., is unnecessary, as insecticide treatment of the hair will provide sufficient protection from re-invasion by the short-lived lice that have strayed from the head.

In community control programs, education and involvement of all participants, parents, education and health professionals, as well as hairdressers, is necessary, and anti-louse preparations should be changed on a regular basis to prevent the emergence of resistance.

PEDICULUS HUMANUS CORPORIS (THE BODY LOUSE)

P. h. corporis is identical to the head louse in appearance, but differs in that it lives on the clothing and only visits the skin to suck blood. The eggs are glued to the clothing, especially the seams, and hatch in about one week to nymphs, which like those of the head louse, develop into adults in 7–10 days.

Pediculosis corporis may be characterized by the presence of feeding punctures appearing as small papules which, in sensitized patients, may become swollen, pigmented and hardened, a condition formerly known as vagabond's disease or *morbus errorum*.

Body lice are more limited to areas of overcrowding and poorer standards of living but may reach epidemic proportions during periods of social upheaval and unrest such as war, earthquakes and floods. They are the vectors of epidemic typhus (*Rickettsia prowazekii*) and epidemic relapsing fever (*Borrelia recurrentis*).

Transmission of body lice is directly from person to person and from shared clothing and blankets. Control is with 0.5% malathion lotion or 5% carbaryl dust and treatment of clothing, blankets, etc., with methyl bromide fumigation, washing in hot water at 60 °C or higher by heating in a domestic tumble drier for at least 5 min.

PTHIRUS PUBIS (THE CRAB OR PUBIC LOUSE)

Pth. pubis has a distinctive appearance and is usually found in the pubic region of humans only. It may also be found tightly attached to the hairs of the leg, the axilla or the beard (Fig. 28.92). Eggs are laid attached to hairs or even eyelashes (Fig. 28.93). It is usually transmitted during sexual intercourse and because of this, it is mostly found infesting

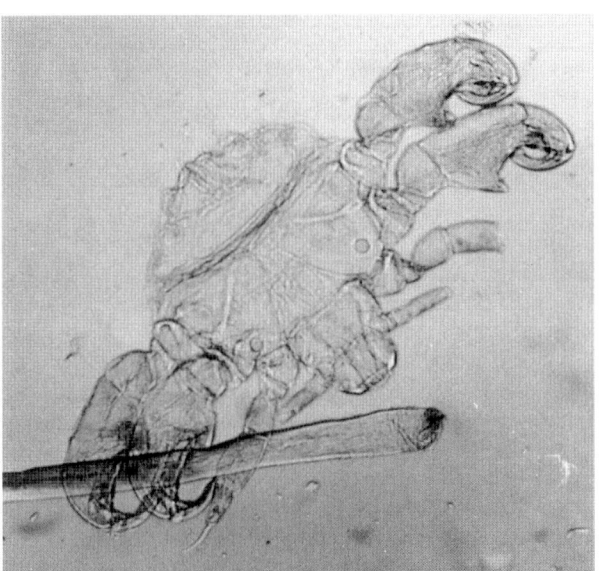

Fig. 28.92 Photomicrograph of nymph of *Pthirus pubis* tightly attached to hair (approx. × 100).

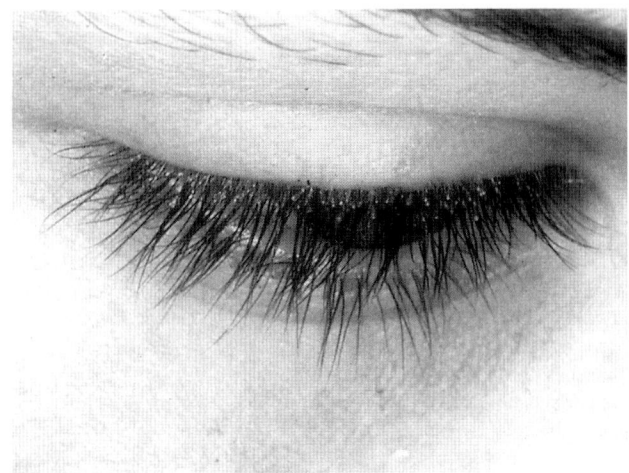

Fig. 28.93 Eggs of pubic louse on eyelashes.

adults. However, children can harbor the lice and even young children may become infected from heavily infested parents through close nonsexual contact. Thus, toddlers are at times found to have phthiriasis, the lice being found attached to the eyelashes and even the hair of the forehead. The lice can survive for 9–44 h off the host, and infestation from clothing and toilet seats is thus feasible, although unlikely.

Heavy infestations may result in itching and, rarely, *maculae cerulae* or bluish spots due to repeated biting may be found.

Treatment is similar to that for head lice, using insecticides such as gamma-benzene hexachloride (lindane) as a lotion, shampoo or powder. This insecticide is toxic and treatment needs to be repeated, as it is not ovicidal. 0.5% malathion or carbaryl are safer and, being ovicidal, are more effective, but spirit base preparations should not be used. Pyrethroids are also effective and are widely used.

When on the eyelashes (Fig. 28.93), *Pth. pubis* should be dealt with by removal of individual lice or by treating each egg individually with a paint brush dipped in an ovicidal insecticide. Alternatively, the thick application of Vaseline twice daily for 8 days may be effective.[1014] Laundering of clothing, sheets, etc., in hot water is advisable to prevent spread.

DISEASES TRANSMITTED BY ANIMALS

These are summarized in Table 28.48.[1029]

CAT-SCRATCH DISEASE (CSD)

Cat-scratch disease is a relatively benign, widely encountered infection characterized by malaise, low grade fever and lymphadenopathy. About half of the patients with CSD develop a nonpruritic, erythematous primary lesion 3–30 days after getting a scratch. This lesion may form a small pustule but overall the infection usually resolves spontaneously in a few weeks. Rarely, complications can occur such as encephalitis, conjunctivitis (Parinaud's oculoglandular syndrome), neuroretinitis and thrombocytopenic purpura.[1029–1031] Contact with cats followed by skin lesions associated with a scratch or bite are found in the majority of cases. There may be a maculopapular rash. Chronic lymphadenitis may occur with the cervical lymph nodes frequently involved. Murano et al[1032] reported a giant hepatic granuloma as associated with *Bartonella henselae* infection and suggested that this infection should be considered in the differential diagnosis of a large hepatic mass. Overall, systemic symptoms are unusual in CSD, but severe disease may occur in HIV positive patients. Isada et al[1033] reported that in the USA, 22 000 cases of CSD occur annually with 10% requiring hospitalization.

Table 28.48   Diseases transmitted/harbored by dogs, cats and rodents*

Dogs	Cats	Rodents
Rabies	Rabies	Lassa fever
Ringworm	Cat-scratch fever (*Bartonella henselae*)	Hantavirus disease
Scabies	Ringworm	S. American arenavirus hemorrhagic fevers
Echinococcus granulosus infection	Scabies	Omsk hemorrhagic fever
Toxocara canis infection (larva migrans)	*Toxocara cati* (larva migrans)	Kyasanur forest disease
Leptospirosis	Pasteurellosis (*Pasteurella multocida*)	Group C virus disease
Canicola fever (*Leptospira canicola*)	Cutaneous larva migrans	E. Hemisphere sandfly fever
Leishmaniasis	Toxoplasmosis	Vesicular stomatitis fever
Dipylidium caninum	*Bartonella clarridgeiae*	Venezuelan equine encephalitis
Cutaneous larva migrans	*Capillaria aerophila*	Lymphocytic choriomeningitis
Dirofilaria immitis	Cutaneous dirofilariasis	Rat bite fever (*Spirillum minor*)
Capnocytophaga canimorsus (DF-2)	Paragonimiasis	Haverhill fever (*Streptobacillus moniliformis*)
Bartonella clarridgeiae	Q fever	Bubonic plague (*Yersinia pestis*)
Bartonella vinsonii	*Ctenocephalides felis*	Campylobacteriosis
Spotted fever (some forms)	Salmonellosis (gastroenteritis)	Salmonellosis (gastroenteritis)
Ehrlichiosis	Giardiasis	Leptospirosis (e.g. Weil disease)
Cutaneous dirofilariasis	*Strongyloides* sp.	Endemic relapsing fever
Paragonimiasis	*Tunga penetrans*	Scrub typhus
Q fever		Murine typhus
Salmonellosis (gastroenteritis)		Rickettsialpox
Ctenocephalides canis		Spotted fever (some forms)
Giardiasis		Q fever
Diphyllobothrium latum		*Bartonella* spp.
Fasciola hepatica		*Babesia microti*
Lyme disease		Toxoplasmosis (where rodents are eaten)
Trichuris vulpis		Cutaneous leishmaniasis (some forms)
Strongyloides sp.		Clonorchis sinensis
Tunga penetrans		*Schistosoma japonicum*
Eosinophilic enteritis		Multilocular hydatid
		Hymenolepis nana
		Hymenolepis diminuta
		Inermicapsifer madagascariensis
		Angiostrongyliasis
		Capillaria hepatica
		Moniliformis moniliformis
		Cordylobia anthropophaga
		Xenopsylla cheopis
		Tunga penetrans
		Dermanyssid mites
		Trombiculid mites

*Not all of these infections are directly transmissible to humans from the animal reservoir and in some cases the animal may only be an occasional reservoir for the infection. For details of these and other infectious diseases relating especially to control, the reference edited by Chin[1029] is strongly recommended.

ETIOLOGY

The bacterium *Bartonella* (formerly *Rochalimaea*) *henselae* is considered the cause of CSD and the role of *Afipia felis* in the causation of CSD (if it has one) is small.[1029,1034,1035] Kordick et al,[1036] however, have described *B. clarridgeiae* as causing a cat-scratch disease-like syndrome.

Other species of the genus *Bartonella* can infect humans but are not involved in causing CSD. The species of *Bartonella* and their disease associations are summarized in Table 28.49.

DIAGNOSIS

The diagnosis of CSD is confirmed if the history of cat contact and a primary skin lesion is associated with typical silver-staining bacteria identified on histopathological sections of lymph nodes, skin or eye lesions. A skin test for cat-scratch disease is available, but this is being superseded by serology using an indirect fluorescent antibody test for *B. henselae* which is said to be more sensitive.

TREATMENT

As most patients with this disease are not ill and spontaneous recovery is common, treatment is usually symptomatic. Antibiotics should be reserved for patients with severe disease. The most commonly used antibiotics are not effective and a recent review indicated that only four antimicrobial drugs are useful, with the oral drugs in decreasing order of efficacy being rifampicin (87%), ciprofloxacin (84%) and trimethoprim–sulfamethoxazole (58%). Intramuscular gentamicin was 73% effective.[1037] Isada et al,[1033] while admitting that no controlled trials have been carried out in the treatment of CSD, report that erythromycin, doxycycline or co-trimoxazole, in that order, might be effective.

CAT-SCRATCH ENCEPHALOPATHY

CNS complications may develop from a few days to some weeks after the first evidence of illness, usually a mildly tender lymphadenopathy. Fever is not characteristic and may occur in only 50% of cases. Convulsions

Table 28.49 Disease associations in the genus *Bartonella* in humans

Species	Disease association	Comments
B. henselae	Cat-scratch disease (CSD) Bacillary angiomatosis	From cat bite/lick
B. quintana	Trench fever Bacillary angiomatosis	From body lice
B. bacilliformis	Oroya fever, verruga peruana	*Lutzomyia* flies
B. elizabethae	Subacute endocarditis Neuroretinitis	
B. clarridgeiae	Subacute endocarditis CSD-like syndrome	From cats/dogs
B. vinsonii	Subacute endocarditis	Various subspecies From cats, dogs, rodents

of varying severity will also affect about 50% of the children with encephalopathy, and they may remain lethargic or even comatose for several weeks. In the recovery phase, 'transient combative behavior' seems to be a characteristic feature of this particular type of encephalopathy. Changes in the CSF are neither consistent nor characteristic and peripheral blood counts are not helpful. In addition to the control of convulsions and supportive measures, the most important aspect is to establish the diagnosis and differentiate it from other causes of encephalopathy as quickly as possible to avoid extensive and invasive investigations. The prognosis is excellent with no evidence of lasting neurological impairment.[1038]

RAT-BITE FEVERS

Rat-bite fevers comprise two separate and distinct infections, both of which are characterized by a relapsing fever usually following a rat bite. They are particularly prevalent in rat-infested communities of low socioeconomic status. Children living in such areas are at especial risk and may even be bitten by rats while asleep. Children may also become infected following a bite from a pet mouse or rat. *Streptobacillus moniliformis* (streptobacillary rat-bite fever; Haverhill fever; erythema arthriticum epidemicum) has been recorded worldwide, including from Europe and the USA; *Spirillum minus* (spirillary rat-bite fever; sodoku or sokosha) has also been reported worldwide, but mostly from Japan.[1029] Streptobacillary rat-bite fever is a more common cause of fever following a rat bite than is the spirillary form.

STREPTOBACILLUS MONILIFORMIS (STREPTOBACILLOSIS)

Streptobacillus moniliformis is a commensal in the rat nasopharynx and has also occasionally been recorded from other small mammal species such as squirrels, weasels and gerbils.[1029,1031,1039] While transmission is usually through a rat bite, epidemic outbreaks in humans are believed to have resulted from ingestion of raw milk or water contaminated with rat urine or saliva.[1029,1031] The incubation period is usually 3–10 days,

occasionally longer, during which a gastroenteritis may be present. The infected bite usually heals rapidly but a fever develops which is often relapsing and, although usually subsiding within 10 days or so, may continue for months if untreated. A generalized erythematous, morbilliform or even purpuric rash, particularly on the hands and feet, may develop and arthralgia (especially of the large joints) and sore throat, extreme prostration and headache may occur. Complications may include infective endocarditis, pericarditis and abscesses of soft tissue or brain.[1029,1040,1041] The fatality rate may reach 10% if untreated.

Streptobacillary rat-bite fever needs to be differentiated from coxsackie infections, meningococcal septicemia and erythema multiforme but infection can be confirmed by isolation of *S. moniliformis* from blood, infected joint fluid, abscesses or pustules. Serological diagnosis using an agglutination test is available and becomes positive in the second to third week of the infection. Penicillin, given as soon as possible after the bite, is effective,[1031] as are cephalosporins, but strains resistant to penicillin, streptomycin and erythromycin have been recorded.

SPIRILLUM MINUS (SPIRILLOSIS)

Transmission of *Spirillum minus* is most commonly via the bite of an infected rat but can occur following the bite from other mammals including cats, which can serve as healthy reservoirs. Food contaminated by infected rat urine may also presumably cause infection.

The incubation period varies from 7 to 28 (mean 8) days after the bite, which may heal or become necrotic and chancre-like. Recurrent fevers occur at 5–10 day intervals, sometimes continuing for weeks in untreated patients, and may be accompanied by profuse sweating, often with a marked flare up of inflammation at the site of the bite. Regional lymphadenopathy usually develops and a characteristic purplish, papular (or sometimes nodular) rash or urticaria may be present, especially on the chest and arms. Muscle pains, but rarely joint pains and arthritis, hyperesthesia and localized edema are additional signs. In severe cases, a meningoencephalitis with delirium may develop, as may endocarditis and involvement of other organs. In untreated cases, the mortality may reach 10%, being associated with neuronal degeneration of the brain and degenerative changes in the liver and kidneys.

The differential diagnosis should consider other febrile infections, including those caused by spirochetes (such as relapsing fever), viruses, rickettsiae (such as the spotted fevers), bacterial infections (such as plague), tularemia and also malaria, in endemic regions. A puffiness of the face may suggest nephritis and children may present with persistent diarrhea and weight loss, which may further confuse the correct diagnosis. During febrile paroxysms there may be a leukocytosis and occasionally eosinophilia and anemia may be present. CSF pressure may be raised.

Diagnosis of spirillosis can be confirmed by detecting *S. minus* in lesion/tissue exudates, in an enlarged lymph node or, during a febrile episode, in peripheral blood by dark ground microscopy or by inoculation of guinea pigs, mice or laboratory rats. No specific serological tests are available.

Penicillin is the treatment of choice for spirillosis[965,1031] but streptomycin, erythromycin, chloramphenicol and tetracyclines (not during pregnancy or for children under 7–8 years of age) are also effective.

REFERENCES (* Level 1 evidence)

Mortality and Morbidity in Infectious Disease
1. World Bank. Investing in health, World Development Report. Oxford: Oxford University Press; 1993.
2. The United Nations Children's Fund. The state of the world's children 2007. New York: United Nations Children's Fund (UNICEF); 2006.
3. UNAIDS and WHO. AIDS epidemic update 2006. Geneva: United Nations AIDS Program (UNAIDS); 2006.

4. Murray CJL, Lopez AD, Chin B, et al. Estimation of potential global pandemic influenza mortality on the basis of vital registry data from the 1918–20 pandemic: a quantitative analysis. Lancet 2006; 368:2211–2218.
5. Fleming D, Smith GE, Charlton J, et al. Impact of infections on primary care – greater than expected. Commun Dis Public Health 2002; 5:7–12.
6. Murray CJL. Quantifying the burden of disease: the technical basis for disability-adjusted life years. In:

Murray CJL, Lopez AD, eds. Global comparative assessments in the health sector. Geneva: WHO; 1994:3–19.
7. Cliffe S, Tookey P, Nicoll A. Antenatal detection of HIV: national surveillance and unlinked anonymous surveys. BMJ 2001; 325:376–377.
8. The UK Collaborative Group for HIV and STI Surveillance. A complex picture. HIV and other sexually transmitted infections in the United Kingdom: 2006. London: Health Protection Agency, Centre for Infections; 2006.

9.   Trotter CL, Ramsay ME, Slack MP. Rising incidence of *Haemophilus influenza* type b disease in England indicates a need for second catch-up vaccination campaign. Commun Dis Public Health 2003; 6:55–58.

10.   Miller E, Salisbury D, Ramsay ME. Planning, registration and implementation of an immunization campaign against meningococcal C disease in the UK: a success story. Vaccine 2002; 20 Suppl 1:S8–S67.

11.   Ramsay M, Gay N, Miller E, et al. The epidemiology of measles in England and Wales: rationale for the 1994 national vaccination campaign. CDR Rev 1994; 4:R141–R146.

12.   Communicable Disease Surveillance Centre (CDSC). The national measles and rubella campaign – one year on. CDR Rev 1995; 5:237.

13.   Health Protection Agency. Protecting the health of England's children: the benefit of vaccines. First national report of the current status of the national universal vaccination programmes from the Centre for Infections. London: Health Protection Agency Centre for Infections; 2005.

14.   Ramsay ME, Yarwood, Lewis D, et al. Parental confidence in measles, mumps and rubella vaccine: evidence from vaccine coverage and attitudinal surveys. Br J Gen Pract 2002; 52:912–916.

15.   Gangarosa EJ, Galazka AM, Wolfe CR, et al. Impact of anti-vaccine movements on pertussis control. Lancet 1998; 351:356–361.

16.   Nicoll A. Benefits, safety and risks of immunisation programmes. Interdiscip Sci Rev 2001; 26:20–30.

17.   Colditz GA, Brewer TF, Berkey JCS, et al. Efficacy of BCG vaccine in the prevention of tuberculosis. JAMA 1994; 271:698–702.

18.   Elliott EJ, Robins-Browne RM, O'Loughlin EV, et al. Contributors to the Australian Paediatric Surveillance Unit. Nationwide study of haemolytic uraemic syndrome: clinical, microbiological, and epidemiological features. Arch Dis Child 2001; 5:125–131.

19.   Nicoll A, Catchpole M, Cliffe S, et al. Sexual health of teenagers in England and Wales. BMJ 1999; 318:1321–1322.

20.   National Chlamydia Screening Steering Group. New frontiers: Annual report of the National Chlamydia Screening Programme in England 2005/6. London: Health Protection Agency; 2006.

21.   Harling R, Twisselmann B, Asgari-Jihandeh N, et al, for the Deliberate Release Team. Deliberate releases of biological agents: initial lessons for Europe from events in the United States. Euro Surveill 2001; 6:166–171.

22.   World Health Organization, International Health Regulations 2005. http://www.who.int/csr/ihr/en/

23.   Satcher D. Emerging infections: getting ahead of the curve. Emerg Infect Dis 1997; 1:1–6.

24.   Verity CM, Nicoll A, Will RG, et al. Variant Creutzfeldt–Jakob disease in UK children: a national surveillance study. Lancet 2000; 356:1224–1227.

25.   Morse SS. Factors in the emergence of infectious diseases. Emerg Infect Dis 1995; 1:7–15.

26.   Begg N, Nicoll A. Myths in medicine, Immunisation. BMJ 1994; 309:1073–1075.

27.   Gill ON, Sockett PN, Bartlett CLR, et al. Outbreak of *Salmonella napoli* caused by contaminated chocolate bars. Lancet 1983; 2:544–547.

28.   Bell BP, Goldoft M, Griffin PM, et al. A multistate outbreak of *E. coli* O157: H7-associated bloody diarrhea and hemolytic uremic syndrome from hamburgers. JAMA 1994; 272:1349–1353.

29.   Wasserheit JN. Effect of changes in human ecology and behaviour on patterns of sexually transmitted diseases, including immunodeficiency virus infection. Proc Natl Acad Sci USA 1994; 91:2430–2435.

30.   Bobadilla J-L, Cowley P, Musgrove P, et al. Design, content and financing of an essential national package of health services. In: Murray CJL, Lopez AD, eds. Global comparative assessments in the health sector. Geneva: WHO; 1994:171–192.

31.   Hull HF, Ward NA, Hull BF, et al. Paralytic poliomyelitis: seasoned strategies, disappearing disease. Lancet 1994; 343:1331–1337.

32.   Grassly NC, Fraser C, Wenger J, et al. New strategies for the elimination of polio from India. Science 2006; 314:1150–1153.

33.   Nicoll A, Lynn R, Rahi J, et al. Public health outputs from the British Paediatric Surveillance Unit and similar clinician-based systems. J Roy Soc Med 2000; 93:580–585.

34.   Rowland D. Mapping communicable disease control administration in the UK: between devolution and Europe. London: Nuffield Trust; 2006.

The Child with Fever

35.   Wailoo MP, Petersen SA, Whitaker H, et al. Sleeping body temperatures in 3–4 month old infants. Arch Dis Child 1989; 64:596–599.

36.   Morley CJ, Hewson PH, Thornton AJ, et al. Axillary and rectal temperature measurements in infants. Arch Dis Child 1992; 67:122–125.

37.   Davies EG, Elliman DAC, Hart CA, et al. Manual of childhood infections. London: WB Saunders; 2001.

38.   Weinberg GA, D'Angio CT. Laboratory aids for diagnosis of neonatal sepsis. In: Remington J, Klein J, eds. Infectious diseases of the fetus and newborn infant, 6th edn. Philadelphia: Elsevier; 2006:1207–1222.

39.   Bonadio WA, Hegenbarth M, Zachamason M. Correlating reported fever in young infants with subsequent temperature patterns and risk of serious bacterial infections. Pediatr Infect Dis J 1990; 9:158–160.

40.   Bass JW, Steele R, Wittler R, et al. Antimicrobial treatment of occult bacteremia: a multicentre cooperative study. Pediatr Infect Dis J 1993; 12:466–473.

41.   Baraff LJ, Oslund SA, Schriger DL, et al. Probability of bacterial infections in febrile infants less than three months of age: a meta-analysis. Pediatr Infect Dis J 1992; 11:257–265.

42   National Institute for Clinical Excellence. Feverish illness in children. http://guidance.nice.org.uk/CG47

Clinical Problems: Suspected Meningitis

43.   Hargreaves RM, Slack MP, Howard AJ, et al. Changing patterns of invasive *Haemophilus influenzae* disease in England and Wales after introduction of the Hib vaccination programme. BMJ 1996; 312:160–161.

44.   Garg RK. Tuberculosis of the central nervous system. Postgrad Med J 1999; 75:133–140.

45.   Carrol ED, Latif AH, Misbah SA, et al. Lesson of the week: Recurrent bacterial meningitis: the need for sensitive imaging. BMJ 2001; 323:501–503.

46.   van Furth AM, Roord JJ, van Furth R. Roles of proinflammatory and anti-inflammatory cytokines in pathophysiology of bacterial meningitis and effect of adjunctive therapy. Infect Immun 1996; 64:4883–4890.

47.   Heyderman RS, Klein NJ. Emergency management of meningitis. J R Soc Med 2000; 93:225–229.

48.   Tauber MG. To tap or not to tap? Clin Infect Dis 1997; 25:289–291.

49.   Reacher MH, Shah A, Livermore DM, et al. Bacteraemia and antibiotic resistance of its pathogens reported in England and Wales between 1990 and 1998: trend analysis. BMJ 2000; 320:213–216.

50.   Trends in Antimicrobial Resistance in England and Wales, 2004–2005. Health Protection Agency, 2006.

51.   Bradley JS, Scheld WM. The challenge of penicillin-resistant *Streptococcus pneumoniae* meningitis: current antibiotic therapy in the 1990s. Clin Infect Dis 1997; 24:S213–S221.

52.   Tauber MG, Moser B. Cytokines and chemokines in meningeal inflammation: biology and clinical implications. Clin Infect Dis 1999; 28:1–11.

53.   McIntyre PB, Berkey CS, King SM, et al. Dexamethasone as adjunctive therapy in bacterial meningitis. A meta-analysis of randomized clinical trials since 1988. JAMA 1997; 278:925–931.

54.   van de Beek D, de Gans J, McIntyre P, et al. Corticosteroids for acute bacterial meningitis. Cochrane Database Syst Rev 2007; (1): CD004405.

55.   Powell KR, Sugarman LI, Eskenazi AE, et al. Normalization of plasma arginine vasopressin concentrations when children with meningitis are given maintenance plus replacement fluid therapy. J Pediatr 1990; 117:515–522.

56.   Bedford H, de Louvois J, Halket S, et al. Meningitis in infancy in England and Wales: follow up at age 5 years. BMJ 2001; 323:533–536.

Septic Shock

57.   Sprung CL, Bernard GR, Dellinger RP. Guidelines for the management of severe sepsis and septic shock. Intensive Care Med 2001; 27(suppl 1).

58.   Docke WD, Randow F, Syrbe U, et al. Monocyte deactivation in septic patients: restoration by IFN-gamma treatment. Nat Med 1997; 3:678–681.

59.   Levin M, Klein N. Shock in the febrile child. In: Isaacs D, Moxon ER, eds. A practical approach to pediatric infections. New York: Churchill Livingstone; 1996:4425–4444.

60.   Novelli V, Peters M, Dobson S. Infectious disease. In: Macnab A, Macrae D, Henning R, eds. Care of the critically ill child. London: Churchill Livingstone; 1999:281–298.

61.   Minneci PC, Deans KJ, Banks SM, et al. Meta-analysis: the effect of steroids on survival and shock during sepsis depends on the dose. Ann Intern Med 2004; 141:47–56.

62.   Alejandria MM, Lansang MA, Dans LF, et al. Intravenous immunoglobulin for treating sepsis and septic shock. Cochrane Database Syst Rev 2002;(1):CD001090.

63.   Bernard GR, Vincent J-L, Laterre P-F, et al. Efficacy and safety of recombinant human activated protein C for severe sepsis. N Engl J Med 2001; 344:699–709.

64.   Van Den Berghe G, Wouters P, Weekers F, et al. Intensive insulin therapy in critically ill patients. N Engl J Med 2001; 345:1359–1367.

Congenital and Neonatal Infections

65.   Gregg NM. Congenital cataract following German measles in the mother. Trans Ophthalmol Soc Aust 1941; 3:35–46.

66.   Tookey PA, Peckham CS. Surveillance of congenital rubella in Great Britain, 1971–1996. BMJ 1999; 318:769–770.

67.   Rahi J, Adams G, Russell-Eggit I, et al. Epidemiological surveillance of rubella must continue. BMJ 2001; 323:112.

68.   Miller E, Cradock-Watson JE, Pollock TM. Consequences of confirmed maternal rubella at successive stages of pregnancy. Lancet 1982; 2:781–784.

69.   Best JM, Banatvala JE, Morgan-Capner P, et al. Fetal infection after maternal reinfection with rubella: criteria for defining reinfection. BMJ 1989; 299:773–775.

70.   Best JM, Castillo-Solorzano C, Spika JS, et al. Reducing the global burden of congenital rubella syndrome: report of the World Health Organization Steering Committee On Research Related To Measles and Rubella Vaccines and Vaccination, June 2004. J Infect Dis 2005; 192:1890–1897.

71.   MMWR 2005; 54:279–282.

72.   Boppana SB, Fowler KB, Britt WJ, et al. Symptomatic congenital cytomegalovirus infection in infants born to mothers with pre-existing immunity to cytomegalovirus. Pediatrics 1999; 104:55–60.

73.   Boppana SB, Rivera LB, Fowler KB, et al. Intrauterine transmission of cytomegalovirus to infants of women with pre-conceptional immunity. N Engl J Med 2001; 344:1366–1371.

74. Ross SA, Folwer KB, Ashrith G, et al. Hearing loss in children with congenital cytomegalovirus infection born to mothers with pre-existing immunity. J Pediatr 2006; 148:332–336.

75. Noyola DE, Demmler GJ, Nelson CT, et al. Early predictors of neurodevelopmental outcome in symptomatic congenital cytomegalovirus infection. J Pediatr 2001; 138:325–331.

76. Fowler KB, McCollister FP, Dahle AJ, et al. Progressive and fluctuating sensorineural hearing loss in children with asymptomatic congenital cytomegalovirus infection. J Pediatr 1997; 130:624–630.

77. Kylat RI, Kelly EN, Ford-Jones EL. Clinical findings and adverse outcomes in neonates with symptomatic congenital cytomegalovirus (SCCMV) infection. Eur J Pediatr 2006; 165:773–778.

78. Lanari M, Lassarotto T, Venturi V, et al. Neonatal cytomegalovirus blood load and risk of sequelae in symptomatic and asymptomatic congenitally infected newborns. Pediatr 2006; 117:76–83.

79. Paryani SG, Yeager AS, Hosford-Dunn H, et al. Sequelae of acquired cytomegalovirus infection in premature and sick term infants. J Pediatr 1985; 107:451–456.

80. Whitley RJ, Cloud G, Gruber W, et al. Ganciclovir treatment of symptomatic congenital cytomegalovirus infection: results of a phase II study. National Institute of Allergy and Infectious Diseases Collaborative Antiviral Study Group. J Infect 1997; 175:1080–1086.

81. Nigro G, Krzysztofiak A, Bartmann U, et al. Ganciclovir therapy for cytomegalovirus-associated liver disease in immunocompetent or immunocompromised children. Arch Virol 1997; 142:573–580.

82. Smets K, De Coen K, Dhooge I, et al. Selecting neonates with congenital cytomegalovirus infection for ganciclovir therapy. Eur J Pediatr 2006; 165:885–890.

83. Rojo P, Ramos JT. Ganciclovir treatment of children with congenital cytomegalovirus infection. Pediatr Infect Dis J 2004; 23:88–89.

84. Nigro G, Adler SP, La Torre R, et al. Passive immunization during pregnancy for congenital cytomegalovirus infection. N Engl J Med 2005; 353:1350–1362.

85. Enders G, Miller E, Cradock-Watson J, et al. Consequences of varicella and herpes zoster in pregnancy: prospective study of 1739 cases. Lancet 1994; 343:1548–1551.

86. Chant KG, Sullivan EA, Burgess MA, et al. Varicella-zoster virus infection in Australia. Aust N Z J Public Health 1998; 22:413–418.

87. Heuchan AM, Isaacs D. The management of varicella-zoster virus exposure and infection in pregnancy and the newborn period. Australasian Subgroup in Paediatric Infectious Diseases of the Australasian Society for Infectious Diseases. Med J Aust 2001; 174:288–292.

88. Reynolds L, Struik S, Nadel S. Neonatal varicella: varicella zoster immunoglobulin (VZIG) does not prevent disease. Arch Dis Child Fetal Neonatal Ed 1999; 81:F69–F70.

89. Gutierrez KM, Falkovitz HM, Maldonado Y, et al. The epidemiology of neonatal herpes simplex virus infections in California from 1985 to 1995. J Infect Dis 1999; 180:199–202.

90. Tookey P, Peckham CS. Neonatal herpes simplex virus infection in the British Isles. Paediatr Perinat Epidemiol 1996; 10:432–442.

91. Brown ZA, Selke S, Zeh J, et al. The acquisition of herpes simplex virus during pregnancy. N Engl J Med 1997; 337:509–515.

92. Whitley RJ. Herpes simplex virus infections of the central nervous system. A review. Am J Med 1988; 85(suppl 2A):61–67.

93. American Academy of Pediatrics. Herpes simplex. In: Pickering L, ed. Red book report of the Committee on Infectious Diseases, 25th edn. Elk Grove Village: American Academy of Pediatrics; 2000:309–318.

*94 Stanberry LR, Spruance SL, Cunningham AL, et al. Glycoprotein-D-adjuvant vaccine to prevent genital herpes. N Engl J Med 2002; 347:1652–1661.

95. Fowler SL, Dickey M, Kern P, et al. Perceptions of parents seeking an experimental herpes simplex vaccine for their adolescent and preadolescent daughters. Pediatr Infect Dis J 2006; 25:747–748.

96. Sheffield JS, Hill JB, Hollier LM, et al. Valacyclovir prophylaxis to prevent recurrent herpes at delivery: a randomized clinical trial. Obstet Gynecol 2006; 108:141–147.

97. Kurt-Jones EA, Belko J, Yu C, et al. The role of toll-like receptors in herpes simplex infection in neonates. J Infect Dis 2005; 191:746–748.

98. Dunn D, Wallon M, Peyron F, et al. Mother-to-child transmission of toxoplasmosis: risk estimates for clinical counselling. Lancet 1999; 353:1829–1833.

99. Gilbert R, Tan HK, Cliffe S, et al. Symptomatic toxoplasma infection due to congenital and postnatally acquired infection. Arch Dis Child 2006; 91:495–498.

100. Vogel N, Kirisits M, Michael E, et al. Congenital toxoplasmosis transmitted from an immunologically competent mother infected before conception. Clin Infect Dis 1996; 23:1055–1060.

101. Dunn D, Gilbert R, Newell ML, et al. Low incidence of congenital toxoplasmosis in children born to women infected with human immunodeficiency virus. European Collaborative Study and Research Network on Congenital Toxoplasmosis. Eur J Obstet Gynecol Reprod Biol 1996; 68:93–96.

102. McAuley J, Boyer KM, Patel D, et al. Early and longitudinal evaluations of treated infants and children and untreated historical patients with congenital toxoplasmosis: the Chicago Collaborative Treatment Trial. Clin Infect Dis J 1994; 18:38–72.

*103. Peyron F, Wallon M, Liou C, et al. Treatments for toxoplasmosis in pregnancy (Cochrane Review). In: The Cochrane Library, 2. Oxford: Update Software; 2000.

104. McMinn P, Stratov I, Nagarajan L, et al. Neurological manifestations of enterovirus 71 infection in children during an outbreak of hand, foot, and mouth disease in Western Australia. Clin Infect Dis J 2001; 32:236–242.

105. Ho M, Chen ER, Hsu KH, et al. An epidemic of enterovirus 71 infection in Taiwan. Taiwan Enterovirus Epidemic Working Group. N Engl J Med 1999; 341:929–935.

106. Rotbart HA, Webster AD. Treatment of potentially life-threatening enterovirus infections with pleconaril. Clin Infect Dis J 2001; 32:228–235.

Hospital Infection Control

107. Huskins WC, Goldman DA. Nosocomial infections. In: Feigin R, Cherry J, Demmler G, et al, eds. Textbook of pediatric infectious disease, 5th edn. Philadelphia: Saunders; 2004.

108. Centers for Disease Control. Guidelines for hand hygiene in health care settings. MMWR 2002; 51:1–44.

109. Edmond MB, Wenzel RP. Isolation. In: Mandell G, Bennett J, Dolin R, eds. Principles and practice of infectious diseases, 6th edn. Philadelphia: Elsevier; 2005.

110. Tablan OC, Boyyard EA, Shapiro CN, et al. Personnel health services. In: Bennett JV, Brachman PS. Hospital infections, 4th edn. Philadelphia: Lippincott-Raven; 1998.

111. Chamberland ME, Bell DM. Human immunodeficiency virus. In: Bennett JV, Brachman PS. Hospital infections, 4th edn. Philadelphia: Lippincott-Raven; 1998.

112. MacDougall C, Polk RE. Antimicrobial stewardship programs in health care systems. Clin Microbiol Rev 2005; 18:638–656.

113. Jarvis WR. Investigating endemic and epidemic nosocomial infections. In: Bennett JV, Brachman PS. Hospital infections, 4th edn. Philadelphia: Lippincott-Raven; 1998.

The Use of the Bacteriology Laboratory by the Pediatrician

114. Peterson LR, Hamilton JD, Baron EJ, et al. Role of the microbiology laboratory in the management and control of infectious diseases and the delivery of health care. Clin Infect Dis 2001; 32:605–611.

115. O'Grady NP, Alexander M, Delinger P, et al. Guidelines for the prevention of intravascular catheter-related infections. Clin Infect Dis 2002; 35:1281–1307.

116. Bisno AL, Gerbe MA, Gwaltney Jr JM, et al. Practice Guidelines for the Diagnosis and Management of Group A Streptococcal Pharyngitis. Clin Infect Dis 2002; 35:113–125.

117. Carroll KC. Laboratory diagnosis of lower respiratory tract infections: controversy and conundrums. J Clin Microbiol 2002; 40:3115–3120.

118. Thompson RB, Bertram H. Laboratory diagnosis of central nervous system infections. Infect Dis Clin North Am 2001; 15:1047–1071.

119. Hayden R, Pershing DH. Diagnostic molecular microbiology. Curr Clin Top Infect Dis 2001; 21:323–348.

120. Hines J, Nachamkin I. Effective use of the clinical microbiology laboratory for the diagnosis of diarrhoeal diseases. Clin Infect Dis 1996; 23(Supp):S97–S101.

Principles of Antimicrobial Therapy

121 Muller M, delaPena A, Derendorf H. Issues in pharmacokinetic and pharmacodynamics of anti-infective agents: Distribution in tissue. Antimicrob Agents Chemother 2004; 48:1441–1453.

122. Lowy FD. Staphylococcus aureus infections. N Engl J Med 1998; 339:520–532.

123. Jacoby GA, Munoz-Price LS. The new β-lactamases. N Engl J Med 2005; 352:380–391.

124. Bradford PA. Extended spectrum β-lactamases in the 21st century; characterisation, epidemiology and detection of this important resistance threat. Clin Microbiol Rev 2001; 14:933–951.

125. Paterson DL, Bronomo RA. Extended-spectrum β-lactamases: a clinical update. Clin Microbiol Rev 2005; 18:657–686.

126. Philippon A, Arlert G, Jacoby GA. Plasmid-determined AmpC-type β-lactamases. Antimicrob Agents Chemother 2002; 46:1–11.

127. Kotra LP, Haddad J, Mobashery S. Aminoglycosides: Perspectives of action and resistance and strategies to counter resistance. Antimicrob Agents Chemother 2000; 44:3249–3256.

128. Gruchalla RS, Pirmoharmed M. Antibiotic allergy. N Engl J Med 2006; 254:601–609.

129. Kessler RE. Cefapime microbiologic profile and update. Pediatr Infect Dis J 2001; 20:331–336.

130. Kucers A. Vancomycin. In: Kucers A, Crowe S, Grayson ML, et al, eds. The use of antibiotics, 5th edn. Oxford: Butterworth-Heinemann; 1997.

131. Vakulenko SB, Mobashery S. Versatility of aminoglycosides and prospects for their future. Clin Microbiol Rev 2003; 16:430–450.

132. Ruuskanen O. Safety and tolerability of azithromycin in pediatric infectious diseases: 2003 update. Pediatr Infect Dis J 2004; 23:S135–S139.

133. Kucers A, Crowe S, Grayson M, et al. The use of antibiotics. Part IV and part V, 5th edn. Oxford: Butterworth-Heinemann; 1997:1245–1881.

134. Groll AH, Walsh TJ. Antifungal agents. In: Feigin R, Cherry J, Demmler G, et al, eds. Textbook of pediatric infectious disease, 5th edn. Philadelphia: Saunders; 2004.

135. Demmler GJ. Antiviral agents. In: Feigin R, Cherry J, Demmler G, et al, eds. Textbook of pediatric infectious disease, 5th edn. Philadelphia: Saunders; 2004.

Bacterial Infections: Botulism

136. Thomas DG. Infant botulism: a review in South Australia (1980–1989). J Paediatr Child Health 1993; 29:24–26.

137. Spika JS, Shaffer N, Hargrett-Bean N, et al. Risk factors for infant botulism in the United States. Am J Dis Child 1989; 143:828–832.

138. Schreiner MS, Field E, Ruddy R. Infant botulism: a review of 12 years' experience at The Children's Hospital of Philadelphia. Pediatrics 1991; 87:59–165.

139. Frankovich TL, Arnon SS. Clinical trial of botulism immune globulin for infant botulism. West J Med 1991; 154:103.

140. Thompson JA, Filloux FM, Van Orman CB, et al. Infant botulism in the age of botulism immune globulin. Neurology 2005; 64:2029–2032.

141. Tackett CO, Shandera WX, Mann JM, et al. Equine antitoxin use and other factors that predict outcome in type A foodborne botulism. Am J Med 1984; 76:794–798.

142. Arnon SS, Schechter R, Maslanka SE, et al. Human botulism immune globulin for the treatment of infant botulism. N Engl J Med 2006; 354:462–471.

Bacterial Infections: Brucellosis; Undulant Fever
*143. Lubani MM, Dudkin KI, Sharda DC, et al. A multicenter therapeutic study of 1100 children with brucellosis. Pediatr Infect Dis J 1989; 8:75–78.

Bacterial Infections: Cholera
144. World Health Organization. Guidelines for cholera control. Geneva: World Health Organization; 1993.

145. Kalluri P, Naheed A, Rahman S, et al. Evaluation of three rapid diagnostic tests for cholera: does the skill level of the technician matter? Trop Med Int Health 2006; 11:49–55.

146. CHOICE Study Group. Multicenter, randomized, double-blind clinical trial to evaluate the efficacy and safety of a reduced osmolarity oral rehydration salts solution in children with acute watery diarrhea. Pediatrics 2001; 107:613–618.

147. Murphy C, Hahn S, Volmink J. Reduced osmolarity oral rehydration solution for treating cholera. Cochrane Database Syst Rev 2004; 4:CD003754.

148. World Health Organization. Implementing the new recommendations on the clinical management of diarrhoea: guidelines for policy makers and programme managers. Geneva: World Health Organization; 2006.

149. Trach DD, Clemens JD, Ke NT, et al. Field trial of locally produced, killed, oral cholera vaccine in Vietnam. Lancet 1997; 349:231–235.

150. Lucas ME, Deen JL, von Seidlein L, et al. Effectiveness of mass oral cholera vaccination in Beira, Mozambique. N Engl J Med 2005; 352:757–767.

151. Ali M, Emch M, von Seidlen L, et al. Herd immunity conferred by killed oral cholera vaccines in Bangladesh: a reanalysis. Lancet 2005; 366:7–9.

152. Thiem VD, Deen JL, von Seidlein L, et al. Long-term effectiveness against cholera of oral killed whole-cell vaccine produced in Vietnam. Vaccine 2006; 24:4297–4303.

Bacterial Infections: Diphtheria
153. Galazka AM, Robertson SE, Oblapenko GP. Resurgence of diphtheria. Eur J Epidemiol 1995; 11:95–105.

154. Dittmann S, Wharton M, Vitek C, et al. Successful control of epidemic diphtheria in the states of the Former Union of Soviet Socialist Republics: lessons learned. J Infect Dis 2000; 181 Suppl 1: S10–S22.

155. WHO. The World Health Report 2004 – changing history. Geneva: World Health Organization; 2004.

156. Bowler IC, Mandal BK, Schlecht B, et al. Diphtheria – the continuing hazard. Arch Dis Child 1988; 63:194–195.

157. PHLS. A case of diphtheria from Pakistan. CDR Weekly 1994; 4:173.

158. Nuorti P. Fatal case of diphtheria in an unvaccinated infant, Finland 2001. Eurosurveill Weekly 2002; 6:4.

159. Efstratiou A, Engler KH, Mazurova IK, et al. Current approaches to the laboratory diagnosis of diphtheria. J Infect Dis 2000; 181 Suppl 1: S138–S145.

160. Engler KH, Efstratiou A. Rapid enzyme immunoassay for determination of toxigenicity among clinical isolates of corynebacteria. J Clin Microbiol 2000; 38:1385–1389.

161. Mothershed EA, Cassiday PK, Pierson K, et al. Development of a real-time fluorescence PCR assay for rapid detection of the diphtheria toxin gene. J Clin Microbiol 2002; 40:4713–4719.

162. Pappenheimer AM, Jr. Diphtheria toxin. Annu Rev Biochem 1977; 46:69–94.

163. Zuber PL, Gruner E, Altwegg M, et al. Invasive infection with non-toxigenic Corynebacterium diphtheriae among drug users. Lancet 1992; 339:1359.

164. Tiley SM, Kociuba KR, Heron LG, et al. Infective endocarditis due to nontoxigenic Corynebacterium diphtheriae: report of seven cases and review. Clin Infect Dis 1993; 16:271–275.

165. MMWR. Respiratory diphtheria caused by Corynebacterium ulcerans – Terre Haute, Indiana, 1996. Morb Mortal Wkly Rep 1997; 46:330–332.

166. Wagner J, Ignatius R, Voss S, et al. Infection of the skin caused by Corynebacterium ulcerans and mimicking classical cutaneous diphtheria. Clin Infect Dis 2001; 33:1598–1600.

167. Harnisch JP, Tronca E, Nolan CM, et al. Diphtheria among alcoholic urban adults. A decade of experience in Seattle. Ann Intern Med 1989; 111:71–82.

168. de Benoist AC, White JM, Efstratiou A, et al. Imported cutaneous diphtheria, United Kingdom. Emerg Infect Dis 2004; 10:511–513.

169. Loukoushkina EF, Bobko PV, Kolbasova EV, et al. The clinical picture and diagnosis of diphtheritic carditis in children. Eur J Pediatr 1998; 157:528–533.

170. Kneen R, Nguyen MD, Solomon T, et al. Clinical features and predictors of diphtheritic cardiomyopathy in Vietnamese children. Clin Infect Dis 2004; 39:1591–1598.

171. Lumio JT, Groundstroem KW, Melnick OB, et al. Electrocardiographic abnormalities in patients with diphtheria: a prospective study. Am J Med 2004; 116:78–83.

172. Logina I, Donaghy M. Diphtheritic polyneuropathy: a clinical study and comparison with Guillain-Barré syndrome. J Neurol Neurosurg Psychiatry 1999; 67:433–438.

173. Solders G, Nennesmo I, Persson A. Diphtheritic neuropathy, an analysis based on muscle and nerve biopsy and repeated neurophysiological and autonomic function tests. J Neurol Neurosurg Psychiatry 1989; 52:876–880.

174. Bonnet JM, Begg NT. Control of diphtheria: guidance for consultants in communicable disease control. World Health Organization. Commun Dis Public Health 1999; 2:242–249.

175. Kneen R, Pham NG, Solomon T, et al. Penicillin vs. erythromycin in the treatment of diphtheria. Clin Infect Dis 1998; 27:845–850.

176. Bethell DB, Nguyen Minh D, Ha Thi L, et al. Prognostic value of electrocardiographic monitoring of patients with severe diphtheria. Clin Infect Dis 1995; 20:1259–1265.

177. Thisyakorn U, Wongvanich J, Kumpeng V. Failure of corticosteroid therapy to prevent diphtheritic myocarditis or neuritis. Pediatr Infect Dis 1984; 3:126–128.

178. Stockins BA, Lanas FT, Saavedra JG, et al. Prognosis in patients with diphtheric myocarditis and bradyarrhythmias: assessment of results of ventricular pacing. Br Heart J 1994; 72:190–191.

179. Dung NM, Kneen R, Kiem N, et al. Treatment of severe diphtheritic myocarditis by temporary insertion of a cardiac pacemaker. Clin Infect Dis 2002; 35:1425–1429.

180. Quick ML, Sutter RW, Kobaidze K, et al. Epidemic diphtheria in the Republic of Georgia, 1993–1996: risk factors for fatal outcome among hospitalized patients. J Infect Dis 2000; 181 Suppl 1: S130–S137.

181. Galazka A. The changing epidemiology of diphtheria in the vaccine era. J Infect Dis 2000; 181 Suppl 1:S2–S9.

Bacterial Infections: Escherichia coli
182. Blattner FR, Plunkett G, Bloch CA, et al. The complete genome sequence of Escherichia coli K12. Science 1997; 277:1453–1474.

183. Perna NT, Plunkett G, Burland V, et al. Genome sequence of enterohaemorrhagic Escherichia coli O157:H7. Nature 2001; 409:529–533.

184. Reid SD, Herbelin CJ, Bumbaugh AC, et al. Parallel evolution of virulence in pathogenic Escherichia coli. Nature 2000; 406:64–67.

185. Whitfield C, Roberts IS. Structure, assembly and regulation of expression of capsules in Escherichia coli. Mol Microbiol 1999; 31:1307–1319.

186. Kariuki S, Gilks C, Kimari J, et al. Genotypic analysis of Escherichia coli strains isolated from children and chickens living in close priority. Appl Environ Microbiol 1999; 65:472–476.

187. Clermont O, Bonacorsi S, Bingen E. Rapid and simple determination of the Escherichia coli phylogenetic group. Appl Environ Microbiol 2000; 66:4555–4558.

188. Martindale J, Stroud D, Moxon ER, et al. Genetic analysis of Escherichia coli K1 gastrointestinal colonization. Mol Microbiol 2000; 37:1293–1305.

189. Kariuki S, Hart CA. Global aspects of antimicrobial resistant enteric bacteria. Curr Opin Infect Dis 2001; 14:579–586.

Bacterial Infections: Haemophilus influenzae
190. Pitmann M. Variation and type specificity in bacterial species of Haemophilus influenzae. J Exp Med 1931; 53:471–492.

*191. Booy R, Hodgson SA, Slack MPE, et al. Invasive Haemophilus-influenzae-type-b disease in the Oxford region (1985–91). Arch Dis Child 1993; 69:225–228.

*192. Kilpi T, Herva E, Kaijalainen T, et al. Bacteriology of acute otitis media in a cohort of Finnish children followed for the first two years of life. Pediatr Infect Dis J 2001; 20:654–662.

*193. Heath PT, Booy R, Azzopardi HJ, et al. Non-type b Haemophilus influenzae disease: clinical and epidemiologic characteristics in the Haemophilus influenzae type b vaccine era. Pediatr Infect Dis J 2001; 20:300–305.

*194. Shann F, Gratten M, Germer S, et al. Aetiology of pneumonia in children in Goroka hospital, Papua, New Guinea. Lancet 1984; 2:537–541.

*195. Farley MM, Stephens DS, Harvey RC, et al and the CDC Meningitis Surveillance Group. Incidence and clinical characteristics of invasive Haemophilus influenzae disease in adults. J Infect Dis 1992; 165(suppl 1):S42–S43.

196. Moxon ER, Zwahlen A, Rubin LB. Pathogenesis of Haemophilus influenzae meningitis: use of a rat model for studying microbial determinants of virulence. In: Sande M, Smith A, Root R, eds. Bacterial meningitis. Edinburgh: Churchill Livingstone; 1985:23–36.

197. Kauppi M, Saarinen L, Kayhty H. Anti-capsular polysaccharide antibodies reduce nasopharyngeal colonization by Haemophilus influenzae type b in infant rats. J Infect Dis 1993; 167:365–371.

*198. Fernandez J, Levine OS, Sanchez J, et al. Prevention of Haemophilus influenzae type b colonization by vaccination: correlation with serum anti-capsular IgG concentration. J Infect Dis 2000; 182:1553–1556.

*199. Heath PT, Booy R, Griffiths H, et al. Clinical and immunological risk factors associated with *Haemophilus influenzae* type b conjugate vaccine failure in childhood. Clin Infect Dis 2000; 31:973–980.

*200. Schaad U, Lips U, Gnehm H, et al. Dexamethasone therapy for bacterial meningitis. Lancet 1993; 342:457–461.

*201. Peltola H, Kayhty H, Virtanen M, et al. Prevention of *Haemophilus influenzae* type b bacteremic infections with the capsular polysaccharide vaccine. N Engl J Med 1984; 310:1561–1566.

*202. Booy R, Hodgson S, Carpenter L, et al. Efficacy of *Haemophilus-influenzae* type b conjugate vaccine PRP-T. Lancet 1994; 344:362–366.

*203. Adegbola RA, Secka O, Lahai G, et al. Elimination of *Haemophilus influenzae* type b (Hib) disease from The Gambia after the introduction of routine immunisation with a Hib conjugate vaccine: a prospective study. Lancet 2005; 366:144–150.

*204. Cowgill KD, Ndiritu M, Nyiro J, et al. Effectiveness of *Haemophilus influenzae* type b conjugate vaccine introduction into routine childhood immunization in Kenya. JAMA 2006; 296:671–678.

*205. Prymula R, Peeters P, Chrobok V, et al. Pneumococcal capsular polysaccharides conjugated to protein D for prevention of acute otitis media caused by both Streptococcus pneumoniae and non-typable Haemophilus influenzae: a randomised double-blind efficacy study. Lancet 2006; 367:740–748.

Bacterial Infections: Leprosy

206. Selvasekar A, Geetha J, Nisha K, et al. Childhood leprosy in an endemic area. Lepr Rev 1999; 70:21–27.

207. Lockwood DNJ, Reid AJC. The diagnosis of leprosy is delayed in the United Kingdom. Q J Med 2001; 94:207–212.

208. WHO Technical Report Series. WHO Expert Committee on Leprosy. Geneva: World Health Organization; 1998.

209. Jain S, Reddy RG, Osmani SN, et al. Childhood leprosy in an urban clinic-Hyderabad, India: clinical presentation and the role of household contacts. Leprosy review 2002; 73:248–253.

210. Hammond PJ, Rao PS. The tragedy of deformity in childhood leprosy. Lepr Rev 1999; 70:217–220.

211. Department of Health and the Welsh Office. Memorandum on leprosy. London: The Stationery Office; 1997.

Bacterial Infections: Lyme Disease

212. Schmid GP. The global distribution of Lyme disease. Rev Infect Dis 1985; 7:41–50.

213. Steere AC, Hardin JA, Malawista SE. Erythema chronicum migrans and Lyme arthritis. Cryoimmunoglobulins and clinical activity of skin and joints. Science 1977; 196:1121.

214. Muhlemann MF, Wright DJM. Emerging pattern of Lyme disease in the United Kingdom and Irish Republic. Lancet 1987; 1:260–263.

215. Berglund J, Eitrem R, Orristein K, et al. An epidemiological study of Lyme disease in Southern Sweden. N Engl J Med 1995; 333:1319–1324.

216. Anderson JF. Epizootiology of *Borellia* in *Ixodes* tick vectors and reservoir hosts. Rev Infect Dis 1989; 11(suppl 6):S1451–S1459.

217. Steere AC, Dwyer E, Winchester R. Association of chronic Lyme arthritis with HLA-DR4 and HLA-DR2 alleles. N Engl J Med 1990; 323:219–223.

218. Steere AC, Gibofsky A, Patarroyo M, et al. Chronic Lyme arthritis. Ann Intern Med 1979; 90:896–901.

219. Steere AC, Bartenhagen NH, Craft JE, et al. The early clinical manifestations of Lyme disease. Ann Intern Med 1983; 99:76–82.

220. Shapiro ED, Gerber MA. Lyme disease in children study group: Lyme disease in children. Sixth International Conference of Lyme Borreliosis, Bologna, Italy, 1994.

221. O'Neill PM, Wright DJM. Lyme disease. Br J Hosp Med 1988; 40:284–289.

222. Garcia-Monoco JC, Benach JI. Lyme neuroborelliosis. Ann Neurol 1995; 37:691–702.

223. Steere AC, Schoen RT, Taylor E. The clinical evolution of Lyme disease arthritis. Ann Intern Med 1987; 107:725–731.

224. Shapiro ED. Lyme disease in children. Am J Med 1995; 98(suppl 4A):695–735.

225. Feder HM, Hunt MS. Pitfalls in the diagnosis and treatment of Lyme disease in children. JAMA 1995; 274:66–68.

226. Dressler F, Whalen JA, Reinhardt BN, et al. Western blotting in the serodiagnosis of Lyme disease. J Infect Dis 1993; 167:392–400.

227. Steere AC. Lyme disease. N Engl J Med 1989; 321:586–596.

228. Gardner P. Editorial. JAMA 2000; 283:658–659.

229. Lufti BJ, Gardener R, Lightfoot RW JR. Empiric antibiotic treatment of patients who are seropositive for Lyme disease but lack classic features. Clin Infect Dis 1994; 18:112.

230. Steere AC, Hutchinson DJ, Rahn DW, et al. Treatment of the early manifestations of Lyme disease. Ann Intern Med 1983; 99:22.

231. Pal GA, Baker JT, Wright DJM. Penicillin resistant borrelia encephalitis responding to cefotaxime. Lancet 1988; 1:50–51.

Bacterial Infections: Meningococcemia

232. Invasive meningococcal infections, England and Wales: Commun Dis Rep CDR Wkly [serial online] 2001 [cited 22 November] 2001; 11(2).

233. van Deuren M, Brandtzaeg P, van der Meer JW. Update on meningococcal disease with emphasis on pathogenesis and clinical management. Clin Microbiol Rev 2000; 13:144–166.

234. Thompson MJ, Ninis N, Perera R, et al. Clinical recognition of meningococcal disease in children and adolescents. Lancet 2006; 367:397–403.

235. Lala HM, Mills GD, Barratt K, et al. Meningococcal disease deaths and the frequency of antibiotic administration delays. J Infect 2007; 54:551–557.

236. Peters MJ, Ross-Russell RI, White D, et al. Early severe neutropenia and thrombocytopenia identifies the highest risk cases of severe meningococcal disease. Paediatr Crit Care Med 2001; 2:225–231.

Bacterial Infections: *Mycobacterium tuberculosis*

237. Wilkins EGL. Antibody detection in tuberculosis. In: Davies PDO, ed. Clinical tuberculosis. London: Chapman & Hall; 1998:367–380.

238. Pfyffer GE. Nucleic acid amplification for mycobacterial diagnosis. J Infect 1999; 39:21–26.

239. Delacourt C, Poueda J-D, Chureau C, et al. Use of polymerase chain reaction for improved diagnosis of tuberculosis in children. J Pediatr 1995; 126:703–709.

240. Gomez-Pastrana D, Torronteras R, Caro P, et al. Comparison of ampiclor, in-house polymerase chain reaction, and conventional culture for the diagnosis of tuberculosis in children. Clin Infect Dis 2001; 32:17–22.

241. Nelson LJ, Wells CD. Global epidemiology of childhood tuberculosis. Int J Tuberc Lung Dis 2004; 8:636–647.

242. Beyers N, Gie RP, Zietsman H, et al. The use of a geographical information system (GIS) to evaluate the distribution of tuberculosis in a high incidence community. S Afr Med J 1996; 86:40–44.

243. Balasegaram S, Watson JM, Rose AMC, et al. A decade of change: tuberculosis in England and Wales. Arch Dis Child 2003; 88:772–777.

244. American Thoracic Society/Centers for Disease Control and Prevention/Infectious Diseases Society of America: controlling tuberculosis in the United States. Am J Respir Crit Care Med 2005; 172:1169–2227.

245. Sharp D. Bovine tuberculosis and badger blame. Lancet 2006; 367:631–632.

246. Miller FJW. Tuberculosis in children. Edinburgh: Churchill Livingstone; 1982.

247. Dannenberg AM. Immune mechanism in the pathogenesis of pulmonary tuberculosis. Rev Infect Dis 1989; II(suppl 2):369–378.

248. Spellberg B, Edwards JE. Type 1/type 2 immunity in infectious diseases. Clin Infect Dis 2001; 32:76–102.

249. Rook GAW, Herandez-Pando R. The pathogenesis of tuberculosis. Ann Rev Microbiol 1996; 50:259–284.

250. Smith DW, Wiegeshaus EH. What animal models can teach us about the pathogenesis of tuberculosis in humans. Rev Infect Dis 1989; II(suppl 2):385–393.

251. Steiner P, Rao M, Victoria MS, et al. Persistently negative tuberculin reactions. Am J Dis Child 1980; 134:747–750.

252. Pai M, Riley LW, Colford Jr JM. Interferon-γ assays in the immunodiagnosis of tuberculosis: a systematic review. Lancet Infect Dis 2004; 4:761–776.

253. Liebeschuetz S, Bamber S, Ewer K, et al. Diagnosis of tuberculosis in South African children with a T-cell-based assay: a prospective study. Lancet 2004; 364:2196–2203.

254. Department of Health (DoH). Immunization against infectious disease. London: HMSO; 2006.

255. Moss WJ, Clements CJ, Halsey NA. Immunisation of children at risk of infection with human immunodeficiency virus. Bull World Health Org 2003; 81:61–70.

256. Hesseling AC, Rabie H, Marais BJ, et al. Bacille Calmette-Guerin vaccine-induced disease in HIV-infected and HIV-uninfected children. Clin Infect Dis 2006; 42:548–558.

257. Casanova JL, Blanche S, Emile JF, et al. Idiopathic disseminated Bacille Calmette-Guerin infection: a French national retrospective study. Pediatrics 1996; 98:774–778.

258. Kroger L, Korppi M, Brander E, et al. Osteitis caused by Bacille Calmette-Guérin vaccinations: a retrospective analysis of 222 cases. J Infect Dis 1995; 172:574–576.

259. Rodrigues LC, Diwan VK, Wheeler JG. Protective effect of BCG against tuberculous meningitis and miliary tuberculosis: a meta analysis. Int J Epidemiol 1993; 22:1154–1158.

260. Colditz GA, Berkey CS, Mosteller F, et al. The efficacy of Bacillus Calmette-Guérin vaccination of newborns and infants in the prevention of tuberculosis: meta-analyses of the published literature. Pediatrics 1995; 96:29–35.

261. Boudin Trunz B, Fine PEM, Dye C. Effect of BCG vaccination on childhood tuberculous meningitis and miliary tuberculosis worldwide: a meta-analysis and assessment of cost-effectiveness. Lancet 2006; 367:1173–1180.

262. Fine PEM. Variation in protection by BCG: implications of and for heterologous immunity. Lancet 1995; ii:1339–1345.

263. Sutherland I, Springett VH. Effectiveness of BCG vaccination in England and Wales in 1983. Tubercle 1987; 68:81–92.

264. Ormerod LP, Garnett JM. Tuberculin skin reactivity four years after neonatal BCG vaccination. Arch Dis Child 1992; 67:530–531.

265. Teale C, Cundall DB, Pearson SB. Heaf status 12 years after BCG vaccination. Tuber Lung Dis 1992; 73:210–212.

266. Menzies D. What does tuberculin reactivity after Bacille Calmette-Guérin vaccination tell us. Clin Infect Dis 2000; 31(suppl 3):S71–S74.

267. Haile M, Kallenius G. Recent developments in tuberculosis vaccines. Curr Opin Infect Dis 2005; 18:211–215.

268.   NICE guideline. Tuberculosis: clinical diagnosis and management of tuberculosis, and measures for its prevention and control. www.nice.org.uk/CGO33NICEguideline

269.   Swanson DS, Starke JR. Drug-resistant tuberculosis in pediatrics. Pediatr Clin North Am 1995; 42:553–581.

270.   Miller FJW. The natural history of primary tuberculosis. WHO/TB/84.144. Geneva: World Health Organization; 1984.

271.   Delacourt C, Mani TM, Bonnerot V, et al. Computed tomography with normal chest radiograph in tuberculous infection. Arch Dis Child 1993; 69:430–432.

272.   Khan EA, Starke JR. Diagnosis of tuberculosis in children: increased need for better methods. Emerg Infect Dis 1995; 1:115–122.

273.   Vallejo JG, Ong LT, Starke JR. Clinical features, diagnosis and treatment of tuberculosis in infants. Pediatrics 1994; 84:1–7.

274.   Graham SM, Gie RP, Schaaf HS, et al. Childhood tuberculosis: clinical research needs. Int J Tuberc Lung Dis 2004:8:648–657.

275.   Thakur A, Coulter JBS, Zutshi K, et al. Laryngeal swabs for diagnosing tuberculosis. Ann Trop Paediatr 1999; 19:333–336.

276.   Franchi LM, Cama RI, Gilman RH, et al. Detection of Mycobacterium tuberculosis in naso-pharyngeal aspirate samples in children. Lancet 1998; 352:1681–1682.

277.   Montenegro SH, Gilman RH, Sheen P, et al. Improved detection of Mycobacterium tuberculosis in Peruvian children by use of a heminested polymerase chain reaction assay. Clin Infect Dis 2003; 36:16–23.

278.   Shata AMA, Coulter JBS, Parry CM, et al. Sputum induction for the diagnosis of tuberculosis. Arch Dis Child 1996; 74:535–536.

279.   Zar HJ, Hanslo D, Apolles P, et al. Induced sputum versus gastric lavage for microbiological confirmation of pulmonary tuberculosis in infants and young children: a prospective study. Lancet 2005; 365:130–134.

280.   Abadco DL, Steiner P. Gastric lavage is better than bronchoalveolar lavage for isolation of Mycobacterium tuberculosis in childhood pulmonary tuberculosis. Pediatr Infect Dis J 1992; 11:735–738.

281.   Somu N, Swaminathan S, Paramasivan CN, et al. Value of bronchoalveolar lavage and gastric lavage in the diagnosis of pulmonary tuberculosis in children. Tuber Lung Dis 1995; 76:295–299.

282.   American Thoracic Society. Treatment of tuberculosis and tuberculosis infection in adults and children. Am J Respir Crit Care Med 1994; 149:1359–1374.

*283.   Matchaba PT, Volmink J. Steroids for treating tuberculous pleurisy. Cochrane Database Syst Rev 2000; (1):CD001876.

284.   Hugo-Hamman CT, Scher H, De Moor MMA. Tuberculous pericarditis in children: a review of 44 cases. Pediatr Infect Dis J 1994; 13:13–18.

*285.   Mayosi BM, Ntsekhe M, Volmink JA, et al. Interventions for treating tuberculous pericarditis. Cochrane Database Syst Rev 2002; (4):CD000526.

286.   Strang JI, Nunn AJ, Johnson DA, et al. Management of tuberculous constrictive pericarditis and tuberculous pericardial effusion in Transkei: results at 10 years follow-up. QJM 2004; 97:525–535.

287.   Hussey G, Chisholm T, Kibel M. Miliary tuberculosis in children: a review of 94 cases. Pediatr Infect Dis J 1991; 10:832–836.

288.   Starke JR. Tuberculosis of the central nervous system in children. Semin Pediatr Neurol 1999; 6:318–331.

289.   Donald PR, Schoeman JF, Cotton MF, et al. Cerebrospinal fluid investigations in tuberculous meningitis. Ann Trop Paediatr 1991; 11:241–246.

290.   Hejazi N, Hassler W. Multiple intracranial tuberculomas with atypical response to tuberculostatic chemotherapy: literature review and a case report. Infection 1997; 25:233–239.

291.   Ravenscroft A, Schoeman JF, Donald PR. Tuberculous granulomas in childhood tuberculous meningitis: radiological features and course. J Trop Pediatr 2001; 47:5–12.

292.   Jacobs RF, Sunakorn P, Chotpitayasunonah T, et al. Intensive short course chemotherapy for tuberculous meningitis. Pediatr Infect Dis J 1992; 11:194–198.

293.   Donald PR, Schoeman JF, Van Zyl LE, et al. Intensive short course chemotherapy in the management of tuberculous meningitis. Int J Tuber Lung Dis 1998; 2:704–711.

294.   Donald PR, Seifart HI. Cerebrospinal fluid concentration of ethionamide in children with tuberculous meningitis. J Pediatr 1989; 115:483–486.

295.   Humphries M. The management of tuberculous meningitis. Thorax 1992; 47:577–581.

296.   Ellard GA, Humphries MJ, Allen BW. Cerebrospinal drug concentrations and the treatment of tuberculous meningitis. Am Rev Respir Dis 1993; 148:650–655.

297.   Girgis NI, Farid Z, Kilpatrick ME, et al. Dexamethasone adjunctive treatment for tuberculous meningitis. Pediatr Infect Dis J 1991; 10:179–183.

298.   Schoeman JF, Van Zyl LE, Laubscher JA, et al. Effect of corticosteroids on intracranial pressure, computed tomographic findings, and clinical outcome in young children with tuberculous meningitis. Pediatrics 1997; 99:226–231.

299.   Prasad K, Volmink J, Menon GR. Steroids for treating tuberculous meningitis (Cochrane Review). In: The Cochrane Library, 3. Oxford: Update Software; 2000.

300.   Humphries MJ, Teoh R, Lau J, et al. Factors of prognostic significance in Chinese children with tuberculous meningitis. Tubercle 1990; 71:161–168.

301.   Starke J, Correa AG. Management of mycobacterial infection and disease in children. Pediatr Infect Dis J 1995; 14:455–470.

302.   Shribman JH, Eastwood JBJ, Uff J. Immune complex nephritis complicating miliary tuberculosis. BMJ 1983; 287:1593–1594.

303.   Lancet Editorial. Perinatal prophylaxis of tuberculosis. Lancet 1990; ii:1479–1480.

304.   Connolly Smith K. Congenital tuberculosis: a rare manifestation of a common infection. Curr Opin Infect Dis 2002; 15:269–274.

305.   Thomas P, Bornschlegel K, Singh TP, et al. Tuberculosis in human immunodeficiency virus-infected and human immunodeficiency virus-exposed children in New York City. Pediatr Infect Dis J 2000; 19:700–706.

306.   Graham SM, Coulter JBS, Gilks CF. Pulmonary disease in HIV-infected African children. Int J Tuber Lung Dis 2000; 15:12–23.

307.   Cotton MF, Schaaf HS, Hesseling AC, et al. HIV and childhood tuberculosis: the way forward. Int J Tuberc Lung Dis 2004; 8:675–682.

308.   Hesseling AC, Westra AE, Werschkull H, et al. Outcome of HIV-infected children with culture confirmed tuberculosis. Arch Dis Child 2005; 90:1171–1174.

*309.   Woldehanna S, Volmink J. Treatment of latent tuberculosis infection in HIV infected persons. Cochrane Database Syst Rev 2004; (1):CD000171.

310.   British Thoracic Society: Joint Tuberculosis Committee. Chemotherapy and management of tuberculosis in the United Kingdom. Thorax 1998; 53:536–548.

311.   Frieden TR, Sterling TR, Munsiff SS, et al. Tuberculosis. Lancet 2003; 362:887–899.

*312.   Volmink J, Garner P. Directly observed therapy for treating tuberculosis. Cochrane Database of Syst Rev 2006; (2):CD003343.

313.   Reed MD, Blumer JL. Clinical pharmacology of antitubercular drugs. Pediatr Clin North Am 1983; 30:177–193.

314.   Ormerod LP, Skinner C, Wales J. Hepatotoxicity of antituberculosis drugs. Thorax 1996; 51:111–113.

315.   Dooley DP, Carpenter JL, Rademacher S. Adjunctive corticosteroid therapy for tuberculosis: a critical reappraisal of the literature. Clin Infect Dis 1997; 25:872–887.

Bacterial Infections: Mycobacteria – Environmental

316.   Grange JM. Mycobacteria and human disease. London: Edward Arnold; 1988.

317.   Coulter JBS, Lloyd DA, Jones M, et al. Nontuberculous mycobacterial adenitis: effectiveness of chemotherapy following incomplete excision. Acta Paediatr 2006; 95:182–188.

318.   Starke JR. Nontuberculous mycobacterial infections in children. Adv Pediatr Infect Dis 1992; 7:123–159.

319.   Wolinsky E. Mycobacterial diseases other than tuberculosis. Clin Infect Dis 1992; 15:1–12.

320.   Romanus V, Hallander HO, Wahten P, et al. Atypical mycobacteria in extrapulmonary disease among children. Incidence in Sweden from 1969 to 1990 related to changing BCG vaccination coverage. Tuber Lung Dis 1995; 76:300–310.

321.   Jindal N, Devi B, Aggarwal A. Mycobacterial cervical lymphadenitis in childhood. Ind J Med Sci 2003; 57:12–15.

322.   Nylen O, Berg-Kelly K, Andersson B. Cervical lymph node infections with non-tuberculous mycobacteria in preschool children: interferon gamma deficiency as a possible cause of clinical infection. Acta Paediatr 2000; 89:1322–1325.

323.   Wolinsky E. Mycobacterial lymphadenitis in children: a prospective study of 105 non-tuberculous cases with long-term follow-up. Clin Infect Dis 1995; 20:954–963.

324.   Starke JR, Correa AG. Management of mycobacterial infection and disease in children. Pediatr Infect Dis J 1995; 14:455–470.

325.   Wansbrough-Jones M, Phillips R. Buruli ulcer: emerging from obscurity. Lancet 2006; 367:1849–1858.

326.   Dore ND, Le Sou'f PN, Masters B. Atypical mycobacterial pulmonary disease and bronchial obstruction in HIV-negative children. Pediatr Pulmonol 1997; 26:380–388.

327.   Oliver KN, Yankaskas JR, Knowles MR. Non-tuberculous mycobacterial pulmonary disease in cystic fibrosis. Semin Respir Infect 1996; 11:272–284.

*328.   British Thoracic Society. Management of opportunist mycobacterial infections: Joint Tuberculosis Committee Guidelines 1999. Thorax 2000; 55:210–218.

329.   Lammas DA, Casanova JL, Kumararatne DS. Clinical consequences of defects in the IL-12-dependent interferon-gamma (IFN-gamma) pathway. Clin Exp Immunol 2000; 121:417–425.

*330.   Gordin FM, Sullam PM, Shafran SD, et al. A randomised placebo-controlled study of rifabutin added to a regimen of clarithromycin and ethambutol for treatment of disseminated infection with Mycobacterium avium complex. Clin Infect Dis 1999; 28:1080–1085.

Bacterial Infections: Pertussis (Whooping Cough)

331.   Olin P, Rasmussen F, Gustafsson L, et al. Randomised controlled trial of two-component, three-component and five-component acellular pertussis vaccines compared with whole-cell vaccine. Lancet 1997; 350:1569–1577.

Bacterial Infections: *Pneumococcus*

332.   Gray BM, Dillon HC. Natural history of pneumococcal infections. Pediatr Infect Dis J 1989; 8 (suppl):S23–S25.

333. Hussain M, Melegaro A, Pebody RG, et al. A longitudinal household study of *Streptococcus pneumoniae* nasopharyngeal carriage in a UK setting. Epidemiol Infect 2005; 133:891–898.

334. Obaro SK, Monteil MA, Henderson DC. The pneumococcal problem. BMJ 1996; 312:1521–1525.

335. Earley A, Richman S, Ansell BM. Pneumococcal arthritis mimicking juvenile chronic arthritis. Arch Dis Child 1988; 63:1089–1090.

336. Lister PD. Multiply-resistant pneumococcus: therapeutic problems in the management of serious infections. Eur J Clin Microbiol Infect Dis 1995; 14(suppl 1):18–25.

337. Ada G, Isaacs D. Vaccination: the facts, the fears, the future. Sydney: Allen & Unwin; 2000.

*338. Black S, Shinefield H, Fireman B, et al. Efficacy, safety and immunogenicity of heptavalent pneumococcal conjugate vaccine in children. Pediatr Infect Dis J 2000; 19:187–195.

*339. Whitney CG, Farley MM, Hadler J, et al. Decline in invasive pneumococcal disease after the introduction of protein-polysaccharide conjugate vaccine. N Engl J Med 2003; 348:1737–1746.

340. Klugman KP, Madhi SA, Huebner RE, et al. A trial of a 9-valent pneumococcal conjugate vaccine in children with and those without HIV infection. N Engl J Med 2003; 349:1341–1348.

341. Black S, Shinefield H, Baxter R, et al. Impact of the use of heptavalent pneumococcal conjugate vaccine on disease epidemiology in children and adults. Vaccine 2006; 24Suppl 2:S2–79–80.

*342. Whitney CG, Pilishvili T, Farley MM, et al. Effectiveness of seven-valent pneumococcal conjugate vaccine against invasive pneumococcal disease: a matched case-control study. Lancet 2006; 368:1495–1502.

*343. Grijalva CG, Nuorti JP, Arbogast PJ, et al. Decline in pneumonia admissions after routine childhood immunisation with pneumococcal conjugate vaccine in the USA: a time-series analysis. Lancet 2007; 369:1179–1186.

344. Centers for Disease Control and Prevention (CDC). Direct and indirect effects of routine vaccination of children with 7-valent pneumococcal conjugate vaccine on incidence of invasive pneumococcal disease – United States, 1998–2003. MMWR Morb Mortal Wkly Rep 2005; 54:893–897.

345. Poehling KA, Talbot TR, Griffin MR, et al. Invasive pneumococcal disease among infants before and after introduction of pneumococcal conjugate vaccine. JAMA 2006; 295:1668–1674.

346. Abzug MJ, Pelton SI, Song LY, et al. Immunogenicity, safety, and predictors of response after a pneumococcal conjugate and pneumococcal polysaccharide vaccine series in human immunodeficiency virus-infected children receiving highly active antiretroviral therapy. Pediatr Infect Dis J 2006; 25:920–929.

347. Gaston MH, Verter JI, Woods G, et al. Prophylaxis with oral penicillin in children with sickle cell anemia: a randomized trial. N Engl J Med 1986; 314:1593–1599.

Bacterial Infections: Pseudomonas

*348. Boisseau AM, Sarlangue J, Perel Y, et al. Perineal ecthyma gangrenosum in infancy and early childhood: septicaemic and nonsepticaemic forms. J Am Acad Dermatol 1992; 27:415–418.

*349. Henwood CJ, Livermore DM, James D, et al. Antimicrobial susceptibility of *Pseudomonas aeruginosa*: results of a UK survey and evaluation of the British Society for Antimicrobial Chemotherapy disc susceptibility test. J Antimicrob Chemother 2001; 47:789–799.

*350. Mahenthiralingam E, Baldwin A, Vandamme P. *burkholderia cepacia* complex in patients with cystic fibrosis. J Med Microbial 2002; 51:533–538.

*351. Chaowagul W. Recent advances in the treatment of severe melioidosis. Acta Trop 2000; 74:133–137.

Bacterial Infections: Relapsing Fever

352. Mekasha A, Mehari S. Outbreak of louse-borne relapsing fever in Jimma, south Western Ethiopia. East Afr Med J 1996; 73:54–58.

353. Southern PM, Sanford JP. Relapsing fever: Clinical and microbiological review. Medicine 1969; 48:12–49.

354. Mekasha A. Louse-borne relapsing fever in children. J Trop Med Hyg 1992; 95:206–209.

355. Hodes R. Relapsing fever. In: Zein AZ, Kloos H, eds. The ecology of health and disease in Ethiopia. Addis Ababa: Ministry of Health; 1988:177–183.

356. Fekade D, Knox K, Hussein K, et al. Prevention of Jarisch–Herxheimer reaction by treatment with antibodies against tumor necrosis factor alpha. N Engl J Med 1996; 335:311–315.

357. Cox RE, Fekade D, Knox K, et al. The effect of TNFα on cytokine response in Jarisch–Herxheimer reactions of louse-borne relapsing fever. Q J Med 1997; 90:213–221.

358. Daniel E, Beyene H, Tessema T. Relapsing fever in children – demographic, social and clinical features. Ethiop Med J 1992; 30:207–214.

359. Bryceson ADM, Parry EHO, Perine PL, et al. Louse-borne relapsing fever: A clinical and laboratory study of 62 cases in Ethiopia and reconsideration of the literature. Q J Med 1970; 39:129–170.

360. Salih SY, Mustafa D. Louse-borne relapsing fever. II Combined penicillin and tetracycline therapy in 160 Sudanese patients. Trans R Soc Trop Med Hyg 1977; 71:49–50.

361. Teklu B, Habte-michael A, Warrell DA, et al. Meptazinol diminishes the Jarisch–Herxheimer reaction of relapsing fever. Lancet 1983; 1:835–839.

362. Barclay AJG, Coulter JBS. Tick-borne relapsing fever in central Tanzania. Trans R Soc Trop Med Hyg 1990; 84:852–856.

363. Ramos JM, Malmierca E, Reyes F, et al. Characteristics of louse-borne relapsing fever in Ethiopian children and adults. Ann Trop Med Parasitol 2004; 98:191–196.

364. Mitiku K, Mengistu G. Relapsing fever in Gondar, Ethiopia. East Afr Med J 2002; 79:85–87.

Bacterial Infections: Salmonellosis

365. Graham SM. Salmonellosis in children in developing and developed countries and populations. Curr Opin Infect Dis 2002; 15:507–512.

366. Weinberger M, Keller N. Recent trends in the epidemiology of non-typhoid Salmonella and antimicrobial resistance: the Israeli experience and worldwide review. Curr Opin Infect Dis 2005; 18:513–521.

367. Graham SM, Molyneux EM, Walsh AL, et al. Nontyphoidal Salmonella infections of children in tropical Africa. Pediatr Infect Dis J 2000; 19:1189–1196.

368. Brent A, Oundo JO, Mwangi I, et al. Salmonella bacteremia in Kenyan children. Pediatr Infect Dis J 2006; 25:230–236.

369. Saha SK, Baqui AH, Hanif M, et al. Typhoid fever in Bangladesh: implications for vaccination policy. Pediatr Infect Dis J 2001; 20:521–524.

*370. Sirinavin S, Garner P. Antibiotics for treating salmonella gut infections (Cochrane Review). In: The Cochrane Library, 4. Oxford: Update Software; 2001.

*371. Sirinavin S, Thavornuth J, Sakchainanont B, et al. Norfloxacin and azithromycin for treatment of nontyphoidal salmonella carriers. Clin Infect Dis 2003; 37:685–691.

372. St Geme JW, Hodes HL, Marcy SM, et al. Consensus management of *Salmonella* infection in the first year of life. Pediatr Infect Dis J 1988; 7:615–621.

Bacterial Infections: Typhoid Fever

373. Health Protection Agency. Accessed at www.hpa.org.uk/infections/default.htm

374. World Health Organization background document. The diagnosis, treatment and prevention of typhoid fever. WHO/V&B/03.07. Accessed at www.who.int/entity/vaccine-_research/documents/en/typhoid-diagnosis.pdf on 26.04.07

375. Parry CM. Typhoid fever. Curr Infect Dis Rep 2004; 6:27–33.

376. Mahle WT, Levine MM. *Salmonella typhi* infections in children younger than five years of age. Pediatr Infect Dis J 1993; 12:627–631.

*377. Parry CM, Ho VA, Phuong LT, et al. Randomized controlled comparison of ofloxacin, azithromycin, and an ofloxacin-azithromycin combination for treatment of multidrug-resistant and nalidixic acid-resistant typhoid fever. Antimicrob Agents Chemother 2007; 51:819–825.

378. Cooke FJ, Wain J, Threlfall EJ. Fluoroquinolone resistance in *Salmonella* typhi. BMJ 2006; 33: 353–354.

379. Schaad UB. Pediatric use of quinolones. Pediatr Infect Dis J 1999; 18:469–470.

*380. Punjabi NH, Hoffman SL, Edman DC, et al. Treatment of severe typhoid fever in children with high dose dexamethasone. Pediatr Infect Dis J 1988; 7:598–600.

*381. Engels EA, Lau J. Vaccines for preventing typhoid fever (Cochrane Review). In: The Cochrane Library, 4. Oxford: Update Software; 2001.

382. Lin FYC, Ho VA, Khiem HB, et al. The efficacy of a *Salmonella typhi* Vi conjugate vaccine in two-to-five year-old children. N Engl J Med 2001; 344: 1263–1269.

Bacterial Infections: *Shigella* (Bacillary Dysentery)

383 Kotloff KL, Winickoff JP, Ivanoff B, et al. Global burden of Shigella infections: Implications for vaccine development and implementation. Bull WHO 1999; 77:651–656.

384. Goma Epidemiology Group. Public health impact of Rwandan refugee crisis: what happened in Goma, Zaire, in July, 1994? Goma Epidemiology Group. Lancet 1995; 345:339–344.

385. Clemens JD, Stanton B, Stoll B, et al. Breast feeding as a determinant of severity in shigellosis. Evidence for protection throughout the first three years of life in Bangladeshi children. Am J Epidemiol 1986; 123:710–720.

386. Tacket CO, Binion SB, Bostwick E, et al. Efficacy of bovine milk immunoglobulin concentrate in preventing illness after *Shigella flexneri* challenge. Am J Trop Med Hyg 1992; 47:276–283.

387. Levine MM, Kotloff KL, Barry EM, et al. Clinical trials of Shigella vaccines: Two steps forward and one step back on a long, hard road. Nat Rev Microbiol In press 2007.

Bacterial Infections: Staphylococcus

388. Yamasaki O, Yamaguchi T, Sugai M, et al. Clinical manifestations of staphylococcal scalded-skin syndrome depend on serotypes of exfoliative toxins. J Clin Microbiol 2005; 43:1890–1893.

389. Gillet Y, Issartel B, Vanhems P, et al. Association between *Staphylococcus aureus* strains carrying gene for Panton-Valentine leukocidin and highly lethal necrotising pneumonia in young immunocompetent patients. Lancet 2002; 359:753–759.

390. Hiramatsu K. Vancomycin-resistant *Staphylococcus aureus*: a new model of antibiotic resistance. Lancet Infect Dis 2001; 1:147–155.

Bacterial Infections: *Streptococcus* and *Enterococcus*

391. Stevens DL. Invasive group A streptococcus infections. Clin Infect Dis 1992; 14:2–11.

392. Zirakzadeh A, Patel R. Vancomycin-resistant enterococci: colonization, infection, detection, and treatment. Mayo Clin Proc 2006; 81:529–536.

Bacterial Infections: Tetanus

393. Farrar JJ, Yen LM, Cook T, et al. Tetanus. J Neurol Neurosurg Psych 2000; 69:292–301.

394. Whitman C, Belgharbi L, Gasse F, et al. Progress towards the global elimination of neonatal tetanus. World Health Stat Q 1992; 45:248–256.

395. Silveira CM, Caceres VM, Dutra MG, et al. Safety of tetanus toxoid in pregnant women: a hospital-based case control study of congenital anomalies. Bull WHO 1995; 73:605–608.

396. Thwaites CL, Yen LM, Loan HT, et al. Magnesium sulphate for treatment of severe tetanus: a randomised controlled trial. Lancet 2006; 368:1436–1443.

397. Anlar B, Yalaz K, Dizmen R. Long-term prognosis after neonatal tetanus. Develop Med Child Neurol 1989; 31:76–80.

Bacterial Infections: Tularemia

398. Johansson A, Ibrahim A, Goransson I, et al. Evaluation of PCR-based methods for discrimination of *Francisella* species and subspecies and development of a specific PCR that distinguishes the two major subspecies of *Francisella tularensis*. J Clin Microbiol 2000; 38:4180–4185.

*399. Staples JE, Kubota KA, Chalcraft LG, et al. Epidemiologic and molecular analysis of human tularemia, United States, 1964–2004. Emerg Infect Dis 2006; 12:1113–1118.

400. Payne L, Arneborn M, Tegnell A, et al. Endemic tularemia, Sweden, 2003. Emerg Infect Dis 2005; 11:1440–1442.

401. Oyston PC, Sjostedt A, Titball RW. Tularaemia: bioterrorism defence renews interest in Francisella tularensis. Nat Rev Microbiol 2004; 2:967–978.

402. Jacobs RF, Condrey YM, Yamauchi T. Tularemia in adults and children: a changing presentation. Pediatrics 1985; 76:818–822.

403. Enderlin G, Morales L, Jacobs RF, et al. Streptomycin and alternative agents for the treatment of tularemia: review of the literature. Clin Infect Dis 1994; 19:42–47.

404. Johansson A, Berglund L, Gothefors L, et al. Ciprofloxacin for treatment of tularemia in children. Pediatr Infect Dis J 2000; 19:449–453.

405. American Academy of Pediatrics. Tularemia. In: Pickering LK, ed. Red book: Report of the Committee on Infectious Diseases, 25th edn. Elk Grove Village: American Academy of Pediatrics; 2000:618–620.

Bacterial Infections: Yersiniosis and Plague

406. Cover TL, Aber RC. Yersinia enterocolitica. N Engl J Med 1989; 321:16–24.

407. Naktin J, Beavis KG. Yersinia enterocolitica and Yersinia pseudotuberculosis. Clin Lab Med 1999; 19:523–536.

408. Fredriksson-Ahomaa M, Stolle A, Korkeala H. Molecular epidemiology of Yersinia enterocolitica infections. FEMS Immunol Med Microbiol 2006; 47:315–329.

409. Larson JH. The spectrum of clinical manifestations of infections with Yersinia enterocolitica and their pathogenesis. Contrib Microbiol Immunol 1979; 5:257–269.

410. Abdel-Haq NM, Papadopol R, Asmar BI, et al. Antibiotic susceptibilities of Yersinia enterocolitica recovered from children over a 12-year period. Int J Antimicrob Agents 2006; 27:449–452.

411. Perry RD, Fetherston JD. Yersinia pestis – etiologic agent of plague. Clin Microbiol Rev 1997; 10:35–66.

412. Smego RA, Frean J, Koornhof HJ. Yersiniosis I: microbiological and clinicoepidemiological aspects of plague and non-plague Yersinia infections. Eur J Clin Microbiol Infect Dis 1999; 18:1–15.

*413. Mwengee W, Butler T, Mgema S, et al. Treatment of plague with gentamicin or doxycycline in a randomized clinical trial in Tanzania. Clin Infect Dis 2006; 42:614–621.

Use of the Virology Laboratory by The Clinician

414. Fong C, Lee M, Griffith B. Evaluation of R-mix fresh cells in shell vials for detection of respiratory viruses. J Clin Microbiol 2000; 38:4660–4662.

415. Liolios L, Jenney A, Spelman D, et al. Comparison of a multiplex reverse transcription-PCR-enzyme hybridization assay with conventional viral culture and immunofluorescence techniques for the detection of seven viral respiratory pathogens. J Clin Microbiol 2001; 39:2779–2783.

416. Mancini A. Exanthems in childhood: an update. Pediatr Ann 1998; 27:163–170.

417. Sawyer MH. Enterovirus infections; Diagnosis and treatment. Curr Opin Paediatr 2001; 13:65–69.

418. Gubler DJ. Resurgent vector-born diseases as a global health problem. Emerg Infect Dis 1998; 4:442–450.

419. Levy J. Three new human herpes viruses (HHV-6, 7 and 8). Lancet 1997; 349:558–562.

420. Yan SS, Fedoroko DP. Recent advances in laboratory diagnosis of human cytomegalovirus infection. Clin Appl Immunol Rev 2002; 2:155–167.

421. Berger C, Day P, Meier G, et al. Dynamics of Epstein-Barr virus DNA levels in serum during EBV-associated disease. J Med Virol 2001; 64:505–512.

422. Fong IW, Britton CB, Luinstra KL, et al. Diagnostic value of detecting JC virus DNA in cerebrospinal fluid of patients with progressive multifocal leukoencephalopathy. J Clin Microbiol 1995; 33:484–486.

423. van den Hoogen BG, de Jong JC, Groen J, et al. A newly discovered human pneumovirus isolated from young children with respiratory tract disease. Nat Med 2001; 7:719–724.

424. Ksiazek TG, Erdman D, Goldsmith CS, et al. A novel coronavirus associated with severe acute respiratory syndrome. N Engl J Med 2003; 348:1953–1966.

HIV Infection

425. Palella FJ Jr, Delaney KM, Moorman AC, et al. Declining morbidity and mortality among patients with advanced human immunodeficiency virus infection. HIV outpatient study investigators. N Engl J Med 1998; 338:853–860.

426. Gibb DM, Duong T, Tookey PA et al. Decline in mortality, AIDS, and hospital admissions in perinatally HIV-1 infected children in the United Kingdom and Ireland. BMJ 2003; 327:1019–1021.

427. European Collaborative Study. HIV-infected pregnant women and vertical transmission in Europe since 1986. AIDS 2001; 15:761–770.

428. Duong T, Ades AE, Gibb DM, et al. HIV vertical transmission in the British Isles: estimates based on surveillance data. BMJ 1999; 319:1227–1229.

429. Joint United Nations Programme on HIV/AIDS. Report on the global HIV/AIDS epidemic. UNAIDS 2006. Available: http://www.unaids.org.

430. Pedraza MA, del Romero J, Roldan F, et al. Heterosexual transmission of HIV-1 is associated with high plasma viral load levels and a positive viral isolation in the infected partner. J Acquir Immune Defic Syndr 1999; 21:120–125.

431. Struick S, Tudor-Williams G, Taylor GP, et al. 4 Cases of infant HIV due to seroconversion in pregnancy; Should partner screening and/or repeat 3rd trimester HIV screening be recommended in the UK? BHIVA 12th Annual Conference, April 2006, p.68.

432. Judd A, Doerholt K, Sharland M, et al. Morbidity, mortality, and response to treatment in perinatally HIV-infected children in the UK and Ireland, 1996–2006: planning for teenage and adult care. In press BMJ 2007

433. European Collaborative Study. The mother-to-child HIV transmission epidemic in Europe: evolving in the East and established in the West. AIDS 2006; 20:1419–1427.

434. Ades AE, Walker J, Botting B, et al. Effect of the worldwide epidemic on HIV prevalence in the United Kingdom: record linkage in anonymous neonatal seroprevalence surveys. AIDS 1999; 13:2437–2443.

435. Cliffe S, Tookey PA, Nicoll A. Antenatal detection of HIV: national surveillance and unlinked anonymous survey. BMJ 2001; 323:376–377.

436. Supplementary data tables: Unlinked Anonymous Prevalence surveys of Pregnant Women: data to the end of 2004 Surveillance Update: 2005 HPA.

437. Melvin D, Jungmann E, Foster C, et al. Guidance on transition and long term follow up services for adolescents with HIV infection acquired in infancy. CHIVA Guidelines 2005 (updated Feb 2007) Available: http://www.BHIVA.org

438. Peckham C, Gibb DM. Mother-to-child transmission of the human immunodeficiency virus. N Engl J Med 1995; 333:298–302.

439. Dunn DT, Newell ML, Ades AE, et al. Risk of human immunodeficiency virus type 1 transmission through breastfeeding. Lancet 1992; 340:585–588.

440. Fowler MC, Simonds RJ, Roonsgpisuthipong A. Update on perinatal HIV transmission. Pediatr Clin North Am 2000; 47:21–38.

441. Mandelbrot L, Le Chenadec J, Berrebi A, et al. Perinatal HIV-1 transmission. Interaction between zidovudine prophylaxis and mode of delivery in the French perinatal cohort. JAMA 1998; 280:55–60.

442. Connor EM, Mofenson LM. Zidovudine for the reduction of perinatal human immunodeficiency virus transmission: Pediatric AIDS Clinical Trials Group Protocol 076 – results and treatment recommendations. Pediatr Infect Dis J 1995; 14:536–541.

443. Fiscus SA, Adimora AA, Schoenbach VJ, et al. Perinatal HIV infection and the effect of zidovudine therapy on transmission in rural and urban countries. JAMA 1996; 275:1483–1488.

444. Mandelbroot L, Landreau-Mascaro A, Rekacewicz C, et al. Lamivudine-zidovudine combination for prevention of maternal-infant transmission of HIV-1. JAMA 2001; 285:2083–2093.

445. Cooper ER, Charurat M, Mofenson L, et al. Combination antiretroviral strategies for the treatment of pregnant HIV-1-infected women and prevention of perinatal HIV-1 transmission. J Acquir Immune Defic Syndr 2002; 29:484–494.

446. Mofenson LM, Lambert JS, Stiehm ER, et al. Risk factors for perinatal transmission of human immunodeficiency virus type 1 in women treated with zidovudine. Pediatric AIDS Clinical Trials Group Study 185 Team. N Engl J Med 1999; 341:385–393.

447. Ioannidis JP, Abrams EJ, Ammann A, et al. Perinatal transmission of human immunodeficiency virus type 1 by pregnant women with RNA virus loads 1000 copies/ml. J Infect Dis 2001; 183:539–545.

448. Guay LA, Musoke P, Fleming T, et al. Intrapartum and neonatal single-dose nevirapine compared with zidovudine for prevention of mother-to-child transmission of HIV-1 in Kampala, Uganda; HIVNET 012 randomized trial. Lancet 1999; 354:795–802.

449. British HIV Association (BHIVA). Guidelines for the management of HIV infection in pregnant women and the prevention of mother-to-child transmission. 2005. Available: http://www.BHIVA.org

450. Live document a. Public Health Service Task Force recommendations for the use of antiretroviral drugs in pregnant women infected with HIV-1 for maternal health and interventions to reduce perinatal HIV-1 transmission in the United States. 12 October 2006 Available: http://www.hivatis.org.

451. Schaffer N, Chuachoowong R, Mock PA, et al. Short-course zidovudine for perinatal HIV-1 transmission in Bangkok. Collaborative Oriental HIV Transmission Study group. Lancet 1999; 353:773–780.

452. Lallemant M, Jourdain G, Le Coeur S, et al. A trial of shortened zidovudine regimens to prevent mother-to-child transmission of human immunodeficiency virus type 1. N Engl J Med 2000; 343:982–991.

453. The PETRA Study Team. Efficacy of three short-course regimens of zidovudine and lamivudine in preventing early and late transmission of HIV-1 from mother to child in Tanzania, South Africa, and Uganda (Petra Study): a randomised, double-blind, placebo-controlled trial. Lancet 2002; 359:1178–1186.

454. Muro E, Droste JA, Hofstede HT, et al. Nevirapine plasma concentrations are still detectable after more than 2 weeks in the majority of women receiving single-dose nevirapine: implications for intervention studies. J Acquir Immune Defic Syndr 2005; 39:419–421.

455. Johnson JA, Li JF, Morris L, et al. Emergence of drug-resistant HIV-1 after intrapartum administration of single-dose nevirapine is substantially under-estimated. J Infect Dis 2005; 192:16–23.

456. Flys T, Nissley DV, Claasen CW, et al. Sensitive drug-resistance assays reveal long-term persistence of HIV-1 variants with the K103N nevirapine (NVP) resistance mutation in some women and infants after the administration of single-dose NVP: HIVNET 012. J Infect Dis 2005; 192:24–29.

457. Jourdian G, Ngo-Giang-Huong N, et al. Perinatal HIV Prevention Trial Group. Intrapartum exposure to nevirapine and subsequent maternal responses to nevirapine-based antiretroviral therapy. N Engl J Med 2004; 351:229–240.

458. Martinson NA, Morris L, Gray G, et al. Selection and persistence of viral resistance in HIV-infected children after exposure to single-dose nevirapine. J Acquir Immune Defic Syndr 2007; 44:148–153.

459. McIntyre J, Martinson N, Boltz V, et al. Addition of short course Combivir (CBV) to single dose Viramune (sdNVP) for prevention of mother-to-child transmission of HIV-1 can significantly decrease the subsequent development of maternal NNRTI-resistant virus. XV Intl AIDS Conference, Bangkok. LbOrB09.

460. McIntyre JA, Martinson N, Gray GE, et al. Single dose nevirapine combined with a short course of Combivir for prevention of mother to child transmission of HIV-1 can significantly decrease the subsequent development of maternal and infant resistant virus. 14th International HIV Drug Resistance Workshop Quebec June 2005. Abstract 2.

461. Eshleman SH, Hoover DR, Hudelson SE, et al. Development of nevirapine resistance in infants is reduced by use of infant-only single-dose nevirapine plus zidovudine postexposure prophylaxis for the prevention of mother-to-child transmission of HIV-1. J Infect Dis 2006; 193:479–481.

462. Lockman S, Shapiro RL, Smeaton LM, et al. Response to antiretroviral therapy after a single, peripartum dose of nevirapine. N Engl J Med 2007; 356:135–147.

463. European Collaborative Study. Mother-to-child transmission of HIV infection in the era of highly active antiretroviral therapy. Clin Infect Dis 2005; 40:458–465.

464. Suy A, Coll O, Martinez E, et al. Increased risk of pre-eclampsia and foetal death in HIV-infected pregnant women receiving highly active antiretroviral therapy. XV International AIDS Conference, Bangkok, 2004 Abs ThOrB1359.

465. Thorne C, Patel D, Newell ML. Increased risk of adverse pregnancy outcomes in HIV-infected women treated with highly active antiretroviral therapy in Europe. AIDS 2004; 18:2337–2339.

466. Tuomala RE, Shapiro DE, Mofenson LM, et al. Antiretroviral therapy during pregnancy and the risk of an adverse outcome. N Engl J Med 2002; 346:1863–1870.

467. Blanche S, Tardieu M, Rustin P, et al. Persistent mitochondrial dysfunction and perinatal exposure to antiretroviral nucleoside analogues. Lancet 1999; 354:1084–1089.

468. Dominguez K, Bertolli J, Fowler M, et al. Lack of definitive severe mitochondrial signs or symptoms among deceased HIV uninfected and HIV indeterminate children < 5 years of age, Pediatric Spectrum of Disease Project (PSD), USA. Ann N Y Acad Sci 2000; 918:236–246.

469. Le Chenadec J, Mayaux MJ, Guihenneuc-Jouyaux C, et al; Enquete Perinatale Francaise Study Group. Perinatal antiretroviral treatment and hematopoiesis in HIV-uninfected infants. AIDS 2003; 17:2053–2061.

470. International Perinatal HIV Group. Duration of ruptured membranes and vertical transmission of HIV-1: a meta-analysis from 15 prospective cohort studies. AIDS 2001; 15:357–368.

471. European Mode of Delivery Collaboration. Elective caesarean-section versus vaginal delivery in prevention of vertical HIV-1 transmission: a randomised clinical trial. Lancet 1999; 353:1035–1039.

472. International Perinatal HIV Group. Mode of delivery and the risk of vertical transmission of human immunodeficiency virus type 1. A meta-analysis of fifteen prospective cohort studies. N Engl J Med 1999; 340:977–987.

473. Read JS. Caesarean section delivery to prevent vertical transmission of human immunodeficiency virus type 1. Associated risks and other considerations. Ann N Y Acad Sci 2000; 918:115–121.

474. Leroy V, Newell ML, Dabis F, et al. International multicentre pooled analysis of late postnatal mother-to-child transmission of HIV-1 infection. Ghent International Working Group on Mother-to-Child Transmission of HIV. Lancet 1998; 352:597–600.

475. Nduati R, John G, Mhori-Ngacha D, et al. Effect of breast-feeding and formula feeding on transmission of HIV-1: a randomized clinical trial. JAMA 2000; 283:1167–1174.

476. WHO Collaborative Study Team on the role of Breastfeeding on the Prevention of Infant Mortality. Effect of breastfeeding on infant and child mortality due to infectious diseases in less developed countries: a pooled analysis. Lancet 2000; 355:451–455.

477. Coutsoudis A, Pillay K, Kuhn L, et al. Method of feeding and transmission of HIV-1 from mothers to children by 15 months of age: prospective cohort study from Durban, South Africa. AIDS 2001; 15:379–387.

478. Giuliano M, Guidotti G, Andreotti M, et al. Triple antiretroviral prophylaxis administered during pregnancy and after delivery significantly reduces breast milk viral load: a study within the Drug Resource Enhancement Against AIDS and Malnutrition Program. J Acquir Immune Defic Syndr 2007; 44:286–291.

479. Gaillard P, Mwanyumba F, Verhofstede C, et al. Vaginal lavage with chlorhexidine during labour to reduce mother-to-child HIV transmission: clinical trial in Mombasa, Kenya. AIDS 2001; 15:389–396.

480. Read JS, Bethel J, Harris DR, et al. Serum vitamin A concentrations in a North American cohort of human immunodeficiency virus type 1-infected children. National Institute of Child Health and Human Development Intravenous Immunoglobulin Clinical Trial Study Group. Pediatr Infect Dis J 1999; 18:134–142.

481. Fawzi WW, Msamanga G, Hunter D, et al. Randomized trial of vitamin supplements in relation to vertical transmission of HIV-1 in Tanzania. J Acquir Immune Defic Syndr 2000; 23:246–254.

482. Ades AE, Sculpher MJ, Gibb DM, et al. Cost-effectiveness of antenatal HIV screening in the UK. BMJ 1999; 319:1230–1234.

483. Williams AJ, Gibb DM. Pneumocystis carinii pneumonia and CMV infection in HIV infected infants. HIV and AIDS, Current Trends March; 2002:1–5.5.

484. De Cock KM, Fowler MG, Mercier E, et al. Prevention of mother-to-child HIV transmission in resource-poor countries: translating research into policy and practice. JAMA 2002; 283:1175–1182.

485. O'Brien SJ, Moore JP. The effect of genetic variation in chemokines and their receptors on HIV transmission and progression to AIDS. Immunol Rev 2000; 177:99–111.

486. Wasik TJ, Bratosiewicz J, Wierzbicki A, et al. Protective role of beta-chemokines associated with HIV-specific Th responses against perinatal HIV transmission. J Immunol 1999; 162:4355–4364.

487. Hogan CM, Hammer SM. Host determinants in HIV infection and disease. Part 1: cellular and humoral immune responses. Ann Intern Med 2001; 134:761–776.

488. Soudeyns H, Pantaleo G. The moving target: mechanisms of HIV persistence during primary infection. Immunol Today 1999; 20:446–450.

489. Feeney ME, Roosevelt KA, Tang Y, et al. Comprehensive screening reveals strong and broadly directed human immunodeficiency virus type 1-specific CD8 responses in perinatally infected children. J Virol 2003; 77:7492–7501.

490. Sandberg JK, Fast NM, Jordan KA. HIV-specific CD8+ T cell function in children with vertically acquired HIV-1 infection is critically influenced by age and the state of the CD4+ T cell compartment. J Immunol 2003; 170:4403–4410.

491. Shearer WT, Quinn TC, LaRussa P, et al. Viral load and disease progression in infants infected with human immunodeficiency virus type 1. Women and Infants Transmission Study Group. N Engl J Med 1997; 336:1337–1342.

492. Gibb DM, Newberry A, de Rossi A, et al. HIV-1 viral load and CD4 count in untreated children with vertically acquired asymptomatic or mild disease – PENTA 1 Virology. AIDS 1998; 12:F1–F8.

493. De Rossi A, Walker AS, De Forni D, et al. for PENTA. Relationship between changes in thymic emigrants and cell associated HIV-1 DNA in HIV-1-infected children initiating antiretroviral therapy. Antivir Ther 2005; 10:63–71.

494. Honeyborne I, Prendergast A, Pereyra F, et al. Control of HIV-1 is associated with HLA-B9913 and targeting of multiple GAG-specific CD8+ T cell epitopes. J Virol 2007; [Epub ahead of print]

495. Ho DD. Perspectives series: host/pathogen interactions. Dynamics of HIV-1 replication in vivo. J Clin Invest 1997; 99:2565–2567.

496. Zhang L, Ramratnam B, Tenner-Racz K, et al. Quantifying residual HIV-1 replication in patients receiving combination antiretroviral therapy. N Engl J Med 1999; 340:1605–1613.

497. Wade AM, Ades AE. Age-related reference ranges: significance tests for models and confidence intervals for centiles. Stat Med 1994; 13:2359–2367.

498. HIV Paediatric Prognostic Markers Collaborative Study (writing committee Dunn DT, Gibb DM, Duong T et al). Short-term risk of disease progression in HIV-1-infected children receiving no antiretroviral therapy or zidovudine monotherapy: a meta-analysis. Lancet 2003; 362:1605–1611.

499. HIV Paediatric Prognostic Markers Collaborative Study (writing committee Dunn DT, Gibb DM, Duong T et al). Use of total lymphocyte count for informing when to start antiretroviral therapy in HIV-infected children: a meta-analysis of longitudinal data. Lancet 2005; 366:1868–1874.

500. HIV Paediatric Prognostic Markers Collaborative Study (writing committee Dunn DT, Gibb DM, Duong T et al). Predictive value of absolute CD4 cell count for disease progression in untreated HIV-1 infected children. AIDS 2006; 20:1289–1294.

501. WHO case definitions of HIV for surveillance and revised clinical staging and immunological classification of HIV-related disease in adults and children. 7 August 2006. www.who. int/hiv/pub/guidelines.

502. Dunn D, Newell ML, Peckham C, et al. (for the European Collaborative Study Group). CD4 T cell count as a predictor of Pneumocystis carinii pneumonia

in children born to mothers infected with HIV. BMJ 1994; 308:437–440.

503. Galli L, de Martino M, Tovo PA, et al. Predictive value of the HIV paediatric classification system for the long term course of perinatally infected children. Int J Epidemiol 2000; 29:573–578.

504. CDC. 1994 Revised classification system for human immunodeficiency virus infection in children <13 years of age. MMWR 1994; 43(RR-12).

505. Dunn DT, Brandt CD, Krivine A, et al. The sensitivity of HIV-1 DNA polymerase chain reaction in the neonatal period and the relative contributions of intra-uterine and intra-partum transmission. AIDS 1995; 9:F7–11.

506. Tovo PA, De Marino M, Gabiano C, et al. Prognostic factors and survival in children with perinatal HIV-1 infection. Lancet 1992; 339:1249–1253.

507. Blanche S, Newell ML, Mayaux MJ, et al. Morbidity and mortality in European children vertically infected by HIV-1. The French Pediatric HIV Infection Study Group and European Collaborative Study. J Acquir Immune Defic Syndr 1998; 14:442–450.

508. Diaz C, Hanson C, Cooper ER, et al. Disease progression in a cohort of infants with vertically acquired HIV infection observed from birth: the Women and Infants Transmission Study (WITS). J Acquir Immune Defic Syndr 1998; 18:221–228.

509. Gona P, Van Dyke R, Williams P, et al. Incidence of opportunistic and other infections in HIV-infected children in the HAART era. JAMA 2006; 296:292–300.

510. Dankner WM, Lindsey JC, Levin MJ and the Pediatric AIDS Clinical Trials Group 2001. Correlates of opportunistic infections in children infected with the human immunodeficiency virus managed before highly active antiretroviral therapy. Pediatr Infect Dis J 2001; 20:40–48.

511. Simonds RJ, Oxtoby MJ, Caldwell MB, et al. Pneumocystis carinii pneumonia among US children with perinatally acquired HIV infection. JAMA 1993; 270:470–473.

512. Williams AJ, Duong T, McNally LM, et al. Pneumocystis carinii pneumonia and cytomegalovirus infection in children with vertically acquired HIV infection. AIDS 2001; 15:335–339.

513. Chintu C, Bhat GJ, Walker AS, et al. on behalf of the CHAP Trial team. A randomized placebo-controlled trial of cotrimoxazole as prophylaxis against opportunistic infections in HIV-infected Zambian children: the CHAP (Children With HIV Antibiotic Prophylaxis) Trial. Lancet 2004; 364:1865–1871.

514. Chandwani S, Kaul A, Bebenroth D, et al. Cytomegalovirus infection in human immuno-deficiency virus type 1-infected children. Pediatr Infect Dis J 1996; 15:310–314.

515. Gibb DM, Giacomelli A, Masters J, et al. Persistence of antibody responses to Haemophilus influenzae type b polysaccharide conjugate vaccine in children with vertically acquired human immunodeficiency virus infection. Pediatr Infect Dis J 1996; 15:1097–1101.

516. Sharland M, Gibb DM, Holland F. Respiratory morbidity from lymphocytic interstitial pneumonitis (LIP) in vertically acquired HIV-1 infection. Arch Dis Child 1997; 76:334–337.

517. Shanbhag MC, Rutstein RM, Zaoutis T, et al. Neurocognitive functioning in pediatric human immunodeficiency virus infection: effects of combined therapy. Arch Pediatr Adolesc Med 2005; 159:651–656.

518. Chiriboga CA, Fleishman S, Champion S, et al. Incidence and prevalence of HIV encephalopathy in children with HIV infection receiving highly active anti-retroviral therapy (HAART). J Pediatr 2005; 146:402–407.

519. Foster C, Biggs R, Melvin D, et al. Neurodevelopmental outcomes in children with HIV infection under 3 years of age. Dev Med Child Neurol 2006; 48:677–682.

520. Gifford GM, Polesel J, Rickenbach M, et al. Cancer risk in the Swiss HIV Cohort Study: associations with immunodeficiency, smoking, and highly active antiretroviral therapy. J Natl Cancer Inst 2005; 97:407–409.

521. Evans JA, Gibb DM, Holland FJ, et al. Malignancies in children with HIV infection acquired from mother-to-child transmission in the United Kingdom. Arch Dis Child 1997; 76:330–334.

522. Rabkin CS. AIDS and cancer in the era of highly active antiretroviral therapy (HAART). Eur J Cancer 2001; 37:1316–1319.

523. Kest H, Brogly S, McSherry G, et al. Malignancy in perinatally human immunodeficiency virus-infected children in the United States. Pediatr Infect Dis J 2005; 24:237–242.

524. Krishnan A, Molina A, Zaia J, et al. Durable remissions with autologous stem cell transplantation for high-risk HIV-associated lymphomas. Blood 2005; 105:874–878.

525. McCarthy GA, Kampmann G, Novelli V, et al. Vertical transmission of Kaposi's sarcoma. Arch Dis Child 1996; 76:455–457.

526. Walker AS, Mulenga V, Sinyinza F, et al. and the CHAP Trial Team. Determinants of survival without antiretroviral therapy after infancy in HIV-1 infected African children in the CHAP Trial. J Acquir Immune Defic Syndr 2006; 42:637–645.

527. Kinghorn G. A sexual health and HIV strategy for England. BMJ 2001; 323:243–244.

528. British HIV Association Guidelines (BHIVA) for the treatment of HIV-infected adults with antiretroviral therapy 2005. Available: http://www.bhiva.org.

529. Guidelines for the use of antiretroviral agents in HIV infected adults and adolescents Available: http://www.aidsinfo.nih.gov/Guidelines 2006

530. Sharland M, Blanche S, Castelli G, et al; PENTA Steering Committee PENTA guidelines for the use of antiretroviral therapy, 2004. HIV Med 2004:5 Suppl 2:61–86. Available: http://www.bhiva.org and www.pentatrials.org

531. Guidelines for the use of antiretroviral agents in pediatric HIV infection. Working Group on Antiretroviral Therapy and Medical Management of HIV-Infected Children 3rd November 2005. Available: http://AIDSinfo.nih.gov.

532. American Academy of Pediatrics. Committee on Pediatric AIDS, Section on International Child Health. Increasing antiretroviral drug access for children with HIV infection. Policy statement 2007. Pediatrics 2007; 119:838–845.

533. Gortmaker SL, Hughes M, Cervia J, et al. for the PACTG 219 team. Effect of combination therapy including protease inhibitors on mortality among children and adolescents infected with HIV-1. N Engl J Med 2001; 345:1522–1528.

534. Mulenga V, Ford D, Walker AS, et al. and the CHAP Trial Team. Effect of cotrimoxizole on causes of death, hospital admissions and antibiotic use in HIV-infected children in the CHAP trial. AIDS 2007; 21:77–84.

535. Paediatric European Network for Treatment of AIDS (PENTA). Comparison of dual nucleoside-analogue reverse-transcriptase inhibitor regimens with and without nelfinavir in children with HIV-1 who have not previously been treated: the PENTA 5 randomised trial. Lancet 2002; 359:733–739.

536. Walker AS, Doerhalt K, Sharland M, et al. Collaborative HIV Paediatric Study (CHIPS) Steering Committee. Response to highly active antiretroviral therapy varies with age: the UK and Ireland Collaborative HIV Paediatric Study. AIDS 2004: 18:1915–1924.

537. Melvin AJ, Rodrigo AG, Mohan KM, et al. HIV-1 dynamics in children. AIDS 1999; 20:468–473.

538. De Rossi A, Walker AS, Klein N, et al. Increased thymic output after initiation of antiretroviral therapy in human immunodeficiency virus type 1-infected children in the Paediatric European Network for Treatment of AIDS (PENTA) 5 Trial. J Infect Dis 2002; 186:312–320.

539. Lindsey JC, Hughes MD, McKinney RE, et al. Treatment mediated changes in human immunodeficiency virus (HIV) type 1 RNA and CD4 cell counts as predictors of weight growth failure, cognitive decline, and survival in HIV infected children. J Infect Dis 2000; 182:1385–1393.

540. Menson EN, Walker AS, Sharland M, et al. Underdosing of antiretrovirals in UK and Irish children with HIV as an example of problems of prescribing medicines to children, 1997–2005:cohort study. BMJ 2006; 332:1183–1187.

541. Foster C, Mackie N, Seery P, et al. Emerging multi-drug resistance in children with perinatally acquired HIV-1. Eighth International Congress on Drug Therapy in HIV Infection, Glasgow, November 2006 [P360].

542. Paediatric European Network for Treatment of AIDS (PENTA). Five-year follow-up of vertically HIV infected children in a randomised double blind controlled trial of immediate versus deferred zidovudine: the PENTA 1 trial. Arch Dis Child 2001; 84:230–236.

543. Strategies for Management of Antiretroviral Therapy (SMART) Study Group; El-Sadr WM, Lundgren JD, Neaton JD, et al. CD4+ count-guided interruption of antiretroviral treatment. N Engl J Med 2006; 355:2359–2361.

544. Doerholt K, Duong T, Tookey P, et al. Collaborative HIV Paediatric Study. Outcomes for human immunodeficiency virus-1-infected infants in the United Kingdom and Republic of Ireland in the era of effective antiretroviral therapy. Pediatr Infect Dis J 2006; 25:420–426.

545. Luzuriaga K, McManus M, Catalina M, et al. Early therapy of vertical human immunodeficiency virus type-1 (HIV-1) infection: control of viral replication and absence of persistent HIV-1 specific immune responses. J Virol 2000; 74:6984–6991.

546. Aboulker JP, Babiker A, Chaix ML, et al. Highly active antiretroviral therapy started in infants under 3 months of age: 72 week follow-up for CD4 count, viral load and drug resistance outcome. AIDS 2004; 18:237–245.

547. Newell ML, Patel D, Goetghebuer T, et al. European Collaborative Study. CD4 cell response to antiretroviral therapy in children with vertically acquired HIV infection: is it associated with age at initiation? J Infect Dis 2006; 193:954–962.

548. Litalein C, Faye A, Compacnucci A, et al. on behalf of PENTA. Pharmacokinetics of nelfinavir and its active metabolite, hydroxy-tert-butylamide, in infants perinatally infected with HIV-1. Pediatr Infect Dis J 2003; 22:48–55.

549. WHO Antiretroviral therapy of HIV infection in infants and children in resource-limited settings: towards universal access: Recommendations for a public health approach. 7 August 2006. www.who.int/hiv/pub/guidelines.

550. Bergshoeff A, Burger D, Verweij C, et al. PENTA-13 Study Group. Plasma pharmacokinetics of once- versus twice-daily lamivudine and abacavir: simplification of combination treatment in HIV-1-infected children (PENTA-13). Antivir Ther 2005; 10:239–246.

551. LePrevost M, Green H, Flynn J, et al: Pediatric European Network for the Treatment of AIDS 13 Study Group. Adherence and acceptability of once daily Lamivudine and abacavir in human immunodeficiency virus type-1 infected children. Pediatr Infect Dis J 2006; 25:533–537.

552. Bergshoeff A, Burger D, Verweij C, et al, on behalf of the PENTA-13 Study Group. Pharmacokinetics of once versus twice daily lamivudine and abacavir; Simplification of combination treatment in HIV-1 infected children (Penta 13). Antivir Ther 2005; 10:239–246.

553. Reddington C, Cohen J, Baldillo A, et al. Adherence to medication regimens among young children with human immunodeficiency virus infection. Pediatr Infect Dis J 2000; 19:1148–1153.

554. Duong T, McGee L, Sharland M, et al, on behalf of CHIPS. Effects of antiretroviral therapy (ART) on morbidity and mortality of UK and Irish HIV infected children. Arch Dis Child 2002; 86(suppl 1):A69.

555. Martinez J, Bell D, Camacho R, et al. Adherence to antiretroviral drug regimens in HIV-infected adolescent patients engaged in care in a comprehensive adolescent young adult clinic. J Nat Med Assoc 2000; 92:55–61.

556. Cohan D, Feakins C, Wara D et al. Perinatal transmission of multi-drug resistant HIV-1 despite viral suppression on an enfuvirtide based regimen. AIDS 2005; 19:989–990.

557. Giaquinto C, Green H, De Rossi A, et al, on behalf of the PENTA 8 Study Group. A randomised trial of resistance testing versus no resistance testing in children with virological failure: the PERA (PENTA 8) trial. IAS 2005 Abstract no. WeOa0106.

558. European Paediatric Lipodystrophy Group. Antiretroviral therapy, fat redistribution and hyperlipidaemia in HIV-infected children in Europe. AIDS 2004; 18:1443–1451.

559. Beregszaszi M, Dollfus C, Levine M, et al. Longitudinal evaluation and risk factors of lipodystrophy and associated metabolic changes in HIV-infected children. J Acquir Immune Defic Syndr 2005; 40:161–168.

560. Hartman K, Verweel G, de Groot R, et al. Detection of lipoatrophy in human immunodeficiency virus-1-infected children treated with highly active antiretroviral therapy. Pediatr Infect Dis J 2006; 25:427–431.

561. Beregszaszi M, Dollfus C, Levine M et al. Longitudinal evaluation and risk factors of lipodystrophy and associated metabolic changes in HIV-infected children. J Acquir Immune Defic Syndr 2005; 40:161–168.

562. Charakida M, Donald AE, Green H, et al. Early structural and functional changes of the vasculature in HIV-infected children: impact of disease and antiretroviral therapy. Circulation 2005; 112:103–109.

563. Mora S, Zamproni I, Beccio S, et al. Longitudinal changes of bone mineral density and metabolism in antiretroviral-treated human immunodeficiency virus-infected children. J Clin Endocrinol Metab 2004; 89:24–28.

564. Rosso R, Vignolo M, Parodi A, et al. Bone quality in perinatally HIV-infected children: role of age, sex, growth, HIV infection, and antiretroviral therapy. AIDS Res Hum Retroviruses 2005; 21:927–932.

565. Rey C, Prieto S, Medina A, et al. Fatal lactic acidosis during antiretroviral therapy. Pediatr Crit Care Med 2003; 4:485–487.

566. Desai N, Mathur M, Weedon J. Lactate levels in children with HIV/AIDS on highly active antiretroviral therapy. AIDS 2003; 17:1565–1568.

567. Centers for Disease Control and Prevention. Revised guidelines for prophylaxis against Pneumocystis carinii pneumonia for children infected with or perinatally exposed to human immunodeficiency virus. MMWR 1995; 44(RR-4):1–11.

568. Urschel S, Schuster T, Dunsch D, et al. Discontinuation of primary Pneumocystis carinii prophylaxis after reconstitution of CD4 cell counts in HIV-infected children. AIDS 2001; 15:1589–1591.

569. Nachman S, Philimon G, Dankner W, et al. The rate of serious bacterial infections among HIV-infected children with immune reconstitution who have discontinued opportunistic infection prophylaxis. Paediatrics 2005; 115:488–494.

570. Gibb DM, Masters J, Shingadia D, et al. A family clinic – optimising care for HIV infected children and their families. Arch Dis Child 1997; 77:478–482.

Exanthemata

571. Rice AL, Sacco L, Hyder A, et al. Malnutrition as an underlying cause of childhood deaths associated with infectious diseases in developing countries. Bull World Health Organ 2000; 78:1207–1221.

572. Karp CL, Wysocka M, Wahl LM, et al. Mechanism of suppression of cell-mediated immunity by measles virus. Science 1996; 273:228–231.

573. Krugman S, Ward R. Infectious diseases of children. St Louis: Mosby; 1968.

574. Ozanne G, d'Halewyn MA. Performance and reliability of the Enzygnost measles enzyme-linked immuno-sorbent assay for detection of measles virus-specific immunoglobulin M antibody during a large measles epidemic. J Clin Microbiol 1992; 30:564–569.

575. Permar SR, Moss WJ, Ryon JJ, et al. Prolonged measles virus shedding in human immunodeficiency virus-infected children, detected by reverse transcriptase-polymerase chain reaction. J Infect Dis 2001; 183:532–538.

576. Mustafa MM, Weitman SD, Winick NJ, et al. Subacute measles encephalitis in the young immunocompromized host: report of two cases diagnosed by polymerase chain reaction and treated with ribavirin and review of the literature. Clin Infect Dis J 1993; 16:654–660.

*577. Shann F, D'Souza RM, D'Souza R. Antibiotics for preventing pneumonia in children with measles (Cochrane Review). In: The Cochrane Library, 4. Oxford: Update Software; 2001.

578. Noah ND. What can we do about measles? BMJ 1984; 289:1476.

579. Aickin R, Hill D, Kemp A. Measles immunisation in children with allergy to egg. BMJ 1994; 309:223–225.

580. Mulholland EK. Measles in the United States, 2006. N Engl J Med 2006; 355:440–443.

581. Asaria P, MacMahon E. Measles in the United Kingdom: can we eradicate it by 2010? BMJ 2006; 333:890–895.

582. Wildig J, Michon P, Siba P, et al. Parvovirus B19 infection contributes to severe anemia in young children in Papua New Guinea. J Infect Dis 2006; 194:146–153.

583. Smith-Whitley K, Zhao H, Hodinka RL, et al. Epidemiology of human parvovirus B19 in children with sickle cell disease. Blood 2004; 103:422–427.

584. Anand A, Gray ES, Brown T, et al. Human parvovirus infection in pregnancy and hydrops fetalis. N Engl J Med 1987; 316:183–186.

585. Yamanishi K, Okuno T, Shiraki K, et al. Identification of human herpesvirus-6 as a causal agent for exanthem subitum. Lancet 1988; i:1065–1067.

586. Jones CA, Isaacs D. Human herpesvirus-6 infections. Arch Dis Child 1996; 74:98–100.

587. Torigoe S, Kumamoto T, Koide W, et al. Clinical manifestations associated with human herpesvirus 7 infection. Arch Dis Child 1995; 72:518–519.

588. Zerr DM, Meier AS, Selke SS, et al. L. A population-based study of primary human herpesvirus 6 infection. N Engl J Med 2005; 352:768–776.

589. Ward KN, Andrews NJ, Verity CM, et al. Human herpesviruses-6 and -7 each cause significant neurological morbidity in Britain and Ireland. Arch Dis Child 2005; 90:619–623.

Herpesviruses

590. Meyer PA, Seward JF, Jumaan AO, et al. Varicella mortality: trends before vaccine licensure in the United States, 1970–1994. J Infect Dis 2000; 182:383–390.

591. Lopez AS, Guris D, Zimmerman L, et al. One dose of varicella vaccine does not prevent school outbreaks: is it time for a second dose? Pediatrics 2006; 117:1070–1077.

592. Heuchan AM, Isaacs D. The management of varicella-zoster virus exposure and infection in

pregnancy and the newborn period. Australasian Subgroup in Paediatric Infectious Diseases of the Australasian. Med J Aust 2001; 174:288–292.

593. Reynolds L, Struik S, Nadel S. Neonatal varicella: varicella zoster immunoglobulin (VZIG) does not prevent disease. Arch Dis Child Fetal Neonatal Ed 1999; 8:F69–70.

594. Vazquez M, LaRussa PS, Gershon AA, et al. The effectiveness of the varicella vaccine in clinical practice. N Engl J Med 2001; 344:955–960.

*595. Weinberg A, Horslen SP, Kaufman SS, et al. Safety and immunogenicity of varicella-zoster virus vaccine in pediatric liver and intestine transplant recipients. Am J Transplant 2006; 6:565–568.

*596. Levin MJ, Gershon AA, Weinberg A, et al. Administration of live varicella vaccine to HIV-infected children with current or past significant depression of CD4(+) T cells. J Infect Dis 2006; 194:247–255.

597. Asano Y, Yoshikawa T, Suga S, et al. Postexposure prophylaxis of varicella in family contact by oral acyclovir. Pediatrics 1993; 92:219–222.

598. Huang YC, Lin TY, Chiu CH. Acyclovir prophylaxis of varicella after household exposure. Pediatr Infect Dis J 1995; 14:152–154.

599. Goldstein SL, Somers MJ, Lande MB, et al. Acyclovir prophylaxis of varicella in children with renal disease receiving steroids. Pediatr Nephrol 2000; 14:305–308.

600. Ogilvie MM. Antiviral prophylaxis and treatment in chickenpox. A review prepared for the UK Advisory Group on chickenpox on behalf of the British Society for the Study of Infection. J Infect Dis 1998; 36(suppl 1):31–38.

601. Watson B, Seward J, Yang A, et al. Postexposure effectiveness of varicella vaccine. Pediatrics 2000; 105:84–88.

*602. Oxman MN, Levin MJ, Johnson GR, et al. A vaccine to prevent herpes zoster and postherpetic neuralgia in older adults. N Engl J Med 2005; 352:2271–2284.

603. Lafferty WE, Coombs RW, Benedetti J, et al. Recurrences after oral and genital herpes simplex virus infection. Influence of site of infection and viral type. N Engl J Med 1987; 316:1444–1449.

604. Thomas J, Rouse BT. Immunopathogenesis of herpetic ocular disease. Immunol Res 1997; 16:375–386.

605. Casrouge A, Zhang SY, Eidenschenk C, et al. Herpes simplex virus encephalitis in human UNC-93B deficiency. Science 2006; 314:308–312.

606. Schwartz GS, Holland EJ. Oral acyclovir for the management of herpes simplex virus keratitis in children. Ophthalmology 2000; 107:278–282.

607. Kovacs A, Schluchter M, Easley K, et al. Cytomegalovirus infection and HIV-1 disease progression in infants born to HIV-1-infected women. Pediatric Pulmonary and Cardiovascular Complications of Vertically Transmitted HIV Infection Study Group. N Engl J Med 1999; 341:77–84.

608. Sia IG, Wilson JA, Groettum CM, et al. Cytomegalovirus (CMV) DNA load predicts relapsing CMV infection after solid organ transplantation. J Infect Dis 2000; 181:717–720.

609. Meyers JD. Management of cytomegalovirus infection. Am J Med 1988; 85(suppl 2A):102–106.

*610. Hodson EM, Jones CA, Webster AC, et al. Antiviral medications to prevent cytomegalovirus disease and early death in recipients of solid-organ transplants: a systematic review of randomised controlled trials. Lancet 2005; 365:2105–2115.

611. Pondarre C, Kebaili K, Dijoud F, et al. Epstein-Barr virus-related lymphoproliferative disease complicating childhood acute lymphoblastic leukemia: no recurrence after unrelated donor bone marrow transplantation. Bone Marrow Transplant 2001; 27:93–95.

Viral and Allied Infections of the Respiratory Tract

612. World Health Organization. Memorandum: a revision of the system of nomenclature for influenza viruses. Bull World Health Organ 1980; 58:585–591.

613. Beigel JH, Farrar J, Han AM, et al. Avian influenza A (H5N1) infection in humans. N Engl J Med 2005; 353:1374–1385.

614. Lancet Editorial. Reinfection with influenza. Lancet 1986; i:1017–1018.

615. Poehling KA, Edwards KM, Weinberg GA, et al. The underrecognized burden of influenza in young children. N Engl J Med 2006; 355:31–40.

616. Keren R, Zaoutis TE, Bridges CB, et al. Neurological and neuromuscular disease as a risk factor for respiratory failure in children hospitalized with influenza infection. JAMA 2005; 294:2188–2194.

*617. Hayden FG, Treanor JJ, Fritz RS, et al. Use of the oral neuraminidase inhibitor oseltamivir in experimental human influenza: randomized controlled trials for prevention and treatment. JAMA 1999; 282:1240–1246.

*618. Lalezari J, Campion K, Keene O, et al. Zanamivir for the treatment of influenza A and B infection in high-risk patients: a pooled analysis of randomized controlled trials. Arch Int Med 2001; 161:212–217.

*619. Advisory Committee on Immunization Practices. Prevention and control of influenza: recommendations of the Advisory Committee on Immunization Practices (ACIP). MMWR Recomm Rep 2006; 55(RR-10):1–42.

*620. Madhi SA, Cutland C, Zhu Y, et al. Transmissibility, infectivity and immunogenicity of a live human parainfluenza type 3 virus vaccine (HPIV 3cp45) among susceptible infants and toddlers. Vaccine 2006; 24:2432–2439.

621. Broughton S, Bhat R, Roberts A, et al. Diminished lung function, RSV infection, and respiratory morbidity in prematurely born infants. Arch Dis Child 2006; 91:26–30.

622. DeVincenzo JP, El Saleeby CM, Bush AJ. Respiratory syncytial virus load predicts disease severity in previously healthy infants. J Infect Dis 2005; 191:1861–1868.

623. Tal G, Mandelberg A, Dalal I, et al. Association between common Toll-like receptor 4 mutations and severe respiratory syncytial virus disease. J Infect Dis 2004; 189:2057–2063.

624. MacDonald NE, Hall CB, Suffin SC, et al. Respiratory syncytial virus infection in infants with congenital heart disease. N Engl J Med 1982; 307:397–400.

625. Hall CB, Powell KR, McDonald NE, et al. Respiratory syncytial virus infection in children with compromised immune function. N Engl J Med 1986; 315:77–80.

626. Isaacs D, Moxon ER, Harvey D, et al. Ribavirin in respiratory syncytial virus infection. Arch Dis Child 1988; 63:986–990.

*627. The PREVENT Study Group. Reduction of respiratory syncytial virus hospitalization among premature infants and infants with bronchopulmonary dysplasia using respiratory syncytial virus immune globulin prophylaxis. Pediatrics 1997; 99:93–99.

628. The IMpact-RSV Study Group. Palivizumab, a humanized respiratory syncytial virus monoclonal antibody, reduces hospitalization from respiratory syncytial virus infection in high-risk infants. Pediatrics 1998; 102:531–537.

*629. Wang EEL, Tang NK. Immunoglobulin for preventing respiratory syncytial virus infection (Cochrane Review). In: The Cochrane Library, 3. Oxford: Update Software; 2001.

630. Thomas M, Bedford-Russell A, Sharland M. Hospitalisation for RSV infection in ex-preterm infants – implications for use of RSV immune globulin. Arch Dis Child 2000; 83:122–127.

631. van den Hoogen BG, de Jong JC, Groen J, et al. A newly discovered human pneumovirus isolated from young children with respiratory tract disease. Nat Med 2001; 7:719–724.

632. van den Hoogen BG, van Doornum GJ, Fockens JC, et al. Prevalence and clinical symptoms of human metapneumovirus infection in hospitalized patients. J Infect Dis 2003; 188:1571–1577.

633. Williams JV, Harris PA, Tollefson SJ, et al. Human metapneumovirus and lower respiratory tract disease in otherwise healthy infants and children. N Engl J Med 2004; 350:443–450.

634. Sloots TP, Mackay IM, Bialasiewicz S, et al. Human metapneumovirus, Australia, 2001–2004. Emerg Infect Dis 2006; 12:1263–1266.

635. Klein MI, Coviello S, Bauer G, et al. The impact of infection with human metapneumovirus and other respiratory viruses in young infants and children at high risk for severe pulmonary disease. J Infect Dis 2006; 193:1544–1551.

636. Debiaggi M, Canducci F, Sampaolo M, et al. Persistent symptomless human metapneumovirus infection in hematopoietic stem cell transplant recipients. J Infect Dis 2006; 194:474–478.

637. Madhi SA, Ludewick H, Kuwanda L, et al. Pneumococcal coinfection with human metapneumovirus. J Infect Dis 2006; 193:1236–1243.

638. Pham TT, Burchette JLJr, Hale LP. Fatal disseminated adenovirus infections in immunocompromized patients. Am J Clin Pathol 2003; 120:575–583.

639. Peled N, Nakar C, Huberman H, et al. Adenovirus infection in hospitalized immuno-competent children. Clin Pediatr (Phila) 2004; 43:223–229.

640. Brandt CD, Kim HW, Rodriguez WJ, et al. Adenoviruses and pediatric gastroenteritis. J Infect Dis 1985; 151:437–443.

641. Legrand F, Berrebi D, Houhou N, et al. Early diagnosis of adenovirus infection and treatment with cidofovir after bone marrow transplantation in children. Bone Marrow Transplant 2001; 27:621–626.

642. Bloom S, Wharton M. Mumps outbreak among young adults in UK. BMJ 2005; 331:E363–E364.

643. Lemanske RF Jr, Jackson DJ, Gangnon RE, et al. Rhinovirus illnesses during infancy predict subsequent childhood wheezing. J Allergy Clin Immunol 2005; 116:571–577.

644. McIntosh K. Coronavirus. In: Mandell GL, Bennett JE, Dolin R, eds. Principles and practice of infectious diseases. New York: John Wiley; 1995.

645. Isaacs D, Flowers D, Clarke JR, et al. Epidemiology of coronavirus respiratory infections. Arch Dis Child 1983; 58:500–503.

646. WHO. Severe acute respiratory syndrome (SARS). Wkly Epidemiol Rec 2003; 78:81–83.

647. WHO. Severe acute respiratory syndrome (SARS). Wkly Epidemiol Rec 2003; 78:86.

648. Peiris JSM, Lai ST, Poon LLM, et al. Coronavirus as a possible cause of severe acute respiratory distress. Lancet 2003; 362:1–8.

649. Kuiken T, Fouchier RA, Schutten M, et al. Newly discovered coronavirus as the primary cause of severe acute respiratory syndrome. Lancet 2003; 362:263–270.

650. Tai JH, Williams JV, Edwards KM, et al. Prevalence of reovirus-specific antibodies in young children in Nashville, Tennessee. J Infect Dis 2005; 191:1221–1224.

651. Corsaro D, Valassina M, Venditti D. Increasing diversity within Chlamydiae. Crit Rev Microbiol 2003; 29:37–78.

652. Bas S, Muzzin P, Ninet B, et al. Chlamydial serology: comparative diagnostic value of immunoblotting, microimmunofluorescence test, and immunoassays using different recombinant proteins as antigens. J Clin Microbiol 2001; 39:1368–1377.

653. Hammerschlag MR. Chlamydia trachomatis and Chlamydia pneumoniae infections in children and adolescents. Pediatr Rev 2004; 25:43–51.

Viral Infections of the CNS

654. Biggar RJ, Woodall JP, Walter PD, et al. Lymphocytic choriomeningitis outbreak associated with pet hamsters. Fifty-seven cases from New York State. JAMA 1975; 232:494–500.

655. Fishbein DB, Robinson LE. Rabies. N Engl J Med 1993; 329:1632–1638.

656. Bahmanyar M, Fayaz A, Nour-Salehi S, et al. Successful protection of humans exposed to rabies infection: postexposure treatment with the new diploid cell rabies vaccine and antirabies serum. JAMA 1976; 236:2751–2754.

657. Pruisner S. Novel proteinaceous infectious particles cause scrapie. Science 1982; 216:134–144.

658. Whitley RJ, MacDonald N, Asher DM. American Academy of Pediatrics. Technical report: transmissible spongiform encephalopathies: a review for pediatricians. Committee on Infectious Disease. Pediatrics 2000; 106:1160–1165.

659. Will RG, Ironside JW, Zeidler M, et al. A new variant of Creutzfeldt–Jakob disease in the UK. Lancet 1996; 347:921–925.

660. Hill AF, Desbruslais M, Joiner S, et al. The same prion strain causes vCJD and BSE. Nature 1997; 389:448–450, 526.

661. Scott MR, Will R, Ironside J, et al. Compelling transgenetic evidence for transmission of bovine spongiform encephalopathy prions to humans. Proc Natl Acad Sci USA 1999; 96:1537–1542.

662. Cousens S, Smith PG, Ward H, et al. Geographical distribution of variant Creutzfeldt–Jakob disease in Great Britain, 1994–2000. Lancet 2001; 357:1002–1007.

663. Centers for Disease Control and Prevention (CDC). Update on vaccine-derived polioviruses. MMWR Morb Mortal Wkly Rep 2006; 55:1093–1097.

664. Halsey NA, Abramson JS, Chesney PJ, et al. Poliomyelitis prevention: revised recommendations for use of inactivated and live oral poliovirus vaccines. American Academy of Pediatrics Committee on Infectious Diseases. Pediatrics 1999; 103:171–172.

665. Burgess M, McIntyre PB. Vaccine-associated paralytic poliomyelitis. Commun Dis Intel 1999; 23:80–81.

666. Rotbart HA, Webster AD. Treatment of potentially life-threatening enterovirus infections with pleconaril. Clin Infect Dis J 2001; 32:228–235.

Viruses and the Gastrointestinal Tract

667. Isaacs D, Day D, Crook S. Child gastroenteritis: a population study. BMJ 1986; 293:545–546.

668. Morbidity and Mortality Weekly Report. Intussusception among recipients of rotavirus vaccine – United States, 1998–1999. Morbid Mortal Wkly Rep 1999; 48:577–581.

669. Bines JE, Liem NT, Justice FA, et al. Risk factors for intussusception in Vietnam and Australia: adenovirus implicated, but not rotavirus. J Pediatr 2006; 149:452–460.

670. Storch GA. Diagnostic virology. Clin Infect Dis J 2000; 31:739–751.

Viral Infection of the Liver

671. Goilav C, Zuckerman J, Lafrenz M, et al. Immunogenicity and safety of a new inactivated hepatitis A vaccine in a comparative study. J Med Virol 1995; 46:287–292.

672. Boxall EH, Sira J, Standish RA, et al. Natural history of hepatitis B in perinatally infected carriers. Arch Dis Child Fetal Neonatal Ed 2004; 89:F456–F460.

673. Wen WH, Chang MH, Hsu HY, et al. The development of hepatocellular carcinoma among prospectively followed children with chronic hepatitis B virus infection. J Pediatr 2004; 144:397–399.

674. Marx G, Martin SR, Chicoine JF, et al. Long-term follow-up of chronic hepatitis B virus infection in children of different ethnic origins. J Infect Dis 2002; 186:295–301.

*675. Lee C, Gong Y, Brok J, et al. Effect of hepatitis B immunisation in newborn infants of mothers positive for hepatitis B surface antigen: systematic review and meta-analysis. BMJ 2006; 332:328–336.

676. Papatheodoridis GV, Hadziyannis SJ. Diagnosis and management of pre-core mutant chronic hepatitis B. J Viral Hepatol 2001; 8:311–321.

677. Lau GK, Piratvisuth T, Luo KX, et al. Peginterferon Alfa-2a, lamivudine, and the combination for HBeAg-positive chronic hepatitis B. N Engl J Med 2005; 352:2682–2695.

678. Kazim SN, Wakil SM, Khan LA, et al. Vertical transmission of hepatitis B virus despite maternal lamivudine therapy. Lancet 2002; 359:1488–1489.

679. Hartman C, Berkowitz D, Eshach-Adiv O, et al. Long-term lamivudine therapy for chronic hepatitis B infection in children unresponsive to interferon. J Pediatr Gastroenterol Nutr 2006; 43:494–498.

680. Resti M, Azzari C, Mannelli F, et al. Mother to child transmission of hepatitis C virus: prospective study of risk factors and timing of infection in children born to women seronegative for HIV-1. Tuscany Study Group on Hepatitis C Virus Infection. BMJ 1998; 317:437–441.

681. Mast EE, Hwang LY, Seto DS, et al. Risk factors for perinatal transmission of hepatitis C virus (HCV) and the natural history of HCV infection acquired in infancy. J Infect Dis 2005; 192:1880–1889.

682. European Paediatric Hepatitis C Virus Network. A significant sex – but not elective cesarean section – effect on mother-to-child transmission of hepatitis C virus infection. J Infect Dis 2005; 192:1872–1879.

683. Ogasawara S, Kage M, Kosai K, et al. Hepatitis C virus RNA in saliva and breastmilk of hepatitis C carrier mothers. Lancet 1993; 341:561.

684. Jones CA. Maternal transmission of infectious pathogens in breast milk. J Paediatr Child Health 2001; 37:576–582.

685. Dunn D, Gibb DM, Healy M, et al. Timing and interpretation of tests for diagnosing perinatally acquired hepatitis C virus infection. Pediatr Infect Dis J 2001; 20:716–717.

686. England K, Pembrey L, Tovo PA, et al, European Paediatric Hcv Network. Growth in the first 5 years of life is unaffected in children with perinatally-acquired hepatitis C infection. J Pediatr 2005; 147:227–232.

687. Bortolotti F, Resti M, Marcellini M, et al. Hepatitis C virus (HCV) genotypes in 373 Italian children with HCV infection: changing distribution and correlation with clinical features and outcome. Gut 2005; 54:852–857.

688. Jhaveri R, Grant W, Kauf TL, et al. The burden of hepatitis C virus infection in children: estimated direct medical costs over a 10-year period. J Pediatr 2006; 148:353–358.

689. Jonas MM. Treatment of chronic hepatitis C in pediatric patients. Clin Liver Dis 1999; 3:855–867.

690. Hardikar W, Moaven LD, Bowden DS, et al. Hepatitis G: viroprevalence and seroconversion in a high-risk group of children. Viral Hepat 1999; 6:337–341.

Miscellaneous Viral Infections

691. Nishizawa T, Okamoto H, Konishi K, et al. A novel DNA virus (TTV) associated with elevated transaminase levels in posttransfusion hepatitis of unknown etiology. Biochem Biophys Res Commun 1997; 241:92–97.

692. Gerner P, Oettinger R, Gerner W, et al. Mother-to-infant transmission of TT virus: prevalence, extent and mechanism of vertical transmission. Pediatr Infect Dis J 2000; 19:1074–1077.

693. Mostashari F, Bunning ML, Kitsutani PT, et al. Epidemic West Nile encephalitis, New York, 1999: results of a household-based seroepidemiological survey. Lancet 2001; 358:261–264.

694. Monath TP. Yellow fever. In: Warren KA, Mahmoud AA, eds. Tropical and geographical medicine. New York: McGraw Hill; 1984.

695. World Health Organization. Haemorrhagic fever with renal syndrome. Bull World Health Organ 1983; 61:269–275.

Protozoal Infections: Amebic Infections

696. Stanley SL Jr. Amoebiasis. Lancet 2003; 361:1025–1034.

697. Haque R, Huston CD, Hughes M, et al. Amebiasis. N Engl J Med 2003; 348:1565–1573.

698. Stauffer W, Ravdin JI. Entamoeba histolytica. Curr Opin Infect Dis 2003; 16:479–485.

699. Hanna RM, Dahniya MH, Badr SS, et al. Percutaneous catheter drainage in drug-resistant amoebic liver abscess. Trop Med Int Health 2000; 5:578–581.

700. Ma P, Visvesvara GS, Martinez AJ, et al. Naegleria and Acanthamoeba infections: review. Rev Infect Dis 1990; 12:490–513.

701. Singhal T, Bajpai A, Kabra V, et al. Successful treatment of Acanthamoeba meningitis with combination oral antimicrobials. Pediatr Infect Dis J 2001; 20:623–627.

702. Kumar R, Lloyd D. Recent advances in the treatment of Acanthamoeba keratitis. Clin Infect Dis 2002; 35:434–439.

Cryptosporidiosis

703. Nime FA, Burek JD, Page DA, et al. Acute enterocolitis in a human being infected with the protozoon Cryptosporidium. Gastroenterology 1976; 70:592–593.

704. Meisel JC, Perera DA, Meligro C, et al. Overwhelming watery diarrhea associated with Cryptosporidium in an immunosuppressed patient. Gastroenterology 1976; 70:1156–1160.

705. Hart CA. Cryptosporidiosis. In: Gilles HM, ed. Protozoal disease. London: Arnold; 1999: 592–606.

706. Xaio L, Ryan UM. Cryptosporidiosis an update in molecular epidemiology. Curr Opin Infect Dis 2004; 17:483–490.

707. Baxby D, Hart CA, Taylor CJ. Human Cryptosporidiosis: a possible case of hospital cross-infection. Br Med J 1983; 287:1760–1761.

708. Rosales MJ, Cordon GP, Moreno MS, et al. Extracellular gregarine-like stages of Cryptosporidium parvum. Acta Trop 2005; 95:74–78.

709. Xu P, Widmer G, Wang Y, et al. The genome of Cryptosporidium hominis. Nature 2004; 431:1107–1112.

710. Current WL, Garcia LS. Cryptosporidiosis. Clin Microbiol Rev 1991; 4:325–358.

711. Mackenzie WR, Hoxie NJ, Proctor ME, et al. A massive outbreak in Milwaukee of cryptosporidium infection transmitted through public water supply. N Engl J Med 1997; 331:161–167.

712. Gatei W, Wamae CN, Mbae C, et al. Cryptosporidiosis: prevalence, genotype analysis and symptoms associated with infection in children in Kenya. Am J Trop Med Hyg 2006; 75:78–82.

713. Tumwine JK, Kekitiinwa A, Bakeera-Kitaka S, et al. Cryptosporidiosis and microsporidiosis in Uganda children with persistent diarrhea with and without concurrent infection with human immunodeficiency virus. Am J Trop Med Hyg 2005; 73:921–925.

714. Gatei W, Greensill J, Ashford RW, et al. Molecular analysis of the 18S rRNA gene of Cryptosporidium parasites from patients with or without human immunodeficiency virus living in Kenya, Malawi, Brazil and the United Kingdom. J Clin Microbiol 2003; 41:1458–1462.

715. Gatei W, Ashford RW, Beeching NJ, et al. Cryptosporidium muris infection in an HIV-infected adult. Emerg Infect Dis 2002; 8:204–206.

716. Ungar BLP. Cryptosporidiosis in humans (Homo sapiens). In: Dubey JP, Speer CA, Fayer R, eds. Cryptosporidiosis of man and animals. Boca Raton, USA: CRC Press; 1990:59–82.

717. Sallon S, El Showaa R, El Masri M, et al. Cryptosporidiosis in children in Gaza. Ann Trop Paed 1991; 11:277–281.

718. Hojlyng N, Holten-Anderson W, Jepson S. Cryptosporidiosis: a case of airborne transmission. Lancet 1987; 2:271–272.

719. Lahdevirta J, Jokipii AMM, Sammalkoysi K, et al. Perinatal infection with Cryptosporidium and failure to thrive. Lancet 1987; 1:48–49.

720. Jokipii L, Jokipii AMM. Timing of symptoms and oocysts excretion in human cryptosporidiosis. N Engl J Med 1986; 315:1643–1647.

721. Chen XM, Keithly JS, Pava CV, et al. Cryptosporidiosis. N Engl J Med 2002; 346:1723–1731.

722. Baxby D, Hart CA. The incidence of cryptosporidiosis: a two year prospective study in a children's hospital. J Hyg 1985; 96:107–111.

723. Hart CA, Baxby D, Blundell N. Gastroenteritis due to Cryptosporidium: a prospective survey in a children's hospital. J Infect 1984; 9:264–270.

724. Baxby D, Hart CA, Blundell N. Shedding of oocyst by immunocompetent individuals with cryptosporidiosis. J Hyg 1985; 95:705–709.

725. MacFarlane DE, Homer-Bryce J. Cryptosporidiosis in well nourished and malnourished children. Acta Paediatr Scand 1987; 76:474–477.

726. Leav BA, Mackay M, Ward HD. Cryptsporidium species: New insights and old challenges. Clin Infect Dis 2003; 36:903–908.

727. Rossignol JF, Kabil SM, el-Gohary Y et al. Effect of nitozoxanide in diarrhea and enteritis caused by Cryptosporidium species. Clin Gastroenterol Hepatol 2006; 4:320–324.

728. Molbak K, Hojlyng N, Ingholt L, et al. Cryptosporidiosis in infancy and childhood mortality in Guinea Bissau. Br Med J 1993; 307:417–420.

Giardiasis

729. Thompson RCA, Hopkins RM, Homan WL. Nomenclature and genetic groupings of Giardia infecting mammals. Parasitol Today 2000; 16:210–213.

730. Adam RD. Biology of Giardia lamblia. Clin Microbiol Rev 2001; 14:447–475.

731. World Health Organization (WHO). The World Health Report: Fighting disease, fostering development. Geneva: WHO; 1996.

732. Warburton ARE, Jones PH, Bruce J. Zoonotic transmission of giardiasis: a case control study. Commun Dis Rep 1994; 4:R33–R36.

733. Homan WL, Monk TG. Human giardiasis: genotype linked differences in clinical symptomatology. Int J Parasitol 2001; 31:822–826.

734. Farthing MJG. Giardiasis. In: Gilles HM, ed. Protozoal diseases. London: Arnold; 1999:562–584.

735. Eichinger D. Encystation in parasitic protozoa. Curr Opin Microbiol 2001; 4:421–426.

736. Weiland MEL, McArthur AG, Morrison HG, et al. Annexin-like alphas giardins: a new cytoskeletal gene family in Giardia lamblia. Int J Parasitol 2005; 35:617–626.

737. Aziz H, Beck CE, Lux MF, et al. A comparison study of different methods used in the detection of Giardia lamblia. Clin Lab Sci 2001; 14:150–154.

738. Sharp SE, Suarez CA, Duncan Y, et al. Evaluation of the Triage Micro Parasite Panel for detection of Giardia lamblia, Entamoeba histolytica/Entamoeba dispar and Cryptosporidium parvum in patient stool samples. J Clin Microbiol 2001; 39:332–334.

*739. Zaat JO, Monk T, Assendelft WJ. Drugs for treating giardiasis (Cochrane Review). In: The Cochrane Library, 2. Oxford: Update Software; 2000.

740. Olson ME, Ceri H, Morck DW. Giardia vaccination. Parasitol Today 2000; 16:213–217.

Leishmaniasis

741. Lainson R, Shaw JJ. The role of animals in the epidemiology of South American leishmaniasis. In:

Lumsden WHR, Evans DA, eds. The biology of the Kinetoplastida. London: Academic Press; 1979: vol 2:1–116.

742. Lainson R, Shaw JJ. Evolution classification and geographical distribution. In: Peters W, Killick-Kendrick R, eds. The leishmaniases in biology and medicine, biology and epidemiology. London: Academic Press; 1987: vol 1:1–20.

743. Chance ML. The biochemical and immunological taxonomy of leishmania. In: Chang KP, Bray RS, eds. Human parasitic diseases, vol 1. Leishmaniasis. Amsterdam: Elsevier; 1985:93–110.

744. Berman JD. Human leishmaniasis: clinical, diagnostic, and chemotherapeutic developments in the last 10 years. Clin Infect Dis 1997; 24:684–703.

745. Herwaldt BL. Leishmaniasis. Lancet 1999; 354:1191–1199.

746. Aronson NE, Wortmann GW, Johnson SC, et al. Safety and efficacy of intravenous sodium stibogluconate in the treatment of leishmaniasis: recent U.S. military experience. Clin Infect Dis 1998; 27:1457–1464.

747. Maltezou HC, Siafas C, Mavrikou M, et al. Visceral leishmaniasis during childhood in southern Greece. Clin Infect Dis 2000; 31:1139–1143.

748. Cascio A, di Martino L, Occorsio P, et al. A 6 day course of liposomal amphotericin B in the treatment of infantile visceral leishmaniasis: the Italian experience. J Antimicrob Chemother 2004; 54:217–220.

749. Sundar S, Jha TK, Sindermann H, et al. Oral miltefosine treatment in children with mild to moderate Indian visceral leishmaniasis. Pediatr Infect Dis J 2003; 22:434–438.

750. Bhattacharya SK, Jha TK, Sundar S, et al. Efficacy and tolerability of miltefosine for childhood visceral leishmaniasis in India. Clin Infect Dis 2004; 38:217–221.

751. Murray HW, Berman JD, Davies CR, et al. Advances in leishmaniasis. Lancet 2005; 366:1561–1577.

752. Uzun S, Uslular C, Yucel A, et al. Cutaneous leishmaniasis: evaluation of 3,074 cases in the Cukurova region of Turkey. Br J Dermatol 1999; 140:347–350.

753. Soto J, Toledo J, Gutierrez P, et al. Treatment of American cutaneous leishmaniasis with miltefosine, an oral agent. Clin Infect Dis 2001; 33:57–61.

754. Palacios R, Osorio LE, Grajalew LF, et al. Treatment failure in children in a randomized clinical trial with 10 and 20 days of meglumine antimonate for cutaneous leishmaniasis due to Leishmania viannia species. Am J Trop Med Hyg 2001; 64:187–193.

755. Bern C, Joshi AB, Jha SN, et al. Factors associated with visceral leishmaniasis in Nepal: bednet use is strongly protective. Am J Trop Med Hyg 2000; 63:184–188.

Malaria

756. Garnham PCC. Malaria parasites of man: life cycles and morphology (excluding ultrastructure). In: Wernsdorfer WH, McGregor IA, eds. Malaria. The principles and practice of malariology, vol 1. Edinburgh: Churchill Livingstone; 1988:61–96.

757. Breman JG. The ears of the hippopotamus: manifestations, determinants and estimates of the malaria burden. Am J Trop Med Hyg 2001; 64:1–11.

758. Snow RW, Guerra CA, Noor AM, et al. The global distribution of clinical episodes of Plasmodium falciparum malaria. Nature 2005; 434:214–217.

759. Snow RW, Craig M, Deichmann U, et al. Estimating mortality, morbidity and disability due to malaria among Africa's non-pregnant population. Bull World Health Organ 1999; 77:624–640.

760. Trape JF. The public health impact of chloroquine resistance in Africa. Am J Trop Med Hyg 2001; 64(1–2 Suppl):12–17.

761. Molineaux L. The epidemiology of human malaria as an explanation of its distribution, including some implications for its control. In: Wernsdorfer WH, McGregor IA, eds. Malaria. The principles and practice of malariology, vol. II. Edinburgh: Churchill Livingstone; 1988:913–998.

762. Miller LH. Genetically determined human resistance factors. In: Wernsdorfer WH, McGregor IA, eds. Malaria. The principles and practice of malariology. Vol. I. Edinburgh: Churchill Livingstone; 1988:487–500.

763. McGregor IA, Wilson RJM. Specific immunity acquired in man. In: Wernsdorfer WH, McGregor IA, eds. Malaria. The principles and practice of malariology. Vol. I. Edinburgh: Churchill Livingstone; 1988:559–619.

764. Allison AC. The role of cell-mediated immune responses in protection against plasmodia and in the pathogenesis of malaria. In: Wernsdorfer WH, McGregor IA, eds. Malaria. The principles and practice of malariology. Vol. I. Edinburgh: Churchill Livingstone; 1988: 501–513.

765. Weatherall DJ. The anaemia of malaria. In: Wernsdorfer WH, McGregor IA, eds. Malaria. The principles and practice of malariology. Vol. I. Edinburgh: Churchill Livingstone; 1988:735–751.

766. Boonpucknavig V, Boonpucknavig S. The histopathology of malaria. In: Wernsdorfer WH, McGregor IA, eds. Malaria. The principles and practice of malariology. Vol. I. Edinburgh: Churchill Livingstone; 1988:673–734.

767. Berendt AR, Ferguson DJP, Gardner J, et al. Molecular mechanisms of sequestration in malaria. Parasitology 1994; 108 (suppl):S19–S28.

*768. Baruch DI, Pasloske BL, Singh HB, et al. Cloning the P. falciparum gene encoding PfEMP-1, a malarial variant antigen and adherence receptor on the surface of parasitised human erythrocytes. Cell 1995; 82:77–87.

*769. Pain A, Ferguson DJP, Kai O, et al. Platelet-mediated clumping of P. falciparum-infected erythrocytes is a common adhesive phenotype and is associated with severe malaria. Proc Natl Acad Sci USA 2001; 98:1805–1810.

770. Clark IA. Monokines and lymphokines in malarial pathology. Ann Trop Med Parasitol 1987; 81:577–585.

771. Grau GE, Mackenzie CD, Carr RA, et al. Platelet accumulation in brain microvessels in fatal paediatric cerebral malaria. J Infect Dis 2003; 187:461–466.

*772. Molyneux ME, Taylor TE, Wirima JJ, et al. Clinical features and prognostic indicators in pediatric cerebral malaria: a study of 131 comatose Malawian children. Q J Med 1989; 71:441–459.

773. Taylor TE, Fu WN, Carr RA, et al. Differentiating the pathologies of cerebral malaria by post mortem parasite counts. Nat Med 2004; 10:143–145.

*774. Croft A. Malaria: prevention in travellers. Clinical evidence issue 5. BMJ 2001; 505–519.

775. Kublin JG, Patnaik P, Jere CJ, et al. Effect of Plasmodium falciparum malaria on HIV-1 RNA blood concentration in a cohort of adults in rural Malawi. Lancet 2005; 365:233–240.

776. Chintu C, Bhat GJ, Walker AS, et al; CHAP trial team. Co-trimoxazole as prophylaxis against opportunistic infections in HIV-infected Zambian children (CHAP): a double-blind randomised placebo-controlled trial. Lancet 2004; 364:1865–1871.

777. Alonso PL, Sacarlal J, Aponte JJ, et al. Efficacy of the RTS,S/AS02A vaccine against Plasmodium falciparum infection and disease in young African children: randomised controlled trial. Lancet 2004; 364:1411–1420.

778. Alonso PL, Sacarlal J, Aponte JJ, et al. Duration of protection with RTS,S/AS02A malaria vaccine in prevention of Plasmodium falciparum disease in Mozambican children: single-blind extended follow-up of a randomised controlled trial. Lancet 2005; 366:2012–2018.

779. Quinn TC, Jacobs RF, Mertz GJ, et al. Congenital malaria: a report of four cases and a review. J Pediatr 1982; 101:229–232.

*780. Marsh K, Foster D, Waruiru C, et al. Indicators of life-threatening malaria in African children. N Engl J Med 1995; 332:1399–1404.

781. Planche T, Krishna S. Severe malaria: metabolic complications. Curr Mol Med 2006; 6:141–153.

*782. Taylor TE, Molyneux ME, Wirima JJ, et al. Blood glucose levels in Malawian children before and during the administration of intravenous quinine for severe falciparum malaria. N Engl J Med 1988; 319:1040–1047.

*783. Lewallen S, Bakker H, Taylor TE, et al. Retinal findings predictive of outcome in cerebral malaria. Trans R Soc Trop Med Hyg 1996; 90:144–146.

784. Lewallen S, Harding SP, Ajewole J, et al. A review of the spectrum of clinical ocular fundus findings in P. falciparum malaria in African children with a proposed classification and grading system. Trans R Soc Trop Med Hyg 1999; 93:619–622.

785. Beare NA, Southern C, Chalira C, et al. Prognostic significance and course of retinopathy in children with severe malaria. Arch Ophthalmol 2004; 122:1141–1147.

*786. Newton CRJC, Crawley J, Sowumni A, et al. Intracranial hypertension in Africans with cerebral malaria. Arch Dis Child 1997; 76:219–226.

*787. Waller D, Krishna S, Crawley J, et al. Clinical features and outcome of severe malaria in Gambian children. Clin Infect Dis 1995; 21:577–587.

788. White NJ, Miller KD, Marsh K, et al. Hypoglycaemia in African children with severe malaria. Lancet 1987; 1:708–711.

*789. Newton CRJC, Peshu N, Kendall B, et al. Brain swelling and ischaemia in Kenyans with cerebral malaria. Arch Dis Child 1994; 70:281–287.

790. Kihara M, Carter JA, Newton CR. The effect of Plasmodium falciparum on cognition: a systematic review. Trop Med Internat Health 2006; 11:386–397.

791. Casals-Pascual C, Roberts DJ. Severe malarial anaemia. Curr Mol Med 2006; 6:155–168.

*792. English M, Sauerwein R, Waruiru C, et al. Acidosis in severe childhood malaria. Q J Med 1997; 90:263–270.

793. Bates I. Splenomegaly in the tropics. In: Gill G, Beeching N, eds. Tropical medicine, 5th edn. Oxford: Blackwell Science; 2004.

*794. Berkley J, Mwarumba S, Bramham K, et al. Bacteraemia complicating severe malaria in children. Trans R Soc Trop Med Hyg 1999; 93:283–286.

795. World Health Organization. Guidelines for the treatment of malaria. Geneva: WHO/HTM/MAL; 2006.

*796. Meremikwu M, Logan K, Garner P. Antipyretic measures for treating fever in malaria (Cochrane Review). In: The Cochrane Library, 4. Oxford: Update Software; 2001.

*797. Lackritz EM, Campbell CC, Ruebush TKII, et al. Effect of blood transfusion on survival among children in a Kenya hospital. Lancet 1992; 340:524–528.

798. Maitland K, Pamba A, English M, et al. Randomised trial of volume expansion with albumin or saline in children with severe malaria: preliminary evidence of albumin benefit. Clin Infect Dis 2005; 40:538–545.

799. World Health Organization. Severe and complicated malaria. Report of an informal technical meeting in Geneva, 1985. Trans R Soc Trop Med Hyg 1986; 80(suppl):1–50.

800. Dondorp A, Nosten F, Stepniewska K, et al. Artesunate versus quinine for treatment of severe falciparum malaria: a randomised trial. Lancet 2005; 366:717–725.

801. Carrara VI, Sirilak S, Thonglairuam J, et al. Deployment of early diagnosis and mefloquine-artesunate treatment of falciparum malaria in Thailand: the Tak Malaria Initiative. PLoS Medicine 2006; 3:e183.

802. Marsh VM, Mutemi WM, Willetts A. Improving malaria home treatment by training drug retailers in rural Kenya. Trop Med Internat Health 2004; 9:451–460.

803. Barnes KI, Mwenechanya J, Tembo M, et al. Efficacy of artesunate administered by suppository in the initial treatment of moderately severe malaria in African children and adults. Lancet 2004; 363:1598–1605.

*804. Lengeler C. Insecticide-treated bednets and curtains for preventing malaria (Cochrane Review). In: The Cochrane Library, 1. Oxford: Update Software; 2001.

*805. Armstrong Schellenberg JRM, Abdulla S, Nathan R. Effect of large-scale social marketing of insecticide-treated nets on child survival in rural Tanzania. Lancet 2001; 357:1241–1247.

*806. Garner P, Gulmezoglu AM. Prevention versus treatment for malaria in pregnant women (Cochrane Review). In: The Cochrane Library, 3. Oxford: Update Software; 2000.

*807. Schellenberg D, Menendez C, Kahigwa E, et al. Intermittent treatment for malaria and anaemia control at time of routine vaccinations in Tanzanian infants: a randomised, placebo-controlled trial. Lancet 2001; 357:1471–1477.

Toxoplasmosis

*808. Dunn D, Wallon M, Peyron F, et al. Mother-to-child transmission of toxoplasmosis: risk estimates for clinical counselling. Lancet 1999; 353:1829–1833.

809. Dubey JP. Sources of *Toxoplasma gondii* infection in pregnancy. Until rates of congenital toxoplasmosis fall, control measures are essential. BMJ 2000; 321:127–128.

810. Cook AJ, Gilbert RE, Buffolano W, et al. Sources of toxoplasma infection in pregnant women: European multicentre case-control study. European Research Network on Congenital Toxoplasmosis. BMJ 2000; 321:142–147.

811. Michaels MG, Wald ER, Fricker FJ, et al. Toxoplasmosis in pediatric recipients of heart transplants. Clin Infect Dis 1992; 14:847–851.

812. Derouin F, Devergie A, Auber P, et al. Toxoplasmosis in bone marrow-transplant recipients: report of seven cases and review. Clin Infect Dis 1992; 15:267–270.

813. Bonametti AM, Passos JN, Koga da Silva EM, et al. Probable transmission of acute toxoplasmosis through breast feeding. J Trop Pediatr 1997; 43:116.

814. Montoya JG, Remington JS. Toxoplasmic chorioretinitis in the setting of acute acquired toxoplasmosis. Clin Infect Dis 1996; 23:277–282.

815. Petersen E, Pollak A, Reiter-Owona I. Recent trends in research on congenital toxoplasmosis. Int J Parasitol 2001; 31:115–144.

*816. Peyron F, Wallon M, Liou C, et al. Treatments for toxoplasmosis in pregnancy (Cochrane Review). In: The Cochrane Library, 2. Oxford: Update Software; 2000.

Trypanosomiasis

817. Triolo N, Trova P, Fusco C, et al. Report on 17 years of studies of human African trypanosomiasis caused by *T. gambiense* in children 0–6 years of age. Med Trop (Mars) 1985; 45:251–257.

818. Blum J, Schmid C, Burri C. Clinical aspects of 2541 patients with second stage human African trypanosomiasis. Acta Trop 2006; 97:55–64.

819. Chappuis F, Loutan L, Simarro P, et al. Options for field diagnosis of human African trypanosomiasis. Clin Microbiol Rev 2005; 18:133–146.

820. Bailey JW, Smith DH. The use of the acridine orange QBC technique in the diagnosis of African trypanosomiasis. Trans R Soc Trop Med Hyg 1992; 86:630.

821. Lumsden WHR, Kimber CD, Evans DA, et al. *Trypanosoma brucei*: miniature anion-exchange centrifugation technique for detection of low parasitaemias: adaptation for field use. Trans R Soc Trop Med Hyg 1979; 73:312–317.

822. Inojosa WO, Augusto I, Bisoffi Z, et al. Diagnosing human African trypanosomiasis in Angola using a card agglutination test: observational study of active and passive case finding strategies. BMJ 2006; 332:1479.

823. Asonganyi T, Doua F, Kibona SN, et al. A multi-centre evaluation of the card indirect agglutination test for trypanosomiasis (TrypTect CIATT). Ann Trop Med Parasitol 1998; 92:837–844.

824. World Health Organization. Control and surveillance of African trypanosomiasis. Technical Report Series No 881. Geneva: World Health Organization; 1998.

825. Burri C, Nkunku S, Merolle A, et al. Efficacy of new, concise schedule for melarsoprol in treatment of sleeping sickness caused by *Trypanosoma brucei gambiense*: a randomised trial. Lancet 2000; 355:1419–1425.

826. Pepin J, Mpia B. Randomized controlled trial of three regimens of melarsoprol in the treatment of *Trypanosoma brucei gambiense* trypanosomiasis. Trans R Soc Trop Med Hyg 2006; 100:437–441.

827. Pepin J, Milord F, Guern C, et al. Trial of prednisolone for prevention of melarsoprol-induced encephalopathy in gambiense sleeping sickness. Lancet 1989; 1:1246–1250.

*828. Balasegaram M, Harris S, Checchi F, et al. Melarsoprol versus eflornithine for treating late-stage Gambian trypanosomiasis in the Republic of the Congo. Bull World Health Organ 2006; 84:783–791.

*829. Chappuis F, Udayraj N, Stietenroth K, et al. Eflornithine is safer than melarsoprol for the treatment of second-stage *Trypanosoma brucei gambiense* human African trypanosomiasis. Clin Infect Dis 2005; 41:748–751.

*830. Bisser S, N'siesi FX, Lejon V, et al. Equivalence trial of melarsoprol and nifurtimox monotherapy and combination therapy for the treatment of second-stage *Trypanosoma brucei gambiense* sleeping sickness. J Infect Dis 2007; 195:322–329.

831. Kierszenbaum F. Chagas' disease and the autoimmunity hypothesis. Clin Microbiol Rev 1999; 12:210–223.

832. Riarte A, Luna C, Sabatiello R, et al. Chagas' disease in patients with kidney transplants: 7 years of experience 1989–1996. Clin Infect Dis 1999; 29:561–567.

833. Russomando G, de Tomassone MM, de Guillen I, et al. Treatment of congenital Chagas' disease diagnosed and followed up by the polymerase chain reaction. Am J Trop Med Hyg 1998; 59:487–491.

834. Solari A, Ortiz S, Soto A, et al. Treatment of *Trypanosoma cruzi*-infected children with nifurtimox: a 3 year follow-up by PCR. J Antimicrob Chemother 2001; 48:515–519.

*835. Villar JC, Marin-Neto JA, Ebrahim S, et al. Trypanocidal drugs for chronic asymptomatic *Trypanosoma cruzi* infection. Cochrane Database Syst Rev 2002;(1):CD003463.

836. Viotti R, Vigliano C, Lococo B, et al. Long-term cardiac outcomes of treating chronic Chagas disease with benznidazole versus no treatment: a nonrandomized trial. Ann Intern Med 2006; 144:724–734.

837. Apt W, Aguilera X, Arribada A, et al. Treatment of chronic Chagas' disease with itraconazole and allopurinol. Am J Trop Med Hyg 1998; 59:133–138.

838. Apt W, Arribada A, Zulantay I, et al. Itraconazole or allopurinol in the treatment of chronic American trypanosomiasis: the regression and prevention of electrocardiographic abnormalities during 9 years of follow-up. Ann Trop Med Parasitol 2003; 97:23–29.

839. Blanco SB, Segura EL, Cura EN, et al. Congenital transmission of *Trypanosoma cruzi*: an operational outline for detecting and treating infected infants in north-western Argentina. Trop Med Int Health 2000; 5:293–301.

840. Moncayo A. Progress towards interruption of transmission of Chagas disease. Mem Inst Oswaldo Cruz 1999; 94 Suppl 1:401–404.

Fungal Infections

841. Drake DP, Holt RJ. Childhood actinomycosis. Report of 3 recent cases. Arch Dis Child 1976; 51:979–981.

842. Schmidt P, Koltai JL, Weltzien A. Actinomycosis of the appendix in childhood. Pediatr Surg Int 1999; 15:63–65.

843. Hilfiker ML. Disseminated actinomycosis presenting as a renal tumor with metastases. J Pediatr Surg 2001; 36:1577–1578.

844. Goussard P, Gie R, Kling S, et al. Thoracic actinomycosis mimicking primary tuberculosis. Pediatr Infect Dis J 1999; 18:473–475.

845. Rosenberg M, Patterson R, Mintzer R, et al. Clinical and immunological criteria for the diagnosis of allergic bronchopulmonary aspergillosis. Ann Intern Med 1977; 86:405–414.

846. Cunningham S, Madge SL. Dinwiddie R. Survey of criteria used to diagnose allergic bronchopulmonary aspergillosis in cystic fibrosis. Arch Dis Child 2001; 84:89.

847. Baddley JW, Thomas P, Stroud D, et al. Invasive mold infections in allogeneic bone marrow transplant recipients. Clin Infect Dis 2001; 32:1319–1324.

848. Wong-Beringer A, Jacobs RA, Guglielmo BJ. Lipid formulations of amphotericin B: clinical efficacy and toxicities. Clin Infect Dis 1998; 27:603–618.

849. Smith CE, Beard RR, Whiting EG, et al. Variation of coccidioidal infection in relation to the epidemiology and control of the disease. Am J Public Health 1946; 36:1394–1402.

850. Rollot F, Bossi P, Tubiana R, et al. Discontinuation of secondary prophylaxis against cryptococcosis in patients with AIDS receiving highly active antiretroviral therapy. AIDS 2001; 15:1448–1449.

851. Kasuga T, Taylor JW, White TJ. Phylogenetic relationships of varieties and geographical groups of the human pathogenic fungus *Histoplasma capsulatum* Darling. J Clin Microbiol 1999; 37:653–663.

852. Deepe GS. Immune response to early and late *Histoplasma capsulatum* infections. Curr Opin Microbiol 2000; 3:359–362.

853. Kügler S, Sebghati TS, Eissenberg LG, et al. Phenotypic variation and intracellular parasitism by *Histoplasma capsulatum*. Proc Natl Acad Sci USA 2000; 97:8794–8798.

854. Odio CM, Navarrete M, Carrillo JM, et al. Disseminated histoplasmosis in infants. Pediatr Infect Dis J 1999; 18:1065–1068.

855. Fahal AH, Hassan MA. Mycetoma. Br J Surg 1992; 79:1138–1141.

856. Hamid ME, Maldonado L, Eldin S, et al. *Nocardia africana* spp. nov., a new pathogen isolated from patients with pulmonary infections. J Clin Microbiol 2001; 39:625–630.

857. Spargo BJ, Crowe LM, Ioneda T, et al. Cord factor (a,a-trehalose 6,6'-dimycolate) inhibits fusion between phospholipid vesicles. Proc Natl Acad Sci USA 1991; 88:737–740.

858. Black CM, Paliescheckey M, Beaman BL, et al. Acidification of phagosomes in murine macrophages: blockage by *Norcardia asteroides*. J Infect Dis 1986; 54:917–919.

859. Fergie JE, Purcell K. Nocardiosis in South Texas children. Pediatr Infect Dis J 2001; 20:711–714.

860. Duong TA. Infection due to *Penicillium marneffei*, an emerging pathogen: review of 155 reported cases. Clin Infect Dis 1996; 23:125–130.

861. Lopez-Martinez R, Neumann L, Gonzalez-Mendoza A. Case report: cutaneous penicilliosis

due to *Penicillium chrysogenum*. Mycoses 1999; 42:347–349.

862. Bustamante B, Campos PE. Endemic sporotrichosis. Curr Opin Infect Dis 2001; 14:145–149.

863. Fleury RN, Taborda PR, Gupta AK, et al. Zoonotic sporotrichosis. Transmission to humans by infected domestic cat scratching: report of four cases in Sao Paulo, Brazil. Int J Dermatol 2001; 40:318–322.

864. de Lima Barros MB, Schubach TMP, Galhardo MCG, et al. Sporotrichosis: an emergent zoonosis in Rio de Janeiro. Mem Inst Oswaldo Cruz, Rio de Janeiro 2001; 96:777–779.

865. Lortholary O, Denning DW, Dupont B. Endemic mycoses: a treatment update. J Antimicrob Chemother 1999; 43:321–331.

866. Lee JW, Siebel NC, Amantea M, et al. Safety and pharmacokinetics of fluconazole in children with neoplastic diseases. J Pediatr 1992; 120:987–993.

867. Spanakis EK, Aperis G, Mylonakis E. New agents for the treatment of fungal infections: Clinical efficacy and gaps in coverage. Clin Infect Dis 2006; 43:1060–1068.

Helminth Infection

868. McCarthy J, Moore TA. Emerging helminth zoonoses. Int J Parasitol 2000; 30:1351–1360.

869. Rim H-J, Forag HF, Sormani S, et al. Food-borne trematodes: ignored or emerging. Parasitol Today 1994; 10:207–209.

870. Goldsmid JM, Speare R. The parasitology of foods. In: Hocking AD, ed. Foodborne microorganisms of public health significance, 6th edn. Sydney: AIFST; 2003.

871. Goldsmid JM. The deadly legacy. Sydney: University of NSW Press; 1988.

872. Nokes C, Bundy DP. Does helminth infection affect mental processing and educational achievement? Parasitol Today 1994; 10:14–18.

*873. Dickson R, Awasthi S, Demellweek C, et al. Antihelmintic drugs for treating worms in children: effects on growth and cognitive performance (Cochrane Review). In: The Cochrane Library, 4. Oxford: Update Software; 2005.

874. Bettoli S, Goldsmid JM. A case of probable imported *Moniliformis moniliformis* infection in Tasmania. J Travel Med 2000; 7:336–337.

875. Maizels R, Blaxter M, Kennedy M. Parasitic helminths: genomes to vaccines. Parasitol Today 1998; 14:131–132.

876. Flores A, Esteban J-G, Anler R, et al. Soil-transmitted helminth infections at very high altitudes. Trans R Soc Trop Med Hyg 2001; 95:272–277.

877. Janssens PG. Chemotherapy of gastrointestinal nematodiasis in man. In: Vanden Bossche H, Thienpont D, Janssens PG, eds. Chemotherapy of gastrointestinal helminths. Berlin: Springer; 1985:183–406.

878. Lancet Editorial. Ascariasis. Lancet 1989; i:997–998.

879. Crompton D. Chronic ascariasis and malnutrition. Parasitol Today 1985; 1:47–52.

880. Pawlowski ZS. Ascariasis. In: Pawlowski ZS, ed. Baillière's Clinical tropical medicine and communicable diseases. Vol 2.3. London: Baillière Tindall; 1987:595–615.

881. Crompton D. The prevalence of ascariasis. Parasitol Today 1988; 4:162–165.

882. Santra A, Bhattacharya T, Chowdhury A, et al. Serodiagnosis of ascariasis with a specific IgG 4 antibody and its use in an epidemiological study. Trans R Soc Trop Med Hyg 2001; 95:289–292.

883. Schneider J, Hughes J, Henderson A. Infectious diseases: prophylaxis and chemotherapy. Australia: Appleton & Lange; 1990.

884. Lengeler C. Insecticide – treated bed nets and curtains for preventing malaria. *Cochrane Database of Systematic Reviews* 2004, Issue 2. Art. No: CD000363.

885. Gustafsson LL, Beerman B, Abdi YA. Handbook of drugs for tropical parasitic infections. London: Taylor & Francis; 1987.

886. James SL, Gilles HM. Human antiparasitic drugs. Chichester: Wiley; 1985.

887. World Bank. Investing in health. World Development Report. Oxford: Oxford University Press; 1993.

888. Guyatt HL. Mass chemotherapy and school-based anthelmintic delivery. Trans R Soc Trop Med Hyg 1999; 93:12–13.

889. Gillespie SH. The epidemiology of *Toxocara canis*. Parasitol Today 1988; 4:180–182.

890. Shorey M, Walker J, Biggs B-A. Clinical parasitology. Melbourne: Melbourne University Press; 2000.

891. Milstein T, Goldsmid JM. The presence of Giardia and other zoonotic parasites of urban dogs in Hobart, Tasmania. Aust Vet J 1995; 72:154–155.

892. Rochette F. Chemotherapy of gastrointestinal nematodiasis in carnivores. In: Vanden Bossche H, Thienpont D, Janssens PG, eds. Chemotherapy of gastrointestinal helminths. Berlin: Springer; 1985:487–504.

893. Hungerford TG. Hazards from domestic pets. Aust Fam Phys 1977; 6:1503–1507.

894. Pawlowski ZS. Enterobiasis. In: Pawlowski ZS, ed. Baillière's Clinical tropical medicine and communicable diseases. Vol 2.3. London: Baillière Tindall; 1987:667–676.

895. Mills A, Goldsmid JM. Intestinal protozoa. In: Doerr WS, Siefert G, eds. Tropical pathology. Vol. 8. Berlin: Springer; 1995:477–556.

896. Marty AM, Andersen EM. Helminthology. In: Doerr WS, Siefert G, eds. Tropical pathology. Vol. 8. Berlin: Springer; 1995:801–982.

897. Smyth JD. Rare, new and emerging helminth zoonoses. Adv Parasitol 1995; 36:1–47.

898. Crompton DH. Hookworm disease: current status and new directions. Parasitol Today 1989; 5:1–2.

899. Behnke JM. Do hookworms elicit protective immunity in man? Parasitol Today 1987; 3:200–206.

900. Pritchard DI. The survival strategies of hookworms. Parasitol Today 1995; 11:255–259.

901. Goldsmid JM. The African hookworm problem: an overview. In: Macpherson C, Craig P, eds. Parasitic helminths and zoonoses in Africa. London: Unwin & Hyman; 1991.

902. Reynolds JEF, ed. Martindale, the extra pharmacopoeia. London: The Pharmaceutical Press; 1996.

903. Quinell RJ, Griffin J, Nowell MA, et al. Predisposition to hookworm infection in Papua New Guinea. Trans R Soc Trop Med Hyg 2001; 95:139–142.

904. Hotez PJ, Le Trang N, Cerami A. Hookworm antigens: a potential for vaccination. Parasitol Today 1987; 3:247–249.

905. Cooper ES, Bundy D. Trichuriasis. In: Pawlowski ZS, ed. Baillière's Clinical tropical medicine and communicable diseases. Vol 2.3. London: Baillière Tindall; 1987:629–643.

906. Cooper ES, Bundy D. Trichuris is not trivial. Parasitol Today 1988; 4:301–306.

907. Ashford RW, Barnish G. Strongyloidiasis in Papua New Guinea. In: Pawlowski ZS, ed. Baillière's Clinical tropical medicine and communicable diseases. Vol 2.3. London: Baillière Tindall; 1987:765–773.

908. Ashford RW, Barnish G, Viney ME. *Strongyloides fuelleborni*: infection and disease in Papua New Guinea. Parasitol Today 1992; 8:314–318.

909. Genta RM. *Strongyloides stercoralis*. In: Guerrant RL, Walker DH, Weller PF, eds. Essentials of tropical infectious diseases. New York: Churchill Livingstone; 2001:464–468.

910. Oliver NW, Rowbottom DJ, Sexton P, et al. Chronic strongyloidiasis in Tasmanian veterans – clinical diagnosis by use of a screening index. Aust N Z J Med 1990; 19:458–462.

911. Smallman LA, Young JA, Shortland-Webb WR, et al. *Strongyloides stercoralis* hyper-infestation syndrome with *Escherichia coli* meningitis: report of two cases. J Clin Pathol 1986; 39:366–370.

912. Pagliuca A, Layton D, Allen S, et al. Hyperinfection with strongyloides after treatment for adult T-cell leukaemia-lymphoma in an African immigrant. BMJ 1988; 297:1456–1457.

913. Pearson RL, et al. Chemotherapy of tropical infectious diseases. In: Guerrant RL, Walker DH, Weller PF, eds. Essentials of tropical infectious diseases. New York: Churchill Livingstone; 2001:613–637.

914. Grove D. Human strongyloidiasis. Adv Parasitol 1996; 38:252–309.

915. Cross JH. Public health importance of *Angiostrongylus cantonensis* and its relatives. Parasitol Today 1987; 3:367–369.

916. Chin J, ed. Control of communicable diseases manual, 17th edn. Washington: APHA; 2000.

917. Morera P. Abdominal angiostrongyliasis: intestinal helminthic infections. In: Pawlowski ZS, ed. Baillière's Clinical tropical medicine and communicable diseases. Vol 2.3. London: Baillière Tindall; 1987:747–753.

918. Polderman AM, Blotkamp J. *Oesophagostomum* infections in humans. Parasitol Today 1995; 11:451–456.

919. Jozefzoon LM, Oostburg BF. Detection of hookworm and hookworm-like larvae in human fecocultures in Suriname. Am J Trop Med Hyg 1994; 51:501–505.

920. Hemsirichart V. *Ternidens* infection – first pathological report of a human case in Asia. J Med Assoc Thailand 2005; 88:1140–1143.

921. Moore DAJ, Girdwood RWA, Chiodini PL. Treatment of anisakiasis with albendazole. Lancet 2002; 360:54.

922. Bier JW, Deardorff TL, Jackson GJ, et al. Human anisakiasis. In: Pawlowski ZS, ed. Baillière's Clinical tropical medicine and communicable diseases. Vol 2.3. London: Baillière Tindall; 1987:723–733.

923. Oshima T. Anisakis – is the sushi bar guilty? Parasitol Today 1987; 3:44–48.

924. Anonymous. Trichinosis outbreak associated with horsemeat. Parasitol Today 1986; 2:295.

925. Campbell WC. Trichinosis revisited – another look at modes of transmission. Parasitol Today 1988; 4:83–86.

926. Kociecka W. Intestinal trichinellosis. In: Pawlowski ZS, ed. Baillière's Clinical tropical medicine and communicable diseases. Vol 2.3. London: Baillière Tindall; 1987:755–763.

927. Cross JH, Basaca-Sevilla V. Intestinal capillariasis. In: Pawlowski ZS, ed. Baillière's Clinical tropical medicine and communicable diseases. Vol 2.3. London: Baillière Tindall; 1987:735–744.

928. Goldsmid JM. More than meets the eye: artefacts and pseudoparasites in faeces. Aust Microbiol 1995; 16:87–89.

929. Muller R. Guineaworm eradication – the end of another disease? Parasitol Today 1985; 1:39.

930. Nelson GS. Lymphatic filaria. In: Gilles HM, ed. Clinics in tropical medicine and communicable disease. Vol 1, no. 3. London: Saunders; 1986: 671–683.

931. Shelley M, Maia-Herzog M, Calvao-Brito R. The specificity of an ELISA for detection of *Onchocerca volvulus* in Brazil in an area endemic for Mansonella. Trans R Soc Trop Med Hyg 2001; 95:171–173.

932. Cupp EW. Treatment of onchocerciasis with ivermectin in Central America. Parasitol Today 1992; 8:212–214.

933. Whitworth J. Treatment of onchocerciasis with ivermectin in Sierra Leone. Parasitol Today 1992; 8:138–140.

934. Chodakewitz J. Ivermectin and lymphatic filariasis: a clinical update. Parasitol Today 1995; 11:233–235.

935. Gardon J, Boussinesq M, Kamgno J, et al. Effects of standard and high doses of ivermectin on adult worms of *Onchocerca volvulus*: a randomized controlled trial. Lancet 2002; 360:203–210.

936. Unnasch TR. River blindness. Lancet 2002; 360:182.

937. Hoerauf A, Mand S, Adjei O, et al. Depletion of Wolbachia endobacteria in *Onchocerca volvulus* by doxycycline and microfilaria after ivermectin treatment. Lancet 2001; 357:1415–1416.

938. Lockwood D. Dermatology. In: Eddleston M, Davidson R, Wilkinson R, et al, eds. Oxford Handbook of tropical medicine, 2nd edn. Oxford: Oxford University Press; 2005:487–514.

939. Pinder M. *Loa loa* – a neglected filaria. Parasitol Today 1988; 4:279–284.

940. Klion AD, Nutman TB. Loiasis and *Mansonella* infections. In: Guerrant RL, Walker DL, Weller PF, eds. Essentials of tropical infectious diseases. New York: Churchill Livingstone; 2001:404–411.

941. Dreyer G, Medeiros Z, Netto M, et al. Acute attacks in the extremeties of persons living in an area endemic to bancroftian filariasis: differentiation of two syndromes. Trans R Soc Trop Med Hyg 1999; 93:413–417.

942. Hightower AW, Lamine PJ, Eberhard MC. Maternal filarial infections – a persistent risk factor for microfilaraemia in offspring? Parasitol Today 1993; 9:418–429.

943. Partono F. Diagnosis and treatment of lymphatic filariasis. Parasitol Today 1985; 1:52–57.

944. Ganesh B, Kader A, Agarwal G, et al. A simple and inexpensive dot-blot assay using a 66-kDa *Brugia malayi* microfilarial protein antigen for diagnosis of bancroftian filariasis in an endemic area. Trans R Soc Trop Med Hyg 2001; 95:168–169.

945. Kluber S, Supali T, Williams S, et al. Rapid PCR-based detection of *Brugia malayi* DNA from blood spots by DNA detection test. Trans R Soc Trop Med Hyg 2001; 95:169–170.

946. Rahmah N, Lim B, Anuar AK, et al. A recombinant antigen-based IgG4 ELISA for the specific and sensitive detection of *Brugia malayi* infection. Trans R Soc Trop Med Hyg 2001; 95:280–284.

947. Ottesen EA, Vijayasekaran V, Kumaraswami V, et al. A controlled trial of ivermectin and diethylcarbamazine in lymphatic filariasis. N Engl J Med 1990; 322:1113–1117.

948. Molyneaux D, Neira M, Liese B, et al. Elimination of lymphatic filariasis as a public health problem. Trans R Soc Trop Med Hyg 2000; 94:589–591.

949. Alexander N, Bockarie M, Dimber Z, et al. Migration and dispersal of lymphatic filariasis in Papua New Guinea. Trans R Soc Trop Med Hyg 2001; 5:277–279.

950. Molyneaux D. Vector-borne infections in the tropics and health policy issues in the twenty-first century. Trans R Soc Trop Med Hyg 2001; 95:233–238.

951. Muller R. *Dipetalonema* by any other name. Parasitol Today 1987; 3:358.

952. Ito A. Cysticercosis in the Asian-Pacific regions. Parasitol Today 1992; 8:182–183.

953. McManus DP, Bowles J. Asian (Taiwan) *Taenia*: species or strain? Parasitol Today 1994; 10:273–275.

954. McKelvie P, Goldsmid JM. Childhood central nervous system cysticercosis in Australia. Med J Aust 1988; 149:42–44.

955. Jaroonvesama N. Differential diagnosis of eosinophilic meningitis. Parasitol Today 1988; 4:262–266.

956. Tillez-Giron E, Ramos MC, Dufour I. Detection of *Cysticercus cellulosae* antigens in cerebrospinal fluid by DOT enzyme-linked immunosorbent assay (DOT-ELISA) and standard ELISA. Am J Trop Med Hyg 1987; 37:169–173.

957. Hughes AJ, Biggs BA. Parasitic worms of the central nervous system: an Australian perspective. Int Med J 2002; 32:541–553.

958. Craig PS, Rogers M, Alfan J. Detection, screening and community epidemiology of taeniid and cestode zoonoses. Adv Parasitol 1996; 38:169–250.

959. Kociecka W. Intestinal cestodiasis. In: Pawlowski ZS, ed. Baillière's Clinical tropical medicine and communicable diseases. Vol 2.3. London: Baillière Tindall; 1987:677–694.

960. Kammerer WS. Chemotherapy of tapeworm infections in man. In: Vanden Bossche H, Thienpont D, Janssens PG, eds. Chemotherapy of gastrointestinal helminths. Berlin: Springer; 1985.

961. Moodley M, Moosa A. Treatment of neurocysticercosis: is praziquantel the new hope? Lancet 1989; 1:262.

*962. Salinas R, Prasad K. Drugs for treating neurocysticercosis (tapeworm infection of the brain) (Cochrane Review). In: The Cochrane Library, 4. Oxford: Update Software; 2001.

963. Goldsmid JM, Rogers S, Parsons GS, et al. The intestinal protozoa and helminths infecting Africans in the Gatooma region of Rhodesia. Cent Afr J Med 1976; 22:91–95.

964. Schenone H. Praziquantel in the treatment of *Hymenolepis nana* infections in children. Am J Trop Med Hyg 1980; 19:320–321.

965. Bartlett JG. Pocket book of infectious disease therapy. Philadelphia: Lippincott Williams and Wilkins; 2002:184.

966. McManus DP, Smyth JD. Hydatidosis: changing concepts in epidemiology and speciation. Parasitol Today 1986; 2:163–167.

967. Craig PS, Desham L, Zhaoxun D. Hydatid disease in China. Parasitol Today 1991; 7:46–50.

968. Lucius R, Frosch M, Kern P. Alveolar echinococcosis: immunogenics and epidemiology. Parasitol Today 1995; 11:4–5.

969. Goldsmid JM, Pickmere J. Hydatid eradication in Tasmania – point of no return? Aust Fam Phys 1987; 16:1672–1674.

970. Gemmell MA, Lawson JR, Roberts MG. Towards global control of cystic and alveolar hydatid disease. Parasitol Today 1987; 3:144–151.

971. Goldsmid JM, Fleming F. The tapeworm infections of children in Rhodesia. Cent Afr J Med 1977; 23:7–10.

972. Frean J, Dini L. Unusual anoplocephalid tapeworm infections in South Africa. Annals of the ACTM 2004; 5:8–11.

973. Warren KS, Mahmoud AAF. Algorithms in the diagnosis and management of exotic diseases. I. Schistosomiasis. J Infect Dis 1975; 131:614–620.

974. Mahmoud AAF, ed. Baillière's Clinical tropical medicine and communicable diseases: schistosomiasis. Vol. 2.2. London: Baillière Tindall; 1987.

975. Woolhouse MEJ. International Conference on Schistosomiasis. Parasitol Today 1993; 9:235–236.

976. Lancet Editorial. Immunity to schistosomiasis. Lancet 1987; i:1015–1016.

977. Hagan P, Williams HA. Concomitant immunity in schistosomiasis. Parasitol Today 1993; 9:1–6.

978. Terry RJ. Concomitant immunity in schistosomiasis. Parasitol Today 1994; 10:377–378.

979. Butterworth AE. Human immunity to schistosomiasis: some questions. Parasitol Today 1994; 10:378–380.

980. Greyseels B. Human resistance to schistosome infections. Parasitol Today 1994; 10:380–384.

981. Anderson RM. Determinants of infection in human schistosomiasis. In: Mahmoud AAF, ed. Baillière's Clinical tropical medicine and communicable diseases. Vol 2.2. London: Baillière Tindall; 1987:279–300.

982. Colley DG. Dynamics of the human immune response to schistosomes. In: Mahmoud AAF, ed. Baillière's Clinical tropical medicine and communicable diseases. Vol 2.2. London: Baillière Tindall; 1987:315–332.

983. Warren KS. Determinants of disease in human schistosomiasis. In: Mahmoud AAF, ed. Baillière's

Clinical tropical medicine and communicable diseases. Vol 2.2. London: Baillière Tindall; 1987:301–313.

984. Wyler DJ. Why does liver fibrosis occur in schistosomiasis? Parasitol Today 1992; 8:277–279.

985. Phillips SM, Lammie PJ. Immunopathology of granuloma formation and fibrosis in schistosomiasis. Parasitol Today 1986; 3:296–302.

986. Peters PAS, Kazura JW. Update on diagnostic methods for schistosomiasis. In: Mahmoud AAF, ed. Baillière's Clinical tropical medicine and communicable diseases. Vol 2.2. London: Baillière Tindall; 1987:419–433.

987. Webster LT. Update on chemotherapy of schistosomiasis. In: Mahmoud AAF, ed. Baillière's Clinical tropical medicine and communicable diseases. Vol 2.2. London: Baillière Tindall; 1987:435–447.

*988. Saconato H, Atalhah A. Interventions for treating *Schistosomiasis mansoni* (Cochrane Review). In: The Cochrane Library, Issue 2. Chichester: Wiley and Sons; Update 2006.

989. Squares N. Interventions for treating *Schistosomiasis haematobium* (Cochrane Review). In: The Cochrane Library. Issue 2. Chichester: Wiley and Sons; 2006.

990. Jong EC, McMullin R. The tropical and travel medicine manual. Philadelphia: Saunders; 1995.

991. Tchuente LAT, Southgate VR, Webster BL, et al. Impact of installation of a water pump on schistosomiasis transmission in a focus in Cameroon. Trans R Soc Trop Med Hyg 2001; 95:255–256.

992. Capron A. Schistosomiasis: Forty years war on the worm. Parasitol Today 1998; 14:379–384.

993. James SL, Sher A. Prospects for a non-living vaccine against schistosomiasis. Parasitol Today 1986; 2:134–137.

994. Butterworth AE. Potential for vaccines against human schistosomes. In: Mahmoud AAF, ed. Baillière's Clinical tropical medicine and communicable diseases. Vol 2.2. London: Baillière Tindall; 1987:465–483.

995. Butterworth AE, Wilkins HA, Capron A, et al. The control of schistosomiasis – is a vaccine necessary? Parasitol Today 1987; 3:1–3.

996. Coulson P. The radiation-attenuated vaccine against schistosomiasis in animal models. Adv Parasitol 1997; 39:272–336.

997. Haswell-Elkins MR, Sithithawarn P, Elkins D. *Opisthorchis viverrini* and cholangiocarcinoma in northwest Thailand. Parasitol Today 1992; 8:86–89.

998. Gillett JD. The behaviour of *Homo sapiens*, the forgotten factor in the transmission of tropical disease. Trans R Soc Trop Med Hyg 1985; 79:12–20.

999. Harinasuta T, Bunnag D, Radomyos P. Intestinal flukes. In: Pawlowski ZS, ed. Baillière's Clinical tropical medicine and communicable diseases. Vol 2.3. London: Baillière Tindall; 1987:695–721.

1000. Butcher AR, Graham AT, Norton RE, et al. Locally acquired *Brachylaima* sp. (Digenia: Brachylaimidae) intestinal fluke infection in two South Australian infants. Med J Aust 1996; 164: 475–478.

Flies, Fleas, Mites and Lice

1001. Hall M, Wall R. Myiasis of humans and domestic animals. Adv Parasitol 1995; 35:257–334.

1002. Alexander JO'D. Arthropods and human skin. Berlin: Springer; 1984.

1003. Goldsmid JM. The deadly legacy. Sydney: University of NSW Press; 1988.

1004. Dominey A, Rosen T, Tschen J. Papulonodular demodicidosis associated with acquired immuno-deficiency syndrome. J Am Acad Dermatol 1989; 20:197–201.

1005. Christopherson J. Epidemiology of scabies. Parasitol Today 1986; 2:247–248.

1006. Chosidow O. Scabies. N Engl J Med 2006; 354:1718–1726.

1007. Robinson J. Fight the mite, ditch the itch. Parasitol Today 1985; 1:140–142.

1008. Commens CA. The treatment of scabies. Aust Prescriber 2000; 23:33–35.

1009. Burgess I. *Sarcoptes scabiei* and scabies. Adv Parasitol 1994; 33:235–292.

1010. Commens CA. We can get rid of scabies: new treatment available soon. Med J Aust 1994; 160:317–318.

1011. Chin J, ed. Control of communicable diseases manual, 17th edn. Washington: APHA; 2000.

1012. Goldsmid JM. Unusual arthropod ectoparasitic infestations of man. Aust Fam Physician 1985; 14:386–388.

*1013. Walker GJ, Johnstone PW. Interventions for treating scabies (Cochrane Review). In: The Cochrane Library, Issue 2. Chichester; 2006.

1014. Burgess I. Human lice. Adv Parasitol 1995; 36:271–342.

1015. Vander Stichele RH, Gyssels L, Bracke C, et al. Wet combing for head lice: feasibility in mass screening, treatment preference and outcome. J Roy Soc Med 2002; 95:348–350.

1016. Counahan M, Andrews R, Buttner P, et al. Head lice prevalence in primary schools in Victoria, Australia. J Paediatr Child Hlth 2004; 40:616–619.

1017. Meinking TL, Taplin D. Advances in pediculosis, scabies and other mite infestations. Adv Dermatol 1990; 5:131–152.

*1018. Vander Steichele RH, Dezeure EM, Bogaert MG. Systematic review of clinical efficacy of topical treatments for head lice. BMJ 1995; 311:604–608.

1019. Burgess I. Malathion lotions for head lice – a less reliable treatment than commonly believed. Pharmaceutical J 1991; (Nov 9):630–632.

*1020. Dodd CS. Interventions for treating headlice. (Cochrane review). In: The Cochrane Library, Issue 2. Chichester: Wiley and Sons; 2006.

1021. Goldsmid JM. The treatment and control of head lice: a review. Aust J Pharm 1989; 70:1021–1024.

1022. Goldsmid JM, Langley J, Naylor P, et al. Further studies on head lice and their control in Tasmania. Aust Fam Physician 1989; 18:253–255.

1023. Burgess I, Peock S, Brown CM, et al. Headlice resistant to pyrethroid insecticides in Britain. BMJ 1995; 311:752.

1024. Wargon O. Treating head lice. Austr Prescriber 2000; 23:62–63.

1025. Namazi MR. Levamisole: a safe and economical weapon against pediculosis. Int J Dermatol 2001; 40:292–294.

1026. Roberts RJ, Casey D, Morgan DA, et al. Comparison of wet combing with malathion for treatment of head lice in the UK. Lancet 2000; 356:540–544.

1027. Roberts RJ. Clinical practice: Head lice. N Engl J Med 2002; 346:1645–1650.

1028. Hill N, Moor G, Cameron MM, et al. The Bug Buster Kit was better than single dose pediculicide for head lice. Evid Based Med 2006; 11:17.

Diseases Transmitted by Animals

1029. Chin J, ed. Control of communicable diseases manual, 17th edn. Washington: APHA; 2000.

1030. Margileth AM. Cat scratch disease. Adv Pediatr Infect Dis 1993; 8:1–21.

1031. Wilks CR, Humble MW. Zoonoses in New Zealand. Palmeston North: Veterinary Continuing Education; 1997.

1032. Murano I, Yoshii H, Kurashige H, et al. Giant hepatic granuloma caused by *Bartonella henselae*. Pediatr Infect Dis J 2001; 20:319–320.

1033. Isada CM, Kasten BL, Goldman MP, et al. Infectious diseases handbook, 3rd edn. Hudson: American Pharmaceutical Association, Lexi-Comp; 1999.

1034. Brenner DJ, Hollis DG, Moss CW, et al. Proposal of *Afipia* gen. nov., with *Afipia felis* sp. nov. (formerly cat scratch disease bacillus), *Afipia clevelandensis* sp. nov. (formerly the Cleveland Clinic Foundation strain), *Afipia broomeae* sp. nov., and three unnamed genospecies. J Clin Microbiol 1991; 29:2450–2460.

1035. Adal KA, Cockerell CJ, Petri WA Jr. Cat scratch disease, bacillary angiomatosis, and other infections due to *Rochalimaea*. N Engl J Med 1994; 330:1509–1515.

1036. Kordick DL, Hilyard EJ, Hadfield TL, et al. *Bartonella clarridgeiae*, a newly recognized zoonotic pathogen causing inoculation papules, fever and lymphadenopathy (cat scratch disease). J Clin Microbiol 1997; 35:1813–1818.

1037. Margileth AM. Antibiotic therapy for cat-scratch disease: clinical study of therapeutic outcome in 268 patients and a review of the literature. Pediatr Infect Dis J 1992; 11:474–478.

1038. Carithers HA, Margileth AM. Cat scratch disease: acute encephalopathy and other neurologic manifestations. Am J Dis Child 1991; 145:98–101.

1039. Stevenson WJ, Hughes KL. Synopsis of zoonoses in Australia, 2nd edn. Canberra: Commonwealth Dept of Community Services; 1988.

1040. Hockman DE, Pence CD, Whittler RR, et al. Septic arthritis of the hip secondary to rat bite fever: a case report. Clin Orthop 2000; 380:173–176.

1041. Rordorf T, Zuger C, Zbinden R, et al. *Streptobacillus moniliformis* endocarditis in an HIV-positive patient. Infection 2000; 28:393–394.

29

Disorders of bones, joints and connective tissues

Joyce Davidson, Andrew Gavin Cleary, Colin Bruce

Musculoskeletal symptoms are common in children and frequently present to pediatricians. A comprehensive review of all conditions affecting the musculoskeletal system in childhood would not be possible within the scope of a single chapter. We have tried to cover in some detail those conditions most commonly seen in pediatrics while also giving sufficient information to enable consideration of many of the more unusual conditions that may be encountered. We have also endeavoured to highlight areas of recent progress.

ASSESSMENT OF THE MUSCULOSKELETAL SYSTEM

Clinical assessment of the musculoskeletal system should be part of the routine pediatric examination. A few simple screening questions and assessments can be used to determine whether or not an abnormality is likely. If a child has no pain, swelling or stiffness of the joints, walks with a normal gait, and is able to keep up with his or her peers in normal activities then it is unlikely that a significant problem exists. Any suggestion of a musculoskeletal problem merits detailed assessment. It must be remembered that some rheumatic conditions may present with constitutional symptoms such as a rash, fever or fatigue before the development of any musculoskeletal problems. This section describes a general approach to the examination of the musculoskeletal system. The more detailed assessment of individual problems is described in the relevant sections of the chapter.

A meticulous history and clinical examination will lead to the correct diagnosis in the majority of cases. Investigations may be diagnostically helpful but are more usually used to confirm the clinically suspected diagnosis.

When assessing the musculoskeletal system in a child, knowledge of normal development is clearly important as normal findings vary considerably at different ages. For example a significant degree of joint laxity is normal in the young child and should not be confused with abnormal hypermobility.

HISTORY

As with many areas of pediatric practice the clinical history is often the most informative part of the assessment. Information must be gleaned from both the parents/carers and the child, even the very young child contributing to the history when age-appropriate questions are used. Questions must be asked about musculoskeletal symptoms such as joint pain or swelling, muscle pain; functional difficulties and about relevant non-articular symptoms.

Non-articular symptoms

Children with musculoskeletal or rheumatic conditions frequently have prominent constitutional symptoms. Fever, fatigue, anorexia and weight loss are common to many inflammatory conditions but may also occur in infection and malignancy. Rashes may be characteristic of individual conditions and may be helpful diagnostically.

Pain

Pain is the most frequently reported musculoskeletal symptom, and musculoskeletal pain is a frequent cause of presentation in both primary care and pediatric practice.[1] Detailed enquiry should be made into its location and characteristics including severity, precipitating and relieving factors, radiation and diurnal variation. It must be remembered that joint pain (arthralgia) is common in children and that most do not have serious pathology (Table 29.1). It should also be noted that not all children with a significant musculoskeletal problem will complain of pain.

Based on the history of the pain, its characteristics and associated features, musculoskeletal problems can be usefully divided into three broad categories: inflammatory, mechanical and idiopathic.

Inflammatory

Inflammatory pain is characteristic of arthritis but also occurs in other conditions such as myositis, the hallmark being a relationship to immobility. The affected child is frequently worst first thing in the morning (morning stiffness) or after periods of inactivity ('gelling'). A young child with arthritis may be unable to walk first thing in the morning but be running around later in the day. Exercise will generally relieve the pain which is usually described as aching or uncomfortable rather than severe. Occasionally children with acute exacerbations of arthritis experience severe pain, sufficient to disturb sleep.

Table 29.1 The differential diagnosis of joint pain in children

1. **Arthritis**
   Infective and reactive
   Juvenile idiopathic arthritis
   Other: autoimmune rheumatic disorders (e.g. systemic lupus erythematosus, dermatomyositis); vasculitis; miscellaneous

2. **Mechanical/degenerative**
   Trauma: accidental and non-accidental
   Hypermobility
   Avascular necrosis, osteochondritis and apophysitis, including Perthes, Osgood–Schlatter and Scheurmann
   Slipped capital femoral epiphysis
   Anterior knee pain

3. **Non-organic/idiopathic**
   Idiopathic pain syndromes – localized and diffuse
   Benign idiopathic limb pains (growing pains)
   Psychogenic

4. **Other**
   Osteomyelitis
   Tumors:
       Malignant: leukemia, neuroblastoma
       Benign: osteoid osteoma, pigmented villonodular synovitis
   Metabolic abnormalities: rickets, diabetes, hypophosphatemic rickets, hypo/hyperthyroidism
   Genetic disorders: skeletal dysplasias, mucopolysaccharidoses, collagen disorders

Inflammatory pain in arthritis is almost universally accompanied by objective evidence of persistent joint swelling without which the diagnosis of arthritis should not be made.

Mechanical

By contrast, mechanical pain is generally exacerbated by exercise and relieved by rest. It is frequently intermittent rather than persistent and tends to be described as more severe than that associated with arthritis. Mechanical problems are more common in older children and adolescents and frequently affect the joints of the lower limb and the back.

Associated symptoms are common. Joint 'locking' is frequently described. True joint locking, where there is a block to extension, is uncommon and may indicate a meniscal problem or patellar dislocation. Joint instability may occur with ligamentous laxity and a complaint of the knee 'giving way' is common with anterior knee pain. Joint swelling may occur with mechanical problems but is usually intermittent rather than persistent.

Idiopathic

Children and adolescents with the most severe pain frequently fall into this category where there is no identifiable organic pathology. Their pain is severe, unremitting and frequently associated with fatigue, poor sleep and significant functional impairment.[2] Complaints of intermittent joint swelling are common but seldom corroborated on clinical examination, which is usually normal.

Functional difficulties

It is important to enquire about the ability of the child to function normally both in activities of day-to-day living such as dressing and toileting and in more physically demanding activities such as sports. Such questions are informative in determining both the type of problem and its severity. It must be remembered that young children are particularly good at compensating for loss of function in one area by using another and absence of functional impairment does not imply absence of pathology. Conversely, the most functionally disabled children may be those with idiopathic or non-organic problems.

Discriminating questions of function are useful in determining progress of disease and are important in assessing response to treatment in conditions such as juvenile idiopathic arthritis. There are a variety of validated quantitative functional assessment tools available for use in children with rheumatic disorders.[3] The Childhood Health Assessment Questionnaire (CHAQ) is the most widely used and has been validated for use in both juvenile arthritis and dermatomyositis[4] in a number of different countries and languages.

EXAMINATION

As with any system, examination of the musculoskeletal system of a child must be age appropriate.[5] Much information can be gained particularly in the younger child by observing the child at play before attempting any more formal examination. Observing the child's general demeanour, gait and ability to get up and down off the floor is informative. Ideally the musculoskeletal system should be examined in detail, with assessment of all joints and muscle groups. This is frequently impractical in the very young or the child who is in a lot of pain. The examination may need to be opportunistic, focusing initially on problem areas which will have been identified by initial observation of the child.

A simple screening examination (Table 29.2) may be appropriately used to identify children who merit more detailed assessment and can be incorporated into the routine physical examination of any child.

General systemic examination

The child should be examined for evidence of any systemic features that may be relevant to musculoskeletal disorders. Rashes may be useful diagnostically. Growth impairment is common in many chronic disorders and documentation of height and weight is mandatory. Temperature, blood pressure and urinalysis should be measured where systemic involvement may occur.

Gait

Observation of the gait may help identify the nature and site of the problem, particularly in the younger child who may find it difficult to localize pain.

A child who is unable to weight bear may have a serious disorder such as septic arthritis or a malignancy. A child with fixed flexion deformities at the hips will adopt an exaggerated lordosis to compensate. Weak hip and pelvic muscles will result in a waddling gait, while a painful hip or knee will result in an antalgic gait, where the child walks in such a way as to spend as little time as possible on the affected leg.

Examination of joints

Joints should be inspected, palpated and their range of movement determined. Preprinted tables or cartoon figures are available to aid systematic documentation of the results.

Inspection of joints yields useful information. The position of the joint and any limb deformity should be documented. The limb should be inspected for evidence of wasting of surrounding muscles or limb length discrepancy, resulting from overgrowth at an inflamed joint. Erythema or unusual laxity of the skin overlying the joint should be noted. Joint swelling is frequently obvious on inspection.

Table 29.2 The screening musculoskeletal examination in a child

1. Extend the arms straight out in front then make a fist
2. Place palms and fingers together with wrists extended to 90°: 'prayer position'
3. Raise arms straight above the head
4. Turn neck to look over each shoulder
5. Walk normally, on tip-toe and on the heels
6. Sit cross-legged on the floor then jump up

A child who can perform all these actions without difficulty is unlikely to have a significant musculoskeletal problem

Following inspection the joint should be palpated for warmth, swelling or tenderness. Documenting the presence of joint effusions is important in assessing and diagnosing arthritis. It must be remembered that in some joints, e.g. the hips, effusions can not be detected clinically and must be sought in other ways, e.g. using ultrasound (Fig. 29.1).

In many musculoskeletal conditions loss of joint range is one of the earliest objective signs of a problem. Examining for this requires experience, patience and a knowledge of the normal range of movement of the joints. Where the problem is clearly localized to a particular joint, the examination may focus on this area. If the child has evidence of a condition that may affect more than one area, e.g. a polyarthritis, a meticulous assessment of all joints should be made. Arthritis in children is usually asymmetrical enabling the contralateral joint to be used for comparison.

Range of movement should be assessed both actively and passively. Assessment of active joint range involves observing the child moving the joints. Passive range is assessed by the examiner moving the joints through their full range. A useful sign of early arthritis in a joint is pain at the end of the range of passive movement. The child may deny pain but withdraw the limb consistently when pushed to the end of its range.

Joints frequently forgotten, but important in the overall assessment of the child, are the sacroiliac joints, the temporomandibular joint and the cervical spine.

Examination of muscles

Assessment of muscles is also an essential part of the musculoskeletal examination. Muscle tenderness may indicate an underlying inflammatory process, while wasting and weakness may indicate a disorder of the muscle itself, of the surrounding joints or of the nervous system. Gait abnormalities, or an inability to get up off the floor easily, may be indicative of muscle weakness. The well-known Gower sign, where the child uses his/her hands to push off the body when attempting to stand is an indicator of proximal muscle weakness and not specific to any one group of disorders.

Muscle strength should be formally assessed using a standard scale for grading muscle strength. This requires experience in young children ensuring that clear, understandable instructions are given and taking care not to underestimate the strength of the younger child. A five-point scale for grading muscle strength is familiar to most clinicians. A ten-point scale may be more precise and is equally simple to use (Table 29.3).[6]

In children with inflammatory myositis the childhood myositis assessment scale (CMAS)[7] is a validated method of quantitating muscle strength by scoring the child's ability to perform a variety of maneuvers. Its use in conjunction with manual testing of muscle strength gives reproducible scores which can be used to assess a child's response to treatment.

CONGENITAL AND DEVELOPMENTAL PROBLEMS

In broad terms congenital abnormalities can be classified into:
1. failure of formation (transverse or longitudinal);
2. failure of differentiation;
3. duplication;
4. overgrowth (or gigantism);
5. undergrowth (or hypoplasia);
6. congenital constriction band syndrome;
7. generalized skeletal abnormalities.

It is important to bear in mind that, although congenital abnormalities may be isolated, they may also occur in association with other abnormalities, sometimes as part of a recognized syndrome.

SPINAL PROBLEMS
Congenital spinal problems

The child with a vertebral anomaly must be fully assessed for associated abnormalities as in the VATER (Vertebral, Anorectal, Tracheo-Esophageal, Renal, Radial) and VACTERL (Vertebral, Anorectal, Cardiac,

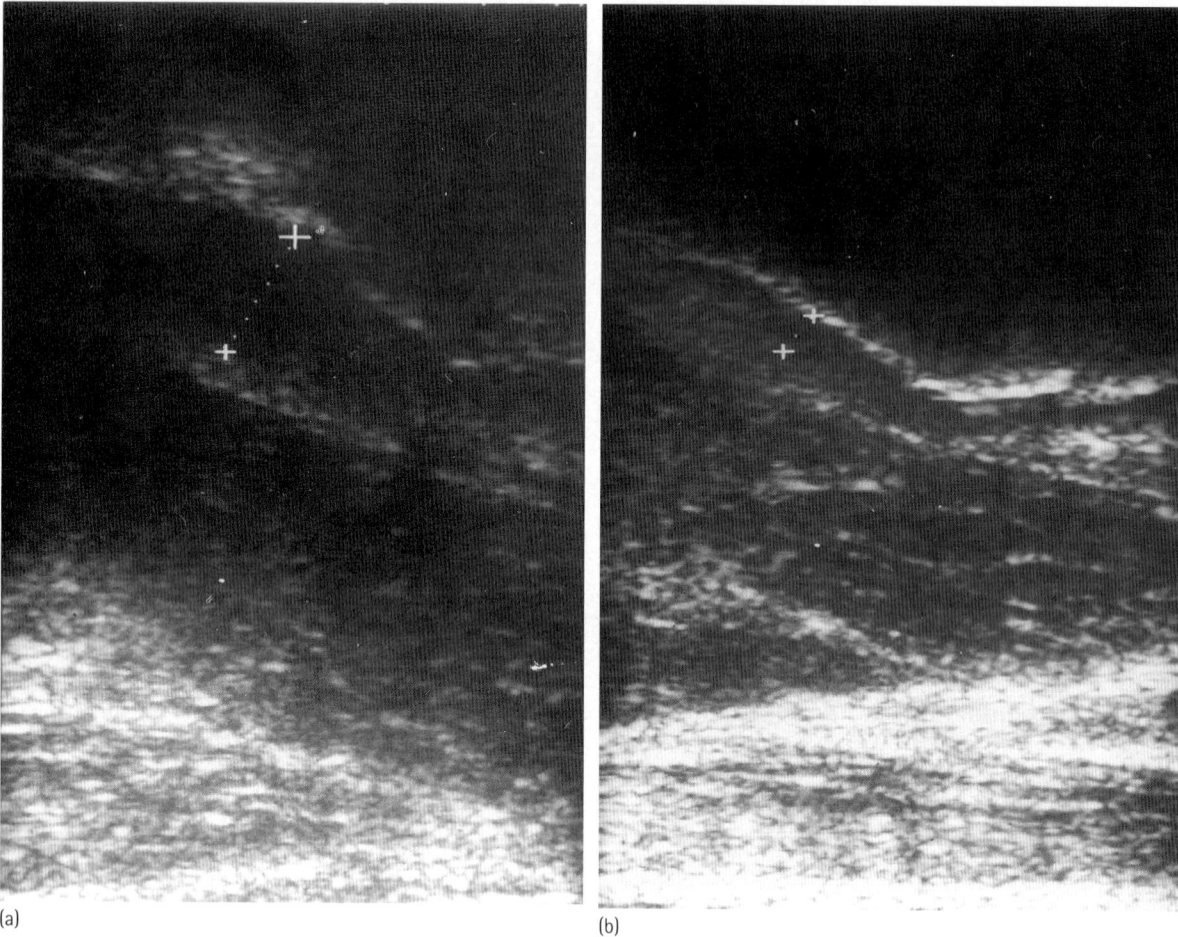

(a)   (b)

Fig. 29.1   (a) Hip ultrasound showing effusion; (b) normal hip for comparison.

Tracheo-Esophageal, Renal, Limb) syndromes. Deformities occurring as result of vertebral anomalies include scoliosis, kyphosis and lordosis.

Congenital spinal anomalies are classified into failure of formation or failure of separation of individual vertebrae or parts of vertebrae. Failure of separation is termed an unsegmented bar, the position of such a bar determining the deformity. With a lateral unsegmented bar the growth of the spinal column is tethered on that side, continued growth on the opposite side leading to a progressive scoliosis. Failure of formation may involve the anterior, posterior or lateral side of a vertebra and once again the site will dictate the deformity. A hemivertebra on one side

of the spinal column leads to extra growth on that side versus the side with the absent segment and a scoliosis may result (Fig. 29.2).

Treatment of the vertebral anomaly depends on its potential to lead to progressive deformity. Some abnormalities have only modest potential and two separate abnormalities may cancel each other out. Other anomalies or combinations have significant potential to progress and will need careful management to prevent progressive deformity.

Idiopathic infantile scoliosis

This usually presents during the first 3 years of life and is distinguished from congenital scoliosis by the absence of a spinal malformation. In contradistinction to adolescent idiopathic scoliosis the condition is more common in boys and the convexity of the thoracic scoliosis is to the left in 90%. The condition is often self-limiting but some cases do progress leading to poor cardiopulmonary development. Prolonged molded plaster jacket treatment is often successful although some may require surgery.

Congenital muscular torticollis

Congenital muscular torticollis, resulting from a contracture of the sternocleidomastoid muscle, is the most common cause of torticollis in the infant. The etiology is unknown. Theories include in-utero crowding and muscle fibrosis following a compartment syndrome within the muscle as a result of compression of the neck during a difficult delivery. Clinically a nontender 'tumor' or swelling can be palpated in the sterno-cleidomastoid muscle in the first 4–6 weeks, but subsequently regresses. Radiographs of the cervical region should be obtained if there is any suspicion of an underlying cervical abnormality.

Left untreated, plagiocephaly and facial asymmetry may develop. Treatment initially consists of passive stretching exercises together with encouragement of head rotation in the restricted direction

Table 29.3   Manual muscle testing: 5- and 10-point scales for grading of muscle strength

5-point scale	10-point scale	
0	0	No evidence of muscle function
1	1	Slight flicker of contractility; no effective function
2	2	Movement with gravity eliminated
3	3	Movement against gravity
	4	Movement against gravity: unable to hold position
	5	Movement against gravity: able to hold position
4	6	Resists slight pressure
	7	Resists slight/moderate pressure
	8	Resists moderate pressure
	9	Resists moderate/strong pressure
5	10	Full power

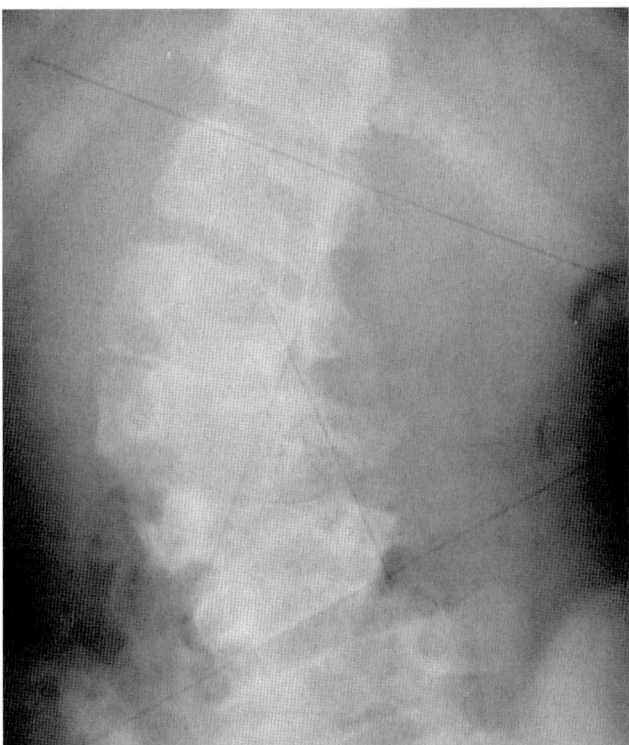

Fig. 29.2   Congenital hemivertebra resulting in scoliosis.

by placing objects of interest toward that side. Passive stretching begun early is successful in 90%.[8] After the age of 1 year surgical treatment may be necessary. This involves division of the tight tendon and is best done before 4 years of age. Established facial deformity or a limitation of more than 30° of rotation usually precludes good results.

Klippel–Feil syndrome

Klippel–Feil syndrome results from failure of the normal segmentation of the cervical vertebrae so that two or more are joined forming block vertebrae. The etiology is unknown. The most consistent clinical finding is limitation of neck motion. Shortening of the neck is subtle.

Associated anomalies include facial asymmetry, torticollis or webbing of the neck in 20%. Sprengel shoulder (a high riding scapula) occurs in up to one third and other associated abnormalities occasionally include ptosis of the eyelid, lateral rectus muscle palsy of the eye, facial nerve palsy, a cleft or high arched palate and abnormalities of the upper limbs including supernumery digits, hypoplasia of the thumb or even the entire upper limb. Abnormalities of the lower limbs are infrequent.[9] Affected patients should be screened for other abnormalities which include scoliosis or kyphosis in up to 60%, renal abnormalities in 30%, cardiovascular abnormalities in 14%, deafness or hearing impairment in 30%. Twenty percent of patients demonstrate mirror motions (synkinesia) or involuntary paired movement of the hands.

UPPER LIMB PROBLEMS

Sprengel shoulder

The scapula develops within the upper limb bud and descends to overlie the second to seventh thoracic vertebrae and ribs. Failure to descend fully gives rise to congenital elevation of the scapula – Sprengel deformity. The condition is usually sporadic but occasionally inherited in an autosomal dominant fashion. It is commoner on the left but can be bilateral. Radiographs of the chest and the cervical spine should be taken to rule out associated rib abnormalities and anomalies of the cervical vertebrae such as Klippel–Feil syndrome.

Shoulder elevation is usually only modestly limited and significant functional problems are rare. Treatment is directed toward maintaining the existing range of movement. Surgical procedures to remove the prominent superomedial tip of the scapula are cosmetic and do not improve shoulder function. Procedures to bring about descent of the whole scapula are associated with significant potential complications and long, sometimes ugly scarring.

Pseudarthrosis of the clavicle

This rare condition presents as a nontender lump at about the midpoint of clavicle. When identified soon after birth it may be mistaken for a fracture, but should be distinguished by the absence of rapid callus formation and persistence of the pseudoarthrosis (Fig. 29.3). It should also be differentiated from cleidocranio-dysostosis where parts of both clavicles are deficient and associated anomalies are found in the skull, facial bones and pelvis. The clavicle develops from medial and lateral ossification centers and the condition may represent a failure of these centers to fuse. Pseudoarthrosis of the clavicle is almost always seen on the right, thought to be a consequence of pressure attrition from the somewhat higher right-sided subclavian vessels.

Shoulder and upper limb function is normally good but the prominent lump is unsightly, and overhead activity may become uncomfortable in maturity. Unlike congenital pseudoarthrosis of the tibia and radius, the condition is not associated with neurofibromatosis and readily unites after excision and bone grafting. Surgery is best performed around the age of 4 years.

Radial club hand (preaxial absence)

Radial dysplasia is the commonest of the major longitudinal failures of formation (Fig. 29.4). It may present as partial or complete absence, bilateral or unilateral. When sporadic the etiology is unknown. The abnormality was seen previously in association with thalidomide when two thirds of cases were bilateral.

Radial dysplasia is always associated with thumb hypoplasia. The spectrum of clinical abnormality can range from mild radial deviation of the wrist and minimal thumb hypoplasia, to complete absence of the preaxial structures including the thumb, the carpal and metacarpal bones and the radius with associated shortening of the ulna and a stiff elbow joint. The deformity is characterized by a weak, radially deviated wrist and a short forearm which grows to only one half to two thirds of normal length. The hand is usually correctable upon the wrist after birth and the elbow lies extended with reduced active and passive flexion.

Early passive stretching and splinting is indicated and should continue until a decision is made regarding surgical treatment. The standard surgical management is centralization of the carpus over the third metacarpal with subsequent pollicization of the index finger.

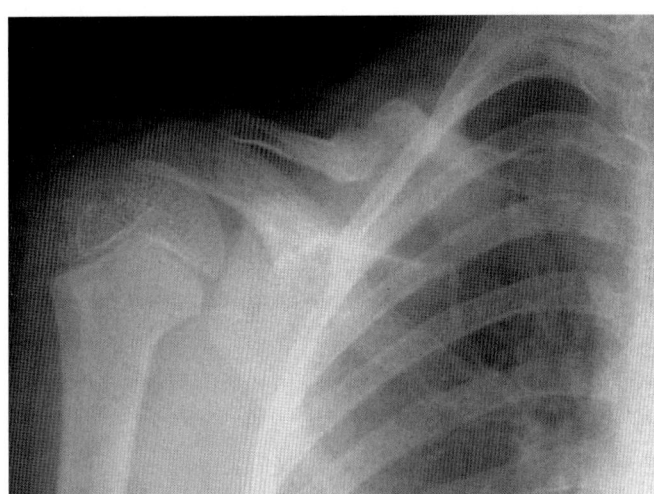

Fig. 29.3   Pseudoarthrosis of the clavicle.

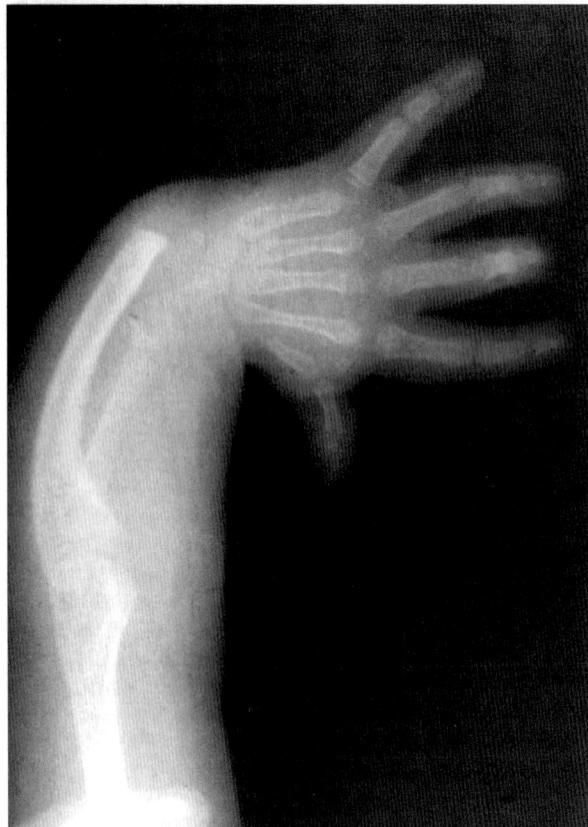

Fig. 29.4   Radial club hand.

Pollicization is the surgical shortening and rotation of an index finger to allow opposition with the other digits, so compensating for the absent thumb. Elbow mobility is a prerequisite for centralization procedures to ensure that hand to mouth movement is possible.

Radial deficiency may occur in isolation. Forty percent of patients with unilateral and 27% with bilateral radial club hand have associated malformations including those of the cardiac, genitourinary, respiratory, skeletal and neurological systems.[10] Syndromes associated with longitudinal radial deficiency include the VATER syndrome; the Holt–Oram syndrome (an autosomal dominantly inherited condition characterized by upper limb and cardiac malformations); thrombocytopenia absent radius (TAR) syndrome (a recessively inherited disorder where thrombocytopenia is present at birth and usually improves with growth); and Fanconi anemia.

Ulna club hand (postaxial absence)

This condition is about ten times less common than absence of the radius. It is usually a partial absence of the lower two thirds of the ulna and sometimes the postaxial rays. The absent bone may be represented by a fibrous remnant which becomes a deforming force during growth, leading to progressive ulnar deviation of the wrist and secondary curvature of the radius. As the forearm grows, the radial bowing increases and the radial head may subluxate or dislocate proximally at the elbow joint.

Complete absence of the ulna is usually associated with a severe flexion contraction of the elbow and surgery has little to offer. In partial absence the deforming fibrous band can be excised to prevent progressive deformity. Other treatment strategies include ulna lengthening procedures as well as procedures to construct a so-called 'one bone forearm' where the proximal ulna is fused to the distal radius.

Congenital dislocation of the radial head

Congenital dislocation of the radial head is rare and usually occurs in isolation (Fig. 29.5). It frequently presents late, often not until school age,

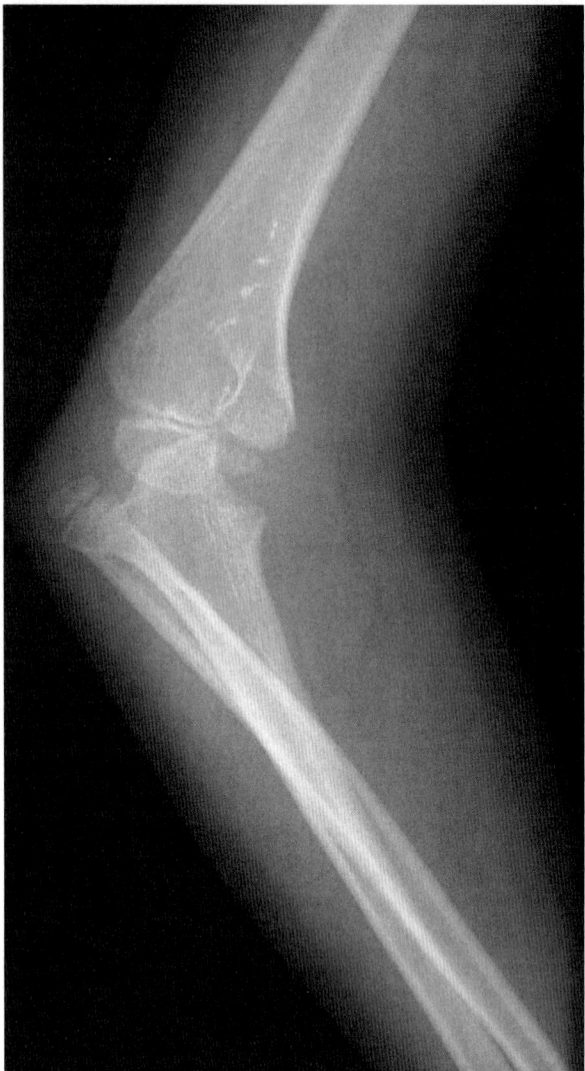

Fig. 29.5   Congenital dislocation of the radial head.

and may be difficult to distinguish from an overlooked post-traumatic dislocation. Radial head dislocation may also be acquired as a result of differential growth disturbance between the radius and ulna or secondary to conditions such as Madelung deformity or familial osteochondromatosis. Features that suggest congenital dislocation include a positive family history, bilateral involvement and the absence of a history of trauma. Radiographic features more typical of congenital dislocation include a small dome-shaped radial head, a hypoplastic capitellum and ulnar bowing.

Children present during school years with limited elbow extension, a palpable mass (the radial head) or pain with athletic activities. The radial head is most commonly dislocated posterolaterally and can be palpated at the lateral side of the elbow joint.

If identified under 2 years, consideration may be given to open surgical reduction of the radial head and anular ligament reconstruction. Though some promise is reported following this procedure the indications are yet to be properly defined, particularly the upper age limit at which surgery might be helpful.[11] Most children present beyond infancy and are best managed conservatively. If significant discomfort occurs, management may include the removal of degenerate fragments of bone or excision of the entire radial head, a procedure to be approached with caution in the immature skeleton because of its association with progressive valgus deformity at the elbow and subsequent elbow, wrist and ulnar nerve problems.

to straighten and adduct the limbs prematurely results in compression forces along the shaft of the femur, pushing the femoral head postero-superiorly, where it is unstable. Cultural swaddling may in part explain the differing incidence of DDH between races. The hips are best allowed to rest in flexion and abduction, the position most infants naturally adopt. Early diagnosis gives the best chance of a satisfactory outcome.

Clinical examination to identify DDH is based on the observations of Ortolani and Barlow. The first part of clinical examination is to determine whether the hip is in or out of joint. Clinical signs sugges-tive of dislocation include limited abduction, limb length asymmetry and asymmetrical skin creases (Fig. 29.10). If the hip is considered to be in joint, its stability is evaluated with a Barlow maneuver. The hip is first placed in a vulnerable position of slight extension and adduction before longitudinal compression is applied along the shaft of the femur (Fig. 29.11a) (the positioning is important because the hip is more sta-ble and resists subluxation or dislocation if held incorrectly in a position of flexion and abduction). If the hip is unstable there is a palpable sen-sation of the femoral head riding posteriorly over the posterior rim of the acetabulum, the so-called 'clunk'. There is a similar sensation when compression is released and the femoral head returns to the acetabu-lum or if an Ortolani maneuver is used to reduce the joint. If the hip is considered to be dislocated, a gentle attempt can be made to return it to the acetabulum using an Ortolani maneuver. Once again positioning is important. The hip is held in 90 degrees of flexion so that the femoral head is directly posterior to the acetabulum. Gentle traction is applied to the leg and the long fingers of the examiner's hand are placed on the greater trochanter where they gently lift the femoral head (Fig. 29.11b). If the dislocation is reducible, the femoral head can be felt passing across the posterior lip of the acetabulum and into the joint. Once in joint, the hip can be gently abducted and flexed to a more stable position so that the reduction can be maintained.

These examinations are difficult and the introduction of clinical screening has not eradicated late presenting dislocations. The sensa-tion of dislocation or reduction is difficult to elicit in the conscious child over about 3–4 months of age and thereafter limited abduction, or limb asymmetry are more reliable. After walking age the child with a uni-lateral dislocated hip stands either with the 'long' leg flexed at the knee or with the 'short' leg standing tiptoe to compensate for the length dis-crepancy. The child will walk with a limp, which can be a simple short leg gait, sometimes with a classic waddle or Trendelenburg gait pattern. Symmetry in bilateral dislocation can make these signs less easily iden-tifiable. Radiographs reveal a subluxed or dislocated femoral head with a small ossific nucleus and a dysplastic acetabulum (Fig. 29.12).

The limitations of clinical examination and the inability of radio-graphs to image the cartilaginous infant hip has led to the development of ultrasound screening. Population ultrasound screening has been intro-duced in Germany and parts of Europe but remains sporadic in the UK.

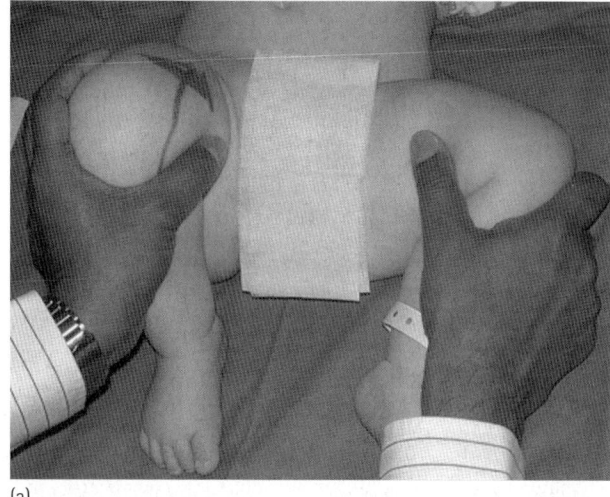

(a)

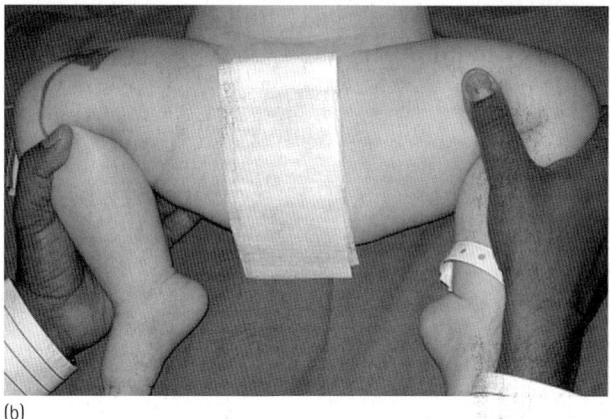

(b)

Fig. 29.11 (a) Barlow and (b) Ortolani maneuvers.

Many units practice selective screening of higher risk infants, i.e. those with a family history, a breech position in utero, a suspicious hip exami-nation or who exhibit other structural examination abnormalities such as metatarsus adductus or torticollis. The investigation can result in false negatives and especially false positives, revealing 'abnormalities' of uncertain significance and resulting in high treatment rates. While it is acknowledged that ultrasound examination is an unequivocally useful tool to evaluate the progress of unstable and dislocated hips, its role as a screening tool for DDH in the UK remains controversial and its cost

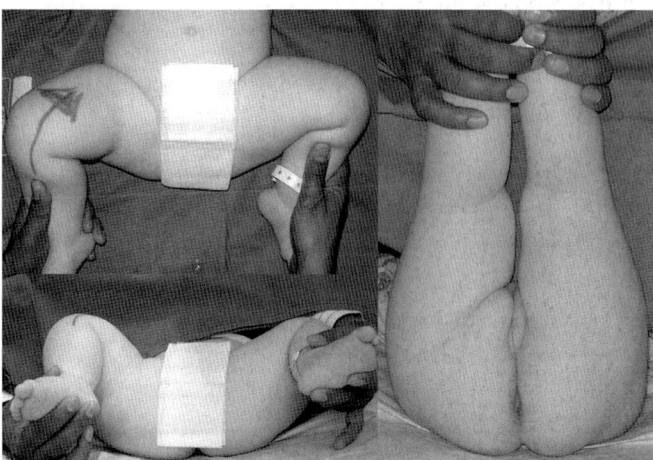

Fig. 29.10 Dislocated right hip showing limited abduction, asymmetrical skin creases and short limb.

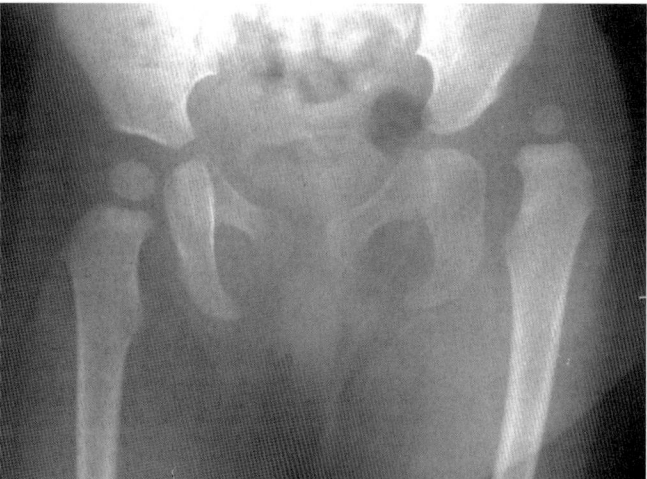

Fig. 29.12 Dislocated left hip with dysplastic acetabulum and small ossific nucleus.

effectiveness is questioned.[14] The National Screening Committee (NSC) in the UK currently recommends that every child should have a clinical examination based on the Ortolani Barlow maneuver within the first week of life and again at 6 weeks.[15] Those with a positive clinical examination should have an ultrasound. In July 2006 the NSC determined that population ultrasound screening should not be offered unless part of an ethically approved and externally funded research project (http://www.library.nhs.uk/screening).

In general terms, reduction of a dislocated hip becomes progressively more difficult the longer it has been dislocated. Treatment involves first reducing the hip and then keeping it in joint until it becomes stable. The chief complications of any treatment are re-dislocation and avascular necrosis (AVN) of the femoral head. The circulation of the femoral head is vulnerable and especially sensitive to pressure. It is known that forceful reduction or positioning of the hip in extreme flexion, abduction or internal rotation can apply excessive pressure to the femoral head and disturb the blood supply leading to AVN. In spite of avoiding these known causes, AVN remains a troublesome complication in the management of hip dislocation (Fig. 29.13).

From birth to about 3–4 months the dislocated or subluxed hip will often reduce with a gentle Ortolani maneuver and should then be maintained in a position of gentle flexion and abduction until it becomes stable when released. There are a wide variety of splints available to maintain this position but the Pavlik harness (Fig. 29.14), a dynamic splint affording the infant some movement within a safe arc, is probably the most widely used. The harness is worn 23–24 hours a day and requires regular scrutiny to ensure proper fitting. Hip development can be followed by repeated ultrasound examination at 2- or 4-weekly intervals until normal with a clinically stable hip. Harness treatment typically lasts 12–16 weeks if the dislocation is identified early. The Pavlik harness is not practical in children older than about 6 months.

When children present between 4 and 6 months of age it can be difficult to be certain of an adequate reduction, in the conscious patient, and these infants are often examined under anaesthesia. Radio-paque contrast is introduced into the hip joint during the examination and the resulting arthrogram outlines the cartilaginous femoral head and acetabulum so that a satisfactory reduction can be confirmed (Fig. 29.15). If there is any obstruction to proper location or extreme force or positioning is required to maintain satisfactory location, closed (nonsurgical) reduction is best abandoned in favor of later open (surgical) reduction when the obstruction or resistance to location can be addressed operatively. If closed reduction is possible, immobilization in a stable position of gentle flexion and abduction can be achieved by a plaster of Paris hip spica cast, once again avoiding extreme or forced positions. The reduction should be confirmed by a later CT scan of the hips in the spica cast. Typically such children remain immobilized for 6–9 months.

When children present after about 12–18 months successful closed reduction becomes unlikely. The later a child presents the more likely they are to require a surgical open reduction and further secondary operations either to the femur or to the acetabulum to correct secondary problems especially persistent acetabular shallowness (dysplasia). Late presentation increases the chance of secondary surgery and complications reducing the chance of a perfect outcome.

Congenital dislocation of the knee

This presents at birth with the knee severely hyperextended instead of in the normal flexed position (Fig. 29.16). The etiology is unknown, but there is a high incidence of breech delivery indicating a role for intrauterine positioning. Associated musculoskeletal abnormalities, especially subluxation or dislocation of the hip, are present in approximately 50%. Plain lateral radiographs reveal anterior subluxation or dislocation of the tibia on the femur.

Treatment begins soon after birth with serial casting to gradually flex the knee and is often successful within a few weeks of birth. If conservative treatment fails, there may be some underlying fibrosis of the quadriceps mechanism and open surgical release early in life can give good long term results.

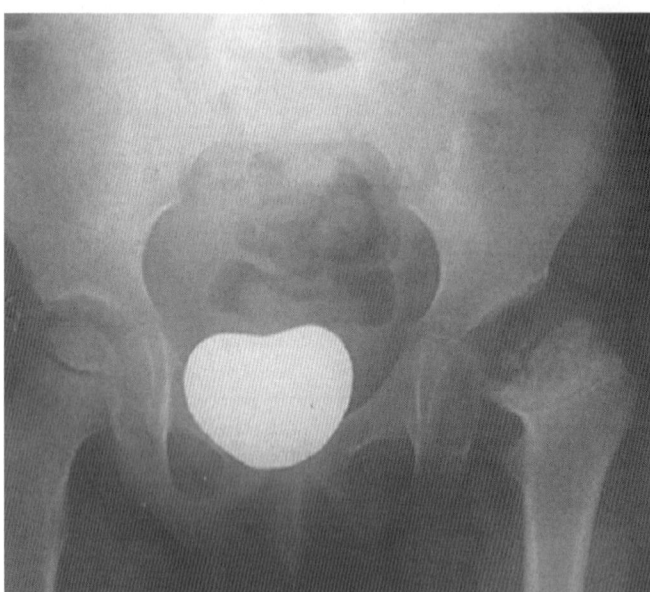

Fig. 29.13 Avascular necrosis after treatment for developmental dislocation of the hip.

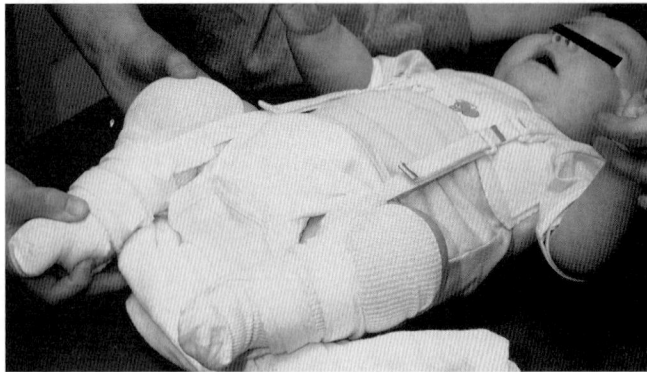

Fig. 29.14 Infant in Pavlik harness.

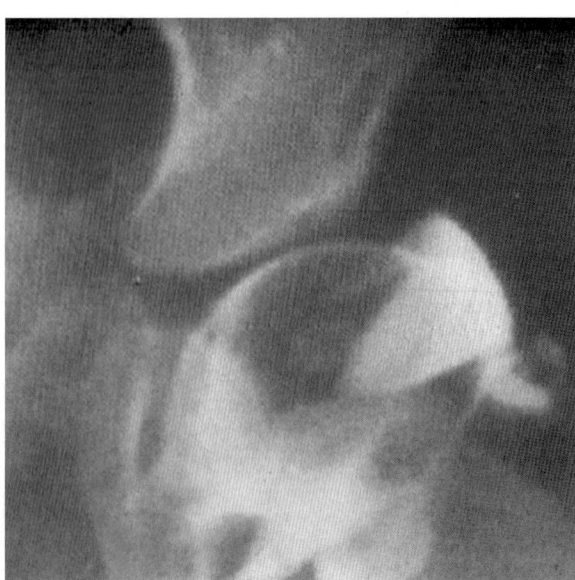

Fig. 29.15 Arthrogram showing a satisfactory closed reduction of a dislocated hip.

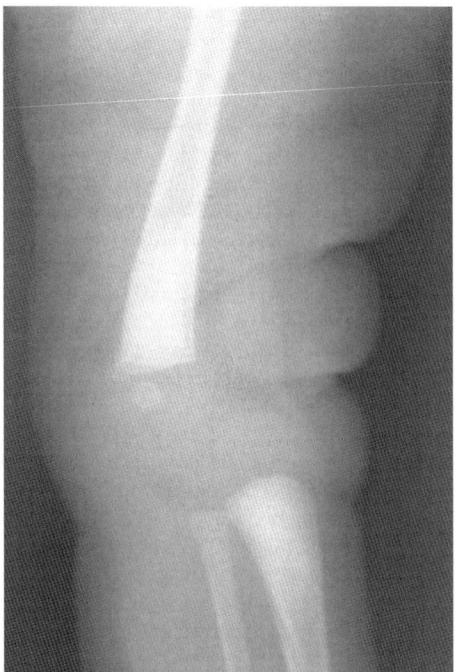

Fig. 29.16   Congenital dislocation of the knee.

Tibial bowing

Tibial bowing at birth can take four characteristic forms. Broadly speaking the convexity of the bow points to the four points of the compass namely anteromedial, anterolateral, posterolateral and posteromedial. The first three directions are associated with relatively severe problems namely fibula hemimelia, pseudoarthrosis of the tibia and tibia hemimelia respectively. Posteromedial bowing of the tibia is relatively benign.

Posteromedial bowing of the tibia

Posteromedial bowing of the tibia is associated with a severe calcaneo-valgus deformity of the foot.[16] The appearance can be alarming at birth. Initial treatment is directed toward passive stretching of the foot deformity, sometimes with the addition of serial casting. The tibial bowing generally corrects in the first year of life, although tibial length inequality may persist and require later orthopedic intervention.

Congenital fibula deficiency (fibula hemimelia)

The fibula is the most frequently congenitally deficient long bone. The deficiency can be modest and isolated. Severe fibula deficiency is more common and is associated with a generally dysplastic limb and other deformities.

The choice of appropriate management can be extremely difficult. Modern prosthetics make amputation more acceptable and new methods of limb reconstruction, especially with the Ilizarov external fixator, make reconstruction more feasible. Amputation is recommended if the foot is nonfunctional, regardless of limb length, and if the length discrepancy is more than 30% even with a functional foot. Application of the appropriate management requires considerable clinical experience and should be tailored to the individual patient.

Congenital tibial deficiency (tibia hemimelia)

The child presents at birth with shortening of the tibia and a rigid equinovarus foot. The leg is bowed convex laterally. Other congenital limb abnormalities occur in up to 75%.[17] The tibia can be completely absent (Type I); absent in its distal portion but with a proximal portion remaining to form an articulation at the knee (Type II) (Fig. 29.17); or present but forming an abnormal distal tibiofibula diastasis or separation at the ankle (Type III).[18]

Management strategies range from prosthetics to reconstruction and once again, as in fibula hemimelia, considerable clinical experience is required to chart an appropriate course for each individual patient.

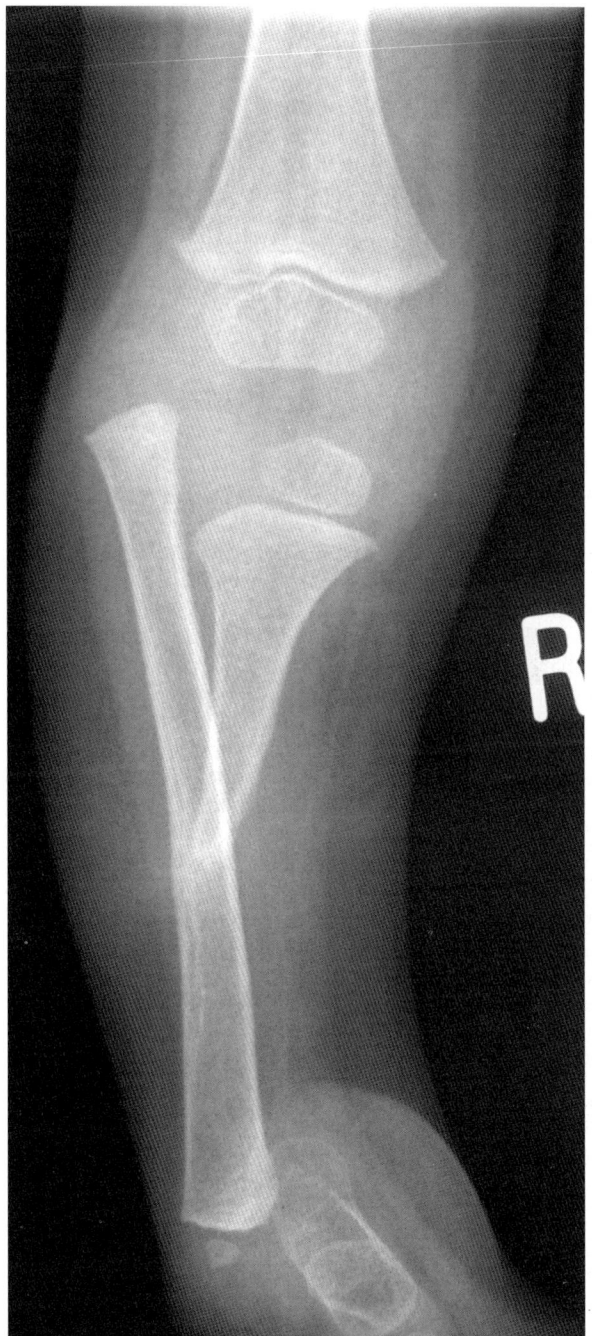

Fig. 29.17   Congenital tibial deficiency.

Congenital pseudoarthrosis of the tibia

Congenital pseudoarthrosis of the tibia presents with anterior or anterolateral bowing at the junction of the proximal two thirds and the distal one third of the tibia. Up to 80% of cases are associated with neurofibromatosis.[19] The bone and its covering periosteum are abnormal at the site of the bowing and the fibula may also be involved in the pathology. Spontaneous fracture at the abnormality can occur and subsequently leads to persistent nonunion or pseudoarthrosis.

Management should include the avoidance of fracture for as long as possible by the use of protective orthoses. Numerous methods have been used to encourage union at the fracture site with modest success. A Syme amputation of the foot followed by a below knee prosthesis remains a satisfactory long term solution, although modern reconstructive techniques especially using the Ilizarov external fixator offer new solutions. The abnormal bone and periosteum at the site of the pathology can be excised and the remaining healthy bone lengthened.

Metatarsus varus

See section on 'Common orthopedic problems in childhood', page 1415.

Congenital talipes calcaneovalgus

This foot posture is frequent in newborns and in the majority of children is within the spectrum of normality. The foot is dorsiflexed so that the dorsum touches the shin. If the foot can be fully plantarflexed the condition is termed postural, requires no treatment and will resolve spontaneously. Occasionally the foot cannot be fully plantarflexed. Physiotherapy and/or splintage should be commenced promptly to stretch the tight anterior structures and should be successful in most cases. In resistant cases, the possibility of an underlying neurological or skeletal abnormality should be considered.

Congenital talipes equinovarus (CTEV; congenital club foot)

Congenital talipes equinovarus is a common foot abnormality with an incidence of 1–2/1000 live births (Fig. 29.18). It is twice as common in boys, bilateral in up to 50% and has a familial predisposition. Unaffected parents with an affected son have a 1:40 chance of having another son with the disorder. The pathogenesis is unknown.

Clinically the hindfoot is in equinus and varus (inversion) and the heel is difficult to feel. The forefoot is adducted and plantarflexed on the hindfoot giving a cavus or high arched appearance, and there is a deep transverse skin crease on the medial border of the foot. Internal tibial torsion is present and the foot and calf are often smaller than the opposite side. The navicular is medially displaced on the head of the talus. Passive correction to a neutral position is not possible.

A complete examination of the child is indicated to rule out potential neurological causes and associated conditions including DDH. Assessment of the severity and rigidity of the deformity at birth is difficult but helpful in determining the likely success of nonoperative treatment such as serial manipulation or casting versus the need for operative surgical correction. According to Harrold and Walker in 1983, if the foot can be passively returned to neutral, conservative treatment can be expected to be successful in 90%.[20] If fixed equinus is 0–20°degrees conservative treatment can be expected to succeed in 50% of cases; but if fixed equinus is more than 20° conservative treatment can only be expected to be successful in 10%.[20]

More recently a serial manipulation and casting technique described by Ignacio Ponseti[21] has become the preferred method of management in many centers. Results indicate a higher success rate for this nonoperative management technique, even in feet that are quite stiff from the outset. Children should be referred soon after delivery so that treatment can begin early. The technique involves a specific series of manipulative maneuvers to correct the underlying deformity followed by the application of a series of holding casts which are changed weekly. Typically after about six cast changes the forefoot and hindfoot are corrected but the foot remains in equinus. A percutaneous Achilles tenotomy is often necessary at this stage to allow correction of the equinus, followed by the application of the final cast which holds the position. The final cast is usually removed about 3–6 weeks later and thereafter the child must wear 'Denis Browne' boots and bar . This consists of boots that are connected by an adjustable bar holding the feet in external rotation, eversion and dorsiflexion. It is important for the success of the method that the patient and family comply with the proper use of this holding device. In the typical program the patient must wear the boots and bar continuously for 3 months following removal of the last holding cast and then for night time and naps for a further 3–4 years.

Although the Ponseti technique has changed the management of CTEV, some cases do not respond favorably and require surgical intervention although this is often less invasive than previously. It is important to warn parents of this potential from the outset and also to explain that some very resistant cases still require a more traditional surgical management. Recurrence of deformity is always a concern during the management of CTEV treated by any means and secondary surgery to correct recurring deformity, especially forefoot varus, is not uncommon. Sometimes repeated recurrence occurs in spite of secondary operations: this can be successfully managed using Ilizarov external fixator techniques.

Congenital vertical talus

This is a rigid foot deformity that presents clinically as a 'rocker bottom' foot. In about 50%[22] the condition is associated with other congenital neuromuscular and genetic disorders like neural tube defects and arthrogryposis. The head of the talus is dislocated from its normal articulation with the navicular and takes on a more vertical position. Diagnosis is made with a lateral radiograph and the foot stressed into maximal plantarflexion. If the navicular remains dorsally dislocated on the talus, the diagnosis is confirmed (Fig. 29.19).

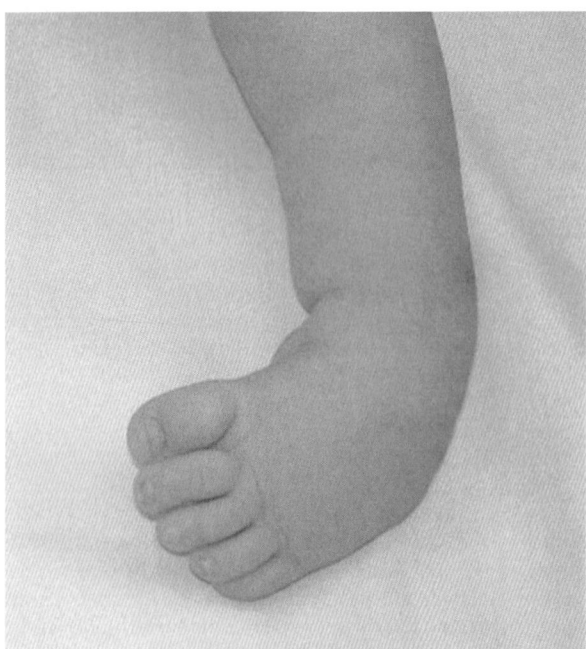

Fig. 29.18   Congenital talipes equinovarus.

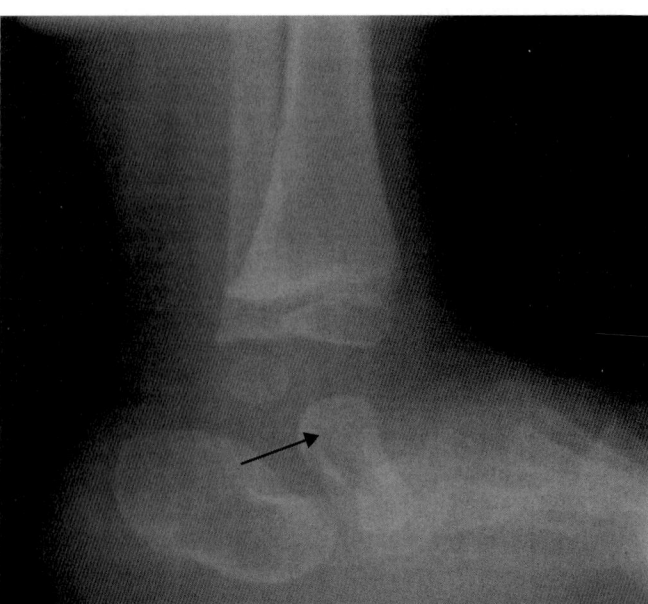

Fig. 29.19   Congenital vertical talus.

In addition to the vertical position of the talus and the tight anterior structures causing dorsal dislocation of the forefoot, the posterior structures are also tight resulting in fixed equinus of the hindfoot as in CTEV. The hindfoot and forefoot are therefore essentially broken over the vertically disposed talus giving the foot the characteristic 'rocker bottom' in severe cases.

Initial treatment is directed toward passive stretching and splinting of the foot into plantarflexion to stretch the tight anterior structures. Surgery is frequently necessary later to lengthen the tight anterior and posterior structures and to restore the normal alignment and relationship of the talus with the other bones of the foot. Favorable results are emerging with a modification of the Ponseti technique used in CTEV.[23]

INHERITED DISORDERS OF BONES AND JOINTS

Inherited disorders of bones and joints are a rare but important source of diagnostic confusion for the unwary as they may be easily confused with other disorders such as juvenile arthritis and Perthes disease. Most present with some combination of joint swelling or deformity; joint hypermobility or stiffness; and short stature. An awareness of these conditions will enable the correct diagnosis to be made, ensuring appropriate advice and genetic counseling is given.

This section is not intended to be an exhaustive review of a very complex area but describes some of the more common primary genetic disorders of bones and connective tissues, as well as identifying other genetic disorders in which bone and joint problems are a dominant feature. Many of these primary disorders of bones and connective tissues have been associated with identifiable genetic defects, particularly of the collagen genes. As these genetic defects are increasingly delineated it seems likely that the classification of these conditions will continually be updated and improved.[24,25]

HYPERMOBILITY

Joint mobility follows a normal distribution in the population and is influenced by factors including age, sex and ethnicity. Infants and young children have joints that are more mobile than older children and adults but there are no good studies defining normal joint ranges in the very young. Females have a greater degree of joint laxity than males and hypermobile joints are much more common in certain ethnic groups, e.g. oriental. Hypermobility of the joints may be generalized or affect only one or two joints. Generalized joint hypermobility may occur as an isolated entity or as part of a number of well-recognized genetic syndromes.

The definition of hypermobility is based on clinical assessment. The criteria most frequently used are those defined by Beighton[26] which assess joint laxity based on a number of clinical maneuvers:

1. passive dorsiflexion of the 5th metacarpophalangeal joint to 90°;
2. apposition of the thumb to the flexor aspect of the forearm (Fig. 29.20a);
3. hyperextension of the elbow to greater than 10° (Fig. 29.20b);
4. hyperextension of the knee to greater than 10°;
5. forward flexion of the trunk to place the palms of the hands flat on the floor with the knees extended.

Those experienced in examining children will immediately realize that these measurements are not appropriate in the very young in whom these degrees of joint laxity are normal. There is a need to define age-related normal values but the Beighton scoring system has been shown to be valid in children over the age of 4 years when interpreted correctly.[27] More recently revised criteria have been developed[28] but have not been extensively used or validated in pediatric practice .

Benign hypermobility syndrome

Joint hypermobility is a normal variant and causes no symptoms in most individuals. In others it is associated with a variety of musculoskeletal symptoms as part of the 'benign joint hypermobility syndrome'(BJHS).[29] Although labeled 'benign', affected individuals may have troublesome symptoms with significant morbidity and it may be impossible to differentiate from the milder variants of some of the genetic disorders such as Ehlers–Danlos syndrome.

BJHS occurs more commonly in females than in males and appears to have an autosomal dominant mode of inheritance. Affected children may have a variety of symptoms including arthralgia, joint effusions, widespread muscle pain, low back pain, flat feet and recurrent dislocations with many reporting significant functional difficulties.[30] Young children with hypermobility should be carefully assessed for associated coordination or proprioceptive difficulties which may contribute to their symptoms. Recurrent sports injuries, back pain and an increase in chronic musculoskeletal pain are reported in older children and adolescents with BJHS.

Despite much interest, the association between hypermobility and symptoms remains poorly understood.[31] Many hypermobile individuals remain asymptomatic while others have significant symptoms. Management consists of explanation of the condition, multidisciplinary input from physiotherapy, occupational therapy and podiatry together with appropriate pain management if required.

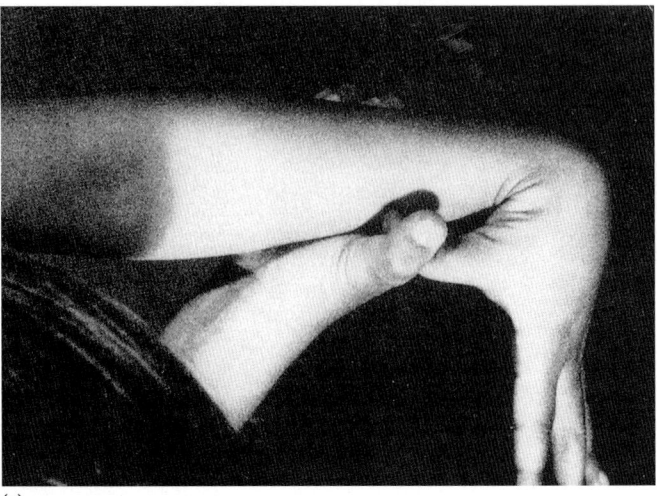

(a)

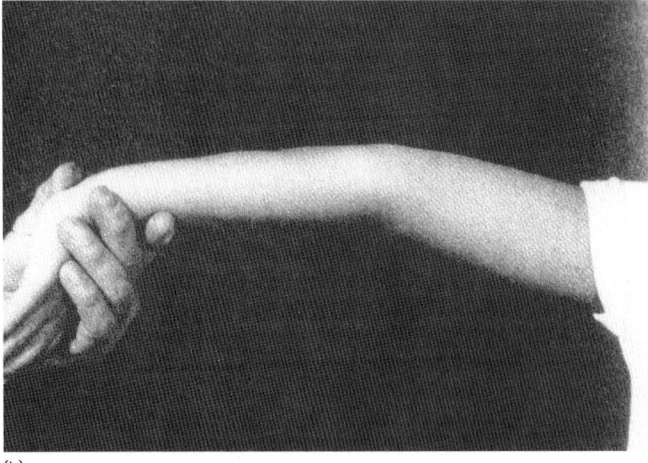

(b)

Fig. 29.20 Hypermobility: (a) apposition of the thumb to the flexor aspect of the forearm; (b) hyperextension of the elbow to greater than 10°.

INHERITED SYNDROMES WITH SIGNIFICANT HYPERMOBILITY

Ehlers–Danlos syndrome

Ehlers–Danlos syndrome (EDS) consists of a group of disorders of connective tissue characterized by joint hypermobility plus fragility and laxity of the skin and other tissues. These conditions are characterized by abnormalities in collagen genes resulting in the production of abnormal collagens III and V and consequent tissue fragility. They vary both in severity and mode of inheritance and an accurate diagnosis is essential if patients are to be offered appropriate advice and counseling.

Over the years, 11 different types of Ehlers–Danlos syndrome have been described. A revised, simplified classification was agreed in 1997[32] with three major types being defined clinically. Although further refinement will occur this classification has been widely accepted and is helpful clinically and prognostically in clearly distinguishing between the vascular, potentially catastrophic, form of the condition and the others. The three major types are defined as follows.

1. 'Classical' EDS (previously types I and II): characterized by the classical skin hyperextensibility and associated joint hypermobility. In many cases this results from abnormalities of the COL5A1 and A2 genes.
2. Hypermobility EDS (previously type III): characterized predominantly by joint hypermobility and very difficult to distinguish from BJHS.
3. Vascular EDS (previously type IV): associated with vascular, intestinal and uterine rupture. This results from mutations in the COL3A1 gene which causes production of abnormal type III collagen. Although the inheritance is autosomal dominant, approximately one third are new mutations. The diagnosis can be confirmed by collagen studies of cultured dermal fibroblasts.

Marfan syndrome

Marfan syndrome, also an inherited disorder of connective tissue, affects approximately 1 in 10 000 of the population. Inherited as an autosomal dominant trait it results from mutations in the genes encoding for the glycoprotein fibrillin, a component of elastin fibrils in the extracellular matrix.[33]

Marfan syndrome is characterized by tall stature, long extremities, fingers and feet, chest deformities, high arched palate and ocular abnormalities including lens dislocation. Joint hypermobility, although not diagnostic, is recognized frequently and there is a high incidence of spinal problems with the development of both scolioses and kyphoses. Mitral valve prolapse is common. Aortic valve disease and a tendency to sudden aortic rupture are of major concern.

Many individuals are only mildly affected and the diagnosis can be difficult. Diagnostic criteria are currently based on clinical features[34] but recent reports suggest that this can now be supported by molecular analysis.[35]

Individuals with type 1 homocystinuria may have tall stature, a high arched palate and resemble Marfan syndrome. Hypotonia occurs but the joints are stiff rather than hypermobile. Severe osteoporosis and mental retardation are characteristic.

Osteogenesis imperfecta

Osteogenesis imperfecta (OI) is a group of autosomal dominantly inherited collagen gene disorders typified by bone fragility and often associated with joint hypermobility.[36] The underlying defect in these conditions lies in the genes COL1A1 and COL1A2[37] which encode the peptide chains of type I collagen, the major structural protein of bone, ligament and tendon. Clinically the important features are those of an inherited osteoporosis. Radiological appearances range from mild osteoporosis with occasional fractures to a widespread skeletal abnormality with multiple fractures. In its most severe form, OI may be lethal in utero.

Types I and IV OI are the mildest forms of the condition, presenting with recurrent fractures in infancy and childhood (Fig. 29.21). Spinal involvement results in short stature which may be marked. There is a

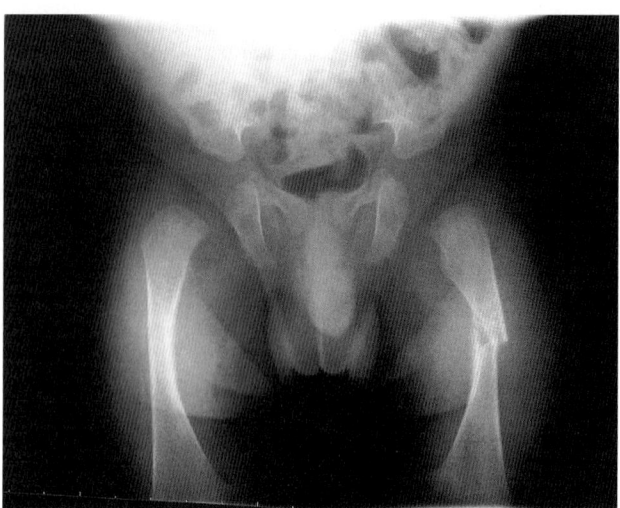

Fig. 29.21   Osteogenesis imperfecta type I.

tendency for the fracture rate to reduce after adolescence but become more severe again in later adult life. Type I is distinguished by the presence of the characteristic blue sclerae. Associated dentinogenesis imperfecta and joint laxity occur with variable frequency.

Type II OI is a severe, crippling and frequently lethal disease. Multiple intrauterine fractures occur and early death results from chest infections and pulmonary restriction caused by the widespread fractures. Type III (Fig. 29.22) is the most severe nonlethal form causing severe bone fragility with marked joint hypermobility. Survivors of infancy are usually significantly disabled.

Until recently there has been no treatment for individuals with OI other than appropriate orthopedic management of fractures and supportive care. Expert physiotherapy and orthopedic input remain critical to optimal management of these children. The development of the bisphosphonate group of drugs offers new possibilities for treatment. Cyclical treatment with intravenous pamidronate has been shown to result in reduced bone pain, a significant increase in bone density, a

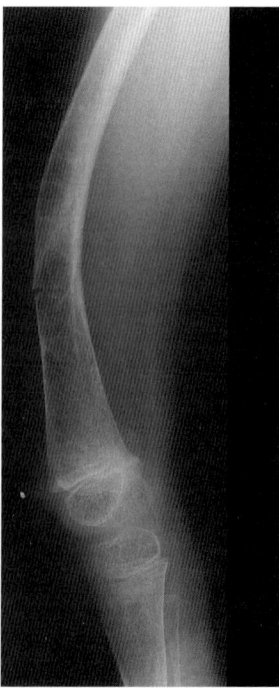

Fig. 29.22   Osteogenesis imperfecta type III showing recent fracture, severe osteoporosis and femoral deformity.

decreased number of fractures and an improved quality of life in many.[38] The role of oral bisphosphates remains unclear.

Stickler syndrome

Stickler syndrome is an inherited disorder of connective tissues characterized by a typical facies with midface hypoplasia, high myopia with early onset, progressive hearing loss and arthropathy. Joint problems include both generalized joint hypermobility and early degenerative joint disease. Retinal detachment is a serious complication. Type I Stickler syndrome, the majority, has been associated with mutations in the COL2A1 gene encoding type II collagen and diagnostic criteria based on clinical features plus genetic confirmation have been developed.[39]

INHERITED SKELETAL DYSPLASIAS

Spondyloepiphyseal dysplasia (SED)

The spondyloepiphyseal dysplasias consist of a group of heritable disorders principally involving the spine and the epiphyses of the long bones. Several forms are described of varying severity. Type II collagen is the main protein component of articular cartilage and mutations of the COL2A1 gene are thought to result not only in the already mentioned Stickler syndrome but also in a number of other disorders including the spondyloepiphyseal dysplasias.

SED congenita is an autosomal dominant condition with its onset at birth. Affected children may have delay in walking, a waddling gait and short stature. Limitation of range of motion affects elbows, knees and hips. Radiological investigation shows flattening of the vertebrae (Fig. 29.23) and coxa vara.

SED tarda results in symptoms which seldom present before adolescence. Although usually X-linked recessive, autosomal recessive and dominant forms have also been described. Spinal and hip involvement occur and the course is usually benign. Early onset of osteoarthritis occurs in adult life.

Progressive pseudorheumatoid arthropathy is a variant of SED (Fig. 29.24) which presents between 3 and 11 years of age with painful, swollen joints especially affecting the hands. Progressive joint contractures and short stature develop and the condition is unresponsive to standard antiinflammatory medication.

Multiple epiphyseal dysplasia

This is one of the more common skeletal dysplasias and is inherited as an autosomal dominant trait. It presents in childhood with pain and stiffness, usually progressing to joint contractures and associated short stature. At first sight it may be confused with juvenile arthritis, but the absence of signs and symptoms of inflammation can distinguish the two. Radiology demonstrates irregularities of the end-plates of the mid-thoracic vertebral bodies, shortening of the metacarpals and flattening, sclerosis and fragmentation of the epiphyses at the hips and knees (Fig. 29.25).

Achondroplasia and hypochondroplasia

These disorders result from mutations of fibroblast growth factor receptor 3 (FGFR3) genes. Although inherited as an autosomal dominant trait, most cases of achondroplasia occur as new mutations. The classic form of achondroplasia causes severe disproportionate short stature. Affected individuals have normal or large heads with shortening of the limbs and an increased lumbar lordosis. The pedicles of the vertebrae are short which may lead to symptomatic spinal stenosis in adult life. Hypochondroplasia is a milder form resulting from different mutations in the FGFR3 gene.

Trichorhinophalangeal dysplasia

This autosomal dominant disorder results from the deletion of multiple genes on chromosome 8. It is characterized by enlargement of the interphalangeal joints with characteristic facial features: a bulbous nose, hyperplastic nares, sparse, brittle hair and short stature.

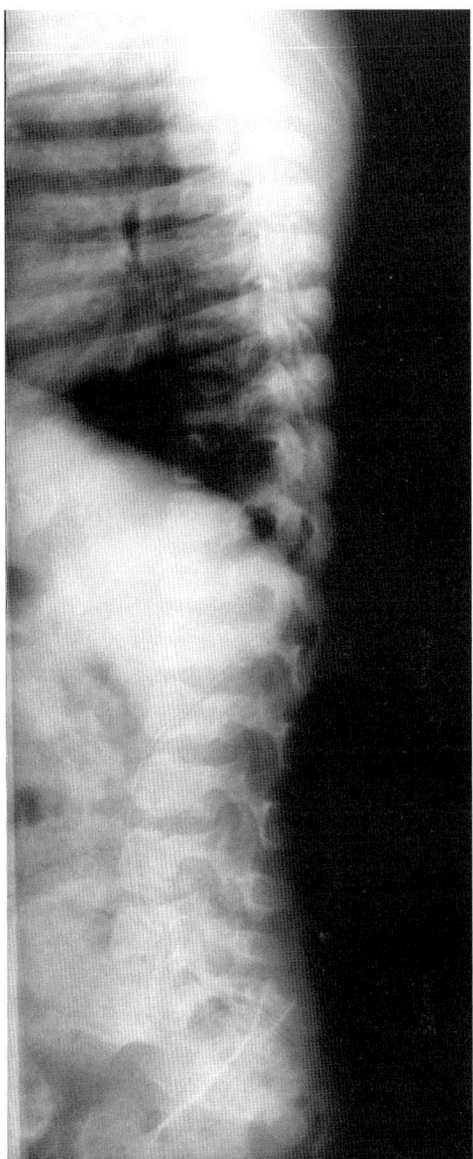

Fig. 29.23 Spondyloepiphyseal dysplasia congenita showing abnormal vertebrae.

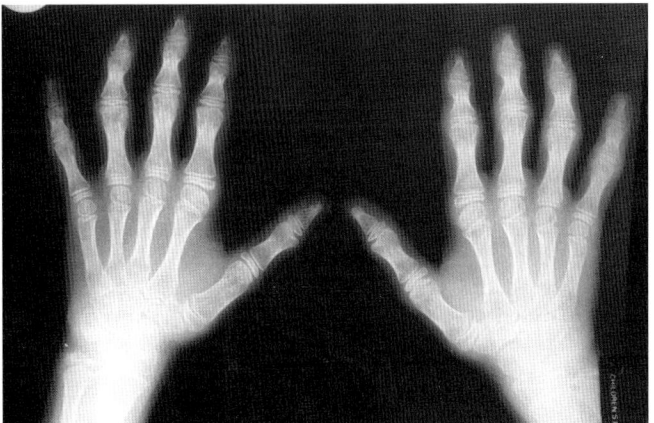

Fig. 29.24 Spondyloepiphyseal dysplasia tarda (progressive pseudorheumatoid arthropathy) affecting hands with obvious swelling of joints and bulbous ends to the phalanges.

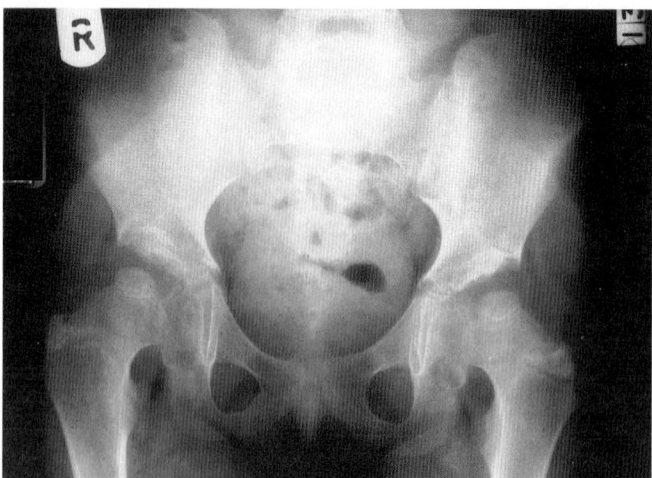

Fig. 29.25 Multiple epiphyseal dysplasia with bilateral hip involvement.

Radiographic features include cone-shaped epiphyses with short metacarpals and metatarsals plus fragmentation of the epiphyses. Fragmentation of the femoral epiphyses may cause confusion with Perthes disease.

Storage disorders: the mucopolysaccharidoses (MPS)

The MPS are genetically determined deficiencies of enzymes involved in the metabolism of glycosaminoglycans. All are inherited as autosomal dominant conditions and a prominent feature of most is a skeletal dysplasia affecting particularly the hands, feet and vertebrae and which may be the presenting feature. In the milder forms such as Scheie and Morquio syndromes the joint problems may dominate the clinical picture. In the more severe forms such as Hurler syndrome the characteristic coarsening of the facial features is striking but may be preceded by flexion deformities of the fingers.

An awareness that these conditions may present with skeletal symptoms will enable their early recognition, allowing appropriate genetic advice and counseling. For more detail see Chapter 26.

OTHER INHERITED DISORDERS PRIMARILY AFFECTING THE MUSCULOSKELETAL SYSTEM

There are many other inherited disorders that primarily affect the musculoskeletal system and are currently difficult to categorize.

Osteopetrosis

This is a rare disorder resulting in frontal bossing, hypertelorism, exophthalmos and nasal obstruction which may be present from birth. It progresses during early childhood resulting in severe bleeding problems, recurrent fractures and early death. The disease is characterized by an increased density of the bones with metaphyseal flaring. Bone marrow transplantation may offer a cure.

Arthrogryposis

This refers to a number of disorders characterized by multiple congenital contractures.

Ollier disease

Ollier disease or multiple enchondromatosis becomes apparent during childhood when it presents with multiple juxta-articular outgrowths.

Idiopathic acro-osteolysis

This is inherited as an autosomal dominant trait and generally presents around 3 years with bony lysis which may affect the carpus or tarsus alone or occur in a more widespread pattern. The condition may

mimic juvenile arthritis in that affected areas are warm and swollen. Radiographs show progressive bone lysis and destruction of affected joints.

Fibrodysplasia ossificans progressiva (FOP)

FOP is a rare autosomal dominant condition now known to result from dysregulation of the BMP-4 signaling pathway.[40] Painful inflammation of muscles and fascia, often triggered by minor trauma, is rapidly followed by fibrosis and calcification and the child presents with swelling in a muscle or the development of a contracture. Radiographs will show calcification in, and eventually ossification of, the muscles (Fig. 29.26a). The condition is characterized by congenitally short great toes (Fig. 29.26b), and sometimes thumbs, which may be diagnostic. The disease progresses to severe disability and to date no treatment has been shown to influence the natural disease progression.

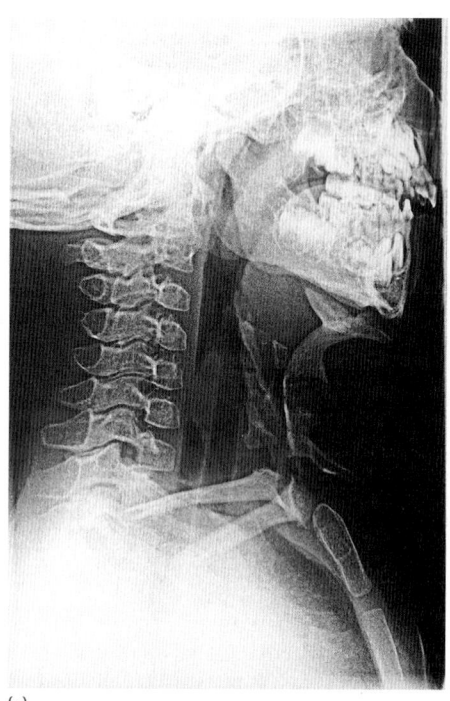

(a)

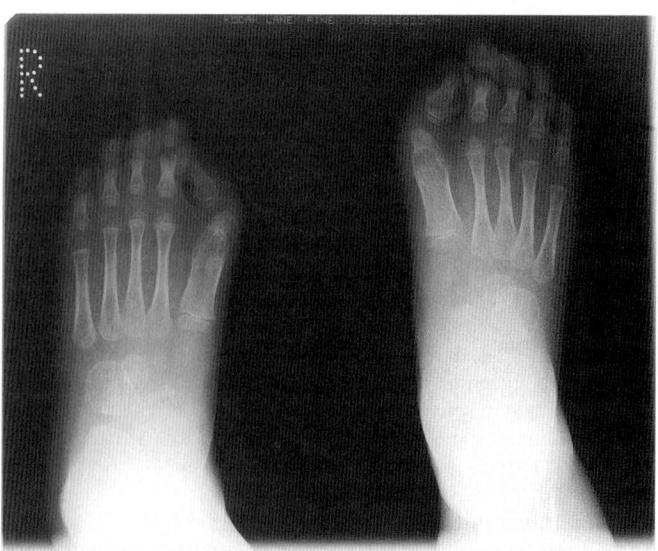

(b)

Fig. 29.26 Fibrodysplasia ossificans progressiva showing (a) ossification of anterior neck muscles and (b) dysplastic great toes.

OTHER INHERITED DISORDERS ASSOCIATED WITH MUSCULOSKELETAL PROBLEMS

Many inherited conditions may result in musculoskeletal problems. Some of the more important are outlined here. All are covered in more detail in other relevant chapters.

Down syndrome (trisomy 21)

Down syndrome is associated with a variety of musculoskeletal problems. In infancy generalized muscular hypotonicity may be striking and many affected individuals remain significantly hypermobile with associated symptoms. Atlantoaxial instability is of major concern. An inflammatory arthropathy of unknown cause is well recognized in affected children.

Velocardiofacial syndrome (22q11 deletion syndrome)

This syndrome is a common cause of congenital cardiac malformations and is associated with a variety of immunological abnormalities, particularly impairment of T cell function. Perhaps as a consequence of this it is now known to be associated with an inflammatory arthritis.[41]

Cystic fibrosis (CF)

Many individuals with CF have arthralgias which may be troublesome but are not associated with any serious joint pathology. A few develop a recurrent acute arthropathy which can be extremely painful and distressing. Although the exact pathology is unclear it seems likely that this results from immune complex deposition and the cutaneous vasculitis that may occur is presumed to have a similar mechanism. Nonsteroidal anti-inflammatory drugs may be inadequate to control these acute symptoms and short courses of oral steroids may be helpful. In severe longstanding cystic fibrosis, hypertrophic pulmonary osteoarthropathy may develop as a cause for joint pain and swelling and should be considered in an individual with marked clubbing of the fingers and severe pulmonary disease. Plain radiography will demonstrate the characteristic periosteal reaction.

Hemophilia

Hemophilia has previously been complicated by a destructive arthritis occurring as a consequence of recurrent intraarticular bleeds. It is a tribute to advances in care in hemophilia and the use of prophylactic factor VIII that chronic hemophilic arthropathy is now seldom seen in resource rich countries. Hemophilia must still be remembered in the differential diagnosis of a young boy presenting for the first time with a tense joint effusion. Joint aspiration demonstrates blood and abnormal coagulation will be found.

Metabolic bone disease

Rickets usually presents with bone pain and bowing of the long bones. The most common cause is vitamin D deficiency (Fig. 29.27), but rickets may also result from a number of inherited disorders. Hypophosphatemic or vitamin D resistant rickets may be inherited as either an X-linked recessive or an autosomal disorder and is characterized by impaired parathormone-dependent proximal renal tubular reabsorption of phosphate. Hypophosphatasia is a rare autosomal recessive disorder characterized by severe rickets and reduced serum levels of alkaline phosphatase.

Gout

Gout may result from either an increased production or a decreased excretion of urate and is extremely rare in childhood. It may result from a number of inherited disorders of purine metabolism; of these, familial juvenile hyperuricemic nephropathy is the most common.[42]

Periodic fever syndromes

Familial Mediterranean fever (FMF) and other periodic fever syndromes may result in musculoskeletal symptoms including myalgia, arthralgia

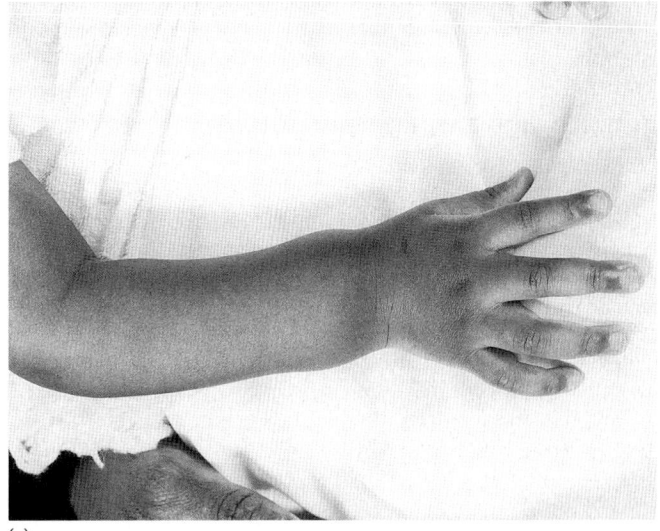

(a)

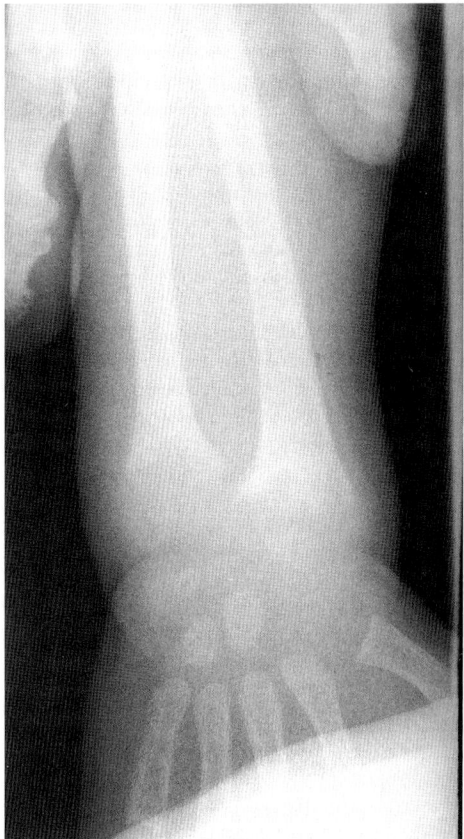

(b)

Fig. 29.27 Dietary rickets in a breast-fed toddler: (a) clinical appearance; (b) radiological features with characteristic metaphyseal fraying.

and arthritis. These conditions are described in more detail in the section on the 'The differential diagnosis of systemic inflammatory disorders' (see p.1434).

INFECTION IN BONES AND JOINTS

Bone and joint infections are relatively rare disorders in children, but may be associated with considerable skeletal morbidity and potential mortality unless rapidly recognized and adequately treated. A multidisciplinary approach to diagnosis and management, with close collaboration between physician, orthopedic surgeon, microbiologist and radiologist, is necessary for optimal management and outcome.

OSTEOMYELITIS AND SEPTIC ARTHRITIS

Frequently the result of hematogenous seeding of bacteria, osteomyelitis may also result from extension of local sepsis, iatrogenic inoculation (rare) or trauma. In osteomyelitis the vascular-rich metaphyses of long bones or vertebral bodies are the commonest sites involved. Fever and pain are frequent symptoms and the differential diagnosis includes trauma, rheumatic fever, septic arthritis, soft tissue infection, rheumatic disease (e.g. juvenile idiopathic arthritis), bone infarction secondary to hemoglobinopathy, leukemia and bony neoplasm.[43] Osteomyelitis may be acute, subacute or chronic. Subacute osteomyelitis has a longer duration than acute and tends to result from infection with less virulent organisms. Chronic osteomyelitis may result from failure to identify or ineffective treatment of acute osteomyelitis.

In neonates the clinical features may be nonspecific and include poor feeding, irritability and poor temperature control. An affected limb may become erythematous, tender and swollen, and there may be a paucity of spontaneous movement ('pseudo-paralysis'). Concomitant septicemia is commoner in this age group. In older children the features tend to be more localized when the peripheral skeleton is affected, but less so in the pelvis or spine.

As with osteomyelitis, the majority of cases of septic arthritis occur as a result of hematogenous seeding of the synovium during an episode of bacteraemia. Septic arthritis occasionally arises from contiguous spread from adjacent osteomyelitis, especially in the younger child in whom the metaphyseal–epiphyseal junction lies adjacent to the joint space.[44]

A septic joint will exhibit the classic features of inflammation: swelling, pain, warmth and erythema. An affected hip is held in flexion and external rotation for comfort; a knee in flexion. All passive movement will be resisted. The hip warrants specific consideration, as increased intracapsular pressure arising from septic arthritis may interrupt blood supply and lead to avascular necrosis of the femoral head.

Fever, malaise and anorexia are usually seen, and progression of symptoms is often rapid. In neonates, as with osteomyelitis, features may be nonspecific. Children with immunodeficiency states, including those on systemic corticosteroid therapy, should be evaluated with great care as clinical signs of inflammation may be masked.

The differential diagnosis includes traumatic effusion, hemarthrosis, transient synovitis, reactive arthritis, JIA, Lyme arthritis, malignant disease, slipper upper femoral epiphysis and Perthes disease. Local spread of infection may result in pyomyositis.

Laboratory investigations

The full blood count may reveal thrombocytosis and neutrophil leucocytosis. Erythrocyte sedimentation rate (ESR) and C-reactive protein (CRP) are both likely to be elevated, the CRP tending to mirror the course of the infection more closely.[45]

Radiological investigations

Plain radiographs remain the primary initial imaging modality for suspected skeletal infections. In osteomyelitis soft tissue swelling and a periosteal reaction may be seen within a few days. Bony changes develop later (Fig. 29.28). In septic arthritis the early features are osteopenia of the epiphysis, increased joint space and soft tissue swelling (Fig. 29.29). Later in the disease destructive changes occur (Fig. 29.30).

Radionuclide bone scanning is sensitive at detecting areas of increased uptake, and may reveal multiple foci within the skeleton. However the specificity of this method is low and the features may not distinguish septic from nonseptic inflammatory lesions.

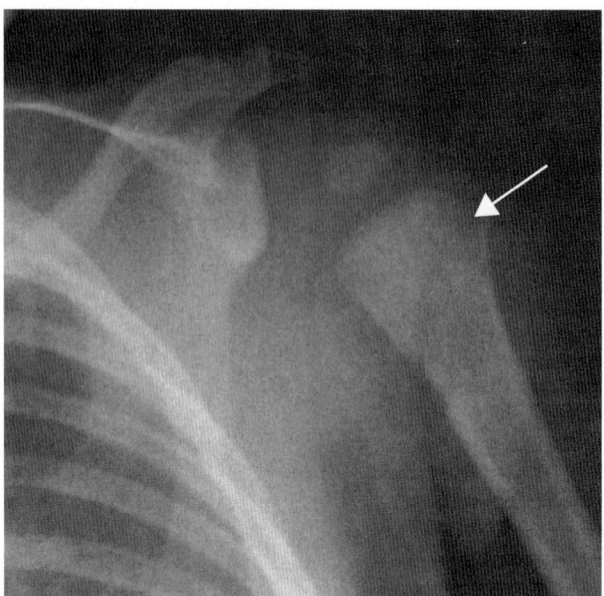

Fig. 29.28   Osteomyelitis of proximal humerus – 'moth eaten' appearance of bone and periosteal reaction.

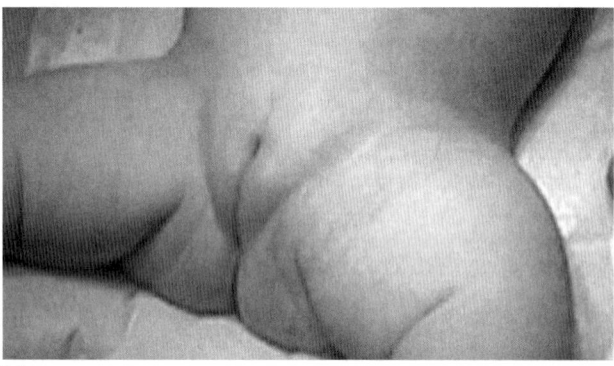

(a)

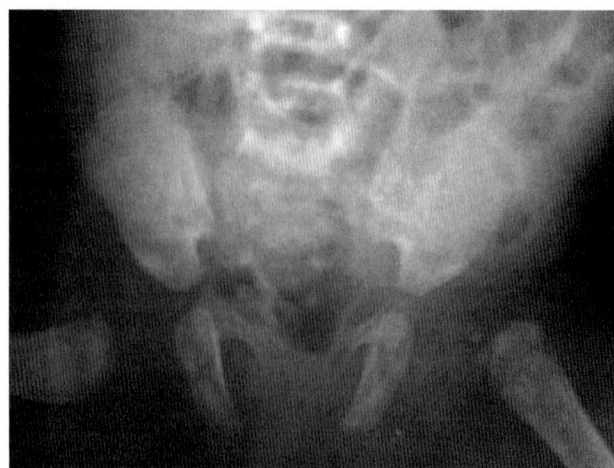

(b)

Fig. 29.29   Septic arthritis of the hip: (a) soft tissue swelling of thigh; (b) subluxation of the hip.

Ultrasound (US) is a rapidly available and sensitive method for detecting effusions in the hip. Magnetic resonance (MR) imaging plays a particular role because of excellent delineation of anatomy including soft tissues and bone. T1-weighted fat-suppressed postcontrast images are recommended in both osteomyelitis and septic arthritis.

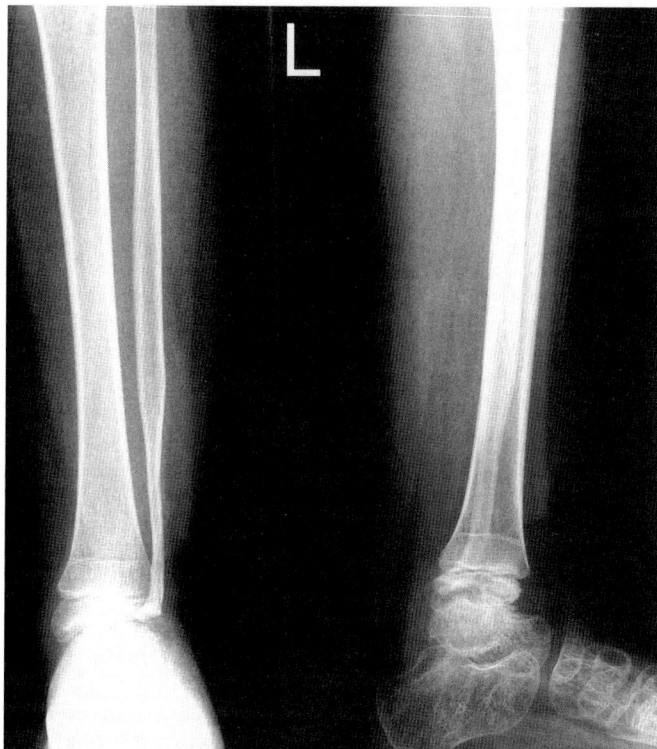

Fig. 29.30 Damage to ankle joint and distal fibula following disseminated staphylococcal sepsis with septic arthritis and osteomyelitis.

Microbiological investigations

Isolation of the infecting organism will allow targetting of appropriate antibiotic therapy, so vigorous microbiological investigation is mandatory. Peripheral blood cultures must be taken. The suspicion of septic arthritis should prompt microbiological analysis of synovial fluid, with joint aspiration also helping to relieve pain. Typical synovial fluid features on microscopy and a comparison with noninfective inflammatory arthritis are shown in Table 29.4.[46] Bone biopsy may reveal the organism in osteomyelitis.

Approximately 75% of bone and joint infection in resource rich countries is currently caused by *Staphylococcus aureus*[47] and the primary source of the infection is rarely clear. The introduction of vaccination against *Haemophilus influenzae* type b (Hib) has virtually eliminated the incidence of septic arthritis caused by this organism in countries where the vaccination is available. In neonates Group B *Streptococcus* and Gram negative enteric bacteria are relatively common cause of skeletal infection. Group A beta-hemolytic streptococci (*Streptococcus pyogenes*) and *Streptococcus pneumoniae* are important causes at all ages. *Kingella kingae* skeletal infections are increasingly recognized and reported, especially in younger children and frequently after upper respiratory tract infections.[48]

Table 29.4 Comparison of synovial fluid analysis in children with infective and inflammatory arthritis. (Adapted from Shetty & Gedalia 1998[46])

Characteristic	Normal	Juvenile idiopathic arthritis	Septic arthritis
Color	Yellow	Yellow	Serosanguinous
Clarity	Clear	Cloudy	Turbid
WBC count/mm³	<200	$15–20 \times 10^3$	$40–300\,000 \times 10^3$
PMN count (%)	<25	60–75	>75

PMN, polymorphic neutrophil; WBC, white blood cell

Tuberculous arthritis is insidious in onset, and there is a tendency to sinus formation. If tuberculosis is suspected, synovial fluid and biopsy of synovial tissue should be sent for specific culture and also for analysis by the polymerase chain reaction (PCR). A Mantoux test should be performed. Gonococcal arthritis must be considered in the adolescent presenting systemically unwell with a very acute arthropathy. Brucellosis and infection with *Mycoplasma pneumoniae* may both cause a low grade septic arthritis.

In the immunocompromised, Gram negative organisms, fungi or atypical mycobacteria need to be considered. Children with hemoglobinopathies are at increased risk of acute recurrent osteomyelitis with Gram negative bacteria such as *Salmonella*, *Shigella sonnei*, *Escherichia coli* and *Serratia* species.

Treatment

Initial therapy is with empirical intravenous antibiotics for both osteomyelitis and septic arthritis. With concomitant septicemia supportive management on the neonatal or pediatric intensive care unit may be necessary.

The septic hip should be drained surgically to relieve pressure in the joint and minimize the risk of subsequent avascular necrosis. Surgical intervention is not always necessary in osteomyelitis[47] but may facilitate microbiological diagnosis. Subperiosteal or soft tissue abscesses and necrotic bone sequestra may need drainage.

The choice of antibiotic will depend upon the clinical context and local guidelines, but in the child with previously normal immune function must include adequate staphylococcal cover. Local incidence of methicillin-resistant *S. aureus* (MRSA) will determine whether antibiotic therapy should cover this possibility, and guidance from an expert microbiologist should be sought. Cefotaxime should be added if the child is not immunized against *Haemophilus influenzae*. A summary of empirical antibiotic therapy, by age, in an immunocompetent child is shown in Table 29.5.

In the immunocompromised, flucloxacillin plus cefotaxime are first line agents to provide adequate Gram positive and Gram negative cover. In the penicillin-allergic child cefradine is an alternative; with cephalosporin allergy vancomycin should be considered. Cefotaxime or ciprofloxacin may be used in *Salmonella* osteomyelitis.[47]

The duration of antibiotic therapy is controversial. There has been a move toward greater use of oral antibiotics beyond the initial stages of treatment in recent years. Intravenous antibiotic therapy should be continued for a minimum of 3 days, and then switched to oral for 3–4 weeks if fever has settled.[49] Switch to oral antibiotics should only be when the clinical condition of the child has improved, the fever has settled and the CRP is falling. Intravenous administration of antibiotics for longer periods is necessary in the immunocompromised or neonate.

Outcome

With early recognition of the diagnosis and prompt treatment, the long term outcome of skeletal sepsis in children is good. Growth disturbance may follow if the epiphysis has been involved and these children will require prolonged follow-up. In the minority with articular damage permanent impairment of joint function and early osteoarthritis may ensue (Fig. 29.30). Inadequate or ineffective treatment of acute osteomyelitis may result in chronic osteomyelitis with necrosis and sequestration of the bone.

DISCITIS

Infection in the intervertebral disc is a condition related to osteomyelitis, with infection arising from the vertebral end-plates, but without resulting in osteomyelitis of the vertebral body. The condition is believed by many to be secondary to infection,[50] the organism most commonly responsible being *S. aureus*. It is considered by others to have a non-infective inflammatory pathogenesis.

Table 29.5 Guidelines for empirical parenteral antibiotic treatment of acute bacterial skeletal sepsis by age

Age	Antibiotic	Notes
Neonate	Cefotaxime and flucloxacillin	Alternative: flucloxacillin with gentamicin
Child < 5 years	Cefotaxime and flucloxacillin or cefuroxime	MRSA* use vancomycin and consider clindamycin if sensitive – beware resistance developing during treatment Flucloxacillin or cefradine monotherapy if methicillin sensitive *Staph. aureus*
Child > 5 years	Cefuroxime or flucloxacillin	MRSA* use vancomycin and *consider* clindamycin if sensitive – beware resistance developing during treatment Flucloxacillin or cefradine monotherapy if methicillin sensitive *Staph. aureus*

* MRSA: Expert microbiologist advice should be sought

The condition is more common in preschool age children and any disc may be involved. The most striking clinical feature is the refusal of the patient to flex the lumbar spine. The older child may have difficulty walking or limp, will have a stiff back and will complain of back pain associated with constitutional upset. The younger child will frequently refuse to walk, often spontaneously adopting a prone position with extension of the lumbar spine for comfort. Discomfort may be reported when the child is traveling in an infant car seat.

The blood picture reveals a leucocytosis and raised ESR. Blood culture is usually negative although *Staph. aureus* may be identified in some. Culture of disc tissue is rarely indicated and frequently negative. Radionuclide bone scanning may highlight a 'hot' spot in the region of a disc space. MRI will demonstrate clearly the inflammatory lesion within the disc (Fig. 29.31a). Plain radiographs eventually reveal disc space narrowing and varying vertebral end-plate damage (Fig. 29.31b).

Most children respond quickly to antibiotic therapy, initially intravenous and then oral, without the need for surgical intervention. Pain is managed symptomatically with analgesics and sometimes a short term removable brace to unload the involved disc. Therapy is usually continued for 6 weeks. Failure to respond after a week or deterioration in spite of treatment should raise concerns regarding the potential of an abscess requiring surgical drainage or an unusual organism such as tuberculosis. The prognosis of juvenile discitis is generally good with no significant long term sequelae in the majority.

VIRAL INFECTION AND ARTHRITIS

Arthralgia is a common symptom of viral infection. In some cases a true septic arthritis results, with virus particles being isolated in the joint fluid. In others arthritis occurs as a reactive process with no evidence of infection in the joint. *Rubella*, particularly 'natural infection' but also post vaccination, is associated with arthritis.[51] *Parvovirus B19* (slapped cheek syndrome or Fifth disease) is occasionally associated with arthritis similar to that of rubella. *Varicella* may be associated with a benign reactive arthritis, but is occasionally complicated by a potentially fatal syndrome of necrotizing fasciitis and toxic shock syndrome as a sequelae of concomitant *Group A streptococcus* infection.[52] *Paromyxovirus* (mumps), *adenovirus*, *ECHO virus* and *Coxsackie B* virus may all be associated with arthritis.

Infection with the human immunodeficiency virus may be associated with a variety of rheumatological problems. These include arthralgias, septic arthritis (frequently fungal in origin), reactive arthritis, Reiter syndrome and a seronegative spondyloarthropathy.

REACTIVE ARTHRITIS
Transient synovitis of the hip
See section on 'Common orthopedic problems in childhood', page 1434.

Reactive arthritis associated with bowel and genitourinary infections
In children, as in adults, a reactive arthritis may develop after enteric infections with *Salmonella*, *Shigella*, *Yersinia* and *Campylobacter*, and posturethritis with *Chlamydia* in sexually active adolescents. The HLA-B27 antigen is commonly identified. There is usually a peripheral, asymmetrical lower limb arthritis. There may be associated dactylitis ('sausage digit' resulting from inflammation of both joints and tendon sheaths), tenosynovitis and involvement of the sacroiliac joints. There is usually a history of enteritis or urethritis within the preceding 4 weeks. Reiter syndrome, a triad of arthritis, conjunctivitis and urethritis, is uncommon in children.

Treatment requires nonsteroidal anti-inflammatory drugs in adequate doses. Occasionally systemic steroids are required to settle an acute arthritis. If the arthritis becomes chronic, intra-articular steroids and second-line agents including sulphasalazine and methotrexate may be considered.

Rheumatic fever and poststreptococcal arthritis
(see Ch. 21)
Acute rheumatic fever remains prevalent in developing areas of the world. The disease arises as a complication of infection (pharyngotonsillitis) with *Group A beta-hemolytic Streptococcus pyogenes*. The modified Jones criteria are the basis for the diagnosis (Table 29.6).

Inflammation in various tissues may result in arthritis, carditis, a typical rash (erythema marginatum), subcutaneous nodules and a characteristic neurological syndrome, Sydenham chorea. Arthritis is a common clinical feature, tends to affect large joints and is flitting and self-limiting in nature. Erythema marginatum is an erythematous macular and nonpruritic lesion with serpiginous margins surrounding areas of normal skin. Sydenham chorea (also known as St Vitus dance) is caused by inflammation of the basal ganglia of the brain. It presents with involuntary movements of the extremities, muscular incoordination and emotional lability. Subcutaneous nodules may be seen on extensor surfaces of joints in the chronic phase of rheumatic heart disease. Rheumatic heart disease is discussed in more detail in Chapter 21.

Arthritis following Group A streptococcal infection is recognized in some children who do not fulfill the criteria for acute rheumatic fever. This poststreptococcal reactive arthritis differs from that of rheumatic fever in that it is nonmigratory and more persistent. As with rheumatic fever recurrent episodes are recognized.

Treatment of both rheumatic fever and poststreptococcal reactive arthritis involves antibiotics to eradicate the streptococcus. Penicillin V is the antibiotic of choice, and should be given as a 10-day course. In penicillin-allergic individuals, erythromycin is a suitable alternative. In rheumatic fever prophylaxis against streptococcal infection is indicated for at least 5 years after the initial attack, and into adulthood in patients with carditis.[53] There is no consensus regarding the use of prophylactic penicillin in those with poststreptococcal arthritis but if attacks are recurrent antibiotic prophylaxis may prove beneficial. Additional prophylaxis for surgical or dental procedures is necessary in the chronic stage of rheumatic heart disease (see Ch. 21).

In the acute illness nonsteroidal anti-inflammatory drugs (NSAIDs) may provide symptomatic relief from the arthritis. Steroids are reserved for patients with pancarditis associated with congestive cardiac failure.

Lyme disease
The infectious spirochaete *Borrelia burgdorferi*, transmitted by the tick *Ixodes*, is responsible for Lyme disease. The regions where Lyme

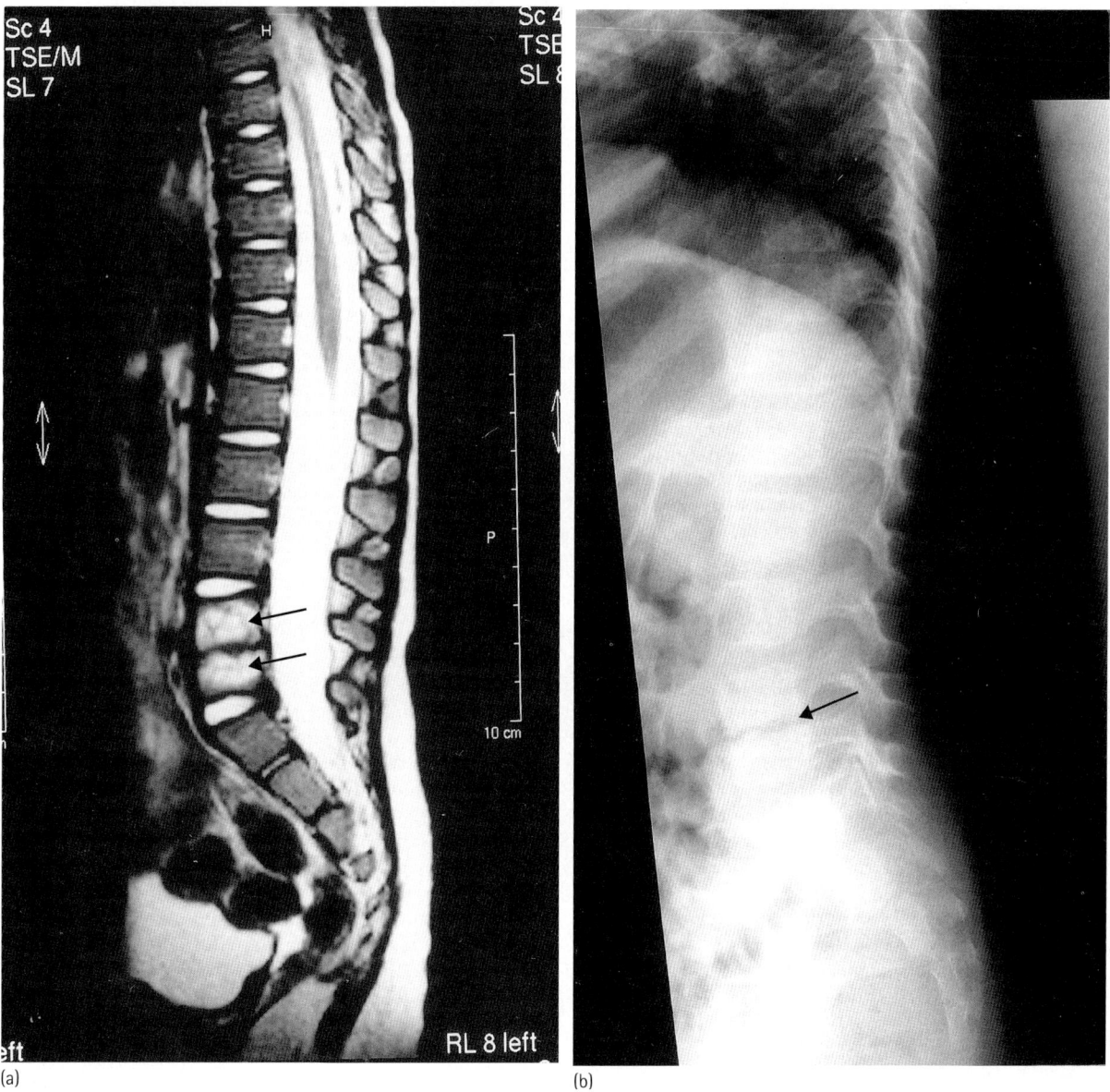

(a) (b)

Fig. 29.31 (a) MRI in discitis – abnormal signal in the L4 and L5 vertebral bodies with destruction of the intervening disc space; (b) plain radiograph showing narrowing of L4/5 disc space following resolution of acute illness.

Table 29.6 Modified Jones criteria for the diagnosis of rheumatic fever

Major criteria	Minor criteria
Polyarthritis common: flitting, large joints	Fever
Carditis common: pancarditis	Arthralgia
Chorea (Sydenham) uncommon: persistent	Prolonged P-R interval
Erythema marginatum uncommon: macules evolving to serpiginous	Elevated ESR/CRP, leucocytosis
Subcutaneous nodules uncommon: extensor surfaces	Previous rheumatic fever

The diagnosis of rheumatic fever is made in the presence of either two major criteria or one major plus two minor criteria together with evidence of recent group A streptococcal infection (positive throat swab, elevated antistreptolysin O titer (ASOT) or other antistreptococcal antibodies).

disease is seen most frequently are central Europe and northeastern United States. The disease is manifest by cutaneous, articular, neurological and other systemic features. The most typical skin manifestation is erythema chronicum migrans. Early lymphocytic meningitis is commoner in children than in adults. The arthritis typically appears months to years after the original infection, and becomes chronic in up to 16%. In the majority there is an episodic monoarthritis, but occasionally polyarthritis develops. Treatment with antibiotics is necessary, with ceftriaxone recommended at a dose of 50 mg/kg/day for 14–28 days.[54] Amoxicillin at a dose of 50 mg/kg/day for 28 days is an alternative, but compliance may be poorer due to the dosage regimen. Some authors recommend doxycycline, but not in children below the age of 8 years. Intra-articular steroids should be avoided until completion of antibiotic therapy.

Arthritis associated with meningococcal infection

Meningococcal disease may be associated with both a true septic arthritis occurring in association with the acute septicemic illness or a reactive arthritis seen in the post-acute phase. With improved survival rates from severe meningococcal septicemia a post-infectious, immune complex mediated arthritis is seen with increasing frequency, often in association with a recrudescence of fever and the development of a vasculitic rash.

JUVENILE IDIOPATHIC ARTHRITIS

Juvenile idiopathic arthritis (JIA) is not a single disease entity, rather a collection of heterogeneous diseases. JIA may be associated with significant morbidity, both articular and extra-articular, and may place a significant burden on child and carers alike. Mortality is rare and largely confined to the systemic onset subtype.

JIA is diagnosed according to a constellation of clinical features supported by the judicious use of relevant investigations (frequently to exclude other causes of arthritis). At the current time there are no pathognomic diagnostic tests for JIA. A number of children with JIA will attain spontaneous remission, although rates vary according to disease subtype. Packham reported follow-up data on 246 adults with all subtypes of JIA and found that 43% had clinically active disease.[55] There is now a realistic expectation of disease control with modern therapeutic regimens delivered by an experienced multidisciplinary team. Future studies reporting the outcome of children treated since the advent of these newer therapeutic approaches are awaited, with an expectation that results will be improved. Nonetheless patients, families and professionals must remain realistic that no fundamental cure yet exists.

Significant advances made during the final decade of the 20th century and beyond include:

- Development and subsequent revision of a new classification system of JIA.
- Preliminary definition of improvement measures to evaluate outcome in drug studies (core set criteria).
- Further understanding of immunogenetic pathways.
- Drug studies exploring both optimal doses and routes of administration for conventional drug therapies such as methotrexate, and the new products of the biotechnology revolution, the so-called 'biologic' agents.
- Online resources: the British Society for Paediatric and Adolescent Rheumatology (BSPAR; www.bspar.org.uk); Paediatric Rheumatology European Society (PReS; www.pres.org); and the Pediatric Rheumatology International Trials Organization (PRINTO;www.printo.it) have all developed websites providing useful sources of information for professionals, patients and parents on childhood rheumatic diseases of childhood with links to other relevant websites.

DEFINITION AND CLASSIFICATION

JIA is defined as arthritis of unknown etiology that begins before the 16th birthday and persists for at least 6 weeks. Other known conditions must be excluded. For the purposes of defining arthritis, an inflamed joint is swollen, or limited in range of joint movement with joint pain or tenderness, which is not due to a primary mechanical disorder or to other identifiable cause.

In the final decade of the 20th century the International League of Associations for Rheumatology (ILAR) proposed and subsequently revised consensus guidelines for the classification of JIA.[56] The goal of this major work was to replace and unify previous historical classification criteria, namely juvenile rheumatoid arthritis and juvenile chronic arthritis. Although the ILAR criteria were proposed with the primary aim of defining and classifying clinically homogeneous subgroups within JIA for research purposes, they have been widely embraced and incorporated into clinical practice and are now in mainstream use as clinical diagnostic criteria despite awaiting full validation in further studies. The ILAR criteria define subtypes according to the onset pattern of the disease and associated clinical features. A summary of the clinical features of the JIA classification system is given in Table 29.7.

DIFFERENTIAL DIAGNOSIS

Juvenile idiopathic arthritis must always be considered a diagnosis of exclusion. Musculoskeletal symptoms are common in childhood, and in many cases are related to simple trauma. It should be possible to make a clinical distinction between inflammatory arthritis and arthralgia. If doubt exists, an expert pediatric rheumatology opinion should be consided before embarking on investigations that may be unpleasant for the child and potentially delay the diagnosis of JIA. As the nature of the differential diagnosis of inflammatory arthritis includes potentially life threatening disorders such as sepsis, malignancy and non-accidental injury, any child presenting requires careful assessment by means of thorough history taking, meticulous clinical examination and prompt, judicious use of appropriate investigations. Etiologies can be considered as follows: infection, trauma, autoimmune, neoplasia,

Table 29.7 Clinical features of juvenile idiopathic arthritis

JIA subtype	Clinical features	Alerts
Systemic arthritis	Arthritis with or preceded by daily ('quotidian') fever for at least 3 days, accompanied by one or more of: evanescent erythematosus rash; lymphadenopathy; hepatomegaly and/or splenomegaly; serositis	Arthritis may not be present early in course Mandatory exclusion of infective and malignant conditions
Oligoarthritis: Persistent Extended	Arthritis of four or fewer joints within the first 6 months Affecting not more than four joints throughout the disease process. Frequently children below the age of 5 years Affecting more than four joints after the first 6 months	High risk of associated uveitis, especially if ANA positive
Polyarthritis RF positive RF negative	Arthritis of five or more joints within the first 6 months. Subdivided according to presence of RF	RF positive disease rare but equivalent to 'adult' rheumatoid arthritis
Psoriatic arthritis	Arthritis and psoriasis OR arthritis with at least two of: dactylitis, nail pitting or onycholysis, psoriasis in first degree relative	Psoriasis and arthritis may not co-exist for many years
Enthesitis-related arthritis	Arthritis and enthesitis OR arthritis or enthesitis with two of: SI joint tenderness or inflammatory lumbosacral pain, HLA B27 antigen, onset after age 6 years in a male, acute (symptomatic) anterior uveitis, history of HLA B27 associated disease in a first degree relative	
Undifferentiated arthritis	Arthritis that fulfils criteria in no or more than two of the above categories	

Abbreviations: ANA, antinuclear antibody; RA, rheumatoid arthritis; RF, rheumatoid factor; SI, sacro-iliac.

hematological, metabolic, genetic, drug reactions, trauma (including non-accidental), mechanical/orthopedic. Such an approach should allow distinction of the many possible causes of arthritis, as shown in Table 29.8.

CORE SET CRITERIA

To facilitate standardization of clinical measures of change in JIA, a core set of criteria have been developed by consensus primarily for the purposes of clinical trials,[57] although they may be useful within routine clinical practice. These criteria comprise:

- physician global assessment of disease activity (10-cm visual analogue scale);
- parent/patient assessment of overall well-being (10-cm visual analogue scale);
- functional ability (Childhood Health Assessment Questionnaire – CHAQ (www.rheumatology.org/sections/pediatric/chaq);
- number of joints with active arthritis;
- number of joints with limited range of movement;
- erythrocyte sedimentation rate.

Table 29.8 Differential diagnosis of inflammatory arthritis in childhood

Infection:
  Acute septic arthritis
  Viral arthritis
  Reactive/post-infectious arthritis

Juvenile idiopathic arthritis.
Arthritis associated with inflammatory bowel disease
Other autoimmune rheumatic disorders:
  Systemic lupus erythematosus
  Juvenile dermatomyositis
  Systemic sclerosis
  Mixed connective tissue disease

Systemic vasculitis:
  Henoch–Schönlein purpura
  Kawasaki disease
  Polyarteritis nodosa

Malignancy:
  Leukemia
  Neuroblastoma

Hematological:
  Sickle cell anemia
  Hemophilia

Immune deficiency syndromes
Genetic disorders:
  Cystic fibrosis
  Velocardiofacial syndrome
  CINCA syndrome
  Down syndrome
  Stickler syndrome

Drug reactions
Trauma including non-accidental injury
Orthopedic:
  Perthe disease
  Pigmented villonodular synovitis
Miscellaneous:
  Sarcoidosis
  SAPHO syndrome
  Familial Mediterranean fever

Abbreviations. SAPHO, synovitis, acne, pustulosis, hyperostosis and osteitis syndrome; CINCA, chronic infantile neurological cutaneous and articular syndrome.

EPIDEMIOLOGY

Data describing incidence and prevalence of JIA are confusing and unclear. A detailed review of 34 studies beginning in 1966 showed the reported prevalence of JIA to vary from 0.07 to 4.01 per 100 000 children, while the reported incidence for JIA over the same period ranged from 0.008 to 0.226 per 1000 children.[58] This study highlights the need for standardization of diagnostic criteria, case definition, and case ascertainment and also the need to consider the clinical qualification and experience of participating researchers, health resources available within the study population, expectation of health and the size of the study cohort. Despite methodological differences between studies there does appear to be a true variability in disease occurrence according to geographical factors.

Overall, girls with JIA outnumber boys by approximately 2:1. There are important variations within disease subtypes with girls outnumbering boys in oligoarthritis, polyarthritis and psoriatic arthritis, but a more even sex distribution in systemic JIA[59] and boys outnumbering girls in the enthesitis-related arthritis subtype. In those with uveitis the ratio of girls to boys is higher, up to 6.6:1.[60]

ETIOLOGY AND PATHOGENESIS

As with all autoimmune disease there is a complex interplay between genetic risk factors and environmental triggers. JIA has been referred to as a 'complex genetic trait', albeit one in which there are now several consistent and strong associations.[61]

Studies of genetic polymorphisms in both adult and childhood chronic arthritis have frequently, but not exclusively, involved the major histocompatibility complex (MHC). The MHC class II loci DR, DQ and DP are particularly associated with JIA. Age-related genetic susceptibility is suggested by the association of early childhood onset oligoarthritis with HLA A2, DR5, DR8 and DPB1*0201.[62] Oligoarthritis in older boys is associated with HLA-B27, and to date this remains the only HLA association with any major relevance to routine clinical practice. Polyarticular JIA with a positive rheumatoid factor is associated with HLA DR4, as in adults with rheumatoid arthritis.

The British Paediatric Rheumatology Study Group demonstrated in a large multicenter study of 521 Caucasian patients with JIA the presence of multiple HLA class II associations. Differences were demonstrated between the seven subtypes defined by the ILAR classification criteria, which encouragingly lends support to this classification approach.[63]

There is growing evidence to support an etiological role for polymorphisms within individual genes coding for pro- and anti-inflammatory cytokines. In studies of synovial tissue from adults with rheumatoid arthritis, proinflammatory cytokines such as interleukin (IL)-1 and tumor necrosis factor (TNF)-alpha are elevated, and induce the release of tissue-destroying metalloproteinases.[64] There has been great interest in the role of cytokines as mediators of the inflammatory response in JIA, both to further the understanding of the pathogenesis of the disease and also as potential targets for biological therapies.

The pro-inflammatory cytokine TNF-alpha (TNFα) occupies a central position in the cytokine network. TNFα is produced by several cells throughout the body, including synovial cells, T lymphocytes and mononuclear phagocytes, but in inflammatory arthritis it is mostly derived from activated macrophages. TNFα, with lymphotoxin-alpha (a related cytokine), is detected in synovial tissue in JIA and may amplify local inflammation and contribute to joint destruction.[65] TNFα stimulates further proinflammatory cytokine production including IL-1 and IL-6.

JIA is a heterogeneous disease. It is not surprising then that studies have revealed differences in cytokine profiles between JIA subtypes. Rooney et al demonstrated an imbalance between TNFα and its soluble receptor (sTNFR) in JIA, with different ratios in different subtypes, which may explain variations in disease patterns and resulting joint damage.[66]

CLINICAL FEATURES
Systemic arthritis

The systemic onset subtype accounts for 11% of all cases of juvenile arthritis, often occurring in younger children with a median age of onset of 4.3 years and a male to female ratio of 1:1.2 (data on percentages of each subclass is taken from Symmons 1996 which uses the historical classification, JCA;[59] percentages using the ILAR classification JIA may differ slightly from these, but data is not yet available).

Systemic JIA is defined as arthritis in one or more joints with or preceded by fever of at least 2 weeks' duration that is documented to be daily ('quotidian') for at least 3 days, and is accompanied by one or more of the following:

- evanescent (nonfixed) erythematous rash;
- generalized lymph node enlargement;
- hepatomegaly and/or splenomegaly;
- serositis.

The systemic features may precede the onset of arthritis. In toddlers, the arthritis may be subtle and difficult to confirm. Many will therefore require detailed workup to exclude sepsis and hematological malignant diseases.

The associated systemic manifestations of the disease are often much worse during the periods of fever, and the children are intensely miserable during these periods, with significant improvement when the fever settles. The rash is pale pink, macular (evanescent) and flitting in nature. It often occurs in linear streaks and it exhibits the Koebner phenomenon (Fig. 29.32). It most commonly occurs on the trunk, but can be generalized. Generalized lymphadenopathy occurs in the majority, and enlarged nodes are painless, rubbery and mobile. Hepatomegaly is common and splenomegaly occurs in approximately 50%. Serum transaminases are frequently elevated, and there is often hypoalbuminemia. Pericardial effusion on echocardiogram is common and usually asymptomatic, but a useful feature to aid diagnosis. Pleural effusion may co-exist with pericardial effusion, and either may occasionally require surgical drainage.

The pattern of arthritis associated with systemic JIA is variable. Approximately one third develop a polyarticular course with joint destruction within 2 years of disease onset (Fig. 29.33). Hepatosplenomegaly, serositis and low serum albumin are recognized as risk factors at disease onset, while later risk factors for an adverse outcome in systemic JIA are thrombocytosis, persistent fever or steroid dependency at 6 months.[67]

Three patterns of disease progression have been described:

1. monocyclic (systemic disease with a single episode);
2. intermittent (recurrent fever and arthritis interspersed with periods of remission);
3. persistent disease activity with systemic and polyarticular phases.

Functional outcome is largely dependent on the course of the arthritis rather than on the systemic features.

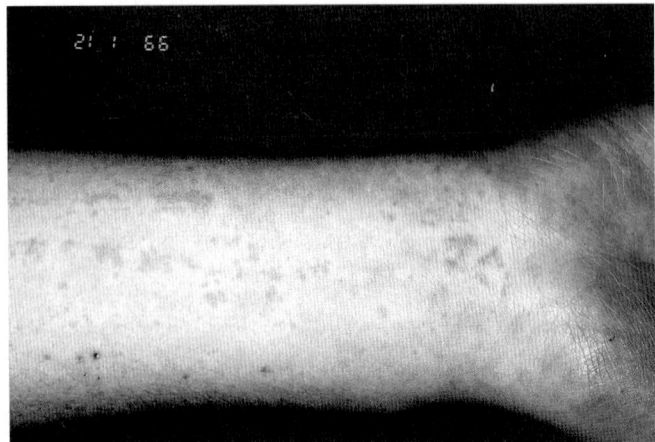

Fig. 29.32   Rash of systemic juvenile idiopathic arthritis.

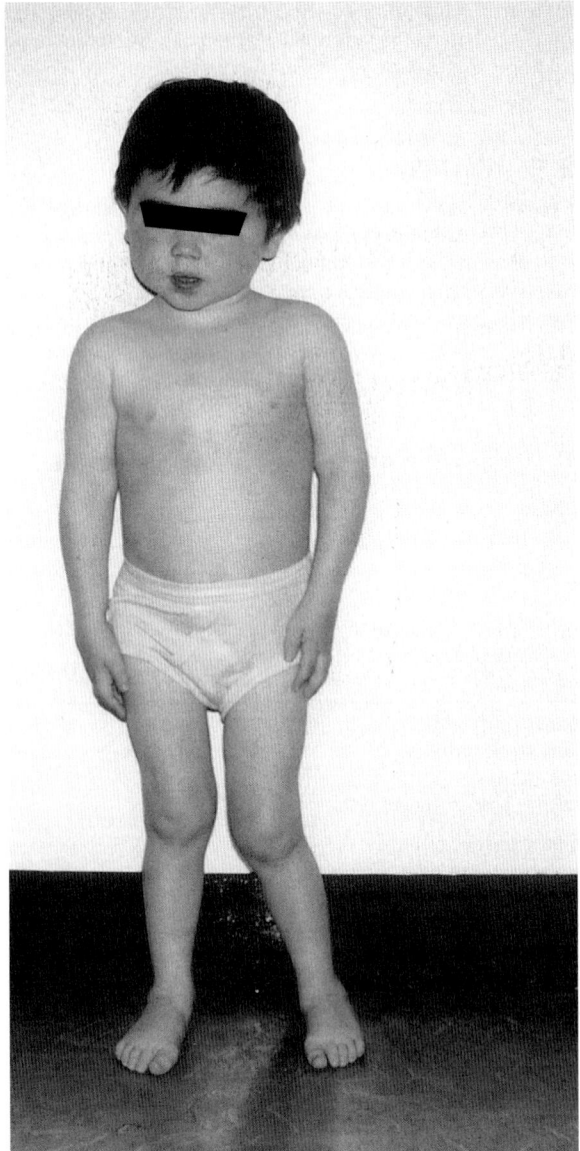

Fig. 29.33   Systemic juvenile idiopathic arthritis with polyarticular course – involvement of knees, ankles, hips, wrists and cervical spine.

Oligoarthritis

This is defined as arthritis affecting between one and four joints during the first 6 months of disease and further subdivided into:

- persistent oligoarthritis: affects no more than four joints throughout the disease course;
- extended oligoarthritis: affects a cumulative total of five joints or more after the first 6 months of disease.

Oligoarthritis is the commonest onset pattern of JIA in Caucasian populations, accounting for approximately 50% of affected children.[59] Persistent oligoarthritis is commonest in preschool age girls (although does occur in boys) and in this age group is frequently associated with positive antinuclear antibodies (ANA) and an increased risk of silent, potentially blinding, uveitis.

Oligoarthritis most frequently develops asymmetrically in large lower limb joints, especially the knee (Fig. 29.34) and the ankle, and occasionally in the upper limb.

Oligoarthritis in preschool children is often insidious, but occasionally manifests acutely. The child may limp, especially after rest. The joint appears swollen and is warm, but rarely painful until passively moved through its full range. Examination of the knee may reveal a palpable effusion. With time, if unrecognized, flexion contractures may occur.

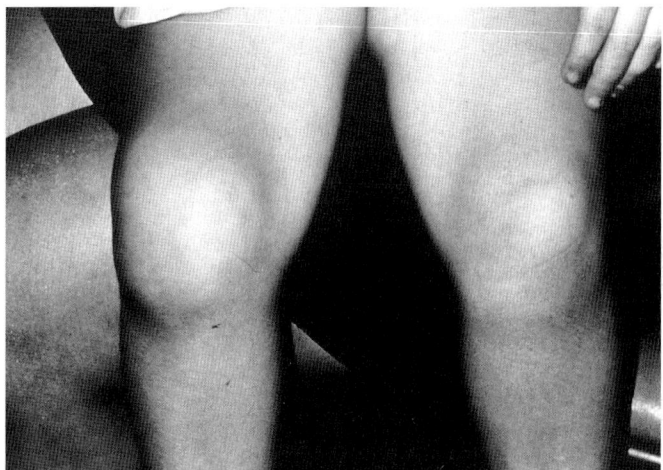

Fig. 29.34   Oligoarthritis showing marked swelling of R knee.

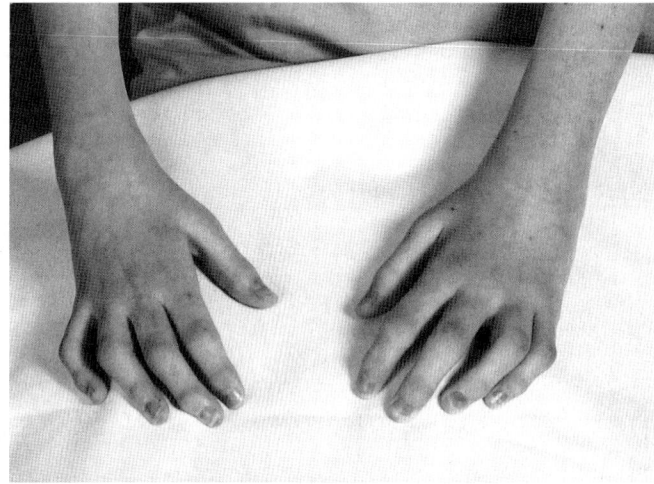

Fig. 29.36   Polyarthritis affecting wrists and the small joints of the hands.

Bony overgrowth of the joint may be seen with leg length discrepancy (Fig. 29.35). Prompt recognition and treatment will prevent the development of such complications.

In a proportion of children with an oligoarticular onset there is an 'adding on' of involved joints beyond 6 months of disease – so-called extended oligoarthritis.

Polyarthritis

This is defined as arthritis affecting five or more joints during the first 6 months of disease. This subtype is further subdivided on the basis of testing for IgM rheumatoid factor into:

- rheumatoid factor positive (seropositive);
- rheumatoid factor negative (seronegative).

Seronegative polyarthritis (Fig. 29.36) has a variable clinical expression ranging from low grade grumbling disease to an aggressive polyarthritis. An early peak age of onset is seen around 2 years, with a later peak around 8 years.[60] It varies in clinical expression ranging from low grade grumbling disease to an aggressive polyarthritis. Joints may be hot and swollen or simply tender with loss of function, without gross synovial swelling or palpable effusions (so-called 'dry synovitis'). Onset may be insidious but joint deformities, of both large and small joints, may develop rapidly.

Seropositive polyarthritis is rare, accounting for 3% of all children with JIA, compared to 17% for seronegative polyarthritis.[59] Children with seropositive polyarthritis typically are girls and develop disease in late childhood and adolescence. The arthritis is usually symmetrical affecting upper and lower limbs, in particular the small joints of the hands and feet. The test for IgM rheumatoid factor should be positive on at least two occasions 3 months apart.

Psoriatic arthritis

Psoriatic arthritis is defined as arthritis and psoriasis (Fig. 29.37), or arthritis and at least two of the following:

- dactylitis;
- nail pitting and onycholysis;
- psoriasis in a first-degree relative.

In the UK, psoriatic arthritis accounts for 7% of all cases of JIA, is commoner in girls (male:female ratio 1:1.6) with a median age of onset 10.1 years.[59] Oligoarticular onset (asymmetrical involvement of large and small joints) is frequent and dactylitis (diffuse swelling of a finger or toe joint and periarticular tissues is a hallmark feature (Fig. 29.38). The arthritis can be highly erosive. Nail abnormalities may be seen, including nail pitting and nail dystrophy (onycholysis). The arthritis precedes the psoriasis in as many as 75% of cases, and 45% of children develop psoriasis within 5 years of onset of arthritis.[68] The outcome in psoriatic arthritis is variable, with both oligo- and polyarticular courses described.

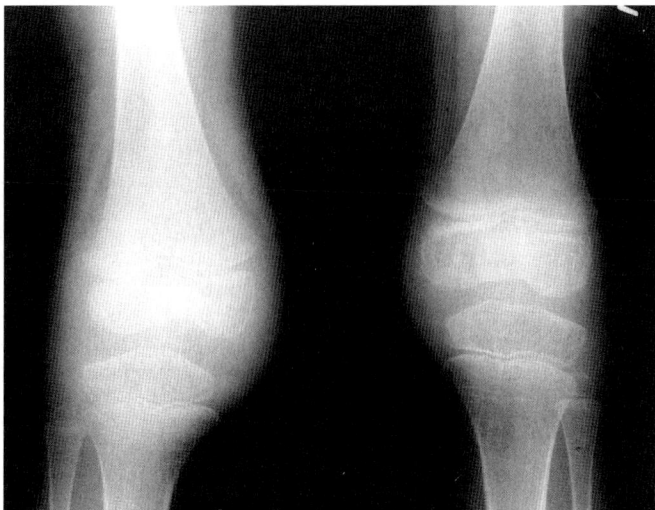

Fig. 29.35   Oligoarthritis – plain radiograph showing overgrowth of right knee.

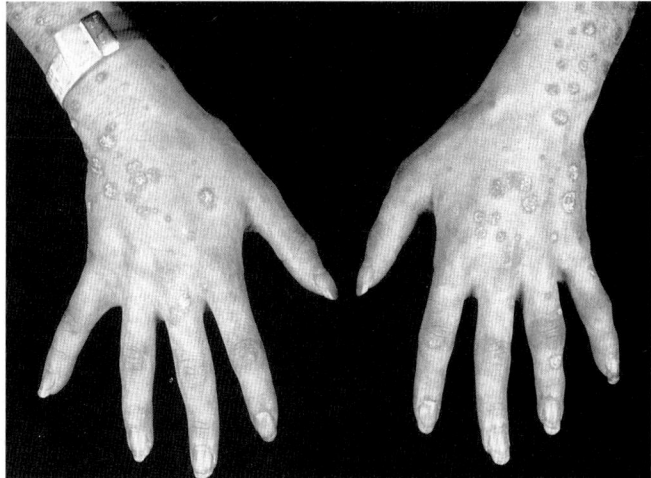

Fig. 29.37   Psoriatic arthritis.

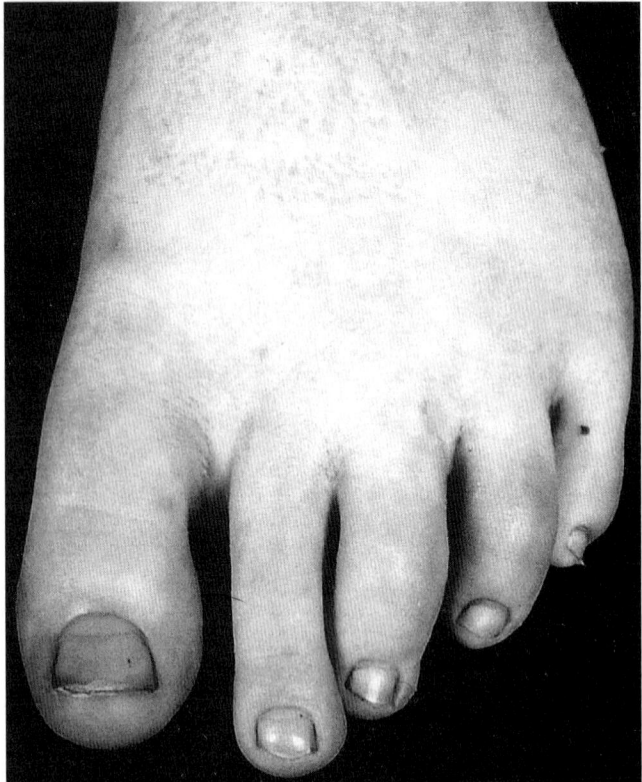

Fig. 29.38   Dactylitis – swelling of third and fourth toes.

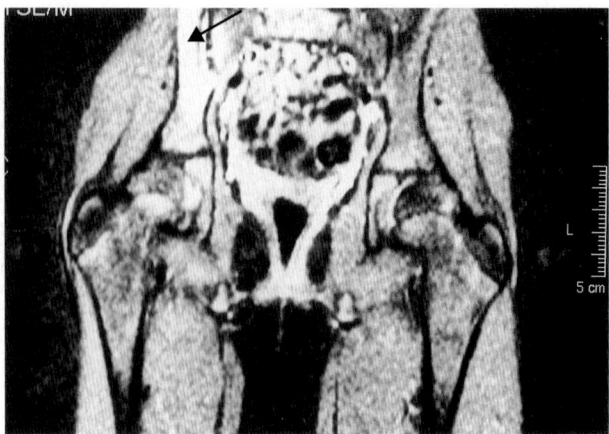

Fig. 29.39   Gadolinium enhanced MRI showing right-sided sacroiliitis (note high signal on right compared to left).

Enthesitis–related arthritis

This is defined as arthritis and enthesitis (inflammation of tendon insertion into bone), or arthritis or enthesitis with at least two of the following:

- sacroiliac joint tenderness and/or inflammatory lumbosacral pain;
- presence of the HLA-B27 antigen;
- onset of arthritis in a male over 6 years of age;
- acute (symptomatic) anterior uveitis;
- history of ankylosing spondylitis, enthesitis-related arthritis, sacroiliitis with inflammatory bowel disease, Reiter syndrome or acute anterior uveitis in a first-degree relative.

This subtype defines those with disease related to the HLA-B27 antigen, and avoids the term juvenile spondyloarthropathy, inaccurate because of the rarity of spinal involvement in children. The commonest joints involved are the peripheral large joints of the lower limb, in an asymmetrical distribution. It is rare for children to present with axial skeleton symptoms or signs, although a minority develops arthritis of the sacroiliac joints in teenage years (Fig. 29.39) and subsequently ankylosing spondylitis in adulthood. There is a marked predominance of boys in this group, presenting after the age of 6 years. Enthesitis is a characteristic feature, often affecting the insertion of the Achilles tendon into the calcaneum, and may be distressingly painful resulting in significant functional impairment. The eye disease associated with enthesitis-related arthritis is an acute painful iritis (in contrast to the asymptomatic uveitis associated with other subtypes of JIA), and occurs in less than 20% of children.

Undifferentiated arthritis

At present children who either fulfill criteria for no category, or who fulfill criteria for more than one of the other categories, are defined as undifferentiated.

INVESTIGATIONS

Judicious investigation may serve to support the diagnosis of JIA. At presentation as a minimum full blood count, liver chemistry and a disease activity measure, preferably erythrocyte sedimentation rate (ESR), are recommended for all JIA subtypes. A positive antinuclear antibody in oligoarthritis is a risk factor for silent uveitis and will help to guide the ophthalmology screening program. Rheumatoid factor is only of clinical significance in the context of those children with a polyarthritis. Serum ferritin may be disproportionately high in systemic JIA. Nonspecific hyperimmunoglobulinemia is often seen in polyarticular and systemic JIA. Hypoalbuminemia is common in systemic JIA, along with elevations of liver enzymes.[67]

Radiological investigations

All imaging modalities may have a potential role in JIA:

- to aid diagnosis – particularly to exclude other musculoskeletal conditions;
- to document and define evidence of joint damage;
- to aid the assessment of complex joints, e.g. hip, subtalar, shoulder and temporomandibular joints;
- to detect subclinical or very early synovitis – magnetic resonance scanning with gadolinium contrast is a very sensitive technique;
- to distinguish synovitis from tenosynovitis;
- to facilitate intra-articular steroid injection.

Three stages of radiigraphic changes are seen on plain radiographs in JIA.[69]

- Early: soft tissue swelling, e.g. blurring of the infrapatellar fat pad on lateral knee radiograph and periarticular osteopenia.
- Intermediate: cortical erosions, joint space narrowing and subchondral cysts.
- Late: destructive joint changes with ankylosis, joint contractures, metaphyseal and diaphyseal changes and growth anomalies (Fig. 29.40).

Radionuclide bone scanning is sensitive in detecting areas of increased uptake within the skeleton, but will not differentiate between inflammation, infection or malignant disease. Ultrasound is a reliable method for detecting effusions, especially in the hip, guiding intra-articular injections and confirmation of popliteal cysts. In expert hands it is also increasingly useful as a method of documenting synovitis of joints and tendons. Intravenous contrast (gadolinium-DPTA) enhanced magnetic resonance sequences are exquisitely sensitive at detecting inflamed synovium and particularly valuable in the assessment of inaccessible joints such as the hip, and complex joints such as the ankle, where it may be difficult to distinguish clinically between the tibiotalar and subtalar joint. T1-weighted images with fat suppression are particularly recommended for demonstrating synovitis (Fig. 29.41).

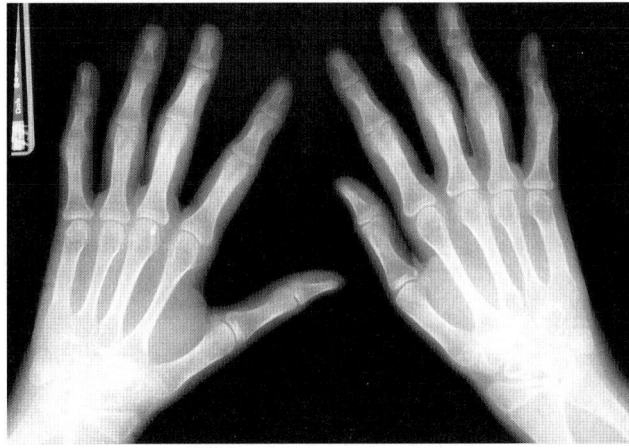

(a)

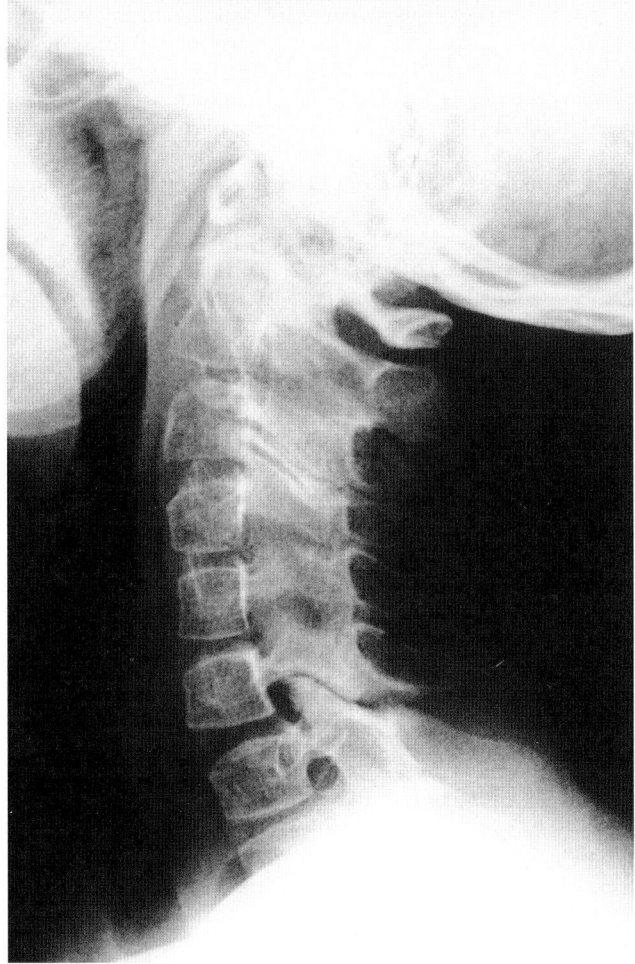

(b)

Fig. 29.40 Plain radiographs in juvenile idiopathic arthritis: (a) destructive changes of wrists with crowding of carpal bones; periarticular osteopenia and loss of joint space at proximal interphalangeal joints; (b) fusion in block of posterior elements of C2–C7.

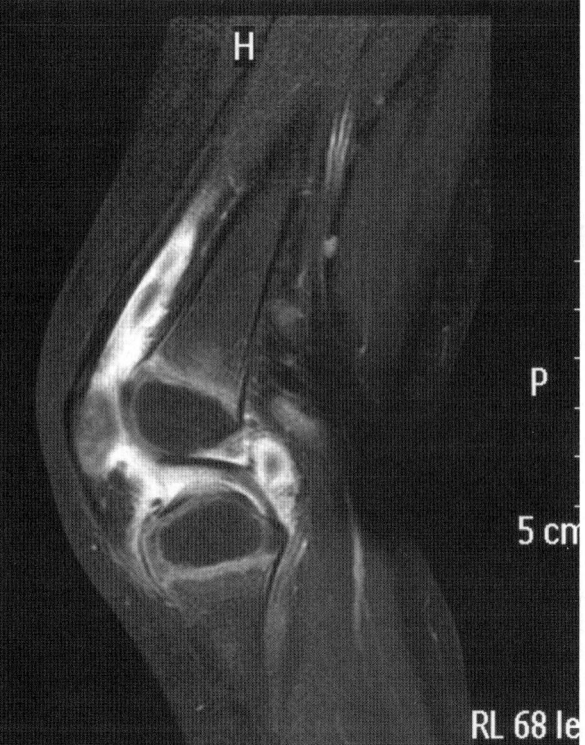

Fig. 29.41 MR scan of left knee with fat suppression and gadolinium contrast. There is a small effusion with synovial thickening and enhancement.

COMPLICATIONS: ARTICULAR

Articular complications are a direct result of synovial inflammation and can generally be minimized or prevented by optimizing control of the inflammatory process. Flexion contractures occur commonly and at a very early stage in JIA and if not treated intensively may become permanent. Overgrowth of affected limbs (Fig. 29.35) is a particular problem of oligoarthritis which may have serious long term complications

e.g. a discrepancy in lower limb length resulting in a pelvic tilt and scoliosis in adult life. The temporomandibular joint (TMJ) may be involved in polyarthritis and specific features such as asymmetrical mouth opening and micrognathia may be noted during clinical examination. TMJ involvement may result in both cosmetic and functional difficulties and appropriate advice from an interested maxillofacial surgeon should be sought.

COMPLICATIONS: EXTRA-ARTICULAR

Uveitis

The incidence of uveitis in JIA overall is approximately 10%, although it is commoner in ANA (antinuclear antibody) positive oligoarthritis.[70] Two patterns of ocular inflammation are seen in JIA. An acute, painful iritis is seen in children with enthesitis-related arthritis, and usually resolves rapidly with topical corticosteroid therapy. Chronic, asymptomatic anterior uveitis that may become sight threatening if not recognized and treated is especially common in preschool age girls with oligoarthritis. It is strongly associated with positive antinuclear antibodies. The diagnosis requires slit-lamp examination by an ophthalmologist.

To date no prospective randomized controlled data exist comparing immunosuppressive therapy in childhood uveitis. Visual complications (synechiae, band keratopathy, cataract or glaucoma) may develop in up to 30%, and significant visual loss has been reported in 11%,[70] highlighting the need for aggressive treatment.

In many cases uveitis in children with JIA can be controlled with topical corticosteroids and short-acting mydriatics. Early steroid-sparing therapy, to reduce the risk of steroid-related complications such as cataract and glaucoma, is indicated if it proves impossible to taper local steroid therapy because of persistent disease activity. Methotrexate is the commonest second line agent in use, with significant reduction in uveitis activity and steroid dependency being shown in a retrospective study.[71] If control cannot be achieved with oral methotrexate alone, parenteral administration of methotrexate, or methotrexate in combination with ciclosporin, should be considered. Data from uncontrolled studies suggest benefit from infliximab in therapy-resistant uveitis.[72] Relapses and first presentation uveitis have been reported in patients receiving etanercept therapy, indicating more studies are needed to define any potential role for the biological agents in treating uveitis.

Nutritional status and growth
Nutritional impairment and growth failure is a recognized complication of all subtypes of JIA. The etiology of nutritional impairment in JIA is not fully understood, nor is it clear how frequently it occurs. It may affect the general well-being of the child and contributes to the growth disturbance that is a serious consequence of JIA in some children.

Osteoporosis
Osteoporosis is a significant long term complication of a variety of rheumatological disorders including JIA and occurs as a consequence of the underlying inflammatory process; of inactivity; and of steroid therapy.

Psychosocial
Long term outcome studies have demonstrated a significant incidence of psychosocial difficulty in young adults with JIA. Attention to rehabilitation and early return to normal activities where possible is essential to minimize this. Families and schools must be encouraged to treat the child as normal and all should be in mainstream schooling. Good transitional care with an early focus on independence and career counseling is essential.

Macrophage activation syndrome (MAS)/secondary hemophagocytic lymphohistiocytosis (HLH)
MAS/HLH is a rare but potentially life threatening complication of systemic JIA. Features in a child raising suspicion of MAS/HLH are fever, lymphadenopathy and hepatosplenomegaly, pancytopenia, low ESR, elevated liver enzymes and coagulopathy.[73] MAS/HLH may be triggered by an intercurrent infection or change in drug therapy. The pathognomic feature, macrophages actively phagocytosing hematopoietic elements, may be seen on the bone marrow aspirate but it must be noted that false negative bone marrow examinations may occur. Other laboratory features include hypertriglyceridemia and hyperferritinemia. Treatment of MAS/HLH consists of high dose corticosteroids and ciclosporin with good supportive care and vigorous treatment of concomitant sepsis. Such patients may require management in a pediatric intensive care setting.

MANAGEMENT
As with all pediatric chronic diseases, optimal management of JIA is delivered by an experienced multidisciplinary team (Table 29.9). Adequate education of the child and family about the disease and possible therapeutic strategies is essential from the outset. The impact of JIA on patient and family may be significant and good results depend on considerable commitment from all. Information and encouragement will empower patients and families to be involved in and committed to their treatment with improved compliance and better results. The provision of appropriate written information is helpful; directing families to appropriate online resources is increasingly important.

Physiotherapy and occupational therapy
The aim of physiotherapy is to maintain and restore joint function, and to increase muscle strength. This can only be achieved in association with medical therapy to control synovitis. An occupational therapist may provide adaptations at home or school. Many different strategies are available, but there is consensus that physical and occupational therapy early in the disease is associated with an improved outcome.[74]

Table 29.9 Members of the multidisciplinary team involved in the care of a child with juvenile idiopathic arthritis

Medical	Professions allied to medicine	Community
Pediatric rheumatologist	Physiotherapist	Family
Pediatrician	Occupational therapist	Friends
Ophthalmologist	Psychologist	School teacher
General practitioner	Social worker	Parental employer
Orthopedic surgeon	Dietitian	
Dental practitioner	Orthotist	
Radiologist	Podiatrist	

Medical management
The pharmacological management of JIA continues to evolve, in terms of specific drugs and strategies for their deployment. Early use of methotrexate (MTX) in polyarthritis, frequently at diagnosis or shortly after, is now standard practice in order to achieve and maintain disease remission. MTX is now regularly used in oligoarthritis resistant to local intra-articular corticosteroid injection therapy. MTX and other systemic immunosuppressive agents are frequently used in uveitis whether or not associated with JIA. Biological agents are now licensed therapies and appear effective and to date safe in treating JIA. There is the likelihood of further advances and new experimental therapies likely to follow rapidly. An algorithm showing an approach to pharmacological management of JIA is shown in Table 29.10.

Nonsteroidal anti-inflammatory drugs (NSAIDs)
NSAIDs are widely used at diagnosis, provide good symptomatic relief and contribute to the control of the inflammatory process although this takes time to achieve. Table 29.11 lists the commonly used NSAIDs and the doses required to achieve anti-inflammatory effect. Drugs with once or twice daily regimens are likely to have better compliance particularly in older children.

Side-effects are uncommon in children. Gastrointestinal upset is uncommon and may be relieved by the addition of a H_2 antagonist or proton pump inhibitor. Naproxen (and occasionally other NSAIDs) may be associated with scarring pseudoporphyria affecting the face and care should be taken in fair skinned children. Mood and behavior disturbances are occasionally reported by parents of young children on NSAIDs.

Corticosteroid therapy
The early use of effective disease-modifying anti-rheumatic drugs (DMARDs), historically methotrexate and more recently anti TNFα agents, has dramatically reduced the dependency upon, and toxicity associated with chronic administration of systemic corticosteroids. Corticosteroids still have a role in the management of JIA, in particular for remission induction, and may be administered systemically by the intravenous and oral route, or locally by intra-articular injection.

Local corticosteroid therapy. Intra-articular steroid injections are effective, with a low risk of complications, in all subtypes of JIA, particularly oligoarthritis.[75] In polyarthritis, multiple intra-articular injections may be used simultaneously with the initiation of methotrexate therapy. The early use of intra-articular steroid injections and rapid resolution of synovitis relieves pain and facilitates early physiotherapy and rehabilitation thus preventing joint contractures. When used early, and if necessary repeatedly, intra-articular steroids may prevent leg length discrepancy in oligoarthritis.[76] Triamcinolone hexacetonide (TH) is the drug of choice for intra-articular injection in JIA, as shown in a randomized controlled trial with the alternative agent triamcinolone acetonide.[77]

A typical regimen for dosage of triamcinolone hexacetonide is 1 mg/kg for large joints (knees, hips and shoulders) to a maximum

Table 29.10 Algorithm for the medical treatment of JIA by onset pattern

Oligoarthritis	Polyarthritis	Systemic JIA
↓	↓	↓ **
NSAIDs IATH	NSAIDs MTX 10-15 mg/m² po Consider: IATH	NSAIDs i.v. MP +/− oral prednisolone
↓		↓
Repeat IATH	↓ **	Disease course
↓ **		↓ ↓
MTX 10-15 mg/m² po	MTX 15 mg/m² sc	Polyarthritis Systemic
↓	↓	↓ ↓
MTX 15 mg/m² sc	Etanercept	MTX MTX +/− corticosteroid
↓		↓
Etanercept		Consider IVIG Etanercept
	↓	↓
	Other biologic agents Infliximab Adalimumab Anakinra	Other biologic agents Infliximab Adalimumab Anakinra/MRA
		↓
		ASCT

Key to algorithm: po—oral, sc—subcutaneous, NSAIDs—nonsteroidal anti-inflammatory drugs, iv MP—iv methylprednisolone, IATH—intra-articular triamcinolone hexacetonide, MTX TNFα methotrexate, IVIG—intravenous immunoglobulin; ASCT—autologous stem cell transplant.
** Indicates stage requiring management in conjunction with regional pediatric rheumatology center.

Table 29.11 Nonsteroidal anti-inflammatory drugs commonly used in children with juvenile idiopathic arthritis

Drug	Dose	Times daily	Notes
Diclofenac sodium	1 mg/kg	2–3	Max 150 mg/day SR available
Naproxen	5–10 mg/kg	2	Max 1 g/day
Ibuprofen	10 mg/kg	3–4	
Indometacin	0.5–1 mg/kg	2	Max 200 mg/day SR available
Piroxicam	<15 kg 5 mg 16–25 kg 10 mg 26–45 kg 15 mg >46 kg 20 mg	Once daily	Sublingual preparation available

SR, slow release.

of 40 mg, 0.5 mg/kg in smaller joints (ankles, wrists and elbows) and 2–4 mg/joint for the small joints of the hands and feet. The dose of triamcinolone acetonide is typically double that of triamcinolone hexacetonide. In young children with JIA or if multiple joints are to be injected, intra-articular injection will be performed using general anesthesia. In older children the procedure can be safely and effectively carried out using a 50/50 mix of nitrous oxide and oxygen (Entonox). Subcutaneous atrophy at the injection site is the only common adverse effect, with the highest incidence in a single study of 8.3% of patients.[78] A transient cushingoid state is reported with the use of triamcinolone acetonide, including occasionally after injection of a single joint.[79]

Systemic corticosteroids. Systemic corticosteroids, administered either as intravenous high dose 'pulses' (methylprednisolone 30 mg/kg usually for 3 consecutive days and repeated as necessary) or oral prednisolone may be considered as an adjunct in a defined course during the 'lag' phase while MTX becomes effective or may be used to control acute disease flares, again in strictly limited courses.

Methotrexate

Methotrexate (MTX) is currently the disease modifying agent of first choice in JIA. MTX is a dihydrofolate reductase inhibitor, although its mechanism of action as an anti-inflammatory agent is not fully understood. In a double-blind placebo-controlled trial, MTX at a dose of $10\,mg/m^2$ was effective in polyarthritis (significant response in 63% of patients).[80] MTX is effective in extended oligoarthritis and systemic JIA.[81] Ruperto and colleagues for PRINTO reported in a randomized controlled trial that 28% of patients failed to respond to an oral dose of 8–12.5 mg/m^2. Of those, a further 62.5% achieved a clinical response to subcutaneous administration at $15\,mg/m^2$/week, but no additional benefit was seen at $30\,mg/m^2$/week.[82]

Subcutaneous administration should be considered if oral administration fails to produce effective control, or is not tolerated. This can be self-administered at home by patients or carers. In the UK the Royal College of Nursing have produced guidelines regarding subcutaneous administration of MTX (http://www.rcn.org.uk/publications/pdf/administering-methotrexate.pdf).

Common side-effects of weekly low dose methotrexate include nausea and vomiting, which in some cases can be overcome by giving the MTX in two doses over 24 hours, use of an antiemetic agent or regular administration of folic acid. Mouth ulcers may also respond to folic acid supplementation. Transient elevations in liver enzymes are common, frequently associated with intercurrent viral infections, and resolving with temporary withdrawal of MTX. Significant liver toxicity and bone marrow suppression is rare.[83] Blood monitoring is mandatory while children take MTX. Monthly full blood count (FBC) and liver function tests (LFTs) initially, reduced to 2–3 monthly thereafter is satisfactory. There is no consensus on the use of folic acid to minimize adverse effects in children on weekly low dose MTX, although weekly administration in doses of 2.5–5 mg per week is standard in some centers.

Immunization with live vaccines is contraindicated during treatment with MTX. If circumstances permit, children known to be varicella zoster (VZ) susceptible should be immunised with VZ vaccine 2 weeks prior to starting MTX. Children known to be VZ susceptible and in contact with VZ, should be treated with either VZ specific immunoglobulin or prophylactic oral aciclovir according to local guidelines. A best practice statement on the immunization of the immunocompromised child is available.[84]

Methotrexate is teratogenic and liver toxicity may be increased with concomitant alcohol ingestion. Adolescents need specific counseling in these areas. A checklist prior to administration of MTX is given in Table 29.12.

Biological therapies

Following publication of the previous edition of this text, there has been rapid growth in this form of therapy in JIA. Acute infection of any type mandates temporary interruption of therapy, and all live vaccines are contraindicated. A summary of anti-TNF agents used to treat JIA is given in Table 29.13.

Etanercept. In a multicenter clinical trial of children with polyarticular JIA who had previously failed to respond to therapy with low dose methotrexate, 74% improved with etanercept.[85] Adverse effects were similar to those in the placebo group, and included injection site

Table 29.12 Information to be discussed prior to commencing methotrexate for JIA

Blood monitoring – FBC and LFTs monthly until dose stable and 2–3 monthly thereafter

Avoid all live vaccines

Miss a dose if acutely unwell with intercurrent infection – contact rheumatology team for advice

Ensure adequate contraception if sexually active

Limit alcohol intake to 5 units per week, and highlight the alcohol content of popular brands

reactions, headaches, minor upper respiratory tract infections, rhinitis, urticarial reactions, nausea and vomiting. Follow-on data have demonstrated safety and efficacy over a 4-year period, with the rate of serious adverse events being 0.13 per patient-year. The rate of serious infections was 0.04 per patient-year, in a total etanercept exposure of 225 patient-years.[86]

Infliximab. Efficacy similar to etanercept has been shown in an open label prospective pilot study of 24 patients.[87] In a randomized controlled trial, comparing infliximab at doses of 3 mg/kg vs 6 mg/kg, 75% of JIA patients responded to a dose of 6 mg/kg. Antibodies to infliximab were higher with the lower dose resulting in a higher incidence of allergic type infusion reactions and serious adverse events in the 3 mg/kg group compared to 6 mg/kg group (19% vs 9% respectively at weeks 14–52 of treatment).[88] Co-administration with weekly methotrexate is recommended to limit autoantibody production.

Adalimumab. Adalimumab is a recombinant human IgG1 monoclonal antibody, specific to human TNF. Theoretically there should be less risk of immunogenic reactions than with infliximab. Efficacy has been demonstrated in in adult rheumatoid arthritis. At the time of writing JIA data are only available in abstract form, albeit with encouraging efficacy and safety at 1-year follow up.[89]

Adverse effects of anti TNF agents. Anti TNF agents have been shown to induce production of antinuclear antibodies, although the incidence of a lupus-like state remains low.[90] There have been reports of lymphoproliferative disease in adult patients with rheumatoid arthritis and Crohn disease treated with anti TNF agents,[91] although a causal link remains to be established. This highlights the need for further long term surveillance studies in JIA and a biologics registry has been established in the UK for this purpose (British Society for Paediatric and Adolescent Rheumatology Biologics and New Drugs Registry: www.bsparreg.org).

At the time of writing, etanercept is the only biological agent licensed for use in JIA in the UK. The National Institute for Health and Clinical Excellence (NICE: www.nice.org.uk) has recommended etanercept for children with active JIA in at least five joints, with inadequate response to MTX, or intolerable side-effects from MTX.

Other biologic agents

Preliminary data suggests a role for two other agents in JIA. IL-1 is now known to play a role in systemic JIA.[92] Anakinra, an IL-1 receptor ana-

Table 29.13 Biologic anti TNF agents for the treatment of JIA

Biologic agent	Structure	Mechanism of action	Administration	Red flags
Etanercept	Soluble fusion molecule of two human p75 TNF receptors	Binds and blocks TNFα and lymphotoxin α	0.4 mg/kg twice weekly s.c. injection, maximum 25 mg per dose	Injection site reactions, infections
Infliximab	Chimeric human-mouse anti TNFα monoclonal antibody	Binds TNFα	6 mg/kg at 0, 2 and 6 weeks, then 8 weekly thereafter by intravenous infusion	Infusion reactions, infection, TB reactivation, ANA and anti-dsDNA antibody formation
Adalimumab	Recombinant human IgG1 anti-TNFα mononclonal antibody	Binds TNFα	24 mg/m² fortnightly by subcutaneous injection	Injection site reactions, infections

tagonist, has been used in adult RA and anecdotal evidence suggests that it may be effective in systemic JIA. An open label phase II clinical trial of anti-IL-6 receptor monoclonal antibody (MRA) has also shown promise in systemic JIA.[93]

Other therapies

Intravenous immunoglobulin may be used in systemic arthritis[94] unresponsive to more conventional therapies. Dose regimens vary between 1 g/kg/day for 2 consecutive days and 400 mg/kg/day for 5 consecutive days, repeated monthly. Hydroxychloroquine may be of benefit in some seropositive patients. Sulphasalazine may be used in enthesitis-related arthritis. Leflunomide, an oral dihydrooratate dehydrogenase inhibitor, has shown efficacy in adults with rheumatoid arthritis. There is anecdotal evidence of benefit in JIA[95] but no controlled studies.

Autologous hemopoietic stem cell transplantation (ASCT) may be a possible option for patients with JIA refractory to conventional treatment and in whom the burden of drug toxicity is unacceptable. Early results have shown the potential for prolonged drug free remission, but a mortality rate of 9% was reported in a preliminary case series highlighting the importance of developing future protocols through collaborative multicenter studies.[96]

Surgical management

Orthopedic surgery has an increasingly limited role in JIA. Joint replacement may ultimately be required in some cases, but should be deferred as long as possible. Newer techniques such as hip resurfacing may have a role in some, but detailed discussion is beyond the scope of this text.

Transitional care

Young people with JIA entering transition into adulthood have specific medical and psychosocial needs, and many advocate that this process should be pro-actively managed. A multicenter study of a coordinated, evidence-based program of transitional care reported encouraging results.[97]

OTHER ARTHROPATHIES IN CHILDHOOD

Infections and JIA are the only common causes of arthritis in childhood. The differential diagnosis of inflammatory arthritis in children (Table 29.8) is wide and other causes must be excluded as necessary. Many of these conditions are described elsewhere in the chapter.

COMMON ORTHOPEDIC PROBLEMS IN CHILDHOOD

Children present to the clinician with a wide spectrum of problems ranging from complaints relating to form, posture and gait to complaints of localized pain at various sites. This section covers the more common orthopedic explanations for such presentations.

COMMON PAINLESS COMPLAINTS

Normal variants

The shape and form of the lower limbs in children cause a great deal of parental anxiety. In spite of such concern, the majority of these children are normal and sound knowledge of normal variation cannot be overemphasized. The most common causes for parental concern are flat feet, bow legs, knock knees, and in-toe gait. The chief objective when presented with such children is to exclude a pathological explanation. In broad terms unilateral 'deformities' are more suspicious of pathology than bilateral which frequently reflect normal physiological variation.

Toe walking

The commonest explanation for this presentation is habitual or idiopathic toe walking although more serious explanations should be considered and excluded. A thorough neuromuscular evaluation is mandatory since toe walking may be a feature of muscular dystrophy, cerebral palsy, a tethered cord or indeed any neuromuscular disorder. Children with habitual or idiopathic toe walking persistently walk on the toes, but can be encouraged to adopt a more normal heel strike. They should be able to stand still with the heels to the ground. Treatment is directed toward constant encouragement to reinforce the normal heel–toe gait pattern, but occasionally serial casting is helpful to break a persistent habit or if true tendo-Achilles shortening develops.

Flat feet

Most children who are brought for assessment of flat feet are normal. The clinician's responsibility is to exclude potential pathological causes such as congenital vertical talus, tarsal coalition or juvenile idiopathic arthritis.

The clinical assessment aims to determine if the flat appearance is flexible or rigid. Rigid flat feet are never normal; flexible flat feet usually are. The feet should be observed weightbearing and walking. Many infants have 'fat feet' rather than flat feet, a pad of fat in the sole of the foot hiding the normal arch. Jack's test should be done. This requires the great toe to be dorsiflexed. As this is done a windlass mechanism tightens the planter fascia and draws the flexible flat foot up into a normal arch (Fig. 29.42). The child should be asked to stand on tiptoe while the foot is observed both from behind and from the medial side. When standing, the heel of the flat foot is in valgus if viewed from behind. On tip toe the heel and hindfoot should swing into a varus posture and when viewed from the medial side an arch should develop. The flexible flat foot has a normal or even an increased range of movement as a result of a degree of ligamentous laxity. Limitation suggests pathology. Radiographs are not necessary in the evaluation of the flexible flat foot but should be included if there is any suspicion of inflexibility or symptoms of pain.

Flexible flat feet are rarely symptomatic and in most individuals represent an anatomical variant. They are occasionally associated with conditions where ligamentous laxity is a feature, such as Ehlers–Danlos and Marfan syndromes when they may persist into adult life. Treatment is rarely necessary. Footwear modifications do not alter the development of the foot although a simple arch support or a heel cup, to prevent the heel collapsing into valgus, can help to reduce symptoms of foot ache or minimize rapid shoe wear. In the rare cases where symptomatic flat foot persists into maturity, surgical correction can be considered.

Bow legs and knock knees

Whilst the majority of children who present with bow legs or knock knees are physiologically normal, both presentations can be a manifestation of metabolic bone disease and consideration of such conditions is important.

Bow legs (genu varum)

Figure 29.43 charts the development of the tibiofemoral angle during growth. Varus angulation is normal in infants but usually resolves by 18–24 months.[98] Valgus angulation is normal in 3- to 5-year-olds, usually resolving by age 7–8 years. Clinical assessment should be made with

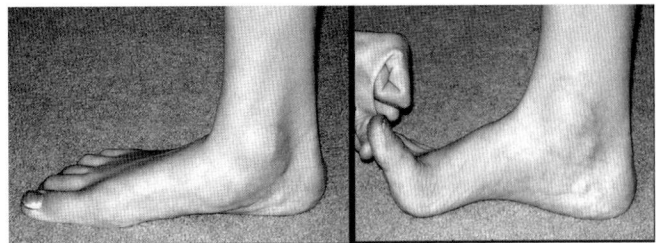

Fig. 29.42 Flexible flat foot – Jack's test.

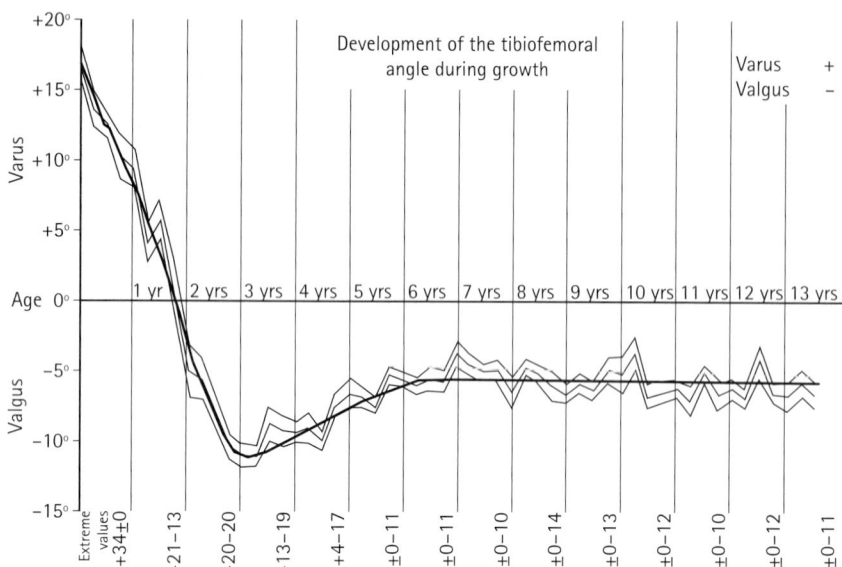

Fig. 29.43   The tibiofemoral angle during growth. (Adapted from Salenius and Vankka 1975[98].)

the child standing, if possible, and both patellae pointing forwards. The tibiofemoral angle can then be measured with a goniometer. This assessment is relatively crude but measurements more than two standard deviations from normal suggest further evaluation, to exclude a pathological explanation.

The principal pathological explanations for bow legs are metabolic bone disease, Blount disease and skeletal dysplasias. Radiographs are not usually helpful under 18 months of age but should be taken if there is a suspicion of pathology. Typical feature of rickets with widening and irregularity of the growth plate and trumpet-like flaring of the metaphysis (Fig. 29.27), or features of Blount disease or some skeletal dysplasia may be seen.

Infantile Blount disease can be difficult to distinguish from physiological bowing but is suggested by bowing that is severe or persisting beyond 24 months. Blount disease is the result of an idiopathic growth disturbance in the posteromedial part of the proximal tibial physis and is most common in people of Scandinavian or West Indian descent. Affected infants are often heavy and walk early and it is thought that increased pressure across the growth plate may play a role in the etiology. Differentiation from physiological bowing can be difficult and it is possible that the two conditions are part of a continuum. Radiographs can be helpful. In physiological bowing there is varus of the whole leg, both the distal femur and the proximal tibia, whereas in Blount disease bowing is principally at the proximal tibia, often with a sharp angulation in the medial metaphyseal region (Fig. 29.44). Early brace treatment may be effective in children under 3 years old.[99] A knee ankle foot orthosis (KAFO) is used to keep the knee in extension for 23 out of 24 hours a day in order to unload the posteromedial physis, but if the deformity continues to progress tibial osteotomy may become necessary.

Knock knees (genu valgum)

As can be seen from Figure 29.43 genu valgum of around 8–10° is normal in 3- to 5-year-old children and gradually returns to adult values of 5–7° by around 7 years of age. Normal children, by definition, fall within two standard deviations of the mean and the normal distribution of the tibiofemoral angle is wide. Treatment of physiological knock knees is not necessary. The underlying cause of pathological cases should be addressed before attending to the limb deformity. Brace treatment is of little benefit and treatment often involves osteotomy or asymmetrical growth plate epiphyseodesis or stapling.

In-toe and out-toe gait

We walk along a straight, imaginary line of progression, which stretches out before us. When the foot is placed on the ground, the line

of its long axis forms an angle with the line of progression and this angle is termed the foot progression angle. In-toe gait (internal foot progression angle) where the toes of each foot point inwards is a common cause for parental concern. Most patients who present with rotational problems in the lower limbs are normal. Occasionally rotational

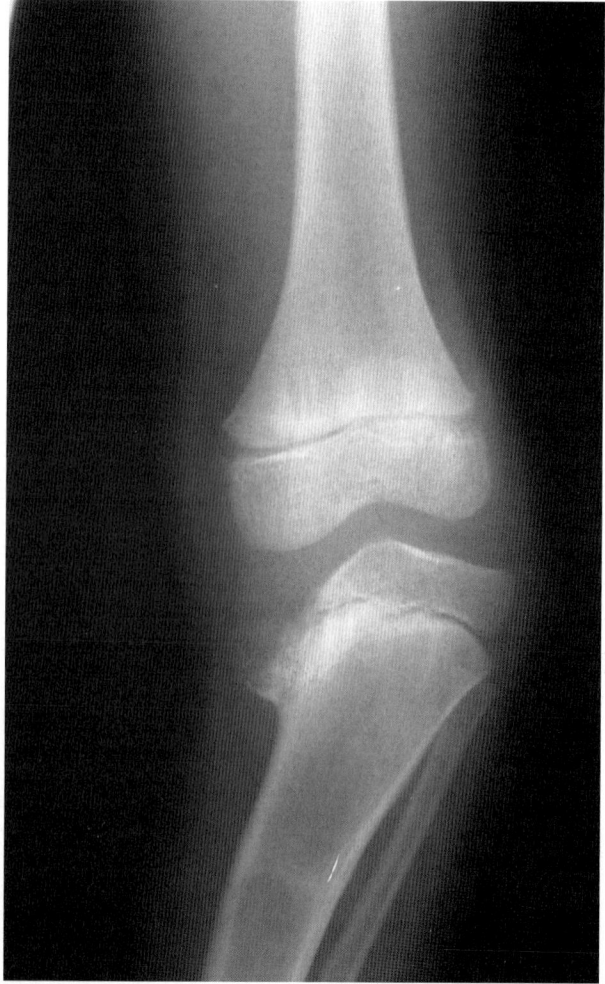

Fig. 29.44   Blount disease.

problems may be pathological, representing part of a bone, joint or neuromuscular disorder.

The foot is at the end of the limb and an in-toe or out-toe gait may result from a twist or torsion in the femur, the tibia or the foot itself. Initial assessment of these children involves determining the site and magnitude of the torsion, by examining the rotational profile of the limb. The child should stand and walk so that the foot progression angle can be estimated. This is very variable in early childhood: most children under 4 years have a degree of in-toeing while most adults have a degree of out-toeing.

The rotational profile of the lower limbs should be evaluated (Fig. 29.45). The hips should be examined with the child prone on the examination couch and the knees flexed to 90°. External and internal rotation at the hip can then be assessed (Fig. 29.45AB,). This gives some indication of torsion within the femur but is also influenced by soft tissue tension about the hip capsule. With the child still prone and the knees flexed to 90° the limb can be viewed from above. The thigh–foot angle is the angle between the long axis of the thigh and the long axis of the foot (Fig. 29.45C). It gives some indication of torsion within the tibia. Care should be taken to encourage the patient to relax the foot for the examination while the examiner gently holds the foot in slight dorsiflexion. Soft tissue laxity about the knee can allow the foot to be twisted into internal or external rotation giving a spurious assessment. The sole of the foot should now be viewed from above. A line bisecting the center of the calcaneum should pass through the second toe or the second web interspace. This assessment helps to determine if deformity in the foot is contributing to the gait pattern.

Femoral torsion

The long axis of the femoral neck is aligned slightly forwards of the transcondylar axis (or coronal plane) of the femur. The angle between the femoral neck axis and the transcondylar axis is the angle of femoral anteversion. At birth, femoral anteversion measures about 40° gradually falling to adult values of 10–15° during development. Infants have

the greatest degree of anteversion but do not normally demonstrate an excessive range of internal rotation at the hips because of soft tissue external rotation contracture which is normal in this age range. Femoral anteversion is the most common explanation for in-toe gait in children over 3–4 years and persistence of immature degrees of femoral anteversion is a frequent cause of in-toe gait in early adolescence particularly in girls. Patients present with various complaints especially awkwardness of gait and tripping. They sit in the 'W' position both because they can and because they find it comfortable.

Treatment is rarely necessary since most cases resolve during development. If the problem persists into late adolescence and is sufficiently severe, derotation osteotomy is effective. Sometimes especially in adolescent girls external tibial torsion coexists: this compensates for the internal femoral torsion so that the feet point forwards but the patellae are left 'squinting' medially toward each other (Fig. 29.46). If treatment proves to be necessary in such patients, it will involve bilateral femoral and tibial osteotomies. This is a considerable undertaking, not to be approached lightly.

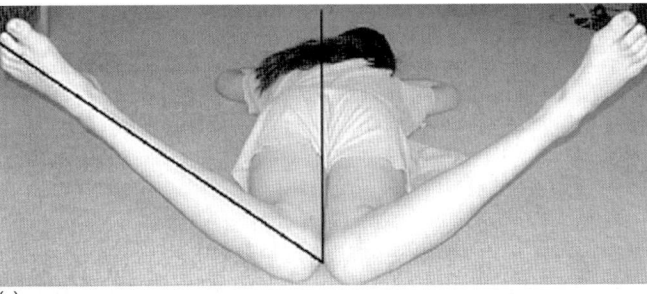

(a)

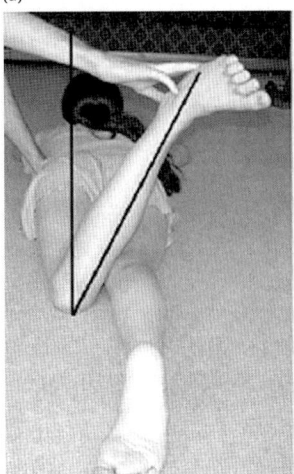

(b)

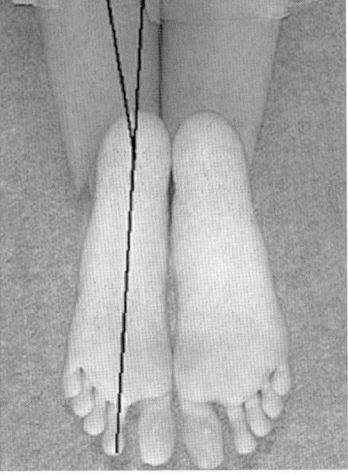

(c)

Fig. 29.45 Assessment of the rotational profile of the lower limbs.

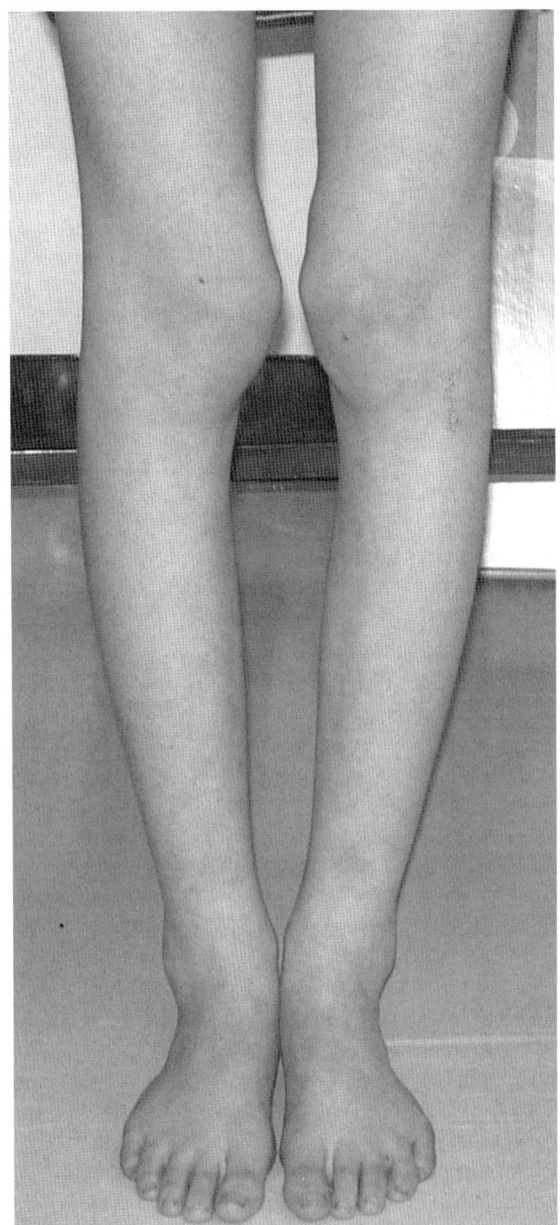

Fig. 29.46 'Squinting' patellae.

Tibial torsion

Internal tibial torsion is a common explanation for in-toe gait in the toddler age range. The degree of tibial torsion is assessed by measuring the thigh–foot axis, as already described, or by measuring the angle between the coronal (or transcondylar) plane and a line joining the tips of medial and lateral malleoli at the ankle. In the term infant at birth, the medial malleolus usually lies behind the lateral malleolus. By walking age the malleoli are level on the coronal plane and by the time walking is well established the lateral malleolus is behind the medial. In other words the infant normally has relative internal tibial torsion, which gradually rotates externally with growth. Internal tibial torsion often coexists with bowing of the legs in infants and young children and may exaggerate the appearance of the bowing. No treatment is necessary or effective for physiological internal tibial torsion.

Excessive external tibial torsion is less common than internal tibial torsion and more likely to persist into adolescence.[100] Once again the only effective treatment for tibial rotational abnormalities is tibial osteotomy. Serious thought needs to be given before offering operative solutions as neither internal nor external tibial torsion have been shown to be risk factors for later degenerative change.

Metatarsus varus

Metatarsus varus or metatarsus adductus is medial deviation of the forefoot on the hindfoot. The subtalar and ankle joints are normal and the hindfoot is in neutral or slight valgus. This distinguishes the condition from clubfoot deformity where the hindfoot is stiff and in varus and equinus. The foot has a concave medial border which can be the cause of, or at least contribute to, an in-toe gait appearance.

The severity of the condition can be classified using the heel bisector as previously described. The condition is described as flexible if the forefoot can be passively overcorrected, partly flexible if it can be passively corrected to the midline and rigid if it cannot be returned to the midline. The natural history is of progressive spontaneous resolution. Consideration can be given to treatment if the deformity is rigid or partly flexible and serial casting has been shown to be effective.[101]

COMMON ORTHOPEDIC EXPLANATIONS FOR MUSCULOSKELETAL PAIN IN CHILDHOOD

Growing pains

Musculoskeletal pain in children is relatively common and usually benign. In evaluating children it is wise to remember that infection and neoplasia are amongst the myriad of potential explanations. Both commonly present in childhood as localized bone pain and must be given due consideration in the differential diagnosis.

The syndrome of benign 'growing pains' is common; usually presenting in children between 4 and 8 years. It can occur in the upper but more frequently the lower limbs. The typical history is of a child who, after a busy day, complains of aching pains in the limbs, frequently in the thighs, shins or around the front or the back of the knees. The pain can be severe, even disturbing sleep, and usually settles after a variable period of parental rubbing of the affected limbs. The next day the child is fine and there are no sequelae. The natural history is of resolution after 18–24 months but the course may be more protracted. The cause remains unknown but growth seems to have little to do with the symptoms. The likely explanation is muscle fatigue or cramp.[102] Treatment is primarily reassurance but can include stretching exercises if muscle fatigue is thought to be a factor.

Neck and back pain

See later section, page 1437.

The painful or irritable hip

The term irritable hip is not a diagnosis but the clinical presentation of hip pathology. The patient may present with symptoms ranging from severe pain with complete inability to weightbear to modest pain, localized to the hip or referred to the knee, with virtually no limp.

The most sensitive sign of hip joint pathology is subtle limitation of internal rotation, which should be carefully sought. Clinical examination of the hip is equally important when patients present with localized hip pain or with isolated thigh or knee pain. The potential for knee pain to be referred from the hip is frequently overlooked.

The commonest cause for an irritable hip in childhood is transient synovitis, but the differential is wide and includes infections, acute and chronic, including septic arthritis and osteomyelitis, Perthes disease and slipped capital femoral epiphysis (SCFE). Less common causes include the inflammatory arthritides such as juvenile idiopathic arthritis, idiopathic chondrolysis and neoplasms. Transient synovitis, Perthes disease, SCFE and chondrolysis will be discussed here. The other disorders are discussed elsewhere in the chapter.

Transient synovitis

This is the commonest cause for hip pain in children: it is estimated that about 3% of children will have at least one episode.[103] It is twice as common in boys and usually occurs between 3 and 8 years with a peak incidence around 6.[104] It is characterized by a transient period of hip joint irritability in a systemically well child. The etiology is unknown but hypotheses include trauma, allergic hypersensitivity or infection. In up to 70% of cases there is a history of either current or antecedent nonspecific upper respiratory infection, and the most widely accepted explanation is that the condition represents a transient reactive synovitis.

Hip joint ultrasonography is the most useful investigation, confirming that the hip joint is the source of complaint. The findings are nonspecific and do not necessarily exclude other causes of an irritable hip. Radiographs and laboratory tests are normal or nonspecific. Transient synovitis is essentially a diagnosis of exclusion and investigations are aimed at excluding other diagnoses. Pyogenic septic arthritis is the most important alternative diagnosis. The child with septic arthritis is usually systemically unwell with a high fever, a high white cell count and ESR and fails to improve with rest. The patient with an effusion due to transient synovitis may have a modest fever and mildy elevated ESR and improves with rest.

Treatment is symptomatic. Skin traction has been popular but is not now recommended because positioning the hip in extension increases intracapsular pressure and pain. If traction is to be used, the leg should be supported with the hip flexed. In practice it is more practical to let the child rest the limb in a position of flexion and external rotation for comfort, provided symptoms settle promptly.

Most cases resolve progressively over 5–10 days. Deterioration is more characteristic of septic arthritis and persistence of moderate or modest symptoms should raise suspicion of alternative explanations such as Perthes disease. Isotope bone scanning can be helpful in these circumstances to distinguish Perthes disease, characterized by reduced uptake, from transient synovitis and other inflammatory conditions where increased uptake is usual. A relationship between transient synovitis and the development of Perthes disease has been suggested but no direct causal correlation has ever been shown. It is safest to conclude that the only relationship is a similar mode of presentation, with an irritable hip.

Perthes disease (Legg–Calvé–Perthes disease)

Perthes disease is avascular necrosis of the femoral head epiphysis due to a disturbance of the epiphyseal blood supply. The disturbance can affect part or all of the femoral epiphysis and the extent of involvement is related to the ultimate prognosis. Despite enthusiasm for the notion that thrombophilia or hypofibrinolysis may be involved in the pathogenesis, more recent work has proved less than encouraging and Perthes disease remains a condition of unknown etiology.[105] Eighty percent of cases occur between the ages of 4 and 9 years and the condition is five times more common in boys.[106] Children present insidiously with an irritable hip syndrome which persists and may deteriorate.

Initial radiographs may be normal. Radionuclide bone scanning shows decreased uptake, distinguishing Perthes from other causes of an irritable hip. MRI can reveal epiphyseal necrosis earlier than plain radiographs as well as defining the extent of involvement. Radiographs will ultimately reveal progressive changes in the hip joint and the femoral epiphysis.

The pathogenesis is reflected in sequential radiological stages. In the initial phase there is increased epiphyseal density which gives way to the fragmentation phase (Fig. 29.47a), sometimes heralded by the appearance of a subchondral radiolucent line or 'crescent sign' (Fig. 29.47b) and eventually characterized by the appearance of lucent areas fragmenting the epiphysis. The reparative or reossification phase supervenes and normal bone density slowly substitutes areas of previous lucency. The process continues from the periphery of the epiphysis to the center until the healed phase is reached. The bony epiphysis once again has the consistency of normal bone but may have become deformed to a greater or lesser degree.

Although Perthes disease can be bilateral in 10–12% of cases[107] radiographs characteristically reveal different stages of disease in the two sides. A similar appearance in both hips is very unususal and should raise suspicion of skeletal dysplasias such as multiple epiphyseal dysplasia (MED) (Fig. 29.25) and spondyloepiphyseal dysplasia (SED).

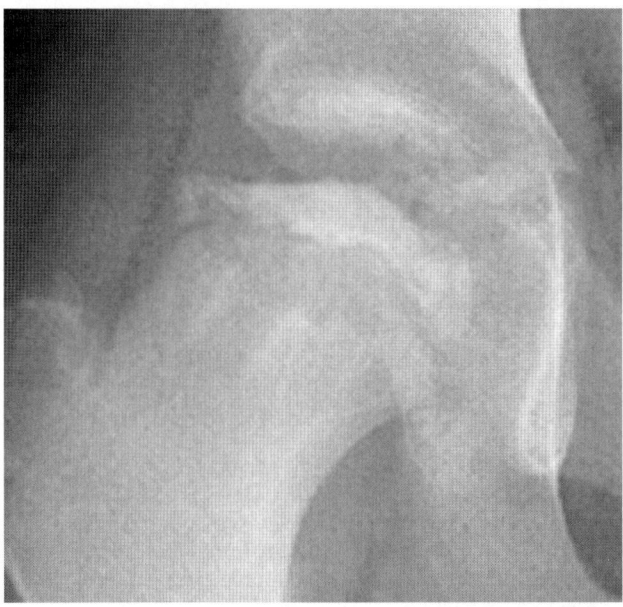

(a)

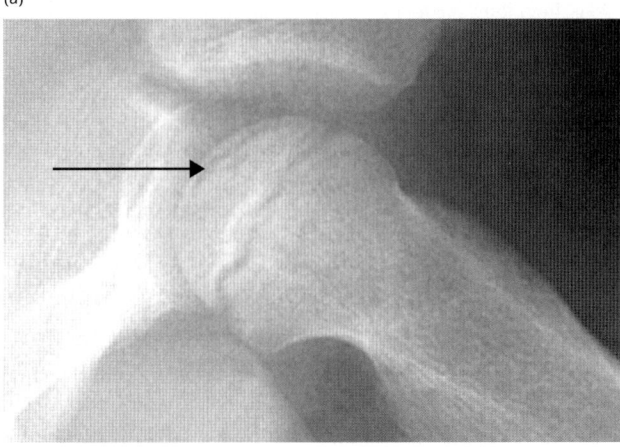

(b)

Fig. 29.47   Perthes disease: (a) stage of fragmentation and collapse; (b) crescent sign.

The progression from the initial phase to the end of the healed phase can take several years. During this time, especially during the fragmentation phase, the cartilaginous femoral head loses the support of its internal bony skeleton and becomes plastic, or able to change shape. The shape the femoral head becomes is determined by the extent of loss of support (or epiphyseal necrosis), and by the mechanical environment in which the plastic femoral head finds itself. The long term prognosis depends on how spherical the femoral head remains and how congruently it fits the acetabulum.

In early Perthes disease, when the femoral head remains plastic, the principle of treatment is the principle of 'containment'. The patient's own acetabulum is used as a template or mold to keep the femoral head spherical, or at least congruent. This can be achieved by the patient themselves if a good range of movement, especially abduction, is maintained. Alternatively, 'containment' treatment with an abduction brace or femoral or pelvic osteotomy is used to position the plastic part of the femoral epiphysis within the acetabulum. Clinical examination is a crucial part of patient assessment. If the patient maintains a good range of movement the soft femoral epiphysis will be constantly moving in and out of the acetabulum during day-to-day activity and will remain congruent. If, on the other hand, range of movement is limited especially abduction, the femoral epiphysis will not be contained within the acetabulum and weightbearing forces will lead to flattening of the epiphysis and incongruity. Loss of range of movement is therefore a sinister clinical sign.

Radiological evaluation is easiest using the Herring grading system. Herring divided the epiphysis as seen on an anteroposterior (AP) radiograph into medial, middle and lateral columns. Only the lateral column is evaluated. The hip is classified as Herring A if there is no necrosis involving the lateral column, Herring B if the lateral column is involved but retains more than 50% of its original height and Herring C if it has lost more than 50% of its original height. The prognosis deteriorates from grades A to C. In concept if the lateral column is intact, the remainder of the femoral head is protected from weightbearing forces, but if the lateral column fails the whole femoral head is exposed to forces from above and will flatten.

Patients under 5 years at the onset of Perthes disease have a good prognosis. In this age group patients frequently maintain an excellent range of movement, even in the face of extensive epiphyseal necrosis on radiographs, and they essentially contain their own femoral head. They rarely require intervention, but should be constantly reviewed to ensure that a good range of movement is maintained. The good prognosis in this age range is also a reflection of the immature acetabulum with much growth remaining. If the femoral head does become aspherical as a result of the Perthes process, the acetabulum will grow to match.

In older children the acetabulum has less growth remaining, is less able to accommodate an aspherical femoral head and incongruity becomes progressively more likely. Clinical signs reflect the radiological extent of epiphyseal necrosis. If there is clinical loss of range of movement in this age group radiographs will usually reveal Herring grade C or B lateral column involvement. These findings usually dictate 'containment' treatment. In the past a wide range of abduction braces have been used but more recent reports question their efficacy.[108] There is a growing inclination to offer surgical containment because of emerging evidence of improved outcome. Surgical containment is usually in the form of a varus femoral or pelvic osteotomy. It is common practice for surgical candidates to undergo an examination of the joint under anesthetic and hip joint arthrography, to ensure that the epiphysis is containable before embarking on surgical treatment. Patients should be followed to maturity, mainly to ensure a significant leg length discrepancy does not develop. A modest leg length discrepancy is common; one requiring treatment unusual.

Once the Perthes disease is over and the femoral epiphysis healed, it is no longer plastic. Hip pain can result if incongruity has developed. The objective of treatment now is restoration of functional congruity. Once again assessment commonly includes examination under anesthesia and arthrography. The principal problem encountered in a deformed incongruent joint is 'hinge abduction'. Because the femoral head is too big to enter the acetabulum during abduction, it levers itself out of the joint with the 'hinge' at the lateral lip of the acetabulum. This limits the patient's functional abduction. The problem can sometimes be helped with a valgus femoral osteotomy.[109]

Slipped capital femoral epiphysis (SCFE)

Slipped capital femoral epiphysis (SCFE) or slipped upper femoral epiphysis (SUFE) is the commonest hip disorder in the adolescent age range and is frequently the subject of medical negligence claims because of delay in diagnosis with potentially disabling consequences for the patient.

The capital femoral epiphysis is fixed to the femoral metaphysis by the proximal femoral growth plate or physis. If the cartilaginous physis is subjected to shear forces it can fail, usually through its hypertrophic zone, and the femoral epiphysis will then 'slip' posteriorly on the metaphysis, either progressively or suddenly. A SCFE occurs when the load applied exceeds the resistance of the physis to slip. This can occur because the load is too great, because the physis is vulnerable or, most often, because of a combination of these factors.

Hormonal events during normal adolescence lead to relative widening of the physis and its hypertrophic zone during periods of rapid growth. The threshold at which the widened physis fails is lower than a normal physis, making the adolescent vulnerable to SCFE. Any condition that widens the growth plate either because of increased growth or decreased ossification predisposes to SCFE and it has been associated with a variety of endocrine abnormalities including hypothyroidism, panhypopituitarism and hypogonadal conditions and treatment of short stature with growth hormone.[110,111] If a vulnerable physis is subjected to increased load, such as might occur in obesity, the risk of SCFE is further increased. Sixty-three percent of affected individuals are over the 90th percentile for weight.

The incidence of SCFE is around 2:100 000 and its peak presentation is 9–15 years in girls and 10–16 years in boys, i.e. during the adolescent growth spurt. The condition is more common in boys than girls in a ratio of 1.5:1.0. If a case presents in a child outside the expected age range or in a child with an unusual body habitus, more serious consideration should be given to an underlying endocrine or metabolic abnormality.

Careful radiographic interpretation is important for early detection. The AP radiograph is insufficiently sensitive and where a slip is considered possible a lateral radiograph should be obtained. Signs on the AP radiograph include subtle blurring and irregularity of the physis and slight loss of epiphyseal height. When the epiphysis slips a little further it is more obvious. A line, Klein's line,[112] drawn along the superior aspect of the femoral neck should cut off the lateral edge of the epiphysis but does not if the epiphysis has slipped. Minor degrees of slip are more easily seen on the lateral radiograph because the epiphysis primarily slips posteriorly (Fig. 29.48).

SCFE is classified into unstable (acute) or stable (chronic).[113] A third category of a stable slip suddenly becoming unstable also exists (acute on chronic). The distinction between the different types of slip is important because the clinical presentation and the prognosis differ significantly.

In the stable slip the femoral epiphysis gradually and progressively slips posteriorly on the femoral metaphysis. The patient may have a limp but can weightbear and the presentation is essentially that of an irritable hip. Referred knee pain may be the patient's only complaint and a futile search for a local explanation at the knee is a common cause for delayed diagnosis. Pain, discomfort or reluctance when the hip is internally rotated is a subtle indicator of hip pathology and should prompt further radiographic evaluation. Stable slips rarely if ever suffer the serious complication of avascular necrosis but can lead to significant proximal femoral deformity, limited range of movement, limb length discrepancy and premature degenerative change. If a stable slip remains undetected an unstable slip may supervene and seriously affect the

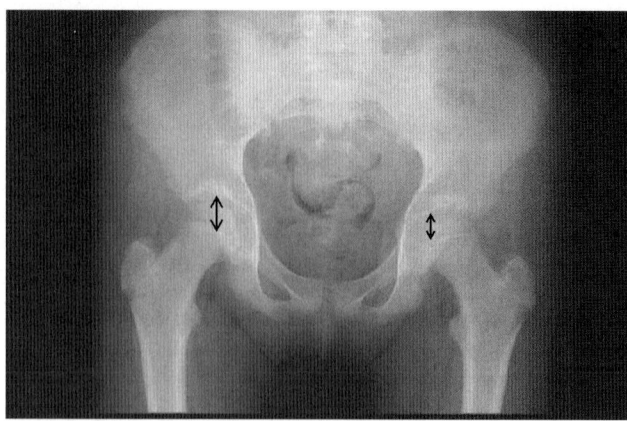

(a)

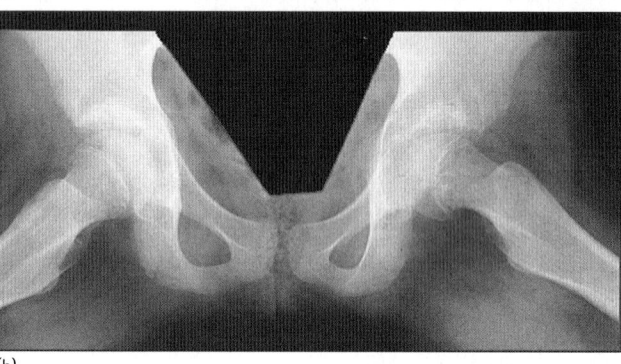

(b)

Fig. 29.48   Slipped capital femoral epiphysis: (a) AP radiograph; (b) frog lateral radiograph. Note the relative insensitivity of the AP radiograph – arrows demonstrate subtle difference in epiphyseal height.

prognosis. The keystone of management is early detection followed in most cases by fixation in situ with a cannulated screw. The principle of this treatment is to promote fusion of the growth plate to prevent further slippage and deformity. Osteotomies to correct deformity are controversial and are usually, though not always, deferred for 18–24 months to allow for remodeling. Persistent difficulties are unlikely to improve spontaneously thereafter.

There is usually no difficulty in diagnosing the unstable slip which occurs when the femoral epiphysis suddenly slips posteriorly off the femoral metaphysis. The patient presents in severe pain, unable to weightbear and the leg is held in external rotation. The rate of avascular necrosis in the unstable slip is around 47%.[113] The blood supply to the femoral epiphysis is vulnerable in the immature hip and the vessels passing along the femoral neck to the epiphysis are suddenly torn or stretched in the unstable slip. The avascular necrosis that follows may not be seen radiographically for some months, but if it occurs it is a devastating complication with no satisfactory treatment. The management of the unstable slip once again involves fixing the slipped epiphysis in situ to promote physeal fusion and to prevent further slippage and damage to the epiphyseal blood supply. No attempt is made to deliberately correct the unstable slip, for fear of further damage to the epiphyseal blood supply, but inadvertent reduction does take place during positioning for fixation in unstable slips and can be accepted. Once again the role of femoral osteotomies in the management of unstable slips is controversial.

The incidence of symptomatic bilateral SCFE averages around 25%, most contralateral slips occurring within 12 months of the original slip. Prophylactic fixation of the opposite side should be considered, especially in the child with an underlying endocrine or metabolic abnormality or some years of growth remaining. If the contralateral hip is not fixed the patient should be warned to return urgently at the first sign of hip or knee symptoms.

Idiopathic chondrolysis

This uncommon condition is characterized by the rapid and progressive destruction of articular cartilage from both sides of the affected joint with subsequent pain and stiffness. It is five times more common in girls than boys and is typically a condition of adolescents. Radiographs reveal narrowing of the affected joint space. Chondrolysis of the hip is of unknown etiology in most cases but has been reported in association with SCFE,[114] trauma, prolonged immobilization and severe burns of the extremities.[115]

The natural history of chondrolysis includes an acute stage lasting 6–18 months with pain, inflammation, loss of range of motion and destruction of articular cartilage. Eventually the chronic stage emerges and can last from 3 to 5 years. During the chronic stage the hip may continue to deteriorate. Ultimately the hip may become pain free but stiff in a poor position, or pain free with partial or rarely complete return of motion and some restoration of the joint space.

The principles of treatment include control of any inflammation with therapeutic doses of NSAIDs and maintenance of motion with an aggressive physiotherapy program. Surgical release of persistent tendon contractures may be necessary in some patients and there are some encouraging results reported following aggressive subtotal capsulotomy and tendon release.[116] Some patients may ultimately come to hip arthrodesis in a functional position for the relief of pain.

Knee pain

Complaints of knee swelling, mechanical symptoms (giving way and locking) or pain are common in both children and adolescents. A knee joint effusion indicates intra-articular pathology and mechanical symptoms often indicate joint instability, loose bodies or meniscal pathology. Pain is either localized or diffuse. There are numerous explanations for localized knee pain in children including a variety of overuse and sport-related problems (see later section, p. 1440). Referred knee pain is common and clinical examination of the hip is important in any patient presenting with unexplained knee pain.

Anterior knee pain (patellofemoral pain syndrome and chondromalacia)

Anterior knee pain is a descriptive term for diffuse pain at the front of the knee. It is a very common complaint in the adolescent age range, typically affecting girls. The complaint is of a diffuse ache around the front of the knee at the patellofemoral joint (patellofemoral pain syndrome), which is worse after activity, after climbing up or down stairs and after sitting for prolonged periods with the knees in a flexed position. Chondromalacia is a term often used to describe this syndrome, but is really a pathological description of cartilage softening and degeneration, rarely present in young patients complaining of anterior knee pain.

The presentation of patellofemoral pain syndrome is fairly typical but evaluation should include reasonable steps to exclude other potential sources of pain. Lateral maltracking or subluxation of the patella is highly correlated with patellofemoral pain syndrome. Because the line of the quadriceps from the anterior superior spine to the tibial tuberosity passes to the lateral side of the knee joint, there is an inherent tendency for the patella to track to the lateral side of the trochlear sulcus in the anterior femur of the patellofemoral articulation. There are mechanisms to prevent such lateral maltracking, but these are sometimes inadequate. Pain at the lateral part of the articular surface of the patella can be a subtle consequence as can more overt subluxation or dislocation. Rotational malalignment also contributes to the problem and many patients will be found to have persistent femoral anteversion in association with compensatory external tibial torsion so that the feet point forwards but the patellae squint medially, the so-called 'miserable malalignment'.[117]

The natural history of anterior knee pain is of slow resolution and most cases respond to non-operative treatment.[118] For many, reassurance is all that is necessary. Physiotherapy is helpful and activity modification, especially the avoidance of provoking sports, may be necessary.

If there is evidence of maltracking some patients find a knee brace with a patella cut out, to hold the patella medially, is useful. An experienced physiotherapist can help with medial taping of the patella in combination with a program to stretch and strengthen quadriceps muscles. If symptoms are persistent and very troublesome in a patient with convincing maltracking, surgical intervention in the form of a lateral retinacular release can be successful in 75% of cases.[119]

Discoid lateral meniscus

This is a congenital abnormality of the meniscus, which is the shape of a disc rather than the usual crescent. The discoid shape can be either complete, covering the whole lateral tibial plateau, or partial forming a rather wider crescent than usual. Children present with mechanical symptoms of giving way, locking or snapping similar to patients with a meniscal tear. Radiographs of the knee sometimes reveal a lateral joint space that is wider than usual, but MRI is the investigation of choice to demonstrate the extensive and thickened meniscus. Asymptomatic discoid menisci found incidentally should be left undisturbed. Symptomatic menisci can be successfully trimmed arthroscopically into a more normal crescent shape.[120]

Popliteal cyst

This common condition presents as a fluctuant transilluminable swelling in the popliteal fossa. The usual reason for referral is parental concern. The cysts are asymptomatic although they may ache with activity and fluctuate in size. They are typically found subcutaneously along the medial side of the popliteal fossa and are simple synovial lined cysts arising from the semimembranosus sheath.

Plain X-rays of the knee are normal and the cyst is best confirmed by ultrasound scan examination. No treatment is required; spontaneous resolution over months or years is usual.

Occasionally, usually in association with an inflammatory arthropathy, popliteal cysts may rupture presenting with calf pain and swelling, the ruptured 'Baker cyst'. Ultrasound and MRI (Fig. 29.49) will distinguish this from other rare causes of calf pain and swelling in children.

Osteochondritis dissecans (OCD)

Osteochondritis dissecans most commonly involves the knee joint, but can affect the articular surface of any joint. For reasons that remain unclear an area of subchondral bone undergoes avascular necrosis. Etiological theories include trauma, ischemia, a genetic predisposition or a combination of these. Symptoms are usually vague and develop insidiously over several months. The overlying cartilage is initially intact but may subsequently develop degenerative change and break into a flap or a loose body causing the onset of mechanical joint symptoms, including locking, snapping or giving way. The most commonly affected part of the knee is the lateral part of the medial femoral condyle, although it can affect any part of the articular surface including the patella.

Radiographs usually reveal a lucent fragmented area in the subchondral bone (Fig. 29.50). In addition to the routine anteroposterior and lateral views of the knee, a tunnel view is useful because it visualizes the intercondylar notch region and the lateral part of the medial femoral condyle where the condition is most common. Magnetic resonance imaging is the investigation of choice and not only delineates the bony abnormality but also provides some indication of whether the overlying cartilage is intact.

The prognosis of the condition is relatively good in young patients when the growth plate remains open but in adults and adolescents with a closed growth plate the prognosis is more guarded. Treatment should include activity modification to limit aggressive sporting activity, which may cause intact overlying cartilage to become loose. If there are no mechanical symptoms and MRI suggests that the overlying cartilage is intact, activity modification to limit symptoms is recommended until resolution which may take months or even years. If there are mechanical symptoms or the MRI suggests the possibility of a breach or flap of the overlying cartilage, arthroscopic examination is recommended. Large flaps, especially on the weightbearing

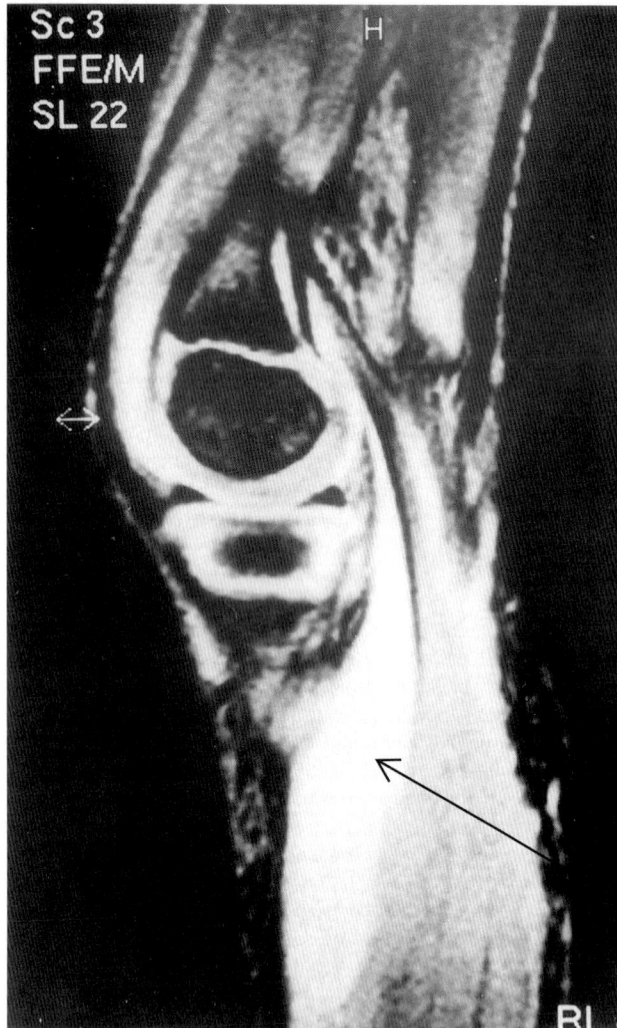

Fig. 29.49   MRI showing ruptured Baker cyst – arrow indicates inflammatory fluid collection extending from the popliteal fossa into the calf.

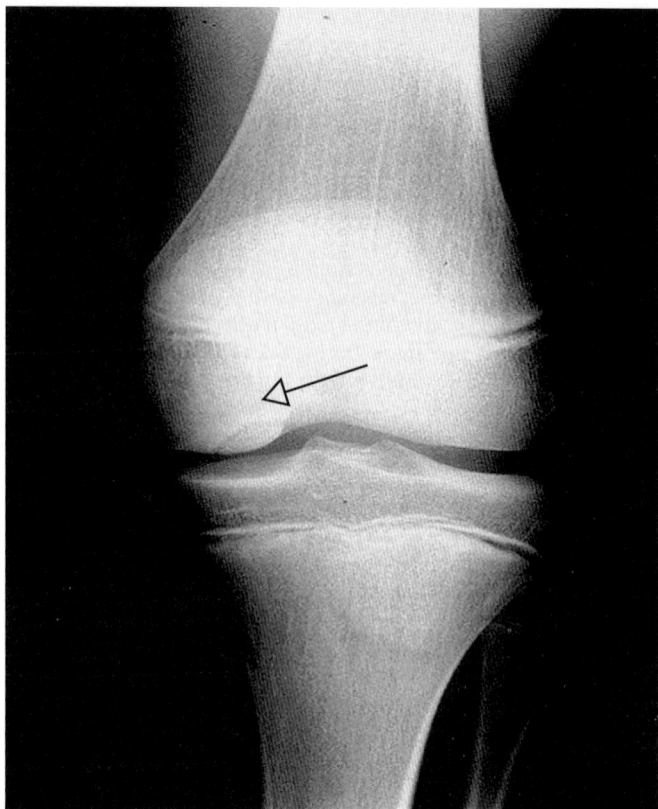

Fig. 29.50   Osteochondritis dissecans of the knee.

surface, should be fixed into position, although loose flaps are usually trimmed flush with the articular surface to prevent further mechanical symptoms and the base of the defect drilled to promote healing with fibrocartilage.

Kohler disease

Kohler disease or osteochondritis of the navicular presents in children around the age of 6 years. The radiographic appearance is that of fragmentation and flattening of the navicular (Fig. 29.51) but this radiological appearance may be a normal variant. The appearance is only considered pathological if there are associated symptoms of localized pain over the bone. Treatment of Kohler disease is symptomatic. There is no evidence of any long term sequelae.

Freiberg disease

Freiberg disease or osteochondritis of the metatarsal head is most common in the second metatarsal. It usually presents in adolescence with localized pain. Radiographs reveal flattening and fragmentation of the metatarsal head. It is believed to be an avascular necrosis developing in a stress fracture and is associated with local trauma as might occur in sport or in dancing. The condition is much commoner in girls. Treatment is initially conservative but persistent local pain and limited dorsiflexion of the metatarsophalangeal joint may necessitate surgical debridement.

Tarsal coalition

Tarsal coalition is an abnormal cartilaginous, fibrous or bony connection between two or more tarsal bones. It is surprisingly common with a reported incidence of 2%. The condition is inherited as an autosomal dominant trait and the incidence in first-degree relatives is 39%.[121] Fortunately the majority of coalitions are asymptomatic. If symptoms develop they usually present during the late juvenile or early adolescent years when the coalition, initially cartilaginous, begins to ossify. The condition is characterized by a painful, rigid valgus foot and peroneal muscle spasm which may be continuous or intermittent, exacerbated by activity and relieved by rest.[122]

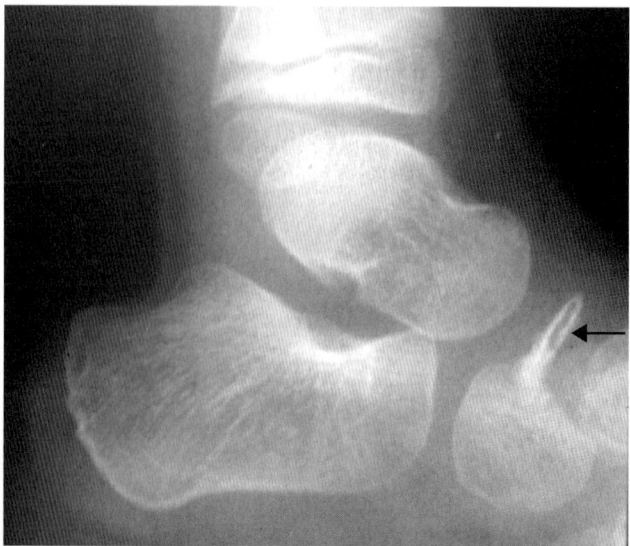

Fig. 29.51   Kohler disease.

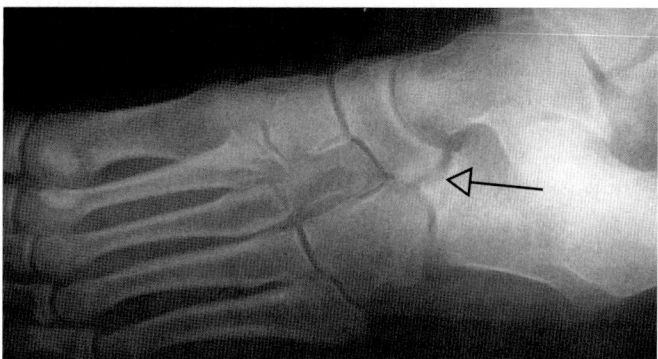

Fig. 29.52 Calcaneonavicular coalition.

The two commonest sites of coalition are between the calcaneus and the navicular (Fig. 29.52) and between the calcaneus and the talus, at the middle facet of the subtalar joint. Sixty percent of calcaneonavicular and 50% of talocalcaneal coalitions are bilateral.[123] Multiple coalitions can rarely coexist in the same foot. Calcaneonavicular coalitions begin to ossify between 8 and 12 years and talocalcaneal coalitions between 12 and 16 years.

Calcaneonavicular coalitions are most easily demonstrated radiographically with a 45° oblique radiograph of the foot. CT best demonstrates talocalcaneal coalitions. Secondary radiographic findings such as talar beaking should suggest the possibility of a tarsal coalition. Treatment is initially symptomatic with analgesia and immobilization. If conservative treatment fails, surgical resection of the abnormal coalition and interposition of fat or muscle to prevent recoalition has been shown to be successful in both calcaneonavicular[124] and talocalcaneal[125] coalitions. Generally, results are less satisfactory after talocalcaneal coalition resection and ultimately some patients come to a triple arthrodesis of the subtalar joint.

Adolescent hallus valgus

Hallux valgus or 'bunions' in adolescents is usually familial rather than the result of poor footwear. It is girls that usually present because of the appearance rather than because of functional problems or pain. There is often an associated bunionette of the fifth toe and patients often have a characteristically broad forefoot with varus of the first metatarsal (metatarsus primus varus). Surgery is best deferred until skeletal maturity is reached. Surgical treatment gives good results for symptomatic feet with a painful bunion but caution should be exercised in the pain free patient who may be disappointed if surgery leaves a better looking but painful foot.

VASCULITIS

Vasculitis is characterized by inflammation and necrosis of vessel walls. This may occur as a primary disorder, where the etiology remains unknown, or as a secondary phenomenon. Within the group of disorders known as the systemic vasculitides there are a variety of different conditions. Categorization of these conditions in childhood has been problematic and it is only recently that a specific pediatric classification system has been proposed[126] (Table 29.14). This is essentially a modification of the Chapel Hill criteria used in adults which classifies the systemic vasculitides based on vessel size.[127] Specific criteria are included for the diagnosis of the main childhood vasculitides.

There remain many children with a systemic vasculitis in whom categorization is difficult due to overlapping clinical features. The importance of attempting to classify these conditions relates to their variable prognosis. While some are self-limiting, others require aggressive immunosuppressive therapy to minimize morbidity and even mortality.

Table 29.14 Classification of childhood vasculitis. (Adapted from Ozen et al 2006[126])

I **Large vessels**
   Takayasu arteritis

II **Medium sized vessels**
   Childhood polyarteritis nodosa
   Cutaneous polyarteritis
   Kawasaki disease

III **Small vessels**
   a. Granulomatous:
      Wegener granulomatosus
      Churg–Strauss syndrome
   b. Nongranulomatous:
      Microscopic polyangiitis
      Henoch–Schönlein purpura
      Other (isolated cutaneous leucocytoclastic vasculitis;
      hypocomplementemic urticarial vasculitis)

IV **Other**
   Behçet disease
   Secondary vasculitis:
      Infection
      Connective tissue disease
   Isolated CNS vasculitis
   Cogan syndrome
   Unclassified

Prompt recognition of those requiring such treatment is perhaps more important than an exact diagnostic label.

PRIMARY VASCULITIS

The only primary vasculitides seen with any frequency in childhood are Henoch–Schönlein purpura and Kawasaki disease.

Henoch–Schönlein purpura

Henoch–Schönlein purpura (HSP) is the most common of the childhood vasculitides with an estimated incidence of 20.4:100 000[128] peaking at around the age of 5. In the majority of affected individuals it is a benign, self-limiting condition but it can be associated with significant morbidity and occasionally mortality if serious organ involvement occurs. It has been estimated that approximately 1% of children with HSP develop persistent renal disease with less than 0.1% having serious disease.[129]

Pathologically HSP causes a leukocytoclastic vasculitis. The etiology remains uncertain but an infectious trigger is postulated in many cases. Although the pathology is poorly understood, there is much interest in the role of IgA. An elevated serum IgA may occur and the renal pathology overlaps with that seen in IgA nephropathy. Abnormalities in glycosylation of IgA1 have been identified in HSP and appear to be associated with renal involvement.[130]

HSP typically involves the skin, joints, GI tract and kidneys. The rash, characteristically a palpable purpura, affects the lower limbs (Fig. 29.53), buttocks, scrotum and elbows. More extensive involvement including rash affecting the face is not uncommon especially in younger children in whom the rash may be atypical.

Arthralgia and an acute, self-limiting arthritis are common. Gastrointestinal involvement with abdominal pain is one of the more troublesome symptoms of HSP and may be complicated by serious gastrointestinal bleeding, intussusception and rarely perforation of the bowel. Renal involvement occurs in around 50%[131] and ranges from mild asymptomatic hematuria and proteinuria to a nephrotic/nephritic picture with hypertension and a rapidly progressive glomerulonephritis. The importance of HSP lies in its potential for long term renal disease, and children with persisting urinary abnormalities require long term follow-up.

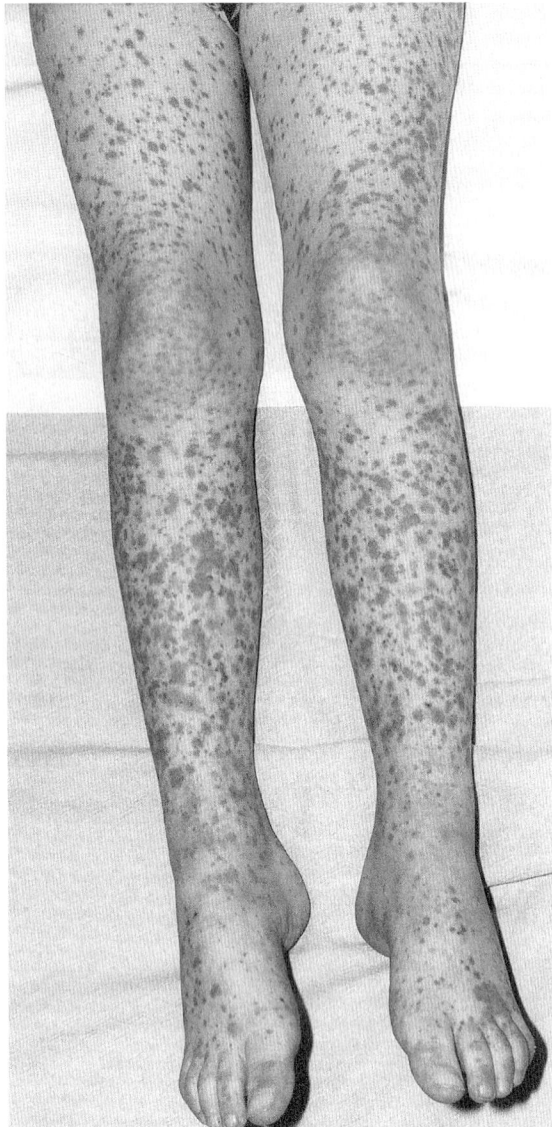

Fig. 29.53   Rash of Henoch–Schönlein purpura.

The diagnosis of HSP is clinical and usually straightforward. With an atypical course, the possibility of some other systemic vasculitis must be considered. Urinalysis should be monitored throughout in all affected children to identify nephritis. Other laboratory investigation is unhelpful and unnecessary in most cases. Abdominal ultrasound may be useful in the assessment of gastrointestinal involvement: characteristic thickening of the bowel wall can be seen and intussusception ruled out where necessary. Evidence of serious or persistent renal involvement may be an indication for renal biopsy to assess the pathology and guide appropriate therapy.

Management of HSP depends on its severity and the particular organ involvement in an individual. In most children it is mild and self-limiting although it may take a few weeks to settle. Recurrent attacks may be seen over a period of a few weeks or months. Most can be managed as outpatients with the parents being taught to test the urine for signs of renal involvement. Simple analgesia such as paracetamol may be adequate for joint and abdominal pain. More significant arthritis may require the use of NSAIDs although these must be used with caution if there is gastrointestinal or renal involvement. There is much anecdotal evidence to support the use of corticosteroids for severe abdominal pain in HSP but no controlled trials. Management of renal involvement depends on its severity. Asymptomatic renal disease requires monitoring but no active

therapy. There is uncontrolled evidence supporting the use of high dose steroids and immunosuppressive therapy where there is a rapidly progressive glomerulonephritis.[132,133] Debate continues around the issue of whether the incidence of serious renal sequelae can be reduced by the earlier administration of steroids. One recent controlled study suggests that in more severe disease early prednisolone therapy while not preventing renal involvement , may shorten its course.[134]

Kawasaki disease

Kawasaki disease or Kawasaki syndrome, first described in Japan in 1967 by Tomisaku Kawasaki, is the other systemic vasculitis seen commonly in childhood, affecting medium sized vessels and with a particular predilection for involvement of the coronary arteries. This may lead to long term sequelae: Kawasaki disease has replaced rheumatic fever as the most common cause of acquired heart disease in children in the resource rich world.[135] Kawasaki disease predominantly affects children under 5 years with most serious sequelae affecting the under twos.

As with all forms of primary vasculitis Kawasaki syndrome is poorly understood and its etiology unclear. Susceptibility to the disease appears to vary with race, children of Asian origin having a higher incidence than Caucasian populations. Recurrence is unusual but reported in around 3%.[136] It occurs in mini-epidemics, its epidemiology suggesting a role for an infectious trigger but no single agent has been consistently associated with Kawasaki disease. There has been interest in the possible role of superantigens in view of clinical similarities to toxic-shock syndrome and the identification of superantigen positive bacteria (both *Staphylococcus aureus* and *Streptococcus*) from a number of individuals with the syndrome.[137] This theory remains unproven. Although the trigger remains uncertain, immunological abnormalities are well documented in Kawasaki disease. Elevated levels of pro-inflammatory cytokines (TNF-α and -β, IL-1 and IL-6); upregulation of adhesion molecules (ELAM-1, ICAM-1 and VCAM-1) and elevated serum levels of macrophage colony-stimulating factor have all been demonstrated.[138]

The diagnosis is based on well-established clinical criteria (Table 29.15).The problem lies with those children, commonly the youngest, who have 'atypical' or 'incomplete' Kawasaki syndrome[139] and are at high risk of coronary artery involvement. The current criteria are insufficiently sensitive for diagnosis in this group and more comprehensive criteria are required.[140] A high index of suspicion is required to ensure that Kawasaki is not missed in the very young child.

The rash in Kawasaki syndrome is polymorphous, usually occurring early in the disease course. Crusting, petechiae and vesicle formation should prompt a search for an alternative diagnosis. An erythematous rash affecting the groin and perineal area and which peels within 48 hours is characteristic (Fig. 29.54a). Involvement of the hands and feet consists of diffuse swelling and/or erythema of the palms and soles. Peeling of the digits (Fig. 29.54b) is well known as a feature of Kawasaki but occurs relatively late in the subacute phase and is not diagnostically helpful. Kawasaki is a multisystem disease and can affect many organ systems. Extreme irritability is very typical of the younger child.

As with most of the vasculitides, laboratory features are nonspecific. Elevation of acute phase reactants, a mild hepatitis and sterile pyuria are common. Thrombocytosis may be marked in the subacute phase.

Table 29.15   Diagnostic criteria for Kawasaki disease

Fever persisting for at least 5 days plus four of the following features:
Changes in peripheral extremities or perineal area
Polymorphous exanthema
Bilateral conjunctival injection
Changes of lips and oral/pharyngeal mucosa
Cervical lymphadenopathy
In the presence of confirmed coronary artery involvement and fever, less than four of the remaining criteria are sufficient to make the diagnosist

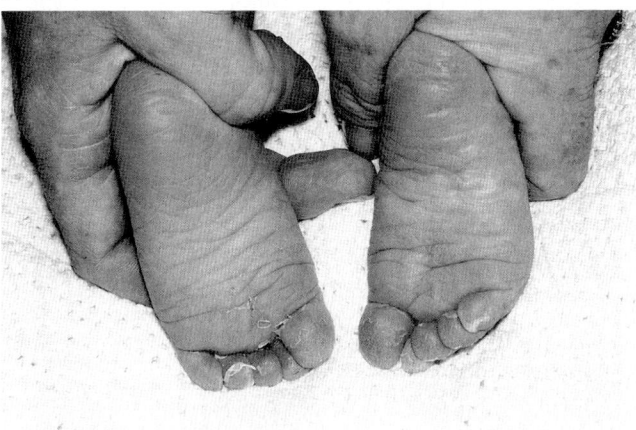

(a)

(b)

Fig. 29.54 Kawasaki disease: (a) typical erythematous groin rash with peeling; (b) peeling of digits

A lumbar puncture may be indicated in the febrile, irritable child and will show a mononuclear pleocytosis.

Untreated Kawasaki disease goes through three phases, acute, subacute and convalescent, the whole process lasting 6–8 weeks. Mortality from coronary artery involvement is 2%. With treatment the process can be switched off in the acute phase and the mortality reduced to 0.3%.

The recognition that the clinical features of Kawasaki disease were the result of an immunologically driven process led to the use of immunoglobulin in treatment with dramatic benefit. Treatment of acute phase Kawasaki disease with intravenous immunoglobulin has been clearly shown to reduce coronary artery involvement and hence mortality and morbidity.[141] A single infusion of 2 g/kg is now known to be the optimal regimen.[142,143] This is given with aspirin in high doses initially with reduction to an antiplatelet dose once defervescence occurs. Up to 20% of children with Kawasaki disease fail to settle following a first dose of intravenous immunoglobulin. Those refractory to a repeat dose are likely to benefit from treatment with high dose steroids.[144] The place of steroids earlier in the therapeutic regimen remains unclear.[145]

All children with a definite diagnosis of Kawasaki disease require cardiac assessment to look for evidence of coronary artery involvement which will necessitate long term cardiology follow-up. Guidelines are available for cardiac assessment and follow-up[146] and the reader is referred to Chapter 21 for further information.

Polyarteritis nodosa

The other primary systemic vasculitides are rare in childhood. Polyarteritis nodosa (PAN) is the least uncommon.

Childhood PAN affects predominantly medium sized arteries. Involved vessels are affected by a necrotizing vasculitis with the formation of aneurysmal nodules in the vessel walls. It frequently presents very nonspecifically and a high index of suspicion is required to make the diagnosis. Presenting symptoms include unexplained malaise and fever, skin rash, abdominal pain, arthropathy and myalgia. Laboratory features are nonspecific with the presence of anemia and raised inflammatory markers. Antineutrophil cytoplasmic antibodies (ANCA) are not associated with classic PAN.

The diagnosis is based on the presence of typical clinical features plus either characteristic abnormalities on biopsy of an affected tissue or abnormal angiography.

Even with correct diagnosis and treatment this condition may have a significant mortality, although this varies considerably in reported series. Prompt treatment is essential in order to minimize damage from the vasculitic process (Fig. 29.55) and improve outcome. Unfortunately the rarity of this condition in childhood means that there are no controlled studies. A combination of high dose steroids plus some other immunosuppressive drug, usually cyclophosphamide, is required. Cyclophosphamide is the drug of choice in most cases and can be used either orally or via intravenous pulses. Once remission has been attained, azathioprine has been shown to be as effective as cyclophosphamide for maintenance and is associated with less long term toxicity. For those children who fail to respond to standard therapy with steroids and cyclophosphamide, anecdotal evidence supports the use of alternatives such as plasmapheresis, new immunosuppressants such as mycophenolate mofetil and biologics (anti-TNFs and rituximab).[147]

Microscopic polyangiitis (MPA)

The microscopic variant of polyarteritis affects the smaller arteries and is less common than classic PAN in childhood. In adults this has a worse prognosis and outcome than classic PAN. It is not clear whether

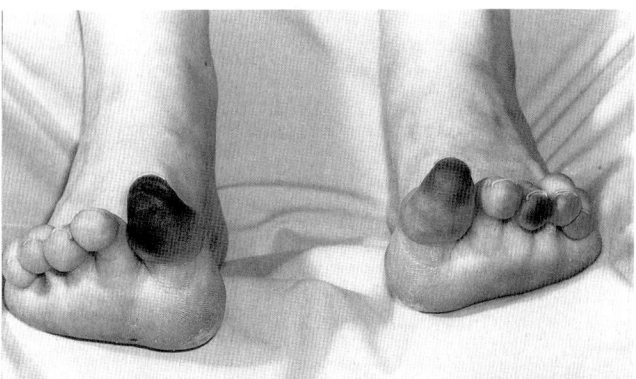

Fig. 29.55 Gangrene of several toes in polyarteritis nodosa.

this applies to pediatric cases. Renal involvement dominates the clinical presentation and course of this condition. As with other small vessel vasculitides, ANCA may be detectable. Management is similar to that of classic PAN.

Cutaneous polyarteritis

There are a group of children who present with a rash identical to that seen in PAN, sometimes associated with systemic upset, but with no evidence of major organ involvement. There is frequently evidence of previous streptococcal infection[148] and this is thought to play a role in the etiology. There is no evidence that this progresses to full blown PAN and it appears to be a separate entity. Prophylaxis with long term penicillin may prevent relapses.

Wegener granulomatosis

Wegener granulomatosis is rare in childhood. Pathologically this is a necrotizing granulomatous vasculitis that affects the small vessels with a predilection for the upper and lower respiratory tract and kidneys. Although the exact pathophysiology is unclear, Wegener granulomatosis is strongly associated with the presence of autoantibodies directed against proteinase 3 (c-ANCA). Whether or not these antibodies play a pathogenic role in the condition remains unclear. Wegener granulomatosis may cause either localized or generalized disease. Steroids and cyclophosphamide are the mainstay of treatment in those with severe disease. With less serious involvement there may be a role for drugs such as methotrexate.

Churg–Strauss syndrome

This vasculitis is exceptionally rare in childhood. The clinical picture is of variable vasculitic features associated with asthma, eosinophilia and infiltrates on chest X-ray.

Takayasu arteritis

Takayasu arteritis, also known as 'pulseless disease', is rare in the UK but worldwide is one of the more common forms of systemic vasculitis affecting younger people. Pathologically it is a chronic giant cell arteritis which segmentally affects the large vessels particularly the aorta and its major branches. Following the initial inflammatory phase, stenosis of vessels leading to ischemia occurs.

During the active inflammatory phase of the disease, affected children may present with features of systemic upset such as fever, weight loss and myalgia. Often the disease presents with evidence of organ ischemia or hypertension.

The etiology of Takayasu arteritis is unclear but genetic factors are important with evidence of racial variations in both incidence and disease expression. Infections and especially tuberculosis have been thought to play a role in triggering the disease but this remains unproven. Management is difficult. Steroids and methotrexate have a role in the active inflammatory phase. Once stricture formation has occurred, angioplasty and reconstructive surgery may be necessary.

Behçet syndrome

Behçet syndrome is an uncommon, poorly understood inflammatory condition in which at least some of the clinical features are the result of a vasculitis which can affect both arteries and veins. Behçet syndrome is characterized by aphthous oral ulceration, genital ulcers and uveitis. Rare in the UK, Behçet syndrome occurs much more commonly in eastern Mediterranean regions.

Behçet syndrome most commonly presents in early adult life and is rare in childhood. The diagnosis is based on clinical features. In children, recurrent oral ulceration may be the only manifestation for some years and until other features become apparent, it may not be possible to confirm the diagnosis. Painful oral ulcers occur in crops lasting up to 2 weeks. Genital ulceration occurs frequently. Uveitis, although common in affected adults, occurs less frequently in children. Arthralgia and arthritis are common in childhood Behçet syndrome as is recurrent fever. Skin lesions seen most frequently in children are folliculitis

and erythema nodosum. Gastrointestinal involvement may cause abdominal pain and diarrhea and is reported in approximately a fifth of affected children. CNS involvement, particularly meningoencephalitis, occurs in approximately 25%. Vascular involvement, which includes both venous and arterial thromboses and aneurysm formation, is potentially the most serious complication of Behçet syndrome. Pulmonary vasculitis, although rare in affected children, is associated with a high mortality.

Significant vascular involvement is associated with a poor outcome and merits treatment with systemic immunosuppressive agents.[149] Colchicine[150] and thalidomide[151] have been shown to be effective for Behçet syndrome where mucocutaneous lesions predominate.

Cogan's syndrome

This systemic vasculitis is extremely rare. It is characterized by the association of vasculitic features with interstitial keratitis and vestibulo-auditory dysfunction.

SECONDARY VASCULITIS

Secondary vasculitis occurs quite commonly in children. It may be seen in the context of a child known to have some other autoimmune rheumatic disorder such as juvenile idiopathic arthritis or systemic lupus erythematosus (Fig. 29.56). Treatment is that of the underlying disorder.

Vasculitis may also occur in association with a variety of infections. These include bacterial infections, viruses such as Epstein–Barr virus and infections such as tuberculosis. Vasculitis is seen not uncommonly in association with meningococcal disease.

Drugs may also be associated with vasculitis which usually remits when the offending agent is withdrawn.

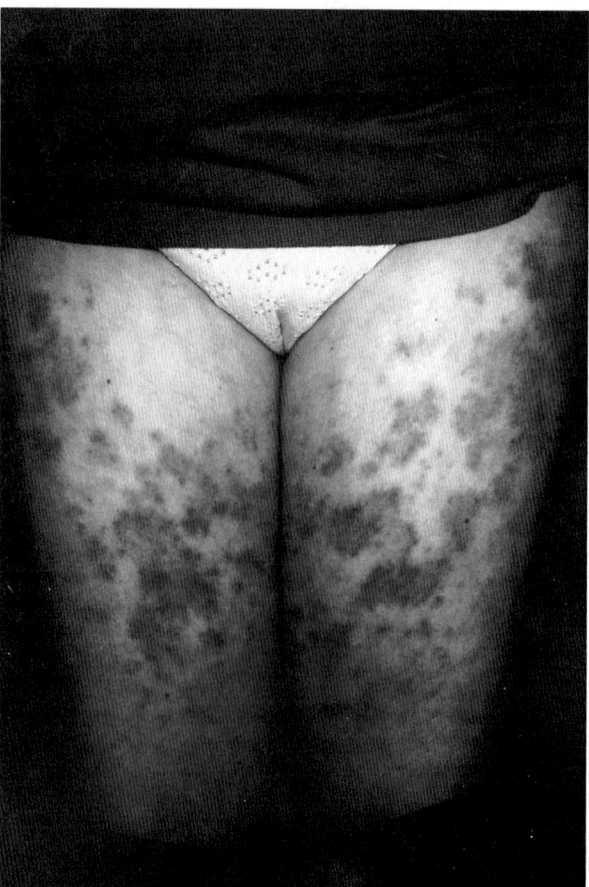

Fig. 29.56 Secondary vasculitis in a child with systemic lupus erythematosus.

ANTINEUTROPHIL CYTOPLASMIC ANTIBODIES (ANCA)

Antineutrophil cytoplasmic antibodies (ANCA) were first described in association with Wegener granulomatosis in 1985 and subsequently with MPA and Churg–Strauss syndrome. Cytoplasmic or c-ANCA gives coarse granular staining of the cytoplasm, is strongly associated with proteinase-3 and is characteristically found in Wegener granulomatosis. Perinuclear or p-ANCA gives staining of the nucleus and perinuclear area, is associated with antimyeloperoxidase and is more commonly seen in MPA. Atypical ANCA staining patterns are seen nonspecifically in many inflammatory conditions. Measurement of these antibodies has become part of the routine workup of a patient with suspected systemic vasculitis. Nonetheless these are not diagnostic tests and results must be interpreted with care. A strongly positive c-ANCA may support the clinical suspicion of a diagnosis of Wegener granulomatosis. A negative ANCA does not rule out the possibility of a systemic vasculitis.

OTHER AUTOIMMUNE RHEUMATIC DISORDERS

SYSTEMIC LUPUS ERYTHEMATOSUS

Systemic lupus erythematosus (SLE) is a multisystem systemic inflammatory disorder most commonly seen in young adult women but well recognized in the pediatric age group. Rare in prepubertal children it occurs more commonly in the teenage years. Most pediatric series show a peak at 11–14 years but this may reflect referral bias, with older teenagers being referred direct to adult clinics. Females predominate in adult series, making up 85–90% of all cases. In childhood males make up a larger percentage of cases with a male to female ratio of 1:4.5. There are no good epidemiological studies of lupus in children: estimates of incidence are in the region of 10–20 per 100 000 children (under 18 years) but vary widely depending on the ethnic mix of the population. Lupus is more common in non-Caucasian races.

SLE has been regarded as the prototype autoimmune disorder with the recognition that one of the hallmarks of the disease is the production of a variety of autoantibodies. The presence of antinuclear antibodies (ANA) is virtually universal in children with lupus, a fact which can aid in making the diagnosis. Despite this recognition, the pathophysiology of lupus remains poorly understood. The presence of antibodies against double-stranded DNA is associated with the development of glomerulonephritis in lupus and the deposition of DNA–anti-DNA immune complexes may play a pathologic role. The role of other autoantibodies remains unclear.

Abnormalities in the functioning of many areas of the immune system have been documented in lupus, with recent interest in the role of dendritic cells[152] and abnormal apoptosis. A genetic predisposition to the development of lupus exists[153] and environmental triggers, including viruses, are thought to be important. Despite progress in our understanding of the widespread immune dysregulation seen in SLE its cause remains unknown. Nonetheless such progress is beginning to open up new therapeutic possibilities.[154]

Lupus is a multisystem disorder which can present in many different ways and with many different features making diagnosis difficult unless a high level of awareness of the condition exists. Delays in making the diagnosis are common, with the mean time to diagnosis being estimated at over a year in most pediatric series. The diagnosis is based on a combination of clinical and laboratory features (Table 29.16). Diagnostic criteria developed for use in adult patients[155] have been validated in a pediatric population.[156]

Lupus is extremely variable in both its clinical presentation and its severity, ranging from a relatively mild condition characterized by a facial rash, joint pains and fatigue to a severe life threatening illness. A wide variety of systems may be affected. General systemic symptoms such as fevers, weight loss, fatigue, arthralgia and general malaise are common throughout the disease course. The fatigue may be profound, disabling and difficult to treat. The characteristic skin rash is the facial butterfly rash which crosses the bridge of the nose and spares the nasolabial folds (Fig. 29.57). Other rashes (e.g. vasculitic)

Table 29.16 Revised American College of Rheumatology criteria for the classification of systemic lupus erythematosus. (Adapted from Hochberg 1997[155])

1. Malar rash
2. Discoid rash
3. Photosensitivity
4. Oral ulceration
5. Arthritis
6. Serositis:
   a. Pleuritis
   b. Pericarditis
7. Renal disorder:
   a. Proteinuria $> 0.5\,g/24\,h$
   b. Cellular casts
8. Neurological disorder:
   a. Seizures
   b. Psychosis (other causes excluded)
9. Hematological disorders:
   a. Hemolytic anemia
   b. Leukopenia $< 4 \times 10^9/L$ (two or more occasions)
   c. Lymphopenia $< 1.510^9/L$ (two or more occasions)
   d. Thrombocytopenia $< 100 \times 10^9/L$
10. Immunological disorders:
    a. Raised antinative DNA antibody binding
    b. Anti-Sm antibody
    c. Antiphospholipid antibodies:
       i. Abnormal serum levels of IgG or IgM anticardiolipin antibodies
       ii. Positive test for lupus anticoagulant
       iii. False positive serological test for syphilis present for at least 3 months
11. Antinuclear antibody present in raised titer

A person shall be said to have SLE if four or more of the 11 criteria are present (serially or simultaneously).

may occur in SLE and many children with lupus exhibit marked photosensitivity. Alopecia is usually mild but can be severe with scarring. Raynaud phenomenon is common. Hematological involvement is frequent in pediatric lupus which may present initially with what appears to be idiopathic thrombocytopenic purpura. CNS lupus is a cause of long term morbidity and may manifest as seizure activity, psychosis, aseptic meningitis or headaches. Mood alteration is common and it

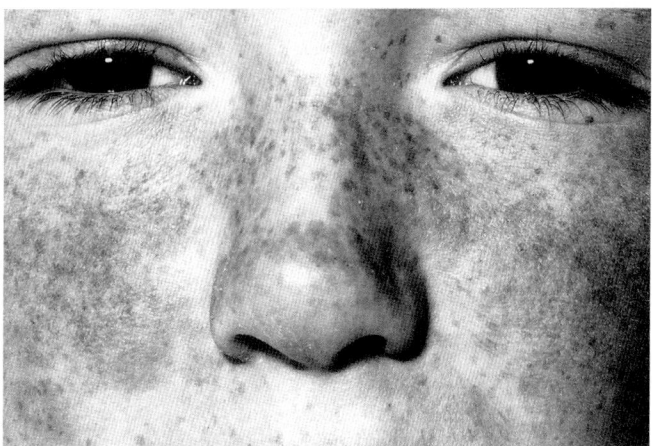

Fig. 29.57 Typical facial rash in systemic lupus erythematosus – crossing the bridge of the nose and sparing the nasolabial folds.

may be difficult to separate organic CNS involvement from reactive symptoms due to coping with a chronic illness. Renal involvement is frequent in childhood lupus and one of the major causes of morbidity. When present it tends to dominate the clinical picture. It may present as asymptomatic hematuria and proteinuria, hypertension, nephrotic syndrome or a rapidly progressing glomerulonephritis. Renal biopsy has an important role to play in determining the severity and therefore the likely outcome of the renal disease. Children with lupus are at particular risk from infection which is now the most common cause of death. This is a result both of the disease process itself and of immunosuppressive treatment regimens. Pneumococcal sepsis is a particular risk and pneumococcal vaccination is recommended.

Laboratory investigations are helpful both in the diagnosis and monitoring of SLE. Anemia occurs as a result of chronic disease or hemolysis. Thrombocytopenia and leukopenia are common. Characteristically the ESR is elevated while the CRP remains normal. Renal function should be monitored in those with renal involvement. A mild transaminitis is common but serious liver abnormalities are rare. Serum complement levels are reduced in most patients while serum immunoglobulin levels are nonspecifically elevated. A positive antinuclear antibody (ANA) is found in virtually all patients and is a useful diagnostic tool. The ANA result must be interpreted in the light of the clinical picture as the specificity for lupus is low and children may have a positive ANA for many reasons. Antibodies against double-stranded DNA and Sm (Smith antigen) are of greater specificity. Other autoantibodies such as anti-Ro, La and RNP may occur.

Management of lupus requires regular monitoring and attention to detail. Optimal management is in a multidisciplinary team setting with input from both a pediatric rheumatologist and a pediatric nephrologist. Drug therapy depends on disease severity and organs involved. Mild lupus can be managed with NSAIDs, hydroxychloroquine and low dose methotrexate. Avoidance of sun exposure and the use of sunblock are important. Thalidomide has been used for severe mucocutaneous disease. More significant organ involvement will require the use of moderate doses of steroids while severe disease which is life or organ threatening will require treatment with high dose steroids and immunosuppressive agents such as azathioprine and cyclophosphamide. Controlled studies in adults have shown the superiority of combinations of steroids and immunosuppressants over steroids alone[157,158] but there are no controlled studies in pediatric SLE. Treatment must be sufficient to suppress disease activity but aim to minimize toxicity. The long term toxicity particularly of high dose steroid regimens is very significant and steroid side-effects are particularly unacceptable to teenage girls who are the group most affected by lupus. Recently there has been interest in the use of mycophenolate mofetil a potentially less toxic alternative to cyclophosphamide.[159] Rituximab, a biologic drug which targets B cells, has been shown to be effective in individuals with disease resistant to more conventional therapies.[160] There are no pediatric studies to date and concern from some anecdotal reports regarding the frequency of side-effects.[161]

The ESR, urine protein level, levels of C3 and C4 and ds-DNA titer may all be used in monitoring disease activity and response to treatment but clinical assessment of disease activity remains the gold standard. A variety of assessment tools have been developed to allow quantitative assessment of disease activity in lupus and have been validated for pediatric use.[162] PRINTO (The Pediatric Rheumatology International Trials Organization) has developed and validated both a disease activity core set and a definition of improvement for use in pediatric lupus.[163,164]

SLE is a serious disease and those who present in childhood have a high incidence of major organ involvement. Current treatment has markedly reduced the mortality but the long term morbidity remains high. Infection is the most common cause of death but renal death with the consequent need for dialysis and transplantation continues to occur in those with aggressive nephritis. Early diagnosis and optimal management should reduce this but the need for improved treatment protocols remains.

As survival rates from childhood lupus have improved it is clear that there is a high incidence of serious long term morbidity.[165] CNS disease results in long term psychological sequelae in many. Osteoporosis results both from the disease and its treatment. Lupus is known to cause a dyslipoproteinemia[166] and early onset coronary artery disease is a major complication of childhood lupus. Whether this can be altered by treatment of the lipid abnormalities is unknown.

Drug-induced lupus

A number of drugs are well known to cause a lupus-like syndrome. The best known in children are the antiepileptic drugs phenytoin and carbamazepine and the antihypertensives hydralazine and captopril. An addition to the list, of importance in teenagers, is minocycline commonly prescribed for acne.[167]

Antiphospholipid syndrome

As with other autoantibodies such as ANA, low titer antiphospholipid antibodies are seen not uncommonly in children, and are frequently thought to be epiphenomena of no clinical significance. Low titer antiphospholipid antibodies occur in around 30% of children with SLE but are of dubious clinical significance. The antiphospholipid syndrome occurs where higher titers of antibodies are associated with coagulation abnormalities and thromboembolic events.

Antiphospholipid syndromes are usually secondary, frequently in association with SLE. Primary antiphospholipid syndromes have been described in childhood but are rare.

These antibodies should be looked for in any child presenting with unexplained thromboembolic phenomena. Anticoagulation is required where there is evidence of an associated thrombotic problem. The role of prophylaxis, with either low dose anticoagulation or aspirin, in children is unclear.

Neonatal lupus erythematosus

The neonatal lupus syndrome is defined by the presence of maternal autoantibodies to Ro and La which cross the placenta causing clinical abnormalities in the fetus and neonate. The characteristic skin rash, thrombocytopenia and hepatic abnormalities are usually self limiting. The importance of the syndrome lies in its association with congenital heart block which may cause intrauterine bradycardia, cardiac failure and death. This syndrome usually affects pregnancies of women with only mild lupus or of healthy women subsequently found to have anti-Ro and La antibodies.

JUVENILE DERMATOMYOSITIS AND POLYMYOSITIS

The idiopathic inflammatory myopathies comprise a group of conditions characterized by unexplained inflammation of the muscles. In childhood, dermatomyositis is ten times more common than polymyositis.

Juvenile dermatomyositis (JDM) is a rare condition with an incidence of 1.9 per million children under 16 years in the UK.[168] Juvenile dermatomyositis occurs at all ages throughout childhood but with two peaks of presentation at 5–9 years and at 11–14 years. The condition is more common in females than males.

The etiology of JDM remains unknown. In children, unlike adults, there is no association with malignancy. Studies have shown a strong association with HLA-DQ1*0501[169] confirming a role for genetic factors. There has been interest in the role of TNF in the inflammatory myopathies and an overrepresentation of TNF-α-308A allele has been demonstrated in a population of children with JDM.[170] A number of epidemiological studies have documented clustering of onset of cases, stimulating interest in the role of infectious agents as triggers. No single agent has been identified.

Once established, a variety of immunological abnormalities occur in children with JDM. Antinuclear antibodies are found in approximately 60%. Their specificity is for the most part unknown and in contrast to adults, myositis-specific antibodies (e.g. Jo-1; Mi) are seldom present. Active disease is associated with elevation of serum immunoglobulin levels, evidence of complement activation, lymphopenia and an increase in the percentage of B lymphocytes.

The diagnosis of JDM is based on criteria published by Bohan and Peters in 1975.[171] A child is considered to have JDM if, having excluded other known causes, they have a characteristic rash plus three of the following four criteria: symmetrical proximal muscle weakness, elevated muscle enzymes, abnormal muscle histology and EMG changes. The increasing use of modalities such as MRI to demonstrate inflammatory muscle changes is replacing more invasive investigations in many patients and there is a need for a revision of these diagnostic criteria.[172]

The rash in JDM is the first symptom in approximately 50%. A further 25% report a simultaneous onset of the rash and weakness while in the last 25% weakness precedes the rash. The typical rash affects the eyelids, knuckles and extensor aspects of the knees and elbows (Fig. 29.58). Erythema affecting the face and upper trunk may also be seen. The eyelid rash is violaceous in hue, while the lesions over the knuckles may have a hypertrophic appearance (Gottron papules) (Fig. 29.59). Marked nailfold erythema occurs and is indicative of the vasculopathy that characterizes JDM. Examination of the nail fold capillaries will show typical changes with capillary dilatation and areas of thrombosis (Fig. 29.59).

The other major feature of JDM is an inflammatory myopathy. This affects the proximal limb muscles, often first noticed by difficulty with climbing stairs or brushing hair. Muscle weakness may be severe and involvement of the neck flexors and abdominal muscles occurs in addition to those in the limbs. Weakness is frequently associated with complaints of muscle pain and tenderness. Myositis is confirmed by documenting abnormalities of muscle enzymes such as creatine kinase, aspartate aminotransferase (AST), alanine aminotransferase (ALT), aldolase and lactate dehydrogenase (LDH). It should be remembered that muscle enzymes may be normal despite active disease. EMG,

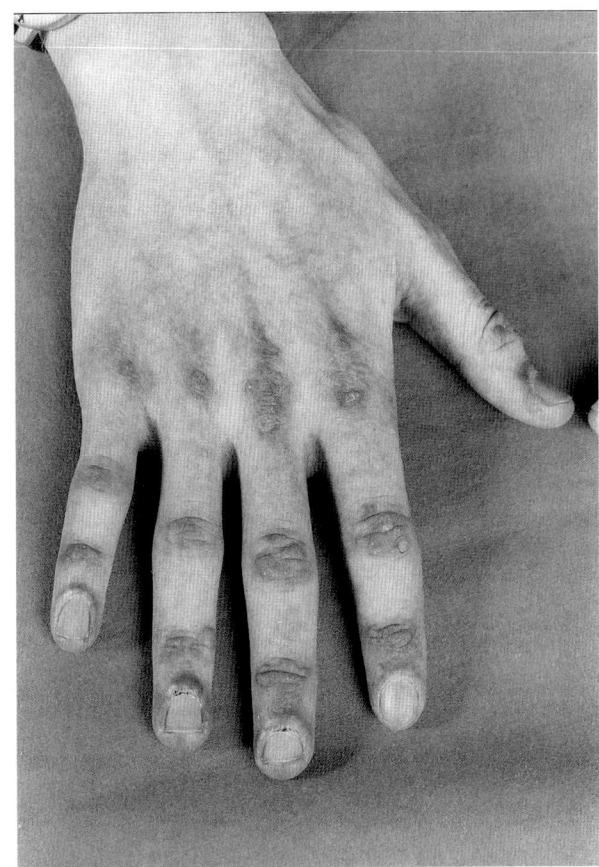

Fig. 29.59 Juvenile dermatomyositis showing Gottron papules and typical nailfold changes.

muscle biopsy and MRI will show characteristic inflammatory change (Fig. 29.60).

JDM is a multisystem disease and although the main features are of skin and muscle involvement, many organ systems can be affected by the widespread vasculopathy. Dysphagia occurs as a result of disease affecting the esophagus, while dysphonia results from involvement of the soft palate. Cardiac abnormalities are reported in up to 50%. Most are minor but cardiomyopathy can occur. Interstitial lung disease is uncommon but carries a poor prognosis.

Before the advent of steroids, JDM had a very poor prognosis. Thirty percent of affected children died, 30% had severe chronic disease and

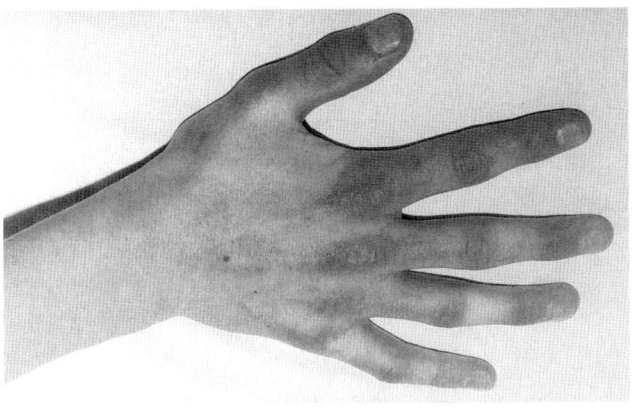

(a)

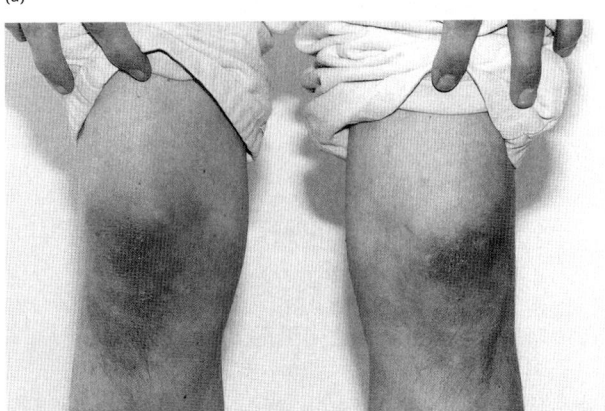

(b)

Fig. 29.58 Typical rash of juvenile dermatomyositis with erythema over: (a) extensor aspects of metacarpophalangeal and proximal interphalangeal joints; (b) knees.

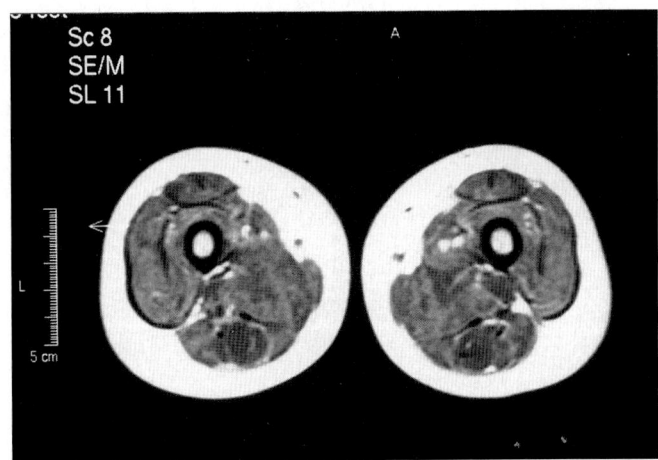

Fig. 29.60 Muscle MRI in juvenile dermatomyositis showing patchy, heterogeneous texture of the muscles typical of an inflammatory myopathy.

only 30% recovered. Steroids and more recent developments in therapy have dramatically changed the outlook but this is still a disease with an associated mortality and significant morbidity. Three characteristic disease courses are recognized. Some children have an acute monocyclic course which resolves with treatment; others a relapsing, remitting course while a third group have severe, unremitting chronic disease. In addition it is now recognized that there is a wide variety of clinical patterns seen within the overall label of JDM. Some children have predominantly muscle disease, others cutaneous. Some have both while a further group have evidence of a widespread vasculopathy with cutaneous ulceration (Fig. 29.61) and serious organ involvement.

Calcinosis of the muscle is a well-recognized complication of JDM (Fig. 29.62). It is at least in part related to disease severity and duration and its incidence can be reduced by prompt and appropriate treatment. Lipodystrophy may complicate JDM (Fig. 29.63) and in some is associated with the development of insulin resistance. As with lupus, osteoporosis is a complication both of the disease and its therapy.

Treatment of JDM remains controversial. There is no consensus on the type, route of administration and duration of treatment and there are no randomized controlled trials. In uncomplicated JDM, oral prednisolone is the most commonly used treatment in a dose of 1–2 mg/kg/day, tapering over 12–18 months. In an attempt to get more rapid disease control and minimize toxicity from oral steroids, many now advocate initial treatment with pulsed intravenous methylprednisolone. Other drugs were traditionally reserved for those with severe or steroid resistant disease but it is now recognized that early use of an additional drug, usually methotrexate,[173] results in reduced morbidity and a reduction

in the total steroid dosage required. Intravenous immunoglobulin may play a role in some patients and cyclophosphamide may be indicated in refractory disease.[174] There is interest in the use of new therapeutic options such as mycophenolate mofetil, the anti-TNF drugs or stem cell transplantation in children who fail to respond to other therapies but these must still be regarded as experimental.

Treatment is adjusted depending on the clinical response but monitoring may be difficult. Levels of muscle enzymes are not a good guide to activity and should not be used to plan treatment. Clinical assessment is the gold standard and there have been various attempts to try and improve methods of doing this. The childhood myositis assessment scale[7] is a useful method for objectively assessing muscle strength, serial scores then being used to quantify changes in the disease process. MRI is being used as a non-invasive method of assessing muscle inflammation and again may be used serially to document progress. A core set of criteria for the assessment of disease activity has been proposed by PRINTO but remains to be validated.[175]

SCLERODERMA IN CHILDHOOD

The scleroderma group of disorders is characterized clinically by thickening of the skin. This can occur in both localized and systemic forms, the former occurring much more commonly in pediatric practice.

Localized scleroderma

Localized scleroderma may be subdivided into morphea and linear scleroderma. Morphea lesions most commonly occur on the trunk

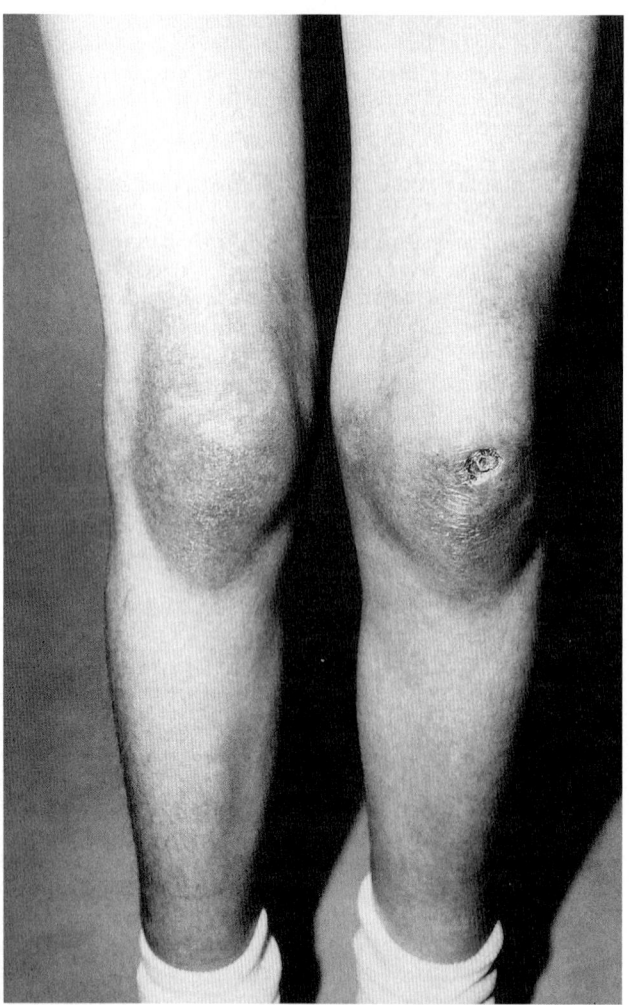

(a)

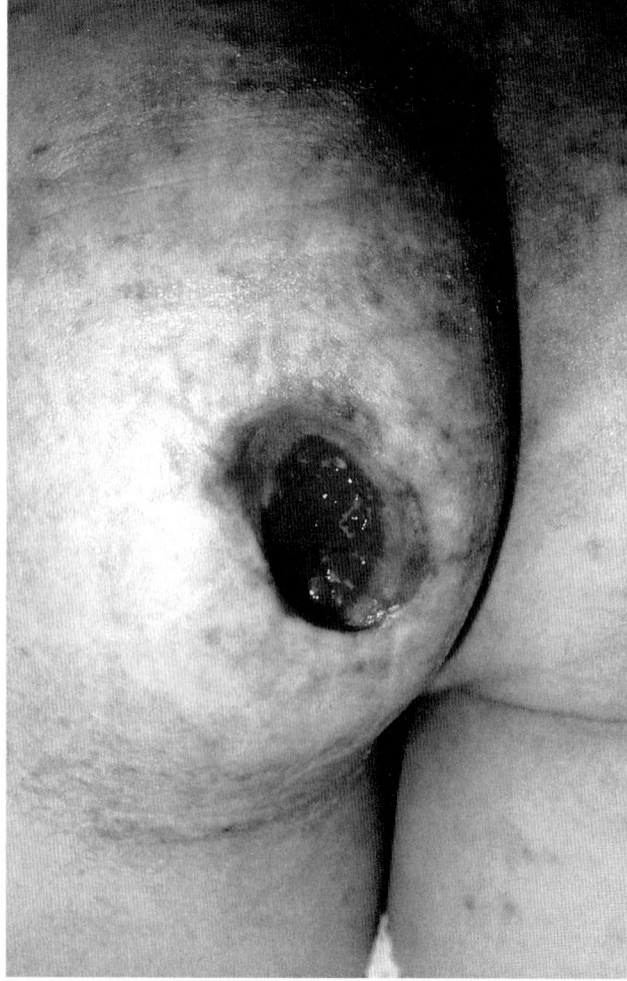

(b)

Fig. 29.61 (a,b) Ulcerative vasculopathy in juvenile dermatomyositis.

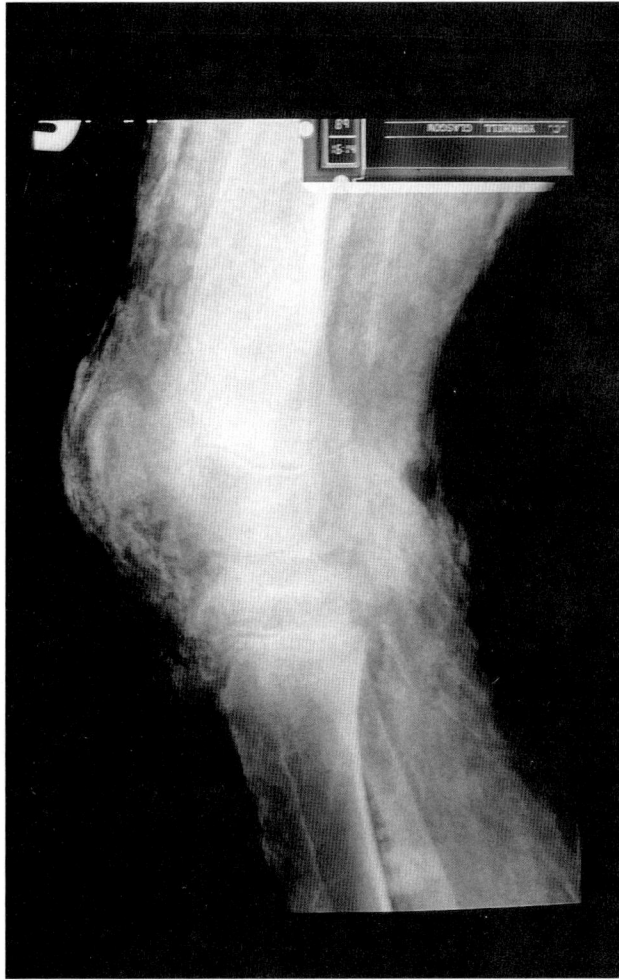

(a)

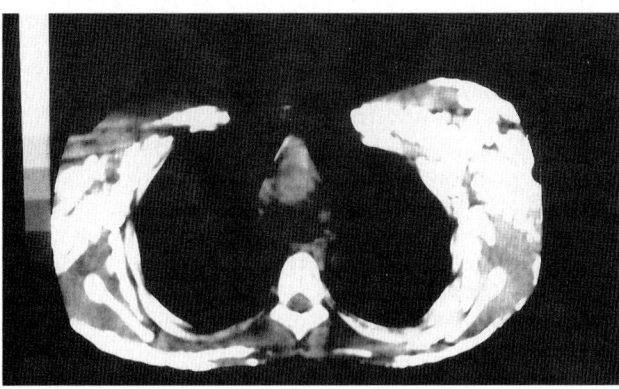

(b)

Fig. 29.62 Juvenile dermatomyositis with extensive calcinosis affecting: (a) lower limb (plain radiograph); (b) chest wall (CT scan).

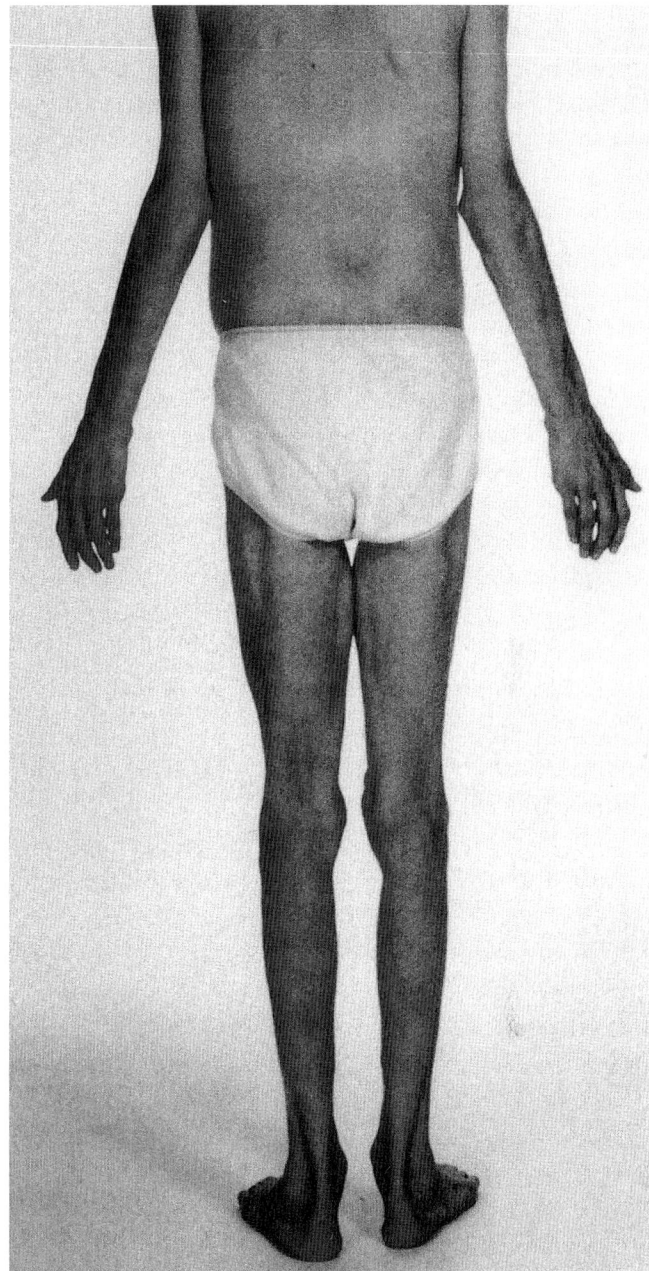

Fig. 29.63 Lipodystrophy in juvenile dermatomyositis – absence of subcutaneous fat in lower limbs.

and present as pale patches of thickened skin. When active there may be surrounding erythema and with time they become hyperpigmented (Fig. 29.64). They usually occur as isolated lesions and, although they may be cosmetically unpleasant, seldom cause other problems.

Linear scleroderma is of much greater concern. In this condition the child or parent may notice a band of skin discoloration in a linear distribution on a limb or on the face/scalp (when it is known as 'en coup de sabre'; Fig. 29.65). These lesions do not follow a dermatomal distribution and they are poorly understood. As with morphea, an erythematous color may indicate an active lesion: with time they become hyperpig-

mented. These lesions may be associated with atrophy and undergrowth of surrounding structures or the affected limb (Fig. 29.66) causing significant cosmetic and functional difficulties.

In a large collaborative data collection, 40% of children with localized scleroderma were found to be ANA positive. In a percentage of affected children extracutaneous manifestations (e.g. arthritis, neurological) occur but progression to systemic sclerosis does not.[176]

Our lack of understanding of the underlying process in these conditions makes treatment difficult. Methotrexate is now widely used to treat active lesions[177] and there is anecdotal evidence supporting the use of steroids and methotrexate in combination. Where a band of scleroderma crosses a joint, vigorous physiotherapy is helpful in maintaining joint range.

Systemic sclerosis

The systemic sclerosis disorders are extremely uncommon in pediatric practice. In adults, systemic sclerosis can be subdivided into

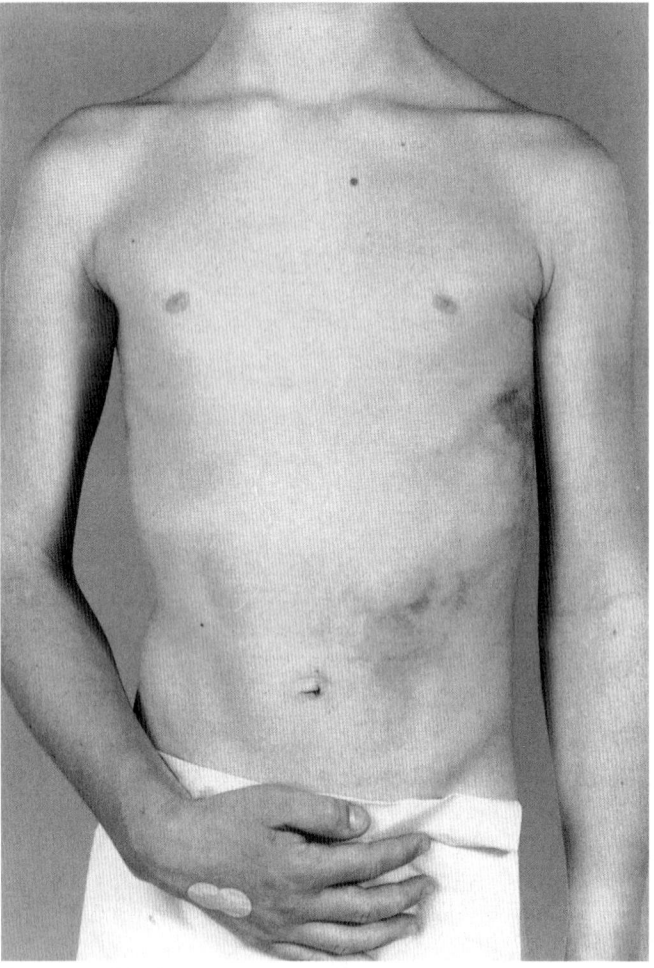

Fig. 29.64   Morphea.

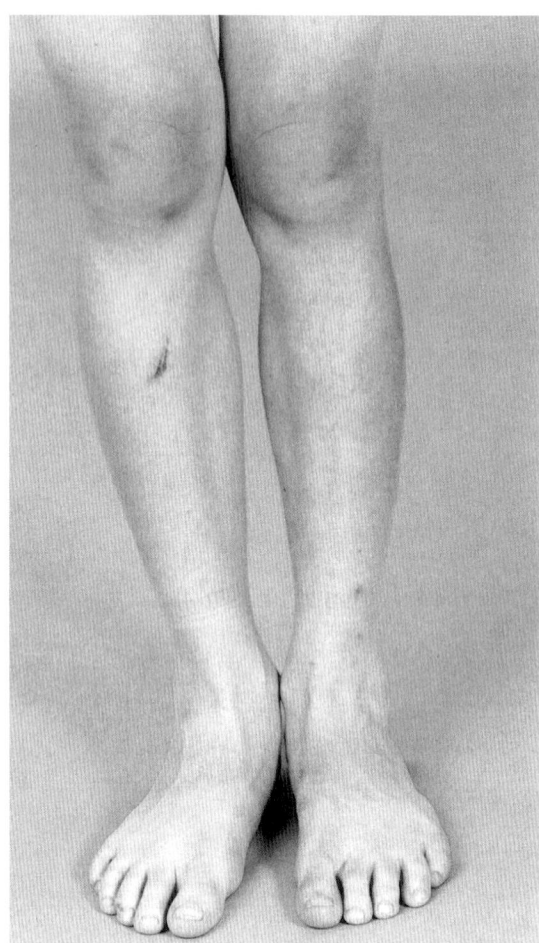

Fig. 29.66   Limb atrophy in linear scleroderma.

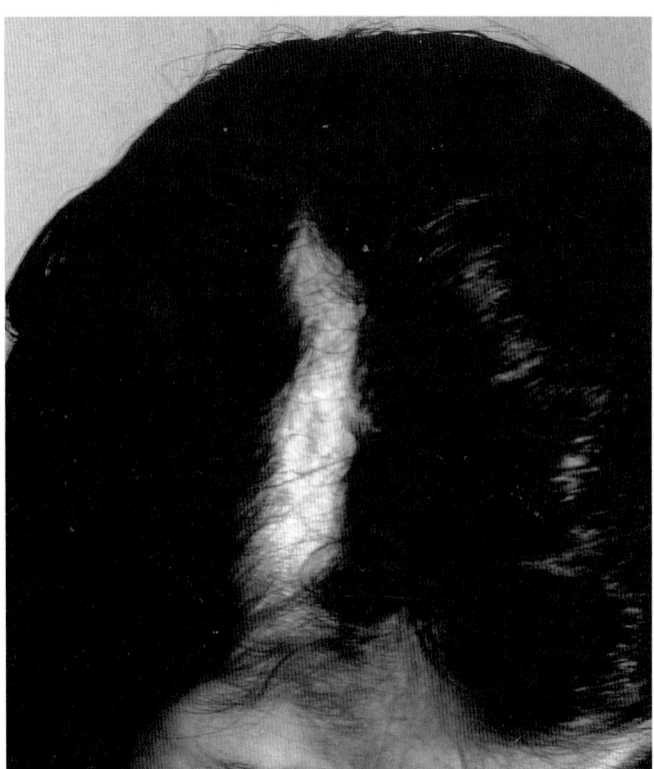

Fig. 29.65   En coup de sabre lesion.

diffuse cutaneous sytemic sclerosis (formerly known as progressive systemic sclerosis) and limited cutaneous systemic sclerosis (formerly CREST syndrome). Diffuse disease, characterized by cutaneous involvement extending to the proximal limbs and trunk, progresses rapidly over the first few years and is associated with the presence of anti-Scl 70 antibodies. The hallmark of limited disease is skin involvement of the distal extremities and face only. These categories appear less clearcut in childhood, many having features that overlap between the two

Raynaud phenomenon is usually the first feature of these conditions and if not present the diagnosis is unlikely. A history of Raynaud phenomenon may be difficult to obtain in a young child. The earliest clinical finding is cutaneous edema usually affecting the hands which consequently feel firm on palpation. Biopsy at this stage will show inflammatory change in the subcutaneous tissue which becomes thicker and tighter. This results in stiffness of the extremities and the characteristic pinched appearance of the face. Joint contractures develop and the skin is very susceptible to minor trauma. Ischemia results in loss of the finger pulp and the typical digital pitting scarring (Fig. 29.67). Severe ischemia may result in the loss of digits. Subcutaneous calcification, pulmonary hypertension and esophageal disease are common in the limited form of the disease. Diffuse disease is characterized by early interstitial lung disease, gastrointestinal involvement, cardiac abnormalities due to small vessel obliteration and renal disease. The scleroderma renal 'crisis' which results from a critical reduction in renal blood flow causing cortical ischemia, activation of the renin–angiotensin system and malignant hypertension, was previously a fatal event but can now be treated with angiotensin converting enzyme (ACE) inhibitors.

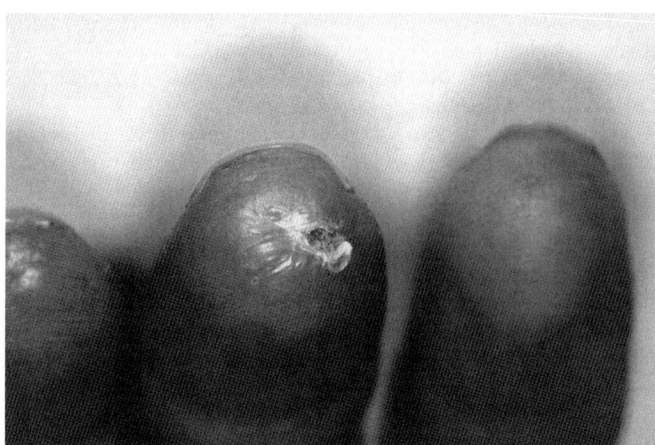

Fig. 29.67   Digital pitting scars in systemic sclerosis.

Renal disease is less common in the childhood form of the disease and the outcome is generally better than in adults.[178] Cardiac disease is the most common cause of death in affected children.

Management requires meticulous attention to detail. Protective measures (avoidance of cold exposure, use of warm mittens and avoidance of smoking) are important in reducing ischemia of the digits. Nifedipine, in a long-acting preparation, is the drug of choice. Occasional patients with severe digital ischemia and impending gangrene will benefit, often impressively, from the use of intravenous prostaglandin. Emollients are helpful for dry skin while physiotherapy and splinting may benefit joint disease. Gastrointestinal symptoms may be helped by the use of omeprazole together with a prokinetic agent such as cisapride. Broad-spectrum antibiotics may help malabsorption secondary to bacterial overgrowth. ACE inhibitors given where there is any evidence of renal involvement will reduce the risk of a scleroderma crisis.

Immunosuppressive therapy is used early where there is evidence of serious organ involvement and may influence the course of the disease. Once fibrosis is well established it is likely to be irreversible. Monitoring to detect signs of early organ involvement is therefore essential. Traditionally, treatment was with d-penicillamine but there is no evidence of benefit and the drug is associated with significant toxicity. Interest now lies in the use of powerful immunosuppressive regimens. Steroids, methotrexate, ciclosporin, cyclophosphamide, mycophenolate mofetil and antithymocyte globulin may all have a role. There is some anecdotal evidence suggesting that if used early, steroids and cyclophosphamide will halt progression of the lung disease which is one of the major determinants of mortality. There are no controlled studies to date and little hard evidence on which to base treatment plans.

MIXED CONNECTIVE TISSUE DISEASE

Mixed connective tissue disease (MCTD) is an entity characterized by Raynaud disease, swollen fingers and hands, myositis and a strongly positive antibody against RNP. Whether this is truly a separate disease or a subset of some other condition such as SLE is a matter of continuing debate. Many individuals with MCTD would also fulfill diagnostic criteria for the diagnosis of SLE.

OVERLAP SYNDROMES

A number of patients are seen with features of more than one autoimmune disorder and are classed as having overlap syndromes. The most commonly seen in pediatric practice are overlaps between JDM or polymyositis and scleroderma.

UNDIFFERENTIATED CONNECTIVE TISSUE DISORDERS

A number of children and adolescents will present with some features of this group of conditions, often associated with a positive antinuclear antibody, but insufficient to be defined as one of the well-characterized conditions already described. Some will evolve with time into one of the clearly defined conditions while others will remain undifferentiated.

SJÖGREN SYNDROME

Sjögren syndrome is a chronic inflammatory disorder characterized by lymphocytic infiltration of the exocrine glands and resulting in sicca symptoms, i.e. dry eyes and dry mouth. Sjögren syndrome may be primary or secondary, occurring in association with some other autoimmune rheumatic disorder. Conditions known to be associated with Sjögren syndrome include SLE, rheumatoid arthritis, MCTD, systemic sclerosis, dermatomyositis and primary biliary cirrhosis. Recognition is important as there is a significant risk of a lymphoid malignancy developing in the affected glands.

Although uncommon in pediatric practice, Sjögren syndrome does occur. Secondary Sjögren syndrome is more common than primary and usually develops in the context of a patient with a known autoimmune rheumatic disorder. Sjögren syndrome in childhood generally presents with parotid swelling which may be troublesome, recurrent and painful (Fig. 29.68a). The most important differential diagnosis is viral sialedinitis. If the problem is recurrent then Sjögren syndrome should be considered.

Although there are established criteria for the diagnosis of Sjögren syndrome in adults these are difficult to apply in children. Parotid imaging may be difficult to interpret. Ultrasound may be the most useful imaging procedure as it is inexpensive, well tolerated and shows characteristic abnormalities (Fig. 29.68b). For the diagnosis to be made the parotid swelling should be accompanied by evidence of dry eyes, dry mouth and the presence of autoantibodies.

Management of Sjögren syndrome consists firstly of management of the underlying disorder. Artificial tears are used for dry eyes and a variety of preparations are available to relieve the dry mouth. Dental care must be meticulous as the lack of saliva predisposes to severe dental caries. Monitoring for the development of malignancy in the salivary glands is important.

RAYNAUD PHENOMENON

Raynaud phenomenon was first described in 1862 as episodic digital ischemia provoked by factors such as cold or emotion. Classically in Raynaud syndrome there is a triphasic color change. The digits initially blanche followed by cyanosis and then erythema on rewarming. For the diagnosis to be considered at least two of these phases must be present. In addition to the digits, changes may be seen in the ear lobes, tip of the nose and around the mouth.

Primary Raynaud syndrome, where the phenomenon occurs in isolation in an otherwise healthy individual, is common in young women and frequently familial. Secondary Raynaud syndrome occurs in conditions such as SLE, systemic sclerosis and MCTD and may be the presenting feature of such illnesses. All young people presenting with Raynaud syndrome should have a careful evaluation to exclude an underlying disorder. Any atypical features (year-round symptoms, digital ulceration) or the presence of antinuclear antibodies raise the possibility of secondary Raynaud syndrome and the child or teenager should be followed up to ensure no further problems develop.

Primary Raynaud syndrome will usually be controlled by symptomatic measures and protection from the cold. Unfortunately the use of warm gloves or mittens is unpopular in teenage years when primary Raynaud syndrome may be troublesome. Nifedipine will often improve symptoms, the dose being titrated to clinical response and the development of side-effects.

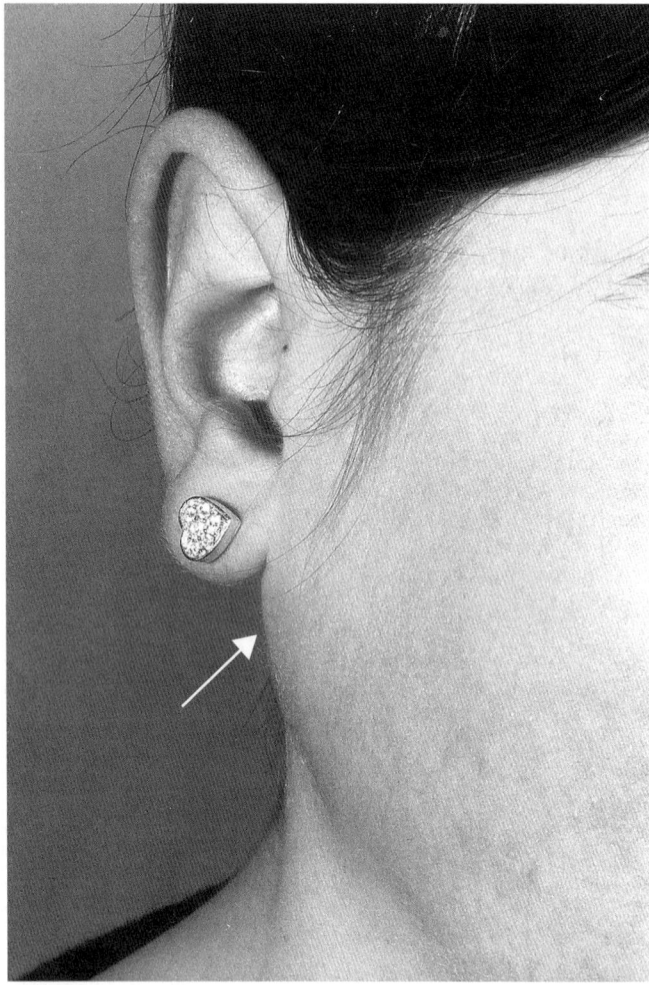

(a)

(b)

Fig. 29.68   Sjögren syndrome: (a) parotid swelling; (b) abnormal echogenicity on ultrasound.

ERYTHEMA NODOSUM

Erythema nodosum is seen not infrequently in children. The typical story is of the sudden onset of one or more tender, erythematous raised nodules or plaques on the anterior surface of the tibia. Pathologically this represents a septal panniculitis (inflammation within the subcutaneous

fat). The nodules lie deep and may be easier to feel than to see. As they resolve they develop an ecchymotic appearance and lesions at varying stages of development are frequently seen. Resolution usually occurs over a 4-to 6-week period.

In the majority of cases, erythema nodosum is an acute process occurring in response to an infectious trigger. Recurrent or chronic erythema nodosum merits investigation for some underlying cause.

Most cases in children occur as a post-streptococcal phenomenon and are associated with markedly raised ASO titers. Other infections such as mycoplasma, viruses and tuberculosis must be remembered. Drugs including antibiotics and oral contraceptive pills may cause erythema nodosum. Rarely, but importantly, it may be the presenting feature of some systemic disorder such as inflammatory bowel disease, sarcoidosis or an autoimmune rheumatic disorder.

THE DIFFERENTIAL DIAGNOSIS OF SYSTEMIC INFLAMMATORY DISORDERS

A chronic systemic inflammatory process in a child may result from chronic infection, malignancy or a rheumatological disorder such as systemic onset juvenile idiopathic arthritis, SLE, JDM or a systemic vasculitis. There are a number of unusual conditions of unknown etiology that may present in this fashion and must be remembered in the differential diagnosis. Some are outlined in this section.

Familial Mediterranean fever and other periodic fever syndromes

The periodic fever syndromes are a group of disorders characterized by unprovoked inflammation. Many have now been associated with gene mutations affecting the IL-1 and TNFα pathways enabling both genetic diagnosis and possible therapeutic options.[179]

Familial Mediterranean fever (FMF) principally affects individuals of eastern Mediterranean origin especially Sephardic and Iraqi Jews, Armenians and Levantine Arabs and is inherited as an autosomal recessive trait. It results from mutations of a gene on chromosome 16 that influences the production of a protein known as pyrin or marenostrum.[180] It is characterized by recurrent episodes of fever, serositis, arthralgia and synovitis of the large joints. Between attacks the joints return to normal. Untreated, it is associated with a high incidence of amyloidosis, the risk of which can be minimized by treating with colchicine.

Other periodic fever syndromes include the hyper-IgD syndrome which is characterized by recurrent fevers and an elevated immunoglobulin-D level. Mutations of the gene encoding mevalonate kinase have been identified in this condition.[181] An autosomal dominant syndrome characterized by periodic fever has been found to result from a mutation of the TNF receptor 1.[182]

Chronic infantile neurological, cutaneous and articular (CINCA) syndrome

This syndrome is characterized by the triad of rash, joint abnormalities and CNS involvement.[183] The rash which is urticarial and migratory appears in the first few months of life. Joint manifestations result from a disordered growth of cartilage (Fig. 29.69) and range from arthralgia and intermittent swelling to severe overgrowth of the epiphyses with loss of range of motion. Severe overgrowth of the patella is characteristic. Abnormalities of the CNS are universal and include chronic meningeal irritation, impairment of cognition and sensorineural deafness. Laboratory examination shows nonspecific elevation of inflammatory markers. Affected individuals have a characteristic facial appearance with frontal bossing, a hypoplastic midface and blond hair. This rare disorder is now known to be associated with dominantly inherited mutations in the CIAS1 gene, involved in the processing of IL-1β.[184] This has led to the therapeutic use of IL-1 blockade in the form of anakinra with dramatic benefit in many patients.

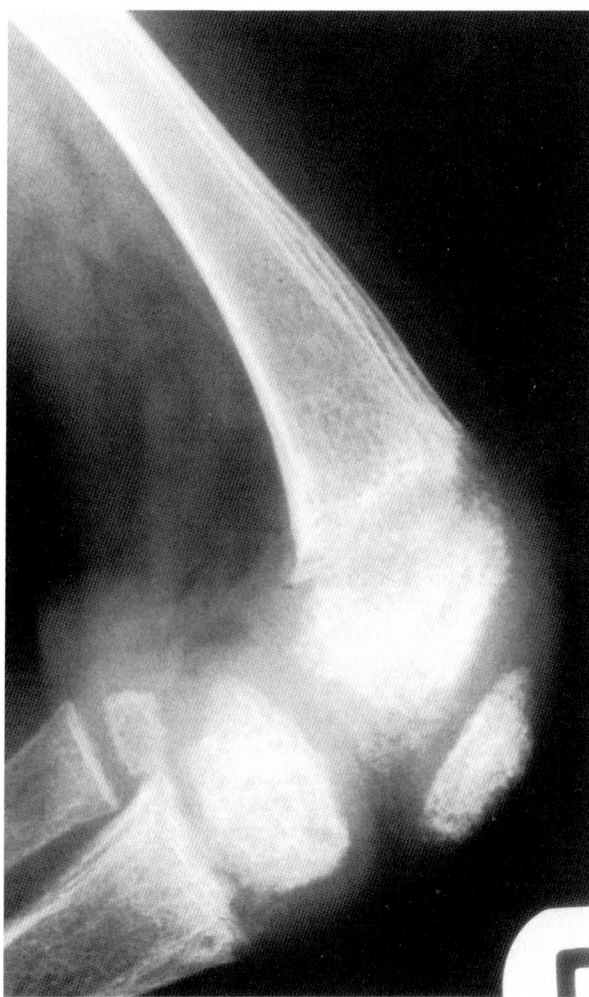

Fig. 29.69 Chronic infantile neurologic cutaneous and articular syndrome showing abnormal bone development.

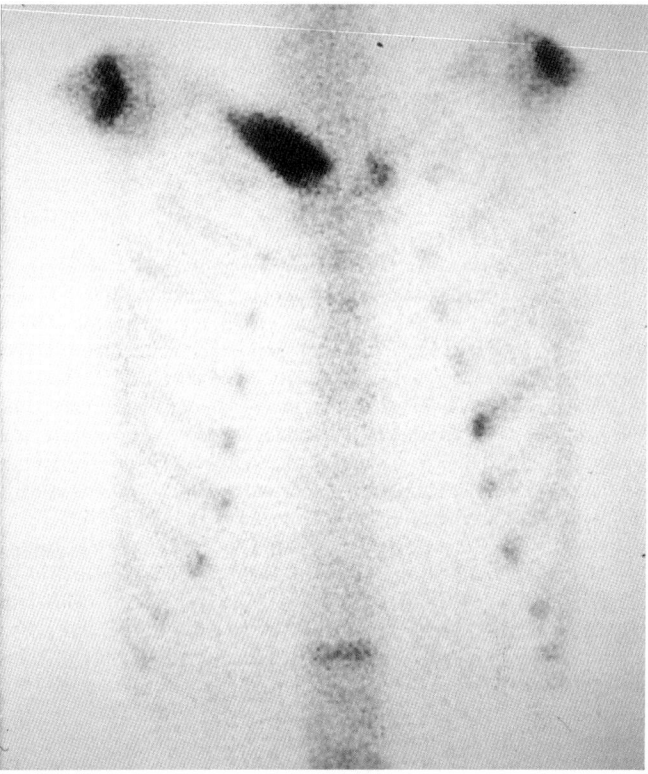

(a)

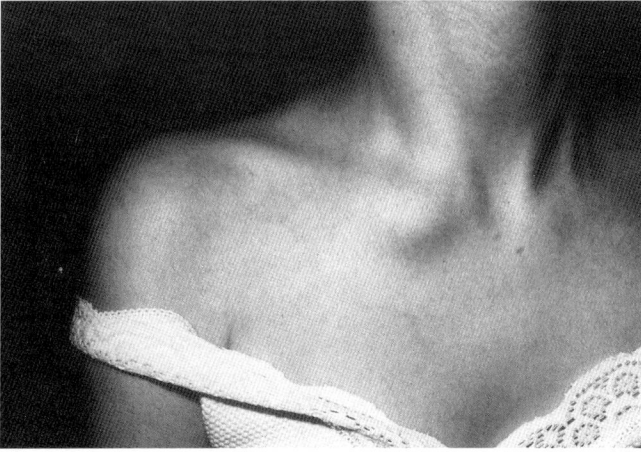

(b)

Fig. 29.70 SAPHO syndrome: (a) radionuclide bone scan demonstrating lesions in clavicle, rib and vertebra; (b) hyperostotic lesion of right clavicle.

Sarcoidosis

Sarcoidosis is an uncommon disorder in children and is characterized by a multisystem inflammatory process of unknown etiology. Two distinct disease patterns are seen although there are many cases where features overlap. In older children the pattern is very similar to that seen in adults with constitutional symptoms, lymphadenopathy and lung disease. In infants and young children a different pattern of disease is described with cutaneous involvement, arthropathy and uveiitis. Histologically the disease may result in the formation of granulomata. There is no single diagnostic test: serum levels of angiotensin converting enzyme are elevated in 80% but it should be remembered that levels are higher in normal children than in adults and pediatric standards are required. The Kveim test is no longer used.

SAPHO syndrome and chronic recurrent multifocal osteomylelitis (CRMO)

The SAPHO syndrome is an inflammatory disorder of unknown etiology characterized by synovitis, acne, pustulosis, hyperostosis and osteitis. Many cases only have a few of these features and CRMO, which is characterized by multifocal osteitic lesions, is thought to be part of the same spectrum of disease. The etiology is unknown. A family history of psoriasis is associated with SAPHO and an infectious trigger has been postulated, although no infecting organism is identified in most individuals. Radionuclide bone scanning is useful for demonstrating the multifocal nature of the problem (Fig. 29.70a). Biopsy may be necessary to exclude infection or malignancy. The hyperostotic clavicular lesions (Fig. 29.70b) may be both painful and cosmetically unsightly. Laboratory investigations may show mildly elevated inflammatory markers. Steroids and methotrexate are used to suppress the inflammatory process and bisphosphonates may also have a role.

CHRONIC PAIN SYNDROMES

Musculoskeletal pain is common in children and adolescents but generally shortlived and easily explained. A small group will develop unexplained disabling chronic musculoskeletal pain which poses a challenging diagnostic and management problem.

Pain is a universal phenomenon and in most cases a useful symptom, alerting the individual to tissue damage. Chronic pain differs in serving no useful function. Chronic pain occurring with no underlying physical disorder, or disproportionate chronic pain where the pain is out of all proportion to any known disease (the idiopathic pain syndromes), are perplexing conditions. Pain is by definition subjective and must therefore be accepted at face value.[185] The International Association for the Study of Pain[186] defines pain as 'an unpleasant sensory and emotional experience associated with actual or potential tissue damage, or described in terms of such damage ... It is unquestionably a sensation in part of the body but is always unpleasant and therefore also an emotional experience.'

In all reported series, idiopathic pain syndromes predominantly affect girls. The age of onset peaks in the early adolescent years and these conditions are uncommon under 8 years.[187] Recent data suggest that the prevalence of these conditions in childhood is increasing.[188]

Children with idiopathic pain syndromes are among the most disabled children seen in pediatric rheumatology and orthopedic clinics. They complain of severe pain unresponsive to standard therapies and frequently have major functional limitations. It is often difficult for both the family and pediatrician to accept that there is no organic pathology and the diagnosis is often delayed while a prolonged series of investigations is undertaken. With the correct diagnosis and management many will do well and it is therefore important to recognize these conditions as early as possible. The diagnosis is by definition one of exclusion of underlying pathology. In most cases this can be done on the basis of a careful history and clinical examination and few investigations are necessary or helpful.

The terminology and classification system used to define the idiopathic pain syndromes in the literature is confusing and generally unhelpful in children. Pain syndromes in children differ in many respects from those described in adults and frequently fail to meet criteria required for clearly defined syndromes. Children with pain syndromes seem to divide into two distinct groups: those with localized pain and those with diffuse or generalized pain.[189]

LOCALIZED IDIOPATHIC PAIN SYNDROMES

The best example of a localized pain syndrome in children is reflex sympathetic dystrophy (RSD) also known as complex regional pain syndrome type 1, reflex neurovascular dystrophy, algodystrophy and Sudeck atrophy. RSD is characterized by localized pain associated with evidence of autonomic dysfunction. In adults this syndrome usually follows immobilization of a limb following trauma. In children any preceding trauma is usually insignificant. It is presumed that the child stops using the limb in response to minor trauma and that subsequent changes are secondary to immobility, but the condition is poorly understood. Psychological factors are thought to be significant in the majority of children with the condition.[190] The child develops severe pain in the affected limb and rapidly becomes unable to use it. Hyperesthesia (an increased sensitivity to stimulation), allodynia (pain due to a stimulus that does not usually cause pain) and dysesthesia (an unpleasant abnormal sensation) are characteristic. The limb becomes cold, blue, diffusely swollen and at times may adopt bizarre postures (Fig. 29.71). Rarely, wasting and trophic changes occur.

The diagnosis in most cases is straightforward as long as the physician is aware of the condition and considers it. The child presents with a single cold, extremely painful limb and complains of severe pain on even light touch. Frequently they are unable to tolerate even a sock on the affected foot. Despite their predicament many seem remarkably unconcerned (la belle indifference) unless asked to touch or use the painful limb. With an atypical history or a younger child, care must be taken to ensure that no underlying pathology (particularly malignancy) is missed. A blood count, ESR, plain radiograph and radionuclide bone scan are usually sufficient, the typical bone scan in established RSD showing reduced uptake in the affected limb (Fig. 29.72).

The management of these children depends on establishing trust. Many have seen multiple health professionals before a diagnosis has been reached;[191] this frequently leads to increasing psychosocial difficulty and a loss of faith in the medical profession. It is essential to successfully reassure both child and family that there is no underlying organic pathology while accepting their pain at face value. Once the diagnosis is made a simple explanation of the effect of immobilization on a limb is usually easily accepted and the role of 'stress' in contributing to this condition can be discussed. A combination of an individualized program of physiotherapy together with attention to psychological factors leads to full recovery in the majority.[187,192] Sympathetic blockade and other treatment modalities used in affected adults are neither necessary nor helpful in the management of children and young people with RSD.

RSD is only one form of localized pain syndrome. Other individuals may have chronic musculoskeletal pain localized to one area of the body but without associated autonomic dysfunction. These syndromes are not clear cut and there is an overlap between such groups of patients.

DIFFUSE CHRONIC PAIN SYNDROMES

Widespread musculoskeletal pain affects a further group of young people, again predominantly female. The mean age tends to be slightly older than those with RSD with a peak at around 15 years. These patients can be subdivided into those with multiple tender points who meet criteria for the diagnosis of fibromyalgia and those without specific tender points. In our experience it is unhelpful to differentiate between

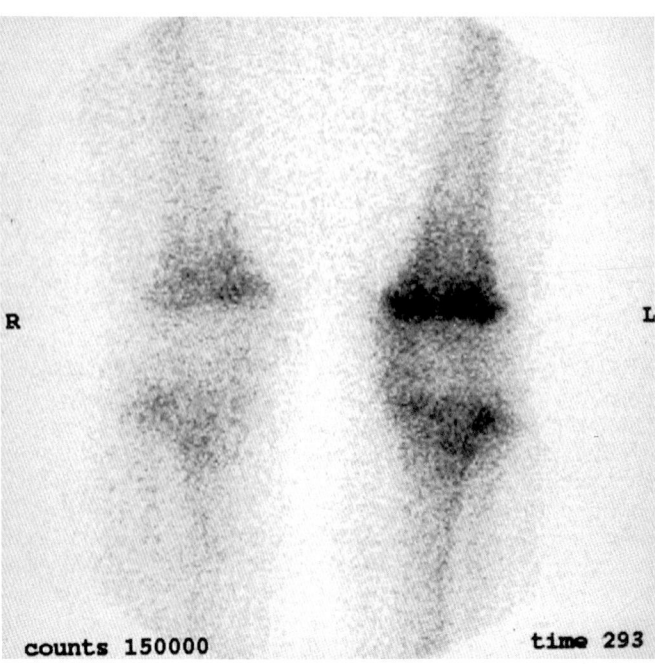

counts 150000   time 293

Fig. 29.72 Radionuclide bone scan in reflex sympathetic dystrophy showing reduced uptake in (R) affected compared to the (L) normal limb.

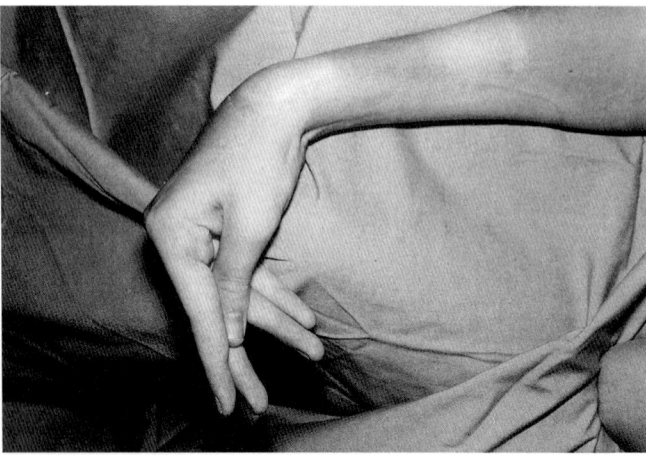

Fig. 29.71 Bizarre posturing of the hand in reflex sympathetic dystrophy.

the two groups. There are no significant differences between them and they differ in many ways from adults with fibromyalgia. It is more helpful to class all as simply having a diffuse chronic pain syndrome.

In association with their pain many of these young people complain of fatigue, poor sleep and, in some, feelings of depression. There appears to be an overlap between this group of teenagers and those with chronic fatigue syndrome, the exact diagnosis depending on whether the pain or the fatigue predominates.

The etiology of this group of disorders is unknown. An association with hypermobility has been noted and psychosocial factors are contributory.[193,194] Management of these young people is similar to those with localized pain, although the outcome is generally less good with a higher incidence of relapse. An exercise regimen will often result in significant improvement but relapse when this is withdrawn is frequent. Attention to psychological factors is essential. In some, particularly those with poor sleep, the use of drugs such as tricyclic antidepressants may be helpful. Recent interest has focussed on improving methods and developing tools for assessing the impact of chronic pain on these young people.[195]

BACK PROBLEMS IN CHILDHOOD AND ADOLESCENCE

Neck or back pain is unusual in the young child and must be taken seriously. Persistent or deteriorating pain is an important complaint and tumors and infections should always be considered in the differential diagnosis. Localized pain is usually more suggestive of significant pathology than ill-defined pain, but young children are often unable to give a history of local pain and some conditions such as discitis may present with odd symptoms such as a gait abnormality or even abdominal pain.

In the adolescent population complaints of ill-defined pain without pathological explanation are common.[196] Nevertheless careful evaluation is important. Additional signs and symptoms such as torticollis, scoliosis or neurological radicular symptoms will direct the approach to appropriate investigations.

As a rule of thumb, while pain, or pain provoking pathology, may cause abnormal spinal postures like torticollis or scoliosis, it is unusual for congenital or developmental explanations for spinal deformity to be responsible for pain.

TUMORS

Malignant neoplasms, primary or secondary, though rare, are a potential source of back pain in children. Primary tumors can arise from the bone, such as Ewing sarcoma; from the hemopoietic tissue, such as the leukemias; or from the contained neurological tissue or its coverings. Only 3% of primary bone tumors occur in the axial skeleton and in children 60% of these are benign.[197] The most common benign lesions include osteoid osteoma or osteoblastoma, eosinophilic granuloma and aneurysmal bone cysts.

Osteoid osteomas typically involve the posterior elements and characteristically present with pain, especially night pain classically relieved by NSAIDs. Radiographs may show an area of sclerosis; radionuclide bone scanning will reveal intense focal uptake in the lesion. Subsequent CT scanning will identify a discrete lesion with a thick sclerotic rim and a lucent nidus of osteoid material at the center. Osteoblastoma is similar histologically to osteoid osteoma but larger. Aneurysmal bone cysts are typically expansile lytic lesions with a thin rim of cortical bone. Once again they usually occur in the posterior elements but may involve the adjacent pedicle or body. Eosinophilic granuloma usually affects the body of the vertebra which subsequently flattens, giving the characteristic vertebra plana of Calvé disease.

INFECTION

See section on 'Infection in bones and joints', page 1401.

TORTICOLLIS

Torticollis secondary to congenital and developmental problems is not usually accompanied by pain. In practice the commonest cause of painful torticollis in children is atlantoaxial rotatory displacement, but it is important to bear in mind that there are other explanations including infections, tumors, CNS abnormalities like syringomyelia, and ocular dysfunction.[198]

Atlantoaxial rotatory displacement

Typically the child awakes with a 'wryneck'. This commonly resolves without treatment over the course of a week but occasionally the posture persists when it is best described as atlantoaxial rotatory fixation. There is often associated muscle spasm of the long sternocleidomastoid muscle because of its attempts to correct the deformity, unlike congenital muscular torticollis where the contracted muscle is responsible for the deformity.

In most cases the etiology is not apparent although the condition can be caused by trauma or occur in association with recent upper respiratory tract infection. When subluxation occurs in association with inflammation of adjacent neck tissues or upper respiratory tract infection it is known as Grisel syndrome. It is postulated that hyperemia of the atlantoaxial joints leads to variable ligament laxity and synovitis. Thickened synovial folds may subsequently impinge during rotation and lead to fixation.

Diagnosis in the acute stage is based on the history. Radiological assessment is difficult because of the head posture, but in the anteroposterior film the anteriorly rotated lateral mass of C1 appears wider and closer to the midline than the posteriorly rotated lateral mass. Because of the difficulty in interpretation of plain radiographs, CT scanning or dynamic MRI is usually of more value for definitive diagnosis.

Atlantoaxial rotatory displacement with minimal subluxation and no encroachment of the vertebral canal is relatively benign. Greater degrees of subluxation are rare but do have potentially serious neurological complications because of increasing encroachment of the vertebral canal. Most cases resolve spontaneously with simple analgesia and a soft collar for support. If persistent the patient should be admitted for halter traction with analgesia and muscle relaxation. Halo traction is occasionally required, especially if presentation is delayed. If the displacement is fixed and significant there is potential compromise of the vertebral canal and surgical fusion is a consideration.

Paroxysmal torticollis of infancy

Paroxysmal torticollis of infancy is a rare episodic torticollis of unknown etiology. Episodes last for minutes to days with eventual spontaneous recovery. Two thirds of affected children are girls, with an average age of onset of 3 months. Attacks usually occur in the morning, occurring 1–4 times each month and can be associated with trunk curvature, eye deviations and torticollis which may alternate sides on different episodes. The condition usually resolves over 12–24 months and requires no treatment.

Sandifer syndrome

This syndrome is the association of infant gastroesophageal reflux with posturing of the neck and trunk. It is believed that the torticollis is the child's attempt to decrease the discomfort resulting from reflux.

JUVENILE DISCITIS

See previous section on 'Infection in bones and joints', page 1401.

Calcific discitis

This condition occurs in children with an average age of onset of 8 years. It is most common in the cervical spine and usually presents with the acute onset of neck pain and sometimes torticollis. Radiographs reveal calcified deposits in the affected nucleus pulposus. The etiology of the condition is unknown and treatment is symptomatic. The calcific deposits disappear in most patients by 6 months.

SCHEUERMANN KYPHOSIS

This condition can be responsible for a painful kyphosis. Patients present either with pain or an increasing round back deformity during adolescence (Fig. 29.73). The condition is more frequent in the thoracic but can also occur in the lumbar spine. There is usually a clear apex to the spinal deformity, which is relatively rigid distinguishing the condition from benign postural round back, which is flexible on extension. Lateral radiographs show vertebral wedging, end-plate irregularity and Schmorl node formation (herniation of intervertebral disc into the end-plate of an adjacent vertebra).

Treatment of the deformity with extension exercises and ocasionally extension bracing is usually successful. Surgical intervention for severe deformities is seldom required.

SPONDYLOLISTHESIS AND SPONDYLOLYSIS

Spondylolisthesis is the slipping forward of a vertebra on its neighbor below. It is classified into five types. Isthmic and dysplastic types are most common in children; degenerative, traumatic and pathological types are unusual.

Isthmic spondylolisthesis occurs when a defect or lysis develops in the pars interarticularis (spondylolysis) and is most common in L5 and L4 (Fig. 29.74). This defect is usually the result of a stress fracture at the pars. Affected patients often give a history of sporting activity. The vertebra concerned, having lost its 'bony hook' on the vertebra below, is able to slip forward, although this probably only occurs in about 20% of cases of spondylolysis. Clinical examination of a significant slip reveals a step on palpation of the lumbar spine and so-called 'heart shaped buttocks' because of the deformity.

Neurological radicular symptoms are rare but there is often associated hamstring spasm. The defect can be seen on oblique radiographs (the classic 'collar on the Scottie dog') but is best seen on reverse gantry CT scanning. If the slip is translated less than 50% symptoms can be treated by activity modification, analgesia and bracing. If symptoms settle the patient can be observed. Persistent symptoms, a slip of more than 50% or progressive slippage are all indications for surgical intervention. There are various surgical techniques but the principle is to fuse the unstable vertebra to its neighbor below.

Dysplastic (or congenital) spondylolisthesis is due to hypoplasia of the L5/S1 facet joint. This leads to instability of the L5 vertebra, which may subsequently slip.

ADOLESCENT DISC PROLAPSE

Disc prolapse is infrequent in children but occurs occasionally in adolescents when its presentation is somewhat different from adults. Stiffness is a more common symptom than back pain. There is commonly severe hamstring spasm with very limited straight leg raising and a spinal list (or tilt) is often present. The majority resolve without need for surgical intervention. If MRI shows a large sequestered fragment of disc material with significant symptoms, surgical excision may be considered.

OSTEOPOROSIS

Osteoporosis is a major health problem in the modern world and of major consequence in terms of its associated morbidity, mortality and health economics. The formation of bone structure occurs primarily during childhood and adolescence, with 90% of the peak bone mass being accumulated during the years of longitudinal growth. At any given age,

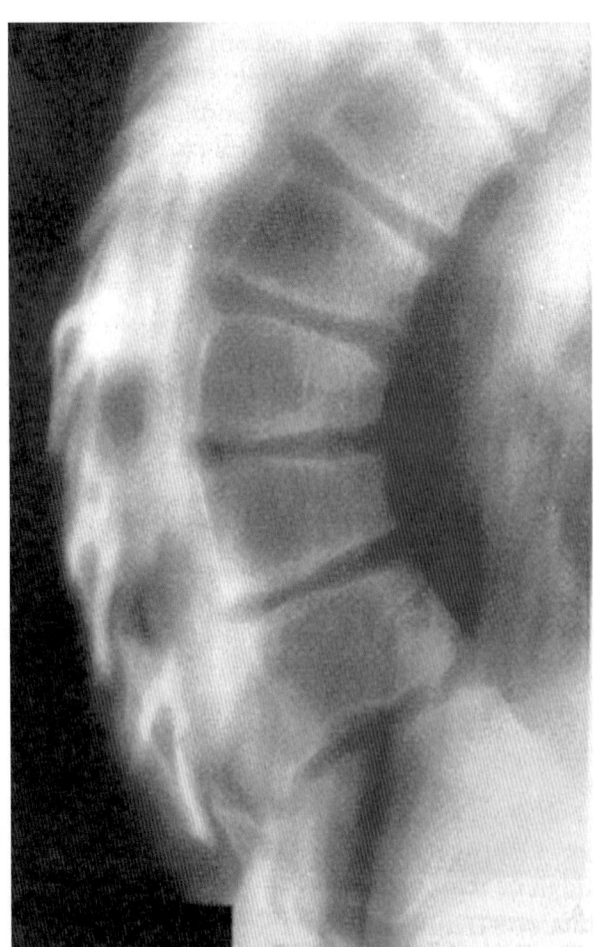

Fig. 29.73   Scheuermann kyphosis.

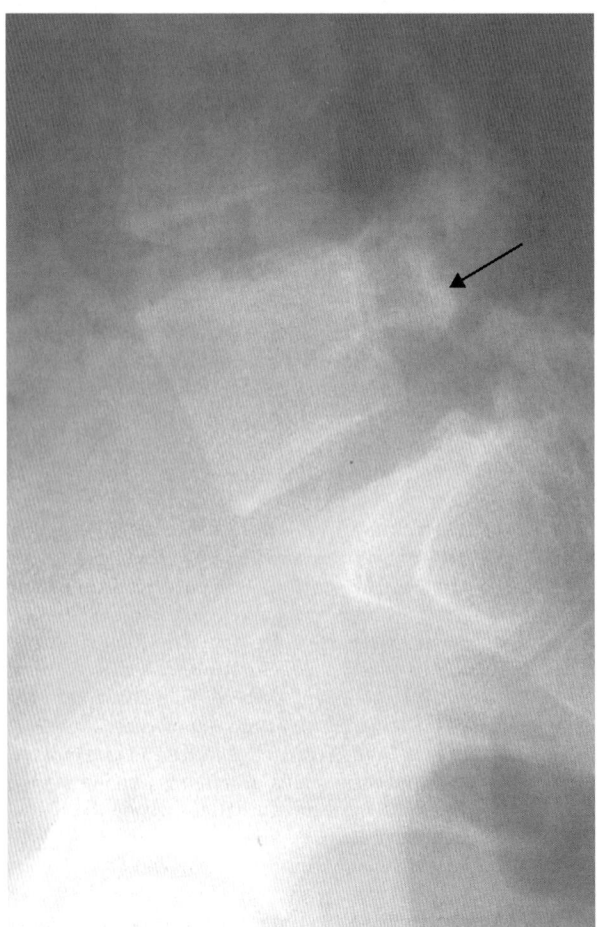

Fig. 29.74   Spondylolysis of L5.

bone mass is the result of both the peak bone mass, i.e. that acquired during the growth years, and the rate of age-related loss which starts from around 30 years and accelerates in women after the menopause. Optimization of skeletal development during childhood and adolescence therefore has a role in the longer term reduction in osteoporosis. This becomes particularly important when caring for children with chronic diseases which may adversely influence bone formation.

Bone exists in a constant state of remodeling during which old bone is removed and replaced by new bone. Bone gain during childhood and adolescence, and bone loss in later life, is therefore the result of a positive or negative balance between these two processes. This balance can be altered or disrupted by a variety of other factors. Bone structure is influenced by both genetic and lifestyle factors. It has been estimated that up to 80% of bone mineral density (BMD) can be accounted for by genetic factors, with gender, race and body size being important determinants. A number of candidate gene polymorphisms have been identified that are significant in relation to bone mass. Of particular importance appear to be polymorphisms of the vitamin D receptor, estrogen receptor and collagen type 1 alpha-1 genes. Other polymorphic genes encoding for bone proteins, hormones and cytokines may prove significant and it seems likely that a great variety of genes are involved in determining bone mass and strength. Lifestyle factors have an important contribution to make, with diet and physical activity being particularly important. There is a relationship between the amounts of muscle and fat in the body and the amount of bone: any dieting that results in an excessive weight loss will be associated with bone loss. Nutritional factors such as dietary calcium and vitamin D are contributory and ensuring an adequate intake will optimize bone development. Physical activity has an importance influence on bone density and an adequate amount of weightbearing activity is essential for optimal bone growth.

The World Health Organization defines osteoporosis as 'a disease characterized by low bone mass and micro-architectural deterioration of bone tissue, leading to enhanced bone fragility and a consequent increased risk in fracture'. Categories of disease are based on the measurement of BMD, with osteoporosis being defined as BMD more than 2.5 SD below the young adult mean value. Severe or established osteoporosis is defined as more than 2.5 SD below the young adult mean value in the presence of one or more low-trauma or fragility fractures.

These diagnostic criteria for osteoporosis have limitations. It must be remembered that they were developed in postmenopausal women and their applicability to other groups such as males and younger patients remains unclear. For such groups the relationship between BMD and fracture risk may be different and it is the fracture risk that is ultimately of importance. There are also difficulties inherent in the measurement of BMD in the growing child (see below) which may make the use of such definitions inappropriate. The definition of osteoporosis where fractures have not yet occurred is therefore somewhat arbitrary at present in children and young people. Further work is needed in this area.

ASSESSMENT OF BONE DENSITY IN PEDIATRIC PRACTICE

Conventional radiography is a relatively insensitive method of assessing bone mass and significant osteoporosis can only be diagnosed confidently when associated with a typical fracture. There has been interest in the use of ultrasound to assess bone density[199] and its acceptibility in pediatric practice may lead to further interest in this method in the future. Quantitative methods of CT scanning can be used to assess bone density but the tool most frequently used now, and generally regarded as the gold standard, is DEXA (dual energy X-ray absorptiometry) scanning.

DEXA scanning can be used to assess muscle mass, total and percent body fat and bone mineral. DEXA measures both the bone mineral content and the bone mineral density. This has a number of pitfalls in pediatric practice and results must be interpreted with care.[200] The amount of bone mineral content is directly related to body size and it is necessary to correlate values with skeletal size. Reference standards for children in different populations are not widely available, while genetic and racial difference in bone density make population-based reference values essential. In addition, machines vary considerably and calibration is important. With these provisos DEXA appears at present to be the method of choice for the assessment of bone density. Measurements are generally taken from the lumbar spine and proximal femur. Results should be expressed in terms of the number of standard deviations above or below the mean of an age-related control population (Z-score). DEXA provides a quantitative method that can be repeated serially to monitor change and assess the effects of treatment, provided the results are interpreted with caution in the growing child or adolescent.

PRIMARY OR IDIOPATHIC JUVENILE OSTEOPOROSIS

Primary osteoporosis is rare in childhood. Juvenile osteoporosis occurs before or around puberty, affects both sexes and is of unknown pathophysiology. The child will present with pain in the back, hips and feet with evidence of fractures including vertebral crush fractures (Fig. 29.75). This is a self-limiting condition which resolves with puberty but treatment with pamidronate to reduce pain and increase bone density during the active phase may be helpful.

SECONDARY OSTEOPOROSIS IN CHILDHOOD

Osteoporosis in children usually occurs in relation to some underlying chronic disease or as a consequence of treatment with glucocorticoids.

Disease related

Osteoporosis is increasingly recognized as an important sequel of a number of chronic childhood disorders, contributing greatly to the long term morbidity. In the childhood rheumatic disorders such as

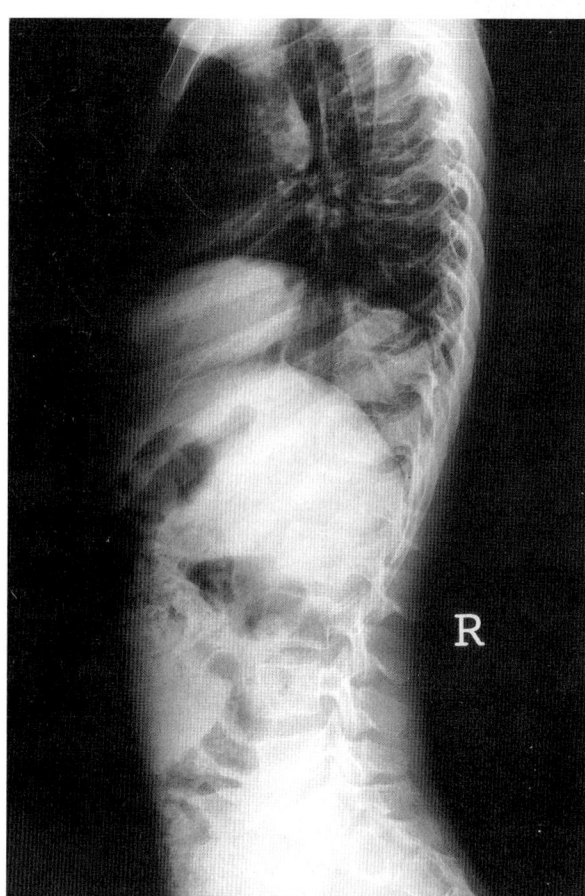

Fig. 29.75 Idiopathic juvenile osteoporosis – plain radiograph showing osteoporotic collapse of thoracic vertebrae.

juvenile idiopathic arthritis, dermatomyositis or systemic lupus erythematosus, osteoporosis occurs as a direct result of the underlying inflammatory process and prevention depends on optimal control of the disease process. Nutritional impairment, immobility or even relative inactivity in children with chronic ill-health are all contributory. Other unknown factors which are disease specific are clearly of importance, e.g. individuals with JDM or SLE appear more vulnerable than those with juvenile arthritis.

Drug related

Glucocorticosteroids are widely used in the treatment of a number of common diseases in childhood including the rheumatic disorders, inflammatory bowel disease, asthma and nephrotic syndrome. Although clearly necessary for treatment their effect on bone mineral density can be significant. The adverse effects of steroids on bone metabolism are well known and result from a variety of actions of these drugs. They are known to induce renal calcium efflux and inhibit calcium uptake from the intestine, leading to a fall in serum calcium and secondary hyperparathyroidism. This increases bone resorption and reduces bone formation and is well documented immediately after commencement of treatment. The increase in bone resorption does not usually continue but the amount of new bone formation is reduced as a result of increased apoptosis of osteoblasts and contributes to ongoing bone loss. The bulk of the bone loss in steroid-induced osteoporosis occurs in the first 6 months of treatment but overall the effect is related both to the total dose used and to the duration of therapy. There is considerable individual variation in the effect of steroids on bone density presumably as a result of genetic factors. Some individuals will tolerate a significant dose with no adverse effect whereas others will become significantly osteoporotic with minimal dosage regimens.

Other drugs such as methotrexate, heparin and thyroxine are known to reduce bone mineral density but none has been shown to have significant clinical effect in pediatric practice.

PROPHYLAXIS OF OSTEOPOROSIS IN CHILDHOOD

There is ongoing debate regarding the use of prophylactic measures to prevent osteoporosis in childhood. General advice regarding exercise and nutrition are important. Weightbearing exercise is clearly beneficial and with an increasingly sedentary lifestyle for many it is important to advise patients regarding this. The avoidance of severe weight loss is also important.

A diet with an adequate calcium intake is frequently lacking in adolescents. There has been much interest in the relationship between calcium intake and bone mineral acquisition and some evidence that calcium supplementation can increase bone mineral density. Any benefit shown in children and adolescents is transient and disappears when the supplementation is discontinued, making it seem unlikely that this is of any longer term benefit. Current evidence supports the use of calcium supplements to improve bone mineralization where the diet is deficient[201] but the benefits of supplementing above the normal dietary recommended intake are unproven.

Current recommendations for adults are that patients on steroids should receive prophylactic treatment for bone loss. There are no recommendations for children. A recent survey of pediatric rheumatology units in the UK (unpublished data) showed no consensus on the use of prophylactic measures in the prevention of steroid-induced osteoporosis. Some units advocate general advice only, some prescribe calcium supplements and others calcium and vitamin D for all children going on to long term steroids. At the moment there is no clear evidence on which to base a decision.

TREATMENT OF OSTEOPOROSIS IN CHILDHOOD

Until relatively recently, no specific treatments were available for osteoporosis. The advent of the bisphosphonates has altered our approach to the investigation and identification of at-risk children as there is now an effective treatment that can be used to reduce fracture risk.[202]

The bisphosphonates are synthetic compounds whose main action consists of the inhibition of osteoclastic bone resorption. The newer bisphosphonates are thought to act directly on the osteoclast to induce apoptosis. There were initial concerns about the use of these drugs in children with rapidly growing bones and in women of child-bearing potential. They are of low molecular weight and therfore likely to be able to cross the placenta. Fetal bone turnover is high and these drugs could potentially cause substantial effects on skeletal development. Nonetheless the cost of untreated osteoporosis is such that these drugs are now well established for use in pediatric practice.

The first generation bisphosphonates such as etidronate have been associated with bone mineralization defects and have generally been superseded in pediatric practice by the newer drugs such as pamidronate and alendronate. Pamidronate is the established treatment for osteoporosis in children and adolescents and is generally well tolerated. It has the disadvantage of requiring to be given by intravenous infusion and there is therefore increasing interest in the use of an oral alternative such as alendronate.[203]

Where there is established osteoporosis with evidence of a fracture there seems little doubt that the use of these drugs is appropriate. With reduced BMD but no fracture, there is no clear agreement as to when children should be treated as the relationship between BMD and fracture risk is not clearly established. Most clinicians would agree that a BMD measurement more than 3 SD below the mean is likely to represent an increased fracture risk and would therefore merit treatment.

OVERUSE AND SPORT-RELATED PROBLEMS IN CHILDREN

Active children frequently present with a variety of musculoskeletal symptoms that are a consequence of their activity. Such overuse syndromes can present in any child but become more common in the participants of organized competitive sport. While children are subject to the same injuries as adults, their immature musculoskeletal system responds somewhat differently. Submaximal loading of musculoskeletal structures leads to tissue damage, followed by repair. Repeated submaximal loading results in tissue hypertrophy. Overuse syndromes are characterized by the development of inflammatory pain when tissue damage exceeds the rate of tissue repair. The structures involved can be the bones, the soft tissues or, most commonly the junctions where they converge. In children these junctions are weaker than either the tendons or ligaments: apophysitis and avulsion fractures are therefore more common than ligament or tendon rupture. In children tendon rupture is also rare because overuse typically results in inflammation of the tendon sheath (tenosynovitis) rather than the tendon itself (tendonitis), and tendon degeneration is rare in the young.

STRESS FRACTURES

Stress fractures are undisplaced fatigue fractures, which develop as a result of repeated loading. The lower limbs are most frequently affected especially the metatarsals (march fractures) and the tibia.

Younger children and even toddlers can present with stress fractures but they are more common in adolescents where the proximal third of the tibia is the most frequent site, and running the most common explanation.[204] Symptoms of localized pain develop insidiously and are usually relieved by rest. Plain radiographs eventually show a localized periosteal reaction and increased density, but are frequently unhelpful at presentation. Radionuclide bone scanning is a more sensitive investigation. Infection and tumors can present with similar features and should always be considered in the differential diagnosis.

Treatment involves protection from further trauma, which sometimes involves immobilization and always involves abstinence from the causative stress, usually running. Once symptoms have resolved a gradual return to activity can be begun.

EPIPHYSEOLYSIS

Repeated traction, compression, torsion and angular stress on the growth plate (physis) can lead to stress injury resulting in localized peri-articular pain. Radiographs reveal widening of the growth plate and irregularity of the metaphyseal margin (Fig. 29.76). Involvement of the proximal humeral physis has been reported in baseball pitchers,[205] while female gymnasts have involvement of the distal radius.[206] Treatment involves modification of activity. Severe cases can be slow to resolve and premature physeal closure with subsequent wrist problems have been reported in gymnasts.[207]

OSTEOCHONDRITIS DISSECANS

See 'Common orthopedic problems in childhood', page 1415.

APOPHYSITIS

In the growing skeleton tendons join long bones at sites of ossification called apophyses. Apophysitis is inflammation at these junctions as a result of traction injury caused by the repeated pull of the attached tendon. Radiographs often reveal fragmentation and sclerosis of the apophysis with small, avulsed ossified fragments. Patients are usually in the adolescent age range from about 10 to 16 years. Symptoms usually begin insidiously, are made worse by activity and better by rest. Eponymous names are associated with the condition at some sites, but all are benign self-limiting conditions. The usual natural history is resolution by maturity. Treatment includes activity modification and symptomatic treatment. Occasionally in young athletes, explosive contraction of a muscle causes a tendon to pull off its whole attachment with a significant fragment of bone.

Pelvic apophysitis and avulsion fractures

The hip and pelvis can be the source of symptoms at the site of several apophyses. Sudden explosive contraction of the attached muscles can result in acute avulsion fractures of these apophyses and repeated submaximal trauma can result in the insidious development of symptoms. The iliac crest is the site of insertion of the abdominal muscles and can become painful as a result of trunk rotation such as when running. Other sites of apophysitis around the hip and pelvis include the insertion of sartorius at the anterior superior iliac spine (Fig. 29.77), the insertion of the rectus femoris at the anterior inferior iliac spine, the insertion of the gluteal muscles at the greater trochanter, the insertion of the psoas muscle at the lesser trochanter and the insertion of the hamstrings at the ischial tuberosity. Each of these conditions can explain pain in and around the hip region, but in the adolescent age range more serious explanations such as a slipped capital femoral epiphysis must be considered.

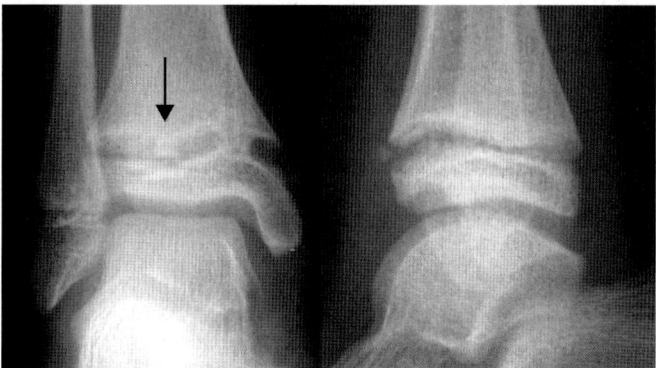

Fig. 29.76   Epiphyseolysis of distal tibia.

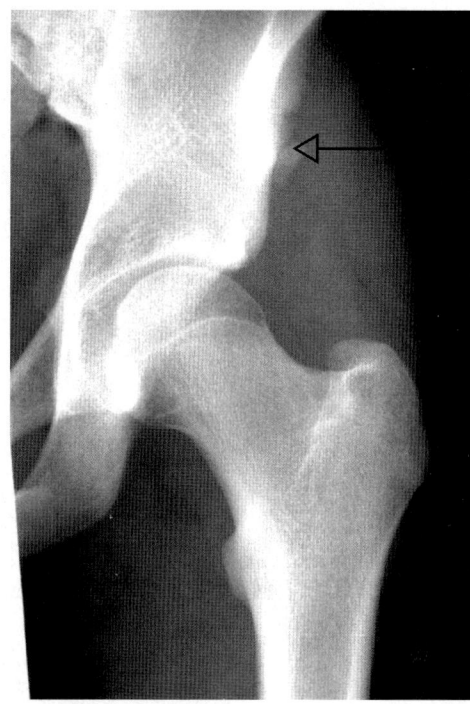

Fig. 29.77   Avulsion of anterior superior iliac spine.

Osgood–Schlatter disease

Osgood–Schlatter disease of the tibial tuberosity is the most common apophysitis, presenting in approximately 15% of teenage boys and 10% of teenage girls.[208] There is localized pain and swelling at the tibial tuberosity. Radiographs typically show fragmentation of the tibial tuberosity with avulsed fragments (Fig. 29.78). Symptoms usually respond to activity modification. In the enthusiastic young athlete sport need not be prevented but simply modified. Occasionally symptoms do persist after maturity with up to 20% of mature patients complaining of discomfort when kneeling.[209] Treatment is seldom required or helpful, except if a loose ossicle persists, when excision can be curative.

Sinding–Larsen–Johansson disease

Sinding–Larsen–Johansson disease is apophysitis at the lower pole of the patella. It is similar to Osgood–Schlatter disease and the two conditions can coexist (Fig. 29.78). Treatment follows a conservative activity modification approach.

Sever disease

Sever disease is inflammation of the calcaneal apophysis, at the insertion of the tendo-Achilles. Radiographs show increased density and fragmentation of the calcaneal apophysis, but this appearance is non-specific and can be seen in asymptomatic subjects. Treatment is conservative and a heel lift is sometimes helpful.

Iselin disease

Iselin disease is apophysitis at the insertion of peroneus brevis at the base of the fifth metatarsal. It should not be confused with fractures in the vicinity, which can follow acute trauma.

VALGUS OVERLOAD OF THE ELBOW

Valgus overload of the elbow occurs in a variety of throwing and batting sports and in activities where the upper limb is required to bear heavy loads such as in gymnastics. Perhaps the best example is the

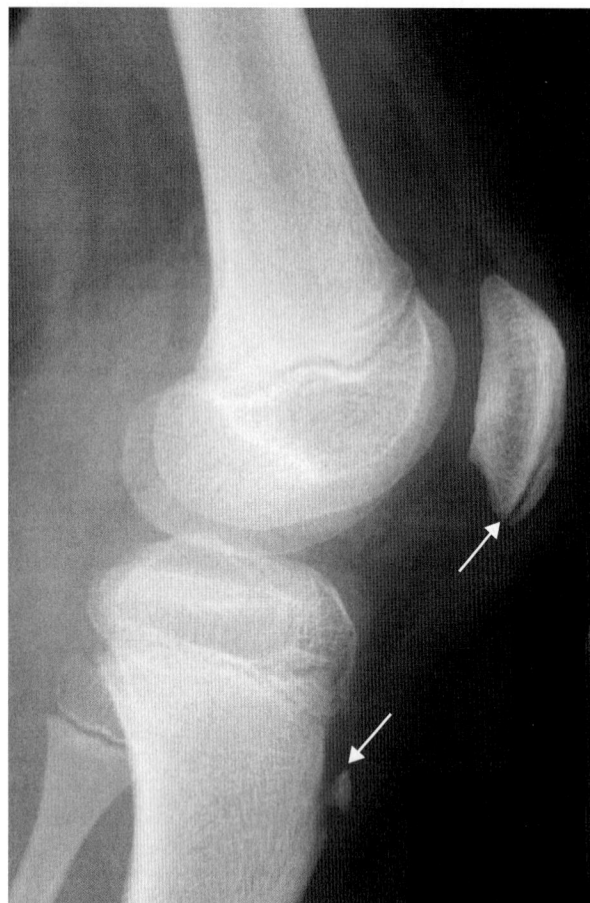

Fig. 29.78   Knee with coincidental Osgood–Schlatter and Sinding–Larsen–Johansson disease.

junior baseball pitcher – 'Little Leaguer's elbow'. Valgus stress of the elbow generates tension and distraction of the medial structures, including the medial collateral ligament and the medial epicondyle and compression of the lateral structures, namely the capitellum and the radial head. The young athlete can develop problems in any of these areas.[210] The medial epicondyle may become painful and prominent in a typical apophysitis-like presentation. Occasionally the medial epicondyle can be completely avulsed and if significantly displaced it should be reduced and fixed. The ossific nucleus of the capitellum may become fragmented with appearances similar to Perthes disease when the condition is referred to as Panner disease. If the patient is young the prognosis for complete resolution is good. Older and adolescent patients can also develop subchondral defects, which are considered to be a form of osteochondritis dissecans. Loose flaps or loose bodies can develop causing mechanical symptoms including elbow locking as well as pain. Treatment of the painful elbow usually involves activity modification but surgical debridement may be necessary if mechanical symptoms secondary to a loose body occur.

SNAPPING TENSOR FASCIA LATA SYNDROME

The iliotibial band is a broad condensation of the fascia on the lateral side of the leg running from the tensor fascia lata muscle at the iliac crest, across the greater trochanter of the hip and across the lateral side of the knee. When the leg is adducted at the hip and internally and externally rotated the iliotibial band can be pushed backward and forward by the passing greater trochanter beneath. The band is put under tension and then suddenly snaps back with a disconcerting clunk. If this occurs repeatedly a tender secondary trochanteric bursitis develops. The condition is more common in girls and the clunking is sometimes

voluntary. Management includes stretching exercises, avoidance of the provoking movements and reassurance because some patients believe that their hip is dislocating. The condition sometimes presents in runners and if refractory to conservative management the iliotibial band can be lengthened by 'Z' plasty.

ILIOTIBIAL BAND FRICTION SYNDROME

This condition is caused by rubbing of the iliotibial band against the lateral epicondyle at the distal femur during repetitive knee flexion and extension. It usually affects runners and most cases are associated with a recent increase in activity.[211] Activity modification sometimes including stretching exercises, is the mainstay of treatment.

ANTERIOR KNEE PAIN, PATELLOFEMORAL PAIN SYNDROME AND CHONDROMALACIA

See 'Common orthopedic problems in childhood', page 1415.

MENISCAL INJURIES OF THE KNEE

Meniscal tears are unusual in young children unless there is an underlying meniscal anomaly such as a discoid meniscus (see 'Common orthopedic problems in childhood', p. 1415). In adolescence the incidence of meniscal tears begins to increase and are usually related to sport. Meniscal tears usually result from a twisting injury when a 'pop' is sometimes heard or felt, followed by knee swelling. There are few specific and reliable clinical tests but the patient may give a history of giving way and 'true' knee locking. 'True' locking specifically implies a block to full extension. If a tear is suspected, MRI is a sensitive investigation. In young patients the meniscus is more vascular than in the adult and is more likely to heal following injury. In recent years the vital role of the meniscus in load distribution and proper knee function has become recognized and preservation or repair of the injured meniscus, especially in young patients, is important. Fortunately children and adolescents have a higher incidence of peripheral tears which, because of a good peripheral blood supply, are more amenable to successful repair.[212]

COLLATERAL AND CRUCIATE LIGAMENT INJURY OF THE KNEE

Ligament injury of the knee, and indeed of other joints, is rare in young children, becoming increasingly common as maturity is approached. Rupture of collateral and cruciate ligaments does sometimes occur, the mechanism of injury being similar to that in the adult. In the child ligaments are stronger than the bone to which they are attached, and mechanisms that would lead to rupture of a ligament in an adult lead to avulsion of the underlying bone. The best example is an avulsion fracture of the tibial eminence, the site of insertion of the anterior cruciate ligament. In general terms if avulsion fractures are significantly displaced from their origin, management includes reduction and sometimes fixation.

BREASTSTROKER'S KNEE

Competitive breaststrokers can develop medial knee pain along the medial collateral ligament. The 'whip kick' technique, a modified frog kick, has been associated with the problem. Rest and avoidance of the technique is helpful.

'SHIN SPLINTS'

'Shin splints' is a term that has emerged to describe exercise-induced shin pain in the athlete. It is a nonspecific clinical presentation with a number of underlying pathological explanations. Radiographs are important to exclude serious explanations for bone pain such as infection or tumor and may identify other explanations such as stress fractures.

Periostitis

Inflammation of the tibial periosteum or periostitis is a common cause for shin splints syndrome. It is characterized by pain along the posteromedial edge of the distal third of the tibia where the soleus muscle and its investing fascia originate. It is presumed to be a traction phenomenon and a variety of anatomical alignment variations such as forefoot pronation, genu valgum, femoral anteversion and external tibial torsion have been implicated as potential causes as well as poor footwear and training regimens.[213]

Radiographs sometimes show periosteal new bone along the posteromedial tibia and radionuclide bone scanning shows increased uptake in a longitudinal distribution in contradistinction to the transverse pattern of increased uptake seen in stress fractures.[214] Management should first involve an attempt to identify the underlying cause followed by conservative measures including footwear and activity modification to address the symptoms. Surgical treatment should only be considered as a last resort.

Chronic compartment syndrome

Chronic compartment syndrome develops when muscle volume increases as a result of increased blood flow during exercise. The relatively unexpandable osseofascial compartment cannot accommodate the extra volume, and pressure within the compartment increases.

When the intracompartmental pressure exceeds capillary filling pressure the muscles within the compartment develop ischemic pain. This usually resolves a short time after exercise stops. Some patients may experience a transient foot drop. Chronic compartment syndrome can present with 'shin splints' symptoms indistinguishable from periostitis.[215] Diagnosis depends on measuring compartment pressures during exercise on a treadmill. All four compartments in the leg should be assessed although the most commonly affected is the anterior compartment. Initial treatment involves a conservative approach with footwear and activity modification. Surgical treatment in the form of fasciotomy is reported to be successful in 90%.[216]

Superficial peroneal nerve compression

Superficial peroneal nerve compression can also give rise to activity-related shin pain. The superficial peroneal nerve emerges from the fascia of the lower third of the anterolateral part of the leg to the subcutaneous plane where it travels distally, to supply sensory innervation to the dorsum of the foot. During exercise increased muscle pressure can compress the superficial peroneal nerve against the edge of the fascial hiatus where it emerges. This leads to exercise-induced leg pain, sometimes with associated local pain at the hiatus in the fascia and altered sensation on the dorsum of the foot. In troublesome cases limited fasciotomy at the fascial hiatus is effective.

REFERENCES (* Level 1 evidence)

1. De Inocencio J. Epidemiology of musculoskeletal pain in primary care. Arch Dis Child 2004; 89:431–434.
2. Konijnenberg AY, Uiterwaal CS, Kimpen JL, et al. Children with unexplained chronic pain: substantial impairment in everyday life. Arch Dis Child 2005; 90:680–686.
3. Duffy CM. Measurement of health status, functional status, and quality of life in children with juvenile idiopathic arthritis: clinical science for the pediatrician. Pediatr Clin North Am 2005; 52:359–372.
4. Huber AM, Hicks JE, Lachenbruch PA, et al. Validation of the Childhood Health Assessment Questionnaire in the juvenile idiopathic myopathies. Juvenile Dermatomyositis Disease Activity Collaborative Study Group. J Rheumatol 2001; 28:1106–1111.
5. Foster HE, Cabral DA. Is musculoskeletal history and examination so different in pediatrics? Best Pract Clin Rheumatol 2006; 20:242–262.
6. Miller FW, Rider LG, Chung YL, et al. Proposed preliminary core set measures for disease outcome assessment in adult and juvenile idiopathic inflammatory myopathies. Rheumatology 2001; 40:1262–1273.
7. Lovell DJ, Lindsley CB, Rennebohm RM, et al. Development of validated disease activity and damage indices in the juvenile idiopathic inflammatory myopathies. II The Childhood Myositis Assessment Scale (CMAS): a quantitative tool for the evaluation of muscle function. The Juvenile Dermatomyositis Disease Activity Collaborative Study Group. Arthritis Rheum 1999; 42:2213–2219.
8. Binder H, Eng GD, Gaiser JF, et al. Congenital muscular torticollis: results of conservative management with long-term follow up in 85 cases. Arch Phys Med Rehabil 1987; 68:222–225.
9. Hensinger RN, Lang JR, MacEwan GD. The Klippel–Feil syndrome: a constellation of related anomalies. J Bone Joint Surg 1974; 56A:1246–1253.
10. Goldberg MJ, Bartoshesky LE. Congenital hand anomaly: etiology and associated malformations. Hand Clin 1985; 1:405–415.
11. Sachar K, Mih A. Congenital radial head dislocations. Hand Clin 1998; 14:39–47.

12. Weighill FJ. The treatment of developmental coxa vara by abduction subtrochanteric and intertrochanteric femoral osteotomy with special reference to the role of adductor tenotomy. Clin Orthop 1976; 116:116–124.
*13. Godward S, Dezateux C. Surgery for congenital dislocation of the hip in the UK as a measure of outcome of screening. MRC working party on congenital dislocation of the hip. Lancet 1998; 351:1149–1152.
14. Jones D. Topic for debate at the crossroads – neonatal detection of developmental dysplasia of the hip. J Bone Joint Surg 2000; 82B:160–164.
15. The National Screening Committee 2006. Online. Available at: http://www.library.nhs.uk/screening/ViewResource.aspx?resID=57180&tabID= 288re
16. Hoffman A, Wenger DR. Posteromedial bowing of the tibia. Progression in leg lengths. J Bone Joint Surg 1981; 63:384–388.
17. Schoenecker PL, Capelli AM, Millar EA, et al. Congenital longitudinal deficiency of the tibia. J Bone Joint Surg 1989; 71A:278–287.
18. Kalamchi A, Dawe RV. Congenital deficiency of the tibia. J Bone Joint Surg 1985; 67B:581–584.
19. Jacobsen ST, Crawford AH, Millar EA, et al. The Symes amputation in patients with congenital pseudoarthrosis of the tibia. J Bone Joint Surg 1983; 65A:533–537.
20. Harrold AJ, Walker CJ. Treatment and prognosis in congenital clubfoot. J Bone Joint Surg 1983; 65B:8–11.
21. Ponseti IV. Congenital clubfoot. Fundamentals of treatment. Oxford: Oxford University Press; 1996.
22. Hamanishi C. Congenital vertical talus: classification with 69 cases and new measurement system. J Pediatr Orthop 1984; 4:318–326.
23. Dobbs MB, Purcell DB, Nunley R, et al. Early results of a new method of treatment for idiopathic congenital vertical talus. J Bone Joint Surg Am 2006; 88:1192–1200.
24. Savariryan R, Rimoin DL. The skeletal dysplasias. Best Pract Clin Endocrinol Metab 2002; 16:547–560.
25. European Skeletal Dysplasia Network. Online. Available at: http://www.esdn.org
26. Beighton P, Solomon L, Soskolne CL. Articular mobility in an African population. Ann Rheum Dis 1973; 32:413–418.

27. van der Giessen LJ, Lickens D, Rutgers KJ, et al. Validation of Beighton score and prevalence of connective tissue signs in 773 Dutch children. J Rheumatol 2001; 28:2726–2730.
28. Grahame R, Bird HA, Child A. The revised (Brighton 1998) criteria for the diagnosis of joint hypermobility syndrome. J Rheumatol 2000; 27:1777–1779.
29. Grahame R. Heritable disorders of connective tissue. Best Pract Res Clin Rheumatol 2000; 14:345–361.
30. Adib N, Davies K, Grahame R, et al. Joint hypermobility syndrome in childhood. A not so benign multisystem disorder? Rheumatol 2005; 44:744–750.
31. Murray KJ. Hypermobility disorders in children and adolescents. Best Pract Res Clin Rheumatol 2006; 20:329–351.
32. Beighton P, De Paepe A, Steinmann B, et al. Ehlers–Danlos syndromes: revised nosology, Villefrance, 1997. Ehlers–Danlos National Foundation (USA) and Ehlers–Danlos Support Group (UK). Am J Med Genet 1998; 77:31–37.
33. Le Parc JM, Molcard S, Tubach F, et al. Marfan syndrome and fibrillin disorders. Joint Bone Spine 2000; 67:401–407.
34. De Paepe A, Devereux RB, Dietz HC, et al. Revised diagnostic criteria for the Marfan syndrome. Am J Med Genet 1996; 62:417–426.
35. Sakai H, Visser R, Ikegawa S, et al. Comprehensive genetic analysis of relevant four genes in 49 patients with Marfan syndrome or Marfan-related phenotypes. Am J Med Genet 2006; 140:1719–1725.
36. Rauch F, Glorieux FH. Osteogenesis imperfecta. Lancet 2004; 363: 1377–1385.
37. Venturi G, Tedeschi E, Mottes M, et al. Osteogenesis imperfecta: clinical, biochemical and molecular findings. Clin Genet 2006; 70:131–139.
38. Rauch F, Glorieux FH. Osteogenesis imperfecta, current and future medical treatment. Am J Med Genet C Semin Med Genet 2005; 139:31–37.
39. Rose PS, Levy HP, Liberfarb RM, et al. Stickler syndrome: clinical characteristics and diagnostic criteria. Am J Med Genet 2005; 138:199–207.
40. Kaplan FS, Fiori J, De La Pena LS, et al. Dysregulation of the BMP-4 signaling pathway in fibrodysplasia ossificans progressiva. Ann NY Acad Sci 2006; 1068:54–65.

41. Davies K, Stiehm ER, Woo P, et al. Juvenile idiopathic polyarticular arthritis and IgA deficiency in the 22q11 deletion syndrome. J Rheumatol 2001; 28:2326–2334.

42. McBride MB, Rigden S, Haycock GB, et al. Presymptomatic detection of familial juvenile hyperuricaemic nephropathy in children. Pediatr Nephrol 1998; 12:357–364.

43. Sonnen GM, Henry NK. Pediatric bone and joint infections. Pediatr Clin North Am 1996; 43:933–947.

44. Dagan R. Management of acute hematogenous osteomyelitis and septic arthritis in the pediatric patient. Pediatr Infect Dis J 1993; 12:88–93.

45. Kallio MJT, Unkila-Kallio L, Aalto K, et al. Serum C-reactive protein, erythrocyte sedimentation rate and white blood cell count in septic arthritis. Pediatr Infect Dis J 1997; 16:411–413.

46. Shetty AK, Gedalia A. Septic arthritis in children. Rheum Dis Clin North Am 1998; 24:287–304.

47. Davies EG, Monsell F. Managing osteoarticular infection in children. Curr Pediatrics 2000; 10:42–48.

48. Frank G, Mahoney HM, Eppes SC. Musculoskeletal infections in children. Pediatr Clin North Am 2005; 52:1083–1106.

49. Peltola H, Kallio-Unkila L, Kallio MJT, et al. Simplified treatment of acute staphylococcal osteomyelitis of childhood. Pediatrics 1997; 99: 846–850.

50. Wenger DR, Bobechko WP, Gilday DL. Spectrum of intervertebal disc space infection in children. J Bone Joint Surg 1978; 60A:100–108.

51. Tingle AJ, Allen M, Petty RE, et al. Rubella-associated arthritis. I. Comparative study of joint manifestations associated with natural rubella infection and RA 27/3 rubella immunization. Ann Rheum Dis 1986; 45:110–114.

52. Wall EJ. Childhood osteomyelitis and septic arthritis. Curr Opin Pediatr 1998; 10:73–76.

53. Dajani A, Taubert K, Ferrieri P, et al. Treatment of acute streptococcal pharyngitis and prevention of rheumatic fever: a statement for health professionals. Pediatrics 1995; 96:758–764.

54. Huppertz HI. Lyme disease in children. Curr Opin Rheumatol 2001; 13:434–439.

55. Packham JC, Hall MA. Long-term follow-up of 246 adults with juvenile idiopathic arthritis: functional outcome. Rheumatology 2002; 41:1428–1435.

56. Petty RE, Southwood TR, Manners P, et al. International League of Associations for Rheumatology classification of juvenile idiopathic arthritis: second revision, Edmonton, 2001. J Rheumatol 2004; 31:390–392.

57. Giannini EH, Ruperto N, Ravelli A, et al. Preliminary definition of improvement in juvenile arthritis. Arthritis Rheum 1997; 40:1202–1209.

58. Manners PJ, Bower C. Worldwide prevalence of juvenile arthritis: why does it vary so much? J Rheumatol 2002; 29:1520–1530.

59. Symmons DM, Jones M, Osborne J, et al. Paediatric rheumatology in the United Kingdom: data from the British Paediatric Rheumatology Group National Diagnostic Register. J Rheumatol 1996; 23:1975–1980.

60. Cassidy JT, Petty RE. 2001 Juvenile rheumatoid arthritis. In: Cassidy JT, Petty RE, eds. Textbook of pediatric rheumatology, 4th edn. Philadelphia: WB Saunders; 2001; 218–322.

61. Glass DN, Giannini EH. Juvenile Rheumatoid Arthritis as a complex genetic trait. Arthritis Rheum 1999; 42:2261–2268.

62. Murray KJ, Moroldo MB, Donnelly P, et al. Age-specific effects of juvenile rheumatoid arthritis-associated alleles. Arthritis Rheum 1999; 42: 1843–1853.

63. Thompson W, Barrett JH, Donn RP, et al. Juvenile idiopathic arthritis classified by the ILAR criteria: HLA associations in UK patients. Rheumatol 2002; 41:1183–1189.

64. Choy ES, Panayi GS. Cytokine pathways and joint inflammation in rheumatoid arthritis. N Engl J Med 2001; 344:907–916.

65. Grom AA, Murray KJ, Luyrink L, et al. Patterns of expression of tumor necrosis factor α, tumor necrosis factor β, and their receptors in the synovia of patients with juvenile rheumatoid arthritis and juvenile spondyloarthropathy. Arthritis Rheum 1996; 39:1703–1710.

66. Rooney M, Varsani H, Martin K, et al. Tumour necrosis factor alpha and its soluble receptors in juvenile chronic arthritis. Rheumatology 2000; 39:432–438.

67. Schneider R, Laxer RM. Systemic onset juvenile rheumatoid arthritis. Ballière Clin Rheum 1998; 12:245–271.

68. Roberton DM, Cabral DA, Malleson PN, et al. Juvenile psoriatic arthritis: Follow up and evaluation of diagnostic criteria. J Rheumatol 1996; 23:166–170.

69. Cohen PA, Job-Deslandre CH, Lalande G, et al. Overview of the radiology of juvenile idiopathic arthritis (JIA). Eur J Radiol 2000; 33:94–101.

70. Chalom EC, Goldsmith DP, Koehler MA, et al. Prevalence and outcome of uveitis in a regional cohort of patients with juvenile rheumatoid arthritis. J Rheumatol 1997; 24:2031–2034.

71. Malik AR, Pavesio C. The use of low dose methotrexate in children with chronic anterior and intermediate uveitis. Br J Ophthalmol 2005; 89:806–808.

72. Khan P, Weiss M, Imundo LF, et al. Favorable response to high-dose infliximab for refractory childhood uveitis. Ophthalmology 2006; 113:864.

73. Sawhney S, Woo P, Murray KJ. Macrophage activation syndrome: a potentially fatal complication of rheumatic disorders. Arch Dis Child 2001; 85:421–426.

74. Hackett J, Johnson B, Parkin A, et al. Physiotherapy and occupational therapy for juvenile chronic arthritis: custom and practice in five centers in the UK, USA and Canada. Br J Rheumatol 1996; 35:695–699.

75. Breit W, Frosch M, Meyer U, et al. A sub-group specific evaluation of the efficacy of intra-articular triamcinolone hexacetonide in juvenile chronic arthritis. J Rheumatol 2000; 27:2696–2702.

76. Sherry DD, Stein LD, Reed AM, et al. Prevention of leg length discrepancy in young children with pauciarticular juvenile rheumatoid arthritis by treatment with intra-articular steroids. Arthritis Rheum 1999; 42:2330–2334.

*77. Zulian F, Martini G, Gobber D, et al. Triamcinolone acetonide and hexacetonide intra-articular treatment of symmetrical joints in juvenile idiopathic arthritis: a double blind trial. Rheumatology 2004; 43:1288–1291.

78. Job-Deslandre C, Menkes CJ. Complications of intra-articular injections of triamcinolone hexacetonide in chronic arthritis in children. Clin Exp Rheumatol 1990; 8:413–416.

79. Gondwe JS, Davidson JE, Deeley S, et al. Secondary Cushing's syndrome in children with juvenile idiopathic arthritis following intra-articular triamcinolone acetonide administration. Rheumatol 2005; 44:1457–1458.

*80. Giannini EH, Brewer EJ, Kuzmina N, et al. Methotrexate in resistant juvenile rheumatoid arthritis. N Engl J Med 1992; 326:1043–1049.

*81. Woo P, Southwood TR, Prieur AM, et al. Randomized, placebo-controlled, crossover trial of low-dose oral methotrexate in children with extended oligoarticular or systemic arthritis. Arthritis Rheum 2000; 43:1849–1857.

*82. Ruperto N, Murray KJ, Gerloni V, et al. A randomized trial of parenteral methotrexate comparing an intermediate dose with a higher dose in children with juvenile idiopathic arthritis who failed to respond to standard doses of methotrexate. Arthritis Rheum 2004; 50:2191–2201.

83. Martini G, Zulian F. Juvenile idiopathic arthritis: current and future treatment options. Expert Opin Pharmacother 2006; 7:387–399.

84. Royal College of Paediatrics and Child Health. Immunization of the Immunocompromised Child. Best Practice Statement. ; February 2002. London: Royal College of Paediatrics and Child Health.

*85. Lovell DJ, Giannini EH, Reiff A. Efficacy and safety of etanercept (tumor necrosis factor receptor p75Fc fusion protein; Enbrel) in children with polyarticular-course juvenile rheumatoid arthritis. N Engl J Med 2000; 342:763–769.

*86. Lovell DJ, Reiff A, Jones OY, et al. Pediatric Rheumatology Collaborative Study Group. Long term safety and efficacy of etanercept in children with polyarticular-course juvenile rheumatoid arthritis. Arthritis Rheum 2006; 54:1987–1994.

87. Gerloni V, Pontikaki I, Gattinara M, et al. Efficacy of repeated infusions of an anti-tumor necrosis factor α monoclonal antibody, Infliximab, in persistently active, refractory juvenile idiopathic arthritis. Arthritis Rheum 2005; 52:548–553.

*88. Lovell DJ, Ruperto N, Cuttica R, et al. Comparison of safety, efficacy and pharmacokinetics for 3 and 6 mg/kg infliximab plus methotrexate therapy in JRA patients. Arthritis Rheum 2005; 52:(suppl):S724.

89. Lovell DJ, Ruperto N, Goodman S, et al. Preliminary data from the study of adalimumab in children with juvenile idiopathic arthritis (JIA). Arthritis Rheum 2004; 50:(suppl):S436–S437.

90. De Rycke L, Baeten D, Kruithof E, et al. The effect of TNFalpha blockade on the antinuclear antibody profile in patients with chronic arthritis: biological and clinical implications. Lupus 2005; 14:931–937.

91. Brown SL, Greene MH, Gershon SK, et al. Tumor necrosis factor antagonist therapy and lymphoma development: twenty-six cases reported to the Food and Drug Administration. Arthritis Rheum 2002; 46:3151–3158.

92. Pascual V, Allantaz F, Arce E, et al. Role of interleukin-1 (IL-1) in the pathogenesis of systemic onset juvenile idiopathic arthritis and clinical response to IL-1 blockade. J Exp Med 2005; 201:1479–1486.

93. Woo P, Wilkinson N, Prieur AM, et al. Open label phase II trial of single, ascending doses of MRA in Caucasian children with severe systemic juvenile idiopathic arthritis: proof of principle of the efficacy of IL-6 receptor blockade in this type of arthritis and demonstration of prolonged clinical improvement. Arthritis Res Ther 2005; 7:R1281–R1288.

94. Uziel Y, Laxer RM, Schneider R, et al. Intravenous immunoglobulin therapy in systemic onset juvenile rheumatoid arthritis: a follow up study. J Rheumatol 1996; 23:910–918.

95. Silverman E, Spiegel L, Hawkins D, et al. Long-term open-label preliminary study of the safety and efficacy of leflunomide in patients with polyarticular-course juvenile rheumatoid arthritis. Arthritis Rheum 2005; 52:554–562.

96. De Kleer IM, Brinkman DM, Ferster A, et al. Autologous stem cell transplantation for refractory juvenile idiopathic arthritis: analysis of clinical effects, mortality, and transplant related morbidity. Ann Rheum Dis 2004; 63:1318–1326.

97. McDonagh JE, Southwood TR, Shaw KL, et al. The impact of a coordinated transitional care program on adolescents with juvenile idiopathic arthritis. Rheumatology 2006; 46:61–68 Jun 20; Epub ahead of print.

98. Salenius P, Vankka E. The development of the tibiofemoral angle in children. J Bone Joint Surg 1975; 57A:259–261.

99. Greene WB. Infantile tibia vara. J Bone Joint Surg 1993; 75A:130–143.

100. Kling TF, Hensinger RN. Angular and torsional deformities of the lower limbs in children. Clin Orthop Rel Res 1983; 176:136–147.

101.   Bleck ED. Metatarsus adductus: classification and relationship to outcome of treatment. J Pediatr Orthop 1983; 3:2–9.

102.   Goodyear-Smith F, Arroll B. Growing pains. BMJ 2006; 333:456–457.

103.   Landin LA, Danielsson LG, Wattsgard C, et al. Transient synovitis of the hip. Its incidence, epidemiology and relation to Perthes disease. J Bone Joint Surg 1987; 69B:238–242.

104.   Haueisen DC, Weiner DS, Weiner SD. The characterization of 'transient synovitis of the hip' in children. J Pediatr Orthop 1986; 6:11–17.

105.   Thomas J, Morgan G, Tayton K. Perthes disease and the relevance of thrombophilia. J Bone Joint Surg 1999; 81B:691–695.

106.   Barker DJP, Hall AJ. The epidemiology of Perthes disease. Clin Orthop 1986; 209:89–94.

107.   Van Den Bogaert G, De Rosa E, Moens P. Bilateral Legg–Calvè–Perthes disease: different from unilateral. Pediatr Orthop 1999; 8B:165–168.

108.   Meehan PL, Angel D, Nelson JM. The Scottish Rite abduction orthosis for the treatment of Legg–Perthes disease: a radiographic analysis. J Bone Joint Surg 1992; 74A:2–12.

109.   Quain S, Catterall A. Hinge abduction of the hip: diagnosis and treatment. J Bone Joint Surg 1986; 68B:61–64.

110.   Loder RT, Wittenberg B, DeSilva G. Slipped capital femoral epiphysis associated with endocrine disorders. J Pediatr Orthop 1995; 15:349–356.

111.   Weiner D. Pathogenesis of slipped capital femoral epiphysis: current concepts. J Pediatr Orthop 1996; 5:67–73.

112.   Klein A, Joplin RJ, Reidy JA, et al. Roentgenographic features of slipped capital femoral epiphysis. Am J Roentgenol 1951; 66:361–374.

113.   Loder RT, Richards BS, Shapiro PS, et al. Acute slipped capital femoral epiphysis: the importance of physeal stability. J Bone Joint Surg 1993; 75A:1134–1140.

114.   Heppenstall RB, Marvel JP, Chung SMK, et al. Chondrolysis of the hip joint. Clin Orthop Rel Res 1974; 103:136–142.

115.   Pellicci PM, Wilson PD. Chondrolysis of the hips associated with severe burns. J Bone and Joint Surg 1979; 61A:592–596.

116.   Roy PR, Crawford AH. Idiopathic chondrolysis of the hip. Management by subtotal capsulectomy and aggressive rehabilitation. J Pediatr Orthop 1988; 8:203–207.

117.   Boucher JP, King MA, Lefebvre R, et al. Quadriceps femoris muscle activity in patellofemoral pain syndrome. Am J Sport Med 1992; 20:527–532.

118.   Yates CK, Granna WA. Patellofemoral pain in children. Clin Orthop Rel Res 1990; 255:36–43.

119.   Granna WA, Hinkley B, Hollingsworth S. Arthroscopic evaluation and treatment of patellar malalignment. Clin Orthop Rel Res 1984; 186:122–128.

120.   Fugikawa K, Iseki F, Mikura Y. Partial resection of the discoid meniscus in the child's knee. J Bone Joint Surg 1981; 63A:391–395.

121.   Leonard MA. The inheritance of tarsal coalition and its relationship to spastic flat foot. J Bone Joint Surg 1974; 56B:520–526.

122.   Mosier KM, Asher M. Tarsal coalitions and peroneal spastic flatfoot. J Bone Joint Surg 1984; 66A:976–984.

123.   Cowell HR. Diagnosis and management of peroneal spastic flatfoot. In: Instructional course lectures, The American Academy of Orthopedic Surgeons. St Louis: Mosby; 1975; 24:94–103.

124.   Gonzalez P, Kumar SJ. Calcaneonavicular coalition treated by resection and interposition of the extensor digitorum brevis muscle. J Bone Joint Surg 1990; 72A:71–77.

125.   Kumar SJ, Guille JT, Lee MS, et al. Osseous and non osseous coalition of the middle facet of the talocalcaneal joint. J Bone Joint Surg 1992; 74A:529–535.

126.   Ozen S, Ruperto N, Dillon MJ, et al. EULAR/PReS endorsed consensus criteria for the classification of childhood vasculitides. Ann Rheum Dis 2006; 65:936–941.

127.   Jenette JC, Falk RJ, Andrassay K, et al. Nomenclature of systemic vasculitides. Proposal of an international consensus conference. Arthritis Rheum 1994; 37:187–192.

128.   Gardner-Medwin JM, Dolezalova P, Cummins C, et al. Incidence of Henoch–Schönlein purpura, Kawasakai disease and rare vasculitides in children of different ethnic origins. Lancet 2002; 360:1197–1202.

129.   Stewart M, Savage JM, Bell B, et al. Long term renal prognosis of Henoch–Schönlein purpura in an unselected childhood population. Eur J Pediatr 1988; 147:113–115.

130.   Allen AC, Willis FR, Beattie TJ, et al. Abnormal IgA glycosylation in Henoch–Schönlein purpura restricted to patients with clinical nephritis. Nephrol Dial Transplant 1998; 13:930–934.

131.   Trapani S, Micheli A, Grisolia F, et al. Henoch–Schönlein Purpura in childhood: epidemiological and clinical analysis of 150 cases over a 5-year period and review of literature. Semin Arthritis Rheum 2005; 35:143–153.

132.   Flynn JT, Smoyer WE, Bunchman TE, et al. Treatment of Henoch–Schönlein purpura with high dose corticosteroids plus oral cyclophosphamide. Am J Nephrol 2001; 21:128–133.

133.   Shin JI, Park JM, Shin YH, et al. Can azathioprine and steroids alter the prognosis of severe Henoch–Schönlein nephritis in children?. Pediatr Nephrol 2005; 20:1087–1092.

*134.   Ronkainen J, Koskimies O, Ala-Houhala M, et al. Early prednisone therapy in Henoch–Schönlein purpura: a randomized, double-blind, placebo-controlled study. J Pediatr 2006; 149:241–247.

135.   Fulton DR, Newburger JW. Long-term sequelae of Kawasaki disease. Curr Rheumatol Rep 2000; 2:324–329.

136.   Yanagawa H, Nakamura Y, Yashiro M, et al. Update of the epidemiology of Kawasaki disease in Japan – from the results of the 1993–1994 nationwide survey. J Epidemiol 1996; 6:148–157.

137.   Leung DYM, Meissner HC, Schlievert PM. The etiology and pathogenesis of Kawasaki disease – how close are we to an answer?. Curr Opin Infect Dis 1997; 10:226–232.

138.   Igarashi H, Hatake K, Shiraishi H, et al. Elevated serum levels of macrophage colony-stimulating factor in patients with Kawasaki disease complicated by cardiac lesions. Clin Exp Rheumatol 2001; 19:751–756.

139.   Chang FY, Hwang B, Chen SJ, et al. Characteristics of Kawasaki disease in infants younger than six months of age. Pediatr Infect Dis 2006; 25:241–244.

140.   Simonini G, Rose CD, Vierucci A, et al. Diagnosing Kawasaki syndrome: the need for a new clinical tool. Rheumatology 2005; 44:959–961.

*141.   Newburger JW, Takahashi M, Burns JC, et al. The treatment of Kawasaki syndrome with intravenous gamma globulin. N Engl J Med 1986; 315:341–347.

*142.   Newburger JW, Takahashi M, Beiser AS, et al. A single intravenous infusion of gamma globulin as compared with four infusions in the treatment of acute Kawasaki syndrome. N Engl J Med 1991; 324:1633–1638.

*143.   Oates-Whitehead RM, Baumer JH, Haines L, et al. Intraveous immunoglobuilin for the treatment of Kawasaki disease in children. Cochrane Database Syst Rev 2003; CD004000.

144.   Lang BA, Yeung RS, Oen KG. Corticosteroid treatment of refractory Kawasaki disease. J Rheumatol 2006; 33:803–809.

145.   Wooditch AC, Aronoff SC. Effect of initial corticosteroid therapy on coronary artery aneurym formation in Kawasaki disease: a meta-analysis of 862 children. Pediatrics 2005; 116:989–995.

146.   Newburger JW, Takahashi M, Gerber MA, et al. Diagnosis, treatment, and long-term management of Kawasaki disease: a statement for health professionals from the Committee on Rheumatic Fever, Endocarditis and Kawasaki disease, Council on Cardiovascular Disease in the Young, American Heart Association. Pediatrics 2004; 114:1708–1733.

147.   Feinstein J, Arroyo R. Successful treatment of childhood onset refractory polyarteritis nodosa with tumor necrosis factor alpha blockade. J Clin Rheumatol 2005; 11:219–222.

148.   David J, Ansell BM, Woo P. Polyarteritis nodosa associated with streptococcus. Arch Dis Child 1993; 69:685–688.

149.   Kaklamani VG, Kaklamanis PG. Treatment of Behçet's disease – an update. Semin Arthritis Rheum 2001; 30:299–312.

*150.   Yurdakul S, Mat C, Tuzun Y, et al. A double-blind trial of colchicine in Behçet's syndrome. Arthritis Rheum 2001; 44:2686–2692.

*151.   Hamuryudan V, Mat C, Saip S, et al. Thalidomide in the treatment of the mucocutaneous lesions of Behçet's syndrome: a randomized, placebo-controlled, double-blind trial. Ann Intern Med 1998; 128:443–450.

152.   Pascual V, Bancherau J, Palucka AK. The central role of dendritic cells and interferon-alpha in SLE. Curr Opinion Rheumatol 2003; 15:548–556.

153.   Smerdel-Ramoya A, Finholt C, Lilleby V, et al. Systemic lupus erythematosus and the extended major histocompatibility complex – evidence for several predisposing loci. Rheumatology 2005; 44:1368–1373.

154.   Stichweh D, Pascual V. Autoimmune mechanisms in children with systemic lupus erythematosus. Curr Rheumatol Rep 2005; 7:421–426.

155.   Hochberg MC. Updating the American College of Rheumatology revised criteria for the classification of systemic lupus erythematosus. Arthritis Rheum 1997; 9:1725.

156.   Ferraz MB, Goldenberg J, Hilario MO, et al. Evaluation of the ARA lupus criteria data set in pediatric patients. Committees of Pediatric Rheumatology of the Brazilian Society of Pediatrics and the Brazilian Society of Rheumatology. Clin Exp Rheumatol 1994; 12:689–690.

*157.   Gourley MF, Austin HA 3rd, Scott D, et al. Methylprednisolone and cyclophosphamide, alone or in combination, in patients with lupus nephritis. A randomized controlled trial. Ann Intern Med 1996; 125:549–557.

*158.   Bansal VK, Beto JA. Treatment of lupus nephritis: a meta-analysis of clinical trials. Am J Kidney Dis 1997; 29:193–199.

159.   Buratti S, Szer IS, Spencer CH, et al. Mycophenolate mofetil treatment of severe renal disease in pediatric onset systemic lupus erythematosus. J Rheumatol 2001; 28:2103–2108.

160.   Leandro MJ, Cambridge G, Edwards JC, et al. B-cell depletion in the treatment of patients with systemic lupus erythematosus: a longitudinal analysis of 24 patients. Rheumatology 2005; 44:1542–1545.

161.   Willems M, Haddad E, Niaudet P, et al. Rituximab therapy for childhood-onset systemic lupus erythematosus. J Pediatr 2006; 148:623–627.

162.   Brunner HI, Feldman BM, Bombardier C, et al. Sensitivity of the Systemic Lupus Erythematosus Disease Activity Index, British Isles Lupus Assessment Group Index and Systemic Lupus Activity Measure in the evaluation of clinical change in childhood-onset systemic lupus erythematosus. Arthritis Rheum 1999; 42:1354–1360.

163.   Ruperto N, Ravelli A, Cuttica R, et al. The Pediatric   Rheumatology   International   Trials

Organization criteria for the evaluation of response to therapy in juvenile systemic lupus erythematosus: prospective validation of the disease activity core set. Arthritis Rheum 2005; 52:2854–2864.

164. Ruperto N, Ravelli A, Oliviera S, et al. The Pediatric Rheumatology International Trials Organization/American College of Rheumatology provisional criteria for the evaluation of response to therapy in juvenile systemic lupus erythematosus: prospective validation of the definition of improvement. Arthritis Rheum 2006; 55:355–363.

165. Ravelli A, Ruperto N, Martini A. Outcome in juvenile systemic lupus erythematosus. Curr Opin Rheumatol 2005; 17:568–573.

166. Sarkissian T, Beyenne J, Feldman B, et al. The complex nature of the interaction between disease activity and therapy on the lipid profile in patients with pediatric systemic lupus erythematosus. Arthritis Rheum 2006; 54:1283–1290.

167. Gough A, Chapman S, Wagstaff K, et al. Minocycline induced autoimmune hepatitis and systemic lupus erythematosus-like syndrome. BMJ 1996; 312:169–172.

168. Symmons DPM, Sills JA, Davis SM. The incidence of juvenile dermatomyositis: results of a nation-wide study. Br J Rheumatol 1995; 43:732–735.

169. Wargula JC. Update on juvenile dermatomyositis: new advances in understanding its etiopathogenesis. Curr Opin Rheumatol 2003; 15:595–601.

170. Pachman LM, Liotta-Davis MR, Hong DK, et al. TNF alpha-308A allele in juvenile dermatomyositis. Association with increased production of tumour necrosis factor, disease duration and pathologic calcifications. Arthritis Rheum 2000; 43:2368–2377.

171. Bohan A, Peter JB. Polymyositis and dermatomyositis. N Engl J Med 1975; 292:344–347.

172. Brown VE, Pilkington CA, Feldman BM, et al. An international consensus survey of the diagnostic criteria for juvenile dermatomyositis. Rheumatology 2006; 45:990–993.

173. Ramanan AV, Campbell-Webster N, Ota S, et al. The effectiveness of treating juvenile dermatomyositis with methotrexate and aggressively tapered corticosteroids. Arthritis Rheum 2005; 52:3570–3578.

174. Riley P, Maillard SM, Wedderburn LR, et al. Intravenous cyclophosphamide pulse therapy in juvenile dermatomyositis. A review of efficacy and safety. Rheumatology 2004; 43:491–496.

175. Ruperto N, Ravelli A, Murray KJ, et al. Preliminary core sets of measures for disease activity and damage assessment in juvenile systemic lupus erythematosus and juvenile dermatomyositis. Rheumatol 2003; 42:1452–1459.

176. Zulian F, Vallongo C, Woo P, et al. Localized scleroderma in childhood is not just a skin disease. Arthritis Rheum 2005; 52:2873–2881.

177. Zulian F, Athreya BH, Laxer R, et al. Juvenile localised scleroderma: clinical and epidemiological features in 750 children. An international study. Rheumatology 2006; 45:614–620.

178. Scalapino K, Arkachaisri T, Lucas M, et al. Childhood onset systemic sclerosis: classification, clinical and serological features and survival in comparison with adult onset disease. J Rheumatol 2006; 33:1004–1013.

179. Samuels J, Ozen S. Familial Mediterranean fever and the other autoinflammatory syndromes: evaluation of the patient with recurrent fever. Curr Opin Rheumatol 2006; 18:108–117.

180. The French FMF Consortium. A candidate gene for familial Mediterranean fever. Nat Genet 1997; 17:25–31.

181. Houten SM, Kuis W, Duran M, et al. Mutations in the gene encoding mevalonate kinase cause hyperimmunoglobulinemia D and periodic fever syndrome. Nat Genet 1999; 22:175–177.

182. McDermott MF, Aksentijevich I, Galen J, et al. Germline mutations in the extracellular domains of the 55 kDa TNF receptor, TNFR1, define a family of dominantly inherited autoinflammatory syndromes. Cell 1999; 9:133–144.

183. Prieur AM, Griscelli C, Lampert F, et al. A chronic, infantile, neurological, articular and cutaneous (CINCA) syndrome. A specific entity analysed in 30 patients. Scand J Rheumatol 1978; 66:57–68.

184. Hawkins PN, Lachmann HJ, Aganna E, et al. Spectrum of clinical features in Muckle–Wells syndrome and response to anakinra. Arthritis Rheum 2004; 50:607–612.

185. Turk DC, Okifuji A. Assessment of patients' reporting of pain: an integrated perspective. Lancet 1999; 353:1784–1788.

186. Merskey H. Pain terms: a list with definitions and notes on usage recommended by the ISAP subcommittee on taxonomy. Pain 1979; 6:249–252.

187. Sherry DD. Diagnosis and treatment of amplified musculoskeletal pain in children. Clin Exp Rheumatol 2001; 19:617–620.

188. Connelly M, Schanberg L. Latest developments in the assessment and management of chronic musculoskeletal pain syndromes in children. Curr Opin Rheumatol 2006; 18:496–502.

189. Malleson PN, Al-Matar M, Petty RE. Idiopathic musculoskeletal pain syndromes in children. J Rheumatol 1992; 19:1786–1789.

190. Sherry DD, Weisman R. Psychologic aspects of childhood reflex neurovascular dystrophy. Pediatrics 1988; 81:572–578.

191. Murray CS, Cohen A, Perkins T, et al. Morbidity in childhood reflex sympathetic dystrophy. Arch Dis Child 2000; 82:231–233.

192. Cleary AG, Sills JA, Davidson JE, et al. Reflex sympathetic dystrophy. Rheumatology 2001; 40:590–591.

193. McBeth J, Macfarlane GJ, Benjamin S, et al. Features of somatization predict the onset of chronic widespread pain: results of a large population-based study. Arthritis Rheum 2001; 44:940–946.

194. Aasland A, Flato B, Vandvik IH. Psychosocial factors in children with idiopathic musculoskeletal pain: a prospective, longitudinal study. Acta Pediatr 1997; 86:740–746.

195. Eccleston C, Jordan A, McCracken LM, et al. The Bath Adolescent Pain Questionnaire (BAPQ): development and preliminary psychometric evaluation of an instrument to assess the impact of chronic pain on adolescents. Pain 2005; 118:263–270.

196. Krist J, Ans D, Ottir G. Prevalence of self-reported back pain in school children: a study of sociodemographic differences. Eur J Pediatr 1996; 155:984–986.

197. Dreghorn CR, Newman RJ, Hardy G, et al. Primary tumours of the axial skeleton; experience of the Leeds Regional Bone Tumour Registry. Proceedings of British Scoliosis Society Meeting. J Bone Joint Surg 1989; 72B:338–339.

198. Williams CRP, O'Flynn E, Clarke NMP, et al. Torticollis secondary to ocular pathology. J Bone Joint Surg 1996; 78B:620–624.

199. Njeh CK, Shaw N, Gardner-Medwin JM, et al. Use of quantitative ultrasound to assess bone status in children with juvenile idiopathic arthritis: a pilot study. J Clin Densitom 2000; 3:251–260.

200. Schonau E. Problems of bone analysis in childhood and adolescence. Pediatr Nephrol 1998; 12:420–429.

201. NIH. Consensus Development Panel on Osteoporosis Prevention, Diagnosis and Therapy. Osteoporosis prevention, diagnosis, and therapy. JAMA 2001; 285:785–795.

202. Thornton J, Ashcroft DM, Mughal MZ, et al. Systematic review of effectiveness of bisphosphonates in treatment of low bone mineral density and fragility fractures in juvenile idiopathic arthritis. Arch Dis Child 2006; 91:753–761.

203. Bianchi ML, Cimaz R, Bardare M, et al. Efficacy and safety of alendronate for the treatment of osteoporosis in diffuse connective tissue diseases in children: a prospective multicenter trial. Arthritis Rheum 2000; 43:1960–1966.

204. Orava S, Jormakka E, Hulkko A. Stress fractures in young athletes. Arch Orthop Trauma Surg 1981; 98:271.

205. Barnett LS. Little league shoulder syndrome: proximal humeral epiphyseolysis in adolescent baseball pitchers. J Bone Joint Surg 1985; 67A:495–496.

206. Roy S, Caine D, Singer KM. Stress changes of the distal radial epiphysis in young gymnasts. Am J Sports Med 1985; 13:301–308.

207. Albanese S, Palmer A, Kerr D. Wrist pain and growth plate closure of the radius in gymnasts. J Pediatr Orthop 1989; 9:23–28.

208. Kujala UM, Kvist M, Heinonen O. Osgood–Schlatter's disease in adolescent athletes. Am J Sports Med 1985; 13:236–241.

209. Krause BL, Williams JPR, Catterral A. Natural history of Osgood–Schlatter's disease. J Pediatr Orthop 1990; 10:65–68.

210. Brogden BG, Crow NE. Little leaguer's elbow. Am J Roentgenol 1960; 83:671–675.

211. Noble CA. Iliotibial band friction syndrome in runners. Am J Sports Med 1980; 8:232–234.

212. Cassidy RE, Schaffer AJ. Repair of peripheral meniscus tears: a preliminary report. Am J Sports Med 1981; 9:209–214.

213. Lutter LD. Runners knee injuries. AAOS Instr Course Lect 1984; 33:258–268.

214. Michael RH, Holder LE. The soleus syndrome. Am J Sports Med 1985; 13:87–94.

215. Mubarak SJ. The medial tibial stress syndrome. Am J Sports Med 1982; 10:201–205.

216. Detmer DE. Chronic compartment syndrome: diagnosis, management and outcomes. Am J Sports Med 1985; 13:162–170.

30

Disorders of the skin

Nigel P Burrows

INTRODUCTION

The skin comprises roughly 15% of the body weight. It is a complex organ which undergoes constant repair. Its main functions are:

1. a barrier to absorption and loss of fluid and electrolytes;
2. a barrier to external injurious agents and mechanical stress;
3. protection against ultraviolet light;
4. protection against pathogenic microorganisms;
5. regulation of body temperature;
6. as a sensory organ;
7. synthesis of vitamin D;
8. social (and sexual) communication.

To perform these functions, the skin requires a complicated structure. It consists of three layers:

1. epidermis, derived from ectoderm;
2. dermis, derived from mesoderm;
3. subcutis, derived from mesoderm.

The main function of the outermost horny layer of the epidermis is to act as a barrier to fluid and electrolyte loss as well as to external injurious agents. Ninety five percent of the epidermis is made up of *keratinocytes* which originate from the basal layer of the epidermis and progress towards the exterior. *Melanocytes* are also found in the basal layer, and are differentiated from keratinocytes by darkly staining nuclei and clear cytoplasm: their main function is protection against ultraviolet radiation by distributing melanin throughout the basal layer. The amount of melanin determines the racial color. The *Langerhans' cell*, located in the mid epidermis, is a dendritic antigen-presenting cell that plays an important role in allergic contact eczema and forms part of the immune defense in the skin. The exact function of a fourth cell, the *Merkel cell*, has not been determined, but present evidence suggests a mechanoreceptor role.

The dermoepidermal junction is the interface between the epidermis and dermis. Its major component, the basement membrane zone, has many functions including adhesion, signaling and barrier.

The dermis is composed of collagen and elastic fibers within a matrix of ground substance. Blood vessels, sensory and autonomic nerves and nerve endings, hair follicles (pilosebaceous units) and sweat glands traverse the dermis. Temperature is regulated mainly by autonomic control of blood shunting between the superficial and deep arteriolar and venular plexuses. Secondary temperature regulation, which is particularly important where the ambient temperature exceeds 37°C, depends on evaporation from the eccrine sweat glands which are under adrenergic control.

The subcutis consists mainly of adipose tissue, whose main function is insulation of the body. In sites such as the sole of the foot, fibrous bands within the subcutis have a buffering and protective effect.

The skin appendages such as hair and nails are largely vestigial in the human; loss of either does not constitute any threat to the survival of the individual.

MANAGEMENT OF A SKIN PROBLEM IN A CHILD

It is important to take a detailed history either from the child or from the parents. History taking is similar to that in internal medicine, though the emphasis is different. Of particular importance are the following:

1. family history – many skin diseases are hereditary;
2. past history of the skin disease – conditions such as psoriasis and atopic eczema tend to be intermittent;
3. general health – some diseases (e.g. connective tissue diseases) are multiorgan problems;
4. previous treatment – both oral and topical: treatment may have modified the clinical picture (for better or for worse).

Examination of the child

The child should be undressed completely to allow full assessment of the condition. A general medical examination should also be performed. If a rash is present, note should be taken of the following points: (1) color, nature and distribution; (2) relationship of the rash to skin appendages, such as hair follicles and sweat ducts; (3) mucous membranes: some skin diseases have a banal appearance in the skin, but a characteristic appearance in mucous membranes, e.g. lichen planus, congenital syphilis; (4) examination of the hair and nails, as changes may give a clue as to the diagnosis.

TREATMENT OF SKIN DISEASES

As the skin is so accessible, it is sensible where possible to treat skin diseases with topical preparations. It is also important to introduce the active agent (e.g. steroid, antibiotic) in a suitable form or vehicle:

1. Lotions (solutions) are very useful for exudative rashes as 'wet dressings', where ointments and creams would 'float off', e.g. potassium permanganate. They are also useful for hairy areas, e.g. scalp. Shake lotions contain insoluble powders. e.g. calamine lotion.
2. Creams (oil–water emulsions). Bases such as cetomacrogol or aqueous cream are very acceptable to the patient, e.g. topical steroid creams.
3. Ointments such as petrolatum have a greasy base. They are useful for dry skin conditions, such as atopic eczema, e.g. steroid and antibiotic ointments.
4. Gels (semicolloids in alcohol base, which dry on the skin). Useful for scalp conditions.
5. Pastes (ointments + 15–30% powdered solids). Used on linen dressings, e.g. tar paste.
6. Powders, e.g. antifungal foot powders, miticides.

Topical corticosteroids

These are useful for treatment of symptoms and signs of inflammatory dermatoses, in particular eczema. Factors to be considered when prescribing include age of child, site of application and type of preparation. The fingertip unit (FTU) technique provides guidance for the quantity of corticosteroid to be applied.[1] One FTU is the amount of topical steroid that is squeezed out from a standard tube along an adult's fingertip. One FTU is used to treat an area of skin on a child equivalent to twice the size of the flat of an adult's hand with the fingers together. The weakest corticosteroid that controls the skin condition should be used. Preparations should be applied no more than twice daily. In general the more potent corticosteroids are not recommended in infants under 1 year but can be used on the trunk and limbs in severe cases for up to 2 weeks.

NEVI AND OTHER DEVELOPMENTAL DEFECTS

MELANOCYTIC NEVI

Congenital melanocytic nevi (CMN)

These occur in 0.5–2% of the population (Figs 30.1 and 30.2). They are arbitrarily classified as small (less than 1.5 cm), medium (1.5–20 cm) or large/giant (greater than 20 cm or 5% or more of body surface), in estimated adult size. They occur at birth as raised, verrucose or lobulated nodules or plaques of varying shades of brown to black, sometimes with blue or pink components. They have an irregular margin and often long dark hairs and may become increasingly lobulated and hairy with time. Giant-sized lesions may produce considerable redundancy of skin and often occur in a 'garment' or 'bathing trunk' distribution on the trunk and adjacent limbs. The very small CMN initially may be difficult to distinguish from café-au-lait macules. In patients with multiple large nevi an eruption of smaller ones (satellite nevi) may occur over the first year of life. Once established, the nevi increase in size in proportion to the patient's growth. Although rare, large CMN on the scalp or dorsal spine, especially with satellite nevi, may be associated with symptomatic leptomeningeal melanocytosis (neurocutaneous melanocytosis) with a median age of onset of neurological symptoms at 2 years.[2] Furthermore, magnetic resonance imaging (MRI) scans detect

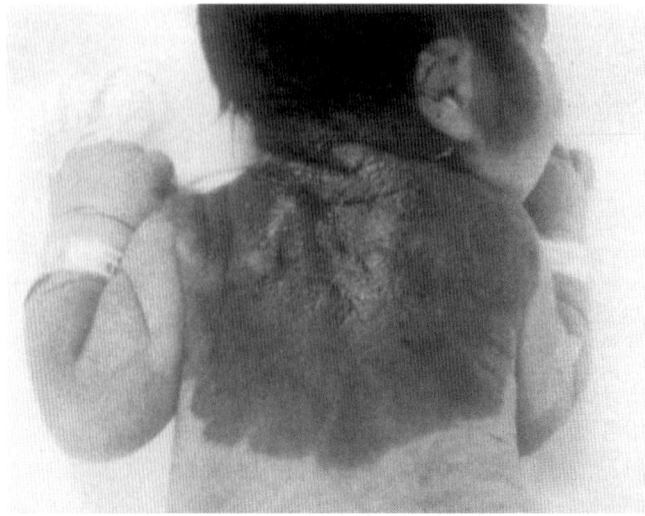

Fig. 30.1 Congenital melanocytic nevus.

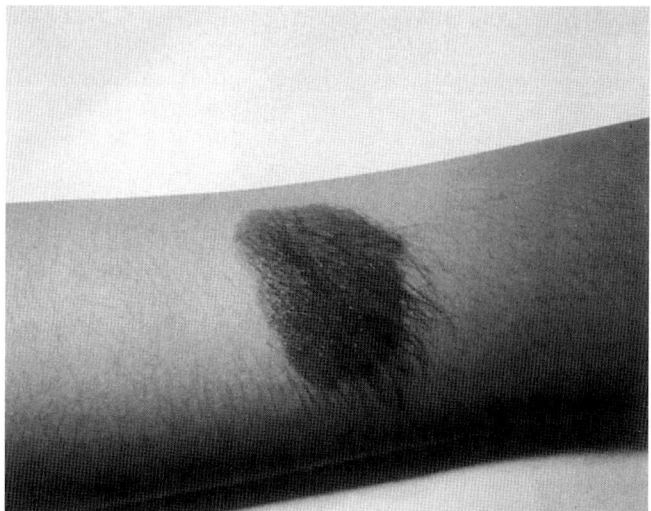

Fig. 30.2 Congenital melanocytic nevus.

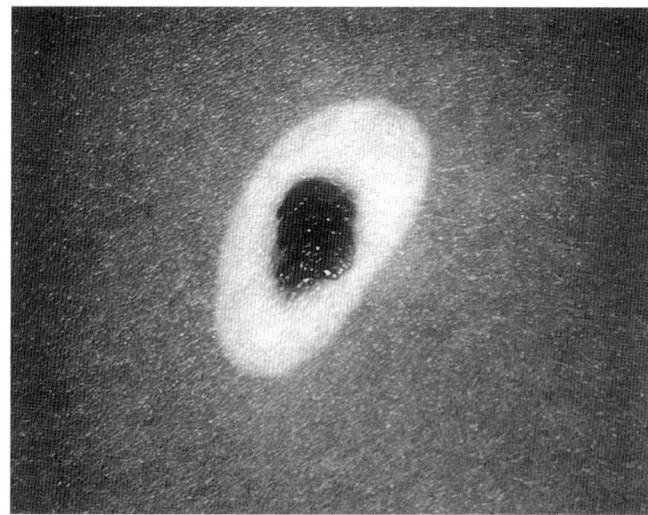

Fig. 30.3 Halo nevus.

leptomeningeal involvement in 5–30% of asymptomatic children with CMN in this distribution.[3–5]

Considerable controversy remains regarding the risk of development of malignant melanoma in CMN and hence the approach to management. Malignancy can arise from the dermal as well as the junctional component of CMN. The incidence of malignancy in large nevi has varied from 2 to 31% in different series but most studies have been retrospective and biased. A long term prospective study based on the Danish birth register is probably the most reliable and a lifetime risk of 4.6% is calculated from it.[6] In a retrospective study which included a review of the world literature primary cutaneous malignant melanoma was diagnosed within a large CMN before the age of 5 years in 50% of cases. No melanoma developed in the satellite nevi. Melanoma also occurs in medium-sized and small CMN[7,8] but the exact incidence for small lesions is not known, though it is definitely lower than for large nevi. A single follow-up study does not support the view of a significantly increased risk of melanoma in banal-appearing, medium-sized CMN, although median follow-up was short at 5.8 years.[9]

While small lesions, in which the malignancy risk is low and is usually postpubertal, can be easily excised, removal of large lesions in which the risk is much more significant is more difficult and with giant lesions may be impossible. In all cases the risk must be weighed against possible functional impairment and the morbidity of multiple operations. Many surgical procedures are available and are chosen depending on the site and extent of the lesions. Dermabrasion and laser therapy may improve the appearance of the nevus by removal of superficial pigment cells but the bulk of the lesion remains and the malignancy risk is not substantially reduced.

Acquired melanocytic nevi (AMN)

In a longitudinal study, 0.5% of babies had a CMN at birth and the number of melanocytic nevi in the same cohort at 1 year had risen to 35%.[10] These nevi continue to increase in number throughout childhood. They commence as brown or black macules, some of which become raised and enlarge laterally as they develop. They are usually of uniform color and well circumscribed. Histologically the flat lesions show clustering of nevus cells at the dermoepidermal junction (junctional nevus) and the raised ones also show intradermal nevus cells (compound nevus). Pure intradermal nevi are rare in children. The risk of melanoma arising from acquired melanocytic nevi is very low (less than 0.1%) and so their prophylactic removal in young patients is not justified.

Halo (Sutton's) nevi

A nevus may develop a depigmented halo (Fig. 30.3). The lesions are often multiple and are relatively common. The nevus may appear inflamed and often disappears leaving a white spot which may repigment years later. This is a completely benign change.

Atypical (dysplastic) nevi

Atypical nevi is the preferred term as dysplasia relates to histological features only. They are a subtype of acquired melanocytic nevi with characteristic clinicopathological features. They are a marker for the development of malignant melanoma, occurring in over 90% of patients with familial melanoma and over 10% of those with sporadic melanoma. These nevi differ from more typical AMNs by being larger (more than 5 mm diameter), having irregular and indistinct margins and irregular tan brown coloration, often with an erythematous component. They are predominantly macular, sometimes with a central elevated portion. They may appear in childhood as small typical appearing nevi which after puberty develop the atypical features. In adolescence and early adult life new atypical lesions may appear de novo. Atypical nevi may appear on the scalp in childhood. The final confirmation is based on the finding of some or all of a constellation of histopathological features of which the most important are nuclear atypia and a lymphocytic infiltrate. Familial atypical nevus syndrome is present when an individual has greater than 50 atypical nevi and a history of melanoma in a first or second degree relative.

Patients with multiple atypical nevi should be monitored with serial photography. Any mole showing significant alteration should be excised. Family members should be checked for the presence of atypical nevi or melanoma.

EPIDERMAL NEVI

Epidermal nevi are hamartomas arising from the basal layer of the embryonic epidermis that gives rise to skin appendages and keratinocytes. These nevi have been conventionally classified according to the main tissue of origin (keratinocytic, sebaceous and follicular) although this is somewhat arbitrary as more than one cell type may be present.

Epidermal nevi can involve any area of skin and may be present at birth (particularly those on the head) or appear in the first few years of life (or exceptionally later). They may simply grow with the patient or can extend well beyond their original distribution over months or years. Extension occurs less often with nevi on the head and with nevi present at birth, whatever their location. It is now clear that the linear and swirled patterns taken by epidermal nevi follow the lines of Blaschko, which define the tracks of clones of genetically identical cells. All epidermal nevi can be explained on the basis of genetic mosaicism[11] with each type of nevus representing the cutaneous manifestation of a different mosaic phenotype. In most patients the nevus is the only detectable manifestation but in some patients there are associated abnormalities in other organ systems, particularly skeletal, neurological and ocular.[12,13] This association has been called the 'epidermal nevus syndrome'.[11]

Keratinocyte nevi often start as lightly pigmented streaks that thicken and darken with time to become verrucous. They usually spare the face and scalp. Up to 10% may show histological features of epidermolytic hyperkeratosis and biopsy is therefore recommended, if possible, due to the risk of parenting a child with bullous ichthyosis. Inflammatory linear verrucous epidermal nevi (ILVEN) usually present after 6 months of age with a linear pruritic and inflamed lesion often on the lower limb.

Sebaceous and verrucous nevi are closely related. The former most commonly occur on the scalp and face and have a yellowish color due to prominent sebaceous glands. They present as a hairless, often solitary linear plaque, usually flat in infancy and childhood and becoming verrucose at puberty. Sebaceous nevi (Fig. 30.4) are rarely (< 5%) complicated in adult life by basal cell or squamous cell carcinoma.

The follicular or comedonal nevus presents as linear plaques with dilated follicular pores with comedones. The face is the commonest site but any involved site can be complicated in adolescence with acne-like cyst formation and scarring.

Skeletal abnormalities occur particularly with nevi of keratinocytic type on the limbs, and neurological and ocular abnormalities with nevi of sebaceous type on the head. The major clinical neurological features are seizures, developmental delay and hemiparesis. All patients with epidermal nevi should have a careful physical examination at presentation. Patients with linear nevi on the head who present in infancy and are normal on initial examination should be followed for several years. Most centers embark on imaging studies only in patients with clinical abnormalities.

Therapy of these lesions is difficult. Topical retinoic acid may temporarily flatten very thick areas. There are a few reports of improvement of gross lesions with oral retinoids but the effect depends on continued use of the drug. Recurrence is almost invariable following diathermy and cryotherapy. Carbon dioxide, argon and more recently erbium:YAG lasers have been used in some cases with good results though these may be temporary. Excision is appropriate for small and linear lesions and for irritating or cosmetically troubling areas of more widespread nevi.

VASCULAR NEVI

These can be divided into hemangiomas, which are proliferative vascular tumors, and vascular malformations which represent fixed collections of dilated abnormal vessels.[14]

Hemangiomas

Hemangiomas (Fig. 30.5) are usually not present at birth, undergo a fast growth phase and then, over a long period, tend to spontaneous

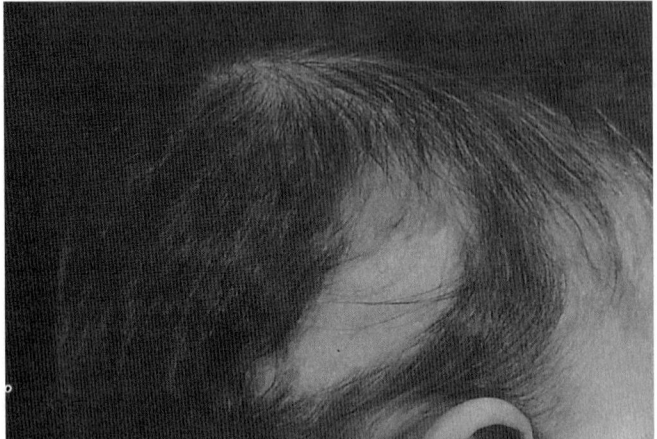

Fig. 30.4　Sebaceous nevus.

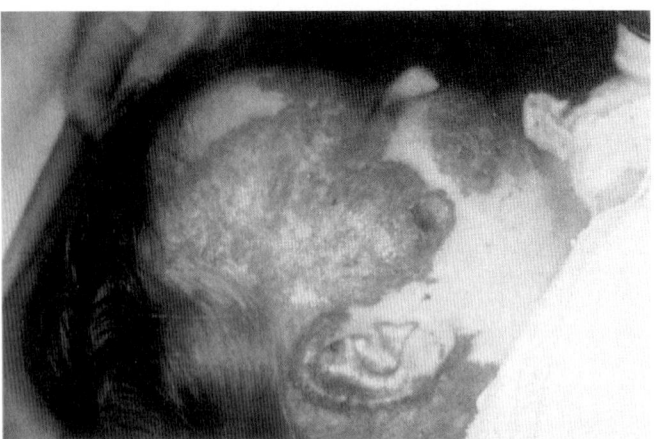

Fig. 30.5　Capillary (strawberry) hemangioma.

resolution. Emerging evidence shows that hemangiomas share unique tissue-specific markers (e.g. GLUT-1) with placental microvessels suggesting a possible common origin.[15] The terms capillary (strawberry), cavernous and capillary–cavernous are misleading and should be abandoned in favor of the simple term hemangioma.

Clinical features

Superficial hemangiomas are usually not present at birth but appear in the first weeks of life as an area of pallor followed by a telangiectatic patch. They then grow rapidly into a lobulated, well-demarcated, bright red tumor. Rapid growth continues over the first 6 months; the growth rate then slows and further growth after 10 months is unusual. After a stationary phase signs of involution appear with the appearance of gray areas which enlarge and coalesce. The tumor becomes softer and less bulky and then disappears in 90% of cases by 9 years of age.

Deeper hemangiomas may occur alone or beneath a superficial lesion. They also usually appear after birth and undergo a growth phase which however may be less striking than that of the more superficial lesions. The overlying skin is normal or bluish in color. As they resolve they soften and shrink and complete disappearance occurs in many cases: occasionally some redundant tissue remains in the place of large lesions. Apparent deep hemangiomas which show no sign of resolution are now recognized as vascular malformations, usually of venous type, and are not hemangiomas at all.

Complications

Ulceration may occur during the rapid growth phase of superficial hemangiomas. If secondary infection is controlled the ulcers usually heal in a few weeks but some scarring is inevitable. Ulceration of lesions on eyelids, lips or ala nasae can lead to full thickness tissue loss. Scarring following ulceration of lesions on or near the eyelids can result in a cicatricial ectropion and alopecia may be permanent after scalp ulceration.

Hemangiomas may encroach on vital structures. A hemangioma closing the eye for as little as 4 weeks in infancy can produce amblyopia. However, even without occluding the pupil an eyelid lesion, by pressing on the eye and producing a refractive error, can lead to failure of development of binocular vision and partial amblyopia. Large hemangiomas around the mouth may interfere with feeding and one blocking both nares can lead to respiratory difficulties while the child is being fed. A large deep hemangioma around the neck may displace the pharynx or trachea; the upper respiratory tract may also be directly involved with the hemangioma. The possibility of laryngeal involvement should be considered whenever there is a fast growing extensive lower face or neck hemangioma, particularly when there is accompanying intraoral involvement, and a lateral airways X-ray or MRI should be arranged. If there is stridor, an urgent laryngoscopy is mandatory. Even when traumatized, uncomplicated hemangiomas rarely bleed significantly.

Management

Simple observation and reassurance while awaiting natural resolution is the ideal approach for most hemangiomas. Serial photography and showing photographs of other resolving lesions are encouraging. Indications for active intervention are: an alarming growth rate; threatening ulceration in areas where serious complications could ensue; interference with vital structures; and severe bleeding. Oral corticosteroids are the treatment of choice. The optimal dose is not known but a meta-analysis suggests that 3 mg/kg or more for 6–8 weeks may give the best response.[16] Repeated courses should be avoided wherever possible. Intralesional steroids may shrink localized hemangiomas which fail to respond to systemic steroids, and interferon-alpha has been effective in some life threatening cases although severe neurotoxicity, including spastic diplegia, has been reported.[17] Laser therapy became an increasingly popular treatment modality for uncomplicated hemangiomas but without good evidence for effectiveness. A randomized, controlled study of early pulsed dye laser treatment has shown no benefit of treatment at 1 year follow-up.[18] Life threatening hemangiomas have been treated with variable success with oral vincristine.[19] Cosmetic surgical procedures can improve the appearance when loose tissue remains.

Congenital hemangioma

Two types of this rare hemangioma are recognized.[20] Both are usually solitary lesions and account for about 3% of all hemangiomas. Rapidly involuting congenital hemangioma (RICH) is similar to infantile hemangioma but differs in that it is fully developed at birth, with subsequent rapid involution and regression. Non-involuting congenital hemangiomas (NICH) are usually plaque-like or bossed and as the name implies do not resolve spontaneously. Unlike infantile hemangiomas they are GLUT1 negative.

PHACE syndrome

PHACE is an acronym to describe a constellation of features: posterior fossa brain malformations, facial hemangioma, arterial anomalies, cardiac anomalies (including aortic coarctation) and eye abnormalities. If ventral developmental defects such as sternal clefting or supraumbilical raphe are present the association is referred to as PHACES. This syndrome should be considered in any infant presenting with an extensive facial hemangioma.[21]

Kasabach–Merritt syndrome (hemangioma – hemorrhage syndrome)

This is the rare association of thrombocytopenia with vascular tumors (Fig. 30.6). In children these are usually either large, deep hemangiomas, especially on limbs and around limb girdles, or diffuse hemangiomatosis. Thrombocytopenia is caused by entrapment of platelets within the lesions and is sometimes followed by disseminated intravascular coagulation (DIC). At first there may be bleeding into the

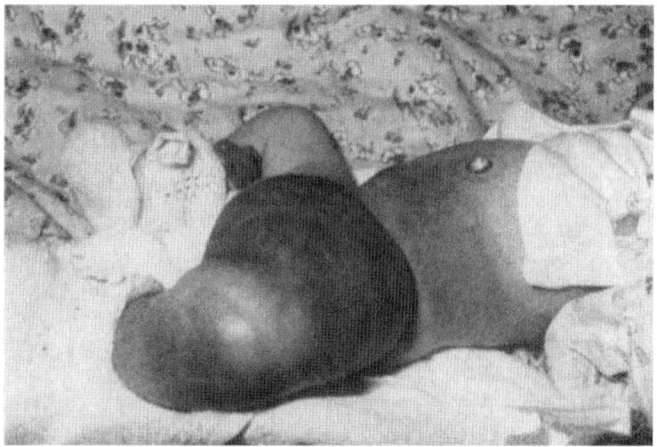

Fig. 30.6 Kasabach–Merritt syndrome.

hemangioma, which rapidly enlarges: widespread life threatening hemorrhage may follow. When bleeding is confined to the hemangiomas the approach should be conservative; in severe cases high dose systemic corticosteroids are indicated together with resuscitation, transfusion, and management of the DIC.

Diffuse infantile hemangiomatosis

This is a condition with multiple small hemangiomas in a widespread distribution. A benign form has lesions limited to the skin but a potentially serious systemic form may occur with lesions in many organs, particularly liver (64%), gastrointestinal tract (52%), lungs (52%) and central nervous system (52%) with or, rarely, without cutaneous lesions.[22] All patients with multiple cutaneous lesions should be carefully assessed with full blood count, chest X-ray, and examination for cardiac failure due to arteriovenous shunts and for bleeding from the gastrointestinal tract. An ultrasound or abdominal computerized tomography (CT) scan should be performed to exclude hepatic involvement and other organs may need to be further investigated. Angiography and technetium-labeled red blood cell scans can delineate further the extent of internal involvement.[23] With severe systemic involvement high dose corticosteroids are required along with management of cardiac failure and other complications, and active surgical intervention may be necessary in selected cases.

Vascular malformations

Vascular malformations are structural abnormalities and as such are present at birth, grow in proportion to the patient's growth and have no tendency at all to resolution. They can be further divided into fast flow, e.g. arteriovenous, or slow flow, e.g. venous, lymphatic or capillary malformations.

Capillary malformation (port-wine stain, nevus flammeus)

This is a vascular malformation composed of dilated mature capillaries. It is present at birth and shows no involution. Lesions may be unilateral or, less often, bilateral, and occur anywhere on the body, though they are most commonly found on the face. They are deep pink in infancy becoming more purple later. After puberty they may become raised and nodular. Good results can be achieved with the pulsed dye laser. Port-wine stains (PWS) must be distinguished from salmon patches at the nape of the neck (stork bite) and lesions on the eyelid or forehead (angel kiss). The vast majority of facial lesions resolve in months whilst the occipital ones persist.

It is important to be aware that, even in the absence of Sturge–Weber syndrome, ocular complications can occur. If the PWS encroaches the upper eyelid glaucoma may occur. The incidence increases to over 30% if the lower eyelid is also involved.[24]

Sturge–Weber syndrome

This is the association of a facial capillary malformation and a vascular malformation of the ipsilateral meninges and cerebral cortex. The cutaneous lesion always involves the skin in the distribution of the first division of the trigeminal nerve.[25] In 20% of infants the neurological manifestations of the syndrome include convulsions, hemiparesis and mental retardation.

Patients presenting with a capillary malformation in the appropriate distribution should have early neurological and ophthalmological consultation and continued close follow-up. A CT scan may demonstrate the intracranial malformations in the first few months of life. Parallel streaks of calcification may be demonstrated radiologically after about 2 years of age.

Vascular malformations with limb hypertrophy

Klippel–Trenaunay syndrome refers to a Parkes–Weber syndrome (PWS), associated with ipsilateral overgrowth of a limb, with soft tissue and/or bony hypertrophy and venous varicosities. The condition arises predominantly due to venous malformations whereas PWS, with similar clinical features, is caused by arteriovenous fistulae. In both instances, deeper lymphatic abnormalities may also be present. In 15% of cases of Klippel–Trenaunay syndrome involvement may be bilateral. Treatment is generally unsatisfactory with few cases being amenable to surgical correction. Compression bandaging may help to some extent with the increased girth of a limb.

CONGENITAL APLASIA CUTIS

Aplasia cutis congenita (ACC) is a congenital absence of skin and in 70% of patients is located as a solitary lesion on the scalp. The commonest form is a localized oval, stellate or linear area at or near the midline of the scalp which presents as an ulcerated area which crusts (Fig. 30.7). Resolution occurs after some months to leave a scar that is usually atrophic but is occasionally hypertrophic. There is permanent alopecia at the site. Rarely the lesion is already scarred at birth. The defect may involve not only skin but also subcutaneous fat and even bone. The bony defect will eventually heal but until it does there is a risk of meningitis. Deep aplasia may erode large vessels producing serious hemorrhage. A skull X-ray should be performed in all cases unless the lesion is obviously very superficial. Early management of scalp ACC is conservative with protection of the area and early treatment of secondary infection. Very deep lesions, however, may require skin and/or bone grafting. In later life scalp reduction techniques can be used to deal with the area of alopecia.

After the scalp the next commonest site is the lower limbs. When multiple lesions occur their distribution is often strikingly symmetrical and they may be covered with a shiny transparent membrane rather than being open erosions. Cases with extensive truncal and limb ACC are often associated with a fetus papyraceus at delivery, indicating the death of a twin early in the second trimester.

ACC-like lesions can occur on the lower limbs of patients with several types of epidermolysis bullosa probably resulting from intrauterine mechanical trauma. ACC may occur in a number of syndromes including trisomy 13, 4p-syndrome, 46XY gonadal dysgenesis and the Johanson–Blizzard syndrome. It may also be associated with a number of morphological abnormalities, particularly those involving the limbs.

DERMOID CYSTS

Congenital inclusion dermoid cysts typically present as asymptomatic subcutaneous swellings. Approximately 40% are present at birth with the rest appearing over the next 5 years. They arise due to entrapment of epithelium along embryonic fusion lines and occur particularly on the head and neck with predilection over the lateral eyebrow and dorsum of the nose. It is essential that adequate imaging investigations are performed prior to surgery as they may form deep tracts into underlying tissue.

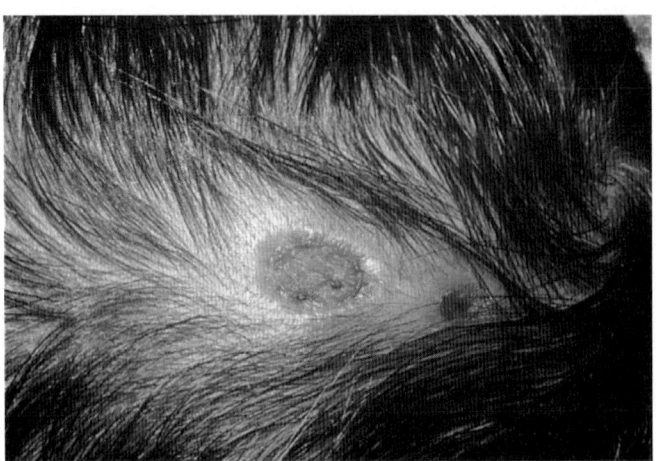

Fig. 30.7 Aplasia cutis.

HEREDITARY DISEASES

THE ICHTHYOSES

These are a group of inherited conditions with dry thickened skin of varying severity. The major ichthyoses comprise:
1. ichthyosis vulgaris (IV);
2. X-linked recessive ichthyosis (XLRI) (Fig. 30.8);
3. lamellar ichthyosis (LI);
4. congenital ichthyosiform erythroderma (CIE) (Fig. 30.9);
5. bullous ichthyosis (BI).

The histopathological and clinical features of the major ichthyoses are listed in Table 30.1. They are life-long disorders with little tendency to spontaneous improvement.

Management

Simple emollients such as aqueous cream may be adequate in IV. Keratolytics containing urea, propylene glycol or alpha-hydroxy acids may be more effective and useful in IV and XLRI but they may sting on fissured skin. The more severe ichthyoses often show little improvement with these topical agents. Oral retinoids may be very helpful in CIE but their effectiveness must always be weighed against their potential

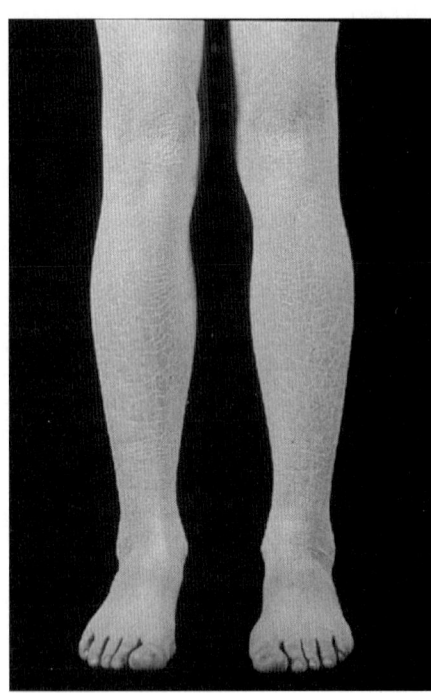

Fig. 30.8 X-linked ichthyosis.

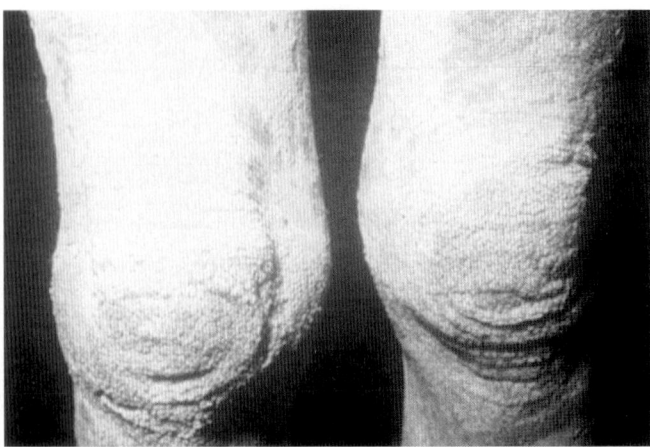

Fig. 30.9 Lamellar ichthyosis (congenital ichthyosiform erythroderma).

Table 30.1   Classification and features of the major ichthyoses

	Onset (and inheritance)	Clinical features	Complications and associations	Chromosomal/gene loci
Ichthyosis vulgaris	After birth but within the first year of life (AD)	Fine pale branny scales especially on extensor surfaces of limbs. Wide sparing of flexures of limbs. Trunk less severely involved. Face usually spared. Hyperlinear palms	Rarely corneal dystrophy, keratosis pilaris, atopy	Loss of function of filaggrin
Recessive X-linked ichthyosis	Appears within the first 3 months of life. Sometimes congenital with a thin shiny covering membrane (XLR)	Large dark adherent scales mainly on extensor surfaces of limbs. Scaling encroaches on limb flexures and axillae with narrow sparing. Trunk is diffusely involved. Sides of face often involved. Usually severe involvement of neck and thick scalp scaling. Palms and soles are uninvolved	Frequent corneal dystrophy (also in carriers). Cryptorchidism. Steroid sulfatase deficiency in most tissues including the amnion (which is derived from fetus). This placental steroid sulfatase deficiency may result in a failure of spontaneous onset of labor	Steroid sulfatase gene deletion (Xp22.3)
Lamellar ichthyosis	Usually at birth as 'collodion baby' (AR/AD)	Large dark plate-like scales. Mild to moderate erythroderma. The whole body surface is involved, including palms and soles	Ectropion. Blockage of external auditory meatus with scale resulting in hearing loss. Block of nares with scale. Pyrexia from sweat duct obstruction. Failure to thrive. Alopecia	TGM1 gene mutations (14q11.2); also 2q33–35, 19p12–q12
Congenital ichthyosiform erythroderma	Usually at birth as 'collodion baby' (AR)	Fine white scale in most areas, sometimes larger and darker on lower legs. Mild to very severe generalized erythroderma. Whole body surface is involved including palms and soles	Similar to those of lamellar ichthyosis but of lesser extent	TGM1 gene mutations (14q11.2); also 3p21
Bullous ichthyosis (epidermolytic hyperkeratosis)	At birth with erythroderma and widespread blistering. After a few days the redness subsides and over early months the blistering tendency reduces (AD)	Thick dark warty scales from time to time to leave denuded areas with a red base. Blistering is rare after 1 year. The condition may be localized to extensor surfaces but is usually widespread although the face is usually spared. Palm and sole involvement is variable	Bacterial superinfection is a recurrent problem. Heavy bacterial colonization is inevitable. Maceration and offensive odor are major problems	K2e gene mutations (12q11–13)

AD, autosomal dominant; AR, autosomal recessive; XLR, X-linked recessive.

side-effects, especially skeletal abnormalities and teratogenicity. In BI their usefulness is limited by their tendency to increase skin fragility. Detection and treatment of secondary bacterial infection is important in BI and topical disinfectants may reduce bacterial colonization and malodor.

Collodion baby

This is a descriptive term for the child who is encased at birth in a shiny tight membrane resembling collodion or plastic skin, producing ectropion and eclabium and fissuring (Fig. 30.10). The skin peels off in days or weeks. This may be a presentation of various conditions, particularly CIE (which overlaps with lamellar ichthyosis), chondrodysplasia punctata, trichothiodystrophy and rarely Netherton syndrome. In approximately 10% of collodion babies the membrane peels off to leave normal skin: this condition is called lamellar ichthyosis of the newborn. Collodion babies show temperature instability and excessive fluid loss. Corneal exposure may result if the eyes are not covered and the eclabium may necessitate squeeze bottle, tube or dropper feeding. As the fissures appear, secondary infection becomes a risk. The child should be nursed in a humidicrib with aseptic handling.

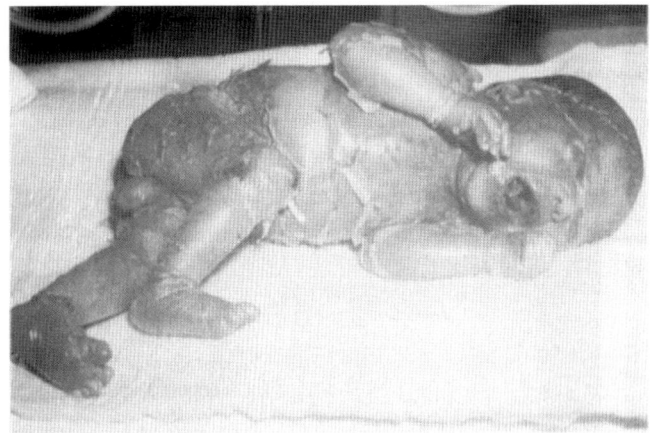

Fig. 30.10   Collodion baby.

Harlequin ichthyosis

This is a rare, potentially lethal, autosomal recesssive disorder. Causative mutations in the ABCA12 gene, which is a member of the ATP-binding (ABC) transporter family, have recently been identified.[26] ABCA12 is an epidermal lipid transporter and loss of the skin lipid barrier is thought to lead to abnormal keratinization.

At birth the child is covered in large dark plates of scale with deep fissures. Severe ectropion and eclabium, deformed ears and claw hands and feet are present. Most used to die as neonates due to secondary infection, anemia, circulatory disturbances or renal failure but the few who have survived have had a severe ichthyosiform erythroderma. (Note – this is different from the harlequin color change.)

Ichthyosis as part of other syndromes

Some of the syndromes of which ichthyosis is a part are listed in Table 30.2.

EPIDERMOLYSIS BULLOSA (EB)

This is a rare group of inherited diseases characterized by trauma-induced blistering of skin and mucosae. The prevalence is between 1/50000 and 1/2000000 for the more common and rarer forms, respectively. Over 20 types are now identified, separated on the basis of inheritance, clinical features, immunohistochemistry, electron microscopic (EM) and molecular pathology. The split may be within the epidermis, at the dermoepidermal junction in the lamina lucida (junctional; Figs 30.11 and 30.12) or in the upper dermis (sublamina densa; Fig. 30.13). A classification is given in Table 30.3. The structure of the cutaneous basement membrane zone and the gene defects in epidermolysis bullosa are shown in Figure 30.14.

A firm diagnosis should be established as soon as possible by EM and immunohistochemical analysis from an unaffected area of skin in which the split is induced by prior rubbing. This enables a prognosis to be given and a management plan to be established for present and future.

Epidermolysis bullosa simplex (EBS)
Localized EBS (Weber – Cockayne)

The blisters are often not noticed until the child starts to walk. It may be so mild that it does not present until adult life. However, morbidity can be such that daily activities are affected. Blisters develop on hands and feet and, as with all forms of EBS, they are often worse with increased temperatures in the summer months. Very occasionally other body sites are affected.

Generalized EBS (Koebner)

The onset of blisters is at birth or early infancy. They may be widespread but affect particularly areas of trauma such as hands, feet, knees and elbows. The oral mucosa is occasionally involved. Nails are not affected and there is no scarring. As with localized EB, secondary infection is the main complication. Life expectancy is normal.

Herpetiform EBS (Dowling – Meara)

Widespread blistering can be present at birth and severe cases may be mistaken for junctional EB. Transient milia develop at sites of grouped blisters. The hands and feet are especially affected, often leading to a palmoplantar keratoderma. Nail thickening is common. Oral, laryngeal and esophageal mucosal involvement is sometimes seen. Although blistering may persist through adult life the tendency is for considerable improvement.

Junctional EB
Generalized severe (Herlitz) EB

Blistering is present at birth and may be relatively minor at first. Slow wound healing is seen particularly on the face and around the nails. Typically affected babies have a hoarse cry due to mucosal involvement which is extensive and severe involving nasal, oral, esophageal as well as anogenital and urinary epithelium. Many infants die due to overwhelming sepsis. Survival to adolescence is rare but older children suffer from chronic sepsis, anemia and growth retardation.

Table 30.2   Syndromes associated with ichthyosis

Syndrome	Inheritance	Type of ichthyosis	Other major features	Molecular defects
Chondrodysplasia punctata	XLR	Onset may be as 'collodion baby'. Initially occurs as a diffuse redness and scaling. Later occurs in a whorled patchy distribution	Epiphyseal dysplasia, cataracts, follicular atrophoderma	XLR: Emopamil binding protein gene mutations
	XLD			XLD: Arylsulfatase E gene mutations
Sjögren–Larsson syndrome	AR	Generalized ichthyosis at birth. Later large dark scales most prominent in flexures	Mental retardation, spasticity	Aldehyde dehydrogenase family mutations
Chanarin–Dorfman syndrome (neutral lipid storage disease with ichthyosis)	AR	Ichthyosis simulating mild to moderate congenital ichthyosiform erythroderma	Lipid vacuoles in almost all cells. Normal serum lipids. Cataracts, deafness, developmental delay	Unknown
Refsum syndrome	AR	Delayed onset of ichthyosis of mild form, simulating ichthyosis vulgaris	Failure to degrade phytanic acid. Retinitis pigmentosa, peripheral neuropathy, cerebellar ataxia	Phytanoyl-CoA hydroxylase gene mutations
Netherton syndrome	AR	Erythroderma at birth. Late development of circinate migratory scaly lesions (ichthyosis linearis circumflexa) in widespread distribution. Some cases simulate congenital ichthyosiform erythroderma	Alopecia due to hair shaft abnormalities, especially trichorrhexis invaginata, atopic diathesis, developmental delay, generalized aminoaciduria	Serine proteinase inhibitor (SPINK 5) gene mutations

AR, autosomal recessive; XLD, X-linked dominant; XLR, X-linked recessive.

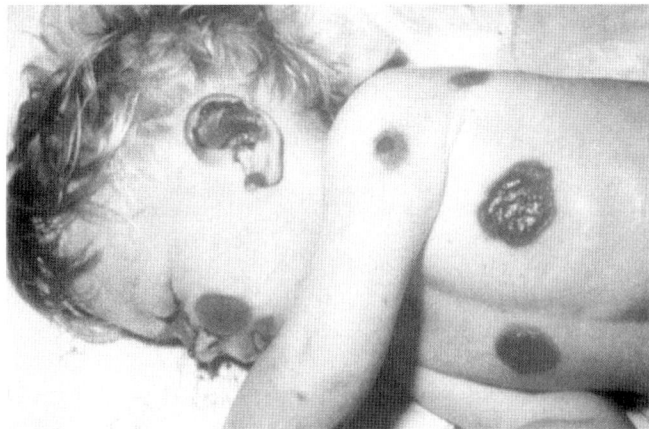

Fig. 30.11   Junctional epidermolysis bullosa.

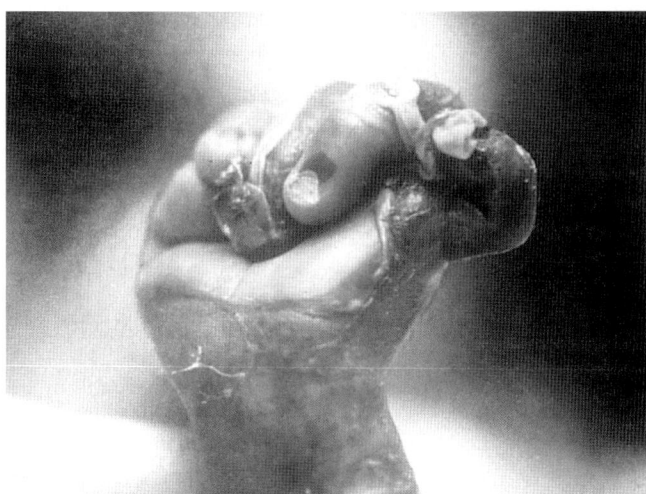

Fig. 30.12   Junctional epidermolysis bullosa.

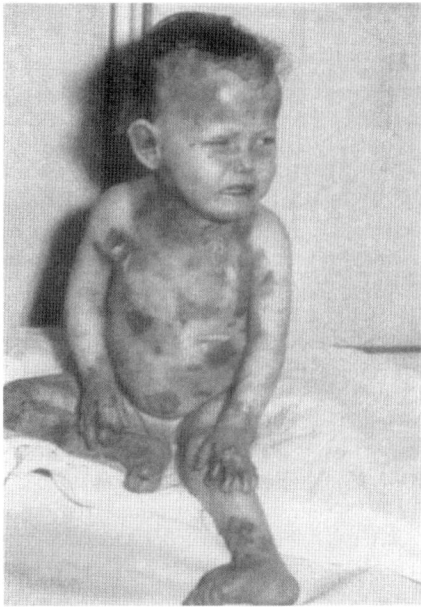

Fig. 30.13   Dystrophic epidermolysis bullosa.

Table 30.3   Classification of major types of hereditary epidermolysis bullosa

	Inheritance
Intraepidermal blister	
Epidermolysis bullosa simplex (EBS)	
Localized (hands and feet) EBS (Weber–Cockayne)	AD
Generalized EBS (Koebner)	AD
Herpetiform EBS (Dowling–Meara)	AD
EBS with muscular dystrophy	AR
Lamina lucida blister	
Junctional epidermolysis bullosa (JEB)	
Generalized severe (Herlitz)	AR
Generalized atrophic benign (GABEB)	AR
JEB with pyloric atresia	AR
Sublamina densa	
Dystrophic epidermolysis bullosa (DEB)	
Dominant DEB	AD
Recessive DEB (Hallopeau)	AR

AD, autosomal dominant; AR, autosomal recessive.

Generalized atrophic benign EB (GABEB)

Although in the initial stages the blistering has a similar pattern to Herlitz EB the child survives with a decreasing tendency to blister. Mucous membranes are involved but less so than the Herlitz form. The major feature of GABEB is alopecia which follows the blistering. Lesions may also heal with hyperpigmentation. The life span of the affected individual is normal.

Dystrophic EB

Dystrophic EB is characterized by skin fragility, blisters, scarring with milia formation and nail changes. The autosomal recessive form is more severe than the dominant disease with greater skin fragility and therefore more widespread blistering. Repeated blistering and scarring can lead to syndactyly of fingers and toes and club-like deformities of hands and feet with several digits encased together in a scar. Severe involvement of oral mucosa may lead to stricture formation in autosomal recessive patients. Laryngeal and tracheal involvement may threaten the airway. Hypoproteinemia is caused by constant loss of protein in blister fluid, malabsorption and malnutrition. In all cases the nails are thickened and often lost. Aggressive squamous cell carcinomas may arise in the scar tissues and metastatic disease is a major cause of death in adult patients with severe disease.

Management

In mild epidermolysis bullosa simplex and dominant dystrophic cases advice is required regarding avoidance of trauma, a reduction of friction, appropriate clothing and footwear. New blisters should be pricked to drain them but not deroofed and various dressings of non-stick material are appropriate. Secondary bacterial infection is treated with topical or oral antibiotics.

In the severe forms with extensive neonatal blistering extreme care is necessary to avoid further skin damage. The infant should initially be nursed naked in a humidicrib lying on non-adherent material with barrier nursing to prevent infection. Blisters should be drained and antibacterial creams such as silver sulfadiazine applied to large erosions. Vaseline gauze or non-adherent plastic dressings should be used as required, secured with tubular gauze or by other means but never taped to the skin with adhesive. A nasogastric tube should never be passed.

Severe complications may require a multidisciplinary approach. In the UK advice, both medical and nursing, should be sought whenever appropriate early in management from regional centers with a particular expertise in EB. Where possible, one physician should coordinate the entire management program to provide stability and continuity. The family should be directed towards support organizations, which can offer practical advice, emotional support and companionship. Finally, genetic counseling of the parents and later the patient should be arranged at an appropriate time.

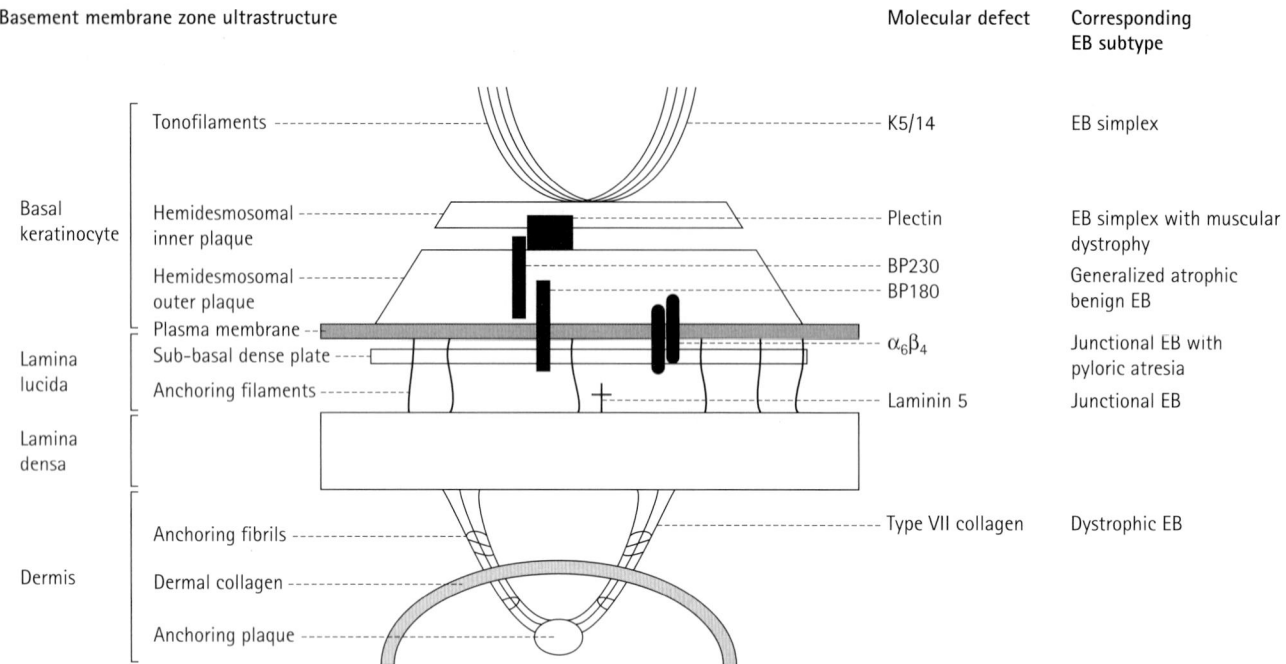

Fig. 30.14   Structure of cutaneous basement membrane zone and gene defects in epidermolysis bullosa.

ECTODERMAL DYSPLASIAS

The ectodermal dysplasias (Fig. 30.15) are a heterogeneous group of inherited conditions with a primary defect in two or more of the following: teeth, nails, hair, sweat glands or abnormalities in tissues of ectodermal origin, including eyes, ears, oral and nasal mucosa, melanocytes and central nervous system. Molecular genetics is increasingly yielding more insight into the abnormal regulatory mechanisms in ectodermal dysplasias and this is leading to revised classifications according to the function of the involved mutated genes.[27]

The major features of some of the more important ectodermal dysplasias are documented in Table 30.4.

Management

As these are disorders manifesting very diverse features, a multidisciplinary approach is essential.

If the scalp hair is very sparse the cosmetic benefit of a good wig may be invaluable. Primary and secondary dentitions can be assessed with dental X-rays in infancy in conjunction with a pediatric dentist experienced in these conditions. Early use of prostheses may prevent development of some of the structural facial abnormalities. Newer techniques include osseous implants into which prosthetic teeth can be fitted.

If hypohidrosis is extreme hyperthermia may result and may be severe and life threatening. Advice regarding activities, clothing and methods of cooling may be required.

Atopic eczema often accompanies hypohidrotic ectodermal dysplasia and will require the usual treatment. Many patients have dry skin and require emollients, and keratolytics may improve palmoplantar keratoderma.

All patients with eye abnormalities should be managed in conjunction with an ophthalmologist. Artificial tears are essential for dry eyes to prevent corneal damage. Reconstructive procedures will be required for atresia of nasolacrimal ducts and canaliculi. Severe respiratory infections complicate some of these syndromes and need antibiotics, physiotherapy and regular pediatric follow-up.

TUBEROUS SCLEROSIS

The tuberous sclerosis complex (TSC) is an autosomal dominant, neurocutaneous disorder characterized by the formation of hamartomata in many organs. Mutations in the hamartin gene (9q34) account for approximately half of the cases (TSC1) and the other half arise due to mutations in the tuberin gene (16p13) (TSC2).[28] Both act as tumor suppressor genes and around 60% arise due to spontaneous mutations. A small number of families are unlinked to either gene. Epilepsy occurs in 80% and mental retardation in 70%. Up to 20% of patients with infantile spasms will have TSC and should therefore have their skin examined. Other systemic abnormalities include retinal phacomata and a variety of hamartomata in renal tract, heart and other organs.

Dermatological features

The most pathognomonic features are angiofibromas (adenoma sebaceum), periungual fibromas, shagreen patches and ash leaf macules (Figs 30.16 and 30.17). The angiofibromas appear as 1–4 mm bright red papules in a centrofacial distribution. Sometimes they coalesce to form cauliflower-like masses. Their onset is usually between the ages of 3 and 10 years and they may become more extensive at puberty. Numbers vary from a few to several hundred. Periungual fibromas appear around puberty as

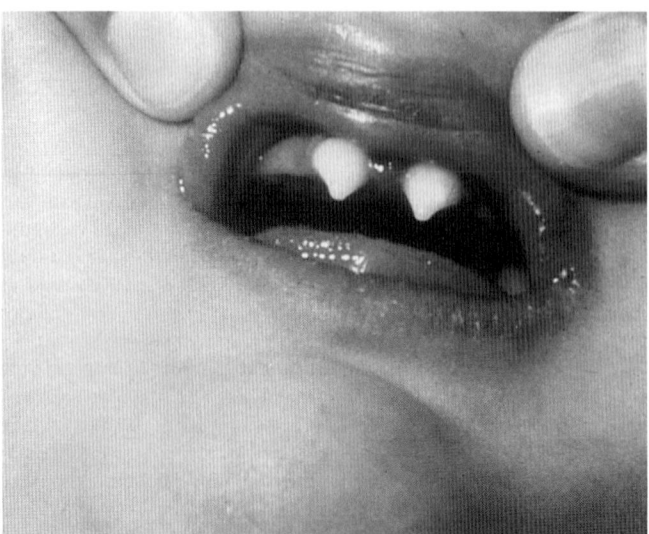

Fig. 30.15   Ectodermal dysplasia.

Table 30.4 The ectodermal dysplasias

	1. Hypohidrotic ectodermal dysplasia (Christ–Siemens–Touraine syndrome)	2. Hidrotic ectodermal dysplasia (Clouson syndrome)	3. Rapp–Hodgkin syndrome	4. EEC syndrome (ectrodactyly, ectodermal dysplasia and clefting)	5. AEC syndrome (ankyloblepharon, ectodermal dysplasia and clefting) (Hay–Wells syndrome)
Inheritance	X-linked recessive*	Autosomal dominant	Autosomal dominant	Autosomal dominant	Autosomal dominant
Hair	Hypotrichosis of scalp, body hair, eyebrows and lashes. Beard normal. Hair fine and fair	Hypotrichosis. Hair fine and dry	Sparse, coarse and stiff with hair shaft abnormalities	Sparse wiry hair	Severe hypotrichosis
Teeth	Hypodontia. Conical teeth	May be normal. Hypodontia, caries, widespaced teeth	Hypodontia, abnormally shaped teeth. Early caries	Hypodontia, abnormally shaped teeth	Variable hypodontia, abnormal shape, delayed eruption
Nails	Often normal. Sometimes fragile and occasionally dystrophic or absent	Thick, striated, discolored. Paronychia and nail loss. Rarely thin and brittle	Small and dysplastic	Thin, pitted and striated	Severe dystrophy. Short due to absence of distal nail plate
Sweating	Hypohidrosis often with hyperthermia	Normal	Hypohidrosis	Occasional hypohidrosis	Variable hypohidrosis
Skin	Smooth and dry, loss of dermatoglyphics, wrinkled and hyperpigmented around eyes, atopic dermatitis	Thick over finger joints, knees and elbows. Palmoplantar keratoderma	Dry and coarse. Thick over elbows and knees. Reduced dermatoglyphics	Dry and thin. Palmoplantar keratoderma	Large weeping areas at birth, later dry and scaly. May be recurrent scalp crusting. Palmoplantar keratoderma
Eyes	Hypoplasia of nasolacrimal duct, decreased lacrimal gland secretion, dry eyes, photophobia and corneal opacities	Usually normal. Occasionally premature cataracts	Atresia of lacrimal puncta producing epiphora, corneal opacities	Nasolacrimal duct stenosis, dacryocystitis, corneal scarring	Ankyloblepharon filiforme adnatum, nasolacrimal duct atresia
Facies	Variable. Thick lips, saddle nose, frontal bossing, maxillary hypoplasia. Occasionally abnormal ears	Normal	Cleft lip, hypoplastic maxilla. Microstomia. Prominent malformed ears	Cleft lip	Cleft lip often, microstomia, broad nasal bridge, sunken maxilla, abnormal pinnae
Mucosae	Poor development of mucous glands in gastrointestinal and respiratory tracts. Atrophic rhinitis, thick nasal secretion, recurrent chest infections, dysphagia. Dry mouth	Normal	Chronic rhinitis	Hoarseness due to abnormality of laryngeal mucosa	Filamentous bands in vagina, anal fissure
Miscellaneous	Absent or supernumerary nipples. Absent breast tissue in carriers. Asthma	Tufting of terminal phalanges with finger clubbing. Thickening of skull bones	Short stature. Cleft palate. Syndactyly	Cleft palate. Ectrodactyly (split hands and feet). Syndactyly	Cleft palate. Syndactyly

* Autosomal recessive variant is difficult to distinguish phenotypically.

firm smooth flesh-colored papules in a periungual or subungual location. The shagreen patch is a connective tissue nevus comprising an accumulation of collagen as an irregularly thickened yellow-white plaque, usually in the lumbosacral area. It develops between the ages of 2 and 5 years. Ash leaf macules are depigmented macules, usually 1–3 cm in diameter but occasionally much larger. They are usually oval in shape, with a minority truly ash leaf shaped. They may be present at birth or appear during the first year. Large numbers may be present and they are best visualized under Wood's (ultraviolet) light.

Other dermatological features include fibromatous plaques on brow or scalp, intraoral fibromas, multiple fibroepithelial polyps around the neck and in the axillae and a variety of other depigmented lesions including numerous guttate macules and large dermatomal lesions. Poliosis and canities may also occur.

Patients who present with these characteristic skin signs should be referred for neurological assessment and computerized axial tomography to demonstrate any intracranial lesions. Laser therapy may improve the cosmetic appearance of the angiofibromas.

INCONTINENTIA PIGMENTI

Incontinentia pigmenti (IP type 2) is a multisystem disorder inherited as an X-linked dominant trait and is usually prenatally lethal in males (Figs 30.18 and 30.19). It arises due to mutations (usually genomic

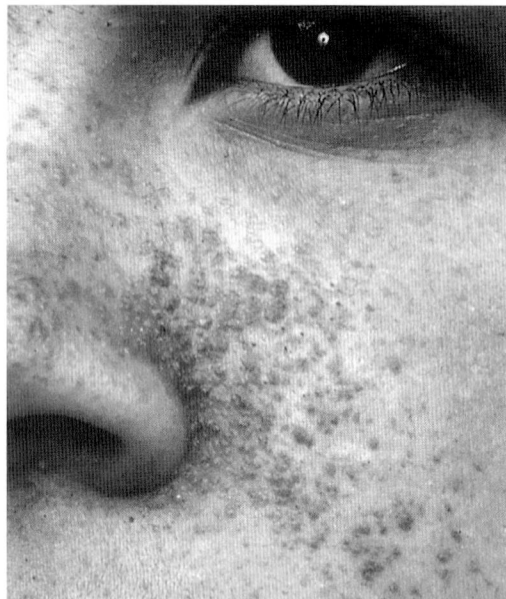

Fig. 30.16   Adenoma sebaceum: tuberous sclerosis.

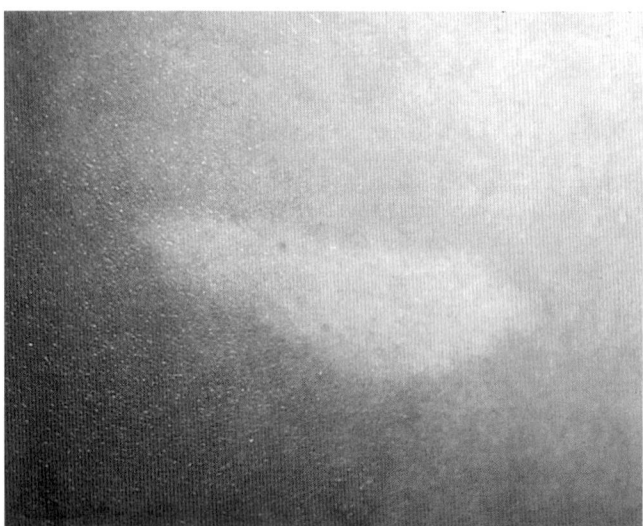

Fig. 30.17   Ash leaf patch: tuberous sclerosis.

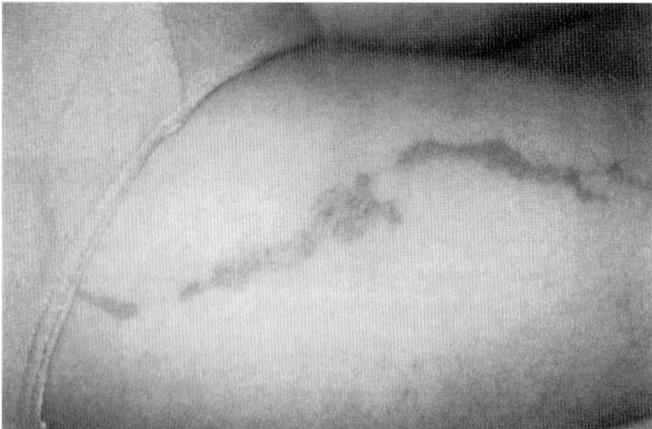

Fig. 30.18   Incontinentia pigmenti: pigmented stage.

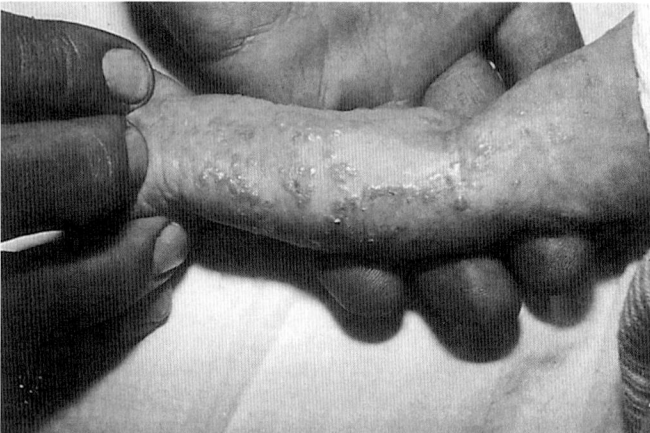

Fig. 30.19   Incontinentia pigmenti: vesicular stage.

rearrangement) in the NEMO gene (Xq28) and lesions probably occur through apoptosis of cells carrying the mutant gene.[29] There is increasing evidence that the 'sporadic type of IP' (IP type 1) represents a distinct disorder, hypomelanosis of Ito (q.v.), linked to Xp11. Neurological abnormalities occur in about 30% of cases and include epilepsy, mental retardation and spastic diplegia and tetraplegia. Ocular abnormalities are seen in 30% and include strabismus, cataracts, retinal vascular proliferation and retinal detachment. Over 80% of patients have dental abnormalities with partial anodontia and peg-shaped or conical teeth. A variety of skeletal abnormalities including limb reduction defects occur, and rarely cardiac abnormalities are seen.

Cutaneous lesions

The four cutaneous stages of this disease may follow each other in an orderly progression; however, overlap may occur, particularly in the earlier stages. Stage one comprises linear groups of vesicles which appear mainly on the limbs at birth or in the first days of life accompanied by a peripheral blood eosinophilia. They clear spontaneously over several weeks. Stage two is the verrucose stage with linear warty lesions appearing between 1 and 4 months of age: they occur particularly on the limbs, especially on dorsa of hands and feet, and resolve spontaneously after

weeks or months. Stage three comprises streaks and whorls and splattered patterns of macular hyperpigmentation which appear on both limbs and trunk at 12–24 months of age. Lesions persist to early adult life. Stage four is typically seen in affected female adults as linear, hypopigmented, atrophic streaks on the lower legs. These lesions are permanent.

Other dermatological features of incontinentia pigmenti are cicatricial alopecia over the vertex of the scalp and nail dystrophy in 40%.

ACRODERMATITIS ENTEROPATHICA AND NUTRITIONAL ZINC DEFICIENCY

Acrodermatitis enteropathica is an autosomal recessive condition in which there is a defective absorption of zinc, possibly due to the absence of a specific carrier protein. An identical condition occurs in infants with nutritional zinc deficiency. This may occur as a result of prematurity with low zinc stores, particularly in bottle-fed babies (as there is a lower bioavailability of zinc in bovine milk as compared to breast milk), or as a result of low breast milk zinc. Zinc deficiency also occurs in acquired immunodeficiency disease, cystic fibrosis and other causes of malabsorption and in infants on parenteral nutrition solutions not containing adequate zinc.

Clinical features

The onset in the primary form occurs usually when the child is weaned or in the first few weeks of life in a bottle-fed infant. In the children with nutritional zinc deficiency the onset is usually at the time of the first growth spurt. Erythematous and crusted, sometimes vesicular and pustular lesions appear in an acral distribution particularly around nose, mouth and eyes (Fig. 30.20) and sometimes on tips of digits and the paronychial areas. An anogenital rash (Fig. 30.21) is also common and psoriasiform

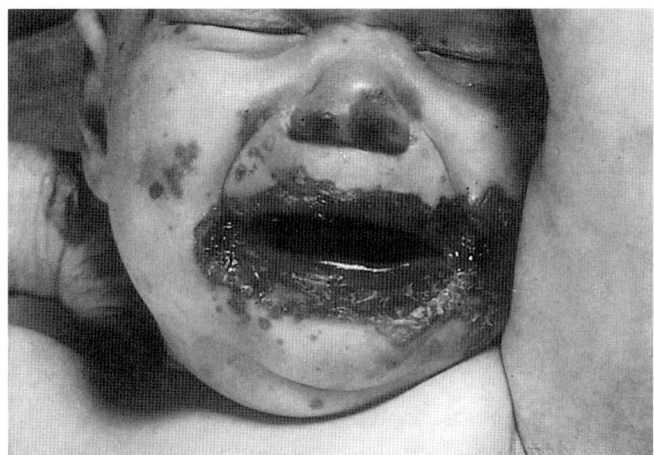

Fig. 30.20 Acrodermatitis enteropathica: mouth.

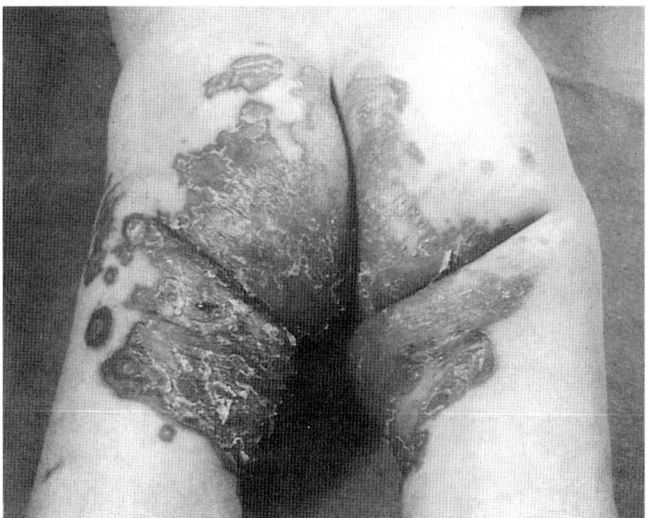

Fig. 30.21 Acrodermatitis enteropathica: buttocks.

lesions may occur on knees and elbows and occasionally elsewhere. Secondary bacterial and candidal infection is common. In the primary form mucosal involvement with glossitis, cheilitis and conjunctivitis may occur, a nail dystrophy is usual, and alopecia and diarrhea may occur.

The diagnosis is confirmed by finding a low serum zinc. The condition responds rapidly to the administration of high doses of oral zinc as either zinc gluconate or zinc sulfate. This is required life-long in the primary form but only for a few weeks in the secondary variety.

NEUROFIBROMATOSIS

Neurofibromatosis is a very variable multisystem disorder which is described in detail in Chapter 22. Only the dermatological features will be considered here.

Pigmented lesions

The café-au-lait macule is the most common of these: most prepubertal individuals with neurofibromatosis have at least six macules of greater than 0.5 cm in diameter increasing to at least 1.5 cm post puberty. Eventually hundreds of macules may be present.

In 20% of cases small freckle-like pigmented macules occur in the axillae. These occur only in the presence of café-au-lait macules and the combination is of great diagnostic significance. Similar small pigmented macules may occur in a widespread distribution, especially in patients with large numbers of café-au-lait spots. Larger pigmented patches 10 cm or more in diameter may overlie plexiform neuromas.

Neurofibromas (mollusca fibrosa)

These are soft pink or skin-colored tumors, often sessile or pedunculated and characteristically indentable. They usually develop after puberty. Their distribution is widespread and up to thousands of tumors half to several centimeters in diameter may occur. Small firmer discrete nodules occur along the course of peripheral nerves. The plexiform neuroma is a larger diffuse elongated neurofibroma along the course of a peripheral nerve. These may be present at birth or develop later. There may be an overgrowth of skin and subcutaneous tissue associated with these lesions producing gross disfigurement as a giant pendulous tumor with a wrinkled surface.

HEREDITARY PHOTOSENSITIVE DISORDERS (Table 30.5)

Photosensitivity is the cardinal feature of most of the porphyrias although some types may present with chronic nonspecific abdominal or musculoskeletal pain.[30] Photosensitivity occurs in other metabolic diseases such as phenylketonuria and Hartnup disease and severe photosensitivity also occurs in oculocutaneous albinism.

SKIN DISEASES OF THE NEONATE

ERYTHEMA TOXICUM NEONATORUM

This is a transient condition of unknown etiology occurring in up to 70% of neonates. The onset is from birth to 14 days but most cases start between day 1 and day 4. The commonest lesions are erythematous macules and papules but in some cases pustules appear. Lesions occur anywhere on the body surface except palms and soles but with a predilection for face and trunk. In cases present at birth, lesions are more acrally distributed and are often pustular. A peripheral blood eosinophilia is present and smears from pustules demonstrate sheets of eosinophils. The condition usually resolves in 2–3 days but, rarely, may persist for several weeks.

Recognition of this entity is important to avoid unnecessary investigations of serious neonatal infections.

TRANSIENT NEONATAL PUSTULAR DERMATOSIS

This is a benign condition in which superficial pustules are present at birth; it is rare for further lesions to develop postnatally. The pustules rupture within 24 h, developing a brown crust that separates after a few days to leave normal skin or a hyperpigmented macule in dark-skinned individuals. Lesions occur mainly on chin, upper anterior trunk, lower back and buttocks. They are asymptomatic and the infant is otherwise well. Lesions are sterile on culture enabling differentiation from important neonatal infections. If hyperpigmented macules occur, they resolve over 3–4 months.

ACROPUSTULOSIS OF INFANCY

This is a benign condition of unknown etiology occurring in otherwise healthy infants. The onset is usually in the neonatal period but may be delayed for some months. Recurrent crops of papules which quickly evolve into 2–4 mm vesicopustules occur, most commonly on the palms and soles and dorsa of hands and feet. Initially each crop takes 1–2 weeks to settle and new crops occur every 2–3 weeks. As time goes on the crops occur less frequently and the episodes are less severe and of shorter duration. Lesions are pruritic and finally resolve by 2–3 years.

The disease must be differentiated from other neonatal pustular conditions including herpes simplex, impetigo, scabies and candidiasis. Cultures of the lesions of infantile acropustulosis are sterile. A clinically identical condition can occur also as a postscabetic reaction in infants who have been successfully treated for scabies.

Topical therapy is usually ineffective. Oral antihistamines can be used if pruritus is severe.

MILIA

These represent retention cysts of the pilosebaceous follicles. They occur in approximately 50% of neonates as firm pearly white 1–2 mm

Table 30.5 Hereditary photosensitivity disorders

	Xeroderma pigmentosa	Bloom syndrome	Cockayne syndrome	Rothmund–Thomson syndrome	Erythropoietic protoporphyria	Congenital erythropoietic porphyria (Gunther disease)
Inheritance	AD	AR	AD	AR	AD	AR
Cutaneous features	Freckling initially, telangiectasia, spider nevi (angioma), subsequently atrophic hypopigmented guttate macules	Reticulate telangiectasia at sun-exposed sites. More than 50% have variable numbers of café-au-lait macules	Scaling and erythema at sun-exposed sites. Subsequently hyperpigmentation and atrophy	Mild photosensitivity only. Poikiloderma of cheeks and hands. Hyperkeratosis of palms and soles in adults	Relatively mild photosensitivity. Burning sensation after exposure to sunlight. Subsequently small scars on nose and cheeks	Severe photosensitivity in infancy. Blistering. Pink urine and brown discoloration of teeth. Hypertrichosis
Other features	Photophobia, conjunctivitis. Short stature, hypogonadism, microcephaly, mental retardation, deafness, ataxia	Dwarfism, hypogammaglobulinemia	Dwarfism. Disproportionately large limbs. Delayed psychomotor development. Optic atrophy, retinal degeneration and progressive deafness	Short stature. Sparse hair, cataracts, hypogonadism	Gallstones and hepatic cirrhosis	
Molecular defect	Defective DNA repair mechanisms	Chromosomal breakage disorder	Pathogenesis unknown	Mutations in RECQL4	Ferrochelatase deficiency	Uroporphyrinogen III synthase deficiency
Malignancy risk	Cutaneous melanoma and non-melanoma skin cancers	Cutaneous squamous cell carcinoma, leukemia, lymphoma, nephroblastoma		Cutaneous squamous cell carcinoma		
Other			Mean age of death 12 years due to renal failure, infections, neurological complications		Diagnosis confirmed by raised erythrocyte protoporphyrin. Beta-carotene may be helpful treatment	Diagnosis confirmed by elevated porphyrins in erythrocytes, urine and feces. Fatal outcome usually by second or third decade due to anemia, hepatic or renal failure. Successful cure following bone marrow/stem cell transplant

AD, autosomal dominant; AR, autosomal recessive.

papules particularly on the face. They usually disappear by 4 weeks of age. Epstein's pearls are epidermal cysts on the palate present in the majority of newborns. Persistent milia may be a marker for certain syndromes including Bazex syndrome, orofaciodigital syndrome type I and Marie–Unna hypotrichosis.

MILIARIA (PRICKLY HEAT)

This is a sweat retention phenomenon common in young infants. Unlike the equivalent condition in older persons it can occur in the absence of fever or significant occlusive factors. An obstruction of unknown etiology occurs within the intraepidermal portion of the eccrine sweat duct with retention of sweat behind the block. Lesions commence as red macules on which are superimposed 2–3 mm papules, vesicles or pustules (Fig. 30.22). Secondary infection can occur but most commonly these pustules are sterile. Characteristically the pattern and severity of the condition alter significantly from day to day enabling differentiation from infantile acne and infective conditions. Lesions occur most commonly on the face but scalp, neck and upper

trunk are other common sites. The condition is also prone to occur under plastic napkins and napkin covers.

Management involves keeping the child as cool as practicable and avoidance of contact with non-porous materials such as nylon and plastic, and of occlusive topical agents. The parents should be reassured that this is a transient condition and is uncommon after 6 months of age.

SUBCUTANEOUS FAT NECROSIS OF THE NEWBORN

This is a necrosis of subcutaneous fat in the newborn probably induced by ischemia. It occurs usually in healthy full-term infants. Often, however, there is a history of a difficult labor and delivery with such complications as prolonged labor, fetal distress, perinatal asphyxia due to meconium aspiration or other cause and forceps delivery. The condition has also been reported in several cases following hypothermic cardiac surgery.

The lesions appear between the second and third weeks of life as non-tender, firm, skin-colored or red–purple nodules or plaques occurring particularly on buttocks, shoulders, upper back, proximal limbs and cheeks. New nodules may develop over several weeks. They usually disappear

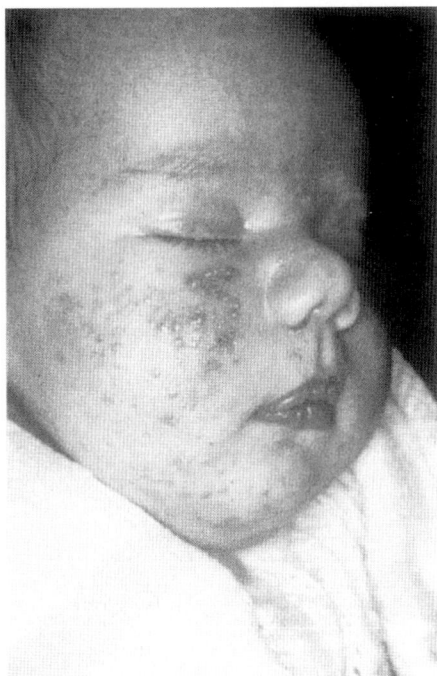

Fig. 30.22   Pustular miliaria (prickly heat).

spontaneously without complication in several months leaving no trace. However, sometimes they become fluctuant, ulcerate or calcify.

Metabolic complications include hypercalcemia, hypoglycemia, thrombocytopenia, anemia and hypertriglyceridemia. Fluctuant lesions should be aspirated, secondary infection should be dealt with if it complicates ulcerated lesions, and serum calcium levels should be monitored, particularly in the presence of calcified lesions, for up to 6 months. Otherwise management involves observation and reassurance.

CUTIS MARMORATA (CONGENITAL LIVEDO RETICULARIS)

This term usually refers to a transient benign physiological vascular reaction occurring in both premature and full-term infants as a response to minor cooling. A blue or purple discoloration in a marbled or reticulate pattern occurs on trunk and limbs. It lasts minutes to hours but reverses quickly on warming the infant. The tendency to the condition lasts for weeks or months.

There are a number of important conditions which may be associated with more severe and persistent cutis marmorata. These include Down syndrome, trisomy 18, homocystinuria, de Lange syndrome, neonatal lupus and congenital hypothyroidism. A nevoid vascular disorder, cutis marmorata telangiectatica congenita (CMTC), presents with reticulate purple lesions but the distribution is often segmental rather than generalized and atrophy and ulceration may occur in the affected areas. Musculoskeletal, neurological and vascular anomalies may be seen with CMTC.[31]

HARLEQUIN COLOR CHANGE

This vascular phenomenon is probably caused by an immature autonomic regulatory mechanism. It does not indicate any significant neural or vascular abnormality. When the neonate lies on one side the lower half of the body is red and the upper half is pale with a clear midline separation. This color change is transient and can be reversed by altering the infant's position. It is rarely seen after the first few days of life.

INFANTILE ACNE

This condition commences at about 3 months of age with lesions particularly on the cheeks. Open comedones predominate but closed comedones,

papules, pustules and even cysts can occur. Deeper lesions may produce significant scarring. Untreated the condition usually lasts 2–3 years. In patients with a strong family history of acne the condition may be more severe and there may be difficult acne at puberty. Hormonal abnormalities are rarely found in these patients and investigation is indicated only in cases which are unusually severe, prolonged or unresponsive to therapy. Most patients with mild acne respond well to topical therapies (benzoyl peroxide, erythromycin or retinoids). Oral antibiotics (erythromycin or trimethoprim) may be required for moderate/severe cases. Isotretinoin has also been successfully used in severe cases.

INFECTIONS AND INFESTATIONS OF THE SKIN

VIRUS INFECTIONS

Herpes simplex

Herpes simplex virus (HSV) infections are extremely common in children, and serological studies confirm that more than 90% of the population have been infected by adulthood (Fig. 30. 23). The commonest type is HSV1, though HSV2 is more important in adulthood, being the cause of genital herpes. Four distinct presentations are recognized in childhood.

Neonatal herpes simplex virus infection

This is a potentially devastating infection usually contracted during delivery from infected vaginal secretions (HSV2) (Fig. 30.24). However, intrauterine and postnatal infection may occur. Approximately 50% of infected infants have skin lesions which are manifested as grouped blisters localized initially on the presenting part, usually the head, with the onset usually between the 4th and 8th days of life. The eruption may

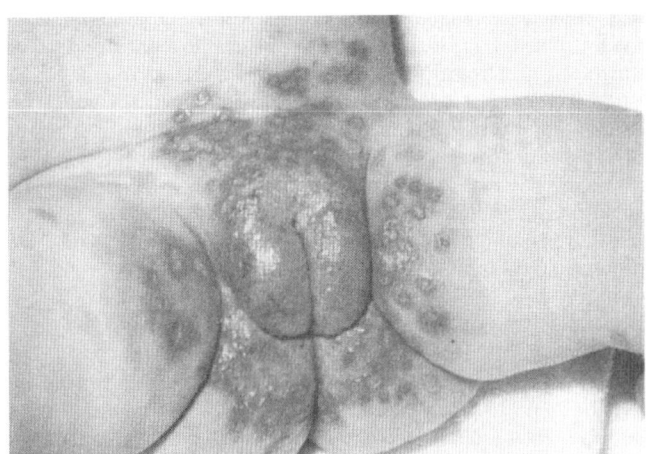

Fig. 30.23   Perineal herpes simplex.

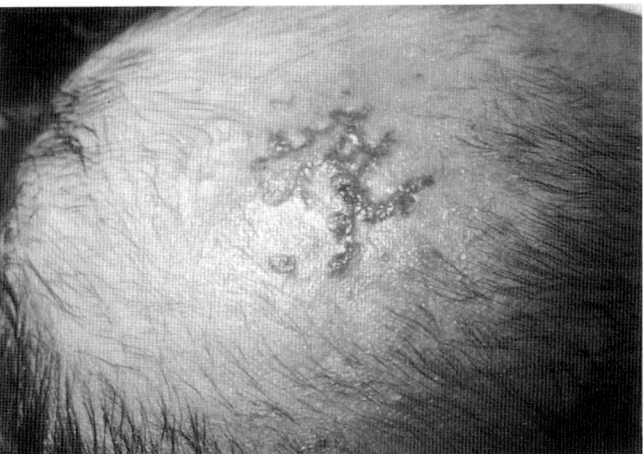

Fig. 30.24   Neonatal herpes on scalp.

become widespread with individual lesions a few millimeters across coalescing to produce large erosions. A rapid immunofluorescence test on material from the blister base enables a diagnosis within a few hours. Culture of the virus takes several days. A rising titer of complement-fixing antibodies can be demonstrated comparing acute and convalescent sera.

The child with cutaneous neonatal herpes should be assessed urgently for the presence and extent of other organ involvement. Immediate treatment with intravenous aciclovir is indicated.

Primary herpetic gingivostomatitis

This is a common presentation of HSV infection in children (Fig. 30.25). The child is systemically unwell with a high fever and there is severe swelling, erosion and bleeding of the gums and the anterior part of the buccal mucosa. Posterior spread is rare but anterior spread to the lips and the facial skin often occurs. There may be considerable soft tissue swelling and prominent lymphadenopathy. The condition is extremely painful and the child often refuses to eat or drink, necessitating parenteral fluids as the condition may take up to 2 weeks to resolve. Oral antibiotics may be required for secondary bacterial infection. Unless the condition is very severe systemic antiviral therapy is not usually required.

Recurrent herpes simplex (herpes labialis)

Recurrent herpes simplex of the face, particularly around the lips (herpes labialis), is common in childhood. As in adults various factors, including fever and sun exposure, may reactivate the virus. Saline bathing of the lesions speeds resolution and prevents secondary infection. Topical antiviral agents are of limited value.

Disseminated herpes simplex (eczema herpeticum)

This occurs as a complication of atopic eczema and in immunosuppressed patients (Fig. 30.26). It may originate from a primary or recurrent infection, or from external reinfection. Spread is both on the surface of the skin and also by hematogenous dissemination. The lesions are vesicles or pustules 2–4 mm across which may spread with alarming rapidity and have a tendency to coalescence to produce extensive punched-out lesions. Topical steroids should be avoided as their application may spread the virus. Secondary bacterial infection should be treated with oral antibiotics. In most cases systemic aciclovir is indicated. Minor recurrences of HSV infection are seen in up to 20% of cases.

Varicella (chickenpox)

Chickenpox (Ch. 28) is caused by the same herpes virus which produces herpes zoster/shingles (the varicella zoster virus). The incubation period is from 9 to 23 days (mean 14–17 days). After a prodrome of 2–3 days a vesicular eruption develops at the sites of erythematous papules. They appear in crops over 2–4 days, initially on the trunk then face and limbs. Vesicles are often seen in the mouth and occasionally affect other

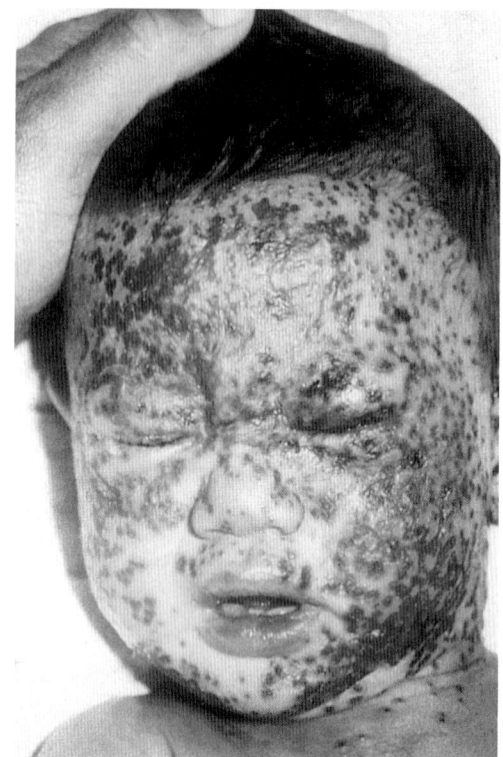

Fig. 30.26   Disseminated herpes simplex (eczema herpeticum).

mucous membranes. Pruritus and pyrexia are variable and resolution takes a little over 2 weeks. Complications (encephalitis, pneumonitis and hepatitis) are rare in otherwise healthy children and routine use of aciclovir is not recommended. A live attenuated vaccine is licensed for prophylactic use in North America.

Herpes zoster

This usually occurs when the virus, which has remained dormant in the cells of dorsal root or cranial nerve ganglia following an attack of chickenpox, reactivates, replicates and spreads along the nerves from these ganglia to infect areas of skin supplied by them (Fig. 30.27). Herpes zoster is much less common in children than in adults but it may occur as early as the first year of life. In children who develop zoster in the first 2 years of life there is rarely a history of previous chickenpox in the child but often a history of maternal chickenpox during pregnancy.

Herpes zoster presents as a segmental blistering eruption on an erythematous base. Usually a single dermatome is affected but spread to

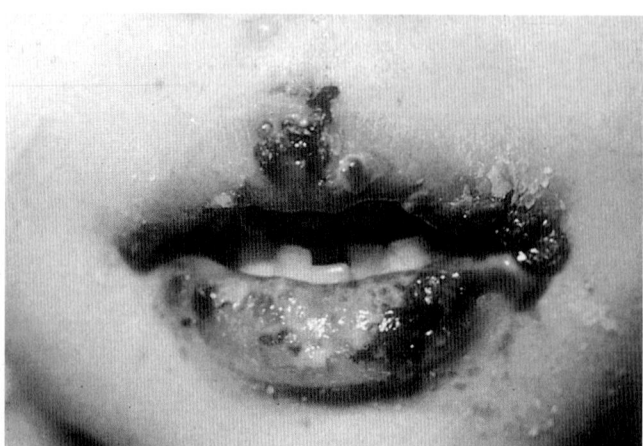

Fig. 30.25   Perioral herpes simplex.

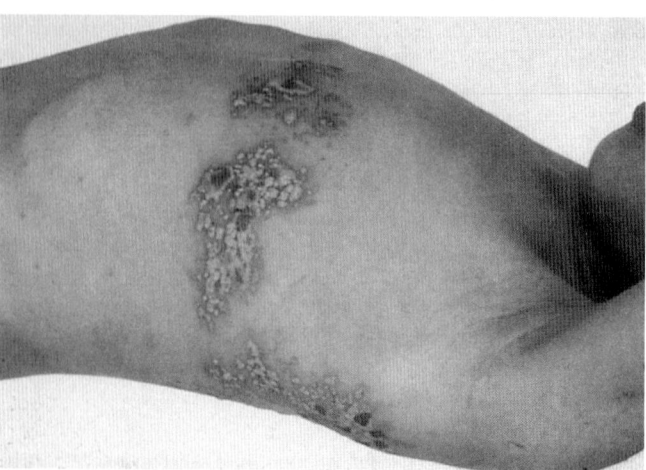

Fig. 30.27   Herpes zoster.

one or two adjoining dermatomes may occur. The eruption is essentially unilateral though there may be minor spread to the opposite side on the trunk or brow. Up to 20 or 30 scattered lesions identical to chickenpox commonly occur. Infection involving the ophthalmic division of the 5th cranial (trigeminal) nerve may produce keratitis and uveitis, threatening vision. An important cutaneous sign of potentially dangerous herpes zoster ophthalmicus is blisters on the nose indicating involvement of the nasociliary branch. Blisters in the oral cavity occur with involvement of maxillary and mandibular divisions of the trigeminal nerve. Anogenital blistering and sometimes disorders of urination and defecation occur with involvement of sacral nerves. Scarring and postherpetic neuralgia are rare complications in children.

Management

This is directed at providing symptomatic treatment with wet compresses and appropriate analgesia, and dealing with any secondary bacterial infection. Early ophthalmological consultation is essential for ophthalmic zoster patients. Intravenous aciclovir is indicated in very severe cases, particularly of ophthalmic zoster and for all immunosuppressed patients.

Molluscum contagiosum

This is a poxvirus infection which is rare under 1 year of age and occurs particularly in the 2–5-year age group (Fig. 30.28). Outbreaks may occur among children who bathe or swim together and in the adolescent age group sexual transmission becomes important. The typical lesion is spherical and pearly white with a central umbilication, but they may vary from tiny 1 mm papules to large nodules over 1 cm in diameter. They occur on any part of the skin surface with common sites being the axillae and sides of the trunk, the lower abdomen and anogenital area. Rarely they occur on the eyelids where they may cause conjunctivitis and punctate keratitis. A secondary eczema often occurs around lesions, particularly in atopics, and scratching of this spreads the mollusca. Hundreds of lesions may be present in an individual patient. Secondary bacterial infection may occur producing crusting, erythema and suppuration. However, these same changes may be seen during spontaneous resolution which occurs in most within 6–9 months leaving normal skin or small varicelliform scars.

Management

With multiple small lesions in a young child spontaneous resolution should be awaited. No controlled trials exist for treatment of mollusca in childhood. However cryotherapy after application of anesthetic cream, topical therapy with salicylic acid, podophyllotoxin, cantharidin and more recently imiquimod or cidofovir have all been reported with variable success. Physical extrusion of the contents of larger lesions can also be undertaken and is usually best after anesthetic cream application. Up

to 10% of cases develop eczema around the lesions which resolves when the mollusca clear. Spontaneous regression may be associated with secondary bacterial infection requiring a topical antibiotic.

Warts

Warts are benign tumors caused by infection with a variety of human papilloma viruses. The common wart (verruca vulgaris) occurs particularly at sites of trauma such as hands, feet, knees and elbows. Plane or flat warts, 1–3 mm pink or brown barely raised papules, occur on the face and often spread along scratch marks or cuts. Plantar warts occur particularly over pressure points on the soles and can be differentiated from calluses by a loss of skin markings over the skin surface. Unlike corns or callosities they tend to be painful on lateral pressure. Warts at mucocutaneous junctions often have a filiform or fronded appearance. Anogenital warts may be acquired from maternal infection during delivery, but their presence should always raise the suspicion of sexual abuse (Fig. 30.29).

Management

Various forms of treatment are available: they depend on the area, the type of wart and the age of the patient. Because spontaneous disappearance is common, aggressive treatment is usually inappropriate. A Cochrane review[32] of local treatments for cutaneous warts shows that there is very little good evidence on which to determine best practice. The best available evidence was for the use of topical salicylic acid preparations. Perhaps surprisingly cryotherapy was not found to be superior. Other currently used topical agents include glutaraldehyde and formaldehyde preparations. Podophyllotoxin is less irritant than podophyllin but both can be used for isolated anogenital warts. Facial plane warts may respond to retinoic acid preparations. Cautery or diathermy is useful for lesions on the lips or anogenital area but elsewhere recurrence is fairly frequent following their use and there is also a risk of producing a painful scar. The initial favorable response to oral cimetidine has not been replicated in double-blind placebo-controlled trials.[33]

Papular acrodermatitis of childhood (Gianotti–Crosti syndrome)

Papular acrodermatitis of childhood was first described by Gianotti as an acrally distributed papular eruption occurring in young children due to the hepatitis B virus (Fig. 30.30). However, a similar eruption may occur with over a dozen different viruses and the condition is best regarded as a reaction pattern with multiple etiologies.[34]

This pattern of exanthem occurs particularly in children between 1 and 4 years of age. The rash comprises discrete firm red papules 1–5 mm in diameter, sometimes surmounted by vesicles. Pruritus is variable but not usually a significant feature. The lesions involve the limbs, particularly distally, and the face, with the trunk being essentially spared. The

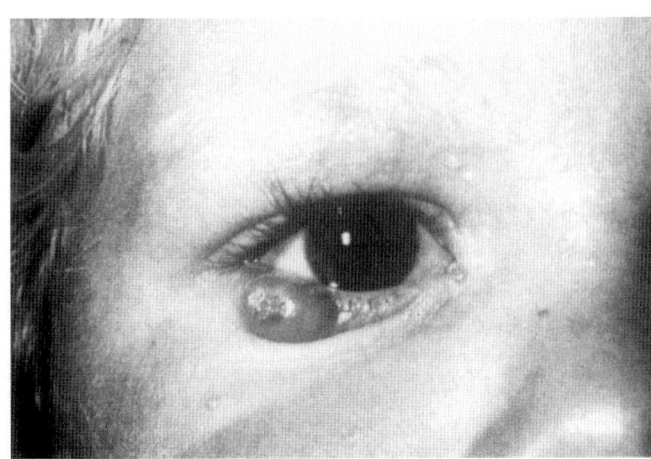

Fig. 30.28 Molluscum contagiosum.

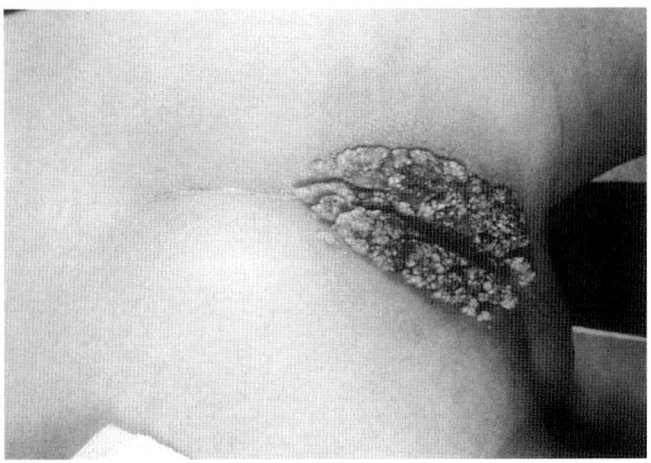

Fig. 30.29 Perianal warts.

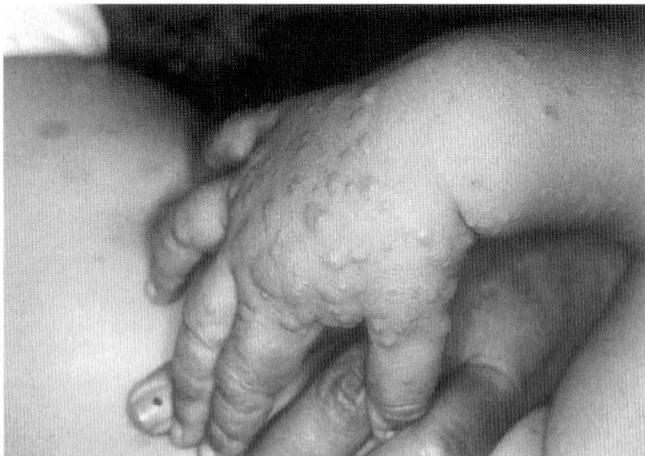

Fig. 30.30   Papular acrodermatitis of childhood.

rash fades within 3–4 weeks. Lymphadenopathy is usually present but the child is often otherwise remarkably well, leading to such misdiagnoses as insect bites and papular eczema.

Investigation should be aimed at excluding the more serious viral etiologies.

Pityriasis rosea

Epidemiological studies suggest a viral origin, now thought to be human herpes virus 7. It occurs in children and young adults and has no sexual or racial predilection (Fig. 30.31).

The eruption commences with the appearance of the so-called herald patch, typically a single round or oval scaly lesion 1–5 cm in diameter, flat or slightly raised with a tendency to clear in the center. It usually occurs on the trunk, neck or proximal limbs. Some 5–15 days later the secondary eruption appears comprising multiple, variably pruritic, dull pink, oval macules with a peripheral collarette of scale. The typical distribution is on trunk and proximal limbs but may be very extensive. The long axis of the lesions on the trunk runs parallel with the ribs giving

a 'Christmas-tree' pattern. Rarer variants have lesions which are papular, urticarial, vesicular, purpuric or pustular but some of the typical lesions are usually intermingled. Lesions crop at 2–3 day intervals for 7–10 days and then spontaneous resolution occurs over several weeks. Sun exposure may speed this resolution and meanwhile symptomatic therapy can be used for the pruritus if this is troublesome.

BACTERIAL INFECTIONS

Staphylococcal and streptococcal infections of the skin are common in childhood. They take the following clinical forms:

Impetigo

This is a bacterial infection caused by *Staphylococcus aureus*, group A beta-hemolytic streptococcus (GABHS) or a combination of these organisms (Fig. 30.32). Recently there has been a worldwide increase in the predominance of staphylococci in the causation of impetigo.[35,36] An increasing proportion of *S. aureus* isolates are resistant to meticillin (MRSA).

Impetigo occurs in two forms, bullous and more commonly non-bullous (or crusted). Bullous impetigo (Fig. 30.33) is always due to staphylococci. Blisters arise on previously normal skin and increase rapidly in size and number, soon rupturing to produce superficial erosions with a peripheral brown crust. The erosions continue to expand, sometimes clearing centrally to produce annular lesions. The condition is usually neither itchy nor painful. Non-bullous impetigo may be due to either organism or to a combination. The lesions begin with a small transient vesicle on an erythematous base. The serum exuding from the ruptured

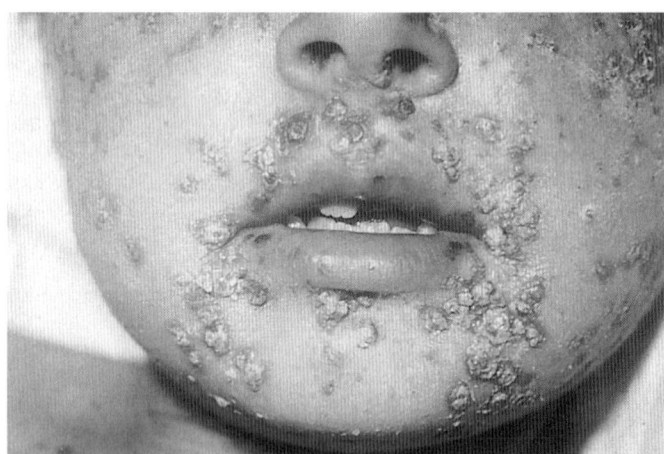

Fig. 30.32   Impetigo.

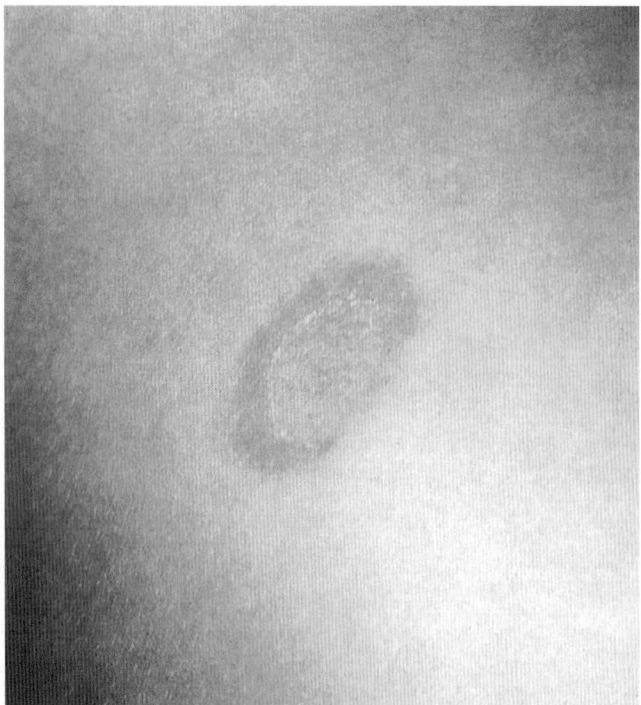

Fig. 30.31   Pityriasis rosea (herald patch).

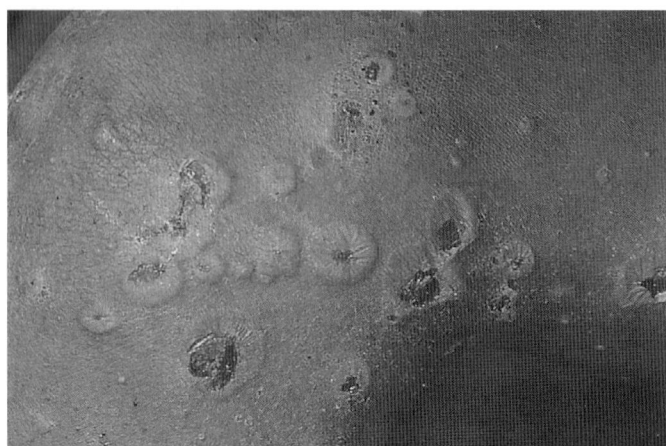

Fig. 30.33   Bullous impetigo.

vesicle produces a thick soft yellow crust, below which there is a moist superficial erosion. The lesions extend slowly and remain much smaller than those of bullous impetigo. Impetigo is often superimposed on other skin diseases such as insect bites, scabies, pediculosis and atopic eczema. As impetigo is an intraepidermal infection, the condition does not scar although postinflammatory pigmentation can occur, particularly in dark-skinned patients.

Management

Impetigo is very contagious and the patient should, if possible, be isolated. A swab for culture and sensitivity testing should always be taken. Topical mupirocin is as successful as oral erythromycin in eradicating both S. aureus and GABHS[37] and a double-blind study has shown hydrogen peroxide cream to be as effective as topical fusidic acid.[38] However, topical therapies will not eradicate bacteria on clinically uninvolved skin and therefore in general oral antibiotics should be used. Because of the rarity in most areas of pure streptococcal impetigo, a penicillinase-resistant penicillin or erythromycin is the treatment of choice while awaiting culture results. In many areas of the world there is an emergence of erythromycin-resistant staphylococci[35,39] and knowledge of the local situation is important in selecting the antibiotic of first choice while awaiting sensitivity testing. Underlying diseases should be sought and treated appropriately if the pattern of impetigo suggests them. If a group A streptococcus is isolated the patient should be watched for 8 weeks for signs of glomerulonephritis.

Folliculitis

Superficial bacterial folliculitis is common in children. It is characterized by inflammation confined to the opening of the hair follicle whereas furuncles or boils are cutaneous abscesses, centered around usually ruptured hair follicles. Both are caused by a wide variety of types and strains of S. aureus and predisposing factors are occlusion (e.g. overuse of very greasy emollients), friction, maceration and sweating. Patients with recurrent attacks are often found to carry the strains of S. aureus in their nose, axillae or perineum, or to be in close contact with another person who is a carrier. Folliculitis commences with perifollicular erythema with pustule formation that often ruptures to form a crust. Pruritus is common. Boils are larger, firm erythematous papules that evolve into fluctuant pus-filled nodules with central necrosis (pointing) and discharge.

Mild folliculitis is often self-limiting but can be treated with topical antiseptics. If the infection is persistent or recurrent, topical or oral antistaphylococcal antibiotics should be given. Swabs should first be taken for culture from affected as well as S. aureus carriage sites. If necessary, other carriers who are in close contact should be identified and treated.

Cellulitis

This is an acute bacterial infection involving the subcutis as well as the dermis. The lesion is erythematous sometimes with a purple or blue hue. It is warm and tender and has a less well-defined edge than erysipelas. Fever and malaise, leukocytosis and lymphadenopathy are usually present. When cellulitis follows a wound or other break in the skin, group A beta-hemolytic streptococcus is the commonest cause. Other organisms involved in cellulitis include *Haemophilus influenzae*, *Streptococcus pneumoniae*, *S. aureus* and *Pseudomonas aeruginosa*. Two special forms are discussed below.

Perianal streptococcal disease

This occurs in children between 1 and 10 years of age (Fig. 30.34). The child may complain of painful defecation or pruritus. Fresh blood is often found on the stool. There is a well-demarcated, very bright red erythema extending out several centimeters from the anus. The anal rim is often macerated and fissured. GABHS is grown from the skin and often also from the patient's throat. The condition may be surprisingly resistant to therapy, recurring after 5–10 days of oral penicillin therapy: an initial course of at least 14 days is advisable. The addition of topical mupirocin may further reduce the risk of recurrence.[40]

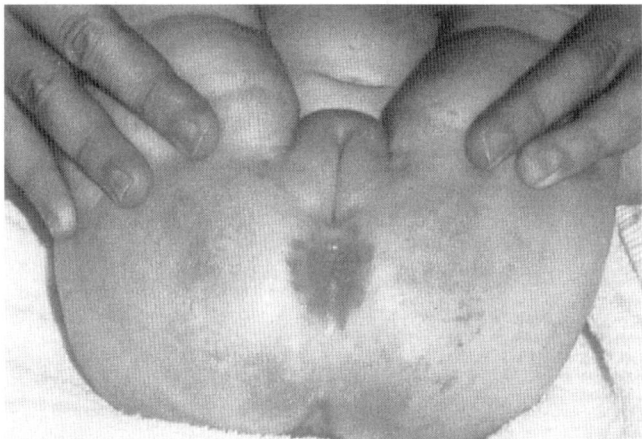

Fig. 30.34 Perianal streptococcal disease.

Facial cellulitis

Facial cellulitis in young children often occurs in the absence of any break in the skin and is due to *H. influenzae* or *S. pneumoniae* accompanying an upper respiratory tract infection or otitis media. Cellulitis due to these bacteria often has a lilac-blue color. The condition may be complicated by bacteremia, septicemia and meningitis. In all cases of facial cellulitis cultures should be taken from nasopharynx, ears, blood and, if indicated, cerebrospinal fluid. Needle aspiration from the lesion after saline injection may provide material from which the organism can be cultured.

Intravenous cefotaxime, a third generation cephalosporin, is the initial treatment of choice until an organism is identified and sensitivity tests performed.

Erysipelas

This is an acute bacterial infection of the dermal connective tissue and superficial lymphatics caused most often by GABHS but occasionally due to other streptococci, *H. influenzae* and *S. aureus*. A brightly erythematous, hot, tender area with a rapidly spreading distinct edge develops. Superimposed bullae may occur. There is accompanying fever and malaise and a leukocytosis. Predisposing factors include lymphatic obstruction and a break in the skin due, for example, to a wound, bite or tinea infection. The episode produces a lymphangitis which further damages the lymphatics, and chronic lymphedema may result from and further predispose to recurrent erysipelas. Treatment involves rest and high doses of the appropriate antibiotic, usually phenoxymethylpenicillin (penicillin V), orally or intravenously depending on the severity.

Staphylococcal scalded skin syndrome
Pathogenesis

The staphylococcal scalded skin syndrome (SSSS) is a widespread blistering disease caused by an epidermolytic toxin produced by certain strains of *S. aureus*, most often of phage group II, but occasionally phage group I or III (Figs 30.35 and 30.36). This toxin produces a superficial splitting of the skin with the level of split being high in the epidermis. Clinical disease occurs when there is sufficient toxin load produced from an infection with these organisms. The commonest sites of infection are the umbilicus (in neonates), the nose, nasopharynx or throat, the conjunctiva and deep wounds.

The condition commences with a macular erythema initially on the face and in the major flexures and then becoming generalized. The skin is exquisitely tender and the child draws back from contact. After 2 days flaccid bullae develop and the skin wrinkles and shears off. The exfoliation is most marked in the groin, neck fold and around the mouth and may involve the entire body surface but mucosae remain uninvolved. The child is usually febrile but because of the superficial level of the split fluid loss is rarely significant. The erosions crust and dry and heal with desquamation over the next 4–8 days leaving no sequelae.

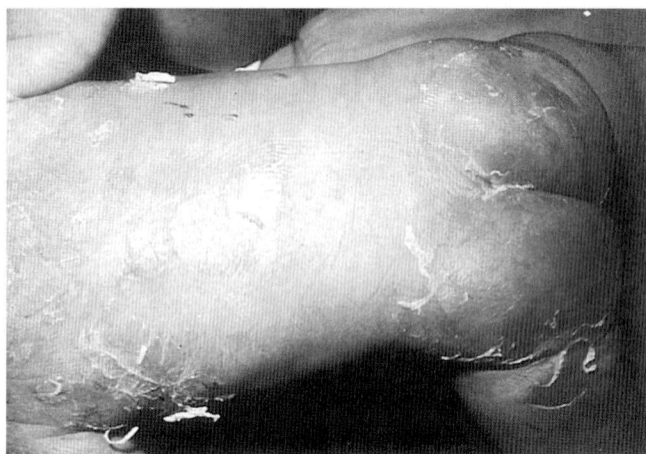

Fig. 30.35 Staphylococcal scalded skin syndrome.

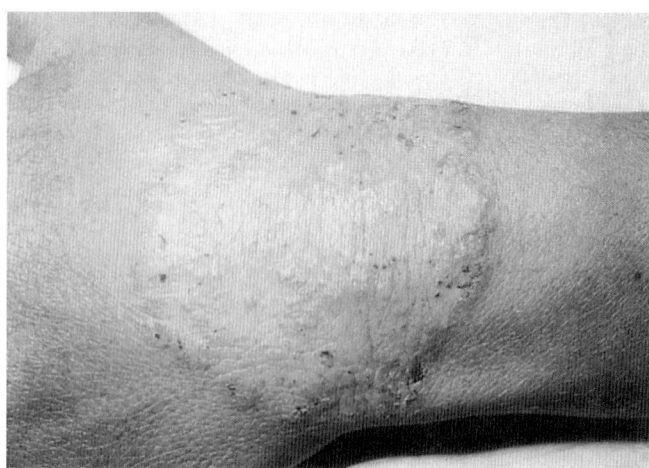

Fig. 30.37   Tinea.

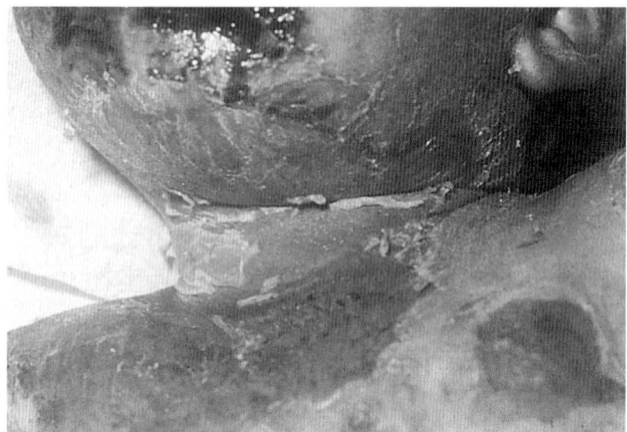

Fig. 30.36 Staphylococcal scalded skin syndrome.

Diagnosis

Cultures from skin and blister fluid are usually negative. Cultures should be obtained from any area of obvious infection but, if none is apparent, from nasopharynx and throat. The most important differential diagnosis is toxic epidermal necrolysis (TEN). In TEN the split is subepidermal and the blisters and erosions are usually hemorrhagic and mucosae are commonly involved. Microscopy of frozen or Giemsa-stained sections of the blister roof can detect the level of the split in the two conditions. Other conditions from which SSSS must be differentiated are scarlet fever, Kawasaki syndrome and toxic shock syndrome, all of which show mucosal involvement and rarely demonstrate frank blistering.

Management

The child should be nursed with as little handling as possible. No topical agents should be applied. A penicillinase-resistant penicillin is the treatment of choice and should be given orally if possible. Insertion and securing of an intravenous line is very painful in these patients and should be performed only if oral antibiotics are refused or if rehydration is required in a child refusing oral fluids. Analgesia is often necessary in the early stages. Emollients are useful once the skin dries and desquamation commences.

FUNGAL INFECTIONS

Tinea

This is an infection due to dermatophyte fungi: the source of the fungus is an animal (e.g. dog, cat, guinea pig, cattle), the soil or another human (Fig. 30.37). Tinea occurs on any part of the skin surface and can involve hair and nails.

The classical features of tinea on the skin are itch, erythema studded with papules or pustules, annular or geographical lesions ('ringworm') with a tendency to central clearing and a superficial scale. Family members or pets are the usual source of infection. On the palms and soles erythema and increased skin markings may be the only signs. Between the toes maceration with a thick white scale is the main finding and an annular lesion may extend onto the dorsum of the foot. On the soles there are deep seated blisters or pustules which dry to produce brown crusts. Tinea is often unilateral and always asymmetrical, whereas eczema and psoriasis, which it may resemble, are often symmetrical in distribution. Nail tinea (onychomycosis) is uncommon in children but increases with age.

In the UK the principal dermatophytes causing tinea capitis are *Microsporum canis* and *Trichophyton tonsurans*. Both cause a combination of alopecia and inflammation with the hair loss being due to breakage of hair shafts. The inflammation varies from mild erythema and a fine dandruff-like scale to a pustular carbuncle-like lesion (kerion), which occurs most commonly with *Trichophyton* species. Other causes of alopecia to be differentiated from tinea are trichotillomania (q.v.) and alopecia areata (q.v). Bright green fluorescence is seen under Wood's (ultraviolet) light in *Microsporum* infection of the scalp. Other varieties of scalp tinea produce no typical fluorescence and the Wood's light has no place in the diagnosis of tinea on the skin surface. The diagnosis of tinea is confirmed by plucking hairs or scraping scales. The fungus can be cultured on appropriate media.

Topical antifungals may be satisfactory for small localized patches of tinea on the skin. Griseofulvin is the only antifungal licensed for oral treatment in children. It is effective against dermatophytes but in general a 3 month course is used with longer courses for nail tinea. Terbinafine is not yet licensed for children but a number of published studies have shown it to be safe and effective for tinea capitis.[41]

Candidiasis (moniliasis)

This is due to a yeast, *Candida albicans*. It occurs on both skin and mucosal surfaces and certain factors predispose to its establishment (Fig. 30.38). General predisposing factors in children include drug therapy with broad spectrum antibiotics, corticosteroids and immunosuppressives, diabetes and any disease which interferes with immunological competence. Local predisposing factors are particularly those which create a warm moist environment. Flexural areas are susceptible, especially in the presence of sweating, obesity and other skin disease. The oral mucosa in infancy also has a particular susceptibility to this infection which is usually acquired during passage through an infected birth canal.

On the general body skin, where candidiasis rarely occurs except in the presence of immunodeficiency, the infection is manifested by small round erythematous lesions with a peripheral overhanging scale.

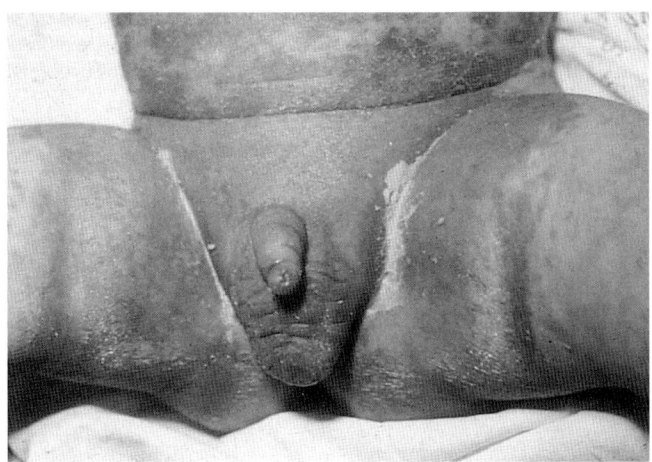

Fig. 30.38 Candidiasis.

Occasionally small papules or superficial pustules occur, especially in the neonate. In flexural areas the typical picture is of a cheesy white material deep in the folds and satellite lesions with the typical peripheral scale. On mucosae a curd-like white material is superimposed on a red base. Acute or chronic paronychia may be seen, particularly in children that suck their fingers.

Chronic mucocutaneous candidiasis is a progressive candidal infection occurring in patients who have an inability to destroy candida due to a severe general immunodeficiency or due to a specific immunological defect. A variety of endocrinopathies may be associated with this syndrome.

The diagnosis of candidiasis is usually a clinical one which may be confirmed by microscopy and culture. Candida is frequently a secondary invader rather than a primary cause of skin disease and local and general predisposing factors should be eliminated. Once predisposing factors have been eliminated most localized infections respond well to topical agents including polyene antibiotics, nystatin and imidazole derivatives. Reduction of intestinal carriage with oral preparations is rarely necessary. Oral ketoconazole is useful in chronic mucocutaneous candidiasis and other candidal infections in the immunosuppressed.

Pityriasis versicolor

This is an infection with *Malassezia* yeasts (*Pityrosporum* species) which are part of the normal skin flora. It occurs mainly in tropical and temperate zones and usually affects adolescents and young adults. It presents as well-demarcated, asymptomatic or slightly itchy macules with a fine branny scale which is often only obvious on light scratching of the lesions. Primary macules 1–10 mm in diameter coalesce into larger patches. They occur in two colors, red–brown especially in the fair skinned and hypopigmented in darker skinned. In a partially tanned individual, lesions of both colors may be found. In young children, unlike adults, approximately 30% present with only facial lesions.[42]

Diagnosis is confirmed by microscopic examination of skin scrapings to which 20% potassium hydroxide has been added. Grape-like clusters of spores and short fragments of thick mycelia are seen. In its hypopigmented forms the condition must be distinguished from: (a) vitiligo, where the depigmentation is total and scale absent; (b) pityriasis alba, where lesions are less well demarcated and some erythema may be seen; and (c) tuberculoid leprosy which is accompanied by anesthesia in the hypopigmented areas. The red-brown form has to be differentiated from seborrheic dermatitis, tinea and psoriasis, all of which lack the very fine branny type of scale.

Untreated the condition is persistent though some improvement may occur in winter. Various treatments are available. The treatment of choice is with topical imidazole creams. Alternatively two overnight applications of 2.5% selenium sulfide may be effective in the short term

but relapse is frequent. With the depigmented form, whatever therapy is used, sun exposure is required for full repigmentation.

ECTOPARASITIC INFESTATIONS

Scabies

This is due to *Sarcoptes scabei*, an eight-legged, oval-shaped mite less than 0.5 mm in length. The disease is transmitted by close physical contact.

A small number of mites burrow into the skin in certain sites, particularly between the fingers, the ulnar border of the hand, around the wrists and elbows, the anterior axillary fold, nipples and penis and, in infants, the palms and soles. The pathognomonic primary lesion, a typical burrow, is a 2–3 mm long curved gray line with a vesicle at the anterior end. Other lesions which mark the sites of burrows are small blisters or papules, larger blisters on the palms and soles of infants, scratch marks, secondary eczema and secondary bacterial infection. Eczema or impetigo in the target areas for scabies should always raise suspicion of this disease as should blisters on the palms and soles of infants.

Often more prominent than the evidence of burrows is the so-called secondary eruption of scabies. This presents as multiple, very pruritic, urticarial papules which are soon excoriated (Fig. 30.39). They occur particularly on the abdomen, thighs and buttocks. Young children may show a striking dermographism in the areas of scratch marks. When dermographism occurs in the first year of life scabies should always be suspected. Large inflammatory nodules may form part of the secondary eruption, occurring particularly on covered areas especially axillae, scrotum, penis and buttocks. They may, however, be very widespread producing diagnostic difficulties. They may persist for months after effective scabies treatment.

The diagnosis of scabies is usually a clinical one but can be confirmed by demonstration of the mite. A burrow is scraped and the material smeared on a slide with potassium hydroxide for microscopic examination. Burrows may be more easily identified by rubbing a thick black marking pen over suspicious areas and wiping with an alcohol swab leaving a burrow outlined with ink.

Management

The patient and all close contacts should be treated simultaneously. The treatment of choice is 5% permethrin cream[43,44]: it should be applied to

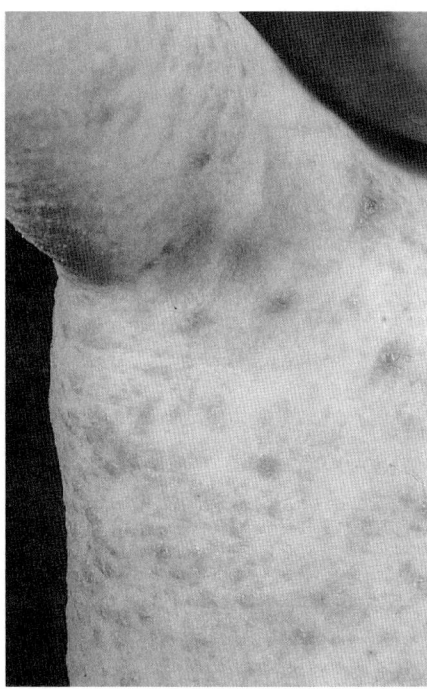

Fig. 30.39 Scabies.

all body surfaces from the neck down and left on overnight. A repeat application should be administered after 1 week. Bedclothes and clothing should be washed in the normal way. An irritant dermatitis may follow scabies treatment, particularly in atopics, and may require emollients and topical steroids once the miticide therapy is fully completed. Persistent nodules may respond to topical corticosteroids and families should be warned that it can take up to 3–4 weeks before the pruritus subsides.

Pediculosis (lice)

Human lice are ectoparasites dependent on man for survival. They are wingless six-legged insects, gray – white in color or red – brown when engorged with blood. The head louse (*Pediculus humanus capitis*) and the body louse (*Pediculus humanus humanus*) have a 24 mm long slim body and three similar pairs of legs. The pubic louse (*Pthirus pubis*, crab louse) has a wider, shorter body 12 mm long and the second and third pairs of legs are larger than the first, producing a crab-like appearance. The nits or ova are seen as oval gray – white 0.5 mm specks firmly attached by a chitinous ring to hairs or clothing.

Pediculosis capitis

This is a very common infection, occurring in epidemics amongst schoolchildren. The infestation is most severe in and may be confined to the occipital area. It is very itchy and excoriations are seen but secondary eczematization and bacterial infection may mask the condition. Nits may be differentiated from epidermal scales and hair casts by their firm attachment and by fluorescence with a Wood's light. Occasionally the head louse infects the eyelashes in children (Fig. 30.40).

Pediculosis corporis

This is rare in children except in conditions of overcrowding and poor hygiene. The louse infects bedding and seams of clothing and nits are not found on the human. With body warmth the pediculi hatch and puncture the skin to produce small urticarial papules with hemorrhagic puncta. Pruritus is extreme and scratch marks are the main clinical sign.

Pediculosis pubis

The pubic hairs are the normal habitat of *Pthirus pubis* but it may also infect facial hair, eyelashes, general body hair and rarely the frontal margin of the scalp. Pubic infestation is usually sexually transmitted but bedding and towels may be responsible. Clinical signs may be minimal, even with severe itching, but excoriated papules and flat blue macules containing altered blood pigment may be seen as may evidence of secondary infection or eczematization. Eyelash infestation in children may occur from innocent close contact with an infected adult but the possibility of sexual abuse must always be considered.

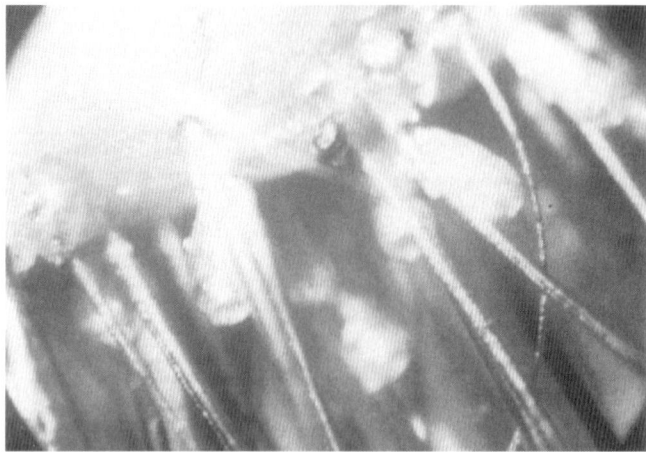

Fig. 30.40   Pediculosis of eyelid.

Management of pediculosis

The management of pediculosis corporis involves removing the infestation from clothing with hot water laundering, hot electric drying, hot ironing or dry cleaning.

Permethrin shampoo is an effective pediculocide for scalp infestations but the efficacy as an ovicide is less certain and repeat application after a few days is recommended. Removal of nits with a fine comb can be facilitated by prior wrapping of the scalp for 1–2 h in a towel soaked in vinegar which softens the chitin.

Pediculosis pubis is treated with 5% permethrin cream applied for 12 h to all hairy areas in the anogenital region, repeated after 1 week. Sexual contacts should be treated simultaneously and all underclothing appropriately laundered.

Pediculosis of eyelashes is best treated with petroleum jelly applied thickly twice a day for a week.

URTICARIA AND ERYTHEMAS

URTICARIA

The most characteristic feature of urticaria (nettle rash or hives) is its transience. Erythematous swellings develop in the skin and last for a few hours before disappearing. The urticarial wheals may be of variable size and may have an obvious annular configuration. Angioedema (giant urticaria) is a variant of urticaria which affects the face and genital region and mainly involves the subcutaneous tissues with resultant gross swelling of the tissues.

Urticaria is common in all age groups, and is particularly so in children. In children, widespread urticaria is often the presenting feature of a number of viral infections, when it is accompanied by fever and malaise. It is due to increased permeability of capillaries or other small vessels, with resultant transudation of fluid. Several chemical mediators are involved, which are mainly released from mast cells: these include histamine, prostaglandins and leukotrienes. Mast cell degranulation results from both immune (IgE, complement) and non-immune mechanisms.

IgE-mediated urticaria and angioedema

Urticaria and angioedema following ingestion of food allergens is quite common in children with atopic eczema and is often IgE mediated (confirmed by positive skin prick tests or radioallergosorbent tests). Swelling of the lips and tongue develops immediately after ingestion of the food, and contact urticaria may be seen if the food is in contact with the skin. If enough food allergen is ingested vomiting and diarrhea may occur, and the child may develop an asthmatic attack: generalized anaphylaxis may occur in a few children, especially with nuts. Widespread urticaria is common, usually occurring within 1 h of ingestion of the food, which may last for a few hours. Common foods involved in such reactions include hens' eggs, cows' milk, fish, nuts and soya. Food allergy is commonly outgrown by the age of 5 years although this is less likely for peanut and nut allergy.[45] IgE-mediated urticaria may also follow drug administration, particularly penicillin, and also insect stings, for example by bees or wasps.

Urticaria due to foods and drugs which is not apparently immunologically mediated

Certain foods such as strawberries, tomatoes and chocolate cause urticaria where no IgE-mediated mechanisms can be demonstrated. It seems likely that this is a direct effect on mast cells and is similar to that caused by tartrazine (a common coloring in foods), benzoates and salicylates. Aspirin and morphine also commonly cause urticaria by a non-immunological mechanism.

Chronic idiopathic urticaria

This type of urticaria is not very common in children. The urticaria may recur repeatedly for a period of years, with often daily exacerbations. It is now recognized that approximately one third of patients with chronic idiopathic urticaria have circulating histamine-releasing autoantibodies directed against the high affinity IgE receptor or less commonly against IgE.[46] The detection of these antibodies, however, is available in only a small number of research laboratories.

Papular urticaria

This is very common in children and results from insect, flea or mite bites. In Britain dog, cat and bird fleas are the usual cause, but human fleas, bed bugs, mosquitoes and dog lice may be implicated. The child presents with papules and blisters on exposed skin such as the legs and arms. Each lasts for about 7–10 days before resolving.

It often takes the parents quite a lot of convincing of the cause of the condition. The family pet should be inspected and treated if necessary.

Treatment of urticaria

The management of a child with urticaria depends on the cause. If a food is implicated, this is usually fairly obvious, except perhaps in infants where skin prick testing may be helpful. Any food implicated should be withdrawn from the diet, though it may be possible to reintroduce it when the child is older. In chronic idiopathic urticaria, by definition no cause is found but certain ingested chemicals in foods (e.g. salicylates, benzoates, food colorings) may make it worse. A non-sedating H1 antihistamine can be given.

MASTOCYTOSIS

This refers to a group of conditions whose signs and symptoms are due to the infiltration of tissues by mast cells and to the release of the chemical mediators contained in these cells. Local effects include erythema and swelling of lesions on rubbing (Darier's sign), dermographism, pruritus, hemorrhage and blistering. General effects include generalized pruritus, fever and flushing; tachycardia and hypotension; headache and irritability; vomiting, diarrhea, increased salivation and peptic ulceration; rhinorrhea and bronchospasm; increased lacrimation; and a generalized hemorrhagic diathesis.

Approximately 65% of patients with mastocytosis present in childhood. A retrospective review of 173 pediatric cases confirms that mastocytomas and urticaria pigmentosa are the commonest presentations in this age group.[47]

Mastocytoma

A round to oval flesh-colored to yellowish nodule or plaque usually presents at birth or appears in the first months of life (Fig. 30.41). Although it is usually solitary, some children develop a number of mastocytomas, particularly on arms or trunk. They usually regress spontaneously over a few years but while present they urticate on rubbing, and blisters, which may be hemorrhagic, often occur in infancy. These children commonly have attacks of generalized flushing but other symptoms and signs of mediator release are rare.

Urticaria pigmentosa

Pigmented multiple macules, with occasional papules, nodules or plaques, occur in a widespread distribution, particularly involving the trunk (Fig. 30.42). Urticaria pigmentosa is the most common form of mastocytosis with an onset usually between 1 and 9 months of age. The lesions erupt over 1–2 months, then become static and finally in most cases resolve by adolescence. They may be pruritic and individual lesions can urticate (Darier's sign) and occasionally blister. There may be dermographism in nearby clinically normal skin. Generalized pruritus and flushing may occur, and less frequently other signs of mediator release.

Diffuse cutaneous mastocytosis

This is a rare form of mastocytosis with the onset usually at birth. Massive mast cell infiltration into the skin produces a diffuse thickening with associated edema, erythema and blistering. The skin may have a leathergrain or peau d'orange appearance or be nodular or verrucose. The color is yellowish or red. Blistering is prominent and may be so severe that the presentation is that of a generalized bullous disease. The full spectrum of local and systemic symptoms and signs of mediator release may be seen. These are usually severe and disabling and may be life threatening. The cutaneous lesions tend to improve with time but some degree of infiltration usually remains.

Systemic mastocytosis

This is defined by infiltration of mast cells into organs other than the skin, and not simply systemic features due to the release of mediators from cutaneous mast cell infiltrates. It is extremely rare in childhood and is almost always associated with diffuse cutaneous involvement in this age group. Hepatosplenomegaly and lymphadenopathy may occur; the cells may infiltrate renal parenchyma and gastrointestinal mucosa; skeletal involvement produces both osteoporotic and osteosclerotic lesions. Mast cell leukemia is a very rare complication.

Management

In general, mastocytosis is a self-limiting disease. If an isolated lesion is producing generalized flushing, excision can be considered. The patient should carry a list of agents (i.e. aspirin, morphine, codeine, d-tubocurarine, scopolamine, quinine, thiamin, procaine, polymixin B, amphotericin B,

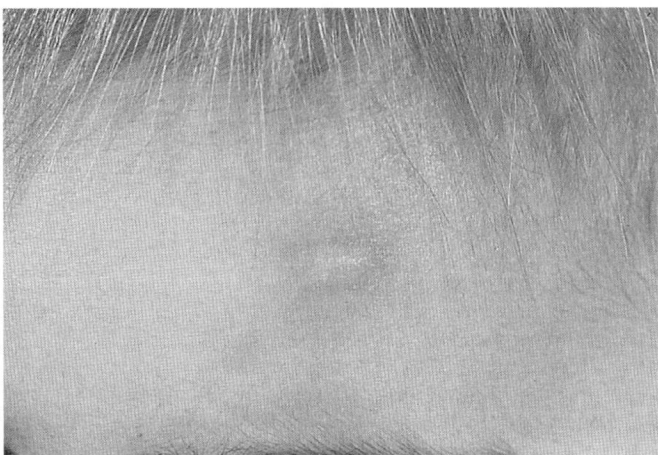

Fig. 30.41 Mastocytoma.

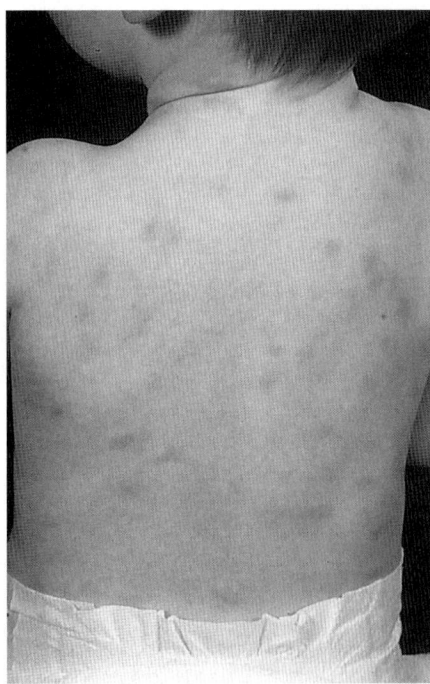

Fig. 30.42 Urticaria pigmentosa.

nonsteroidal anti-inflammatory drugs, and radiographic contrast media) which stimulate mast cell degranulation and avoid these where possible. Physical trauma to the lesions should be avoided.

H1 antihistamines are rarely effective in controlling symptoms and signs of mediator release but combined with H2 blockers they may be more effective. In more severe cases oral disodium cromoglicate, ketotifen and nifedipine may be tried.

A greater understanding of the underlying molecular abnormalities in the systemic mastocytoses is allowing patients to benefit from more specific therapy, for example 'kit-targeting' tyrosine kinase inhibitors.

ERYTHEMA MULTIFORME

This is an uncommon condition in children which tends to follow herpes simplex infection, mycoplasma pneumonia and sulfonamide ingestion (Figs 30.43 and 30.44). Clinically, it is characterized by the formation of circular target lesions on the limbs, with a red periphery and blue (often bullous) center. Stomatitis and genital involvement are common. The rash of erythema multiforme, unlike urticaria, for which it is often mistaken, is fixed with lesions lasting days as compared to hours in urticaria. The lesions may be widespread, and if extensive erosions are present at two or more mucosal sites the diagnosis of Stevens–Johnson syndrome (SJS) can be made. SJS in turn overlaps both clinically and histologically with toxic epidermal necrolysis. The rash of erythema multiforme usually fades within 10 days but may recur, particularly in the case of erythema multiforme following recurrent herpes simplex infections. No randomized controlled trials have been performed for treatment of childhood erythema multiforme and there is therefore no evidence to

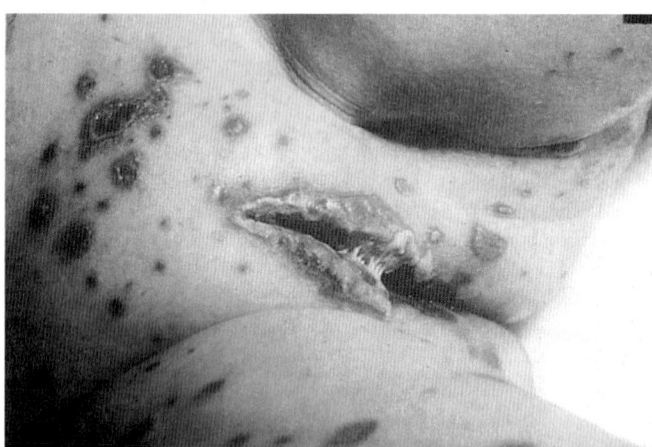

Fig. 30.43   Erythema multiforme, Stevens–Johnson: perineal.

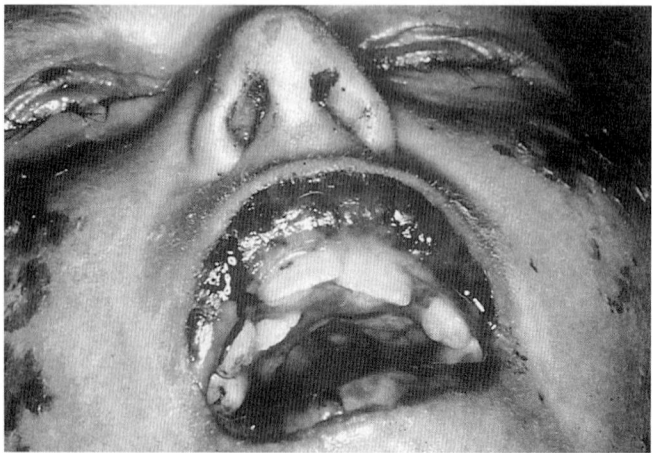

Fig. 30.44   Erythema multiforme, Stevens–Johnson: oral.

recommend oral steroids. However, one double-blind placebo-controlled study in adults found benefit with continuous aciclovir in recurrent erythema multiforme.[48]

VESICOBULLOUS DISORDERS

DERMATITIS HERPETIFORMIS

Dermatitis herpetiformis is associated with gluten-sensitive enteropathy (celiac disease), and in a study of 57 children only 3 (5%) had normal jejunal biopsies.[49] Deposition of IgA in the dermal papillae of skin is the hallmark of the disorder.

It is rare before the age of 2 years, and presents with small intensely itchy blisters symmetrically on the elbows, knees, shoulders and buttocks. The correct treatment is a gluten-free diet, when the blisters, and small bowel mucosa, should resolve (permanently) within 2 years: concomitant treatment with dapsone or sulfapyridine is usually required.

BULLOUS PEMPHIGOID

This rare blistering disease results from the formation of IgG antibodies to the basement membrane zone of the epidermis. The child presents with large and widespread blisters, which may (as in chronic bullous disease of childhood) be most marked on the face and around the genitalia. The hands and feet are more frequently involved in children 1 year or younger compared to older age groups. The diagnosis is confirmed by immunofluorescence of skin biopsy or serum (with appropriate substrate) to demonstrate anti basement membrane zone antibodies. Treatment is with oral steroids, which should be tapered off as the condition allows. In most the disease is self-limiting.

PEMPHIGUS

Pemphigus is also rare in children, the most common types being pemphigus vulgaris and foliaceus. The blistering is less evident than in pemphigoid, though there may be widespread plaques and erosions. Over 50% of children with pemphigus vulgaris present with erosive stomatitis. The diagnosis is confirmed by immunofluorescence studies of skin and serum, which demonstrate IgG antibodies to the intercellular substance of the keratinocytes in the epidermis. Treatment is with oral steroids, as in pemphigoid.

CHRONIC BULLOUS DISEASE OF CHILDHOOD

It is most commonly seen in young children, with blistering around the mouth, neck and genital regions (Fig. 30.45). Genital blistering may be mistaken for herpes simplex infection. Immunofluorescence studies of skin show linear IgA deposition along the basement membrane zone of the epidermis with evidence of circulating IgA antibodies in up to 80%.

Treatment with dapsone or sulfonamides usually clears the blisters very effectively. The disease is self-limiting, after months or years.

VASCULITIS

Vasculitis can be classified according to the size and nature of the vessel and the infiltrate.[50]

HENOCH–SCHÖNLEIN PURPURA

This is a distinct subset within the spectrum of leukocytoclastic (allergic) vasculitis that is relatively common in children (Fig. 30.46). The damage occurs to small blood vessels in the dermis, resulting in the development of purpura (often palpable) over the lower limbs, buttocks and forearms. Other organs involved in the vasculitis are the kidneys and intestinal vessels, resulting in proteinuria and hematuria, abdominal pain and gastrointestinal hemorrhage. In some arthralgia is also

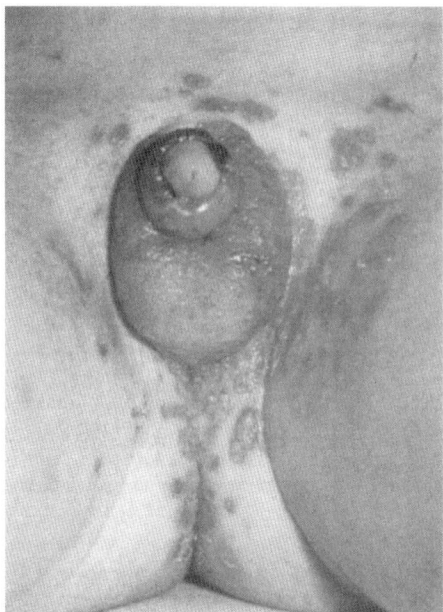

Fig. 30.45 Chronic bullous disease of childhood.

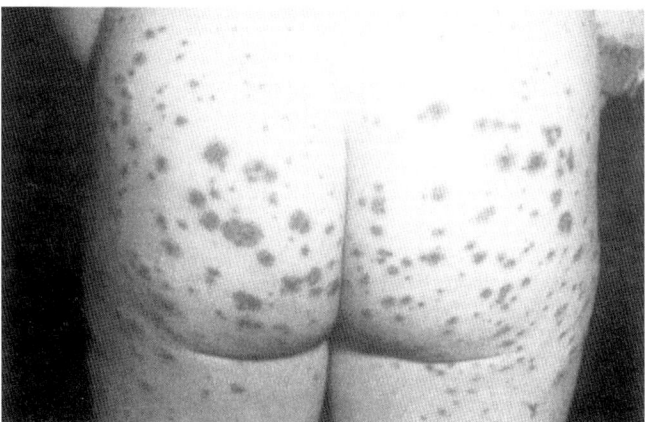

Fig. 30.46 Henoch–Schönlein purpura.

prominent. It usually follows a virus or respiratory infection, the vasculitis resulting from deposition of immune complexes in the vessels of the skin, kidneys and intestines, with complement activation and resultant polymorph infiltration. In Henoch–Schönlein purpura the immunoglobulin deposited is IgA, whereas in other types of vasculitis it is IgG.

The prognosis is very variable. In most children the condition is self-limiting; others may develop renal failure (usually treatable with dialysis or renal transplant) or may die of gastrointestinal hemorrhage.

URTICARIAL VASCULITIS

This is another variant of allergic vasculitis. The urticarial wheals last for several days, unlike those in 'classical' urticaria, where they last for a few hours. Urticarial vasculitis is often accompanied by arthralgia, and skin lesions may resolve with purpura. A skin biopsy shows leukocytoclastic vasculitis, and complement studies may reveal low CH50 and C3 levels. It may result from drug ingestion or viral infection, or may be a feature of lupus erythematosus.

ERYTHEMA NODOSUM

This is rare in young children. It is a type of vasculitis affecting initially deep, dermal venules with subsequent development of a septal panniculitis.

Clinically, erythematous nodules develop, usually on the shins though sometimes on the thighs and forearms. They last for about 2–3 weeks and are characteristically tender. They resolve leaving bruising, but then tend to recur in crops. Causes include streptococcal infections, sarcoidosis, tuberculosis and sulfonamide ingestion: often it occurs without obvious reason. Treatment is of the underlying cause. Usually it resolves spontaneously, but occasionally treatment with oral steroids is indicated.

ECZEMA, DERMATITIS AND PSORIASIS

Eczema and dermatitis are synonymous and are often used interchangeably. Eczema/dermatitis can be subdivided into atopic and non-atopic eczema, contact dermatitis (allergic and irritant) and other types (e.g. discoid, seborrheic, photosensitive).[51]

ATOPIC ECZEMA

Atopy is a genetically determined disorder with an increased tendency to form IgE antibody to inhalants and foods (see Ch. 33). There is increased susceptibility to asthma, allergic rhinitis and atopic eczema (Figs 30.47 and 30.48). Although eczema may begin at any age, in 75% of patients first signs are present by 6 months. Recent evidence has demonstrated that abnormality of the epidermal barrier is a major predisposing factor in atopic disease through loss of function of the epidermal barrier protein filaggrin.[52]

Clinical features

Diagnostic criteria have been defined for atopic eczema but the characteristic clinical features are erythema, generalized dryness and itching

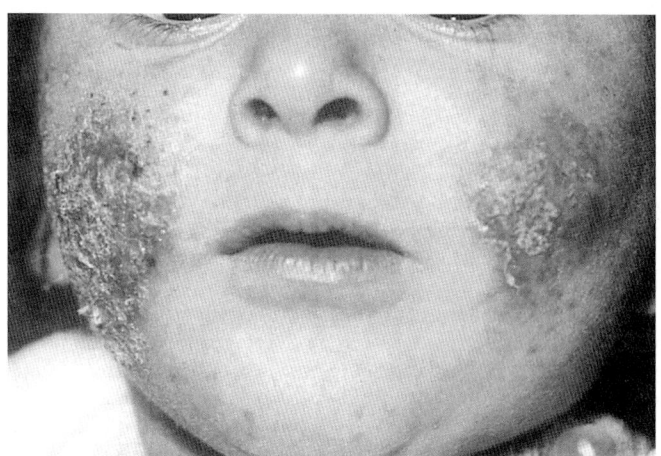

Fig. 30.47 Atopic eczema: facial in young infant.

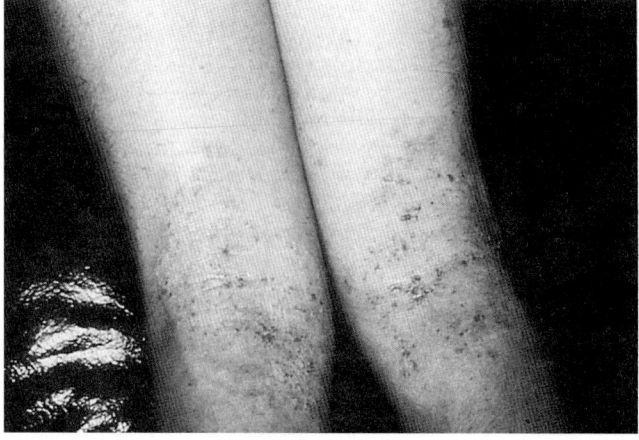

Fig. 30.48 Atopic eczema: flexural in older child.

which leads to excoriations and ultimately lichenification or thickening of the skin, particularly in children older than 2 years.[51] Involvement of the whole cutaneous surface may occur but the predominant areas are the face in infants, extensor aspects of the limbs as the child begins to crawl, and the limb flexures in older children. In severe cases the whole skin may be erythematous and in these patients white dermographism is often a prominent feature: this indicates that the condition is likely to be unstable and difficult.

Complications

Patients with atopic eczema may develop secondary bacterial infection which presents either as impetigo or folliculitis, or simply as worsening eczema. Mollusca contagiosa appear more common, although there are no prevalence studies to confirm this. Atopic patients are at risk of developing severe widespread herpes simplex infections. The usual childhood immunizations are quite safe.

Management

A comprehensive systematic review of all treatments for atopic eczema has been published.[53] This review summarizes the available data from all the randomized controlled trials. It is clear that although emollients and topical steroids are the mainstays of treatment there are very few objective data to recommend their use. Despite this, clinical practice suggests that they are very helpful in the management of atopic eczema.

Time should be taken in discussing factors that act as external irritants. Wool is a major irritant and should never be worn in direct contact with the skin. It is important to warn that wool contact may also occur with the parents' clothing, carpets, car seat and stroller covers, blankets and toys. Cotton material is always safe and cotton polyester combinations rarely irritate, but acrylic may be as troublesome as wool. Perfumed and medicated products, disinfectants and strong cleansers should be avoided. Soap in excess and bubble baths overdry the skin, so soap substitutes should be used.

It should be emphasized to parents that topical steroids are safe as long as these are used only where and when there is active eczema. In general, ointment bases, which are more emollient, are preferred. Only 1% hydrocortisone should be used on the face and in the groin but fluorinated steroids may be used elsewhere for short periods. Patients and parents should be educated regarding the quantities of creams necessary to apply and guidance has been published regarding amount and frequency of application.[1,54]

Second line therapy for severe cases or those not responding to routine treatment includes paste bandages or wet wraps. The latter involves applying two layers of tubular cotton bandages over topical steroids and emollients on the skin. The inner bandage is soaked in warm water prior to application. These dressings increase the hydration of the skin, physically prevent scratching, immediately reduce itching and enhance the penetration of topical steroids. In infants only weak steroids should be used because of the risk of absorption. The use of dressings should be adequately supervised and used for no more than a few days at a time with topical steroids.

Obvious secondary bacterial infection should be treated with oral antibiotics. However, these are indicated in most patients with severe weeping eczema even in the absence of clinically obvious infection. Although current randomized controlled trial evidence does not support the routine use of antihistamines in atopic eczema many parents say that their child appears to be more comfortable at night with less scratching after a nocturnal dose of a sedative antihistamine. Oral steroids should be avoided because a severe rebound can occur on withdrawal and after several courses the eczema is rendered very unstable.

Recently topical tacrolimus and topical pimecrolimus have received approval by the UK National Institute for Clinical Excellence (NICE) as second line treatments for patients greater than 2 years where topical corticosteroids have not worked or there is a serious risk of adverse effects with topical corticosteroids.[55] Concern has been raised about possible cancer risks based on information from animal studies, small numbers of post-marketing reports and how the drugs work. These drugs should therefore be prescribed only by doctors with experience in skin disease.

Third line treatments include phototherapy (narrow band UVB or psoralen plus UVA), ciclosporin (although not yet licensed in the UK for pediatric eczema)[56] and azathioprine. Small studies in children suggest montelukast might be beneficial[57] although a larger study in adults concluded that montelukast is not an effective treatment.[58] Further studies are required in children.

Chinese herbal medicine (CHM) has been evaluated and 1 year follow-up of children treated with CHM showed good, sustained improvement in nearly 50% although 1 out of 37 developed abnormal liver function tests and 14 withdrew due to lack of efficacy or unpalatability.[59]

In the absence of a clear history of worsening of eczema relating to food, no alteration to the child's diet should be considered unless the eczema has failed to respond to conventional topical therapy. Dietary manipulation in the management of refractory eczema is covered in Chapter 33. The role of the dust mite in these severe cases is covered in the same section.

There is increasing interest in the primary prevention of atopic disease. Probiotics are cultures of potentially beneficial bacteria and a randomized controlled trial of *Lactobacillus* GG was effective in reducing the frequency, but not severity, of atopic eczema.[60] At present, evidence is lacking to show the benefit of probiotics in established eczema.

As a child becomes older discussion about future careers is important as certain occupations are likely to aggravate the skin, such as hairdressing or car mechanics. It is important to develop a trusting and cooperative relationship with the patient and his parents as they will require much encouragement to help them cope with this distressing condition.

DISCOID ECZEMA (NUMMULAR ECZEMA)

In children this is often a manifestation of the atopic state. Well-defined patches of acute eczema occur in a strikingly symmetrical distribution (Fig. 30.49). In infants the commonest sites are the upper back and the tops of the shoulders; in older patients the extensor aspects of the limbs are particularly involved. The lesions may be very thick and exudative and they are very itchy. They have to be distinguished from tinea and impetigo which are less symmetrical and psoriasis which is rarely moist. The management involves emollients and topical steroids as for atopic dermatitis, with the continued use of emollient helping to prevent recurrences.

PITYRIASIS ALBA

This condition appears as poorly defined, slightly scaly, hypopigmented patches occurring particularly on the face and the upper

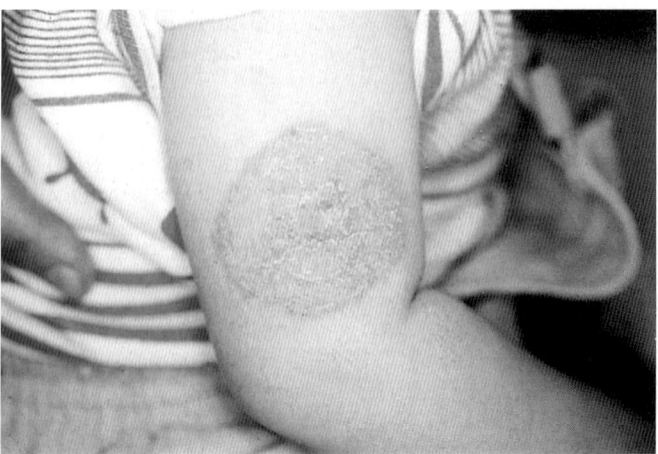

Fig. 30.49   Discoid eczema.

arms. It probably represents a very mild eczema which, however, produces a striking postinflammatory hypopigmentation. Occasionally some areas will show erythema and more definite eczematous changes. The condition is more common in atopics. The mild irritation and signs of mild eczema respond to emollients and weak topical corticosteroids but the hypopigmentation may be very persistent and require sun exposure over a prolonged period before repigmentation is complete. Most lesions clear by puberty. The condition should be differentiated from vitiligo where there is total depigmentation and no scale and from tinea versicolor which has very well demarcated lesions with very fine branny scaling.

SEBORRHEIC DERMATITIS

This condition usually presents between weeks 2 and 6 of infancy with a second peak in adult life; whilst in adults the dermatitis relates to sites of greatest sebum production, this relationship is less clear in infants.

The rash has an erythematous background and a greasy yellow scale. In the proximal flexures the scale may be absent and a glazed erythema the only sign. Scaling is particularly prominent on the scalp, producing the so-called 'cradle cap'. The main areas of involvement are scalp, glabella, behind and inside the ears, nasolabial folds, axillae and groin and in infants the neck and limb flexures. In the flexural areas candidiasis is commonly superimposed. The rash is usually asymptomatic.

Various conditions mimic seborrheic dermatitis including drug reactions (in children particularly due to phenytoin sodium), early psoriasis and Langerhans' cell histiocytosis. These should be considered when what appears to be a seborrheic dermatitis occurs at an unexpected age or fails to respond to therapy.

Seborrheic dermatitis usually responds quickly to weak topical corticosteroid preparations with the addition of an anticandidal agent for the flexural areas. On the scalp, sulfur and salicylic acid preparations left on overnight are usually more effective than corticosteroids. If the scale is very thick, warmed olive or paraffin oil can be used to soften it before the cream is applied. It should be emphasized that the disorder will tend to recur through infancy.

NAPKIN DERMATITIS

Napkin dermatitis encompasses various skin diseases of different etiologies. Irritant contact dermatitis is the most common due to damage to skin integrity through friction, occlusion, excessive moisture and irritants under the nappy. Secondary infection (bacterial and candidal) usually occurs. Seborrheic dermatitis and psoriasis may also affect the napkin area

The newer superabsorbent disposable napkins are often preferable to cloth napkins. A combination cream of 1% hydrocortisone and anticandidal agent is usually effective and a silicone or zinc barrier cream may be added to protect the skin against moisture. There will usually be a quick response to therapy but recurrences are to be expected.

ALLERGIC CONTACT ECZEMA

Allergic contact eczema is one of the main examples of delayed type hypersensitivity in the skin. It is much less common in children than in adults, probably due to lack of contact with sensitizing chemicals. The commonest allergen in children is nickel, which is contained in metal clips and studs (e.g. jeans studs) and in non-gold earrings. It seems likely that a number of children are sensitized following piercing of the ears and by wearing costume jewelry earrings. Other contact allergens in children include plants such as *Rhus* (particularly in the USA and Australia) (Fig. 30.50), chemicals used in rubber production and topical medications such as neomycin and gentamicin.

Identification of the allergen is essential, and this is carried out by patch testing the child. Interpretation requires expertise, as not all reactions are necessarily specific delayed type hypersensitivity reactions.

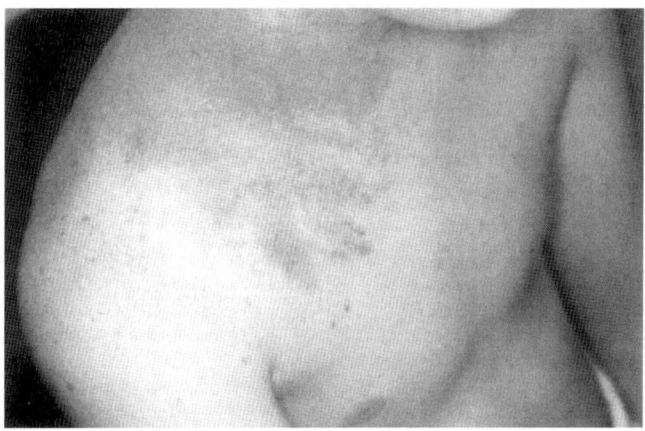

Fig. 30.50   Plant (*Rhus*) dermatitis.

PHYTOPHOTODERMATITIS

This is a cutaneous phototoxic inflammatory response resulting from direct contact to naturally occurring plant psoralen followed by ultraviolet (UVA) sensitization. It typically manifests in spring or summer months as painful streaky/linear erythema on exposed sites that may blister and subsequently heal with postinflammatory hyperpigmentation. The most common plants to cause this reaction are in the Umbelliferae family.

JUVENILE PLANTAR DERMATOSIS

This condition affects mainly children aged 3–14 years and is characterized by a shiny, smooth erythema affecting the plantar aspect of the weightbearing area on the foot. The forefoot and toes are typically commonly involved and the heels in about a quarter of patients. The feet are affected symmetrically and the toe webs are spared helping differentiate juvenile plantar dermatosis from tinea pedis. Pain from cracks and fissures is a major symptom. Rarely a similar pattern can be seen on the fingertips.

The exact cause is unknown but hot humid conditions caused by less porous, synthetic materials in socks and shoes are thought to contribute to the maceration process. Most cases will clear by adolescence but some are helped by changing footwear and use of emollients.

PSORIASIS

A combination of epidemiological, family and human leukocyte antigen (HLA) studies indicate that psoriasis is a genetic condition. Its mode of inheritance is probably autosomal dominant with variable penetrance. Psoriasis appears by the age of 15 years in 30% of patients. Children may present with typical adult large erythematous plaques, with a thick silvery white scale, predominantly on the knees, elbows, buttocks and scalp, but usually the plaques are smaller and with a finer scale. A common presentation is acute guttate psoriasis with the eruption of small papules in a widespread distribution, often following an intercurrent illness, particularly a streptococcal throat infection. A micropapular form of psoriasis occurs particularly in dark-skinned children with 1–2 mm papules most marked on the extensor aspects of the limbs. These lesions are usually skin colored until scratching demonstrates the white scale.

The face and intertriginous sites, such as retroauricular areas, axillae, groin, genital and perianal area, are commonly affected in children. Children presenting with vulvitis, balanitis and perianal itching may be found to have psoriasis. In these areas the typical scale is absent and the condition presents as a glazed erythema often with fissuring. Generalized pustular psoriasis is rare in children and has an explosive onset with sheets of pustules on a background of bright erythema accompanied by severe systemic toxicity. It may be the first presentation of psoriasis and settle spontaneously in a few weeks leaving

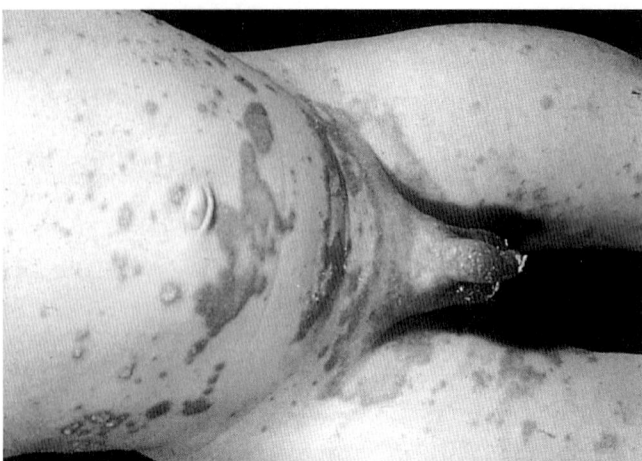

Fig. 30.51 Napkin psoriasis.

normal skin. It often recurs and usually more typical psoriasis eventually supervenes. Pustular psoriasis of the palms and soles is also very rare in children. Acropustulosis, a glazed erythema studded with pustules followed by thick scaling and fissuring, involving one or more digits, is an occasional childhood presentation. Nail involvement is usually absent or minimal with minor pitting, and psoriatic arthropathy is extremely uncommon in children.

Controversy exists over whether or not the condition called 'napkin psoriasis' or 'sebopsoriasis' (Fig. 30.51) is in fact a form of psoriasis. It occurs in the first 3 months of life with a nonspecific napkin dermatitis suddenly becoming more severe and extensive with bright, well-demarcated erythema involving most of the napkin area including the folds. Lesions resembling typical psoriasis then erupt elsewhere, usually first on face and scalp, then neck fold and axillae and finally trunk and limbs. In the scalp the lesions may appear similar to seborrhea. Evidence for this representing a form of psoriasis rather than dermatitis comes from the work of Andersen & Thomsen[61] who found a family history of psoriasis in 26% of patients compared with 4.9% of controls, and of Neville & Finn[62] who, on review of these patients at 5–13 years, found psoriasis in 17% with the expected rate being 0.4%.

In any child with a difficult napkin dermatitis responding poorly to conventional measures psoriasis should be considered, particularly if the lesions have well-defined margins and remain fairly fixed in position.

Management

Many systemic therapies (e.g. retinoids, methotrexate and ciclosporin) used in adults are inappropriate in children. As a general rule, psoriasis in children is better treated with tars than topical corticosteroids. They are often more effective, are safer for long term use, and rebound on their cessation is less of a problem. Tars may be irritant in infants, as they may be at any age when applied to the face or intertriginous areas. Useful preparations for guttate or small plaque psoriasis are coal tar and salicylic acid mixtures (equal parts 2–4%) in an aqueous cream base applied twice a day. A prospective, multicenter, double-blind study in children showed that the topical vitamin D analogue calcipotriol is effective and safe when applied to less than 30% of the body surface area.[63] Whilst oral antibiotics and tonsillectomy have been advocated for patients with recurrent guttate psoriasis following recent streptococcal infection, there are no data to show they are beneficial.[64] For large plaque psoriasis in older children the adult regimens of topical dithranol with or without ultraviolet B (UVB) (preferably narrow band) are usually tolerated.

Patients with generalized pustular psoriasis require urgent hospitalization and close monitoring of fluid and electrolyte balance and evidence of infection. Wet compresses give symptomatic relief while awaiting spontaneous recovery. Tars are contraindicated and topical steroids must be used very cautiously due to the risk of considerable absorption.

Palmoplantar pustulosis and acropustulosis usually respond slowly to tar preparations. Napkin psoriasis often clears quickly with hydrocortisone and anticandidal agents for the flexural areas and a weak corticosteroid elsewhere.

It is essential for the parents, and the child if old enough, to appreciate that psoriasis is a capricious, recurrent disease which will require varying treatments depending on the site, nature and severity of the condition at different stages. Long term follow-up, preferably with the same practitioner, is important.

CONNECTIVE TISSUE DISEASES (Ch. 29)

LUPUS ERYTHEMATOSUS (LE)

This is rare in children but neonatal lupus erythematosus is of considerable importance.

Neonatal lupus erythematosus

This occurs due to the passage of maternal antibodies through the placenta (Fig. 30.52), where the mother suffers from systemic LE, subacute cutaneous LE or the sicca syndrome. In 50% of cases the mother is asymptomatic but the vast majority have SS-A (anti-Ro) antibodies. The most important feature of neonatal LE is heart block of varying degrees. This is usually permanent, and without pacing there is a significant mortality (Ch. 21). Other features include autoimmune hemolytic anemia, thrombocytopenia, hepatitis, pneumonitis and splenomegaly.

The skin lesions resemble those of subacute cutaneous LE in the adult, occurring on the face, neck and scalp, with erythematous macules or plaques with scaling. They are often present at birth and disappear within the first year of life. There may also be photosensitivity. Treatment of the skin is with 1% hydrocortisone cream and protection from the sun.

Lupus erythematosus in the older child

This takes two main forms: systemic LE and discoid LE. It is thought that this is a spectrum of disease, as sometimes patients with discoid LE will progress to systemic LE and a proportion of those with discoid LE have circulating antinuclear antibodies, anemia, leukopenia and thrombocytopenia and other features such as Raynaud's phenomenon and arthralgia.

Discoid lupus erythematosus

This usually affects girls, who develop erythematous plaques on the face, the arms and dorsum of the hands. The most commonly affected parts of the face are the nose and the cheeks. Involvement of the scalp usually leads to scarring alopecia.

There may be mild anemia, leukopenia or thrombocytopenia and some children will have circulating antinuclear antibodies.

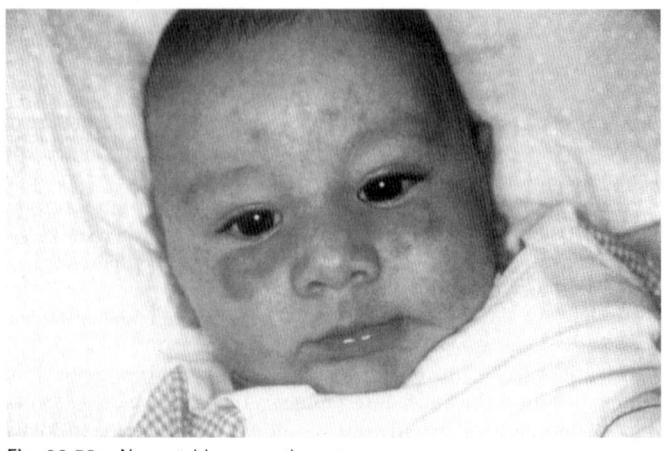

Fig. 30.52 Neonatal lupus erythematosus.

The prognosis is variable, as in some the plaques will resolve spontaneously whereas in others they tend to be persistent. Avoidance of sun exposure by the use of sunscreens and a hat is important.

Systemic lupus erythematosus

As in discoid LE, the systemic form is more common in girls. It is a multisystem connective tissue disease which often carries a poor prognosis, due to renal involvement. This is discussed fully in Chapter 29 (see p. 1427). The skin manifestations include a butterfly rash on the face, which characteristically spares the nasolabial folds, discoid plaques usually on the face, reticulate livedo most marked on the legs, panniculitis, vasculitic ulcers, cuticular hemorrhages at the fingernail folds, and alopecia. Almost half of patients will have mouth ulcers.

DERMATOMYOSITIS

This is a rare connective tissue disease affecting the skin, muscle and blood vessels. Its etiology is unknown, though in some adults there is an association with carcinomas of internal viscera and lymphomas. The histological changes in the skin may resemble those of LE, though the dermal edema is more marked. In the later stages the dermis becomes sclerotic, and the picture may be similar to the changes in scleroderma.

The clinical manifestations are extremely variable. In some children the skin signs may be very prominent with minimal myositis, whereas in others there is polymyositis with little evidence of skin involvement. Myositis is manifested by a proximal muscular weakness with difficulty in flexing the neck, climbing stairs and raising the arms above the shoulder girdle, and by a raised serum creatine phosphokinase. There may be concomitant fever and malaise.

The rash when present is very characteristic. A heliotrope (purplish-red) rash occurs on the face involving the eyelids, the forehead and upper cheeks. There may be marked edema of the hands and arms with an erythematous linear rash over the dorsum of the hands with nail fold telangiectasia. Erythema of the scalp may develop and there may be marked alopecia. Reticulate livedo is seen in some, and may lead to ulceration of the skin.

Calcification is common in children, affecting more than 50% of cases. It primarily involves the muscles, particularly around the pelvic and shoulder girdles, and may cause marked functional disability. It also occurs in the subcutaneous tissues, and there may be extrusion through the skin with ulceration.

The course of the disease is variable, but there is generally a good prognosis in children. Death may occur due to respiratory failure, difficulty in swallowing, or the side-effects of steroid therapy.

Treatment with methotrexate is now considered first line therapy in an attempt to reduce the cumulative dose of oral coricosteroids.[65] Therapy is usually necessary for months or years until the serum creatine phosphokinase returns to normal and the signs of the disease have disappeared. Physiotherapy may be useful to prevent contractures.

SCLERODERMA

In children this may take two forms: morphea (localized scleroderma), which is relatively common, and systemic sclerosis which is very rare.

Morphea

This is a localized and benign form of scleroderma, though it can cause quite marked disfigurement. On histological examination, the dermis is at first edematous with swelling and degeneration of the collagen fibrils, with later thickening of the dermis and loss of appendages. The etiology of the condition is unknown.

The areas of morphea occur usually as either plaques or linear lesions of sclerosis in the skin. These are at first purplish in color, and later become white and waxy. Hairs are lost within the area, with loss of sweating. They occur on the trunk and limbs. When they involve a limb (usually linear lesions), they may involve muscles and bone leading to shortening of the limb.

A particular disfigurement which results from morphea is the so-called 'coup de sabre', which occurs in the frontoparietal area. This starts with contraction of the skin over the affected area with development of an ivory plaque with hyperpigmentation at the edge and telangiectatic vessels coursing over it. The resulting groove may extend downwards, affecting the mouth and mandible. The tongue may be atrophic on the affected side, and there may be marked alopecia. There is marked facial asymmetry with consequent disfigurement.

A prospective, nonrandomized, open pilot study suggests that combined low dose methotrexate and high dose pulsed corticosteroids is an effective treatment (see Kreuter et al. Arch Dermatol 2005 – reference 66).[66]

Systemic sclerosis

This is very rare in children. The etiology is unknown, but as similar changes may be seen in graft versus host reactions, it may be some sort of rejection phenomenon.

In the majority of patients the condition starts with Raynaud's phenomenon which may continue for several years before other manifestations occur. These include: swelling of the hands; sclerodactyly with atrophy of the pulps of the fingers; calcinosis of the finger pulps which may be prominent; ulceration; and gangrene. In some, terminal phalangeal absorption also occurs.

Later, other features occur with beaking of the nose, radial furrowing around the mouth which becomes smaller, macroglossia, esophageal dilatation and stricture, and abnormal colonic peristalsis.

The prognosis is variable and depends on internal organ involvement, though most patients continue with the condition for many years with increasing deformity. No formal trials have evaluated the wide range of potential immunosuppressive therapies.

LICHEN SCLEROSUS

Although the precise etiology of lichen sclerosus is unknown, evidence for an autoimmune basis to the disorder is emerging. Circulating IgG autoantibodies to the glycoprotein extracellular matrix protein 1 (ECM1) have been demonstrated in the sera of about 75% of affected individuals.[67] Lichen sclerosus has a predilection for genital and perianal skin. It is more common in females and usually presents with itch although in children it may be asymptomatic. Erythema and excoriations appear in the early stages with subsequent development of well-defined pale atrophic areas. The lesions often occur in a figure of eight pattern around the vulva and anal region. Lichen sclerosus may be misdiagnosed as sexual abuse. In approximately 10% extragenital lesions are also present. In boys, the usual history is of balanitis and tightening of the foreskin which can progress to phimosis (balanitis xerotica obliterans). Potent topical steroids are the treatment of choice.[68] A Cochrane review of topical therapies is currently underway. The overall prognosis is good but for cases that persist long term follow-up is recommended because of the risk of malignant change in adults.

IDIOPATHIC PHOTOSENSITIVITY ERUPTIONS

Before considering a child to have an idiopathic photosensitivity eruption, it is important to exclude one of the hereditary diseases (q.v.), and photosensitive drug eruptions which are common and may be caused by a number of drugs (notably sulfonamides, tetracyclines and phenothiazines).

POLYMORPHIC LIGHT ERUPTION (PLE)

About 20% of patients with PLE present before the age of 10 years. A delayed reaction occurring several hours or the next day after exposure to the sun results in erythema, burning and itching, followed by papule and plaque formation. With avoidance of sun exposure this reaction will settle but will usually relapse when the child is exposed to the sun again. It usually presents during the summer, but in some children it is most marked in the spring and early summer, with remission of the symptoms in midsummer with 'hardening' of the skin. Juvenile spring eruption is probably a localized variant of PLE with papules and vesicles confined to the helices of the ears.

Most children with PLE continue into adulthood with it. Action spectrum studies are usually normal, and are therefore unhelpful. Prevention of PLE depends on adequate topical photoprotection with sunscreens. In those children with severe PLE, photochemotherapy with oral psoralen and UVA light (PUVA) may be helpful.

ACTINIC PRURIGO

This condition is clinically similar to PLE but is now recognized to be a separate entity. It is significantly associated with the haplotype HLA-DR4/DRB1*0407.[69] Actinic prurigo nearly always develops in early childhood and 80% of patients are female. There is usually progressive improvement in adolescence.

Clinically all exposed sites are affected, including face, lips, neck, ears, arms, dorsum of hands and lower legs. In the majority there is also involvement of covered skin, though to a lesser extent. It is worse during summer months but very often persists even in winter. In most cases there is a family history and there is also a strong association with atopy.

Action spectrum studies are abnormal in the majority with sensitivity to both UVA and UVB; however, in some children these studies are normal. Treatment is similar to that of PLE, but thalidomide has also been found to be particularly effective in this condition.

HYDROA VACCINIFORME

This is a very rare condition which invariably starts in childhood. On exposure to sunlight the child develops tingling and erythema followed by blistering and umbilicated papules on the face, ears, arms and dorsum of hands. These lead to crusting and varioliform scars.

Action spectrum studies are abnormal with sensitivity mainly involving UVA. Treatment is generally unsatisfactory, though broad spectrum topical sunscreens may be helpful.

DISORDERS OF HYPOPIGMENTATION

HEREDITARY DISORDERS OF HYPOPIGMENTATION

Pigmentary disorders may indicate a more serious systemic disease and the hereditary disorders of hypopigmentation are summarized in Table 30.6.

VITILIGO

This is possibly an autoimmune disease. Though specific antimelanocyte antibodies cannot be demonstrated by immunofluorescence, complement-fixing antibody to melanocytes has been shown in some patients. It is well recognized that patients with vitiligo frequently have thyroid, gastric and adrenal autoantibodies (Fig. 30.53). Vitiligo causes complete depigmentation of the skin (unlike tinea versicolor and pityriasis alba) due to absence of melanocytes and melanin in the epidermis. Vitiligo is common in adults, and is not rare in children. The depigmentation is usually symmetrical but localized, although in some patients the condition progresses to involve almost the whole body. Spontaneous repigmentation occurs more in children than in adults. In those that do not repigment topical corticosteroids can be tried although fluorinated steroids should not be used for prolonged periods. Photochemotherapy with topical or oral psoralen may be helpful in the older child although complete repigmentation rates are disappointing. The efficacy of PUVA (oral administration of psoralen and subsequent exposure to UVA) has been shown in adults to be enhanced by concurrent topical calcipotriol.[70] Several small studies and case reports have shown variable responses to topical immunomodulators (tacrolimus). Otherwise cosmetic camouflage may be applied to the depigmented skin to minimize disfiguration.

NEVUS DEPIGMENTOSUS

Usually solitary, nevoid patches of hypopigmentation are present at birth and can involve any body site. A decrease but not absence of pigment helps differentiate nevus depigmentosus (achromic nevus) from vitiligo. Furthermore, unlike vitiligo, slight darkening may be seen in the affected site following ultraviolet light exposure. The differential diagnosis also includes ash leaf macules seen in tuberous sclerosus but these are often multiple and smaller. Systemic abnormalities have only been rarely reported.[71]

HYPOMELANOSIS OF ITO

There is convincing evidence that hypomelanosis of Ito does not represent a distinct entity but is rather a symptom of many different states of mosaicism.[72] Incontinentia pigmenti type 1, which was subsequently shown to be hypomelanosis of Ito, is a sporadic condition associated with an X/autosome translocation involving Xp11.

Unilateral or bilateral macular hypopigmented whorls, streaks, and patches of hypopigmentation present at birth along the lines of Blaschko. Although some features are similar to those of classic incontinentia pigmenti the preceding inflammatory stage is absent. Abnormalities of the eyes and the musculoskeletal and central nervous systems occur in some.

DISORDERS OF HAIR LOSS

The normal transition from vellus to terminal hair in the newborn may be delayed up to 1 year giving the false impression of diffuse congenital alopecia. Genuine inability to grow normal hair can be seen in a number of genetic conditions including the ectodermal dysplasias and hair shaft abnormalities. The latter group may be detected by light microscopy of the affected hair and includes trichorrhexis nodosa which occurs as an isolated problem or in Menkes syndrome; trichothiodystrophy, characterized by sulfur-deficient, brittle hair; trichorrhexis invaginata (bamboo hair) usually associated with Netherton syndrome; monilethrix (beaded hairs due to keratin mutations); and pili torti which describes flattened and twisted hairs.

LOOSE ANAGEN SYNDROME

Diffuse or occasionally patchy hair loss is seen typically in fair-haired girls aged 2–9 years. The hair is a little unruly. Loose anagen syndrome is often familial and is diagnosed by an increased number of anagen hairs present when plucked from the scalp. The features become less prominent into adult life.

TELOGEN EFFLUVIUM

This refers to hair loss following the abrupt transformation of anagen hairs to the telogen phase during which they are shed. Normally 80–90% of hairs are in anagen but up to half may change in synchronization to telogen. This results in hair loss 3–4 months after the initiating event which may be 'stress', severe illness or certain drugs, e.g. anticoagulants, retinoids, etc.

ALOPECIA AREATA

It seems likely that at least in some patients with this condition the process is due to autoimmunity, though conclusive proof is lacking (Fig. 30.54). There is an increased incidence of autoantibodies and autoimmune diseases. There is also an increased incidence of atopy, and atopic children are more likely to develop total alopecia. A family history of alopecia areata is present in 5–25% of cases.

Most children develop discoid areas of alopecia in the scalp with peripheral exclamation hairs, and these areas regrow hair normally in due course. In some children, however, particularly those with an ophiasiform distribution of hair loss (involving the temples and occipital region), the condition is progressive to become total, and regrowth is much less likely. There are also nail changes with fine pitting and horizontal depressions known as Beau's lines. Although alopecia areata is not a life threatening condition it is obviously distressing for children and parents.

Table 30.6   Hereditary syndromes associated with hypopigmentation

	Oculocutaneous albinism (OCA types I and II)	Chediak–Higashi syndrome	Hermansky–Pudlak syndrome	Piebald trait	Waardenburg syndrome (types I–III)	Cross syndrome
Inheritance	AR	AR	AR	AD	AD	AR
Pigment loss	Type I: total, hair white. Type II: freckles in sun-exposed sites, hair yellow	Variable (patchy) oculocutaneous albinism. Silvery hair which may be sparse	Tyrosinase-positive oculocutaneous albinism	White forelock, absent pigmentation (leukoderma) ventral chest, abdomen and midportion of limbs. Pigmented macules often within affected areas	Piebaldism	Reduction in skin pigment. Variable loss of hair color
Ocular features	Nystagmus, visual loss. Type I: photophobia	Nystagmus, visual loss, photophobia pale retinae, and translucent irides	Blindness, nystagmus, strabismus, iris transillumination, foveal hypoplasia, and albinotic retinal midperiphery	Heterochromia iridis	Type I: dystopia canthorum Type II: more frequently heterochromia iridis	Nystagmus, reduced eye color
Other features		Frequent and severe pyogenic infections. Progressive neuropathy and neurodegeneration Lymphadenopathy	Bleeding tendency due to poor platelet aggregation. Cellular storage problems lead to pulmonary fibrosis, granulomatous enteropathic disease, and renal failure		Sensorineural deafness more common in type II Type III: additional severe musculoskeletal abnormalities	Mental and growth retardation, spasticity, athetoid movements
Molecular defect	Type I: tyrosinase (TYR) gene Type II: transmembrane protein (P gene)	Lysosomal trafficking regulator gene (CHS1)	Seven gene defects are associated with the four known subtypes	KIT protooncogene and occasionally zinc finger transcription factor SNA12	Types I and III: paired box homeotic gene-3 (PAX-3). Type IIA: microphthalmia-associated transcription factor gene (MITF)	Unknown
Other	Type II most common type of OCA (types I–VI) OCAIII due to TRP-1 mutations. Individuals have reddish hair and reddish-brown skin		HPS type 2 patients also have immunodeficiency	Hirschsprung disease occasionally associated	Hirschsprung disease occasionally associated	Very rare. Also referred to as oculocerebral syndrome with hypopigmentation

AR; autosomal recessive. AD; autosomal dominant.

There is no effective treatment for alopecia areata at present. Intralesional steroids may cause some local hair growth but this has no permanent effect on the course of the alopecia. In older children, short contact dithranol treatment may induce hair growth but the result is rarely cosmetically acceptable. There is no evidence as yet that topical minoxidil is helpful.

TRICHOTILLOMANIA (HAIR PULLING)

Trichotillomania is more common in girls. The alopecia is patchy with variable hair lengths in the affected region usually located on the contralateral side to the child's handedness. Hair ingestion may lead to bowel symptoms. Trichotillomania is most often an isolated symptom with a good prognosis following appropriate psychological support. However, follow-up until resolution is important to avoid missing more severe psychological disease.

THE HISTIOCYTOSES

Histiocytes include circulating monocytes and tissue macrophages as well as the dendritic cell system (antigen presenting cells). The histiocytoses

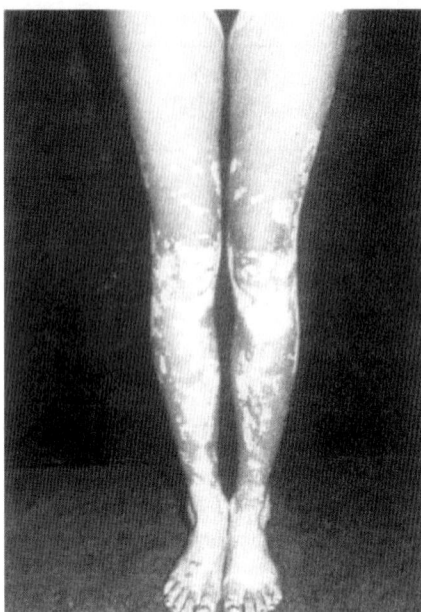

Fig. 30.53   Vitiligo.

have been classified into class I (Langerhans' cell histiocytosis), class II (proliferative histiocytoses of mononuclear phagocytes other than Langerhans' cell) and class III (malignant histiocyte disorders).[73]

CLASS I LANGERHANS' CELL HISTIOCYTOSIS (HISTIOCYTOSIS X)

This condition is rare (Ch. 24, pp. 1030) and the cells involved are Langerhans' cells which contain Birbeck granules and express the common thymocyte antigen CD1 markers. Although historically four types are recognized on the basis of clinical organ involvement, the presentations may overlap and the disease may progress from one subtype to another.[74]

Letterer–Siwe disease

This usually presents in the first year of life (Fig. 30.55). Discrete yellow–brown papules develop on the scalp, face, upper trunk and flexures, with a distribution mimicking seborrheic eczema. Purpura and crusting of the lesion may become evident. In some children mucous membranes are also involved, with gingivitis and oral and genital ulceration.

Signs of systemic involvement become manifest, with hepatosplenomegaly, lymphadenopathy and anemia. Chest X-ray shows miliary shadowing and bone scans may show osteolytic areas. Treatment with steroids and cytotoxic drugs has reduced the mortality and slowed the progression.

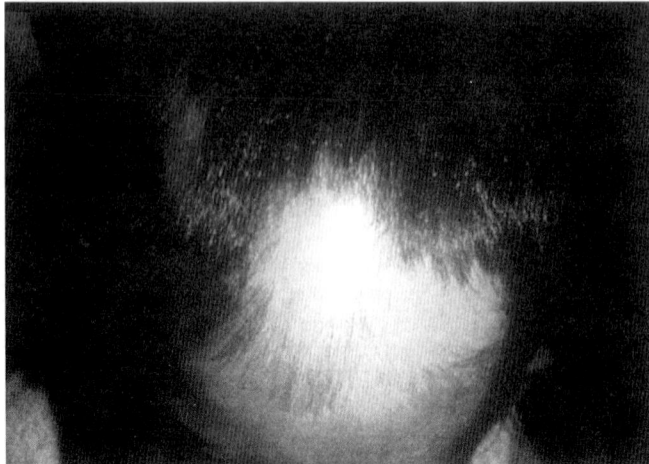

Fig. 30.54   Alopecia areata.

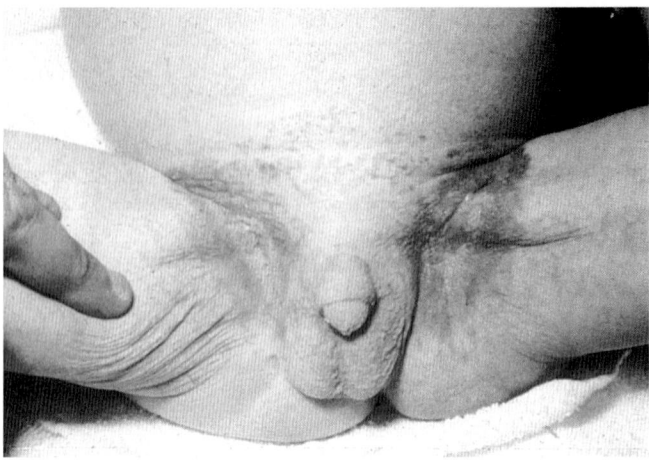

Fig. 30.55   Letterer–Siwe disease.

Hand–Schüller–Christian disease

This is a more benign form of histiocytosis X, which usually presents within the first 5 years of life and follows a chronic non-fatal course. The usual manifestations are radiological bone defects, exophthalmos and diabetes insipidus. Skin lesions similar to those in Letterer–Siwe disease are present in 30%.

Eosinophilic granuloma

This is the most benign form of histiocytosis X. It commonly presents within the first 5 years of life, and skin involvement is rare. When it does occur, yellowish or brownish papules are found on the scalp and trunk in a distribution similar to the other forms of histiocytosis X. Spontaneous resolution usually occurs.

Congenital self-healing histiocytosis

This usually affects skin only with lesions that are nodular or may mimic chickenpox. If this is the case spontaneous resolution occurs within months.

JUVENILE XANTHOGRANULOMA (JXG)

JXG is an example of a benign self-limiting non-Langerhans' cell histiocytosis (class II) (Fig. 30.56). Histologically lesions are characterized by histiocytes with foamy macrophages and multinucleated giant cells. Despite its name and appearance JXG is not associated with lipid disorders. Lesions are occasionally present at birth but typically before 1 year. They are dome-shaped nodules with a red and then orange color often located on the head and neck. Single lesions are more common but if multiple lesions are present up to 10% have ocular involvement which may lead to glaucoma.

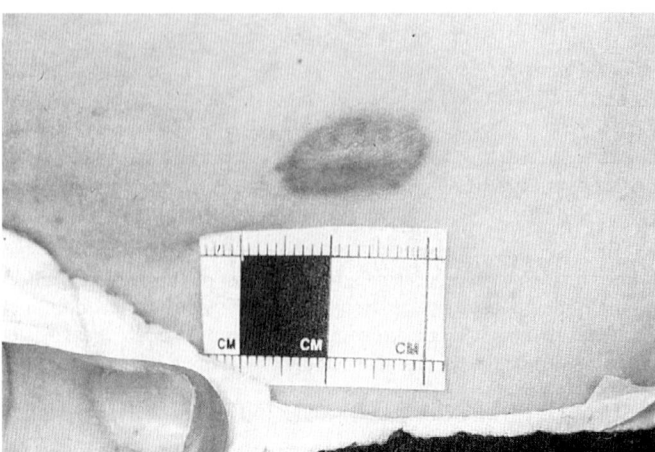

Fig. 30.56   Juvenile xanthogranuloma (XTG).

REFERENCES (* Level 1 evidence)

1. Long CC, Mills CM, Finlay AY. A practical guide to topical therapy in children. Br J Dermatol 1998; 138:293–296.
2. DeDavid M, Orlow SJ, Provost N, et al. Neurocutaneous melanosis: clinical features of large congenital melanocytic nevi in patients with manifest central nervous system melanosis. J Am Acad Dermatol 1996; 35:529–538.
3. Foster RD, Williams ML, Barkovich AJ, et al. Giant congenital melanocytic nevi: the significance of neurocutaneous melanosis in neurologically asymptomatic children. Plast Reconstr Surg 2001; 107:933–941.
4. Agero AL, Benvenuto-Andrade C, Dusza SW, et al. Asymptomatic neurocutaneous melanocytosis in patients with large congenital melanocytic nevi. A study of cases from an internet-based registry. J Am Acad Dermatol 2005; 53:959–965.
5. Bett BJ. Large or multiple congenital melanocytic nevi: Occurrence of neurocutaneous melanocytosis in 1008 persons. J Am Acad Dermatol 2006; 54:767–777.
6. Lorentzen M, Pers M, Bretteville Jensen G. The incidence of malignant transformation in giant pigmented nevi. Scand J Plast Reconstr Surg 1977; II:163–167.
7. Illig W, Weidner F, Hundeeker M, et al. Congenital nevi < 10cms as precursors to melanoma. Arch Dermatol 1985; 121:1274–1281.
8. Rhodes AR, Sober AJ, Calvin L, et al. The malignant potential of small congenital nevocellular nevi. J Am Acad Dermatol 1982; 6:230–241.
9. Sahin S, Levin L, Kopf AW, et al. Risk of melanoma in medium-sized congenital melanocytic nevi: a follow-up study. J Am Acad Dermatol 1998; 39:428–433.
10. Goss BD, Ansell PE, Bennett V, et al. The prevalence and characteristics of congenital pigmented lesions in the newborn babies in Oxford. Paediatr Perinatal Epidemiol 1990; 4:448–457.
11. Happle R. How many epidermal nevus syndromes exist?. J Am Acad Dermatol 1991; 25:550–556.
12. Solomon LM, Esterly NM. Epidermal and other organoid nevi. Curr Probl Pediatr 1975; 6:1–56.
13. Rogers M. Epidermal nevi and the epidermal nevus syndromes: a review of 233 cases. Pediatr Dermatol 1992; 9:342–344.
14. Enjolras O, Mulliken JB. The current management of vascular birthmarks. Pediatr Dermatol 1993; 10:311–333.
15. North PE, Waner M, Mizeracki A, et al. A unique microvascular phenotype shared by juvenile hemangiomas and human placenta. Arch Dermatol 2001; 137:559–570.
*16. Bennett ML, Fleischer AB, Chamlin SL, et al. Oral corticosteroid use is effective for cutaneous hemangiomas. Arch Dermatol 2001; 137:1208–1213.
17. Dubois J, Hershon L, Carmant L, et al. Toxicity profile of interferon alfa-2b in children: a prospective evaluation. J Pediatr 1999; 135:782–785.
*18. Batta K, Goodyear HM, Moss C, et al. Randomised controlled study of early pulsed dye laser treatment of uncomplicated childhood haemangiomas: results of a 1-year analysis. Lancet 2002; 360:521–527.
19. Payarols J, Masferrer J, Gomez Bellvert C. . Treatment of life-threatening infantile hemangiomas with vincristine. N Engl J Med 1995; 333:69.
20. Krol A, MacArthur CJ. Congenital hemangiomas: rapidly involuting and noninvoluting congenital hemangiomas. Arch Facial Plast Surg 2005; 7:307–311.
21. Metry DW, Dowd CF, Barkovich AJ, et al. The many faces of PHACE syndrome. J Pediatr 2001; 139:117–123.
22. Golitz LE, Rudikoff J, O'Meara OP. Diffuse neonatal hemangiomatosis. Pediatr Dermatol 1986; 3:145–152.
23. Esterly NB, Margileth AM, Kahn G. The management of disseminated eruptive haemangiomata in infants: special symposium. Pediatr Dermatol 2001; 1:312–317.
24. Stevenson RF, Thompson HG, Marin JD. Unrecognized ocular problems associated with port wine stain of the face in children. Can Med Assoc J 1974; 11:953–955.
25. Enjolras O, Riche MC, Merland JJ. Facial port wine stains and Sturge Weber syndrome. Pediatrics 1985; 76:48–51.
26. Kelsell DP, Norgett EE, Unsworth H, et al. Mutations in ABCA12 underlie the severe congenital skin disease harlequin ichthyosis. Am J Hum Genet 2005; 76:794–803.
27. Itin PH, Fistarol SK. Ectodermal dysplasias. Am J Med Genet C Semin Med Genet 2004; 131C:45–51.
28. Cheadle JP, Reeve MP, Sampson JR, et al. Molecular genetic advances in tuberose sclerosis. Hum Genet 2000; 107:97–114.
29. Smahi A, Courtois G, Vabres P, et al. Genomic rearrangement in NEMO impairs NF-kappaB activation and is a cause of incontinentia pigmenti. The International Incontinentia Pigmenti (IP) Consortium. Nature 2000; 405:466–472.
30. Peters TJ, Sarkany R. Porphyria for the general physician. Clin Med 2005; 5:275–281.
31. Gelmetti C, Schianchi R, Ermacora E. Cutis marmorata telangiectatica congenita. 4 new cases and review of the literature. Ann Dermatol Venereol 1987; 114:1517–1528.
*32. Gibbs S, Harvey I, Sterling JC, et al. Local treatments for cutaneous warts: systematic review. Br Med J 2002; 325:461–464.
33. Karabulut AA, Sahin S. Is cimetidine effective for nongenital warts: a double-blind, placebo-controlled study. Arch Dermatol 1997; 133:533–534.
34. Caputo R, Gelmetti C, Ermacora E, et al. Gianotti-Crosti syndrome: a retrospective analysis of 308 cases. J Am Acad Dermatol 1992; 26:207–210.
35. Coskey RJ, Coskey LA. Diagnosis and treatment of impetigo. J Am Acad Dermatol 1987; 17:62–63.
*36. Barton LL, Friedman AD, Portilla MG. Impetigo contagiosa: a comparison of erythromycin and dicloxacillin therapy. Pediatr Dermatol 1988; 5:88–91.
*37. McLinn S. Topical mupirocin vs. systemic erythromycin treatment for pyoderma. Pediatr Infect Dis J 1988; 7:785–790.
*38. Christensen OB, Anehus S. Hydrogen peroxide cream: an alternative to topical antibiotics in the treatment of impetigo contagiosa. Acta Derm Venereol 1994; 74:460–462.
39. Rogers M, Dorman DC, Gapes M, et al. A three year study of impetigo in Sydney. Med J Aust 1987; 147:59–62.
40. Krol AL. Perianal streptococcal dermatitis. Pediatr Dermatol 1990; 7:97–100.
41. Jones TC. Overview of the use of terbinafine (Lamisil) in children. Br J Dermatol 1995; 132:683–689.
42. Terragni L, Lasagni A, Oriani A, et al. Pityriasis versicolor in the pediatric age. Pediatr Dermatol 1991; 8:9–12.
*43. Schultz MW, Gomez M, Hansen RC, et al. Comparative study of 5% permethrin cream and 1% lindane lotion for the treatment of scabies. Arch Dermatol 1990; 126:167–170.
*44. Taplin D, Meinking TL, Chen JA, et al. Comparison on crotamiton 10% cream (Eurax) and permethrin 5% cream (Elimite) for the treatment of scabies in children. Pediatr Dermatol 1990; 7:67–73.
45. Hourihane JO, Roberts SA, Warner JO. Resolution of peanut allergy: a case control study. BMJ 1998; 316:1271–1275.
46. Sabroe RA, Greaves MW. Chronic idiopathic urticaria with functional autoantibodies: 12 years on. Br J Dermatol 2006; 154:813–819.
47. Hannaford R, Rogers M. Presentation of cutaneous mastocytosis in 173 children. Australas J Dermatol 2001; 42:15–21.
*48. Tatnall FM, Schofield JK, Leigh IM. A double-blind, placebo-controlled trial of continuous acyclovir therapy in recurrent erythema multiforme. Br J Dermatol 1995; 132:267–270.
49. Reunala T, Kosnai I, Karparti S, et al. Dermatitis herpetiformis: jejunal findings and skin response to gluten free diet. Arch Dis Child 1984; 59:517–522.
50. Barham KL, Jorizzo JL, Grattan B, et al. Vasculitis and neutrophilic vascular reactions. In: Burns DA, Breatnach S, Cox N, et al, eds. Textbook of dermatology. Oxford: Blackwell Science; 2004.49.1.
51. Brown S, Reynolds NJ. Atopic and non-atopic eczema. BMJ 2006; 332:584–588.
52. Palmer CN, Irvine AD, Terron-Kwiatkowski A, et al. Common loss-of-function variants of the epidermal barrier protein filaggrin are a major predisposing factor for atopic dermatitis. Nat Genet 2006; 38:441–446.
53. Hoare C, Li Wan Po A, Williams H. Systematic review of treatments of atopic eczema. Health Technol Assess 2000; 4:37.
54. Frequency of application of topical corticosteroids for eczema. www.nice.org.uk/TA081guidance
55. Tacrolimus and pimecrolimus for atopic eczema. www.nice.org.uk/TA082guidance
56. Zaki I, Emerson R, Allen BR. Treatment of severe atopic dermatitis in childhood with cyclosporin. Br J Dermatol 1996; 135:(suppl 48):21–24.
*57. Pei AY, Chan HH, Leung TF. Montelukast in the treatment of children with moderate-to-severe atopic dermatitis: a pilot study. Pediatr Allergy Immunol 2001; 12:154–158.
*58. Tewary M, Friedmann PS, Hotchkiss K, et al. A double blind, placebo-controlled trial of montelukast in adult atopic dermatitis. [PO02.37], EADV meeting, Rhods, October 2006.
*59. Sheehan MP, Atherton DJ. One-year follow up of children treated with Chinese medicinal herbs for atopic eczema. Br J Dermatol 1994; 130:488–493.
60. Kalliomaki M, Salminen S, Arvilommi H, et al. Probiotics in primary prevention of atopic disease: a randomised placebo-controlled trial. Lancet 2001; 357:1076–1079.
61. Andersen SL, Thomsen K. Psoriasiform napkin dermatitis. Br J Dermatol 1971; 84:316–319.
62. Neville EA, Finn OA. Psoriasiform napkin dermatitis – a follow up study. Br J Dermatol 1975; 92:279–285.
*63. Oranje AP, Marcoux D, Svensson A, et al. Topical calcipotriol in childhood psoriasis. J Am Acad Dermatol 1997; 36:203–208.
*64. Owen CM, Chalmers RJG, O'Sullivan T, et al. Antistreptococcal interventions for guttate and chronic plaque psoriasis (Cochrane review). In: The Cochrane Library. 3. Oxford: Update Software; 2001.
65. Ramanan AV, Campbell-Webster N, Ota S, et al. The effectiveness of treating juvenile dermatomyositis with methotrexate and aggressively tapered corticosteroids. Arthritis Rheum 2005; 52:3570–3578.
66. Kreuter A, Gambichler T, Breuckmann F, et al. Arch Dermatol. 2005; 141:847–852.
67. Oyama N, Chan I, Neill SM, et al. Autoantibodies to extracellular matrix protein 1 in lichen sclerosus. Lancet 2004; 362:118–123.
68. Dalziel K, Millard PR, Wojnarowska F. The treatment of vulvar lichen sclerosus with a very potent corticosteroid (clobetasol proprionate 0.05%) cream. Br J Dermatol 1991; 124:461–464.

69. Grabczynska SA, McGregor JM, Kondeatis E, et al. Actinic prurigo and polymorphic light eruption: common pathogenesis and the importance of HLA-DR4/DRB1*0407. Br J Dermatol 1999; 140:232–236.

*70. Ermis O, Alpsoy E, Cetin L, et al. Is the efficacy of psoralen plus ultraviolet A therapy for vitiligo enhanced by concurrent topical calcipotriol? A placebo-controlled double-blind study. Br J Dermatol 2001; 145:472–475.

71. Dahr S, Kanwar AJ, Kaur S. Nevus depigmentation in India: experience with 50 patients. Pediatr Dermatol 1993; 10:299–300.

72. Donnai D, Read AP, McKeown C, et al. Hypomelanosis of Ito: a manifestation of mosaicism or chimerism. J Med Genet 1988; 25:809–818.

73. Chu T, D'Angio GJ, Favara B, et al. Histiocytosis syndromes in children. Lancet 1987; i:208–209.

74. Komp DM. Concepts in staging and clinical studies for treatment of Langerhans' cell histiocytosis. Semin Oncol 1991; 18:18–23.

31

Disorders of the eye

Brian W Fleck, Alan O Mulvihill

NORMAL VISUAL DEVELOPMENT

At around 6 weeks an infant will smile in response to visual stimuli; delay of this developmental stage is significant. Visually directed reaching commences at age 2–3 months.

Preferential looking grating measurements of vision reach 6/6 level at 3 years[1] however this test is dependent on complex sensory and motor responses. Cortical VEP estimates of visual acuity give a 6/6 response by age 6–8 months.[2] Stereopsis develops between the ages of 2 and 6 months.[3]

CRITICAL PERIOD OF VISUAL DEVELOPMENT

Early visual experience is critical to the development of synaptic connections in the primary visual cortex.[4] Input from each eye 'competes' for cortical connections.[5] The visual outcome of congenital cataract surgery is poor if visual rehabilitation is delayed beyond 3 months of age. The visual outcome of surgery for uniocular cataract is less satisfactory than that for binocular cataract[6] as the normal eye dominates synaptic development.

PLASTIC PERIOD OF VISUAL DEVELOPMENT

While the critical period of visual development is at age 0–3 months, the visual system remains plastic until at least the age of 8–12 years, and probably longer.[7] Interrupted visual development below the age of about 6 years[8] may lead to permanent reduction of visual acuity even after the causative abnormality has been removed. This is termed 'amblyopia'. The younger the age at which developmental interruption happens, the greater the degree of amblyopia that may occur. Once again uniocular defects produce a greater effect than binocular defects, because of competition effects at the occipital cortex. Amblyopia may be treated during the critical and plastic period of visual development – up to approximately age 8–12 years.[7]

CLINICAL ASSESSMENT

CLINICAL HISTORY

Symptoms related to visual functions cover a wide spectrum of difficulties. Progressive bilateral visual loss in young children may go unnoticed until a relatively late stage, and may present with impairment of a wide spectrum of visually dependent behaviors. Symptoms related to consistently bumping into doorways may indicate visual field reduction on one side. Symptoms related to difficulties coming down stairs or frequent tripping may indicate inferior visual field restriction. Increased sensitivity to light (photophobia) may indicate ocular inflammation or retinal cone dysfunction. Difficulties in dim light (night blindness) may indicate poor retinal rod function. The prenatal history, birth history, developmental history, drug history, family history and educational history should always be taken.

In older children perceptual visual difficulties related to central nervous system (CNS) disease may go undetected unless a careful history is taken. Useful screening questions include:

- Does the child have difficulty identifying objects within a 'busy' or 'fast-moving' environment?
- Does the child have difficulty with coordination and movement in three-dimensional space?
- Does the child have difficulty recognizing familiar faces?
- Does the child have difficulty with orientation in familiar environments?

VISION ASSESSMENT

In infants and very young children, observed visual behavior will give useful qualitative information about visual function. A visually alert infant will fixate on and follow the movement of small objects of interest held by an examiner. Each eye is tested separately by covering one eye with a hand or eye patch. If a child will not tolerate uniocular testing then some useful information may be obtained from binocular testing. However, poor vision in one eye will not be detected by binocular testing.

QUANTITATIVE MEASUREMENTS OF VISUAL ACUITY

'Visibility' refers to the ability to identify a single object such as a sweet, thread on a carpet, or airplane in the sky. 'Resolution' refers to the ability to distinguish between two points or lines. Visual acuity tests measure resolution. Clinical tests of visibility such as Stycar balls, Catford drum, etc. may significantly overestimate results obtained with resolution tests and should be interpreted with caution.

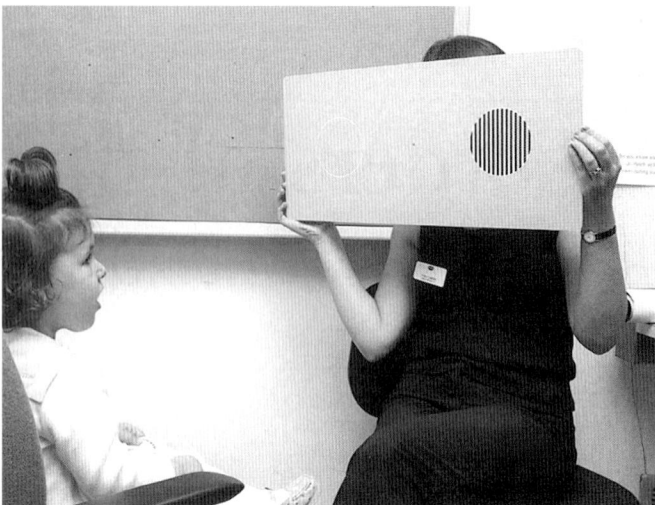

Fig. 31.1 Forced choice preferential looking test (Keeler cards). The tester looks through a hole in the card and chooses which target area the child looks at.

PREFERENTIAL LOOKING ACUITY CARDS

An infant will 'prefer' to look at an object of interest rather than at a blank background. Black and white stripes (gratings) of varying widths ('spatial frequency') are used as the stimulus (Fig. 31.1). The tester uses a series of test cards, each of which has two test areas – one blank and one a test grating. The tester observes the area the infant looks at. The test is repeated a number of times, using various stripe widths. The narrowest stripe width (lowest spatial frequency) consistently looked at by the infant is a measure of the infant's visual resolution. Preferential looking tests may be successfully used in most infants, but are of less interest to 18–24-month-old children.

Cardiff cards use black and white lines shaped into interesting pictures (Fig. 31.2). These are useful in children aged 1–3 years. The child will look at the picture if the black and white stripes are sufficiently wide to be observed (resolved).

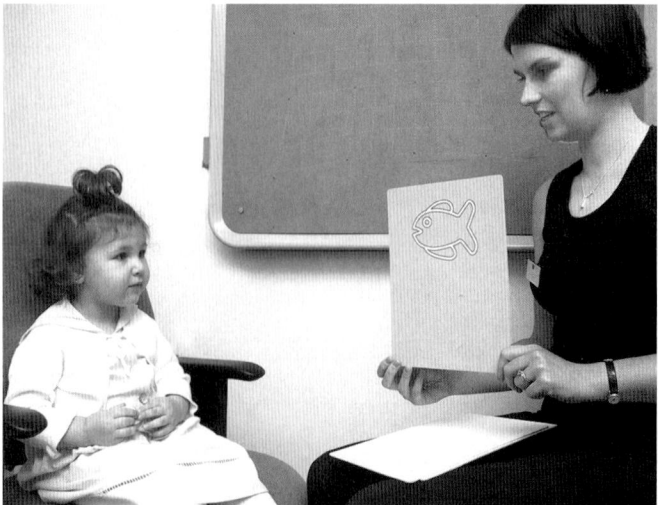

Fig. 31.2 The tester observes whether the child looks at the top or bottom half of the test card. The images are randomly distributed to the top halves and bottom halves of the test cards. The test is normally performed at 50 cm or 100 cm.

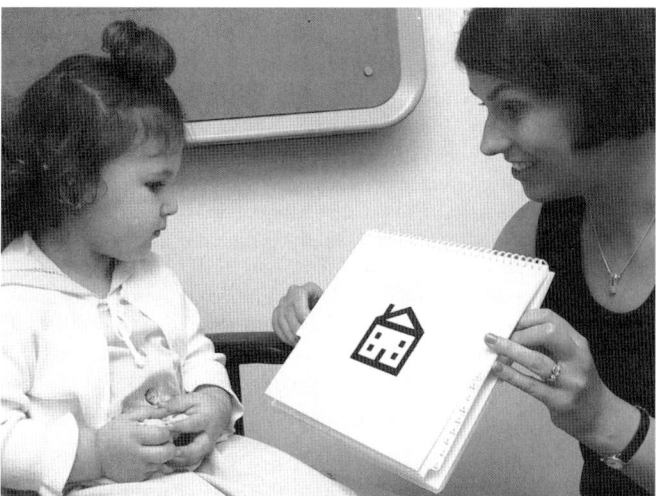

Fig. 31.3 Kay picture optotypes. The test is normally performed at 3 m or 6 m.

OPTOTYPE TESTS

From the age of 3 years upward more traditional 'optotype' visual acuity symbols may be used. Kay pictures use simple line drawings (Fig. 31.3). The Sheridan Gardiner test uses letters. A limited range of letters is used so that the child may match the shape of the letter rather than name it (Fig. 31.4). A letter placed among a line of other letters is less easily observed than a single letter. Charts that use lines of letters arranged in log unit size are preferred in children aged 4–5 years and upwards – LogMAR charts (Fig. 31.5).

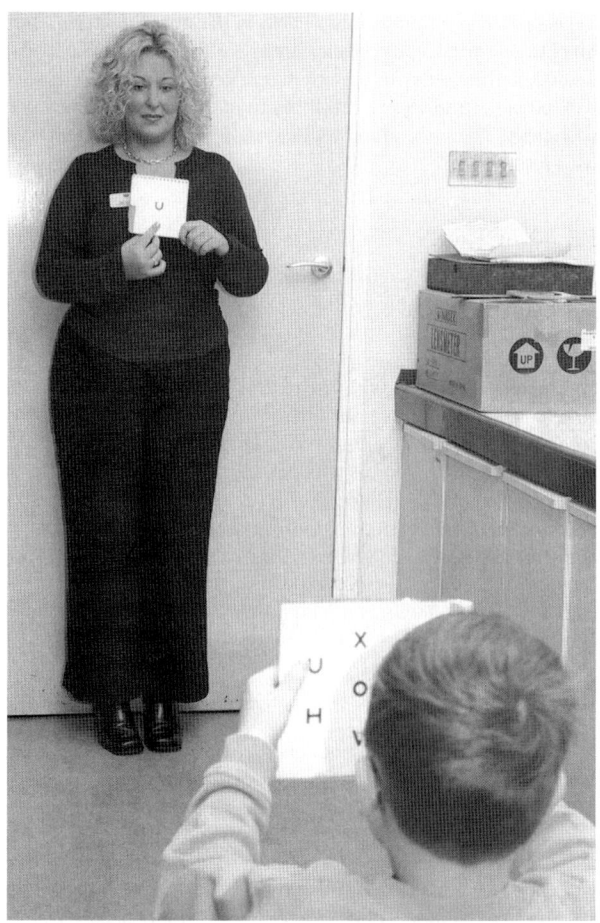

Fig. 31.4 Sheridan Gardiner optotypes. The test is usually performed at 6 m and the child matches the test letter to the key card.

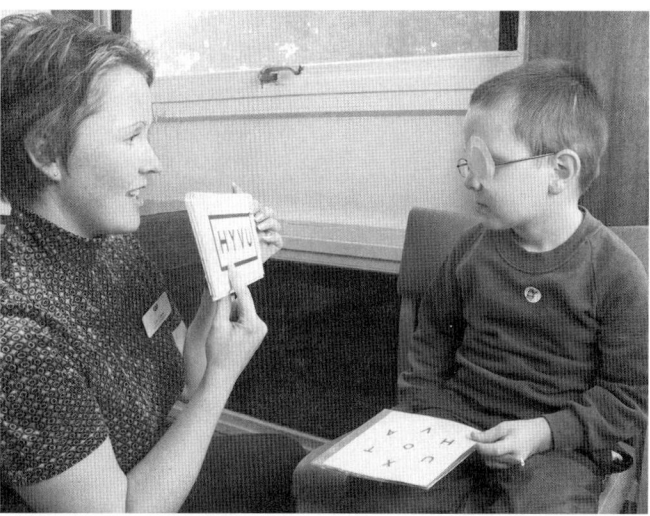

Fig. 31.5 LogMAR optotypes (Glasgow cards). The test is usually performed at 6 m and the child matches the test letter to the key card. Reduced vision due to 'crowding' is detected as the test letter is placed within a row of letters.

VISUAL FIELDS

Visual field testing may be undertaken in infants and young children by introducing an object of interest from either side and observing the response. Two observers are required (Fig. 31.6). The child sits on the lap of a carer. An observer sits approximately 1–2 m in front of the child. A second observer stands behind the parent and child. The second observer slowly brings an object of interest into the field of vision of the child. The child will turn to look at the object when it comes into the observable visual field. Binocular testing is more easily performed than uniocular testing, and will adequately detect a significant binocular visual field defect such as homonymous hemianopia or inferior visual field restriction.

In children aged 6 years upwards, Goldman visual field testing may be possible. This type of detailed visual field testing requires considerable

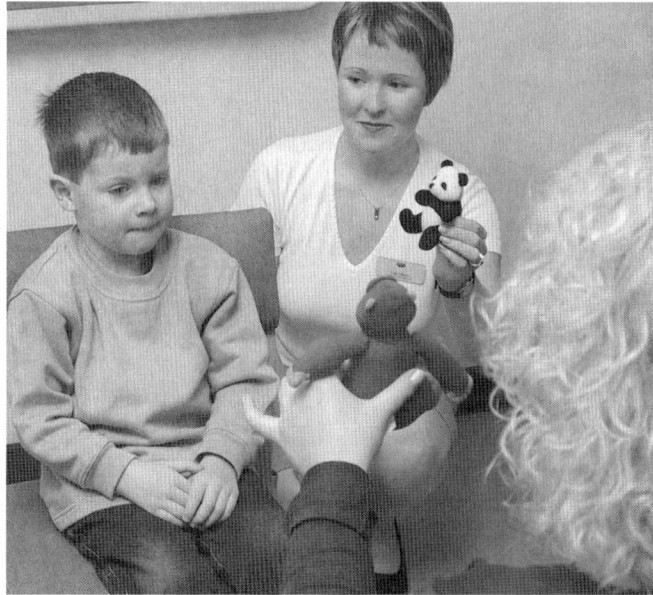

Fig. 31.6 Binocular visual field testing. Observer 1 maintains interest while observer 2 brings the test object (panda) into the child's visual field from behind. The child turns to look at the test object when it becomes visible.

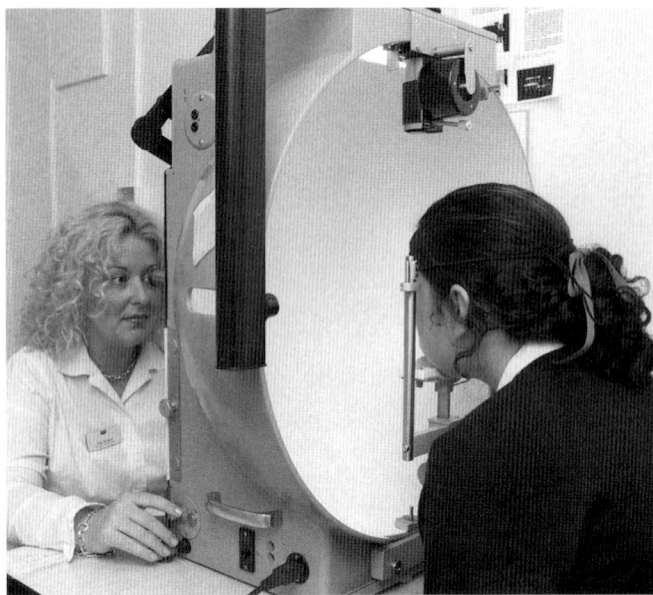

Fig. 31.7 Goldman visual field testing. The tester observes the eye fixing behavior of the child. The child fixes on the center target within the bowl and presses a buzzer when the test spot of light becomes visible in the peripheral visual field.

cooperation from the child. The child must fix on a central point in the testing bowl and a spot of light is brought in from the peripheral field of vision (Fig. 31.7). The child presses a buzzer when the spot of light comes into view. The test is very operator dependent. Testing is normally performed uniocularly, and accurate and reproducible charting of visual field defects related to optic nerve and CNS disease may be obtained.

CLINICAL EYE MOVEMENT TESTING

The cover test may be performed in order to detect a strabismus. When the straight eye is covered the strabismic eye quickly moves in order to take up fixation (Figs 31.8 and 31.9).

The range of eye movements may then be observed. The child is asked to observe an interesting target moved by the examiner. The examiner may use his or her face as the target and move from side to side and up

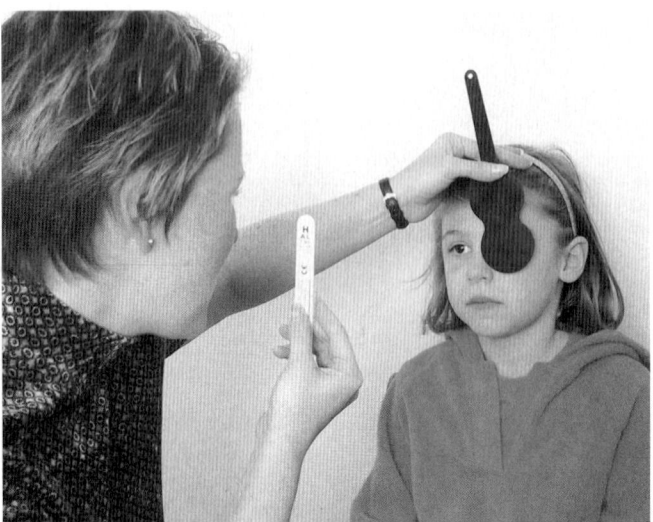

Fig. 31.8 Cover test. The child fixes on a test target at 6 m or 50 cm. The normal eye is covered. The strabismic eye then moves in order to take up fixation. Small flicks of movement may be easily detected, allowing diagnosis of small angled deviations.

and down in front of the child. Limitations of movements and changes in palpebral fissure width are observed.

Nystagmus may be described using the mnemonic 'DWARF':
Direction (horizontal or vertical)
Wave form (jerk or pendular)
Amplitude (large amplitude or small amplitude oscillations)
Rest (primary position (at rest/gaze euoked))
Frequency (rapid movements or slow movements).
The direction of nystagmus movements is recorded as the direction of the fast phase (jerk) of the oscillation.

While some information on nystagmus movements may be obtained by clinical observation, more detailed information may be obtained by analysis in an eye movement laboratory.

EXTERNAL EYE EXAMINATION

The eyelids, conjunctiva, cornea and iris may be observed using a torch. Ophthalmologists use magnification in the form of a slit lamp microscope to allow detailed examination of these structures (Fig. 31.10). Where there is a suspicion of a corneal epithelial abrasion or other corneal epithelial disease a drop of fluorescein dye may be instilled and the corneal epithelium may be observed using a blue light (Fig. 31.11). Any defects in the corneal epithelium will absorb fluorescein and these areas will fluoresce yellow.

Corneal signs such as posterior embryotoxon may be visualized with a slit lamp (Fig. 31.12).

PUPIL RED REFLEX

The transparency of the 'media' of the eye may be observed by observing the red reflex. When the media are transparent a beam of light directed from a direct ophthalmoscope will be observed to produce an orange–red reflection of the fundus, observable in the pupil area (Fig. 31.13). When cataract or vitreous opacity is present the red reflex will be dark or absent. A white reflex in the pupil area (leukocoria) is an important sign of possible underlying retinoblastoma or other significant ocular pathology. The normal red reflex is more difficult to detect in dark brown eyes.

PUPIL REACTIONS

The relative size of the pupils should be observed. Slight asymmetry of pupil size (anisocoria) may be physiological and the difference in pupil size is constant in light or dark. A torchlight may then be shone in each eye and the direct response to light observed. The light is then alternately shone in each eye, with the torch swinging backwards and forwards from eye to eye; this tests for relative afferent pupil defect. When the torch is shone in the healthy eye, the pupil constricts. However when the torch is then swung across to the eye with a sensory defect the pupil of this eye paradoxically dilates. This is because limited neural stimulation is produced by light shining in the defective eye and the dominant effect is the withdrawal of light from the healthy eye. Pupil dilatation in both eyes results and is observed in the defective eye. Motor pupil defects such as those seen following anticholinergic eye drop instillation or a III nerve palsy result in an absent pupil reaction to any stimulus.

RETINOSCOPY

The focusing of the eyes may be measured at any age using a streak retinoscope. Anticholinergic eye drops are instilled to dilate the pupil and relax the ciliary muscle so that there is no accommodation. In Caucasians cyclopentolate 1% eyedrops may be used, with measurements performed 30 min after instillation. In children with dark brown eyes it may be necessary to use atropine 1% eyedrops or ointment, instilled on two or more occasions a number of hours before the examination. A streak of light is directed into the pupil area and movement of the pupil light reflex is observed when the streak of light is moved from

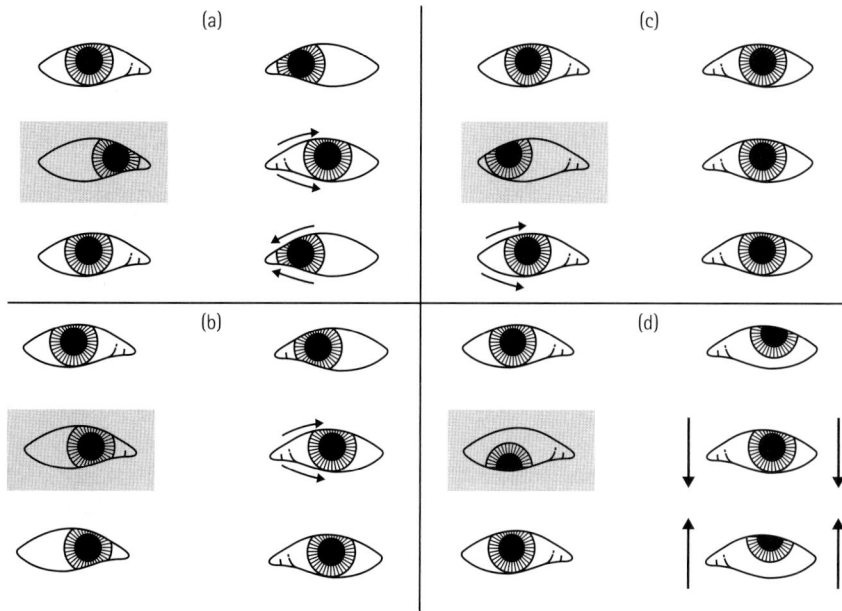

Fig. 31.9 The cover test for squint. Where there is no squint and there is normal binocular vision, both eyes maintain steady fixation on a distant object. There will be no deviation when one or other eye is covered and this is the basis of a cover test. When there is a latent or manifest squint some deviation will be observed on occluding one or other eye. (a) In manifest convergent squint the squinting eye is turned in and the nonsquinting eye maintains fixation. If the squinting eye is occluded in the cover test there will be no variation in the angle of squint, but when the nonsquinting eye ('fixing eye') is occluded it converges and the squinting eye takes up fixation. When the occluder is removed the original position of the eyes is resumed. (b) In alternating convergent squint either eye can maintain fixation while the other eye is turned in. If the squinting eye is occluded there is no alteration in the angle of deviation, but when the 'fixing eye' is occluded the opposite eye fixes the distant object and the previously straight eye converges. The former position is not resumed when the occluder is removed and the previously squinting eye maintains fixation (and the previously straight eye converges) until the occluder covers the originally squinting eye, when the originally fixing eye takes up position. (c) In latent squint both eyes will fix on a distant object but when one eye is covered it deviates. When the cover is removed the eye with the latent squint resumes fixation. The other eye does not shift or lose fixation while the opposite eye is being covered or uncovered. (d) The cover test is used to diagnose vertical squint as in horizontal squint, e.g. in left hypertropia the left eye is elevated (or the right eye depressed) and when the fixing eye is covered the opposite eye moves vertically to take up fixation.

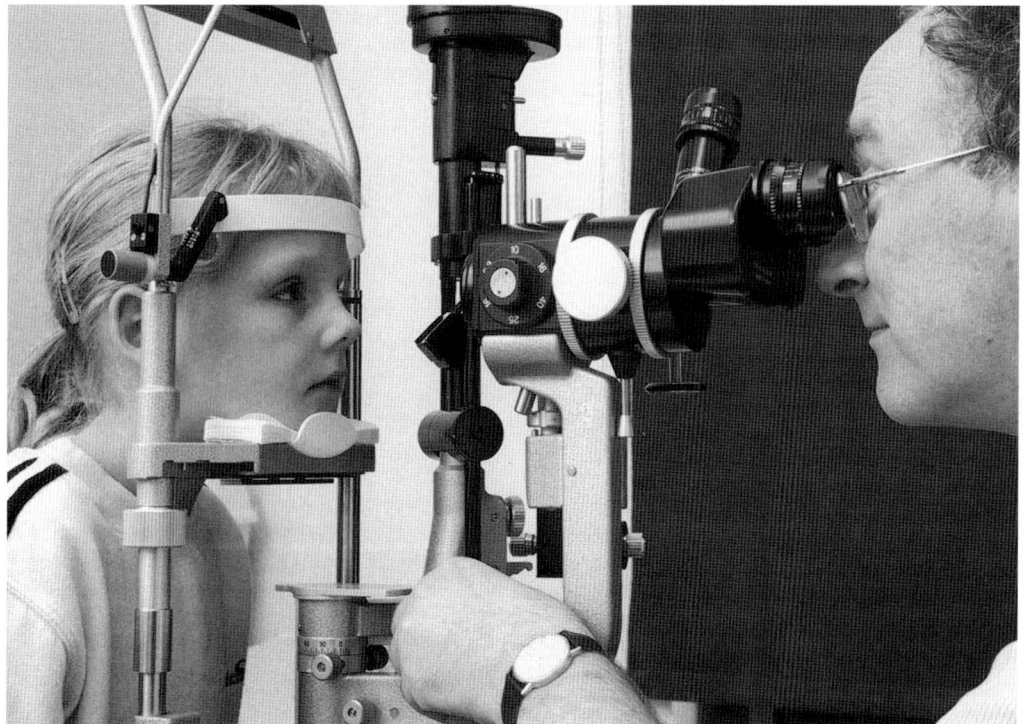

Fig. 31.10 The slit lamp is a binocular microscope with an illuminating light in the form of a slit. This enhances stereoscopic viewing of tissues.

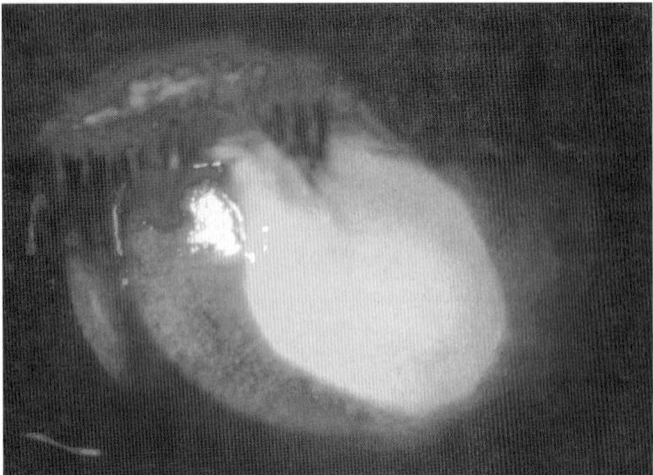

Fig. 31.11   Yellow/green fluorescein staining of an area of cornea abrasion visualized using blue light.

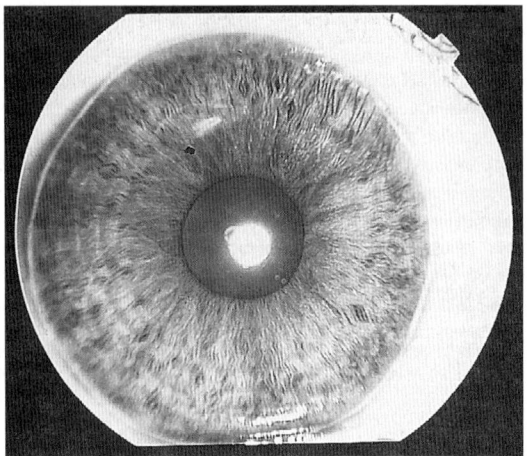

Fig. 31.12   Posterior embryotoxon. The edge of the basement membrane of the corneal endothelium is visible as a fine white line just inside the edge of the cornea. This is termed 'posterior embryotoxon'. This line is normally more peripheral, and therefore not visible.

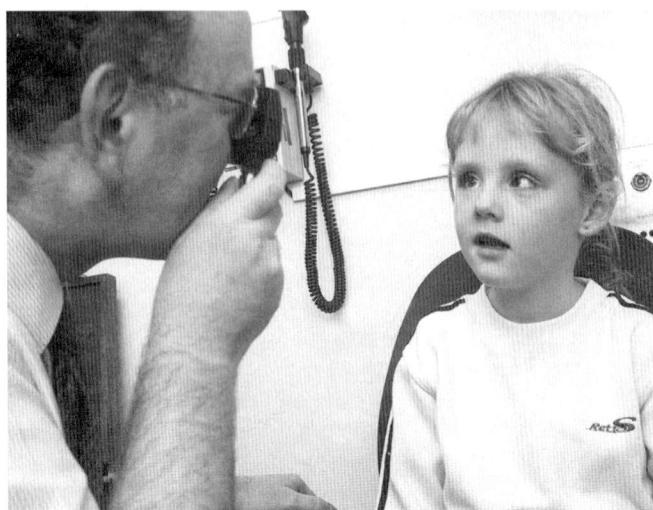

Fig. 31.13   Pupil red reflex testing using a direct ophthalmoscope. This is normally performed in a dimly lit room.

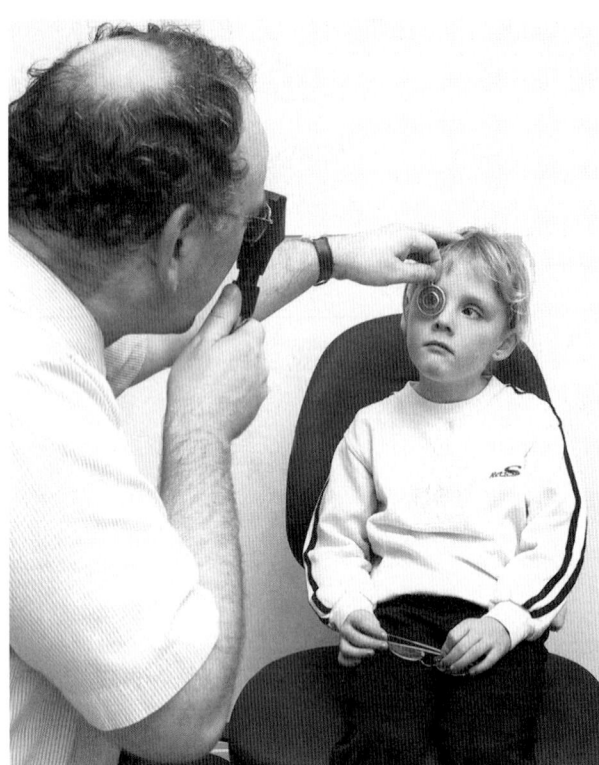

Fig. 31.14   Retinoscopy measurement of eye focusing.

side to side. A test spectacle lens is then held in front of the eye and the process is repeated (Fig. 31.14). The power of the lens that neutralizes movements of the pupil light reflex gives a measure of the focusing of the eye.

OPHTHALMOSCOPY

The fundi may be examined with the pupils dilated. Fundus examination of infants and young children is difficult with a direct ophthalmoscope. Ophthalmologists prefer to use an indirect ophthalmoscope. The light source is worn on the head and a convex lens is held in front of the eye in order to produce a focused image of the fundus (Fig. 31.15). The optic disc, macula, retinal vessels and retinal periphery may be examined. In older children, more detailed examination of the optic disc may be performed using a slit lamp microscope, in conjunction with a high powered convex lens. This allows detailed stereoscopic examination of the optic disc.

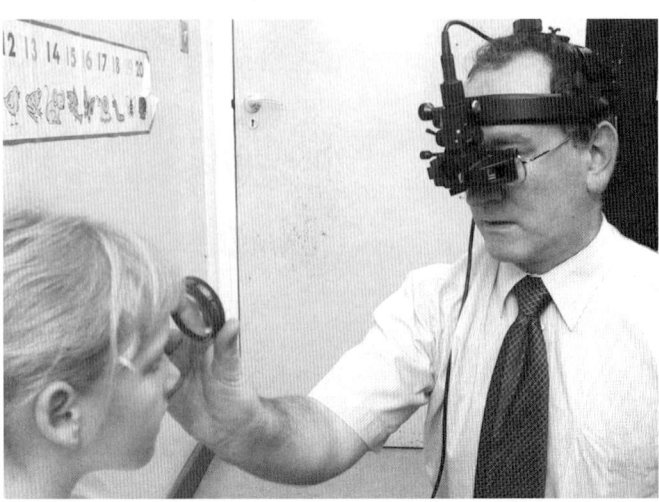

Fig. 31.15   Binocular indirect ophthalmoscope examination of the fundus.

SPECIALIZED METHODS OF EXAMINATION

ULTRASOUND

Ultrasound imaging may be used to examine the retina when the media are opaque due to cataract or other pathology (Fig. 31.16). The diameter of tumors such as retinoblastoma may be measured. High-definition ultrasound scans may be used to image the optic nerve head and optic nerve. Optic nerve head drusen may be detected. Widening of the cerebrospinal fluid (CSF) space around the optic nerve may be helpful in the diagnosis of raised intracranial pressure with papilledema.[9]

FUNDUS FLUORESCEIN ANGIOGRAPHY

Angiogram photographs of the retinal blood vessels may be obtained using i.v. or oral fluorescein dye (Fig. 31.17). This technique may be of value in assessing retinal vascular disease, retinal inflammatory disease and optic disc abnormalities. In the presence of optic disc edema, capillaries on the surface of the optic disc are dilated and leaky (Fig. 31.18). Optic nerve head drusen 'autofluoresce'–angiogram fluorescence is seen in the absence of fluorescein dye.

ELECTROPHYSIOLOGY STUDIES

Studies of the visual system using visually evoked potentials (VEPs) and of the retina using the electroretinogram may be of great diagnostic value in infants and young children with reduced vision. The stimulus for a VEP is a flash of light or a reversing pattern of black and white squares (Fig. 31.19). Pattern onset stimulation may be used as an

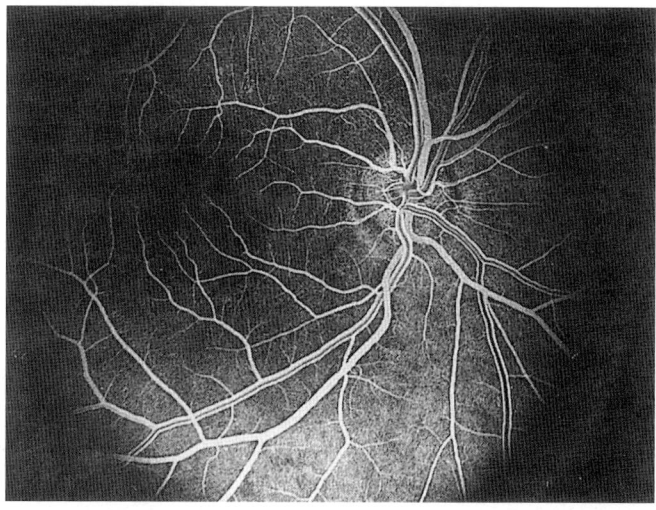

Fig. 31.18   Fluorescein dye is seen in the retinal arteries and capillaries 12 s after i.v. injection. Dye is starting to return to the veins.

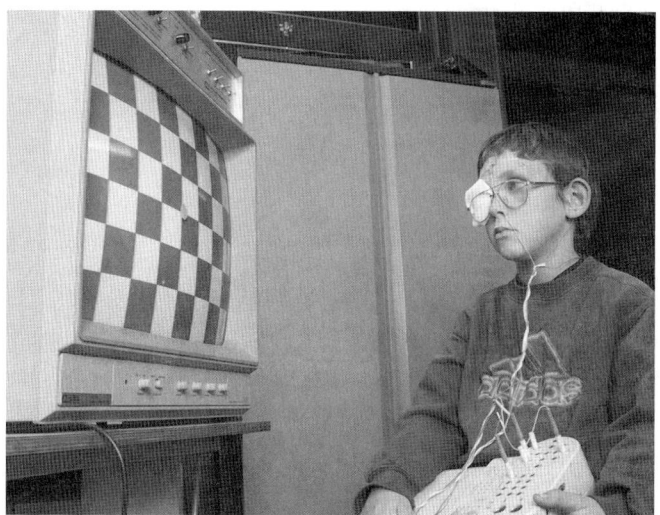

Fig. 31.19   Visually evoked potential examination using a reversing checker pattern stimulus.

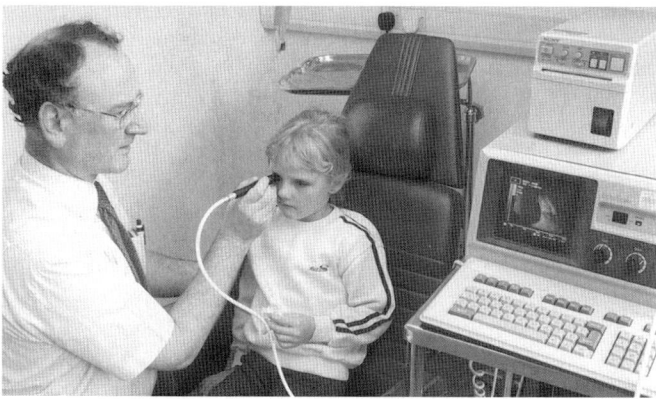

Fig. 31.16   Ocular ultrasound examination.

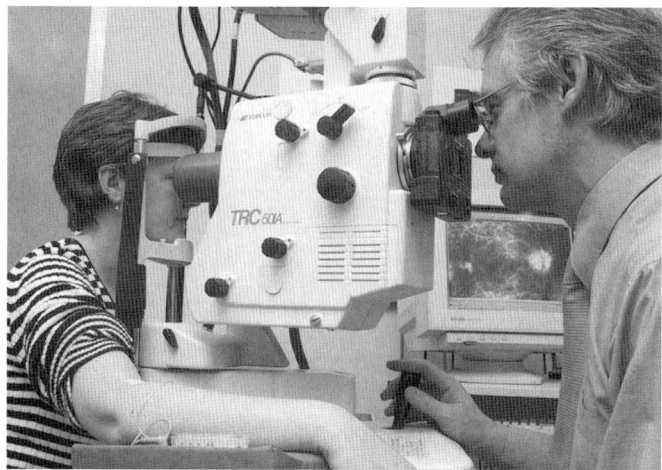

Fig. 31.17   A digital fundus camera images the retina following i.v. injection of fluorescein dye.

alternative to pattern reversal. Uniocular testing and hemifield testing may be performed. The occipital cortex response is detected using electroencephalogram (EEG) electrodes. Delayed VEP response following stimulation of one eye may indicate optic nerve demyelination on that side, while reduced amplitude may indicate reduced axonal function as in optic nerve hypoplasia (Fig. 31.20). In albinism there is increased chiasmal nerve crossing, which produces asymmetrical occipital cortex responses to uniocular stimuli.

VEPs may be used to measure visual acuity in infants. Statistical analysis of a rapid sequence ('sweep') of checker pattern sizes is used to produce an estimate of visual acuity.

The electroretinogram (ERG) gives information about retinal function. The stimulus is a flash of light. The response is detected by skin electrodes on the eyelids or by ocular contact electrodes.[10] The electrical response is generated in the retina – the 'a' wave by the photoreceptors and the 'b' wave by the inner retina. Cone function and rod function may be analyzed separately by using a range of test strategies in which the background illumination is varied and the light flash stimulation is varied. Rod responses are measured using dim flash stimuli after dark adaptation (scotopic responses). Cone responses are measured in normal lighting conditions (photopic responses) (Fig. 31.21). 30 Hz flicker stimuli are used to isolate cone responses. The individual components of

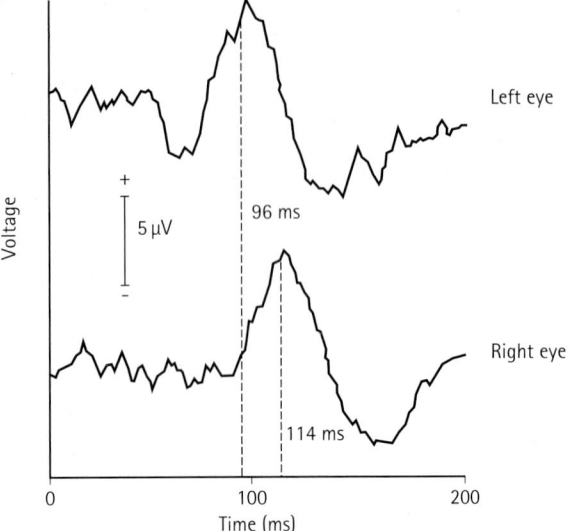

Fig. 31.20 Pattern reversal visual evoked response. The VER of two eyes where the left eye (upper trace) shows a normal pattern and there is a slight delay in the right eye (lower trace).

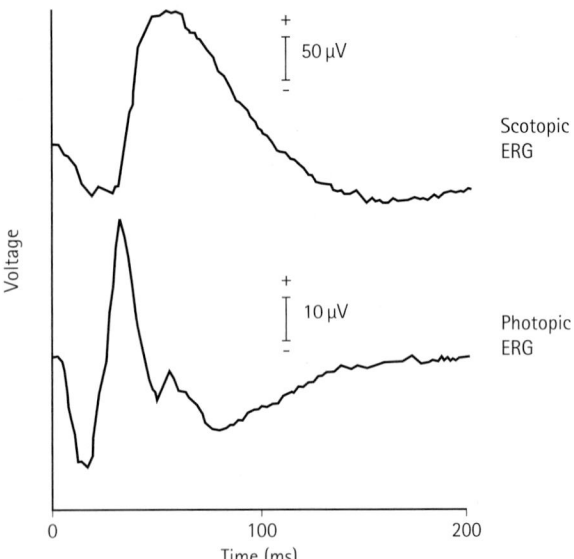

Fig. 31.21 A normal electroretinogram (ERG) showing the typical wave pattern and amplitude. The electroretinogram is taken under photopic (light adapted) conditions and scotopic (dark adapted) conditions. The wave pattern is reduced or abolished in various pathological conditions of the retina.

the ERG are best seen in the bright flash response following dark adaptation. Diseases that predominantly affect rod function produce abnormal scotopic ERG responses. Diseases that predominantly affect cone function produce abnormal photopic and 30 Hz flicker ERG responses. Diseases that predominantly affect the inner retina produce abnormal ERG b-wave responses.

REFRACTIVE ERRORS AND AMBLYOPIA

REFRACTIVE ERRORS

Refractive errors may be treated with spectacles. However the presence of a refractive error may also be of diagnostic importance. Leber's congenital amaurosis is often associated with hypermetropia,[11] and Marfan syndrome[12] with myopia.

In hypermetropia, additional accommodation is used to maintain clear focus. This may lead to excessive convergence of the eyes and is a common cause of convergent squint. In myopia, distance vision is blurred but near vision is in focus. Astigmatism causes irregular focusing due to the toric (oval) curvature of the corneal surface.

Most infants are slightly hypermetropic, which normally resolves by age 2 years – 'emmetropization'.[13] Hypermetropia present after the age of 2 years normally persists into adult life. Myopia is rare in young children. When high degrees of myopia do occur an underlying disease such as homocystinuria,[14] Marfan syndrome[12] or Stickler syndrome[15] should be considered. While refractive errors are relatively uncommon among schoolchildren in resource limited countries,[16] the incidence of myopia among schoolchildren is rapidly increasing in resource rich countries.[17,18]

AMBLYOPIA

When one eye is more hypermetropic than the other, accommodation produces a clear image in the more normal eye. However the retinal image in the more hypermetropic eye remains blurred, as accommodation amplitude is under bilateral neural drive. Untreated, occipital cortex synaptic connections related to the hypermetropic eye will remain underdeveloped.[19] This is termed 'anisometropic amblyopia'.

When a squint develops, the brain suppresses vision from the squinting eye in order to avoid diplopia. However continued suppression leads to failure of development of synaptic connections in the occipital cortex and once again the affected eye becomes amblyopic – strabismic amblyopia.[19] Anisometropic and strabismic amblyopia may coexist.[20]

The treatment of amblyopia is to first treat the underlying cause with glasses.[21] Occlusion of the normal eye is then used to drive development of synaptic connections relating to the amblyopic eye (Fig. 31.22). Atropine eyedrops may be used to blur vision in the normal eye, as an alternative to occlusion (atropine penalization).[21]

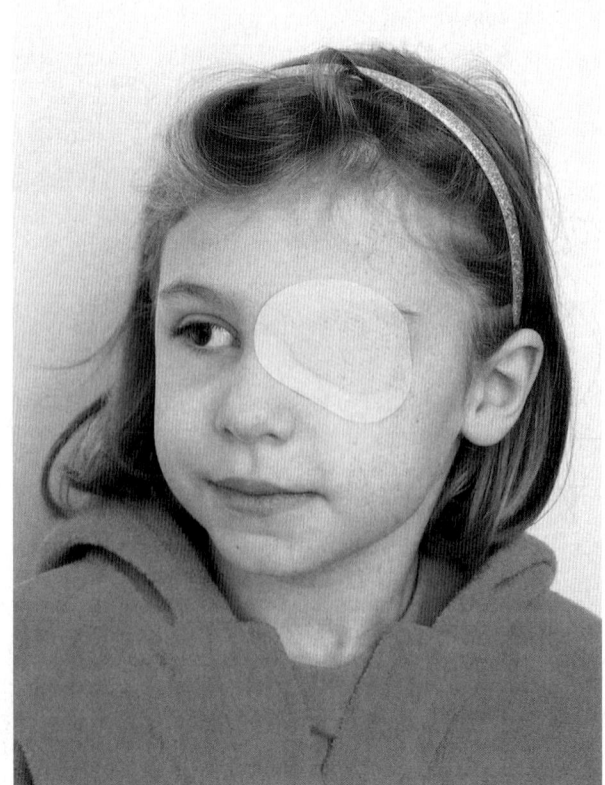

Fig. 31.22 Occlusion treatment.

Community visual screening programs are used to detect amblyopia. These are particularly necessary for the detection of anisometropic amblyopia, which is generally asymptomatic. Visual acuity measurements in each eye detect reduced vision in the amblyopic eye and lead to referral for assessment and treatment.[22] Screening may also detect small angled strabismus with amblyopia. Photographic techniques, which use pupil light reflex patterns to measure refractive errors, are an alternative approach to community screening.[23]

CEREBRAL VISUAL IMPAIRMENT

CNS disease is the most common cause of visual impairment in children.[24,25] Causes of cerebral visual impairment (CVI) in children are given in Table 31.1. A wide spectrum of severity and type of impairment may occur. Damage to the anterior visual pathways, optic radiations and occipital cortex lead to reduced visual acuity and limited visual fields. Damage to visual association areas also causes significant impairment in children, which is often under-recognized. Two key pathways associated with visual processing are the 'ventral stream' and the 'dorsal stream.'[26]

The ventral stream connects the primary visual cortex with the fusiform gyri of the inferior temporal lobes. An 'archive' of learned images is held in this area. Children with ventral stream dysfunction may have difficulty recognizing faces, shapes and objects. They may also have difficulty with orientation in familiar environments.

The dorsal stream connects the primary visual pathway with the posterior parietal lobes, and associated pathways. Dorsal stream structures subserve visual attention and visually guided motor functions. Visual attention refers to the ability to analyze complex visual scenes, concentrate on specific elements of these scenes, and suppress other elements in order to avoid distraction. Ability to suppress auditory and tactile input is an additional requirement of visual attention.

Dorsal stream structures also provide information about orientation in three-dimensional space. Connections to the motor cortex guide limb movements and connections to the frontal eye fields guide saccadic eye movements.

Timing of insult

The pattern of CVI impairment in an individual child is largely determined by the timing of the insult. Preterm infants typically sustain ischemic injury to the periventricular white matter and associated pathways (periventricular leukomalacia – PVL) following neonatal periventricular haemorrhage.[27] Symptoms emerge at about the age of 2–5 years. Reduced visual acuity, inferior visual field defects, nystagmus, and diplegia may be present. Dorsal and ventral stream impairments frequently occur. The optic discs show an enlarged physiological cup, which may be due to transsynaptic degeneration of fibers synapsing in the lateral geniculate bodies.

Damage to the visual pathways and to the dorsal and ventral streams occurs in relation to perinatal or antenatal insult in term infants. A variable combination of visual acuity, visual field and dorsal and ventral stream impairments occur. Optic atrophy may occur as a result of the primary insult or secondary to posterior visual pathway damage. Many of these infants also develop cerebral palsy.

Ischemic injury in children after infancy typically results in watershed infarcts of the cerebral cortex, especially the occipital cortex. The pupil responses are preserved. Variable degrees of optic atrophy may be present. Nystagmus is usually not present.[28] The VEP may be normal or abnormal. The visual defect may be total initially, but there is variable improvement with time, dependent on etiology and severity. Most children achieve some navigational vision. Recovery when it does occur may take from a few hours to 2 years. Full recovery has been reported after head injury and cardiac arrest, but is less likely after bacterial meningitis and does not occur in children with neurodegenerative disorders.

Ocular motor defects and CVI

Impaired eye movement control causes further visual difficulties for children with CVI. Strabismus, nystagmus, dystonic movements, impaired pursuit movements and impaired saccadic movement control may occur. In addition poor control of accommodation may lead to significant blurring of vision, especially for near tasks. Spectacles to correct hypermetropia and accommodation deficits are often helpful.[29]

Coping strategies for children with CVI

Educational approaches to help children with visual impairment are given in the section entitled 'Education of visually impaired children'. Symptoms due to inferior visual field loss may be aided by using a tilted work board so that the child may look directly at written material rather than looking down. An awareness of reduced visual field to one side will ensure that parents and teachers introduce objects of interest (including themselves) in seeing areas.

Dutton has developed behavioral strategies to reduce the impact of dorsal and ventral stream impairments, and these are given in Table 31.2.[26]

Table 31.1 Causes of cerebral visual impairment

Prenatal	Brain malformations
	Intrauterine infections
	Placental dysfunction
Preterm neonatal	Preterm neonatal periventricular haemorrhage
Perinatal	Neonatal asphyxia
	Intracerebral hemorrhage
	Meningitis
	Encephalitis
Postnatal	Trauma (accidental and non-accidental)
	Cardiac arrest
	Meningitis
	Encephalitis
	Neurodegenerative disorders

Table 31.2 Cerebral visual impairment – ventral stream and dorsal stream defects and suggested coping strategies (modified from Dutton et al.[26])

Defects	Suggested coping strategies
Ventral stream	
Impaired recognition of familiar faces	Verbal introduction; wear color/shape identifiers
Impaired orientation in familiar environment	Orientation training using cues and pathway markers
Dorsal stream	
Confused by complex ('busy') visual scenes	Store toys separately
	Store clothes separately (in transparent containers)
	Use plain carpets, bed covers and wall decoration
Difficulty identifying an individual in a group	Wave and speak
Disorientation in crowded environment	Train to use landmarks
	Visit shops when they are quiet
Reading	Mask surrounding text
Visually guide movements – upper limbs	Occupational therapy training strategies for reaching
Visually guide movements – lower limbs	Use tactile guide to height of ground – push a toy pram or bicycle, hold elbow or clothing of accompanying person
Distraction, leading to frustration at school and home	Limit visual and auditory 'clutter' in order to enhance concentration
Lose visual attention and bump or trip when talking or listening while walking	Keep quiet while walking

STRABISMUS

TERMINOLOGY

The term 'strabismus' and 'squint' are used interchangeably. 'Strabismus' is preferred. The prefix 'eso' is used for convergent deviations, and 'exo' for divergent deviations. 'Hyper' refers to upward deviation of an eye and 'hypo' to downward deviation. A 'tropia' is a manifest strabismus, which is present in binocular viewing conditions and is detected using the cover test. A 'phoria' is a latent strabismus, which is only apparent when binocular viewing is disrupted. The word 'deviation' is used to include both tropias and phorias. In 'concomitant' strabismus the deviation angle is the same in all directions of gaze. In 'incomitant' strabismus the deviation angle may be greater in one direction of gaze – for example in the direction of action of a paretic muscle. Adduction refers to medial movement of one eye, towards the nose, and abduction to lateral movement of one eye. 'Primary position' refers to the straight-ahead viewing position.

'Pseudosquint' refers to the appearance of apparent esotropia due to wide epicanthic skin folds. No true ocular deviation is present when a cover test is performed.

There are three common types of concomitant strabismus in childhood.

INFANTILE ESOTROPIA

This type of convergent strabismus becomes apparent at age 3–4 months (Fig. 31.23). Infants who have developmental neurological problems are at increased risk of developing infantile esotropia. The typical characteristics of infantile esotropia are a large angled convergent strabismus, which alternates between the eyes. There is no amblyopia as each eye is alternately used. There is no significant refractive error in most cases. Hypermetropia is present in some cases. The lateral recti may appear to be weak, as the infant habitually tends to use the right eye to look to the left side and vice versa ('cross fixation'). This may lead to the suspicion of bilateral VI cranial nerve weakness. Occlusion of one or other eye for 20–30 min will usually reveal normal abduction of the uncovered eye rather than VI palsy.

A characteristic type of nystagmus may be present, termed 'manifest latent nystagmus'. In this form of nystagmus, the nystagmus is exaggerated by covering one eye. The uncovered eye develops a jerking nystagmus with the jerk towards the side of the fixing eye.

When present, hypermetropia should be treated with spectacles.[30] Very early surgery, performed during infancy, improves binocular function outcome.[31]

ACQUIRED ESOTROPIA

Children who are hypermetropic habitually use extra accommodation in order to maintain clear focus. As accommodation and convergence reflexes are linked, this may lead to excessive convergence. Loss of control of convergence will lead to a convergent strabismus. The treatment is to promptly provide full spectacle correction.[32] This may reverse the condition. However if the strabismus does not fully reverse, occlusion treatment for amblyopia and surgical treatment may be needed. The use of preoperative prism spectacles improves the accuracy of surgical outcome.[33]

A late onset acquired esotropia may be mistakenly diagnosed as an acute VI nerve palsy. Patients with acute onset of esotropia should be assessed by an ophthalmologist as this may lead to prompt curative spectacle treatment rather than to a series of neurological investigations. Conversely concomitant convergent strabismus may be a presenting feature of VI nerve weakness due to a brainstem glioma, raised intracranial pressure or other pathology. A high index of suspicion for underlying neurological disease must therefore be maintained.

INTERMITTENT EXOTROPIA

The third common cause of strabismus in children is intermittent exotropia. In this condition binocular control is maintained at times but at other times one eye deviates laterally. The child may close the deviating eye in order to concentrate when using the straight eye. Vision is normal in each eye. Usually there is no significant refractive error and no treatment is needed unless the child is significantly symptomatic, in which case surgical correction may be undertaken.[34]

CONVERGENCE WEAKNESS

Weakness of convergence is usually an isolated abnormality, and can be treated with orthoptic convergence exercises.

STRABISMUS AS A SIGN OF UNDERLYING ORGANIC DISEASE

All cases of strabismus should be promptly assessed, as both convergent and divergent strabismus may be a presenting feature of underlying neurological disease (Table 31.3). Mild VI cranial nerve weakness can cause apparently concomitant strabismus.

INCOMITANT STRABISMUS

Weak lateral rectus function is the most common cause of incomitant strabismus. VI cranial nerve weakness should be considered in all cases (Table 31.4).

Table 31.3   Conditions that may present with (apparent) concomitant strabismus

Retinoblastoma
Optic nerve hypoplasia
Optic atrophy:
Primary
Secondary to neoplasm
Unilateral cataract
Persistent fetal vasculature
VI cranial nerve weakness

Table 31.4   Causes of true or apparent VI nerve weakness in children

VI cranial nerve paresis:
Raised intracranial pressure
Brainstem glioma
Moebius syndrome
Duane's syndrome
Esotropia (abduction is usually normal)

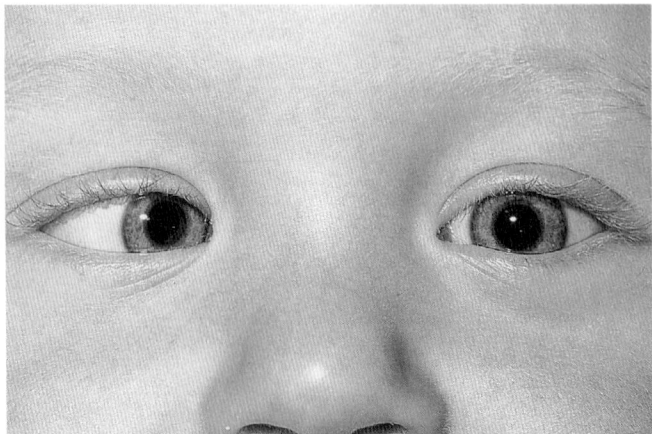

Fig. 31.23   Infantile esotropia. The right eye was converging when the photograph was taken.

Incomitant strabismus syndromes
Duane syndrome
In Duane syndrome VI cranial nerve innervation of the lateral rectus muscle is variably defective, and an anomalous branch of the III cranial nerve supplies the lateral rectus muscle. On attempted abduction there is variable lateral rectus weakness, which may be mistaken for VI cranial nerve palsy caused by acquired neurological disease. On attempted adduction of the eye the medial rectus and lateral rectus muscle co-contract and the eye retracts into the orbit, with narrowing of the palpebral aperture. A number of associated neurological deficits, including partial sensorineural deafness, are associated with Duane syndrome.

Surgical treatment is reserved for those children who develop a significant compensatory head turn (towards the side of the affected eye), or strabismus in primary position.[35]

Moebius syndrome
Moebius syndrome consists of congenital absence of cranial nerve nuclei, including the VI and VII nerve nuclei. Abduction is absent in each eye, and there is bilateral facial palsy.

Brown syndrome
In Brown syndrome there is a congenital anomaly of superior oblique tendon and trochlea function. When the affected eye is adducted it shoots downwards. The condition is usually treated conservatively as some spontaneous recovery may occur. In severe cases superior oblique tendon surgery may be performed.

Congenital superior oblique tendon laxity
Weakness of superior oblique function in children (and adults) is more commonly caused by congenital laxity of the superior oblique tendon than by IV cranial nerve paresis. Typically there is a compensatory head tilt to the opposite side. This may be mistaken for sternomastoid muscle induced torticollis. Eye movement examination reveals weakness of the affected superior oblique, with secondary overaction of inferior oblique function. Surgery may be performed if there is a significant compensatory head posture, or strabismus in primary position. The lax tendon may be tucked, or the overactive inferior oblique muscle may be weakened by recession surgery.

PUPIL ABNORMALITIES

Children presenting with unequal pupil size (anisocoria) tend to cause great concern to both the parents/carers and clinicians. In practice, intracranial pathology is uncommon. The most common cause is physiological anisocoria; other causes include III nerve palsy, Horner syndrome, previous blunt trauma or dilating eye drops.

The examination should be directed at determining the presence or absence of ptosis, eye movement abnormalities such as III palsy and other cranial and peripheral nerve palsies. In physiological anisocoria, the difference in pupil size is proportionately the same in bright or dim lighting.

III (OCULOMOTOR) PALSY

There is usually a marked or complete ptosis and restriction of eye movements. The eye is typically turned down and outwards. The pupil on the affected side may be enlarged. Causes include congenital (usually idiopathic), head injury, and tumors. Prompt neuroimaging is indicated in acquired cases.

HORNER SYNDROME

Horner syndrome is caused by reduced sympathetic nerve supply to the eye and comprises a partial ptosis with a small (miosed) pupil. Most cases in children are congenital. Acquired cases require prompt investigation for possible abdominal neuroblastoma. In Horner syndrome, the anisocoria is more pronounced in dim light due to failure of the affected pupil to dilate.

NYSTAGMUS
CONGENITAL IDIOPATHIC NYSTAGMUS

In congenital idiopathic nystagmus the onset of nystagmus occurs between the ages of 2 and 3 months. Some cases are familial – dominant, recessive and X-linked inheritance has been described. An underlying vision defect should be excluded. Typically the nystagmus is horizontal and the amplitude is greater on looking to one side and less on looking to the other side (null zone). Head nodding may be present. Ocular examination is otherwise normal and there are no neurological abnormalities. The ERG and VEPs are normal. On follow up, near vision develops to a relatively normal level. There is moderate reduction of distance vision and some modification of the classroom environment is often helpful. Treatment consists of spectacle correction of refractive errors. Surgical treatment may produce some benefit in selected cases,[36] and medical treatment with gabapentin is currently under investigation.[37]

SENSORY DEFECT NYSTAGMUS

Infants with congenital nystagmus may have an underlying vision defect. In most cases an ocular abnormality is present and a systematic approach to ocular and electrophysiological examination is required. A differential diagnosis is given in Table 31.5. In general, posterior visual pathway defects do not result in nystagmus.[28] Periventricular leukomalacia is an exception to this rule.[27]

ALBINISM

Albinism refers to a group of conditions that may be divided into oculocutaneous albinism (OCA) and ocular albinism (OA). The ocular abnormalities found are common to all forms of albinism. In addition to defective iris and fundus pigmentation, abnormalities include: reduced vision and photophobia; nystagmus; strabismus; delayed visual maturation; foveal hypoplasia and abnormal chiasmal crossing. More than 90% of fibers cross at the chiasm, resulting in cortical asymmetry of VEP responses. Iris translucency varies in severity and relatively minor defects of iris pigmentation may only be detected by slit lamp transillumination performed in a dark room. Most forms of OCA are autosomal recessive. Two rare forms of OCA are associated with systemic disease – increased susceptibility to infection in Chediak–Higashi disease[38] and frequent bruising due to platelet dysfunction in Hermansky–Pudlak syndrome.[39]

In ocular albinism typical ocular abnormalities are present, but skin and hair color are normal.

Refractive errors should be corrected with spectacles, and photophobia reduced with tinted spectacles and peaked hats. Mainstream education, with some attention to the classroom environment, and normal educational attainment may be anticipated in almost all cases.

ANIRIDIA

Aniridia is an autosomal dominant condition caused by mutations in the PAX 6 homeobox gene. About 30% of cases are sporadic, with deletions at 11p13. Sporadic cases have a high incidence of associated abnormalities, including Wilms tumor,[40] genitourinary abnormalities and mental retardation. Abdominal palpation and/or abdominal ultrasound examination should be performed in all new cases and as part of follow up.

Table 31.5 Causes of sensory congenital nystagmus

Albinism
Leber's amaurosis
Aniridia
Optic nerve hypoplasia
Retinal cone dystrophy

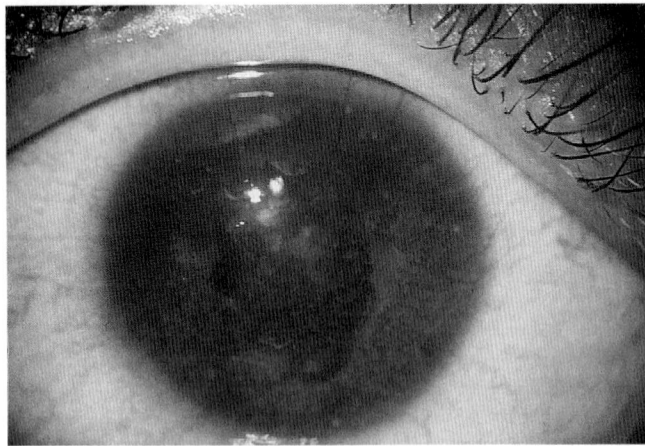

Fig. 31.24 Aniridia. No iris tissue is seen. There is fibrovascular pannus covering the peripheral cornea in this case.

Aniridia represents a defect of neural crest cell development. In addition to the striking absence of iris tissue, with only very rudimentary stubs of iris tissue present, the following ocular abnormalities are frequently seen: nystagmus, fibrovascular corneal pannus, refractive errors, glaucoma, cataract, foveal hypoplasia and optic nerve hypoplasia (Fig. 31.24). Foveal hypoplasia refers to poorly differentiated foveal structures; in extreme cases major retinal blood vessels may cross the normally avascular fovea. Corneal disease is due to defective limbal stem cell function, and responds to stem cell transplant surgery. Glaucoma surgery outcomes are limited by conjunctival scarring. Cataract surgery is also complicated, because of absent iris tissue and weak lens zonules. Progressive loss of vision over decades is usual in aniridia patients.

ACQUIRED NYSTAGMUS

Acquired nystagmus in childhood always requires prompt ophthalmic and neurological assessment. A differential diagnosis is given in Table 31.6. Vertical nystagmus may consist of downbeat nystagmus, associated with craniocervical junction abnormalities, or more rarely upbeat nystagmus, associated with brainstem and cerebellar lesions. Urgent neurological investigation, including brain imaging, is required in all cases of acquired nystagmus.

SPASMUS NUTANS

Spasmus nutans is a syndrome of infancy with nystagmus, head nodding and torticollis. Investigation to exclude an intracranial tumor is required. The syndrome resolves after 12–18 months and the diagnosis is one of exclusion, made retrospectively.

THE APPARENTLY BLIND INFANT

A carer's concern for an infant's vision is usually reliable. Infants with poor visual behavior require urgent assessment by an ophthalmologist. Treatable disease such as cataract must be dealt with promptly in order to avoid the development of irreversible amblyopia. In most cases the

Table 31.6   Causes of acquired nystagmus in children

Suprasellar tumor
Posterior fossa tumor or malformation
Neurodegenerative diseases such as:
Batten's disease
Neurolipososes
Peroxisomal disorders

Table 31.7   Ocular defects that may cause bilateral congenital blindness

Whole globe	Anophthalmos
	Microphthalmos
Cornea	Sclerocornea
	Peter's anomaly
Lens	Cataract
Retina	Retinal detachment (e.g. following retinopathy of prematurity)
	Retinal dysplasia (e.g. Norrie's disease)
	Chorioretinal coloboma
	Chorioretinitis scarring
	Cherry red spot in storage diseases (e.g. Tay–Sachs disease)
Optic atrophy	Prenatal:
	Infection
	Asphyxia
	Cerebral malformations
	Perinatal:
	Asphyxia
	Postnatal:
	Meningitis/encephalitis
	Compression (e.g. hydrocephalus, craniopharyngioma)
	Genetic (e.g. autosomal dominant optic atrophy)
	Secondry to retinal disease
Optic nerve hypoplasia	
Optic disc colobomas	

Table 31.8   The blind infant with apparently normal eyes

Delayed visual maturation
Cerebral visual impairment
Leber's congenital amaurosis
Retinal cone dystrophy
Optic nerve hypoplasia
Oculomotor praxia

cause is apparent following ophthalmic examination. Ocular defects that may cause bilateral congenital blindness are given in Table 31.7.

In some cases there may be no ocular abnormality evident, or only very subtle defects are found (Table 31.8). In these cases electrophysiological and neurological investigations may be required.

DELAYED VISUAL MATURATION

Delayed visual maturation (DVM) refers to visual unresponsiveness from birth that subsequently improves.[41] The diagnosis is one of exclusion and is always retrospective. The onset of visually stimulated smiling is delayed; clinical pupil responses are normal and there is no nystagmus.

LEBER'S CONGENITAL AMAUROSIS

Leber's congenital amaurosis (LCA, isolated infantile rod–cone dystrophy) is an autosomal recessive congenital retinal dystrophy.[42] Vision is absent or severely reduced from birth and the ERG is markedly reduced or absent. The pupils may show a sluggish afferent response. Refraction usually shows significant hypermetropia. The fundus appearances are normal or near normal. The term 'Leber's congenital amaurosis' should be reserved for cases of isolated infantile rod–cone dystrophy, and the diagnosis of Leber's congenital amaurosis should only be made after

Table 31.9 Syndromes associated with infantile rod–cone dystrophy

Cerebellar vermis hypoplasia, e.g. Joubert's syndrome
Deafness, e.g. Usher's syndrome type 1
Renal disease, e.g. nephronophthisis
Skeletal abnormalities
Peroxisomal disorders, e.g. Zellweger syndrome
Mitochondrial cytopathies, e.g. hydroxyacyl-CoA
   dehydrogenase deficiency
Amino acid disorders, e.g. methylmalonic aciduria

exclusion of other recognized syndromes (Table 31.9). Hearing, neurological, renal and metabolic abnormalities should be sought.

While no active treatment for LCA is possible at present, gene therapy trials are under development.[43] Genetic counseling and molecular diagnosis are therefore required.

OPTIC NERVE HYPOPLASIA

Optic nerve hypoplasia (ONH) is not inherited, and most cases are idiopathic. Insults in early embryonic development have been associated with ONH – maternal diabetes, maternal alcohol and other substance abuse. ONH may occur in isolation or in association with failure of development of the anterior midline structures of the brain (septo-optic dysplasia [SOD]), hydranencephaly, porencephaly, cerebral atrophy or leukomalacia. ONH also occurs in aniridia. A genetic basis has been identified in a small number of cases of SOD.[44] Severe bilateral cases are associated with neuroendocrine dysfunction. Hypoglycemia may occur in the neonatal period. Sudden infant death may occur as a result of an abnormal stress response to febrile illness. All cases should be referred for endocrine investigation. In addition to abnormal cortisol response, growth, thyroid and gonadotrophic hormones may be defective. Magnetic resonance imaging (MRI) is useful as a predictor of neuroendocrine dysfunction and allows assessment of optic nerve size.

There is a spectrum of severity ranging from complete blindness with very tiny optic nerve structures to virtually normal vision with very minor degrees of ONH. Cases may be unilateral, bilateral or asymmetric.

Mild cases present later in childhood. The optic disc appearances vary (Fig. 31.25) and include:
- variably small optic disc;
- peripapillary pigmented ring (double ring sign);
- slightly tortuous retinal vessels;
- associated optic atrophy;
- segmental disc hypoplasia.

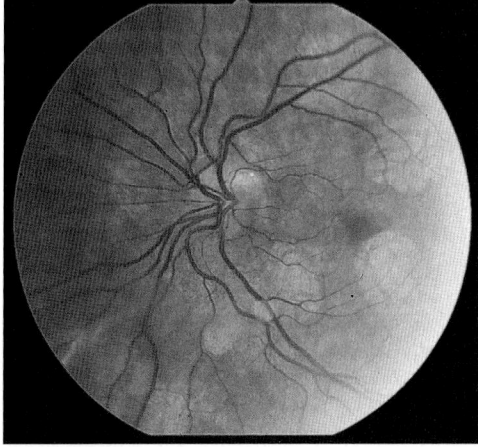

Fig. 31.25 Hypoplastic disc. Optic nerve hypoplasia. The optic disc is anatomically very small in this case, with severely reduced vision.

Mild cases present with reduced vision in one or both eyes, or with strabismus. Mild degrees of optic nerve hypoplasia may be misdiagnosed as amblyopia, and cases of amblyopia that do not respond well to occlusion treatment should always be carefully examined for the presence of subtle optic nerve hypoplasia.

OCULOMOTOR APRAXIA

Absent saccadic eye movements may be mistakenly interpreted as defective visual function. The ERG is reduced in some cases,[45] further increasing the possibility of misdiagnosing Leber's congenital amaurosis. Once the child is able to support and move their head, characteristic side-to-side head thrusting movements develop. These head movements are used as a substitute for voluntary saccadic eye movements.

ACQUIRED VISUAL LOSS IN CHILDREN

Acquired visual loss at any age requires urgent investigation. Uniocular visual loss may result in the development of strabismus. Binocular visual loss will lead to impaired visual behavior and, in older children, a complaint of reduced vision. In most cases, acquired visual loss is due to retinal, optic nerve or neurological disease (Table 31.10). When the cause is not evident on ophthalmic examination, neurological, electrophysiological, and neuro-imaging assessment will be needed.

CATARACT

Bilateral cataract developing in later childhood is rare. Metabolic disorders such as diabetes mellitus and disorders of galactose metabolism should be excluded.[46]

RETINAL DYSTROPHIES

This term refers to genetic abnormalities of the retina or retinal pigment epithelium that lead to reduced retinal function. Rod dysfunction presents with reduced vision, especially in dim lighting conditions. Cone dysfunction presents with reduced vision, photophobia, and reduced color vision. Fundus examination may show pigmentary disturbance. When the rods are predominantly affected, black spiky

Table 31.10 Causes of visual loss in children evident on ophthalmic examination.

Cataract	Metabolic disease		
Retina	Retinal dystrophies	Rod–cone dystrophies X-linked juvenile retinoschisis Stargardt's disease	
Optic atrophy	External compression	Hydrocephalus Tumor	Craniopharyngioma Other suprasellar tumors
	Intrinsic tumor	Glioma	Neurofibromatosis type 1
	Retinal diseases		
	Genetic	Autosomal dominant optic atrophy	
	Demyelinating diseases		

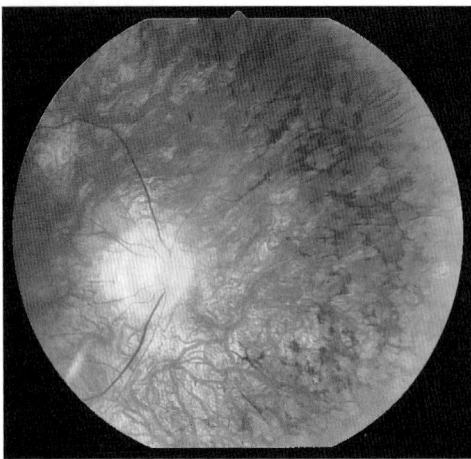

Fig. 31.26   Retinitis pigmentosa. Typical 'bone spicule' pigmentation is seen in the mid-periphery of the fundus.

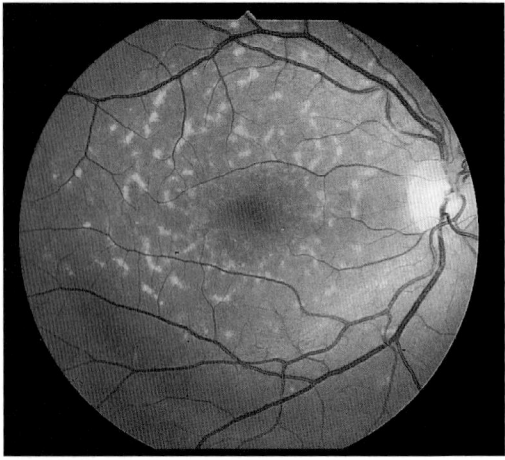

Fig. 31.28   Stargardt disease. Typical creamy fishtail-shaped flecks are seen in the fundus. There are no macular pigment changes in this case.

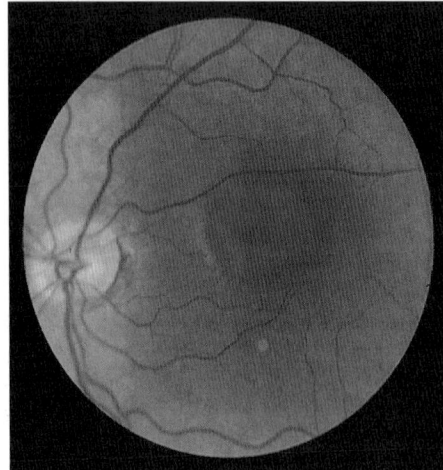

Fig. 31.27   Retinal cone dystrophy with typical 'bull's eye' pigmentation at the center of the macula.

blotches of pigment are seen in the retinal periphery (bone spicule pigmentation) (Fig. 31.26). This appearance leads to the historical term 'retinitis pigmentosa'. When the cones are affected pigmentation may be present at the macula, often in a ring shape (bull's eye) (Fig. 31.27). The diagnosis is made on clinical grounds, supported by electroretinogram abnormalities of rod and cone functions.

Most types of retinal dystrophy are currently not treatable. Two rare forms of rod-cone dystrophy of childhood are amenable to treatment. In Refsum disease serum phytanic acid levels are raised. Dietary intervention will improve the prognosis for vision and also reduce morbidity due to other systemic features of the disease. In abetalipoproteinemia, vitamin and dietary treatment improve the prognosis.

STARGARDT DISEASE

Stargardt disease is an autosomal recessive disease with onset in late childhood. Symptoms are limited to reduced visual acuity, with no symptoms of night blindness or of photophobia. Typically there are creamy fishtail-shaped flecks in the retina (fundus flavimaculatus) with additional retinal pigment epithelium atrophy at the macula (Fig. 31.28). The disease progresses until visual acuity is reduced to about 6/60.[47]

AUTOSOMAL DOMINANT OPTIC ATROPHY

The finding of reduced vision and optic atrophy should lead to prompt neurological and neuroimaging investigations. In autosomal dominant optic atrophy neurological investigations are normal. The condition is associated with defects in the OPA1 gene.[48] There is reduced visual acuity, some reduction of color vision, reduced visual field sensitivity between fixation and the blind spot ('centrocaecal scotoma'), reduced amplitude pattern VEP, and variable pallor of the temporal part of the optic disc. Visual loss is not severe, and progression is very slow.

CHILDHOOD VISUAL LOSS WITH NO ABNORMALITY ON OPHTHALMIC EXAMINATION

BATTEN DISEASE (JUVENILE NEURONAL CEROID LIPOFUSCINOSIS)

The neuronal ceroid lipofuscinoses (NCLs) are a group of autosomal recessive neurodegenerative lysosomal storage diseases. While classification by age of disease onset has been helpful in the past, more precise molecular genetic diagnosis is now possible.[49] The majority of cases of juvenile NCL have a mutation in the CLN3 gene. These cases may present with visual loss.[50] Neurological degenerative symptoms may not develop for up to 3 years later. The diagnosis must therefore be considered in any child aged 4–10 years with visual loss that cannot be explained on ophthalmic examination. The fundi may initially appear normal. The ERG is reduced, and typically shows an electronegative waveform. Later a pigmentary disturbance develops at the macula. The disease is progressive, with epileptic seizures and dementia. No treatment is currently available.

FUNCTIONAL VISUAL LOSS

A relatively common cause of apparent reduction of vision in young teenagers is 'functional' visual loss. Symptoms are precipitated by stress. Typically the child complains of blurred vision. On examination there are no objective abnormalities. The diagnosis can be made if the child is 'tricked' into giving normal visual acuity test results by using neutralizing combinations of spectacle lenses or other means. Having made the diagnosis, psychological counseling may be helpful. Underlying problems at school or in the home may be detected. The prognosis is usually good, as the underlying psychological disturbance tends to be relatively minor. When a positive diagnosis cannot be made, follow up and investigations to exclude other causes of visual loss are necessary.

DISEASES OF ORBITAL AND OCULAR TISSUES

ORBITAL DISEASE

Congenital abnormalities of skull development

A number of craniosynostoses have ocular features. Crouzon, Apert and Pfeiffer syndromes result in shallow orbits, which can lead to corneal exposure. Hydrocephalus is common in these conditions and regular optic disc examination is required. Visual loss may also occur because of amblyopia secondary to refractive errors and strabismus.[51] Complex horizontal and vertical strabismus patterns are frequently present. Strabismus surgery may be considered after corrective skull surgery has been performed.

Symptoms and signs of orbital disease

Symptoms of orbital disease include reduced vision, diplopia and altered appearance. Signs include proptosis, which may be axial (forward protrusion of the eye in the axis of the orbit) or non-axial. The pattern of non-axial proptosis gives useful clues to the site of orbital disease. For instance, if the eye is deviated laterally, it is likely that the site of orbital disease will be medial. Eye movements may be reduced. Visual acuity may be reduced and there may be sensory abnormalities of pupil reactions.

Preseptal cellulites

Preseptal cellulitis refers to eyelid cellulitis that does not extend beyond the orbital septum into the orbit. The eye appears normal and vision remains normal. While the infection may be related to local skin infection or local skin trauma, this form of cellulitis is commonly secondary to sinus infection with *Haemophilus influenzae* or *Streptococcus aureus* and is part of the spectrum of orbital cellulitis.[52] An orbital computerized tomography (CT) scan may be indicated when severe eyelid swelling prevents adequate eye examination. Treatment is with i.v. antibiotics.

Orbital cellulitis

True orbital cellulitis is much less common than preseptal cellulitis. The orbit becomes inflamed with proptosis of the eye, reduced eye movement and reduced vision. Prompt and effective treatment must be instituted as orbital cellulitis may lead to orbital or even brain abscess. Most cases are secondary to ethmoidal sinusitis. Since the advent of *H. influenzae* vaccination, streptococci sp. have become the most common organisms responsible.[53] Blood cultures should be performed and an orbital CT scan should be performed. Treatment is with broad-spectrum i.v. antibiotics covering Gram positive, Gram negative and anaerobic organisms. Visual acuity should be monitored regularly. An otolaryngologist should be involved in all cases as urgent sinus drainage may be needed in order to protect vision.[54]

Orbital tumors

Capillary hemangioma, venous-lymphatic malformations and dermoid cysts are the most common orbital masses in infants and children under the age of 2 years.

Capillary hemangiomas grow rapidly during the first 6 months of life, stabilize, and then regress at age 3–8 years. Superficial lesions are a typical 'strawberry' color (Fig. 31.29); deeper lesions have a bluish appearance. The diagnosis may be made clinically, and CT or MRI scans may be used to delineate the extent of the lesion. Visual loss is usually related to amblyopia,[55] but can be due to optic nerve compression or corneal exposure. Amblyopia may be due to occlusion of the pupil, or astigmatism in the axis of the lesion. Treatment is conservative when there is no threat of amblyopia. However lesions that occlude the pupil or cause significant astigmatism may require early intervention to prevent amblyopia. Intralesional depot steroids or even systemic steroids may be used.[55] Surgery is normally deferred until maximal spontaneous regression has occurred at about age 8 years.

Venous-lymphatic malformations present with proptosis in childhood, which may be abrupt if bleeding occurs into a cystic space. While the

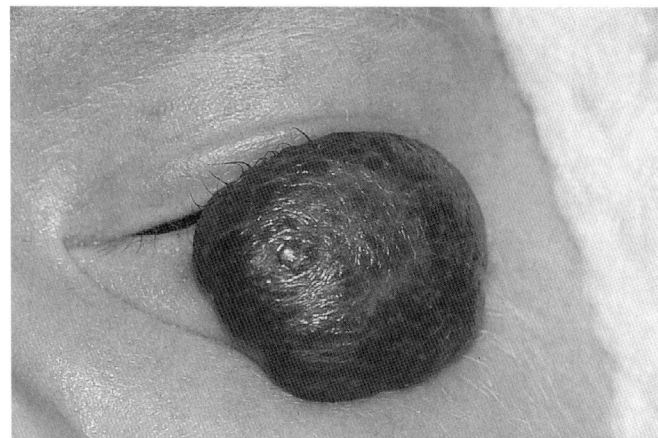

Fig. 31.29   Capillary hemangioma of the lower eyelid.

lesions consist of venous-like vascular channels they are not directly connected to the venous system.[56] They may be delineated by CT or MRI scan. Unlike capillary hemangiomas they do not regress with age. Surgical intervention is unsatisfactory and most lesions are best treated conservatively.

Dermoid cysts may be superficial or deep. Superficial lesions are most often found at the upper outer angle of the orbit. Having excluded a deeper component of the lesion by clinical examination, ultrasound examination, MRI or CT scan, excision may be performed. Deeper lesions tend to present with proptosis, at a later age. Conservative treatment is often appropriate.[57]

Rhabdomyosarcoma is the commonest malignant orbital tumor of childhood and usually develops between the ages of 4 and 12 years. The tumor enlarges rapidly with increasing proptosis, mild redness and edema of the eyelids and reduced eye movements.[58] The diagnosis is made by biopsy, and as much tissue as possible should be removed for examination. A direct approach to the lesion should be performed, as tumor seeding may occur in the biopsy track. Depending on clinical stage, chemotherapy with or without radiotherapy is the initial treatment. Orbital exenteration may be needed if primary treatment fails.

EYELID ABNORMALITIES

Epiblepharon refers to the presence of a fold of skin near the lower eyelid margin, which may cause inturning eyelashes (Fig. 31.30), most commonly affecting oriental infants. The natural history is spontaneous resolution during the first 1–2 years of life and surgery is reserved for severe cases.

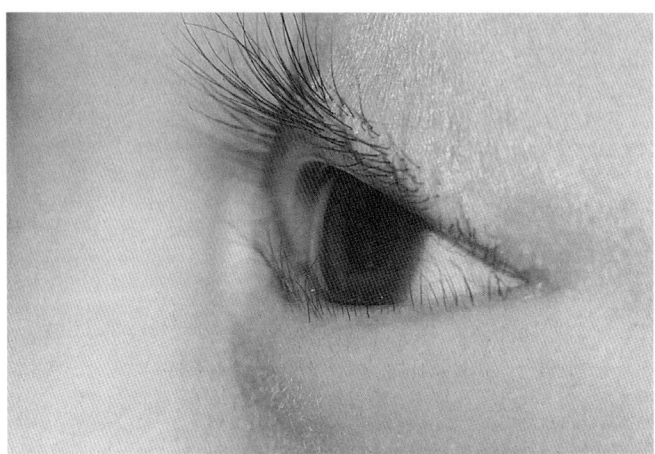

Fig. 31.30   Epiblepharon.

Blepharitis refers to inflammation of the eyelid margins. This is a relatively common condition in older children and in adults. Hot bathing and eyelid margin toilet using cotton tipped buds may be effective. When secondary staphylococcal infection is present, treatment with topical fucidic acid cream is indicated. In a small number of cases corneal inflammation with vascularization and scarring may develop, and topical steroid therapy may be needed to control this process.

A *tarsal cyst* is a retention cyst of an oil-producing meibomian gland of an eyelid. These cysts resolve spontaneously over a period of months. Surgical drainage is indicated in the minority of cases in which significant eye discomfort is present.

CONGENITAL PTOSIS

Dystrophic changes of the levator muscle of one or both upper eyelids will result in drooping of the upper eyelid, termed 'ptosis' (Fig. 31.31). Congenital III nerve palsy and Horner syndrome should be excluded. Congenital Horner syndrome is associated with neuroblastoma.[59] The jaw winking (Marcus Gunn) phenomenon should be sought – lateral movements of the jaw produce synkinetic movements of the ipsilateral upper eyelid.

If the pupil is occluded by ptosis, prompt surgery is indicated in order to prevent amblyopia. However in milder cases corrective surgery is best deferred until teenage years, when cooperation with surgery under local anesthetic may be obtained, leading to a better cosmetic result. Surgery generally involves advancement or resection of the levator aponeurosis.

LACRIMAL SYSTEM

CONGENITAL NASOLACRIMAL DUCT OBSTRUCTION

The nasolacrimal duct commonly has a persistent membranous occlusion at the distal end of the duct. This leads to watering (epiphora) of the affected eye or eyes. Epiphora is almost always first noticed during the first month of life. The fluorescein dye disappearance test is useful in diagnosis. A drop of fluorescein dye is placed in the conjunctival sac and the time taken for dye to clear is observed. Delayed drainage implies that the nasolacrimal duct is not patent. The natural history is spontaneous resolution of watering during the first 1–2 years of life. If watering persists beyond the age of 2 years, probing of the nasolacrimal duct may be undertaken.[60] While waiting for spontaneous resolution, the eyes should be bathed if they become sticky. Topical antibiotics need only be used if signs of active tissue inflammation are present.

LACRIMAL OBSTRUCTION IN OLDER CHILDREN

In some children, epiphora persists despite probing. In these cases intranasal anatomical abnormalities may be found.[61] Endoscopic exploration, with silicone intubation of the lacrimal system, is effective in 80% of cases.[62] Where severe anatomical occlusion of the nasolacrimal duct is present, dacryocystorhinostomy surgery may be required. However epiphora in older children is more often due to allergy or upper respiratory tract infection than to nasolacrimal duct occlusion.[63]

CONGENITAL ABNORMALITIES OF EYE DEVELOPMENT

The whole eye may be absent at birth (anophthalmos) (Fig. 31.32) or may be small (microphthalmos).

Orbital growth is partly stimulated by the volume effect of the eye. Orbital growth is reduced if an eye is removed during early childhood. Hydrophilic tissue expanders are therefore used to enhance orbital growth in cases of anophthalmos or severe microphthalmos.

Microphthalmos is commonly associated with coloboma due to embryonic optic fissure closure defects. Typically the inferior part of the iris is absent along with the inferior choroid and retina (Fig. 31.33). The optic disc may or may not be involved. Microphthalmos and coloboma may be isolated abnormalities, associated with chromosomal syndromes such as trisomy 13, or associated with a single gene defect such as choanal atresia with ear, eye, heart and genital defects (CHARGE) syndrome.[64]

CONJUNCTIVITIS

Neonatal conjunctivitis has been discussed in Chapter 12. Bacterial infection, viral infection, chlamydial infection and allergy may cause conjunctivitis in older infants and in children.

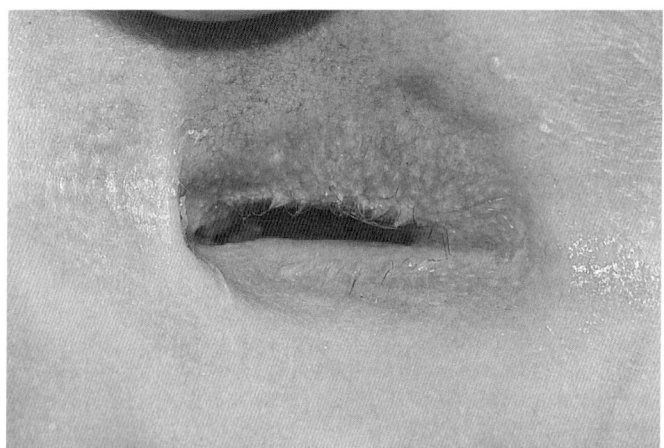

Fig. 31.32 Anophthalmos. No identifiable ocular structures are apparent.

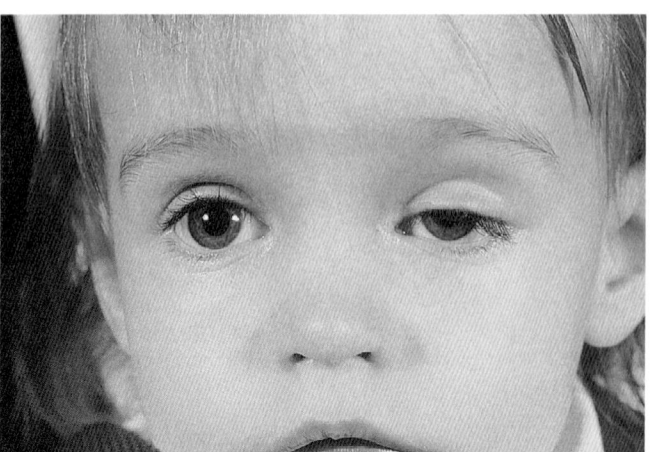

Fig. 31.31 Congenital ptosis of the left upper eyelid due to levator muscle dystrophy.

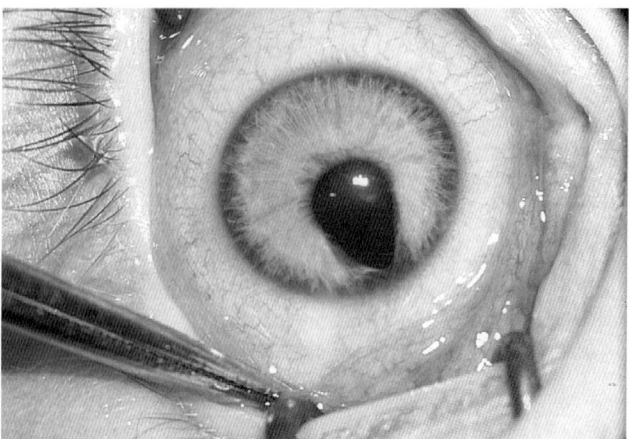

Fig. 31.33 Coloboma of the inferior iris.

Bacterial conjunctivitis produces a purulent discharge and is generally self-limiting – topical antibiotics are generally not indicated.[65] Viral conjunctivitis produces a watery discharge with a mucous component and is generally self-limiting. Chlamydial neonatal infection has been discussed in Chapter 12. In hot, dry countries with limited water supplies flies cause endemic chlamydial conjunctivitis – trachoma. Conjunctival scarring leads to dry eyes and eyelid scarring. Secondary corneal scarring follows, and remains a common avoidable cause of blindness worldwide. Prevention is by improved water supply and hygiene, and treatment of acute infection by community use of oral azithromycin.[66]

Chronic allergy in the form of vernal keratoconjunctivitis results in morbidity due to ocular discomfort and visual loss. Corneal scarring may be present along with papillary inflammation of the tarsal conjunctiva. Treatment is with mast cell stabilizers such as sodium cromoglycate, steroid eye drops, and topical cyclosporin eye drops. Topical steroid eye drops may cause glaucoma and cataract. Close supervision by an ophthalmologist is required.

Conjunctival dryness (xerosis) and corneal melting are features of vitamin A deficiency. Acute deficiency signs may be precipitated by intercurrent respiratory or gastrointestinal infection and urgent treatment with high doses of vitamin A is then needed.

CORNEAL DISEASE

Corneal scarring due to trachoma and vitamin A deficiency remains a leading cause of childhood blindness in resource poor countries.

In wealthy countries herpes simplex corneal infection is a relatively frequent cause of morbidity. Prompt treatment with topical antiviral drops or ointment (e.g. aciclovir) is usually sufficient to clear the infection, but in some cases areas of chronic inflammation and scarring of the cornea develop. Epidemics of adenovirus keratoconjunctivitis occur from time to time. While the condition is limited to viral conjunctivitis in most cases, some individuals develop inflammatory infiltrates deep to the corneal epithelium. Cautious use of topical steroids reduces symptoms, and reduces scarring.

Congenital corneal opacities due to dystrophies or as part of Peter's anomaly or sclerocornea are relatively rare. In bilateral cases corneal transplant surgery may be indicated. As with congenital cataracts, surgical treatment must be undertaken early if visual loss due to amblyopia is to be avoided. Corneal transplant surgery in infants, and the necessary intensive aftercare, are very demanding of the surgeon and the family and treatment is best undertaken in specialized referral departments.

Congenital limbal dermoids (Fig. 31.34) may occur in isolation or as part of a number of syndromes. They may be excised later in childhood. Surgery in infancy is generally not required.

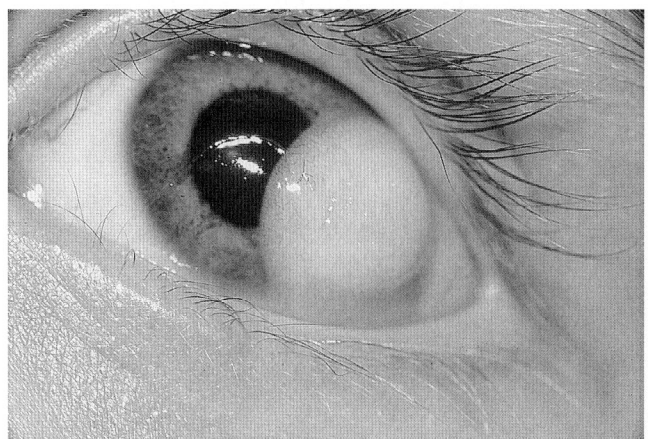

Fig. 31.34   Limbal dermoid.

UVEITIS

Uveitis screening is necessary in children with juvenile idiopathic arthritis (JIA) (Fig. 31.35). This is because the intraocular inflammation may be asymptomatic in its early stages, but untreated, may lead to glaucoma and cataract development. Slit lamp screening examination should be performed urgently when a diagnosis of JIA has been made. The groups at highest risk are those with oligoarticular disease and those who are antinuclear factor positive.[67] These children should be screened every 2–3 months initially. The children at lowest risk are children with systemic onset JIA, juvenile spondyloarthropathy and juvenile-onset rheumatoid factor positive arthritis. In these cases, screening is only required once, at disease onset. Children with other categories of JIA are at intermediate risk and should be examined every 3–4 months. Screening may generally be discontinued at age 12 years. Detailed guidelines for screening have been published by the American Academy of Pediatrics, and these are summarized in Table 31.11.[68] When iritis is detected, topical steroids and mydriatics may be used. Supervision of treatment by an ophthalmologist is needed because of the risks of glaucoma and cataract development due to steroid treatment. In more severe cases, or when there is a persisting topical steroid requirement, treatment with low-dose methotrexate, with mycophenolate or with the anti-TNF alpha agent infliximab may be required in order to reduce exposure to glucocorticoids and their side-effects.[69]

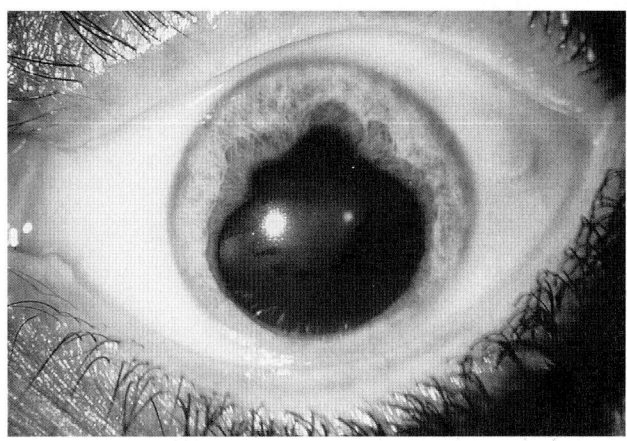

Fig. 31.35   Iritis. The pupil has been dilated and adhesions between the iris and lens (posterior synechiae) are seen.

Table 31.11   Guidelines for screening for uveitis in juvenile arthritis (taken from American Academy of Pediatrics guidelines.[68]

Juvenile arthritis subtype at onset	Age onset < 7 years	Age onset >/= 7 years
Oligoarticular, ANA positive	High	Medium
Oligoarticular, ANA negative	Medium	Medium
Polyarticular, ANA positive	High	Medium
Polyarticular, ANA negative	Medium	Medium
Systemic	Low	Low

Rules:
High risk = examinations 3–4 monthly
Medium risk = examinations 6 monthly
Low risk = examinations 12 monthly
Onset age < 7 years – risk becomes low 7 years after disease onset
Onset age >/= 7 years – risk becomes low 4 years after disease onset
All 'high risk' becomes 'Medium risk' 4 years after disease onset

CATARACT

Congenital cataract remains a major cause of childhood blindness worldwide (Fig. 31.36). In resource rich countries severe visual handicap due to congenital cataract is now rare because of improvements in surgical management.[24] The key to a satisfactory outcome is early detection and early surgery in order to avoid amblyopia.[70–72]

Two thirds of cases of congenital cataract are bilateral and one third unilateral.[73] Underlying causes or associated risk factors were present in 62% of bilateral and 8% of unilateral cases in a national UK study.[74] The causes of congenital cataract are given in Table 31.12. Every infant with congenital cataract should be examined for dysmorphic features or

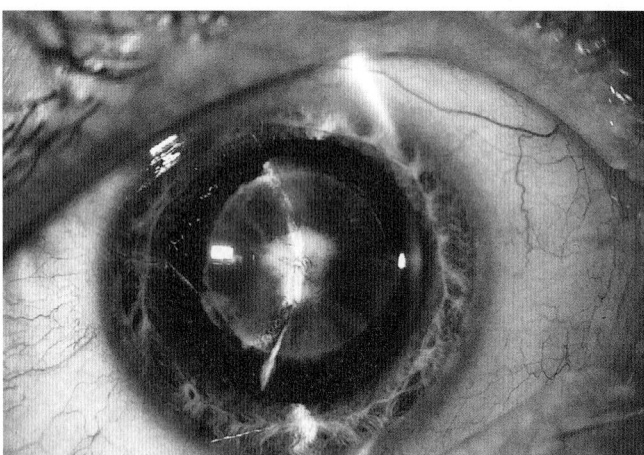

Fig. 31.36   Congenital cataract. This is a partial, lamellar cataract with relatively good vision. Surgery in infancy was not needed in this case.

Table 31.12   Causes of congenital cataracts

Idiopathic		
Isolated inherited	Dominant, recessive, X-linked	
Inherited syndrome	Chromosomal	Trisomy 21,13,18 Turner's Translocation 3;4 and 2;14 Cri du chat 5q15.2
	Mitochondrial diseases Lowe's oculocerebrorenal syndrome Ectodermal dysplasia	
Metabolic	Galactosemia Galactokinase deficiency Hypocalcemia Hypoglycemia Mannosidosis	
Prenatal infection	Rubella Toxoplasma Herpes simplex Varicella	
Trauma	Accidental Non-accidental	
Ocular associations	Microphthalmos Aniridia Persistent fetal vasculature Peter's anomaly Endophthalmitis	

evidence of metabolic disease. The parents should be examined for evidence of cataract as autosomal dominant cataracts may vary in disease expression.

Surgery should be performed within the first 6 weeks of life in order to ensure that optical rehabilitation has been completed by the age of 8–10 weeks.[73] Delayed detection and treatment will lead to irreversible visual loss due to amblyopia.[74] In bilateral cases the surgery is performed on one eye initially, with surgery to the second eye a few days later. There is uncertainty as to whether intraocular lens implants should be used at primary surgery.[76] An alternative to primary intraocular lens implantation is the use of contact lenses for primary optical correction, followed by secondary lens implantation at approximately age 2 years.

LENS SUBLUXATION

The most common cause of lens subluxation (Fig. 31.37) in children is Marfan syndrome.[75] The lenses tend to be subluxed from an early age and there is rarely any significant progression with time.[75] For this reason a single screening examination in early childhood is sufficient to detect lens subluxation and regular follow up is generally not required. The differential diagnosis includes homocystinuria.[76]

When lens subluxation occurs, treatment may be either optical or surgical. Surgical treatment generally involves removing the whole lens and using contact lenses or sutured intraocular lens implants for optical correction.[78]

GLAUCOMA

PRIMARY CONGENITAL GLAUCOMA

Primary congenital glaucoma typically occurs in boys between the age of birth and 2 years. Some cases are autosomal recessive and there is a one in 20 empirical recurrence risk in siblings. The presenting signs may be present in one or both eyes. Watering, photophobia and enlargement of the corneas occur (Fig. 31.38). The diagnosis is made by performing an examination under anesthetic and measuring the intraocular pressure; i.v. or i.m. ketamine sedation is preferred for these examinations as ketamine produces a small, predictable rise in intraocular pressure. In contrast inhalational anesthetics produce a variable lowering of intraocular pressure. Treatment is surgical and demanding. Multiple operations may be required and surgical treatment is better undertaken in a pediatric glaucoma referral center.

SECONDARY GLAUCOMAS

Glaucoma may be secondary to other congenital ocular abnormalities. These include Reiger syndrome (Fig. 31.39) and aniridia. Glaucoma may develop secondary to iritis and steroid therapy in patients with JIA.

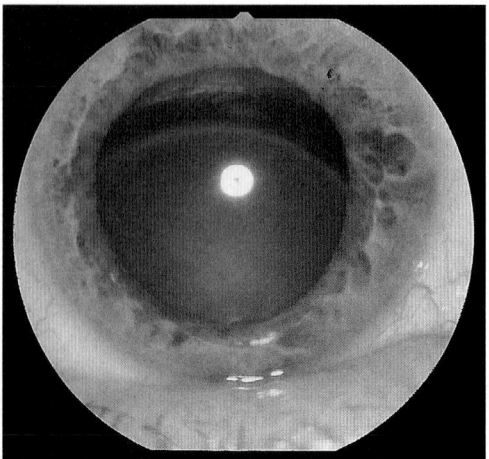

Fig. 31.37   Subluxed lens.

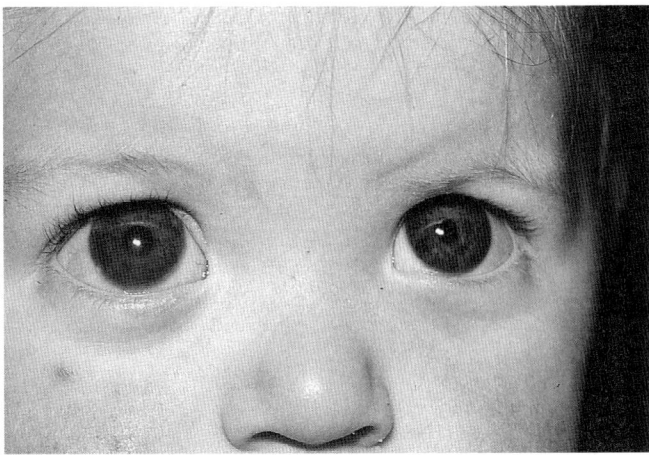

Fig. 31.38 Congenital glaucoma. Note enlarged corneas. This child had goniotomy surgery performed in infancy, which satisfactorily controlled the intraocular pressures.

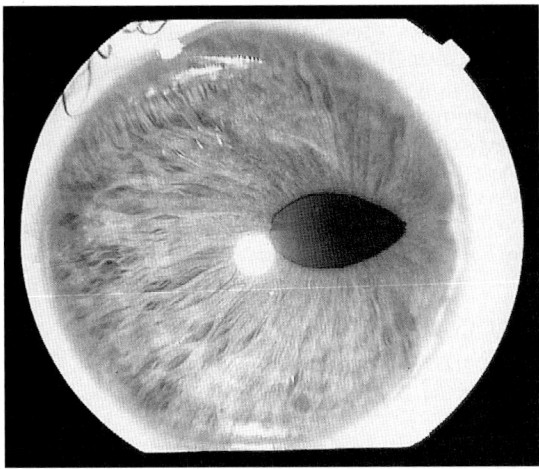

Fig. 31.39 Reiger syndrome. Note posterior embryotoxon and abnormal pupil shape and position (corectopia).

A particularly difficult form of childhood glaucoma is aphakic glaucoma in children who have had congenital cataract surgery.[79] Complex surgical treatment may be required.

Glaucoma may develop in Sturge–Weber syndrome, especially if the upper eyelid has a port wine stain lesion (Fig. 31.40).

RETINAL DISEASES

Retinal disorders, which cause bilateral visual loss in children, have been described earlier. Causes of unilateral retinal disease include those following.

COATS DISEASE

Coats disease is a primary retinal telangiectatic disease in which leaky vessels cause progressive accumulation of fatty deposits in the subretinal space (Fig. 31.41). Mutations in the gene for Norrie disease have been identified as the underlying cause.[81] The condition is diagnosed at a median age of 5 years, is more common in males and is almost always unilateral.[81] There are no systemic associations. Treatment with laser therapy or cryotherapy can reduce serous leakage and improve visual prognosis.[82]

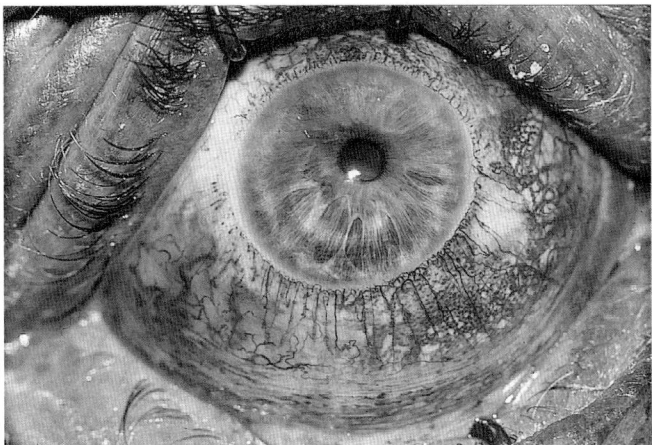

Fig. 31.40 Sturge–Weber syndrome. Note eyelid port wine stain, and abnormal scleral blood vessels.

RETINOBLASTOMA

Retinoblastoma (RB) is a malignant neuroblastic tumor of the retina, which normally develops during the first 2 years of life. Presenting signs include leukocoria (white pupil) and strabismus. Approximately 50% of cases are heritable, with a mutation of the RB1 tumor suppressor gene. In these cases, additional somatic mutations of allelic RB1 genes in retinal cells lead to loss of tumor suppressor function and neoplasia occurs. Tumors are usually multiple. Approximately 50% of heritable cases have a family history of retinoblastoma; the remainder represent new germline mutations.

In cases in which there is no germ-cell mutation, two mutations are needed to produce neoplasia in a retinal cell.[83] In these cases, the tumor is almost always solitary, with slightly later onset than heritable cases (median age 24 months compared to 12 months). However 15% of cases with solitary tumors have an underlying germ-cell mutation.

The diagnosis is made clinically. Typically the tumors have a creamy white appearance, are moderately vascular, and have areas of calcification (Fig. 31.42). The tumors tend to grow out from the retina into the vitreous ('endophytic') or grow underneath the retina ('exophytic'). Rarely the tumor diffusely infiltrates the retina. A relatively benign form of retinoblastoma – 'retinoma' – also exists. The age of onset is older, retinal pigment epithelium changes are seen surrounding the elevated gray retinal mass, and the tumor remains nonprogressive.

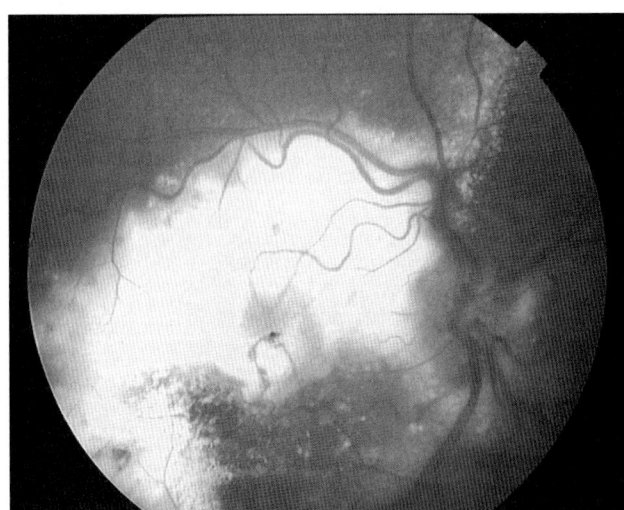

Fig. 31.41 Coats disease. Massive subretinal lipid exudation is seen at the macula, with severely reduced visual acuity.

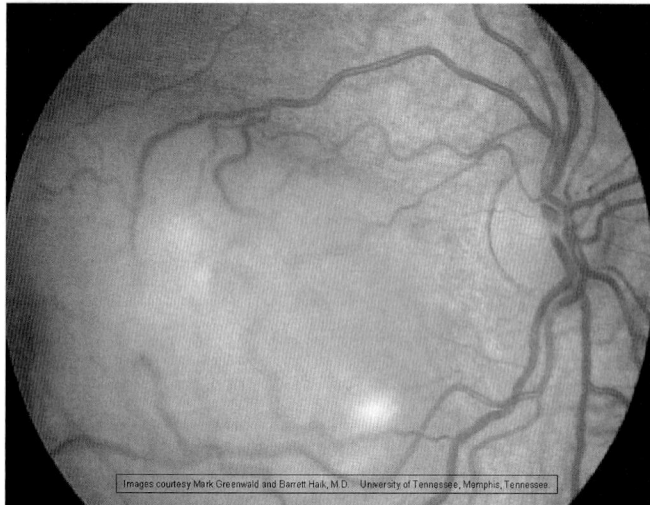

Fig. 31.42 Retinoblastoma. Creamy white tumor. Image taken with 'Retcam' digital fundus camera.

The differential diagnosis includes Coats disease, tuberous sclerosis, retinal hamartomas, Norrie disease, *Toxocara* infection, and, in diffuse cases, endophthalmitis. When the optic nerve is clinically in contact with retinoblastoma tissue, assessment will include examination of the CSF and imaging of the brain and orbits. The scan will delineate the extent of the tumor, and exclude a coexisting pineal tumor ('trilateral retinoblastoma'). The most common route of spread is along the optic nerve. In advanced cases blood spread to bone marrow may occur.

An ocular oncology team in specialized referral centers should undertake management.

A range of treatment modalities may be used. Primary enucleation surgery is indicated for advanced disease (Fig. 31.43). A long length of optic nerve should be removed with the eye, and a primary orbital implant placed within the muscle cone.

Chemotherapy is now the first-line treatment for bilateral cases, though it is often necessary to enucleate one eye later. Unilateral cases that have been detected at an early stage may also be treated with chemotherapy. Six cycles of cisplatin, etoposide and vincristine are given.[84] Additional treatment modalities are required in some cases. These include retinal laser therapy, retinal cryotherapy, plaque brachytherapy and external beam radiotherapy.[85]

Frequent follow-up examinations are performed in order to detect tumor regression, and to look for new tumors, which develop in 10% of cases.[86] If there has been no evidence of local or metastatic disease for 3 years after local disease control, cure is very likely. Long-term survival is over 95%.

Heritable cases will transmit the defective RB1 gene to 50% of offspring, with 90% penetrance. The risk of disease is therefore 45%. All cases should have molecular genetic testing for an RB1 gene mutation.[88] This includes cases of solitary tumor, as 15% of these cases have an underlying germline mutation. The siblings of cases and the offspring of cases should also have molecular genetic testing.[87] If a defect is detected, or when there is uncertainty about the genetic status of an individual, regular retinal examinations must be performed. The initial examination may be performed without general anesthetic soon after birth. Examinations under anesthetic are then performed every 2–4 months until age 2 years. At each examination the peripheral retina must be fully visualized using scleral indentation. Further examinations without anesthetic are then performed 4–6 monthly until age 5 years.

All heritable cases require long-term oncology follow up. The product of the RB1 gene is the retinoblastoma protein pRB. RB1 mutations normally result in no detectable pRB production. pRB is a phosphoprotein that is involved in cell cycle control and inhibits cell proliferation. Its function is tissue specific – RB1 mutations increase the risk of retinoblastoma, pineal tumors (which presents with hydrocephalus), osteogenic sarcoma (especially in the orbit following ocular radiotherapy for retinoblastoma),[88] other sarcomas, and some carcinomas. However the RB1 gene does not predispose to other childhood neoplasias such as leukemia.

TOXOCARA INFECTION

Toxocara infection of the retina may occur in early childhood either in subclinical infection or as part of a systemic illness. The nematode dies

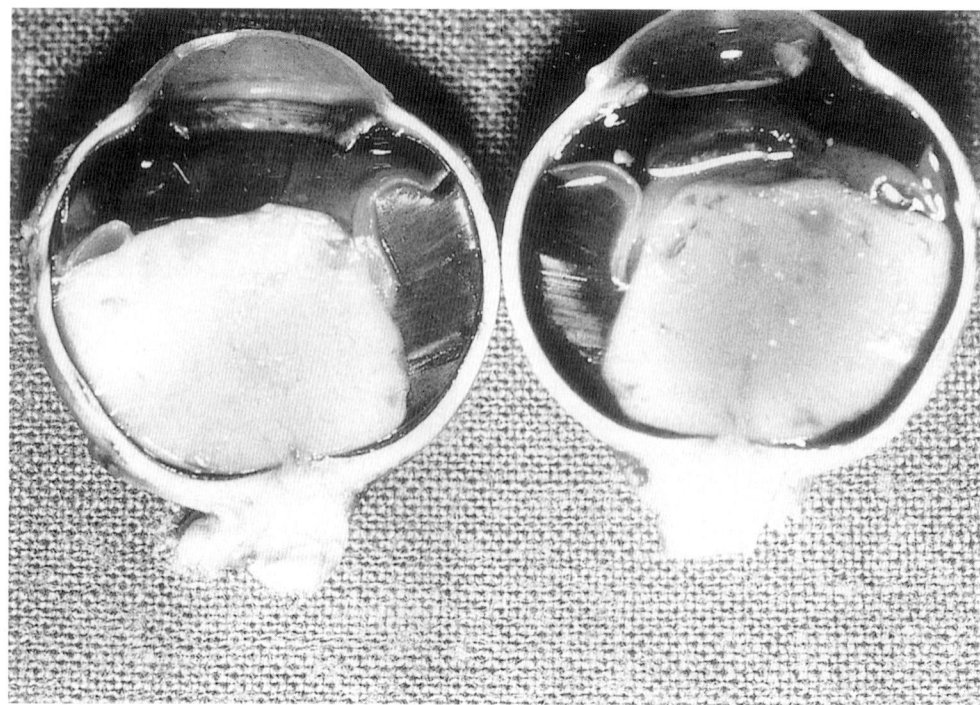

Fig. 31.43 An enucleated eye showing a large retinoblastoma causing detachment of the retina and almost filling the vitreous cavity.

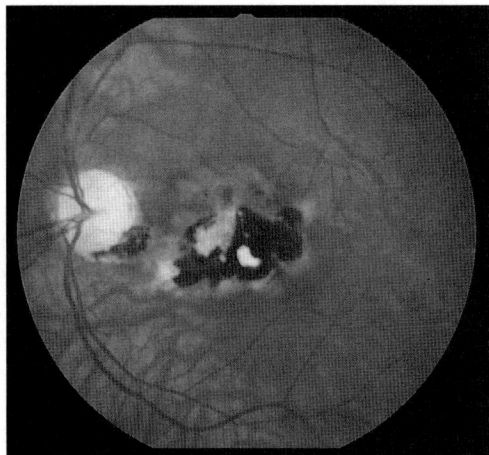

Fig. 31.44 Toxoplasmosis. Pigmented scar at macula. No active inflammation present.

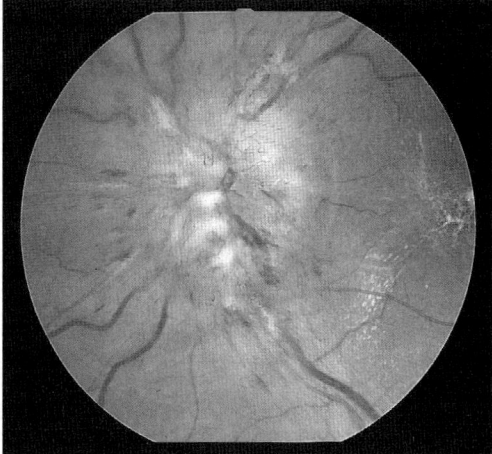

Fig. 31.45 Severe papilledema with hemorrhages and exudates.

within the eye and antigen release incites a profound inflammatory reaction. This leads to an isolated area of fibrosis with associated retinal traction. No active treatment is possible.

TOXOPLASMA INFECTION

The congenital toxoplasmosis syndrome includes chorioretinitis, intracranial calcification, seizures, hydrocephalus, microcephaly, hepatosplenomegaly, jaundice, anemia and fever.

However *Toxoplasma* infection acquired in the late prenatal period, or postnatally may remain quiescent for many years and then reactivate. The individual may have no neurological or systemic features of *Toxoplasma* infection. At the time of infection recurrence, an area of scarring of the choroid and retina is seen, with an adjacent area of retinal and vitreous inflammation (Fig. 31.44). The symptoms are reduced vision and floaters. A number of antimicrobial treatments have been used. Controlled trial evidence of efficacy is lacking.[89] Azithromycin has been used as monotherapy. Triple therapy with sulfadiazine, pyrimethamine and folinic acid has also been used. When antimicrobial therapy is given, very close follow-up is needed as death of the organisms may lead to increased inflammation due to antigen release. For this reason oral steroid treatment is often given 24–48 h after commencement of antimicrobial treatment.

DISEASES OF THE OPTIC NERVE

OPTIC ATROPHY

The causes of optic atrophy have been discussed earlier. Significant optic atrophy leads to reduced visual acuity, reduced color vision, and constricted visual fields.

OPTIC DISC EDEMA
Optic disc edema with severe visual loss

Optic disc edema due to inflammatory diseases (optic neuritis) results in profound visual loss. In children the most common pattern is bilateral optic neuritis. The discs are swollen, but hemorrhages and exudates are rare. Afferent pupil defects are present. Spontaneous, complete recovery over a period of days is usual. A neurological assessment should be carried out, including neuroimaging. There are usually no long-term neurological sequelae and the condition should be regarded as an entity separate from multiple sclerosis.

Optic disc edema without severe visual loss

The most significant cause of optic disc edema is raised intracranial pressure and the term 'papilledema' is normally used in these cases.

Papilledema may cause no visual symptoms. However in more severe cases brief periods of visual disturbance (visual obscurations) occur, and urgent investigation and control of intracranial pressure is required. Visual field examination shows enlarged blind spots in almost all cases. Paracentral scotomas may also be found. Poor intracranial pressure control leads to progressive loss of axons, with progressive constriction of the visual fields and visual impairment.

In its mildest form, papilledema causes slight blurring of the optic disc margins superiorly and inferiorly. As severity increases a larger portion of the optic disc circumference becomes blurred and the optic disc develops a pink appearance. The normal 'physiological' optic disc cup is lost, and normal venous pulsation is lost. In severe cases hemorrhages and exudates (nerve fiber layer infarcts) are seen (Fig. 31.45).

In mild cases the diagnosis may be aided by fluorescein angiography. In mild optic disc edema the capillaries on the surface of the optic disc are dilated and leak fluorescein dye (Fig. 31.46). High definition ultrasound examination of the optic disc and orbital optic nerve may allow detection of enlargement of the CSF space within the optic nerve sheath.

The differential diagnosis of papilledema includes hypermetropia and optic disc drusen. Moderately severe hypermetropia leads to small 'crowded' optic discs, which may have blurred edges and may be elevated. Optic disc drusen are deposits of amyloid tissue deep within the optic discs, leading to apparent swelling of the optic discs (Fig. 31.47). Drusen may be diagnosed using fluorescence photography or ultrasound examination.

THE EYE IN RELATION TO MEDICAL PEDIATRICS AND CLINICAL GENETICS

DIABETES MELLITUS

Diabetic retinopathy is exceptionally rare before puberty. Retinal screening examinations should be carried out annually from puberty. Cataract may develop as an acute feature of diabetes mellitus.

NEUROMETABOLIC STORAGE DISEASES – EYE SIGNS
Cherry red spot

In Tay–Sachs disease (GM2 type1) ganglioside accumulation in retinal ganglion cells leads to a 'cherry red spot' appearance (Fig. 31.48). The central fovea has no overlying ganglion cells and remains a red color due to the underlying choroidal circulation. The surrounding retina is a milky white color due to ganglioside storage in the ganglion cells. The ERG is normal, but the VEP is reduced. A cherry red spot is also seen in Niemann–Pick disease type A (sphingomyelinase deficiency) and neuraminidase deficiency (sialidosis types 1 and 2). With disease progression the cherry red spot fades as ganglion cells die and optic atrophy develops.

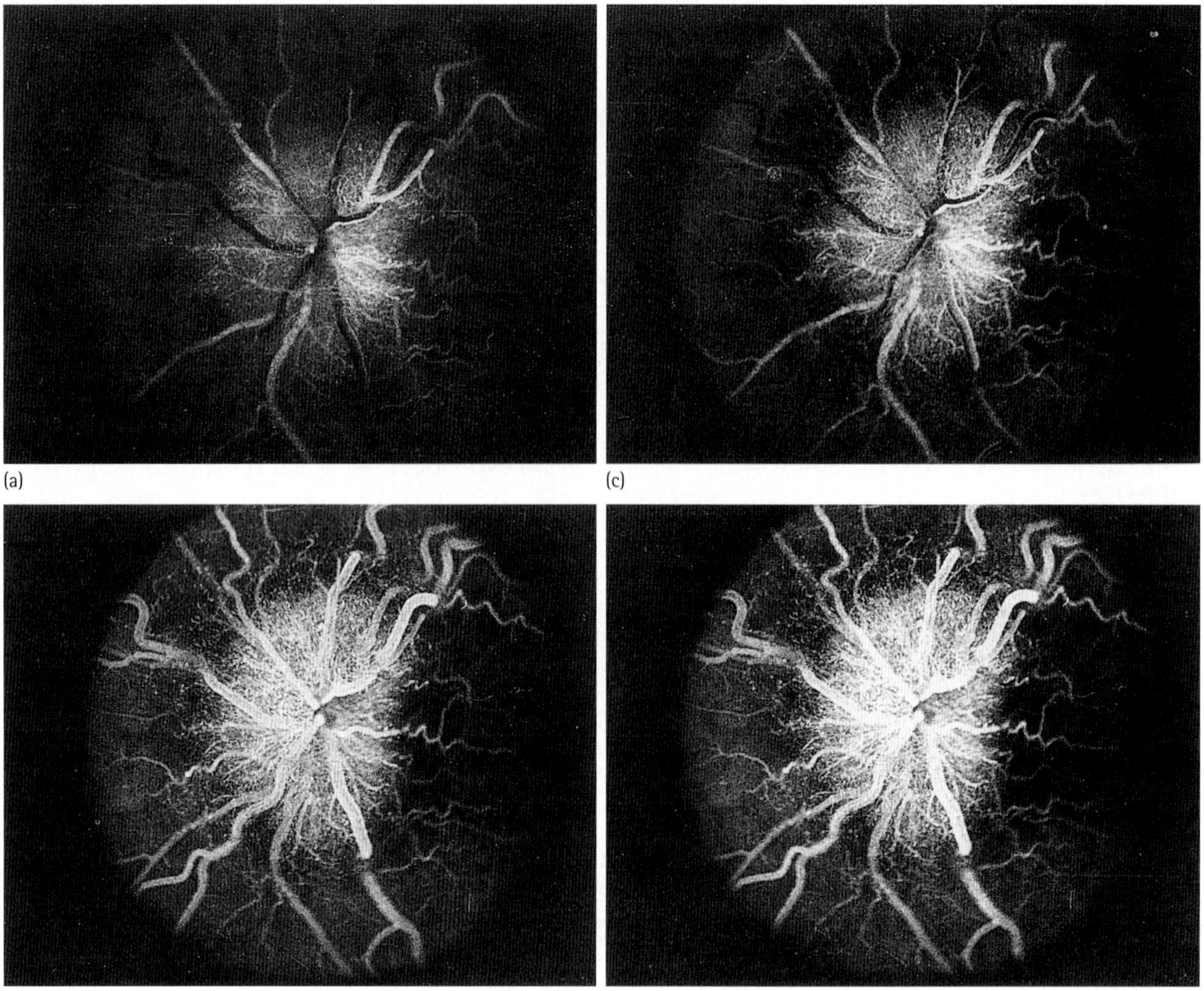

(a)

(c)

(b)

(d)

Fig. 31.46 (a–d) Fundus fluorescein angiogram showing dilated capillaries on the optic disc surface.

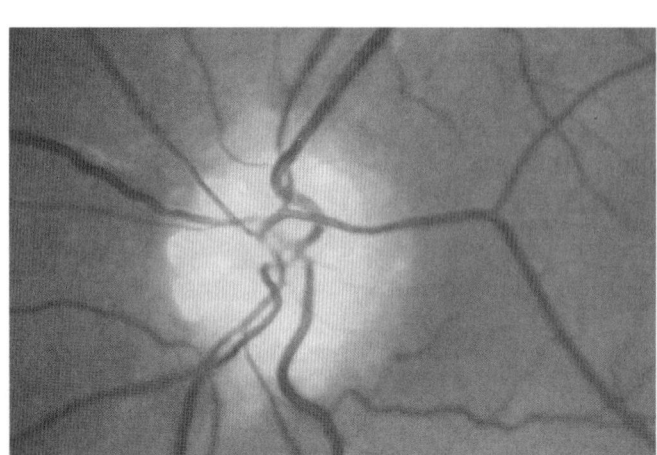

Fig. 31.47 Optic disc drusen.

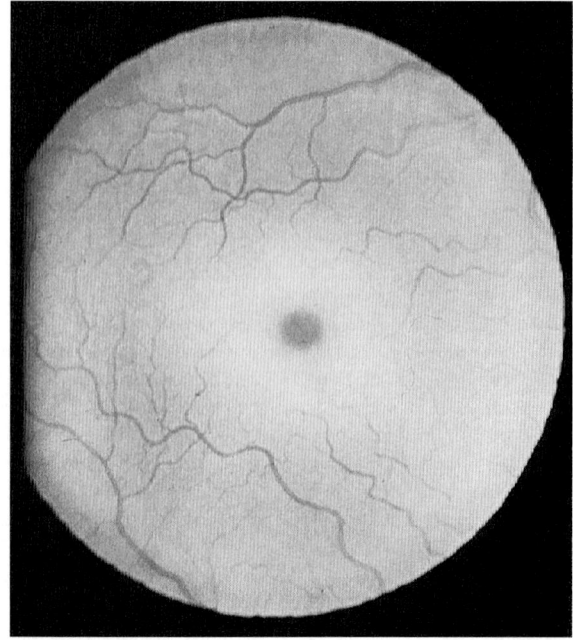

Fig. 31.48 Cherry red spot due to Tay–Sachs disease.

Corneal clouding

Corneal clouding develops in:

- mucopolysaccharidoses, all of which show corneal clouding, except MPSII and MPSIII;
- mucolipidoses;
- fucosidosis;
- mannosidosis.

WILSON DISEASE

Copper deposition in the peripheral cornea may be detected on slit lamp examination.[90]

OPHTHALMOLOGY CHANGES IN LEUKEMIA

Retinal hemorrhages may be found in severe anemia and leukemia (Fig. 31.49). The iris may act as a sanctuary site following chemotherapy for lymphoblastic leukemia. During remission periods, disease recurrence may occur in the iris, with clinical effects similar to those seen in iritis. Clinical suspicion and, if necessary, iris biopsy, will allow the correct diagnosis to be made. Treatment with further chemotherapy, and with radiotherapy to the irises, is indicated.

Opportunistic infections occur in immunosuppressed children. Infections commonly seen include herpes zoster and herpes simplex infections of the cornea or retina; and cytomegalovirus, *Toxoplasma* or *Candida* infections of the retina.

OPHTHALMOLOGY AND THE CLINICAL GENETICIST

The ophthalmologist may be asked to look for diagnostic signs in a range of inherited syndromes.

Marfan syndrome

Screening for lens subluxation may be requested. A single examination in early childhood is usually sufficient as lens subluxation develops early in life and there is rarely any significant progression with time.[78]

Neurofibromatosis

The ophthalmologist may provide diagnostic information in cases of suspected neurofibromatosis types 1 and 2 (NF1, NF2). Lisch nodules of the iris will be present in over 90% of children aged 8 years or older who have NF1 (Fig. 31.50), but are less frequent in younger children.[91] Symptomatic optic nerve gliomas are normally diagnosed by age 3 years.[91] Vision may fluctuate, deteriorate or remain stable for many years. When there is consistent deterioration of visual function, active treatment may be considered, such as chemotherapy using etoposide and cisplatin. Children with confirmed NF1 should have regular

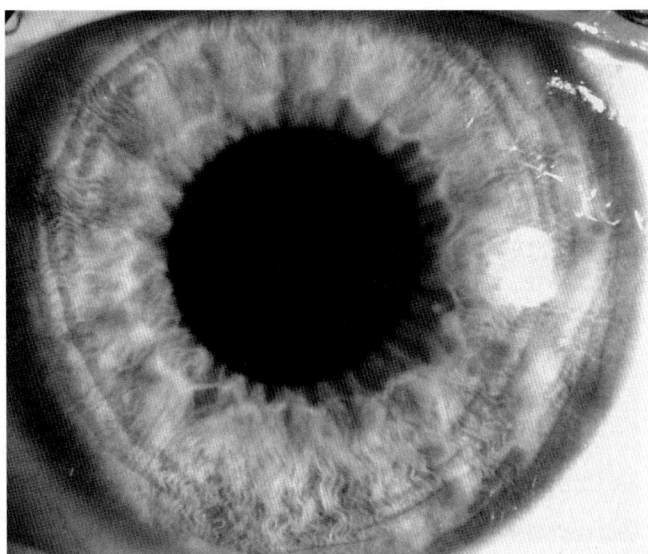

Fig. 31.50 Lisch nodules of the iris. Multiple pigmented nodules are easily visualized against the background of a lightly pigmented iris in this case.

screening examinations for anterior optic pathway gliomas. Screening examinations include measurement of visual acuity, color vision, pupil reactions, visual field measurements and optic disc examination (Fig. 31.51). Neurofibromas of the upper eyelid are associated with glaucoma in the ipsilateral eye.

In NF2, posterior subcapsular cataract is present in more than 50% of cases and is a useful diagnostic sign.[92]

Tuberous sclerosis

Fundus examination for retinal hamartomas should be performed in children with seizures and delayed cognitive development, as part of the diagnostic work-up for tuberous sclerosis. Hamartomas are found in the majority of patients with tuberous sclerosis.[93] These may appear as minimally elevated smooth translucent retinal lesions anywhere in the fundus, or as yellowish multinodular masses near the optic disc (Fig. 31.52). The lesions usually do not change significantly with time and do not cause significant visual defects, however occasional exceptions to this rule have been reported.[94]

Von Hippel–Lindau disease

Retinal angiomas are the earliest and most common clinical features of von Hippel–Lindau disease. Careful annual fundus examination is required in order to detect early lesions, which are most often found in the mid periphery.[95] The lesions tend to grow, and larger lesions leak serous fluid, which may lead to visual impairment. Early lesions should therefore be treated with laser or cryotherapy.[96]

Screening retinal examinations are needed for patients with known von Hippel–Lindau disease, and for presymptomatic family members who are known to have a mutation of the von Hippel–Lindau gene (3p25–26).

OCULAR TRAUMA

Significant ocular trauma remains a relatively common occurrence in children. Examination of an injured child requires patience, and examination under anesthetic is often preferred, especially when there is a suspicion of ocular perforation. Foreign bodies tend to lodge in the corneal epithelium, or become trapped underneath the upper eyelid. Corneal abrasions may be more easily detected by instilling a drop of fluorescein dye. A prophylactic topical broad-spectrum antibiotic should be prescribed when the corneal epithelium has been damaged. Eyelid lacerations should be carefully repaired, with particular attention to correct apposition of lacerations that involve the eyelid margins. Small ocular

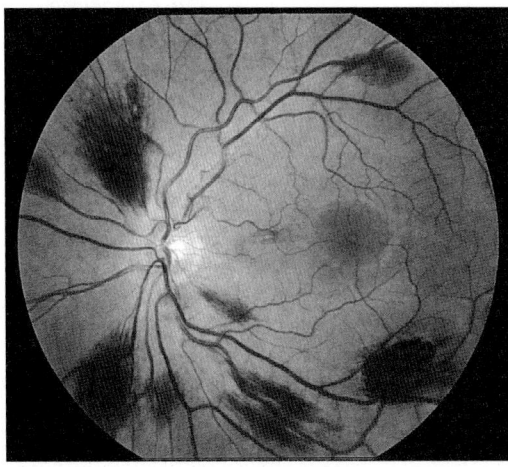

Fig. 31.49 Retinal hemorrhages related to leukemia.

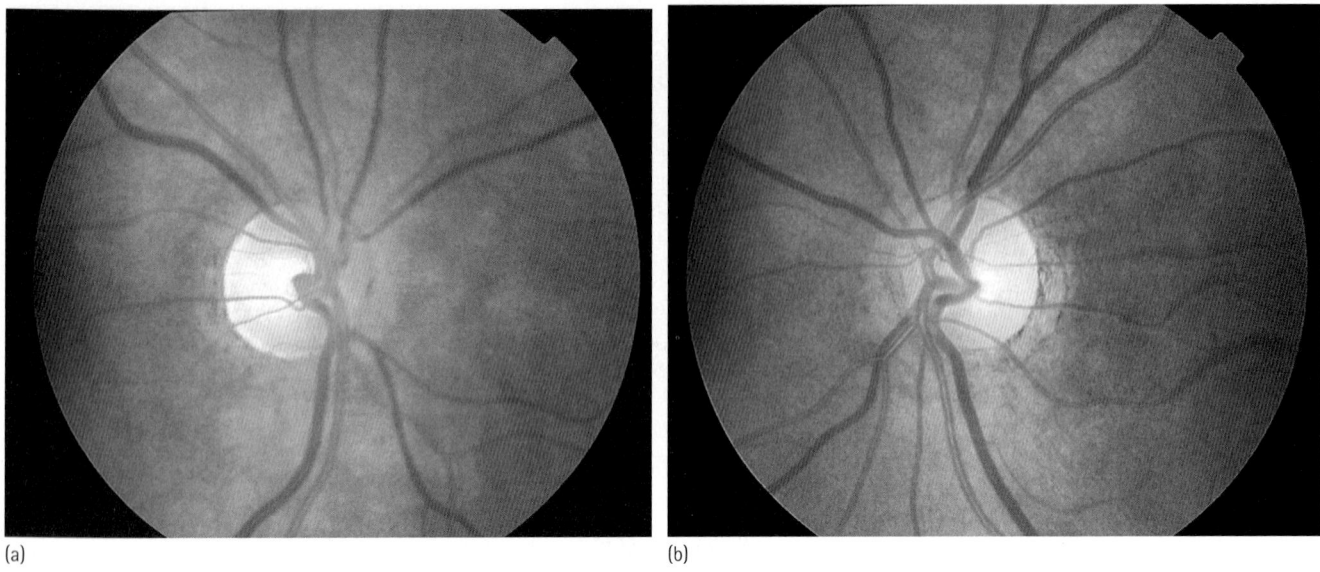

(a)   (b)

Fig. 31.51   (a) Right optic disc showing pallor on the temporal side. MRI scan showed optic nerve glioma. (b) Normal left optic disc.

lacerations may result in a distorted pupil, with prolapse of iris tissue at the perforation site.

Nonperforating blunt injuries most frequently present with hyphema – blood within the anterior chamber (Fig. 31.53). The intraocular pressure should be measured, and treated if elevated. Topical steroid and mydriatic eyedrops are given to treat associated iritis. Follow-up examinations are required in order to detect fundus abnormalities and traumatic glaucoma. Permanent visual loss is most often due to choroidal rupture (Fig. 31.54) or retinal detachment.

SHAKING INJURIES

Shaking injuries commonly produce extensive retinal hemorrhages and an ophthalmologist should be involved early in the diagnostic process.[97,98] Possible mechanisms include raised venous pressure and direct shearing forces within the retina and at the vitreoretinal interface. Typically hemorrhages are extensive, covering the whole retina from the optic disc to the ora serrata (Fig. 31.55). The hemorrhages are present deep within the retina (dot and blot hemorrhages), on the surface of the retina (flame-shaped hemorrhages within the nerve fiber layer) and on the surface of the retina (preretinal hemorrhages). Vitreous hemorrhage and traction retinal detachment may be present in more severe cases.

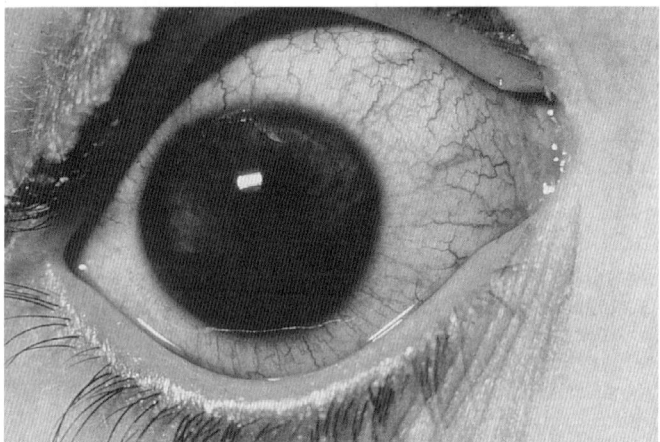

Fig. 31.53   Hyphema. Blood in the anterior chamber obscures the iris.

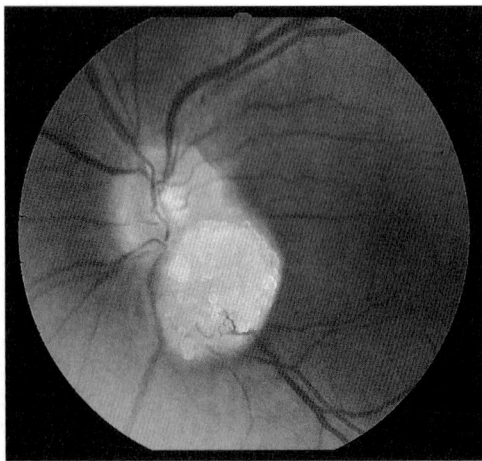

Fig. 31.52   Large multinodular retinal hamartoma adjacent to optic disc in a case of tuberous sclerosis.

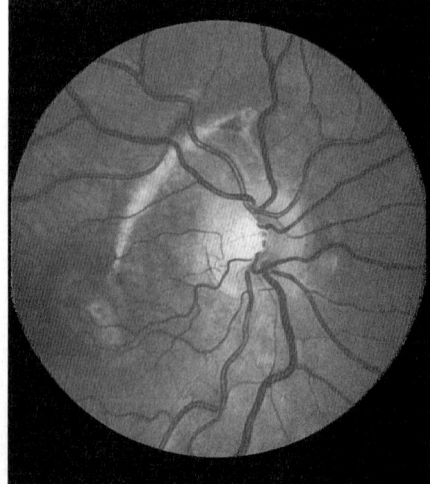

Fig. 31.54   Choroidal rupture. Blunt force has caused a curved tear in Bruch's membrane deep to the retinal pigment epithelium. There is additional pigment scarring at the macula.

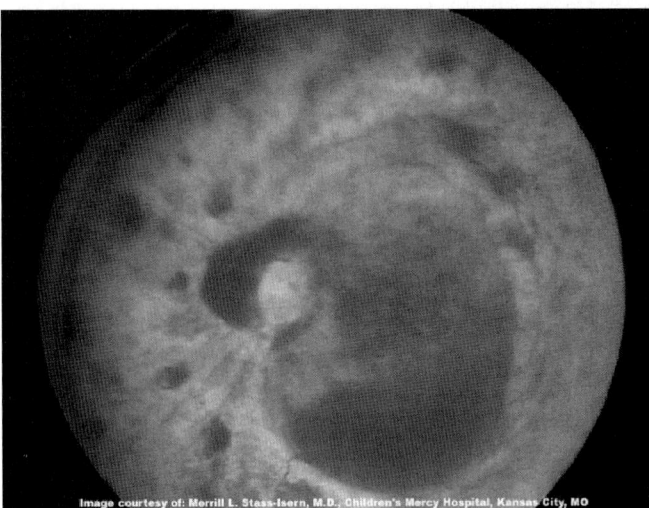

Image courtesy of: Merrill L. Stass-Isern, M.D., Children's Mercy Hospital, Kansas City, MO

Fig. 31.55 Retinal hemorrhages following non-accidental shaking injury in an infant. Image taken with 'Retcam' digital fundus camera.

Flame-shaped surface retinal hemorrhages tend to clear within 1–2 weeks, although deep retinal hemorrhages and pre-retinal and vitreous hemorrhages may persist for a number of weeks. The differential diagnosis is given in Table 31.13 and includes birth hemorrhages and retinal hemorrhages secondary to blood clotting disorders. Retinal hemorrhages do not occur as a part of accidental head injury unless trauma is severe.[99] A few small retinal hemorrhages have been found in case series following seizures, and following cardiopulmonary resuscitation.[100]

No specific treatment is indicated for retinal hemorrhages secondary to shaking injury. On follow-up, long-term visual loss is more often due to associated brain and optic nerve injury than to retinal injury.[101]

MANAGEMENT OF THE VISUALLY IMPAIRED CHILD AND THEIR FAMILY

The diagnosis of visual impairment in an infant or child may be devastating for a family. Parents are often in a state of shock when bad news is

Table 31.13 Differential diagnosis of retinal hemorrhages in an infant with suspected shaking injury (not exhaustive).

Non-accidental shaking injury
Accidental injury (severe trauma)
Leukemia
Coagulation disorders
Birth hemorrhages
Meningococcal meningitis
Glutaric aciduria type 1
Severe papilledema with raised intracranial pressure
Copper deficiency

given and an early review consultation is helpful in order to further discuss the implications of the diagnosis. Visual impairment in infants has secondary effects on general development, and appropriate use of sound and tactile stimuli by the parents will improve developmental progress. Considerable social and educational support will be needed in addition to medical interventions. Local and national parent support groups are available and should be used. Useful information may be obtained at *www.viscotland.org.uk*.

EDUCATION OF VISUALLY IMPAIRED CHILDREN

Many children with visual impairment may be satisfactorily educated in a mainstream school, provided that adequate additional teaching resources are made available. Simple measures such as satisfactory positioning of the child within the room and satisfactory lighting should be considered. Impairment due to reduced visual acuity may be helped in a wide range of ways, which include: allowing the child to observe objects of interest and text very close to their face; the use of large text (produced by photocopying with enlargement if necessary); the use of optical magnification devices and the use of computer-based technology. Braille supplemented by audiotape and speech recognition computer software enables many severely visually impaired children to progress to tertiary education. Strategies related to cerebral visual impairments are given in Table 31.2.

REFERENCES (* Level 1 evidence)

1. Teller DM. Assessment of visual acuity in infants and children: the acuity card procedure. Dev Med Child Neurol 1986; 28:770–790.

2. Norcia AM, Tyler CW. Spatial frequency sweep VEP: visual acuity during the first year of life. Vision Res 1985; 25:1399–1408.

3. Fawcett SL, Wang YZ, Birch EE. The critical period for susceptibility of human stereopsis. Invest Ophthalmol Vis Sci 2005; 46:521–525.

4. Wiesel TN, Hubel DH. Single-cell responses in striate cortex of kittens deprived of vision in one eye. J Neurophysiol 1963; 26:1003–1017.

5. Wiesel TN, Hubel DH. Comparison of the effects of unilateral and bilateral eye closure on cortical unit responses in kittens. J Neurophysiol 1965; 28:1029–1040.

6. Vaegan, Taylor D. Critical period for deprivation amblyopia in children. Trans Ophthalmol Soc UK 1979; 99:432–439.

7. Scheiman MM, Hertle RW, Beck RW, et al. Randomized trial of treatment of amblyopia in children aged 7 to 17 years. Arch Ophthalmol 2005; 123:437–447.

8. Keech RV, Kutschke PJ. Upper age limit for the development of amblyopia. J Pediatr Ophthalmol Strabismus 1995; 32:89–93.

9. Newman WD, Hollman AS, Dutton GN, et al. Measurement of optic nerve sheath diameter by ultrasound: a means of detecting acute raised intracranial pressure in hydrocephalus. Br J Ophthalmol 2002; 86:1109–1113.

10. Kriss A. Skin ERGs: their effectiveness in paediatric visual assessment, confounding factors, and comparison with ERGs recorded using various types of corneal electrode. Int J Psychophysiol 1994; 16:137–146.

11. Dagi LR, Leys MJ, Hansen RM, et al. Hyperopia in complicated Leber's congenital amaurosis. Arch Ophthalmol 1990; 108:709–712.

12. Izquierdo NJ, Traboulsi EI, Enger C, et al. Strabismus in the Marfan syndrome. Am J Ophthalmol 1994; 117:632–635.

13. Watanabe S, Yamashita T, Ohba N. A longitudinal study of cycloplegic refraction in a cohort of 350 Japanese schoolchildren. Cycloplegic refraction. Ophthalmic Physiol Opt 1999; 19:22–29.

14. Mulvihill A, O'Keeffe M, Yap S, et al. Ocular axial length in homocystinuria patients with and without ocular changes: effects of early treatment and biochemical control. J AAPOS 2004; 8:254–258.

15. Logan NS, Gilmartin B, Marr JE, et al. Community-based study of the association of high myopia in children with ocular and systemic disease. Optom Vis Sci 2004; 81:11–13.

16. Pokharel GP, Negrel AD, Munoz SR, et al. Refractive Error Study in Children: results from Mechi Zone, Nepal. Am J Ophthalmol 2000; 129:436–444.

17. Saw SM, Shankar A, Tan SB, et al. A cohort study of incident myopia in Singaporean children. Invest Ophthalmol Vis Sci 2006; 47:1839–1844.

18. Rose K, Smith W, Morgan I, et al. The increasing prevalence of myopia: implications for Australia. Clin Experiment Ophthalmol 2001; 29:116–120.

19. Choi MY, Lee KM, Hwang JM, et al. Comparison between anisometropic and strabismic amblyopia using functional magnetic resonance imaging. Br J Ophthalmol 2001; 85:1052–1056.

20. Weakley DR Jr, Birch E, Kip K. The role of anisometropia in the development of accommodative esotropia. J AAPOS 2001; 5:153–157.

21. Holmes JM, Clarke MP. Amblyopia. Lancet 2006; 367:1343–1351.

22. Williams C, Northstone K, Harrad RA, et al. Amblyopia treatment outcomes after preschool screening v school entry screening: observational data from a prospective cohort study. Br J Ophthalmol 2003; 87:988–993.

23. Salcido AA, Bradley J, Donahue SP. Predictive value of photoscreening and traditional screening of preschool children. J AAPOS 2005; 9:114–120.

24. Fleck BW, Dangata Y. Causes of visual handicap in the Royal Blind School, Edinburgh, 1991–2. Br J Ophthalmol 1994; 78:421.

25. Bamashmus MA, Matlhaga B, Dutton GN. Causes of blindness and visual impairment in the West of Scotland. Eye 2004; 18:257–261.

26. Dutton GN, McKillop ECA, Saidkasimova S. Visual problems as a result of brain damage in children. Br J Ophthalmol 2006; 90:932–933.

27. Jacobson LK, Dutton GN. Periventricular leukomalacia: an important cause of visual and ocular motility dysfunction in children. Surv Ophthalmol 2000; 45:1–13.

28. Fielder AR, Evans NM. Is the geniculostriate system a prerequisite for nystagmus?. Eye 1988; 2:(Pt 6):628–635.

29. Ross LM, Heron G, Mackie R, et al. Reduced accommodative function in dyskinetic cerebral palsy: a novel management strategy. Dev Med Child Neurol 2000; 42:701–703.

30. Koc F, Ozal H, Firat E. Is it possible to differentiate early-onset accommodative esotropia from early-onset essential esotropia?. Eye 2003; 17:707–710.

31. Birch EE, Fawcett S, Stager DR. Why does early surgical alignment improve stereoacuity outcomes in infantile esotropia?. J AAPOS 2000; 4:10–14.

32. Mulvihill A, MacCann A, Flitcroft I, et al. Outcome in refractive accommodative esotropia. Br J Ophthalmol 2000; 84:746–749.

33. Efficacy of prism adaptation in the surgical management of acquired esotropia. Prism Adaptation Study Research Group. Arch Ophthalmol 1990; 108:1248–1256.

34. Hatt S, Gnanaraj L. Interventions for intermittent exotropia. Cochrane Database Syst Rev 2006; 3:CD003737.

35. Rosenbaum AL. Costenbader Lecture. The efficacy of rectus muscle transposition surgery in esotropic Duane syndrome and VI nerve palsy. J AAPOS 2004; 8:409–419.

36. Bagheri A, Farahi A, Yazdani S. The effect of bilateral horizontal rectus recession on visual acuity, ocular deviation or head posture in patients with nystagmus. J AAPOS 2005; 9:433–437.

37. Shery T, Proudlock FA, Sarvananthan N, et al. The effects of gabapentin and memantine in acquired and congenital nystagmus: a retrospective study. Br J Ophthalmol 2006; 90:839–843.

38. Introne W, Boissy RE, Gahl WA. Clinical, molecular, and cell biological aspects of Chediak–Higashi syndrome. Mol Genet Metab 1999; 68:283–303.

39. Wei ML. Hermansky–Pudlak syndrome: a disease of protein trafficking and organelle function. Pigment Cell Res 2006; 19:19–42.

40. Craft AW, Parker L, Stiller C, et al. Screening for Wilms' tumour in patients with aniridia, Beckwith syndrome, or hemihypertrophy. Med Pediatr Oncol 1995; 24:231–234.

41. Lambert SR, Kriss A, Taylor D. Delayed visual maturation. A longitudinal clinical and electrophysiological assessment. Ophthalmology 1989; 96:524–528.

42. Foxman SG, Heckenlively JR, Bateman JB, et al. Classification of congenital and early onset retinitis pigmentosa. Arch Ophthalmol 1985; 103:1502–1506.

43. Preising MN, Heegard S. Recent advances in early-onset severe retinal degeneration: more than just basic research. Trends Mol Med 2004; 10:51–54.

44. Rainbow LA, Rees SA, Shaikh MG, et al. Mutation analysis of POUF-1, PROP-1 and HESX-1 show low frequency of mutations in children with sporadic forms of combined pituitary hormone deficiency and septo-optic dysplasia. Clin Endocrinol (Oxf) 2005; 62:163–168.

45. Moore AT, Taylor DS. A syndrome of congenital retinal dystrophy and saccade palsy – a subset of Leber's amaurosis. Br J Ophthalmol 1984; 68:421–431.

46. Falck A, Laatikainen L. Diabetic cataract in children. Acta Ophthalmol Scand 1998; 76:238–240.

47. Kim LS, Fishman GA. Comparison of visual acuity loss in patients with different stages of Stargardt's disease. Ophthalmology 2006; 113:1748–1751

48. Wang AG, Fann MJ, Yu HY, et al. OPA1 expression in the human retina and optic nerve. Exp Eye Res 2006; 83:1171–1178

49. Ju W, Wronska A, Moroziewicz DN, et al. Genotype-phenotype analyses of classic neuronal ceroid lipofuscinosis (NCLs): genetic predictions from clinical and pathological findings. Beijing Da Xue Xue Bao 2006; 38:41–48.

50. Collins J, Holder GE, Herbert H, et al. Batten disease: features to facilitate early diagnosis. Br J Ophthalmol 2006; 90:1119–1124.

51. Newman SA. Ophthalmic features of craniosynostosis. Neurosurg Clin N Am 1991; 2:587–610.

52. Jackson K, Baker SR. Periorbital cellulitis. Head Neck Surg 1987; 9:227–234.

53. Starkey CR, Steele RW. Medical management of orbital cellulitis. Pediatr Infect Dis J 2001; 20:1002–1005.

54. Nageswaran S, Woods CR, Benjamin DK Jr, et al. Orbital cellulitis in children. Pediatr Infect Dis J 2006; 25:695–699.

55. O'Keefe M, Lanigan B, Byrne SA. Capillary haemangioma of the eyelids and orbit: a clinical review of the safety and efficacy of intralesional steroid. Acta Ophthalmol Scand 2003; 81:294–298.

56. Rootman J. Vascular malformations of the orbit: hemodynamic concepts. Orbit 2003; 22:103–120.

57. Shields JA, Shields CL. Orbital cysts of childhood – classification, clinical features, and management. Surv Ophthalmol 2004; 49:281–299.

58. Shields CL, Shields JA, Honavar SG, et al. Clinical spectrum of primary ophthalmic rhabdomyosarcoma. Ophthalmology 2001; 108:2284–2292.

59. Jeffery AR, Ellis FJ, Repka MX, et al. Pediatric Horner syndrome. J AAPOS 1998; 2:159–167.

60. Young JD, MacEwen CJ, Ogston SA. Congenital nasolacrimal duct obstruction in the second year of life: a multicentre trial of management. Eye 1996; 10(Pt 4):485–491.

61. MacEwen CJ, Young JD, Barras CW, et al. Value of nasal endoscopy and probing in the diagnosis and management of children with congenital epiphora. Br J Ophthalmol 2001; 85:314–318.

62. Lim CS, Martin F, Beckenham T, et al. Nasolacrimal duct obstruction in children: outcome of intubation. J AAPOS 2004; 8:466–472.

63. Maini R, MacEwen CJ, Young JD. The natural history of epiphora in childhood. Eye 1998; 12:(Pt 4):669–671.

64. Morrison D, FitzPatrick D, Hanson I, et al. National study of microphthalmia, anophthalmia, and coloboma (MAC) in Scotland: investigation of genetic aetiology. J Med Genet 2002; 39:16–22.

65. Everitt HA, Little PS, Smith PW. A randomised controlled trial of management strategies for acute infective conjunctivitis in general practice. BMJ 2006; 333:321.

66. Solomon AW, Mohammed Z, Massae PA, et al. Impact of mass distribution of azithromycin on the antibiotic susceptibilities of ocular Chlamydia trachomatis. Antimicrob Agents Chemother 2005; 49:4804–4806.

67. Kanski JJ. Screening for uveitis in juvenile chronic arthritis. Br J Ophthalmol 1989; 73:225–228.

68. American Academy of Pediatrics Section on Rheumatology and Section on Ophthalmology. Guidelines for ophthalmologic examinations in children with juvenile rheumatoid arthritis. Pediatrics 1993; 92:295–296.

69. Saurenmann RK, Levin AV, Rose JB, et al. Tumour necrosis factor alpha inhibitors in the treatment of childhood uveitis. Rheumatology (Oxford) 2006; 45:982–989.

70. Watts P, Abdolell M, Levin AV. Complications in infants undergoing surgery for congenital cataract in the first 12 weeks of life: is early surgery better? J AAPOS 2003; 7:81–85.

71. Lloyd IC, Goss-Sampson M, Jeffrey BG, et al. Neonatal cataract: aetiology, pathogenesis and management. Eye 1992; 6:(Pt 2):184–196.

72. Rahi JS, Dezateux C. National cross sectional study of detection of congenital and infantile cataract in the United Kingdom: role of childhood screening and surveillance. The British Congenital Cataract Interest Group. BMJ 1999; 318:362–365.

73. Rahi JS, Dezateux C. Congenital and infantile cataract in the United Kingdom: underlying or associated factors. British Congenital Cataract Interest Group. Invest Ophthalmol Vis Sci 2000; 41:2108–2014.

74. Rahi JS, Dezateux C. Congenital and infantile cataract in the United Kingdom: underlying or associated factors. British Congenital Cataract Interest Group. Invest Ophthalmol Vis Sci 2000; 41: 2108–2114.

75. Lambert SR, Lynn M, Drews-Botsch C, et al. Intraocular lens implantation during infancy: perceptions of parents and the American Association for Pediatric Ophthalmology and Strabismus members. J AAPOS 2003; 7:400–405.

76. Fuchs J. Marfan syndrome and other systemic disorders with congenital ectopia lentis. A Danish national survey. Acta Paediatr 1997; 86:947–952.

77. Maumenee IH. The eye in the Marfan syndrome. Birth Defects Orig Artic Ser 1982; 18:515–524.

78. Vadala P, Capozzi P, Fortunato M, et al. Intraocular lens implantation in Marfan's syndrome. J Pediatr Ophthalmol Strabismus 2000; 37:206–208.

79. Trivedi RH, Wilson ME Jr, Golub RL. Incidence and risk factors for glaucoma after pediatric cataract surgery with and without intraocular lens implantation. J AAPOS 2006; 10:117–123.

80. Black GC, Perveen R, Bonshek R, et al. Coats' disease of the retina (unilateral retinal telangiectasis) caused by somatic mutation in the NDP gene: a role for norrin in retinal angiogenesis. Hum Mol Genet 1999; 8:2031–2035.

81. Shields JA, Shields CL, Honavar SG, et al. Clinical variations and complications of Coats' disease in 150 cases: the 2000 Sanford Gifford Memorial Lecture. Am J Ophthalmol 2001; 131:561–571.

82. Budning AS, Heon E, Gallie BL. Visual prognosis of Coats' disease. J AAPOS 1998; 2:356–359.

83. Knudson AG Jr. Mutation and cancer: statistical study of retinoblastoma. Proc Natl Acad Sci USA 1971; 68:820–823.

84. Demirci H, Shields CL, Meadows AT, et al. Long-term visual outcome following chemoreduction for retinoblastoma. Arch Ophthalmol 2005; 123: 1525–1530.

85. McDaid C, Hartley S, Bagnall AM, et al. Systematic review of effectiveness of different treatments for childhood retinoblastoma. Health Technol Assess 2005; 9:145.

86. Schueler AO, Anastassiou G, Jurklies C, et al. De novo intraocular retinoblastoma development after chemotherapy in patients with hereditary retinoblastoma. Retina 2006; 26:425–431.

87. Tsai T, Fulton L, Smith BJ, et al. Rapid identification of germline mutations in retinoblastoma by protein truncation testing. Arch Ophthalmol 2004; 122:239–248.

88. Koshy M, Paulino AC, Mai WY, et al. Radiation-induced osteosarcomas in the pediatric population. Int J Radiat Oncol Biol Phys 2005; 63:1169–1174.

89. Stanford MR, See SE, Jones LV, et al. Antibiotics for toxoplasmic retinochoroiditis: an evidence-based systematic review. Ophthalmology 2003; 110:926–931.

90. Yuce A, Kocak N, Demir H, et al. Evaluation of diagnostic parameters of Wilson's disease in childhood. Indian J Gastroenterol 2003; 22:4–6.

91. DeBella K, Szudek J, Friedman JM. Use of the national institutes of health criteria for diagnosis of neurofibromatosis 1 in children. Pediatrics 2000; 105:608–614.

92. Ragge NK, Baser ME, Riccardi VM, et al. The ocular presentation of neurofibromatosis 2. Eye 1997; 11:(Pt 1):12–18.

93. Kiribuchi K, Uchida Y, Fukuyama Y, et al. High incidence of fundus hamartomas and clinical significance of a fundus score in tuberous sclerosis. Brain Dev 1986; 8:509–517.

94. Shields JA, Eagle RC Jr, Shields CL, et al. Aggressive retinal astrocytomas in four patients with tuberous sclerosis complex. Trans Am Ophthalmol Soc 2004; 102:139–147.

95. Kreusel KM, Bechrakis NE, Heinichen T, et al. Retinal angiomatosis and von Hippel–Lindau disease. Graefes Arch Clin Exp Ophthalmol 2000; 238:916–921.

96. Schmidt D, Natt E, Neumann HP. Long-term results of laser treatment for retinal angiomatosis in von Hippel–Lindau disease. Eur J Med Res 2000; 5:47–58.

97. Biron D, Shelton D. Perpetrator accounts in infant abusive head trauma brought about by a shaking event. Child Abuse Negl 2005; 29:1347–1358.

98. Adams G, Ainsworth J, Butler L, et al. Update from the ophthalmology child abuse working party: Royal College Ophthalmologists. Eye 2004; 18:795–798.

99. Pierre-Kahn V, Roche O, Dureau P, et al. Ophthalmologic findings in suspected child abuse victims with subdural hematomas. Ophthalmology 2003; 110:1718–1723.

100. Odom A, Christ E, Kerr N, et al. Prevalence of retinal hemorrhages in pediatric patients after in-hospital cardiopulmonary resuscitation: a prospective study. Pediatrics 1997; 99:E3.

101. Kivlin JD, Simons KB, Lazoritz S, et al. Shaken baby syndrome. Ophthalmology 2000; 107:1246–1254.

32

Disorders of the ear, nose and throat
Alastair IG Kerr

THE EAR

CONGENITAL ABNORMALITIES

Microtia/anotia/meatal atresia
The auricle forms from the six tubercles of His. Malformations include microtia, a misshapen auricle, or anotia, the absence of the auricle. Both may be associated with accessory auricles, which are small residual tubercles that may lie sometimes over the cheek without function. Either of these congenital abnormalities of the auricle may be associated with meatal atresia, the absence of the bony meatus. They are commonly associated together in a variety of congenital conditions and syndromes. They may present as a unilateral problem, e.g. first arch syndrome, or as a bilateral problem, e.g. craniofacial dysostosis or Treacher Collins syndrome. If the deformity is a unilateral one it is extremely important to investigate the normal ear to ensure that the hearing is normal on the unaffected side. Assuming the contralateral ear has normal hearing, then surgical or other intervention on the affected side becomes purely cosmetic. If the condition is bilateral, then the degree of conductive hearing loss should be established and, in the first instance, a bone conduction hearing aid fixed by a head band should be fitted at an early age. With the advent of osseointegrated implants, this bone conduction hearing aid should be replaced by an osseointegrated, bone-anchored hearing aid (BAHA) when the skull is thick enough to sustain this (usually ages 3–4 years). Surgical attempts to construct a patent meatus have not been successful and have been largely abandoned but reconstruction of the pinna using sculpted rib graft is becoming increasingly popular. An alternative to this is an osseointegrated prosthesis.

Meatal stenosis
Meatal stenosis may occur either as a congenital abnormality or as a result of chronic otitis externa. Down syndrome children have very narrow external auditory meati and they often have middle ear problems. This sometimes makes the fitting of grommet tubes difficult and hence careful monitoring of their hearing is important.

Ossicular abnormalities
Congenital abnormalities of the ear ossicles are rarely seen in isolation and are usually associated with some other manifest congenital abnormality. Attempts at surgical repair of ossicles in children are not normally advisable and any bilateral hearing deficit should be treated by a hearing aid.

TRAUMA AND INJURIES
Direct trauma to the auricle may produce a hematoma and is commonly seen in sporting injuries. The hematoma should be aspirated and a pressure bandage applied to avoid the cosmetic abnormality known as 'cauliflower ear'.

Perforation of tympanic membrane
This can be caused either by an object inserted into the ear or alternatively by pressure, e.g. in non-accidental injury, where a slap across the ear can cause a perforation of the drum due to the pressure of the air column in the narrow meatus. This form of injury is also seen in explosions or in diving accidents. Head injuries may be associated with perforation of the eardrum and also leakage of cerebrospinal fluid.

Treatment of perforation of the eardrum is conservative; the ear is kept dry and in the great majority of traumatic perforations the eardrum will heal spontaneously. This healing may take several months but no attempt at surgical intervention should be considered for at least 6 months.

Ninety-five percent of traumatic tympanic membrane perforations will close spontaneously and return to normal.

Foreign bodies
Aural foreign bodies are quite common and can present at any age. They usually are found in those aged 4 years or older who have the manual dexterity to put objects into their ears. They are best removed; this often requires a general anesthesia. Syringing is not recommended as this can push the object, often a bead or plastic toy, further in, potentially damaging the tympanic membrane.

Wax
It is normal for wax to be present in ears and this causes no problems unless it has been pushed into the external auditory meatus usually by the use of cotton buds. The superficial squamous epithelial cells in the external meatus have a natural flow pattern outwards, so that wax will be naturally

extruded from the ear and hence, if the wax is kept soft by the use of simple olive or almond oil drops, syringing of the ears should not be required. As a general rule it is preferable not to syringe children's ears as they will find it uncomfortable and it will interfere with the natural extrusion process.

INFECTIONS OF THE EARS
Otitis externa
This condition does not occur commonly in children. The basis of treatment is aural toilet and the application of a topical antibiotic, with or without steroids, either on a small gauze dressing, which is preferable, or, alternatively, administered as eardrops. The skin of the meatus is often swollen and extremely tender and aural toilet may have to be carried out under a general anesthetic.

Furunculosis
A furuncle, or boil, in the external meatus will produce an acutely painful ear that is tender to the touch. It is often associated with a tender lymph node over the mastoid and hence the combination is often mistaken as an acute mastoiditis. The swelling in the latter is more widespread and the child is systemically unwell. Treatment of furunculosis is with oral antibiotics, usually flucloxacillin, and local dressings.

Acute otitis media
This occurs more commonly in those in the 6–36-month age range than in any other group. This is probably due to immaturity of the immune system, which can be slow in developing antibodies against bacteria with polysaccharides in their capsules, e.g. *Streptococcus pneumoniae* and *Haemophilus influenzae*. Infants also have short, wide horizontal Eustachian tubes that may allow easier passage of bacteria from the nasopharynx. Acute otitis media may occur as an accompaniment to an upper respiratory tract infection[1] but it can also occur on its own.

Clinically it will present with acute otalgia, sometimes bilateral, and the child will be fevered and may have a febrile convulsion. The eardrum, if inspected, will appear either acutely inflamed or bulging, with obvious pus behind it, the pain being due to the build-up of mucopurulent secretions in the middle ear. The first-line treatment is analgesics/antipyretics. Antibiotics provide only a small benefit for acute otitis media in children.[2] A Cochrane review[3] compared the outcome of antibiotics for 5 d with antibiotics for 8–10 d and concluded that 5 d of antibiotics (ceftriaxone or azithromycin) is effective. If the eardrum perforates, the pain will subside. In the vast majority of patients the drum will heal once the infection has settled. The treatment of infants and children with recurrent attacks of acute otitis media is either by repeated use of antibiotics or by surgical intervention. In young children, whose adenoids have not developed, the insertion of ventilation tubes (grommets) in the tympanic membranes will prevent recurrent attacks of acute otitis media. In older children who have significant adenoids, their removal may reduce further attacks of otitis media.

Acute otitis media is the commonest cause of otalgia with fever in children.

Acute mastoiditis
Acute mastoiditis still occurs but not nearly as frequently as it used to. This may be due to the use of antibiotics for acute otitis media but is more likely to be a reflection of a healthier population. Clinically, the child with acute mastoiditis will present with an acutely tender swelling in the postauricular region with the area of maximum tenderness being over the surface marking of the mastoid antrum, which is at the level of the top of the tragus. If looked at from behind, the auricle will be seen to be projecting outwards from the skull due to the loss of the postauricular sulcus and this is most commonly due to the collection of subperiosteal pus. The ear may or may not be discharging. The child will usually be in considerable pain and will be febrile. Treatment is admission, administration of i.v. antibiotics and analgesics and careful monitoring of the pulse and temperature for 24–48 h. If the postauricular

swelling is increasing or if the temperature is not settling in that time, then surgical drainage of the subperiosteal pus and drilling away of the diseased cortical bone should be undertaken under general anesthesia. Acute mastoiditis rarely becomes a recurrent problem nor does it lead to chronic otitis media or cholesteatoma formation.

Postaural subperiosteal swelling with a protruding pinna is pathognomonic of acute mastoiditis.

Chronic otitis media
Chronic otitis media is associated with a permanent perforation of the tympanic membrane. There are two quite distinct groups: tubotympanic disease and attico/antral disease.

Tubotympanic disease
Usually such children have had recurrent attacks of otitis media that have either been inappropriately treated or that have resulted in a permanent residual anterior central perforation of the tympanic membrane. The clinical presentation is of intermittent, quite profuse painless mucopurulent discharge from the ear. The profuse discharge occurs in association with an upper respiratory tract infection or following the child swimming or getting the ear wet. If treated with oral antibiotics, the discharge should cease. The hearing loss will be minimal. Effective antibiotic treatment of tubotympanic disease is required and the child should keep the ear dry. Closure of the perforation by myringoplasty using a temporalis fascia graft is not advisable until the child has gone at least 6 months without any discharge from the ear and this will rarely be before the age of 8 or 9 years.

Attico/antral disease
These children have a continuous painless moderate purulent or blood-stained discharge from the ear. There may be middle ear granulations. This discharge will often be foul-smelling as the commonest organism is *Pseudomonas pyocyaneus*. This form of chronic otitis media does not usually respond to antibiotics and is more serious as it is usually associated with cholesteatoma in the mastoid antrum or mastoid air cell system, which may erode the ossicles and cause a significant hearing loss. If cholesteatoma is identified in the ear by suction clearance, under general anesthesia, then mastoid surgery is indicated as facial nerve palsy or cerebral complications can occur if the cholesteatoma is not cleared completely from the mastoid system.

REFERRED OTALGIA
Referred pain in the ear may be from the tonsils, nasopharynx or teeth, all of which must be considered in a child who has unexplained otalgia.

Otitis media with effusion
This is a very common condition in childhood that can occur at any age but is found most commonly between the ages of 4 and 6 years. It is commoner in boys. It is alternatively called 'serous otitis media', secretory otitis media, or simply 'glue ear'. Children with otitis media with effusion (OME) commonly present with a hearing loss due to the collection of fluid in their middle ears. The fluid contains polymorphonuclear leukocytes, macrophages and cell debris but no ciliated columnar cells or eosinophils. The fluid is invariably sterile and various searches for viruses have proved negative. The fluid contains glycoproteins and nucleoproteins and this gives the fluid its thick, tenacious quality.

Clinical presentation
Classically, a child with secretory OME will present with painless insidious bilateral conductive deafness that should not be greater than 40 dB. Fluid will collect without prior middle ear infections and often the child does not remark on the loss of hearing. The problem may not be identified until routine audiometric testing is done at school. The fluid collects secondary to functional blockage of the Eustachian tube. If children are left for up to 12 weeks in 30–40% of them the fluid will disappear and their hearing will return to normal. Other children present as having recurrent

episodes or otalgia and hearing loss not responding completely to antibiotics or analgesics. Occasionally the ear drum may perforate. Some children can develop behavioral problems, becoming withdrawn or naughty presumably as they cannot hear properly. Others, especially toddlers, can become unsteady on their feet and start falling over, due it is thought to the vestibular system being affected by fluid in the middle ear.

Prevalence

At any one time, one child in 100 will have OME and approximately 10% of children under 10 years will have had OME.

Otitis media with effusion is the commonest cause of conductive deafness in childhood.

Diagnosis

Diagnosis is usually made by taking a careful history from the parents and/or the teachers, who are seeing the child on an everyday basis. Otoscopic examination will reveal an abnormal eardrum that may be retracted, bulging, dull, blue/yellow in color, or have an air–fluid level or bubbles visible behind it. Puretone audiometry will reveal a conductive hearing loss that is usually bilateral and worse in the lower frequencies than the higher frequencies but never greater than 40 dB. Impedance audiometry will give a flat tympanogram with a negative middle ear pressure and a greatly reduced tympanic membrane compliance.

Etiology

The underlying cause is believed to be Eustachian tube dysfunction, and certainly children with cleft palate and hence impaired Eustachian tube opening have a greatly increased risk of having OME. Children with chronic OME do have persistent negative middle ear pressure and this results in the loss of the middle fibrous layer of the tympanic membrane with atelectasis or atrophy of the membrane. Adenoids blocking the Eustachian tube orifice in the nasopharynx have long been associated with this condition and so their removal is often undertaken as a form of treatment. However, children without adenoids still get OME and therefore there must be more complex factors involved. Attempts to associate nasal allergy with OME have never been substantiated and apart from the already mentioned age and sex factors, the only other recently proven etiologic factor is passive smoking within the home environment.[4] Because the Eustachian tube is situated so centrally, it is extremely difficult to investigate its function in these children, and hence the etiology remains obscure.

Treatment

Management of OME remains controversial. The policy of 'watchful waiting' is the mainstay of treatment as over 50% of cases will spontaneously resolve in 12 weeks.[5] Medical treatment using antibiotics decongestants or nasal steroids have been shown to be ineffective.[6] Grommets offer a short-term hearing improvement only and therefore surgery is reserved for those with persisting hearing loss or those who are at increased risk of persistence at presentation.[7–9] These include those presenting in July to December and those whose hearing thresholds are worse than 30 dB in the better ear.

Surgery consists of myringotomy (drainage of the fluid) and insertion of ventilation tubes (grommets). This should be combined with adenoidectomy if a child presents with symptoms of enlarged adenoids (chronic mouth breathing, snoring, etc.) Adenoids are very small at birth but grow to a maximum size between the ages of 4 and 8 and it is in this group that adenoidectomy may be required. By ventilating the middle ear, grommet tubes reduce negative middle ear pressure and prevent the development of an effusion.

Children who have grommets can go swimming but are advised not to dive. It is sensible however to wear earplugs either customized or held in place by a headband. Grommets stay in place for 6–15 months and can cause minor scarring of the ear drums. Occasionally infections occur requiring antibiotic or removal of the grommet(s) and about 1% are associated with persisting perforations.

Surgery for otitis media with effusion should only follow 3 months of watchful waiting.

DEAFNESS

OME will produce a conductive deafness of up to 40 dB, which can affect speech and language development. If a child has a hearing loss it is important to identify whether it is conductive, sensorineural or a combination of the two. In conductive deafness the disability is not so severe and often there may be a surgical or medical method of treating it.

Sensorineural deafness in children is not uncommon. In resource rich countries, the incidence of bilateral significant sensorineural deafness is one in 1000 live births. 'Significant loss' is a loss of between 25 and 35 dB in the better ear. It is the high-frequency component of the loss that is usually important. If the loss in the better ear is at a level of 30 dB when averaged over the four frequencies 500 Hz, 1 kHz, 2 kHz and 4 kHz, then the child will require some kind of amplification to attain normal speech and language.

Significant bilateral sensorineural deafness has an incidence of one in 1000 live births.

Causes of sensorineural deafness

Only about 50% of children with significant bilateral sensorineural loss have an identifiable cause.

Hereditary prenatal causes

There are large numbers of syndromes in which deafness is a recognized factor:

Waardenburg syndrome. This autosomal dominant condition with variable expression consists of some or all of the following characteristics: unilateral or bilateral sensorineural deafness (20% of cases); hypertrichosis of the eyebrows that meet in the midline; heterochromia of the irises; or a white forelock.

Klippel–Feil syndrome. These children have short necks, which limits head movements. The hairline is low at the back, there may be paralysis of the external rectus muscle in one or both eyes and there is sensorineural hearing loss, which may be severe.

Alport syndrome. This is X-linked dominant and affects boys more severely than girls. There is severe progressive glomerulonephritis and a progressive sensorineural hearing loss, which does not show itself until the boy is about 10 years old.

Pendred syndrome. This is autosomal recessive and causes simple goiter at about the age of 4–5 years. There is an associated deafness that is often severe.

Refsum syndrome. This consists of ichthyosis, ataxia, retinitis pigmentosa, night blindness, mental retardation and sensorineural deafness.

Usher syndrome. This is autosomal recessive. There is retinitis pigmentosa with contraction of the visual fields and a severe sensorineural hearing loss that may be progressive.

Jervell and Lange–Nielsen syndrome. This is autosomal recessive with a cardiac arrhythmia secondary to a prolonged QT period, and a profound sensorineural deafness. These children may present with syncopal attacks and if untreated, these attacks can be fatal.

The inheritance of deafness is well recognized and in some children with recessive inheritance, the sensorineural hearing loss may be progressive. Nonhereditary prenatal deafness may be due to maternal illness, especially in the first trimester of pregnancy. Cytomegalovirus infections, toxoplasmosis, glandular fever and rubella are the most common, but parental syphilis and the taking of certain ototoxic drugs by the mother may also cause deafness in the baby.

Ototoxic drugs that should be specifically avoided during pregnancy are the aminoglycosides, quinine and to a lesser extent salicylates and alcohol.

Perinatal causes of deafness are usually related to prematurity or hypoxia. With the advances in neonatology, when extremely immature babies with complex neonatal problems are now surviving, the number of children with significant bilateral deafness sometimes associated with other abnormalities, and often related to hypoxia, is increasing. The cochlea is particularly sensitive to lack of oxygen. As neonatology improves further, the numbers of children with perinatal deafness will hopefully reduce.

Early diagnosis of sensorineural deafness is vital for acquisition of speech and language.

Postnatal causes

Middle ear problems cause conductive deafness and the causes of these have already been discussed. Sensorineural loss may result from head injury, from the use of ototoxic drugs and as a result of specific infections. Parents whose children get repeated attacks of acute otitis media are often concerned that significant sensorineural loss may result, but this is extremely rare.

Measles and mumps. Measles and mumps remain the specific infections that can cause significant sensorineural hearing loss. Mumps, although it will sometimes cause a profound sensorineural loss, is generally only a unilateral loss. The increasing use of the measles/mumps/rubella (MMR) vaccine will reduce the incidence of deafness from these infections.

Meningitis. Meningococcal or pneumococcal meningitis may give severe bilateral sensorineural hearing loss that will be permanent and may progress in severity following recovery from the meningitis. All children who have recovered from bacterial meningitis should have their hearing tested and monitored.

Diagnosis of deafness

The first 2 years of life are vital for the acquisition of speech and language and hence the early detection of significant hearing loss in a baby is extremely important.

Neonatal hearing screening

Programs for this are now in place throughout the UK. They are based around maternity units, the aim being to test all newborns before they leave hospital. Techniques used are otoacoustic emissions then going on to automated brainstem audiometry, if necessary

Only 50% of children with sensorineural deafness have an identifiable cause.

Subjective audiometry

Distraction audiometry

This is still a reliable, efficient method of testing that requires the minimum of equipment. The disadvantage is that it cannot be performed until the child is holding his head up unsupported. In the UK this is carried out by the health visitor as one of the routine screening tests at 7 or 8 months.

Conditioned audiometry

As the child gets older, he can be conditioned to perform a specific task in response to the input of sound.

Puretone audiometry

This is the main method of testing but cannot be done until the child will tolerate wearing headphones and can be relied upon to respond accurately to puretone sounds.

Objective audiometry

Brainstem evoked response audiometry

This is the most reliable form of objective audiometry and can be performed at any age. It is not, however frequency specific and young children, apart from neonates, require sedation or anesthetic.

Otoacoustic emissions

This test is based on the cochlear echo, which is an acoustic response of the cochlea when it is exposed to sound. It is easily done very quickly and gives a qualitative result as to whether the child's cochlea is working normally or not. Its disadvantage is that it does not distinguish between conductive deafness and sensorineural deafness, and any children who fail the otoacoustic emission test usually have to then progress to brainstem-evoked response audiometry.

Impedance audiometry or tympanometry

This is a simple test that measures the compliance of the eardrum and the pressure of the air in the middle ear. It is ideally suited for identifying otitis media with effusion and is useful in screening those who have failed their routine school audiometric testing.

Treatment of deafness

Treatment of conductive deafness has been discussed elsewhere in this chapter. There is no medical treatment for sensorineural deafness and management is based on prophylaxis. Genetic counseling and preventive measures such as immunization are important to avoid some causes of sensorineural hearing loss. As neonatology advances and hypoxia becomes less common, the incidence of deafness amongst ex-premature infants will be reduced. Sensorineural hearing loss is not normally progressive but in some congenital conditions it is, and so careful monitoring of the child's hearing is vital once the diagnosis has been made.

The mainstay of treatment remains amplification by some form of hearing aid. A large range of hearing aids is now available for children with sensorineural hearing loss and it is extremely important that the degree of handicap and the shape of the audiogram is known before the hearing aid is prescribed. Nowadays the hearing aid can be customized to the individual child's specific hearing loss.

The phonic ear

Teaching the deaf has been revolutionized by the advent of the phonic ear. This is a radio-aid type of hearing device where the mother or the teacher wears a microphone and a transmitter and the child wears the radio receiver. This means the child can sit anywhere in the class and be in direct radio contact with the teacher and hence the degree of amplification can be greatly enhanced. Many children with quite severe hearing handicap can therefore now be educated in their own local school rather than having to go to specific schools for the hearing impaired.

Cochlear implants

These have been used in children for nearly 20 years and are now established as the most effective way of enabling children to develop speech and language where hearing aids are not providing adequate amplification of sound. They are considered only after a thorough trial of hearing aids but experience is showing that the younger the child is implanted the better the outcome in terms of speech and language. The devices are expensive and are only available in specialized centers. Implantation is then followed by programming of the device and an intensive ongoing process of habilitation involving audiologists, teachers of the deaf, speech and language therapists, social and community workers as well as medical staff.

Cochlear implants are only required for a very small number of profoundly deaf children.

THE NOSE, SINUSES AND THROAT

THE NOSE

The nose functions as an air conditioner for the lower respiratory tract. It achieves this by cleaning, warming and humidifying the inspired air. The turbinates (Fig. 32.1) project from the lateral wall, increasing the surface area and causing turbulence. This allows heat and fluid exchange and causes any particles to be deposited on the lining of the nose in the sticky mucus, which then passes posteriorly and is swallowed. The function of the paranasal sinuses is unknown.

Foreign bodies

These present as foul-smelling, sometimes bloodstained unilateral nasal discharge. They occur most often in children between the ages of 2 and 4 years, and are usually bits of foam rubber or toys that

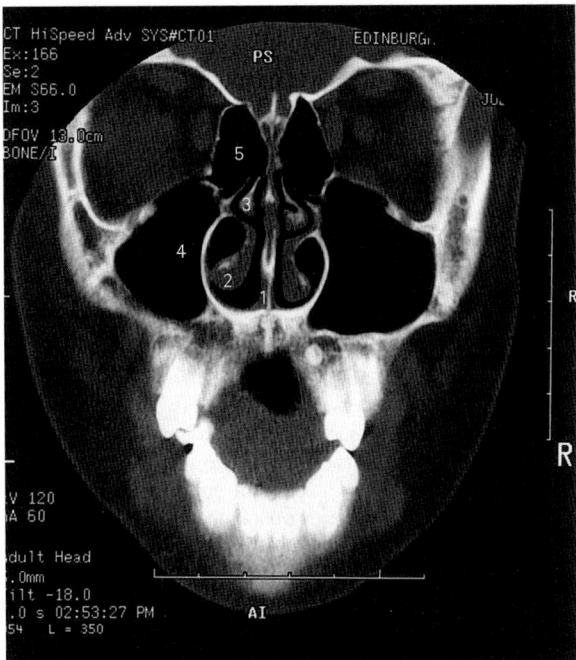

Fig. 32.1 Normal coronal CT scan of an 11-year-old boy showing: (1) nasal septum; (2) inferior turbinates; (3) middle turbinates; (4) maxillary sinuses; (5) ethmoid sinuses.

they have inserted themselves. It is rare for them to cause lower respiratory tract infections and the treatment is removal of the foreign body.

This can be done in a treatment or outpatient area sometimes by a 'parental kiss', where the parent blows into the child's mouth, the aim being to blow the foreign body out of the nose. If this is unsuccessful, and a headlight and appropriate instruments are available, and the child is cooperative, they can be removed under direct vision. Often, however, it has to be done under a general anesthetic.

Unilateral foul-smelling nasal discharge in a young child is pathognomic of a nasal foreign body.

Fracture of the nose

The nose is the commonest bone in the body to be broken. In children nasal fractures are less common than in adults as the nasal bones are smaller and the tissues more pliant.

Nasal fractures result from direct trauma. Initially, there is swelling over the bridge of the nose and around the eyes, which takes 5–7 d to subside. It is then possible to see whether the nasal bones are deviated, when manipulation under general anesthetic to straighten them is usually advised. Manipulation must be carried out within 21 d of the injury otherwise the bones become fixed.

Hematoma of the septum presents as severe blockage of the nose after an injury. This inevitably becomes infected, resulting in development of a septal abscess and destruction of cartilage and requires surgical drainage and a broad-spectrum antibiotic for 10 d.

Epistaxis

This is common after infancy. The bleeding can be spontaneous or secondary to mild trauma and usually arises from Little's area, in the anterior part of the nasal septum. Epistaxis can occur in leukemia or patients with bleeding disorders (e.g. hemophilia or thrombocytopenia) but is rarely the presenting feature of these conditions. First-aid treatment consisting of pinching the anterior cartilaginous portion of the nose with the child upright is usually successful. If there are repeated episodes, nasal cautery is indicated.

Epistaxis in a child usually comes from Little's area at the front of the nose and can be controlled by local pressure.

After identifying the source of bleeding, local anesthetic, 5% topical lidocaine (lignocaine) with 0.5% phenylephrine hydrochloride (co-phenylcaine) is applied using cotton wool or a spray. The area is then cauterized using a silver nitrate stick. In rare cases not responding to cautery, admission with nasal packing and i.v. fluid replacement may be required.

Epistaxis or oronasal hemorrhage in the first year of life is rare; coagulation disorder needs to be ruled out, and in the absence of this or obvious trauma, suffocatory child abuse should be considered.

Rhinitis

This is extremely common and is characterized by swelling and inflammation of the lining of the nose, often accompanied by clear or purulent rhinorrhea.

Viral rhinitis (the common cold or coryza)

This occurs very commonly with a pyrexial illness, runny nose, throat discomfort, sneezing and occasional earache. Treatment is symptomatic – analgesics and antipyretics as required. There is no proven place for decongestants in this condition. Viruses that have been identified as causing the common cold include rhinovirus, reovirus and adenovirus.

Viral rhinitis may be the precursor of laryngotracheobronchitis or pneumonia. A simple cold will normally last for 7–10 d and the child will not be unwell.

Bacterial rhinitis

This usually presents as purulent discharge following acute rhinitis. Antibiotics are rarely required unless the nasal blockage becomes worse or systemic symptoms such as fever and headaches occur, when adenoiditis or sinusitis should be suspected. In some children there is a constant low-grade bacterial rhinitis variable in severity, where no definitive underlying cause can be found. This can be associated with poor diet, damp housing and parental smoking. The underlying problem is thought to be lowered local nasal immunity. Antibiotics can sometimes stop persistent runny noses in children but there is no evidence of long-term benefit.[10] Most children with this condition will improve spontaneously from about the age of 8 years onwards. Immotile cilia syndrome is a rare cause and will often be associated with lower respiratory tract disease.

Allergic rhinitis

This usually occurs in children older than 5 years old. It presents as sneezing, associated with clear rhinorrhea and nasal blockage, and can be accompanied by conjunctivitis and sore throat. Seasonal rhinitis usually occurs in the summer and is caused by allergy to pollens. Perennial rhinitis can occur at any time of the year and can be associated with exposure to extrinsic allergens such as animals (e.g. cats or dogs) or housedust mite.

The diagnosis is made from the history. On examination, the nasal lining will usually be slightly pale and swollen. Confirmation of the allergic basis can be made by carrying out skin testing or serum immunoglobulin E assay.

Treatment is, if possible, by removal of the allergen but if this is not possible (e.g. seasonal rhinitis), a nonsedating antihistamine such as loratidine, supplemented by occasional use of a nasal steroid spray such as beclometasone may be helpful. Allergy to the housedust mite and housedust is increasingly recognized as a cause of rhinitis and allergic asthma. Treatment consists of cutting down the allergen in the bedroom by use of sprays or antiallergic sheeting. Nonsedating antihistamines and sometimes a short course of steroid sprays are also useful in combating this condition.

Non-allergic rhinitis (vasomotor rhinitis)

This presents as nasal blockage and catarrh and is differentiated from allergic rhinitis by negative allergy testing. Treatment is by antihistamine and decongestant combinations, and occasionally by steroid sprays for 2 months. Where there is no response to medical treatment, surgical diathermy or laser reduction of the inferior turbinate can be carried out.

NASAL SEPTAL DEVIATION

This can be traumatic but is more commonly developmental. Slight deviation is common and causes no symptoms, but more severe deviation will cause nasal obstruction, sometimes on both sides, occasionally with external nasal deformity. There may be associated allergic or vasomotor rhinitis. Surgery is only indicated for significant nasal blockage and is usually performed only in older children as surgery in young children can cause deformity, which increases with age.

DISEASES OF THE PARANASAL SINUSES

The paranasal sinuses (maxillary, ethmoid, frontal and sphenoid; Fig. 32.1) are all derived from the nasal cavity and are lined by respiratory epithelium. The maxillary sinuses are small at birth and do not attain significant size until 4 or 5 years of age. The ethmoid sinuses are well developed at birth, but the frontal sinuses do not develop until 9 or 10 years of age. The sphenoid sinuses rarely cause symptoms in childhood.

There is slight inflammation of the sinus mucosa in all forms of rhinitis and when the ostium to the sinus gets blocked, secretions are retained and purulent sinusitis develops. Treatment with antibiotics and local decongestants opens up the ostium and allows the sinuses to drain.

Maxillary sinusitis

This is rare under the age of 6 and it usually follows influenza or parainfluenza. The nose becomes very congested, there is copious purulent catarrh and there may be associated headache and fever. The commonest organisms found are *Pneumococcus* and *Haemophilus influenzae*. Diagnosis is on suspicion and the finding of purulent catarrh in the nose and throat. Treatment is by ephedrine nosedrops, combined with a broad-spectrum antibiotic such as amoxicillin or erythromycin for 1 week. X-rays are indicated only if there is no response to the appropriate antibiotics, at which time surgical drainage may occasionally be required.

Ethmoiditis

This is a potentially serious condition that occurs in children from 3 years upwards. It usually follows an upper respiratory tract infection. The symptoms are of frontal headache and pain around the eye with fever and nasal blockage. Examination shows periorbital swelling and tenderness with marked inflammation. If there is abscess formation it is usually subperiosteal and this causes lateral displacement of the globe. The clinical diagnosis is now confirmed by a computerized tomography (CT) scan. Urgent treatment with a parenteral broad-spectrum antibiotic and ephedrine nose drops is required with surgical drainage if there is abscess formation.[11] If the condition is not treated or inadequately treated, extension of the infection can result in the serious complication of cavernous sinus thrombosis or intracranial abscess.[12]

Periorbital infection often arises from infection of the ethmoid or frontal sinuses and should be treated vigorously.

Frontal sinusitis

This is less common than ethmoiditis and presents in children over 10. Like ethmoiditis, it is potentially serious with a risk of spread to involve the orbit or intracranial structures. It usually occurs after a cold or flu and causes severe frontal headache associated with inflammation and tenderness over the frontal sinus. Nasal symptoms are often minimal. Diagnosis and treatment are similar to that for ethmoiditis. Spread can occur inferiorly to involve the eye.

NASAL POLYPS

These present as unilateral or bilateral nasal blockage. Examination of the nose will show a pale, fleshy, usually mobile structure. Most common

is a unilateral antrochoanal polyp arising from the maxillary antra. These grow into the nose and down into the nasopharynx, often causing total obstruction of one side with purulent catarrh. They are benign and treatment is removal.

Ethmoidal polyps are less common and cause nasal blockage and catarrh. Ethmoidal polyps occur in children with cystic fibrosis, when the histology is different from the usual 'allergic type'. Treatment is removal under general anesthetic.

CHOANAL ATRESIA

This rare anomaly is due to failure of breakdown of the nasobuccal membrane, which normally occurs at 6 weeks' fetal development. The incidence bilaterally is one in 8000 but unilateral atresia is more common. Of these cases, 50% are associated with the choanal atresia with ear, eye, heart and genital defects (CHARGE) syndrome.

Gasping respiration in a neonate is suggestive of choanal atresia.

Bilateral choanal atresia is a neonatal emergency. The nose-breathing neonate may gasp and make significant respiratory efforts but soon becomes hypoxic and requires airway support. Some cases may mouth breathe, but then have difficulty when feeding. The diagnosis is by suspicion, by inability to pass a catheter along the nose and confirmation by endoscopic examination. The treatment consists of establishment of either an oral or orotracheal airway. A CT scan is carried out to determine the characteristics and extent of the atresia. Reviews using CT studies suggest that most atresias contain both bony and membranous components. Corrective endoscopic surgery is carried out as soon as is practicable.[13]

DISEASES OF THE NASOPHARYNX

Adenoids (nasopharyngeal tonsil)

These are part of the Waldeyer's ring of lymphoid tissue, which protects the upper airway. Adenoids are normally small at birth but enlarge from 18 months and regress normally at 8–9 years.

Adenoid hypertrophy

Since all children have adenoids, obstruction is a result of either a relatively small nasopharynx or large adenoids. Persistent enlargement causes snoring and often results in children having upper respiratory tract infections that last for 3–4 weeks instead of for 7–10 d. Such children usually mouth breathe and have hyponasal speech. There is an association between enlarged or infected adenoids and middle ear disease.

Adenoid hypertrophy is suspected with the above history and on the finding of a patent anterior nasal airway. Confirmation of adenoid size can be carried out by a lateral soft tissue X-ray of the neck (Fig. 32.2). In mild or intermittent cases, treatment is reassurance that the adenoids will go away. Surgery should be reserved for more persistent problems.

Adenoiditis

Adenoiditis occurs with viral infections and exacerbates nasal blockage. It can be quite severe in a small child with fever and purulent nasal discharge. A broad-spectrum antibiotic for 5 d is indicated in severe cases.

Adenoidectomy

Removal of the adenoids is indicated for:
1. airway obstruction in a small child (see airway obstruction, tonsillitis);
2. severe persistent nasal obstruction;
3. recurrent acute otitis media;
4. otitis media with effusion.

Primary or secondary hemorrhage occurs in about one case in 200.

Angiofibroma

This is a benign tumor of the back of the nose and nasopharynx that presents in males in their early teens. Its symptoms are of nasal blockage

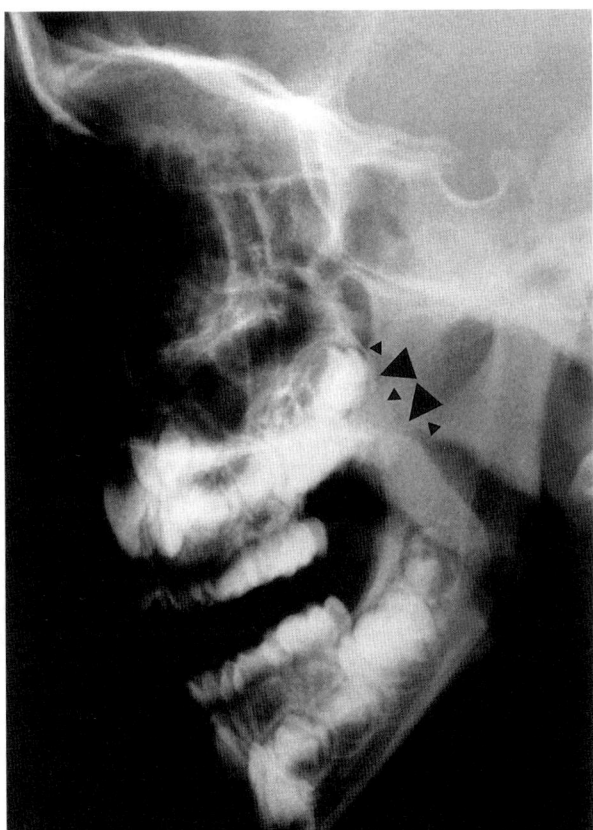

Fig. 32.2   Lateral soft tissue X-ray of a 4-year-old boy showing enlarged adenoids occluding the postnasal airway (arrowed).

with epistaxis. If expansion is rapid, cranial nerve compression can occur. The diagnosis is confirmed by endoscopy and a CT scan. Treatment is by surgery initially, radiotherapy being reserved for intracranial extension.

DISEASES OF THE PHARYNX

Pharyngitis

This is very common and usually of viral origin. It is a common presenting symptom of many upper respiratory tract infections, including the common cold, and may also precede the exanthemata of rubella or measles. There is generalized inflammation of the pharynx and often rhinitis. Treatment is supportive with antipyretics and analgesics as necessary.

Tonsils

The palatine tonsils, like the adenoids, are part of the body's defensive mechanism and serve to protect the upper airway from infection. Their removal, however, causes no subsequent immunological problems, nor is it associated with any deleterious long-term effect.

Acute tonsillitis

This is commonest between the ages of 3 and 8, but can occur at any age. Of these cases, 50% are viral and 50% are bacterial, with the beta-hemolytic streptococcus being commonest, although *Staphylococcus aureus*, *Pneumococcus* and *H. influenzae* are also implicated.

The onset is abrupt, with pain in the throat, associated shivering and a pyrexia up to 39°C. The pain may be severe and radiate to the ears. Swallowing is acutely sore and solid food is refused, although fluids may be accepted. The disease progresses over 48 h, even with antibiotic therapy, and the swelling of the throat and the tonsils results in dysphagia for fluids and even for saliva that may dribble from the mouth. Speech may become thick and muffled and there is often painful enlargement of cervical glands.

On examination, the mucosa of the pillars of the fauces and soft palate are congested and as the disease progresses the tongue becomes coated and the breath become offensive. The tonsils are swollen and inflamed, with a purulent exudate. In severe cases, edema of the palate and the uvula may make the voice muffled and thick. Sometimes in streptococcal infections a scarlatiniform rash appears over the body.

Investigation

Throat cultures showing Group A beta-hemolytic *Streptococcus* may confirm the diagnosis but a negative culture does not rule it out. There is also a high asymptomatic carrier rate of this *Streptococcus*.[14] Throat swabs should not be carried out routinely in sore throats according to the Scottish Intercollegiate Guidelines Network (SIGN) guidelines.[15]

Rapid antigen testing, e.g. antistreptolysin O titer, although widely used and although showing a high specificity, shows a low sensitivity compared both with throat culture and clinical assessment.[16,17] Rapid antigen testing should therefore not be carried out routinely in the case of a sore throat.[15]

Differential diagnosis

1. *Infectious mononucleosis.* This occurs in older children and is often accompanied by marked lymphadenopathy in the neck and other areas. The child is miserable with throat discomfort due to generalized congestion of the throat and swelling of the tonsils. Serological confirmation can resolve doubt and treatment is supportive with analgesia and fluids.
2. *Viral pharyngitis.* In this condition, the child is less ill and has other symptoms, e.g. a blocked-up nose.
3. *Herpangina.* This self-limiting condition due to Coxsackie virus has papular, vesicular and ulcerative lesions on the anterior pillars of the fauces, palate and tonsils.
4. *Herpes simplex stomatitis.* This may be quite severe although it is self-limiting in the toddler, with severe pain and drooling of saliva from the pain of swallowing.
5. *Moniliasis.* White patches are present on the tongue and on the tonsils and pharynx. This is usually associated with immunodeficiency but can occur after antibiotic therapy.

Treatment

In mild tonsillitis, analgesia, usually paracetamol, and adequate fluid intake is all that is required. Antibiotics are of limited use in most people with sore throats[18] but it has been traditional in more severe cases to give penicillin V for 7–10 d. Erythromycin has been used where there is penicillin sensitivity. Amoxicillin or co-amoxiclav if given to a child with mononucleosis will result in an extensive skin rash. Parenteral penicillin may be required in persistent cases. The child should be encouraged to drink and eat a soft diet if possible. There is no clear evidence that the use of antibiotics in tonsillitis expedites symptomatic improvement, prevents rheumatic fever or glomerulonephritis or reduces the occurrence of suppurative complications, e.g. quinsy.[15]

> There is no good evidence that antibiotics for tonsillitis alter the course or severity of the acute episode.

Complications of tonsillitis

1. *Peritonsillitis.* Inflammation spreads outwith the tonsillar area and the child develops increasing pain and fever, often with significant swelling of the soft palate. Parenteral penicillin for 3–4 d can be changed to oral medication as the fever and pain subside.
2. *Peritonsillar abscess (quinsy).* When peritonsillitis localizes, an abscess can form. Although this condition is less common in children, it still presents as a serious and potentially lethal complication. It occurs during or just after an acute attack of tonsillitis, presenting with increasing pain and swelling, usually on one side of the throat, with marked dysphagia and often otalgia. The child will have difficulty in opening his mouth. Examination can be difficult because of trismus but will show the affected tonsil to be very red, covered in pus and pushed medially. In addition,

there will be gross swelling and redness of the palate and marked cervical lymphadenopathy on the ipsilateral side. If untreated, the abscess can spread to give rise to a parapharyngeal abscess with the risk of spread to the base of the skull or even into the superior mediastinum. The treatment is drainage under general anesthetic and can be a hazardous procedure. If it is not certain that pus is present, i.v. penicillin or erythromycin is given with fluids and analgesics.

3. *Airway obstruction.* This usually occurs in children aged 2–3 as a result of chronic hypertrophy of the adenoids and tonsils. The child breathes noisily at night and often during the day. Occasionally the parents will volunteer that the child stops breathing for short periods during the night and this can cause them some understandable alarm. At other times more direct questioning is required to elicit this symptom. If untreated, this relatively common complication of tonsillitis can lead to chronic hypoxia, pulmonary hypertension and, in severe cases, cor pulmonale. Where there is any suggestion of airway obstruction, the child should undergo a sleep study with monitoring of the oxygen saturation. If there are episodes of desaturation, indicative of sleep apnea, and there is no other cause for the airway obstruction, adenotonsillectomy usually cures the condition.[19] Such children should be admitted to the high-dependency unit on the night of surgery and their breathing pattern should be monitored. In some more severe cases the respiratory drive is depressed. Oxygen may be needed until the respiratory drive returns to normal.

4. *Rheumatic fever and glomerulonephritis.* These are very rarely seen now as a complication of tonsillitis.

Indications for tonsillectomy

The following are indications for tonsillectomy (enlargement of the tonsils on their own is not an indication for their removal):

1. Airway obstruction in small children with persistent noisy breathing and suspected or proven sleep apnea. The adenoids will also be removed.
2. Suspicion of other pathology, e.g. lymphoma, is also an absolute indication. There is usually a change in the architecture of the tonsil that would suggest lymphoma.
3. Two or more attacks of peritonsillar abscess.[20]
4. Recurrent acute tonsillitis. By this is meant five or six attacks of definite tonsillitis in 1 year.[15] This number has been arrived at arbitrarily.[21] Mild symptoms do not benefit from surgery.[22]

Complications of tonsillectomy

A primary hemorrhage occurs within the first 24 h in 0.5–1.0% of children. Usually this is in the first 6 h after surgery and the child will start coughing up blood or, if unrecognized, may vomit a variable quantity of blood. After fluid replacement the child is returned to the operating room, where the bleeding vessels are identified and controlled by diathermy or ligature. A secondary hemorrhage occurs after 7–10 d. Often the child's throat will have started to become sore again and he then becomes aware of blood coming into his mouth. These children should be admitted, cross-matched and i.v. access obtained.

A broad-spectrum antibiotic such as amoxicillin is administered and local treatment consisting of hydrogen peroxide gargles and, occasionally, local adrenaline swabs can be carried out. If the bleeding persists, return to theater for ligature of the vessels or in rare cases packing of the tonsillar fossa.

DISORDERS OF PHONATION
Dysphonia

Dysphonia, or difficulty in producing sound, is usually associated with laryngeal disease (hoarseness). Some children have weakness or roughness of their voice in the course of an upper respiratory tract infection, this being a manifestation of laryngitis. Following recovery the voice usually returns to normal and no further investigation is required. Persistent hoarseness should be investigated and this can only be done by visualization of the larynx with a fiberoptic endoscope passed along the nose, into the nasopharynx. This can be done in the clinic where the child is cooperative but where this is not possible, examination under a general anesthetic is indicated to define the pathology.

The causes of hoarseness in children are as follows:

1. *Vocal nodules.* These occur at the junction between the anterior third and posterior two thirds of the vocal cords. They are usually secondary to voice abuse and in loud and noisy children are known as 'screamers' nodes. Small nodules can improve with speech therapy or if the nodules grow, surgery involving microscopic dissection is indicated. Histology shows hypertrophic squamous epithelium with underlying edema of Reinke's space.
2. *Polyps of the larynx.* These occur spontaneously or following intubation and cause variable hoarseness. They are removed under general anesthetic.
3. *Laryngeal papillomas.* These are a rare cause of hoarseness associated with maternal genital warts (papilloma virus). They present as persistent hoarseness, sometimes with aphonia and occasionally airway obstruction. Treatment is by removal and multiple operations may be required. They do not become malignant but can spread into the trachea and in rare cases, into the bronchus.
4. *Unilateral vocal cord paralysis.* This can follow surgical or nonsurgical trauma to the neck, or occur following viral infections including mononucleosis. The voice may be breathy if the cord is abducted or well maintained if the cord is medialized. The diagnosis is usually made on fiberoptic endoscopy, and treatment consists of speech therapy.

Aphonia

Complete loss of voice can occasionally occur with laryngeal pathology, e.g. papillomas, and in most cases the larynx should be visualized. Complete aphonia in an otherwise healthy child should be viewed with suspicion. Functional or 'hysterical' aphonia occurs after emotional or physical trauma, e.g. tonsillectomy. It usually affects older children and in most cases is self-correcting. Occasionally a laryngoscopy may have to be carried out to establish the diagnosis, but usually explanation of the problem together with counseling will suffice.

REFERENCES (* Level 1 evidence)

The ear

*1. Uhari M, Niemala M, Hietala J. Prediction of acute otitis media with symptoms and signs. Acta Paediatrics 1995; 84:90–92.

*2. Glasziou PP, DelMar CB, Sanders SL, et al. Antibiotics for acute otitis media in children (Cochrane Review). In: The Cochrane Library, Issue 4 Oxford: Update Software; 2002.

*3. Kozyrskyj AL, Hildes-Ripstein GE, Longstaffe SEA, et al. Short course antibiotics for otitis media (Cochrane Review). In: The Cochrane Library, 1. Oxford: Update Software; 2001.

*4. Maw AR, Parker AJ, Lance GN, et al. The effects of parental smoking on outcome after treatment for glue ear in children. Clin Otolaryngol 1992; 17:411–414.

*5. SIGN – Scottish Intercollegiate Guidelines Network. Diagnosis and management of childhood otitis media in primary care. Sign publication 66; 2003.

*6. Butler CC, van der Voort JH. Oral or topical nasal steroids for hearing loss associated with otitis media with effusion in children. In: Cochrane Library 1. Oxford; 2001.

*7. Lous J, Burton MJ, Felding JV, et al. Grommets (ventilation tubes) for hearing loss associated with otitis media with effusion in children. Cochrane Database Syst Rev. 2005. Jan 25; (1): CD001801.

*8. MRC Multicentre Otitis Media Study group. Risk factors for persistence of bilateral otitis media with effusion. Clin Otol. 2001; 26:147–156.

*9. Rovers MM, Black N, Browning GG, et al. Grommets in otitis media with effusion; an individual patient meta analysis. Arch Dis Child 2005; 90: 480–485.

The nose, sinuses and throat

*10. Morris P, Leach A. Antibiotics for persistent nasal discharge (rhonosinusitis) in children. Oxford: Cochrane Library; 2006.

*11. Arjmand EM, Lusk RP, Muntz HR. Acute sinusitis, children and the eye. Otolaryngol Head Neck Surgery 1993; 109:886–894.

*12. Bluestone CD, Stool SE. Paediatric otolaryngology. WB Saunders; 1982; 793–796.

*13. Brown OE, Pownell P, Manning SC. Choanal atresia: a new anatomic classification and clinical management applications. Laryngoscope 1996; 106: 97–101.

*14. Feery BJ, Forsell P, Guylasekharam M. Streptococcal sore throat in general practice – a controlled study. Med J Aust 1976; 1:989–991.

*15. SIGN – Scottish Intercollegiate Guidelines Network. Management of sore throat and indications for tonsillectomy. SIGN publication 34; 1999.

*16. Lewey S, White GB, Lieberman MM, et al. Evaluation of the throat culture as a follow up for an initially negative enzyme immunosorbent assay rapid streptococcal antigen detection test. Paediatr Infect Dis J 1988; 7:765–769.

*17. Burke P, Bain J, Lowes A, et al. Rational decisions in managing sore throat: evaluation of a rapid test. Br Med J 1988; 296:1646–1649.

*18. Del Mar CB, Glasziou PP, Spinks AB. Antibiotics for sore throat. Oxford: Cochrane Library; 2006.

*19. Strading JR, Thomas G, Warley ARH, et al. Effect of adeno-tonsillectomy, on nocturnal hyponaemia, sleep disturbance and symptoms in snoring children. Lancet 1990; 335:249–253.

*20. Wolf M, Euen-Chen I, Talmi YP, et al. Tonsillectomy following peritonsillar abscess. Int J Paediatr Otolaryngol 1995; 31:43–46.

*21. Paradise JL, Bluestone CD, Bachman RZ, et al. Efficacy of tonsillectomy for recurrent throat infection in severely affected children. Results of parallel randomised and non-randomised clinical trials. N Engl J Med 1984; 310:674–683.

*22. van Staaij BK, van den Akker EH, Rovers MM, et al. Effectiveness of adenotonsillectomy in children with mild symptoms of throat infections or adenotonsillar hypertrophy; open randomized trial. Br Med J 2004; 329:651–654.

33

Allergic disorders

Peter D Arkwright, Timothy J David

DEFINITIONS AND EXPLANATION OF TERMS

The widespread misuse of the word 'allergy' causes confusion. It is essential to have a definition or explanation of terms as follows.

ALLERGY

Allergy is a reproducible adverse reaction to an extrinsic substance mediated by an immunological response, irrespective of the precise mechanism. The substance provoking the reaction may have been ingested, injected, inhaled or may merely have come into contact with the skin or mucous membranes. The terms 'allergy' and 'hypersensitivity' have the same meaning and are interchangeable.

ATOPY

There is no good definition of atopy. The term was introduced to describe the 'asthma and hay fever group' of diseases. Subsequently, atopy has been redefined as a hereditary predisposition to the production of IgE antibody, an unsatisfactory oversimplification. The atopic diseases comprise atopic dermatitis, asthma, allergic rhinoconjunctivitis and some cases of urticaria. The association between food allergy and these atopic diseases is so strong that there is a case for considering food allergy as an atopic disease.[1]

ANAPHYLAXIS

The term 'anaphylaxis' is usually reserved for an allergic reaction associated with severe, life-threatening circulatory and/or respiratory compromise.

FOOD INTOLERANCE

Food intolerance is a reproducible adverse reaction to a specific food or food ingredient, and it is not psychologically based. Food intolerance occurs even when the subject cannot identify the type of food that has been given. This definition does not take into account dosage. Clearly any food in vast excess will cause a reproducible adverse reaction. Such events are not generally covered by the term 'food intolerance'.

IMMUNE MECHANISMS AND TIMING OF THE ALLERGIC RESPONSE

When the skin, airways, or conjunctivae are challenged by a single dose of allergen, an allergic reaction can be classified as immediate, delayed or dual (that is both immediate and delayed). Two main immune mechanisms determine the timing of these allergic responses (see Table 33.1). Immediate (acute) reactions usually occur within

Table 33.1 Immune mechanisms leading to allergic reactions

Mechanism	Clinical characteristics
Direct, IgE- or IgG-mediated **mast cell degranulation** with release of proinflammatory mediators (e.g. histamine, bradykinin, leukotrienes, platelet-activating factor)	Immediate/acute hypersensitivity reactions
RAST and SPT only useful if IgE mediated	Rapid onset (usually minutes) Urticaria/angioedema, rhinoconjunctivitis/pharyngeal edema/bronchospasm, hypotension, vomiting/diarrhea, anaphylaxis Mainstay of pharmacological treatment: antihistamines, adrenaline for anaphylaxis
T-lymphocyte-mediated, release of cytokines and chemokines	Delayed hypersensitivity reactions
RAST and SPT not indicated	Slower onset over hours/days Contact dermatitis/atopic dermatitis, chronic asthma, allergic enterocolitis Mainstay of pharmacological treatment: topical/local corticosteroids

minutes of contact with the allergen and are caused by mast cell degranulation usually triggered by antigen cross-linking IgE on the mast cell surface. Delayed hypersensitivity reactions may occur hours after contact with the allergen and are mediated by T-lymphocytes and the inflammatory cytokines they release. Although IgE-based allergy (skin prick tests and serum-specific IgE [RAST]) tests may be useful in the diagnostic workup of some immediate-type allergic reactions, they are not useful in delayed reactions, which are typically not IgE mediated. A summary of the types of the clinical spectrum of diseases is given in Table 33.2. The pathogenesis and mechanisms of allergic disorders are reviewed in more detail elsewhere.[2,3] It should be noted that some allergic reactions, for example reversible airway obstruction (asthma) may be mediated by both humoral and cellular immune mechanisms.

Table 33.2 Clinical spectrum of allergic disease based and immune responses aimed at allergen avoidance and removal

Body interface		
Skin	Respiratory tract	Gastrointestinal tract
A. Diseases		
Urticaria (humoral)	Rhinoconjunctivitis (humoral)	Food intolerance (humoral/cellular)
Atopic eczema (cellular)	Asthma (humoral/cellular)	
B. Protective responses against allergens		
Pruritus (rubbing/ scratching)	Copious secretions Sneezing and coughing	Vomiting and diarrhea
Hyperkeratosis (barrier)	Bronchospasm (prevent/reduce further exposure)	

HYGIENE HYPOTHESIS

The hygiene hypothesis is derived from the notion that infections and unhygienic contact might confer protection against the development of allergic illness.[4-6] The hypothesis attempts to reconcile the following facts:

- **Increase in the prevalence of atopic diseases over the last few decades:** The prevalence of atopic diseases (atopic dermatitis, asthma and allergic rhinitis) has doubled over the last few generations.[7] These diseases are largely a problem of developed countries such as the UK, USA, Australasia and Canada. Within these countries, the affluent within these communities (social classes I and II) are most commonly affected. Because this increase in prevalence has occurred over only a few generations, it must be due to environmental rather than genetic causes.[8]
- **Increase in certain autoimmune conditions over the last few decades:** What is often less appreciated is that as well as a rise in allergic diseases, there has been a parallel increase in some autoimmune conditions, such as multiple sclerosis, Crohn's disease and insulin-dependent diabetes mellitus. Other autoimmune diseases have either shown little change in prevalence (ulcerative colitis) or a reduced prevalence (rheumatoid arthritis).
- **Reduction in exposure to certain environmental microbes, particularly those spread via the orofecal route, over the same time period:** This evidence comes from two main sources. Firstly, a Japanese study of 867 children over the age of 12 years showed a clear negative relationship between delayed hypersensitivity responses to tuberculin and the presence of asthma.[9] Secondly, a number of studies performed in Switzerland, Austria and Germany have provided convincing evidence that growing up on a farm with regular contact with farm animals protects against allergic sensitization and the development of childhood allergic diseases.[10-12]

Based on these observations, the hygiene hypothesis proposes that certain environmental viruses and bacteria help to induce immune tolerance to normally innocuous environmental antigens (allergens) and self (autoantigens). The hypothesis is that reduced exposure to these environmental microbes, associated with modern western living has led to a lack of immune tolerance and thus an increase in immune hypersensitivity, atopy and autoimmunity.

GENETICS OF ALLERGY AND ALLERGIC DISORDERS

As well as environmental factors, there is no doubt that genetic factors are also important in the development of atopic diseases. Evidence for this comes from a number of sources:

- **Epidemiology: family history and twin studies:** Strong family history of atopic disease in many affected individuals, as well as twin studies point to a strong genetic influence.[13] For instance, the risk of atopic disease in the general community is approximately 10%, but this increases to 50% if one parent is affected and up to 75% if both parents are affected. Twin studies suggest that the genetic component accounts for approximately 80% of the predisposition to atopic dermatitis, asthma, allergic rhinoconjunctivitis and peanut allergy.
- **Polygenic disease:** In most cases, predisposition to allergic diseases is thought to be due to not one but the additive or synergistic effect of a number of genes. Rarely single gene mutations may cause allergic symptoms such as the FoxP3 gene in IPEX and the WASP gene in Wiskott–Aldrich syndrome (see Chapter 27).
- **Specific genes largely unknown:** The specific genes causing allergic disease in most patients are still unknown. Although numerous candidate genes have been implicated in the development of atopy, definitive evidence linking any one of these genes as a major cause of clinical atopy is lacking.[14]
- **Candidate genes now thought to relate to molecules sensing foreign antigens and those involved in immune tolerance induction:** Current research is focusing on genes that regulate the

innate and acquired immune responses, particularly genes that code for receptors on dendritic cells and T-lymphocytes recognizing foreign microbes (e.g. CD14, TLR 2, 4, 6, 10, TIM3).[15-17] Genetic factors that are important in regulatory immune cell function (FoxP3, TGF-β, IL-10) are also being studied.[18]

CLINICAL SPECTRUM OF DISEASE

Clinical features of allergic disease occur mainly at the three major interfaces between the body and its environment: the skin, upper and lower respiratory tract and gastrointestinal system. This subdivision, although paralleling the types of pediatric specialists to whom such patients will be referred (namely dermatologists, respiratory physicians and gastroenterologists), is artificial. Moreover in some ways it may be unhelpful to characterize allergic diseases in this way. For instance, acute allergic reactions to ingested food may manifest not only as vomiting and diarrhea, but in some cases solely as cutaneous urticaria and in others as acute pharyngeal angioedema or bronchospasm, or in yet other cases with clinical features related to all three systems. Allergic disease is primarily a systemic illness with many overlapping features.

SKIN

URTICARIA
Acute urticaria

Acute urticaria is the result of a variety of causes (often not identified) and mechanisms. The proportion of cases in which a cause is found varies; in childhood the most common is viral infection. Urticaria may develop during an illness or within 1–2 weeks after the illness, and remain a problem for a few days or weeks. Immediate allergic reactions to foods are the other major cause of acute urticaria. A parent notices, for example, that whenever a child eats fish his lips swell and he develops an urticarial rash. Fish is avoided, and the problem disappears. Occasional lapses of avoidance either demonstrate continued intolerance or, with time, loss of symptoms. Cases that come to medical attention are mostly severe (e.g. associated with pharyngeal edema), atypical, or associated with other disorders, notably atopic eczema. The common foods incriminated (cows' milk, egg, nuts, fish, tomatoes and fruit) are similar to those that cause allergic contact urticaria (see later), the difference being that children are in general more likely to touch raw foods than to eat them, and raw foods are on the whole more likely to trigger urticaria than cooked foods.

Allergic contact urticaria

This is an immediate allergic reaction, and should not be confused with contact dermatitis, which represents a delayed reaction. Although certain foods, such as cows' milk, raw eggs, raw potatoes, raw fish, apples and nuts are particularly common causes, any food containing protein could in theory cause allergic contact urticaria. The tissues and secretions of pet mammals are also common causes of allergic contact urticaria in childhood. Other causes are grass pollen, chemicals, a number of drugs applied topically, and a few vehicles contained in topical medicaments.

Irritant contact urticaria

Common causes are plants such as stinging nettles or creatures such as jellyfish, moths and caterpillars. Chemicals are a major cause of irritant contact urticaria, and the relevant chemicals are widely used in food, medicines and cosmetics.

Chronic urticaria

Chronic urticaria is defined as urticaria that has persisted for more than 6 weeks and affects the patient for several days each week. The condition can be associated with serious adverse effects on quality of life, sleep and daily activities, but is rarely associated with systemic features or life-threatening anaphylaxis.[19,20] Of these patients, 40% also have angioedema. Very few cases are caused by allergy and therefore allergy testing is rarely indicated. One half are associated with physical triggers such as cold, heat, sunlight, or stress (home or school). An autoimmune etiology should be considered, particularly in teenage girls and where there is a personal or family history of autoimmune disease, especially thyroid disease. In these cases IgG autoantibodies bind specifically to Fcε receptors on mast cells triggering degranulation. Thyroid function should be monitored in this subgroup of children, as up to one third of patients are at risk of autoimmune thyroid disease. In younger children viral or bacterial infections may also trigger the condition. Salicylates in drugs and sometimes foods can also provoke urticaria.[21] Rarely chronic urticaria may be a manifestation of cutaneous mastocytosis and therefore a careful examination of the skin is required. The natural history varies with the cause. Urticaria caused by infection or drugs is most likely to resolve, while physical and autoimmune urticaria often persists for years. Most cases respond to avoidance of obvious triggers and oral antihistamines. For refractory or more urticarial vasculitis as detailed later, immunosuppressive drugs may be required and referral to a specialist is indicated.

If urticaria persists in one location for over 48 h, or leaves residue (e.g. hyperpigmentation), or is associated with purpura or systemic manifestations (arthritis, fever, etc.) an underlying vasculitis (urticarial vasculitis) should be considered.[22,23] Skin manifestations are typically recurrent episodes of urticaria-like weals, often associated with arthralgia (50%) and angioedema (40%). In addition to the skin, the respiratory (20%), renal (5–10%) and gastrointestinal (20%) systems are most frequently involved in the disease. Urticarial vasculitis is most commonly an acquired idiopathic phenomenon but may occur in association with other disorders, most often systemic lupus erythematosus (SLE), Sjögren syndrome and serum sickness. Of these patients, 60–80% is female. Investigations should include a skin biopsy with immunofluorescent staining for immunoglobulin deposits. The most common laboratory abnormalities reported are an elevated ESR, hypocomplementemia and circulating immune complexes. Measurement of serum complement is useful prognostically, as hypocomplementemia is associated with more serious systemic involvement. There is no universally effective therapy for urticarial vasculitis but commencing treatment with antihistamines and proceeding through nonsteroidal anti-inflammatory drugs (NSAIDs), to colchicine, dapsone or hydroxychloroquine. If these medications do not achieve control, systemic steroids and azathioprine can be tried. The causes of urticaria and angioedema (see later) are listed in Table 33.3.

Table 33.3 Classification of urticaria and angioedema

Urticaria

1. Local irritants:
   plants, jellyfish, chemicals
2. Direct mast cell activation:
   opiates, antibiotics, curare, contrast media physical (cold: consider cryoglobulinemia, solar: consider SLE and porphyria, exercise, cholinergic, vibration)
3. Agents altering arachidonic acid metabolism:
   aspirin/NSAIDs, benzoates
4. IgE mediated:
   allergen mediated (pollens, dander, foods, worms, molds, *Hymenoptera* venom, drugs)
5. IgG mediated:
   viral infections, autoimmune (associated with other autoimmune diseases, especially thyroid disease), urticarial vasculitis
6. Idiopathic

Angioedema

1. Complement inhibitor deficiency:
   hereditary angioedema
2. Complement activation:
   vasculitis, infections, serum sickness
3. Angiotensin-converting enzyme (ACE) inhibitors

ANGIOEDEMA

Unlike urticaria, where the inflammatory edema is in the superficial dermis, in angioedema the swelling is mainly in the deeper subcutaneous and submucosal layers. Angioedema may be painful rather than pruritic, and commonly affects the face and extremities. In the upper respiratory tract it is associated with swelling of the lips, tongue, and pharyngeal tissues, which may rarely lead to life-threatening upper airway obstruction. Angioedema of the gastrointestinal tract usually manifests as abdominal pain. The major mediators of angioedema are plasma kinins (e.g. bradykinin), the activation of which is inhibited by C1 inhibitor and other protease inhibitors. Angioedema is associated with urticaria in 80% of cases; in the remaining 20% of cases angioedema occurs without any urticaria.

Hereditary angioedema

The most important differential diagnosis of allergy-induced angioedema is hereditary angioedema, because the prognosis and management of this condition is different.[24] In the past, the mortality rate for attacks involving the upper airways were around one third of patients. Subcutaneous, respiratory and gastrointestinal tract angioedema characteristic of hereditary angioedema is due to an autosomal dominantly inherited deficiency of C1 esterase inhibitor.[25] Swelling of the gastrointestinal mucosa results in nausea, vomiting, diarrhea and severe pain that can mimic a surgical emergency. The subcutaneous swellings are disfiguring but not erythematous, pruritic or painful. The angioedema is solely mediated by kinins and never associated with urticaria. That is why angioedema in combination with urticaria rules out a diagnosis of hereditary angioedema. Interestingly the pulmonary vascular tree is spared, probably because the cells lining the pulmonary vessels have surface enzymes that inactivate bradykinin and other kinins. Symptoms can last from 1–4 d. Symptom frequency may vary from very few, if any, particularly in prepubertal children, to frequent daily or weekly episodes.

The diagnosis of hereditary angioedema should be considered if: (1) angioedema occurs without urticaria; (2) there is an atypical pattern of angioedema (hands, feet, abdomen rather than face); (3) there is a family history (but 20% of cases are sporadic); (4) there are abdominal symptoms. There are two types of disease: type 1 (85% of cases) due to absent C1 inhibitor and type 2 (15% of cases) where there are normal or elevated levels of C1 inhibitor antigen, but the protein is dysfunctional.

Diagnosis in suspected cases is made by measuring C1 inhibitor levels and function as well as C4, which may be low only during acute attacks.

Unlike allergen-mediated urticaria and angioedema, antihistamines, adrenaline (epinephrine) and steroids are of little or no use in the treatment of hereditary angioedema. C1 esterase inhibitor concentrate, which should be available in all hospital emergency departments, is the treatment of choice for pharyngeal edema and severe abdominal attacks. If the concentrate is not available, fresh-frozen plasma may be used. Danazol can be used as prophylaxis in postpubertal children and non-pregnant adults. In younger children the plasmin inhibitor tranexamic acid is an alternative. Angiotensin-converting enzyme (ACE) inhibitors may precipitate attacks by blocking bradykinin degradation and should be avoided, as should estrogen-based contraceptives.

ALLERGIC ASPECTS OF ATOPIC DERMATITIS

Approximately 10% of infants attending community clinics and up to 30% of infants and young children attending specialist allergy clinics may benefit from antigen avoidance regimens.[26,27] Older children are less likely to respond to dietary manipulation, and avoidance of aero-allergens that might influence their disease is often not practical. Thus the first-line management (see also Chapter 30) is usually symptomatic treatment with emollients and topical steroids, recognition and treatment of bacterial and viral skin infection, and use of sedating H_1 antihistamines at night. The situations in which antigen avoidance should be considered are:

1. **Severe disease.** Exclusion diets are highly disruptive to family life, and are potentially nutritionally hazardous, so it makes little sense to employ a diet when the condition is mild (< 10% of the skin surface area affected) and easily controlled with simple topical therapy. Such diets are more appropriate if 25% or more of the skin surface area is affected.
2. **History.** A history of immediate urticarial or gastrointestinal reactions to foods is common. It is sensible to avoid foods for which there is a clear history of an immediate allergic reaction.
3. **Multiple atopic disorders in infancy.** The occurrence of more than one atopic disorder appears to increase the possibility of an important allergic element. This is especially true if atopic features such as eczema, asthma or rhinitis are accompanied by gastrointestinal symptoms such as persistent loose stools or vomiting.
4. **Age.** Elimination diets are simpler to administer and control in infancy and results are better at this age.
5. **Severe eczema in exclusively breast-fed infants.** In one study, in six of 37 breast-fed infants eczema improved when the mother avoided cows' milk protein and egg and relapsed when these were reintroduced.[28] It is often difficult to predict which baby would respond to maternal dietary exclusion. It is reasonable to try maternal avoidance of cows' milk and egg in an infant with eczema who is being exclusively breast-fed. Other foods can provoke eczema in this way, but their detection relies on the suspicions of a parent or doctor followed by avoidance and later challenge.

ANTIGEN AVOIDANCE IN ATOPIC DERMATITIS

Diets

The important principles underlying any elimination diet are:
1. The diet should in the first instance be tried for a defined period of time (e.g. 6 weeks in patients with eczema) and not just imposed indefinitely.
2. At the end of this period the patient should be reassessed to see if the diet has been helpful. If it has not, then the diet should be discontinued. If the diet has helped, and the parents and doctor feel that the therapeutic benefit outweighs the inconvenience of the diet, then the items omitted should be reintroduced one by one (in eczema at the rate of about one new food every 5–7 d).
3. The help of a dietitian is important to ensure that specific food items have been properly excluded from the diet, and to ensure the nutritional adequacy of the diet.

There are a variety of exclusion diets available. Infants and toddlers are far more likely to benefit than older children.

Half-hearted attempts to 'have a go'

The very small quantity of food that can provoke an adverse reaction means that the 'try cutting down his milk' type of tinkering with the diet is most unlikely to succeed. The advantage of a carefully conducted diet is that even if it fails, at least the parents will be satisfied in the knowledge that it was tried properly.

Complete avoidance of known triggers

A trial of rigorous avoidance of known or suspected triggers is a logical first step. It is common to see a child with a clear history of intolerance to a food, but where the food is being incompletely avoided. In infants with eczema, specific avoidance of cows' milk, egg and/or wheat are most often considered. These diets are unlikely to be successful in the absence of history of the eczema being made worse by these foods.

Avoidance of 10 common food triggers

The patient avoids approximately 10 common food triggers, plus foods for which there is a history of intolerance. The foods usually chosen for exclusion are cows' milk, egg, wheat, fish, legumes (pea, bean, soya, lentil), tomato, nuts, berries and currants, citrus fruit and food additives

Table 33.4 Measures that kill the house dust mite and reduce levels of mite antigen in the home

1. Reducing indoor relative humidity below 50%
   High-efficiency dehumidifiers
2. Removal of dust mites and allergens
   Washing bed linen in hot water (≥55 °C)
   Adding benzyl benzoate (0.03%) to wash cycle
   Tumble drying bed linen ((≥55 °C for more than 10 min)
   Dry cleaning
   Replace carpets, draperies and upholstery
   Vacuuming carpets
   Freezing toys and small items (< 17 °C for 24 h), then wash
   Dust with damp cloth
3. Encasements
   Mattress and pillow dust mite proof encasements

(for a discussion of these see separate section later). The chances of a useful clinical benefit are small.

The few-foods diet (so-called oligoantigenic diet)

This consists of exclusion of all foods except for five or six items. These items should not include a food for which there is a history of intolerance. Such diets comprise a meat (usually lamb or turkey), three vegetables (e.g. potato, rice, and carrot or a brassica – cauliflower, cabbage, broccoli or sprouts), a fruit (usually pear) and possibly a breakfast cereal (e.g. Rice Krispies). There are scanty data on the outcome of few-foods diets. In one study, a few-foods diet was associated with marked improvement in 50% of patients (median age 2.9 years, range 0.4–14.8) with atopic eczema, but after 12 months' follow-up, the results were the same (marked improvement) in the group that improved, the group that failed to improve, and the group that tried a diet but were unable to cope.[29] In another study, 85 children (median age 2.3 years, range 0.3–13.3 years) with atopic eczema were randomly allocated to receive a few-foods diet supplemented with either a whey hydrolysate or a casein hydrolysate formula, or to remain on their usual diet and act as controls, for a 6-week period.[30] After 6 weeks, there was a significant reduction in all three groups in the percentage of surface area involved and skin severity score. Of those who participated, 16 (73%) of the 22 controls and 15 (58%) of the 24 who received the diet showed a greater than 20% improvement in the skin severity score. This is the only controlled study of a few-foods diet, and it failed to show benefit. However, the drawback to these two studies is the relatively high median age and the wide age range, which is important because it is general experience that the best results for elimination diets are in infants. Given the tendency for most children with food hypersensitivity to grow out of the problem by the age of 3 years, the inclusion of substantial numbers of older children in these studies unintentionally biased the results against finding benefit from a diet.

Elemental diet

The application of an inpatient regimen of 4–6 weeks of a so-called elemental diet (e.g. Elemental 028, Vivonex or Tolerex) is the ultimate test of whether food intolerance is relevant or not, but until more data are available this approach must be regarded as experimental.[31] The drawbacks comprise the lack of a guarantee of success, family disruption associated with 2–3 months' hospitalization, loose stools (due to hyperosmolarity of the formula), weight loss and hypoalbuminemia.

House dust mite and pet avoidance

House dust mites and pets can trigger atopic eczema. However, the number of patients who experience benefit solely from the avoidance of pets or mites appears to be small. As with elimination diets, there is no test that predicts benefit from avoidance measures. In some children, particularly those with troublesome facial eczema and periocular irritation worse first thing in the morning, the house dust mite in pillow cases and

mattresses may be a significant factor. Even though previous trials have not shown dust-proof covers to be useful in unselected patients with eczema, they may be helpful in these selected cases. A number of additional measures are recommended to kill house dust mites and remove mite antigen from homes (Table 33.4)[32] but none of these measures have been found to significantly affect the clinical severity of eczema. Some patients with atopic eczema are worse during the pollen season or after grass has been cut, but avoidance is impossible.

RESPIRATORY TRACT

ALLERGIC ASPECTS OF ASTHMA

There is no doubt that exposure to various triggers can provoke or worsen asthma in certain patients. Observations of children with unusually severe asthma who are sent to alpine resorts, where the exposure to house dust mites and pets is greatly reduced or abolished, are that somewhere between one and two thirds become completely asymptomatic and can discontinue all therapy. Return home is followed by relapse in most patients. In the past it was believed that this improvement was due to separation from parents and 'family tension', but the current doctrine is that the benefit is due to the avoidance of inhaled allergens. A history may help identify intermittent triggers that provoke attacks (e.g. cat dander), but may not identify allergens to which the patient is regularly exposed and which are responsible for maintaining the asthmatic state (e.g. house dust mites). However, there is a lack of objective investigations to establish the qualitative importance of allergy. For example, it is impossible to state, for asthmatic children of any specific age, in what proportion exposure to an animal provokes an attack of asthma, or what proportion will benefit from removal of a household pet. Some triggers are allergens, but others are not, so it is misleading to think of asthma solely as an allergic disease. Non-allergic triggers are discussed in Chapter 20.

Trigger avoidance

It is impossible to avoid triggers such as cold weather, exercise, laughing and crying. Viral infections, pollens and fungal spores are ubiquitous, and total avoidance is impossible without unacceptable restrictions.

Avoidance of pets and pet antigens is theoretically possible but often unpopular or unacceptable to the family. Removal of the animal itself is insufficient, and if the level of pet antigen in the household is to be adequately reduced then also required are intensive carpet and furniture cleaning. Complete removal of cat antigen is especially difficult (if not impossible), and because of its adhesion to wall surfaces requires washing of the walls.

Role of antigen avoidance in management of asthma

There are no objective data upon which to base clear recommendations, with the result that there are differences of opinion about the relevance of antigen avoidance. The cornerstone of the treatment of asthma is drug therapy, supplemented where possible or relevant by the avoidance of triggers. Even with the most enthusiastic approach to the identification and avoidance of triggers, it is rare for this alone to abolish symptoms. The major triggers that are at least potentially avoidable are house dust mites and pets. Since there is no clinical or laboratory test that can accurately identify those patients who will benefit from antigen avoidance, the only logical approach is to attempt a defined trial period of avoidance, including an assessment after an agreed period of time (e.g. 3 months) as to whether there has been any benefit.

ALLERGIC RHINOCONJUCTIVITIS

Allergic rhinoconjunctivitis may be either perennial or seasonal. Important triggers of perennial disease are house dust mite and pet danders. Seasonal rhinoconjunctivitis is most frequently caused by allergy to tree (spring), grass (summer) pollens or less frequently mould spores (*Cladosporium*, *Alternaria* and *Aspergillus*). Salicylate sensitivity occurs mainly in adults and may start with symptoms of perennial rhinitis and then progress to include chronic sinusitis, nasal polyposis and asthma, which may be severe.[21]

Over 50% of patients have a combination of nasal and ocular symptoms. Nasal symptoms include sneezing, rhinorrhea and nasal blockage. Eye symptoms include itching, watering, redness, swelling and stinging. A severe seasonal form associated with cobblestoning of the conjunctiva, more common in boys is sometimes called 'vernal (spring) conjunctivitis'. During an exacerbation keratitis is common, causing photophobia and reduced visual acuity, and sometimes leading to an ulcer that may in turn cause permanent loss of vision. Asthmatic symptoms sometimes coexist with attacks of hay fever.

Avoidance of allergens is often not possible and therefore the mainstay of treatment is using medication to reduce the inflammatory effects of mast cell degranulation, particularly histamine. Nonsedating H_1 antihistamines are by far the simplest and most useful treatment for mild and moderate cases, given prophylactically during the pollen season. An advantage of H_1 antihistamines is that they help to prevent both nasal and eye symptoms.

Additional prophylactic medication for more troublesome nasal symptoms is mainly topical nasal corticosteroids. Systemic nasal decongestants are not recommended in children. Sodium cromoglycate nasal spray and oral montelukast are sometimes used, but are less effective than topical corticosteroids.

For allergic conjunctivitis, eye drops are often more effective than oral antihistamines but in more troublesome cases a combination should be used. Drops containing antihistamine, mast cell stabilizer (sodium cromoglycate), nonsteroidal anti-inflammatory agents and a combination of the above are available. Sodium cromoglycate works best if applied four times a day, which is demanding.

An exceptionally severe form of allergic conjunctivitis is known as vernal conjunctivitis, and for this steroid or cyclosporine drops may be justifiable, but these can only be prescribed under the supervision of an ophthalmologist, who can monitor for complications or adverse events side-effects such as corneal abrasions, glaucoma or cataracts.

Immunotherapy in selected children with severe allergic rhinoconjunctivitis due to grass pollen allergy can alleviate symptoms. It is worth considering where there is a poor response to oral antihistamines and topical treatments, and where the illness is having a major impact on the child's life. Referral to a specialist center for allergy testing and treatment is required.

ADVERSE REACTIONS TO FOODS AND THE GASTROINTESTINAL TRACT

All eating causes reactions, for example satiety, the urge to defecate, a feeling of warmth, and weight gain. The mechanisms for food intolerance may be immunological (food allergy), metabolic (e.g. lactase deficiency), pharmacological (e.g. vasoactive amines), toxic (e.g. lectins in red kidney beans), irritant (e.g. curry) or unknown. Individuals vary in their tolerance of events.

The prevalence of reported food intolerance in children ranges widely from 6–18%,[33,34] a problem with these figures being that only about one third of parental reports of food intolerance can be confirmed when tested by blind food challenge. Intolerance to most other foods can occur; these are mainly responsible for immediate allergic reactions. Where there is doubt about a specific food intolerance, the only reliable way to confirm or refute the diagnosis is to perform a food challenge. The management consists of avoidance. The prognosis for food intolerance in young children is good. A prospective study showed that the offending food or fruit was back in the diet after only 9 months in half the cases, and virtually all the offending foods were back in the diet by the third birthday.[35]

IgE–MEDIATED GASTROINTESTINAL HYPERSENSITIVITY DISORDERS

Symptoms of immediate gastrointestinal hypersensitivity are acute – usually occurring within minutes of consuming the food. Nausea and vomiting is very common in IgE-mediated food allergy and help to rid the body of the triggering allergen. Diarrhea may follow several hours after the initial symptoms. The usual offenders are milk, egg, peanut, soy, wheat and seafood. Similar to other IgE-dependent allergic disorders, allergy to milk, egg, wheat and soy general resolve, whereas allergies to peanuts, tree nuts and seafood are more likely to persist. Allergens that are enzymes, for example in some fruit and vegetables, are rapidly degrading by salivary and gastric enzymes and therefore symptoms are often localized to the lips and oral cavity (oral allergy syndrome).[36] Oral allergy syndrome may be preceded by the onset of pollen-induced allergic rhinoconjunctivitis and is sometimes secondary to cross-reactivity between allergens of similar structure (see Table 33.5). These include oral pruritus, angioedema of the lips, tongue and palate. In around 9% of cases symptoms are systemic and in 1% of cases they may be severe.

EOSINOPHILIC GASTROINTESTINAL DISORDERS

Eosinophilic gastrointestinal disorders (EGIDs) are defined as disorders that selectively effect the gut with eosinophil-rich inflammation in the absence of known causes for eosinophilia.[37,38] They need to be distinguished from drug reactions, parasitic infections (particularly strongyloides and ancylostoma), malignancies and inflammatory bowel disease. A family history of EGID was present in 10% of patients and 75% of cases are atopic. The prevalence is hard to estimate but seems to be as common as inflammatory bowel disease.

EGID is thought to have an allergic basis and the pathophysiology may involve either IgE or cell-mediated allergic responses. Clinical features and management vary depending on the segment of bowel affected (esophagus, stomach, small intestine, colon). Milk, egg, wheat, peanut and soy may trigger these disorders but in many cases multiple food allergies are involved. In 50% of cases there is a peripheral blood eosinophilia. Endoscopic appearance may be normal and the disease is often patchy. Diagnosis is dependent on the presence of an excessive eosinophilic infiltrate evaluated on multiple gut biopsies.

Eosinophilic esophagitis is associated with gastroesophageal reflux, vomiting, epigastric or chest pain, respiratory obstructive problems and dysphagia. The dysphagia, occurring in 85% of cases, may be severe enough to lead to impaction of food. Strictures and Barrett's esophagus may occur in chronic cases. Two thirds of patients are males and there is a high rate of atopic disease, particularly asthma. The condition has been thought of 'asthma of the esophagus'. Food allergens play a pathological role as dietary restriction or hydrolyzed formulae are associated with an improvement in 98% of children. Topical corticosteroids (the patient is instructed to swallow the dose from a metered-dose inhaler delivered without a spacer) provide long-term control but systemic steroids may be required for acute flares.

Eosinophilic gastritis and *gastroenteritis* are less well-defined entities and may present with vomiting, abdominal pain, anemia, failure to thrive and diarrhea, which may mimic Celiac disease. In such cases a jejunal biopsy usually shows some degree of villous atrophy. Treatment is similar to eosinophilic esophagitis with dietary restrictions and topical steroids (oral budesonide). The condition is often chronic waxing and waning.

Table 33.5   Common food allergy syndromes

Birch	Apples, cherries, peach, pear, nectarine, plum, apricot, hazelnut, walnut, almond, pecan, brazil (i.e. tree nuts), kiwi, carrot, celery, tomato, coconut, turnip, parsnip
Ragwood	Watermelon, cucumber, zucchini, banana
Mugwood	Celery, carrot, caraway, dill, parsley, fennel, green pepper
Grass	Potato, tomato, melon, peanut, orange, celery, kiwi
Latex	Banana, avocado, chestnut, kiwi

Eosinophilic colitis (including cows' milk protein intolerance) is the most common cause of bloody stools in infancy, is often due to cows' milk protein allergy and less commonly soy. Frequent loose stools occur in 25–75% of patients. In an uncommon but florid picture, infants can present with heavily bloodstained loose stools, sometimes accompanied by mucus. Acute abdominal pain (often but not always accompanied by vomiting or loose stools) can be a striking symptom. The acute presentation of blood in the stools and abdominal pain may mimic intussusception. Discomfort, crying or irritability are common and major features in infancy.

In contrast to eosinophilic esophagitis, eosinophilic colitis is a non-IgE mediated disease and thus RAST and skin prink tests are usually negative. In infants, exclusion of the offending food usually leads to resolution of the bloody diarrhea within 72 h and thus endoscopy and biopsy are reserved for refractory cases. The vast majority of infants outgrow the food intolerance by 1–3 years of age and therefore intermittent trials of reintroduction of the milk at 12 months old and then 6 monthly is advised. In older children the prognosis is similar to eosinophilic gastroenteritis with a chronic course.

Celiac disease

Celiac disease represents an immune response to a food protein (gluten in wheat, rye and barley) and therefore may be considered a food-allergic disorder.[39] Its prevalence is 1% in western populations. Symptoms include vomiting, diarrhea, anorexia and growth failure but are now recognized as often being more subtle or nonspecific. Thus the mean age of diagnosis has shifted from the first few years of life to middle adulthood. The α-gliadin peptide of gluten is presented particularly well by dendritic cells expressing HLA-DQ2 and/or DQ8 and > 95% of patients have these HLA types. α-gliadin cross-react with tissue transglutaminase 2 and stimulates the γδT lymphocytic infiltrate and villous atrophy characteristic of this inflammatory enteropathy. Avoidance of dietary gluten leads to resolution of the disease, but this dietary restriction needs to be continued lifelong to prevent recurrences. Delay in removing gluten from the diet may be associated with an increased risk of other autoimmune diseases, particularly type I diabetes mellitus and autoimmune thyroid disease, as well as intestinal lymphoma. A detailed appraisal is given in Chapter 19.

BEHAVIORAL PROBLEMS

Both hospital and community-based double-blind placebo-controlled studies have repeatedly failed to confirm any validity in the idea that food or food additives cause severe behavioral problems in otherwise healthy individuals. The avoidance of food additives seems to have only a very short-lived beneficial effect on hyperkinesis and other behavior problems, and any benefit from additive avoidance diets is likely to be a placebo response. One source of confusion has been the presence of atopic disease. If a food additive makes eczema or asthma worse, then the concentration span and behavior may also be expected to suffer, but there is no evidence that this is anything other than an indirect effect.

IMPORTANT ALLERGENS IN CHILDREN

COWS' MILK PROTEIN

Cows' milk protein intolerance is a heterogeneous disorder and may present with symptoms of immediate (acute allergy, rarely even anaphylaxis) or delayed hypersensitivity reactions (EGID) (see section on the gastrointestinal tract earlier). Prevalence studies of intolerance to cows' milk protein vary from 1.9–7.5%. A most detailed study estimated a point prevalence of cows' milk protein intolerance in children with parentally perceived reactions at the age of 2.5 years at 1.1% (CI 0.8–1.6).[40]

The most common antigens in cows' milk are α-lactoglobulin, casein, α-lactalbumin, bovine serum albumin and bovine α-globulin. Digestion may result in the production of additional antigens. The marked antigenic similarity between cows' and goats' milk proteins explains why most children with cows' milk protein intolerance are intolerant to goats' milk. Intolerance to carbohydrates present in cows' milk and milk formulae is dealt with in Chapter 16.

The quantity of cows' milk required to produce an adverse reaction varies. Some patients develop anaphylaxis after ingestion of less than 1 mg of casein, α-lactoglobulin or α-lactalbumin. In contrast, Goldman et al[41] showed that 29 out of 89 children (33%) with cows' milk intolerance did not react to 100 ml of milk but only to 200 ml or more. The median reaction onset time in those who reacted to 100 ml milk challenges was 2 h, but the median reaction onset time in those who required larger amounts of milk to elicit reactions was 24 h.

Most cows' milk formula-fed infants with cows' milk protein intolerance develop symptoms in the first 3 months of life. The age of onset of the first symptoms in breast-fed babies depends on the age at which cows' milk is first introduced. A proportion of infants with cows' milk protein intolerance react adversely to traces of cows' milk protein in their mother's milk. Patients with cows' milk protein intolerance may be intolerant to other foods. In one hospital-based series of 100 children with cows' milk protein intolerance, over 50% exhibited intolerance to one or more other foods.[42] Approximately 8–14% of children with intolerance to cows' milk protein are also intolerant to soya protein.

Clues to the diagnosis of cows' milk protein intolerance in the history

1. Symptoms occur, or are made worse, soon after ingestion of cows' milk protein. Multiple affected systems (e.g. gut, chest and skin) make the diagnosis more likely; single symptoms make it most unlikely.
2. Symptoms date from the time, or soon after the time, that breast-feeding was stopped or cows' milk protein was first introduced into the diet. (NB feeding changes often coincide with the onset of atopic disease, and do not prove a cause-and-effect relationship)
3. There is a family history of cows' milk protein intolerance.
4. The presence of severe atopic disease in an infant under the age of 12 months.
5. The observation that spilling cows' milk onto non-eczematous skin causes an urticarial rash.

Making the diagnosis of cows' milk protein intolerance

Most patients whose symptoms commence within 20–30 min of cows' milk ingestion have a positive skin prick test, but most of those whose symptoms occur more slowly have negative skin prick tests. Skin prick tests and RAST tests are usually unhelpful, particularly if symptoms are delayed. A jejunal biopsy is unnecessary because it cannot replace the need for milk elimination and challenge, and the histological changes seen in the small intestine are not diagnostic for cows' milk protein intolerance.

The procedure required to diagnose cows' milk protein intolerance is:

1. a period of avoidance (2 d for those with symptoms occurring within 1 h of milk ingestion; 14–28 d for those with delayed-onset symptoms) causing loss of symptoms;
2. recurrence of symptoms on reintroduction of cows' milk protein;
3. loss of symptoms after second withdrawal of cows' milk protein;
4. Continued abatement of symptoms with continued avoidance of cows' milk protein.

This strategy must be accompanied by regular attempts to reintroduce cows' milk protein, for example yearly, to see if the patient has grown out of the intolerance.

Failure of cows' milk exclusion

The reasons why a trial period of cows' milk elimination may fail are:

1. The patient has an alternative cause for the reported symptoms.
2. The period of elimination was too short.
3. Foods containing cows' milk protein have not been fully excluded from the diet.

4. The patient is intolerant to the cows' milk substitute that has been given. This is common with goat's milk or sheep's milk. About 8–14% of patients with cows' milk protein intolerance are also intolerant to soya. An unknown proportion are intolerant to whey hydrolysate formulae (these vary in their antigenicity), and there are rare cases of intolerance to casein hydrolysate formulae (Pregestimil or Nutramigen).

5. The patient has a coexisting or intercurrent disease, e.g. gastroenteritis.

6. The patient is intolerant to other items that have not been withdrawn from the diet or the environment.

7. The patient's symptoms are trivial and have been exaggerated, or alternatively do not exist at all and have either been imagined or fabricated by the parents. Complete fabrication of symptoms by parents is rare, but the mistaken belief that a child's symptoms are attributable to food intolerance is common.

Milk challenge procedure

A challenge with cows' milk protein is carried out either to confirm the diagnosis or to see if the patient has grown out of the intolerance. If it is known that the child can tolerate small amounts of cows' milk at home then a formal challenge in hospital is not required, and the parents can continue to increase the quantity of cows' milk given at home.

It is vital to remember that during cows' milk protein challenge, symptoms may appear that had not been present previously, the most serious being anaphylactic shock. In Goldman et al's original study, three of 89 patients developed anaphylactic shock as a new symptom during milk challenge.[42] In a further five patients, anaphylaxis had been noted prior to milk challenge. Any strategy for cows' milk protein challenges has to take into account the risk of anaphylaxis.

Milk challenge procedure for patients with no history of anaphylaxis after cows' milk ingestion

The first step, prior to the oral administration of cows' milk, is the topical application of milk to the child's skin, using the back. Some cows' milk is firmly rubbed onto the patient's skin with a piece of gauze or cotton wool, and the skin observed for 15 min. A positive reaction comprises a weal, surrounded by a red flare; redness without a weal is a negative response. If there is a positive response, the challenge procedure is halted, and cows' milk protein should be avoided for a further 12 months before repeating the test.

It is acknowledged that a positive rub test may sometimes be a false positive, but the above strategy is designed to protect the child, and the need to minimize the risks of anaphylaxis. A small number of centers bypass the application of milk (or other foods) to the skin as part of the challenge procedure, and as a precaution conduct the challenge in a high dependency or intensive care facility, with an i.v. line inserted and i.v. fluids running. Reasons for the former more cautious approach are: (1) if there is a significant risk of a life-threatening adverse reaction then it is safer to avoid doing the food challenge altogether, (2) the first-line treatment of anaphylaxis is intramuscular adrenaline, and (3) i.v. fluids are not an immediate requirement.

For the first 60 min of the procedure, a nurse, doctor or parent should be present; the patient must not be left alone. The observer is looking for signs of an adverse reaction, which are:

- rash around the mouth;
- urticarial rash;
- sneezing;
- vomiting;
- irritability and pallor;
- wheezing or coughing;
- loose stools;
- **stridor;**
- **collapse**.

After the first 60 min, the patient should be checked half hourly, provided a parent is present, or quarter hourly if no parent is present. The observer needs to know that the signs above are being sought, and that it is just as important to remove the clothes and look for an urticarial rash as it is to perform the usual nursing observations of the temperature, pulse and respiration rate.

If any of the above signs appear, no further cows' milk should be given, and in the event of a rash, wheezing, stridor or collapse a doctor should be summoned.

The oral challenge procedure itself is:

1. Place one drop of ordinary cows' milk on the patient's tongue, and observe for 15 min.
2. If no reaction, give 5 ml of cows' milk and observe for 15 min.
3. If no reaction, give 10 ml of cows' milk and observe for 15 min.
4. If no reaction, give 30 ml of cows' milk and observe for 15 min.
5. If no reaction, give cows' milk freely, and give cows' milk protein-free solids as normal at meal times. Provided this does not exceed the usual intake volume, ensure the patient has taken at least 200 ml of cows' milk.

It is unclear how long observation in hospital should be continued. Rare cases are described in which severe reactions have developed late (e.g. 6 h after starting challenge) so parents must be warned that a reaction may develop later in the day, when the child is at home.

If any adverse reaction occurs, as well as stopping further cows' milk it is essential to monitor the patient very closely, as such patients are at special risk of suffering severe and possibly fatal collapse without warning. One may need to keep an infant in hospital overnight where a challenge has had to be stopped because of an adverse reaction. Such infants require close monitoring, including the use of an apnea alarm.

Procedure for patients with previous history of anaphylaxis after cows' milk ingestion

Serious consideration should be given to whether a cows' milk challenge is really necessary. If it is being carried out to confirm the diagnosis it is best omitted, because the risks of misdiagnosis are likely to be outweighed by the hazards of the challenge procedure. If the challenge is being carried out to see if the patient has grown out of cows' milk protein intolerance, then it is recommended that at least 12 months have elapse since the previous positive challenge or anaphylactic reaction. The challenge procedure is the same as detailed earlier.

Natural history of cows' milk protein intolerance

Cows' milk protein intolerance often lasts only a few months, and in many cases it has disappeared completely by the age of 12 months, hence the need for milk challenge at the age of 12 months in patients who were diagnosed in infancy. Most children become tolerant to cows' milk protein by the age of 3 years, although some degree of intolerance persists, occasionally into adult life, in a small number of patients.

Cows' milk-free diets

Cows' milk exclusion means the avoidance of all foods that contain cows' milk protein. A dietitian will be able to provide an appropriate diet sheet containing an up-to-date list of milk-free manufactured foods. Beef avoidance is unnecessary as the coexistence of intolerance to cows' milk and beef is unusual. Infants on a cows' milk-free diet require a cows' milk substitute. The choice is between formulae based on soya (bearing in mind that 8–14% of infants with cows' milk protein intolerance will also be intolerant to soya), casein hydrolysate (Pregestimil or Nutramigen) or amino acids (Neocate). The main drawback to casein hydrolysates or formulae based on amino acid is their poor palatability. The milks of other animals (goat, sheep) are inadvisable because of the high incidence of cross-sensitivity with cows' milk protein, their high solute content, and the risk of serious gastrointestinal infections due to unhygienic methods of collection and distribution. Non-infant formulae soya-based milks are unsuitable because of their low calcium, vitamin and energy content. In 2003, the UK Scientific Advisory Committee on Nutrition advised against the use of infant soya-based formulae because of their content of phytoestrogens, specifically isoflavones, which may theoretically affect reproductive health and fertility. There is currently no direct evidence from human studies to support this concern. If an infant who has not been weaned is intolerant to both soya and casein hydrolysate, the options are donated human milk, an elemental diet, or in exceptional circumstances i.v. nutrition. After weaning has commenced, if milk substitutes are unsuitable then supplementation with calcium and maybe other nutrients will be required. Even where a soya or casein hydrolysate infant milk formula is provided, the calcium intake may fall below the recommended requirements. The importance of such low intakes of calcium is unknown, but there may be special risks for patients with atopic eczema. In these children intestinal absorption may be impaired because of an associated enteropathy, the absence of lactose from the diet may impair calcium absorption, and there is a risk of vitamin D deficiency and consequently diminished gastrointestinal calcium absorption in children with atopic eczema who are kept out of sunlight.

EGG

The major allergens in egg white are ovalbumin, ovomucoid and ovotransferrin, and all three are also present in much smaller quantities in egg yolk. Cooking reduces the allergenicity of eggs by 70%. Almost all children with egg intolerance can tolerate cooked chicken. The eggs of turkeys, duck and goose contain similar allergens to hen's eggs.

Egg intolerance is very common, and one population-based study found the estimated point prevalence of intolerance to egg in children aged 2½ years was 1.6% (CI 1.3–2.0%), with an upper estimate of the cumulative incidence by this age of 2.6% (CI 1.6–3.6).[43] It is particularly common in infants with atopic dermatitis. It is most common in the first 6 months of life, and the most frequent presentation is the rapid onset of symptoms minutes after an infant is given egg for the first time. Reactions mostly occur within minutes of eating egg, and consist of an erythematous rash around the mouth, swelling and urticaria of the oral mucosa and angioedema of the face, sometimes with wheezing, stridor, conjunctivitis, rhinitis, vomiting, loose stools and in severe cases anaphylaxis. Those with immediate reactions also exhibit urticaria after skin contact with egg.

The diagnosis of egg intolerance is made from the history. Skin prick tests and RAST tests, although providing information as to whether the child is allergic to raw egg protein, may be falsely positive (e.g. in children who can tolerate cooked egg contained in cake or biscuits, and in children who have outgrown their egg allergy). When the diagnosis is in doubt it can be confirmed by challenge, which would normally comprise ingestion of increasing quantities of egg-containing biscuit, and where this is tolerated hard-boiled egg. The management is to exclude egg in a form that leads to reactions (e.g. raw egg only, partly cooked egg, or all egg) from the diet.

Egg intolerance is not a contraindication to measles or measles–mumps–rubella (MMR) vaccination because modern measles vaccines are grown on fibroblasts and do not contain detectable quantities of egg protein. The MMR vaccine can be safely given to children with egg allergy. The majority of life-threatening allergic reactions to the MMR vaccine have been reported in children who are not allergic to eggs, and these are mainly explained by IgE-mediated gelatin allergy.[44] The same may not apply to other vaccines such as the influenza vaccine, which is grown in the allantoic cavity of chick eggs and which does contain traces of egg protein.

In the majority of cases, egg intolerance has disappeared by the age of 3 years. Where the presentation is after the age of 12 months, which is unusual, the duration of intolerance may be longer, and is occasionally life-long.

SOYA

Soya protein is a permitted ingredient of flour in the UK, and this is not usually declared on manufactured food labels listing ingredients. Soya protein is widely distributed in manufactured foods including bread, pastry and sausages. Soya protein is also commonly employed as a meat extender and found in sausages, hamburgers and pie fillings.

Soya protein intolerance is less common than cows' milk protein intolerance. The clinical features and management of the two disorders are the same, but the widespread use of soya in manufactured foods means that soya protein avoidance is more difficult than cows' milk protein avoidance.

Soya and other beans can cause flatulence, abdominal pain and loose stools, which are due to the action of intestinal bacteria on poorly digestible oligosaccharides, mainly raffinose and stachyose.

FISH AND SHELLFISH

Fish allergy is common in children, whereas shellfish allergy appears to be more prevalent in adults. Fish allergens are highly cross-reactive on in vitro testing with the exception of tuna fish, in keeping with the clinical association between codfish allergy and allergy to hake, carp, pike and whiting but not tuna.

Although most reactions to fish are caused by ingestion, reactions can also occur as a result of inhalation of fish aeroallergens at fish markets or when fish is being cooked. Reactions to food aeroallergens are either respiratory (asthma) or in the skin (urticaria). The latter has been labeled as *osmylogenic urticaria*; 'osmyls' are minute particles given off by odoriferous substances. Aas has reported from Norway that fish antigens could be found in house dust in most homes where fish is often eaten, and he suggested that this was a possible source for sensitization to fish.[45]

Anaphylaxis caused by the unexpected presence of casein after consuming salmon has been reported. Casein has been used in the processing of salmon, posing a threat to individuals who are intolerant to cows' milk protein.

PEANUT AND TREE NUTS

What is a nut?

There is much confusion as to what does or does not constitute a nut. Whereas most nuts come from trees, peanut, the most common nut to cause allergic reactions, is in fact a legume, and the seed pod grows underground (hence an alternative name, 'groundnut'). As far as allergic reactions are concerned, the key information is not the precise botanical origin or plant family but the degree to which the nut does or does not provoke allergic reactions. Allergic reactions to peanuts, walnuts, pecans, brazil nuts, hazelnuts, cashew nuts, pistachio nuts, almonds (strictly speaking a fruit) and macadamia nuts are all well recognized. In contrast, allergic reactions to coconuts, pine nuts, oyster nuts, sweet chestnuts and horse chestnuts are only very rarely reported, and these items do not need to be avoided in children with peanut allergy.

Epidemiology and importance

Peanuts are a major cause of allergic reactions. The prevalence of peanut intolerance in western countries is approximately 0.5%. In a US survey[46] it was estimated that the prevalence of peanut and/or tree nut intolerance was 1.1% (95% CI, 1.0–1.4%). In another US survey, it was noted that peanuts and tree nuts accounted for 20 out of 32 (72%) total fatalities due to food-induced anaphylaxis.[47] Similar trends have been found in the UK.[48]

The main source of exposure to peanut and its products is consumption, but peanut oil (also known as arachis oil) has been used in some injectable, oral and topically applied pharmaceutical preparations. Because of concern that percutaneous absorption of peanut protein could cause sensitization to peanut, efforts have been made in recent years to remove arachis oil from topically applied pharmaceutical products.

The incidence of peanut intolerance is higher in siblings of affected individuals; in one study, three out of 39 siblings (7%) had peanut intolerance.[49] The concordance rate for peanut allergy in monozygotic twins is 64% compared with 7% in dizygotic twins, providing evidence for a strong genetic predisposition.[1] Nearly all patients who have had fatal or near-fatal reactions to nuts have other atopic diseases, especially asthma, but often also atopic dermatitis and allergic rhinitis. The severity of the asthma in these fatalities is variable and may be relatively mild. Asthma has in the past been thought of as a risk factor for the development of potentially severe reactions, but this is probably misleading and it is likely that asthma and peanut allergy are simply different manifestations of the same atopic disease process.

Peanut processing and its effects

The prevalence of peanut intolerance in China is low despite a high rate of peanut consumption. The method of frying or boiling peanuts, as practiced in China, reduces the allergenicity of peanuts compared with the method of dry roasting practiced widely in western countries.[50] Roasting uses higher temperatures that apparently increase the allergenic property of peanut proteins, and this may help to explain the difference in prevalence of peanut allergy observed in the two countries.

Untreated peanut oil contains peanut protein and consumption risks provoking adverse reactions in individuals with peanut intolerance. However processed and refined peanut oil, which has been subjected to degumming (separation of oil and water by centrifugation at 30–50 °C), refining with alkali and further centrifugation at 60–70 °C, bleaching with filters at 110 °C, and deodorization with steam under vacuum at 230–260 °C, does not contain peanut protein, and in one study refined peanut oil failed to provoke a reaction in any of 60 individuals with peanut intolerance.[51] However the marked variation in the degree of processing of peanut and other nut oils means that there will be marked variation in the nut protein content of various different types of refined nut oils.[52] It is worth noting that peanut oil may be used in the pharmaceutical industry, and has been used, for example, in vitamin A and D solutions.

Different cultivars of peanut are grown in many different parts of the world, but peanuts of different varieties from different parts of the world all appear to contain similar antigenic proteins.

Cross-reactivity

In a study of 122 children with allergic reactions to peanuts and tree nuts, 68 had reactions to peanuts alone, 20 to tree nuts alone, and 34 had reactions to both peanuts and at least one tree nut.[53] Of those reacting to tree nuts, 34 had reactions to one, 12 to two, and 8 to three or more different tree nuts, the most common being walnut, almond and pecan. Although there is extensive cross-reactivity between peanuts and other legumes on skin prick testing and RAST testing, clinically important cross-reactivity is uncommon. Nevertheless the risk of confusion between different nuts provides an argument for the avoidance of all nuts in a child known to be allergic to one type of nut. On the other hand, in a clear allergy to a single nut in patients known to be tolerant to others, avoidance of all nuts is not required.

Clinical features

Reactions can involve the skin (urticaria, angioedema), the respiratory tract (wheezing, throat tightness, coughing, dyspnea), and the gastrointestinal tract. Multiple organ systems may be affected. Accidental ingestion is common (30–50% over a 5-year period). In general the symptoms after accidental exposure are similar to those at an initial reaction.[54]

Modes of accidental ingestion include sharing food, hidden food ingredients,[55] cross-contamination (in kitchen utensils or in food manufacturing), and school craft projects using peanut butter.

The threshold dose required to produce a reaction varies. In one study of 14 individuals with peanut intolerance, the lowest dose of peanut to produce a convincing reaction was 2 mg, although individuals with peanut intolerance sometimes report short-lived symptoms after doses as low at 100 µg.[56] It is not uncommon for peanut-intolerant individuals to experience local urticaria after being kissed by someone who has eaten peanut. This is not specific for peanut intolerance; the same phenomenon is seen in individuals who are intolerant to other foods.

Acute allergic reactions to peanuts have been seen in neonates, and thus in some children, sensitization must occur in utero. At present there is no definitive evidence to suggest that avoidance of peanuts during pregnancy and lactation will prevent the development of peanut allergy in the child. The severity of any reaction is in part related to the quantity of nut eaten. When patients with peanut intolerance are followed-up, and experience a further reaction resulting from accidental ingestion, most follow-up reactions are less severe than the index reaction.[57]

Diagnosis

Although skin prick tests and RAST tests may provide useful supportive evidence of a peanut allergy in the absence of a clinical history, they should not be used to diagnose an allergy to peanut or any other food as false-positive reactions do occur and may inappropriately lead to children being labeled as food allergic when they are not. Furthermore, these tests cannot indicate the severity of symptoms. If the history suggests a nonlife-threatening allergy to a food but the skin prick test is negative then a food challenge should be considered as the definitive test of an allergy. If a life-threatening reaction to a food has occurred then food challenges should be avoided.

Natural history

Whilst most children fairly rapidly grow out of some food intolerances, nut allergy has always been regarded as an exception, being lifelong in most cases. Recent claims that up to 20% of patients outgrow peanut allergy have often been based on studies of patients whose original diagnosis was questionable. There probably are a few genuine cases in which nut allergy is not permanent, but they are uncommon.

Management

The management of nut allergy consists of education on avoiding the allergen, common traps being 'groundnut' (another name for peanut) and arachis oil (derived from peanuts). There are three additional treatment options – antihistamine for mild reactions, antihistamine plus inhaled adrenaline for moderate reactions, and antihistamine, adrenaline inhaler and adrenaline autoinjector for severe reactions. In the UK adrenaline inhalers (Medihaler Epi) are unavailable, and this means that adrenaline autoinjectors may need to be considered for some UK patients who have had moderately severe reactions.

Peanuts are cheap, readily available and are often used as a substitute for other nuts. For these reasons, even if there are no features of clinical cross-reactivity, patients who have peanut intolerance should in general avoid all tree nuts. Treatment of peanut allergy by immunotherapy using injections of peanut extract is not currently recommended.

FOOD-PROVOKED EXERCISE-INDUCED ANAPHYLAXIS

Exercise-induced anaphylaxis is usually associated with a combination of cholinergic urticaria (widespread tiny 1–3 mm wheals with variable erythema that last 30–60 min and occur in association with sweating) often starting in the palms and soles before spreading. Signs of autonomic dysfunction such as nausea, vomiting and diarrhea, dilated pupils and hypotension may follow. Attacks may occur spontaneously, or in association with ingestion of specific foods such as celery, shellfish, peaches or wheat.[58,59] The mechanism of this uncommon exercise-induced anaphylaxis is obscure. Management includes warm-up and moderation in exercise, avoidance of food and NSAIDs prior to exercise and making sure the patient is with someone who knows of their condition. Nonsedating antihistamines are often helpful. Hypotension should be treated by lying the patient down with their feet raised.

FOOD ADDITIVES

Food additives include coloring agents, preservatives, antioxidants, emulsifiers, stabilizers, sweeteners, other flavor modifiers and a large miscellaneous group of other agents. An obsession with food that is natural overlooks both the large number of toxic substances naturally occurring in food and the fact that most substances that provoke food intolerance are naturally occurring, such as eggs, cows' milk and nuts. There is an enormous discrepancy between the public's perception of food additive intolerance and objectively verified intolerance.[60]

Tartrazine and benzoic acid

Tartrazine is a yellow coloring agent, and one of the group of azo dyes. It is used as a coloring agent in a wide range of foods and medicines. Benzoic acid and the related benzoates retard the growth of bacteria and yeasts, and are used as food preservatives. Double-blind placebo-controlled studies have demonstrated that tartrazine can provoke urticaria, asthma or rhinitis in a small number of atopic subjects.[61] Similar studies have shown that benzoates can provoke urticaria. There is a lack of objective information about whether benzoates can provoke asthma. Tartrazine or benzoate intolerance can be identified by history (particularly unreliable in suspected food additive intolerance), elimination and challenge. It is possible that repeated administration of tartrazine or the benzoates leads to tolerance, and the severity of adverse reaction may not always be severe enough to warrant avoidance.

Sulfites

Sulfur dioxide and the sodium or potassium salts of sulfite or metabisulfite are widely used as food preservatives. Dried fruit is commonly treated with sulfur dioxide, and high levels of sulfite are sometimes found in wine, beer and salads in restaurants. Sulfites are sometimes used as preservatives in parenteral preparations of drugs, including several drugs used for the i.v. or inhalational treatment of asthma. Double-blind placebo-controlled studies have demonstrated that the oral administration of sulfite solutions can provoke bronchoconstriction in 35–70% of children with asthma.

A history of worsening of pre-existing asthma after consuming artificial drinks, eating in a restaurant or inhalation or injection of a drug containing sulfite raises the possibility of sulfite intolerance. Skin tests are unhelpful, and the diagnosis can only be confirmed by challenge, employing increasing doses of sulfite so as to establish the patient's threshold dose that can provoke asthma. Knowledge of the threshold enables the patient to avoid only those foods with a relatively high sulfite level, making a very restrictive diet unnecessary.

HOUSE DUST
House dust mites

The predominant allergens are digestive enzymes entrapped in mite fecal pellets, which are of a similar size to pollen grains. The main species of house dust mite in Europe is *Dermatophagoides pteronyssinus* and in the USA it is *Dermatophagoides farinae*. Mites feed on desquamated human skin scales, which are mainly shed in the bed and bedroom, where they can be found in mattresses, pillow cases, carpets, cuddly toys and upholstered furniture. The decisive factors that influence the number of mites are air humidity and temperature. Optimum conditions for mites are 70–80% relative humidity and an ambient temperature of 26°C. Mites cannot reproduce when the relative humidity falls below 60%, and cannot survive for more than a few days in a relative humidity of below 40% if the temperature is above 25°C. The relationship between the season and mite density in houses is attributable to seasonal changes in the ambient indoor humidity. In temperate areas, the number of mites is lowest in the winter, when central heating dries the indoor air. Lack of mites at higher altitudes (e.g. alpine resorts) is due to the lower relative humidity. Skin prick and RAST tests may be useful as supportive evidence where there is a history suggestive of an immediate-type hypersensitivity to house dust mite. Although it is possible to reduce levels of the house dust mite in the home (Table 33.4), these measures do not usually lead to an improvement in symptoms of eczema or asthma.

LATEX

Natural latex is produced by nearly 2000 species of plants, although only the rubber tree *Hevea brasiliensis* is commercially valuable as a source of natural rubber. Proteins or peptides, which make up 1–2% of latex are responsible for allergic reactions and different patients appear to be sensitized to different groups of latex proteins.[62] The major rubber proteins are hevamines (proteins with chitinase and lysozyme properties),

and hevein, a fungotoxic protein with considerable structural homology with wheat germ agglutinin and other plant lectins.

Latex is used in the manufacture of a number of products in general and medical use, including gloves, catheters, condoms, balloons, rubber bands, toys and tyres. About 90% of harvested rubber is processed by acid coagulation at pH 4.5–4.8 into dry sheets or crumbled particles for manufacture of extruded rubber products (rubber thread); compression, transfer, or injection molded goods (rubber seals or diaphragms); or pneumatic tyres. The remaining 10% of harvested rubber is noncoagulated and ammoniated; it is used in the manufacture of rubber gloves and other 'dipped' products, such as condoms and balloons and it is these products that are responsible for most allergic reactions to natural rubber latex (see Table 33.6).

Latex antigens can be leached from rubber gloves by normal skin moisture, with subsequent adsorption onto corn starch powder inside the gloves. Latex allergen can also be adsorbed to powder inside gloves that have not been worn. When the gloves are donned or discarded, the corn starch particles with adsorbed latex allergens become airborne and can sensitize nearby persons by inhalation or can evoke symptoms in previously sensitized persons.

Predisposing factors

Atopy is a significant risk factor in the development of latex allergy with two thirds of affected patients being atopic. Latex allergy is one disease that may affect providers of health care services more frequently than patients themselves. Other high-risk workers include housekeepers, doll manufacturers and tyre plant workers. High-risk patient groups are those requiring multiple surgical procedures, such as individuals with spina bifida, where the prevalence is reported as 18–64%.

Reasons for increased prevalence of latex allergy

Other than increased awareness, possible explanations are: (1) the increased use of gloves during medical, dental and surgical procedures, owing to the risk of hepatitis and AIDS; (2) the replacement of mineral talc powder by cornstarch powder. Mineral talc is heavy and only transiently airborne, and has a high capacity to act as an allergen eliminator by binding firmly to latex allergens.

Cross-reactions

Cross-reactions may occur between proteins in latex and various foods such as avocado, bananas, kiwi and chestnut; the so-called 'latex-fruit syndrome' (see Table 33.5).[63,64] Cross-reactions may also occur with the

Table 33.6 Relative risk of latex-containing products

High risk
Medical latex rubber gloves with powder
Latex rubber gloves for use at home
Balloons
Latex for modeling, dental impressions, etc.

Medium risk
Unpowdered gloves
Catheters
Rubber bands
Teats, dummies
Pencil erasers
Some medicines for injection in multi-dose vials

Lower risk
Tyres
Shoe soles
Hot water bottles
Squash balls, other rubber balls
Red or black rubber tubing or sheet
Condoms
Elastic threads in elasticated clothing

weeping fig *Ficus benjamani*, which is increasingly used for indoor decoration. The existence of cross-reacting allergenic structures in plant-derived products such as latex, fruit and enzymes may explain extensive allergenic reactivity.

Clinical manifestations

The most common reaction to latex products is non-immunological, *irritant contact dermatitis*, the development of dry, irritated areas on the skin caused by the effects of repeated hand washing, detergents or sanitizers, or powders added to gloves. *Allergic contact dermatitis* appears 1–2 d after contact with the offending product such as rubber gloves, shoes, sports equipment and medical devices. The dermatitis is a cell-mediated delayed-type hypersensitivity reaction to low molecular weight accelerators and antioxidants in the rubber product. Examples of rubber product components that cause contact dermatitis are thiurams, carbamates, benzothiazoles, thioureas and amine derivatives. Patients may also present with acute urticaria. Inhalation of latex allergen-coated cornstarch particles from powdered gloves can cause *rhinitis* and *asthma* in latex-allergic individuals, mainly adults who manufacture gloves and health care workers. Latex-allergic individuals can rarely experience *anaphylaxis*, occasionally fatal in a variety of medical care situations and as a result of blowing into balloons or using rubber-handled squash racquets. Finally, latex-allergic individuals can react to food that has been contaminated by latex, for example by food handlers wearing latex gloves.

Diagnosis of latex allergy

Diagnosis depends on the clinical history, coupled with examination and laboratory tests. Latex-specific IgE tests result in up to 25% false-negative and 27% false-positive results and must be interpreted with caution.

Management

The mainstay of management is avoidance, especially of powdered latex gloves, which are the major contributors of transferable allergen.[65]

STINGING INSECT VENOM

Stinging insect allergy has a prevalence of 0.3–3% within the general population. It is more common in adults than in children, and males than females. Insects of the order *Hymenoptera* (vespids [wasps] and apids [bees]) sting and these insects are most active in summer and early autumn. The venoms contain proteins such as phospholipase and hyaluronidase.

Normal local reactions consist of pain, swelling and erythema. Larger local reactions can be confused with cellulitis, which is uncommon after insect stings. These are more extensive and may peak at 48 h and last as long as 1–2 weeks. Malaise and nausea may also develop. Symptomatic treatment is with NSAIDs and antihistamines. Oral prednisolone for 2–3 d may also be helpful. People who develop large local reactions to stings typically continue to have similar reactions after subsequent stings. The risk of anaphylaxis following large local reactions is < 5% and patients do not require venom skin tests and are not candidates for immunotherapy.

The most common symptoms of acute systemic IgE-mediated reactions are dermal (urticaria and angioedema). Life-threatening symptoms include edema of the upper airway, circulatory collapse and shock, which can occur at any age.[66] There have been no deaths from insect stings in children and young adults (< 20 years old) in the UK. Deaths are most likely to occur in adults with concurrent pathology (e.g. coronary vascular disease) or those on certain drugs (ACE inhibitors; beta-blockers, tricyclic antidepressants). Just over half of deaths in the UK have been from shock, one third from upper airway obstruction, 10% from asthma.

The risk of systemic IgE-mediated reactions is highest if the second sting occurs 2–8 weeks after the first and decreases with time, being very low > 5 years after the last sting. Children who have had systemic IgE-mediated reactions (skin, respiratory or cardiovascular symptoms) should have blood taken for specific IgE to the insect and be referred to a pediatric allergist. These children should be prescribed an injectable adrenaline device and appropriate training given. They should be told that early adrenaline administration after a sting is important, as patients in established shock are unlikely to respond to this treatment. First-aid should concentrate on lying the patient down with their legs up and calling an ambulance. Venom immunotherapy typically involves a 3–5-year course of desensitizing injections and is rarely indicated in children.

DRUGS
Epidemiology

Prospective studies have estimated that the incidence of serious adverse drug reactions in hospitalized patients is 6.7% and the incidence of fatal drug reactions is 0.32%. Whereas most adverse drug reactions are non-allergic in nature, 6–10% may be attributed to an immune mechanism involving either antibodies or T cells. Drug reactions that are immunologically mediated: (1) require a period of sensitization, (2) occur in a small proportion of the population, (3) are elicited at drug doses far below the therapeutic range, and (4) in most instances subside after drug discontinuation.

The mean age of allergic drug reactions is approximately 40 years, allergic drug reactions in childhood being much less common than in adulthood. Many patients who are said to have drug allergies are not allergic to the drug. For instance, 80–90% of patients who report a penicillin allergy are not truly allergic when assessed by skin testing, and virtually all patients with a negative skin test result can take penicillin without serious sequelae.[67] In children, most of the reactions that coincide with drug administration are exanthema, which are usually due to the underlying disease.

Clinical spectrum of disease

True allergic reactions are restricted to a limited number of syndromes that are generally accepted as allergic in nature, such as anaphylaxis, Stevens–Johnson syndrome, angioedema and urticaria, contact sensitivity and various exanthema, among others. Skin reactions are the most frequent symptoms of adverse drug reactions, occurring in nearly 80% of patients and are most commonly observed with ampicillin, amoxicillin and co-trimoxazole. Beta-lactam antibiotics are the most frequent pharmacological group involved in allergic drug reactions. NSAIDs, minor analgesics and other antibiotics (e.g. co-trimoxazole) are other drugs implicated. Anesthetic agents may cause immediate-type allergic reactions: muscle relaxants are implicated in 60% of cases, suxamethonium being responsible for 39% of these.[68]

Drug antigenicity

Only a few drugs such as large peptides (e.g. insulin), papain, streptokinase and foreign antisera can directly induce an immune response. The majority of drugs are simple chemicals of low molecular weight that are not immunogenic unless combined with serum or tissue proteins to form an immunogenic complex. Thus most drugs that cause hypersensitivity reactions must first be made immunogenic by being haptenated onto proteins, a process that occurs as the drug is metabolized. The cytochrome P450-dependent oxidation pathway in the liver is an important enzyme involved in the production of these reactive drug intermediates that covalently bind to serum and membrane proteins. Penicillin is an exception, as it may haptenate proteins directly without previous metabolism. Acylation of serum proteins results from an amine bond formed from the hydrolyzed beta-lactam ring of the antibiotic.

Diagnosis and management

Diagnosis of drug allergy is largely based on history (Table 33.7) and examination. Although diagnostic testing methods exist, overall they are still of limited practical value for the clinician who is evaluating a patient with suspected drug allergy. One major problem that affects the use of diagnostic tests for drug allergies is that, except for penicillin,

Table 33.7 Important questions to ask in the history of a patient with suspected drug allergy

1. What drugs were administered, by what route and at what dose?
2. For what reason was the drug administered?
3. How long after starting the drug did the reaction commence?
4. What was the nature of the reaction?
5. What treatment if any was required for the reaction?
6. What happened when the drug was discontinued?
7. Has the patient taken the drug (or similar drugs) before and after the reaction? If so, what was the result?
8. How old was the patient at the time of the reaction?

the immunochemistry of most drugs is still not known. In most instances the definitive test for drug allergy is rechallenge; this must be approached with caution as it may precipitate anaphylactic reactions.

In children where the use of a particular drug is essential and there are no alternatives, hyposensitization can be used to induce tolerance in a highly sensitized patient.[69] The procedure is performed by the cautious administration of incremental doses of the drug to the patient over a period of hours to days. The drug can be administered either by oral or i.v. route. The starting dose for the procedure can be determined by performing intradermal skin tests with the native drug at a dose that does not cause a nonspecific reaction. Typically, doses are doubled every 15–30 min and vital signs, physical examination, and peak flow values are regularly monitored. It is critical that the individuals involved with the hyposensitization procedure understand that it can have serious consequences. While anaphylactic reactions rarely occur if conservative protocols are used, health care personnel must be prepared to treat anaphylaxis if it does happen.

Penicillin and cephalosporin allergy

Anaphylactic reactions occur in approximately 1 per 10 000 penicillin or cephalosporin courses and are mostly seen in adults between the ages of 20 and 49 years. Only 2–6% of patients with a history of acute penicillin allergy are also allergic to cephalosporins. A history of atopy does not generally place an individual at increased risk for an IgE-mediated penicillin reaction.

Degradation products of penicillin may bind with tissue or serum proteins to form an immunogenic complex that can elicit an immune response. Penicillin allergy is attributed either to the benzylpenicilloyl hapten (the so-called 'major' determinant because 95% of tissue-bound penicillin is in this form), or to a group of compounds collectively called the 'minor' determinants, which are paradoxically responsible for many of the most severe allergic reactions. Adverse reactions to penicillin can be most simply classified by the timing of their occurrence. Immediate reactions occur within 1 h of administration and are usually directed against the minor determinant antigens. Life-threatening reactions occurring beyond 1 h of penicillin administration are rare.

The clinical features include urticaria, laryngeal edema, bronchospasm and anaphylactic shock. Accelerated reactions occur 1–72 h after penicillin administration, have the same clinical features as immediate reactions, and are usually directed against the major determinant. Late reactions, the mechanisms of which are generally less well understood, occur more than 72 h after drug administration. They comprise such disorders as a maculopapular (measles-like) rash, urticaria, serum sickness, erythema multiforme, hemolytic anemia, thrombocytopenia and neutropenia. Rarely, late reactions are due to the new development of an immediate or accelerated reaction. Only 3.5% of patients with a maculopapular rash associated with penicillin administration had adverse reactions to oral challenge with penicillin.[70] Maculopapular eruptions caused by penicillin may subside spontaneously despite continuing use of the drug and may not recur on re-exposure, presumably as many of these exanthema are due to the infectious disease rather than the antibiotic.

Ampicillin can provoke the same allergic reactions as other penicillins, but in addition is associated with a particularly high incidence of a non-allergic maculopapular rash, beginning a week or more after starting therapy.

An inquiry about possible penicillin allergy is mandatory prior to an injection of penicillin. However, not all patients with penicillin allergy give a history of previous penicillin administration. In these patients either the history is incorrect and the patient has received penicillin therapy, or sensitization has occurred through inadvertent exposure to penicillin in other sources such as food, milk or even soft drinks. Almost all deaths from anaphylaxis have resulted from injection of the drug, and the oral route has only been associated with a handful of fatal cases.

The penicillin skin test has no place in the management of patients without a clinical history of an IgE-mediated penicillin allergy, and is unnecessary in the face of a bona fide history of a life-threatening acute reaction, in which case the drug should be avoided. In cases where the history is suggestive of a milder acute hypersensitivity reaction, a negative result to skin testing is associated with tolerance to penicillin in 98% of cases. In contrast, a positive skin test result should lead to avoidance of this antibiotic, or use only after hyposensitization. There are no clinically useful skin tests or IgE tests for use in patients with suspected cephalosporin allergy. On the rare occasions in childhood (e.g. endocarditis) when treatment with penicillin is essential, then it is possible to hyposensitize the patient by oral and then continuous i.v. administration, but this procedure carries a risk of fatal anaphylaxis. The protection from hyposensitization is short lived, although it is possible to maintain a state of hyposensitization by long-term administration of a low dose.

Aspirin – nonsteroidal anti-inflammatory drug intolerance

The prevalence of aspirin intolerance is around 5–6%. Up to 20% of the asthmatic population is sensitive to aspirin and other NSAIDs and present with a triad of perennial rhinitis, sinusitis and asthma when exposed to the offending drug. Chronic persistent inflammation is the hallmark of patients with aspirin-induced allergy.[21] Of the patients with aspirin-induced intolerance 50% have chronic, severe, corticosteroid-dependent asthma, 30% have moderate asthma that can be controlled with inhaled steroids, and the remaining 20% of patients have mild and intermittent asthma. Up to 25% of hospital admissions for acute asthma requiring mechanical ventilation may be due to NSAID ingestion.

Aspirin intolerance is now thought to be at least partly due to a deviation of the arachidonic acid metabolic pathway towards the production of excessive inflammatory leukotrienes (especially LTC_4 and away from the production of anti-inflammatory prostaglandins (PGE_2). Leukotriene-modifying drugs (montelukast, zileuton) have been found to attenuate but not abolish aspirin-induced bronchial reactions in aspirin-induced intolerant patients. Salmeterol, a long-acting alpha$_2$-agonist has also been found useful in the management of aspirin-induced intolerance.

Local anesthetic agents

Older amino-ester LA (e.g. cocaine) are documented to cause allergic reactions, including contact dermatitis and redness or edema of the skin or mucous membranes. These compounds are no longer used as injectable local anesthetics and modern amide anesthetics (lidocaine [Xylocaine]), mepicaine [Carbocaine], bupivacaine [Marcain], prilocaine [Citanest] and articaine [Septanest] rarely if ever cause such reactions. Symptoms suggestive of an allergic reaction may be due to vasovagal reactions, adrenaline responses, 'panic attacks' and systemic toxic reactions. These effects are compounded by the fact that patients presenting for minor surgical and dental procedures under local anesthetics are usually anxious to start with, and up to 6% of patients have a problematic fear of needles. Infrequently, reactions may be to confounding factors such as latex or the preservative in preloaded syringes. In the latter case this is due to an irritant rather than allergic reaction to benzalkonium chloride, a quaternary ammonia cationic surfactant that is also present in some skin disinfectants. If suspected, further reactions can be prevented by using preservative-free vials of the drug.

Local anesthetic agents are too small to be antigenic by themselves but are sufficiently alien to bind as haptens to tissues with antigenic properties. Large series including hundreds or thousands of patients have consistently shown that both skin prick tests and intradermal tests are negative in almost all patients referred with an adverse reaction.[71] Furthermore specific IgE in the few cases where there are reactions have been negative.

ANAPHYLAXIS

In this chapter, and in the clinical situation, the term 'anaphylaxis' or 'anaphylactic shock' is taken to mean a severe life-threatening reaction of rapid onset, with circulatory collapse or respiratory compromise. In the past the term 'anaphylaxis' was used to describe any immediate allergic reaction caused by IgE antibodies, however mild, but such usage fails to distinguish between, for example, trivial urticaria and a life-threatening event. The mechanisms are believed to be IgE mediated (e.g. penicillin or insulin allergy), the generation of immune complexes (e.g. reactions to blood products), a direct (not involving antigens or antibodies) effect on mast cells or basophils causing inflammatory mediator release (e.g. reactions to radiocontrast media) and presumed abnormalities of arachidonic acid metabolism (e.g. anaphylactoid reactions to aspirin). It is possible to theoretically differentiate between anaphylaxis (immunologically mediated reactions) and anaphylactoid (non-immunologically mediated) reactions.[72] Previous sensitization is required for the former but not the latter.

The major causes of anaphylactic shock are drugs (e.g. penicillin, muscle relaxants), heterologous antisera (used for the prophylaxis and treatment of tetanus, diphtheria, rabies, snake bites and botulism), radiographic contrast media, the administration of blood products, hyposensitization injections, venoms from stinging insects (honeybee, wasp, hornet, yellow jacket) and foods (especially nuts, cows' milk, fish, shellfish and egg).[73] Death from anaphylaxis to medicines given intravenously usually occurs within a few minutes, while in the case of stinging insect stings it is usually delayed by 15 min and with foods by 30 min, although rarely it may be delayed for up to 6 h.[73] In general, the sooner the symptoms occur the more severe is the reaction. The first symptoms are feeling unwell, feeling warm, generalized pruritus, fear, faintness and sneezing. In severe cases these early symptoms are quickly (in seconds or minutes) followed by loss of consciousness, and death from severe bronchospasm, suffocation (edema of the larynx, epiglottis and pharynx) or shock and cardiac arrhythmia.[74]

DIAGNOSIS OF ALLERGY – TAKING A HISTORY

The lack of really useful laboratory tests for allergy (see later) means that there is no substitute for a careful history.

IMPORTANT QUESTIONS WHEN TAKING A HISTORY FOR ALLERGY

The history should include questions about:
1. when symptoms occur (e.g. day or night, time of year – tree pollen allergy occurs in early spring; grass pollen allergy in summer);
2. where symptoms occur (e.g. particular place);
3. when or where the patient is free of symptoms;
4. the presence of other allergic symptoms;
5. family history of allergy or atopic disease;
6. nature and quantity of substance thought to be causing reaction;
7. timing of reaction (e.g. immediate versus delayed);
8. severity of reaction (e.g. skin, respiratory, gut, circulatory, anaphylaxis);
9. time to resolution (e.g. hours, days, weeks);
10. response to treatment (e.g. no treatment required, antihistamines, intramuscular adrenaline);
11. previous contact with trigger and reactions (e.g. has a food previously been tolerated or previously caused a similar reaction?);
12. effect of changes in environment (e.g. if it is worse in a playground this might suggest a grass pollen allergy; if it resolves on holidays this might suggest house dust mite or pet allergy).

OTHER CLUES FROM THE HISTORY

1. **The symptoms are worse at night.** Both asthma and eczema are often worse at night, but it is wrong to equate all nocturnal symptoms with house dust mite allergy, as there are other possible explanations. Circadian rhythms affecting airway caliber, bronchial reactivity[75] and cortisol secretion may account for some of the increase in symptoms at night in asthma. In eczema, heat, tiredness and low cortisol secretion may contribute to nocturnal symptoms. In theory a high concentration of house dust mite antigen found in some bedrooms could contribute to nocturnal symptoms in asthma, rhinitis or atopic eczema, but in one large study there was no association between worsening at night or on waking and the presence of house dust mite allergy.[76] Only improvement in the symptoms following the complete avoidance of house dust mites in the bedroom (very difficult to achieve – see later), and recurrence of symptoms on re-exposure, will prove the point. A study of the symptoms associated with house dust mite allergy showed that a history of symptoms being provoked during domestic activity that stirs up house dust (bed making, dusting, vacuuming, emptying a vacuum cleaner bag, sweeping, shaking out bedding) when house dust mite antigen becomes airborne, is probably the only reliable pointer to house dust mite allergy.[76]

2. **The symptoms are worse at certain times of the year.** The usual inference is that the symptoms are attributable to a seasonal allergen. Sometimes the history is convincing. For example, where sneezing and conjunctivitis occur each year in June and July on sunny days when the grass pollen count is high, it is highly probable that the symptoms are attributable to allergy to grass pollen. Often, the history is not so easy to interpret. For example, a worsening of asthma in August, September or October is often difficult to explain. Possibilities include allergy to inhaled molds, an increase in the number of house dust mites in the autumn, changes in the weather, or catching viral respiratory infections when returning to school after the summer holidays.[77,78]

3. **The symptoms are worse in certain weather conditions.** The reasons for attacks of asthma after a thunderstorm or heavy rainfall are not fully understood. Allergy to inhaled fungal spores, a fall in the barometric pressure, a sudden fall in air temperature, and release of allergenic starch granules from ruptured pollen grains are all possible explanations.

4. **The symptoms improve when the patient is away from home (e.g. on holiday).** Improvement in atopic eczema when the patient goes on holiday is frequently noted, but the reason is usually obscure. In one study[79] there was a significant correlation between improvement in eczema and a more southerly holiday location; improvement was common in holidays taken in the Mediterranean or further south (63/92 – 69%), while holidays in northern Britain were more likely to be associated with deterioration (27/100 – 27%) than improvement (13/100 – 13%). The absence of pets or house dust mites may be the explanation in some cases, although the improvement that occurs on holidays (the disease often virtually disappears) is far greater than the modest improvement that can be seen after admission to hospital in the same patients. Exposure to sea water, sunlight or lack of stress are believed by some parents to be the explanation for such improvement, but there is no evidence to support these ideas. The improvement or complete disappearance of asthma at high-altitude resorts, seen in some patients, is generally attributed to the absence of house dust mite and pet animal antigens.

5. ***The presence or absence of a family history of atopic disease.***
Patients with atopic disease often have a positive family history of atopic disease, though atopy is so common in the normal population (wheezing in 21%, eczema in 12% and hay fever in 4% of all children in the UK by the age of 5 years)[80] that a positive family history is a rather nonspecific finding. In an apparently atopic child, the absence of a positive family history is more important, and should make the physician reconsider a diagnosis of atopic disease.

6. ***Multiplicity of symptoms.*** Allergic symptoms are usually multiple. It is important to inquire if the patient has other symptoms or signs that may be allergic in origin, in addition to the presenting complaint, and these features are: wheezing, sneezing, pruritus, urticaria, perioral erythema, eczema and conjunctivitis. Several symptoms may coexist. Unilateral symptoms, whether nasal, ocular or respiratory suggest the presence of a non-allergic condition.

7. ***Symptoms occurring after exposure to pets.*** Several situations cause confusion:
   a. The patient who is noted to have an immediate allergic reaction when stroking or being licked by, for example, a dog, but who is otherwise apparently able to live in the same house as the animal without obvious immediate allergic reactions; delayed reactions or enhanced bronchial reactivity may be overlooked.
   b. The patient who apparently experiences an immediate allergic reaction to, for example, certain cats but not others; again, delayed reactions or enhanced bronchial reactivity may be overlooked.
   c. The patient whose atopic disease predates the acquisition of a pet animal; the animal could still be an important trigger continuing to provoke the disease.
   d. The patient who had a pet animal some years before the onset of symptoms; the animal could still be an important trigger.
   e. The patient's symptoms did not improve when the pet was sent to live elsewhere for a few weeks; sufficient pet antigen to provoke disease may still be present in the household.

A major source of confusion is that parents equate allergy with immediate reactions and are unaware that constant exposure to pet antigen in the home tends to cause chronic rather than acute symptoms. Many patients who are allergic to pets react to minute traces of the animal, for example a few hairs on someone's clothing, and this explains why the disease in question fails to improve after the pet is removed from the household. For therapeutic trials to be meaningful, extensive cleaning of carpets, upholstered furniture, clothing and bedding is necessary to remove the allergen.

8. ***Food intolerance.*** Food intolerance is generally associated with multiple symptoms, and it is rare for a single symptom (e.g. asthma, rhinitis, abdominal pain) to be caused by food intolerance. Parents commonly overvalue food intolerance as a cause of symptoms.
   In one study, double-blind food challenges provoked symptoms in only 27 of 81 (33%) of children whose parents had reported food intolerance.[81]

UNQUALIFIED REPORTS OF ALLERGY

It is unhelpful to write 'allergy' in a patient's notes without any description of the evidence for the diagnosis. Many untoward events are wrongly labeled as allergies. For example, there are several reasons why penicillin administration may be followed by an adverse event, but few justify a diagnosis of penicillin allergy. A rash during antibiotic therapy may be caused by an underlying infection, or by a coloring agent or preservative included in a liquid preparation of the antibiotic. Loose stools are likely to be due to an underlying viral infection or a disturbance of the gut flora, but it is common to find this described by parents as an allergy to the antibiotic. The incorrect and careless labeling of a child as having penicillin allergy may rob the patient of penicillin treatment for life. Common and similar examples are the patient said to be allergic to cows' milk, in whom inquiry reveals that this is based not on observation of the patient but on the fact that someone has placed the child on a cows' milk-free diet, or the patient said to be allergic to something solely on the basis of skin or blood tests.

SIMPLE CAUSE AND EFFECT

The interpretation of the observation that exposure to a single item (e.g. a cat) is followed within minutes by an obvious adverse event (e.g. sneezing and orbital edema) should be quite simple, but there are pitfalls. The history is more reliable if it is based on the parents' unprompted original observations. The parents' observations may be especially unreliable because:

1. There is a strong emotional underlay, e.g. strong attachment to a family pet, leading to underdiagnosis of allergy because the family members do not want to part with the animal.
2. In the case of food intolerance, double-blind studies have repeatedly shown parental histories to be particularly unreliable (see later).
3. In the case of behavioral symptoms, there is a widespread but mistaken belief in the importance of adverse reactions to foods or food additives.[61]
4. A parent's report of alleged allergic reactions may have been fabricated (factitious illness).

In general, the quicker the onset of the allergic reaction, the more reliable is the history. A history of the same allergic symptoms after repeated exposure to an allergen is more reliable than a report of a single episode.

DIAGNOSTIC TESTING FOR ALLERGY

There is no ideal test that will predict with certainty whether avoidance of a specific allergen will improve or abolish symptoms in an individual. Some of the problems are due to difficulties intrinsic to the test, but some are inherent in the complex nature of atopic disease. Take, for example, a child with asthma who develops sneezing, conjunctivitis and angioedema of the orbit immediately after playing with a cat, and who has a positive skin prick test and positive RAST test to cat dander. Clearly it is logical that the child should avoid cats, but there is no guarantee that cat avoidance will help the patient's asthma. The reasons for the failure of allergen avoidance are discussed later, but can be summarized as:

1. The allergen was incompletely avoided.
2. The allergen was only one of several factors provoking the patient's disease.
3. The allergen was irrelevant to the patient's symptoms.

It is unrealistic to expect any clinical or laboratory test to cope with the first two of these problems. The best that can be hoped for is that a test will help establish the potential clinical relevance of a particular allergy. Regrettably, the currently available tests, described later, all suffer from serious limitations.

SCRATCH, PRICK AND INTRADERMAL SKIN TESTS

The principle of these skin tests is that the skin wheal and flare reaction to an allergen demonstrates the presence of mast-cell-fixed antibody. This is mainly IgE antibody, although in theory it could also be IgG4 antibody. IgE is produced by plasma cells primarily in lymphoid tissue in the respiratory and gastrointestinal tract, and is distributed via the circulation to all parts of the body, so that the sensitization is generalized and therefore can be demonstrated by skin testing. Age influences the reaction, and a child under 2 years of age produces much less reaction than an older child.

Short-acting antihistamines (H₁ receptor antagonists) must be discontinued at least 5 d prior to skin testing. Because of the variability of cutaneous reactivity, it is necessary to include positive and negative controls whenever skin prick tests are performed. The negative control solution should consist of the diluent used to preserve the allergen extracts. The positive control solution usually consists of histamine, and is mainly used to detect suppression of reactivity, for example caused by H₁ antihistamine medication.

Scratch testing

A drop of allergen solution is placed on the skin, which is then scratched so as to superficially penetrate the skin. The scratch test introduces an inconstant amount of allergen through the skin and is therefore poorly standardized and produces results that are too variable for routine clinical use.[82,83]

Prick testing

A drop of allergen solution is placed on the skin, which is then pricked with a plastic lance, and the result read after 15 min. The negative control should be negative, unless the patient has dermographism. The histamine control should be positive, unless the patient has recently received H_1 antihistamines, which would invalidate negative skin test results. The flare is ignored, and the diameter of the wheal is measured. Later reactions may occur, but their significance is unclear. Prick tests can also produce variable results, but the introduction of standardized precision lances for prick testing has made the method potentially more reproducible.

The interpretation of skin prick tests is difficult. There is a lack of agreed definition about what constitutes a positive reaction.[84] Most definitions of a positive reaction are based on the absolute diameter of the wheal, with arbitrary cutoff points for positivity at 1 mm, 2 mm or 3 mm. The problems with the interpretation of prick test results in an individual patient are:

1. Skin prick test reactivity may be present in subjects with no clinical evidence of allergy.[85,86]
2. Skin prick test reactivity may persist after clinical evidence of allergy has subsided.[87]
3. Skin prick tests may be negative in some patients with allergies. For example, skin prick tests are negative in 13–17% of those with rhinitis provoked by pollen.[88]
4. False-negative results may occur in infants and toddlers. The whealing capacity of the skin is diminished in early infancy, and when wheals are produced they are smaller than in later life, so that the criteria for a positive wheal must be adjusted.[86] There are no age-related guidelines for what constitutes a positive reaction.
5. There is a poor correlation between the results of provocation tests and prick tests.
6. Skin prick tests for foods are especially unreliable.[60] A positive result using a raw food antigen does not necessarily mean that the cooked food will cause a reaction.
7. False-negative skin prick tests can occur after anaphylaxis.[89]

The results of skin tests cannot be taken alone, but need to account for the history and physical findings.[86,90] From a carefully taken history one might suspect a particular allergen, and the finding of a positive prick test would increase the likelihood that the allergen was causing symptoms. Few people, however, would be prepared to ignore a strong history of allergy in the face of a negative prick test, yet it is illogical to regard the prick test as significant when it confirms the history and to disregard it when it fails to do so. The contentious issues in clinical practice are whether a child with atopic disease will benefit from attempts to avoid household pets, house dust mites or certain foods, but skin prick tests are unreliable predictors of response to such measures.

Intradermal testing

Intradermal testing is painful, can cause fatal anaphylaxis, and is only performed for limited reasons and then only if a preliminary skin prick test is negative.[91] Intradermal tests are more sensitive than skin prick testing, and also produce more false-positive reactions. As with skin prick testing, there is a lack of agreement as to what constitutes a positive reaction. The number of false-positive reactions makes the interpretation of the results of intradermal testing even more difficult than skin prick testing.

Skin patch testing

Patch testing is used to identify causative allergens in suspected allergic contact dermatitis, and is discussed elsewhere.[92]

Measurement of circulating IgE antibody

In vitro tests for circulating allergen-specific IgE antibody (e.g. RAST tests) avoid possible confounding variables in skin testing, namely IgE affinity for mast cells, their tendency for degranulation, and skin reactivity to released mediators. Thus, in theory, the in vitro test should be more reliable than skin testing. However, the clinical interpretation of in vitro IgE antibody tests is subject to most of the same pitfalls as the interpretation of skin prick testing. Additional problems with IgE antibody tests are:

1. Cost.
2. The IgE antibody concentration in the plasma varies with allergen exposure. A few patients with allergic rhinitis are RAST negative before the pollen season, but become positive after the pollen season.
3. A very high level of total circulating IgE (e.g. in children with severe atopic eczema) may cause a false-positive result.
4. A very low level of circulating IgE may be associated with false-negative results.
5. A very high level of IgG antibody with the same allergen specificity as IgE antibody can cause a false-negative result.
6. For each allergen, the test differs in the degree to which it is influenced by elevated total serum IgE.
7. In vitro IgE assays are slightly less sensitive than skin testing.

In vitro tests for IgE antibody are only preferable to skin testing where the patient has had a very severe reaction to the allergen in question (because of the small risk of anaphylaxis with skin testing), where the patient has widespread skin disease (e.g. atopic eczema), where the skin shows dermographism, or when H_1 antihistamines cannot be discontinued.

Provocation challenge tests

With the exception of food challenges in patients with suspected food intolerance, provocation tests (bronchial, nasal, conjunctival) have little place in routine clinical practice but have been helpful in the study of the pathophysiology and pharmacology of atopic disease. The results suffer from the same major limitation as the results of skin or IgE antibody testing, which is that a positive result from an allergen challenge by no means proves that the allergen is contributing to the patient's disease.

Blinded oral food challenge

The test comprises the oral administration of a challenge substance, which is either the item under investigation or an indistinguishable inactive (placebo) substance. Neither the child, the parents nor the observers know the identity of the administered material at the time of the challenge. Food challenges are subject to a number of pitfalls:

1. There is a danger of producing anaphylactic shock, even if anaphylactic shock had not occurred on previous exposure to the food.
2. Difficulties arise if a cooked food is used for testing and the patient is only sensitive to a raw food, or vice versa. Cooking reduces the sensitizing capacity of cows' milk, and intolerance to raw but not cooked egg, potato and fish are well described.
3. It is unclear what dosage of different foods is required to exclude food intolerance. The dosage used in studies employing encapsulated foods is inevitably limited. Larger quantities of food may cause an adverse reaction when smaller quantities do not. For example, Hill et al[91] found that whereas 8–10 g of milk powder (corresponding to 60–70 ml of milk) was adequate to provoke a response in some patients with cows' milk protein intolerance, other patients (with late-onset symptoms) required up to 10 times this volume of milk daily for more than 48 h before symptoms developed.
4. Failure to randomize the order of placebo with active substance or to employ a double-blind placebo-controlled methodology are errors common to many studies, especially those of food additives in chronic urticaria.

5. A food challenge performed during a quiescent phase of the disease may fail to provoke an adverse reaction. For example, in chronic urticaria intolerance to salicylates is confined to patients with active disease.

6. The regular administration of salicylates to patients with salicylate intolerance quickly leads to a state of tolerance to salicylate. It is possible, although unproven, that a similar phenomenon occurs with certain food additives. Thus a double-blind challenge performed while a patient is regularly consuming a foodstuff may fail to provoke an adverse reaction.

7. Where food intolerance exists in children with atopic dermatitis, it is common for the patient to be intolerant to several foods. The removal of only one offending item may fail to help the patient and reintroduction may not provoke deterioration.

8. In some situations, factors other than a food are necessary for positive challenges to occur. For example, in a subgroup of patients with exercise-induced anaphylaxis, symptoms only occur if exercise follows the ingestion of a particular food.[94] Exercise or the food alone fail to provoke symptoms.

DRUG TREATMENT OF ANAPHYLAXIS AND ACUTE ALLERGIES

Anaphylaxis not associated with circulatory failure/arrest

Adrenaline 10μg/kg (0.01 ml/kg of a 1:1000 solution), given intramuscularly is the drug and route of choice for most patients with anaphylaxis associated with life-threatening respiratory compromise (Project Team of the Resuscitation Council [UK] 1999). Subcutaneous administration results in slower rates of systemic absorption than via the intramuscular route and is therefore not recommended.

Preloaded adrenaline syringes are available for use in the community. Min-I-jet 1 ml 1:1000 epinephrine with a 6 mm needle is for s.c. injection, requires assembly before use and the dose will need to be adjusted before administration. Thus it is less suitable than the EpiPen or the Anapen, which are spring-loaded devices with a concealed needle giving a single dose of 0.3 ml of 1:1000 or 1:2000 adrenaline (0.15 or 0.30 mg) as a deep i.m. injection. The simplicity of use and concealed needle makes this the most popular option with many patients.

The junior EpiPen or Anapen (0.15 mg) are suitable for children weighing 15–30 kg; above this weight the adult EpiPen or Anapen (0.3 mg) should be used. It will rarely be appropriate to issue epinephrine for children weighing less than 15 kg.

Adrenaline has a short half-life, and if necessary the i.m. injection is repeated at 5-minute intervals. Repeated (i.e. more than one) adrenaline injections are required in approximately 10–40% of patients with anaphylaxis, and therefore it is advisable to prescribe two preloaded adrenaline syringes per patient. I.v. administration of adrenaline has been associated with acute strokes and is therefore to be avoided in most situations.

Only 20% of fatal/near-fatal anaphylactic reactions to foods occur at home. The remainder occurs at the home of friends, at school and at restaurants[95] and thus it is essential that if a pre-loaded adrenaline syringe is prescribed, it is available where the patient is and that there is someone around who is trained in its use. Thus for schoolchildren it is important that two preloaded adrenaline syringes are available at the school and that teachers have appropriate training in the recognition of anaphylaxis and the use of the adrenaline syringe.

Indications for use of preloaded adrenaline syringes

A major factor predisposing to fatalities in cases of food anaphylaxis was the delay in recognition and instigation of medical treatment. In general it is recommended that a preloaded adrenaline syringe should be given at the first signs of upper airway obstruction, wheeziness not relieved by a bronchodilator inhaler or if there is any faintness. Allergic reactions are frightening and are often associated with panic attacks, which may mimic or exacerbate the symptoms and signs of anaphylaxis. This often makes it difficult to differentiate between clinical features of allergy and acute anxiety.

Indications for preloaded adrenaline syringe prescribing

The indications for prescribing preloaded adrenaline syringes vary from center to center.[96] Some authorities recommend, for example, that all children with peanut intolerance should be issued with adrenaline syringes, however mild the previous reactions, on the basis that the next reaction could be life threatening. Others are concerned that adrenaline syringes are vastly overprescribed, and should only be used in very selected cases.[97] Unfortunately it is not possible to predict which individuals are likely to get severe reactions, except to say that those who have had previous severe reactions are those at greatest risk. The possible role of asthma as a risk factor has already been discussed earlier in relation to peanut allergy. Fatal or near-fatal anaphylactic reactions are rare (approximately 1 per million per year), often occur in places where the prescribed preloaded adrenaline syringe is not available, where there is no one trained in its use, or in some cases the reaction occurs so rapidly as to lead to circulatory arrest that is unlikely to respond to i.m. adrenaline (see section on Anaphylaxis associated with circulatory failure/arrest later).[98] Most nonvenom- and non-medication-induced allergic reactions respond to antihistamines. There is no guarantee that treatment with adrenaline will be life saving, and there are well-documented cases in which death has occurred despite the correct use of adrenaline syringes.

Preloaded adrenaline syringes
Advantages
Efficacy: most effective acute treatment for anaphylaxis not associated with circulatory failure/arrest;
Provides reassurance for the patient and relatives.

Disadvantages
Rarity: risk of death from anaphylaxis is approximately 1/million/y.
May not work: Anaphylaxis associated with circulatory failure is not likely to respond, and some cases of anaphylaxis will prove fatal, even if adrenaline is given early.
Can cause anxiety: having to carry an adrenaline syringe everywhere causes considerable anxiety to some patients, relatives, carers and teachers. Exclusion from school trips and social outings have in some cases been associated directly with prescription of a preloaded adrenaline syringe to children.
Lack of warning signs: fatal reactions are sometimes not associated with warning signs.
Side-effects: preloaded adrenaline syringe use for anaphylaxis has caused death from arrhythmias and strokes.
Availability: preloaded adrenaline syringes are often not available at the emergency (i.e. reactions away from home, patient not carrying adrenaline).
Need for training: inadequate training may prevent adequate recognition of anaphylaxis or use of preloaded adrenaline syringe.

Based on the current difficulties associated with the use of a preloaded adrenaline syringe, if it is prescribed, it is recommended that the following conditions are met:

- Appropriate training should be given to the patient, their relatives, teachers and work colleagues (see later).
- Preloaded adrenaline syringes should be available at all times, not just at home but also at school, when visiting friends and during all leisure activities.
- All trainees should undergo periodic retraining and reassessment.

Information that should be given to users of preloaded adrenaline syringes

As mentioned earlier, training of patients and their relatives in the correct use and safe handling of the preloaded adrenaline syringe as well as regular annual review of technique is essential. Table 33.8 lists the information that should be covered at training sessions.

Table 33.8 Information that should be covered at preloaded adrenaline syringe training sessions

A. Instructions should be given to the parents and if old enough the patient on the following:
How to recognize an anaphylactic reaction
When to use the preloaded adrenaline syringe(s)
Where and how to inject the adrenaline
How to dispose of the used preloaded adrenaline syringe
What to do if the adrenaline is injected incorrectly
When to use other medicines
Always to seek medical help if having a reaction
When to replace the preloaded adrenaline syringe

B. The preloaded adrenaline syringe should be checked and the parents/patient told:
To keep the preloaded adrenaline syringe in the original pack
Label with the patient's name
Store safely
Store at room temperature
Always keep accessible for an emergency

Table 33.9 H₁ Antihistamines used in the treatment of allergic reactions

Antihistamine	Route of administration
Sedating	
Chlorpheniramine (Piriton)	Oral/parenteral
Promethazine (Phenergan)	Oral/parenteral
Trimeprazine (Vallergan)	Oral
Non-sedating	
Loratadine (Clarityn)	Oral
Desloratadine (Neoclarityn)	Oral
Fexofenadine (Telfast)	Oral
Cetirizine (Zirtek)	Oral
Mizolastine (Mistamine)	Oral
Antazoline (Otrivine-Antistin)	Eye drops
Azelastine (Optilast)	Eye drops
Levocabastine (Livostin)	Eye drops
Azelastine (Rhinolast)	Nasal spray
Levocabastine (Livostin)	Nasal spray
Antazoline (Wasp-Eze)	Topical skin ointment
Mepyramine (Anthisan)	Topical skin ointment

The date on which training was given, the people trained, the adrenaline dose and a list of the information given to the patient and the relatives should be documented in the clinical notes. Allergy clinics might use a standardized preloaded adrenaline syringe checklist form, signed and dated by the prescribing doctor, with copies added to the clinical notes, sent to the GP and given to the patient.

Nebulized adrenaline and other treatment modalities

Nebulized adrenaline is no longer recommended as treatment of anaphylaxis in the UK because the metered-dose aerosol (Medihaler-epi) has been withdrawn from the market. Bronchoconstriction is best treated with a nebulized alpha₂-agonist (e.g. salbutamol or terbutaline). I.v. fluid boluses are often required in addition to adrenaline for treatment of hypotension. A number of 20 ml/kg boluses may be required. After injection of adrenaline, an H₁ antihistamine, for example chlorphenamine should be administered, and may be continued for 48 h to prevent recurrences of the reaction. Steroids take some hours to be effective and are unhelpful in the immediate treatment of anaphylaxis, but are of possible benefit in preventing a secondary relapse. Further management consists of avoidance of the cause, and in the case of insect venom stings consideration of hyposensitization.

Anaphylaxis associated with circulatory failure/arrest

If the patient has life-threatening circulatory compromise with no palpable peripheral pulse, then i.m. adrenaline is unlikely to be effective, as it will not be adequately absorbed. In patients with circulatory failure, basic life support must be commenced, followed by the injection of i.v. adrenaline (at an initial dose of 0.1 ml/kg of a 1:10 000 solution) as per the asystole protocol for advanced pediatric life support (APLS). Great vigilance is needed to ensure that the correct strength of adrenaline is used; anaphylactic shock kits need to make a very clear distinction between the 1 in 10 000 strength normally used for i.v. use and 1 in 1000 strength used for i.m. use. I.v. administration of adrenaline for treatment of patients with anaphylaxis has been associated with death from acute strokes and ventricular fibrillation, and is therefore to be avoided in anaphylaxis not associated with circulatory failure.

Medication for nonlife-threatening allergic reactions

H₁ antihistamines are very useful in controlling symptoms of nonlife-threatening allergic reactions such as acute and chronic urticaria and allergic rhinitis and conjunctivitis. Antihistamines can be divided into two groups (Table 33.9). The older sedating antihistamines are very effective, but because they cross the blood–brain barrier they are sedative and therefore may adversely affect children's learning ability. In an effort to reduce the sedative side-effects of these drugs, a new generation of nonsedating antihistamines has been developed. Some of these nonsedating antihistamines (in particular astemizole, terfenadine) are associated with life-threatening arrhythmias (torsades de pointes) by inhibiting potassium ion channels in cardiac tissue. Astemizole and terfenadine are therefore no longer available. Mizolastine, which is still available, has been associated with an increased risk of ventricular fibrillation when given together with other drugs (analgesics, antiarrhythmics, sotalol).

Doxepin is classed as a tricyclic antidepressant, but also has anti-H₁ and H₂ antihistamine activity (75× more potent than diphenhydramine and 6× more potent than cimetidine). It may be a useful therapeutic adjunct in older children with urticaria not controlled with traditional antihistamines.

HYPOSENSITIZATION

Hyposensitization comprises the regular administration of allergen with the objective of reducing or abolishing the patient's reaction to the allergen. The basis of allergy or 'immune hypersensitivity' is increasingly recognized as an imbalance between the proinflammatory and regulatory immune responses. Although desensitization or more precisely hyposensitization, as the allergy is rarely completely abrogated, has been used for many decades, it is only now appreciated that it works by resetting the immune balance by increasing the regulatory immune response.[99] All antigens can stimulate both effector and regulatory arms of the immune system. Hyposensitization is the method of presenting the allergen in a way that the regulatory response predominates. The induction of regulatory cell memory is less robust than for proinflammatory responses and therefore regular prolonged exposure to the allergen is usually required to maintain immune tolerance. Prematurely discontinuing immunotherapy prematurely risks development of allergic reactions to the allergen, which may be severe.

Allergy immunotherapy involves exposing the patient to increasing amounts of allergen starting at a low enough dose that does not provoke a proinflammatory response (induction phase), before maintaining tolerance with continuing exposure to the allergen (maintenance phase). Allergen may be given subcutaneously (SCIT), orally, or most recently the possibility of giving it sublingually (SLIT) has been explored. There is no doubt that SCIT and oral hyposensitization can be very effective in patients where the symptoms are being provoked by specific allergens. SCIT is limited by the availability of licensed allergens, and in the UK is largely used for patients with grass and tree pollen allergen, as well as bee and wasp allergen. As SCIT requires regular injections, initially weekly and then monthly for up to 3–5 years, hyposensitization is not commonly used in children. Oral hyposensitization is almost exclusively used for drug hyposensitization.

SUBCUTANEOUS IMMUNOTHERAPY (SCIT)

Since Noon's report in 1911, controlled studies have shown that allergen immunotherapy is effective in patients with allergic rhinoconjunctivitis and allergic reactions to *Hymenoptera* venoms. Patients may be considered for immunotherapy if they have well-defined, clinically relevant allergic triggers that markedly affect their quality of life or daily function and if they do not attain adequate symptom relief with avoidance measures and pharmacotherapy. Because of the risk of death from anaphylaxis (26 deaths in the UK between 1967 and 1986), the Committee for Safety of Medicines (CSM) in the UK has concluded that SCIT should only be used for: (1) life-threatening allergy to bee or wasp venom (rare in childhood); and (2) seasonal allergic hay fever (which has not responded to anti-allergy drugs), caused by grass or tree pollen, using licensed products only. In patients with hay fever, those who also have asthma should not be treated with hyposensitizing vaccines as they are more likely to develop severe adverse reactions. Hyposensitization must only be performed in hospitals or clinics with full facilities for cardiopulmonary resuscitation, and patients need to be monitored for 30–60 min after injections. Induction of tolerance requires weekly injections of increasing doses of allergen to reach a maintenance dose of 5–20 mcg over 6 or more weeks. This is often followed by monthly injections of this maintenance dose for 3–5 years.

ORAL HYPOSENSITIZATION

Oral hyposensitization is used to induce tolerance to essential medication required and can be used for most drugs including antibiotics, anti-epilepsy medication, chemotherapeutic agents and protein, e.g. insulin. Children can be hyposensitized to most drugs using this method. This form of hyposensitization is thought to work through controlled degranulation of mast cells.[100] Clinical reactivity returns within a few days of discontinuing drug administration, implying that continuous presence of the antigen is required for continuing mast cell degranulation and thus maintaining tolerance. Oral hyposensitization has also been achieved in asthmatic patients with aspirin-exacerbated respiratory disease,[101] and in a small number of children with food intolerance, e.g. to milk, but at present must be regarded as experimental.[102,103]

The procedure is performed by the cautious administration of incremental doses of the drug to the patient over a period of hours to days. The drug can be administered either by oral or i.v. route. The starting dose for the procedure can be determined by performing intradermal skin tests with the native drug at a dose that does not cause a nonspecific reaction and may be one hundredth to one thousandth of the usual therapeutic dose. Typically, the dose is doubled every 15–30 min and vital signs, physical examination, and peak flow values are regularly monitored. It is critical that the individuals involved with the desensitization procedure understand that it can have serious consequences. While anaphylactic reactions rarely occur if conservative protocols are used, health care personnel must be prepared to treat anaphylaxis if it does occur.

SUBLINGUAL IMMUNOTHERAPY

Sublingual immunotherapy (SLIT) has been used with increasing frequency in Europe as a possible means of hyposensitization in hay fever and asthma.[104] The allergen solution or tablet is kept under the tongue for 1–2 min before either spitting it out or swallowing it. This method appears safe in that there are to date no reported severe allergic reactions, although 75% of patients may experience local symptoms in the oral cavity. At present there is no standardization of dose, timing and duration of treatment, which has varied considerably between studies.

In terms of efficacy, a 2006 Cochrane review of SLIT for hay fever concluded that in 22 double-blinded, placebo-controlled trials involving 979 patients (6 house dust mite, 5 grass pollen, 5 *Parietaria*, 2 olive, 5 other) there was a 15–69% reduction of symptoms ($P = 0.002$) and a 23–63% reduction in mediation required ($P = 0.00003$).[105] However a larger independent American review of the European studies found that in 47 randomized, controlled studies, although there was a significant improvement in symptom and medication scores in 14 (35%) of 39 studies where data was available, there was no significant improvement in either parameter in 15 (38%) trials. Of the 43 trials that provided symptom scores, 20 (46%) demonstrated no significant improvement, and a total of 20 (51%) of 39 studies that provided medication scores demonstrated no significant improvement.[82] The Cochrane review of the five studies conducted in only children found no benefit. Based on these data, routine use of SLIT cannot be recommended in children at the present time.

NOVEL TREATMENT APPROACHES

There are a number of novel approaches currently under investigation for the management of allergic diseases. These include reduction of IgE by the infusion of anti-IgE antibodies, attempts to induce tolerance by stimulating regulatory pathways with plasmid DNA, immunostimulatory sequences, cytokines and bacterial agents, as well as complementary medicines such as Chinese herbs.

ANTI-IGE THERAPY

Anti-IgE (omalizumab and TNX-901) are humanized monoclonal anti-IgE antibodies that bind to the Fc region of IgE at the same epitope that binds FcεR1. They are given subcutaneously at a dose of 0.016 mg/kg body weight 3–4 weekly. They have been well tolerated in the trials that have so far been conducted in patients over the age of 12 years and there is so far little evidence for the development of antibodies and thus resistance with repeated use. As complete neutralizing of circulating IgE is required for clinical efficacy, their use has so far been restricted to patients with total serum IgE concentrations of < 700–1000 IU/ml. Trials have shown efficacy in seasonal allergic rhinitis and moderate (but not severe) allergic asthma, significantly reducing symptoms and medication use.[83,106] In peanut-allergic patients and at a dose of 450 mg, tolerance to peanuts increases from an average of 1 peanut to 6–8 peanuts.[56] With the restrictions in use to patients with only moderately raised serum IgE levels, and an estimated average annual cost of 4–5 times that of standard asthma therapy, and the need to long-term injections, its place in the management of allergic diseases in adults and particularly children is unclear at the present time.

CHINESE HERBAL REMEDIES

Chinese herbal medicines may have a role in the treatment of allergies and atopic diseases. However the complexity of traditional Chinese herbal formulae containing many constituents makes standardization and therefore licensing of herbal products problematic. A 2005 Cochrane review of the four published randomized controlled trials of Chinese herbal remedies for eczema involving 159 participants aged 1–60 years, suggested some clinical benefit, but the conclusion was that further well-designed large-scale trials are required.[107] Attempts are ongoing to reduce the number of components within these remedies to those that are most active and least toxic but these studies are currently in the preclinical or early clinical trial stage. For example, in a murine model of peanut allergy, pretreatment of mice with a modified Chinese herbal formulae was associated with complete abrogation of clinical anaphylaxis.[108] At the present time however, patients should be warned that currently available Chinese herbal remedies are non-standardized and unlicensed and although may be efficacious have also been associated with liver and renal toxicity and therefore must be used with caution.

PREVENTION OF ATOPIC DISEASE

Since 1930, when Grulee and Sanford reported a significantly lower incidence of eczema in infants who were breast-fed babies,[109] further research has been unable to provide the definitive answer whether the development of allergic disease can be prevented by breast-feeding.[110] One explanation may be that food antigens can pass to the infant via both human milk and also via the placenta prior to birth, but breast-feeding does not necessarily lead to complete avoidance of potentially sensitizing allergens. An alternative explanation is that more children at increased risk of allergic disease may be breast-fed by their mothers.[111] Studies using hydrolyzed formulae would avoid some of these factors and may provide more conclusive data. However a Cochrane review of studies provide no support to the idea that hydrolyzed formula prevents the development of allergy any more than breast-feeding.[112]

With the recognition that early exposure to potential allergens in the gut normally induces and maintains tolerance in young children, and complete avoidance may increase the risk of allergic reactions,[113] advice on avoidance should currently be given with caution.[114] Studies looking at potential aeroallergens show that ownership of cats and dogs in early childhood may protect against rather than promote the later development of asthma. In one study of 224 28-year-olds, those who owned a cat prior to the age of 18 years had a relative risk of having asthma of 0.08 (0.01–0.46) while those who acquired a cat after the age of 18 years had a relative risk of asthma of 2.62 (0.34–19.97) compared with participants who had never owned a cat.[115,116]

The induction of oral tolerance to food allergens may be augmented by certain bacterial (e.g. environmental mycobacteria) and viral (hepatitis A virus) antigens in the gut, a concept that may help to explain the epidemiological data leading to the development of the Hygiene hypothesis.[8] There is growing interest in supplementing people's diet with normal bacterial flora, particularly *Lactobacillus* and *Bifidobacterium* strains in the form of 'probiotics' to try and prevent or treat atopic diseases. Most studies to date using probiotics have looked at their effect in children with established atopic eczema rather than the prevention[117] of the condition and therefore it is not possible to draw any firm conclusions as to the usefulness of probiotics in the prevention of atopic disease.[118] However, overall the studies detailed earlier suggest that augmentation of intestinal regulatory cell activity in early infancy might possibly help to protect against immune hypersensitivity diseases in later life.

REFERENCES (* Level 1 evidence)

*1. Sicherer SH, Furlong TJ, Maes HH, et al. Genetics of peanut allergy: a twin study. J Allergy Clin Immunol 2000; 106:53–56.

2. Church MK, Holgate ST, Lichtenstein LM. Allergy. St Louis: Elsevier Health Sciences; 2006.

3. Sampson HA, Geha RS, Leung DY. Pediatric allergy: Principles and practice. St Louis: C. V. Mosby Co.; 2003.

4. Schaub B, Lauener R, von Mutius E. The many faces of the hygiene hypothesis. J Allergy Clin Immunol 2006; 117:969–977.

5. Liu AH, Leung DYM. Renaissance of the hygiene hypothesis. J Allergy Clin Immunol 2006; 117:1063–1066.

6. Lau S, Matricardi PM. Worms, asthma, and the hygiene hypothesis. Lancet 2006; 367:1556–1558.

*7. Strachan DR. Hayfever, hygiene and household size. BMJ 1989; 299:1259–1260.

8. Arkwright PD, David TJ. Eat dirt – the hygiene hypothesis of atopic diseases. In: David TJ (ed.) Recent advances in paediatrics, vol.21. Roy Soc Med Press 2004: 197–213.

*9. Shirakawa T, Enomoto T, Shimazu S, et al. The inverse association between tuberculin responses and atopic disorder. Science 1997; 275:77–79.

*10. von Ehrenstein OS, von Mutius E, Illi SL, et al. Reduced risk of hay fever and asthma among children of farmers. Clin Exp Allergy 2000; 30:187–193.

*11. Riedler J, Braun-Fahrlander C, Eder W, et al. Exposure to farming in early life and development of asthma and allergy: a cross-sectional survey. Lancet 2001; 358:1129–1133.

*12. Braun-Fahrlander C, Riedler J, Herz U, et al. Environmental exposure to endotoxin and its relation to asthma in school-age children. N Engl J Med 2002; 347:869–877.

13. Schultz, Larsen F. Atopic dermatitis: a genetic-epidemiologic study in a population-based twin sample. J Am Acad Dermatol 1993; 28:719–723.

14. Ober C, Hoffjan S. Asthma genetics 2006: the long and winding road to gene discovery. Genes Immun 2006; 7:95–100.

*15. Arbour NC, Lorenz E, Schutte BC, et al. TLR4 mutations are associated with endotoxin hyporesponsiveness in humans. Nat Genet 2000; 25:187–191.

*16. Eder W, Klimecki W, Yu L, et al. Toll-like receptor 2 as a major gene for asthma in children of European farmers. J Allergy Clin Immunol 2004; 113:482–488.

*17. Umetsu SE, Lee WL, McIntyre JJ, et al. TIM-1 induces T cell activation and inhibits the development of peripheral tolerance. Nat Immunol 2005; 6:447–454.

18. Akbari O, Umetsu DT. Role of regulatory dendritic cells in allergy and asthma. Curr Opin Allergy Clin Immunol 2004; 4:533–538.

19. Boguniewicz M. Chronic urticaria in children. Allergy Asthma Proc 2005; 26:13–17.

20. Kaplan AP. Chronic urticaria: pathogenesis and treatment. J Allergy Clin Immunol 2004; 114:465–474.

21. Picado C. Mechanisms of aspirin sensitivity. Curr Allergy Asthma Rep 2006; 6:198–202.

22. Black AK. Urticarial vasculitis. Clinics Dermatol 1999; 17:565–569.

23. Venzor J, Lee WL, Huston DP. Urticarial vasculitis. Clin Rev Allergy Immunology 2002; 23:201–216.

24. Gompels MM, Lock RJ, Abinun M, et al. C1 inhibitor deficiency: consensus document. Clin Exp Immunol 2005; 141:189–190.

25. Davis AE. The pathophysiology of hereditary angioedema. Clin Immunol 2005; 114:3–9.

*26. Langan SM, Williams HC. What causes worsening of eczezma? A systematic review. Br J Dermatol 2006; 155:504–514.

*27. Hoare C, Li Wan Po A, Williams H. Systematic review of treatments for atopic eczema. Health Technol Assess 2000; 4:1–191.

*28. Cant AJ, Bailes JA, Marsden RA, et al. Effect of maternal dietary exclusion on breast fed infants with eczema: two controlled studies. BMJ 1986; 293:231–233.

*29. Devlin J, David TJ, Stanton RHJ. Six food diet for childhood atopic dermatitis. Acta Dermatovenereologica 1991; 71:20–24.

*30. Mabin DC, Sykes AE, David TJ. Controlled trial of a few foods diet in severe atopic dermatitis. Arch Dis Child 1995; 73:202–207.

31. Devlin J, David TJ, Stanton RHJ. Elemental diet for refractory atopic eczema. Arch Dis Child 1991; 66:93–99.

32. Arlian LG, Platts-Mills TAE. The biology of dust mites and the remediation of mite allergens in allergic disease. J Allergy Clin Immunol 2001; 107:S406–S413.

33. Devereux G. Epidemiology of food intolerance and food allergy. In: Buttriss J, (ed.) Adverse reactions to food. The report of a British Nutrition Foundation task force. Oxford: Blackwell Science; 2002.57–65.

34. Venter C, Pereira B, Grundy J, et al. Incidence of parentally reported and clinically diagnosed food hypersensitivity in the first year of life. J Allergy Clin Immunol 2006; 117:1118–1124.

35. Bock SA. Prospective appraisal of complaints of adverse reactions to foods in children during the first three years of life. Pediatrics 1987; 79:683–688.

36. Mari A, Ballmer-Weber BK, Vieths S. The oral allergy syndrome: improved diagnostic and treatment methods. Curr Opin Allergy Clin Immunol 2005; 5:267–273.

37. Rothenberg ME. Eosinophilic gastrointestinal disorders (EGID). J Allergy Clin Immunol 2004; 113:11–28.

38. Liacouras CA, Spergel JM, Ruchelli E, et al. Eosinophilic esophagitis: a 10-year experience in 381 children. Clin Gastroenterol Hepatol 2005; 3:1198–1206.

39. Farrell RJ, Kelly CP. Celiac sprue. N Engl J Med 2002; 346:180–188.

40. Eggesbø M, Botten G, Halvorsen R, et al. The prevalence of CMA/CMPI in young children: the validity of parentally perceived reactions in a population-based study. Allergy 2001; 56:393–402.

41. Goldman AS, Anderson DW, Sellers WA, et al. Oral challenge with milk and isolated milk proteins in allergic children. Pediatrics 1963; 32:425–443.

42. Hill DJ, Ford RP, Shelton MJ, et al. A study of 100 infants and young children with cow's milk allergy. Clin Rev Allergy 1984; 2:125–142.

43. Eggesbø M, Botten G, Halvorsen R, et al. The prevalence of allergy to egg: a population-based study in young children. Allergy 2001; 56:403–411.

44. Khakoo GA, Lack G. Recommendations for using MMR vaccine in children allergic to eggs. BMJ 2000; 320:929–932.

45. Aas K. Fish allergy and the codfish model. In: Brostoff J, Challacombe SJ (eds). Food allergy and intolerance. London: Baillière Tindall; 1987.356–366.

46. Sicherer SH, Munoz-Furlong A, Burks AW, et al. Prevalence of peanut and tree nut allergy in the US determined by a random digit telephone survey. J Allergy Clin Immunol 1999; 103:559–562.

47. Bock SA, Munoz-Furlong A, Sampson HA. Fatalities due to anaphylactic reactions to foods. J Allergy Clin Immunol 2001; 107:191–193.

48. Pumphrey RSH, Stanworth SJ. The clinical spectrum of anaphylaxis in north-west England. Clin Exp Allergy 1996; 26:1364–1370.

49. Hourihane JOB, Dean TP, Warner JO. Peanut allergy in relation to heredity, maternal diet, and other atopic diseases: results of a questionnaire survey,

skin prick testing, and food challenges. BMJ 1996; 313:518–521.

50. Beyer K, Morrow E, Li XM, et al. Effects of cooking methods on peanut allergenicity. J Allergy Clin Immunol 2001; 107:1077–1081.

*51. Hourihane JOB, Bedwani SJ, Dean TP, et al. Randomised, double blind, crossover challenge study of allergenicity of peanut oils in subjects allergic to peanuts. BMJ 1997; 314:1084–1088.

52. Teuber SS, Brown RL, Haapanen LA. Allergenicity of gourmet nut oils processed by different methods. J Allergy Clin Immunol 1997; 99:502–506.

53. Sicherer SH, Burks AW, Sampson HA. Clinical features of acute allergic reactions to peanut and tree nuts in children. Pediatrics 1998; 102:e6.

54. Bernhisel-Broadbent J, Sampson HA. Cross-allergenicity in the legume botanical family in children with food hypersensitivity. J Allergy Clin Immunol 1989; 83:435–440.

55. Yu JW, Kagan R, Verreault N. Accidental ingestion in children with peanut allergy 2006; 118:466–472.

*56. Leung DY, Sampson HA, Yunginger JW, et al. Effect of anti-IgE therapy in patients with peanut allergy. N Engl J Med 2003; 348:986–993.

57. Ewan PW, Clark AT. Long-term prospective observational study of patients with peanut and nut allergy after participation in a management plan. Lancet 2001; 357:111–115.

58. Hosey RG, Carek PJ, Goo A. Exercise-induced anaphylaxis and urticaria. Am Fam Physician 2001; 64:1367–1372.

59. Tewari A, Du Toit G, Lack G. The difficulties of diagnosing food-dependent exercise-induced anaphylaxis in childhood – a case study and review. Pediatr Allergy Immunol 2006; 17:157–160.

60. David TJ. Food and food additive intolerance in childhood. Oxford: Blackwell Scientific; 1993.

*61. David TJ. Reactions to dietary tartrazine. Arch Dis Child 1987; 62:119–122.

62. Cullinan P, Brown R, Field A, et al. Latex allergy. A position paper of the British Society of Allergy and Clinical Immunology. Clin Exp Allergy 2003; 33:1484–1499.

63. Brehler R, Theissen U, Mohr C, et al. 'Latex-fruit syndrome'. Frequency of cross-reacting IgE antibodies. Allergy 1997; 52:404–410.

*64. Chen Z, Posch A, Cremer R, et al. Identification of hevein (Hev b 6.02) in Hevea latex as a major cross-reacting allergen with avocado fruit in patients with latex allergy. J Allergy Clin Immunol 1998; 102:476–481.

65. Heilman DK, Jones RT, Swanson MC, et al. A prospective controlled study showing that rubber gloves are the major contributor to latex aeroallergen levels in the operating room. J Allergy Clin Immunol 1996; 98:325–330.

66. Reisman RE. Stinging insect allergy. Med Clin North Am 1992; 76:883–894.

*67. Salkind AR, Cuddy PG, Foxworth JW. Is this patient allergic to penicillin? An evidence-based analysis of the likelihood of penicillin allergy. JAMA 2001; 285:2498–2505.

68. Gueant JL, Aimone-Gastin I, Namour F. Diagnosis and pathogenesis of the anaphylactic and anaphylactoid reactions to anesthetics. Clin Exp Allergy 1998; 28:(Suppl 4):65–70.

69. Gruchalla RS. Acute drug desensitization. Clin Exp Allergy 1998; 28:(Suppl 4):63–64.

70. Green GR, Rosenblum AH, Sweet LC. Evaluation of penicillin hypersensitivity: value of clinical history and skin testing with penicilloyl-polyserine and penicillin G. J Allergy Clin Immunol 1977; 60:339–345.

71. Gall H, Kaufman R, Kalveram CM. Adverse reactions to local anesthetics: analysis of 197 cases. J Allergy Clin Immunol 1996; 97:933–937.

72. Kemp SF, Lockey RF. Anaphylaxis: a review of causes and mechanisms. J Allergy Clin Immunol 2002; 110:341–38l.

73. Pumphrey RS. Lessons for management of anaphylaxis from a study of fatal reactions. Clin Exp Allergy 2000; 30:1144–1150.

74. Pumphrey RS, Roberts IS. Postmortem findings after fatal anaphylactic reactions. J Clin Pathol 2000; 53:273–276.

75. Sly PD, Landau LI. Diurnal variation in bronchial responsiveness in asthmatic children. Pediatr Pulmonol 1986; 2:344–352.

76. Murray AB, Ferguson AC, Morrison BJ. Diagnosis of house dust mite allergy in asthmatic children: what constitutes a positive history?. J Allergy Clin Immunol 1983; 71:21–28.

77. Khot A, Burn R, Evans N, et al. Biometeorological triggers in childhood asthma. Clin Allergy 1988; 18:351–358.

78. Storr J, Lenney W. School holidays and admissions with asthma. Arch Dis Child 1989; 64:103–107.

79. Turner MA, Devlin J, David TJ. Holidays and atopic eczema. Arch Dis Child 1991; 66:212–215.

80. Butler NR, Golding J. A study of the health and behaviour of Britain's 5-year-olds. Oxford: Pergamon; 1986.

81. May CD, Bock SA. A modern clinical approach to food hypersensitivity. Allergy 1978; 33:166–188.

82. Lessof MH, Buisseret PD, Merrett J, et al. Assessing the value of skin tests. Clin Allergy 1980; 10:115–120.

83. Lessof MH. Skin tests. In: Lessof MH, Lee TH, Kemeny DM (eds) Allergy: An international textbook. Chichester: John Wiley; 1987:281–287.

84. Bousquet J, Michel FB. In vivo methods for study of allergy. Skin tests, techniques, and interpretation. In: Middleton E, Reed CE, Ellis EF, et al, (eds) Allergy. Principles and practice. St Louis: Mosby; 1993.573–627.

85. Ford RPK, Taylor B. Natural history of egg hypersensitivity. Arch Dis Child 1982; 57:649–652.

86. Pepys J. Skin testing. Br J Hosp Med 1975; 14:412–417.

87. Aalto-Korte K, Mökinen-Kiljunen S. False negative SPT after anaphylaxis. Allergy 2001; 56:461–462.

88. Patterson R. Allergic diseases. Diagnosis and management. 3rd edn. Philadelphia: Lippincott; 1985.

89. Bernstein IL. Proceedings of the task force guidelines for standardizing old and new techniques used for the diagnosis and treatment of allergic diseases. J Allergy Clin Immunol 1988; 82:(Suppl):487–526.985.

90. Wilkinson JD, Rycroft RJG. Contact dermatitis. In: Champion RH, Burton JL, Ebling FJG (eds) Rook/ Wilkinson/Ebling textbook of dermatology. Oxford: Blackwell Scientific; 1992.611–715.

91. Hill DJ, Ball G, Hosking CS. Clinical manifestations of cows' milk allergy in childhood. I. Associations with in-vitro cellular immune responses. Clin Allergy 1988; 18:469–479.

92. Kidd JM, Cohen SH, Sosman AJ, et al. Food-dependent exercise-induced anaphylaxis. J Allergy Clin Immunol 1983; 71:407–411.

93. McLean-Tooke AP, Bethune CA, Fay AC, et al. Adrenaline in the treatment of anaphylaxis: what is the evidence?. BMJ 2003; 327:1332–1335.

94. Colver A, Hourihane J. For and against. Are the dangers of childhood food allergy exaggerated? BMJ 2006; 333:494–498.

95. Unsworth DJ. Adrenaline syringes are vastly over prescribed. Arch Dis Child 2001; 84:410–411.

96. Arkwright PD, Farragher AJ. Factors determining the ability of parents to effectively administer intramuscular adrenaline to food allergic children. Pediatr Allergy Immunol 2006; 17:227–229.

97. Jutel M, Akdis M, Blaser K, et al. Mechanisms of allergen specific immunotherapy-T-cell tolerance and more. Allergy 2006; 61:796–807.

98. Thien FC. Drug hypersensitivity. Med J Aust 2006; 185:333–338.

99. Pfaar O, Klimek L. Aspirin desensitization in aspirin intolerance: update on current standards and recent improvements. Curr Opin Allergy Clin Immunol 2006; 6:161–166.

100. Meglio P, Bartone E, Plantamura M, et al. A protocol for oral desensitization in children with IgE-mediated cow's milk allergy. Allergy 2004; 59:980–987.

101. Rolinck-Werninghaus C, Staden U, Mehl A, et al. Specific oral tolerance induction with food in children: transient or persistent effect on food allergy?. Allergy 2005; 60:1320–1322.

102. Cox LS, Linnemann DL, Nolte H, et al. Sublingual immunotherapy: a comprehensive review. J Allergy Clin Immunol 2006; 117:1021–1035.

*103. Wilson DR, Torres Lima M, et al. Sublingual immunotherapy for allergic rhinitis. Cochrane Database Systemic Rev 2006, Issue 2.

*104. Cox LS, Linnemann DL, Nolte H, et al. Sublingual immunotherapy: A comprehensive review. J Allergy Clin Immunol 2006; 117:1021–1035.

*105. Casale TB. Anti-immunoglobulin E (omali-zumab) therapy in seasonal allergic rhinitis. Am J Respir Crit Care Med 2001; 164:S18–S21.

*106. Strunk RC, Bloomberg GR. Omalizumab for asthma. N Engl J Med 2006; 354:2689–2695.

*107. Zhang W, Leonard T, Bath-Hextall F, et al. Chinese herbal medicine for atopic eczema. Cochrane Database Syst Rev 2005; 2:CD002291.

108. Srivastava KD, Kattan JD, Zou ZM, et al. The Chinese herbal medicine formula FAHF-2 completely blocks anaphylactic reactions in a murine model of peanut allergy. J Allergy Clin Immunol 2005; 115:171–178.

109. Grulee CG, Sanford HN. The influence of breast and artificial feeding on infantile eczema. J Pediatr 1930; 9:223–225.

110. Chan-Yeung M, Becker A. Primary prevention of childhood asthma and allergic disorders. Curr Opin Allergy Clin Immunol 2006; 6:146–151.

111. Lowe AJ, Carlin JB, Bennett CM, et al. Atopic disease and breast-feeding – cause or consequence? J Allergy Clin Immunol 2006; 117:682–687.

*112. Osborn DA, Sinn J. Formulas containing hydrolysed protein for prevention of allergy and food intolerance in infants. Cochrane Database Syst Rev 2003; CD003664.

113. Barbi E, Gerarduzzi T, Longo G, et al. Fatal allergy as a possible consequence of long-term elimination diet. Allergy 2004; 59:668–672.

114. Strobel S, Mowat AM. Oral tolerance and allergic responses to food proteins. Curr Opin Allergy Clin Immunol 2006; 6:207–213.

*115. deMeer G, Toelle BG, Ng K, et al. Presence and timing of cat ownership by age 18 and the effect on atopy and asthma at age 28. J Allergy Clin Immunol 2004; 113:433–438.

*116. Ownby DR, Johnson CC, Peterson EL. Exposure to dogs and cats in the first year of life and risk of allergic sensitization at 6 to 7 years of age. JAMA 2002; 28:963–972.

117. Kalliomaki M, Salminen S, Poussa T, et al. Probiotics and prevenation of atopic disease: 4-year follow-up of a randomised placebo-controlled trial. Lancet 2003; 361:1869–1871.

118. Boyle RJ, Tang ML. The role of probiotics in the management of allergic disease. Clin Exp Allergy 2006; 36:568–576.

34

Psychiatric disorders in childhood

Peter Hoare

INTRODUCTION

Child psychiatry is concerned with the assessment and treatment of children's emotional and behavioral problems. These problems are common with prevalence rates of 10–20% reported in community studies. The majority of disturbed children are not seen by specialist psychiatric services, but by general practitioners, community doctors and pediatricians along with other professionals such as teachers and residential care staff. Consequently, knowledge about the range and variety of emotional and behavioral problems shown by children is important for all doctors involved in the care of children. The everyday work of the pediatrician provides clear evidence of the stressful effects of illness on the children and family's psychological well-being and adjustment.

Psychiatric disturbance in childhood is most usefully defined as an abnormality in at least one of three areas: emotions, behavior or relationships. It is *not* helpful to regard these abnormalities as strictly defined disease entities with a precise etiology, treatment and prognosis. Rather, it is preferable to regard them as deviations or departures from the norm,

1541

which are distressing to the child or to those involved with his care (the male gender is used throughout the chapter for ease of presentation rather than from any bias or discrimination). Although child psychiatric disorders do not conform to a strict medical model of illness, it does not mean that these disorders are trivial or unimportant. Some disorders such as autism or conduct disorder have major implications for the child's development and adjustment in adult life.

In childhood, the distinction between disturbance and normality is imprecise. Isolated symptoms are common and not pathological. For example, many children will occasionally feel sad, unhappy or have temper tantrums. This does not mean that they are disturbed. Disturbance is characterized by the number, frequency, severity and duration of symptoms rather than by the type of symptomatology. In addition, disturbed children rarely present with unequivocal pathological symptoms such as hallucinations or delusions, whereas symptoms such as unhappiness and lying are common and not diagnostic. In clinical practice, it is often more important to establish why the child is the focus for concern rather than to adopt the more narrow perspective of whether the child is disturbed or not.

Another important feature of psychiatric disturbance in childhood is that several, as opposed to single, factors contribute to the development of disturbance. This makes assessment and treatment more difficult, so that an essential prerequisite for successful treatment is the correct evaluation of the relative contribution of the different etiological factors. Etiological factors are usually categorized into two groups: constitutional and environmental. The former includes heredity factors, intelligence and temperament. The three major environmental influences are the family, schooling and the community. Another factor, physical illness or disability, if present, can have a profound effect on the child's development and on his vulnerability to disturbance.

Three other considerations are of general importance in understanding children's behavior: the situation-specific nature of behavior, the impact of current stressful events, and the role of family. Children's behavior varies markedly in different situations, that is, it is situation specific. For instance, a child may be a major problem at school but not at home, or vice versa. Consequently, there may well be an apparent discrepancy between accounts of the child's behavior from the parents and from the teachers. The most likely explanation for this discrepancy is that the demands and expectations upon the child in the two situations are different. It is therefore essential to obtain several independent accounts about the child's behavior wherever possible in order to derive a more accurate and realistic assessment of the problem. This situation-specific nature of the behavior has implications for treatment, as it is important to explain to parents and to teachers the reasons for the discrepancy, thereby lessening the likelihood of misunderstanding.

Children are immature and developing individuals whose capacities and coping skills change markedly during childhood. Childhood is also a period of life characterized by change, challenge and the necessity for adaptation. Consequently it is not surprising that symptoms of disturbance may arise at times of stress when the demands on the child are excessive. Research has shown that life events are associated with an increased psychiatric morbidity among children,[1] a finding similar to that reported for adults. Some stresses such as the birth of a sibling or starting school are of course normal and inevitable, whereas others, such as marital break-up or life-threatening illness, are serious with long term implications for the child's well-being.

The child may, however, cope successfully with the stress, thereby enhancing their self-esteem and confidence. Alternatively, the child may be overwhelmed, responding with the development of symptomatic behavior. The latter may involve regressive behavior (i.e. behaving in a more immature, dependent fashion), or more specifically maladaptive (e.g. aggression, excessive anxiety or withdrawal). A crucial feature of assessment is the identification of stressful factors that may be contributing to the problem, as this will influence treatment strategies and the prognosis.

The family is the most potent force for the promotion of health as well as for the development of disturbance in the child's life. Assessment of parenting qualities, the marital relationship and the quality of family interaction are essential components of child psychiatric practice. It is a frequent observation that it is the parents who are disturbed and not the child. One consequence of this observation is that in many cases the focus of treatment is likely to be the parents, or the whole family, rather than the child. Indeed, in many instances the main emphasis of treatment is the promotion of normal healthy family interaction as much as in the amelioration of disturbed behavior.

Finally, many disturbed children do not complain about their distress nor admit to problems, but rather it is their parents or other adults involved with their care who bring the child to the attention of professionals. Disturbed children more commonly manifest their distress or unhappiness indirectly through symptoms such as abdominal pain, aggression or withdrawal. Direct questioning of the child during the initial interview is unlikely to reveal the true extent of the child's feelings or the degree of his distress. Sensitive observations during the interview and the use of indirect techniques such as play are necessary to elicit a more accurate view of the child's feelings. This is only likely to be successful once a relationship of trust has been established between the child and the clinician.

NORMAL AND ABNORMAL PSYCHOLOGICAL DEVELOPMENT

Children are developing individuals. They are not small adults. A 2-year-old is very different to a 12-year-old, whereas an adult aged 25 may not differ that much from a 35-year-old. During childhood, the child undergoes a remarkable transformation from a helpless, dependent infant to an independent self-sufficient individual with his own views and outlook, capable of embarking on a career and living separately from his family. Knowledge about the *mechanisms, processes* and the *sequences* underlying these events is necessary in order to understand the nature of psychological disturbance in childhood. This knowledge also helps to define more clearly what age-appropriate behavior is and to distinguish the pathological from the normal. This section has three parts: developmental theories, developmental psychopathology and personality development.

DEVELOPMENTAL THEORIES (Table 34.1)

It is useful to define some terms at the outset, as they are often used interchangeably. *Growth* refers to the incremental increase of a characteristic; *maturation* is those phases and products of development that are mainly due to innate or endogenous factors; *development* is those changes in the nature and organization of an organism's structure and behavior that are systematically related to age. Many behaviors (for example walking and talking) have a substantial maturational component, whereas others (for instance emotional and social development) are strongly influenced by environmental factors. The continuous interaction between maturational and environmental factors throughout childhood helps to mold the personality development of the child.

Developmental theories tend to focus on at least one of the following areas: cognitive, emotional or social. They differ widely in theoretical orientation, in supporting empirical evidence and in the relative importance attributed to experience in influencing development. No single theory is satisfactory, so that most clinicians utilize some parts of the various theories to explain different aspects of development. The theories are usually described as stage theories, implying that they regard development as a series of recognizable phases of increasing complexity through which the child progresses.

COGNITIVE DEVELOPMENT

In 1929, the Swiss psychologist Piaget proposed a comprehensive theory of cognitive development. Many of his conclusions were based on experiments conducted on his own children over a number of years. Piaget has had a tremendous impact on educational concepts and teaching, particularly in primary schools over the last 30 years. More recently, the

Table 34.1   Summary of cognitive, emotional and social development

	Age in years				
	0	2	6	9	12+ upwards
Cognitive (Piaget)	*Sensori-motor*	*Pre-operational*	*Concrete operational*		*Formal operational*
	Differentiates self from objects	Learns to use language and to represent objects by image and words	Thinking is more logical and less egocentric		Able to think in abstract manner about propositions and hypotheses
	Begins to act intentionally	Thinking is egocentric (unable to see other viewpoint) and animistic (everything has feelings including inanimate objects)	Achieves conservation of number (age 6), volume (age 7) mass (age 8) Able to arrange objects in rank order		
	Achieves object permanence				
Emotional (Freud)	*Oral*	*Anal*	*Phallic*	*Latency*	*Genital*
	Main concern is initially with satisfaction of basic needs such as hunger	Co-operative activity with caregiver	Learns to interact with peers, often leads to rivalry	Reduced sexual interest with main concerns about peer relationships and position within peer group	Revival of earlier conflict, especially sexual conflict
	Later on, attachment to care giver	Satisfaction with increased self-control and achievement	Aware of own sexuality causing Oedipal conflict, resolved by identification with the same sex parent Conscience begins to form		Four main tasks: separation from parents, sexual role, career choice, identity
Social & personality development	Social smiling (8 weeks) Attachment (6 months) Stranger anxiety (10 months)	Cooperative play (3 years)	Strong preference for same-sex friends with stereotyped expectations (6–7 years)	Enduring relationships (8 years onwards)	
	Erikson's stage of trust vs. mistrust	*Erikson's stage of autonomy vs. shame and doubt*	*Erikson's stage of initiative vs. guilt*	*Erikson's stage of industry vs. inferiority*	*Erikson's stage of identity vs. role diffusion*

theoretical basis and validity of Piaget's conclusions have been questioned by further empirical studies.[2] Despite these criticisms, his views remain the most useful account of cognitive development.

Piaget's theory is set within a biological framework. In order to survive, the individual must have the capacity to adapt to the demands of the environment. Cognitive development is the result of interaction between the individual and the environment. Four factors influence cognitive development: increased neurological maturation, enabling the child to appreciate new aspects of experience and to apply more complex reasoning as he gets older; the opportunity to practice newly acquired skills; the opportunity for social interaction and to benefit from schooling; and the emergence of internal psychological mechanisms or *structures* that allow the child to construct a successively more complex cognitive model based on maturation and experience.

Piaget describes two types of intellectual structure: *schemas* and *operations*. The former are present at birth, the latter arise during childhood. *Schemas* are internal representations of some specific action, for instance sucking or grasping, whereas *operations* are internal rules of a higher order that have the distinctive feature that they are *reversible*, as, for example, multiplication is reversible by division. There are two ways whereby the child adapts his cognitive structure to the demands of the environment: *assimilation* and *accommodation*. The former refers to the incorporation of new objects, thoughts and behavior into existing structures, whereas the latter describes the change of existing structures in response to novel experiences. The child attends and learns most when his environment has a degree of novelty that challenges his curiosity but is not so strange that it becomes too confusing.

Piaget describes four main phases: *sensorimotor, pre-operational, concrete operational* and *formal operational*. The age range given for each stage is the average, though this can vary considerably depending upon intelligence, cultural background and socioeconomic factors. However, the order is assumed to be the same for all children. Schemas predominate in the sensorimotor and pre-operational stages, whereas operations predominate in the concrete operational and formal operational stages.

Sensorimotor (birth–2 years). Initially, behavior is dominated by innate reflexes such as feeding, sucking and following, hence the name for this period. Gradually, the infant realizes the distinction between *self* and *non-self*, namely where his body ends and the world outside begins. The infant also realizes that his behavior can influence the environment, so that intentional and purposeful behavior begins. Finally, the infant achieves *object permanence* whereby he recognizes that an object still exists even although it is no longer visible.

Pre-operational period (2–7 years). Language development greatly facilitates cognition, so that the individual begins to represent objects by symbols and words. Thinking is, however, *egocentric* and *animistic*. The former refers to the child's tendency to regard the world solely from his own position along with an inability to see a situation from another point of view. Animistic thinking describes the child's tendency to regard everything in the world as endowed with feelings, thoughts and wishes. For instance, the moon is watching over you when you sleep, the child says 'naughty door' when he bangs into the door.

The child has problems with the principles of conservation for number, volume and mass. The essential principle underlying conservation is that the number, volume or mass of an object are not changed by any visual alteration in their display or appearance. For instance, the child readily believes that the more widely spaced of two rows of counters has more counters than a denser packed row, or that there is more water in a tall beaker when it has been poured there from a shorter, more squat beaker.

The child also believes that every event has a preceding cause, rejecting the concept of chance or coincidence. Again, the child's moral sense is rigid and inflexible, so that punishment is invariable, irrespective of the circumstances. The child's concept of illness is radically different to that of the adult, with illness seen as a consequence for misdeeds, a punishment for a misdemeanor.

Concrete operational (7–12 years). Thinking becomes more logical and less dominated by immediate perceptual experience or by changes in appearance. Conservation of number, volume and mass is successively achieved during this period. The child becomes less egocentric, capable of seeing events from another person's standpoint. The child is able to appreciate and utilize reversibility, for example if 2 and 2 equals 4, then 4 minus 2 must equal 2.

Formal operational (12 years and upwards). This stage represents the most complex mode of thinking. Its main characteristics are the ability to think in an abstract fashion, to formulate general rules and principles and to devise and test hypotheses, an approach similar to that used in mathematics or in a scientific investigation. An example of such reasoning is the following: Joan is fairer than Susan; Joan is darker than Anne. Who is the darkest? (Answer: Susan). Prior to the formal operational stage, the child would require the aid of dolls to solve this problem. It should be pointed out that not everyone achieves this stage of thinking, even as an adult! The content of thinking also alters markedly with an emphasis on the hypothetical, the future and ideological issues.

CRITICAL COMMENT ON PIAGET

Recently, the Piagetian model has been criticized extensively for the lack of evidence to support the existence of the internal structures necessary for the concrete and formal operational stages. Alternative nonPiagetian explanations for a child's inability to carry out conservation tasks successfully before a certain age have also been put forward.[3] These criticisms are substantial, but they do not detract from the major conceptual contribution that Piaget has made to knowledge about cognitive development in children.

RECENT DEVELOPMENTS IN COGNITIVE THEORY

Psychologists and psychiatrists have become increasingly interested in the development and application of cognitive theory to the understanding and treatment of psychiatric disorders.[4,5] The main principles underlying this theory are that an individual's beliefs about (1) himself, (2) the future and (3) the world influence his mood and behavior, an idea similar in some ways to the Piagetian concept of schemas. When a person is depressed, his thoughts are self-defeating and he commits certain cognitive errors. Two common types of cognitive error are *personalization* and *dichotomous thinking*. The following two statements are examples of these two errors, respectively: 'The reason my parents separated is all because of me' and 'I'm no good at tennis, so I'm bound to be useless at any other sport'.

A major extension of these ideas in childhood is the notion of the *self-concept*. By the age of 6 or 7 years, most children have very definite and clear ideas about themselves and their qualities. For example, they are able to compare themselves to other children with respect to popularity, attractiveness, scholastic ability, and so on. Self-concept is a construct similar to that of a schema in Piaget's theory. Another important facet of self-concept is the favorable or unfavorable evaluation that the child makes of himself, an aspect called *self-esteem*. Children with high self-esteem appear to do better in school, regard themselves as in control of their own destiny, have more friends and get along better with their families.[2]

EMOTIONAL AND SOCIAL DEVELOPMENT

Sigmund Freud developed the most comprehensive theory about emotional development while Erikson,[6] also a psychoanalyst, applied psychoanalytic concepts within a social and cultural framework. Freudian theory emphasizes the biological and maturational components of development with an invariable sequence to development for everyone. Like Piaget, it is a stage or phase theory with the individual progressing successively through each phase. A major criticism of Freudian theory is that its concepts do not lend themselves readily to scientific investigation, so that it is difficult to prove or disprove the validity of the theory.

Freud proposed that an individual goes through five stages prior to adulthood, namely *oral, anal, phallic, latency* and *genital*. These terms refer to the major developmental task or potential conflict that the individual has to achieve or resolve during this period. Table 34.1 describes the important features of the different stages, e.g. during the phallic stage, the Oedipal crisis arises. At this time (around 3–4 years), the child becomes aware of his own sexual feelings and also that he is attracted in a sexual manner to the parent of the opposite sex. Moreover, the child is simultaneously aware that the parent of the same sex is a rival for the attention of the other parent. The conflict arises because the child is caught between the desire for one parent and the wrath of the other. The conflict is successfully resolved by the child identifying with the parent of the same sex, thereby eliminating the rivalrous feelings.

Erikson's major contribution has been to place psychoanalytic concepts in a social and cultural dimension (see Table 34.1). For Erikson, the most important task for the individual is to achieve a coherent sense of identity, a balanced and mature appraisal of one's abilities and limitations, with recognition of the importance of previous experience and with realistic expectations for the future. Such a task occupies the individual throughout his lifetime. The individual passes through a series of developmental stages, all of which are polarized into two extremes, one successful and adaptive and the other unsuccessful and maladaptive. The two poles of the first stage are *trust* and *mistrust*. The former refers to the child's belief that the world is safe, predictable, and that he can influence events towards a favorable outcome, whereas a sense of mistrust implies a world that is cruel, erratic and unable to meet his needs. The role of the caregiver, usually the mother, is crucial to the achievement of a successful outcome. Erikson also believed that the individual carries forward the residues of earlier stages into the present, thereby giving the past an influence on contemporary behavior. Erikson's writings are a compelling and coherent account of development. A major weakness is, however, the lack of empirical evidence to support the conclusions.

Development of social relationships[2]

A characteristic of human beings is their predisposition to establish and maintain social relationships. Although Freud and Erikson refer to social relationships, it is only with the recent elaboration of *attachment theory* by Bowlby[7] and by Ainsworth[8] that a plausible theory for this phenomenon has been described. Attachment theory proposes that social relationships develop in response to the mutual biological and psychological needs of the mother and the infant. Mother–infant interaction promotes social relationships. Each member of the dyad has a repertoire of behavior that facilitates interaction: (1) the infant by crying, smiling and vocalization; (2) the mother by facial expression, vocalization and gaze. A mother can regulate the infant's state of alertness, for instance rocking or stroking to soothe the child, whilst talking or facial expressions stimulate the child.

The term *attachment* describes the infant's predisposition to seek proximity to certain people and to be more secure in their presence. Bowlby maintained that there is a biological basis for this behavior, as it has been found extensively in other primates as well as in most human societies. It has considerable survival and adaptive value for the species, as it enables the dependent infant to explore from a secure base and also to use the base as a place of safety at times of distress. From the age of 6 months onwards, infants develop selective attachment to people, usually the mother initially, but not exclusively to her. This first relationship is regarded as the prototype for subsequent relationships, so that its success or failure may have long term consequences. Clinicians distinguish between *secure attachment* and *anxious attachment*, with the former referring to healthy and the latter to potentially unsatisfactory relationships.

Bonding refers to the persistence of relationships over time, namely the child's capacity to retain the relationship despite the absence of the other individual. Much of the infant's behavior promotes the development of attachments by ensuring close proximity and interaction with the mother. These ideas have many implications for obstetric and pediatric practice, for the reduction of stress associated with hospitalization and for possibly explaining the origins of non-accidental injury to children.

Other aspects of development
Gender and sex role concepts
Gender identity is a part of self-concept, but the development of the child's understanding about 'boyness' or 'girlness', the sex role concept, is a more elaborate process. Children usually acquire *gender identity* (correctly labeling themselves and others) by about age 2 or 3 followed by *gender stability* (permanence of gender identity) by about 4. *Gender constancy* (gender identity unalterable by change in appearance) appears around 6 years, similar to other conservation-like concepts. Children show clear evidence of sex role stereotyping from an early age, with an excessively rigid concept for a brief period around 6 or 7 years. Freudian theory explains these findings on the basis of identification whereby the child imitates the same-sex parent, thus acquiring appropriate sex-typed behavior. Alternative explanations emphasize the importance of social reinforcement and of cognition whereby the child acquires a schema about the respective roles and behavior of boys and girls.

Moral development
The acquisition of moral or ethical values is an important aspect of the socialization of children. Freud and Piaget have both described how this process happens. Freudian theory maintains that the superego or conscience develops during the phallic stage around 4–5 years. At this time, the child is identifying strongly with the same-sex parent in order to resolve the Oedipal conflict and in consequence acquires parental values and prohibitions. In contrast, Piaget hypothesizes a much more gradual or stage-like sequence to the acquisition of moral values. The child around 3 years old bases his judgment on the outcome rather than the intention of an act, with an emphasis on punishment following on from a misdemeanor. Subsequently, the child adopts a more conventional morality based upon conformity with family values. Finally, the adolescent derives a personal value system that combines his own idiosyncratic values with those of his family and of society with the intention of achieving the 'greatest good for the greatest number'.

DEVELOPMENTAL PSYCHOPATHOLOGY

This long-winded phrase refers to two important dimensions necessary to evaluate children's behavior: first, whether the behavior is age appropriate (the developmental aspect); and second, whether the behavior is abnormal (the psychopathological). For example, separation anxiety is a normal phenomenon among children between 9 months and 4 years approximately, whereas it would be abnormal in a child aged 6 years.

The threefold division of disturbance into abnormalities of behavior, emotions or relationships provides a useful way to analyze disturbance. Many behavioral problems can be conceptualized in terms of deficits or excesses. For instance, children with encopresis or enuresis can be regarded as having failed to acquire the skills necessary for toileting. Similarly, the aggressive child is showing excessive belligerent or assertive behavior at an inappropriate time. This approach also has implications for treatment, as the latter is often based on behavioral techniques designed to increase certain behaviors or alternatively to eliminate others.

Anxiety is central to the understanding of emotional disturbance. It has physical manifestations such as palpitations or dry mouth as well as psychological such as fear or apprehension. Anxiety is a normal, indeed essential, part of growing up. It may occur in many situations: in response to external threat, new or strange situations, and in response to the operation of conscience. Anna Freud[9] developed the concept of *defense mechanisms* to explain how an individual dealt with excessive anxiety. This response is entirely healthy and appropriate in many situations, only becoming maladaptive when it is used exclusively or excessively, thereby preventing the individual from learning how to cope with a normal amount of anxiety. Common defense mechanisms include *denial, rationalization, regression, and displacement*. Denial is the process where the child refuses to accept the psychological implications of a particular event or situation. For instance, a child refuses to admit to stealing, even when the theft is obvious, as the resultant loss of self-esteem and the sense of guilt make this impossible. Rationalization is when the child attempts to justify or minimize the psychological consequences of an event. 'I don't really like football, so that I am not bothered about playing for the team' is an example of the way in which the child may deal with a failure to gain selection for the school team. Regression occurs when a child behaves in a more developmentally immature manner, often at times of stress, for example becoming enuretic at the start of primary school. Displacement is the transfer of hostile or aggressive feelings from their original source on to another person, for instance getting angry with a sibling rather than with an adult.

Social relationships are often impaired among disturbed children. This may be a primary failure in some instances, such as autism, or more commonly a secondary phenomenon. Children with neurotic or conduct disorders are usually isolated and unpopular with their peer group as they have either excluded themselves or have alternatively been excluded as a result of their deviant behavior. In addition, the behavior usually brings them into conflict with parents or other adults such as teachers.

PERSONALITY DEVELOPMENT

Childhood is the time during which personality is formed. Wordsworth's aphorism 'the child is father to the man' is substantially true. Personality is a broad concept referring to the enduring and uniquely individual constellation of attributes that distinguish one person from another. It comprises cognitive, emotional, motivational and temperamental attributes that determine the individual's view about himself, his world and the future. Throughout childhood, the various elements interact with each other to mold the child's personality. Moreover, this process occurs in the context of the child's life experiences, particularly within the family, and also subsequently in the world outside the family. Healthy personality formation is an important prerequisite for satisfactory adjustment during childhood and also during adult life.

Personality is influenced by two main factors – constitutional and environmental – whilst a third, illness or disability, if present, can have a profound effect on the child. Constitutional factors include intelligence and temperament. The former describes the individual's ability to think rationally about himself and his environment, while the latter refers to the individual's characteristic style or approach to new people or situations, his level of activity and prevailing mood. These temperamental traits influence the child's response to his environment and also shape the range and variety of his experiences.

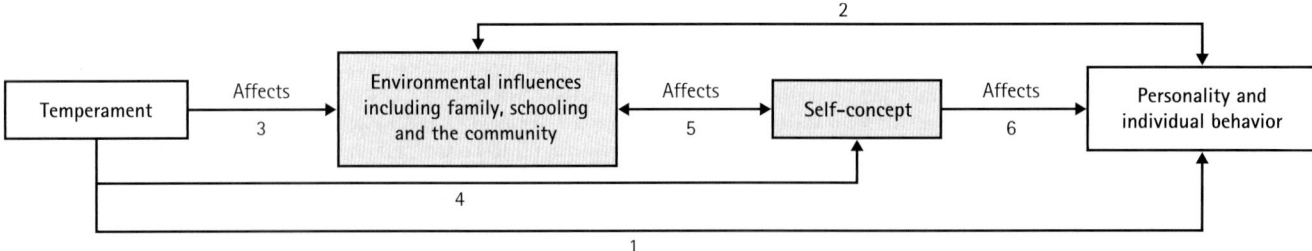

Fig. 34.1   Interactive model of personality development.

The main environmental influences are the family, schooling and the community. The family is the most powerful force for promoting healthy development as well as for causing severe disturbance in a child's life. Families fulfil many functions for children including: (1) the satisfaction of basic physical needs such as food and shelter; (2) the provision of love and security; (3) the development of social relationships with adults and peers; (4) the promotion of cognitive and language skills; (5) the experience of appropriate role models and socialization; and (6) the acquisition of ethical and moral values.

Schooling has three main roles for children: (1) the attainment of scholastic skills; (2) the promotion of peer relationships; and (3) the acceptance of adult authority outside the family. The community through the quality of housing and the availability of resources also has a considerable influence on the child's development. Finally, physical disability or illness, when present, exerts a major effect on personality development. This arises not only from the direct restrictions or limitations that they may impose on the child's abilities or activities, but more commonly and importantly, through indirect effects on the child's self-esteem, from overprotectiveness by the parents and from poor social relationships with siblings and peers.

Figure 34.1 is a diagrammatic representation of an interactive model of personality development that incorporates these ideas discussed in this section. As shown in Figure 34.1, constitutionally determined temperamental traits have a direct effect on personality and behavior, with the environment also exerting a similar impact. Environmental and temperamental factors also have direct effects on the self-concept, which in turn shapes and modifies the personality as well as the environment. These interactive processes continue throughout childhood in a dynamic manner to produce a final product, an individual.

GENERAL FEATURES OF PSYCHIATRIC DISTURBANCE

DIAGNOSTIC CLASSIFICATION

A single cause is rarely responsible for the development of disturbance. The usual pattern is for several factors to be involved with a broad distinction into constitutional and environmental factors. The important constitutional factors are intelligence and temperament, whilst current life circumstances, the family, schooling and the community are the major environmental influences. One consequence of this multiple causation is that it is not possible to devise a diagnostic classification on the basis of etiology, as the relative contribution of each factor is often unclear.

Diagnostic practice is therefore descriptive or phenomenological, with three main categories of abnormality: *emotions*, *behavior* and *relationships*. In addition, these abnormalities should be of sufficient severity that they impair the individual in his daily activities and/or cause distress to the individual or to those responsible for his well-being. A commonly used definition of disturbance is as follows: an abnormality of emotions, behavior or relationships that is sufficiently severe and persistent to handicap the child in his social or personal functioning and/or to cause distress to the child, his parents or to people in the community.

The two commonest systems are the ICD-10[10] and DSM-IV.[11] DSM-IV is used extensively in North America, whereas ICD-10 is popular in the

UK. The two systems have similar underlying principles with an emphasis on a clinical-descriptive approach to diagnosis. An important difference between ICD-10 and DSM-IV is that the latter allows for more than one diagnosis, whereas ICD-10 prefers a single diagnosis. The following list shows a convenient way to classify the important psychiatric syndromes in childhood:

1. conduct disorders;
2. emotional disorders;
3. mixed disorders of conduct and emotions;
4. hyperkinetic disorders (ICD-10) or attention deficit hyperactivity disorder (DSM-IV);
5. disorders of social functioning;
6. tic disorders;
7. pervasive developmental disorders;
8. Miscellaneous disorders – encopresis, enuresis, sleep disorders and eating disorders.

Conduct disorder is characterized by severe, persistent, socially disapproved of behavior such as aggression or stealing that often involves damage to or destruction of property and is unresponsive to normal sanctions. The main feature of emotional disorder is a subjective sense of distress, often arising in response to stress. This group is further divided into phobic, anxiety, obsessional, conversion states and severe reactions to stress. Many disturbed children show a mixture of emotional and behavioral symptoms, so that a mixed category is clinically useful. An important source of confusion between the two classification systems is the terminology relating to hyperkinetic disorders in ICD-10 and attention deficit hyperactivity disorder (ADHD) in DSM-IV. Although both systems have the same core features (overactivity, impulsivity and inattention), the different names imply the two systems regard the main abnormality differently, namely hyperactivity for ICD-10 and inattention for DSM-IV. The situation is further complicated by the popular usage of another term to describe this group of disorders: ADHD. Disorders of social functioning comprise conditions such as selective mutism and attachment disorders. Pervasive developmental disorders include autistic spectrum disorder, Rett syndrome and childhood disintegrative disorder. The miscellaneous group contains a diverse group of problems such as encopresis, enuresis and developmental disorders. Other important but uncommon conditions such as schizophrenia and mood disorders are categorized in a similar fashion to that for adults, providing that the diagnostic criteria are fulfilled.

EPIDEMIOLOGY OF DISTURBANCE

Epidemiological research has been an important research interest in the UK for the past 30 years. It has provided accurate information about the frequency and distribution of disturbance throughout childhood and adolescence,[12] the differences between urban and rural areas,[13] the effects of illness and disability on vulnerability to disturbance[14] as well as providing clues about the relative importance of various etiological factors.[13]

Most studies have shown prevalence rates of between 10% and 20% depending on the criteria for deviance. The first and most influential study was the Isle of Wight (IOW) study carried out by Rutter and colleagues.[12] Using a strict definition of disorder, they found rates of approximately 7% among 10–11-year-old children. Follow-up of these children into adolescence indicated a prevalence rate of around 7% with more than 40% of the children with conduct disorder still having major problems. Disorders arising for the first time during adolescence were more adult like in presentation, with a preponderance of females. Over 80% of the disorders were in the emotional, conduct or mixed categories. Emotional disorders were more common among girls, with anxiety the commonest type. By contrast, conduct disorders, and to an important extent mixed disorder, were more common among boys with an association with specific reading retardation. A comparative study of 10-year-olds living in London[13] showed a rate of disturbance over twice that on the IOW. This study also showed that the difference in prevalence rate was entirely accounted for by the increased frequency of predisposing factors among children and their families in London compared with those on the IOW. These factors were family discord, parental psychiatric disorder, social disadvantage and inferior quality of schooling.

The IOW study[14] also showed that children with chronic illness or disability had much higher rates of disturbance than healthy children. For instance, children with a central nervous disease such as epilepsy or cerebral palsy had a rate over five times that of the general population, while children with other illnesses such as asthma or diabetes were twice as likely to be disturbed as healthy children. A more recent epidemiological study carried out by the Department of Health in the UK[15] on 10 000 children aged 5–15 years found a very similar prevalence rate and range of disturbance as the IOW study, namely an overall prevalence rate of 10% with conduct disorder (5%), emotional disorder (4%) and attention deficit disorder (ADD) (1%) the main diagnostic categories. The survey also confirmed that adverse social circumstance, chronic illness and learning difficulties were still important risk factors for disturbance.

Studies of pre-school children, most notably by Richman et al,[16] have found that about 20% of children have significant behavior problems, with 7% classified as severe. Follow-up studies of these children indicated that about 60% persisted, most commonly among overactive boys of low ability. An important association was found between language delay and disturbed behavior. Finally, problems were more likely to persist when there was marital discord, maternal psychiatric ill health and psychosocial disadvantage such as poor housing or large family size.

ASSESSMENT PROCEDURES

Assessment is more time consuming in child psychiatry than in other branches of pediatrics. It has three components: history taking and examination, psychological assessment, and information about the child and family from other professionals.

HISTORY TAKING AND EXAMINATION

This has many similarities to traditional methods, though with important modifications. Interview skills are essential to the elucidation, understanding and treatment of emotional and behavioral problems in children. Points of general importance include: (1) clarification about the nature of the problem and the reason for referral; (2) obtaining adequate factual information; (3) observing and eliciting emotional responses and attitudes about past events and about behavior during the interview; (3) establishing trust and confidence of the child and family; and (4) providing the parents with a summary of problems and a provisional treatment plan at the end of the initial interview.

There are no absolute rules about interviewing, indeed flexibility is essential. However, the following guidelines are useful:

1. The interview room should be large enough to seat the family comfortably and also to allow the children to use the play material in a relaxed manner.
2. Avoid having a desk between the interviewer and the family, i.e. put the desk against the wall of the interview room.
3. Do not spend the interview writing down notes but rather encourage eye-to-eye contact, taking the minimal notes necessary.
4. The play material must be suitable for a wide age range and include crayons and paper, jigsaws, simple games, books (provides a rough estimate of reading ability), doll's house, play telephones and miniature domestic and zoo animals.
5. The play material should be gradually introduced as appropriate and not left around in a haphazard manner.
6. Interview parents and young children together.
7. Older children and adolescents like to be seen separately from parents at some point during interview.
8. Older children and adolescents are able to talk about problems openly once trust in the interviewer has been established.
9. Too direct questions usually elicit denial from the child, so that open-ended questions are much more preferable.

The interview should provide information about the following (bold type indicates essential facts):

1. **Presenting problem(s). Frequency. Severity. Onset. Course. Exacerbating/ameliorating factors. Effect on family. Help given so far.**
2. Other problems or complaints:
   - general health: eating, sleeping, elimination, physical complaints, fits or faints;
   - interests, activities and hobbies;
   - **relationship with parents and siblings**;
   - relationship with other children, special friends
   - mood – happy, sad, anxious
   - level of activity, attention span, concentration
   - antisocial behavior
   - **schooling: attainments, attendance, friendships, relationship with teachers**
   - sexual knowledge, interests and behavior (when relevant).
3. **Any other problems not previously mentioned**
4. Family structure:
   a. **Parents: ages**, occupations, Current physical and psychiatric state. Previous physical and psychiatric history;
   b. siblings, ages, problems;
   c. home circumstances.
5. Family function:
   a. quality of parenting: mutual support and help, level of communication and ability to resolve problems;
   b. parent–child relationship: warmth, affection and acceptance, level of criticism, hostility and rejection;
   c. siblings' relationship;
   d. pattern of family relationships.
6. Personal history:
   a. pregnancy and delivery;
   b. early mother–child relationship, postpartum depression, early feeding patterns;
   c. temperamental characteristics: easy or difficult, irregular, restless baby and toddler;
   d. developmental milestones;
   e. **past illnesses and injuries, hospitalization;**
   f. separations greater than 1 week;
   g. Previous schooling.
7. observation of child's behavior and emotional state:
   a. appearance: nutritional state, signs of neglect or injury;
   b. activity level: involuntary movements, concentration;
   c. mood: expressions or signs of sadness, misery, anxiety;
   d. reaction to and relationship with the doctor: eye contact, spontaneous talk, inhibition and disinhibition;
   e. relationship with parents: affection/resentment, ease of separation;
   f. habits and mannerisms;
   g. presence of delusions, hallucinations, thought disorder.
8. observation of family relationships:
   a. patterns of interaction;
   b. clarity of boundaries between parents and child;
   c. communication;
   d. emotional atmosphere of family: mutual warmth/tension, criticisms.

9. physical examination:
   a. screening neurological examination:
      i. note any facial asymmetry;
      ii. eye movements. Ask child to follow a moving finger and observe eye movement for jerkiness, uncoordination;
      iii. finger–thumb apposition. Ask child to press the tip of each finger against the thumb in rapid succession. Observe clumsiness, weakness;
      iv. copying pattern: drawing a man;
      v. observe grip and dexterity in drawing;
      vi. observe visual competence when drawing;
      vii. jumping up and down on the spot;
      viii. hopping;
      ix. hearing. Capacity of child to repeat numbers whispered 2 m behind him.
   b. further medical examination (if relevant).

FORMULATION

At completion of the assessment, the clinician should be able to make a formulation. This is a succinct summary of the important features of the individual case. The formulation consists of the following: (1) statement of main problems; (2) diagnosis and differential diagnosis; (3) relative contribution of constitutional and environmental factors to the etiology; (4) probable short term and long term outcome; further information required (including special investigations); and (5) initial treatment plan. The formulation should be included in the case notes, thereby providing the clinician with a record of his views at referral.

PSYCHOLOGICAL ASSESSMENT

Psychological assessment carried out by a child psychologist is a valuable part of the overall assessment of a child's problems in some situations. It can provide information about three aspects of development: general intelligence, educational attainments and special skills. Assessment is usually based upon the administration of standardized assessment tests. These are either norm referenced or criterion referenced. The former compares the child's ability with other children of the same age, whereas the latter is on a pass/fail basis, for instance whether he can tie his shoelaces. Ideally, the test items should have good discriminatory value (distinguish between children of different ability), be reliable (give similar results when repeated) and valid (in agreement with other independent evidence). An important aspect of the assessment is that the tasks are carried out in a standardized fashion, thereby increasing reliability and validity.

INTELLECTUAL ABILITY

Developmental assessment in infancy and early childhood

The commonly used tests are the Bailey's Scales,[17] Griffiths Mental Development Scales[18] and the Kaufman Assessment Battery for Children (K-ABC).[19]

Assessment of general intelligence amongst school-age children

The most popular test is the Wechsler Intelligence Scale for Children – Revised Form (WISC-R).[20] This covers an age range from 6–16 years. Ten sub tests are usually used, measuring different aspects of the child's ability. Commonly, the tests are divided into 'verbal' and 'performance' categories, yielding a 'verbal IQ' and a 'performance IQ'. The 'verbal' subtests commonly used are information, comprehension, arithmetic, similarities and vocabulary, whilst the 'performance' tests are picture completion, picture arrangement, block design, object assembly and coding. Each subtest has a mean score of 10, so that combining the 10 tests gives a 'full scale' intelligence quotient (IQ) of 100 with a standard deviation of 15. The 'normal' distribution of the test scores means that it is possible to state that 66% of children will

be within the IQ range 85–115, 95% within IQ range 70–130, 99% within IQ range 55–145. Other tests used include the Stanford-Binet[21] and the British Ability Scales (BAS).[22]

EDUCATIONAL ATTAINMENT

There are two commonly used reading tests, the WORD (Wechsler Objective Reading Test)[23] and the Neale Analysis of Reading Ability.[24] The former measures basic reading, comprehension and spelling skills, whilst the latter provides information about speed, accuracy and comprehension of reading. The scores on the Neale test can be transformed into reading ages of so many years and months, for instance 6 years 11 months. The subtest scores of the WISC-R or the BAS can be used as a guide to mathematical ability.

Specific skills

Reynell development language scale,[25] Bender Motor Gestalt Test and the Vineland Social Maturity Scale are examples of tests to assess the child's acquisition of certain abilities and skills. These are often helpful with some specific problems.

Limitations of assessment

Caution should always be exercised in the interpretation of test results. It is wrong to attribute undue significance to a single result, most often done with the IQ score. Many factors influence test results including fatigue, poor testing conditions and the use of inappropriate tests. The results should be evaluated in the context of the overall assessment and the report from the child psychologist. A great deal of harm, upset and distress can arise for a child when he is incorrectly classified or labeled as too able or too dull on the basis of an unreliable psychological assessment.

Additional information

A distinctive feature of child psychiatry practice is the importance attached to obtaining independent evidence about the child's behavior. This is for two reasons: firstly, a child's behavior varies from one situation to another, so that it is helpful to have information about the child's behavior in several contexts; secondly, parental accounts of the child's behavior are likely to be distorted in many cases, as it is the parents who are disturbed rather than the child. Consequently, an important part of assessment is to obtain reports from other professionals involved with the family such as schools, health visitors or general practitioners. Another common practice is the use of questionnaires to supplement information provided by referrers and other more formal reports. Several questionnaires[16,26] have been devised to assess different age ranges and have satisfactory psychometric properties. Until recently, the most extensively used questionnaires for school-age children in the UK have been the Rutter parents' and teachers' scales, also known as Rutter A and Rutter B, respectively. These scales have established reliability and validity as well as classifying children into neurotic or emotional, conduct or antisocial and mixed categories. Over the past 5 years, the Strengths and Difficulties Questionnaire (SDQ)[27] has become more popular, as it assesses pro-social behavior as well as disturbed behavior.

DISORDERS IN PRESCHOOL CHILDREN

Except for rare but severe disorders such as childhood autism, psychiatric disorders in this age group are mostly deviations or delays from normality rather than a psychiatric illness as such. Moreover, the child's behavior and development are so influenced by the immediate surroundings that it is often the environment rather than the child that is responsible for the problems.

ETIOLOGY

Four types of factors contribute to problems in varying degrees in the individual case: temperamental factors, physical illness or handicap, family psychopathology and social disadvantage. The New York

Longitudinal Study[28] showed clearly that children with certain types of temperamental characteristics, the so-called 'difficult child' and the 'slow to warm up child' profiles, were more likely to develop problems. Again, physical illness or disability can reduce activity, directly or indirectly affect developmental progress and increase parental anxiety, all of which potentate the likelihood of behavioral disturbance. Parental psychiatric illness, marital disharmony and poor parenting skills are examples when disturbance in the parents adversely affects the child's behavior. Several authors[16,29] have shown high rates of depression among mothers with pre-school children. Social disadvantage such as poor housing or inadequate recreational facilities increases the risk of disturbance among pre-school children.[16]

FREQUENCY OF PROBLEMS

Table 34.2 shows the prevalence of common problems among 3- and 4-year-olds in the general population.[30]

Problems are mainly about eating, sleeping and elimination, with a marked decrease in wetting and soiling over the 1-year period. Affective symptoms such as unhappiness and relationship problems are much less common, but probably more significant. Community studies[16] indicate that 20% of children are regarded by their mothers as having problems, with 7% rated as severe.

COMMON PROBLEMS

This section discusses those problems that are particularly frequent among the pre-school child, whilst others such as soiling, which occur in older children as well are discussed later in the chapter.

Temper tantrums

They usually arise when the child is thwarted, angry or has hurt himself. They can occur in isolation or as part of a wider problem. They comprise a variety of behaviors, including screaming, crying, often with collapse onto the floor and banging of feet. A child can be aggressive towards other people around him, but the child rarely injures himself. Most tantrums 'burn themselves out', so that specific intervention is not necessary. If it is, then the following points are useful: if necessary, restrain from behind by folding arms around child's body; minimize any additional attention to the child; and only respond and praise when behavior is back to normal.

Feeding problems

They range in severity from a minor problem such as the finicky child to the severe disabling problem of non-organic failure to thrive. Minor problems will usually respond to patient and attentive listening to the

parents' concerns, counseling and specific advice. Severe non-organic failure to thrive (prevalence 2%) is a complex problem requiring comprehensive assessment and a large amount of time and resources to remedy.[31] Several factors are responsible in most cases including a poor mother–child relationship, often in the context of more widespread emotional and social deprivation, and factors in the child, including temperamental factors and an aversion to feeding. *Pica*, the ingestion of inedible material such as dirt or rubbish, is a normal transitory phenomenon during the toddler period. Persistent ingestion is found amongst mentally retarded, psychotic or socially deprived children. Lead poisoning, though always mentioned, is a possible but uncommon danger from pica.

Sleep problems (sleep problems in older children are discussed in the miscellaneous disorders section)

These are common with up to 20% of 2-year-olds, waking at least five times per week.[16,32] The two most frequent problems are reluctance to settle at night and persistent waking up during the night. Several factors contribute to the problem including adverse temperamental characteristics in the child, perinatal problems and maternal anxiety. It is also important to distinguish between those factors responsible for the onset of the problem and those for maintaining the problem. Medication such as trimeprazine and promethazine are frequently prescribed, but side-effects often outweigh any advantages. The only real indication is to provide a brief respite for the parents as well as ensuring that the child has an uninterrupted night's sleep. The most successful management is a behavioral strategy (see Treatment section). Richman & Landsdown[30] provide a useful summary of these techniques. More recently, there have been case reports[33] suggesting the successful use of melatonin to treat sleep disorders among visually and neurologically impaired children and substantial randomized controlled trials are currently underway.

PSYCHIATRIC ASPECTS OF CHILD ABUSE[34]

Originally this was restricted to the 'battered baby syndrome', but it has now been extended to include physical abuse, sexual abuse, emotional abuse and neglect. This section will concentrate on the psychiatric aspects in childhood as other sections discuss diagnostic (see Ch. 6) and adolescent issues (see later in the chapter). It is also important to remember that the different aspects of child abuse are frequently present in the same child and family and that many comments about the detection, management and treatment apply equally to all aspects of child abuse.

PHYSICAL ABUSE

Diagnostic awareness and suspicion are the key elements in the detection and recognition of physical abuse. The following list summarizes the common characteristics of abused children and their families, although the most important factor to recognize is that child abuse can occur in any family irrespective of social class, ethnic group or religious affiliation.

Common characteristics of abused children and their families

Risk characteristics of the abused child:

1. product of unwanted pregnancy;
2. unwanted child in the family;
3. low birth weight;
4. separation from mother in neonatal period;
5. mental or physical disability;
6. habitually restless, sleeplessness or incessantly crying;
7. physically unattractive.

Risk characteristics of the parent(s):

1. single parent;
2. young;
3. abused themselves as a child;

Table 34.2 Problem behaviors in 3- and 4-year-olds[30]

Behavior	3-year-olds (%)	4-year-olds (%)
Poor appetite	19	20
Faddy eater	15	24
Difficulty settling at night	16	15
Waking at night	14	12
Overactive and restless	17	13
Poor concentration	9	6
Difficult to control	11	10
Temper	5	6
Unhappy mood	4	7
Worries	4	1
Fears	10	12
Poor relationships with siblings	10	15
Poor relationships with peers	4	6
Regular day wetting	26	8
Regular night wetting	33	19
Regular soiling	16	3

4. low self-esteem;
5. unrealistic expectations of the child and his development;
6. inconsistent or punishment-orientated discipline.

Risk characteristics of social circumstances:

1. low income or unemployment;
2. social isolation;
3. current stress such as housing crisis, domestic friction, exhaustion or ill-health;
4. large family.

Management

Most cases of child abuse do not require the involvement of a child psychiatrist, as the principal concerns are the protection of the child, practical support for the family and help with parenting skills. The child psychiatrist can make a useful contribution in two ways: firstly, to act as an outside consultant on various aspects of management and treatment to the other professionals and agencies working with the family; and secondly to provide individual and or family therapy for the child, the parents or the family depending upon the assessment.

In addition to the immediate effects, child abuse may have medium term and long term sequelae. Many abused children continue to be exposed to emotional abuse and neglect throughout their childhood, so that they often show symptoms of disturbance such as unhappiness, wariness, untrusting, low self-esteem and poor peer relationships. This childhood experience in turn predisposes abused children to become abusing parents when adults.

SEXUAL ABUSE

This has become a major public and pediatric concern over the past decade. Several factors have contributed to the increased concern: it is a common event affecting 12–17% of females and 5–8% males according to several epidemiological surveys.[35] It is traumatic for the child, giving rise to major distress at the time of its occurrence, but equally importantly acts as a predisposing factor for psychiatric disorder later on in life. Indeed, a history of sexual abuse in childhood is a very common finding among women referred to adult psychiatric services.

Complex psychological processes contribute to the development of psychopathology, as attitudes to sexuality are shaped in a dysfunctional manner by the abuse. Also, the individual has a sense of betrayal, powerlessness and stigmatization leading to shame, guilt and low self-esteem. One consequence of this process is that sexual abuse can present in a wide variety of ways from the physical, e.g. vaginal discharge to the psychological such as anxiety, aggression or encopresis. It is therefore crucial to be aware that unexplained or atypical symptoms may be the presenting complaint for a child with a current or past history of sexual abuse.

The child psychiatry team has a more clearly defined role in the management of sexual abuse, as interviewing skills, psychotherapeutic expertise and the use of specialist equipment (anatomically accurate dolls) are often necessary at the detection and also during the treatment stage of management. Detailed accounts of this work, including the use of the anatomical dolls, are well described in the several books (the Great Ormond Street child sex abuse team[36]) and the APSAC Handbook.[34]

EMOTIONAL ABUSE

This term has been introduced to describe the severe impairment of social and emotional development resulting from repeated and persistent criticism, lack of affection, rejection, verbal abuse and other similar behavior by the parent(s) to the child. Affected children display a variety of symptoms: low self-esteem; limited capacity for enjoyment; severe aggression; and impulsive behavior.

NEGLECT

This varies markedly, ranging from relative inadequacy and incompetence in providing basic shelter, love and security for the child, to a severe failure in the provision of basic essentials, often combined with emotional and social deprivation.

FACTITIOUS OR INDUCED ILLNESS[37]

This remarkable variant of physical abuse (previously called Munchausen syndrome by proxy) often occurs against the same background of parental psychopathology and social disadvantage as other forms of abuse. The role of the child psychiatrist is usually confined in most cases to offering counseling for the parents and/or family therapy when indicated.

PERVASIVE DEVELOPMENTAL DISORDERS[38,39]

Historically, these disorders were classified under childhood psychoses, as they are severe and disabling with clear-cut abnormalities. However, autistic children do not experience hallucinations or delusions, key features of a psychotic disorder, and moreover have had the abnormalities from early infancy. For these reasons, ICD-10 and DSM-IV have separated out childhood autism and related conditions from other psychotic conditions in childhood into a new diagnostic category called pervasive developmental disorders. In clinical practice, most people recognize that autistic disorders comprise a spectrum of disabilities (autistic spectrum disorders) with childhood autism at the severe end and Asperger syndrome at the mild end. Rett syndrome and disintegrative disorder are also included in the pervasive developmental disorders category.

CHILDHOOD AUTISM

Kanner's[40] original description of 11 children with 'an extreme autistic aloneness' has not been improved upon with its astute observation of 'inability to relate in an ordinary way to people and to situations' and 'an anxiously obsessive desire for the maintenance of sameness'. Subsequently, opinions have fluctuated about the diagnosis, etiology and treatment. Most authorities now agree that three features are essential to the diagnosis: general and profound failure to develop social relationships; language retardation; and ritualistic and compulsive behavior. Additionally, these abnormalities should be manifest before 30 months.

Prevalence

Previous epidemiological studies in childhood have found prevalence rates of four per 10 000 increasing to 20/10 000 when individuals with severe mental retardation and some autistic features are included. Boys are three times more affected than girls. However, a more recent study[41] reported a rate of 16 per 10 000 for autistic disorder and 64 per 10 000 for other pervasive developmental disorders. It remains to be seen whether these new findings are replicated elsewhere.

Clinical features
Impaired social relationships
Parental recollections of infancy often reveal that as an infant the child was slow to smile, unresponsive and passive with a dislike of physical contact and affection. Contemporary social deficits include the failure to use eye-to-eye gaze and facial expression for social interaction, rarely seeking others for comfort or affection, rarely initiating interaction with others, a lack of empathy (the ability to understand how others feel and think) and of cooperative play. The children are aloof and indifferent to people.

Language abnormalities
Language acquisition is delayed and deviant with many autistic children never developing language (approximately 50%). When present, language abnormalities are many and varied, including immediate and delayed echolalia (repetition of spoken word(s) or phrase(s)), poor comprehension and use of gesture, pronominal reversal (the use of the third person when 'I' is meant) and abnormalities in intonation, rhythm and pitch.

Ritualistic and compulsive behavior

Common abnormalities are rigid and restricted patterns of play, intense attachments to unusual objects such as stones, unusual preoccupations and interests (timetables, bus routes) to the exclusion of other pursuits and a marked resistance to any change in the environment or daily routine. Tantrums and explosive outbursts often occur when any change is attempted.

Other features

Autistic children often exhibit a variety of stereotypies including rocking, finger twirling, spinning and tiptoe walking. They are often overactive with a short attention span. Of autistic children 70% are in the retarded range of intelligence with only 5% having an IQ above 100. Occasionally, some have remarkable abilities in isolated areas, for instance computation, music or rote memory. About 20% will develop epilepsy during adolescence, though not usually severe.

Association with other conditions

Autistic behavior occurs in some patients with a diverse group of conditions including the fragile X syndrome, congenital rubella, phenylketonuria, tuberous sclerosis, neurolipoidoses and infantile spasms.[43] More recently, Rett syndrome, with its marked autistic features, has been described.[44]

Etiology

Most people favor an organic basis as neurological abnormalities are common, the association with epilepsy and various neurological syndromes, the increased rate of perinatal complications and a greater concordance rate among monozygotic compared with dizygotic twins.[43,45] Application of new investigative techniques such as CAT scan, MRI and positron emission tomography are beginning to reveal abnormalities in the frontal lobe region, with distinctive deficits on tests of executive function.[46] The relationship between autism and the fragile X syndrome is also unclear, as the different rates in the various studies may be a reflection of the degree of mental handicap rather than of any etiological significance. A most interesting psychological perspective on the autistic deficit is provided by the work of Baron-Cohen[47] and Hobson.[48] On the basis of sophisticated cognitive experiments with autistic children, they propose that the primary deficit in autism is a lack of empathy, namely an inability to perceive and interpret emotional cues in social situations.

Treatment

The explanation of the diagnosis is a vital first step in helping parents to accept the presence of handicap with the consequent lessening of the parental guilt about etiology. Counseling and advice are likely to be necessary throughout childhood. Lord & Rutter[43] suggested that treatment aims should have four components: (1) the promotion of normal development, (2) the reduction of rigidity and stereotypies, (3) the removal of maladaptive behavior, and (4) the alleviation of family stress. Behavioral methods, including operant conditioning and shaping (see behavioral treatment section), are the most likely ways to achieve some success with the first three aims, whilst counseling is important for the fourth. Special schooling, where the child's special social and educational needs are recognized, is very beneficial, sometimes on a residential basis. Drugs do not have an important part in management.

Outcome

Many autistic individuals are unable to live independently with only 15% looking after and supporting themselves as adults. Many were placed previously in institutions for the mentally handicapped, though government policy now favors community care. Autistic children with an IQ of at least 70, receiving proper education and coming from middle-class families do better than those in other groups. In most individuals there is some improvement in social relationships, though many are still handicapped. Parents often find it helpful to join a voluntary society such as the National Society for Autistic Children.

OTHER PERVASIVE DEVELOPMENTAL DISORDERS

Asperger syndrome/schizoid personality

This condition, originally described by Asperger,[49] shows some similarities to childhood autism in that there is an impairment of social relationships with a lack of reciprocal social interaction and a restricted repertoire of interests and activities. However, the children differ diagnostically from those with childhood autism in two important respects: there is no general intellectual retardation, and the language development is normal. Other characteristics include male preponderance and poor motor coordination with marked clumsiness. The condition is now regarded as one of the autistic spectrum disorders[39] with the impairment in social relationships persisting into adult life.

The term 'schizoid' personality of childhood was coined by Wolff & Chick[50] to describe a small number of children with unusual but distinctive personality characteristics, similar in some ways to children with Asperger syndrome. These 'schizoid' children were described as aloof, distant and lacking in empathy. Other features include: obstinate and aggressive outbursts when under pressure to conform, often at school; undue rigidity; sensitivity to criticism; and unusual interests to the exclusion of everything else. More recently, Wolff[51] has argued from follow-up studies of these children that they form a separate diagnostic category, the schizoid personality of childhood, similar to but distinct from childhood autism and Asperger syndrome. As adults, Wolff[51] found that they showed features of the schizotypal disorder.

Rett syndrome

In 1966 Rett described 22 mentally handicapped children, all girls, who had a history of regression in development and displayed strikingly repetitive movements of the hands. He thought that the children were autistic with progressive spasticity, and proposed that diffuse cerebral atrophy was the underlying cause. A more recent review[44] has indicated this syndrome is more common than previously thought with a prevalence rate of 1 per 15 000 girls.

Clinical features

The condition, which has only been described in girls, shows a characteristic clinical picture: a period of normal development up to around 18 months followed by a rapid decline in developmental progress and the rapid deterioration of higher brain functions.

Over the following 18 months, there is evidence of severe dementia, a loss of purposeful hand movements, jerky ataxia and acquired microcephaly. After this rapid decline, the condition may stabilize with no further progression for some time. Subsequently, more neurological abnormalities appear including spastic paraplegia and epilepsy.

Etiology

Rett originally believed that high levels of ammonia were responsible for the condition, though subsequent studies have not confirmed this observation. The most commonly proposed explanation is that it is due to a dominant mutation on one X chromosome, and that the condition is nonviable in the male. Genetic studies indicate that the disorder is associated with the MECP2 gene at Xq28.

Prognosis

The majority of children are left profoundly retarded with severe neurological impairments. Many succumb to intermittent infections or to the underlying neuropathological disorder.

Disintegrative disorder

Clinical features[43,52]

This term refers to a group of conditions characterized by normal development until around 4 years of age followed by profound regression and behavioral disintegration, loss of language and other skills, impairment of social relationships and the development of stereotypies. It can follow on from a minor illness or from more definite neurological disease such as measles encephalitis. The prognosis is poor due to the underlying degenerative pathology in many cases. Most individuals are left with severe learning disability.

Other related conditions

Many children with learning disabilities show some autistic features. In clinical practice, it is often difficult to know whether they fulfil the criteria for pervasive developmental disorder in addition to that for intellectual retardation. It is clear that there is a wide diversity in the severity of these 'autistic features', so that it is often arbitrary whether the label 'childhood autism' is applied to these children. Many of them also show features of hyperactivity and aggression. For these reasons, ICD-10 has made two additional categories: (1) overactive disorder associated with mental retardation and stereotyped movements and (2) pervasive developmental disorder unspecified.

EMOTIONAL DISORDERS

The primary abnormality is a subjective sense of distress due to anxiety that can be expressed overtly as in anxiety disorders or covertly as in somatization or conversion disorders. This group of disorders is similar in many respects to neurotic disorders in adults. They are further divided into the following categories: anxiety and phobic states; obsessional disorders; conversion disorders, dissociative states and somatization disorders; and reaction to severe stress and adjustment disorders. Many children often show a mixed pattern of symptoms, so that a clear-cut distinction into a single category is not possible. The DOH 2000 study[15] found a prevalence rate of 4.0% with an equal gender prevalence. Prognosis is generally favorable as many problems arise from an acute stress, so that the problems should resolve once the stressful effects lessen.

ANXIETY STATES
Clinical features

This is the commonest type of emotional disorder. Anxiety has physical and psychological components, with the former referring to palpitations and dry mouth, while the latter to the subjective sense of fear and apprehension. Somatic symptoms, particularly abdominal pain, are common. Again, many symptoms represent the persistence or exaggeration of normal developmental fears, ranging in severity from an acute panic attack to a chronic anxiety state over several months. Predisposing factors include temperamental characteristics, overinvolved and over-concerned parents and the 'special child syndrome'. The latter refers to children who are treated differently by their parents. This may arise in several circumstances, for instance the child is much wanted and previous ill health during pregnancy or infancy has resulted in an 'anxious' attachment between the child and parents. In turn, 'anxious' attachment may lead the parents to inadvertently reinforce normal fears and anxieties.

Treatment

Several approaches, including individual, behavioral and family therapy, are used, often in combination depending upon the assessment and formulation. The newer serotonin re-uptake inhibitors (SRIs) such as buspirone have been shown to be effective in clinical trials, and are preferable to benzodiazepines.

PHOBIC STATES
Clinical features

Phobias are common and normal among children. For instance, toddlers are fearful of strangers, whereas adolescents are anxious about their appearance or weight. Pathological fears often arise from ordinary fears that are exacerbated by parental and/or social reinforcement. A phobia is defined as 'a fear of specific object or situation', for instance dogs or heights. Its characteristics are that it is out of proportion to the situation, is irrational, is beyond voluntary control and leads to avoidance of the feared situation. This avoidance behaviour is the main reason the fear is maladaptive as it leads to increasing restriction and limitation of the child's activities.

Treatment

A behavioural approach using graded exposure to the feared situation is the most commonly used treatment. The rationale for this approach is that continued exposure to the feared stimulus reduces the anxiety associated with the stimulus, thereby decreasing avoidance behaviour. The success of this method often depends on the ability of the therapist to devise a treatment program that combines gradual exposure without inducing too much anxiety. Occasionally, anxiolytic drugs are used in conjunction with this behavioral approach.

SCHOOL REFUSAL[53]

This term, also known as school phobia, refers to the child's irrational rear about school attendance. It is also known as the 'masquerade syndrome' as it can present in a variety of disguises, including abdominal pain, headaches or a viral infection. The child is reluctant to leave home in the morning to attend school, in contrast to the truant who leaves home but not arrive at school. It occurs most commonly at the commencement of schooling, change of school, or the beginning of secondary school.

Most cases can be understood in terms of the following three mechanisms, often in combination: firstly, separation anxiety, whereby the child and/or the parent are fearful of separation, of which school is an example; secondly, a specific phobia about some aspect of school such as traveling to school, mixing with other children, or some part of the school routine, for instance some subjects, gym, or assembly; and thirdly, an indication of a more general psychiatric disturbance such as depression or low self-esteem. The latter is more frequent among adolescents. Typically, most school refusers have good academic attainments and are conformist at school, but oppositional at home. School refusal can present acutely or insidiously, often becoming a chronic problem in adolescence.

Treatment

The initial essential step is to recognize the condition itself, namely to avoid unnecessary and extensive investigations for minor somatic symptoms or to advise prolonged convalescence following a minor illness. For the acute case, early return to school with firm support for the parents and liaison with the school is the most successful approach. For the more intractable cases, extensive work with the child and parents, along with a graded return to school is advisable. A specific behavioral program for the phobic aspects may be necessary as well as the use of anxiolytic drugs in some instances. The chronic problem often requires a concerted approach, sometimes involving a period of assessment and treatment at a child psychiatric day or inpatient unit. Many clinicians use family therapy to tackle the major relationship problems that exist in some cases.

Outcome

Two thirds usually return to school regularly, whilst the remainder, usually adolescents from disturbed families, only achieve erratic attendance at school at best. Follow-up studies have found that approximately one third continue with neurotic symptoms and social impairment into adult life.

OBSESSIVE–COMPULSIVE DISORDERS[54] (Fig. 34.2)
Definition

An obsession is a recurrent, intrusive thought that the individual recognizes is irrational but cannot ignore. A compulsion or ritual is the behavior(s) accompanying these ideas, the aim of which is to reduce the associated anxiety.

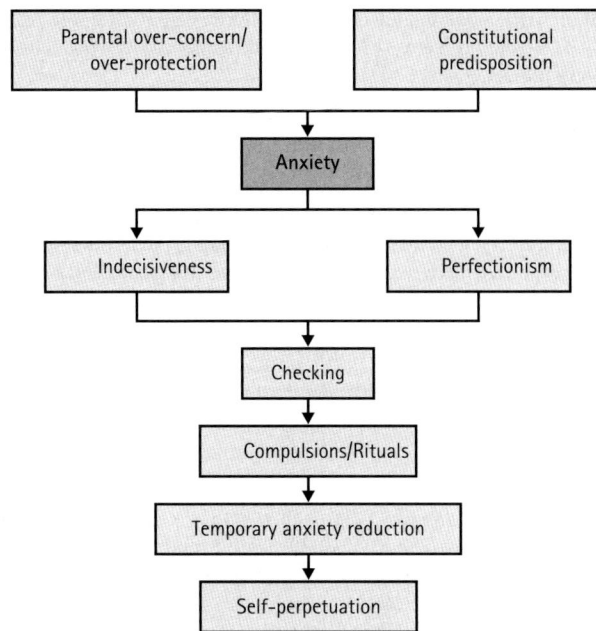

Fig. 34.2 Development of obsessional systems.

Clinical features

Most children display obsessional symptoms to a minor degree at some time, for instance avoiding cracks on paving stones or walking under ladders. They have no significance. It is when the behavior interferes with ordinary activities that it amounts to a disorder. Common obsessional rituals are hand washing and dressing. Obsessional thoughts often have a foreboding quality, for instance that 'something could happen' to a parent or sibling, that he might die, or get run over. The rituals are maintained, though maladaptive, because they produce a temporary reduction in anxiety. Commonly, the child involves other members of the family in the performance of rituals, so that the child assumes a controlling role within the family. The disorder is rare (community prevalence 0.3%) but commoner among older children and adolescents with an acute or gradual onset. In addition to anxiety symptoms, many children have depressive features.

Treatment

Behavioral methods, particularly response prevention, are successful in eliminating the obsessive–compulsive behavior. Response prevention consists of training the child to become aware of the cues that trigger the symptom and then using distraction techniques to make the performance of the ritual impossible. Recent clinical trials[54] have shown that SRIs such as paroxetine or sertraline are effective in their own right, but more importantly are very valuable as part of a combined medication – behavioral treatment package. Involvement of other members of the family, whether specifically in family therapy or to assist the child in the elimination of rituals, is necessary. Some cases require inpatient admission.

Outcome

Two thirds do well and the remainder continue to have problems, usually in a fluctuating fashion.

CONVERSION DISORDERS AND DISSOCIATIVE STATES

Clinical features

These are rare in childhood. Conversion disorder is the development of physical symptoms, usually of the special senses or limbs, without any pathological basis in the presence of identifiable stress and/or affective disturbance. The emotional conflict is said to be 'converted' into physical symptoms, which is less threatening to the individual than the under-

lying psychological conflict. A dissociative state is the restriction or narrowing of consciousness due to psychological causes, for example amnesic or fugue states. It is, however, extremely dangerous to diagnose the condition solely by the exclusion of organic disease, as follow-up studies have found that a minority subsequently develop definite organic illness. There should always be positive psychological reasons to explain the development of the symptoms. Common reasons include major life events or stresses for the child, a similar illness among other family members/peers or an underlying depressive disorder.

Minor degrees of these disorders are extremely common and frequently occur as a transitory phenomenon during the course of many illnesses. The more general term 'abnormal illness behavior', similar to the physician's phrase 'functional overlay', has been coined to describe the situation when the individual persists with or exaggerates symptoms following on from an illness.

Treatment

Successful treatment depends upon the recognition that the symptoms are 'real' for the child. Psychic pain is just as distressing as physical pain. Anger and confrontation are unhelpful. A firm sympathetic approach with little attention to the symptom per se as well as avoiding rewarding the symptom is the best strategy. Allow the child to give up the symptoms with good grace, often providing the child with some face-saving reason for improvement. Identify and treat any affective disturbance. The outcome is good for the individual episode, though other psychological problems may persist.

SOMATOFORM DISORDERS[55] (see adolescent section for chronic fatigue syndrome)

Clinical features and management

Many children complain of somatic symptoms that do not have a pathological basis. Common symptoms are abdominal pain, headaches and limb pains with community prevalence rates of approximately 10%. This condition is usually managed by general practitioners, though it sometimes results in a referral for a specialist opinion. Management involves the minimum necessary investigation to exclude any pathology, the identification of any stressful circumstances and a sensitive explanation of the basis for the symptoms. The prevention of restrictions and the active encouragement of normal activities are essential.

When the somatic symptoms are persistent, chronic and involve several systems of the body, ICD and DSM use the term *somatization disorder*. Whilst it is doubtful whether this disorder occurs in childhood, there is no doubt that persistent unexplained physical complaints are a common reason for children being taken to see the doctor. In many cases, there is clear evidence of underlying anxiety or recent stressful events.

REACTION TO SEVERE STRESS AND ADJUSTMENT DISORDERS

This group of disorders arises in response to an exceptionally stressful event or to a significantly adverse life change. The clinical features of the different syndromes vary considerably with a preponderance of affective symptoms in most cases.

Adjustment disorder

Definition

This is a maladaptive response occurring within 3 months of an identifiable psychosocial stressor. The maladaptive response must be of sufficient severity to impair daily activities such as schooling, hamper social relationships and be greater than expected given the nature of the stressor. Finally, the reaction must not last longer than 6 months.

Clinical features

By definition, the symptoms vary with ICD and DSM recognizing more than six categories. Clinical practice shows that anxiety and depressive symptoms, often combined, are the most frequent categories. Common stressors include parental divorce, unemployment, family illness or family move.

Predisposing factors

Age has different effects depending on the type of stressor. For instance, separation is more upsetting for a younger child than for an adolescent, whereas a loss of or change in a heterosexual relationship is far more important for an adolescent than for a younger child. Boys are also more vulnerable to the adverse effects of stress than girls. Temperamental characteristics such as 'difficult' or 'slow to warm up' style probably influence susceptibility as well. Again, the child's previous experience and repertoire of coping skills affect the response to the current stressor. For instance, if the child has successfully coped with adversity in the past, resilience and ability to withstand the present situation are enhanced. Finally, the family, particularly the parents, can magnify or minimize the impact of a stressor, dependent on their resourcefulness and coping style.

Outcome

By definition, the disorder can only last for 6 months, after which time the diagnostic category must change. The more important clinical consideration is not the change in diagnostic category, but the adverse effect that chronic or repeated stresses can have on the child's long term adjustment.

Post-traumatic stress disorder (PTSD)[56]

The 'epidemic' of disasters that some British children have been involved with over the past 20 years (the capsize of the Herald of Free Enterprise, the sinking of the cruise ship Jupiter, the PanAm Lockerbie air crash and the crushing disaster at the Hillsborough football stadium) have made clinicians acutely aware of this syndrome. Clinicians are now familiar with the wide symptomatology often found, and have also become involved in treatment programs to reduce the distress both in the immediate aftermath and also in the long term.

Definition

This disorder arises following exposure to a stressful event of an exceptionally threatening or catastrophic nature that would cause pervasive distress in almost anyone. The events include accidents or disasters as well as more personal traumas such as witnessing a murder, a rape or torture. In clinical practice, children who have been sexually abused commonly present with symptoms falling within the diagnostic category of PTSD.

Clinical features

These include 'flashbacks' (the repeated re-enactment of the event with intrusive memories, dreams or nightmares); a sense of detachment, 'numbness' and emotional blunting; irritability, poor concentration and memory problems. Following disasters, many survivors often experience an increased awareness of danger, a foreshortened view of the future ('only plan for today'), a feeling of 'survivor' guilt (self-reproach about own survival, whilst companions died) and acute panic reactions.

Yule[56] indicates that 30–50% of children show significant psychological morbidity following disasters with symptoms persisting for several months.

Individual vulnerability factors

Important modifying factors are probably age, previous experiences, current life situation and the availability of help. Though cognitive immaturity may protect the child from appreciating the implications of a disaster, it may also be a disadvantage, as the child may not be given the opportunity to talk about the event. The child's previous experience of stressful events and their outcome, successful or otherwise, are likely to influence the response to the disaster.

Similarly, co-existing adverse circumstances such as family disharmony or school problems reduce the child's capacity to cope with the new situation.

Management

Though most research is anecdotal rather than systematic, the available evidence[56] suggests that post-disaster 'debriefing' sessions on an individual or group basis are helpful. Specific counseling sessions to help a child deal with phobic, anxiety or depressive symptoms are frequently necessary as well. Cognitive/behavioral approaches are particularly suitable for this pattern of symptoms.

MOOD DISORDERS (See adolescent section)

CONDUCT DISORDER

Clinical features

This is usually defined as persistent antisocial or socially disapproved of behavior that often involves damage to property and is unresponsive to normal sanctions. The IOW study[14] found a prevalence rate of 4% when the mixed disorder category was included as well, with a marked male predominance (at least 3:1). There is no independent criterion for deviancy as social and cultural values determine the seriousness or otherwise attached to antisocial behavior. Consequently, most clinicians would include the criterion of impairment, namely an adverse effect on the child's daily life or development, before applying the diagnostic label of 'conduct disorder'.

Common symptoms include temper tantrums, oppositional behavior, overactivity, irritability, aggression, stealing, lying, truancy, bullying and wandering away from home/school. Delinquency (a legal term for someone committing an offence against the law) is a frequent feature among older children and adolescents. Stealing, vandalism, arson and fire setting are common forms of delinquency (male:female 10:1).

Traditionally, a distinction has been made between socialized and unsocialized behavior. The former describes behavior that is in accord with peer group values, but contrary to those of society, for instance antisocial gang behavior such as stealing and vandalism. Unsocialized antisocial behavior implies more disturbed behavior as it is often done alone against a background of parental rejection or neglect and poor peer relationships. Learning difficulties, especially specific reading retardation, occur more commonly among children with conduct disorders. This is a further reason why schooling is unpopular and a source of discouragement for these children. Additionally, many children with conduct disorder have affective symptoms such as anxiety or unhappiness, as well as low self-esteem and poor peer relationships. When these symptoms are prominent, it is often appropriate to classify the disorder as mixed, implying both emotional and behavioral symptomatology.

Etiology

Four factors – the family, the peer group, the neighborhood and constitutional – make some contribution in most cases, but the family is usually the most important. Families of children with conduct disorder are characterized by having a lack of affection and rejection, marital disharmony, inconsistent and ineffective discipline, parental violence and aggression. The families are often of large size, which aggravates the problems of supervision and care. Constitutional factors present in some cases include low intelligence and learning difficulties, along with adverse temperamental features such as overactivity and impulsiveness. Oppositional peer group values are an important feature in older children and adolescents. Many children with conduct disorder live in areas of urban deprivation with poor schooling. The intractable and chronic nature of these problems is a major reason for the continuation of conduct disorder into adolescence and adult life.

Treatment

Help for the family, either by counseling for the parents or by family therapy, is often used. More recently, specific intervention programs aimed at promoting positive parenting have been developed with good outcomes in the short term at least.[57] Educational support through remedial teaching or the provision of special education can be important in some cases. For many families however, the role of psychiatric services is limited, with practical support with rehousing in order to alleviate social disadvantage the most important contribution.

Prognosis

Continuity into adult life is common, with over 50% having problems as adults. Bad prognostic features are many and varied symptoms, problems at home and in the community, and anti-authority and aggressive attitudes.

HYPERACTIVITY AND ATTENTION DEFICIT SYNDROMES[39,58]

Clinical features

Considerable controversy surrounds the diagnostic terms hyperkinetic disorder (HKD), ADHD and ADD. HKD is the category used by ICD-10, which is the diagnostic system mainly used in the UK. This emphasizes the importance of pervasive overactivity (i.e. present in all situations) as a diagnostic feature. By contrast, North American psychiatrists use DSM-IV, which has the diagnostic category of ADHD. The latter stresses inattentiveness as a key symptom rather than overactivity. The different diagnostic practices probably explain the wide variation in prevalence rates (1–10%) found in epidemiological studies. Despite the difference in terminology, the two systems agree upon the same three core features: *overactivity*, *impulsivity* and *inattentiveness*.

Current UK practice has changed radically over the past 10 years, so that most UK psychiatrists use the term ADHD rather than HKD. One consequence of this change has been the dramatic increase in the prescription of methylphenidate with the annual rate in England rising from 220 000 in 1998 to 418 000 in 2004.[59]

Another controversy concerns the existence of co-morbidity among children with ADHD symptoms, which in turn is linked to the conceptual argument about whether disorders are categorical or dimensional. Traditional UK clinical practice prefers a single as opposed to several concurrent diagnoses. For instance, if a child was overactive, they would be classified as having HKD or conduct disorder, but not both. By contrast, North American practice allows, or even encourages, more than one diagnosis, namely the overactive child could have ADHD and conduct disorder. Unfortunately, current evidence is unable to provide a definite answer about the best approach. This difference in diagnostic approach is another reason for the divergent prevalence rates in epidemiological studies.

In conclusion, it is probably best to regard overactivity as a symptom rather than a diagnostic term that can occur in many clinical situations: a symptom of ADHD, HKD or ADD; a feature of many children with conduct disorder; a reflection of developmental delay on its own or in association with general intellectual retardation; one extreme of normal temperamental variation; an uncommon response to high anxiety or tension; a symptom of childhood autism; and rarely, as a reaction to some drugs, for example barbiturates or benzodiazepines.

Treatment of attention deficit hyperactivity disorder

The recent MTA Study[60] and the NICE Report[59] have provided the clearest evidence and guidance, respectively, about the most effective treatment package. Most people would advocate a multi-modal approach involving drug treatment, psycho-educational, parenting skills program and individual or group work with the child. The MTA Study showed that 80% of children improved significantly on methylphenidate with improvement persisting over the 14-month trial period. There appeared little convincing evidence that a combined approach involving drug and behavioral treatments significantly improved the outcome, but it must be remembered that the MTA study was carried out in the USA, where diagnostic practices are different.

Methylphenidate (up to 60 mg/d in divided doses) is the commonest prescribed drug in the UK, whereas dexamphetamine (up to 30 mg/d) is more popular in the USA and Australasia. Both drugs are equally effective with a similar side-effect profile, but dexamphetamine has a longer time course of effect. Stimulant drugs seem to work through an increase in dopamine levels in the frontal lobes. The common side-effects of both drugs are loss of appetite and night-time insomnia, with abdominal pain, headache, tearfulness and tics less common. It is debatable whether stimulants have any long term effect on growth or the exacerbation of tics, but careful monitoring is advisable. The last 5 years have seen important advances in the range of medications available with the licensing of extended-release preparations of methylphenidate such as Concerta XL or Equasym XL and also the availability of a once-a-day noradrenergic compound, atomoxetine. Comparative trials with these new preparations are currently underway in the UK.

Tricyclic antidepressants such as imipramine or nortriptyline are also an effective alternative treatment, and are used when the child is unresponsive to stimulants, side-effects are disabling or there is a depressive component to the child's symptoms. There are also open-label studies with clonidine, particularly for aggressive symptoms, but there have been case reports of sudden death due to cardiac arrhythmias, so that an ECG prior to commencement of treatment is essential. Pemoline, which has the considerable advantage as a once-daily dosage, has now been withdrawn in the UK on account of fears about hepatic toxicity.

Behavioral techniques, parental counseling and the alteration and manipulation of the child's environment, particularly at school, to reduce and minimize distraction are important components of most treatment programs. An alternative approach adopted by some clinicians has been the use of exclusion diets on the basis that the child is allergic to certain substances, commonly tartrazine. Evidence for the efficacy of these exclusion diets other than as a placebo response is unconvincing, though Egger et al,[61] using a sophisticated methodological design, showed that children with severe hyperactivity and mental retardation did respond. It is, however, unclear whether these results would apply to children of normal intelligence with less severe problems, who make up the majority of children with ADHD.

Outcome

Hyperactivity and attention deficits lessen considerably by adolescence, though other major problems such as learning difficulties and behavior problems persist. A substantial minority continue to have problems in adult life, mainly of an antisocial nature. There is also increasing evidence for the efficacy of methylphenidate in adults in whom the diagnosis of ADD had been missed in childhood or who have continued on treatment from childhood.[62,63]

DISORDERS OF ELIMINATION

ENURESIS

This term refers to the involuntary passage of urine in the absence of physical abnormality after the age of 5 years. It may be nocturnal and/or diurnal. Bed wetting continuously, though not usually every night, since birth is termed *primary enuresis*, whereas when there has been a 6-month period of dry beds at some stage, recurrence of bed wetting is termed *secondary* or *onset enuresis*. Diurnal enuresis is much less common than nocturnal, but more common among girls and among children who are psychiatrically disturbed. Depending upon definition, approximately 10% of 5-year-olds, 5% of 10-year-olds and 1% of 18-year-olds will have nocturnal enuresis. The majority of children with nocturnal enuresis are not psychiatrically ill, though a substantial minority, approximately 25%, have signs of psychiatric disturbance.

Etiology

A combination of individual factors such as positive family history (approximately 70%), low intelligence, psychiatric disturbance and small bladder capacity along with environmental factors such as recent stressful life events, large family size and social disadvantage are present in most cases.

Treatment

It is important to exclude any physical basis for the enuresis by history, examination and, if necessary, investigation of the renal tract. Assuming no physical pathology, the most important initial step is to minimize the handicap, namely to point out to the parents the very favorable natural outcome of the condition, and to re-label the child's enuresis as immaturity rather than laziness or wilfulness. A star chart, the accurate recording of enuresis plus positive reinforcement for dry nights, provides an accurate baseline as well as a successful treatment in its own right. An enuresis alarm is successful with older cooperative children. The success of this approach is probably because the child becomes more aware of the sensation of a full bladder along with the encouragement from parents for dry nights. The modern alarms are extremely compact and do not require a pad placed between the sheets, thereby increasing patient compliance considerably. It is useful to combine a buzzer with a star chart. Drugs such as desmopressin and imipramine are very effective at stopping enuresis, though their major limitation is that the enuresis returns when they are stopped. Most pediatricians believe it is wrong to prescribe potentially lethal drugs such as imipramine for a benign condition such as enuresis, so that desmopressin is the preferred drug treatment.

SOILING AND ENCOPRESIS

Most children are continent of feces and clean by their 4th birthday. Encopresis is usually defined as the inappropriate passage of formed feces, usually onto the underwear, in the absence of any physical pathology after 4 years of age. Soiling, the passage of semi-solid feces, is often used synonymously with encopresis. Symptoms vary widely in severity, ranging from slight staining of underwear to encopresis with the smearing of feces onto the walls. It is uncommon with a community prevalence among 8-year-olds of 1.8% for boys and of 0.7% for girls. Psychiatric disturbance is common among children with encopresis. Enuresis may also be present.

Clinical features

Figure 34.3 shows a convenient way to classify encopresis with a broad distinction between children who retain feces with eventual overflow incontinence and those who deposit feces inappropriately on a regular basis. Some children have never achieved continence, a situation called 'continuous' or 'primary encopresis', whilst others have had periods of cleanliness followed by relapse, the so-called 'discontinuous' or 'secondary encopresis'. Figure 34.3 also lists the common different patterns of interaction found among children with encopresis and their parents. For instance, children with retentive encopresis have often been subjected to coercive and obsessional toilet training practices, so that the encopresis is seen as a reaction, often of anger or aggression, towards this practice. Similarly, many children with continuous nonretentive encopresis come from disorganized, chaotic families where regular training and toileting are not the norm. Again, encopresis can arise in some children as a response to a stressful situation. Finally, encopresis can reflect poor parent–child relationship, often longstanding and usually associated with other aspects of psychiatric disturbance. The clinical picture is often, however, not as clear-cut, with the different elements each making some contribution. There may be a previous history of constipation and occasionally of anal fissure.

Treatment

A physical etiology such as Hirschsprung disease must be excluded before commencement of psychiatric treatment. The assessment must include an account of previous treatments and most importantly, the current attitude of the parents and the child to the problem. Treatment has two aims: the promotion of a normal bowel habit and the improvement of the parent–child relationship. Initially, a bowel washout and/

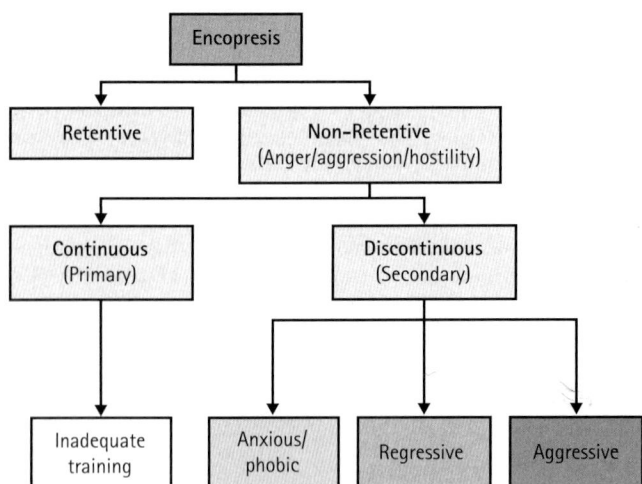

Fig. 34.3 Types of encopresis and their psychopathology. Three patterns are common in children: primary encopresis, retentive encopresis and secondary encopresis.

or microenemata may be necessary to clear out the bowel. Judicious use of bowel smooth muscle stimulants (Senokot), stool softeners (Dioctyl) and bulk agents (macrogol, lactulose) is helpful for the child with retention. Again, suppositories may be useful from time to time. This should also be combined with parent and child education about the dietary importance of fiber. The psychological component includes behavioral (star chart) and individual psychotherapy to gain the cooperation and trust of the child along with parental counseling or family therapy to modify attitudes and hostile interactions between the child and his parents.

Prognosis

It usually resolves by adolescence, though other problems may persist. Occasional case reports of persistence into adult life have been published.

MISCELLANEOUS DISORDERS

DEVELOPMENTAL DISORDERS

Language disorders (see also Ch. 23)

Children with language disorders are more vulnerable to disturbance, mainly because of the associated anxiety and embarrassment caused by the disorder. Specific language delay (5–6/1000) is twice as common in boys as in girls, with a strong association with large family size and lower social class. Richman et al[16] found that approximately 25% of 3-year-olds with specific language delay had behavioral problems.

Stuttering, an abnormality of speech rhythm consisting of hesitations and repetitions at the beginning of syllables and words is a normal, though transitory phenomenon, occurring at around 3–4 years of age. When it persists (approximately 3% of the general population), often due to inadvertent parental attention, it leads to anxiety and low self-esteem.

Selective mutism

This is not strictly a language disorder, as the main problem is the child's refusal to talk in certain situations, most commonly at school, rather than an inability to speak. Mild forms of the disorder are common but transitory, usually at the commencement of schooling, while the severe form has a prevalence rate of about 1 in 1000. Other features include a previous history of speech delay, excessively shy but stubborn temperament and parental overprotectiveness.

A combination of behavioral and family therapy techniques to promote communication and the use of speech is most commonly used, though some cases require inpatient assessment. Fluoxetine had been shown to be effective in an open trial of children with selective mutism and co-morbid anxiety disorder.[64] Prognosis is good for approximately 50%, with failure to improve by the age of 10 years a poor prognostic sign.

Reading difficulties

Though mainly of educational concern, the pediatrician or child psychiatrist may get involved because of the associated behavioral or emotional problems. The two main types are first, general reading backwardness, when the retardation is a reflection of generalized intellectual delay, and second, specific reading retardation when the attainment in reading is significantly behind the expected level after controlling for age and intelligence. The problem is 'significant' when the delay is at least 2 years. Dyslexia is a concept similar to specific reading retardation, implying a neuropsychological substrate for the specific reading difficulties. The use of this term is contentious, so that the more bland expression, 'specific reading retardation', is preferred by many clinical psychologists.

The etiology is multifactorial, involving genetic, social, perceptual and language deficits. A noteworthy feature is the strong association between specific reading retardation and conduct disorder with the behavior problem most likely arising secondary to the frustration and disillusionment associated with the reading difficulty. Treatment involves detailed psychometric assessment of the problem by a psychologist followed by an individualized remedial program carried out by a specialized teacher in collaboration with the psychologist. Help with the behavioral problem is also necessary in order to prevent more serious problems arising during adolescence.

HABIT DISORDERS

Tics and Tourette syndrome

Tics are rapid, involuntary, repetitive muscular movements, usually involving the face and neck, for instance blinks, grimaces and throat clearing. Simple tics occur as a transitory phenomenon in about 10% of the population with boys outnumbering girls three to one and with a mean age of onset around 7 years. They range in severity from simple tics involving head and neck through to complex tics extending to the limbs and trunk and finally to Tourette syndrome. The latter comprises complex tics accompanied by coprolalia (uttering obscene words and phrases) and echolalia (the repetition of sounds or words). Like stammering, tics are made worse at times of stress and may be exacerbated by undue parental concern. The differential diagnosis of tics in childhood is principally from chorea, where the movements are less coordinated and predictable, not stereotypic in form and cannot be suppressed.

Other features of tics are a positive family history and a previous history of neurodevelopmental delay. Many tics resolve spontaneously, but those that persist can be extremely disabling and difficult to treat.

Treatment

Several approaches are used singly or in combination, depending on assessment. Medication is effective, but should be reserved for severe cases. Haloperidol is the most common drug used for Tourette syndrome, but pimozide and clonidine are alternative drugs. Many children with simple tics respond to explanation and reassurance along with advice for the parents. Individual and/or family therapy may be indicated when anxiety and tension are clearly making important contributions to the problem. Behavior therapy in the form of relaxation and/or massed practice can also be helpful.

Prognosis

Simple tics have a good outcome with complete remission, whereas in Tourette syndrome the condition fluctuates in a chronic manner with 50% continuing with symptoms into adult life.

SLEEP DISORDERS (see preschool children section)

Night terrors

The usual pattern is for the child to wake up in a frightened, even terrified state, not to respond when spoken to, nor appear to see objects or people. Instead, he appears to be hallucinating, talking to and looking at people/things not actually present. The child may be difficult to comfort with the period of disturbed behavior and altered consciousness lasting up to 15 min, occasionally longer. Eventually the behavior settles, with or without comfort, and the child goes back to sleep, awakening in the morning with no recollection of the episode. The latter point is invaluable in helping to allay parental anxiety about the episodes. Night terrors arise from stage 4 or deep sleep. The peak incidence is between 4 and 7 years with a continuation of 1–3% into older children. It is also helpful to identify and ameliorate any identifiable stresses that may occasionally contribute to the problem. Lask[65] has described an apparently successful novel behavioral approach relying on waking the child 15 min prior to the expected time of the night terror. Drugs such as benzodiazepines or tricyclics have also been used successfully.

Nightmares

These are frightening or unpleasant dreams, occurring during REM (rapid eye movement) sleep. The child may or may not wake up but there will be a clear recollection of the dream if he does wake up and also in the morning. There is no period of altered consciousness or inaccessibility as in night terrors. Again, daytime anxieties and/or frightening television programs in the evening may be contributory factors.

Sleep walking (somnambulism)

The child, usually aged between 8 and 14 years, calmly arises from his bed with a blank facial expression, does not respond to attempts at communication and can only be awakened with difficulty. The child is in a state of altered consciousness at the deep level of sleep (stages 3 or 4). Any contributory anxiety should be treated as well as giving the parents some advice about the safety and protection of the child during these episodes.

PSYCHOLOGICAL EFFECTS OF ILLNESS AND DISABILITY

Approximately 15% of children have some form of chronic illness or disability. The IOW study[14] showed clearly that this group of children was much more at risk for disturbance, namely a rate of 33% for children with chronic illness affecting the central nervous system and of 12% for children with chronic illness not affecting the central nervous system compared with 7% among the general population. The IOW study also reported that children with chronic illness or handicap had the same range of disorders as other disturbed children, thereby implying that the mechanisms involved with this increased morbidity are probably indirect and nonspecific rather than direct and specific to each illness or disability. Illness or disability imposes psychological stress on the child and family not only at the time of diagnosis but also in the long term. These effects are now discussed with regard to the child himself and to other family members, though the two effects interact with each other.

Effects on the child

Three aspects are important: the acquisition of skills and outside interests, the development of self-concept, and the development of adaptive coping behavior. Many illnesses or disabilities inevitably restrict the child's ability or opportunity to acquire everyday skills and to develop interests and hobbies. For example, the child with cerebral palsy is by definition motor impaired, having the dietary restrictions of diabetes, the exercise limitations of asthma and the avoidance by children with epilepsy of some activities such as cycling or swimming. Additionally, educational problems are common among this group of children for a variety of reasons including increased absence from school, specific learning difficulties, especially among children with epilepsy, and low expectations of parents and teachers.

Illness and disability can adversely affect the child's self-concept in several ways through the effects on the child's body image and self-esteem. Many children have a distorted view of their body, believing the disability to be very prominent or disfiguring. These ideas can be reinforced by comments from parents or peers. Self-esteem can also be impaired due to a faulty cognitive appraisal of the situation and to a pessimistic attitude to the situation. This leads the child to have low self-esteem with a gloomy view about his illness and the outlook for the future. This is particularly likely and also potentially very disabling among older children and adolescents.

Successful adaptation to a disability depends on the acquisition of a range of coping behaviors and defense mechanisms to lessen anxiety to an acceptable level. Effective coping strategies include regulating the amount of stress into containable amounts, obtaining information, rehearsing the possible outcomes of treatment and assessing the situation from several viewpoints. Parents, nursing staff and pediatricians have an important role in promoting this repertoire of skills for children with a disability. Additionally, defense mechanisms such as denial, rationalization and displacement can be helpful for the child during the initial stages of adjustment to the illness or disability.

Effects on the parents

The parents can respond in various ways in the short term and also in the long term. Most parents eventually achieve some degree of adaptation, though for a minority maladaptive behavior patterns emerge and are prominent. The common reaction is overprotection whereby the parent(s) is unable to allow the child to experience the normal disappointments and upsets inevitable during childhood, so that the child leads a 'cotton wool' existence. Less frequently, the parent(s) may be rejecting and indifferent to the child because the child's disability is so damaging to the parents' self-esteem or because the disability has exacerbated an already precarious parent–child relationship. Overprotection and rejection are sometimes combined in the parental reaction.

The parents may also find it difficult to provide appropriate discipline and control, as they irrationally fear that such control may aggravate the child's illness. For example, parents of children with epilepsy may think that thwarting the child's wishes may induce an epileptic fit.

Finally, the stress of coping with the child's illness may exacerbate parental marital disharmony, though in a minority it may paradoxically unite them as they face the adversity together.

Effect on siblings

This can manifest itself in several ways: the oldest sibling may be given excessive responsibility such as looking after the disabled sibling; the siblings may lose friendships because they are reluctant to bring their friends home in case their disabled sibling is an embarrassment; and finally, the sibling's own developmental needs may be neglected with consequent resentment and frustration.

BREAKING BAD NEWS TO PARENTS

This distressing but inevitable aspect of pediatrics comes in various guises such as the birth of a child with Down syndrome or with the diagnosis of cystic fibrosis. Unfortunately, most undergraduate and postgraduate training includes very little teaching about this important subject. Though the details vary for each case, the following general principles are important:

1. Information should be given by the most senior and experienced doctor involved with the child's care.
2. Both parents must be seen together if at all possible, as this reduces misinformation and allows the parents to be mutually supportive from the outset.
3. Allow adequate time for the interview (not 10 min at the end of a ward round).
4. Privacy is essential not only as a matter of courtesy and dignity but also because it allows parents to express their emotions more freely.
5. Begin the interview by asking the parents to tell you what they know about the problems.
6. Tell parents frankly and honestly in simple and non-technical language the nature of the problem, explaining the reasons for the investigations and the basis for the diagnosis.
7. Encourage the parents to ask questions (by asking them some open-ended questions).
8. Emphasize the positive as well as the negative aspects of the diagnosis, for instance the child will be able to have physiotherapy and special equipment, will be able to go to school and to receive effective control for pain.
9. Facilitate the expression of emotions by the parents, namely respond sympathetically and sensitively to the parent(s)' distress and crying.
10. Make a definite offer of a further appointment to talk things over again.
11. Many parents find it helpful to continue the discussion with a nurse or social worker after the interview.

REACTIONS TO HOSPITALIZATION

Admission to hospital is a common experience during childhood with approximately 25% admitted by the age of 4 years. For most children, this is a short admission for a brief treatable illness, whilst a minority (approximately 4%) remains in hospital for at least 1 month. While most parents and their children cope successfully with the admission, some, particularly those with repeated admissions for minor illnesses, show evidence of disturbance that may in turn have been the reason why the child was admitted in the first place.

Admission to hospital can have adverse short term and long term effects. The contributory factors can be grouped under three headings: (1) the child and family, (2) the nature of the illness, and (3) the attitudes and practices of the hospital and its staff. Important factors within the child and family include age, temperament of the child, previous experience of hospital, previous parent–child relationship and current family circumstances. Children aged between 1 and 4 years are particularly stressed by separation from familiar figures. Similarly, children with adverse temperamental characteristics, such as poor adaptability or irregularity of habits, are more vulnerable. If the child had a favorable experience when in hospital previously, this will ease the burden for any subsequent admission. If the parent–child relationship was poor prior to admission, hospitalization is likely to exacerbate this problem because of the additional stress. Adverse family circumstances, for instance financial, may also be aggravated by admission.

The nature of the illness, particularly the associated pain or the necessity for painful procedures, influences the child's response. Again, an acute admission is likely to be more stressful than an elective procedure.

The attitudes of the staff and hospital practices can minimize the distress for the child. Helpful and favorable aspects include good rooming-in facilities, adequate preparation for painful or unpleasant procedures, and nursing and medical staff trained to minimize distress and to offer comfort when required. The ward should be organized so that parents and siblings are encouraged to visit as well as ensuring the ready availability of play leaders and teachers. Medical and nursing staff should also have access to social work resources as well as to psychological and psychiatric services. Finally, joint liaison between the medical and psychiatric team and the establishment of a staff support group to enable staff to discuss their own anxieties about working in a stressful environment are likely to be beneficial.

TREATMENT METHODS

Several factors are usually responsible for the development of disturbance, so that it is unlikely that one treatment method will resolve the problem. All treatment approaches also rely upon common elements that are not only necessary but also essential for a successful outcome.

Table 34.3 Drug treatment in child psychiatry

Drug	Usage	Comment
Anxiolytics	Anxiety / phobic conditions	Short-term adjunct to behavior treatment
Neuroleptics	Phenothiazines (e.g. chlorpromazine)	Butyrophenones (e.g. haloperidol)
Newer antipsychotics	Schizophrenia/ADHD	Extrapyramidal side-effects common
(e.g. risperidone/olanzapine)	Complex tics/Tourette syndrome	Extrapyramidal side-effects common
	Schizophrenia	Fewer side-effects
Tricyclics		
Imipramine / nortriptyline	Second-line treatment for ADHD	Useful when an affective component present
clomipramine	Obsessional–compulsive disorder	Long-term usage often necessary
SRIs (fluoxetine, paroxetine, sertraline)	Probably first choice for depressive disorder	Better compliance with fewer side-effects
Stimulants		
Methylphenidate/dexamphetamine	ADHD	80% effective. Side-effects closely monitored
Hypnotics (melatonin) with ADHD	Persistent sleep disorder	Sometimes used for sleep problems associated
Lithium	Recurrent bipolar affective disorder	Close supervision of blood level and for signs of toxicity
Laxatives (e.g. bulk-forming (methylcellulose), stimulants (senna), softener (dioctyl)	Encopresis with constipation	Facilitates formation and passage of feces
Central α-agonist (e.g. clonidine)	Unresponsive Tourette syndrome	Sedation and rebound hypertension

SRIs, serotonin reuptake inhibitors.

These elements include active cooperation between the therapist and the child and family, agreement between them about the aims of treatment, and a mutual trust to enable these aims to be achieved. Again, the relative efficacy of different treatments is not clearly established, so that the choice of treatment is often a reflection of the therapist(s)' training and experience rather than an absolute indication in any particular instance. Careful analysis of the following elements is therefore necessary in order to devise an effective treatment program:

1. Individual:
   - physical illness or disability;
   - intellectual ability;
   - type of symptomatology.
2. Family
   - developmental stage (for instance a family with pre-school children or one with adolescents);
   - psychiatric health of parents;
   - marital relationship;
   - parenting qualities;
   - communication patterns within the family;
   - ability to resolve conflict;
   - support network, for instance availability of the extended family.
3. School:
   - scholastic attainments;
   - child and parents' attitude to the authority of the school;
   - peer relationships.
4. Community:
   - quality of peer relationships and of role models;
   - neighborhood and community resources.

The formulation of the problem along these four dimensions provides the basis to decide the suitable treatment program.

The three main types of treatment approach available are: (1) drug treatment, (2) the psychotherapies and (3) liaison or consultation work. The latter refers to the common practice whereby the child psychiatrist or a member of the psychiatric team does not have direct contact with the referred child, but rather helps those involved with the child to understand and modify the child's behavior. Psychotherapies are those treatments that use a variety of psychological techniques to ameliorate disturbance. They include individual therapy, behavior therapy, family therapy and group therapy as well as counseling and advice for parents.

Drug treatment[66]

This has increasing importance in child psychiatry. Table 34.3 summarizes the important indications and side-effects of various drugs used in child psychiatry.

Psychotherapies

These are a very common treatment approach in child psychiatric practice.

Individual psychotherapy[67]

Though there are several theoretical orientations, including psychoanalytic[68] and Rogerian,[69] the therapist has nevertheless the same therapeutic tasks. These are: (1) to develop a trusting, nonjudgmental relationship with the child; (2) to enable the child to express his feelings and thoughts; (3) to understand the meaning of the child's symptoms, including his behavior during the therapeutic session; and finally (4) to provide the child with some understanding and explanation for his behavior. The indications for individual psychotherapy are not clearly established, though most usually it is for children with a neurotic or reactive disorder rather than for those with a constitutionally based disorder. For younger children the medium for communication is play such as sand play or through drawing, whilst for older children verbal exchange and discussion are possible.

Behavioral psychotherapy[70]

This approach is based upon the application of the findings from experimental psychology, particularly learning theory, to a wide range of problems such as enuresis, encopresis, tantrums and aggression. Its characteristics are as follows:

1. Define problem(s) objectively with reference to the Antecedents, the Behavior itself and the Consequences (the ABC approach).
2. Place emphasis on the current behavior rather than on past events.
3. Set up hypotheses to account for the behavior.
4. Set pre-treatment baseline to determine the frequency and severity of the problem.
5. Devise behavioral program on an individual basis to test the hypothesis.
6. Evaluate outcome of treatment program.
7. Tackle one problem at a time.

As with other psychotherapies, success depends upon the establishment of a trusting relationship with the patient and the close supervision of the treatment program together with the involvement of teachers and parents in many cases.

Cognitive behavioral therapy (CBT)[71]

This is used increasingly with older children and adolescents for a variety of conditions including anxiety, depression and anorexia nervosa. The central premise is that the individual's cognitive distortions are responsible for the symptoms and the disorder, so that therapy is designed to change cognitions through a collaborative approach between the therapist and the patient. Usually the treatment lasts about 12 sessions. The early part of the treatment is devoted to teaching the patient to recognize their cognitive distortions, and then training them to devise alternative and more healthy interpretations of the situation. This is combined with 'homework tasks' between sessions in order to put into practice the new ideas or responses to situations that they find difficult.

Family therapy[72]

This is a popular treatment approach now. The rationale underlying family therapy is that the child's disturbed behavior is symptomatic of the disturbance within the family as a group. There are many different theoretical approaches and techniques,[72] but all usually involve interviewing the whole family on each occasion for about 1 h. Most family work is short term, lasting about 6 months, with approximately monthly sessions. The emphasis is on current behavior, verbal and nonverbal, observed during the session rather than on past events. The main aim is to improve communication within the family, so that dysfunctional patterns of behavior are replaced by more healthy and adaptive behavior.

Group therapy

Older children and adolescents often benefit from group therapy when the aim is to improve interpersonal relationships, particularly with the peer group, using a variety of theoretical models (for instance psychodynamic and social skills).

Supportive psychotherapy and counseling

The former is frequently used for the child with chronic illness or handicap when the focus may be the child or the parents. It is especially beneficial at the time of diagnosis and also in the long term, when the implications of the disability become more evident. Parental counseling is also used to help the parents understand their child's behavioral problems, the factors that may have led to them and that are responsible for their continuation, along with an emphasis on the parent–child relationship and the improvement of parenting skills. Counseling may therefore help the parents to devise and implement a behavioral program to modify the child's behavior as well as to promote normal development.

Liaison and consultation psychiatry[73]

This is a collaborative approach between the child psychiatry team and the professionals directly involved with the child, for instance hospital staff, teachers or residential care staff, in order to help these professionals to understand the child's disturbed behavior, their own possible contribution to the problem and to suggest ways to improve the situation. Although the child psychiatrist may see the referred child in the first instance, subsequent contact is usually with the staff rather than with the child. This approach can also include the establishment and supervision of a staff support group whose aim is to look at the attitudes and emotional responses of the staff towards the behavior shown by the children under their care.

PSYCHIATRIC DISORDERS IN ADOLESCENCE

This section has two parts: adolescent psychological development and adolescent psychiatric syndromes.

ADOLESCENT DEVELOPMENT

Adolescence is the transition between childhood and adult life. Four maturational tasks must be accomplished successfully to ensure a favorable outcome:
- attainment of independence;
- establishment of a sexual role and orientation;
- self-control of aggressive and oppositional impulses;
- achievement of self-identity.

Though these tasks are not necessarily complete nor entirely resolved by the end of adolescence, the adolescent should have made substantial progress with these tasks. Three tasks – independence, sex role and orientation, self-control of aggressive and oppositional impulses – refer to specific aspects of psychological development, whereas the fourth – self-identity – is a global term referring to that sense of uniqueness or individuality that distinguishes one person from another. Erikson[6] believed that the attainment of a stable self-identity during adolescence is the prerequisite for successful adult adjustment. Important components of self-identity for Erikson are 'sexual identity' and 'career identity'. The Eriksonian unsuccessful outcome of adolescent conflict is 'identity diffusion', with the person lacking clear goals and direction in the fulfilment of individual ambition.

Adolescent development is commonly divided into four phases:
- pre-adolescent phase (11–13 years);
- early adolescence (13–15 years);
- mid adolescence (15–17 years);
- late adolescence (18 years onwards).

The main features of the pre-adolescent phase are the onset of biological puberty and an increased interest in peer relationships and teenage pursuits. Early adolescence is characterized by the critical questioning of parental values combined with an uncritical acceptance of peer group views. The establishment of a separate sexual and social identity occurs during mid-adolescence. The individual explores and develops their own gender and sexual role. The development of social relationships outside the family enables the individual to have their own social network as well as altering the basis of their relationship with their parents. Later adolescence is focused on the career or work choice along with the expression of the sexual role through more satisfying and enduring relationships.

DETERMINANTS OF ADOLESCENT ADJUSTMENT

Though the same general factors influence development and adjustment in adolescence as in earlier periods, brief mention will be made of those that are of particular relevance.

Previous childhood experience(s)

Unsatisfactory earlier experience(s) and relationships, particularly the child–parent(s) relationship, are major factors affecting predisposition to adjustment during adolescence. The individual's capacity to withstand the inevitable stresses of adolescence and also their resilience are greatly impaired when the outcome of earlier experiences was unsatisfactory. Adverse childhood experience is an important vulnerability factor in adolescent breakdown.

Family psychopathology

Parental psychopathology such as marital disharmony or parental psychiatric illness has a powerful influence on children's behavior throughout childhood, but even more so during adolescence, when conflicts over discipline, control and autonomy are normal and unavoidable. Parental disagreements and disunity on these matters greatly exacerbate the difficulties.

Schooling

Common problems are: academic failure with scholastic subjects, poor motivation and disillusionment with schooling, conflicts over authority with teaching staff.

Peer group

Peer group values and pressure exert enormous influence on the adolescent, so that contact with and membership of a deviant peer group can lead to major problems in school, for instance truancy, or in the community, for instance delinquency or vandalism.

Chronic illness or disability

The normal adolescent drive for self-appraisal and self-identity leaves the disabled or disabled adolescent feeling isolated and different from their peers, a most distressing experience. Early childhood feelings of acceptance and tolerance by peers are replaced by those of exclusion and separateness with a reluctance or inability to gain peer group acceptance. The adolescent often deals with these feelings of anger and frustration by denial or minimalization of the seriousness of his condition. This can result in poor compliance with medication or reckless exposure to dangerous situations.

INTERVIEWING AND ASSESSMENT OF ADOLESCENTS

Though the earlier part of the chapter discussed the general principles of interviewing and assessment, it is helpful to mention some specific points relating to adolescence. Flexibility in approach is essential for successful interviewing. In general, the older the adolescent and the more serious or intimate the problem, the greater the necessity for a separate interview with the adolescent. Usually, this is combined with a family interview in order to complete the assessment.

Many adolescents are reluctant, confused or anxious attenders, so that the clinician must clarify and explain the purpose, sequence and duration of the assessment procedures at the outset. Respect for the adolescent's maturity, the right to privacy and confidentiality must be acknowledged clearly. The distinction between 'family business' and 'individual business' must be emphasized to the adolescent and to the parents. Adolescent anxieties about 'seeing the shrink' or being 'treated like a child' must be addressed and talked through. The individual interview may allow the clinician to conduct a thorough assessment of the mental state, though careful phrasing of questions about sexual or psychotic phenomena is essential in order to avoid a dismissive denial and a further increase in anxiety and confusion.

Silence and refusal to talk during the interview are common and often difficult to overcome. The clinician can use three tactics to deal with this problem: (1) it can be pointed out that the silence is just as difficult for the interviewer as it is for the adolescent; (2) there will be the opportunity and time to talk through difficult topics now or alternatively on another occasion; and finally, (3) to terminate the interview when necessary to prevent prolonged or undue tension.

Family interviews are often not only part of the assessment procedure but also of the treatment plan. Sometimes however, it is more appropriate to interview the parents and the child together rather than the whole family.

ADOLESCENT PSYCHIATRIC SYNDROMES

These are divided into three categories: those disorders persisting from earlier childhood; new disorders arising during adolescence; and those disorders with features special to adolescence. Prior to the discussion of these topics, brief comment will be made about the prevalence of psychiatric disorders in adolescence.

Prevalence

This varies widely from 10–20% depending upon the population studied, the diagnostic criteria and the age group. Most studies do however show a consistent pattern with respect to gender ratio, urban vs. rural differences and the range of clinical syndromes. In contrast to earlier childhood, when psychiatric disorder is more common among boys, the adolescent period shows a shift towards an equal gender ratio in early adolescence followed by a subsequent female preponderance in late adolescence and adult life. Prevalence rates in urban populations are at least twice that for rural populations. Schizophrenia, major affective disorder, suicide and attempted suicide, anorexia and substance abuse all begin to appear with some frequency during adolescence, whereas encopresis or enuresis decrease markedly.

PERSISTENT CHILDHOOD DISORDERS

Childhood disorders are more likely to continue into adolescence when one or more of the following are present: a major constitutional factor to the syndrome, the adverse circumstances responsible for the onset of the disorder are still present and perpetuating or maintaining factors are prominent. The follow-up study of 10-year-old children in the IOW study[13] showed that 40% of the disorders had persisted into adolescence with a strong continuity for boys with conduct disorder and associated educational problems. This section now discusses the factors responsible for the persistence of some disorders into adolescence from earlier childhood.

Conduct disorder

The oppositional and defiant character of conduct disorder means that it is very likely to be exacerbated by the rebellious and anti-authoritarian nature of ordinary adolescent behavior. Childhood predictors of persistent conduct disorder are: early onset of symptoms, extensive and varied symptomatology, and the severity of aggressive behavior. Adverse temperamental characteristics combined with continued exposure to deviant family psychopathology such as deficient and ineffective parenting, marital disharmony or parental psychiatric illness are thought to be important factors maintaining the conduct disorder. The persistence of the frequently associated learning disorders is another source of frustration and disillusionment for the adolescent, producing conflict with the teachers and reluctance to attend school.

Emotional disorders

Generally, emotional disorders have a good prognosis, often because they arise in response to some identifiable but remedial stress. Consequently, emotional disorder persisting into adolescence implies a more serious underlying cause. The school refusal syndrome is the most likely condition to show continuity from early childhood. It may reappear at the transfer from primary to secondary school, or early on during secondary schooling. Previous history of separation difficulties, for instance at the start of nursery or primary school and/or an overdependent relationship between the child and parent(s), are commonly found. The increased necessity for independence, autonomy and assertiveness at secondary school may prove too much for the vulnerable adolescent.

Childhood autism

The overt autistic-like behavior and overactivity prominent in younger children with the disorder often decrease during adolescence, but the majority are still profoundly impaired in social and communication skills with a marked apathy and lack of empathy. Educational and learning disabilities are very evident. Epilepsy also develops in about 15% of individuals with a greater risk when severe mental retardation is also present.

Attention deficit hyperactivity disorder

The overactivity usually decreases during adolescence, but persistent problems with antisocial behavior, impulsivity, recklessness, distractibility and learning disorders mean that the adolescent with ADHD is likely to remain disturbed.

NEW DISORDERS ARISING DURING ADOLESCENCE

These can be divided into two categories: those related to the stress of adolescence and major adult-like disorders arising in adolescence.

Stress-related adolescent disorders

During adolescence, the distinction between normal and abnormal behavior is often imprecise, so that it is more important to understand why the adolescent's behavior is such a cause of concern rather than whether the behavior fulfils the criteria for a disorder in a diagnostic classification system. In many cases, conflict often arises between the adolescent and the parents' overindependence and control issues. Allied with the pressure from peers, this often leads the adolescent to engage in antisocial or conduct-disordered behavior. Delinquency, vandalism and out-of-control behavior are common, sometimes mixed with a pattern of alcohol or drug abuse. Persistent antisocial disorder often culminates in criminal behavior and arrest by the police. Co-existent family problems with a limited capacity to resolve issues also contribute to the severity of the disorder. Eventually, it may be necessary for the adolescent to leave the family home and to provide him with alternative care arrangements, for instance with foster parents or community carers. Another solution sometimes adopted by the adolescent is to run away from home. Although the majority of runaways eventually return home, a minority stay away and become involved with the homeless subculture found in large cities.

The common neurotic or emotional responses to adolescent stress are affective symptoms such as irritability, liability of mood and anxiety symptoms, particularly related to social situations or mixing with peers. The latter may sometimes lead to marked social withdrawal. School refusal may sometimes present for the first time during early adolescence, when it represents a combination of adolescent stress and the revival of an earlier overdependent parent–child relationship. The increased need for independence and autonomy posed by the demands of secondary school precipitates an avoidance response to school attendance from the adolescent. The anxiety symptoms often masquerade themselves as physical complaints such as headaches or abdominal pain. The prompt exclusion of organic pathology with a minimum amount of investigation is essential in order to prevent the secondary elaboration of physical symptomatology. Delay in the recognition of the underlying psychological basis for the problem greatly exacerbates the difficulties. The prognosis is not good for a significant minority of adolescents with up to one third failing to maintain regular school attendance. Poor prognosis is usually a sign of more serious underlying family psychopathology. Follow-up studies into adult life have shown that anxiety or agoraphobic symptoms are present in about 20%.[53]

Obsessive–compulsive disorder sometimes begins during adolescence, when its occurrence can be seen as a maladaptive response to the stress of adolescence. There is often a history of earlier childhood obsessional and anxiety traits. The key element in the maintenance and exacerbation of the disorder is usually the willingness of the family to participate in the ritualistic behavior. SRIs such as sertraline and fluvoxamine have been shown to be effective in reducing OCD symptoms, but more importantly are particularly effective when combined with cognitive-behavior therapy.[74]

Major adult–like disorders arising in adolescence

Three categories of disorder – schizophrenia, mood disorders and anorexia nervosa – begin to occur with increasing frequency during adolescence.

Schizophrenia[75]

This is a rare disease during childhood. Even during adolescence, it has a frequency of less than 3 per 10 000. Symptoms are usually classified into two groups: positive and negative. Positive symptoms comprise delusions (fixed, false beliefs), hallucinations (a perceptual experience in the absence of the relevant sensory stimulus) and distortions of thinking (thought insertion and withdrawal). Negative symptoms include social withdrawal, emotional blunting, apathy, lack of motivation, poverty of speech and slowness of thought. The usual presentation is insidious rather than florid with a gradual social withdrawal and increased internal preoccupation. Dysphoric symptoms are common, so that a diagnosis of affective disorder is sometimes made. The adolescent is often able to conceal his bizarre ideas from parents and peers. However, it is the presence of increasingly unpredictable and

erratic behavior that indicates something more serious is occurring. The possibility of drug misuse is an important alternative diagnostic possibility.

Etiology

There is good evidence of a genetic component with approximately 20% of relatives having the disease.[75] The Maudsley long term follow-up study of early-onset psychosis[75] showed that one third had significant premorbid social difficulties affecting the ability to make and retain friends. There was also a downward shift in intelligence with a mean IQ of 85. The disorder tends to run a chronic course with only a minority making a full symptomatic recovery – only 12% of patients in the Maudsley study were in remission at 6 months. The best prognostic indicator was the clinical state at that time.

Treatment

It must be comprehensive including drug treatment with antipsychotics, individual and family therapy as well as help with education. Traditional antipsychotics such as chlorpromazine and haloperidol are effective, particularly for positive symptoms, but side-effects such as extrapyramidal side-effects and drowsiness adversely affect compliance. Consequently, the newer antipsychotics such as risperidone and olanzapine, with their low side-effect profile, are now the drugs of first choice. When treatment with first-line drugs is ineffective, serious consideration should be given to clozapine. This drug has been shown to be effective for treatment-resistant schizophrenia in adults, and promising case reports have been published for adolescents. There must be careful screening and monitoring for side-effects, particularly for blood dyscrasias, when clozapine is used.

Finally, bad prognostic features include poor premorbid functioning, negative symptoms and a long period of untreated illness.

MOOD DISORDERS[76,77]

This section has the following parts: depression as a symptom, depressive disorders, bipolar affective disorder, and suicide and attempted suicide.

Depression as a symptom/syndrome

Depression has been recognized as a syndrome in adults for a long time because of its characteristic constellation of symptoms, response to treatment and outcome. The depressed mood or dysphoria has qualities other than just simple sadness or unhappiness. Rather, it is the inability to derive pleasure or satisfaction from daily life (anhedonia) or to be able to respond emotionally to ordinary events. Other features of the syndrome are cognitive disturbances, behavioral changes and alterations in physiological functions. The cognitive disturbances are primarily cognitive distortions around oneself (self-blame, self-reproach, guilt and worthlessness), the world (helplessness and despair about one's life situation) and the future (hopelessness and despondency about the future). The behavioral changes range from marked agitation to withdrawal and stupor, while the physiological changes are poor appetite, weight loss and disturbed sleep pattern.

In adolescence, depression can present in the following ways: as a transient mood state; as a symptom in other psychiatric disorders, for instance anxiety states; as a symptom in physical illnesses, for instance infectious mononucleosis; and as part of a symptom complex in major depressive disorder. Epidemiological studies have shown an increasing prevalence of depressive symptomatology from childhood to adolescence. Rutter et al[78] found that many adolescents had experienced feelings of misery and depression (40%), self-deprecation (20%) and suicidal thoughts (7%) at one time or another.

Depressive disorders

Both the ICD and DSM classifications now state that depression in children and adolescents should have the same features as that in adults. They recognize the following core features: abnormal depressed mood for at least 2 weeks, marked loss of interest or pleasure in almost all activities, decreased energy or increased fatigue. Additional features include: loss of confidence and self-esteem, unreasonable feelings of guilt or self-reproach, suicidal thoughts, poor concentration and indecisiveness, psychomotor agitation or retardation, sleep disturbance, and loss of appetite.

Etiology

The etiology of child and adolescent depression is not clear but there is some support for the two main theories: genetic and environmental. Evidence for a genetic component comes from twin studies, adoption and family studies, though the size of the effect is not known. Environmental theories range from the traditional psychoanalytic perspective, to the adverse impact of life events and to the cognitive theory of Beck et al.[79] The latter regards the individual's negative view of himself, the world and the future as the cause of the depression, though clearly these cognitions could be seen as a consequence of the depressed mood rather than the cause.

Assessment

This involves detailed and sensitive interviewing of the adolescent, usually alone, as well assessment of the adolescent and the family. Family assessment is useful for two reasons: the adolescent's behavior can be seen in the context of current family functioning, and other sources of stress for the adolescent or family may be identified. Physical symptoms are frequently found among depressed adolescents, though the findings are not specific as anxious adolescents often have physical symptoms as well. The differential diagnosis must involve the distinction between normal sadness or unhappiness, other psychiatric conditions with depressive symptomatology, for instance anorexia nervosa, or physical illnesses such as infectious mononucleosis or influenza.

Treatment

A comprehensive treatment package is most likely to be most effective. Components include drug treatment, individual and family therapy and the reduction or lessening of stressful circumstances. The relative emphasis and sequence of treatments are dependent upon assessment.

Drug treatment is most likely to be effective for adolescents who are most severely affected and have a disturbance of physiological functions such as appetite, sleep or weight. Emslie et al[80] have reported the superiority of fluoxetine to placebo in a well-conducted randomized control trial. Fluoxetine is currently the only recommended SRI for the treatment of depression. This advice arose from a review of published clinical trial data of SRIs that reported that evidence of efficacy was lacking for most SRIs in this age group and they were associated with increased suicidality, namely suicidal thoughts and behavior.

The purpose of individual therapy varies widely depending on the assessment and therapeutic style of the clinician. The common aims of an individual approach are: to establish a trusting relationship with the adolescent, to enable the adolescent to feel understood and accepted, and to allow the adolescent to disclose their concerns and anxieties including suicidal thoughts. Beyond these core aims, the therapeutic approach is varied, ranging from the psychodynamically insight-orientated psychotherapy to the cognitive–behavioral.

Work with the family is often undertaken more to improve communication between members of the family rather than to specifically treat family dysfunction. Family sessions are extremely useful at the start of treatment as a way to discuss events of emotional significance that may have happened recently but have not been talked through, for instance a family illness or a bereavement. These sessions also provide the opportunity to discuss ways to reduce any overt source of stress or anxiety for the adolescent. Common sources of stress include lack of friends, bullying or teasing at school and the adolescent's sense, usually distorted, of academic failure.

Bipolar disorder or manic-depressive psychosis

ICD and DSM use similar criteria for the diagnosis of bipolar disorder whether in adolescents or adults. The following points summarize the main diagnostic criteria of ICD and DSM:

- A disorder characterized by repeated episodes (two or more) in which the subject's mood and activity are significantly disturbed. This disturbance consists on some occasions of an elevation of mood with increased energy and activity (mania or hypomania), and on others of a lowering of mood with decreased energy and activity (depression).
- Recovery is characteristically complete between episodes.
- Manic episodes usually begin abruptly, lasting from 2 weeks to 4 or 5 months, whilst depressive episodes often last longer.

Clinical features

A hypomanic or depressive episode is equally common as the first manifestation of a bipolar illness with subsequent episodes more likely to be hypomanic than depressive. A depressive episode shows similar features to other depressive illnesses except that it tends to be more severe with a pronounced disturbance in physiological functioning and frequent suicidal thoughts.

The main feature of the hypomanic episode is an elevated, expansive or irritable mood with the other aspects understandable in terms of the elevated mood. The common features are: increased physical activity or physical restlessness, increased talkativeness, difficulty in concentration and distractibility, less need for sleep, increased sexual energy, mild spending sprees or other types of reckless behavior, and increased sociability or overfamiliarity. A manic episode causes severe disruption to the individual's life. The increased talkativeness becomes a 'pressure of speech' with flight of ideas (rapid switching of ideas based on a literal rather than a logical association, for instance rhyming or punning). The social disinhibition and recklessness can have a devastating effect on the individual's life. Cases with early onset have a worse prognosis with more frequent episodes, rapid cycling and a greater risk of suicide.

Though uncommon, several organic conditions can mimic a hypomanic episode. These include infections (encephalitis), endocrine (hyperthyroidism), neurological (repeated seizures, head trauma), brain tumor (meningioma, glioma), medication (steroids) and substance misuse (alcohol and amphetamine/LSD misuse).

Management

A depressive episode should be managed in a similar manner to other depressive episodes: that is SRIs, individual and family support. ECT may need to be considered for a severely depressed and/or suicidal patient.

The hypomanic episode is often harder to manage, as it usually requires inpatient admission, measures to ensure the safety and protection of the patient and drug treatment. The most useful drug for an acute episode is haloperidol (dosage 0.05 mg/kg/d in three divided doses). It is usually necessary to supplement this medication with antiparkinsonian drugs such as benzhexol or orphenadrine. An acute dystonic reaction such as an oculogyric crisis or acute torticollis can occur when treatment is commenced. Consequently, it is essential to observe closely the initiation of the medication.

Lithium carbonate is also effective in the acute episode, though its effect has a slower onset. Lithium is more useful as a prophylactic medication for individuals who have had several episodes. Its introduction should be carefully supervised and monitored. There have however been no controlled trials of the effectiveness of lithium in the prevention of further episodes in children or adolescents. Lithium has however been shown to be less effective among individuals with a rapid cycling disorder, features common among adolescents with bipolar disorder. Other drugs such as carbamazepine and sodium valproate have been used in the treatment of previously drug-resistant manic episodes in adults, but there is insufficient evidence to evaluate their efficacy for adolescents with bipolar disorder.

Prognosis

Most individuals usually recover from an acute episode. For individuals with repeated episodes, poor prognostic features include the absence of a precipitating factor, a family history of recurrent illness and the continuation of some symptoms between acute episodes.

SUICIDE

This is extremely rare below the age of 12 years with an increase during adolescence to approximately 30 cases per million per year.[81] It is more common in males with no trend in social class. Males tend to use violent methods such as hanging or jumping from high buildings or bridges, whilst females have a preference for self-poisoning. Shaffer & Piancentini[81] identified four types of personality characteristics among adolescents who commit suicide: irritable and oversensitive to criticism; impulsive and volatile; withdrawn and uncommunicative; and perfectionist and self-critical. They also found that some evidence for an increased psychiatric disturbance in the family and that a 'disciplinary crisis' was the most common reason precipitating the suicide.

Attempted suicide

This is common with a rate of 4 per 1000 per year among 15–19-year-olds. Females are three times more likely than males to make an attempt with an excess among lower socioeconomic groups. Not surprisingly, the families show evidence of marital disharmony, maternal psychiatric ill health, particularly depression, and paternal personality disorder. About 50% of adolescents show some evidence of psychiatric disorder, usually depression. In older adolescents, there is often a history of alcohol or drug misuse and running away from home. Social isolation and poor peer relationships are also common.

The most common method is an overdose of non-opiate analgesics such as aspirin or paracetamol, probably related to their easy availability. The severity of the overdose varies markedly from a few tablets taken impulsively to swallowing the contents of a bottle of analgesics. The attempt often follows a row with a boyfriend or a serious dispute with the parents over discipline. The adolescent may have threatened to take an overdose on previous occasions, and about 50% have consulted their general practitioner in the month prior to the overdose.

A crucial part of management is the assessment of future suicide risk. This depends on three factors: the circumstances of the attempt, the patient's current mental state and their attitude to the future. Detailed questioning about events prior to the attempt are necessary as well as a 'blow-by-blow' account of the attempt. The latter includes information about the degree of planning, whether anybody else was present and any action taken after the attempt. The identification of any difficulties at home or at school is also important.

The presence of significant depressive symptoms and pessimism about the future are predictors of continued suicide risk. It is important to enquire whether the overdose has altered the adolescent's or family's attitude to their current difficulties and their resolve to improve the situation. An assessment of the coping strategies and the capacity for change within the family is important in order to make a more realistic judgment about the future. Finally, there should be some agreement about future plans and any further contact between the adolescent, the family and the relevant professional agencies.

Treatment depends on the assessment and clinical judgment. The majority of adolescents do not require specialist psychiatric follow-up, though clearly they must know how to access psychiatric services in order to arrange further help when necessary. The indications for more specialized help include: (1) the seriousness of the attempt; (2) the presence of definite depressive disorder or persistent suicidal ideas; (3) poor family circumstances and social support; and (4) the limited capacity of the family for change. A small number may require inpatient psychiatric care, particularly the older adolescent. Follow-up psychiatric contact often involves individual counseling for the adolescent as well as family sessions to improve communication and the capacity to resolve disagreements.

There have been few systematic follow-up studies, though clinical impression suggests that those with definite psychiatric disorder or adverse social or family circumstances are more likely to be 'repeaters'.

ANOREXIA NERVOSA AND RELATED DISORDERS[82]

Anorexia nervosa is a disorder of older female adolescents with a prevalence rate of 1% among 15–19-year-olds. It does however occur among prepubertal children. The core features are:

- self-induced starvation and weight loss;
- a strong desire to be thinner with a marked fear of weight gain;
- a distorted body image (for instance feeling fat when emaciated);
- a body mass index (BMI) < 17.5.

Clinical features

The presentation is varied, sometimes mimicking physical illness or the consequences of weight loss and starvation. The history is of prolonged self-imposed starvation. Dieting often begins following a chance remark about size or shape, or alternatively as a group behavior with other adolescent girls. Food portions at mealtimes are reduced, and some meals such as breakfast or lunch are skipped entirely with the total elimination of high calorific foods such as sweets, puddings or cakes. The individual derives satisfaction from the weight loss, which in turn is a further incentive for weight loss. Parents and other adults are often complimentary and pleased at this initial weight loss. More extreme and rigid dieting is then self-imposed to meet the target for further weight reduction. Appetite and hunger pains are prominent, but the prospect of further weight loss is a powerful motivator. Only when the illness is well established does the anorexia and nausea over food become apparent. Interest and participation in exercise and athletic activities often parallel the dieting in the belief that these activities will enhance weight loss. Later on, excessive laxative use begins in order to reduce weight further.

Despite an increasingly thin physique, the adolescent refuses to accept her emaciated status, still believing and perceiving herself as fat or overweight. The distorted body image is often the first indication to the parents that the adolescent has a serious illness. Increasing arguments over food and its consumption combined with an implacable refusal to eat convince the parents that urgent medical help is required. Often, the adolescent is initially referred to a pediatrician or an endocrinologist in order to exclude a physical basis to the problem rather than accepting a psychological basis for the weight loss.

Physical examination usually shows an individual who is bright and alert despite the evident emaciation. Prominent cheekbones, sunken eyes, bones protruding through the skin, dry skin and hair with blue cold hands and feet are common features. Severe emaciation is accompanied by the appearance of fine downy hair or lanugo hair on the face, limbs and trunk with a slow pulse rate, low blood pressure and hypothermia. Most biochemical investigations are normal, but low gonadotrophin levels with high growth hormone and cortisol levels are sometimes found. Although anorexia is the most likely diagnosis, other psychiatric such as depression, obsessive–compulsive disorder or schizophrenia may need to be excluded.

Etiology

Almost as many theories have been proposed as the number of people who have researched the condition with individual, family or societal factors prominent in most explanations. Review of the premorbid personality characteristics of anorexics shows them to be conformist, conscientious, compliant and high achieving. Issues over autonomy and independence are core issues for anorexics with control over food intake the only available means to preserve self-identity and independence. Similar conflicts over autonomy and independence have been observed among families with an anorectic member, but whether this is cause or effect is unclear. Again, over the past 40 years, society's view about female attractiveness has veered towards the thin end of the spectrum, so that the 'pursuit of thinness' is a major issue for many women.

Management

The severity of the condition varies widely, so that treatment includes outpatient and inpatient management with an emphasis on a 'multimodal' approach. The latter implies that a variety of treatment strategies such as individual, family or cognitive therapies are used, often concurrently or sequentially, dependent on assessment. Recognition and acknowledgement of the problem are the first crucial steps in management. The nature and seriousness of the condition highlighted by the avoidance of food and the irrational ideas about eating must be explored thoroughly in order to establish a therapeutic alliance with the adolescent and the family. Only when the latter has occurred is it possible to commence a specific treatment program.

The next stage is the alteration of eating habits in order to restore weight loss and to correct nutritional deficiencies. Advice and collaboration with the dietician are important from the outset, particularly for any nutritional deficiencies. A target weight, usually around the average for the age and height, should be agreed upon along with the appropriate daily calorific intake to ensure its attainment. Only minimal concessions to food fads or preferences should be allowed with a standard protocol for regular weight checks.

If the patient is in hospital, the nursing care and support are the most important aspects of management. The nursing staff members have to win the cooperation of the adolescent for the treatment plan. They must also be vigilant about food hoarding and surreptitious vomiting. Treatment programs usually involve a graded series of privileges dependent upon satisfactory weight gain. Once the target weight is attained, the diet should be modified, so that age-appropriate weight gain continues. Inpatient programs often involve nursing staff supervising family meals at home during weekend leave.

Working with the family has two aims: to provide educational advice about the disorder and to improve communication patterns within the family. Individual and group work is also useful, but drug treatment is not indicated unless there is a specific treatable disorder such as co-morbid depression. Russell et al[83] in a randomized intervention study reported that family therapy was better than individual therapy in the prevention of relapse among anorexics under 18 years of age who had had the illness for less than 3 years. An important limitation of this study was that only 65% of the 80 patients completed the intervention program.

In many ways, the easiest part of the treatment program, particularly with inpatients, is the restoration of weight loss. A more challenging aspect is the restructuring of the adolescent's and family's attitude to food and their pattern of interaction. Regular supervision, support and contact are essential to maintain progress and keep up morale. Very often a compromise has to be made between an ideal resolution of the problem and a realistic appraisal of the adolescent's and family's capacity to change.

Outcome

Results from follow-up studies vary widely according to inclusion criteria, outcome measures and length of follow-up. Despite these problems, outcome appears to fall into three categories, one third good, one third intermediate and one third poor. There is a 10% mortality in the long term with malnutrition and suicide accounting for most deaths. Poor prognostic factors are an early age of onset, co-existent psychiatric disorder and poor family functioning.

BULIMIA NERVOSA

This has three key features: (1) recurrent binges and purges, (2) a lack of control and (3) a morbid preoccupation with weight and shape. It is rare in the prepubertal period, but becomes increasingly common in older adolescents and young adults, when it is often associated with depression. Most patients are of normal weight. The most serious medical concern is potassium depletion from frequent vomiting. The patient's lifestyle is often chaotic, so that the first aim of treatment is to establish some structure and boundaries for the patient. Dependent on assessment, a combination of individual, cognitive – behavioral and family work is appropriate in most cases.

Two new types of eating disorder have recently been described: *food avoidance emotional disorder* and *pervasive refusal syndrome*. The former is a disorder of emotions in which food avoidance is a prominent symptom along with other affective symptoms such as depression, anxiety or phobias. There is often a previous history of food fads or food restrictions, but the symptoms do not meet the criteria for anorexia nervosa. The validity and independence of this syndrome has however not yet been established.

Pervasive refusal syndrome is a severe life-threatening syndrome characterized by pervasive refusal to eat, drink, talk, walk or engage in any self-care skills. The patients are markedly underweight with an adamant refusal to eat or drink, which ultimately becomes life threatening. Although they fulfil some criteria for anorexia nervosa, the pervasiveness of the symptomatology makes this diagnosis inappropriate. They require prolonged and extensive inpatient nursing care in order to maintain vital body functions. Most patients have been girls with some suggestion that previous traumatic sexual abuse, often involving violence, may have been responsible for the precipitation of the disorder. Most make a satisfactory physical recovery, but the long term psychiatric adjustment is not yet known.

SPECIAL TOPICS

CHRONIC FATIGUE SYNDROME[84]

This has attracted widespread media coverage because of the controversy surrounding etiology and treatment. It is usually defined as a severe disabling fatigue affecting physical and mental functioning accompanied by myalgia, mood and/or sleep disturbance. Accurate prevalence figures are difficult to obtain, but are probably about 1 in 2000. Clinic samples tend to be adolescents aged between 11–15 years, with more girls and from a higher socioeconomic grouping.

Two thirds of patients have had a previous viral infection, but not usually of the Epstein–Barr type. This leads to fatigue, which results in a reduction in physical activity, leading to more fatigue on undertaking any physical activity. The situation is reinforced by parental and personal beliefs about causation, so that a state of inactivity and fatigue become established.

Management involves a thorough assessment to exclude co-morbid psychiatric disorder such as depression, but keeping investigations to an agreed minimum. The establishment of mutual trust and a collaborative approach with the adolescent and the parents are essential to a good outcome. Individual cognitive and family work combined with a structured incremental rehabilitation strategy (a graded exercise program) are the best way to make progress and limit further incapacity. A coordinated plan for school and social reintegration is also necessary.

Outcome varies depending on the initial severity, but three quarters have made a reasonable recovery after 2 years.

SUBSTANCE MISUSE

This ranges from the readily available and legal substances such as tobacco or alcohol to the more uncommon and illegal substances such as heroin or cocaine. Though the latter give rise to more public concern, there is little doubt that cigarette smoking and excessive alcohol consumption have a far more deleterious effect on the health of the population as a whole. A recent survey of over 7000 15- and 16-year-olds in the UK[85] found that almost everyone had drunk alcohol, 30% had smoked cigarettes in the previous 30 d and 43% had at some time used illicit drugs. High levels of smoking were associated with a poorer school performance, and smoking was more common among girls. Adolescents are however only rarely referred to psychiatric services because of their smoking or alcohol habits.

Solvent abuse (glue sniffing)

Ashton[86] reviewing the available literature, estimated that 5–10% of adolescents have at some time inhaled solvents, with 0.5–1% regular users. Since 1971, the death rate from solvent overdose has risen from 2 per annum to over a 100 per annum recently. Solvent abusers have the following characteristics: male gender; peak adolescent usage between 13–15 years; and more common among lower socioeconomic groupings, minority ethnic groups and disrupted families.

Inhaled substances include many everyday items such as adhesives, aerosols, dry cleaning fluids and cigarette lighter fuel. The substances are inhaled through paper bags, saturated rags or direct inhalation. It is often done as a group activity in the socioeconomically disadvantaged areas of large cities, with regular solitary sniffing a cause for more serious concern. The immediate effect is euphoria followed by confusion, perceptual distortion, hallucinations and delusions. The regular user is often able to titrate the 'sniffs', so that a pleasantly euphoric state is maintained for several hours. The characteristic appearance of red spots around the mouth is highly suggestive of solvent abuse.

Sudden death during inhalation can occur from anoxia, respiratory depression, trauma or cardiac arrhythmia. The latter accounts for over half the deaths, whilst anoxia, usually from inhalation of vomit, is responsible for over 10% of deaths. Accidents or suicide attempts during the intoxication are another cause of death, particularly with toluene adhesives. Long term effects include neurological damage (peripheral neuropathy, encephalopathy, dementia and fits) as well as renal and liver damage.

Most solvent abusers do not come into contact with psychiatric services, unless they are referred following hospital admission with acute intoxication. School-based educational program and community-resource initiatives are more likely to be beneficial in the long term. The encouragement of retailers and shop owners to enforce the restrictions on the sale of solvents is also useful. A number of solvent abusers are referred for psychiatric assessment, usually when the abuse is seen as part of more widespread individual or family psychopathology. In the long term, most adolescents do not persist with the habit, but a minority progresses onto more addictive drugs such as heroin or cocaine.

Other substances

These include 'soft' drugs such as cannabis (marijuana) or 'hard' drugs such as amphetamines, cocaine, heroin, lysergic acid diethylamide (LSD) and designer drugs such as 'Ecstasy'. The effects are euphoric and relaxing in the short term, but apathy and inertia occur with chronic use. Most individuals do not progress from cannabis to other more seriously addictive drugs, and its consumption is not indicative of underlying psychological disturbance.

Hard drug consumption is a far more serious problem with deleterious effects on physical and psychological well-being and also from the risk of physical or psychological dependence. In addition to euphoric and pleasurable effects, most of these drugs can produce acutely distressing symptoms such as panic, fright or hallucinations. This can result in suicidal behavior or an increased risk of accidents. Long term use, for example with amphetamine or cocaine, can precipitate a florid psychotic episode with hallucinations, usually visual, and paranoid delusions. Psychological withdrawal symptoms such as an unbearable craving for a 'fix' and physical withdrawal symptoms such as nausea, vomiting and diarrhea make stopping the drug extremely difficult. Physical neglect and malnutrition are also common and exacerbate the problems. The necessity for a regular supply of the drug means that the individual resorts frequently to stealing or crime to support the addiction. The practice of needle-sharing is a major health hazard with human immunodeficiency virus (HIV) infection a strong possibility. Referral of the adolescent to a specialist treatment center and support for the parents are essential to prevent the serious social and psychological problems inevitable with long term drug misuse.

SEXUAL PROBLEMS

Two topics are discussed: sexual abuse and sexual offenders in adolescence; and gender identity disorders.

Sexual abuse and sexual offenders in adolescence[34]

Sexual abuse can present in two ways, direct disclosure of abuse or indirect manifestations of abuse. The same principles of practice and management apply to adolescents as to children (see child section of the chapter), but some special features are important. Open disclosure by the adolescent is often accompanied by the plea for complete confidentiality and no further action. Clearly this guarantee cannot be given, and the adolescent must be counseled about the necessity for an open investigation and the need for a child protection conference.

Indirect manifestations of abuse are twofold, sexually related behavior and psychiatric symptomatology. Sexually related manifestations include pregnancy, venereal disease and promiscuity. The latter often arises because the adolescent relates too readily to adults in a sexual manner as a result of the earlier experience of sexual abuse by an adult. Paradoxically, the promiscuous behavior may also lead some adults to disbelieve the adolescent's claims of abuse or believe that the adolescent was responsible for the initiation of the sexual contact. Psychiatric presentations of abuse are numerous with distress a prominent feature. Common presentations include depression, deteriorating school performance or attendance, suicidal behavior and running away from home.

Help for the sexually abused adolescent has two aims: the protection of the adolescent from further abuse and the provision of therapy to lessen the psychological trauma of the abuse. The first aim is usually achieved by ensuring that the perpetrator is no longer living at home and/or does not have contact with the adolescent. A wide range of therapies is used including individual counseling and support, family therapy or group therapy. Group therapy has become extremely popular recently. This approach has several advantages: the adolescent realizes that other adolescents have had a similar experience, the adolescent has the opportunity to discuss and share their feelings with other adolescents who are in a similar predicament, and they may feel less stigmatized. The group approach is probably less successful when the predominant feeling of the adolescent is betrayal. In this instance, it is more useful to offer individual psychotherapy to enable the adolescent to establish trust with the therapist, so that disclosure and discussion can occur in a confidential setting.

A more recent development has been the provision of treatment strategies for adolescents who have committed sexual offences. The latter include exhibitionism or indecent exposure as well as sexual abuse of other, usually younger, children. The treatment program involves an assessment of the offender's sexual knowledge and attitudes as well as their social skills and relationships. Treatment programs use a variety of approaches, often in combination, including social skills training, sex education and cognitive – behavioral approaches.

GENDER IDENTITY DISORDERS[87]

Society's attitudes towards sexuality have been changing in recent years, so that a more open discussion about sexual values and behavior is possible with greater tolerance and less stigma associated with homosexuality whether in males or females. Homosexual behavior in some form or another is quite common during the pre-adolescent and adolescent years, occurring in approximately 20% of boys and 10% of girls. It appears to be a transitory pattern of behavior as adult estimates of male and female homosexuality are 3% and 1.5%, respectively. Whilst homosexuality per se is most unlikely to be a reason for psychiatric referral, occasionally anxiety and depression associated with doubts about the homosexual role are sufficiently severe to warrant referral.

Clinicians are more likely to be involved with children or adolescents who have a gender identity disorder. A core distinction is made between individuals who display anomalous gender role behavior and those with gender identity disorder. Anomalous gender role behavior is the individual's preference for interests, activities and clothes normally associated with the opposite gender. For example, effeminate boys prefer girls' style of clothing and to play with dolls, whilst 'tomboy' girls like aggressive contact games and boys' style of clothing.

By contrast, the essential feature of the gender identity disorder is the persistent wish to be of the opposite gender. This is confirmed by the frequent expression of this wish and by extensive anomalous gender role behavior including cross-dressing. During adolescence, referral is often sought for problems associated with cross-dressing, homosexual behavior and social ostracism from peers. Trans-sexualism or the wish for permanent change of gender assignment can also become an issue.

The search for etiological factors in gender identity disorder has not been fruitful with no convincing evidence for chromosomal, physiological or endocrine abnormalities. Most clinicians believe that several psychosocial factors acting in combination are responsible. The initial parental tolerance of the anomalous sexual behavior followed by subsequent acceptance and reinforcement is a common finding among referred patients together with an overdependent mother–child relationship.

Treatment strategies for gender identity disorder include individual and family therapy, parental counseling and behavior therapy. The most important aspect of treatment is to define and agree goals with the parents and the child. Clinic studies[88] indicate that the earlier treatment is commenced the better the prognosis. Behavioral programs with attainable short term goals are much more likely to be successful than more ambitious plans. Minimizing anomalous gender behavior such as cross-dressing and the promotion of gender-appropriate behavior are the basis for intervention strategies. Treatment of co-existing individual and family psychopathology is also beneficial. Finally, the long term follow-up of 66 effeminate boys[88] found that three quarters were bisexual or homosexual as adults.

PSYCHIATRIC ASPECTS OF LEARNING DISABILITY IN CHILDHOOD

INTRODUCTION
Child psychiatrists are likely to become involved with children who have learning disability in several different ways. Sometimes they are responsible for the provision of the specialist medical care for these children, but more commonly they are asked for advice from other professionals about the emotional and behavioral problems that are quite frequent in this group of children.

TERMINOLOGY
Many terms such as mental *subnormality* or/and *mental handicap* have been used in the past. ICD and DSM use IQ or mental age as the basis for classification. IQ is defined as: mental age/chronological age × 100. The mean or average IQ is therefore 100 with a standard deviation of 15. The normal or Gaussian distribution of intelligence means that approximately 2.5% of individuals are two standard deviations below the mean, corresponding to an IQ of 70. This is usually taken as the dividing point between the normal range of intelligence and learning disability/mental retardation. ICD and DSM have four categories of mental retardation: mild (IQ 50–69 approximately); moderate (IQ 35–49 approximately); severe (IQ 20–34 approximately); profound (IQ less than 20). The other important defining criterion is that there should be evidence of social impairment and limitation in the individual's daily activities and self-care skills.

PSYCHIATRIC DISORDER IN CHILDREN WITH LEARNING DISABILITY
Prevalence
The IOW study[14] found that approximately one third of children with learning disability showed signs of disturbance with the rate rising to 50% among moderate to severely learning disabled children. The children exhibited the same range of disturbance as children of normal ability but in addition three disorders were much more frequent: childhood autism, pervasive hyperkinetic disorder and severe stereotyped movement disorder. Self-injurious behavior and pica were also more frequent.

Etiology
It is important to distinguish between the factors responsible for disorders occurring in mildly learning-disabled children and those with moderate to severe learning disability. The former probably have the same risk factors as children of average ability, but to a greater extent, that is adverse temperamental characteristics, specific learning disorders and family psychopathology. The latter is particularly important, as parents of children with mild learning disability are also likely to be within the lower range of intellectual ability. Consequently, their parenting capacity may be limited with inconsistent discipline and control prominent features. In addition, this may be combined with marital disharmony

and socioeconomic disadvantage, so that the vulnerability to psychiatric disturbance is considerably increased among this group of children.

By contrast, brain damage is an important causative factor among children with severe learning disability. Several studies[12,14] have reported that half the children with moderate to severe learning disability have demonstrable brain damage. This increases the risk of psychiatric disturbance in several ways: loss of specific functions or skills; active disruption or dysfunction of normal brain activity; and the increased risk of epilepsy. These children are also more likely to have specific learning difficulties that further increase vulnerability. In addition, adverse temperamental characteristics such as impulsivity, distractibility or overactivity are more common among this group of children. The psychosocial consequences of disability for the child and the family also make a factor in some cases, though its importance is difficult to quantify.

PSYCHIATRIC SYNDROMES SPECIFICALLY ASSOCIATED WITH MODERATE TO SEVERE LEARNING DISABILITY
Childhood autism
80% of children with childhood autism have an IQ less than 70. Many clinicians distinguish between individuals who have classical childhood autism from those with severe learning disability and some autistic features. The latter include stereotypies, mannerisms and deficits in comprehension and expressive language. These symptoms, which are quite common among many retarded children, tend to occur in isolation, so that the individual does not fulfil the diagnostic criteria for childhood autism. Clinical practice and research findings do not however provide clear-cut criteria to decide the dividing line between childhood autism and severe learning disability with autistic features. Consequently, clinicians tend to have their own personal preferences in terminology and classification.

Autistic behaviors are also features of some syndromes associated with learning disability such as tuberous sclerosis, congenital rubella, fragile X syndrome and infantile spasms. In some cases, for instance congenital rubella, the autistic behavior seems to be a response to the co-existing sensory deficit rather than the separate occurrence of childhood autism. Finally, individuals with the extremely uncommon neurodegenerative diseases such as subacute sclerosing panencephalitis or with disintegrative disorder often show autistic-like stereotypic behavior.

Hyperkinetic syndrome/attention deficit hyperactivity disorder
Like autistic behavior, overactive or hyperkinetic behavior is common among children with severe learning disability. In most cases, the overactivity occurs in some situations but not others with the overactivity reflecting an immaturity in behavior and language skills. A much smaller but nevertheless significant number do show pervasive hyperactivity with other features of that syndrome including distractibility, impulsivity and aggressive behavior.

Stereotypic and self-injurious behavior
Stereotypic movements such as body rocking or hand-flapping have been reported as frequently as 40% in mild to severely learning-disabled children. Self-injurious behavior such as head banging, biting of limbs or eye gauging is much less common but more potentially harmful and also difficult to eradicate. It often arises in an individual of very limited ability whose surroundings and immediate environment provide little or minimal stimulation. The Lesch–Nyhan syndrome is particularly associated with the development of self-mutilating behavior.

Murphy[89] reviewed the treatment methods for these intractable and destructive behaviors. Protective devices such as helmets, treatment with major tranquillizers such as haloperidol and behavioral approaches have all been used with some success. A real disadvantage with drug treatment is that once started it is difficult to stop, so that the individual can remain on a drug for several years, often with an increasing dose over time. A behavioral approach is more likely to produce long-lasting benefits, but it is more time consuming to carry out and more demanding of staff cooperation.

Pica

The ingestion of inedible substances is a transitory phenomenon among normal toddlers and is even more common among children with severe learning disability. The main adverse consequence of this behavior is lead intoxication from the licking of objects. Fecal smearing and ingestion can occur among some children, particularly those with an additional sensory handicap such as blindness.

LEARNING DISABILITY SYNDROMES ASSOCIATED WITH SPECIFIC BEHAVIORAL CHARACTERISTICS

Traditionally, children with certain learning disability syndromes have been said to show a characteristic behavioral or personality profile, though contemporary opinion is more sceptical about such association.

Down syndrome

Children with this syndrome are often described as sociable, musical, contented and easy going, features they share with their siblings. Overall, these children have a slightly increased rate of disturbance with a minority showing aggressive and oppositional behavior, usually associated with Down syndrome due to a translocation trisomy.

Phenylketonuria

Untreated, these children develop severe learning disability with autistic and hyperkinetic behavior prominent. Successful dietary treatment usually results in normal growth and development, but treated children have a greater risk of psychiatric disturbance with overactivity, distractibility and restlessness common.

Lesch – Nyhan syndrome

This sex-linked disorder of purine metabolism, occurring only in boys, is associated with an extrapyramidal movement disorder including chorea and athetosis, severe mental retardation and self-injurious behavior. The latter is extremely difficult to treat and eliminate.

Prader–Willi syndrome

The main behavioral feature is the explosive outbursts associated with dietary restriction frequently imposed to control the voracious appetite and accompanying obesity.

Hydrocephalus

Children with hydrocephalus were previously described as showing the 'cocktail party' syndrome. This is characterized by a verbosity to their speech and a superficiality or shallowness to the content of their conversation. The early detection and treatment of hydrocephalus has now produced a reduction in morbidity, so that these features are less commonly seen.

Management

Many professionals including pediatricians, teachers and psychologists are likely to be involved in the provision of care for children with learning disabilities and their families. A multidisciplinary approach to assessment and treatment is vital. Different aspects of management are important at various stages during the child's life.

Breaking the news

This topic is discussed more fully in the child section of the chapter, so that only brief comments are made here. The ability to communicate bad news in a sensitive manner is a skill rarely taught to medical students or junior doctors. Many parents complain justifiably that the initial interview with the doctor was unsatisfactory and distressing. Tact, sympathy and time are essential to enable the parent(s) to begin to grasp and understand the implications of the situation. Honest discussion combined with an emphasis on the hopeful aspects are the important prerequisites for a satisfactory interview.

Promotion of normal development

Parents should be encouraged from the outset to develop the social, self-care and educational skills of their child to the maximum. A 'normalization' and 'optimalization' strategy is the basis to the approach. Specific treatment packages, for example the Portage scheme, are helpful in enabling the parents to set realistic targets for their child.

Treatment of medical and behavioral problems

Advice from neurologists, physiotherapists and occupational therapists is important in the management of the neurological deficits frequently present among this group of children. Behavioral problems are managed in a variety of ways including medication (for hyperactivity and aggressive outbursts), protective devices (for excessive head-banging) and operant or time-out procedures (for maladaptive behavior).

Educational needs

Parents need advice from an early stage about the most appropriate educational provision. A specialized pre-school nursery is vital, and should be combined with a plan for later special educational placement. Some children may benefit from attendance at schools for children with communication or autistic-like disorders.

Genetic counseling

This is clearly essential for all parents, especially when a specific syndrome is identified.

Long term casework and support

Clinical experience and practice suggest that many families find this type of help invaluable in the long term. The identification of a key professional worker who coordinates the care plan for the child is very useful. A social worker or a professional from a voluntary organization with counseling skills is often the person best placed to fulfil this role.

Outcome

Treatment programs with an emphasis on maximizing potential, minimizing adverse effects and integrating the child into the community are the best approach. Despite cognitive impairment, behavioral problems can be reduced by the treatment program, and families learn to adapt satisfactorily. The policy of the UK Government is to close institutions for individuals with learning disability and to integrate them into the community in order to promote better long term adjustment.

REFERENCES

1. Goodyer I. Life experiences. Development and childhood psychopathology. Chichester: Wiley; 1990.
2. Bee H. The developing child. 9th edn. New York: Harper; 1999.
3. Matthews S. Cognitive development. In: Bryant P, Colman A, eds. Developmental psychology. London: Longman; 1994.
4. Hawton K, Salkovskis P, Kirk J, et al. Cognitive behaviour therapy for psychiatric problems: a practical guide. 2nd edn. Oxford: Oxford University Press; 1995.

5. Johnstone E, Owens D, Lawrie S, et al. Companion to psychiatric studies. 7th edn. Edinburgh: Churchill Livingstone; 2004.
6. Erikson E. Childhood and society. London: Penguin; 1965.
7. Bowlby J. Attachment and loss, vol. 1: Attachment London: Hogarth Press; 1969.
8. Ainsworth M. Attachment: retrospect and prospect. In: Parkes CM, Stevenson-Hinde J, eds. The place of attachment in human behaviour. New York: Basic Books; 1982.
9. Freud A. The ego and the mechanisms of defence. London: Hogarth Press; 1936.

10. World Health Organization. The ICD-10 classification of mental and behaviour disorders: clinical descriptions and diagnostic guidelines. Geneva: World Health Organization; 1992.
11. American Psychiatric Association. Diagnostic and statistical manual of mental disorders. 4th edn. Washington DC: American Psychiatric Association; 1994.
12. Rutter M, Tizard J, Whitmore K. Education, health and behaviour. London: Longmans; 1970.
13. Rutter M, Yule B, Quinton D, et al. Attainment and adjustment in two geographical areas. III. Some factors accounting for area differences. Br J Psychiatry 1975; 126:520–533.

14. Rutter M, Graham P, Yule W. A neuropsychiatric study of childhood. Clinics in developmental medicine, nos. 35/36, London: SIMP/Heinemann; 1970.

15. Meltzer H, Gatward R. Mental health of children and adolescents in Great Britain. London: The Stationary Office; 2000.

16. Richman N, Stevenson J, Graham P. Pre-school to school: a behavioural study. London: Academic Press; 1982.

17. Bailey N. Bailey's Scales II. San Antonio: Psychological Corporation; 1993.

18. Huntley M. Griffiths mental development scales from birth to two years. London: Association for Research on Infant and Child Development; 1996.

19. Kaufman A, Kaufman N. Kaufman Assessment Battery for Children (K-ABC). Circle Pines: American Guidance Service; 1983.

20. Wechsler D. Manual for the Wechsler Intelligence Scale for Children – Third UK Edition (WISC-III UK). Kent: Psychological Corporation; 1992.

21. Thorndike R, Hagen E, Sattler J. Stanford Binet Intelligence Scale. 4th edn. San Antonio: Psychological Corporation; 1986.

22. Elliott C. British Ability Scales Second Edition (BASI II). Windsor: National Foundation for Educational Research/Nelson; 1996.

23. Rust J. Wechsler Individual Achievement Tests. San Antonio: Psychological Corporation; 1995.

24. Neale MD. Neale Analysis of Reading Ability Test. 2nd edn. Windsor: National Foundation for Educational Research/Nelson; 1989.

25. Reynell J. Reynell Developmental Language Scales. Windsor: Second Revision NFER; 1985.

26. Achenbach T. Integrative Guide for the 1991 CBCL/4–18, YSR and TRF Profiles. Burlington: University of Vermont; 1991.

27. Goodman R. The Strengths and Difficulties Questionnaire: a research note. J Child Psychol Psychiatry 1997; 38:581–586.

28. Thomas A, Chess S, Birch H. Temperament and behaviour disorders in childhood. New York: New York University Press; 1968.

29. Brown G, Harris T. Social origins of depression. London: Tavistock; 1978.

30. Richman N, Lansdown R. Problems of pre-school children. Chichester: Wiley; 1988.

31. Skuse D, Wolke D, Reilly S. Failure to thrive. Clinical and developmental aspects. In: Remschmidt H, Schmidt M, eds. Child and youth psychiatry, European perspectives. vol. II: Developmental psychopathology. Stuttgart: Hans Huber; 1992.

32. Morrell J. The infant sleep questionnaire: a new tool to assess infant sleep problems for clinical and research purposes. Child Psychol Psychiatry Rev 1999; 4:20–26.

33. Jan J, Espezel H, Appleton P. The treatment of sleep disorders. Develop Med Child Neurol 1994; 36:97–107.

34. Briere J, Berliner L, Buckley J, et al. The ASPAC Handbook on Child Maltreatment. Thousand Oaks: Sage Publications; 1996.

35. Stevenson J. Treatment of sequelae of child abuse. J Child Psychol Psychiatry 1999; 40:89–112.

36. Bentovim A, Elton A, Hildebrand J, et al. Sexual abuse within the family. London: Wright; 1988.

37. Eminson M, Postlethwaite R. Munchausen by proxy: a practical approach. Oxford: Butterworth-Heinemann; 1999.

38. Cohen D, Volkmar F. A handbook of autism and pervasive developmental disorders. Chichester: Wiley; 1997.

39. Gillberg C. Clinical child neuropsychiatry. Cambridge: Cambridge University Press; 1995.

40. Kanner L. Autistic disturbances of affective contact. The Nervous Child 1943; 2:217–250.

41. Chakrabarti S, Fombonne E. Pervasive developmental disorders in pre-school children. J Am Med Assoc 2001; 285:3094–3098.

42. Farrington CP, Miller E, Taylor B. MMR and autism: further evidence against a causal association. Vaccine 2001; 19:3632–3635.

43. Lord C, Rutter M. Autism and other pervasive developmental disorders. In: Rutter M, Taylor E, Hersov L, eds. Child and adolescent psychiatry: Modern approaches. 3rd edn. Oxford: Blackwell; 1994.

44. Hagberg B. Rett syndrome – clinical and biological aspects. London: MacKeith Press; 1993.

45. Rutter M, Schopler E, eds. Autism: a reappraisal of concepts and treatment. New York: Plenum Press; 1988.

46. Pennington B, Ozonoff. Executive functions and developmental psychopathology. J Child Psychol Psychiatry 1996; 37:51–88.

47. Baron-Cohen S. Mindblindness. London: MIT Press; 1995.

48. Hobson P. Autism and the development of mind. Hove: Lawrence Erlbaum Associates; 1993.

49. Asperger H. 'Die Autistischen psychopathen' im kindesalter. Archive für Psychiatrie und Nervenkrankheiten 1944; 117:76–136.

50. Wolff S, Chick J. Schizoid personality in childhood: a controlled follow-up study. Psychol Med 1980; 10:85–100.

51. Wolff S. Schizoid personality in childhood and adult life III: The childhood picture. Br J Psychiatry 1991; 159:629–635.

52. Corbett J, Harris R, Taylor E, et al. Progressive disintegrative psychosis of childhood. J Child Psychol Psychiatry 1977; 18:211–219.

53. Berg I. Absence from school and mental health. Br J Psychiatry 1992; 161:154–166.

54. Shafran R. Obsessive–compulsive disorders in children and adolescents. Child Psychology Psychiatry Rev 2001; 6:50–58.

55. Garralda E. Somatisation in children. J Child Psychol Psychiatry 1996; 37:13–33.

56. Yule W. Posttraumatic stress disorder. In: Rutter M, Taylor E, Hersov L, eds. Child and adolescent psychiatry: Modern approaches. 3rd edn. Oxford: Blackwell; 1994.

57. Webster-Stratton C, Herbert M. Troubled families – Problem children. Chichester: Wiley; 1993.

58. Taylor E, Sergeant J, Doepfner M, et al. Clinical guidelines for hyperkinetic disorder. Eur Child Adolesc Psychiatry 1998; 7:184–200.

59. NIHCE Report. Methylphenidate, atomoxetine and dexamfhetamine for attention deficit hyperactivity disorder in children and adolescents. London: NIHCE; 2006. 2006.

60. MTA Co-operative Group. Fourteen-month randomized clinical trial of treatment strategies for attention deficit hyperactivity disorder. Arch Gen Psychiatry 1999; 56:1073–1086.

61. Egger J, Stolla A, McEwan L. Controlled trial of hyposensitisation in children with food-induced hyperkinetic syndrome. Lancet 1992; 339:1150–1153.

62. Bierderman J, Faraone S, Spencer T, et al. Patterns of comorbidity, cognition, and psychosocial functioning in adults with attention deficit hyperactivity disorder. Am J Psychiatry 1993; 150:1792–1798.

63. Spencer T, Wilens T, Biederman J, et al. A double-blind crossover comparison of methylphenidate in adults with childhood-onset attention deficit hyperactivity disorder. Arch Gen Psychiatry 1995; 52:434–443.

64. Dummit E, Klein R, Tancer N, et al. Fluoxetine treatment of children with selective mutism. J Am Acad Child Adolesc Psychiatry 1996; 35:615–621.

65. Lask B. Novel and non-toxic treatment for night terrors. BMJ 1988; 297:592.

66. Kutcher S. Practical child & adolescent psychopharmacology. Cambridge: Cambridge University Press; 2002.

67. Lanyardo M, Horne A. A handbook of child and adolescent psychotherapy. London: Routledge; 1999.

68. Freud A. The psychological treatment of children. London: Imago; 1946.

69. Reisman JM. Principles of psychotherapy with children. 2nd edn. New York: Wiley; 1973.

70. Herbert M. ABC of behavioural methods. Leicester: British Psychological Society; 1996.

71. Kendall P. Child and adolescent therapy: cognitive-behavioural procedures. New York: Guilford Press; 1999.

72. Gorrell Barnes G. Family therapy. In: Rutter M, Taylor E, Hersov L, eds. Child and adolescent psychiatry: Modern approaches. 3rd edn. Oxford: Blackwell; 1994.

73. Lask B. Paediatric liaison work. In: Rutter M, Taylor E, Hersov L, eds. Child and adolescent psychiatry: Modern approaches. 3rd edn. Oxford: Blackwell; 1994.

74. King R, Leonard H, March J, et al. Practice parameters for the assessment and treatment of children and adolescents with obsessive–compulsive disorder. J Am Acad Child Adolesc Psychiatry 1998; 39 (Suppl):27S–47S.

75. Hollis C. Adolescent schizophrenia. Advances in Psychiatric Treatment 2000; 6:83–92.

76. Goodyer I. The depressed child and adolescent: developmental and clinical perspectives. Cambridge: Cambridge University Press; 1995.

77. Park R, Goodyer I. Clinical guidelines for depressive disorders in childhood and adolescence. Eur Child Adolesc Psychiatry 2000; 9:147–161.

78. Rutter M, Graham P, Chadwick O, et al. Adolescent turmoil: fact or fiction? J Child Psychol Psychiatr 1976; 17:35–56.

79. Beck A, Rush A, Shaw B, et al. Cognitive therapy of depression. New York: Wiley; 1979.

80. Emslie G, Rush J, Weinberg W, et al. A double blind, randomized, placebo-controlled trial of fluoxetine in child and adolescents with depression. Arch Gen Psychiatr 1997; 54:1031–1037.

81. Shaffer D, Piancentini J. Suicide and attempted suicide. In: Rutter M, Taylor E, Hersov L, eds. Child and adolescent psychiatry: Modern approaches. 3rd edn. Oxford: Blackwell; 1994.

82. Gowers S, Bryant-Waugh R. Management of child and adolescent eating disorders: the current evidence-base and future directions. J Child Psychol Psychiatry 2004; 45:63–83.

83. Russell G, Szmulker G, Dare C, et al. An evaluation of family therapy in anorexia nervosa and bulimia nervosa. Arch Gen Psychiatry 1987; 44:1047–1056.

84. Gorralda E, Chalder T. Chronic fatigue in childwood. J Child Psychol Psychiatry 2005; 46:1143–1151.

85. Miller P, Platt M. Drinking, smoking and illicit drug use among 15 and 16 year olds in the United Kingdom. BMJ 1996; 313:394–397.

86. Ashton C. Solvent abuse: little progress after twenty years. BMJ 1990; 300:135–136.

87. Di Ceglie D. Gender identity disorder in young people. Advances in Psychiatric Treatment 2000; 6:458–467.

88. Zucker K, Bradley S. Gender identity disorder and psychosexual problems in children and adolescents. New York: Plenum Press; 1995.

89. Murphy G. Update—self-injuring behaviour in the mentally handicapped. Assoc Child Psychol Psychiatry Newsletter 1985; 7:2–11.

35

Adolescent medicine

Russell Viner

WHAT IS ADOLESCENCE?

Strictly speaking, adolescence is the period between childhood and adulthood. But finding a useful definition of adolescence is difficult. Biologically it is the time of sexual maturation and the completion of growth. More than mere biology, adolescence is psychosocially the period between childhood dependency and being a functionally independent autonomous adult. Theorists have viewed adolescence in different ways; Freud saw adolescence as the period of recapitulation of the childhood Oedipal complex, while Erickson claimed that the struggle between Identity and Role Confusion typified the adolescent stage of development.[1]

Chronological definitions abound and are more pragmatic for allowing us to identify who is or is not an 'adolescent'. The World Health Organization for example defines adolescence as the second decade of life, from 10 to 20 years of age, but also defines a category of 'youth' as being 10–25 years.[2] However, chronological definitions take little account of the developmental changes of adolescence and their temporal variation, failing to apply to certain cultures or to those who are early or late developers. Because of this, some have suggested that adolescence is merely a social construct, a rite of passage that is culturally and socially invented.[3] These claims ignore the biological changes of puberty and the psychological developments driven by increasing CNS maturation and myelination. The most useful definition of adolescence is that it is a period of biopsychosocial maturation between the ages of 10 and 20 years, leading to functional independence in adult life. This definition has been adopted by the Royal Medical Colleges in the UK.[4]

WHY IS A SPECIAL MEDICAL APPROACH NEEDED FOR ADOLESCENTS?

Adolescence, the period between childhood and adulthood, is increasingly recognized as a life period that poses specific challenges for treating disease and promoting health. In working with adolescents, the treatment of disease, the prevention of ill-health and the promotion of healthy behaviors are played out against a background of rapid physical, psychological and social developmental changes – changes that produce specific disease patterns, unusual symptom presentations, and above all, unique communication and management challenges. At no other time of life are the physical and the psychosocial elements of illness and behavior so inextricably intertwined as in adolescence. This can make working with adolescents difficult. However given the right skills (which can be learned!), practicing medicine with young people can be extremely rewarding and fruitful. These skills are not only for those who deal solely with young people, but are needed by all in pediatric practice. Specific skills in adolescent health are recognized as being necessary for the practice of pediatrics in the UK,[5] the USA and other countries.

The reasons for a distinct approach to medicine with adolescents are outlined below.

ADOLESCENTS ARE A LARGE CLIENT GROUP

One argument for considering adolescents differently to children is sheer numbers; young people between 10 and 20 years of age make up between 12% and 15% of the population in most resource rich countries (13% in the UK), a client group as large as children under 10 in the UK. Projections suggest that the adolescent population will grow by 8.5% between 1998 and 2011.[6] While adolescence is generally considered to be a healthy period, health resource use by young people is higher than in late childhood.[7] Most adolescents visit their general practitioner (GP) each year,[8] around 30% have a chronic condition that requires some health resource utilization,[9] mental health resource use is higher than in childhood[10] and hospital bed use is higher during adolescence than in late childhood.[11]

ADOLESCENTS HAVE A UNIQUE EPIDEMIOLOGY OF DISEASE AND HEALTH RISK

The second argument for a special approach to adolescent health is that young people have a distinct epidemiology of disease and health risk. The diseases that are unique to adolescence are small in number (Table 35.1). But both disease and health behaviors in adolescents present a unique constellation of symptoms and problems not found in children or adults. **1571**

Table 35.1   Disorders unique to adolescence or with onset predominantly in adolescence

Disorders of puberty and pubertal growth
Adolescent idiopathic scoliosis
Juvenile idiopathic arthritis – subtypes
Adolescent acne
Eating disoders (anorexia nervosa; bulimia nervosa)
Mental disorders, e.g. conduct disorder; adolescent psychosis

Those practicing with adolescents must be familiar with both persistent or late-onset 'pediatric' diseases and with early-onset 'adult' diseases. In each, ongoing adolescent development produces characteristic symptom patterns and management problems that meld the biological with the psychosocial in unique ways. For example, type 1 diabetes has its peak age of incidence around 12–14 years, and the growth hormone excess of puberty and the psychosocial challenges of chronic illness self-management produces poorer metabolic control during adolescence than at any other age.[12] Furthermore, puberty itself accelerates the progression of diabetic complications such as nephropathy.[13] Cancer during adolescence is remarkable for its threats of mortality to a personality with a newly developing sense of identity and place in the world, but also in its combination of 'late' presentations of pediatric type cancers (e.g. rhabdomyosarcoma, medulloblastoma), 'age-specific' cancers of adolescence (e.g. bone tumors) and early onset 'adult-type' carcinomas.[14]

INCREASING SURVIVAL FROM AND INCIDENCE OF CHRONIC ILLNESS IN YOUNG PEOPLE

The increase in the prevalence of chronic illness among adolescents is changing the pattern of pediatric practice, and it is likely that young people will in the future make up a larger part of the pediatric workload. This has been driven by an increasing incidence of common chronic illnesses such as asthma and diabetes, but also by increasing survival from congenital diseases previously fatal in childhood. Cohort studies in the UK report a 70% increase in the prevalence of wheezing illness at age 16 years between 1974 and 1986, with further rises apparent in the 1990s.[15] It has been reported that almost 20% of UK 12–14 year olds used asthma medications in the past 12 months.[15] Diabetes in 10–14 year olds has increased by almost 24% Europe-wide during the past 10 years,[16] and the incidence of type 2 diabetes has risen dramatically in adolescents, particularly in minority ethnic populations.[17]

Advances in the last 20 years in the treatment of metabolic conditions, cystic fibrosis and congenital heart disease has produced new cohorts of young people surviving into adolescence and early adulthood.[18–21] The prevalence of cystic fibrosis over 15 years of age in the UK more than doubled between 1977 and 1985,[21] and currently over 85% of children with chronic illness survive to adult life.[20]

HEALTH BEHAVIORS ARE LAID DOWN IN ADOLESCENCE AND CONTINUE INTO ADULT LIFE

One of the most compelling arguments for a focus on adolescent health is that adolescence is a time when new health behaviors are laid down, behaviors that track into adulthood and will influence health and morbidity life-long. Health behaviors in childhood are dominated by parental instruction and shared family values. During adolescence young people begin to explore alternative or 'adult' health behaviors, including smoking, drinking, drug use, violence and sexual intimacy. The continuities between adolescent initiation of health behaviors and adult behavior are well documented. Regular smoking rates rise from 1% at 11 years to 24% at 15 years,[22] and over 90% of adult smokers began in the teenage years.[23] Depression and its related mental health problems are rare in childhood, but rise through puberty to adult levels in late adolescence.[24]

Equally importantly, health behaviors around exercise and food are laid down in adolescence and track into adult life. Adolescent obesity

predicts adult obesity,[25] which is strongly and independently predictive of cardiovascular risk,[26,27] and cardiovascular risk in young adulthood is highly related to the degree of adiposity as early as age 13 years.[25]

ADOLESCENTS HAVE UNIQUE NEEDS IN THE MANAGEMENT OF HEALTH AND ILLNESS

Dynamic and continued development in every aspect of a young person's life during adolescence means that young people have distinct needs in the management of illness and health. In clinical interactions with younger children, management decisions are made 'adult to adult' by health professionals in consultation with parents, and day-to-day disease management is generally undertaken directly by parents. When working with adolescents, the wishes, desires, knowledge base, capabilities and rights of the young person involved must also be taken into account – as must the fact that these wishes, desires, knowledge, capabilities and rights are constantly evolving and changing! Different approaches are required to all aspects of the doctor–patient relationship. Specialized clinical communication skills are needed to take an accurate history, bearing in mind new life domains not applicable to children (sex and drugs) and adding communication and engagement of the young person to the standard pediatric communication with the family. Physical examinations of adolescents require consideration of privacy and personal integrity as well as requiring additional skills such as pubertal assessment, breast examination and possibly genital examinations. The effective treatment of illness in adolescence requires adept management of the issues regarding adherence (compliance), consent and confidentiality, and relationships between the young person and their family.

INCREASING SOCIAL MORBIDITIES AND MORTALITY LEVELS

Perhaps the most cogent argument for specific attention to adolescent health lies in the public health arena. The causes of mortality and morbidity in adolescents are distinct from both children and adults, as environmental or social causes of mortality (e.g. accidents and suicide) make up a larger proportion of total adolescent mortality than at any other age. In most public health priority areas, including cardiovascular risk (obesity, diabetes, smoking), mental health (suicide) and sexual health (teenage pregnancy and sexually transmitted diseases (STI)), the extent of problems in young people is stable or increasing rather than diminishing (Table 35.2).

Suicide rates among older male teenagers doubled over the last three decades of the 20th century and remain high.[28] Obesity has doubled among teenagers in the past 10 years, leading to the emergence of type 2 diabetes as a significant clinical and public health problem.[29,30] While smoking rates have fallen among teenage boys, rates among teenage girls have risen over the past 20 years. Earlier sexual debut and increased rates of high-risk sexual activity have lead to high rates of teenage pregnancy and STIs in countries with poor sexual and relationship education such as the UK and USA. Given explicit evidence of the continuities between adolescent and adult health risk behaviors, adolescent morbidity trends argue strongly for urgent attention to adolescent health and the development of targeted adolescent-specific interventions.

ADOLESCENT DEVELOPMENT

All clinical interactions with adolescents must be seen against the dynamic background of continued development. For example, chronic illness management issues can be quite different between a 13-year-old boy in very early puberty who has poorly developed abstract thinking and a 16-year-old girl who is sexually mature, at final height and has well-developed adult cognitive skills. The developmental tasks or events of adolescence are outlined in Table 35.3. While we group development for convenience into early, mid- and late adolescence, it

Table 35.2 Trends in indicators of adolescent health over the past two decades. (Adapted from Viner & Barker 2005[78])

Key indicator area	Outcome	Direction of change in past 30 years	Detail
Cardiovascular risk	Obesity	⬆	The prevalence of adolescent obesity (defined as BMI ≥95th centile) has quadrupled in representative samples since 1970s, rising from 4–5% in 1972[72] to 8% in the mid-1990s[73] and 21–23% in 2002
	Smoking	⬅	There has been no significant change in prevalence of regular smoking among adolescents aged 11–15 years since 1982,[74] while smoking among adults declined significantly during the 1980s and early 1990s[75]
Sexual health	Teenage pregnancy	⬅	Live birth rates to women aged 15–19 years in the UK have changed little since the late 1970s, while rates have declined markedly in the same period in other European countries such as Germany and the Netherlands[76]
	STIs	⬆	Rates of uncomplicated *Chlamydia* infections among 16- to 19-year-old females doubled during the 1990s in the UK (PHLS)
Mental health	Suicide	⬆	In contrast to dramatic declines in suicide rates among men and women over 45 years of age between 1950 and 1998, among 15–24 year olds, suicide rates doubled in young men and remained stable in young women[28,77]

is important to remember that the timing and tempo of biological, psychological and social development each proceed independently in each individual, although each strand can influence the others. Those who are pubertally early developers may be late in developing cognitive skills or vice versa, and it is imperative to assess biological and psychosocial maturity separately. Gender issues are important here, as the timing of biological and psychosocial maturation is subtly different in boys and girls.

BIOLOGICAL CHANGES

The biological changes of adolescence are puberty, the pubertal growth spurt, and accompanying maturational changes in other organ systems. The processes and timing of puberty and pubertal assessment skills are outlined in Chapter 15. The defining event of puberty in girls is menarche. The mean age at menarche showed a dramatic decline in most resource rich countries through the first half of the 20th century, stabilizing in the 1960s at 12.8 years in the USA and 13.2 years in the

Table 35.3 Developmental tasks of adolescence

	Biological	Psychological	Social
Early adolescence	Early puberty *Girls:* Breast bud and pubic hair development (Tanner Stage II); initiation of growth spurt *Boys:* Testicular enlargement; beginning of genital growth (Stage II)	Thinking remains concrete but with development of early moral concepts Progression of sexual identity development: development of sexual orientation – possibly by experimentation Possible homosexual peer interest Reassessment and restructuring of body image in face of rapid growth	Realization of differences from parents Beginning of strong peer identification Early exploratory behaviors (smoking, violence)
Mid-adolescence	*Girls:* Mid to late puberty (Stages IV–V) and completion of growth Menarche (Stage IV event) Development of female body shape with fat deposition *Boys:* Mid-puberty (Stages III and IV) Spermarche and nocturnal emissions Voice breaking Initiation of growth spurt (Stages III–IV)	Emergence of abstract thinking although ability to imagine future applies to others rather than self (self seen as 'bullet-proof') Growing verbal abilities; adaptation to increasing educational demands Conventional morality (identification of law with morality) Development of fervently held ideology (religious/political)	Establishment of emotional separation from parents Strong peer group identification Increased health risk behaviors (smoking, alcohol, drugs, sexual exploration) Heterosexual peer interests develop Early vocational plans Development of an educational trajectory; early notions of vocational future
Late adolescence	*Boys:* Completion of pubertal development (Stage V) Continued androgenic effects on muscle bulk and body hair	Complex abstract thinking Postconventional morality (ability to recognize difference between law and morality) Increased impulse control Further completion of personal identity Further development or rejection of ideology and religion – often fervently	Further separation from parents and development of social autonomy Development of intimate relationships – initially within peer group, then separation of couples from peer group Development of vocational capability, potential or real financial independence

UK.[31] Despite recent controversy, the evidence is clear that there has been no change in the age of menarche in the USA or the UK over the past 40 years.[31]

As well as completion of linear growth and sexual maturation, other biological systems develop their final adult form during adolescence. These include maturation of enzyme systems such as cytochrome P450 systems, accretion of peak bone mass, and the development of sexually dimorphic adult patterns in blood lipids, haemoglobin and red cell indices.

PSYCHOLOGICAL DEVELOPMENT

Psychological changes in thought patterns and cognitive ability are driven by increasing maturation and myelination of the adolescent brain.[32] Between the ages of 6 and 11 years, children generally think concretely, understanding only the immediate and short-term consequence of actions or events. Ideas and concepts can only be manipulated through using concrete representations. From the age of 12 years onwards, thought patterns begin to change to formal operational or abstract thought, the ability to manipulate ideas rather than things, imagine the future, and conceive of multiple outcomes of actions. These capacities are important for the development of a settled personal and sexual identity.[33] These psychological changes, like the biological changes of puberty, are universal to all races and cultures. However, the majority of psychological and social development is culture specific, varying with social and cultural norms regarding the roles of children and adults in society.

SOCIAL DEVELOPMENT

The social changes of adolescence are outlined in Table 35.3. Biological and psychological changes occur within the context of an individual's social environment. The essential social tasks of adolescence are developing a sense of personal identity, moving from dependence to independence, and developing mature relationship with peers. These challenges exist across all cultures; however the timing of changes and the point at which successful completion is expected varies greatly between cultures.[34] In Western societies, adolescence commonly extends over many years, with its endpoints marked by relative financial independence after the completion of education. By contrast, in some societies, the social rights and responsibilities of adulthood are conferred at initiation ceremonies or rites.

IMPLICATIONS OF ADOLESCENT DEVELOPMENT FOR HEALTH

It is the reciprocal impacts of adolescent development on disease management and health-related quality of life that pose the greatest challenges of adolescent medicine. This is especially true in chronic conditions (Table 35.4). A chronic illness or disability of any type may retard normal adolescent development, producing pubertal and growth delay, delayed social independence, poor body and sexual self-image and educational and vocational failure. Doctors, including both pediatricians and adult physicians, are poor at monitoring growth and pubertal development in adolescents with chronic illness, and attention is required to growth in chronic illness well into the early twenties.[35]

Being chronically ill, having a visible disability or being required to adhere to difficult treatment regimens is difficult at all ages – but particularly so during adolescence. Alienation from the peer group and absence from school cause social isolation, failure of socialization and ultimately, educational and vocational failure. The importance of thinking proactively about helping young people with chronic illness or disability develop independent adult living and vocational skills has been shown in longitudinal follow-up studies.[36]

Conversely, adolescent development issues impact upon the management of illness and disability. Poor adherence to medical regimens and poor disease management are virtually developmentally 'appropriate' in adolescence. Immature abilities to imagine future consequences allied with a concept of themselves as 'bullet-proof' means that the prevention of long-term complications of illness is a poor motivator for compliance. Additionally, medical advice may be rejected as part of a young person's growing independence from parents, particularly in chronic pediatric illnesses where medical staff have become medical 'parents'. Adherence and disease control are also put at risk by the developmental need to explore possible modes of future behavior, no matter how dangerous (usually derogatively referred to as 'adolescent risk-taking'). Health risk behaviors such as smoking, alcohol and drug use are as common in adolescents with chronic illness or disability as in the general population.[37]

Developmental issues in adolescent medicine are becoming more important, as the burden of chronic illness in adolescence increases as larger numbers of chronically ill children survive into the second and third decades.

Table 35.4   Reciprocal effects of chronic illness or disability and adolescent development

Effects of chronic illness or disability on development	Effects of developmental issues on chronic illness or disability
Biological: Delayed puberty Short stature Reduced bone mass accretion	*Biologically:* Increased caloric requirement for growth may negatively impact on disease parameters Pubertal hormones may impact upon disease parameters (e.g. growth hormone impairs metabolic control in diabetes)
Psychological: Infantilization Adoption of sick role as personal identifier Egocentricity persists into late adolescence Impaired development of sense of sexual or attractive self	*Poor adherence and poor disease control due to:* Poorly developed abstract thinking and planning (reduced ability to plan and prepare using abstract concepts) Difficulty in imagining the future; self-concept as being 'bullet-proof' Rejection of medical professionals as part of separation from parents Exploratory (risk-taking) behaviors
Social: Reduced independence at a time when independence is normally developing Failure of peer relationships then intimate (couple) relationships Social isolation Educational failure and then vocational failure; failure of development of independent living ability	*Associated health risk behaviors:* Chaotic eating habits may result in poor nutrition Smoking, alcohol and drug use often in excess of normal population rates Sexual risk-taking, possibly in view of realization of limited life span

RESILIENCE AND RISK IN ADOLESCENT HEALTH

Morbidity in adolescence is generally understood to result from 'risk-taking', impulsivity, the rejection of parental values and the testing of boundaries. But the standard conceptions of adolescents as risk-takers with poor future thinking abilities have been shown to be largely false.[38] Most adults take as many risks and have equally poor future thinking abilities as the majority of young people. Indeed, mental health problems, drug use and sexual risk-taking is co-morbid in the same way in adults as occurs in adolescents.[39,40] That adults seem to take fewer risks is largely because they have learned to more effectively manage the consequences of their risk-taking. It is more helpful to understand so-called 'risk-taking' behaviors in young people as developmentally appropriate 'exploratory behaviors'; i.e. young people exploring the diversity of possible adult behaviors open to them – behaviors that they may or may not continue as adults.

Once these behaviors are understood to be largely developmentally motivated, it becomes unsurprising that interventions based upon education about 'risk' behaviors show very poor results.[41] Large studies of adolescent behavior and health show convincingly that health risk behaviors of all types (substance misuse, sexual risk, suicide, injuries and violence) occur together, and are strongly associated with deprivation and ethnicity.[42] Conversely, high family, community and school support ('connectedness' or 'social capital') are protective against most health risk behaviors in adolescents.[42] Identifying such 'resilience' or protective factors is now the focus of public health interventions with young people, and known protective factors for different behaviors are outlined in Table 35.5.

The search for protective factors applies equally to clinical management of acute or chronic illness in young people. In young people with poor control of a chronic illness, it is traditional to search for causes of poor control and why things go wrong. In a young person with recurrent hospital admissions with asthma, for example, causes of exacerbations may be a lack of education or lack of a crisis plan, or psychological problems including non-adherence and manipulation of the treatment regimen. In some cases, it may be more fruitful to examine 'what has helped' and what has kept the young person out of hospital between admissions. This 'solution-focused' approach, asking young people what resources they have used to stay well between exacerbations, can be very effective in treating poor chronic illness control.[42]

THE MANAGEMENT OF ILL-HEALTH IN ADOLESCENCE

Most doctors (with the notable exceptions of neonatologists and geriatricians) have adolescents in their practice. But many are not comfortable or skilled in dealing with adolescents. American studies suggest that only around a third of physicians and pediatricians actually like working with adolescents and that around another third have very little interest in adolescent care.[43]

The effective management of young people with acute or chronic illnesses requires a nonjudgemental communication style, knowledge of adolescent development and an awareness of consent and confidentiality issues, and an ethnographic approach which aims at understanding the health beliefs and contexts in which the young person manages their disease.

COMMUNICATION WITH YOUNG PEOPLE

Consultations with adolescents differ from pediatric consultations in that the young person forms a more important and more problematic third party in the decision-making process. In working with young people, we must communicate not with another adult, but with a personality undergoing rapid psychological and social changes who may or may not share an adult's understanding of society nor adult cognitive abilities to decide between treatment alternatives in the light of future risk.

Effective clinical communication is a basic health right for young people, as well as being necessary for effective disease management. Yet adolescents report that they frequently find communication with doctors unsatisfactory, with doctors often seen as remote and judgmental figures whose confidentiality cannot be trusted.[44] Communication with adolescents requires an understanding of the cognitive and social developmental level of the young person and a nonjudgmental understanding of the social contexts of that individual's health behaviors. Important elements of effective communication with young people are outlined in Table 35.6.

Table 35.5 Identified risk and protective factors for adolescent morbidities and health behaviors

Behavior	Risk factors	Protective factors
Smoking	Depression[61] Alcohol use[59] Disconnectedness from school or family[59] Difficulty talking with parents[59] Minority ethnicity[62,63] Low school achievement[42] Peer smoking and high peer popularity[64]	Family connectedness[42] Perceived healthiness[59] Higher parental expectations[42] Low school smoking prevalence[64]
Alcohol and substance use	Depression[62] Low self-esteem[42] Easy family access to alcohol[42] Ethnicity[62] Working outside school[42] Difficulty talking with parents[59] Risk factors for transition from occasional to regular use are cigarette smoking, availability, peer use and other risk behaviors[65]	Connectedness with school and family[42] Religious affiliation[42]
Teenage pregnancy	Disadvantage Urbanicity Low educational expectations[66,67] Lack of access to sexual health services[68,69] Drug and alcohol use[70]	Religious affiliation[71] Parental connectedness and expectations[42,67,68]
Sexually transmitted infections (STI)	Psychological disturbance[40] Substance use[40]	

Table 35.6 Practical points for communicating and working with adolescents

Assure confidentiality – both in the clinical interaction and in the clinical/hospital set up

See young people by themselves as well as with their parents. The best strategy for getting the parents out of the room is warning families when you first see them that you routinely see adolescents by themselves as a way of respecting their rights as a young person

Be empathic, respectful and nonjudgemental and try to avoid taking the 'expert' position. Treat the young person as the expert in their own condition, with the doctor as the medical advisor. Find out what the young person's goals are for their treatment and health, and negotiate matching treatments to their health goals

Try to communicate and explain concepts in a developmentally appropriate fashion. This is particularly important in health promotion. For young adolescents, concentrate on concrete 'here-and-now' issues and avoid abstract discussions, particularly about possible future health risks. You may need to repeat the information in a different form as they mature cognitively

Be yourself and don't be 'cool' or use youth language. Young people don't want you as a friend, they want a knowledgeable doctor whom they can respect and trust

Provide an emotionally and physically safe environment. A gender balance among staff is important, particularly where physical examinations are undertaken

Take a full psychosocial history when seeing young people for the first time, for example using the HEADSS protocol (see Table 35.7)

Table 35.7 HEADSS psychosocial assessment interview[46]

H	Home life including relationship with parents
E	Education or employment, including achievements and financial issues
A	Activities: particularly friendships and social relationships and the existence of close friends that the young person can rely on and talk to. Also participation in sports and exercise
D	Drug use, including cigarettes and alcohol
S	Sex: information on intimate relationships and sexual risk behaviors may be important in both acute and chronic illnesses in adolescents
S	Suicide: this is short-hand for depression and other mood disturbances and self-harming behavior

The standard pediatric consultation (doctor communicates with parents) and the standard adult consultation (doctor communications solely with patient) are both inappropriate in dealing with adolescents. Best practice is to see young people both together with their parents and by themselves. While this is time consuming, it is essential for taking an accurate history, understanding the young person's motivations and goals, and for getting accurate information on health risk behaviors such as smoking, drinking, drugs and unsafe sex.[45]

Frameworks have been developed for best practice in clinical settings with young people, the most well known being the HEADSS approach which reminds clinicians to cover the important domains of Home life, Education, Activities, Drugs, Sexuality and Suicide (depression and self-harming) when interviewing any young person (Table 35.7).[46] But having a framework is not enough; the key skills required for effective communication with young people are to understand adolescent development, to be empathic, respectful and nonjudgmental, to understand the link between physical and emotional well-being, and to provide a physically and emotionally safe environment for the clinical interaction. The good news is that these skills can be learned.[47]

EXAMINING YOUNG PEOPLE

While the bulk of physical examination of adolescents is similar to that of children, new types of examinations may provide a challenge to the pediatrician, including pubertal assessments, pelvic examinations and breast and testicular examinations. Regardless of the examination, adolescents require more attention to privacy and confidentiality than children. Ensuring personal privacy is essential, and it is appropriate to ask all young people whether or not they wish their parents to be present during physical examination, especially of the genitals. Be sensitive that they may not wish their parent to be present but may have difficulty saying this in front of their parent. This can be dealt with by suggesting to the parent that the young person may now be old enough to want their privacy and then asking the young person what they wish.

The issue of the gender of the doctor and chaperones for intimate examinations is important. Many but not all adolescents prefer to be examined by a same-sex doctor, and providing a gender balance and choice of examiner is useful if this is possible. Having a chaperone for examination of adolescents of the opposite sex is obviously mandatory to protect both the patient and the doctor.

Assessment of pubertal stage is important for the management of all chronic illnesses in adolescents as well as in the assessment of endocrine disorders. These skills are easily learned, and pubertal stage should be assessed at least annually in young people with chronic illnesses during early adolescence. For those who refuse direct genital examination, pubertal self-assessment using standard Tanner photographs or drawings offers a less accurate alternative.[48] Pediatricians in most medical systems will rarely be required to undertake pelvic examinations on adolescents, although in others this is routine.

CONFIDENTIALITY AND CONSENT ISSUES

Confidentiality and consent issues are central to the management and examination of young people, who are potentially legally underage. Adolescents are very clear that the major things they want from clinicians are confidentiality, respect and clinical excellence.[49,50] Services that are not considered to be confidential are less likely to be used by young people.[51,52] Full confidentiality (including keeping confidentiality from parents) should be assured to young people unless they are found to be at risk from suicide, sexual abuse or reveal plans to harm others.[44]

In relation to issues of consent to treatment, adolescents can fall into a no-mans' land between parental rights over minors and adult rights. In most countries including the UK, adolescents are now deemed to have adult rights to consent to treatment themselves if they are legally competent, regardless of their parents' wishes. The legal criteria for competence differ between countries, but usually require the ability to give informed consent and understand the benefits and risks of treatment or nontreatment. In the UK, competence is presumed over the age of 18 years, and adolescents between 16 and 18 years can consent to treatment but cannot refuse life-saving treatment. Under 16 years of age, adolescents are legally presumed incompetent unless they show otherwise.[53] Of course, many young people under this age are competent, so in a practical sense, it is appropriate to treat adolescents from 12 to 14 years upwards as if they have full adult medical rights and responsibilities.

ADHERENCE (COMPLIANCE) AND THE CONTROL OF CHRONIC ILLNESS IN ADOLESCENCE

Adolescents are frequently poor clinic attenders and adolescence is a time of poor disease control in many chronic conditions. Because of this, adolescents are frequently labeled as 'noncompliant',[54] although there is very little evidence that young people adhere more poorly to medical regimens than adults. Many young people struggle with the organizational responsibility of managing difficult regimens; others manipulate their regimen as part of ongoing conflict with parents; but most are faithfully adherent, but adherent to a regimen of their own choosing – one that may have little relationship to that prescribed by their doctor!

Practical measures to improve adherence to medical regimens are outlined in Table 35.8. The most important aspect is to 'decriminalize' non-adherence by recognizing that some non-adherence is universal, and working with the adolescent to tailor the regimen to meet their health goals. The most effective medical regimen for adolescents is one that ensures its own success by being tailored to meet the health goals of the young person. Finding out what the young person is most worried about, what would motivate them to take their treatments, and what they would like to change about their illness, their appearance and their life, allows doctors to start a negotiation with a young person about a regimen that would maximize adherence.

When thinking about disease 'control' in adolescence, we cannot assume that control means the same thing for the young person as it does for health professionals. In diabetes for example, good medical control is defined as a low HbA1c, few hypoglycemic episodes and no admissions to hospital in diabetic ketoacidosis. But from a young person's point of view, good 'control' may mean minimizing the impact and appearance of diabetes in their lives – which may manifest as carefully running blood sugars moderately high to avoid embarrassing 'hypos' but not high enough to cause ketosis, eating a normal diet (dietary non-adherence) and doing very few blood sugar levels. Good 'control' for the young person may also include withholding insulin to control weight. This phenotype of 'careful poor control' is common in many diseases

in adolescence, and is a product of young people's health goals being focused on the here-and-now and on living a normal teenage life rather than on future disease complications. The management of this form of poor control focuses on exploring the motivations and aims of the behavior, and negotiating with the young person to fulfill their aims while also producing good medical control.

Other phenotypes of poor disease control in adolescence may result from psychological problems associated with chronic illness. Perhaps more than at any other time, the developmental changes during adolescence means that the psyche and soma are inextricably interrelated. Many young people with chronic medical conditions suffer adverse psychological sequelae, particularly depression and anxiety and adjustment disorders, as well as delayed psychosocial development.[55] This can manifest as poor disease control, frequent hospital admissions and long term school absence. Assessment and management of the reciprocal psychosocial impacts of adolescence and chronic illness (Table 35.4) are a central part of medicine for adolescents. Severe or chronic illness in adolescence should be managed in the context of multidisciplinary teams that include mental health professionals, social workers, youth workers and teachers, as well as doctors and nurses. As noted above, taking a 'solution-focused' approach may help. A young person admitted for an asthma exacerbation every month has 25 days per month when their asthma is well controlled. Find out what helped them do this and identify resiliency factors that can be worked upon to help keep the young person well and their disease better controlled.

TRANSITION

The transition of adolescents with chronic illness from pediatric to adult services is now a central part of chronic illness management (Table 35.9). This transition means more than just a transfer from one clinic to another.[56] It entails a significant change from the family-centred and developmentally focused pediatric paradigm (which frequently infantilizes the adolescent) to an adult medical culture which acknowledges patient autonomy and reproduction and employment issues but neglects growth, development and family concerns. It also entails the loss of well-known and valued pediatric care-givers and the necessity of trusting new and unknown adult carers. Because this change is so significant for the young person and their family, traditional methods of transfer of care by referral letter can lead to adolescents settling poorly into the new adult service or even dropping out of medical supervision altogether for a period.[57]

This transition period is particularly dangerous in those diseases where adult services or skills are poorly developed, such as in 'pediatric' metabolic diseases or congenital heart disease. It is important for all pediatric specialist clinics to have transition guidelines and those where larger numbers of adolescents are transferring should develop an active transition program with the receiving adult service. Preparation for transition should begin in early

Table 35.8 Practical measures to improve adherence and disease control in adolescents

'Decriminalize' non-adherence. Ask: 'Most young people have trouble taking medications. How many days a week do you manage to take them all?'

Involve the adolescent as much as possible in planning the regimen, choosing the drugs (if there are alternatives), and deciding on dose timing. Young people are more likely to adhere to programs they feel responsible for

Search for motivating factors that will help the young person stick with treatment. Issues about growth, weight and appearance are often useful in chronic illness

Make a contract with the young person where each side agrees to fulfill certain conditions

Provide written instructions (in adolescent-friendly language) about the treatment regimen

Focus the regimen on the least chaotic time in the adolescent's daily life. This is usually the morning but is different for different adolescents

For complex regimens, don't assume adherence is the same for each drug. Adolescents may faithfully adhere to some and never take others because of beliefs about the drug or side-effects. Discuss compliance with each medication separately and explore beliefs and knowledge about the drug

Find ways to involve the family in ways that do not increase parent–adolescent conflict about independence; e.g. assign the parents 'check-points' every 2–3 days but forbid constant nagging (which usually reduces compliance!)

Don't believe that non-adherence is because of ignorance or that education will improve compliance

Take a 'solution-focused' approach. Find out when things have gone well and try to work out why. Use these

Table 35.9 Transition recommendations

Transition preparation must be seen as an essential component of high quality health care in adolescence

Every pediatric general and speciality clinic should have a specific transition policy. More formal transition programs are necessary where large numbers of young people are being transferred to adult care

Young people should not be transferred to adult services until they have the necessary skills to function in an adult service and have finished growth and puberty

An identified person within the pediatric and adult teams must be responsible for transition arrangements. The most suitable persons are nurse specialists

Management links must be developed between the two hospitals

Evaluation of transition arrangements must be undertaken

adolescence, and young people should only move to adult care when they have the necessary skill-set to survive independently in the adult service.[58]

HEALTH PROMOTION FOR YOUNG PEOPLE

The most serious health problems affecting young people are primary care issues including teenage pregnancy, drug misuse, mental health problems and violence. By 15 years of age, around 24% of adolescents in the UK are regular smokers, 38% will be regular alcohol consumers[59] and around 25% are sexually active.[60] While these problems are generally the province of general practitioners and others in primary care, all health professionals who deal with young people should possess basic health promotion skills. Over 70% of adolescents visit a doctor every year[8] and each clinical interaction with an adolescent should provide an opportunity for health promotion.

As noted above, young people with chronic illness have similar rates of risk behaviors to the general population,[37] although few pediatricians address smoking, alcohol or sex in clinical interactions with young people with chronic conditions. Health behaviors begun in adolescence continue into adult life, and health promotion during adolescence can positively influence smoking, drug use and sexual exploratory behaviors. Those looking after young people with chronic illness must begin to address smoking, alcohol and drug use and sexual health in early adolescence as this is when exploration with health behaviors begins. This is often best done by other members of the multidisciplinary team, or by the inclusion of consultation with sexual health workers, etc. as part of the multidisciplinary management of adolescents with chronic illness.

CONCLUSIONS

Adolescent health is of increasing importance in both pediatric practice and in public health. Young people require and benefit from a distinct clinical approach based upon knowledge of adolescent development in biological, psychological and social domains and the search for resiliency factors that promote health and healthy behaviors. Although chronic illness control is frequently poorer during adolescence, concepts of the 'non-adherent' or 'difficult' adolescent are based on a lack of understanding of the disparity between traditional medical goals and the health and life goals of the young person. The most effective ways to foster healthy behavior and improve disease control during adolescence are to aim for concordance between the treatment regimen and the health goals of the young person, and to focus on factors the young person finds helpful in maintaining good health/disease control.

REFERENCES

1. Cooklin A. Psychological changes of adolescence. In Brook CDG, ed. The practice of medicine in adolescence. London: Edward Arnold; 1993: 8–24.
2. World Health Organization. The health of young people. WHO: Geneva; 1993.
3. Rutter M. Changing youth in a changing society. Cambridge MA: Harvard University Press; 1980.
4. Bridging the gaps: Healthcare for adolescents. Report of the joint working party on adolescent health of the Royal medical and nursing colleges of the UK. London: Royal College of Paediatrics & Child Health; 2003.
5. Department of Health, Department for Education and Skills. National service framework for children, young people and maternity services. Gateway Ref: 3779. London: Department of Health; 2004.
6. National Statistics 2000. Social focus on young people. London: The Stationery Office; 2000.
7. MacFaul R,. Werneke U. Recent trends in hospital use by children in England. Arch Dis Child 2001; 85:203–207.
8. Kari J, Donovan C, Li J, et al. Adolescents' attitudes to general practice in North London. Br J Gen Pract 1997; 47:109–110.
9. Health Survey for England: The Health of Young People '95–97. London: Stationery Office; 1998.
10. College Research Unit, Royal College of Psychiatrists. National In-patient Child and Adolescent Psychiatry Study (NICAPS). 2001.
11. Viner RM. National survey of use of hospital beds by adolescents aged 12 to 19 in the United Kingdom. BMJ 2001; 322:957–958.
12. Greene S. Diabetes in the young: Current challenges in their management. Balliere Clin Pediatr 1996; 4:563–575.
13. Lawson ML, Sochett EB, Chait PG, et al. JW, Daneman D. Effect of puberty on markers of glomerular hypertrophy and hypertension in IDDM. Diabetes 1996; 45:51–55.
14. Michelagnoli M, Viner RM. Commentary: care of the adolescent with cancer. Eur J Cancer 2001; 37:1523–1530.
15. Kaur B, Anderson HR, Austin J, et al. Prevalence of asthma symptoms, diagnosis, and treatment in 12–14 year old children across Great Britain (international study of asthma and allergies in childhood, IS AAC UK). BMJ 1998; 316:118–124.
16. Variation and trends in incidence of childhood diabetes in Europe. EURODIAB ACE Study Group. Lancet 2000; 355:873–876.
17. Fagot-Campagna A, Pettitt DJ, Engelgau MM, et al. Type 2 diabetes among North American children and adolescents: an epidemiologic review and a public health perspective. J Pediatr 2000; 136:664–672.
18. Siegel D. Adolescents and chronic illness. JAMA 1987; 257:3396–3399.
19. Newacheck P, Taylor W. Childhood chronic illness: prevalence, severity and impact. Am J Public Health 1992; 82:364–371.
20. Gortmaker S, Sappenfield W. Chronic childhood disorders: prevalence and impact. Pediatr Clin North Am 1984; 31:3–18.
21. British Paediatric Association. Working Party on Cystic Fibrosis. Report on cystic fibrosis. 1988.
22. Goddard E, Higgins V. Smoking, drinking and drug use among young teenagers in 1998. London: The Stationery Office; 1999.
23. US Department of Health and Human Services. Preventing tobacco use among young people: A report of the Surgeon General. Washington DC: US Department of Health & Human Services, Centers for Disease Control & Prevention; 1994.
24. Harrington R, Fudge H, Rutter M. et al. Adult outcomes of childhood and adolescent depression. Arch Gen Psychiatry 1990; 47:465–473.
25. Steinberger J, Moran A, Hong CP, et al. Adiposity in childhood predicts obesity and insulin resistance in young adulthood. J Pediatr 2001; 138:469–473.
26. Hubert HB, Feinleib M, McNamara PM, et al. Obesity as an independent risk factor for cardiovascular disease: a 26-year follow-up of participants in the Framingham Heart Study. Circulation 1983; 67:968–977.
27. Osmond C, Barker DJ. Fetal, infant, and childhood growth are predictors of coronary heart disease, diabetes, and hypertension in adult men and women. Environ Health Perspect 2000; 108 (suppl 3): 545–553.
28. McClure GM. Suicide in children and adolescents in England and Wales 1970–1998. Br J Psychiatry 2001; 178:469–474.
29. Reilly JJ, Dorosty AR. Epidemic of obesity in UK children. Lancet 1999; 354:1874–1875.
30. Fagot-Campagna A, Narayan KM, Imperatore G. Type 2 diabetes in children. BMJ 2001; 322:377–378.
31. Eveleth P, Tanner J. Worldwide variation in human growth. Cambridge: Cambridge University Press; 1990.
32. Paus T, Collins DL, Evans AC, et al. Maturation of white matter in the human brain: a review of magnetic resonance studies. Brain Res Bull 2001; 54:255–266.
33. Leffert N, Petersen AC. Patterns of development during adolescence. In: Rutter M, Smith DJ, eds. Psychosocial disorders in young people. London: John Wiley; 1995:67–103.
34. Muuss RE. Theories of adolescence. New York: McGraw Hill; 1996.
35. Ghosh S, Drummond H, Ferguson A. Neglect of growth and development in the clinical monitoring of children and teenagers with inflammatory bowel disease: review of case records. BMJ 1998; 317:120–121.
36. White PD. Transition to adulthood. Curr Opin Rheumatol 1999; 11:408–411.
37. Hargrave DR, McMaster C, O'Hare MM, et al Tobacco smoke exposure in children and adolescents with diabetes mellitus. Diabet Med 1999; 16:31–34.
38. Males M. Adolescents: daughters or alien sociopaths? Lancet 1997; 349 (suppl 1):I13–I16.
39. Cohen ED. An exploratory attempt to distinguish subgroups among crack-abusing African-American women. J Addict Dis 1999; 18:41–54.
40. Ramrakha S, Avshalom C, Dickson N, et al. Psychiatric disorders and risky sexual behavior in young adulthood: cross-sectional study in birth cohort. BMJ 2000; 321:66.
41. Lister-Sharp D, Chapman S, Stewart-Brown S, et al. Health promoting schools and health promotion in schools: two systematic reviews. Health Technol Assessment 2001; 3:1–6.
42. Christie D, Fredman G. Working systemically in an adolescent medical unit: collaborating with the network. Clin Psychol 2001; 3:8–11.
43. Klitsner I, Borok G, Neintstein L, et al. Adolescent health care in a large multispecialty prepaid group practice: Who provides it and how well are they doing? West J Med 1992; 156:628–632.

44. Royal College of General Practitioners and Brook. Confidentiality and young people. London: Royal College of General Practitioners; 2000.

45. MacKenzie RG. Approach to the adolescent in the clinical setting. Med Clin North Am 1990; 74:1085–1095.

46. Goldenring JM, Cohen E. Getting into adolescent heads. Contemp Pediatr 1988; July:75–90.

47. Sanci LA, Coffey CM, Veit FC, et al. Evaluation of the effectiveness of an educational intervention for general practitioners in adolescent health care: randomised controlled trial. BMJ 2000; 320:224–230.

48. Taylor SJ, Whincup PH, Hindmarsh PC, et al. Performance of a new pubertal self-assessment questionnaire: a preliminary study. Pediatr Perinat Epidemiol 2001; 15:88–94.

49. Oppong-Odiseng ACK, Heycock EG. Adolescent health services–through their eyes. Arch Dis Child 1997; 77:115–119.

50. Burack R. Young teenagers' attitudes towards general practitioners and their provision of sexual health care. Br J Gen Pract 2000; 50:550–554.

51. Ford CA, Millstein SG, Halpern-Felsher BL, et al. Influence of physician confidentiality assurances on adolescents' willingness to disclose information and seek future health care. A randomized controlled trial. JAMA 1997; 278:1029–1034.

52. Churchill R, Allen J, Denman S, et al. Do the attitudes and beliefs of young teenagers towards general practice influence actual consultation behavior? Br J Gen Pract 2000; 50:953–957.

53. British Medical Association. Consent, rights and choices in health care for children and young people. London: BMJ; 2001.

54. Kyngas HA, Kroll T, Duffy ME. Compliance in adolescents with chronic diseases: a review. J Adolesc Health 2000; 26:379–388.

55. Eiser C. Psychological effects of chronic disease. J Child Psychol Psychiatry 1990; 31:85–98.

56. Sawyer S, Blair S, Bowes G. et al. Chronic illness in adolescents: transfer or transition to adult services?. J Pediatr Child Health 1997; 33:88–90.

57. Rosen D. Between two worlds: bridging the cultures of child health and adult medicine. J Adolesc Health 1995; 17:10–16.

58. Viner RM. Transition from pediatric to adult care. Bridging the gaps or passing the buck? Arch Dis Child 1999; 81:271–275.

59. Health and health behavior among young people. Health behavior in school-aged children: A WHO cross-national study (HSBC) international report. Copenhagen: WHO; 2000.

60. Coleman J. Key data on adolescence. Brighton: Trust for the Study of Adolescence; 1999.

61. Windle M, Windle RC. Depressive symptoms and cigarette smoking among middle adolescents: prospective associations and intrapersonal and interpersonal influences. J Consult Clin Psychol 2001; 69:215–226.

62. Kelder SH, Murray NG, Orpinas P, et al. Depression and substance use in minority middle-school students. Am J Public Health 2001; 91: 761–766.

63. Alexander CS, Allen P, Crawford MA, et al. Taking a first puff: cigarette smoking experiences among ethnically diverse adolescents. Ethn Health 1999; 4:245–257.

64. Alexander C, Piazza M, Mekos D, et al. Peers, schools, and adolescent cigarette smoking. J Adolesc Health 2001; 29:22–30.

65. Coffey C, Lynskey M, Wolfe R, et al. Initiation and progression of cannabis use in a population-based Australian adolescent longitudinal study. Addiction 2000; 95:1679–1690.

66. Hogan DP, Sun R, Cornwell GT. et al. Sexual and fertility behaviors of American females aged 15–19 years: 1985, 1990, and 1995. Am J Public Health 2000; 90:1421–1425.

67. Lammers C, Ireland M, Resnick M, et al. Influences on adolescents' decision to postpone onset of sexual intercourse: a survival analysis of virginity among youths aged 13 to 18 years. J Adolesc Health 2000; 26:42–48.

68. DuRant RH, Jay S, Seymore C. Contraceptive and sexual behavior of black female adolescents. A test of a social-psychological theoretical model. J Adolesc Health Care 1990; 11:326–334.

69. Porter LE, Ku L. Use of reproductive health services among young men, 1995. J Adolesc Health 2000; 27:186–194.

70. Raine TR, Jenkins R, Aarons SJ, et al. Sociodemographic correlates of virginity in seventh-grade black and Latino students. J Adolesc Health 1999; 24:304–312.

71. Coyne-Beasley T, Schoenbach VJ. The African-American church: a potential forum for adolescent comprehensive sexuality education. J Adolesc Health 2000; 26:289–294.

72. UK Data Archive. National Study of Health and Growth, Phase I: 1972–1976 (Years 1–5). Colchester: University of Essex, 2004.

73. UK Data Archive National Study of Health and Growth, Phase III : 1982–1994 (Years 11–23). Colchester: University of Essex, 1994.

74. Boreham R, Shaw A. Drug use, smoking and drinking among young people in England in 2001. London, ONS; 2002.

75. Statistics on smoking. England, 1978 onwards. Statistical Bulletin (National Statistics, UK) 2000; 17:1–36.

76. Social Exclusion Unit. Teenage pregnancy. London: Stationery Office; 1999.

77. Gunnell D, Middleton N, Whitley E, et al. Why are suicide rates rising in young men but falling in the elderly? – a time-series analysis of trends in England and Wales 1950–1998. Soc Sci Med 2003; 57:595–611.

78. Viner RM, Barker M. Young people's health: the need for action. BMJ 2005; 330 (7496):901–903.

36

Emergency care

Thomas F Beattie, Gale A Pearson

PEDIATRIC INJURY AND EMERGENCY CARE

A PEDIATRIC EMERGENCY MEDICAL SERVICE (PEMS)

Most children become critically ill or are injured in their own environment. In order to provide optimum care for these children a seamless structure of continuous care, from environment to hospital, is essential. There are few centers in the world where this seamless care exists. Where it has been achieved however, outcomes for critically ill and injured children have been positively influenced.[1,2]

The continuum of pediatric emergency care is best summarized in Figure 36.1. Within this there should be the desire to keep as many children as possible out of hospital and maintain their care within the home and community environment for as much of the time as possible.

THE HOME SETTING

For the first 5 years of life most children spend the bulk of their time within the home and local community. The majority of children coming into contact with emergency medical services do so as a result of infection or injury.

Most children will experience upper and lower respiratory tract infection with considerable frequency between the ages of 0 and 5 years. After this age it is much less frequent. Much of this illness can be treated within the home providing parents have sufficient confidence and education. Most illness in this age group will be viral and will require little more than supportive measures such as antipyretic therapy and encouraging fluid intake. However, there is an increasing demand for this type of treatment to be obtained from family doctors or emergency departments. The disintegration of the nuclear family is one factor increasing this demand on medical time, particularly in primary care. Recent evidence has indicated that attenders at emergency departments for minor illness and injury come from deprived areas of the community.[3] The reasons for this are complex but probably relate to coping mechanisms and education.

In a small number of cases bacterial infections will be present that require antibiotic therapy. In an even smaller number significant infectious disease such as meningitis, septicemia and osteomyelitis will be present. A small number of children with viral illness will get further complications such as a febrile seizure, or superimposed bacterial infection may supervene. If parents are unaware of these problems they will lose confidence in managing illness within the community.

One way to tackle such issues is to develop an educational program aimed at developing competence in minor illness and injury management. Such an education program must also alert parents to the dangers of significant illness or injury that may require further treatment with or without a stay in hospital. Within this education program it is important to differentiate the needs of the infant younger than 3 months of age from those older than 3 months of age. The response of the younger child to infection is totally different from that of older children and adults and parents should be aware of how to get advice for these children should the need arise.[4] This is a difficult task as even health professionals using clinical decision tools cannot reliably detect children with significant infection.[5–7] Similarly injury in the infant may be a harbinger of child abuse or neglect.

Despite the frequency of infections, injuries are still the leading cause of morbidity and mortality between the ages of 1 and 5 years. Most of these injuries occur within the home setting, which includes the garden and its surroundings. Burns and scalds, poisonings, falls from a height, finger tip injuries and near drowning account for the majority.

One of the means to tackle the toll wrought by injury in this age group is an integrated injury prevention program within an emergency medical system. The components of such a system include:

1. injury surveillance;
2. data analysis;
3. identification of problems;
4. development of strategies;
5. implementation of strategies;
6. injury surveillance.

In many ways this is a typical audit cycle. It relies on collaboration among emergency physicians, general practice, public health medicine, educationalists and health promotion agencies. Their respective skills should be brought together in a coordinated fashion.

At present injury surveillance is patchy with much information being derived from inpatient databases. These are inaccurate and only reflect 10% of total injuries that occur.[8] Without meaningful measures of injury severity these data are at best a reflection of current medical practice. A good example of this is the documentation of poisoning. Many children who are poisoned can be safely dealt with in the home without ever coming to hospital provided adequate medical advice can be given and monitored by telephone. If this advice is not available then many children will present to hospital. They will present to the emergency room, where their treatment will depend on the experience and confidence of the staff working in that department. Junior staff, insecure or ill taught will tend to admit because they are unsure of what to do. Senior staff, experienced and confident will be able to manage many of these children on an outpatient basis. In an institution staffed in the former manner poisonings determined from inpatient stay will be at a high level whereas those in an institution managed in the latter manner will be lower. This has nothing to do with the incidence of the poisoning but all to do with medical practice. Simply by changing medical practice an apparent fall in the incidence of poisoning can be demonstrated when in fact the incidence remains high. Failure to take cognizance of these matters when developing injury surveillance will lead to inappropriate preventive measures.[9]

Effective data surveillance should start with a minimum data set. This minimum data set should aim to capture a small, important amount of information on every child who presents.[10] If too much information is to be documented staff members will tend not to collect it and parents will get irritated because they feel that their child should be treated rather than them answering questions. Typically it should include age, sex, postcode and proxies for social class and/or deprivation. Some idea as to the causation should also be included. One way of doing this is to use international classification of disease E codes;[11] this is universally accepted and is adequate for most things. This could be further

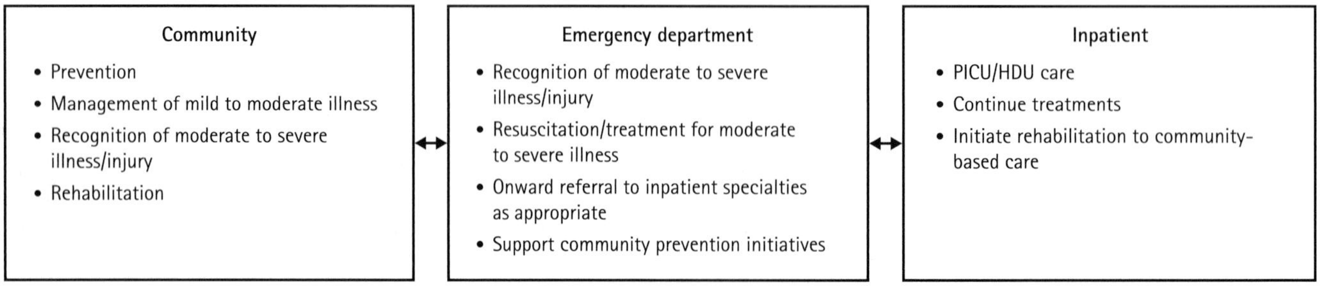

Community	Emergency department	Inpatient
• Prevention • Management of mild to moderate illness • Recognition of moderate to severe illness/injury • Rehabilitation	• Recognition of moderate to severe illness/injury • Resuscitation/treatment for moderate to severe illness • Onward referral to inpatient specialties as appropriate • Support community prevention initiatives	• PICU/HDU care • Continue treatments • Initiate rehabilitation to community-based care

Fig. 36.1 Continuum of emergency care.

refined to having the most common injuries already precoded. Similarly some ideas to the most common diagnoses using a system such as the International Classification of Disease codes (ICD) could also be included on discharge. If this information were to be collected on all children a very suitable injury surveillance system would very rapidly be developed that could be expanded as the need arose.

DATA ANALYSIS AND PROBLEM IDENTIFICATION

Once an accurate database is in place that gathers details on a substantial proportion of injury occurring within the community then problem areas can be identified. This can be on the basis of deprivation or need; clustering; type of injury, e.g. fall, poisoning; type of injury, e.g. fracture or head injury. Once analyzed this information can then be made available to the relevant health education agencies, who can then implement parts three and four of the audit cycle.

DEVISING A STRATEGY

Before any strategy can be devised to protect against childhood injury three components have to be addressed:
1. the child;
2. the family;
3. the environment.

Tackling any of these on their own will fail if it does not concomitantly address the problems inherent in the other two areas. It is well recognized that some children are more injury prone than others. Is this because the family is poor or the environment is poor? Or is it that that child is inherently more prone to injury for reasons of clumsiness, poor eyesight/coordination? Attention deficit and hyperactivity disorder is an example of a behavioral problem that might be expected to be associated with injury and this is the case.[12] To date many injury prevention programs have been simplistic with individuals working in isolation without the complete umbrella of a PEMS.

IMPLEMENTING A STRATEGY

Before a strategy can be successful the lessons from commercial advertisers have to be learned. Simply repeating the same message ad infinitum leads to message fatigue. The message must be appropriate to the target audience and must take note of all the above factors. In addition the audience must be identified and targeted effectively.

RE-AUDIT

It is important to measure any effect of the prevention campaigns against the initial database. Failure to do so may lead to inappropriate and ineffective campaigning being continued indefinitely. If there has been no diminution in the levels of injury that one has targeted then the strategies need to be re-evaluated in the light of the data analysis and message.

COMMUNITY EDUCATION

In order for the child to be cared for within the home as effectively as possible, ideally not accessing emergency medical services, a substantial amount of effort must be paid to community education. However, the target audience has not been well defined. Does the practitioner, for instance, tackle children in junior school or senior school in an effort to help future generations? Should the practitioner address the problem at antenatal classes, where there is a substantial chance of reaching an interested mother and perhaps the father? Is it appropriate to address the issue of safety in the postnatal period, when the father is almost certainly not going to be present? These issues need to be addressed as a matter of urgency if child injury prevention is to be taken forward in a meaningful manner.

COMMUNITY CARE

Within the context of a PEMS, community care should be directed at disease prevention. There will however be a significant proportion of children who have transient episodes of acute illness requiring medical intervention. Interspersed with these will be children with chronic disability who will have more sophisticated needs for emergency care than their able-bodied peers.

To work effectively there needs to be a network of experienced general practitioners and community pediatricians working alongside health visitors, district nurses, midwives and other paramedical staff. The public health system working alongside ensures good sanitation and maintenance of water supplies. Attention to housing and overcrowding is also all-important in the prevention of disease and illness. Surveillance by public health physicians and public health laboratories can identify trends in disease. Many infectious diseases, e.g. *Mycoplasma* infection, occur in a cyclical fashion over a period of years. Croup will present 2–3 times per year, one being significantly greater than the others.[13] Disease reporting can help identify when these infections are imminent and serological testing can help confirm that they have actually arrived. This will alert practitioners to the common disease that may be in the community setting at any given time and may help avoid unnecessary hospital admissions by the correct use of antibiotics.

The health professionals within the community have several roles. The first is disease prevention, primarily in terms of immunization and injury prevention. Where immunization has been effective many diseases have all but been eradicated. This is in danger of disappearing with recent changes in attitude to immunization. The recent scare regarding possible links with autism and bowel disease has led to concern about the safety of the combined measles/mumps/rubella (MMR) vaccination.[14] That this link has been convincingly disproved has not yet convinced a section of the public. This has led to a small but significant decrease in herd immunity, opening the way for a measles epidemic in particular.[15–17]

Health professionals in the community should be able to give advice to parents on disease and injury prevention. They should also be able to recognize situations where family dynamics are breaking down, making injury and child abuse more common.

Within the community one of the more vital functions is recognition of the child who has a disease process that is not suitable for treatment in the community but needs further care within a hospital setting. A good example of this is bronchiolitis. Many cases of bronchiolitis will be cared for in the community with children getting supportive care and advice. However, family practitioners should be in the position to identify the child at risk from significant airway distress, e.g. not feeding, a respiratory rate over 55 or apneic attacks.[18] In this situation the child needs to get to hospital for further treatment that may include high-dependency and/or intensive care. Equally the community services should be able to identify the child who may not be so ill but where the family circumstances mean that the child is not going to be capably looked after at home. Situations where this may occur include poverty, a mother who is not coping because of two or three other small children, and single parents or families of drug abusers. In these situations even though the child may not warrant admission for medical reasons, the social factors may indicate the child needs to be transferred for inpatient care. Community practitioners are much better placed to identify these problems than hospital-based staff.

PREHOSPITAL CARE

Prehospital care is a link between home and the community on one hand and the hospital-based services of emergency and tertiary level care on the other. The function of prehospital care is to transfer ill or injured children to places of either advanced or definitive care. Two issues predominate within the prehospital care setting:
1. access;
2. education.

To be effective prehospital care has to be easily accessed by all members of the community, e.g. in the UK dialling '999' gains access to the ambulance service. This universal national access code available to all and free of charge is probably the most effective component in the prehospital setting.

Education is also vital. The role of practitioners in prehospital care has got to be fully defined. It must be relevant to the PEMS within which the prehospital care is practiced. It will differ between urban and rural areas in terms of decisions to 'stay and play' and 'scoop and run'. It must be remembered that the absolute numbers of true pediatric emergencies (illness or trauma) is relatively rare, particularly compared to the adult population. The skills needed to carry out emergency care effectively require time to attain and practice to maintain.[19] An integrated PEMS can best evaluate the needs of its catchment area and train the prehospital care staff accordingly. Where short distances are envisaged and transfer times are rapid then training needs may be less demanding with concentration on simple airway, breathing and circulation skills. In rural areas where transport times may be prolonged advanced life support skills may be necessary.[20] Where land-based transport is adequate, training in driving skills may be required. However, should air medical transport by helicopter or fixed-wing aircraft be necessary as a routine then training in aviation medicine and the associated problems will need to be included in the training package.

There is increasing evidence that prehospital life support should include effective, simple measures. Gausche et al showed that prehospital intubation had no benefit on outcome, and worryingly might increase mortality and morbidity.[21-23] This poses a dilemma for rural practitioners in particular. Urban and semiurban situations have clear guidance that in an emergency intubation should not be attempted in the field. Rather they should concentrate on bag–valve–mask ventilation with good, simple airway-opening maneuvers and transport of the child to the nearest pediatric unit. In rural and remote areas or in situations where weather or geography make transport impossible, advanced airway care may be needed. The rarities of this, combined with the complexity of skills needed, make maintenance of skills difficult. Innovative and practical solutions have to be found, but there is no doubt that this will lead to increasing costs. Similarly the value of i.v. access has been questioned.[24] In particular the value of delaying at scene must be set against potential benefits. In this study Teach et al found no such benefit and some possible harm, either from delay at scene or inappropriate fluid administration.

Inner city areas with significant drugs problems may well have a high incidence of penetrating trauma, which will require an emphasis to be placed on treatment of such injuries within that setting.[25]

THE EMERGENCY DEPARTMENT SERVICES

Pediatric emergency departments fall into three broad categories:
1. those attached to specialist pediatric hospitals that treat only children;
2. those attached to large district or teaching hospitals that have combined pediatric and adult populations;
3. those attached to small community or cottage hospitals treating relatively small numbers of patients overall.

Within each of these three settings various problems exist.

The dedicated pediatric unit is usually situated in a large conurbation, often attached to a university or medical school. It will provide child- and family-centered care of an exceptionally high order. Major injury and illness will often be much less than that in a comparable adult population so there will have to be significant emphasis on education directed at the recognition of illness and the development of resuscitation skills to facilitate optimum care of ill and injured children. Retention of these skills is also a major issue that needs to be addressed.[26,27]

In a unit that combines pediatric and adult patients, general resuscitation skills and teamwork will be much more practiced but in contrast recognition of pediatric illness and skill in treatment may be deficient.

The ability to provide a child- and family-centered approach is often more difficult than in the purely pediatric setting.

The cottage hospital may benefit from being able to provide care closer to the patient's home but illness recognition and resuscitation skills may be poor unless teaching programs are available. This may require that staff rotate to busy units at regular intervals to update and recertify in pediatric skills.

A computer-based model of a typical region with various types of hospital postulates that all types of hospital are necessary to enable children to receive optimal care. This presupposes that skills are present and are updated regularly in each setting and that facilities for children are maintained.[28]

In all settings with the regular turnover of staff inherent with movement of junior doctors and nursing staff, regular resuscitation updates (e.g. pediatric advanced life support courses) are essential. Staffing and training in departments that have children attending should build in adequate time for training and staff development to ensure that skills are maintained at an optimum level. Within these settings certain basic concepts need to be addressed.

There should always be dedicated facilities for the reception and treatment of children, removed from the sights and sounds of the adult world. Children are often already frightened and distressed by being in hospital and every effort should be made to keep them as calm and content as possible. An attractive child-friendly environment should facilitate this. Examination rooms should have sufficient toys and pictures to enable efficient distraction therapy to be practiced. Play leaders are an invaluable resource to aid this process.

Resuscitation rooms should be fully equipped with all the various equipment that is required for pediatric resuscitation. Children change shape and size with age. A full knowledge of how this occurs and the clinical implications are important. It is almost impossible to accurately recall all the weights of children at various age groups. Drug and fluid therapy is usually done on a dose-per-weight basis. It is important to avoid calculations in 'the heat of the moment'. It is all too easy to place a decimal point in the wrong place and either over- or underdose children. For this reason charts should be available or tapes laid out on beds so that rapid determination of dosage depending on the weight/length of the child can be established. These charts will also have details of the correct size of endotracheal tube, the length to which the tube should be cut and various other parameters necessary for effective pediatric resuscitation.[29,30]

Typical equipment required in the resuscitation room is shown in Table 36.1.

The staff working within such an environment must be familiar with recognition of the sick child and similarly be comfortable with all aspects of pediatric care.

Parents often arrive at the emergency department with other siblings. The presence of play leaders will help entertain these children and enable the distressed relatives to be with the sick or injured child. Quiet rooms should be laid aside so that bereaved or distressed relatives can be alone in their time of distress though a staff member should always be available for this if required. Facilities should be available to enable nappy changing and breast-feeding to occur in private.

The function of staff in the emergency department is to receive all ill and injured children and to institute treatment in a timely and appropriate fashion depending on the urgency of the condition (triage).

The nursing staff members usually perform triage but medical staff could also perform this task. Objective triage is difficult in the pediatric population. There are few objective pediatric scales that can be related to all types of presenting problems, medical, surgical, trauma or other. Much triage therefore is subjective and will in part depend upon the volume of work. A well child presenting at a quiet time will very often get through the system more rapidly than an ill child presenting at a busy time. It is imperative that staff members working within the emergency department are able to recognize the child who has a disease process which, if left untreated, will lead to serious incapacity or death. Key recognition skills relate to respiratory and circulatory compromise.

Table 36.1 Equipment to provide emergency care for children: equipment for the resuscitation room

Airway

Guedel airways – 000→3
Endotracheal tubes – 2.5→8 uncuffed, 7→10.5 cuffed
Introducers
Laryngoscope handles
Laryngoscope blades – straight and curved
Yankauer suction catheters
Argyle suction catheters
Suction device (with backup)
Cricothyroid puncture set (this may be commercial or 'homemade')
Jet insufflation system

Breathing

Round masks
Triangular masks
Bag–valve–mask device with pressure-limiting device set at 30–40 cmH$_2$O
Reservoir bag
O$_2$ supply (with backup)
Ayres T-piece circuit (or equivalent)
Chest drains 10→32G
Drainage tubing and jars for underwater seal

Circulation

I.v. cannulae 24→14F
Central venous cannulae and Seldinger introducer wire
Intraosseous cannulae 17F
Giving sets
Blood warmer
Infusion pumps
Defibrillator with facility for synchronized DC version capable of variable energy delivery

Disability

Cervical collars
Spinal boards
Arm and leg splints

Monitoring equipment

Pulse oximeter
Cardiac monitor
Blood glucose test machines
Blood gas analyzer

Other

Tapes for i.v. lines, ETT tubes, chest drains
Syringes 1 ml, 2 ml, 5 ml, 10 ml
3-way taps
Connection tubing
Suture material

Suture packs
Chest drain packs
Urinary catheters
Nasogastric tubes
Clock
Warmth

Drugs

Epinephrine (adrenaline) – 1:10 000 and 1:1000
Atropine
Lidocaine – 1%, 2%
Sodium bicarbonate – 1.84%, 4.2%, 8.4%
Morphine
Naloxone
Glucose – 50%, 25%
Glucagon
Diazepam (as emulsion) or lorazepam
Midazolam
Phenytoin
Adenosine
Disopyramide
Beta-blocker
Thiopental
Suxamethonium
Atracurium
Mannitol – 10%, 20%
Beta 2-agonists – nebulizer solution
Ipratropium – nebulizer solution
Beta agonists – i.v. solution
Aminophylline
Hydrocortisone
Procyclidine

Fluids

Normal saline
Plasma

If neonates are expected the following equipment should also be available in addition:

Resuscitaire
Heat source
Warm towels/wraps
Umbilical catheters

In parallel, skills are needed to:

1. open and secure an airway;
2. ensure that oxygenation is maintained;
3. ensure that circulation is maintained.

The frequency with which these skills are practiced will depend on the population served and the effectiveness of the home, community and pre-hospital services. Communities that have poor home safety, poor community immunization rates and primitive public sanitation can expect to deal with large numbers of ill or injured children.

Where numbers are small maintenance of recognition skills can only be maintained by appropriate teaching programs, for example pediatric advanced life support (PALS). PALS courses were introduced into the UK in the early 1990s. Roberts et al[31] have demonstrated increased survival since these were introduced. Cause and effect have still to be reconciled.

Once a child has been received into the emergency department and the airway, breathing and circulation have been stabilized, the child needs to be transferred to a place of definitive treatment. Often this will be via an imaging facility to surgery, and from there to an intensive care setting. To complete the emergency medical system, a system of safe

transfer to and from each of these areas needs to be established. Even if the emergency department is within the tertiary care center, transfer to the scanning suite or the intensive care unit can be fraught with danger if not performed expertly and efficiently. For this reason transfers should be kept to a minimum.

A transport team should be a priority development in any pediatric emergency care system so that there can be safe transfer to the tertiary care center for definitive treatment.

Both within the injury and emergency setting and the tertiary care unit rehabilitation is important. This will enable the ill or injured child to regain his place as effectively as possible within the home/community setting.

APPROACH TO THE MANAGEMENT OF THE SEVERELY ILL OR INJURED CHILD IN THE EMERGENCY DEPARTMENT

Most ill children will be brought to hospital by the prehospital services. In these situations airway care and circulatory support will have been instituted according to local training and policy guidelines. In addition there will be an element of warning so that the resuscitation team can be gathered and tasks allocated.

As it is very easy for parents or bystanders to pick up smaller children, children who are severely ill or injured will often be brought to hospital unannounced and unexpected in private transport.

Consequently the components of the resuscitation team should be established in advance. It is important that one doctor is in charge to coordinate the resuscitation and decide on the priorities for care, with other staff in complementary roles.

INITIAL ASSESSMENT

Rapid assessment of the airway, breathing and circulation is mandatory (primary survey).

AIRWAY

The airway can be described as open, maintainable or unmaintainable. An open airway is defined as one with no obstruction present. This includes the absence of secretions, stridor, gurgling or other noises. An open airway needs no further management at this stage but this should be kept under review.[32,33]

A maintainable airway is defined as one that can be kept open with simple measures such as positioning; chin lift/head tilt (or jaw-thrust only, if trauma to the cervical spine is a possibility); the use of an oropharyngeal airway or the use of gentle suction.

An unmaintainable airway is one that is still at risk despite these simple measures necessitating either intubation or the creation of a surgical airway (cricothyrotomy).

The airway should be maintained at this stage by the simplest effective measures available. Intubation must only be carried out by experienced operators who can intubate with skill in a timely fashion. Any attempt taking longer than 30 s should be abandoned and the child oxygenated with a bag–valve–mask device pending a second attempt.

All sick or injured children require high flow oxygen. This should be administered using a facemask if the airway is open and maintainable. Otherwise artificial ventilation should be established using a bag–valve–mask device (see later).

BREATHING

The efficacy of breathing can be assessed only after the airway has been opened. The rate, volume and symmetry of respiration should be assessed by observation and auscultation.

Respiratory compromise can be characterized by either an increasing or decreasing work of breathing.

Increased work of breathing
Increasing respiratory rate
Increasing heart rate
Use of accessory muscles in respiration
Flared nostrils
Intercostal/sternal recession
Grunting
Decreasing level of consciousness

Decreased work of breathing
Decreasing respiratory rate
Poor respiratory effort
Poor lung expansion

If breathing is absent or diminished, ventilation using a bag–valve–mask device should be instituted as soon as possible. Absent breath sounds and hyper-resonance to percussion on one side should lead one to consider a pneumothorax. This should be immediately drained using a needle thoracostomy. The needle should be inserted into the midclavicular line in the second intercostal space pending the insertion of a formal chest drain. Once inserted the needle should be left in place until the chest drain is working properly. If signs of respiratory compromise are present supplemental oxygen should be administered in the highest rate available.

CIRCULATION

The adequacy of the circulation should only be assessed when Airway and Breathing are adequate. A central pulse should be palpated at this stage. The carotid pulse should be palpated lateral to the thyroid cartilage and medial to the sternocleidomastoid muscle in a child. In an infant the brachial pulse should be palpated in the upper arm.

If there is no pulse palpable (or pulse is less than 60 beats/min) cardiac massage should be started at a rate of 80–100 b.p.m. If a pulse is palpable look for other signs of circulatory embarrassment.

Physical signs of circulatory embarrassment
Rising pulse
Tachypnea
Weakening peripheral pulses
Increasing delay of capillary return (greater than 2 s)
Increasing peripheral core temperature difference
Decreased urine output
Altered level of consciousness

All children with circulatory embarrassment (and all children who are severely ill or injured) should have i.v. access established as soon as possible. Failure to establish peripheral i.v. access within a few minutes in children who are in circulatory distress should lead one to insert an intraosseous needle into the tibia or femur. If signs of circulatory embarrassment or shock are present, fluid should be administered as a 20 ml/kg bolus. Recent meta-analysis has suggested that crystalloid fluids are to be preferred.[34] Certainly UK practice has been to use colloid, e.g. plasma, but crystalloid has been widely used elsewhere. The quality of the literature makes it difficult to make a definitive decision as to best initial fluid resuscitation, but the Cochrane database review recommends avoiding albumin outwith controlled studies.

Blood pressure (BP) is an unreliable sign of circulatory compromise in children. Up to 40% of the circulating blood volume needs to be lost before the blood pressure will fall. A falling blood pressure is a late sign and indicates a failure of compensatory mechanisms to maintain perfusion to vital areas. Once BP falls, early and urgent treatment is indicated if permanent harm is to be avoided.

While the medical staff are assessing the airway, breathing and circulation, the nursing staff should help get the child undressed and should attach a cardiac monitor and a pulse oximeter.

As a result of this initial assessment, the practitioner should be dealing with one of the following:
1. a child in cardiac arrest;
2. a traumatized child who requires further trauma-orientated resuscitation; or
3. an unstable child with continuing airway, breathing or circulatory compromise associated with underlying pathology.

CARDIAC ARREST

Cardiac arrest is rare in the pediatric population. Common causes include sudden infant death syndrome, trauma, drowning and asphyxia.[35]

Cardiac arrest in children is primarily asystolic in nature. Occasionally pulseless electrical activity ([PEA] also known as electromechanical dissociation [EMD]) or ventricular fibrillation (VF) is present.[35] It is important to begin resuscitation as above but consider definitive drug and fluid therapies as indicated by the underlying rhythm.

The outcome of cardiac arrest in children is dismal, particularly when it occurs in the community.[36] Children who sustain cardiac arrest in the emergency department have a better outcome than those who arrest in the community, but worse than those who arrest in hospital.[37] Prolonged hypoxia, hypoglycemia and acidosis in addition to the underlying disease process, all contribute to cell death particularly in the myocardium and brain, making restoration of vital functions difficult. Even if cardiac function is restored the prolonged insult to the brain usually leaves the child with permanent and usually profound neurological deficit.

ASYSTOLE

Asystole is characterized by a pulseless, apneic child associated with no complexes on the cardiac monitor. It is important to confirm that this is so by going through the following procedure:
1. turning up the gain on the cardiac monitor;
2. ensuring that all the connections are made;
3. checking that the monitor is not connected to 'paddles'.

The recommended sequence for dealing with asystole is found in Figure 36.2.[38]

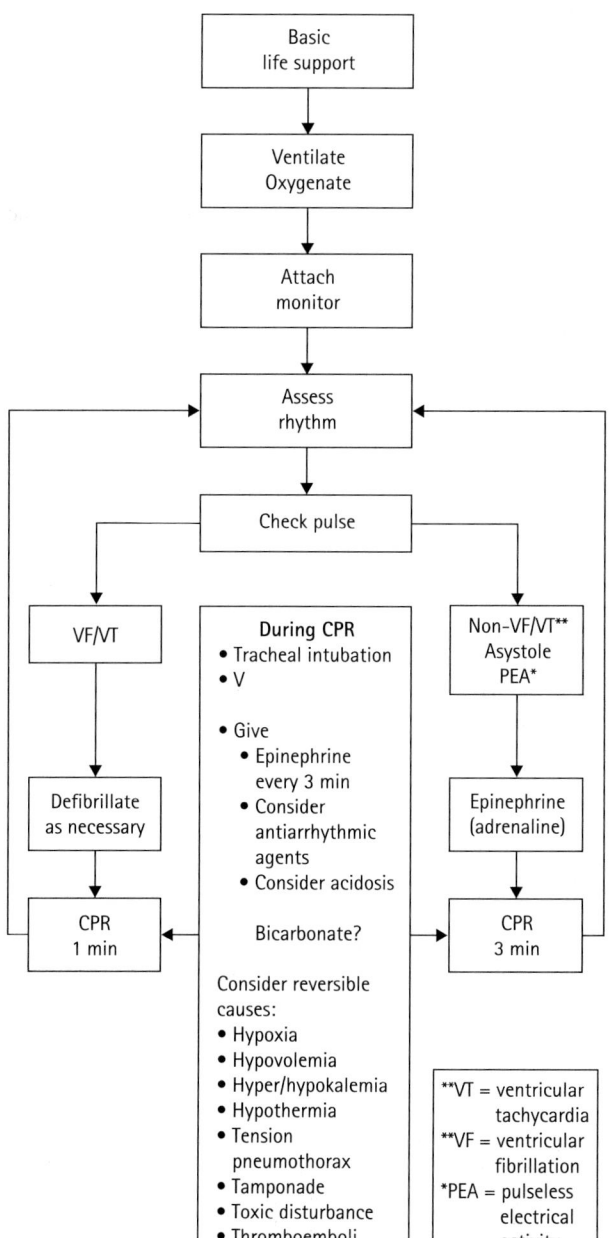

Fig. 36.2 Algorithm for management of pediatric cardiac arrest. (Adapted from Resuscitation Council (UK)[38] with permission)

PULSELESS ELECTRICAL ACTIVITY (PEA) (PREVIOUSLY KNOWN AS ELECTROMECHANICAL DISSOCIATION [EMD])

PEA is associated with a pulseless, apneic child and often bizarre complexes on a cardiac monitor. This may be associated with underlying pathology such as pneumothorax, cardiac tamponade, electrolyte imbalance, hypovolemia and hypothermia. Treatment should be aimed at correcting these underlying disorders. An algorithm for treating EMD can be seen in Figure 36.2.

VENTRICULAR FIBRILLATION

VF is much rarer in children than in adults. Recent reports have indicated that it might be more frequent than once suspected.[39,40] An algorithm for treating VF can be found in Figure 36.2.

STOPPING RESUSCITATION

The decision to terminate resuscitation can be difficult. Children who have been poisoned, drowned or who are hypothermic should have active resuscitation continued for considerable time. This will usually occur within the intensive care setting with continuing resuscitation during transit. Post-traumatic cardiac arrest has a very poor prognosis and prolonged attempts at resuscitation should be avoided. Similarly sudden infant death syndrome should not lead to unduly prolonged resuscitation attempts.

APPROACH TO THE SEVERELY INJURED CHILD

Major trauma is a relatively rare occurrence in the pediatric population compared to the adult population. Of children who die, 80% will be dead on arrival of the paramedical team at the scene, a fact which makes injury prevention all the more important. The role of paramedical intervention at the scene is crucial.

As with other forms of illness care of the airway, breathing and circulation are of paramount importance. *One of the major differences however, is that traumatized children are at risk of having damage to the spinal column, particularly the cervical spine, without radiological evidence of such injury (SCIWORA – see later).* In particular this means that one has to be able to perform airway-opening maneuvers without excessive movement being involved in the cervical spine area. Measures such as chin lift *without* head tilt are important. Oropharyngeal airways are important adjuncts to the process.

SCIWORA

SCIWORA is an acronym for *S*pinal *C*ord *I*njury *W*ith*O*ut *R*adiological *A*bnormality. This is a rare finding but has a potentially horrendous outcome.[41]

PATHOPHYSIOLOGY

Relative laxity of spinal ligaments associated with underdevelopment of the articular facets of the vertebrae in the spinal column allow excessive movement to take place during severe hyperflexion/extension injuries. This results in compression of the spinal cord with subsequent damage. The column will return to its normal anatomy without any evidence of fracture or subluxation being present. Normal X-rays therefore in an unconscious child should not lead one to assume that there is no possibility of spinal cord injury.

IMPLICATIONS FOR CLINICAL PRACTICE

If the child is awake and is able to move all four limbs then SCIWORA is unlikely to be present.[41] However, in those children who have an altered level of consciousness, SCIWORA must be suspected. In these children full spinal column immobilization measures must be implemented until such time as the spine can be cleared either radiologically or clinically. Simple measures to immobilize the spine will include: use of sand bags or other similar sized objects to immobilize the head, taping the head to a spinal board and immobilizing the head on the shoulders using hands and arms. The airway should be assessed and opened in the simplest way possible and this should be carried out without moving the cervical spine (see earlier).

BREATHING

Breathing abnormalities are common following trauma. Causes include pneumothorax, hemothorax, rib fractures and gastric dilatation. Children with traumatic injuries should be given supplemental oxygen and any specific underlying disease treated as appropriate. A pneumothorax should be decompressed by needle thoracostomy (above). Gastric dilatation should be decompressed by a gastric tube. If a basal skull fracture is suspected the gastric tube should be passed orally rather than nasally to avoid inadvertent placement in the brain!

CIRCULATION

Problems with circulation may be due to hypovolemia, tension pneumothorax or cardiac tamponade. Hypovolemia is the most common, particularly after intra-abdominal injuries. Small babies may become hypovolemic from an intracerebral bleed but this is unusual and other causes must be sought first. Some of the signs of hypovolemia are mimicked by trauma, in particular altered level of consciousness and poor peripheral pulses. A low blood pressure is a sign of great importance, indicating the need for urgent fluid replacement.

I.v. cannulae should be inserted into large veins, ideally avoiding fractured limbs. At the same time blood should be taken for laboratory analysis. If the child is stable and blood is not required urgently a simple 'group and save serum' is all that is required. Where the child is unstable blood will be required urgently. Ideally this blood should be fully grouped and cross-matched but occasionally O-negative blood will be needed. If sufficient blood is obtained the rest can be sent for full blood count, serum amylase and possibly urea and electrolytes. The value of each in managing the child will depend on the nature of the injury, underlying illness and local laboratory policies.

DISABILITY

Most head injuries are minor with the incidence of intracranial bleed being much less in the pediatric population than in the adult population.[42] As part of the first assessment the complete coma score, e.g. the Glasgow Coma Scale, does not need to be assessed. It is sufficient to document whether the child is Awake, responding to Verbal stimuli, responding to Painful stimuli or Unresponsive (the AVPU scale). Pupillary reflexes may be documented but at this stage they will not alter management significantly. Indeed papillary responses are often confusing. While the medical team are assessing airway, breathing, circulation and disability the nursing team should undress the child, apply a cardiac monitor and a pulse oximeter and prepare to assist with airway and i.v. access procedures. Surgical trays should be made available if required.

SECONDARY SURVEY

Once the airway, breathing and circulation have been addressed a full secondary survey of the child should be carried out. Every part of the body will be examined both visually and by palpation. Judicious use of plain X-ray, ultrasound and computed tomography (CT) will aid the diagnostic process. Minor injuries that may have been missed on the first brief survey will be detected and will lead to further treatment and investigation. Injuries that are commonly detected during the secondary survey include bleeding from the ear and nose, small pneumothoraces, gastric dilatation and minor fractures to the peripheries.

HEAD INJURY

Head injury is a significant cause of morbidity and mortality in the pediatric population.[43] The relatively large head changes the center of gravity and the head is one of the most commonly injured parts of the body in the pediatric population.

The causes of significant head injury include falls from a height, motor vehicle collisions and child abuse.

While most children who sustain significant head injury will lose consciousness it should be borne in mind that hypoxia, hypovolemia or both are significant causes of altered level of consciousness. Sharples et al[44] have shown that children transferred to a central neurosurgical unit with head injury were more likely to die as a result of associated hypoxia and/or hypovolemia due to respiratory or circulatory distress than death from the head injury. It must be questioned whether these children actually needed to be transferred at all as the head injury was often a relatively minor part of the problem. It is extremely important to exclude respiratory or circulatory problems before diagnosing intracranial problems as the cause of the altered level of consciousness.

The role of the emergency department in managing head injury is straightforward but it is important to grasp the concept of primary and secondary brain injury.

Primary brain injury occurs at the time of impact. Any damage done at this stage is usually irreversible. Secondary brain injury occurs early due to an extra insult, commonly hypoxia, hypovolemia and brain edema. Later infection, hydrocephalus and seizures may contribute substantially. The management of these later problems will fall to inpatient teams, but emergency staff members need to be aware of their role in identifying circumstances where and when they are likely to occur. There is a complex relationship between the primary injury and these other secondary factors. As a result of the initial injury there will be a degree of swelling secondary to a normal inflammatory response. Localized brain injury, which might occur if the child has been hit with a hard object such as a golf club or hammer, will result in a reasonably localized injury. Here the inflammation will be localized and will not cause generalized brain edema. At the other extreme is the small baby who is exposed to vigorous shaking (non-accidental injury). Here there will be diffuse brain injury with generalized inflammation throughout the brain. Postmortem examinations in this situation reveal multiple hemorrhages and diffuse brain edema that is often progressive and unstoppable. This malignant cerebral edema is almost impossible to treat and is usually the cause of significant morbidity and mortality associated with 'shaken baby syndrome'.[45,46] Most cases of head injury fall between these two extremes.

If the initial insult is associated with loss of consciousness then hypoxia will almost certainly follow as a result of an obstructed airway, usually from the tongue obstructing the oropharynx, or from vomitus entering the lungs. This will in turn cause cerebral anoxia with resultant cell damage and death and lead to a generalized inflammatory response with a variable degree of cerebral edema being present. The same situation will occur with other causes of hypoxia, e.g. pneumothorax, pulmonary contusion.

A decrease in perfusion pressure to the brain secondary to hemorrhage or other cause of hypovolemia will result in failure to deliver glucose and oxygen to the brain leading to an equivalent situation. Again as the inflammation increases the intracranial pressure also increases and unless there is adequate circulatory drive to perfuse the brain, a vicious circle ensues.

The primary role of the emergency department therefore is to ensure that the airway is open, that ventilation is maximized and that oxygen saturations are maintained between 95% and 100%, and to maintain circulation to enable cerebral perfusion to be normalized.

By the time the child gets to the emergency department a degree of intracranial swelling may already have taken place. In the early stages this will usually be due to an intracranial hematoma. Extradural, acute subdural or intracranial bleeds can all produce considerable pressure effects. It is important to recognize that children can sustain an extradural hematoma in the absence of fractures to the middle meningeal region, in contrast to the adult population, and normal skull X-rays therefore can be misleading.[47] The role of the emergency department is to ensure the airway, breathing and circulation are maximized and that any other life-threatening injury is identified and controlled. Only then should the child be transferred to the scanning suite, when the formal diagnosis can be made. There will often be a dilemma between surgical hemostasis (e.g. from a ruptured liver or spleen) and management of significant intracranial hematoma. It is imperative in these situations to control the circulation and to ensure brain perfusion is maximized to reduce the effect of secondary brain injury from hypoxia and/or hypovolemia. This tension is not easy to resolve and takes considerable experience and seniority to ensure the optimum sequence of events occurs.

With CT there is often evidence of raised intracranial pressure and no evidence of intracranial bleed. In this situation the practitioner is dealing with cerebral edema and several mechanisms exist to try to reduce the pressure including: hyperventilation to maintain a $PaCO_2$ of about 4 kPa, use of mannitol or furosemide (frusemide) (or other loop diuretic) and sedative techniques such as barbiturate anesthesia. It should be noted that most of these measures only work on a normal brain and are of little benefit at best. Use of these agents should be discussed with the neurosurgeon.

The emergency department is responsible for identifying basal skull fractures by clinical examination. Physical signs that indicate a basal skull fracture include 'panda eyes' (raccoon eyes), blood or cerebrospinal fluid from the nose or ears or 'Battle's sign' (bruising over the mastoid process). Basal skull fractures are open fractures and there is a high risk that infection will supervene between 12 h and 24 h, or possibly later. The use of antibiotics for the management of basal skull fractures is controversial. There is no clear evidence that antibiotics will reduce the chance of meningitis but this should be discussed with the local neurosurgical unit.[48] Many children will have seizures subsequent to the head injury. This can result in hypoxia with the inherent risks discussed earlier. After supplying oxygen and assisting ventilation the fit should be stopped using diazepam 0.2 mg/kg. Assessment of the level of consciousness is now difficult and these children should undergo CT scanning. Phenytoin 15 mg/kg may be used to reduce subsequent seizures after discussion with the neurosurgical unit.

Once a child has had a secure airway established, oxygenation is maximized and circulation and perfusion restored to normal, the child should be transferred for definitive diagnosis to the CT suite under stringent transfer conditions. Transfer from the safety of the resuscitation room should not start until full transfer protocols have been instituted. Transfer from the emergency setting to the scanning suite is just as dangerous as traveling from one center to another.

THORACOABDOMINAL INJURIES

Thoracoabdominal injury is relatively rare in the pediatric population compared with the adolescent and adult population. Most injuries are blunt although increase of firearms has meant that penetrating thoracoabdominal trauma is rising.[25] Many children with major thoracic injuries will die before reaching hospital although improvements in pre-hospital care may mean that an increasing number may survive. Injuries that fall into this category include traumatic dissection of the aorta and massive tension pneumothorax.

Traumatic dissection of the thoracic aorta is typically caused by rapid deceleration injury and most children will die in the pre-hospital phase. If they survive to reach hospital the diagnosis can be suspected by the presence of a widened mediastinum on a chest film associated with fractures of the upper ribs. It is best confirmed by either arteriography or CT. If suspected the child should be transferred to a thoracic surgical center.

Tension pneumothorax is treated by the insertion of a large-bore needle into the second intercostal space on the affected side. Signs of tension pneumothorax include signs of respiratory distress, distended neck veins and absent breath sounds on the affected side. Once the pneumothorax is drained using the needle a formal chest drain should

be inserted and connected to an underwater seal as soon as possible. Drainage of a pneumothorax on one side may reveal the presence of a lesion on the other side and this should be treated appropriately.

MODERATE CHEST INJURY

The use of seat belts and seat restraints has led to an increase in chest wall bruising due to the seat belt physically restraining the child. Children who have seat belt abrasions to the chest and abdomen have been subjected to quite considerable deceleration forces. While the mostly likely thoracic injuries will be a fractured clavicle with or without a fractured sternum, it should be borne in mind that underlying myocardial contusion is possible. This is extremely difficult to detect clinically. The presence of slightly abnormal electrocardiograms (ECGs) and raised cardiac enzymes are unreliable. If there is any doubt the child should be admitted for a period of observation with continuous cardiac monitoring.

Fractured ribs are rare in the pediatric population. If seen in the infant or toddler group non-accidental injury should be suspected. Management is required for relief of pain. If there are more than three ribs fractured on one side the child should to be admitted to a high-dependency care unit for intercostal blocks to be administered. Bilateral rib fractures may lead to a flail chest but this is rare in children.

ABDOMINAL INJURY

Blunt trauma is the usual cause. Penetrating trauma increases in frequency as children get older. Blunt trauma can result in hemorrhage and loss of perfusion from rupture to solid organs such as spleen, kidney and liver; or peritonitis from injury to the bowel and pancreas. With each of these a strong index of suspicion is needed as early on the child can have minimal abdominal signs, but will subsequently develop significant problems. This is particularly so of pancreatitis and bowel perforation, where peritonitis can take between 6 h and 12 h to develop.

Intra-abdominal hemorrhage should be considered in any child who shows evidence of circulatory collapse following trauma. Clinical diagnosis is unreliable and imaging is almost certainly indicated, particularly if the child is stable. Ultrasound is a useful screening tool. In skilled hands even small amounts of free fluid can be detected. Most skilled ultrasonographers will be able to identify the site of bleeding if due to damage to solid organs, i.e. liver, spleen and kidney. If free fluid is present but no solid organ damage is identified then CT with contrast is indicated. Children who are unstable should have intra-abdominal bleeding suspected and treated according to the accompanying diagram (Fig. 36.3). Hepatic and splenic trauma will usually be treated conservatively provided the child remains stable.[49]

SEAT BELT INJURY

A seat belt ideally involves three-point fixation with a lap belt and harness. If children are restrained using a lap belt alone and are involved in a high-speed collision there is a reasonable chance they will sustain a hyperflexion injury of the torso. This will usually result in intra-abdominal injury with a significant hepatic or splenic component. This will often be associated with a degree of spinal instability with fractures occurring in the L_1, L_2 region of the lumbar spine.[50] Any child who has a significant lap belt injury to the midabdominal region should have spinal injury suspected and should have full spinal immobilization carried out until the spine has been fully cleared both radiologically and clinically (see SCIWORA as earlier).

ORTHOPEDIC INJURY

It should be stressed that orthopedic injuries are a long way down the order of treatment. Priority should be given to airway, breathing and circulation prior to doing anything with orthopedic injuries.

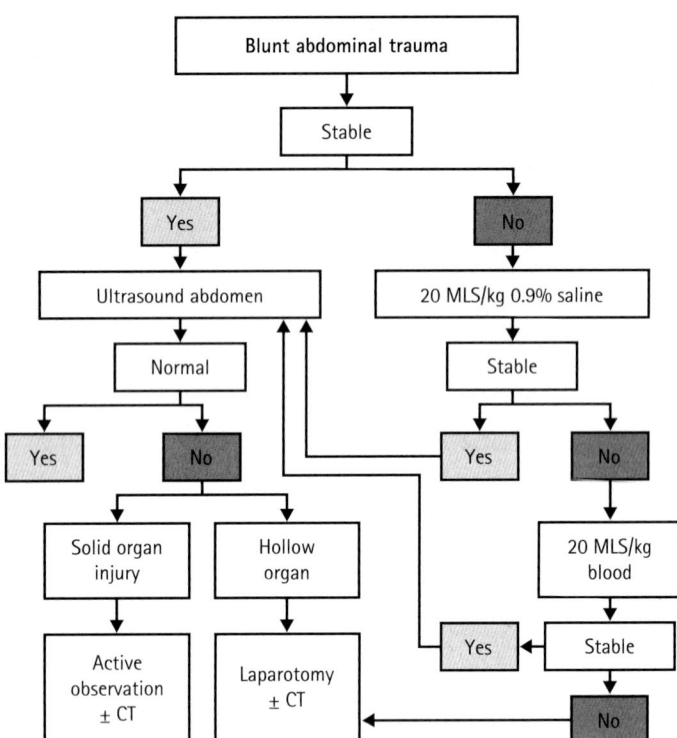

Fig. 36.3 Management of blunt abdominal trauma.

Orthopedic injury following trauma is common. Within the emergency department there are three aspects that should be considered:
1. recognition of the fracture;
2. identification of associated soft tissue injury that may cause compromise to the limb;
3. splintage and analgesia.

RECOGNITION OF THE FRACTURE

If a bone is bent, it is broken! Of more concern is the occult undisplaced fracture. Such fractures can bleed into tight fascial compartments with subsequent compartment syndrome. Vascular compromise is particularly common with fractures of the elbow, where the brachial artery may be involved, and the tibia. If there is any concern about the presence of an occult fracture the area should be X-rayed to either confirm it or rule it out.

With all fractures the distal pulses should be palpated and distal neurological function should be checked. If the perfusion is adequate distal to the fracture site then all that is needed is for the limb to be splinted until life-threatening conditions such hypoxia or hypovolemia are corrected. Nerve injuries need to be noted and examined further when the child is stable.

IDENTIFICATION OF ASSOCIATED SOFT TISSUE INJURY

Soft tissue injuries associated with fractures include:
1. tissue loss;
2. open wounds;
3. vascular damage;
4. nerve damage;
5. tendon damage.

Tissue loss and open wounds associated with fracture will lead to infection in the bone if not adequately treated and debrided. The emergency department is not the place to start this process but the wound should not be ignored. It is sufficient to assess the distal pulses and neurological function and as long as these are intact, dress the wound with a disinfectant dressing and leave further management to the orthopedic department. Broad-spectrum antibiotics effective against Gram positive, Gram negative and anaerobic organisms are important. Local policies determine which antibiotics are given. Tetanus prophylaxis is also important if the patient is not fully immunized.

ANALGESIA

Pain with a long bone fracture is severe and analgesia is greatly underused. There is often a fear of masking intra-abdominal injury or of aggravating conscious level with head injury. Both of these are inadequate reasons to withhold analgesia in a child who is in considerable pain. Two methods of analgesia exist in this situation:
1. local and peripheral nerve block;
2. i.v. opiate.

LOCAL AND PERIPHERAL NERVE BLOCK

The femur is most amenable to this management strategy. Successful block can be obtained by infiltrating a long-acting anesthetic such as levobupivacaine around the femoral nerve where it passes under the inguinal ligament lateral to the femoral artery. This will take 5–10 min to work (and can be preceded by a more fast-acting local anesthetic such as lidocaine or prilocaine). If epinephrine (adrenaline) is used great care must be taken not to inject epinephrine (adrenaline) into the femoral artery, which is adjacent to the nerve. Some authors advocate the use of sciatic nerve block for tibial fractures. To be effective however, this requires sophisticated equipment that is not always available within the emergency setting.

INTRAVENOUS OPIATE

In trauma situations opiate analgesia should always be given intravenously. Recent reports on the efficacy of intranasal diamorphine should be treated cautiously. These reports compared intranasal diamorphine against intramuscular.[51,52] There is no place for the intramuscular route as absorption is unreliable. Whether i.v. opiate will be replaced by intranasal has yet to be established.

The weight of the child should be estimated by whatever means possible and the appropriate dose of opiate obtained. This should be further diluted to 10 ml. This can then be titrated 1 ml at a time over a period of 10 min to maximal effect. As soon as the child becomes settled the administration can be stopped and a further bolus given at intervals to maintain analgesia. Usually at this stage the pain drive will be sufficient to keep the child awake and to counteract any possible diminution of level of consciousness. If there is any concern subsequently about the ability to assess either level of consciousness or the abdomen then naloxone can be used to reverse the opiate. This is rarely necessary.

Once analgesia has been administered then the fractured limb should be splinted until the child can be brought to theater by the orthopedic surgeons. Splintage is an important consideration for analgesia in injured children. One of the major challenges for pediatric emergency departments is the absence of commercially available splints suitable for all the different shapes of children. Often these have to be fashioned on an ad hoc basis from plaster of Paris or some other newer synthetic casting material.

BURN CARE

Burns are a common problem in children. Two broad issues need to be addressed:
1. the burn injury (by whatever cause);
2. complications such as smoke inhalation, hypothermia, toxic shock syndrome.

Although both issues can occur together, usually one or the other is the main problem on initial presentation to the emergency department. There are many etiologies for burn injury (Table 36.2). No matter what the cause, the approach to a burn injury is the same. The airway, breathing and circulation should be assessed and looked after as in all previous circumstances. Once these have been addressed it is important to identify the size of the burn. Management of the burn will depend on the following factors:
1. area involved;
2. depth of the burn;
3. site of the burn.

AREA OF THE BURN

Small burns, i.e. less than 5% of total body surface area (TBSA), can be managed on an outpatient basis provided that the burn is superficial, does not involve a significant area and there are no complications present.

Treatment will consist of analgesia, usually oral, and dressings according to local policy. One method of dressing the burn is to use tulle gras impregnated with mupirocin, which is an effective anti-staphylococcal agent. Once the burn is greater than 5% TBSA analgesia requirements will usually necessitate admission and an i.v. opiate will be required. Whether the wounds are dressed or left open is dependent on local practice. Once the burn is greater than 10% TBSA then the child will need i.v. rehydration according to local formulae, e.g. Parkland formula.

DEPTH OF THE BURN

Burns can be classified as superficial, partial thickness and full thickness. Superficial burns include those with erythema only or with small amounts of blistering. Partial-thickness burns are those that have a significant area of blistering, with either blisters intact or spontaneously

Table 36.2 Causes of burn injury

1. Wet heat	Scald
2. Dry heat	Flame
	Hot surface
3. Radiation	Ultraviolet (sunburn)
	Iatrogenic (as radiation treatment in oncology)
4. Chemical	Acid
	Alkali
	Corrosive
5. Electrical	

burst. Full-thickness burns present as white avascular areas that are insensitive to touch (it is unkind to touch burns in children and inspection is usually all that is required for diagnosis).

In reality a mixture of superficial, partial thickness and full thickness is usually present depending on the burning agent and the duration it has been in contact with the skin. In general all full-thickness burns should be referred to a plastic surgeon for immediate assessment and treatment. Partial-thickness burns may be suitable for outpatient care if they do not extend over a large surface area. Treatment is as discussed earlier.

SITE OF THE BURN

Burns to the face, airway, mouth, pharynx, buttock and perineum, hands and feet and any circumferential burn to either the trunk or a limb need to be treated with a great deal of caution. Burns in any of these areas need to be referred to a burns specialist for inpatient treatment. Burns to the face and airway in particular, may require admission to an intensive care unit as the risk to the airway is quite considerable.

COMPLICATIONS OF BURNS

In the emergency department it is important to identify those children with complications such as smoke inhalation, hypothermia or those with burns possibly from non-accidental injury.

SMOKE INHALATION

Smoke inhalation is a complex entity with several mechanisms:
1. inhalation of toxic fumes such as carbon monoxide and/or cyanide;
2. local action of soot and other organic particles;
3. chemical burns from acids and other compounds.

Carbon monoxide poisoning and cyanide lead to asphyxia due to red cells being unable to release oxygen. It is the leading cause of death following house fires. Children who are suspected of having carbon monoxide poisoning should be resuscitated with 100% oxygen. If cyanide poisoning is suspected then treatment with standard cyanide kits is suggested either with dicobalt edetate if the child is comatose or hydroxycobalamin if the child is comatose but still perfusing.

Bronchial lavage may be considered if particulate matter or acids are considered to be present in the airway.

The net result of the contamination is a fulminant inflammatory process leading to significant pulmonary edema. This can be of insidious onset and consequently all children who are suspected of having had smoke inhalation should be admitted for a period of observation until such time as they are proved normal.

TOXIC SHOCK

Toxic shock is a rare but significant complication of burn injury (and occasionally other minor wounds including those following minor surgery). Typically caused by staphylococcal toxins, streptococci have also been implicated. Usually the wound/burn will be colonized rather than overtly infected by the bacteria. Symptoms include fever > 38.5°C, erythematous rash, vomiting, diarrhea and malaise. If a child presents within 2–3 days of sustaining a burn/wound with any or all of these signs or symptoms toxic shock should be suspected.

Treatment consists of identifying the cause (wound swab, blood for blood culture and serology), urgent resuscitation with fluids and antibiotics (which should reflect local streptococcal and staphylococcal antibiotic sensitivities) and local wound care as appropriate. Affected children should be admitted to a critical care area for further care.

MANAGEMENT OF THE UNSTABLE CHILD WITH UNDERLYING PATHOLOGY

After securing the airway, breathing and circulation, the real challenge is to identify the actual disease process and the etiological factors that have led to the presentation so that the most appropriate therapy can be given.

The standard approach of taking a history and then doing a physical examination is often inappropriate. The history available at this stage can be scrappy and imprecise. Most information will be gained from a detailed physical examination. This is best done in a systematic fashion, excluding groups of illnesses in turn. Patterns of illness include:

1. infection and life-threatening infection;
2. seizure disorder and coma;
3. metabolic abnormalities;
4. cardiac lesions;
5. respiratory disorders;
6. surgical pathology;
7. poisoning.

INFECTION

Life-threatening infection is relatively rare in the western world where vaccination and immunization are widespread. Diseases such as diphtheria and epiglottitis have been almost eradicated with effective vaccination but in areas where vaccination is less good or has waned these diseases continue to form important causes of mortality. Meningococcemia continues to be one of the most important life-threatening infections to appear acutely to the emergency department.

When dealing with infection three broad age groups have to be considered:

1. 0–3 months;
2. 3 months–3 years;
3. 3 years and over.

Children aged 0–3 months

Neonates and young infants have many of the problems related to infection. The symptoms with which these children present are many and varied.[53,54] They include going off feeds, failure to thrive, jitteriness and irritability. While many of these children will have an infection, other causes have to be considered. These include congenital anomalies such as congenital heart disease or inborn errors of metabolism or surgical causes such as intussusception and obstructed hernia.

Physical signs such as neck stiffness and bulging fontanelles are unreliable in this age group as are blood parameters such as white cell count and preponderance of neutrophils to lymphocytes. Clinical suspicion therefore is the mainstay of diagnosis and if there is any doubt children should have blood cultures taken and antibiotic treatment started. These children are usually admitted until such time as the diagnosis is reached.

Children aged 3 months–3 years

The children at the lower end of this spectrum will still be prone to neonatal illness. Viral illness is more common than bacterial illness in this age group but underlying bacterial illness or bacteremia should still be considered. However, it is still important to recognize the child who is toxic, and who is 'not right'.[55,56] Physical signs are more precise, with these children often being pyrexial, tachycardiac and tachypneic. Signs such as neck stiffness are more reliable in the diagnosis of meningitis. Signs of chest infection, osteomyelitis and septic arthritis may be easier to detect.

Children aged 3 years and over

Significant bacterial disease is relatively rare in this age group but includes chest infection, septicemia, urinary tract infection and orthopedic infection. Meningitis and meningococcal septicemia are still relatively rare. Abdominal conditions are easier to diagnose in these children because these children are better able to communicate symptoms.

Meningococcal disease

Infection with *Neisseria meningitidis* is one of the most significant reasons for a child to be critically ill. Often starting as a vague nonspecific illness at any age this infection can kill within hours. The florid purpuric rash is often not present initially, more often developing from a subtle finding in the early stages. Limb pains are common. (In the community, treatment should consist of intramuscular benzyl penicillin and urgent transfer to hospital with supplemental oxygen by mask. In the emergency department i.v. access and fluid replacement will be added. Fluid volumes of 60 ml/kg may be needed (in 10–20 ml/kg bolus) to restore perfusion. A cephalosporin (e.g. ceftriaxone, cefuroxime or cefotaxime) will be added to penicillin to control infection. Prompt transfer to the intensive care unit should be arranged when inotropic agents may be added to the management. It is helpful to complete an assessment of the Glasgow Meningococcal Prognostic score as soon as sufficient clinical data is available.

Management of life-threatening infection

These children should be resuscitated and blood taken for full blood count, urea and electrolytes, blood glucose and culture. Capillary blood gas analysis may also help determine initial status of the child and monitor early response to resuscitation. Chest X-ray, urine culture and lumbar puncture may also be indicated. Care should be taken not to perform lumbar puncture on children who are unconscious as this may produce herniation of the brain through the tentorium with resultant brain death.

I.v. antibiotics should be administered according to local sensitivity patterns and protocols. Children should be admitted to a high dependency or intensive care unit where inotropic support may be needed.

SEIZURE DISORDER

The list of underlying pathologies for patients presenting with seizure disorders is vast. Most will either be due to idiopathic epilepsy, a febrile seizure disorder or secondary to metabolic defects such as hypoglycemia or electrolyte disorder. Trauma should also be considered. Treatment should be aimed at stopping the seizure and at the same time trying to identify underlying treatable causes such as hypoglycemia and electrolyte imbalance. If fever is present this should be reduced as rapidly as possible.

Management of seizure disorder in the emergency situation

First-line treatment is i.v. diazepam, 0.2 mg/kg to a maximum 0.6 mg/kg intravenously. Lorazepam 0.1 mg/kg is also acceptable. If i.v. access is not readily available then rectal diazepam (2.5–10 mg depending on age) or intranasal midazolam (0.2 mg/kg) are acceptable treatments. This should be followed (if the seizure is not stopped) by a slow i.v. administration of phenytoin 10–15 mg/kg under ECG control. At this stage if the child is still fitting then consideration must be given to reducing intracranial pressure, paralysis and ventilation in order to control the seizure with additional anticonvulsants. Such management will need an intensive care/high dependency unit.

Blood sugar should always be tested by strip testing. If the blood sugar is low this may reveal an underlying metabolic disorder. Further blood should be taken along with urine to help diagnose metabolic anomalies if present and the child given 10% glucose 3–5 ml/kg.

COMA

Comatose children are particularly at risk of obstructing their airway so great care must be given to maintaining this. Once the airway is secured the underlying causes such as poisoning, epilepsy, head injury or other trauma, hypoglycemia or intracranial infection should be investigated. Treatable causes should be identified and treated appropriately and the child transferred to a high-dependency area as soon as possible. This may involve transfer via CT scanning if intracranial lesion is suspected. If trauma is suspected, particularly non-accidental injury, the child should be treated as with any other trauma victim and resuscitated aggressively prior to transfer.

METABOLIC ABNORMALITIES

Diabetic abnormalities, either hypo- or hyperglycemia, are the commonest. Small babies may present critically ill as a result of an inborn error of metabolism. While these are relatively rare they should be suspected in any child who presents close to the neonatal period, particularly if there is an intercurrent infection suspected. A strong clue to this might be the presence of hypoglycemia. Diabetic emergencies should be treated as detailed under the diabetic section (Ch. 15).

CARDIAC LESIONS

Children with cardiac lesions present in one of two ways:
1. in heart failure;
2. in cardiac arrest.

Heart failure is often due to progression of cardiac abnormalities. Underlying disease processes such as renal failure with hyperkalemia may have to be considered. Previously well children may have developed myocarditis. Supraventricular tachycardia is the commonest underlying cardiac dysrhythmia to cause heart failure, particularly in the younger age groups. The treatment of heart failure should be aimed towards maximizing oxygenation and reducing the fluid load. Any underlying dysrhythmia should be treated appropriately according to local guidelines. The child should be transferred to a high dependency area as soon as possible where future treatment can be monitored and inotropic support given if necessary.

The management of cardiac arrest is described earlier (p. 1586). The underlying causes may include hypertrophic cardiomyopathy or dysrhythmia.

RESPIRATORY DISORDERS

Common respiratory disorders to present include asthma, bronchiolitis, croup and foreign body in the airway. Recognition of respiratory distress/failure has been considered earlier. All children with respiratory disease should have oxygen delivery maximized and treatment directed to the underlying cause.

If it is suspected that a foreign body is wedged in the airway, the Heimlich maneuver or chest thrust maneuver may be necessary depending on the level of consciousness of the child.

SURGICAL CAUSES

Surgical causes of collapse are often forgotten in the emergency department, particularly in those in the younger age group. Intussusception and obstructed herniae commonly cause symptoms such as vomiting. This vomiting is not typical of that of gastroenteritis; it may only consist of one or two vomits. After that the child becomes unduly collapsed. Intussusception in particular can present with a child who is deathly pale but without much else in the way of physical signs. The classic signs of redcurrant jelly stool and a palpable mass are often absent.[56]

Pyloric stenosis may present with a dehydrated alkalotic child if the vomiting has been profuse.

If a pubertal girl presents in a collapsed state, two diagnoses should be considered – drug overdose (either intentional or accidental) and ectopic pregnancy. These may be related, i.e. the pregnancy is the reason for the overdose. In both situations resuscitation is vital. Pregnancy may be the result of child sexual abuse and this should be treated, if suspected, along local guidelines.

POISONING (see Ch. 6)

Poisoning in children is commonest between the second and third year of life. Children who are poisoned usually present with minimal signs or symptoms. The role of the emergency department is to identify the child who is at risk of either airway or circulatory collapse and to deal with these problems accordingly. All doctors working in emergency departments should have a good working knowledge of pharmacology of medications that are both prescribed and bought over the counter. The knowledge of the potential side-effects will help in determining which children can be discharged and those that need to be admitted for further care.

The role of gastric decontamination in this age group is difficult. The current trend is to move away from gastric lavage, which is a particularly unpleasant process. The role of syrup of ipecacuanha has also been challenged. There is evidence to suggest that it will only be effective (if at all) if administered within 1 h of the ingestion. The current vogue is for decontamination using charcoal. Most children will actually drink charcoal despite it looking unpleasant and this probably is the method of choice for all children who actually require gastric decontamination.

Specific antidotes are available for only a few poisons. Staff working within the emergency department should be familiar with these and their usage.

CONCLUSION

The pediatric emergency medical system has many facets, all of which need to be coordinated to provide for the streamlined care of sick or injured children. The aim should be prevention if at all possible. If prevention is not possible then facilities must exist for the efficient care of all children within a seamless emergency medical structure capable of providing all aspects of emergency care and rehabilitation back to the community.

PEDIATRIC INTENSIVE CARE

INTRODUCTION

Intensive care is distinguished from high-dependency or ward care by the level of observation and the level of intervention required by the patients. Close observation is assured by:

- The numbers of staff: at least one nurse per patient and at least one doctor awake and working on the unit at all times;
- The skill level of staff: only experienced pediatric intensive care nurses are allowed to work at the bedside and the resident medical staff members have to have advanced resuscitation and airway skills. There are high levels of supervision from senior staff. Higher levels of intervention take the form of:
- Continuous physiological monitoring: this will often involve additional circulatory access such as arterial and central venous lines but may also include a variety of other techniques, for example more invasive hemodynamic monitoring, indwelling oximetric catheters, intracranial pressure monitoring;
- Intensive care dependent techniques of organ–system support: the term 'intensive care dependent' meaning that it would be inappropriate to contemplate undertaking such support for a critically ill child without the level of monitoring and supervision available on the pediatric intensive care unit. Examples include mechanical ventilation, inotropic or mechanical circulatory support and renal replacement therapies such as hemofiltration.

Pediatric intensive care units cater for critically ill children from birth to 16 years of age but the age distribution is heavily skewed towards the lower age range. The median age of admissions is frequently less than 1 year and the mean is usually around 3 years. The units are predominantly geared towards emergency admissions since typically only about 30% of admissions are booked in advance in association with elective surgery or other procedures. The case mix bears comparison with the predominant causes of death in pediatrics, which themselves change with age. Infections and congenital abnormalities along with their attendant surgery figure prominently in young patients, whereas malignancy and trauma are commoner in older patients. Of admissions, 40% occur in the context of congenital heart disease whether they are new presentations, elective admissions after surgery or emergency admissions for other causes such as respiratory infection complicating pulmonary edema. Otherwise primary respiratory problems account for about 20% of admissions with strong seasonal and geographical variations. Major trauma also displays seasonal variation (lower in winter and highest during summer holidays) but accounts for up to 15% of admissions overall. Neurological problems (other than trauma) make up less than 10%.

The contribution of other diagnostic categories is more varied, depending upon the allocation of neonatal surgical patients and other services. Survival rates amongst critically ill children are generally high (about 92% of admissions) compared to the intensive care of other age groups. The length of intensive care stay is another skewed distribution (most are of very short duration, median circa 24 h) but the mean varies from 2 to 4 d depending principally on the quality of local 'step down' (high-dependency) facilities. This average length of stay is comparatively short compared to neonatal and adult intensive care.

Many intensive care admissions are critical emergencies and decisions to admit the patient under these circumstances are not difficult or often disputed. However, the apparently abrupt decline in a patient's condition is frequently the manifest decompensation of a process or processes that have been proceeding for some time and hence could, at least in theory, have been identified in advance. The final common pathway of cellular hypoxia/ischemia and organ dysfunction that leads to death in children is initiated by circulatory or respiratory failure and ends in asystole. The potential benefits of intensive care are therefore best realized by pre-emptive intervention to avert probable further deterioration.

Hence it is important to learn to recognize the sick child. Firstly, recognize ominous diagnoses for which the likely course of the disease is known (e.g. purpura fulminans in meningococcal septicemia). Alternatively, try to realize the severity of illness from basic clinical signs. Work on a system-by-system basis taking respiration and circulation first. The two key questions are:

1. How much work is being done? Which then indicates a second question: how sustainable is this level of physiological effort? and
2. How effective is it? (since ineffective effort will need to be supplemented sooner rather than later).

For example the work of breathing can be assessed by the respiratory rate, tidal volume and the apparent ease or otherwise of chest expansion. Look for the use of accessory muscles and the strain involved. Breathing may be difficult due to poor compliance or airway obstruction (listen for inspiratory stridor or expiratory wheeze) and there may be subcostal, intercostal, costal or sternal recession, tracheal tug or head bobbing, etc. Assess the effectiveness of breathing by the adequacy of chest expansion, the amount of oxygen required to avoid desaturation, conscious level, heart rate, presence of sweating and adequacy of peripheral perfusion as well as measurements of oxygen saturation and formal blood gases. Remember that cyanosis is a preterminal sign in respiratory failure and that premature infants respond to stress (including hypoxia) with bradycardia rather than the tachycardia otherwise expected first.

Once compensatory mechanisms have been exceeded, a precipitate and rapid deterioration occurs. Hence it is also very important to use recent *trends* in physiological observations as an indication of the patient's current condition and likely progress. Early intervention is far more likely to be successful and the use of thresholds for action usually causes delay even if they are based upon age-appropriate norms and reference ranges.

In the acute presentation of critical illness, the ultimate cause (i.e. the diagnosis) may not be apparent. Hence a treatment plan may have to be devised that addresses all the possibilities until further information becomes available. The sequence of priorities is to Resuscitate, then Diagnose and Treat, i.e. *Resuscitation comes first*. If immediate resuscitation is not necessary, still concentrate on physiology/pathophysiology (in terms of work and effectiveness) to decide how and when to instigate specific organ system support and monitoring. Then proceed with investigations that may lead to more specific treatment. The ultimate diagnosis may be made over a broad timeframe and the patient may sometimes have left intensive care before the whole clinical picture is apparent.

POST-RESUSCITATION STABILIZATION AND TRANSFER

The initial resuscitation of acutely ill children is often described as being followed by a period of 'postresuscitation stabilization'. This may be prolonged and it may be found necessary to defer some aspects of care depending upon the resuscitation priorities. For example in severe trauma the resuscitation can involve emergency surgery after which the patient is moved to the intensive care unit. At this point reassess the patient and complete a secondary survey. The resuscitation may have also created problems that need to be identified and dealt with. Studies suggest that medically significant complications due to cardiopulmonary resuscitation are rare in children (< 3%). Those complications that have been reported include retroperitoneal hemorrhage, pneumothorax, pulmonary hemorrhage, epicardial hematoma, and gastric perforation.

Once resuscitation is complete or nearing completion, prepare the patient for longer term intensive care by revision/augmentation of airway and vascular access. For example oral intubation may need changing to nasal and if necessary replace intraosseous access with a central venous line and peripheral i.v. cannulae. An arterial line may be required. Good intensive care is about doing simple things well. Hence procedures such as the style of intubation, the manner of endotracheal tube fixation and the method of securing drips should all be controlled by unit protocol unless otherwise contraindicated. For example routine, non-essential revision of the intubation is unwise if the airway was precarious initially or if intubation was difficult to achieve. But in all other circumstances, especially if the patient is to be transferred, the most stable and familiar techniques should be employed.

Oxygenation is the highest priority but adequate minute volume must be provided to clear carbon dioxide. Assess both by serial measurements of arterial blood gases. Acidosis may have metabolic consequences such as hyperkalemia (a compartment shift) or pharmacological effects such as failure to respond to catecholamines. It may aggravate symptoms of poisoning with drugs that are weak acids. Correct any respiratory acidosis by increasing minute volume particularly if the $[H^+] > 63$ nmol/L (pH < 7.2). Treat the cause of any metabolic acidosis in preference to giving bicarbonate, since without treatment of the cause the acidosis will recur. I.v. bicarbonate may be indicated to compensate for recognized bicarbonate losses (e.g. ileostomy fluid) or to recruit a pharmacodynamic response (e.g. if there is a poor response to inotrope therapy due to acidosis) but otherwise runs the risk of increasing the work of breathing (through CO_2 production) and aggravating intracellular acidosis ($CO_{2(aq)}$ and H^+ ions diffuse into cells more rapidly than bicarbonate).

A normal blood pressure is not a sufficient assessment of the cardiovascular system. Determine the adequacy of the circulation by assessing end organ (cellular) function using markers like urine output, mental state, degree of metabolic acidosis or serum lactate levels. Remember that resuscitation may have compensated for the presenting problem rather than resolved it. Furthermore a variety of other problems are common after acute resuscitation. Look for dilutional anemia, which can arise as a consequence of large intravascular volume boluses having been given during resuscitation. Give red cell transfusion priority if oxygen delivery is critical or compromised (one possible cause of metabolic acidosis). Also establish an appropriate ongoing i.v. fluid and electrolyte regime at this point that includes maintenance requirements, metered replacement of any deficit and comprehensive replacement of ongoing losses. If inotropic or chronotropic support is required then use titratable infusions of short-acting agents in preference over longer acting agents whose effects may persist when the current hemodynamic state changes. Measure the blood glucose level since hypoglycemia is common and not detectable by clinical observation in the obtunded, sedated or otherwise critically ill child. The risk of hypoglycemia is increased in smaller and younger patients as a consequence of low glycogen reserves and a high basal metabolic rate. The dose of glucose in acute hypoglycemia is 0.5 g/kg. This dose must be followed by repeated assessment of the blood glucose level to check that a therapeutic effect has been achieved and that the resulting level is maintained. The normal maintenance requirement for babies is 6 mg/kg/min.

For all but the most straightforward of resuscitation scenarios the patient then requires further management on an intensive care unit. For all but the simplest cases this should be a specialist pediatric intensive care unit particularly if it is difficult to anticipate what the length of intensive care unit stay will be or if it is likely to be more than 24 h. Transfers within hospital or between hospitals usually occur after stabilization and are conducted without undue haste by a retrieval team from the pediatric intensive care unit. The use of a skilled and trained transfer team substantially reduces critical incidents and morbidity. The need for such transfer is entirely predictable and so detailed protocols should be prepared in advance including specified indications and provision for more urgent movement. Training in intensive care transport must be practical and is best provided by supervised episodes accompanying a skilled team. Trainees must become familiar with the modes of transport used and must attain higher levels of proficiency in equipment maintenance and repair than are necessary for clinical staff within a hospital environment. This is because technical backup is not available during transfers.

RESPIRATORY SYSTEM

INDICATIONS FOR MECHANICAL VENTILATION

One of the commonest reasons for arranging intensive care admission is a decision to start mechanical ventilation. Infants and children have less respiratory reserve than adults, which leads to a relatively high incidence of respiratory failure during severe illness. Respiratory support may be indicated:

- to secure the upper airway;
- to reduce the work of spontaneous breathing;
- to supplement gas exchange in respiratory disease;
- to achieve desirable hemodynamic effects;
- as an incidental requirement during sedation or anesthesia;
- due to neurological disease with or without respiratory complications.

If the patient has adequate airway protection reflexes it may be possible to provide mechanical support with minimal sedation and without intubation.[57] Select such patients carefully on their own merits. Successful nose mask or face mask ventilation requires a degree of patient cooperation and a pressure controlled device with the capacity to deliver high flows to compensate for any leak. Negative pressure devices, whether tank or cuirass, have the disadvantage of obstructing access to the patient. So-called 'non-invasive' ventilation should only be provided in an environment where anesthetic and airway skills are readily available.

TECHNIQUE OF INTUBATION

The purpose of recognizing sick children is to enable appropriate early intervention. Hence intubation is usually performed as part of the induction of anesthesia. There are two basic approaches to the administration of an anesthetic: i.v. (usually a rapid sequence induction) and inhalation. Anesthetic skills, equipment and assistants are required for both. Rapid sequence induction is the preferred approach for most situations especially when regurgitation and aspiration of stomach contents are potential problems. It is contraindicated when the airway is compromised or when intubation may be difficult, in which case inhaled anesthetics are used.

Use a straight-bladed laryngoscope to view the larynx in infants because its position is high (at the level of the C4 vertebra) and anterior compared to the adult. The large, soft, sigma-shaped epiglottis can be kept under the blade if it obscures the laryngeal inlet. In older children, use a curved blade and lift away from you (as opposed to rotating) for a better view of the vocal cords. Once beyond puberty the larynx has assumed its adult position.

Use noncuffed tubes in prepubertal children because the larynx has a gradually tapering shape narrowest in the subglottic region (behind the cricoid cartilage). The tube should be small enough to permit a small leak of air under pressure, giving reassurance that excessive pressure is not being exerted on the subglottic tracheal mucosa where damage would otherwise lead to scarring and subsequent stenosis. After puberty the vocal cords are the narrowest part of the airway so use cuffed tubes in more mature children. The ideal position of an endotracheal tube tip is at the level of the sternoclavicular junction on the chest X-ray. In infants

the trachea bifurcates at the level of T2. The tip of the tube will move significantly when the neck is flexed (moves down) or extended (moves up).

Always attempt to preoxygenate the patient and make sure that you are proficient in airway intervention techniques because any interruption in ventilation in babies and infants very quickly leads to hypoxemia. Their high metabolic rate means faster consumption of oxygen and greater carbon dioxide production. Furthermore normal ventilator settings must include the routine use of positive end expiratory pressure because atelectasis occurs early and at a higher volume relative to the functional residual capacity of older children and adults.

CHOICE OF VENTILATOR

Ventilators differ in relation to their power source, cycling characteristics, method of generating gas flow and the provision of gas supply for spontaneous breaths. The 'cycling' label is attached to the parameter (pressure, time, volume or flow) that determines when inspiration stops and expiration starts.

The choice of cycling method will affect the behavior of the ventilator as the patient's condition changes (Table 36.3).

The method by which gas flow is generated affects the choice of 'control' mode (e.g. pressure control and volume control) and hence the pattern of pressure and flow over time during inspiration. The terms 'support' or 'assist' are applied to modes where the breath is initiated by the patient then detected and supported by the ventilator. 'Mandatory' or 'control' breaths are initiated by the ventilator and may be blended with 'support' (e.g. synchronized intermittent mandatory ventilation with pressure support).

For neonates there is a historical preference for using continuous flow, pressure-regulated, time-cycled ventilators. They are less susceptible to the fluctuations in tidal volume that are generated by the disparity between tidal volume and total gas volume in the ventilator circuit. They also do not generate large pressure fluctuations when the patient is uncoordinated with the ventilator and can function in the presence of a modest leak around the endotracheal tube. However, when compliance changes (e.g. as muscle relaxants wear off, or disease severity worsens) large changes in delivered tidal volume occur. Despite being intrinsically sensitive in the detection of circuit disruption, older models may not be capable of detecting absent tidal volume (endotracheal tube blockage). They must therefore be used in combination with an apnea monitor.

For older patients there is a historical preference for volume-controlled ventilation. Nevertheless improved technology is making it easier and sometimes more appropriate to ventilate smaller patients with such devices. However, even with newer models, when compliance changes or airway obstruction develops, airway pressure escalates and the effective tidal volume is reduced as gas is compressed in the ventilator tubing.

VENTILATOR SETTINGS

Oxygenation is critical. Since oxygen is poorly soluble in water, the important factors in oxygen uptake across the lung are:

- the amount of blood flow (e.g. the cardiac output);
- the hemoglobin concentration;

Table 36.3 Ventilator cycling

	Low compliance/high airways resistance	High compliance/low airways resistance
Volume cycled	V_T becomes a smaller % of cycled volume	i.t. becomes short
	PIP increases	PIP falls
Pressure cycled	i.t. and V_T both fall	i.t. becomes very long V_T increases
Flow cycled	i.t. and V_T both fall	i.t. and V_T both rise
Time cycled	No effect	No effect

i.t., inspiratory time; PIP, peak inspiratory pressure; V_T, tidal volume.

- the effective surface area of the lung (after the effects of shunt, deadspace and ventilation–perfusion matching);
- the diffusion gradient for oxygen.

All of the above can be manipulated independently but the ventilator is only used for the last two. To increase the diffusion gradient for oxygen, increase the inspired oxygen concentration. The effective surface area of the lung can be increased (within limits) by increases in tidal volume and mean airway pressure. Some components of shunt may be relatively fixed and not respond to changes in ventilation. It is important not to overventilate under these circumstances. Deadspace is proportionately more significant at low tidal volumes. Ventilation–perfusion matching changes with posture and positioning of the patient as well as other changes in ventilation technique.

Carbon dioxide diffuses easily across respiratory membranes and comes in and out of solution easily. Hence the rate-limiting step in removal across the lung is the speed with which equilibrated (alveolar) gas is replaced with fresh gas, i.e. the alveolar minute ventilation. Use tidal volume and respiratory rate to influence the minute volume and create responses in arterial carbon dioxide level. At low tidal volumes deadspace is more significant and reduces the effectiveness of each tidal volume in clearing carbon dioxide. There are therefore limits to how much a reduction in tidal volume can be compensated by increasing respiratory rate.

Wherever possible, choose ventilator settings that can be considered therapeutic, such as the use of higher levels of positive end expiratory pressure in pulmonary edema to reduce alveolar water content or in bronchomalacia to maintain patency of the conductance airways. Lung volume and $[H^+]$ (via carbon dioxide partial pressure; PCO_2) can also be used to manipulate pulmonary vascular resistance. The amount of work required to breathe is increased when compliance is poor or when airway resistance is high. Try to adapt ventilator settings to match the disease state and avoid complications such as gas trapping (dynamic hyperinflation), for example allow a long expiratory time if the patient has bronchospasm.

CONSEQUENCES OF VENTILATION

Endotracheal intubation and mechanical ventilation are not natural processes and are associated with hazards that can be minimized by appropriate attention to detail. Choose the correct size and length endotracheal tube. Take care to ensure that the inhaled gases are humidified to 100% relative humidity at body temperature. Avoid high pressures and tidal volumes. Any ventilator settings that induce overinflation are likely to induce or aggravate lung injury although the specific settings involved will differ between restrictive and obstructive diseases. Peak pressure is far more dangerous than end expiratory pressure and many of the problems previously associated with peak pressure are as much to do with the associated high end inflation lung volume and tidal volume as anything else. Previously injured lungs are more susceptible to ventilator-induced lung injury and if the disease is not homogenous it may be the less severely diseased segments that receive the greater insult.

NEWER VENTILATION STRATEGIES

In recent times the concept of minimizing the stress of mechanical ventilation has become pivotal in the ventilation of patients with respiratory disease. The appeal of novel approaches to ventilation is often based upon their potential (even if unproven) abilities in this respect. The simplest approaches include improved coordination between the ventilator and the patient. More complex approaches are aimed at providing increasing degrees of 'lung rest'. The conventional and best validated method of providing lung rest is extracorporeal membrane oxygenation (ECMO), which is a modified form of cardiopulmonary bypass. ECMO can be used to achieve total lung rest (gas exchange during prolonged apnea) and the circuit can be configured to provide pulmonary (venovenous cannulation) or cardiopulmonary support (venoarterial cannulation).

Examples of ventilation strategies with proposed benefits in terms of reducing ventilator-associated lung injury include:

- Permissive hypercarbia: where (pressure-limited) minute ventilation is minimized in the hope of reducing lung stress. To perform this technique, once hypoxia is overcome, allow arterial carbon dioxide levels to rise to limits dictated by the associated rise in hydrogen ion concentration (e.g. ≤ 63 nmol/L correlating with pH ≥ 7.2). Over time, metabolic compensation allows higher and higher carbon dioxide levels to be tolerated.[57-60]
- High-frequency oscillation: these devices use the continuous distending pressure (mean airway pressure) to recruit and maintain lung volume. Gas exchange is achieved by a high-frequency vibration (6–12 Hz). Minimal tidal volumes (less than deadspace) result from the amplitude of the vibration, which itself is highly attenuated within the respiratory tract, hence minimizing shearing forces.[58] Use the amplitude (ΔP) preferentially to control the partial pressure of carbon dioxide in arterial blood ($PaCO_2$). The fall in tidal volume as frequency increases attenuates carbon dioxide removal, which is otherwise highly efficient.
- Inhaled nitric oxide[61-63]: in responsive patients, ventilation perfusion mismatch can be reduced by NO, which causes vasodilatation in ventilated areas. Some cases of pulmonary hypertension may also respond.
- Liquid ventilation (usually in the form of perfluorocarbon-assisted gas exchange)[64]: this technique involves first gradually replacing the functional residual capacity of the lung by slow instillation of perfluorocarbon during conventional ventilation. This causes bulk distention of the alveoli and considerable recruitment of lung volume. Subsequent tidal ventilation with 100% oxygen is more effective as the low surface tension at the perfluorocarbon:gas interface improves compliance.
- Intratracheal pressure release ventilation[63,65]: where expiratory flows are augmented increasing respiratory efficiency at lower tidal volumes and lower mean pressures.

WEANING VENTILATION

Improving respiratory function is reflected in the behavior of the patient and the ventilator. In the latter case the effects depend upon the mode of ventilation employed at the time. Improved compliance or airways resistance during volume-controlled ventilation causes airway pressures to fall. With pressure-controlled ventilation under the same circumstances, tidal volumes increase and the partial pressure of oxygen in arterial blood (PaO_2) may rise as the $PaCO_2$ falls. Effective tidal volume can be usefully expressed in relation to deadspace using end tidal carbon dioxide measurements. In flow-cycled ventilator modes such as pressure support, the inspiratory time decreases as compliance improves. Close observation of the patient and regular blood gas measurement allows you to respond to these changes.

Start to deliberately wean patients from mechanical ventilation when the pathology or indication for ventilation is resolving or finished. The speed of successful weaning is dictated by the adequacy of the response and the skill lies in getting the best performance out of the partially dependent patient. The patient must be able to take over ventilation without excess energy expenditure, and there must be adequate respiratory muscle strength, hemodynamic stability and a good nutritional state. Only extubate electively when the patient:

- is hemodynamically and metabolically stable;
- is making effective efforts to breathe;
- is sufficiently awake and alert;
- has protective airway reflexes.

Prior to extubation, always ensure that there is adequate provision of equipment, medication and staff to deal with complications such as laryngospasm, which might require urgent reintubation.

CARDIOVASCULAR SYSTEM

Another common reason to arrange intensive care admission is the need to perform invasive monitoring of the circulation using arterial or central venous lines. This need arises:

- as a wise precaution in case of potential instability, e.g. after major surgery or other trauma;
- in the treatment of shock such as during large volume fluid losses/replacement;
- when blood pressure is excessively high or low;
- when vasoactive drugs are being administered by infusion.

RECOGNITION OF SHOCK

Do not rely on blood pressure in the first instance or alone to assess the circulation. Shock is defined as inadequate perfusion of tissues (in particular oxygenation) and its severity is assessed in terms of end-organ function. When flow measurements are available, the global delivery of oxygen to the tissues can be calculated as the product of the oxygen content of arterial blood and the cardiac output; but not all of this oxygen is available to the tissues. Factors that influence the distribution of blood also apply and may be particularly affected by disease. The two most sensitive and clinically useful organs in the assessment of the circulation are the brain and the kidney. Altered conscious level is an important sign of shock and up to the point of acute renal failure urine output is a good marker of renal perfusion. The patient with severe cardiovascular dysfunction (shock) generally has peripheral pulses that are difficult to feel, poor capillary refill, cool extremities, decreased urine output and altered sensorium. A *low blood pressure* is a preterminal *sign* since blood pressure can be maintained by intense vasoconstriction even in the presence of a markedly reduced circulating volume. The fall in blood pressure thus represents decompensation and indicates that the patient is out of control.

It is important to monitor fluid losses and replacement accurately. In the short term this can be approximated by the fluid balance but remember to extend the comparison over days. Weigh the patient regularly and match your impressions with clinical and laboratory observations.

RECOGNITION OF HEART FAILURE

Heart failure is distinguishable from shock. It is a more chronic condition in which the heart fails to respond adequately to its preload and hence fails to obey its normal Starling relation. There may be diastolic or systolic dysfunction or both and the problem may apply to specific ventricles or regions of myocardium. Fluid retention results from 'back pressure' as well as humoral responses to a reduced cardiac output. Although true heart failure can occur in children, most patients with signs that would represent heart 'failure' in an adult are in fact displaying the manifestations of a left-to-right shunt. These patients may have positively athletic cardiac function.

RECOGNITION OF CONGENITAL HEART DISEASE

Suspect congenital heart disease especially and most importantly in neonates with shock or cyanosis but also in patients with:

- murmurs;
- pulmonary edema;
- rhythm disturbances;
- abnormally severe symptoms from respiratory disease;
- failure to thrive.

Right-to-left shunts cause cyanosis and rarely cause murmurs because they are relatively low volume shunts occurring at low pressure. Left-to-right shunts cause pulmonary and ventricular volume overload. The loudness of the murmur is to some extent inversely proportional to the size of the shunt. Sustained high pulmonary blood flow causes pulmonary hypertension. Ventricular outflow tract obstruction (pressure overload) tends to cause ventricular hypertrophy. Ventricular hypertrophy is associated with decreased ventricular compliance (diastolic dysfunction).

Congenital heart disease can produce many combinations of defects, which also evolve according to the loading forces they create.

It is essential to recognize duct-dependent lesions. These present early in the neonatal period. Duct-dependent pulmonary flow presents with cyanosis and duct-dependent systemic flow with heart failure and/or shock in the first week of life. Both require an infusion of prostaglandin (typically 20 ng/kg/min) and urgent evaluation by a pediatric cardiologist.

TREATMENT OF SHOCK

The first line in cardiovascular resuscitation and support is an intravascular volume bolus of 20 ml/kg. Such preload augmentation should increase stroke volume and therefore blood pressure even if heart failure is suspected as well as shock. The most common cause of an inadequate response to this treatment is that the magnitude of the problem has been underestimated and inadequate fluid volumes have been used, hence the protocol for repeating the boluses of i.v. fluid at least twice if there is an inadequate response. However, do not give excessive amounts of intravascular volume if heart failure is present. In rapid large volume resuscitations the central venous pressure is a useful guide to how the volume is being handled by the circulation. Palpating the liver edge can also help; hepatic engorgement suggests right ventricular volume overload.

Both myocardial contractility (and hence stroke volume) and heart rate are increased by catecholamines. The first-line inotropic support started after the second or third fluid bolus is usually adrenaline (0.05–0.5 mcg/kg/min) or dopamine (2–10 mcg/kg/min). Cardiac output can also be influenced by manipulation of afterload (end systolic ventricular wall tension) for example by agents that affect the systemic vascular resistance. The term 'systemic vascular resistance' refers to a global approximation of the resistance of the circulation to blood flow. It is calculated after measuring cardiac output by dividing the pressure drop across the circulation by the measured blood flow. Reduction of afterload may improve cardiac output in conditions where there is a left-to-right shunt. Increases in afterload (e.g. using alpha adrenergic agents) are an important component of support in shock states such as septic shock when characterized by a low systemic vascular resistance.

The intrinsic response of the cardiovascular system both to disease and resuscitation depends upon the age of the patient and the nature and stage of palliation of any congenital heart disease as well as any intercurrent disease. The fetal circulation is characterized by the fetal connections, a high pulmonary vascular resistance and a low systemic vascular resistance. The neonatal (transitional) circulation is characterized by the potential persistence of all the fetal connections other than the umbilical vessels, reactive pulmonary vasculature and limited inotropic and chronotropic reserve; that is to say reduced capacity to increase contractility in response to catecholamines and a poor return in terms of cardiac output for increases in heart rate (despite a rate-dependent cardiac output in bradycardia). The neonatal heart also displays muted (e.g. to potassium) or accentuated (e.g. to calcium) responses to various electrolytes and drugs compared to later life. In infancy and childhood the myocardium adapts progressively to its new loading conditions and develops an increased reserve to beta adrenergic stimulation.

In refractory shock, i.e. failure to respond to intravascular volume loading, it is crucially important to get accurate monitoring of the circulation. Then consider the following possible explanations:

- Overestimation of the filling pressures: both central venous and pulmonary capillary wedge pressures are heavily influenced by thoracic pressure and hence positive pressure ventilation. Use the end expiratory values in your evaluation.
- Systolic cardiac dysfunction: depression of the contractile state of the myocardium can occur with a range of common disorders, for example sepsis, acidosis, hypoglycemia, hypoxia or hypocalcemia. In addition, drugs (especially antiarrhythmics) can also decrease the contractile state. A hydrogen ion concentration greater than 63 (pH < 7.2) can decrease the effectiveness of catecholamines and may need to be corrected.

37

Surgical pediatrics

Gordon A MacKinlay

INTRODUCTION

Pediatric surgery encompasses a wider range of surgery than any other surgical specialty. It is confined to an age group rather than an organ system. In the older child, adult surgeons may deal with some commoner problems.

Congenital problems presenting in the neonatal period or later, together with other conditions peculiar to childhood, should be treated in a specialist center by trained pediatric surgeons backed by pediatric anesthetists, pediatric radiologists, pediatric pathologists and experienced nursing staff specifically trained in the care of children. In a general hospital the child should be nursed on a children's ward and if there is no pediatric surgeon, care should be provided by the surgeon who is treating the child *together* with a pediatrician.

In the case of the neonate, a particular surgical challenge is encountered not only in the requirement for a meticulous surgical technique but also in careful pre- and postoperative management. The reward is the prospect of a full three score years and ten survival compared with the commonly sought 5-year survival in many aspects of adult surgery.

The presence of an anomaly requiring surgery is often detected antenatally by ultrasound, enabling discussion with the parents, obstetrician, pediatric surgeon and neonatologist. The parents can thus be prepared and reassured, where possible, that although an abnormality has been detected it can be treated. They can visit the surgical neonatal unit, meet the staff and, where appropriate, the timing of delivery may be planned to facilitate optimal transfer of the baby to the awaiting surgical unit or direct to the operating theater. Pregnancy is a time of potential parental stress and unless great care is taken in explaining the possible consequences of an antenatally diagnosed anomaly their anxiety will be increased.

The most significant development in pediatric surgery in the last decade has been the adoption of minimally invasive surgical techniques – mainly laparoscopy and thoracoscopy. The majority of major operations in children can be accomplished through 'keyhole surgery', which results in less postoperative pain, less analgesia, less ileus, earlier postoperative feeding, fewer wound infections and reduced hospital stay.

NEONATAL SURGERY

RESPIRATORY PROBLEMS

Whilst respiratory distress in the newborn is primarily the domain of the neonatologist some causes may be surgical and early referral to a pediatric surgeon may be of lifesaving importance.

CAUSES OF RESPIRATORY DISTRESS IN THE NEWBORN

1. Upper airway:
    a. choanal atresia;
    b. nasal encephalocele;
    c. tumors of the nasopharynx;
    d. Pierre Robin syndrome;
    e. macroglossia;
    f. hemangio/lymphangiomata of oral cavity;
    g. laryngotracheoesophageal cleft;
    h. laryngeal web;
    i. laryngeal stenosis;
    j. hemangioma of larynx;
    k. laryngomalacia;

    l. tracheomalacia;
    m. tracheal stenosis;
    n. cystic hygroma;
    o. cervical teratoma;
2. Intrathoracic:
    a. congenital lobar emphysema;
    b. cystic adenomatoid lung malformation;
    c. bronchogenic and lung cysts;
    d. enterogenous cysts;
    e. pneumothorax;
    f. sequestration of lung;
    g. vascular ring;
    h. congenital heart disease;
    i. Diaphragmatic hernia;
    j. eventration of the diaphragm;
    k. esophageal atresia and tracheoesophageal fistula.

Choanal atresia is obstruction of the posterior nares by a bony or occasionally membranous septum. If bilateral it is a neonatal emergency, as babies are obligate nasal breathers. An oral airway will overcome this problem until the obstruction is relieved.

An oral airway is also of benefit in *Pierre Robin syndrome*, where there is a hypoplastic mandible and central cleft palate, the tongue falling posteriorly to occlude both the oropharynx and the nasopharynx. An airway can be maintained in position for several weeks, the baby being fed nasogastrically or via a gastrostomy. A tracheostomy may be easier to manage and is maintained until the mandible grows. It also facilitates repair of the cleft palate, which is associated in the majority of cases.

A *laryngeal web*, if complete, leads to death in utero. If partial, the symptoms may merit emergency tracheostomy. *Laryngomalacia* leads to inspiratory stridor, which usually resolves in the first 2.5 years of life. *Tracheomalacia* is commonly associated with esophageal atresia. It has been postulated that the hypertrophied upper pouch, containing swallowed liquor, compresses the developing trachea, preventing the normal growth of tracheal rings. The problem increases postoperatively, sometimes making it impossible to extubate these babies. The diagnosis may be confirmed radiologically by lateral screening of the neck, observing the anteroposterior narrowing of the trachea with inspiration. Aortopexy, suturing the aorta to the back of the sternum, thus pulling the pretracheal fascia and hence the anterior tracheal wall forward, is sometimes of benefit. Prolonged intubation may allow time for the tracheal rings to become more supportive but may itself lead to subglottic stenosis. Tracheostomy is required in some cases.

Congenital lobar emphysema leads to overexpansion of a lung lobe with compromise of ventilation. Half the cases present within days of birth, the remainder in the first few months of life. The most common cause is bronchomalacia of the associated bronchus although some cases may be caused by external compression. The baby may present with feeding difficulties due to dyspnea. The diagnosis is made radiologically and the most commonly affected lobes are the left upper lobe or the right middle lobe. Treatment is lobectomy in severe cases but in many conservative management is appropriate.

Cystic adenomatoid lung and *congenital lung cysts* can present in much the same way as lobar emphysema. Their expansion produces respiratory distress. Congenital cysts tend to be unilocular and solitary. *Cystic adenomatoid malformation* is due to excessive overgrowth of bronchioles with multiple cysts lined by cuboidal and ciliated pseudostratified columnar epithelium. The left lower lobe is commonly affected and the appearance may antenatally or even postnatally be mistaken for a diaphragmatic hernia. Treatment is resection of the affected lobe, which can now be safely performed thoracoscopically.

Pulmonary sequestration is a mass of lung tissue not communicating with the bronchial tree and which receives its blood supply from an anomalous systemic vessel. It may be within the substance of the lung (intralobar sequestration) or completely separate (extralobar). Areas of sequestration are thought to arise from an extra bronchopulmonary bud of the foregut. They most commonly occur in the left lower lobe and the blood supply comes direct from the aorta, above or below the diaphragm. The anomalous blood supply may be identified by ultrasound techniques, avoiding the need for angiography. The condition usually presents with respiratory infections, more commonly after the neonatal period. The treatment is resection.[1]

Diaphragmatic hernia

Diaphragmatic hernia may be congenital or acquired, the latter usually being traumatic in origin. Congenital diaphragmatic hernia arises due to an abnormality in the formation of the diaphragm between the fourth and tenth weeks of fetal life.

The commonest herniation is the Bochdalek type, a posterolateral defect, possibly a failure of closure of the pleuroperitoneal canal. It has been postulated that the primary anomaly is in the developing lungs that fail to induce diaphragmatic closure and this may explain hypoplasia in the contralateral lung. A hernia through the foramen of Morgagni is less common in neonates. This defect is retrosternal, to the right or left of the midline. The third site for herniation is the esophageal hiatus – the so-called hiatus hernia.

The true incidence of congenital diaphragmatic hernia is difficult to ascertain as so many die at birth; others present as live births and others after the neonatal period. This lesion represents 8% of major fatal congenital anomalies noted in a British perinatal mortality survey (present in one in 2200 of all births). In Edinburgh the incidence is one in 7000 live births, other series report 1:4000–1:10 000.

Some cases are now detected antenatally by ultrasound but the majority present with respiratory distress – cyanosis, dyspnea and tachypnea – either immediately after birth or within a few hours. Occasionally, particularly on the right side, the presentation may be later, the defect being present at birth but actual herniation of abdominal content occurring as a postnatal event. The later the onset of symptoms, the better the prognosis. Examination reveals a scaphoid abdomen, bowel sounds on auscultation of the affected side of the chest and a shift of the apex beat to the right in the case of a left-sided hernia. The right side is less common, perhaps due to plugging by the liver, but if a defect is present here it tends to be large with herniation of the liver as well as bowel.

Once air has been swallowed after birth a chest X-ray confirms the diagnosis, showing gas-filled loops of bowel on the affected side of the chest with displacement of the mediastinum to the opposite side (Fig. 37.1).

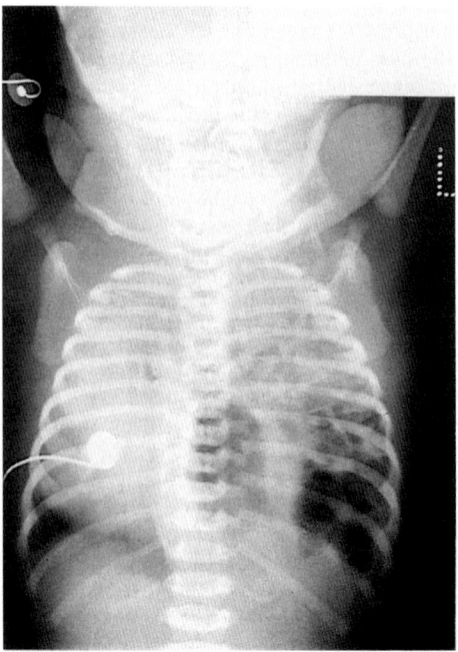

Fig. 37.1 Diaphragmatic hernia (left-sided Bochdalek defect).

Treatment

A nasogastric tube is passed to reduce the gaseous distention of the bowel with air. In the past the surgical repair of the hernia was a true emergency, it being felt that the sooner the hernia was reduced the more easily the lungs could expand. Babies were operated on virtually regardless of condition and the survival rates were poor. It has been shown that respiratory mechanics, far from improving, frequently deteriorate as a result of repair of the hernia. The role of urgent surgery has thus been re-evaluated. It has always been known that the babies with the least hypoplastic lungs fared better. These also tend to be the cases that present after hours rather than immediately at birth. Now an initial, non-surgical approach to diaphragmatic hernia has been adopted in most centers with the aim of improving pulmonary function and reducing pulmonary vascular resistance.[2,3] After diagnosis the baby is intubated and hyperventilated to reduce the $PaCO_2$ to < 4.7 kPa (< 35 mmHg) and paralyzed. Metabolic acidosis is corrected with bicarbonate therapy. A chest X-ray is taken to verify the endotracheal tube position and exclude a pneumothorax. A preductal arterial line (radial) is sited for blood gas and pressure monitoring. The ventilatory index (mean airway pressure × respiratory rate) is calculated and this should be < 1000 with a $PaCO_2$ < 5.3 (< 40 mmHg) prior to surgery. If the index is higher, high-frequency oscillatory ventilation is instituted. Tolazoline may be administered to reduce pulmonary vascular resistance and prevent shunting through the ductus arteriosus. In some centers extracorporeal membrane oxygenation (ECMO) is used for prolonged support with variable results. Whatever the method of stabilization preoperatively, it must be carried out in a surgical unit as it is the pediatric surgeon who must be in a position to determine the timing of surgery.

Operative treatment

An abdominal approach is usually preferred with a transverse upper abdominal incision on the side of the hernia. The bowel and other organs are reduced and the defect in the diaphragm examined. If the defect is large a patch of prosthetic material may be used. Repairing a defect under tension merely reduces lung compliance. An underwater seal drain is positioned prior to completion of the repair. If the baby's condition is very stable the repair may be accomplished thoracoscopically.

Postoperatively, support is maintained until the baby can be weaned from the ventilator. A few patients who require little or no ventilatory support preoperatively may be extubated immediately. Of the remainder the mortality rate still remains around 50%, although it is hoped that the change in preoperative management will improve the outlook.

Eventration of the diaphragm

This is due to a deficiency in the muscle of the diaphragm. The thin layer becomes attenuated and bulges up into the thorax. Extensive eventrations are similar to diaphragmatic hernia presenting in the neonatal period. Smaller eventrations present later and require localized plication.

Esophageal atresia

Atresia is absence or closure of a normal body orifice or passage (Greek *a* = negative, *tresis* = hole). A fistula is an abnormal communication between two epithelial surfaces.

Esophageal atresia is a congenital defect of unknown etiology, the great majority of cases being associated with a tracheoesophageal fistula. The incidence is approximately 1 per 3000 live births. Many babies with esophageal atresia are premature and of low birth weight. The lower the birth weight, the greater the mortality. More than half the babies presenting with esophageal atresia have associated congenital abnormalities, commonly associated with vertebral, anorectal, cardiac, tracheoesophageal, renal and limb anomalies (VACTERL). This was formerly known as the VATER complex. The anatomical varieties of esophageal atresia and related disorders are illustrated in Figure 37.2.

Clinical features

Maternal hydramnios is so common that all babies born to a mother with hydramnios should have a tube passed to assess the patency of the esophagus. In cases with esophageal atresia the tube will be arrested about 10 cm from the lips. If the diagnosis is not made in this manner then the baby will be noted to froth at the mouth, choke, cough or become dyspneic and cyanosed. These symptoms will be exacerbated by attempts to feed the baby. The patency of the esophagus should then be tested by a firm tube of at least 10 or 12 FG, which should be passed orally. Acid secretions aspirated from the tube may have refluxed through the fistula so radiological confirmation of the position of the tube is necessary if suspicion is high.

A Replogle tube is a double lumen plastic catheter that can be passed via the nose into the upper esophageal pouch, enabling continuous suction to be applied without causing damage to the mucosa. Suction is applied to the end of the catheter, air passing along the finer of the two lumina as secretions are aspirated. If the latter are particularly thick, careful irrigation may be carried out via the finer lumen tube.

A plain chest X-ray with gentle pressure on the Replogle tube enables the distal extent of the pouch to be ascertained. The presence of air in the stomach and bowel confirms the presence of a distal tracheoesophageal fistula (TEF) (Fig. 37.3). In the case of atresia without a fistula there

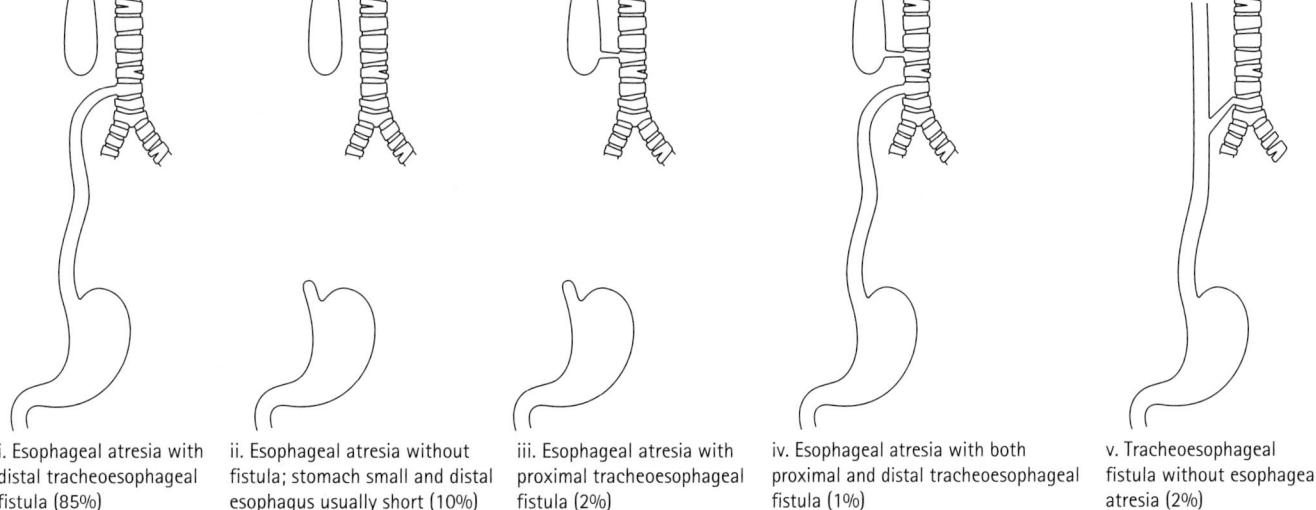

i. Esophageal atresia with distal tracheoesophageal fistula (85%)

ii. Esophageal atresia without fistula; stomach small and distal esophagus usually short (10%)

iii. Esophageal atresia with proximal tracheoesophageal fistula (2%)

iv. Esophageal atresia with both proximal and distal tracheoesophageal fistula (1%)

v. Tracheoesophageal fistula without esophageal atresia (2%)

Fig. 37.2 Esophageal atresia and tracheoesophageal fistula.

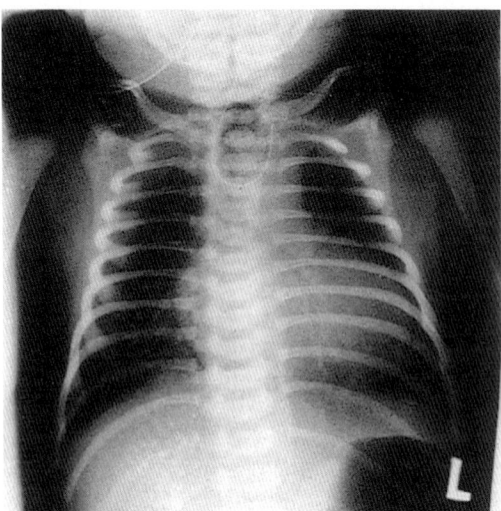

Fig. 37.3 Esophageal atresia with distal tracheoesophageal fistula.

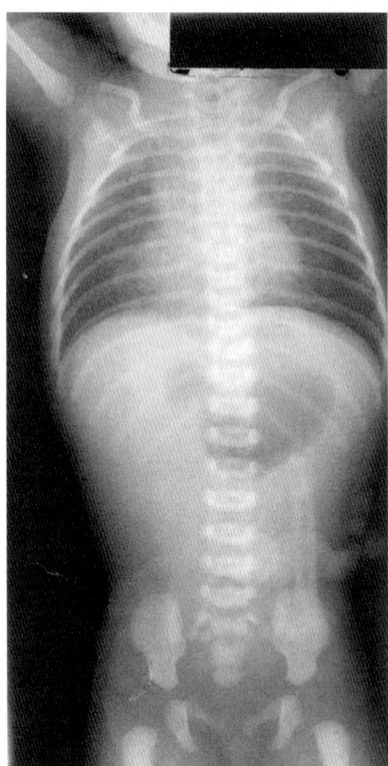

Fig. 37.5 Esophageal atresia with duodenal atresia.

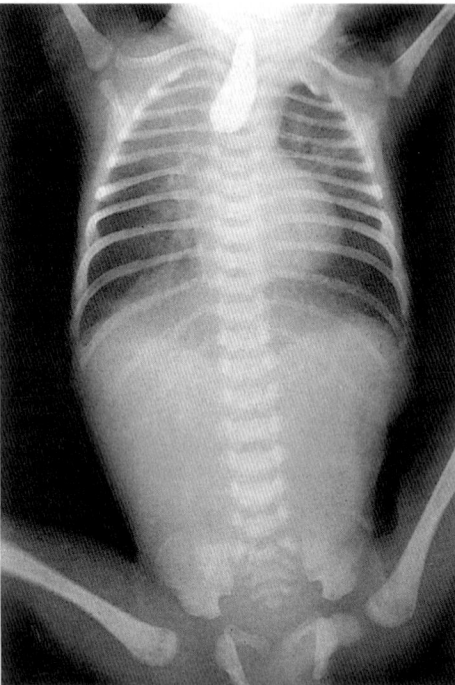

Fig. 37.4 Esophageal atresia without TEF.

is absence of air in the stomach (Fig. 37.4). Occasionally there may be associated duodenal atresia, but providing there is a TEF, then the gas pattern should clarify this (Fig. 37.5).

Some surgeons like to use 1–2 ml of contrast to define the upper pouch but there is great danger of spillage into the tracheobronchial tree and the procedure is unnecessary. Preoperatively, apart from adequate aspiration of the upper pouch, opinions differ as to the best position in which to nurse the baby. Some advocate the Trendelenburg (head down) position to prevent aspiration of secretions but this may lead to reflux of gastric content via the fistula into the lungs (especially the right upper lobe). Others, to prevent this, advise a head up position. A horizontal and semiprone position reduces the incidence of right upper lobe collapse and seems satisfactory.

Treatment

In the commonest type of anomaly (with a distal TEF), surgery does not have to be performed immediately in the middle of the night but can be safely left until the following day. If pneumonitis is present, it is

justifiable to delay treatment for 24 h or more to allow chest physiotherapy and appropriate antibiotics to be administered. A right posterolateral thoracotomy is made and, via an extrapleural approach, the fistula is divided and repaired and an end-to-end anastomosis between the proximal and distal esophagus is made in a single layer. A fine transanastomotic silastic tube is passed nasogastrically prior to completion of the anastomosis so that early nasogastric feeding can be instituted. In some centers the operation can be safely performed thoracoscopically.

On the fifth postoperative day a contrast swallow is performed to confirm patency of the anastomosis and exclude leakage at this site. If leakage is present it can usually be safely managed conservatively. Anastomotic stricture, if it occurs, is treated by esophagoscopy and bougienage or balloon dilation under X-ray control. Most children, following a successful repair, have a persistent brassy cough or 'seal bark' that may last for a few years. This is probably due to a degree of tracheomalacia.

Dysphagia due to abnormal motility in the esophagus both above and below the anastomosis may be due to vagal nerve damage or, more probably, an intrinsic abnormality associated with the lesion. This, like the seal bark, usually resolves by the age of 2 years.

Cases of esophageal atresia without a fistula are best managed initially by gastrostomy and aspiration of the upper pouch via a Replogle tube. In my experience, delayed primary anastomosis can be achieved after 3 months of regular stretching of the upper pouch by the nursing staff using a Nelaton catheter at feed times. Once there is radiological evidence of a gap of less than 3 cm, as visualized with a metal bougie in the lower pouch (passed per gastrostomy) and a radiopaque tube in the upper pouch, surgery can be carried out thoracoscopically or via thoracotomy. Postoperatively, the infants are electively paralyzed and ventilated for up to 7 d to relieve the tension on the anastomosis, a technique also of value in tight anastomosis in the common type of atresia with a distal fistula.[4] Others favor construction of a cervical esophagostomy followed by gastric transposition, jejunal or colonic interposition to bridge the gap between the upper pouch and the stomach.

H-type tracheoesophageal fistula

These occasionally present in the first few weeks of life with coughing or cyanosis on feeding. More commonly they present much later with recurrent chest infections, a history of coughing on feeds, and sometimes abdominal distention. Because the fistula runs obliquely upwards from esophagus to trachea, the flow of esophageal content into the trachea is limited and intermittent. The diagnosis is made at a contrast swallow under screening. Treatment is surgical division of the fistula, usually via a cervical approach.

DUODENAL OBSTRUCTION

Duodenal obstruction may be intrinsic (atresia, membrane, stenosis or anular pancreas) or extrinsic (Ladd's bands with or without volvulus of the midgut).

Intrinsic duodenal obstruction (Fig. 37.6)

The etiology of duodenal atresias and other intrinsic duodenal obstructions differs from that of intrinsic obstructions in the remainder of the small intestine. It appears to be a failure of luminal development due to an early insult and there are often associated abnormalities. Down syndrome is present in 30% of cases. In 10% there is esophageal atresia, and a further 10% have anorectal anomalies. Cardiac and renal anomalies may also be associated. Cardiac abnormalities are particularly common in those with Down syndrome.

Atresia or stenosis usually affects the second or occasionally the third part of the duodenum.

Complete obstructions present with vomiting within 24 h after birth. The vomitus may or may not be bile stained, depending on whether the obstruction is proximal or distal to the ampulla of Vater. In those with bile-stained vomitus the meconium, if passed, may also be normally bile stained as there may be openings of the bile duct proximal and distal to the obstruction via Wirsung's and Santorini's ducts.

In maternity units where passage of a nasogastric tube is a routine soon after birth, aspiration of more than 20 ml of fluid may be indicative of a duodenal or small bowel obstruction.

Abdominal distention, if any, is confined to the upper abdomen due to obstruction of the stomach and duodenum.

The diagnosis is confirmed by a plain erect X-ray that demonstrates the characteristic 'double bubble' appearance of air–fluid levels in the stomach and duodenum (Fig. 37.7). The double bubble may also be detected antenatally, ultrasound detecting fluid distention of the stomach and duodenum.[5] An incomplete obstruction, stenosis, or membrane with a small hole in it may allow air to pass through to the rest of the bowel, thus masking the double bubble (Fig. 37.8), but a contrast study confirms the presence of obstruction (Fig. 37.9). Sometimes the diagnosis may be delayed several months or even a year or two if sufficient food can pass through.

Treatment

If there is any delay in diagnosis of a duodenal obstruction then any resulting metabolic disturbance must be corrected preoperatively. At laparotomy a duodenoduodenostomy is the procedure of choice (Fig. 37.10), or for a stenosis or membrane a duodenoplasty may be performed,

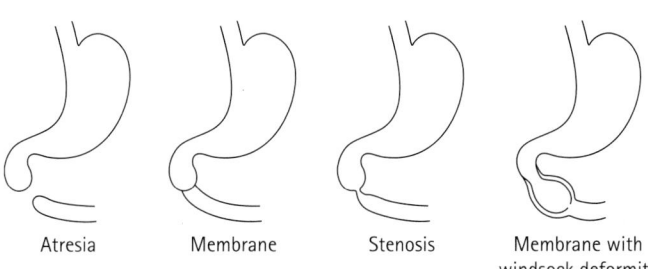

Atresia   Membrane   Stenosis   Membrane with windsock deformity

Fig. 37.6 Duodenal anomalies.

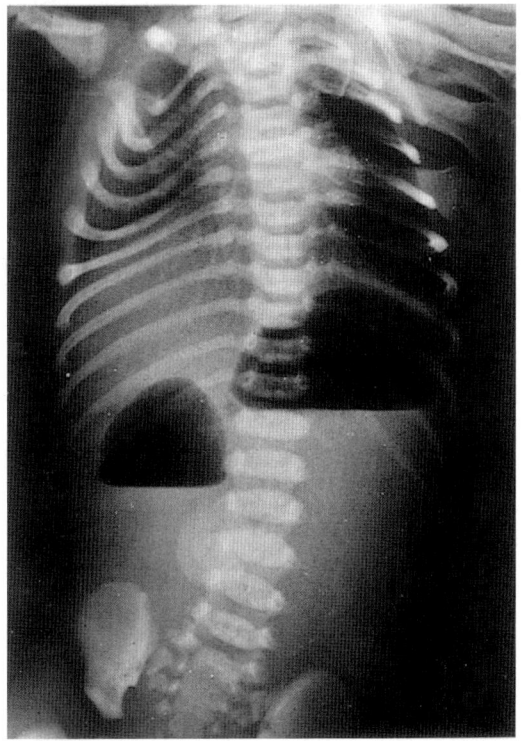

Fig. 37.7 'Double bubble' in duodenal atresia.

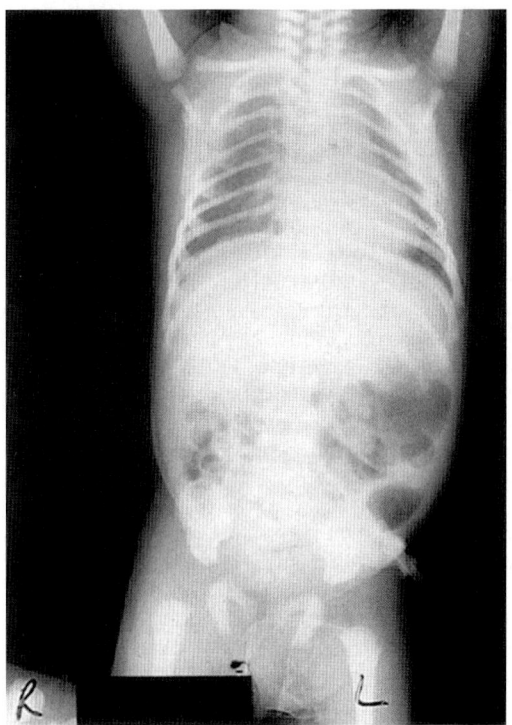

Fig. 37.8 Plain film of baby soon after birth.

opening the duodenum lengthways across the obstruction and closing it transversely. Resection of a diaphragm must be undertaken cautiously to avoid damage to the ampulla of Vater.

An anular pancreas (Fig. 37.10a) is caused by the failure of the normal migration of the ventral bud to join the dorsal one. It is rarely a true ring around the duodenum but more commonly associated with an intrinsic obstruction within the duodenum (membrane or stenosis). A duodenoduodenostomy is performed with no attempt to divide the pancreas for fear of fistula formation.

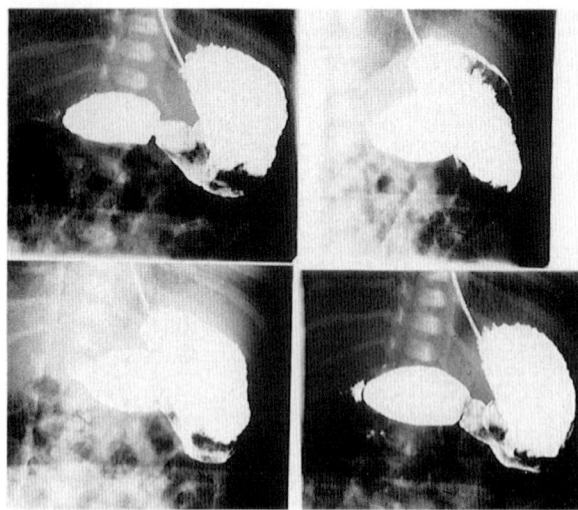

Fig. 37.9 Upper gastrointestinal contrast study on same baby as Figure 37.8.

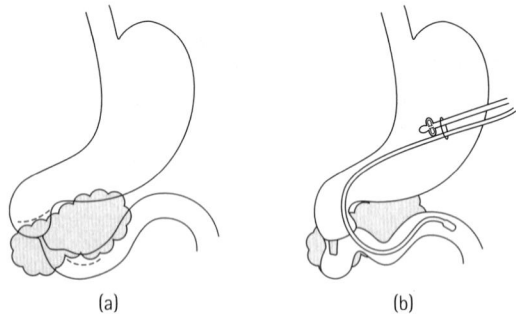

(a) (b)

Fig. 37.10 (a) Anular pancreas with intrinsic duodenal membrane. (b) Duodenoduodenostomy with gastrostomy and transanastomotic silastic feeding tube.

Extrinsic duodenal obstruction

Ladd's bands may obstruct the duodenum, occasionally alone but more commonly in association with a midgut volvulus (volvulus neonatorum). Such a volvulus may present in the neonatal period or at any age and arises due to an incomplete, or malrotation of the bowel. By the sixth week of intrauterine life the gut tube elongates to a greater extent than can be accommodated in the developing abdominal cavity and thus herniation through the umbilical ring occurs. During the next month the bowel undergoes an anticlockwise rotation returning to the abdominal cavity by the tenth week. By the time the stomach has rotated to the left, the duodenal C-loop has formed and the small bowel, followed by the large bowel, returns to the abdomen. The cecum and ascending colon pass to the right of the abdomen, the latter becoming retroperitoneal. The small bowel mesentery is then fixed between the duodenojejunal flexure and the ileocecal region. Failure of the cecum and ascending colon to reach their normal position results in a short base to the midgut mesentery and peritoneal bands passing from the cecum (in the midline or to the left side) to the right posterior abdominal wall. These bands (Ladd's bands) obstruct the duodenum. In addition, the short base to the mesentery allows a midgut volvulus to arise, the bowel rotating in a clockwise direction, and resulting in duodenal obstruction. A plain X-ray will show a double bubble and usually a small amount of gas in the bowel more distally. Contrast studies may confirm the diagnosis. An upper gastrointestinal study may show a duodenal obstruction and a typical coiled spring sign. An enema may show an anomalous position of the cecum.

Once any electrolyte or acid–base disturbance is corrected, laparotomy must be performed without delay to avoid ischemia of the midgut.

SMALL BOWEL OBSTRUCTION

This may arise due to an abnormality directly associated with the bowel itself (intrinsic), pressure from without (extrinsic), or obstruction within the lumen (intraluminal).

Intrinsic anomalies

These are mainly atresias, membranes, stenoses and duplications of the bowel. Atresias may arise anywhere along the length of the bowel, being most common in the distal ileum and rarely seen in the colon. Their likely cause is an interruption of the mesenteric vessels in utero. These vary from membranous obstruction in continuity, those with or without an associated gap in the mesentery and multiple atresias, to the so-called apple-peel type deformity with extensive loss of mesentery and bowel, the distal small bowel receiving its blood supply from the middle colic vessels through a precarious continuity between marginal arcades (Fig. 37.11).

The bowel proximal to the obstruction is distended and hypertrophied and distally the bowel is collapsed, often with a microcolon (unused) although babies with obstructions of this kind may pass meconium of normal appearance. The latter is dependent on the timing of the vascular accident in utero.

The diagnosis is confirmed by plain X-ray, which will show a number of distended loops of small bowel with air–fluid levels in an erect view (Fig. 37.12). The level of obstruction can be estimated by the number of distended loops. There will be absence of air distal to a complete obstruction.

Contrast studies have a limited role in the diagnosis of such obstructions unless to exclude intraluminal or functional conditions.

Treatment

Preoperative treatment involves passage of a nasogastric tube and correction of electrolyte imbalance by appropriate administration of i.v. fluids. If the diagnosis is established early there is little or no requirement for i.v. resuscitation.

Operative treatment involves laparotomy, resection or tapering of grossly dilated bowel proximal to the atresia (to prevent problems of postoperative peristaltic inertia) and then anastomosis between the dilated proximal bowel and the collapsed distal bowel.

Duplications

Duplications of the alimentary tract can occur at any level from mouth to anus. A length of bowel may be duplicated, the two segments sharing a common blood supply and muscular wall yet having separate mucosal

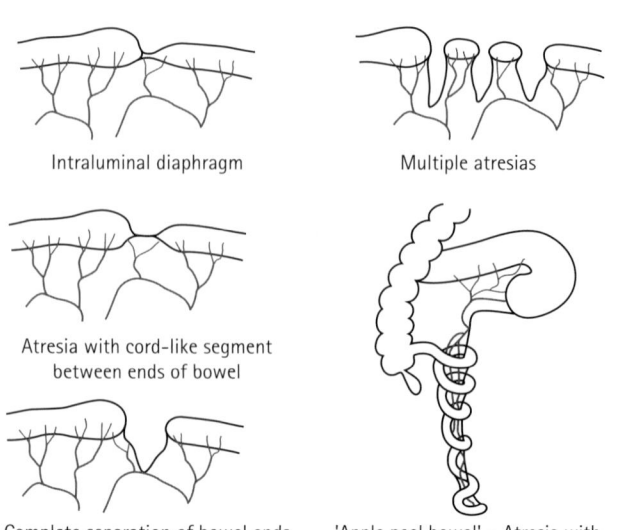

Intraluminal diaphragm

Multiple atresias

Atresia with cord-like segment between ends of bowel

Complete separation of bowel ends with mesenteric defect

'Apple peel bowel' – Atresia with extensive mesenteric defect and tenuous blood supply to distal ileum

Fig. 37.11 Small bowel atresias.

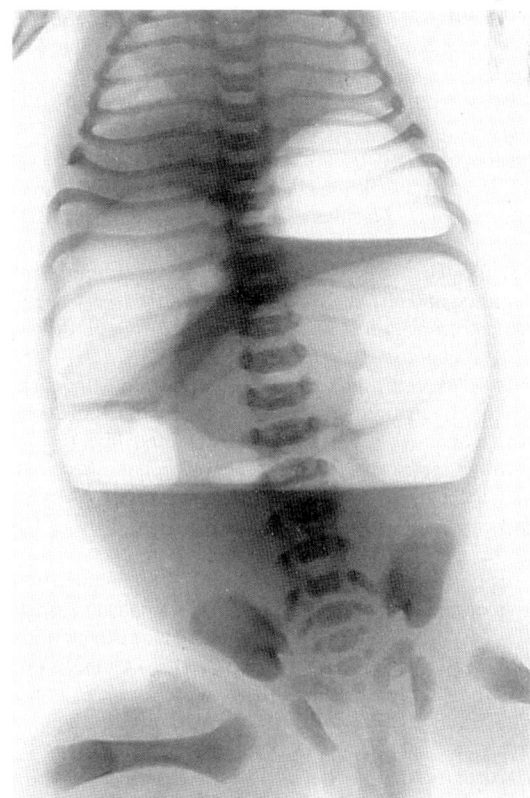

Fig. 37.12 Jejunal atresia.

linings. They may or may not communicate, and it is the noncommunicating type that tends to form a short cystic segment which, by accumulation of secretions within it, leads to intestinal obstruction. Such duplications may be palpable as a cystic intra-abdominal mass that together with the signs of intestinal obstruction lead to the diagnosis. Ultrasound and contrast studies may be of value.

Treatment. The treatment usually involves a localized bowel resection but if the duplication is extensive in length or at a site such as the ileocecal junction, the mucosa of the duplicated segment should be dissected out, thus avoiding extensive resection or loss of the ileocecal valve.

Extrinsic anomalies

Extrinsic anomalies leading to intestinal obstruction include hernias (inguinal or internal), localized volvulus, bands, vitellointestinal remnants and mesenteric cysts.

An incarcerated inguinal hernia is the commonest cause of intestinal obstruction at any age. The inguinal region must thus be carefully examined when any patient, neonate or older, presents with intestinal obstruction. Internal hernias are rare and can only be identified at laparotomy.

Localized volvulus may arise in relation to bands, duplication cysts and vitellointestinal remnants. Treatment at laparotomy varies according to the causative factor and the condition of the affected bowel. Mesenteric cysts may lead to local volvulus or may present as a palpable cystic mass. They are treated by resection.

Intraluminal anomalies

Intraluminal causes of intestinal obstruction include meconium ileus, milk curd obstruction and meconium plug syndrome.

Around 10–15% of patients with cystic fibrosis present in the neonatal period with obstruction of the distal ileum (meconium ileus). The distal few centimeters of ileum contain pale grey 'rabbit pellets' of inspissated meconium proximal to which is a segment containing hard green–black meconium and, more proximally still, distended loops containing tarry fluid meconium and air. Distal to the obstruction is a microcolon

and usually no meconium is passed, presenting signs being abdominal distention and bile-stained vomiting within a few days of birth.

Plain abdominal films show gross abdominal distention with few fluid levels and often a ground glass appearance (of air bubbles in the viscid meconium) in the right iliac fossa. Sometimes there are signs of calcification from perforation and leakage of meconium antenatally.

Volvulus of the hypertrophied distended bowel may also lead to atresia, or perforation may occur after birth.

The presence of meconium ileus has no relationship to the subsequent 'severity' of the cystic fibrosis.

Conservative management

Treatment can be either conservative or operative. Conservative management involves the administration of a Gastrografin enema under fluoroscopic control. Gastrografin with 0.1% Tween 80, a detergent, added as a wetting agent has a high osmolarity of 1900 mOsm/L and acts by drawing fluid into the bowel, thus freeing the inspissated meconium in the distal ileum. It is essential, therefore, that the baby is adequately hydrated and an i.v. infusion must be in progress. If necessary the procedure may be repeated after 24 h. If there is calcification the procedure is best avoided for fear of reperforation.

Surgical management

For cases in which there are complications such as perforation or signs of meconium peritonitis (calcification) or after failed Gastrografin enema, operative treatment is required. Laparotomy is performed via an upper transverse abdominal incision. Intestinal resection is necessary for bowel that is grossly dilated or of doubtful viability. A Bishop Koop ileostomy may be performed. This is a Roux-en-Y anastomosis between the end of the proximal limb of ileum and the side of the distal limb, bringing the end of the latter out of the abdomen as an end ileostomy in the right iliac fossa. This acts as a safety valve through which the distal ileum can be irrigated. In the case of continued obstruction the stoma will function. Once it is relieved, bowel contents pass the natural way.

Milk plug or mild curd obstruction also occurs in the distal ileum and may be due to the administration of inappropriately concentrated artificial milk feeds, or possibly a transient low bile acid excretion. The management is similar to that described earlier.

MECONIUM PLUG SYNDROME/SMALL LEFT COLON SYNDROME

Meconium plug syndrome must not be confused with meconium ileus. It is sometimes described as small left colon syndrome. The distal colon or rectum is plugged by sticky grey–white mucus distally with sticky meconium above it. The presentation is usually at about 2 d with a history of failure to pass meconium. There is evidence of low intestinal obstruction with generalized abdominal distention, frequently with a history of bile-stained vomiting and X-ray showing gaseous distention. There are multiple fluid levels present in the majority of cases.

The diagnosis is made by contrast enema. Initially barium is used to exclude Hirschsprung disease, but then changed to water-soluble contrast when the appearance of a meconium plug is seen in a narrowed left colon. The colon is usually narrow up to the splenic flexure, where it becomes dilated (Fig. 37.13). It has been postulated that there is a discrepancy in the activity of the parasympathetic supply from the vagus nerve (supplying the bowel to two thirds of the way across the transverse colon to the splenic flexure) and the sacral parasympathetics that supply the remainder. Whatever the etiology, the enema invariably proves to be therapeutic with satisfactory evacuation of meconium. The abdomen in most cases decompresses over 24 h and feeds can then be introduced. If bowel evacuation is not normal then Hirschsprung disease must be excluded.

HIRSCHSPRUNG DISEASE[6]

Hirschsprung, a Danish pediatrician, described two patients who died at 7 and 11 months from constipation associated with gross abdominal

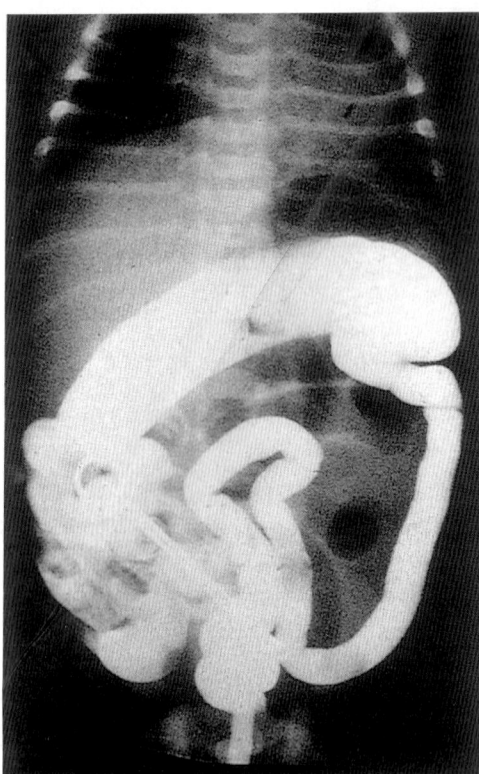

Fig. 37.13 Small left colon syndrome.

distention and a highly dilated hypertrophied colon full of feces. There is absence of ganglion cells in the myenteric plexuses (both Auerbach's and Meissner's) of the most distal bowel and extending proximally for a variable distance. Aganglionosis involving only the rectum or rectosigmoid is often termed 'short segment' Hirschsprung disease and affects males five times more commonly than females. 'Long segment' Hirschsprung disease, extending above the sigmoid, has an equal sex incidence and a greater likelihood of siblings being affected. In short segment disease there is a 1 in 20 risk that brothers will be affected and a 1 in 100 risk for sisters. In long segment disease the risk to all siblings is 1 in 10.

In a few cases there is total colonic aganglionosis with disease extending into the small bowel and in extremely rare cases involving the whole alimentary canal. At least 70% of cases are short segment, 25% long segment and about 5% total colonic.

Hirschsprung disease differs from many other alimentary tract abnormalities in that the birth weight is usually within the normal range. It is uncommon in premature and low birth weight babies. Associated congenital anomalies are uncommon apart from Down syndrome, which affects 1 in 20. The cause of the disease is unknown. It has been postulated that it is due to a failure of migration of ganglion cells from the neural crest, which normally proceeds in a craniocaudal direction having entered the upper end of the alimentary tract.[7] Differentiation of ganglion cells occurs in the wall of the gut between the seventh and eighth week of intrauterine life and proceeds in a craniocaudal direction.

Clinical features

Usually the symptoms of Hirschsprung disease are manifest within the first few days of life. This is certainly the case in all long segment or total colonic cases but some short segment cases and especially 'ultrashort' segment cases may present later, even into old age.

Failure to pass meconium within the first 24 h, abdominal distention, bile-stained vomiting and reluctance to feed are the main symptoms. Diarrhea may be the presenting feature of Hirschsprung enterocolitis, a devastating complication of the condition that has a high mortality. The etiology of Hirschsprung enterocolitis is unknown but apart from

diarrhea it is associated with gross abdominal distention and circulatory collapse. A rectal examination results in the explosive passage of flatus and loose stool, deflating the abdomen.

Diagnosis

A plain abdominal X-ray shows distended small and large bowel, sometimes with multiple fluid levels on an erect film. A barium enema is best carried out without a previous rectal examination as then the narrow aganglionic bowel with dilation proximally is demonstrated. A delayed film at 24 h, again avoiding an invasive rectal examination, shows retained barium and often a clear indication of the level of disease with a cone-shaped transition zone between normal bowel above and the narrowed aganglionic distal segment.

Definitive diagnosis is by rectal biopsy. A suction biopsy is adequate to confirm the absence of ganglion cells in the submucosal plexus, specimens being taken at 1 and 3 cm above the dentate line. Histochemical staining will demonstrate excessive acetyl cholinesterase activity in abnormal nerve trunks and absence of ganglion cells.

Treatment

Once the diagnosis is made, bowel washouts may be sufficient to maintain bowel decompression prior to a laparoscopically assisted 'pull through' procedure. Others prefer a defunctioning stoma, proximal to the diseased bowel. A definitive procedure is then carried out when the infant is 3–12 months of age, depending on the surgeon's preference. It usually consists of excision of the aganglionic bowel and a pull through procedure.

If enterocolitis supervenes (and it can even happen after a definitive procedure, especially if an aganglionic segment remains), then rapid replacement of lost fluid by a suitable electrolyte solution, often preceded by plasma, is required. This should be combined with saline bowel washouts using a two tube technique, one to run saline in, preferably above the aganglionic segment, the other at a slightly lower level to allow evacuation. Broad-spectrum antibiotics are usually administered prophylactically although infection has not been shown to be the precipitating factor. Enterocolitis is the most lethal complication of Hirschsprung disease.

UROLOGICAL PROBLEMS IN THE NEONATE

Posterior urethral valves

The commonest obstructive uropathy in male children is valvular obstruction of the posterior urethra. Occasionally the diagnosis is made on antenatal ultrasound. A large proportion of cases present in the first 2 weeks of life, the majority in the first 6 months and the remainder, whilst usually becoming apparent in the first few years, may present as late as early adult life.

The neonate may present with retention of urine or dribbling and a palpably distended bladder with or without infection or uremia. Later presentation is usually with incontinence or infection.

The valves are classically folds of mucosa attached just below the verumontanum and attempts to void lead to apposition of the valves. The obstruction leads to dilation of the posterior urethra, the bladder, the ureter and renal pelvis.

As micturition commences in the fetus in the first trimester, the back pressure on the kidneys may lead antenatally to severe damage – renal dysplasia. Occasionally the bladder hypertrophy is such that reflux no longer occurs but the ureters remain dilated and tortuous.

Diagnosis

A micturating cystourethrogram (MCU) is diagnostic in this anomaly, demonstrating the gross dilation of the posterior urethra and usually the refluxing dilated ureters and bilateral hydronephrosis.

Treatment

Disruption of the valves is required. This may be effected by pulling the inflated balloon of a Fogarty catheter across the valves or by delicately disrupting them with a Whitaker hook. A resectoscope can be used transurethrally and the valves either fulgurated or, to avoid a deep destruction of tissue, cut with a cold knife. If renal function is particularly poor, temporary drainage via bilateral cutaneous ureterostomies (preferably ring ureterostomies) may be required.

Prune belly syndrome (triad syndrome)

This consists of deficiency of the anterior abdominal wall muscles, cryptorchidism and urinary tract deformities. The abdominal muscular deficiency is mainly in the lower abdomen, the whole abdominal wall taking on the wrinkled appearance of a prune (Fig. 37.14). The ribs may be flared outwards at the lower costal margin and respiratory infections are common.

Surgery is best avoided unless there is significant renal impairment. In severe cases ring ureterostomies may be required, followed at a later date by tapering and reimplantation of the ureters, trimming of the bladder, orchidopexies and excision and repair of the lower anterior abdominal wall. Some cases have a functional urethral obstruction, which may require urethrotomy. Other cases show urethral stricture or even a diverticulum at the site of the prostatic utricle.

Urachal anomalies

The urachus in the embryo connects the bladder to the allantois. It is normally obliterated to form the median umbilical ligament. It may, however, persist as a patent urachus in the neonate, requiring repair. Occasionally the two extremities of the urachus close, leaving a cyst in the middle that becomes filled with secretions and may present as a mass or more commonly, when it becomes infected, as an abscess.

Bladder exstrophy (ectopia vesicae)

This is part of a range of lower abdominal wall defects, ranging from epispadias, through exstrophy of the bladder, to the even more catastrophic vesicointestinal fissure or cloacal exstrophy.

In bladder exstrophy there is a lower abdominal wall anomaly in which there is wide separation of the pubic bones, the bladder surface

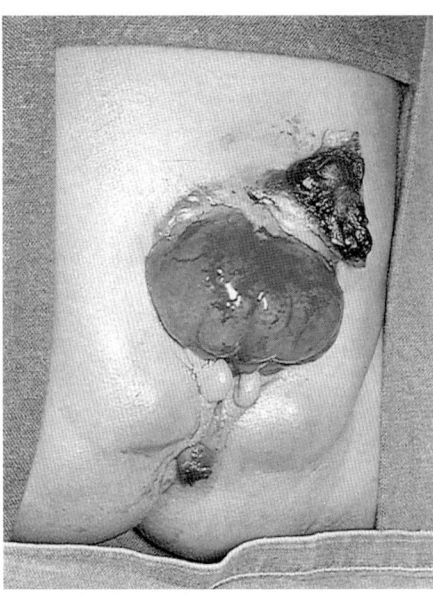

Fig. 37.15   Ectopic vesicae.

being flat and exposed with the two ureteric orifices clearly visible (Fig. 37.15). In the male there is complete epispadias with a strip of urethral mucosa on the dorsum of a short broadened, flattened penis. In the female there is also an epispadiac urethra with a bifid clitoris and separation of the labia anteriorly at the level of the vaginal orifice.

The bladder is best repaired soon after birth. If necessary, bilateral iliac osteotomies enable the pubic bones to be better approximated thus facilitating the repair. Careful construction of the bladder neck is vital to achieve subsequent continence, and in the male later repair of the severe epispadiac deformity is required. If the bladder repair is unsuccessful it may be necessary to carry out a urinary diversion procedure.

EXOMPHALOS AND GASTROSCHISIS

These are two distinct conditions of different etiology. Although formerly exomphalos was believed to be more common, gastroschisis is now seen more frequently. Antenatal diagnosis of both conditions by ultrasound examination is now almost routine. Gastroschisis also gives rise to an elevated maternal serum alpha-fetoprotein and distinction from other anomalies such as neural tube defects is by ultrasonography. Gastroschisis is not an indication for termination of pregnancy whilst exomphalos major, with its high incidence (30–40%) of associated anomalies, may be.

Exomphalos

Exomphalos (omphalocele) is a herniation of intra-abdominal contents through the umbilical ring into the umbilical cord. Defects less than 4 cm in diameter are classified as *exomphalos minor* (Fig. 37.16). There are rarely associated abnormalities in this group.

Exomphalos major (Fig. 37.17), on the other hand, commonly has coexisting abnormalities and a defect greater than 4 cm in diameter, presumably arising through failure of development of the anterior abdominal wall prior to herniation of the midgut loop. In a large defect, not only the intestines (small and large) herniate but also the liver, spleen, stomach, bladder and even ovaries and fallopian tubes in the female. Incomplete or malrotation of the bowel is common and the associated abnormalities often include cardiac defects; 20% of cases are anencephalic. In the *Beckwith–Wiedemann* syndrome there is exomphalos, macroglossia and gigantism. The baby is large for his gestational age with an exomphalos, a big tongue and large solid viscera. There is also a facial nevus flammeus in the center of the forehead and odd indentations in the ear lobe (Fig. 37.18). There may also be pancreatic hyperplasia leading to severe neonatal hypoglycemia.

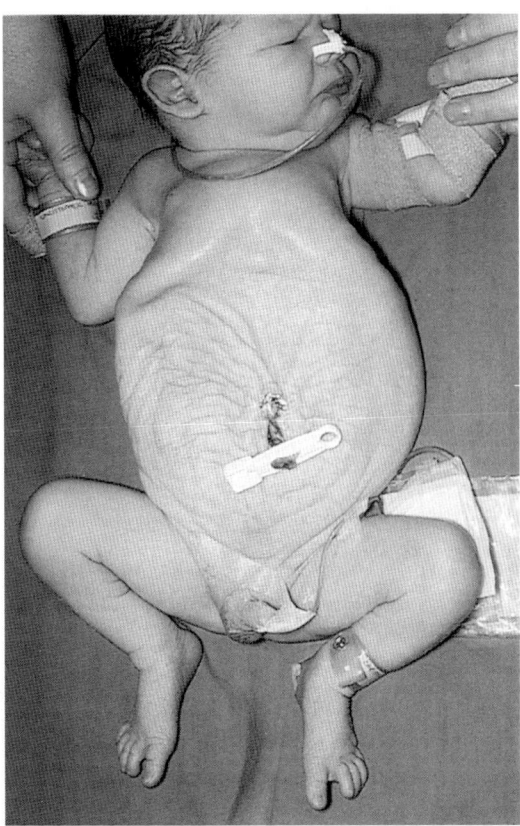

Fig. 37.14   Prune belly syndrome.

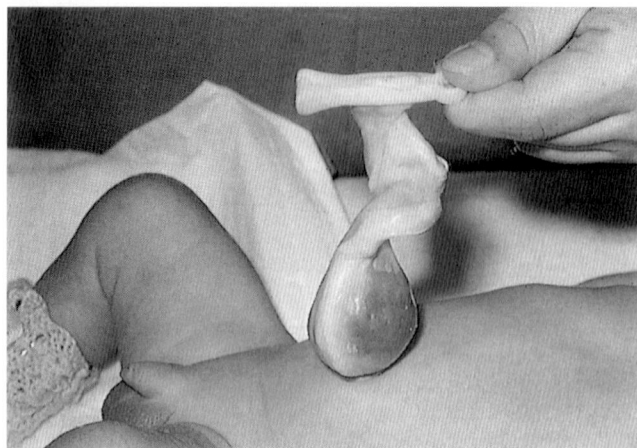

Fig. 37.16 Exomphalos minor.

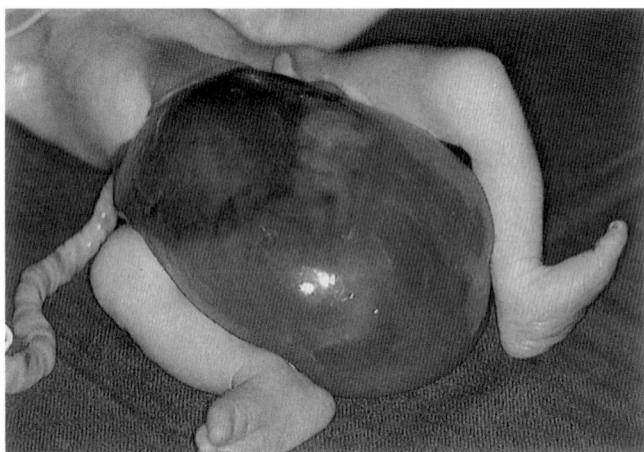

Fig. 37.17 Exomphalos major.

An *omphalocele* is usually covered by a sac composed of the fused layers of amniotic membrane and peritoneum. The sac may rupture ante-, intra- or postpartum.

Treatment

In a large omphalocele, conservative management may be appropriate in the neonatal period. Silver sulfadiazine dessings[8] or simple alcohol solution should be applied daily until an eschar forms. Epithelialization of the sac from the periphery results over the ensuing weeks. It may take 3–4 months before the infant can be discharged home, returning for later surgical repair of the ventral hernia. Other methods of treatment include mobilization of skin around the defect and skin coverage or coverage with prosthetic material and later repair of the ventral hernia. If the defect is small enough, with stretching of the anterior abdominal wall, primary repair may be possible as in gastroschisis (see later). In cases with an apparently simple herniation through a small defect into the umbilical cord it is tempting to twist the cord to reduce the contained bowel into the abdominal cavity, then simply ligate the cord. Such a temptation must be strongly resisted as all too frequently there is a Meckel's diverticulum or another cause of adherence of the bowel to the sac and serious damage may result. Formal surgical repair is always indicated.

Gastroschisis

Gastroschisis is a complete defect through all layers of the anterior abdominal wall extending up to about 3 cm in length and usually lying to the right of a normally attached umbilical cord (Fig. 37.19). It is almost as though a short transverse incision had been made with a scalpel antenatally. The etiology is unknown. Almost all the small and large bowel are eviscerated through the small defect – in most instances from stomach to rectum inclusive. Other organs are rarely apparent. The eviscerated bowel is markedly thickened, apparently foreshortened, matted together and often covered with a confluent gelatinous layer like 'gut in aspic'.

If possible, delivery should be in a perinatal center close to the regional pediatric surgical center. The decision whether to deliver the baby with exomphalos or gastroschisis by Cesarean section or vaginally is an obstetric one. The results of treatment of the baby are not significantly improved by cesarean delivery.

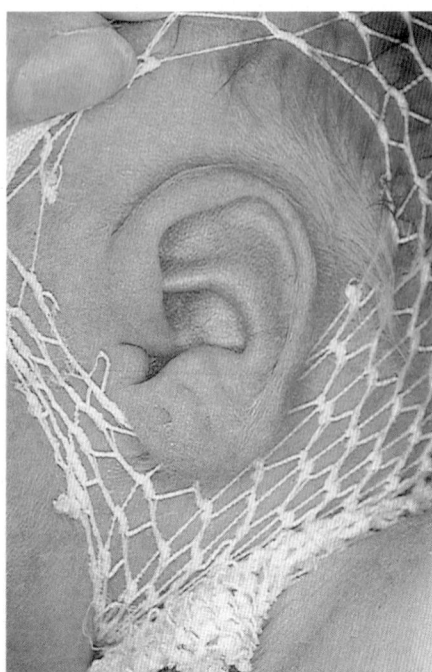

Fig. 37.18 Earlobe indentations in Beckwith–Wiedemann syndrome.

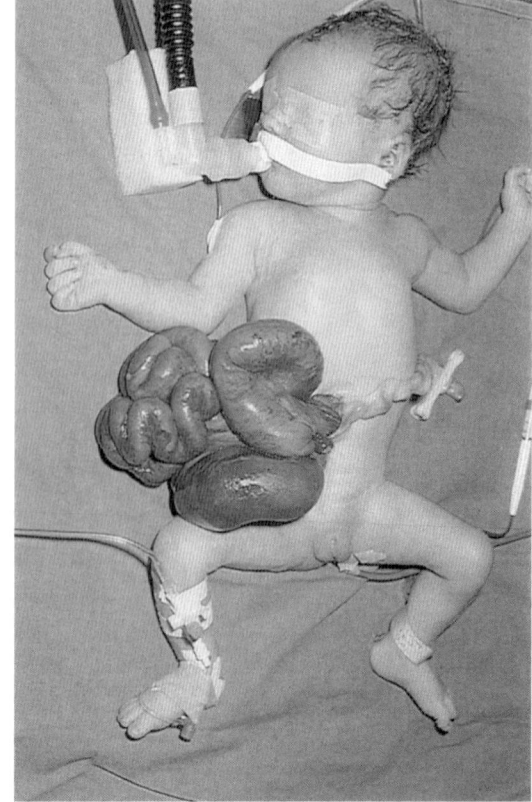

Fig. 37.19 Gastroschisis.

At delivery it is essential that the baby is placed in a plastic bag extending to above the level of the defect and leaving the head and, if necessary, the upper limbs exposed. The bowel must not be allowed to become contaminated, the baby being transferred in a transport incubator directly to the pediatric surgical operating table and the baby extracted from the bag aseptically, by the surgeon, once anesthesia is induced. The passage of a nasogastric tube prior to transfer reduces bowel distention and resulting ischemia if the anterior abdominal wall defect is very small. Transport in a polyethylene bag helps reduce hypothermia, which would otherwise result from heat loss by evaporation. These babies rapidly drop their temperature from 37°C to 35°C when exposed for even a few minutes to site an i.v. infusion. The application of warm saline soaked swabs is not a good idea as they rapidly cool, increasing the heat loss.

Treatment

Recently bedside reduction with or without a preformed silo have changed the immediate management of gastroschisis.[9,10] Providing the temperature has been adequately maintained and no significant fluid loss has occurred, direct transfer to the surgical neonatal unit and direct reduction or application of a preformed silo achieve the best results. If the bowel is particularly matted then surgical reduction in theater may be required. Leaving the cord intact and not enlarging the defect with either technique gives the best cosmetic result. The defect is usually so small that the umbilicus is not eccentric in position.

Postoperatively, no ventilatory support is required for ward reductions. A prolonged ileus however necessitates i.v. nutrition for days or in some cases even weeks. The prognosis in gastroschisis cases treated in this manner is excellent.

SACROCOCCYGEAL TERATOMA

The sacrococcygeal teratoma is the commonest teratoma presenting in the neonatal period. They tend to be large and protrude from the space between the anus and the coccyx (Fig. 37.20). The lesion is usually covered in skin but the most protuberant part may be necrotic due to vascular compromise. The tumor may also extend up into the pelvis and a large retrorectal component is palpable in all cases. In a presacral teratoma there is no protrusion behind the anus and the presentation may be later in the first year of life.

The tumor may be both solid and cystic in nature. A very large tumor may give rise to dystocia and if diagnosed antenatally is best delivered by Cesarean section.

Treatment is excision within the first few days of life. A double 'chevron' incision is made with the baby in a prone position and with careful excision and reconstruction of the pelvic floor which, despite its gross stretching, recovers normal function (Fig. 37.21). Excision of the coccyx is an essential component of the operation as failing to do so may predispose to the development of a yolk sac tumor.

There is usually an elevated alpha-fetoprotein level in the baby at birth and this should decline appropriately following excision. Even benign tumors should be followed up into adulthood as recurrence of benign or malignant elements may occur.

ANORECTAL ANOMALIES

Congenital anomalies of the anus and rectum are reported to occur in 1 in 1800 to 1 in 10 000 live births. In Edinburgh the incidence is 1 in 3100. There is a wide spectrum of anomalies and many attempts have been made to classify them. Recently a new international diagnostic classification system, operative groupings and a method of postoperative assessment of continence was developed by a large contingent of participants experienced in the management of anorectal malformations[11].

An anatomical approach simplifies matters (Table 37.1).[12] The lesions are grouped according to whether the end of the rectum is above levator ani, *high* (supralevator), or below, *low* (translevator). There is also an *intermediate*, partially translevator group. The essential component of the levator ani in these malformations is the puborectalis sling, which is the key to fecal continence.

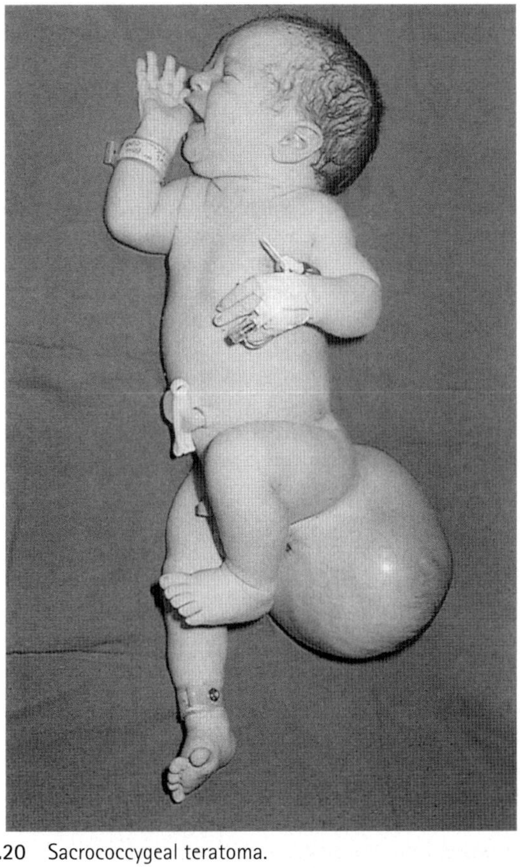

Fig. 37.20   Sacrococcygeal teratoma.

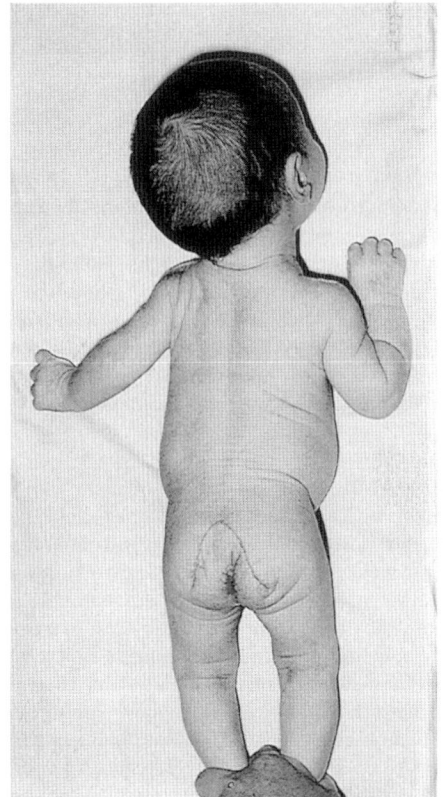

Fig. 37.21   Postoperative appearance of Figure 37.20.

Table 37.1   Classification of anorectal malformations (Stephens 1984[12])

Female	Male
High	*High*
Anorectal agenesis:	Anorectal agenesis:
With rectovaginal fistula	With recto–prostatic–urethral fistula
Without fistula	Without fistula
Intermediate	*Intermediate*
Rectovestibular fistula	Rectobulbar urethral fistula
Rectovaginal fistula	
Anal agenesis without fistula	Anal agenesis without fistula
Low	*Low*
Anovestibular fistula	
Anocutaneous fistula	Anocutaneous fistula
Anal stenosis	Anal stenosis
Cloacal malformations	
Rare malformations	Rare malformations

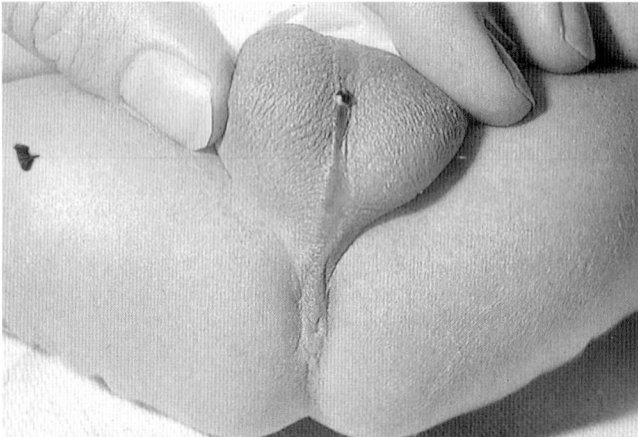

Fig. 37.22   Low anorectal anomaly.

In the male a high lesion commonly communicates with the urethra whereas in the female, with the genital tract intervening, the fistula is to the vagina. A low lesion may open onto the skin of the perineum, or in the male, track forwards along the median raphe of the scrotum (Fig. 37.22), or in the female, towards the vestibule. In addition, a severe cloacal anomaly may arise in girls with urethra, vagina and rectum opening into a common channel. Anal stenosis may arise in either sex and presents with the passage of toothpaste-like motions.

Treatment

Anal stenosis is treated by graduated anal dilation with Hegar's dilators. A low lesion with a long subcutaneous tract should have the latter opened and an anoplasty performed. An anovestibular fistula can also be managed by a cutback procedure. This may result in rather close proximity of anal and vaginal openings (shotgun perineum) but the perineum develops as the child grows, separating the orifices. To avoid this appearance some prefer to transpose the anal opening to a more normal site.

High and intermediate lesions, and low lesions where the diagnosis is not at first obvious, require a defunctioning colostomy in the neonatal period. A sigmoid colostomy will enable subsequent adequate washouts of the distal loop, a procedure that is especially important in lesions communicating with the urinary tract. Prophylactic antibiotics are also required in such cases.

Once the colostomy is established, formal contrast studies via the distal loop (distal loopogram) define the level of the lesion accurately. Definitive repair is then deferred for a few weeks or months depending on the preference of the surgeon. The procedure of choice is the posterior sagittal anorectoplasty described by de Vries and Pena,[13] requiring meticulous technique and a thorough understanding of the anatomy. Some now perform a laparoscopically assisted pull through.

NEONATAL NECROTIZING ENTEROCOLITIS (NEC)

This condition is described in detail in Chapter 12. Presenting as it does with abdominal distention and bile-stained vomiting, it is occasionally considered that the baby has intestinal obstruction but the presence of blood in the stool and pneumatosis intestinalis, often with portal venous gas, are pathognomonic of NEC. The management is conservative, wherever possible with nasogastric decompression, i.v. feeding and broad-spectrum antibiotics. The criteria for surgical management include pneumoperitoneum, persistent and increasing abdominal tenderness and continued clinical deterioration despite appropriate medical management. Operative management includes resection of necrotic bowel and stoma formation. Occasionally localized drainage under local anesthesia is of value in extremely ill babies, with appropriate intervention at a later date. Conservatively managed survivors often develop intestinal strictures requiring later resection. Asymptomatic strictures identified on contrast studies are best kept under review, reserving surgery for symptomatic cases.

BILIARY ATRESIA

Biliary atresia is a condition in which the extrahepatic bile ducts are grossly nonpatent. The condition is characterized by obstructive jaundice. There has traditionally been a division into 'correctable' biliary atresia, where only the distal ducts are occluded, and 'noncorrectable', in which the proximal ducts are occluded.

Presentation is with jaundice persisting beyond the first 2 weeks of life. Appropriate tests are carried out to exclude causes of hepatocellular disease (hepatitis A, hepatitis B, toxoplasmosis, rubella, cytomegalovirus, herpes, syphilis, listeriosis, galactosemia, fructosemia, alpha1-antitrypsin deficiency, etc.) It is vital not to waste too much time awaiting the results of all tests as delay in treatment of biliary atresia will adversely affect the progress. Suspected cases must therefore be referred early to a center capable of undertaking the necessary investigation and surgery. Ultrasound will rarely show a gallbladder and may show increased hepatic parenchymal echoes in biliary atresia. An isotope liver scan using a ^{99m}Tc iminodiacetic acid (IDA) radiopharmaceutical will demonstrate good hepatic uptake but no excretion into the bowel at 24 h. In hepatocellular jaundice there is a decrease in hepatocyte clearance.

Some surgeons prefer to do a percutaneous liver biopsy, which may be strongly indicative of biliary atresia, but others proceed directly to operative cholangiography if there is a positive IDA scan. This is carried out through a small transverse right upper abdominal incision. The gallbladder is often small and fibrotic, making a cholangiogram impossible. Occasionally patency of the cystic duct and common bile duct may be identified and, rarely, biliary hypoplasia.

Treatment

The procedure of choice for extrahepatic biliary atresia is Kasai's hepatic portoenterostomy. This was first described in Japanese in 1959 and only in 1968 in English.[14]

Kasai reports satisfactory bile drainage in 80% of cases. In other series this ranges from 35 to 75% (personal small series 75%). Many will develop portal hypertension and cholangitis (various modifications of Kasai's procedure are carried out to reduce this complication). Liver transplantation is of great value in cases that fail to achieve or maintain bile drainage following the Kasai procedure.

SURGERY OF THE INFANT AND CHILD

HEAD AND NECK, FACE AND MOUTH
Embryological abnormalities
Branchial arch–abnormalities

Sinuses, fistulae, cysts and cartilaginous elements may be apparent at birth or may be noted in infancy or later in childhood. These anomalies arise from the first and second pharyngeal arches and clefts. First cleft remnants are rare and include a tract from the external auditory canal to the upper lateral neck. They may present with recurrent abscesses in the neck, and treatment involves excision of the whole tract, usually a sinus, being blind ending at the external auditory canal. Abnormal development of the first arch results in cleft lip and palate, abnormal shape of the pinna, and deafness due to malformation of the malleus and incus.

Second branchial remnants are more common. In theory sinuses should be more common than fistulae but the reverse is true and cysts are the least common, often presenting in adult life. Fistulae have a skin opening over the anterior border of the lower third of the sternomastoid. This may be noted to discharge clear mucus. The tract passes upwards between the internal and external carotid arteries to open in the tonsillar fossa.

The length of this tract often necessitates two incisions to facilitate its removal, one being at the skin opening and the other parallel to it, at a higher level, to follow the tract through the carotid bifurcation.

Branchial cysts manifest themselves as they slowly enlarge with secretions, appearing in late childhood or young adulthood. They tend to lie deep to the anterior border of the upper third of the sternocleidomastoid muscle. They may become infected. The treatment is excision.

Cartilaginous branchial remnants may appear along the anterior border of sternocleidomastoid. They do not usually have an associated tract and are excised purely for cosmetic reasons.

Thyroglossal cysts

These are more common than branchial remnants. The thyroid develops as a diverticulum from the floor of the pharynx, leaving it attached to the foramen cecum (at the junction of the anterior two thirds, and posterior one third of the tongue) by a stalk, the thyroglossal duct, which is normally completely reabsorbed. The tract of a persistent thyroglossal duct should developmentally be ventral to the hyoid bone but differential growth results in part of the duct reaching its deep surface. A thyroglossal cyst arises typically in the midline of the neck anteriorly, or occasionally just to one or other side of the midline. By virtue of its attachment to the thyroglossal duct the cyst moves on swallowing or protrusion of the tongue (Fig. 37.23a–c). The cyst is usually at the level of or just below the hyoid bone but can be anywhere along the line of the duct. Surgery is best performed when the lesion is diagnosed, as infection may arise and lead to difficulty in complete excision. The operation involves not only removal of the cyst but the body of the hyoid and the tract must be followed up to the level of the foramen cecum. Failure to do this is likely to lead to recurrence.

Dermoid cysts

These usually occur at sites of embryological fusion. These may be in the midline. A dermoid cyst in the neck may be mistaken for a thyroglossal cyst although it will not move on swallowing or protrusion of the tongue. A common site is the external angular dermoid cyst in the eyebrow area at the outer angle of the eye. Occasionally there may be a dumbbell extension intracranially. They occur if ectodermal cells become buried beneath the skin surface during development. An inclusion dermoid cyst may similarly arise secondary to trauma.

Cystic hygroma

Commonly arising in the neck, these fluid-filled lesions of lymphatic origin may be found elsewhere, including the axilla and groin or, rarely, on the trunk. They are either present at birth, sometimes being diagnosed on antenatal ultrasonography, or may appear within the first 2 years or sometimes later. Usually arising in the posterior triangle of the neck,

they may sometimes be very large indeed, extending into the floor of the mouth and tongue, where complete excision may prove difficult, leading to disfigurement and occasionally the need for a tracheostomy. Infection leads to difficulty with subsequent surgery, which is thus best performed soon after diagnosis. Aspiration of the cysts and injection of a streptococcal derivative 'OK432' (Picibanil) is a treatment that is proving to be an effective alternative to surgery.[15]

Salivary gland enlargement

This may arise secondary to a calculus in a duct (the submandibular duct in particular). Parotid duct calculi are rare but recurrent swelling of the gland may be due to sialectasis, seen on a sialogram as dilated duct radicles. The treatment is to advise the sucking of acid drop sweets to promote salivary flow and at the same time massaging the gland from back to front. If infection supervenes then antibiotics must be administered.

Ranula (Latin rana = frog)

This is a sublingual cyst that may be small or may fill the floor of the mouth. It may be related to a salivary or mucus gland. It is thin walled and contains clear viscid fluid. Care is required not to damage the submandibular duct during its excision and marsupialization is often safer.

Tongue tie

A short lingual frenum leads to maternal anxiety regarding future problems with speech. Speech therapists confirm that there will be no speech problem and others that the anterior third of the tongue will grow and a normal appearance will result. Tongue tie may lead to difficulty with breast-feeding. Division of the tongue tie in a baby prior to appearance of dentition is a simple procedure for a surgeon in the outpatient clinic. In the older child, general anesthesia is required. Tongue tie may occasionally present beyond the first 2 years and the current author personally believes in division, as all children deserve to be able to stick their tongue out – if only to lick an ice cream!

Cervical lymphadenopathy

Cervical lymph nodes are readily palpable in most children. Lymphoma is rare, but persistent painless enlargement of a cervical node is best diagnosed by excision biopsy although it is reasonable to administer an antibiotic in doubtful cases and re-examine the child in 2 weeks. Cat scratch disease, *Toxoplasma* and both tuberculosis and atypical mycobacterial infections may occur and usually affect jugulodigastric and submandibular nodes.

In mycobacterial infections, nodes may feel fixed to deeper tissues and to skin and may caseate and discharge. Sinus formation may result from abscess rupture or incomplete excision. Antituberculous chemotherapy is necessary once the diagnosis has become established.

Acute suppurative cervical lymphadenitis usually results from an upper respiratory tract infection. Early administration of antibiotics may lead to resolution without abscess formation but if an abscess does form it should be allowed to point before drainage. Kaolin poultices seem old fashioned but are still of value in this process.

Sternomastoid tumor

This is the commonest cause of torticollis in childhood (other causes include hemivertebrae, acute fasciitis, cervical adenitis and ocular muscle imbalance). The cause of this lesion is unknown. It is more common in babies born by breech presentation and was considered to be a result of trauma to the muscle during delivery. It seems likely, however, that it arises in utero, resulting in breech presentation. Within the muscle there is an area of endomysial fibrosis with atrophied muscle fibers surrounded by collagen and fibroblasts. The infant presents usually at 2–3 weeks of age with a hard swelling within the substance of sternocleidomastoid. The shortening of the muscle makes the infant look upwards and to the opposite side. It is important to commence physiotherapy as soon as the diagnosis is made. The parents are taught how to stretch the muscle by rotating the head towards the side of the tumor. These stretching exercises should be carried out twice daily and must continue

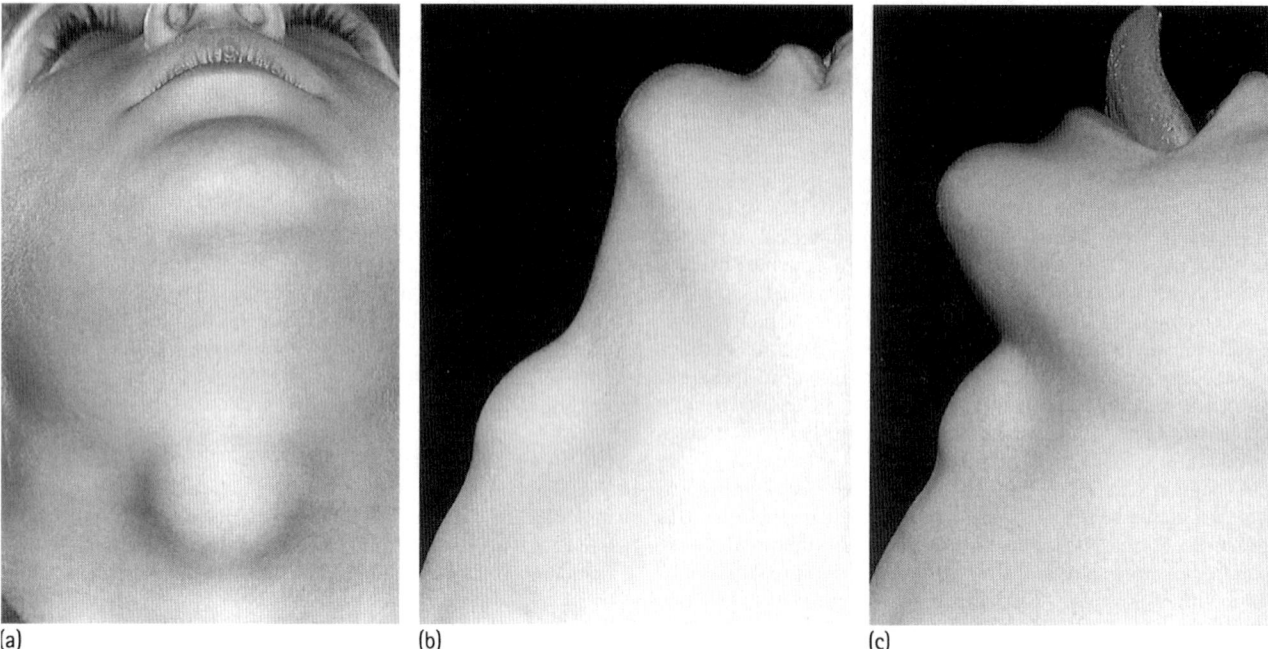

(a)   (b)   (c)

Fig. 37.23 (a) Thyroglossal cyst; (b) and (c) show elevation on tongue protrusion.

for at least the first year, diminishing in frequency thereafter. Failure to treat adequately leads to shortening of deeper cervical structures and craniofacial asymmetry. Surgical division of the muscle and deeper strictures is necessary in cases that fail to respond or are missed in the neonatal period.

Thyroid swellings
(see Chapter 15).

PYLORIC STENOSIS

Though often called congenital, hypertrophic pyloric stenosis only very rarely has its onset of symptoms at birth and has never been described in a stillbirth. Vomiting normally commences around 2–3 weeks of age, becoming more frequent and projectile. The vomitus is of gastric content (milk) and is never bile stained. It may become brownish or visibly bloodstained due either to an accompanying gastritis or to rupture of capillaries in the gastric mucosa from frequent vomiting. The baby fails to thrive, becomes constipated and dehydrated, developing a hypochloremic alkalosis from the loss of gastric acid.

Examination reveals a hungry, worried looking baby and if recently fed, visible gastric peristalsis, and a wave traveling from the left hypochondrium towards the right may be apparent (Fig. 37.24). The diagnosis is confirmed during a test feed. For this the surgeon and the nurse or mother sit facing in opposite directions, the surgeon to the left of the nurse (Fig. 37.25). The baby is fed with the bottle in the right hand or at the left breast of the nursing mother. The surgeon palpates the tumor with the left hand. It is felt as an olive-shaped mass that lies just to the right of the midline, in the right hypochondrium. Contraction of the tumor is noted with variation in palpability, thus confirming that it is not confused with a Riedel's lobe of liver, or similar anomaly. If difficulty is encountered in palpating the tumor, the passage of a nasogastric tube to wash out the stomach may facilitate the procedure (it may be that the filled gastric antrum has previously obscured the pylorus). This seemingly ritual routine not only enhances the chance of palpating the tumor but avoids the calamity of the baby vomiting over the examiner's trousers!

Most surgeons will only operate if they can palpate the tumor but if difficulty is encountered in palpation, ultrasound examination is now the diagnostic investigation of choice.

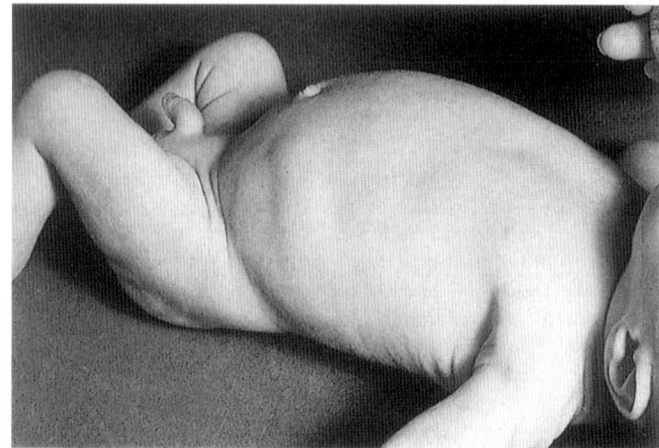

Fig. 37.24 Pyloric stenosis: visible peristalsis.

Treatment

First the hypochloremic alkalosis together with any associated hypokalemia is corrected by administering 5% dextrose in 0.45% saline with added potassium chloride if required. Although the use of 0.45% saline takes twice as long to correct the deficit as normal saline would, it is safer to administer. Preoperative gastric lavage is also performed and the nasogastric tube left in situ.

Once the electrolyte and acid–base deficit is corrected, surgery is performed under general anesthesia. The universally accepted operation of choice is the pyloromyotomy attributed to Ramstedt.[16] Actually the first recorded use of this procedure was by Sir Harold Stiles[17] in the Royal Hospital for Sick Children, Edinburgh on 3 February 1910, a year prior to Ramstedt's operation performed on 28 July 1911 and published in 1912. Unfortunately Stiles' patient died on the fourth postoperative day, either from gastroenteritis or delayed chloroform poisoning!

The pylorus can be delivered through a right transverse upper abdominal or a periumbilical incision, and an incision is made from the pyloroduodenal junction well onto the antrum of the stomach. The incision extends down into the muscle, which is then spread bluntly, all muscle fibers being ruptured, allowing the intact mucosa to bulge. The pylorus is returned to the abdomen and the wound closed.

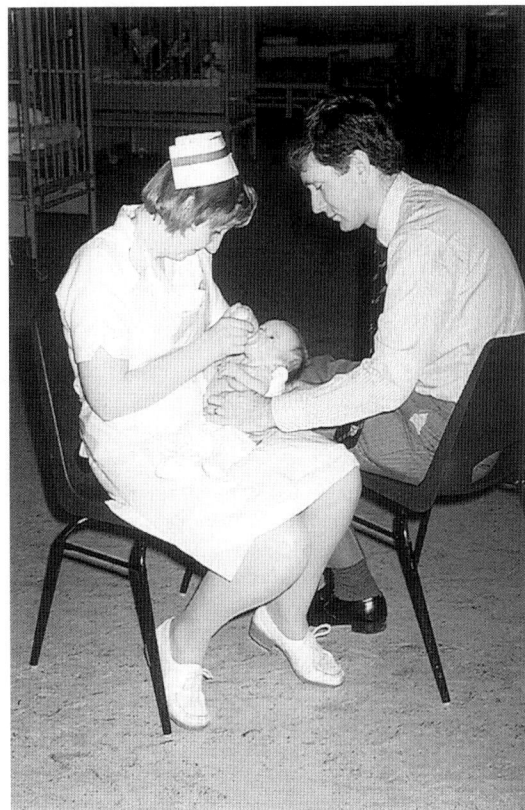

Fig. 37.25   Pyloric stenosis: test feed.

A laparoscopic approach is preferred in centers where the surgeons have the appropriate skills and is already proving to have better results with less postoperative gastric paresis.

Oral feeding can be commenced within 4 h. Some choose a graduated feeding regime of dextrose, half strength, then full strength milk introduced over 24–48 h. Others advise a more rapid return to normal feeds. Certainly breast-fed infants come to no harm from being returned to the breast initially for a short time, gradually increasing to normal feeding time.

Vomiting in the first 24 h postoperatively is not unusual and is presumably related to preoperative gastritis. If persistent it usually settles after gastric lavage. Most babies will be fit for discharge within 24–72 h after surgery.

GASTROESOPHAGEAL REFLUX

This is due to incompetence at the cardia and is another cause of vomiting that may commence as early as the neonatal period. The condition may or may not be associated with a hiatus hernia. The infant vomits effortlessly at any time, and usually appears unconcerned about the problem. The vomiting need not be related to feed times. The vomitus may be coffee ground or streaked with bright red blood if there is associated peptic esophagitis. The diagnosis is confirmed by barium studies and pH studies together with endoscopy, if indicated. Most cases respond to conservative management of thickening the feeds, sitting the baby up at all times (although there is dispute about this) and the administration of an antacid such as Gaviscon. In more severe cases an H_2 antagonist or a proton pump inhibitor is used. If, however, the infant fails to thrive, has persistent peptic esophagitis, recurrent aspiration pneumonitis or a proven large 'sliding' hiatus hernia, then a surgical antireflux procedure is required. If an esophageal stricture has already developed it will usually resolve after surgery but in some cases bougienage or balloon dilation is required. Various antireflux operations have been devised, the most popular being the Nissen fundoplication. The esophagus and the gastric fundus is mobilized, the right crus of the diaphragm tightened and wrapped around the abdominal esophagus. This operation is now best performed laparoscopically,[18] reducing postoperative discomfort and length of hospital stay.

Children with severe neurological handicap are especially prone to gastroesophageal reflux and hiatus hernia. Usually their parents or carers welcome the surgical treatment of these children, as their well-being is so obviously improved. Presumably they suffer a great deal of discomfort related to esophagitis and their frustration is increased by their inability to complain. The results of surgery in such cases is invariably rewarding.

INTUSSUSCEPTION

Intussusception is the invagination of part of the intestine into itself. An intussusception arising in the ileum may pass all the way round the large bowel to appear at the anus. The lead point is known as the *intussusceptum*, the sheath as the *intussuscipiens* and between these are the entering and returning layers of the bowel. Naturally, the mesentery with its vessels is drawn between the entering and returning layers, leading to engorgement of the vessels and diapedesis of red cells into the lumen of the bowel. Mucus is produced by the engorgement of the mucosal cells and, mixed with the red cells, creates the classic redcurrant jelly stool. Eventually a strangulating obstruction occurs and gangrene of the intussusceptum may result.

In infants the lead point is presumed to be an enlarged Peyer's patch, the lymphoid tissue presumably responding to a viral stimulant. This becomes the apex of the intussusception, which then proceeds for a variable distance into the colon. The peak incidence is in infants 3–9 months of age. The timing has been attributed to a change in the bowel flora associated with weaning. In older children the lead point may be an invaginated Meckel's diverticulum, a polyp, an enteric cyst, or hemorrhage into the bowel wall in Henoch–Schönlein purpura or leukemia. It is more common in boys than in girls, some reporting a ratio as high as 5:1, but in Edinburgh the ratio is only 1.2:1. Some report seasonal variation, possibly related to infectious agents.

The presentation is with a painful cry, drawing up the knees and going pale, presumably in relation to colic (88% in our series). The colicky pain is intermittent and occurs with increasing frequency as the condition progresses, rather like labor pains. Vomiting is a common symptom (86%) and the passage of redcurrant jelly stools is frequent (56%).

On examination, between attacks of colic, an abdominal mass is usually palpable. This is typically sausage shaped and commonly palpable in the ascending or transverse colon. A small percentage of intussusceptions present at the anus.

Investigation

Plain abdominal X-ray will often show a filling defect corresponding to the intussusception and will demonstrate any obstruction by the presence of fluid levels within the bowel. Ultrasound can identify a 'target sign' corresponding to the layers of the intussusception. Occasionally a contrast enema may be used diagnostically in frankly obstructed cases.

Treatment

First an i.v. infusion is set up. Some collapsed infants require blood or plasma for primary resuscitation, others only require isotonic fluids. A nasogastric tube may be passed, especially if vomiting has been a marked symptom at presentation. Preparation is as for a surgical reduction; the operating room is arranged in case it is required but in most cases non-operative reduction is first attempted. The only contraindications to non-operative management are a seriously ill child with a prolonged history, marked intestinal obstruction or evidence of peritonitis (rare).

Hydrostatic reduction has been intermittently popular since first advocated by Hirschsprung in 1876. A barium enema under X-ray screening is used as a therapeutic technique and is frequently successful. Recently air has been used for reduction rather than barium. (The method has for centuries found favor in China, where fire bellows have traditionally been used.) Air is an excellent contrast medium and scientific control of the pressure is by attaching the rectal Foley catheter to a sphygmomanometer, increasing the pressure to 100 mmHg if necessary. This method appears to have a greater success rate than barium and in the rare occurrence of perforation, proves safer.

Surgical reduction is required for those in whom non-operative reduction fails. The intussusception is reduced manually by stripping it back from the point the apex has reached. Pulling on the entering layer of bowel can lead to serosal splitting or rupture of the bowel. Once the intussusception is reduced appendectomy is usually performed. This may help to prevent recurrence by adherence of the cecum in the right iliac fossa. If reduction proves impossible then a limited bowel resection may be required.

Recurrence rates of 2–4% have been recorded and seem unrelated to the method of reduction.

APPENDICITIS

This is the most common condition for which emergency abdominal surgery is required in childhood. Its symptomatology and management are similar to those in adults although in the very young child there may be difficulty in making the appropriate diagnosis. Appendicitis is still a condition with significant morbidity and mortality. In a recent series, reporting on the last 5 years of the 1970s, there were four deaths related to appendicitis in children in Scotland. Delay in diagnosis can thus convert an eminently treatable condition into a lethal one.

Classically the condition presents with pain, vomiting and fever. The pain commences periumbilically, the distended appendix causing dull and poorly localized midgut pain via visceral nerve fibers to the tenth thoracic nerve root. The pathology of appendicitis is of spreading inflammation from the mucosa through the wall to the serosa. Serosal inflammation leads to peritoneal inflammation and the pain is accurately localized to the right iliac fossa – classically at McBurney's point (two thirds along a line from the umbilicus to the anterior superior iliac spine). Atypical presentation leads to difficulty in diagnosis, especially in the very young. Neonatal appendicitis is exceedingly rare and the mortality rate is high. In the preschool child the diagnosis is also difficult and a high perforation rate is encountered. The preschool child may present with anorexia, listlessness, fever, vomiting and diarrhea.

Care must be taken in the examination of the child with suspected appendicitis. The tongue may be coated and there is a classic 'fetor oris', a sweet smell on the breath perhaps partly related to ketones. The child is reluctant to climb onto the examination couch. The chest is examined to exclude a right lower lobe pneumonia, which may easily lead to a mistaken diagnosis of appendicitis. Examination of the abdomen must be very gentle, starting in the left lower quadrant and gradually working round each quadrant to finish in the right iliac fossa. Clumsy technique can lose a child's confidence and lead to voluntary guarding. Tenderness at McBurney's point remains the cardinal sign of appendicitis.

Involuntary guarding and rigidity are reliable signs of peritonism or peritonitis. There is no excuse in endeavoring to elicit rebound tenderness as, if present, the child's confidence is immediately lost, the pain being so severe, thus precluding subsequent examination. Likewise, rectal examination should be reserved for cases with negative or equivocal abdominal findings, where it may be the only means of diagnosis of a pelvic appendicitis. It may otherwise confirm a diagnosis of constipation or, in females, gynecological disease. It must be remembered that the appendix can adopt a variety of intra-abdominal positions circumferentially around the attachment to the cecum. A retrocecal appendix may have few abdominal signs initially, although psoas spasm may be apparent.

There are no investigations that can prove the presence of appendicitis. The white cell count need not be raised and an X-ray, whilst occasionally showing a fecolith, is generally unhelpful. Ultrasound is now of value in recognizing a thickened appendix with surrounding edema.

The differential diagnosis includes intestinal diseases such as gastroenteritis, Crohn disease and other causes of terminal ileitis such as

Yersinia infection, Meckel's diverticulitis and leukemic typhlitis, mesenteric adenitis and deep iliac adenitis. In addition, gynecological problems such as salpingitis and ovarian cysts must be considered. Urinary tract infection may also be confused with appendicitis, the situation being further complicated by the possible occurrence of pyuria when an inflamed appendix is adjacent to the bladder. Finally, medical disorders such as right basal pneumonia, diabetes mellitus, Henoch–Schönlein purpura and sickle cell disease have all been misdiagnosed as appendicitis. In fact almost all causes of acute abdominal pain in childhood must be considered but appendicitis is the commonest surgical emergency.

Treatment

If necessary, preliminary resuscitation of the patient by administration of i.v. fluids should be considered. Once the patient has been adequately hydrated then appendectomy is carried out through a skin crease incision an inch or more below McBurney's point to leave a neat scar well below the 'bikini line' or preferably a laparoscopic approach is used. At induction of anesthesia a single dose of broad-spectrum antibiotics such as an aminoglycoside and metronidazole, to cover bowel flora including *Escherichia coli* and *Bacteroides fragilis*, is administered to endeavor to prevent postoperative complications such as wound infections and intra-abdominal abscesses, especially pelvic and subphrenic. If an appendix mass is palpated some prefer conservative management with bed rest, i.v. fluids and antibiotics with an interval appendectomy at 3 months. Others proceed to appendectomy appropriately covered by antibiotic therapy.

PRIMARY PERITONITIS

This has a similar presentation to appendicitis but without a history of central pain moving to the right iliac fossa. The abdominal signs are those of peritonitis especially in the lower abdomen. At operation diffuse peritonitis is found with peritoneal exudate, yet no obvious focus of infection. The commonest causative organisms are pneumococci and streptococci. The source of infection has been thought to be the genital tract, the condition being commoner in girls, but the occasional occurrence in boys leads one to suspect blood-borne spread. There may be a preceding or coexisting upper respiratory tract infection. The management is appropriate antibiotic therapy (usually penicillin).

MECKEL'S DIVERTICULUM

Meckel's diverticulum arises from the vitellointestinal duct, which leads from the primitive gut to the yolk sac. Persistence of the proximal end of the duct occurs in 2% of the population (the 2 ft from the ileocecal valve, 2 in long story is erroneous: it may be a variable length and variable distance from the ileocecal valve).

The vitellointestinal duct can lead to a number of anomalies if it persists (Fig. 37.26). The duct itself may remain patent to the umbilicus and thus present as a fistula in neonates. Partial obliteration may give rise to cyst formation or a persistent fibrous cord from the umbilicus to the ileum may act as an axis for localized volvulus or lead to bowel obstruction.

A Meckel's diverticulum may become inflamed, lead to hemorrhage or invaginate into the ileum and cause intussusception. Meckel's diverticulitis has an identical presentation to acute appendicitis and must always be considered if a normal appendix is identified at surgery.

Bleeding in relation to a Meckel's diverticulum arises because the lining often contains heterotopic gastric mucosa (35–49%). This leads to peptic ulceration of the adjacent normal ileal mucosa (Fig. 37.27). Bleeding usually occurs in preschool children, especially toddlers. It may be intermittent passage of a small amount of altered blood in the stool, although massive hemorrhage with the passage of maroon or even bright red blood is more common. After adequate resuscitation, with blood replacement, a Meckel's scan should be performed. This is a ^{99m}Tc pertechnetate isotope scan that has an affinity for parietal cells. The stomach is visualized on the scan image, together with the bladder,

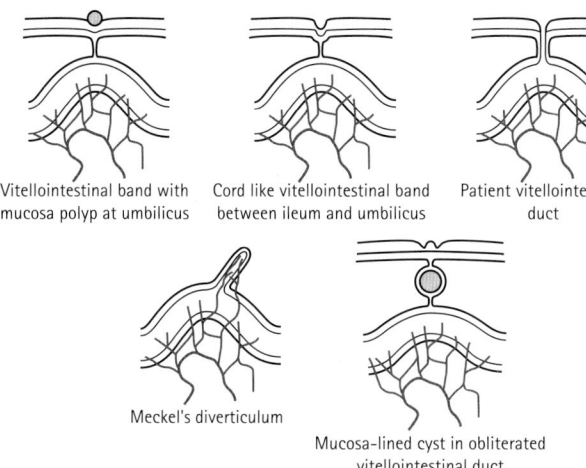

Vitellointestinal band with mucosa polyp at umbilicus

Cord like vitellointestinal band between ileum and umbilicus

Patient vitellointestinal duct

Meckel's diverticulum

Mucosa-lined cyst in obliterated vitellointestinal duct

Fig. 37.26   Vitellointestinal remnants.

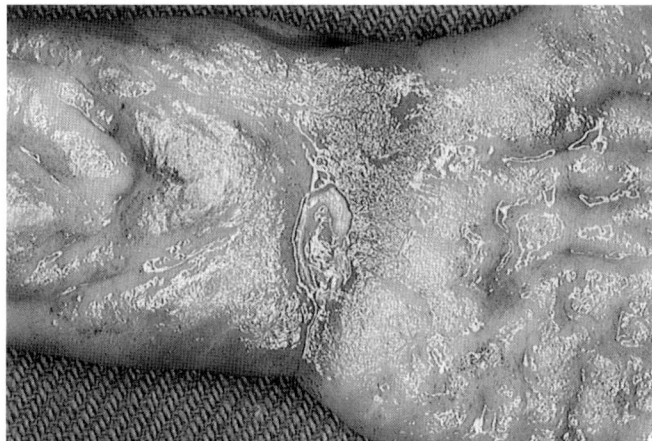

Fig. 37.27   Peptic ulcer at junction of gastric and ileal mucosa in Meckel's diverticulum.

as the isotope is excreted through the kidneys. A third 'blob' of isotope is likely to indicate ectopic gastric mucosa in a Meckel's diverticulum (or rarely in a duplicated segment of bowel). Priming the patient with cimetidine for a few days enhances the scan image. Laparoscopy can avoid the need for a scan and even in the absence of a Meckel's demonstrate the presence or absence of blood in the upper small bowel. An appropriate upper or lower gastrointestinal endoscopy can then be performed under the same anesthetic.

The treatment is in all cases Meckel's diverticulectomy, the diverticulum being found on the antimesenteric aspect of the ileum 40–100 cm proximal to the ileocecal valve.

SUPERIOR MESENTERIC ARTERY SYNDROME

This syndrome, a cause of acute and chronic abdominal pain in childhood, is due to obstruction of the third part of the duodenum by the superior mesenteric artery. It has variously been called 'Cast syndrome', 'Wilkie's syndrome', 'chronic duodenal ileus' and 'arteriomesenteric duodenal compression syndrome'. It may be congenital or acquired, the latter being due to rapid growth without associated weight gain, rapid weight loss or from hyperextension of the vertebral column in a plaster cast. The presentation may be acute or chronic with acute obstructive symptoms or intermittent abdominal pain and vomiting. Contrast studies, if performed between attacks, may show little but if performed in an acute episode will demonstrate obstruction of the third part of the duodenum. The superior mesenteric artery normally subtends an angle of 45 degrees with the aorta but under the conditions described earlier

the angle may decrease to 15 degrees, thus occluding the underlying duodenum.

Management is conservative or surgical, the former being alteration of diet, nursing prone and removing or windowing a plaster cast if present. Surgical management entails division of the ligament of Treitz and transposition of the small bowel to the right side in a position of nonrotation.[19]

CHOLEDOCHAL CYST

This is a cystic dilation of the choledochus (the common bile duct). The etiology is unknown but some believe it to be related to the reflux of pancreatic secretions into the common duct. The presentation may be in infancy with obstructive jaundice suggestive of biliary atresia, or in the older child with intermittent jaundice, abdominal pain and vomiting often associated with fever suggestive of ascending cholangitis. The diagnosis is by ultrasonography. Treatment consists of excision of the cyst and a Roux-en-Y choledochojejunostomy or hepaticojejunostomy. Failure to excise the entire cyst may result in carcinoma of the cyst wall in the long term.

CHOLELITHIASIS

Gallstones are uncommon in childhood but must be considered in children with hereditary spherocytosis. If metabolic stones develop then cholecystectomy is required, but in hemolytic disease the gallbladder is usually normal and simple cholecystotomy and removal of the stones is all that is required. This procedure should always be considered at the time of splenectomy in these children.

INGUINAL HERNIA AND HYDROCELE

These conditions have the same origin in childhood – the presence of a patent processus vaginalis. The only difference between them is the caliber of the processus (Fig. 37.28). If wide a hernia is produced, if narrow then peritoneal fluid may tract down to the tunica vaginalis. This explains the use of the term 'hydrocele' from the Greek *hydro* = water, *kele* = hernia. (A similar derivation applies to encephalocele, omphalocele, ureterocele, etc.) Frequently hydrocele is spelt, erroneously, 'coele', even in textbooks: it is not derived from coelom (Greek *koiloma* = hollow).

The processus vaginalis is an outpouching of peritoneum drawn down by the descent of the testis. The distal portion persists as the tunica

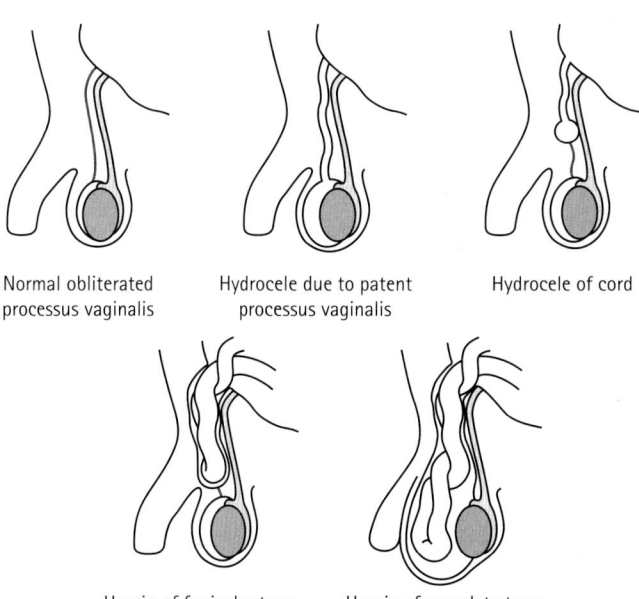

Normal obliterated processus vaginalis

Hydrocele due to patent processus vaginalis

Hydrocele of cord

Hernia of funicular type

Hernia of complete type

Fig. 37.28   Inguinal herniae and hydroceles.

vaginalis but the intervening communication with the peritoneal cavity is normally obliterated. Persistence of a widely patent processus along its whole length results in a hernia of the 'complete' type – a scrotal hernia. Obliteration of the distal portion results in a 'funicular' hernial sac. Similarly, a hydrocele of the cord can arise, the distal portion being obliterated and the proximal communication narrowed.

These conditions are more common on the right side than the left, presumably related to the later descent of the right testis. They may also arise in girls, although hernias are less common. Occasionally an ovary may prolapse into a hernia – at surgery it must be inspected to confirm that it is indeed an ovary and not a testis in testicular feminization syndrome (Fig. 37.29). Chromosomal analysis may be of value in excluding this condition in girls with bilateral hernias but the incidence is extremely low. The hydrocele equivalent in a female is a hydrocele of the canal of Nuck – a small diverticulum of peritoneum accompanying the round ligament of the uterus through the inguinal canal.

In general, hydroceles are only treated surgically if they persist beyond the age of 1 year, the majority resolving spontaneously prior to that. In toddlers there is often a history of a hydrocele increasing in size towards the end of the day – the fluid slowly returns to the peritoneum through the narrow processus when the child is recumbent at night. Surgery consists of ligation and division of the patent processus vaginalis through a small inguinal incision.

Inguinal hernias are treated with a similar operation. If the hernia is not obvious on examination, despite a typical history, tickling may increase the intra-abdominal pressure to demonstrate the hernia, but its presence can be confirmed by rolling the spermatic cord over the pubic bone with the index finger, thickening being apparent in the presence of a hernia.

If a scrotal swelling is present, a hydrocele can usually be distinguished from a hernia by the fact that the surgeon can get above it. Rarely does a hydrocele extend up into the inguinal canal. Transillumination may be misleading, as the thin bowel wall with intraluminal fluid in a young infant will also transilluminate. The surgery is a semi-urgent herniotomy. There is no requirement for herniorrhaphy (repair).

Incarceration of an inguinal hernia implies irreducibility, which will lead to strangulation of the bowel if left untreated. Gentle reduction is attempted. Force must not be applied and unless reduction is easy the child should be sedated with i.m. morphine and tipped head down; occasionally gallows traction is of benefit. If reduction is unsuccessful, immediate surgical reduction and herniotomy are necessary. If it is successfully reduced then herniotomy must be performed before the infant is discharged.

Confirmation of the previous incarceration may be made by observing an increase in testicular size on the affected side (a positive Robarts' sign). This results from venous obstruction of the pampiniform plexus, which can result in testicular infarction in cases where the hernia is not urgently reduced.

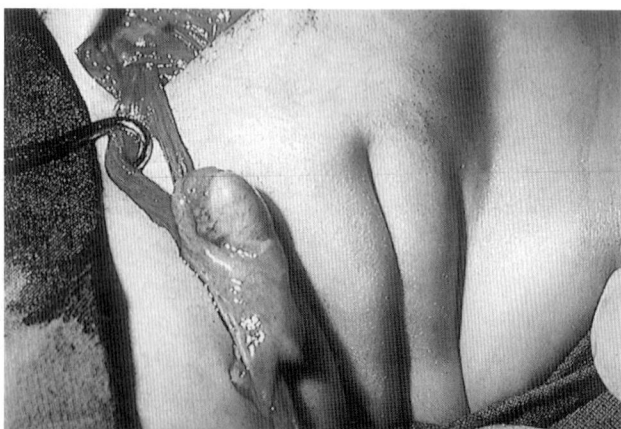

Fig. 37.29   External female genitalia and normal testis in testicular feminization syndrome.

FEMORAL HERNIA

This is uncommon in children but, as in adults, is recognized by the swelling lying below the inguinal ligament and lateral to the pubic tubercle. Femoral herniorrhaphy is required.

UMBILICAL HERNIA

By the time the umbilical cord has separated in the newborn the umbilical ring has usually closed but in a proportion of children a defect is left, resulting in an umbilical hernia. There is a higher incidence of this condition in blacks than in whites. Umbilical hernia occurs in Beckwith syndrome, Hurler syndrome, trisomy 18, and trisomy 13.

The vast majority of umbilical hernias will resolve spontaneously within the first 2 years of life. Incarceration and strangulation in umbilical hernias in childhood are so rare that they need not cause concern. Persistence of the hernia beyond the age of 2 years merits surgical repair, provided that care is taken to ensure that the incision lies within the umbilical folds.

A *paraumbilical hernia* usually lies in the linea alba immediately above the umbilical ring. This will not close spontaneously and surgical repair is required.

EPIGASTRIC HERNIA

An epigastric hernia occurs through the linea alba, usually midway between the xiphisternum and the umbilicus. It presents as a pea-sized swelling occasionally associated with pain and results from herniation of extraperitoneal fat through the defect. It is best treated surgically although it can safely be left alone.

SURGICAL ASPECTS OF THE GENITOURINARY TRACT

ANOMALIES OF TESTICULAR DESCENT

It is best to consider the following distinct entities: the testis arrested in the normal line of descent (true undescended), ectopic testes and retractile testes. In addition, testes may be atrophic or absent (anorchia).

Testes arrested along the normal line of descent

The term *cryptorchidism* (Greek *cryptos* = hidden, *orchis* = testis) should be reserved for impalpable, usually abdominal, testes. There is a higher incidence of undescended testes in premature than in full-term babies. Two thirds of undescended testes in newborn infants will descend, usually by 6 weeks in term and 3 months in preterm babies. There is an increased incidence of cryptorchidism in anencephalics and other cerebral anomalies.

Ectopic testes

These have descended as far as the external inguinal ring and then become deviated into the superficial inguinal, perineal (Fig. 37.30), suprapubic or femoral ectopic sites. The commonest by far is the superficial inguinal pouch, above and lateral to the external inguinal ring.

Retractile testes

The cremasteric reflex in young children will draw the testes into the region of the superficial inguinal pouch very readily but they can be manipulated back down to the bottom of the scrotum. The testis would normally reside in the scrotum if such a child is in a warm bath or relaxed in bed.

Anorchia

Anorchia may be on one or both sides. If on one side alone there may be ipsilateral renal agenesis. If the baby is fully masculinized but both testes are absent it must be assumed that they have atrophied subsequent to torsion or infarction during development. Absence of testicular tissue

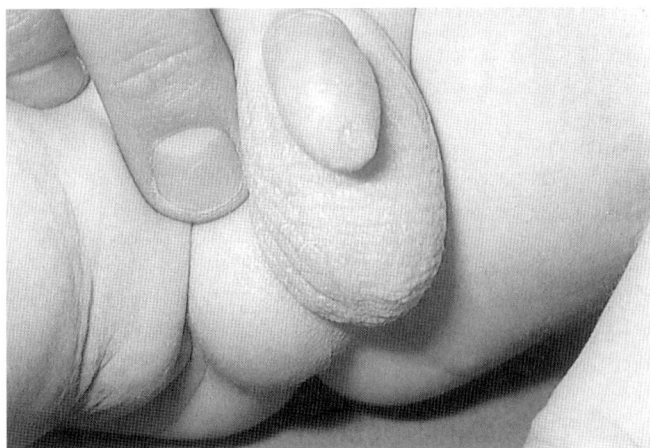

Fig. 37.30 Perineal ectopic testis.

and therefore lack of Müllerian inhibitory hormone during early gestation can lead to Müllerian development along female lines. The lack of androgenic stimulation (testosterone) from the testes leads to failure of Wolffian duct development.

'Ascending testis'

Some boys with recorded testicular descent at routine clinic checks in infancy may be found later at preschool or school medicals to have an undescended testis. This phenomenon of the 'ascending testis' was noted first by Atwell.[20] It has been suggested that this is caused by failure of elongation of the spermatic cord during differential body growth, so that the testis is drawn up by absorption of the processus vaginalis.

Treatment

It has been shown that adverse morphological changes occur in undescended testes from the second year of life onwards with a statistically significant reduction of spermatogonia and tubular growth. Most surgeons therefore choose to perform orchidopexies between 2 and 3 years of age. An associated hernia is an indication for earlier surgery. There is no place now for delaying surgery until 9 or 10 years of age. Any testis that has not descended in the first year of life will not appear later.

The treatment of the true undescended testis and the ectopic testis is orchidopexy, the testis and cord being mobilized via an inguinal approach and usually fixed in the scrotum in a subdartos pouch. Intra-abdominal testes may best be treated laparoscopically in a staged Fowler–Stephens procedure where in the first stage the testicular vessels are divided and 3–6 months later the testis may be advanced to the scrotum supplied by the artery to the vas, which has had time to hypertrophy.

Malignancy in the undescended testis

Testicular malignancy occurs in 0.0021% of adult males. Undescended testes occur in 0.28% of the population and 12% of cases of testicular malignancy are reported to occur in testes known to have been undescended. There is thus a 40 times greater incidence of malignancy in cryptorchid patients than in the general population. Orchidopexy probably does not eradicate the problem but at least the testis is placed in a position where early malignancy may be detected. In unilateral undescended testes there is also an increased risk of malignancy in the contralateral testis.

Fertility

Only one third of those following bilateral orchidopexy and two thirds of those after unilateral orchidopexy appear to have a sperm count sufficient to be potentially fertile. It is hoped, however, that these figures will be improved by the change in policy over the past few years to operate on the majority of cases in the second year of life.

THE ACUTE SCROTUM

This may result from torsion of the testis, torsion of a testicular appendage, epididymo-orchitis or idiopathic scrotal edema or, rarely, a testicular tumor.

Torsion of the testis

Torsion of the testis most commonly occurs in the neonatal period or at puberty, with a few cases presenting in the intervening years. In the neonate the torsion occurs outside the tunica vaginalis. In the neonatal period there is a plane of mobility between the tunica vaginalis and the outer layer of the scrotum. Presentation is with a reddened hemiscrotum with a hard, swollen, often indurated testis. This is not infrequently noted 24 h after birth although the torsion may have occurred at delivery. On exploration, through a groin incision, the testis is often black and infarcted but usually it is 'given the benefit of the doubt', untwisted and replaced in the scrotum, although the majority will atrophy.

After the newborn period, torsion occurs secondary to an abnormally high investment of the tunica, the testis often being described as having bell-clapper fixation. Presentation is with pain, which is usually testicular in position but theoretically, as testicular innervation is from T10, it should be felt centrally in the abdomen. Examination reveals a swollen hemiscrotum often with edema and erythema, depending on the length of history. There is exquisite tenderness on palpation. The treatment is emergency surgery as delay will affect the viability of the testis.

Preoperative isotope scanning or Doppler probing to confirm the diagnosis merely wastes time. The scrotum is explored, the testis derotated and, providing surgery is carried out within 6 h, the testis is likely to become pink under warm towels. It is then fixed in the scrotum. As the anomalous tunical attachment is likely to be bilateral, orchidopexy is also performed on the other side.

Torsion of testicular appendages

Embryological remnants are commonly attached to the testis. The hydatid of Morgagni is attached to the upper pole and is a Müllerian duct remnant. It varies in size from a pinhead to a pea or may be absent. Other remnants include the appendix epididymis (a Wolffian tubercle remnant), the paradidymis or organ of Giraldés (another mesonephric remnant) and the vas aberrans of Haller. The hydatid of Morgagni is the most common to undergo torsion, which leads to less acute pain than testicular torsion, the pain being usually at the upper pole of the testis where occasionally a bluish nodule is seen through the scrotal skin. An infarcted hydatid can give rise to considerable swelling and inflammation and doubtful cases are best explored (Fig. 37.31) to exclude testicular torsion. In any case, the necrotic hydatid is best excised as an emergency, giving instant pain relief. If treated conservatively the pain lingers on for up to 2 weeks.

Epididymo-orchitis

This is rare in children unless there is an associated renal tract anomaly. If the latter has already been established then it is safe to treat with antibiotic therapy. If, however, the clinical picture cannot be distinguished from torsion of the testis, exploration is mandatory to establish the diagnosis.

Idiopathic scrotal edema

This is a fascinating entity presenting with erythema and edema of the scrotum suggestive of a possible underlying torsion. The erythema and edema spread beyond the scrotum however into the groin and perineum (Fig. 37.32). Usually the process is confined to one side of the scrotum and the adjacent groin and perineum.

The etiology is unknown. It may be an allergic phenomenon; it is occasionally associated with an eosinophilia and may respond to antihistamine therapy. Some suggest it may be caused by an insect bite. The testis is nontender and the condition settles within a few days.

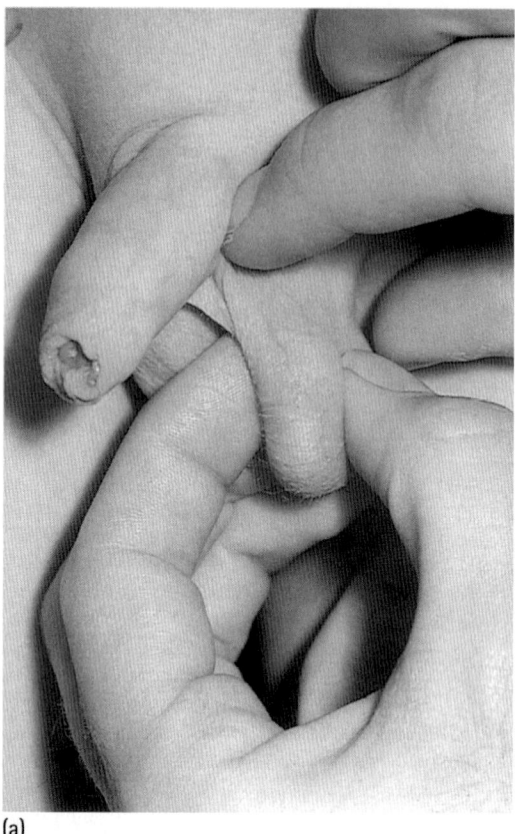

(a)

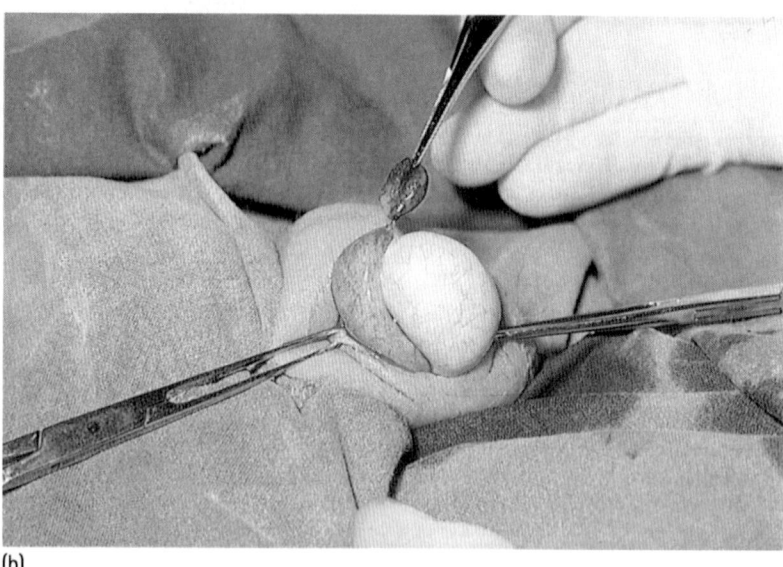

(b)

Fig. 37.31   Hydatid of Morgagni: (a) clinical appearance; (b) at operation.

CIRCUMCISION

Routine circumcision of the newborn as commonly practiced in the USA is to be condemned, the incidence of complications, including death, far outweighing the supposed advantage of avoiding such problems as carcinoma of the penis. The latter is virtually unknown in those who practice adequate hygiene. The fact that it is 'more hygienic' is often used as an excuse for circumcision but one does not chop off the ears to save washing them, or the feet because they may smell! It has been suggested that lack of carcinoma of the cervix in Jewish women is related to male circumcision but Aitken-Swan & Baird[21] showed no difference in incidence in wives of circumcised and uncircumcised men. In 1975 a committee of the American Academy of Pediatrics stated: 'There is no absolute medical indication for the routine circumcision of the newborn. A program of good penile hygiene, simply retracting the foreskin to wash away accumulated smegma on a daily basis, would appear to offer all the advantages of circumcision without the attendant surgical risks or the increased risk of meatal stenosis'.[22]

Nonretractability of the prepuce, in childhood, should not be used as an excuse for 'lopping off an innocent and useful appendage'. Bokai[23] in 1869 was the first to draw attention to the physiological adherence

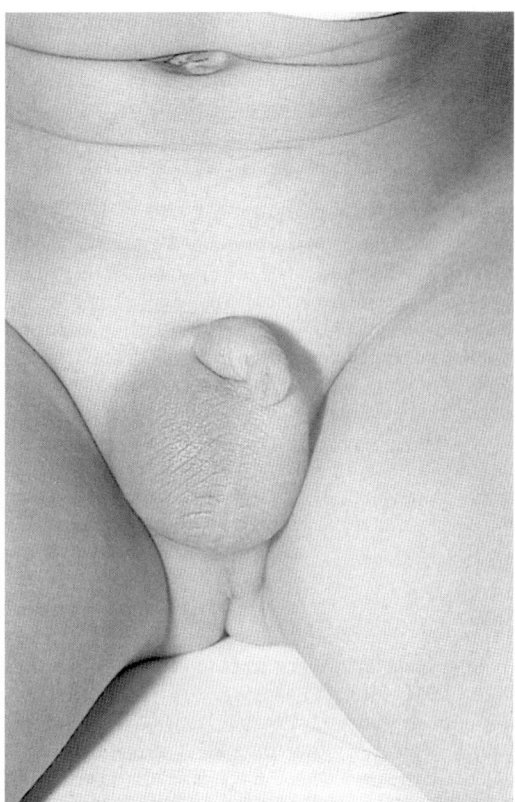

Fig. 37.32   Idiopathic scrotal edema.

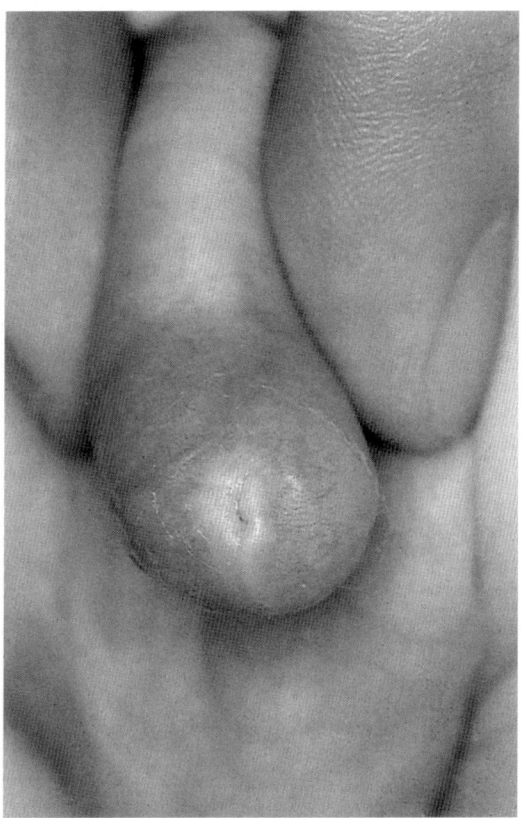

Fig. 37.33   Fibrous phimosis (balanitis xerotica obliterans).

of the foreskin, there being fusion of the glans and the prepuce developmentally. Diebert,[24] in 1933, showed that separation of the prepuce in the human penis is due to keratinization of the subpreputial epithelium, a process not complete at birth but accomplished during early childhood. Phimosis (a muzzling, from Greek *phimos* = muzzle) is thus physiological at birth.

Apart from religious or tribal reasons there are few indications for circumcision. The only valid one is a fibrous phimosis (Fig. 37.33). This may be due to inappropriate attempts at retraction at an early age, causing splitting and scarring of the preputial meatus, or perhaps is related to recurrent infections. In its most severe form it presents as balanitis xerotica obliterans with scarring of the underlying glans and urethral meatus. Meatal strictures also arise after neonatal circumcision secondary to meatitis, which arises in the absence of the protective covering of the foreskin. Ballooning of the foreskin is often seen as an indication for circumcision but it will usually resolve in time. Recurrent balanitis or balanoposthitis is possibly related to partial separation of preputial adhesion and infection of inadequately draining secretions. This can readily be resolved by separation of the adhesions. Previously this was normally carried out under general anesthesia but with the advent of EMLA cream (eutectic mixture of local anesthetics) the separation can readily be carried out painlessly and simply in the outpatient clinic or GP surgery.[25] Daily retraction with application of petroleum jelly for a few days to prevent readherence followed subsequently by normal preputial hygiene is all that is required.

In examination of the foreskin in small boys it often appears tight on attempted retraction. The simple technique advocated in 1950 by Sir James Spence[26] should be adopted: 'Retract the prepuce and you will see a pinpoint opening, but draw it forward and you will see a channel wide enough for all the purposes for which the infant needs the organ at that early age. What looks like a pinpoint opening at 7 months will become a wide channel of communication at 17 years.'

Operation

Circumcision is thus performed either for religious or tribal reasons, for fibrous phimosis or, perhaps most frequently, for remuneration! Hypospadias is a contraindication for neonatal circumcision, as is a buried penis. Neonatal circumcision is practiced, often without anesthesia using a Plastibell or a Gomco clamp. In the former, a plastic ring is placed under the foreskin and a string tied round the foreskin in a groove in the plastic device. Redundant skin together with the device separates off within a few days, leaving a very neat cosmetic result. A Gomco clamp has a similar action but rather than the string, a cutting device removes the prepuce and compresses the skin edges causing them to fuse and prevent hemorrhage. In older children a surgical cutting technique with absorbable sutures is used. In many cases of phimosis a foreskin preserving preputioplasty is sufficient.

PARAPHIMOSIS

This occurs when a narrowed foreskin is retracted behind the corona glandis penis and cannot be returned. The constriction leads to engorgement of the glans and of a cuff of foreskin distal to the tight band but behind the corona (Fig. 37.34). Firm manual compression with gauze and EMLA cream will usually reduce the edema and facilitate return of the foreskin. If this fails, injection of hyaluronidase into the swollen ring of prepuce, under general anesthesia, followed by compression, allows reduction (Fig. 37.35). Occasionally the tight constricting band needs to be incised. Circumcision is frequently advocated following paraphimosis but, surprisingly, the foreskin is usually easily retractable a fortnight after the event and recurrence is exceptional.

HYPOSPADIAS (Greek *hypo* = below, *spadon* = rent)

This is one of the commonest congenital anomalies, occurring in 1 in 400 live male births. The meatus lies in an abnormal position on the ventral aspect of the penile shaft or even scrotally or perineally. The

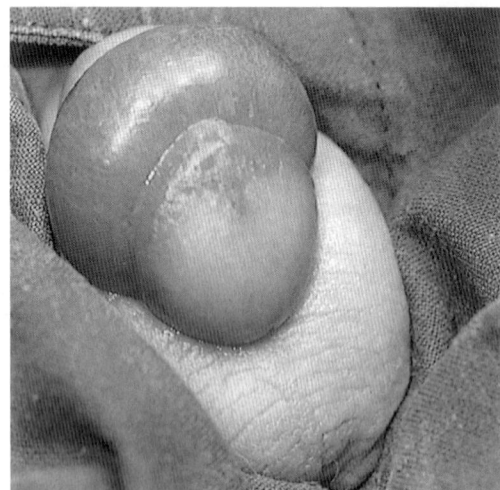

Fig. 37.34   Paraphimosis.

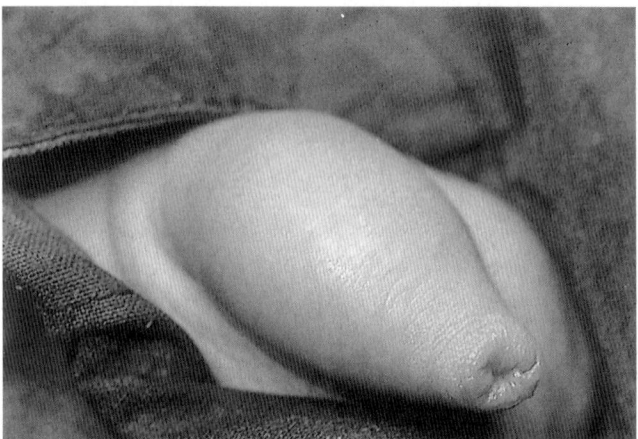

Fig. 37.35   Reduced paraphimosis.

foreskin tends to be deficient in its ventral aspect and thus is described as 'hooded'. Thirdly, there is chordee, a ventral flexion of the penis, the incidence and degree of which increases as the meatus is more proximally placed. The meatus itself may be narrowed leading to potential problems of back pressure. In the majority of cases the meatus is coronal in position; rarely it is glandular. Of the remainder, most are on the penile shaft but a few lie more proximally still in the scrotum or perineum. It is often thought that hypospadias is frequently associated with upper renal tract anomalies but in fact the incidence of these is much the same as in the general population, except perhaps in the most severe types of the deformity. In those penoscrotal and perineal types there may be associated undescended testes and the possibility of an intersex state must be investigated.

There are over 200 operations described in the literature for the correction of hypospadias. This gives some indication of the complication rate, each newly described repair aiming to be an improvement in this regard. The age for surgery is mainly the surgeon's preference. It has always been agreed that, where possible, correction should be complete by the time the boy starts school so that he may stand and pee like his peers! The more distally placed the meatus the easier it is to achieve a successful result. The essential components to the repair of the more severe varieties are release of the chordee and urethral reconstruction. The chordee is related to tight fibrous bands distal to the meatus and thought possibly to relate to atrophy of that portion of the corpus spongiosum. It is, however, possible to have chordee without hypospadias so the etiology is uncertain. Fistula formation is unfortunately common

following hypospadias repair and a few unfortunate cases require multiple interventions to achieve successful closure. The aim of all modern repairs is to create a terminal meatus on a well-formed glans and a penile shaft that is straight on erection together with a good cosmetic result (a good 'body image').

EPISPADIAS

In its most extreme form this is associated with bladder exstrophy. Otherwise it may be balanic, penile or penopubic. It may also occur in girls. In epispadias the urethra is deficient dorsally. The penis is flattened with a splayed glans and shortened, the crura being attached to often separated pubic bones. The prepuce is deficient dorsally with a ventral hood prepuce and there is dorsal chordee. Occasionally the problem is not obvious, the foreskin being complete and phimotic and the penis buried, but once the prepuce is retractable the condition is revealed. In the female the clitoris is duplicated on either side of the wide open urethra, defective dorsally (Fig. 37.36). The treatment is likewise dependent on sex and severity and the degree of continence and the success rate is variable.

URINARY TRACT INFECTION – SURGICAL ASPECTS

Medical management of urinary tract infections in neonates and in older children is discussed in Chapter 18.

The commonest cause of infection is *vesicoureteric reflux*. There remains much controversy over the role of surgery in vesicoureteric reflux.[27] Reflux in the presence of infection leads to pyelonephritis, the extension of the intrarenal reflux, if present, leading to scarring. If the child can be kept free of infection, the reflux may improve or resolve. Severe reflux should be treated surgically. This entails a transvesical operation to lengthen the submucosal tunnel of the ureter. It has a high rate of success but in a few cases leads to stenosis. More recently, a new technique involving the endoscopic injection of Teflon submucosally[28] beneath the ureteric orifice has been devised (STING – subureteric Teflon injection). This has proved very successful but long-term results have yet to be evaluated. Other substances such as Bioplastique, collagen or 'Deflux' may be used as concern has been raised that Teflon may migrate to the brain or elsewhere, although the original authors refute this concept. Deflux, a polysaccharide gel of a dextranomer and hyaluronic acid, is now the most widely used substance for this purpose.[29]

Stenosis of the lower end of the ureter requires reimplantation, the stenotic segment being excised.

Duplex ureters may be an incidental finding without causing problems in the majority of cases. If detected in investigation of a urinary tract infection, there is usually an associated anomaly. The ureter from the upper pole tends to enter the bladder at a lower level. Thus the lower pole ureter has a shorter intramural course and a tendency to reflux. The upper pole ureter has a tendency to stenosis, an association with a ureterocele and a possible tendency to open below the bladder neck, leading to incontinence. It may even open ectopically into the vagina.

If there is reflux of both ureters, reimplantation of both, in their common sheath, is usually the treatment of choice. Occasionally they join at a higher level leading to yo-yo reflux between the two and a predisposition to infection. This is treated either by heminephroureterectomy if one moiety is shown to have poor function on isotope studies, or else anastomosis at the level of the pelves may be advocated.

A *ureterocele* may arise in relation to the upper pole ureter. It represents herniation of the intramural portion of the ureter into the bladder. Its meatus may be stenosed, may open below the bladder neck or may even on occasion allow reflux. The ureterocele may obstruct the lower ureter or even lead to bladder outlet obstruction by prolapsing across the internal urethral meatus. The ureterocele may be incised endoscopically to relieve an acute problem, especially of value in the infant, or may be excised with ureteric reimplantation,

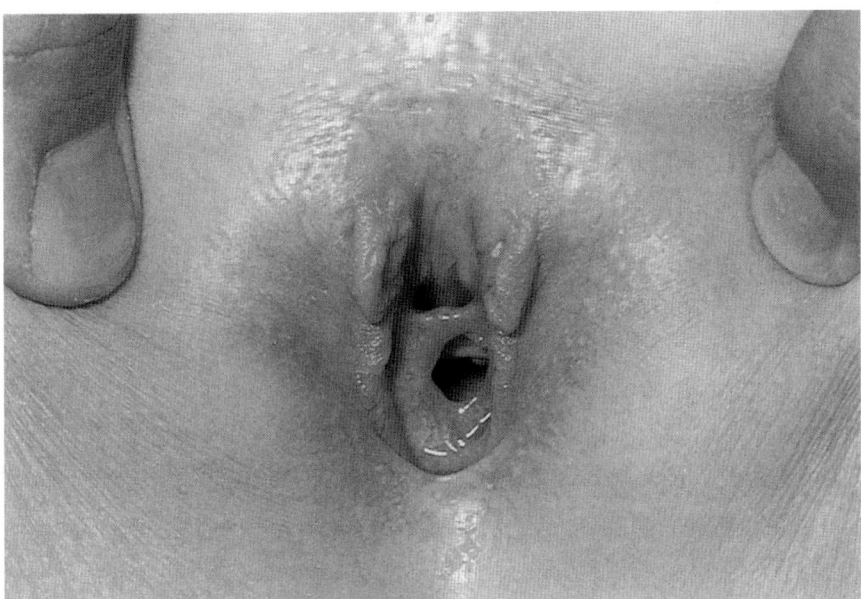

Fig. 37.36 Female epispadias.

if appropriate. If an isotope scan shows minimal function in the affected moiety then partial nephroureterectomy may be the treatment of choice.

Hydronephrosis may be due to obstruction at the pelviureteric junction (PUJ) or, if the ureter is also dilated, to vesicoureteric obstruction or vesicoureteric reflux. Obstruction at the PUJ may be due to congenital narrowing, high insertion of the ureter, or aberrant renal vessels. The presentation is usually with investigation of a urinary tract infection. It may be diagnosed antenatally or in the older child may present with a Dietl's crisis, acute obstruction at the PUJ secondary to kinking after an abnormal fluid load. This may not present until the first beer-drinking spree in a young adult! In the neonate, antenatally diagnosed hydronephrosis may be a stable condition that can be monitored with serial ultrasound examinations and isotope studies as some infants will acquire normal drainage across the PUJ as they grow. At any age an isotope study will indicate whether the kidney has already suffered major damage. If its contribution to total renal function is less than 10% then nephrectomy is the treatment of choice. If there is doubt in an acute presentation, a percutaneous nephrostomy tube may be inserted under ultrasound guidance and further isotope studies, after draining for 1–2 weeks, may show improvement. If there is reasonable function but a definite PUJ obstruction then the treatment of choice is a pyeloplasty. This involves excision of the redundant extra renal pelvis and pelviureteric junction with reanastomosis of the proximal ureter to the dependent portion of the repaired pelvis.

CONGENITAL VASCULAR MALFORMATIONS

Hemangiomas
These are malformations of developing blood vessels. They commonly appear in the skin but may develop in any organ.

Strawberry nevus
These usually appear at about a week of age and may rapidly enlarge in the first few months of life. They then stop growing and usually resolve spontaneously by intravascular thrombosis. This process is normally complete by 5–7 years of age, leaving only a minor blemish or none at all. Unless they are causing a problem such as occlusion of the eyelids, which can lead to permanent visual impairment, surgery is best avoided. The parents must be reassured that even the most unsightly

facial lesions will resolve within a year or two of the child starting school. A few involute so rapidly that they become ulcerated. This is most common in lesions subject to trauma as on the perineum or back. Scarring will result from ulceration.

Stork mark
This is a superficial capillary hemangioma that may be seen on the forehead, bridge of the nose and upper eyelids. The lesion is often v-shaped, pointing down to the nose and there is a corresponding mark on the nape of the neck. These marks presumably arise from the stork suspending the baby by the head in its beak! Again the parents can be reassured that the frontal lesion will resolve spontaneously although the nuchal one will commonly persist throughout life, usually hidden by the hair.

Port wine stain (nevus flammeus)
Unlike a strawberry nevus this is present at birth and may be very disfiguring, as it becomes darker and increasingly nodular with age. In recent years laser treatment with a pulsed tuneable dye laser has considerably improved the appearance of these lesions in childhood.[30]

Sturge–Weber syndrome is a severe form of port wine stain on the scalp and face, in the distribution of one of the branches of the trigeminal nerve, associated with an underlying vascular anomaly of the arachnoid covering the cerebral hemisphere. This leads to epilepsy, hemiplegia and mental retardation.

Cavernous hemangioma
These may occur alone or in association with a capillary lesion in the overlying skin. They increase in size after birth but usually in proportion to the growth of the infant. Most resolve spontaneously but some persist, requiring excision, if appropriate, or injection with sclerosants. Care must be taken in the latter option not to lead to ulceration of the skin. Very large lesions may lead to high output cardiac failure due to arteriovenous shunting. Embolization under radiological control may be required although some lesions regress on oral corticosteroid therapy.

Kasabach–Merritt syndrome
In the neonate, large or multiple hemangiomas are occasionally associated with a generalized bleeding disorder caused by the trapping of platelets within them, which produces a profound thrombocyto-

penia. A course of prednisone, 2–4 mg/kg per 24 h can effect dramatic improvement, or, if this fails, embolization of the hemangioma can be considered.

Lymphangioma

These are similar to hemangiomas but involve lymphatics. They may also occur anywhere in the body but in particular they may present as a *cystic hygroma* most commonly arising in the cervical region (see earlier under 'Head and neck').

Mixed *hamartomatous* lesions may contain hemangiomatous and lymphangiomatous elements.

CLEFT LIP AND PALATE

The main etiological factor in these anomalies is genetic. In about one third of patients there is a family history. The incidence is about 1 in 700 births. The ratio of cleft lip (with or without cleft palate) to cleft palate alone is about 2:1.

The lip, alveolus and the portion of the hard palate anterior to the incisive foramen are derived from the maxillary and medial nasal processes. These fuse by the sixth week. The remainder of the palate forms from the palatine shelves. These grow from the maxillary swellings and fuse from anterior to posterior in the ninth to twelfth weeks. At the same time the nasal septum grows down to meet the palate.

Clefts result from failure of these lines of fusion. They vary in severity from a notch in the margin of the lip to a complete cleft in the maxilla. They may be unilateral or bilateral. Figure 37.37 illustrates the major types of cleft lip and palate.

Treatment is aimed at both a good cosmetic result with normal growth as well as a functional closure to facilitate swallowing and speech. The repair of the lip and alveolus is usually performed at around 3 months of age and the palatal defect between 6 and 15 months to give the best chance of normal speech. A multidisciplinary approach is required including a plastic surgeon, orthodontist, speech therapist, ENT surgeon, audiologist, etc.

BURNS

Thermal injury is a common childhood accident in all countries. Predisposing factors include primitive, poor or overcrowded housing, families under stress, flammable clothing, ignorance and lack of insight in parents.

The toddler, exploring his world on hands and knees or with unsteady gait, is a ready victim and boys are burned more often than girls. Scalding with hot liquids is by far the commonest cause of injury in this age group. Flame burns are less common than they were, but house fires still claim victims with the added risk of smoke inhalation injury. Other causes include contact with hot objects, chemicals, friction and electric current.

Severity of injury

This depends on three main factors:

1. **Extent.** Heat damages the underlying capillaries, causing them to leak protein-rich fluid. The resulting loss from the circulation reaches a critical level when the extent of the burn exceeds about 10% of the body surface area, and the child will require i.v. resuscitation. Extent is measured by using a chart (Fig. 37.38) or by taking the area of the hand as about 1%. Erythema should be discounted when making this measurement.

2. **Depth.** Healing depends on whether epithelial elements survive in the dermis. Partial-thickness burns will heal by outgrowth of epithelial cells from hair follicles and sweat glands; they can be subdivided into superficial, which heal in less than 3 weeks and do not cause scars, and deep dermal, which take longer to heal and cause hypertrophic scars. Deep or full-thickness burns can heal only from the margins. The depth of tissue destruction is determined by the temperature of the agent, the duration of its contact, the skin thickness and the victim's age.

3. **Site.** Burns of the face and hands are particularly serious, and those of the perineum cause problems in management. While the skin is the site of injury in most instances, the epithelial linings of the respiratory and upper alimentary tracts may be damaged separately or together with a skin burn.

Pathophysiology

Local

The fluid loss from the circulation is at its maximum immediately after the burn and decreases over the following 48 h. A deep burn destroys significant numbers of red cells. The insulating and protective functions of skin are lost, and body heat, water and electrolytes pass from the body in much increased amounts. Nitrogen losses also rise.

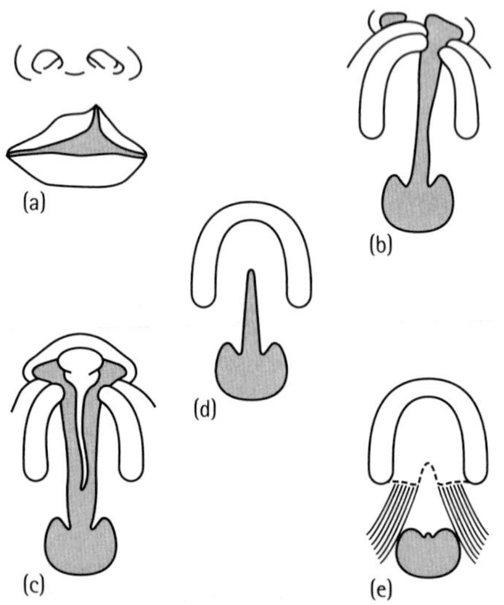

Fig. 37.37 (a) Incomplete unilateral cleft lip. (b) Complete unilateral cleft lip and palate. (c) Complete bilateral cleft lip and palate. (d) Isolated cleft of soft palate. (e) Submucous cleft palate.

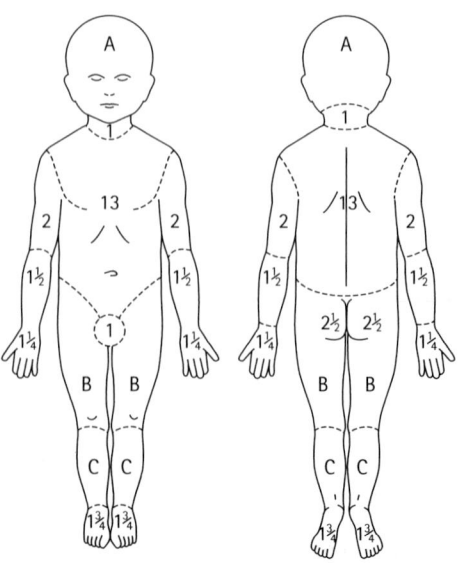

Fig. 37.38 Chart for calculating percentage area burned in childhood. A = ½ of head; B = ½ of one thigh; C = ½ of one leg. The percentages of these areas vary with age.

General

There is a massive rise in the secretion of stress hormones.[31] Urinary water and sodium excretion fall and potassium and nitrogen losses increase. The larger the burn, the more profound the reaction tends to be. The catabolic phase lasts until the burn is healed.

Treatment

First aid

After separating the child from the source of the injury, clothing should be removed and the burn cooled by immersion in lukewarm water or by use of a wet cloth (the risk of hypothermia must be remembered). The burn can then be covered with a clean cloth or clingfilm until definitive local treatment is possible.

Pain

A partial-thickness burn is very painful, while deeply burned skin is anesthetic. Potent analgesia by the i.m. or i.v. route is essential. Throughout treatment, attention must be focused on the avoidance of pain during practical procedures; analgesic or anesthetic drugs should be selected and used with precision.

Shock

Where the area burned exceeds 10% of the body surface, an i.v. infusion will be required. The restoration and maintenance of an effective circulation can be achieved with plasma, purified protein solution, dextran or balanced salt solutions. The quantities to be given vary with the weight of the child and the extent of the burn. The rate of administration is rapid initially and usually lasts for 36–48 h. Close patient observation, hourly urinary output measurement by an indwelling urethral catheter and serial hemoglobin and hematocrit estimations provide adequate control data. A central venous pressure line can be helpful in the severe case, but it has been indicted as a major source of infection if maintained for days in the burned patient.

System management

Respiratory system

Where a child has been rescued from a burning building or where clothing has burned over the face, airway problems can be anticipated. Arterial blood gases should be monitored and intubation and assisted ventilation may be necessary. Bronchopneumonia is a frequent later complication of large burns.

Central nervous system

Toddlers with even minor scalds are liable to convulse in the first 2 d with serious or even fatal outcome. The cause is thought to lie with early fluid shifts and the lag that occurs within the brain and its meninges. Papilledema is not always present. Diazepam and mannitol (1 g/kg i.v. over 20 min) gain quick control of fits and brain swelling, and phenytoin sodium and dexamethasone prolong the effect. Focal neurological deficits may occur at any time, probably as a result of septic emboli.

Urinary system

In the first 2 d after injury increased levels of antidiuretic hormone limit urinary output. Infusion should be used circumspectly and a serum sodium level of not less than 130 mmol/L should be maintained.

In deep burns, thermal damage to red blood cells causes hemoglobinuria, which may lead to tubular necrosis and renal failure. If rapid restoration of circulating fluid volume does not clear the urine, a solute diuretic such as 20% mannitol should be given without delay. A catheter may be required to monitor urine output or avoid contamination of the burn. It should be removed as soon as possible.

Cardiovascular system

Electrical current injury may cause cardiac damage and an ECG examination is advisable after such an injury. General anesthesia is best avoided until the tracing has returned to normal.

Tachycardia persists throughout recovery from a large burn and is largely a product of a high metabolic rate to offset the high evaporative heat losses. Heat regulation is disturbed and the child must be kept warm to avoid hypothermia.

Hemopoietic system

Loss of red cells, destroyed by a deep burn, must be replaced by early transfusion. Further losses take place during surgery and erythropoiesis remains depressed until a large burn has healed. The red cell mass must be maintained by transfusion if the body is to achieve quick healing.

Alimentary system

Gastric stasis is common in the early hours after a large burn but oral intake should be started as soon as possible. Ranitidine has reduced the incidence of hemorrhagic gastritis and Curling's ulcer is now rarely seen.

Accurate naked weights, obtained twice weekly from admission, guide the clinician through the early weight gain of fluid retention, diuresis, the catabolic phase, and the anabolic phase that comes more quickly and strongly in the child.

Nutrition

Daily fluid intake must take account of increased losses through the burn wound. A high calorie intake is needed to balance heat loss and minimize lean tissue breakdown. A protein intake at the upper end of the normal range is adequate. Iron and vitamins C and B complex are supplemented to combat anemia and aid wound healing. The seriously burned child cannot take food in solid form and it is kinder and more effective to give most of this as a fortified liquid feed. A fine-bore nasogastric feeding tube for this purpose should be passed in all children with burns over 15%. The planned intake should be achieved stepwise over the first 1–2 weeks. Early forcing of high food intake may predispose to a post-stress diabetes that may be resistant to insulin. Neglect of food intake will result in a profound weight loss, hypoproteinemia, and failure of the burn to heal.

Musculoskeletal system

While immobilization may be unavoidable for practical reasons, its use will increase muscle wasting and delay the recovery of an effective musculature. Regular active exercises should be performed wherever possible. Joint positioning and joint movement require constant attention if severe, and possibly permanent, joint contracture is to be avoided.

Local care

Infection is the major complication of all but the smallest burn. It can destroy surviving epithelium and penetrate a deep burn, with a risk of invasive infection. The commonest organism is *Staphylococcus aureus* but the beta-hemolytic streptococcus is feared for its destructive capabilities and *Pseudomonas aeruginosa* can be dangerous on extensive burns. Constant monitoring, scrupulous hygiene and prevention of overcrowding are essential to control infection. Large burns should be isolated. Where appropriate, early excision and grafting can lead to healing before infection can occur. Local antibacterial agents are valuable but systemic antibiotics must be used with care as they can easily lead to superinfection with resistant organisms or fungi.

A superficial burn will, if protected from infection and trauma, heal in less than 3 weeks and is usually dressed with a well-padded gauze and cotton wool dressing with a Vaseline gauze inner layer. Deeper burns need skin grafting, unless very small.

Toxic shock syndrome

This can follow even very minor burns in the child[32] and can have a mortality rate of 11%.[33] It is therefore essential to recognize and treat it on suspicion. Signs are of an unwell, irritable child, 3 d or longer after a burn, with pyrexia and three or more of the following: rash, hypotension, diarrhea or vomiting, inflamed mucous membranes, *Staphylococcus aureus* on wound swabs and occlusive dressings.

Treatment is with i.v. fluids, gammaglobulins (0.4 g/kg) or fresh blood or fresh frozen plasma (10 ml/kg over 4 h), exposure of the burn, topical antibacterial agent and i.v. antibiotics.

Scarring

A superficial burn should leave little physical trace; the healed skin will be dry and should be creamed several times a day. With deeper injuries, scarring is unavoidable. The hypertrophic scar reaction is most intense in childhood. On the face, it disfigures and distorts features. On the flexures, it limits joint movement. Unrelieved scar contracture impedes growth of that part and deforms the growing skeleton. Spontaneous resolution of the hypertrophic scar is slow, variable and incomplete. Its full development may be cut short and its regression accelerated by elastic compression, intralesional injection of steroid hormones, or application of silicone gel. Secondary surgical procedures are often required to replace the worst scars, their timing and scope being dictated by the physical, psychological and educational needs of the child.

Psychological support

A close rapport between child, nurse, parents and doctor is fundamental in such a taxing hospital stay, which can extend over months. The child deserves explanation, occupation, and freedom from recurring pain. The parents, whose guilt feelings should be appreciated, should be incorporated into the therapeutic effort. The help of an interested and experienced psychiatrist may be invaluable.

Prognosis

Intensive early therapy can resuscitate a child with the gravest of surface burns. However, long-term survival is rare where 70% or more of the skin is destroyed. A child who survives a burn with significant scarring faces the prospect of physical and psychological problems that will probably become worse during adolescence. Continued longterm support is needed for patient and family for many years.

REFERENCES (* Level 1 evidence)

1. Clements BS, Warner JO. Pulmonary sequestration and related bronchopulmonary vascular malformations: nomenclature and classification based on anatomical and embryological considerations. Thorax 1987; 42:401–408.
2. Bohn D, Tamura M, Perrin D, et al. Ventilatory predictors of pulmonary hypoplasia in congenital diaphragmatic hernia, confirmed by morphologic assessment. J Pediatr 1987; 111:423–431.
3. Sakai H, Tamura M, Hosokawa Y, et al. Effect of surgical repair on respiratory mechanics in congenital diaphragmatic hernia. J Pediatr 1987; 111:432–438.
4. MacKinlay GA, Burtles R. Oesophageal atresia: paralysis and ventilation in management of the wide gap. Pediatr Surg Int 1987; 2:10–12.
5. Hancock BJ, Wiseman NE. Congenital duodenal obstruction: the impact of an antenatal diagnosis. J Pediatr Surg 1989; 24:1027–1031.
6. Hirschsprung H. Stuhlragheit Neugeborener in Fotge von Dilation und Hypertrophie des Colons. Jahreb Kinderheilk 1887; 27:1–7.
7. Bodian M, Carter CO. A family study of Hirschsprung's disease. Ann Hum Genet 1963; 26:261–277.
8. Lee SL, Beyer TD, Kim SS, et al. Initial nonoperative management and delayed closure for treatment of giant omphaloceles. J Pediatr Surg 2006; 41:1846–1849.
9. Bianchi A, Dickson AP and Alizai NK. Elective delayed midgut reduction – No Anesthesia for Gastroschisis: Selection and Conversion criteria. J Pediatr Surg 2002; 37:1334–1336.
10. Owen A, Marven S, Jackson L, et al. Experience of bedside preformed silo staged reduction and closure for gastroschisis. J Pediatr Surg 2006; 41:1830–1835.
11. Holschneider A, Hutson J, Pena A, et al. Preliminary report on the International Conference for the Development of Standards for the Treatment of Anorectal Malformations. J Pediatr Surg 2005; 40:1521–1526.
12. Stephens FD. Wingspread Conference on Anorectal Malformations. Racine: Wisconsin; 1984.
13. de Vries PA, Pena A. Posterior sagittal anorectoplasty. J Pediatr Surg 1982; 17:638–643.
14. Kasai M, Kimura S, Asakura Y. Surgical treatment of biliary atresia. J Pediatr Surg 1968; 3:665–675.
15. Ogita S, Tsuto T, Nakamura K, et al. OK-432 therapy for lymphangioma in children: why and how does it work?. J Pediatr Surg 1996; 31:477–480.
16. Ramstedt C. Zur Operation der angeborenen Pylorusstenose. Medizinische Klinik (Berlin) 1912; 8:1702–1705.
17. Stiles HJ. (original operation note 3 February 1910 – personal possession) 1910.
18. Rothenburg SS. Experience with 220 consecutive laparoscopic Nissen fundoplications in infants and children. J Pediatr Surg 1998; 33:297–305.
19. Wilson-Storey D, MacKinlay GA. The superior mesenteric artery syndrome. J R Coll Surg Edin 1986; 31:175–178.
20. Atwell JD. Ascent of the testis: fact or fiction. Br J Urol 1985; 57:474–477.
21. Aitken-Swan J, Baird D. Circumcision and cancer of the cervix. Br J Cancer 1965; 19:217–227.
22. Report of the Ad Hoc Task Force on Circumcision. Pediatrics 1975; 56:610–611.
23. Bokai J. A fitma (preputium) sejtes adatapadasa a makkoz gyermakelnel. Orvosi Hetil 1869; 4:583–587.
24. Diebert GA. The separation of the prepuce in the human penis. Anatomical Records 1933; 54:387–393.
25. MacKinlay GA. Save the prepuce. Painless separation of preputial adhesions in the outpatient clinic. BMJ 1988; 297:590–591.
26. Spence, Sir James (1950). Spence on circumcision. Lancet 1964; ii:902.
27. White RHR, O'Donnell B. Controversies in therapeutics Management of urinary tract infection and vesico-ureteric reflux in children. 1. Operative treatment has no advantage over medical management (RHRW). 2. The case for surgery (BO'D). BMJ 1990; 300:1391–1394.
28. Puri P, Ninan GK, Sirana R. Subureteric Teflon injection (STING) Result of a European Survey. Eur Urol 1995; 27:71–73.
29. Puri P, Chertin B, Velaydham M, et al. Treatment of vesicoureteric reflux by endoscopic injection of dextranomer/hyaluronic acid copolymer: preliminary results. J Urol 2003; 170:1541–1544.
30. Tan OT, Sherwood K, Gilchrist BA. Treatment of children with port-wine stains using the flashlamp-pulsed tuneable dye laser. N Engl J Med 1989; 320:416–442.
31. Smith A, McIntosh N, Thomson M, et al. The stress effect of thermal injury on the hormones controlling fluid balance. Baillière's Clinical Paediatrics. London: Baillière; 1995.
32. Cole RP, Shakespeare PG. Toxic shock syndrome in scalded children. Burns 1990; 16:221–224.
33. de Saxe MJ, Hawtin P, Wieneke AA. Toxic shock syndrome in Britain – epidemiology and microbiology. Postgrad Med J 1985; 61:5–8.

38

Pain and palliative care

Richard F Howard, Finella Craig

INTRODUCTION

Relief from pain and suffering is a basic human right no matter what age, level of cognitive development or ability to communicate. Although children's pain is still often under-recognized around the world, in recent years there have been enormous advances in our understanding of pain in childhood.[1] Today, in the twenty-first century, it seems incredible to think that less than 20 years ago there was considerable debate about whether newborn infants were capable of feeling pain, and whether the benefits of potent analgesics outweighed their risks in young children. Since that time the study of the developmental neurobiology of pain has left little doubt that even the youngest and most premature infant is capable of pain perception, and we have learned to safely manage pain at all ages.[1,2]

Pain is a subjective experience, not necessarily proportional to any underlying physiological damage and is powerfully influenced by psychological, social and cultural factors. A common definition is that adopted by the IASP (International Association for the Study of Pain), the largest multidisciplinary international professional organization concerned with pain research and practice:

> 'Pain is an unpleasant sensory and emotional experience associated with actual or potential tissue damage, or described in terms of such damage. Note: The inability to communicate verbally does not negate the possibility that an individual is experiencing pain and is in need of appropriate pain-relieving treatment.'

Children may experience pain for many reasons, and because of its complex nature a rigid system of classification is not possible. For clinical purposes it can be helpful to consider painful experiences as acute, chronic and recurrent. Acute pain, lasting days or weeks is often clearly related to causes such as trauma or common illnesses, like accidents, ear and throat infections, appendicitis and sickle cell disease. Medical interventions are also an important cause of acute pain including immunization, diagnostic procedures and postoperative pain. Chronic pain, lasting months or years may also be associated with obvious underlying disease such as chronic rheumatological disorders, orthopedic problems in cerebral palsy and progressive malignant disease. However a large group of children with chronic pain, which may be constant but is often recurrent, have much less obvious tissue damage or have pain persisting far beyond the expected normal of period recovery from injury. These pains may occur in a wide range of sites, may be associated with other diffuse symptoms including sympathetically mediated changes and are frequently associated with prominent and sometimes extreme behavioral changes.

Physiologically, pain can also be classified as either 'nociceptive' or 'neuropathic' according to the underlying neural mechanism. Nociceptive pain is that which results from a normal, intact, nervous system. It is usually self-limiting, resolving as the underlying injury resolves, and it will respond to the 'classical' analgesics such as nonsteroidal anti-inflammatory drugs (NSAIDs) and opioids. In contrast, neuropathic pain is due to damage or malfunction of the nervous system, it is particularly characterized by spontaneous pain, unpleasant abnormal painful sensations or dysesthesias and sometimes associated sensory deficits. Neuropathic pain may persist despite treatment for considerable periods, sometimes the underlying injury is not obvious, and crucially it does not respond well to classical analgesics and may require alternative treatment strategies. Both nociceptive and neuropathic pain may co-exist in the same patient, and accurate diagnosis will assist in the selection of appropriate therapy.

ASSESSMENT

A thorough assessment of pain forms the foundation for its prevention and management. There is substantial literature on pain assessment in children, and the subject has been extensively reviewed.[3-7] Children's age, developmental level and also the type of pain they are experiencing will influence the approach to assessment, and in all situations a broad picture acknowledging the complex nature of pain and the multiple factors which influence it needs to be constructed. The majority of available pain assessment tools are designed to measure pain intensity in developmentally normal individuals, mostly in acute settings. Recently tools have also been developed for use in children with severe neurological disability.[8,9] Questionnaires designed to measure functional impairment due to chronic pain are also available; see later sections of this chapter for more detail.[10,11]

SELF-ASSESSMENT

Since pain is a subjective experience the ideal or 'gold standard' approach is one of self-reporting with as much information as possible about the pain coming directly from the child. A detailed history is especially important when the pain is chronic or the cause unknown and aims to discover the sites of the pain, its nature, frequency, severity, precipitating and relieving factors and other associated symptoms. Additional wider aspects to consider include the effect of the pain on the child and family's daily life, their coping skills and the meaning of the pain for them and within their culture. A variety of formal self-report tools to measure pain intensity have now been developed and validated; the majority of these have been designed to help children quantify acute pain usually on a numerical scale, typically in the range 0–10, where 0 equals no pain and 10 the worst pain imaginable. They can also be valuable in the wider assessment of long-term pain and also to monitor the effectiveness of treatment. The type of self-report scale used will depend on age, developmental level and setting. No scale can be universally recommended and each has its advantages and limitations.[12] However there are many children in whom self-reporting cannot be used, and in whom one or more proxy measures such as behaviors or physiological parameters have to be used.

ADOLESCENTS AND SCHOOL-AGE CHILDREN

Older children are usually able to use classical visual analogue scale (VAS), and numerical rating scales (Fig. 38.1). More user-friendly scales such as those using drawings of faces depicting different degrees of pain are suitable for this age group and can also be used for pre-school children down to the age of about 4 years.[13,14]

TODDLERS AND YOUNG CHILDREN

Toddlers and young children can provide simple information about their pain and its site but may not have the abstract concepts or verbal ability to describe its nature or intensity.[3–5] Young children tend to choose the extreme ends of the scales, and the type of face and the way it is depicted may also influence their ratings.[15,16] Another example is the poker chip tool, which uses small plastic blocks to represent 'pieces of hurt' with options of picking up between 1 and 4 to indicate pain severity.[17]

BEHAVIORAL AND MULTIDIMENSIONAL ASSESSMENT

Infants, preverbal children and children with severe developmental delay are unable to report their own pain. Assessment depends on observation of the child and knowing them well. Health care workers consistently underestimate children's pain compared with children's own self-reports and although parents' ratings are closer to the children's own they still tend to underestimate the pain.[18]

In infants indicators for pain that have been studied include facial expression, cry, motor movements and changes in behavioral state and patterns.[5] Preterm infants' responses appear to be less vigorous than those of full-term infants and their expression of pain cues are more subtle. Evaluation of pain through facial expression is best established and typical characteristics that express pain include eyes tightly closed, furrowed brows, broadened nasal root and deepened nasolabial furrow with a squared mouth and taut tongue.[19] A variety of tools to measure pain in neonates and infants are available; some 'multidimensional scales' combine behaviors and physiological parameters.[5] A number of behavioral scales have also been developed for preverbal children that may also be used in older children unable or unwilling to self-report. Two have been used extensively for postoperative pain are FLACC (Fig. 38.1), and CHEOPS, which use observation of verbal and facial

FLACC   Behavioral pain assessment

Categories	Scoring		
	0	1	2
Face	No particular expression or smile	Occasional grimace or frown, withdrawn, disinterested	Frequent to constant quivering chin, clenched jaw
Legs	Normal position or relaxed	Uneasy, restless, tense	Kicking, or legs drawn up
Activity	Lying quietly, normal position, moves easily	Squirming, shifting back and forth, tense	Arched, rigid or jerking
Cry	No cry (awake or asleep)	Moans or whimpers, occasional complaint	Crying steadily, screams or sobs, frequent complaints
Consolability	Content, relaxed	Reassured by occasional touching, hugging or being talked to, distractible	Difficult to console or comfort

Each of the five categories: (F) Face; (L) Legs; (A) Activity; (C) Cry; (C) Consolability; is scored from 0–2 which results in a total score between 0 and 10

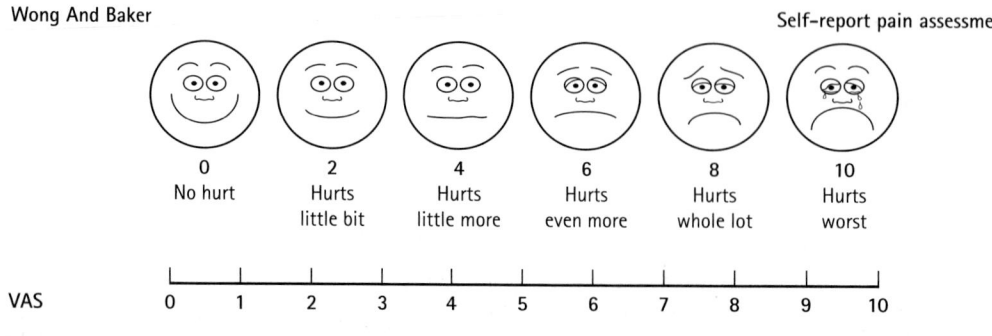

Wong And Baker   Self-report pain assessment

| 0 | 2 | 4 | 6 | 8 | 10 |
| No hurt | Hurts little bit | Hurts little more | Hurts even more | Hurts whole lot | Hurts worst |

VAS   0   1   2   3   4   5   6   7   8   9   10

Fig. 38.1 Behavioral and self-report pain scales (Adapted from [13,21]).

expressions of pain, behaviors, changes in muscle tone, and movement.[20,21] In intensive care settings the multi-dimensional COMFORT score has become popular.[22]

Assessment of pain in children with severe developmental delay poses a complex problem that has only recently been addressed by researchers. One approach is to document 'normal' and 'pain-related' behaviors in individual children over a period of time in order to estimate pain intensity associated with painful events such as surgery.[9]

PHYSIOLOGICAL RESPONSES

Physiological responses to pain are activated by the autonomic nervous system and include tachycardia, sweating, increasing secretion of catecholamines and adrenocorticoid hormones. These have not proved to be clinically reliable or useful as they are part of a global response to stress and not specific to pain; also, measurement of hormonal changes is invasive and slow.

CLINICAL MANAGEMENT OF PAIN

Both nonpharmacological and drug treatments of pain have a place in clinical pain management, the balance depending on the mechanism, source and circumstances of pain.

NONPHARMACOLOGICAL APPROACHES

Psychological
The unpleasant nature of pain and the many factors influencing it mean that all pain and pain management is immersed in a psychological context that needs to be taken into account.

Some approaches are very simple. Parents offer children the support children value most at times of stress, but they are still sometimes mistakenly excluded from their child's presence and care. Clinical staff need to be aware of the distress and anxiety that pain causes children, particularly in the Accident and Emergency unit, postoperatively and on the wards. Simple and honest explanations of disease processes and thorough preparation for procedures and surgery can help reassure children and families, enhance feelings of control and so reduce anxiety.[23]

A variety of more formal techniques have also been used effectively and well validated in a wide range of clinical situations, including the use of relaxation, cognitive approaches including distraction, imagery and thought blocking, and hypnosis.[24–28] Children are often very willing and co-operative subjects and enjoy the novelty of these techniques and the sense of control they engender. Such techniques are very effective for procedural pain management, and they are also used in a variety of chronic pain conditions to improve pain coping skills, with particular success in children with headache.[29]

Physiotherapy
Physiotherapy has a range of useful techniques that can contribute to pain management and are particularly important for children with chronic pain. These aim to restore optimal physical function by promoting strength and mobility, as well as to decrease pain. They include the use of active and passive exercise, often combined with goal setting and close monitoring. A number of other physical pain reduction techniques are frequently used concurrently such as desensitization of cutaneous hypersensitivity, local heat and cooling, hydrotherapy, ultrasound and TENS (transcutaneous electrical nerve stimulation).[30,31]

PHARMACOLOGICAL APPROACHES

Selection of analgesics: multi-modal analgesia
A relatively small range of analgesics is used in children. Selection of the most appropriate depends upon the cause and severity of the pain, the age and general condition of the patient, the setting and the facilities for supervision, monitoring and treatment of any side-effects. The underlying neural mechanisms responsible for the clinical characteris-

tics of both acute and chronic pain, and the influence of development on pain processing are becoming better understood. Increased pain sensitivity and tenderness (hyperalgesia and allodynia) at and near the site of injury are known to be the result of multiple changes within the CNS involving many neural and chemical mediators. The individual components of these 'pain pathways' can be targeted by combining different analgesics in order to compound their effects, thereby increasing efficacy.[32] A combination of analgesic drugs and techniques, with complimentary modes of action, maximizes the therapeutic advantage of each whilst keeping the doses and side effects to a minimum. This is the rationale underpinning the 'pain ladder' concept, in which new and more potent drugs are added as pain increases (Fig. 38.2). Whenever possible, analgesic pharmacotherapy is also combined with suitable nonpharmacological techniques in order to further reduce the pain response.

Mild analgesics
Paracetamol
Paracetamol is one of the most widely used drugs in children; it is available in oral, i.v. and rectal preparations. It is regarded as a safe and effective analgesic for mild and moderately severe pain; it can be used at all ages, including the neonate. Traditionally, paracetamol is thought to act centrally. Analgesia is attributed to inhibition of cyclo-oxygenase and thereby prostaglandin production in the CNS; other mechanisms have also been proposed including antagonism of serotonin (5HT) and possibly N-methyl D-aspartate (NMDA) receptors.[33,34]

Although several systematic reviews have demonstrated the analgesic efficacy of paracetamol for mild pain in the adult, few studies have been performed in children.[35–40] The analgesic efficacy of paracetamol is probably low; the correct dosage is important and for moderate or severe pain is probably best combined with other agents, typically opioids and nonsteroidal anti-inflammatory drugs (NSAIDs). Paracetamol does not reduce the pain response to heel lance or to circumcision in neonates although it does appear to have a small effect on late post-circumcision pain.[41,42]

Paracetamol is conjugated to glucuronide, sulphate or cysteine and excreted. In normal circumstances less than 10% is metabolized to a potentially hepatotoxic metabolite, N acetyl P amino benzoquinone imine (NAPQI). NAPQI is neutralized by combination with hepatic glutathione or with N acetyl cysteine and excreted harmlessly unless this pathway is saturated due to overdose or conjugates are in reduced supply. The p450 isoenzyme responsible for metabolism of paracetamol is developmentally regulated, with lower activity in the neonate, and this may confer some protection. However reduced clearance in neonates may lead to accumulation of the drug and its metabolites and so a reduced daily dose is usually recommended. Paracetamol hepatotoxicity is a well recognized dose-dependent complication associated with acute ingestion of more than 150 mg/kg. Long-term paracetamol treatment can also lead to toxicity at lower doses and it has been suggested that the maximum recommended dose should not be given for more than

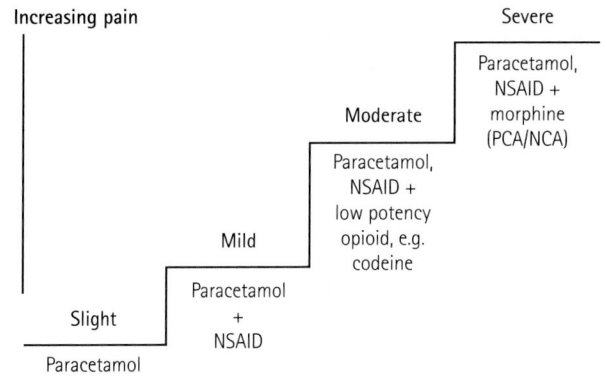

Fig. 38.2 Analgesic ladder. NCA, nurse-controlled analgesia. PCA, patient-controlled analgesia.

5 d.[43] Risk factors for toxicity include: chronic ingestion, especially in the malnourished due to reduced hepatic glutathione stores; pre-existing liver impairment (single doses are reasonably safe); hepatic enzyme induction and miscalculation or misinterpretation of commercial package labeling leading to accidental overdose.

The recommended total daily oral dose is 30 mg/kg in pre-term neonates 28–32 weeks' postmenstrual age, 60 mg/kg up to 3 months and 90 mg/kg in infants and older children.[44] This is usually given in divided doses 3 or 4 times daily. Absorption after oral paracetamol is excellent, rectal bio-availability is lower and more variable at 25–98% of the administered dose. In order to achieve therapeutic plasma levels a higher initial rectal dose is recommended (of the order of 30–40 mg/kg) followed by regular doses as above but not exceeding recommended maximum daily doses. The introduction of i.v. paracetamol has been a considerable advance, currently the recommended dose is 60 mg/kg/d for children weighing 10–50 kg and 4 g/d for those > 50 kg.[44]

Propacetamol

Propacetamol is an intravenously injectable pro-drug which is hydrolyzed to paracetamol 2:1 (1 g propacetamol yields 0.5 g paracetamol). It is useful when other preparations/routes of administration for paracetamol are not available; it is important that this preparation is not confused with i.v. paracetamol. The pharmacokinetics of propacetamol have been studied in neonates and children, and it has been used for postoperative pain.[45-47] Transient but mild platelet dysfunction after propacetamol has been described; contact dermatitis in health care workers may also occur.

Nonsteroidal anti-inflammatory drugs

This group of drugs is thought to exert their effects mainly peripherally by cyclo-oxygenase inhibition (cf paracetamol); they also inhibit the release of inflammatory mediators from neutrophils and macrophages. Cyclo-oxygenase helps to catalyze the conversion of arachidonic acid to prostaglandins, which modulate many auto-regulatory physiological processes including sensitization of normally high threshold nociceptors at sites of inflammation. The NSAIDs ibuprofen, diclofenac and ketorolac are used widely for pain due to injury, surgery and many acute and chronic disease processes. These three drugs are used interchangeably in clinical practice, but their effect and side-effect profiles may differ at an individual patient level. Table 38.1 shows doses and routes; ibuprofen is available 'over the counter' in the UK, diclofenac is presented in a convenient rectal formulation, and ketorolac is available parenterally. Piroxicam, a long-acting NSAID which can be given once daily, is useful in long-term treatment and if compliance with multiple-dosing is a problem (Table 38.1).

Side-effects and toxicity

Asthma: caution is advised in the use of NSAIDs in the presence of wheezing as they are known to be cross-reactive with aspirin-induced asthma. The risks may have been overemphasized in children and short-term ibuprofen treatment appears to pose very little risk.[48] Aspirin is not used in children apart from special circumstances such as Kawasaki syndrome (see Ch. 19, p. 649) because of the risk of Reye's syndrome. Aspirin-induced asthma is very rare in the young and one study in children with asthma found no deterioration in respiratory function after diclofenac administration.[49]

Renal: kidney function is regulated by prostaglandins and two mechanisms of NSAID nephrotoxicity have been described. Functional renal failure can occur in a dose-dependent fashion, disappearing on withdrawal of the drug. Pre-existing poor function and dehydration may be contributing factors. Dose-independent interstitial nephritis with or without nephritic syndrome is rare; treatment is conservative or with corticosteroids.[50,51]

Coagulopathy: Platelet function is altered by NSAIDs due to their reversible inhibition of thromboxane A2 and platelet endoperoxides. Gastrointestinal blood loss can occur particularly associated with peptic ulceration. Increased intraoperative and postoperative blood loss, which is not usually clinically significant, has also been described. Simultaneous prescription of H_2-receptor antagonists can help reduce the risk of gastrointestinal problems.[52,53]

Infants and neonates: NSAIDs are rarely given to those under the age of 3 months and are not usually used for pain indications in neonates due to fears of possible interference with cerebral blood flow auto-regulation and risk to immature renal function.

Gastrointestinal: the normal protective function of the gastric mucosa is reduced by NSAIDs and this can lead to peptic ulceration. It is not usually a problem in short-term use; some newer drugs may be beneficial (see later).

NSAIDs and cyclo-oxygenase

Cyclo-oxygenase exists in two isoforms: COX-1 and COX-2. COX-1 is found in virtually all cell types; COX-2 is expressed in some organs, notably the brain and lung, but is specifically induced in inflammation in conjunction with a rapid rise in prostaglandin levels. The traditional NSAIDs are nonselective for these isoforms but individual drugs may differ slightly in their ability to depress activity. Selective COX-2 inhibitors have reputedly fewer gastrointestinal side-effects in comparison with nonselective NSAIDs and may therefore widen the indications for NSAIDs. However the exact consequences of this selectivity is not yet fully understood; for example their use in the adult has been found to be associated with increased risk of adverse cardiovascular events and the incidence of renal complications may be similar to nonselective inhibitors. The use of COX-2 selective NSAIDs has not been adequately studied in children so at present there is little evidence upon which to evaluate their use.

Opioids and related drugs

Opioids exert their effects by acting at opioid receptors primarily in the spinal cord and brain. Despite the fact that morphine is one of the oldest and most widely used analgesics, opioid pharmacology is still not fully understood and many important questions remain unanswered. Opioids are the most powerful analgesics available with high efficacy for many types of acute and chronic pain, with the notable exception of neuropathic pain. Important considerations when prescribing opioids include their unpleasant and potentially dangerous side-effects and the development of tolerance, which can be troublesome. Neonates in particular appear clinically to be more susceptible to the depressant effects of opioids; the causes of this are probably multifactorial but have not been fully explained (see later).

The doses and possible routes of administration of the commonly used opioids for children are shown in Table 38.2. Morphine has a fairly direct relationship between dose, efficacy and side effects. The same is not true for all other opioids; partial agonist drugs such as buprenorphine have a ceiling effect and others such as codeine and pethidine have unacceptable side-effect profiles at high doses, which limit their use.

Table 38.1 Nonsteroidal analgesics

Drug	Routes of administration	Doses	Notes
Ibuprofen (above 5 kg)	Oral	30 mg/kg/d (3–4 divided doses)	Max. 2.4 g/d
Diclofenac	Oral or rectal	3 mg/kg/d (3 divided doses)	Max. 150 mg/d
Ketorolac	Oral I.v.	0.5–1 mg/kg (4 times daily) 0.5 mg/kg (4 times daily)	Dosage restrictions apply in some countries. Max. 40 mg/d
Piroxicam	Oral	0.3–0.5 mg/kg/d	Maximum dose 20 mg in children > 6 years

Table 38.2   Opioids

Drug	Routes of administration	Doses	
Codeine	Oral	1 mg/kg (4 times daily)	
	Rectal	1–1.5 mg/kg (4 times daily)	
Oxycodone/hydrocodone	Oral	0.2 mg/kg (4 times daily)	
Morphine	Oral	0.2–0.4 mg/kg (4 times daily)	Long-acting oral preparations available
	Intravenous	0.05 mg/kg	
	Subcutaneous	0.05 mg/kg	
	Epidural	0.02–0.05 mg/kg	
Fentanyl	OTFC (oral transmucosal)	1–10 μg/kg	See relevant product
	Transdermal	1–3 μg/kg	See relevant product
	Intravenous	0.5–1.5 μg/kg/h	Loading dose (if required)
		1 μg/kg/h	Incremental dose
	Epidural		Infusion
			Infusion
Pethidine	Oral	2 mg/kg (4 times daily)	Incremental/loading dose
	Intravenous	0.5–1 mg/kg	Incremental/loading dose
	Subcutaneous	0.5–1 mg/kg	
Methadone	Oral	0.2 mg/kg (3 times daily)	Useful long acting opioid
	Intravenous	0.1–0.2 mg/kg	

Morphine

Morphine is the prototype, high potency opioid and enormous experience in its use often makes it the drug of choice for severe pain. The pharmacokinetics and clinical use of morphine in children have been studied extensively.[54,55] The pharmacokinetics and efficacy of morphine are developmentally regulated, although outside the neonatal period, which is characterized by high variability, efficacy is largely predictable and dose related.[56]

Morphine is well absorbed orally; formulations of morphine include a suspension and a slow-release compound (MST). Parenteral morphine is usually given intravenously either by intermittent dosing, continuous infusion or in a patient-controlled analgesia (PCA) or nurse-controlled analgesia (NCA) regimen see Table 38.3. Subcutaneous infusion of morphine is also used, particularly in palliative care and when i.v. access is difficult or precious. Preservative-free (as a precaution against chemical toxicity) morphine is also effective in the epidural space, usually combined with local anesthetic.

Nausea and vomiting, sedation, and respiratory depression are the most frequently seen acute adverse effects of morphine; itching also

Table 38.3   Protocols for i.v. morphine administration

1. Morphine infusion
Preparation:	Morphine sulphate 1 mg/kg in 50 ml solution	
Concentration:	20 μg/kg/ml	
Initial dose:	2.5–5.0 ml (50–100 μg/kg)	
Infusion:	0.5–1.5 ml/h (10–30 μg/kg/h)	

2. PCA
Preparation:	Morphine sulphate 1 mg/kg in 50 ml solution	
Concentration:	20 μg/kg/ml	
Initial dose:	2.5–5.0 ml (50–100 μg/kg)	
Programming	Background infusion:	0–0.2 ml/h (0–4 μg/kg/h)
	PCA dose	0.5–1.0 ml (10–20 μg/kg/h)
	Lockout interval:	5 min

3. NCA
Preparation:	Morphine sulphate 1 mg/kg in 50 ml solution	
Concentration:	20 μg/kg/ml	
Initial dose:	2.5–5.0 ml (50–100 μg/kg)	
Programming	Background infusion:	0.5–1.0 ml/h (10–20 μg/kg/h)
	NCA dose	0.5–1.0 ml (10–20 μg/kg/h)
	Lockout interval:	20 min

4. Subcutaneous morphine
Preparation:	Morphine sulphate 1 mg/kg in 20 ml solution	
Concentration:	50 μg/kg/ml	
Initial dose:	Infusion:	1–2.0 ml (50–100 μg/kg)
Programming		0.2–0.4 ml/h (10–20 μg/kg/h)

Source: Pain control service, Great Ormond Street Hospital for Children.

occurs, especially after epidural morphine. Depression of gastrointestinal motility and constipation are a problem with prolonged use. In clinical practice, non-life-threatening side-effects can be treated by reducing the dosage of morphine, often in palliative care by waiting for tolerance to the side-effect to develop – drowsiness almost always wears off in a few days, or with appropriate therapy, e.g. anti-emetics, anti-pruritics and laxatives. In an emergency, adverse effects of morphine can be reversed with the opioid antagonist, naloxone 4–10 mcg/kg.

Fentanyl

Fentanyl is a synthetic, high potency (100 × morphine) lipid soluble opioid. Its main use is during general anesthesia, where its efficacy, rapid onset and short initial half-life are an advantage. Fentanyl is usually given intravenously; it is also a popular choice for ventilated neonates and infants on ICUs (see later). Postoperatively fentanyl is commonly infused into the epidural space as its high lipid solubility may limit rostral spread and reduce the incidence of some complications, notably respiratory depression, retention of urine, and itching, in comparison with morphine. Fentanyl is available as oral (transmucosal) and transdermal (fentanyl patch) preparations which can be used for procedural pain and pain in chronic conditions and palliative care.

Fentanyl is very potent with a fast onset after i.v. administration. Opioid related side-effects of sedation, respiratory depression and itching are to be expected. High doses, > 5 mcg/kg, have also been associated with chest wall rigidity and are usually only given when respiration is controlled.[57,58]

Codeine

Codeine is a low potency opioid used for mild to moderate pain including some postoperative pain and cancer pain. It is often combined with other analgesics for best effect, particularly paracetamol and NSAIDs (Fig. 38.2). Codeine is a morphine prodrug; the response to codeine is more variable than that to morphine and this may be due to genetic (and possibly developmental) differences in metabolizing capacity.[59] Of individuals from some populations, 10% or more will not benefit from codeine analgesia; despite this they may experience some adverse effects as codeine can produce these without metabolism to morphine.[60] Codeine should not be administered intravenously as it causes hypotension.

Oxycodone and hydrocodone

Oxycodone and hydrocodone are semi-synthetic opioids suitable for moderate to severe pain, especially in combination with paracetamol or NSAIDs. Oxycodone is active by oral, buccal, sublingual and i.v. routes.[61] Sustained-release formulations have also been used in children.[62]

Tramadol

Tramadol is a synthetic moderate potency analgesic which has a novel dual mode of action by a combination of inhibition of serotonin and norepinephrine reuptake and μ-opioid receptor agonism by its active metabolite o-desmethyltramadol. Metabolism of tramadol is by the same cytochrome P450 enzyme subgroup responsible for codeine metabolism, and therefore may be subject to the same drawbacks (see earlier). Tramadol has been used for early postoperative analgesia in children with good effect. It has also been used in the caudal epidural space, where it appears to have a slow onset (about 1 h) and moderate potency.

Pethidine

Pethidine is a synthetic opioid which has few advantages over morphine. Pethidine is metabolized to norpethidine, which is neurotoxic, causing tremor, twitching, agitation and even convulsions. Norpethidine is probably also the cause of abnormal neurobehavioral tests in the neonate following maternal pethidine for labor pain. High and repeated dosage and renal impairment are risk factors, but convulsions have been reported with low doses in the therapeutic range. The traditional use of pethidine in acute sickle cell pain has declined subsequent to reports of convulsions in children.

Pethidine was originally considered to induce less nausea and vomiting and to be less depressant to the respiratory center of the fetus and neonate than morphine. If it is administered in equi-analgesic dosage these differences are not apparent, although it remains popular in some centers.

Pethidine has also been recommended for use in pancreatitis as it was thought to be less likely to precipitate spasm of the sphincter of Oddi than morphine or other opioids. Evidence from adult literature does not support this hypothesis as all opioids including pethidine appear to elevate intrabiliary pressures; the question has not been examined in children.[63]

Novel systemic analgesics

Clonidine

Clonidine is an alpha-2 adrenoceptor agonist with multiple effects including analgesia, sedation, anti-hypertension, anti-sialogogue, and others. Clonidine has a direct effect on spinal pre- and postsynaptic adrenoceptors in the dorsal horn; it also has many supraspinal effects which may also contribute to analgesia. The pharmacology, use and advantages of clonidine and other alpha-2 adrenoceptor agonists appear to be particularly useful in managing postoperative pain although moderate dose-independent reductions in blood pressure have been found at doses within the therapeutic range 0.625–2.5 mg/kg. The efficacy of clonidine in the neonate is not established; severe respiratory depression after a single dose of 2 μg/kg caudal clonidine has been reported.

Ketamine

Ketamine is an antagonist at the glutamate NMDA receptor. The receptor is important in the generation of hyperalgesia and ketamine may therefore be helpful in controlling nociceptive and neuropathic pain. High doses of 1–2 mg/kg have been used for many years as a general anesthetic. At 'low dose', < 1 mg/kg, ketamine has been found to be an effective analgesic both systemically and epidurally. The use of low-dose ketamine for postoperative pain in adults is fairly commonplace, although its efficacy has not been clearly ascertained.[64] There are many reports of its use in children, including analgesia–sedation in the pediatric ICU, and for procedural pain and postoperative pain. Ketamine in high doses induces neurobehavioral and cognitive depression sometimes accompanied by psychotomimetic effects characterized by bizarre dreams or hallucinations. Ketamine has been shown to have toxic effects to the infant mouse brain, and this observation together with the potential for abuse is has lead to a reappraisal of its use in humans.[65]

Local anesthesia

Local anesthesia has a particularly important role in pediatric pain management as it is often extremely effective and avoids many of the complications of systemic analgesics.

Bupivacaine and levobupivacaine

The amide-type local anesthetic bupivacaine and its isomer levobupivacaine are popular because of their long duration of action. Bupivacaine has been used widely for most types of local anesthetic procedure in children: following trauma, wound infiltration after surgery, peripheral nerve blocks and epidural analgesia. It is almost universally the drug of choice for epidural analgesia, where it can be infused for several days for postoperative pain, and sometimes longer for other indications. The pharmacokinetics of bupivacaine and levobupivacaine in children have been studied. Neurotoxicity and cardiotoxicity have been reported, with a slightly less risk with levobupivacaine. However the incidence of these adverse events appears to be low with both drugs if dosage recommendations are not exceeded.

Local anesthetic creams and gels are widely used for procedural pain and are discussed in the relevant sections.

MANAGEMENT OF ACUTE AND POSTOPERATIVE PAIN

Pain after surgery is a largely predictable event and therefore analgesia should be planned in advance according to the expected pain and postoperative setting. Pediatric anesthetists have special training in the use of systemic analgesics and local anesthetic techniques for surgery and they should also take some responsibility for postoperative pain management. Many of the principles and techniques used for postoperative pain may also be applied to other sources of acute or acute on chronic pain. Examples are post-traumatic injury, acute sickle cell crisis, mucositis (ulceration at a mucosal surface) and many others.

ANALGESIA FOR MINOR AND AMBULATORY OR DAY-CARE SURGERY

Most routine surgery in children is relatively minor and very often undertaken on a day-case or day-stay basis. Analgesia for day surgery should be effective and not delay discharge from hospital. The objective is to maximize comfort and mobility with little sedation or other side-effects. Postoperative nausea and vomiting (PONV) is a particular problem. In practice, this means limiting or avoiding the use of sedatives and opioids whilst encouraging the use of local anesthetic techniques. Health care workers need education and training to ensure that all runs smoothly and patients are pain free at discharge. Further analgesia will usually need to be continued at home for several days managed by parents who will need information and support in order to be able to do this effectively. Postoperative pain should be mostly treatable with 'over-the-counter' analgesics, which are safe and easily obtainable by parents at home, otherwise the suitability of a procedure for day surgery must be questioned. Take home 'packs' containing analgesics and written information are often supplied to families at day-surgery centers.

Local anesthetic techniques

Infiltration of the surgical wound can be used in many situations, especially for very superficial surgery, its utility being limited mainly by the need for large volumes of local anesthetic and dosage restrictions. Infiltration is effective for a number of common pediatric procedures including herniotomy, eye surgery, dental surgery and tonsillectomy. A range of peripheral nerve blocks are frequently used. The ilioinguinal and iliohypogastric nerves, which supply the sensory innervation to the groin area, are easy to locate and block. Surgical exploration of the inguinal region includes hernia repair, ligation of patent processus vaginalis and orchidopexy. Recognized complications include quadriceps weakness due to spread of local anesthetic to the femoral nerve. The distal third of the penis is supplied by the dorsal nerves, which are easily blocked by an injection of local anesthetic at the base of the penis. Analgesia is suitable for circumcision, minor hypospadias repair and surgery on the urethral meatus. Dorsal nerve block has also been particularly advocated for neonatal circumcision, which is performed in some countries without general anesthesia.

Caudal block

There is an enormous literature extending back at least 30 years describing caudal epidural local anesthesia in children. Caudal block is effective for most operations below the level of the umbilicus; bupivacaine lasts 4–6 h by this route. Opioids, ketamine and clonidine have also been used either alone or in combination with local anesthetic, prolonging analgesia to 12 h or longer. The complications of caudal analgesia are rare but include temporary leg weakness, delayed micturition, vascular puncture, dural puncture, and inadvertent intravascular or intradural injection of local anesthetic. Epidural infection or neurological sequelae have not been reported after single caudal local anesthetic injections.

Systemic analgesia

Potent analgesia is likely to be necessary in the early postoperative period, even after minor surgery. Institution of systemic analgesia after surgery should be planned to ensure a smooth and comfortable transition from the immediate postoperative and post-anesthesia recovery phase. Drugs, timing and routes of administration selected are important. Reactive, p.r.n. or 'as required' dosing schedules are not appropriate during the period of expected postoperative pain, and if used they are likely to lead to avoidable painful intervals while drugs are taking effect.[66]

Postoperative nausea and vomiting

Nausea and vomiting is a common cause of morbidity after minor and day-care surgery; its causes are multifactorial, and it is associated with poor analgesia and not with preoperative anxiety. Risk factors for PONV include a previous history of PONV, general anesthesia, the use of opioids, early resumption of oral fluids and certain surgical procedures, notably tonsillectomy and strabismus surgery. 5HT antagonists (e.g. ondansetron) are popular for prophylaxis and first-line treatment, the synthetic corticosteroid dexamethasone, either alone or in combination has potent anti-emetic effects. Combination anti-emetic therapy is probably the most effective treatment (Table 38.4).[67]

ANALGESIA AFTER MAJOR SURGERY

As the oral route is rarely available after major surgery for at least the first postoperative day, and often much longer after gastrointestinal operations, other options must be utilized. Local anesthetic techniques, performed under general anesthesia before or after surgery can reduce analgesic requirements in the early postoperative period.[68,69] After major operations further analgesia can be accomplished by infusion of local anesthetic through a catheter located at the site of the block, e.g. continuous epidural analgesia. More commonly pain after major surgery is managed with morphine or other opioids. Paracetamol, NSAIDs, codeine and morphine are all readily available in rectal formulations, which are popular. Rectal absorption for many drugs is known to be erratic and unpredictable, and a fatality following rectal morphine in a child has been reported. Nevertheless rectal administration of less potent drugs appears to be safe and is still widespread for paracetamol and NSAIDs.

Parenteral opioid infusions

Morphine infusion has been used safely for postoperative analgesia in children for more than 20 years, the dose range in nonventilated children in general ward areas is around 10–30 mcg/kg/h. Either i.v. or s.c. routes can be used for morphine infusions, although the latter requires more concentrated solutions (Table 38.3). A wide range of morphine requirements after surgery in children has been observed and inadequate analgesia on the first postoperative day is more frequent at infusion rates < 20 mcg/kg/h.[70] Patient-controlled analgesia (PCA) is popular for children 5 years or older; there is a substantial literature describing its use and efficacy.[71–73] Nurse-controlled analgesia (NCA) is a modified continuous morphine infusion suitable for children who are unable to operate the PCA handset. Nursing staff can administer extra doses of morphine on the basis of pain assessments or before painful care or movement by operating the PCA handset. NCA increases flexibility, total morphine consumption and parent and nurse satisfaction with analgesia.[74] Protocols for morphine infusion, PCA and NCA are given in Table 38.3. Inadequate analgesia, nausea and vomiting, excessive sedation and respiratory depression can be troublesome problems in the postoperative period. Better pain assessment, appropriate dosing, multi-modal analgesia and

Table 38.4 Drug treatment of opioid side-effects

1. Respiratory depression		
Naloxone*	(Infant–12 years)	10 μg/kg i.v.
	(12–18 years)	1.5–3 μg/kg i.g.
2. Nausea and vomiting		
Cyclizine	1 mg/kg	Oral/i.v.
	3 times daily	(< 6 years max. 25 mg)
		(> 6 years max. 50 mg)
Ondansetron	0.1 mg/kg	Oral/i.v.
		(< 12 years max. 4 mg)
		(> 12 years max. 8 mg)
Dexamethasone	0.1 mg/kg	I.v.

Larger doses may be required for severe overdose. Lower doses should be used postoperatively with titration to obtain respiratory response while maintaining adequate analgesia.

clear protocols should minimize poor efficacy and side-effects. Naloxone should always be available when opioids are being infused.

MANAGEMENT OF NEONATAL PAIN

Pain in the neonatal period requires special consideration because the immaturity of many body systems has profound and often unpredictable effects on both the response to pain and analgesics. Advances in perinatal care have meant that many younger and smaller patients undergo diagnostic and therapeutic procedures and present for surgery in early life. The management of these painful situations is hindered by our inability to accurately measure pain in this group and a lack of information on the precise effects of many analgesics during early postnatal development. Research in the fields of pain assessment and the developmental neurobiology and pharmacology of pain may soon influence practice, but for the present pharmacological neonatal pain management is largely based on the empirical and judicious use of, opioids (principally codeine, morphine, and fentanyl), paracetamol, and local anesthesia.

OPIOIDS

Despite the fact that opioids are widely used in the neonatal period both for pain and sedation little is known of the thresholds for treatment or response in the term or preterm neonate.[75] The pharmacokinetics of morphine and other opioids have been investigated and clear relationships between age and volume of distribution and plasma clearance have been established.[16] Underlying medical condition is probably also important as the maturation in morphine clearance observed in infants in the first few months of life is delayed in those undergoing corrective cardiac surgery in comparison with age-matched controls after other surgical procedures.[76] The lack of sensitive pain measurement tools and failure to correlate plasma morphine levels with analgesia has led some authors to use the emergence of side-effects such as respiratory depression to quantify the response to morphine.[77] Although there is no clear dose–response relationship between plasma morphine and respiratory depression, a common threshold in neonates and infants of around 15–20 ng/ml has been suggested.[77,78] Based on this finding, the dose of morphine to reach this target level has been investigated and found to be 5–15 mcg/kg/h in the neonate, some 25–50% lower than in older children; suggested protocols are shown in Table 38.5.[54,78] Clearly, determination of the analgesic dose–response for opioids in the neonate still remains an important priority for further research.

PARACETAMOL

Paracetamol is considered to be safe and effective in the neonatal period although, as with adults and older children, the plasma level associated with analgesia is not known.

The majority of pharmacokinetic studies have assumed plasma levels associated with the antipyretic effect of paracetamol to be therapeutic, and therefore a guide to dosing schedules. The pharmacokinetics of paracetamol have been shown to be age dependent; neonates have a higher volume of distribution (174%) and lower clearance (62%) in comparison with older children.[79] Paracetamol is metabolized in the liver, where it is conjugated to glucuronide, a small amount being oxidized by cytochrome P450 to a potentially hepatotoxic product (see earlier) which is conjugated to glutathione. Both these pathways are immature in the neonate and show high variability; enhanced sulfation of paracetamol has been demonstrated, which may compensate for reduced glucuronidation.[80] The current recommended oral dose of paracetamol in the term neonate is 60 mg/kg/d, with 30–45 mg/kg/d suggested for pre-term infants; there are variations between different countries regarding this. The route of administration is important as bioavailability is very variable; in term neonates 20 mg/kg rectal paracetamol 6 hourly (80 mg/kg/d) does not reliably achieve therapeutic plasma levels and an initial dose of 30 mg/kg is recommended.[81] In pre-term neonates 20 mg/kg is effective but prolonged elimination results in accumulation if the dosing interval is less than 8 h.[81] I.v. paracetamol has not yet been adequately investigated in the neonate but reports of its use are starting to appear.[82] Propacetamol, the paracetamol pro-drug has been used in the neonate; at less than 10 d old, 30 mg/kg/d of paracetamol (60 mg/kg/d of propacetamol) maintained plasma levels between 4 and 10 mg/L, whereas after 10 d double this dose was required.[45]

LOCAL ANESTHESIA IN THE NEONATE

Local anesthesia is popular in the neonate as it avoids many of the problems associated with systemic drugs. Topical local anesthesia, infiltration and nerve blocks including epidural anesthesia can be used in the newborn. Neonates may be more susceptible to toxic effects of local anesthetics so lower doses are generally recommended. Local anesthetics are extensively protein bound, the free (unbound) fraction is considered to be pharmacologically active and therefore also important for toxicity. The protein A-acid glycoprotein (AAG) and albumin are the most important plasma proteins involved and AAG levels are lower in neonates. Prilocaine is a constituent of the topical formulation eutectic mixture of local anesthetics (EMLA) and its use in the neonate has been a cause for concern. A metabolite of prilocaine, orthotoluidine is produced, which leads to the development of methemoglobin, (oxidized hemoglobin), which has a reduced oxygen carrying capacity. Methemoglobin is reduced to hemoglobin by the enzyme methemoglobin reductase, which is developmentally regulated. Neonates are also particularly susceptible because fetal hemoglobin is more easily oxidized than adult hemoglobin. Studies have shown that EMLA can be used safely in neonates provided the dose is limited proportionally.[83,84] In a systematic review of analgesia for neonatal circumcision, local anesthetic techniques were found to be the most effective and were recommended for this procedure.[85]

SUCROSE AND NONPHARMACOLOGICAL PAIN MANAGEMENT

Sweet tasting solutions such as glucose and sucrose have been found to reduce pain responses to brief procedures in the neonate.[86–88] Sucrose has become popular, and there are commercially available preparations for clinical use. The analgesic effect of sucrose is thought to be related to the release of endogenous endorphins, however administration of naloxone did not decrease the analgesic effect in one trial.[89] Non-nutritive sucking using a pacifier, breast-feeding, and tactile stimulation have all been found to reduce pain associated responses in neonates.[90–93]

MANAGEMENT OF PAIN IN THE ICU

In the intensive care unit (ICU) sources of pain include the underlying condition, the presence of endotracheal and other tubes, drains and catheters and also the many procedures which such patients frequently undergo. See section on neonatal pain for details of techniques.

Table 38.5 Suggested morphine infusion protocols in the neonate*

Neonatal morphine infusion		
Preparation:	Morphine sulphate 1.0 mg/kg in 50 ml solution	
Concentration:	20 μg/kg/ml	
Initial dose:	0.5–5.0 ml (10–100 μg/kg)	
Infusion:	0.1–0.7 ml/h (2– 14 μg/kg/h)	
Neonatal NCA		
Preparation:	Morphine sulphate	1 mg/kg in 50 ml solution.
Concentration:		20 μg/kg/ml
Initial dose:		0.5–5.0 ml (10–100 μg/kg)
Programming	Background infusion:	0.0–0.5 ml/h (0–10 μg/kg/h)
NCA dose		0.5–1.0 ml (10–20 μg/kg/h)
Lockout interval:		20 min

* With full cardiorespiratory monitoring in intensive care areas, higher doses may be appropriate when respiration is supported.

OPIOID INFUSIONS, TOLERANCE AND WITHDRAWAL

Opioid infusions provide background analgesia, sedation, improve comfort and facilitate synchronization of respiration with artificial ventilation in neonates and older children.[94,95] Morphine is the drug of choice, although fentanyl is a useful alternative, particularly if pulmonary hypertension is a concern.[96]

A characteristic feature of opioid infusions for more than a few days is progressive tolerance to both the analgesic and sedative effects and it is not uncommon for patients to receive doses far in excess of what is normally considered therapeutic. Intermittent administration is less likely to cause tolerance than continuous infusion but this can be impractical. Use of a background infusion with intermittent doses when necessary, e.g. for routine care, blood sampling, endotracheal suction and other procedures may reduce the likelihood of tolerance. This is very similar in concept to NCA (see earlier). Multi-modal analgesia may also be helpful and the use of agents such as clonidine and low-dose ketamine may reduce tolerance.

Abrupt withdrawal of opioids after 5 or more days of continuous use is very likely to result in the appearance of symptoms and signs of withdrawal. Gradual reduction of infusion rates by 10–20% per day should not delay tracheal extubation of the airway or discharge from ICU and will usually prevent unpleasant and distressing symptoms and potentially dangerous cerebral excitatory phenomena including convulsions. If necessary oral preparations can be used and weaning from high doses continued in low dependency areas, even at home. Clonidine and benzodiazepines ameliorate the withdrawal syndrome associated with opioids. High-dose infusions of benzodizepines, such as midazolam, may result in benzodizepine withdrawal, which can be avoided by substituting a long-acting benzodiazepine such as lorazepam with subsequent gradual withdrawal.

CHRONIC PAIN

There is no precise definition of when a pain becomes chronic as it is strongly influenced by patient perception. In acute pain the prevailing mood tends toward anxiety, whereas in chronic pain withdrawal from daily life and even depression can predominate. Hope remains strong in acute pain whereas despair can dominate the chronic situation. In acute pain the person is able to focus on the pain itself but with chronic pain it becomes all pervasive.[97]

Effective management depends on recognizing the need to tackle both the underlying cause for the pain and its wider manifestations. Pain may be constant, such as in progressive cancer or related to exacerbations, such as in rheumatoid and connective tissue disorders. In other disorders a combination of background chronic pain interspersed with acute episodes including from procedures such as in sickle cell disease, osteogenesis imperfecta and epidermolysis bullosa. Specific treatment aimed at reversing or relieving the underlying illness is the most effective approach accompanied by short- or long-term analgesia. Analgesics are chosen according to the severity of the pain and whether it appears to be primarily related to tissue damage to inflammatory or neuropathic elements. Psychological assessment may identify a role for cognitive and behavioral pain management skills.

SICKLE CELL DISEASE

The dual aspects of acute and chronic pain are vividly represented by sickle cell disease, where the severe pain of sickle cell crises exemplifies acute pain whereas the recurrent nature of the crises, their unpredictable nature and the lifelong and incurable nature of the disease results in aspects characteristic of chronic intractable pain.[98] Management of pain for these children and young people has a poor record, with inappropriate fears of addiction and misunderstanding of cultural aspects of the illness, resulting in analgesics being under used. Current approaches recognize the need to give patients more credence and con-

trol, by enabling a more rapid response at the start of a crisis including i.v. opioids by PCA and using nonpharmacological approaches.

CHRONIC PAIN SYNDROMES

A significant number of children present with symptoms of pain but where a physical cause is not evident, where the pain seems disproportionate to the tissue damage or where pain persists after previous damage appears to have healed.

Complex regional pain syndrome

One common picture, often occurring with limb pains is that of increasing disability and associated sympathetically mediated features such as edema, decreased temperature and pallor or cyanotic coloring of the affected part, hyper-esthesia of the skin, muscle wasting and eventually osteoporosis and atrophy. This has been called reflex sympathetic dystrophy (RSD) in the past but is now considered part of the spectrum of chronic regional pain syndrome (CRPS). Although sympathetic nervous system involvement is not invariable fatigue, widely disseminated pains and other features such as malaise, disability, school absence and family disruption are common. Significant analgesic use is usual and reported as rarely effective in relieving the pain. Sometimes these children are labeled as malingering or disbelieved, resulting in anger and frustration. CRPS is more common in girls, and in contrast to adult presentations, the lower limb is usually involved.[99] A confident diagnosis of CRPS depends on careful exclusion of an observable underlying pathology and effective intervention begins with acknowledging the reality of the pain and symptoms, of the impact on the child and family and a recognition of the complex and ill-understood nature of the problem. The causes are not clearly understood and appear to involve features of neuropathic pain, with a persistent and inappropriate upregulation of pain perception, in the wider context of a bio-behavioral response to the pain. Early diagnosis of CRPS is thought to improve prognosis, immobilization of the affected limb is strongly contraindicated and a regimen of desensitization treatment with active and passive movement should be introduced as soon as possible.[100] The most successful management is multidisciplinary.[99,100] As well as medical and nursing input it involves physiotherapy, psychological and pharmaceutical assessment followed by the development of a comprehensive treatment program, with the involvement of the child and family. Interventions should be outpatient based, but in severe situations intensive inpatient programs may be needed.[31] Care includes the gradual withdrawal of inappropriate analgesics, and cautious use of medications effective in neuropathic pain such as the sodium channel blockers gabapentin and the tricyclic antidepressants; there is little evidence to support the use of sympathetic blocks for CRPS.[99] Learning coping skills, cognitive-behavioral therapy, graded exercise, goal setting and regular support and monitoring are the mainstays of treatment. The course may be one of improvement and relapses.

PALLIATIVE CARE

Pediatric palliative care is a holistic approach to the care of children with life-limiting and life-threatening illness, where symptom management is addressed alongside the provision of practical, psychological, social and spiritual support for the whole family. It should be provided from the time of diagnosis of a life-limiting or life-threatening condition and should continue though life, death and bereavement. It is not confined to the terminal phase of an illness and can co-exist alongside life-prolonging and life-saving treatments.

WHO NEEDS PALLIATIVE CARE?

Many of the relevant illnesses are specific to children, are very rare and have a protracted course. Some are familial and may affect several children in the same family, with genetic implications for the parents and healthy siblings.

Children who may benefit from a palliative care referral can be considered in four broad groups:[101]

1. life-threatening conditions where curative treatment may be possible but may fail. Palliative care is needed in times of prognostic uncertainty or when cure becomes impossible. Cancer is an example;
2. conditions where there are long periods of intensive treatment aimed at prolonging life, but where life expectancy is significantly reduced. Cystic fibrosis and acquired immune deficiency syndrome (AIDS) fit this pattern;
3. progressive conditions where treatment is entirely palliative and may extend over many years. Neurodegenerative diseases and many inborn errors of metabolism are examples;
4. irreversible but nonprogressive conditions causing severe disability, such as severe cerebral palsy.

PROVIDING SERVICES FOR THE FAMILY

The overall needs for children and their families have been summarized in the Association for Children with life-threatening or terminal conditions and their families (ACT) Charter (Fig. 38.3).[102] These must be considered when planning and delivering palliative care services.

An increasing recognition of the need for pediatric palliative care services has resulted in an increase in the number of children's hospices and community teams and medical and nursing specialists providing these services.

- Every child shall be treated with dignity and respect and shall be afforded privacy whatever the child's physical or intellectual ability.
- Parents shall be acknowledged as the primary carers and involved as partners in all care and decisions involving their child.
- Every child shall be given the opportunity to participate in decisions affecting his or her care, according to age and understanding.
- An honest and open approach shall be the basis of all communication.
- Information shall be provided for the parent, the child, the siblings and other relatives, appropriate to age and understanding.
- The family home shall remain the center of caring whenever possible. Care away from home shall be provided in a child-centered environment by staff trained in the care of children.
- Every child shall have access to a 24-hour multidisciplinary children's palliative care team for flexible support in the home, and be in the care of a local pediatrician.
- Every child and family shall receive emotional, psychological and spiritual support to meet their needs. This shall begin at diagnosis and continue throughout the child's lifetime, death and in bereavement.
- Every family shall be entitled to a named keyworker who will enable the family to build up and maintain access to an appropriate network of support.
- Every family shall be given the opportunity of a consultation with a pediatric specialist who has particular knowledge of the child's condition.
- Every family shall have access to flexible short-term breaks (respite care) both in their own home and away from home, with appropriate children's nursing and medical support.
- Every child shall have access to education and other appropriate childhood activities.
- The needs of adolescents and young people shall be addressed and planned for well in advance.
- Every family shall have timely access to practical support, including clinical equipment, financial grants, suitable housing and domestic help.

Fig. 38.3   ACT Charter.[102]

LOCATION OF CARE

It is important that families are given choices as to where their child receives care. Many will prefer to care for their child at home,[103] whereas others will prefer hospital or hospice care. Families must be brought to a realistic expectation with regard to the needs of their child as their health deteriorates and the support that is available, particularly if they choose to be at home. They will also need access to advice and support 24 hours a day from professionals with palliative care expertise, or supported by professionals with this specialist knowledge. There should be sufficient flexibility to enable the family to move between home and/or hospice, as they choose, without care being compromised.

SYMPTOM MANAGEMENT

As parents frequently worry that their child will experience symptoms that will be difficult to control it is important to provide them with detailed and honest information about the management of their child's current and anticipated symptoms. Both they and their child need to take an active part in planning a practical and acceptable regimen of care, in order to instill a level of competence and confidence in controlling pain and discomfort and in understanding their child's management.

As death approaches parents will need and value further information, including knowledge of the possible modes of death and the physical signs that suggest death is imminent. Knowing what to expect and having a clear plan of action as the situation changes can enable families to cope better.

Almost all families can be reassured that death will be peaceful, but if there are concerns about the possibility of sudden distressing symptoms (such as convulsions, acute agitation, or bleeding) these should be discussed openly. Emergency drugs (e.g. anticonvulsants, analgesics and sedatives) should be accessible in suitable doses via appropriate routes.

PATTERN OF SYMPTOMS

Although many unpleasant and distressing symptoms are common to a number of different illnesses, their underlying cause (and therefore the approach to symptom management) may be different. For rare conditions anticipation of possible symptoms will require input from specialist pediatricians and nursing staff.

Children with malignant disease often have a relatively short final illness, lasting weeks or months, with pain from tumor progression as a predominant feature whereas in nonmalignant conditions onset may be more insidious with less prominence of pain and greater likelihood of muscle spasms, gastroesophageal reflux, seizures and respiratory distress.

ASSESSMENT OF SYMPTOMS

Thorough assessment of any symptom is essential before developing a plan of management. As much information as possible should be elicited, and this can be particularly challenging in nonverbal children and those with severe developmental impairment.[104] A range of tools are available to assess pain in children of different ages and developmental levels, but similar tools are not yet sufficiently developed to aid the assessment of other symptoms. Parents and carers should also be asked to contribute their observations to the assessment, as they will notice subtle changes that may not be apparent to health care professionals. Psychological and social factors affecting the child and family are often significant and should be considered as part of an assessment.

ROUTES OF DRUG ADMINISTRATION

The preferences of the child and family need to be taken into account. Taking a lot of medication can be difficult and complex regimens should be avoided. It is important to find the most acceptable route for the child and to be flexible to changing situations, such as a deteriorating swallow or an increasing reluctance to comply with medication regimens. Key issues in deciding routes of administration include:

- The oral route is often preferable and the child should be allowed to choose between liquids capsules and whole or crushed tablets.
- Long-acting preparations are more convenient and less intrusive.
- As the condition deteriorates the treatment plan often has to be simplified, routes of administration altered and priority given to those drugs that contribute most to the child's comfort.
- Some children prefer rectal medication to needles when the oral route is not possible and rectal preparations can also be helpful in the final hours when the child's level of consciousness has deteriorated.
- If parenteral drugs are needed they are usually given by continuous s.c. infusion, not as boluses. An i.v. line can be used if it is already in place. The transdermal route should also be considered.
- Intramuscular drugs are painful and should be avoided.

NON-DRUG MANAGEMENT

Adopting a holistic approach that addresses the psychological, social and spiritual concerns of the child and family is likely to achieve better symptom management than medication alone. Explaining the reason for the symptom agreeing a logical step-wise approach and reassuring the child and family that the situation is not going to be allowed to go 'out of control' are the foundations of successful management. Other measures that can be used alongside or in place of drug therapy include careful positioning of the child, maintaining a calm environment, distraction, imagery and relaxation techniques, play, art and music therapy.

PAIN

Pain management will include treating the underlying cause of the pain, where possible. For example, bony metastases may be treated with radiotherapy and painful muscle spasms with muscle relaxants rather than analgesics. Where treatment of the underlying cause is not possible, or does not relieve pain sufficiently, analgesics should be used alongside psychological and practical approaches. The WHO ladder of analgesia has been widely adopted, although recent evidence has shed some doubt on the routine use of codeine as up to 10% of the population may be poor metabolizers of the drug to morphine (the active metabolite). Poor efficacy is also a feature in infants because of immature enzyme systems.[105]

Opioid-sensitive pain
Strong opioids
These are used extensively in managing pain in pediatric palliative care. When prescribing strong opioids for children, the following points should be considered:
- long-acting morphine preparations are effective and convenient;
- short-acting preparations will be needed for breakthrough pain;
- where oral administration is difficult or impossible the use of transdermal patches (e.g. fentanyl) has proved invaluable;[106]
- sudden onset of severe pain may require break-through analgesia with a faster onset of action than oral morphine. Fentanyl lozenges, buccal or intranasal morphine may be appropriate in these situations.[107,108]
- studies of the pharmacokinetics of oral opioids and their metabolites suggest that in young children metabolism is more rapid than in adults and they may require relatively higher doses;
- neonates and children under 6 months old usually require a lower starting dose of opioids because of their reduced metabolism and increased sensitivity.[109]

Side-effects of opioids
Many doctors lack experience of using strong opioids in children, which can lead to unnecessary caution, underdosing and inadequate pain control. Respiratory depression with strong opioids is not usually a problem in children with severe pain and in general the side-effects from opioids tend

to be less marked than in adults. Nausea and vomiting are rare and routine anti-emetics are often not needed. Constipation is the most common side-effect of opiates and regular laxatives should always be prescribed.

Parents and children should be warned that they may become drowsy during the first few days of starting opioids but reassured that this will resolve. Itching usually responsive to antihistamines may also be a problem within the first few days. If either somnolence or pruritus remain troublesome, switching to an alternative preparation, such as fentanyl or hydromorphone is usually effective.[110]

Parental concerns about opioids

Parents may express concern that opioids will precipitate death, or worry that if they are started 'too early' they will lose efficacy as the illness and symptoms progress. Others find the transition to opioids difficult from a psychological and emotional perspective and that by agreeing to use opioids they are acknowledging that their child is going to die imminently.

Parental concerns require sensitive discussion and support. Parents must be assured that:

- their child will receive appropriate analgesia in the lowest dose needed to relieve pain;
- opioids do not precipitate death when used appropriately;
- there is no upper or ceiling dose for effective pain relief.

Musculoskeletal pain

Nonsteroidal anti-inflammatory drugs (NSAIDs) are often helpful for musculoskeletal pain, although caution is needed in the presence of bone marrow infiltration because of the increased risk of bleeding. Bisphosphonates should also be considered, particularly in children with long-term conditions associated with immobility, such as osteogenesis imperfecta.[111] Oral chemotherapy may be helpful in reducing tumor-related musculoskeletal pain.

Headaches in malignant disease

Headaches from central nervous system leukemia respond well to intrathecal methotrexate whereas those associated with raised intracranial pressure, are best managed with gradually increasing analgesics. Although steroids may seem helpful initially, the symptoms will inevitably recur as the tumor increases in size, necessitating increased doses of steroids with associated side-effects that almost always outweigh the benefits.[112]

Neuropathic pain

Neuropathic pain can often be helped by antiepileptic and antidepressant drugs. Ketamine can also be helpful, either orally or by continuous infusion.[113,114] For severe pain unresponsive to these drugs, intrathecal, epidural anesthesia and nerve blocks should be considered.

Muscle spasm and dystonia

These can be particularly problematic in children with neurological conditions and untreated can cause considerable pain and discomfort. An assessment of seating should be a priority as simple changes can have significant benefits. Muscle relaxants such as diazepam, baclofen and dantrolene may also be required.[115]

Gastro-esophageal reflux

A significant proportion of children with neurological impairment and/or disorders affecting muscle tone experience pain associated with gastro-esophageal reflux. Management should include a combination of approaches, such as attention to the feeding regimen, posture during and after feeds, as well as medical approaches including drugs to reduce acid production and to increase gastric emptying. Surgical management should also be considered for some children[116] (see Chapter 19: gastro- and hepatology chapter section GOR pp 605)

Nausea and vomiting

Nausea and vomiting can be a significant symptom in children with raised intracranial pressure and in a variety of other diseases causing metabolic disturbance or impaired gastrointestinal function. Anti-emetics

that work well in one situation (e.g. ondansetron in cancer patients undergoing chemotherapy) may be far less useful in other situations (e.g. cancer patients not having chemotherapy), so must be selected according to their site of action and the presumed cause of symptoms. This is summarized in Table 38.6.

Seizures

Children with neurodegenerative diseases often develop seizures as part of their ongoing disease with increasing problems in seizure control as the disease progresses. Other children may only develop seizures towards or during the terminal phase of their illness. Sudden acute onset of seizures can be treated with rectal diazepam or buccal midazolam.[117] Repeated severe or continuous seizures in a terminally ill child can be treated at home with a continuous subcutaneous infusion of midazolam and/or phenobarbitone.

Agitation and anxiety

Agitation and anxiety may reflect a child's need to talk about his or her fears and distress. Open communication should be encouraged throughout the child's illness, so that anxiety and fears can be addressed while the child is still able to communicate easily. If additional drugs are needed, benzodiazepines, haloperidol and levomepromazine can provide relief, especially in the final stages of life.

Respiratory symptoms

Dyspnea, cough, and excess secretions can all cause distress to children and anxiety for their parents. If the underlying cause of the symptom can be relieved, even temporarily, this may be appropriate. Palliative radiotherapy, for example, can bring good symptomatic relief to some children with primary or secondary thoracic tumors.

Breathlessness

Where treatment of the underlying cause is unlikely to be beneficial, symptom relief can be addressed by combining drugs with practical and supportive approaches. Fear is often an important element in dyspnea and reassurance and management of anxiety may help to relieve symptoms. Simple practical measures include finding the optimum body position, using a fan, and relaxation exercises. Opioids can help to relieve the sensation of breathlessness and small doses of sedatives, such as diazepam or midazolam, can relieve the associated anxiety.

Increasing hypoxemia may result in headaches, nausea, daytime drowsiness, and poor-quality sleep. Intermittent oxygen may help relieve these symptoms and can be given relatively easily at home.

Secretions

Excess secretions may occur during the terminal phase and are often a problem for children with chronic neurodegenerative diseases as they become less able to cough and swallow. Oral glycopyrronium bromide, or hyoscine hydrobromide (given transdermally or subcutaneously) can often help to reduce the secretions. For children in the terminal stage of an illness, altering the child's position to allow secretions to

Table 38.6   Medical management of nausea and vomiting

Cause of vomiting	Recommended drugs
Drug induced and metabolic	Haloperidol Levomepromazine Ondansetron
Poor gastric outflow	Metoclopramide Domperidone
Gastric outflow obstruction	Octreotide Hyoscine butylbromide
Raised intracranial pressure	Cyclizine Hyoscine Dexamethasone (in short courses of 3–5 d)

drain orally may provide temporary relief. Suction equipment may be helpful in some situations, but can stimulate increased production of secretions and also increase the burden of nursing care for the parents.

ANEMIA AND BLEEDING

The treatment of anemia by blood transfusion in the late stages of a child's life should only be used in the relief of symptoms.

Florid bleeding (e.g. severe hemoptysis or hematemesis) is extremely frightening for a child and their carers and when this occurs death is usually very rapid. If this is a serious risk both an analgesic and a sedative, such as morphine and midazolam should be readily available. In an emergency, parents can give these drugs by the buccal route and should repeat the dose every 15 min until the child is calm. Medication should be continued by continuous s.c. or i.v. infusion.

Many children with malignant diseases have widespread bone marrow infiltration and low platelets. Petechiae and minor gum bleeding are common although significant bleeding is unusual. Minor gum and nose bleeding can be managed by direct application of tranexamic acid to the bleeding point. Platelet transfusions should only be used to manage bleeding that is severe or that interferes with the child's quality of life.

IMPAIRED APPETITE AND POOR FEEDING

For many children, disease progression is associated with impaired appetite, which parents often find extremely distressing. For children, constant attempts by parents to encourage them to eat are similarly distressing.

Reasons for reduced feeding should be explored and reversible causes treated where possible. Assisted feeding, via a nasogastric tube or gastrostomy, may be necessary for children with slowly progressive disease, especially where this is associated with a declining ability to swallow but not a reduced appetite. For children with a poor appetite and rapidly progressive disease, nasogastric or gastrostomy feeding is usually inappropriate and can cause increased nausea and vomiting.

Where a child has a poor appetite or cannot tolerate amounts of food that parents consider acceptable, parents should be encouraged to relax nutritional goals and to provide only small amounts of food that the child enjoys, throughout the day. It is important to explain to parents that a reduced appetite is part of the disease progression and encouraging the child to eat more than they can manage may make them feel more unwell.

PSYCHOSOCIAL AND SPIRITUAL SUPPORT

All children and young people facing death or with a reduced life expectancy deserve help in maintaining as much normal life as possible, ensuring good access to play, education and social experiences and assistance in focusing on and achieving appropriate goals. A number of themes facing the sick child and family have been identified and these occur at diagnosis and then recur at different critical points throughout the course of the illness. Awareness and attention to these difficulties and common themes can provide valuable support for families:

- the need to be given appropriate information;
- the importance of enabling children and families to identify and express their emotions and spiritual needs;
- recognition that emotional and spiritual needs and ways of coping vary between different members of the family and at different times during the illness;
- awareness of the difficulty for families of living with uncertainty;
- acknowledging the benefits of and enabling open and honest communication both within families and between families and professionals;
- the value of empowering families and enabling them to retain choices and a sense of control.

For the parents and siblings of children with nonmalignant diseases, the prolonged time course and enormous nursing demands will increase the stress and practical difficulties. Throughout the course of a child's illness and death family members are likely to experience a huge range of feelings, such as sadness, despair, depression, hopelessness, anger, guilt, resentment of the sick child and isolation. Siblings often feel a sense of exclusion and neglect, although those who are very involved in caring for the sibling may also express positive experiences.[118,119]

Talking openly with families and with the sick child, however difficult, is usually helpful in reducing the child's level of anxiety and improving the family's later adjustment.[120] Most children are already aware, through their own interpretation of verbal and nonverbal cues, of much more about their illness and situation than most adults expect. Listening to their cues, exploring their fears and worries, responding honestly but gradually and using a range of nonverbal approaches (play, stories, art) are all skills that can help and which members of the multidisciplinary palliative care team can bring to the family and child.[121] Factors which need to be taken into account when talking with children include the child's age and developmental level, their likely understanding of their illness and of death, the child and family's past experiences and the family's normal communication pattern and culture.[122,123]

THE BEREAVED FAMILY

It is essential that the emotional support provided throughout the child's life is continued through the family's bereavement. The grief suffered after the loss of a child has been described as the most painful, enduring and difficult to survive and is associated with a high risk of pathological grief. Parents lose not only the child they have loved, but their hopes for the future and their confidence in themselves as parents. It puts an additional stress on their own relationship and alters the whole family structure. The brothers and sisters who are grieving may continue to feel isolated and neglected as their parents can spare little time or emotion for them. Ideally the professionals who know the family well and have been involved throughout the sick child's life should continue to be available through their bereavement. Grief is likely to continue over many years, and its depth and persistence is often underestimated. Parents value continuing contact with professionals who have known their child and the opportunity to talk about the child and their grief when others in the community expect them to 'have come to terms with it'.[124] This support, initially more frequent and gradually decreasing, helps facilitate the normal tasks of mourning. Most families will not need formal counseling but it is important to be able to recognize when there are signs of abnormal grief that may require referral for specialist help.

Helping to care for a child with a life-threatening illness, and for the family of such a child, is rarely easy. It presents many challenges both in terms of the professional tasks that may be required and to our own emotional resources. Though the task may seem daunting, families greatly value professionals who stay alongside them throughout their journey, providing practical help and support in an almost intolerable situation. Parents will have a lasting memory of their child's death and as professionals we have the opportunity to ensure this memory is as good as it can be.

CONCLUSION

Knowledge and skills in pain management and palliative care have been increasing in recent years. It will be essential to continue to these developments, to challenge misinformation and to work towards enhancing pain management and reducing suffering for children, throughout the world. Although little evidence-based information is available to date it is likely that employing the basic principles of pain and relief and control and good communication with children and families will ensure optimal management.

REFERENCES (* LEVEL 1 EVIDENCE)

1. Howard RF. Current status of pain management in children. JAMA 2003; 290:2464–2469.

2. Fitzgerald M. The development of nociceptive circuits. Nat Rev Neurosci 2005; 6:507–520.

3. Finley GA, McGrath PJ. Measurement of pain in infants and children. Seattle: IASP Press; 1998.

4. Clinical guidelines for the recognition and assessment of acute pain in children. London: Royal College of Nursing Institute; 1999.

5. Franck LS, Greenberg CS, Stevens B. Pain assessment in infants and children. Pediatr Clin North Am 2000; 47:487–512.

*6. Duhn LJ, Medves JM. A systematic integrative review of infant pain assessment tools. Adv Neonatal Care 2004; 4:126–140.

*7. Stinson JN, Kavanagh T, Yamada J, et al. Systematic review of the psychometric properties, interpretability and feasibility of self-report pain intensity measures for use in clinical trials in children and adolescents. Pain 2006; 125:143–157.

8. Breau LM, McGrath PJ, Camfield C, et al. Preliminary validation of an observational pain checklist for persons with cognitive impairments and inability to communicate verbally. Dev Med Child Neurol 2000; 42:609–616.

9. Hunt A, Goldman A, Seers K, et al. Clinical validation of the paediatric pain profile. Dev Med Child Neurol 2004; 46:9–18.

10. Varni JW, Thompson KL, Hanson V. The Varni/Thompson Pediatric Pain Questionnaire. I. Chronic musculoskeletal pain in juvenile rheumatoid arthritis. Pain 1987; 28:27–38.

11. Palermo TM, Witherspoon D, Valenzuela D, et al. Development and validation of the Child Activity Limitations Interview: a measure of pain-related functional impairment in school-age children and adolescents. Pain 2004; 109:461–470.

*12. von Baeyer CL, Spagrud LJ. Systematic review of observational (behavioral) measures of pain for children and adolescents aged 3 to 18 years. Pain 2007; 127:140–150.

13. Wong DL, Baker CM. Pain in children: comparison of assessment scales. Pediatr Nurs 1988; 14:9–17.

14. Hicks CL, von BCL, Spafford PA, et al. The Faces Pain Scale-Revised: toward a common metric in pediatric pain measurement. Pain 2001; 93:173–183.

15. Stanford EA, Chambers CT, Craig KD. The role of developmental factors in predicting young children's use of a self-report scale for pain. Pain 2006; 120:16–23.

16. Chambers CT, Craig KD. An intrusive impact of anchors in children's faces pain scales. Pain 1998; 78:27–37.

17. Hester NO. The preoperational child's reaction to immunizations. Nurs Res 1979; 28:250–255.

18. Chambers CT, Reid GJ, Craig KD, et al. Agreement between child and parent reports of pain. Clin J Pain 1998; 14:336–342.

19. Grunau RE, Oberlander T, Holsti L, et al. Bedside application of the Neonatal Facial Coding System in pain assessment of premature neonates. Pain 1998; 76:277–286.

20. McGrath PJ, Johnson G, Goodman JT, et al. CHEOPS: A behavioral scale for rating postoperative pain in children. Adv Pain Res Ther 1985; 9:395–402.

21. Merkel SI, Voepel-Lewis T, Shayevitz JR, et al. The FLACC: a behavioral scale for scoring postoperative pain in young children. Pediatr Nurs 1997; 23:293–227.

22. van Dijk M, Peters JW, van Deventer P, et al. The COMFORT Behavior Scale: a tool for assessing pain and sedation in infants. Am J Nurs 2005; 105:33–36.

23. Kolk AM, van Hoof R, Fiedeldij Dop MJ. Preparing children for venepuncture. The effect of an integrated intervention on distress before and during venepuncture. Child Care Health Dev 2000; 26:251–260.

24. Chen E, Joseph MH, Zeltzer L. Behavioral and cognitive interventions in the treatment of acute pain in children. Pediatr Clin North Am 2000; 47:513–525.

25. Liossi C, Hatira P. Clinical hypnosis in the alleviation of procedure-related pain in pediatric oncology patients. Int J Clin Exp Hypn 2003; 51:4–28.

26. Butler LD, Symons BK, Henderson SL, et al. Hypnosis reduces distress and duration of an invasive medical procedure for children. Pediatrics 2005; 115:e77–e85.

27. Rusy LM, Weisman SJ. Complementary therapies for acute pediatric pain management. Pediatr Clin North Am 2000; 47:589–599.

*28. Uman LS, Chambers CT, McGrath PJ, et al. Psychological interventions for needle-related procedural pain and distress in children and adolescents. Cochrane Database Syst Rev 2006; 4:CD005179.

29. Eccleston C, Yorke L, Morley S, et al. Psychological therapies for the management of chronic and recurrent pain in children and adolescents. Cochrane Database Syst Rev 2003; 1:CD003968.

30. Sherry DD, Wallace CA, Kelley C, et al. Short- and long-term outcomes of children with complex regional pain syndrome type I treated with exercise therapy. Clin J Pain 1999; 15:218–223.

31. Maillard SM, Davies K, Khubchandani R, et al. Reflex sympathetic dystrophy: a multidisciplinary approach. Arthritis Rheum 2004; 51:284–290.

32. Fitzgerald M, Howard RF. Schechter N L, Berde CB, Yaster M, eds. The neurobiologic basis of paediatric pain. In: 2nd edn. Philadelphia, PA: Lippincott Williams and Wilkins; 2003.19–42.

33. Koppert W, Wehrfritz A, Korber N, et al. The cyclooxygenase isozyme inhibitors parecoxib and paracetamol reduce central hyperalgesia in humans. Pain 2004; 108:148–153.

34. Bonnefont J, Daulhac L, Etienne M, et al. Acetaminophen recruits spinal p42/p44 MAPKs and GH/IGF-1 receptors to produce analgesia via the serotonergic system. Mol Pharmacol 2007; 71:407–415.

*35. Moore A, Collins S, Carroll D, et al. Single dose paracetamol (acetaminophen), with and without codeine, for postoperative pain. Cochrane Database Syst Rev 2000; CD001547.

36. Zhang WY, Li Wan Po A. Analgesic efficacy of paracetamol and its combination with codeine and caffeine in surgical pain – a meta-analysis. J Clin Pharm Ther 1996; 21:261–282.

37. Anderson B, Kanagasundarum S, Woollard G. Analgesic efficacy of paracetamol in children using tonsillectomy as a pain model. Anaesth Intensive Care 1996; 24:669–673.

38. Bean-Lijewski JD, Stinson JC. Acetaminophen or ketorolac for post myringotomy pain in children? A prospective, double-blinded comparison. Paediatr Anaesth 1997; 7:131–137.

*39. de Craen AJ, DiGiulio G, Lampe-Schoenmaeckers JE, et al. Analgesic efficacy and safety of paracetamol-codeine combinations versus paracetamol alone: a systematic review. BMJ 1996; 313:321–325.

40. Morton NS, O'Brien K. Analgesic efficacy of paracetamol and diclofenac in children receiving PCA morphine. Br J Anaesth 1999; 82:715–717.

41. Shah V, Taddio A, Ohlsson A. Randomised controlled trial of paracetamol for heel prick pain in neonates. Arch Dis Child Fetal Neonatal Ed 1998; 79:F209–F211.

42. Howard CR, Howard FM, Weitzman ML. Acetaminophen analgesia in neonatal circumcision: the effect on pain. Pediatrics 1994; 93:641–646.

43. Hynson JL, South M. Childhood hepatotoxicity with paracetamol doses less than 150 mg/kg per day. Med J Aust 1999; 171:497.

44. BNFC. The British National Formulary for Children. London: BMJ Publishing Group Ltd.; 2006.

45. Autret E, Dutertre JP, Breteau M, et al. Pharmacokinetics of paracetamol in the neonate and infant after administration of propacetamol chlorhydrate. Dev Pharmacol Ther 1993; 20:129–134.

46. Granry JC, Rod B, Monrigal JP, et al. The analgesic efficacy of an injectable prodrug of acetaminophen in children after orthopaedic surgery. Paediatr Anaesth 1997; 7:445–449.

47. Rod B, Monrigal JP, Lepoittevin L, et al. Treatment of postoperative pain in children in the recovery room. Use of morphine and propacetamol by the intravenous route. Cah Anesthesiol 1989; 37:525–530.

48. Lesko SM, Louik C, Vezina RM, et al. Asthma morbidity after the short-term use of ibuprofen in children. Pediatrics 2002; 109:E20.

49. Short JA, Barr CA, Palmer CD, et al. Use of diclofenac in children with asthma. Anaesthesia 2000; 55:334–337.

50. Clive DM, Stoff JS. Renal syndromes associated with nonsteroidal antiinflammatory drugs. N Engl J Med 1984; 310:563–572.

51. Robinson J, Malleson P, Lirenman D, et al. Nephrotic syndrome associated with nonsteroidal anti-inflammatory drug use in two children. Pediatrics 1990; 85:844–847.

52. Chan FK, Sung JJ. Role of acid suppressants in prophylaxis of NSAID damage. Best Pract Res Clin Gastroenterol 2001; 15:433–445.

*53. Rostom A, Wells G, Tugwell P, et al. The prevention of chronic NSAID induced upper gastrointestinal toxicity: a Cochrane collaboration metaanalysis of randomized controlled trials. J Rheumatol 2000; 27:2203–2214.

54. Kart T, Christrup LL, Rasmussen M. Recommended use of morphine in neonates, infants and children based on a literature review: Part 2 – Clinical use. Paediatr Anaesth 1997; 7:93–101.

55. Kart T, Christrup LL, Rasmussen M. Recommended use of morphine in neonates, infants and children based on a literature review: Part 1 – Pharmacokinetics. Paediatr Anaesth 1997; 7:5–11.

56. Hartley R, Levine MI. Opioid pharmacology in the newborn. In: Aynsley-Green A A, Ward Platt M P, AR L-T, eds. 3:3. London: Baillière Tindall; 1995.467–494.

57. Fahnenstich H, Steffan J, Kau N, Bartmann P. Fentanyl-induced chest wall rigidity and laryngospasm in preterm and term infants. Crit Care Med 2000; 28:836–839.

58. Streisand JB, Bailey PL, LeMaire L, et al. Fentanyl-induced rigidity and unconsciousness in human volunteers. Incidence, duration, and plasma concentrations. Anesthesiology 1993; 78:629–634.

59. William DG, Hatch DJ, Howard RF. Codeine phosphate in paediatric medicine. Br J Anaesth 2001; 86:413–421.

60. Williams DG, Patel A, Howard RF. Pharmacogenetics of codeine metabolism in an urban population of children and its implications for analgesic reliability. Br J Anaesth 2002; 89:839–845.

61. Kokki H, Rasanen I, Lasalmi M, et al. Comparison of oxycodone pharmacokinetics after buccal and sublingual administration in children. Clin Pharmacokinet 2006; 45:745–754.

62. Czarnecki ML, Jandrisevits MD, Theiler SC, et al. Controlled-release oxycodone for the management of pediatric postoperative pain. J Pain Symptom Manage 2004; 27:379–386.

63. Thompson DR. Narcotic analgesic effects on the sphincter of Oddi: a review of the data and

therapeutic implications in treating pancreatitis. Am J Gastroenterol 2001; 96:1266–1272.

64. Elia N, Tramer MR. Ketamine and postoperative pain – a quantitative systematic review of randomised trials. Pain 2005; 113:61–70.

65. Young C, Jevtovic-Todorovic V, Qin YQ, et al. Potential of ketamine and midazolam, individually or in combination, to induce apoptotic neurodegeneration in the infant mouse brain. Br J Pharmacol 2005; 146:189–197.

66. Howard RF. Planning for pain relief. In: Lindahl S G E, ed. Clinical anesthesiology: Pediatric anesthesia. London: Baillière Tindall; 1997.657–676.

67. Rose JB, Watcha MF. Postoperative nausea and vomiting in paediatric patients. Br J Anaesth 1999; 83:104–117.

68. Conroy JM, Othersen HBJ, Dorman BH, et al. A comparison of wound instillation and caudal block for analgesia following pediatric inguinal herniorrhaphy. J Pediatr Surg 1993; 28:565–567.

69. Markakis DA. Regional anesthesia in pediatrics. Anesthesiol Clin North America 2000; 18:355–381.

70. Esmail Z, Montgomery C, Courtrn C, et al. Efficacy and complications of morphine infusions in postoperative paediatric patients. Paediatr Anaesth 1999; 9:321–327.

71. Berde CB, Lehn BM, Yee JD, et al. Patient-controlled analgesia in children and adolescents: a randomized, prospective comparison with intramuscular administration of morphine for postoperative analgesia. J Pediatr 1991; 118:460–466.

72. Bray RJ, Woodhams AM, Vallis CJ, et al. Morphine consumption and respiratory depression in children receiving postoperative analgesia from continuous morphine infusion or patient controlled analgesia. Paediatr Anaesth 1996; 6:129–134.

73. Collins JJ, Geake J, Grier HE, et al. Patient-controlled analgesia for mucositis pain in children: a three-period crossover study comparing morphine and hydromorphone. J Pediatr 1996; 129:722–728.

74. Lloyd-Thomas AR, Howard RF. A pain service for children. Paediatric Anaesthesia 1994; 4:3–15.

75. Choonara I. Why do babies cry? We still know too little about what will ease babies' pain. BMJ 1999; 319:1381.

76. Lynn A, Nespeca MK, Bratton SL, et al. Clearance of morphine in postoperative infants during intravenous infusion: the influence of age and surgery. Anesth Analg 1998; 86:958–963.

77. Lynn AM, Nespeca MK, Opheim KE, et al. Respiratory effects of intravenous morphine infusions in neonates, infants, and children after cardiac surgery. Anesth Analg 1993; 77:695–701.

78. Bouwmeester NJ, van den Anker JN, Hop WC, et al. Age- and therapy-related effects on morphine requirements and plasma concentrations of morphine and its metabolites in postoperative infants. Br J Anaesth 2003; 90:642–652.

79. Anderson BJ, Woollard GA, Holford NH. A model for size and age changes in the pharmacokinetics of paracetamol in neonates, infants and children. Br J Clin Pharmacol 2000; 50:125–134.

80. Allegaert K, de Hoon J, Verbesselt R, et al. Intra- and interindividual variability of glucuronidation of paracetamol during repeated administration of propacetamol in neonates. Acta Paediatr 2005; 94:1273–1279.

81. van Lingen RA, Deinum HT, Quak CM, et al. Multiple-dose pharmacokinetics of rectally administered acetaminophen in term infants. Clin Pharmacol Ther 1999; 66:509–515.

82. Agrawal S, Fitzsimons JJ, Horn V, et al. Intravenous paracetamol for postoperative analgesia in a 4-day-old term neonate. Paediatr Anaesth 2007; 17:70–71.

83. Brisman M, Ljung BM, Otterbom I, et al. Methaemoglobin formation after the use of EMLA cream in term neonates. Acta Paediatr 1998; 87:1191–1194.

84. Taddio A, Ohlsson A, Einarson TR, et al. A systematic review of lidocaine-prilocaine cream (EMLA) in the treatment of acute pain in neonates. Pediatrics 1998; 101:E1.

85. Brady-Fryer B, Wiebe N, Lander J. Pain relief for neonatal circumcision. Cochrane Database Syst Rev 2004; 4:CD004217.

86. Stevens B, Yamada J, Ohlsson A. Sucrose for analgesia in newborn infants undergoing painful procedures. Cochrane Database Syst Rev 2004; 3:CD001069.

87. Bucher HU, Baumgartner R, Bucher N, et al. Artificial sweetener reduces nociceptive reaction in term newborn infants. Early Hum Dev 2000; 59:51–60.

88. Skogsdal Y, Eriksson M, Schollin J. Analgesia in newborns given oral glucose. Acta Paediatr 1997; 86:217–220.

89. Gradin M, Schollin J. The role of endogenous opioids in mediating pain reduction by orally administered glucose among newborns. Pediatrics 2005; 115:1004–1007.

90. Bellieni CV, Bagnoli F, Perrone S, et al. Effect of multisensory stimulation on analgesia in term neonates: a randomized controlled trial. Pediatr Res 2002; 51:460–463.

91. Shah PS, Aliwalas LI, Shah V. Breastfeeding or breast milk for procedural pain in neonates. Cochrane Database Syst Rev 2006; 3:CD004950.

92. Carbajal R, Veerapen S, Couderc S, et al. Analgesic effect of breast feeding in term neonates: randomised controlled trial. BMJ 2003; 326:313.

93. Carbajal R, Chauvet X, Couderc S, et al. Randomised trial of analgesic effects of sucrose, glucose, and pacifiers in term neonates. BMJ 1999; 319:1393–1397.

94. Tobias JD, Rasmussen GE. Pain management and sedation in the pediatric intensive care unit. Pediatr Clin North Am 1994; 41:1269–1292.

95. Dyke MP, Kohan R, Evans S. Morphine increases synchronous ventilation in preterm infants. J Paediatr Child Health 1995; 31:176–179.

96. Hickey PR, Hansen DD, Wessel DL, et al. Pulmonary and systemic hemodynamic responses to fentanyl in infants. Anesth Analg 1985; 64:483–486.

97. Palermo TM. Impact of recurrent and chronic pain on child and family daily functioning: a critical review of the literature. J Dev Behav Pediatr 2000; 21:58–69.

98. Yaster M, Kost-Byerly S, Maxwell LG. The management of pain in sickle cell disease. Pediatr Clin North Am 2000; 47:699–710.

99. Wilder RT. Management of pediatric patients with complex regional pain syndrome. Clin J Pain 2006; 22:443–448.

100. Finniss DG, Murphy PM, Brooker C, et al. Complex regional pain syndrome in children and adolescents. Eur J Pain 2006; 10:767–770.

101. Association for Children with Life-Threatening or Terminal Conditions and Their Families, and the Royal College of Paediatrics and Child Health. A guide to the development of children's palliative care services. London: RCPCH; 2003.

102. Association for Children with Life-Threatening or Terminal Conditions and their Families. ACT Charter. 1998. www.act.org.uk/dmdocuments/act_charter.pdf

103. Goldman A. Care of the dying child. Oxford: Oxford University Press; 1994.

104. Hunt A, Mastroyannopoulou K, Goldman A, et al. Not knowing – the problem of pain in children with severe neurological impairment. Int J Nurs Stud 2003; 40:171–183.

105. Williams DG, Hatch DJ, Howard RF. Codeine phosphate in paediatric medicine. Br J Anaesth 2001; 86:421–427.

106. Hunt A, Goldman A, Devine T, et al. Transdermal fentanyl for pain relief in a paediatric palliative care population. Palliat Med 2001; 15:405–412.

107. Wheeler M, Birmingham PK, Dsida RM, et al. Uptake pharmacokinetics of the Fentanyl Oralet in children scheduled for central venous access removal: implications for the timing of initiating painful procedures. Paediatr Anaesth 2002; 12:594–599.

108. Fitzgibbon D, Morgan D, Dockter D, et al. Initial pharmacokinetic, safety and efficacy evaluation of nasal morphine gluconate for breakthrough pain in cancer patients. Pain 2003; 106:309–315.

109. McGrath P, Brown S, Collins J. Paediatric palliative medicine. In: Oxford Textbook of palliative medicine, 3rd edn Oxford: Oxford University Press; 2004.775–797.

110. Goodarzi M. Comparison of epidural morphine, hydromorphone and fentanyl for postoperative pain control in children undergoing orthopaedic surgery. Paediatr Anaesth 1999; 9:419–422.

111. Devogelaer JP, Coppin C. Osteogenesis imperfecta: current treatment options and future prospects. Treat Endocrinol 2006; 5:229–242.

112. Watterson G, Goldman A, Michalski A. Corticosteroids in the palliative phase of peadiatric brain tumours. Arch Dis Child 2002; 86:A76.

113. Fitzgibbon EJ, Viola R. Parenteral ketamine as an analgesic adjuvant for severe pain: development and retrospective audit of a protocol for a palliative care unit. J Palliat Med 2005; 8:49–57.

114. Kronenberg RH. Ketamine as an analgesic: parenteral, oral, rectal, subcutaneous, transdermal and intranasal administration. J Pain Palliat Care Pharmacother 2002; 16:27–35.

115. Krach LE. Pharmacotherapy of spasticity: oral medications and intrathecal baclofen. J Child Neurol 2001; 16:31–36.

116. Hassall E. Decisions in diagnosing and managing chronic gastroesophageal reflux disease in children. J Pediatr 2005; 146:S3–S12.

117. Scott RC, Besag FM, Neville BG. Buccal midazolam and rectal diazepam for treatment of prolonged seizures in childhood and adolescence: a randomised trial. Lancet 1999; 353:623–626.

118. Foster C, Eiser C, Oades P, et al. Treatment demands and differential treatment of patients with cystic fibrosis and their siblings: patient, parent and sibling accounts. Child Care Health Dev 2001; 27:349–364.

119. Pettle Michael SA, Lansdown RG. Adjustment to the death of a sibling. Arch Dis Child 1986; 61:278–283.

120. Whittam EH. Terminal care of the dying child. Psychosocial implications of care. Cancer 1993; 71:3450–3462.

121. Wellings T. Drawings by dying and bereaved children. Paediatr Nurs 2001; 13:30–36.

122. Bluebond-Langner M. The private worlds of the dying child. Princeton: Princeton University Press; 1978.

123. Stevens M. Psychological adaptation of the dying child, 3rd edn. Oxford: Oxford University Press; 2004.775–797.

124. Laakso H, Paunonen-Ilmonen M. Mothers' experience of social support following the death of a child. J Clin Nurs 2002; 11:176–185.

Appendix

Anne Green, Rachel Webster, IA Auchterlonie, Anita MacDonald

REFERENCE RANGES FOR BIOCHEMICAL LABORATORY TESTS

INTRODUCTION

It is important to note that there are no internationally accepted worldwide reference ranges available for laboratory data. It should also be noted that it is difficult for individual laboratories to collect their own data on 'normal' subjects for ethical and logistical reasons. This problem is highlighted particularly with neonatal and pediatric reference ranges and hence many of the data available today still originate from historical studies. There are many variables which affect particular biochemical parameters and must be considered before specific data from an individual patient can be reliably used. These variables are summarized below as a prompt when considering reference data. The values detailed in this chapter are therefore a **guide only** to interpreting laboratory data for neonates, infants and children and must never be considered as absolute. They apply to the specific laboratory methods used by the individual laboratories and centers from which the assembled data has been sourced and will not necessarily apply to methods used in other laboratories.

In addition to reference ranges, many laboratories have defined 'action limits' for a number of analytes, e.g. sodium, potassium, glucose, calcium and C-reactive protein (CRP). Action limits are usually concentrations which could indicate medical emergencies and therefore need acting on promptly; values are usually agreed between laboratories and medical staff in individual units. The laboratory will usually have in place a telephoning protocol to the clinician in charge of that patient. Action limits should be differentiated from reference ranges.

Methodology

Measurement of an analyte using different technologies may significantly affect the result and hence reference ranges. This is because different methods use different characteristics of a compound to quantify the amount: this may be a chemical reaction with another molecule to produce a product which can be measured, an immunological feature or parameters based on fluorescence, light absorption or electrical activity. For example, sodium can be measured using the principle of light absorption by flame photometry or electrical activity by ion selective electrodes (ISEs). Values derived from ISEs are lower than those from flame photometry. Interference from other molecules is another factor which may be a problem for some methods used – such an example is interference by ketones in creatinine measurement. Bilirubin measurement may be interfered with by hemoglobin in some methods and therefore capillary blood samples, in which there is a greater risk of hemolysis compared to venous samples, require special attention when choosing a suitable method. Due attention must be given when a patient is referred from one hospital or clinic to another if laboratories use different analytical methods. In such circumstances apparent differences in the value of analytes may be due to the different methodologies and not to physiological changes.

Neonatal reference ranges

Providing reference range data for the neonatal period is even more difficult than for other age ranges in view of the number of physiological processes that the newborn undergoes. The birth process and subsequent rapid growth and maturation result in significant changes during the first four weeks of life for many analytes such as cortisol, TSH and thyroxine, which are all elevated immediately after birth in order to provide the newborn with the hormonal stimulation it requires to adapt to life outside the womb. Biochemical changes are also seen with different feeding regimens. Two notable examples include higher values of urea in bottle fed compared with breast fed infants, and significant differences in some amino acid levels associated with the use of formula milks.

Patient variables

Reference range data can also differ between gender, gestation, age and ethnicity. There can be marked differences in values for certain analytes, obvious examples between male and female being hormones, and differences across age range are highlighted by alkaline phosphatase. It must therefore be remembered that the cohorts of patients used to derive the reference ranges detailed in this chapter may not directly relate to the population from which the individual patient under consideration has been drawn. Where significant differences occur this has been annotated in the tables with specific text.

Specimen type

The specimen type used in the collection of the reference range data is stated in the tables where appropriate. The use of different types (plasma vs. serum) or anticoagulants (lithium heparin vs. EDTA) can greatly affect the results obtained by certain methodologies and this must be taken into account. For some analytes, such as glucose, triglycerides and amino acids, fasting is of particular importance. These features are noted in the tables where relevant.

Measurement and units

In this chapter, reference values are generally given in SI units and, where considered appropriate, a conversion factor has been given to convert from weight units. This is the number by which weight units need to be multiplied in order to convert weight units into SI (Système International d'Unités) units.

The SI unit of quantity is the mole (the molecular weight of a substance expressed in grams) and the unit of volume is the liter, therefore the SI unit used in these tables is moles/Liter or mol/L. Smaller multiples of this SI unit are generally used to convert the figure into a whole number or to reduce decimal points:

Millimole/L (mmol/L) $\times$) 10^{-3}
Micromole/L (µmol/L) $\times$) 10^{-6}
Nanomole/L (nmol/L) $\times$) 10^{-9}
Picomole/L (pmol/L) $\times$) 10^{-12}

LABORATORY REFERENCE VALUES

For enzyme measurements, where the weight and therefore molarity is often unknown, activity is measured rather than the absolute quantity of the enzyme. The International Union of Biochemistry recommended in 1964 that enzymes should be expressed in international units (IU). In this scheme 1 IU is the amount of enzyme that will catalyze the transformation of 1 micromole of substrate per minute. In addition to IU of measurement, units/liter or U/L is now in common use.

Data interpretation

The correct interpretation of laboratory results from an individual patient can only be carried out with adequate liaison with the local laboratory which should be able to provide the appropriate reference ranges taking into consideration the patient variables, methodology and sample type used.

The ranges provided in this chapter are based on literature sources, our own studies, unpublished data from specialist groups, and in some cases a combination of sources.[1-36]

Key: y = year
     m = month
     d = day

Table A.1   Blood and plasma reference ranges (common 20 analytes)

Analyte	Age	Reference range		Weight unit (where applicable)	Conversion factor	Comments
Alanine aminotransferase (ALT)	Neonate Infants Children	0–40 U/L 10–80 U/L 10–40 U/L				Gross hemolysis will cause false elevation
Alkaline phosphatase (ALP)	Preterm Neonate Infants 2–5 y 6–7 y 8–9 y 10–11 y 12–13 y 14–15 y 16–18 y	Up to 1500 U/L Up to 700 U/L 250–1000 U/L 250–850 U/L 250–1000 U/L 250–750 U/L *Male* 250–730 U/L 275–875 U/L 170–970 U/L 125–720 U/L	*Female* 250–950 U/L 200–730 U/L 170–460 U/L 75–270 U/L			Alkaline phosphatase activity changes markedly through life and reference ranges are highly method dependent. These ranges should be used as a guide only and you should refer to your local laboratory for their reference ranges
Ammonia	Neonate Infants/ children Preterm or sick neonate	< 100 µmol/L < 40 µmol/L < 150 µmol/L		µg/100 ml	0.54	Venous samples are preferred. Capillary concentrations are generally higher. Venous ranges are shown
Aspartate aminotransferase (AST)	Neonate Infants Children	< 120 U/L < 80 U/L 15–50 U/L				Gross hemolysis will cause false elevation
Bilirubin, total	Neonate 2–6 d Neonate 6–10 d > 1 m	Up to 217 µmol/L Up to 230 µmol/L 1.7–26 µmol/L		mg/100 ml	17.1	
Bilirubin, unconjugated	0–10 d 11 d–20 y	10–180 µmol/L 3–17 µmol/L				Conjugated and unconjugated values are method dependent; older methods may measure direct and indirect bilirubin which is different

Analyte	Age	Reference range		Weight unit (where applicable)	Conversion factor	Comments
Calcium	0–5 d 5 d – 1 y 2–5 y > 5 y	1.95–2.75 mmol/L 2.15–2.75 mmol/L 2.15–2.65 mmol/L 2.20–2.60 mmol/L		mg/100 ml	0.25	Interpretation of calcium concentration should take into account the albumin concentration as hypoalbuminemia reduces the total calcium concentration. An equation for 'adjusted calcium', which takes into account the albumin concentration, should be available from your local hospital
Chloride		95–106 mmol/L		mEq/L	1	
Cholesterol	Birth 1 w 1–3 y 4–6 y 7–9 y 10–11 y 12–13 y 14–15 y	0.5–3.2 mmol/L 1.7–4.2 mmol/L 1.2–4.7 mmol/L 2.8–4.8 mmol/L 2.9–5.3 mmol/L *Male* 3.3–6.0 mmol/L 3.3–6.0 mmol/L 2.8–5.8 mmol/L	*Female* 3.3–6.3 mmol/L 3.3–5.6 mmol/L 3.4–5.6 mmol/L	mg/100 ml	0.026	Cholesterol rises rapidly after birth and levels are higher when fed on human rather than cows' milk
Cortisol	At 9 am At midnight	180–550 nmol/L < 130 nmol/L		μg/100 ml	27.6	Stress raises cortisol levels. Cortisol levels are lower in neonates but reach near adult levels by 2 m of age. Hydrocortisone and prednisolone cross react with many assays, but dexamethasone generally does not
Creatine kinase (CK)	Newborn Infant 4–6 y 7–9 y 10–11 y 12–13 y 14–15 y 16–19 y	160–1230 U/L 60–305 U/L *Male* 75–230 U/L 60–365 U/L 55–215 U/L 60–330 U/L 60–335 U/L 55–370 U/L	 *Female* 75–230 U/L 60–365 U/L 80–230 U/L 50–295 U/L 50–240 U/L 45–230 U/L			Activity increases after exercise or muscle trauma
Creatinine	Neonate > 1 m and up to 2 y Up to 5 y 5 y and over	20–100 μmol/L 20–60 μmol/L 20–70 μmol/L 20–80 μmol/L		mg/100 ml	88.4	Levels rise gradually with age, are dependent on muscle mass and are very method dependent. Values shown are based on a Jaffe method and should be used as a guide only. Contact your local laboratory for its method-related reference ranges
Glucose	Neonate 12–24 h 25–48 h 4–7 d Over 7 d	 2.4–5.4 mmol/L 2.9–5.2 mmol/L 3.2–5.9 mmol/L 3.9–6.0 mmol/L		mg/100 ml	0.055	Symptomatic hypoglycemia is usually associated with concentrations < 2.5 mmol/L. It is recommended that fasting glucose results > 6.0 mmol/L should be further investigated by WHO criteria. Ranges shown are for a fasting sample
γ-Glutamyl-transferase (γGT)	Newborns Infants Children	< 200 U/L < 120 U/L < 35 U/L				
Magnesium	Neonate > 1 m	0.48–1.05 mmol/L 0.6–0.95 mmol/L		mg/100 ml	0.411	
Osmolality		275–295 mmol/kg		mosmol/kg	1	
Phosphate	Neonate 1–3 y 4–6 y 7–11 y 12–13 y 14–15 y 16–19 y	1.55–2.65 mmol/L 1.25–2.10 mmol/L 1.3–1.75 mmol/L 1.20–1.80 mmol/L 1.05–1.75 mmol/L 0.95–1.75 mmol/L 0.90–1.50 mmol/L		mg/100 ml	0.323	Hemolysis and capillary samples give elevated results

(Continued)

Table A.1 Blood and plasma reference ranges (common 20 analytes)—Cont'd

Analyte	Age	Reference range		Weight unit (where applicable)	Conversion factor	Comments
Potassium	Neonate 1 w – 1 m 1–6 m 6 m – 1 y > 1 y	3.2–5.5 mmol/L 3.4–6.0 mmol/L 3.5–5.6 mmol/L 3.5–5.1 mmol/L 3.3–4.6 mmol/L		mEq/L	1	Hemolysis and delayed separation can give falsely elevated results. Ranges shown are for venous samples
Total protein	Neonate 1–3 y > 3 y	54–70 g/L 60–70 g/L 60–80 g/L		g/100 ml	10.0	
Triglyceride	1–3 y 4–6 y 7–9 y *Male* 10–11 y 12–13 y 14–15 y	0.33–1.48 mmol/L 0.38–1.38 mmol/L 0.34–1.53 mmol/L 0.28–1.63 mmol/L 0.28–1.72 mmol/L 0.40–1.95 mmol/L	*Female* 0.46–1.66 mmol/L 0.44–1.54 mmol/L 0.43–1.60 mmol/L	mg/100 ml	0.011	Ranges shown are for a fasting sample
Sodium	Neonate > 1 m	132–145 mmol/L 135–145 mmol/L		mEq/L	1	Pseudohyponatremia can occur due to gross lipemia or hypoproteinemia when indirect ISE and flame photometry methods are used
Standard bicarbonate	Newborns > 1 m	18–25 mmol/L 21–25 mmol/L		mEq/L	1	
Urea		2.5–6.6 mmol/L		mg/100 ml	0.357	Values in neonates and breast-fed infants may be lower

Table A.2 Blood and plasma reference ranges

Analyte	Age	Reference ranges		Comments
Albumin	Newborn	25–50 g/L		Albumin concentrations in the preterm infant are *normally* lower than in the term infant and are not indicative of protein deficiency
	1 y	35–50 g/L		
	4 y and older	37–50 g/L		
Adrenocorticotropic hormone (ACTH)		< 46 ng/L		There is diurnal variation with levels being higher in the morning. Samples should be taken at 10 am with a serum cortisol
Aldosterone	Infants	165–2930 pmol/L		Patients should be on a normal salt diet and recumbent before blood collection
	1–4 y	70–950 pmol/L		
	5–9 y	30–620 pmol/L		
	10–15 y	70–580 pmol/L		
Amino acids		(µmol/L)		Many laboratories perform qualitative amino acid investigations looking for an abnormal pattern before undertaking quantitative investigation
Taurine		20–120		These are approximate ranges for children and are only a guide; values for the neonate and infant will differ
Aspartic acid		1.0–20		Reference values will vary with age and feeding/fasting states – consult your specialized laboratory
Threonine		40–200		
Serine		70–200		
Asparagine		15–85		
Glutamic acid		15–80		
Glutamine		330–810		
Proline		40–330		
Glycine		110–340		
Alanine		120–600		
Citrulline		10–50		
Valine		130–350		
Cystine		25–70		
Methionine		5.0–40		
Isoleucine		30–100		
Leucine		50–200		
Tyrosine		30–100		
Phenylalanine		25–100		
Ornithine		20–135		
Lysine		70–270		
Histidine		45–120		
Arginine		10–110		
Amylase	Neonates	< 50 U/L		
	> 1 m	30–100 U/L		
Androstenedione	Neonates	1.3–16.5 nmol/L		
	Prepubertal	2.0–4.2 nmol/L		
	Post puberty: male	2.8–10.5 nmol/L		
	Post puberty: female	1.7–12.9 nmol/L		
α1-antitrypsin		1.8–4.0 g/L		α1-antitrypsin is an acute phase protein
Base excess		± 2.5–2.5 mmol/L		
Bicarbonate or total CO_2	Neonates	18–23 mmol/L		
	> 1 m	20–26 mmol/L		
PCO_2		4.7–6.0 kPa		
Carboxyhemoglobin		Up to 1.5% of total Hb		
Carotenes		0.9–3.7 µmol/L		
Catecholamines (plasma)				
Noradrenaline		591–2364 pmol/L	Supine	
		1773–5320 pmol/L	Standing	
Adrenaline		< 382 pmol/L	Supine	
		< 546 pmol/L	Standing	
Dopamine		< 196 pmol/L	Supine and standing	
Ceruloplasmin	< 4 m	0.09–0.27 g/L		
	4 m – 1 y	0.14–0.41 g/L		
	1–10 y	0.24–0.47 g/L		
	10–13 y	0.18–0.27 g/L		
	> 13 y	0.24–0.71 g/L		

(Continued)

Table A.2   Blood and plasma reference ranges—Cont'd

Analyte	Age	Reference ranges		Comments
Copper	0–5 d	1.4–7.2 µmol/L		
	5 d – 6 m	4.0–11.0 µmol/L		
	>6 m	11.0–22 µmol/L		
Dehydroepiandrosterone sulfate (DHAS)		*Male*	*Female*	
	1–3 y	0.2–0.6 µmol/L	0.2–2.1 µmol/L	
	4–6 y	0.1–5.1 µmol/L	0.2–1.0 µmol/L	
	7–8 y	0.3–2.6 µmol/L	0.4–1.9 µmol/L	
	9–10 y	0.4–2.0 µmol/L	0.4–4.3 µmol/L	
	11 y	0.5–4.1 µmol/L	0.4–2.7 µmol/L	
	12 y	0.5–9.4 µmol/L	0.8–4.8 µmol/L	
	13 y	0.6–6.6 µmol/L	0.6–4.5 µmol/L	
	14 y	0.5–7.8 µmol/L	0.8–8.2 µmol/L	
	15 y	1.6–8.4 µmol/L	1.1–7.8 µmol/L	
	16 y	1.3–9.7 µmol/L	1.6–9.6 µmol/L	
Estradiol				Estradiol levels in children should only be interpreted on an individual patient basis. Reference ranges are therefore not quoted. Refer to your local laboratory for interpretation and guidance
α1-fetoprotein	>8 m	< 10 KIU/L		Falls with time and should be less than 10 KU/L by 8 m. Since a single AFP result is difficult to interpret, it is advisable to repeat the test in 2–3 weeks to look for an appropriate fall in concentration
Follicle-stimulating hormone (FSH)		*Male*	*Female*	Girls at menarche show similar typical cycle variation to adult females
	0–15 d	< 1 IU/L	0.2–3.0 IU/L	
	15 d – 6 y	0.2–3.0 IU/L	0.2–6.0 IU/L	
	7–10 y	0.2–4.0 IU/L		
	10–14 y	0.5–7.0 IU/L		
	Follicular		2–24.0 IU/L	
	Mid-cycle		0.6–11.0 IU/L	
	Luteal		0.6–9.0 IU/L	
Free fatty acids		100–300 µmol/L	If FFA > 1000 FFA:3HB < 2	Fasting sample
3-hydroxy butyrate		0–300 µmol/L		Fasting sample
Galactose-1-phosphate		Not detected in normal children Treated galactosemics < 150 µmol/L Untreated > 1000 µmol/L		
Growth hormone (GH)	Insulin stress test	> 17 mIU/L		Random GH is of little value. Provocative tests should be used
	GTT	< 1.0 mIU/L		
HBA1c		4.7–7.9% of total Hb		
Haptoglobins		0.3–2.0 g/L		
17 hydroxyprogesterone	Infants (unstressed)	< 13 nmol/L		There is a rapid fall from very high levels of 17-OHP (maternal source) in the first 24–48 h of life making interpretation difficult. Premature and sick infants also have 2–3 fold higher levels of 17-OHP compared with values quoted for full term well infants. Concentrations in neonates with untreated CAH are usually > 60 nmol/L
	Infants (stressed)	< 40 nmol/L		
25 OH Vitamin D		12.5–75 nmol/L		
1,25-dihydroxy vitamin D		48–120 pmol/L		

Analyte	Age	Reference ranges		Comments
Immunoglobulins				
IgG	Neonates	6.5–14.5 g/L		
	1–3 m	2.0–6.5 g/L		
	4–6 m	1.5–8.0 g/L		
	1 y	3.0–12.0 g/L		
	3 y and older	5.0–15.0 g/L		
IgA	Neonates	0–0.1 g/L		
	1–3 m	0.05–0.4 g/L		
	4–6 m	0.1–0.6 g/L		
	1 y	0.2–0.8 g/L		
	3 y and older	0.3–3.0 g/L		
IgM	Neonates	0–0.3 g/L		
	1–3 m	0.1–1.0 g/L		
	4–6 m	0.1–1.0 g/L		
	1 y	0.4–2.0 g/L		
	3 y and older	0.4–2.0 g/L		
Insulin				Insulin cannot be interpreted without a paired glucose and c-peptide result. Please refer to your local laboratory for guidance
Iron	0–4 w	10–30.0 µmol/L		The value of plasma iron is of little value in the investigation of iron deficiency as there is much within-individual variation. In addition, many conditions such as infection, trauma and chronic inflammation are associated with low plasma iron concentration but normal total body iron stores
	4 w–5 y	5–25.0 µmol/L		
	6–9 y	7–25.0 µmol/L		
		Male	*Female*	
	10–14 y	5–24.0 µmol/L	8–26.0 µmol/L	
	15–19 y	6–29.0 µmol/L	5–33.0 µmol/L	
Iron-binding capacity		*Male*	*Female*	
	1–5 y	48–79 µmol/L	48–79 µmol/L	
	6–9 y	43–91 µmol/L	43–91 µmol/L	
	10–14 y	54–91 µmol/L	57–103 µmol/L	
	14–19 y	52–102 µmol/L	52–101 µmol/L	
Lactate (plasma)	Neonates	Up to 3.0 mmol/L		Plasma lactate measurements are usually carried out as part of a timed profile and need to be interpreted with respect to glucose and other metabolites. CSF lactate: plasma lactate ratio should be calculated if a respiratory chain defect is suspected
	>1 m	1.0–1.8 mmol/L		
Lactate dehydrogenase	0–5 d	730–1650 U/L		
	1–3 y	400–720 U/L		
	4–6 y	375–700 U/L		
	7–9 y	335–590 U/L		
		Male	*Female*	
	10–11 y	345–550 U/L	305–605 U/L	
	12–13 y	375–590 U/L	305–505 U/L	
	14–15 y	290–570 U/L	315–460 U/L	
	16–19 y	275–525 U/L	275–525 U/L	
Lead		<0.5 µmol/L		
Luteinizing hormone (LH)		*Male*	*Female*	
	0–15 d	<1 I/U	<1 I/U	
	15 d–10 y	0.7–2.2 I/U	0.7–2.2 I/U	
	10–13 y	0.3–5.0 I/U		
	13–60 y	0.5–8.0 I/U		
	Follicular		1–11.0 I/U	
	Mid-cycle		15–96 I/U	
	Luteal		1–11.0 I/U	
Oxygen saturation	Umbilical artery	0.32%		
	Umbilical vein	26–73%		
	Children	86–101%		
	Newborns	30–80%		
	Older children	60–85%		

(Continued)

Table A.2 Blood and plasma reference ranges—Cont'd

Analyte	Age	Reference ranges		Comments
Parathyroid hormone (PTH)	2–15 y	13–29 ng/L		Intact PTH ranges
	> 16 y	12–65.0 ng/L		
pH		7.35–7.45		
PO$_2$	Neonates	9.3–13.3 kPa		
	> 1 m	11.3–14.0 kPa		
Progesterone	Male	< 2 nmol/L		
	Female	< 90 nmol/L		
Prolactin	Neonates	< 4000 mU/L		Values may rise to above the quoted ranges in response to stress
	Children	60–390 mU/L		
Renin	0–6 d	2.8–79.0 nmol/L/h		Values shown are for a recumbent patient on a normal sodium diet
	6 d – 1 y	6.4–27.2 nmol/L/h		
	2–4 y	1.5–22.6 nmol/L/h		
	5–9 y	1.8–7.2 nmol/L/h		
	10–15 y	0.7–7.8 nmol/L/h		
Testosterone	1–6 d	2.0–7.0 nmol/L	Male	
	1–9 w	< 13 nmol/L	Male	
	9–12 w	Up to 3.5 nmol/L	Male	
	12–16 w	10.0–30.0 nmol/L	Male	
	Prepubertal > 16 w	< 1 nmol/L	Male	
	Pubertal stage 2	< 8 nmol/L	Male	
	Pubertal stage 3	1.0–18 nmol/L	Male	
	Pubertal stage 4/5	4.5–25 nmol/L	Male	
	Female	< 3.5 nmol/L		
Thyroid stimulating hormone (TSH)	0–5 d	0.5–7.9 mU/L		
	5 d – 9 y	0.4–3.5 mU/L		
	10–13 y male	0.4–3.5 mU/L		
	10–13 y female	0.6–4.8 mU/L		
	14–15 y	0.4–3.5 mU/L		
	> 15 y	0.5–5.0 mU/L		
Free T4	0–5 d	21–52 pmol/L		
	5 d – 11 y	12.0–25 pmol/L		
	12–18 y	11.0–22 pmol/L		
	> 18 y	10.0–24 pmol/L		
Free T3	1–15 d	3.0–15.0 pmol/L		
	15 d – 12 y	3.6–8.5 pmol/L		
	13–19 y	3.7–7.3 pmol/L		
	> 19 y	2.7–6.5 pmol/L		
Uric acid		*Male*	*Female*	
	1–3 y	105–300 μmol/L	105–300 μmol/L	
	4–6 y	130–280 μmol/L	130–280 μmol/L	
	7–9 y	120–295 μmol/L	120–295 μmol/L	
	10–11 y	135–320 μmol/L	180–280 μmol/L	
	12–13 y	160–400 μmol/L	180–345 μmol/L	
	14–15 y	140–465 μmol/L	180–345 μmol/L	
	16–19 y	235–510 μmol/L	180–350 μmol/L	
Vitamin A	1–6 y	0.7–1.5 μmol/L		
	7–12 y	0.9–1.7 μmol/L		
	13–19 y	0.9–2.5 μmol/L		
Vitamin E	Newborn infants	5–14 μmol/L		
	2 y and older	12–28 μmol/L		
Zinc	Children	11.0–24.0 μmol/L		

Table A.3 Normal constituents of urine

Analyte	Age	Reference ranges			Comments
Amino acids					Urine amino acid concentrations vary widely with age, with high concentrations in the neonatal period and early infancy. Concentrations fall particularly over the first 6 months as the renal tubules mature
					Many laboratories perform qualitative amino acid investigations looking for an abnormal pattern before undertaking quantitative investigation
δ-aminolevulinic acid		< 5.2 μmol/mmol Creat			
Calcium	< 7 m	< 2.4 mmol/mmol Creat			These values refer to a random, spot urine taken when the overnight urine has been voided
	7–18 m	< 1.7 mmol/mmol Creat			
	19 m – 6 y	< 1.2 mmol/mmol Creat			
	> 6 y	< 0.7 mmol/mmol Creat			
Catecholamines		*Noradrenaline*	*Dopamine*	*HMMA*	These values refer to a random, spot urine
	0–6 m	0.32 mmol/mol Creat	2.2 mmol/mmol Creat	19 mmol/mmol Creat	
	6 m – 1 y	0.3 mmol/mol Creat	2 mmol/mmol Creat	16 mmol/mmol Creat	
	12–18 m	0.25 mmol/mmol Creat	1.8 mmol/mmol Creat	14 mmol/mmol Creat	
	18 m – 2 y	0.2 mmol/mmol Creat	1.6 mmol/mmol Creat	12 mmol/mmol Creat	
	2–3 y	0.17 mmol/mmol Creat	1.4 mmol/mmol Creat	11 mmol/mmol Creat	
	3–4 y	0.14 mmol/mmol Creat	1.25 mmol/mmol Creat	9 mmol/mmol Creat	
	4–5 y	0.125 mmol/mmol Creat	1.05 mmol/mmol Creat	8 mmol/mmol Creat	
	5–6 y	0.11 mmol/mmol Creat	0.9 mmol/mmol Creat	7 mmol/mmol Creat	
	6–8 y	0.09 mmol/mmol Creat	0.75 mmol/mmol Creat	6.5 mmol/mmol Creat	
	8–10 y	0.085 mmol/mmol Creat	0.65 mmol/mmol Creat	6 mmol/mmol Creat	
	10–12 y	0.08 mmol/mmol Creat	0.55 mmol/mmol Creat	5 mmol/mmol Creat	
	12–14 y	0.075 mmol/mmol Creat	0.5 mmol/mmol Creat	4.5 mmol/mmol Creat	
	14–16 y	0.07 mmol/mmol Creat	0.5 mmol/mmol Creat	4.5 mmol/mmol Creat	
	> 16 y	0.07 mmol/mmol Creat	0.5 mmol/mmol Creat	4.5 mmol/mmol Creat	
Copper		< 50 μg/24 h			Random urines are not useful as results are not interpretable in most cases
Homovanillic acid (HVA)	0–6 m	25 mmol/mol Creat			
	6 m – 1 y	25 mmol/mmol Creat			
	12–18 m	22 mmol/mmol Creat			
	18 m – 2 y	19 mmol/mmol Creat			
	2–3 y	16 mmol/mmol Creat			
	3–4 y	13 mmol/mmol Creat			
	4–5 y	12 mmol/mmol Creat			
	5–6 y	11 mmol/mmol Creat			
	6–8 y	9 mmol/mmol Creat			
	8–10 y	8 mmol/mmol Creat			
	10–12 y	7 mmol/mmol Creat			
	12–14 y	6 mmol/mmol Creat			
	14–16 y	6 mmol/mmol Creat			
	> 16 y	4.5 mmol/mmol Creat			

(Continued)

Table A.3 Normal constituents of urine—Cont'd

Analyte	Age	Reference ranges		Comments
5-hydroxyindole acetic acid (5HIAA)		<50 μmol/24 h		
Lead		<10 μg/24 h		
Magnesium	1–6 m	0.006–0.105 mmol/kg/24 h	Breast fed	
		0.006–0.132 mmol/kg/24 h	Formula fed	
	1–15 y	0.051–0.181 mmol/kg/24 h		
Magnesium/creatinine ratio	2–15 y	<1.05 mmol/mmol Creat		These values refer to a random, spot urine taken when the overnight urine has been voided
Osmolality	Newborns delivery urine	79–118 mmol/kg		
	Maximum in neonatal period	600 mmol/kg		
pH	Newborns	5.0 or higher		
	Older children	5.3–7.2		
Phosphate	% Tubular reabsorption of phosphate (TRP)	>80%		Values may be much different in the neonate
Porphobilinogen		0–10.7 μmol/L		
Potassium	Neonate	<5 mmol/kg/d		These values refer to a 24 h urine collection and are dependent on potassium intake and gestational age
	Child	25–125 mmol/24 h		
Sodium		0.08–0.16 mmol/kg/24 h		These values refer to a 24 h urine collection
Aldosterone		6–60 nmol/24 h		In children, excretion rates would increase during childhood from <1 mg/24 h in the first year
17-hydroxycorticosteroids		*Male*	*Female*	
	Adult	4.0–14 mg/24 h	2.0–12 mg/24 h	
	Children			
17-ketosteroids		*Male*	*Female*	Serum DHAS is a much better measurement
	Adult	8–20 mg/24 h	6–12 mg/24 h	
	0–1 y	0–1.0 mg/24 h	0–1.0 mg/24 h	
	1–5 y	1.0–2.0 mg/24 h	1.0–2.0 mg/24 h	
	6–10 y	1–4.4 mg/24 h	1.4–3.9 mg/24 h	
	11–12 y	1.3–8.5 mg/24 h	3.8–9.5 mg/24 h	
	13–16 y	3.4–9.8 mg/24 h	4.5–17.1 mg/24 h	
Pregnanediol			*Female*	Not a useful marker in pediatrics, measure serum progesterone
	>10 y		<50 μg/24 h	
	12 y		20–600 mg/24 h	
Pregnanetriol			*Female*	17-hydroxyprogesterone has superseded this assay
	>10 y		<50 μg/24 h	
	12 y		20–100 mg/24 h	
Vanillylmandelic acid (VMA)	0–1 y	0–18 mg/g Creat		
	2–4 y	0–11.0 mg/g Creat		
	5–9 y	0–8.3 mg/g Creat		
	10–19 y	0–8.2 mg/g Creat		
Total porphyrin		20–320 nmol/L		

Table A.4 Normal cerebrospinal fluid (CSF) values

Analyte	Age	Reference ranges	
WBC	Neonate	0–15/mm³	
	Child	0–5/mm³	
Glucose		2.5–4.5 mmol/L	
Lactate		0.8–2.4 mmol/L	CSF lactate:plasma lactate ratio should be calculated if a respiratory chain defect is suspected
Protein	0–2 m	< 1.2 g/L	
	2–4 m	<0.6 g/L	
	5 m –10 y	<0.25 g/L	
	10–18 y	<0.3 g/L	

Table A.5 Normal constituents of stools

Analyte	Reference ranges
Porphyrins	0–200 nmol/g dry weight
α1-antitrypsin (AAT)	0–0.48 mg AAT/g wet weight
Elastase	
Normal exocrine function	>200 µg/g
Mild exocrine insufficiency	100–200 µg/g
Severe exocrine deficiency	< 100 µg/g

Table A.6 Therapeutic ranges of medicines commonly used in children

Drug	Therapeutic range in blood	Comments
Caffeine	12–36.0 mg/L	1–2 h post dose
Carbamazepine	4–12.0 mg/L	Pre-dose
Digoxin	0.8–2.0 µg/L	6–24 h post dose
Ethosuximide	40–100 mg/L	Pre-dose
Gentamicin	5–10 mg/L	
Lithium	0.4–1.0 mmol/L	
Paracetamol	> 1300 µmol/L	Toxic value at 4 h
	>650 µmol/L	Toxic value at 8 h
	>300 µmol/L	Toxic value at 12 h
Phenobarbital	15–40 mg/L	Pre-dose
Phenytoin	10–20.0 mg/L	Pre-dose
Theophylline		
Neonates	5–10.0 mg/L	2–4 h post dose
Children	10–20.0 mg/L	
Sodium valproate	< 100 mg/L	Pre-dose
Salicylate	< 400 mg/L	Rarely causes symptoms
	>400 mg/L	Toxic level
	>1200 mg/L	Usually lethal

Table A.7a Normal blood count values from birth to 18 years

Age	Hb (g/dl)	RBC (×10¹²/L)	Hct	MCV (fl)	WBC (×10⁹/L)	Neutrophils (×10⁹/L)	Lympho-cytes (×10⁹/L)	Monocytes (×10⁹/L)	Eosinophils (×10⁹/L)	Basophils (×10⁹/L)	Platelets (×10⁹/L)	Reticulo-cytes (×10⁹/L)
Birth (term/ infants)	14.9–23.7	3.7–6.5	0.47–0.75	100–125	10–26	2.7–14.4	2.0–7.3	0–1.9	0–0.85	0–0.1	150–450	110–450
2 weeks	13.4–19.8	3.9–5.9	0.41–0.65	88–110	6–21	1.5–5.4	2.8–9.1	0.1–1.7	0–0.85	0–0.1	170–500	10–80
2 months	9.4–13.0	3.1–4.3	0.28–0.42	84–98	5–15	0.7–4.8	3.3–10.3	0.4–1.2	0.05–0.9	0.02–0.13	210–650	35–200
6 months	10.0–13.0	3.8–4.9	0.3–0.38	73–84	6–17	1–6	3.3–11.5	0.2–1.3	0.1–1.1	0.02–0.2	210–560	15–110
1 y	10.1–13.0	3.9–5.1	0.3–0.38	70–82	6–16	1–8	3.4–10.5	0.2–0.9	0.05–0.9	0.02–0.13	200–550	
2–6 y	11.0–13.8	3.9–5.0	0.32–0.4	72–87	6–17	1.5–8.5	1.8–8.4	0.15–1.3	0.05–1.1	0.02–0.12	210–490	
6–12 y	11.1–14.7	3.9–5.2	0.32–0.43	76–90	4.5–14.5	1.5–8.0	1.5–5.0	0.15–1.3	0.05–1.0	0.02–0.12	170–450	50–130
12–18 y												
Female	12.1–15.1	4.1–5.1	0.35–0.44	77–94	4.5–13	1.5–6	1.5–4.5	0.15–1.3	0.05–0.8	0.02–0.12	180–430	
Male	12.1–16.6	4.2–5.6	0.35–0.49	77–92								

Red cell values at birth derived from skin puncture blood; most other data from venous blood.
Adapted from Hinchliffe.[37]

Table A.7b Reference values for coagulation tests in healthy children aged 1–16 years compared with adults

Coagulation tests	Age			
	1–5 years Mean (boundary)	6–10 years Mean (boundary)	11–16 years Mean (boundary)	Adult mean (boundary)
PT (s)	11 (10.6–11.4)	11.1 (10.1–12.1)	11.2 (10.2–12.0)	12 (11.0–14.0)
INR	1.0 (0.96–1.04)	1.01 (0.91–1.11)	1.02 (0.93–1.10)	1.10 (1.0–1.3)
APTT (s)	30 (24–36)	31 (26–36)	32 (26–37)	33 (27–40)
Fibrinogen (g/L)	2.76 (1.70–4.05)	2.79 (1.57–4.0)	3.0 (1.54–4.48)	2.78 (1.56–4.0)
Bleeding time (min)	6 (2.5–10)*	7 (2.5–13)*	5 (3–8)*	4 (1–7)
II (unit/ml)	0.94 (0.71–1.16)*	0.88 (0.67–1.07)*	0.83 (0.61–1.04)*	1.08 (0.70–1.46)
V (unit/ml)	1.03 (0.79–1.27)	0.90 (0.63–1.16)*	0.77 (0.55–0.99)*	1.06 (0.62–1.50)
VII (unit/ml)	0.82 (0.55–1.16)*	0.85 (0.52–1.20)*	0.83 (0.58–1.15)*	1.05 (0.67–1.43)
VIII (unit/ml)	0.90 (0.59–1.42)	0.95 (0.58–1.32)	0.92 (0.53–1.31)	0.99 (0.50–1.49)
vWF (unit/ml)	0.82 (0.60–1.20)	0.95 (0.44–1.44)	1.00 (0.46–1.53)	0.92 (0.50–1.58)
IX (unit/ml)	0.73 (0.47–1.04)*	0.75 (0.63–0.89)*	0.82 (0.59–1.22)*	1.09 (0.55–1.63)
X (unit/ml)	0.88 (0.58–1.16)*	0.75 (0.55–1.01)*	0.79 (0.50–1.17)*	1.06 (0.70–1.52)
XI (unit/ml)	0.97 (0.56–1.50)	0.86 (0.52–1.20)	0.74 (0.50–0.97)*	0.97 (0.67–1.27)
XII (unit/ml)	0.93 (0.64–1.29)	0.92 (0.60–1.40)	0.81 (0.34–1.37)*	1.08 (0.52–1.64)
PK (unit/ml)	0.95 (0.65–1.30)	0.99 (0.66–1.31)	0.99 (0.53–1.45)	1.12 (0.62–1.62)
HMWK (unit/ml)	0.98 (0.64–1.32)	0.93 (0.60–1.30)	0.91 (0.63–1.19)	0.92 (0.50–1.36)
XIIIa (unit/ml)	1.08 (0.72–1.43)*	1.09 (0.65–1.51)*	0.99 (0.57–1.40)	1.05 (0.55–1.55)
XIIIs (unit/ml)	1.13 (0.69–1.56)*	1.16 (0.77–1.54)*	1.02 (0.60–1.43)	0.97 (0.57–1.37)

All factors except fibrinogen are expressed as unit/ml, where pooled plasma contains 1.0 unit/ml. All data are expressed as the mean, followed by the upper and lower boundary encompassing 95% of the population. Between 20 and 50 samples were assayed for each value for each age group. Some measurements were skewed due to a disproportionate number of high values. The lower limit, which excludes the lower 2.5% of the population, is given.
APTT, activated partial thromboplastin time; HMWK, high molecular weight kininogen; INR, international normalized ratio; PK, prekallikrein; PT, prothrombin time; VIII, factor VIII procoagulant; vWF, von Willebrand factor. *Values that are significantly different from adults. From Chalmers & Gibson.[38]

NUTRIENTS AND FORMULA FEEDS

Introduction
Normal infants and children

Infant (0–12 months). Term infants with normal gastrointestinal function are fed either human breast milk or normal infant formula during the first year of life. Normal infant formula is defined as 'a food intended for nutritional use by infants in good health for the first year of life, and satisfying, by itself the nutritional requirements of such infants'. It is based on whey- or casein-dominant protein, lactose ± maltodextrin and amylose, vegetable oil and milk fat. Whey-dominant milks are the closest in composition to breast milk. Although some infant formulas contain novel nutrients such as long chain fatty acids (docosahexaenoic acid and arachidonic acid), nucleotides and prebiotics, the composition of all normal and soya infant formulas has to meet the UK's *The Infant Formula and Follow-on Formula Regulations 1995,*[39] which enact the European Community Regulations 91/321/EC.[40] The energy content by law must not be less than 60 kcal (250 kJ) and not more than 70 kcal (295 kJ) per 100 ml.

Infant (over 6 months of age). 'Follow-on formulas' are feeds designed for infants over the age of 6 months and 'constitute the principal liquid element in a progressively diversified diet'.[40] They are based on modified cows' milk. They contain less protein, calcium and phosphorus than cows' milk, but more than standard infant formula, and are fortified with other nutrients.

Children over 1 year: Growing up milk is fortified formula designed for children over 1 year. It is based on cows' milk.

Special infant formulas

It is essential that any infant or child who is intolerant of breast milk or normal infant formula, or whose condition requires nutrient specific adaptation, is prescribed a nutritional complete replacement formula in adequate volume. The composition of special infant formula has to meet the Commission Directive (1999/21/EC) on Dietary Foods for Special Medical Purposes.[41]

Soya formula. Soya infant formula is based on soya-protein isolate supplemented with L-methionine, taurine and carnitine. These formulas support normal growth, protein status and mineralization. Although they are suitable for cows' milk protein and lactose intolerance, the Committee on Toxicity of Chemicals in Food, Consumer Products and the Environment (COT) has expressed concern about the use of soya infant formula in infancy.[42] Soya infant formula contains 18–41 mg/L of phytoestrogens. This is several times higher than the quantity in human breast milk. Although the COT report concluded that there is no direct evidence that soya infant formula affects the health of infants, particularly fertility, it is believed that soya infant formula may be a potential risk to the infant. Therefore it is not recommended that soya-based infant formula is used as the first choice formula for infants with cows' milk sensitivity or lactose intolerance, but it is widely used for infants with galactosemia because of the residual lactose content of low lactose formula and protein hydrolysate formula which are both derived from cows' milk.

Protein hydrolysate formula. Based on casein, whey, meat and soya, these formulas are suitable for infants with disaccharide and/or whole protein intolerance. Protein hydrolysates are the result of heat treatment and/or enzymatic cleavage, which is used in order to produce peptides of minor antigenic activity, with a molecular weight of less than 1200 daltons. Some of the formulas contain a significant proportion of their fat source in the form of medium chain triglyceride (MCT) oil.

Low lactose formula. This type of formula is based on whole cows' milk protein. Although suitable for lactose intolerance they contain residual lactose in very small quantities. They are unsuitable for infants with cows' milk protein intolerance.

Elemental (amino acid based formula). There is only one elemental nutritionally complete formula available for infants in the UK. There is evidence to demonstrate that the feed tolerance and growth of infants taking this formula is satisfactory.

Other specialist formula. A number of specialized formulas are available for liver and renal indications. High medium chain fat based formulas for conditions such as chylothorax and long chain fatty acid disorders are available. Ketogenic, low calcium and protein free feeds are also available. These should always be used under dietetic supervision.

Complete enteral feeds

The composition of all enteral feeds has to meet the Commission Directive (1999/21/EC) on Dietary Foods for Special Medical Purposes.[41]

Infant (0–12 months). An infant with faltering growth may be given a high energy and nutrient dense feed containing between 9 and 11% energy from protein. Concentrating or supplementing normal infant formula should not be attempted without the advice of a pediatric dietitian.

Children 1–6 years (8–20 kg). A number of nutritionally complete 0.75 kcal/ml, 1.0 kcal/ml and over 1.0 kcal/ml (± fiber) ready to use feeds designed for the 1–6-year age group are available. They are all based on caseinates, maltodextrin and vegetable oils ± added medium chain triglyceride oil (MCT) and contain residual lactose only. These products were originally designed for 1–6-year-old (8–20 kg) children, but some products have had Advisory Committee on Borderline Substances (ACBS) extensions for children weighing up to 30 kg (approximately 10 years of age).

Children 7–12 years. Nutritionally complete 1.0 kcal/ml and 1.5 kcal/ml (± fiber) ready to use feeds designed for this age group are available. They are also based on caseinates, maltodextrin and vegetable oils and contain residual lactose only. Their formulation is in between pediatric and adult feeds.

Children 13 years and over. There are no standard enteral feeds designed for teenagers, so adult feeds are given. The intake of protein, electrolytes, vitamins and trace minerals should be carefully assessed and monitored.

Other dietary supplements

A number of dietary supplements, either based on carbohydrates, fat and/or protein, which can be used to enhance the nutrient density of the diet or nutritionally complete supplements are available. The amount and timing of supplements is important so as not to impair appetite. Ideally supplements should be administered after meals or at bedtime. Many supplements are high in sugar or maltodextrin. Care should be taken to prevent prolonged contact with teeth.

Products for phenylketonuria

There is a wide range of phenylalanine-free protein substitutes for PKU. They have a high osmolality so should be administered with extra water. Some are nutritionally incomplete and require vitamin and/or other nutrient supplementation. Protein substitutes should be taken at least 3 times daily equally distributed throughout the day.

Useful website

www.foodstandards.gov.uk/multimedia/pdfs/phtoreport0503

Notes

The Advisory Committee on Borderline Substances (ACBS) advises GPs on prescription of products that are not drugs or medical devices. The committee is an advisory nondepartmental public body (NDPB), non-statutory and UK-wide. The approved list consists of foodstuffs such as enteral feeds or foods formulated for people with medical conditions.

Table A.8a Standard infant formulas (whey dominant)

	Aptamil First	Cow and Gate First Infant Milk	Farley's First Infant Milk	Hipp Organic First Infant Milk	SMA Gold
Manufacturer	Milupa	Cow and Gate	Heinz	Hipp	SMA
kcal/100 ml	67	67*	68	68	67
kJ/100 ml	275	280	284	283	281
Protein source	Whey and skimmed milk	Whey and skimmed milk	Whey and skimmed milk	Organic whey and skimmed milk	Whey and skimmed milk
Casein: whey ratio	40:60	40:60	40:60	40:60	40:60
Protein g/100 ml	1.3	1.4	1.45	1.6	1.4
Fat source	Vegetable oils, fish oil	Vegetable oils (contains soya), fish oil	Vegetable oils, fish oil	Palm, rapeseed, sunflower oils	Vegetable fats
Fat g/100 ml	3.5	3.5	3.8	3.3	3.6
Contains LCPs	Yes	Yes	Yes	No	Yes
Carbohydrate source	Lactose	Lactose	Lactose	Lactose	Lactose
Carbohydrate g/100 ml	7.3	7.4	7.0	7.9	7.3
Fiber g/100 ml	0.8	0.8	0	0	0
Sodium mmol/100 ml	0.8	0.9	0.7	0.9	0.7
Potassium mmol/100 ml	1.6	1.6	1.5	1.7	1.7
Calcium mg/100 ml	50	50	39	65	42
Iron mg/100 ml	0.53	0.7	0.65	0.7	0.8
Nutritionally complete	Yes	Yes	Yes	Yes	Yes
% Dilution	13.7	13.9	13	13.5	12.7
Presentation	900 g powder; 200 ml carton	400 g, 900 g powder. 200 and 500 ml carton	900 g powder; 250 ml cartons	900 g powder	450 g, 900 g powder, sachets. 250 ml and 1 liter cartons
Other information	Contains prebiotics and nucleotides	Contains prebiotics and nucleotides	Contains nucleotides		Contains nucleotides, alpha-lactalbumin

*Analysis powder only.

Table A.8b   Standard infant formulas (casein dominant)

	Aptamil Extra Hungry	Cow and Gate Infant Milk for Hungrier Babies	Farley's Second Milk	SMA White
Manufacturer	Milupa	Cow and Gate	Heinz	SMA
kcal/100 ml	66*	67*	69*	67*
kJ/100 ml	275	280	289	280
Protein source	Skimmed milk	Skimmed milk	Skimmed milk	Skimmed milk
Protein g/100 ml	1.6	1.7	1.7	1.6
Casein: whey ratio	80:20	80:20	80:20	80:20
Fat source	Vegetable oils	Vegetable oils	Vegetable oils, fish oil	Vegetable oils
Fat g/100 ml	3.2	3.3	3.5	3.6
Contains LCPs	Yes	No	Yes	No
Carbohydrate source	Lactose	Lactose	Lactose	Lactose
Carbohydrate g/100 ml	7.7	7.7	7.7	7
Fiber g/100 ml	0.8	0.8	0	0
Sodium mmol/100 ml	0.9	0.9	0.8	0.90
Potassium mmol/100 ml	2.1	2.1	2.0	2.1
Calcium mg/100 ml	70	79	56	56
Iron mg/100 ml	0.53	0.68	0.73	0.8
Nutritionally complete	Yes	Yes	Yes	Yes
% Dilution	14.1	14.2	13.7	12.7
Presentation	900 g powder. 200 ml cartons	400 g, 900 g powder. 200 and 500 ml cartons	900 g; 250 ml cartons	450 g, 900 g powder. 250 ml and 500 ml cartons
Other information	Contains prebiotics and nucleotides	Contains prebiotics and nucleotides		Contains nucleotides

*Analysis powder only.

Table A.8c   Standard infant formulas (Follow-on)

	Aptamil Follow on	Cow and Gate Follow on for Hungrier Babies 6 Months	Farley's Follow on Milk	Hipp Organic Follow on Milk	SMA Progress
Manufacturer	Milupa	Cow and Gate	Heinz	Hipp	SMA
kcal/100 ml	70*	70*	68*	69	67*
kJ/100 ml	295	295	285	287	280
Protein source	Skimmed milk	Skimmed milk	Whey, skimmed milk	Organic whey and skimmed milk	Skimmed milk
Casein:whey ratio	80:20	80:20	62:38	55:45	80:20
Protein g/100 ml	1.8	1.8	1.8	2.1	1.9
Fat source	Vegetable oils	Vegetable oils (contains soya)	Vegetable oils	Palm, rapeseed, sunflower oils	Vegetable oils
Fat g/100 ml	3.4	3.4	3.4	3.5	3.3
Contains LCPs	No	No	No	No	No
Carbohydrate source	Lactose	Lactose	Lactose	Lactose	Lactose
Carbohydrate g/100 ml	8.1	8.1	7.6	7.2	7.4
Fiber g/100 ml	0.8	0.8	0	0	0
Sodium mmol/100 ml	0.9	0.95	1.3	1.6	1.3
Potassium mmol/100 ml	2.2	2.2	2.3	3.4	2.3
Calcium mg/100 ml	83	83	72	99	90
Iron mg/100 ml	1.3	1.3	1.2	1.2	1.3
Nutritionally complete	Yes	Yes	Yes	Yes	Yes
% Dilution	14.9	14.9	13.8	13.5	13.1
Presentation	900 g powder. 200 ml cartons	400 g, 900 g powder. 200 and 500 ml cartons	900 g powder; 250 ml cartons	900 g powder; 27 g sachet	450 g, 900 g powder; 250 ml, 500 ml cartons
Other information		Contains prebiotics		900 g carton	

*Analysis powder only.

Table A.8d   Growing up milk

	Aptamil Growing Up Milk	Cow and Gate Growing Up Milk	Hipp Growing Up Milk
Manufacturer	Milupa	Cow and Gate	Hipp
kcal/100 ml	67	67*	79*
kJ/100 ml	280	280	330
Protein source	Skimmed milk	Skimmed milk	Organic whey and skimmed milk
Protein g/100 ml	1.9	1.9	2.5
Fat source	Canola, sunflower, and corn oil	Vegetable oils	Vegetable oil
Fat g/100 ml	3.0	3.0	3.5
Contains LCPs	No	No	No
Carbohydrate source	Lactose	Lactose	Starch, glucose, glucose syrup
Carbohydrate g/100 ml	8.1	8.1	9.2
Fiber g/100 ml	0.8	0.8	0
Sodium mmol/100 ml	1.1	1.3	1.7
Potassium mmol/100 ml	2.6	2.6	3.1
Calcium mg/100 ml	91	91	107
Iron mg/100 ml	1.2	1.2	1.0
Nutritionally complete	Yes	Yes	Yes
% Dilution	Ready made	Ready made	16.5
Presentation	200 and 500 ml bottles Contains prebiotics	200 and 500 ml bottles Contains prebiotics	600 g, 500 ml bottle 250 ml bottle

*Analysis powder only.

Table A.9a Special infant formulas

	Pre-thickened infant formula					Infant soya formula				
	Comfort First Infant Milk from Birth	Comfort Follow-on Milk from 6 Months	Enfamil AR with Lipil	SMA Staydown	Aptamil Easy Digest	Farley's Soya Formula	InfaSoy	Isomil	Prosobee	Wysoy
Manufacturer	Cow & Gate	Cow & Gate	Mead Johnson Nutritionals	SMA	Milupa	Heinz	Cow & Gate	Abbott Laboratories	Mead Johnson Nutritionals	SMA
kcal/100 ml	70	72	68	67	70	70	66	68	68	67
kJ/100 ml	295	300	285	279	295	293	275	284	285	280
Protein source	Hydrolysed whey protein	Hydrolysed whey protein	Skimmed milk	Skimmed milk	Hydrolysed whey protein	Soya protein isolate	Soya protein isolate	Soya protein isolate	Soya protein isolate	Soya protein isolate
Protein g/100 ml	1.7	1.9	1.7	1.6	1.7	1.95	1.8	1.8	1.8	1.8
Fat source	Structured vegetable oils	Structured vegetable oils	Palm olein, coconut, soya, sunflower oil	Coconut, palm, soya, sunflower oil	Structured vegetables oils	Sunflower, palm kernel, rapeseed oil, palm olein oil	Palm, sunflower, rapeseed, coconut oil	Sunflower, coconut, soya oil	Palm olein, coconut, soya, and sunflower oil	Palm, coconut, sunflower, soya oil
Fat g/100 ml	3.3	3.3	3.5	3.6	3.3	3.8	3.6	3.7	3.7	3.6
Contains LCPs	No	No	Yes	No	No	No	No	No	No	No
Carbohydrate source	Glucose syrup, starch, lactose	Glucose syrup Starch, lactose	Glucose polymers, lactose, rice starch	Lactose, glucose syrup, corn starch	Glucose syrup, starch, lactose	Glucose syrup	Glucose syrup	Corn syrup, sucrose	Glucose syrup	Glucose syrup
Carbohydrate g/100 ml	8.4	8.7	7.6	7	8.4	7.0	6.6	6.9	6.8	6.9
Fiber g/100 ml	0.8	0.8	0	0	0.8	0	0	0	0	0
Sodium mmol/100 ml	1.0	1.6	1.0	1.0	1	1.1	0.9	1.4	1.1	0.8
Potassium mmol/100 ml	2.1	2.2	2.2	2.1	2.1	1.9	1.7	2.0	2.0	1.9
Calcium mg/100 ml	53	91	55	56	53	56	54	70	66	67
Iron mg/100 ml	0.5	1.2	0.74	0.8	0.5	0.7	0.8	1.0	1.2	0.8
Nutritionally complete	Yes	Yes	Yes	Yes	Y	Yes	Yes	Yes	Yes	Yes
Suitable for vegans	No	No	No	No	No	Yes	No	No	No	No
Lactose free	No	No	No	No	No	Yes	Yes	Yes	Yes	Yes
% Dilution	15.2	15.9	13.5	13.5	15.2	15.1	12.7	13.2	12.9	13.5
Presentation	900 g powder	900 g powder	400 g powder	900 g powder	900 g powder	450 g; 900 g powder	900 g powder	400 g powder	400 g powder	430 g, 860 g powder
ACBS listed	No	No	Yes[a]	Yes[a]	No	Yes[b]	Yes[b]	Yes[b]	Yes[b]	Yes[b]
Other information	Contains prebiotics	Contains prebiotics			Contains prebiotics					

[a] Thickened formula is ACBS listed for use in the management of significant reflux. Not for use in excess of a 6 month period. Do not use in combination with other feed thickeners or antacid products.

[b] Infant soya formula ACBS listed for proven lactose intolerance in pre-school children, galactokinase deficiency, galactosemia, and proven whole cows' milk sensitivity

Table A.9b   Special infant formulas

	Infant protein hydrolysate							Infant amino acid formula	Child amino acid formula
	Nutramigen 1	Nutramigen 2	Pepti-Junior	Pepti	Pepdite	Pregestimil	Prejomin	Neocate	Neocate Advance
Manufacturer	Mead Johnson Nutritionals	Mead Johnson Nutritionals	Cow and Gate	Cow and Gate	SHS International	Mead Johnson Nutritionals	Milupa	SHS International	SHS International
kcal/100 ml	68	68	66	66	71	68	75	71	100
kJ/100 ml	280	285	275	275	297	283	315	298	420
Protein source	Enzymatically hydrolysed casein	Enzymatically hydrolysed casein	Hydrolysed whey protein	Hydrolysed whey protein	Hydrolysed pork and soya, amino acids	Enzymatically hydrolysed casein	Porcine collagen, soya hydrolysate	L-amino acids	L-amino acids
Protein g/100 ml	1.9	1.7	1.8	1.6	2.1	1.9	2.0	1.95	2.5
Fat source	Palm olein, coconut, soya, sunflower oil	Palm olein, coconut, sunflower, soya oil	MCT oil, soya, rapeseed, sunflower oil	Palm, coconut, rapeseed, sunflower oil single cell oil	Coconut, safflower, soya oil	MCT oil, corn, soya, sunflower oil	Palm, sunflower, rape seed, coconut oil	Safflower, coconut, soya oil	Safflower, coconut, canola oil
Fat g/100 ml	3.4	2.9	3.5 (50% of fat is MCT)	3.3	3.5	3.8 (55% of fat is MCT)	3.6	3.5	3.5
Contains LCPs	No	No	Yes	Yes	No	No	No	No	No
Carbohydrate source	Glucose polymer, modified corn starch	Glucose polymer, modified corn starch, fructose	Glucose syrup	Maltodextrin	Glucose syrup	Glucose polymer, dextrose, maltodextrin, modified corn starch	Maltodextrin, pre-cooked starch	Dried glucose syrup	Dried glucose syrup (glucose in flavored Neocate Advance)
Carbohydrate g/100 ml	7.5	8.6	6.8	7.1	7.8	6.9	8.6	8.1	14.6
Sodium mmol/100 ml	1.39	1.1	0.8	0.9	1.5	1.26	1.4	0.78	2.6
Potassium mmol/100 ml	2.1	2.1	1.7	1.9	1.5	1.9	2.0	1.6	3
Calcium mg/100 ml	64	94	50	47	45	78	63	49	50
Iron mg/100 ml	1.22	1.2	0.77	0.5	1	1.2	1	1.1	0.62
Nutritionally complete	Yes	Yes	Yes	Yes	Yes	Yes	Yes	Yes	Yes
Suitable for vegans	No	No	No	No	No	No	No	No, may include amino acids of animal origin. Contains fish gelatin	No, may include amino acids of animal origin. Contains fish gelatin
Lactose free	Residual lactose only	Residual lactose only	Residual lactose only	Low lactose	Yes	Residual lactose only	Yes	Yes	Yes
% Dilution	13.5	14.7	12.8	13.6	15	13.5	15	15	25
Presentation	425 g powder	425 g powder	450 g powder	900 g powder	400 g powder	450 g powder	400 g powder	400 g powder	Sachets: 100 g (unflavored); 400 g powder
ACBS listed	Yes	Yes	Yes	Yes	Yes	Yes	Yes	Yes	Yes

Nutramigen is ACBS listed for disaccharide and/or whole protein intolerance where additional medium chain triglycerides are not indicated. Nutramigen Stage 2 is ACBS listed for the same indications but for infants from 6 months onwards. Pepti-Junior and Pregestimil are ACBS listed for disaccharide and/or whole protein intolerance or where amino acids are indicated. Pepti may be prescribed for cows' milk protein intolerance with/without secondary lactose intolerance. Neocate and Neocate Advance is ACBS listed for disaccharide or dietary protein intolerance where an elemental formula is specifically indicated.

Table A.9c　Special infant formulas

	Low lactose infant formula			MCT infant formula			Other special infant formula	
	Enfamil Lactofree	Galactomin 17	SMA LF	Caprilon	MCT Pepdite	Monogen	Galactomin 19	Locasol
Manufacturer	Mead Johnson Nutritionals	SNS International	SMA Nutrition	SHS International	SHS International	SHS International	SHS Inter-national	SHS International
kcal/100ml	68	70	67	66	68	74	69	66
kJ/100ml	280	295	281	277	286	313	288	278
Protein source	Milk protein (isolate)	Caseinate	69% whey 40% casein	Skimmed milk powder, whey	Hydrolyzed pork and soya, amino acids	Whey protein, amino acids	Caseinate, L amino acids	Demineralized whey, caseinate
Protein g/100ml	1.4	1.7	1.5	1.5	2.0	2.0	1.9	1.9
Fat source	Palm olein, coconut, soya, sunflower oil	Palm, safflower, rapeseed, and coconut oil	Palm, coconut, soya, sunflower oil	MCT oil, soya oil	Walnut, palm kernel, coconut, maize oil	Coconut oil, walnut oil	Safflower, palm, rapeseed, coconut oil	Palm, sunflower, rapeseed, coconut oil
Fat g/100ml	3.7	3.7	3.6	3.6 (75% MCT)	2.7 (75%) MCT	2.1 (90% MCT)	4	3.4
Contains LCPs	No	No	No	No	No	No	No	No
Carbohydrate source	Glucose polymers	Glucose syrup	Glucose syrup	Glucose syrup	Glucose syrup	Glucose syrup	Fructose	Lactose, dried glucose syrup
Carbohydrate g/100ml	7.2	7.5	7.2	7	8.8	12	6.4	7
Sodium mmol/100ml	1.35	0.9	0.7	0.88	1.5	1.5	0.9	1.2
Potassium mmol/100ml	2.0	1.8	1.8	1.7	1.5	1.6	1.5	2
Calcium mg/100ml	78	55	55	53	45	45	55	<7
Iron mg/100ml	0.8	0.9	0.8	0.5	1	0.74	0.5	0.5
Nutritionally complete	Yes	Yes	Yes	Yes	Yes	Yes	Yes	Very low in calcium and vitamin D
Suitable for vegans	No	No	No	No	No	No	No	No
Lactose free	Contains residual lactose	Contains residual lactose	Contains residual lactose	No	Yes	No	Residual lactose only	No
% Dilution	12.9	13.6	13	12.7	15	17.5	12.9	13.1
Presentation	400g powder	400g powder	430g powder	420g powder	400g powder	400g powder	400g powder	400g
ACBS listed	Yes	Yes	Yes	Yes	Yes	Yes	Yes	Yes
								Prepare with distilled water as tap water may contain calcium. Monitor vitamin D levels.

Galactomin 17 is ACBS listed for proven lactose intolerance in pre-school children, galactosemia, and galactokinase deficiency. SMA LF and Enfamil Lactofree are ACBS listed for proven lactose intolerance. Caprilon and MCT Pepdite are ACBS listed for disorders in which a high intake of MCT is beneficial. Monogen ACBS listed for long chain acyl-COA dehydrogenase deficiency, carnitine palmitoyl transferase deficiency, primary and secondary lipoprotein lipase deficiency. Locasol is ACBS listed for hypercalcemia and other conditions which require extreme calcium restriction in the diet. Galactomin 19 is ACBS listed for glucose–galactose intolerance.

Table A.10a Enteral feeds for infants and children

| | Infant enteral feeds | | Post-discharge preterm formula |
	Infatrini	SMA High Energy Formula	Nutriprem 2
Manufacturer	Nutricia	SMA	Cow and Gate
kcal/100 ml	100	91	75
kJ/100 ml	420	382	315
Protein source	Skimmed milk, whey protein	60% whey, 40% casein	Whey protein, skimmed milk
Protein g/100 ml	2.6	2	2
Fat source	Vegetable oils	Coconut, palm, soya oil	Vegetable oils, egg lipid, milk fat, fish oil, sunflower oils
Fat g/100 ml	5.4	4.9	4.1
Contains LCPs	Yes	Yes	Yes
Carbohydrate source	Lactose, Maltodextrin	Lactose	Lactose, glucose syrup
Carbohydrate g/100 ml	10.3	9.8	7.4
Fiber g/100 ml	0.8 (Prebioticmix)	0	0.8 (Prebiotic mix)
Sodium mmol/100 ml	1.1	1.0	1.13
Potassium mmol/100 ml	2.4	2.3	2.0
Calcium mg/100 ml	80	57	94
Iron mg/100 ml	1.0	1.1	1.2
Nutritionally complete	Yes	Yes	Yes
Suitable for vegans	No	No	No
Lactose free	No	No	No
% Dilution	N/a	N/a	15.4
Presentation	200 ml bottle/100 ml glass bottle	200 ml carton	900 g, 200 ml carton, 100 ml glass bottle
ACBS listed	Yes	Yes	Yes
Other information			Contains prebiotics

Infant enteral feeds ACBS listed for disease-related malnutrition, malabsorption and growth failure in infancy. Both feeds are suitable for enteral and oral feeds.
Post-discharge formula ACBS listed for catch-up growth in pre-term (i.e. less than 35 weeks at birth) and small for gestational age infants, up to 6 months corrected age.

Table A10b Enteral feeds for children

	Enteral feeds: children; standard 1 kcal/ml or less					Enteral feeds: children; standard >1 kcal/ml feeds			
	Clinutren Junior	Frebini Original	Nutrini	Paediasure	Nutrini Low Energy Multi fibre	Frebini Energy	Isosource Junior	Nutrini Energy	Paediasure Plus
Manufacturer	Nestle Clinical	Fresenius Kabi	Nutricia	Abbott	Nutricia	Fresenius Kabi	Novartis	Nutricia	Abbott
kcal/100 ml	100*	100	100	101	75	150	122	150	151
kJ/100 ml	420	420	420	422	315	630	512	630	632
Protein source	Caseinate, whey	Milk proteins	Milk proteins	Milk protein	Milk proteins	Milk proteins	Milk proteins	Milk proteins	Sodium and calcium caseinates, whey protein.
Protein g/100 ml	2.97	2.5	2.8	2.8	2.1	3.75	2.7	4.1	4.2
Fat source	MCT oil, rapeseed, corn, sunflower oil	Vegetable oils (with soya oil), MCT oil, fish oil	Vegetable oils	Sunflower, soya, MCT oil	Vegetable oils	Vegetable oils (with soya oil), MCT oil, fish oil	Rapeseed, sunflower, MCT oil	Vegetable oils	Sunflower, soya, MCT oil
Fat g/100 ml	3.9	4.4	4.4	5.0	3.3	6.7	4.7	6.7	7.5
Contains LCPs	No	Yes	No	No	No	Yes	No	No	No
Carbohydrate source	Sucrose and maltodextrin (corn syrup in powder only)	Maltodextrin	Malto-dextrin	Malto-dextrin, sucrose	Malto-dextrin	Malto-dextrin	Malto-dextrin	Malto-dextrin	Malto-dextrin, sucrose
Carbohydrate g/100 ml	13.3	12.5	12.3	11.2	9.3	18.8	17	18.5	16.7
Fiber g/100 ml	0	0	0	0	0.8	0	0	0	0
Sodium mmol/100 ml	2.1	2.2	2.6	2.61	2.6	3.3	2.6	3.9	2.61
Potassium mmol/100 ml	2.8	2.6	2.8	2.8	3.4	3.8	3.0	4.2	3.5
Calcium mg/100 ml	89	60	60	56	60	90	66	90	83
Iron mg/100 ml	1	0.9	1.0	1.0	1.0	1.35	0.8	1.5	1.5
Nutritionally complete	Yes	Yes	Yes	Yes	Yes	Yes	Yes	Yes	Yes
Suitable for vegans	No	No	No	No	No	No	No	No	No
Lactose free	Residual lactose only	Residual lactose only	Residual lactose only	Residual lactose only	Residual lactose only	Residual lactose only	Residual lactose only	Residual lactose only	Residual lactose only
% Dilution	For 1 kcal per ml: 22 g powder + 85 ml water	N/a	N/a	N/a	N/a	N/a	N/a	N/a	N/a
Presentation	400 g powder	500 ml packs	200 ml bottle; 500 ml packs	250 ml cans; 500 ml packs	200 ml bottle; 500 ml packs	500 ml packs	500 ml packs	200 ml bottle; 500 ml packs	500 ml packs
ACBS listed	Yes	Yes	Yes	Yes	Yes	Yes	Yes	Yes	Yes

All children's enteral feeds are ACBS listed for the following indications: short bowel syndrome, intractable malabsorption, preoperative preparation of patients who are undernourished, dysphagia, bowel fistulas, and disease-related malnutrition and/or growth failure.
*Clinotren Junior powder can also be made up to a concentration of 1.5 kcal/ml (32 g powder; 80 ml water).

Table A.10c Enteral feeds for children

	Enteral feeds: children; fiber enriched					Enteral feeds: children aged 7–12 years (21–45 kg)				
	Frebini Original Fibre	Frebini Energy Fibre	Nutrini Multi Fibre	Nutrini Energy Multi Fibre	Paediasure Fibre	Paediasure Plus Fibre	Tentrini	Tentrini Multi Fibre	Tentrini Energy	Tentrini Energy Multi-fibre
Manufacturer	Fresenius Kabi	Fresenius Kabi	Nutricia	Nutricia	Abbott	Abbott	Nutricia	Nutricia	Nutricia	Nutricia
kcal/100 ml	100	150	100	150	100	150	100	100	150	150
kJ/100 ml	420	630	420	630	420	629	420	420	630	630
Protein source	Milk proteins	Milk proteins	Milk proteins	Milk proteins	Milk protein	Sodium and calcium caseinate, whey protein	Milk proteins	Milk proteins	Milk proteins	Milk proteins
Protein g/100 ml	2.5	3.75	2.8	4.1	2.8	4.2	3.3	3.3	4.9	4.9
Fat source	Vegetable oils (with soya oil), MCT oil, fish oil	Vegetable oils (with soya oil), MCT oil, fish oil	Vegetable oils	Vegetable oil	Sunflower, soya, MCT oil	Sunflower, soya, MCT oil	Vegetable oils	Vegetable oils	Vegetable oils	Vegetable oils
Fat g/100 ml	4.4	6.7	4.4	6.7	5.0	7.5	4.2	4.2	6.3	6.3
Contains LCPs	Yes	Yes	No	No	No	No	No	No	No	No
Carbohydrate source	Malto-dextrin	Malto-dextrin	Malto-dextrin	Malto-dextrin	Malto-dextrin, sucrose	Malto-dextrin, sucrose	Malto-dextrin	Malto-dextrin	Malto-dextrin	Malto-dextrin
Carbohydrate g/100 ml	12.5	18.8	12.3	18.5	10.9	16.4	12.3	12.3	18.5	18.5
Fiber g/100 ml	0.75	1.13	0.8	0.8	0.73	1.1	0	1.1	0	1.1
Sodium mmol/100 ml	2.2	3.3	2.6	3.9	2.61	2.61	3.5	3.5	4.6	4.6
Potassium mmol/100 ml	2.6	3.8	2.8	4.2	2.8	3.5	3.3	3.3	4.4	4.4
Calcium mmol/100 ml	60	90	60	90	56	83	70	70	95	95
Iron mg/100 ml	0.9	1.35	1.0	1.5	1.0	1.5	1.3	1.3	2	2
Nutritionally complete	Yes	Yes	Yes	Yes	Yes	Yes	Yes	Yes	Yes	Yes
Suitable for vegans	No	No	No	No	No	No	No	No	No	No
Lactose free	Residual lactose	Residual lactose	Residual lactose	Residual lactose	Residual lactose	Residual lactose	Residual lactose	Residual lactose	Residual lactose	Residual lactose
% Dilution	N/a	N/a	N/a	N/a	N/a	N/a	N/a	N/a	N/a	N/a
Presentation	500 ml packs	500 ml packs	200 ml bottle; 500 ml packs	200 ml bottle; 500 ml packs	250 ml cans; 500 ml packs	500 ml packs	500 ml bottle; 500 ml packs	500 ml bottle; 500 ml packs	500 ml bottle; 500 ml packs	500 ml bottle; 500 ml packs
ACBS listed	Yes	Yes	Yes	Yes	Yes	Yes	Yes	Yes	Yes	Yes

All children's enteral feeds are ACBS listed for the following indications: short bowel syndrome, intractable malabsorption, preoperative preparation of patients who are undernourished, dysphagia, bowel fistulas, and disease-related malnutrition and/or growth failure.

Table A.11a   Protein substitutes for phenylketonuria (PKU)

Analysis per 100 ml/100 g	Infant protein substitutes for PKU				Protein substitutes for PKU				
	PKU Start	XP Analog LCP	XP Analog	Easiphen	Minaphlex	Lophlex	Lophlex LQ	Phlexy 10 Drink Mix	Phlexy 10 Bar
	100 ml	100 ml	100 ml	100 ml	100 g	100 g	100 ml	100 g	100 g
Manufacturer	Vitaflo International Ltd	SHS International	SHS International	SHS International	SHS International	SHS International	SHS International	SHS International	SHS International
kcal	68	72	72	65	390	326	92	343	355
kJ	282	300	300	275	1639	1384	391	1456	1496
Protein source	L-amino acids	L-amino acids	L-amino acids	L-amino acids	L-amino acids	L-amino acids	L-amino acids	L-amino acids	L-amino acids
Protein g	2.0	1.95	1.95	6.7	29	72	16	41.7	19.8
Fat source	Walnut, palm, and rapeseed oil.	Walnut, olive, coconut, tuna oil	Safflower, coconut, and soy oil	Canola, sunflower, walnut oil	Canola, safflower, coconut oil	None	None	None	Soy, palm, and peanut oil
Fat g	2.9	3.5	3.5	2	13.5	0.2	0	Nil	8.9
Contains LCPs	Yes	Yes	No	No	No	No	No	No	No
Contains essential fatty acids	Yes	Yes	Yes	Yes	Yes	No	No	No	Yes
Carbohydrate source	Maltodextrin, lactose	Glucose syrup	Glucose syrup	Glucose syrup	Glucose syrup, sugar	Glucose syrup	Maltodextrin, sugar	Glucose syrup	Glucose syrup sucrose
Carbohydrate g	8.3	8.1	8.1	5.1	38	9	7	44	48.8
Sodium mmol	1.0	0.78	0.78	4.1	30	<0.87	<5	<1	<1
Potassium mmol	1.5	1.62	1.62	3.1	25	<10	<5	<1	–
Calcium mg	60	49	49	160	945	1280	285	–	–
Iron mg	0.8	1.05	1.05	4	14	19.2	4.2	–	–

Needs vitamin and mineral supplementation	No	No	No	No	No	No	No	Yes	Yes
Suitable for vegans	No	No	No	No	No	No	No	No	No
Lactose free	No	Yes	Yes	Yes	Yes	Yes	Yes	Yes	Yes
% Dilution	N/a	15	15	N/a	N/a	N/a	N/a	N/a	N/a
Presentation	500 ml	400 g powder	400 g powder	250 ml	29 g sachet	28 g sachet	125 ml pack	20 g sachet	42 g bar
ACBS listed	Yes	Yes	Yes	Yes	Yes	Yes	Yes	Yes	Yes
Other information				Available in Forest Berries and Grapefruit flavors	Available unflavored and flavored: pineapple and vanilla flavor, chocolate, tropical twist	Available in Berry and Orange flavors	Available in Citrus, Berry and Orange flavors	Available in Citrus, Berry and Orange flavors	Available in Citrus Burst, Apple and Blackcurrant, and tropical surprise flavors

All of these products are ACBS listed for phenylketonuria.

Table A.11b Protein substitutes

	Other protein substitutes										
	Phlexy 10 Capsules	Phlexy 10 Tablets	PK Aid 4	PKU 2	PKU 3	PKU Cooler 10	PKU Cooler 15	PKU Cooler 20	PKU Express	PKU Gel	XP Maxamaid
Analysis per 100 ml/100 g or as specified	Per 200 capsules	Per 100 capsules	Per 100 g	Per 100 g	Per 100 g	Per 100 ml	Per 100 ml	Per 100 ml	Per 100 g	Per 100 g	100 g
Manufacturer	SHS International	SHS International	SHS International	Milupa	Milupa	Vitaflo International	Vitaflo International	Vitaflo International	Vitaflo International	Vitaflo International	SHS International
kcal	333	377	334	300	288	71	71	71	302	342	309
kJ	1416	1601	1420	1275	1222	297	297	297	1260	1428	1311
Protein source	L-amino acids	L-amino acids	L-amino acids	L-amino acids	L-amino acids	L-amino acids	L-amino acids	L-amino acids	L-amino acids	L-amino acids	L-amino acids
Protein g	83.3	83.3	79	66.8	68	11.5	11.5	11.5	60	42	25
Fat source	None	Vegetable oil	0	0	0	0	0	0	0	0	0
Fat g	Nil	2	No	No	No	Trace	Trace	Trace	<0.5	<0.5	<0.5
Contains LCPs	No	No	No	No	No	No	No	No	No	No	No
Contains essential fatty acids	No	No	No	No	No	No	No	No	No	No	No
Carbohydrate source	None	Maize starch	Glucose syrup	Malto-dextrin	Malto-dextrin	Sugar, modified maize starch	Sugar, modified maize starch	Sugar, modified maize starch	Glucose syrup, maize starch	Maltodextrin, maize starch	Glucose syrup, sugar
Carbohydrate g	None	6.5	4.5	8.2	3.9	5.9	5.9	5.9	15	43	51
Sodium mmol	–	–	–	27.8	27.8	4.7	4.7	4.7	24.4	16.3	25.2
Potassium mmol	–	–	–	34.1	34.1	5.2	5.2	5.2	27.2	24.3	21.5
Calcium mg	–	–	–	1310	1310	215	215	215	1116	1085	810
Iron mg	–	–	–	15	21	4.2	4.2	4.2	21.6	10.5	12
Needs vitamin and mineral supplementation	Yes	Yes	Yes	No but does not contain selenium	No but does not contain selenium	No	No	No	No	No	No
Suitable for vegans	No	No	No	No	No	No	No	No	No	No	No
Lactose free	Yes	Yes	Yes	Yes	Yes	Yes	Yes	Yes	Yes	Yes	Yes
% Dilution	N/a	N/a	N/a	N/a	N/a	N/a	N/a	N/a	N/a	N/a	N/a
Presentation	200 capsules	75 tablets	500 g	500 g	500 g	87 ml pouch	130 ml pouch	174 ml pouch	25 g sachet	20 g sachet	500 g powder
ACBS listed	Yes	Yes	Yes	Yes	Yes	Yes	Yes	Yes	Yes	Yes	Yes
Other information						Purple and orange flavors	Purple and orange flavors	Purple and orange flavors	Orange, lemon, tropical and unflavored	Orange, raspberry, unflavored	Orange, unflavored

Table A.11c   Protein substitutes

	Other protein substitutes for PKU			Other useful special formulas		
Analysis per 100 ml/100 g	XP Maxamaid Concentrate	XP Maxamum	Kindergen	Ketocal	Heparon Junior	Energivit
	Per 100 g	Per 100 g	Per 100 ml	Per 100 ml	Per 100 ml	Per 100 ml
Manufacturer	SHS International	SHS International	SHS International	SHS International	SHS International	SHS International
kcal	239	297	101	146	86	74
kJ	1013	1260	421	602	363	309
Protein source	L-amino acids	L-amino acids	Whey protein, amino acids	Milk protein	Whey protein, skimmed milk powder	N/a
Protein g	53.5	39	1.5	3.1	2.0	0
Fat source	None	None	Safflower, coconut, soya oil.	Soya, milk fat	MCT oil, soya oil.	Safflower, coconut, and soya oil
Fat g	<0.5	<0.5	5.3	14.6	3.6	3.75
Contains LCPs	No	No	No	No	No	No
Contains essential fatty acids	No	No	Yes	Yes	Yes	Yes
Carbohydrate source	Glucose syrup, sugar	Glucose syrup, sugar	Glucose syrup	Glucose syrup, lactose	Glucose syrup	Glucose syrup
Carbohydrate g	5	34	11.8	0.6	11.6	10
Sodium mmol	54	24.3	2	4.3	0.56	0.78
Potassium mmol	46.1	17.9	0.6	4.1	1.9	1.62
Calcium mg	1733	670	22.4	86	92	48.8
Iron mg	25.7	23.5	4.8	1.5	1.3	1.05
Needs vitamin and mineral supplementation	Yes	Yes	Yes	Yes	Yes	Yes
Suitable for vegans	No	No	No	No	No	
Lactose free	Yes	Yes	No	No	No	Yes
% Dilution	N/a	N/a	20%	20%	18%	15%
Presentation	500 g powder	500 g powder	400 g powder	300 g powder	400 g powder	400 g powder
ACBS listed	Yes	Yes	Yes	No	Yes	Yes
Other information	Available orange and unflavored		Low in calcium and phosphorus	High fat feed (73% fat calories). Can be used for classical 4:1 ketogenic diet	Nutritionally complete in recommended dilution	

Kindergen is ACBS listed for complete nutritional support or supplementary feeding for infants and children with chronic renal failure who are receiving rapid overnight peritoneal dialysis. Energivit is ACBS listed for infants with disorders of amino acid and protein metabolism on a protein-restricted diet.

Table A.12a   Milk based nutritional supplements

	Frebini Energy Drink	Frebini Energy Fibre Drink	Fortini	Fortini Multi Fibre	Children 8–30 kg				
					Paediasure Tetrapak	Paediasure Fibre Tetrapak	Paediasure Plus Tetrapak	Paediasure Plus Fibre Tetrapak	Resource Junior
Manufacturer	Fresenius Kabi	Fresenius Kabi	Nutricia	Nutricia	Abbott Nutrition	Abbott Nutrition	Abbott Nutrition	Abbott Nutrition	Novartis
kcal/100 ml	150	150	150	150	101	100	151	150	150
kJ/100 ml	630	630	630	630	422	420	632	626	630
Protein source	Milk proteins	Milk proteins	Milk proteins	Milk proteins	Whey protein, calcium caseinate	Whey protein, calcium caseinate	Whey protein, calcium caseinate	Whey protein, calcium caseinate	Skimmed milk
Protein g/100 ml	3.75	3.75	3.4	3.4	2.8	2.8	4.2	4.2	3.0
Fat source	Vegetable oils (with soya oil), MCT oil, fish oil	Vegetable oils (with soya oil), MCT oil, fish oil	Veg oils	Veg oils	Sunflower oil, soya oil, MCT oil	Sunflower oil, soya oil, MCT oil	Sunflower oil, soya oil, MCT oil	Sunflower oil, soya oil, MCT oil	Cream, corn oil, rapeseed oil
Fat g/100 ml	6.7	6.7	6.8	6.8	5	5	7.5	7.5	6.2
Carbohydrate source	Maltodextrin	Maltodextrin, inulin, soya polysaccharide	Maltodextrin, sucrose	Maltodextrin, sucrose	Maltodextrin, sucrose	Maltodextrin, sucrose	Maltodextrin, sucrose	Maltodextrin, sucrose	Maltodextrin, sucrose
Carbohydrate g/100 ml	18.8	18.8	18.8	18.8	11.2	10.9	16.7	16.4	20.6
Fiber g/100 ml	0	1.1	0	1.5	0	0.73	0	1.1	–
Nutritionally complete	Yes	Yes	Yes	Yes	Yes	Yes	Yes	Yes	Yes
Presentation	Carton: 200 ml	Carton: 200 ml	Bottle 200 ml	Bottle 200 ml	Carton: 200 ml Can: 250 ml	Carton: 200 ml	Carton: 200 ml	Carton: 200 ml	Carton: 200 ml
ACBS listed	Yes	Yes	Yes	Yes	Yes	Yes	Yes	Yes	Yes
Flavors	Strawberry, banana	Chocolate	Vanilla, strawberry	Vanilla, strawberry, chocolate, banana	Carton: vanilla, strawberry, chocolate, banana Can: vanilla	Carton: vanilla, strawberry, banana	Carton: vanilla, strawberry, banana Can: vanilla	Carton: vanilla	Carton: chocolate, strawberry, vanilla

All children's nutritional supplements are ACBS listed for the following indications: short bowel syndrome, intractable malabsorption, preoperative preparation of patients who are undernourished, dysphagia, bowel fistulas, disease-related malnutrition and/or growth failure.

Table A.12b Carbohydrate based nutritional supplements

	Caloreen	Maxijul liquid	Maxijul Super Soluble	Polycal liquid	Polycal powder	Polycose powder	Vitajoule
Analysis per 100 ml/100 g	Per 100 g	Per 100 ml	Per 100 g	Per 100 ml	Per 100 g	Per 100 g	Per 100 g
Manufacturer	Nestle Clinical Nutrition	SHS International	SHS International	Nutricia	Nutricia	Abbott	Vitaflo
kcal	390	200	380	247	384	376	380
kJ	1638	850	1615	1050	1630	1598	1610
Carbohydrate source	Glucose polymer	Glucose syrup	Dried glucose syrup	Maltodextrin, glucose syrup	Maltodextrin	Glucose polymer	Glucose polymer
Carbohydrate g		50	95	61.9	96	94	96
Pack size	Can: 500 g	Carton: 200 ml	Can: 200 g Sachets: 4 × 132 g 2.5 kg tub 25 kg drum	Carton: 200 ml	Can: 400 g	Can: 350 g	Tub: 500 g 2.5 kg 25 kg
ACBS listed	Yes	Yes	Yes	Yes	Yes	Yes	Yes
Flavors	Unflavored	Orange and natural	Unflavored	Neutral, orange	Unflavored	Unflavored	Unflavored

All carbohydrate supplements are ACBS listed for disease-related malnutrition, malabsorption states, and other conditions requiring fortification with high energy or readily available carbohydrate supplements. Caution: flavored glucose polymer syrups are not suitable for use in children < 12 months of age. Liquid preparations should always be diluted at least 50% for children < 5 years of age.

Table A.12c Fat based nutritional supplements

	Calogen	Liquigen	MCT oil
Manufacturer	nutricia	SHS International	SHS International
kcal/100 ml	450	450	855
kJ/100 ml	1850	1850	3515
Fat source	Canola, sunflower	Coconut, palm kernel	Coconut oil and palm kernel oil
Fat g/100 ml	50	50 (MCT)	95 (MCT)
Pack size	Bottles: 200 ml, 500 ml ≤C14:0; 0.01% C16; 6.3% C18: 3.4% C18:1; 59.1% C18:2; 23.7% C18:3; 4.8% >C20; 2.4%	Bottles: 250 ml C6; 0.97% C8: 80.3% C10; 14.52% C12; 0.97% C14; 0.03% C16; 1.59%	Bottle: 500 ml C6; <2% C8; 58% C10; 38% C12; <2% C14; <1%
ACBS listed	Yes	Yes	Yes
Flavors	Strawberry, banana and unflavored	C18; 1.52% C20; 0.03%	

All products ACBS listed for disease-related malnutrition, malabsorption states, and other conditions requiring fortification with a high fat supplement, with or without fluid and electrolyte restrictions. MCT oil and Liquigen also ACBS listed for ketogenic diets in the management of epilepsy and type 1 hyperlipoproteinemia.

Table A.12d Combined nutritional supplements

	Combined fat and carbohydrate supplements					Combined protein, fat and carbohydrate supplements		
	Duobar	Liquid Duocal	Super Soluble Duocal Powder	MCT Duocal Powder	Vitabite	Pro-cal	Quickcal	Pro-cal shot
Analysis per 100 ml/100 g	Per 100 g	Per 100 ml	Per 100 g	Per 100 g	Per 100 g	Per 100 g	Per 100 g	Per 100 ml
Manufacturer	SHS International	SHS International	SHS International	SHS International	Vitaflo International	Vitaflo International	Vitaflo International	Vitaflo International
kcal	648	166	492	497	547	667	780	334
kJ	2692	605	2061	2082	2284	2788	3260	1385
Protein source	N/a	N/a	N/a	N/a	0.12	Skimmed milk powder	N/a	Skimmed milk powder sodium carbonate
Protein g	N/a	N/a	N/a	N/a	N/a	13.5	4.6	6.7
Fat source	Palm oil, shea fat, ilipe oil	Coconut, maize, palm kernel oil	Coconut, safflower, canola oil	Coconut, walnut maize, palm kernal oil	Soya, rapeseed, and palm oil	Hydrogenated vegetable oil	Hydrogenated vegetable oil	High oleic sunflower MCT oil
Fat g	49.9	7.9	22.3	23.2 (75% MCT)	334	56	77	28.2 (17.4% MCT)
Carbohydrate source	Sucrose	Glucose syrup	Glucose syrup	Glucose syrup	Lactose, sucrose, carob flour	Lactose	Lactose	Lactose
Carbohydrate g	49.9	23.7	72.7	72	61.4	27	17	13.4
Presentation	8 × 45 g bars	Bottles: 250 ml	Can: 400 g	Can: 400 g	Bars: 7 × 25 g	25 × 15 g sachets, 200 × 15 g sachets, 510 g, 1.5 kg, 12.5 kg, 25 kg	25 × 13 g sachets	6 × 250 ml bottles
ACBS listed	Yes	Yes	Yes	Yes	Yes	Yes	Yes	Yes
Flavors	Strawberry, toffee, natural							

All combined fat and carbohydrate products ACBS listed for disease-related malnutrition, malabsorption states, and other conditions requiring fortification with fat/carbohydrate supplement.
All combined protein, fat and carbohydrate products ACBS listed for disease-related malnutrition, malabsorption states, and other conditions requiring fortification with a protein, fat and carbohydrate supplement.

Table A.12e Protein supplements

	Casilan 90	ProMod	Protifar	Vitapro
Manufacturer	Heinz	Abbott	Nutricia	Vitaflo
kcal/100 g	370	426	373	360
kJ/100 g	1572	1798	1580	1506
Protein source	Calcium caseinate	Whey protein	Milk protein	Whey protein
Protein g/100 g	90	75.8	88.5	75
Presentation	Carton: 500 g	Can: 275 g	Can: 225 g	250 g; 2 kg
ACBS listed	Yes	Yes	Yes	Yes

All protein supplements are ACBS listed for biochemically proven hypoproteinemia.

Table A.13 Feed thickeners

Name	Instant Carobel	Nestargel	Thick and Easy	Thixo D	Vitaquick
Manufacturer	Cow and Gate	Nestle Clinical Nutrition	Fresenius Kabi	Sutherland Health	Vitaflo International
Ingredients	Carob bean gum with maltodextrin and calcium lactate	Carob seed flour and calcium lactate. It contains no metabolizable carbohydrate	Modified food starch (maize), maltodextrin	Modified waxy maize, food starch (E1442)	Modified maize starch, (E1442)
Energy kcal/100 g	251	38	373	392	380
kJ/100 g	1065	158	1567	1635	1590
CHO g/100 g	59	0	92.6	97	96
Sodium mg/100 g	8	5	175	125	< 200
Potassium mg/100 g	240	350	0	10	< 1.0
Calcium mg/100 g	130	640	4.5	Not declared	Not declared
Phosphorus mg/100 g	20	Not declared	24	13	20
Reconstitution	Bottle feed: add 2–3 level scoops of Carobel for every 60–90 ml (2–3 fl oz) hand-warm infant formula. Shake well and leave to thicken for 3–4 minutes. Breast feeds: add 6–7 level scoops of Carobel to 60 ml (2 fl oz) hand-warm water to form a thick gel. Feed in small quantities by spoon before and during the breast feed	Recommended concentration 0.5–1%. Bottle feed: add Nestargel in the quantity of cold water required for the feed; gently bring to the boil, stir and simmer for 1 minute; cool and add the formula powder; mix until smooth. Breast feeds: give 1 tablespoon of thickened Nestargel water (1% concentration) pre-feeds	No specific instructions given for infants. 1–3% concentration suggested.[45]		
Comments	An instant thickener 1 scoop = 0.7 g Carobel	An effective thickener; produces a smooth and stable thickened liquid. 1 scoop = 1 g Nestargel	Effective thickeners. Unsuitable for infants under 1 year, unless failing to thrive		An effective thickener. Unsuitable for infants under 1 year, unless failing to thrive. Each tub contains a 5 g scoop
Presentation	Box: 135 g	Can: 125 g	Can: 225 g, Sachets: 9 g	Tub: 375 g	Tube: 300 g, 12 kg, 6 kg
ACBS listed	Yes, for thickening feeds in the treatment of vomiting	Yes, for thickening feeds in the treatment of vomiting	Yes, for thickening of foods in the treatment of dysphagia	Yes, for thickening of foods in the treatment of dysphagia	Yes, for thickening of foods in the treatment of dysphagia
Side-effects	A minority of infants may develop loose stools. If used in galactosemia, the red cell galactose 1-phosphate should be monitored	A minority of infants may develop loose stools. If used in galactosemia, the red cell galactose 1-phosphate should be monitored	–	–	–

Table A.14 Miscellaneous

Product	Manufacturer	Description	ACBS Prescribable
Cornflour/cornstarch	Various	Maize starch BP-maize starch powder	Hypoglycemia associated with glycogen storage disease
Fructose	Various	Fructose BP Laevulose powder. 500 g	Glucose-galactose intolerance
Glucose/dextrose	Various	Glucose BP Dextrose monohydrate powder	Glycogen storage disease. Sucrose-isomaltose intolerance
SHS Module Flavour System	SHS International	Blackcurrant, orange, pineapple, tomato, *grapefruit, *cherry vanilla, *lemon and lime. Contains maltodextrin ±lactose, modified starch, sugar according to flavor. Presentation: 100 g tubs or *5 g sachets	For flavoring unflavored amino acid/peptide based products
Vitaflo Flavour Pac	Vitaflo International	Blackcurrant, lemon, orange, raspberry, tropical fruit. On a carbohydrate base containing sugar and sweeteners. Presentation 30 × 4 g sachets	For flavouring unflavoured amino acid products

Table A.15 Dietary reference values for the UK. Estimated average requirements (EARs) for energy

MJ/d (kcal/d)	Males		Females	
0–3 m	2.28	(545)	2.16	(515)
4–6 m	2.89	(690)	2.69	(645)
7–9 m	3.44	(825)	3.20	(765)
10–12 m	3.85	(920)	3.61	(865)
1–3 y	5.15	(1230)	4.86	(1165)
4–6 y	7.16	(1715)	6.46	(1545)
7–10 y	8.24	(1970)	7.28	(1740)
11–14 y	9.27	(2220)	7.72	(1845)
15–18 y	11.51	(2755)	8.83	(2110)
19–50 y	10.60	(2550)	8.10	(1940)
51–59 y	10.60	(2550)	8.00	(1900)
60–64 y	9.93	(2380)	7.99	(1900)
65–74 y	9.71	(2330)	7.96	(1900)
75+ y	8.77	(2100)	7.61	(1810)
Pregnancy			+0.80[a]	(200)
Lactation:				
1 m			+1.90	(450)
2 m			+2.20	(530)
3 m			+2.40	(570)
4–6 m (Group 1)[b]			+2.00	(480)
4–6 m (Group 2)			+2.40	(570)
>6 m (Group 1)			+1.00	(240)
>6 m (Group 2)			+2.30	(550)

Extracted from Dietary Reference Values for Food Energy and Nutrients for the United Kingdom.[46]
[a]Last trimester only.

Table A.16 Reference nutrient intakes for protein

Age	Reference nutrient intake[a] g/d
0–3 m	12.5[b]
0–4 m	12.7
7–9 m	13.7
10–12 m	14.9
1–3 y	14.5
4–6 y	19.7
7–10 y	28.3
Males	
11–14 y	42.1
15–18 y	55.2
19–50 y	55.5
51+ y	53.3
Females	
11–14 y	41.2
15–18 y	45.0
19–50 y	45.0
51+ y	46.5
Pregnancy[c]	+6
Lactation[c]	
0–4 m	+11
4+ m	+8

Extracted from Dietary Reference Values for Food Energy and Nutrients for the United Kingdom.[46]
[a]These figures, based on egg and milk protein, assume complete digestibility.
[b]No values for infants 0–3 months are given by WHO. The RNI is calculated from the recommendations of COMA.
[c]To be added to adult requirement through all stages of pregnancy and lactation.

Table A.17 Reference nutrient Intakes for vitamins

Age	Thiamin mg/d	Riboflavin mg/d	Niacin (nicotinic acid equivalent) mg/d	Vitamin B_6 mg/d[a]	Vitamin B_{12} µg/d	Folate µg/d	Vitamin C mg/d	Vitamin A µg/d	Vitamin D µg/d
0–3 m	0.2	0.4	3	0.2	0.3	50	25	350	8.5
0–4 m	0.2	0.4	3	0.2	0.3	50	25	350	8.5
7–9 m	0.2	0.4	4	0.3	0.4	50	25	350	7
10–12 m	0.3	0.4	5	0.4	0.4	50	25	350	7
1–3 y	0.5	0.6	8	0.7	0.5	70	30	400	7
4–6 y	0.7	0.8	11	0.9	0.8	100	30	400	–
7–10 y	0.7	1.0	12	1.0	1.0	150	30	500	–
Males									
11–14 y	0.9	1.2	15	1.2	1.2	200	35	600	–
15–18 y	1.1	1.3	18	1.5	1.5	200	40	700	–
19–50 y	1.0	1.3	17	1.4	1.5	200	40	700	–
50+ y	0.9	1.3	16	1.4	1.5	200	40	700	b
Females									
11–14 y	0.7	1.1	12	1.0	1.2	200	35	600	–
15–18 y	0.8	1.1	14	1.2	1.5	200	40	600	–
19–50 y	0.8	1.1	13	1.2	1.5	200	40	600	–
51+ y	0.8	1.1	12	1.2	1.5	200	40	600	b
Pregnancy	+0.1[c]	+0.3	d	d	d	+100	+10[c]	+100	10
Lactation:									
0–4 m	+0.2	+0.5	+2	d	+0.5	+600	+30	+350	10
4+ m	+0.2	+0.5	+2	d	+0.5	+600	+30	+350	10

Extracted from Dietary Reference Values for Food Energy and Nutrients for the United Kingdom.[46]
[a]Based on protein providing 14.7 per cent of EAR for energy.
[b]After age 65 the RNI µg/d for men and women.
[c]For last trimester only.
[d]No increment.

Table A.18a Reference nutrient intakes for minerals (SI units)

Age	Calcium mmol/d	Phosphorus[a] mmol/d	Magnesium mmol/d	Sodium mmol/d[b]	Potassium mmol/d[c]	Chloride[d] mmol/d	Iron mmol/d	Zinc μmol/d	Copper μmol/d	Selenium μmol/d	Iodine μmol/d
0–3 m	13.1	13.1	2.2	9	20	9	30	60	5	0.1	0.4
0–4 m	13.1	13.1	2.5	12	22	12	80	60	5	0.2	0.5
7–9 m	13.1	13.1	3.2	14	18	14	140	75	5	0.1	0.5
10–12 m	13.1	13.1	3.3	15	18	15	140	75	5	0.1	0.5
1–3 y	8.8	8.8	3.5	22	20	22	120	75	6	0.2	0.6
4–6 y	11.3	11.3	4.8	30	28	30	110	100	9	0.3	0.8
7–10 y	13.8	13.8	8.0	50	50	50	160	110	11	0.4	0.9
Males											
11–14 y	25.0	25.0	11.5	70	80	70	200	140	13	0.6	1.0
15–18 y	25.0	25.0	12.3	70	90	70	200	145	16	0.9	1.0
19–50 y	17.5	17.50	12.3	70	90	70	160	145	19	0.9	1.0
50+ y	17.5	17.50	12.3	70	90	70	160	145	19	0.9	1.0
Females											
11–14 y	20.0	20.0	11.5	70	80	70	260[e]	140	13	0.6	1.0
15–18 y	20.0	20.0	12.3	70	90	70	260[e]	110	16	0.8	1.1
19–50 y	17.5	17.5	10.9	70	90	70	260[e]	110	19	0.8	1.1
51+ y	17.5	17.5	10.9	70	90	70	160	110	19	0.8	1.1
Pregnancy[f]	[g]	[g]	[g]	[g]	[g]	[g]	[g]	[g]	[g]	[g]	[g]
Lactation[f]											
0–4 m	+14.3	+14.3	+2.1	[g]	[g]	[g]	[g]	+90	+5	+0.2	[g]
4+ m	+14.3	+14.3	+2.1	[g]	[g]	[g]	[g]	+40	+5	+0.2	[g]

Extracted from Dietary Reference Values for Food Energy and Nutrients for the United Kingdom.[46]
[a]Phosphorus RNI is set equal to calcium in molar terms.
[b]1 mmol sodium = 23 mg.
[c]1 mmol potassium = 39 mg.
[d]Corresponds to sodium 1 mmol = 35.5 mg.
[e]Insufficient for women with high menstrual losses where the most practical way of meeting iron requirements is to take iron supplements.
[f]To be added to adult requirement through all stages of pregnancy and lactation.
[g]No increment.

Table A.18b   Reference nutrient intakes for minerals

Age	Calcium mg/d	Phosphorus mg/d[a]	Magnesium mg/d	Sodium mg/d[b]	Potassium mg/d[c]	Chloride[d] mg/d	Iron mg/d	Zinc mg/d	Copper mg/d	Selenium µg/d	Iodine µg/d
0–3 m	525	400	55	210	800	320	1.7	4.0	0.2	10	50
0–4 m	525	400	60	280	850	400	4.3	4.0	0.3	13	60
7–9 m	525	400	75	320	700	500	7.8	5.0	0.3	10	60
10–12 m	525	400	80	350	700	500	7.8	5.0	0.3	10	60
1–3 y	350	270	85	500	800	800	6.9	5.0	0.4	15	70
4–6 y	450	350	120	700	1100	1100	6.1	6.5	0.6	20	100
7–10 y	550	450	200	1200	2000	1800	8.7	0.7	0.7	30	110
Males											
11–14 y	1000	775	280	1600	3100	2500	11.3	9.0	0.8	45	130
15–18 y	1000	775	300	1600	3500	2500	11.3	9.5	1.0	70	140
19–50 y	700	550	300	1600	3500	2500	8.7	9.5	1.2	75	140
50+ y	700	550	300	1600	3500	2500	8.7	9.5	1.2	75	140
Females											
11–14 y	800	625	280	1600	3100	2500	14.8[e]	9.0	0.8	45	130
15–18 y	800	625	300	1600	3500	2500	14.8[e]	7.0	1.0	60	140
19–50 y	700	550	270	1600	3500	2500	14.8[e]	7.0	1.2	60	140
51+ y	700	550	270	1600	3500	2500	8.7	7.0	1.2	60	140
Pregnancy[f]	g	g	g	g	g	g	g	g	g	g	g
Lactation[f]											
0–4 m	+550	+440	+50	g	g	g	g	+6.0	+0.3	+15	g
4+ m	+550	+440	+50	g	g	g	g	+2.5	+0.3	+15	g

Extracted from Dietary Reference Values for Food Energy and Nutrients for the United Kingdom.[46]
[a]Phosphorus RNI is set equal to calcium in molar terms.
[b]1 mmol sodium = 23 mg.
[c]1 mmol potassium = 39 mg.
[d]Corresponds to sodium 1 mmol = 35.5 mg.
[e]Insufficient for women with high menstrual losses where the most practical way of meeting iron requirements is to take iron supplements.
[f]To be added to adult requirement through all stages of pregnancy and lactation.
[g]No increment.

Table A.19   Safe intakes of vitamins and minerals

Nutrient	Safe intake
Vitamins	
Pantothenic acid	
Adults	3–7 mg/d
Infants	1.7 mg/d
Biotin	10–200 µg/d
Vitamin E	
Men	Above 4 mg/d
Women	Above 3 mg/d
Infants	0.4 mg/d polyunsaturated fatty acids
Vitamin K	
Adults	1 µg/kg/d
Infants	10 µg/d
Minerals	
Manganese	
Adults	Above 1.4 mg/dN (26 µmol/d)
Infants and children	Above 16 µg/kg/d (0.3 µmol/kg/d)
Molybdenum	
Adults	50–400 µg/d
Infants, children and adolescents	0.5–1.5 µg/kg/d
Chromium	
Adults	Above 25 µg (0.5 µmol/d)
Children and adolescents	0.1–1.0 µg (2–20 nmol/kg/d)
Fluoride	
Children over 6 years and adults	0.5 mg/kg/d (3 µmol/kg/d)
Children over 6 months	0.12 mg/kg/d (6 µmol/kg/d)
Infants under 6 months	0.22 mg/kg/d (12 µmol/kg/d)

Extracted from Dietary Reference Values for Food Energy and Nutrients for the United Kingdom.[46]

Table A.20 Multiple values proposed for adults. (Amounts per day, unless given in other items. If that for women is different from that for men, it is in parentheses)

Nutrient	Average requirement	Population reference intake	Lowest threshold intake
Protein (g)	0.6/kg body wt	0.75/kg body wt	0.45/kg body wt
Vitamin A (μg)	500 (400)	700 (600)	300 (250)
Thiamin (μg)	72/MJ	100/MJ	50/MJ
Riboflavin (mg)	1.3 (1.1)	1.6 (1.3)	0.6
Niacin (mg niacin equivalents)	1.3/MJ	1.6/MJ	1.0/MJ
Vitamin B6 (μg)	13/g protein	15/g protein	–
Folate (μg)	140	200	85
Vitamin B_{12} (μg)	1.0	1.4	0.6
Vitamin C (mg)	30	45	12
Vitamin E (mg α-tocopherol equivalents)		0.4/g PUFA	4 (3)/d regardless of PUFA intakes
n-6 PUFA (as percentage of dietary energy)	1	2	0.5
n-3 PUFA (as percentage of dietary energy)	0.2	0.5	0.1
Calcium (mg)	550	700	400
Phosphorus (mg)	400	550	300
Potassium (mg)	–	3100	1600
Iron (mg)	7 (10, 6[a])	9 (16[b], 8[a])	5 (7, 4[a])
Zinc (mg)	7.5 (5.5)	9.5 (7)	5 (4)
Copper (mg)	0.8	1.1	0.6
Selenium (μg)	40	55	20
Iodine (μg)	100	130	70
For the following, acceptable ranges of intake are given:			
Pantothenic acid (mg)	3–12		
Biotin (μg)	15–100		
Vitamin D (μg)	0–10		
Sodium (g)	0.575–3.5		
Magnesium (mg)	150–500		
Manganese (mg)	1–10		

PUFA, polyunsaturated fatty acids.
[a]Postmenopausal.
[b]PRI to cover 90% of women.
Reproduced from Nutrient and Energy Intakes for the European Community.[47]

Table A.21 EU reference intakes

Age group	Protein (g/kg body weight/d)	n-6 PUFA (% of dietary energy)	n-3 PUFA (% of dietary energy)	Vitamin A (μg/d)	Thiamin (μg/MJ)	Riboflavin (mg/d)	Niacin (mg/MJ)	Vitamin B_6 (μg/g protein)	Folate (μg/d)	Vitamin B_{12} (μg/d)	Vitamin C (mg/d)
6–11 months	1.6	4.5	0.5	350	100	0.4	1.6	15	50	0.5	20
1–3 yr	1.1	3	0.5	400	100	0.8	1.6	15	100	0.7	25
4–6 yr	1.0	2	0.5	400	100	1.0	1.6	15	130	0.9	25
7–10 yr	1.0	2	0.5	500	100	1.2	1.6	15	150	1.0	30
Males											
11–14 yr	1.0	2	0.5	600	100	1.4	1.6	15	180	1.3	35
15–17 yr	0.9	2	0.5	700	100	1.6	1.6	15	200	1.4	40
18+ yr	0.75	2	0.5	700	100	1.6	1.6	15	200	1.4	45
Females											
11–14 yr	0.95	2	0.5	600	100	1.2	1.6	15	180	1.3	35
15–17 yr	0.85	2	0.5	600	100	1.3	1.6	15	200	1.4	40
18+ yr	0.75	2	0.5	600	100	1.3	1.6	15	200[c]	1.4	45
Pregnancy	0.75 (+10 g/d)	2	0.5	700	100	1.6	1.6	15	400	1.6	55
Lactation	0.75 (+16 g/d)	2	0.5	950	100	1.7	1.6 (+2 mg/day)	15	350	1.9	70

(Continued)

Index